ICD-10-CM Official Guidelines for Coding and Reporting

> Note: The 2017 *ICD-10-CM Official Guidelines for Coding and Reporting* have been included as the 2018 guidelines were not available at the time of printing. As soon as the 2018 guidelines become available a downloadable PDF version will be posted to our website. You will also receive a booklet containing the updated 2018 ICD-10-CM guidelines in a separate shipment.

Narrative changes appear in **bold** text

Items underlined have been moved within the guidelines since the FY 2017 version

Italics are used to indicate revisions to heading changes

The Centers for Medicare and Medicaid Services (CMS) and the National Center for Health Statistics (NCHS), two departments within the U.S. Federal Government's Department of Health and Human Services (DHHS) provide the following guidelines for coding and reporting using the International Classification of Diseases, 10th Revision, Clinical Modification (ICD-10-CM). These guidelines should be used as a companion document to the official version of the ICD-10-CM as published on the NCHS website. The ICD-10-CM is a morbidity classification published by the United States for classifying diagnoses and reason for visits in all health care settings. The ICD-10-CM is based on the ICD-10, the statistical classification of disease published by the World Health Organization (WHO).

These guidelines have been approved by the four organizations that make up the Cooperating Parties for the ICD-10-CM: the American Hospital Association (AHA), the American Health Information Management Association (AHIMA), CMS, and NCHS.

These guidelines are a set of rules that have been developed to accompany and complement the official conventions and instructions provided within the ICD-10-CM itself. The instructions and conventions of the classification take precedence over guidelines. These guidelines are based on the coding and sequencing instructions in the Tabular List and Alphabetic Index of ICD-10-CM, but provide additional instruction. Adherence to these guidelines when assigning ICD-10-CM diagnosis codes is required under the Health Insurance Portability and Accountability Act (HIPAA). The diagnosis codes (Tabular List and Alphabetic Index) have been adopted under HIPAA for all healthcare settings. A joint effort between the healthcare provider and the coder is essential to achieve complete and accurate documentation, code assignment, and reporting of diagnoses and procedures. These guidelines have been developed to assist both the healthcare provider and the coder in identifying those diagnoses that are to be reported. The importance of consistent, complete documentation in the medical record cannot be overemphasized. Without such documentation accurate coding cannot be achieved. The entire record should be reviewed to determine the specific reason for the encounter and the conditions treated.

The term encounter is used for all settings, including hospital admissions. In the context of these guidelines, the term provider is used throughout the guidelines to mean physician or any qualified health care practitioner who is legally accountable for establishing the patient's diagnosis. Only this set of guidelines, approved by the Cooperating Parties, is official.

The guidelines are organized into sections. Section I includes the structure and conventions of the classification and general guidelines that apply to the entire classification, and chapter-specific guidelines that correspond to the chapters as they are arranged in the classification. Section II includes guidelines for selection of principal diagnosis for non-outpatient settings. Section III includes guidelines for reporting additional diagnoses in non-outpatient settings. Section IV is for outpatient coding and reporting. It is necessary to review all sections of the guidelines to fully understand all of the rules and instructions needed to code properly.

Section I. Conventions, general coding guidelines and chapter specific guidelines

The conventions, general guidelines and chapter-specific guidelines are applicable to all health care settings unless otherwise indicated. The conventions and instructions of the classification take precedence over guidelines.

A. Conventions for the ICD-10-CM

The conventions for the ICD-10-CM are the general rules for use of the classification independent of the guidelines. These conventions are incorporated within the Alphabetic Index and Tabular List of the ICD-10-CM as instructional notes.

1. The Alphabetic Index and Tabular List
The ICD-10-CM is divided into the Alphabetic Index, an alphabetical list of terms and their corresponding code, and the Tabular List, a structured list of codes divided into chapters based on body system or condition. The Alphabetic Index consists of the following parts: the Index of Diseases and Injury, the Index of External Causes of Injury, the Table of Neoplasms and the Table of Drugs and Chemicals.

See Section I.C2. General guidelines

See Section I.C.19. Adverse effects, poisoning, underdosing and toxic effects

2. Format and Structure:
The ICD-10-CM Tabular List contains categories, subcategories and codes. Characters for categories, subcategories and codes may be either a letter or a number. All categories are 3 characters. A three-character category that has no further subdivision is equivalent to a code. Subcategories are either 4 or 5 characters. Codes may be 3, 4, 5, 6 or 7 characters. That is, each level of subdivision after a category is a subcategory. The final level of subdivision is a code. Codes that have applicable 7th characters are still referred to as codes, not subcategories. A code that has an applicable 7th character is considered invalid without the 7th character.

The ICD-10-CM uses an indented format for ease in reference.

3. Use of codes for reporting purposes
For reporting purposes only codes are permissible, not categories or subcategories, and any applicable 7th character is required.

4. Placeholder character
The ICD-10-CM utilizes a placeholder character "X". The "X" is used as a placeholder at certain codes to allow for future expansion. An example of this is at the poisoning, adverse effect and underdosing codes, categories T36-T50.

Where a placeholder exists, the X must be used in order for the code to be considered a valid code.

5. 7th Characters
Certain ICD-10-CM categories have applicable 7th characters. The applicable 7th character is required for all codes within the category, or as the notes in the Tabular List instruct. The 7th character must always be the 7th character in the data field. If a code that requires a 7th character is not 6 characters, a placeholder X must be used to fill in the empty characters.

6. Abbreviations
  a. Alphabetic Index abbreviations
    NEC   "Not elsewhere classifiable"

This abbreviation in the Alphabetic Index represents "other specified." When a specific code is not available for a condition, the Alphabetic Index directs the coder to the "other specified" code in the Tabular List.

    NOS   "Not otherwise specified"

This abbreviation is the equivalent of unspecified.

  b. Tabular List abbreviations
    NEC   "Not elsewhere classifiable"

This abbreviation in the Tabular List represents "other specified". When a specific code is not available for a condition, the Tabular List includes an NEC entry under a code to identify the code as the "other specified" code.

    NOS   "Not otherwise specified"

This abbreviation is the equivalent of unspecified.

7. Punctuation
  [ ]   Brackets are used in the Tabular List to enclose synonyms, alternative wording or explanatory phrases. Brackets are used in the Alphabetic Index to identify manifestation codes.

  ( )   Parentheses are used in both the Alphabetic Index and Tabular List to enclose supplementary words that may be present or absent in the statement of a disease or procedure without affecting the code number to which it is assigned. The terms within the parentheses are referred to as nonessential modifiers. The nonessential modifiers in the Alphabetic Index to Diseases apply to subterms following a main term except when a nonessential modifier and a subentry are mutually exclusive, the subentry takes precedence. For example, in the ICD-10-CM Alphabetic Index under the main term Enteritis, "acute" is a nonessential modifier and "chronic" is a subentry. In this case, the nonessential modifier "acute" does not apply to the subentry "chronic".

  :   Colons are used in the Tabular List after an incomplete term which needs one or more of the modifiers following the colon to make it assignable to a given category.

8. Use of "and".
See Section I.A.14. Use of the term "And"

9. Other and Unspecified codes
  a. "Other" codes
Codes titled "other" or "other specified" are for use when the information in the medical record provides detail for which a specific code does not exist. Alphabetic Index entries with NEC in the line designate "other" codes in the Tabular List. These Alphabetic Index entries represent specific disease entities for which no specific code exists so the term is included within an "other" code.

  b. "Unspecified" codes
Codes titled "unspecified" are for use when the information in the medical record is insufficient to assign a more specific code. For those categories for which an unspecified code is not provided, the "other specified" code may represent both other and unspecified.

See Section I.B.18 Use of Signs/Symptom/Unspecified Codes

10. Includes Notes
This note appears immediately under a three character code title to further define, or give examples of, the content of the category.

11. Inclusion terms
List of terms is included under some codes. These terms are the conditions for which that code is to be used. The terms may be synonyms of the code title, or, in the case of "other specified" codes, the terms are a list of the various conditions assigned to that code. The inclusion terms are not necessarily exhaustive. Additional terms found only in the Alphabetic Index may also be assigned to a code.

12. Excludes Notes
The ICD-10-CM has two types of excludes notes. Each type of note has a different definition for use but they are all similar in that they indicate that codes excluded from each other are independent of each other.

  a. Excludes1
A type 1 Excludes note is a pure excludes note. It means "NOT CODED HERE!" An Excludes1 note indicates that the code excluded should never be used at the same time as the code above the Excludes1 note. An Excludes1 is used when two conditions cannot occur together, such as a congenital form versus an acquired form of the same condition.

An exception to the Excludes1 definition is the circumstance when the two conditions are unrelated to each other. If it is not clear whether the two conditions involving an Excludes1 note are related or not, query the provider. For example, code F45.8, Other somatoform disorders, has an Excludes1 note for "sleep related teeth grinding (G47.63)," because "teeth grinding" is an inclusion term under F45.8. Only one of these two codes should be assigned for teeth grinding. However psychogenic dysmenorrhea is also an inclusion term under F45.8, and a patient could have both this condition and sleep related teeth grinding. In this case, the two conditions are clearly unrelated to each other, and so it would be appropriate to report F45.8 and G47.63 together.

b. Excludes2

A type 2 Excludes note represents "Not included here." An excludes2 note indicates that the condition excluded is not part of the condition represented by the code, but a patient may have both conditions at the same time. When an Excludes2 note appears under a code, it is acceptable to use both the code and the excluded code together, when appropriate.

13. Etiology/manifestation convention ("code first", "use additional code" and "in diseases classified elsewhere" notes)

Certain conditions have both an underlying etiology and multiple body system manifestations due to the underlying etiology. For such conditions, the ICD-10-CM has a coding convention that requires the underlying condition be sequenced first, if applicable, followed by the manifestation. Wherever such a combination exists, there is a "use additional code" note at the etiology code, and a "code first" note at the manifestation code. These instructional notes indicate the proper sequencing order of the codes, etiology followed by manifestation.

In most cases the manifestation codes will have in the code title, "in diseases classified elsewhere." Codes with this title are a component of the etiology/ manifestation convention. The code title indicates that it is a manifestation code. "In diseases classified elsewhere" codes are never permitted to be used as first-listed or principal diagnosis codes. They must be used in conjunction with an underlying condition code and they must be listed following the underlying condition. See category F02, Dementia in other diseases classified elsewhere, for an example of this convention.

There are manifestation codes that do not have "in diseases classified elsewhere" in the title. For such codes, there is a "use additional code" note at the etiology code and a "code first" note at the manifestation code, and the rules for sequencing apply.

In addition to the notes in the Tabular List, these conditions also have a specific Alphabetic Index entry structure. In the Alphabetic Index both conditions are listed together with the etiology code first followed by the manifestation codes in brackets. The code in brackets is always to be sequenced second.

An example of the etiology/manifestation convention is dementia in Parkinson's disease. In the Alphabetic Index, code G20 is listed first, followed by code F02.80 or F02.81 in brackets. Code G20 represents the underlying etiology, Parkinson's disease, and must be sequenced first, whereas codes F02.80 and F02.81 represent the manifestation of dementia in diseases classified elsewhere, with or without behavioral disturbance.

"Code first" and "Use additional code" notes are also used as sequencing rules in the classification for certain codes that are not part of an etiology/ manifestation combination.

See Section I.B.7. Multiple coding for a single condition.

14. "And"

The word "and" should be interpreted to mean either "and" or "or" when it appears in a title.

For example, cases of "tuberculosis of bones", "tuberculosis of joints" and "tuberculosis of bones and joints" are classified to subcategory A18.0, Tuberculosis of bones and joints.

15. "With"

The word "with" should be interpreted to mean "associated with" or "due to" when it appears in a code title, the Alphabetic Index, or an instructional note in the Tabular List. The classification presumes a causal relationship between the two conditions linked by these terms in the Alphabetic Index or Tabular List. These conditions should be coded as related even in the absence of provider documentation explicitly linking

them, unless the documentation clearly states the conditions are unrelated. For conditions not specifically linked by these relational terms in the classification, provider documentation must link the conditions in order to code them as related. The word "with" in the Alphabetic Index is sequenced immediately following the main term, not in alphabetical order.

16. "See" and "See Also"

The "see" instruction following a main term in the Alphabetic Index indicates that another term should be referenced. It is necessary to go to the main term referenced with the "see" note to locate the correct code.

A "see also" instruction following a main term in the Alphabetic Index instructs that there is another main term that may also be referenced that may provide additional Alphabetic Index entries that may be useful. It is not necessary to follow the "see also" note when the original main term provides the necessary code.

17. "Code also" note

A "code also" note instructs that two codes may be required to fully describe a condition, but this note does not provide sequencing direction.

18. Default codes

A code listed next to a main term in the ICD-10-CM Alphabetic Index is referred to as a default code. The default code represents that condition that is most commonly associated with the main term, or is the unspecified code for the condition. If a condition is documented in a medical record (for example, appendicitis) without any additional information, such as acute or chronic, the default code should be assigned.

19. Code assignment and Clinical Criteria

The assignment of a diagnosis code is based on the provider's diagnostic statement that the condition exists. The provider's statement that the patient has a particular condition is sufficient. Code assignment is not based on clinical criteria used by the provider to establish the diagnosis.

B. General Coding Guidelines

1. Locating a code in the ICD-10-CM

To select a code in the classification that corresponds to a diagnosis or reason for visit documented in a medical record, first locate the term in the Alphabetic Index, and then verify the code in the Tabular List. Read and be guided by instructional notations that appear in both the Alphabetic Index and the Tabular List.

It is essential to use both the Alphabetic Index and Tabular List when locating and assigning a code. The Alphabetic Index does not always provide the full code. Selection of the full code, including laterality and any applicable 7th character can only be done in the Tabular List. A dash (-) at the end of an Alphabetic Index entry indicates that additional characters are required. Even if a dash is not included at the Alphabetic Index entry, it is necessary to refer to the Tabular List to verify that no 7th character is required.

2. Level of Detail in Coding

Diagnosis codes are to be used and reported at their highest number of characters available.

ICD-10-CM diagnosis codes are composed of codes with 3, 4, 5, 6 or 7 characters. Codes with three characters are included in ICD-10-CM as the heading of a category of codes that may be further subdivided by the use of fourth and/or fifth characters and/or sixth characters, which provide greater detail.

A three-character code is to be used only if it is not further subdivided. A code is invalid if it has not been coded to the full number of characters required for that code, including the 7th character, if applicable.

3. Code or codes from A00.0 through T88.9, Z00-Z99.8

The appropriate code or codes from A00.0 through T88.9, Z00-Z99.8 must be used to identify diagnoses, symptoms, conditions, problems, complaints or other reason(s) for the encounter/visit.

4. Signs and symptoms

Codes that describe symptoms and signs, as opposed to diagnoses, are acceptable for reporting purposes when a related definitive diagnosis has not been established (confirmed) by the provider. Chapter 18 of ICD-10-CM, Symptoms, Signs, and Abnormal Clinical and Laboratory Findings, Not Elsewhere Classified (codes R00.0 - R99) contains many, but not all, codes for symptoms.

See Section I.B.18 Use of Signs/Symptom/Unspecified Codes

5. Conditions that are an integral part of a disease process
Signs and symptoms that are associated routinely with a disease process should not be assigned as additional codes, unless otherwise instructed by the classification.

6. Conditions that are not an integral part of a disease process
Additional signs and symptoms that may not be associated routinely with a disease process should be coded when present.

7. Multiple coding for a single condition
In addition to the etiology/manifestation convention that requires two codes to fully describe a single condition that affects multiple body systems, there are other single conditions that also require more than one code. "Use additional code" notes are found in the Tabular List at codes that are not part of an etiology/manifestation pair where a secondary code is useful to fully describe a condition. The sequencing rule is the same as the etiology/manifestation pair, "use additional code" indicates that a secondary code should be added.

For example, for bacterial infections that are not included in chapter 1, a secondary code from category B95, Streptococcus, Staphylococcus, and Enterococcus, as the cause of diseases classified elsewhere, or B96, Other bacterial agents as the cause of diseases classified elsewhere, may be required to identify the bacterial organism causing the infection. A "use additional code" note will normally be found at the infectious disease code, indicating a need for the organism code to be added as a secondary code.

"Code first" notes are also under certain codes that are not specifically manifestation codes but may be due to an underlying cause. When there is a "code first" note and an underlying condition is present, the underlying condition should be sequenced first.

"Code, if applicable, any causal condition first" notes indicate that this code may be assigned as a principal diagnosis when the causal condition is unknown or not applicable. If a causal condition is known, then the code for that condition should be sequenced as the principal or first-listed diagnosis.

Multiple codes may be needed for sequela, complication codes and obstetric codes to more fully describe a condition. See the specific guidelines for these conditions for further instruction.

8. Acute and Chronic Conditions
If the same condition is described as both acute (subacute) and chronic, and separate subentries exist in the Alphabetic Index at the same indentation level, code both and sequence the acute (subacute) code first.

9. Combination Code
A combination code is a single code used to classify:
Two diagnoses, or
A diagnosis with an associated secondary process (manifestation)
A diagnosis with an associated complication

Combination codes are identified by referring to subterm entries in the Alphabetic Index and by reading the inclusion and exclusion notes in the Tabular List.

Assign only the combination code when that code fully identifies the diagnostic conditions involved or when the Alphabetic Index so directs. Multiple coding should not be used when the classification provides a combination code that clearly identifies all of the elements documented in the diagnosis. When the combination code lacks necessary specificity in describing the manifestation or complication, an additional code should be used as a secondary code.

10. Sequela (Late Effects)
A sequela is the residual effect (condition produced) after the acute phase of an illness or injury has terminated. There is no time limit on when a sequela code can be used. The residual may be apparent early, such as in cerebral infarction, or it may occur months or years later, such as that due to a previous injury. Examples of sequela include: scar formation resulting from a burn, deviated septum due to a nasal fracture, and infertility due to tubal occlusion from old tuberculosis. Coding of sequela generally requires two codes sequenced in the following order: the condition or nature of the sequela is sequenced first. The sequela code is sequenced second.

An exception to the above guidelines are those instances where the code for the sequela is followed by a manifestation code identified in the Tabular List and title, or the sequela code has been expanded (at the

fourth, fifth or sixth character levels) to include the manifestation(s). The code for the acute phase of an illness or injury that led to the sequela is never used with a code for the late effect.

See Section I.C.9. Sequelae of cerebrovascular disease

See Section I.C.15. Sequelae of complication of pregnancy, childbirth and the puerperium

See Section I.C.19. Application of 7th characters for Chapter 19

11. Impending or Threatened Condition
Code any condition described at the time of discharge as "impending" or "threatened" as follows:

If it did occur, code as confirmed diagnosis.
If it did not occur, reference the Alphabetic Index to determine if the condition has a subentry term for "impending" or "threatened" and also reference main term entries for "Impending" and for "Threatened." If the subterms are listed, assign the given code.
If the subterms are not listed, code the existing underlying condition(s) and not the condition described as impending or threatened.

12. Reporting Same Diagnosis Code more than Once
Each unique ICD-10-CM diagnosis code may be reported only once for an encounter. This applies to bilateral conditions when there are no distinct codes identifying laterality or two different conditions classified to the same ICD-10-CM diagnosis code.

13. Laterality
Some ICD-10-CM codes indicate laterality, specifying whether the condition occurs on the left, right or is bilateral. If no bilateral code is provided and the condition is bilateral, assign separate codes for both the left and right side. If the side is not identified in the medical record, assign the code for the unspecified side.

When a patient has a bilateral condition and each side is treated during separate encounters, assign the "bilateral" code (as the condition still exists on both sides), including for the encounter to treat the first side. For the second encounter for treatment after one side has previously been treated and the condition no longer exists on that side, assign the appropriate unilateral code for the side where the condition still exists (e.g., cataract surgery performed on each eye in separate encounters). The bilateral code would not be assigned for the subsequent encounter, as the patient no longer has the condition in the previously-treated site. If the treatment on the first side did not completely resolve the condition, then the bilateral code would still be appropriate.

14. Documentation for BMI, Depth of Non-pressure ulcers, Pressure Ulcer Stages, Coma Scale, and NIH Stroke Scale
For the Body Mass Index (BMI), depth of non-pressure chronic ulcers, pressure ulcer stage, coma scale, and NIH stroke scale (NIHSS) codes, code assignment may be based on medical record documentation from clinicians who are not the patient's provider (i.e., physician or other qualified healthcare practitioner legally accountable for establishing the patient's diagnosis), since this information is typically documented by other clinicians involved in the care of the patient (e.g., a dietitian often documents the BMI, a nurse often documents the pressure ulcer stages, and an emergency medical technician often documents the coma scale). However, the associated diagnosis (such as overweight, obesity, acute stroke, or pressure ulcer) must be documented by the patient's provider. If there is conflicting medical record documentation, either from the same clinician or different clinicians, the patient's attending provider should be queried for clarification.

The BMI, coma scale, and NIHSS codes should only be reported as secondary diagnoses.

15. Syndromes
Follow the Alphabetic Index guidance when coding syndromes. In the absence of Alphabetic Index guidance, assign codes for the documented manifestations of the syndrome. Additional codes for manifestations that are not an integral part of the disease process may also be assigned when the condition does not have a unique code.

16. Documentation of Complications of Care
Code assignment is based on the provider's documentation of the relationship between the condition and the care or procedure, unless otherwise instructed by the classification. The guideline extends to any complications of care, regardless of the chapter the code is located in. It is important to note that not all conditions that occur during or following medical care or surgery are classified as complications. There must be a cause-and-effect relationship between the care provided and

the condition, and an indication in the documentation that it is a complication. Query the provider for clarification, if the complication is not clearly documented.

17. Borderline Diagnosis

If the provider documents a "borderline" diagnosis at the time of discharge, the diagnosis is coded as confirmed, unless the classification provides a specific entry (e.g., borderline diabetes). If a borderline condition has a specific index entry in ICD-10-CM, it should be coded as such. Since borderline conditions are not uncertain diagnoses, no distinction is made between the care setting (inpatient versus outpatient). Whenever the documentation is unclear regarding a borderline condition, coders are encouraged to query for clarification.

18. Use of Sign/Symptom/Unspecified Codes

Sign/symptom and "unspecified" codes have acceptable, even necessary, uses. While specific diagnosis codes should be reported when they are supported by the available medical record documentation and clinical knowledge of the patient's health condition, there are instances when signs/symptoms or unspecified codes are the best choices for accurately reflecting the healthcare encounter. Each healthcare encounter should be coded to the level of certainty known for that encounter.

If a definitive diagnosis has not been established by the end of the encounter, it is appropriate to report codes for sign(s) and/or symptom(s) in lieu of a definitive diagnosis. When sufficient clinical information isn't known or available about a particular health condition to assign a more specific code, it is acceptable to report the appropriate "unspecified" code (e.g., a diagnosis of pneumonia has been determined, but not the specific type). Unspecified codes should be reported when they are the codes that most accurately reflect what is known about the patient's condition at the time of that particular encounter. It would be inappropriate to select a specific code that is not supported by the medical record documentation or conduct medically unnecessary diagnostic testing in order to determine a more specific code.

C. Chapter-Specific Coding Guidelines

In addition to general coding guidelines, there are guidelines for specific diagnoses and/or conditions in the classification. Unless otherwise indicated, these guidelines apply to all health care settings. Please refer to Section II for guidelines on the selection of principal diagnosis.

1. Chapter 1: Certain Infectious and Parasitic Diseases (A00-B99)

a. Human Immunodeficiency Virus (HIV) Infections

1) Code only confirmed cases

Code only confirmed cases of HIV infection/illness. This is an exception to the hospital inpatient guideline Section II, H.

In this context, "confirmation" does not require documentation of positive serology or culture for HIV; the provider's diagnostic statement that the patient is HIV positive, or has an HIV-related illness is sufficient.

2) Selection and sequencing of HIV codes

(a) Patient admitted for HIV-related condition

If a patient is admitted for an HIV-related condition, the principal diagnosis should be B20, Human immunodeficiency virus [HIV] disease followed by additional diagnosis codes for all reported HIV-related conditions.

(b) Patient with HIV disease admitted for unrelated condition

If a patient with HIV disease is admitted for an unrelated condition (such as a traumatic injury), the code for the unrelated condition (e.g., the nature of injury code) should be the principal diagnosis. Other diagnoses would be B20 followed by additional diagnosis codes for all reported HIV-related conditions.

(c) Whether the patient is newly diagnosed

Whether the patient is newly diagnosed or has had previous admissions/encounters for HIV conditions is irrelevant to the sequencing decision.

(d) Asymptomatic human immunodeficiency virus

Z21, Asymptomatic human immunodeficiency virus [HIV] infection status, is to be applied when the patient without any documentation of symptoms is listed as being "HIV

positive," "known HIV," "HIV test positive," or similar terminology. Do not use this code if the term "AIDS" is used or if the patient is treated for any HIV-related illness or is described as having any condition(s) resulting from his/her HIV positive status; use B20 in these cases.

(e) Patients with inconclusive HIV serology

Patients with inconclusive HIV serology, but no definitive diagnosis or manifestations of the illness, may be assigned code R75, Inconclusive laboratory evidence of human immunodeficiency virus [HIV].

(f) Previously diagnosed HIV-related illness

Patients with any known prior diagnosis of an HIV-related illness should be coded to B20. Once a patient has developed an HIV-related illness, the patient should always be assigned code B20 on every subsequent admission/encounter. Patients previously diagnosed with any HIV illness (B20) should never be assigned to R75 or Z21, Asymptomatic human immunodeficiency virus [HIV] infection status.

(g) HIV Infection in Pregnancy, Childbirth and the Puerperium

During pregnancy, childbirth or the puerperium, a patient admitted (or presenting for a health care encounter) because of an HIV-related illness should receive a principal diagnosis code of O98.7-, Human immunodeficiency [HIV] disease complicating pregnancy, childbirth and the puerperium, followed by B20 and the code(s) for the HIV-related illness(es). Codes from Chapter 15 always take sequencing priority.

Patients with asymptomatic HIV infection status admitted (or presenting for a health care encounter) during pregnancy, childbirth, or the puerperium should receive codes of O98.7- and Z21.

(h) Encounters for testing for HIV

If a patient is being seen to determine his/her HIV status, use code Z11.4, Encounter for screening for human immunodeficiency virus [HIV]. Use additional codes for any associated high risk behavior.

If a patient with signs or symptoms is being seen for HIV testing, code the signs and symptoms. An additional counseling code Z71.7, Human immunodeficiency virus [HIV] counseling, may be used if counseling is provided during the encounter for the test.

When a patient returns to be informed of his/her HIV test results and the test result is negative, use code Z71.7, Human immunodeficiency virus [HIV] counseling.

If the results are positive, see previous guidelines and assign codes as appropriate.

b. Infectious agents as the cause of diseases classified to other chapters

Certain infections are classified in chapters other than Chapter 1 and no organism is identified as part of the infection code. In these instances, it is necessary to use an additional code from Chapter 1 to identify the organism. A code from category B95, Streptococcus, Staphylococcus, and Enterococcus as the cause of diseases classified to other chapters, B96, Other bacterial agents as the cause of diseases classified to other chapters, or B97, Viral agents as the cause of diseases classified to other chapters, is to be used as an additional code to identify the organism. An instructional note will be found at the infection code advising that an additional organism code is required.

c. Infections resistant to antibiotics

Many bacterial infections are resistant to current antibiotics. It is necessary to identify all infections documented as antibiotic resistant. Assign a code from category Z16, Resistance to antimicrobial drugs, following the infection code only if the infection code does not identify drug resistance.

d. **Sepsis, Severe Sepsis, and Septic Shock**

1) **Coding of Sepsis and Severe Sepsis**

(a) **Sepsis**

For a diagnosis of sepsis, assign the appropriate code for the underlying systemic infection. If the type of infection or causal organism is not further specified, assign code A41.9, Sepsis, unspecified organism.

A code from subcategory R65.2, Severe sepsis, should not be assigned unless severe sepsis or an associated acute organ dysfunction is documented.

(i) Negative or inconclusive blood cultures and sepsis

Negative or inconclusive blood cultures do not preclude a diagnosis of sepsis in patients with clinical evidence of the condition; however, the provider should be queried.

(ii) Urosepsis

The term urosepsis is a nonspecific term. It is not to be considered synonymous with sepsis. It has no default code in the Alphabetic Index. Should a provider use this term, he/she must be queried for clarification.

(iii) Sepsis with organ dysfunction

If a patient has sepsis and associated acute organ dysfunction or multiple organ dysfunction (MOD), follow the instructions for coding severe sepsis.

(iv) Acute organ dysfunction that is not clearly associated with the sepsis

If a patient has sepsis and an acute organ dysfunction, but the medical record documentation indicates that the acute organ dysfunction is related to a medical condition other than the sepsis, do not assign a code from subcategory R65.2, Severe sepsis. An acute organ dysfunction must be associated with the sepsis in order to assign the severe sepsis code. If the documentation is not clear as to whether an acute organ dysfunction is related to the sepsis or another medical condition, query the provider.

(b) **Severe sepsis**

The coding of severe sepsis requires a minimum of 2 codes: first a code for the underlying systemic infection, followed by a code from subcategory R65.2, Severe sepsis. If the causal organism is not documented, assign code A41.9, Sepsis, unspecified organism, for the infection. Additional code(s) for the associated acute organ dysfunction are also required.

Due to the complex nature of severe sepsis, some cases may require querying the provider prior to assignment of the codes.

2) **Septic shock**

(a) Septic shock generally refers to circulatory failure associated with severe sepsis, and therefore, it represents a type of acute organ dysfunction.

For cases of septic shock, the code for the systemic infection should be sequenced first, followed by code R65.21, Severe sepsis with septic shock or code T81.12, Postprocedural septic shock. Any additional codes for the other acute organ dysfunctions should also be assigned. As noted in the sequencing instructions in the Tabular List, the code for septic shock cannot be assigned as a principal diagnosis.

3) **Sequencing of severe sepsis**

If severe sepsis is present on admission, and meets the definition of principal diagnosis, the underlying systemic infection should be assigned as principal diagnosis followed by the appropriate code from subcategory R65.2 as required by the sequencing rules in the Tabular List. A code from subcategory R65.2 can never be assigned as a principal diagnosis.

When severe sepsis develops during an encounter (it was not present on admission), the underlying systemic infection and the appropriate code from subcategory R65.2 should be assigned as secondary diagnoses.

Severe sepsis may be present on admission, but the diagnosis may not be confirmed until sometime after admission. If the documentation is not clear whether severe sepsis was present on admission, the provider should be queried.

4) **Sepsis and severe sepsis with a localized infection**

If the reason for admission is both sepsis or severe sepsis and a localized infection, such as pneumonia or cellulitis, a code(s) for the underlying systemic infection should be assigned first and the code for the localized infection should be assigned as a secondary diagnosis. If the patient has severe sepsis, a code from subcategory R65.2 should also be assigned as a secondary diagnosis. If the patient is admitted with a localized infection, such as pneumonia, and sepsis/severe sepsis doesn't develop until after admission, the localized infection should be assigned first, followed by the appropriate sepsis/severe sepsis codes.

5) **Sepsis due to a postprocedural infection**

(a) **Documentation of causal relationship**

As with all postprocedural complications, code assignment is based on the provider's documentation of the relationship between the infection and the procedure.

(b) **Sepsis due to a postprocedural infection**

For such cases, the postprocedural infection code, such as T80.2, Infections following infusion, transfusion, and therapeutic injection, T81.4, Infection following a procedure, T88.0, Infection following immunization, or O86.0, Infection of obstetric surgical wound, should be coded first, followed by the code for the specific infection. If the patient has severe sepsis, the appropriate code from subcategory R65.2 should also be assigned with the additional code(s) for any acute organ dysfunction.

(c) **Postprocedural infection and postprocedural septic shock**

In cases where a postprocedural infection has occurred and has resulted in severe sepsis the code for the precipitating complication such as code T81.4, Infection following a procedure, or O86.0, Infection of obstetrical surgical wound should be coded first followed by code R65.20, Severe sepsis without septic shock. A code for the systemic infection should also be assigned.

If a postprocedural infection has resulted in postprocedural septic shock, the code for the precipitating complication such as code T81.4, Infection following a procedure, or O86.0, Infection of obstetrical surgical wound should be coded first followed by code T81.12-, Postprocedural septic shock. A code for the systemic infection should also be assigned.

6) **Sepsis and severe sepsis associated with a noninfectious process (condition)**

In some cases a noninfectious process (condition), such as trauma, may lead to an infection which can result in sepsis or severe sepsis. If sepsis or severe sepsis is documented as associated with a noninfectious condition, such as a burn or serious injury, and this condition meets the definition for principal diagnosis, the code for the noninfectious condition should be sequenced first, followed by the code for the resulting infection. If severe sepsis is present, a code from subcategory R65.2 should also be assigned with any associated organ dysfunction(s) codes. It is not necessary to assign a code from subcategory R65.1, Systemic inflammatory response syndrome (SIRS) of non-infectious origin, for these cases.

If the infection meets the definition of principal diagnosis, it should be sequenced before the non-infectious condition. When both the associated non-infectious condition and the infection meet the definition of principal diagnosis, either may be assigned as principal diagnosis.

Only one code from category R65, Symptoms and signs specifically associated with systemic inflammation and infection, should be assigned. Therefore, when a non-infectious condition leads to an infection resulting in severe sepsis, assign the appropriate code from subcategory R65.2, Severe sepsis. Do not additionally assign a code from subcategory R65.1, Systemic inflammatory response syndrome (SIRS) of non-infectious origin.

See Section I.C.18. SIRS due to non-infectious process

7) Sepsis and septic shock complicating abortion, pregnancy, childbirth, and the puerperium
See Section I.C.15. Sepsis and septic shock complicating abortion, pregnancy, childbirth and the puerperium

8) Newborn sepsis
See Section I.C.16. f. Bacterial sepsis of Newborn

e. Methicillin Resistant *Staphylococcus aureus* (MRSA) Conditions

1) Selection and sequencing of MRSA codes

(a) Combination codes for MRSA infection
When a patient is diagnosed with an infection that is due to methicillin resistant *Staphylococcus aureus* (MRSA), and that infection has a combination code that includes the causal organism (e.g., sepsis, pneumonia) assign the appropriate combination code for the condition (e.g., code A41.02, Sepsis due to Methicillin resistant Staphylococcus aureus or code J15.212, Pneumonia due to Methicillin resistant Staphylococcus aureus). Do not assign code B95.62, Methicillin resistant Staphylococcus aureus infection as the cause of diseases classified elsewhere, as an additional code, because the combination code includes the type of infection and the MRSA organism. Do not assign a code from subcategory Z16.11, Resistance to penicillins, as an additional diagnosis.

See Section C.1. for instructions on coding and sequencing of sepsis and severe sepsis.

(b) Other codes for MRSA infection
When there is documentation of a current infection (e.g., wound infection, stitch abscess, urinary tract infection) due to MRSA, and that infection does not have a combination code that includes the causal organism, assign the appropriate code to identify the condition along with code B95.62, Methicillin resistant Staphylococcus aureus infection as the cause of diseases classified elsewhere for the MRSA infection. Do not assign a code from subcategory Z16.11, Resistance to penicillins.

(c) Methicillin susceptible Staphylococcus aureus (MSSA) and MRSA colonization
The condition or state of being colonized or carrying MSSA or MRSA is called colonization or carriage, while an individual person is described as being colonized or being a carrier. Colonization means that MSSA or MSRA is present on or in the body without necessarily causing illness. A positive MRSA colonization test might be documented by the provider as "MRSA screen positive" or "MRSA nasal swab positive".

Assign code Z22.322, Carrier or suspected carrier of Methicillin resistant Staphylococcus aureus, for patients documented as having MRSA colonization. Assign code Z22.321, Carrier or suspected carrier of Methicillin susceptible Staphylococcus aureus, for patient documented as having MSSA colonization. Colonization is not necessarily indicative of a disease process or as the cause of a specific condition the patient may have unless documented as such by the provider.

(d) MRSA colonization and infection
If a patient is documented as having both MRSA colonization and infection during a hospital admission, code Z22.322, Carrier or suspected carrier of Methicillin resistant Staphylococcus aureus, and a code for the MRSA infection may both be assigned.

f. Zika virus infections

1) Code only confirmed cases
Code only a confirmed diagnosis of Zika virus (A92.5, Zika virus disease) as documented by the provider. This is an exception to the hospital inpatient guideline Section II, H.

In this context, "confirmation" does not require documentation of the type of test performed; the physician's diagnostic

statement that the condition is confirmed is sufficient. This code should be assigned regardless of the stated mode of transmission.

If the provider documents "suspected", "possible" or "probable" Zika, do not assign code A92.5. Assign a code(s) explaining the reason for encounter (such as fever, rash, or joint pain) or Z20.828, Contact with and (suspected) exposure to other viral communicable diseases.

2. Chapter 2: Neoplasms (C00-D49)

General guidelines
Chapter 2 of the ICD-10-CM contains the codes for most benign and all malignant neoplasms. Certain benign neoplasms, such as prostatic adenomas, may be found in the specific body system chapters. To properly code a neoplasm it is necessary to determine from the record if the neoplasm is benign, in-situ, malignant, or of uncertain histologic behavior. If malignant, any secondary (metastatic) sites should also be determined.

Primary malignant neoplasms overlapping site boundaries

A primary malignant neoplasm that overlaps two or more contiguous (next to each other) sites should be classified to the subcategory/code .8 ('overlapping lesion'), unless the combination is specifically indexed elsewhere. For multiple neoplasms of the same site that are not contiguous such as tumors in different quadrants of the same breast, codes for each site should be assigned.

Malignant neoplasm of ectopic tissue

Malignant neoplasms of ectopic tissue are to be coded to the site of origin mentioned, e.g., ectopic pancreatic malignant neoplasms involving the stomach are coded to pancreas, unspecified (C25.9).

The neoplasm table in the Alphabetic Index should be referenced first. However, if the histological term is documented, that term should be referenced first, rather than going immediately to the Neoplasm Table, in order to determine which column in the Neoplasm Table is appropriate. For example, if the documentation indicates "adenoma," refer to the term in the Alphabetic Index to review the entries under this term and the instructional note to "see also neoplasm, by site, benign." The table provides the proper code based on the type of neoplasm and the site. It is important to select the proper column in the table that corresponds to the type of neoplasm. The Tabular List should then be referenced to verify that the correct code has been selected from the table and that a more specific site code does not exist.

See Section I.C.21. Factors influencing health status and contact with health services, Status, for information regarding Z15.0, codes for genetic susceptibility to cancer.

a. Treatment directed at the malignancy
If the treatment is directed at the malignancy, designate the malignancy as the principal diagnosis.

The only exception to this guideline is if a patient admission/encounter is solely for the administration of chemotherapy, immunotherapy or radiation therapy, assign the appropriate Z51.-- code as the first-listed or principal diagnosis, and the diagnosis or problem for which the service is being performed as a secondary diagnosis.

b. Treatment of secondary site
When a patient is admitted because of a primary neoplasm with metastasis and treatment is directed toward the secondary site only, the secondary neoplasm is designated as the principal diagnosis even though the primary malignancy is still present.

c. Coding and sequencing of complications
Coding and sequencing of complications associated with the malignancies or with the therapy thereof are subject to the following guidelines:

1) Anemia associated with malignancy
When admission/encounter is for management of an anemia associated with the malignancy, and the treatment is only for anemia, the appropriate code for the malignancy is sequenced as the principal or first-listed diagnosis followed by the appropriate code for the anemia (such as code D63.0, Anemia in neoplastic disease).

2) **Anemia associated with chemotherapy, immunotherapy and radiation therapy**
When the admission/encounter is for management of an anemia associated with an adverse effect of the administration of chemotherapy or immunotherapy and the only treatment is for the anemia, the anemia code is sequenced first followed by the appropriate codes for the neoplasm and the adverse effect (T45.1X5, Adverse effect of antineoplastic and immunosuppressive drugs).

When the admission/encounter is for management of an anemia associated with an adverse effect of radiotherapy, the anemia code should be sequenced first, followed by the appropriate neoplasm code and code Y84.2, Radiological procedure and radiotherapy as the cause of abnormal reaction of the patient, or of later complication, without mention of misadventure at the time of the procedure.

3) **Management of dehydration due to the malignancy**
When the admission/encounter is for management of dehydration due to the malignancy and only the dehydration is being treated (intravenous rehydration), the dehydration is sequenced first, followed by the code(s) for the malignancy.

4) **Treatment of a complication resulting from a surgical procedure**
When the admission/encounter is for treatment of a complication resulting from a surgical procedure, designate the complication as the principal or first-listed diagnosis if treatment is directed at resolving the complication.

d. **Primary malignancy previously excised**
When a primary malignancy has been previously excised or eradicated from its site and there is no further treatment directed to that site and there is no evidence of any existing primary malignancy, a code from category Z85, Personal history of malignant neoplasm, should be used to indicate the former site of the malignancy. Any mention of extension, invasion, or metastasis to another site is coded as a secondary malignant neoplasm to that site. The secondary site may be the principal or first-listed with the Z85 code used as a secondary code.

e. **Admissions/Encounters involving chemotherapy, immunotherapy and radiation therapy**

1) **Episode of care involves surgical removal of neoplasm**
When an episode of care involves the surgical removal of a neoplasm, primary or secondary site, followed by adjunct chemotherapy or radiation treatment during the same episode of care, the code for the neoplasm should be assigned as principal or first-listed diagnosis.

2) **Patient admission/encounter solely for administration of chemotherapy, immunotherapy and radiation therapy**
If a patient admission/encounter is solely for the administration of chemotherapy, immunotherapy or radiation therapy assign code Z51.0, Encounter for antineoplastic radiation therapy, or Z51.11, Encounter for antineoplastic chemotherapy, or Z51.12, Encounter for antineoplastic immunotherapy as the first-listed or principal diagnosis. If a patient receives more than one of these therapies during the same admission more than one of these codes may be assigned, in any sequence.

The malignancy for which the therapy is being administered should be assigned as a secondary diagnosis.

3) **Patient admitted for radiation therapy, chemotherapy or immunotherapy and develops complications**
When a patient is admitted for the purpose of radiotherapy, immunotherapy or chemotherapy and develops complications such as uncontrolled nausea and vomiting or dehydration, the principal or first-listed diagnosis is Z51.0, Encounter for antineoplastic radiation therapy, or Z51.11, Encounter for antineoplastic chemotherapy, or Z51.12, Encounter for antineoplastic immunotherapy followed by any codes for the complications.

f. **Admission/encounter to determine extent of malignancy**
When the reason for admission/encounter is to determine the extent of the malignancy, or for a procedure such as paracentesis or thoracentesis, the primary malignancy or appropriate metastatic site is designated as the principal or first-listed diagnosis, even though chemotherapy or radiotherapy is administered.

g. **Symptoms, signs, and abnormal findings listed in Chapter 18 associated with neoplasms**
Symptoms, signs, and ill-defined conditions listed in Chapter 18 characteristic of, or associated with, an existing primary or secondary site malignancy cannot be used to replace the malignancy as principal or first-listed diagnosis, regardless of the number of admissions or encounters for treatment and care of the neoplasm.

See section I.C.21. Factors influencing health status and contact with health services, Encounter for prophylactic organ removal.

h. **Admission/encounter for pain control/management**
See Section I.C.6. for information on coding admission/encounter for pain control/management.

i. **Malignancy in two or more noncontiguous sites**
A patient may have more than one malignant tumor in the same organ. These tumors may represent different primaries or metastatic disease, depending on the site. Should the documentation be unclear, the provider should be queried as to the status of each tumor so that the correct codes can be assigned.

j. **Disseminated malignant neoplasm, unspecified**
Code C80.0, Disseminated malignant neoplasm, unspecified, is for use only in those cases where the patient has advanced metastatic disease and no known primary or secondary sites are specified. It should not be used in place of assigning codes for the primary site and all known secondary sites.

k. **Malignant neoplasm without specification of site**
Code C80.1, Malignant (primary) neoplasm, unspecified, equates to Cancer, unspecified. This code should only be used when no determination can be made as to the primary site of a malignancy. This code should rarely be used in the inpatient setting.

l. **Sequencing of neoplasm codes**

1) **Encounter for treatment of primary malignancy**
If the reason for the encounter is for treatment of a primary malignancy, assign the malignancy as the principal/first-listed diagnosis. The primary site is to be sequenced first, followed by any metastatic sites.

2) **Encounter for treatment of secondary malignancy**
When an encounter is for a primary malignancy with metastasis and treatment is directed toward the metastatic (secondary) site(s) only, the metastatic site(s) is designated as the principal/first-listed diagnosis. The primary malignancy is coded as an additional code.

3) **Malignant neoplasm in a pregnant patient**
When a pregnant woman has a malignant neoplasm, a code from subcategory O9A.1-, Malignant neoplasm complicating pregnancy, childbirth, and the puerperium, should be sequenced first, followed by the appropriate code from Chapter 2 to indicate the type of neoplasm.

4) **Encounter for complication associated with a neoplasm**
When an encounter is for management of a complication associated with a neoplasm, such as dehydration, and the treatment is only for the complication, the complication is coded first, followed by the appropriate code(s) for the neoplasm.

The exception to this guideline is anemia. When the admission/encounter is for management of an anemia associated with the malignancy, and the treatment is only for anemia, the appropriate code for the malignancy is sequenced as the principal or first-listed diagnosis followed by code D63.0, Anemia in neoplastic disease.

5) **Complication from surgical procedure for treatment of a neoplasm**
When an encounter is for treatment of a complication resulting from a surgical procedure performed for the treatment of the neoplasm, designate the complication as the principal/first-listed diagnosis. See guideline regarding the coding of a current malignancy versus personal history to determine if the code for the neoplasm should also be assigned.

6) Pathologic fracture due to a neoplasm

When an encounter is for a pathological fracture due to a neoplasm, and the focus of treatment is the fracture, a code from subcategory M84.5, Pathological fracture in neoplastic disease, should be sequenced first, followed by the code for the neoplasm.

If the focus of treatment is the neoplasm with an associated pathological fracture, the neoplasm code should be sequenced first, followed by a code from M84.5 for the pathological fracture.

m. Current malignancy versus personal history of malignancy

When a primary malignancy has been excised but further treatment, such as an additional surgery for the malignancy, radiation therapy or chemotherapy is directed to that site, the primary malignancy code should be used until treatment is completed.

When a primary malignancy has been previously excised or eradicated from its site, there is no further treatment (of the malignancy) directed to that site, and there is no evidence of any existing primary malignancy, a code from category Z85, Personal history of malignant neoplasm, should be used to indicate the former site of the malignancy.

See Section I.C.21. Factors influencing health status and contact with health services, History (of)

n. Leukemia, Multiple Myeloma, and Malignant Plasma Cell Neoplasms in remission versus personal history

The categories for leukemia, and category C90, Multiple myeloma and malignant plasma cell neoplasms, have codes indicating whether or not the leukemia has achieved remission. There are also codes Z85.6, Personal history of leukemia, and Z85.79, Personal history of other malignant neoplasms of lymphoid, hematopoietic and related tissues. If the documentation is unclear as to whether the leukemia has achieved remission, the provider should be queried.

See Section I.C.21. Factors influencing health status and contact with health services, History (of)

o. Aftercare following surgery for neoplasm

See Section I.C.21. Factors influencing health status and contact with health services, Aftercare

p. Follow-up care for completed treatment of a malignancy

See Section I.C.21. Factors influencing health status and contact with health services, Follow-up

q. Prophylactic organ removal for prevention of malignancy

See Section I.C. 21, Factors influencing health status and contact with health services, Prophylactic organ removal

r. Malignant neoplasm associated with transplanted organ

A malignant neoplasm of a transplanted organ should be coded as a transplant complication. Assign first the appropriate code from category T86.-, Complications of transplanted organs and tissue, followed by code C80.2, Malignant neoplasm associated with transplanted organ. Use an additional code for the specific malignancy.

3. Chapter 3: Disease of the blood and blood-forming organs and certain disorders involving the immune mechanism (D50-D89)

Reserved for future guideline expansion

4. Chapter 4: Endocrine, Nutritional, and Metabolic Diseases (E00-E89)

a. Diabetes mellitus

The diabetes mellitus codes are combination codes that include the type of diabetes mellitus, the body system affected, and the complications affecting that body system. As many codes within a particular category as are necessary to describe all of the complications of the disease may be used. They should be sequenced based on the reason for a particular encounter. Assign as many codes from categories E08 – E13 as needed to identify all of the associated conditions that the patient has.

1) Type of diabetes

The age of a patient is not the sole determining factor, though most type 1 diabetics develop the condition before reaching puberty. For this reason type 1 diabetes mellitus is also referred to as juvenile diabetes.

2) Type of diabetes mellitus not documented

If the type of diabetes mellitus is not documented in the medical record the default is E11.-, Type 2 diabetes mellitus.

3) Diabetes mellitus and the use of insulin and oral hypoglycemics

If the documentation in a medical record does not indicate the type of diabetes but does indicate that the patient uses insulin, code E11, Type 2 diabetes mellitus, should be assigned. Code Z79.4, Long-term (current) use of insulin, or Z79.84, Long term (current) use of oral hypoglycemic drugs, should also be assigned to indicate that the patient uses insulin or hypoglycemic drugs. Code Z79.4 should not be assigned if insulin is given temporarily to bring a type 2 patient's blood sugar under control during an encounter.

4) Diabetes mellitus in pregnancy and gestational diabetes

See Section I.C.15. Diabetes mellitus in pregnancy.

See Section I.C.15. Gestational (pregnancy induced) diabetes

5) Complications due to insulin pump malfunction

(a) Underdose of insulin due to insulin pump failure

An underdose of insulin due to an insulin pump failure should be assigned to a code from subcategory T85.6, Mechanical complication of other specified internal and external prosthetic devices, implants and grafts, that specifies the type of pump malfunction, as the principal or first-listed code, followed by code T38.3X6-, Underdosing of insulin and oral hypoglycemic [antidiabetic] drugs. Additional codes for the type of diabetes mellitus and any associated complications due to the underdosing should also be assigned.

(b) Overdose of insulin due to insulin pump failure

The principal or first-listed code for an encounter due to an insulin pump malfunction resulting in an overdose of insulin, should also be T85.6-, Mechanical complication of other specified internal and external prosthetic devices, implants and grafts, followed by code T38.3X1-, Poisoning by insulin and oral hypoglycemic [antidiabetic] drugs, accidental (unintentional).

6) Secondary diabetes mellitus

Codes under categories E08, Diabetes mellitus due to underlying condition, E09, Drug or chemical induced diabetes mellitus, and E13, Other specified diabetes mellitus, identify complications/manifestations associated with secondary diabetes mellitus. Secondary diabetes is always caused by another condition or event (e.g., cystic fibrosis, malignant neoplasm of pancreas, pancreatectomy, adverse effect of drug, or poisoning).

(a) Secondary diabetes mellitus and the use of insulin or hypoglycemic drugs

For patients who routinely use insulin or hypoglycemic drugs, code Z79.4, Long-term (current) use of insulin, or Z79.84, Long term (current) use of oral hypoglycemic drugs should also be assigned. Code Z79.4 should not be assigned if insulin is given temporarily to bring a patient's blood sugar under control during an encounter.

(b) Assigning and sequencing secondary diabetes codes and its causes

The sequencing of the secondary diabetes codes in relationship to codes for the cause of the diabetes is based on the Tabular List instructions for categories E08, E09 and E13.

(i) Secondary diabetes mellitus due to pancreatectomy

For postpancreatectomy diabetes mellitus (lack of insulin due to the surgical removal of all or part of the pancreas), assign code E89.1, Postprocedural hypoinsulinemia. Assign a code from category E13 and a code from subcategory Z90.41-, Acquired absence of pancreas, as additional codes.

(ii) Secondary diabetes due to drugs
Secondary diabetes may be caused by an adverse effect of correctly administered medications, poisoning or sequela of poisoning.
See section I.C.19.e for coding of adverse effects and poisoning, and section I.C.20 for external cause code reporting.

5. **Chapter 5: Mental, Behavioral and Neurodevelopmental disorders (F01-F99)**

a. **Pain disorders related to psychological factors**
Assign code F45.41, for pain that is exclusively related to psychological disorders. As indicated by the Excludes 1 note under category G89, a code from category G89 should not be assigned with code F45.41.

Code F45.42, Pain disorders with related psychological factors, should be used with a code from category G89, Pain, not elsewhere classified, if there is documentation of a psychological component for a patient with acute or chronic pain.

See Section I.C.6. Pain

b. **Mental and behavioral disorders due to psychoactive substance use**

1) **In Remission**
Selection of codes for "in remission" for categories F10-F19, Mental and behavioral disorders due to psychoactive substance use (categories F10-F19 with -.21) requires the provider's clinical judgment. The appropriate codes for "in remission" are assigned only on the basis of provider documentation (as defined in the Official Guidelines for Coding and Reporting).

2) **Psychoactive Substance Use, Abuse And Dependence**
When the provider documentation refers to use, abuse and dependence of the same substance (e.g. alcohol, opioid, cannabis, etc.), only one code should be assigned to identify the pattern of use based on the following hierarchy:

- If both use and abuse are documented, assign only the code for abuse
- If both abuse and dependence are documented, assign only the code for dependence
- If use, abuse and dependence are all documented, assign only the code for dependence
- If both use and dependence are documented, assign only the code for dependence.

3) **Psychoactive Substance Use**
As with all other diagnoses, the codes for psychoactive substance use (F10.9-, F11.9-, F12.9-, F13.9-, F14.9-, F15.9-, F16.9-) should only be assigned based on provider documentation and when they meet the definition of a reportable diagnosis (see Section III, Reporting Additional Diagnoses). The codes are to be used only when the psychoactive substance use is associated with a mental or behavioral disorder, and such a relationship is documented by the provider.

6. **Chapter 6: Diseases of the Nervous System (G00-G99)**

a. **Dominant/nondominant side**
Codes from category G81, Hemiplegia and hemiparesis, and subcategories G83.1, Monoplegia of lower limb, G83.2, Monoplegia of upper limb, and G83.3, Monoplegia, unspecified, identify whether the dominant or nondominant side is affected. Should the affected side be documented, but not specified as dominant or nondominant, and the classification system does not indicate a default, code selection is as follows:

- For ambidextrous patients, the default should be dominant.
- If the left side is affected, the default is non-dominant.
- If the right side is affected, the default is dominant.

b. **Pain - Category G89**

1) **General coding information**
Codes in category G89, Pain, not elsewhere classified, may be used in conjunction with codes from other categories and chapters to provide more detail about acute or chronic pain and neoplasm-related pain, unless otherwise indicated below.

If the pain is not specified as acute or chronic, post-thoracotomy, postprocedural, or neoplasm-related, do not assign codes from category G89.

A code from category G89 should not be assigned if the underlying (definitive) diagnosis is known, unless the reason for the encounter is pain control/ management and not management of the underlying condition.

When an admission or encounter is for a procedure aimed at treating the underlying condition (e.g., spinal fusion, kyphoplasty), a code for the underlying condition (e.g., vertebral fracture, spinal stenosis) should be assigned as the principal diagnosis. No code from category G89 should be assigned.

(a) **Category G89 Codes as Principal or First-Listed Diagnosis**
Category G89 codes are acceptable as principal diagnosis or the first-listed code:

- When pain control or pain management is the reason for the admission/encounter (e.g., a patient with displaced intervertebral disc, nerve impingement and severe back pain presents for injection of steroid into the spinal canal). The underlying cause of the pain should be reported as an additional diagnosis, if known.
- When a patient is admitted for the insertion of a neurostimulator for pain control, assign the appropriate pain code as the principal or first-listed diagnosis. When an admission or encounter is for a procedure aimed at treating the underlying condition and a neurostimulator is inserted for pain control during the same admission/encounter, a code for the underlying condition should be assigned as the principal diagnosis and the appropriate pain code should be assigned as a secondary diagnosis.

(b) **Use of Category G89 Codes in Conjunction with Site Specific Pain Codes**

(i) **Assigning Category G89 and Site-Specific Pain Codes**
Codes from category G89 may be used In conjunction with codes that identify the site of pain (including codes from chapter 18) if the category G89 code provides additional information. For example, if the code describes the site of the pain, but does not fully describe whether the pain is acute or chronic, then both codes should be assigned.

(ii) **Sequencing of Category G89 Codes with Site-Specific Pain Codes**
The sequencing of category G89 codes with site-specific pain codes (including chapter 18 codes), is dependent on the circumstances of the encounter/admission as follows:

- If the encounter is for pain control or pain management, assign the code from category G89 followed by the code identifying the specific site of pain (e.g., encounter for pain management for acute neck pain from trauma is assigned code G89.11, Acute pain due to trauma, followed by code M54.2, Cervicalgia, to identify the site of pain).
- If the encounter is for any other reason except pain control or pain management, and a related definitive diagnosis has not been established (confirmed) by the provider, assign the code for the specific site of pain first, followed by the appropriate code from category G89.

2) **Pain due to devices, implants and grafts**
See Section I.C.19. Pain due to medical devices

3) **Postoperative Pain**
The provider's documentation should be used to guide the coding of postoperative pain, as well as *Section III. Reporting Additional Diagnoses* and *Section IV. Diagnostic Coding and Reporting in the Outpatient Setting.*

The default for post-thoracotomy and other postoperative pain not specified as acute or chronic is the code for the acute form.

Routine or expected postoperative pain immediately after surgery should not be coded.

(a) **Postoperative pain not associated with specific postoperative complication**
Postoperative pain not associated with a specific postoperative complication is assigned to the appropriate postoperative pain code in category G89.

(b) **Postoperative pain associated with specific postoperative complication**
Postoperative pain associated with a specific postoperative complication (such as painful wire sutures) is assigned to the appropriate code(s) found in Chapter 19, Injury, poisoning, and certain other consequences of external causes. If appropriate, use additional code(s) from category G89 to identify acute or chronic pain (G89.18 or G89.28).

4) **Chronic pain**
Chronic pain is classified to subcategory G89.2. There is no time frame defining when pain becomes chronic pain. The provider's documentation should be used to guide use of these codes.

5) **Neoplasm Related Pain**
Code G89.3 is assigned to pain documented as being related, associated or due to cancer, primary or secondary malignancy, or tumor. This code is assigned regardless of whether the pain is acute or chronic.

This code may be assigned as the principal or first-listed code when the stated reason for the admission/encounter is documented as pain control/pain management. The underlying neoplasm should be reported as an additional diagnosis.

When the reason for the admission/encounter is management of the neoplasm and the pain associated with the neoplasm is also documented, code G89.3 may be assigned as an additional diagnosis. It is not necessary to assign an additional code for the site of the pain.

See Section I.C.2 for instructions on the sequencing of neoplasms for all other stated reasons for the admission/encounter (except for pain control/pain management).

6) **Chronic pain syndrome**
Central pain syndrome (G89.0) and chronic pain syndrome (G89.4) are different than the term "chronic pain," and therefore codes should only be used when the provider has specifically documented this condition.

See Section I.C.5. Pain disorders related to psychological factors

7. **Chapter 7: Diseases of the Eye and Adnexa (H00-H59)**
a. **Glaucoma**
1) **Assigning Glaucoma Codes**
Assign as many codes from category H40, Glaucoma, as needed to identify the type of glaucoma, the affected eye, and the glaucoma stage.

2) **Bilateral glaucoma with same type and stage**
When a patient has bilateral glaucoma and both eyes are documented as being the same type and stage, and there is a code for bilateral glaucoma, report only the code for the type of glaucoma, bilateral, with the seventh character for the stage.

When a patient has bilateral glaucoma and both eyes are documented as being the same type and stage, and the classification does not provide a code for bilateral glaucoma (i.e. subcategories H40.10, H40.11 and H40.20) report only one code for the type of glaucoma with the appropriate seventh character for the stage.

3) **Bilateral glaucoma stage with different types or stages**
When a patient has bilateral glaucoma and each eye is documented as having a different type or stage, and the classification distinguishes laterality, assign the appropriate code for each eye rather than the code for bilateral glaucoma.

When a patient has bilateral glaucoma and each eye is documented as having a different type, and the classification does not distinguish laterality (i.e. subcategories H40.10, H40.11 and H40.20), assign one code for each type of glaucoma with the appropriate seventh character for the stage.

When a patient has bilateral glaucoma and each eye is documented as having the same type, but different stage, and the classification does not distinguish laterality (i.e. subcategories H40.10, H40.11 and H40.20), assign a code for the type of glaucoma for each eye with the seventh character for the specific glaucoma stage documented for each eye.

4) **Patient admitted with glaucoma and stage evolves during the admission**
If a patient is admitted with glaucoma and the stage progresses during the admission, assign the code for highest stage documented.

5) **Indeterminate stage glaucoma**
Assignment of the seventh character "4" for "indeterminate stage" should be based on the clinical documentation. The seventh character "4" is used for glaucomas whose stage cannot be clinically determined. This seventh character should not be confused with the seventh character "0", unspecified, which should be assigned when there is no documentation regarding the stage of the glaucoma.

8. **Chapter 8: Diseases of the Ear and Mastoid Process (H60-H95)**
Reserved for future guideline expansion

9. **Chapter 9: Diseases of the Circulatory System (I00-I99)**
a. **Hypertension**
The classification presumes a causal relationship between hypertension and heart involvement and between hypertension and kidney involvement, as the two conditions are linked by the term "with" in the Alphabetic Index. These conditions should be coded as related even in the absence of provider documentation explicitly linking them, unless the documentation clearly states the conditions are unrelated.

For hypertension and conditions not specifically linked by relational terms such as "with," "associated with" or "due to" in the classification, provider documentation must link the conditions in order to code them as related.

1) **Hypertension with Heart Disease**
Hypertension with heart conditions classified to I50.- or I51.4-I51.9, are assigned to a code from category I11, Hypertensive heart disease. Use an additional code from category I50, Heart failure, to identify the type of heart failure in those patients with heart failure.

The same heart conditions (I50.-, I51.4-I51.9) with hypertension are coded separately if the provider has specifically documented a different cause. Sequence according to the circumstances of the admission/encounter.

2) **Hypertensive Chronic Kidney Disease**
Assign codes from category I12, Hypertensive chronic kidney disease, when both hypertension and a condition classifiable to category N18, Chronic kidney disease (CKD), are present. CKD should not be coded as hypertensive if the physician has specifically documented a different cause.

The appropriate code from category N18 should be used as a secondary code with a code from category I12 to identify the stage of chronic kidney disease.

See Section I.C.14. Chronic kidney disease.

If a patient has hypertensive chronic kidney disease and acute renal failure, an additional code for the acute renal failure is required.

3) **Hypertensive Heart and Chronic Kidney Disease**
Assign codes from combination category I13, Hypertensive heart and chronic kidney disease, when there is hypertension with both heart and kidney involvement. If heart failure is present, assign an additional code from category I50 to identify the type of heart failure.

The appropriate code from category N18, Chronic kidney disease, should be used as a secondary code with a code from category I13 to identify the stage of chronic kidney disease.

See Section I.C.14. Chronic kidney disease.

The codes in category I13, Hypertensive heart and chronic kidney disease, are combination codes that include hypertension, heart disease and chronic kidney disease. The

Includes note at I13 specifies that the conditions included at I11 and I12 are included together in I13. If a patient has hypertension, heart disease and chronic kidney disease, then a code from I13 should be used, not individual codes for hypertension, heart disease and chronic kidney disease, or codes from I11 or I12.

For patients with both acute renal failure and chronic kidney disease, an additional code for acute renal failure is required.

4) Hypertensive Cerebrovascular Disease
For hypertensive cerebrovascular disease, first assign the appropriate code from categories I60-I69, followed by the appropriate hypertension code.

5) Hypertensive Retinopathy
Subcategory H35.0, Background retinopathy and retinal vascular changes, should be used with a code from category I10 – I15, Hypertensive disease to include the systemic hypertension. The sequencing is based on the reason for the encounter.

6) Hypertension, Secondary
Secondary hypertension is due to an underlying condition. Two codes are required: one to identify the underlying etiology and one from category I15 to identify the hypertension. Sequencing of codes is determined by the reason for admission/encounter.

7) Hypertension, Transient
Assign code R03.0, Elevated blood pressure reading without diagnosis of hypertension, unless patient has an established diagnosis of hypertension. Assign code O13.-, Gestational [pregnancy-induced] hypertension without significant proteinuria, or O14.-, Pre-eclampsia, for transient hypertension of pregnancy.

8) Hypertension, Controlled
This diagnostic statement usually refers to an existing state of hypertension under control by therapy. Assign the appropriate code from categories I10-I15, Hypertensive diseases.

9) Hypertension, Uncontrolled
Uncontrolled hypertension may refer to untreated hypertension or hypertension not responding to current therapeutic regimen. In either case, assign the appropriate code from categories I10-I15, Hypertensive diseases.

10) Hypertensive Crisis
Assign a code from category I16, Hypertensive crisis, for documented hypertensive urgency, hypertensive emergency or unspecified hypertensive crisis. Code also any identified hypertensive disease (I10-I15). The sequencing is based on the reason for the encounter.

b. Atherosclerotic Coronary Artery Disease and Angina
ICD-10-CM has combination codes for atherosclerotic heart disease with angina pectoris. The subcategories for these codes are I25.11, Atherosclerotic heart disease of native coronary artery with angina pectoris and I25.7, Atherosclerosis of coronary artery bypass graft(s) and coronary artery of transplanted heart with angina pectoris.

When using one of these combination codes it is not necessary to use an additional code for angina pectoris. A causal relationship can be assumed in a patient with both atherosclerosis and angina pectoris, unless the documentation indicates the angina is due to something other than the atherosclerosis.

If a patient with coronary artery disease is admitted due to an acute myocardial infarction (AMI), the AMI should be sequenced before the coronary artery disease.

See Section I.C.9. Acute myocardial infarction (AMI)

c. Intraoperative and Postprocedural Cerebrovascular Accident
Medical record documentation should clearly specify the cause-and-effect relationship between the medical intervention and the cerebrovascular accident in order to assign a code for intraoperative or postprocedural cerebrovascular accident.

Proper code assignment depends on whether it was an infarction or hemorrhage and whether it occurred intraoperatively or postoperatively. If it was a cerebral hemorrhage, code assignment depends on the type of procedure performed.

d. Sequelae of Cerebrovascular Disease
1) Category I69, Sequelae of Cerebrovascular disease
Category I69 is used to indicate conditions classifiable to categories I60-I67 as the causes of sequela (neurologic deficits), themselves classified elsewhere. These "late effects" include neurologic deficits that persist after initial onset of conditions classifiable to categories I60-I67. The neurologic deficits caused by cerebrovascular disease may be present from the onset or may arise at any time after the onset of the condition classifiable to categories I60-I67.

Codes from category I69, Sequelae of cerebrovascular disease, that specify hemiplegia, hemiparesis and monoplegia identify whether the dominant or nondominant side is affected. Should the affected side be documented, but not specified as dominant or nondominant, and the classification system does not indicate a default, code selection is as follows:

- For ambidextrous patients, the default should be dominant.
- If the left side is affected, the default is non-dominant.
- If the right side is affected, the default is dominant.

2) Codes from category I69 with codes from I60-I67
Codes from category I69 may be assigned on a health care record with codes from I60-I67, if the patient has a current cerebrovascular disease and deficits from an old cerebrovascular disease.

3) Codes from category I69 and Personal history of transient ischemic attack (TIA) and cerebral infarction (Z86.73)
Codes from category I69 should not be assigned if the patient does not have neurologic deficits.

See Section I.C.21. 4. History (of) for use of personal history codes

e. Acute myocardial infarction (AMI)
1) ST elevation myocardial infarction (STEMI) and non ST elevation myocardial infarction (NSTEMI)
The ICD-10-CM codes for acute myocardial infarction (AMI) identify the site, such as anterolateral wall or true posterior wall. Subcategories I21.0-I21.2 and code I21.3 are used for ST elevation myocardial infarction (STEMI). Code I21.4, Non-ST elevation (NSTEMI) myocardial infarction, is used for non ST elevation myocardial infarction (NSTEMI) and nontransmural MIs.

If NSTEMI evolves to STEMI, assign the STEMI code. If STEMI converts to NSTEMI due to thrombolytic therapy, it is still coded as STEMI.

For encounters occurring while the myocardial infarction is equal to, or less than, four weeks old, including transfers to another acute setting or a postacute setting, and the myocardial infarction meets the definition for "other diagnoses" (see Section III, Reporting Additional Diagnoses), codes from category I21 may continue to be reported. For encounters after the 4 week time frame and the patient is still receiving care related to the myocardial infarction, the appropriate aftercare code should be assigned, rather than a code from category I21. For old or healed myocardial infarctions not requiring further care, code I25.2, Old myocardial infarction, may be assigned.

2) Acute myocardial infarction, unspecified
Code I21.3, ST elevation (STEMI) myocardial infarction of unspecified site, is the default for unspecified acute myocardial infarction. If only STEMI or transmural MI without the site is documented, assign code I21.3.

3) AMI documented as nontransmural or subendocardial but site provided
If an AMI is documented as nontransmural or subendocardial, but the site is provided, it is still coded as a subendocardial AMI.

See Section I.C.21.3 for information on coding status post administration of tPA in a different facility within the last 24 hours.

4) Subsequent acute myocardial infarction
A code from category I22, Subsequent ST elevation (STEMI) and non ST elevation (NSTEMI) myocardial infarction, is to be used when a patient who has suffered an AMI has a new AMI within the 4 week time frame of the initial AMI. A code from category I22 must be used in conjunction with a code from category I21.

The sequencing of the I22 and I21 codes depends on the circumstances of the encounter.

10. Chapter 10: Diseases of the Respiratory System (J00-J99)

a. Chronic Obstructive Pulmonary Disease [COPD] and Asthma

1) Acute exacerbation of chronic obstructive bronchitis and asthma

The codes in categories J44 and J45 distinguish between uncomplicated cases and those in acute exacerbation. An acute exacerbation is a worsening or a decompensation of a chronic condition. An acute exacerbation is not equivalent to an infection superimposed on a chronic condition, though an exacerbation may be triggered by an infection.

b. Acute Respiratory Failure

1) Acute respiratory failure as principal diagnosis

A code from subcategory J96.0, Acute respiratory failure, or subcategory J96.2, Acute and chronic respiratory failure, may be assigned as a principal diagnosis when it is the condition established after study to be chiefly responsible for occasioning the admission to the hospital, and the selection is supported by the Alphabetic Index and Tabular List. However, chapter-specific coding guidelines (such as obstetrics, poisoning, HIV, newborn) that provide sequencing direction take precedence.

2) Acute respiratory failure as secondary diagnosis

Respiratory failure may be listed as a secondary diagnosis if it occurs after admission, or if it is present on admission, but does not meet the definition of principal diagnosis.

3) Sequencing of acute respiratory failure and another acute condition

When a patient is admitted with respiratory failure and another acute condition, (e.g., myocardial infarction, cerebrovascular accident, aspiration pneumonia), the principal diagnosis will not be the same in every situation. This applies whether the other acute condition is a respiratory or nonrespiratory condition. Selection of the principal diagnosis will be dependent on the circumstances of admission. If both the respiratory failure and the other acute condition are equally responsible for occasioning the admission to the hospital, and there are no chapter-specific sequencing rules, the guideline regarding two or more diagnoses that equally meet the definition for principal diagnosis *(Section II, C.)* may be applied in these situations.

If the documentation is not clear as to whether acute respiratory failure and another condition are equally responsible for occasioning the admission, query the provider for clarification.

c. Influenza due to certain identified influenza viruses

Code only confirmed cases of influenza due to certain identified influenza viruses (category J09), and due to other identified influenza virus (category J10). This is an exception to the hospital inpatient guideline Section II, H. (Uncertain Diagnosis).

In this context, "confirmation" does not require documentation of positive laboratory testing specific for avian or other novel influenza A or other identified influenza virus. However, coding should be based on the provider's diagnostic statement that the patient has avian influenza, or other novel influenza A, for category J09, or has another particular identified strain of influenza, such as H1N1 or H3N2, but not identified as novel or variant, for category J10.

If the provider records "suspected" or "possible" or "probable" avian influenza, or novel influenza, or other identified influenza, then the appropriate influenza code from category J11, Influenza due to unidentified influenza virus, should be assigned. A code from category J09, Influenza due to certain identified influenza viruses, should not be assigned nor should a code from category J10, Influenza due to other identified influenza virus.

d. Ventilator associated Pneumonia

1) Documentation of Ventilator associated Pneumonia

As with all procedural or postprocedural complications, code assignment is based on the provider's documentation of the relationship between the condition and the procedure.

Code J95.851, Ventilator associated pneumonia, should be assigned only when the provider has documented ventilator

associated pneumonia (VAP). An additional code to identify the organism (e.g., Pseudomonas aeruginosa, code B96.5) should also be assigned. Do not assign an additional code from categories J12-J18 to identify the type of pneumonia.

Code J95.851 should not be assigned for cases where the patient has pneumonia and is on a mechanical ventilator and the provider has not specifically stated that the pneumonia is ventilator-associated pneumonia. If the documentation is unclear as to whether the patient has a pneumonia that is a complication attributable to the mechanical ventilator, query the provider.

2) Ventilator associated Pneumonia Develops after Admission

A patient may be admitted with one type of pneumonia (e.g., code J13, Pneumonia due to Streptococcus pneumonia) and subsequently develop VAP. In this instance, the principal diagnosis would be the appropriate code from categories J12-J18 for the pneumonia diagnosed at the time of admission. Code J95.851, Ventilator associated pneumonia, would be assigned as an additional diagnosis when the provider has also documented the presence of ventilator associated pneumonia.

11. Chapter 11: Diseases of the Digestive System (K00-K95)

Reserved for future guideline expansion

12. Chapter 12: Diseases of the Skin and Subcutaneous Tissue (L00-L99)

a. Pressure ulcer stage codes

1) Pressure ulcer stages

Codes from category L89, Pressure ulcer, identify the site of the pressure ulcer as well as the stage of the ulcer.

The ICD-10-CM classifies pressure ulcer stages based on severity, which is designated by stages 1-4, unspecified stage and unstageable.

Assign as many codes from category L89 as needed to identify all the pressure ulcers the patient has, if applicable.

2) Unstageable pressure ulcers

Assignment of the code for unstageable pressure ulcer (L89.--0) should be based on the clinical documentation. These codes are used for pressure ulcers whose stage cannot be clinically determined (e.g., the ulcer is covered by eschar or has been treated with a skin or muscle graft) and pressure ulcers that are documented as deep tissue injury but not documented as due to trauma. This code should not be confused with the codes for unspecified stage (L89.--9). When there is no documentation regarding the stage of the pressure ulcer, assign the appropriate code for unspecified stage (L89.--9).

3) Documented pressure ulcer stage

Assignment of the pressure ulcer stage code should be guided by clinical documentation of the stage or documentation of the terms found in the Alphabetic Index. For clinical terms describing the stage that are not found in the Alphabetic Index, and there is no documentation of the stage, the provider should be queried.

4) Patients admitted with pressure ulcers documented as healed

No code is assigned if the documentation states that the pressure ulcer is completely healed.

5) Patients admitted with pressure ulcers documented as healing

Pressure ulcers described as healing should be assigned the appropriate pressure ulcer stage code based on the documentation in the medical record. If the documentation does not provide information about the stage of the healing pressure ulcer, assign the appropriate code for unspecified stage.

If the documentation is unclear as to whether the patient has a current (new) pressure ulcer or if the patient is being treated for a healing pressure ulcer, query the provider.

For ulcers that were present on admission but healed at the time of discharge, assign the code for the site and stage of the pressure ulcer at the time of admission.

6) Patient admitted with pressure ulcer evolving into another stage during the admission

If a patient is admitted with a pressure ulcer at one stage and it progresses to a higher stage, two separate codes should be assigned: one code for the site and stage of the ulcer on admission and a second code for the same ulcer site and the highest stage reported during the stay.

13. Chapter 13: Diseases of the Musculoskeletal System and Connective Tissue (M00-M99)

a. Site and laterality

Most of the codes within Chapter 13 have site and laterality designations. The site represents the bone, joint or the muscle involved. For some conditions where more than one bone, joint or muscle is usually involved, such as osteoarthritis, there is a "multiple sites" code available. For categories where no multiple site code is provided and more than one bone, joint or muscle is involved, multiple codes should be used to indicate the different sites involved.

1) Bone versus joint

For certain conditions, the bone may be affected at the upper or lower end, (e.g., avascular necrosis of bone, M87, Osteoporosis, M80, M81). Though the portion of the bone affected may be at the joint, the site designation will be the bone, not the joint.

b. Acute traumatic versus chronic or recurrent musculoskeletal conditions

Many musculoskeletal conditions are a result of previous injury or trauma to a site, or are recurrent conditions. Bone, joint or muscle conditions that are the result of a healed injury are usually found in chapter 13. Recurrent bone, joint or muscle conditions are also usually found in chapter 13. Any current, acute injury should be coded to the appropriate injury code from chapter 19. Chronic or recurrent conditions should generally be coded with a code from chapter 13. If it is difficult to determine from the documentation in the record which code is best to describe a condition, query the provider.

c. Coding of Pathologic Fractures

7th character A is for use as long as the patient is receiving active treatment for the fracture. While the patient may be seen by a new or different provider over the course of treatment for a pathological fracture, assignment of the 7th character is based on whether the patient is undergoing active treatment and not whether the provider is seeing the patient for the first time.

7th character D is to be used for encounters after the patient has completed active treatment. The other 7th characters, listed under each subcategory in the Tabular List, are to be used for subsequent encounters for routine care of fractures during the healing and recovery phase as well as treatment of problems associated with the healing, such as malunions, nonunions, and sequelae.

Care for complications of surgical treatment for fracture repairs during the healing or recovery phase should be coded with the appropriate complication codes.

See Section I.C.19. Coding of traumatic fractures.

d. Osteoporosis

Osteoporosis is a systemic condition, meaning that all bones of the musculoskeletal system are affected. Therefore, site is not a component of the codes under category M81, Osteoporosis without current pathological fracture. The site codes under category M80, Osteoporosis with current pathological fracture, identify the site of the fracture, not the osteoporosis.

1) Osteoporosis without pathological fracture

Category M81, Osteoporosis without current pathological fracture, is for use for patients with osteoporosis who do not currently have a pathologic fracture due to the osteoporosis, even if they have had a fracture in the past. For patients with a history of osteoporosis fractures, status code Z87.310, Personal history of (healed) osteoporosis fracture, should follow the code from M81.

2) Osteoporosis with current pathological fracture

Category M80, Osteoporosis with current pathological fracture, is for patients who have a current pathologic fracture at the time of an encounter. The codes under M80 identify the site of the fracture. A code from category M80, not a traumatic fracture code, should be used for any patient with known osteoporosis who suffers a fracture, even if the patient had a minor fall or trauma, if that fall or trauma would not usually break a normal, healthy bone.

14. Chapter 14: Diseases of Genitourinary System (N00-N99)

a. Chronic kidney disease

1) Stages of chronic kidney disease (CKD)

The ICD-10-CM classifies CKD based on severity. The severity of CKD is designated by stages 1-5. Stage 2, code N18.2, equates to mild CKD; stage 3, code N18.3, equates to moderate CKD; and stage 4, code N18.4, equates to severe CKD. Code N18.6, End stage renal disease (ESRD), is assigned when the provider has documented end-stage-renal disease (ESRD).

If both a stage of CKD and ESRD are documented, assign code N18.6 only.

2) Chronic kidney disease and kidney transplant status

Patients who have undergone kidney transplant may still have some form of chronic kidney disease (CKD) because the kidney transplant may not fully restore kidney function. Therefore, the presence of CKD alone does not constitute a transplant complication. Assign the appropriate N18 code for the patient's stage of CKD and code Z94.0, Kidney transplant status. If a transplant complication such as failure or rejection or other transplant complication is documented, see section I.C.19.g for information on coding complications of a kidney transplant. If the documentation is unclear as to whether the patient has a complication of the transplant, query the provider.

3) Chronic kidney disease with other conditions

Patients with CKD may also suffer from other serious conditions, most commonly diabetes mellitus and hypertension. The sequencing of the CKD code in relationship to codes for other contributing conditions is based on the conventions in the Tabular List.

See I.C.9. Hypertensive chronic kidney disease.

See I.C.19. Chronic kidney disease and kidney transplant complications.

15. Chapter 15: Pregnancy, Childbirth, and the Puerperium (O00-O9A)

a. General Rules for Obstetric Cases

1) Codes from chapter 15 and sequencing priority

Obstetric cases require codes from chapter 15, codes in the range O00-O9A, Pregnancy, Childbirth, and the Puerperium. Chapter 15 codes have sequencing priority over codes from other chapters. Additional codes from other chapters may be used in conjunction with chapter 15 codes to further specify conditions. Should the provider document that the pregnancy is incidental to the encounter, then code Z33.1, Pregnant state, incidental, should be used in place of any chapter 15 codes. It is the provider's responsibility to state that the condition being treated is not affecting the pregnancy.

2) Chapter 15 codes used only on the maternal record

Chapter 15 codes are to be used only on the maternal record, never on the record of the newborn.

3) Final character for trimester

The majority of codes in Chapter 15 have a final character indicating the trimester of pregnancy. The timeframes for the trimesters are indicated at the beginning of the chapter. If trimester is not a component of a code, it is because the condition always occurs in a specific trimester, or the concept of trimester of pregnancy is not applicable. Certain codes have characters for only certain trimesters because the condition does not occur in all trimesters, but it may occur in more than just one. Assignment of the final character for trimester should be based on the provider's documentation of the trimester (or number of weeks) for the current admission/encounter. This applies to the assignment of trimester for pre-existing conditions as well as those that develop during or are due to the pregnancy. The provider's documentation of the number of weeks may be used to assign the appropriate code identifying the trimester.

Whenever delivery occurs during the current admission, and there is an "in childbirth" option for the obstetric complication being coded, the "in childbirth" code should be assigned.

4) Selection of trimester for inpatient admissions that encompass more than one trimester

In instances when a patient is admitted to a hospital for complications of pregnancy during one trimester and remains in the hospital into a subsequent trimester, the trimester character for the antepartum complication code should be assigned on the basis of the trimester when the complication developed, not the trimester of the discharge. If the condition developed prior to the current admission/encounter or represents a pre-existing condition, the trimester character for the trimester at the time of the admission/encounter should be assigned.

5) Unspecified trimester

Each category that includes codes for trimester has a code for "unspecified trimester." The "unspecified trimester" code should rarely be used, such as when the documentation in the record is insufficient to determine the trimester and it is not possible to obtain clarification.

6) 7th character for Fetus Identification

Where applicable, a 7th character is to be assigned for certain categories (O31, O32, O33.3 - O33.6, O35, O36, O40, O41, O60.1, O60.2, O64, and O69) to identify the fetus for which the complication code applies.

Assign 7th character "0":

- For single gestations
- When the documentation in the record is insufficient to determine the fetus affected and it is not possible to obtain clarification.
- When it is not possible to clinically determine which fetus is affected.

b. Selection of OB Principal or First-listed Diagnosis

1) Routine outpatient prenatal visits

For routine outpatient prenatal visits when no complications are present, a code from category Z34, Encounter for supervision of normal pregnancy, should be used as the first-listed diagnosis. These codes should not be used in conjunction with chapter 15 codes.

2) Supervision of High-Risk Pregnancy

Codes from category O09, Supervision of high-risk pregnancy, are intended for use only during the prenatal period. For complications during the labor or delivery episode as a result of a high-risk pregnancy, assign the applicable complication codes from Chapter 15. If there are no complications during the labor or delivery episode, assign code O80, Encounter for full-term uncomplicated delivery.

For routine prenatal outpatient visits for patients with high-risk pregnancies, a code from category O09, Supervision of high-risk pregnancy, should be used as the first-listed diagnosis. Secondary chapter 15 codes may be used in conjunction with these codes if appropriate.

3) Episodes when no delivery occurs

In episodes when no delivery occurs, the principal diagnosis should correspond to the principal complication of the pregnancy which necessitated the encounter. Should more than one complication exist, all of which are treated or monitored, any of the complications codes may be sequenced first.

4) When a delivery occurs

When an obstetric patient is admitted and delivers during that admission, the condition that prompted the admission should be sequenced as the principal diagnosis. If multiple conditions prompted the admission, sequence the one most related to the delivery as the principal diagnosis. A code for any complication of the delivery should be assigned as an additional diagnosis. In cases of cesarean delivery, if the patient was admitted with a condition that resulted in the performance of a cesarean procedure, that condition should be selected as the principal diagnosis. If the reason for the admission was unrelated to the condition resulting in the cesarean delivery, the condition related to the reason for the admission should be selected as the principal diagnosis.

5) Outcome of delivery

A code from category Z37, Outcome of delivery, should be included on every maternal record when a delivery has occurred. These codes are not to be used on subsequent records or on the newborn record.

c. Pre-existing conditions versus conditions due to the pregnancy

Certain categories in Chapter 15 distinguish between conditions of the mother that existed prior to pregnancy (pre-existing) and those that are a direct result of pregnancy. When assigning codes from Chapter 15, it is important to assess if a condition was pre-existing prior to pregnancy or developed during or due to the pregnancy in order to assign the correct code.

Categories that do not distinguish between pre-existing and pregnancy-related conditions may be used for either. It is acceptable to use codes specifically for the puerperium with codes complicating pregnancy and childbirth if a condition arises postpartum during the delivery encounter.

d. Pre-existing hypertension in pregnancy

Category O10, Pre-existing hypertension complicating pregnancy, childbirth and the puerperium, includes codes for hypertensive heart and hypertensive chronic kidney disease. When assigning one of the O10 codes that includes hypertensive heart disease or hypertensive chronic kidney disease, it is necessary to add a secondary code from the appropriate hypertension category to specify the type of heart failure or chronic kidney disease.

See Section I.C.9. Hypertension.

e. Fetal Conditions Affecting the Management of the Mother

1) Codes from categories O35 and O36

Codes from categories O35, Maternal care for known or suspected fetal abnormality and damage, and O36, Maternal care for other fetal problems, are assigned only when the fetal condition is actually responsible for modifying the management of the mother, i.e., by requiring diagnostic studies, additional observation, special care, or termination of pregnancy. The fact that the fetal condition exists does not justify assigning a code from this series to the mother's record.

2) In utero surgery

In cases when surgery is performed on the fetus, a diagnosis code from category O35, Maternal care for known or suspected fetal abnormality and damage, should be assigned identifying the fetal condition. Assign the appropriate procedure code for the procedure performed.

No code from Chapter 16, the perinatal codes, should be used on the mother's record to identify fetal conditions. Surgery performed in utero on a fetus is still to be coded as an obstetric encounter.

f. HIV Infection in Pregnancy, Childbirth and the Puerperium

During pregnancy, childbirth or the puerperium, a patient admitted because of an HIV-related illness should receive a principal diagnosis from subcategory O98.7-, Human immunodeficiency [HIV] disease complicating pregnancy, childbirth and the puerperium, followed by the code(s) for the HIV-related illness(es).

Patients with asymptomatic HIV infection status admitted during pregnancy, childbirth, or the puerperium should receive codes of O98.7- and Z21, Asymptomatic human immunodeficiency virus [HIV] infection status.

g. Diabetes mellitus in pregnancy

Diabetes mellitus is a significant complicating factor in pregnancy. Pregnant women who are diabetic should be assigned a code from category O24, Diabetes mellitus in pregnancy, childbirth, and the puerperium, first, followed by the appropriate diabetes code(s) (E08-E13) from Chapter 4.

h. Long term use of insulin and oral hypoglycemics

Code Z79.4, Long-term (current) use of insulin, or code Z79.84, Long-term (current) use of oral hypoglycemic drugs, should also be assigned if the diabetes mellitus is being treated with insulin or oral medications. If the patient is treated with both oral medications and insulin, only the code for insulin-controlled should be assigned.

i. **Gestational (pregnancy induced) diabetes**
    Gestational (pregnancy induced) diabetes can occur during the second and third trimester of pregnancy in women who were not diabetic prior to pregnancy. Gestational diabetes can cause complications in the pregnancy similar to those of pre-existing diabetes mellitus. It also puts the woman at greater risk of developing diabetes after the pregnancy. Codes for gestational diabetes are in subcategory O24.4, Gestational diabetes mellitus. No other code from category O24, Diabetes mellitus in pregnancy, childbirth, and the puerperium, should be used with a code from O24.4.

    The codes under subcategory O24.4 include diet controlled, insulin controlled, and controlled by oral hypoglycemic drugs. If a patient with gestational diabetes is treated with both diet and insulin, only the code for insulin-controlled is required. If a patient with gestational diabetes is treated with both diet and oral hypoglycemic medications, only the code for "controlled by oral hypoglycemic drugs" is required. Code Z79.4, Long-term (current) use of insulin or code Z79.84, Long-term (current) use of oral hypoglycemic drugs, should not be assigned with codes from subcategory O24.4.

    An abnormal glucose tolerance in pregnancy is assigned a code from subcategory O99.81, Abnormal glucose complicating pregnancy, childbirth, and the puerperium.

j. **Sepsis and septic shock complicating abortion, pregnancy, childbirth and the puerperium**
    When assigning a chapter 15 code for sepsis complicating abortion, pregnancy, childbirth, and the puerperium, a code for the specific type of infection should be assigned as an additional diagnosis. If severe sepsis is present, a code from subcategory R65.2, Severe sepsis, and code(s) for associated organ dysfunction(s) should also be assigned as additional diagnoses.

k. **Puerperal sepsis**
    Code O85, Puerperal sepsis, should be assigned with a secondary code to identify the causal organism (e.g., for a bacterial infection, assign a code from category B95-B96, Bacterial infections in conditions classified elsewhere). A code from category A40, Streptococcal sepsis, or A41, Other sepsis, should not be used for puerperal sepsis. If applicable, use additional codes to identify severe sepsis (R65.2-) and any associated acute organ dysfunction.

l. **Alcohol and tobacco use during pregnancy, childbirth and the puerperium**
    1) **Alcohol use during pregnancy, childbirth and the puerperium**
        Codes under subcategory O99.31, Alcohol use complicating pregnancy, childbirth, and the puerperium, should be assigned for any pregnancy case when a mother uses alcohol during the pregnancy or postpartum. A secondary code from category F10, Alcohol related disorders, should also be assigned to identify manifestations of the alcohol use.

    2) **Tobacco use during pregnancy, childbirth and the puerperium**
        Codes under subcategory O99.33, Smoking (tobacco) complicating pregnancy, childbirth, and the puerperium, should be assigned for any pregnancy case when a mother uses any type of tobacco product during the pregnancy or postpartum. A secondary code from category F17, Nicotine dependence, should also be assigned to identify the type of nicotine dependence.

m. **Poisoning, toxic effects, adverse effects and underdosing in a pregnant patient**
    A code from subcategory O9A.2, Injury, poisoning and certain other consequences of external causes complicating pregnancy, childbirth, and the puerperium, should be sequenced first, followed by the appropriate injury, poisoning, toxic effect, adverse effect or underdosing code, and then the additional code(s) that specifies the condition caused by the poisoning, toxic effect, adverse effect or underdosing.

    See Section I.C.19. Adverse effects, poisoning, underdosing and toxic effects.

n. **Normal Delivery, Code O80**
    1) **Encounter for full term uncomplicated delivery**
        Code O80 should be assigned when a woman is admitted for a full-term normal delivery and delivers a single, healthy infant without any complications antepartum, during the delivery, or postpartum during the delivery episode. Code O80 is always a principal diagnosis. It is not to be used if any other code from chapter 15 is needed to describe a current complication of the antenatal, delivery, or perinatal period. Additional codes from other chapters may be used with code O80 if they are not related to or are in any way complicating the pregnancy.

    2) **Uncomplicated delivery with resolved antepartum complication**
        Code O80 may be used if the patient had a complication at some point during the pregnancy, but the complication is not present at the time of the admission for delivery.

    3) **Outcome of delivery for O80**
        Z37.0, Single live birth, is the only outcome of delivery code appropriate for use with O80.

o. **The Peripartum and Postpartum Periods**
    1) **Peripartum and Postpartum periods**
        The postpartum period begins immediately after delivery and continues for six weeks following delivery. The peripartum period is defined as the last month of pregnancy to five months postpartum.

    2) **Peripartum and postpartum complication**
        A postpartum complication is any complication occurring within the six-week period.

    3) **Pregnancy-related complications after 6 week period**
        Chapter 15 codes may also be used to describe pregnancy-related complications after the peripartum or postpartum period if the provider documents that a condition is pregnancy related.

    4) **Admission for routine postpartum care following delivery outside hospital**
        When the mother delivers outside the hospital prior to admission and is admitted for routine postpartum care and no complications are noted, code Z39.0, Encounter for care and examination of mother immediately after delivery, should be assigned as the principal diagnosis.

    5) **Pregnancy associated cardiomyopathy**
        Pregnancy associated cardiomyopathy, code O90.3, is unique in that it may be diagnosed in the third trimester of pregnancy but may continue to progress months after delivery. For this reason, it is referred to as peripartum cardiomyopathy. Code O90.3 is only for use when the cardiomyopathy develops as a result of pregnancy in a woman who did not have pre-existing heart disease.

p. **Code O94, Sequelae of complication of pregnancy, childbirth, and the puerperium**
    1) **Code O94**
        Code O94, Sequelae of complication of pregnancy, childbirth, and the puerperium, is for use in those cases when an initial complication of a pregnancy develops a sequelae requiring care or treatment at a future date.

    2) **After the initial postpartum period**
        This code may be used at any time after the initial postpartum period.

    3) **Sequencing of Code O94**
        This code, like all sequela codes, is to be sequenced following the code describing the sequelae of the complication.

q. **Termination of Pregnancy and Spontaneous abortions**
    1) **Abortion with Liveborn Fetus**
        When an attempted termination of pregnancy results in a liveborn fetus, assign code Z33.2, Encounter for elective termination of pregnancy and a code from category Z37, Outcome of Delivery.

    2) **Retained Products of Conception following an abortion**
        Subsequent encounters for retained products of conception following a spontaneous abortion or elective termination of pregnancy are assigned the appropriate code from category

O03, Spontaneous abortion, or codes O07.4, Failed attempted termination of pregnancy without complication and Z33.2, Encounter for elective termination of pregnancy. This advice is appropriate even when the patient was discharged previously with a discharge diagnosis of complete abortion.

3) Complications leading to abortion

Codes from Chapter 15 may be used as additional codes to identify any documented complications of the pregnancy in conjunction with codes in categories in O07 and O08.

r. Abuse in a pregnant patient

For suspected or confirmed cases of abuse of a pregnant patient, a code(s) from subcategories O9A.3, Physical abuse complicating pregnancy, childbirth, and the puerperium, O9A.4, Sexual abuse complicating pregnancy, childbirth, and the puerperium, and O9A.5, Psychological abuse complicating pregnancy, childbirth, and the puerperium, should be sequenced first, followed by the appropriate codes (if applicable) to identify any associated current injury due to physical abuse, sexual abuse, and the perpetrator of abuse.

See Section I.C.19. Adult and child abuse, neglect and other maltreatment.

16. Chapter 16: Certain Conditions Originating in the Perinatal Period (P00-P96)

For coding and reporting purposes the perinatal period is defined as before birth through the 28th day following birth. The following guidelines are provided for reporting purposes.

a. General Perinatal Rules

1) Use of Chapter 16 Codes

Codes in this chapter are never for use on the maternal record. Codes from Chapter 15, the obstetric chapter, are never permitted on the newborn record. Chapter 16 codes may be used throughout the life of the patient if the condition is still present.

2) Principal Diagnosis for Birth Record

When coding the birth episode in a newborn record, assign a code from category Z38, Liveborn infants according to place of birth and type of delivery, as the principal diagnosis. A code from category Z38 is assigned only once, to a newborn at the time of birth. If a newborn is transferred to another institution, a code from category Z38 should not be used at the receiving hospital.

A code from category Z38 is used only on the newborn record, not on the mother's record.

3) Use of Codes from other Chapters with Codes from Chapter 16

Codes from other chapters may be used with codes from chapter 16 if the codes from the other chapters provide more specific detail. Codes for signs and symptoms may be assigned when a definitive diagnosis has not been established. If the reason for the encounter is a perinatal condition, the code from chapter 16 should be sequenced first.

4) Use of Chapter 16 Codes after the Perinatal Period

Should a condition originate in the perinatal period, and continue throughout the life of the patient, the perinatal code should continue to be used regardless of the patient's age.

5) Birth process or community acquired conditions

If a newborn has a condition that may be either due to the birth process or community acquired and the documentation does not indicate which it is, the default is due to the birth process and the code from Chapter 16 should be used. If the condition is community-acquired, a code from Chapter 16 should not be assigned.

6) Code all clinically significant conditions

All clinically significant conditions noted on routine newborn examination should be coded. A condition is clinically significant if it requires:

- clinical evaluation; or
- therapeutic treatment; or
- diagnostic procedures; or
- extended length of hospital stay; or

- increased nursing care and/or monitoring; or
- has implications for future health care needs

Note: The perinatal guidelines listed above are the same as the general coding guidelines for "additional diagnoses", except for the final point regarding implications for future health care needs. Codes should be assigned for conditions that have been specified by the provider as having implications for future health care needs.

b. Observation and Evaluation of Newborns for Suspected Conditions not Found

1) Assign a code from category Z05, Observation and evaluation of newborns and infants for suspected conditions ruled out, to identify those instances when a healthy newborn is evaluated for a suspected condition that is determined after study not to be present. Do not use a code from category Z05 when the patient has identified signs or symptoms of a suspected problem; in such cases code the sign or symptom.

2) A code from category Z05 may also be assigned as a principal or first-listed code for readmissions or encounters when the code from category Z38 code no longer applies. Codes from category Z05 are for use only for healthy newborns and infants for which no condition after study is found to be present.

3) Z05 on a birth record

A code from category Z05 is to be used as a secondary code after the code from category Z38, Liveborn infants according to place of birth and type of delivery.

c. Coding Additional Perinatal Diagnoses

1) Assigning codes for conditions that require treatment

Assign codes for conditions that require treatment or further investigation, prolong the length of stay, or require resource utilization.

2) Codes for conditions specified as having implications for future health care needs

Assign codes for conditions that have been specified by the provider as having implications for future health care needs.

Note: This guideline should not be used for adult patients.

d. Prematurity and Fetal Growth Retardation

Providers utilize different criteria in determining prematurity. A code for prematurity should not be assigned unless it is documented. Assignment of codes in categories P05, Disorders of newborn related to slow fetal growth and fetal malnutrition, and P07, Disorders of newborn related to short gestation and low birth weight, not elsewhere classified, should be based on the recorded birth weight and estimated gestational age. Codes from category P05 should not be assigned with codes from category P07.

When both birth weight and gestational age are available, two codes from category P07 should be assigned, with the code for birth weight sequenced before the code for gestational age.

e. Low birth weight and immaturity status

Codes from category P07, Disorders of newborn related to short gestation and low birth weight, not elsewhere classified, are for use for a child or adult who was premature or had a low birth weight as a newborn and this is affecting the patient's current health status.

See Section I.C.21. Factors influencing health status and contact with health services, Status.

f. Bacterial Sepsis of Newborn

Category P36, Bacterial sepsis of newborn, includes congenital sepsis. If a perinate is documented as having sepsis without documentation of congenital or community acquired, the default is congenital and a code from category P36 should be assigned. If the P36 code includes the causal organism, an additional code from category B95, Streptococcus, Staphylococcus, and Enterococcus as the cause of diseases classified elsewhere, or B96, Other bacterial agents as the cause of diseases classified elsewhere, should not be assigned. If the P36 code does not include the causal organism, assign an additional code from category B96. If applicable, use additional codes to identify severe sepsis (R65.2-) and any associated acute organ dysfunction.

g. Stillbirth

Code P95, Stillbirth, is only for use in institutions that maintain separate records for stillbirths. No other code should be used with P95. Code P95 should not be used on the mother's record.

17. Chapter 17: Congenital malformations, deformations, and chromosomal abnormalities (Q00-Q99)

Assign an appropriate code(s) from categories Q00-Q99, Congenital malformations, deformations, and chromosomal abnormalities when a malformation/deformation or chromosomal abnormality is documented. A malformation/deformation/or chromosomal abnormality may be the principal/first-listed diagnosis on a record or a secondary diagnosis.

When a malformation/deformation or chromosomal abnormality does not have a unique code assignment, assign additional code(s) for any manifestations that may be present.

When the code assignment specifically identifies the malformation/deformation or chromosomal abnormality, manifestations that are an inherent component of the anomaly should not be coded separately. Additional codes should be assigned for manifestations that are not an inherent component.

Codes from Chapter 17 may be used throughout the life of the patient. If a congenital malformation or deformity has been corrected, a personal history code should be used to identify the history of the malformation or deformity. Although present at birth, malformation/deformation/or chromosomal abnormality may not be identified until later in life. Whenever the condition is diagnosed by the physician, it is appropriate to assign a code from codes Q00-Q99.For the birth admission, the appropriate code from category Z38, Liveborn infants, according to place of birth and type of delivery, should be sequenced as the principal diagnosis, followed by any congenital anomaly codes, Q00- Q99.

18. Chapter 18: Symptoms, signs, and abnormal clinical and laboratory findings, not elsewhere classified (R00-R99)

Chapter 18 includes symptoms, signs, abnormal results of clinical or other investigative procedures, and ill-defined conditions regarding which no diagnosis classifiable elsewhere is recorded. Signs and symptoms that point to a specific diagnosis have been assigned to a category in other chapters of the classification.

a. Use of symptom codes

Codes that describe symptoms and signs are acceptable for reporting purposes when a related definitive diagnosis has not been established (confirmed) by the provider.

b. Use of a symptom code with a definitive diagnosis code

Codes for signs and symptoms may be reported in addition to a related definitive diagnosis when the sign or symptom is not routinely associated with that diagnosis, such as the various signs and symptoms associated with complex syndromes. The definitive diagnosis code should be sequenced before the symptom code.

Signs or symptoms that are associated routinely with a disease process should not be assigned as additional codes, unless otherwise instructed by the classification.

c. Combination codes that include symptoms

ICD-10-CM contains a number of combination codes that identify both the definitive diagnosis and common symptoms of that diagnosis. When using one of these combination codes, an additional code should not be assigned for the symptom.

d. Repeated falls

Code R29.6, Repeated falls, is for use for encounters when a patient has recently fallen and the reason for the fall is being investigated.

Code Z91.81, History of falling, is for use when a patient has fallen in the past and is at risk for future falls. When appropriate, both codes R29.6 and Z91.81 may be assigned together.

e. Coma scale

The coma scale codes (R40.2-) can be used in conjunction with traumatic brain injury codes, acute cerebrovascular disease or sequelae of cerebrovascular disease codes. These codes are primarily for use by trauma registries, but they may be used in any setting where this information is collected. The coma scale may also be used to assess the status of the central nervous system for other non-trauma conditions, such as monitoring patients in the intensive care unit regardless of medical condition. The coma scale codes should be sequenced after the diagnosis code(s).

These codes, one from each subcategory, are needed to complete the scale. The 7th character indicates when the scale was recorded. The 7th character should match for all three codes.

At a minimum, report the initial score documented on presentation at your facility. This may be a score from the emergency medicine technician (EMT) or in the emergency department. If desired, a facility may choose to capture multiple coma scale scores.

Assign code R40.24, Glasgow coma scale, total score, when only the total score is documented in the medical record and not the individual score(s).

f. Functional quadriplegia

Functional quadriplegia (code R53.2) is the lack of ability to use one's limbs or to ambulate due to extreme debility. It is not associated with neurologic deficit or injury, and code R53.2 should not be used for cases of neurologic quadriplegia. It should only be assigned if functional quadriplegia is specifically documented in the medical record.

g. SIRS due to Non-Infectious Process

The systemic inflammatory response syndrome (SIRS) can develop as a result of certain non-infectious disease processes, such as trauma, malignant neoplasm, or pancreatitis. When SIRS is documented with a noninfectious condition, and no subsequent infection is documented, the code for the underlying condition, such as an injury, should be assigned, followed by code R65.10, Systemic inflammatory response syndrome (SIRS) of non-infectious origin without acute organ dysfunction, or code R65.11, Systemic inflammatory response syndrome (SIRS) of non-infectious origin with acute organ dysfunction. If an associated acute organ dysfunction is documented, the appropriate code(s) for the specific type of organ dysfunction(s) should be assigned in addition to code R65.11. If acute organ dysfunction is documented, but it cannot be determined if the acute organ dysfunction is associated with SIRS or due to another condition (e.g., directly due to the trauma), the provider should be queried.

h. Death NOS

Code R99, Ill-defined and unknown cause of mortality, is only for use in the very limited circumstance when a patient who has already died is brought into an emergency department or other healthcare facility and is pronounced dead upon arrival. It does not represent the discharge disposition of death.

i. NIHSS Stroke Scale

The NIH stroke scale (NIHSS) codes (R29.7- -) can be used in conjunction with acute stroke codes (I63) to identify the patient's neurological status and the severity of the stroke. The stroke scale codes should be sequenced after the acute stroke diagnosis code(s).

At a minimum, report the initial score documented. If desired, a facility may choose to capture multiple stroke scale scores.

See Section I.B.14. for information concerning the medical record documentation that may be used for assignment of the NIHSS codes.

19. Chapter 19: Injury, poisoning, and certain other consequences of external causes (S00-T88)

a. Application of 7th Characters in Chapter 19

Most categories in chapter 19 have a 7th character requirement for each applicable code. Most categories in this chapter have three 7th character values (with the exception of fractures): A, initial encounter, D, subsequent encounter and S, sequela. Categories for traumatic fractures have additional 7th character values. While the patient may be seen by a new or different provider over the course of treatment for an injury, assignment of the 7th character is based on whether the patient is undergoing active treatment and not whether the provider is seeing the patient for the first time.

For complication codes, active treatment refers to treatment for the condition described by the code, even though it may be related to an earlier precipitating problem. For example, code T84.50XA, Infection and inflammatory reaction due to unspecified internal joint prosthesis, initial encounter, is used when active treatment is provided for the infection, even though the condition relates to the prosthetic device, implant or graft that was placed at a previous encounter.

7th character "A", initial encounter is used for each encounter where the patient is receiving active treatment for the condition.

7th character "D" subsequent encounter is used for encounters after the patient has completed active treatment of the condition and is receiving routine care for the condition during the healing or recovery phase.

The aftercare Z codes should not be used for aftercare for conditions such as injuries or poisonings, where 7th characters are provided to identify subsequent care. For example, for aftercare of an injury, assign the acute injury code with the 7th character "D" (subsequent encounter).

7th character "S", sequela, is for use for complications or conditions that arise as a direct result of a condition, such as scar formation after a burn. The scars are sequelae of the burn. When using 7th character "S", it is necessary to use both the injury code that precipitated the sequela and the code for the sequela itself. The "S" is added only to the injury code, not the sequela code. The 7th character "S" identifies the injury responsible for the sequela. The specific type of sequela (e.g. scar) is sequenced first, followed by the injury code.

See Section I.B.10 Sequelae, (Late Effects)

b. Coding of Injuries

When coding injuries, assign separate codes for each injury unless a combination code is provided, in which case the combination code is assigned. Code T07, Unspecified multiple injuries should not be assigned in the inpatient setting unless information for a more specific code is not available. Traumatic injury codes (S00-T14.9) are not to be used for normal, healing surgical wounds or to identify complications of surgical wounds.

The code for the most serious injury, as determined by the provider and the focus of treatment, is sequenced first.

1) Superficial injuries

Superficial injuries such as abrasions or contusions are not coded when associated with more severe injuries of the same site.

2) Primary injury with damage to nerves/blood vessels

When a primary injury results in minor damage to peripheral nerves or blood vessels, the primary injury is sequenced first with additional code(s) for injuries to nerves and spinal cord (such as category S04), and/or injury to blood vessels (such as category S15). When the primary injury is to the blood vessels or nerves, that injury should be sequenced first.

c. Coding of Traumatic Fractures

The principles of multiple coding of injuries should be followed in coding fractures. Fractures of specified sites are coded individually by site in accordance with both the provisions within categories S02, S12, S22, S32, S42, S49, S52, S59, S62, S72, S79, S82, S89, S92 and the level of detail furnished by medical record content.

A fracture not indicated as open or closed should be coded to closed. A fracture not indicated whether displaced or not displaced should be coded to displaced.

More specific guidelines are as follows:

1) Initial vs. Subsequent Encounter for Fractures

Traumatic fractures are coded using the appropriate 7th character for initial encounter (A, B, C) for each encounter where the patient is receiving active treatment for the fracture. The appropriate 7th character for initial encounter should also be assigned for a patient who delayed seeking treatment for the fracture or nonunion.

Fractures are coded using the appropriate 7th character for subsequent care for encounters after the patient has completed active treatment of the fracture and is receiving routine care for the fracture during the healing or recovery phase.

Care for complications of surgical treatment for fracture repairs during the healing or recovery phase should be coded with the appropriate complication codes.

Care of complications of fractures, such as malunion and nonunion, should be reported with the appropriate 7th character for subsequent care with nonunion (K, M, N,) or subsequent care with malunion (P, Q, R).

Malunion/nonunion: The appropriate 7th character for initial encounter should also be assigned for a patient who delayed seeking treatment for the fracture or nonunion.

The open fracture designations in the assignment of the 7th character for fractures of the forearm, femur and lower leg, including ankle are based on the Gustilo open fracture classification. When the Gustilo classification type is not specified for an open fracture, the 7th character for open fracture type I or II should be assigned (B, E, H, M, Q).

A code from category M80, not a traumatic fracture code, should be used for any patient with known osteoporosis who suffers a fracture, even if the patient had a minor fall or trauma, if that fall or trauma would not usually break a normal, healthy bone.

See Section I.C.13. Osteoporosis.

The aftercare Z codes should not be used for aftercare for traumatic fractures. For aftercare of a traumatic fracture, assign the acute fracture code with the appropriate 7th character.

2) Multiple fractures sequencing

Multiple fractures are sequenced in accordance with the severity of the fracture.

d. Coding of Burns and Corrosions

The ICD-10-CM makes a distinction between burns and corrosions. The burn codes are for thermal burns, except sunburns, that come from a heat source, such as a fire or hot appliance. The burn codes are also for burns resulting from electricity and radiation. Corrosions are burns due to chemicals. The guidelines are the same for burns and corrosions.

Current burns (T20-T25) are classified by depth, extent and by agent (X code). Burns are classified by depth as first degree (erythema), second degree (blistering), and third degree (full-thickness involvement). Burns of the eye and internal organs (T26-T28) are classified by site, but not by degree.

1) Sequencing of burn and related condition codes

Sequence first the code that reflects the highest degree of burn when more than one burn is present.

a. When the reason for the admission or encounter is for treatment of external multiple burns, sequence first the code that reflects the burn of the highest degree.

b. When a patient has both internal and external burns, the circumstances of admission govern the selection of the principal diagnosis or first-listed diagnosis.

c. When a patient is admitted for burn injuries and other related conditions such as smoke inhalation and/or respiratory failure, the circumstances of admission govern the selection of the principal or first-listed diagnosis.

2) Burns of the same local site

Classify burns of the same local site (three-character category level, T20-T28) but of different degrees to the subcategory identifying the highest degree recorded in the diagnosis.

3) Non-healing burns

Non-healing burns are coded as acute burns.

Necrosis of burned skin should be coded as a non-healed burn.

4) Infected Burn

For any documented infected burn site, use an additional code for the infection.

5) Assign separate codes for each burn site

When coding burns, assign separate codes for each burn site. Category T30, Burn and corrosion, body region unspecified is extremely vague and should rarely be used.

6) Burns and Corrosions Classified According to Extent of Body Surface Involved

Assign codes from category T31, Burns classified according to extent of body surface involved, or T32, Corrosions classified according to extent of body surface involved, when the site of the burn is not specified or when there is a need for additional data. It is advisable to use category T31 as additional coding when needed to provide data for evaluating burn mortality, such as that needed by burn units. It is also advisable to use category T31 as an additional code for reporting purposes when there is mention of a third-degree burn involving 2Ø percent or more of the body surface.

Categories T31 and T32 are based on the classic "rule of nines" in estimating body surface involved: head and neck are assigned nine percent, each arm nine percent, each leg 18 percent, the anterior trunk 18 percent, posterior trunk 18 percent, and genitalia one percent. Providers may change these percentage assignments where necessary to accommodate infants and children who have proportionately larger heads than adults, and patients who have large buttocks, thighs, or abdomen that involve burns.

7) Encounters for treatment of sequela of burns
Encounters for the treatment of the late effects of burns or corrosions (i.e., scars or joint contractures) should be coded with a burn or corrosion code with the 7th character "S" for sequela.

8) Sequelae with a late effect code and current burn
When appropriate, both a code for a current burn or corrosion with 7th character "A" or "D" and a burn or corrosion code with 7th character "S" may be assigned on the same record (when both a current burn and sequelae of an old burn exist). Burns and corrosions do not heal at the same rate and a current healing wound may still exist with sequela of a healed burn or corrosion.

See Section I.B.10 Sequela (Late Effects)

9) Use of an external cause code with burns and corrosions
An external cause code should be used with burns and corrosions to identify the source and intent of the burn, as well as the place where it occurred.

e. Adverse Effects, Poisoning, Underdosing and Toxic Effects
Codes in categories T36-T65 are combination codes that include the substance that was taken as well as the intent. No additional external cause code is required for poisonings, toxic effects, adverse effects and underdosing codes.

1) Do not code directly from the Table of Drugs
Do not code directly from the Table of Drugs and Chemicals. Always refer back to the Tabular List.

2) Use as many codes as necessary to describe
Use as many codes as necessary to describe completely all drugs, medicinal or biological substances.

3) If the same code would describe the causative agent
If the same code would describe the causative agent for more than one adverse reaction, poisoning, toxic effect or underdosing, assign the code only once.

4) If two or more drugs, medicinal or biological substances
If two or more drugs, medicinal or biological substances are reported, code each individually unless a combination code is listed in the Table of Drugs and Chemicals.

5) The occurrence of drug toxicity is classified in ICD-10-CM as follows:
(a) Adverse Effect
When coding an adverse effect of a drug that has been correctly prescribed and properly administered, assign the appropriate code for the nature of the adverse effect followed by the appropriate code for the adverse effect of the drug (T36-T5Ø). The code for the drug should have a 5th or 6th character "5" (for example T36.ØX5-) Examples of the nature of an adverse effect are tachycardia, delirium, gastrointestinal hemorrhaging, vomiting, hypokalemia, hepatitis, renal failure, or respiratory failure.

(b) Poisoning
When coding a poisoning or reaction to the improper use of a medication (e.g., overdose, wrong substance given or taken in error, wrong route of administration), first assign the appropriate code from categories T36-T5Ø. The poisoning codes have an associated intent as their 5th or 6th character (accidental, intentional self-harm, assault and undetermined. If the intent of the poisoning is unknown or unspecified, code the intent as accidental intent. The

undetermined intent is only for use if the documentation in the record specifies that the intent cannot be determined. Use additional code(s) for all manifestations of poisonings.

If there is also a diagnosis of abuse or dependence of the substance, the abuse or dependence is assigned as an additional code.

Examples of poisoning include:

(i) Error was made in drug prescription

Errors made in drug prescription or in the administration of the drug by provider, nurse, patient, or other person.

(ii) Overdose of a drug intentionally taken

If an overdose of a drug was intentionally taken or administered and resulted in drug toxicity, it would be coded as a poisoning.

(iii) Nonprescribed drug taken with correctly prescribed and properly administered drug

If a nonprescribed drug or medicinal agent was taken in combination with a correctly prescribed and properly administered drug, any drug toxicity or other reaction resulting from the interaction of the two drugs would be classified as a poisoning.

(iv) Interaction of drug(s) and alcohol

When a reaction results from the interaction of a drug(s) and alcohol, this would be classified as poisoning.

See Section I.C.4. if poisoning is the result of insulin pump malfunctions.

(c) Underdosing
Underdosing refers to taking less of a medication than is prescribed by a provider or a manufacturer's instruction. For underdosing, assign the code from categories T36-T5Ø (fifth or sixth character "6").

Codes for underdosing should never be assigned as principal or first-listed codes. If a patient has a relapse or exacerbation of the medical condition for which the drug is prescribed because of the reduction in dose, then the medical condition itself should be coded.

Noncompliance (Z91.12-, Z91.13-) or complication of care (Y63.6-Y63.9) codes are to be used with an underdosing code to indicate intent, if known.

(d) Toxic Effects
When a harmful substance is ingested or comes in contact with a person, this is classified as a toxic effect. The toxic effect codes are in categories T51-T65.

Toxic effect codes have an associated intent: accidental, intentional self-harm, assault and undetermined.

f. Adult and child abuse, neglect and other maltreatment
Sequence first the appropriate code from categories T74.- (Adult and child abuse, neglect and other maltreatment, confirmed) or T76.- (Adult and child abuse, neglect and other maltreatment, suspected) for abuse, neglect and other maltreatment, followed by any accompanying mental health or injury code(s).

If the documentation in the medical record states abuse or neglect it is coded as confirmed (T74.-). It is coded as suspected if it is documented as suspected (T76.-).

For cases of confirmed abuse or neglect an external cause code from the assault section (X92-YØ9) should be added to identify the cause of any physical injuries. A perpetrator code (YØ7) should be added when the perpetrator of the abuse is known. For suspected cases of abuse or neglect, do not report external cause or perpetrator code.

If a suspected case of abuse, neglect or mistreatment is ruled out during an encounter code ZØ4.71, Encounter for examination and observation following alleged physical adult abuse, ruled out, or code ZØ4.72, Encounter for examination and observation following alleged child physical abuse, ruled out, should be used, not a code from T76.

If a suspected case of alleged rape or sexual abuse is ruled out during an encounter code Z04.41, Encounter for examination and observation following alleged adult rape or code Z04.42, Encounter for examination and observation following alleged child rape, should be used, not a code from T76.

See Section I.C.15. Abuse in a pregnant patient.

g. Complications of care

1) General guidelines for complications of care

(a) Documentation of complications of care
See Section I.B.16. for information on documentation of complications of care.

2) Pain due to medical devices
Pain associated with devices, implants or grafts left in a surgical site (for example painful hip prosthesis) is assigned to the appropriate code(s) found in Chapter 19, Injury, poisoning, and certain other consequences of external causes. Specific codes for pain due to medical devices are found in the T code section of the ICD-10-CM. Use additional code(s) from category G89 to identify acute or chronic pain due to presence of the device, implant or graft (G89.18 or G89.28).

3) Transplant complications

(a) Transplant complications other than kidney
Codes under category T86, Complications of transplanted organs and tissues, are for use for both complications and rejection of transplanted organs. A transplant complication code is only assigned if the complication affects the function of the transplanted organ. Two codes are required to fully describe a transplant complication: the appropriate code from category T86 and a secondary code that identifies the complication.

Pre-existing conditions or conditions that develop after the transplant are not coded as complications unless they affect the function of the transplanted organs.

See I.C.21. for transplant organ removal status

See I.C.2. for malignant neoplasm associated with transplanted organ.

(b) Kidney transplant complications
Patients who have undergone kidney transplant may still have some form of chronic kidney disease (CKD) because the kidney transplant may not fully restore kidney function. Code T86.1- should be assigned for documented complications of a kidney transplant, such as transplant failure or rejection or other transplant complication. Code T86.1- should not be assigned for post kidney transplant patients who have chronic kidney (CKD) unless a transplant complication such as transplant failure or rejection is documented. If the documentation is unclear as to whether the patient has a complication of the transplant, query the provider.

Conditions that affect the function of the transplanted kidney, other than CKD, should be assigned a code from subcategory T86.1, Complications of transplanted organ, Kidney, and a secondary code that identifies the complication.

For patients with CKD following a kidney transplant, but who do not have a complication such as failure or rejection, *see section I.C.14. Chronic kidney disease and kidney transplant status.*

4) Complication codes that include the external cause
As with certain other T codes, some of the complications of care codes have the external cause included in the code. The code includes the nature of the complication as well as the type of procedure that caused the complication. No external cause code indicating the type of procedure is necessary for these codes.

5) Complications of care codes within the body system chapters
Intraoperative and postprocedural complication codes are found within the body system chapters with codes specific to the organs and structures of that body system. These codes

should be sequenced first, followed by a code(s) for the specific complication, if applicable.

20. Chapter 20: External Causes of Morbidity (V00-Y99)
The external causes of morbidity codes should never be sequenced as the first-listed or principal diagnosis.

External cause codes are intended to provide data for injury research and evaluation of injury prevention strategies. These codes capture how the injury or health condition happened (cause), the intent (unintentional or accidental; or intentional, such as suicide or assault), the place where the event occurred the activity of the patient at the time of the event, and the person's status (e.g., civilian, military).

There is no national requirement for mandatory ICD-10-CM external cause code reporting. Unless a provider is subject to a state-based external cause code reporting mandate or these codes are required by a particular payer, reporting of ICD-10-CM codes in Chapter 20, External Causes of Morbidity, is not required. In the absence of a mandatory reporting requirement, providers are encouraged to voluntarily report external cause codes, as they provide valuable data for injury research and evaluation of injury prevention strategies.

a. General External Cause Coding Guidelines

1) Used with any code in the range of A00.0-T88.9, Z00-Z99
An external cause code may be used with any code in the range of A00.0-T88.9, Z00-Z99, classification that is a health condition due to an external cause. Though they are most applicable to injuries, they are also valid for use with such things as infections or diseases due to an external source, and other health conditions, such as a heart attack that occurs during strenuous physical activity.

2) External cause code used for length of treatment
Assign the external cause code, with the appropriate 7th character (initial encounter, subsequent encounter or sequela) for each encounter for which the injury or condition is being treated.

Most categories In chapter 20 have a 7th character requirement for each applicable code. Most categories in this chapter have three 7th character values: A, initial encounter, D, subsequent encounter and S, sequela. While the patient may be seen by a new or different provider over the course of treatment for an injury or condition, assignment of the 7th character for external cause should match the 7th character of the code assigned for the associated injury or condition for the encounter.

3) Use the full range of external cause codes
Use the full range of external cause codes to completely describe the cause, the intent, the place of occurrence, and if applicable, the activity of the patient at the time of the event, and the patient's status, for all injuries, and other health conditions due to an external cause.

4) Assign as many external cause codes as necessary
Assign as many external cause codes as necessary to fully explain each cause. If only one external code can be recorded, assign the code most related to the principal diagnosis.

5) The selection of the appropriate external cause code
The selection of the appropriate external cause code is guided by the Alphabetic Index of External Causes and by Inclusion and Exclusion notes in the Tabular List.

6) External cause code can never be a principal diagnosis
An external cause code can never be a principal (first-listed) diagnosis.

7) Combination external cause codes
Certain of the external cause codes are combination codes that identify sequential events that result in an injury, such as a fall which results in striking against an object. The injury may be due to either event or both. The combination external cause code used should correspond to the sequence of events regardless of which caused the most serious injury.

8) No external cause code needed in certain circumstances
No external cause code from Chapter 20 is needed if the external cause and intent are included in a code from another chapter (e.g. T36.0X1- Poisoning by penicillins, accidental (unintentional)).

b. **Place of Occurrence Guideline**
Codes from category Y92, Place of occurrence of the external cause, are secondary codes for use after other external cause codes to identify the location of the patient at the time of injury or other condition.

Generally, a place of occurrence code is assigned only once, at the initial encounter for treatment. However, in the rare instance that a new injury occurs during hospitalization, an additional place of occurrence code may be assigned. No 7th characters are used for Y92.

Do not use place of occurrence code Y92.9 if the place is not stated or is not applicable.

c. **Activity Code**
Assign a code from category Y93, Activity code, to describe the activity of the patient at the time the injury or other health condition occurred.

An activity code is used only once, at the initial encounter for treatment. Only one code from Y93 should be recorded on a medical record.

The activity codes are not applicable to poisonings, adverse effects, misadventures or sequela.

Do not assign Y93.9, Unspecified activity, if the activity is not stated.

A code from category Y93 is appropriate for use with external cause and intent codes if identifying the activity provides additional information about the event.

d. **Place of Occurrence, Activity, and Status Codes Used with other External Cause Code**
When applicable, place of occurrence, activity, and external cause status codes are sequenced after the main external cause code(s). Regardless of the number of external cause codes assigned, generally there should be only one place of occurrence code, one activity code, and one external cause status code assigned to an encounter. However, in the rare instance that a new injury occurs during hospitalization, an additional place of occurrence code may be assigned.

e. **If the Reporting Format Limits the Number of External Cause Codes**
If the reporting format limits the number of external cause codes that can be used in reporting clinical data, report the code for the cause/intent most related to the principal diagnosis. If the format permits capture of additional external cause codes, the cause/intent, including medical misadventures, of the additional events should be reported rather than the codes for place, activity, or external status.

f. **Multiple External Cause Coding Guidelines**
More than one external cause code is required to fully describe the external cause of an illness or injury. The assignment of external cause codes should be sequenced in the following priority:

If two or more events cause separate injuries, an external cause code should be assigned for each cause. The first-listed external cause code will be selected in the following order:

External codes for child and adult abuse take priority over all other external cause codes.

See Section I.C.19., Child and Adult abuse guidelines.

External cause codes for terrorism events take priority over all other external cause codes except child and adult abuse.

External cause codes for cataclysmic events take priority over all other external cause codes except child and adult abuse and terrorism.

External cause codes for transport accidents take priority over all other external cause codes except cataclysmic events, child and adult abuse and terrorism.

Activity and external cause status codes are assigned following all causal (intent) external cause codes.

The first-listed external cause code should correspond to the cause of the most serious diagnosis due to an assault, accident, or self-harm, following the order of hierarchy listed above.

g. **Child and Adult Abuse Guideline**
Adult and child abuse, neglect and maltreatment are classified as assault. Any of the assault codes may be used to indicate the external cause of any injury resulting from the confirmed abuse.

For confirmed cases of abuse, neglect and maltreatment, when the perpetrator is known, a code from Y07, Perpetrator of maltreatment and neglect, should accompany any other assault codes.

See Section I.C.19. Adult and child abuse, neglect and other maltreatment

h. **Unknown or Undetermined Intent Guideline**
If the intent (accident, self-harm, assault) of the cause of an injury or other condition is unknown or unspecified, code the intent as accidental intent. All transport accident categories assume accidental intent.

1) **Use of undetermined intent**
External cause codes for events of undetermined intent are only for use if the documentation in the record specifies that the intent cannot be determined.

i. **Sequelae (Late Effects) of External Cause Guidelines**
1) **Sequelae external cause codes**
Sequela are reported using the external cause code with the 7th character "S" for sequela. These codes should be used with any report of a late effect or sequela resulting from a previous injury.

See Section I.B.10 Sequela (Late Effects)

2) **Sequela external cause code with a related current injury**
A sequela external cause code should never be used with a related current nature of injury code.

3) **Use of sequela external cause codes for subsequent visits**
Use a late effect external cause code for subsequent visits when a late effect of the initial injury is being treated. Do not use a late effect external cause code for subsequent visits for follow-up care (e.g., to assess healing, to receive rehabilitative therapy) of the injury when no late effect of the injury has been documented.

j. **Terrorism Guidelines**
1) **Cause of injury identified by the Federal Government (FBI) as terrorism**
When the cause of an injury is identified by the Federal Government (FBI) as terrorism, the first-listed external cause code should be a code from category Y38, Terrorism. The definition of terrorism employed by the FBI is found at the inclusion note at the beginning of category Y38. Use additional code for place of occurrence (Y92.-). More than one Y38 code may be assigned if the injury is the result of more than one mechanism of terrorism.

2) **Cause of an injury is suspected to be the result of terrorism**
When the cause of an injury is suspected to be the result of terrorism a code from category Y38 should not be assigned. Suspected cases should be classified as assault.

3) **Code Y38.9, Terrorism, secondary effects**
Assign code Y38.9, Terrorism, secondary effects, for conditions occurring subsequent to the terrorist event. This code should not be assigned for conditions that are due to the initial terrorist act.

It is acceptable to assign code Y38.9 with another code from Y38 if there is an injury due to the initial terrorist event and an injury that is a subsequent result of the terrorist event.

k. **External cause status**
A code from category Y99, External cause status, should be assigned whenever any other external cause code is assigned for an encounter, including an Activity code, except for the events noted below. Assign a code from category Y99, External cause status, to indicate the work status of the person at the time the event occurred. The status code indicates whether the event occurred during military activity, whether a non-military person was at work, whether an individual including a student or volunteer was involved in a non-work activity at the time of the causal event.

A code from Y99, External cause status, should be assigned, when applicable, with other external cause codes, such as transport accidents and falls. The external cause status codes are not applicable to poisonings, adverse effects, misadventures or late effects.

Do not assign a code from category Y99 if no other external cause codes (cause, activity) are applicable for the encounter.

An external cause status code is used only once, at the initial encounter for treatment. Only one code from Y99 should be recorded on a medical record.

Do not assign code Y99.9, Unspecified external cause status, if the status is not stated.

21. Chapter 21: Factors influencing health status and contact with health services (Z00-Z99)

Note: The chapter specific guidelines provide additional information about the use of Z codes for specified encounters.

a. Use of Z codes in any healthcare setting

Z codes are for use in any healthcare setting. Z codes may be used as either a first-listed (principal diagnosis code in the inpatient setting) or secondary code, depending on the circumstances of the encounter. Certain Z codes may only be used as first-listed or principal diagnosis.

b. Z Codes indicate a reason for an encounter

Z codes are not procedure codes. A corresponding procedure code must accompany a Z code to describe any procedure performed.

c. Categories of Z Codes

1) Contact/Exposure

Category Z20 indicates contact with, and suspected exposure to, communicable diseases. These codes are for patients who do not show any sign or symptom of a disease but are suspected to have been exposed to it by close personal contact with an infected individual or are in an area where a disease is epidemic.

Category Z77, Other contact with and (suspected) exposures hazardous to health, indicates contact with and suspected exposures hazardous to health.

Contact/exposure codes may be used as a first-listed code to explain an encounter for testing, or, more commonly, as a secondary code to identify a potential risk.

2) Inoculations and vaccinations

Code Z23 is for encounters for inoculations and vaccinations. It indicates that a patient is being seen to receive a prophylactic inoculation against a disease. Procedure codes are required to identify the actual administration of the injection and the type(s) of immunizations given. Code Z23 may be used as a secondary code if the inoculation is given as a routine part of preventive health care, such as a well-baby visit.

3) Status

Status codes indicate that a patient is either a carrier of a disease or has the sequelae or residual of a past disease or condition. This includes such things as the presence of prosthetic or mechanical devices resulting from past treatment. A status code is informative, because the status may affect the course of treatment and its outcome. A status code is distinct from a history code. The history code indicates that the patient no longer has the condition.

A status code should not be used with a diagnosis code from one of the body system chapters, if the diagnosis code includes the information provided by the status code. For example, code Z94.1, Heart transplant status, should not be used with a code from subcategory T86.2, Complications of heart transplant. The status code does not provide additional information. The complication code indicates that the patient is a heart transplant patient.

For encounters for weaning from a mechanical ventilator, assign a code from subcategory J96.1, Chronic respiratory failure, followed by code Z99.11, Dependence on respirator [ventilator] status.

The status Z codes/categories are:

Z14   Genetic carrier

Genetic carrier status indicates that a person carries a gene, associated with a particular disease, which may be passed to offspring who may develop that disease. The person does not have the disease and is not at risk of developing the disease.

Z15   Genetic susceptibility to disease

Genetic susceptibility indicates that a person has a gene that increases the risk of that person developing the disease.

Codes from category Z15 should not be used as principal or first-listed codes. If the patient has the condition to which he/she is susceptible, and that condition is the reason for the encounter, the code for the current condition should be sequenced first. If the patient is being seen for follow-up after completed treatment for this condition, and the condition no longer exists, a follow-up code should be sequenced first, followed by the appropriate personal history and genetic susceptibility codes. If the purpose of the encounter is genetic counseling associated with procreative management, code Z31.5, Encounter for genetic counseling, should be assigned as the first-listed code, followed by a code from category Z15. Additional codes should be assigned for any applicable family or personal history.

Z16   Resistance to antimicrobial drugs

This code indicates that a patient has a condition that is resistant to antimicrobial drug treatment. Sequence the infection code first.

Z17   Estrogen receptor status

Z18   Retained foreign body fragments

Z19   Hormone sensitivity malignancy status

Z21   Asymptomatic HIV infection status

This code indicates that a patient has tested positive for HIV but has manifested no signs or symptoms of the disease.

Z22   Carrier of infectious disease

Carrier status indicates that a person harbors the specific organisms of a disease without manifest symptoms and is capable of transmitting the infection.

Z28.3   Underimmunization status

Z33.1   Pregnant state, incidental

This code is a secondary code only for use when the pregnancy is in no way complicating the reason for visit. Otherwise, a code from the obstetric chapter is required.

Z66   Do not resuscitate

This code may be used when it is documented by the provider that a patient is on do not resuscitate status at any time during the stay.

Z67   Blood type

Z68   Body mass index (BMI)

As with all other secondary diagnosis codes, the BMI codes should only be assigned when they meet the definition of a reportable diagnosis (see Section III, Reporting Additional Diagnoses).

Z74.01   Bed confinement status

Z76.82   Awaiting organ transplant status

Z78   Other specified health status

Code Z78.1, Physical restraint status, may be used when it is documented by the provider that a patient has been put in restraints during the current encounter. Please note that this code should not be reported when it is documented by the provider that a patient is temporarily restrained during a procedure.

Z79   Long-term (current) drug therapy

Codes from this category indicate a patient's continuous use of a prescribed drug (including such things as aspirin therapy) for the long-term treatment of a condition or for prophylactic use. It is not for use for patients who have addictions to drugs. This subcategory is not for use of medications for detoxification or maintenance programs to prevent withdrawal symptoms in patients with drug dependence (e.g., methadone maintenance for opiate dependence). Assign the appropriate code for the drug dependence instead.

Assign a code from Z79 if the patient is receiving a medication for an extended period as a prophylactic measure (such as for the prevention of deep vein thrombosis) or as treatment of a chronic condition (such as arthritis) or a disease requiring a lengthy course of treatment (such as cancer). Do not assign a code from category Z79 for medication being administered for a brief period of time to treat an acute illness or injury (such as a course of antibiotics to treat acute bronchitis).

Z88   Allergy status to drugs, medicaments and biological substances

Except: Z88.9, Allergy status to unspecified drugs, medicaments and biological substances status

Z89   Acquired absence of limb

Z90   Acquired absence of organs, not elsewhere classified

Z91.0- Allergy status, other than to drugs and biological substances

Z92.82 Status post administration of tPA (rtPA) in a different facility within the last 24 hours prior to admission to a current facility

Assign code Z92.82, Status post administration of tPA (rtPA) in a different facility within the last 24 hours prior to admission to current facility, as a secondary diagnosis when a patient is received by transfer into a facility and documentation indicates they were administered tissue plasminogen activator (tPA) within the last 24 hours prior to admission to the current facility.

This guideline applies even if the patient is still receiving the tPA at the time they are received into the current facility.

The appropriate code for the condition for which the tPA was administered (such as cerebrovascular disease or myocardial infarction) should be assigned first.

Code Z92.82 is only applicable to the receiving facility record and not to the transferring facility record.

Z93   Artificial opening status

Z94   Transplanted organ and tissue status

Z95   Presence of cardiac and vascular implants and grafts

Z96   Presence of other functional implants

Z97   Presence of other devices

Z98   Other postprocedural states

Assign code Z98.85, Transplanted organ removal status, to indicate that a transplanted organ has been previously removed. This code should not be assigned for the encounter in which the transplanted organ is removed. The complication necessitating removal of the transplant organ should be assigned for that encounter.

See section I.C19. for information on the coding of organ transplant complications.

Z99   Dependence on enabling machines and devices, not elsewhere classified

Note: Categories Z89-Z90 and Z93-Z99 are for use only if there are no complications or malfunctions of the organ or tissue replaced, the amputation site or the equipment on which the patient is dependent.

4) **History (of)**

There are two types of history Z codes, personal and family. Personal history codes explain a patient's past medical condition that no longer exists and is not receiving any treatment, but that has the potential for recurrence, and therefore may require continued monitoring.

Family history codes are for use when a patient has a family member(s) who has had a particular disease that causes the patient to be at higher risk of also contracting the disease.

Personal history codes may be used in conjunction with follow-up codes and family history codes may be used in conjunction with screening codes to explain the need for a test or procedure. History codes are also acceptable on any medical record regardless of the reason for visit. A history of an illness, even if no longer present, is important information that may alter the type of treatment ordered.

The history Z code categories are:

Z80   Family history of primary malignant neoplasm

Z81   Family history of mental and behavioral disorders

Z82   Family history of certain disabilities and chronic diseases (leading to disablement)

Z83   Family history of other specific disorders

Z84   Family history of other conditions

Z85   Personal history of malignant neoplasm

Z86   Personal history of certain other diseases

Z87   Personal history of other diseases and conditions

Z91.4- Personal history of psychological trauma, not elsewhere classified

Z91.5   Personal history of self-harm

Z91.8- Other specified personal risk factors, not elsewhere classified

Exception: Z91.83, Wandering in diseases classified elsewhere

Z92   Personal history of medical treatment

Except: Z92.0, Personal history of contraception

Except: Z92.82, Status post administration of tPA (rtPA) in a different facility within the last 24 hours prior to admission to a current facility

5) **Screening**

Screening is the testing for disease or disease precursors in seemingly well individuals so that early detection and treatment can be provided for those who test positive for the disease (e.g., screening mammogram).

The testing of a person to rule out or confirm a suspected diagnosis because the patient has some sign or symptom is a diagnostic examination, not a screening. In these cases, the sign or symptom is used to explain the reason for the test.

A screening code may be a first-listed code if the reason for the visit is specifically the screening exam. It may also be used as an additional code if the screening is done during an office visit for other health problems. A screening code is not necessary if the screening is inherent to a routine examination, such as a pap smear done during a routine pelvic examination.

Should a condition be discovered during the screening then the code for the condition may be assigned as an additional diagnosis.

The Z code indicates that a screening exam is planned. A procedure code is required to confirm that the screening was performed.

The screening Z codes/categories:

Z11   Encounter for screening for infectious and parasitic diseases

Z12   Encounter for screening for malignant neoplasms

Z13   Encounter for screening for other diseases and disorders

Except: Z13.9, Encounter for screening, unspecified

Z36   Encounter for antenatal screening for mother

6)   Observation

There are three observation Z code categories. They are for use in very limited circumstances when a person is being observed for a suspected condition that is ruled out. The observation codes are not for use if an injury or illness or any signs or symptoms related to the suspected condition are present. In such cases the diagnosis/symptom code is used with the corresponding external cause code.

The observation codes are to be used as principal diagnosis only. The only exception to this is when the principal diagnosis is required to be a code from category Z38, Liveborn infants according to place of birth and type of delivery. Then a code from category Z05, Encounter for observation and evaluation of newborn for suspected diseases and conditions ruled out, is sequenced after the Z38 code. Additional codes may be used in addition to the observation code, but only if they are unrelated to the suspected condition being observed.

Codes from subcategory Z03.7, Encounter for suspected maternal and fetal conditions ruled out, may either be used as a first-listed or as an additional code assignment depending on the case. They are for use in very limited circumstances on a maternal record when an encounter is for a suspected maternal or fetal condition that is ruled out during that encounter (for example, a maternal or fetal condition may be suspected due to an abnormal test result). These codes should not be used when the condition is confirmed. In those cases, the confirmed condition should be coded. In addition, these codes are not for use if an illness or any signs or symptoms related to the suspected condition or problem are present. In such cases the diagnosis/symptom code is used.

Additional codes may be used in addition to the code from subcategory Z03.7, but only if they are unrelated to the suspected condition being evaluated.

Codes from subcategory Z03.7 may not be used for encounters for antenatal screening of mother. *See Section I.C.21. Screening.*

For encounters for suspected fetal condition that are inconclusive following testing and evaluation, assign the appropriate code from category O35, O36, O40 or O41.

The observation Z code categories:

Z03   Encounter for medical observation for suspected diseases and conditions ruled out

Z04   Encounter for examination and observation for other reasons

   Except: Z04.9, Encounter for examination and observation for unspecified reason

Z05   Encounter for observation and evaluation of newborn for suspected diseases and conditions ruled out

7)   Aftercare

Aftercare visit codes cover situations when the initial treatment of a disease has been performed and the patient requires continued care during the healing or recovery phase, or for the long-term consequences of the disease. The aftercare Z code should not be used if treatment is directed at a current, acute disease. The diagnosis code is to be used in these cases. Exceptions to this rule are codes Z51.0, Encounter for antineoplastic radiation therapy, and codes from subcategory Z51.1, Encounter for antineoplastic chemotherapy and immunotherapy. These codes are to be first-listed, followed by the diagnosis code when a patient's encounter is solely to receive radiation therapy, chemotherapy, or immunotherapy for the treatment of a neoplasm. If the reason for the encounter is more than one type of antineoplastic therapy, code Z51.0 and a code from subcategory Z51.1 may be assigned together, in which case one of these codes would be reported as a secondary diagnosis.

The aftercare Z codes should also not be used for aftercare for injuries. For aftercare of an injury, assign the acute injury code with the appropriate 7th character (for subsequent encounter).

The aftercare codes are generally first-listed to explain the specific reason for the encounter. An aftercare code may be used as an additional code when some type of aftercare is provided in addition to the reason for admission and no diagnosis code is applicable. An example of this would be the closure of a colostomy during an encounter for treatment of another condition.

Aftercare codes should be used in conjunction with other aftercare codes or diagnosis codes to provide better detail on the specifics of an aftercare encounter visit, unless otherwise directed by the classification. Should a patient receive multiple types of antineoplastic therapy during the same encounter, code Z51.0, Encounter for antineoplastic radiation therapy, and codes from subcategory Z51.1, Encounter for antineoplastic chemotherapy and immunotherapy, may be used together on a record. The sequencing of multiple aftercare codes depends on the circumstances of the encounter.

Certain aftercare Z code categories need a secondary diagnosis code to describe the resolving condition or sequelae. For others, the condition is included in the code title.

Additional Z code aftercare category terms include fitting and adjustment, and attention to artificial openings.

Status Z codes may be used with aftercare Z codes to indicate the nature of the aftercare. For example code Z95.1, Presence of aortocoronary bypass graft, may be used with code Z48.812, Encounter for surgical aftercare following surgery on the circulatory system, to indicate the surgery for which the aftercare is being performed. A status code should not be used when the aftercare code indicates the type of status, such as using Z43.0, Encounter for attention to tracheostomy, with Z93.0, Tracheostomy status.

The aftercare Z category/codes:

Z42   Encounter for plastic and reconstructive surgery following medical procedure or healed injury

Z43   Encounter for attention to artificial openings

Z44   Encounter for fitting and adjustment of external prosthetic device

Z45   Encounter for adjustment and management of implanted device

Z46   Encounter for fitting and adjustment of other devices

Z47   Orthopedic aftercare

Z48   Encounter for other postprocedural aftercare

Z49   Encounter for care involving renal dialysis

Z51   Encounter for other aftercare and medical care

8)   Follow-up

The follow-up codes are used to explain continuing surveillance following completed treatment of a disease, condition, or injury. They imply that the condition has been fully treated and no longer exists. They should not be confused with aftercare codes, or injury codes with a 7th character for subsequent encounter, that explain ongoing care of a healing condition or its sequelae. Follow-up codes may be used in conjunction with history codes to provide the full picture of the healed condition and its treatment. The follow-up code is sequenced first, followed by the history code.

A follow-up code may be used to explain multiple visits. Should a condition be found to have recurred on the follow-up visit, then the diagnosis code for the condition should be assigned in place of the follow-up code.

The follow-up Z code categories:

Z08   Encounter for follow-up examination after completed treatment for malignant neoplasm

Z09   Encounter for follow-up examination after completed treatment for conditions other than malignant neoplasm

Z39   Encounter for maternal postpartum care and examination

9)   Donor

Codes in category Z52, Donors of organs and tissues, are used for living individuals who are donating blood or other body tissue. These codes are only for individuals donating for others, not for self-donations. They are not used to identify cadaveric donations.

10) Counseling

Counseling Z codes are used when a patient or family member receives assistance in the aftermath of an illness or injury, or when support is required in coping with family or social problems. They are not used in conjunction with a diagnosis code when the counseling component of care is considered integral to standard treatment.

The counseling Z codes/categories:

Z30.0- Encounter for general counseling and advice on contraception

Z31.5 Encounter for genetic counseling

Z31.6- Encounter for general counseling and advice on procreation

Z32.2 Encounter for childbirth instruction

Z32.3 Encounter for childcare instruction

Z69 Encounter for mental health services for victim and perpetrator of abuse

Z70 Counseling related to sexual attitude, behavior and orientation

Z71 Persons encountering health services for other counseling and medical advice, not elsewhere classified

Z76.81 Expectant mother prebirth pediatrician visit

11) Encounters for Obstetrical and Reproductive Services

See Section I.C.15. Pregnancy, Childbirth, and the Puerperium, for further instruction on the use of these codes.

Z codes for pregnancy are for use in those circumstances when none of the problems or complications included in the codes from the Obstetrics chapter exist (a routine prenatal visit or postpartum care). Codes in category Z34, Encounter for supervision of normal pregnancy, are always first-listed and are not to be used with any other code from the OB chapter.

Codes in category Z3A, Weeks of gestation, may be assigned to provide additional information about the pregnancy. Category Z3A codes should not be assigned for pregnancies with abortive outcomes (categories O00-O08), elective termination of pregnancy (code Z33.32), nor for postpartum conditions, as category Z3A is not applicable to these conditions. The date of the admission should be used to determine weeks of gestation for inpatient admissions that encompass more than one gestational week.

The outcome of delivery, category Z37, should be included on all maternal delivery records. It is always a secondary code. Codes in category Z37 should not be used on the newborn record.

Z codes for family planning (contraceptive) or procreative management and counseling should be included on an obstetric record either during the pregnancy or the postpartum stage, if applicable.

Z codes/categories for obstetrical and reproductive services:

Z30 Encounter for contraceptive management

Z31 Encounter for procreative management

Z32.2 Encounter for childbirth instruction

Z32.3 Encounter for childcare instruction

Z33 Pregnant state

Z34 Encounter for supervision of normal pregnancy

Z36 Encounter for antenatal screening of mother

Z3A Weeks of gestation

Z37 Outcome of delivery

Z39 Encounter for maternal postpartum care and examination

Z76.81 Expectant mother prebirth pediatrician visit

12) Newborns and Infants

See Section I.C.16. Newborn (Perinatal) Guidelines, for further instruction on the use of these codes.

Newborn Z codes/categories:

Z76.1 Encounter for health supervision and care of foundling

Z00.1- Encounter for routine child health examination

Z38 Liveborn infants according to place of birth and type of delivery

13) Routine and administrative examinations

The Z codes allow for the description of encounters for routine examinations, such as, a general check-up, or, examinations for administrative purposes, such as, a pre-employment physical. The codes are not to be used if the examination is for diagnosis of a suspected condition or for treatment purposes. In such cases the diagnosis code is used. During a routine exam, should a diagnosis or condition be discovered, it should be coded as an additional code. Pre-existing and chronic conditions and history codes may also be included as additional codes as long as the examination is for administrative purposes and not focused on any particular condition.

Some of the codes for routine health examinations distinguish between "with" and "without" abnormal findings. Code assignment depends on the information that is known at the time the encounter is being coded. For example, if no abnormal findings were found during the examination, but the encounter is being coded before test results are back, it is acceptable to assign the code for "without abnormal findings." When assigning a code for "with abnormal findings," additional code(s) should be assigned to identify the specific abnormal finding(s).

Pre-operative examination and pre-procedural laboratory examination Z codes are for use only in those situations when a patient is being cleared for a procedure or surgery and no treatment is given.

The Z codes/categories for routine and administrative examinations:

Z00 Encounter for general examination without complaint, suspected or reported diagnosis

Z01 Encounter for other special examination without complaint, suspected or reported diagnosis

Z02 Encounter for administrative examination

Except: Z02.9, Encounter for administrative examinations, unspecified

Z32.0- Encounter for pregnancy test

14) Miscellaneous Z codes

The miscellaneous Z codes capture a number of other health care encounters that do not fall into one of the other categories. Certain of these codes identify the reason for the encounter; others are for use as additional codes that provide useful information on circumstances that may affect a patient's care and treatment.

Prophylactic Organ Removal

For encounters specifically for prophylactic removal of an organ (such as prophylactic removal of breasts due to a genetic susceptibility to cancer or a family history of cancer), the principal or first-listed code should be a code from category Z40, Encounter for prophylactic surgery, followed by the appropriate codes to identify the associated risk factor (such as genetic susceptibility or family history).

If the patient has a malignancy of one site and is having prophylactic removal at another site to prevent either a new primary malignancy or metastatic disease, a code for the malignancy should also be assigned in addition to a code from subcategory Z40.0, Encounter for prophylactic surgery for risk factors related to malignant neoplasms. A Z40.0 code should not be assigned if the patient is having organ removal for treatment of a malignancy, such as the removal of the testes for the treatment of prostate cancer.

Miscellaneous Z codes/categories:

Z28	Immunization not carried out
	Except: Z28.3, Underimmunization status
Z29	Encounter for other prophylactic measures
Z40	Encounter for prophylactic surgery
Z41	Encounter for procedures for purposes other than remedying health state
	Except: Z41.9, Encounter for procedure for purposes other than remedying health state, unspecified
Z53	Persons encountering health services for specific procedures and treatment, not carried out
Z55	Problems related to education and literacy
Z56	Problems related to employment and unemployment
Z57	Occupational exposure to risk factors
Z58	Problems related to physical environment
Z59	Problems related to housing and economic circumstances
Z60	Problems related to social environment
Z62	Problems related to upbringing
Z63	Other problems related to primary support group, including family circumstances
Z64	Problems related to certain psychosocial circumstances
Z65	Problems related to other psychosocial circumstances
Z72	Problems related to lifestyle
	Note: These codes should be assigned only when the documentation specifies that the patient has an associated problem
Z73	Problems related to life management difficulty
Z74	Problems related to care provider dependency
	Except: Z74.01, Bed confinement status
Z75	Problems related to medical facilities and other health care
Z76.0	Encounter for issue of repeat prescription
Z76.3	Healthy person accompanying sick person
Z76.4	Other boarder to healthcare facility
Z76.5	Malingerer [conscious simulation]
Z91.1-	Patient's noncompliance with medical treatment and regimen
Z91.83	Wandering in diseases classified elsewhere
Z91.89	Other specified personal risk factors, not elsewhere classified

15) Nonspecific Z codes

Certain Z codes are so non-specific, or potentially redundant with other codes in the classification, that there can be little justification for their use in the inpatient setting. Their use in the outpatient setting should be limited to those instances when there is no further documentation to permit more precise coding. Otherwise, any sign or symptom or any other reason for visit that is captured in another code should be used.

Nonspecific Z codes/categories:

Z02.9	Encounter for administrative examinations, unspecified
Z04.9	Encounter for examination and observation for unspecified reason
Z13.9	Encounter for screening, unspecified
Z41.9	Encounter for procedure for purposes other than remedying health state, unspecified
Z52.9	Donor of unspecified organ or tissue
Z86.59	Personal history of other mental and behavioral disorders
Z88.9	Allergy status to unspecified drugs, medicaments and biological substances status
Z92.0	Personal history of contraception

16) Z Codes That May Only be Principal/First-Listed Diagnosis

The following Z codes/categories may only be reported as the principal/first-listed diagnosis, except when there are multiple encounters on the same day and the medical records for the encounters are combined:

Z00	Encounter for general examination without complaint, suspected or reported diagnosis
	Except: Z00.6
Z01	Encounter for other special examination without complaint, suspected or reported diagnosis
Z02	Encounter for administrative examination
Z03	Encounter for medical observation for suspected diseases and conditions ruled out
Z04	Encounter for examination and observation for other reasons
Z33.2	Encounter for elective termination of pregnancy
Z31.81	Encounter for male factor infertility in female patient
Z31.83	Encounter for assisted reproductive fertility procedure cycle
Z31.84	Encounter for fertility preservation procedure
Z34	Encounter for supervision of normal pregnancy
Z39	Encounter for maternal postpartum care and examination
Z38	Liveborn infants according to place of birth and type of delivery
Z42	Encounter for plastic and reconstructive surgery following medical procedure or healed injury
Z51.0	Encounter for antineoplastic radiation therapy
Z51.1-	Encounter for antineoplastic chemotherapy and immunotherapy
Z52	Donors of organs and tissues
	Except: Z52.9, Donor of unspecified organ or tissue
Z76.1	Encounter for health supervision and care of foundling
Z76.2	Encounter for health supervision and care of other healthy infant and child
Z99.12	Encounter for respirator [ventilator] dependence during power failure

Section II. Selection of Principal Diagnosis

The circumstances of inpatient admission always govern the selection of principal diagnosis. The principal diagnosis is defined in the Uniform Hospital Discharge Data Set (UHDDS) as "that condition established after study to be chiefly responsible for occasioning the admission of the patient to the hospital for care."

The UHDDS definitions are used by hospitals to report inpatient data elements in a standardized manner. These data elements and their definitions can be found in the July 31, 1985, Federal Register (Vol. 50, No, 147), pp. 31038-40.

Since that time the application of the UHDDS definitions has been expanded to include all non-outpatient settings (acute care, short term, long term care and psychiatric hospitals; home health agencies; rehab facilities; nursing homes, etc). The UHDDS definitions also apply to hospice services (all levels of care).

In determining principal diagnosis, coding conventions in the ICD-10-CM, the Tabular List and Alphabetic Index take precedence over these official coding guidelines.

(See Section I.A., Conventions for the ICD-10-CM)

The importance of consistent, complete documentation in the medical record cannot be overemphasized. Without such documentation the application of all coding guidelines is a difficult, if not impossible, task.

A. Codes for symptoms, signs, and ill-defined conditions

Codes for symptoms, signs, and ill-defined conditions from Chapter 18 are not to be used as principal diagnosis when a related definitive diagnosis has been established.

B. Two or more interrelated conditions, each potentially meeting the definition for principal diagnosis.

When there are two or more interrelated conditions (such as diseases in the same ICD-10-CM chapter or manifestations characteristically associated with a certain disease) potentially meeting the definition of principal diagnosis, either condition may be sequenced first, unless the circumstances of the admission, the therapy provided, the Tabular List, or the Alphabetic Index indicate otherwise.

C. Two or more diagnoses that equally meet the definition for principal diagnosis

In the unusual instance when two or more diagnoses equally meet the criteria for principal diagnosis as determined by the circumstances of admission, diagnostic workup and/or therapy provided, and the Alphabetic Index, Tabular List, or another coding guidelines does not provide sequencing direction, any one of the diagnoses may be sequenced first.

D. Two or more comparative or contrasting conditions

In those rare instances when two or more contrasting or comparative diagnoses are documented as "either/or" (or similar terminology), they are coded as if the diagnoses were confirmed and the diagnoses are sequenced according to the circumstances of the admission. If no further determination can be made as to which diagnosis should be principal, either diagnosis may be sequenced first.

E. A symptom(s) followed by contrasting/comparative diagnoses

GUIDELINE HAS BEEN DELETED EFFECTIVE OCTOBER 1, 2014

F. Original treatment plan not carried out

Sequence as the principal diagnosis the condition, which after study occasioned the admission to the hospital, even though treatment may not have been carried out due to unforeseen circumstances.

G. Complications of surgery and other medical care

When the admission is for treatment of a complication resulting from surgery or other medical care, the complication code is sequenced as the principal diagnosis. If the complication is classified to the T80-T88 series and the code lacks the necessary specificity in describing the complication, an additional code for the specific complication should be assigned.

H. Uncertain Diagnosis

If the diagnosis documented at the time of discharge is qualified as "probable", "suspected", "likely", "questionable", "possible", or "still to be ruled out", or other similar terms indicating uncertainty, code the condition as if it existed or was established. The bases for these guidelines are the diagnostic workup, arrangements for further workup or observation, and initial therapeutic approach that correspond most closely with the established diagnosis.

Note: This guideline is applicable only to inpatient admissions to short-term, acute, long-term care and psychiatric hospitals.

I. Admission from Observation Unit

1. Admission Following Medical Observation

When a patient is admitted to an observation unit for a medical condition, which either worsens or does not improve, and is subsequently admitted as an inpatient of the same hospital for this same medical condition, the principal diagnosis would be the medical condition which led to the hospital admission.

2. Admission Following Post-Operative Observation

When a patient is admitted to an observation unit to monitor a condition (or complication) that develops following outpatient surgery, and then is subsequently admitted as an inpatient of the same hospital, hospitals should apply the Uniform Hospital Discharge Data Set (UHDDS) definition of principal diagnosis as "that condition established after study to be chiefly responsible for occasioning the admission of the patient to the hospital for care."

J. Admission from Outpatient Surgery

When a patient receives surgery in the hospital's outpatient surgery department and is subsequently admitted for continuing inpatient care at the same hospital, the following guidelines should be followed in selecting the principal diagnosis for the inpatient admission:

- If the reason for the inpatient admission is a complication, assign the complication as the principal diagnosis.

- If no complication, or other condition, is documented as the reason for the inpatient admission, assign the reason for the outpatient surgery as the principal diagnosis.

- If the reason for the inpatient admission is another condition unrelated to the surgery, assign the unrelated condition as the principal diagnosis.

K. Admissions/Encounters for Rehabilitation

When the purpose for the admission/encounter is rehabilitation, sequence first the code for the condition for which the service is being performed. For example, for an admission/encounter for rehabilitation for right-sided dominant hemiplegia following a cerebrovascular infarction, report code I69.351, Hemiplegia and hemiparesis following cerebral infarction affecting right dominant side, as the first-listed or principal diagnosis. If the condition for which the rehabilitation service is no longer present, report the appropriate aftercare code as the first-listed or principal diagnosis. For example, if a patient with severe degenerative osteoarthritis of the hip, underwent hip replacement and the current encounter/admission is for rehabilitation, report code Z47.1, Aftercare following joint replacement surgery, as the first-listed or principal diagnosis.

See Section I.C.21.c.7, Factors influencing health states and contact with health services, Aftercare.

Section III. Reporting Additional Diagnoses

GENERAL RULES FOR OTHER (ADDITIONAL) DIAGNOSES

For reporting purposes the definition for "other diagnoses" is interpreted as additional conditions that affect patient care in terms of requiring:

clinical evaluation; or

therapeutic treatment; or

diagnostic procedures; or

extended length of hospital stay; or

increased nursing care and/or monitoring.

The UHDDS item #11-b defines Other Diagnoses as "all conditions that coexist at the time of admission, that develop subsequently, or that affect the treatment received and/or the length of stay. Diagnoses that relate to an earlier episode which have no bearing on the current hospital stay are to be excluded." UHDDS definitions apply to inpatients in acute care, short-term, long term care and psychiatric hospital setting. The UHDDS definitions are used by acute care short-term hospitals to report inpatient data elements in a standardized manner. These data elements and their definitions can be found in the July 31, 1985, Federal Register (Vol. 50, No, 147), pp. 31038-40.

Since that time the application of the UHDDS definitions has been expanded to include all non-outpatient settings (acute care, short term, long term care and psychiatric hospitals; home health agencies; rehab facilities; nursing homes, etc). The UHDDS definitions also apply to hospice services (all levels of care).

The following guidelines are to be applied in designating "other diagnoses" when neither the Alphabetic Index nor the Tabular List in ICD-10-CM provide direction. The listing of the diagnoses in the patient record is the responsibility of the attending provider.

A. Previous conditions

If the provider has included a diagnosis in the final diagnostic statement, such as the discharge summary or the face sheet, it should ordinarily be coded. Some providers include in the diagnostic statement resolved conditions or diagnoses and status-post procedures from previous admission that have no bearing on the current stay. Such conditions are not to be reported and are coded only if required by hospital policy.

However, history codes (categories Z80-Z87) may be used as secondary codes if the historical condition or family history has an impact on current care or influences treatment.

B. Abnormal findings

Abnormal findings (laboratory, x-ray, pathologic, and other diagnostic results) are not coded and reported unless the provider indicates their clinical significance. If the findings are outside the normal range and the attending provider has ordered other tests to evaluate the condition or prescribed treatment, it is appropriate to ask the provider whether the abnormal finding should be added.

Please note: This differs from the coding practices in the outpatient setting for coding encounters for diagnostic tests that have been interpreted by a provider.

C. Uncertain Diagnosis

If the diagnosis documented at the time of discharge is qualified as "probable", "suspected", "likely", "questionable", "possible", or "still to be ruled out" or other similar terms indicating uncertainty, code the condition as if it existed or was established. The bases for these guidelines are the diagnostic workup, arrangements for further workup or observation, and initial therapeutic approach that correspond most closely with the established diagnosis.

Note: This guideline is applicable only to inpatient admissions to short-term, acute, long-term care and psychiatric hospitals.

Section IV. Diagnostic Coding and Reporting Guidelines for Outpatient Services

These coding guidelines for outpatient diagnoses have been approved for use by hospitals/ providers in coding and reporting hospital-based outpatient services and provider-based office visits. Guidelines in Section I, Conventions, general coding guidelines and chapter-specific guidelines, should also be applied for outpatient services and office visits.

Information about the use of certain abbreviations, punctuation, symbols, and other conventions used in the ICD-10-CM Tabular List (code numbers and titles), can be found in Section IA of these guidelines, under "Conventions Used in the Tabular List." Section I.B. contains general guidelines that apply to the entire classification. Section I.C. contains chapter-specific guidelines that correspond to the chapters as they are arranged in the classification. Information about the correct sequence to use in finding a code is also described in Section I.

The terms encounter and visit are often used interchangeably in describing outpatient service contacts and, therefore, appear together in these guidelines without distinguishing one from the other.

Though the conventions and general guidelines apply to all settings, coding guidelines for outpatient and provider reporting of diagnoses will vary in a number of instances from those for inpatient diagnoses, recognizing that:

The Uniform Hospital Discharge Data Set (UHDDS) definition of principal diagnosis does not apply to hospital-based outpatient services and provider-based office visits.

Coding guidelines for inconclusive diagnoses (probable, suspected, rule out, etc.) were developed for inpatient reporting and do not apply to outpatients.

A. Selection of first-listed condition

In the outpatient setting, the term first-listed diagnosis is used in lieu of principal diagnosis.

In determining the first-listed diagnosis the coding conventions of ICD-10-CM, as well as the general and disease specific guidelines take precedence over the outpatient guidelines.

Diagnoses often are not established at the time of the initial encounter/visit. It may take two or more visits before the diagnosis is confirmed.

The most critical rule involves beginning the search for the correct code assignment through the Alphabetic Index. Never begin searching initially in the Tabular List as this will lead to coding errors.

1. Outpatient Surgery

When a patient presents for outpatient surgery (same day surgery), code the reason for the surgery as the first-listed diagnosis (reason for the encounter), even if the surgery is not performed due to a contraindication.

2. Observation Stay

When a patient is admitted for observation for a medical condition, assign a code for the medical condition as the first-listed diagnosis.

When a patient presents for outpatient surgery and develops complications requiring admission to observation, code the reason for the surgery as the first reported diagnosis (reason for the encounter), followed by codes for the complications as secondary diagnoses.

B. Codes from A00.0 through T88.9, Z00-Z99

The appropriate code(s) from A00.0 through T88.9, Z00-Z99 must be used to identify diagnoses, symptoms, conditions, problems, complaints, or other reason(s) for the encounter/visit.

C. Accurate reporting of ICD-10-CM diagnosis codes

For accurate reporting of ICD-10-CM diagnosis codes, the documentation should describe the patient's condition, using terminology which includes specific diagnoses as well as symptoms, problems, or reasons for the encounter. There are ICD-10-CM codes to describe all of these.

D. Codes that describe symptoms and signs

Codes that describe symptoms and signs, as opposed to diagnoses, are acceptable for reporting purposes when a diagnosis has not been established (confirmed) by the provider. Chapter 18 of ICD-10-CM, Symptoms, Signs, and Abnormal Clinical and Laboratory Findings Not Elsewhere Classified (codes R00-R99) contain many, but not all codes for symptoms.

E. Encounters for circumstances other than a disease or injury

ICD-10-CM provides codes to deal with encounters for circumstances other than a disease or injury. The Factors Influencing Health Status and Contact with Health Services codes (Z00-Z99) are provided to deal with occasions when circumstances other than a disease or injury are recorded as diagnosis or problems.

See Section I.C.21. Factors influencing health status and contact with health services.

F. Level of Detail in Coding

1. ICD-10-CM codes with 3, 4, 5, 6 or 7 characters

ICD-10-CM is composed of codes with 3, 4, 5, 6 or 7 characters. Codes with three characters are included in ICD-10-CM as the heading of a category of codes that may be further subdivided by the use of fourth, fifth, sixth or seventh characters to provide greater specificity.

2. Use of full number of characters required for a code

A three-character code is to be used only if it is not further subdivided. A code is invalid if it has not been coded to the full number of characters required for that code, including the 7th character, if applicable.

G. ICD-10-CM code for the diagnosis, condition, problem, or other reason for encounter/visit

List first the ICD-10-CM code for the diagnosis, condition, problem, or other reason for encounter/visit shown in the medical record to be chiefly responsible for the services provided. List additional codes that describe any coexisting conditions. In some cases the first-listed diagnosis may be a symptom when a diagnosis has not been established (confirmed) by the physician.

H. Uncertain diagnosis

Do not code diagnoses documented as "probable", "suspected," "questionable," "rule out," or "working diagnosis" or other similar terms indicating uncertainty. Rather, code the condition(s) to the highest degree of certainty for that encounter/visit, such as symptoms, signs, abnormal test results, or other reason for the visit.

Please note: This differs from the coding practices used by short-term, acute care, long-term care and psychiatric hospitals.

I. Chronic diseases

Chronic diseases treated on an ongoing basis may be coded and reported as many times as the patient receives treatment and care for the condition(s)

J. Code all documented conditions that coexist

Code all documented conditions that coexist at the time of the encounter/visit, and require or affect patient care treatment or management. Do not code conditions that were previously treated and no longer exist. However, history codes (categories Z80-Z87) may be used as secondary codes if the historical condition or family history has an impact on current care or influences treatment.

K. Patients receiving diagnostic services only

For patients receiving diagnostic services only during an encounter/visit, sequence first the diagnosis, condition, problem, or other reason for encounter/visit shown in the medical record to be chiefly responsible for the outpatient services provided during the encounter/visit. Codes for other diagnoses (e.g., chronic conditions) may be sequenced as additional diagnoses.

For encounters for routine laboratory/radiology testing in the absence of any signs, symptoms, or associated diagnosis, assign Z01.89, Encounter for other specified special examinations. If routine testing is performed during the same encounter as a test to evaluate a sign, symptom, or diagnosis, it is appropriate to assign both the Z code and the code describing the reason for the non-routine test.

For outpatient encounters for diagnostic tests that have been interpreted by a physician, and the final report is available at the time of coding, code any confirmed or definitive diagnosis(es) documented in the interpretation. Do not code related signs and symptoms as additional diagnoses.

Please note: This differs from the coding practice in the hospital inpatient setting regarding abnormal findings on test results.

L. Patients receiving therapeutic services only
For patients receiving therapeutic services only during an encounter/visit, sequence first the diagnosis, condition, problem, or other reason for encounter/visit shown in the medical record to be chiefly responsible for the outpatient services provided during the encounter/visit. Codes for other diagnoses (e.g., chronic conditions) may be sequenced as additional diagnoses.

The only exception to this rule is that when the primary reason for the admission/encounter is chemotherapy or radiation therapy, the appropriate Z code for the service is listed first, and the diagnosis or problem for which the service is being performed listed second.

M. Patients receiving preoperative evaluations only
For patients receiving preoperative evaluations only, sequence first a code from subcategory Z01.81, Encounter for pre-procedural examinations, to describe the pre-op consultations. Assign a code for the condition to describe the reason for the surgery as an additional diagnosis. Code also any findings related to the pre-op evaluation.

N. Ambulatory surgery
For ambulatory surgery, code the diagnosis for which the surgery was performed. If the postoperative diagnosis is known to be different from the preoperative diagnosis at the time the diagnosis is confirmed, select the postoperative diagnosis for coding, since it is the most definitive.

O. Routine outpatient prenatal visits
See Section I.C.15. Routine outpatient prenatal visits.

P. Encounters for general medical examinations with abnormal findings
The subcategories for encounters for general medical examinations, Z00.0-, provide codes for with and without abnormal findings. Should a general medical examination result in an abnormal finding, the code for general medical examination with abnormal finding should be assigned as the first-listed diagnosis. An examination with abnormal findings refers to a condition/diagnosis that is newly identified or a change in severity of a chronic condition (such as uncontrolled hypertension, or an acute exacerbation of chronic obstructive pulmonary disease) during a routine physical examination. A secondary code for the abnormal finding should also be coded.

Q. Encounters for routine health screenings
See Section I.C.21. Factors influencing health status and contact with health services, Screening

Appendix I. Present on Admission Reporting Guidelines

Introduction
These guidelines are to be used as a supplement to the *ICD-10-CM Official Guidelines for Coding and Reporting* to facilitate the assignment of the Present on Admission (POA) indicator for each diagnosis and external cause of injury code reported on claim forms (UB-04 and 837 Institutional).

These guidelines are not intended to replace any guidelines in the main body of the *ICD-10-CM Official Guidelines for Coding and Reporting*. The POA guidelines are not intended to provide guidance on when a condition should be coded, but rather, how to apply the POA indicator to the final set of diagnosis codes that have been assigned in accordance with Sections I, II, and III of the official coding guidelines. Subsequent to the assignment of the ICD-10-CM codes, the POA indicator should then be assigned to those conditions that have been coded.

As stated in the Introduction to the ICD-10-CM Official Guidelines for Coding and Reporting, a joint effort between the healthcare provider and the coder is essential to achieve complete and accurate documentation, code assignment, and reporting of diagnoses and procedures. The importance of consistent, complete documentation in the medical record cannot be overemphasized.

Medical record documentation from any provider involved in the care and treatment of the patient may be used to support the determination of whether a condition was present on admission or not. In the context of the official coding guidelines, the term "provider" means a physician or any qualified healthcare practitioner who is legally accountable for establishing the patient's diagnosis.

These guidelines are not a substitute for the provider's clinical judgment as to the determination of whether a condition was/was not present on admission. The provider should be queried regarding issues related to the linking of signs/symptoms, timing of test results, and the timing of findings.

Please see the CDC website for the detailed list of ICD-10-CM codes that do not require the use of a POA indicator (ftp://ftp.cdc.gov/pub/Health_Statistics/NCHS/Publications/ICD10CM/2017/). The conditions on this exempt list represent categories and/or codes for circumstances regarding the healthcare encounter or factors influencing health status that do not represent a current disease or injury or are always present on admission.

General Reporting Requirements
All claims involving inpatient admissions to general acute care hospitals or other facilities that are subject to a law or regulation mandating collection of present on admission information.

Present on admission is defined as present at the time the order for inpatient admission occurs -- conditions that develop during an outpatient encounter, including emergency department, observation, or outpatient surgery, are considered as present on admission.

POA indicator is assigned to principal and secondary diagnoses (as defined in Section II of the Official Guidelines for Coding and Reporting) and the external cause of injury codes.

Issues related to inconsistent, missing, conflicting or unclear documentation must still be resolved by the provider.

If a condition would not be coded and reported based on UHDDS definitions and current official coding guidelines, then the POA indicator would not be reported.

Reporting Options

    Y - Yes

    N - No

    U - Unknown

    W – Clinically undetermined

    Unreported/Not used – (Exempt from POA reporting)

Reporting Definitions

    Y = present at the time of inpatient admission

    N = not present at the time of inpatient admission

    U = documentation is insufficient to determine if condition is present on admission

    W = provider is unable to clinically determine whether condition was present on admission or not

Timeframe for POA Identification and Documentation
There is no required timeframe as to when a provider (per the definition of "provider" used in these guidelines) must identify or document a condition to be present on admission. In some clinical situations, it may not be possible for a provider to make a definitive diagnosis (or a condition may not be recognized or reported by the patient) for a period of time after admission. In some cases it may be several days before the provider arrives at a definitive diagnosis. This does not mean that the condition was not present on admission. Determination of whether the condition was present on admission or not will be based on the applicable POA guideline as identified in this document, or on the provider's best clinical judgment.

If at the time of code assignment the documentation is unclear as to whether a condition was present on admission or not, it is appropriate to query the provider for clarification.

Assigning the POA Indicator

Condition is on the "Exempt from Reporting" list

Leave the "present on admission" field blank if the condition is on the list of ICD-10-CM codes for which this field is not applicable. This is the only circumstance in which the field may be left blank.

POA Explicitly Documented

Assign Y for any condition the provider explicitly documents as being present on admission.

Assign N for any condition the provider explicitly documents as not present at the time of admission.

Conditions diagnosed prior to inpatient admission

Assign "Y" for conditions that were diagnosed prior to admission (example: hypertension, diabetes mellitus, asthma)

Conditions diagnosed during the admission but clearly present before admission

Assign "Y" for conditions diagnosed during the admission that were clearly present but not diagnosed until after admission occurred.

Diagnoses subsequently confirmed after admission are considered present on admission if at the time of admission they are documented as suspected, possible, rule out, differential diagnosis, or constitute an underlying cause of a symptom that is present at the time of admission.

Condition develops during outpatient encounter prior to inpatient admission

Assign Y for any condition that develops during an outpatient encounter prior to a written order for inpatient admission.

Documentation does not indicate whether condition was present on admission

Assign "U" when the medical record documentation is unclear as to whether the condition was present on admission. "U" should not be routinely assigned and used only in very limited circumstances. Coders are encouraged to query the providers when the documentation is unclear.

Documentation states that it cannot be determined whether the condition was or was not present on admission

Assign "W" when the medical record documentation indicates that it cannot be clinically determined whether or not the condition was present on admission.

Chronic condition with acute exacerbation during the admission

If a single code identifies both the chronic condition and the acute exacerbation, see POA guidelines pertaining to codes that contain multiple clinical concepts.

If a single code only identifies the chronic condition and not the acute exacerbation (e.g., acute exacerbation of chronic leukemia), assign "Y."

Conditions documented as possible, probable, suspected, or rule out at the time of discharge

If the final diagnosis contains a possible, probable, suspected, or rule out diagnosis, and this diagnosis was based on signs, symptoms or clinical findings suspected at the time of inpatient admission, assign "Y."

If the final diagnosis contains a possible, probable, suspected, or rule out diagnosis, and this diagnosis was based on signs, symptoms or clinical findings that were not present on admission, assign "N".

Conditions documented as impending or threatened at the time of discharge

If the final diagnosis contains an impending or threatened diagnosis, and this diagnosis is based on symptoms or clinical findings that were present on admission, assign "Y".

If the final diagnosis contains an impending or threatened diagnosis, and this diagnosis is based on symptoms or clinical findings that were not present on admission, assign "N".

Acute and Chronic Conditions

Assign "Y" for acute conditions that are present at time of admission and N for acute conditions that are not present at time of admission.

Assign "Y" for chronic conditions, even though the condition may not be diagnosed until after admission.

If a single code identifies both an acute and chronic condition, see the POA guidelines for codes that contain multiple clinical concepts.

Codes That Contain Multiple Clinical Concepts

Assign "N" if at least one of the clinical concepts included in the code was not present on admission (e.g., COPD with acute exacerbation and the exacerbation was not present on admission; gastric ulcer that does not start bleeding until after admission; asthma patient develops status asthmaticus after admission).

Assign "Y" if all of the clinical concepts included in the code were present on admission (e.g., duodenal ulcer that perforates prior to admission).

For infection codes that include the causal organism, assign "Y" if the infection (or signs of the infection) were present on admission, even though the culture results may not be known until after admission (e.g., patient is admitted with pneumonia and the provider documents Pseudomonas as the causal organism a few days later).

Same Diagnosis Code for Two or More Conditions

When the same ICD-10-CM diagnosis code applies to two or more conditions during the same encounter (e.g. two separate conditions classified to the same ICD-10-CM diagnosis code):

Assign "Y" if all conditions represented by the single ICD-10-CM code were present on admission (e.g. bilateral unspecified age-related cataracts).

Assign "N" if any of the conditions represented by the single ICD-10-CM code was not present on admission (e.g. traumatic secondary and recurrent hemorrhage and seroma is assigned to a single code T79.2, but only one of the conditions was present on admission).

Obstetrical conditions

Whether or not the patient delivers during the current hospitalization does not affect assignment of the POA indicator. The determining factor for POA assignment is whether the pregnancy complication or obstetrical condition described by the code was present at the time of admission or not.

If the pregnancy complication or obstetrical condition was present on admission (e.g., patient admitted in preterm labor), assign "Y".

If the pregnancy complication or obstetrical condition was not present on admission (e.g., 2nd degree laceration during delivery, postpartum hemorrhage that occurred during current hospitalization, fetal distress develops after admission), assign "N".

If the obstetrical code includes more than one diagnosis and any of the diagnoses identified by the code were not present on admission assign "N".

(e.g., Category O11, Pre-existing hypertension with pre-eclampsia)

Perinatal conditions

Newborns are not considered to be admitted until after birth. Therefore, any condition present at birth or that developed in utero is considered present at admission and should be assigned "Y". This includes conditions that occur during delivery (e.g., injury during delivery, meconium aspiration, exposure to streptococcus B in the vaginal canal).

Congenital conditions and anomalies

Assign "Y" for congenital conditions and anomalies except for categories Q00-Q99, Congenital anomalies, which are on the exempt list. Congenital conditions are always considered present on admission.

External cause of injury codes

Assign "Y" for any external cause code representing an external cause of morbidity that occurred prior to inpatient admission (e.g., patient fell out of bed at home, patient fell out of bed in emergency room prior to admission)

Assign "N" for any external cause code representing an external cause of morbidity that occurred during inpatient hospitalization (e.g., patient fell out of hospital bed during hospital stay, patient experienced an adverse reaction to a medication administered after inpatient admission)

A

Aarskog's syndrome Q87.1
Abandonment — *see* Maltreatment
Abasia (-astasia) (hysterical) F44.4
Abderhalden-Kaufmann-Lignac syndrome (cystinosis) E72.04
Abdomen, abdominal (*see also* condition)
    acute R10.0
    angina K55.1
    muscle deficiency syndrome Q79.4
Abdominalgia — *see* Pain, abdominal
Abduction contracture, hip or other joint — *see* Contraction, joint
Aberrant (congenital) (*see also* Malposition, congenital)
    adrenal gland Q89.1
    artery (peripheral) Q27.8
        basilar NEC Q28.1
        cerebral Q28.3
        coronary Q24.5
        digestive system Q27.8
        eye Q15.8
        lower limb Q27.8
        precerebral Q28.1
        pulmonary Q25.79
        renal Q27.2
        retina Q14.1
        specified site NEC Q27.8
        subclavian Q27.8
        upper limb Q27.8
        vertebral Q28.1
    breast Q83.8
    endocrine gland NEC Q89.2
    hepatic duct Q44.5
    pancreas Q45.3
    parathyroid gland Q89.2
    pituitary gland Q89.2
    sebaceous glands, mucous membrane, mouth, congenital Q38.6
    spleen Q89.09
    subclavian artery Q27.8
    thymus (gland) Q89.2
    thyroid gland Q89.2
    vein (peripheral) NEC Q27.8
        cerebral Q28.3
        digestive system Q27.8
        lower limb Q27.8
        precerebral Q28.1
        specified site NEC Q27.8
        upper limb Q27.8
Aberration
    distantial — *see* Disturbance, visual
    mental F99
Abetalipoproteinemia E78.6
Abiotrophy R68.89
Ablatio, ablation
    retinae — *see* Detachment, retina
Ablepharia, ablepharon Q10.3
Abnormal, abnormality, abnormalities (*see also* Anomaly)
    acid-base balance (mixed) E87.4
    albumin R77.0
    alphafetoprotein R77.2
    alveolar ridge K08.9
    anatomical relationship Q89.9
    apertures, congenital, diaphragm Q79.1
    auditory perception H93.29- ☑
        diplacusis — *see* Diplacusis
        hyperacusis — *see* Hyperacusis
        recruitment — *see* Recruitment, auditory
        threshold shift — *see* Shift, auditory threshold
    autosomes Q99.9
        fragile site Q95.5
    basal metabolic rate R94.8
    biosynthesis, testicular androgen E29.1
    bleeding time R79.1
    blood level (of)
        cobalt R79.0
        copper R79.0
        iron R79.0
        lithium R78.89
        magnesium R79.0

Abnormal, abnormality, abnormalities — *continued*
    blood level — *continued*
        mineral NEC R79.0
        zinc R79.0
    blood pressure
        elevated R03.0
        low reading (nonspecific) R03.1
    blood sugar R73.09
    blood-gas level R79.81
    bowel sounds R19.15
        absent R19.11
        hyperactive R19.12
    brain scan R94.02
    breathing R06.9
    caloric test R94.138
    cerebrospinal fluid R83.9
        cytology R83.6
        drug level R83.2
        enzyme level R83.0
        hormones R83.1
        immunology R83.4
        microbiology R83.5
        nonmedicinal level R83.3
        specified type NEC R83.8
    chemistry, blood R79.9
        C-reactive protein R79.82
        drugs — *see* Findings, abnormal, in blood
        gas level R79.81
        minerals R79.0
        pancytopenia D61.818
        PTT R79.1
        specified NEC R79.89
        toxins — *see* Findings, abnormal, in blood
    chest sounds (friction) (rales) R09.89
    chromosome, chromosomal Q99.9
        with more than three X chromosomes, female Q97.1
        analysis result R89.8
            bronchial washings R84.8
            cerebrospinal fluid R83.8
            cervix uteri NEC R87.89
            nasal secretions R84.8
            nipple discharge R89.8
            peritoneal fluid R85.89
            pleural fluid R84.8
            prostatic secretions R86.8
            saliva R85.89
            seminal fluid R86.8
            sputum R84.8
            synovial fluid R89.8
            throat scrapings R84.8
            vagina R87.89
            vulva R87.89
            wound secretions R89.8
        dicentric replacement Q93.2
        ring replacement Q93.2
        sex Q99.8
            female phenotype Q97.9
                specified NEC Q97.8
            male phenotype Q98.9
                specified NEC Q98.8
            structural male Q98.6
        specified NEC Q99.8
    clinical findings NEC R68.89
    coagulation D68.9
        newborn, transient P61.6
        profile R79.1
        time R79.1
    communication — *see* Fistula
    conjunctiva, vascular H11.41- ☑
    coronary artery Q24.5
    cortisol-binding globulin E27.8
    course, eustachian tube Q17.8
    creatinine clearance R94.4
    cytology
        anus R85.619
            atypical squamous cells cannot exclude high grade squamous intraepithelial lesion (ASC-H) R85.611
            atypical squamous cells of undetermined significance (ASC-US) R85.610
            cytologic evidence of malignancy R85.614

Abnormal, abnormality, abnormalities — *continued*
    cytology — *continued*
        anus — *continued*
            high grade squamous intraepithelial lesion (HGSIL) R85.613
            human papillomavirus (HPV) DNA test
                high risk positive R85.81
                low risk postive R85.82
            inadequate smear R85.615
            low grade squamous intraepithelial lesion (LGSIL) R85.612
            satisfactory anal smear but lacking transformation zone R85.616
            specified NEC R85.618
            unsatisfactory smear R85.615
        female genital organs — *see* Abnormal, Papanicolaou (smear)
    dark adaptation curve H53.61
    dentofacial NEC — *see* Anomaly, dentofacial
    development, developmental Q89.9
        central nervous system Q07.9
    diagnostic imaging
        abdomen, abdominal region NEC R93.5
        biliary tract R93.2
        bladder R93.41
        breast R92.8
        central nervous system NEC R90.89
        cerebrovascular NEC R90.89
        coronary circulation R93.1
        digestive tract NEC R93.3
        gastrointestinal (tract) R93.3
        genitourinary organs R93.8
        head R93.0
        heart R93.1
        intrathoracic organ NEC R93.8
        kidney R93.42- ☑
        limbs R93.6
        liver R93.2
        lung (field) R91.8
        musculoskeletal system NEC R93.7
        renal pelvis R93.41
        retroperitoneum R93.5
        site specified NEC R93.8
        skin and subcutaneous tissue R93.8
        skull R93.0
        ureter R93.41
        urinary organs specified NEC R93.49
    direction, teeth, fully erupted M26.30
    ear ossicles, acquired NEC H74.39- ☑
        ankylosis — *see* Ankylosis, ear ossicles
        discontinuity — *see* Discontinuity, ossicles, ear
        partial loss — *see* Loss, ossicles, ear (partial)
    Ebstein Q22.5
    echocardiogram R93.1
    echoencephalogram R90.81
    echogram — *see* Abnormal, diagnostic imaging
    electrocardiogram [ECG] [EKG] R94.31
    electroencephalogram [EEG] R94.01
    electrolyte — *see* Imbalance, electrolyte
    electromyogram [EMG] R94.131
    electro-oculogram [EOG] R94.110
    electrophysiological intracardiac studies R94.39
    electroretinogram [ERG] R94.111
    erythrocytes
        congenital, with perinatal jaundice D58.9
    feces (color) (contents) (mucus) R19.5
    finding — *see* Findings, abnormal, without diagnosis
    fluid
        amniotic — *see* Abnormal, specimen, specified
        cerebrospinal — *see* Abnormal, cerebrospinal fluid
        peritoneal — *see* Abnormal, specimen, digestive organs
        pleural — *see* Abnormal, specimen, respiratory organs
        synovial — *see* Abnormal, specimen, specified
        thorax (bronchial washings) (pleural fluid) — *see* Abnormal, specimen, respiratory organs
        vaginal — *see* Abnormal, specimen, female genital organs
    form
        teeth K00.2
        uterus — *see* Anomaly, uterus

Abnormal, abnormality, abnormalities —
    continued
    function studies
      auditory R94.120
      bladder R94.8
      brain R94.09
      cardiovascular R94.30
      ear R94.128
      endocrine NEC R94.7
      eye NEC R94.118
      kidney R94.4
      liver R94.5
      nervous system
        central NEC R94.09
        peripheral NEC R94.138
      pancreas R94.8
      placenta R94.8
      pulmonary R94.2
      special senses NEC R94.128
      spleen R94.8
      thyroid R94.6
      vestibular R94.121
    gait — *see* Gait
      hysterical F44.4
    gastrin secretion E16.4
    globulin R77.1
      cortisol-binding E27.8
      thyroid-binding E07.89
    glomerular, minor (*see also* N00-N07 with fourth
      character .0) N05.0
    glucagon secretion E16.3
    glucose tolerance (test) (non-fasting) R73.09
    gravitational (G) forces or states (effect of) T75.81 ☑
    hair (color) (shaft) L67.9
      specified NEC L67.8
    hard tissue formation in pulp (dental) K04.3
    head movement R25.0
    heart
      rate R00.9
        specified NEC R00.8
      shadow R93.1
      sounds NEC R01.2
    hemoglobin (disease) (*see also* Disease, hemoglobin)
      D58.2
      trait — *see* Trait, hemoglobin, abnormal
    histology NEC R89.7
    immunological findings R89.4
      in serum R76.9
        specified NEC R76.8
    increase in appetite R63.2
    involuntary movement — *see* Abnormal, movement,
      involuntary
    jaw closure M26.51
    karyotype R89.8
    kidney function test R94.4
    knee jerk R29.2
    leukocyte (cell) (differential) NEC D72.9
    liver function test R94.5
    loss of
      height R29.890
      weight R63.4
    mammogram NEC R92.8
      calcification (calculus) R92.1
      microcalcification R92.0
    Mantoux test R76.11
    movement (disorder) (*see also* Disorder, movement)
      head R25.0
      involuntary R25.9
        fasciculation R25.3
        of head R25.0
        spasm R25.2
        specified type NEC R25.8
        tremor R25.1
    myoglobin (Aberdeen) (Annapolis) R89.7
    neonatal screening P09
    oculomotor study R94.113
    palmar creases Q82.8
    Papanicolaou (smear)
      anus R85.619
        atypical squamous cells cannot exclude high
          grade squamous intraepithelial lesion
          (ASC-H) R85.611
        atypical squamous cells of undetermined signif-
          icance (ASC-US) R85.610
        cytologic evidence of malignancy R85.614
        high grade squamous intraepithelial lesion
          (HGSIL) R85.613
        human papillomavirus (HPV) DNA test
          high risk positive R85.81

Abnormal, abnormality, abnormalities —
    continued
    Papanicolaou — *continued*
      anus — *continued*
        human papillomavirus DNA test — *contin-
          ued*
          low risk postive R85.82
        inadequate smear R85.615
        low grade squamous intraepithelial lesion
          (LGSIL) R85.612
        satisfactory anal smear but lacking transforma-
          tion zone R85.616
        specified NEC R85.618
        unsatisfactory smear R85.615
      bronchial washings R84.6
      cerebrospinal fluid R83.6
      cervix R87.619
        atypical squamous cells cannot exclude high
          grade squamous intraepithelial lesion
          (ASC-H) R87.611
        atypical squamous cells of undetermined signif-
          icance (ASC-US) R87.610
        cytologic evidence of malignancy R87.614
        high grade squamous intraepithelial lesion
          (HGSIL) R87.613
        inadequate smear R87.615
        low grade squamous intraepithelial lesion
          (LGSIL) R87.612
        non-atypical endometrial cells R87.618
        satisfactory cervical smear but lacking transfor-
          mation zone R87.616
        specified NEC R87.618
        thin preparaton R87.619
        unsatisfactory smear R87.615
      nasal secretions R84.6
      nipple discharge R89.6
      peritoneal fluid R85.69
      pleural fluid R84.6
      prostatic secretions R86.6
      saliva R85.69
      seminal fluid R86.6
      sites NEC R89.6
      sputum R84.6
      synovial fluid R89.6
      throat scrapings R84.6
      vagina R87.629
        atypical squamous cells cannot exclude high
          grade squamous intraepithelial lesion
          (ASC-H) R87.621
        atypical squamous cells of undetermined signif-
          icance (ASC-US) R87.620
        cytologic evidence of malignancy R87.624
        high grade squamous intraepithelial lesion
          (HGSIL) R87.623
        inadequate smear R87.625
        low grade squamous intraepithelial lesion
          (LGSIL) R87.622
        specified NEC R87.628
        thin preparation R87.629
        unsatisfactory smear R87.625
      vulva R87.69
      wound secretions R89.6
    partial thromboplastin time (PTT) R79.1
    pelvis (bony) — *see* Deformity, pelvis
    percussion, chest (tympany) R09.89
    periods (grossly) — *see* Menstruation
    phonocardiogram R94.39
    plantar reflex R29.2
    plasma
      protein R77.9
        specified NEC R77.8
      viscosity R70.1
    pleural (folds) Q34.0
    posture R29.3
    product of conception O02.9
      specified type NEC O02.89
    prothrombin time (PT) R79.1
    pulmonary
      artery, congenital Q25.79
      function, newborn P28.89
      test results R94.2
    pulsations in neck R00.2
    pupillary H21.56- ☑
      function (reaction) (reflex) — *see* Anomaly, pupil,
      function
    radiological examination — *see* Abnormal, diagnostic
      imaging
    red blood cell(s) (morphology) (volume) R71.8
    reflex — *see* Reflex

Abnormal, abnormality, abnormalities —
    continued
    renal function test R94.4
    response to nerve stimulation R94.130
    retinal correspondence H53.31
    retinal function study R94.111
    rhythm, heart (*see also* Arrhythmia)
    saliva — *see* Abnormal, specimen, digestive organs
    scan
      kidney R94.4
      liver R93.2
      thyroid R94.6
    secretion
      gastrin E16.4
      glucagon E16.3
    semen, seminal fluid — *see* Abnormal, specimen, male
      genital organs
    serum level (of)
      acid phosphatase R74.8
      alkaline phosphatase R74.8
      amylase R74.8
      enzymes R74.9
        specified NEC R74.8
      lipase R74.8
      triacylglycerol lipase R74.8
    shape
      gravid uterus — *see* Anomaly, uterus
    sinus venosus Q21.1
    size, tooth, teeth K00.2
    spacing, tooth, teeth, fully erupted M26.30
    specimen
      digestive organs (peritoneal fluid) (saliva) R85.9
        cytology R85.69
        drug level R85.2
        enzyme level R85.0
        histology R85.7
        hormones R85.1
        immunology R85.4
        microbiology R85.5
        nonmedicinal level R85.3
        specified type NEC R85.89
      female genital organs (secretions) (smears) R87.9
        cytology R87.69
          cervix R87.619
            human papillomavirus (HPV) DNA test
              high risk positive R87.810
              low risk positive R87.820
            inadequate (unsatisfactory) smear
              R87.615
            non-atypical endometrial cells R87.618
            specified NEC R87.618
          vagina R87.629
            human papillomavirus (HPV) DNA test
              high risk positive R87.811
              low risk positive R87.821
            inadequate (unsatisfactory) smear
              R87.625
          vulva R87.69
        drug level R87.2
        enzyme level R87.0
        histological R87.7
        hormones R87.1
        immunology R87.4
        microbiology R87.5
        nonmedicinal level R87.3
        specified type NEC R87.89
      male genital organs (prostatic secretions) (semen)
        R86.9
        cytology R86.6
        drug level R86.2
        enzyme level R86.0
        histological R86.7
        hormones R86.1
        immunology R86.4
        microbiology R86.5
        nonmedicinal level R86.3
        specified type NEC R86.8
      nipple discharge — *see* Abnormal, specimen,
        specified
      respiratory organs (bronchial washings) (nasal se-
        cretions) (pleural fluid) (sputum) R84.9
        cytology R84.6
        drug level R84.2
        enzyme level R84.0
        histology R84.7
        hormones R84.1
        immunology R84.4
        microbiology R84.5
        nonmedicinal level R84.3

☑ **Additional Character Required — Refer to the Tabular List for Character Selection**   ▽ **Subterms under main terms may continue to next column or page**

Abnormal, abnormality, abnormalities — *continued*
　specimen — *continued*
　　respiratory organs — *continued*
　　　specified type NEC R84.8
　　specified organ, system and tissue NOS R89.9
　　　cytology R89.6
　　　drug level R89.2
　　　enzyme level R89.0
　　　histology R89.7
　　　hormones R89.1
　　　immunology R89.4
　　　microbiology R89.5
　　　nonmedicinal level R89.3
　　　specified type NEC R89.8
　　synovial fluid — *see* Abnormal, specimen, specified
　　thorax (bronchial washings) (pleural fluids) — *see* Abnormal, specimen, respiratory organs
　　vagina (secretion) (smear) R87.629
　　vulva (secretion) (smear) R87.69
　　wound secretion — *see* Abnormal, specimen, specified
　spermatozoa — *see* Abnormal, specimen, male genital organs
　sputum (amount) (color) (odor) R09.3
　stool (color) (contents) (mucus) R19.5
　　bloody K92.1
　　guaiac positive R19.5
　synchondrosis Q78.8
　thermography (*see also* Abnormal, diagnostic imaging) R93.8
　thyroid-binding globulin E07.89
　tooth, teeth (form) (size) K00.2
　toxicology (findings) R78.9
　transport protein E88.09
　tumor marker NEC R97.8
　ultrasound results — *see* Abnormal, diagnostic imaging
　umbilical cord complicating delivery O69.9 ☑
　urination NEC R39.198
　urine (constituents) R82.90
　　bile R82.2
　　cytological examination R82.8
　　drugs R82.5
　　fat R82.0
　　glucose R81
　　heavy metals R82.6
　　hemoglobin R82.3
　　histological examination R82.8
　　ketones R82.4
　　microbiological examination (culture) R82.79
　　myoglobin R82.1
　　positive culture R82.79
　　protein — *see* Proteinuria
　　specified substance NEC R82.99
　　　chromoabnormality NEC R82.91
　　substances nonmedical R82.6
　uterine hemorrhage — *see* Hemorrhage, uterus
　vectorcardiogram R94.39
　visually evoked potential (VEP) R94.112
　white blood cells D72.9
　　specified NEC D72.89
　X-ray examination — *see* Abnormal, diagnostic imaging
Abnormity (any organ or part) — *see* Anomaly
Abocclusion M26.29
　hemolytic disease (newborn) P55.1
　incompatibility reaction ABO — *see* Complication(s), transfusion, incompatibility reaction, ABO
Abolition, language R48.8
Aborter, habitual or recurrent — *see* Loss (of), pregnancy, recurrent
Abortion (complete) (spontaneous) O03.9
　with
　　retained products of conception — *see* Abortion, incomplete
　attempted (elective) (failed) O07.4
　　complicated by O07.30
　　　afibrinogenemia O07.1
　　　cardiac arrest O07.36
　　　chemical damage of pelvic organ(s) O07.34
　　　circulatory collapse O07.31
　　　cystitis O07.38
　　　defibrination syndrome O07.1
　　　electrolyte imbalance O07.33
　　　embolism (air) (amniotic fluid) (blood clot) (fat) (pulmonary) (septic) (soap) O07.2
　　　endometritis O07.0

Abortion — *continued*
　attempted — *continued*
　　complicated by — *continued*
　　　genital tract and pelvic infection O07.0
　　　hemolysis O07.1
　　　hemorrhage (delayed) (excessive) O07.1
　　　infection
　　　　genital tract or pelvic O07.0
　　　　urinary tract tract O07.38
　　　intravascular coagulation O07.1
　　　laceration of pelvic organ(s) O07.34
　　　metabolic disorder O07.33
　　　oliguria O07.32
　　　oophoritis O07.0
　　　parametritis O07.0
　　　pelvic peritonitis O07.0
　　　perforation of pelvic organ(s) O07.34
　　　renal failure or shutdown O07.32
　　　salpingitis or salpingo-oophoritis O07.0
　　　sepsis O07.37
　　　shock O07.31
　　　specified condition NEC O07.39
　　　tubular necrosis (renal) O07.32
　　　uremia O07.32
　　　urinary tract infection O07.38
　　　venous complication NEC O07.35
　　　　embolism (air) (amniotic fluid) (blood clot) (fat) (pulmonary) (septic) (soap) O07.2
　complicated (by) (following) O03.80
　　afibrinogenemia O03.6
　　cardiac arrest O03.86
　　chemical damage of pelvic organ(s) O03.84
　　circulatory collapse O03.81
　　cystitis O03.88
　　defibrination syndrome O03.6
　　electrolyte imbalance O03.83
　　embolism (air) (amniotic fluid) (blood clot) (fat) (pulmonary) (septic) (soap) O03.7
　　endometritis O03.5
　　genital tract and pelvic infection O03.5
　　hemolysis O03.6
　　hemorrhage (delayed) (excessive) O03.6
　　infection
　　　genital tract or pelvic O03.5
　　　urinary tract O03.88
　　intravascular coagulation O03.6
　　laceration of pelvic organ(s) O03.84
　　metabolic disorder O03.83
　　oliguria O03.82
　　oophoritis O03.5
　　parametritis O03.5
　　pelvic peritonitis O03.5
　　perforation of pelvic organ(s) O03.84
　　renal failure or shutdown O03.82
　　salpingitis or salpingo-oophoritis O03.5
　　sepsis O03.87
　　shock O03.81
　　specified condition NEC O03.89
　　tubular necrosis (renal) O03.82
　　uremia O03.82
　　urinary tract infection O03.88
　　venous complication NEC O03.85
　　　embolism (air) (amniotic fluid) (blood clot) (fat) (pulmonary) (septic) (soap) O03.7
　failed — *see* Abortion, attempted
　habitual or recurrent N96
　　with current abortion — *see* categories O03-O04
　　without current pregnancy N96
　　care in current pregnancy O26.2- ☑
　incomplete (spontaneous) O03.4
　　complicated (by) (following) O03.30
　　　afibrinogenemia O03.1
　　　cardiac arrest O03.36
　　　chemical damage of pelvic organ(s) O03.34
　　　circulatory collapse O03.31
　　　cystitis O03.38
　　　defibrination syndrome O03.1
　　　electrolyte imbalance O03.33
　　　embolism (air) (amniotic fluid) (blood clot) (fat) (pulmonary) (septic) (soap) O03.2
　　　endometritis O03.0
　　　genital tract and pelvic infection O03.0
　　　hemolysis O03.1
　　　hemorrhage (delayed) (excessive) O03.1
　　　infection
　　　　genital tract or pelvic O03.0
　　　　urinary tract O03.38
　　　intravascular coagulation O03.1
　　　laceration of pelvic organ(s) O03.34

Abortion — *continued*
　incomplete — *continued*
　　complicated — *continued*
　　　metabolic disorder O03.33
　　　oliguria O03.32
　　　oophoritis O03.0
　　　parametritis O03.0
　　　pelvic peritonitis O03.0
　　　perforation of pelvic organ(s) O03.34
　　　renal failure or shutdown O03.32
　　　salpingitis or salpingo-oophoritis O03.0
　　　sepsis O03.37
　　　shock O03.31
　　　specified condition NEC O03.39
　　　tubular necrosis (renal) O03.32
　　　uremia O03.32
　　　urinary infection O03.38
　　　venous complication NEC O03.35
　　　　embolism (air) (amniotic fluid) (blood clot) (fat) (pulmonary) (septic) (soap) O03.2
　induced (encounter for) Z33.2
　　complicated by O04.80
　　　afibrinogenemia O04.6
　　　cardiac arrest O04.86
　　　chemical damage of pelvic organ(s) O04.84
　　　circulatory collapse O04.81
　　　cystitis O04.88
　　　defibrination syndrome O04.6
　　　electrolyte imbalance O04.83
　　　embolism (air) (amniotic fluid) (blood clot) (fat) (pulmonary) (septic) (soap) O04.7
　　　endometritis O04.5
　　　genital tract and pelvic infection O04.5
　　　hemolysis O04.6
　　　hemorrhage (delayed) (excessive) O04.6
　　　infection
　　　　genital tract or pelvic O04.5
　　　　urinary tract O04.88
　　　intravascular coagulation O04.6
　　　laceration of pelvic organ(s) O04.84
　　　metabolic disorder O04.83
　　　oliguria O04.82
　　　oophoritis O04.5
　　　parametritis O04.5
　　　pelvic peritonitis O04.5
　　　perforation of pelvic organ(s) O04.84
　　　renal failure or shutdown O04.82
　　　salpingitis or salpingo-oophoritis O04.5
　　　sepsis O04.87
　　　shock O04.81
　　　specified condition NEC O04.89
　　　tubular necrosis (renal) O04.82
　　　uremia O04.82
　　　urinary tract infection O04.88
　　　venous complication NEC O04.85
　　　　embolism (air) (amniotic fluid) (blood clot) (fat) (pulmonary) (septic) (soap) O04.7
　missed O02.1
　spontaneous — *see* Abortion (complete) (spontaneous)
　　threatened O20.0
　threatened (spontaneous) O20.0
　tubal O00.10- ☑
　　with intrauterine pregnancy O00.11- ☑
Abortus fever A23.1
Aboulomania F60.7
Abrami's disease D59.8
Abramov-Fiedler myocarditis (acute isolated myocarditis) I40.1
Abrasion T14.8 ☑
　abdomen, abdominal (wall) S30.811 ☑
　alveolar process S00.512 ☑
　ankle S90.51- ☑
　antecubital space — *see* Abrasion, elbow
　anus S30.817 ☑
　arm (upper) S40.81- ☑
　auditory canal — *see* Abrasion, ear
　auricle — *see* Abrasion, ear
　axilla — *see* Abrasion, arm
　back, lower S30.810 ☑
　breast S20.11- ☑
　brow S00.81 ☑
　buttock S30.810 ☑
　calf — *see* Abrasion, leg
　canthus — *see* Abrasion, eyelid
　cheek S00.81 ☑
　　internal S00.512 ☑
　chest wall — *see* Abrasion, thorax

Abrasion — *continued*
- chin S00.81 ☑
- clitoris S30.814 ☑
- cornea S05.0- ☑
- costal region — *see* Abrasion, thorax
- dental K03.1
- digit(s)
  - foot — *see* Abrasion, toe
  - hand — *see* Abrasion, finger
- ear S00.41- ☑
- elbow S50.31- ☑
- epididymis S30.813 ☑
- epigastric region S30.811 ☑
- epiglottis S10.11 ☑
- esophagus (thoracic) S27.818 ☑
  - cervical S10.11 ☑
- eyebrow — *see* Abrasion, eyelid
- eyelid S00.21- ☑
- face S00.81 ☑
- finger(s) S60.41- ☑
  - index S60.41- ☑
  - little S60.41- ☑
  - middle S60.41- ☑
  - ring S60.41- ☑
- flank S30.811 ☑
- foot (except toe(s) alone) S90.81- ☑
  - toe — *see* Abrasion, toe
- forearm S50.81- ☑
  - elbow only — *see* Abrasion, elbow
- forehead S00.81 ☑
- genital organs, external
  - female S30.816 ☑
  - male S30.815 ☑
- groin S30.811 ☑
- gum S00.512 ☑
- hand S60.51- ☑
- head S00.91 ☑
  - ear — *see* Abrasion, ear
  - eyelid — *see* Abrasion, eyelid
  - lip S00.511 ☑
  - nose S00.31 ☑
  - oral cavity S00.512 ☑
  - scalp S00.01 ☑
  - specified site NEC S00.81 ☑
- heel — *see* Abrasion, foot
- hip S70.21- ☑
- inguinal region S30.811 ☑
- interscapular region S20.419 ☑
- jaw S00.81 ☑
- knee S80.21- ☑
- labium (majus) (minus) S30.814 ☑
- larynx S10.11 ☑
- leg (lower) S80.81- ☑
  - knee — *see* Abrasion, knee
  - upper — *see* Abrasion, thigh
- lip S00.511 ☑
- lower back S30.810 ☑
- lumbar region S30.810 ☑
- malar region S00.81 ☑
- mammary — *see* Abrasion, breast
- mastoid region S00.81 ☑
- mouth S00.512 ☑
- nail
  - finger — *see* Abrasion, finger
  - toe — *see* Abrasion, toe
- nape S10.81 ☑
- nasal S00.31 ☑
- neck S10.91 ☑
  - specified site NEC S10.81 ☑
  - throat S10.11 ☑
- nose S00.31 ☑
- occipital region S00.01 ☑
- oral cavity S00.512 ☑
- orbital region — *see* Abrasion, eyelid
- palate S00.512 ☑
- palm — *see* Abrasion, hand
- parietal region S00.01 ☑
- pelvis S30.810 ☑
- penis S30.812 ☑
- perineum
  - female S30.814 ☑
  - male S30.810 ☑
- periocular area — *see* Abrasion, eyelid
- phalanges
  - finger — *see* Abrasion, finger
  - toe — *see* Abrasion, toe

Abrasion — *continued*
- pharynx S10.11 ☑
- pinna — *see* Abrasion, ear
- popliteal space — *see* Abrasion, knee
- prepuce S30.812 ☑
- pubic region S30.810 ☑
- pudendum
  - female S30.816 ☑
  - male S30.815 ☑
- sacral region S30.810 ☑
- scalp S00.01 ☑
- scapular region — *see* Abrasion, shoulder
- scrotum S30.813 ☑
- shin — *see* Abrasion, leg
- shoulder S40.21- ☑
- skin NEC T14.8 ☑
- sternal region S20.319 ☑
- submaxillary region S00.81 ☑
- submental region S00.81 ☑
- subungual
  - finger(s) — *see* Abrasion, finger
  - toe(s) — *see* Abrasion, toe
- supraclavicular fossa S10.81 ☑
- supraorbital S00.81 ☑
- temple S00.81 ☑
- temporal region S00.81 ☑
- testis S30.813 ☑
- thigh S70.31- ☑
- thorax, thoracic (wall) S20.91 ☑
  - back S20.41- ☑
  - front S20.31- ☑
- throat S10.11 ☑
- thumb S60.31- ☑
- toe(s) (lesser) S90.416 ☑
  - great S90.41- ☑
- tongue S00.512 ☑
- tooth, teeth (dentifrice) (habitual) (hard tissues) (occupational) (ritual) (traditional) K03.1
- trachea S10.11 ☑
- tunica vaginalis S30.813 ☑
- tympanum, tympanic membrane — *see* Abrasion, ear
- uvula S00.512 ☑
- vagina S30.814 ☑
- vocal cords S10.11 ☑
- vulva S30.814 ☑
- wrist S60.81- ☑

Abrism — *see* Poisoning, food, noxious, plant

Abruptio placentae O45.9- ☑
- with
  - afibrinogenemia O45.01- ☑
  - coagulation defect O45.00- ☑
    - specified NEC O45.09- ☑
  - disseminated intravascular coagulation O45.02- ☑
  - hypofibrinogenemia O45.01- ☑
  - specified NEC O45.8- ☑

Abruption, placenta — *see* Abruptio placentae

Abscess (connective tissue) (embolic) (fistulous) (infective) (metastatic) (multiple) (pernicious) (pyogenic) (septic) L02.91
- with
  - diverticular disease (intestine) K57.80
    - with bleeding K57.81
    - large intestine K57.20
      - with
        - bleeding K57.21
        - small intestine K57.40
          - with bleeding K57.41
    - small intestine K57.00
      - with
        - bleeding K57.01
        - large intestine K57.40
          - with bleeding K57.41
  - lymphangitis — *code by* site under Abscess
- abdomen, abdominal
  - cavity K65.1
  - wall L02.211
- abdominopelvic K65.1
- accessory sinus — *see* Sinusitis
- adrenal (capsule) (gland) E27.8
- alveolar K04.7
  - with sinus K04.6
- amebic A06.4
  - brain (and liver or lung abscess) A06.6
  - genitourinary tract A06.82
  - liver (without mention of brain or lung abscess) A06.4

Abscess — *continued*
- amebic — *continued*
  - lung (and liver) (without mention of brain abscess) A06.5
  - specified site NEC A06.89
  - spleen A06.89
- anerobic A48.0
- ankle — *see* Abscess, lower limb
- anorectal K61.2
- antecubital space — *see* Abscess, upper limb
- antrum (chronic) (Highmore) — *see* Sinusitis, maxillary
- anus K61.0
- apical (tooth) K04.7
  - with sinus (alveolar) K04.6
- appendix K35.3
- areola (acute) (chronic) (nonpuerperal) N61.1
  - puerperal, postpartum or gestational — *see* Infection, nipple
- arm (any part) — *see* Abscess, upper limb
- artery (wall) I77.89
- atheromatous I77.2
- auricle, ear — *see* Abscess, ear, external
- axilla (region) L02.41- ☑
  - lymph gland or node L04.2
- back (any part, except buttock) L02.212
- Bartholin's gland N75.1
  - with
    - abortion — *see* Abortion, by type complicated by, sepsis
    - ectopic or molar pregnancy O08.0
  - following ectopic or molar pregnancy O08.0
- Bezold's — *see* Mastoiditis, acute
- bilharziasis B65.1
- bladder (wall) — *see* Cystitis, specified type NEC
- bone (subperiosteal) (*see also* Osteomyelitis, specified type NEC)
  - accessory sinus (chronic) — *see* Sinusitis
  - chronic or old — *see* Osteomyelitis, chronic
  - jaw (lower) (upper) M27.2
  - mastoid — *see* Mastoiditis, acute, subperiosteal
  - petrous — *see* Petrositis
  - spinal (tuberculous) A18.01
    - nontuberculous — *see* Osteomyelitis, vertebra
- bowel K63.0
- brain (any part) (cystic) (otogenic) G06.0
  - amebic (with abscess of any other site) A06.6
  - gonococcal A54.82
  - pheomycotic (chromomycotic) B43.1
  - tuberculous A17.81
- breast (acute) (chronic) (nonpuerperal) N61.1
  - newborn P39.0
  - puerperal, postpartum, gestational — *see* Mastitis, obstetric, purulent
- broad ligament N73.2
  - acute N73.0
  - chronic N73.1
- Brodie's (localized) (chronic) M86.8X- ☑
- bronchi J98.09
- buccal cavity K12.2
- bulbourethral gland N34.0
- bursa M71.00
  - ankle M71.07- ☑
  - elbow M71.02- ☑
  - foot M71.07- ☑
  - hand M71.04- ☑
  - hip M71.05- ☑
  - knee M71.06- ☑
  - multiple sites M71.09
  - pharyngeal J39.1
  - shoulder M71.01- ☑
  - specified site NEC M71.08
  - wrist M71.03- ☑
- buttock L02.31
- canthus — *see* Blepharoconjunctivitis
- cartilage — *see* Disorder, cartilage, specified type NEC
- cecum K35.3
- cerebellum, cerebellar G06.0
  - sequelae G09
- cerebral (embolic) G06.0
  - sequelae G09
- cervical (meaning neck) L02.11
  - lymph gland or node L04.0
- cervix (stump) (uteri) — *see* Cervicitis
- cheek (external) L02.01
  - inner K12.2
- chest J86.9
  - with fistula J86.0
  - wall L02.213

Abscess — *continued*
chin L02.01
choroid — *see* Inflammation, chorioretinal
circumtonsillar J36
cold (lung) (tuberculous) (*see also* Tuberculosis, abscess, lung)
    articular — *see* Tuberculosis, joint
colon (wall) K63.0
colostomy K94.02
conjunctiva — *see* Conjunctivitis, acute
cornea H16.31- ☑
corpus
    cavernosum N48.21
    luteum — *see* Oophoritis
Cowper's gland N34.0
cranium G06.0
cul-de-sac (Douglas') (posterior) — *see* Peritonitis, pelvic, female
cutaneous — *see* Abscess, by site
dental K04.7
    with sinus (alveolar) K04.6
dentoalveolar K04.7
    with sinus K04.6
diaphragm, diaphragmatic K65.1
Douglas' cul-de-sac or pouch — *see* Peritonitis, pelvic, female
Dubois A50.59
ear (middle) (*see also* Otitis, media, suppurative)
    acute — *see* Otitis, media, suppurative, acute
    external H60.0- ☑
entamebic — *see* Abscess, amebic
enterostomy K94.12
epididymis N45.4
epidural G06.2
    brain G06.0
    spinal cord G06.1
epiglottis J38.7
epiploon, epiploic K65.1
erysipelatous — *see* Erysipelas
esophagus K20.8
ethmoid (bone) (chronic) (sinus) J32.2
external auditory canal — *see* Abscess, ear, external
extradural G06.2
    brain G06.0
        sequelae G09
    spinal cord G06.1
extraperitoneal K68.19
eye — *see* Endophthalmitis, purulent
eyelid H00.03- ☑
face (any part, except ear, eye and nose) L02.01
fallopian tube — *see* Salpingitis
fascia M72.8
fauces J39.1
fecal K63.0
femoral (region) — *see* Abscess, lower limb
filaria, filarial — *see* Infestation, filarial
finger (any) (*see also* Abscess, hand)
    nail — *see* Cellulitis, finger
foot L02.61- ☑
forehead L02.01
frontal sinus (chronic) J32.1
gallbladder K81.0
genital organ or tract
    female (external) N76.4
    male N49.9
        multiple sites N49.8
        specified NEC N49.8
gestational mammary O91.11- ☑
gestational subareolar O91.11- ☑
gingival — *see* Peridontitis, aggressive, localized
gland, glandular (lymph) (acute) — *see* Lymphadenitis, acute
gluteal (region) L02.31
gonorrheal — *see* Gonococcus
groin L02.214
gum — *see* Peridontitis, aggressive, localized
hand L02.51- ☑
head NEC L02.811
    face (any part, except ear, eye and nose) L02.01
heart — *see* Carditis
heel — *see* Abscess, foot
helminthic — *see* Infestation, helminth
hepatic (cholangitic) (hematogenic) (lymphogenic) (pylephlebitic) K75.0
    amebic A06.4
hip (region) — *see* Abscess, lower limb
ileocecal K35.3
ileostomy (bud) K94.12

Abscess — *continued*
iliac (region) L02.214
    fossa K35.3
infraclavicular (fossa) — *see* Abscess, upper limb
inguinal (region) L02.214
    lymph gland or node L04.1
intestine, intestinal NEC K63.0
    rectal K61.1
intra-abdominal (*see also* Abscess, peritoneum) K65.1
    postprocedural T81.4 ☑
        retroperitoneal K68.11
intracranial G06.0
intramammary — *see* Abscess, breast
intraorbital — *see* Abscess, orbit
intraperitoneal K65.1
intrasphincteric (anus) K61.4
intraspinal G06.1
intratonsillar J36
ischiorectal (fossa) K61.3
jaw (bone) (lower) (upper) M27.2
joint — *see* Arthritis, pyogenic or pyemic
    spine (tuberculous) A18.01
        nontuberculous — *see* Spondylopathy, infective
kidney N15.1
    with calculus N20.0
        with hydronephrosis N13.6
    puerperal (postpartum) O86.21
knee (*see also* Abscess, lower limb)
    joint M00.9
labium (majus) (minus) N76.4
lacrimal
    caruncle — *see* Inflammation, lacrimal, passages, acute
    gland — *see* Dacryoadenitis
    passages (duct) (sac) — *see* Inflammation, lacrimal, passages, acute
lacunar N34.0
larynx J38.7
lateral (alveolar) K04.7
    with sinus K04.6
leg (any part) — *see* Abscess, lower limb
lens H27.8
lingual K14.0
    tonsil J36
lip K13.0
Littre's gland N34.0
liver (cholangitic) (hematogenic) (lymphogenic) (pylephlebitic) (pyogenic) K75.0
    amebic (due to Entamoeba histolytica) (dysenteric) (tropical) A06.4
    with
        brain abscess (and liver or lung abscess) A06.6
        lung abscess A06.5
loin (region) L02.211
lower limb L02.41- ☑
lumbar (tuberculous) A18.01
    nontuberculous L02.212
lung (miliary) (putrid) J85.2
    with pneumonia J85.1
        due to specified organism (see Pneumonia, in (due to))
    amebic (with liver abscess) A06.5
    with
        brain abscess A06.6
        pneumonia A06.5
lymph, lymphatic, gland or node (acute) (*see also* Lymphadenitis, acute)
    mesentery I88.0
malar M27.2
mammary gland — *see* Abscess, breast
marginal, anus K61.0
mastoid — *see* Mastoiditis, acute
maxilla, maxillary M27.2
    molar (tooth) K04.7
        with sinus K04.6
    premolar K04.7
    sinus (chronic) J32.0
mediastinum J85.3
meibomian gland — *see* Hordeolum
meninges G06.2
mesentery, mesenteric K65.1
mesosalpinx — *see* Salpingitis
mons pubis L02.215
mouth (floor) K12.2
muscle — *see* Myositis, infective
myocardium I40.0

Abscess — *continued*
nabothian (follicle) — *see* Cervicitis
nasal J32.9
nasopharyngeal J39.1
navel L02.216
    newborn P38.9
        with mild hemorrhage P38.1
        without hemorrhage P38.9
neck (region) L02.11
    lymph gland or node L04.0
nephritic — *see* Abscess, kidney
nipple N61.1
    associated with
        lactation — *see* Pregnancy, complicated by
        pregnancy — *see* Pregnancy, complicated by
nose (external) (fossa) (septum) J34.0
    sinus (chronic) — *see* Sinusitis
omentum K65.1
operative wound T81.4 ☑
orbit, orbital — *see* Cellulitis, orbit
otogenic G06.0
ovary, ovarian (corpus luteum) — *see* Oophoritis
oviduct — *see* Oophoritis
palate (soft) K12.2
    hard M27.2
palmar (space) — *see* Abscess, hand
pancreas (duct) — *see* Pancreatitis, acute
parafrenal N48.21
parametric, parametrium N73.2
    acute N73.0
    chronic N73.1
paranephric N15.1
parapancreatic — *see* Pancreatitis, acute
parapharyngeal J39.0
pararectal K61.1
parasinus — *see* Sinusitis
parauterine (*see also* Disease, pelvis, inflammatory) N73.2
paravaginal — *see* Vaginitis
parietal region (scalp) L02.811
parodontal — *see* Peridontitis, aggressive, localized
parotid (duct) (gland) K11.3
    region K12.2
pectoral (region) L02.213
pelvis, pelvic
    female — *see* Disease, pelvis, inflammatory
    male, peritoneal K65.1
penis N48.21
    gonococcal (accessory gland) (periurethral) A54.1
perianal K61.0
periapical K04.7
    with sinus (alveolar) K04.6
periappendicular K35.3
pericardial I30.1
pericecal K35.3
pericemental — *see* Peridontitis, aggressive, localized
pericholecystic — *see* Cholecystitis, acute
pericoronal — *see* Peridontitis, aggressive, localized
peridental — *see* Peridontitis, aggressive, localized
perimetric (*see also* Disease, pelvis, inflammatory) N73.2
perinephric, perinephritic — *see* Abscess, kidney
perineum, perineal (superficial) L02.215
    urethra N34.0
periodontal (parietal) — *see* Peridontitis, aggressive, localized
    apical K04.7
periosteum, periosteal (*see also* Osteomyelitis, specified type NEC)
    with osteomyelitis (*see also* Osteomyelitis, specified type NEC)
        acute — *see* Osteomyelitis, acute
        chronic — *see* Osteomyelitis, chronic
peripharyngeal J39.0
peripleuritic J86.9
    with fistula J86.0
periprostatic N41.2
perirectal K61.1
perirenal (tissue) — *see* Abscess, kidney
perisinuous (nose) — *see* Sinusitis
peritoneum, peritoneal (perforated) (ruptured) K65.1
    with appendicitis K35.3
    pelvic
        female — *see* Peritonitis, pelvic, female
        male K65.1
    postoperative T81.4 ☑
    puerperal, postpartum, childbirth O85
    tuberculous A18.31

Abscess — *continued*
- peritonsillar J36
- perityphlic K35.3
- periureteral N28.89
- periurethral N34.0
  - gonococcal (accessory gland) (periurethral) A54.1
- periuterine (*see also* Disease, pelvis, inflammatory) N73.2
- perivesical — *see* Cystitis, specified type NEC
- petrous bone — *see* Petrositis
- phagedenic NOS L02.91
  - chancroid A57
- pharynx, pharyngeal (lateral) J39.1
- pilonidal L05.01
- pituitary (gland) E23.6
- pleura J86.9
  - with fistula J86.0
- popliteal — *see* Abscess, lower limb
- postcecal K35.3
- postlaryngeal J38.7
- postnasal J34.0
- postoperative (any site) T81.4 ☑
  - retroperitoneal K68.11
- postpharyngeal J39.0
- posttonsillar J36
- post-typhoid A01.09
- pouch of Douglas — *see* Peritonitis, pelvic, female
- premammary — *see* Abscess, breast
- prepatellar — *see* Abscess, lower limb
- prostate N41.2
  - gonococcal (acute) (chronic) A54.22
- psoas muscle K68.12
- puerperal — *code by* site under Puerperal, abscess
- pulmonary — *see* Abscess, lung
- pulp, pulpal (dental) K04.01
  - irreversible K04.02
  - reversible K04.01
- rectovaginal septum K63.0
- rectovesical — *see* Cystitis, specified type NEC
- rectum K61.1
- renal — *see* Abscess, kidney
- retina — *see* Inflammation, chorioretinal
- retrobulbar — *see* Abscess, orbit
- retrocecal K65.1
- retrolaryngeal J38.7
- retromammary — *see* Abscess, breast
- retroperitoneal NEC K68.19
  - postprocedural K68.11
- retropharyngeal J39.0
- retrouterine — *see* Peritonitis, pelvic, female
- retrovesical — *see* Cystitis, specified type NEC
- root, tooth K04.7
  - with sinus (alveolar) K04.6
- round ligament (*see also* Disease, pelvis, inflammatory) N73.2
- rupture (spontaneous) NOS L02.91
- sacrum (tuberculous) A18.01
  - nontuberculous M46.28
- salivary (duct) (gland) K11.3
- scalp (any part) L02.811
- scapular — *see* Osteomyelitis, specified type NEC
- sclera — *see* Scleritis
- scrofulous (tuberculous) A18.2
- scrotum N49.2
- seminal vesicle N49.0
- septal, dental K04.7
  - with sinus (alveolar) K04.6
- serous — *see* Periostitis
- shoulder (region) — *see* Abscess, upper limb
- sigmoid K63.0
- sinus (accessory) (chronic) (nasal) (*see also* Sinusitis)
  - intracranial venous (any) G06.0
- Skene's duct or gland N34.0
- skin — *see* Abscess, by site
- specified site NEC L02.818
- spermatic cord N49.1
- sphenoidal (sinus) (chronic) J32.3
- spinal cord (any part) (staphylococcal) G06.1
  - tuberculous A17.81
- spine (column) (tuberculous) A18.01
  - epidural G06.1
  - nontuberculous — *see* Osteomyelitis, vertebra
- spleen D73.3
  - amebic A06.89
- stitch T81.4 ☑
- subarachnoid G06.2
  - brain G06.0
  - spinal cord G06.1

Abscess — *continued*
- subareolar — *see* Abscess, breast
- subcecal K35.3
- subcutaneous (*see also* Abscess, by site)
  - pheomycotic (chromomycotic) B43.2
- subdiaphragmatic K65.1
- subdural G06.2
  - brain G06.0
    - sequelae G09
  - spinal cord G06.1
- subgaleal L02.811
- subhepatic K65.1
- sublingual K12.2
  - gland K11.3
- submammary — *see* Abscess, breast
- submandibular (region) (space) (triangle) K12.2
  - gland K11.3
- submaxillary (region) L02.01
  - gland K11.3
- submental L02.01
  - gland K11.3
- subperiosteal — *see* Osteomyelitis, specified type NEC
- subphrenic K65.1
  - postoperative T81.4 ☑
- suburethral N34.0
- sudoriparous L75.8
- supraclavicular (fossa) — *see* Abscess, upper limb
- suprapelvic, acute N73.0
- suprarenal (capsule) (gland) E27.8
- sweat gland L74.8
- tear duct — *see* Inflammation, lacrimal, passages, acute
- temple L02.01
- temporal region L02.01
- temporosphenoidal G06.0
- tendon (sheath) M65.00
  - ankle M65.07- ☑
  - foot M65.07- ☑
  - forearm M65.03- ☑
  - hand M65.04- ☑
  - lower leg M65.06- ☑
  - pelvic region M65.05- ☑
  - shoulder region M65.01- ☑
  - specified site NEC M65.08
  - thigh M65.05- ☑
  - upper arm M65.02- ☑
- testis N45.4
- thigh — *see* Abscess, lower limb
- thorax J86.9
  - with fistula J86.0
- throat J39.1
- thumb (*see also* Abscess, hand)
  - nail — *see* Cellulitis, finger
- thymus (gland) E32.1
- thyroid (gland) E06.0
- toe (any) (*see also* Abscess, foot)
  - nail — *see* Cellulitis, toe
- tongue (staphylococcal) K14.0
- tonsil(s) (lingual) J36
- tonsillopharyngeal J36
- tooth, teeth (root) K04.7
  - with sinus (alveolar) K04.6
  - supporting structures NEC — *see* Peridontitis, aggressive, localized
- trachea J39.8
- trunk L02.219
  - abdominal wall L02.211
  - back L02.212
  - chest wall L02.213
  - groin L02.214
  - perineum L02.215
  - umbilicus L02.216
- tubal — *see* Salpingitis
- tuberculous — *see* Tuberculosis, abscess
- tubo-ovarian — *see* Salpingo-oophoritis
- tunica vaginalis N49.1
- umbilicus L02.216
- upper
  - limb L02.41- ☑
  - respiratory J39.8
- urethral (gland) N34.0
- urinary N34.0
- uterus, uterine (wall) (*see also* Endometritis)
  - ligament (*see also* Disease, pelvis, inflammatory) N73.2
  - neck — *see* Cervicitis
- uvula K12.2
- vagina (wall) — *see* Vaginitis

Abscess — *continued*
- vaginorectal — *see* Vaginitis
- vas deferens N49.1
- vermiform appendix K35.3
- vertebra (column) (tuberculous) A18.01
  - nontuberculous — *see* Osteomyelitis, vertebra
- vesical — *see* Cystitis, specified type NEC
- vesico-uterine pouch — *see* Peritonitis, pelvic, female
- vitreous (humor) — *see* Endophthalmitis, purulent
- vocal cord J38.3
- von Bezold's — *see* Mastoiditis, acute
- vulva N76.4
- vulvovaginal gland N75.1
- web space — *see* Abscess, hand
- wound T81.4 ☑
- wrist — *see* Abscess, upper limb

Absence (of) (organ or part) (complete or partial)
- adrenal (gland) (congenital) Q89.1
  - acquired E89.6
- albumin in blood E88.09
- alimentary tract (congenital) Q45.8
  - upper Q40.8
- alveolar process (acquired) — *see* Anomaly, alveolar
- ankle (acquired) Z89.44- ☑
- anus (congenital) Q42.3
  - with fistula Q42.2
- aorta (congenital) Q25.41
- appendix, congenital Q42.8
- arm (acquired) Z89.20- ☑
  - above elbow Z89.22- ☑
    - congenital (with hand present) — *see* Agenesis, arm, with hand present
    - and hand — *see* Agenesis, forearm, and hand
  - below elbow Z89.21- ☑
    - congenital (with hand present) — *see* Agenesis, arm, with hand present
    - and hand — *see* Agenesis, forearm, and hand
  - congenital — *see* Defect, reduction, upper limb
  - shoulder (following explantation of shoulder joint prosthesis) (joint) (with or without presence of antibiotic-Impregnated cement spacer) Z89.23- ☑
    - congenital (with hand present) — *see* Agenesis, arm, with hand present
- artery (congenital) (peripheral) Q27.8
  - brain Q28.3
  - coronary Q24.5
  - pulmonary Q25.79
  - specified NEC Q27.8
  - umbilical Q27.0
- atrial septum (congenital) Q21.1
- auditory canal (congenital) (external) Q16.1
- auricle (ear), congenital Q16.0
- bile, biliary duct, congenital Q44.5
- bladder (acquired) Z90.6
  - congenital Q64.5
- bowel sounds R19.11
- brain Q00.0
  - part of Q04.3
- breast(s) (and nipple(s)) (acquired) Z90.1- ☑
  - congenital Q83.8
- broad ligament Q50.6
- bronchus (congenital) Q32.4
- canaliculus lacrimalis, congenital Q10.4
- cerebellum (vermis) Q04.3
- cervix (acquired) (with uterus) Z90.710
  - with remaining uterus Z90.712
  - congenital Q51.5
- chin, congenital Q18.8
- cilia (congenital) Q10.3
  - acquired — *see* Madarosis
- clitoris (congenital) Q52.6
- coccyx, congenital Q76.49
- cold sense R20.8
- congenital
  - lumen — *see* Atresia
  - organ or site NEC — *see* Agenesis
  - septum — *see* Imperfect, closure
- corpus callosum Q04.0
- cricoid cartilage, congenital Q31.8
- diaphragm (with hernia), congenital Q79.1
- digestive organ(s) or tract, congenital Q45.8
  - acquired NEC Z90.49
  - upper Q40.8
- ductus arteriosus Q28.8
- duodenum (acquired) Z90.49

Absence — *continued*
  duodenum — *continued*
    congenital Q41.0
  ear, congenital Q16.9
    acquired H93.8- ☑
    auricle Q16.0
    external Q16.0
    inner Q16.5
    lobe, lobule Q17.8
    middle, except ossicles Q16.4
      ossicles Q16.3
    ossicles Q16.3
  ejaculatory duct (congenital) Q55.4
  endocrine gland (congenital) NEC Q89.2
    acquired E89.89
  epididymis (congenital) Q55.4
    acquired Z90.79
  epiglottis, congenital Q31.8
  esophagus (congenital) Q39.8
    acquired (partial) Z90.49
  eustachian tube (congenital) Q16.2
  extremity (acquired) Z89.9
    congenital Q73.0
    knee (following explanation of knee joint prosthe-
        sis) (joint) (with or without presence of an-
        tibiotic-impregnated cement spacer)
        Z89.52- ☑
    lower (above knee) Z89.619
      below knee Z89.51- ☑
    upper — *see* Absence, arm
  eye (acquired) Z90.01
    congenital Q11.1
    muscle (congenital) Q10.3
  eyeball (acquired) Z90.01
  eyelid (fold) (congenital) Q10.3
    acquired Z90.01
  face, specified part NEC Q18.8
  fallopian tube(s) (acquired) Z90.79
    congenital Q50.6
  family member (causing problem in home) NEC (*see
      also* Disruption, family) Z63.32
  femur, congenital — *see* Defect, reduction, lower limb,
      longitudinal, femur
  fibrinogen (congenital) D68.2
    acquired D65
  finger(s) (acquired) Z89.02- ☑
    congenital — *see* Agenesis, hand
  foot (acquired) Z89.43- ☑
    congenital — *see* Agenesis, foot
  forearm (acquired) — *see* Absence, arm, below elbow
  gallbladder (acquired) Z90.49
    congenital Q44.0
  gamma globulin in blood D80.1
    hereditary D80.0
  genital organs
    acquired (female) (male) Z90.79
    female, congenital Q52.8
      external Q52.71
      internal NEC Q52.8
    male, congenital Q55.8
  genitourinary organs, congenital NEC
    female Q52.8
    male Q55.8
  globe (acquired) Z90.01
    congenital Q11.1
  glottis, congenital Q31.8
  hand and wrist (acquired) Z89.11- ☑
    congenital — *see* Agenesis, hand
  head, part (acquired) NEC Z90.09
  heat sense R20.8
  hip (following explanation of hip joint prosthesis)
      (joint) (with or without presence of antibiotic-
      impregnated cement spacer) Z89.62- ☑
  hymen (congenital) Q52.4
  ileum (acquired) Z90.49
    congenital Q41.2
  immunoglobulin, isolated NEC D80.3
    IgA D80.2
    IgG D80.3
    IgM D80.4
  incus (acquired) — *see* Loss, ossicles, ear
    congenital Q16.3
  inner ear, congenital Q16.5
  intestine (acquired) (small) Z90.49
    congenital Q41.9
      specified NEC Q41.8
    large Z90.49
      congenital Q42.9

Absence — *continued*
  intestine — *continued*
    large — *continued*
      congenital — *continued*
        specified NEC Q42.8
  iris, congenital Q13.1
  jejunum (acquired) Z90.49
    congenital Q41.1
  joint
    acquired
      hip (following explantation of hip joint prosthe-
          sis) (with or without presence of antibiot-
          ic-impregnated cement spacer)
          Z89.62- ☑
      knee (following explantation of knee joint
          prosthesis) (with or without presence of
          antibiotic-impregnated cement spacer)
          Z89.52- ☑
      shoulder (following explantation of shoulder
          joint prosthesis) (with or without pres-
          ence of antibiotic-impregnated cement
          spacer) Z89.23- ☑
    congenital NEC Q74.8
  kidney(s) (acquired) Z90.5
    congenital Q60.2
      bilateral Q60.1
      unilateral Q60.0
  knee (following explantation of knee joint prosthesis)
      (joint) (with or without presence of antibiotic-
      impregnated cement spacer) Z89.52- ☑
  labyrinth, membranous Q16.5
  larynx (congenital) Q31.8
    acquired Z90.02
  leg (acquired) (above knee) Z89.61- ☑
    below knee (acquired) Z89.51- ☑
    congenital — *see* Defect, reduction, lower limb
  lens (acquired) (*see also* Aphakia)
    congenital Q12.3
    post cataract extraction Z98.4- ☑
  limb (acquired) — *see* Absence, extremity
  lip Q38.6
  liver (congenital) Q44.7
  lung (fissure) (lobe) (bilateral) (unilateral) (congenital)
      Q33.3
    acquired (any part) Z90.2
  menstruation — *see* Amenorrhea
  muscle (congenital) (pectoral) Q79.8
    ocular Q10.3
  neck, part Q18.8
  neutrophil — *see* Agranulocytosis
  nipple(s) (with breast(s)) (acquired) Z90.1- ☑
    congenital Q83.2
  nose (congenital) Q30.1
    acquired Z90.09
  organ
    of Corti, congenital Q16.5
    or site, congenital NEC Q89.8
      acquired NEC Z90.89
  osseous meatus (ear) Q16.4
  ovary (acquired)
    bilateral Z90.722
    congenital
      bilateral Q50.02
      unilateral Q50.01
    unilateral Z90.721
  oviduct (acquired)
    bilateral Z90.722
    congenital Q50.6
    unilateral Z90.721
  pancreas (congenital) Q45.0
    acquired Z90.410
      complete Z90.410
      partial Z90.411
      total Z90.410
  parathyroid gland (acquired) E89.2
    congenital Q89.2
  patella, congenital Q74.1
  penis (congenital) Q55.5
    acquired Z90.79
  pericardium (congenital) Q24.8
  pituitary gland (congenital) Q89.2
    acquired E89.3
  prostate (acquired) Z90.79
    congenital Q55.4
  pulmonary valve Q22.0
  punctum lacrimale (congenital) Q10.4
  radius, congenital — *see* Defect, reduction, upper limb,
      longitudinal, radius

Absence — *continued*
  rectum (congenital) Q42.1
    with fistula Q42.0
    acquired Z90.49
  respiratory organ NOS Q34.9
  rib (acquired) Z90.89
    congenital Q76.6
  sacrum, congenital Q76.49
  salivary gland(s), congenital Q38.4
  scrotum, congenital Q55.29
  seminal vesicles (congenital) Q55.4
    acquired Z90.79
  septum
    atrial (congenital) Q21.1
    between aorta and pulmonary artery Q21.4
    ventricular (congenital) Q20.4
  sex chromosome
    female phenotype Q97.8
    male phenotype Q98.8
  skull bone (congenital) Q75.8
    with
      anencephaly Q00.0
      encephalocele — *see* Encephalocele
      hydrocephalus Q03.9
        with spina bifida — *see* Spina bifida, by site,
            with hydrocephalus
      microcephaly Q02
  spermatic cord, congenital Q55.4
  spine, congenital Q76.49
  spleen (congenital) Q89.01
    acquired Z90.81
  sternum, congenital Q76.7
  stomach (acquired) (partial) Z90.3
    congenital Q40.2
  superior vena cava, congenital Q26.8
  teeth, tooth (congenital) K00.0
    acquired (complete) K08.109
      class I K08.101
      class II K08.102
      class III K08.103
      class IV K08.104
      due to
        caries K08.139
          class I K08.131
          class II K08.132
          class III K08.133
          class IV K08.134
        periodontal disease K08.129
          class I K08.121
          class II K08.122
          class III K08.123
          class IV K08.124
        specified NEC K08.199
          class I K08.191
          class II K08.192
          class III K08.193
          class IV K08.194
        trauma K08.119
          class I K08.111
          class II K08.112
          class III K08.113
          class IV K08.114
      partial K08.409
        class I K08.401
        class II K08.402
        class III K08.403
        class IV K08.404
        due to
          caries K08.439
            class I K08.431
            class II K08.432
            class III K08.433
            class IV K08.434
          periodontal disease K08.429
            class I K08.421
            class II K08.422
            class III K08.423
            class IV K08.424
          specified NEC K08.499
            class I K08.491
            class II K08.492
            class III K08.493
            class IV K08.494
          trauma K08.419
            class I K08.411
            class II K08.412
            class III K08.413
            class IV K08.414
  tendon (congenital) Q79.8

Absence — *continued*
  testis (congenital) Q55.0
    acquired Z90.79
  thumb (acquired) Z89.01- ☑
    congenital — *see* Agenesis, hand
  thymus gland Q89.2
  thyroid (gland) (acquired) E89.0
    cartilage, congenital Q31.8
    congenital E03.1
  toe(s) (acquired) Z89.42- ☑
    with foot — *see* Absence, foot and ankle
    congenital — *see* Agenesis, foot
    great Z89.41- ☑
  tongue, congenital Q38.3
  trachea (cartilage), congenital Q32.1
  transverse aortic arch, congenital Q25.49
  tricuspid valve Q22.4
  umbilical artery, congenital Q27.0
  upper arm and forearm with hand present, congenital — *see* Agenesis, arm, with hand present
  ureter (congenital) Q62.4
    acquired Z90.6
  urethra, congenital Q64.5
  uterus (acquired) Z90.710
    with cervix Z90.710
    with remaining cervical stump Z90.711
    congenital Q51.0
  uvula, congenital Q38.5
  vagina, congenital Q52.0
  vas deferens (congenital) Q55.4
    acquired Z90.79
  vein (peripheral) congenital NEC Q27.8
    cerebral Q28.3
    digestive system Q27.8
    great Q26.8
    lower limb Q27.8
    portal Q26.5
    precerebral Q28.1
    specified site NEC Q27.8
    upper limb Q27.8
  vena cava (inferior) (superior), congenital Q26.8
  ventricular septum Q20.4
  vertebra, congenital Q76.49
  vulva, congenital Q52.71
  wrist (acquired) Z89.12- ☑
Absorbent system disease I87.8
Absorption
  carbohydrate, disturbance K90.49
  chemical — *see* Table of Drugs and Chemicals
    through placenta (newborn) P04.9
      environmental substance P04.6
      nutritional substance P04.5
      obstetric anesthetic or analgesic drug P04.0
  drug NEC — *see* Table of Drugs and Chemicals
    addictive
      through placenta (newborn) P04.49
        cocaine P04.41
    medicinal
      through placenta (newborn) P04.1
    through placenta (newborn) P04.1
      obstetric anesthetic or analgesic drug P04.0
  fat, disturbance K90.49
    pancreatic K90.3
  noxious substance — *see* Table of Drugs and Chemicals
  protein, disturbance K90.49
  starch, disturbance K90.49
  toxic substance — *see* Table of Drugs and Chemicals
  uremic — *see* Uremia
Abstinence symptoms, syndrome
  alcohol F10.239
    with delirium F10.231
  cocaine F14.23
  neonatal P96.1
  nicotine — *see* Dependence, drug, nicotine, with, withdrawal
  opioid F11.93
    with dependence F11.23
  psychoactive NEC F19.939
    with
      delirium F19.931
      dependence F19.239
        with
          delirium F19.231
          perceptual disturbance F19.232
        uncomplicated F19.230
      perceptual disturbance F19.932
    uncomplicated F19.930

Abstinence symptoms, syndrome — *continued*
  sedative F13.939
    with
      delirium F13.931
      dependence F13.239
        with
          delirium F13.231
          perceptual disturbance F13.232
        uncomplicated F13.230
      perceptual disturbance F13.932
    uncomplicated F13.930
  stimulant NEC F15.93
    with dependence F15.23
Abulia R68.89
Abulomania F60.7
Abuse
  adult — *see* Maltreatment, adult
    as reason for
      couple seeking advice (including offender) Z63.0
  alcohol (non-dependent) F10.10
    with
      anxiety disorder F10.180
      intoxication F10.129
        with delirium F10.121
        uncomplicated F10.120
      mood disorder F10.14
      other specified disorder F10.188
      psychosis F10.159
        delusions F10.150
        hallucinations F10.151
      sexual dysfunction F10.181
      sleep disorder F10.182
      unspecified disorder F10.19
    counseling and surveillance Z71.41
    in remission (early) (sustained) F10.11
  amphetamine (or related substance) — *see* Abuse, drug, stimulant NEC
  analgesics (non-prescribed) (over the counter) F55.8
  antacids F55.0
  antidepressants — *see* Abuse, drug, psychoactive NEC
  anxiolytic — *see* Abuse, drug, sedative
  barbiturates — *see* Abuse, drug, sedative
  caffeine — *see* Abuse, drug, stimulant NEC
  cannabis, cannabinoids — *see* Abuse, drug, cannabis
  child — *see* Maltreatment, child
  cocaine — *see* Abuse, drug, cocaine
  drug NEC (non-dependent) F19.10
    with sleep disorder F19.182
    amphetamine type — *see* Abuse, drug, stimulant NEC
    analgesics (non-prescribed) (over the counter) F55.8
    antacids F55.0
    antidepressants — *see* Abuse, drug, psychoactive NEC
    anxiolytics — *see* Abuse, drug, sedative
    barbiturates — *see* Abuse, drug, sedative
    caffeine — *see* Abuse, drug, stimulant NEC
    cannabis F12.10
      with
        anxiety disorder F12.180
        intoxication F12.129
          with
            delirium F12.121
            perceptual disturbance F12.122
          uncomplicated F12.120
        other specified disorder F12.188
        psychosis F12.159
          delusions F12.150
          hallucinations F12.151
        unspecified disorder F12.19
      in remission (early) (sustained) F12.11
    cocaine F14.10
      with
        anxiety disorder F14.180
        intoxication F14.129
          with
            delirium F14.121
            perceptual disturbance F14.122
          uncomplicated F14.120
        mood disorder F14.14
        other specified disorder F14.188
        psychosis F14.159
          delusions F14.150
          hallucinations F14.151
        sexual dysfunction F14.181
        sleep disorder F14.182

Abuse — *continued*
  drug — *continued*
    cocaine — *continued*
      with — *continued*
        unspecified disorder F14.19
      in remission (early) (sustained) F14.11
      counseling and surveillance Z71.51
    hallucinogen F16.10
      with
        anxiety disorder F16.180
        flashbacks F16.183
        intoxication F16.129
          with
            delirium F16.121
            perceptual disturbance F16.122
          uncomplicated F16.120
        mood disorder F16.14
        other specified disorder F16.188
        perception disorder, persisting F16.183
        psychosis F16.159
          delusions F16.150
          hallucinations F16.151
        unspecified disorder F16.19
      in remission (early) (sustained) F16.11
    hashish — *see* Abuse, drug, cannabis
    herbal or folk remedies F55.1
    hormones F55.3
    hypnotics — *see* Abuse, drug, sedative
    in remission (early) (sustained) F19.11
    inhalant F18.10
      with
        anxiety disorder F18.180
        dementia, persisting F18.17
        intoxication F18.129
          with delirium F18.121
          uncomplicated F18.120
        mood disorder F18.14
        other specified disorder F18.188
        psychosis F18.159
          delusions F18.150
          hallucinations F18.151
        unspecified disorder F18.19
      in remission (early) (sustained) F18.11
    laxatives F55.2
    LSD — *see* Abuse, drug, hallucinogen
    marihuana — *see* Abuse, drug, cannabis
    morphine type (opioids) — *see* Abuse, drug, opioid
    opioid F11.10
      with
        intoxication F11.129
          with
            delirium F11.121
            perceptual disturbance F11.122
          uncomplicated F11.120
        mood disorder F11.14
        other specified disorder F11.188
        psychosis F11.159
          delusions F11.150
          hallucinations F11.151
        sexual dysfunction F11.181
        sleep disorder F11.182
        unspecified disorder F11.19
      in remission (early) (sustained) F11.11
    PCP (phencyclidine) (or related substance) — *see* Abuse, drug, hallucinogen
    psychoactive NEC F19.10
      with
        amnestic disorder F19.16
        anxiety disorder F19.180
        dementia F19.17
        intoxication F19.129
          with
            delirium F19.121
            perceptual disturbance F19.122
          uncomplicated F19.120
        mood disorder F19.14
        other specified disorder F19.188
        psychosis F19.159
          delusions F19.150
          hallucinations F19.151
        sexual dysfunction F19.181
        sleep disorder F19.182
        unspecified disorder F19.19
    sedative, hypnotic or anxiolytic F13.10
      with
        anxiety disorder F13.180
        intoxication F13.129
          with delirium F13.121
          uncomplicated F13.120

Abuse — *continued*
  drug — *continued*
    sedative, hypnotic or anxiolytic — *continued*
      with — *continued*
        mood disorder F13.14
        other specified disorder F13.188
        psychosis F13.159
          delusions F13.150
          hallucinations F13.151
        sexual dysfunction F13.181
        sleep disorder F13.182
        unspecified disorder F13.19
      in remission (early) (sustained) F13.11
    solvent — *see* Abuse, drug, inhalant
    steroids F55.3
    stimulant NEC F15.10
      with
        anxiety disorder F15.180
        intoxication F15.129
          with
            delirium F15.121
            perceptual disturbance F15.122
          uncomplicated F15.120
        mood disorder F15.14
        other specified disorder F15.188
        psychosis F15.159
          delusions F15.150
          hallucinations F15.151
        sexual dysfunction F15.181
        sleep disorder F15.182
        unspecified disorder F15.19
      in remission (early) (sustained) F15.11
    tranquilizers — *see* Abuse, drug, sedative
    vitamins F55.4
    hallucinogens — *see* Abuse, drug, hallucinogen
    hashish — *see* Abuse, drug, cannabis
    herbal or folk remedies F55.1
    hormones F55.3
    hypnotic — *see* Abuse, drug, sedative
    inhalant — *see* Abuse, drug, inhalant
    laxatives F55.2
    LSD — *see* Abuse, drug, hallucinogen
    marihuana — *see* Abuse, drug, cannabis
    morphine type (opioids) — *see* Abuse, drug, opioid
    non-psychoactive substance NEC F55.8
      antacids F55.0
      folk remedies F55.1
      herbal remedies F55.1
      hormones F55.3
      laxatives F55.2
      steroids F55.3
      vitamins F55.4
    opioids — *see* Abuse, drug, opioid
    PCP (phencyclidine) (or related substance) — *see* Abuse, drug, hallucinogen
    physical (adult) (child) — *see* Maltreatment
    psychoactive substance — *see* Abuse, drug, psychoactive NEC
    psychological (adult) (child) — *see* Maltreatment
    sedative — *see* Abuse, drug, sedative
    sexual — *see* Maltreatment
    solvent — *see* Abuse, drug, inhalant
    steroids F55.3
    vitamins F55.4
Acalculia R48.8
  developmental F81.2
Acanthamebiasis (with) B60.10
  conjunctiva B60.12
  keratoconjunctivitis B60.13
  meningoencephalitis B60.11
  other specified B60.19
Acanthocephaliasis B83.8
Acanthocheilonemiasis B74.4
Acanthocytosis E78.6
Acantholysis L11.9
Acanthosis (acquired) (nigricans) L83
  benign Q82.8
  congenital Q82.8
  seborrheic L82.1
    inflamed L82.0
  tongue K14.3
Acapnia E87.3
Acarbia E87.2
Acardia, acardius Q89.8
Acardiacus amorphus Q89.8
Acardiotrophia I51.4
Acariasis B88.0
  scabies B86

Acarodermatitis (urticarioides) B88.0
Acarophobia F40.218
Acatalasemia, acatalasia E80.3
Acathisia (drug induced) G25.71
Accelerated atrioventricular conduction I45.6
Accentuation of personality traits (type A) Z73.1
Accessory (congenital)
  adrenal gland Q89.1
  anus Q43.4
  appendix Q43.4
  atrioventricular conduction I45.6
  auditory ossicles Q16.3
  auricle (ear) Q17.0
  biliary duct or passage Q44.5
  bladder Q64.79
  blood vessels NEC Q27.9
    coronary Q24.5
  bone NEC Q79.8
  breast tissue, axilla Q83.1
  carpal bones Q74.0
  cecum Q43.4
  chromosome(s) NEC (nonsex) Q92.9
    with complex rearrangements NEC Q92.5
      seen only at prometaphase Q92.8
    13 — *see* Trisomy, 13
    18 — *see* Trisomy, 18
    21 — *see* Trisomy, 21
    partial Q92.9
    sex
      female phenotype Q97.8
  coronary artery Q24.5
  cusp(s), heart valve NEC Q24.8
    pulmonary Q22.3
  cystic duct Q44.5
  digit(s) Q69.9
  ear (auricle) (lobe) Q17.0
  endocrine gland NEC Q89.2
  eye muscle Q10.3
  eyelid Q10.3
  face bone(s) Q75.8
  fallopian tube (fimbria) (ostium) Q50.6
  finger(s) Q69.0
  foreskin N47.8
  frontonasal process Q75.8
  gallbladder Q44.1
  genital organ(s)
    female Q52.8
      external Q52.79
      internal NEC Q52.8
    male Q55.8
  genitourinary organs NEC Q89.8
    female Q52.8
    male Q55.8
  hallux Q69.2
  heart Q24.8
    valve NEC Q24.8
      pulmonary Q22.3
  hepatic ducts Q44.5
  hymen Q52.4
  intestine (large) (small) Q43.4
  kidney Q63.0
  lacrimal canal Q10.6
  leaflet, heart valve NEC Q24.8
  ligament, broad Q50.6
  liver Q44.7
    duct Q44.5
  lobule (ear) Q17.0
  lung (lobe) Q33.1
  muscle Q79.8
  navicular of carpus Q74.0
  nervous system, part NEC Q07.8
  nipple Q83.3
  nose Q30.8
  organ or site not listed — *see* Anomaly, by site
  ovary Q50.31
  oviduct Q50.6
  pancreas Q45.3
  parathyroid gland Q89.2
  parotid gland (and duct) Q38.4
  pituitary gland Q89.2
  preauricular appendage Q17.0
  prepuce N47.8
  renal arteries (multiple) Q27.2
  rib Q76.6
    cervical Q76.5
  roots (teeth) K00.2
  salivary gland Q38.4
  sesamoid bones Q74.8

Accessory — *continued*
  sesamoid bones — *continued*
    foot Q74.2
    hand Q74.0
  skin tags Q82.8
  spleen Q89.09
  sternum Q76.7
  submaxillary gland Q38.4
  tarsal bones Q74.2
  teeth, tooth K00.1
  tendon Q79.8
  thumb Q69.1
  thymus gland Q89.2
  thyroid gland Q89.2
  toes Q69.2
  tongue Q38.3
  tooth, teeth K00.1
  tragus Q17.0
  ureter Q62.5
  urethra Q64.79
  urinary organ or tract NEC Q64.8
  uterus Q51.2
  vagina Q52.10
  valve, heart NEC Q24.8
    pulmonary Q22.3
  vertebra Q76.49
  vocal cords Q31.8
  vulva Q52.79
Accident
  birth — *see* Birth, injury
  cardiac — *see* Infarct, myocardium
  cerebral I63.9
  cerebrovascular (embolic) (ischemic) (thrombotic) I63.9
    aborted I63.9
    hemorrhagic — *see* Hemorrhage, intracranial, intracerebral
    old (without sequelae) Z86.73
      with sequelae (of) — *see* Sequelae, infarction, cerebral
  coronary — *see* Infarct, myocardium
  craniovascular I63.9
  vascular, brain I63.9
Accidental — *see* condition
Accommodation (disorder) (*see also* condition)
  hysterical paralysis of F44.89
  insufficiency of H52.4
  paresis — *see* Paresis, of accommodation
  spasm — *see* Spasm, of accommodation
Accouchement — *see* Delivery
Accreta placenta O43.21- ☑
Accretio cordis (nonrheumatic) I31.0
Accretions, tooth, teeth K03.6
Acculturation difficulty Z60.3
Accumulation secretion, prostate N42.89
Acephalia, acephalism, acephalus, acephaly Q00.0
Acephalobrachia monster Q89.8
Acephalochirus monster Q89.8
Acephalogaster Q89.8
Acephalostomus monster Q89.8
Acephalothorax Q89.8
Acerophobia F40.298
Acetonemia R79.89
  in Type 1 diabetes E10.10
    with coma E10.11
Acetonuria R82.4
Achalasia (cardia) (esophagus) K22.0
  congenital Q39.5
  pylorus Q40.0
  sphincteral NEC K59.8
Ache(s) — *see* Pain
Acheilia Q38.6
Achillobursitis — *see* Tendinitis, Achilles
Achillodynia — *see* Tendinitis, Achilles
Achlorhydria, achlorhydric (neurogenic) K31.83
  anemia D50.8
  diarrhea K31.83
  psychogenic F45.8
  secondary to vagotomy K91.1
Achluophobia F40.228
Acholia K82.8
Acholuric jaundice (familial) (splenomegalic) (*see also* Spherocytosis)
  acquired D59.8
Achondrogenesis Q77.0
Achondroplasia (osteosclerosis congenita) Q77.4
Achroma, cutis L80

Achromat (ism), achromatopsia (acquired) (congenital) H53.51
Achromia, congenital — see Albinism
Achromia parasitica B36.0
Achylia gastrica K31.89
  psychogenic F45.8
Acid
  burn — see Corrosion
  deficiency
    amide nicotinic E52
    ascorbic E54
    folic E53.8
    nicotinic E52
    pantothenic E53.8
  intoxication E87.2
  peptic disease K30
  phosphatase deficiency E83.39
  stomach K30
    psychogenic F45.8
Acidemia E87.2
  argininosuccinic E72.22
  isovaleric E71.110
  metabolic (newborn) P19.9
    first noted before onset of labor P19.0
    first noted during labor P19.1
    noted at birth P19.2
  methylmalonic E71.120
  pipecolic E72.3
  propionic E71.121
Acidity, gastric (high) K30
  psychogenic F45.8
Acidocytopenia — see Agranulocytosis
Acidocytosis D72.1
Acidopenia — see Agranulocytosis
Acidosis (lactic) (respiratory) E87.2
  in Type 1 diabetes E10.10
    with coma E10.11
  kidney, tubular N25.89
  lactic E87.2
  metabolic NEC E87.2
    with respiratory acidosis E87.4
    late, of newborn P74.0
  mixed metabolic and respiratory, newborn P84
  newborn P84
  renal (hyperchloremic) (tubular) N25.89
  respiratory E87.2
    complicated by
      metabolic
        acidosis E87.4
        alkalosis E87.4
Aciduria
  argininosuccinic E72.22
  glutaric (type I) E72.3
    type II E71.313
    type III E71.5- ☑
  orotic (congenital) (hereditary) (pyrimidine deficiency) E79.8
    anemia D53.0
Acladiosis (skin) B36.0
Aclasis, diaphyseal Q78.6
Acleistocardia Q21.1
Aclusion — see Anomaly, dentofacial, malocclusion
Acne L70.9
  artificialis L70.8
  atrophica L70.2
  cachecticorum (Hebra) L70.8
  conglobata L70.1
  cystic L70.0
  decalvans L66.2
  excoriée (des jeunes filles) L70.5
  frontalis L70.2
  indurata L70.0
  infantile L70.4
  keloid L73.0
  lupoid L70.2
  necrotic, necrotica (miliaris) L70.2
  neonatal L70.4
  nodular L70.0
  occupational L70.8
  picker's L70.5
  pustular L70.0
  rodens L70.2
  rosacea L71.9
  specified NEC L70.8
  tropica L70.3
  varioliformis L70.2
  vulgaris L70.0
Acnitis (primary) A18.4

Acosta's disease T70.29 ☑
Acoustic — see condition
Acousticophobia F40.298
Acquired (see also condition)
  immunodeficiency syndrome (AIDS) B20
Acrania Q00.0
Acroangiodermatitis I78.9
Acroasphyxia, chronic I73.89
Acrobystitis N47.7
Acrocephalopolysyndactyly Q87.0
Acrocephalosyndactyly Q87.0
Acrocephaly Q75.0
Acrochondrohyperplasia — see Syndrome, Marfan's
Acrocyanosis I73.8 ☑
  newborn P28.2
    meaning transient blue hands and feet — omit code
Acrodermatitis L30.8
  atrophicans (chronica) L90.4
  continua (Hallopeau) L40.2
  enteropathica (hereditary) E83.2
  Hallopeau's L40.2
  infantile papular L44.4
  perstans L40.2
  pustulosa continua L40.2
  recalcitrant pustular L40.2
Acrodynia — see Poisoning, mercury
Acromegaly, acromegalia E22.0
Acromelalgia I73.81
Acromicria, acromikria Q79.8
Acronyx L60.0
Acropachy, thyroid — see Thyrotoxicosis
Acroparesthesia (simple) (vasomotor) I73.89
Acropathy, thyroid — see Thyrotoxicosis
Acrophobia F40.241
Acroposthitis N47.7
Acroscleriasis, acroscleroderma, acrosclerosis — see Sclerosis, systemic
Acrosphacelus I96
Acrospiroma, eccrine — see Neoplasm, skin, benign
Acrostealgia — see Osteochondropathy
Acrotrophodynia — see Immersion
ACTH ectopic syndrome E24.3
Actinic — see condition
Actinobacillosis, actinobacillus A28.8
  mallei A24.0
  muris A25.1
Actinomyces israelii (infection) — see Actinomycosis
Actinomycetoma (foot) B47.1
Actinomycosis, actinomycotic A42.9
  with pneumonia A42.0
  abdominal A42.1
  cervicofacial A42.2
  cutaneous A42.89
  gastrointestinal A42.1
  pulmonary A42.0
  sepsis A42.7
  specified site NEC A42.89
Actinoneuritis G62.82
Action, heart
  disorder I49.9
  irregular I49.9
    psychogenic F45.8
Activated protein C resistance D68.51
Activation
  mast cell (disorder) (syndrome) D89.40
    idiopathic D89.42
    monoclonal D89.41
    secondary D89.43
    specified type NEC D89.49
Active — see condition
Acute (see also condition)
  abdomen R10.0
  gallbladder — see Cholecystitis, acute
Acyanotic heart disease (congenital) Q24.9
Acystia Q64.5
Adair-Dighton syndrome (brittle bones and blue sclera, deafness) Q78.0
Adamantinoblastoma — see Ameloblastoma
Adamantinoma (see also Cyst, calcifying odontogenic)
  long bones C40.90
    lower limb C40.2- ☑
    upper limb C40.0- ☑
  malignant C41.1
    jaw (bone) (lower) C41.1
      upper C41.0
  tibial C40.2- ☑

Adamantoblastoma — see Ameloblastoma
Adams-Stokes (-Morgagni) disease or syndrome I45.9
Adaption reaction — see Disorder, adjustment
Addiction (see also Dependence) F19.20
  alcohol, alcoholic (ethyl) (methyl) (wood) (without remission) F10.20
    with remission F10.21
  drug — see Dependence, drug
  ethyl alcohol (without remission) F10.20
    with remission F10.21
  heroin — see Dependence, drug, opioid
  methyl alcohol (without remission) F10.20
    with remission F10.21
  methylated spirit (without remission) F10.20
    with remission F10.21
  morphine (-like substances) — see Dependence, drug, opioid
  nicotine — see Dependence, drug, nicotine
  opium and opioids — see Dependence, drug, opioid
  tobacco — see Dependence, drug, nicotine
Addison-Biermer anemia (pernicious) D51.0
Addisonian crisis E27.2
Addison's
  anemia (pernicious) D51.0
  disease (bronze) or syndrome E27.1
    tuberculous A18.7
  keloid L94.0
Addison-Schilder complex E71.528
Additional (see also Accessory)
  chromosome(s) Q99.8
    21 — see Trisomy, 21
    sex — see Abnormal, chromosome, sex
Adduction contracture, hip or other joint — see Contraction, joint
Adenitis (see also Lymphadenitis)
  acute, unspecified site L04.9
  axillary I88.9
    acute L04.2
    chronic or subacute I88.1
  Bartholin's gland N75.8
  bulbourethral gland — see Urethritis
  cervical I88.9
    acute L04.0
    chronic or subacute I88.1
  chancroid (Hemophilus ducreyi) A57
  chronic, unspecified site I88.1
  Cowper's gland — see Urethritis
  due to Pasteurella multocida (P. septica) A28.0
  epidemic, acute B27.09
  gangrenous L04.9
  gonorrheal NEC A54.89
  groin I88.9
    acute L04.1
    chronic or subacute I88.1
  infectious (acute) (epidemic) B27.09
  inguinal I88.9
    acute L04.1
    chronic or subacute I88.1
  lymph gland or node, except mesenteric I88.9
    acute — see Lymphadenitis, acute
    chronic or subacute I88.1
  mesenteric (acute) (chronic) (nonspecific) (subacute) I88.0
  parotid gland (suppurative) — see Sialoadenitis
  salivary gland (any) (suppurative) — see Sialoadenitis
  scrofulous (tuberculous) A18.2
  Skene's duct or gland — see Urethritis
  strumous, tuberculous A18.2
  subacute, unspecified site I88.1
  sublingual gland (suppurative) — see Sialoadenitis
  submandibular gland (suppurative) — see Sialoadenitis
  submaxillary gland (suppurative) — see Sialoadenitis
  tuberculous — see Tuberculosis, lymph gland
  urethral gland — see Urethritis
  Wharton's duct (suppurative) — see Sialoadenitis
Adenoacanthoma — see Neoplasm, malignant, by site
Adenoameloblastoma — see Cyst, calcifying odontogenic
Adenocarcinoid (tumor) — see Neoplasm, malignant, by site
Adenocarcinoma (see also Neoplasm, malignant, by site)
  acidophil
    specified site — see Neoplasm, malignant, by site
    unspecified site C75.1
  adrenal cortical C74.0- ☑
  alveolar — see Neoplasm, lung, malignant

Adenocarcinoma — *continued*
  apocrine
    breast — *see* Neoplasm, breast, malignant
    in situ
      breast D05.8- ☑
      specified site NEC — *see* Neoplasm, skin, in situ
      unspecified site D04.9
    specified site NEC — *see* Neoplasm, skin, malignant
    unspecified site C44.99
  basal cell
    specified site — *see* Neoplasm, skin, malignant
    unspecified site C08.9
  basophil
    specified site — *see* Neoplasm, malignant, by site
    unspecified site C75.1
  bile duct type C22.1
    liver C22.1
    specified site NEC — *see* Neoplasm, malignant, by site
    unspecified site C22.1
  bronchiolar — *see* Neoplasm, lung, malignant
  bronchioloalveolar — *see* Neoplasm, lung, malignant
  ceruminous C44.29- ☑
  cervix, in situ (*see also* Carcinoma, cervix uteri, in situ) D06.9
  chromophobe
    specified site — *see* Neoplasm, malignant, by site
    unspecified site C75.1
  diffuse type
    specified site — *see* Neoplasm, malignant, by site
    unspecified site C16.9
  duct
    infiltrating
      with Paget's disease — *see* Neoplasm, breast, malignant
      specified site — *see* Neoplasm, malignant, by site
      unspecified site (female) C50.91- ☑
        male C50.92- ☑
    specified site — *see* Neoplasm, malignant, by site
    unspecified site
      female C56.9
      male C61
  eosinophil
    specified site — *see* Neoplasm, malignant, by site
    unspecified site C75.1
  follicular
    with papillary C73
    moderately differentiated C73
    specified site — *see* Neoplasm, malignant, by site
    trabecular C73
    unspecified site C73
    well differentiated C73
  Hurthle cell C73
  in
    adenomatous
      polyposis coli C18.9
  infiltrating duct
    with Paget's disease — *see* Neoplasm, breast, malignant
    specified site — *see* Neoplasm, by site, malignant
    unspecified site (female) C50.91- ☑
      male C50.92- ☑
  inflammatory
    specified site — *see* Neoplasm, by site, malignant
    unspecified site (female) C50.91- ☑
      male C50.92- ☑
  intestinal type
    specified site — *see* Neoplasm, by site, malignant
    unspecified site C16.9
  intracystic papillary
  intraductal
    breast D05.1- ☑
    noninfiltrating
      breast D05.1- ☑
      papillary
        with invasion
          specified site — *see* Neoplasm, by site, malignant
          unspecified site (female) C50.91- ☑
            male C50.92- ☑
        breast D05.1- ☑
        specified site NEC — *see* Neoplasm, in situ, by site
        unspecified site D05.1- ☑
    specified site NEC — *see* Neoplasm, in situ, by site

Adenocarcinoma — *continued*
  intraductal — *continued*
    noninfiltrating — *continued*
      unspecified site D05.1- ☑
    papillary
      with invasion
        specified site — *see* Neoplasm, malignant, by site
        unspecified site (female) C50.91- ☑
          male C50.92- ☑
      breast D05.1- ☑
      specified site — *see* Neoplasm, in situ, by site
      unspecified site D05.1- ☑
    specified site NEC — *see* Neoplasm, in situ, by site
    unspecified site D05.1- ☑
  islet cell
    with exocrine, mixed
      specified site — *see* Neoplasm, malignant, by site
      unspecified site C25.9
    pancreas C25.4
    specified site NEC — *see* Neoplasm, malignant, by site
    unspecified site C25.4
  lobular
    in situ
      breast D05.0- ☑
      specified site NEC — *see* Neoplasm, in situ, by site
      unspecified site D05.0- ☑
    specified site — *see* Neoplasm, malignant, by site
    unspecified site (female) C50.91- ☑
      male C50.92- ☑
  mucoid (*see also* Neoplasm, malignant, by site)
    cell
      specified site — *see* Neoplasm, malignant, by site
      unspecified site C75.1
  nonencapsulated sclerosing C73
  papillary
    with follicular C73
    follicular variant C73
    intraductal (noninfiltrating)
      with invasion
        specified site — *see* Neoplasm, malignant, by site
        unspecified site (female) C50.91- ☑
          male C50.92- ☑
      breast D05.1- ☑
      specified site NEC — *see* Neoplasm, in situ, by site
      unspecified site D05.1- ☑
    serous
      specified site — *see* Neoplasm, malignant, by site
      unspecified site C56.9
  papillocystic
    specified site — *see* Neoplasm, malignant, by site
    unspecified site C56.9
  pseudomucinous
    specified site — *see* Neoplasm, malignant, by site
    unspecified site C56.9
  renal cell C64- ☑
  sebaceous — *see* Neoplasm, skin, malignant
  serous (*see also* Neoplasm, malignant, by site)
    papillary
      specified site — *see* Neoplasm, malignant, by site
      unspecified site C56.9
  sweat gland — *see* Neoplasm, skin, malignant
  water-clear cell C75.0
Adenocarcinoma-in-situ (*see also* Neoplasm, in situ, by site)
  breast D05.9- ☑
Adenofibroma
  clear cell — *see* Neoplasm, benign, by site
  endometrioid D27.9
    borderline malignancy D39.10
    malignant C56- ☑
  mucinous
    specified site — *see* Neoplasm, benign, by site
    unspecified site D27.9
  papillary
    specified site — *see* Neoplasm, benign, by site
    unspecified site D27.9
  prostate — *see* Enlargement, enlarged, prostate

Adenofibroma — *continued*
  serous
    specified site — *see* Neoplasm, benign, by site
    unspecified site D27.9
  specified site — *see* Neoplasm, benign, by site
  unspecified site D27.9
Adenofibrosis
  breast — *see* Fibroadenosis, breast
  endometrioid N80.0
Adenoiditis (chronic) J35.02
  with tonsillitis J35.03
  acute J03.90
    recurrent J03.91
    specified organism NEC J03.80
      recurrent J03.81
    staphylococcal J03.80
      recurrent J03.81
    streptococcal J03.00
      recurrent J03.01
Adenoids — *see* condition
Adenolipoma — *see* Neoplasm, benign, by site
Adenolipomatosis, Launois-Bensaude E88.89
Adenolymphoma
  specified site — *see* Neoplasm, benign, by site
  unspecified site D11.9
Adenoma (*see also* Neoplasm, benign, by site)
  acidophil
    specified site — *see* Neoplasm, benign, by site
    unspecified site D35.2
  acidophil-basophil, mixed
    specified site — *see* Neoplasm, benign, by site
    unspecified site D35.2
  adrenal (cortical) D35.00
    clear cell D35.00
    compact cell D35.00
    glomerulosa cell D35.00
    heavily pigmented variant D35.00
    mixed cell D35.00
  alpha-cell
    pancreas D13.7
    specified site NEC — *see* Neoplasm, benign, by site
    unspecified site D13.7
  alveolar D14.30
  apocrine
    breast D24- ☑
    specified site NEC — *see* Neoplasm, skin, benign, by site
    unspecified site D23.9
  basal cell D11.9
  basophil
    specified site — *see* Neoplasm, benign, by site
    unspecified site D35.2
  basophil-acidophil, mixed
    specified site — *see* Neoplasm, benign, by site
    unspecified site D35.2
  beta-cell
    pancreas D13.7
    specified site NEC — *see* Neoplasm, benign, by site
    unspecified site D13.7
  bile duct D13.4
    common D13.5
    extrahepatic D13.5
    intrahepatic D13.4
    specified site NEC — *see* Neoplasm, benign, by site
    unspecified site D13.4
  black D35.00
  bronchial D38.1
    cylindroid type — *see* Neoplasm, lung, malignant
  ceruminous D23.2- ☑
  chief cell D35.1
  chromophobe
    specified site — *see* Neoplasm, benign, by site
    unspecified site D35.2
  colloid
    specified site — *see* Neoplasm, benign, by site
    unspecified site D34
  duct
  eccrine, papillary — *see* Neoplasm, skin, benign
  endocrine, multiple
    single specified site — *see* Neoplasm, uncertain behavior, by site
    two or more specified sites D44- ☑
    unspecified site D44.9
  endometrioid (*see also* Neoplasm, benign)
    borderline malignancy — *see* Neoplasm, uncertain behavior, by site
  eosinophil
    specified site — *see* Neoplasm, benign, by site

Subterms under main terms may continue to next column or page   ☑ Additional Character Required — Refer to the Tabular List for Character Selection   11

Adenocarcinoma — Adenoma

Adenoma — *continued*
  eosinophil — *continued*
    unspecified site D35.2
  fetal
    specified site — *see* Neoplasm, benign, by site
    unspecified site D34
  follicular
    specified site — *see* Neoplasm, benign, by site
    unspecified site D34
  hepatocellular D13.4
  Hurthle cell D34
  islet cell
    pancreas D13.7
    specified site NEC — *see* Neoplasm, benign, by site
    unspecified site D13.7
  liver cell D13.4
  macrofollicular
    specified site — *see* Neoplasm, benign, by site
    unspecified site D34
  malignant, malignum — *see* Neoplasm, malignant, by site
  microcystic
    pancreas D13.6
    specified site NEC — *see* Neoplasm, benign, by site
    unspecified site D13.6
  microfollicular
    specified site — *see* Neoplasm, benign, by site
    unspecified site D34
  mucoid cell
    specified site — *see* Neoplasm, benign, by site
    unspecified site D35.2
  multiple endocrine
    single specified site — *see* Neoplasm, uncertain behavior, by site
    two or more specified sites D44- ☑
    unspecified site D44.9
  nipple D24- ☑
  papillary (*see also* Neoplasm, benign, by site)
    eccrine — *see* Neoplasm, skin, benign, by site
  Pick's tubular
    specified site — *see* Neoplasm, benign, by site
    unspecified site
      female D27.9
      male D29.20
  pleomorphic
    carcinoma in — *see* Neoplasm, salivary gland, malignant
      specified site — *see* Neoplasm, malignant, by site
      unspecified site C08.9
  polypoid (*see also* Neoplasm, benign)
    adenocarcinoma in — *see* Neoplasm, malignant, by site
    adenocarcinoma in situ — *see* Neoplasm, in situ, by site
  prostate — *see* Neoplasm, benign, prostate
  rete cell D29.20
  sebaceous — *see* Neoplasm, skin, benign
  Sertoli cell
    specified site — *see* Neoplasm, benign, by site
    unspecified site
      female D27.9
      male D29.20
  skin appendage — *see* Neoplasm, skin, benign
  sudoriferous gland — *see* Neoplasm, skin, benign
  sweat gland — *see* Neoplasm, skin, benign
  testicular
    specified site — *see* Neoplasm, benign, by site
    unspecified site
      female D27.9
      male D29.20
  tubular (*see also* Neoplasm, benign, by site)
    adenocarcinoma in — *see* Neoplasm, malignant, by site
    adenocarcinoma in situ — *see* Neoplasm, in situ, by site
    Pick's
      specified site — *see* Neoplasm, benign, by site
      unspecified site
        female D27.9
        male D29.20
  tubulovillous (*see also* Neoplasm, benign, by site)
    adenocarcinoma in — *see* Neoplasm, malignant, by site
    adenocarcinoma in situ — *see* Neoplasm, in situ, by site
  villous — *see* Neoplasm, uncertain behavior, by site

Adenoma — *continued*
  villous — *see* Neoplasm, uncertain behavior, by site — *continued*
    adenocarcinoma in — *see* Neoplasm, malignant, by site
    adenocarcinoma in situ — *see* Neoplasm, in situ, by site
  water-clear cell D35.1
Adenomatosis
  endocrine (multiple) E31.20
    single specified site — *see* Neoplasm, uncertain behavior, by site
  erosive of nipple D24- ☑
  pluriendocrine — *see* Adenomatosis, endocrine
  pulmonary D38.1
    malignant — *see* Neoplasm, lung, malignant
  specified site — *see* Neoplasm, benign, by site
  unspecified site D12.6
Adenomatous
  goiter (nontoxic) E04.9
    with hyperthyroidism — *see* Hyperthyroidism, with, goiter, nodular
    toxic — *see* Hyperthyroidism, with, goiter, nodular
Adenomyoma (*see also* Neoplasm, benign, by site)
  prostate — *see* Enlarged, prostate
Adenomyometritis N80.0
Adenomyosis N80.0
Adenopathy (lymph gland) R59.9
  generalized R59.1
  inguinal R59.0
  localized R59.0
  mediastinal R59.0
  mesentery R59.0
  syphilitic (secondary) A51.49
  tracheobronchial R59.0
    tuberculous A15.4
      primary (progressive) A15.7
  tuberculous (*see also* Tuberculosis, lymph gland)
    tracheobronchial A15.4
      primary (progressive) A15.7
Adenosalpingitis — *see* Salpingitis
Adenosarcoma — *see* Neoplasm, malignant, by site
Adenosclerosis I88.8
Adenosis (sclerosing) breast — *see* Fibroadenosis, breast
Adenovirus, as cause of disease classified elsewhere B97.0
Adentia (complete) (partial) — *see* Absence, teeth
Adherent (*see also* Adhesions)
  labia (minora) N90.89
  pericardium (nonrheumatic) I31.0
    rheumatic I09.2
  placenta (with hemorrhage) O72.0
    without hemorrhage O73.0
  prepuce, newborn N47.0
  scar (skin) L90.5
  tendon in scar L90.5
Adhesions, adhesive (postinfective) K66.0
  with intestinal obstruction K56.50
    complete K56.52
    incomplete K56.51
    partial K56.51
  abdominal (wall) — *see* Adhesions, peritoneum
  appendix K38.8
  bile duct (common) (hepatic) K83.8
  bladder (sphincter) N32.89
  bowel — *see* Adhesions, peritoneum
  cardiac I31.0
    rheumatic I09.2
  cecum — *see* Adhesions, peritoneum
  cervicovaginal N88.1
    congenital Q52.8
    postpartal O90.89
    old N88.1
  cervix N88.1
  ciliary body NEC — *see* Adhesions, iris
  clitoris N90.89
  colon — *see* Adhesions, peritoneum
  common duct K83.8
  congenital (*see also* Anomaly, by site)
    fingers — *see* Syndactylism, complex, fingers
    omental, anomalous Q43.3
    peritoneal Q43.3
    tongue (to gum or roof of mouth) Q38.3
  conjunctiva (acquired) H11.21- ☑
    congenital Q15.8
  cystic duct K82.8
  diaphragm — *see* Adhesions, peritoneum
  due to foreign body — *see* Foreign body

Adhesions, adhesive — *continued*
  duodenum — *see* Adhesions, peritoneum
  ear
    middle H74.1- ☑
  epididymis N50.89
  epidural — *see* Adhesions, meninges
  epiglottis J38.7
  eyelid H02.59
  female pelvis N73.6
  gallbladder K82.8
  globe H44.89
  heart I31.0
    rheumatic I09.2
  ileocecal (coil) — *see* Adhesions, peritoneum
  ileum — *see* Adhesions, peritoneum
  intestine (*see also* Adhesions, peritoneum)
    with obstruction K56.50
      complete K56.52
      incomplete K56.51
      partial K56.51
  intra-abdominal — *see* Adhesions, peritoneum
  iris H21.50- ☑
    anterior H21.51- ☑
    goniosynechiae H21.52- ☑
    posterior H21.54- ☑
    to corneal graft T85.898 ☑
  joint — *see* Ankylosis
    knee M23.8X ☑
    temporomandibular M26.61- ☑
  labium (majus) (minus), congenital Q52.5
  liver — *see* Adhesions, peritoneum
  lung J98.4
  mediastinum J98.59
  meninges (cerebral) (spinal) G96.12
    congenital Q07.8
    tuberculous (cerebral) (spinal) A17.0
  mesenteric — *see* Adhesions, peritoneum
  nasal (septum) (to turbinates) J34.89
  ocular muscle — *see* Strabismus, mechanical
  omentum — *see* Adhesions, peritoneum
  ovary N73.6
    congenital (to cecum, kidney or omentum) Q50.39
  paraovarian N73.6
  pelvic (peritoneal)
    female N73.6
      postprocedural N99.4
    male — *see* Adhesions, peritoneum
    postpartal (old) N73.6
    tuberculous A18.17
  penis to scrotum (congenital) Q55.8
  periappendiceal (*see also* Adhesions, peritoneum)
  pericardium (nonrheumatic) I31.0
    focal I31.8
    rheumatic I09.2
    tuberculous A18.84
  pericholecystic K82.8
  perigastric — *see* Adhesions, peritoneum
  periovarian N73.6
  periprostatic N42.89
  perirectal — *see* Adhesions, peritoneum
  perirenal N28.89
  peritoneum, peritoneal (postinfective)
    with obstruction (intestinal) K56.50
      complete K56.52
      incomplete K56.51
      partial K56.51
    congenital Q43.3
    pelvic, female N73.6
      postprocedural N99.4
    postpartal, pelvic N73.6
    postprocedural K66.0
    to uterus N73.6
  peritubal N73.6
  periureteral N28.89
  periuterine N73.6
  perivesical N32.89
  perivesicular (seminal vesicle) N50.89
  pleura, pleuritic J94.8
    tuberculous NEC A15.6
  pleuropericardial J94.8
  postoperative (gastrointestinal tract) K66.0
    with obstruction (*see also* Obstruction, intestine, postoperative) K91.30
    due to foreign body accidentally left in wound — *see* Foreign body, accidentally left during a procedure
  pelvic peritoneal N99.4
  urethra — *see* Stricture, urethra, postprocedural

☑ **Additional Character Required** — Refer to the Tabular List for Character Selection   ▽ Subterms under main terms may continue to next column or page

Adhesions, adhesive — *continued*
  postoperative — *continued*
    vagina N99.2
  postpartal, old (vulva or perineum) N90.89
  preputial, prepuce N47.5
  pulmonary J98.4
  pylorus — *see* Adhesions, peritoneum
  sciatic nerve — *see* Lesion, nerve, sciatic
  seminal vesicle N50.89
  shoulder (joint) — *see* Capsulitis, adhesive
  sigmoid flexure — *see* Adhesions, peritoneum
  spermatic cord (acquired) N50.89
    congenital Q55.4
  spinal canal G96.12
  stomach — *see* Adhesions, peritoneum
  subscapular — *see* Capsulitis, adhesive
  temporomandibular M26.61- ☑
  tendinitis (*see also* Tenosynovitis, specified type NEC)
    shoulder — *see* Capsulitis, adhesive
  testis N44.8
  tongue, congenital (to gum or roof of mouth) Q38.3
    acquired K14.8
  trachea J39.8
  tubo-ovarian N73.6
  tunica vaginalis N44.8
  uterus N73.6
    internal N85.6
    to abdominal wall N73.6
  vagina (chronic) N89.5
    postoperative N99.2
  vitreomacular H43.82- ☑
  vitreous H43.89
  vulva N90.89
Adiaspiromycosis B48.8
Adie (-Holmes) **pupil or syndrome** — *see* Anomaly, pupil, function, tonic pupil
Adiponecrosis neonatorum P83.88
Adiposis (*see also* Obesity)
  cerebralis E23.6
  dolorosa E88.2
Adiposity (*see also* Obesity)
  heart — *see* Degeneration, myocardial
  localized E65
Adiposogenital dystrophy E23.6
Adjustment
  disorder — *see* Disorder, adjustment
  implanted device — *see* Encounter (for), adjustment (of)
  prosthesis, external — *see* Fitting
  reaction — *see* Disorder, adjustment
Administration of tPA (rtPA) in a different facility within the last 24 hours prior to admission to current facility Z92.82
Admission (for) (*see also* Encounter (for))
  adjustment (of)
    artificial
      arm Z44.00- ☑
        complete Z44.01- ☑
        partial Z44.02- ☑
      eye Z44.2 ☑
      leg Z44.10- ☑
        complete Z44.11- ☑
        partial Z44.12- ☑
    brain neuropacemaker Z46.2
      implanted Z45.42
    breast
      implant Z45.81 ☑
      prosthesis (external) Z44.3 ☑
    colostomy belt Z46.89
    contact lenses Z46.0
    cystostomy device Z46.6
    dental prosthesis Z46.3
    device NEC
      abdominal Z46.89
      implanted Z45.89
        cardiac Z45.09
          defibrillator (with synchronous cardiace pacemaker) Z45.02
          pacemaker (cardiac resynchronization therapy (CRT-P)) Z45.018
          pulse generator Z45.010
          resynchronization therapy defibrillator (CRT-D) Z45.02
        hearing device Z45.328
          bone conduction Z45.320
          cochlear Z45.321
        infusion pump Z45.1
        nervous system Z45.49

Admission — *continued*
  adjustment — *continued*
    device — *continued*
      implanted — *continued*
        nervous system — *continued*
          CSF drainage Z45.41
          hearing device — *see* Admission, adjustment, device, implanted, hearing device
          neuropacemaker Z45.42
          visual substitution Z45.31
        specified NEC Z45.89
        vascular access Z45.2
        visual substitution Z45.31
      nervous system Z46.2
        implanted — *see* Admission, adjustment, device, implanted, nervous system
      orthodontic Z46.4
      prosthetic Z44.9
        arm — *see* Admission, adjustment, artificial, arm
        breast Z44.3 ☑
        dental Z46.3
        eye Z44.2 ☑
        leg — *see* Admission, adjustment, artificial, leg
        specified type NEC Z44.8
      substitution
        auditory Z46.2
          implanted — *see* Admission, adjustment, device, implanted, hearing device
        nervous system Z46.2
          implanted — *see* Admission, adjustment, device, implanted, nervous system
        visual Z46.2
          implanted Z45.31
      urinary Z46.6
    hearing aid Z46.1
      implanted — *see* Admission, adjustment, device, implanted, hearing device
    ileostomy device Z46.89
    intestinal appliance or device NEC Z46.89
    neuropacemaker (brain) (peripheral nerve) (spinal cord) Z46.2
      implanted Z45.42
    orthodontic device Z46.4
    orthopedic (brace) (cast) (device) (shoes) Z46.89
    pacemaker (cardiac resynchronization therapy (CRT-P))
      cardiac Z45.018
        pulse generator Z45.010
      nervous system Z46.2
        implanted Z45.42
    portacath (port-a-cath) Z45.2
    prosthesis Z44.9
      arm — *see* Admission, adjustment, artificial, arm
      breast Z44.3 ☑
      dental Z46.3
      eye Z44.2 ☑
      leg — *see* Admission, adjustment, artificial, leg
      specified NEC Z44.8
    spectacles Z46.0
  aftercare (*see also* Aftercare) Z51.89
    postpartum
      immediately after delivery Z39.0
      routine follow-up Z39.2
    radiation therapy (antineoplastic) Z51.0
  attention to artificial opening (of) Z43.9
    artificial vagina Z43.7
    colostomy Z43.3
    cystostomy Z43.5
    enterostomy Z43.4
    gastrostomy Z43.1
    ileostomy Z43.2
    jejunostomy Z43.4
    nephrostomy Z43.6
    specified site NEC Z43.8
      intestinal tract Z43.4
      urinary tract Z43.6
    tracheostomy Z43.0
    ureterostomy Z43.6
    urethrostomy Z43.6
  breast augmentation or reduction Z41.1
  breast reconstruction following mastectomy Z42.1

Admission — *continued*
  change of
    dressing (nonsurgical) Z48.00
    neuropacemaker device (brain) (peripheral nerve) (spinal cord) Z46.2
      implanted Z45.42
    surgical dressing Z48.01
  circumcision, ritual or routine (in absence of diagnosis) Z41.2
  clinical research investigation (control) (normal comparison) (participant) Z00.6
  contraceptive management Z30.9
  cosmetic surgery NEC Z41.1
  counseling (*see also* Counseling)
    dietary Z71.3
    gestational carrier Z31.7
    HIV Z71.7
    human immunodeficiency virus Z71.7
    nonattending third party Z71.0
    procreative management NEC Z31.69
  delivery, full-term, uncomplicated O80
    cesarean, without indication O82
  desensitization to allergens Z51.6
  dietary surveillance and counseling Z71.3
  ear piercing Z41.3
  examination at health care facility (adult) (*see also* Examination) Z00.00
    with abnormal findings Z00.01
    clinical research investigation (control) (normal comparison) (participant) Z00.6
    dental Z01.20
      with abnormal findings Z01.21
    donor (potential) Z00.5
    ear Z01.10
      with abnormal findings NEC Z01.118
    eye Z01.00
      with abnormal findings Z01.01
    general, specified reason NEC Z00.8
    hearing Z01.10
      with abnormal findings NEC Z01.118
    postpartum checkup Z39.2
    psychiatric (general) Z00.8
      requested by authority Z04.6
    vision Z01.00
      with abnormal findings Z01.01
  fitting (of)
    artificial
      arm — *see* Admission, adjustment, artificial, arm
      eye Z44.2 ☑
      leg — *see* Admission, adjustment, artificial, leg
    brain neuropacemaker Z46.2
      implanted Z45.42
    breast prosthesis (external) Z44.3 ☑
    colostomy belt Z46.89
    contact lenses Z46.0
    cystostomy device Z46.6
    dental prosthesis Z46.3
    dentures Z46.3
    device NEC
      abdominal Z46.89
      nervous system Z46.2
        implanted — *see* Admission, adjustment, device, implanted, nervous system
      orthodontic Z46.4
      prosthetic Z44.9
        breast Z44.3 ☑
        dental Z46.3
        eye Z44.2 ☑
      substitution
        auditory Z46.2
          implanted — *see* Admission, adjustment, device, implanted, hearing device
        nervous system Z46.2
          implanted — *see* Admission, adjustment, device, implanted, nervous system
        visual Z46.2
          implanted Z45.31
    hearing aid Z46.1
    ileostomy device Z46.89
    intestinal appliance or device NEC Z46.89
    neuropacemaker (brain) (peripheral nerve) (spinal cord) Z46.2
      implanted Z45.42
    orthodontic device Z46.4
    orthopedic device (brace) (cast) (shoes) Z46.89

◣ Subterms under main terms may continue to next column or page   ☑ Additional Character Required — Refer to the Tabular List for Character Selection   **13**

Adhesions, adhesive — Admission

Admission — *continued*
fitting — *continued*
prosthesis Z44.9
arm — *see* Admission, adjustment, artificial, arm
breast Z44.3 ☑
dental Z46.3
eye Z44.2 ☑
leg — *see* Admission, adjustment, artificial, leg
specified type NEC Z44.8
spectacles Z46.0
follow-up examination Z09
intrauterine device management Z30.431
initial prescription Z30.014
mental health evaluation Z00.8
requested by authority Z04.6
observation — *see* Observation
Papanicolaou smear, cervix Z12.4
for suspected malignant neoplasm Z12.4
plastic and reconstructive surgery following medical procedure or healed injury NEC Z42.8
plastic surgery, cosmetic NEC Z41.1
postpartum observation
immediately after delivery Z39.0
routine follow-up Z39.2
poststerilization (for restoration) Z31.0
aftercare Z31.42
procreative management Z31.9
prophylactic (measure) — (*see also* Encounter, prophylactic measures)
organ removal Z40.00
breast Z40.01
fallopian tube(s) Z40.03
with ovary(s) Z40.02
ovary(s) Z40.02
specified organ NEC Z40.09
testes Z40.09
vaccination Z23
psychiatric examination (general) Z00.8
requested by authority Z04.6
radiation therapy (antineoplastic) Z51.0
reconstructive surgery following medical procedure or healed injury NEC Z42.8
removal of
cystostomy catheter Z43.5
drains Z48.03
dressing (nonsurgical) Z48.00
implantable subdermal contraceptive Z30.46
intrauterine contraceptive device Z30.432
neuropacemaker (brain) (peripheral nerve) (spinal cord) Z46.2
implanted Z45.42
staples Z48.02
surgical dressing Z48.01
sutures Z48.02
ureteral stent Z46.6
respirator [ventilator] use during power failure Z99.12
restoration of organ continuity (poststerilization) Z31.0
aftercare Z31.42
sensitivity test (*see also* Test, skin)
allergy NEC Z01.82
Mantoux Z11.1
tuboplasty following previous sterilization Z31.0
aftercare Z31.42
vasoplasty following previous sterilization Z31.0
aftercare Z31.42
vision examination Z01.00
with abnormal findings Z01.01
waiting period for admission to other facility Z75.1
Adnexitis (suppurative) — *see* Salpingo-oophoritis
Adolescent X-linked adrenoleukodystrophy E71.521
Adrenal (gland) — *see* condition
Adrenalism, tuberculous A18.7
Adrenalitis, adrenitis E27.8
autoimmune E27.1
meningococcal, hemorrhagic A39.1
Adrenarche, premature E27.0
Adrenocortical syndrome — *see* Cushing's, syndrome
Adrenogenital syndrome E25.9
acquired E25.8
congenital E25.0
salt loss E25.0
Adrenogenitalism, congenital E25.0
Adrenoleukodystrophy E71.529
neonatal E71.511
X-linked E71.529
Addison only phenotype E71.528
Addison-Schilder E71.528

Adrenoleukodystrophy — *continued*
X-linked — *continued*
adolescent E71.521
adrenomyeloneuropathy E71.522
childhood cerebral E71.520
other specified E71.528
Adrenomyeloneuropathy E71.522
Adventitious bursa — *see* Bursopathy, specified type NEC
Adverse effect — *see* Table of Drugs and Chemicals, categories T36-T50, with 6th character 5
Advice — *see* Counseling
Adynamia (episodica) (hereditary) (periodic) G72.3
Aeration lung imperfect, newborn — *see* Atelectasis
Aerobullosis T70.3 ☑
Aerocele — *see* Embolism, air
Aerodermectasia
subcutaneous (traumatic) T79.7 ☑
Aerodontalgia T70.29 ☑
Aeroembolism T70.3 ☑
Aerogenes capsulatus infection A48.0
Aero-otitis media T70.0 ☑
Aerophagy, aerophagia (psychogenic) F45.8
Aerophobia F40.228
Aerosinusitis T70.1 ☑
Aerotitis T70.0 ☑
Affection — *see* Disease
Afibrinogenemia (*see also* Defect, coagulation) D68.8
acquired D65
congenital D68.2
following ectopic or molar pregnancy O08.1
in abortion — *see* Abortion, by type, complicated by, afibrinogenemia
puerperal O72.3
African
sleeping sickness B56.9
tick fever A68.1
trypanosomiasis B56.9
gambian B56.0
rhodesian B56.1
Aftercare (*see also* Care) Z51.89
following surgery (for) (on)
amputation Z47.81
attention to
drains Z48.03
dressings (nonsurgical) Z48.00
surgical Z48.01
sutures Z48.02
circulatory system Z48.812
delayed (planned) wound closure Z48.1
digestive system Z48.815
explantation of joint prosthesis (staged procedure)
hip Z47.32
knee Z47.33
shoulder Z47.31
genitourinary system Z48.816
joint replacement Z47.1
neoplasm Z48.3
nervous system Z48.811
oral cavity Z48.814
organ transplant
bone marrow Z48.290
heart Z48.21
heart-lung Z48.280
kidney Z48.22
liver Z48.23
lung Z48.24
multiple organs NEC Z48.288
specified NEC Z48.298
orthopedic NEC Z47.89
planned wound closure Z48.1
removal of internal fixation device Z47.2
respiratory system Z48.813
scoliosis Z47.82
sense organs Z48.810
skin and subcutaneous tissue Z48.817
specified body system
circulatory Z48.812
digestive Z48.815
genitourinary Z48.816
nervous Z48.811
oral cavity Z48.814
respiratory Z48.813
sense organs Z48.810
skin and subcutaneous tissue Z48.817
teeth Z48.814
specified NEC Z48.89
spinal Z47.89

Aftercare — *continued*
following surgery — *continued*
teeth Z48.814
fracture — *code to* fracture with seventh character D
involving
removal of
drains Z48.03
dressings (nonsurgical) Z48.00
staples Z48.02
surgical dressings Z48.01
sutures Z48.02
neuropacemaker (brain) (peripheral nerve) (spinal cord) Z46.2
implanted Z45.42
orthopedic NEC Z47.89
postprocedural — *see* Aftercare, following surgery
After-cataract — *see* Cataract, secondary
Agalactia (primary) O92.3
elective, secondary or therapeutic O92.5
Agammaglobulinemia (acquired) (secondary) (nonfamilial) D80.1
with
immunoglobulin-bearing B-lymphocytes D80.1
lymphopenia D81.9
autosomal recessive (Swiss type) D80.0
Bruton's X-linked D80.0
common variable (CVAgamma) D80.1
congenital sex-linked D80.0
hereditary D80.0
lymphopenic D81.9
Swiss type (autosomal recessive) D80.0
X-linked (with growth hormone deficiency) (Bruton) D80.0
Aganglionosis (bowel) (colon) Q43.1
Age (old) — *see* Senility
Agenesis
adrenal (gland) Q89.1
alimentary tract (complete) (partial) NEC Q45.8
upper Q40.8
anus, anal (canal) Q42.3
with fistula Q42.2
aorta Q25.41
appendix Q42.8
arm (complete) Q71.0- ☑
with hand present Q71.1- ☑
artery (peripheral) Q27.9
brain Q28.3
coronary Q24.5
pulmonary Q25.79
specified NEC Q27.8
umbilical Q27.0
auditory (canal) (external) Q16.1
auricle (ear) Q16.0
bile duct or passage Q44.5
bladder Q64.5
bone Q79.9
brain Q00.0
part of Q04.3
breast (with nipple present) Q83.8
with absent nipple Q83.0
bronchus Q32.4
canaliculus lacrimalis Q10.4
carpus — *see* Agenesis, hand
cartilage Q79.9
cecum Q42.8
cerebellum Q04.3
cervix Q51.5
chin Q18.8
cilia Q10.3
circulatory system, part NOS Q28.9
clavicle Q74.0
clitoris Q52.6
coccyx Q76.49
colon Q42.9
specified NEC Q42.8
corpus callosum Q04.0
cricoid cartilage Q31.8
diaphragm (with hernia) Q79.1
digestive organ(s) or tract (complete) (partial) NEC Q45.8
upper Q40.8
ductus arteriosus Q28.8
duodenum Q41.0
ear Q16.9
auricle Q16.0
lobe Q17.8
ejaculatory duct Q55.4
endocrine (gland) NEC Q89.2

☑ **Additional Character Required** — **Refer to the Tabular List for Character Selection** ▽ **Subterms under main terms may continue to next column or page**

Agenesis — *continued*
  epiglottis Q31.8
  esophagus Q39.8
  eustachian tube Q16.2
  eye Q11.1
    adnexa Q15.8
  eyelid (fold) Q10.3
  face
    bones NEC Q75.8
    specified part NEC Q18.8
  fallopian tube Q50.6
  femur — *see* Defect, reduction, lower limb, longitudinal, femur
  fibula — *see* Defect, reduction, lower limb, longitudinal, fibula
  finger (complete) (partial) — *see* Agenesis, hand
  foot (and toes) (complete) (partial) Q72.3- ☑
  forearm (with hand present) — *see* Agenesis, arm, with hand present
    and hand Q71.2- ☑
  gallbladder Q44.0
  gastric Q40.2
  genitalia, genital (organ(s))
    female Q52.8
      external Q52.71
      internal NEC Q52.8
    male Q55.8
  glottis Q31.8
  hair Q84.0
  hand (and fingers) (complete) (partial) Q71.3- ☑
  heart Q24.8
    valve NEC Q24.8
      pulmonary Q22.0
  hepatic Q44.7
  humerus — *see* Defect, reduction, upper limb
  hymen Q52.4
  ileum Q41.2
  incus Q16.3
  intestine (small) Q41.9
    large Q42.9
      specified NEC Q42.8
  iris (dilator fibers) Q13.1
  jaw M26.09
  jejunum Q41.1
  kidney(s) (partial) Q60.2
    bilateral Q60.1
    unilateral Q60.0
  labium (majus) (minus) Q52.71
  labyrinth, membranous Q16.5
  lacrimal apparatus Q10.4
  larynx Q31.8
  leg (complete) Q72.0- ☑
    with foot present Q72.1- ☑
      lower leg (with foot present) — *see* Agenesis, leg, with foot present
        and foot Q72.2- ☑
  lens Q12.3
  limb (complete) Q73.0
    lower — *see* Agenesis, leg
    upper — *see* Agenesis, arm
  lip Q38.0
  liver Q44.7
  lung (fissure) (lobe) (bilateral) (unilateral) Q33.3
  mandible, maxilla M26.09
  metacarpus — *see* Agenesis, hand
  metatarsus — *see* Agenesis, foot
  muscle Q79.8
    eyelid Q10.3
    ocular Q15.8
  musculoskeletal system NEC Q79.8
  nail(s) Q84.3
  neck, part Q18.8
  nerve Q07.8
  nervous system, part NEC Q07.8
  nipple Q83.2
  nose Q30.1
  nuclear Q07.8
  organ
    of Corti Q16.5
    or site not listed — *see* Anomaly, by site
  osseous meatus (ear) Q16.1
  ovary
    bilateral Q50.02
    unilateral Q50.01
  oviduct Q50.6
  pancreas Q45.0
  parathyroid (gland) Q89.2
  parotid gland(s) Q38.4

Agenesis — *continued*
  patella Q74.1
  pelvic girdle (complete) (partial) Q74.2
  penis Q55.5
  pericardium Q24.8
  pituitary (gland) Q89.2
  prostate Q55.4
  punctum lacrimale Q10.4
  radioulnar — *see* Defect, reduction, upper limb
  radius — *see* Defect, reduction, upper limb, longitudinal, radius
  rectum Q42.1
    with fistula Q42.0
  renal Q60.2
    bilateral Q60.1
    unilateral Q60.0
  respiratory organ NEC Q34.8
  rib Q76.6
  roof of orbit Q75.8
  round ligament Q52.8
  sacrum Q76.49
  salivary gland Q38.4
  scapula Q74.0
  scrotum Q55.29
  seminal vesicles Q55.4
  septum
    atrial Q21.1
    between aorta and pulmonary artery Q21.4
    ventricular Q20.4
  shoulder girdle (complete) (partial) Q74.0
  skull (bone) Q75.8
    with
      anencephaly Q00.0
      encephalocele — *see* Encephalocele
      hydrocephalus Q03.9
        with spina bifida — *see* Spina bifida, by site, with hydrocephalus
      microcephaly Q02
  spermatic cord Q55.4
  spinal cord Q06.0
  spine Q76.49
  spleen Q89.01
  sternum Q76.7
  stomach Q40.2
  submaxillary gland(s) (congenital) Q38.4
  tarsus — *see* Agenesis, foot
  tendon Q79.8
  testicle Q55.0
  thymus (gland) Q89.2
  thyroid (gland) E03.1
    cartilage Q31.8
  tibia — *see* Defect, reduction, lower limb, longitudinal, tibia
  tibiofibular — *see* Defect, reduction, lower limb, specified type NEC
  toe (and foot) (complete) (partial) — *see* Agenesis, foot
  tongue Q38.3
  trachea (cartilage) Q32.1
  ulna — *see* Defect, reduction, upper limb, longitudinal, ulna
  upper limb — *see* Agenesis, arm
  ureter Q62.4
  urethra Q64.5
  urinary tract NEC Q64.8
  uterus Q51.0
  uvula Q38.5
  vagina Q52.0
  vas deferens Q55.4
  vein(s) (peripheral) Q27.9
    brain Q28.3
    great NEC Q26.8
    portal Q26.5
  vena cava (inferior) (superior) Q26.8
  vermis of cerebellum Q04.3
  vertebra Q76.49
  vulva Q52.71
Ageusia R43.2
Agitated — *see* condition
Agitation R45.1
Aglossia (congenital) Q38.3
Aglossia-adactylia syndrome Q87.0
Aglycogenosis E74.00
Agnosia (body image) (other senses) (tactile) R48.1
  developmental F88
  verbal R48.1
    auditory R48.1
      developmental F80.2

Agnosia — *continued*
  verbal — *continued*
    developmental F80.2
  visual (object) R48.3
Agoraphobia F40.00
  with panic disorder F40.01
  without panic disorder F40.02
Agrammatism R48.8
Agranulocytopenia — *see* Agranulocytosis
Agranulocytosis (chronic) (cyclical) (genetic) (infantile) (periodic) (pernicious) (*see also* Neutropenia) D70.9
  congenital D70.0
  cytoreductive cancer chemotherapy sequela D70.1
  drug-induced D70.2
    due to cytoreductive cancer chemotherapy D70.1
  due to infection D70.3
  secondary D70.4
    drug-induced D70.2
      due to cytoreductive cancer chemotherapy D70.1
Agraphia (absolute) R48.8
  with alexia R48.0
  developmental F81.81
Ague (dumb) — *see* Malaria
Agyria Q04.3
Ahumada-del Castillo syndrome E23.0
Aichomophobia F40.298
AIDS (related complex) B20
Ailment heart — *see* Disease, heart
Ailurophobia F40.218
AIN — *see* Neoplasia, intraepithelial, anal
Ainhum (disease) L94.6
AIPHI (acute idiopathic pulmonary hemorrhage in infants (over 28 days old)) R04.81
Air
  anterior mediastinum J98.2
  compressed, disease T70.3 ☑
  conditioner lung or pneumonitis J67.7
  embolism (artery) (cerebral) (any site) T79.0 ☑
    with ectopic or molar pregnancy O08.2
    due to implanted device NEC — *see* Complications, by site and type, specified NEC
    following
      abortion — *see* Abortion by type, complicated by, embolism
      ectopic or molar pregnancy O08.2
    infusion, therapeutic injection or transfusion T80.0 ☑
    in pregnancy, childbirth or puerperium — *see* Embolism, obstetric
    traumatic T79.0 ☑
  hunger, psychogenic F45.8
  rarefied, effects of — *see* Effect, adverse, high altitude
  sickness T75.3 ☑
Airplane sickness T75.3 ☑
Akathisia (drug-induced) (treatment-induced) G25.71
  neuroleptic induced (acute) G25.71
  tardive G25.71
Akinesia R29.898
Akinetic mutism R41.89
Akureyri's disease G93.3
Alactasia, congenital E73.0
Alagille's syndrome Q44.7
Alastrim B03
Albers-Schönberg syndrome Q78.2
Albert's syndrome — *see* Tendinitis, Achilles
Albinism, albino E70.30
  with hematologic abnormality E70.339
    Chédiak-Higashi syndrome E70.330
    Hermansky-Pudlak syndrome E70.331
    other specified E70.338
  I E70.320
  II E70.321
  ocular E70.319
    autosomal recessive E70.311
    other specified E70.318
    X-linked E70.310
  oculocutaneous E70.329
    other specified E70.328
    tyrosinase (ty) negative E70.320
    tyrosinase (ty) positive E70.321
  other specified E70.39
Albinismus E70.30
Albright (-McCune)(-Sternberg) syndrome Q78.1
Albuminous — *see* condition
Albuminuria, albuminuric (acute) (chronic) (subacute) (*see also* Proteinuria) R80.9

Albuminuria, albuminuric — *continued*
- complicating pregnancy — *see* Proteinuria, gestational
  - with
    - gestational hypertension — *see* Pre-eclampsia
    - pre-existing hypertension — *see* Hypertension, complicating pregnancy, pre-existing, with, pre-eclampsia
  - gestational — *see* Proteinuria, gestational
    - with
      - gestational hypertension — *see* Pre-eclampsia
      - pre-existing hypertension — *see* Hypertension, complicating pregnancy, pre-existing, with, pre-eclampsia
- orthostatic R80.2
- postural R80.2
- pre-eclamptic — *see* Pre-eclampsia
- scarlatinal A38.8

Albuminurophobia F40.298
Alcaptonuria E70.29
Alcohol, alcoholic, alcohol-induced
- addiction (without remission) F10.20
  - with remission F10.21
- amnestic disorder, persisting F10.96
  - with dependence F10.26
- anxiety disorder F10.980
- bipolar and related disorder F10.94
- brain syndrome, chronic F10.97
  - with dependence F10.27
- cardiopathy I42.6
- counseling and surveillance Z71.41
  - family member Z71.42
- delirium (acute) (tremens) (withdrawal) F10.231
  - with intoxication F10.921
    - in
      - abuse F10.121
      - dependence F10.221
- dementia F10.97
  - with dependence F10.27
- depressive disorder F10.94
- deterioration F10.97
  - with dependence F10.27
- hallucinosis (acute) F10.951
  - in
    - abuse F10.151
    - dependence F10.251
- insanity F10.959
- intoxication (acute) (without dependence) F10.129
  - with
    - delirium F10.121
    - dependence F10.229
      - with delirium F10.221
      - uncomplicated F10.220
    - uncomplicated F10.120
- jealousy F10.988
- Korsakoff's, Korsakov's, Korsakow's F10.26
- liver K70.9
  - acute — *see* Disease, liver, alcoholic, hepatitis
- major neurocognitive disorder, amnestic-confabulatory type F10.96
- major neurocognitive disorder, nonamnestic-confabulatory type F10.97
- mania (acute) (chronic) F10.959
- mild neurocognitive disorder F10.988
- paranoia, paranoid (type) psychosis F10.950
- pellagra E52
- poisoning, accidental (acute) NEC — *see* Table of Drugs and Chemicals, alcohol, poisoning
- psychosis — *see* Psychosis, alcoholic
- psychotic disorder F10.959
- sexual dysfunction F10.981
- sleep disorder F10.982
- withdrawal (without convulsions) F10.239
  - with delirium F10.231

Alcoholism (chronic) (without remission) F10.20
- with
  - psychosis — *see* Psychosis, alcoholic
  - remission F10.21
- Korsakov's F10.96
  - with dependence F10.26

Alder (-Reilly) **anomaly or syndrome** (leukocyte granulation) D72.0
Aldosteronism E26.9
- familial (type I) E26.02
- glucocorticoid-remediable E26.02
- primary (due to (bilateral) adrenal hyperplasia) E26.09
- primary NEC E26.09
- secondary E26.1
- specified NEC E26.89

Aldosteronoma D44.10
Aldrich (-Wiskott) **syndrome** (eczema-thrombocytopenia) D82.0
Alektorophobia F40.218
Aleppo boil B55.1
Aleukemic — *see* condition
Aleukia
- congenital D70.0
- hemorrhagica D61.9
  - congenital D61.09
- splenica D73.1

Alexia R48.0
- developmental F81.0
- secondary to organic lesion R48.0

Algoneurodystrophy M89.00
- ankle M89.07- ☑
- foot M89.07- ☑
- forearm M89.03- ☑
- hand M89.04- ☑
- lower leg M89.06- ☑
- multiple sites M89.0- ☑
- shoulder M89.01- ☑
- specified site NEC M89.08
- thigh M89.05- ☑
- upper arm M89.02- ☑

Algophobia F40.298
Alienation, mental — *see* Psychosis
Alkalemia E87.3
Alkalosis E87.3
- metabolic E87.3
  - with respiratory acidosis E87.4
- respiratory E87.3

Alkaptonuria E70.29
Allen-Masters syndrome N83.8
Allergy, allergic (reaction) (to) T78.40 ☑
- air-borne substance NEC (rhinitis) J30.89
- alveolitis (extrinsic) J67.9
  - due to
    - Aspergillus clavatus J67.4
    - Cryptostroma corticale J67.6
    - organisms (fungal, thermophilic actinomycete) growing in ventilation (air conditioning) systems J67.7
  - specified type NEC J67.8
- anaphylactic reaction or shock T78.2 ☑
- angioneurotic edema T78.3 ☑
- animal (dander) (epidermal) (hair) (rhinitis) J30.81
- bee sting (anaphylactic shock) — *see* Toxicity, venom, arthropod, bee
- biological — *see* Allergy, drug
- colitis (*see also* Colitis, allergic) K52.29
- dander (animal) (rhinitis) J30.81
- dandruff (rhinitis) J30.81
- dental restorative material (existing) K08.55
- dermatitis — *see* Dermatitis, contact, allergic
- diathesis — *see* History, allergy
- drug, medicament & biological (any) (external) (internal) T78.40 ☑
  - correct substance properly administered — *see* Table of Drugs and Chemicals, by drug, adverse effect
  - wrong substance given or taken NEC (by accident) — *see* Table of Drugs and Chemicals, by drug, poisoning
- due to pollen J30.1
- dust (house) (stock) (rhinitis) J30.89
  - with asthma — *see* Asthma, allergic extrinsic
- eczema — *see* Dermatitis, contact, allergic
- epidermal (animal) (rhinitis) J30.81
- feathers (rhinitis) J30.89
- food (any) (ingested) NEC T78.1 ☑
  - anaphylactic shock — *see* Shock, anaphylactic, due to food
  - dermatitis — *see* Dermatitis, due to, food
  - dietary counseling and surveillance Z71.3
  - in contact with skin L23.6
  - rhinitis J30.5
  - status (without reaction) Z91.018
    - eggs Z91.012
    - milk products Z91.011
    - peanuts Z91.010
    - seafood Z91.013
    - specified NEC Z91.018
- gastrointestinal — *see also* specific type of allergic reaction
  - meaning colitis (*see also* Colitis, allergic) K52.29

Allergy, allergic — *continued*
- gastrointestinal — *see also* specific type of allergic reaction — *continued*
  - meaning gastroenteritis (*see also* Gastroenteritis, allergic) K52.29
  - meaning other adverse food reaction not elsewhere classified T78.1 ☑
- grain J30.1
- grass (hay fever) (pollen) J30.1
  - asthma — *see* Asthma, allergic extrinsic
- hair (animal) (rhinitis) J30.81
- history (of) — *see* History, allergy
- horse serum — *see* Allergy, serum
- inhalant (rhinitis) J30.89
  - pollen J30.1
- kapok (rhinitis) J30.89
- medicine — *see* Allergy, drug
- milk protein (*see also* Allergy, food) Z91.011
  - anaphylactic reaction T78.07 ☑
  - dermatitis L27.2
  - enterocolitis syndrome K52.21
  - enteropathy K52.22
  - gastroenteritis K52.29
  - gastroesophageal reflux (*see also* Reaction, adverse, food) K21.9
    - with esophagitis K21.0
  - proctocolitis K52.82
- nasal, seasonal due to pollen J30.1
- pneumonia J82
- pollen (any) (hay fever) J30.1
  - asthma — *see* Asthma, allergic extrinsic
- primrose J30.1
- primula J30.1
- proctocolitis K52.82
- purpura D69.0
- ragweed (hay fever) (pollen) J30.1
  - asthma — *see* Asthma, allergic extrinsic
- rose (pollen) J30.1
- seasonal NEC J30.2
- Senecio jacobae (pollen) J30.1
- serum (*see also* Reaction, serum) T80.69 ☑
  - anaphylactic shock T80.59 ☑
- shock (anaphylactic) T78.2 ☑
  - due to
    - administration of blood and blood products T80.51 ☑
    - adverse effect of correct medicinal substance properly administered T88.6 ☑
    - immunization T80.52 ☑
    - serum NEC T80.59 ☑
    - vaccination T80.52 ☑
- specific NEC T78.49 ☑
- tree (any) (hay fever) (pollen) J30.1
  - asthma — *see* Asthma, allergic extrinsic
- upper respiratory J30.9
- urticaria L50.0
- vaccine — *see* Allergy, serum
- wheat — *see* Allergy, food

Allescheriasis B48.2
Alligator skin disease Q80.9
Allocheiria, allochiria R20.8
Almeida's disease — *see* Paracoccidioidomycosis
Alopecia (hereditaria) (seborrheica) L65.9
- androgenic L64.9
  - drug-induced L64.0
  - specified NEC L64.8
- areata L63.9
  - ophiasis L63.2
  - specified NEC L63.8
  - totalis L63.0
  - universalis L63.1
- cicatricial L66.9
  - specified NEC L66.8
- circumscripta L63.9
- congenital, congenitalis Q84.0
- due to cytotoxic drugs NEC L65.8
- mucinosa L65.2
- postinfective NEC L65.8
- postpartum L65.0
- premature L64.8
- specific (syphilitic) A51.32
- specified NEC L65.8
- syphilitic (secondary) A51.32
- totalis (capitis) L63.0
- universalis (entire body) L63.1
- X-ray L58.1

Alpers' disease G31.81
Alpine sickness T70.29 ☑

Alport syndrome Q87.81
ALTE (apparent life threatening event) **in newborn and infant** R68.13
Alteration (of), **Altered**
  awareness
    transient R40.4
    unintended under general anesthesia, during procedure T88.53 ☑
  mental status R41.82
  pattern of family relationships affecting child Z62.898
  sensation
    following
      cerebrovascular disease I69.998
        cerebral infarction I69.398
        intracerebral hemorrhage I69.198
        nontraumatic intracranial hemorrhage NEC I69.298
        specified disease NEC I69.898
        subarachnoid hemorrhage I69.098
Alternating — *see* condition
Altitude, high (effects) — *see* Effect, adverse, high altitude
Aluminosis (of lung) J63.0
Alveolitis
  allergic (extrinsic) — *see* Pneumonitis, hypersensitivity
  due to
    Aspergillus clavatus J67.4
    Cryptostroma corticale J67.6
  fibrosing (cryptogenic) (idiopathic) J84.112
  jaw M27.3
  sicca dolorosa M27.3
Alveolus, alveolar — *see* condition
Alymphocytosis D72.810
  thymic (with immunodeficiency) D82.1
Alymphoplasia, thymic D82.1
Alzheimer's disease or sclerosis — *see* Disease, Alzheimer's
Amastia (with nipple present) Q83.8
  with absent nipple Q83.0
Amathophobia F40.228
Amaurosis (acquired) (congenital) (*see also* Blindness)
  fugax G45.3
  hysterical F44.6
  Leber's congenital H35.50
  uremic — *see* Uremia
Amaurotic idiocy (infantile) (juvenile) (late) E75.4
Amaxophobia F40.248
Ambiguous genitalia Q56.4
Amblyopia (congenital) (ex anopsia) (partial) (suppression) H53.00- ☑
  anisometropic — *see* Amblyopia, refractive
  deprivation H53.01- ☑
  hysterical F44.6
  nocturnal (*see also* Blindness, night)
    vitamin A deficiency E50.5
  refractive H53.02- ☑
  strabismic H53.03- ☑
  suspect H53.04- ☑
  tobacco H53.8
  toxic NEC H53.8
  uremic — *see* Uremia
Ameba, amebic (histolytica) (*see also* Amebiasis)
  abscess (liver) A06.4
Amebiasis A06.9
  with abscess — *see* Abscess, amebic
  acute A06.0
  chronic (intestine) A06.1
    with abscess — *see* Abscess, amebic
  cutaneous A06.7
  cutis A06.7
  cystitis A06.81
  genitourinary tract NEC A06.82
  hepatic — *see* Abscess, liver, amebic
  intestine A06.0
  nondysenteric colitis A06.2
  skin A06.7
  specified site NEC A06.89
Ameboma (of intestine) A06.3
Amelia Q73.0
  lower limb — *see* Agenesis, leg
  upper limb — *see* Agenesis, arm
Ameloblastoma (*see also* Cyst, calcifying odontogenic)
  long bones C40.9-
    lower limb C40.2- ☑
    upper limb C40.0- ☑
  malignant C41.1
    jaw (bone) (lower) C41.1

Ameloblastoma — *continued*
  malignant — *continued*
    jaw — *continued*
      upper C41.0
    tibial C40.2- ☑
Amelogenesis imperfecta K00.5
  nonhereditaria (segmentalis) K00.4
Amenorrhea N91.2
  hyperhormonal E28.8
  primary N91.0
  secondary N91.1
Amentia — *see* Disability, intellectual
  Meynert's (nonalcoholic) F04
American
  leishmaniasis B55.2
  mountain tick fever A93.2
Ametropia — *see* Disorder, refraction
AMH (asymptomatic microscopic hematuria) R31.21
Amianthosis J61
Amimia R48.8
Amino-acid disorder E72.9
  anemia D53.0
Aminoacidopathy E72.9
Aminoaciduria E72.9
Amnesia R41.3
  anterograde R41.1
  auditory R48.8
  dissociative F44.0
    with dissociative fugue F44.1
  hysterical F44.0
  postictal in epilepsy — *see* Epilepsy
  psychogenic F44.0
  retrograde R41.2
  transient global G45.4
Amnes(t)ic syndrome (post-traumatic) F04
  induced by
    alcohol F10.96
      with dependence F10.26
    psychoactive NEC F19.96
      with
        abuse F19.16
        dependence F19.26
    sedative F13.96
      with dependence F13.26
Amnion, amniotic — *see* condition
Amnionitis — *see* Pregnancy, complicated by
Amok F68.8
Amoral traits F60.89
Amphetamine (or other stimulant) -**induced**
  anxiety disorder F15.980
  bipolar and related disorder F15.94
  delirium F15.921
  depressive disorder F15.94
  obsessive-compulsive and related disorder F15.988
  psychotic disorder F15.959
  sexual dysfunction F15.981
  sleep disorder F15.982
  stimulant withdrawal F15.23
Ampulla
  lower esophagus K22.8
  phrenic K22.8
Amputation (*see also* Absence, by site, acquired)
  neuroma (postoperative) (traumatic) — *see* Complications, amputation stump, neuroma
  stump (surgical)
    abnormal, painful, or with complication (late) — *see* Complications, amputation stump
    healed or old NOS Z89.9
  traumatic (complete) (partial)
    arm (upper) (complete) S48.91- ☑
      at
        elbow S58.01- ☑
          partial S58.02- ☑
        shoulder joint (complete) S48.01- ☑
          partial S48.02- ☑
      between
        elbow and wrist (complete) S58.11- ☑
          partial S58.12- ☑
        shoulder and elbow (complete) S48.11- ☑
          partial S48.12- ☑
      partial S48.92- ☑
    breast (complete) S28.21- ☑
      partial S28.22- ☑
    clitoris (complete) S38.211 ☑
      partial S38.212 ☑
    ear (complete) S08.11- ☑
      partial S08.12- ☑

Amputation — *continued*
  traumatic — *continued*
    finger (complete) (metacarpophalangeal)
      S68.11- ☑
      index S68.11- ☑
      little S68.11- ☑
      middle S68.11- ☑
      partial S68.12- ☑
        index S68.12- ☑
        little S68.12- ☑
        middle S68.12- ☑
        ring S68.12- ☑
      ring S68.11- ☑
      thumb — *see* Amputation, traumatic, thumb
      transphalangeal (complete) S68.61- ☑
        index S68.61- ☑
        little S68.61- ☑
        middle S68.61- ☑
        partial S68.62- ☑
          index S68.62- ☑
          little S68.62- ☑
          middle S68.62- ☑
          ring S68.62- ☑
        ring S68.61- ☑
    foot (complete) S98.91- ☑
      at ankle level S98.01- ☑
        partial S98.02- ☑
      midfoot S98.31- ☑
        partial S98.32- ☑
      partial S98.92- ☑
    forearm (complete) S58.91- ☑
      at elbow level (complete) S58.01- ☑
        partial S58.02- ☑
      between elbow and wrist (complete) S58.11- ☑
        partial S58.12- ☑
      partial S58.92- ☑
    genital organ(s) (external)
      female (complete) S38.211 ☑
        partial S38.212 ☑
      male
        penis (complete) S38.221 ☑
          partial S38.222 ☑
        scrotum (complete) S38.231 ☑
          partial S38.232 ☑
        testes (complete) S38.231 ☑
          partial S38.232 ☑
    hand (complete) (wrist level) S68.41- ☑
      finger(s) alone — *see* Amputation, traumatic, finger
      partial S68.42- ☑
      thumb alone — *see* Amputation, traumatic, thumb
      transmetacarpal (complete) S68.71- ☑
        partial S68.72- ☑
    head
      ear — *see* Amputation, traumatic, ear
      nose (partial) S08.812 ☑
        complete S08.811 ☑
      part S08.89 ☑
        scalp S08.0 ☑
    hip (and thigh) (complete) S78.91- ☑
      at hip joint (complete) S78.01- ☑
        partial S78.02- ☑
      between hip and knee (complete) S78.11- ☑
        partial S78.12- ☑
      partial S78.92- ☑
    labium (majus) (minus) (complete) S38.21- ☑
      partial S38.21- ☑
    leg (lower) S88.91- ☑
      at knee level S88.01- ☑
        partial S88.02- ☑
      between knee and ankle S88.11- ☑
        partial S88.12- ☑
      partial S88.92- ☑
    nose (partial) S08.812 ☑
      complete S08.811 ☑
    penis (complete) S38.221 ☑
      partial S38.222 ☑
    scrotum (complete) S38.231 ☑
      partial S38.232 ☑
    shoulder — *see* Amputation, traumatic, arm
      at shoulder joint — *see* Amputation, traumatic, arm, at shoulder joint
    testes (complete) S38.231 ☑
      partial S38.232 ☑
    thigh — *see* Amputation, traumatic, hip

Amputation — continued
  traumatic — continued
    thorax, part of S28.1 ☑
      breast — see Amputation, traumatic, breast
    thumb (complete) (metacarpophalangeal)
        S68.01- ☑
      partial S68.02- ☑
      transphalangeal (complete) S68.51- ☑
        partial S68.52- ☑
    toe (lesser) S98.13- ☑
      great S98.11- ☑
        partial S98.12- ☑
      more than one S98.21- ☑
        partial S98.22- ☑
      partial S98.14- ☑
    vulva (complete) S38.211 ☑
      partial S38.212 ☑
Amputee (bilateral) (old) Z89.9
Amsterdam dwarfism Q87.1
Amusia R48.8
  developmental F80.89
Amyelencephalus, amyelencephaly Q00.0
Amyelia Q06.0
Amygdalitis — see Tonsillitis
Amygdalolith J35.8
Amyloid heart (disease) E85.4 [I43]
Amyloidosis (generalized) (primary) E85.9
  with lung involvement E85.4 [J99]
  familial E85.2
  genetic E85.2
  heart E85.4 [I43]
  hemodialysis-associated E85.3
  light chain (AL) E85.81
  liver E85.4 [K77]
  localized E85.4
  neuropathic heredofamilial E85.1
  non-neuropathic heredofamilial E85.0
  organ limited E85.4
  Portuguese E85.1
  pulmonary E85.4 [J99]
  secondary systemic E85.3
  senile systemic (SSA) E85.82
  skin (lichen) (macular) E85.4 [L99]
  specified NEC E85.89
  subglottic E85.4 [J99]
  wild-type transthyretin-related (ATTR) E85.82
Amylopectinosis (brancher enzyme deficiency) E74.03
Amylophagia — see Pica
Amyoplasia congenita Q79.8
Amyotonia M62.89
  congenita G70.2
Amyotrophia, amyotrophy, amyotrophic G71.8
  congenita Q79.8
  diabetic — see Diabetes, amyotrophy
  lateral sclerosis G12.21
  neuralgic G54.5
  spinal progressive G12.25
Anacidity, gastric K31.83
  psychogenic F45.8
Anaerosis of newborn P28.89
Analbuminemia E88.09
Analgesia — see Anesthesia
Analphalipoproteinemia E78.6
Anaphylactic
  purpura D69.0
  shock or reaction — see Shock, anaphylactic
Anaphylactoid shock or reaction — see Shock, anaphylactic
Anaphylactoid syndrome of pregnancy O88.01- ☑
Anaphylaxis — see Shock, anaphylactic
Anaplasia cervix (see also Dysplasia, cervix) N87.9
Anaplasmosis, human A77.49
Anarthria R47.1
Anasarca R60.1
  cardiac — see Failure, heart, congestive
  lung J18.2
  newborn P83.2
  nutritional E43
  pulmonary J18.2
  renal N04.9
Anastomosis
  aneurysmal — see Aneurysm
  arteriovenous ruptured brain I60.8
  intestinal K63.89
    complicated NEC K91.89
      involving urinary tract N99.89
  retinal and choroidal vessels (congenital) Q14.8

Anatomical narrow angle H40.03- ☑
Ancylostoma, ancylostomiasis (braziliense) (caninum) (ceylanicum) (duodenale) B76.0
  Necator americanus B76.1
Andersen's disease (glycogen storage) E74.09
Anderson-Fabry disease E75.21
Andes disease T70.29 ☑
Andrews' disease (bacterid) L08.89
Androblastoma
  benign
    specified site — see Neoplasm, benign, by site
    unspecified site
      female D27.9
      male D29.20
  malignant
    specified site — see Neoplasm, malignant, by site
    unspecified site
      female C56.9
      male C62.90
  specified site — see Neoplasm, uncertain behavior, by site
  tubular
    with lipid storage
      specified site — see Neoplasm, benign, by site
      unspecified site
        female D27.9
        male D29.20
    specified site — see Neoplasm, benign, by site
    unspecified site
      female D27.9
      male D29.20
  unspecified site
    female D39.10
    male D40.10
Androgen insensitivity syndrome (see also Syndrome, androgen insensitivity) E34.50
Androgen resistance syndrome (see also Syndrome, androgen insensitivity) E34.50
Android pelvis Q74.2
  with disproportion (fetopelvic) O33.3 ☑
    causing obstructed labor O65.3
Androphobia F40.290
Anectasis, pulmonary (newborn) — see Atelectasis
Anemia (essential) (general) (hemoglobin deficiency) (infantile) (primary) (profound) D64.9
  with (due to) (in)
    disorder of
      anaerobic glycolysis D55.2
      pentose phosphate pathway D55.1
    koilonychia D50.9
  achlorhydric D50.8
  achrestic D53.1
  Addison (-Biermer) (pernicious) D51.0
  agranulocytic — see Agranulocytosis
  amino-acid-deficiency D53.0
  aplastic D61.9
    congenital D61.09
    drug-induced D61.1
    due to
      drugs D61.1
      external agents NEC D61.2
      infection D61.2
      radiation D61.2
    idiopathic D61.3
    red cell (pure) D60.9
      chronic D60.0
      congenital D61.01
      specified type NEC D60.8
      transient D60.1
    specified type NEC D61.89
    toxic D61.2
  aregenerative
    congenital D61.09
  asiderotic D50.9
  atypical (primary) D64.9
  Baghdad spring D55.0
  Balantidium coli A07.0
  Biermer's (pernicious) D51.0
  blood loss (chronic) D50.0
    acute D62
  bothriocephalus B70.0 [D63.8]
  brickmaker's B76.9 [D63.8]
  cerebral I67.89
  childhood D58.9
  chlorotic D50.8
  chronic
    blood loss D50.0
    hemolytic D58.9

Anemia — continued
  chronic — continued
    hemolytic — continued
      idiopathic D59.9
    simple D53.9
  chronica congenita aregenerativa D61.09
  combined system disease NEC D51.0 [G32.0]
    due to dietary vitamin B12 deficiency D51.3 [G32.0]
  complicating pregnancy, childbirth or puerperium — see Pregnancy, complicated by (management affected by), anemia
  congenital P61.4
    aplastic D61.09
    due to isoimmunization NOS P55.9
    dyserythropoietic, dyshematopoietic D64.4
    following fetal blood loss P61.3
    Heinz body D58.2
    hereditary hemolytic NOS D58.9
    pernicious D51.0
    spherocytic D58.0
  Cooley's (erythroblastic) D56.1
  cytogenic D51.0
  deficiency D53.9
    6-PGD D55.1
    2, 3 diphosphoglycurate mutase D55.2
    2, 3 PG D55.2
    6 phosphogluconate dehydrogenase D55.1
    amino-acid D53.0
    combined B12 and folate D53.1
    enzyme D55.9
      drug-induced (hemolytic) D59.2
      glucose-6-phosphate dehydrogenase (G6PD) D55.0
      glycolytic D55.2
      nucleotide metabolism D55.3
      related to hexose monophosphate (HMP) shunt pathway NEC D55.1
      specified type NEC D55.8
    erythrocytic glutathione D55.1
    folate D52.9
      dietary D52.0
      drug-induced D52.1
    folic acid D52.9
      dietary D52.0
      drug-induced D52.1
    G SH D55.1
    G6PD D55.0
    GGS-R D55.1
    glucose-6-phosphate dehydrogenase D55.0
    glutathione reductase D55.1
    glyceraldehyde phosphate dehydrogenase D55.2
    hexokinase D55.2
    iron D50.9
      secondary to blood loss (chronic) D50.0
    nutritional D53.9
      with
        poor iron absorption D50.8
        specified deficiency NEC D53.8
    phosphofructo-aldolase D55.2
    phosphoglycerate kinase D55.2
    PK D55.2
    protein D53.0
    pyruvate kinase D55.2
    transcobalamin II D51.2
    triose-phosphate isomerase D55.2
    vitamin B12 NOS D51.9
      dietary D51.3
      due to
        intrinsic factor deficiency D51.0
        selective vitamin B12 malabsorption with proteinuria D51.1
      pernicious D51.0
      specified type NEC D51.8
  Diamond-Blackfan (congenital hypoplastic) D61.01
  dibothriocephalus B70.0 [D63.8]
  dimorphic D53.1
  diphasic D53.1
  Diphyllobothrium (Dibothriocephalus) B70.0 [D63.8]
  due to (in) (with)
    antineoplastic chemotherapy D64.81
    blood loss (chronic) D50.0
      acute D62
    chemotherapy, antineoplastic D64.81
    chronic disease classified elsewhere NEC D63.8
    chronic kidney disease D63.1
    deficiency
      amino-acid D53.0
      copper D53.8
      folate (folic acid) D52.9

18

☑ Additional Character Required — Refer to the Tabular List for Character Selection   ▽ Subterms under main terms may continue to next column or page

Anemia — *continued*
  due to — *continued*
    deficiency — *continued*
      folate — *continued*
        dietary D52.0
        drug-induced D52.1
      molybdenum D53.8
      protein D53.0
      zinc D53.8
    dietary vitamin B12 deficiency D51.3
    disorder of
      glutathione metabolism D55.1
      nucleotide metabolism D55.3
    drug — *see* Anemia, by type (*see also* Table of Drugs and Chemicals)
    end stage renal disease D63.1
    enzyme disorder D55.9
    fetal blood loss P61.3
    fish tapeworm (D.latum) infestation B70.0 [D63.8]
    hemorrhage (chronic) D50.0
      acute D62
    impaired absorption D50.9
    loss of blood (chronic) D50.0
      acute D62
    myxedema E03.9 [D63.8]
    Necator americanus B76.1 [D63.8]
    prematurity P61.2
    selective vitamin B12 malabsorption with proteinuria D51.1
    transcobalamin II deficiency D51.2
  Dyke-Young type (secondary) (symptomatic) D59.1
  dyserythropoietic (congenital) D64.4
  dyshematopoietic (congenital) D64.4
  Egyptian B76.9 [D63.8]
  elliptocytosis — *see* Elliptocytosis
  enzyme-deficiency, drug-induced D59.2
  epidemic (*see also* Ancylostomiasis) B76.9 [D63.8]
  erythroblastic
    familial D56.1
    newborn (*see also* Disease, hemolytic) P55.9
    of childhood D56.1
  erythrocytic glutathione deficiency D55.1
  erythropoietin-resistant anemia (EPO resistant anemia) D63.1
  Faber's (achlorhydric anemia) D50.9
  factitious (self-induced blood letting) D50.0
  familial erythroblastic D56.1
  Fanconi's (congenital pancytopenia) D61.09
  favism D55.0
  fish tapeworm (D. latum) infestation B70.0 [D63.8]
  folate (folic acid) deficiency D52.9
  glucose-6-phosphate dehydrogenase (G6PD) deficiency D55.0
  glutathione-reductase deficiency D55.1
  goat's milk D52.0
  granulocytic — *see* Agranulocytosis
  Heinz body, congenital D58.2
  hemolytic D58.9
    acquired D59.9
      with hemoglobinuria NEC D59.6
      autoimmune NEC D59.1
      infectious D59.4
      specified type NEC D59.8
      toxic D59.4
    acute D59.9
      due to enzyme deficiency specified type NEC D55.8
      Lederer's D59.1
    autoimmune D59.1
      drug-induced D59.0
    chronic D58.9
      idiopathic D59.9
    cold type (secondary) (symptomatic) D59.1
    congenital (spherocytic) — *see* Spherocytosis
    due to
      cardiac conditions D59.4
      drugs (nonautoimmune) D59.2
        autoimmune D59.0
      enzyme disorder D55.9
        drug-induced D59.2
      presence of shunt or other internal prosthetic device D59.4
    familial D58.9
    hereditary D58.9
      due to enzyme disorder D55.9
        specified type NEC D55.8
      specified type NEC D58.8
    idiopathic (chronic) D59.9
    mechanical D59.4

Anemia — *continued*
  hemolytic — *continued*
    microangiopathic D59.4
    nonautoimmune D59.4
      drug-induced D59.2
    nonspherocytic
      congenital or hereditary NEC D55.8
        glucose-6-phosphate dehydrogenase deficiency D55.0
        pyruvate kinase deficiency D55.2
        type
          I D55.1
          II D55.2
      type
        I D55.1
        II D55.2
    secondary D59.4
      autoimmune D59.1
    specified (hereditary) type NEC D58.8
    Stransky-Regala type (*see also* Hemoglobinopathy) D58.8
    symptomatic D59.4
      autoimmune D59.1
    toxic D59.4
    warm type (secondary) (symptomatic) D59.1
  hemorrhagic (chronic) D50.0
    acute D62
  Herrick's D57.1
  hexokinase deficiency D55.2
  hookworm B76.9 [D63.8]
  hypochromic (idiopathic) (microcytic) (normoblastic) D50.9
    due to blood loss (chronic) D50.0
      acute D62
    familial sex-linked D64.0
    pyridoxine-responsive D64.3
    sideroblastic, sex-linked D64.0
  hypoplasia, red blood cells D61.9
    congenital or familial D61.01
  hypoplastic (idiopathic) D61.9
    congenital or familial (of childhood) D61.01
  hypoproliferative (refractive) D61.9
  idiopathic D64.9
    aplastic D61.3
    hemolytic, chronic D59.9
  in (due to) (with)
    chronic kidney disease D63.1
    end stage renal disease D63.1
    failure, kidney (renal) D63.1
    neoplastic disease (*see also* Neoplasm) D63.0
  intertropical (*see also* Ancylostomiasis) D63.8
  iron deficiency D50.9
    secondary to blood loss (chronic) D50.0
      acute D62
    specified type NEC D50.8
  Joseph-Diamond-Blackfan (congenital hypoplastic) D61.01
  Lederer's (hemolytic) D59.1
  leukoerythroblastic D61.82
  macrocytic D53.9
    nutritional D52.0
    tropical D52.8
  malarial (*see also* Malaria) B54 [D63.8]
  malignant (progressive) D51.0
  malnutrition D53.9
  marsh (*see also* Malaria) B54 [D63.8]
  Mediterranean (with other hemoglobinopathy) D56.9
  megaloblastic D53.1
    combined B12 and folate deficiency D53.1
    hereditary D51.1
    nutritional D52.0
    orotic aciduria D53.0
    refractory D53.1
    specified type NEC D53.1
  megalocytic D53.1
  microcytic (hypochromic) D50.9
    due to blood loss (chronic) D50.0
      acute D62
    familial D56.8
  microdrepanocytosis D57.40
  microelliptopoikilocytic (Rietti-Greppi- Micheli) D56.9
  miner's B76.9 [D63.8]
  myelodysplastic D46.9
  myelofibrosis D75.81
  myelogenous D64.89
  myelopathic D64.89
  myelophthisic D61.82
  myeloproliferative D47.Z9 (*following* D47.4)
  newborn P61.4

Anemia — *continued*
  newborn — *continued*
    due to
      ABO (antibodies, isoimmunization, maternal/fetal incompatibility) P55.1
      Rh (antibodies, isoimmunization, maternal/fetal incompatibility) P55.0
    following fetal blood loss P61.3
    posthemorrhagic (fetal) P61.3
  nonspherocytic hemolytic — *see* Anemia, hemolytic, nonspherocytic
  normocytic (infectional) D64.9
    due to blood loss (chronic) D50.0
      acute D62
    myelophthisic D61.82
  nutritional (deficiency) D53.9
    with
      poor iron absorption D50.8
      specified deficiency NEC D53.8
    megaloblastic D52.0
  of prematurity P61.2
  orotaciduric (congenital) (hereditary) D53.0
  osteosclerotic D64.89
  ovalocytosis (hereditary) — *see* Elliptocytosis
  paludal (*see also* Malaria) B54 [D63.8]
  pernicious (congenital) (malignant) (progressive) D51.0
  pleochromic D64.89
    of sprue D52.8
  posthemorrhagic (chronic) D50.0
    acute D62
    newborn P61.3
  postoperative (postprocedural)
    due to (acute) blood loss D62
      chronic blood loss D50.0
    specified NEC D64.9
  postpartum O90.81
  pressure D64.89
  progressive D64.9
    malignant D51.0
    pernicious D51.0
  protein-deficiency D53.0
  pseudoleukemica infantum D64.89
  pure red cell D60.9
    congenital D61.01
  pyridoxine-responsive D64.3
  pyruvate kinase deficiency D55.2
  refractory D46.4
    with
      excess of blasts D46.20
        1 (RAEB 1) D46.21
        2 (RAEB 2) D46.22
        in transformation (RAEB T) — *see* Leukemia, acute myeloblastic
      hemochromatosis D46.1
      sideroblasts (ring) (RARS) D46.1
    without ring sideroblasts, so stated D46.0
    without sideroblasts without excess of blasts D46.0
    megaloblastic D53.1
    sideroblastic D46.1
    sideropenic D50.9
  Rietti-Greppi-Micheli D56.9
  scorbutic D53.2
  secondary to
    blood loss (chronic) D50.0
      acute D62
    hemorrhage (chronic) D50.0
      acute D62
  semiplastic D61.89
  sickle-cell — *see* Disease, sickle-cell
  sideroblastic D64.3
    hereditary D64.0
    hypochromic, sex-linked D64.0
    pyridoxine-responsive NEC D64.3
    refractory D46.1
    secondary (due to)
      disease D64.1
      drugs and toxins D64.2
    specified type NEC D64.3
  sideropenic (refractory) D50.9
    due to blood loss (chronic) D50.0
      acute D62
  simple chronic D53.9
  specified type NEC D64.89
  spherocytic (hereditary) — *see* Spherocytosis
  splenic D64.89
  splenomegalic D64.89
  stomatocytosis D58.8
  syphilitic (acquired) (late) A52.79 [D63.8]
  target cell D64.89

Anemia — *continued*
  thalassemia D56.9
  thrombocytopenic — *see* Thrombocytopenia
  toxic D61.2
  tropical B76.9 [D63.8]
    macrocytic D52.8
  tuberculous A18.89 [D63.8]
  vegan D51.3
  vitamin
    B6-responsive D64.3
    B12 deficiency (dietary) pernicious D51.0
  von Jaksch's D64.89
  Witts' (achlorhydric anemia) D50.8
Anemophobia F40.228
Anencephalus, anencephaly Q00.0
Anergasia — *see* Psychosis, organic
Anesthesia, anesthetic R20.0
  complication or reaction NEC (*see also* Complications, anesthesia) T88.59 ☑
    due to
      correct substance properly administered — *see* Table of Drugs and Chemicals, by drug, adverse effect
      overdose or wrong substance given — *see* Table of Drugs and Chemicals, by drug, poisoning
      unintended awareness under general anesthesia during procedure T88.53 ☑
        personal history of Z92.84
  cornea H18.81- ☑
  dissociative F44.6
  functional (hysterical) F44.6
  hyperesthetic, thalamic G89.0
  hysterical F44.6
  local skin lesion R20.0
  sexual (psychogenic) F52.1
  shock (due to) T88.2 ☑
  skin R20.0
  testicular N50.9
Anetoderma (maculosum) (of) L90.8
  Jadassohn-Pellizzari L90.2
  Schweniger-Buzzi L90.1
Aneurin deficiency E51.9
Aneurysm (anastomotic) (artery) (cirsoid) (diffuse) (false) (fusiform) (multiple) (saccular) I72.9
  abdominal (aorta) I71.4
    ruptured I71.3
    syphilitic A52.01
  aorta, aortic (nonsyphilitic) I71.9
    abdominal I71.4
      ruptured I71.3
    arch I71.2
      ruptured I71.1
    arteriosclerotic I71.9
      ruptured I71.8
    ascending I71.2
      ruptured I71.1
    congenital Q25.43
    descending I71.9
      abdominal I71.4
        ruptured I71.3
      ruptured I71.8
      thoracic I71.2
        ruptured I71.1
    root Q25.43
    ruptured I71.8
    sinus, congenital Q25.43
    syphilitic A52.01
    thoracic I71.2
      ruptured I71.1
    thoracoabdominal I71.6
      ruptured I71.5
    thorax, thoracic (arch) I71.2
      ruptured I71.1
    transverse I71.2
      ruptured I71.1
    valve (heart) (*see also* Endocarditis, aortic) I35.8
  arteriosclerotic I72.9
    cerebral I67.1
      ruptured — *see* Hemorrhage, intracranial, subarachnoid
  arteriovenous (congenital) (*see also* Malformation, arteriovenous)
    acquired I77.0
      brain I67.1
      coronary I25.41
      pulmonary I28.0
    brain Q28.2

Aneurysm — *continued*
  arteriovenous (*see also* Malformation, arteriovenous) — *continued*
    brain — *continued*
      ruptured I60.8
      peripheral — *see* Malformation, arteriovenous, peripheral
    precerebral vessels Q28.0
    specified site NEC (*see also* Malformation, arteriovenous)
      acquired I77.0
  basal — *see* Aneurysm, brain
  basilar (trunk) I72.5
  berry (congenital) (nonruptured) I67.1
    ruptured I60.7
  brain I67.1
    arteriosclerotic I67.1
      ruptured — *see* Hemorrhage, intracranial, subarachnoid
    arteriovenous (congenital) (nonruptured) Q28.2
      acquired I67.1
        ruptured I60.8
      ruptured I60.8
    berry (congenital) (nonruptured) I67.1
      ruptured (*see also* Hemorrhage, intracranial, subarachnoid) I60.7
    congenital Q28.3
      ruptured I60.7
    meninges I67.1
      ruptured I60.8
    miliary (congenital) (nonruptured) I67.1
      ruptured (*see also* Hemorrhage, intracranial, subarachnoid) I60.7
    mycotic I33.0
    ruptured — *see* Hemorrhage, intracranial, subarachnoid
    syphilitic (hemorrhage) A52.05
  cardiac (false) (*see also* Aneurysm, heart) I25.3
  carotid artery (common) (external) I72.0
    internal (intracranial) I67.1
      extracranial portion I72.0
    ruptured into brain I60.0- ☑
    syphilitic A52.09
      intracranial A52.05
  cavernous sinus I67.1
    arteriovenous (congenital) (nonruptured) Q28.3
      ruptured I60.8
  celiac I72.8
  central nervous system, syphilitic A52.05
  cerebral — *see* Aneurysm, brain
  chest — *see* Aneurysm, thorax
  circle of Willis I67.1
    congenital Q28.3
      ruptured I60.6
    ruptured I60.6
  common iliac artery I72.3
  congenital (peripheral) Q27.8
    aorta (root) (sinus) Q25.43
    brain Q28.3
      ruptured I60.7
    coronary Q24.5
    digestive system Q27.8
    lower limb Q27.8
    pulmonary Q25.79
    retina Q14.1
    specified site NEC Q27.8
    upper limb Q27.8
  conjunctiva — *see* Abnormality, conjunctiva, vascular
  conus arteriosus — *see* Aneurysm, heart
  coronary (arteriosclerotic) (artery) I25.41
    arteriovenous, congenital Q24.5
    congenital Q24.5
    ruptured — *see* Infarct, myocardium
    syphilitic A52.06
    vein I25.89
  cylindroid (aorta) I71.9
    ruptured I71.8
    syphilitic A52.01
  ductus arteriosus Q25.0
  endocardial, infective (any valve) I33.0
  femoral (artery) (ruptured) I72.4
  gastroduodenal I72.8
  gastroepiploic I72.8
  heart (wall) (chronic or with a stated duration of over 4 weeks) I25.3
    valve — *see* Endocarditis
  hepatic I72.8
  iliac (common) (artery) (ruptured) I72.3

Aneurysm — *continued*
  infective I72.9
    endocardial (any valve) I33.0
  innominate (nonsyphilitic) I72.8
    syphilitic A52.09
  interauricular septum — *see* Aneurysm, heart
  interventricular septum — *see* Aneurysm, heart
  intrathoracic (nonsyphilitic) I71.2
    ruptured I71.1
    syphilitic A52.01
  lower limb I72.4
  lung (pulmonary artery) I28.1
  mediastinal (nonsyphilitic) I72.8
    syphilitic A52.09
  miliary (congenital) I67.1
    ruptured — *see* Hemorrhage, intracerebral, subarachnoid, intracranial
  mitral (heart) (valve) I34.8
  mural — *see* Aneurysm, heart
  mycotic I72.9
    endocardial (any valve) I33.0
    ruptured, brain — *see* Hemorrhage, intracerebral, subarachnoid
  myocardium — *see* Aneurysm, heart
  neck I72.0
  pancreaticoduodenal I72.8
  patent ductus arteriosus Q25.0
  peripheral NEC I72.8
    congenital Q27.8
      digestive system Q27.8
      lower limb Q27.8
      specified site NEC Q27.8
      upper limb Q27.8
  popliteal (artery) (ruptured) I72.4
  precerebral
    congenital (nonruptured) Q28.1
    specified site, NEC I72.5
  pulmonary I28.1
    arteriovenous Q25.72
      acquired I28.0
    syphilitic A52.09
    valve (heart) — *see* Endocarditis, pulmonary
  racemose (peripheral) I72.9
    congenital — *see* Aneurysm, congenital
  radial I72.1
  Rasmussen NEC A15.0
  renal (artery) I72.2
  retina (*see also* Disorder, retina, microaneurysms)
    congenital Q14.1
    diabetic — *see* Diabetes, microaneurysms, retinal
  sinus of Valsalva Q25.49
  specified NEC I72.8
  spinal (cord) I72.8
    syphilitic (hemorrhage) A52.09
  splenic I72.8
  subclavian (artery) (ruptured) I72.8
    syphilitic A52.09
  superior mesenteric I72.8
  syphilitic (aorta) A52.01
    central nervous system A52.05
    congenital (late) A50.54 [I79.0]
    spine, spinal A52.09
  thoracoabdominal (aorta) I71.6
    ruptured I71.5
    syphilitic A52.01
  thorax, thoracic (aorta) (arch) (nonsyphilitic) I71.2
    ruptured I71.1
    syphilitic A52.01
  traumatic (complication) (early), specified site — *see* Injury, blood vessel
  tricuspid (heart) (valve) I07.8
  ulnar I72.1
  upper limb (ruptured) I72.1
  valve, valvular — *see* Endocarditis
  venous (*see also* Varix) I86.8
    congenital Q27.8
      digestive system Q27.8
      lower limb Q27.8
      specified site NEC Q27.8
      upper limb Q27.8
  ventricle — *see* Aneurysm, heart
  vertebral artery I72.6
  visceral NEC I72.8
Angelman syndrome Q93.5
Anger R45.4
Angiectasis, angiectopia I99.8
Angiitis I77.6
  allergic granulomatous M30.1

Angiitis — *continued*
- hypersensitivity M31.0
- necrotizing M31.9
  - specified NEC M31.8
- nervous system, granulomatous I67.7

Angina (attack) (cardiac) (chest) (heart) (pectoris) (syndrome) (vasomotor) I20.9
- with
  - atherosclerotic heart disease — *see* Arteriosclerosis, coronary (artery),
  - documented spasm I20.1
- abdominal K55.1
- accelerated — *see* Angina, unstable
- agranulocytic — *see* Agranulocytosis
- angiospastic — *see* Angina, with documented spasm
- aphthous B08.5
- crescendo — *see* Angina, unstable
- croupous J05.0
- cruris I73.9
- de novo effort — *see* Angina, unstable
- diphtheritic, membranous A36.0
- equivalent I20.8
- exudative, chronic J37.0
- following acute myocardial infarction I23.7
- gangrenous diphtheritic A36.0
- intestinal K55.1
- Ludovici K12.2
- Ludwig's K12.2
- malignant diphtheritic A36.0
- membranous J05.0
  - diphtheritic A36.0
  - Vincent's A69.1
- mesenteric K55.1
- monocytic — *see* Mononucleosis, infectious
- of effort — *see* Angina, specified NEC
- phlegmonous J36
  - diphtheritic A36.0
- post-infarctional I23.7
- pre-infarctional — *see* Angina, unstable
- Prinzmetal — *see* Angina, with documented spasm
- progressive — *see* Angina, unstable
- pseudomembranous A69.1
- pultaceous, diphtheritic A36.0
- spasm-induced — *see* Angina, with documented spasm
- specified NEC I20.8
- stable I20.8
- stenocardia — *see* Angina, specified NEC
- stridulous, diphtheritic A36.2
- tonsil J36
- trachealis J05.0
- unstable I20.0
- variant — *see* Angina, with documented spasm
- Vincent's A69.1
- worsening effort — *see* Angina, unstable

Angioblastoma — *see* Neoplasm, connective tissue, uncertain behavior
Angiocholecystitis — *see* Cholecystitis, acute
Angiocholitis (*see also* Cholecystitis, acute) K83.0
Angiodysgenesis spinalis G95.19
Angiodysplasia (cecum) (colon) K55.20
- with bleeding K55.21
- duodenum (and stomach) K31.819
  - with bleeding K31.811
- stomach (and duodenum) K31.819
  - with bleeding K31.811
Angioedema (allergic) (any site) (with urticaria) T78.3 ☑
- hereditary D84.1
Angioendothelioma — *see* Neoplasm, uncertain behavior, by site
- benign D18.00
  - intra-abdominal D18.03
  - intracranial D18.02
  - skin D18.01
  - specified site NEC D18.09
- bone — *see* Neoplasm, bone, malignant
- Ewing's — *see* Neoplasm, bone, malignant
Angioendotheliomatosis C85.8- ☑
Angiofibroma (*see also* Neoplasm, benign, by site)
- juvenile
  - specified site — *see* Neoplasm, benign, by site
  - unspecified site D10.6
Angiohemophilia (A) (B) D68.0
Angioid streaks (choroid) (macula) (retina) H35.33
Angiokeratoma — *see* Neoplasm, skin, benign
- corporis diffusum E75.21
Angioleiomyoma — *see* Neoplasm, connective tissue, benign

Angiolipoma (*see also* Lipoma)
- infiltrating — *see* Lipoma
Angioma (*see also* Hemangioma, by site)
- capillary I78.1
- hemorrhagicum hereditaria I78.0
- intra-abdominal D18.03
- intracranial D18.02
- malignant — *see* Neoplasm, connective tissue, malignant
- plexiform D18.00
  - intra-abdominal D18.03
  - intracranial D18.02
  - skin D18.01
  - specified site NEC D18.09
- senile I78.1
- serpiginosum L81.7
- skin D18.01
- specified site NEC D18.09
- spider I78.1
- stellate I78.1
- venous Q28.3
Angiomatosis Q82.8
- bacillary A79.89
- encephalotrigeminal Q85.8
- hemorrhagic familial I78.0
- hereditary familial I78.0
- liver K76.4
Angiomyolipoma — *see* Lipoma
Angiomyoliposarcoma — *see* Neoplasm, connective tissue, malignant
Angiomyoma — *see* Neoplasm, connective tissue, benign
Angiomyosarcoma — *see* Neoplasm, connective tissue, malignant
Angiomyxoma — *see* Neoplasm, connective tissue, uncertain behavior
Angioneurosis F45.8
Angioneurotic edema (allergic) (any site) (with urticaria) T78.3 ☑
- hereditary D84.1
Angiopathia, angiopathy I99.9
- cerebral I67.9
  - amyloid E85.4 [I68.0]
- diabetic (peripheral) — *see* Diabetes, angiopathy
- peripheral I73.9
  - diabetic — *see* Diabetes, angiopathy
  - specified type NEC I73.89
- retinae syphilitica A52.05
- retinalis (juvenilis)
  - diabetic — *see* Diabetes, retinopathy
  - proliferative — *see* Retinopathy, proliferative
Angiosarcoma (*see also* Neoplasm, connective tissue, malignant)
- liver C22.3
Angiosclerosis — *see* Arteriosclerosis
Angiospasm (peripheral) (traumatic) (vessel) I73.9
- brachial plexus G54.0
- cerebral G45.9
- cervical plexus G54.2
- nerve
  - arm — *see* Mononeuropathy, upper limb
    - axillary G54.0
    - median — *see* Lesion, nerve, median
    - ulnar — *see* Lesion, nerve, ulnar
  - axillary G54.0
  - leg — *see* Mononeuropathy, lower limb
  - median — *see* Lesion, nerve, median
  - plantar — *see* Lesion, nerve, plantar
  - ulnar — *see* Lesion, nerve, ulnar
Angiospastic disease or edema I73.9
Angiostrongyliasis
- due to
  - Parastrongylus
    - cantonensis B83.2
    - costaricensis B81.3
- intestinal B81.3
Anguillulosis — *see* Strongyloidiasis
Angulation
- cecum — *see* Obstruction, intestine
- coccyx (acquired) (*see also* subcategory) M43.8 ☑
  - congenital NEC Q76.49
- femur (acquired) (*see also* Deformity, limb, specified type NEC, thigh)
  - congenital Q74.2
- intestine (large) (small) — *see* Obstruction, intestine
- sacrum (acquired) (*see also* subcategory) M43.8 ☑
  - congenital NEC Q76.49
- sigmoid (flexure) — *see* Obstruction, intestine

Angulation — *continued*
- spine — *see* Dorsopathy, deforming, specified NEC
- tibia (acquired) (*see also* Deformity, limb, specified type NEC, lower leg)
  - congenital Q74.2
- ureter N13.5
  - with infection N13.6
- wrist (acquired) (*see also* Deformity, limb, specified type NEC, forearm)
  - congenital Q74.0
Angulus infectiosus (lips) K13.0
Anhedonia R45.84
- sexual F52.0
Anhidrosis L74.4
Anhydration E86.0
Anhydremia E86.0
Anidrosis L74.4
Aniridia (congenital) Q13.1
Anisakiasis (infection) (infestation) B81.0
Anisakis larvae infestation B81.0
Aniseikonia H52.32
Anisocoria (pupil) H57.02
- congenital Q13.2
Anisocytosis R71.8
Anisometropia (congenital) H52.31
Ankle — *see* condition
Ankyloblepharon (eyelid) (acquired) (*see also* Blepharophimosis)
- filiforme (adnatum) (congenital) Q10.3
- total Q10.3
Ankyloglossia Q38.1
Ankylosis (fibrous) (osseous) (joint) M24.60
- ankle M24.67- ☑
- arthrodesis status Z98.1
- cricoarytenoid (cartilage) (joint) (larynx) J38.7
- dental K03.5
- ear ossicles H74.31- ☑
- elbow M24.62- ☑
- foot M24.67- ☑
- hand M24.64- ☑
- hip M24.65- ☑
- incostapedial joint (infectional) — *see* Ankylosis, ear ossicles
- jaw (temporomandibular) M26.61- ☑
- knee M24.66- ☑
- lumbosacral (joint) M43.27
- postoperative (status) Z98.1
- produced by surgical fusion, status Z98.1
- sacro-iliac (joint) M43.28
- shoulder M24.61- ☑
- spine (joint) (*see also* Fusion, spine)
  - spondylitic — *see* Spondylitis, ankylosing
- surgical Z98.1
- temporomandibular M26.61- ☑
- tooth, teeth (hard tissues) K03.5
- wrist M24.63- ☑
Ankylostoma — *see* Ancylostoma
Ankylostomiasis — *see* Ancylostomiasis
Ankylurethria — *see* Stricture, urethra
Annular (*see also* condition)
- detachment, cervix N88.8
- organ or site, congenital NEC — *see* Distortion
- pancreas (congenital) Q45.1
Anodontia (complete) (partial) (vera) K00.0
- acquired K08.10 ☑
Anomaly, anomalous (congenital) (unspecified type) Q89.9
- abdominal wall NEC Q79.59
- acoustic nerve Q07.8
- adrenal (gland) Q89.1
- Alder (-Reilly) (leukocyte granulation) D72.0
- alimentary tract Q45.9
  - upper Q40.9
- alveolar M26.70
  - hyperplasia M26.79
    - mandibular M26.72
    - maxillary M26.71
  - hypoplasia M26.79
    - mandibular M26.74
    - maxillary M26.73
  - ridge (process) M26.79
  - specified NEC M26.79
- ankle (joint) Q74.2
- anus Q43.9
- aorta (arch) NEC Q25.40
  - coarctation (preductal) (postductal) Q25.1
- aortic cusp or valve Q23.9

▽ Subterms under main terms may continue to next column or page   ☑ Additional Character Required — Refer to the Tabular List for Character Selection   **21**

Angiitis — Anomaly, anomalous

Anomaly, anomalous — *continued*
- appendix Q43.8
- apple peel syndrome Q41.1
- aqueduct of Sylvius Q03.0
  - with spina bifida — *see* Spina bifida, with hydrocephalus
- arm Q74.0
- arteriovenous NEC
  - coronary Q24.5
  - gastrointestinal Q27.33
    - acquired — *see* Angiodysplasia
- artery (peripheral) Q27.9
  - basilar NEC Q28.1
  - cerebral Q28.3
  - coronary Q24.5
  - digestive system Q27.8
  - eye Q15.8
  - great Q25.9
    - specified NEC Q25.8
  - lower limb Q27.8
  - peripheral Q27.9
    - specified NEC Q27.8
  - pulmonary NEC Q25.79
  - renal Q27.2
  - retina Q14.1
  - specified site NEC Q27.8
  - subclavian Q27.8
    - origin Q25.48
  - umbilical Q27.0
  - upper limb Q27.8
  - vertebral NEC Q28.1
- aryteno-epiglottic folds Q31.8
- atrial
  - bands or folds Q20.8
  - septa Q21.1
- atrioventricular
  - excitation I45.6
  - septum Q21.0
- auditory canal Q17.8
- auricle
  - ear Q17.8
    - causing impairment of hearing Q16.9
  - heart Q20.8
- Axenfeld's Q15.0
- back Q89.9
- band
  - atrial Q20.8
  - heart Q24.8
  - ventricular Q24.8
- Bartholin's duct Q38.4
- biliary duct or passage Q44.5
- bladder Q64.70
  - absence Q64.5
  - diverticulum Q64.6
  - exstrophy Q64.10
    - cloacal Q64.12
    - extroversion Q64.19
    - specified type NEC Q64.19
    - supravesical fissure Q64.11
  - neck obstruction Q64.31
  - specified type NEC Q64.79
- bone Q79.9
  - arm Q74.0
  - face Q75.9
  - leg Q74.2
  - pelvic girdle Q74.2
  - shoulder girdle Q74.0
  - skull Q75.9
    - with
      - anencephaly Q00.0
      - encephalocele — *see* Encephalocele
      - hydrocephalus Q03.9
        - with spina bifida — *see* Spina bifida, by site, with hydrocephalus
      - microcephaly Q02
- brain (multiple) Q04.9
  - vessel Q28.3
- breast Q83.9
- broad ligament Q50.6
- bronchus Q32.4
- bulbus cordis Q21.9
- bursa Q79.9
- canal of Nuck Q52.4
- canthus Q10.3
- capillary Q27.9
- cardiac Q24.9
  - chambers Q20.9
    - specified NEC Q20.8
  - septal closure Q21.9

Anomaly, anomalous — *continued*
- cardiac — *continued*
  - septal closure — *continued*
    - specified NEC Q21.8
  - valve NEC Q24.8
    - pulmonary Q22.3
- cardiovascular system Q28.8
- carpus Q74.0
- caruncle, lacrimal Q10.6
- cascade stomach Q40.2
- cauda equina Q06.3
- cecum Q43.9
- cerebral Q04.9
  - vessels Q28.3
- cervix Q51.9
- Chédiak-Higashi (-Steinbrinck) (congenital gigantism of peroxidase granules) E70.330
- cheek Q18.9
- chest wall Q67.8
  - bones Q76.9
- chin Q18.9
- chordae tendineae Q24.8
- choroid Q14.3
  - plexus Q07.8
- chromosomes, chromosomal Q99.9
  - D (1) — *see* condition, chromosome 13
  - E (3) — *see* condition, chromosome 18
  - G — *see* condition, chromosome 21
  - sex
    - female phenotype Q97.8
    - gonadal dysgenesis (pure) Q99.1
    - Klinefelter's Q98.4
    - male phenotype Q98.9
    - Turner's Q96.9
  - specified NEC Q99.8
- cilia Q10.3
- circulatory system Q28.9
- clavicle Q74.0
- clitoris Q52.6
- coccyx Q76.49
- colon Q43.9
- common duct Q44.5
- communication
  - coronary artery Q24.5
  - left ventricle with right atrium Q21.0
- concha (ear) Q17.3
- connection
  - portal vein Q26.5
  - pulmonary venous Q26.4
    - partial Q26.3
    - total Q26.2
  - renal artery with kidney Q27.2
- cornea (shape) Q13.4
- coronary artery or vein Q24.5
- cranium — *see* Anomaly, skull
- cricoid cartilage Q31.8
- cystic duct Q44.5
- dental
  - alveolar — *see* Anomaly, alveolar
  - arch relationship M26.20
    - specified NEC M26.29
- dentofacial M26.9
  - alveolar — *see* Anomaly, alveolar
  - dental arch relationship M26.20
    - specified NEC M26.29
  - functional M26.50
    - specified NEC M26.59
  - jaw size M26.00
    - macrogenia M26.05
    - mandibular
      - hyperplasia M26.03
      - hypoplasia M26.04
    - maxillary
      - hyperplasia M26.01
      - hypoplasia M26.02
    - microgenia M26.06
    - specified type NEC M26.09
  - jaw-cranial base relationship M26.10
    - asymmetry M26.12
      - maxillary M26.11
    - specified type NEC M26.19
  - malocclusion M26.4
    - dental arch relationship NEC M26.29
    - jaw size — *see* Anomaly, dentofacial, jaw size
    - jaw-cranial base relationship — *see* Anomaly, dentofacial, jaw-cranial base relationship
  - specified type NEC M26.89
  - temporomandibular joint M26.60- ☑

Anomaly, anomalous — *continued*
- dentofacial — *continued*
  - temporomandibular joint — *continued*
    - adhesions M26.61- ☑
    - ankylosis M26.61- ☑
    - arthralgia M26.62- ☑
    - articular disc M26.63- ☑
    - specified type NEC M26.69
  - tooth position, fully erupted M26.30
    - specified NEC M26.39
- dermatoglyphic Q82.8
- diaphragm (apertures) NEC Q79.1
- digestive organ(s) or tract Q45.9
  - lower Q43.9
  - upper Q40.9
- distance, interarch (excessive) (inadequate) M26.25
- distribution, coronary artery Q24.5
- ductus
  - arteriosus Q25.0
  - botalli Q25.0
- duodenum Q43.9
- dura (brain) Q04.9
  - spinal cord Q06.9
- ear (external) Q17.9
  - causing impairment of hearing Q16.9
  - inner Q16.5
  - middle (causing impairment of hearing) Q16.4
    - ossicles Q16.3
- Ebstein's (heart) (tricuspid valve) Q22.5
- ectodermal Q82.9
- Eisenmenger's (ventricular septal defect) Q21.8
- ejaculatory duct Q55.4
- elbow Q74.0
- endocrine gland NEC Q89.2
- epididymis Q55.4
- epiglottis Q31.8
- esophagus Q39.9
- eustachian tube Q17.8
- eye Q15.9
  - anterior segment Q13.9
    - specified NEC Q13.89
  - posterior segment Q14.9
    - specified NEC Q14.8
  - ptosis (eyelid) Q10.0
  - specified NEC Q15.8
- eyebrow Q18.8
- eyelid Q10.3
  - ptosis Q10.0
- face Q18.9
  - bone(s) Q75.9
- fallopian tube Q50.6
- fascia Q79.9
- femur NEC Q74.2
- fibula NEC Q74.2
- finger Q74.0
- fixation, intestine Q43.3
- flexion (joint) NOS Q74.9
  - hip or thigh Q65.89
- foot NEC Q74.2
  - varus (congenital) Q66.3
- foramen
  - Botalli Q21.1
  - ovale Q21.1
- forearm Q74.0
- forehead Q75.8
- form, teeth K00.2
- fovea centralis Q14.1
- frontal bone — *see* Anomaly, skull
- gallbladder (position) (shape) (size) Q44.1
- Gartner's duct Q52.4
- gastrointestinal tract Q45.9
- genitalia, genital organ(s) or system
  - female Q52.9
    - external Q52.70
    - internal NOS Q52.9
  - male Q55.9
    - hydrocele P83.5
    - specified NEC Q55.8
- genitourinary NEC
  - female Q52.9
  - male Q55.9
- Gerbode Q21.0
- glottis Q31.8
- granulation or granulocyte, genetic (constitutional) (leukocyte) D72.0
- gum Q38.6
- gyri Q07.9
- hair Q84.2
- hand Q74.0

Anomaly, anomalous — *continued*
- hard tissue formation in pulp K04.3
- head — *see* Anomaly, skull
- heart Q24.9
  - auricle Q20.8
  - bands or folds Q24.8
  - fibroelastosis cordis I42.4
  - obstructive NEC Q22.6
  - patent ductus arteriosus (Botalli) Q25.0
  - septum Q21.9
    - auricular Q21.1
    - interatrial Q21.1
    - interventricular Q21.0
      - with pulmonary stenosis or atresia, dextra-position of aorta and hypertrophy of right ventricle Q21.3
    - specified NEC Q21.8
    - ventricular Q21.0
      - with pulmonary stenosis or atresia, dextra-position of aorta and hypertrophy of right ventricle Q21.3
  - tetralogy of Fallot Q21.3
  - valve NEC Q24.8
    - aortic
      - bicuspid valve Q23.1
      - insufficiency Q23.1
      - stenosis Q23.0
        - subaortic Q24.4
    - mitral
      - insufficiency Q23.3
      - stenosis Q23.2
    - pulmonary Q22.3
      - atresia Q22.0
      - insufficiency Q22.2
      - stenosis Q22.1
        - infundibular Q24.3
        - subvalvular Q24.3
    - tricuspid
      - atresia Q22.4
      - stenosis Q22.4
  - ventricle Q20.8
- heel NEC Q74.2
- Hegglin's D72.0
- hemianencephaly Q00.0
- hemicephaly Q00.0
- hemicrania Q00.0
- hepatic duct Q44.5
- hip NEC Q74.2
- hourglass stomach Q40.2
- humerus Q74.0
- hydatid of Morgagni
  - female Q50.5
  - male (epididymal) Q55.4
    - testicular Q55.29
- hymen Q52.4
- hypersegmentation of neutrophils, hereditary D72.0
- hypophyseal Q89.2
- ileocecal (coil) (valve) Q43.9
- ileum Q43.9
- ilium NEC Q74.2
- integument Q84.9
  - specified NEC Q84.8
- interarch distance (excessive) (inadequate) M26.25
- intervertebral cartilage or disc Q76.49
- intestine (large) (small) Q43.9
  - with anomalous adhesions, fixation or malrotation Q43.3
- iris Q13.2
- ischium NEC Q74.2
- jaw — *see* Anomaly, dentofacial
  - alveolar — *see* Anomaly, alveolar
- jaw-cranial base relationship — *see* Anomaly, dentofacial, jaw-cranial base relationship
- jejunum Q43.8
- joint Q74.9
  - specified NEC Q74.8
- Jordan's D72.0
- kidney(s) (calyx) (pelvis) Q63.9
  - artery Q27.2
  - specified NEC Q63.8
- Klippel-Feil (brevicollis) Q76.1
- knee Q74.1
- labium (majus) (minus) Q52.70
- labyrinth, membranous Q16.5
- lacrimal apparatus or duct Q10.6
- larynx, laryngeal (muscle) Q31.9
  - web (bed) Q31.0
- lens Q12.9
- leukocytes, genetic D72.0

Anomaly, anomalous — *continued*
- leukocytes, genetic — *continued*
  - granulation (constitutional) D72.0
- lid (fold) Q10.3
- ligament Q79.9
  - broad Q50.6
  - round Q52.8
- limb Q74.9
  - lower NEC Q74.2
    - reduction deformity — *see* Defect, reduction, lower limb
  - upper Q74.0
- lip Q38.0
- liver Q44.7
  - duct Q44.5
- lower limb NEC Q74.2
- lumbosacral (joint) (region) Q76.49
  - kyphosis — *see* Kyphosis, congenital
  - lordosis — *see* Lordosis, congenital
- lung (fissure) (lobe) Q33.9
- mandible — *see* Anomaly, dentofacial
- maxilla — *see* Anomaly, dentofacial
- May (-Hegglin) D72.0
- meatus urinarius NEC Q64.79
- meningeal bands or folds Q07.9
  - constriction of Q07.8
  - spinal Q06.9
- meninges Q07.9
  - cerebral Q04.8
  - spinal Q06.9
- meningocele Q05.9
- mesentery Q45.9
- metacarpus Q74.0
- metatarsus NEC Q74.2
- middle ear Q16.4
  - ossicles Q16.3
- mitral (leaflets) (valve) Q23.9
  - insufficiency Q23.3
  - specified NEC Q23.8
  - stenosis Q23.2
- mouth Q38.6
- Müllerian (*see also* Anomaly, by site)
  - uterus NEC Q51.818
- multiple NEC Q89.7
- muscle Q79.9
  - eyelid Q10.3
- musculoskeletal system, except limbs Q79.9
- myocardium Q24.8
- nail Q84.6
- narrowness, eyelid Q10.3
- nasal sinus (wall) Q30.8
- neck (any part) Q18.9
- nerve Q07.9
  - acoustic Q07.8
  - optic Q07.8
- nervous system (central) Q07.9
- nipple Q83.9
- nose, nasal (bones) (cartilage) (septum) (sinus) Q30.9
  - specified NEC Q30.8
- ocular muscle Q15.8
- omphalomesenteric duct Q43.0
- opening, pulmonary veins Q26.4
- optic
  - disc Q14.2
  - nerve Q07.8
- opticociliary vessels Q13.2
- orbit (eye) Q10.7
- organ Q89.9
  - of Corti Q16.5
- origin
  - artery
    - innominate Q25.8
    - pulmonary Q25.79
    - renal Q27.2
    - subclavian Q25.48
- osseous meatus (ear) Q16.1
- ovary Q50.39
- oviduct Q50.6
- palate (hard) (soft) NEC Q38.5
- pancreas or pancreatic duct Q45.3
- papillary muscles Q24.8
- parathyroid gland Q89.2
- paraurethral ducts Q64.79
- parotid (gland) Q38.4
- patella Q74.1
- Pelger-Huët (hereditary hyposegmentation) D72.0
- pelvic girdle NEC Q74.2
- pelvis (bony) NEC Q74.2
  - rachitic E64.3

Anomaly, anomalous — *continued*
- penis (glans) Q55.69
- pericardium Q24.8
- peripheral vascular system Q27.9
- Peter's Q13.4
- pharynx Q38.8
- pigmentation L81.9
  - congenital Q82.8
- pituitary (gland) Q89.2
- pleural (folds) Q34.0
- portal vein Q26.5
  - connection Q26.5
- position, tooth, teeth, fully erupted M26.30
  - specified NEC M26.39
- precerebral vessel Q28.1
- prepuce Q55.69
- prostate Q55.4
- pulmonary Q33.9
  - artery NEC Q25.79
  - valve Q22.3
    - atresia Q22.0
    - insufficiency Q22.2
    - specified type NEC Q22.3
    - stenosis Q22.1
      - infundibular Q24.3
      - subvalvular Q24.3
  - venous connection Q26.4
    - partial Q26.3
    - total Q26.2
- pupil Q13.2
  - function H57.00
    - anisocoria H57.02
    - Argyll Robertson pupil H57.01
    - miosis H57.03
    - mydriasis H57.04
    - specified type NEC H57.09
    - tonic pupil H57.05- ☑
- pylorus Q40.3
- radius Q74.0
- rectum Q43.9
- reduction (extremity) (limb)
  - femur (longitudinal) — *see* Defect, reduction, lower limb, longitudinal, femur
  - fibula (longitudinal) — *see* Defect, reduction, lower limb, longitudinal, fibula
  - lower limb — *see* Defect, reduction, lower limb
  - radius (longitudinal) — *see* Defect, reduction, upper limb, longitudinal, radius
  - tibia (longitudinal) — *see* Defect, reduction, lower limb, longitudinal, tibia
  - ulna (longitudinal) — *see* Defect, reduction, upper limb, longitudinal, ulna
  - upper limb — *see* Defect, reduction, upper limb
- refraction — *see* Disorder, refraction
- renal Q63.9
  - artery Q27.2
  - pelvis Q63.9
  - specified NEC Q63.8
- respiratory system Q34.9
  - specified NEC Q34.8
- retina Q14.1
- rib Q76.6
  - cervical Q76.5
- Rieger's Q13.81
- rotation — *see* Malrotation
  - hip or thigh Q65.89
- round ligament Q52.8
- sacroiliac (joint) NEC Q74.2
- sacrum NEC Q76.49
  - kyphosis — *see* Kyphosis, congenital
  - lordosis — *see* Lordosis, congenital
- saddle nose, syphilitic A50.57
- salivary duct or gland Q38.4
- scapula Q74.0
- scrotum — *see* Malformation, testis and scrotum
- sebaceous gland Q82.9
- seminal vesicles Q55.4
- sense organs NEC Q07.8
- sex chromosomes NEC (*see also* Anomaly, chromosomes)
  - female phenotype Q97.8
  - male phenotype Q98.9
- shoulder (girdle) (joint) Q74.0
- sigmoid (flexure) Q43.9
- simian crease Q82.8
- sinus of Valsalva Q25.49
- skeleton generalized Q78.9
- skin (appendage) Q82.9

Anomaly, anomalous — *continued*
  skull Q75.9
    with
      anencephaly Q00.0
      encephalocele — *see* Encephalocele
      hydrocephalus Q03.9
        with spina bifida — *see* Spina bifida, by site,
          with hydrocephalus
      microcephaly Q02
  specified organ or site NEC Q89.8
  spermatic cord Q55.4
  spine, spinal NEC Q76.49
    column NEC Q76.49
      kyphosis — *see* Kyphosis, congenital
      lordosis — *see* Lordosis, congenital
    cord Q06.9
    nerve root Q07.8
  spleen Q89.09
    agenesis Q89.01
  stenonian duct Q38.4
  sternum NEC Q76.7
  stomach Q40.3
  submaxillary gland Q38.4
  tarsus NEC Q74.2
  tendon Q79.9
  testis — *see* Malformation, testis and scrotum
  thigh NEC Q74.2
  thorax (wall) Q67.8
    bony Q76.9
  throat Q38.8
  thumb Q74.0
  thymus gland Q89.2
  thyroid (gland) Q89.2
    cartilage Q31.8
  tibia NEC Q74.2
    saber A50.56
  toe Q74.2
  tongue Q38.3
  tooth, teeth K00.9
    eruption K00.6
    position, fully erupted M26.30
    spacing, fully erupted M26.30
  trachea (cartilage) Q32.1
  tragus Q17.9
  tricuspid (leaflet) (valve) Q22.9
    atresia or stenosis Q22.4
    Ebstein's Q22.5
  Uhl's (hypoplasia of myocardium, right ventricle) Q24.8
  ulna Q74.0
  umbilical artery Q27.0
  union
    cricoid cartilage and thyroid cartilage Q31.8
    thyroid cartilage and hyoid bone Q31.8
    trachea with larynx Q31.8
  upper limb Q74.0
  urachus Q64.4
  ureter Q62.8
    obstructive NEC Q62.39
      cecoureterocele Q62.32
      orthotopic ureterocele Q62.31
  urethra Q64.70
    absence Q64.5
    double Q64.74
    fistula to rectum Q64.73
    obstructive Q64.39
      stricture Q64.32
    prolapse Q64.71
    specified type NEC Q64.79
  urinary tract Q64.9
  uterus Q51.9
    with only one functioning horn Q51.4
  uvula Q38.5
  vagina Q52.4
  valleculae Q31.8
  valve (heart) NEC Q24.8
    coronary sinus Q24.5
    inferior vena cava Q24.8
    pulmonary Q22.3
    sinus coronario Q24.5
    venae cavae inferioris Q24.8
  vas deferens Q55.4
  vascular Q27.9
    brain Q28.3
    ring Q25.45
  vein(s) (peripheral) Q27.9
    brain Q28.3
    cerebral Q28.3
    coronary Q24.5
    developmental Q28.3

Anomaly, anomalous — *continued*
  vein(s) — *continued*
    great Q26.9
      specified NEC Q26.8
  vena cava (inferior) (superior) Q26.9
  venous — *see* Anomaly, vein(s)
  venous return Q26.8
  ventricular
    bands or folds Q24.8
    septa Q21.0
  vertebra Q76.49
    kyphosis — *see* Kyphosis, congenital
    lordosis — *see* Lordosis, congenital
  vesicourethral orifice Q64.79
  vessel(s) Q27.9
    optic papilla Q14.2
    precerebral Q28.1
  vitelline duct Q43.0
  vitreous body or humor Q14.0
  vulva Q52.70
  wrist (joint) Q74.0
Anomia R48.8
Anonychia (congenital) Q84.3
  acquired L60.8
Anophthalmos, anophthalmus (congenital) (globe)
    Q11.1
  acquired Z90.01
Anopia, anopsia H53.46- ☑
  quadrant H53.46- ☑
Anorchia, anorchism, anorchidism Q55.0
Anorexia R63.0
  hysterical F44.89
  nervosa F50.00
    atypical F50.9
    binge-eating type F50.2
      with purging F50.02
    restricting type F50.01
Anorgasmy, psychogenic (female) F52.31
  male F52.32
Anosmia R43.0
  hysterical F44.6
  postinfectional J39.8
Anosognosia R41.89
Anosteoplasia Q78.9
Anovulatory cycle N97.0
Anoxemia R09.02
  newborn P84
Anoxia (pathological) R09.02
  altitude T70.29 ☑
  cerebral G93.1
    complicating
      anesthesia (general) (local) or other sedation
        T88.59 ☑
      in labor and delivery O74.3
      in pregnancy O29.21- ☑
      postpartum, puerperal O89.2
    delivery (cesarean) (instrumental) O75.4
    during a procedure G97.81
    newborn P84
    resulting from a procedure G97.82
  due to
    drowning T75.1 ☑
    high altitude T70.29 ☑
  heart — *see* Insufficiency, coronary
  intrauterine P84
  myocardial — *see* Insufficiency, coronary
  newborn P84
  spinal cord G95.11
  systemic (by suffocation) (low content in atmosphere)
    — *see* Asphyxia, traumatic
Anteflexion — *see* Anteversion
Antenatal
  care (normal pregnancy) Z34.90
  screening (encounter for) of mother (*see also* En-
    counter, antenatal screening) Z36.9
Antepartum — *see* condition
Anterior — *see* condition
Antero-occlusion M26.220
Anteversion
  cervix — *see* Anteversion, uterus
  femur (neck), congenital Q65.89
  uterus, uterine (cervix) (postinfectional) (postpartal)
    (old) N85.4
    congenital Q51.818
    in pregnancy or childbirth — *see* Pregnancy,
      complicated by
Anthophobia F40.228
Anthracosilicosis J60

Anthracosis (lung) (occupational) J60
  lingua K14.3
Anthrax A22.9
  with pneumonia A22.1
  cerebral A22.8
  colitis A22.2
  cutaneous A22.0
  gastrointestinal A22.2
  inhalation A22.1
  intestinal A22.2
  meningitis A22.8
  pulmonary A22.1
  respiratory A22.1
  sepsis A22.7
  specified manifestation NEC A22.8
Anthropoid pelvis Q74.2
  with disproportion (fetopelvic) O33.0
Anthropophobia F40.10
  generalized F40.11
Antibodies, maternal (blood group) — *see* Isoimmu-
    nization, affecting management of pregnancy
  anti-D — *see* Isoimmunization, affecting management
    of pregnancy, Rh
  newborn P55.0
Antibody
  anticardiolipin R76.0
    with
      hemorrhagic disorder D68.312
      hypercoagulable state D68.61
  antiphosphatidylglycerol R76.0
    with
      hemorrhagic disorder D68.312
      hypercoagulable state D68.61
  antiphosphatidylinositol R76.0
    with
      hemorrhagic disorder D68.312
      hypercoagulable state D68.61
  antiphosphatidylserine R76.0
    with
      hemorrhagic disorder D68.312
      hypercoagulable state D68.61
  antiphospholipid R76.0
    with
      hemorrhagic disorder D68.312
      hypercoagulable state D68.61
Anticardiolipin syndrome D68.61
Anticoagulant, circulating (intrinsic) (*see also* Disorder,
    hemorrhagic) D68.318
  drug-induced (extrinsic) (*see also* Disorder, hemorrhag-
    ic) D68.32
  iatrogenic D68.32
Antidiuretic hormone syndrome E22.2
Antimonial cholera — *see* Poisoning, antimony
Antiphospholipid
  antibody
    with hemorrhagic disorder D68.312
    syndrome D68.61
Antisocial personality F60.2
Antithrombinemia — *see* Circulating anticoagulants
Antithromboplastinemia D68.318
Antithromboplastinogenemia D68.318
Antitoxin complication or reaction — *see* Complica-
    tions, vaccination
Antlophobia F40.228
Antritis J32.0
  maxilla J32.0
    acute J01.00
      recurrent J01.01
  stomach K29.60
    with bleeding K29.61
Antrum, antral — *see* condition
Anuria R34
  calculous (impacted) (recurrent) (*see also* Calculus,
    urinary) N20.9
  following
    abortion — *see* Abortion by type complicated by,
      renal failure
    ectopic or molar pregnancy O08.4
  newborn P96.0
  postprocedural N99.0
  postrenal N13.8
  traumatic (following crushing) T79.5 ☑
Anus, anal — *see* condition
Anusitis K62.89
Anxiety F41.9
  depression F41.8
  episodic paroxysmal F41.0
  generalized F41.1

Anxiety — *continued*
hysteria F41.8
neurosis F41.1
panic type F41.0
reaction F41.1
separation, abnormal (of childhood) F93.0
specified NEC F41.8
state F41.1
Aorta, aortic — *see* condition
Aortectasia — *see* Ectasia, aorta
with aneurysm — *see* Aneurysm, aorta
Aortitis (nonsyphilitic) (calcific) I77.6
arteriosclerotic I70.0
Doehle-Heller A52.02
luetic A52.02
rheumatic — *see* Endocarditis, acute, rheumatic
specific (syphilitic) A52.02
syphilitic A52.02
congenital A50.54 [I79.1]
Apathetic thyroid storm — *see* Thyrotoxicosis
Apathy R45.3
Apeirophobia F40.228
Apepsia K30
psychogenic F45.8
Aperistalsis, esophagus K22.0
Apertognathia M26.29
Apert's syndrome Q87.0
Aphagia R13.0
psychogenic F50.9
Aphakia (acquired) (postoperative) H27.0- ☑
congenital Q12.3
Aphasia (amnestic) (global) (nominal) (semantic) (syntactic) R47.01
acquired, with epilepsy (Landau-Kleffner syndrome)
— *see* Epilepsy, specified NEC
auditory (developmental) F80.2
developmental (receptive type) F80.2
expressive type F80.1
Wernicke's F80.2
following
cerebrovascular disease I69.920
cerebral infarction I69.320
intracerebral hemorrhage I69.120
nontraumatic intracranial hemorrhage NEC
I69.220
specified disease NEC I69.820
subarachnoid hemorrhage I69.020
primary progressive G31.01 [F02.80]
with behavioral disturbance G31.01 [F02.81]
progressive isolated G31.01 [F02.80]
with behavioral disturbance G31.01 [F02.81]
sensory F80.2
syphilis, tertiary A52.19
Wernicke's (developmental) F80.2
Aphonia (organic) R49.1
hysterical F44.4
psychogenic F44.4
Aphthae, aphthous (*see also* condition)
Bednar's K12.0
cachectic K14.0
epizootic B08.8
fever B08.8
oral (recurrent) K12.0
stomatitis (major) (minor) K12.0
thrush B37.0
ulcer (oral) (recurrent) K12.0
genital organ(s) NEC
female N76.6
male N50.89
larynx J38.7
Apical — *see* condition
Apiphobia F40.218
Aplasia (*see also* Agenesis)
abdominal muscle syndrome Q79.4
alveolar process (acquired) — *see* Anomaly, alveolar
congenital Q38.6
aorta (congenital) Q25.41
axialis extracorticalis (congenita) E75.29
bone marrow (myeloid) D61.9
congenital D61.01
brain Q00.0
part of Q04.3
bronchus Q32.4
cementum K00.4
cerebellum Q04.3
cervix (congenital) Q51.5
congenital pure red cell D61.01
corpus callosum Q04.0

Aplasia — *continued*
cutis congenita Q84.8
erythrocyte congenital D61.01
extracortical axial E75.29
eye Q11.1
fovea centralis (congenital) Q14.1
gallbladder, congenital Q44.0
iris Q13.1
labyrinth, membranous Q16.5
limb (congenital) Q73.8
lower — *see* Defect, reduction, lower limb
upper — *see* Agenesis, arm
lung, congenital (bilateral) (unilateral) Q33.3
pancreas Q45.0
parathyroid-thymic D82.1
Pelizaeus-Merzbacher E75.29
penis Q55.5
prostate Q55.4
red cell (with thymoma) D60.9
acquired D60.9
due to drugs D60.9
adult D60.9
chronic D60.0
congenital D61.01
constitutional D61.01
due to drugs D60.9
hereditary D61.01
of infants D61.01
primary D61.01
pure D61.01
due to drugs D60.9
specified type NEC D60.8
transient D60.1
round ligament Q52.8
skin Q84.8
spermatic cord Q55.4
spleen Q89.01
testicle Q55.0
thymic, with immunodeficiency D82.1
thyroid (congenital) (with myxedema) E03.1
uterus Q51.0
ventral horn cell Q06.1
Apnea, apneic (of) (spells) R06.81
newborn NEC P28.4
obstructive P28.4
sleep (central) (obstructive) (primary) P28.3
prematurity P28.4
sleep G47.30
central (primary) G47.31
idiopathic G47.31
in conditions classified elsewhere G47.37
obstructive (adult) (pediatric) G47.33
hypopnea G47.33
primary central G47.31
specified NEC G47.39
Apneumatosis, newborn P28.0
Apocrine metaplasia (breast) — *see* Dysplasia, mammary, specified type NEC
Apophysitis (bone) (*see also* Osteochondropathy)
calcaneus M92.8
juvenile M92.9
Apoplectiform convulsions (cerebral ischemia) I67.82
Apoplexia, apoplexy, apoplectic
adrenal A39.1
heart (auricle) (ventricle) — *see* Infarct, myocardium
heat T67.0 ☑
hemorrhagic (stroke) — *see* Hemorrhage, intracranial
meninges, hemorrhagic — *see* Hemorrhage, intracranial, subarachnoid
uremic N18.9 [I68.8]
Appearance
bizarre R46.1
specified NEC R46.89
very low level of personal hygiene R46.0
Appendage
epididymal (organ of Morgagni) Q55.4
intestine (epiploic) Q43.8
preauricular Q17.0
testicular (organ of Morgagni) Q55.29
Appendicitis (pneumococcal) (retrocecal) K37
with
perforation or rupture K35.2
peritoneal abscess K35.3
peritonitis NEC K35.3
generalized (with perforation or rupture) K35.2
localized (with perforation or rupture) K35.3
acute (catarrhal) (fulminating) (gangrenous) (obstructive) (retrocecal) (suppurative) K35.80

Appendicitis — *continued*
acute — *continued*
with
peritoneal abscess K35.3
peritonitis NEC K35.3
generalized (with perforation or rupture) K35.2
localized (with perforation or rupture) K35.3
specified NEC K35.89
amebic A06.89
chronic (recurrent) K36
exacerbation — *see* Appendicitis, acute
gangrenous — *see* Appendicitis, acute
healed (obliterative) K36
interval K36
neurogenic K36
obstructive K36
recurrent K36
relapsing K36
subacute (adhesive) K36
subsiding K36
suppurative — *see* Appendicitis, acute
tuberculous A18.32
Appendicopathia oxyurica B80
Appendix, appendicular (*see also* condition)
epididymis Q55.4
Morgagni
female Q50.5
male (epididymal) Q55.4
testicular Q55.29
testis Q55.29
Appetite
depraved — *see* Pica
excessive R63.2
lack or loss (*see also* Anorexia) R63.0
nonorganic origin F50.89
psychogenic F50.89
perverted (hysterical) — *see* Pica
Apple peel syndrome Q41.1
Apprehension state F41.1
Apprehensiveness, abnormal F41.9
Approximal wear K03.0
Apraxia (classic) (ideational) (ideokinetic) (ideomotor) (motor) (verbal) R48.2
following
cerebrovascular disease I69.990
cerebral infarction I69.390
intracerebral hemorrhage I69.190
nontraumatic intracranial hemorrhage NEC
I69.290
specified disease NEC I69.890
subarachnoid hemorrhage I69.090
oculomotor, congenital H51.8
Aptyalism K11.7
Apudoma — *see* Neoplasm, uncertain behavior, by site
Aqueous misdirection H40.83- ☑
Arabicum elephantiasis — *see* Infestation, filarial
Arachnitis — *see* Meningitis
Arachnodactyly — *see* Syndrome, Marfan's
Arachnoiditis (acute) (adhesive) (basal) (brain) (cerebrospinal) — *see* Meningitis
Arachnophobia F40.210
Arboencephalitis, Australian A83.4
Arborization block (heart) I45.5
ARC (AIDS-related complex) B20
Arch
aortic Q25.49
bovine Q25.49
Arches — *see* condition
Arcuate uterus Q51.810
Arcuatus uterus Q51.810
Arcus (cornea) senilis — *see* Degeneration, cornea, senile
Arc-welder's lung J63.4
Areflexia R29.2
Areola — *see* condition
Argentaffinoma (*see also* Neoplasm, uncertain behavior, by site)
malignant — *see* Neoplasm, malignant, by site
syndrome E34.0
Argininemia E72.21
Arginosuccinic aciduria E72.22
Argyll Robertson phenomenon, pupil or syndrome (syphilitic) A52.19
atypical H57.09
nonsyphilitic H57.09
Argyria, argyriasis
conjunctival H11.13- ☑

Argyria, argyriasis — *continued*
  from drug or medicament — *see* Table of Drugs and Chemicals, by substance
Argyrosis, conjunctival H11.13- ☑
Arhinencephaly Q04.1
Ariboflavinosis E53.0
Arm — *see* condition
Arnold-Chiari disease, obstruction or syndrome (type II) Q07.00
  with
    hydrocephalus Q07.02
      with spina bifida Q07.03
    spina bifida Q07.01
      with hydrocephalus Q07.03
  type III — *see* Encephalocele
  type IV Q04.8
Aromatic amino-acid metabolism disorder E70.9
  specified NEC E70.8
Arousals, confusional G47.51
Arrest, arrested
  cardiac I46.9
    complicating
      abortion — *see* Abortion, by type, complicated by cardiac arrest
      anesthesia (general) (local) or other sedation — *see* Table of Drugs and Chemicals, by drug
        in labor and delivery O74.2
        in pregnancy O29.11- ☑
        postpartum, puerperal O89.1
      delivery (cesarean) (instrumental) O75.4
    due to
      cardiac condition I46.2
      specified condition NEC I46.8
    intraoperative I97.71- ☑
    newborn P29.81
    personal history, successfully resuscitated Z86.74
    postprocedural I97.12- ☑
      obstetric procedure O75.4
  cardiorespiratory — *see* Arrest, cardiac
  circulatory — *see* Arrest, cardiac
  deep transverse O64.0 ☑
  development or growth
    bone — *see* Disorder, bone, development or growth
    child R62.50
    tracheal rings Q32.1
  epiphyseal
    complete
      femur M89.15- ☑
      humerus M89.12- ☑
      tibia M89.16- ☑
      ulna M89.13- ☑
      forearm M89.13- ☑
        specified NEC M89.13- ☑
      ulna — *see* Arrest, epiphyseal, by type, ulna
      lower leg M89.16- ☑
        specified NEC M89.168
      tibia — *see* Arrest, epiphyseal, by type, tibia
    partial
      femur M89.15- ☑
      humerus M89.12- ☑
      tibia M89.16- ☑
      ulna M89.13- ☑
    specified NEC M89.18
  granulopoiesis — *see* Agranulocytosis
  growth plate — *see* Arrest, epiphyseal
  heart — *see* Arrest, cardiac
  legal, anxiety concerning Z65.3
  physeal — *see* Arrest, epiphyseal
  respiratory R09.2
    newborn P28.81
  sinus I45.5
  spermatogenesis (complete) — *see* Azoospermia
    incomplete — *see* Oligospermia
  transverse (deep) O64.0 ☑
Arrhenoblastoma
  benign
    specified site — *see* Neoplasm, benign, by site
    unspecified site
      female D27.9
      male D29.20
  malignant
    specified site — *see* Neoplasm, malignant, by site
    unspecified site
      female C56.9
      male C62.90

Arrhenoblastoma — *continued*
  specified site — *see* Neoplasm, uncertain behavior, by site
  unspecified site
    female D39.10
    male D40.10
Arrhythmia (auricle) (cardiac) (juvenile) (nodal) (reflex) (sinus) (supraventricular) (transitory) (ventricle) I49.9
  block I45.9
  extrasystolic I49.49
  newborn
    bradycardia P29.12
      occurring before birth P03.819
        before onset of labor P03.810
        during labor P03.811
    tachycardia P29.11
  psychogenic F45.8
  specified NEC I49.8
  vagal R55
  ventricular re-entry I47.0
Arrillaga-Ayerza syndrome (pulmonary sclerosis with pulmonary hypertension) I27.0
Arsenical pigmentation L81.8
  from drug or medicament — *see* Table of Drugs and Chemicals
Arsenism — *see* Poisoning, arsenic
Arterial — *see* condition
Arteriofibrosis — *see* Arteriosclerosis
Arteriolar sclerosis — *see* Arteriosclerosis
Arteriolith — *see* Arteriosclerosis
Arteriolitis I77.6
  necrotizing, kidney I77.5
  renal — *see* Hypertension, kidney
Arteriolosclerosis — *see* Arteriosclerosis
Arterionephrosclerosis — *see* Hypertension, kidney
Arteriopathy I77.9
Arteriosclerosis, arteriosclerotic (diffuse) (obliterans) (of) (senile) (with calcification) I70.90
  aorta I70.0
  arteries of extremities — *see* Arteriosclerosis, extremities
  brain I67.2
  bypass graft
    coronary — *see* Arteriosclerosis, coronary, bypass graft
    extremities — *see* Arteriosclerosis, extremities, bypass graft
  cardiac — *see* Disease, heart, ischemic, atherosclerotic
  cardiopathy — *see* Disease, heart, ischemic, atherosclerotic
  cardiorenal — *see* Hypertension, cardiorenal
  cardiovascular — *see* Disease, heart, ischemic, atherosclerotic
  carotid (*see also* Occlusion, artery, carotid) I65.2- ☑
  central nervous system I67.2
  cerebral I67.2
  cerebrovascular I67.2
  coronary (artery) I25.10
    bypass graft I25.810
      with
        angina pectoris I25.709
          with documented spasm I25.701
          specified type NEC I25.708
          unstable I25.700
        ischemic chest pain I25.709
      autologous artery I25.810
        with
          angina pectoris I25.729
            with documented spasm I25.721
            specified type I25.728
            unstable I25.720
          ischemic chest pain I25.729
      autologous vein I25.810
        with
          angina pectoris I25.719
            with documented spasm I25.711
            specified type I25.718
            unstable I25.710
          ischemic chest pain I25.719
      nonautologous biological I25.810
        with
          angina pectoris I25.739
            with documented spasm I25.731
            specified type I25.738
            unstable I25.730
          ischemic chest pain I25.739
      specified type NEC I25.810

Arteriosclerosis, arteriosclerotic — *continued*
  coronary — *continued*
    bypass graft — *continued*
      specified type — *continued*
        with
          angina pectoris I25.799
            with documented spasm I25.791
            specified type I25.798
            unstable I25.790
          ischemic chest pain I25.799
    due to
      calcified coronary lesion (severely) I25.84
      lipid rich plaque I25.83
    native vessel
      with
        angina pectoris I25.119
          with documented spasm I25.111
          specified type NEC I25.118
          unstable I25.110
        ischemic chest pain I25.119
    transplanted heart I25.811
      bypass graft I25.812
        with
          angina pectoris I25.769
            with documented spasm I25.761
            specified type I25.768
            unstable I25.760
          ischemic chest pain I25.769
      native coronary artery I25.811
        with
          angina pectoris I25.759
            with documented spasm I25.751
            specified type I25.758
            unstable I25.750
          ischemic chest pain I25.759
  extremities (native arteries) I70.209
    bypass graft I70.309
      autologous vein graft I70.409
        leg I70.409
          with
            gangrene (and intermittent claudication, rest pain and ulcer) I70.469
            intermittent claudication I70.419
            rest pain (and intermittent claudication) I70.429
        bilateral I70.403
          with
            gangrene (and intermittent claudication, rest pain and ulcer) I70.463
            intermittent claudication I70.463
            rest pain (and intermittent claudication) I70.423
            specified type NEC I70.493
        left I70.402
          with
            gangrene (and intermittent claudication, rest pain and ulcer) I70.462
            intermittent claudication I70.412
            rest pain (and intermittent claudication) I70.422
            ulceration (and intermittent claudication and rest pain) I70.449
              ankle I70.443
              calf I70.442
              foot site NEC I70.445
              heel I70.444
              lower leg NEC I70.448
              midfoot I70.444
              thigh I70.441
            specified type NEC I70.492
        right I70.401
          with
            gangrene (and intermittent claudication, rest pain and ulcer) I70.461
            intermittent claudication I70.411
            rest pain (and intermittent claudication) I70.421
            ulceration (and intermittent claudication and rest pain) I70.439
              ankle I70.433
              calf I70.432
              foot site NEC I70.435
              heel I70.434

Arteriosclerosis, arteriosclerotic — *continued*
  extremities — *continued*
    bypass graft — *continued*
      autologous vein graft — *continued*
        leg — *continued*
          right — *continued*
            with — *continued*
              ulceration — *continued*
                lower leg NEC I70.438
                midfoot I70.434
                thigh I70.431
              specified type NEC I70.491
            specified type NEC I70.499
          specified NEC I70.408
            with
              gangrene (and intermittent claudication, rest pain and ulcer) I70.468
              intermittent claudication I70.418
              rest pain (and intermittent claudication) I70.428
              ulceration (and intermittent claudication and rest pain) I70.45
            specified type NEC I70.498
        leg I70.309
          with
            gangrene (and intermittent claudication, rest pain and ulcer) I70.369
            intermittent claudication I70.319
            rest pain (and intermittent claudication) I70.329
          bilateral I70.303
            with
              gangrene (and intermittent claudication, rest pain and ulcer) I70.363
              intermittent claudication I70.313
              rest pain (and intermittent claudication) I70.323
            specified type NEC I70.393
          left I70.302
            with
              gangrene (and intermittent claudication, rest pain and ulcer) I70.362
              intermittent claudication I70.312
              rest pain (and intermittent claudication) I70.322
              ulceration (and intermittent claudication and rest pain) I70.349
                ankle I70.343
                calf I70.342
                foot site NEC I70.345
                heel I70.344
                lower leg NEC I70.348
                midfoot I70.344
                thigh I70.341
            specified type NEC I70.392
          right I70.301
            with
              gangrene (and intermittent claudication, rest pain and ulcer) I70.361
              intermittent claudication I70.311
              rest pain (and intermittent claudication) I70.321
              ulceration (and intermittent claudication and rest pain I70.339
                ankle I70.333
                calf I70.332
                foot site NEC I70.335
                heel I70.334
                lower leg NEC I70.338
                midfoot I70.334
                thigh I70.331
            specified type NEC I70.391
        specified type NEC I70.399
      nonautologous biological graft I70.509
        leg I70.509
          with
            gangrene (and intermittent claudication, rest pain and ulcer) I70.569
            intermittent claudication I70.519
            rest pain (and intermittent claudication) I70.529
          bilateral I70.503

Arteriosclerosis, arteriosclerotic — *continued*
  extremities — *continued*
    bypass graft — *continued*
      nonautologous biological graft — *continued*
        leg — *continued*
          bilateral — *continued*
            with
              gangrene (and intermittent claudication, rest pain and ulcer) I70.563
              intermittent claudication I70.513
              rest pain (and intermittent claudication) I70.523
            specified type NEC I70.593
          left I70.502
            with
              gangrene (and intermittent claudication, rest pain and ulcer) I70.562
              intermittent claudication I70.512
              rest pain (and intermittent claudication) I70.522
              ulceration (and intermittent claudication and rest pain) I70.549
                ankle I70.543
                calf I70.542
                foot site NEC I70.545
                heel I70.544
                lower leg NEC I70.548
                midfoot I70.544
                thigh I70.541
            specified type NEC I70.592
          right I70.501
            with
              gangrene (and intermittent claudication, rest pain and ulcer) I70.561
              intermittent claudication I70.511
              rest pain (and intermittent claudication) I70.521
              ulceration (and intermittent claudication and rest pain) I70.539
                ankle I70.533
                calf I70.532
                foot site NEC I70.535
                heel I70.534
                lower leg NEC I70.538
                midfoot I70.534
                thigh I70.531
            specified type NEC I70.591
        specified type NEC I70.599
        specified NEC I70.508
          with
            gangrene (and intermittent claudication, rest pain and ulcer) I70.568
            intermittent claudication I70.518
            rest pain (and intermittent claudication) I70.528
            ulceration (and intermittent claudication and rest pain) I70.55
        specified type NEC I70.598
      nonbiological graft I70.609
        leg I70.609
          with
            gangrene (and intermittent claudication, rest pain and ulcer) I70.669
            intermittent claudication I70.619
            rest pain (and intermittent claudication) I70.629
          bilateral I70.603
            with
              gangrene (and intermittent claudication, rest pain and ulcer) I70.663
              intermittent claudication I70.613
              rest pain (and intermittent claudication) I70.623
            specified type NEC I70.693
          left I70.602
            with
              gangrene (and intermittent claudication, rest pain and ulcer) I70.662
              intermittent claudication I70.612

Arteriosclerosis, arteriosclerotic — *continued*
  extremities — *continued*
    bypass graft — *continued*
      nonbiological graft — *continued*
        leg — *continued*
          left — *continued*
            with — *continued*
              rest pain (and intermittent claudication) I70.622
              ulceration (and intermittent claudication and rest pain) I70.649
                ankle I70.643
                calf I70.642
                foot site NEC I70.645
                heel I70.644
                lower leg NEC I70.648
                midfoot I70.644
                thigh I70.641
            specified type NEC I70.692
          right I70.601
            with
              gangrene (and intermittent claudication, rest pain and ulcer) I70.661
              intermittent claudication I70.611
              rest pain (and intermittent claudication) I70.621
              ulceration (and intermittent claudication and rest pain) I70.639
                ankle I70.633
                calf I70.632
                foot site NEC I70.635
                heel I70.634
                lower leg NEC I70.638
                midfoot I70.634
                thigh I70.631
            specified type NEC I70.691
        specified type NEC I70.699
        specified NEC I70.608
          with
            gangrene (and intermittent claudication, rest pain and ulcer) I70.668
            intermittent claudication I70.618
            rest pain (and intermittent claudication) I70.628
            ulceration (and intermittent claudication and rest pain) I70.65
        specified type NEC I70.698
      specified graft NEC I70.709
        leg I70.709
          with
            gangrene (and intermittent claudication, rest pain and ulcer) I70.769
            intermittent claudication I70.719
            rest pain (and intermittent claudication) I70.729
          bilateral I70.703
            with
              gangrene (and intermittent claudication, rest pain and ulcer) I70.763
              intermittent claudication I70.713
              rest pain (and intermittent claudication) I70.723
            specified type NEC I70.793
          left I70.702
            with
              gangrene (and intermittent claudication, rest pain and ulcer) I70.762
              intermittent claudication I70.712
              rest pain (and intermittent claudication) I70.722
              ulceration (and intermittent claudication and rest pain) I70.749
                ankle I70.743
                calf I70.742
                foot site NEC I70.745
                heel I70.744
                lower leg NEC I70.748
                midfoot I70.744
                thigh I70.741
            specified type NEC I70.792
          right I70.701

Arteriosclerosis, arteriosclerotic — *continued*
  extremities — *continued*
    bypass graft — *continued*
      specified graft — *continued*
        leg — *continued*
          right — *continued*
            with
              gangrene (and intermittent claudication, rest pain and ulcer) I70.761
              intermittent claudication I70.711
              rest pain (and intermittent claudication) I70.721
              ulceration (and intermittent claudication and rest pain) I70.739
                ankle I70.733
                calf I70.732
                foot site NEC I70.735
                heel I70.734
                lower leg NEC I70.738
                midfoot I70.734
                thigh I70.731
            specified type NEC I70.791
        specified type NEC I70.799
      specified NEC I70.708
        with
          gangrene (and intermittent claudication, rest pain and ulcer) I70.768
          intermittent claudication I70.718
          rest pain (and intermittent claudication) I70.728
          ulceration (and intermittent claudication and rest pain) I70.75
          specified type NEC I70.798
    specified NEC I70.308
      with
        gangrene (and intermittent claudication, rest pain and ulcer) I70.368
        intermittent claudication I70.318
        rest pain (and intermittent claudication) I70.328
        ulceration (and intermittent claudication and rest pain) I70.35
        specifiec type NEC I70.398
  leg I70.209
    with
      gangrene (and intermittent claudication, rest pain and ulcer) I70.269
      intermittent claudication I70.219
      rest pain (and intermittent claudication) I70.229
    bilateral I70.203
      with
        gangrene (and intermittent claudication, rest pain and ulcer) I70.263
        intermittent claudication I70.213
        rest pain (and intermittent claudication) I70.223
      specified type NEC I70.293
    left I70.202
      with
        gangrene (and intermittent claudication, rest pain and ulcer) I70.262
        intermittent claudication I70.212
        rest pain (and intermittent claudication) I70.222
        ulceration (and intermittent claudication and rest pain) I70.249
          ankle I70.243
          calf I70.242
          foot site NEC I70.245
          heel I70.244
          lower leg NEC I70.248
          midfoot I70.244
          thigh I70.241
      specified type NEC I70.292
    right I70.201
      with
        gangrene (and intermittent claudication, rest pain and ulcer) I70.261
        intermittent claudication I70.211
        rest pain (and intermittent claudication) I70.221
        ulceration (and intermittent claudication and rest pain) I70.239
          ankle I70.233
          calf I70.232

Arteriosclerosis, arteriosclerotic — *continued*
  extremities — *continued*
    leg — *continued*
      right — *continued*
        with — *continued*
          ulceration — *continued*
            foot site NEC I70.235
            heel I70.234
            lower leg NEC I70.238
            midfoot I70.234
            thigh I70.231
          specified type NEC I70.291
      specified type NEC I70.299
    specified site NEC I70.208
      with
        gangrene (and intermittent claudication, rest pain and ulcer) I70.268
        intermittent claudication I70.218
        rest pain (and intermittent claudication) I70.228
        ulceration (and intermittent claudication and rest pain) I70.25
      specified type NEC I70.298
  generalized I70.91
  heart (disease) — *see* Arteriosclerosis, coronary (artery),
  kidney — *see* Hypertension, kidney
  medial — *see* Arteriosclerosis, extremities
  mesenteric (artery) K55.1
  Mönckeberg's — *see* Arteriosclerosis, extremities
  myocarditis I51.4
  peripheral (of extremities) — *see* Arteriosclerosis, extremities
  pulmonary (idiopathic) I27.0
  renal (arterioles) (*see also* Hypertension, kidney)
    artery I70.1
  retina (vascular) I70.8 [H35.0-] ☑
  specified artery NEC I70.8
  spinal (cord) G95.19
  vertebral (artery) I67.2
Arteriospasm I73.9
Arteriovenous — *see* condition
Arteritis I77.6
  allergic M31.0
  aorta (nonsyphilitic) I77.6
    syphilitic A52.02
  aortic arch M31.4
  brachiocephalic M31.4
  brain I67.7
    syphilitic A52.04
  cerebral I67.7
    in systemic lupus erythematosus M32.19
    listerial A32.89
    syphilitic A52.04
    tuberculous A18.89
  coronary (artery) I25.89
    rheumatic I01.8
      chronic I09.89
    syphilitic A52.06
  cranial (left) (right), giant cell M31.6
  deformans — *see* Arteriosclerosis
  giant cell NEC M31.6
    with polymyalgia rheumatica M31.5
  necrosing or necrotizing M31.9
    specified NEC M31.8
  nodosa M30.0
  obliterans — *see* Arteriosclerosis
  pulmonary I28.8
  rheumatic — *see* Fever, rheumatic
  senile — *see* Arteriosclerosis
  suppurative I77.2
  syphilitic (general) A52.09
    brain A52.04
    coronary A52.06
    spinal A52.09
  temporal, giant cell M31.6
  young female aortic arch syndrome M31.4
Artery, arterial (*see also* condition)
  abscess I77.89
  single umbilical Q27.0
Arthralgia (allergic) (*see also* Pain, joint)
  in caisson disease T70.3 ☑
  temporomandibular M26.62- ☑
Arthritis, arthritic (acute) (chronic) (nonpyogenic) (subacute) M19.90
  allergic — *see* Arthritis, specified form NEC
  ankylosing (crippling) (spine) (*see also* Spondylitis, ankylosing)

Arthritis, arthritic — *continued*
  ankylosing (*see also* Spondylitis, ankylosing) — *continued*
    sites other than spine — *see* Arthritis, specified form NEC
  atrophic — *see* Osteoarthritis
    spine — *see* Spondylitis, ankylosing
  back — *see* Spondylopathy, inflammatory
  blennorrhagic (gonococcal) A54.42
  Charcot's — *see* Arthropathy, neuropathic
    diabetic — *see* Diabetes, arthropathy, neuropathic
    syringomyelic G95.0
  chylous (filarial) (*see also* category M01) B74.9
  climacteric (any site) NEC — *see* Arthritis, specified form NEC
  crystal (-induced) — *see* Arthritis, in, crystals
  deformans — *see* Osteoarthritis
  degenerative — *see* Osteoarthritis
  due to or associated with
    acromegaly E22.0
    brucellosis — *see* Brucellosis
    caisson disease T70.3 ☑
    diabetes — *see* Diabetes, arthropathy
    dracontiasis (*see also* category M01) B72
    enteritis NEC
      regional — *see* Enteritis, regional
    erysipelas (*see also* category M01) A46
    erythema
      epidemic A25.1
      nodosum L52
    filariasis NOS B74.9
    glanders A24.0
    helminthiasis (*see also* category M01) B83.9
    hemophilia D66 [M36.2]
    Henoch- (Schönlein) purpura D69.0 [M36.4]
    human parvovirus (*see also* category M01) B97.6
    infectious disease NEC M01 ☑
    leprosy (*see also* category M01) (*see also* Leprosy) A30.9
    Lyme disease A69.23
    mycobacteria (*see also* category M01) A31.8
    parasitic disease NEC (*see also* category M01) B89
    paratyphoid fever (*see also* category M01) (*see also* Fever, paratyphoid) A01.4
    rat bite fever (*see also* category M01) A25.1
    regional enteritis — *see* Enteritis, regional
    respiratory disorder NOS J98.9
    serum sickness (*see also* Reaction, serum) T80.69 ☑
    syringomyelia G95.0
    typhoid fever A01.04
  epidemic erythema A25.1
  febrile — *see* Fever, rheumatic
  gonococcal A54.42
  gouty (acute) — *see* Gout
  in (due to)
    acromegaly (*see also* subcategory M14.8-) E22.0
    amyloidosis (*see also* subcategory M14.8-) E85.4
    bacterial disease (*see also* subcategory M01) A49.9
    Behçet's syndrome M35.2
    caisson disease (*see also* subcategory M14.8-) T70.3 ☑
    coliform bacilli (Escherichia coli) — *see* Arthritis, in, pyogenic organism NEC
    crystals M11.9
      dicalcium phosphate — *see* Arthritis, in, crystals, specified type NEC
      hydroxyapatite M11.0- ☑
      pyrophosphate — *see* Arthritis, in, crystals, specified type NEC
      specified type NEC M11.80
        ankle M11.87- ☑
        elbow M11.82- ☑
        foot joint M11.87- ☑
        hand joint M11.84- ☑
        hip M11.85- ☑
        knee M11.86- ☑
        multiple sites M11.8- ☑
        shoulder M11.81- ☑
        vertebrae M11.88
        wrist M11.83- ☑
    dermatoarthritis, lipoid E78.81
    dracontiasis (dracunculiasis) (*see also* category M01) B72
    endocrine disorder NEC (*see also* subcategory M14.8-) E34.9
    enteritis, infectious NEC (*see also* category M01) A09

Arthritis, arthritic — *continued*
  in — *continued*
    enteritis, infectious (*see also* category M01) — *continued*
      specified organism NEC (*see also* category M01) A08.8
    erythema
      multiforme (*see also* subcategory M14.8-) L51.9
      nodosum (*see also* subcategory M14.8-) L52
    gout — *see* Gout
    helminthiasis NEC (*see also* category M01) B83.9
    hemochromatosis (*see also* subcategory M14.8-) E83.118
    hemoglobinopathy NEC D58.2 [M36.3]
    hemophilia NEC D66 [M36.2]
    Hemophilus influenzae M00.8- ☑ [B96.3]
    Henoch (-Schönlein) purpura D69.0 [M36.4]
    hyperparathyroidism NEC (*see also* subcategory M14.8-) E21.3
    hypersensitivity reaction NEC T78.49 ☑ [M36.4]
    hypogammaglobulinemia (*see also* subcategory M14.8-) D80.1
    hypothyroidism NEC (*see also* subcategory M14.8-) E03.9
    infection — *see* Arthritis, pyogenic or pyemic
      spine — *see* Spondylopathy, infective
    infectious disease NEC M01 ☑
    leprosy (*see also* category M01) A30.9
    leukemia NEC C95.9- ☑ [M36.1]
    lipoid dermatoarthritis E78.81
    Lyme disease A69.23
    Mediterranean fever, familial (*see also* subcategory M14.8-) M04.1
    Meningococcus A39.83
    metabolic disorder NEC (*see also* subcategory M14.8-) E88.9
    multiple myelomatosis C90.0- ☑ [M36.1]
    mumps B26.85
    mycosis NEC (*see also* category M01) B49
    myelomatosis (multiple) C90.0- ☑ [M36.1]
    neurological disorder NEC G98.0
    ochronosis (*see also* subcategory M14.8-) E70.29
    O'nyong-nyong (*see also* category M01) A92.1
    parasitic disease NEC (*see also* category M01) B89
    paratyphoid fever (*see also* category M01) A01.4
    Pseudomonas — *see* Arthritis, pyogenic, bacterial NEC
    psoriasis L40.50
    pyogenic organism NEC — *see* Arthritis, pyogenic, bacterial NEC
    Reiter's disease — *see* Reiter's disease
    respiratory disorder NEC (*see also* subcategory M14.8-) J98.9
    reticulosis, malignant (*see also* subcategory M14.8-) C86.0
    rubella B06.82
    Salmonella (arizonae) (cholerae-suis) (enteritidis) (typhimurium) A02.23
    sarcoidosis D86.86
    specified bacteria NEC — *see* Arthritis, pyogenic, bacterial NEC
    sporotrichosis B42.82
    syringomyelia G95.0
    thalassemia NEC D56.9 [M36.3]
    tuberculosis — *see* Tuberculosis, arthritis
    typhoid fever A01.04
    urethritis, Reiter's — *see* Reiter's disease
    viral disease NEC (*see also* category M01) B34.9
  infectious or infective (*see also* Arthritis, pyogenic or pyemic)
    spine — *see* Spondylopathy, infective
  juvenile M08.90
    with systemic onset — *see* Still's disease
    ankle M08.97- ☑
    elbow M08.92- ☑
    foot joint M08.97- ☑
    hand joint M08.94- ☑
    hip M08.95- ☑
    knee M08.96- ☑
    multiple site M08.99
    pauciarticular M08.40
      ankle M08.47- ☑
      elbow M08.42- ☑
      foot joint M08.47- ☑
      hand joint M08.44- ☑
      hip M08.45- ☑
      knee M08.46- ☑

Arthritis, arthritic — *continued*
  juvenile — *continued*
    pauciarticular — *continued*
      shoulder M08.41- ☑
      vertebrae M08.48
      wrist M08.43- ☑
    psoriatic L40.54
    rheumatoid — *see* Arthritis, rheumatoid, juvenile
    shoulder M08.91- ☑
    specified type NEC M08.80
      ankle M08.87- ☑
      elbow M08.82- ☑
      foot joint M08.87- ☑
      hand joint M08.84- ☑
      hip M08.85- ☑
      knee M08.86- ☑
      multiple site M08.89
      shoulder M08.81- ☑
      specified joint NEC M08.88
      vertebrae M08.88
      wrist M08.83- ☑
    wrist M08.93- ☑
  meaning osteoarthritis — *see* Osteoarthritis
  meningococcal A39.83
  menopausal (any site) NEC — *see* Arthritis, specified form NEC
  mutilans (psoriatic) L40.52
  mycotic NEC (*see also* category M01) B49
  neuropathic (Charcot) — *see* Arthropathy, neuropathic
    diabetic — *see* Diabetes, arthropathy, neuropathic
    nonsyphilitic NEC G98.0
    syringomyelic G95.0
  ochronotic (*see also* subcategory M14.8-) E70.29
  palindromic (any site) — *see* Rheumatism, palindromic
  pneumococcal M00.10
    ankle M00.17- ☑
    elbow M00.12- ☑
    foot joint — *see* Arthritis, pneumococcal, ankle
    hand joint M00.14- ☑
    hip M00.15- ☑
    knee M00.16- ☑
    multiple site M00.19
    shoulder M00.11- ☑
    vertebra M00.18
    wrist M00.13- ☑
  postdysenteric — *see* Arthropathy, postdysenteric
  postmeningococcal A39.84
  postrheumatic, chronic — *see* Arthropathy, postrheumatic, chronic
  primary progressive (*see also* Arthritis, specified form NEC)
    spine — *see* Spondylitis, ankylosing
  psoriatic L40.50
  purulent (any site except spine) — *see* Arthritis, pyogenic or pyemic
    spine — *see* Spondylopathy, infective
  pyogenic or pyemic (any site except spine) M00.9
    bacterial NEC M00.80
      ankle M00.87- ☑
      elbow M00.82- ☑
      foot joint — *see* Arthritis, pyogenic, bacterial NEC, ankle
      hand joint M00.84- ☑
      hip M00.85- ☑
      knee M00.86- ☑
      multiple site M00.89
      shoulder M00.81- ☑
      vertebra M00.88
      wrist M00.83- ☑
    pneumococcal — *see* Arthritis, pneumococcal
    spine — *see* Spondylopathy, infective
    staphylococcal — *see* Arthritis, staphylococcal
    streptococcal — *see* Arthritis, streptococcal NEC
      pneumococcal — *see* Arthritis, pneumococcal
  reactive — *see* Reiter's disease
  rheumatic (*see also* Arthritis, rheumatoid)
    acute or subacute — *see* Fever, rheumatic
  rheumatoid M06.9
    with
      carditis — *see* Rheumatoid, carditis
      endocarditis — *see* Rheumatoid, carditis
      heart involvement NEC — *see* Rheumatoid, carditis
      lung involvement — *see* Rheumatoid, lung
      myocarditis — *see* Rheumatoid, carditis
      myopathy — *see* Rheumatoid, myopathy
      pericarditis — *see* Rheumatoid, carditis

Arthritis, arthritic — *continued*
  rheumatoid — *continued*
    with — *continued*
      polyneuropathy — *see* Rheumatoid, polyneuropathy
      rheumatoid factor — *see* Arthritis, rheumatoid, seropositive
      splenoadenomegaly and leukopenia — *see* Felty's syndrome
      vasculitis — *see* Rheumatoid, vasculitis
      visceral involvement NEC — *see* Rheumatoid, arthritis, with involvement of organs NEC
    juvenile (with or without rheumatoid factor) M08.00
      ankle M08.07- ☑
      elbow M08.02- ☑
      foot joint M08.07- ☑
      hand joint M08.04- ☑
      hip M08.05- ☑
      knee M08.06- ☑
      multiple site M08.09
      shoulder M08.01- ☑
      vertebra M08.08
      wrist M08.03- ☑
    seronegative M06.00
      ankle M06.07- ☑
      elbow M06.02- ☑
      foot joint M06.07- ☑
      hand joint M06.04- ☑
      hip M06.05- ☑
      knee M06.06- ☑
      multiple site M06.09
      shoulder M06.01- ☑
      vertebra M06.08
      wrist M06.03- ☑
    seropositive M05.9
      without organ involvement M05.70
        ankle M05.77- ☑
        elbow M05.72- ☑
        foot joint M05.77- ☑
        hand joint M05.74- ☑
        hip M05.75- ☑
        knee M05.76- ☑
        multiple sites M05.79
        shoulder M05.71- ☑
        vertebra — *see* Spondylitis, ankylosing
        wrist M05.73- ☑
      specified NEC M05.80
        ankle M05.87- ☑
        elbow M05.82- ☑
        foot joint M05.87- ☑
        hand joint M05.84- ☑
        hip M05.85- ☑
        knee M05.86- ☑
        multiple sites M05.89
        shoulder M05.81- ☑
        vertebra — *see* Spondylitis, ankylosing
        wrist M05.83- ☑
    specified type NEC M06.80
      ankle M06.87- ☑
      elbow M06.82- ☑
      foot joint M06.87- ☑
      hand joint M06.84- ☑
      hip M06.85- ☑
      knee M06.86- ☑
      multiple site M06.89
      shoulder M06.81- ☑
      vertebra M06.88
      wrist M06.83- ☑
    spine — *see* Spondylitis, ankylosing
  rubella B06.82
  scorbutic (*see also* subcategory M14.8-) E54
  senile or senescent — *see* Osteoarthritis
  septic (any site except spine) — *see* Arthritis, pyogenic or pyemic
    spine — *see* Spondylopathy, infective
  serum (nontherapeutic) (therapeutic) — *see* Arthropathy, postimmunization
  specified form NEC M13.80
    ankle M13.87- ☑
    elbow M13.82- ☑
    foot joint M13.87- ☑
    hand joint M13.84- ☑
    hip M13.85- ☑
    knee M13.86- ☑
    multiple site M13.89

Arthritis, arthritic — *continued*
  specified form — *continued*
    shoulder M13.81- ☑
    specified joint NEC M13.88
    wrist M13.83- ☑
  spine (*see also* Spondylopathy, inflammatory)
    infectious or infective NEC — *see* Spondylopathy, infective
    Marie-Strümpell — *see* Spondylitis, ankylosing
    pyogenic — *see* Spondylopathy, infective
    rheumatoid — *see* Spondylitis, ankylosing
    traumatic (old) — *see* Spondylopathy, traumatic
    tuberculous A18.01
  staphylococcal M00.00
    ankle M00.07- ☑
    elbow M00.02- ☑
    foot joint — *see* Arthritis, staphylococcal, ankle
    hand joint M00.04- ☑
    hip M00.05- ☑
    knee M00.06- ☑
    multiple site M00.09
    shoulder M00.01- ☑
    vertebra M00.08
    wrist M00.03- ☑
  streptococcal NEC M00.20
    ankle M00.27- ☑
    elbow M00.22- ☑
    foot joint — *see* Arthritis, streptococcal, ankle
    hand joint M00.24- ☑
    hip M00.25- ☑
    knee M00.26- ☑
    multiple site M00.29
    shoulder M00.21- ☑
    vertebra M00.28
    wrist M00.23- ☑
  suppurative — *see* Arthritis, pyogenic or pyemic
  syphilitic (late) A52.16
    congenital A50.55 [M12.80]
  syphilitica deformans (Charcot) A52.16
  temporomandibular M26.69
  toxic of menopause (any site) — *see* Arthritis, specified form NEC
  transient — *see* Arthropathy, specified form NEC
  traumatic (chronic) — *see* Arthropathy, traumatic
  tuberculous A18.02
    spine A18.01
  uratic — *see* Gout
  urethritica (Reiter's) — *see* Reiter's disease
  vertebral — *see* Spondylopathy, inflammatory
  villous (any site) — *see* Arthropathy, specified form NEC
Arthrocele — *see* Effusion, joint
Arthrodesis status Z98.1
Arthrodynia (*see also* Pain, joint)
Arthrodysplasia Q74.9
Arthrofibrosis, joint — *see* Ankylosis
Arthrogryposis (congenital) Q68.8
  multiplex congenita Q74.3
Arthrokatadysis M24.7
Arthropathy (*see also* Arthritis) M12.9
  Charcot's — *see* Arthropathy, neuropathic
    diabetic — *see* Diabetes, arthropathy, neuropathic
    syringomyelic G95.0
  cricoarytenoid J38.7
  crystal (-induced) — *see* Arthritis, in, crystals
  diabetic NEC — *see* Diabetes, arthropathy
  distal interphalangeal, psoriatic L40.51
  enteropathic M07.60
    ankle M07.67- ☑
    elbow M07.62- ☑
    foot joint M07.67- ☑
    hand joint M07.64- ☑
    hip M07.65- ☑
    knee M07.66- ☑
    multiple site M07.69
    shoulder M07.61- ☑
    vertebra M07.68
    wrist M07.63- ☑
  following intestinal bypass M02.00
    ankle M02.07- ☑
    elbow M02.02- ☑
    foot joint M02.07- ☑
    hand joint M02.04- ☑
    hip M02.05- ☑
    knee M02.06- ☑
    multiple site M02.09
    shoulder M02.01- ☑

Arthropathy — *continued*
  following intestinal bypass — *continued*
    vertebra M02.08
    wrist M02.03- ☑
  gouty (*see also* Gout)
    in (due to)
      Lesch-Nyhan syndrome E79.1 [M14.8-] ☑
      sickle-cell disorders D57- [M14.8-] ☑
  hemophilic NEC D66 [M36.2]
    in (due to)
      hyperparathyroidism NEC E21.3 [M14.8-] ☑
      metabolic disease NOS E88.9 [M14.8-] ☑
  in (due to)
    acromegaly E22.0 [M14.8-] ☑
    amyloidosis E85.4 [M14.8-] ☑
    blood disorder NOS D75.9 [M36.3]
    diabetes — *see* Diabetes, arthropathy
    endocrine disease NOS E34.9 [M14.8-] ☑
    erythema
      multiforme L51.9 [M14.8-] ☑
      nodosum L52 [M14.8-] ☑
    hemochromatosis E83.118 [M14.8-] ☑
    hemoglobinopathy NEC D58.2 [M36.3]
    hemophilia NEC D66 [M36.2]
    Henoch-Schönlein purpura D69.0 [M36.4]
    hyperthyroidism E05.90 [M14.8-] ☑
    hypothyroidism E03.9 [M14.8-] ☑
    infective endocarditis I33.0 [M12.80]
    leukemia NEC C95.9- ☑ [M36.1]
    malignant histiocytosis C96.A [M36.1]
    metabolic disease NOS E88.9 [M14.8-] ☑
    multiple myeloma C90.0- ☑ [M36.1]
    neoplastic disease NOS (*see also* Neoplasm) D49.9 [M36.1]
    nutritional deficiency (*see also* subcategory M14.8-) E63.9
    psoriasis NOS L40.50
    sarcoidosis D86.86
    syphilis (late) A52.77
      congenital A50.55 [M12.80]
    thyrotoxicosis (*see also* subcategory M14.8-) E05.90
    ulcerative colitis K51.90 [M07.60]
    viral hepatitis (postinfectious) NEC B19.9 [M12.80]
    Whipple's disease (*see also* subcategory M14.8-) K90.81
  Jaccoud — *see* Arthropathy, postrheumatic, chronic
  juvenile — *see* Arthritis, juvenile
    psoriatic L40.54
  mutilans (psoriatic) L40.52
  neuropathic (Charcot) M14.60
    ankle M14.67- ☑
    diabetic — *see* Diabetes, arthropathy, neuropathic
    elbow M14.62- ☑
    foot joint M14.67- ☑
    hand joint M14.64- ☑
    hip M14.65- ☑
    knee M14.66- ☑
    multiple site M14.69
    nonsyphilitic NEC G98.0
    shoulder M14.61- ☑
    syringomyelic G95.0
    vertebra M14.68
    wrist M14.63- ☑
  osteopulmonary — *see* Osteoarthropathy, hypertrophic, specified NEC
  postdysenteric M02.10
    ankle M02.17- ☑
    elbow M02.12- ☑
    foot joint M02.17- ☑
    hand joint M02.14- ☑
    hip M02.15- ☑
    knee M02.16- ☑
    multiple site M02.19
    shoulder M02.11- ☑
    vertebra M02.18
    wrist M02.13- ☑
  postimmunization M02.20
    ankle M02.27- ☑
    elbow M02.22- ☑
    foot joint M02.27- ☑
    hand joint M02.24- ☑
    hip M02.25- ☑
    knee M02.26- ☑
    multiple site M02.29
    shoulder M02.21- ☑
    vertebra M02.28
    wrist M02.23- ☑

Arthropathy — *continued*
  postinfectious NEC B99 ☑ [M12.80]
    in (due to)
      enteritis due to Yersinia enterocolitica A04.6 [M12.80]
      syphilis A52.77
      viral hepatitis NEC B19.9 [M12.80]
  postrheumatic, chronic (Jaccoud) M12.00
    ankle M12.07- ☑
    elbow M12.02- ☑
    foot joint M12.07- ☑
    hand joint M12.04- ☑
    hip M12.05- ☑
    knee M12.06- ☑
    multiple site M12.09
    shoulder M12.01- ☑
    specified joint NEC M12.08
    vertebrae M12.08
    wrist M12.03- ☑
  psoriatic NEC L40.59
    interphalangeal, distal L40.51
  reactive M02.9
    in (due to)
      infective endocarditis I33.0 [M02.9]
    specified type NEC M02.80
      ankle M02.87- ☑
      elbow M02.82- ☑
      foot joint M02.87- ☑
      hand joint M02.84- ☑
      hip M02.85- ☑
      knee M02.86- ☑
      multiple site M02.89
      shoulder M02.81- ☑
      vertebra M02.88
      wrist M02.83- ☑
  specified form NEC M12.80
    ankle M12.87- ☑
    elbow M12.82- ☑
    foot joint M12.87- ☑
    hand joint M12.84- ☑
    hip M12.85- ☑
    knee M12.86- ☑
    multiple site M12.89
    shoulder M12.81- ☑
    specified joint NEC M12.88
    vertebrae M12.88
    wrist M12.83- ☑
  syringomyelic G95.0
  tabes dorsalis A52.16
  tabetic A52.16
  transient — *see* Arthropathy, specified form NEC
  traumatic M12.50
    ankle M12.57- ☑
    elbow M12.52- ☑
    foot joint M12.57- ☑
    hand joint M12.54- ☑
    hip M12.55- ☑
    knee M12.56- ☑
    multiple site M12.59
    shoulder M12.51- ☑
    specified joint NEC M12.58
    vertebrae M12.58
    wrist M12.53- ☑
Arthropyosis — *see* Arthritis, pyogenic or pyemic
Arthrosis (deformans) (degenerative) (localized) (*see also* Osteoarthritis) M19.90
  spine — *see* Spondylosis
Arthus' phenomenon or reaction T78.41 ☑
  due to
    drug — *see* Table of Drugs and Chemicals, by drug
Articular — *see* condition
Articulation, reverse (teeth) M26.24
Artificial
  insemination complication — *see* Complications, artificial, fertilization
  opening status (functioning) (without complication) Z93.9
    anus (colostomy) Z93.3
    colostomy Z93.3
    cystostomy Z93.50
      appendico-vesicostomy Z93.52
      cutaneous Z93.51
      specified NEC Z93.59
    enterostomy Z93.4
    gastrostomy Z93.1
    ileostomy Z93.2
    intestinal tract NEC Z93.4

Artificial — *continued*
  opening status — *continued*
    jejunostomy Z93.4
    nephrostomy Z93.6
    specified site NEC Z93.8
    tracheostomy Z93.0
    ureterostomy Z93.6
    urethrostomy Z93.6
    urinary tract NEC Z93.6
    vagina Z93.8
    vagina status Z93.8
Arytenoid — *see* condition
Asbestosis (occupational) J61
Ascariasis B77.9
  with
    complications NEC B77.89
    intestinal complications B77.0
    pneumonia, pneumonitis B77.81
Ascaridosis, ascaridiasis — *see* Ascariasis
Ascaris (infection) (infestation) (lumbricoides) — *see* Ascariasis
Ascending — *see* condition
ASC-H (atypical squamous cells cannot exclude high grade squamous intraepithelial lesion on cytologic smear)
  anus R85.611
  cervix R87.611
  vagina R87.621
Aschoff's bodies — *see* Myocarditis, rheumatic
Ascites (abdominal) R18.8
  cardiac (*see also* Failure, heart, right) I50.810
  chylous (nonfilarial) I89.8
    filarial — *see* Infestation, filarial
  due to
    cirrhosis, alcoholic K70.31
    hepatitis
      alcoholic K70.11
      chronic active K71.51
    S. japonicum B65.2
  heart (*see also* Failure, heart, right) I50.810
  malignant R18.0
  pseudochylous R18.8
  syphilitic A52.74
  tuberculous A18.31
ASC-US (atypical squamous cells of undetermined significance on cytologic smear)
  anus R85.610
  cervix R87.610
  vagina R87.620
Aseptic — *see* condition
Asherman's syndrome N85.6
Asialia K11.7
Asiatic cholera — *see* Cholera
Asimultagnosia (simultanagnosia) R48.3
Askin's tumor — *see* Neoplasm, connective tissue, malignant
Asocial personality F60.2
Asomatognosia R41.4
Aspartylglucosaminuria E77.1
Asperger's disease or syndrome F84.5
Aspergilloma — *see* Aspergillosis
Aspergillosis (with pneumonia) B44.9
  bronchopulmonary, allergic B44.81
  disseminated B44.7
  generalized B44.7
  pulmonary NEC B44.1
    allergic B44.81
    invasive B44.0
  specified NEC B44.89
  tonsillar B44.2
Aspergillus (flavus) (fumigatus) (infection) (terreus) — *see* Aspergillosis
Aspermatogenesis — *see* Azoospermia
Aspermia (testis) — *see* Azoospermia
Asphyxia, asphyxiation (by) R09.01
  antenatal P84
  birth P84
  bunny bag — *see* Asphyxia, due to, mechanical threat to breathing, trapped in bed clothes
  crushing S28.0 ☑
  drowning T75.1 ☑
  gas, fumes, or vapor — *see* Table of Drugs and Chemicals
  inhalation — *see* Inhalation
  intrauterine P84
  local I73.00
    with gangrene I73.01

Asphyxia, asphyxiation — *continued*
  mucus (*see also* Foreign body, respiratory tract, causing asphyxia)
  newborn P84
  pathological R09.01
  postnatal P84
    mechanical — *see* Asphyxia, due to, mechanical threat to breathing
  prenatal P84
  reticularis R23.1
  strangulation — *see* Asphyxia, due to, mechanical threat to breathing
  submersion T75.1 ☑
  traumatic T71.9 ☑
    due to
      crushed chest S28.0 ☑
      foreign body (in) — *see* Foreign body, respiratory tract, causing asphyxia
      low oxygen content of ambient air T71.20 ☑
        due to
          being trapped in
            low oxygen environment T71.29 ☑
            in car trunk T71.221 ☑
              circumstances undetermined T71.224 ☑
              done with intent to harm by
                another person T71.223 ☑
                self T71.222 ☑
            in refrigerator T71.231 ☑
              circumstances undetermined T71.234 ☑
              done with intent to harm by
                another person T71.233 ☑
                self T71.232 ☑
        cave-in T71.21 ☑
      mechanical threat to breathing (accidental) T71.191 ☑
        circumstances undetermined T71.194 ☑
        done with intent to harm by
          another person T71.193 ☑
          self T71.192 ☑
        hanging T71.161 ☑
          circumstances undetermined T71.164 ☑
          done with intent to harm by
            another person T71.163 ☑
            self T71.162 ☑
        plastic bag T71.121 ☑
          circumstances undetermined T71.124 ☑
          done with intent to harm by
            another person T71.123 ☑
            self T71.122 ☑
        smothering
          in furniture T71.151 ☑
            circumstances undetermined T71.154 ☑
            done with intent to harm by
              another person T71.153 ☑
              self T71.152 ☑
          under
            another person's body T71.141 ☑
              circumstances undetermined T71.144 ☑
              done with intent to harm T71.143 ☑
            pillow T71.111 ☑
              circumstances undetermined T71.114 ☑
              done with intent to harm by
                another person T71.113 ☑
                self T71.112 ☑
        trapped in bed clothes T71.131 ☑
          circumstances undetermined T71.134 ☑
          done with intent to harm by
            another person T71.133 ☑
            self T71.132 ☑
  vomiting, vomitus — *see* Foreign body, respiratory tract, causing asphyxia
Aspiration
  amniotic (clear) fluid (newborn) P24.10
    with
      pneumonia (pneumonitis) P24.11
      respiratory symptoms P24.11
  blood
    newborn (without respiratory symptoms) P24.20
      with
        pneumonia (pneumonitis) P24.21
        respiratory symptoms P24.21

Aspiration — *continued*
  blood — *continued*
    specified age NEC — *see* Foreign body, respiratory tract
  bronchitis J69.0
  food or foreign body (with asphyxiation) — *see* Asphyxia, food
  liquor (amnii) (newborn) P24.10
    with
      pneumonia (pneumonitis) P24.11
      respiratory symptoms P24.11
  meconium (newborn) (without respiratory symptoms) P24.00
    with
      pneumonitis (pneumonitis) P24.01
      respiratory symptoms P24.01
  milk (newborn) (without respiratory symptoms) P24.30
    with
      pneumonia (pneumonitis) P24.31
      respiratory symptoms P24.31
    specified age NEC — *see* Foreign body, respiratory tract
  mucus (*see also* Foreign body, by site, causing asphyxia)
    newborn P24.10
      with
        pneumonia (pneumonitis) P24.11
        respiratory symptoms P24.11
  neonatal P24.9
    specific NEC (without respiratory symptoms) P24.80
      with
        pneumonia (pneumonitis) P24.81
        respiratory symptoms P24.81
  newborn P24.9
    specific NEC (without respiratory symptoms) P24.80
      with
        pneumonia (pneumonitis) P24.81
        respiratory symptoms P24.81
  pneumonia J69.0
  pneumonitis J69.0
  syndrome of newborn — *see* Aspiration, by substance, with pneumonia
  vernix caseosa (newborn) P24.80
    with
      pneumonia (pneumonitis) P24.81
      respiratory symptoms P24.81
  vomitus (*see also* Foreign body, respiratory tract)
    newborn (without respiratory symptoms) P24.30
      with
        pneumonia (pneumonitis) P24.31
        respiratory symptoms P24.31
Asplenia (congenital) Q89.01
  postsurgical Z90.81
Assam fever B55.0
Assault, sexual — *see* Maltreatment
Assmann's focus NEC A15.0
Astasia (-abasia) (hysterical) F44.4
Asteatosis cutis L85.3
Astereognosia, astereognosis R48.1
Asterixis R27.8
  in liver disease K71.3
Asteroid hyalitis — *see* Deposit, crystalline
Asthenia, asthenic R53.1
  cardiac (*see also* Failure, heart) I50.9
    psychogenic F45.8
  cardiovascular (*see also* Failure, heart) I50.9
    psychogenic F45.8
  heart (*see also* Failure, heart) I50.9
    psychogenic F45.8
  hysterical F44.4
  myocardial (*see also* Failure, heart) I50.9
    psychogenic F45.8
  nervous F48.8
  neurocirculatory F45.8
  neurotic F48.8
  psychogenic F48.8
  psychoneurotic F48.8
  psychophysiologic F48.8
  reaction (psychophysiologic) F48.8
  senile R54
Asthenopia (*see also* Discomfort, visual)
  hysterical F44.6
  psychogenic F44.6
Asthenospermia — *see* Abnormal, specimen, male genital organs
Asthma, asthmatic (bronchial) (catarrh) (spasmodic) J45.909

Asthma, asthmatic — *continued*
with
  chronic obstructive bronchitis J44.9
    with
      acute lower respiratory infection J44.0
      exacerbation (acute) J44.1
  chronic obstructive pulmonary disease J44.9
    with
      acute lower respiratory infection J44.0
      exacerbation (acute) J44.1
  exacerbation (acute) J45.901
  hay fever — *see* Asthma, allergic extrinsic
  rhinitis, allergic — *see* Asthma, allergic extrinsic
  status asthmaticus J45.902
allergic extrinsic J45.909
  with
    exacerbation (acute) J45.901
    status asthmaticus J45.902
atopic — *see* Asthma, allergic extrinsic
cardiac — *see* Failure, ventricular, left
cardiobronchial I50.1
childhood J45.909
  with
    exacerbation (acute) J45.901
    status asthmaticus J45.902
chronic obstructive J44.9
  with
    acute lower respiratory infection J44.0
    exacerbation (acute) J44.1
collier's J60
cough variant J45.991
detergent J69.8
due to
  detergent J69.8
  inhalation of fumes J68.3
eosinophilic J82
extrinsic, allergic — *see* Asthma, allergic extrinsic
grinder's J62.8
hay — *see* Asthma, allergic extrinsic
heart I50.1
idiosyncratic — *see* Asthma, nonallergic
intermittent (mild) J45.20
  with
    exacerbation (acute) J45.21
    status asthmaticus J45.22
intrinsic, nonallergic — *see* Asthma, nonallergic
Kopp's E32.8
late-onset J45.909
  with
    exacerbation (acute) J45.901
    status asthmaticus J45.902
mild intermittent J45.20
  with
    exacerbation (acute) J45.21
    status asthmaticus J45.22
mild persistent J45.30
  with
    exacerbation (acute) J45.31
    status asthmaticus J45.32
Millar's (laryngismus stridulus) J38.5
miner's J60
mixed J45.909
  with
    exacerbation (acute) J45.901
    status asthmaticus J45.902
moderate persistent J45.40
  with
    exacerbation (acute) J45.41
    status asthmaticus J45.42
nervous — *see* Asthma, nonallergic
nonallergic (intrinsic) J45.909
  with
    exacerbation (acute) J45.901
    status asthmaticus J45.902
persistent
  mild J45.30
    with
      exacerbation (acute) J45.31
      status asthmaticus J45.32
  moderate J45.40
    with
      exacerbation (acute) J45.41
      status asthmaticus J45.42
  severe J45.50
    with
      exacerbation (acute) J45.51
      status asthmaticus J45.52
platinum J45.998

Asthma, asthmatic — *continued*
pneumoconiotic NEC J64
potter's J62.8
predominantly allergic J45.909
psychogenic F54
pulmonary eosinophilic J82
red cedar J67.8
Rostan's I50.1
sandblaster's J62.8
sequoiosis J67.8
severe persistent J45.50
  with
    exacerbation (acute) J45.51
    status asthmaticus J45.52
specified NEC J45.998
stonemason's J62.8
thymic E32.8
tuberculous — *see* Tuberculosis, pulmonary
Wichmann's (laryngismus stridulus) J38.5
wood J67.8
Astigmatism (compound) (congenital) H52.20- ☑
irregular H52.21- ☑
regular H52.22- ☑
Astraphobia F40.220
Astroblastoma
specified site — *see* Neoplasm, malignant, by site
unspecified site C71.9
Astrocytoma (cystic)
anaplastic
  specified site — *see* Neoplasm, malignant, by site
  unspecified site C71.9
fibrillary
  specified site — *see* Neoplasm, malignant, by site
  unspecified site C71.9
fibrous
  specified site — *see* Neoplasm, malignant, by site
  unspecified site C71.9
gemistocytic
  specified site — *see* Neoplasm, malignant, by site
  unspecified site C71.9
juvenile
  specified site — *see* Neoplasm, malignant, by site
  unspecified site C71.9
pilocytic
  specified site — *see* Neoplasm, malignant, by site
  unspecified site C71.9
piloid
  specified site — *see* Neoplasm, malignant, by site
  unspecified site C71.9
protoplasmic
  specified site — *see* Neoplasm, malignant, by site
  unspecified site C71.9
specified site NEC — *see* Neoplasm, malignant, by site
subependymal D43.2
  giant cell
    specified site — *see* Neoplasm, uncertain be-
      havior, by site
    unspecified site D43.2
  specified site — *see* Neoplasm, uncertain behavior,
    by site
  unspecified site D43.2
unspecified site C71.9
Astroglioma
specified site — *see* Neoplasm, malignant, by site
unspecified site C71.9
Asymbolia R48.8
Asymmetry (*see also* Distortion)
between native and reconstructed breast N65.1
face Q67.0
jaw (lower) — *see* Anomaly, dentofacial, jaw-cranial
  base relationship, asymmetry
Asynergia, asynergy R27.8
ventricular I51.89
Asystole (heart) — *see* Arrest, cardiac
At risk
for
  dental caries Z91.849
    high Z91.843
    low Z91.841
    moderate Z91.842
  falling Z91.81
Ataxia, ataxy, ataxic R27.0
acute R27.8
brain (hereditary) G11.9
cerebellar (hereditary) G11.9
  with defective DNA repair G11.3
  alcoholic G31.2
  early-onset G11.1

Ataxia, ataxy, ataxic — *continued*
cerebellar — *continued*
  in
    alcoholism G31.2
    myxedema E03.9 [G13.2]
    neoplastic disease (*see also* Neoplasm)
      D49.9 [G32.81]
    specified disease NEC G32.81
  late-onset (Marie's) G11.2
cerebral (hereditary) G11.9
congenital nonprogressive G11.0
family, familial — *see* Ataxia, hereditary
following
  cerebrovascular disease I69.993
    cerebral infarction I69.393
    intracerebral hemorrhage I69.193
    nontraumatic intracranial hemorrhage NEC
      I69.293
    specified disease NEC I69.893
    subarachnoid hemorrhage I69.093
Friedreich's (heredofamilial) (cerebellar) (spinal) G11.1
gait R26.0
  hysterical F44.4
general R27.8
gluten M35.9 [G32.81]
  with celiac disease K90.0 [G32.81]
hereditary G11.9
  with neuropathy G60.2
  cerebellar — *see* Ataxia, cerebellar
  spastic G11.4
  specified NEC G11.8
  spinal (Friedreich's) G11.1
heredofamilial — *see* Ataxia, hereditary
Hunt's G11.1
hysterical F44.4
locomotor (progressive) (syphilitic) (partial) (spastic)
  A52.11
  diabetic — *see* Diabetes, ataxia
Marie's (cerebellar) (heredofamilial) (late- onset) G11.2
nonorganic origin F44.4
nonprogressive, congenital G11.0
psychogenic F44.4
Roussy-Lévy G60.0
Sanger-Brown's (hereditary) G11.2
spastic hereditary G11.4
spinal
  hereditary (Friedreich's) G11.1
  progressive (syphilitic) A52.11
spinocerebellar, X-linked recessive G11.1
telangiectasia (Louis-Bar) G11.3
Ataxia-telangiectasia (Louis-Bar) G11.3
Atelectasis (massive) (partial) (pressure) (pulmonary)
  J98.11
newborn P28.10
  due to resorption P28.11
  partial P28.19
  primary P28.0
  secondary P28.19
primary (newborn) P28.0
tuberculous — *see* Tuberculosis, pulmonary
Atelocardia Q24.9
Atelomyelia Q06.1
Atheroembolism
of
  extremities
    lower I75.02- ☑
    upper I75.01- ☑
  kidney I75.81
  specified NEC I75.89
Atheroma, atheromatous (*see also* Arteriosclerosis)
  I70.90
aorta, aortic I70.0
  valve (*see also* Endocarditis, aortic) I35.8
aorto-iliac I70.0
artery — *see* Arteriosclerosis
basilar (artery) I67.2
carotid (artery) (common) (internal) I67.2
cerebral (arteries) I67.2
coronary (artery) I25.10
  with angina pectoris — *see* Arteriosclerosis, coro-
    nary (artery),
degeneration — *see* Arteriosclerosis
heart, cardiac — *see* Disease, heart, ischemic,
  atherosclerotic
mitral (valve) I34.8
myocardium, myocardial — *see* Disease, heart, ischemic, atherosclerotic

☑ Additional Character Required — Refer to the Tabular List for Character Selection   ▽ Subterms under main terms may continue to next column or page

Atheroma, atheromatous — *continued*
- pulmonary valve (heart) (*see also* Endocarditis, pulmonary) I37.8
- tricuspid (heart) (valve) I36.8
- valve, valvular — *see* Endocarditis
- vertebral (artery) I67.2

Atheromatosis — *see* Arteriosclerosis

Atherosclerosis (*see also* Arteriosclerosis)
- coronary
  - artery I25.10
    - with angina pectoris — *see* Arteriosclerosis, coronary (artery),
    - due to
      - calcified coronary lesion (severely) I25.84
      - lipid rich plaque I25.83
  - transplanted heart I25.811
    - bypass graft I25.812
      - with angina pectoris — *see* Arteriosclerosis, coronary (artery),
    - native coronary artery I25.811
      - with angina pectoris — *see* Arteriosclerosis, coronary (artery),

Athetosis (acquired) R25.8
- bilateral (congenital) G80.3
- congenital (bilateral) (double) G80.3
- double (congenital) G80.3
- unilateral R25.8

Athlete's
- foot B35.3
- heart I51.7

Athrepsia E41

Athyrea (acquired) (*see also* Hypothyroidism)
- congenital E03.1

Atonia, atony, atonic
- bladder (sphincter) (neurogenic) N31.2
- capillary I78.8
- cecum K59.8
  - psychogenic F45.8
- colon — *see* Atony, intestine
- congenital P94.2
- esophagus K22.8
- intestine K59.8
  - psychogenic F45.8
- stomach K31.89
  - neurotic or psychogenic F45.8
- uterus (during labor) O62.2
  - with hemorrhage (postpartum) O72.1
  - postpartum (with hemorrhage) O72.1
    - without hemorrhage O75.89

Atopy — *see* History, allergy

Atransferrinemia, congenital E88.09

Atresia, atretic
- alimentary organ or tract NEC Q45.8
  - upper Q40.8
- ani, anus, anal (canal) Q42.3
  - with fistula Q42.2
- aorta (ring) Q25.29
- aortic (orifice) (valve) Q23.0
  - arch Q25.21
  - congenital with hypoplasia of ascending aorta and defective development of left ventricle (with mitral stenosis) Q23.4
  - in hypoplastic left heart syndrome Q23.4
- aqueduct of Sylvius Q03.0
  - with spina bifida — *see* Spina bifida, with hydrocephalus
- artery NEC Q27.8
  - cerebral Q28.3
  - coronary Q24.5
  - digestive system Q27.8
  - eye Q15.8
  - lower limb Q27.8
  - pulmonary Q25.5
  - specified site NEC Q27.8
  - umbilical Q27.0
  - upper limb Q27.8
- auditory canal (external) Q16.1
- bile duct (common) (congenital) (hepatic) Q44.2
  - acquired — *see* Obstruction, bile duct
- bladder (neck) Q64.39
  - obstruction Q64.31
- bronchus Q32.4
- cecum Q42.8
- cervix (acquired) N88.2
  - congenital Q51.828
  - in pregnancy or childbirth — *see* Anomaly, cervix, in pregnancy or childbirth
    - causing obstructed labor O65.5

Atresia, atretic — *continued*
- choana Q30.0
- colon Q42.9
  - specified NEC Q42.8
- common duct Q44.2
- cricoid cartilage Q31.8
- cystic duct Q44.2
  - acquired K82.8
    - with obstruction K82.0
- digestive organs NEC Q45.8
- duodenum Q41.0
- ear canal Q16.1
- ejaculatory duct Q55.4
- epiglottis Q31.8
- esophagus Q39.0
  - with tracheoesophageal fistula Q39.1
- eustachian tube Q17.8
- fallopian tube (congenital) Q50.6
  - acquired N97.1
- follicular cyst N83.0- ☑
- foramen of
  - Luschka Q03.1
    - with spina bifida — *see* Spina bifida, with hydrocephalus
  - Magendie Q03.1
    - with spina bifida — *see* Spina bifida, with hydrocephalus
- gallbladder Q44.1
- genital organ
  - external
    - female Q52.79
    - male Q55.8
  - internal
    - female Q52.8
    - male Q55.8
- glottis Q31.8
- gullet Q39.0
  - with tracheoesophageal fistula Q39.1
- heart valve NEC Q24.8
  - pulmonary Q22.0
  - tricuspid Q22.4
- hymen Q52.3
  - acquired (postinfective) N89.6
- ileum Q41.2
- intestine (small) Q41.9
  - large Q42.9
    - specified NEC Q42.8
- iris, filtration angle Q15.0
- jejunum Q41.1
- lacrimal apparatus Q10.4
- larynx Q31.8
- meatus urinarius Q64.33
- mitral valve Q23.2
  - in hypoplastic left heart syndrome Q23.4
- nares (anterior) (posterior) Q30.0
- nasopharynx Q34.8
- nose, nostril Q30.0
  - acquired J34.89
- organ or site NEC Q89.8
- osseous meatus (ear) Q16.1
- oviduct (congenital) Q50.6
  - acquired N97.1
- parotid duct Q38.4
  - acquired K11.8
- pulmonary (artery) Q25.5
  - valve Q22.0
- pulmonic Q22.0
- pupil Q13.2
- rectum Q42.1
  - with fistula Q42.0
- salivary duct Q38.4
  - acquired K11.8
- sublingual duct Q38.4
  - acquired K11.8
- submandibular duct Q38.4
  - acquired K11.8
- submaxillary duct Q38.4
  - acquired K11.8
- thyroid cartilage Q31.8
- trachea Q32.1
- tricuspid valve Q22.4
- ureter Q62.10
  - pelvic junction Q62.11
  - vesical orifice Q62.12
- ureteropelvic junction Q62.11
- ureterovesical orifice Q62.12
- urethra (valvular) Q64.39
  - stricture Q64.32
- urinary tract NEC Q64.8

Atresia, atretic — *continued*
- uterus Q51.818
  - acquired N85.8
- vagina (congenital) Q52.4
  - acquired (postinfectional) (senile) N89.5
- vas deferens Q55.3
- vascular NEC Q27.8
  - cerebral Q28.3
  - digestive system Q27.8
  - lower limb Q27.8
  - specified site NEC Q27.8
  - upper limb Q27.8
- vein NEC Q27.8
  - digestive system Q27.8
  - great Q26.8
  - lower limb Q27.8
  - portal Q26.5
  - pulmonary Q26.4
    - partial Q26.3
    - total Q26.2
  - specified site NEC Q27.8
  - upper limb Q27.8
- vena cava (inferior) (superior) Q26.8
- vesicourethral orifice Q64.31
- vulva Q52.79
  - acquired N90.5

Atrichia, atrichosis — *see* Alopecia

Atrophia (*see also* Atrophy)
- cutis senilis L90.8
  - due to radiation L57.8
- gyrata of choroid and retina H31.23
- senilis R54
  - dermatological L90.8
    - due to radiation (nonionizing) (solar) L57.8
- unguium L60.3
  - congenita Q84.6

Atrophie blanche (en plaque) (de Milian) L95.0

Atrophoderma, atrophodermia (of) L90.9
- diffusum (idiopathic) L90.4
- maculatum L90.8
  - et striatum L90.8
    - due to syphilis A52.79
  - syphilitic A51.39
- neuriticum L90.8
- Pasini and Pierini L90.3
- pigmentosum Q82.1
- reticulatum symmetricum faciei L66.4
- senile L90.8
  - due to radiation (nonionizing) (solar) L57.8
- vermiculata (cheeks) L66.4

Atrophy, atrophic (of)
- adrenal (capsule) (gland) E27.49
  - primary (autoimmune) E27.1
- alveolar process or ridge (edentulous) K08.20
- anal sphincter (disuse) N81.84
- appendix K38.8
- arteriosclerotic — *see* Arteriosclerosis
- bile duct (common) (hepatic) K83.8
- bladder N32.89
  - neurogenic N31.8
- blanche (en plaque) (of Milian) L95.0
- bone (senile) NEC (*see also* Disorder, bone, specified type NEC)
  - due to
    - tabes dorsalis (neurogenic) A52.11
- brain (cortex) (progressive) G31.9
  - frontotemporal circumscribed G31.01 [F02.80]
    - with behavioral disturbance G31.01 [F02.81]
  - senile NEC G31.1
- breast N64.2
  - obstetric — *see* Disorder, breast, specified type NEC
- buccal cavity K13.79
- cardiac — *see* Degeneration, myocardial
- cartilage (infectional) (joint) — *see* Disorder, cartilage, specified NEC
- cerebellar — *see* Atrophy, brain
- cerebral — *see* Atrophy, brain
- cervix (mucosa) (senile) (uteri) N88.8
  - menopausal N95.8
- Charcot-Marie-Tooth G60.0
- choroid (central) (macular) (myopic) (retina) H31.10- ☑
  - diffuse secondary H31.12- ☑
  - gyrate H31.23
  - senile H31.11- ☑
- ciliary body — *see* Atrophy, iris
- conjunctiva (senile) H11.89
- corpus cavernosum N48.89

Atrophy, atrophic — *continued*
- cortical — *see* Atrophy, brain
- cystic duct K82.8
- Déjérine-Thomas G23.8
- disuse NEC — *see* Atrophy, muscle
- Duchenne-Aran G12.21
- ear H93.8- ☑
- edentulous alveolar ridge K08.20
- endometrium (senile) N85.8
  - cervix N88.8
- enteric K63.89
- epididymis N50.89
- eyeball — *see* Disorder, globe, degenerated condition, atrophy
- eyelid (senile) — *see* Disorder, eyelid, degenerative
- facial (skin) L90.9
- fallopian tube (senile) N83.32- ☑
  - with ovary N83.33- ☑
- fascioscapulohumeral (Landouzy- Déjérine) G71.0
- fatty, thymus (gland) E32.8
- gallbladder K82.8
- gastric K29.40
  - with bleeding K29.41
- gastrointestinal K63.89
- glandular I89.8
- globe H44.52- ☑
- gum — *see* Recession, gingival
- hair L67.8
- heart (brown) — *see* Degeneration, myocardial
- hemifacial Q67.4
  - Romberg G51.8
- infantile E41
  - paralysis, acute — *see* Poliomyelitis, paralytic
- intestine K63.89
- iris (essential) (progressive) H21.26- ☑
  - specified NEC H21.29
- kidney (senile) (terminal) (*see also* Sclerosis, renal) N26.1
  - congenital or infantile Q60.5
    - bilateral Q60.4
    - unilateral Q60.3
  - hydronephrotic — *see* Hydronephrosis
- lacrimal gland (primary) H04.14- ☑
  - secondary H04.15- ☑
- Landouzy-Déjérine G71.0
- laryngitis, infective J37.0
- larynx J38.7
- Leber's optic (hereditary) H47.22
- lip K13.0
- liver (yellow) K72.90
  - with coma K72.91
  - acute, subacute K72.00
    - with coma K72.01
  - chronic K72.10
    - with coma K72.11
- lung (senile) J98.4
- macular (dermatological) L90.8
  - syphilitic, skin A51.39
    - striated A52.79
- mandible (edentulous) K08.20
  - minimal K08.21
  - moderate K08.22
  - severe K08.23
- maxilla K08.20
  - minimal K08.24
  - moderate K08.25
  - severe K08.26
- muscle, muscular (diffuse) (general) (idiopathic) (primary) M62.50
  - ankle M62.57- ☑
  - Duchenne-Aran G12.21
  - foot M62.57- ☑
  - forearm M62.53- ☑
  - hand M62.54- ☑
  - infantile spinal G12.0
  - lower leg M62.56- ☑
  - multiple sites M62.59
  - myelopathic — *see* Atrophy, muscle, spinal
  - myotonic G71.11
  - neuritic G58.9
  - neuropathic (peroneal) (progressive) G60.0
  - pelvic (disuse) N81.84
  - peroneal G60.0
  - progressive (bulbar) G12.21
    - adult G12.1
    - infantile (spinal) G12.0
    - spinal G12.25
      - adult G12.1

Atrophy, atrophic — *continued*
- muscle, muscular — *continued*
  - progressive — *continued*
    - spinal — *continued*
      - infantile G12.0
  - pseudohypertrophic G71.0
  - shoulder region M62.51- ☑
  - specified site NEC M62.58
  - spinal G12.9
    - adult form G12.1
    - Aran-Duchenne G12.21
    - childhood form, type II G12.1
    - distal G12.1
    - hereditary NEC G12.1
    - infantile, type I (Werdnig-Hoffmann) G12.0
    - juvenile form, type III (Kugelberg- Welander) G12.1
    - progressive G12.25
    - scapuloperoneal form G12.1
    - specified NEC G12.8
  - syphilitic A52.78
  - thigh M62.55- ☑
  - upper arm M62.52- ☑
- myocardium — *see* Degeneration, myocardial
- myometrium (senile) N85.8
  - cervix N88.8
- myopathic NEC — *see* Atrophy, muscle
- myotonia G71.11
- nail L60.3
- nasopharynx J31.1
- nerve (*see also* Disorder, nerve)
  - abducens — *see* Strabismus, paralytic, sixth nerve
  - accessory G52.8
  - acoustic or auditory H93.3 ☑
  - cranial G52.9
    - eighth (auditory) H93.3 ☑
    - eleventh (accessory) G52.8
    - fifth (trigeminal) G50.8
    - first (olfactory) G52.0
    - fourth (trochlear) — *see* Strabismus, paralytic, fourth nerve
    - second (optic) H47.20
    - sixth (abducens) — *see* Strabismus, paralytic, sixth nerve
    - tenth (pneumogastric) (vagus) G52.2
    - third (oculomotor) — *see* Strabismus, paralytic, third nerve
    - twelfth (hypoglossal) G52.3
  - hypoglossal G52.3
  - oculomotor — *see* Strabismus, paralytic, third nerve
  - olfactory G52.0
  - optic (papillomacular bundle)
    - syphilitic (late) A52.15
    - congenital A50.44
  - pneumogastric G52.2
  - trigeminal G50.8
  - trochlear — *see* Strabismus, paralytic, fourth nerve
  - vagus (pneumogastric) G52.2
- neurogenic, bone, tabetic A52.11
- nutritional E41
- old age R54
- olivopontocerebellar G23.8
- optic (nerve) H47.20
  - glaucomatous H47.23- ☑
  - hereditary H47.22
  - primary H47.21- ☑
  - specified type NEC H47.29- ☑
  - syphilitic (late) A52.15
    - congenital A50.44
- orbit H05.31- ☑
- ovary (senile) N83.31- ☑
  - with fallopian tube N83.33- ☑
- oviduct (senile) — *see* Atrophy, fallopian tube
- palsy, diffuse (progressive) G12.22
- pancreas (duct) (senile) K86.89
- parotid gland K11.0
- pelvic muscle N81.84
- penis N48.89
- pharynx J39.2
- pluriglandular E31.8
  - autoimmune E31.0
- polyarthritis M15.9
- prostate N42.89
- pseudohypertrophic (muscle) G71.0
- renal (*see also* Sclerosis, renal) N26.1
- retina, retinal (postinfectional) H35.89
- rhinitis J31.0

Atrophy, atrophic — *continued*
- salivary gland K11.0
- scar L90.5
- sclerosis, lobar (of brain) G31.09 [F02.80]
  - with behavioral disturbance G31.09 [F02.81]
- scrotum N50.89
- seminal vesicle N50.89
- senile R54
  - due to radiation (nonionizing) (solar) L57.8
- skin (patches) (spots) L90.9
  - degenerative (senile) L90.8
  - due to radiation (nonionizing) (solar) L57.8
  - senile L90.8
- spermatic cord N50.89
- spinal (acute) (cord) G95.89
  - muscular — *see* Atrophy, muscle, spinal
  - paralysis G12.20
    - acute — *see* Poliomyelitis, paralytic
    - meaning progressive muscular atrophy G12.21
- spine (column) — *see* Spondylopathy, specified NEC
- spleen (senile) D73.0
- stomach K29.40
  - with bleeding K29.41
- striate (skin) L90.6
  - syphilitic A52.79
- subcutaneous L90.9
- sublingual gland K11.0
- submandibular gland K11.0
- submaxillary gland K11.0
- Sudeck's — *see* Algoneurodystrophy
- suprarenal (capsule) (gland) E27.49
  - primary E27.1
- systemic affecting central nervous system
  - in
    - myxedema E03.9 [G13.2]
    - neoplastic disease (*see also* Neoplasm) D49.9 [G13.1]
    - specified disease NEC G13.8
- tarso-orbital fascia, congenital Q10.3
- testis N50.0
- thenar, partial — *see* Syndrome, carpal tunnel
- thymus (fatty) E32.8
- thyroid (gland) (acquired) E03.4
  - with cretinism E03.1
  - congenital (with myxedema) E03.1
- tongue (senile) K14.8
  - papillae K14.4
- trachea J39.8
- tunica vaginalis N50.89
- turbinate J34.89
- tympanic membrane (nonflaccid) H73.82- ☑
  - flaccid H73.81- ☑
- upper respiratory tract J39.8
- uterus, uterine (senile) N85.8
  - cervix N88.8
  - due to radiation (intended effect) N85.8
    - adverse effect or misadventure N99.89
- vagina (senile) N95.2
- vas deferens N50.89
- vascular I99.8
- vertebra (senile) — *see* Spondylopathy, specified NEC
- vulva (senile) N90.5
- Werdnig-Hoffmann G12.0
- yellow — *see* Failure, hepatic

Attack, attacks
- with alteration of consciousness (with automatisms) — *see* Epilepsy, localization-related, symptomatic, with complex partial seizures
- without alteration of consciousness — *see* Epilepsy, localization-related, symptomatic, with simple partial seizures
- Adams-Stokes I45.9
- akinetic — *see* Epilepsy, generalized, specified NEC
- angina — *see* Angina
- atonic — *see* Epilepsy, generalized, specified NEC
- benign shuddering G25.83
- cataleptic — *see* Catalepsy
- coronary — *see* Infarct, myocardium
- cyanotic, newborn P28.2
- drop NEC R55
- epileptic — *see* Epilepsy
- heart — *see* infarct, myocardium
- hysterical F44.9
- jacksonian — *see* Epilepsy, localization-related, symptomatic, with simple partial seizures
- myocardium, myocardial — *see* Infarct, myocardium
- myoclonic — *see* Epilepsy, generalized, specified NEC
- panic F41.0

Attack, attacks — *continued*
psychomotor — *see* Epilepsy, localization-related, symptomatic, with complex partial seizures
salaam — *see* Epilepsy, spasms
schizophreniform, brief F23
shuddering, benign G25.83
Stokes-Adams I45.9
syncope R55
transient ischemic (TIA) G45.9
specified NEC G45.8
unconsciousness R55
hysterical F44.89
vasomotor R55
vasovagal (paroxysmal) (idiopathic) R55
Attention (to)
artificial
opening (of) Z43.9
digestive tract NEC Z43.4
colon Z43.3
ilium Z43.2
stomach Z43.1
specified NEC Z43.8
trachea Z43.0
urinary tract NEC Z43.6
cystostomy Z43.5
nephrostomy Z43.6
ureterostomy Z43.6
urethrostomy Z43.6
vagina Z43.7
colostomy Z43.3
cystostomy Z43.5
deficit disorder or syndrome F98.8
with hyperactivity — *see* Disorder, attention-deficit hyperactivity
gastrostomy Z43.1
ileostomy Z43.2
jejunostomy Z43.4
nephrostomy Z43.6
surgical dressings Z48.01
sutures Z48.02
tracheostomy Z43.0
ureterostomy Z43.6
urethrostomy Z43.6
Attrition
gum — *see* Recession, gingival
tooth, teeth (excessive) (hard tissues) K03.0
Atypical, atypism (*see also* condition)
cells (on cytolgocial smear) (endocervical) (endometrial) (glandular)
cervix R87.619
vagina R87.629
cervical N87.9
endometrium N85.9
hyperplasia N85.00
parenting situation Z62.9
Auditory — *see* condition
Aujeszky's disease B33.8
Aurantiasis, cutis E67.1
Auricle, auricular (*see also* condition)
cervical Q18.2
Auriculotemporal syndrome G50.8
Austin Flint murmur (aortic insufficiency) I35.1
Australian
Q fever A78
X disease A83.4
Autism, autistic (childhood) (infantile) F84.0
atypical F84.9
spectrum disorder F84.0
Autodigestion R68.89
Autoerythrocyte sensitization (syndrome) D69.2
Autographism L50.3
Autoimmune
disease (systemic) M35.9
inhibitors to clotting factors D68.311
lymphoproliferative syndrome [ALPS] D89.82
thyroiditis E06.3
Autointoxication R68.89
Automatism G93.89
with temporal sclerosis G93.81
epileptic — *see* Epilepsy, localization-related, symptomatic, with complex partial seizures
paroxysmal, idiopathic — *see* Epilepsy, localization-related, symptomatic, with complex partial seizures
Autonomic, autonomous
bladder (neurogenic) N31.2
hysteria seizure F44.5
Autosensitivity, erythrocyte D69.2

Autosensitization, cutaneous L30.2
Autosome — *see* condition by chromosome involved
Autotopagnosia R48.1
Autotoxemia R68.89
Autumn — *see* condition
Avellis' syndrome G46.8
Aversion
oral R63.3
newborn P92.-✓
nonorganic origin F98.2 ✓
sexual F52.1
Aviator's
disease or sickness — *see* Effect, adverse, high altitude
ear T70.0 ✓
Avitaminosis (multiple) (*see also* Deficiency, vitamin) E56.9
B E53.9
with
beriberi E51.11
pellagra E52
B2 E53.0
B6 E53.1
B12 E53.8
D E55.9
with rickets E55.0
G E53.0
K E56.1
nicotinic acid E52
AVNRT (atrioventricular nodal re-entrant tachycardia) I47.1
AVRT (atrioventricular nodal re-entrant tachycardia) I47.1
Avulsion (traumatic)
blood vessel — *see* Injury, blood vessel
bone — *see* Fracture, by site
cartilage (*see also* Dislocation, by site)
symphyseal (inner), complicating delivery O71.6
external site other than limb — *see* Wound, open, by site
eye S05.7-
head (intracranial)
external site NEC S08.89 ✓
scalp S08.0 ✓
internal organ or site — *see* Injury, by site
joint (*see also* Dislocation, by site)
capsule — *see* Sprain, by site
kidney S37.06-✓
ligament — *see* Sprain, by site
limb (*see also* Amputation, traumatic, by site)
skin and subcutaneous tissue — *see* Wound, open, by site
muscle — *see* Injury, muscle
nerve (root) — *see* Injury, nerve
scalp S08.0 ✓
skin and subcutaneous tissue — *see* Wound, open, by site
spleen S36.032 ✓
symphyseal cartilage (inner), complicating delivery O71.6
tendon — *see* Injury, muscle
tooth S03.2 ✓
Awareness of heart beat R00.2
Axenfeld's
anomaly or syndrome Q15.0
degeneration (calcareous) Q13.4
Axilla, axillary (*see also* condition)
breast Q83.1
Axonotmesis — *see* Injury, nerve
Ayerza's disease or syndrome (pulmonary artery sclerosis with pulmonary hypertension) I27.0
Azoospermia (organic) N46.01
due to
drug therapy N46.021
efferent duct obstruction N46.023
infection N46.022
radiation N46.024
specified cause NEC N46.029
systemic disease N46.025
Azotemia R79.89
meaning uremia N19
Aztec ear Q17.3
Azygos
continuation inferior vena cava Q26.8
lobe (lung) Q33.1

B

Baastrup's disease — *see* Kissing spine

Babesiosis B60.0
Babington's disease (familial hemorrhagic telangiectasia) I78.0
Babinski's syndrome A52.79
Baby
crying constantly R68.11
floppy (syndrome) P94.2
Bacillary — *see* condition
Bacilluria R82.71
Bacillus (*see also* Infection, bacillus)
abortus infection A23.1
anthracis infection A22.9
coli infection (*see also* Escherichia coli) B96.20
Flexner's A03.1
mallei infection A24.0
Shiga's A03.0
suipestifer infection — *see* Infection, salmonella
Back — *see* condition
Backache (postural) M54.9
sacroiliac M53.3
specified NEC M54.89
Backflow — *see* Reflux
Backward reading (dyslexia) F81.0
Bacteremia R78.81
with sepsis — *see* Sepsis
Bactericholia — *see* Cholecystitis, acute
Bacterid, bacteride (pustular) L40.3
Bacterium, bacteria, bacterial
agent NEC, as cause of disease classified elsewhere B96.89
in blood — *see* Bacteremia
in urine — *see* Bacteriuria
Bacteriuria, bacteruria R82.71
asymptomatic R82.71
Bacteroides
fragilis, as cause of disease classified elsewhere B96.6
Bad
heart — *see* Disease, heart
trip
due to drug abuse — *see* Abuse, drug, hallucinogen
due to drug dependence — *see* Dependence, drug, hallucinogen
Baelz's disease (cheilitis glandularis apostematosa) K13.0
Baerensprung's disease (eczema marginatum) B35.6
Bagasse disease or pneumonitis J67.1
Bagassosis J67.1
Baker's cyst — *see* Cyst, Baker's
Bakwin-Krida syndrome (metaphyseal dysplasia) Q78.5
Balancing side interference M26.56
Balanitis (circinata) (erosiva) (gangrenosa) (phagedenic) (vulgaris) N48.1
amebic A06.82
candidal B37.42
due to Haemophilus ducreyi A57
gonococcal (acute) (chronic) A54.09
xerotica obliterans N48.0
Balanoposthitis N47.6
gonococcal (acute) (chronic) A54.09
ulcerative (specific) A63.8
Balanorrhagia — *see* Balanitis
Balantidiasis, balantidiosis A07.0
Bald tongue K14.4
Baldness (*see also* Alopecia)
male-pattern — *see* Alopecia, androgenic
Balkan grippe A78
Balloon disease — *see* Effect, adverse, high altitude
Balo's disease (concentric sclerosis) G37.5
Bamberger-Marie disease — *see* Osteoarthropathy, hypertrophic, specified type NEC
Bancroft's filariasis B74.0
Band(s)
adhesive — *see* Adhesions, peritoneum
anomalous or congenital (*see also* Anomaly, by site)
heart (atrial) (ventricular) Q24.8
intestine Q43.3
omentum Q43.3
cervix N88.1
constricting, congenital Q79.8
gallbladder (congenital) Q44.1
intestinal (adhesive) — *see* Adhesions, peritoneum
obstructive
intestine K56.50
complete K56.52
incomplete K56.51
partial K56.51
peritoneum K56.50

Band(s) — *continued*
  obstructive — *continued*
   peritoneum — *continued*
    complete K56.52
    incomplete K56.51
    partial K56.51
  periappendiceal, congenital Q43.3
  peritoneal (adhesive) — *see* Adhesions, peritoneum
  uterus N73.6
   internal N85.6
   vagina N89.5
Bandemia D72.825
Bandl's ring (contraction), complicating delivery O62.4
Bangkok hemorrhagic fever A91
Bang's disease (brucella abortus) A23.1
Bankruptcy, anxiety concerning Z59.8
Bannister's disease T78.3 ☑
  hereditary D84.1
Banti's disease or syndrome (with cirrhosis) (with portal hypertension) K76.6
Bar, median, prostate — *see* Enlargement, enlarged, prostate
Barcoo disease or rot — *see* Ulcer, skin
Barlow's disease E54
Barodontalgia T70.29 ☑
Baron Münchausen syndrome — *see* Disorder, factitious
Barosinusitis T70.1 ☑
Barotitis T70.0 ☑
Barotrauma T70.29 ☑
  odontalgia T70.29 ☑
  otitic T70.0 ☑
  sinus T70.1 ☑
Barraquer (-Simons) **disease or syndrome** (progressive lipodystrophy) E88.1
Barré-Guillain disease or syndrome G61.0
Barrel chest M95.4
Barré-Liéou syndrome (posterior cervical sympathetic) M53.0
Barrett's
  disease — *see* Barrett's, esophagus
  esophagus K22.70
   with dysplasia K22.719
    high grade K22.711
    low grade K22.710
   without dysplasia K22.70
  syndrome — *see* Barrett's, esophagus
  ulcer K22.10
   with bleeding K22.11
   without bleeding K22.10
Bársony (-Polgár) (-Teschendorf) **syndrome** (corkscrew esophagus) K22.4
Barth syndrome E78.71
Bartholinitis (suppurating) N75.8
  gonococcal (acute) (chronic) (with abscess) A54.1
Bartonellosis A44.9
  cutaneous A44.1
  mucocutaneous A44.1
  specified NEC A44.8
  systemic A44.0
Barton's fracture S52.56- ☑
Bartter's syndrome E26.81
Basal — *see* condition
Basan's (hidrotic) ectodermal dysplasia Q82.4
Baseball finger — *see* Dislocation, finger
Basedow's disease (exophthalmic goiter) — *see* Hyperthyroidism, with, goiter
Basic — *see* condition
Basilar — *see* condition
Bason's (hidrotic) ectodermal dysplasia Q82.4
Basopenia — *see* Agranulocytosis
Basophilia D72.824
Basophilism (cortico-adrenal) (Cushing's) (pituitary) E24.0
Bassen-Kornzweig disease or syndrome E78.6
Bat ear Q17.5
Bateman's
  disease B08.1
  purpura (senile) D69.2
Bathing cramp T75.1 ☑
Bathophobia F40.248
Batten (-Mayou) **disease** E75.4
  retina E75.4 [H36]
Batten-Steinert syndrome G71.11
Battered — *see* Maltreatment
Battey Mycobacterium infection A31.0
Battle exhaustion F43.0

Battledore placenta O43.19- ☑
Baumgarten-Cruveilhier cirrhosis, disease or syndrome K74.69
Bauxite fibrosis (of lung) J63.1
Bayle's disease (general paresis) A52.17
Bazin's disease (primary) (tuberculous) A18.4
Beach ear — *see* Swimmer's, ear
Beaded hair (congenital) Q84.1
Béal conjunctivitis or syndrome B30.2
Beard's disease (neurasthenia) F48.8
Beat(s)
  atrial, premature I49.1
  ectopic I49.49
  elbow — *see* Bursitis, elbow
  escaped, heart I49.49
  hand — *see* Bursitis, hand
  knee — *see* Bursitis, knee
  premature I49.40
   atrial I49.1
   auricular I49.1
   supraventricular I49.1
Beau's
  disease or syndrome — *see* Degeneration, myocardial
  lines (transverse furrows on fingernails) L60.4
Bechterev's syndrome — *see* Spondylitis, ankylosing
Becker's
  cardiomyopathy I42.8
  disease
   idiopathic mural endomyocardial disease I42.3
   myotonia congenita, recessive form G71.12
  dystrophy G71.0
  pigmented hairy nevus D22.5
Beck's syndrome (anterior spinal artery occlusion) I65.8
Beckwith(-Wiedemann) syndrome Q87.3
Bed confinement status Z74.01
Bed sore — *see* Ulcer, pressure, by site
Bedbug bite(s) — *see* Bite(s), by site, superficial, insect
Bedclothes, asphyxiation or suffocation by — *see* Asphyxia, traumatic, due to, mechanical, trapped
Bednar's
  aphthae K12.0
  tumor — *see* Neoplasm, malignant, by site
Bedridden Z74.01
Bedsore — *see* Ulcer, pressure, by site
Bedwetting — *see* Enuresis
Bee sting (with allergic or anaphylactic shock) — *see* Toxicity, venom, arthropod, bee
Beer drinker's heart (disease) I42.6
Begbie's disease (exophthalmic goiter) — *see* Hyperthyroidism, with, goiter
Behavior
  antisocial
   adult Z72.811
   child or adolescent Z72.810
  disorder, disturbance — *see* Disorder, conduct
  disruptive — *see* Disorder, conduct
  drug seeking Z76.5
  inexplicable R46.2
  marked evasiveness R46.5
  obsessive-compulsive R46.81
  overactivity R46.3
  poor responsiveness R46.4
  self-damaging (life-style) Z72.89
  sleep-incompatible Z72.821
  slowness R46.4
  specified NEC R46.89
  strange (and inexplicable) R46.2
  suspiciousness R46.5
  type A pattern Z73.1
  undue concern or preoccupation with stressful events R46.6
  verbosity and circumstantial detail obscuring reason for contact R46.7
Behçet's disease or syndrome M35.2
Behr's disease — *see* Degeneration, macula
Beigel's disease or morbus (white piedra) B36.2
Bejel A65
Bekhterev's syndrome — *see* Spondylitis, ankylosing
Belching — *see* Eructation
Bell's
  mania F30.8
  palsy, paralysis G51.0
   infant or newborn P11.3
  spasm G51.3
Bence Jones albuminuria or proteinuria NEC R80.3
Bends T70.3 ☑
Benedikt's paralysis or syndrome G46.3

Benign (*see also* condition)
  prostatic hyperplasia — *see* Hyperplasia, prostate
Bennett's fracture (displaced) S62.21- ☑
Benson's disease — *see* Deposit, crystalline
Bent
  back (hysterical) F44.4
  nose M95.0
   congenital Q67.4
Bereavement (uncomplicated) Z63.4
Bergeron's disease (hysterical chorea) F44.4
Berger's disease — *see* Nephropathy, IgA
Beriberi (dry) E51.11
  heart (disease) E51.12
  polyneuropathy E51.11
  wet E51.12
   involving circulatory system E51.11
Berlin's disease or edema (traumatic) S05.8X- ☑
Berlock (berloque) **dermatitis** L56.2
Bernard-Horner syndrome G90.2
Bernard-Soulier disease or thrombopathia D69.1
Bernhardt (-Roth) **disease** — *see* Mononeuropathy, lower limb, meralgia paresthetica
Bernheim's syndrome — *see* Failure, heart, right
Bertielliasis B71.8
Berylliosis (lung) J63.2
Besnier-Boeck (-Schaumann) **disease** — *see* Sarcoidosis
Besnier's
  lupus pernio D86.3
  prurigo L20.0
Bestiality F65.89
Best's disease H35.50
Betalipoproteinemia, broad or floating E78.2
Beta-mercaptolactate-cysteine disulfiduria E72.09
Betting and gambling Z72.6
  pathological (compulsive) F63.0
Bezoar T18.9 ☑
  intestine T18.3 ☑
  stomach T18.2 ☑
Bezold's abscess — *see* Mastoiditis, acute
Bianchi's syndrome R48.8
Bicornate or bicornis uterus Q51.3
  in pregnancy or childbirth O34.00
   causing obstructed labor O65.5
Bicuspid aortic valve Q23.1
Biedl-Bardet syndrome Q87.89
Bielschowsky (-Jansky) **disease** E75.4
Biermer's (pernicious) anemia or disease D51.0
Biett's disease L93.0
Bifid (congenital)
  apex, heart Q24.8
  clitoris Q52.6
  kidney Q63.8
  nose Q30.2
  patella Q74.1
  scrotum Q55.29
  toe NEC Q74.2
  tongue Q38.3
  ureter Q62.8
  uterus Q51.3
  uvula Q35.7
Biforis uterus (suprasimplex) Q51.3
Bifurcation (congenital)
  gallbladder Q44.1
  kidney pelvis Q63.8
  renal pelvis Q63.8
  rib Q76.6
  tongue, congenital Q38.3
  trachea Q32.1
  ureter Q62.8
  urethra Q64.74
  vertebra Q76.49
Big spleen syndrome D73.1
Bigeminal pulse R00.8
Bilateral — *see* condition
Bile
  duct — *see* condition
  pigments in urine R82.2
Bilharziasis (*see also* Schistosomiasis)
  chyluria B65.0
  cutaneous B65.3
  galacturia B65.0
  hematochyluria B65.0
  intestinal B65.1
  lipemia B65.9
  lipuria B65.0
  oriental B65.2
  piarhemia B65.9

☑ Additional Character Required — Refer to the Tabular List for Character Selection   ▽ Subterms under main terms may continue to next column or page

Bilharziasis — *continued*
  pulmonary NOS B65.9 [J99]
    pneumonia B65.9 [J17]
  tropical hematuria B65.0
  vesical B65.0
Biliary — *see* condition
Bilirubin metabolism disorder E80.7
  specified NEC E80.6
Bilirubinemia, familial nonhemolytic E80.4
Bilirubinuria R82.2
Biliuria R82.2
Bilocular stomach K31.2
Binswanger's disease I67.3
Biparta, bipartite
  carpal scaphoid Q74.0
  patella Q74.1
  vagina Q52.10
Bird
  face Q75.8
  fancier's disease or lung J67.2
Birth
  complications in mother — *see* Delivery, complicated
  compression during NOS P15.9
  defect — *see* Anomaly
  immature (less than 37 completed weeks) — *see* Preterm, newborn
    extremely (less than 28 completed weeks) — *see* Immaturity, extreme
  inattention, at or after — *see* Maltreatment, child, neglect
  injury NOS P15.9
    basal ganglia P11.1
    brachial plexus NEC P14.3
    brain (compression) (pressure) P11.2
    central nervous system NOS P11.9
    cerebellum P11.1
    cerebral hemorrhage P10.1
    external genitalia P15.5
    eye P15.3
    face P15.4
    fracture
      bone P13.9
        specified NEC P13.8
      clavicle P13.4
      femur P13.2
      humerus P13.3
      long bone, except femur P13.3
      radius and ulna P13.3
      skull P13.0
      spine P11.5
      tibia and fibula P13.3
    intracranial P11.2
      laceration or hemorrhage P10.9
        specified NEC P10.8
    intraventricular hemorrhage P10.2
    laceration
      brain P10.1
      by scalpel P15.8
      peripheral nerve P14.9
    liver P15.0
    meninges
      brain P11.1
      spinal cord P11.5
    nerve
      brachial plexus P14.3
      cranial NEC (except facial) P11.4
      facial P11.3
      peripheral P14.9
      phrenic (paralysis) P14.2
    paralysis
      facial nerve P11.3
      spinal P11.5
    penis P15.5
    rupture
      spinal cord P11.5
    scalp P12.9
    scalpel wound P15.8
    scrotum P15.5
    skull NEC P13.1
      fracture P13.0
    specified type NEC P15.8
    spinal cord P11.5
    spine P11.5
    spleen P15.1
    sternomastoid (hematoma) P15.2
    subarachnoid hemorrhage P10.3
    subcutaneous fat necrosis P15.6
    subdural hemorrhage P10.0

Birth — *continued*
  injury — *continued*
    tentorial tear P10.4
    testes P15.5
    vulva P15.5
  lack of care, at or after — *see* Maltreatment, child, neglect
  neglect, at or after — *see* Maltreatment, child, neglect
  palsy or paralysis, newborn, NOS (birth injury) P14.9
  premature (infant) — *see* Preterm, newborn
  shock, newborn P96.89
  trauma — *see* Birth, injury
  weight
    4000 grams to 4499 grams P08.1
    4500 grams or more P08.0
    low (2499 grams or less) — *see* Low, birthweight
      extremely (999 grams or less) — *see* Low, birthweight, extreme
Birthmark Q82.5
Birt-Hogg-Dube syndrome Q87.89
Bisalbuminemia E88.09
Biskra's button B55.1
Bite(s) (animal) (human)
  abdomen, abdominal
    wall S31.159 ☑
      with penetration into peritoneal cavity S31.659 ☑
      epigastric region S31.152 ☑
        with penetration into peritoneal cavity S31.652 ☑
      left
        lower quadrant S31.154 ☑
          with penetration into peritoneal cavity S31.654 ☑
        upper quadrant S31.151 ☑
          with penetration into peritoneal cavity S31.651 ☑
      periumbilic region S31.155 ☑
        with penetration into peritoneal cavity S31.655 ☑
      right
        lower quadrant S31.153 ☑
          with penetration into peritoneal cavity S31.653 ☑
        upper quadrant S31.150 ☑
          with penetration into peritoneal cavity S31.650 ☑
    superficial NEC S30.871 ☑
      insect S30.861 ☑
  alveolar (process) — *see* Bite, oral cavity
  amphibian (venomous) — *see* Venom, bite, amphibian
  animal (*see also* Bite, by site)
    venomous — *see* Venom
  ankle S91.05- ☑
    superficial NEC S90.57- ☑
      insect S90.56- ☑
  antecubital space — *see* Bite, elbow
  anus S31.835 ☑
    superficial NEC S30.877 ☑
      insect S30.867 ☑
  arm (upper) S41.15- ☑
    lower — *see* Bite, forearm
    superficial NEC S40.87- ☑
      insect S40.86- ☑
  arthropod NEC — *see* Venom, bite, arthropod
  auditory canal (external) (meatus) — *see* Bite, ear
  auricle, ear — *see* Bite, ear
  axilla — *see* Bite, arm
  back (*see also* Bite, thorax, back)
    lower S31.050 ☑
      with penetration into retroperitoneal space S31.051 ☑
      superficial NEC S30.870 ☑
        insect S30.860 ☑
  bedbug — *see* Bite(s), by site, superficial, insect
  breast S21.05- ☑
    superficial NEC S20.17- ☑
      insect S20.16- ☑
  brow — *see* Bite, head, specified site NEC
  buttock S31.805 ☑
    left S31.825 ☑
    right S31.815 ☑
    superficial NEC S30.870 ☑
      insect S30.860 ☑
  calf — *see* Bite, leg
  canaliculus lacrimalis — *see* Bite, eyelid

Bite(s) — *continued*
  canthus, eye — *see* Bite, eyelid
  centipede — *see* Toxicity, venom, arthropod, centipede
  cheek (external) S01.45- ☑
    internal — *see* Bite, oral cavity
    superficial NEC S00.87 ☑
      insect S00.86 ☑
  chest wall — *see* Bite, thorax
  chigger B88.0
  chin — *see* Bite, head, specified site NEC
  clitoris — *see* Bite, vulva
  costal region — *see* Bite, thorax
  digit(s)
    hand — *see* Bite, finger
    toe — *see* Bite, toe
  ear (canal) (external) S01.35- ☑
    superficial NEC S00.47- ☑
      insect S00.46- ☑
  elbow S51.05- ☑
    superficial NEC S50.37- ☑
      insect S50.36- ☑
  epididymis — *see* Bite, testis
  epigastric region — *see* Bite, abdomen
  epiglottis — *see* Bite, neck, specified site NEC
  esophagus, cervical S11.25 ☑
    superficial NEC S10.17 ☑
      insect S10.16 ☑
  eyebrow — *see* Bite, eyelid
  eyelid S01.15- ☑
    superficial NEC S00.27- ☑
      insect S00.26- ☑
  face NEC — *see* Bite, head, specified site NEC
  finger(s) S61.259 ☑
    with
      damage to nail S61.359 ☑
    index S61.258 ☑
      with
        damage to nail S61.358 ☑
      left S61.251 ☑
        with
          damage to nail S61.351 ☑
      right S61.250 ☑
        with
          damage to nail S61.350 ☑
      superficial NEC S60.478 ☑
        insect S60.46- ☑
    little S61.25- ☑
      with
        damage to nail S61.35- ☑
      superficial NEC S60.47- ☑
        insect S60.46- ☑
    middle S61.25- ☑
      with
        damage to nail S61.35- ☑
      superficial NEC S60.47- ☑
        insect S60.46- ☑
    ring S61.25- ☑
      with
        damage to nail S61.35- ☑
      superficial NEC S60.47- ☑
        insect S60.46- ☑
    superficial NEC S60.479 ☑
      insect S60.469 ☑
    thumb — *see* Bite, thumb
  flank — *see* Bite, abdomen, wall
  flea — *see* Bite, by site, superficial, insect
  foot (except toe(s) alone) S91.35- ☑
    superficial NEC S90.87- ☑
      insect S90.86- ☑
    toe — *see* Bite, toe
  forearm S51.85- ☑
    elbow only — *see* Bite, elbow
    superficial NEC S50.87- ☑
      insect S50.86- ☑
  forehead — *see* Bite, head, specified site NEC
  genital organs, external
    female S31.552 ☑
      superficial NEC S30.876 ☑
        insect S30.866 ☑
      vagina and vulva — *see* Bite, vulva
    male S31.551 ☑
      penis — *see* Bite, penis
      scrotum — *see* Bite, scrotum
      superficial NEC S30.875 ☑
        insect S30.865 ☑

Bite(s) — *continued*
genital organs, external — *continued*
male — *continued*
testes — *see* Bite, testis
groin — *see* Bite, abdomen, wall
gum — *see* Bite, oral cavity
hand S61.45- ☑
finger — *see* Bite, finger
superficial NEC S60.57- ☑
insect S60.56- ☑
thumb — *see* Bite, thumb
head S01.95 ☑
cheek — *see* Bite, cheek
ear — *see* Bite, ear
eyelid — *see* Bite, eyelid
lip — *see* Bite, lip
nose — *see* Bite, nose
oral cavity — *see* Bite, oral cavity
scalp — *see* Bite, scalp
specified site NEC S01.85 ☑
superficial NEC S00.87 ☑
insect S00.86 ☑
superficial NEC S00.97 ☑
insect S00.96 ☑
temporomandibular area — *see* Bite, cheek
heel — *see* Bite, foot
hip S71.05- ☑
superficial NEC S70.27- ☑
insect S70.26- ☑
hymen S31.45 ☑
hypochondrium — *see* Bite, abdomen, wall
hypogastric region — *see* Bite, abdomen, wall
inguinal region — *see* Bite, abdomen, wall
insect — *see* Bite, by site, superficial, insect
instep — *see* Bite, foot
interscapular region — *see* Bite, thorax, back
jaw — *see* Bite, head, specified site NEC
knee S81.05- ☑
superficial NEC S80.27- ☑
insect S80.26- ☑
labium (majus) (minus) — *see* Bite, vulva
lacrimal duct — *see* Bite, eyelid
larynx S11.015 ☑
superficial NEC S10.17 ☑
insect S10.16 ☑
leg (lower) S81.85- ☑
ankle — *see* Bite, ankle
foot — *see* Bite, foot
knee — *see* Bite, knee
superficial NEC S80.87- ☑
insect S80.86- ☑
toe — *see* Bite, toe
upper — *see* Bite, thigh
lip S01.551 ☑
superficial NEC S00.571 ☑
insect S00.561 ☑
lizard (venomous) — *see* Venom, bite, reptile
loin — *see* Bite, abdomen, wall
lower back — *see* Bite, back, lower
lumbar region — *see* Bite, back, lower
malar region — *see* Bite, head, specified site NEC
mammary — *see* Bite, breast
marine animals (venomous) — *see* Toxicity, venom, marine animal
mastoid region — *see* Bite, head, specified site NEC
mouth — *see* Bite, oral cavity
nail
finger — *see* Bite, finger
toe — *see* Bite, toe
nape — *see* Bite, neck, specified site NEC
nasal (septum) (sinus) — *see* Bite, nose
nasopharynx — *see* Bite, head, specified site NEC
neck S11.95 ☑
involving
cervical esophagus — *see* Bite, esophagus, cervical
larynx — *see* Bite, larynx
pharynx — *see* Bite, pharynx
thyroid gland S11.15
trachea — *see* Bite, trachea
specified site NEC S11.85 ☑
superficial NEC S10.87 ☑
insect S10.86 ☑
superficial NEC S10.97 ☑
insect S10.96 ☑
throat S11.85 ☑

Bite(s) — *continued*
neck — *continued*
throat — *continued*
superficial NEC S10.17 ☑
insect S10.16 ☑
nose (septum) (sinus) S01.25 ☑
superficial NEC S00.37 ☑
insect S00.36 ☑
occipital region — *see* Bite, scalp
oral cavity S01.552 ☑
superficial NEC S00.572 ☑
insect S00.562 ☑
orbital region — *see* Bite, eyelid
palate — *see* Bite, oral cavity
palm — *see* Bite, hand
parietal region — *see* Bite, scalp
pelvis S31.050 ☑
with penetration into retroperitoneal space S31.051 ☑
superficial NEC S30.870 ☑
insect S30.860 ☑
penis S31.25 ☑
superficial NEC S30.872 ☑
insect S30.862 ☑
perineum
female — *see* Bite, vulva
male — *see* Bite, pelvis
periocular area (with or without lacrimal passages) — *see* Bite, eyelid
phalanges
finger — *see* Bite, finger
toe — *see* Bite, toe
pharynx S11.25 ☑
superficial NEC S10.17 ☑
insect S10.16 ☑
pinna — *see* Bite, ear
poisonous — *see* Venom
popliteal space — *see* Bite, knee
prepuce — *see* Bite, penis
pubic region — *see* Bite, abdomen, wall
rectovaginal septum — *see* Bite, vulva
red bug B88.0
reptile NEC (*see also* Venom, bite, reptile)
nonvenomous — *see* Bite, by site
snake — *see* Venom, bite, snake
sacral region — *see* Bite, back, lower
sacroiliac region — *see* Bite, back, lower
salivary gland — *see* Bite, oral cavity
scalp S01.05 ☑
superficial NEC S00.07 ☑
insect S00.06 ☑
scapular region — *see* Bite, shoulder
scrotum S31.35 ☑
superficial NEC S30.873 ☑
insect S30.863 ☑
sea-snake (venomous) — *see* Toxicity, venom, snake, sea snake
shin — *see* Bite, leg
shoulder S41.05- ☑
superficial NEC S40.27- ☑
insect S40.26- ☑
snake (*see also* Venom, bite, snake)
nonvenomous — *see* Bite, by site
spermatic cord — *see* Bite, testis
spider (venomous) — *see* Toxicity, venom, spider
nonvenomous — *see* Bite, by site, superficial, insect
sternal region — *see* Bite, thorax, front
submaxillary region — *see* Bite, head, specified site NEC
submental region — *see* Bite, head, specified site NEC
subungual
finger(s) — *see* Bite, finger
toe — *see* Bite, toe
superficial — *see* Bite, by site, superficial
supraclavicular fossa S11.85 ☑
supraorbital — *see* Bite, head, specified site NEC
temple, temporal region — *see* Bite, head, specified site NEC
temporomandibular area — *see* Bite, cheek
testis S31.35 ☑
superficial NEC S30.873 ☑
insect S30.863 ☑
thigh S71.15- ☑
superficial NEC S70.37- ☑
insect S70.36- ☑
thorax, thoracic (wall) S21.95 ☑

Bite(s) — *continued*
thorax, thoracic — *continued*
back S21.25- ☑
with penetration into thoracic cavity S21.45- ☑
breast — *see* Bite, breast
front S21.15- ☑
with penetration into thoracic cavity S21.35- ☑
superficial NEC S20.97 ☑
back S20.47- ☑
front S20.37- ☑
insect S20.96 ☑
back S20.46- ☑
front S20.36- ☑
throat — *see* Bite, neck, throat
thumb S61.05- ☑
with
damage to nail S61.15- ☑
superficial NEC S60.37- ☑
insect S60.36- ☑
thyroid S11.15 ☑
superficial NEC S10.87 ☑
insect S10.86 ☑
toe(s) S91.15- ☑
with
damage to nail S91.25- ☑
great S91.15- ☑
with
damage to nail S91.25- ☑
lesser S91.15- ☑
with
damage to nail S91.25- ☑
superficial NEC S90.47- ☑
great S90.47- ☑
insect S90.46- ☑
great S90.46- ☑
tongue S01.552 ☑
trachea S11.025 ☑
superficial NEC S10.17 ☑
insect S10.16 ☑
tunica vaginalis — *see* Bite, testis
tympanum, tympanic membrane — *see* Bite, ear
umbilical region S31.155 ☑
uvula — *see* Bite, oral cavity
vagina — *see* Bite, vulva
venomous — *see* Venom
vocal cords S11.035 ☑
superficial NEC S10.17 ☑
insect S10.16 ☑
vulva S31.45 ☑
superficial NEC S30.874 ☑
insect S30.864 ☑
wrist S61.55- ☑
superficial NEC S60.87- ☑
insect S60.86- ☑

Biting, cheek or lip K13.1
Biventricular failure (heart) I50.82
Björck (-Thorson) **syndrome** (malignant carcinoid) E34.0
Black
death A20.9
eye S00.1- ☑
hairy tongue K14.3
heel (foot) S90.3- ☑
lung (disease) J60
palm (hand) S60.22- ☑
Blackfan-Diamond anemia or syndrome (congenital hypoplastic anemia) D61.01
Blackhead L70.0
Blackout R55
Bladder — *see* condition
Blast (air) (hydraulic) (immersion) (underwater)
blindness S05.8X- ☑
injury
abdomen or thorax — *see* Injury, by site
ear (acoustic nerve trauma) — *see* Injury, nerve, acoustic, specified type NEC
syndrome NEC T70.8 ☑
Blastoma — *see* Neoplasm, malignant, by site
pulmonary — *see* Neoplasm, lung, malignant
Blastomycosis, blastomycotic B40.9
Brazilian — *see* Paracoccidioidomycosis
cutaneous B40.3
disseminated B40.7
European — *see* Cryptococcosis
generalized B40.7
keloidal B48.0
North American B40.9

☑ Additional Character Required — Refer to the Tabular List for Character Selection ▽ Subterms under main terms may continue to next column or page

Blastomycosis, blastomycotic — *continued*
- primary pulmonary B40.0
- pulmonary B40.2
  - acute B40.0
  - chronic B40.1
- skin B40.3
- South American — *see* Paracoccidioidomycosis
- specified NEC B40.89

Bleb(s) R23.8
- emphysematous (lung) (solitary) J43.9
- endophthalmitis H59.43
- filtering (vitreous), after glaucoma surgery Z98.83
- inflamed (infected), postprocedural H59.40
  - stage 1 H59.41
  - stage 2 H59.42
  - stage 3 H59.43
- lung (ruptured) J43.9
  - congenital — *see* Atelectasis
  - newborn P25.8
- subpleural (emphysematous) J43.9

Blebitis, postprocedural H59.40
- stage 1 H59.41
- stage 2 H59.42
- stage 3 H59.43

Bleeder (familial) (hereditary) — *see* Hemophilia

Bleeding (*see also* Hemorrhage)
- anal K62.5
- anovulatory N97.0
- atonic, following delivery O72.1
- capillary I78.8
  - puerperal O72.2
- contact (postcoital) N93.0
- due to uterine subinvolution N85.3
- ear — *see* Otorrhagia
- excessive, associated with menopausal onset N92.4
- familial — *see* Defect, coagulation
- following intercourse N93.0
- gastrointestinal K92.2
- hemorrhoids — *see* Hemorrhoids
- intermenstrual (regular) N92.3
  - irregular N92.1
- intraoperative — *see* Complication, intraoperative, hemorrhage
- irregular N92.6
- menopausal N92.4
- newborn, intraventricular — *see* Newborn, affected by, hemorrhage, intraventricular
- nipple N64.59
- nose R04.0
- ovulation N92.3
- postclimacteric N95.0
- postcoital N93.0
- postmenopausal N95.0
- postoperative — *see* Complication, postprocedural, hemorrhage
- preclimacteric N92.4
- pre-pubertal vaginal N93.1
- puberty (excessive, with onset of menstrual periods) N92.2
- rectum, rectal K62.5
  - newborn P54.2
- tendencies — *see* Defect, coagulation
- throat R04.1
- tooth socket (post-extraction) K91.840
- umbilical stump P51.9
- uterus, uterine NEC N93.9
  - climacteric N92.4
  - dysfunctional or functional N93.8
  - menopausal N92.4
  - preclimacteric or premenopausal N92.4
  - unrelated to menstrual cycle N93.9
- vagina, vaginal (abnormal) N93.9
  - dysfunctional or functional N93.8
  - newborn P54.6
  - pre-pubertal N93.1
- vicarious N94.89

Blennorrhagia, blennorrhagic — *see* Gonorrhea

Blennorrhea (acute) (chronic) (*see also* Gonorrhea)
- inclusion (neonatal) (newborn) P39.1
- lower genitourinary tract (gonococcal) A54.00
- neonatorum (gonococcal ophthalmia) A54.31

Blepharelosis — *see* Entropion

Blepharitis (angularis) (ciliaris) (eyelid) (marginal) (nonulcerative) H01.009
- herpes zoster B02.39
- left H01.006
  - lower H01.005
  - upper H01.004

Blepharitis — *continued*
- right H01.003
  - lower H01.002
  - upper H01.001
- squamous H01.029
  - left H01.026
    - lower H01.025
    - upper H01.024
  - right H01.023
    - lower H01.022
    - upper H01.021
- ulcerative H01.019
  - left H01.016
    - lower H01.015
    - upper H01.014
  - right H01.013
    - lower H01.012
    - upper H01.011

Blepharochalasis H02.30
- congenital Q10.0
- left H02.36
  - lower H02.35
  - upper H02.34
- right H02.33
  - lower H02.32
  - upper H02.31

Blepharoclonus H02.59

Blepharoconjunctivitis H10.50- ☑
- angular H10.52- ☑
- contact H10.53- ☑
- ligneous H10.51- ☑

Blepharophimosis (eyelid) H02.529
- congenital Q10.3
- left H02.526
  - lower H02.525
  - upper H02.524
- right H02.523
  - lower H02.522
  - upper H02.521

Blepharoptosis H02.40- ☑
- congenital Q10.0
- mechanical H02.41- ☑
- myogenic H02.42- ☑
- neurogenic H02.43- ☑
- paralytic H02.43- ☑

Blepharopyorrhea, gonococcal A54.39

Blepharospasm G24.5
- drug induced G24.01

Blighted ovum O02.0

Blind (*see also* Blindness)
- bronchus (congenital) Q32.4
- loop syndrome K90.2
  - congenital Q43.8
- sac, fallopian tube (congenital) Q50.6
- spot, enlarged — *see* Defect, visual field, localized, scotoma, blind spot area
- tract or tube, congenital NEC — *see* Atresia, by site

Blindness (acquired) (congenital) (both eyes) H54.0X- ☑
- blast S05.8X- ☑
- color — *see* Deficiency, color vision
- concussion S05.8X- ☑
- cortical H47.619
  - left brain H47.612
  - right brain H47.611
- day H53.11
- due to injury (current episode) S05.9- ☑
  - sequelae — *code to* injury with seventh character S
- eclipse (total) — *see* Retinopathy, solar
- emotional (hysterical) F44.6
- face H53.16
- hysterical F44.6
- legal (both eyes) (USA definition) H54.8
- mind R48.8
- night H53.60
  - abnormal dark adaptation curve H53.61
  - acquired H53.62
  - congenital H53.63
  - specified type NEC H53.69
  - vitamin A deficiency E50.5
- one eye (other eye normal) H54.40
  - left (normal vision on right) H54.42- ☑
    - low vision on right H54.12- ☑
  - low vision, other eye H54.10
  - right (normal vision on left) H54.41- ☑
    - low vision on left H54.11- ☑
- psychic R48.8
- river B73.01

Blindness — *continued*
- snow — *see* Photokeratitis
- sun, solar — *see* Retinopathy, solar
- transient — *see* Disturbance, vision, subjective, loss, transient
- traumatic (current episode) S05.9- ☑
- word (developmental) F81.0
  - acquired R48.0
  - secondary to organic lesion R48.0

Blister (nonthermal)
- abdominal wall S30.821 ☑
- alveolar process S00.522 ☑
- ankle S90.52- ☑
- antecubital space — *see* Blister, elbow
- anus S30.827 ☑
- arm (upper) S40.82- ☑
- auditory canal — *see* Blister, ear
- auricle — *see* Blister, ear
- axilla — *see* Blister, arm
- back, lower S30.820 ☑
- beetle dermatitis L24.89
- breast S20.12- ☑
- brow S00.82 ☑
- calf — *see* Blister, leg
- canthus — *see* Blister, eyelid
- cheek S00.82 ☑
  - internal S00.522 ☑
- chest wall — *see* Blister, thorax
- chin S00.82 ☑
- costal region — *see* Blister, thorax
- digit(s)
  - foot — *see* Blister, toe
  - hand — *see* Blister, finger
- due to burn — *see* Burn, by site, second degree
- ear S00.42- ☑
- elbow S50.32- ☑
- epiglottis S10.12 ☑
- esophagus, cervical S10.12 ☑
- eyebrow — *see* Blister, eyelid
- eyelid S00.22- ☑
- face S00.82 ☑
- fever B00.1
- finger(s) S60.429 ☑
  - index S60.42- ☑
  - little S60.42- ☑
  - middle S60.42- ☑
  - ring S60.42- ☑
- foot (except toe(s) alone) S90.82- ☑
  - toe — *see* Blister, toe
- forearm S50.82- ☑
  - elbow only — *see* Blister, elbow
- forehead S00.82 ☑
- fracture — *omit code*
- genital organ
  - female S30.826 ☑
  - male S30.825 ☑
- gum S00.522 ☑
- hand S60.52- ☑
- head S00.92 ☑
  - ear — *see* Blister, ear
  - eyelid — *see* Blister, eyelid
  - lip S00.521 ☑
  - nose S00.32 ☑
  - oral cavity S00.522 ☑
  - scalp S00.02 ☑
  - specified site NEC S00.82 ☑
- heel — *see* Blister, foot
- hip S70.22- ☑
- interscapular region S20.429 ☑
- jaw S00.82 ☑
- knee S80.22- ☑
- larynx S10.12 ☑
- leg (lower) S80.82- ☑
  - knee — *see* Blister, knee
  - upper — *see* Blister, thigh
- lip S00.521 ☑
- malar region S00.82 ☑
- mammary — *see* Blister, breast
- mastoid region S00.82 ☑
- mouth S00.522 ☑
- multiple, skin, nontraumatic R23.8
- nail
  - finger — *see* Blister, finger
  - toe — *see* Blister, toe
- nasal S00.32 ☑
- neck S10.92 ☑

▽ **Subterms under main terms may continue to next column or page**   ☑ **Additional Character Required** — Refer to the Tabular List for Character Selection   **39**

Blastomycosis, blastomycotic — Blister

Index

Blister — Body, bodies

Blister — *continued*
- neck — *continued*
  - specified site NEC S10.82 ☑
    - throat S10.12 ☑
  - nose S00.32 ☑
  - occipital region S00.02 ☑
  - oral cavity S00.522 ☑
  - orbital region — *see* Blister, eyelid
  - palate S00.522 ☑
  - palm — *see* Blister, hand
  - parietal region S00.02 ☑
  - pelvis S30.820 ☑
  - penis S30.822 ☑
  - periocular area — *see* Blister, eyelid
  - phalanges
    - finger — *see* Blister, finger
    - toe — *see* Blister, toe
  - pharynx S10.12 ☑
  - pinna — *see* Blister, ear
  - popliteal space — *see* Blister, knee
  - scalp S00.02 ☑
  - scapular region — *see* Blister, shoulder
  - scrotum S30.823 ☑
  - shin — *see* Blister, leg
  - shoulder S40.22- ☑
  - sternal region S20.329 ☑
  - submaxillary region S00.82 ☑
  - submental region S00.82 ☑
  - subungual
    - finger(s) — *see* Blister, finger
    - toe(s) — *see* Blister, toe
  - supraclavicular fossa S10.82 ☑
  - supraorbital S00.82 ☑
  - temple S00.82 ☑
  - temporal region S00.82 ☑
  - testis S30.823 ☑
  - thermal — *see* Burn, second degree, by site
  - thigh S70.32- ☑
  - thorax, thoracic (wall) S20.92 ☑
    - back S20.42- ☑
    - front S20.32- ☑
  - throat S10.12 ☑
  - thumb S60.32- ☑
  - toe(s) S90.42- ☑
    - great S90.42- ☑
  - tongue S00.522 ☑
  - trachea S10.12 ☑
  - tympanum, tympanic membrane — *see* Blister, ear
  - upper arm — *see* Blister, arm (upper)
  - uvula S00.522 ☑
  - vagina S30.824 ☑
  - vocal cords S10.12 ☑
  - vulva S30.824 ☑
  - wrist S60.82- ☑

Bloating R14.0
Bloch-Sulzberger disease or syndrome Q82.3
Block, blocked
- alveolocapillary J84.10
- arborization (heart) I45.5
- arrhythmic I45.9
- atrioventricular (incomplete) (partial) I44.30
  - with atrioventricular dissociation I44.2
  - complete I44.2
    - congenital Q24.6
  - congenital Q24.6
  - first degree I44.0
  - second degree (types I and II) I44.1
  - specified NEC I44.39
  - third degree I44.2
  - types I and II I44.1
- auriculoventricular — *see* Block, atrioventricular
- bifascicular (cardiac) I45.2
- bundle-branch (complete) (false) (incomplete) I45.4
  - bilateral I45.2
  - left I44.7
    - with right bundle branch block I45.2
    - hemiblock I44.60
      - anterior I44.4
      - posterior I44.5
    - incomplete I44.7
      - with right bundle branch block I45.2
  - right I45.10
    - with
      - left bundle branch block I45.2
      - left fascicular block I45.2
    - specified NEC I45.19
  - Wilson's type I45.19

Block, blocked — *continued*
- cardiac I45.9
- conduction I45.9
  - complete I44.2
- fascicular (left) I44.60
  - anterior I44.4
  - posterior I44.5
  - right I45.0
  - specified NEC I44.69
- foramen Magendie (acquired) G91.1
  - congenital Q03.1
    - with spina bifida — *see* Spina bifida, by site, with hydrocephalus
- heart I45.9
  - bundle branch I45.4
    - bilateral I45.2
  - complete (atrioventricular) I44.2
  - congenital Q24.6
  - first degree (atrioventricular) I44.0
  - second degree (atrioventricular) I44.1
  - specified type NEC I45.5
  - third degree (atrioventricular) I44.2
- hepatic vein I82.0
- intraventricular (nonspecific) I45.4
  - bundle branch
    - bilateral I45.2
- kidney N28.9
  - postcystoscopic or postprocedural N99.0
- Mobitz (types I and II) I44.1
- myocardial — *see* Block, heart
- nodal I45.5
- organ or site, congenital NEC — *see* Atresia, by site
- portal (vein) I81
- second degree (types I and II) I44.1
- sinoatrial I45.5
- sinoauricular I45.5
- third degree I44.2
- trifascicular I45.3
- tubal N97.1
- vein NOS I82.90
- Wenckebach (types I and II) I44.1

Blockage — *see* Obstruction
Blocq's disease F44.4
Blood
- constituents, abnormal R78.9
- disease D75.9
- donor — *see* Donor, blood
- dyscrasia D75.9
  - with
    - abortion — *see* Abortion, by type, complicated by, hemorrhage
    - ectopic pregnancy O08.1
    - molar pregnancy O08.1
  - following ectopic or molar pregnancy O08.1
  - newborn P61.9
  - puerperal, postpartum O72.3
- flukes NEC — *see* Schistosomiasis
- in
  - feces K92.1
    - occult R19.5
  - urine — *see* Hematuria
- mole O02.0
- occult in feces R19.5
- pressure
  - decreased, due to shock following injury T79.4 ☑
  - examination only Z01.30
  - fluctuating I99.8
  - high — *see* Hypertension
    - borderline R03.0
    - incidental reading, without diagnosis of hypertension R03.0
  - low (*see also* Hypotension)
    - incidental reading, without diagnosis of hypotension R03.1
- spitting — *see* Hemoptysis
- staining cornea — *see* Pigmentation, cornea, stromal
- transfusion
  - reaction or complication — *see* Complications, transfusion
- type
  - A (Rh positive) Z67.10
    - Rh negative Z67.11
  - AB (Rh positive) Z67.30
    - Rh negative Z67.31
  - B (Rh positive) Z67.20
    - Rh negative Z67.21
  - O (Rh positive) Z67.40
    - Rh negative Z67.41

Blood — *continued*
- type — *continued*
  - Rh (positive) Z67.90
    - negative Z67.91
- vessel rupture — *see* Hemorrhage
- vomiting — *see* Hematemesis

Blood-forming organs, disease D75.9
Bloodgood's disease — *see* Mastopathy, cystic
Bloom (-Machacek)(-Torre) **syndrome** Q82.8
Blount's disease or osteochondrosis — *see* Osteochondrosis, juvenile, tibia
Blue
- baby Q24.9
- diaper syndrome E72.09
- dome cyst (breast) — *see* Cyst, breast
- dot cataract Q12.0
- nevus D22.9
- sclera Q13.5
  - with fragility of bone and deafness Q78.0
- toe syndrome I75.02- ☑
Blueness — *see* Cyanosis
Blues, postpartal O90.6
- baby O90.6
Blurring, visual H53.8
Blushing (abnormal) (excessive) R23.2
BMI — *see* Body, mass index
Boarder, hospital NEC Z76.4
- accompanying sick person Z76.3
- healthy infant or child Z76.2
  - foundling Z76.1
Bockhart's impetigo L01.02
Bodechtel-Guttman disease (subacute sclerosing panencephalitis) A81.1
Boder-Sedgwick syndrome (ataxia-telangiectasia) G11.3
Body, bodies
- Aschoff's — *see* Myocarditis, rheumatic
- asteroid, vitreous — *see* Deposit, crystalline
- cytoid (retina) — *see* Occlusion, artery, retina
- drusen (degenerative) (macula) (retinal) (*see also* Degeneration, macula, drusen)
  - optic disc — *see* Drusen, optic disc
- foreign — *see* Foreign body
- loose
  - joint, except knee — *see* Loose, body, joint
    - knee M23.4- ☑
  - sheath, tendon — *see* Disorder, tendon, specified type NEC
- mass index (BMI)
  - adult
    - 19.9 or less Z68.1
    - 20.0-20.9 Z68.20
    - 21.0-21.9 Z68.21
    - 22.0-22.9 Z68.22
    - 23.0-23.9 Z68.23
    - 24.0-24.9 Z68.24
    - 25.0-25.9 Z68.25
    - 26.0-26.9 Z68.26
    - 27.0-27.9 Z68.27
    - 28.0-28.9 Z68.28
    - 29.0-29.9 Z68.29
    - 30.0-30.9 Z68.30
    - 31.0-31.9 Z68.31
    - 32.0-32.9 Z68.32
    - 33.0-33.9 Z68.33
    - 34.0-34.9 Z68.34
    - 35.0-35.9 Z68.35
    - 36.0-36.9 Z68.36
    - 37.0-37.9 Z68.37
    - 38.0-38.9 Z68.38
    - 39.0-39.9 Z68.39
    - 40.0-44.9 Z68.41
    - 45.0-49.9 Z68.42
    - 50.0-59.9 Z68.43
    - 60.0-69.9 Z68.44
    - 70 and over Z68.45
  - pediatric
    - 5th percentile to less than 85th percentile for age Z68.52
    - 85th percentile to less than 95th percentile for age Z68.53
    - less than fifth percentile for age Z68.51
    - greater than or equal to ninety-fifth percentile for age Z68.54
- Mooser's A75.2
- rice (*see also* Loose, body, joint)
  - knee M23.4- ☑
- rocking F98.4

Boeck's
  disease or sarcoid — *see* Sarcoidosis
  lupoid (miliary) D86.3
Boerhaave's syndrome (spontaneous esophageal rupture) K22.3
Boggy
  cervix N88.8
  uterus N85.8
Boil (*see also* Furuncle, by site)
  Aleppo B55.1
  Baghdad B55.1
  Delhi B55.1
  lacrimal
    gland — *see* Dacryoadenitis
    passages (duct) (sac) — *see* Inflammation, lacrimal, passages, acute
  Natal B55.1
  orbit, orbital — *see* Abscess, orbit
  tropical B55.1
Bold hives — *see* Urticaria
Bombé, iris — *see* Membrane, pupillary
Bone — *see* condition
Bonnevie-Ullrich syndrome (*see also* Turner's syndrome) Q87.1
Bonnier's syndrome H81.8 ☑
Bonvale dam fever T73.3 ☑
Bony block of joint — *see* Ankylosis
BOOP (bronchiolitis obliterans organized pneumonia) J84.89
Borderline
  diabetes mellitus R73.03
  hypertension R03.0
  osteopenia M85.8- ☑
  pelvis, with obstruction during labor O65.1
  personality F60.3
Borna disease A83.9
Bornholm disease B33.0
Boston exanthem A88.0
Botalli, ductus (patent) (persistent) Q25.0
Bothriocephalus latus infestation B70.0
Botulism (foodborne intoxication) A05.1
  infant A48.51
  non-foodborne A48.52
  wound A48.52
Bouba — *see* Yaws
Bouchard's nodes (with arthropathy) M15.2
Bouffée délirante F23
Bouillaud's disease or syndrome (rheumatic heart disease) I01.9
Bourneville's disease Q85.1
Boutonniere deformity (finger) — *see* Deformity, finger, boutonniere
Bouveret (-Hoffmann) **syndrome** (paroxysmal tachycardia) I47.9
Bovine heart — *see* Hypertrophy, cardiac
Bowel — *see* condition
Bowen's
  dermatosis (precancerous) — *see* Neoplasm, skin, in situ
  disease — *see* Neoplasm, skin, in situ
  epithelioma — *see* Neoplasm, skin, in situ
  type
    epidermoid carcinoma-in-situ — *see* Neoplasm, skin, in situ
    intraepidermal squamous cell carcinoma — *see* Neoplasm, skin, in situ
Bowing
  femur (*see also* Deformity, limb, specified type NEC, thigh)
    congenital Q68.3
  fibula (*see also* Deformity, limb, specified type NEC, lower leg)
    congenital Q68.4
  forearm — *see* Deformity, limb, specified type NEC, forearm
  leg(s), long bones, congenital Q68.5
  radius — *see* Deformity, limb, specified type NEC, forearm
  tibia (*see also* Deformity, limb, specified type NEC, lower leg)
    congenital Q68.4
Bowleg(s) (acquired) M21.16- ☑
  congenital Q68.5
  rachitic E64.3
Boyd's dysentery A03.2
Brachial — *see* condition
Brachycardia R00.1

Brachycephaly Q75.0
Bradley's disease A08.19
Bradyarrhythmia, cardiac I49.8
Bradycardia (sinoatrial) (sinus) (vagal) R00.1
  neonatal P29.12
  reflex G90.09
  tachycardia syndrome I49.5
Bradykinesia R25.8
Bradypnea R06.89
Bradytachycardia I49.5
Brailsford's disease or osteochondrosis — *see* Osteochondrosis, juvenile, radius
Brain (*see also* condition)
  death G93.82
  syndrome — *see* Syndrome, brain
Branched-chain amino-acid disorder E71.2
Branchial — *see* condition
  cartilage, congenital Q18.2
Branchiogenic remnant (in neck) Q18.0
Brandt's syndrome (acrodermatitis enteropathica) E83.2
Brash (water) R12
Bravais-jacksonian epilepsy — *see* Epilepsy, localization-related, symptomatic, with simple partial seizures
Braxton Hicks contractions — *see* False, labor
Brazilian leishmaniasis B55.2
BRBPR K62.5
Break, retina (without detachment) H33.30- ☑
  with retinal detachment — *see* Detachment, retina
  horseshoe tear H33.31- ☑
  multiple H33.33- ☑
  round hole H33.32- ☑
Breakdown
  device, graft or implant (*see also* Complications, by site and type, mechanical) T85.618 ☑
    arterial graft NEC — *see* Complication, cardiovascular device, mechanical, vascular
    breast (implant) T85.41 ☑
    catheter NEC T85.618 ☑
      cystostomy T83.010 ☑
      dialysis (renal) T82.41 ☑
        intraperitoneal T85.611 ☑
      Hopkins T83.018 ☑
      ileostomy T83.018 ☑
      infusion NEC T82.514 ☑
        cranial T85.610- ☑
        epidural T85.610 ☑
        intrathecal T85.610 ☑
        spinal T85.610 ☑
        subarachnoid T85.610 ☑
        subdural T85.610 ☑
      nephrostomy T83.012 ☑
      urethral indwelling T83.011 ☑
      urinary NEC T83.018 ☑
      urostomy T83.018 ☑
    electronic (electrode) (pulse generator) (stimulator)
      bone T84.310 ☑
      cardiac T82.119 ☑
        electrode T82.110 ☑
        pulse generator T82.111 ☑
        specified type NEC T82.118 ☑
      nervous system — *see* Complication, prosthetic device, mechanical, electronic nervous system stimulator
      urinary — *see* Complication, genitourinary, device, urinary, mechanical
    fixation, internal (orthopedic) NEC — *see* Complication, fixation device, mechanical
    gastrointestinal — *see* Complications, prosthetic device, mechanical, gastrointestinal device
    genital NEC T83.418 ☑
      intrauterine contraceptive device T83.31 ☑
      penile prosthesis (cylinder) (implanted) (pump) (resevoir) T83.410 ☑
      testicular prosthesis T83.411 ☑
    heart NEC — *see* Complication, cardiovascular device, mechanical
    intrathecal infusion pump T85.615 ☑
    joint prosthesis — *see* Complications..., joint prosthesis,internal, mechanical, by site
    nervous system, specified device NEC T85.615 ☑
    ocular NEC — *see* Complications, prosthetic device, mechanical, ocular device
    orthopedic NEC — *see* Complication, orthopedic, device, mechanical
    specified NEC T85.618 ☑

Breakdown — *continued*
  device, graft or implant (*see also* Complications, by site and type, mechanical) — *continued*
    subcutaneous device pocket
      nervous system prosthetic device, implant, or graft T85.890 ☑
      other internal prosthetic device, implant, or graft T85.898 ☑
    sutures, permanent T85.612 ☑
      used in bone repair — *see* Complications, fixation device, internal (orthopedic), mechanical
    urinary NEC T83.118 ☑
      graft T83.21 ☑
      sphincter, implanted T83.111 ☑
      stent (ileal conduit) (nephroureteral) T83.113 ☑
        ureteral indwelling T83.112 ☑
    vascular NEC — *see* Complication, cardiovascular device, mechanical
    ventricular intracranial shunt T85.01 ☑
  nervous F48.8
  perineum O90.1
  respirator J95.850
    specified NEC J95.859
  ventilator J95.850
    specified NEC J95.859
Breast (*see also* condition)
  buds E30.1
    in newborn P96.89
  dense R92.2
  nodule (*see also* Lump, breast) N63.0
Breath
  foul R19.6
  holder, child R06.89
  holding spell R06.89
  shortness R06.02
Breathing
  labored — *see* Hyperventilation
  mouth R06.5
    causing malocclusion M26.5
  periodic R06.3
    high altitude G47.32
Breathlessness R06.81
Breda's disease — *see* Yaws
Breech presentation (mother) O32.1 ☑
  causing obstructed labor O64.1 ☑
  footling O32.8 ☑
    causing obstructed labor O64.8 ☑
  incomplete O32.8 ☑
    causing obstructed labor O64.8 ☑
Breisky's disease N90.4
Brennemann's syndrome I88.0
Brenner
  tumor (benign) D27.9
    borderline malignancy D39.1- ☑
    malignant C56 ☑
    proliferating D39.1- ☑
Bretonneau's disease or angina A36.0
Breus' mole O02.0
Brevicollis Q76.49
Brickmakers' anemia B76.9 [D63.8]
Bridge, myocardial Q24.5
Bright red blood per rectum (BRBPR) K62.5
Bright's disease (*see also* Nephritis)
  arteriosclerotic — *see* Hypertension, kidney
Brill (-Zinsser) **disease** (recrudescent typhus) A75.1
  flea-borne A75.2
  louse-borne A75.1
Brill-Symmers' disease C82.90
Brion-Kayser disease — *see* Fever, parathyroid
Briquet's disorder or syndrome F45.0
Brissaud's
  infantilism or dwarfism E23.0
  motor-verbal tic F95.2
Brittle
  bones disease Q78.0
  nails L60.3
    congenital Q84.6
Broad (*see also* condition)
  beta disease E78.2
  ligament laceration syndrome N83.8
Broad- or floating-betalipoproteinemia E78.2
Brock's syndrome (atelectasis due to enlarged lymph nodes) J98.19
Brocq-Duhring disease (dermatitis herpetiformis) L13.0
Brodie's abscess or disease M86.8X- ☑

Broken
- arches (see also Deformity, limb, flat foot)
- arm (meaning upper limb) — see Fracture, arm
- back — see Fracture, vertebra
- bone — see Fracture
- implant or internal device — see Complications, by site and type, mechanical
- leg (meaning lower limb) — see Fracture, leg
- nose S02.2 ☑
- tooth, teeth — see Fracture, tooth

Bromhidrosis, bromidrosis L75.0

Bromidism, bromism G92
- chronic (dependence) F13.20
- due to
  - correct substance properly administered — see Table of Drugs and Chemicals, by drug, adverse effect
  - overdose or wrong substance given or taken — see Table of Drugs and Chemicals, by drug, poisoning

Bromidrosiphobia F40.298

Bronchi, bronchial — see condition

Bronchiectasis (cylindrical) (diffuse) (fusiform) (localized) (saccular) J47.9
- with
  - acute
    - bronchitis J47.0
    - lower respiratory infection J47.0
    - exacerbation (acute) J47.1
- congenital Q33.4
- tuberculous NEC — see Tuberculosis, pulmonary

Bronchiolectasis — see Bronchiectasis

Bronchiolitis (acute) (infective) (subacute) J21.9
- with
  - bronchospasm or obstruction J21.9
  - influenza, flu or grippe — see Influenza, with, respiratory manifestations NEC
- chemical (chronic) J68.4
  - acute J68.0
- chronic (fibrosing) (obliterative) J44.9
- due to
  - external agent — see Bronchitis, acute, due to
  - human metapneumovirus J21.1
  - respiratory syncytial virus J21.0
  - specified organism NEC J21.8
- fibrosa obliterans J44.9
- influenzal — see Influenza, with, respiratory manifestations NEC
- obliterans J42
  - with organizing pneumonia (BOOP) J84.89
- obliterative (chronic) (subacute) J44.9
  - due to chemicals, gases, fumes or vapors (inhalation) J68.4
  - due to fumes or vapors J68.4
- respiratory, interstitial lung disease J84.115

Bronchitis (diffuse) (fibrinous) (hypostatic) (infective) (membranous) J40
- with
  - influenza, flu or grippe — see Influenza, with, respiratory manifestations NEC
  - obstruction (airway) (lung) J44.9
  - tracheitis (15 years of age and above) J40
    - acute or subacute J20.9
    - chronic J42
    - under 15 years of age J20.9
- acute or subacute (with bronchospasm or obstruction) J20.9
  - with
    - bronchiectasis J47.0
    - chronic obstructive pulmonary disease J44.0
  - chemical (due to gases, fumes or vapors) J68.0
  - due to
    - fumes or vapors J68.0
    - Haemophilus influenzae J20.1
    - Mycoplasma pneumoniae J20.0
    - radiation J70.0
    - specified organism NEC J20.8
    - Streptococcus J20.2
    - virus
      - coxsackie J20.3
      - echovirus J20.7
      - parainfluenzae J20.4
      - respiratory syncytial J20.5
      - rhinovirus J20.6
  - viral NEC J20.8
- allergic (acute) J45.909
  - with
    - exacerbation (acute) J45.901

Bronchitis — continued
- allergic — continued
  - with — continued
    - status asthmaticus J45.902
- arachidic T17.528 ☑
- aspiration (due to fumes or vapors) J68.0
- asthmatic J45.9 ☑
  - chronic J44.9
    - with
      - acute lower respiratory infection J44.0
      - exacerbation (acute) J44.1
- capillary — see Pneumonia, broncho
- caseous (tuberculous) A15.5
- Castellani's A69.8
- catarrhal (15 years of age and above) J40
  - acute — see Bronchitis, acute
  - chronic J41.0
  - under 15 years of age J20.9
- chemical (acute) (subacute) J68.0
  - chronic J68.4
  - due to fumes or vapors J68.0
    - chronic J68.4
- chronic J42
  - with
    - airways obstruction J44.9
    - tracheitis (chronic) J42
  - asthmatic (obstructive) J44.9
  - catarrhal J41.0
  - chemical (due to fumes or vapors) J68.4
  - due to
    - chemicals, gases, fumes or vapors (inhalation) J68.4
    - radiation J70.1
    - tobacco smoking J41.0
  - emphysematous J44.9
  - mucopurulent J41.1
  - non-obstructive J41.0
  - obliterans J44.9
  - obstructive J44.9
  - purulent J41.1
  - simple J41.0
- croupous — see Bronchitis, acute
- due to gases, fumes or vapors (chemical) J68.0
- emphysematous (obstructive) J44.9
- exudative — see Bronchitis, acute
- fetid J41.1
- grippal — see Influenza, with, respiratory manifestations NEC
- in those under 15 years age — see Bronchitis, acute
  - chronic — see Bronchitis, chronic
- influenzal — see Influenza, with, respiratory manifestations NEC
- mixed simple and mucopurulent J41.8
- moulder's J62.8
- mucopurulent (chronic) (recurrent) J41.1
  - acute or subacute J20.9
  - simple (mixed) J41.8
- obliterans (chronic) J44.9
- obstructive (chronic) (diffuse) J44.9
- pituitous J41.1
- pneumococcal, acute or subacute J20.2
- pseudomembranous, acute or subacute — see Bronchitis, acute
- purulent (chronic) (recurrent) J41.1
  - acute or subacute — see Bronchitis, acute
- putrid J41.1
- senile (chronic) J42
- simple and mucopurulent (mixed) J41.8
- smokers' J41.0
- spirochetal NEC A69.8
- subacute — see Bronchitis, acute
- suppurative (chronic) J41.1
  - acute or subacute — see Bronchitis, acute
- tuberculous A15.5
- under 15 years of age — see Bronchitis, acute
  - chronic — see Bronchitis, chronic
- viral NEC, acute or subacute (see also Bronchitis, acute) J20.8

Bronchoalveolitis J18.0

Bronchoaspergillosis B44.1

Bronchocele meaning goiter E04.0

Bronchocholithiasis J98.09
- tuberculous NEC A15.5

Bronchomalacia J98.09
- congenital Q32.2

Bronchomycosis NOS B49 [J99]
- candidal B37.1

Bronchopleuropneumonia — see Pneumonia, broncho

Bronchopneumonia — see Pneumonia, broncho

Bronchopneumonitis — see Pneumonia, broncho

Bronchopulmonary — see condition

Bronchopulmonitis — see Pneumonia, broncho

Bronchorrhagia (see Hemoptysis)

Bronchorrhea J98.09
- acute J20.9
- chronic (infective) (purulent) J42

Bronchospasm (acute) J98.01
- with
  - bronchiolitis, acute J21.9
  - bronchitis, acute (conditions in J20) — see Bronchitis, acute
- due to external agent — see condition, respiratory, acute, due to
- exercise induced J45.990

Bronchospirochetosis A69.8
- Castellani A69.8

Bronchostenosis J98.09

Bronchus — see condition

Brontophobia F40.220

Bronze baby syndrome P83.88

Brooke's tumor — see Neoplasm, skin, benign

Brown enamel of teeth (hereditary) K00.5

Brown's sheath syndrome H50.61- ☑

Brown-Séquard disease, paralysis or syndrome G83.81

Bruce sepsis A23.0

Brucellosis (infection) A23.9
- abortus A23.1
- canis A23.3
- dermatitis A23.9
- melitensis A23.0
- mixed A23.8
- sepsis A23.9
  - melitensis A23.0
  - specified NEC A23.8
- suis A23.2

Bruck-de Lange disease Q87.1

Bruck's disease — see Deformity, limb

BRUE (brief resolved unexplained event) R68.13

Brugsch's syndrome Q82.8

Bruise (skin surface intact) (see also Contusion)
- with
  - open wound — see Wound, open
  - internal organ — see Injury, by site
- newborn P54.5
- scalp, due to birth injury, newborn P12.3
- umbilical cord O69.5 ☑

Bruit (arterial) R09.89
- cardiac R01.1

Brush burn — see Abrasion, by site

Bruton's X-linked agammaglobulinemia D80.0

Bruxism
- psychogenic F45.8
- sleep related G47.63

Bubbly lung syndrome P27.0

Bubo I88.8
- blennorrhagic (gonococcal) A54.89
- chancroidal A57
- climatic A55
- due to Haemophilus ducreyi A57
- gonococcal A54.89
- indolent (nonspecific) I88.8
- inguinal (nonspecific) I88.8
  - chancroidal A57
  - climatic A55
  - due to H. ducreyi A57
  - infective I88.8
- scrofulous (tuberculous) A18.2
- soft chancre A57
- suppurating — see Lymphadenitis, acute
- syphilitic (primary) A51.0
  - congenital A50.07
- tropical A55
- virulent (chancroidal) A57

Bubonic plague A20.0

Bubonocele — see Hernia, inguinal

Buccal — see condition

Buchanan's disease or osteochondrosis M91.0

Buchem's syndrome (hyperostosis corticalis) M85.2

Bucket-handle fracture or tear (semilunar cartilage) — see Tear, meniscus

Budd-Chiari syndrome (hepatic vein thrombosis) I82.0

Budgerigar fancier's disease or lung J67.2

Buds
- breast E30.1

Buds — *continued*
  breast — *continued*
    in newborn P96.89
Buerger's disease (thromboangiitis obliterans) I73.1
Bulbar — *see* condition
Bulbus cordis (left ventricle) (persistent) Q21.8
Bulimia (nervosa) F50.2
  atypical F50.9
  normal weight F50.9
Bulky
  stools R19.5
  uterus N85.2
Bulla (e) R23.8
  lung (emphysematous) (solitary) J43.9
    newborn P25.8
Bullet wound (*see also* Wound, open)
  fracture — *code as* Fracture, by site
  internal organ — *see* Injury, by site
Bundle
  branch block (complete) (false) (incomplete) — *see*
      Block, bundle-branch
  of His — *see* condition
Bunion M21.61- ☑
  tailor's M21.62- ☑
Bunionette M21.62- ☑
Buphthalmia, buphthalmos (congenital) Q15.0
Burdwan fever B55.0
Bürger-Grütz disease or syndrome E78.3
Buried
  penis (congenital) Q55.64
    acquired N48.83
  roots K08.3
Burke's syndrome K86.89
Burkitt
  cell leukemia C91.0- ☑
  lymphoma (malignant) C83.7- ☑
    small noncleaved, diffuse C83.7- ☑
    spleen C83.77
    undifferentiated C83.7- ☑
  tumor C83.7- ☑
  type
    acute lymphoblastic leukemia C91.0- ☑
    undifferentiated C83.7- ☑
Burn (electricity) (flame) (hot gas, liquid or hot object)
    (radiation) (steam) (thermal) T30.0
  abdomen, abdominal (muscle) (wall) T21.02 ☑
    first degree T21.12 ☑
    second degree T21.22 ☑
    third degree T21.32 ☑
  above elbow T22.039 ☑
    first degree T22.139 ☑
    left T22.032 ☑
      first degree T22.132 ☑
      second degree T22.232 ☑
      third degree T22.332 ☑
    right T22.031 ☑
      first degree T22.131 ☑
      second degree T22.231 ☑
      third degree T22.331 ☑
    second degree T22.239 ☑
    third degree T22.339 ☑
  acid (caustic) (external) (internal) — *see* Corrosion, by
      site
  alimentary tract NEC T28.2 ☑
    esophagus T28.1 ☑
    mouth T28.0 ☑
    pharynx T28.0 ☑
  alkaline (caustic) (external) (internal) — *see* Corrosion,
      by site
  ankle T25.019 ☑
    first degree T25.119 ☑
    left T25.012 ☑
      first degree T25.112 ☑
      second degree T25.212 ☑
      third degree T25.312 ☑
    multiple with foot — *see* Burn, lower, limb, multi-
        ple, ankle and foot
    right T25.011 ☑
      first degree T25.111 ☑
      second degree T25.211 ☑
      third degree T25.311 ☑
    second degree T25.219 ☑
    third degree T25.319 ☑
  anus — *see* Burn, buttock
  arm (lower) (upper) — *see* Burn, upper, limb
  axilla T22.049 ☑

Burn — *continued*
  axilla — *continued*
    first degree T22.149 ☑
    left T22.042 ☑
      first degree T22.142 ☑
      second degree T22.242 ☑
      third degree T22.342 ☑
    right T22.041 ☑
      first degree T22.141 ☑
      second degree T22.241 ☑
      third degree T22.341 ☑
    second degree T22.249 ☑
    third degree T22.349 ☑
  back (lower) T21.04 ☑
    first degree T21.14 ☑
    second degree T21.24 ☑
    third degree T21.34 ☑
    upper T21.03 ☑
      first degree T21.13 ☑
      second degree T21.23 ☑
      third degree T21.33 ☑
  blisters — *code as* Burn, second degree, by site
  breast(s) — *see* Burn, chest wall
  buttock(s) T21.05 ☑
    first degree T21.15 ☑
    second degree T21.25 ☑
    third degree T21.35 ☑
  calf T24.039 ☑
    first degree T24.139 ☑
    left T24.032 ☑
      first degree T24.132 ☑
      second degree T24.232 ☑
      third degree T24.332 ☑
    right T24.031 ☑
      first degree T24.131 ☑
      second degree T24.231 ☑
      third degree T24.331 ☑
    second degree T24.239 ☑
    third degree T24.339 ☑
  canthus (eye) — *see* Burn, eyelid
  caustic acid or alkaline — *see* Corrosion, by site
  cervix T28.3 ☑
  cheek T20.06 ☑
    first degree T20.16 ☑
    second degree T20.26 ☑
    third degree T20.36 ☑
  chemical (acids) (alkalines) (caustics) (external) (inter-
      nal) — *see* Corrosion, by site
  chest wall T21.01 ☑
    first degree T21.11 ☑
    second degree T21.21 ☑
    third degree T21.31 ☑
  chin T20.03 ☑
    first degree T20.13 ☑
    second degree T20.23 ☑
    third degree T20.33 ☑
  colon T28.2 ☑
  conjunctiva (and cornea) — *see* Burn, cornea
  cornea (and conjunctiva) T26.1- ☑
    chemical — *see* Corrosion, cornea
  corrosion (external) (internal) — *see* Corrosion, by site
  deep necrosis of underlying tissue — *code as* Burn,
      third degree, by site
  dorsum of hand T23.069 ☑
    first degree T23.169 ☑
    left T23.062 ☑
      first degree T23.162 ☑
      second degree T23.262 ☑
      third degree T23.362 ☑
    right T23.061 ☑
      first degree T23.161 ☑
      second degree T23.261 ☑
      third degree T23.361 ☑
    second degree T23.269 ☑
    third degree T23.369 ☑
  due to ingested chemical agent — *see* Corrosion, by
      site
  ear (auricle) (external) (canal) T20.01 ☑
    first degree T20.11 ☑
    second degree T20.21 ☑
    third degree T20.31 ☑
  elbow T22.029 ☑
    first degree T22.129 ☑
    left T22.022 ☑
      first degree T22.122 ☑
      second degree T22.222 ☑

Burn — *continued*
  elbow — *continued*
    left — *continued*
      third degree T22.322 ☑
    right T22.021 ☑
      first degree T22.121 ☑
      second degree T22.221 ☑
      third degree T22.321 ☑
    second degree T22.229 ☑
    third degree T22.329 ☑
  epidermal loss — *code as* Burn, second degree, by site
  erythema, erythematous — *code as* Burn, first degree,
      by site
  esophagus T28.1 ☑
  extent (percentage of body surface)
    less than 10 percent T31.0
    10-19 percent T31.10
      with 0-9 percent third degree burns T31.10
      with 10-19 percent third degree burns T31.11
    20-29 percent T31.20
      with 0-9 percent third degree burns T31.20
      with 10-19 percent third degree burns T31.21
      with 20-29 percent third degree burns T31.22
    30-39 percent T31.30
      with 0-9 percent third degree burns T31.30
      with 10-19 percent third degree burns T31.31
      with 20-29 percent third degree burns T31.32
      with 30-39 percent third degree burns T31.33
    40-49 percent T31.40
      with 0-9 percent third degree burns T31.40
      with 10-19 percent third degree burns T31.41
      with 20-29 percent third degree burns T31.42
      with 30-39 percent third degree burns T31.43
      with 40-49 percent third degree burns T31.44
    50-59 percent T31.50
      with 0-9 percent third degree burns T31.50
      with 10-19 percent third degree burns T31.51
      with 20-29 percent third degree burns T31.52
      with 30-39 percent third degree burns T31.53
      with 40-49 percent third degree burns T31.54
      with 50-59 percent third degree burns T31.55
    60-69 percent T31.60
      with 0-9 percent third degree burns T31.60
      with 10-19 percent third degree burns T31.61
      with 20-29 percent third degree burns T31.62
      with 30-39 percent third degree burns T31.63
      with 40-49 percent third degree burns T31.64
      with 50-59 percent third degree burns T31.65
      with 60-69 percent third degree burns T31.66
    70-79 percent T31.70
      with 0-9 percent third degree burns T31.70
      with 10-19 percent third degree burns T31.71
      with 20-29 percent third degree burns T31.72
      with 30-39 percent third degree burns T31.73
      with 40-49 percent third degree burns T31.74
      with 50-59 percent third degree burns T31.75
      with 60-69 percent third degree burns T31.76
      with 70-79 percent third degree burns T31.77
    80-89 percent T31.80
      with 0-9 percent third degree burns T31.80
      with 10-19 percent third degree burns T31.81
      with 20-29 percent third degree burns T31.82
      with 30-39 percent third degree burns T31.83
      with 40-49 percent third degree burns T31.84
      with 50-59 percent third degree burns T31.85
      with 60-69 percent third degree burns T31.86
      with 70-79 percent third degree burns T31.87
      with 80-89 percent third degree burns T31.88
    90 percent or more T31.90
      with 0-9 percent third degree burns T31.90
      with 10-19 percent third degree burns T31.91
      with 20-29 percent third degree burns T31.92
      with 30-39 percent third degree burns T31.93
      with 40-49 percent third degree burns T31.94
      with 50-59 percent third degree burns T31.95
      with 60-69 percent third degree burns T31.96
      with 70-79 percent third degree burns T31.97
      with 80-89 percent third degree burns T31.98
      with 90 percent or more third degree burns
          T31.99
  extremity — *see* Burn, limb
  eye(s) and adnexa T26.4- ☑
    with resulting rupture and destruction of eyeball
        T26.2- ☑
    conjunctival sac — *see* Burn, cornea
    cornea — *see* Burn, cornea
    lid — *see* Burn, eyelid
    periocular area — *see* Burn, eyelid

Burn — *continued*
  eye(s) and adnexa — *continued*
    specified site NEC T26.3- ✓
  eyeball — *see* Burn, eye
  eyelid(s) T26.0- ✓
    chemical — *see* Corrosion, eyelid
  face — *see* Burn, head
  finger T23.029 ✓
    first degree T23.129 ✓
    left T23.022 ✓
      first degree T23.122 ✓
      second degree T23.222 ✓
      third degree T23.322 ✓
    multiple sites (without thumb) T23.039 ✓
      with thumb T23.049 ✓
        first degree T23.149 ✓
        left T23.042 ✓
          first degree T23.142 ✓
          second degree T23.242 ✓
          third degree T23.342 ✓
        right T23.041 ✓
          first degree T23.141 ✓
          second degree T23.241 ✓
          third degree T23.341 ✓
      second degree T23.249 ✓
      third degree T23.349 ✓
    first degree T23.139 ✓
    left T23.032 ✓
      first degree T23.132 ✓
      second degree T23.232 ✓
      third degree T23.332 ✓
    right T23.031 ✓
      first degree T23.131 ✓
      second degree T23.231 ✓
      third degree T23.331 ✓
    second degree T23.239 ✓
    third degree T23.339 ✓
    right T23.021 ✓
      first degree T23.121 ✓
      second degree T23.221 ✓
      third degree T23.321 ✓
    second degree T23.229 ✓
    third degree T23.329 ✓
  flank — *see* Burn, abdominal wall
  foot T25.029 ✓
    first degree T25.129 ✓
    left T25.022 ✓
      first degree T25.122 ✓
      second degree T25.222 ✓
      third degree T25.322 ✓
    multiple with ankle — *see* Burn, lower, limb, multiple, ankle and foot
    right T25.021 ✓
      first degree T25.121 ✓
      second degree T25.221 ✓
      third degree T25.321 ✓
    second degree T25.229 ✓
    third degree T25.329 ✓
  forearm T22.019 ✓
    first degree T22.119 ✓
    left T22.012 ✓
      first degree T22.112 ✓
      second degree T22.212 ✓
      third degree T22.312 ✓
    right T22.011 ✓
      first degree T22.111 ✓
      second degree T22.211 ✓
      third degree T22.311 ✓
    second degree T22.219 ✓
    third degree T22.319 ✓
  forehead T20.06 ✓
    first degree T20.16 ✓
    second degree T20.26 ✓
    third degree T20.36 ✓
  fourth degree — *code as* Burn, third degree, by site
  friction — *see* Burn, by site
  from swallowing caustic or corrosive substance NEC — *see* Corrosion, by site
  full thickness skin loss — *code as* Burn, third degree, by site
  gastrointestinal tract NEC T28.2 ✓
    from swallowing caustic or corrosive substance T28.7 ✓
  genital organs
    external
      female T21.07 ✓

Burn — *continued*
  genital organs — *continued*
    external — *continued*
      female — *continued*
        first degree T21.17 ✓
        second degree T21.27 ✓
        third degree T21.37 ✓
      male T21.06 ✓
        first degree T21.16 ✓
        second degree T21.26 ✓
        third degree T21.36 ✓
    internal T28.3 ✓
      from caustic or corrosive substance T28.8 ✓
  groin — *see* Burn, abdominal wall
  hand(s) T23.009 ✓
    back — *see* Burn, dorsum of hand
    finger — *see* Burn, finger
    first degree T23.109 ✓
    left T23.002 ✓
      first degree T23.102 ✓
      second degree T23.202 ✓
      third degree T23.302 ✓
    multiple sites with wrist T23.099 ✓
      first degree T23.199 ✓
      left T23.092 ✓
        first degree T23.192 ✓
        second degree T23.292 ✓
        third degree T23.392 ✓
      right T23.091 ✓
        first degree T23.191 ✓
        second degree T23.291 ✓
        third degree T23.391 ✓
      second degree T23.299 ✓
      third degree T23.399 ✓
    palm — *see* Burn, palm
    right T23.001 ✓
      first degree T23.101 ✓
      second degree T23.201 ✓
      third degree T23.301 ✓
    second degree T23.209 ✓
    third degree T23.309 ✓
    thumb — *see* Burn, thumb
  head (and face) (and neck) T20.00 ✓
    cheek — *see* Burn, cheek
    chin — *see* Burn, chin
    ear — *see* Burn, ear
    eye(s) only — *see* Burn, eye
    first degree T20.10 ✓
    forehead — *see* Burn, forehead
    lip — *see* Burn, lip
    multiple sites T20.09 ✓
      first degree T20.19 ✓
      second degree T20.29 ✓
      third degree T20.39 ✓
    neck — *see* Burn, neck
    nose — *see* Burn, nose
    scalp — *see* Burn, scalp
    second degree T20.20 ✓
    third degree T20.30 ✓
  hip(s) — *see* Burn, thigh
  inhalation — *see* Burn, respiratory tract
    caustic or corrosive substance (fumes) — *see* Corrosion, respiratory tract
  internal organ(s) T28.40 ✓
    alimentary tract T28.2 ✓
      esophagus T28.1 ✓
    eardrum T28.41 ✓
    esophagus T28.1 ✓
      from caustic or corrosive substance (swallowing) NEC — *see* Corrosion, by site
    genitourinary T28.3 ✓
    mouth T28.0 ✓
    pharynx T28.0 ✓
    respiratory tract — *see* Burn, respiratory tract
    specified organ NEC T28.49 ✓
  interscapular region — *see* Burn, back, upper
  intestine (large) (small) T28.2 ✓
  knee T24.029 ✓
    first degree T24.129 ✓
    left T24.022 ✓
      first degree T24.122 ✓
      second degree T24.222 ✓
      third degree T24.322 ✓
    right T24.021 ✓
      first degree T24.121 ✓
      second degree T24.221 ✓

Burn — *continued*
  knee — *continued*
    right — *continued*
        third degree T24.321 ✓
      second degree T24.229 ✓
      third degree T24.329 ✓
  labium (majus) (minus) — *see* Burn, genital organs, external, female
  lacrimal apparatus, duct, gland or sac — *see* Burn, eye, specified site NEC
  larynx T27.0 ✓
    with lung T27.1 ✓
  leg(s) (lower) (upper) — *see* Burn, lower, limb
  lightning — *see* Burn, by site
  limb(s)
    lower (except ankle or foot alone) — *see* Burn, lower, limb
    upper — *see* Burn, upper limb
  lip(s) T20.02 ✓
    first degree T20.12 ✓
    second degree T20.22 ✓
    third degree T20.32 ✓
  lower
    back — *see* Burn, back
    limb T24.009 ✓
      ankle — *see* Burn, ankle
      calf — *see* Burn, calf
      first degree T24.109 ✓
      foot — *see* Burn, foot
      hip — *see* Burn, thigh
      knee — *see* Burn, knee
      left T24.002 ✓
        first degree T24.102 ✓
        second degree T24.202 ✓
        third degree T24.302 ✓
      multiple sites, except ankle and foot T24.099 ✓
        ankle and foot T25.099 ✓
          first degree T25.199 ✓
          left T25.092 ✓
            first degree T25.192 ✓
            second degree T25.292 ✓
            third degree T25.392 ✓
          right T25.091 ✓
            first degree T25.191 ✓
            second degree T25.291 ✓
            third degree T25.391 ✓
          second degree T25.299 ✓
          third degree T25.399 ✓
        first degree T24.199 ✓
        left T24.092 ✓
          first degree T24.192 ✓
          second degree T24.292 ✓
          third degree T24.392 ✓
        right T24.091 ✓
          first degree T24.191 ✓
          second degree T24.291 ✓
          third degree T24.391 ✓
        second degree T24.299 ✓
        third degree T24.399 ✓
      right T24.001 ✓
        first degree T24.101 ✓
        second degree T24.201 ✓
        third degree T24.301 ✓
      second degree T24.209 ✓
      thigh — *see* Burn, thigh
      third degree T24.309 ✓
      toe — *see* Burn, toe
  lung (with larynx and trachea) T27.1 ✓
  mouth T28.0 ✓
  neck T20.07 ✓
    first degree T20.17 ✓
    second degree T20.27 ✓
    third degree T20.37 ✓
  nose (septum) T20.04 ✓
    first degree T20.14 ✓
    second degree T20.24 ✓
    third degree T20.34 ✓
  ocular adnexa — *see* Burn, eye
  orbit region — *see* Burn, eyelid
  palm T23.059 ✓
    first degree T23.159 ✓
    left T23.052 ✓
      first degree T23.152 ✓
      second degree T23.252 ✓
      third degree T23.352 ✓
    right T23.051 ✓

✓ **Additional Character Required** — Refer to the Tabular List for Character Selection   ▽ **Subterms under main terms may continue to next column or page**

Burn — continued
  palm — continued
    right — continued
      first degree T23.151 ☑
      second degree T23.251 ☑
      third degree T23.351 ☑
    second degree T23.259 ☑
    third degree T23.359 ☑
  partial thickness — code as Burn, unspecified degree, by site
  pelvis — see Burn, trunk
  penis — see Burn, genital organs, external, male
  perineum
    female — see Burn, genital organs, external, female
    male — see Burn, genital organs, external, male
  periocular area — see Burn, eyelid
  pharynx T28.0 ☑
  rectum T28.2 ☑
  respiratory tract T27.3 ☑
    larynx — see Burn, larynx
    specified part NEC T27.2 ☑
    trachea — see Burn, trachea
  sac, lacrimal — see Burn, eye, specified site NEC
  scalp T20.05 ☑
    first degree T20.15 ☑
    second degree T20.25 ☑
    third degree T20.35 ☑
  scapular region T22.069 ☑
    first degree T22.169 ☑
    left T22.062 ☑
      first degree T22.162 ☑
      second degree T22.262 ☑
      third degree T22.362 ☑
    right T22.061 ☑
      first degree T22.161 ☑
      second degree T22.261 ☑
      third degree T22.361 ☑
    second degree T22.269 ☑
    third degree T22.369 ☑
  sclera — see Burn, eye, specified site NEC
  scrotum — see Burn, genital organs, external, male
  shoulder T22.059 ☑
    first degree T22.159 ☑
    left T22.052 ☑
      first degree T22.152 ☑
      second degree T22.252 ☑
      third degree T22.352 ☑
    right T22.051 ☑
      first degree T22.151 ☑
      second degree T22.251 ☑
      third degree T22.351 ☑
    second degree T22.259 ☑
    third degree T22.359 ☑
  stomach T28.2 ☑
  temple — see Burn, head
  testis — see Burn, genital organs, external, male
  thigh T24.019 ☑
    first degree T24.119 ☑
    left T24.012 ☑
      first degree T24.112 ☑
      second degree T24.212 ☑
      third degree T24.312 ☑
    right T24.011 ☑
      first degree T24.111 ☑
      second degree T24.211 ☑
      third degree T24.311 ☑
    second degree T24.219 ☑
    third degree T24.319 ☑
  thorax (external) — see Burn, trunk
  throat (meaning pharynx) T28.0 ☑
  thumb(s) T23.019 ☑
    first degree T23.119 ☑
    left T23.012 ☑
      first degree T23.112 ☑
      second degree T23.212 ☑
      third degree T23.312 ☑
    multiple sites with fingers T23.049 ☑
      first degree T23.149 ☑
      left T23.042 ☑
        first degree T23.142 ☑
        second degree T23.242 ☑
        third degree T23.342 ☑
      right T23.041 ☑
        first degree T23.141 ☑
        second degree T23.241 ☑
        third degree T23.341 ☑

Burn — continued
  thumb(s) — continued
    multiple sites with fingers — continued
      second degree T23.249 ☑
      third degree T23.349 ☑
    right T23.011 ☑
      first degree T23.111 ☑
      second degree T23.211 ☑
      third degree T23.311 ☑
    second degree T23.219 ☑
    third degree T23.319 ☑
  toe T25.039 ☑
    first degree T25.139 ☑
    left T25.032 ☑
      first degree T25.132 ☑
      second degree T25.232 ☑
      third degree T25.332 ☑
    right T25.031 ☑
      first degree T25.131 ☑
      second degree T25.231 ☑
      third degree T25.331 ☑
    second degree T25.239 ☑
    third degree T25.339 ☑
  tongue T28.0 ☑
  tonsil(s) T28.0 ☑
  trachea T27.0 ☑
    with lung T27.1 ☑
  trunk T21.00 ☑
    abdominal wall — see Burn, abdominal wall
    anus — see Burn, buttock
    axilla — see Burn, upper limb
    back — see Burn, back
    breast — see Burn, chest wall
    buttock — see Burn, buttock
    chest wall — see Burn, chest wall
    first degree T21.10 ☑
    flank — see Burn, abdominal wall
    genital
      female — see Burn, genital organs, external, female
      male — see Burn, genital organs, external, male
    groin — see Burn, abdominal wall
    interscapular region — see Burn, back, upper
    labia — see Burn, genital organs, external, female
    lower back — see Burn, back
    penis — see Burn, genital organs, external, male
    perineum
      female — see Burn, genital organs, external, female
      male — see Burn, genital organs, external, male
    scapula region — see Burn, scapular region
    scrotum — see Burn, genital organs, external, male
    second degree T21.20 ☑
    specified site NEC T21.09 ☑
      first degree T21.19 ☑
      second degree T21.29 ☑
      third degree T21.39 ☑
    testes — see Burn, genital organs, external, male
    third degree T21.30 ☑
    upper back — see Burn, back, upper
    vulva — see Burn, genital organs, external, female
  unspecified site with extent of body surface involved specified
    less than 10 percent T31.0
    10-19 percent (0-9 percent third degree) T31.10
      with 10-19 percent third degree T31.11
    20-29 percent (0-9 percent third degree) T31.20
      with
        10-19 percent third degree T31.21
        20-29 percent third degree T31.22
    30-39 percent (0-9 percent third degree) T31.30
      with
        10-19 percent third degree T31.31
        20-29 percent third degree T31.32
        30-39 percent third degree T31.33
    40-49 percent (0-9 percent third degree) T31.40
      with
        10-19 percent third degree T31.41
        20-29 percent third degree T31.42
        30-39 percent third degree T31.43
        40-49 percent third degree T31.44
    50-59 percent (0-9 percent third degree) T31.50
      with
        10-19 percent third degree T31.51
        20-29 percent third degree T31.52
        30-39 percent third degree T31.53
        40-49 percent third degree T31.54

Burn — continued
  unspecified site with extent of body surface involved specified — continued
    50-59 percent — continued
      with — continued
        50-59 percent third degree T31.55
    60-69 percent (0-9 percent third degree) T31.60
      with
        10-19 percent third degree T31.61
        20-29 percent third degree T31.62
        30-39 percent third degree T31.63
        40-49 percent third degree T31.64
        50-59 percent third degree T31.65
        60-69 percent third degree T31.66
    70-79 percent (0-9 percent third degree) T31.70
      with
        10-19 percent third degree T31.71
        20-29 percent third degree T31.72
        30-39 percent third degree T31.73
        40-49 percent third degree T31.74
        50-59 percent third degree T31.75
        60-69 percent third degree T31.76
        70-79 percent third degree T31.77
    80-89 percent (0-9 percent third degree) T31.80
      with
        10-19 percent third degree T31.81
        20-29 percent third degree T31.82
        30-39 percent third degree T31.83
        40-49 percent third degree T31.84
        50-59 percent third degree T31.85
        60-69 percent third degree T31.86
        70-79 percent third degree T31.87
        80-89 percent third degree T31.88
    90 percent or more (0-9 percent third degree) T31.90
      with
        10-19 percent third degree T31.91
        20-29 percent third degree T31.92
        30-39 percent third degree T31.93
        40-49 percent third degree T31.94
        50-59 percent third degree T31.95
        60-69 percent third degree T31.96
        70-79 percent third degree T31.97
        80-89 percent third degree T31.98
        90-99 percent third degree T31.99
  upper limb T22.00 ☑
    above elbow — see Burn, above elbow
    axilla — see Burn, axilla
    elbow — see Burn, elbow
    first degree T22.10 ☑
    forearm — see Burn, forearm
    hand — see Burn, hand
    interscapular region — see Burn, back, upper
    multiple sites T22.099 ☑
      first degree T22.199 ☑
      left T22.092 ☑
        first degree T22.192 ☑
        second degree T22.292 ☑
        third degree T22.392 ☑
      right T22.091 ☑
        first degree T22.191 ☑
        second degree T22.291 ☑
        third degree T22.391 ☑
      second degree T22.299 ☑
      third degree T22.399 ☑
    scapular region — see Burn, scapular region
    second degree T22.20 ☑
    shoulder — see Burn, shoulder
    third degree T22.30 ☑
    wrist — see Burn, wrist
  uterus T28.3 ☑
  vagina T28.3 ☑
  vulva — see Burn, genital organs, external, female
  wrist T23.079 ☑
    first degree T23.179 ☑
    left T23.072 ☑
      first degree T23.172 ☑
      second degree T23.272 ☑
      third degree T23.372 ☑
    multiple sites with hand T23.099 ☑
      first degree T23.199 ☑
      left T23.092 ☑
        first degree T23.192 ☑
        second degree T23.292 ☑
        third degree T23.392 ☑
      right T23.091 ☑
        first degree T23.191 ☑

☟ Subterms under main terms may continue to next column or page   ☑ Additional Character Required — Refer to the Tabular List for Character Selection   45

Burn — Burn

Burn — *continued*
  wrist — *continued*
    multiple sites with hand — *continued*
      right — *continued*
        second degree T23.291 ☑
        third degree T23.391 ☑
      second degree T23.299 ☑
      third degree T23.399 ☑
      right T23.071 ☑
        first degree T23.171 ☑
        second degree T23.271 ☑
        third degree T23.371 ☑
      second degree T23.279 ☑
      third degree T23.379 ☑
Burnett's syndrome E83.52
Burning
  feet syndrome E53.9
  sensation R20.8
  tongue K14.6
Burn-out (state) Z73.0
Burns' disease or osteochondrosis — *see* Osteochondrosis, juvenile, ulna
Bursa — *see* condition
Bursitis M71.9
  Achilles — *see* Tendinitis, Achilles
  adhesive — *see* Bursitis, specified NEC
  ankle — *see* Enthesopathy, lower limb, ankle, specified type NEC
  calcaneal — *see* Enthesopathy, foot, specified type NEC
  collateral ligament, tibial — *see* Bursitis, tibial collateral
  due to use, overuse, pressure (*see also* Disorder, soft tissue, due to use, specified type NEC)
    specified NEC — *see* Disorder, soft tissue, due to use, specified NEC
  Duplay's M75.0 ☑
  elbow NEC M70.3- ☑
    olecranon M70.2- ☑
  finger — *see* Disorder, soft tissue, due to use, specified type NEC, hand
  foot — *see* Enthesopathy, foot, specified type NEC
  gonococcal A54.49
  gouty — *see* Gout
  hand M70.1- ☑
  hip NEC M70.7- ☑
    trochanteric M70.6- ☑
  infective NEC M71.10
    abscess — *see* Abscess, bursa
    ankle M71.17- ☑
    elbow M71.12- ☑
    foot M71.17- ☑
    hand M71.14- ☑
    hip M71.15- ☑
    knee M71.16- ☑
    multiple sites M71.19
    shoulder M71.11- ☑
    specified site NEC M71.18
    wrist M71.13- ☑
  ischial — *see* Bursitis, hip
  knee NEC M70.5- ☑
    prepatellar M70.4- ☑
  occupational NEC (*see also* Disorder, soft tissue, due to, use)
  olecranon — *see* Bursitis, elbow, olecranon
  pharyngeal J39.1
  popliteal — *see* Bursitis, knee
  prepatellar M70.4- ☑
  radiohumeral M77.8
  rheumatoid M06.20
    ankle M06.27- ☑
    elbow M06.22- ☑
    foot joint M06.27- ☑
    hand joint M06.24- ☑
    hip M06.25- ☑
    knee M06.26- ☑
    multiple site M06.29
    shoulder M06.21- ☑
    vertebra M06.28
    wrist M06.23- ☑
  scapulohumeral — *see* Bursitis, shoulder
  semimembranous muscle (knee) — *see* Bursitis, knee
  shoulder M75.5- ☑
    adhesive — *see* Capsulitis, adhesive
  specified NEC M71.50
    ankle M71.57- ☑

Bursitis — *continued*
  specified — *continued*
    due to use, overuse or pressure — *see* Disorder, soft tissue, due to, use
    elbow M71.52- ☑
    foot M71.57- ☑
    hand M71.54- ☑
    hip M71.55- ☑
    knee M71.56- ☑
    shoulder — *see* Bursitis, shoulder
    specified site NEC M71.58
    tibial collateral M76.4- ☑
    wrist M71.53- ☑
  subacromial — *see* Bursitis, shoulder
  subcoracoid — *see* Bursitis, shoulder
  subdeltoid — *see* Bursitis, shoulder
  syphilitic A52.78
  Thornwaldt, Tornwaldt J39.2
  tibial collateral M76.4- ☑
  toe — *see* Enthesopathy, foot, specified type NEC
  trochanteric (area) — *see* Bursitis, hip, trochanteric
  wrist — *see* Bursitis, hand
Bursopathy M71.9
  specified type NEC M71.80
    ankle M71.87- ☑
    elbow M71.82- ☑
    foot M71.87- ☑
    hand M71.84- ☑
    hip M71.85- ☑
    knee M71.86- ☑
    multiple sites M71.89
    shoulder M71.81- ☑
    specified site NEC M71.88
    wrist M71.83- ☑
Burst stitches or sutures (complication of surgery) T81.31 ☑
  external operation wound T81.31 ☑
  internal operation wound T81.32 ☑
Buruli ulcer A31.1
Bury's disease L95.1
Buschke's
  disease B45.3
  scleredema — *see* Sclerosis, systemic
Busse-Buschke disease B45.3
Buttock — *see* condition
Button
  Biskra B55.1
  Delhi B55.1
  oriental B55.1
Buttonhole deformity (finger) — *see* Deformity, finger, boutonniere
Bwamba fever A92.8
Byssinosis J66.0
Bywaters' syndrome T79.5 ☑

C

Cachexia R64
  cancerous R64
  cardiac — *see* Disease, heart
  dehydration E86.0
  due to malnutrition R64
  exophthalmic — *see* Hyperthyroidism
  heart — *see* Disease, heart
  hypophyseal E23.0
  hypopituitary E23.0
  lead — *see* Poisoning, lead
  malignant R64
  marsh — *see* Malaria
  nervous F48.8
  old age R54
  paludal — *see* Malaria
  pituitary E23.0
  renal N28.9
  saturnine — *see* Poisoning, lead
  senile R54
  Simmonds' E23.0
  splenica D73.0
  strumipriva E03.4
  tuberculous NEC — *see* Tuberculosis
Café, au lait spots L81.3
Caffeine-induced
  anxiety disorder F15.980
  sleep disorder F15.982
Caffey's syndrome Q78.8
Caisson disease T70.3 ☑
Cake kidney Q63.1

Caked breast (puerperal, postpartum) O92.79
Calabar swelling B74.3
Calcaneal spur — *see* Spur, bone, calcaneal
Calcaneo-apophysitis M92.8
Calcareous — *see* condition
Calcicosis J62.8
Calciferol (vitamin D) deficiency E55.9
  with rickets E55.0
Calcification
  adrenal (capsule) (gland) E27.49
    tuberculous E35 [B90.8]
  aorta I70.0
  artery (annular) — *see* Arteriosclerosis
  auricle (ear) — *see* Disorder, pinna, specified type NEC
  basal ganglia G23.8
  bladder N32.89
    due to Schistosoma hematobium B65.0
  brain (cortex) — *see* Calcification, cerebral
  bronchus J98.09
  bursa M71.40
    ankle M71.47- ☑
    elbow M71.42- ☑
    foot M71.47- ☑
    hand M71.44- ☑
    hip M71.45- ☑
    knee M71.46- ☑
    multiple sites M71.49
    shoulder M75.3- ☑
    specified site NEC M71.48
    wrist M71.43- ☑
  cardiac — *see* Degeneration, myocardial
  cerebral (cortex) G93.89
    artery I67.2
  cervix (uteri) N88.8
  choroid plexus G93.89
  conjunctiva — *see* Concretion, conjunctiva
  corpora cavernosa (penis) N48.89
  cortex (brain) — *see* Calcification, cerebral
  dental pulp (nodular) K04.2
  dentinal papilla K00.4
  fallopian tube N83.8
  falx cerebri G96.19
  gallbladder K82.8
  general E83.59
  heart (*see also* Degeneration, myocardial)
    valve — *see* Endocarditis
  idiopathic infantile arterial (IIAC) Q28.8
  intervertebral cartilage or disc (postinfective) — *see* Disorder, disc, specified NEC
  intracranial — *see* Calcification, cerebral
  joint — *see* Disorder, joint, specified type NEC
  kidney N28.89
    tuberculous N29 [B90.1]
  larynx (senile) J38.7
  lens — *see* Cataract, specified NEC
  lung (active) (postinfectional) J98.4
    tuberculous B90.9
  lymph gland or node (postinfectional) I89.8
    tuberculous (*see also* Tuberculosis, lymph gland) B90.8
  mammographic R92.1
  massive (paraplegic) — *see* Myositis, ossificans, in, quadriplegia
  medial — *see* Arteriosclerosis, extremities
  meninges (cerebral) (spinal) G96.19
  metastatic E83.59
  Mönckeberg's — *see* Arteriosclerosis, extremities
  muscle M61.9
    due to burns — *see* Myositis, ossificans, in, burns
    paralytic — *see* Myositis, ossificans, in, quadriplegia
    specified type NEC M61.40
      ankle M61.47- ☑
      foot M61.47- ☑
      forearm M61.43- ☑
      hand M61.44- ☑
      lower leg M61.46- ☑
      multiple sites M61.49
      pelvic region M61.45- ☑
      shoulder region M61.41- ☑
      specified site NEC M61.48
      thigh M61.45- ☑
      upper arm M61.42- ☑
  myocardium, myocardial — *see* Degeneration, myocardial
  ovary N83.8
  pancreas K86.89
  penis N48.89

Calcification — *continued*
    periarticular — *see* Disorder, joint, specified type NEC
    pericardium (*see also* Pericarditis) I31.1
    pineal gland E34.8
    pleura J94.8
        postinfectional J94.8
        tuberculous NEC B90.9
    pulpal (dental) (nodular) K04.2
    sclera H15.89
    spleen D73.89
    subcutaneous L94.2
    suprarenal (capsule) (gland) E27.49
    tendon (sheath) (*see also* Tenosynovitis, specified type NEC)
        with bursitis, synovitis or tenosynovitis — *see* Tendinitis, calcific
    trachea J39.8
    ureter N28.89
    uterus N85.8
    vitreous — *see* Deposit, crystalline
Calcified — *see* Calcification
Calcinosis (interstitial) (tumoral) (universalis) E83.59
    with Raynaud's phenomenon, esophageal dysfunction, sclerodactyly, telangiectasia (CREST syndrome) M34.1
    circumscripta (skin) L94.2
    cutis L94.2
Calciphylaxis (*see also* Calcification, by site) E83.59
Calcium
    deposits — *see* Calcification, by site
    metabolism disorder E83.50
    salts or soaps in vitreous — *see* Deposit, crystalline
Calciuria R82.99
Calculi — *see* Calculus
Calculosis, intrahepatic — *see* Calculus, bile duct
Calculus, calculi, calculous
    ampulla of Vater — *see* Calculus, bile duct
    anuria (impacted) (recurrent) (*see also* Calculus, urinary) N20.9
    appendix K38.1
    bile duct (common) (hepatic) K80.50
      with
        calculus of gallbladder — *see* Calculus, gallbladder and bile duct
        cholangitis K80.30
          with
            cholecystitis — *see* Calculus, bile duct, with cholecystitis
            obstruction K80.31
          acute K80.32
            with
              chronic cholangitis K80.36
                with obstruction K80.37
              obstruction K80.33
          chronic K80.34
            with
              acute cholangitis K80.36
                with obstruction K80.37
              obstruction K80.35
        cholecystitis (with cholangitis) K80.40
          with obstruction K80.41
          acute K80.42
            with
              chronic cholecystitis K80.46
                with obstruction K80.47
              obstruction K80.43
          chronic K80.44
            with
              acute cholecystitis K80.46
                with obstruction K80.47
              obstruction K80.45
    biliary (*see also* Calculus, gallbladder)
      specified NEC K80.80
        with obstruction K80.81
    bilirubin, multiple — *see* Calculus, gallbladder
    bladder (encysted) (impacted) (urinary) (diverticulum) N21.0
    bronchus J98.09
    calyx (kidney) (renal) — *see* Calculus, kidney
    cholesterol (pure) (solitary) — *see* Calculus, gallbladder
    common duct (bile) — *see* Calculus, bile duct
    conjunctiva — *see* Concretion, conjunctiva
    cystic N21.0
      duct — *see* Calculus, gallbladder
    dental (subgingival) (supragingival) K03.6
    diverticulum
        bladder N21.0
        kidney N20.0

Calculus, calculi, calculous — *continued*
    epididymis N50.89
    gallbladder K80.20
      with
        bile duct calculus — *see* Calculus, gallbladder and bile duct
        cholecystitis K80.10
          with obstruction K80.11
          acute K80.00
            with
              chronic cholecystitis K80.12
                with obstruction K80.13
              obstruction K80.01
          chronic K80.10
            with
              acute cholecystitis K80.12
                with obstruction K80.13
              obstruction K80.11
        specified NEC K80.18
          with obstruction K80.19
      obstruction K80.21
    gallbladder and bile duct K80.70
      with
        cholecystitis K80.60
          with obstruction K80.61
          acute K80.62
            with
              chronic cholecystitis K80.66
                with obstruction K80.67
              obstruction K80.63
          chronic K80.64
            with
              acute cholecystitis K80.66
                with obstruction K80.67
              obstruction K80.65
      obstruction K80.71
    hepatic (duct) — *see* Calculus, bile duct
    ileal conduit N21.8
    intestinal (impaction) (obstruction) K56.49
    kidney (impacted) (multiple) (pelvis) (recurrent) (staghorn) N20.0
      with calculus, ureter N20.2
      congenital Q63.8
    lacrimal passages — *see* Dacryolith
    liver (impacted) — *see* Calculus, bile duct
    lung J98.4
    mammographic R92.1
    nephritic (impacted) (recurrent) — *see* Calculus, kidney
    nose J34.89
    pancreas (duct) K86.89
    parotid duct or gland K11.5
    pelvis, encysted — *see* Calculus, kidney
    prostate N42.0
    pulmonary J98.4
    pyelitis (impacted) (recurrent) N20.0
      with hydronephrosis N13.2
    pyelonephritis (impacted) (recurrent) N20 ☑
      with hydronephrosis N13.2
    renal (impacted) (recurrent) — *see* Calculus, kidney
    salivary (duct) (gland) K11.5
    seminal vesicle N50.89
    staghorn — *see* Calculus, kidney
    Stensen's duct K11.5
    stomach K31.89
    sublingual duct or gland K11.5
      congenital Q38.4
    submandibular duct, gland or region K11.5
    submaxillary duct, gland or region K11.5
    suburethral N21.8
    tonsil J35.8
    tooth, teeth (subgingival) (supragingival) K03.6
    tunica vaginalis N50.89
    ureter (impacted) (recurrent) N20.1
      with calculus, kidney N20.2
        with hydronephrosis N13.2
          with infection N13.6
    urethra (impacted) N21.1
    urinary (duct) (impacted) (passage) (tract) N20.9
      with hydronephrosis N13.2
        with infection N13.6
      in (due to)
        lower N21.9
          specified NEC N21.8
    vagina N89.8
    vesical (impacted) N21.0
    Wharton's duct K11.5
    xanthine E79.8 [N22]
Calicectasis N28.89

Caliectasis N28.89
California
    disease B38.9
    encephalitis A83.5
Caligo cornea — *see* Opacity, cornea, central
Callositas, callosity (infected) L84
Callus (infected) L84
    bone — *see* Osteophyte
      excessive, following fracture — *code as* Sequelae of fracture
CALME (childhood asymmetric labium majus enlargement) N90.61
Calorie deficiency or malnutrition (*see also* Malnutrition) E46
Calvé-Perthes disease — *see* Legg-Calvé-Perthes disease
Calvé's disease — *see* Osteochondrosis, juvenile, spine
Calvities — *see* Alopecia, androgenic
Cameroon fever — *see* Malaria
Camptocormia (hysterical) F44.4
Camurati-Engelmann syndrome Q78.3
Canal (*see also* condition)
    atrioventricular common Q21.2
Canaliculitis (lacrimal) (acute) (subacute) H04.33- ☑
    Actinomyces A42.89
    chronic H04.42- ☑
Canavan's disease E75.29
Canceled procedure (surgical) Z53.9
    because of
      contraindication Z53.09
        smoking Z53.01
      left against medical advice (AMA) Z53.21
      patient's decision Z53.20
        for reasons of belief or group pressure Z53.1
        specified reason NEC Z53.29
      specified reason NEC Z53.8
Cancer (*see also* Neoplasm, by site, malignant)
    bile duct type liver C22.1
    blood — *see* Leukemia
    breast (*see also* Neoplasm, breast, malignant) C50.91- ☑
    hepatocellular C22.0
    lung (*see also* Neoplasm, lung, malignant) C34.90
    ovarian (*see also* Neoplasm ovary, malignant) C56.9
    unspecified site (primary) C80.1
Cancer (o)**phobia** F45.29
Cancerous — *see* Neoplasm, malignant, by site
Cancrum oris A69.0
Candidiasis, candidal B37.9
    balanitis B37.42
    bronchitis B37.1
    cheilitis B37.83
    congenital P37.5
    cystitis B37.41
    disseminated B37.7
    endocarditis B37.6
    enteritis B37.82
    esophagitis B37.81
    intertrigo B37.2
    lung B37.1
    meningitis B37.5
    mouth B37.0
    nails B37.2
    neonatal P37.5
    onychia B37.2
    oral B37.0
    osteomyelitis B37.89
    otitis externa B37.84
    paronychia B37.2
    perionyxis B37.2
    pneumonia B37.1
    proctitis B37.82
    pulmonary B37.1
    pyelonephritis B37.49
    sepsis B37.7
    skin B37.2
    specified site NEC B37.89
    stomatitis B37.0
    systemic B37.7
    urethritis B37.41
    urogenital site NEC B37.49
    vagina B37.3
    vulva B37.3
    vulvovaginitis B37.3
Candidid L30.2
Candidosis — *see* Candidiasis
Candiru infection or infestation B88.8
Canities (premature) L67.1

▽ Subterms under main terms may continue to next column or page   ☑ Additional Character Required — Refer to the Tabular List for Character Selection   47

Calcification — Canities

Canities — *continued*
  congenital Q84.2
Canker (mouth) (sore) K12.0
  rash A38.9
Cannabinosis J66.2
Cannabis induced
  anxiety disorder F12.980
  psychotic disorder F12.959
  sleep disorder F12.988
Canton fever A75.9
Cantrell's syndrome Q87.89
Capillariasis (intestinal) B81.1
  hepatic B83.8
Capillary — *see* condition
Caplan's syndrome — *see* Rheumatoid, lung
Capsule — *see* condition
Capsulitis (joint) (*see also* Enthesopathy)
  adhesive (shoulder) M75.0- ☑
  hepatic K65.8
  labyrinthine — *see* Otosclerosis, specified NEC
  thyroid E06.9
Caput
  crepitus Q75.8
  medusae I86.8
  succedaneum P12.81
Car sickness T75.3 ☑
Carapata (disease) A68.0
Carate — *see* Pinta
Carbon lung J60
Carbuncle L02.93
  abdominal wall L02.231
  anus K61.0
  auditory canal, external — *see* Abscess, ear, external
  auricle ear — *see* Abscess, ear, external
  axilla L02.43- ☑
  back (any part) L02.232
  breast N61.1
  buttock L02.33
  cheek (external) L02.03
  chest wall L02.233
  chin L02.03
  corpus cavernosum N48.21
  ear (any part) (external) (middle) — *see* Abscess, ear, external
  external auditory canal — *see* Abscess, ear, external
  eyelid — *see* Abscess, eyelid
  face NEC L02.03
  femoral (region) — *see* Carbuncle, lower limb
  finger — *see* Carbuncle, hand
  flank L02.231
  foot L02.63- ☑
  forehead L02.03
  genital — *see* Abscess, genital
  gluteal (region) L02.33
  groin L02.234
  hand L02.53- ☑
  head NEC L02.831
  heel — *see* Carbuncle, foot
  hip — *see* Carbuncle, lower limb
  kidney — *see* Abscess, kidney
  knee — *see* Carbuncle, lower limb
  labium (majus) (minus) N76.4
  lacrimal
    gland — *see* Dacryoadenitis
    passages (duct) (sac) — *see* Inflammation, lacrimal, passages, acute
  leg — *see* Carbuncle, lower limb
  lower limb L02.43- ☑
  malignant A22.0
  navel L02.236
  neck L02.13
  nose (external) (septum) J34.0
  orbit, orbital — *see* Abscess, orbit
  palmar (space) — *see* Carbuncle, hand
  partes posteriores L02.33
  pectoral region L02.233
  penis N48.21
  perineum L02.235
  pinna — *see* Abscess, ear, external
  popliteal — *see* Carbuncle, lower limb
  scalp L02.831
  seminal vesicle N49.0
  shoulder — *see* Carbuncle, upper limb
  specified site NEC L02.838
  temple (region) L02.03
  thumb — *see* Carbuncle, hand
  toe — *see* Carbuncle, foot

Carbuncle — *continued*
  trunk L02.239
    abdominal wall L02.231
    back L02.232
    chest wall L02.233
    groin L02.234
    perineum L02.235
    umbilicus L02.236
  umbilicus L02.236
  upper limb L02.43- ☑
  urethra N34.0
  vulva N76.4
Carbunculus — *see* Carbuncle
Carcinoid (tumor) — *see* Tumor, carcinoid
Carcinoidosis E34.0
Carcinoma (malignant) (*see also* Neoplasm, by site, malignant)
  acidophil
    specified site — *see* Neoplasm, malignant, by site
    unspecified site C75.1
  acidophil-basophil, mixed
    specified site — *see* Neoplasm, malignant, by site
    unspecified site C75.1
  adnexal (skin) — *see* Neoplasm, skin, malignant
  adrenal cortical C74.0- ☑
  alveolar — *see* Neoplasm, lung, malignant
    cell — *see* Neoplasm, lung, malignant
  ameloblastic C41.1
    upper jaw (bone) C41.0
  apocrine
    breast — *see* Neoplasm, breast, malignant
    specified site NEC — *see* Neoplasm, skin, malignant
    unspecified site C44.99
  basal cell (pigmented) (*see also* Neoplasm, skin, malignant) C44.91
    fibro-epithelial — *see* Neoplasm, skin, malignant
    morphea — *see* Neoplasm, skin, malignant
    multicentric — *see* Neoplasm, skin, malignant
  basaloid
  basal-squamous cell, mixed — *see* Neoplasm, skin, malignant
  basophil
    specified site — *see* Neoplasm, malignant, by site
    unspecified site C75.1
  basophil-acidophil, mixed
    specified site — *see* Neoplasm, malignant, by site
    unspecified site C75.1
  basosquamous — *see* Neoplasm, skin, malignant
  bile duct
    with hepatocellular, mixed C22.0
    liver C22.1
    specified site NEC — *see* Neoplasm, malignant, by site
    unspecified site C22.1
  branchial or branchiogenic C10.4
  bronchial or bronchogenic — *see* Neoplasm, lung, malignant
  bronchiolar — *see* Neoplasm, lung, malignant
  bronchioloalveolar — *see* Neoplasm, lung, malignant
  C cell
    specified site — *see* Neoplasm, malignant, by site
    unspecified site C73
  ceruminous C44.29- ☑
  cervix uteri
    in situ D06.9
      endocervix D06.0
      exocervix D06.1
      specified site NEC D06.7
  chorionic
    specified site — *see* Neoplasm, malignant, by site
    unspecified
      female C58
      male C62.90
  chromophobe
    specified site — *see* Neoplasm, malignant, by site
    unspecified site C75.1
  cloacogenic
    specified site — *see* Neoplasm, malignant, by site
    unspecified site C21.2
  diffuse type
    specified site — *see* Neoplasm, malignant, by site
    unspecified site C16.9
  duct (cell)
    with Paget's disease — *see* Neoplasm, breast, malignant

Carcinoma — *continued*
  duct — *continued*
    infiltrating
      with lobular carcinoma (in situ)
        specified site — *see* Neoplasm, malignant, by site
        unspecified site (female) C50.91- ☑
          male C50.92- ☑
      specified site — *see* Neoplasm, malignant, by site
      unspecified site (female) C50.91- ☑
        male C50.92- ☑
  ductal
    with lobular
      specified site — *see* Neoplasm, malignant, by site
      unspecified site (female) C50.91- ☑
        male C50.92- ☑
  ductular, infiltrating
    specified site — *see* Neoplasm, malignant, by site
    unspecified site (female) C50.91- ☑
      male C50.92- ☑
  embryonal
    liver C22.7
  endometrioid
    specified site — *see* Neoplasm, malignant, by site
    unspecified site
      female C56.9
      male C61
  eosinophil
    specified site — *see* Neoplasm, malignant, by site
    unspecified site C75.1
  epidermoid (*see also* Neoplasm, skin, malignant)
    in situ, Bowen's type — *see* Neoplasm, skin, in situ
  fibroepithelial, basal cell — *see* Neoplasm, skin, malignant
  follicular
    with papillary (mixed) C73
    moderately differentiated C73
    pure follicle C73
    specified site — *see* Neoplasm, malignant, by site
    trabecular C73
    unspecified site C73
    well differentiated C73
  generalized, with unspecified primary site C80.0
  glycogen-rich — *see* Neoplasm, breast, malignant
  granulosa cell C56- ☑
  hepatic cell C22.0
  hepatocellular C22.0
    with bile duct, mixed C22.0
    fibrolamellar C22.0
  hepatocholangiolitic C22.0
  Hurthle cell C73
  in
    adenomatous
      polyposis coli C18.9
    pleomorphic adenoma — *see* Neoplasm, salivary glands, malignant
    situ — *see* Carcinoma-in-situ
  infiltrating
    duct
      with lobular
        specified site — *see* Neoplasm, malignant, by site
        unspecified site (female) C50.91- ☑
          male C50.92- ☑
      with Paget's disease — *see* Neoplasm, breast, malignant
      specified site — *see* Neoplasm, malignant
      unspecified site (female) C50.91- ☑
        male C50.92- ☑
    ductular
      specified site — *see* Neoplasm, malignant
      unspecified site (female) C50.91- ☑
        male C50.92- ☑
    lobular
      specified site — *see* Neoplasm, malignant
      unspecified site (female) C50.91- ☑
        male C50.92- ☑
  inflammatory
    specified site — *see* Neoplasm, malignant
    unspecified site (female) C50.91- ☑
      male C50.92- ☑
  intestinal type
    specified site — *see* Neoplasm, malignant, by site
    unspecified site C16.9

Carcinoma — *continued*
  intracystic
    noninfiltrating — *see* Neoplasm, in situ, by site
  intraductal (noninfiltrating)
    with Paget's disease — *see* Neoplasm, breast, malignant
    breast D05.1- ☑
    papillary
      with invasion
        specified site — *see* Neoplasm, malignant, by site
        unspecified site (female) C50.91- ☑
          male C50.92- ☑
      breast D05.1- ☑
      specified site NEC — *see* Neoplasm, in situ, by site
      unspecified site (female) D05.1- ☑
    specified site NEC — *see* Neoplasm, in situ, by site
    unspecified site (female) D05.1- ☑
  intraepidermal — *see* Neoplasm, in situ
    squamous cell, Bowen's type — *see* Neoplasm, skin, in situ
  intraepithelial — *see* Neoplasm, in situ, by site
    squamous cell — *see* Neoplasm, in situ, by site
  intraosseous C41.1
    upper jaw (bone) C41.0
  islet cell
    with exocrine, mixed
      specified site — *see* Neoplasm, malignant, by site
      unspecified site C25.9
    pancreas C25.4
    specified site NEC — *see* Neoplasm, malignant, by site
    unspecified site C25.4
  juvenile, breast — *see* Neoplasm, breast, malignant
  large cell
    small cell
      specified site — *see* Neoplasm, malignant, by site
      unspecified site C34.90
  Leydig cell (testis)
    specified site — *see* Neoplasm, malignant, by site
    unspecified site
      female C56.9
      male C62.90
  lipid-rich (female) C50.91- ☑
    male C50.92- ☑
  liver cell C22.0
  liver NEC C22.7
  lobular (infiltrating)
    with intraductal
      specified site — *see* Neoplasm, malignant, by site
      unspecified site (female) C50.91- ☑
        male C50.92- ☑
    noninfiltrating
      breast D05.0- ☑
      specified site NEC — *see* Neoplasm, in situ, by site
      unspecified site D05.0- ☑
    specified site — *see* Neoplasm, malignant, by site
    unspecified site (female) C50.91- ☑
      male C50.92- ☑
  medullary
    with
      amyloid stroma
        specified site — *see* Neoplasm, malignant, by site
        unspecified site C73
      lymphoid stroma
        specified site — *see* Neoplasm, malignant, by site
        unspecified site (female) C50.91- ☑
          male C50.92- ☑
  Merkel cell C4A.9 (*following* C43)
    anal margin C4A.51 (*following* C43)
    anal skin C4A.51 (*following* C43)
    canthus C4A.1- ☑ (*following* C43)
    ear and external auricular canal C4A.2- ☑ (*following* C43)
    external auricular canal C4A.2- ☑ (*following* C43)
    eyelid, including canthus C4A.1- ☑ (*following* C43)
    face C4A.30 (*following* C43)
      specified NEC C4A.39 (*following* C43)
    hip C4A.7- ☑ (*following* C43)
    lip C4A.0 (*following* C43)

Carcinoma — *continued*
  Merkel cell — *continued*
    lower limb, including hip C4A.7- ☑ (*following* C43)
    neck C4A.4 (*following* C43)
    nodal presentation C7B.1 (*following* C75)
    nose C4A.31 (*following* C43)
    overlapping sites C4A.8 (*following* C43)
    perianal skin C4A.51 (*following* C43)
    scalp C4A.4 (*following* C43)
    secondary C7B.1 (*following* C75)
    shoulder C4A.6- ☑ (*following* C43)
    skin of breast C4A.52 (*following* C43)
    trunk NEC C4A.59 (*following* C43)
    upper limb, including shoulder C4A.6- ☑ (*following* C43)
    visceral metastatic C7B.1 (*following* C75)
  metastatic — *see* Neoplasm, secondary, by site
  metatypical — *see* Neoplasm, skin, malignant
  morphea, basal cell — *see* Neoplasm, skin, malignant
  mucoid
    cell
      specified site — *see* Neoplasm, malignant, by site
      unspecified site C75.1
  neuroendocrine (*see also* Tumor, neuroendocrine)
    high grade, any site C7A.1 (*following* C75)
    poorly differentiated, any site C7A.1 (*following* C75)
  nonencapsulated sclerosing C73
  noninfiltrating
    intracystic — *see* Neoplasm, in situ, by site
    intraductal
      breast D05.1- ☑
      papillary
        breast D05.1- ☑
        specified site NEC — *see* Neoplasm, in situ, by site
        unspecified site D05.1- ☑
      specified site — *see* Neoplasm, in situ, by site
      unspecified site D05.1- ☑
    lobular
      breast D05.0- ☑
      specified site NEC — *see* Neoplasm, in situ, by site
      unspecified site (female) D05.0- ☑
  oat cell
    specified site — *see* Neoplasm, malignant, by site
    unspecified site C34.90
  odontogenic C41.1
    upper jaw (bone) C41.0
  papillary
    with follicular (mixed) C73
    follicular variant C73
    intraductal (noninfiltrating)
      with invasion
        specified site — *see* Neoplasm, malignant, by site
        unspecified site (female) C50.91- ☑
          male C50.92- ☑
      breast D05.1- ☑
      specified site NEC — *see* Neoplasm, in situ, by site
      unspecified site D05.1- ☑
    serous
      specified site — *see* Neoplasm, malignant, by site
      surface
        specified site — *see* Neoplasm, malignant, by site
        unspecified site C56.9
      unspecified site C56.9
  papillocystic
    specified site — *see* Neoplasm, malignant, by site
    unspecified site C56.9
  parafollicular cell
    specified site — *see* Neoplasm, malignant, by site
    unspecified site C73
  pilomatrix — *see* Neoplasm, skin, malignant
  pseudomucinous
    specified site — *see* Neoplasm, malignant, by site
    unspecified site C56.9
  renal cell C64- ☑
  Schmincke — *see* Neoplasm, nasopharynx, malignant
  Schneiderian
    specified site — *see* Neoplasm, malignant, by site
    unspecified site C30.0
  sebaceous — *see* Neoplasm, skin, malignant

Carcinoma — *continued*
  secondary (*see also* Neoplasm, secondary, by site)
    Merkel cell C7B.1 (*following* C75)
  secretory, breast — *see* Neoplasm, breast, malignant
  serous
    papillary
      specified site — *see* Neoplasm, malignant, by site
      unspecified site C56.9
    surface, papillary
      specified site — *see* Neoplasm, malignant, by site
      unspecified site C56.9
  Sertoli cell
    specified site — *see* Neoplasm, malignant, by site
    unspecified site C62.90
      female C56.9
      male C62.90
  skin appendage — *see* Neoplasm, skin, malignant
  small cell
    fusiform cell
      specified site — *see* Neoplasm, malignant, by site
      unspecified site C34.90
    intermediate cell
      specified site — *see* Neoplasm, malignant, by site
      unspecified site C34.90
    large cell
      specified site — *see* Neoplasm, malignant, by site
      unspecified site C34.90
  solid
    with amyloid stroma
      specified site — *see* Neoplasm, malignant, by site
      unspecified site C73
    microinvasive
      specified site — *see* Neoplasm, malignant, by site
      unspecified site C53.9
  sweat gland — *see* Neoplasm, skin, malignant
  theca cell C56.- ☑
  thymic C37
  unspecified site (primary) C80.1
  water-clear cell C75.0
Carcinoma-in-situ (*see also* Neoplasm, in situ, by site)
  breast NOS D05.9- ☑
    specified type NEC D05.8- ☑
  epidermoid (*see also* Neoplasm, in situ, by site)
    with questionable stromal invasion
      cervix D06.9
      specified site NEC — *see* Neoplasm, in situ, by site
      unspecified site D06.9
    Bowen's type — *see* Neoplasm, skin, in situ
  intraductal
    breast D05.1- ☑
    specified site NEC — *see* Neoplasm, in situ, by site
    unspecified site D05.1- ☑
  lobular
    with
      infiltrating duct
        breast (female) C50.91- ☑
          male C50.92- ☑
        specified site NEC — *see* Neoplasm, malignant
        unspecified site (female) C50.91- ☑
          male C50.92- ☑
      intraductal
        breast D05.8- ☑
        specified site NEC — *see* Neoplasm, in situ, by site
        unspecified site (female) D05.8- ☑
    breast D05.0- ☑
    specified site NEC — *see* Neoplasm, in situ, by site
    unspecified site D05.0- ☑
  squamous cell (*see also* Neoplasm, in situ, by site)
    with questionable stromal invasion
      cervix D06.9
      specified site NEC — *see* Neoplasm, in situ, by site
      unspecified site D06.9
Carcinomaphobia F45.29
Carcinomatosis C80.0
  peritonei C78.6

Carcinomatosis — *continued*
  unspecified site (primary) (secondary) C80.0
Carcinosarcoma — *see* Neoplasm, malignant, by site
  embryonal — *see* Neoplasm, malignant, by site
Cardia, cardial — *see* condition
Cardiac (*see also* condition)
  death, sudden — *see* Arrest, cardiac
  pacemaker
    in situ Z95.0
      management or adjustment Z45.018
    tamponade I31.4
Cardialgia — *see* Pain, precordial
Cardiectasis — *see* Hypertrophy, cardiac
Cardiochalasia K21.9
Cardiomalacia I51.5
Cardiomegalia glycogenica diffusa E74.02 [I43]
Cardiomegaly (*see also* Hypertrophy, cardiac)
  congenital Q24.8
  glycogen E74.02 [I43]
  idiopathic I51.7
Cardiomyolipossis I51.5
Cardiomyopathy (familial) (idiopathic) I42.9
  alcoholic I42.6
  amyloid E85.4 [I43]
    transthyretin-related (ATTR) familial E85.4
  arteriosclerotic — *see* Disease, heart, ischemic, atherosclerotic
  beriberi E51.12
  cobalt-beer I42.6
  congenital I42.4
  congestive I42.0
  constrictive NOS I42.5
  dilated I42.0
  due to
    alcohol I42.6
    beriberi E51.12
    cardiac glycogenosis E74.02 [I43]
    drugs I42.7
    external agents NEC I42.7
    Friedreich's ataxia G11.1
    myotonia atrophica G71.11 [I43]
    progressive muscular dystrophy G71.0 [I43]
  glycogen storage E74.02 [I43]
  hypertensive — *see* Hypertension, heart
  hypertrophic (nonobstructive) I42.2
    obstructive I42.1
      congenital Q24.8
  in
    Chagas' disease (chronic) B57.2
      acute B57.0
    sarcoidosis D86.85
  ischemic I25.5
  metabolic E88.9 [I43]
    thyrotoxic E05.90 [I43]
      with thyroid storm E05.91 [I43]
  newborn I42.8
    congenital I42.4
  nutritional E63.9 [I43]
    beriberi E51.12
  obscure of Africa I42.8
  peripartum O90.3
  postpartum O90.3
  restrictive NEC I42.5
  rheumatic I09.0
  secondary I42.9
  stress induced I51.81
  takotsubo I51.81
  thyrotoxic E05.90 [I43]
    with thyroid storm E05.91 [I43]
  toxic NEC I42.7
  transthyretin-related (ATTR) familial amyloid E85.4
  tuberculous A18.84
  viral B33.24
Cardionephritis — *see* Hypertension, cardiorenal
Cardionephropathy — *see* Hypertension, cardiorenal
Cardionephrosis — *see* Hypertension, cardiorenal
Cardiopathia nigra I27.0
Cardiopathy (*see also* Disease, heart) I51.9
  idiopathic I42.9
  mucopolysaccharidosis E76.3 [I52]
Cardiopericarditis — *see* Pericarditis
Cardiophobia F45.29
Cardiorenal — *see* condition
Cardiorrhexis — *see* Infarct, myocardium
Cardiosclerosis — *see* Disease, heart, ischemic, atherosclerotic
Cardiosis — *see* Disease, heart
Cardiospasm (esophagus) (reflex) (stomach) K22.0

Cardiospasm — *continued*
  congenital Q39.5
    with megaesophagus Q39.5
Cardiostenosis — *see* Disease, heart
Cardiosymphysis I31.0
Cardiovascular — *see* condition
Carditis (acute) (bacterial) (chronic) (subacute) I51.89
  meningococcal A39.50
  rheumatic — *see* Disease, heart, rheumatic
  rheumatoid — *see* Rheumatoid, carditis
  viral B33.20
Care (of) (for) (following)
  child (routine) Z76.2
  family member (handicapped) (sick)
    creating problem for family Z63.6
    provided away from home for holiday relief Z75.5
    unavailable, due to
      absence (person rendering care) (sufferer) Z74.2
      inability (any reason) of person rendering care Z74.2
  foundling Z76.1
  holiday relief Z75.5
  improper — *see* Maltreatment
  lack of (at or after birth) (infant) — *see* Maltreatment, child, neglect
  lactating mother Z39.1
  palliative Z51.5
  postpartum
    immediately after delivery Z39.0
    routine follow-up Z39.2
  respite Z75.5
  unavailable, due to
    absence of person rendering care Z74.2
    inability (any reason) of person rendering care Z74.2
  well-baby Z76.2
Caries
  bone NEC A18.03
  dental (dentino enamel junction) (early childhood) (of dentine) (pre-eruptive) (recurrent) (to the pulp) K02.9
    arrested (coronal) (root) K02.3
    chewing surface
      limited to enamel K02.51
      penetrating into dentin K02.52
      penetrating into pulp K02.53
    coronal surface
      chewing surface
        limited to enamel K02.51
        penetrating into dentin K02.52
        penetrating into pulp K02.53
      pit and fissure surface
        limited to enamel K02.51
        penetrating into dentin K02.52
        penetrating into pulp K02.53
      smooth surface
        limited to enamel K02.61
        penetrating into dentin K02.62
        penetrating into pulp K02.63
    pit and fissure surface
      limited to enamel K02.51
      penetrating into dentin K02.52
      penetrating into pulp K02.53
    primary, cervical origin K02.52
    root K02.7
    smooth surface
      limited to enamel K02.61
      penetrating into dentin K02.62
      penetrating into pulp K02.63
  external meatus — *see* Disorder, ear, external, specified type NEC
  hip (tuberculous) A18.02
  initial (tooth)
    chewing surface K02.51
    pit and fissure surface K02.51
    smooth surface K02.61
  knee (tuberculous) A18.02
  labyrinth H83.8 ✔
  limb NEC (tuberculous) A18.03
  mastoid process (chronic) — *see* Mastoiditis, chronic
    tuberculous A18.03
  middle ear H74.8 ✔
  nose (tuberculous) A18.03
  orbit (tuberculous) A18.03
  ossicles, ear — *see* Abnormal, ear ossicles
  petrous bone — *see* Petrositis
  root (dental) (tooth) K02.7
  sacrum (tuberculous) A18.01

Caries — *continued*
  spine, spinal (column) (tuberculous) A18.01
  syphilitic A52.77
    congenital (early) A50.02 [M90.80]
  tooth, teeth — *see* Caries, dental
  tuberculous A18.03
  vertebra (column) (tuberculous) A18.01
Carious teeth — *see* Caries, dental
Carneous mole O02.0
Carnitine insufficiency E71.40
Carotid body or sinus syndrome G90.01
Carotidynia G90.01
Carotinemia (dietary) E67.1
Carotinosis (cutis) (skin) E67.1
Carpal tunnel syndrome — *see* Syndrome, carpal tunnel
Carpenter's syndrome Q87.0
Carpopedal spasm — *see* Tetany
Carr-Barr-Plunkett syndrome Q97.1
Carrier (suspected) of
  amebiasis Z22.1
  bacterial disease NEC Z22.39
    diphtheria Z22.2
    intestinal infectious NEC Z22.1
      typhoid Z22.0
    meningococcal Z22.31
    sexually transmitted Z22.4
    specified NEC Z22.39
    staphylococcal (Methicillin susceptible) Z22.321
      Methicillin resistant Z22.322
    streptococcal Z22.338
      group B Z22.330
        complicating pregnancy or delivery O99.82- ✔
  typhoid Z22.0
  cholera Z22.1
  diphtheria Z22.2
  gastrointestinal pathogens NEC Z22.1
  genetic Z14.8
    cystic fibrosis Z14.1
    hemophilia A (asymptomatic) Z14.01
      symptomatic Z14.02
  gestational, pregnant Z33.1
  gonorrhea Z22.4
  HAA (hepatitis Australian-antigen) B18.8
  HB (c)(s)-AG B18.1
  hepatitis (viral) B18.9
    Australia-antigen (HAA) B18.8
    B surface antigen (HBsAg) B18.1
      with acute delta- (super)infection B17.0
    C B18.2
    specified NEC B18.8
  human T-cell lymphotropic virus type-1 (HTLV-1) infection Z22.6
  infectious organism Z22.9
    specified NEC Z22.8
  meningococci Z22.31
  Salmonella typhosa Z22.0
  serum hepatitis — *see* Carrier, hepatitis
  staphylococci (Methicillin susceptible) Z22.321
    Methicillin resistant Z22.322
  streptococci Z22.338
    group B Z22.330
      complicating pregnancy or delivery O99.82- ✔
  syphilis Z22.4
  typhoid Z22.0
  venereal disease NEC Z22.4
Carrion's disease A44.0
Carter's relapsing fever (Asiatic) A68.1
Cartilage — *see* condition
Caruncle (inflamed)
  conjunctiva (acute) — *see* Conjunctivitis, acute
  labium (majus) (minus) N90.89
  lacrimal — *see* Inflammation, lacrimal, passages
  myrtiform N89.8
  urethral (benign) N36.2
Cascade stomach K31.2
Caseation lymphatic gland (tuberculous) A18.2
Cassidy (-Scholte) syndrome (malignant carcinoid) E34.0
Castellani's disease A69.8
Castration, traumatic, male S38.231 ✔
Casts in urine R82.99
Cat
  cry syndrome Q93.4
  ear Q17.3
  eye syndrome Q92.8
Catabolism, senile R54
Catalepsy (hysterical) F44.2
  schizophrenic F20.2

Cataplexy (idiopathic) — *see* Narcolepsy
Cataract (cortical) (immature) (incipient) H26.9
  with
    neovascularization — *see* Cataract, complicated
  age-related — *see* Cataract, senile
  anterior
    and posterior axial embryonal Q12.0
    pyramidal Q12.0
  associated with
    galactosemia E74.21 [H28]
    myotonic disorders G71.19 [H28]
  blue Q12.0
  central Q12.0
  cerulean Q12.0
  complicated H26.20
    with
      neovascularization H26.21- ☑
      ocular disorder H26.22- ☑
    glaucomatous flecks H26.23- ☑
  congenital Q12.0
  coraliform Q12.0
  coronary Q12.0
  crystalline Q12.0
  diabetic — *see* Diabetes, cataract
  drug-induced H26.3- ☑
  due to
    ocular disorder — *see* Cataract, complicated
    radiation H26.8
  electric H26.8
  extraction status Z98.4- ☑
  glass-blower's H26.8
  heat ray H26.8
  heterochromic — *see* Cataract, complicated
  hypermature — *see* Cataract, senile, morgagnian type
  in (due to)
    chronic iridocyclitis — *see* Cataract, complicated
    diabetes — *see* Diabetes, cataract
    endocrine disease E34.9 [H28]
    eye disease — *see* Cataract, complicated
    hypoparathyroidism E20.9 [H28]
    malnutrition-dehydration E46 [H28]
    metabolic disease E88.9 [H28]
    myotonic disorders G71.19 [H28]
    nutritional disease E63.9 [H28]
  infantile — *see* Cataract, presenile
  irradiational — *see* Cataract, specified NEC
  juvenile — *see* Cataract, presenile
  malnutrition-dehydration E46 [H28]
  morgagnian — *see* Cataract, senile, morgagnian type
  myotonic G71.19 [H28]
  myxedema E03.9 [H28]
  nuclear
    embryonal Q12.0
    sclerosis — *see* Cataract, senile, nuclear
  presenile H26.00- ☑
    combined forms H26.06- ☑
    cortical H26.01- ☑
    lamellar — *see* Cataract, presenile, cortical
    nuclear H26.03- ☑
    specified NEC H26.09
    subcapsular polar (anterior) H26.04- ☑
      posterior H26.05- ☑
    zonular — *see* Cataract, presenile, cortical
  secondary H26.40
    Soemmering's ring H26.41- ☑
    specified NEC H26.49- ☑
    to eye disease — *see* Cataract, complicated
  senile H25.9
    brunescens — *see* Cataract, senile, nuclear
    combined forms H25.81- ☑
    coronary — *see* Cataract, senile, incipient
    cortical H25.01- ☑
    hypermature — *see* Cataract, senile, morgagnian
      type
    incipient (mature) (total) H25.09- ☑
      cortical — *see* Cataract, senile, cortical
      subcapsular — *see* Cataract, senile, subcapsular
    morgagnian type (hypermature) H25.2- ☑
    nuclear (sclerosis) H25.1- ☑
    polar subcapsular (anterior) (posterior) — *see*
      Cataract, senile, incipient
    punctate — *see* Cataract, senile, incipient
    specified NEC H25.89
    subcapsular polar (anterior) H25.03- ☑
      posterior H25.04- ☑
  snowflake — *see* Diabetes, cataract
  specified NEC H26.8

Cataract — *continued*
  toxic — *see* Cataract, drug-induced
  traumatic H26.10- ☑
    localized H26.11- ☑
    partially resolved H26.12- ☑
    total H26.13- ☑
  zonular (perinuclear) Q12.0
Cataracta (*see also* Cataract)
  brunescens — *see* Cataract, senile, nuclear
  centralis pulverulenta Q12.0
  cerulea Q12.0
  complicata — *see* Cataract, complicated
  congenita Q12.0
  coralliformis Q12.0
  coronaria Q12.0
  diabetic — *see* Diabetes, cataract
  membranacea
    accreta — *see* Cataract, secondary
    congenita Q12.0
  nigra — *see* Cataract, senile, nuclear
  sunflower — *see* Cataract, complicated
Catarrh, catarrhal (acute) (febrile) (infectious) (inflam-
    mation) (*see also* condition) J00
  bronchial — *see* Bronchitis
  chest — *see* Bronchitis
  chronic J31.0
  due to congenital syphilis A50.03
  enteric — *see* Enteritis
  eustachian H68.009
  fauces — *see* Pharyngitis
  gastrointestinal — *see* Enteritis
  gingivitis K05.00
    nonplaque induced K05.01
    plaque induced K05.00
  hay — *see* Fever, hay
  intestinal — *see* Enteritis
  larynx, chronic J37.0
  liver B15.9
    with hepatic coma B15.0
  lung — *see* Bronchitis
  middle ear, chronic — *see* Otitis, media, nonsuppura-
    tive, chronic, serous
  mouth K12.1
  nasal (chronic) — *see* Rhinitis
  nasobronchial J31.1
  nasopharyngeal (chronic) J31.1
    acute J00
  pulmonary — *see* Bronchitis
  spring (eye) (vernal) — *see* Conjunctivitis, acute, atopic
  summer (hay) — *see* Fever, hay
  throat J31.2
  tubotympanal (*see also* Otitis, media, nonsuppurative)
    chronic — *see* Otitis, media, nonsuppurative,
      chronic, serous
Catatonia (schizophrenic) F20.2
Catatonic
  disorder due to known physiologic condition F06.1
  schizophrenia F20.2
  stupor R40.1
Cat-scratch (*see also* Abrasion)
  disease or fever A28.1
Cauda equina — *see* condition
Cauliflower ear M95.1- ☑
Causalgia (upper limb) G56.4- ☑
  lower limb G57.7- ☑
Cause
  external, general effects T75.89 ☑
Caustic burn — *see* Corrosion, by site
Cavare's disease (familial periodic paralysis) G72.3
Cave-in, injury
  crushing (severe) — *see* Crush
  suffocation — *see* Asphyxia, traumatic, due to low
    oxygen, due to cave-in
Cavernitis (penis) N48.29
Cavernositis N48.29
Cavernous — *see* condition
Cavitation of lung (*see also* Tuberculosis, pulmonary)
  nontuberculous J98.4
Cavities, dental — *see* Caries, dental
Cavity
  lung — *see* Cavitation of lung
  optic papilla Q14.2
  pulmonary — *see* Cavitation of lung
Cavovarus foot, congenital Q66.1
Cavus foot (congenital) Q66.7
  acquired — *see* Deformity, limb, foot, specified NEC
Cazenave's disease L10.2

Cecitis K52.9
  with perforation, peritonitis, or rupture K65.8
Cecum — *see* condition
Celiac
  artery compression syndrome I77.4
  disease (with steatorrhea) K90.0
  infantilism K90.0
Cell(s), **cellular** (*see also* condition)
  in urine R82.99
Cellulitis (diffuse) (phlegmonous) (septic) (suppurative)
    L03.90
  abdominal wall L03.311
  anaerobic A48.0
  ankle — *see* Cellulitis, lower limb
  anus K61.0
  arm — *see* Cellulitis, upper limb
  auricle (ear) — *see* Cellulitis, ear
  axilla L03.11- ☑
  back (any part) L03.312
  breast (acute) (nonpuerperal) (subacute) N61.0
    nipple N61.0
  broad ligament
    acute N73.0
  buttock L03.317
  cervical (meaning neck) L03.221
  cervix (uteri) — *see* Cervicitis
  cheek (external) L03.211
    internal K12.2
  chest wall L03.313
  chronic L03.90
  clostridial A48.0
  corpus cavernosum N48.22
  digit
    finger — *see* Cellulitis, finger
    toe — *see* Cellulitis, toe
  Douglas' cul-de-sac or pouch
    acute N73.0
  drainage site (following operation) T81.4 ☑
  ear (external) H60.1- ☑
  eosinophilic (granulomatous) L98.3
  erysipelatous — *see* Erysipelas
  external auditory canal — *see* Cellulitis, ear
  eyelid — *see* Abscess, eyelid
  face NEC L03.211
  finger (intrathecal) (periosteal) (subcutaneous) (subcu-
    ticular) L03.01- ☑
  foot — *see* Cellulitis, lower limb
  gangrenous — *see* Gangrene
  genital organ NEC
    female (external) N76.4
    male N49.9
      multiple sites N49.8
      specified NEC N49.8
  gluteal (region) L03.317
  gonococcal A54.89
  groin L03.314
  hand — *see* Cellulitis, upper limb
  head NEC L03.811
    face (any part, except ear, eye and nose) L03.211
  heel — *see* Cellulitis, lower limb
  hip — *see* Cellulitis, lower limb
  jaw (region) L03.211
  knee — *see* Cellulitis, lower limb
  labium (majus) (minus) — *see* Vulvitis
  lacrimal passages — *see* Inflammation, lacrimal, pas-
    sages
  larynx J38.7
  leg — *see* Cellulitis, lower limb
  lip K13.0
  lower limb L03.11- ☑
    toe — *see* Cellulitis, toe
  mouth (floor) K12.2
  multiple sites, so stated L03.90
  nasopharynx J39.1
  navel L03.316
    newborn P38.9
      with mild hemorrhage P38.1
      without hemorrhage P38.9
  neck (region) L03.221
  nipple (acute) (nonpuerperal) (subacute) N61.0
  nose (septum) (external) J34.0
  orbit, orbital H05.01- ☑
  palate (soft) K12.2
  pectoral (region) L03.313
  pelvis, pelvic (chronic)
    female (*see also* Disease, pelvis, inflammatory)
      N73.2
      acute N73.0

Cellulitis — *continued*
pelvis, pelvic — *continued*
following ectopic or molar pregnancy O08.0
male K65.0
penis N48.22
perineal, perineum L03.315
periorbital L03.213
perirectal K61.1
peritonsillar J36
periurethral N34.0
periuterine (*see also* Disease, pelvis, inflammatory) N73.2
acute N73.0
pharynx J39.1
preseptal L03.213
rectum K61.1
retroperitoneal K68.9
round ligament
acute N73.0
scalp (any part) L03.811
scrotum N49.2
seminal vesicle N49.0
shoulder — *see* Cellulitis, upper limb
specified site NEC L03.818
submandibular (region) (space) (triangle) K12.2
gland K11.3
submaxillary (region) K12.2
gland K11.3
thigh — *see* Cellulitis, lower limb
thumb (intrathecal) (periosteal) (subcutaneous) (sub-cuticular) — *see* Cellulitis, finger
toe (intrathecal) (periosteal) (subcutaneous) (subcutic-ular) L03.03- ☑
tonsil J36
trunk L03.319
abdominal wall L03.311
back (any part) L03.312
buttock L03.317
chest wall L03.313
groin L03.314
perineal, perineum L03.315
umbilicus L03.316
tuberculous (primary) A18.4
umbilicus L03.316
upper limb L03.11- ☑
axilla — *see* Cellulitis, axilla
finger — *see* Cellulitis, finger
thumb — *see* Cellulitis, finger
vaccinal T88.0 ☑
vocal cord J38.3
vulva — *see* Vulvitis
wrist — *see* Cellulitis, upper limb
Cementoblastoma, benign — *see* Cyst, calcifying odontogenic
Cementoma — *see* Cyst, calcifying odontogenic
Cementoperiostitis — *see* Periodontitis
Cementosis K03.4
Central auditory processing disorder H93.25
Central pain syndrome G89.0
Cephalematocele, cephal (o)hematocele
newborn P52.8
birth injury P10.8
traumatic — *see* Hematoma, brain
Cephalematoma, cephalhematoma (calcified)
newborn (birth injury) P12.0
traumatic — *see* Hematoma, brain
Cephalgia, cephalalgia (*see also* Headache)
histamine G44.009
intractable G44.001
not intractable G44.009
trigeminal autonomic (TAC) NEC G44.099
intractable G44.091
not intractable G44.099
Cephalic — *see* condition
Cephalitis — *see* Encephalitis
Cephalocele — *see* Encephalocele
Cephalomenia N94.89
Cephalopelvic — *see* condition
Cerclage (with cervical incompetence) in pregnancy — *see* Incompetence, cervix, in pregnancy
Cerebellitis — *see* Encephalitis
Cerebellum, cerebellar — *see* condition
Cerebral — *see* condition
Cerebritis — *see* Encephalitis
Cerebro-hepato-renal syndrome Q87.89
Cerebromalacia — *see* Softening, brain
sequelae of cerebrovascular disease I69.398
Cerebroside lipidosis E75.22

Cerebrospasticity (congenital) G80.1
Cerebrospinal — *see* condition
Cerebrum — *see* condition
Ceroid-lipofuscinosis, neuronal E75.4
Cerumen (accumulation) (impacted) H61.2- ☑
Cervical (*see also* condition)
auricle Q18.2
dysplasia in pregnancy — *see* Abnormal, cervix, in pregnancy or childbirth
erosion in pregnancy — *see* Abnormal, cervix, in pregnancy or childbirth
fibrosis in pregnancy — *see* Abnormal, cervix, in pregnancy or childbirth
fusion syndrome Q76.1
rib Q76.5
shortening (complicating pregnancy) O26.87- ☑
Cervicalgia M54.2
Cervicitis (acute) (chronic) (nonvenereal) (senile (atroph-ic)) (subacute) (with ulceration) N72
with
abortion — *see* Abortion, by type complicated by genital tract and pelvic infection
ectopic pregnancy O08.0
molar pregnancy O08.0
chlamydial A56.09
gonococcal A54.03
herpesviral A60.03
puerperal (postpartum) O86.11
syphilitic A52.76
trichomonal A59.09
tuberculous A18.16
Cervicocolpitis (emphysematosa) (see also Cervicitis) N72
Cervix — *see* condition
Cesarean delivery, previous, affecting management of pregnancy O34.219
classical (vertical) scar O34.212
low transverse scar O34.211
Céstan (-Chenais) paralysis or syndrome G46.3
Céstan-Raymond syndrome I65.8
Cestode infestation B71.9
specified type NEC B71.8
Cestodiasis B71.9
Chabert's disease A22.9
Chacaleh E53.8
Chafing L30.4
Chagas' (-Mazza) disease (chronic) B57.2
with
cardiovascular involvement NEC B57.2
digestive system involvement B57.30
megacolon B57.32
megaesophagus B57.31
other specified B57.39
megacolon B57.32
megaesophagus B57.31
myocarditis B57.2
nervous system involvement B57.40
meningitis B57.41
meningoencephalitis B57.42
other specified B57.49
specified organ involvement NEC B57.5
acute (with) B57.1
cardiovascular NEC B57.0
myocarditis B57.0
Chagres fever B50.9
Chairridden Z74.09
Chalasia (cardiac sphincter) K21.9
Chalazion H00.19
left H00.16
lower H00.15
upper H00.14
right H00.13
lower H00.12
upper H00.11
Chalcosis (*see also* Disorder, globe, degenerative, chalco-sis)
cornea — *see* Deposit, cornea
crystalline lens — *see* Cataract, complicated
retina H35.89
Chalicosis (pulmonum) J62.8
Chancre (any genital site) (hard) (hunterian) (mixed) (primary) (seronegative) (seropositive) (syphilitic) A51.0
congenital A50.07
conjunctiva NEC A51.2
Ducrey's A57
extragenital A51.2
eyelid A51.2

Chancre — *continued*
lip A51.2
nipple A51.2
Nisbet's A57
of
carate A67.0
pinta A67.0
yaws A66.0
palate, soft A51.2
phagedenic A57
simple A57
soft A57
bubo A57
palate A51.2
urethra A51.0
yaws A66.0
Chancroid (anus) (genital) (penis) (perineum) (rectum) (urethra) (vulva) A57
Chandler's disease (osteochondritis dissecans, hip) — *see* Osteochondritis, dissecans, hip
Change(s) (in) (of) (*see also* Removal)
arteriosclerotic — *see* Arteriosclerosis
bone (*see also* Disorder, bone)
diabetic — *see* Diabetes, bone change
bowel habit R19.4
cardiorenal (vascular) — *see* Hypertension, cardiorenal
cardiovascular — *see* Disease, cardiovascular
circulatory I99.9
cognitive (mild) (organic) R41.89
color, tooth, teeth
during formation K00.8
posteruptive K03.7
contraceptive device Z30.433
corneal membrane H18.30
Bowman's membrane fold or rupture H18.31- ☑
Descemet's membrane
fold H18.32- ☑
rupture H18.33- ☑
coronary — *see* Disease, heart, ischemic
degenerative, spine or vertebra — *see* Spondylosis
dental pulp, regressive K04.2
dressing (nonsurgical) Z48.00
surgical Z48.01
heart — *see* Disease, heart
hip joint — *see* Derangement, joint, hip
hyperplastic larynx J38.7
hypertrophic
nasal sinus J34.89
turbinate, nasal J34.3
upper respiratory tract J39.8
indwelling catheter Z46.6
inflammatory (*see also* Inflammation)
sacroiliac M46.1
job, anxiety concerning Z56.1
joint — *see* Derangement, joint
life — *see* Menopause
mental status R41.82
minimal (glomerular) (*see also* N00-N07 with fourth character .0) N05.0
myocardium, myocardial — *see* Degeneration, myocar-dial
of life — *see* Menopause
pacemaker Z45.018
pulse generator Z45.010
personality (enduring) F68.8
due to (secondary to)
general medical condition F07.0
secondary (nonspecific) F60.89
regressive, dental pulp K04.2
renal — *see* Disease, renal
retina H35.9
myopic (*see also* Myopia, degenerative) H44.2- ☑
sacroiliac joint M53.3
senile (*see also* condition) R54
sensory R20.8
skin R23.9
acute, due to ultraviolet radiation L56.9
specified NEC L56.8
chronic, due to nonionizing radiation L57.9
specified NEC L57.8
cyanosis R23.0
flushing R23.2
pallor R23.1
petechiae R23.3
specified change NEC R23.8
swelling — *see* Mass, localized
texture R23.4

Change(s) — *continued*
 trophic
  arm — *see* Mononeuropathy, upper limb
  leg — *see* Mononeuropathy, lower limb
 vascular I99.9
 vasomotor I73.9
 voice R49.9
  psychogenic F44.4
  specified NEC R49.8
Changing sleep-work schedule, affecting sleep
 G47.26
Changuinola fever A93.1
Chapping skin T69.8 ☑
Charcot-Marie-Tooth disease, paralysis or syndrome
 G60.0
Charcot's
 arthropathy — *see* Arthropathy, neuropathic
 cirrhosis K74.3
 disease (tabetic arthropathy) A52.16
 joint (disease) (tabetic) A52.16
  diabetic — *see* Diabetes, with, arthropathy
  syringomyelic G95.0
 syndrome (intermittent claudication) I73.9
CHARGE association Q89.8
Charley-horse (quadriceps) M62.831
 traumatic (quadriceps) S76.11- ☑
Charlouis' disease — *see* Yaws
Cheadle's disease E54
Checking (of)
 cardiac pacemaker (battery) (electrode(s)) Z45.018
  pulse generator Z45.010
 implantable subdermal contraceptive Z30.46
 intrauterine contraceptive device Z30.431
 wound Z48.0- ☑
  due to injury — code to Injury, by site, using appropriate seventh character for subsequent encounter
Check-up — *see* Examination
Chédiak-Higashi (-Steinbrinck) **syndrome** (congenital
 gigantism of peroxidase granules) E70.330
Cheek — *see* condition
Cheese itch B88.0
Cheese-washer's lung J67.8
Cheese-worker's lung J67.8
Cheilitis (acute) (angular) (catarrhal) (chronic) (exfoliative)
 (gangrenous) (glandular) (infectional) (suppurative)
 (ulcerative) (vesicular) K13.0
 actinic (due to sun) L56.8
  other than from sun L59.8
 candidal B37.83
Cheilodynia K13.0
Cheiloschisis — *see* Cleft, lip
Cheilosis (angular) K13.0
 with pellagra E52
 due to
  vitamin B2 (riboflavin) deficiency E53.0
Cheiromegaly M79.89
Cheiropompholyx L30.1
Cheloid — *see* Keloid
Chemical burn — *see* Corrosion, by site
Chemodectoma — *see* Paraganglioma, nonchromaffin
Chemosis, conjunctiva — *see* Edema, conjunctiva
Chemotherapy (session) (for)
 cancer Z51.11
 neoplasm Z51.11
Cherubism M27.8
Chest — *see* condition
Cheyne-Stokes breathing (respiration) R06.3
Chiari's
 disease or syndrome (hepatic vein thrombosis) I82.0
 malformation
  type I G93.5
  type II — *see* Spina bifida
 net Q24.8
Chicago disease B40.9
Chickenpox — *see* Varicella
Chiclero ulcer or sore B55.1
Chigger (infestation) B88.0
Chignon (disease) B36.8
 newborn (from vacuum extraction) (birth injury) P12.1
Chilaiditi's syndrome (subphrenic displacement, colon)
 Q43.3
Chilblain(s) (lupus) T69.1 ☑
Child
 custody dispute Z65.3
Childbirth — *see* Delivery

Childhood
 cerebral X-linked adrenoleukodystrophy E71.520
 period of rapid growth Z00.2
Chill(s) R68.83
 with fever R50.9
 without fever R68.83
 congestive in malarial regions B54
Chilomastigiasis A07.8
Chimera 46,XX/46,XY Q99.0
Chin — *see* condition
Chinese dysentery A03.9
Chionophobia F40.228
Chitral fever A93.1
Chlamydia, chlamydial A74.9
 cervicitis A56.09
 conjunctivitis A74.0
 cystitis A56.01
 endometritis A56.11
 epididymitis A56.19
 female
  pelvic inflammatory disease A56.11
  pelviperitonitis A56.11
 orchitis A56.19
 peritonitis A74.81
 pharyngitis A56.4
 proctitis A56.3
 psittaci (infection) A70
 salpingitis A56.11
 sexually-transmitted infection NEC A56.8
 specified NEC A74.89
 urethritis A56.01
 vulvovaginitis A56.02
Chlamydiosis — *see* Chlamydia
Chloasma (skin) (idiopathic) (symptomatic) L81.1
 eyelid H02.719
  hyperthyroid E05.90 [H02.719]
   with thyroid storm E05.91 [H02.719]
  left H02.716
   lower H02.715
   upper H02.714
  right H02.713
   lower H02.712
   upper H02.711
Chloroma C92.3- ☑
Chlorosis D50.9
 Egyptian B76.9 [D63.8]
 miner's B76.9 [D63.8]
Chlorotic anemia D50.8
Chocolate cyst (ovary) N80.1
Choked
 disc or disk — *see* Papilledema
 on food, phlegm, or vomitus NOS — *see* Foreign body,
  by site
 while vomiting NOS — *see* Foreign body, by site
Chokes (resulting from bends) T70.3 ☑
Choking sensation R09.89
Cholangiectasis K83.8
Cholangiocarcinoma
 with hepatocellular carcinoma, combined C22.0
 liver C22.1
 specified site NEC — *see* Neoplasm, malignant, by site
 unspecified site C22.1
Cholangiohepatitis K83.8
 due to fluke infestation B66.1
Cholangiohepatoma C22.0
Cholangiolitis (acute) (chronic) (extrahepatic) (gangrenous) (intrahepatic) K83.0
 paratyphoidal — *see* Fever, paratyphoid
 typhoidal A01.09
Cholangioma D13.4
 malignant — *see* Cholangiocarcinoma
Cholangitis (ascending) (primary) (recurrent) (sclerosing)
 (secondary) (stenosing) (suppurative) K83.0
 with calculus, bile duct — *see* Calculus, bile duct, with
  cholangitis
 chronic nonsuppurative destructive K74.3
Cholecystectasia K82.8
Cholecystitis K81.9
 with
  calculus, stones in
   bile duct (common) (hepatic) — *see* Calculus,
    bile duct, with cholecystitis
   cystic duct — *see* Calculus, gallbladder, with
    cholecystitis
   gallbladder — *see* Calculus, gallbladder, with
    cholecystitis
  choledocholithiasis — *see* Calculus, bile duct, with
   cholecystitis

Cholecystitis — *continued*
 with — *continued*
  cholelithiasis — *see* Calculus, gallbladder, with
   cholecystitis
 acute (emphysematous) (gangrenous) (suppurative)
  K81.0
  with
   calculus, stones in
    cystic duct — *see* Calculus, gallbladder, with
     cholecystitis, acute
    gallbladder — *see* Calculus, gallbladder,
     with cholecystitis, acute
   choledocholithiasis — *see* Calculus, bile duct,
    with cholecystitis, acute
   cholelithiasis — *see* Calculus, gallbladder, with
    cholecystitis, acute
   chronic cholecystitis K81.2
    with gallbladder calculus K80.12
     with obstruction K80.13
 chronic K81.1
  with acute cholecystitis K81.2
   with gallbladder calculus K80.12
    with obstruction K80.13
 emphysematous (acute) — *see* Cholecystitis, acute
 gangrenous — *see* Cholecystitis, acute
 paratyphoidal, current A01.4
 suppurative — *see* Cholecystitis, acute
 typhoidal A01.09
Cholecystolithiasis — *see* Calculus, gallbladder
Choledochitis (suppurative) K83.0
Choledocholith — *see* Calculus, bile duct
Choledocholithiasis (common duct) (hepatic duct) —
 see Calculus, bile duct
 cystic — *see* Calculus, gallbladder
 typhoidal A01.09
Cholelithiasis (cystic duct) (gallbladder) (impacted)
 (multiple) — *see* Calculus, gallbladder
 bile duct (common) (hepatic) — *see* Calculus, bile duct
 hepatic duct — *see* Calculus, bile duct
 specified NEC K80.80
  with obstruction K80.81
Cholemia (*see also* Jaundice)
 familial (simple) (congenital) E80.4
 Gilbert's E80.4
Choleperitoneum, choleperitonitis K65.3
Cholera (Asiatic) (epidemic) (malignant) A00.9
 antimonial — *see* Poisoning, antimony
 classical A00.0
 due to Vibrio cholerae 01 A00.9
  biovar cholerae A00.0
  biovar eltor A00.1
  el tor A00.1
 el tor A00.1
Cholerine — *see* Cholera
Cholestasis NEC K83.1
 with hepatocyte injury K71.0
 due to total parenteral nutrition (TPN) K76.89
 pure K71.0
Cholesteatoma (ear) (middle) (with reaction) H71.9- ☑
 attic H71.0- ☑
 external ear (canal) H60.4- ☑
 mastoid H71.2- ☑
 postmastoidectomy cavity (recurrent) — *see* Complications, postmastoidectomy, recurrent
  cholesteatoma
 recurrent (postmastoidectomy) — *see* Complications,
  postmastoidectomy, recurrent cholesteatoma
 tympanum H71.1- ☑
Cholesteatosis, diffuse H71.3- ☑
Cholesteremia E78.00
Cholesterin in vitreous — *see* Deposit, crystalline
Cholesterol
 deposit
  retina H35.89
  vitreous — *see* Deposit, crystalline
 elevated (high) E78.00
  with elevated (high) triglycerides E78.2
  screening for Z13.220
 imbibition of gallbladder K82.4
Cholesterolemia (essential) (pure) E78.00
 familial E78.01
 hereditary E78.01
Cholesterolosis, cholesterosis (gallbladder) K82.4
 cerebrotendinous E75.5
Cholocolic fistula K82.3
Choluria R82.2
Chondritis M94.8X9

Chondritis — *continued*
  aural H61.03- ☑
  costal (Tietze's) M94.0
  external ear H61.03- ☑
  patella, posttraumatic — *see* Chondromalacia, patella
  pinna H61.03- ☑
  purulent M94.8X- ☑
  tuberculous NEC A18.02
    intervertebral A18.01
Chondroblastoma (*see also* Neoplasm, bone, benign)
  malignant — *see* Neoplasm, bone, malignant
Chondrocalcinosis M11.20
  ankle M11.27- ☑
  elbow M11.22- ☑
  familial M11.10
    ankle M11.17- ☑
    elbow M11.12- ☑
    foot joint M11.17- ☑
    hand joint M11.14- ☑
    hip M11.15- ☑
    knee M11.16- ☑
    multiple site M11.19
    shoulder M11.11- ☑
    vertebrae M11.18
    wrist M11.13- ☑
  foot joint M11.27- ☑
  hand joint M11.24- ☑
  hip M11.25- ☑
  knee M11.26- ☑
  multiple site M11.29
  shoulder M11.21- ☑
  specified type NEC M11.20
    ankle M11.27- ☑
    elbow M11.22- ☑
    foot joint M11.27- ☑
    hand joint M11.24- ☑
    hip M11.25- ☑
    knee M11.26- ☑
    multiple site M11.29
    shoulder M11.21- ☑
    vertebrae M11.28
    wrist M11.23- ☑
  vertebrae M11.28
  wrist M11.23- ☑
Chondrodermatitis nodularis helicis or anthelicis
  — *see* Perichondritis, ear
Chondrodysplasia Q78.9
  with hemangioma Q78.4
  calcificans congenita Q77.3
  fetalis Q77.4
  metaphyseal (Jansen's) (McKusick's) (Schmid's) Q78.8
  punctata Q77.3
Chondrodystrophy, chondrodystrophia (familial)
  (fetalis) (hypoplastic) Q78.9
  calcificans congenita Q77.3
  myotonic (congenital) G71.13
  punctata Q77.3
Chondroectodermal dysplasia Q77.6
Chondrogenesis imperfecta Q77.4
Chondrolysis M94.35- ☑
Chondroma (*see also* Neoplasm, cartilage, benign)
  juxtacortical — *see* Neoplasm, bone, benign
  periosteal — *see* Neoplasm, bone, benign
Chondromalacia (systemic) M94.20
  acromioclavicular joint M94.21- ☑
  ankle M94.27- ☑
  elbow M94.22- ☑
  foot joint M94.27- ☑
  glenohumeral joint M94.21- ☑
  hand joint M94.24- ☑
  hip M94.25- ☑
  knee M94.26- ☑
    patella M22.4- ☑
  multiple sites M94.29
  patella M22.4- ☑
  rib M94.28
  sacroiliac joint M94.259
  shoulder M94.21- ☑
  sternoclavicular joint M94.21- ☑
  vertebral joint M94.28
  wrist M94.23- ☑
Chondromatosis (*see also* Neoplasm, cartilage, uncertain behavior)
  internal Q78.4
Chondromyxosarcoma — *see* Neoplasm, cartilage, malignant

Chondro-osteodysplasia (Morquio-Brailsford type) E76.219
Chondro-osteodystrophy E76.29
Chondro-osteoma — *see* Neoplasm, bone, benign
Chondropathia tuberosa M94.0
Chondrosarcoma — *see* Neoplasm, cartilage, malignant
  juxtacortical — *see* Neoplasm, bone, malignant
  mesenchymal — *see* Neoplasm, connective tissue, malignant
  myxoid — *see* Neoplasm, cartilage, malignant
Chordee (nonvenereal) N48.89
  congenital Q54.4
  gonococcal A54.09
Chorditis (fibrinous) (nodosa) (tuberosa) J38.2
Chordoma — *see* Neoplasm, vertebral (column), malignant
Chorea (chronic) (gravis) (posthemiplegic) (senile) (spasmodic) G25.5
  with
    heart involvement I02.0
      active or acute (conditions in I01-) I02.0
        rheumatic I02.9
          with valvular disorder I02.0
      rheumatic heart disease (chronic) (inactive)(quiescent) — *code to* rheumatic heart condition involved
  drug-induced G25.4
  habit F95.8
  hereditary G10
  Huntington's G10
  hysterical F44.4
  minor I02.9
    with heart involvement I02.0
  progressive G25.5
    hereditary G10
  rheumatic (chronic) I02.9
    with heart involvement I02.0
  Sydenham's I02.9
    with heart involvement — *see* Chorea, with rheumatic heart disease
  nonrheumatic G25.5
Choreoathetosis (paroxysmal) G25.5
Chorioadenoma (destruens) D39.2
Chorioamnionitis O41.12- ☑
Chorioangioma D26.7
Choriocarcinoma — *see* Neoplasm, malignant, by site
  combined with
    embryonal carcinoma — *see* Neoplasm, malignant, by site
    other germ cell elements — *see* Neoplasm, malignant, by site
    teratoma — *see* Neoplasm, malignant, by site
  specified site — *see* Neoplasm, malignant, by site
  unspecified site
    female C58
    male C62.90
Chorioencephalitis (acute) (lymphocytic) (serous) A87.2
Chorioepithelioma — *see* Choriocarcinoma
Choriomeningitis (acute) (lymphocytic) (serous) A87.2
Chorionepithelioma — *see* Choriocarcinoma
Chorioretinitis (*see also* Inflammation, chorioretinal)
  disseminated (*see also* Inflammation, chorioretinal, disseminated)
    in neurosyphilis A52.19
  Egyptian B76.9 [D63.8]
  focal (*see also* Inflammation, chorioretinal, focal)
  histoplasmic B39.9 [H32]
  in (due to)
    histoplasmosis B39.9 [H32]
    syphilis (secondary) A51.43
      late A52.71
    toxoplasmosis (acquired) B58.01
      congenital (active) P37.1 [H32]
    tuberculosis A18.53
  juxtapapillary, juxtapapillaris — *see* Inflammation, chorioretinal, focal, juxtapapillary
  leprous A30.9 [H32]
  miner's B76.9 [D63.8]
  progressive myopia (degeneration) (*see also* Myopia, degenerative) H44.2- ☑
  syphilitic (secondary) A51.43
    congenital (early) A50.01 [H32]
      late A50.32
    late A52.71
  tuberculous A18.53
Chorioretinopathy, central serous H35.71- ☑
Choroid — *see* condition
Choroideremia H31.21

Choroiditis — *see* Chorioretinitis
Choroidopathy — *see* Disorder, choroid
Choroidoretinitis — *see* Chorioretinitis
Choroidoretinopathy, central serous — *see* Chorioretinopathy, central serous
Christian-Weber disease M35.6
Christmas disease D67
Chromaffinoma (*see also* Neoplasm, benign, by site)
  malignant — *see* Neoplasm, malignant, by site
Chromatopsia — *see* Deficiency, color vision
Chromhidrosis, chromidrosis L75.1
Chromoblastomycosis — *see* Chromomycosis
Chromoconversion R82.91
Chromomycosis B43.9
  brain abscess B43.1
  cerebral B43.1
  cutaneous B43.0
  skin B43.0
  specified NEC B43.8
  subcutaneous abscess or cyst B43.2
Chromophytosis B36.0
Chromosome — *see* Anomaly, by chromosome involved
  D (1) — *see* Anomaly, chromosome 13
  E (3) — *see* Anomaly, chromosome 18
  G — *see* Anomaly, chromosome 21
Chromotrichomycosis B36.8
Chronic — *see* condition
  fracture — *see* Fracture, pathological
Churg-Strauss syndrome M30.1
Chyle cyst, mesentery I89.8
Chylocele (nonfilarial) I89.8
  filarial (*see also* Infestation, filarial) B74.9 [N51]
  tunica vaginalis N50.89
    filarial (*see also* Infestation, filarial) B74.9 [N51]
Chylomicronemia (fasting) (with hyperprebetalipoproteinemia) E78.3
Chylopericardium I31.3
  acute I30.9
Chylothorax (nonfilarial) I89.8
  filarial (*see also* Infestation, filarial) B74.9 [J91.8]
Chylous — *see* condition
Chyluria (nonfilarial) R82.0
  due to
    bilharziasis B65.0
    Brugia (malayi) B74.1
      timori B74.2
    schistosomiasis (bilharziasis) B65.0
    Wuchereria (bancrofti) B74.0
  filarial — *see* Infestation, filarial
Cicatricial (deformity) — *see* Cicatrix
Cicatrix (adherent) (contracted) (painful) (vicious) (*see also* Scar) L90.5
  adenoid (and tonsil) J35.8
  alveolar process M26.79
  anus K62.89
  auricle — *see* Disorder, pinna, specified type NEC
  bile duct (common) (hepatic) K83.8
  bladder N32.89
  bone — *see* Disorder, bone, specified type NEC
  brain G93.89
  cervix (postoperative) (postpartal) N88.1
  common duct K83.8
  cornea H17.9
    tuberculous A18.59
  duodenum (bulb), obstructive K31.5
  esophagus K22.2
  eyelid — *see* Disorder, eyelid function
  hypopharynx J39.2
  lacrimal passages — *see* Obstruction, lacrimal
  larynx J38.7
  lung J98.4
  middle ear H74.8 ☑
  mouth K13.79
  muscle M62.89
    with contracture — *see* Contraction, muscle NEC
  nasopharynx J39.2
  palate (soft) K13.79
  penis N48.89
  pharynx J39.2
  prostate N42.89
  rectum K62.89
  retina — *see* Scar, chorioretinal
  semilunar cartilage — *see* Derangement, meniscus
  seminal vesicle N50.89
  skin L90.5
    infected L08.89
    postinfective L90.5

Cicatrix — *continued*
  skin — *continued*
    tuberculous B90.8
    specified site NEC L90.5
  throat J39.2
  tongue K14.8
  tonsil (and adenoid) J35.8
  trachea J39.8
  tuberculous NEC B90.9
  urethra N36.8
  uterus N85.8
  vagina N89.8
    postoperative N99.2
  vocal cord J38.3
  wrist, constricting (annular) L90.5
CIDP (chronic inflammatory demyelinating polyneuropathy) G61.81
CIN — *see* Neoplasia, intraepithelial, cervix
CINCA (chronic infantile neurological, cutaneous and articular syndrome) M04.2
Cinchonism — *see* Deafness, ototoxic
  correct substance properly administered — *see* Table of Drugs and Chemicals, by drug, adverse effect
  overdose or wrong substance given or taken — *see* Table of Drugs and Chemicals, by drug, poisoning
Circle of Willis — *see* condition
Circular — *see* condition
Circulating anticoagulants (*see also* Disorder, hemorrhagic) D68.318
  due to drugs (*see also* Disorder, hemorrhagic) D68.32
  following childbirth O72.3
Circulation
  collateral, any site I99.8
  defective (lower extremity) I99.9
    congenital Q28.9
  embryonic Q28.9
  failure (peripheral) R57.9
    newborn P29.89
  fetal, persistent P29.38
  heart, incomplete Q28.9
Circulatory system — *see* condition
Circulus senilis (cornea) — *see* Degeneration, cornea, senile
Circumcision (in absence of medical indication) (ritual) (routine) Z41.2
Circumscribed — *see* condition
Circumvallate placenta O43.11- ☑
Cirrhosis, cirrhotic (hepatic) (liver) K74.60
  alcoholic K70.30
    with ascites K70.31
  atrophic — *see* Cirrhosis, liver
  Baumgarten-Cruveilhier K74.69
  biliary (cholangiolitic) (cholangitic) (hypertrophic) (obstructive) (pericholangiolitic) K74.5
    due to
      Clonorchiasis B66.1
      flukes B66.3
    primary K74.3
    secondary K74.4
  cardiac (of liver) K76.1
  Charcot's K74.3
  cholangiolitic, cholangitic, cholostatic (primary) K74.3
  congestive K76.1
  Cruveilhier-Baumgarten K74.69
  cryptogenic (liver) K74.69
  due to
    hepatolenticular degeneration E83.01
    Wilson's disease E83.01
    xanthomatosis E78.2
  fatty K76.0
    alcoholic K70.0
  Hanot's (hypertrophic) K74.3
  hepatic — *see* Cirrhosis, liver
  hypertrophic K74.3
  Indian childhood K74.69
  kidney — *see* Sclerosis, renal
  Laennec's K70.30
    with ascites K70.31
    alcoholic K70.30
      with ascites K70.31
    nonalcoholic K74.69
  liver K74.60
    alcoholic K70.30
      with ascites K70.31
      fatty K70.0
    congenital P78.81
    syphilitic A52.74

Cirrhosis, cirrhotic — *continued*
  lung (chronic) J84.10
  macronodular K74.69
    alcoholic K70.30
      with ascites K70.31
  micronodular K74.69
    alcoholic K70.30
      with ascites K70.31
  mixed type K74.69
  monolobular K74.3
  nephritis — *see* Sclerosis, renal
  nutritional K74.69
    alcoholic K70.30
      with ascites K70.31
  obstructive — *see* Cirrhosis, biliary
  ovarian N83.8
  pancreas (duct) K86.89
  pigmentary E83.110
  portal K74.69
    alcoholic K70.30
      with ascites K70.31
  postnecrotic K74.69
    alcoholic K70.30
      with ascites K70.31
  pulmonary J84.10
  renal — *see* Sclerosis, renal
  spleen D73.2
  stasis K76.1
  Todd's K74.3
  unilobar K74.3
  xanthomatous (biliary) K74.5
    due to xanthomatosis (familial) (metabolic) (primary) E78.2
Cistern, subarachnoid R93.0
Citrullinemia E72.23
Citrullinuria E72.23
Civatte's disease or poikiloderma L57.3
Clam digger's itch B65.3
Clammy skin R23.1
Clap — *see* Gonorrhea
Clarke-Hadfield syndrome (pancreatic infantilism) K86.89
Clark's paralysis G80.9
Clastothrix L67.8
Claude Bernard-Horner syndrome G90.2
  traumatic — *see* Injury, nerve, cervical sympathetic
Claude's disease or syndrome G46.3
Claudicatio venosa intermittens I87.8
Claudication (intermittent) I73.9
  cerebral (artery) G45.9
  spinal cord (arteriosclerotic) G95.19
    syphilitic A52.09
  venous (axillary) I87.8
Claustrophobia F40.240
Clavus (infected) L84
Clawfoot (congenital) Q66.89
  acquired — *see* Deformity, limb, clawfoot
Clawhand (acquired) (*see also* Deformity, limb, clawhand)
  congenital Q68.1
Clawtoe (congenital) Q66.89
  acquired — *see* Deformity, toe, specified NEC
Clay eating — *see* Pica
Cleansing of artificial opening — *see* Attention to, artificial, opening
Cleft (congenital) — *see also* Imperfect, closure
  alveolar process M26.79
  branchial (persistent) Q18.2
    cyst Q18.0
      fistula Q18.0
      sinus Q18.0
  cricoid cartilage, posterior Q31.8
  cyst Q18.0
    fistula Q18.0
    sinus Q18.0
  foot Q72.7 ☑
  hand Q71.6 ☑
  lip (unilateral) Q36.9
    with cleft palate Q37.9
      hard Q37.1
        with soft Q37.5
      soft Q37.3
        with hard Q37.5
    bilateral Q36.0
      with cleft palate Q37.8
        hard Q37.0
          with soft Q37.4
        soft Q37.2
          with hard Q37.4

Cleft — *continued*
  lip — *continued*
    median Q36.1
  nose Q30.2
  palate Q35.9
    with cleft lip (unilateral) Q37.9
      bilateral Q37.8
    hard Q35.1
      with
        cleft lip (unilateral) Q37.1
          bilateral Q37.0
        soft Q35.5
          with cleft lip (unilateral) Q37.5
            bilateral Q37.4
    medial Q35.5
    soft Q35.3
      with
        cleft lip (unilateral) Q37.3
          bilateral Q37.2
        hard Q35.5
          with cleft lip (unilateral) Q37.5
            bilateral Q37.4
  penis Q55.69
  scrotum Q55.29
  thyroid cartilage Q31.8
  uvula Q35.7
Cleidocranial dysostosis Q74.0
Cleptomania F63.2
Clicking hip (newborn) R29.4
Climacteric (female) (*see also* Menopause)
  arthritis (any site) NEC — *see* Arthritis, specified form NEC
  depression (single episode) F32.89
    recurrent episode F33.8
  male (symptoms) (syndrome) NEC N50.89
  melancholia (single episode) F32.89
    recurrent episode F33.8
  paranoid state F22
  polyarthritis NEC — *see* Arthritis, specified form NEC
  symptoms (female) N95.1
Clinical research investigation (clinical trial) (control subject) (normal comparison) (participant) Z00.6
Clitoris — *see* condition
Cloaca (persistent) Q43.7
Clonorchiasis, clonorchis infection (liver) B66.1
Clonus R25.8
Closed bite M26.29
Clostridium (C.) **perfringens, as cause of disease classified elsewhere** B96.7
Closure
  congenital, nose Q30.0
  cranial sutures, premature Q75.0
  defective or imperfect NEC — *see* Imperfect, closure
  fistula, delayed — *see* Fistula
  foramen ovale, imperfect Q21.1
  hymen N89.6
  interauricular septum, defective Q21.1
  interventricular septum, defective Q21.0
  lacrimal duct (*see also* Stenosis, lacrimal, duct)
    congenital Q10.5
  nose (congenital) Q30.0
    acquired M95.0
  of artificial opening — *see* Attention to, artificial, opening
  vagina N89.5
  valve — *see* Endocarditis
  vulva N90.5
Clot (blood) (*see also* Embolism)
  artery (obstruction) (occlusion) — *see* Embolism
  bladder N32.89
  brain (intradural or extradural) — *see* Occlusion, artery, cerebral
  circulation I74.9
  heart (*see also* Infarct, myocardium)
    not resulting in infarction I51.3
  vein — *see* Thrombosis
Clouded state R40.1
  epileptic — *see* Epilepsy, specified NEC
  paroxysmal — *see* Epilepsy, specified NEC
Cloudy antrum, antra J32.0
Clouston's (hidrotic) **ectodermal dysplasia** Q82.4
Clubbed nail pachydermoperiostosis M89.40 [L62]
Clubbing of finger(s) (nails) R68.3
Clubfinger R68.3
  congenital Q68.1
Clubfoot (congenital) Q66.89
  acquired — *see* Deformity, limb, clubfoot
  equinovarus Q66.0

Clubfoot — continued
  paralytic — see Deformity, limb, clubfoot
Clubhand (congenital) (radial) Q71.4- ☑
  acquired — see Deformity, limb, clubhand
Clubnail R68.3
  congenital Q84.6
Clump, kidney Q63.1
Clumsiness, clumsy child syndrome F82
Cluttering F80.81
Clutton's joints A50.51 [M12.80]
Coagulation, intravascular (diffuse) (disseminated)
    (see also Defibrination syndrome)
  complicating abortion — see Abortion, by type, com-
    plicated by, intravascular coagulation
  following ectopic or molar pregnancy O08.1
Coagulopathy (see also Defect, coagulation)
  consumption D65
  intravascular D65
    newborn P60
Coalition
  calcaneo-scaphoid Q66.89
  tarsal Q66.89
Coalminer's
  elbow — see Bursitis, elbow, olecranon
  lung or pneumoconiosis J60
Coalworker's lung or pneumoconiosis J60
Coarctation
  aorta (preductal) (postductal) Q25.1
  pulmonary artery Q25.71
Coated tongue K14.3
Coats' disease (exudative retinopathy) — see
    Retinopathy, exudative
Cocaine-induced
  anxiety disorder F14.980
  bipolar and related disorder F14.94
  depressive disorder F14.94
  obsessive-compulsive and related disorder F14.988
  psychotic disorder F14.959
  sexual dysfunction F14.981
  sleep disorder F14.982
Cocainism — see Disorder, cocaine use
Coccidioidomycosis B38.9
  cutaneous B38.3
  disseminated B38.7
  generalized B38.7
  meninges B38.4
  prostate B38.81
  pulmonary B38.2
    acute B38.0
    chronic B38.1
  skin B38.3
  specified NEC B38.89
Coccidioidosis — see Coccidioidomycosis
Coccidiosis (intestinal) A07.3
Coccydynia, coccygodynia M53.3
Coccyx — see condition
Cochin-China diarrhea K90.1
Cockayne's syndrome Q87.1
Cocked up toe — see Deformity, toe, specified NEC
Cock's peculiar tumor L72.3
Codman's tumor — see Neoplasm, bone, benign
Coenurosis B71.8
Coffee-worker's lung J67.8
Cogan's syndrome H16.32- ☑
  oculomotor apraxia H51.8
Coitus, painful (female) N94.10
  male N53.12
  psychogenic F52.6
Cold J00
  with influenza, flu, or grippe — see Influenza, with,
    respiratory manifestations NEC
  agglutinin disease or hemoglobinuria (chronic) D59.1
  bronchial — see Bronchitis
  chest — see Bronchitis
  common (head) J00
  effects of T69.9 ☑
    specified effect NEC T69.8 ☑
  excessive, effects of T69.9 ☑
    specified effect NEC T69.8 ☑
  exhaustion from T69.8 ☑
  exposure to T69.9 ☑
    specified effect NEC T69.8 ☑
  head J00
  injury syndrome (newborn) P80.0
  on lung — see Bronchitis
  rose J30.1
  sensitivity, auto-immune D59.1

Cold — continued
  symptoms J00
  virus J00
Coldsore B00.1
Colibacillosis A49.8
  as the cause of other disease (see also Escherichia coli)
    B96.20
  generalized A41.50
Colic (bilious) (infantile) (intestinal) (recurrent) (spasmod-
    ic) R10.83
  abdomen R10.83
    psychogenic F45.8
  appendix, appendicular K38.8
  bile duct — see Calculus, bile duct
  biliary — see Calculus, bile duct
  common duct — see Calculus, bile duct
  cystic duct — see Calculus, gallbladder
  Devonshire NEC — see Poisoning, lead
  gallbladder — see Calculus, gallbladder
  gallstone — see Calculus, gallbladder
    gallbladder or cystic duct — see Calculus, gallblad-
      der
  hepatic (duct) — see Calculus, bile duct
  hysterical F45.8
  kidney N23
  lead NEC — see Poisoning, lead
  mucous K58.9
    with diarrhea K58.0
    psychogenic F54
  nephritic N23
  painter's NEC — see Poisoning, lead
  pancreas K86.89
  psychogenic F45.8
  renal N23
  saturnine NEC — see Poisoning, lead
  ureter N23
  urethral N36.8
    due to calculus N21.1
  uterus NEC N94.89
    menstrual — see Dysmenorrhea
  worm NOS B83.9
Colicystitis — see Cystitis
Colitis (acute) (catarrhal) (chronic) (noninfective) (hemor-
    rhagic) (see also Enteritis) K52.9
  allergic K52.29
    with
      food protein-induced enterocolitis syndrome
        K52.21
      proctocolitis K52.82
  amebic (acute) (see also Amebiasis) A06.0
    nondysenteric A06.2
  anthrax A22.2
  bacillary — see Infection, Shigella
  balantidial A07.0
  Clostridium difficile
    not specified as recurrent A04.72
    recurrent A04.71
  coccidial A07.3
  collagenous K52.831
  cystica superficialis K52.89
  dietary counseling and surveillance (for) Z71.3
  dietetic (see also Colitis, allergic) K52.29
  drug-induced K52.1
  due to radiation K52.0
  eosinophilic K52.82
  food hypersensitivity (see also Colitis, allergic) K52.29
  giardial A07.1
  granulomatous — see Enteritis, regional, large intes-
    tine
  indeterminate, so stated K52.3
  infectious — see Enteritis, infectious
  ischemic K55.9
    acute (subacute) (see also Ischemia, intestine,
      acute) K55.039
    chronic K55.1
    due to mesenteric artery insufficiency K55.1
    fulminant (acute) (see also Ischemia, intestine,
      acute) K55.039
  left sided K51.50
    with
      abscess K51.514
      complication K51.519
        specified NEC K51.518
      fistula K51.513
      obstruction K51.512
      rectal bleeding K51.511
  lymphocytic K52.832

Colitis — continued
  membranous
    psychogenic F54
  microscopic K52.839
    specified NEC K52.838
  mucous — see Syndrome, irritable, bowel
    psychogenic F54
  noninfective K52.9
    specified NEC K52.89
  polyposa — see Polyp, colon, inflammatory
  protozoal A07.9
  pseudomembranous
    not specified as recurrent A04.72
    recurrent A04.71
  pseudomucinous — see Syndrome, irritable, bowel
  regional — see Enteritis, regional, large intestine
    infectious A09
  segmental — see Enteritis, regional, large intestine
  septic — see Enteritis, infectious
  spastic K58.9
    with diarrhea K58.0
    psychogenic F54
  staphylococcal A04.8
    foodborne A05.0
  subacute ischemic (see also Ischemia, intestine, acute)
    K55.039
  thromboulcerative (see also Ischemia, intestine, acute)
    K55.039
  toxic NEC K52.1
    due to Clostridium difficile
      not specified as recurrent A04.72
      recurrent A04.71
  transmural — see Enteritis, regional, large intestine
  trichomonal A07.8
  tuberculous (ulcerative) A18.32
  ulcerative (chronic) K51.90
    with
      complication K51.919
        abscess K51.914
        fistula K51.913
        obstruction K51.912
        rectal bleeding K51.911
        specified complication NEC K51.918
    enterocolitis — see Enterocolitis, ulcerative
    ileocolitis — see Ileocolitis, ulcerative
    mucosal proctocolitis — see Proctocolitis, mucosal
    proctitis — see Proctitis, ulcerative
    pseudopolyposis — see Polyp, colon, inflammatory
    psychogenic F54
    rectosigmoiditis — see Rectosigmoiditis, ulcerative
    specified type NEC K51.80
      with
        complication K51.819
          abscess K51.814
          fistula K51.813
          obstruction K51.812
          rectal bleeding K51.811
          specified complication NEC K51.818
Collagenosis, collagen disease (nonvascular) (vascular)
    M35.9
  cardiovascular I42.8
  reactive perforating L87.1
  specified NEC M35.8
Collapse R55
  adrenal E27.2
  cardiorespiratory R57.0
  cardiovascular R57.0
    newborn P29.89
  circulatory (peripheral) R57.9
    during or after labor and delivery O75.1
    following ectopic or molar pregnancy O08.3
    newborn P29.89
  during or
    after labor and delivery O75.1
    resulting from a procedure, not elsewhere classified
      T81.10 ☑
  external ear canal — see Stenosis, external ear canal
  general R55
  heart — see Disease, heart
  heat T67.1 ☑
  hysterical F44.89
  labyrinth, membranous (congenital) Q16.5
  lung (massive) (see also Atelectasis) J98.19
    pressure due to anesthesia (general) (local) or
      other sedation T88.2 ☑
      during labor and delivery O74.1
      in pregnancy O29.02- ☑
      postpartum, puerperal O89.09

☑ **Additional Character Required** — Refer to the Tabular List for Character Selection   ⌖ Subterms under main terms may continue to next column or page

Collapse — *continued*
  myocardial — *see* Disease, heart
  nervous F48.8
  neurocirculatory F45.8
  nose M95.0
  postoperative T81.10 ☑
  pulmonary (*see also* Atelectasis) J98.19
    newborn — *see* Atelectasis
  trachea J39.8
  tracheobronchial J98.09
  valvular — *see* Endocarditis
  vascular (peripheral) R57.9
    during or after labor and delivery O75.1
    following ectopic or molar pregnancy O08.3
    newborn P29.89
  vertebra M48.50-
    cervical region M48.52- ☑
    cervicothoracic region M48.53- ☑
    in (due to)
        metastasis — *see* Collapse, vertebra, in, speci-
          fied disease NEC
        osteoporosis (*see also* Osteoporosis) M80.88 ☑
          cervical region M80.88 ☑
          cervicothoracic region M80.88 ☑
          lumbar region M80.88 ☑
          lumbosacral region M80.88 ☑
          multiple sites M80.88 ☑
          occipito-atlanto-axial region M80.88 ☑
          sacrococcygeal region M80.88 ☑
          thoracic region M80.88 ☑
          thoracolumbar region M80.88 ☑
        specified disease NEC M48.50- ☑
          cervical region M48.52- ☑
          cervicothoracic region M48.53- ☑
          lumbar region M48.56- ☑
          lumbosacral region M48.57- ☑
          occipito-atlanto-axial region M48.51- ☑
          sacrococcygeal region M48.58- ☑
          thoracic region M48.54- ☑
          thoracolumbar region M48.55- ☑
    lumbar region M48.56- ☑
    lumbosacral region M48.57- ☑
    occipito-atlanto-axial region M48.51- ☑
    sacrococcygeal region M48.58- ☑
    thoracic region M48.54- ☑
    thoracolumbar region M48.55- ☑
Collateral (*see also* condition)
  circulation (venous) I87.8
  dilation, veins I87.8
Colles' fracture S52.53- ☑
Collet (-Sicard) syndrome G52.7
Collier's asthma or lung J60
Collodion baby Q80.2
Colloid nodule (of thyroid) (cystic) E04.1
Coloboma (iris) Q13.0
  eyelid Q10.3
  fundus Q14.8
  lens Q12.2
  optic disc (congenital) Q14.2
    acquired H47.31- ☑
Coloenteritis — *see* Enteritis
Colon — *see* condition
Colonization
  MRSA (Methicillin resistant Staphylococcus aureus) Z22.322
  MSSA (Methicillin susceptible Staphylococcus aureus) Z22.321
  status — *see* Carrier (suspected) of
Coloptosis K63.4
Color blindness — *see* Deficiency, color vision
Colostomy
  attention to Z43.3
  fitting or adjustment Z46.89
  malfunctioning K94.03
  status Z93.3
Colpitis (acute) — *see* Vaginitis
Colpocele N81.5
Colpocystitis — *see* Vaginitis
Colpospasm N94.2
Column, spinal, vertebral — *see* condition
Coma R40.20
  with
    motor response (none) R40.231 ☑
      abnormal extensor posturing to pain or noxious stimuli (< 2 years of age) R40.232 ☑
      abnormal flexure posturing to pain or noxious stimuli (0-5 years of age) R40.233 ☑

Coma — *continued*
  with — *continued*
    motor response — *continued*
      extensor posturing to pain or noxious stimuli (2-5 years of age) R40.232 ☑
      flexion/decorticate posturing (< 2 years of age) R40.233 ☑
      localizes pain (2-5 years of age) R40.235 ☑
      normal or spontaneous movement (< 2 years of age) R40.236 ☑
      obeys commands (2-5 years of age) R40.236 ☑
      withdraws from pain or noxious stimuli (0-5 years of age) R40.234 ☑
      withdraws to touch (< 2 years of age) R40.235 ☑
    opening of eyes (never) R40.211 ☑
      in response to
        pain R40.212 ☑
        sound R40.213 ☑
      spontaneous R40.214 ☑
    verbal response (none) R40.221 ☑
      confused conversation R40.224 ☑
      cooing or babbling or crying appropriately (< 2 years of age) R40.225 ☑
      inappropriate crying or screaming (< 2 years of age) R40.223 ☑
      inappropriate words (2-5 years of age) R40.224 ☑
      incomprehensible sounds (2-5 years of age) R40.222 ☑
      incomprehensible words R40.222 ☑
      irritable cries (< 2 years of age) R40.224 ☑
      moans/grunts to pain; restless (< 2 years old) R40.222 ☑
      oriented R40.225 ☑
      screaming (2-5 years of age) R40.223 ☑
      uses appropriate words (2-5 years of age) R40.225 ☑
  eclamptic — *see* Eclampsia
  epileptic — *see* Epilepsy
  Glasgow, scale score — *see* Glasgow coma scale
  hepatic — *see* Failure, hepatic, by type, with coma
  hyperglycemic (diabetic) — *see* Diabetes, by type, with hyperosmolarity, with coma
  hyperosmolar (diabetic) — *see* Diabetes, by type, with hyperosmolarity, with coma
  hypoglycemic (diabetic) — *see* Diabetes, by type, with hypoglycemia, with coma
    nondiabetic E15
  in diabetes — *see* Diabetes, coma
  insulin-induced — *see* Coma, hypoglycemic
  ketoacidotic (diabetic) — *see* Diabetes, by type, with ketoacidosis, with coma
  myxedematous E03.5
  newborn P91.5
  persistent vegetative state R40.3
  specified NEC, without documented Glasgow coma scale score, or with partial Glasgow coma scale score reported R40.244 ☑
Comatose — *see* Coma
Combat fatigue F43.0
Combined — *see* condition
Comedo, comedones (giant) L70.0
Comedocarcinoma (*see also* Neoplasm, breast, malignant)
  noninfiltrating
    breast D05.8- ☑
    specified site — *see* Neoplasm, in situ, by site
    unspecified site D05.8- ☑
Comedomastitis — *see* Ectasia, mammary duct
Comminuted fracture — *code as* Fracture, closed
Common
  arterial trunk Q20.0
  atrioventricular canal Q21.2
  atrium Q21.1
  cold (head) J00
  truncus (arteriosus) Q20.0
  variable immunodeficiency — *see* Immunodeficiency, common variable
  ventricle Q20.4
Commotio, commotion (current)
  brain — *see* Injury, intracranial, concussion
  cerebri — *see* Injury, intracranial, concussion
  retinae S05.8X- ☑
  spinal cord — *see* Injury, spinal cord, by region
  spinalis — *see* Injury, spinal cord, by region

Communication
  between
    base of aorta and pulmonary artery Q21.4
    left ventricle and right atrium Q20.5
    pericardial sac and pleural sac Q34.8
    pulmonary artery and pulmonary vein, congenital Q25.72
  congenital between uterus and digestive or urinary tract Q51.7
Compartment syndrome (deep) (posterior) (traumatic) T79.A0 ☑ (*following* T79.7)
  abdomen T79.A3 ☑ (*following* T79.7)
  lower extremity (hip, buttock, thigh, leg, foot, toes) T79.A2 ☑ (*following* T79.7)
  nontraumatic
    abdomen M79.A3 (*following* M79.7)
    lower extremity (hip, buttock, thigh, leg, foot, toes) M79.A2- ☑ (*following* M79.7)
    specified site NEC M79.A9 (*following* M79.7)
    upper extremity (shoulder, arm, forearm, wrist, hand, fingers) M79.A1- ☑ (*following* M79.7)
  specified site NEC T79.A9 ☑ (*following* T79.7)
  upper extremity (shoulder, arm, forearm, wrist, hand, fingers) T79.A1- ☑ (*following* T79.7)
Compensation
  failure — *see* Disease, heart
  neurosis, psychoneurosis — *see* Disorder, factitious
Complaint (*see also* Disease)
  bowel, functional K59.9
    psychogenic F45.8
  intestine, functional K59.9
    psychogenic F45.8
  kidney — *see* Disease, renal
  miners' J60
Complete — *see* condition
Complex
  Addison-Schilder E71.528
  cardiorenal — *see* Hypertension, cardiorenal
  Costen's M26.69
  disseminated mycobacterium avium- intracellulare (DMAC) A31.2
  Eisenmenger's (ventricular septal defect) I27.83
  hypersexual F52.8
  jumped process, spine — *see* Dislocation, vertebra
  primary, tuberculous A15.7
  Schilder-Addison E71.528
  subluxation (vertebral) M99.19
    abdomen M99.19
    acromioclavicular M99.17
    cervical region M99.11
    cervicothoracic M99.11
    costochondral M99.18
    costovertebral M99.18
    head region M99.10
    hip M99.15
    lower extremity M99.16
    lumbar region M99.13
    lumbosacral M99.13
    occipitocervical M99.10
    pelvic region M99.15
    pubic M99.15
    rib cage M99.18
    sacral region M99.14
    sacrococcygeal M99.14
    sacroiliac M99.14
    specified NEC M99.19
    sternochondral M99.18
    sternoclavicular M99.17
    thoracic region M99.12
    thoracolumbar M99.12
    upper extremity M99.17
  Taussig-Bing (transposition, aorta and overriding pulmonary artery) Q20.1
Complication(s) (from) (of)
  accidental puncture or laceration during a procedure (of) — *see* Complications, intraoperative (intraprocedural), puncture or laceration
  amputation stump (surgical) (late) NEC T87.9
    dehiscence T87.81
    infection or inflammation T87.40
      lower limb T87.4- ☑
      upper limb T87.4- ☑
    necrosis T87.50
      lower limb T87.5- ☑
      upper limb T87.5- ☑
    neuroma T87.30
      lower limb T87.3- ☑
      upper limb T87.3- ☑

Complication(s) — *continued*
- amputation stump — *continued*
  - specified type NEC T87.89
- anastomosis (and bypass) (*see also* Complications, prosthetic device or implant)
  - intestinal (internal) NEC K91.89
    - involving urinary tract N99.89
  - urinary tract (involving intestinal tract) N99.89
  - vascular — *see* Complications, cardiovascular device or implant
- anesthesia, anesthetic (*see also* Anesthesia, complication) T88.59
  - brain, postpartum, puerperal O89.2
  - cardiac
    - in
      - labor and delivery O74.2
      - pregnancy O29.19- ☑
    - postpartum, puerperal O89.1
  - central nervous system
    - in
      - labor and delivery O74.3
      - pregnancy O29.29- ☑
    - postpartum, puerperal O89.2
  - difficult or failed intubation T88.4 ☑
    - in pregnancy O29.6- ☑
  - failed sedation (conscious) (moderate) during procedure T88.52 ☑
  - general, unintended awareness during procedure T88.53 ☑
  - hyperthermia, malignant T88.3 ☑
  - hypothermia T88.51 ☑
  - intubation failure T88.4 ☑
  - malignant hyperthermia T88.3 ☑
  - pulmonary
    - in
      - labor and delivery O74.1
      - pregnancy NEC O29.09- ☑
    - postpartum, puerperal O89.09
  - shock T88.2 ☑
  - spinal and epidural
    - in
      - labor and delivery NEC O74.6
        - headache O74.5
      - pregnancy NEC O29.5X- ☑
    - postpartum, puerperal NEC O89.5
      - headache O89.4
  - unintended awareness under general anesthesia during procedure T88.53 ☑
- anti-reflux device — *see* Complications, esophageal anti-reflux device
- aortic (bifurcation) graft — *see* Complications, graft, vascular
- aortocoronary (bypass) graft — *see* Complications, coronary artery (bypass) graft
- aortofemoral (bypass) graft — *see* Complications, extremity artery (bypass) graft
- arteriovenous
  - fistula, surgically created T82.9 ☑
    - embolism T82.818 ☑
    - fibrosis T82.828 ☑
    - hemorrhage T82.838 ☑
    - infection or inflammation T82.7 ☑
    - mechanical
      - breakdown T82.510 ☑
      - displacement T82.520 ☑
      - leakage T82.530 ☑
      - malposition T82.520 ☑
      - obstruction T82.590 ☑
      - perforation T82.590 ☑
      - protrusion T82.590 ☑
    - pain T82.848 ☑
    - specified type NEC T82.898 ☑
    - stenosis T82.858 ☑
    - thrombosis T82.868 ☑
  - shunt, surgically created T82.9 ☑
    - embolism T82.818 ☑
    - fibrosis T82.828 ☑
    - hemorrhage T82.838 ☑
    - infection or inflammation T82.7 ☑
    - mechanical
      - breakdown T82.511 ☑
      - displacement T82.521 ☑
      - leakage T82.531 ☑
      - malposition T82.521 ☑
      - obstruction T82.591 ☑
      - perforation T82.591 ☑
      - protrusion T82.591 ☑

Complication(s) — *continued*
- arteriovenous — *continued*
  - shunt, surgically created — *continued*
    - pain T82.848 ☑
    - specified type NEC T82.898 ☑
    - stenosis T82.858 ☑
    - thrombosis T82.868 ☑
- arthroplasty — *see* Complications, joint prosthesis
- artificial
  - fertilization or insemination N98.9
    - attempted introduction (of)
      - embryo in embryo transfer N98.3
      - ovum following in vitro fertilization N98.2
    - hyperstimulation of ovaries N98.1
    - infection N98.0
    - specified NEC N98.8
  - heart T82.9
    - embolism T82.817 ☑
    - fibrosis T82.827 ☑
    - hemorrhage T82.837 ☑
    - infection or inflammation T82.7 ☑
    - mechanical
      - breakdown T82.512 ☑
      - displacement T82.522 ☑
      - leakage T82.532 ☑
      - malposition T82.522 ☑
      - obstruction T82.592 ☑
      - perforation T82.592 ☑
      - protrusion T82.592 ☑
    - pain T82.847 ☑
    - specified type NEC T82.897 ☑
    - stenosis T82.857 ☑
    - thrombosis T82.867 ☑
  - opening
    - cecostomy — *see* Complications, colostomy
    - colostomy — *see* Complications, colostomy
    - cystostomy — *see* Complications, cystostomy
    - enterostomy — *see* Complications, enterostomy
    - gastrostomy — *see* Complications, gastrostomy
    - ileostomy — *see* Complications, enterostomy
    - jejunostomy — *see* Complications, enterostomy
    - nephrostomy — *see* Complications, stoma, urinary tract
    - tracheostomy — *see* Complications, tracheostomy
    - ureterostomy — *see* Complications, stoma, urinary tract
    - urethrostomy — *see* Complications, stoma, urinary tract
- balloon implant or device
  - gastrointestinal T85.9 ☑
    - embolism T85.818 ☑
    - fibrosis T85.828 ☑
    - hemorrhage T85.838 ☑
    - infection and inflammation T85.79 ☑
    - pain T85.848 ☑
    - specified type NEC T85.898 ☑
    - stenosis T85.858 ☑
    - thrombosis T85.868 ☑
  - vascular (counterpulsation) T82.9 ☑
    - embolism T82.818 ☑
    - fibrosis T82.828 ☑
    - hemorrhage T82.838 ☑
    - infection or inflammation T82.7 ☑
    - mechanical
      - breakdown T82.513 ☑
      - displacement T82.523 ☑
      - leakage T82.533 ☑
      - malposition T82.523 ☑
      - obstruction T82.593 ☑
      - perforation T82.593 ☑
      - protrusion T82.593 ☑
    - pain T82.848 ☑
    - specified type NEC T82.898 ☑
    - stenosis T82.858 ☑
    - thrombosis T82.868 ☑
- bariatric procedure
  - gastric band procedure K95.09
    - infection K95.01
  - specified procedure NEC K95.89
    - infection K95.81
- bile duct implant (prosthetic) T85.9 ☑
  - embolism T85.818 ☑
  - fibrosis T85.828 ☑
  - hemorrhage T85.838 ☑

Complication(s) — *continued*
- bile duct implant — *continued*
  - infection and inflammation T85.79 ☑
  - mechanical
    - breakdown T85.510 ☑
    - displacement T85.520 ☑
    - malfunction T85.510 ☑
    - malposition T85.520 ☑
    - obstruction T85.590 ☑
    - perforation T85.590 ☑
    - protrusion T85.590 ☑
    - specified NEC T85.590 ☑
  - pain T85.848 ☑
  - specified type NEC T85.898 ☑
  - stenosis T85.858 ☑
  - thrombosis T85.868 ☑
- bladder device (auxiliary) — *see* Complications, genitourinary, device or implant, urinary system
- bleeding (postoperative) — *see* Complication, postoperative, hemorrhage
  - intraoperative — *see* Complication, intraoperative, hemorrhage
- blood vessel graft — *see* Complications, graft, vascular
- bone
  - device NEC T84.9 ☑
    - embolism T84.81 ☑
    - fibrosis T84.82 ☑
    - hemorrhage T84.83 ☑
    - infection or inflammation T84.7 ☑
    - mechanical
      - breakdown T84.318 ☑
      - displacement T84.328 ☑
      - malposition T84.328 ☑
      - obstruction T84.398 ☑
      - perforation T84.398 ☑
      - protrusion T84.398 ☑
    - pain T84.84 ☑
    - specified type NEC T84.89 ☑
    - stenosis T84.85 ☑
    - thrombosis T84.86 ☑
  - graft — *see* Complications, graft, bone
  - growth stimulator (electrode) — *see* Complications, electronic stimulator device, bone
  - marrow transplant — *see* Complications, transplant, bone, marrow
- brain neurostimulator (electrode) — *see* Complications, electronic stimulator device, brain
- breast implant (prosthetic) T85.9 ☑
  - capsular contracture T85.44 ☑
  - embolism T85.818 ☑
  - fibrosis T85.828 ☑
  - hemorrhage T85.838 ☑
  - infection and inflammation T85.79 ☑
  - mechanical
    - breakdown T85.41 ☑
    - displacement T85.42 ☑
    - leakage T85.43 ☑
    - malposition T85.42 ☑
    - obstruction T85.49 ☑
    - perforation T85.49 ☑
    - protrusion T85.49 ☑
    - specified NEC T85.49 ☑
  - pain T85.848 ☑
  - specified type NEC T85.898 ☑
  - stenosis T85.858 ☑
  - thrombosis T85.868 ☑
- bypass (*see also* Complications, prosthetic device or implant)
  - aortocoronary — *see* Complications, coronary artery (bypass) graft
  - arterial (*see also* Complications, graft, vascular)
    - extremity — *see* Complications, extremity artery (bypass) graft
- cardiac (*see also* Disease, heart)
  - device, implant or graft T82.9 ☑
    - embolism T82.817 ☑
    - fibrosis T82.827 ☑
    - hemorrhage T82.837 ☑
    - infection or inflammation T82.7 ☑
      - valve prosthesis T82.6 ☑
    - mechanical
      - breakdown T82.519 ☑
        - specified device NEC T82.518 ☑
      - displacement T82.529 ☑
        - specified device NEC T82.528 ☑
      - leakage T82.539 ☑

Complication(s) — *continued*
  cardiac (*see also* Disease, heart) — *continued*
    device, implant or graft — *continued*
      mechanical — *continued*
        leakage — *continued*
          specified device NEC T82.538 ☑
        malposition T82.529 ☑
          specified device NEC T82.528 ☑
        obstruction T82.599 ☑
          specified device NEC T82.598 ☑
        perforation T82.599 ☑
          specified device NEC T82.598 ☑
        protrusion T82.599 ☑
          specified device NEC T82.598 ☑
      pain T82.847 ☑
      specified type NEC T82.897 ☑
      stenosis T82.857 ☑
      thrombosis T82.867 ☑
  cardiovascular device, graft or implant T82.9 ☑
    aortic graft — *see* Complications, graft, vascular
    arteriovenous
      fistula, artificial — *see* Complication, arteriovenous, fistula, surgically created
      shunt — *see* Complication, arteriovenous, shunt, surgically created
    artificial heart — *see* Complication, artificial, heart
    balloon (counterpulsation) device — *see* Complication, balloon implant, vascular
    carotid artery graft — *see* Complications, graft, vascular
    coronary bypass graft — *see* Complication, coronary artery (bypass) graft
    dialysis catheter (vascular) — *see* Complication, catheter, dialysis
    electronic T82.9 ☑
      electrode T82.9 ☑
        embolism T82.817 ☑
        fibrosis T82.827 ☑
        hemorrhage T82.837 ☑
        infection T82.7 ☑
        mechanical
          breakdown T82.110 ☑
          displacement T82.120 ☑
          leakage T82.190 ☑
          obstruction T82.190 ☑
          perforation T82.190 ☑
          protrusion T82.190 ☑
          specified type NEC T82.190 ☑
        pain T82.847 ☑
        specified NEC T82.897 ☑
        stenosis T82.857 ☑
        thrombosis T82.867 ☑
      embolism T82.817 ☑
      fibrosis T82.827 ☑
      hemorrhage T82.837 ☑
      infection T82.7 ☑
      mechanical
        breakdown T82.119 ☑
        displacement T82.129 ☑
        leakage T82.199 ☑
        obstruction T82.199 ☑
        perforation T82.199 ☑
        protrusion T82.199 ☑
        specified type NEC T82.199 ☑
      pain T82.847 ☑
      pulse generator T82.9 ☑
        embolism T82.817 ☑
        fibrosis T82.827 ☑
        hemorrhage T82.837 ☑
        infection T82.7 ☑
        mechanical
          breakdown T82.111 ☑
          displacement T82.121 ☑
          leakage T82.191 ☑
          obstruction T82.191 ☑
          perforation T82.191 ☑
          protrusion T82.191 ☑
          specified type NEC T82.191 ☑
        pain T82.847 ☑
        specified NEC T82.897 ☑
        stenosis T82.857 ☑
        thrombosis T82.867 ☑
      specified condition NEC T82.897 ☑
      specified device NEC T82.9 ☑
        embolism T82.817 ☑
        fibrosis T82.827 ☑

Complication(s) — *continued*
  cardiovascular device, graft or implant — *continued*
    electronic — *continued*
      specified device — *continued*
        hemorrhage T82.837 ☑
        infection T82.7 ☑
        mechanical
          breakdown T82.118 ☑
          displacement T82.128 ☑
          leakage T82.198 ☑
          obstruction T82.198 ☑
          perforation T82.198 ☑
          protrusion T82.198 ☑
          specified type NEC T82.198 ☑
        pain T82.847 ☑
        specified NEC T82.897 ☑
        stenosis T82.857 ☑
        thrombosis T82.867 ☑
      stenosis T82.857 ☑
      thrombosis T82.867 ☑
    extremity artery graft — *see* Complication, extremity artery (bypass) graft
    femoral artery graft — *see* Complication, extremity artery (bypass) graft
    heart
      transplant — *see* Complication, transplant, heart
      valve — *see* Complication, prosthetic device, heart valve
        graft — *see* Complication, heart, valve, graft
    heart-lung transplant — *see* Complication, transplant, heart, with lung
    infection or inflammation T82.7 ☑
    umbrella device — *see* Complication, umbrella device, vascular
    vascular graft (or anastomosis) — *see* Complication, graft, vascular
  carotid artery (bypass) graft — *see* Complications, graft, vascular
  catheter (device) NEC (*see also* Complications, prosthetic device or implant)
    cranial infusion
      infection and inflammation T85.735 ☑
      mechanical
        breakdown T85.610 ☑
        displacement T85.620 ☑
        leakage T85.630 ☑
        malfunction T85.690 ☑
        malposition T85.620 ☑
        obstruction T85.690 ☑
        perforation T85.690 ☑
        protrusion T85.690 ☑
        specified NEC T85.690 ☑
    cystostomy T83.9 ☑
      embolism T83.81 ☑
      fibrosis T83.82 ☑
      hemorrhage T83.83 ☑
      infection and inflammation T83.510 ☑
      mechanical
        breakdown T83.010 ☑
        displacement T83.020 ☑
        leakage T83.030 ☑
        malposition T83.020 ☑
        obstruction T83.090 ☑
        perforation T83.090 ☑
        protrusion T83.090 ☑
        specified NEC T83.090 ☑
      pain T83.84 ☑
      specified type NEC T83.89 ☑
      stenosis T83.85 ☑
      thrombosis T83.86 ☑
    dialysis (vascular) T82.9 ☑
      embolism T82.818 ☑
      fibrosis T82.828 ☑
      hemorrhage T82.838 ☑
      infection and inflammation T82.7 ☑
      intraperitoneal — *see* Complications, catheter, intraperitoneal
      mechanical
        breakdown T82.41 ☑
        displacement T82.42 ☑
        leakage T82.43 ☑
        malposition T82.42 ☑
        obstruction T82.49 ☑
        perforation T82.49 ☑

Complication(s) — *continued*
  catheter (*see also* Complications, prosthetic device or implant) — *continued*
    dialysis — *continued*
      mechanical — *continued*
        protrusion T82.49 ☑
      pain T82.848 ☑
      specified type NEC T82.898 ☑
      stenosis T82.858 ☑
      thrombosis T82.868 ☑
    epidural infusion T85.9 ☑
      embolism T85.810 ☑
      fibrosis T85.820 ☑
      hemorrhage T85.830 ☑
      infection and inflammation T85.735 ☑
      mechanical
        breakdown T85.610 ☑
        displacement T85.620 ☑
        leakage T85.630 ☑
        malfunction T85.610 ☑
        malposition T85.620 ☑
        obstruction T85.690 ☑
        perforation T85.690 ☑
        protrusion T85.690 ☑
        specified NEC T85.690 ☑
      pain T85.840 ☑
      specified type NEC T85.890 ☑
      stenosis T85.850 ☑
      thrombosis T85.860 ☑
    intraperitoneal dialysis T85.9 ☑
      embolism T85.818 ☑
      fibrosis T85.828 ☑
      hemorrhage T85.838 ☑
      infection and inflammation T85.71 ☑
      mechanical
        breakdown T85.611 ☑
        displacement T85.621 ☑
        leakage T85.631 ☑
        malfunction T85.611 ☑
        malposition T85.621 ☑
        obstruction T85.691 ☑
        perforation T85.691 ☑
        protrusion T85.691 ☑
        specified NEC T85.691 ☑
      pain T85.848 ☑
      specified type NEC T85.898 ☑
      stenosis T85.858 ☑
      thrombosis T85.868 ☑
    intrathecal infusion
      infection and inflammation T85.735 ☑
      mechanical
        breakdown T85.610 ☑
        displacement T85.620 ☑
        leakage T85.630 ☑
        malfunction T85.690 ☑
        malposition T85.620 ☑
        obstruction T85.690 ☑
        perforation T85.690 ☑
        protrusion T85.690 ☑
        specified NEC T85.690 ☑
    intravenous infusion T82.9 ☑
      embolism T82.818 ☑
      fibrosis T82.828 ☑
      hemorrhage T82.838 ☑
      infection or inflammation T82.7 ☑
      mechanical
        breakdown T82.514 ☑
        displacement T82.524 ☑
        leakage T82.534 ☑
        malposition T82.524 ☑
        obstruction T82.594 ☑
        perforation T82.594 ☑
        protrusion T82.594 ☑
      pain T82.848 ☑
      specified type NEC T82.898 ☑
      stenosis T82.858 ☑
      thrombosis T82.868 ☑
    spinal infusion
      infection and inflammation T85.735 ☑
      mechanical
        breakdown T85.610 ☑
        displacement T85.620 ☑
        leakage T85.630 ☑
        malfunction T85.690 ☑
        malposition T85.620 ☑
        obstruction T85.690 ☑

Complication(s) — *continued*
　catheter (*see also* Complications, prosthetic device or
　　implant) — *continued*
　　spinal infusion — *continued*
　　　mechanical — *continued*
　　　　perforation T85.690 ☑
　　　　protrusion T85.690 ☑
　　　　specified NEC T85.690 ☑
　　　subarachnoid infusion
　　　　infection and inflammation T85.735 ☑
　　　　mechanical
　　　　　breakdown T85.610 ☑
　　　　　displacement T85.620 ☑
　　　　　leakage T85.630 ☑
　　　　　malfunction T85.690 ☑
　　　　　malposition T85.620 ☑
　　　　　obstruction T85.690 ☑
　　　　　perforation T85.690 ☑
　　　　　protrusion T85.690 ☑
　　　　　specified NEC T85.690 ☑
　　　subdural infusion T85.9 ☑
　　　　embolism T85.810 ☑
　　　　fibrosis T85.820 ☑
　　　　hemorrhage T85.830 ☑
　　　　infection and inflammation T85.735 ☑
　　　　mechanical
　　　　　breakdown T85.610 ☑
　　　　　displacement T85.620 ☑
　　　　　leakage T85.630 ☑
　　　　　malfunction T85.610 ☑
　　　　　malposition T85.620 ☑
　　　　　obstruction T85.690 ☑
　　　　　perforation T85.690 ☑
　　　　　protrusion T85.690 ☑
　　　　　specified NEC T85.690 ☑
　　　　pain T85.840 ☑
　　　　specified type NEC T85.890 ☑
　　　　stenosis T85.850 ☑
　　　　thrombosis T85.860 ☑
　　urethral T83.9 ☑
　　　displacement T83.028 ☑
　　　embolism T83.81 ☑
　　　fibrosis T83.82 ☑
　　　hemorrhage T83.83 ☑
　　　indwelling
　　　　breakdown T83.011 ☑
　　　　displacement T83.021 ☑
　　　　infection and inflammation T83.511 ☑
　　　　leakage T83.031 ☑
　　　　specified complication NEC T83.091 ☑
　　　infection and inflammation T83.511 ☑
　　　leakage T83.038 ☑
　　　malposition T83.028 ☑
　　　mechanical
　　　　breakdown T83.011 ☑
　　　obstruction (mechanical) T83.091 ☑
　　　pain T83.84 ☑
　　　perforation T83.091 ☑
　　　protrusion T83.091 ☑
　　　specified type NEC T83.091 ☑
　　　stenosis T83.85 ☑
　　　thrombosis T83.86 ☑
　　urinary NEC
　　　breakdown T83.018 ☑
　　　displacement T83.028 ☑
　　　infection and inflammation T83.518 ☑
　　　leakage T83.038 ☑
　　　specified complication NEC T83.098 ☑
　cecostomy (stoma) — *see* Complications, colostomy
　cesarean delivery wound NEC O90.89
　　disruption O90.0
　　hematoma O90.2
　　infection (following delivery) O86.0
　chemotherapy (antineoplastic) NEC T88.7 ☑
　chin implant (prosthetic) — *see* Complication, pros-
　　thetic device or implant, specified NEC
　circulatory system I99.8
　　intraoperative I97.88
　　postprocedural I97.89
　　　following cardiac surgery (*see also* Infarct, my-
　　　　ocardium, associated with revasculariza-
　　　　tion procedure) I97.19- ☑
　　　　postcardiotomy syndrome I97.0
　　　hypertension I97.3
　　　lymphedema after mastectomy I97.2
　　　postcardiotomy syndrome I97.0

Complication(s) — *continued*
　circulatory system — *continued*
　　postprocedural — *continued*
　　　specified NEC I97.89
　colostomy (stoma) K94.00
　　hemorrhage K94.01
　　infection K94.02
　　malfunction K94.03
　　mechanical K94.03
　　specified complication NEC K94.09
　contraceptive device, intrauterine — *see* Complica-
　　tions, intrauterine, contraceptive device
　cord (umbilical) — *see* Complications, umbilical cord
　corneal graft — *see* Complications, graft, cornea
　coronary artery (bypass) graft T82.9 ☑
　　atherosclerosis — *see* Arteriosclerosis, coronary
　　　(artery),
　　embolism T82.818 ☑
　　fibrosis T82.828 ☑
　　hemorrhage T82.838 ☑
　　infection and inflammation T82.7 ☑
　　mechanical
　　　breakdown T82.211 ☑
　　　displacement T82.212 ☑
　　　leakage T82.213 ☑
　　　malposition T82.212 ☑
　　　obstruction T82.218 ☑
　　　perforation T82.218 ☑
　　　protrusion T82.218 ☑
　　　specified NEC T82.218 ☑
　　pain T82.848 ☑
　　specified type NEC T82.898 ☑
　　stenosis T82.858 ☑
　　thrombosis T82.868 ☑
　counterpulsation device (balloon), intra- aortic — *see*
　　Complications, balloon implant, vascular
　cystostomy (stoma) N99.518
　　catheter — *see* Complications, catheter, cystosto-
　　　my
　　hemorrhage N99.510
　　infection N99.511
　　malfunction N99.512
　　specified type NEC N99.518
　delivery (*see also* Complications, obstetric) O75.9
　　procedure (instrumental) (manual) (surgical) O75.4
　　specified NEC O75.89
　dialysis (peritoneal) (renal) (*see also* Complications,
　　infusion)
　　catheter (vascular) — *see* Complication, catheter,
　　　dialysis
　　peritoneal, intraperitoneal — *see* Complica-
　　　tions, catheter, intraperitoneal
　dorsal column (spinal) neurostimulator — *see* Compli-
　　cations, electronic stimulator device, spinal cord
　drug NEC T88.7 ☑
　ear procedure (*see also* Disorder, ear)
　　intraoperative H95.88
　　　hematoma — *see* Complications, intraopera-
　　　　tive, hemorrhage (hematoma) (of), ear
　　　hemorrhage — *see* Complications, intraopera-
　　　　tive, hemorrhage (hematoma) (of), ear
　　　laceration — *see* Complications, intraoperative,
　　　　puncture or laceration..., ear
　　　specified NEC H95.88
　　postoperative H95.89
　　　external ear canal stenosis H95.81- ☑
　　　hematoma — *see* Complications, postprocedu-
　　　　ral, hematoma (of), ear
　　　hemorrhage — *see* Complications, postproce-
　　　　dural, hemorrhage (of), ear
　　　postmastoidectomy — *see* Complications,
　　　　postmastoidectomy
　　　seroma — *see* Complications, postprocedural,
　　　　seroma (of), mastoid process
　　　specified NEC H95.89
　ectopic pregnancy O08.9
　　damage to pelvic organs O08.6
　　embolism O08.2
　　genital infection O08.0
　　hemorrhage (delayed) (excessive) O08.1
　　metabolic disorder O08.5
　　renal failure O08.4
　　shock O08.3
　　specified type NEC O08.0
　　venous complication NEC O08.7

Complication(s) — *continued*
　electronic stimulator device
　　bladder (urinary) — *see* Complications, electronic
　　　stimulator device, urinary
　　bone T84.9 ☑
　　　breakdown T84.310 ☑
　　　displacement T84.320 ☑
　　　embolism T84.81 ☑
　　　fibrosis T84.82 ☑
　　　hemorrhage T84.83 ☑
　　　infection or inflammation T84.7 ☑
　　　malfunction T84.310 ☑
　　　malposition T84.320 ☑
　　　mechanical NEC T84.390 ☑
　　　obstruction T84.390 ☑
　　　pain T84.84 ☑
　　　perforation T84.390 ☑
　　　protrusion T84.390 ☑
　　　specified type NEC T84.89 ☑
　　　stenosis T84.85 ☑
　　　thrombosis T84.86 ☑
　　brain T85.9 ☑
　　　embolism T85.810 ☑
　　　fibrosis T85.820 ☑
　　　hemorrhage T85.830 ☑
　　　infection and inflammation T85.731 ☑
　　　mechanical
　　　　breakdown T85.110 ☑
　　　　displacement T85.120 ☑
　　　　leakage T85.190 ☑
　　　　malposition T85.120 ☑
　　　　obstruction T85.190 ☑
　　　　perforation T85.190 ☑
　　　　protrusion T85.190 ☑
　　　　specified NEC T85.190 ☑
　　　pain T85.840 ☑
　　　specified type NEC T85.890 ☑
　　　stenosis T85.850 ☑
　　　thrombosis T85.860 ☑
　　cardiac (defibrillator) (pacemaker) — *see* Compli-
　　　cations, cardiovascular device or implant,
　　　electronic
　　generator (brain) (gastric) (peripheral) (sacral)
　　　(spinal)
　　　breakdown T85.113 ☑
　　　displacement T85.123 ☑
　　　leakage T85.193 ☑
　　　malposition T85.123 ☑
　　　obstruction T85.193 ☑
　　　perforation T85.193 ☑
　　　protrusion T85.193 ☑
　　　specified type NEC T85.193 ☑
　　muscle T84.9 ☑
　　　breakdown T84.418 ☑
　　　displacement T84.428 ☑
　　　embolism T84.81 ☑
　　　fibrosis T84.82 ☑
　　　hemorrhage T84.83 ☑
　　　infection or inflammation T84.7 ☑
　　　mechanical NEC T84.498 ☑
　　　pain T84.84 ☑
　　　specified type NEC T84.89 ☑
　　　stenosis T84.85 ☑
　　　thrombosis T84.86 ☑
　　nervous system T85.9 ☑
　　　brain — *see* Complications, electronic stimula-
　　　　tor device, brain
　　　cranial nerve — *see* Complications, electronic
　　　　stimulator device, peripheral nerve
　　　embolism T85.810 ☑
　　　fibrosis T85.820 ☑
　　　gastric nerve — *see* Complications, electronic
　　　　stimulator device, peripheral nerve
　　　hemorrhage T85.830 ☑
　　　infection and inflammation T85.738 ☑
　　　mechanical
　　　　breakdown T85.118 ☑
　　　　displacement T85.128 ☑
　　　　leakage T85.199 ☑
　　　　malposition T85.128 ☑
　　　　obstruction T85.199 ☑
　　　　perforation T85.199 ☑
　　　　protrusion T85.199 ☑
　　　　specified NEC T85.199 ☑
　　　pain T85.840 ☑

☑ **Additional Character Required — Refer to the Tabular List for Character Selection**　　▽ **Subterms under main terms may continue to next column or page**

Complication(s) — *continued*
 electronic stimulator device — *continued*
  nervous system — *continued*
   peripheral nerve — *see* Complications, electronic stimulator device, peripheral nerve
   sacral nerve — *see* Complications, electronic stimulator device, peripheral nerve
   specified type NEC T85.890 ☑
   spinal cord — *see* Complications, electronic stimulator device, spinal cord
   stenosis T85.850 ☑
   thrombosis T85.860 ☑
   vagal nerve — *see* Complications, electronic stimulator device, peripheral nerve
  peripheral nerve T85.9 ☑
   embolism T85.810 ☑
   fibrosis T85.820 ☑
   hemorrhage T85.830 ☑
   infection and inflammation T85.732 ☑
   mechanical
    breakdown T85.111 ☑
    displacement T85.121 ☑
    leakage T85.191 ☑
    malposition T85.121 ☑
    obstruction T85.191 ☑
    perforation T85.191 ☑
    protrusion T85.191 ☑
    specified NEC T85.191 ☑
   pain T85.840 ☑
   specified type NEC T85.890 ☑
   stenosis T85.850 ☑
   thrombosis T85.860 ☑
  spinal cord T85.9 ☑
   embolism T85.810 ☑
   fibrosis T85.820 ☑
   hemorrhage T85.830 ☑
   infection and inflammation T85.733 ☑
   mechanical
    breakdown T85.112 ☑
    displacement T85.122 ☑
    leakage T85.192 ☑
    malposition T85.122 ☑
    obstruction T85.192 ☑
    perforation T85.192 ☑
    protrusion T85.192 ☑
    specified NEC T85.192 ☑
   pain T85.840 ☑
   specified type NEC T85.890 ☑
   stenosis T85.850 ☑
   thrombosis T85.860 ☑
  urinary T83.9 ☑
   embolism T83.81 ☑
   fibrosis T83.82 ☑
   hemorrhage T83.83 ☑
   infection and inflammation T83.598 ☑
   mechanical
    breakdown T83.110 ☑
    displacement T83.120 ☑
    malposition T83.120 ☑
    perforation T83.190 ☑
    protrusion T83.190 ☑
    specified NEC T83.190 ☑
   pain T83.84 ☑
   specified type NEC T83.89 ☑
   stenosis T83.85 ☑
   thrombosis T83.86 ☑
 electroshock therapy T88.9 ☑
  specified NEC T88.8 ☑
 endocrine E34.9
  postprocedural
   adrenal hypofunction E89.6
   hypoinsulinemia E89.1
   hypoparathyroidism E89.2
   hypopituitarism E89.3
   hypothyroidism E89.0
   ovarian failure E89.40
    asymptomatic E89.40
    symptomatic E89.41
   specified NEC E89.89
   testicular hypofunction E89.5
 endodontic treatment NEC M27.59
 enterostomy (stoma) K94.10
  hemorrhage K94.11
  infection K94.12
  malfunction K94.13
  mechanical K94.13

Complication(s) — *continued*
 enterostomy — *continued*
  specified complication NEC K94.19
 episiotomy, disruption O90.1
 esophageal anti-reflux device T85.9 ☑
  embolism T85.818 ☑
  fibrosis T85.828 ☑
  hemorrhage T85.838 ☑
  infection and inflammation T85.79 ☑
  mechanical
   breakdown T85.511 ☑
   displacement T85.521 ☑
   malfunction T85.511 ☑
   malposition T85.521 ☑
   obstruction T85.591 ☑
   perforation T85.591 ☑
   protrusion T85.591 ☑
   specified NEC T85.591 ☑
  pain T85.848 ☑
  specified type NEC T85.898 ☑
  stenosis T85.858 ☑
  thrombosis T85.868 ☑
 esophagostomy K94.30
  hemorrhage K94.31
  infection K94.32
  malfunction K94.33
  mechanical K94.33
  specified complication NEC K94.39
 extracorporeal circulation T80.90 ☑
 extremity artery (bypass) graft T82.9 ☑
  arteriosclerosis — *see* Arteriosclerosis, extremities, bypass graft
  embolism T82.818 ☑
  fibrosis T82.828 ☑
  hemorrhage T82.838 ☑
  infection and inflammation T82.7 ☑
  mechanical
   breakdown T82.318 ☑
    femoral artery T82.312 ☑
   displacement T82.328 ☑
    femoral artery T82.322 ☑
   leakage T82.338 ☑
    femoral artery T82.332 ☑
   malposition T82.328 ☑
    femoral artery T82.322 ☑
   obstruction T82.398 ☑
    femoral artery T82.392 ☑
   perforation T82.398 ☑
    femoral artery T82.392 ☑
   protrusion T82.398 ☑
    femoral artery T82.392 ☑
  pain T82.848 ☑
  specified type NEC T82.898 ☑
  stenosis T82.858 ☑
  thrombosis T82.868 ☑
 eye H57.9
  corneal graft — *see* Complications, graft, cornea
  implant (prosthetic) T85.9 ☑
   embolism T85.818 ☑
   fibrosis T85.828 ☑
   hemorrhage T85.838 ☑
   infection and inflammation T85.79 ☑
   mechanical
    breakdown T85.318 ☑
    displacement T85.328 ☑
    leakage T85.398 ☑
    malposition T85.328 ☑
    obstruction T85.398 ☑
    perforation T85.398 ☑
    protrusion T85.398 ☑
    specified NEC T85.398 ☑
   pain T85.848 ☑
   specified type NEC T85.898 ☑
   stenosis T85.858 ☑
   thrombosis T85.868 ☑
  intraocular lens — *see* Complications, intraocular lens
  orbital prosthesis — *see* Complications, orbital prosthesis
 female genital N94.9
  device, implant or graft NEC — *see* Complications, genitourinary, device or implant, genital tract
 femoral artery (bypass) graft — *see* Complication, extremity artery (bypass) graft
 fixation device, internal (orthopedic) T84.9 ☑
  infection and inflammation T84.60 ☑

Complication(s) — *continued*
 fixation device, internal — *continued*
  infection and inflammation — *continued*
   arm T84.61- ☑
    humerus T84.61- ☑
    radius T84.61- ☑
    ulna T84.61- ☑
   leg T84.629 ☑
    femur T84.62- ☑
    fibula T84.62- ☑
    tibia T84.62- ☑
   specified site NEC T84.89 ☑
   spine T84.63 ☑
  mechanical
   breakdown
    limb T84.119 ☑
     carpal T84.210 ☑
     femur T84.11- ☑
     fibula T84.11- ☑
     humerus T84.11- ☑
     metacarpal T84.210 ☑
     metatarsal T84.213 ☑
     phalanx
      foot T84.213 ☑
      hand T84.210 ☑
     radius T84.11- ☑
     tarsal T84.213 ☑
     tibia T84.11- ☑
     ulna T84.11- ☑
    specified bone NEC T84.218 ☑
    spine T84.216 ☑
   displacement
    limb T84.129 ☑
     carpal T84.220 ☑
     femur T84.12- ☑
     fibula T84.12- ☑
     humerus T84.12- ☑
     metacarpal T84.220 ☑
     metatarsal T84.223 ☑
     phalanx
      foot T84.223 ☑
      hand T84.220 ☑
     radius T84.12- ☑
     tarsal T84.223 ☑
     tibia T84.12- ☑
     ulna T84.12- ☑
    specified bone NEC T84.228 ☑
    spine T84.226 ☑
   malposition — *see* Complications, fixation device, internal, mechanical, displacement
   obstruction — *see* Complications, fixation device, internal, mechanical, specified type NEC
   perforation — *see* Complications, fixation device, internal, mechanical, specified type NEC
   protrusion — *see* Complications, fixation device, internal, mechanical, specified type NEC
   specified type NEC
    limb T84.199 ☑
     carpal T84.290 ☑
     femur T84.19- ☑
     fibula T84.19- ☑
     humerus T84.19- ☑
     metacarpal T84.290 ☑
     metatarsal T84.293 ☑
     phalanx
      foot T84.293 ☑
      hand T84.290 ☑
     radius T84.19- ☑
     tarsal T84.293 ☑
     tibia T84.19- ☑
     ulna T84.19- ☑
    specified bone NEC T84.298 ☑
    vertebra T84.296 ☑
  specified type NEC T84.89 ☑
   embolism T84.81 ☑
   fibrosis T84.82 ☑
   hemorrhage T84.83 ☑
   pain T84.84 ☑
   specified complication NEC T84.89 ☑
   stenosis T84.85 ☑
   thrombosis T84.86 ☑
 following
  acute myocardial infarction NEC I23.8

Complication(s) — *continued*
  following — *continued*
    acute myocardial infarction — *continued*
      aneurysm (false) (of cardiac wall) (of heart wall) (ruptured) I23.3
      angina I23.7
      atrial
        septal defect I23.1
        thrombosis I23.6
      cardiac wall rupture I23.3
      chordae tendinae rupture I23.4
      defect
        septal
          atrial (heart) I23.1
          ventricular (heart) I23.2
      hemopericardium I23.0
      papillary muscle rupture I23.5
      rupture
        cardiac wall I23.3
          with hemopericardium I23.0
        chordae tendineae I23.4
        papillary muscle I23.5
      specified NEC I23.8
      thrombosis
        atrium I23.6
        auricular appendage I23.6
        ventricle (heart) I23.6
      ventricular
        septal defect I23.2
        thrombosis I23.6
    ectopic or molar pregnancy O08.9
      cardiac arrest O08.81
      sepsis O08.82
      specified type NEC O08.89
      urinary tract infection O08.83
    termination of pregnancy — *see* Abortion
  gastrointestinal K92.9
    bile duct prosthesis — *see* Complications, bile duct implant
    esophageal anti-reflux device — *see* Complications, esophageal anti-reflux device
    postoperative
      colostomy — *see* Complications, colostomy
      dumping syndrome K91.1
      enterostomy — *see* Complications, enterostomy
      gastrostomy — *see* Complications, gastrostomy
      malabsorption NEC K91.2
      obstruction (*see also* Obstruction, intestine, postoperative) K91.30
      postcholecystectomy syndrome K91.5
      specified NEC K91.89
      vomiting after GI surgery K91.0
    prosthetic device or implant
      bile duct prosthesis — *see* Complications, bile duct implant
      esophageal anti-reflux device — *see* Complications, esophageal anti-reflux device
      specified type NEC
        embolism T85.818 ☑
        fibrosis T85.828 ☑
        hemorrhage T85.838 ☑
        mechanical
          breakdown T85.518 ☑
          displacement T85.528 ☑
          malfunction T85.518 ☑
          malposition T85.528 ☑
          obstruction T85.598 ☑
          perforation T85.598 ☑
          protrusion T85.598 ☑
          specified NEC T85.598 ☑
        pain T85.848 ☑
        specified complication NEC T85.898 ☑
        stenosis T85.858 ☑
        thrombosis T85.868 ☑
  gastrostomy (stoma) K94.20
    hemorrhage K94.21
    infection K94.22
    malfunction K94.23
    mechanical K94.23
    specified complication NEC K94.29
  genitourinary
    device or implant T83.9 ☑
      genital tract T83.9 ☑
        infection or inflammation T83.69 ☑
        intrauterine contraceptive device — *see* Complications, intrauterine, contraceptive device

Complication(s) — *continued*
  genitourinary — *continued*
    device or implant — *continued*
      genital tract — *continued*
        mechanical — *see* Complications, by device, mechanical
        mesh — *see* Complications, mesh
        penile prosthesis — *see* Complications, prosthetic device, penile
        specified type NEC T83.89 ☑
          embolism T83.81 ☑
          fibrosis T83.82 ☑
          hemorrhage T83.83 ☑
          pain T83.84 ☑
          specified complication NEC T83.89 ☑
          stenosis T83.85 ☑
          thrombosis T83.86 ☑
        vaginal mesh — *see* Complications, mesh
      urinary system T83.9 ☑
        cystostomy catheter — *see* Complication, catheter, cystostomy
        electronic stimulator — *see* Complications, electronic stimulator device, urinary
        indwelling urethral catheter — *see* Complications, catheter, urethral, indwelling
        infection or inflammation T83.598 ☑
          indwelling urethral catheter T83.511 ☑
        kidney transplant — *see* Complication, transplant, kidney
        organ graft — *see* Complication, graft, urinary organ
        specified type NEC T83.89 ☑
          embolism T83.81 ☑
          fibrosis T83.82 ☑
          hemorrhage T83.83 ☑
          mechanical T83.198 ☑
            breakdown T83.118 ☑
            displacement T83.128 ☑
            malfunction T83.118 ☑
            malposition T83.128 ☑
            obstruction T83.198 ☑
            perforation T83.198 ☑
            protrusion T83.198 ☑
            specified NEC T83.198 ☑
          sphincter implant — *see* Complications, implant, urinary sphincter
          sphincter, implanted T83.191 ☑
          stent (ileal conduit) (nephroureteral) T83.193 ☑
          pain T83.84 ☑
          specified complication NEC T83.89 ☑
          stenosis T83.85 ☑
          thrombosis T83.86 ☑
          ureteral indwelling T83.192 ☑
    postprocedural
      pelvic peritoneal adhesions N99.4
      renal failure N99.0
      specified NEC N99.89
      stoma — *see* Complications, stoma, urinary tract
      urethral stricture — *see* Stricture, urethra, postprocedural
      vaginal
        adhesions N99.2
        vault prolapse N99.3
  graft (bypass) (patch) (*see also* Complications, prosthetic device or implant)
    aorta — *see* Complications, graft, vascular
    arterial — *see* Complication, graft, vascular
    bone T86.839
      failure T86.831
      infection T86.832
      mechanical T84.318 ☑
        breakdown T84.318 ☑
        displacement T84.328 ☑
        protrusion T84.398 ☑
        specified type NEC T84.398 ☑
      rejection T86.830
      specified type NEC T86.838
    carotid artery — *see* Complications, graft, vascular
    cornea T86.849
      failure T86.841
      infection T86.842
      mechanical T85.398 ☑
        breakdown T85.318 ☑
        displacement T85.328 ☑
        protrusion T85.398 ☑

Complication(s) — *continued*
  graft (*see also* Complications, prosthetic device or implant) — *continued*
    cornea — *continued*
      mechanical — *continued*
        specified type NEC T85.398 ☑
      rejection T86.840
      retroprosthetic membrane T85.398 ☑
      specified type NEC T86.848
    femoral artery (bypass) — *see* Complication, extremity artery (bypass) graft
    genital organ or tract — *see* Complications, genitourinary, device or implant, genital tract
    muscle T84.9 ☑
      breakdown T84.410 ☑
      displacement T84.420 ☑
      embolism T84.81 ☑
      fibrosis T84.82 ☑
      hemorrhage T84.83 ☑
      infection and inflammation T84.7 ☑
      mechanical NEC T84.490 ☑
      pain T84.84 ☑
      specified type NEC T84.89 ☑
      stenosis T84.85 ☑
      thrombosis T84.86 ☑
    nerve — *see* Complication, prosthetic device or implant, specified NEC
    skin — *see* Complications, prosthetic device or implant, skin graft
    tendon T84.9 ☑
      breakdown T84.410 ☑
      displacement T84.420 ☑
      embolism T84.81 ☑
      fibrosis T84.82 ☑
      hemorrhage T84.83 ☑
      infection and inflammation T84.7 ☑
      mechanical NEC T84.490 ☑
      pain T84.84 ☑
      specified type NEC T84.89 ☑
      stenosis T84.85 ☑
      thrombosis T84.86 ☑
    urinary organ T83.9 ☑
      embolism T83.81 ☑
      fibrosis T83.82 ☑
      hemorrhage T83.83 ☑
      infection and inflammation T83.598 ☑
        indwelling urethral catheter T83.511 ☑
      mechanical
        breakdown T83.21 ☑
        displacement T83.22 ☑
        erosion T83.24 ☑
        exposure T83.25 ☑
        leakage T83.23 ☑
        malposition T83.22 ☑
        obstruction T83.29 ☑
        perforation T83.29 ☑
        protrusion T83.29 ☑
        specified NEC T83.29 ☑
      pain T83.84 ☑
      specified type NEC T83.89 ☑
      stenosis T83.85 ☑
      thrombosis T83.86 ☑
    vascular T82.9 ☑
      embolism T82.818 ☑
      femoral artery — *see* Complication, extremity artery (bypass) graft
      fibrosis T82.828 ☑
      hemorrhage T82.838 ☑
      mechanical
        breakdown T82.319 ☑
          aorta (bifurcation) T82.310 ☑
          carotid artery T82.311 ☑
          specified vessel NEC T82.318 ☑
        displacement T82.329 ☑
          aorta (bifurcation) T82.320 ☑
          carotid artery T82.321 ☑
          specified vessel NEC T82.328 ☑
        leakage T82.339 ☑
          aorta (bifurcation) T82.330 ☑
          carotid artery T82.331 ☑
          specified vessel NEC T82.338 ☑
        malposition T82.329 ☑
          aorta (bifurcation) T82.320 ☑
          carotid artery T82.321 ☑
          specified vessel NEC T82.328 ☑
        obstruction T82.399 ☑

☑ **Additional Character Required — Refer to the Tabular List for Character Selection**   ▽ **Subterms under main terms may continue to next column or page**

Complication(s) — *continued*
graft (*see also* Complications, prosthetic device or implant) — *continued*
  vascular — *continued*
    mechanical — *continued*
      obstruction — *continued*
        aorta (bifurcation) T82.390 ☑
        carotid artery T82.391 ☑
        specified vessel NEC T82.398 ☑
      perforation T82.399
        aorta (bifurcation) T82.390 ☑
        carotid artery T82.391 ☑
        specified vessel NEC T82.398 ☑
      protrusion T82.399
        aorta (bifurcation) T82.390 ☑
        carotid artery T82.391 ☑
        specified vessel NEC T82.398 ☑
    pain T82.848 ☑
    specified complication NEC T82.898 ☑
    stenosis T82.858 ☑
    thrombosis T82.868 ☑
heart I51.9
  assist device
    infection and inflammation T82.7 ☑
  following acute myocardial infarction — *see* Complications, following, acute myocardial infarction
  postoperative — *see* Complications, circulatory system
  transplant — *see* Complication, transplant, heart and lung(s) — *see* Complications, transplant, heart, with lung
  valve
    graft (biological) T82.9 ☑
      embolism T82.817 ☑
      fibrosis T82.827 ☑
      hemorrhage T82.837 ☑
      infection and inflammation T82.7 ☑
      mechanical T82.228 ☑
        breakdown T82.221 ☑
        displacement T82.222 ☑
        leakage T82.223 ☑
        malposition T82.222 ☑
        obstruction T82.228 ☑
        perforation T82.228 ☑
        protrusion T82.228 ☑
      pain T82.847 ☑
      specified type NEC T82.897 ☑
      stenosis T82.857 ☑
      thrombosis T82.867 ☑
    prosthesis T82.9 ☑
      embolism T82.817 ☑
      fibrosis T82.827 ☑
      hemorrhage T82.837 ☑
      infection or inflammation T82.6 ☑
      mechanical T82.09 ☑
        breakdown T82.01 ☑
        displacement T82.02 ☑
        leakage T82.03 ☑
        malposition T82.02 ☑
        obstruction T82.09 ☑
        perforation T82.09 ☑
        protrusion T82.09 ☑
      pain T82.847 ☑
      specified type NEC T82.897 ☑
        mechanical T82.09 ☑
      stenosis T82.857 ☑
      thrombosis T82.867 ☑
hematoma
  intraoperative — *see* Complication, intraoperative, hemorrhage
  postprocedural — *see* Complication, postprocedural, hematoma
hemodialysis — *see* Complications, dialysis
hemorrhage
  intraoperative — *see* Complication, intraoperative, hemorrhage
  postprocedural — *see* Complication, postprocedural, hemorrhage
ileostomy (stoma) — *see* Complications, enterostomy
immunization (procedure) — *see* Complications, vaccination
implant (*see also* Complications, by site and type)
  urinary sphincter T83.9 ☑
    embolism T83.81 ☑
    fibrosis T83.82 ☑

Complication(s) — *continued*
implant (*see also* Complications, by site and type) — *continued*
  urinary sphincter — *continued*
    hemorrhage T83.83 ☑
    infection and inflammation T83.591 ☑
    mechanical
      breakdown T83.111 ☑
      displacement T83.121 ☑
      leakage T83.191 ☑
      malposition T83.121 ☑
      obstruction T83.191 ☑
      perforation T83.191 ☑
      protrusion T83.191 ☑
      specified NEC T83.191 ☑
    pain T83.84 ☑
    specified type NEC T83.89 ☑
    stenosis T83.85 ☑
    thrombosis T83.86 ☑
infusion (procedure) T80.90 ☑
  air embolism T80.0 ☑
  blood — *see* Complications, transfusion
  catheter — *see* Complications, catheter
  infection T80.29 ☑
  pump — *see* Complications, cardiovascular, device or implant
  sepsis T80.29 ☑
  serum reaction (*see also* Reaction, serum) T80.69 ☑
    anaphylactic shock (*see also* Shock, anaphylactic) T80.59 ☑
  specified type NEC T80.89 ☑
inhalation therapy NEC T81.81 ☑
injection (procedure) T80.90 ☑
  drug reaction — *see* Reaction, drug
  infection T80.29 ☑
  sepsis T80.29 ☑
  serum (prophylactic) (therapeutic) — *see* Complications, vaccination
  specified type NEC T80.89 ☑
  vaccine (any) — *see* Complications, vaccination
inoculation (any) — *see* Complications, vaccination
insulin pump
  infection and inflammation T85.72 ☑
  mechanical
    breakdown T85.614 ☑
    displacement T85.624 ☑
    leakage T85.633 ☑
    malposition T85.624 ☑
    obstruction T85.694 ☑
    perforation T85.694 ☑
    protrusion T85.694 ☑
    specified NEC T85.694 ☑
intestinal pouch NEC K91.858
intraocular lens (prosthetic) T85.9 ☑
  embolism T85.818 ☑
  fibrosis T85.828 ☑
  hemorrhage T85.838 ☑
  infection and inflammation T85.79 ☑
  mechanical
    breakdown T85.21 ☑
    displacement T85.22 ☑
    malposition T85.22 ☑
    obstruction T85.29 ☑
    perforation T85.29 ☑
    protrusion T85.29 ☑
    specified NEC T85.29 ☑
  pain T85.848 ☑
  specified type NEC T85.898 ☑
  stenosis T85.858 ☑
  thrombosis T85.868 ☑
intraoperative (intraprocedural)
  cardiac arrest (*see also* Infarct, myocardium, associated with revascularization procedure)
    during cardiac surgery I97.710
    during other surgery I97.711
  cardiac functional disturbance NEC (*see also* Infarct, myocardium, associated with revascularization procedure)
    during cardiac surgery I97.790
    during other surgery I97.791
  hemorrhage (hematoma) (of)
    circulatory system organ or structure
      during cardiac bypass I97.411
      during cardiac catheterization I97.410
      during other circulatory system procedure I97.418

Complication(s) — *continued*
intraoperative — *continued*
  hemorrhage — *continued*
    circulatory system organ or structure — *continued*
      during other procedure I97.42
    digestive system organ
      during procedure on digestive system K91.61
      during procedure on other organ K91.62
    ear
      during procedure on ear and mastoid process H95.21
      during procedure on other organ H95.22
    endocrine system organ or structure
      during procedure on endocrine system organ or structure E36.01
      during procedure on other organ E36.02
    eye and adnexa
      during ophthalmic procedure H59.11- ☑
      during other procedure H59.12- ☑
    genitourinary organ or structure
      during procedure on genitourinary organ or structure N99.61
      during procedure on other organ N99.62
    mastoid process
      during procedure on ear and mastoid process H95.21
      during procedure on other organ H95.22
    musculoskeletal structure
      during musculoskeletal surgery M96.810
      during non-orthopedic surgery M96.811
      during orthopedic surgery M96.810
    nervous system
      during a nervous system procedure G97.31
      during other procedure G97.32
    respiratory system
      during other procedure J95.62
      during procedure on respiratory system organ or structure J95.61
    skin and subcutaneous tissue
      during a dermatologic procedure L76.01
      during a procedure on other organ L76.02
    spleen
      during a procedure on other organ D78.02
      during a procedure on the spleen D78.01
  puncture or laceration (accidental) (unintentional) (of)
    brain
      during a nervous system procedure G97.48
      during other procedure G97.49
    circulatory system organ or structure
      during circulatory system procedure I97.51
      during other procedure I97.52
    digestive system
      during procedure on digestive system K91.71
      during procedure on other organ K91.72
    ear
      during procedure on ear and mastoid process H95.31
      during procedure on other organ H95.32
    endocrine system organ or structure
      during procedure on endocrine system organ or structure E36.11
      during procedure on other organ E36.12
    eye and adnexa
      during ophthalmic procedure H59.21- ☑
      during other procedure H59.22- ☑
    genitourinary organ or structure
      during procedure on genitourinary organ or structure N99.71
      during procedure on other organ N99.72
    mastoid process
      during procedure on ear and mastoid process H95.31
      during procedure on other organ H95.32
    musculoskeletal structure
      during musculoskeletal surgery M96.820
      during non-orthopedic surgery M96.821
      during orthopedic surgery M96.820
    nervous system
      during a nervous system procedure G97.48
      during other procedure G97.49
    respiratory system
      during other procedure J95.72
      during procedure on respiratory system organ or structure J95.71

Complication(s) — *continued*
  intraoperative — *continued*
    puncture or laceration — *continued*
      skin and subcutaneous tissue
        during a dermatologic procedure L76.11
        during a procedure on other organ L76.12
      spleen
        during a procedure on other organ D78.12
        during a procedure on the spleen D78.11
    specified NEC
      circulatory system I97.88
      digestive system K91.81
      ear H95.88
      endocrine system E36.8
      eye and adnexa H59.88
      genitourinary system N99.81
      mastoid process H95.88
      musculoskeletal structure M96.89
      nervous system G97.81
      respiratory system J95.88
      skin and subcutaneous tissue L76.81
      spleen D78.81
  intraperitoneal catheter (dialysis) (infusion) — *see* Complications, catheter, intraperitoneal
  intrathecal infusion pump
    infection and inflammation T85.738 ☑
    mechanical
      breakdown T85.615 ☑
      displacement T85.625 ☑
      leakage T85.635 ☑
      malfunction T85.695 ☑
      malposition T85.625 ☑
      obstruction T85.695 ☑
      perforation T85.695 ☑
      protrusion T85.695 ☑
      specified NEC T85.695 ☑
  intrauterine
    contraceptive device
      embolism T83.81 ☑
      fibrosis T83.82 ☑
      hemorrhage T83.83 ☑
      infection and inflammation T83.69 ☑
      mechanical
        breakdown T83.31 ☑
        displacement T83.32 ☑
        malposition T83.32 ☑
        obstruction T83.39 ☑
        perforation T83.39 ☑
        protrusion T83.39 ☑
        specified NEC T83.39 ☑
      pain T83.84 ☑
      specified type NEC T83.89 ☑
      stenosis T83.85 ☑
      thrombosis T83.86 ☑
    procedure (fetal), to newborn P96.5
  jejunostomy (stoma) — *see* Complications, enterostomy
  joint prosthesis, internal T84.9 ☑
    breakage (fracture) T84.01- ☑
    dislocation T84.02- ☑
    fracture T84.01- ☑
    infection or inflammation T84.50 ☑
      hip T84.5- ☑
      knee T84.5- ☑
      specified joint NEC T84.59 ☑
    instability T84.02- ☑
    malposition — *see* Complications, joint prosthesis, mechanical, displacement
    mechanical
      breakage, broken T84.01- ☑
      dislocation T84.02- ☑
      fracture T84.01- ☑
      instability T84.02- ☑
      leakage — *see* Complications, joint prosthesis, mechanical, specified NEC
      loosening T84.039 ☑
        hip T84.03- ☑
        knee T84.03- ☑
        specified joint NEC T84.038 ☑
      obstruction — *see* Complications, joint prosthesis, mechanical, specified NEC
      perforation — *see* Complications, joint prosthesis, mechanical, specified NEC
        osteolysis T84.059 ☑
          hip T84.05- ☑
          knee T84.05- ☑
          other specified joint T84.058 ☑

Complication(s) — *continued*
  joint prosthesis, internal — *continued*
    mechanical — *continued*
      protrusion — *see* Complications, joint prosthesis, mechanical, specified NEC
      specified complication NEC T84.099 ☑
        hip T84.09- ☑
        knee T84.09- ☑
        other specified joint T84.098 ☑
      subluxation T84.02- ☑
      wear of articular bearing surface T84.069 ☑
        hip T84.06- ☑
        knee T84.06- ☑
        other specified joint T84.068 ☑
      specified joint NEC T84.89 ☑
        embolism T84.81 ☑
        fibrosis T84.82 ☑
        hemorrhage T84.83 ☑
        pain T84.84 ☑
        specified complication NEC T84.89 ☑
        stenosis T84.85 ☑
        thrombosis T84.86 ☑
      subluxation T84.02- ☑
  kidney transplant — *see* Complications, transplant, kidney
  labor O75.9
    specified NEC O75.89
  liver transplant (immune or nonimmune) — *see* Complications, transplant, liver
  lumbar puncture G97.1
    cerebrospinal fluid leak G97.0
    headache or reaction G97.1
  lung transplant — *see* Complications, transplant, lung
    and heart — *see* Complications, transplant, lung, with heart
  male genital N50.9
    device, implant or graft — *see* Complications, genitourinary, device or implant, genital tract
    postprocedural or postoperative — *see* Complications, genitourinary, postprocedural
    specified NEC N99.89
  mastoid (process) procedure
    intraoperative H95.88
      hematoma — *see* Complications, intraoperative, hemorrhage (hematoma) (of), mastoid process
      hemorrhage — *see* Complications, intraoperative, hemorrhage (hematoma) (of), mastoid process
      laceration — *see* Complications, intraoperative, puncture or laceration, mastoid process
      specified NEC H95.88
    postmastoidectomy — *see* Complications, postmastoidectomy
    postoperative H95.89
      external ear canal stenosis H95.81 ☑
      hematoma — *see* Complications, postprocedural, hematoma (of), mastoid process
      hemorrhage — *see* Complications, postprocedural, hemorrhage (of), mastoid process
      postmastoidectomy — *see* Complications, postmastoidectomy
      seroma — *see* Complications, postprocedural, seroma (of), mastoid process
      specified NEC H95.89
  mastoidectomy cavity — *see* Complications, postmastoidectomy
  mechanical — *see* Complications, by site and type, mechanical
  medical procedures (*see also* Complication(s), intraoperative) T88.9 ☑
  metabolic E88.9
    postoperative E89.89
      specified NEC E89.89
  molar pregnancy NOS O08.9
    damage to pelvic organs O08.6
    embolism O08.2
    genital infection O08.0
    hemorrhage (delayed) (excessive) O08.1
    metabolic disorder O08.5
    renal failure O08.4
    shock O08.3
    specified type NEC O08.0
    venous complication NEC O08.7

Complication(s) — *continued*
  musculoskeletal system (*see also* Complication, intraoperative (intraprocedural), by site)
    device, implant or graft NEC — *see* Complications, orthopedic, device or implant
      internal fixation (nail) (plate) (rod) — *see* Complications, fixation device, internal
      joint prosthesis — *see* Complications, joint prosthesis
    post radiation M96.89
      kyphosis M96.2
      scoliosis M96.5
      specified complication NEC M96.89
    postoperative (postprocedural) M96.89
      with osteoporosis — *see* Osteoporosis
      fracture following insertion of device — *see* Fracture, following insertion of orthopedic implant, joint prosthesis or bone plate
      joint instability after prosthesis removal M96.89
      lordosis M96.4
      postlaminectomy syndrome NEC M96.1
        kyphosis M96.3
      pseudarthrosis M96.0
      specified complication NEC M96.89
  nephrostomy (stoma) — *see* Complications, stoma, urinary tract, external NEC
  nervous system G98.8
    central G96.9
    device, implant or graft (*see also* Complication, prosthetic device or implant, specified NEC)
      electronic stimulator (electrode(s)) — *see* Complications, electronic stimulator device
      specified NEC
        infection and inflammation T85.738 ☑
        mechanical T85.695 ☑
          breakdown T85.615 ☑
          displacement T85.625 ☑
          leakage T85.635 ☑
          malfunction T85.695 ☑
          malposition T85.625 ☑
          obstruction T85.695 ☑
          perforation T85.695 ☑
          protrusion T85.695 ☑
          specified NEC T85.695 ☑
      ventricular shunt — *see* Complications, ventricular shunt
    electronic stimulator (electrode(s)) — *see* Complications, electronic stimulator device
    postprocedural G97.82
      intracranial hypotension G97.2
      specified NEC G97.82
      spinal fluid leak G97.0
  newborn, due to intrauterine (fetal) procedure P96.5
  nonabsorbable (permanent) sutures — *see* Complication, sutures, permanent
  obstetric O75.9
    procedure (instrumental) (manual) (surgical)
      specified NEC O75.4
    specified NEC O75.89
    surgical wound NEC O90.89
      hematoma O90.2
      infection O86.0
  ocular lens implant — *see* Complications, intraocular lens
  ophthalmologic
    postprocedural bleb — *see* Blebitis
  orbital prosthesis T85.9 ☑
    embolism T85.818 ☑
    fibrosis T85.828 ☑
    hemorrhage T85.838 ☑
    infection and inflammation T85.79 ☑
    mechanical
      breakdown T85.31- ☑
      displacement T85.32- ☑
      malposition T85.32- ☑
      obstruction T85.39- ☑
      perforation T85.39- ☑
      protrusion T85.39- ☑
      specified NEC T85.39- ☑
    pain T85.848 ☑
    specified type NEC T85.898 ☑
    stenosis T85.858 ☑
    thrombosis T85.868 ☑
  organ or tissue transplant (partial) (total) — *see* Complications, transplant

Complication(s) — *continued*

orthopedic (*see also* Disorder, soft tissue)

device or implant T84.9 ☑
bone
device or implant — *see* Complication, bone, device NEC
graft — *see* Complication, graft, bone
breakdown T84.418 ☑
displacement T84.428 ☑
electronic bone stimulator — *see* Complications, electronic stimulator device, bone
embolism T84.81 ☑
fibrosis T84.82 ☑
fixation device — *see* Complication, fixation device, internal
hemorrhage T84.83 ☑
infection or inflammation T84.7 ☑
joint prosthesis — *see* Complication, joint prosthesis, internal
malfunction T84.418 ☑
malposition T84.428 ☑
mechanical NEC T84.498 ☑
muscle graft — *see* Complications, graft, muscle
obstruction T84.498 ☑
pain T84.84 ☑
perforation T84.498 ☑
protrusion T84.498 ☑
specified complication NEC T84.89 ☑
stenosis T84.85 ☑
tendon graft — *see* Complications, graft, tendon
thrombosis T84.86 ☑
fracture (following insertion of device) — *see* Fracture, following insertion of orthopedic implant, joint prosthesis or bone plate
postprocedural M96.89
fracture — *see* Fracture, following insertion of orthopedic implant, joint prosthesis or bone plate
postlaminectomy syndrome NEC M96.1
kyphosis M96.3
lordosis M96.4
postradiation
kyphosis M96.2
scoliosis M96.5
pseudarthrosis post-fusion M96.0
specified type NEC M96.89
pacemaker (cardiac) — *see* Complications, cardiovascular device or implant, electronic
pancreas transplant — *see* Complications, transplant, pancreas
penile prosthesis (implant) — *see* Complications, prosthetic device, penile
perfusion NEC T80.90 ☑
perineal repair (obstetrical) NEC O90.89
disruption O90.1
hematoma O90.2
infection (following delivery) O86.0
phototherapy T88.9 ☑
specified NEC T88.8 ☑
postmastoidectomy NEC H95.19- ☑
cyst, mucosal H95.13- ☑
granulation H95.12- ☑
inflammation, chronic H95.11- ☑
recurrent cholesteatoma H95.0- ☑
postoperative — *see* Complications, postprocedural
circulatory — *see* Complications, circulatory system
ear — *see* Complications, ear
endocrine — *see* Complications, endocrine
eye — *see* Complications, eye
lumbar puncture G97.1
cerebrospinal fluid leak G97.0
nervous system (central) (peripheral) — *see* Complications, nervous system
respiratory system — *see* Complications, respiratory system
postprocedural (*see also* Complications, surgical procedure)
cardiac arrest (*see also* Infarct, myocardium, associated with revascularization procedure)
following cardiac surgery I97.120
following other surgery I97.121
cardiac functional disturbance NEC (*see also* Infarct, myocardium, associated with revascularization procedure)
following cardiac surgery I97.190

Complication(s) — *continued*

postprocedural (*see also* Complications, surgical procedure) — *continued*
cardiac functional disturbance (*see also* Infarct, myocardium, associated with revascularization procedure) — *continued*
following other surgery I97.191
cardiac insufficiency
following cardiac surgery I97.110
following other surgery I97.111
chorioretinal scars following retinal surgery H59.81- ☑
following cataract surgery
cataract (lens) fragments H59.02- ☑
cystoid macular edema H59.03- ☑
specified NEC H59.09- ☑
vitreous (touch) syndrome H59.01- ☑
heart failure
following cardiac surgery I97.130
following other surgery I97.131
hematoma (of)
circulatory system organ or structure
following cardiac bypass I97.631
following cardiac catheterization I97.630
following other circulatory system procedure I97.638
following other procedure I97.621
digestive system
following procedure on digestive system K91.870
following procedure on other organ K91.871
ear
following other procedure H95.52
following procedure on ear and mastoid process H95.51
endocrine system
following endocrine system procedure E89.820
following other procedure E89.821
eye and adnexa
following ophthalmic procedure H59.33- ☑
following other procedure H59.34- ☑
genitourinary organ or structure
following procedure on genitourinary organ or structure N99.840
following procedure on other organ N99.841
mastoid process
following other procedure H95.52
following procedure on ear and mastoid process H95.51
musculoskeletal structure
following musculoskeletal surgery M96.840
following non-orthopedic surgery M96.841
following orthopedic surgery M96.840
nervous system
following nervous system procedure G97.61
following other procedure G97.62
respiratory system
following other procedure J95.861
following procedure on respiratory system organ or structure J95.860
skin and subcutaneous tissue
following dermatologic procedure L76.31
following procedure on other organ L76.32
spleen
following procedure on other organ D78.32
following procedure on the spleen D78.31
hemorrhage (of)
circulatory system organ or structure
following cardiac bypass I97.611
following cardiac catheterization I97.610
following other circulatory system procedure I97.618
following other procedure I97.620
digestive system
following procedure on digestive system K91.840
following procedure on other organ K91.841
ear
following other procedure H95.42
following procedure on ear and mastoid process H95.41
endocrine system
following endocrine system procedure E89.810
following other procedure E89.811

Complication(s) — *continued*

postprocedural (*see also* Complications, surgical procedure) — *continued*
hemorrhage — *continued*
eye and adnexa
following ophthalmic procedure H59.31- ☑
following other procedure H59.32- ☑
genitourinary organ or structure
following procedure on genitourinary organ or structure N99.820
following procedure on other organ N99.821
mastoid process
following other procedure H95.42
following procedure on ear and mastoid process H95.41
musculoskeletal structure
following musculoskeletal surgery M96.830
following non-orthopedic surgery M96.831
following orthopedic surgery M96.830
nervous system
following nervous system procedure G97.51
following other procedure G97.52
respiratory system
following a respiratory system procedure J95.830
following other procedure J95.831
skin and subcutaneous tissue
following a procedure on other organ L76.22
following dermatologic procedure L76.21
spleen
following procedure on other organ D78.22
following procedure on the spleen D78.21
seroma (of)
circulatory system organ or structure
following cardiac bypass I97.641
following cardiac catheterization I97.640
following other circulatory system procedure I97.648
following other procedure I97.622
digestive system
following procedure on digestive system K91.872
following procedure on other organ K91.873
ear
following other procedure H95.54
following procedure on ear and mastoid process H95.53
endocrine system
following endocrine system procedure E89.822
following other procedure E89.823
eye and adnexa
following ophthalmic procedure H59.35- ☑
following other procedure H59.36- ☑
genitourinary organ or structure
following procedure on genitourinary organ or structure N99.842
following procedure on other organ N99.843
mastoid process
following other procedure H95.54
following procedure on ear and mastoid process H95.53
musculoskeletal structure
following musculoskeletal surgery M96.842
following non-orthopedic surgery M96.843
following orthopedic surgery M96.842
nervous system
following nervous system procedure G97.63
following other procedure G97.64
respiratory system
following other procedure J95.863
following procedure on respiratory system organ or structure J95.862
skin and subcutaneous tissue
following dermatologic procedure L76.33
following procedure on other organ L76.34
spleen
following procedure on other organ D78.34
following procedure on the spleen D78.33
specified NEC
circulatory system I97.89
digestive K91.89
ear H95.89
endocrine E89.89
eye and adnexa H59.89
genitourinary N99.89

Complication(s) — *continued*
  postprocedural (*see also* Complications, surgical procedure) — *continued*
    specified — *continued*
      mastoid process H95.89
      metabolic E89.89
      musculoskeletal structure M96.89
      nervous system G97.82
      respiratory system J95.89
      skin and subcutaneous tissue L76.82
      spleen D78.89
  pregnancy NEC — *see* Pregnancy, complicated by
  prosthetic device or implant T85.9 ☑
    bile duct — *see* Complications, bile duct implant
    breast — *see* Complications, breast implant
    bulking agent
      ureteral
        erosion T83.714 ☑
        exposure T83.724 ☑
      urethral
        erosion T83.713 ☑
        exposure T83.723 ☑
    cardiac and vascular NEC — *see* Complications, cardiovascular device or implant
    corneal transplant — *see* Complications, graft, cornea
    electronic nervous system stimulator — *see* Complications, electronic stimulator device
    epidural infusion catheter — *see* Complications, catheter, epidural
    esophageal anti-reflux device — *see* Complications, esophageal anti-reflux device
    genital organ or tract — *see* Complications, genitourinary, device or implant, genital tract
      specified NEC T83.79-
    heart valve — *see* Complications, heart, valve, prosthesis
    infection or inflammation T85.79 ☑
      intestine transplant T86.892
      liver transplant T86.43
      lung transplant T86.812
      pancreas transplant T86.892
      skin graft T86.822
    intraocular lens — *see* Complications, intraocular lens
    intraperitoneal (dialysis) catheter — *see* Complications, catheter, intraperitoneal
    joint — *see* Complications, joint prosthesis, internal
    mechanical NEC T85.698 ☑
      dialysis catheter (vascular) (*see also* Complication, catheter, dialysis, mechanical)
        peritoneal — *see* Complication, catheter, intraperitoneal, mechanical
      gastrointestinal device T85.598 ☑
      ocular device T85.398 ☑
      subdural (infusion) catheter T85.690 ☑
      suture, permanent T85.692 ☑
        that for bone repair — *see* Complications, fixation device, internal (orthopedic), mechanical
      ventricular shunt
        breakdown T85.01 ☑
        displacement T85.02 ☑
        leakage T85.03 ☑
        malposition T85.02 ☑
        obstruction T85.09 ☑
        perforation T85.09 ☑
        protrusion T85.09 ☑
        specified NEC T85.09 ☑
    mesh
      erosion (to surrounding organ or tissue) T83.718 ☑
        urethral (into pelvic floor muscles) T83.712 ☑
        vaginal (into pelvic floor muscles) T83.711 ☑
      exposure (into surrounding organ or tissue) T83.728 ☑
        urethral (through urethral wall) T83.722 ☑
        vaginal (into vagina) (through vaginal wall) T83.721 ☑
    orbital — *see* Complications, orbital prosthesis
    penile T83.9 ☑
      embolism T83.81 ☑
      fibrosis T83.82 ☑
      hemorrhage T83.83 ☑
      infection and inflammation T83.61 ☑

Complication(s) — *continued*
  prosthetic device or implant — *continued*
    penile — *continued*
      mechanical
        breakdown T83.410 ☑
        displacement T83.420 ☑
        leakage T83.490 ☑
        malposition T83.420 ☑
        obstruction T83.490 ☑
        perforation T83.490 ☑
        protrusion T83.490 ☑
        specified NEC T83.490 ☑
      pain T83.84 ☑
      specified type NEC T83.89 ☑
      stenosis T83.85 ☑
      thrombosis T83.86 ☑
    prosthetic materials NEC
      erosion (to surrounding organ or tissue) T83.718 ☑
      exposure (into surrounding organ or tissue) T83.728 ☑
    skin graft T86.829
      artificial skin or decellularized allodermis
        embolism T85.818 ☑
        fibrosis T85.828 ☑
        hemorrhage T85.838 ☑
        infection and inflammation T85.79 ☑
        mechanical
          breakdown T85.613 ☑
          displacement T85.623 ☑
          malfunction T85.613 ☑
          malposition T85.623 ☑
          obstruction T85.693 ☑
          perforation T85.693 ☑
          protrusion T85.693 ☑
          specified NEC T85.693 ☑
        pain T85.848 ☑
        specified type NEC T85.898 ☑
        stenosis T85.858 ☑
        thrombosis T85.868 ☑
      failure T86.821
      infection T86.822
      rejection T86.820
      specified NEC T86.828
    sling
      urethral (female) (male)
        erosion T83.712 ☑
        exposure T83.722 ☑
    specified NEC T85.9 ☑
      embolism T85.818 ☑
      fibrosis T85.828 ☑
      hemorrhage T85.838 ☑
      infection and inflammation T85.79 ☑
      mechanical
        breakdown T85.618 ☑
        displacement T85.628 ☑
        leakage T85.638 ☑
        malfunction T85.618 ☑
        malposition T85.628 ☑
        obstruction T85.698 ☑
        perforation T85.698 ☑
        protrusion T85.698 ☑
        specified NEC T85.698 ☑
      pain T85.848 ☑
      specified type NEC T85.898 ☑
      stenosis T85.858 ☑
      thrombosis T85.868 ☑
    subdural infusion catheter — *see* Complications, catheter, subdural
    sutures — *see* Complications, sutures
    urinary organ or tract NEC — *see* Complications, genitourinary, device or implant, urinary system
    vascular — *see* Complications, cardiovascular device or implant
    ventricular shunt — *see* Complications, ventricular shunt (device)
  puerperium — *see* Puerperal
  puncture, spinal G97.1
    cerebrospinal fluid leak G97.0
    headache or reaction G97.1
  pyelogram N99.89
  radiation
    kyphosis M96.2
    scoliosis M96.5

Complication(s) — *continued*
  reattached
    extremity (infection) (rejection)
      lower T87.1X- ☑
      upper T87.0X- ☑
    specified body part NEC T87.2
  reconstructed breast
    asymmetry between native and reconstructed breast N65.1
    deformity N65.0
    disproportion between native and reconstructed breast N65.1
    excess tissue N65.0
    misshappen N65.0
  reimplant NEC (*see also* Complications, prosthetic device or implant)
    limb (infection) (rejection) — *see* Complications, reattached, extremity
    organ (partial) (total) — *see* Complications, transplant
    prosthetic device NEC — *see* Complications, prosthetic device
  renal N28.9
    allograft — *see* Complications, transplant, kidney
    dialysis — *see* Complications, dialysis
  respirator
    mechanical J95.850
      specified NEC J95.859
  respiratory system J98.9
    device, implant or graft — *see* Complication, prosthetic device or implant, specified NEC
    lung transplant — *see* Complications, prosthetic device or implant, lung transplant
    postoperative J95.89
      air leak J95.812
      Mendelson's syndrome (chemical pneumonitis) J95.4
      pneumothorax J95.811
      pulmonary insufficiency (acute) (after nonthoracic surgery) J95.2
        chronic J95.3
        following thoracic surgery J95.1
      respiratory failure (acute) J95.821
        acute and chronic J95.822
      specified NEC J95.89
      subglottic stenosis J95.5
      tracheostomy complication — *see* Complications, tracheostomy
    therapy T81.89 ☑
  sedation during labor and delivery O74.9
    cardiac O74.2
    central nervous system O74.3
    pulmonary NEC O74.1
  shunt (*see also* Complications, prosthetic device or implant)
    arteriovenous — *see* Complications, arteriovenous, shunt
    ventricular (communicating) — *see* Complications, ventricular shunt
  skin
    graft T86.829
      failure T86.821
      infection T86.822
      rejection T86.820
      specified type NEC T86.828
  spinal
    anesthesia — *see* Complications, anesthesia, spinal
    catheter (epidural) (subdural) — *see* Complications, catheter
    puncture or tap G97.1
      cerebrospinal fluid leak G97.0
      headache or reaction G97.1
  stent
    bile duct — *see* Complications, bile duct prosthesis
    ureteral indwelling
      breakdown T83.112 ☑
      displacement T83.122 ☑
      leakage T83.192 ☑
      malposition T83.122 ☑
      obstruction T83.192 ☑
      perforation T83.192 ☑
      protrusion T83.192 ☑
      specified NEC T83.192 ☑
    urinary NEC (ileal conduit) (nephroureteral) T83.193 ☑
      embolism T83.81 ☑
      fibrosis T83.82 ☑
      hemorrhage T83.83 ☑

  ☑ **Additional Character Required — Refer to the Tabular List for Character Selection**   ▽ Subterms under main terms may continue to next column or page

Complication(s) — *continued*
  stent — *continued*
    urinary — *continued*
      infection and inflammation T83.593 ☑
      mechanical
        breakdown T83.113 ☑
        displacement T83.123 ☑
        leakage T83.193 ☑
        malposition T83.123 ☑
        obstruction T83.193 ☑
        perforation T83.193 ☑
        protrusion T83.193 ☑
        specified type NEC T83.193 ☑
      pain T83.84 ☑
      specified type NEC T83.89 ☑
      stenosis T83.85 ☑
      thrombosis T83.86 ☑
    vascular
      end stent stenosis — *see* Restenosis, stent
      in stent stenosis — *see* Restenosis, stent
  stoma
    digestive tract
      colostomy — *see* Complications, colostomy
      enterostomy — *see* Complications, enterostomy
      esophagostomy — *see* Complications, esophagostomy
      gastrostomy — *see* Complications, gastrostomy
    urinary tract N99.528
      continent N99.538
        hemorrhage N99.530
        herniation N99.533
        infection N99.531
        malfunction N99.532
        specified type NEC N99.538
        stenosis N99.534
      cystostomy — *see* Complications, cystostomy
      external NOS N99.528
      hemorrhage N99.520
      herniation N99.523
      incontinent N99.528
        hemorrhage N99.520
        herniation N99.523
        infection N99.521
        malfunction N99.522
        specified type NEC N99.528
        stenosis N99.524
      infection N99.521
      malfunction N99.522
      specified type NEC N99.528
      stenosis N99.524
  stomach banding — *see* Complication(s), bariatric procedure
  stomach stapling — *see* Complication(s), bariatric procedure
  surgical material, nonabsorbable — *see* Complication, suture, permanent
  surgical procedure (on) T81.9 ☑
    amputation stump (late) — *see* Complications, amputation stump
    cardiac — *see* Complications, circulatory system
    cholesteatoma, recurrent — *see* Complications, postmastoidectomy, recurrent cholesteatoma
    circulatory (early) — *see* Complications, circulatory system
    digestive system — *see* Complications, gastrointestinal
    dumping syndrome (postgastrectomy) K91.1
    ear — *see* Complications, ear
    elephantiasis or lymphedema I97.89
      postmastectomy I97.2
    emphysema (surgical) T81.82 ☑
    endocrine — *see* Complications, endocrine
    eye — *see* Complications, eye
    fistula (persistent postoperative) T81.83 ☑
    foreign body inadvertently left in wound (sponge) (suture) (swab) — *see* Foreign body, accidentally left during a procedure
    gastrointestinal — *see* Complications, gastrointestinal
    genitourinary NEC N99.89
    hematoma
      intraoperative — *see* Complication, intraoperative, hemorrhage
      postprocedural — *see* Complication, postprocedural, hematoma

Complication(s) — *continued*
  surgical procedure — *continued*
    hemorrhage
      intraoperative — *see* Complication, intraoperative, hemorrhage
      postprocedural — *see* Complication, postprocedural, hemorrhage
    hepatic failure K91.82
    hyperglycemia (postpancreatectomy) E89.1
    hypoinsulinemia (postpancreatectomy) E89.1
    hypoparathyroidism (postparathyroidectomy) E89.2
    hypopituitarism (posthypophysectomy) E89.3
    hypothyroidism (post-thyroidectomy) E89.0
    intestinal obstruction (*see also* Obstruction, intestine, postoperative) K91.30
    intracranial hypotension following ventricular shunting (ventriculostomy) G97.2
    lymphedema I97.89
      postmastectomy I97.2
    malabsorption (postsurgical) NEC K91.2
      osteoporosis — *see* Osteoporosis, postsurgical malabsorption
    mastoidectomy cavity NEC — *see* Complications, postmastoidectomy
    metabolic E89.89
      specified NEC E89.89
    musculoskeletal — *see* Complications, musculoskeletal system
    nervous system (central) (peripheral) — *see* Complications, nervous system
    ovarian failure E89.40
      asymptomatic E89.40
      symptomatic E89.41
    peripheral vascular — *see* Complications, surgical procedure, vascular
    postcardiotomy syndrome I97.0
    postcholecystectomy syndrome K91.5
    postcommissurotomy syndrome I97.0
    postgastrectomy dumping syndrome K91.1
    postlaminectomy syndrome NEC M96.1
      kyphosis M96.3
    postmastectomy lymphedema syndrome I97.2
    postmastoidectomy cholesteatoma — *see* Complications, postmastoidectomy, recurrent cholesteatoma
    postvagotomy syndrome K91.1
    postvalvulotomy syndrome I97.0
    pulmonary insufficiency (acute) J95.2
      chronic J95.3
      following thoracic surgery J95.1
    reattached body part — *see* Complications, reattached
    respiratory — *see* Complications, respiratory system
    shock (hypovolemic) T81.19 ☑
    spleen (postoperative) D78.89
      intraoperative D78.81
    stitch abscess T81.4 ☑
    subglottic stenosis (postsurgical) J95.5
    testicular hypofunction E89.5
    transplant — *see* Complications, organ or tissue transplant
    urinary NEC N99.89
    vaginal vault prolapse (posthysterectomy) N99.3
    vascular (peripheral)
      artery T81.719 ☑
        mesenteric T81.710 ☑
        renal T81.711 ☑
        specified NEC T81.718 ☑
      vein T81.72 ☑
    wound infection T81.4 ☑
  suture, permanent (wire) NEC T85.9 ☑
    with repair of bone — *see* Complications, fixation device, internal
    embolism T85.818 ☑
    fibrosis T85.828 ☑
    hemorrhage T85.838 ☑
    infection and inflammation T85.79 ☑
    mechanical
      breakdown T85.612 ☑
      displacement T85.622 ☑
      malfunction T85.612 ☑
      malposition T85.622 ☑
      obstruction T85.692 ☑
      perforation T85.692 ☑
      protrusion T85.692 ☑

Complication(s) — *continued*
  suture, permanent — *continued*
    mechanical — *continued*
      specified NEC T85.692 ☑
    pain T85.848 ☑
    specified type NEC T85.898 ☑
    stenosis T85.858 ☑
    thrombosis T85.868 ☑
  tracheostomy J95.00
    granuloma J95.09
    hemorrhage J95.01
    infection J95.02
    malfunction J95.03
    mechanical J95.03
    obstruction J95.03
    specified type NEC J95.09
    tracheo-esophageal fistula J95.04
  transfusion (blood) (lymphocytes) (plasma) T80.92 ☑
    air embolism T80.0 ☑
    circulatory overload E87.71
    febrile nonhemolytic transfusion reaction R50.84
    hemochromatosis E83.111
    hemolysis T80.89 ☑
    hemolytic reaction (antigen unspecified) T80.919 ☑
    incompatibility reaction (antigen unspecified) T80.919 ☑
      ABO T80.30 ☑
        delayed serologic (DSTR) T80.39 ☑
        hemolytic transfusion reaction (HTR) (unspecified time after transfusion) T80.319 ☑
          acute (AHTR) (less than 24 hours after transfusion) T80.310 ☑
          delayed (DHTR) (24 hours or more after transfusion) T80.311 ☑
        specified NEC T80.39 ☑
      acute (antigen unspecified) T80.910 ☑
      delayed (antigen unspecified) T80.911 ☑
      delayed serologic (DSTR) T80.89 ☑
      non-ABO (minor antigens (Duffy) (Kell) (Kidd) (Lewis) (M) (N) (P) (S)) T80.A0 ☑ (*following* T80.4)
        delayed serologic (DSTR) T80.A9 ☑ (*following* T80.4)
        hemolytic transfusion reaction (HTR) (unspecified time after transfusion) T80.A19 ☑ (*following* T80.4)
          acute (AHTR) (less than 24 hours after transfusion) T80.A10 ☑ (*following* T80.4)
          delayed (DHTR) (24 hours or more after transfusion) T80.A11 ☑ (*following* T80.4)
        specified NEC T80.A9 ☑ (*following* T80.4)
      Rh (antigens (C) (c) (D) (E) (e)) (factor) T80.40 ☑
        delayed serologic (DSTR) T80.49 ☑
        hemolytic transfusion reaction (HTR) (unspecified time after transfusion) T80.419 ☑
          acute (AHTR) (less than 24 hours after transfusion) T80.410 ☑
          delayed (DHTR) (24 hours or more after transfusion) T80.411 ☑
        specified NEC T80.49 ☑
    infection T80.29 ☑
      acute T80.22- ☑
    reaction NEC T80.89 ☑
    sepsis T80.29 ☑
    shock T80.89 ☑
  transplant T86.90
    bone T86.839
      failure T86.831
      infection T86.832
      rejection T86.830
      specified type NEC T86.838
    bone marrow T86.00
      failure T86.02
      infection T86.03
      rejection T86.01
      specified type NEC T86.09
    cornea T86.849
      failure T86.841
      infection T86.842
      rejection T86.840
      specified type NEC T86.848
    failure T86.92

▽ Subterms under main terms may continue to next column or page   ☑ Additional Character Required — Refer to the Tabular List for Character Selection   67

Complication — Complication

Complication(s) — *continued*
  transplant — *continued*
    heart T86.20
      with lung T86.30
        cardiac allograft vasculopathy T86.290
          failure T86.32
          infection T86.33
          rejection T86.31
          specified type NEC T86.39
        failure T86.22
        infection T86.23
        rejection T86.21
        specified type NEC T86.298
      infection T86.93
      intestine T86.859
        failure T86.851
        infection T86.852
        rejection T86.850
        specified type NEC T86.858
      kidney T86.10
        failure T86.12
        infection T86.13
        rejection T86.11
        specified type NEC T86.19
      liver T86.40
        failure T86.42
        infection T86.43
        rejection T86.41
        specified type NEC T86.49
      lung T86.819
        with heart T86.30
          failure T86.32
          infection T86.33
          rejection T86.31
          specified type NEC T86.39
        failure T86.811
        infection T86.812
        rejection T86.810
        specified type NEC T86.818
      malignant neoplasm C80.2
      pancreas T86.899
        failure T86.891
        infection T86.892
        rejection T86.890
        specified type NEC T86.898
      peripheral blood stem cells T86.5
      post-transplant lymphoproliferative disorder (PTLD) D47.Z1 (*following* D47.4)
      rejection T86.91
      skin T86.829
        failure T86.821
        infection T86.822
        rejection T86.820
        specified type NEC T86.828
      specified
        tissue T86.899
          failure T86.891
          infection T86.892
          rejection T86.890
          specified type NEC T86.898
        type NEC T86.99
      stem cell (from peripheral blood) (from umbilical cord) T86.5
      umbilical cord stem cells T86.5
  trauma (early) T79.9 ☑
    specified NEC T79.8 ☑
  ultrasound therapy NEC T88.9 ☑
  umbilical cord NEC
    complicating delivery O69.9 ☑
      specified NEC O69.89 ☑
  umbrella device, vascular T82.9 ☑
    embolism T82.818 ☑
    fibrosis T82.828 ☑
    hemorrhage T82.838 ☑
    infection or inflammation T82.7 ☑
    mechanical
      breakdown T82.515 ☑
      displacement T82.525 ☑
      leakage T82.535 ☑
      malposition T82.525 ☑
      obstruction T82.595 ☑
      perforation T82.595 ☑
      protrusion T82.595 ☑
    pain T82.848 ☑
    specified type NEC T82.898 ☑
    stenosis T82.858 ☑
    thrombosis T82.868 ☑

Complication(s) — *continued*
  urethral catheter — *see* Complications, catheter, urethral, indwelling
  vaccination T88.1 ☑
    anaphylaxis NEC T80.52 ☑
    arthropathy — *see* Arthropathy, postimmunization
    cellulitis T88.0 ☑
    encephalitis or encephalomyelitis G04.02
    infection (general) (local) NEC T88.0 ☑
    meningitis G03.8
    myelitis G04.02
    protein sickness T80.62 ☑
    rash T88.1 ☑
    reaction (allergic) T88.1 ☑
      serum T80.62 ☑
    sepsis T88.0 ☑
    serum intoxication, sickness, rash, or other serum reaction NEC T80.62 ☑
      anaphylactic shock T80.52 ☑
    shock (allergic) (anaphylactic) T80.52 ☑
    vaccinia (generalized) (localized) T88.1 ☑
  vas deferens device or implant — *see* Complications, genitourinary, device or implant, genital tract
  vascular I99.9
    device or implant T82.9 ☑
      embolism T82.818 ☑
      fibrosis T82.828 ☑
      hemorrhage T82.838 ☑
      infection or inflammation T82.7 ☑
      mechanical
        breakdown T82.519 ☑
          specified device NEC T82.518 ☑
        displacement T82.529 ☑
          specified device NEC T82.528 ☑
        leakage T82.539 ☑
          specified device NEC T82.538 ☑
        malposition T82.529 ☑
          specified device NEC T82.528 ☑
        obstruction T82.599 ☑
          specified device NEC T82.598 ☑
        perforation T82.599 ☑
          specified device NEC T82.598 ☑
        protrusion T82.599 ☑
          specified device NEC T82.598 ☑
      pain T82.848 ☑
      specified type NEC T82.898 ☑
      stenosis T82.858 ☑
      thrombosis T82.868 ☑
    dialysis catheter — *see* Complication, catheter, dialysis
    following infusion, therapeutic injection or transfusion T80.1 ☑
    graft T82.9 ☑
      embolism T82.818 ☑
      fibrosis T82.828 ☑
      hemorrhage T82.838 ☑
      mechanical
        breakdown T82.319 ☑
          aorta (bifurcation) T82.310 ☑
          carotid artery T82.311 ☑
          specified vessel NEC T82.318 ☑
        displacement T82.329 ☑
          aorta (bifurcation) T82.320 ☑
          carotid artery T82.321 ☑
          specified vessel NEC T82.328 ☑
        leakage T82.339 ☑
          aorta (bifurcation) T82.330 ☑
          carotid artery T82.331 ☑
          specified vessel NEC T82.338 ☑
        malposition T82.329 ☑
          aorta (bifurcation) T82.320 ☑
          carotid artery T82.321 ☑
          specified vessel NEC T82.328 ☑
        obstruction T82.399 ☑
          aorta (bifurcation) T82.390 ☑
          carotid artery T82.391 ☑
          specified vessel NEC T82.398 ☑
        perforation T82.399 ☑
          aorta (bifurcation) T82.390 ☑
          carotid artery T82.391 ☑
          specified vessel NEC T82.398 ☑
        protrusion T82.399 ☑
          aorta (bifurcation) T82.390 ☑
          carotid artery T82.391 ☑
          specified vessel NEC T82.398 ☑
      pain T82.848 ☑

Complication(s) — *continued*
  vascular — *continued*
    graft — *continued*
      specified complication NEC T82.898 ☑
      stenosis T82.858 ☑
      thrombosis T82.868 ☑
    postoperative — *see* Complications, postoperative, circulatory
  vena cava device (filter) (sieve) (umbrella) — *see* Complications, umbrella device, vascular
  ventilation therapy NEC T81.81 ☑
  ventilator
    mechanical J95.850
      specified NEC J95.859
  ventricular (communicating) shunt (device) T85.9 ☑
    embolism T85.810 ☑
    fibrosis T85.820 ☑
    hemorrhage T85.830 ☑
    infection and inflammation T85.730 ☑
    mechanical
      breakdown T85.01 ☑
      displacement T85.02 ☑
      leakage T85.03 ☑
      malposition T85.02 ☑
      obstruction T85.09 ☑
      perforation T85.09 ☑
      protrusion T85.09 ☑
      specified NEC T85.09 ☑
    pain T85.840 ☑
    specified type NEC T85.890 ☑
    stenosis T85.850 ☑
    thrombosis T85.860 ☑
  wire suture, permanent (implanted) — *see* Complications, suture, permanent
Compressed air disease T70.3 ☑
Compression
  with injury — *code by* Nature of injury
  artery I77.1
    celiac, syndrome I77.4
  brachial plexus G54.0
  brain (stem) G93.5
    due to
      contusion (dIffuse) — *see* Injury, intracranial, diffuse
        focal — *see* Injury, intracranial, focal
      injury NEC — *see* Injury, intracranial, diffuse
      traumatic — *see* Injury, intracranial, diffuse
  bronchus J98.09
  cauda equina G83.4
  celiac (artery) (axis) I77.4
  cerebral — *see* Compression, brain
  cervical plexus G54.2
  cord
    spinal — *see* Compression, spinal
    umbilical — *see* Compression, umbilical cord
  cranial nerve G52.9
    eighth H93.3 ☑
    eleventh G52.8
    fifth G50.8
    first G52.0
    fourth — *see* Strabismus, paralytic, fourth nerve
    ninth G52.1
    second — *see* Disorder, nerve, optic
    seventh G51.8
    sixth — *see* Strabismus, paralytic, sixth nerve
    tenth G52.2
    third — *see* Strabismus, paralytic, third nerve
    twelfth G52.3
  diver's squeeze T70.3 ☑
  during birth (newborn) P15.9
  esophagus K22.2
  eustachian tube — *see* Obstruction, eustachian tube, cartilaginous
  facies Q67.1
  fracture
    nontraumatic NOS — *see* Collapse, vertebra
    pathological — *see* Fracture, pathological
    traumatic — *see* Fracture, traumatic
  heart — *see* Disease, heart
  intestine — *see* Obstruction, intestine
  laryngeal nerve, recurrent G52.2
    with paralysis of vocal cords and larynx J38.00
      bilateral J38.02
      unilateral J38.01
  lumbosacral plexus G54.1
  lung J98.4
  lymphatic vessel I89.0

Compression — *continued*
　　medulla — *see* Compression, brain
　　nerve (*see also* Disorder, nerve) G58.9
　　　arm NEC — *see* Mononeuropathy, upper limb
　　　axillary G54.0
　　　cranial — *see* Compression, cranial nerve
　　　leg NEC — *see* Mononeuropathy, lower limb
　　　median (in carpal tunnel) — *see* Syndrome, carpal tunnel
　　　optic — *see* Disorder, nerve, optic
　　　plantar — *see* Lesion, nerve, plantar
　　　posterior tibial (in tarsal tunnel) — *see* Syndrome, tarsal tunnel
　　　root or plexus NOS (in) G54.9
　　　　intervertebral disc disorder NEC — *see* Disorder, disc, with, radiculopathy
　　　　with myelopathy — *see* Disorder, disc, with, myelopathy
　　　　neoplastic disease (*see also* Neoplasm) D49.9 [G55]
　　　　spondylosis — *see* Spondylosis, with radiculopathy
　　　sciatic (acute) — *see* Lesion, nerve, sciatic
　　　sympathetic G90.8
　　　traumatic — *see* Injury, nerve
　　　ulnar — *see* Lesion, nerve, ulnar
　　　upper extremity NEC — *see* Mononeuropathy, upper limb
　　spinal (cord) G95.20
　　　by displacement of intervertebral disc NEC (*see also* Disorder, disc, with, myelopathy)
　　　nerve root NOS G54.9
　　　　due to displacement of intervertebral disc NEC — *see* Disorder, disc, with, radiculopathy
　　　　with myelopathy — *see* Disorder, disc, with, myelopathy
　　　specified NEC G95.29
　　　spondylogenic (cervical) (lumbar, lumbosacral) (thoracic) — *see* Spondylosis, with myelopathy NEC
　　　anterior — *see* Syndrome, anterior, spinal artery, compression
　　　traumatic — *see* Injury, spinal cord, by region
　　subcostal nerve (syndrome) — *see* Mononeuropathy, upper limb, specified NEC
　　sympathetic nerve NEC G90.8
　　syndrome T79.5 ☑
　　trachea J39.8
　　ulnar nerve (by scar tissue) — *see* Lesion, nerve, ulnar
　　umbilical cord
　　　complicating delivery O69.2 ☑
　　　cord around neck O69.1 ☑
　　　prolapse O69.0 ☑
　　　specified NEC O69.2 ☑
　　ureter N13.5
　　vein I87.1
　　vena cava (inferior) (superior) I87.1
Compulsion, compulsive
　　gambling F63.0
　　neurosis F42.8
　　personality F60.5
　　states F42.8
　　swearing F42.8
　　　in Gilles de la Tourette's syndrome F95.2
　　tics and spasms F95.9
Concato's disease (pericardial polyserositis) A19.9
　　nontubercular I31.1
　　pleural — *see* Pleurisy, with effusion
Concavity chest wall M95.4
Concealed penis Q55.69
Concern (normal) **about sick person in family** Z63.6
Concrescence (teeth) K00.2
Concretio cordis I31.1
　　rheumatic I09.2
Concretion (*see also* Calculus)
　　appendicular K38.1
　　canaliculus — *see* Dacryolith
　　clitoris N90.89
　　conjunctiva H11.12- ☑
　　eyelid — *see* Disorder, eyelid, specified type NEC
　　lacrimal passages — *see* Dacryolith
　　prepuce (male) N47.8
　　salivary gland (any) K11.5
　　seminal vesicle N50.89
　　tonsil J35.8
Concussion (brain) (cerebral) (current) S06.0X9 ☑

Concussion — *continued*
　　with
　　　loss of consciousness of 30 minutes or less S06.0X1 ☑
　　　loss of consciousness of unspecified duration S06.0X9 ☑
　　　without loss of consciousness S06.0X0 ☑
　　blast (air) (hydraulic) (immersion) (underwater)
　　　abdomen or thorax — *see* Injury, blast, by site
　　　ear with acoustic nerve injury — *see* Injury, nerve, acoustic, specified type NEC
　　cauda equina S34.3 ☑
　　conus medullaris S34.02 ☑
　　ocular S05.8X- ☑
　　spinal (cord)
　　　cervical S14.0 ☑
　　　lumbar S34.01 ☑
　　　sacral S34.02 ☑
　　　thoracic S24.0 ☑
　　syndrome F07.81
Condition — *see* Disease
Conditions arising in the perinatal period — *see* Newborn, affected by
Conduct disorder — *see* Disorder, conduct
Condyloma A63.0
　　acuminatum A63.0
　　gonorrheal A54.09
　　latum A51.31
　　syphilitic A51.31
　　　congenital A50.07
　　venereal, syphilitic A51.31
Conflagration (*see also* Burn)
　　asphyxia (by inhalation of gases, fumes or vapors) (*see also* Table of Drugs and Chemicals) T59.9- ☑
Conflict (with) (*see also* Discord)
　　family Z73.9
　　marital Z63.0
　　　involving divorce or estrangement Z63.5
　　parent-child Z62.820
　　　parent-adopted child Z62.821
　　　parent-biological child Z62.820
　　　parent-foster child Z62.822
　　social role NEC Z73.5
Confluent — *see* condition
Confusion, confused R41.0
　　epileptic F05
　　mental state (psychogenic) F44.89
　　psychogenic F44.89
　　reactive (from emotional stress, psychological trauma) F44.89
Confusional arousals G47.51
Congelation T69.9 ☑
Congenital (*see also* condition)
　　aortic septum Q25.49
　　intrinsic factor deficiency D51.0
　　malformation — *see* Anomaly
Congestion, congestive
　　bladder N32.89
　　bowel K63.89
　　brain G93.89
　　breast N64.59
　　bronchial J98.09
　　catarrhal J31.0
　　chest R09.89
　　chill, malarial — *see* Malaria
　　circulatory NEC I99.8
　　duodenum K31.89
　　eye — *see* Hyperemia, conjunctiva
　　facial, due to birth injury P15.4
　　general R68.89
　　glottis J37.0
　　heart — *see* Failure, heart, congestive
　　hepatic K76.1
　　hypostatic (lung) — *see* Edema, lung
　　intestine K63.89
　　kidney N28.89
　　labyrinth H83.8 ☑
　　larynx J37.0
　　liver K76.1
　　lung R09.89
　　　active or acute — *see* Pneumonia
　　malaria, malarial — *see* Malaria
　　nasal R09.81
　　nose R09.81
　　orbit, orbital (*see also* Exophthalmos)
　　　inflammatory (chronic) — *see* Inflammation, orbit
　　ovary N83.8

Congestion, congestive — *continued*
　　pancreas K86.89
　　pelvic, female N94.89
　　pleural J94.8
　　prostate (active) N42.1
　　pulmonary — *see* Congestion, lung
　　renal N28.89
　　retina H35.81
　　seminal vesicle N50.1
　　spinal cord G95.19
　　spleen (chronic) D73.2
　　stomach K31.89
　　trachea — *see* Tracheitis
　　urethra N36.8
　　uterus N85.8
　　　with subinvolution N85.3
　　venous (passive) I87.8
　　viscera R68.89
Congestive — *see* Congestion
Conical
　　cervix (hypertrophic elongation) N88.4
　　cornea — *see* Keratoconus
　　teeth K00.2
Conjoined twins Q89.4
Conjugal maladjustment Z63.0
　　involving divorce or estrangement Z63.5
Conjunctiva — *see* condition
Conjunctivitis (staphylococcal) (streptococcal) NOS H10.9
　　Acanthamoeba B60.12
　　acute H10.3- ☑
　　　atopic H10.1- ☑
　　　chemical (*see also* Corrosion, cornea) H10.21- ☑
　　　mucopurulent H10.02- ☑
　　　　follicular H10.01- ☑
　　　pseudomembranous H10.22- ☑
　　　serous except viral H10.23- ☑
　　　　viral — *see* Conjunctivitis, viral
　　　toxic H10.21- ☑
　　adenoviral (acute) (follicular) B30.1
　　allergic (acute) — *see* Conjunctivitis, acute, atopic
　　　chronic H10.45
　　　　vernal H10.44
　　anaphylactic — *see* Conjunctivitis, acute, atopic
　　Apollo B30.3
　　atopic (acute) — *see* Conjunctivitis, acute, atopic
　　Béal's B30.2
　　blennorrhagic (gonococcal) (neonatorum) A54.31
　　chemical (acute) (*see also* Corrosion, cornea) H10.21- ☑
　　chlamydial A74.0
　　　due to trachoma A71.1
　　　neonatal P39.1
　　chronic (nodosa) (petrificans) (phlyctenular) H10.40- ☑
　　　allergic H10.45
　　　　vernal H10.44
　　　follicular H10.43- ☑
　　　giant papillary H10.41- ☑
　　　simple H10.42- ☑
　　　vernal H10.44
　　coxsackievirus 24 B30.3
　　diphtheritic A36.86
　　due to
　　　dust — *see* Conjunctivitis, acute, atopic
　　　filariasis B74.9
　　　mucocutaneous leishmaniasis B55.2
　　enterovirus type 70 (hemorrhagic) B30.3
　　epidemic (viral) B30.9
　　　hemorrhagic B30.3
　　gonococcal (neonatorum) A54.31
　　granular (trachomatous) A71.1
　　　sequelae (late effect) B94.0
　　hemorrhagic (acute) (epidemic) B30.3
　　herpes zoster B02.31
　　in (due to)
　　　Acanthamoeba B60.12
　　　adenovirus (acute) (follicular) B30.1
　　　Chlamydia A74.0
　　　coxsackievirus 24 B30.3
　　　diphtheria A36.86
　　　enterovirus type 70 (hemorrhagic) B30.3
　　　filariasis B74.9
　　　gonococci A54.31
　　　herpes (simplex) virus B00.53
　　　　zoster B02.31
　　　infectious disease NEC B99 ☑
　　　meningococci A39.89
　　　mucocutaneous leishmaniasis B55.2

Conjunctivitis — continued
 in — continued
  rosacea L71.9
  syphilis (late) A52.71
  zoster B02.31
 inclusion A74.0
 infantile P39.1
  gonococcal A54.31
 Koch-Weeks' — see Conjunctivitis, acute, mucopurulent
 light — see Conjunctivitis, acute, atopic
 ligneous — see Blepharoconjunctivitis, ligneous
 meningococcal A39.89
 mucopurulent — see Conjunctivitis, acute, mucopurulent
 neonatal P39.1
  gonococcal A54.31
 Newcastle B30.8
 of Béal B30.2
 parasitic
  filariasis B74.9
  mucocutaneous leishmaniasis B55.2
 Parinaud's H10.89
 petrificans H10.89
 rosacea L71.9
 specified NEC H10.89
 swimming-pool B30.1
 trachomatous A71.1
  acute A71.0
  sequelae (late effect) B94.0
 traumatic NEC H10.89
 tuberculous A18.59
 tularemic A21.1
 tularensis A21.1
 viral B30.9
  due to
   adenovirus B30.1
   enterovirus B30.3
  specified NEC B30.8
Conjunctivochalasis H11.82- ☑
Connective tissue — see condition
Conn's syndrome E26.01
Conradi (-Hunermann) **disease** Q77.3
Consanguinity Z84.3
 counseling Z71.89
Conscious simulation (of illness) Z76.5
Consecutive — see condition
Consolidation lung (base) — see Pneumonia, lobar
Constipation (atonic) (neurogenic) (simple) (spastic)
   K59.00
 chronic K59.09
  idiopathic K59.04
 drug-induced K59.03
 functional K59.04
 outlet dysfunction K59.02
 psychogenic F45.8
 slow transit K59.01
 specified NEC K59.09
Constitutional (see also condition)
 substandard F60.7
Constitutionally substandard F60.7
Constriction (see also Stricture)
 auditory canal — see Stenosis, external ear canal
 bronchial J98.09
 duodenum K31.5
 esophagus K22.2
 external
  abdomen, abdominal (wall) S30.841 ☑
  alveolar process S00.542 ☑
  ankle S90.54- ☑
  antecubital space — see Constriction, external,
    forearm
  arm (upper) S40.84- ☑
  auricle — see Constriction, external, ear
  axilla — see Constriction, external, arm
  back, lower S30.840 ☑
  breast S20.14- ☑
  brow S00.84 ☑
  buttock S30.840 ☑
  calf — see Constriction, external, leg
  canthus — see Constriction, external, eyelid
  cheek S00.84 ☑
   internal S00.542 ☑
  chest wall — see Constriction, external, thorax
  chin S00.84 ☑
  clitoris S30.844 ☑
  costal region — see Constriction, external, thorax

Constriction — continued
 external — continued
  digit(s)
   foot — see Constriction, external, toe
   hand — see Constriction, external, finger
  ear S00.44- ☑
  elbow S50.34- ☑
  epididymis S30.843 ☑
  epigastric region S30.841 ☑
  esophagus, cervical S10.14 ☑
  eyebrow — see Constriction, external, eyelid
  eyelid S00.24- ☑
  face S00.84 ☑
  finger(s) S60.44- ☑
   index S60.44- ☑
   little S60.44- ☑
   middle S60.44- ☑
   ring S60.44- ☑
  flank S30.841 ☑
  foot (except toe(s) alone) S90.84- ☑
   toe — see Constriction, external, toe
  forearm S50.84- ☑
   elbow only — see Constriction, external, elbow
  forehead S00.84 ☑
  genital organs, external
   female S30.846 ☑
   male S30.845 ☑
  groin S30.841 ☑
  gum S00.542 ☑
  hand S60.54- ☑
  head S00.94 ☑
   ear — see Constriction, external, ear
   eyelid — see Constriction, external, eyelid
   lip S00.541 ☑
   nose S00.34 ☑
   oral cavity S00.542 ☑
   scalp S00.04 ☑
   specified site NEC S00.84 ☑
  heel — see Constriction, external, foot
  hip S70.24- ☑
  inguinal region S30.841 ☑
  interscapular region S20.449 ☑
  jaw S00.84 ☑
  knee S80.24- ☑
  labium (majus) (minus) S30.844 ☑
  larynx S10.14 ☑
  leg (lower) S80.84- ☑
   knee — see Constriction, external, knee
   upper — see Constriction, external, thigh
  lip S00.541 ☑
  lower back S30.840 ☑
  lumbar region S30.840 ☑
  malar region S00.84 ☑
  mammary — see Constriction, external, breast
  mastoid region S00.84 ☑
  mouth S00.542 ☑
  nail
   finger — see Constriction, external, finger
   toe — see Constriction, external, toe
  nasal S00.34 ☑
  neck S10.94 ☑
   specified site NEC S10.84 ☑
   throat S10.14 ☑
  nose S00.34 ☑
  occipital region S00.04 ☑
  oral cavity S00.542 ☑
  orbital region — see Constriction, external, eyelid
  palate S00.542 ☑
  palm — see Constriction, external, hand
  parietal region S00.04 ☑
  pelvis S30.840 ☑
  penis S30.842 ☑
  perineum
   female S30.844 ☑
   male S30.840 ☑
  periocular area — see Constriction, external, eyelid
  phalanges
   finger — see Constriction, external, finger
   toe — see Constriction, external, toe
  pharynx S10.14 ☑
  pinna — see Constriction, external, ear
  popliteal space — see Constriction, external, knee
  prepuce S30.842 ☑
  pubic region S30.840 ☑
  pudendum
   female S30.846 ☑

Constriction — continued
 external — continued
  pudendum — continued
   male S30.845 ☑
  sacral region S30.840 ☑
  scalp S00.04 ☑
  scapular region — see Constriction, external,
    shoulder
  scrotum S30.843 ☑
  shin — see Constriction, external, leg
  shoulder S40.24- ☑
  sternal region S20.349 ☑
  submaxillary region S00.84 ☑
  submental region S00.84 ☑
  subungual
   finger(s) — see Constriction, external, finger
   toe(s) — see Constriction, external, toe
  supraclavicular fossa S10.84 ☑
  supraorbital S00.84 ☑
  temple S00.84 ☑
  temporal region S00.84 ☑
  testis S30.843 ☑
  thigh S70.34- ☑
  thorax, thoracic (wall) S20.94 ☑
   back S20.44- ☑
   front S20.34- ☑
  throat S10.14 ☑
  thumb S60.34- ☑
  toe(s) (lesser) S90.44- ☑
   great S90.44- ☑
  tongue S00.542 ☑
  trachea S10.14 ☑
  tunica vaginalis S30.843 ☑
  uvula S00.542 ☑
  vagina S30.844 ☑
  vulva S30.844 ☑
  wrist S60.84- ☑
 gallbladder — see Obstruction, gallbladder
 intestine — see Obstruction, intestine
 larynx J38.6
  congenital Q31.8
   specified NEC Q31.8
   subglottic Q31.1
 organ or site, congenital NEC — see Atresia, by site
 prepuce (acquired) (congenital) N47.1
 pylorus (adult hypertrophic) K31.1
  congenital or infantile Q40.0
  newborn Q40.0
 ring dystocia (uterus) O62.4
 spastic (see also Spasm)
  ureter N13.5
 ureter N13.5
  with infection N13.6
 urethra — see Stricture, urethra
 visual field (peripheral) (functional) — see Defect, visual field
Constrictive — see condition
Consultation
 without complaint or sickness Z71.9
  feared complaint unfounded Z71.1
   specified reason NEC Z71.89
 medical — see Counseling, medical
 religious Z71.81
 specified reason NEC Z71.89
 spiritual Z71.81
Consumption — see Tuberculosis
Contact (with) (see also Exposure (to))
 acariasis Z20.7
 AIDS virus Z20.6
 air pollution Z77.110
 algae and algae toxins Z77.121
 algae bloom Z77.121
 anthrax Z20.810
 aromatic amines Z77.020
 aromatic (hazardous) compounds NEC Z77.028
 aromatic dyes NOS Z77.028
 arsenic Z77.010
 asbestos Z77.090
 bacterial disease NEC Z20.818
 benzene Z77.021
 blue-green algae bloom Z77.121
 body fluids (potentially hazardous) Z77.21
 brown tide Z77.121
 chemicals (chiefly nonmedicinal) (hazardous) NEC
   Z77.098
 cholera Z20.09
 chromium compounds Z77.018

Contact — *continued*
- communicable disease Z20.9
  - bacterial NEC Z20.818
    - specified NEC Z20.89
  - viral NEC Z20.828
- cyanobacteria bloom Z77.121
- dyes Z77.098
- Escherichia coli (E. coli) Z20.01
- fiberglass — *see* Table of Drugs and Chemicals, fiber-glass
- German measles Z20.4
- gonorrhea Z20.2
- hazardous metals NEC Z77.018
- hazardous substances NEC Z77.29
- hazards in the physical environment NEC Z77.128
- hazards to health NEC Z77.9
- HIV Z20.6
- HTLV-III/LAV Z20.6
- human immunodeficiency virus (HIV) Z20.6
- infection Z20.9
  - specified NEC Z20.89
- infestation (parasitic) NEC Z20.7
- intestinal infectious disease NEC Z20.09
  - Escherichia coli (E. coli) Z20.01
- lead Z77.011
- meningococcus Z20.811
- mold (toxic) Z77.120
- nickel dust Z77.018
- noise Z77.122
- parasitic disease Z20.7
- pediculosis Z20.7
- pfiesteria piscicida Z77.121
- poliomyelitis Z20.89
- pollution
  - air Z77.110
  - environmental NEC Z77.118
  - soil Z77.112
  - water Z77.111
- polycyclic aromatic hydrocarbons Z77.028
- rabies Z20.3
- radiation, naturally occurring NEC Z77.123
- radon Z77.123
- red tide (Florida) Z77.121
- rubella Z20.4
- sexually-transmitted disease Z20.2
- smallpox (laboratory) Z20.89
- syphilis Z20.2
- tuberculosis Z20.1
- uranium Z77.012
- varicella Z20.820
- venereal disease Z20.2
- viral disease NEC Z20.828
- viral hepatitis Z20.5
- water pollution Z77.111

Contamination, food — *see* Intoxication, foodborne
Contraception, contraceptive
- advice Z30.09
- counseling Z30.09
- device (intrauterine) (in situ) Z97.5
  - causing menorrhagia T83.83 ☑
  - checking Z30.431
  - complications — *see* Complications, intrauterine, contraceptive device
  - in place Z97.5
  - initial prescription Z30.014
  - reinsertion Z30.433
  - removal Z30.432
  - replacement Z30.433
- emergency (postcoital) Z30.012
- initial prescription Z30.019
  - barrier Z30.018
  - diaphragm Z30.018
  - injectable Z30.013
  - intrauterine device Z30.014
  - pills Z30.011
  - postcoital (emergency) Z30.012
  - specified type NEC Z30.018
  - subdermal implantable Z30.017
  - transdermal patch hormonal Z30.016
  - vaginal ring hormonal Z30.015
- maintenance Z30.40
  - barrier Z30.49
  - diaphragm Z30.49
  - examination Z30.8
  - injectable Z30.42
  - intrauterine device Z30.431
  - pills Z30.41
  - specified type NEC Z30.49
  - subdermal implantable Z30.46

Contraception, contraceptive — *continued*
- maintenance — *continued*
  - transdermal patch hormonal Z30.45
  - vaginal ring hormonal Z30.44
- management Z30.9
  - specified NEC Z30.8
- postcoital (emergency) Z30.012
- prescription Z30.019
  - repeat Z30.40
- sterilization Z30.2
- surveillance (drug) — *see* Contraception, maintenance

Contraction(s), contracture, contracted
- Achilles tendon (*see also* Short, tendon, Achilles)
  - congenital Q66.89
- amputation stump (surgical) (flexion) (late) (next proximal joint) T87.89
- anus K59.8
- bile duct (common) (hepatic) K83.8
- bladder N32.89
  - neck or sphincter N32.0
- bowel, cecum, colon or intestine, any part — *see* Obstruction, intestine
- Braxton Hicks — *see* False, labor
- breast implant, capsular T85.44 ☑
- bronchial J98.09
- burn (old) — *see* Cicatrix
- cervix — *see* Stricture, cervix
- cicatricial — *see* Cicatrix
- conjunctiva, trachomatous, active A71.1
  - sequelae (late effect) B94.0
- Dupuytren's M72.0
- eyelid — *see* Disorder, eyelid function
- fascia (lata) (postural) M72.8
  - Dupuytren's M72.0
  - palmar M72.0
  - plantar M72.2
- finger NEC (*see also* Deformity, finger)
  - congenital Q68.1
  - joint — *see* Contraction, joint, hand
- flaccid — *see* Contraction, paralytic
- gallbladder K82.0
- heart valve — *see* Endocarditis
- hip — *see* Contraction, joint, hip
- hourglass
  - bladder N32.89
    - congenital Q64.79
  - gallbladder K82.0
    - congenital Q44.1
  - stomach K31.89
    - congenital Q40.2
    - psychogenic F45.8
  - uterus (complicating delivery) O62.4
- hysterical F44.4
- internal os — *see* Stricture, cervix
- joint (abduction) (acquired) (adduction) (flexion) (rotation) M24.50
  - ankle M24.57- ☑
  - congenital NEC Q68.8
    - hip Q65.89
  - elbow M24.52- ☑
  - foot joint M24.57- ☑
  - hand joint M24.54- ☑
  - hip M24.55- ☑
    - congenital Q65.89
  - hysterical F44.4
  - knee M24.56- ☑
  - shoulder M24.51- ☑
  - wrist M24.53- ☑
- kidney (granular) (secondary) N26.9
  - congenital Q63.8
  - hydronephritic — *see* Hydronephrosis
  - Page N26.2
  - pyelonephritic — *see* Pyelitis, chronic
  - tuberculous A18.11
- ligament (*see also* Disorder, ligament)
  - congenital Q79.8
- muscle (postinfective) (postural) NEC M62.40
  - with contracture of joint — *see* Contraction, joint
  - ankle M62.47- ☑
  - congenital Q79.8
    - sternocleidomastoid Q68.0
  - extraocular — *see* Strabismus
  - eye (extrinsic) — *see* Strabismus
  - foot M62.47- ☑
  - forearm M62.43- ☑
  - hand M62.44- ☑
  - hysterical F44.4

Contraction(s), contracture, contracted — *continued*
- muscle — *continued*
  - ischemic (Volkmann's) T79.6 ☑
  - lower leg M62.46- ☑
  - multiple sites M62.49
  - pelvic region M62.45- ☑
  - posttraumatic — *see* Strabismus, paralytic
  - psychogenic F45.8
    - conversion reaction F44.4
  - shoulder region M62.41- ☑
  - specified site NEC M62.48
  - thigh M62.45- ☑
  - upper arm M62.42- ☑
- neck — *see* Torticollis
- ocular muscle — *see* Strabismus
- organ or site, congenital NEC — *see* Atresia, by site
- outlet (pelvis) — *see* Contraction, pelvis
- palmar fascia M72.0
- paralytic
  - joint — *see* Contraction, joint
  - muscle (*see also* Contraction, muscle NEC)
    - ocular — *see* Strabismus, paralytic
- pelvis (acquired) (general) M95.5
  - with disproportion (fetopelvic) O33.1
    - causing obstructed labor O65.1
  - inlet O33.2
  - mid-cavity O33.3 ☑
  - outlet O33.3 ☑
- plantar fascia M72.2
- premature
  - atrium I49.1
  - auriculoventricular I49.49
  - heart I49.49
  - junctional I49.2
  - supraventricular I49.1
  - ventricular I49.3
- prostate N42.89
- pylorus NEC (*see also* Pylorospasm)
  - psychogenic F45.8
- rectum, rectal (sphincter) K59.8
- ring (Bandl's) (complicating delivery) O62.4
- scar — *see* Cicatrix
- spine — *see* Dorsopathy, deforming
- sternocleidomastoid (muscle), congenital Q68.0
- stomach K31.89
  - hourglass K31.89
    - congenital Q40.2
    - psychogenic F45.8
  - psychogenic F45.8
- tendon (sheath) M62.40
  - with contracture of joint — *see* Contraction, joint
  - Achilles — *see* Short, tendon, Achilles
  - ankle M62.47- ☑
    - Achilles — *see* Short, tendon, Achilles
  - foot M62.47- ☑
  - forearm M62.43- ☑
  - hand M62.44- ☑
  - lower leg M62.46- ☑
  - multiple sites M62.49
  - neck M62.48
  - pelvic region M62.45- ☑
  - shoulder region M62.41- ☑
  - specified site NEC M62.48
  - thigh M62.45- ☑
  - thorax M62.48
  - trunk M62.48
  - upper arm M62.42- ☑
- toe — *see* Deformity, toe, specified NEC
- ureterovesical orifice (postinfectional) N13.5
  - with infection N13.6
- urethra (*see also* Stricture, urethra)
  - orifice N32.0
- uterus N85.8
  - abnormal NEC O62.9
  - clonic (complicating delivery) O62.4
  - dyscoordinate (complicating delivery) O62.4
  - hourglass (complicating delivery) O62.4
  - hypertonic O62.4
  - hypotonic NEC O62.2
  - inadequate
    - primary O62.0
    - secondary O62.1
  - incoordinate (complicating delivery) O62.4
  - poor O62.2
  - tetanic (complicating delivery) O62.4
- vagina (outlet) N89.5
- vesical N32.89

Contraction(s), contracture, contracted —
continued
  vesical — *continued*
    neck or urethral orifice N32.0
  visual field — *see* Defect, visual field, generalized
  Volkmann's (ischemic) T79.6 ☑
Contusion (skin surface intact) T14.8 ☑
  abdomen, abdominal (muscle) (wall) S30.1 ☑
  adnexa, eye NEC S05.8X- ☑
  adrenal gland S37.812 ☑
  alveolar process S00.532 ☑
  ankle S90.0- ☑
  antecubital space — *see* Contusion, forearm
  anus S30.3 ☑
  arm (upper) S40.02- ☑
    lower (with elbow) — *see* Contusion, forearm
  auditory canal — *see* Contusion, ear
  auricle — *see* Contusion, ear
  axilla — *see* Contusion, arm, upper
  back (*see also* Contusion, thorax, back)
    lower S30.0 ☑
  bile duct S36.13 ☑
  bladder S37.22 ☑
  bone NEC T14.8 ☑
  brain (diffuse) — *see* Injury, intracranial, diffuse
    focal — *see* Injury, intracranial, focal
  brainstem S06.38- ☑
  breast S20.0- ☑
  broad ligament S37.892 ☑
  brow S00.83 ☑
  buttock S30.0 ☑
  canthus, eye S00.1- ☑
  cauda equina S34.3 ☑
  cerebellar, traumatic S06.37- ☑
  cerebral S06.33- ☑
    left side S06.32- ☑
    right side S06.31- ☑
  cheek S00.83 ☑
    internal S00.532 ☑
  chest (wall) — *see* Contusion, thorax
  chin S00.83 ☑
  clitoris S30.23 ☑
  colon — *see* Injury, intestine, large, contusion
  common bile duct S36.13 ☑
  conjunctiva S05.1- ☑
    with foreign body (in conjunctival sac) — *see* Foreign body, conjunctival sac
  conus medullaris (spine) S34.139 ☑
  cornea — *see* Contusion, eyeball
    with foreign body — *see* Foreign body, cornea
  corpus cavernosum S30.21 ☑
  cortex (brain) (cerebral) — *see* Injury, intracranial, diffuse
    focal — *see* Injury, intracranial, focal
  costal region — *see* Contusion, thorax
  cystic duct S36.13 ☑
  diaphragm S27.802 ☑
  duodenum S36.420 ☑
  ear S00.43- ☑
  elbow S50.0- ☑
    with forearm — *see* Contusion, forearm
  epididymis S30.22 ☑
  epigastric region S30.1 ☑
  epiglottis S10.0 ☑
  esophagus (thoracic) S27.812 ☑
    cervical S10.0 ☑
  eyeball S05.1- ☑
  eyebrow S00.1- ☑
  eyelid (and periocular area) S00.1- ☑
  face NEC S00.83 ☑
  fallopian tube S37.529 ☑
    bilateral S37.522 ☑
    unilateral S37.521 ☑
  femoral triangle S30.1 ☑
  finger(s) S60.00 ☑
    with damage to nail (matrix) S60.10 ☑
    index S60.02- ☑
      with damage to nail S60.12- ☑
    little S60.05- ☑
      with damage to nail S60.15- ☑
    middle S60.03- ☑
      with damage to nail S60.13- ☑
    ring S60.04- ☑
      with damage to nail S60.14- ☑
    thumb — *see* Contusion, thumb
  flank S30.1 ☑

Contusion — *continued*
  foot (except toe(s) alone) S90.3- ☑
    toe — *see* Contusion, toe
  forearm S50.1- ☑
    elbow only — *see* Contusion, elbow
  forehead S00.83 ☑
  gallbladder S36.122 ☑
  genital organs, external
    female S30.202 ☑
    male S30.201 ☑
  globe (eye) — *see* Contusion, eyeball
  groin S30.1 ☑
  gum S00.532 ☑
  hand S60.22- ☑
    finger(s) — *see* Contusion, finger
    wrist — *see* Contusion, wrist
  head S00.93 ☑
    ear — *see* Contusion, ear
    eyelid — *see* Contusion, eyelid
    lip S00.531 ☑
    nose S00.33 ☑
    oral cavity S00.532 ☑
    scalp S00.03 ☑
    specified part NEC S00.83 ☑
  heart (*see also* Injury, heart) S26.91 ☑
  heel — *see* Contusion, foot
  hepatic duct S36.13 ☑
  hip S70.0- ☑
  ileum S36.428 ☑
  iliac region S30.1 ☑
  inguinal region S30.1 ☑
  interscapular region S20.229 ☑
  intra-abdominal organ S36.92 ☑
    colon — *see* Injury, intestine, large, contusion
    liver S36.112 ☑
    pancreas — *see* Contusion, pancreas
    rectum S36.62 ☑
    small intestine — *see* Injury, intestine, small, contusion
    specified organ NEC S36.892 ☑
    spleen — *see* Contusion, spleen
    stomach S36.32 ☑
  iris (eye) — *see* Contusion, eyeball
  jaw S00.83 ☑
  jejunum S36.428 ☑
  kidney S37.01- ☑
    major (greater than 2 cm) S37.02- ☑
    minor (less than 2 cm) S37.01- ☑
  knee S80.0- ☑
  labium (majus) (minus) S30.23 ☑
  lacrimal apparatus, gland or sac S05.8X- ☑
  larynx S10.0 ☑
  leg (lower) S80.1- ☑
    knee — *see* Contusion, knee
  lens — *see* Contusion, eyeball
  lip S00.531 ☑
  liver S36.112 ☑
  lower back S30.0 ☑
  lumbar region S30.0 ☑
  lung S27.329 ☑
    bilateral S27.322 ☑
    unilateral S27.321 ☑
  malar region S00.83 ☑
  mastoid region S00.83 ☑
  membrane, brain — *see* Injury, intracranial, diffuse
    focal — *see* Injury, intracranial, focal
  mesentery S36.892 ☑
  mesosalpinx S37.892 ☑
  mouth S00.532 ☑
  muscle — *see* Contusion, by site
  nail
    finger — *see* Contusion, finger, with damage to nail
    toe — *see* Contusion, toe, with damage to nail
  nasal S00.33 ☑
  neck S10.93 ☑
    specified site NEC S10.83 ☑
    throat S10.0 ☑
  nerve — *see* Injury, nerve
  newborn P54.5
  nose S00.33 ☑
  occipital
    lobe (brain) — *see* Injury, intracranial, diffuse
      focal — *see* Injury, intracranial, focal
    region (scalp) S00.03 ☑
  orbit (region) (tissues) S05.1- ☑

Contusion — *continued*
  ovary S37.429 ☑
    bilateral S37.422 ☑
    unilateral S37.421 ☑
  palate S00.532 ☑
  pancreas S36.229 ☑
    body S36.221 ☑
    head S36.220 ☑
    tail S36.222 ☑
  parietal
    lobe (brain) — *see* Injury, intracranial, diffuse
      focal — *see* Injury, intracranial, focal
    region (scalp) S00.03 ☑
  pelvic organ S37.92 ☑
    adrenal gland S37.812 ☑
    bladder S37.22 ☑
    fallopian tube — *see* Contusion, fallopian tube
    kidney — *see* Contusion, kidney
    ovary — *see* Contusion, ovary
    prostate S37.822 ☑
    specified organ NEC S37.892 ☑
    ureter S37.12 ☑
    urethra S37.32 ☑
    uterus S37.62 ☑
  pelvis S30.0 ☑
  penis S30.21 ☑
  perineum
    female S30.23 ☑
    male S30.0 ☑
  periocular area S00.1- ☑
  peritoneum S36.81 ☑
  periurethral tissue — *see* Contusion, urethra
  pharynx S10.0 ☑
  pinna — *see* Contusion, ear
  popliteal space — *see* Contusion, knee
  prepuce S30.21 ☑
  prostate S37.822 ☑
  pubic region S30.1 ☑
  pudendum
    female S30.202 ☑
    male S30.201 ☑
  quadriceps femoris — *see* Contusion, thigh
  rectum S36.62 ☑
  retroperitoneum S36.892 ☑
  round ligament S37.892 ☑
  sacral region S30.0 ☑
  scalp S00.03 ☑
    due to birth injury P12.3
  scapular region — *see* Contusion, shoulder
  sclera — *see* Contusion, eyeball
  scrotum S30.22 ☑
  seminal vesicle S37.892 ☑
  shoulder S40.01- ☑
  skin NEC T14.8 ☑
  small intestine — *see* Injury, intestine, small, contusion
  spermatic cord S30.22 ☑
  spinal cord — *see* Injury, spinal cord, by region
    cauda equina S34.3 ☑
    conus medullaris S34.139 ☑
  spleen S36.029 ☑
    major S36.021 ☑
    minor S36.020 ☑
  sternal region S20.219 ☑
  stomach S36.32 ☑
  subconjunctival S05.1- ☑
  subcutaneous NEC T14.8 ☑
  submaxillary region S00.83 ☑
  submental region S00.83 ☑
  subperiosteal NEC T14.8 ☑
  subungual
    finger — *see* Contusion, finger, with damage to nail
    toe — *see* Contusion, toe, with damage to nail
  supraclavicular fossa S10.83 ☑
  supraorbital S00.83 ☑
  suprarenal gland S37.812 ☑
  temple (region) S00.83 ☑
  temporal
    lobe (brain) — *see* Injury, intracranial, diffuse
      focal — *see* Injury, intracranial, focal
    region S00.83 ☑
  testis S30.22 ☑
  thigh S70.1- ☑
  thorax (wall) S20.20 ☑
    back S20.22- ☑
    front S20.21- ☑

Corrosion — *continued*
  extent — *continued*
    40-49 percent — *continued*
      with — *continued*
        20-29 percent third degree T32.42
        30-39 percent third degree T32.43
        40-49 percent third degree T32.44
    50-59 percent (0-9 percent third degree) T32.50
      with
        10-19 percent third degree T32.51
        20-29 percent third degree T32.52
        30-39 percent third degree T32.53
        40-49 percent third degree T32.54
        50-59 percent third degree T32.55
    60-69 percent (0-9 percent third degree) T32.60
      with
        10-19 percent third degree T32.61
        20-29 percent third degree T32.62
        30-39 percent third degree T32.63
        40-49 percent third degree T32.64
        50-59 percent third degree T32.65
        60-69 percent third degree T32.66
    70-79 percent (0-9 percent third degree) T32.70
      with
        10-19 percent third degree T32.71
        20-29 percent third degree T32.72
        30-39 percent third degree T32.73
        40-49 percent third degree T32.74
        50-59 percent third degree T32.75
        60-69 percent third degree T32.76
        70-79 percent third degree T32.77
    80-89 percent (0-9 percent third degree) T32.80
      with
        10-19 percent third degree T32.81
        20-29 percent third degree T32.82
        30-39 percent third degree T32.83
        40-49 percent third degree T32.84
        50-59 percent third degree T32.85
        60-69 percent third degree T32.86
        70-79 percent third degree T32.87
        80-89 percent third degree T32.88
    90 percent or more (0-9 percent third degree) T32.90
      with
        10-19 percent third degree T32.91
        20-29 percent third degree T32.92
        30-39 percent third degree T32.93
        40-49 percent third degree T32.94
        50-59 percent third degree T32.95
        60-69 percent third degree T32.96
        70-79 percent third degree T32.97
        80-89 percent third degree T32.98
        90-99 percent third degree T32.99
  extremity — *see* Corrosion, limb
  eye(s) and adnexa T26.9-
    with resulting rupture and destruction of eyeball T26.7-
    conjunctival sac — *see* Corrosion, cornea
    cornea — *see* Corrosion, cornea
    lid — *see* Corrosion, eyelid
    periocular area — *see* Corrosion eyelid
    specified site NEC T26.8-
  eyeball — *see* Corrosion, eye
  eyelid(s) T26.5-
  face — *see* Corrosion, head
  finger T23.429 ☑
    first degree T23.529 ☑
    left T23.422 ☑
      first degree T23.522 ☑
      second degree T23.622 ☑
      third degree T23.722 ☑
      multiple sites (without thumb) T23.439 ☑
        with thumb T23.449 ☑
          first degree T23.549 ☑
          left T23.442 ☑
            first degree T23.542 ☑
            second degree T23.642 ☑
            third degree T23.742 ☑
          right T23.441 ☑
            first degree T23.541 ☑
            second degree T23.641 ☑
            third degree T23.741 ☑
          second degree T23.649 ☑
          third degree T23.749 ☑
        first degree T23.539 ☑
        left T23.432 ☑
          first degree T23.532 ☑

Corrosion — *continued*
  finger — *continued*
    multiple sites — *continued*
      left
        second degree T23.632 ☑
        third degree T23.732 ☑
      right T23.431 ☑
        first degree T23.531 ☑
        second degree T23.631 ☑
        third degree T23.731 ☑
      second degree T23.639 ☑
      third degree T23.739 ☑
    right T23.421 ☑
      first degree T23.521 ☑
      second degree T23.621 ☑
      third degree T23.721 ☑
    second degree T23.629 ☑
    third degree T23.729 ☑
  flank — *see* Corrosion, abdomen
  foot T25.429 ☑
    first degree T25.529 ☑
    left T25.422 ☑
      first degree T25.522 ☑
      second degree T25.622 ☑
      third degree T25.722 ☑
    multiple with ankle — *see* Corrosion, lower, limb, multiple, ankle and foot
    right T25.421 ☑
      first degree T25.521 ☑
      second degree T25.621 ☑
      third degree T25.721 ☑
    second degree T25.629 ☑
    third degree T25.729 ☑
  forearm T22.419 ☑
    first degree T22.519 ☑
    left T22.412 ☑
      first degree T22.512 ☑
      second degree T22.612 ☑
      third degree T22.712 ☑
    right T22.411 ☑
      first degree T22.511 ☑
      second degree T22.611 ☑
      third degree T22.711 ☑
    second degree T22.619 ☑
    third degree T22.719 ☑
  forehead T20.46 ☑
    first degree T20.56 ☑
    second degree T20.66 ☑
    third degree T20.76 ☑
  fourth degree — *code as* Corrosion, third degree, by site
  full thickness skin loss — *code as* Corrosion, third degree, by site
  gastrointestinal tract NEC T28.7 ☑
  genital organs
    external
      female T21.47 ☑
        first degree T21.57 ☑
        second degree T21.67 ☑
        third degree T21.77 ☑
      male T21.46 ☑
        first degree T21.56 ☑
        second degree T21.66 ☑
        third degree T21.76 ☑
    internal T28.8 ☑
  groin — *see* Corrosion, abdominal wall
  hand(s) T23.409 ☑
    back — *see* Corrosion, dorsum of hand
    finger — *see* Corrosion, finger
    first degree T23.509 ☑
    left T23.402 ☑
      first degree T23.502 ☑
      second degree T23.602 ☑
      third degree T23.702 ☑
    multiple sites with wrist T23.499 ☑
      first degree T23.599 ☑
      left T23.492 ☑
        first degree T23.592 ☑
        second degree T23.692 ☑
        third degree T23.792 ☑
      right T23.491 ☑
        first degree T23.591 ☑
        second degree T23.691 ☑
        third degree T23.791 ☑
    second degree T23.699 ☑
    third degree T23.799 ☑

Corrosion — *continued*
  hand(s) — *continued*
    palm — *see* Corrosion, palm
    right T23.401 ☑
      first degree T23.501 ☑
      second degree T23.601 ☑
      third degree T23.701 ☑
    second degree T23.609 ☑
    third degree T23.709 ☑
    thumb — *see* Corrosion, thumb
  head (and face) (and neck) T20.40 ☑
    cheek — *see* Corrosion, cheek
    chin — *see* Corrosion, chin
    ear — *see* Corrosion, ear
    eye(s) only — *see* Corrosion, eye
    first degree T20.50 ☑
    forehead — *see* Corrosion, forehead
    lip — *see* Corrosion, lip
    multiple sites T20.49 ☑
      first degree T20.59 ☑
      second degree T20.69 ☑
      third degree T20.79 ☑
    neck — *see* Corrosion, neck
    nose — *see* Corrosion, nose
    scalp — *see* Corrosion, scalp
    second degree T20.60 ☑
    third degree T20.70 ☑
  hip(s) — *see* Corrosion, lower, limb
  inhalation — *see* Corrosion, respiratory tract
  internal organ(s) (*see also* Corrosion, by site) T28.90 ☑
    alimentary tract T28.7 ☑
      esophagus T28.6 ☑
    esophagus T28.6 ☑
    genitourinary T28.8 ☑
    mouth T28.5 ☑
    pharynx T28.5 ☑
    specified organ NEC T28.99 ☑
  interscapular region — *see* Corrosion, back, upper
  intestine (large) (small) T28.7 ☑
  knee T24.429 ☑
    first degree T24.529 ☑
    left T24.422 ☑
      first degree T24.522 ☑
      second degree T24.622 ☑
      third degree T24.722 ☑
    right T24.421 ☑
      first degree T24.521 ☑
      second degree T24.621 ☑
      third degree T24.721 ☑
    second degree T24.629 ☑
    third degree T24.729 ☑
  labium (majus) (minus) — *see* Corrosion, genital organs, external, female
  lacrimal apparatus, duct, gland or sac — *see* Corrosion, eye, specified site NEC
  larynx T27.4 ☑
    with lung T27.5 ☑
  leg(s) (meaning lower limb(s)) — *see* Corrosion, lower limb
  limb(s)
    lower — *see* Corrosion, lower, limb
    upper — *see* Corrosion, upper limb
  lip(s) T20.42 ☑
    first degree T20.52 ☑
    second degree T20.62 ☑
    third degree T20.72 ☑
  lower
    back — *see* Corrosion, back
    limb T24.409 ☑
      ankle — *see* Corrosion, ankle
      calf — *see* Corrosion, calf
      first degree T24.509 ☑
      foot — *see* Corrosion, foot
      knee — *see* Corrosion, knee
      left T24.402 ☑
        first degree T24.502 ☑
        second degree T24.602 ☑
        third degree T24.702 ☑
      multiple sites, except ankle and foot T24.499 ☑
        ankle and foot T25.499 ☑
          first degree T25.599 ☑
          left T25.492 ☑
            first degree T25.592 ☑
            second degree T25.692 ☑
            third degree T25.792 ☑
          right T25.491 ☑

Corrosion — *continued*
lower — *continued*
  limb — *continued*
    multiple sites, except ankle and foot — *continued*
      ankle and foot — *continued*
        right — *continued*
          first degree T25.591 ☑
          second degree T25.691 ☑
          third degree T25.791 ☑
        second degree T25.699 ☑
        third degree T25.799 ☑
      first degree T24.599 ☑
      left T24.492 ☑
        first degree T24.592 ☑
        second degree T24.692 ☑
        third degree T24.792 ☑
      right T24.491 ☑
        first degree T24.591 ☑
        second degree T24.691 ☑
        third degree T24.791 ☑
      second degree T24.699 ☑
      third degree T24.799 ☑
      right T24.401 ☑
        first degree T24.501 ☑
        second degree T24.601 ☑
        third degree T24.701 ☑
      second degree T24.609 ☑
      thigh — *see* Corrosion, thigh
      third degree T24.709 ☑
lung (with larynx and trachea) T27.5 ☑
mouth T28.5 ☑
neck T20.47 ☑
  first degree T20.57 ☑
  second degree T20.67 ☑
  third degree T20.77 ☑
nose (septum) T20.44 ☑
  first degree T20.54 ☑
  second degree T20.64 ☑
  third degree T20.74 ☑
ocular adnexa — *see* Corrosion, eye
orbit region — *see* Corrosion, eyelid
palm T23.459 ☑
  first degree T23.559 ☑
  left T23.452 ☑
    first degree T23.552 ☑
    second degree T23.652 ☑
    third degree T23.752 ☑
  right T23.451 ☑
    first degree T23.551 ☑
    second degree T23.651 ☑
    third degree T23.751 ☑
  second degree T23.659 ☑
  third degree T23.759 ☑
partial thickness — *code as* Corrosion, unspecified degree, by site
pelvis — *see* Corrosion, trunk
penis — *see* Corrosion, genital organs, external, male
perineum
  female — *see* Corrosion, genital organs, external, female
  male — *see* Corrosion, genital organs, external, male
periocular area — *see* Corrosion, eyelid
pharynx T28.5 ☑
rectum T28.7 ☑
respiratory tract T27.7 ☑
  larynx — *see* Corrosion, larynx
  specified part NEC T27.6 ☑
  trachea — *see* Corrosion, larynx
sac, lacrimal — *see* Corrosion, eye, specified site NEC
scalp T20.45 ☑
  first degree T20.55 ☑
  second degree T20.65 ☑
  third degree T20.75 ☑
scapular region T22.469 ☑
  first degree T22.569 ☑
  left T22.462 ☑
    first degree T22.562 ☑
    second degree T22.662 ☑
    third degree T22.762 ☑
  right T22.461 ☑
    first degree T22.561 ☑
    second degree T22.661 ☑
    third degree T22.761 ☑
  second degree T22.669 ☑

Corrosion — *continued*
scapular region — *continued*
  third degree T22.769 ☑
sclera — *see* Corrosion, eye, specified site NEC
scrotum — *see* Corrosion, genital organs, external, male
shoulder T22.459 ☑
  first degree T22.559 ☑
  left T22.452 ☑
    first degree T22.552 ☑
    second degree T22.652 ☑
    third degree T22.752 ☑
  right T22.451 ☑
    first degree T22.551 ☑
    second degree T22.651 ☑
    third degree T22.751 ☑
  second degree T22.659 ☑
  third degree T22.759 ☑
stomach T28.7 ☑
temple — *see* Corrosion, head
testis — *see* Corrosion, genital organs, external, male
thigh T24.419 ☑
  first degree T24.519 ☑
  left T24.412 ☑
    first degree T24.512 ☑
    second degree T24.612 ☑
    third degree T24.712 ☑
  right T24.411 ☑
    first degree T24.511 ☑
    second degree T24.611 ☑
    third degree T24.711 ☑
  second degree T24.619 ☑
  third degree T24.719 ☑
thorax (external) — *see* Corrosion, trunk
throat (meaning pharynx) T28.5 ☑
thumb(s) T23.419 ☑
  first degree T23.519 ☑
  left T23.412 ☑
    first degree T23.512 ☑
    second degree T23.612 ☑
    third degree T23.712 ☑
  multiple sites with fingers T23.449 ☑
    first degree T23.549 ☑
    left T23.442 ☑
      first degree T23.542 ☑
      second degree T23.642 ☑
      third degree T23.742 ☑
    right T23.441 ☑
      first degree T23.541 ☑
      second degree T23.641 ☑
      third degree T23.741 ☑
    second degree T23.649 ☑
    third degree T23.749 ☑
  right T23.411 ☑
    first degree T23.511 ☑
    second degree T23.611 ☑
    third degree T23.711 ☑
  second degree T23.619 ☑
  third degree T23.719 ☑
toe T25.439 ☑
  first degree T25.539 ☑
  left T25.432 ☑
    first degree T25.532 ☑
    second degree T25.632 ☑
    third degree T25.732 ☑
  right T25.431 ☑
    first degree T25.531 ☑
    second degree T25.631 ☑
    third degree T25.731 ☑
  second degree T25.639 ☑
  third degree T25.739 ☑
tongue T28.5 ☑
tonsil(s) T28.5 ☑
total body — *see* Corrosion, multiple body regions
trachea T27.4 ☑
  with lung T27.5 ☑
trunk T21.40 ☑
  abdominal wall — *see* Corrosion, abdominal wall
  anus — *see* Corrosion, buttock
  axilla — *see* Corrosion, upper limb
  back — *see* Corrosion, back
  breast — *see* Corrosion, chest wall
  buttock — *see* Corrosion, buttock
  chest wall — *see* Corrosion, chest wall
    first degree T21.50 ☑
  flank — *see* Corrosion, abdominal wall

Corrosion — *continued*
trunk — *continued*
  genital
    female — *see* Corrosion, genital organs, external, female
    male — *see* Corrosion, genital organs, external, male
  groin — *see* Corrosion, abdominal wall
  interscapular region — *see* Corrosion, back, upper
  labia — *see* Corrosion, genital organs, external, female
  lower back — *see* Corrosion, back
  penis — *see* Corrosion, genital organs, external, male
  perineum
    female — *see* Corrosion, genital organs, external, female
    male — *see* Corrosion, genital organs, external, male
  scapular region — *see* Corrosion, upper limb
  scrotum — *see* Corrosion, genital organs, external, male
  second degree T21.60 ☑
  shoulder — *see* Corrosion, upper limb
  specified site NEC T21.49 ☑
    first degree T21.59 ☑
    second degree T21.69 ☑
    third degree T21.79 ☑
  testes — *see* Corrosion, genital organs, external, male
  third degree T21.70 ☑
  upper back — *see* Corrosion, back, upper
  vagina T28.8 ☑
  vulva — *see* Corrosion, genital organs, external, female
unspecified site with extent of body surface involved specified
  less than 10 percent T32.0
  10-19 percent (0-9 percent third degree) T32.10
    with 10-19 percent third degree T32.11
  20-29 percent (0-9 percent third degree) T32.20
    with
      10-19 percent third degree T32.21
      20-29 percent third degree T32.22
  30-39 percent (0-9 percent third degree) T32.30
    with
      10-19 percent third degree T32.31
      20-29 percent third degree T32.32
      30-39 percent third degree T32.33
  40-49 percent (0-9 percent third degree) T32.40
    with
      10-19 percent third degree T32.41
      20-29 percent third degree T32.42
      30-39 percent third degree T32.43
      40-49 percent third degree T32.44
  50-59 percent (0-9 percent third degree) T32.50
    with
      10-19 percent third degree T32.51
      20-29 percent third degree T32.52
      30-39 percent third degree T32.53
      40-49 percent third degree T32.54
      50-59 percent third degree T32.55
  60-69 percent (0-9 percent third degree) T32.60
    with
      10-19 percent third degree T32.61
      20-29 percent third degree T32.62
      30-39 percent third degree T32.63
      40-49 percent third degree T32.64
      50-59 percent third degree T32.65
      60-69 percent third degree T32.66
  70-79 percent (0-9 percent third degree) T32.70
    with
      10-19 percent third degree T32.71
      20-29 percent third degree T32.72
      30-39 percent third degree T32.73
      40-49 percent third degree T32.74
      50-59 percent third degree T32.75
      60-69 percent third degree T32.76
      70-79 percent third degree T32.77
  80-89 percent (0-9 percent third degree) T32.80
    with
      10-19 percent third degree T32.81
      20-29 percent third degree T32.82
      30-39 percent third degree T32.83
      40-49 percent third degree T32.84
      50-59 percent third degree T32.85
      60-69 percent third degree T32.86
      70-79 percent third degree T32.87

Corrosion — *continued*
  unspecified site with extent of body surface involved
      specified — *continued*
    80-89 percent — *continued*
      with — *continued*
        80-89 percent third degree T32.88
      90 percent or more (0-9 percent third degree)
          T32.90
        with
          10-19 percent third degree T32.91
          20-29 percent third degree T32.92
          30-39 percent third degree T32.93
          40-49 percent third degree T32.94
          50-59 percent third degree T32.95
          60-69 percent third degree T32.96
          70-79 percent third degree T32.97
          80-89 percent third degree T32.98
          90-99 percent third degree T32.99
  upper limb (axilla) (scapular region) T22.40 ☑
    above elbow — *see* Corrosion, above elbow
    axilla — *see* Corrosion, axilla
    elbow — *see* Corrosion, elbow
    first degree T22.50 ☑
    forearm — *see* Corrosion, forearm
    hand — *see* Corrosion, hand
    interscapular region — *see* Corrosion, back, upper
    multiple sites T22.499 ☑
      first degree T22.599 ☑
      left T22.492 ☑
        first degree T22.592 ☑
        second degree T22.692 ☑
        third degree T22.792 ☑
      right T22.491 ☑
        first degree T22.591 ☑
        second degree T22.691 ☑
        third degree T22.791 ☑
      second degree T22.699 ☑
      third degree T22.799 ☑
    scapular region — *see* Corrosion, scapular region
    second degree T22.60 ☑
    shoulder — *see* Corrosion, shoulder
    third degree T22.70 ☑
    wrist — *see* Corrosion, hand
  uterus T28.8 ☑
  vagina T28.8 ☑
  vulva — *see* Corrosion, genital organs, external, female
  wrist T23.479 ☑
    first degree T23.579 ☑
    left T23.472 ☑
      first degree T23.572 ☑
      second degree T23.672 ☑
      third degree T23.772 ☑
    multiple sites with hand T23.499 ☑
      first degree T23.599 ☑
      left T23.492 ☑
        first degree T23.592 ☑
        second degree T23.692 ☑
        third degree T23.792 ☑
      right T23.491 ☑
        first degree T23.591 ☑
        second degree T23.691 ☑
        third degree T23.791 ☑
      second degree T23.699 ☑
      third degree T23.799 ☑
    right T23.471 ☑
      first degree T23.571 ☑
      second degree T23.671 ☑
      third degree T23.771 ☑
    second degree T23.679 ☑
    third degree T23.779 ☑
Corrosive burn — *see* Corrosion
Corsican fever — *see* Malaria
Cortical — *see* condition
Cortico-adrenal — *see* condition
Coryza (acute) J00
  with grippe or influenza — *see* Influenza, with, respiratory manifestations NEC
  syphilitic
    congenital (chronic) A50.05
Costen's syndrome or complex M26.69
Costiveness — *see* Constipation
Costochondritis M94.0
Cot death R99
Cotard's syndrome F22
Cotia virus B08.8
Cotton wool spots (retinal) H35.81

Cotungo's disease — *see* Sciatica
Cough (affected) (chronic) (epidemic) (nervous) R05
  with hemorrhage — *see* Hemoptysis
  bronchial R05
    with grippe or influenza — *see* Influenza, with, respiratory manifestations NEC
  functional F45.8
  hysterical F45.8
  laryngeal, spasmodic R05
  psychogenic F45.8
  smokers' J41.0
  tea taster's B49
Counseling (for) Z71.9
  abuse NEC
    perpetrator Z69.82
    victim Z69.81
  alcohol abuser Z71.41
    family Z71.42
  child abuse
    nonparental
      perpetrator Z69.021
      victim Z69.020
    parental
      perpetrator Z69.011
      victim Z69.010
  consanguinity Z71.89
  contraceptive Z30.09
  dietary Z71.3
  drug abuser Z71.51
    family member Z71.52
  exercise Z71.82
  family Z71.89
  fertility preservation (prior to cancer therapy) (prior to removal of gonads) Z31.62
  for non-attending third party Z71.0
    related to sexual behavior or orientation Z70.2
  genetic
    nonprocreative Z71.83
    procreative NEC Z31.5
  gestational carrier Z31.7
  health (advice) (education) (instruction) — *see* Counseling, medical
  human immunodeficiency virus (HIV) Z71.7
  impotence Z70.1
  insulin pump use Z46.81
  medical (for) Z71.9
    boarding school resident Z59.3
    consanguinity Z71.89
    feared complaint and no disease found Z71.1
    human immunodeficiency virus (HIV) Z71.7
    institutional resident Z59.3
    on behalf of another Z71.0
      related to sexual behavior or orientation Z70.2
    person living alone Z60.2
    specified reason NEC Z71.89
  natural family planning
    procreative Z31.61
    to avoid pregnancy Z30.02
  perpetrator (of)
    abuse NEC Z69.82
    child abuse
      non-parental Z69.021
      parental Z69.011
    rape NEC Z69.82
    spousal abuse Z69.12
  procreative NEC Z31.69
    fertility preservation (prior to cancer therapy) (prior to removal of gonads) Z31.62
    using natural family planning Z31.61
  promiscuity Z70.1
  rape victim Z69.81
  religious Z71.81
  sex, sexual (related to) Z70.9
    attitude(s) Z70.0
    behavior or orientation Z70.1
    combined concerns Z70.3
    non-responsiveness Z70.1
    on behalf of third party Z70.2
    specified reason NEC Z70.8
  specified reason NEC Z71.89
  spiritual Z71.81
  spousal abuse (perpetrator) Z69.12
    victim Z69.11
  substance abuse Z71.89
    alcohol Z71.41
    drug Z71.51
    tobacco Z71.6
  tobacco use Z71.6

Counseling — *continued*
  use (of)
    insulin pump Z46.81
  victim (of)
    abuse Z69.81
    child abuse
      by parent Z69.010
      non-parental Z69.020
    rape NEC Z69.81
Coupled rhythm R00.8
Couvelaire syndrome or uterus (complicating delivery) O45.8X- ☑
Cowperitis — *see* Urethritis
Cowper's gland — *see* condition
Cowpox B08.010
  due to vaccination T88.1 ☑
Coxa
  magna M91.4- ☑
  plana M91.2- ☑
  valga (acquired) (*see also* Deformity, limb, specified type NEC, thigh)
    congenital Q65.81
    sequelae (late effect) of rickets E64.3
  vara (acquired) (*see also* Deformity, limb, specified type NEC, thigh)
    congenital Q65.82
    sequelae (late effect) of rickets E64.3
Coxalgia, coxalgic (nontuberculous) (*see also* Pain, joint, hip)
  tuberculous A18.02
Coxitis — *see* Monoarthritis, hip
Coxsackie (virus) (infection) B34.1
  as cause of disease classified elsewhere B97.11
  carditis B33.20
  central nervous system NEC A88.8
  endocarditis B33.21
  enteritis A08.39
  meningitis (aseptic) A87.0
  myocarditis B33.22
  pericarditis B33.23
  pharyngitis B08.5
  pleurodynia B33.0
  specific disease NEC B33.8
Crabs, meaning pubic lice B85.3
Crack baby P04.41
Cracked nipple N64.0
  associated with
    lactation O92.13
    pregnancy O92.11- ☑
    puerperium O92.12
Cracked tooth K03.81
Cradle cap L21.0
Craft neurosis F48.8
Cramp(s) R25.2
  abdominal — *see* Pain, abdominal
  bathing T75.1 ☑
  colic R10.83
    psychogenic F45.8
  due to immersion T75.1 ☑
  fireman T67.2 ☑
  heat T67.2 ☑
  immersion T75.1 ☑
  intestinal — *see* Pain, abdominal
    psychogenic F45.8
  leg, sleep related G47.62
  limb (lower) (upper) NEC R25.2
    sleep related G47.62
  linotypist's F48.8
    organic G25.89
  muscle (limb) (general) R25.2
    due to immersion T75.1 ☑
    psychogenic F45.8
  occupational (hand) F48.8
    organic G25.89
  salt-depletion E87.1
  sleep related, leg G47.62
  stoker's T67.2 ☑
  swimmer's T75.1 ☑
  telegrapher's F48.8
    organic G25.89
  typist's F48.8
    organic G25.89
  uterus N94.89
    menstrual — *see* Dysmenorrhea
  writer's F48.8
    organic G25.89
Cranial — *see* condition

☑ **Additional Character Required** — Refer to the Tabular List for Character Selection   ▽ **Subterms under main terms may continue to next column or page**

Craniocleidodysostosis Q74.0
Craniofenestria (skull) Q75.8
Craniolacunia (skull) Q75.8
Craniopagus Q89.4
Craniopathy, metabolic M85.2
Craniopharyngeal — *see* condition
Craniopharyngioma D44.4
Craniorachischisis (totalis) Q00.1
Cranioschisis Q75.8
Craniostenosis Q75.0
Craniosynostosis Q75.0
Craniotabes (cause unknown) M83.8
  neonatal P96.3
  rachitic E64.3
  syphilitic A50.56
Cranium — *see* condition
Craw-craw — *see* Onchocerciasis
Creaking joint — *see* Derangement, joint, specified type NEC
Creeping
  eruption B76.9
  palsy or paralysis G12.22
Crenated tongue K14.8
Creotoxism A05.9
Crepitus
  caput Q75.8
  joint — *see* Derangement, joint, specified type NEC
Crescent or conus choroid, congenital Q14.3
CREST syndrome M34.1
Cretin, cretinism (congenital) (endemic) (nongoitrous) (sporadic) E00.9
  pelvis
    with disproportion (fetopelvic) O33.0
      causing obstructed labor O65.0
  type
    hypothyroid E00.1
    mixed E00.2
    myxedematous E00.1
    neurological E00.0
Creutzfeldt-Jakob disease or syndrome (with dementia) A81.00
  familial A81.09
  iatrogenic A81.09
  specified NEC A81.09
  sporadic A81.09
  variant (vCJD) A81.01
Crib death R99
Cribriform hymen Q52.3
Cri-du-chat syndrome Q93.4
Crigler-Najjar disease or syndrome E80.5
Crime, victim of Z65.4
Crimean hemorrhagic fever A98.0
Criminalism F60.2
Crisis
  abdomen R10.0
  acute reaction F43.0
  addisonian E27.2
  adrenal (cortical) E27.2
  celiac K90.0
  Dietl's N13.8
  emotional (*see also* Disorder, adjustment)
    acute reaction to stress F43.0
    specific to childhood and adolescence F93.8
  glaucomatocyclitic — *see* Glaucoma, secondary, inflammation
  heart — *see* Failure, heart
  nitritoid I95.2
    correct substance properly administered — *see* Table of Drugs and Chemicals, by drug, adverse effect
    overdose or wrong substance given or taken — *see* Table of Drugs and Chemicals, by drug, poisoning
  oculogyric H51.8
    psychogenic F45.8
  Pel's (tabetic) A52.11
  psychosexual identity F64.2
  renal N28.0
  sickle-cell D57.00
    with
      acute chest syndrome D57.01
      splenic sequestration D57.02
  state (acute reaction) F43.0
  tabetic A52.11
  thyroid — *see* Thyrotoxicosis with thyroid storm
  thyrotoxic — *see* Thyrotoxicosis with thyroid storm
Crocq's disease (acrocyanosis) I73.89

Crohn's disease — *see* Enteritis, regional
Crooked septum, nasal J34.2
Cross syndrome E70.328
Crossbite (anterior) (posterior) M26.24
Cross-eye — *see* Strabismus, convergent concomitant
Croup, croupous (catarrhal) (infectious) (inflammatory) (nondiphtheritic) J05.0
  bronchial J20.9
  diphtheritic A36.2
  false J38.5
  spasmodic J38.5
    diphtheritic A36.2
  stridulous J38.5
    diphtheritic A36.2
Crouzon's disease Q75.1
Crowding, tooth, teeth, fully erupted M26.31
CRST syndrome M34.1
Cruchet's disease A85.8
Cruelty in children (*see also* Disorder, conduct)
Crural ulcer — *see* Ulcer, lower limb
Crush, crushed, crushing T14.8 ☑
  abdomen S38.1 ☑
  ankle S97.0- ☑
  arm (upper) (and shoulder) S47.- ☑
  axilla — *see* Crush, arm
  back, lower S38.1 ☑
  buttock S38.1 ☑
  cheek S07.0 ☑
  chest S28.0 ☑
  cranium S07.1 ☑
  ear S07.0 ☑
  elbow S57.0- ☑
  extremity
    lower
      ankle — *see* Crush, ankle
      below knee — *see* Crush, leg
      foot — *see* Crush, foot
      hip — *see* Crush, hip
      knee — *see* Crush, knee
      thigh — *see* Crush, thigh
      toe — *see* Crush, toe
    upper
      below elbow S67.9- ☑
      elbow — *see* Crush, elbow
      finger — *see* Crush, finger
      forearm — *see* Crush, forearm
      hand — *see* Crush, hand
      thumb — *see* Crush, thumb
      upper arm — *see* Crush, arm
      wrist — *see* Crush, wrist
  face S07.0 ☑
  finger(s) S67.1- ☑
    with hand (and wrist) — *see* Crush, hand, specified site NEC
    index S67.19- ☑
    little S67.19- ☑
    middle S67.19- ☑
    ring S67.19- ☑
    thumb — *see* Crush, thumb
  foot S97.8- ☑
    toe — *see* Crush, toe
  forearm S57.8- ☑
  genitalia, external
    female S38.002 ☑
      vagina S38.03 ☑
      vulva S38.03 ☑
    male S38.001 ☑
      penis S38.01 ☑
      scrotum S38.02 ☑
      testis S38.02 ☑
  hand (except fingers alone) S67.2- ☑
    with wrist S67.4- ☑
  head S07.9 ☑
    specified NEC S07.8 ☑
  heel — *see* Crush, foot
  hip S77.0- ☑
    with thigh S77.2- ☑
  internal organ (abdomen, chest, or pelvis) NEC T14.8 ☑
  knee S87.0- ☑
  labium (majus) (minus) S38.03 ☑
  larynx S17.0 ☑
  leg (lower) S87.8- ☑
    knee — *see* Crush, knee
  lip S07.0 ☑

Crush, crushed, crushing — *continued*
  lower
    back S38.1 ☑
    leg — *see* Crush, leg
  neck S17.9 ☑
  nerve — *see* Injury, nerve
  nose S07.0 ☑
  pelvis S38.1 ☑
  penis S38.01 ☑
  scalp S07.8 ☑
  scapular region — *see* Crush, arm
  scrotum S38.02 ☑
  severe, unspecified site T14.8 ☑
  shoulder (and upper arm) — *see* Crush, arm
  skull S07.1 ☑
  syndrome (complication of trauma) T79.5 ☑
  testis S38.02 ☑
  thigh S77.1- ☑
    with hip S77.2- ☑
  throat S17.8 ☑
  thumb S67.0- ☑
    with hand (and wrist) — *see* Crush, hand, specified site NEC
  toe(s) S97.10- ☑
    great S97.11- ☑
    lesser S97.12- ☑
  trachea S17.0 ☑
  vagina S38.03 ☑
  vulva S38.03 ☑
  wrist S67.3- ☑
    with hand S67.4- ☑
Crusta lactea L21.0
Crusts R23.4
Crutch paralysis — *see* Injury, brachial plexus
Cruveilhier-Baumgarten cirrhosis, disease or syndrome K74.69
Cruveilhier's atrophy or disease G12.8
Crying (constant) (continuous) (excessive)
  child, adolescent, or adult R45.83
  infant (baby) (newborn) R68.11
Cryofibrinogenemia D89.2
Cryoglobulinemia (essential) (idiopathic) (mixed) (primary) (purpura) (secondary) (vasculitis) D89.1
  with lung involvement D89.1 [J99]
Cryptitis (anal) (rectal) K62.89
Cryptococcosis, cryptococcus (infection) (neoformans) B45.9
  bone B45.3
  cerebral B45.1
  cutaneous B45.2
  disseminated B45.7
  generalized B45.7
  meningitis B45.1
  meningocerebralis B45.1
  osseous B45.3
  pulmonary B45.0
  skin B45.2
  specified NEC B45.8
Cryptopapillitis (anus) K62.89
Cryptophthalmos Q11.2
  syndrome Q87.0
Cryptorchid, cryptorchism, cryptorchidism Q53.9
  bilateral Q53.20
    abdominal Q53.211
    perineal Q53.22
  unilateral Q53.10
    abdominal Q53.111
    perineal Q53.12
Cryptosporidiosis A07.2
  hepatobiliary B88.8
  respiratory B88.8
Cryptostromosis J67.6
Crystalluria R82.99
Cubitus
  congenital Q68.8
  valgus (acquired) M21.0- ☑
    congenital Q68.8
    sequelae (late effect) of rickets E64.3
  varus (acquired) M21.1- ☑
    congenital Q68.8
    sequelae (late effect) of rickets E64.3
Cultural deprivation or shock Z60.3
Curling esophagus K22.4
Curling's ulcer — *see* Ulcer, peptic, acute
Curschmann (-Batten) (-Steinert) **disease or syndrome** G71.11
Curse, Ondine's — *see* Apnea, sleep

Curvature
organ or site, congenital NEC — *see* Distortion
penis (lateral) Q55.61
Pott's (spinal) A18.01
radius, idiopathic, progressive (congenital) Q74.0
spine (acquired) (angular) (idiopathic) (incorrect)
(postural) — *see* Dorsopathy, deforming
congenital Q67.5
due to or associated with
Charcot-Marie-Tooth disease (*see also* subcategory M49.8) G60.0
osteitis
deformans M88.88
fibrosa cystica (*see also* subcategory M49.8)
E21.0
tuberculosis (Pott's curvature) A18.01
sequelae (late effect) of rickets E64.3
tuberculous A18.01
Cushingoid due to steroid therapy E24.2
correct substance properly administered — *see* Table
of Drugs and Chemicals, by drug, adverse effect
overdose or wrong substance given or taken — *see*
Table of Drugs and Chemicals, by drug, poisoning
Cushing's
syndrome or disease E24.9
drug-induced E24.2
iatrogenic E24.2
pituitary-dependent E24.0
specified NEC E24.8
ulcer — *see* Ulcer, peptic, acute
Cusp, Carabelli — *omit code*
Cut (external) (*see also* Laceration)
muscle — *see* Injury, muscle
Cutaneous (*see also* condition)
hemorrhage R23.3
larva migrans B76.9
Cutis (*see also* condition)
hyperelastica Q82.8
acquired L57.4
laxa (hyperelastica) — *see* Dermatolysis
marmorata R23.8
osteosis L94.2
pendula — *see* Dermatolysis
rhomboidalis nuchae L57.2
verticis gyrata Q82.8
acquired L91.8
Cyanosis R23.0
due to
patent foramen botalli Q21.1
persistent foramen ovale Q21.1
enterogenous D74.8
paroxysmal digital — *see* Raynaud's disease
with gangrene I73.01
retina, retinal H35.89
Cyanotic heart disease I24.9
congenital Q24.9
Cycle
anovulatory N97.0
menstrual, irregular N92.6
Cyclencephaly Q04.9
Cyclical vomiting (*see also* Vomiting, cyclical) G43.A0
(*following* G43.7)
psychogenic F50.89
Cyclitis (*see also* Iridocyclitis) H20.9
chronic — *see* Iridocyclitis, chronic
Fuchs' heterochromic H20.81- ☑
granulomatous — *see* Iridocyclitis, chronic
lens-induced — *see* Iridocyclitis, lens-induced
posterior H30.2- ☑
Cycloid personality F34.0
Cyclophoria H50.54
Cyclopia, cyclops Q87.0
Cyclopism Q87.0
Cyclosporiasis A07.4
Cyclothymia F34.0
Cyclothymic personality F34.0
Cyclotropia H50.41- ☑
Cylindroma (*see also* Neoplasm, malignant, by site)
eccrine dermal — *see* Neoplasm, skin, benign
skin — *see* Neoplasm, skin, benign
Cylindruria R82.99
Cynanche
diphtheritic A36.2
tonsillaris J36
Cynophobia F40.218
Cynorexia R63.2

Cyphosis — *see* Kyphosis
Cyprus fever — *see* Brucellosis
Cyst (colloid) (mucous) (simple) (retention)
adenoid (infected) J35.8
adrenal gland E27.8
congenital Q89.1
air, lung J98.4
allantoic Q64.4
alveolar process (jaw bone) M27.40
amnion, amniotic O41.8X- ☑
aneurysmal M27.49
anterior
chamber (eye) — *see* Cyst, iris
nasopalatine K09.1
antrum J34.1
anus K62.89
apical (tooth) (periodontal) K04.8
appendix K38.8
arachnoid, brain (acquired) G93.0
congenital Q04.6
arytenoid J38.7
Baker's M71.2- ☑
ruptured M66.0
tuberculous A18.02
Bartholin's gland N75.0
bile duct (common) (hepatic) K83.5
bladder (multiple) (trigone) N32.89
blue dome (breast) — *see* Cyst, breast
bone (local) NEC M85.60
aneurysmal M85.50
ankle M85.57- ☑
foot M85.57- ☑
forearm M85.53- ☑
hand M85.54- ☑
jaw M27.49
lower leg M85.56- ☑
multiple site M85.59
neck M85.58
rib M85.58
shoulder M85.51- ☑
skull M85.58
specified site NEC M85.58
thigh M85.55- ☑
toe M85.57- ☑
upper arm M85.52- ☑
vertebra M85.58
solitary M85.40
ankle M85.47- ☑
fibula M85.46- ☑
foot M85.47- ☑
hand M85.44- ☑
humerus M85.42- ☑
jaw M27.49
neck M85.48
pelvis M85.45- ☑
radius M85.43- ☑
rib M85.48
shoulder M85.41- ☑
skull M85.48
specified site NEC M85.48
tibia M85.46- ☑
toe M85.47- ☑
ulna M85.43- ☑
vertebra M85.48
specified type NEC M85.60
ankle M85.67- ☑
foot M85.67- ☑
forearm M85.63- ☑
hand M85.64- ☑
jaw M27.40
developmental (nonodontogenic) K09.1
odontogenic K09.0
latent M27.0
lower leg M85.66- ☑
multiple site M85.69
neck M85.68
rib M85.68
shoulder M85.61- ☑
skull M85.68
specified site NEC M85.68
thigh M85.65- ☑
toe M85.67- ☑
upper arm M85.62- ☑
vertebra M85.68
brain (acquired) G93.0
congenital Q04.6
hydatid B67.99 [G94]

Cyst — *continued*
brain — *continued*
third ventricle (colloid), congenital Q04.6
branchial (cleft) Q18.0
branchiogenic Q18.0
breast (benign) (blue dome) (pedunculated) (solitary)
N60.0- ☑
involution — *see* Dysplasia, mammary, specified
type NEC
sebaceous — *see* Dysplasia, mammary, specified
type NEC
broad ligament (benign) N83.8
bronchogenic (mediastinal) (sequestration) J98.4
congenital Q33.0
buccal K09.8
bulbourethral gland N36.8
bursa, bursal NEC M71.30
with rupture — *see* Rupture, synovium
ankle M71.37- ☑
elbow M71.32- ☑
foot M71.37- ☑
hand M71.34- ☑
hip M71.35- ☑
multiple sites M71.39
pharyngeal J39.2
popliteal space — *see* Cyst, Baker's
shoulder M71.31- ☑
specified site NEC M71.38
wrist M71.33- ☑
calcifying odontogenic D16.5
upper jaw (bone) (maxilla) D16.4
canal of Nuck (female) N94.89
congenital Q52.4
canthus — *see* Cyst, conjunctiva
carcinomatous — *see* Neoplasm, malignant, by site
cauda equina G95.89
cavum septi pellucidi — *see* Cyst, brain
celomic (pericardium) Q24.8
cerebellopontine (angle) — *see* Cyst, brain
cerebellum — *see* Cyst, brain
cerebral — *see* Cyst, brain
cervical lateral Q18.0
cervix NEC N88.8
embryonic Q51.6
nabothian N88.8
chiasmal optic NEC — *see* Disorder, optic, chiasm
chocolate (ovary) N80.1
choledochus, congenital Q44.4
chorion O41.8X- ☑
choroid plexus G93.0
ciliary body — *see* Cyst, iris
clitoris N90.7
colon K63.89
common (bile) duct K83.5
congenital NEC Q89.8
adrenal gland Q89.1
epiglottis Q31.8
esophagus Q39.8
fallopian tube Q50.4
kidney Q61.00
more than one (multiple) Q61.02
specified as polycystic Q61.3
adult type Q61.2
infantile type NEC Q61.19
collecting duct dilation Q61.11
solitary Q61.01
larynx Q31.8
liver Q44.6
lung Q33.0
mediastinum Q34.1
ovary Q50.1
oviduct Q50.4
periurethral (tissue) Q64.79
prepuce Q55.69
salivary gland (any) Q38.4
sublingual Q38.6
submaxillary gland Q38.6
thymus (gland) Q89.2
tongue Q38.3
ureterovesical orifice Q62.8
vulva Q52.79
conjunctiva H11.44- ☑
cornea H18.89- ☑
corpora quadrigemina G93.0
corpus
albicans N83.29- ☑
luteum (hemorrhagic) (ruptured) N83.1- ☑
Cowper's gland (benign) (infected) N36.8

☑ **Additional Character Required** — Refer to the Tabular List for Character Selection
🖤 **Subterms under main terms may continue to next column or page**

Cyst — *continued*
- cranial meninges G93.0
- craniobuccal pouch E23.6
- craniopharyngeal pouch E23.6
- cystic duct K82.8
- Cysticercus — *see* Cysticercosis
- Dandy-Walker Q03.1
  - with spina bifida — *see* Spina bifida
- dental (root) K04.8
  - developmental K09.0
  - eruption K09.0
  - primordial K09.0
- dentigerous (mandible) (maxilla) K09.0
- dermoid — *see* Neoplasm, benign, by site
  - with malignant transformation C56.- ☑
  - implantation
    - external area or site (skin) NEC L72.0
    - iris — *see* Cyst, iris, implantation
    - vagina N89.8
    - vulva N90.7
  - mouth K09.8
  - oral soft tissue K09.8
  - sacrococcygeal — *see* Cyst, pilonidal
- developmental K09.1
  - odontogenic K09.0
  - oral region (nonodontogenic) K09.1
  - ovary, ovarian Q50.1
- dura (cerebral) G93.0
  - spinal G96.19
- ear (external) Q18.1
- echinococcal — *see* Echinococcus
- embryonic
  - cervix uteri Q51.6
  - fallopian tube Q50.4
  - vagina Q52.4
- endometrium, endometrial (uterus) N85.8
  - ectopic — *see* Endometriosis
- enterogenous Q43.8
- epidermal, epidermoid (inclusion) (*see also* Cyst, skin) L72.0
  - mouth K09.8
  - oral soft tissue K09.8
- epididymis N50.3
- epiglottis J38.7
- epiphysis cerebri E34.8
- epithelial (inclusion) L72.0
- epoophoron Q50.5
- eruption K09.0
- esophagus K22.8
- ethmoid sinus J34.1
- external female genital organs NEC N90.7
- eyelid (sebaceous) H02.829
  - infected — *see* Hordeolum
  - left H02.826
    - lower H02.825
    - upper H02.824
  - right H02.823
    - lower H02.822
    - upper H02.821
- eye NEC H57.8
  - congenital Q15.8
- fallopian tube N83.8
  - congenital Q50.4
- fimbrial (twisted) Q50.4
- fissural (oral region) K09.1
- follicle (graafian) (hemorrhagic) N83.0- ☑
  - nabothian N88.8
- follicular (atretic) (hemorrhagic) (ovarian) N83.0- ☑
  - dentigerous K09.0
  - odontogenic K09.0
  - skin L72.9
    - specified NEC L72.8
- frontal sinus J34.1
- gallbladder K82.8
- ganglion — *see* Ganglion
- Gartner's duct Q52.4
- gingiva K09.0
- gland of Moll — *see* Cyst, eyelid
- globulomaxillary K09.1
- graafian follicle (hemorrhagic) N83.0- ☑
- granulosal lutein (hemorrhagic) N83.1- ☑
- hemangiomatous D18.00
  - intra-abdominal D18.03
  - intracranial D18.02
  - skin D18.01
  - specified site NEC D18.09
- hemorrhagic M27.49
- hydatid (*see also* Echinococcus) B67.90

Cyst — *continued*
- hydatid (*see also* Echinococcus) — *continued*
  - brain B67.99 [G94]
  - liver (*see also* Cyst, liver, hydatid) B67.8
  - lung NEC B67.99 [J99]
  - Morgagni
    - female Q50.5
    - male (epididymal) Q55.4
      - testicular Q55.29
  - specified site NEC B67.99
- hymen N89.8
  - embryonic Q52.4
- hypopharynx J39.2
- hypophysis, hypophyseal (duct) (recurrent) E23.6
  - cerebri E23.6
- implantation (dermoid)
  - external area or site (skin) NEC L72.0
  - iris — *see* Cyst, iris, implantation
  - vagina N89.8
  - vulva N90.7
- incisive canal K09.1
- inclusion (epidermal) (epithelial) (epidermoid) (squamous) L72.0
  - not of skin — *code under* Cyst, by site
- intestine (large) (small) K63.89
- intracranial — *see* Cyst, brain
- intraligamentous (*see also* Disorder, ligament)
  - knee — *see* Derangement, knee
- intrasellar E23.6
- iris H21.309
  - exudative H21.31- ☑
  - idiopathic H21.30- ☑
  - implantation H21.32- ☑
  - parasitic H21.33- ☑
  - pars plana (primary) H21.34- ☑
    - exudative H21.35- ☑
- jaw (bone) M27.40
  - aneurysmal M27.49
  - developmental (odontogenic) K09.0
  - fissural K09.1
  - hemorrhagic M27.49
  - traumatic M27.49
- joint NEC — *see* Disorder, joint, specified type NEC
- kidney (acquired) N28.1
  - calyceal — *see* Hydronephrosis
  - congenital Q61.00
  - more than one (multiple) Q61.02
    - specified as polycystic Q61.3
      - adult type (autosomal dominant) Q61.2
      - infantile type (autosomal recessive) NEC Q61.19
        - collecting duct dilation Q61.11
  - pyelogenic — *see* Hydronephrosis
  - simple N28.1
  - solitary (single) Q61.01
    - acquired N28.1
- labium (majus) (minus) N90.7
  - sebaceous N90.7
- lacrimal (*see also* Disorder, lacrimal system, specified NEC)
  - gland H04.13- ☑
  - passages or sac — *see* Disorder, lacrimal system, specified NEC
- larynx J38.7
- lateral periodontal K09.0
- lens H27.8
  - congenital Q12.8
- lip (gland) K13.0
- liver (idiopathic) (simple) K76.89
  - congenital Q44.6
  - hydatid B67.8
    - granulosus B67.0
    - multilocularis B67.5
- lung J98.4
  - congenital Q33.0
  - giant bullous J43.9
- lutein N83.1- ☑
- lymphangiomatous D18.1
- lymphoepithelial, oral soft tissue K09.8
- macula — *see* Degeneration, macula, hole
- malignant — *see* Neoplasm, malignant, by site
- mammary gland — *see* Cyst, breast
- mandible M27.40
  - dentigerous K09.0
  - radicular K04.8
- maxilla M27.40
  - dentigerous K09.0
  - radicular K04.8

Cyst — *continued*
- medial, face and neck Q18.8
- median
  - anterior maxillary K09.1
  - palatal K09.1
- mediastinum, congenital Q34.1
- meibomian (gland) — *see* Chalazion
  - infected — *see* Hordeolum
- membrane, brain G93.0
- meninges (cerebral) G93.0
  - spinal G96.19
- meniscus, knee — *see* Derangement, knee, meniscus, cystic
- mesentery, mesenteric K66.8
  - chyle I89.8
- mesonephric duct
  - female Q50.5
  - male Q55.4
- milk N64.89
- Morgagni (hydatid)
  - female Q50.5
  - male (epididymal) Q55.4
    - testicular Q55.29
- mouth K09.8
- Müllerian duct Q50.4
  - appendix testis Q55.29
  - cervix Q51.6
  - fallopian tube Q50.4
  - female Q50.4
  - male Q55.29
  - prostatic utricle Q55.4
  - vagina (embryonal) Q52.4
- multilocular (ovary) D39.10
  - benign — *see* Neoplasm, benign, by site
- myometrium N85.8
- nabothian (follicle) (ruptured) N88.8
- nasoalveolar K09.1
- nasolabial K09.1
- nasopalatine (anterior) (duct) K09.1
- nasopharynx J39.2
- neoplastic — *see* Neoplasm, uncertain behavior, by site
  - benign — *see* Neoplasm, benign, by site
- nervous system NEC G96.8
- neuroenteric (congenital) Q06.8
- nipple — *see* Cyst, breast
- nose (turbinates) J34.1
  - sinus J34.1
- odontogenic, developmental K09.0
- omentum (lesser) K66.8
  - congenital Q45.8
- ora serrata — *see* Cyst, retina, ora serrata
- oral
  - region K09.9
    - developmental (nonodontogenic) K09.1
    - specified NEC K09.8
  - soft tissue K09.9
    - specified NEC K09.8
- orbit H05.81- ☑
- ovary, ovarian (twisted) N83.20- ☑
  - adherent N83.20- ☑
  - chocolate N80.1
  - corpus
    - albicans N83.29- ☑
    - luteum (hemorrhagic) N83.1- ☑
  - dermoid D27.9
  - developmental Q50.1
  - due to failure of involution NEC N83.20- ☑
  - endometrial N80.1
  - follicular (graafian) (hemorrhagic) N83.0- ☑
  - hemorrhagic N83.20- ☑
  - in pregnancy or childbirth O34.8- ☑
    - with obstructed labor O65.5
  - multilocular D39.10
  - pseudomucinous D27.9
  - retention N83.29- ☑
  - serous N83.20- ☑
  - specified NEC N83.29- ☑
  - theca lutein (hemorrhagic) N83.1- ☑
  - tuberculous A18.18
- oviduct N83.8
- palate (median) (fissural) K09.1
- palatine papilla (jaw) K09.1
- pancreas, pancreatic (hemorrhagic) (true) K86.2
  - congenital Q45.2
  - false K86.3
- paralabral
  - hip M24.85- ☑

Cyst — *continued*
paralabral — *continued*
   shoulder S43.43- ☑
  paramesonephric duct Q50.4
   female Q50.4
   male Q55.29
  paranephric N28.1
  paraphysis, cerebri, congenital Q04.6
  parasitic B89
  parathyroid (gland) E21.4
  paratubal N83.8
  paraurethral duct N36.8
  paroophoron Q50.5
  parotid gland K11.6
  parovarian Q50.5
  pelvis, female N94.89
   in pregnancy or childbirth O34.8- ☑
    causing obstructed labor O65.5
  penis (sebaceous) N48.89
  periapical K04.8
  pericardial (congenital) Q24.8
   acquired (secondary) I31.8
  pericoronal K09.0
  periodontal K04.8
   lateral K09.0
  peripelvic (lymphatic) N28.1
  peritoneum K66.8
   chylous I89.8
  periventricular, acquired, newborn P91.1
  pharynx (wall) J39.2
  pilar L72.11
  pilonidal (infected) (rectum) L05.91
   with abscess L05.01
   malignant C44.59- ☑
  pituitary (duct) (gland) E23.6
  placenta O43.19- ☑
  pleura J94.8
  popliteal — *see* Cyst, Baker's
  porencephalic Q04.6
   acquired G93.0
  postanal (infected) — *see* Cyst, pilonidal
  postmastoidectomy cavity (mucosal) — *see* Complications, postmastoidectomy, cyst
  preauricular Q18.1
  prepuce N47.4
   congenital Q55.69
  primordial (jaw) K09.0
  prostate N42.83
  pseudomucinous (ovary) D27.9
  pupillary, miotic H21.27- ☑
  radicular (residual) K04.8
  radiculodental K04.8
  ranular K11.8
  Rathke's pouch E23.6
  rectum (epithelium) (mucous) K62.89
  renal — *see* Cyst, kidney
  residual (radicular) K04.8
  retention (ovary) N83.29- ☑
   salivary gland K11.6
  retina H33.19- ☑
   ora serrata H33.11- ☑
   parasitic H33.12- ☑
  retroperitoneal K68.9
  sacrococcygeal (dermoid) — *see* Cyst, pilonidal
  salivary gland or duct (mucous extravasation or retention) K11.6
  Sampson's N80.1
  sclera H15.89
  scrotum L72.9
   sebaceous L72.3
  sebaceous (duct) (gland) L72.3
   breast — *see* Dysplasia, mammary, specified type NEC
   eyelid — *see* Cyst, eyelid
   genital organ NEC
    female N94.89
    male N50.89
   scrotum L72.3
  semilunar cartilage (knee) (multiple) — *see* Derangement, knee, meniscus, cystic
  seminal vesicle N50.89
  serous (ovary) N83.20- ☑
  sinus (accessory) (nasal) J34.1
  Skene's gland N36.8
  skin L72.9
   breast — *see* Dysplasia, mammary, specified type NEC
   epidermal, epidermoid L72.0

Cyst — *continued*
skin — *continued*
   epithelial L72.0
   eyelid — *see* Cyst, eyelid
   genital organ NEC
    female N90.7
    male N50.89
   inclusion L72.0
   scrotum L72.9
   sebaceous L72.3
   sweat gland or duct L74.8
  solitary
   bone — *see* Cyst, bone, solitary
   jaw M27.40
   kidney N28.1
  spermatic cord N50.89
  sphenoid sinus J34.1
  spinal meninges G96.19
  spleen NEC D73.4
   congenital Q89.09
   hydatid (*see also* Echinococcus) B67.99 [D77]
  Stafne's M27.0
  subarachnoid intrasellar R93.0
  subcutaneous, pheomycotic (chromomycotic) B43.2
  subdural (cerebral) G93.0
   spinal cord G96.19
  sublingual gland K11.6
  submandibular gland K11.6
  submaxillary gland K11.6
  suburethral N36.8
  suprarenal gland E27.8
  suprasellar — *see* Cyst, brain
  sweat gland or duct L74.8
  synovial (*see also* Cyst, bursa)
   ruptured — *see* Rupture, synovium
  tarsal — *see* Chalazion
  tendon (sheath) — *see* Disorder, tendon, specified type NEC
  testis N44.2
   tunica albuginea N44.1
  theca lutein (ovary) N83.1- ☑
  Thornwaldt's J39.2
  thymus (gland) E32.8
  thyroglossal duct (infected) (persistent) Q89.2
  thyroid (gland) E04.1
  thyrolingual duct (infected) (persistent) Q89.2
  tongue K14.8
  tonsil J35.8
  tooth — *see* Cyst, dental
  Tornwaldt's J39.2
  trichilemmal (proliferating) L72.12
  trichodermal L72.12
  tubal (fallopian) N83.8
   inflammatory — *see* Salpingitis, chronic
  tubo-ovarian N83.8
   inflammatory N70.13
  tunica
   albuginea testis N44.1
   vaginalis N50.89
  turbinate (nose) J34.1
  Tyson's gland N48.89
  urachus, congenital Q64.4
  ureter N28.89
  ureterovesical orifice N28.89
  urethra, urethral (gland) N36.8
  uterine ligament N83.8
  uterus (body) (corpus) (recurrent) N85.8
   embryonic Q51.818
   cervix Q51.6
  vagina, vaginal (implantation) (inclusion) (squamous cell) (wall) N89.8
   embryonic Q52.4
  vallecula, vallecular (epiglottis) J38.7
  vesical (orifice) N32.89
  vitreous body H43.89
  vulva (implantation) (inclusion) N90.7
   congenital Q52.79
   sebaceous gland N90.7
  vulvovaginal gland N90.7
  wolffian
   female Q50.5
   male Q55.4

Cystadenocarcinoma — *see* Neoplasm, malignant, by site
  bile duct C22.1
  endometrioid — *see* Neoplasm, malignant, by site
   specified site — *see* Neoplasm, malignant, by site

Cystadenocarcinoma — *continued*
endometrioid — *see* Neoplasm, malignant, by site — *continued*
   unspecified site
    female C56.9
    male C61
  mucinous
   papillary
    specified site — *see* Neoplasm, malignant, by site
    unspecified site C56.9
   specified site — *see* Neoplasm, malignant, by site
   unspecified site C56.9
  papillary
   mucinous
    specified site — *see* Neoplasm, malignant, by site
    unspecified site C56.9
   pseudomucinous
    specified site — *see* Neoplasm, malignant, by site
    unspecified site C56.9
   serous
    specified site — *see* Neoplasm, malignant, by site
    unspecified site C56.9
   specified site — *see* Neoplasm, malignant, by site
   unspecified site C56.9
  pseudomucinous
   papillary
    specified site — *see* Neoplasm, malignant, by site
    unspecified site C56.9
   specified site — *see* Neoplasm, malignant, by site
   unspecified site C56.9
  serous
   papillary
    specified site — *see* Neoplasm, malignant, by site
    unspecified site C56.9
   specified site — *see* Neoplasm, malignant, by site
   unspecified site C56.9

Cystadenofibroma
  clear cell — *see* Neoplasm, benign, by site
  endometrioid D27.9
   borderline malignancy D39.1- ☑
   malignant C56.- ☑
  mucinous
   specified site — *see* Neoplasm, benign, by site
   unspecified site D27.9
  serous
   specified site — *see* Neoplasm, benign, by site
   unspecified site D27.9
  specified site — *see* Neoplasm, benign, by site
  unspecified site D27.9

Cystadenoma (*see also* Neoplasm, benign, by site)
  bile duct D13.4
  endometrioid — *see* Neoplasm, benign, by site
   borderline malignancy — *see* Neoplasm, uncertain behavior, by site
   malignant — *see* Neoplasm, malignant, by site
  mucinous
   borderline malignancy
    ovary C56.- ☑
    specified site NEC — *see* Neoplasm, uncertain behavior, by site
    unspecified site C56.9
   papillary
    borderline malignancy
     ovary C56.- ☑
     specified site NEC — *see* Neoplasm, uncertain behavior, by site
     unspecified site C56.9
    specified site — *see* Neoplasm, benign, by site
    unspecified site D27.9
   specified site — *see* Neoplasm, benign, by site
   unspecified site D27.9
  papillary
   borderline malignancy
    ovary C56.- ☑
    specified site NEC — *see* Neoplasm, uncertain behavior, by site
    unspecified site C56.9
   lymphomatosum
    specified site — *see* Neoplasm, benign, by site
    unspecified site D11.9

☑ Additional Character Required — Refer to the Tabular List for Character Selection   ▽ Subterms under main terms may continue to next column or page

Cystadenoma — *continued*
  papillary — *continued*
    mucinous
      borderline malignancy
        ovary C56.- ☑
        specified site NEC — *see* Neoplasm, uncertain behavior, by site
        unspecified site C56.9
      specified site — *see* Neoplasm, benign, by site
      unspecified site D27.9
    pseudomucinous
      borderline malignancy
        ovary C56.- ☑
        specified site NEC — *see* Neoplasm, uncertain behavior, by site
        unspecified site C56.9
      specified site — *see* Neoplasm, benign, by site
      unspecified site D27.9
    serous
      borderline malignancy
        ovary C56.- ☑
        specified site NEC — *see* Neoplasm, uncertain behavior, by site
        unspecified site C56.9
      specified site — *see* Neoplasm, benign, by site
      unspecified site D27.9
  specified site — *see* Neoplasm, benign, by site
  unspecified site D27.9
  pseudomucinous
    borderline malignancy
      ovary C56.- ☑
      specified site NEC — *see* Neoplasm, uncertain behavior, by site
      unspecified site C56.9
    papillary
      borderline malignancy
        ovary C56.- ☑
        specified site NEC — *see* Neoplasm, uncertain behavior, by site
        unspecified site C56.9
      specified site — *see* Neoplasm, benign, by site
      unspecified site D27.9
    specified site — *see* Neoplasm, benign, by site
    unspecified site D27.9
  serous
    borderline malignancy
      ovary C56.- ☑
      specified site NEC — *see* Neoplasm, uncertain behavior, by site
      unspecified site C56.9
    papillary
      borderline malignancy
        ovary C56.- ☑
        specified site NEC — *see* Neoplasm, uncertain behavior, by site
        unspecified site C56.9
      specified site — *see* Neoplasm, benign, by site
      unspecified site D27.9
    specified site — *see* Neoplasm, benign, by site
    unspecified site D27.9
Cystathionine synthase deficiency E72.11
Cystathioninemia E72.19
Cystathioninuria E72.19
Cystic (*see also* condition)
  breast (chronic) — *see* Mastopathy, cystic
  corpora lutea (hemorrhagic) N83.1- ☑
  duct — *see* condition
  eyeball (congenital) Q11.0
  fibrosis — *see* Fibrosis, cystic
  kidney (congenital) Q61.9

Cystic — *continued*
  kidney — *continued*
    adult type Q61.2
    infantile type NEC Q61.19
      collecting duct dilatation Q61.11
    medullary Q61.5
  liver, congenital Q44.6
  lung disease J98.4
    congenital Q33.0
  mastitis, chronic — *see* Mastopathy, cystic
  medullary, kidney Q61.5
  meniscus — *see* Derangement, knee, meniscus, cystic
  ovary N83.20- ☑
Cysticercosis, cysticerciasis B69.9
  with
    epileptiform fits B69.0
    myositis B69.81
  brain B69.0
  central nervous system B69.0
  cerebral B69.0
  ocular B69.1
  specified NEC B69.89
Cysticercus cellulose infestation — *see* Cysticercosis
Cystinosis (malignant) E72.04
Cystinuria E72.01
Cystitis (exudative) (hemorrhagic) (septic) (suppurative) N30.90
  with
    fibrosis — *see* Cystitis, chronic, interstitial
    hematuria N30.91
    leukoplakia — *see* Cystitis, chronic, interstitial
    malakoplakia — *see* Cystitis, chronic, interstitial
    metaplasia — *see* Cystitis, chronic, interstitial
    prostatitis N41.3
  acute N30.00
    with hematuria N30.01
    of trigone N30.30
      with hematuria N30.31
  allergic — *see* Cystitis, specified type NEC
  amebic A06.81
  bilharzial B65.9 [N33]
  blennorrhagic (gonococcal) A54.01
  bullous — *see* Cystitis, specified type NEC
  calculous N21.0
  chlamydial A56.01
  chronic N30.20
    with hematuria N30.21
    interstitial N30.10
      with hematuria N30.11
    of trigone N30.30
      with hematuria N30.31
    specified NEC N30.20
      with hematuria N30.21
  cystic (a) — *see* Cystitis, specified type NEC
  diphtheritic A36.85
  echinococcal
    granulosus B67.39
    multilocularis B67.69
  emphysematous — *see* Cystitis, specified type NEC
  encysted — *see* Cystitis, specified type NEC
  eosinophilic — *see* Cystitis, specified type NEC
  follicular — *see* Cystitis, of trigone
  gangrenous — *see* Cystitis, specified type NEC
  glandularis — *see* Cystitis, specified type NEC
  gonococcal A54.01
  incrusted — *see* Cystitis, specified type NEC
  interstitial (chronic) — *see* Cystitis, chronic, interstitial
  irradiation N30.40
    with hematuria N30.41
  irritation — *see* Cystitis, specified type NEC

Cystitis — *continued*
  malignant — *see* Cystitis, specified type NEC
  of trigone N30.30
    with hematuria N30.31
  panmural — *see* Cystitis, chronic, interstitial
  polyposa — *see* Cystitis, specified type NEC
  prostatic N41.3
  puerperal (postpartum) O86.22
  radiation — *see* Cystitis, irradiation
  specified type NEC N30.80
    with hematuria N30.81
  subacute — *see* Cystitis, chronic
  submucous — *see* Cystitis, chronic, interstitial
  syphilitic (late) A52.76
  trichomonal A59.03
  tuberculous A18.12
  ulcerative — *see* Cystitis, chronic, interstitial
Cystocele (-urethrocele)
  female N81.10
    with prolapse of uterus — *see* Prolapse, uterus
    lateral N81.12
    midline N81.11
    paravaginal N81.12
  in pregnancy or childbirth O34.8- ☑
    causing obstructed labor O65.5
  male N32.89
Cystolithiasis N21.0
Cystoma (*see also* Neoplasm, benign, by site)
  endometrial, ovary N80.1
  mucinous
    specified site — *see* Neoplasm, benign, by site
    unspecified site D27.9
  serous
    specified site — *see* Neoplasm, benign, by site
    unspecified site D27.9
  simple (ovary) N83.29- ☑
Cystoplegia N31.2
Cystoptosis N32.89
Cystopyelitis — *see* Pyelonephritis
Cystorrhagia N32.89
Cystosarcoma phyllodes D48.6- ☑
  benign D24- ☑
  malignant — *see* Neoplasm, breast, malignant
Cystostomy
  attention to Z43.5
  complication — *see* Complications, cystostomy
  status Z93.50
    appendico-vesicostomy Z93.52
    cutaneous Z93.51
    specified NEC Z93.59
Cystourethritis — *see* Urethritis
Cystourethrocele (*see also* Cystocele)
  female N81.10
    with uterine prolapse — *see* Prolapse, uterus
    lateral N81.12
    midline N81.11
    paravaginal N81.12
  male N32.89
Cytomegalic inclusion disease
  congenital P35.1
Cytomegalovirus infection B25.9
Cytomycosis (reticuloendothelial) B39.4
Cytopenia D75.9
  refractory
    with multilineage dysplasia D46.A (*following* D46.2)
    and ring sideroblasts (RCMD RS) D46.B (*following* D46.2)
Czerny's disease (periodic hydrarthrosis of the knee) — *see* Effusion, joint, knee

D

Da Costa's syndrome F45.8
Daae (-Finsen) **disease** (epidemic pleurodynia) B33.0
Dabney's grip B33.0
Dacryoadenitis, dacryadenitis H04.00- ☑
  acute H04.01- ☑
  chronic H04.02- ☑
Dacryocystitis H04.30- ☑
  acute H04.32- ☑
  chronic H04.41- ☑
  neonatal P39.1
  phlegmonous H04.31- ☑
  syphilitic A52.71
    congenital (early) A50.01
  trachomatous, active A71.1
    sequelae (late effect) B94.0
Dacryocystoblenorrhea — *see* Inflammation, lacrimal, passages, chronic
Dacryocystocele — *see* Disorder, lacrimal system, changes
Dacryolith, dacryolithiasis H04.51- ☑
Dacryoma — *see* Disorder, lacrimal system, changes
Dacryopericystitis — *see* Dacryocystitis
Dacryops H04.11- ☑
Dacryostenosis (*see also* Stenosis, lacrimal)
  congenital Q10.5
Dactylitis
  bone — *see* Osteomyelitis
  sickle-cell D57.00
    Hb C D57.219
    Hb SS D57.00
    specified NEC D57.819
  skin L08.9
  syphilitic A52.77
  tuberculous A18.03
Dactylolysis spontanea (ainhum) L94.6
Dactylosymphysis Q70.9
  fingers — *see* Syndactylism, complex, fingers
  toes — *see* Syndactylism, complex, toes
Damage
  arteriosclerotic — *see* Arteriosclerosis
  brain (nontraumatic) G93.9
    anoxic, hypoxic G93.1
      resulting from a procedure G97.82
    child NEC G80.9
    due to birth injury P11.2
  cardiorenal (vascular) — *see* Hypertension, cardiorenal
  cerebral NEC — *see* Damage, brain
  coccyx, complicating delivery O71.6
  coronary — *see* Disease, heart, ischemic
  eye, birth injury P15.3
  liver (nontraumatic) K76.9
    alcoholic K70.9
    due to drugs — *see* Disease, liver, toxic
    toxic — *see* Disease, liver, toxic
  medication T88.7 ☑
  pelvic
    joint or ligament, during delivery O71.6
    organ NEC
      during delivery O71.5
      following ectopic or molar pregnancy O08.6
  renal — *see* Disease, renal
  subendocardium, subendocardial — *see* Degeneration, myocardial
  vascular I99.9
Dana-Putnam syndrome (subacute combined sclerosis with pernicious anemia) — *see* Degeneration, combined
Danbolt (-Cross) **syndrome** (acrodermatitis enteropathica) E83.2
Dandruff L21.0
Dandy-Walker syndrome Q03.1
  with spina bifida — *see* Spina bifida
Danlos' syndrome Q79.6
Darier (-White) **disease** (congenital) Q82.8
  meaning erythema annulare centrifugum L53.1
Darier-Roussy sarcoid D86.3
Darling's disease or histoplasmosis B39.4
Darwin's tubercle Q17.8
Dawson's (inclusion body) **encephalitis** A81.1

De Beurmann (-Gougerot) **disease** B42.1
De la Tourette's syndrome F95.2
De Lange's syndrome Q87.1
De Morgan's spots (senile angiomas) I78.1
De Quervain's
  disease (tendon sheath) M65.4
  syndrome E34.51
  thyroiditis (subacute granulomatous thyroiditis) E06.1
De Toni-Fanconi (-Debré) **syndrome** E72.09
  with cystinosis E72.04
Dead
  fetus, retained (mother) O36.4 ☑
    early pregnancy O02.1
  labyrinth H83.2 ☑
  ovum, retained O02.0
Deaf nonspeaking NEC H91.3
Deafmutism (acquired) (congenital) NEC H91.3
  hysterical F44.6
  syphilitic, congenital (*see also* subcategory) H94.8 A50.09
Deafness (acquired) (complete) (hereditary) (partial) H91.9- ☑
  with blue sclera and fragility of bone Q78.0
  auditory fatigue — *see* Deafness, specified type NEC
  aviation T70.0 ☑
    nerve injury — *see* Injury, nerve, acoustic, specified type NEC
  boilermaker's H83.3 ☑
  central — *see* Deafness, sensorineural
  conductive H90.2
    and sensorineural
      mixed H90.8
        bilateral H90.6
    bilateral H90.0
    unilateral H90.1- ☑
      with restricted hearing on the contralateral side H90.A- ☑
  congenital H90.5
    with blue sclera and fragility of bone Q78.0
  due to toxic agents — *see* Deafness, ototoxic
  emotional (hysterical) F44.6
  functional (hysterical) F44.6
  high frequency H91.9- ☑
  hysterical F44.6
  low frequency H91.9- ☑
  mental R48.8
  mixed conductive and sensorineural H90.8
    bilateral H90.6
    unilateral H90.7- ☑
  nerve — *see* Deafness, sensorineural
  neural — *see* Deafness, sensorineural
  noise-induced (*see also* subcategory) H83.3 ☑
    nerve injury — *see* Injury, nerve, acoustic, specified type NEC
  nonspeaking H91.3
  ototoxic H91.0 ☑
  perceptive — *see* Deafness, sensorineural
  psychogenic (hysterical) F44.6
  sensorineural H90.5
    and conductive
      bilateral H90.6
      mixed H90.8
        bilateral H90.6
    bilateral H90.3
    unilateral H90.4- ☑
      with restricted hearing on the contralateral side H90.A- ☑
  sensory — *see* Deafness, sensorineural
  specified type NEC H91.8 ☑
  sudden (idiopathic) H91.2- ☑
  syphilitic A52.15
  transient ischemic H93.01- ☑
  traumatic — *see* Injury, nerve, acoustic, specified type NEC
  word (developmental) H93.25
Death (cause unknown) (of) (unexplained) (unspecified cause) R99
  brain G93.82
  cardiac (sudden) (with successful resuscitation) — *code to* underlying disease
    family history of Z82.41
    personal history of Z86.74

Death — *continued*
  family member (assumed) Z63.4
Debility (chronic) (general) (nervous) R53.81
  congenital or neonatal NOS P96.9
  nervous R53.81
  old age R54
  senile R54
Débove's disease (splenomegaly) R16.1
Decalcification
  bone — *see* Osteoporosis
  teeth K03.89
Decapsulation, kidney N28.89
Decay
  dental — *see* Caries, dental
  senile R54
  tooth, teeth — *see* Caries, dental
Deciduitis (acute)
  following ectopic or molar pregnancy O08.0
Decline (general) — *see* Debility
  cognitive, age-associated R41.81
Decompensation
  cardiac (acute) (chronic) — *see* Disease, heart
  cardiovascular — *see* Disease, cardiovascular
  heart — *see* Disease, heart
  hepatic — *see* Failure, hepatic
  myocardial (acute) (chronic) — *see* Disease, heart
  respiratory J98.8
Decompression sickness T70.3 ☑
Decrease (d)
  absolute neutrophile count — *see* Neutropenia
  blood
    platelets — *see* Thrombocytopenia
    pressure R03.1
      due to shock following
        injury T79.4 ☑
        operation T81.19 ☑
  estrogen E28.39
    postablative E89.40
      asymptomatic E89.40
      symptomatic E89.41
  fragility of erythrocytes D58.8
  function
    lipase (pancreatic) K90.3
    ovary in hypopituitarism E23.0
    parenchyma of pancreas K86.89
    pituitary (gland) (anterior) (lobe) E23.0
      posterior (lobe) E23.0
  functional activity R68.89
  glucose R73.09
  hematocrit R71.0
  hemoglobin R71.0
  leukocytes D72.819
    specified NEC D72.818
  libido R68.82
  lymphocytes D72.810
  platelets D69.6
  respiration, due to shock following injury T79.4 ☑
  sexual desire R68.82
  tear secretion NEC — *see* Syndrome, dry eye
  tolerance
    fat K90.49
    glucose R73.09
    pancreatic K90.3
    salt and water E87.8
  vision NEC H54.7
  white blood cell count D72.819
    specified NEC D72.818
Decubitus (ulcer) — *see* Ulcer, pressure, by site
  cervix N86
Deepening acetabulum — *see* Derangement, joint, specified type NEC, hip
Defect, defective Q89.9
  3-beta-hydroxysteroid dehydrogenase E25.0
  11-hydroxylase E25.0
  21-hydroxylase E25.0
  abdominal wall, congenital Q79.59
  antibody immunodeficiency D80.9
  aorticopulmonary septum Q21.4
  atrial septal (ostium secundum type) Q21.1
    following acute myocardial infarction (current complication) I23.1
    ostium primum type Q21.2

☑ Additional Character Required — Refer to the Tabular List for Character Selection ▽ Subterms under main terms may continue to next column or page

Defect, defective — *continued*

atrioventricular
  canal Q21.2
  septum Q21.2
auricular septal Q21.1
bilirubin excretion NEC E80.6
biosynthesis, androgen (testicular) E29.1
bulbar septum Q21.0
catalase E80.3
cell membrane receptor complex (CR3) D71
circulation I99.9
  congenital Q28.9
  newborn Q28.9
coagulation (factor) (*see also* Deficiency, factor) D68.9
  with
    ectopic pregnancy O08.1
    molar pregnancy O08.1
  acquired D68.4
  antepartum with hemorrhage — *see* Hemorrhage,
    antepartum, with coagulation defect
  due to
    liver disease D68.4
    vitamin K deficiency D68.4
  hereditary NEC D68.2
  intrapartum O67.0
  newborn, transient P61.6
  postpartum O99.13
    with hemorrhage O72.3
  specified type NEC D68.8
complement system D84.1
conduction (heart) I45.9
  bone — *see* Deafness, conductive
congenital, organ or site not listed — *see* Anomaly,
  by site
coronary sinus Q21.1
cushion, endocardial Q21.2
degradation, glycoprotein E77.1
dental bridge, crown, fillings — *see* Defect, dental
  restoration
dental restoration K08.50
  specified NEC K08.59
dentin (hereditary) K00.5
Descemet's membrane, congenital Q13.89
developmental (*see also* Anomaly)
  cauda equina Q06.3
diaphragm
  with elevation, eventration or hernia — *see* Hernia,
    diaphragm
  congenital Q79.1
    with hernia Q79.0
    gross (with hernia) Q79.0
ectodermal, congenital Q82.9
Eisenmenger's Q21.8
enzyme
  catalase E80.3
  peroxidase E80.3
esophagus, congenital Q39.9
extensor retinaculum M62.89
fibrin polymerization D68.2
filling
  bladder R93.41
  kidney R93.42- ☑
  renal pelvis R93.41
  stomach R93.3
  ureter R93.41
  urinary organs, specified NEC R93.49
Gerbode Q21.0
glycoprotein degradation E77.1
Hageman (factor) D68.2
hearing — *see* Deafness
high grade F70
interatrial septal Q21.1
interauricular septal Q21.1
interventricular septal Q21.0
  with dextroposition of aorta, pulmonary stenosis
    and hypertrophy of right ventricle Q21.3
  in tetralogy of Fallot Q21.3
learning (specific) — *see* Disorder, learning
lymphocyte function antigen-1 (LFA-1) D84.0
lysosomal enzyme, post-translational modification
  E77.0
major osseous M89.70
  ankle M89.77- ☑
  carpus M89.74- ☑
  clavicle M89.71- ☑
  femur M89.75- ☑
  fibula M89.76- ☑
  fingers M89.74- ☑

Defect, defective — *continued*

major osseous — *continued*
  foot M89.77- ☑
  forearm M89.73- ☑
  hand M89.74- ☑
  humerus M89.72- ☑
  lower leg M89.76- ☑
  metacarpus M89.74- ☑
  metatarsus M89.77- ☑
  multiple sites M89.79
  pelvic region M89.75- ☑
  pelvis M89.75- ☑
  radius M89.73- ☑
  scapula M89.71- ☑
  shoulder region M89.71- ☑
  specified NEC M89.78
  tarsus M89.77- ☑
  thigh M89.75- ☑
  tibia M89.76- ☑
  toes M89.77- ☑
  ulna M89.73- ☑
mental — *see* Disability, intellectual
modification, lysosomal enzymes, post-translational
  E77.0
obstructive, congenital
  renal pelvis Q62.39
  ureter Q62.39
    atresia — *see* Atresia, ureter
    cecoureterocele Q62.32
    megaureter Q62.2
    orthotopic ureterocele Q62.31
osseous, major M89.70
  ankle M89.77- ☑
  carpus M89.74- ☑
  clavicle M89.71- ☑
  femur M89.75- ☑
  fibula M89.76- ☑
  fingers M89.74- ☑
  foot M89.77- ☑
  forearm M89.73- ☑
  hand M89.74- ☑
  humerus M89.72- ☑
  lower leg M89.76- ☑
  metacarpus M89.74- ☑
  metatarsus M89.77- ☑
  multiple sites M89.9
  pelvic region M89.75- ☑
  pelvis M89.75- ☑
  radius M89.73- ☑
  scapula M89.71- ☑
  shoulder region M89.71- ☑
  specified NEC M89.78
  tarsus M89.77- ☑
  thigh M89.75- ☑
  tibia M89.76- ☑
  toes M89.77- ☑
  ulna M89.73- ☑
osteochondral NEC (*see also* Deformity) M95.8
ostium
  primum Q21.2
  secundum Q21.1
peroxidase E80.3
placental blood supply — *see* Insufficiency, placental
platelets, qualitative D69.1
  constitutional D68.0
postural NEC, spine — *see* Dorsopathy, deforming
reduction
  limb Q73.8
    lower Q72.9- ☑
      absence — *see* Agenesis, leg
        foot — *see* Agenesis, foot
      longitudinal
        femur Q72.4- ☑
        fibula Q72.6- ☑
        tibia Q72.5- ☑
      specified type NEC Q72.89- ☑
      split foot Q72.7- ☑
    specified type NEC Q73.8
    upper Q71.9- ☑
      absence — *see* Agenesis, arm
        forearm — *see* Agenesis, forearm
        hand — *see* Agenesis, hand
      lobster-claw hand Q71.6- ☑
      longitudinal
        radius Q71.4- ☑
        ulna Q71.5- ☑

Defect, defective — *continued*

reduction — *continued*
  limb — *continued*
    upper — *continued*
      specified type NEC Q71.89- ☑
renal pelvis Q63.8
  obstructive Q62.39
respiratory system, congenital Q34.9
restoration, dental K08.50
  specified NEC K08.59
retinal nerve bundle fibers H35.89
septal (heart) NOS Q21.9
  acquired (atrial) (auricular) (ventricular) (old) I51.0
  atrial Q21.1
    concurrent with acute myocardial infarction —
      see Infarct, myocardium
    following acute myocardial infarction (current
      complication) I23.1
  ventricular (*see also* Defect, ventricular septal)
    Q21.0
sinus venosus Q21.1
speech R47.9
  developmental F80.9
  specified NEC R47.89
Taussig-Bing (aortic transposition and overriding pulmonary artery) Q20.1
teeth, wedge K03.1
vascular (local) I99.9
  congenital Q27.9
ventricular septal Q21.0
  concurrent with acute myocardial infarction — *see*
    Infarct, myocardium
  following acute myocardial infarction (current
    complication) I23.2
  in tetralogy of Fallot Q21.3
vision NEC H54.7
visual field H53.40
  bilateral
    heteronymous H53.47
    homonymous H53.46- ☑
  generalized contraction H53.48- ☑
  localized
    arcuate H53.43- ☑
    scotoma (central area) H53.41- ☑
      blind spot area H53.42- ☑
    sector H53.43- ☑
    specified type NEC H53.45- ☑
voice R49.9
  specified NEC R49.8
wedge, tooth, teeth (abrasion) K03.1

Deferentitis N49.1
  gonorrheal (acute) (chronic) A54.23

Defibrination (syndrome) D65
  antepartum — *see* Hemorrhage, antepartum, with
    coagulation defect, disseminated intravascular
    coagulation
  following ectopic or molar pregnancy O08.1
  intrapartum O67.0
  newborn P60
  postpartum O72.3

Deficiency, deficient
3-beta hydroxysteroid dehydrogenase E25.0
5-alpha reductase (with male pseudohermaphroditism) E29.1
11-hydroxylase E25.0
21-hydroxylase E25.0
abdominal muscle syndrome Q79.4
AC globulin (congenital) (hereditary) D68.2
  acquired D68.4
accelerator globulin (Ac G) (blood) D68.2
acid phosphatase E83.39
activating factor (blood) D68.2
adenosine deaminase (ADA) D81.3
aldolase (hereditary) E74.19
alpha-1-antitrypsin E88.01
amino-acids E72.9
anemia — *see* Anemia
aneurin E51.9
antibody with
  hyperimmunoglobulinemia D80.6
  near-normal immunoglobins D80.6
antidiuretic hormone E23.2
anti-hemophilic
  factor (A) D66
    B D67
    C D68.1
  globulin (AHG) NEC D66
antithrombin (antithrombin III) D68.59

Deficiency, deficient — *continued*
ascorbic acid E54
attention (disorder) (syndrome) F98.8
   with hyperactivity — *see* Disorder, attention-deficit hyperactivity
autoprothrombin
   C D68.2
   I D68.2
   II D67
beta-glucuronidase E76.29
biotin E53.8
biotin-dependent carboxylase D81.819
biotinidase D81.810
brancher enzyme (amylopectinosis) E74.03
C1 esterase inhibitor (C1-INH) D84.1
calciferol E55.9
   with
      adult osteomalacia M83.8
      rickets — *see* Rickets
calcium (dietary) E58
calorie, severe E43
   with marasmus E41
      and kwashiorkor E42
cardiac — *see* Insufficiency, myocardial
carnitine E71.40
   due to
      hemodialysis E71.43
      inborn errors of metabolism E71.42
      Valproic acid therapy E71.43
   iatrogenic E71.43
   muscle palmityltransferase E71.314
   primary E71.41
   secondary E71.448
carotene E50.9
central nervous system G96.8
ceruloplasmin (Wilson) E83.01
choline E53.8
Christmas factor D67
chromium E61.4
clotting (blood) (*see also* Deficiency, coagulation factor) D68.9
clotting factor NEC (hereditary) (*see also* Deficiency, factor) D68.2
coagulation NOS D68.9
   with
      ectopic pregnancy O08.1
      molar pregnancy O08.1
   acquired (any) D68.4
   antepartum hemorrhage — *see* Hemorrhage, antepartum, with coagulation defect
   clotting factor NEC (*see also* Deficiency, factor) D68.2
   due to
      hyperprothrombinemia D68.4
      liver disease D68.4
      vitamin K deficiency D68.4
   newborn, transient P61.6
   postpartum O72.3
   specified NEC D68.8
cognitive F09
color vision H53.50
   achromatopsia H53.51
   acquired H53.52
   deuteranomaly H53.53
   protanomaly H53.54
   specified type NEC H53.59
   tritanomaly H53.55
combined glucocorticoid and mineralocorticoid E27.49
contact factor D68.2
copper (nutritional) E61.0
corticoadrenal E27.40
   primary E27.1
craniofacial axis Q75.0
cyanocobalamin E53.8
debrancher enzyme (limit dextrinosis) E74.03
dehydrogenase
   long chain/very long chain acyl CoA E71.310
   medium chain acyl CoA E71.311
   short chain acyl CoA E71.312
diet E63.9
dihydropyrimidine dehydrogenase (DPD) E88.89
disaccharidase E73.9
edema — *see* Malnutrition, severe
endocrine E34.9
energy-supply — *see* Malnutrition
enzymes, circulating NEC E88.09
ergosterol E55.9

Deficiency, deficient — *continued*
ergosterol — *continued*
   with
      adult osteomalacia M83.8
      rickets — *see* Rickets
essential fatty acid (EFA) E63.0
factor (*see also* Deficiency, coagulation)
   Hageman D68.2
   I (congenital) (hereditary) D68.2
   II (congenital) (hereditary) D68.2
   IX (congenital) (functional) (hereditary) (with functional defect) D67
   multiple (congenital) D68.8
      acquired D68.4
   V (congenital) (hereditary) D68.2
   VII (congenital) (hereditary) D68.2
   VIII (congenital) (functional) (hereditary) (with functional defect) D66
      with vascular defect D68.0
   X (congenital) (hereditary) D68.2
   XI (congenital) (hereditary) D68.1
   XII (congenital) (hereditary) D68.2
   XIII (congenital) (hereditary) D68.2
femoral, proximal focal (congenital) — *see* Defect, reduction, lower limb, longitudinal, femur
fibrinase D68.2
fibrinogen (congenital) (hereditary) D68.2
   acquired D65
fibrin-stabilizing factor (congenital) (hereditary) D68.2
   acquired D68.4
folate E53.8
folic acid E53.8
foreskin N47.3
fructokinase E74.11
fructose 1,6-diphosphatase E74.19
fructose-1-phosphate aldolase E74.19
galactokinase E74.29
galactose-1-phosphate uridyl transferase E74.29
gammaglobulin in blood D80.1
   hereditary D80.0
glass factor D68.2
glucocorticoid E27.49
   mineralocorticoid E27.49
glucose-6-phosphatase E74.01
glucose-6-phosphate dehydrogenase anemia D55.0
glucuronyl transferase E80.5
glycogen synthetase E74.09
gonadotropin (isolated) E23.0
growth hormone (idiopathic) (isolated) E23.0
Hageman factor D68.2
hemoglobin D64.9
hepatophosphorylase E74.09
homogentisate 1,2-dioxygenase E70.29
hormone
   anterior pituitary (partial) NEC E23.0
      growth E23.0
   growth (isolated) E23.0
   pituitary E23.0
   testicular E29.1
hypoxanthine- (guanine)-phosphoribosyltransferase (HG- PRT) (total H-PRT) E79.1
immunity D84.9
   cell-mediated D84.8
      with thrombocytopenia and eczema D82.0
   combined D81.9
   humoral D80.9
   IgA (secretory) D80.2
   IgG D80.3
   IgM D80.4
immuno — *see* Immunodeficiency
immunoglobulin, selective
   A (IgA) D80.2
   G (IgG) (subclasses) D80.3
   M (IgM) D80.4
inositol (B complex) E53.8
intrinsic
   factor (congenital) D51.0
   sphincter N36.42
      with urethral hypermobility N36.43
iodine E61.8
   congenital syndrome — *see* Syndrome, iodine-deficiency, congenital
iron E61.1
   anemia D50.9
kalium E87.6
kappa-light chain D80.8
labile factor (congenital) (hereditary) D68.2
   acquired D68.4

Deficiency, deficient — *continued*
lacrimal fluid (acquired) (*see also* Syndrome, dry eye)
   congenital Q10.6
lactase
   congenital E73.0
   secondary E73.1
Laki-Lorand factor D68.2
lecithin cholesterol acyltransferase E78.6
lipocaic K86.89
lipoprotein (familial) (high density) E78.6
liver phosphorylase E74.09
lysosomal alpha-1, 4 glucosidase E74.02
magnesium E61.2
major histocompatibility complex
   class I D81.6
   class II D81.7
manganese E61.3
menadione (vitamin K) E56.1
   newborn P53
mental (familial) (hereditary) — *see* Disability, intellectual
methylenetetrahydrofolate reductase (MTHFR) E72.12
mevalonate kinase M04.1
mineralocorticoid E27.49
   with glucocorticoid E27.49
mineral NEC E61.8
molybdenum (nutritional) E61.5
moral F60.2
multiple nutrient elements E61.7
muscle
   carnitine (palmityltransferase) E71.314
   phosphofructokinase E74.09
myoadenylate deaminase E79.2
myocardial — *see* Insufficiency, myocardial
myophosphorylase E74.04
NADH diaphorase or reductase (congenital) D74.0
NADH-methemoglobin reductase (congenital) D74.0
natrium E87.1
niacin (amide) (-tryptophan) E52
nicotinamide E52
nicotinic acid E52
number of teeth — *see* Anodontia
nutrient element E61.9
   multiple E61.7
   specified NEC E61.8
nutrition, nutritional E63.9
   sequelae — *see* Sequelae, nutritional deficiency
   specified NEC E63.8
of interleukin 1 receptor antagonist [DIRA] M04.8
ornithine transcarbamylase E72.4
ovarian E28.39
oxygen — *see* Anoxia
pantothenic acid E53.8
parathyroid (gland) E20.9
perineum (female) N81.89
phenylalanine hydroxylase E70.1
phosphoenolpyruvate carboxykinase E74.4
phosphofructokinase E74.19
phosphomannomutase E74.8
phosphomannose isomerase E74.8
phosphomannosyl mutase E74.8
phosphorylase kinase, liver E74.09
pituitary hormone (isolated) E23.0
plasma thromboplastin
   antecedent (PTA) D68.1
   component (PTC) D67
platelet NEC D69.1
   constitutional D68.0
polyglandular E31.8
   autoimmune E31.0
potassium (K) E87.6
prepuce N47.3
proaccelerin (congenital) (hereditary) D68.2
   acquired D68.4
proconvertin factor (congenital) (hereditary) D68.2
   acquired D68.4
protein (*see also* Malnutrition) E46
   anemia D53.0
   C D68.59
   S D68.59
prothrombin (congenital) (hereditary) D68.2
   acquired D68.4
Prower factor D68.2
pseudocholinesterase E88.09
PTA (plasma thromboplastin antecedent) D68.1
PTC (plasma thromboplastin component) D67
purine nucleoside phosphorylase (PNP) D81.5

Deficiency, deficient — *continued*
  pyracin (alpha) (beta) E53.1
  pyridoxal E53.1
  pyridoxamine E53.1
  pyridoxine (derivatives) E53.1
  pyruvate
    carboxylase E74.4
    dehydrogenase E74.4
  riboflavin (vitamin B2) E53.0
  salt E87.1
  secretion
    ovary E28.39
    salivary gland (any) K11.7
    urine R34
  selenium (dietary) E59
  serum antitrypsin, familial E88.01
  short stature homeobox gene (SHOX)
    with
      dyschondrosteosis Q78.8
      short stature (idiopathic) E34.3
      Turner's syndrome Q96.9
  sodium (Na) E87.1
  SPCA (factor VII) D68.2
  sphincter, intrinsic N36.42
    with urethral hypermobility N36.43
  stable factor (congenital) (hereditary) D68.2
    acquired D68.4
  Stuart-Prower (factor X) D68.2
  sucrase E74.39
  sulfatase E75.29
  sulfite oxidase E72.19
  thiamin, thiaminic (chloride) E51.9
    beriberi (dry) E51.11
      wet E51.12
  thrombokinase D68.2
    newborn P53
  thyroid (gland) — *see* Hypothyroidism
  tocopherol E56.0
  tooth bud K00.0
  transcobalamine II (anemia) D51.2
  vanadium E61.6
  vascular I99.9
  vasopressin E23.2
  vertical ridge K06.8
  viosterol — *see* Deficiency, calciferol
  vitamin (multiple) NOS E56.9
    A E50.9
      with
        Bitot's spot (corneal) E50.1
        follicular keratosis E50.8
        keratomalacia E50.4
        manifestations NEC E50.8
        night blindness E50.5
        scar of cornea, xerophthalmic E50.6
        xeroderma E50.8
        xerophthalmia E50.7
        xerosis
          conjunctival E50.0
            and Bitot's spot E50.1
          cornea E50.2
            and ulceration E50.3
      sequelae E64.1
    B (complex) NOS E53.9
      with
        beriberi (dry) E51.11
          wet E51.12
        pellagra E52
    B1 NOS E51.9
      beriberi (dry) E51.11
        with circulatory system manifestations E51.11
        wet E51.12
    B2 (riboflavin) E53.0
    B6 E53.1
    B12 E53.8
    C E54
      sequelae E64.2
    D E55.9
      with
        adult osteomalacia M83.8
        rickets — *see* Rickets
      25-hydroxylase E83.32
    E E56.0
    folic acid E53.8
    G E53.0
    group B E53.9
      specified NEC E53.8
    H (biotin) E53.8
    K E56.1

Deficiency, deficient — *continued*
  vitamin — *continued*
    K — *continued*
      of newborn P53
    nicotinic E52
    P E56.8
    PP (pellagra-preventing) E52
    specified NEC E56.8
    thiamin E51.9
      beriberi — *see* Beriberi
  zinc, dietary E60
Deficit (*see also* Deficiency)
  attention and concentration R41.840
    disorder — *see* Attention, deficit
    following
      cerebral infarction I69.310
      cerebrovascular disease I69.910
        specified disease NEC I69.810
      nontraumatic
        intracerebral hemorrhage I69.110
        specified intracranial hemorrhage NEC I69.210
        subarachnoid hemorrhage I69.010
  cognitive
    communication R41.841
    emotional
      following
        cerebral infarction I69.315
        cerebrovascular disease I69.915
          specified disease NEC I69.815
        nontraumatic
          intracerebral hemorrhage I69.115
          specified intracranial hemorrhage NEC I69.215
          subarachnoid hemorrhage I69.015
    following
      cerebral infarction I69.319
      cerebrovascular disease I69.919
        specified disease NEC I69.819
      nontraumatic
        intracerebral hemorrhage I69.119
        specified intracranial hemorrhage NEC I69.219
        subarachnoid hemorrhage I69.019
    social
      following
        cerebral infarction I69.315
        cerebrovascular disease I69.915
          specified disease NEC I69.815
        nontraumatic
          intracerebral hemorrhage I69.115
          specified intracranial hemorrhage NEC I69.215
          subarachnoid hemorrhage I69.015
  cognitive NEC R41.89
    following
      cerebral infarction I69.318
      cerebrovascular disease I69.918
        specified disease NEC I69.818
      nontraumatic
        intracerebral hemorrhage I69.118
        specified intracranial hemorrhage NEC I69.218
        subarachnoid hemorrhage I69.018
  concentration R41.840
  executive function R41.844
    following
      cerebral infarction I69.314
      cerebrovascular disease I69.914
        specified disease NEC I69.814
      nontraumatic
        intracerebral hemorrhage I69.114
        specified intracranial hemorrhage NEC I69.214
        subarachnoid hemorrhage I69.014
  frontal lobe R41.844
    following
      cerebral infarction I69.314
      cerebrovascular disease I69.914
        specified disease NEC I69.814
      nontraumatic
        intracerebral hemorrhage I69.114
        specified intracranial hemorrhage NEC I69.214
        subarachnoid hemorrhage I69.014
  memory
    following
      cerebral infarction I69.311
      cerebrovascular disease I69.911

Deficit — *continued*
  memory — *continued*
    following — *continued*
      cerebrovascular disease — *continued*
        specified disease NEC I69.811
      nontraumatic
        intracerebral hemorrhage I69.111
        specified intracranial hemorrhage NEC I69.211
        subarachnoid hemorrhage I69.011
  neurologic NEC R29.818
    ischemic
      reversible (RIND) I63.9
        prolonged (PRIND) I63.9
  oxygen R09.02
  prolonged reversible ischemic neurologic (PRIND) I63.9
  psychomotor R41.843
    following
      cerebral infarction I69.313
      cerebrovascular disease I69.913
        specified disease NEC I69.813
      nontraumatic
        intracerebral hemorrhage I69.113
        specified intracranial hemorrhage NEC I69.213
        subarachnoid hemorrhage I69.013
  visuospatial R41.842
    following
      cerebral infarction I69.312
      cerebrovascular disease I69.912
        specified disease NEC I69.812
      nontraumatic
        intracerebral hemorrhage I69.112
        specified intracranial hemorrhage NEC I69.212
        subarachnoid hemorrhage I69.012

Deflection
  radius — *see* Deformity, limb, specified type NEC, forearm
  septum (acquired) (nasal) (nose) J34.2
  spine — *see* Curvature, spine
  turbinate (nose) J34.2
Defluvium
  capillorum — *see* Alopecia
  ciliorum — *see* Madarosis
  unguium L60.8
Deformity Q89.9
  abdomen, congenital Q89.9
  abdominal wall
    acquired M95.8
    congenital Q79.59
  acquired (unspecified site) M95.9
  adrenal gland Q89.1
  alimentary tract, congenital Q45.9
    upper Q40.9
  ankle (joint) (acquired) (*see also* Deformity, limb, lower leg)
    abduction — *see* Contraction, joint, ankle
    congenital Q68.8
    contraction — *see* Contraction, joint, ankle
    specified type NEC — *see* Deformity, limb, foot, specified NEC
  anus (acquired) K62.89
    congenital Q43.9
  aorta (arch) (congenital) Q25.40
    acquired I77.89
  aortic
    arch, acquired I77.89
    cusp or valve (congenital) Q23.8
      acquired (*see also* Endocarditis, aortic) I35.8
  arm (acquired) (upper) (*see also* Deformity, limb, upper arm)
    congenital Q68.8
    forearm — *see* Deformity, limb, forearm
  artery (congenital) (peripheral) NOS Q27.9
    acquired I77.89
    coronary (acquired) I25.9
      congenital Q24.5
    umbilical Q27.0
  atrial septal Q21.1
  auditory canal (external) (congenital) (*see also* Malformation, ear, external)
    acquired — *see* Disorder, ear, external, specified type NEC
  auricle
    ear (congenital) (*see also* Malformation, ear, external)
      acquired — *see* Disorder, pinna, deformity

Deformity — *continued*
  limb — *continued*
    specified type NEC M21.80
      forearm M21.83- ☑
      lower leg M21.86- ☑
      thigh M21.85- ☑
      upper arm M21.82- ☑
    thigh M21.95- ☑
    unequal length M21.70
      short site is
        femur M21.75- ☑
        fibula M21.76- ☑
        humerus M21.72- ☑
        radius M21.73- ☑
        tibia M21.76- ☑
        ulna M21.73- ☑
    upper arm M21.92- ☑
    valgus — *see* Deformity, valgus
    varus — *see* Deformity, varus
    wrist drop M21.33- ☑
  lip (acquired) NEC K13.0
    congenital Q38.0
  liver (congenital) Q44.7
    acquired K76.89
  lumbosacral (congenital) (joint) (region) Q76.49
    acquired — *see* subcategory M43.8 ☑
    kyphosis — *see* Kyphosis, congenital
    lordosis — *see* Lordosis, congenital
  lung (congenital) Q33.9
    acquired J98.4
  lymphatic system, congenital Q89.9
  Madelung's (radius) Q74.0
  mandible (acquired) (congenital) M26.9
  maxilla (acquired) (congenital) M26.9
  meninges or membrane (congenital) Q07.9
    cerebral Q04.8
      acquired G96.19
    spinal cord (congenital) G96.19
      acquired G96.19
  metacarpus (acquired) — *see* Deformity, limb, forearm
    congenital Q74.0
  metatarsus (acquired) — *see* Deformity, foot
    congenital Q66.9
  middle ear (congenital) Q16.4
    ossicles Q16.3
  mitral (leaflets) (valve) I05.8
    parachute Q23.2
    stenosis, congenital Q23.2
  mouth (acquired) K13.79
    congenital Q38.6
  multiple, congenital NEC Q89.7
  muscle (acquired) M62.89
    congenital Q79.9
      sternocleidomastoid Q68.0
  musculoskeletal system (acquired) M95.9
    congenital Q79.9
    specified NEC M95.8
  nail (acquired) L60.8
    congenital Q84.6
  nasal — *see* Deformity, nose
  neck (acquired) M95.3
    congenital Q18.9
      sternocleidomastoid Q68.0
  nervous system (congenital) Q07.9
  nipple (congenital) Q83.9
    acquired N64.89
  nose (acquired) (cartilage) M95.0
    bone (turbinate) M95.0
    congenital Q30.9
      bent or squashed Q67.4
    saddle M95.0
      syphilitic A50.57
    septum (acquired) J34.2
      congenital Q30.8
    sinus (wall) (congenital) Q30.8
      acquired M95.0
    syphilitic (congenital) A50.57
      late A52.73
  ocular muscle (congenital) Q10.3
    acquired — *see* Strabismus, mechanical
  opticociliary vessels (congenital) Q13.2
  orbit (eye) (acquired) H05.30
    atrophy — *see* Atrophy, orbit
    congenital Q10.7
    due to
      bone disease NEC H05.32- ☑
      trauma or surgery H05.33- ☑
    enlargement — *see* Enlargement, orbit

Deformity — *continued*
  orbit — *continued*
    exostosis — *see* Exostosis, orbit
  organ of Corti (congenital) Q16.5
  ovary (congenital) Q50.39
    acquired N83.8
  oviduct, acquired N83.8
  palate (congenital) Q38.5
    acquired M27.8
    cleft (congenital) — *see* Cleft, palate
  pancreas (congenital) Q45.3
    acquired K86.89
  parathyroid (gland) Q89.2
  parotid (gland) (congenital) Q38.4
    acquired K11.8
  patella (acquired) — *see* Disorder, patella, specified NEC
  pelvis, pelvic (acquired) (bony) M95.5
    with disproportion (fetopelvic) O33.0
      causing obstructed labor O65.0
    congenital Q74.2
    rachitic sequelae (late effect) E64.3
  penis (glans) (congenital) Q55.69
    acquired N48.89
  pericardium (congenital) Q24.8
    acquired — *see* Pericarditis
  pharynx (congenital) Q38.8
    acquired J39.2
  pinna, acquired (*see also* Disorder, pinna, deformity)
    congenital Q17.9
  pituitary (congenital) Q89.2
  posture — *see* Dorsopathy, deforming
  prepuce (congenital) Q55.69
    acquired N47.8
  prostate (congenital) Q55.4
    acquired N42.89
  pupil (congenital) Q13.2
    acquired — *see* Abnormality, pupillary
  pylorus (congenital) Q40.3
    acquired K31.89
  rachitic (acquired), old or healed E64.3
  radius (acquired) (*see also* Deformity, limb, forearm)
    congenital Q68.8
  rectum (congenital) Q43.9
    acquired K62.89
  reduction (extremity) (limb), congenital (*see also* condition and site) Q73.8
    brain Q04.3
    lower — *see* Defect, reduction, lower limb
    upper — *see* Defect, reduction, upper limb
  renal — *see* Deformity, kidney
  respiratory system (congenital) Q34.9
  rib (acquired) M95.4
    congenital Q76.6
    cervical Q76.5
  rotation (joint) (acquired) — *see* Deformity, limb, specified site NEC
    congenital Q74.9
    hip — *see* Deformity, limb, specified type NEC, thigh
      congenital Q65.89
  sacroiliac joint (congenital) — *see* subcategory Q74.2
    acquired — *see* subcategory M43.8 ☑
  sacrum (acquired) — *see* subcategory M43.8 ☑
  saddle
    back — *see* Lordosis
    nose M95.0
      syphilitic A50.57
  salivary gland or duct (congenital) Q38.4
    acquired K11.8
  scapula (acquired) M95.8
    congenital Q68.8
  scrotum (congenital) (*see also* Malformation, testis and scrotum)
    acquired N50.89
  seminal vesicles (congenital) Q55.4
    acquired N50.89
  septum, nasal (acquired) J34.2
  shoulder (joint) (acquired) — *see* Deformity, limb, upper arm
    congenital Q74.0
    contraction — *see* Contraction, joint, shoulder
  sigmoid (flexure) (congenital) Q43.9
    acquired K63.89
  skin (congenital) Q82.9
  skull (acquired) M95.2
    congenital Q75.8

Deformity — *continued*
  skull — *continued*
    congenital — *continued*
      with
        anencephaly Q00.0
        encephalocele — *see* Encephalocele
        hydrocephalus Q03.9
          with spina bifida — *see* Spina bifida, by site, with hydrocephalus
        microcephaly Q02
  soft parts, organs or tissues (of pelvis)
    in pregnancy or childbirth NEC O34.8- ☑
      causing obstructed labor O65.5
  spermatic cord (congenital) Q55.4
    acquired N50.89
    torsion — *see* Torsion, spermatic cord
  spinal — *see* Dorsopathy, deforming
    column (acquired) — *see* Dorsopathy, deforming
    congenital Q67.5
    cord (congenital) Q06.9
      acquired G95.89
    nerve root (congenital) Q07.9
  spine (acquired) (*see also* Dorsopathy, deforming)
    congenital Q67.5
    rachitic E64.3
    specified NEC — *see* Dorsopathy, deforming, specified NEC
  spleen
    acquired D73.89
    congenital Q89.09
  Sprengel's (congenital) Q74.0
  sternocleidomastoid (muscle), congenital Q68.0
  sternum (acquired) M95.4
    congenital NEC Q76.7
  stomach (congenital) Q40.3
    acquired K31.89
  submandibular gland (congenital) Q38.4
  submaxillary gland (congenital) Q38.4
    acquired K11.8
  talipes — *see* Talipes
  testis (congenital) (*see also* Malformation, testis and scrotum)
    acquired N44.8
    torsion — *see* Torsion, testis
  thigh (acquired) (*see also* Deformity, limb, thigh)
    congenital NEC Q68.8
  thorax (acquired) (wall) M95.4
    congenital Q67.8
    sequelae of rickets E64.3
  thumb (acquired) (*see also* Deformity, finger)
    congenital NEC Q68.1
  thymus (tissue) (congenital) Q89.2
  thyroid (gland) (congenital) Q89.2
    cartilage Q31.8
      acquired J38.7
  tibia (acquired) (*see also* Deformity, limb, specified type NEC, lower leg)
    congenital NEC Q68.8
    saber (syphilitic) A50.56
  toe (acquired) M20.6- ☑
    congenital Q66.9
    hallux rigidus M20.2- ☑
    hallux valgus M20.1- ☑
    hallux varus M20.3- ☑
    hammer toe M20.4- ☑
    specified NEC M20.5X- ☑
  tongue (congenital) Q38.3
    acquired K14.8
  tooth, teeth K00.2
  trachea (rings) (congenital) Q32.1
    acquired J39.8
  transverse aortic arch (congenital) Q25.49
  tricuspid (leaflets) (valve) I07.8
    atresia or stenosis Q22.4
    Ebstein's Q22.5
  trunk (acquired) M95.8
    congenital Q89.9
  ulna (acquired) (*see also* Deformity, limb, forearm)
    congenital NEC Q68.8
  urachus, congenital Q64.4
  ureter (opening) (congenital) Q62.8
    acquired N28.89
  urethra (congenital) Q64.79
    acquired N36.8
  urinary tract (congenital) Q64.9
    urachus Q64.4
  uterus (congenital) Q51.9
    acquired N85.8

Deformity — continued
 uvula (congenital) Q38.5
 vagina (acquired) N89.8
  congenital Q52.4
 valgus NEC M21.00
  ankle M21.07- ✓
  elbow M21.02- ✓
  hip M21.05- ✓
  knee M21.06- ✓
 valve, valvular (congenital) (heart) Q24.8
  acquired — see Endocarditis
 varus NEC M21.10
  ankle M21.17- ✓
  elbow M21.12- ✓
  hip M21.15 ✓
  knee M21.16- ✓
  tibia — see Osteochondrosis, juvenile, tibia
 vas deferens (congenital) Q55.4
  acquired N50.89
 vein (congenital) Q27.9
  great Q26.9
 vertebra — see Dorsopathy, deforming
 vertical talus (congenital) Q66.80
  left foot Q66.82
  right foot Q66.81
 vesicourethral orifice (acquired) N32.89
  congenital NEC Q64.79
 vessels of optic papilla (congenital) Q14.2
 visual field (contraction) — see Defect, visual field
 vitreous body, acquired H43.89
 vulva (congenital) Q52.79
  acquired N90.89
 wrist (joint) (acquired) (see also Deformity, limb, forearm)
  congenital Q68.8
  contraction — see Contraction, joint, wrist

Degeneration, degenerative
 adrenal (capsule) (fatty) (gland) (hyaline) (infectional) E27.8
 amyloid (see also Amyloidosis) E85.9
 anterior cornua, spinal cord G12.29
 anterior labral S43.49- ✓
 aorta, aortic I70.0
  fatty I77.89
 aortic valve (heart) — see Endocarditis, aortic
 arteriovascular — see Arteriosclerosis
 artery, arterial (atheromatous) (calcareous) (see also Arteriosclerosis)
  cerebral, amyloid E85.4 [I68.0]
  medial — see Arteriosclerosis, extremities
 articular cartilage NEC — see Derangement, joint, articular cartilage, by site
 atheromatous — see Arteriosclerosis
 basal nuclei or ganglia G23.9
  specified NEC G23.8
 bone NEC — see Disorder, bone, specified type NEC
 brachial plexus G54.0
 brain (cortical) (progressive) G31.9
  alcoholic G31.2
  arteriosclerotic I67.2
  childhood G31.9
   specified NEC G31.89
  cystic G31.89
   congenital Q04.6
  in
   alcoholism G31.2
   beriberi E51.2
   cerebrovascular disease I67.9
   congenital hydrocephalus Q03.9
    with spina bifida (see also Spina bifida)
   Fabry-Anderson disease E75.21
   Gaucher's disease E75.22
   Hunter's syndrome E76.1
   lipidosis
    cerebral E75.4
    generalized E75.6
   mucopolysaccharidosis — see Mucopolysaccharidosis
   myxedema E03.9 [G32.89]
   neoplastic disease (see also Neoplasm) D49.6 [G32.89]
   Niemann-Pick disease E75.249 [G32.89]
   sphingolipidosis E75.3 [G32.89]
   vitamin B12 deficiency E53.8 [G32.89]
  senile NEC G31.1
 breast N64.89
 Bruch's membrane — see Degeneration, choroid
 capillaries (fatty) I78.8

Degeneration, degenerative — continued
 capillaries — continued
  amyloid E85.89 [I79.8]
 cardiac (see also Degeneration, myocardial)
  valve, valvular — see Endocarditis
 cardiorenal — see Hypertension, cardiorenal
 cardiovascular (see also Disease, cardiovascular)
  renal — see Hypertension, cardiorenal
 cerebellar NOS G31.9
  alcoholic G31.2
  primary (hereditary) (sporadic) G11.9
 cerebral — see Degeneration, brain
 cerebrovascular I67.9
  due to hypertension I67.4
 cervical plexus G54.2
 cervix N88.8
  due to radiation (intended effect) N88.8
   adverse effect or misadventure N99.89
 chamber angle H21.21- ✓
 changes, spine or vertebra — see Spondylosis
 chorioretinal (see also Degeneration, choroid)
  hereditary H31.20
 choroid (colloid) (drusen) H31.10- ✓
  atrophy — see Atrophy, choroidal
  hereditary — see Dystrophy, choroidal, hereditary
 ciliary body H21.22- ✓
 cochlear — see subcategory H83.8 ✓
 combined (spinal cord) (subacute) E53.8 [G32.0]
  with anemia (pernicious) D51.0 [G32.0]
   due to dietary vitamin B12 deficiency D51.3 [G32.0]
  in (due to)
   vitamin B12 deficiency E53.8 [G32.0]
    anemia D51.9 [G32.0]
 conjunctiva H11.10
  concretions — see Concretion, conjunctiva
  deposits — see Deposit, conjunctiva
  pigmentations — see Pigmentation, conjunctiva
  pinguecula — see Pinguecula
  xerosis — see Xerosis, conjunctiva
 cornea H18.40
  calcerous H18.43
   band keratopathy H18.42- ✓
  familial, hereditary — see Dystrophy, cornea
  hyaline (of old scars) H18.49
  keratomalacia — see Keratomalacia
  nodular H18.45- ✓
  peripheral H18.46- ✓
  senile H18.41- ✓
  specified type NEC H18.49
 cortical (cerebellar) (parenchymatous) G31.89
  alcoholic G31.2
  diffuse, due to arteriopathy I67.2
 corticobasal G31.85
 cutis L98.8
  amyloid E85.4 [L99]
 dental pulp K04.2
 disc disease — see Degeneration, intervertebral disc NEC
 dorsolateral (spinal cord) — see Degeneration, combined
 extrapyramidal G25.9
 eye, macular (see also Degeneration, macula)
  congenital or hereditary — see Dystrophy, retina
 facet joints — see Spondylosis
 fatty
  liver NEC K76.0
   alcoholic K70.0
 grey matter (brain) (Alpers') G31.81
 heart (see also Degeneration, myocardial)
  amyloid E85.4 [I43]
  atheromatous — see Disease, heart, ischemic, atherosclerotic
  ischemic — see Disease, heart, ischemic
 hepatolenticular (Wilson's) E83.01
 hepatorenal K76.7
 hyaline (diffuse) (generalized)
  localized — see Degeneration, by site
 infrapatellar fat pad M79.4
 intervertebral disc NOS
  with
   myelopathy — see Disorder, disc, with, myelopathy
   radiculitis or radiculopathy — see Disorder, disc, with, radiculopathy
  cervical, cervicothoracic — see Disorder, disc, cervical, degeneration

Degeneration, degenerative — continued
 intervertebral disc — continued
  cervical, cervicothoracic — see Disorder, disc, cervical, degeneration — continued
   with
    myelopathy — see Disorder, disc, cervical, with myelopathy
    neuritis, radiculitis or radiculopathy — see Disorder, disc, cervical, with neuritis
  lumbar region M51.36
   with
    myelopathy M51.06
    neuritis, radiculitis, radiculopathy or sciatica M51.16
  lumbosacral region M51.37
   with
    neuritis, radiculitis, radiculopathy or sciatica M51.17
  sacrococcygeal region M53.3
  thoracic region M51.34
   with
    myelopathy M51.04
    neuritis, radiculitis, radiculopathy M51.14
  thoracolumbar region M51.35
   with
    myelopathy M51.05
    neuritis, radiculitis, radiculopathy M51.15
 intestine, amyloid E85.4
 iris (pigmentary) H21.23- ✓
 ischemic — see Ischemia
 joint disease — see Osteoarthritis
 kidney N28.89
  amyloid E85.4 [N29]
  cystic, congenital Q61.9
  fatty N28.89
  polycystic Q61.3
   adult type (autosomal dominant) Q61.2
   infantile type (autosomal recessive) NEC Q61.19
    collecting duct dilatation Q61.11
 Kuhnt-Junius (see also Degeneration, macula) H35.32- ✓
 lens — see Cataract
 lenticular (familial) (progressive) (Wilson's) (with cirrhosis of liver) E83.01
 liver (diffuse) NEC K76.89
  amyloid E85.4 [K77]
  cystic K76.89
   congenital Q44.6
  fatty NEC K76.0
   alcoholic K70.0
  hypertrophic K76.89
  parenchymatous, acute or subacute K72.00
   with coma K72.01
  pigmentary K76.89
  toxic (acute) K71.9
 lung J98.4
 lymph gland I89.8
  hyaline I89.8
 macula, macular (acquired) (age-related) (senile) H35.30
  angioid streaks H35.33
  atrophic age-related H35.31- ✓
  congenital or hereditary — see Dystrophy, retina
  cystoid H35.35- ✓
  drusen H35.36- ✓
  dry age-related H35.31- ✓
  exudative H35.32- ✓
  hole H35.34- ✓
  nonexudative H35.31- ✓
  puckering H35.37- ✓
  toxic H35.38- ✓
  wet age-related H35.32- ✓
 membranous labyrinth, congenital (causing impairment of hearing) Q16.5
 meniscus — see Derangement, meniscus
 mitral — see Insufficiency, mitral
 Mönckeberg's — see Arteriosclerosis, extremities
 motor centers, senile G31.1
 multi-system G90.3
 mural — see Degeneration, myocardial
 muscle (fatty) (fibrous) (hyaline) (progressive) M62.89
  heart — see Degeneration, myocardial
 myelin, central nervous system G37.9
 myocardial, myocardium (fatty) (hyaline) (senile) I51.5
  with rheumatic fever (conditions in I00) I09.0
   active, acute or subacute I01.2
    with chorea I02.0
   inactive or quiescent (with chorea) I09.0

✓ **Additional Character Required** — Refer to the Tabular List for Character Selection   ⚠ **Subterms under main terms may continue to next column or page**

Degeneration, degenerative — *continued*
  myocardial, myocardium — *continued*
    hypertensive — *see* Hypertension, heart
    rheumatic — *see* Degeneration, myocardial, with
        rheumatic fever
    syphilitic A52.06
  nasal sinus (mucosa) J32.9
    frontal J32.1
    maxillary J32.0
  nerve — *see* Disorder, nerve
  nervous system G31.9
    alcoholic G31.2
    amyloid E85.4 [G99.8]
    autonomic G90.9
    fatty G31.89
    specified NEC G31.89
  nipple N64.89
  olivopontocerebellar (hereditary) (familial) G23.8
  osseous labyrinth — *see* subcategory H83.8 ☑
  ovary N83.8
    cystic N83.20- ☑
    microcystic N83.20- ☑
  pallidal pigmentary (progressive) G23.0
  pancreas K86.89
    tuberculous A18.83
  penis N48.89
  pigmentary (diffuse) (general)
    localized — *see* Degeneration, by site
    pallidal (progressive) G23.0
  pineal gland E34.8
  pituitary (gland) E23.6
  popliteal fat pad M79.4
  posterolateral (spinal cord) — *see* Degeneration,
      combined
  pulmonary valve (heart) I37.8
  pulp (tooth) K04.2
  pupillary margin H21.24- ☑
  renal — *see* Degeneration, kidney
  retina H35.9
    hereditary (cerebroretinal) (congenital) (juvenile)
        (macula) (peripheral) (pigmentary) — *see*
        Dystrophy, retina
    Kuhnt-Junius (*see also* Degeneration, macula)
        H35.32- ☑
    macula (cystic) (exudative) (hole) (nonexudative)
        (pseudohole) (senile) (toxic) — *see* Degener-
        ation, macula
    peripheral H35.40
        lattice H35.41- ☑
        microcystoid H35.42- ☑
        paving stone H35.43- ☑
        secondary
            pigmentary H35.45- ☑
            vitreoretinal H35.46- ☑
        senile reticular H35.44- ☑
    pigmentary (primary) (*see also* Dystrophy, retina)
        secondary — *see* Degeneration, retina, periph-
            eral, secondary
    posterior pole — *see* Degeneration, macula
  saccule, congenital (causing impairment of hearing)
      Q16.5
  senile R54
    brain G31.1
    cardiac, heart or myocardium — *see* Degeneration,
        myocardial
    motor centers G31.1
    vascular — *see* Arteriosclerosis
  sinus (cystic) (*see also* Sinusitis)
    polypoid J33.1
  skin L98.8
    amyloid E85.4 [L99]
    colloid L98.8
  spinal (cord) G31.89
    amyloid E85.4 [G32.89]
    combined (subacute) — *see* Degeneration, com-
        bined
    dorsolateral — *see* Degeneration, combined
    familial NEC G31.89
    fatty G31.89
    funicular — *see* Degeneration, combined
    posterolateral — *see* Degeneration, combined
    subacute combined — *see* Degeneration, com-
        bined
    tuberculous A17.81
  spleen D73.0
    amyloid E85.4 [D77]
  stomach K31.89
  striatonigral G23.2

Degeneration, degenerative — *continued*
  suprarenal (capsule) (gland) E27.8
  synovial membrane (pulpy) — *see* Disorder, synovium,
      specified type NEC
  tapetoretinal — *see* Dystrophy, retina
  thymus (gland) E32.8
    fatty E32.8
  thyroid (gland) E07.89
  tricuspid (heart) (valve) I07.9
  tuberculous NEC — *see* Tuberculosis
  turbinate J34.89
  uterus (cystic) N85.8
  vascular (senile) — *see* Arteriosclerosis
    hypertensive — *see* Hypertension
  vitreoretinal, secondary — *see* Degeneration, retina,
      peripheral, secondary, vitreoretinal
  vitreous (body) H43.81- ☑
  Wallerian — *see* Disorder, nerve
  Wilson's hepatolenticular E83.01
Deglutition
  paralysis R13.0
    hysterical F44.4
  pneumonia J69.0
Degos' disease I77.89
Dehiscence (of)
  amputation stump T87.81
  cesarean wound O90.0
  closure of
    cornea T81.31 ☑
    craniotomy T81.32 ☑
    fascia (muscular) (superficial) T81.32 ☑
    internal organ or tissue T81.32 ☑
    laceration (external) (internal) T81.33 ☑
    ligament T81.32 ☑
    mucosa T81.31 ☑
    muscle or muscle flap T81.32 ☑
    ribs or rib cage T81.32 ☑
    skin and subcutaneous tissue (full-thickness) (su-
        perficial) T81.31 ☑
    skull T81.32 ☑
    sternum (sternotomy) T81.32 ☑
    tendon T81.32 ☑
    traumatic laceration (external) (internal) T81.33 ☑
  episiotomy O90.1
  operation wound NEC T81.31 ☑
    external operation wound (superficial) T81.31 ☑
    internal operation wound (deep) T81.32 ☑
  perineal wound (postpartum) O90.1
  traumatic injury wound repair T81.33 ☑
  wound T81.30 ☑
    traumatic repair T81.33 ☑
Dehydration E86.0
  newborn P74.1
Déjérine-Roussy syndrome G89.0
Déjérine-Sottas disease or neuropathy (hypertrophic)
    G60.0
Déjérine-Thomas atrophy G23.8
Delay, delayed
  any plane in pelvis
    complicating delivery O66.9
  birth or delivery NOS O63.9
  closure, ductus arteriosus (Botalli) P29.38
  coagulation — *see* Defect, coagulation
  conduction (cardiac) (ventricular) I45.9
  delivery, second twin, triplet, etc O63.2
  development R62.50
    global F88
    intellectual (specific) F81.9
    language F80.9
        due to hearing loss F80.4
    learning F81.9
    pervasive F84.9
    physiological R62.50
        specified stage NEC R62.0
    reading F81.0
    sexual E30.0
    speech F80.9
        due to hearing loss F80.4
    spelling F81.81
  ejaculation F52.32
  gastric emptying K30
  menarche E30.0
  menstruation (cause unknown) N91.0
  milestone R62.0
  passage of meconium (newborn) P76.0
  primary respiration P28.9
  puberty (constitutional) E30.0

Delay, delayed — *continued*
  separation of umbilical cord P96.82
  sexual maturation, female E30.0
  sleep phase syndrome G47.21
  union, fracture — *see* Fracture, by site
  vaccination Z28.9
Deletion(s)
  autosome Q93.9
    identified by fluorescence in situ hybridization
        (FISH) Q93.89
    identified by in situ hybridization (ISH) Q93.89
  chromosome
    with complex rearrangements NEC Q93.7
    part of NEC Q93.5
    seen only at prometaphase Q93.89
    short arm
        22q11.2 Q93.81
        4 Q93.3
        5p Q93.4
    specified NEC Q93.89
  long arm chromosome 18 or 21 Q93.89
    with complex rearrangements NEC Q93.7
  microdeletions NEC Q93.88
Delhi boil or button B55.1
Delinquency (juvenile) (neurotic) F91.8
  group Z72.810
Delinquent immunization status Z28.3
Delirium, delirious (acute or subacute) (not alcohol- or
    drug-induced) (with dementia) R41.0
  alcoholic (acute) (tremens) (withdrawal) F10.921
    with intoxication F10.921
        in
            abuse F10.121
            dependence F10.221
  due to (secondary to)
    alcohol
        intoxication F10.921
            in
                abuse F10.121
                dependence F10.221
        withdrawal F10.231
    amphetamine intoxication F15.921
        in
            abuse F15.121
            dependence F15.221
    anxiolytic
        intoxication F13.921
            in
                abuse F13.121
                dependence F13.221
        withdrawal F13.231
    cannabis intoxication (acute) F12.921
        in
            abuse F12.121
            dependence F12.221
    cocaine intoxication (acute) F14.921
        in
            abuse F14.121
            dependence F14.221
    general medical condition F05
    hallucinogen intoxication F16.921
        in
            abuse F16.121
            dependence F16.221
    hypnotic
        intoxication F13.921
            in
                abuse F13.121
                dependence F13.221
        withdrawal F13.231
    inhalant intoxication (acute) F18.921
        in
            abuse F18.121
            dependence F18.221
    multiple etiologies F05
    opioid intoxication (acute) F11.921
        in
            abuse F11.121
            dependence F11.221
    other (or unknown) substance F19.921
    phencyclidine intoxication (acute) F16.921
        in
            abuse F16.121
            dependence F16.221
    psychoactive substance NEC intoxication (acute)
        F19.921
        in
            abuse F19.121
            dependence F19.221

Delirium, delirious — *continued*
- due to — *continued*
  - sedative
    - intoxication F13.921
      - in
        - abuse F13.121
        - dependence F13.221
    - withdrawal F13.231
  - unknown etiology F05
- exhaustion F43.0
- hysterical F44.89
- postprocedural (postoperative) F05
- puerperal F05
- thyroid — *see* Thyrotoxicosis with thyroid storm
- traumatic — *see* Injury, intracranial
- tremens (alcohol-induced) F10.231
  - sedative-induced F13.231

Delivery (childbirth) (labor)
- arrested active phase O62.1
- cesarean (for)
  - without indication O82
  - abnormal
    - pelvis (bony) (deformity) (major) NEC with disproportion (fetopelvic) O33.0
      - with obstructed labor O65.0
    - presentation or position O32.9 ☑
  - abruptio placentae (*see also* Abruptio placentae) O45.9- ☑
  - acromion presentation O32.2 ☑
  - atony, uterus O62.2
  - breech presentation O32.1 ☑
    - incomplete O32.8 ☑
  - brow presentation O32.3 ☑
  - cephalopelvic disproportion O33.9
  - cerclage O34.3- ☑
  - chin presentation O32.3 ☑
  - cicatrix of cervix O34.4- ☑
  - contracted pelvis (general)
    - inlet O33.2
    - outlet O33.3 ☑
  - cord presentation or prolapse O69.0 ☑
  - cystocele O34.8- ☑
  - deformity (acquired) (congenital)
    - pelvic organs or tissues NEC O34.8- ☑
    - pelvis (bony) NEC O33.0
  - disproportion NOS O33.9
  - eclampsia — *see* Eclampsia
  - face presentation O32.3 ☑
  - failed
    - forceps O66.5
    - induction of labor O61.9
      - instrumental O61.1
      - mechanical O61.1
      - medical O61.0
      - specified NEC O61.8
      - surgical O61.1
    - trial of labor NOS O66.40
      - following previous cesarean delivery O66.41
    - vacuum extraction O66.5
    - ventouse O66.5
  - fetal-maternal hemorrhage O43.01- ☑
  - hemorrhage (intrapartum) O67.9
    - with coagulation defect O67.0
    - specified cause NEC O67.8
  - high head at term O32.4 ☑
  - hydrocephalic fetus O33.6 ☑
  - incarceration of uterus O34.51- ☑
  - incoordinate uterine action O62.4
  - increased size, fetus O33.5 ☑
  - inertia, uterus O62.2
    - primary O62.0
    - secondary O62.1
  - lateroversion, uterus O34.59- ☑
  - mal lie O32.9 ☑
  - malposition
    - fetus O32.9 ☑
    - pelvic organs or tissues NEC O34.8- ☑
    - uterus NEC O34.59- ☑
  - malpresentation NOS O32.9 ☑
  - oblique presentation O32.2 ☑
  - occurring after 37 completed weeks of gestation but before 39 completed weeks gestation due to (spontaneous) onset of labor O75.82
  - oversize fetus O33.5 ☑
  - pelvic tumor NEC O34.8- ☑
  - placenta previa O44.0- ☑
    - complete O44.0- ☑

Delivery — *continued*
- cesarean — *continued*
  - placenta previa — *continued*
    - complete — *continued*
      - with hemorrhage O44.1- ☑
  - placental insufficiency O36.51- ☑
  - planned, occurring after 37 completed weeks of gestation but before 39 completed weeks gestation due to (spontaneous) onset of labor O75.82
  - polyp, cervix O34.4- ☑
    - causing obstructed labor O65.5
  - poor dilatation, cervix O62.0
  - pre-eclampsia O14.94
    - mild O14.04
    - moderate O14.04
    - severe O14.14
      - with hemolysis, elevated liver enzymes and low platelet count (HELLP) O14.24
  - previous
    - cesarean delivery O34.219
      - classical (vertical) scar O34.212
      - low transverse scar O34.211
    - surgery (to)
      - cervix O34.4- ☑
      - gynecological NEC O34.8- ☑
      - rectum O34.7- ☑
      - uterus O34.29
      - vagina O34.6- ☑
  - prolapse
    - arm or hand O32.2 ☑
    - uterus O34.52- ☑
  - prolonged labor NOS O63.9
  - rectocele O34.8- ☑
  - retroversion
    - uterus O34.53- ☑
  - rigid
    - cervix O34.4- ☑
    - pelvic floor O34.8- ☑
    - perineum O34.7- ☑
    - vagina O34.6- ☑
    - vulva O34.7- ☑
  - sacculation, pregnant uterus O34.59- ☑
  - scar(s)
    - cervix O34.4- ☑
    - cesarean delivery O34.219
      - classical (vertical) O34.212
      - low transverse O34.211
    - transmural uterine O34.29
    - uterus O34.29
  - Shirodkar suture in situ O34.3- ☑
  - shoulder presentation O32.2 ☑
  - stenosis or stricture, cervix O34.4- ☑
  - streptococcus group B (GBS) carrier state O99.824
  - transmural uterine scar O34.29
  - transverse presentation or lie O32.2 ☑
  - tumor, pelvic organs or tissues NEC O34.8- ☑
    - cervix O34.4- ☑
  - umbilical cord presentation or prolapse O69.0 ☑
- completely normal case O80
- complicated O75.9
  - by
    - abnormal, abnormality (of)
      - forces of labor O62.9
        - specified type NEC O62.8
      - glucose O99.814
      - uterine contractions NOS O62.9
    - abruptio placentae (*see also* Abruptio placentae) O45.9- ☑
    - abuse
      - physical O9A.32 (*following* O99)
      - psychological O9A.52 (*following* O99)
      - sexual O9A.42 (*following* O99)
    - adherent placenta O72.0
      - without hemorrhage O73.0
    - alcohol use O99.314
    - anemia (pre-existing) O99.02
    - anesthetic death O74.8
    - annular detachment of cervix O71.3
    - atony, uterus O62.2
    - attempted vacuum extraction and forceps O66.5
    - Bandl's ring O62.4
    - bariatric surgery status O99.844
    - biliary tract disorder O26.62
    - bleeding — *see* Delivery, complicated by, hemorrhage
    - blood disorder NEC O99.12

Delivery — *continued*
- complicated — *continued*
  - by — *continued*
    - cervical dystocia (hypotonic) O62.2
      - primary O62.0
      - secondary O62.1
    - circulatory system disorder O99.42
    - compression of cord (umbilical) NEC O69.2 ☑
    - condition NEC O99.89
    - contraction, contracted ring O62.4
    - cord (umbilical)
      - around neck
        - with compression O69.1 ☑
        - without compression O69.81 ☑
      - bruising O69.5 ☑
      - complication O69.9 ☑
        - specified NEC O69.89 ☑
      - compression NEC O69.2 ☑
      - entanglement O69.2 ☑
        - without compression O69.82 ☑
      - hematoma O69.5 ☑
      - presentation O69.0 ☑
      - prolapse O69.0 ☑
      - short O69.3 ☑
      - thrombosis (vessels) O69.5 ☑
      - vascular lesion O69.5 ☑
    - Couvelaire uterus O45.8X- ☑
    - damage to (injury to) NEC
      - perineum O71.82
      - periurethral tissue O71.82
      - vulva O71.82
    - delay following rupture of membranes (spontaneous) — *see* Pregnancy, complicated by, premature rupture of membranes
    - depressed fetal heart tones O76
    - diabetes O24.92
      - gestational O24.429
        - diet controlled O24.420
        - insulin controlled O24.424
        - oral drug controlled (antidiabetic) (hypoglycemic) O24.425
      - pre-existing O24.32
        - specified NEC O24.82
        - type 1 O24.02
        - type 2 O24.12
    - diastasis recti (abdominis) O71.89
    - dilatation
      - bladder O66.8
      - cervix incomplete, poor or slow O62.0
    - disease NEC O99.89
    - disruptio uteri — *see* Delivery, complicated by, rupture, uterus
    - drug use O99.324
    - dysfunction, uterus NOS O62.9
      - hypertonic O62.4
      - hypotonic O62.2
        - primary O62.0
        - secondary O62.1
      - incoordinate O62.4
    - eclampsia O15.1
    - embolism (pulmonary) — *see* Embolism, obstetric
    - endocrine, nutritional or metabolic disease NEC O99.284
    - failed
      - attempted vaginal birth after previous cesarean delivery O66.41
      - induction of labor O61.9
        - instrumental O61.1
        - mechanical O61.1
        - medical O61.0
        - specified NEC O61.8
        - surgical O61.1
      - trial of labor O66.40
    - female genital mutilation O65.5
    - fetal
      - abnormal acid-base balance O68
      - acidemia O68
      - acidosis O68
      - alkalosis O68
      - death, early O02.1
      - deformity O66.3
      - heart rate or rhythm (abnormal) (non-reassuring) O76
      - hypoxia O77.8
      - stress O77.9
        - due to drug administration O77.1
        - electrocardiographic evidence of O77.8

Delivery — *continued*
  complicated — *continued*
    by — *continued*
      fetal — *continued*
        stress — *continued*
          specified NEC O77.8
          ultrasound evidence of O77.8
      fever during labor O75.2
      gastric banding status O99.844
      gastric bypass status O99.844
      gastrointestinal disease NEC O99.62
      gestational
        diabetes O24.429
          diet controlled O24.420
          insulin (and diet) controlled O24.424
          oral drug controlled (antidiabetic) (hypo-glycemic) O24.425
        edema O12.04
          with proteinuria O12.24
        proteinuria O12.14
      gonorrhea O98.22
      hematoma O71.7
        ischial spine O71.7
        pelvic O71.7
        vagina O71.7
        vulva or perineum O71.7
      hemorrhage (uterine) O67.9
        associated with
          afibrinogenemia O67.0
          coagulation defect O67.0
          hyperfibrinolysis O67.0
          hypofibrinogenemia O67.0
        due to
          low implantation of placenta O44.5- ☑
          low-lying placenta O44.5- ☑
          placenta previa O44.1- ☑
            marginal O44.3- ☑
            partial O44.3- ☑
          premature separation of placenta (nor-mally implanted) (*see also* Abruptio placentae) O45.9- ☑
          retained placenta O72.0
          uterine leiomyoma O67.8
        placenta NEC O67.8
        postpartum NEC (atonic) (immediate) O72.1
          with retained or trapped placenta O72.0
          delayed O72.2
          secondary O72.2
          third stage O72.0
      hourglass contraction, uterus O62.4
      hypertension, hypertensive (pre-existing) — *see* Hypertension, complicated by, child-birth (labor)
      hypotension O26.5- ☑
      incomplete dilatation (cervix) O62.0
      incoordinate uterus contractions O62.4
      inertia, uterus O62.2
        during latent phase of labor O62.0
        primary O62.0
        secondary O62.1
      infection (maternal) O98.92
        carrier state NEC O99.834
        gonorrhea O98.22
        human immunodeficiency virus (HIV) O98.72
        sexually transmitted NEC O98.32
        specified NEC O98.82
        syphilis O98.12
        tuberculosis O98.02
        viral hepatitis O98.42
        viral NEC O98.52
      injury (to mother) (*see also* Delivery, complicat-ed, by, damage to) O71.9
        nonobstetric O9A.22 (*following* O99)
          caused by abuse — *see* Delivery, compli-cated by, abuse
      intrauterine fetal death, early O02.1
      inversion, uterus O71.2
      laceration (perineal) O70.9
        anus (sphincter) O70.4
          with third degree laceration (*see also* Delivery, complicated, by, lacera-tion, perineum, third degree) O70.20
            with mucosa O70.3
          without third degree laceration O70.2 ☑
        bladder (urinary) O71.5
        bowel O71.5

Delivery — *continued*
  complicated — *continued*
    by — *continued*
      laceration — *continued*
        cervix (uteri) O71.3
        fourchette O70.0
        hymen O70.0
        labia O70.0
        pelvic
          floor O70.1
          organ NEC O71.5
        perineum, perineal O70.9
          first degree O70.0
          fourth degree O70.3
          muscles O70.1
          second degree O70.1
          skin O70.0
          slight O70.0
          third degree O70.20
            with
              less than 50% of external anal sphincter (EAS) thickness torn (IIIa) O70.21
              both external anal sphincter (EAS) and internal anal sphincter (IAS) torn (IIIc) O70.23
              more than 50% external anal sphincter (EAS) thickness torn (IIIb) O70.22
            IIIa O70.21
            IIIb O70.22
            IIIc O70.23
        peritoneum (pelvic) O71.5
        rectovaginal (septum) (without perineal laceration) O71.4
          with perineum (*see also* Delivery, compli-cated, by, laceration, perineum, third degree)
          with anal or rectal mucosa O70.3
        specified NEC O71.89
        sphincter ani — *see* Delivery, complicated, by, laceration, anus (sphincter)
        urethra O71.5
        uterus O71.81
          before labor O71.81
        vagina, vaginal (deep) (high) (without per-ineal laceration) O71.4
          with perineum O70.0
          muscles, with perineum O70.1
        vulva O70.0
      liver disorder O26.62
      malignancy O9A.12 (*following* O99)
      malnutrition O25.2
      malposition, malpresentation
        without obstruction (*see also* Delivery, complicated by, obstruction) O32.9 ☑
          breech O32.1 ☑
          compound O32.6 ☑
          face (brow) (chin) O32.3 ☑
          footling O32.8 ☑
          high head O32.4 ☑
          oblique O32.2 ☑
          specified NEC O32.8 ☑
          transverse O32.2 ☑
          unstable lie O32.0 ☑
        placenta O44.0- ☑
          with hemorrhage O44.1- ☑
        uterus or cervix O65.5
      meconium in amniotic fluid O77.0
      mental disorder NEC O99.344
      metrorrhexis — *see* Delivery, complicated by, rupture, uterus
      nervous system disorder O99.354
      obesity (pre-existing) O99.214
      obesity surgery status O99.844
      obstetric trauma O71.9
        specified NEC O71.89
      obstructed labor
        due to
          breech (complete) (frank) presentation O64.1 ☑
            incomplete O64.8 ☑
          brow presenation O64.3 ☑
          buttock presentation O64.1 ☑
          chin presentation O64.2 ☑
          compound presentation O64.5 ☑
          contracted pelvis O65.1
          deep transverse arrest O64.0 ☑

Delivery — *continued*
  complicated — *continued*
    by — *continued*
      obstructed labor — *continued*
        due to — *continued*
          deformed pelvis O65.0
          dystocia (fetal) O66.9
            due to
              conjoined twins O66.3
              fetal
                abnormality NEC O66.3
                ascites O66.3
                hydrops O66.3
                meningomyelocele O66.3
                sacral teratoma O66.3
                tumor O66.3
             hydrocephalic fetus O66.3
            shoulder O66.0
          face presentation O64.2 ☑
          fetopelvic disproportion O65.4
          footling presentation O64.8 ☑
          impacted shoulders O66.0
          incomplete rotation of fetal head O64.0 ☑
          large fetus O66.2
          locked twins O66.1
          malposition O64.9 ☑
            specified NEC O64.8 ☑
          malpresentation O64.9 ☑
            specified NEC O64.8 ☑
          multiple fetuses NEC O66.6
          pelvic
            abnormality (maternal) O65.9
              organ O65.5
              specified NEC O65.8
            contraction
              inlet O65.2
              mid-cavity O65.3
              outlet O65.3
          persistent (position)
            occipitoiliac O64.0 ☑
            occipitoposterior O64.0 ☑
            occipitosacral O64.0 ☑
            occipitotransverse O64.0 ☑
          prolapsed arm O64.4 ☑
          shoulder presentation O64.4 ☑
        specified NEC O66.8
      pathological retraction ring, uterus O62.4
      penetration, pregnant uterus by instrument O71.1
      perforation — *see* Delivery, complicated by, laceration
      placenta, placental
        ablatio (*see also* Abruptio placentae) O45.9- ☑
        abnormality O43.9- ☑
          specified NEC O43.89- ☑
        abruptio (*see also* Abruptio placentae) O45.9- ☑
        accreta O43.21- ☑
        adherent (with hemorrhage) O72.0
          without hemorrhage O73.0
        detachment (premature) (*see also* Abruptio placentae) O45.9- ☑
        disorder O43.9- ☑
          specified NEC O43.89- ☑
        hemorrhage NEC O67.8
        increta O43.22- ☑
        low (implantation) (lying) O44.4- ☑
          with hemorrhage O44.5- ☑
        malformation O43.10- ☑
        malposition O44.0- ☑
          without hemorrhage O44.1- ☑
        percreta O43.23- ☑
        previa (central) (complete) (lateral) (total) O44.0- ☑
          with hemorrhage O44.1- ☑
          marginal O44.2- ☑
            with hemorrhage O44.3- ☑
          partial O44.2- ☑
            with hemorrhage O44.3- ☑
        retained (with hemorrhage) O72.0
          without hemorrhage O73.0
        separation (premature) O45.9- ☑
          specified NEC O45.8X- ☑
        vicious insertion O44.1- ☑
      precipitate labor O62.3

Subterms under main terms may continue to next column or page   ☑ Additional Character Required — Refer to the Tabular List for Character Selection   91

Delivery — Delivery

Delivery — continued
  complicated — continued
    by — continued
      premature rupture, membranes (see also Pregnancy, complicated by, premature rupture of membranes) O42.90
      prolapse
        arm or hand O32.2 ☑
        cord (umbilical) O69.0 ☑
        foot or leg O32.8 ☑
        uterus O34.52- ☑
      prolonged labor O63.9
        first stage O63.0
        second stage O63.1
      protozoal disease (maternal) O98.62
      respiratory disease NEC O99.52
      retained membranes or portions of placenta O72.2
        without hemorrhage O73.1
      retarded birth O63.9
      retention of secundines (with hemorrhage) O72.0
        without hemorrhage O73.0
        partial O72.2
          without hemorrhage O73.1
      rupture
        bladder (urinary) O71.5
        cervix O71.3
        pelvic organ NEC O71.5
        urethra O71.5
        uterus (during or after labor) O71.1
          before labor O71.0- ☑
      separation, pubic bone (symphysis pubis) O71.6
      shock O75.1
      shoulder presentation O64.4 ☑
      skin disorder NEC O99.72
      spasm, cervix O62.4
      stenosis or stricture, cervix O65.5
      streptococcus group B (GBS) carrier state O99.824
      subluxation of symphysis (pubis) O26.72
      syphilis (maternal) O98.12
      tear — see Delivery, complicated by, laceration
      tetanic uterus O62.4
      trauma (obstetrical) (see also Delivery, complicated, by, damage to) O71.9
        non-obstetric O9A.22 (following O99)
        periurethral O71.82
        specified NEC O71.89
      tuberculosis (maternal) O98.02
      tumor, pelvic organs or tissues NEC O65.5
      umbilical cord around neck
        with compression O69.1 ☑
        without compression O69.81 ☑
      uterine inertia O62.2
        during latent phase of labor O62.0
        primary O62.0
        secondary O62.1
      vasa previa O69.4 ☑
      velamentous insertion of cord O43.12- ☑
    specified complication NEC O75.89
  delayed NOS O63.9
    following rupture of membranes artificial O75.5
  second twin, triplet, etc. O63.2
  forceps, low following failed vacuum extraction O66.5
  missed (at or near term) O36.4 ☑
  normal O80
  obstructed — see Delivery, complicated by, obstructed labor
  precipitate O62.3
  preterm (see also Pregnancy, complicated by, preterm labor) O60.10 ☑
  spontaneous O80
  term pregnancy NOS O80
  uncomplicated O80
  vaginal, following previous cesarean delivery O34.219
    classical (vertical) scar O34.212
    low transverse scar O34.211
Delusions (paranoid) — see Disorder, delusional
Dementia (degenerative (primary)) (old age) (persisting) F03.90
  with
    aggressive behavior F03.91
    behavioral disturbance F03.91
    combative behavior F03.91
    Lewy bodies G31.83 [F02.80]
      with behavioral disturbance G31.83 [F02.81]

Dementia — continued
  with — continued
    Parkinsonism G31.83 [F02.80]
      with behavioral disturbance G31.83 [F02.81]
    Parkinson's disease G20 [F02.80]
      with behavioral disturbance G20 [F02.81]
    violent behavior F03.91
  alcoholic F10.97
    with dependence F10.27
  Alzheimer's type — see Disease, Alzheimer's
  arteriosclerotic — see Dementia, vascular
  atypical, Alzheimer's type — see Disease, Alzheimer's, specified NEC
  congenital — see Disability, intellectual
  frontal (lobe) G31.09 [F02.80]
    with behavioral disturbance G31.09 [F02.81]
  frontotemporal G31.09 [F02.80]
    with behavioral disturbance G31.09 [F02.81]
    specified NEC G31.09 [F02.80]
      with behavioral disturbance G31.09 [F02.81]
  Huntington's disease or chorea G10
    with dementia G10 [F02.80]
  in (due to)
    with behavioral disturbance G31.83 [F02.81]
    alcohol F10.97
      with dependence F10.27
    Alzheimer's disease — see Disease, Alzheimer's
    arteriosclerotic brain disease — see Dementia, vascular
    cerebral lipidoses E75.- ☑ [F02.80]
      with behavioral disturbance E75.- ☑ [F02.81]
    Creutzfeldt-Jakob disease (see also Creutzfeldt-Jakob disease or syndrome (with dementia)) A81.00
    epilepsy G40.- ☑ [F02.80]
      with behavioral disturbance G40.- ☑ [F02.81]
    hepatolenticular degeneration E83.01 [F02.80]
      with behavioral disturbance E83.01 [F02.81]
    human immunodeficiency virus (HIV) disease B20 [F02.80]
      with behavioral disturbance B20 [F02.81]
    Huntington's disease or chorea G10 [F02.80]
      with behavioral disturbance G10 [F02.81]
    hypercalcemia E83.52 [F02.80]
      with behavioral disturbance E83.52 [F02.81]
    hypothyroidism, acquired E03.9 [F02.80]
      with behavioral disturbance E03.9 [F02.81]
      due to iodine deficiency E01.8 [F02.80]
        with behavioral disturbance E01.8 [F02.81]
    inhalants F18.97
      with dependence F18.27
    multiple
      etiologies F03 ☑
      sclerosis G35 [F02.80]
        with behavioral disturbance G35 [F02.81]
    neurosyphilis A52.17 [F02.80]
      with behavioral disturbance A52.17 [F02.81]
      juvenile A50.49 [F02.80]
        with behavioral disturbance A50.49 [F02.81]
    niacin deficiency E52 [F02.80]
      with behavioral disturbance E52 [F02.81]
    paralysis agitans G20 [F02.80]
      with behavioral disturbance G20 [F02.81]
    Parkinson's disease G20 [F02.80]
    pellagra E52 [F02.80]
      with behavioral disturbance E52 [F02.81]
    Pick's G31.01 [F02.80]
      with behavioral disturbance G31.01 [F02.81]
    polyarteritis nodosa M30.0 [F02.80]
      with behavioral disturbance M30.0 [F02.81]
    psychoactive drug F19.97
      with dependence F19.27
      inhalants F18.97
        with dependence F18.27
      sedatives, hypnotics or anxiolytics F13.97
        with dependence F13.27
    sedatives, hypnotics or anxiolytics F13.97
      with dependence F13.27
    systemic lupus erythematosus M32.- ☑ [F02.80]
      with behavioral disturbance M32.- ☑ [F02.81]
    trypanosomiasis
      African B56.9 [F02.80]
        with behavioral disturbance B56.9 [F02.81]
    unknown etiology F03 ☑
    vitamin B12 deficiency E53.8 [F02.80]
      with behavioral disturbance E53.8 [F02.81]
    volatile solvents F18.97
      with dependence F18.27

Dementia — continued
  infantile, infantilis F84.3
  Lewy body G31.83 [F02.80]
    with behavioral disturbance G31.83 [F02.81]
  multi-infarct — see Dementia, vascular
  paralytica, paralytic (syphilitic) A52.17 [F02.80]
    with behavioral disturbance A52.17 [F02.81]
    juvenilis A50.45
  paretic A52.17
  praecox — see Schizophrenia
  presenile F03 ☑
    Alzheimer's type — see Disease, Alzheimer's, early onset
  primary degenerative F03 ☑
  progressive, syphilitic A52.17
  senile F03 ☑
    with acute confusional state F05
    Alzheimer's type — see Disease, Alzheimer's, late onset
    depressed or paranoid type F03 ☑
  vascular (acute onset) (mixed) (multi-infarct) (subcortical) F01.50
    with behavioral disturbance F01.51
Demineralization, bone — see Osteoporosis
Demodex folliculorum (infestation) B88.0
Demophobia F40.248
Demoralization R45.3
Demyelination, demyelinization
  central nervous system G37.9
    specified NEC G37.8
  corpus callosum (central) G37.1
  disseminated, acute G36.9
    specified NEC G36.8
  global G35
  in optic neuritis G36.0
Dengue (classical) (fever) A90
  hemorrhagic A91
  sandfly A93.1
Dennie-Marfan syphilitic syndrome A50.45
Dens evaginatus, in dente or invaginatus K00.2
Dense breasts R92.2
Density
  increased, bone (disseminated) (generalized) (spotted) — see Disorder, bone, density and structure, specified type NEC
  lung (nodular) J98.4
Dental (see also condition)
  examination Z01.20
    with abnormal findings Z01.21
  restoration
    aesthetically inadequate or displeasing K08.56
    defective K08.50
      specified NEC K08.59
    failure of marginal integrity K08.51
    failure of periodontal anatomical integrity K08.54
Dentia praecox K00.6
Denticles (pulp) K04.2
Dentigerous cyst K09.0
Dentin
  irregular (in pulp) K04.3
  opalescent K00.5
  secondary (in pulp) K04.3
  sensitive K03.89
Dentinogenesis imperfecta K00.5
Dentinoma — see Cyst, calcifying odontogenic
Dentition (syndrome) K00.7
  delayed K00.6
  difficult K00.7
  precocious K00.6
  premature K00.6
  retarded K00.6
Dependence (on) (syndrome) F19.20
  with remission F19.21
  alcohol (ethyl) (methyl) (without remission) F10.20
    with
      amnestic disorder, persisting F10.26
      anxiety disorder F10.280
      dementia, persisting F10.27
      intoxication F10.229
        with delirium F10.221
        uncomplicated F10.220
      mood disorder F10.24
      psychotic disorder F10.259
        with
          delusions F10.250
          hallucinations F10.251
      remission F10.21
      sexual dysfunction F10.281

Dependence — *continued*
   alcohol — *continued*
      with — *continued*
         sleep disorder F10.282
         specified disorder NEC F10.288
         withdrawal F10.239
            with
               delirium F10.231
               perceptual disturbance F10.232
            uncomplicated F10.230
      counseling and surveillance Z71.41
   amobarbital — *see* Dependence, drug, sedative
   amphetamine(s) (type) — *see* Dependence, drug, stimulant NEC
   amytal (sodium) — *see* Dependence, drug, sedative
   analgesic NEC F55.8
   anesthetic (agent) (gas) (general) (local) NEC — *see* Dependence, drug, psychoactive NEC
   anxiolytic NEC — *see* Dependence, drug, sedative
   barbital(s) — *see* Dependence, drug, sedative
   barbiturate(s) (compounds) (drugs classifiable to T42) — *see* Dependence, drug, sedative
   benzedrine — *see* Dependence, drug, stimulant NEC
   bhang — *see* Dependence, drug, cannabis
   bromide(s) NEC — *see* Dependence, drug, sedative
   caffeine — *see* Dependence, drug, stimulant NEC
   cannabis (sativa) (indica) (resin) (derivatives) (type) — *see* Dependence, drug, cannabis
   chloral (betaine) (hydrate) — *see* Dependence, drug, sedative
   chlordiazepoxide — *see* Dependence, drug, sedative
   coca (leaf) (derivatives) — *see* Dependence, drug, cocaine
   cocaine — *see* Dependence, drug, cocaine
   codeine — *see* Dependence, drug, opioid
   combinations of drugs F19.20
   dagga — *see* Dependence, drug, cannabis
   demerol — *see* Dependence, drug, opioid
   dexamphetamine — *see* Dependence, drug, stimulant NEC
   dexedrine — *see* Dependence, drug, stimulant NEC
   dextromethorphan — *see* Dependence, drug, opioid
   dextromoramide — *see* Dependence, drug, opioid
   dextro-nor-pseudo-ephedrine — *see* Dependence, drug, stimulant NEC
   dextrorphan — *see* Dependence, drug, opioid
   diazepam — *see* Dependence, drug, sedative
   dilaudid — *see* Dependence, drug, opioid
   D-lysergic acid diethylamide — *see* Dependence, drug, hallucinogen
   drug NEC F19.20
      with sleep disorder F19.282
      cannabis F12.20
         with
            anxiety disorder F12.280
            intoxication F12.229
               with
                  delirium F12.221
                  perceptual disturbance F12.222
               uncomplicated F12.220
            other specified disorder F12.288
            psychosis F12.259
               delusions F12.250
               hallucinations F12.251
            unspecified disorder F12.29
         in remission F12.21
      cocaine F14.20
         with
            anxiety disorder F14.280
            intoxication F14.229
               with
                  delirium F14.221
                  perceptual disturbance F14.222
               uncomplicated F14.220
            mood disorder F14.24
            other specified disorder F14.288
            psychosis F14.259
               delusions F14.250
               hallucinations F14.251
            sexual dysfunction F14.281
            sleep disorder F14.282
            unspecified disorder F14.29
            withdrawal F14.23
         in remission F14.21
         withdrawal symptoms in newborn P96.1
      counseling and surveillance Z71.51
      hallucinogen F16.20

Dependence — *continued*
   drug — *continued*
      hallucinogen — *continued*
         with
            anxiety disorder F16.280
            flashbacks F16.283
            intoxication F16.229
               with delirium F16.221
               uncomplicated F16.220
            mood disorder F16.24
            other specified disorder F16.288
            perception disorder, persisting F16.283
            psychosis F16.259
               delusions F16.250
               hallucinations F16.251
            unspecified disorder F16.29
         in remission F16.21
      in remission F19.21
      inhalant F18.20
         with
            anxiety disorder F18.280
            dementia, persisting F18.27
            intoxication F18.229
               with delirium F18.221
               uncomplicated F18.220
            mood disorder F18.24
            other specified disorder F18.288
            psychosis F18.259
               delusions F18.250
               hallucinations F18.251
            unspecified disorder F18.29
         in remission F18.21
      nicotine F17.200
         with disorder F17.209
            in remission F17.201
            specified disorder NEC F17.208
            withdrawal F17.203
         chewing tobacco F17.220
            with disorder F17.229
               in remission F17.221
               specified disorder NEC F17.228
               withdrawal F17.223
         cigarettes F17.210
            with disorder F17.219
               in remission F17.211
               specified disorder NEC F17.218
               withdrawal F17.213
         specified product NEC F17.290
            with disorder F17.299
               remission F17.291
               specified disorder NEC F17.298
               withdrawal F17.293
      opioid F11.20
         with
            intoxication F11.229
               with
                  delirium F11.221
                  perceptual disturbance F11.222
               uncomplicated F11.220
            mood disorder F11.24
            other specified disorder F11.288
            psychosis F11.259
               delusions F11.250
               hallucinations F11.251
            sexual dysfunction F11.281
            sleep disorder F11.282
            unspecified disorder F11.29
            withdrawal F11.23
         in remission F11.21
      psychoactive NEC F19.20
         with
            amnestic disorder F19.26
            anxiety disorder F19.280
            dementia F19.27
            intoxication F19.229
               with
                  delirium F19.221
                  perceptual disturbance F19.222
               uncomplicated F19.220
            mood disorder F19.24
            other specified disorder F19.288
            psychosis F19.259
               delusions F19.250
               hallucinations F19.251
            sexual dysfunction F19.281
            sleep disorder F19.282
            unspecified disorder F19.29
            withdrawal F19.239

Dependence — *continued*
   drug — *continued*
      psychoactive — *continued*
         with — *continued*
            withdrawal — *continued*
               with
                  delirium F19.231
                  perceptual disturbance F19.232
               uncomplicated F19.230
      sedative, hypnotic or anxiolytic F13.20
         with
            amnestic disorder F13.26
            anxiety disorder F13.280
            dementia, persisting F13.27
            intoxication F13.229
               with delirium F13.221
               uncomplicated F13.220
            mood disorder F13.24
            other specified disorder F13.288
            psychosis F13.259
               delusions F13.250
               hallucinations F13.251
            sexual dysfunction F13.281
            sleep disorder F13.282
            unspecified disorder F13.29
            withdrawal F13.239
               with
                  delirium F13.231
                  perceptual disturbance F13.232
               uncomplicated F13.230
         in remission F13.21
      stimulant NEC F15.20
         with
            anxiety disorder F15.280
            intoxication F15.229
               with
                  delirium F15.221
                  perceptual disturbance F15.222
               uncomplicated F15.220
            mood disorder F15.24
            other specified disorder F15.288
            psychosis F15.259
               delusions F15.250
               hallucinations F15.251
            sexual dysfunction F15.281
            sleep disorder F15.282
            unspecified disorder F15.29
            withdrawal F15.23
         in remission F15.21
   ethyl
      alcohol (without remission) F10.20
         with remission F10.21
      bromide — *see* Dependence, drug, sedative
      carbamate F19.20
      chloride F19.20
      morphine — *see* Dependence, drug, opioid
   ganja — *see* Dependence, drug, cannabis
   glue (airplane) (sniffing) — *see* Dependence, drug, inhalant
   glutethimide — *see* Dependence, drug, sedative
   hallucinogenics — *see* Dependence, drug, hallucinogen
   hashish — *see* Dependence, drug, cannabis
   hemp — *see* Dependence, drug, cannabis
   heroin (salt) (any) — *see* Dependence, drug, opioid
   hypnotic NEC — *see* Dependence, drug, sedative
   Indian hemp — *see* Dependence, drug, cannabis
   inhalants — *see* Dependence, drug, inhalant
   khat — *see* Dependence, drug, stimulant NEC
   laudanum — *see* Dependence, drug, opioid
   LSD (-25) (derivatives) — *see* Dependence, drug, hallucinogen
   luminal — *see* Dependence, drug, sedative
   lysergic acid — *see* Dependence, drug, hallucinogen
   maconha — *see* Dependence, drug, cannabis
   marihuana — *see* Dependence, drug, cannabis
   meprobamate — *see* Dependence, drug, sedative
   mescaline — *see* Dependence, drug, hallucinogen
   methadone — *see* Dependence, drug, opioid
   methamphetamine(s) — *see* Dependence, drug, stimulant NEC
   methaqualone — *see* Dependence, drug, sedative
   methyl
      alcohol (without remission) F10.20
         with remission F10.21
      bromide — *see* Dependence, drug, sedative
      morphine — *see* Dependence, drug, opioid

Dependence — continued
  methyl — continued
    phenidate — see Dependence, drug, stimulant
      NEC
    sulfonal — see Dependence, drug, sedative
  morphine (sulfate) (sulfite) (type) — see Dependence,
    drug, opioid
  narcotic (drug) NEC — see Dependence, drug, opioid
  nembutal — see Dependence, drug, sedative
  neraval — see Dependence, drug, sedative
  neravan — see Dependence, drug, sedative
  neurobarb — see Dependence, drug, sedative
  nicotine — see Dependence, drug, nicotine
  nitrous oxide F19.20
  nonbarbiturate sedatives and tranquilizers with similar
    effect — see Dependence, drug, sedative
  on
    artificial heart (fully implantable) (mechanical)
      Z95.812
    aspirator Z99.0
    care provider (because of) Z74.9
      impaired mobility Z74.09
      need for
        assistance with personal care Z74.1
        continuous supervision Z74.3
      no other household member able to render
        care Z74.2
      specified reason NEC Z74.8
    machine Z99.89
      enabling NEC Z99.89
      specified type NEC Z99.89
    renal dialysis (hemodialysis) (peritoneal) Z99.2
    respirator Z99.11
    ventilator Z99.11
    wheelchair Z99.3
  opiate — see Dependence, drug, opioid
  opioids — see Dependence, drug, opioid
  opium (alkaloids) (derivatives) (tincture) — see Depen-
    dence, drug, opioid
  oxygen (long-term) (supplemental) Z99.81
  paraldehyde — see Dependence, drug, sedative
  paregoric — see Dependence, drug, opioid
  PCP (phencyclidine) (or related substance) — see De-
    pendence, drug, hallucinogen
  pentobarbital — see Dependence, drug, sedative
  pentobarbitone (sodium) — see Dependence, drug,
    sedative
  pentothal — see Dependence, drug, sedative
  peyote — see Dependence, drug, hallucinogen
  phencyclidine (PCP) (or related substance) — see De-
    pendence, drug, hallucinogen
  phenmetrazine — see Dependence, drug, stimulant
    NEC
  phenobarbital — see Dependence, drug, sedative
  polysubstance F19.20
  psilocibin, psilocin, psilocyn, psilocyline — see Depen-
    dence, drug, hallucinogen
  psychostimulant NEC — see Dependence, drug, stim-
    ulant NEC
  secobarbital — see Dependence, drug, sedative
  seconal — see Dependence, drug, sedative
  sedative NEC — see Dependence, drug, sedative
  specified drug NEC — see Dependence, drug
  stimulant NEC — see Dependence, drug, stimulant
    NEC
  substance NEC — see Dependence, drug
  supplemental oxygen Z99.81
  tobacco — see Dependence, drug, nicotine
    counseling and surveillance Z71.6
  tranquilizer NEC — see Dependence, drug, sedative
  vitamin B6 E53.1
  volatile solvents — see Dependence, drug, inhalant
Dependency
  care-provider Z74.9
  passive F60.7
  reactions (persistent) F60.7
Depersonalization (in neurotic state) (neurotic) (syndrome) F48.1
Depletion
  extracellular fluid E86.9
  plasma E86.1
  potassium E87.6
    nephropathy N25.89
  salt or sodium E87.1
    causing heat exhaustion or prostration T67.4 ☑
    nephropathy N28.9
  volume NOS E86.9

Deployment (current) (military) status Z56.82
  in theater or in support of military war, peacekeeping
    and humanitarian operations Z56.82
  personal history of Z91.82
    military war, peacekeeping and humanitarian de-
      ployment (current or past conflict) Z91.82
  returned from Z91.82
Depolarization, premature I49.40
  atrial I49.1
  junctional I49.2
  specified NEC I49.49
  ventricular I49.3
Deposit
  bone in Boeck's sarcoid D86.89
  calcareous, calcium — see Calcification
  cholesterol
    retina H35.89
    vitreous (body) (humor) — see Deposit, crystalline
  conjunctiva H11.11- ☑
  cornea H18.00- ☑
    argentous H18.02- ☑
    due to metabolic disorder H18.03- ☑
    Kayser-Fleischer ring H18.04- ☑
    pigmentation — see Pigmentation, cornea
  crystalline, vitreous (body) (humor) H43.2- ☑
  hemosiderin in old scars of cornea — see Pigmenta-
    tion, cornea, stromal
  metallic in lens — see Cataract, specified NEC
  skin R23.8
  tooth, teeth (betel) (black) (green) (materia alba) (or-
    ange) (tobacco) K03.6
  urate, kidney — see Calculus, kidney
Depraved appetite — see Pica
Depressed
  HDL cholesterol E78.6
Depression (acute) (mental) F32.9
  agitated (single episode) F32.2
  anaclitic — see Disorder, adjustment
  anxiety F41.8
    persistent F34.1
  arches (see also Deformity, limb, flat foot)
  atypical (single episode) F32.89
    recurrent episode F33.8
  basal metabolic rate R94.8
  bone marrow D75.89
  central nervous system R09.2
  cerebral R29.818
    newborn P91.4
  cerebrovascular I67.9
  chest wall M95.4
  climacteric (single episode) F32.89
    recurrent episode F33.8
  endogenous (without psychotic symptoms) F33.2
    with psychotic symptoms F33.3
  functional activity R68.89
  hysterical F44.89
  involutional (single episode) F32.89
    recurrent episode F33.8
  major F32.9
    with psychotic symptoms F32.3
    recurrent — see Disorder, depressive, recurrent
  manic-depressive — see Disorder, depressive, recur-
    rent
  masked (single episode) F32.89
  medullary G93.89
  menopausal (single episode) F32.89
    recurrent episode F33.8
  metatarsus — see Depression, arches
  monopolar F33.9
  nervous F34.1
  neurotic F34.1
  nose M95.0
  postnatal F53
  postpartum F53
  post-psychotic of schizophrenia F32.89
  post-schizophrenic F32.89
  psychogenic (reactive) (single episode) F32.9
  psychoneurotic F34.1
  psychotic (single episode) F32.3
    recurrent F33.3
  reactive (psychogenic) (single episode) F32.9
    psychotic (single episode) F32.3
  recurrent — see Disorder, depressive, recurrent
  respiratory center G93.89
  seasonal — see Disorder, depressive, recurrent
  senile F03 ☑
  severe, single episode F32.2
  situational F43.21

Depression — continued
  skull Q67.4
  specified NEC (single episode) F32.89
  sternum M95.4
  visual field — see Defect, visual field
  vital (recurrent) (without psychotic symptoms) F33.2
    with psychotic symptoms F33.3
    single episode F32.2
Deprivation
  cultural Z60.3
  effects NOS T73.9 ☑
    specified NEC T73.8 ☑
  emotional NEC Z65.8
    affecting infant or child — see Maltreatment, child,
      psychological
  food T73.0 ☑
  protein — see Malnutrition
  sleep Z72.820
  social Z60.4
    affecting infant or child — see Maltreatment, child,
      psychological
  specified NEC T73.8 ☑
  vitamins — see Deficiency, vitamin
  water T73.1 ☑
Derangement
  ankle (internal) — see Derangement, joint, ankle
  cartilage (articular) NEC — see Derangement, joint,
    articular cartilage, by site
    recurrent — see Dislocation, recurrent
  cruciate ligament, anterior, current injury — see
    Sprain, knee, cruciate, anterior
  elbow (internal) — see Derangement, joint, elbow
  hip (joint) (internal) (old) — see Derangement, joint,
    hip
  joint (internal) M24.9
    ankylosis — see Ankylosis
    articular cartilage M24.10
      ankle M24.17- ☑
      elbow M24.12- ☑
      foot M24.17- ☑
      hand M24.14- ☑
      hip M24.15- ☑
      knee NEC M23.9- ☑
      loose body — see Loose, body
      shoulder M24.11- ☑
      wrist M24.13- ☑
    contracture — see Contraction, joint
    current injury (see also Dislocation)
      knee, meniscus or cartilage — see Tear, menis-
        cus
    dislocation
      pathological — see Dislocation, pathological
      recurrent — see Dislocation, recurrent
    knee — see Derangement, knee
    ligament — see Disorder, ligament
    loose body — see Loose, body
    recurrent — see Dislocation, recurrent
    specified type NEC M24.80
      ankle M24.87- ☑
      elbow M24.82- ☑
      foot joint M24.87- ☑
      hand joint M24.84- ☑
      hip M24.85- ☑
      shoulder M24.81- ☑
      wrist M24.83- ☑
    temporomandibular M26.69
  knee (recurrent) M23.9- ☑
    ligament disruption, spontaneous M23.60- ☑
      anterior cruciate M23.61- ☑
      capsular M23.67- ☑
      instability, chronic M23.5- ☑
      lateral collateral M23.64- ☑
      medial collateral M23.63- ☑
      posterior cruciate M23.62- ☑
    loose body M23.4- ☑
    meniscus M23.30- ☑
      cystic M23.00- ☑
        lateral M23.002
          anterior horn M23.04- ☑
          posterior horn M23.05- ☑
          specified NEC M23.06- ☑
        medial M23.005
          anterior horn M23.01- ☑
          posterior horn M23.02- ☑
          specified NEC M23.03- ☑

Derangement — continued
　knee — continued
　　meniscus — continued
　　　degenerate — see Derangement, knee, menis-
　　　　cus, specified NEC
　　　detached — see Derangement, knee, meniscus,
　　　　specified NEC
　　　due to old tear or injury M23.20- ☑
　　　　lateral M23.20- ☑
　　　　　anterior horn M23.24- ☑
　　　　　posterior horn M23.25- ☑
　　　　　specified NEC M23.26- ☑
　　　　medial M23.20- ☑
　　　　　anterior horn M23.21- ☑
　　　　　posterior horn M23.22- ☑
　　　　　specified NEC M23.23- ☑
　　　retained — see Derangement, knee, meniscus,
　　　　specified NEC
　　　specified NEC M23.30- ☑
　　　　lateral M23.30- ☑
　　　　　anterior horn M23.34- ☑
　　　　　posterior horn M23.35- ☑
　　　　　specified NEC M23.36- ☑
　　　　medial M23.30- ☑
　　　　　anterior horn M23.31- ☑
　　　　　posterior horn M23.32- ☑
　　　　　specified NEC M23.33- ☑
　　old M23.8X- ☑
　　specified NEC — see subcategory M23.8 ☑
　low back NEC — see Dorsopathy, specified NEC
　meniscus — see Derangement, knee, meniscus
　mental — see Psychosis
　patella, specified NEC — see Disorder, patella, derange-
　　ment NEC
　semilunar cartilage (knee) — see Derangement, knee,
　　meniscus, specified NEC
　shoulder (internal) — see Derangement, joint, shoul-
　　der
Dercum's disease E88.2
Derealization (neurotic) F48.1
Dermal — see condition
Dermaphytid — see Dermatophytosis
Dermatitis (eczematous) L30.9
　ab igne L59.0
　acarine B88.0
　actinic (due to sun) L57.8
　　other than from sun L59.8
　allergic — see Dermatitis, contact, allergic
　ambustionis, due to burn or scald — see Burn
　amebic A06.7
　ammonia L22
　arsenical (ingested) L27.8
　artefacta L98.1
　　psychogenic F54
　atopic L20.9
　　psychogenic F54
　　specified NEC L20.89
　autoimmune progesterone L30.8
　berlock, berloque L56.2
　blastomycotic B40.3
　blister beetle L24.89
　bullous, bullosa L13.9
　　mucosynechial, atrophic L12.1
　　seasonal L30.8
　　specified NEC L13.8
　calorica L59.0
　　due to burn or scald — see Burn
　caterpillar L24.89
　cercarial B65.3
　combustionis L59.0
　　due to burn or scald — see Burn
　congelationis T69.1 ☑
　contact (occupational) L25.9
　　allergic L23.9
　　　due to
　　　　adhesives L23.1
　　　　cement L23.5
　　　　chemical products NEC L23.5
　　　　chromium L23.0
　　　　cosmetics L23.2
　　　　dander (cat) (dog) L23.81
　　　　drugs in contact with skin L23.3
　　　　dyes L23.4
　　　　food in contact with skin L23.6
　　　　hair (cat) (dog) L23.81
　　　　insecticide L23.5
　　　　metals L23.0

Dermatitis — continued
　contact — continued
　　allergic — continued
　　　due to — continued
　　　　nickel L23.0
　　　　plants, non-food L23.7
　　　　plastic L23.5
　　　　rubber L23.5
　　　　specified agent NEC L23.89
　　　due to
　　　　cement L25.3
　　　　chemical products NEC L25.3
　　　　cosmetics L25.0
　　　　dander (cat) (dog) L23.81
　　　　drugs in contact with skin L25.1
　　　　dyes L25.2
　　　　food in contact with skin L25.4
　　　　hair (cat) (dog) L23.81
　　　　plants, non-food L25.5
　　　　specified agent NEC L25.8
　　irritant L24.9
　　　due to
　　　　cement L24.5
　　　　chemical products NEC L24.5
　　　　cosmetics L24.3
　　　　detergents L24.0
　　　　drugs in contact with skin L24.4
　　　　food in contact with skin L24.6
　　　　oils and greases L24.1
　　　　plants, non-food L24.7
　　　　solvents L24.2
　　　　specified agent NEC L24.89
　contusiformis L52
　diabetic — see E08-E13 with .620
　diaper L22
　diphtheritica A36.3
　dry skin L85.3
　due to
　　acetone (contact) (irritant) L24.2
　　acids (contact) (irritant) L24.5
　　adhesive(s) (allergic) (contact) (plaster) L23.1
　　　irritant L24.5
　　alcohol (irritant) (skin contact) (substances in cate-
　　　gory T51) L24.2
　　　taken internally L27.8
　　alkalis (contact) (irritant) L24.5
　　arsenic (ingested) L27.8
　　carbon disulfide (contact) (irritant) L24.2
　　caustics (contact) (irritant) L24.5
　　cement (contact) L25.3
　　cereal (ingested) L27.2
　　chemical(s) NEC L25.3
　　　taken internally L27.8
　　chlorocompounds L24.2
　　chromium (contact) (irritant) L24.81
　　coffee (ingested) L27.2
　　cold weather L30.8
　　cosmetics (contact) L25.0
　　　allergic L23.2
　　　irritant L24.3
　　cyclohexanes L24.2
　　dander (cat) (dog) L23.81
　　Demodex species B88.0
　　Dermanyssus gallinae B88.0
　　detergents (contact) (irritant) L24.0
　　dichromate L24.81
　　drugs and medicaments (generalized) (internal
　　　use) L27.0
　　　external — see Dermatitis, due to, drugs, in
　　　　contact with skin
　　　in contact with skin L25.1
　　　　allergic L23.3
　　　　irritant L24.4
　　　localized skin eruption L27.1
　　　specified substance — see Table of Drugs and
　　　　Chemicals
　　dyes (contact) L25.2
　　　allergic L23.4
　　　irritant L24.89
　　epidermophytosis — see Dermatophytosis
　　esters L24.2
　　external irritant NEC L24.9
　　fish (ingested) L27.2
　　flour (ingested) L27.2
　　food (ingested) L27.2
　　　in contact with skin L25.4
　　fruit (ingested) L27.2
　　furs (allergic) (contact) L23.81
　　glues — see Dermatitis, due to, adhesives

Dermatitis — continued
　due to — continued
　　glycols L24.2
　　greases NEC (contact) (irritant) L24.1
　　hair (cat) (dog) L23.81
　　hot
　　　objects and materials — see Burn
　　　weather or places L59.0
　　hydrocarbons L24.2
　　infrared rays L59.8
　　ingestion, ingested substance L27.9
　　　chemical NEC L27.8
　　　drugs and medicaments — see Dermatitis, due
　　　　to, drugs
　　　food L27.2
　　　specified NEC L27.8
　　insecticide in contact with skin L24.5
　　internal agent L27.9
　　　drugs and medicaments (generalized) — see
　　　　Dermatitis, due to, drugs
　　　food L27.2
　　irradiation — see Dermatitis, due to, radioactive
　　　substance
　　ketones L24.2
　　lacquer tree (allergic) (contact) L23.7
　　light (sun) NEC L57.8
　　　acute L56.8
　　　other L59.8
　　Liponyssoides sanguineus B88.0
　　low temperature L30.8
　　meat (ingested) L27.2
　　metals, metal salts (contact) (irritant) L24.81
　　milk (ingested) L27.2
　　nickel (contact) (irritant) L24.81
　　nylon (contact) (irritant) L24.5
　　oils NEC (contact) (irritant) L24.1
　　paint solvent (contact) (irritant) L24.2
　　petroleum products (contact) (irritant) (substances
　　　in T52.0) L24.2
　　plants NEC (contact) L25.5
　　　allergic L23.7
　　　irritant L24.7
　　plasters (adhesive) (any) (allergic) (contact) L23.1
　　　irritant L24.5
　　plastic (contact) L25.3
　　preservatives (contact) — see Dermatitis, due to,
　　　chemical, in contact with skin
　　primrose (allergic) (contact) L23.7
　　primula (allergic) (contact) L23.7
　　radiation L59.8
　　　nonionizing (chronic exposure) L57.8
　　　sun NEC L57.8
　　　　acute L56.8
　　radioactive substance L58.9
　　　acute L58.0
　　　chronic L58.1
　　radium L58.9
　　　acute L58.0
　　　chronic L58.1
　　ragweed (allergic) (contact) L23.7
　　Rhus (allergic) (contact) (diversiloba) (radicans)
　　　(toxicodendron) (venenata) (verniciflua)
　　　L23.7
　　rubber (contact) L24.5
　　Senecio jacobaea (allergic) (contact) L23.7
　　solvents (contact) (irritant) (substances in category
　　　T52) L24.2
　　specified agent NEC (contact) L25.8
　　　allergic L23.89
　　　irritant L24.89
　　sunshine NEC L57.8
　　　acute L56.8
　　tetrachlorethylene (contact) (irritant) L24.2
　　toluene (contact) (irritant) L24.2
　　turpentine (contact) L24.2
　　ultraviolet rays (sun NEC) (chronic exposure) L57.8
　　　acute L56.8
　　vaccine or vaccination L27.0
　　　specified substance — see Table of Drugs and
　　　　Chemicals
　　varicose veins — see Varix, leg, with, inflammation
　　X-rays L58.9
　　　acute L58.0
　　　chronic L58.1
　dyshidrotic L30.1
　dysmenorrheica N94.6
　escharotica — see Burn
　exfoliative, exfoliativa (generalized) L26

Dermatitis — *continued*
exfoliative, exfoliativa — *continued*
  neonatorum L00
eyelid (*see also* Dermatosis, eyelid)
  allergic H01.119
    left H01.116
      lower H01.115
      upper H01.114
    right H01.113
      lower H01.112
      upper H01.111
    contact — *see* Dermatitis, eyelid, allergic
    due to
      Demodex species B88.0
      herpes (zoster) B02.39
        simplex B00.59
    eczematous H01.139
      left H01.136
        lower H01.135
        upper H01.134
      right H01.133
        lower H01.132
        upper H01.131
facta, factitia, factitial L98.1
  psychogenic F54
flexural NEC L20.82
friction L30.4
fungus B36.9
  specified type NEC B36.8
gangrenosa, gangrenous infantum L08.0
harvest mite B88.0
heat L59.0
herpesviral, vesicular (ear) (lip) B00.1
herpetiformis (bullous) (erythematous) (pustular)
    (vesicular) L13.0
  juvenile L12.2
  senile L12.0
hiemalis L30.8
hypostatic, hypostatica — *see* Varix, leg, with, inflammation
infectious eczematoid L30.3
infective L30.3
irritant — *see* Dermatitis, contact, irritant
Jacquet's (diaper dermatitis) L22
Leptus B88.0
lichenified NEC L28.0
medicamentosa (generalized) (internal use) — *see*
    Dermatitis, due to drugs
mite B88.0
multiformis L13.0
  juvenile L12.2
napkin L22
neurotica L13.0
nummular L30.0
papillaris capillitii L73.0
pellagrous E52
perioral L71.0
photocontact L56.2
polymorpha dolorosa L13.0
pruriginosa L13.0
pruritic NEC L30.8
psychogenic F54
purulent L08.0
pustular
  contagious B08.02
  subcorneal L13.1
pyococcal L08.0
pyogenica L08.0
repens L40.2
Ritter's (exfoliativa) L00
Schamberg's L81.7
schistosome B65.3
seasonal bullous L30.8
seborrheic L21.9
  infantile L21.1
  specified NEC L21.8
sensitization NOS L23.9
septic L08.0
solare L57.8
specified NEC L30.8
stasis I87.2
  with
    varicose ulcer — *see* Varix, leg, with ulcer, with
        inflammation
    varicose veins — *see* Varix, leg, with, inflammation
  due to postthrombotic syndrome — *see* Syndrome,
      postthrombotic

Dermatitis — *continued*
suppurative L08.0
traumatic NEC L30.4
trophoneurotica L13.0
ultraviolet (sun) (chronic exposure) L57.8
  acute L56.8
varicose — *see* Varix, leg, with, inflammation
vegetans L10.1
veget, vesicular, herpesviral B00.1
verrucosa B43.0
vesicular, herpesviral B00.1
Dermatoarthritis, lipoid E78.81
Dermatochalasis, eyelid H02.839
  left H02.836
    lower H02.835
    upper H02.834
  right H02.833
    lower H02.832
    upper H02.831
Dermatofibroma (lenticulare) — *see* Neoplasm, skin,
    benign
  protuberans — *see* Neoplasm, skin, uncertain behavior
Dermatofibrosarcoma (pigmented) (protuberans) —
    see Neoplasm, skin, malignant
Dermatographia L50.3
Dermatolysis (exfoliativa) (congenital) Q82.8
  acquired L57.4
  eyelids — *see* Blepharochalasis
  palpebrarum — *see* Blepharochalasis
  senile L57.4
Dermatomegaly NEC Q82.8
Dermatomucosomyositis M33.10
  with
    myopathy M33.12
    respiratory involvement M33.11
    specified organ involvement NEC M33.19
Dermatomycosis B36.9
  furfuracea B36.0
  specified type NEC B36.8
Dermatomyositis (acute) (chronic) (*see also* Dermatopolymyositis)
  adult (*see also* Dermatomyositis, specified NEC) M33.10
  in (due to) neoplastic disease (*see also* Neoplasm)
      D49.9 [M36.0]
  juvenile M33.00
    with
      myopathy M33.02
      respiratory involvement M33.01
      specified organ involvement NEC M33.09
    without myopathy M33.03
  specified NEC M33.10
    with
      myopathy M33.12
      respiratory involvement M33.11
      specified organ involvement NEC M33.19
    without myopathy M33.13
Dermatoneuritis of children — *see* Poisoning, mercury
Dermatophilosis A48.8
Dermatophytid L30.2
Dermatophytide — *see* Dermatophytosis
Dermatophytosis (epidermophyton) (infection) (Microsporum) (tinea) (Trichophyton) B35.9
  beard B35.0
  body B35.4
  capitis B35.0
  corporis B35.4
  deep-seated B35.8
  disseminated B35.8
  foot B35.3
  granulomatous B35.8
  groin B35.6
  hand B35.2
  nail B35.1
  perianal (area) B35.6
  scalp B35.0
  specified NEC B35.8
Dermatopolymyositis M33.90
  with
    myopathy M33.92
    respiratory involvement M33.91
    specified organ involvement NEC M33.99
  without myopathy M33.93
  in neoplastic disease (*see also* Neoplasm)
      D49.9 [M36.0]
  juvenile M33.00
    with
      myopathy M33.02
      respiratory involvement M33.01
      specified organ involvement NEC M33.09

Dermatopolymyositis — *continued*
  specified NEC M33.10
    myopathy M33.12
    respiratory involvement M33.11
    specified organ involvement NEC M33.19
Dermatopolyneuritis — *see* Poisoning, mercury
Dermatorrhexis Q79.6
  acquired L57.4
Dermatosclerosis (*see also* Scleroderma)
  localized L94.0
Dermatosis L98.9
  Andrews' L08.89
  Bowen's — *see* Neoplasm, skin, in situ
  bullous L13.9
    specified NEC L13.8
  exfoliativa L26
  eyelid (noninfectious)
    dermatitis — *see* Dermatitis, eyelid
    discoid lupus erythematosus — *see* Lupus, erythematosus, eyelid
    xeroderma — *see* Xeroderma, acquired, eyelid
  factitial L98.1
  febrile neutrophilic L98.2
  gonococcal A54.89
  herpetiformis L13.0
    juvenile L12.2
  linear IgA L13.8
  menstrual NEC L98.8
  neutrophilic, febrile L98.2
  occupational — *see* Dermatitis, contact
  papulosa nigra L82.1
  pigmentary L81.9
    progressive L81.7
    Schamberg's L81.7
  psychogenic F54
  purpuric, pigmented L81.7
  pustular, subcorneal L13.1
  transient acantholytic L11.1
Dermographia, dermographism L50.3
Dermoid (cyst) (*see also* Neoplasm, benign, by site)
  with malignant transformation C56- ☑
  due to radiation (nonionizing) L57.8
Dermopathy
  infiltrative with thyrotoxicosis — *see* Thyrotoxicosis
  nephrogenic fibrosing L90.8
Dermophytosis — *see* Dermatophytosis
Descemetocele H18.73- ☑
Descemet's membrane — *see* condition
Descending — *see* condition
Descensus uteri — *see* Prolapse, uterus
Desert
  rheumatism B38.0
  sore — *see* Ulcer, skin
Desertion (newborn) — *see* Maltreatment
Desmoid (extra-abdominal) (tumor) — *see* Neoplasm,
    connective tissue, uncertain behavior
  abdominal D48.1
Despondency F32.9
Desquamation, skin R23.4
Destruction, destructive (*see also* Damage)
  articular facet (*see also* Derangement, joint, specified
      type NEC)
    knee M23.8X- ☑
    vertebra — *see* Spondylosis
  bone (*see also* Disorder, bone, specified type NEC)
    syphilitic A52.77
  joint (*see also* Derangement, joint, specified type NEC)
    sacroiliac M53.3
  rectal sphincter K62.89
  septum (nasal) J34.89
  tuberculous NEC — *see* Tuberculosis
  tympanum, tympanic membrane (nontraumatic) —
      see Disorder, tympanic membrane, specified
      NEC
  vertebral disc — *see* Degeneration, intervertebral disc
Destructiveness (*see also* Disorder, conduct)
  adjustment reaction — *see* Disorder, adjustment
Desultory labor O62.2
Detachment
  cartilage — *see* Sprain
  cervix, annular N88.8
    complicating delivery O71.3
  choroid (old) (postinfectional) (simple) (spontaneous)
      H31.40- ☑
    hemorrhagic H31.41- ☑
    serous H31.42- ☑
  ligament — *see* Sprain

☑ **Additional Character Required** — Refer to the Tabular List for Character Selection   ▽ Subterms under main terms may continue to next column or page

Detachment — *continued*
  meniscus (knee) (*see also* Derangement, knee, meniscus, specified NEC)
    current injury — *see* Tear, meniscus
    due to old tear or injury — *see* Derangement, knee, meniscus, due to old tear
  retina (without retinal break) (serous) H33.2- ☑
    with retinal:
      break H33.00- ☑
        giant H33.03- ☑
        multiple H33.02- ☑
        single H33.01- ☑
      dialysis H33.04- ☑
    pigment epithelium — *see* Degeneration, retina, separation of layers, pigment epithelium detachment
    rhegmatogenous — *see* Detachment, retina, with retinal, break
    specified NEC H33.8
    total H33.05- ☑
    traction H33.4- ☑
  vitreous (body) H43.81 ☑
Detergent asthma J69.8
Deterioration
  epileptic F06.8
  general physical R53.81
  heart, cardiac — *see* Degeneration, myocardial
  mental — *see* Psychosis
  myocardial, myocardium — *see* Degeneration, myocardial
  senile (simple) R54
Deuteranomaly (anomalous trichromat) H53.53
Deuteranopia (complete) (incomplete) H53.53
Development
  abnormal, bone Q79.9
  arrested R62.50
    bone — *see* Arrest, development or growth, bone
    child R62.50
    due to malnutrition E45
  defective, congenital (*see also* Anomaly, by site)
    cauda equina Q06.3
    left ventricle Q24.8
      in hypoplastic left heart syndrome Q23.4
    valve Q24.8
      pulmonary Q22.3
  delayed (*see also* Delay, development) R62.50
    arithmetical skills F81.2
    language (skills) (expressive) F80.1
    learning skill F81.9
    mixed skills F88
    motor coordination F82
    reading F81.0
    specified learning skill NEC F81.89
    speech F80.9
    spelling F81.81
    written expression F81.81
  imperfect, congenital (*see also* Anomaly, by site)
    heart Q24.9
    lungs Q33.6
  incomplete
    bronchial tree Q32.4
    organ or site not listed — *see* Hypoplasia, by site
    respiratory system Q34.9
  sexual, precocious NEC E30.1
  tardy, mental (*see also* Disability, intellectual) F79
Developmental — *see* condition
  testing, infant or child — *see* Examination, child
Devergie's disease (pityriasis rubra pilaris) L44.0
Deviation (in)
  conjugate palsy (eye) (spastic) H51.0
  esophagus (acquired) K22.8
  eye, skew H51.8
  midline (jaw) (teeth) (dental arch) M26.29
    specified site NEC — *see* Malposition
  nasal septum J34.2
    congenital Q67.4
  opening and closing of the mandible M26.53
  organ or site, congenital NEC — *see* Malposition, congenital
  septum (nasal) (acquired) J34.2
    congenital Q67.4
  sexual F65.9
    bestiality F65.89
    erotomania F52.8
    exhibitionism F65.2
    fetishism, fetishistic F65.0
      transvestism F65.1
    frotteurism F65.81

Deviation — *continued*
  sexual — *continued*
    masochism F65.51
    multiple F65.89
    necrophilia F65.89
    nymphomania F52.8
    pederosis F65.4
    pedophilia F65.4
    sadism, sadomasochism F65.52
    satyriasis F52.8
    specified type NEC F65.89
    transvestism F64.1
    voyeurism F65.3
  teeth, midline M26.29
  trachea J39.8
  ureter, congenital Q62.61
Device
  cerebral ventricle (communicating) in situ Z98.2
  contraceptive — *see* Contraceptive, device
  drainage, cerebrospinal fluid, in situ Z98.2
Devic's disease G36.0
Devil's
  grip B33.0
  pinches (purpura simplex) D69.2
Devitalized tooth K04.99
Devonshire colic — *see* Poisoning, lead
Dextraposition, aorta Q20.3
  in tetralogy of Fallot Q21.3
Dextrinosis, limit (debrancher enzyme deficiency) E74.03
Dextrocardia (true) Q24.0
  with
    complete transposition of viscera Q89.3
    situs inversus Q89.3
Dextrotransposition, aorta Q20.3
d-glycericacidemia E72.59
Dhat syndrome F48.8
Dhobi itch B35.6
Di George's syndrome D82.1
Di Guglielmo's disease C94.0- ☑
Diabetes, diabetic (mellitus) (sugar) E11.9
  with
    amyotrophy E11.44
    arthropathy NEC E11.618
    autonomic (poly)neuropathy E11.43
    cataract E11.36
    Charcot's joints E11.610
    chronic kidney disease E11.22
    circulatory complication NEC E11.59
    complication E11.8
      specified NEC E11.69
    dermatitis E11.620
    foot ulcer E11.621
    gangrene E11.52
    gastroparalysis E11.43
    gastroparesis E11.43
    glomerulonephrosis, intracapillary E11.21
    glomerulosclerosis, intercapillary E11.21
    hyperglycemia E11.65
    hyperosmolarity E11.00
      with coma E11.01
    hypoglycemia E11.649
      with coma E11.641
    ketoacidosis E11.10
      with coma E11.11
    kidney complications NEC E11.29
    Kimmelstiel-Wilson disease E11.21
    loss of protective sensation (LOPS) — *see* Diabetes, by type, with neuropathy
    mononeuropathy E11.41
    myasthenia E11.44
    necrobiosis lipoidica E11.620
    nephropathy E11.21
    neuralgia E11.42
    neurologic complication NEC E11.49
    neuropathic arthropathy E11.610
    neuropathy E11.40
    ophthalmic complication NEC E11.39
    oral complication NEC E11.638
    osteomyelitis E11.69
    periodontal disease E11.630
    peripheral angiopathy E11.51
      with gangrene E11.52
    polyneuropathy E11.42
    renal complication NEC E11.29
    renal tubular degeneration E11.29
    retinopathy E11.319
      with macular edema E11.311

Diabetes, diabetic — *continued*
  with — *continued*
    retinopathy — *continued*
      with macular edema — *continued*
        resolved following treatment E11.37 ☑
      nonproliferative E11.329 ☑
        with macular edema E11.321 ☑
        mild E11.329 ☑
          with macular edema E11.321 ☑
        moderate E11.339 ☑
          with macular edema E11.331 ☑
        severe E11.349 ☑
          with macular edema E11.341 ☑
      proliferative E11.359 ☑
        with
          combined traction retinal detachment and rhegmatogenous retinal detachment E11.354 ☑
          macular edema E11.351 ☑
          stable proliferative diabetic retinopathy E11.355 ☑
          traction retinal detachment involving the macula E11.352 ☑
          traction retinal detachment not involving the macula E11.353 ☑
    skin complication NEC E11.628
    skin ulcer NEC E11.622
  brittle — *see* Diabetes, type 1
  bronzed E83.110
  complicating pregnancy — *see* Pregnancy, complicated by, diabetes
  dietary counseling and surveillance Z71.3
  due to
    autoimmune process — *see* Diabetes, type 1
    immune mediated pancreatic islet beta-cell destruction — *see* Diabetes, type 1
  due to drug or chemical E09.9
    with
      amyotrophy E09.44
      arthropathy NEC E09.618
      autonomic (poly)neuropathy E09.43
      cataract E09.36
      Charcot's joints E09.610
      chronic kidney disease E09.22
      circulatory complication NEC E09.59
      complication E09.8
        specified NEC E09.69
      dermatitis E09.620
      foot ulcer E09.621
      gangrene E09.52
      gastroparalysis E09.43
      gastroparesis E09.43
      glomerulonephrosis, intracapillary E09.21
      glomerulosclerosis, intercapillary E09.21
      hyperglycemia E09.65
      hyperosmolarity E09.00
        with coma E09.01
      hypoglycemia E09.649
        with coma E09.641
      ketoacidosis E09.10
        with coma E09.11
      kidney complications NEC E09.29
      Kimmelstiel-Wilson disease E09.21
      mononeuropathy E09.41
      myasthenia E09.44
      necrobiosis lipoidica E09.620
      nephropathy E09.21
      neuralgia E09.42
      neurologic complication NEC E09.49
      neuropathic arthropathy E09.610
      neuropathy E09.40
      ophthalmic complication NEC E09.39
      oral complication NEC E09.638
      periodontal disease E09.630
      peripheral angiopathy E09.51
        with gangrene E09.52
      polyneuropathy E09.42
      renal complication NEC E09.29
      renal tubular degeneration E09.29
      retinopathy E09.319
        with macular edema E09.311
        nonproliferative E09.329 ☑
          with macular edema E09.321 ☑
          mild E09.329 ☑
            with macular edema E09.321 ☑
          moderate E09.339 ☑
            with macular edema E09.331 ☑
          severe E09.349 ☑

Diabetes, diabetic — *continued*
 due to drug or chemical — *continued*
  with — *continued*
   retinopathy — *continued*
    nonproliferative — *continued*
     severe — *continued*
      with macular edema E09.341 ☑
    proliferative E09.359 ☑
     with
      combined traction retinal detach-
        ment and rhegmatogenous
        retinal detachment E09.354 ☑
      macular edema E09.351 ☑
      stable proliferative diabetic
        retinopathy E09.355 ☑
      traction retinal detachment involving
        the macula E09.352 ☑
      traction retinal detachment not in-
        volving the macula E09.353 ☑
    resolved following treatment E09.37 ☑
   skin complication NEC E09.628
   skin ulcer NEC E09.622
 due to underlying condition E08.9
  with
   amyotrophy E08.44
   arthropathy NEC E08.618
   autonomic (poly)neuropathy E08.43
   cataract E08.36
   Charcot's joints E08.610
   chronic kidney disease E08.22
   circulatory complication NEC E08.59
   complication E08.8
    specified NEC E08.69
   dermatitis E08.620
   foot ulcer E08.621
   gangrene E08.52
   gastroparalysis E08.43
   gastroparesis E08.43
   glomerulonephrosis, intracapillary E08.21
   glomerulosclerosis, intercapillary E08.21
   hyperglycemia E08.65
   hyperosmolarity E08.00
    with coma E08.01
   hypoglycemia E08.649
    with coma E08.641
   ketoacidosis E08.10
    with coma E08.11
   kidney complications NEC E08.29
   Kimmelsteil-WIlson disease E08.21
   mononeuropathy E08.41
   myasthenia E08.44
   necrobiosis lipoidica E08.620
   nephropathy E08.21
   neuralgia E08.42
   neurologic complication NEC E08.49
   neuropathic arthropathy E08.610
   neuropathy E08.40
   ophthalmic complication NEC E08.39
   oral complication NEC E08.638
   periodontal disease E08.630
   peripheral angiopathy E08.51
    with gangrene E08.52
   polyneuropathy E08.42
   renal complication NEC E08.29
   renal tubular degeneration E08.29
   retinopathy E08.319
    with macular edema E08.311
    nonproliferative E08.329 ☑
     with macular edema E08.321 ☑
     mild E08.329 ☑
      with macular edema E08.321 ☑
     moderate E08.339 ☑
      with macular edema E08.331 ☑
     severe E08.349 ☑
      with macular edema E08.341 ☑
    proliferative E08.359 ☑
     with
      combined traction retinal detach-
        ment and rhegmatogenous
        retinal detachment E08.354 ☑
      macular edema E08.351 ☑
      stable proliferative diabetic
        retinopathy E08.355 ☑
      traction retinal detachment involving
        the macula E08.352 ☑
      traction retinal detachment not in-
        volving the macula E08.353 ☑
    resolved following treatment E08.37 ☑

Diabetes, diabetic — *continued*
 due to underlying condition — *continued*
  with — *continued*
   skin complication NEC E08.628
   skin ulcer NEC E08.622
 gestational (in pregnancy) O24.419
  affecting newborn P70.0
  diet controlled O24.410
  in childbirth O24.429
   diet controlled O24.420
   insulin (and diet) controlled O24.424
   oral drug controlled (antidiabetic) (hypo-
     glycemic) O24.425
  insulin (and diet) controlled O24.414
  oral drug controlled (antidiabetic) (hypoglycemic)
    O24.415
  puerperal O24.439
   diet controlled O24.430
   insulin (and diet) controlled O24.434
   oral drug controlled (antidiabetic) (hypo-
     glycemic) O24.435
 hepatogenous E13.9
 idiopathic — *see* Diabetes, type 1
 inadequately controlled — *code to* Diabetes, by type,
   with hyperglycemia
 insipidus E23.2
  nephrogenic N25.1
  pituitary E23.2
  vasopressin resistant N25.1
 insulin dependent — *code to* type of diabetes
 juvenile-onset — *see* Diabetes, type 1
 ketosis-prone — *see* Diabetes, type 1
 latent R73.03
 neonatal (transient) P70.2
 non-insulin dependent — *code to* type of diabetes
 out of control — *code to* Diabetes, by type, with hyperglycemia
 phosphate E83.39
 poorly controlled — *code to* Diabetes, by type, with
   hyperglycemia
 postpancreatectomy — *see* Diabetes, specified type
   NEC
 postprocedural — *see* Diabetes, specified type NEC
 secondary diabetes mellitus NEC — *see* Diabetes,
   specified type NEC
 specified type NEC E13.9
  with
   amyotrophy E13.44
   arthropathy NEC E13.618
   autonomic (poly)neuropathy E13.43
   cataract E13.36
   Charcot's joints E13.610
   chronic kidney disease E13.22
   circulatory complication NEC E13.59
   complication E13.8
    specified NEC E13.69
   dermatitis E13.620
   foot ulcer E13.621
   gangrene E13.52
   gastroparalysis E13.43
   gastroparesis E13.43
   glomerulonephrosis, intracapillary E13.21
   glomerulosclerosis, intercapillary E13.21
   hyperglycemia E13.65
   hyperosmolarity E13.00
    with coma E13.01
   hypoglycemia E13.649
    with coma E13.641
   ketoacidosis E13.10
    with coma E13.11
   kidney complications NEC E13.29
   Kimmelsteil-Wilson disease E13.21
   mononeuropathy E13.41
   myasthenia E13.44
   necrobiosis lipoidica E13.620
   nephropathy E13.21
   neuralgia E13.42
   neurologic complication NEC E13.49
   neuropathic arthropathy E13.610
   neuropathy E13.40
   ophthalmic complication NEC E13.39
   oral complication NEC E13.638
   periodontal disease E13.630
   peripheral angiopathy E13.51
    with gangrene E13.52
   polyneuropathy E13.42
   renal complication NEC E13.29
   renal tubular degeneration E13.29

Diabetes, diabetic — *continued*
 specified type — *continued*
  with — *continued*
   retinopathy E13.319
    with macular edema E13.311
    nonproliferative E13.329 ☑
     with macular edema E13.321 ☑
     mild E13.329 ☑
      with macular edema E13.321 ☑
     moderate E13.339 ☑
      with macular edema E13.331 ☑
     severe E13.349 ☑
      with macular edema E13.341 ☑
    proliferative E13.359 ☑
     with
      combined traction retinal detach-
        ment and rhegmatogenous
        retinal detachment E13.354 ☑
      macular edema E13.351 ☑
      stable proliferative diabetic
        retinopathy E13.355 ☑
      traction retinal detachment involving
        the macula E13.352 ☑
      traction retinal detachment not in-
        volving the macula E13.353 ☑
    resolved following treatment E13.37 ☑
   skin complication NEC E13.628
   skin ulcer NEC E13.622
 steroid-induced — *see* Diabetes, due to, drug or
   chemical
 type 1 E10.9
  with
   amyotrophy E10.44
   arthropathy NEC E10.618
   autonomic (poly)neuropathy E10.43
   cataract E10.36
   Charcot's joints E10.610
   chronic kidney disease E10.22
   circulatory complication NEC E10.59
   complication E10.8
    specified NEC E10.69
   dermatitis E10.620
   foot ulcer E10.621
   gangrene E10.52
   gastroparalysis E10.43
   gastroparesis E10.43
   glomerulonephrosis, intracapillary E10.21
   glomerulosclerosis, intercapillary E10.21
   hyperglycemia E10.65
   hypoglycemia E10.649
    with coma E10.641
   ketoacidosis E10.10
    with coma E10.11
   kidney complications NEC E10.29
   Kimmelsteil-Wilson disease E10.21
   mononeuropathy E10.41
   myasthenia E10.44
   necrobiosis lipoidica E10.620
   nephropathy E10.21
   neuralgia E10.42
   neurologic complication NEC E10.49
   neuropathic arthropathy E10.610
   neuropathy E10.40
   ophthalmic complication NEC E10.39
   oral complication NEC E10.638
   osteomyelitis E10.69
   periodontal disease E10.630
   peripheral angiopathy E10.51
    with gangrene E10.52
   polyneuropathy E10.42
   renal complication NEC E10.29
   renal tubular degeneration E10.29
   retinopathy E10.319
    with macular edema E10.311
    nonproliferative E10.329 ☑
     with macular edema E10.321 ☑
     mild E10.329 ☑
      with macular edema E10.321 ☑
     moderate E10.339 ☑
      with macular edema E10.331 ☑
     severe E10.349 ☑
      with macular edema E10.341 ☑
    proliferative E10.359 ☑
     with
      combined traction retinal detach-
        ment and rhegmatogenous
        retinal detachment E10.354 ☑
      macular edema E10.351 ☑

Diabetes, diabetic — *continued*
  type 1 — *continued*
    with — *continued*
      retinopathy — *continued*
        proliferative — *continued*
          with — *continued*
            stable proliferative diabetic
              retinopathy E10.355 ☑
            traction retinal detachment involving
              the macula E10.352 ☑
            traction retinal detachment not in-
              volving the macula E10.353 ☑
        resolved following treatment E10.37 ☑
    skin complication NEC E10.628
    skin ulcer NEC E10.622
  type 2 E11.9
    with
      amyotrophy E11.44
      arthropathy NEC E11.618
      autonomic (poly)neuropathy E11.43
      cataract E11.36
      Charcot's joints E11.610
      chronic kidney disease E11.22
      circulatory complication NEC E11.59
      complication E11.8
        specified NEC E11.69
      dermatitis E11.620
      foot ulcer E11.621
      gangrene E11.52
      gastroparalysis E11.43
      gastroparesis E11.43
      glomerulonephrosis, intracapillary E11.21
      glomerulosclerosis, intercapillary E11.21
      hyperglycemia E11.65
      hyperosmolarity E11.00
        with coma E11.01
      hypoglycemia E11.649
        with coma E11.641
      ketoacidosis E11.10
        with coma E11.11
      kidney complications NEC E11.29
      Kimmelstiel-Wilson disease E11.21
      mononeuropathy E11.41
      myasthenia E11.44
      necrobiosis lipoidica E11.620
      nephropathy E11.21
      neuralgia E11.42
      neurologic complication NEC E11.49
      neuropathic arthropathy E11.610
      neuropathy E11.40
      ophthalmic complication NEC E11.39
      oral complication NEC E11.638
      osteomyelitis E11.69
      periodontal disease E11.630
      peripheral angiopathy E11.51
        with gangrene E11.52
      polyneuropathy E11.42
      renal complication NEC E11.29
      renal tubular degeneration E11.29
      retinopathy E11.319
        with macular edema E11.311
        nonproliferative E11.329 ☑
          with macular edema E11.321 ☑
          mild E11.329 ☑
            with macular edema E11.321 ☑
          moderate E11.339 ☑
            with macular edema E11.331 ☑
          severe E11.349 ☑
            with macular edema E11.341 ☑
        proliferative E11.359 ☑
          with
            combined traction retinal detach-
              ment and rhegmatogenous
              retinal detachment E11.354 ☑
            macular edema E11.351 ☑
            stable proliferative diabetic
              retinopathy E11.355 ☑
            traction retinal detachment involving
              the macula E11.352 ☑
            traction retinal detachment not in-
              volving the macula E11.353 ☑
        resolved following treatment E11.37 ☑
    skin complication NEC E11.628
    skin ulcer NEC E11.622
  uncontrolled
    meaning
      hyperglycemia — *see* Diabetes, by type, with,
        hyperglycemia

Diabetes, diabetic — *continued*
  uncontrolled — *continued*
    meaning — *continued*
      hypoglycemia — *see* Diabetes, by type, with,
        hypoglycemia
Diacyclothrombopathia D69.1
Diagnosis deferred R69
Dialysis (intermittent) (treatment)
  noncompliance (with) Z91.15
  renal (hemodialysis) (peritoneal), status Z99.2
  retina, retinal — *see* Detachment, retina, with retinal,
    dialysis
Diamond-Blackfan anemia (congenital hypoplastic)
  D61.01
Diamond-Gardener syndrome (autoerythrocyte sensi-
  tization) D69.2
Diaper rash L22
Diaphoresis (excessive) R61
Diaphragm — *see* condition
Diaphragmalgia R07.1
Diaphragmatitis, diaphragmitis J98.6
Diaphysial aclasis Q78.6
Diaphysitis — *see* Osteomyelitis, specified type NEC
Diarrhea, diarrheal (disease) (infantile) (inflammatory)
  R19.7
  achlorhydric K31.83
  allergic K52.29
    due to
      colitis — *see* Colitis, allergic
      enteritis — *see* Enteritis, allergic
  amebic (*see also* Amebiasis) A06.0
    with abscess — *see* Abscess, amebic
    acute A06.0
    chronic A06.1
    nondysenteric A06.2
  bacillary — *see* Dysentery, bacillary
  balantidial A07.0
  cachectic NEC K52.89
  Chilomastix A07.8
  choleriformis A00.1
  chronic (noninfectious) K52.9
  coccidial A07.3
  Cochin-China K90.1
    strongyloidiasis B78.0
  Dientamoeba A07.8
  dietetic (*see also* Diarrhea, allergic) K52.29
  drug-induced K52.1
  due to
    bacteria A04.9
      specified NEC A04.8
    Campylobacter A04.5
    Capillaria philippinensis B81.1
    Clostridium difficile
      not specified as recurrent A04.72
      recurrent A04.71
    Clostridium perfringens (C) (F) A04.8
    Cryptosporidium A07.2
    drugs K52.1
    Escherichia coli A04.4
      enteroaggregative A04.4
      enterohemorrhagic A04.3
      enteroinvasive A04.2
      enteropathogenic A04.0
      enterotoxigenic A04.1
      specified NEC A04.4
    food hypersensitivity (*see also* Diarrhea, allergic)
      K52.29
    Necator americanus B76.1
    S. japonicum B65.2
    specified organism NEC A08.8
      bacterial A04.8
      viral A08.39
    Staphylococcus A04.8
    Trichuris trichiuria B79
    virus — *see* Enteritis, viral
    Yersinia enterocolitica A04.6
  dysenteric A09
  endemic A09
  epidemic A09
  flagellate A07.9
  Flexner's (ulcerative) A03.1
  functional K59.1
    following gastrointestinal surgery K91.89
    psychogenic F45.8
  Giardia lamblia A07.1
  giardial A07.1
  hill K90.1
  infectious A09

Diarrhea, diarrheal — *continued*
  malarial — *see* Malaria
  mite B88.0
  mycotic NEC B49
  neonatal (noninfectious) P78.3
  nervous F45.8
  neurogenic K59.1
  noninfectious K52.9
  postgastrectomy K91.1
  postvagotomy K91.1
  protozoal A07.9
    specified NEC A07.8
  psychogenic F45.8
  specified
    bacterium NEC A04.8
    virus NEC A08.39
  strongyloidiasis B78.0
  toxic K52.1
  trichomonal A07.8
  tropical K90.1
  tuberculous A18.32
  viral — *see* Enteritis, viral
Diastasis
  cranial bones M84.88
    congenital NEC Q75.8
  joint (traumatic) — *see* Dislocation
  muscle M62.00
    ankle M62.07- ☑
    congenital Q79.8
    foot M62.07- ☑
    forearm M62.03- ☑
    hand M62.04- ☑
    lower leg M62.06- ☑
    pelvic region M62.05- ☑
    shoulder region M62.01- ☑
    specified site NEC M62.08
    thigh M62.05- ☑
    upper arm M62.02- ☑
  recti (abdomen)
    complicating delivery O71.89
    congenital Q79.59
Diastema, tooth, teeth, fully erupted M26.32
Diastematomyelia Q06.2
Diataxia, cerebral G80.4
Diathesis
  allergic — *see* History, allergy
  bleeding (familial) D69.9
  cystine (familial) E72.00
  gouty — *see* Gout
  hemorrhagic (familial) D69.9
    newborn NEC P53
  spasmophilic R29.0
Diaz's disease or osteochondrosis (juvenile) (talus) —
  see Osteochondrosis, juvenile, tarsus
Dibothriocephalus, dibothriocephaliasis (latus) (infection) (Infestation) B70.0
  larval B70.1
Dicephalus, dicephaly Q89.4
Dichotomy, teeth K00.2
Dichromat, dichromatopsia (congenital) — *see* Deficiency, color vision
Dichuchwa A65
Dicroceliasis B66.2
Didelphia, didelphys — *see* Double uterus
Didymytis N45.1
  with orchitis N45.3
Dietary
  inadequacy or deficiency E63.9
  surveillance and counseling Z71.3
Dietl's crisis N13.8
Dieulafoy lesion (hemorrhagic)
  duodenum K31.82
  esophagus K22.8
  intestine (colon) K63.81
  stomach K31.82
Difficult, difficulty (in)
  acculturation Z60.3
  feeding R63.3
    newborn P92.9
      breast P92.5
      specified NEC P92.8
    nonorganic (infant or child) F98.29
  intubation, in anesthesia T88.4 ☑
  mechanical, gastroduodenal stoma K91.89
    causing obstruction (*see also* Obstruction, intestine,
      postoperative) K91.30
  micturition
    need to immediately re-void R39.191

Difficult, difficulty — *continued*
  micturition — *continued*
    position dependent R39.192
    specified NEC R39.198
  reading (developmental) F81.0
    secondary to emotional disorders F93.9
  spelling (specific) F81.81
    with reading disorder F81.89
    due to inadequate teaching Z55.8
  swallowing — *see* Dysphagia
  walking R26.2
  work
    conditions NEC Z56.5
    schedule Z56.3
Diffuse — *see* condition
Digestive — *see* condition
Dihydropyrimidine dehydrogenase disease (DPD)
    E88.89
Diktyoma — *see* Neoplasm, malignant, by site
Dilaceration, tooth K00.4
Dilatation
  anus K59.8
    venule — *see* Hemorrhoids
  aorta (focal) (general) — *see* Ectasia, aorta
    with aneuysm — *see* Aneurysm, aorta
    congenital Q25.44
  artery — *see* Aneurysm
  bladder (sphincter) N32.89
    congenital Q64.79
  blood vessel I99.8
  bronchial J47.9
    with
      exacerbation (acute) J47.1
      lower respiratory infection J47.0
  calyx (due to obstruction) — *see* Hydronephrosis
  capillaries I78.8
  cardiac (acute) (chronic) (*see also* Hypertrophy, cardiac)
    congenital Q24.8
      valve NEC Q24.8
        pulmonary Q22.3
    valve — *see* Endocarditis
  cavum septi pellucidi Q06.8
  cervix (uteri) (*see also* Incompetency, cervix)
    incomplete, poor, slow complicating delivery O62.0
  colon K59.39
    congenital Q43.1
    psychogenic F45.8
    toxic K59.31
  common duct (acquired) K83.8
    congenital Q44.5
  cystic duct (acquired) K82.8
    congenital Q44.5
  duct, mammary — *see* Ectasia, mammary duct
  duodenum K59.8
  esophagus K22.8
    congenital Q39.5
    due to achalasia K22.0
  eustachian tube, congenital Q17.8
  gallbladder K82.8
  gastric — *see* Dilatation, stomach
  heart (acute) (chronic) (*see also* Hypertrophy, cardiac)
    congenital Q24.8
    valve — *see* Endocarditis
  ileum K59.8
    psychogenic F45.8
  jejunum K59.8
    psychogenic F45.8
  kidney (calyx) (collecting structures) (cystic)
      (parenchyma) (pelvis) (idiopathic) N28.89
  lacrimal passages or duct — *see* Disorder, lacrimal
      system, changes
  lymphatic vessel I89.0
  mammary duct — *see* Ectasia, mammary duct
  Meckel's diverticulum (congenital) Q43.0
    malignant — *see* Table of Neoplasms, small intes-
        tine, malignant
  myocardium (acute) (chronic) — *see* Hypertrophy,
      cardiac
  organ or site, congenital NEC — *see* Distortion
  pancreatic duct K86.89
  pericardium — *see* Pericarditis
  pharynx J39.2
  prostate N42.89
  pulmonary
    artery (idiopathic) I28.8
    valve, congenital Q22.3
  pupil H57.04
  rectum K59.39

Dilatation — *continued*
  saccule, congenital Q16.5
  salivary gland (duct) K11.8
  sphincter ani K62.89
  stomach K31.89
    acute K31.0
    psychogenic F45.8
  submaxillary duct K11.8
  trachea, congenital Q32.1
  ureter (idiopathic) N28.82
    congenital Q62.2
    due to obstruction N13.4
  urethra (acquired) N36.8
  vasomotor I73.9
  vein I86.8
  ventricular, ventricle (acute) (chronic) (*see also* Hyper-
      trophy, cardiac)
    cerebral, congenital Q04.8
  venule NEC I86.8
  vesical orifice N32.89
Dilated, dilation — *see* Dilatation
Diminished, diminution
  hearing (acuity) — *see* Deafness
  sense or sensation (cold) (heat) (tactile) (vibratory)
      R20.8
  vision NEC H54.7
  vital capacity R94.2
Diminuta taenia B71.0
Dimitri-Sturge-Weber disease Q85.8
Dimple
  congenital sacral Q82.6
  parasacral Q82.6
  pilonidal or postanal — *see* Cyst, pilonidal
Dioctophyme renalis (infection) (infestation) B83.8
Dipetalonemiasis B74.4
Diphallus Q55.69
Diphtheria, diphtheritic (gangrenous) (hemorrhagic)
    A36.9
  carrier (suspected) Z22.2
  cutaneous A36.3
  faucial A36.0
  infection of wound A36.3
  laryngeal A36.2
  myocarditis A36.81
  nasal, anterior A36.89
  nasopharyngeal A36.1
  neurological complication A36.89
  pharyngeal A36.0
  specified site NEC A36.89
  tonsillar A36.0
Diphyllobothriasis (intestine) B70.0
  larval B70.1
Diplacusis H93.22- ☑
Diplegia (upper limbs) G83.0
  congenital (cerebral) G80.8
  facial G51.0
  lower limbs G82.20
  spastic G80.1
Diplococcus, diplococcal — *see* condition
Diplopia H53.2
Dipsomania F10.20
  with
    psychosis — *see* Psychosis, alcoholic
    remission F10.21
Dipylidiasis B71.1
DIRA (deficiency of interleukin 1 receptor antagonist)
    M04.8
Direction, teeth, abnormal, fully erupted M26.30
Dirofilariasis B74.8
Dirt-eating child F98.3
Disability, disabilities
  heart — *see* Disease, heart
  intellectual F79
    with
      autistic features F84.9
      mild (I.Q. 50-69) F70
      moderate (I.Q. 35-49) F71
      profound (I.Q. under 20) F73
      severe (I.Q. 20-34) F72
      specified level NEC F78
  knowledge acquisition F81.9
  learning F81.9
  limiting activities Z73.6
  spelling, specific F81.81
Disappearance of family member Z63.4
Disarticulation — *see* Amputation
  meaning traumatic amputation — *see* Amputation,
      traumatic

Discharge (from)
  abnormal finding in — *see* Abnormal, specimen
  breast (female) (male) N64.52
  diencephalic autonomic idiopathic — *see* Epilepsy,
      specified NEC
  ear (*see also* Otorrhea)
    blood — *see* Otorrhagia
  excessive urine R35.8
  nipple N64.52
  penile R36.9
  postnasal R09.82
  prison, anxiety concerning Z65.2
  urethral R36.9
    without blood R36.0
    hematospermia R36.1
  vaginal N89.8
Discitis, diskitis M46.40
  cervical region M46.42
  cervicothoracic region M46.43
  lumbar region M46.46
  lumbosacral region M46.47
  multiple sites M46.49
  occipito-atlanto-axial region M46.41
  pyogenic — *see* Infection, intervertebral disc, pyogenic
  sacrococcygeal region M46.48
  thoracic region M46.44
  thoracolumbar region M46.45
Discoid
  meniscus (congenital) Q68.6
  semilunar cartilage (congenital) — *see* Derangement,
      knee, meniscus, specified NEC
Discoloration
  nails L60.8
  teeth (posteruptive) K03.7
    during formation K00.8
Discomfort
  chest R07.89
  visual H53.14- ☑
Discontinuity, ossicles, ear H74.2- ☑
Discord (with)
  boss Z56.4
  classmates Z55.4
  counselor Z64.4
  employer Z56.4
  family Z63.8
  fellow employees Z56.4
  in-laws Z63.1
  landlord Z59.2
  lodgers Z59.2
  neighbors Z59.2
  probation officer Z64.4
  social worker Z64.4
  teachers Z55.4
  workmates Z56.4
Discordant connection
  atrioventricular (congenital) Q20.5
  ventriculoarterial Q20.3
Discrepancy
  centric occlusion maximum intercuspation M26.55
  leg length (acquired) — *see* Deformity, limb, unequal
      length
    congenital — *see* Defect, reduction, lower limb
  uterine size date O26.84- ☑
Discrimination
  ethnic Z60.5
  political Z60.5
  racial Z60.5
  religious Z60.5
  sex Z60.5
Disease, diseased (*see also* Syndrome)
  absorbent system I87.8
  acid-peptic K30
  Acosta's T70.29 ☑
  Adams-Stokes (-Morgagni) (syncope with heart block)
      I45.9
  Addison's anemia (pernicious) D51.0
  adenoids (and tonsils) J35.9
  adrenal (capsule) (cortex) (gland) (medullary) E27.9
    hyperfunction E27.0
    specified NEC E27.8
  ainhum L94.6
  airway
    obstructive, chronic J44.9
      due to
        cotton dust J66.0
        specific organic dusts NEC J66.8
    reactive — *see* Asthma
  akamushi (scrub typhus) A75.3

Disease, diseased — *continued*
Albers-Schönberg (marble bones) Q78.2
Albert's — *see* Tendinitis, Achilles
alimentary canal K63.9
alligator-skin Q80.9
  acquired L85.0
alpha heavy chain C88.3
alpine T70.29 ☑
altitude T70.20 ☑
alveolar ridge
  edentulous K06.9
    specified NEC K06.8
alveoli, teeth K08.9
Alzheimer's G30.9 [F02.80]
  with behavioral disturbance G30.9 [F02.81]
  early onset G30.0 [F02.80]
    with behavioral disturbance G30.0 [F02.81]
  late onset G30.1 [F02.80]
    with behavioral disturbance G30.1 [F02.81]
  specified NEC G30.8 [F02.80]
    with behavioral disturbance G30.8 [F02.81]
amyloid — *see* Amyloidosis
Andersen's (glycogenosis IV) E74.09
Andes T70.29 ☑
Andrews' (bacterid) L08.89
angiospastic I73.9
  cerebral G45.9
  vein I87.8
anterior
  chamber H21.9
  horn cell G12.29
antiglomerular basement membrane (anti- GBM) antibody M31.0
  tubulo-interstitial nephritis N12
antral — *see* Sinusitis, maxillary
anus K62.9
  specified NEC K62.89
aorta (nonsyphilitic) I77.9
  syphilitic NEC A52.02
aortic (heart) (valve) I35.9
  rheumatic I06.9
Apollo B30.3
aponeuroses — *see* Enthesopathy
appendix K38.9
  specified NEC K38.8
aqueous (chamber) H21.9
Arnold-Chiari — *see* Arnold-Chiari disease
arterial I77.9
  occlusive — *see* Occlusion, by site
    due to stricture or stenosis I77.1
arteriocardiorenal — *see* Hypertension, cardiorenal
arteriolar (generalized) (obliterative) I77.9
arteriorenal — *see* Hypertension, kidney
arteriosclerotic (*see also* Arteriosclerosis)
  cardiovascular — *see* Disease, heart, ischemic, atherosclerotic
  coronary (artery) — *see* Disease, heart, ischemic, atherosclerotic
  heart — *see* Disease, heart, ischemic, atherosclerotic
artery I77.9
  cerebral I67.9
  coronary I25.10
    with angina pectoris — *see* Arteriosclerosis, coronary (artery)
arthropod-borne NOS (viral) A94
  specified type NEC A93.8
atticoantral, chronic H66.20
  left H66.22
    with right H66.23
  right H66.21
    with left H66.23
auditory canal — *see* Disorder, ear, external
auricle, ear NEC — *see* Disorder, pinna
Australian X A83.4
autoimmune (systemic) NOS M35.9
  hemolytic (cold type) (warm type) D59.1
    drug-induced D59.0
  thyroid E06.3
aviator's — *see* Effect, adverse, high altitude
Ayerza's (pulmonary artery sclerosis with pulmonary hypertension) I27.0
Babington's (familial hemorrhagic telangiectasia) I78.0
bacterial A49.9
  specified NEC A48.8
  zoonotic A28.9
    specified type NEC A28.8
Baelz's (cheilitis glandularis apostematosa) K13.0

Disease, diseased — *continued*
bagasse J67.1
balloon — *see* Effect, adverse, high altitude
Bang's (brucella abortus) A23.1
Bannister's T78.3 ☑
barometer makers' — *see* Poisoning, mercury
Barraquer (-Simons') (progressive lipodystrophy) E88.1
Barrett's — *see* Barrett's, esophagus
Bartholin's gland N75.9
basal ganglia G25.9
  degenerative G23.9
    specified NEC G23.8
  specified NEC G25.89
Basedow's (exophthalmic goiter) — *see* Hyperthyroidism, with, goiter (diffuse)
Bateman's B08.1
Batten-Steinert G71.11
Battey A31.0
Beard's (neurasthenia) F48.8
Becker
  idiopathic mural endomyocardial I42.3
  myotonia congenita G71.12
Begbie's (exophthalmic goiter) — *see* Hyperthyroidism, with, goiter (diffuse)
behavioral, organic F07.9
Beigel's (white piedra) B36.2
Benson's — *see* Deposit, crystalline
Bernard-Soulier (thrombopathy) D69.1
Bernhardt (-Roth) — *see* Mononeuropathy, lower limb, meralgia paresthetica
Biermer's (pernicious anemia) D51.0
bile duct (common) (hepatic) K83.9
  with calculus, stones — *see* Calculus, bile duct
  specified NEC K83.8
biliary (tract) K83.9
  specified NEC K83.8
Billroth's — *see* Spina bifida
bird fancier's J67.2
black lung J60
bladder N32.9
  in (due to)
    schistosomiasis (bilharziasis) B65.0 [N33]
  specified NEC N32.89
bleeder's D66
blood D75.9
  forming organs D75.9
  vessel I99.9
Bloodgood's — *see* Mastopathy, cystic
Bodechtel-Guttmann (subacute sclerosing panencephalitis) A81.1
bone (*see also* Disorder, bone)
  aluminum M83.4
  fibrocystic NEC
    jaw M27.49
bone-marrow D75.9
Borna A83.9
Bornholm (epidemic pleurodynia) B33.0
Bouchard's (myopathic dilatation of the stomach) K31.0
Bouillaud's (rheumatic heart disease) I01.9
Bourneville (-Brissaud) (tuberous sclerosis) Q85.1
Bouveret (-Hoffmann) (paroxysmal tachycardia) I47.9
bowel K63.9
  functional K59.9
    psychogenic F45.8
brain G93.9
  arterial, artery I67.9
  arteriosclerotic I67.2
  congenital Q04.9
  degenerative — *see* Degeneration, brain
  inflammatory — *see* Encephalitis
  organic G93.9
    arteriosclerotic I67.2
  parasitic NEC B71.9 [G94]
  senile NEC G31.1
  specified NEC G93.89
breast (*see also* Disorder, breast) N64.9
  cystic (chronic) — *see* Mastopathy, cystic
  fibrocystic — *see* Mastopathy, cystic
  Paget's
    female, unspecified side C50.91- ☑
    male, unspecified side C50.92- ☑
  specified NEC N64.89
Breda's — *see* Yaws
Bretonneau's (diphtheritic malignant angina) A36.0
Bright's — *see* Nephritis
  arteriosclerotic — *see* Hypertension, kidney
Brill's (recrudescent typhus) A75.1

Disease, diseased — *continued*
Brill-Zinsser (recrudescent typhus) A75.1
Brion-Kayser — *see* Fever, paratyphoid
broad
  beta E78.2
  ligament (noninflammatory) N83.9
    inflammatory — *see* Disease, pelvis, inflammatory
    specified NEC N83.8
Brocq-Duhring (dermatitis herpetiformis) L13.0
Brocq's
  meaning
    dermatitis herpetiformis L13.0
    prurigo L28.2
bronchopulmonary J98.4
bronchus NEC J98.09
bronze Addison's E27.1
  tuberculous A18.7
budgerigar fancier's J67.2
Buerger's (thromboangiitis obliterans) I73.1
bullous L13.9
  chronic of childhood L12.2
  specified NEC L13.8
Bürger-Grütz (essential familial hyperlipemia) E78.3
bursa — *see* Bursopathy
caisson T70.3 ☑
California — *see* Coccidioidomycosis
capillaries I78.9
  specified NEC I78.8
Carapata A68.0
cardiac — *see* Disease, heart
cardiopulmonary, chronic I27.9
cardiorenal (hepatic) (hypertensive) (vascular) — *see* Hypertension, cardiorenal
cardiovascular (atherosclerotic) I25.10
  with angina pectoris — *see* Arteriosclerosis, coronary (artery),
  congenital Q28.9
  hypertensive — *see* Hypertension, heart
  newborn P29.9
    specified NEC P29.89
  renal (hypertensive) — *see* Hypertension, cardiorenal
  syphilitic (asymptomatic) A52.00
cartilage — *see* Disorder, cartilage
Castellani's A69.8
Castleman (unicentric) (multicentric) D47.Z2
  HHV-8-associated (*see also* Herpesvirus, human, 8) D47.Z2
cat-scratch A28.1
Cavare's (familial periodic paralysis) G72.3
cecum K63.9
celiac (adult) (infantile) (with steatorrhea) K90.0
cellular tissue L98.9
central core G71.2
cerebellar, cerebellum — *see* Disease, brain
cerebral (*see also* Disease, brain)
  degenerative — *see* Degeneration, brain
cerebrospinal G96.9
cerebrovascular I67.9
  acute I67.89
    embolic I63.4- ☑
    thrombotic I63.3- ☑
  arteriosclerotic I67.2
  specified NEC I67.89
cervix (uteri) (noninflammatory) N88.9
  inflammatory — *see* Cervicitis
  specified NEC N88.8
Chabert's A22.9
Chandler's (osteochondritis dissecans, hip) — *see* Osteochondritis, dissecans, hip
Charlouis — *see* Yaws
Chédiak-Steinbrinck (-Higashi) (congenital gigantism of peroxidase granules) E70.330
chest J98.9
Chiari's (hepatic vein thrombosis) I82.0
Chicago B40.9
Chignon B36.8
chigo, chigoe B88.1
childhood granulomatous D71
Chinese liver fluke B66.1
chlamydial A74.9
  specified NEC A74.89
cholecystic K82.9
choroid H31.9
  specified NEC H31.8
Christmas D67
chronic bullous of childhood L12.2

Disease, diseased — continued
  chylomicron retention E78.3
  ciliary body H21.9
    specified NEC H21.89
  circulatory (system) NEC I99.8
    newborn P29.9
    syphilitic A52.00
      congenital A50.54
  coagulation factor deficiency (congenital) — see Defect, coagulation
  coccidioidal — see Coccidioidomycosis
  cold
    agglutinin or hemoglobinuria D59.1
      paroxysmal D59.6
    hemagglutinin (chronic) D59.1
  collagen NOS (nonvascular) (vascular) M35.9
    specified NEC M35.8
  colon K63.9
    functional K59.9
      congenital Q43.2
    ischemic (see also Ischemia, intestine, acute) K55.039
  colonic inflammatory bowel, unclassified (IBDU) K52.3
  combined system — see Degeneration, combined
  compressed air T70.3 ☑
  Concato's (pericardial polyserositis) A19.9
    nontubercular I31.1
    pleural — see Pleurisy, with effusion
  conjunctiva H11.9
    chlamydial A74.0
    specified NEC H11.89
    viral B30.9
      specified NEC B30.8
  connective tissue, systemic (diffuse) M35.9
    in (due to)
      hypogammaglobulinemia D80.1 [M36.8]
      ochronosis E70.29 [M36.8]
    specified NEC M35.8
  Conor and Bruch's (boutonneuse fever) A77.1
  Cooper's — see Mastopathy, cystic
  Cori's (glycogenosis III) E74.03
  corkhandler's or corkworker's J67.3
  cornea H18.9
    specified NEC H18.89- ☑
  coronary (artery) — see Disease, heart, ischemic, atherosclerotic
    congenital Q24.5
    ostial, syphilitic (aortic) (mitral) (pulmonary) A52.03
  corpus cavernosum N48.9
    specified NEC N48.89
  Cotugno's — see Sciatica
  coxsackie (virus) NEC B34.1
  cranial nerve NOS G52.9
  Creutzfeldt-Jakob — see Creutzfeldt-Jakob disease or syndrome
  Crocq's (acrocyanosis) I73.89
  Crohn's — see Enteritis, regional
  Curschmann G71.11
  cystic
    breast (chronic) — see Mastopathy, cystic
    kidney, congenital Q61.9
    liver, congenital Q44.6
    lung J98.4
      congenital Q33.0
  cytomegalic inclusion (generalized) B25.9
    with pneumonia B25.0
    congenital P35.1
  cytomegaloviral B25.9
    specified NEC B25.8
  Czerny's (periodic hydrarthrosis of the knee) — see Effusion, joint, knee
  Daae (-Finsen) (epidemic pleurodynia) B33.0
  Darling's — see Histoplasmosis capsulati
  de Quervain's (tendon sheath) M65.4
    thyroid (subacute granulomatous thyroiditis) E06.1
  Débove's (splenomegaly) R16.1
  deer fly — see Tularemia
  Degos' I77.89
  demyelinating, demyelinizating (nervous system) G37.9
    multiple sclerosis G35
    specified NEC G37.8
  dense deposit (see also N00-N07 with fourth character .6) N05.6
  deposition, hydroxyapatite — see Disease, hydroxyapatite deposition
  Devergie's (pityriasis rubra pilaris) L44.0
  Devic's G36.0

Disease, diseased — continued
  diaphorase deficiency D74.0
  diaphragm J98.6
  diarrheal, infectious NEC A09
  digestive system K92.9
    specified NEC K92.89
  disc, degenerative — see Degeneration, intervertebral disc
  discogenic (see also Displacement, intervertebral disc NEC)
    with myelopathy — see Disorder, disc, with, myelopathy
  diverticular — see Diverticula
  Dubois (thymus) A50.59 [E35]
  Duchenne-Griesinger G71.0
  Duchenne's
    muscular dystrophy G71.0
    pseudohypertrophy, muscles G71.0
  ductless glands E34.9
  Duhring's (dermatitis herpetiformis) L13.0
  duodenum K31.9
    specified NEC K31.89
  Dupré's (meningism) R29.1
  Dupuytren's (muscle contracture) M72.0
  Durand-Nicholas-Favre (climatic bubo) A55
  Duroziez's (congenital mitral stenosis) Q23.2
  ear — see Disorder, ear
  Eberth's — see Fever, typhoid
  Ebola (virus) A98.4
  Ebstein's heart Q22.5
  Echinococcus — see Echinococcus
  echovirus NEC B34.1
  Eddowes' (brittle bones and blue sclera) Q78.0
  edentulous (alveolar) ridge K06.9
    specified NEC K06.8
  Edsall's T67.2 ☑
  Eichstedt's (pityriasis versicolor) B36.0
  Eisenmenger's (irreversible) I27.83
  Ellis-van Creveld (chondroectodermal dysplasia) Q77.6
  end stage renal (ESRD) N18.6
    due to hypertension I12.0
  endocrine glands or system NEC E34.9
  endomyocardial (eosinophilic) I42.3
  English (rickets) E55.0
  enteroviral, enterovirus NEC B34.1
    central nervous system NEC A88.8
  epidemic B99.9
    specified NEC B99.8
  epididymis N50.9
  Erb (-Landouzy) G71.0
  Erdheim-Chester (ECD) E88.89
  esophagus K22.9
    functional K22.4
    psychogenic F45.8
    specified NEC K22.8
  Eulenburg's (congenital paramyotonia) G71.19
  eustachian tube — see Disorder, eustachian tube
  external
    auditory canal — see Disorder, ear, external
    ear — see Disorder, ear, external
  extrapyramidal G25.9
    specified NEC G25.89
  eye H57.9
    anterior chamber H21.9
    inflammatory NEC H57.8
    muscle (external) — see Strabismus
    specified NEC H57.8
    syphilitic — see Oculopathy, syphilitic
  eyeball H44.9
    specified NEC H44.89
  eyelid — see Disorder, eyelid
    specified NEC — see Disorder, eyelid, specified type NEC
  eyeworm of Africa B74.3
  facial nerve (seventh) G51.9
    newborn (birth injury) P11.3
  Fahr (of brain) G23.8
  Fahr Volhard (of kidney) I12.- ☑
  fallopian tube (noninflammatory) N83.9
    inflammatory — see Salpingo-oophoritis
    specified NEC N83.8
  familial periodic paralysis G72.3
  Fanconi's (congenital pancytopenia) D61.09
  fascia NEC (see also Disorder, muscle)
    inflammatory — see Myositis
    specified NEC M62.89
  Fauchard's (periodontitis) — see Periodontitis
  Favre-Durand-Nicolas (climatic bubo) A55

Disease, diseased — continued
  Fede's K14.0
  Feer's — see Poisoning, mercury
  female pelvic inflammatory (see also Disease, pelvis, inflammatory) N73.9
    syphilitic (secondary) A51.42
    tuberculous A18.17
  Fernels' (aortic aneurysm) I71.9
  fibrocaseous of lung — see Tuberculosis, pulmonary
  fibrocystic — see Fibrocystic disease
  Fiedler's (leptospiral jaundice) A27.0
  fifth B08.3
  file-cutter's — see Poisoning, lead
  fish-skin Q80.9
    acquired L85.0
  Flajani (-Basedow) (exophthalmic goiter) — see Hyperthyroidism, with, goiter (diffuse)
  flax-dresser's J66.1
  fluke — see Infestation, fluke
  foot and mouth B08.8
  foot process N04.9
  Forbes' (glycogenosis III) E74.03
  Fordyce-Fox (apocrine miliaria) L75.2
  Fordyce's (ectopic sebaceous glands) (mouth) Q38.6
  Forestier's (rhizomelic pseudopolyarthritis) M35.3
    meaning ankylosing hyperostosis — see Hyperostosis, ankylosing
  Fothergill's
    neuralgia — see Neuralgia, trigeminal
    scarlatina anginosa A38.9
  Fournier (gangrene) N49.3
    female N76.89
  fourth B08.8
  Fox (-Fordyce) (apocrine miliaria) L75.2
  Francis' — see Tularemia
  Franklin C88.2
  Frei's (climatic bubo) A55
  Friedreich's
    combined systemic or ataxia G11.1
    myoclonia G25.3
  frontal sinus — see Sinusitis, frontal
  fungus NEC B49
  Gaisböck's (polycythemia hypertonica) D75.1
  gallbladder K82.9
    calculus — see Calculus, gallbladder
    cholecystitis — see Cholecystitis
    cholesterolosis K82.4
    fistula — see Fistula, gallbladder
    hydrops K82.1
    obstruction — see Obstruction, gallbladder
    perforation K82.2
    specified NEC K82.8
  gamma heavy chain C88.2
  Gamna's (siderotic splenomegaly) D73.2
  Gamstorp's (adynamia episodica hereditaria) G72.3
  Gandy-Nanta (siderotic splenomegaly) D73.2
  ganister J62.8
  gastric — see Disease, stomach
  gastroesophageal reflux (GERD) K21.9
    with esophagitis K21.0
  gastrointestinal (tract) K92.9
    amyloid E85.4
    functional K59.9
      psychogenic F45.8
    specified NEC K92.89
  Gee (-Herter) (-Heubner) (-Thaysen) (nontropical sprue) K90.0
  genital organs
    female N94.9
    male N50.9
  Gerhardt's (erythromelalgia) I73.81
  Gibert's (pityriasis rosea) L42
  Gierke's (glycogenosis I) E74.01
  Gilles de la Tourette's (motor-verbal tic) F95.2
  gingiva K06.9
    plaque induced K05.00
    specified NEC K06.8
  gland (lymph) I89.9
  Glanzmann's (hereditary hemorrhagic thrombasthenia) D69.1
  glass-blower's (cataract) — see Cataract, specified NEC
  salivary gland hypertrophy K11.1
  Glisson's — see Rickets
  globe H44.9
    specified NEC H44.89
  glomerular (see also Glomerulonephritis)
    with edema — see Nephrosis
    acute — see Nephritis, acute

Disease, diseased — *continued*
- glomerular (*see also* Glomerulonephritis) — *continued*
    - chronic — *see* Nephritis, chronic
    - minimal change N05.0
    - rapidly progressive N01.9
- glycogen storage E74.00
    - Andersen's E74.09
    - Cori's E74.03
    - Forbes' E74.03
    - generalized E74.00
    - glucose-6-phosphatase deficiency E74.01
    - heart E74.02 [I43]
    - hepatorenal E74.09
    - Hers' E74.09
    - liver and kidney E74.09
    - McArdle's E74.04
    - muscle phosphofructokinase E74.09
    - myocardium E74.02 [I43]
    - Pompe's E74.02
    - Tauri's E74.09
    - type 0 E74.09
    - type I E74.01
    - type II E74.02
    - type III E74.03
    - type IV E74.09
    - type V E74.04
    - type VI-XI E74.09
    - Von Gierke's E74.01
- Goldstein's (familial hemorrhagic telangiectasia) I78.0
- gonococcal NOS A54.9
- graft-versus-host (GVH) D89.813
    - acute D89.810
    - acute on chronic D89.812
    - chronic D89.811
- grainhandler's J67.8
- granulomatous (childhood) (chronic) D71
- Graves' (exophthalmic goiter) — *see* Hyperthyroidism, with, goiter (diffuse)
- Griesinger's — *see* Ancylostomiasis
- Grisel's M43.6
- Gruby's (tinea tonsurans) B35.0
- Guillain-Barré G61.0
- Guinon's (motor-verbal tic) F95.2
- gum K06.9
- gynecological N94.9
- H (Hartnup's) E72.02
- Haff — *see* Poisoning, mercury
- Hageman (congenital factor XII deficiency) D68.2
- hair (color) (shaft) L67.9
    - follicles L73.9
        - specified NEC L73.8
- Hamman's (spontaneous mediastinal emphysema) J98.2
- hand, foot and mouth B08.4
- Hansen's — *see* Leprosy
- Hantavirus, with pulmonary manifestations B33.4
    - with renal manifestations A98.5
- Harada's H30.81- ☑
- Hartnup (pellagra-cerebellar ataxia-renal aminoaciduria) E72.02
- Hart's (pellagra-cerebellar ataxia-renal aminoaciduria) E72.02
- Hashimoto's (struma lymphomatosa) E06.3
- Hb — *see* Disease, hemoglobin
- heart (organic) I51.9
    - with
        - pulmonary edema (acute) (*see also* Failure, ventricular, left) I50.1
        - rheumatic fever (conditions in I00)
            - active I01.9
                - with chorea I02.0
                - specified NEC I01.8
            - inactive or quiescent (with chorea) I09.9
                - specified NEC I09.89
    - amyloid E85.4 [I43]
    - aortic (valve) I35.9
    - arteriosclerotic or sclerotic (senile) — *see* Disease, heart, ischemic, atherosclerotic
    - artery, arterial — *see* Disease, heart, ischemic, atherosclerotic
    - beer drinkers' I42.6
    - beriberi (wet) E51.12
    - black I27.0
    - congenital Q24.9
        - cyanotic Q24.9
        - specified NEC Q24.8
    - coronary — *see* Disease, heart, ischemic

Disease, diseased — *continued*
- heart — *continued*
    - cryptogenic I51.9
    - fibroid — *see* Myocarditis
    - functional I51.89
        - psychogenic F45.8
    - glycogen storage E74.02 [I43]
    - gonococcal A54.83
    - hypertensive — *see* Hypertension, heart
    - hyperthyroid (*see also* Hyperthyroidism)
        - E05.90 [I43]
        - with thyroid storm E05.91 [I43]
    - ischemic (chronic or with a stated duration of over 4 weeks) I25.9
        - atherosclerotic (of) I25.10
            - with angina pectoris — *see* Arteriosclerosis, coronary (artery)
            - coronary artery bypass graft — *see* Arteriosclerosis, coronary (artery),
            - cardiomyopathy I25.5
            - diagnosed on ECG or other special investigation, but currently presenting no symptoms I25.6
            - silent I25.6
        - specified form NEC I25.89
    - kyphoscoliotic I27.1
    - meningococcal A39.50
        - endocarditis A39.51
        - myocarditis A39.52
        - pericarditis A39.53
    - mitral I05.9
        - specified NEC I05.8
    - muscular — *see* Degeneration, myocardial
    - psychogenic (functional) F45.8
    - pulmonary (chronic) I27.9
        - in schistosomiasis B65.9 [I52]
        - specified NEC I27.89
    - rheumatic (chronic) (inactive) (old) (quiescent) (with chorea) I09.9
        - active or acute I01.9
            - with chorea (acute) (rheumatic) (Sydenham's) I02.0
        - specified NEC I09.89
    - senile — *see* Myocarditis
    - syphilitic A52.06
        - aortic A52.03
            - aneurysm A52.01
        - congenital A50.54 [I52]
    - thyrotoxic (*see also* Thyrotoxicosis) E05.90 [I43]
        - with thyroid storm E05.91 [I43]
    - valve, valvular (obstructive) (regurgitant) (*see also* Endocarditis)
        - congenital NEC Q24.8
        - pulmonary Q22.3
    - vascular — *see* Disease, cardiovascular
- heavy chain NEC C88.2
    - alpha C88.3
    - gamma C88.2
    - mu C88.2
- Hebra's
    - pityriasis
        - maculata et circinata L42
        - rubra pilaris L44.0
    - prurigo L28.2
- hematopoietic organs D75.9
- hemoglobin or Hb
    - abnormal (mixed) NEC D58.2
        - with thalassemia D56.9
    - AS genotype D57.3
    - Bart's D56.0
    - C (Hb-C) D58.2
        - with other abnormal hemoglobin NEC D58.2
        - elliptocytosis D58.1
        - Hb-S D57.2- ☑
        - sickle-cell D57.2- ☑
        - thalassemia D56.8
    - Constant Spring D58.2
    - D (Hb-D) D58.2
    - E (Hb-E) D58.2
    - E-beta thalassemia D56.5
    - elliptocytosis D58.1
    - H (Hb-H) (thalassemia) D56.0
        - with other abnormal hemoglobin NEC D56.9
        - Constant Spring D56.0
    - I thalassemia D56.9
    - M D74.0
    - S or SS D57.1
    - SC D57.2- ☑

Disease, diseased — *continued*
- hemoglobin or Hb — *continued*
    - SD D57.8- ☑
    - SE D57.8- ☑
    - spherocytosis D58.0
    - unstable, hemolytic D58.2
- hemolytic (newborn) P55.9
    - autoimmune (cold type) (warm type) D59.1
    - drug-induced D59.0
    - due to or with
        - incompatibility
            - ABO (blood group) P55.1
            - blood (group) (Duffy) (K(ell)) (Kidd) (Lewis) (M) (S) NEC P55.8
            - Rh (blood group) (factor) P55.0
            - Rh negative mother P55.0
    - specified type NEC P55.8
    - unstable hemoglobin D58.2
- hemorrhagic D69.9
    - newborn P53
- Henoch (-Schönlein) (purpura nervosa) D69.0
- hepatic — *see* Disease, liver
- hepatolenticular E83.01
- heredodegenerative NEC
    - spinal cord G95.89
- herpesviral, disseminated B00.7
- Hers' (glycogenosis VI) E74.09
- Herter (-Gee) (-Heubner) (nontropical sprue) K90.0
- Heubner-Herter (nontropical sprue) K90.0
- high fetal gene or hemoglobin thalassemia D56.9
- Hildenbrand's — *see* Typhus
- hip (joint) M25.9
    - congenital Q65.89
    - suppurative M00.9
    - tuberculous A18.02
- His (-Werner) (trench fever) A79.0
- Hodgson's I71.2
    - ruptured I71.1
- Holla — *see* Spherocytosis
- hookworm B76.9
    - specified NEC B76.8
- host-versus-graft D89.813
    - acute D89.810
    - acute on chronic D89.812
    - chronic D89.811
- human immunodeficiency virus (HIV) B20
- Huntington's G10
    - with dementia G10 [F02.80]
- Hutchinson's (cheiropompholyx) — *see* Hutchinson's disease
- hyaline (diffuse) (generalized)
    - membrane (lung) (newborn) P22.0
    - adult J80
- hydatid — *see* Echinococcus
- hydroxyapatite deposition M11.00
    - ankle M11.07- ☑
    - elbow M11.02- ☑
    - foot joint M11.07- ☑
    - hand joint M11.04- ☑
    - hip M11.05- ☑
    - knee M11.06- ☑
    - multiple site M11.09
    - shoulder M11.01- ☑
    - vertebra M11.08
    - wrist M11.03- ☑
- hyperkinetic — *see* Hyperkinesia
- hypertensive — *see* Hypertension
- hypophysis E23.7
- Iceland G93.3
- I-cell E77.0
- immune D89.9
- immunoproliferative (malignant) C88.9
    - small intestinal C88.3
    - specified NEC C88.8
- inclusion B25.9
    - salivary gland B25.9
- infectious, infective B99.9
    - congenital P37.9
        - specified NEC P37.8
    - viral P35.9
        - specified type NEC P35.8
    - specified NEC B99.8
- inflammatory
    - penis N48.29
        - abscess N48.21
        - cellulitis N48.22
    - prepuce N47.7
        - balanoposthitis N47.6

Disease, diseased — *continued*
  inflammatory — *continued*
    tubo-ovarian — *see* Salpingo-oophoritis
  intervertebral disc (*see also* Disorder, disc)
    with myelopathy — *see* Disorder, disc, with, myelopathy
    cervical, cervicothoracic — *see* Disorder, disc, cervical
    with
      myelopathy — *see* Disorder, disc, cervical, with myelopathy
      neuritis, radiculitis or radiculopathy — *see* Disorder, disc, cervical, with neuritis
      specified NEC — *see* Disorder, disc, cervical, specified type NEC
    lumbar (with)
      myelopathy M51.06
      neuritis, radiculitis, radiculopathy or sciatica M51.16
      specified NEC M51.86
    lumbosacral (with)
      neuritis, radiculitis, radiculopathy or sciatica M51.17
      specified NEC M51.87
    specified NEC — *see* Disorder, disc, specified NEC
    thoracic (with)
      myelopathy M51.04
      neuritis, radiculitis or radiculopathy M51.14
      specified NEC M51.84
    thoracolumbar (with)
      myelopathy M51.05
      neuritis, radiculitis or radiculopathy M51.15
      specified NEC M51.85
  intestine K63.9
    functional K59.9
      psychogenic F45.8
      specified NEC K59.8
    organic K63.9
    protozoal A07.9
    specified NEC K63.89
  iris H21.9
    specified NEC H21.89
  iron metabolism or storage E83.10
  island (scrub typhus) A75.3
  itai-itai — *see* Poisoning, cadmium
  Jakob-Creutzfeldt — *see* Creutzfeldt-Jakob disease or syndrome
  jaw M27.9
    fibrocystic M27.49
    specified NEC M27.8
  jigger B88.1
  joint (*see also* Disorder, joint)
    Charcot's — *see* Arthropathy, neuropathic (Charcot)
    degenerative — *see* Osteoarthritis
      multiple M15.9
      spine — *see* Spondylosis
    hypertrophic — *see* Osteoarthritis
    sacroiliac M53.3
    specified NEC — *see* Disorder, joint, specified type NEC
    spine NEC — *see* Dorsopathy
    suppurative — *see* Arthritis, pyogenic or pyemic
  Jourdain's (acute gingivitis) K05.00
    nonplaque induced K05.01
    plaque induced K05.00
  Kaschin-Beck (endemic polyarthritis) M12.10
    ankle M12.17- ☑
    elbow M12.12- ☑
    foot joint M12.17- ☑
    hand joint M12.14- ☑
    hip M12.15- ☑
    knee M12.16- ☑
    multiple site M12.19
    shoulder M12.11- ☑
    vertebra M12.18
    wrist M12.13- ☑
  Katayama B65.2
  Kedani (scrub typhus) A75.3
  Keshan E59
  kidney (functional) (pelvis) N28.9
    chronic N18.9
      hypertensive — *see* Hypertension, kidney
      stage 1 N18.1
      stage 2 (mild) N18.2
      stage 3 (moderate) N18.3
      stage 4 (severe) N18.4
      stage 5 N18.5

Disease, diseased — *continued*
  kidney — *continued*
    complicating pregnancy — *see* Pregnancy, complicated by, renal disease
    cystic (congenital) Q61.9
    fibrocystic (congenital) Q61.8
    hypertensive — *see* Hypertension, kidney
    in (due to)
      schistosomiasis (bilharziasis) B65.9 [N29]
    multicystic Q61.4
    polycystic Q61.3
      adult type Q61.2
      childhood type NEC Q61.19
        collecting duct dilatation Q61.11
  Kimmelstiel (-Wilson) (intercapillary polycystic (congenital) glomerulosclerosis) — *see* E08-E13 with .21
  Kinnier Wilson's (hepatolenticular degeneration) E83.01
  kissing — *see* Mononucleosis, infectious
  Klebs' (*see also* Glomerulonephritis) N05- ☑
  Klippel-Feil (brevicollis) Q76.1
  Köhler-Pellegrini-Stieda (calcification, knee joint) — *see* Bursitis, tibial collateral
  Kok Q89.8
  König's (osteochondritis dissecans) — *see* Osteochondritis, dissecans
  Korsakoff's (nonalcoholic) F04
    alcoholic F10.96
      with dependence F10.26
  Kostmann's (infantile genetic agranulocytosis) D70.0
  kuru A81.81
  Kyasanur Forest A98.2
  labyrinth, ear — *see* Disorder, ear, inner
  lacrimal system — *see* Disorder, lacrimal system
  Lafora's — *see* Epilepsy, generalized, idiopathic
  Lancereaux-Mathieu (leptospiral jaundice) A27.0
  Landry's G61.0
  Larrey-Weil (leptospiral jaundice) A27.0
  larynx J38.7
  legionnaires' A48.1
    nonpneumonic A48.2
  Lenegre's I44.2
  lens H27.9
    specified NEC H27.8
  Lev's (acquired complete heart block) I44.2
  Lewy body (dementia) G31.83 [F02.80]
    with behavioral disturbance G31.83 [F02.81]
  Lichtheim's (subacute combined sclerosis with pernicious anemia) D51.0
  Lightwood's (renal tubular acidosis) N25.89
  Lignac's (cystinosis) E72.04
  lip K13.0
  lipid-storage E75.6
    specified NEC E75.5
  Lipschütz's N76.6
  liver (chronic) (organic) K76.9
    alcoholic (chronic) K70.9
      acute — *see* Disease, liver, alcoholic, hepatitis
      cirrhosis K70.30
        with ascites K70.31
      failure K70.40
        with coma K70.41
      fatty liver K70.0
      fibrosis K70.2
      hepatitis K70.10
        with ascites K70.11
      sclerosis K70.2
    cystic, congenital Q44.6
    drug-induced (idiosyncratic) (toxic) (predictable) (unpredictable) — *see* Disease, liver, toxic
    end stage K72.90
      due to hepatitis — *see* Hepatitis
    fatty, nonalcoholic (NAFLD) K76.0
      alcoholic K70.0
    fibrocystic (congenital) Q44.6
    fluke
      Chinese B66.1
      oriental B66.1
      sheep B66.3
    gestational alloimmune (GALD) P78.84
    glycogen storage E74.09 [K77]
    in (due to)
      schistosomiasis (bilharziasis) B65.9 [K77]
    inflammatory K75.9
      alcoholic K70.1 ☑
      specified NEC K75.89
    polycystic (congenital) Q44.6

Disease, diseased — *continued*
  liver — *continued*
    toxic K71.9
      with
        cholestasis K71.0
        cirrhosis (liver) K71.7
        fibrosis (liver) K71.7
        focal nodular hyperplasia K71.8
        hepatic granuloma K71.8
        hepatic necrosis K71.10
          with coma K71.11
        hepatitis NEC K71.6
          acute K71.2
          chronic
            active K71.50
              with ascites K71.51
            lobular K71.4
            persistent K71.3
        lupoid K71.50
          with ascites K71.51
        peliosis hepatis K71.8
        veno-occlusive disease (VOD) of liver K71.8
    veno-occlusive K76.5
  Lobo's (keloid blastomycosis) B48.0
  Lobstein's (brittle bones and blue sclera) Q78.0
  Ludwig's (submaxillary cellulitis) K12.2
  lumbosacral region M53.87
  lung J98.4
    black J60
    congenital Q33.9
    cystic J98.4
      congenital Q33.0
    fibroid (chronic) — *see* Fibrosis, lung
    fluke B66.4
      oriental B66.4
    in
      amyloidosis E85.4 [J99]
      sarcoidosis D86.0
      Sjögren's syndrome M35.02
      systemic
        lupus erythematosus M32.13
        sclerosis M34.81
    interstitial J84.9
      of childhood, specified NEC J84.848
      respiratory bronchiolitis J84.115
      specified NEC J84.89
    obstructive (chronic) J44.9
      with
        acute
          bronchitis J44.0
          exacerbation NEC J44.1
          lower respiratory infection J44.0
        alveolitis, allergic J67.9
        asthma J44.9
        bronchiectasis J47.9
          with
            exacerbation (acute) J47.1
            lower respiratory infection J47.0
        bronchitis J44.9
          with
            exacerbation (acute) J44.1
            lower respiratory infection J44.0
        emphysema J43.9
        hypersensitivity pneumonitis J67.9
      decompensated J44.1
        with
          exacerbation (acute) J44.1
    polycystic J98.4
      congenital Q33.0
    rheumatoid (diffuse) (interstitial) — *see* Rheumatoid, lung
  Lutembacher's (atrial septal defect with mitral stenosis) Q21.1
  Lyme A69.20
  lymphatic (gland) (system) (channel) (vessel) I89.9
  lymphoproliferative D47.9
    specified NEC D47.Z9 (*following* D47.4)
    T-gamma D47.Z9 (*following* D47.4)
    X-linked D82.3
  Magitot's M27.2
  malarial — *see* Malaria
  malignant (*see also* Neoplasm, malignant, by site)
  Manson's B65.1
  maple bark J67.6
  maple-syrup-urine E71.0
  Marburg (virus) A98.3
  Marion's (bladder neck obstruction) N32.0
  Marsh's (exophthalmic goiter) — *see* Hyperthyroidism, with, goiter (diffuse)

Disease, diseased — *continued*

mastoid (process) — *see* Disorder, ear, middle
Mathieu's (leptospiral jaundice) A27.Ø
Maxcy's A75.2
McArdle (-Schmid-Pearson) (glycogenosis V) E74.Ø4
mediastinum J98.59
medullary center (idiopathic) (respiratory) G93.89
Meige's (chronic hereditary edema) Q82.Ø
meningococcal — *see* Infection, meningococcal
mental F99
    organic FØ9
mesenchymal M35.9
mesenteric embolic (*see also* Ischemia, intestine, acute)
    K55.Ø39
metabolic, metabolism E88.9
    bilirubin E8Ø.7
metal-polisher's J62.8
metastatic (*see also* Neoplasm, secondary, by site)
    C79.9
microvascular - code to condition
microvillus
    atrophy Q43.8
    inclusion (MVD) Q43.8
middle ear — *see* Disorder, ear, middle
Mikulicz' (dryness of mouth, absent or decreased
    lacrimation) K11.8
Milroy's (chronic hereditary edema) Q82.Ø
Minamata — *see* Poisoning, mercury
minicore G71.2
Minor's G95.19
Minot's (hemorrhagic disease, newborn) P53
Minot-von Willebrand-Jürgens (angiohemophilia)
    D68.Ø
Mitchell's (erythromelalgia) I73.81
mitral (valve) IØ5.9
    nonrheumatic I34.9
mixed connective tissue M35.1
moldy hay J67.Ø
Monge's T7Ø.29 ☑
Morgagni-Adams-Stokes (syncope with heart block)
    I45.9
Morgagni's (syndrome) (hyperostosis frontalis interna)
    M85.2
Morton's (with metatarsalgia) — *see* Lesion, nerve,
    plantar
Morvan's G6Ø.8
motor neuron (bulbar) (mixed type) (spinal) G12.2Ø
    amyotrophic lateral sclerosis G12.21
    familial G12.24
    progressive bulbar palsy G12.22
    specified NEC G12.29
moyamoya I67.5
mu heavy chain disease C88.2
multicore G71.2
muscle (*see also* Disorder, muscle)
    inflammatory — *see* Myositis
    ocular (external) — *see* Strabismus
musculoskeletal system, soft tissue — *see also* Disor-
    der, soft tissue
    specified NEC — *see* Disorder, soft tissue, specified
        type NEC
mushroom workers' J67.5
mycotic B49
myelodysplastic, not classified C94.6
myeloproliferative, not classified C94.6
    chronic D47.1
myocardial, myocardium (*see also* Degeneration, my-
    ocardial) I51.5
    primary (idiopathic) I42.9
myoneural G7Ø.9
Naegeli's D69.1
nails L6Ø.9
    specified NEC L6Ø.8
Nairobi (sheep virus) A93.8
nasal J34.9
nemaline body G71.2
nerve — *see* Disorder, nerve
nervous system G98.8
    autonomic G9Ø.9
    central G96.9
        specified NEC G96.8
    congenital QØ7.9
    parasympathetic G9Ø.9
    specified NEC G98.8
    sympathetic G9Ø.9
    vegetative G9Ø.9
neuromuscular system G7Ø.9
Newcastle B3Ø.8

Disease, diseased — *continued*

Nicolas (-Durand)-Favre (climatic bubo) A55
nipple N64.9
    Paget's C5Ø.Ø1- ☑
        female C5Ø.Ø1- ☑
        male C5Ø.Ø2- ☑
Nishimoto (-Takeuchi) I67.5
nonarthropod-borne NOS (viral) B34.9
    enterovirus NEC B34.1
nonautoimmune hemolytic D59.4
    drug-induced D59.2
Nonne-Milroy-Meige (chronic hereditary edema) Q82.Ø
nose J34.9
nucleus pulposus — *see* Disorder, disc
nutritional E63.9
oast-house-urine E72.19
    ocular
        herpesviral BØØ.5Ø
        zoster BØ2.3Ø
obliterative vascular I77.1
Ohara's — *see* Tularemia
Opitz's (congestive splenomegaly) D73.2
Oppenheim-Urbach (necrobiosis lipoidica diabetico-
    rum) — *see* EØ8-E13 with .62Ø
optic nerve NEC — *see* Disorder, nerve, optic
orbit — *see* Disorder, orbit
Oriental liver fluke B66.1
Oriental lung fluke B66.4
Ormond's N13.5
Oropouche virus A93.Ø
Osler-Rendu (familial hemorrhagic telangiectasia) I78.Ø
osteofibrocystic E21.Ø
Otto's M24.7
outer ear — *see* Disorder, ear, external
ovary (noninflammatory) N83.9
    cystic N83.2Ø- ☑
    inflammatory — *see* Salpingo-oophoritis
    polycystic E28.2
    specified NEC N83.8
Owren's (congenital) — *see* Defect, coagulation
pancreas K86.9
    cystic K86.2
    fibrocystic E84.9
    specified NEC K86.89
panvalvular IØ8.9
    specified NEC IØ8.8
parametrium (noninflammatory) N83.9
parasitic B89
    cerebral NEC B71.9 [G94]
    intestinal NOS B82.9
    mouth B37.Ø
    skin NOS B88.9
    specified type — *see* Infestation
    tongue B37.Ø
parathyroid (gland) E21.5
    specified NEC E21.4
Parkinson's G2Ø
parodontal KØ5.6
Parrot's (syphilitic osteochondritis) A5Ø.Ø2
Parry's (exophthalmic goiter) — *see* Hyperthyroidism,
    with, goiter (diffuse)
Parson's (exophthalmic goiter) — *see* Hyperthyroidism,
    with, goiter (diffuse)
Paxton's (white piedra) B36.2
pearl-worker's — *see* Osteomyelitis, specified type
    NEC
Pellegrini-Stieda (calcification, knee joint) — *see* Bur-
    sitis, tibial collateral
pelvis, pelvic
    female NOS N94.9
        specified NEC N94.89
    gonococcal (acute) (chronic) A54.24
    inflammatory (female) N73.9
        acute N73.Ø
        chlamydial A56.11
        chronic N73.1
        specified NEC N73.8
        syphilitic (secondary) A51.42
            late A52.76
        tuberculous A18.17
    organ, female N94.9
    peritoneum, female NEC N94.89
penis N48.9
    inflammatory N48.29
        abscess N48.21
        cellulitis N48.22
    specified NEC N48.89
periapical tissues NOS KØ4.9Ø

Disease, diseased — *continued*

periodontal KØ5.6
    specified NEC KØ5.5
periosteum — *see* Disorder, bone, specified type NEC
peripheral
    arterial I73.9
    autonomic nervous system G9Ø.9
    nerves — *see* Polyneuropathy
    vascular NOS I73.9
peritoneum K66.9
    pelvic, female NEC N94.89
    specified NEC K66.8
persistent mucosal (middle ear) H66.2Ø
    left H66.22
        with right H66.23
    right H66.21
        with left H66.23
Petit's — *see* Hernia, abdomen, specified site NEC
pharynx J39.2
    specified NEC J39.2
Phocas' — *see* Mastopathy, cystic
photochromogenic (acid-fast bacilli) (pulmonary)
    A31.Ø
    nonpulmonary A31.9
Pick's G31.Ø1 [FØ2.8Ø]
    with behavioral disturbance G31.Ø1 [FØ2.81]
    brain G31.Ø1 [FØ2.8Ø]
        with behavioral disturbance G31.Ø1 [FØ2.81]
    of pericardium (pericardial pseudocirrhosis of liver)
        I31.1
pigeon fancier's J67.2
pineal gland E34.8
pink — *see* Poisoning, mercury
Pinkus' (lichen nitidus) L44.1
pinworm B8Ø
Piry virus A93.8
pituitary (gland) E23.7
pituitary-snuff-taker's J67.8
pleura (cavity) J94.9
    specified NEC J94.8
pneumatic drill (hammer) T75.21 ☑
Pollitzer's (hidradenitis suppurativa) L73.2
polycystic
    kidney or renal Q61.3
        adult type Q61.2
        childhood type NEC Q61.19
            collecting duct dilatation Q61.11
    liver or hepatic Q44.6
    lung or pulmonary J98.4
        congenital Q33.Ø
    ovary, ovaries E28.2
    spleen Q89.Ø9
polyethylene T84.Ø5- ☑
Pompe's (glycogenosis II) E74.Ø2
Posadas-Wernicke B38.9
Potain's (pulmonary edema) — *see* Edema, lung
prepuce N47.8
    inflammatory N47.7
        balanoposthitis N47.6
Pringle's (tuberous sclerosis) Q85.1
prion, central nervous system A81.9
    specified NEC A81.89
prostate N42.9
    specified NEC N42.89
protozoal B64
    acanthamebiasis — *see* Acanthamebiasis
    African trypanosomiasis — *see* African trypanoso-
        miasis
    babesiosis B6Ø.Ø
    Chagas disease — *see* Chagas disease
    intestine, intestinal AØ7.9
    leishmaniasis — *see* Leishmaniasis
    malaria — *see* Malaria
    naegleriasis B6Ø.2
    pneumocystosis B59
    specified organism NEC B6Ø.8
    toxoplasmosis — *see* Toxoplasmosis
pseudo-Hurler's E77.Ø
psychiatric F99
psychotic — *see* Psychosis
Puente's (simple glandular cheilitis) K13.Ø
puerperal (*see also* Puerperal) O9Ø.89
pulmonary (*see also* Disease, lung)
    artery I28.9
    chronic obstructive J44.9
        with
            acute bronchitis J44.Ø
            exacerbation (acute) J44.1

Disease, diseased — continued
  pulmonary (see also Disease, lung) — continued
    chronic obstructive — continued
      with — continued
        lower respiratory infection (acute) J44.0
      decompensated J44.1
        with
          exacerbation (acute) J44.1
    heart I27.9
      specified NEC I27.89
    hypertensive (vascular) (see also Hypertension, pulmonary) I27.20
      primary (idiopathic) I27.0
      NEC I27.2 ☑
    valve I37.9
      rheumatic I09.89
  pulp (dental) NOS K04.90
  pulseless M31.4
  Putnam's (subacute combined sclerosis with pernicious anemia) D51.0
  Pyle (-Cohn) (metaphyseal dysplasia) Q78.5
  ragpicker's or ragsorter's A22.1
  Raynaud's — see Raynaud's disease
  reactive airway — see Asthma
  Reclus' (cystic) — see Mastopathy, cystic
  rectum K62.9
    specified NEC K62.89
  Refsum's (heredopathia atactica polyneuritiformis) G60.1
  renal (functional) (pelvis) (see also Disease, kidney) N28.9
    with
      edema — see Nephrosis
      glomerular lesion — see Glomerulonephritis
        with edema — see Nephrosis
      interstitial nephritis N12
    acute N28.9
    chronic (see also Disease, kidney, chronic) N18.9
    cystic, congenital Q61.9
    diabetic — see E08-E13 with .22
    end-stage (failure) N18.6
      due to hypertension I12.0
    fibrocystic (congenital) Q61.8
    hypertensive — see Hypertension, kidney
    lupus M32.14
    phosphate-losing (tubular) N25.0
    polycystic (congenital) Q61.3
      adult type Q61.2
      childhood type NEC Q61.19
        collecting duct dilatation Q61.11
    rapidly progressive N01.9
    subacute N01.9
  Rendu-Osler-Weber (familial hemorrhagic telangiectasia) I78.0
  renovascular (arteriosclerotic) — see Hypertension, kidney
  respiratory (tract) J98.9
    acute or subacute NOS J06.9
      due to
        chemicals, gases, fumes or vapors (inhalation) J68.3
        external agent J70.9
          specified NEC J70.8
        radiation J70.0
        smoke inhalation J70.5
      noninfectious J39.8
    chronic NOS J98.9
      due to
        chemicals, gases, fumes or vapors J68.4
        external agent J70.9
          specified NEC J70.8
        radiation J70.1
      newborn P27.9
        specified NEC P27.8
    due to
      chemicals, gases, fumes or vapors J68.9
        acute or subacute NEC J68.3
        chronic J68.4
      external agent J70.9
        specified NEC J70.8
    newborn P28.9
      specified type NEC P28.89
    upper J39.9
      acute or subacute J06.9
      noninfectious NEC J39.8
      specified NEC J39.8
      streptococcal J06.9
  retina, retinal H35.9

Disease, diseased — continued
  retina, retinal — continued
    Batten's or Batten-Mayou E75.4 [H36]
    specified NEC H35.89
  rheumatoid — see Arthritis, rheumatoid
  rickettsial NOS A79.9
    specified type NEC A79.89
  Riga (-Fede) (cachectic aphthae) K14.0
  Riggs' (compound periodontitis) — see Periodontitis
  Ritter's L00
  Rivalta's (cervicofacial actinomycosis) A42.2
  Robles' (onchocerciasis) B73.01
  Roger's (congenital interventricular septal defect) Q21.0
  Rosenthal's (factor XI deficiency) D68.1
  Ross River B33.1
  Rossbach's (hyperchlorhydria) K30
  Rotes Quérol — see Hyperostosis, ankylosing
  Roth (-Bernhardt) — see Mononeuropathy, lower limb, meralgia paresthetica
  Runeberg's (progressive pernicious anemia) D51.0
  sacroiliac NEC M53.3
  salivary gland or duct K11.9
    inclusion B25.9
    specified NEC K11.8
    virus B25.9
  sandworm B76.9
  Schimmelbusch's — see Mastopathy, cystic
  Schmorl's — see Schmorl's disease or nodes
  Schönlein (-Henoch) (purpura rheumatica) D69.0
  Schottmüller's — see Fever, paratyphoid
  Schultz's (agranulocytosis) — see Agranulocytosis
  Schwalbe-Ziehen-Oppenheim G24.1
  Schwartz-Jampel G71.13
  sclera H15.9
    specified NEC H15.89
  scrofulous (tuberculous) A18.2
  scrotum N50.9
  sebaceous glands L73.9
  semilunar cartilage, cystic (see also Derangement, knee, meniscus, cystic)
  seminal vesicle N50.9
  serum NEC (see also Reaction, serum) T80.69 ☑
  sexually transmitted A64
    anogenital
      herpesviral infection — see Herpes, anogenital
      warts A63.0
    chancroid A57
    chlamydial infection — see Chlamydia
    gonorrhea — see Gonorrhea
    granuloma inguinale A58
    specified organism NEC A63.8
    syphilis — see Syphilis
    trichomoniasis — see Trichomoniasis
  Sézary C84.1- ☑
  shimamushi (scrub typhus) A75.3
  shipyard B30.0
  sickle-cell D57.1
    with crisis (vasoocclusive pain) D57.00
      with
        acute chest syndrome D57.01
        splenic sequestration D57.02
    elliptocytosis D57.8- ☑
    Hb-C D57.20
      with crisis (vasoocclusive pain) D57.219
        with
          acute chest syndrome D57.211
          splenic sequestration D57.212
      without crisis D57.20
    Hb-SD D57.80
      with crisis D57.819
        with
          acute chest syndrome D57.811
          splenic sequestration D57.812
    Hb-SE D57.80
      with crisis D57.819
        with
          acute chest syndrome D57.811
          splenic sequestration D57.812
    specified NEC D57.80
      with crisis D57.819
        with
          acute chest syndrome D57.811
          splenic sequestration D57.812
    spherocytosis D57.80
      with crisis D57.819
        with
          acute chest syndrome D57.811

Disease, diseased — continued
  sickle-cell — continued
    spherocytosis — continued
      with crisis — continued
        with — continued
          splenic sequestration D57.812
    thalassemia D57.40
      with crisis (vasoocclusive pain) D57.419
        with
          acute chest syndrome D57.411
          splenic sequestration D57.412
      without crisis D57.40
  silo-filler's J68.8
    bronchitis J68.0
    pneumonitis J68.0
    pulmonary edema J68.1
  simian B B00.4
  Simons' (progressive lipodystrophy) E88.1
  sin nombre virus B33.4
  sinus — see Sinusitis
  Sirkari's B55.0
  sixth B08.20
    due to human herpesvirus 6 B08.21
    due to human herpesvirus 7 B08.22
  skin L98.9
    due to metabolic disorder NEC E88.9 [L99]
    specified NEC L98.8
  slim (HIV) B20
  small vessel I73.9
  Sneddon-Wilkinson (subcorneal pustular dermatosis) L13.1
  South African creeping B88.0
  spinal (cord) G95.9
    congenital Q06.9
    specified NEC G95.89
  spine (see also Spondylopathy)
    joint — see Dorsopathy
    tuberculous A18.01
  spinocerebellar (hereditary) G11.9
    specified NEC G11.8
  spleen D73.9
    amyloid E85.4 [D77]
    organic D73.9
    polycystic Q89.09
    postinfectional D73.89
  sponge-diver's — see Toxicity, venom, marine animal, sea anemone
  Startle Q89.8
  Steinert's G71.11
  Sticker's (erythema infectiosum) B08.3
  Stieda's (calcification, knee joint) — see Bursitis, tibial collateral
  Stokes' (exophthalmic goiter) — see Hyperthyroidism, with, goiter (diffuse)
  Stokes-Adams (syncope with heart block) I45.9
  stomach K31.9
    functional, psychogenic F45.8
    specified NEC K31.89
  stonemason's J62.8
  storage
    glycogen — see Disease, glycogen storage
    mucopolysaccharide — see Mucopolysaccharidosis
  striatopallidal system NEC G25.89
  Stuart-Prower (congenital factor X deficiency) D68.2
  Stuart's (congenital factor X deficiency) D68.2
  subcutaneous tissue — see Disease, skin
  supporting structures of teeth K08.9
    specified NEC K08.89
  suprarenal (capsule) (gland) E27.9
    hyperfunction E27.0
    specified NEC E27.8
  sweat glands L74.9
    specified NEC L74.8
  Sweeley-Klionsky E75.21
  Swift (-Feer) — see Poisoning, mercury
  swimming-pool granuloma A31.1
  Sylvest's (epidemic pleurodynia) B33.0
  sympathetic nervous system G90.9
  synovium — see Disorder, synovium
  syphilitic — see Syphilis
  systemic tissue mast cell C96.20
  tanapox (virus) B08.71
  Tangier E78.6
  Tarral-Besnier (pityriasis rubra pilaris) L44.0
  Tauri's E74.09
  tear duct — see Disorder, lacrimal system
  tendon, tendinous (see also Disorder, tendon)
    nodular — see Trigger finger

☑ Additional Character Required — Refer to the Tabular List for Character Selection   ▽ Subterms under main terms may continue to next column or page

Disease, diseased — *continued*
- terminal vessel I73.9
- testis N50.9
- thalassemia Hb-S — *see* Disease, sickle-cell, thalassemia
- Thaysen-Gee (nontropical sprue) K90.0
- Thomsen G71.12
- throat J39.2
  - septic J02.0
- thromboembolic — *see* Embolism
- thymus (gland) E32.9
  - specified NEC E32.8
- thyroid (gland) E07.9
  - heart (*see also* Hyperthyroidism) E05.90 [I43]
    - with thyroid storm E05.91 [I43]
  - specified NEC E07.89
- Tietze's M94.0
- tongue K14.9
  - specified NEC K14.8
- tonsils, tonsillar (and adenoids) J35.9
- tooth, teeth K08.9
  - hard tissues K03.9
    - specified NEC K03.89
  - pulp NEC K04.99
  - specified NEC K08.89
- Tourette's F95.2
- trachea NEC J39.8
- tricuspid I07.9
  - nonrheumatic I36.9
- triglyceride-storage E75.5
- trophoblastic — *see* Mole, hydatidiform
- tsutsugamushi A75.3
- tube (fallopian) (noninflammatory) N83.9
  - inflammatory — *see* Salpingitis
  - specified NEC N83.8
- tuberculous NEC — *see* Tuberculosis
- tubo-ovarian (noninflammatory) N83.9
  - inflammatory — *see* Salpingo-oophoritis
  - specified NEC N83.8
- tubotympanic, chronic — *see* Otitis, media, suppurative, chronic, tubotympanic
- tubulo-interstitial N15.9
  - specified NEC N15.8
- tympanum — *see* Disorder, tympanic membrane
- Uhl's Q24.8
- Underwood's (sclerema neonatorum) P83.0
- Unverricht (-Lundborg) — *see* Epilepsy, generalized, idiopathic
- Urbach-Oppenheim (necrobiosis lipoidica diabeticorum) — *see* E08-E13 with .620
- ureter N28.9
  - in (due to)
    - schistosomiasis (bilharziasis) B65.0 [N29]
- urethra N36.9
  - specified NEC N36.8
- urinary (tract) N39.9
  - bladder N32.9
    - specified NEC N32.89
  - specified NEC N39.8
- uterus (noninflammatory) N85.9
  - infective — *see* Endometritis
  - inflammatory — *see* Endometritis
  - specified NEC N85.8
- uveal tract (anterior) H21.9
  - posterior H31.9
- vagabond's B85.1
- vagina, vaginal (noninflammatory) N89.9
  - inflammatory NEC N76.89
  - specified NEC N89.8
- valve, valvular I38
  - multiple I08.9
    - specified NEC I08.8
- van Creveld-von Gierke (glycogenosis I) E74.01
- vas deferens N50.9
- vascular I99.9
  - arteriosclerotic — *see* Arteriosclerosis
  - ciliary body NEC — *see* Disorder, iris, vascular
  - hypertensive — *see* Hypertension
  - iris NEC — *see* Disorder, iris, vascular
  - obliterative I77.1
    - peripheral I73.9
  - occlusive I99.8
  - peripheral (occlusive) I73.9
    - in diabetes mellitus — *see* E08-E13 with .51
- vasomotor I73.9
- vasospastic I73.9
- vein I87.9
- venereal (*see also* Disease, sexually transmitted) A64

Disease, diseased — *continued*
- venereal (*see also* Disease, sexually transmitted) — *continued*
  - chlamydial NEC A56.8
    - anus A56.3
    - genitourinary NOS A56.2
    - pharynx A56.4
    - rectum A56.3
  - fifth A55
  - sixth A55
  - specified nature or type NEC A63.8
- vertebra, vertebral (*see also* Spondylopathy)
  - disc — *see* Disorder, disc
- vibration — *see* Vibration, adverse effects
- viral, virus (*see also* Disease, by type of virus) B34.9
  - arbovirus NOS A94
  - arthropod-borne NOS A94
  - congenital P35.9
    - specified NEC P35.8
  - Hanta (with renal manifestations) (Dobrava) (Puumala) (Seoul) A98.5
    - with pulmonary manifestations (Andes) (Bayou) (Bermejo) (Black Creek Canal) (Choclo) (Juquitiba) (Laguna negra) (Lechiguanas) (New York) (Oran) (Sin nombre) B33.4
  - Hantaan (Korean hemorrhagic fever) A98.5
  - human immunodeficiency (HIV) B20
  - Kunjin A83.4
  - nonarthropod-borne NOS B34.9
  - Powassan A84.8
  - Rocio (encephalitis) A83.6
  - Sin nombre (Hantavirus) (cardio)-pulmonary syndrome) B33.4
  - Tahyna B33.8
  - vesicular stomatitis A93.8
- vitreous H43.9
  - specified NEC H43.89
- vocal cord J38.3
- Volkmann's, acquired T79.6 ☑
- von Eulenburg's (congenital paramyotonia) G71.19
- von Gierke's (glycogenosis I) E74.01
- von Graefe's — *see* Strabismus, paralytic, ophthalmoplegia, progressive
- von Willebrand (-Jürgens) (angiohemophilia) D68.0
- Vrolik's (osteogenesis imperfecta) Q78.0
- vulva (noninflammatory) N90.9
  - inflammatory NEC N76.89
  - specified NEC N90.89
- Wallgren's (obstruction of splenic vein with collateral circulation) I87.8
- Wassilieff's (leptospiral jaundice) A27.0
- wasting NEC R64
  - due to malnutrition E41
- Waterhouse-Friderichsen A39.1
- Wegner's (syphilitic osteochondritis) A50.02
- Weil's (leptospiral jaundice of lung) A27.0
- Weir Mitchell's (erythromelalgia) I73.81
- Werdnig-Hoffmann G12.0
- Wermer's E31.21
- Werner-His (trench fever) A79.0
- Werner-Schultz (neutropenic splenomegaly) D73.81
- Wernicke-Posadas B38.9
- whipworm B79
- white blood cells D72.9
  - specified NEC D72.89
- white matter R90.82
- white-spot, meaning lichen sclerosus et atrophicus L90.0
  - penis N48.0
  - vulva N90.4
- Wilkie's K55.1
- Wilkinson-Sneddon (subcorneal pustular dermatosis) L13.1
- Willis' — *see* Diabetes
- Wilson's (hepatolenticular degeneration) E83.01
- woolsorter's A22.1
- yaba monkey tumor B08.72
- yaba pox (virus) B08.72
- Zika virus A92.5
- zoonotic, bacterial A28.9
  - specified type NEC A28.8

Disfigurement (due to scar) L90.5
Disgerminoma — *see* Dysgerminoma
DISH (diffuse idiopathic skeletal hyperostosis) — *see* Hyperostosis, ankylosing
Disinsertion, retina — *see* Detachment, retina
Dislocatable hip, congenital Q65.6

Dislocation (articular)
- with fracture — *see* Fracture
- acromioclavicular (joint) S43.10- ☑
  - with displacement
    - 100%-200% S43.12- ☑
    - more than 200% S43.13- ☑
  - inferior S43.14- ☑
  - posterior S43.15- ☑
- ankle S93.0- ☑
- astragalus — *see* Dislocation, ankle
- atlantoaxial S13.121 ☑
- atlantooccipital S13.111 ☑
- atloidooccipital S13.111 ☑
- breast bone S23.29 ☑
- capsule, joint — *code by* site under Dislocation
- carpal (bone) — *see* Dislocation, wrist
- carpometacarpal (joint) NEC S63.05- ☑
  - thumb S63.04- ☑
- cartilage (joint) — *code by* site under Dislocation
- cervical spine (vertebra) — *see* Dislocation, vertebra, cervical
- chronic — *see* Dislocation, recurrent
- clavicle — *see* Dislocation, acromioclavicular joint
- coccyx S33.2 ☑
- congenital NEC Q68.8
- coracoid — *see* Dislocation, shoulder
- costal cartilage S23.29 ☑
- costochondral S23.29 ☑
- cricoarytenoid articulation S13.29 ☑
- cricothyroid articulation S13.29 ☑
- dorsal vertebra — *see* Dislocation, vertebra, thoracic
- ear ossicle — *see* Discontinuity, ossicles, ear
- elbow S53.10- ☑
  - congenital Q68.8
  - pathological — *see* Dislocation, pathological NEC, elbow
  - radial head alone — *see* Dislocation, radial head
  - recurrent — *see* Dislocation, recurrent, elbow
  - traumatic S53.10- ☑
    - anterior S53.11- ☑
    - lateral S53.14- ☑
    - medial S53.13- ☑
    - posterior S53.12- ☑
    - specified type NEC S53.19- ☑
- eye, nontraumatic — *see* Luxation, globe
- eyeball, nontraumatic — *see* Luxation, globe
- femur
  - distal end — *see* Dislocation, knee
  - proximal end — *see* Dislocation, hip
- fibula
  - distal end — *see* Dislocation, ankle
  - proximal end — *see* Dislocation, knee
- finger S63.25- ☑
  - index S63.25- ☑
  - Interphalangeal S63.27- ☑
    - distal S63.29- ☑
      - index S63.29- ☑
      - little S63.29- ☑
      - middle S63.29- ☑
      - ring S63.29- ☑
    - index S63.27- ☑
    - little S63.27- ☑
    - middle S63.27- ☑
    - proximal S63.28- ☑
      - index S63.28- ☑
      - little S63.28- ☑
      - middle S63.28- ☑
      - ring S63.28- ☑
  - little S63.25- ☑
  - metacarpophalangeal S63.26- ☑
    - index S63.26- ☑
    - little S63.26- ☑
    - middle S63.26- ☑
    - ring S63.26- ☑
  - middle S63.25- ☑
  - recurrent — *see* Dislocation, recurrent, finger
  - ring S63.25- ☑
  - thumb — *see* Dislocation, thumb
- foot S93.30- ☑
  - recurrent — *see* Dislocation, recurrent, foot
  - specified site NEC S93.33- ☑
  - tarsal joint S93.31- ☑
  - tarsometatarsal joint S93.32- ☑
  - toe — *see* Dislocation, toe
- fracture — *see* Fracture

▽ **Subterms under main terms may continue to next column or page**   ☑ **Additional Character Required — Refer to the Tabular List for Character Selection**   **107**

Disease, diseased — Dislocation

Dislocation — *continued*
- glenohumeral (joint) — *see* Dislocation, shoulder
- glenoid — *see* Dislocation, shoulder
- habitual — *see* Dislocation, recurrent
- hip S73.00- ☑
  - anterior S73.03- ☑
    - obturator S73.02- ☑
  - central S73.04- ☑
  - congenital (total) Q65.2
    - bilateral Q65.1
    - partial Q65.5
      - bilateral Q65.4
      - unilateral Q65.3- ☑
    - unilateral Q65.0- ☑
  - developmental M24.85- ☑
  - pathological — *see* Dislocation, pathological NEC, hip
  - posterior S73.01- ☑
  - recurrent — *see* Dislocation, recurrent, hip
- humerus, proximal end — *see* Dislocation, shoulder
- incomplete — *see* Subluxation, by site
- incus — *see* Discontinuity, ossicles, ear
- infracoracoid — *see* Dislocation, shoulder
- innominate (pubic junction) (sacral junction) S33.39 ☑
  - acetabulum — *see* Dislocation, hip
- interphalangeal (joint(s))
  - finger S63.279 ☑
    - distal S63.29- ☑
      - index S63.29- ☑
      - little S63.29- ☑
      - middle S63.29- ☑
      - ring S63.29- ☑
    - index S63.27- ☑
    - little S63.27- ☑
    - middle S63.27- ☑
    - proximal S63.28- ☑
      - index S63.28- ☑
      - little S63.28- ☑
      - middle S63.28- ☑
      - ring S63.28- ☑
    - ring S63.27- ☑
  - foot or toe — *see* Dislocation, toe
  - thumb S63.12- ☑
    - distal joint S63.14- ☑
    - proximal joint S63.13- ☑
- jaw (cartilage) (meniscus) S03.0- ☑
- joint prosthesis — *see* Complications, joint prosthesis, mechanical, displacement, by site
- knee S83.106 ☑
  - cap — *see* Dislocation, patella
  - congenital Q68.2
  - old M23.8X- ☑
  - patella — *see* Dislocation, patella
  - pathological — *see* Dislocation, pathological NEC, knee
  - proximal tibia
    - anteriorly S83.11- ☑
    - laterally S83.14- ☑
    - medially S83.13- ☑
    - posteriorly S83.12- ☑
  - recurrent (*see also* Derangement, knee, specified NEC)
  - specified type NEC S83.19- ☑
- lacrimal gland H04.16- ☑
- lens (complete) H27.10
  - anterior H27.12- ☑
  - congenital Q12.1
  - ocular implant — *see* Complications, intraocular lens
  - partial H27.11- ☑
  - posterior H27.13- ☑
  - traumatic S05.8X- ☑
- ligament — *code by* site under Dislocation
- lumbar (vertebra) — *see* Dislocation, vertebra, lumbar
- lumbosacral (vertebra) (*see also* Dislocation, vertebra, lumbar)
  - congenital Q76.49
- mandible S03.0- ☑
- meniscus (knee) — *see* Tear, meniscus
  - other sites - code by site under Dislocation
- metacarpal (bone)
  - distal end — *see* Dislocation, finger
  - proximal end S63.06- ☑
- metacarpophalangeal (joint)
  - finger S63.26- ☑
    - index S63.26- ☑

Dislocation — *continued*
- metacarpophalangeal — *continued*
  - finger — *continued*
    - little S63.26- ☑
    - middle S63.26- ☑
    - ring S63.26- ☑
    - thumb S63.11- ☑
- metatarsal (bone) — *see* Dislocation, foot
- metatarsophalangeal (joint(s)) — *see* Dislocation, toe
- midcarpal (joint) S63.03- ☑
- midtarsal (joint) — *see* Dislocation, foot
- neck S13.20 ☑
  - specified site NEC S13.29 ☑
  - vertebra — *see* Dislocation, vertebra, cervical
- nose (septal cartilage) S03.1 ☑
- occipitoatloid S13.111 ☑
- old — *see* Derangement, joint, specified type NEC
- ossicles, ear — *see* Discontinuity, ossicles, ear
- partial — *see* Subluxation, by site
- patella S83.006 ☑
  - congenital Q74.1
  - lateral S83.01- ☑
  - recurrent (nontraumatic) M22.0- ☑
    - incomplete M22.1- ☑
  - specified type NEC S83.09- ☑
- pathological NEC M24.30
  - ankle M24.37- ☑
  - elbow M24.32- ☑
  - foot joint M24.37- ☑
  - hand joint M24.34- ☑
  - hip M24.35- ☑
  - knee M24.36- ☑
  - lumbosacral joint — *see* subcategory M53.2
  - pelvic region — *see* Dislocation, pathological, hip
  - sacroiliac — *see* subcategory M53.2
  - shoulder M24.31- ☑
  - wrist M24.33- ☑
- pelvis NEC S33.30 ☑
  - specified NEC S33.39 ☑
- phalanx
  - finger or hand — *see* Dislocation, finger
  - foot or toe — *see* Dislocation, toe
- prosthesis, internal — *see* Complications, prosthetic device, by site, mechanical
- radial head S53.006 ☑
  - anterior S53.01- ☑
  - posterior S53.02- ☑
  - specified type NEC S53.09- ☑
- radiocarpal (joint) S63.02- ☑
- radiohumeral (joint) — *see* Dislocation, radial head
- radioulnar (joint)
  - distal S63.01- ☑
  - proximal — *see* Dislocation, elbow
- radius
  - distal end — *see* Dislocation, wrist
  - proximal end — *see* Dislocation, radial head
- recurrent M24.40
  - ankle M24.47- ☑
  - elbow M24.42- ☑
  - finger M24.44- ☑
  - foot joint M24.47- ☑
  - hand joint M24.44- ☑
  - hip M24.45- ☑
  - knee M24.46- ☑
    - patella — *see* Dislocation, patella, recurrent
  - patella — *see* Dislocation, patella, recurrent
  - sacroiliac — *see* subcategory M53.2
  - shoulder M24.41- ☑
  - toe M24.47- ☑
  - vertebra (*see also* subcategory) M43.5 ☑
    - atlantoaxial M43.4
      - with myelopathy M43.3
  - wrist M24.43- ☑
- rib (cartilage) S23.29 ☑
- sacrococcygeal S33.2 ☑
- sacroiliac (joint) (ligament) S33.2 ☑
  - congenital Q74.2
  - recurrent — *see* subcategory M53.2
- sacrum S33.2 ☑
- scaphoid (bone) (hand) (wrist) — *see* Dislocation, wrist
  - foot — *see* Dislocation, foot
- scapula — *see* Dislocation, shoulder, girdle, scapula
- semilunar cartilage, knee — *see* Tear, meniscus
- septal cartilage (nose) S03.1 ☑
- septum (nasal) (old) J34.2

Dislocation — *continued*
- sesamoid bone — *code by* site under Dislocation
- shoulder (blade) (ligament) (joint) (traumatic) S43.006 ☑
  - acromioclavicular — *see* Dislocation, acromioclavicular
  - chronic — *see* Dislocation, recurrent, shoulder
  - congenital Q68.8
  - girdle S43.30- ☑
    - scapula S43.31- ☑
    - specified site NEC S43.39- ☑
  - humerus S43.00- ☑
    - anterior S43.01- ☑
    - inferior S43.03- ☑
    - posterior S43.02- ☑
  - pathological — *see* Dislocation, pathological NEC, shoulder
  - recurrent — *see* Dislocation, recurrent, shoulder
  - specified type NEC S43.08- ☑
- spine
  - cervical — *see* Dislocation, vertebra, cervical
  - congenital Q76.49
  - due to birth trauma P11.5
  - lumbar — *see* Dislocation, vertebra, lumbar
  - thoracic — *see* Dislocation, vertebra, thoracic
- spontaneous — *see* Dislocation, pathological
- sternoclavicular (joint) S43.206 ☑
  - anterior S43.21- ☑
  - posterior S43.22- ☑
- sternum S23.29 ☑
- subglenoid — *see* Dislocation, shoulder
- symphysis pubis S33.4 ☑
- talus — *see* Dislocation, ankle
- tarsal (bone(s)) (joint(s)) — *see* Dislocation, foot
- tarsometatarsal (joint(s)) — *see* Dislocation, foot
- temporomandibular (joint) S03.0- ☑
- thigh, proximal end — *see* Dislocation, hip
- thorax S23.20 ☑
  - specified site NEC S23.29 ☑
  - vertebra — *see* Dislocation, vertebra
- thumb S63.10- ☑
  - interphalangeal joint — *see* Dislocation, interphalangeal (joint), thumb
  - metacarpophalangeal joint — *see* Dislocation, metacarpophalangeal (joint), thumb
- thyroid cartilage S13.29 ☑
- tibia
  - distal end — *see* Dislocation, ankle
  - proximal end — *see* Dislocation, knee
- tibiofibular (joint)
  - distal — *see* Dislocation, ankle
  - superior — *see* Dislocation, knee
- toe(s) S93.106 ☑
  - great S93.10- ☑
    - interphalangeal joint S93.11- ☑
    - metatarsophalangeal joint S93.12- ☑
  - interphalangeal joint S93.119 ☑
  - lesser S93.106 ☑
    - interphalangeal joint S93.11- ☑
    - metatarsophalangeal joint S93.12- ☑
  - metatarsophalangeal joint S93.12- ☑
- tooth S03.2 ☑
- trachea S23.29 ☑
- ulna
  - distal end S63.07- ☑
  - proximal end — *see* Dislocation, elbow
- ulnohumeral (joint) — *see* Dislocation, elbow
- vertebra (articular process) (body) (traumatic)
  - cervical S13.101 ☑
    - atlantoaxial joint S13.121 ☑
    - atlantooccipital joint S13.111 ☑
    - atloidooccipital joint S13.111 ☑
    - joint between
      - C0 and C1 S13.111 ☑
      - C1 and C2 S13.121 ☑
      - C2 and C3 S13.131 ☑
      - C3 and C4 S13.141 ☑
      - C4 and C5 S13.151 ☑
      - C5 and C6 S13.161 ☑
      - C6 and C7 S13.171 ☑
      - C7 and T1 S13.181 ☑
    - occipitoatloid joint S13.111 ☑
    - congenital Q76.49
  - lumbar S33.101 ☑
    - joint between
      - L1 and L2 S33.111 ☑

Dislocation — *continued*
  vertebra — *continued*
    lumbar — *continued*
      joint between — *continued*
        L2 and L3 S33.121 ☑
        L3 and L4 S33.131 ☑
        L4 and L5 S33.141 ☑
      nontraumatic — *see* Displacement, intervertebral disc
      partial — *see* Subluxation, by site
      recurrent NEC — *see* subcategory M43.5 ☑
    thoracic S23.101 ☑
      joint between
        T1 and T2 S23.111 ☑
        T2 and T3 S23.121 ☑
        T3 and T4 S23.123 ☑
        T4 and T5 S23.131 ☑
        T5 and T6 S23.133 ☑
        T6 and T7 S23.141 ☑
        T7 and T8 S23.143 ☑
        T8 and T9 S23.151 ☑
        T9 and T10 S23.153 ☑
        T10 and T11 S23.161 ☑
        T11 and T12 S23.163 ☑
        T12 and L1 S23.171 ☑
  wrist (carpal bone) S63.006 ☑
    carpometacarpal joint — *see* Dislocation, carpometacarpal (joint)
    distal radioulnar joint — *see* Dislocation, radioulnar (joint), distal
    metacarpal bone, proximal — *see* Dislocation, metacarpal (bone), proximal end
    midcarpal — *see* Dislocation, midcarpal (joint)
    radiocarpal joint — *see* Dislocation, radiocarpal (joint)
    recurrent — *see* Dislocation, recurrent, wrist
    specified site NEC S63.09- ☑
    ulna — *see* Dislocation, ulna, distal end
  xiphoid cartilage S23.29 ☑
Disorder (of) (*see also* Disease)
  acantholytic L11.9
    specified NEC L11.8
  acute
    psychotic — *see* Psychosis, acute
    stress F43.0
  adjustment (grief) F43.20
    with
      anxiety F43.22
        with depressed mood F43.23
      conduct disturbance F43.24
        with emotional disturbance F43.25
      depressed mood F43.21
        with anxiety F43.23
      other specified symptom F43.29
  adrenal (capsule) (gland) (medullary) E27.9
    specified NEC E27.8
  adrenogenital E25.9
    drug-induced E25.8
    iatrogenic E25.8
    idiopathic E25.8
  adult personality (and behavior) F69
    specified NEC F68.8
  affective (mood) — *see* Disorder, mood
  aggressive, unsocialized F91.1
  alcohol use
    mild F10.10
      with
        alcohol intoxication F10.129
          delirium F10.121
        alcohol-induced
          anxiety disorder F10.180
          bipolar and related disorder F10.14
          depressive disorder F10.14
          psychotic disorder F10.159
          sexual dysfunction F10.181
          sleep disorder F10.182
      in remission (early) (sustained) F10.11
    moderate or severe F10.20
      with
        alcohol intoxication F10.229
          delirium F10.221
        alcohol-induced
          anxiety disorder F10.280
          bipolar and related disorder F10.24
          depressive disorder F10.24
          major neurocognitive disorder, amnestic-confabulatory type F10.26

Disorder — *continued*
  alcohol use — *continued*
    moderate or severe — *continued*
      with — *continued*
        alcohol-induced — *continued*
          major neurocognitive disorder, non-amnestic-confabulatory type F10.27
          mild neurocognitive disorder F10.288
          psychotic disorder F10.259
          sexual dysfunction F10.281
          sleep disorder F10.282
      in remission (early) (sustained) F10.21
  alcohol-related F10.99
    with
      amnestic disorder, persisting F10.96
      anxiety disorder F10.980
      dementia, persisting F10.97
      intoxication F10.929
        with delirium F10.921
        uncomplicated F10.920
      mood disorder F10.94
      other specified F10.988
      psychotic disorder F10.959
        with
          delusions F10.950
          hallucinations F10.951
      sexual dysfunction F10.981
      sleep disorder F10.982
  allergic — *see* Allergy
  alveolar NEC J84.09
  amino-acid
    cystathioninuria E72.19
    cystinosis E72.04
    cystinuria E72.01
    glycinuria E72.09
    homocystinuria E72.11
    metabolism — *see* Disturbance, metabolism, amino-acid
    specified NEC E72.8
    neonatal, transitory P74.8
    renal transport NEC E72.09
    transport NEC E72.09
  amnesic, amnestic
    alcohol-induced F10.96
      with dependence F10.26
    due to (secondary to) general medical condition F04
    psychoactive NEC-induced F19.96
      with
        abuse F19.16
        dependence F19.26
    sedative, hypnotic or anxiolytic-induced F13.96
      with dependence F13.26
  amphetamine (or other stimulant) use
    mild
      with
        amphetamine, cocaine, or other stimulant intoxication
          with perceptual disturbances F15.122
          without perceptual disturbances F15.129
        amphetamine (or other stimulant) -induced
          anxiety disorder F15.180
          bipolar and related disorder F15.14
          depressive disorder F15.14
          obsessive-compulsive and related disorder F15.188
          psychotic disorder F15.159
          sexual dysfunction F15.181
        intoxication delirium F15.121
    moderate or severe
      with
        amphetamine, cocaine, or other stimulant intoxication
          with perceptual disturbances F15.222
          without perceptual disturbances F15.229
        amphetamine (or other stimulant) -induced
          anxiety disorder F15.280
          bipolar and related disorder F15.24
          depressive disorder F15.24
          obsessive-compulsive and related disorder F15.288
          psychotic disorder F15.259
          sexual dysfunction F15.281
        intoxication delirium F15.221
  amphetamine-type substance use
    mild F15.10
      in remission (early) (sustained) F15.11
    moderate F15.20

Disorder — *continued*
  amphetamine-type substance use — *continued*
    moderate — *continued*
      in remission (early) (sustained) F15.21
    severe F15.20
      in remission (early) (sustained) F15.21
  anaerobic glycolysis with anemia D55.2
  anxiety F41.9
    due to (secondary to)
      alcohol F10.980
        in
          abuse F10.180
          dependence F10.280
      amphetamine F15.980
        in
          abuse F15.180
          dependence F15.280
      anxiolytic F13.980
        in
          abuse F13.180
          dependence F13.280
      caffeine F15.980
        in
          abuse F15.180
          dependence F15.280
      cannabis F12.980
        in
          abuse F12.180
          dependence F12.280
      cocaine F14.980
        in
          abuse F14.180
          dependence F14.180
      general medical condition F06.4
      hallucinogen F16.980
        in
          abuse F16.180
          dependence F16.280
      hypnotic F13.980
        in
          abuse F13.180
          dependence F13.280
      inhalant F18.980
        in
          abuse F18.180
          dependence F18.280
      phencyclidine F16.980
        in
          abuse F16.180
          dependence F16.280
      psychoactive substance NEC F19.980
        in
          abuse F19.180
          dependence F19.280
      sedative F13.980
        in
          abuse F13.180
          dependence F13.280
      volatile solvents F18.980
        in
          abuse F18.180
          dependence F18.280
    generalized F41.1
    illness F45.21
    mixed
      with depression (mild) F41.8
      specified NEC F41.3
    organic F06.4
    phobic F40.9
      of childhood F40.8
    specified NEC F41.8
  aortic valve — *see* Endocarditis, aortic
  aromatic amino-acid metabolism E70.9
    specified NEC E70.8
  arteriole NEC I77.89
  artery NEC I77.89
  articulation — *see* Disorder, joint
  attachment (childhood)
    disinhibited F94.2
    reactive F94.1
  attention-deficit hyperactivity (adolescent) (adult) (child) F90.9
    combined
      presentation F90.2
      type F90.2
    hyperactive
      impulsive presentation F90.1
      type F90.1

Disorder — *continued*
  attention-deficit hyperactivity — *continued*
    inattentive
      presentation F90.0
      type F90.0
    specified type NEC F90.8
  attention-deficit without hyperactivity (adolescent) (adult) (child) F98.8
  auditory processing (central) H93.25
  autism spectrum F84.0
  autistic F84.0
  autoimmune D89.89
  autonomic nervous system G90.9
    specified NEC G90.8
  avoidant
    child or adolescent F40.10
    restrictive food intake F50.82
  balance
    acid-base E87.8
      mixed E87.4
    electrolyte E87.8
    fluid NEC E87.8
  behavioral (disruptive) — *see* Disorder, conduct
  beta-amino-acid metabolism E72.8
  bile acid and cholesterol metabolism E78.70
    Barth syndrome E78.71
    other specified E78.79
    Smith-Lemli-Opitz syndrome E78.72
  bilirubin excretion E80.6
  binge eating F50.81
  binocular
    movement H51.9
      convergence
        excess H51.12
        insufficiency H51.11
      internuclear ophthalmoplegia — *see* Ophthalmoplegia, internuclear
      palsy of conjugate gaze H51.0
      specified type NEC H51.8
    vision NEC — *see* Disorder, vision, binocular
  bipolar (I) (type I) F31.9
    and related due to a known physiological condition
      with
        manic features F06.33
        manic- or hypomanic-like episodes F06.33
        mixed features F06.34
    current (or most recent) episode
      depressed F31.9
        with psychotic features F31.5
        without psychotic features F31.30
          mild F31.31
          moderate F31.32
          severe (without psychotic features) F31.4
            with psychotic features F31.5
      hypomanic F31.0
      manic F31.9
        with psychotic features F31.2
        without psychotic features F31.10
          mild F31.11
          moderate F31.12
          severe (without psychotic features) F31.13
            with psychotic features F31.2
      mixed F31.60
        mild F31.61
        moderate F31.62
        severe (without psychotic features) F31.63
          with psychotic features F31.64
      severe depression (without psychotic features) F31.4
        with psychotic features F31.5
    in remission (currently) F31.70
      in full remission
        most recent episode
          depressed F31.76
          hypomanic F31.72
          manic F31.74
          mixed F31.78
      in partial remission
        most recent episode
          depressed F31.75
          hypomanic F31.71
          manic F31.73
          mixed F31.77
    organic F06.30
    single manic episode F30.9
      mild F30.11
      moderate F30.12
      severe (without psychotic symptoms) F30.13

Disorder — *continued*
  bipolar — *continued*
    single manic episode — *continued*
      severe — *continued*
        with psychotic symptoms F30.2
      specified NEC F31.89
  bipolar II (type 2) F31.81
  bladder N32.9
    functional NEC N31.9
    in schistosomiasis B65.0 [N33]
    specified NEC N32.89
  bleeding D68.9
  blood D75.9
    in congenital early syphilis A50.09 [D77]
  body dysmorphic F45.22
  bone M89.9
    continuity M84.9
      specified type NEC M84.80
        ankle M84.87- ☑
        fibula M84.86- ☑
        foot M84.87- ☑
        hand M84.84- ☑
        humerus M84.82- ☑
        neck M84.88
        pelvis M84.859
        radius M84.83- ☑
        rib M84.88
        shoulder M84.81- ☑
        skull M84.88
        thigh M84.85- ☑
        tibia M84.86- ☑
        ulna M84.83- ☑
        vertebra M84.88
    density and structure M85.9
      cyst (*see also* Cyst, bone, specified type NEC)
        aneurysmal — *see* Cyst, bone, aneurysmal
        solitary — *see* Cyst, bone, solitary
      diffuse idiopathic skeletal hyperostosis — *see* Hyperostosis, ankylosing
      fibrous dysplasia (monostotic) — *see* Dysplasia, fibrous, bone
      fluorosis — *see* Fluorosis, skeletal
      hyperostosis of skull M85.2
      osteitis condensans — *see* Osteitis, condensans
      specified type NEC M85.8- ☑
        ankle M85.87- ☑
        foot M85.87- ☑
        forearm M85.83- ☑
        hand M85.84- ☑
        lower leg M85.86- ☑
        multiple sites M85.89
        neck M85.88
        rib M85.88
        shoulder M85.81- ☑
        skull M85.88
        thigh M85.85- ☑
        upper arm M85.82- ☑
        vertebra M85.88
    development and growth NEC M89.20
      carpus M89.24- ☑
      clavicle M89.21- ☑
      femur M89.25- ☑
      fibula M89.26- ☑
      finger M89.24- ☑
      humerus M89.22- ☑
      ilium M89.259
      ischium M89.259
      metacarpus M89.24- ☑
      metatarsus M89.27- ☑
      multiple sites M89.29
      neck M89.28
      radius M89.23- ☑
      rib M89.28
      scapula M89.21- ☑
      skull M89.28
      tarsus M89.27- ☑
      tibia M89.26- ☑
      toe M89.27- ☑
      ulna M89.23- ☑
      vertebra M89.28
    specified type NEC M89.8X- ☑
  brachial plexus G54.0
  branched-chain amino-acid metabolism E71.2
    specified NEC E71.19
  breast N64.9
    agalactia — *see* Agalactia

Disorder — *continued*
  breast — *continued*
    associated with
      lactation O92.70
        specified NEC O92.79
      pregnancy O92.20
        specified NEC O92.29
      puerperium O92.20
        specified NEC O92.29
    cracked nipple — *see* Cracked nipple
    galactorrhea — *see* Galactorrhea
    hypogalactia O92.4
    lactation disorder NEC O92.79
    mastitis — *see* Mastitis
    nipple infection — *see* Infection, nipple
    retracted nipple — *see* Retraction, nipple
    specified type NEC N64.89
  Briquet's F45.0
  bullous, in diseases classified elsewhere L14
  caffeine use
    mild
      with
        caffeine-induced
          anxiety disorder F15.180
          sleep disorder F15.182
    moderate or severe
      with
        caffeine-induced
          anxiety disorder F15.280
          sleep disorder F15.282
  cannabis use
    mild F12.10
      with
        cannabis intoxication delirium F12.121
          with perceptual disturbances F12.122
          without perceptual disturbances F12.129
        cannabis-induced
          anxiety disorder F12.180
          psychotic disorder F12.159
          sleep disorder F12.188
      in remission (early) (sustained) F12.11
    moderate or severe F12.20
      with
        cannabis Intoxication
          with perceptual disturbances F12.222
          without perceptual disturbances F12.229
        cannabis-induced
          anxiety disorder F12.280
          psychotic disorder F12.259
          sleep disorder F12.288
        delirium F12.221
      in remission (early) (sustained) F12.21
  carbohydrate
    absorption, intestinal NEC E74.39
    metabolism (congenital) E74.9
      specified NEC E74.8
  cardiac, functional I51.89
  carnitine metabolism E71.40
  cartilage M94.9
    articular NEC — *see* Derangement, joint, articular cartilage
    chondrocalcinosis — *see* Chondrocalcinosis
    specified type NEC M94.8X- ☑
      articular — *see* Derangement, joint, articular cartilage
      multiple sites M94.8X0
  catatonia (due to known physiological condition) (with another mental disorder) F06.1
  catatonic
    due to (secondary to) known physiological condition F06.1
    organic F06.1
  central auditory processing H93.25
  cervical
    region NEC M53.82
    root (nerve) NEC G54.2
  character NOS F60.9
  childhood disintegrative NEC F84.3
  cholesterol and bile acid metabolism E78.70
    Barth syndrome E78.71
    other specified E78.79
    Smith-Lemli-Opitz syndrome E78.72
  choroid H31.9
    atrophy — *see* Atrophy, choroid
    degeneration — *see* Degeneration, choroid
    detachment — *see* Detachment, choroid
    dystrophy — *see* Dystrophy, choroid
    hemorrhage — *see* Hemorrhage, choroid

☑ **Additional Character Required** — Refer to the Tabular List for Character Selection   ▽ **Subterms under main terms may continue to next column or page**

Disorder — *continued*
  choroid — *continued*
    rupture — *see* Rupture, choroid
    scar — *see* Scar, chorioretinal
    solar retinopathy — *see* Retinopathy, solar
    specified type NEC H31.8
  ciliary body — *see* Disorder, iris
    degeneration — *see* Degeneration, ciliary body
  coagulation (factor) (*see also* Defect, coagulation)
    D68.9
    newborn, transient P61.6
  cocaine use
    mild F14.10
      with
        amphetamine, cocaine, or other stimulant
          intoxication
          with perceptual disturbances F14.122
          without perceptual disturbances F14.129
        cocaine intoxication delirium F14.121
        cocaine-induced
          anxiety disorder F14.180
          bipolar and related disorder F14.14
          depressive disorder F14.14
          obsessive-compulsive and related disor-
            der F14.188
          psychotic disorder F14.159
          sexual dysfunction F14.181
          sleep disorder F14.182
      in remission (early) (sustained) F14.11
    moderate or severe F14.20
      with
        amphetamine, cocaine, or other stimulant
          intoxication
          with perceptual disturbances F14.222
          without perceptual disturbances F14.229
        cocaine intoxication delirium F14.221
        cocaine-induced
          anxiety disorder F14.280
          bipolar and related disorder F14.24
          depressive disorder F14.24
          obsessive-compulsive and related disor-
            der F14.288
          psychotic disorder F14.259
          sexual dysfunction F14.281
          sleep disorder F14.282
      in remission (early) (sustained) F14.21
  coccyx NEC M53.3
  cognitive F09
    due to (secondary to) general medical condition
      F09
    persisting R41.89
      due to
        alcohol F10.97
          with dependence F10.27
        anxiolytics F13.97
          with dependence F13.27
        hypnotics F13.97
          with dependence F13.27
        sedatives F13.97
          with dependence F13.27
        specified substance NEC F19.97
          with
            abuse F19.17
            dependence F19.27
  communication F80.9
    social pragmatic F80.82
  conduct (childhood) F91.9
    adjustment reaction — *see* Disorder, adjustment
    adolescent onset type F91.2
    childhood onset type F91.1
    compulsive F63.9
    confined to family context F91.0
    depressive F91.8
    group type F91.2
    hyperkinetic — *see* Disorder, attention-deficit hy-
      peractivity
    oppositional defiance F91.3
    socialized F91.2
    solitary aggressive type F91.1
    specified NEC F91.8
    unsocialized (aggressive) F91.1
  conduction, heart I45.9
  congenital glycosylation (CDG) E74.8
  conjunctiva H11.9
    infection — *see* Conjunctivitis
  connective tissue, localized L94.9
    specified NEC L94.8

Disorder — *continued*
  conversion (functional neurological symptom disorder)
    with
      abnormal movement F44.4
      anesthesia or sensory loss F44.6
      attacks or seizures F44.5
      mixed symptoms F44.7
      special sensory symptoms F44.6
      speech symptoms F44.4
      swallowing symptoms F44.4
      weakness or paralysis F44.4
  convulsive (secondary) — *see* Convulsions
  cornea H18.9
    deformity — *see* Deformity, cornea
    degeneration — *see* Degeneration, cornea
    deposits — *see* Deposit, cornea
    due to contact lens H18.82- ☑
      specified as edema — *see* Edema, cornea
    edema — *see* Edema, cornea
    keratitis — *see* Keratitis
    keratoconjunctivitis — *see* Keratoconjunctivitis
    membrane change — *see* Change, corneal mem-
      brane
    neovascularization — *see* Neovascularization,
      cornea
    scar — *see* Opacity, cornea
    specified type NEC H18.89- ☑
    ulcer — *see* Ulcer, cornea
  corpus cavernosum N48.9
  cranial nerve — *see* Disorder, nerve, cranial
  cyclothymic F34.0
  defiant oppositional F91.3
  delusional (persistent) (systematized) F22
    induced F24
  depersonalization F48.1
  depressive F32.9
    due to known physiological condition
      with
        depressive features F06.31
        major depressive-like episode F06.32
        mixed features F06.34
    major F32.9
      with psychotic symptoms F32.3
      in remission (full) F32.5
        partial F32.4
      recurrent F33.9
        with psychotic features F33.3
      single episode F32.9
        mild F32.0
        moderate F32.1
        severe (without psychotic symptoms) F32.2
          with psychotic symptoms F32.3
    organic F06.31
    persistent F34.1
    recurrent F33.9
      current episode
        mild F33.0
        moderate F33.1
        severe (without psychotic symptoms) F33.2
          with psychotic symptoms F33.3
      in remission F33.40
        full F33.42
        partial F33.41
      specified NEC F33.8
    single episode — *see* Episode, depressive
    specified NEC F32.89
  developmental F89
    arithmetical skills F81.2
    coordination (motor) F82
    expressive writing F81.81
    language F80.9
      expressive F80.1
      mixed receptive and expressive F80.2
      receptive type F80.2
      specified NEC F80.89
    learning F81.9
      arithmetical F81.2
      reading F81.0
    mixed F88
    motor coordination or function F82
    pervasive F84.9
      specified NEC F84.8
    phonological F80.0
    reading F81.0
    scholastic skills (*see also* Disorder, learning)
      mixed F81.89
    specified NEC F88
    speech F80.9

Disorder — *continued*
  developmental — *continued*
    speech — *continued*
      articulation F80.0
      specified NEC F80.89
      written expression F81.81
  diaphragm J98.6
  digestive (system) K92.9
    newborn P78.9
      specified NEC P78.89
    postprocedural — *see* Complication, gastrointesti-
      nal
    psychogenic F45.8
  disc (intervertebral) M51.9
    with
      myelopathy
        cervical region M50.00
        cervicothoracic region M50.03
        high cervical region M50.01
        lumbar region M51.06
        mid-cervical region M50.020
        sacrococcygeal region M53.3
        thoracic region M51.04
        thoracolumbar region M51.05
      radiculopathy
        cervical region M50.10
        cervicothoracic region M50.13
        high cervical region M50.11
        lumbar region M51.16
        lumbosacral region M51.17
        mid-cervical region M50.120
        sacrococcygeal region M53.3
        thoracic region M51.14
        thoracolumbar region M51.15
    cervical M50.90
      with
        myelopathy M50.00
          C2-C3 M50.01
          C3-C4 M50.01
          C4-C5 M50.021
          C5-C6 M50.022
          C6-C7 M50.023
          C7-T1 M50.03
          cervicothoracic region M50.03
          high cervical region M50.01
          mid-cervical region M50.020
        neuritis, radiculitis or radiculopathy M50.10
          C2-C3 M50.11
          C3-C4 M50.11
          C4-C5 M50.121
          C5-C6 M50.122
          C6-C7 M50.123
          C7-T1 M50.13
          cervicothoracic region M50.13
          high cervical region M50.11
          mid-cervical region M50.120
      C2-C3 M50.91
      C3-C4 M50.91
      C4-C5 M50.921
      C5-C6 M50.922
      C6-C7 M50.923
      C7-T1 M50.93
      cervicothoracic region M50.93
      degeneration M50.30
        C2-C3 M50.31
        C3-C4 M50.31
        C4-C5 M50.321
        C5-C6 M50.322
        C6-C7 M50.323
        C7-T1 M50.33
        cervicothoracic region M50.33
        high cervical region M50.31
        mid-cervical region M50.320
      displacement M50.20
        C2-C3 M50.21
        C3-C4 M50.21
        C4-C5 M50.221
        C5-C6 M50.222
        C6-C7 M50.223
        C7-T1 M50.23
        cervicothoracic region M50.23
        high cervical region M50.21
        mid-cervical region M50.220
      high cervical region M50.91
      mid-cervical region M50.920
      specified type NEC M50.80
        C2-C3 M50.81
        C3-C4 M50.81
        C4-C5 M50.821

⛉ **Subterms under main terms may continue to next column or page**   ☑ **Additional Character Required — Refer to the Tabular List for Character Selection**   **111**

Disorder — Disorder

Disorder — *continued*
  disc — *continued*
    cervical — *continued*
      specified type — *continued*
        C5-C6 M50.822
        C6-C7 M50.823
        C7-T1 M50.83
        cervicothoracic region M50.83
        high cervical region M50.81
        mid-cervical region M50.820
    specified NEC
      lumbar region M51.86
      lumbosacral region M51.87
      sacrococcygeal region M53.3
      thoracic region M51.84
      thoracolumbar region M51.85
  disinhibited attachment (childhood) F94.2
  disintegrative, childhood NEC F84.3
  disruptive F91.9
    mood dysregulation F34.81
    specified NEC F91.8
  disruptive behavior — *see* Disorder, conduct
  dissocial personality F60.2
  dissociative F44.9
    affecting
      motor function F44.4
        and sensation F44.7
      sensation F44.6
        and motor function F44.7
    brief reactive F43.0
    due to (secondary to) general medical condition
        F06.8
    mixed F44.7
    organic F06.8
    other specified NEC F44.89
  double heterozygous sickling — *see* Disease, sickle-cell
  dream anxiety F51.5
  drug induced hemorrhagic D68.32
  drug related F19.99
    abuse — *see* Abuse, drug
    dependence — *see* Dependence, drug
  dysmorphic body F45.22
  dysthymic F34.1
  ear H93.9- ☑
    bleeding — *see* Otorrhagia
    deafness — *see* Deafness
    degenerative H93.09- ☑
    discharge — *see* Otorrhea
    external H61.9- ☑
      auditory canal stenosis — *see* Stenosis, external ear canal
      exostosis — *see* Exostosis, external ear canal
      impacted cerumen — *see* Impaction, cerumen
      otitis — *see* Otitis, externa
      perichondritis — *see* Perichondritis, ear
      pinna — *see* Disorder, pinna
      specified type NEC H61.89- ☑
    inner H83.9- ☑
      vestibular dysfunction — *see* Disorder, vestibular function
    middle H74.9- ☑
      adhesive H74.1- ☑
      ossicle — *see* Abnormal, ear ossicles
      polyp — *see* Polyp, ear (middle)
      specified NEC, in diseases classified elsewhere H75.8- ☑
    postprocedural — *see* Complications, ear, procedure
    specified NEC, in diseases classified elsewhere H94.8- ☑
  eating (adult) (psychogenic) F50.9
    anorexia — *see* Anorexia
    binge F50.81
    bulimia F50.2
    child F98.29
      pica F98.3
      rumination disorder F98.21
    pica F50.89
      childhood F98.3
  electrolyte (balance) NEC E87.8
    with
      abortion — *see* Abortion by type complicated by specified condition NEC
      ectopic pregnancy O08.5
      molar pregnancy O08.5
    acidosis (metabolic) (respiratory) E87.2
    alkalosis (metabolic) (respiratory) E87.3

Disorder — *continued*
  elimination, transepidermal L87.9
    specified NEC L87.8
  emotional (persistent) F34.9
    of childhood F93.9
      specified NEC F93.8
  endocrine E34.9
    postprocedural E89.89
    specified NEC E89.89
  erectile (male) (organic) (*see also* Dysfunction, sexual, male, erectile) N52.9
    nonorganic F52.21
  erythematous — *see* Erythema
  esophagus K22.9
    functional K22.4
    psychogenic F45.8
  eustachian tube H69.9- ☑
    infection — *see* Salpingitis, eustachian
    obstruction — *see* Obstruction, eustachian tube
    patulous — *see* Patulous, eustachian tube
    specified NEC H69.8- ☑
  exhibitionistic F65.2
  extrapyramidal G25.9
    in deseases classified elsewhere — *see* category G26
    specified type NEC G25.89
  eye H57.9
    postprocedural — *see* Complication, postprocedural, eye
  eyelid H02.9
    cyst — *see* Cyst, eyelid
    degenerative H02.70
      chloasma — *see* Chloasma, eyelid
      madarosis — *see* Madarosis
      specified type NEC H02.79
      vitiligo — *see* Vitiligo, eyelid
      xanthelasma — *see* Xanthelasma
    dermatochalasis — *see* Dermatochalasis
    edema — *see* Edema, eyelid
    elephantiasis — *see* Elephantiasis, eyelid
    foreign body, retained — *see* Foreign body, retained, eyelid
    function H02.59
      abnormal innervation syndrome — *see* Syndrome, abnormal innervation
      blepharochalasis — *see* Blepharochalasis
      blepharoclonus — *see* Blepharoclonus
      blepharophimosis — *see* Blepharophimosis
      blepharoptosis — *see* Blepharoptosis
      lagophthalmos — *see* Lagophthalmos
      lid retraction — *see* Retraction, lid
    hypertrichosis — *see* Hypertrichosis, eyelid
    specified type NEC H02.89
    vascular H02.879
      left H02.876
        lower H02.875
        upper H02.874
      right H02.873
        lower H02.872
        upper H02.871
  factitious F68.10
    with predominantly
      physical symptoms F68.12
        with psychological symptoms F68.13
      psychological symptoms F68.11
        with physical symptoms F68.13
  factor, coagulation — *see* Defect, coagulation
  fatty acid
    metabolism E71.30
      specified NEC E71.39
    oxidation
      LCAD E71.310
      MCAD E71.311
      SCAD E71.312
      specified deficiency NEC E71.318
  feeding (infant or child) (*see also* Disorder, eating) R63.3
    or eating disorder F50.9
    specified NEC F50.9
  feigned (with obvious motivation) Z76.5
    without obvious motivation — *see* Disorder, factitious
  female
    hypoactive sexual desire F52.0
    orgasmic F52.31
    sexual interest/arousal F52.22
  fetishistic F65.0
  fibroblastic M72.9

Disorder — *continued*
  fibroblastic — *continued*
    specified NEC M72.8
  fluency
    adult onset F98.5
    childhood onset F80.81
    following
      cerebral infarction I69.323
      cerebrovascular disease I69.923
        specified disease NEC I69.823
      intracerebral hemorrhage I69.123
      nontraumatic intracranial hemorrhage NEC I69.223
      subarachnoid hemorrhage I69.023
    in conditions classified elsewhere R47.82
  fluid balance E87.8
  follicular (skin) L73.9
    specified NEC L73.8
  frotteuristic F65.81
  fructose metabolism E74.10
    essential fructosuria E74.11
    fructokinase deficiency E74.11
    fructose-1, 6-diphosphatase deficiency E74.19
    hereditary fructose intolerance E74.12
    other specified E74.19
  functional polymorphonuclear neutrophils D71
  gallbladder, biliary tract and pancreas in diseases classified elsewhere K87
  gambling F63.0
  gamma-glutamyl cycle E72.8
  gastric (functional) K31.9
    motility K30
    psychogenic F45.8
    secretion K30
  gastrointestinal (functional) NOS K92.9
    newborn P78.9
    psychogenic F45.8
  gender-identity or -role F64.9
    childhood F64.2
    effect on relationship F66
    of adolescence or adulthood F64.0
      nontranssexual F64.8
    specified NEC F64.8
    uncertainty F66
  genito-pelvic pain penetration F52.6
  genitourinary system
    female N94.9
    male N50.9
    psychogenic F45.8
  globe H44.9
    degenerated condition H44.50
      absolute glaucoma H44.51- ☑
      atrophy H44.52- ☑
      leucocoria H44.53- ☑
    degenerative H44.30
      chalcosis H44.31- ☑
      myopia (*see also* Myopia, degenerative) H44.2- ☑
      siderosis H44.32- ☑
      specified type NEC H44.39- ☑
    endophthalmitis — *see* Endophthalmitis
    foreign body, retained — *see* Foreign body, intraocular, old, retained
    hemophthalmos — *see* Hemophthalmos
    hypotony H44.40
      due to
        ocular fistula H44.42- ☑
        specified disorder NEC H44.43- ☑
      flat anterior chamber H44.41- ☑
      primary H44.44- ☑
    luxation — *see* Luxation, globe
    specified type NEC H44.89
  glomerular (in) N05.9
    amyloidosis E85.4 [N08]
    cryoglobulinemia D89.1 [N08]
    disseminated intravascular coagulation D65 [N08]
    Fabry's disease E75.21 [N08]
    familial lecithin cholesterol acyltransferase deficiency E78.6 [N08]
    Goodpasture's syndrome M31.0
    hemolytic-uremic syndrome D59.3
    Henoch (-Schönlein) purpura D69.0 [N08]
    malariae malaria B52.0
    microscopic polyangiitis M31.7 [N08]
    multiple myeloma C90.0- ☑ [N08]
    mumps B26.83
    schistosomiasis B65.9 [N08]
    sepsis NEC A41.- ☑ [N08]

☑ **Additional Character Required** — Refer to the Tabular List for Character Selection   ▽ **Subterms under main terms may continue to next column or page**

Disorder — continued
  glomerular — continued
    sepsis — continued
      streptococcal A40.- ☑ [N08]
    sickle-cell disorders D57.- ☑ [N08]
    strongyloidiasis B78.9 [N08]
    subacute bacterial endocarditis I33.0 [N08]
    syphilis A52.75
    systemic lupus erythematosus M32.14
    thrombotic thrombocytopenic purpura
      M31.1 [N08]
    Waldenström macroglobulinemia C88.0 [N08]
    Wegener's granulomatosis M31.31
  gluconeogenesis E74.4
  glucosaminoglycan metabolism — see Disorder,
    metabolism, glucosaminoglycan
  glycine metabolism E72.50
    d-glycericacidemia E72.59
    hyperhydroxyprolinemia E72.59
    hyperoxaluria E72.53
    hyperprolinemia E72.59
    non-ketotic hyperglycinemia E72.51
    oxalosis E72.53
    oxaluria E72.53
    sarcosinemia E72.59
    trimethylaminuria E72.52
  glycoprotein metabolism E77.9
    specified NEC E77.8
  habit (and impulse) F63.9
    involving sexual behavior NEC F65.9
    specified NEC F63.89
  hallucinogen use
    mild F16.10
      with
        hallucinogen intoxication delirium F16.121
        hallucinogen-induced
          anxiety disorder F16.180
          bipolar and related disorder F16.14
          depressive disorder F16.14
          psychotic disorder F16.159
        other hallucinogen intoxication F16.129
      in remission (early) (sustained) F16.11
    moderate or severe F16.20
      with
        hallucinogen intoxication delirium F16.221
        hallucinogen-induced
          anxiety disorder F16.280
          bipolar and related disorder F16.24
          depressive disorder F16.24
          psychotic disorder F16.259
        other hallucinogen intoxication F16.229
      in remission (early) (sustained) F16.21
  heart action I49.9
  hematological D75.9
    newborn (transient) P61.9
      specified NEC P61.8
  hematopoietic organs D75.9
  hemorrhagic NEC D69.9
    drug-induced D68.32
    due to
      extrinsic circulating anticoagulants D68.32
      increase in
        anti-IIa D68.32
        anti-Xa D68.32
      intrinsic
        circulating anticoagulants D68.318
        increase in
          anti-IXa D68.318
          antithrombin D68.318
          anti-VIIIa D68.318
          anti-XIa D68.318
    following childbirth O72.3
  hemostasis — see Defect, coagulation
  histidine metabolism E70.40
    histidinemia E70.41
    other specified E70.49
  hoarding F42.3
  hyperkinetic — see Disorder, attention-deficit hyper-
    activity
  hyperleucine-isoleucinemia E71.19
  hypervalinemia E71.19
  hypoactive sexual desire F52.0
  hypochondriacal F45.20
    body dysmorphic F45.22
    neurosis F45.21
    other specified F45.29
  identity
    dissociative F44.81
    illness anxiety F45.21

Disorder — continued
  identity — continued
    of childhood F93.8
  immune mechanism (immunity) D89.9
    specified type NEC D89.89
  impaired renal tubular function N25.9
    specified NEC N25.89
  impulse (control) F63.9
  inflammatory
    pelvic, in diseases classified elsewhere — see cate-
      gory N74
    penis N48.29
      abscess N48.21
      cellulitis N48.22
  inhalant use
    mild F18.10
      with
        inhalant intoxication F18.129
        inhalant intoxication delirium F18.121
        inhalant-induced
          anxiety disorder F18.180
          depressive disorder F18.14
          major neurocognitive disorder F18.17
          mild neurocognitive disorder F18.188
          psychotic disorder F18.159
      in remission (early) (sustained) F18.11
    moderate or severe F18.20
      with
        inhalant intoxication F18.229
        inhalant intoxication delirium F18.221
        inhalant-induced
          anxiety disorder F18.280
          depressive disorder F18.24
          major neurocognitive disorder F18.27
          mild neurocognitive disorder F18.288
          psychotic disorder F18.259
      in remission (early) (sustained) F18.21
  integument, newborn P83.9
    specified NEC P83.88
  intermittent explosive F63.81
  internal secretion pancreas — see Increased, secretion,
    pancreas, endocrine
  intestine, intestinal
    carbohydrate absorption NEC E74.39
      postoperative K91.2
    functional NEC K59.9
      postoperative K91.89
    psychogenic F45.8
    vascular K55.9
      chronic K55.1
      specified NEC K55.8
  intraoperative (intraprocedural) — see Complications,
    intraoperative
  involuntary emotional expression (IEED) F07.89
  iris H21.9
    adhesions — see Adhesions, iris
    atrophy — see Atrophy, iris
    chamber angle recession — see Recession, cham-
      ber angle
    cyst — see Cyst, iris
    degeneration — see Degeneration, iris
    in diseases classified elsewhere H22
    iridodialysis — see Iridodialysis
    iridoschisis — see Iridoschisis
    miotic pupillary cyst — see Cyst, pupillary
    pupillary
      abnormality — see Abnormality, pupillary
      membrane — see Membrane, pupillary
    specified type NEC H21.89
    vascular NEC H21.1X- ☑
  iron metabolism E83.10
    specified NEC E83.19
  isovaleric acidemia E71.110
  jaw, developmental M27.0
    temporomandibular (see also Anomaly, dentofacial,
      temporomandibular joint) M26.60- ☑
  joint M25.9
    derangement — see Derangement, joint
    effusion — see Effusion, joint
    fistula — see Fistula, joint
    hemarthrosis — see Hemarthrosis
    instability — see Instability, joint
    osteophyte — see Osteophyte
    pain — see Pain, joint
    psychogenic F45.8
    specified type NEC M25.80
      ankle M25.87- ☑
      elbow M25.82- ☑

Disorder — continued
  joint — continued
    specified type — continued
      foot joint M25.87- ☑
      hand joint M25.84- ☑
      hip M25.85- ☑
      knee M25.86- ☑
      shoulder M25.81- ☑
      wrist M25.83- ☑
    stiffness — see Stiffness, joint
  ketone metabolism E71.32
  kidney N28.9
    functional (tubular) N25.9
    in
      schistosomiasis B65.9 [N29]
    tubular function N25.9
      specified NEC N25.89
  lacrimal system H04.9
    changes H04.69
      fistula — see Fistula, lacrimal
    gland H04.19
      atrophy — see Atrophy, lacrimal gland
      cyst — see Cyst, lacrimal, gland
      dacryops — see Dacryops
      dislocation — see Dislocation, lacrimal gland
      dry eye syndrome — see Syndrome, dry eye
      infection — see Dacryoadenitis
      granuloma — see Granuloma, lacrimal
      inflammation — see Inflammation, lacrimal
      obstruction — see Obstruction, lacrimal
    specified NEC H04.89
  lactation NEC O92.79
  language (developmental) F80.9
    expressive F80.1
    mixed receptive and expressive F80.2
    receptive F80.2
  late luteal phase dysphoric N94.89
  learning (specific) F81.9
    acalculia R48.8
    alexia R48.0
    mathematics F81.2
    reading F81.0
    specified
      with impairment in
        mathematics F81.2
        reading F81.0
        written expression F81.81
    specified NEC F81.89
    spelling F81.81
    written expression F81.81
  lens H27.9
    aphakia — see Aphakia
    cataract — see Cataract
    dislocation — see Dislocation, lens
    specified type NEC H27.8
  ligament M24.20
    ankle M24.27- ☑
    attachment, spine — see Enthesopathy, spinal
    elbow M24.22- ☑
    foot joint M24.27- ☑
    hand joint M24.24- ☑
    hip M24.25- ☑
    knee — see Derangement, knee, specified NEC
    shoulder M24.21- ☑
    vertebra M24.28
    wrist M24.23- ☑
  ligamentous attachments (see also Enthesopathy)
    spine — see Enthesopathy, spinal
  lipid
    metabolism, congenital E78.9
    storage E75.6
      specified NEC E75.5
  lipoprotein
    deficiency (familial) E78.6
    metabolism E78.9
      specified NEC E78.89
  liver K76.9
    malarial B54 [K77]
  low back (see also Dorsopathy, specified NEC)
  lumbosacral
    plexus G54.1
    root (nerve) NEC G54.4
  lung, interstitial, drug-induced J70.4
    acute J70.2
    chronic J70.3
  lymphoproliferative, post-transplant (PTLD) D47.Z1
    (following D47.4)
  lysine and hydroxylysine metabolism E72.3

Disorder — *continued*
- major neurocognitive — *see* Dementia, in (due to)
- male
  - erectile (organic) (*see also* Dysfunction, sexual, male, erectile) N52.9
    - nonorganic F52.21
  - hypoactive sexual desire F52.0
  - orgasmic F52.32
- manic F30.9
  - organic F06.33
- mast cell activation — *see* Activation, mast cell
- mastoid (*see also* Disorder, ear, middle)
  - postprocedural — *see* Complications, ear, procedure
- meniscus — *see* Derangement, knee, meniscus
- menopausal N95.9
  - specified NEC N95.8
- menstrual N92.6
  - psychogenic F45.8
  - specified NEC N92.5
- mental (or behavioral) (nonpsychotic) F99
  - due to (secondary to)
    - amphetamine
      - due to drug abuse — *see* Abuse, drug, stimulant
      - due to drug dependence — *see* Dependence, drug, stimulant
    - brain disease, damage and dysfunction F09
    - caffeine use
      - due to drug abuse — *see* Abuse, drug, stimulant
      - due to drug dependence — *see* Dependence, drug, stimulant
    - cannabis use
      - due to drug abuse — *see* Abuse, drug, cannabis
      - due to drug dependence — *see* Dependence, drug, cannabis
    - general medical condition F09
    - sedative or hypnotic use
      - due to drug abuse — *see* Abuse, drug, sedative
      - due to drug dependence — *see* Dependence, drug, sedative
    - tobacco (nicotine) use — *see* Dependence, drug, nicotine
  - following organic brain damage F07.9
    - frontal lobe syndrome F07.0
    - personality change F07.0
    - postconcussional syndrome F07.81
    - specified NEC F07.89
  - infancy, childhood or adolescence F98.9
  - neurotic — *see* Neurosis
  - organic or symptomatic F09
  - presenile, psychotic F03 ☑
  - problem NEC
  - psychoneurotic — *see* Neurosis
  - psychotic — *see* Psychosis
  - puerperal F53
  - senile, psychotic NEC F03 ☑
- metabolic, amino acid, transitory, newborn P74.8
- metabolism NOS E88.9
  - amino-acid E72.9
    - aromatic E70.9
      - albinism — *see* Albinism
      - histidine E70.40
        - histidinemia E70.41
        - other specified E70.49
      - hyperphenylalaninemia E70.1
        - classical phenylketonuria E70.0
      - other specified E70.8
      - tryptophan E70.5
      - tyrosine E70.20
        - hypertyrosinemia E70.21
        - other specified E70.29
    - branched chain E71.2
      - 3-methylglutaconic aciduria E71.111
      - hyperleucine-isoleucinemia E71.19
      - hypervalinemia E71.19
      - isovaleric acidemia E71.110
      - maple syrup urine disease E71.0
      - methylmalonic acidemia E71.120
      - organic aciduria NEC E71.118
      - other specified E71.19
      - proprionate NEC E71.128
      - proprionic acidemia E71.121
    - glycine E72.50
      - d-glycericacidemia E72.59

Disorder — *continued*
- metabolism — *continued*
  - amino-acid — *continued*
    - glycine — *continued*
      - hyperhydroxyprolinemia E72.59
      - hyperoxaluria E72.53
      - hyperprolinemia E72.59
      - non-ketotic hyperglycinemia E72.51
      - other specified E72.59
      - sarcosinemia E72.59
      - trimethylaminuria E72.52
    - hydroxylysine E72.3
    - lysine E72.3
    - ornithine E72.4
    - other specified E72.8
      - beta-amino acid E72.8
      - gamma-glutamyl cycle E72.8
    - straight-chain E72.8
    - sulfur-bearing E72.10
      - homocystinuria E72.11
      - methylenetetrahydrofolate reductase deficiency E72.12
      - other specified E72.19
  - bile acid and cholesterol metabolism E78.70
  - bilirubin E80.7
    - specified NEC E80.6
  - calcium E83.50
    - hypercalcemia E83.52
    - hypocalcemia E83.51
    - other specified E83.59
  - carbohydrate E74.9
    - specified NEC E74.8
  - cholesterol and bile acid metabolism E78.70
  - congenital E88.9
  - copper E83.00
    - specified type NEC E83.09
    - Wilson's disease E83.01
  - cystinuria E72.01
  - fructose E74.10
  - galactose E74.20
  - glucosaminoglycan E76.9
    - mucopolysaccharidosis — *see* Mucopolysaccharidosis
    - specified NEC E76.8
  - glutamine E72.8
  - glycine E72.50
  - glycogen storage (hepatorenal) E74.09
  - glycoprotein E77.9
    - specified NEC E77.8
  - glycosaminoglycan E76.9
    - specified NEC E76.8
  - in labor and delivery O75.89
  - iron E83.10
  - isoleucine E71.19
  - leucine E71.19
  - lipoid E78.9
  - lipoprotein E78.9
    - specified NEC E78.89
  - magnesium E83.40
    - hypermagnesemia E83.41
    - hypomagnesemia E83.42
    - other specified E83.49
  - mineral E83.9
    - specified NEC E83.89
  - mitochondrial E88.40
    - MELAS syndrome E88.41
    - MERRF syndrome (myoclonic epilepsy associated with ragged-red fibers) E88.42
    - other specified E88.49
  - ornithine E72.4
  - phosphatases E83.30
  - phosphorus E83.30
    - acid phosphatase deficiency E83.39
    - hypophosphatasia E83.39
    - hypophosphatemia E83.39
      - familial E83.31
    - other specified E83.39
    - pseudovitamin D deficiency E83.32
  - plasma protein NEC E88.09
  - porphyrin — *see* Porphyria
  - postprocedural E89.89
    - specified NEC E89.89
  - purine E79.9
    - specified NEC E79.8
  - pyrimidine E79.9
    - specified NEC E79.8
  - pyruvate E74.4
  - serine E72.8
  - sodium E87.8

Disorder — *continued*
- metabolism — *continued*
  - specified NEC E88.89
  - threonine E72.8
  - valine E71.19
  - zinc E83.2
  - methylmalonic acidemia E71.120
  - micturition NEC (*see also* Difficulty, micturition) R39.198
    - feeling of incomplete emptying R39.14
    - hesitancy R39.11
    - poor stream R39.12
    - psychogenic F45.8
    - split stream R39.13
    - straining R39.16
    - urgency R39.15
- mild neurocognitive G31.84
- mitochondrial metabolism E88.40
- mitral (valve) — *see* Endocarditis, mitral
- mixed
  - anxiety and depressive F41.8
  - of scholastic skills (developmental) F81.89
  - receptive expressive language F80.2
- mood F39
  - bipolar — *see* Disorder, bipolar
  - depressive — *see* Disorder, depressive
  - due to (secondary to)
    - alcohol F10.94
    - amphetamine F15.94
      - in
        - abuse F15.14
        - dependence F15.24
    - anxiolytic F13.94
      - in
        - abuse F13.14
        - dependence F13.24
    - cocaine F14.94
      - in
        - abuse F14.14
        - dependence F14.24
    - general medical condition F06.30
    - hallucinogen F16.94
      - in
        - abuse F16.14
        - dependence F16.24
    - hypnotic F13.94
      - in
        - abuse F13.14
        - dependence F13.24
    - inhalant F18.94
      - in
        - abuse F18.14
        - dependence F18.24
    - opioid F11.94
      - in
        - abuse F11.14
        - dependence F11.24
    - phencyclidine (PCP) F16.94
      - in
        - abuse F16.14
        - dependence F16.24
    - physiological condition F06.30
      - with
        - depressive features F06.31
        - major depressive-like episode F06.32
        - manic features F06.33
        - mixed features F06.34
    - psychoactive substance NEC F19.94
      - in
        - abuse F19.14
        - dependence F19.24
    - sedative F13.94
      - in
        - abuse F13.14
        - dependence F13.24
    - volatile solvents F18.94
      - in
        - abuse F18.14
        - dependence F18.24
  - manic episode F30.9
    - with psychotic symptoms F30.2
    - without psychotic symptoms F30.10
      - mild F30.11
      - moderate F30.12
      - severe F30.13
    - in remission (full) F30.4
      - partial F30.3
    - specified type NEC F30.8
  - organic F06.30

☑ **Additional Character Required** — Refer to the Tabular List for Character Selection ▽ **Subterms under main terms may continue to next column or page**

Disorder — *continued*
  mood — *continued*
    organic — *continued*
      right hemisphere F07.89
    persistent F34.9
      cyclothymia F34.0
      dysthymia F34.1
      specified type NEC F34.89
    recurrent F39
    right hemisphere organic F07.89
  movement G25.9
    drug-induced G25.70
      akathisia G25.71
      specified NEC G25.79
    hysterical F44.4
    in diseases classified elsewhere — *see* category
      G26
    periodic limb G47.61
      sleep related G47.61
    sleep related NEC G47.69
    specified NEC G25.89
    stereotyped F98.4
    treatment-induced G25.9
  multiple personality F44.81
  muscle M62.9
    attachment, spine — *see* Enthesopathy, spinal
    in trichinellosis — *see* Trichinellosis, with muscle
      disorder
    psychogenic F45.8
    specified type NEC M62.89
    tone, newborn P94.9
      specified NEC P94.8
  muscular
    attachments (*see also* Enthesopathy)
      spine — *see* Enthesopathy, spinal
    urethra N36.44
  musculoskeletal system, soft tissue — *see* Disorder,
      soft tissue
    postprocedural M96.89
    psychogenic F45.8
  myoneural G70.9
    due to lead G70.1
    specified NEC G70.89
    toxic G70.1
  myotonic NEC G71.19
  nail, in diseases classified elsewhere L62
  neck region NEC — *see* Dorsopathy, specified NEC
  neonatal onset multisystemic inflammatory (NOMID)
      M04.2
  nerve G58.9
    abducent NEC — *see* Strabismus, paralytic, sixth
      nerve
    accessory G52.8
    acoustic — *see* subcategory H93.3 ☑
    auditory — *see* subcategory H93.3 ☑
    auriculotemporal G50.8
    axillary G54.0
    cerebral — *see* Disorder, nerve, cranial
    cranial G52.9
      eighth — *see* subcategory H93.3 ☑
      eleventh G52.8
      fifth G50.9
      first G52.0
      fourth NEC — *see* Strabismus, paralytic, fourth
        nerve
      multiple G52.7
      ninth G52.1
      second NEC — *see* Disorder, nerve, optic
      seventh NEC G51.8
      sixth NEC — *see* Strabismus, paralytic, sixth
        nerve
      specified NEC G52.8
      tenth G52.2
      third NEC — *see* Strabismus, paralytic, third
        nerve
      twelfth G52.3
    entrapment — *see* Neuropathy, entrapment
    facial G51.9
      specified NEC G51.8
    femoral — *see* Lesion, nerve, femoral
    glossopharyngeal NEC G52.1
    hypoglossal G52.3
    intercostal G58.0
    lateral
      cutaneous of thigh — *see* Mononeuropathy,
        lower limb, meralgia paresthetica
      popliteal — *see* Lesion, nerve, popliteal
    lower limb — *see* Mononeuropathy, lower limb

Disorder — *continued*
  nerve — *continued*
    medial popliteal — *see* Lesion, nerve, popliteal,
      medial
    median NEC — *see* Lesion, nerve, median
    multiple G58.7
    oculomotor NEC — *see* Strabismus, paralytic, third
      nerve
    olfactory G52.0
    optic NEC H47.09- ☑
      hemorrhage into sheath — *see* Hemorrhage,
        optic nerve
      ischemic H47.01- ☑
    peroneal — *see* Lesion, nerve, popliteal
    phrenic G58.8
    plantar — *see* Lesion, nerve, plantar
    pneumogastric G52.2
    posterior tibial — *see* Syndrome, tarsal tunnel
    radial — *see* Lesion, nerve, radial
    recurrent laryngeal G52.2
    root G54.9
      cervical G54.2
      lumbosacral G54.1
      specified NEC G54.8
      thoracic G54.3
    sciatic NEC — *see* Lesion, nerve, sciatic
    specified NEC G58.8
      lower limb — *see* Mononeuropathy, lower limb,
        specified NEC
      upper limb — *see* Mononeuropathy, upper
        limb, specified NEC
    sympathetic G90.9
    tibial — *see* Lesion, nerve, popliteal, medial
    trigeminal G50.9
      specified NEC G50.8
    trochlear NEC — *see* Strabismus, paralytic, fourth
      nerve
    ulnar — *see* Lesion, nerve, ulnar
    upper limb — *see* Mononeuropathy, upper limb
    vagus G52.2
  nervous system G98.8
    autonomic (peripheral) G90.9
      specified NEC G90.8
    central G96.9
      specified NEC G96.8
    parasympathetic G90.9
    specified NEC G98.8
    sympathetic G90.9
    vegetative G90.9
  neurocognitive R41.9
    major
      with
        aggressive behavior F01.51
        combative behavior F01.51
        violent behavior F01.51
      without behavioral disturbance F01.50
      due to vascular disease, with behavioral distur-
        bance F01.51
      in (due to) (other diseases classified elsewhere)
        (*see also* Dementia, in (due to)) F02.80
        with
          aggressive behavior F02.81
          combative behavior F02.81
          violent behavior F02.81
    mild G31.84
  neurodevelopmental F89
    specified NEC F88
  neurohypophysis NEC E23.3
  neurological NEC R29.818
  neuromuscular G70.9
    hereditary NEC G71.9
    specified NEC G70.89
    toxic G70.1
  neurotic F48.9
    specified NEC F48.8
  neutrophil, polymorphonuclear D71
  nicotine use — *see* Dependence, drug, nicotine
  nightmare F51.5
  non-rapid eye movement sleep arousal
    sleep terror type F51.4
    sleepwalking type F51.3
  nose J34.9
    specified NEC J34.89
  obsessive-compulsive F42.9
    and related disorder due to a known physiological
      condition F06.8
  odontogenesis NOS K00.9

Disorder — *continued*
  opioid use
    with
      opioid-induced psychotic disorder F11.959
        with
          delusions F11.950
          hallucinations F11.951
    due to drug abuse — *see* Abuse, drug, opioid
    due to drug dependence — *see* Dependence, drug,
      opioid
    mild F11.10
      with
        opioid intoxication
          with perceptual disturbances F11.122
          without perceptual disturbances F11.129
          delirium F11.121
        opioid-induced
          anxiety disorder F11.188
          depressive disorder F11.14
          sexual dysfunction F11.181
      in remission (early) (sustained) F11.11
    moderate or severe F11.20
      with
        opioid intoxication
          with perceptual disturbances F11.222
          without perceptual disturbances F11.229
          delirium F11.221
        opioid-induced
          anxiety disorder F11.288
          anxiety disorder F11.988
          depressive disorder F11.24
          depressive disorder F11.94
          sexual dysfunction F11.281
          sexual dysfunction F11.981
      in remission (early) (sustained) F11.21
  oppositional defiant F91.3
  optic
    chiasm H47.49
      due to
        inflammatory disorder H47.41
        neoplasm H47.42
        vascular disorder H47.43
    disc H47.39- ☑
      coloboma — *see* Coloboma, optic disc
      drusen — *see* Drusen, optic disc
      pseudopapilledema — *see* Pseudopapilledema
    radiations — *see* Disorder, visual, pathway
    tracts — *see* Disorder, visual, pathway
  orbit H05.9
    cyst — *see* Cyst, orbit
    deformity — *see* Deformity, orbit
    edema — *see* Edema, orbit
    enophthalmos — *see* Enophthalmos
    exophthalmos — *see* Exophthalmos
    hemorrhage — *see* Hemorrhage, orbit
    inflammation — *see* Inflammation, orbit
    myopathy — *see* Myopathy, extraocular muscles
    retained foreign body — *see* Foreign body, orbit,
      old
    specified type NEC H05.89
  organic
    anxiety F06.4
    catatonic F06.1
    delusional F06.2
    dissociative F06.8
    emotionally labile (asthenic) F06.8
    mood (affective) F06.30
    schizophrenia-like F06.2
  orgasmic (female) F52.31
    male F52.32
  ornithine metabolism E72.4
  overanxious F41.1
    of childhood F93.8
  pain
    with related psychological factors F45.42
    exclusively related to psychological factors F45.41
    genito-pelvic penetration disorder F52.6
  pancreatic internal secretion E16.9
    specified NEC E16.8
  panic F41.0
    with agoraphobia F40.01
  papulosquamous L44.9
    in diseases classified elsewhere L45
    specified NEC L44.8
  paranoid F22
    induced F24
    shared F24
  paraphilic F65.9

☜ Subterms under main terms may continue to next column or page   ☑ Additional Character Required — Refer to the Tabular List for Character Selection   115

Disorder — Disorder

Disorder — *continued*

paraphilic — *continued*
  specified NEC F65.89
parathyroid (gland) E21.5
  specified NEC E21.4
parietoalveolar NEC J84.09
paroxysmal, mixed R56.9
patella M22.9- ☑
  chondromalacia — *see* Chondromalacia, patella
  derangement NEC M22.3X- ☑
  recurrent
    dislocation — *see* Dislocation, patella, recurrent
    subluxation — *see* Dislocation, patella, recurrent, incomplete
  specified NEC M22.8X- ☑
patellofemoral M22.2X- ☑
pedophilic F65.4
pentose phosphate pathway with anemia D55.1
perception, due to hallucinogens F16.983
  in
    abuse F16.183
    dependence F16.283
peripheral nervous system NEC G64
peroxisomal E71.50
  biogenesis
    neonatal adrenoleukodystrophy E71.511
    specified disorder NEC E71.518
    Zellweger syndrome E71.510
  rhizomelic chondrodysplasia punctata E71.540
  specified form NEC E71.548
    group 1 E71.518
    group 2 E71.53
    group 3 E71.542
  X-linked adrenoleukodystrophy E71.529
    adolescent E71.521
    adrenomyeloneuropathy E71.522
    childhood E71.520
    specified form NEC E71.528
  Zellweger-like syndrome E71.541
persistent
  (somatoform) pain F45.41
  affective (mood) F34.9
personality (*see also* Personality) F60.9
  affective F34.0
  aggressive F60.3
  amoral F60.2
  anankastic F60.5
  antisocial F60.2
  anxious F60.6
  asocial F60.2
  asthenic F60.7
  avoidant F60.6
  borderline F60.3
  change (secondary) due to general medical condition F07.0
  compulsive F60.5
  cyclothymic F34.0
  dependent (passive) F60.7
  depressive F34.1
  dissocial F60.2
  emotional instability F60.3
  expansive paranoid F60.0
  explosive F60.3
  following organic brain damage F07.9
  histrionic F60.4
  hyperthymic F34.0
  hypothymic F34.1
  hysterical F60.4
  immature F60.89
  inadequate F60.7
  labile F60.3
  mixed (nonspecific) F60.89
  moral deficiency F60.2
  narcissistic F60.81
  negativistic F60.89
  obsessional F60.5
  obsessive (-compulsive) F60.5
  organic F07.9
  overconscientious F60.5
  paranoid F60.0
  passive (-dependent) F60.7
  passive-aggressive F60.89
  pathological NEC F60.9
  pseudosocial F60.2
  psychopathic F60.2
  schizoid F60.1
  schizotypal F21
  self-defeating F60.7

Disorder — *continued*

personality (*see also* Personality) — *continued*
  specified NEC F60.89
  type A F60.5
  unstable (emotional) F60.3
pervasive, developmental F84.9
phencyclidine use
  mild F16.10
    with
      phencyclidine intoxication F16.129
      phencyclidine intoxication delirium F16.121
      phencyclidine-induced
        anxiety disorder F16.180
        bipolar and related disorder F16.14
        depressive disorder F16.14
        psychotic disorder F16.159
    in remission (early) (sustained) F16.11
  moderate or severe F16.20
    with
      phencyclidine intoxication F16.229
      phencyclidine intoxication delirium F16.221
      phencyclidine-induced
        anxiety disorder F16.280
        bipolar and related disorder F16.14
        depressive disorder F16.24
        psychotic disorder F16.259
    in remission (early) (sustained) F16.21
phobic anxiety, childhood F40.8
phosphate-losing tubular N25.0
pigmentation L81.9
  choroid, congenital Q14.3
  diminished melanin formation L81.6
  iron L81.8
  specified NEC L81.8
pinna (noninfective) H61.10- ☑
  deformity, acquired H61.11- ☑
  hematoma H61.12- ☑
  perichondritis — *see* Perichondritis, ear
  specified type NEC H61.19- ☑
pituitary gland E23.7
  iatrogenic (postprocedural) E89.3
  specified NEC E23.6
platelets D69.1
plexus G54.9
  specified NEC G54.8
polymorphonuclear neutrophils D71
porphyrin metabolism — *see* Porphyria
postconcussional F07.81
posthallucinogen perception F16.983
  in
    abuse F16.183
    dependence F16.283
postmenopausal N95.9
  specified NEC N95.8
postprocedural (postoperative) — *see* Complications, postprocedural
post-transplant lymphoproliferative D47.Z1 (*following* D47.4)
post-traumatic stress (PTSD) F43.10
  acute F43.11
  chronic F43.12
premenstrual dysphoric (PMDD) F32.81
prepuce N47.8
propionic acidemia E71.121
prostate N42.9
  specified NEC N42.89
psychogenic NOS (*see also* condition) F45.9
  anxiety F41.8
  appetite F50.9
  asthenic F48.8
  cardiovascular (system) F45.8
  compulsive F42.8
  cutaneous F54
  depressive F32.9
  digestive (system) F45.8
  dysmenorrheic F45.8
  dyspneic F45.8
  endocrine (system) F54
  eye NEC F45.8
  feeding — *see* Disorder, eating
  functional NEC F45.8
  gastric F45.8
  gastrointestinal (system) F45.8
  genitourinary (system) F45.8
  heart (function) (rhythm) F45.8
  hyperventilatory F45.8
  hypochondriacal — *see* Disorder, hypochondriacal
  intestinal F45.8

Disorder — *continued*

psychogenic (*see also* condition) — *continued*
  joint F45.8
  learning F81.9
  limb F45.8
  lymphatic (system) F45.8
  menstrual F45.8
  micturition F45.8
  monoplegic NEC F44.4
  motor F44.4
  muscle F45.8
  musculoskeletal F45.8
  neurocirculatory F45.8
  obsessive F42.8
  occupational F48.8
  organ or part of body NEC F45.8
  paralytic NEC F44.4
  phobic F40.9
  physical NEC F45.8
  rectal F45.8
  respiratory (system) F45.8
  rheumatic F45.8
  sexual (function) F52.9
  skin (allergic) (eczematous) F54
  sleep F51.9
  specified part of body NEC F45.8
  stomach F45.8
psychological F99
  associated with
    disease classified elsewhere F54
    sexual
      development F66
      relationship F66
    uncertainty about gender identity F64.9
psychomotor NEC F44.4
  hysterical F44.4
psychoneurotic (*see also* Neurosis)
  mixed NEC F48.8
psychophysiologic — *see* Disorder, somatoform
psychosexual F65.9
  development F66
  identity of childhood F64.2
psychosomatic NOS — *see* Disorder, somatoform
  multiple F45.0
  undifferentiated F45.1
psychotic — *see* Psychosis
  transient (acute) F23
puberty E30.9
  specified NEC E30.8
pulmonary (valve) — *see* Endocarditis, pulmonary
purine metabolism E79.9
pyrimidine metabolism E79.9
pyruvate metabolism E74.4
reactive attachment (childhood) F94.1
reading R48.0
  developmental (specific) F81.0
receptive language F80.2
receptor, hormonal, peripheral (*see also* Syndrome, androgen insensitivity) E34.50
recurrent brief depressive F33.8
reflex R29.2
refraction H52.7
  aniseikonia H52.32
  anisometropia H52.31
  astigmatism — *see* Astigmatism
  hypermetropia — *see* Hypermetropia
  myopia — *see* Myopia
  presbyopia H52.4
  specified NEC H52.6
relationship F68.8
  due to sexual orientation F66
REM sleep behavior G47.52
renal function, impaired (tubular) N25.9
resonance R49.9
  specified NEC R49.8
respiratory function, impaired (*see also* Failure, respiration)
  postprocedural — *see* Complication, postoperative, respiratory system
  psychogenic F45.8
retina H35.9
  angioid streaks H35.33
  changes in vascular appearance H35.01- ☑
  degeneration — *see* Degeneration, retina
  dystrophy (hereditary) — *see* Dystrophy, retina
  edema H35.81
  hemorrhage — *see* Hemorrhage, retina
  ischemia H35.82

☑ Additional Character Required — Refer to the Tabular List for Character Selection ▽ Subterms under main terms may continue to next column or page

Disorder — *continued*
retina — *continued*
macular degeneration — *see* Degeneration, macula
microaneurysms H35.04- ☑
microvascular abnormality NEC H35.09
neovascularization — *see* Neovascularization,
retina
retinopathy — *see* Retinopathy
separation of layers H35.70
central serous chorioretinopathy H35.71- ☑
pigment epithelium detachment (serous)
H35.72- ☑
hemorrhagic H35.73- ☑
specified type NEC H35.89
telangiectasis — *see* Telangiectasis, retina
vasculitis — *see* Vasculitis, retina
retroperitoneal K68.9
right hemisphere organic affective F07.89
rumination (infant or child) F98.21
sacrum, sacrococcygeal NEC M53.3
schizoaffective F25.9
bipolar type F25.0
depressive type F25.1
manic type F25.0
mixed type F25.0
specified NEC F25.8
schizoid of childhood F84.5
schizophrenia spectrum and other psychotic disorder
F29
specified NEC F28
schizophreniform F20.81
brief F23
schizotypal (personality) F21
secretion, thyrocalcitonin E07.0
sedative, hypnotic, or anxiolytic use
mild F13.10
with
sedative, hypnotic, or anxiolytic intoxication
F13.129
sedative, hypnotic, or anxiolytic intoxication
delirium F13.121
sedative, hypnotic, or anxiolytic-induced
anxiety disorder F13.180
bipolar and related disorder F13.14
depressive disorder F13.14
psychotic disorder F13.159
sexual dysfunction F13.181
in remission (early) (sustained) F13.11
moderate or severe F13.20
with
sedative, hypnotic, or anxiolytic intoxication
F13.229
sedative, hypnotic, or anxiolytic intoxication
delirium F13.221
sedative, hypnotic, or anxiolytic-induced
anxiety disorder F13.280
bipolar and related disorder F13.24
depressive disorder F13.24
major neurocognitive disorder F13.27
mild neurocognitive disorder F13.288
psychotic disorder F13.259
sexual dysfunction F13.281
in remission (early) (sustained) F13.21
seizure (*see also* Epilepsy) G40.909
intractable G40.919
with status epilepticus G40.911
semantic pragmatic F80.89
with autism F84.0
sense of smell R43.1
psychogenic F45.8
separation anxiety, of childhood F93.0
sexual
aversion F52.1
function, psychogenic F52.9
interest/arousal, female F52.22
masochism F65.51
maturation F66
nonorganic F52.9
preference (*see also* Deviation, sexual) F65.9
fetishistic transvestism F65.1
relationship F66
sadism F65.52
shyness, of childhood and adolescence F40.10
sibling rivalry F93.8
sickle-cell (sickling) (homozygous) — *see* Disease,
sickle-cell
heterozygous D57.3
specified type NEC D57.8- ☑

Disorder — *continued*
sickle-cell — *see* Disease, sickle-cell — *continued*
trait D57.3
sinus (nasal) J34.9
specified NEC J34.89
skin L98.9
atrophic L90.9
specified NEC L90.8
granulomatous L92.9
specified NEC L92.8
hypertrophic L91.9
specified NEC L91.8
infiltrative NEC L98.6
newborn P83.9
specified NEC P83.88
picking F42.4
psychogenic (allergic) (eczematous) F54
sleep G47.9
breathing-related — *see* Apnea, sleep
circadian rhythm G47.20
advance sleep phase type G47.22
delayed sleep phase type G47.21
due to
alcohol
abuse F10.182
dependence F10.282
use F10.982
amphetamines
abuse F15.182
dependence F15.282
use F15.982
caffeine
abuse F15.182
dependence F15.282
use F15.982
cocaine
abuse F14.182
dependence F14.282
use F14.982
drug NEC
abuse F19.182
dependence F19.282
use F19.982
opioid
abuse F11.182
dependence F11.282
use F11.982
psychoactive substance NEC
abuse F19.182
dependence F19.282
use F19.982
sedative, hypnotic, or anxiolytic
abuse F13.182
dependence F13.282
use F13.982
stimulant NEC
abuse F15.182
dependence F15.282
use F15.982
free running type G47.24
in conditions classified elsewhere G47.27
irregular sleep wake type G47.23
jet lag type G47.25
non-24-hour sleep-wake type G47.24
shift work type G47.26
specified NEC G47.29
due to
alcohol
abuse F10.182
dependence F10.282
use F10.982
amphetamine
abuse F15.182
dependence F15.282
use F15.982
anxiolytic
abuse F13.182
dependence F13.282
use F13.982
caffeine
abuse F15.182
dependence F15.282
use F15.982
cocaine
abuse F14.182
dependence F14.282
use F14.982
drug NEC
abuse F19.182

Disorder — *continued*
sleep — *continued*
due to — *continued*
drug — *continued*
dependence F19.282
use F19.982
hypnotic
abuse F13.182
dependence F13.282
use F13.982
opioid
abuse F11.182
dependence F11.282
use F11.982
psychoactive substance NEC
abuse F19.182
dependence F19.282
use F19.982
sedative
abuse F13.182
dependence F13.282
use F13.982
stimulant NEC
abuse F15.182
dependence F15.282
use F15.982
emotional F51.9
excessive somnolence — *see* Hypersomnia
hypersomnia type — *see* Hypersomnia
initiating or maintaining — *see* Insomnia
nightmares F51.5
nonorganic F51.9
specified NEC F51.8
parasomnia type G47.50
specified NEC G47.8
terrors F51.4
walking F51.3
sleep-wake pattern or schedule (*see also* Disorder,
sleep, circadian rhythm) G47.9
specified NEC G47.8
social
anxiety (of childhood) F40.10
generalized F40.11
functioning in childhood F94.9
specified NEC F94.8
pragmatic F80.82
soft tissue M79.9
ankle M79.9
due to use, overuse and pressure M70.90
ankle M70.97- ☑
bursitis — *see* Bursitis
foot M70.97- ☑
forearm M70.93- ☑
hand M70.94- ☑
lower leg M70.96- ☑
multiple sites M70.99
pelvic region M70.95- ☑
shoulder region M70.91- ☑
specified site NEC M70.98
specified type NEC M70.80
ankle M70.87- ☑
foot M70.87- ☑
forearm M70.83- ☑
hand M70.84- ☑
lower leg M70.86- ☑
multiple sites M70.89
pelvic region M70.85- ☑
shoulder region M70.81- ☑
specified site NEC M70.88
thigh M70.85- ☑
upper arm M70.82- ☑
thigh M70.95- ☑
upper arm M70.92- ☑
foot M79.9
forearm M79.9
hand M79.9
lower leg M79.9
multiple sites M79.9
occupational — *see* Disorder, soft tissue, due to
use, overuse and pressure
pelvic region M79.9
shoulder region M79.9
specified type NEC M79.89
thigh M79.9
upper arm M79.9
somatic symptom F45.1
somatization F45.0
somatoform F45.9

☟ **Subterms under main terms may continue to next column or page**   ☑ **Additional Character Required — Refer to the Tabular List for Character Selection**   **117**

Disorder — Disorder

Disorder — *continued*
somatoform — *continued*
pain (persistent) F45.41
somatization (multiple) (long-lasting) F45.0
specified NEC F45.8
undifferentiated F45.1
somnolence, excessive — *see* Hypersomnia
specific
arithmetical F81.2
developmental, of motor F82
reading F81.0
speech and language F80.9
spelling F81.81
written expression F81.81
speech R47.9
articulation (functional) (specific) F80.0
developmental F80.9
specified NEC R47.89
speech-sound F80.0
spelling (specific) F81.81
spine (*see also* Dorsopathy)
ligamentous or muscular attachments, peripheral
— *see* Enthesopathy, spinal
specified NEC — *see* Dorsopathy, specified NEC
stereotyped, habit or movement F98.4
stimulant use (other) (unspecified)
mild F15.10
in remission (early) (sustained) F15.11
moderate or severe F15.20
in remission (early) (sustained) F15.21
stomach (functional) — *see* Disorder, gastric
stress F43.9
acute F43.0
post-traumatic F43.10
acute F43.11
chronic F43.12
substance use (other) (unknown)
mild F19.10
with substance-induced
anxiety disorder F19.180
bipolar and related disorder F19.14
depressive disorder F19.14
major neurocognitive disorder F19.17
mild neurocognitive disorder F19.188
obsessive-compulsive and related disorder
F19.188
sexual dysfunction F19.181
substance intoxication F19.129
substance intoxication delirium F19.121
moderate or severe F19.20
with substance-induced
anxiety disorder F19.280
bipolar and related disorder F19.24
depressive disorder F19.24
major neurocognitive disorder F19.27
mild neurocognitive disorder F19.288
obsessive-compulsive and related disorder
F19.288
sexual dysfunction F19.281
in remission (early) (sustained) F19.21
substance intoxication F19.229
substance intoxication delirium F19.221
sulfur-bearing amino-acid metabolism E72.10
sweat gland (eccrine) L74.9
apocrine L75.9
specified NEC L75.8
specified NEC L74.8
synovium M67.90
acromioclavicular M67.91- ☑
ankle M67.97- ☑
elbow M67.92- ☑
foot M67.97- ☑
forearm M67.93- ☑
hand M67.94- ☑
hip M67.95- ☑
knee M67.96- ☑
multiple sites M67.99
rupture — *see* Rupture, synovium
shoulder M67.91- ☑
specified type NEC M67.80
acromioclavicular M67.81- ☑
ankle M67.87- ☑
elbow M67.82- ☑
foot M67.87- ☑
hand M67.84- ☑
hip M67.85- ☑
knee M67.86- ☑
multiple sites M67.89

Disorder — *continued*
synovium — *continued*
specified type — *continued*
wrist M67.83- ☑
synovitis — *see* Synovitis
upper arm M67.92- ☑
wrist M67.93- ☑
temperature regulation, newborn P81.9
specified NEC P81.8
temporomandibular joint M26.60- ☑
tendon M67.90
acromioclavicular M67.91- ☑
ankle M67.97- ☑
contracture — *see* Contracture, tendon
elbow M67.92- ☑
foot M67.97- ☑
forearm M67.93- ☑
hand M67.94- ☑
hip M67.95- ☑
knee M67.96- ☑
multiple sites M67.99
rupture — *see* Rupture, tendon
shoulder M67.91- ☑
specified type NEC M67.80
acromioclavicular M67.81- ☑
ankle M67.87- ☑
elbow M67.82- ☑
foot M67.87- ☑
hand M67.84- ☑
hip M67.85- ☑
knee M67.86- ☑
multiple sites M67.89
trunk M67.88
wrist M67.83- ☑
synovitis — *see* Synovitis
tendinitis — *see* Tendinitis
tenosynovitis — *see* Tenosynovitis
trunk M67.98
upper arm M67.92- ☑
wrist M67.93- ☑
thoracic root (nerve) NEC G54.3
thyrocalcitonin hypersecretion E07.0
thyroid (gland) E07.9
function NEC, neonatal, transitory P72.2
iodine-deficiency related E01.8
specified NEC E07.89
tic — *see* Tic
tobacco use
chewing tobacco (mild) (moderate) (severe)
in remission (early) (sustained) F17.221
cigarettes (mild) (moderate) (severe)
in remission (early) (sustained) F17.211
mild Z72.0
in remission (early) (sustained) F17.201
moderate F17.200
in remission (early) (sustained) F17.201
severe F17.200
in remission (early) (sustained) F17.201
specified product NEC (mild) (moderate) (severe)
in remission (early) (sustained) F17.291
tooth K08.9
development K00.9
specified NEC K00.8
eruption K00.6
Tourette's F95.2
trance and possession F44.89
transvestic F65.1
trauma and stressor-related F43.9
other specified F43.8
tricuspid (valve) — *see* Endocarditis, tricuspid
tryptophan metabolism E70.5
tubular, phosphate-losing N25.0
tubulo-interstitial (in)
brucellosis A23.9 [N16]
cystinosis E72.04
diphtheria A36.84
glycogen storage disease E74.00 [N16]
leukemia NEC C95.9- ☑ [N16]
lymphoma NEC C85.9- ☑ [N16]
mixed cryoglobulinemia D89.1 [N16]
multiple myeloma C90.0- ☑ [N16]
Salmonella infection A02.25
sarcoidosis D86.84
sepsis A41.9 [N16]
streptococcal A40.9 [N16]
systemic lupus erythematosus M32.15
toxoplasmosis B58.83

Disorder — *continued*
tubulo-interstitial — *continued*
transplant rejection T86.91 [N16]
Wilson's disease E83.01 [N16]
tubulo-renal function, impaired N25.9
specified NEC N25.89
tympanic membrane H73.9- ☑
atrophy — *see* Atrophy, tympanic membrane
infection — *see* Myringitis
perforation — *see* Perforation, tympanum
specified NEC H73.89- ☑
unsocialized aggressive F91.1
urea cycle metabolism E72.20
argininemia E72.21
argininosuccinic aciduria E72.22
citrullinemia E72.23
ornithine transcarbamylase deficiency E72.4
other specified E72.29
ureter (in) N28.9
schistosomiasis B65.0 [N29]
tuberculosis A18.11
urethra N36.9
specified NEC N36.8
urinary system N39.9
specified NEC N39.8
valve, heart
aortic — *see* Endocarditis, aortic
mitral — *see* Endocarditis, mitral
pulmonary — *see* Endocarditis, pulmonary
rheumatic
aortic — *see* Endocarditis, aortic, rheumatic
mitral — *see* Endocarditis, mitral
pulmonary — *see* Endocarditis, pulmonary,
rheumatic
tricuspid — *see* Endocarditis, tricuspid
tricuspid — *see* Endocarditis, tricuspid
vestibular function H81.9- ☑
specified NEC — *see* subcategory H81.8 ☑
in diseases classified elsewhere H82.- ☑
vertigo — *see* Vertigo
vision, binocular H53.30
abnormal retinal correspondence H53.31
diplopia H53.2
fusion with defective stereopsis H53.32
simultaneous perception H53.33
suppression H53.34
visual
cortex
blindness H47.619
left brain H47.612
right brain H47.611
due to
inflammatory disorder H47.629
left brain H47.622
right brain H47.621
neoplasm H47.639
left brain H47.632
right brain H47.631
vascular disorder H47.649
left brain H47.642
right brain H47.641
pathway H47.9
due to
inflammatory disorder H47.51- ☑
neoplasm H47.52- ☑
vascular disorder H47.53- ☑
optic chiasm — *see* Disorder, optic, chiasm
vitreous body H43.9
crystalline deposits — *see* Deposit, crystalline
degeneration — *see* Degeneration, vitreous
hemorrhage — *see* Hemorrhage, vitreous
opacities — *see* Opacity, vitreous
prolapse — *see* Prolapse, vitreous
specified type NEC H43.89
voice R49.9
specified type NEC R49.8
volatile solvent use
due to drug abuse — *see* Abuse, drug, inhalant
due to drug dependence — *see* Dependence, drug,
inhalant
voyeuristic F65.3
white blood cells D72.9
specified NEC D72.89
withdrawing, child or adolescent F40.10
Disorientation R41.0
Displacement, displaced
acquired traumatic of bone, cartilage, joint, tendon
NEC — *see* Dislocation

☑ **Additional Character Required** — **Refer to the Tabular List for Character Selection**   ▽ **Subterms under main terms may continue to next column or page**

Displacement, displaced — *continued*
adrenal gland (congenital) Q89.1
appendix, retrocecal (congenital) Q43.8
auricle (congenital) Q17.4
bladder (acquired) N32.89
   congenital Q64.19
brachial plexus (congenital) Q07.8
brain stem, caudal (congenital) Q04.8
canaliculus (lacrimalis), congenital Q10.6
cardia through esophageal hiatus (congenital) Q40.1
cerebellum, caudal (congenital) Q04.8
cervix — *see* Malposition, uterus
colon (congenital) Q43.3
device, implant or graft (*see also* Complications, by
   site and type, mechanical) T85.628 ☑
   arterial graft NEC — *see* Complication, cardiovas-
     cular device, mechanical, vascular
   breast (implant) T85.42 ☑
   catheter NEC T85.628 ☑
     dialysis (renal) T82.42 ☑
       intraperitoneal T85.621 ☑
     infusion NEC T82.524 ☑
       spinal (epidural) (subdural) T85.620 ☑
     urinary
       cystostomy T83.020 ☑
       Hopkins T83.028 ☑
       ileostomy T83.028 ☑
       indwelling T83.021 ☑
       nephrostomy T83.022 ☑
       specified NEC T83.028 ☑
       urostomy T83.028 ☑
   electronic (electrode) (pulse generator) (stimulator)
     — *see* Complication, electronic stimulator
   fixation, internal (orthopedic) NEC — *see* Compli-
     cation, fixation device, mechanical
   gastrointestinal — *see* Complications, prosthetic
     device, mechanical, gastrointestinal device
   genital NEC T83.428 ☑
     intrauterine contraceptive device (string)
       T83.32 ☑
     penile prosthesis (cylinder) (implanted) (pump)
       (reservoir) T83.420 ☑
     testicular prosthesis T83.421 ☑
   heart NEC — *see* Complication, cardiovascular de-
     vice, mechanical
   joint prosthesis — *see* Complications, joint prosthe-
     sis, mechanical
   ocular — *see* Complications, prosthetic device,
     mechanical, ocular device
   orthopedic NEC — *see* Complication, orthopedic,
     device or graft, mechanical
   specified NEC T85.628 ☑
   urinary NEC T83.128 ☑
     graft T83.22 ☑
     sphincter, implanted T83.121 ☑
     stent (ileal conduit) (nephroureteral) T83.123 ☑
     ureteral indwelling T83.122 ☑
   vascular NEC — *see* Complication, cardiovascular
     device, mechanical
   ventricular intracranial shunt T85.02 ☑
electronic stimulator
   bone T84.320 ☑
   cardiac — *see* Complications, cardiac device, elec-
     tronic
   nervous system — *see* Complication, prosthetic
     device, mechanical, electronic nervous sys-
     tem stimulator
   urinary — *see* Complications, electronic stimulator,
     urinary
esophageal mucosa into cardia of stomach, congenital
   Q39.8
esophagus (acquired) K22.8
   congenital Q39.8
eyeball (acquired) (lateral) (old) — *see* Displacement,
   globe
   congenital Q15.8
   current — *see* Avulsion, eye
fallopian tube (acquired) N83.4- ☑
   congenital Q50.6
   opening Q50.6
gallbladder (congenital) Q44.1
gastric mucosa (congenital) Q40.2
globe (acquired) (old) (lateral) H05.21- ☑
   current — *see* Avulsion, eye
heart (congenital) Q24.8
   acquired I51.89
hymen (upward) (congenital) Q52.4

Displacement, displaced — *continued*
intervertebral disc NEC
   with myelopathy — *see* Disorder, disc, with,
     myelopathy
   cervical, cervicothoracic (with) M50.20
     myelopathy — *see* Disorder, disc, cervical, with
       myelopathy
     neuritis, radiculitis or radiculopathy — *see* Dis-
       order, disc, cervical, with neuritis
   due to trauma — *see* Dislocation, vertebra
   lumbar region M51.26
     with
       myelopathy M51.06
       neuritis, radiculitis, radiculopathy or sciatica
        M51.16
   lumbosacral region M51.27
     with
       neuritis, radiculitis, radiculopathy or sciatica
        M51.17
   sacrococcygeal region M53.3
   thoracic region M51.24
     with
       myelopathy M51.04
       neuritis, radiculitis, radiculopathy M51.14
   thoracolumbar region M51.25
     with
       myelopathy M51.05
       neuritis, radiculitis, radiculopathy M51.15
intrauterine device (string) T83.32 ☑
kidney (acquired) N28.83
   congenital Q63.2
lachrymal, lacrimal apparatus or duct (congenital)
   Q10.6
lens, congenital Q12.1
macula (congenital) Q14.1
Meckel's diverticulum Q43.0
   malignant — *see* Table of Neoplasms, small intes-
     tine, malignant
nail (congenital) Q84.6
   acquired L60.8
opening of Wharton's duct in mouth Q38.4
organ or site, congenital NEC — *see* Malposition,
   congenital
ovary (acquired) N83.4- ☑
   congenital Q50.39
   free in peritoneal cavity (congenital) Q50.39
   into hernial sac N83.4- ☑
oviduct (acquired) N83.4- ☑
   congenital Q50.6
parathyroid (gland) E21.4
parotid gland (congenital) Q38.4
punctum lacrimale (congenital) Q10.6
sacro-iliac (joint) (congenital) Q74.2
   current injury S33.2 ☑
   old — *see* subcategory M53.2 ☑
salivary gland (any) (congenital) Q38.4
spleen (congenital) Q89.09
stomach, congenital Q40.2
sublingual duct Q38.4
tongue (downward) (congenital) Q38.3
tooth, teeth, fully erupted M26.30
   horizontal M26.33
   vertical M26.34
trachea (congenital) Q32.1
ureter or ureteric opening or orifice (congenital)
   Q62.62
uterine opening of oviducts or fallopian tubes Q50.6
uterus, uterine — *see* Malposition, uterus
ventricular septum Q21.0
   with rudimentary ventricle Q20.4
Disproportion
between native and reconstructed breast N65.1
fiber-type G71.2
Disruptio uteri — *see* Rupture, uterus
Disruption (of)
ciliary body NEC H21.89
closure of
   cornea T81.31 ☑
   craniotomy T81.32 ☑
   fascia (muscular) (superficial) T81.32 ☑
   internal organ or tissue T81.32 ☑
   laceration (external) (internal) T81.33 ☑
   ligament T81.32 ☑
   mucosa T81.31 ☑
   muscle or muscle flap T81.32 ☑
   ribs or rib cage T81.32 ☑
   skin and subcutaneous tissue (full-thickness) (su-
     perficial) T81.31 ☑

Disruption — *continued*
closure of — *continued*
   skull T81.32 ☑
   sternum (sternotomy) T81.32 ☑
   tendon T81.32 ☑
   traumatic laceration (external) (internal) T81.33 ☑
family Z63.8
   due to
     absence of family member due to military de-
       ployment Z63.31
     absence of family member NEC Z63.32
     alcoholism and drug addiction in family Z63.72
     bereavement Z63.4
     death (assumed) or disappearance of family
       member Z63.4
     divorce or separation Z63.5
     drug addiction in family Z63.72
     return of family member from military deploy-
       ment (current or past conflict) Z63.71
     stressful life events NEC Z63.79
iris NEC H21.89
ligament(s) (*see also* Sprain)
   knee
     current injury — *see* Dislocation, knee
     old (chronic) — *see* Derangement, knee, insta-
       bility
     spontaneous NEC — *see* Derangement, knee,
       disruption ligament
ossicular chain — *see* Discontinuity, ossicles, ear
pelvic ring (stable) S32.810 ☑
   unstable S32.811 ☑
traumatic injury wound repair T81.33 ☑
wound T81.30 ☑
   episiotomy O90.1
   operation T81.31 ☑
     cesarean O90.0
     external operation wound (superficial)
       T81.31 ☑
     internal operation wound (deep) T81.32 ☑
   perineal (obstetric) O90.1
   traumatic injury repair T81.33 ☑
Dissatisfaction with
employment Z56.9
school environment Z55.4
Dissecting — *see* condition
Dissection
aorta I71.00
   abdominal I71.02
   thoracic I71.01
   thoracoabdominal I71.03
artery I77.70
   basilar (trunk) I77.75
   carotid I77.71
   cerebral (nonruptured) I67.0
     ruptured — *see* Hemorrhage, intracranial,
       subarachnoid
   coronary I25.42
   extremity
     lower I77.77
     upper I77.76
   iliac I77.72
   precerebral
     congenital (nonruptured) Q28.1
     specified site NEC I77.75
   renal I77.73
   specified NEC I77.79
   vertebral I77.74
precerbral artery, congenital (nonruptured) Q28.1
Heartland A93.8
traumatic — *see* Wound, open, by site
vascular I99.8
wound — *see* Wound, open
Disseminated — *see* condition
Dissociation
auriculoventricular or atrioventricular (AV) (any degree) (isorhythmic) I45.89
   with heart block I44.2
interference I45.89
Dissociative reaction, state F44.9
Dissolution, vertebra — *see* Osteoporosis
Distension, distention
abdomen R14.0
bladder N32.89
cecum K63.89
colon K63.89
gallbladder K82.8
intestine K63.89
kidney N28.89

Distension, distention — *continued*
  liver K76.89
  seminal vesicle N50.89
  stomach K31.89
    acute K31.0
    psychogenic F45.8
  ureter — *see* Dilatation, ureter
  uterus N85.8
Distoma hepaticum infestation B66.3
Distomiasis B66.9
  bile passages B66.3
  hemic B65.9
  hepatic B66.3
    due to Clonorchis sinensis B66.1
  intestinal B66.5
  liver B66.3
    due to Clonorchis sinensis B66.1
  lung B66.4
  pulmonary B66.4
Distomolar (fourth molar) K00.1
Disto-occlusion (Division I) (Division II) M26.212
Distortion(s) (congenital)
  adrenal (gland) Q89.1
  arm NEC Q68.8
  bile duct or passage Q44.5
  bladder Q64.79
  brain Q04.9
  cervix (uteri) Q51.9
  chest (wall) Q67.8
    bones Q76.8
  clavicle Q74.0
  clitoris Q52.6
  coccyx Q76.49
  common duct Q44.5
  coronary Q24.5
  cystic duct Q44.5
  ear (auricle) (external) Q17.3
    inner Q16.5
    middle Q16.4
      ossicles Q16.3
  endocrine NEC Q89.2
  eustachian tube Q17.8
  eye (adnexa) Q15.8
  face bone(s) NEC Q75.8
  fallopian tube Q50.6
  femur NEC Q68.8
  fibula NEC Q68.8
  finger(s) Q68.1
  foot Q66.9
  genitalia, genital organ(s)
    female Q52.8
      external Q52.79
      internal NEC Q52.8
  gyri Q04.8
  hand bone(s) Q68.1
  heart (auricle) (ventricle) Q24.8
    valve (cusp) Q24.8
  hepatic duct Q44.5
  humerus NEC Q68.8
  hymen Q52.4
  intrafamilial communications Z63.8
  jaw NEC M26.89
  labium (majus) (minus) Q52.79
  leg NEC Q68.8
  lens Q12.8
  liver Q44.7
  lumbar spine Q76.49
    with disproportion O33.8
      causing obstructed labor O65.0
  lumbosacral (joint) (region) Q76.49
    kyphosis — *see* Kyphosis, congenital
    lordosis — *see* Lordosis, congenital
  nerve Q07.8
  nose Q30.8
  organ
    of Corti Q16.5
    or site not listed — *see* Anomaly, by site
  ossicles, ear Q16.3
  oviduct Q50.6
  pancreas Q45.3
  parathyroid (gland) Q89.2
  pituitary (gland) Q89.2
  radius NEC Q68.8
  sacroiliac joint Q74.2
  sacrum Q76.49
  scapula Q74.0
  shoulder girdle Q74.0
  skull bone(s) NEC Q75.8

Distortion(s) — *continued*
  skull bone(s) — *continued*
    with
      anencephalus Q00.0
      encephalocele — *see* Encephalocele
      hydrocephalus Q03.9
        with spina bifida — *see* Spina bifida, with
          hydrocephalus
      microcephaly Q02
  spinal cord Q06.8
  spine Q76.49
    kyphosis — *see* Kyphosis, congenital
    lordosis — *see* Lordosis, congenital
  spleen Q89.09
  sternum NEC Q76.7
  thorax (wall) Q67.8
    bony Q76.8
  thymus (gland) Q89.2
  thyroid (gland) Q89.2
  tibia NEC Q68.8
  toe(s) Q66.9
  tongue Q38.3
  trachea (cartilage) Q32.1
  ulna NEC Q68.8
  ureter Q62.8
  urethra Q64.79
    causing obstruction Q64.39
  uterus Q51.9
  vagina Q52.4
  vertebra Q76.49
    kyphosis — *see* Kyphosis, congenital
    lordosis — *see* Lordosis, congenital
  visual (*see also* Disturbance, vision)
    shape and size H53.15
  vulva Q52.79
  wrist (bones) (joint) Q68.8
Distress
  abdomen — *see* Pain, abdominal
  acute respiratory R06.03
    syndrome (adult) (child) J80
  epigastric R10.13
  fetal P84
    complicating pregnancy — *see* Stress, fetal
  gastrointestinal (functional) K30
    psychogenic F45.8
  intestinal (functional) NOS K59.9
    psychogenic F45.8
  maternal, during labor and delivery O75.0
  relationship, with spouse or intimate partner Z63.0
  respiratory (adult) (child) R06.03
    newborn P22.9
      specified NEC P22.8
    orthopnea R06.01
    psychogenic F45.8
    shortness of breath R06.02
    specified type NEC R06.09
Distribution vessel, atypical Q27.9
  coronary artery Q24.5
  precerebral Q28.1
Districhiasis L68.8
Disturbance(s) (*see also* Disease)
  absorption K90.9
    calcium E58
    carbohydrate K90.49
    fat K90.49
      pancreatic K90.3
    protein K90.49
    starch K90.49
    vitamin — *see* Deficiency, vitamin
  acid-base equilibrium E87.8
    mixed E87.4
  activity and attention (with hyperkinesis) — *see* Disor-
    der, attention-deficit hyperactivity
  amino acid transport E72.00
  assimilation, food K90.9
  auditory nerve, except deafness — *see* subcategory
    H93.3 ☑
  behavior — *see* Disorder, conduct
  blood clotting (mechanism) (*see also* Defect, coagula-
    tion) D68.9
  cerebral
    nerve — *see* Disorder, nerve, cranial
    status, newborn P91.9
      specified NEC P91.88
  circulatory I99.9
  conduct (*see also* Disorder, conduct) F91.9
    adjustment reaction — *see* Disorder, adjustment
    compulsive F63.9

Disturbance(s) — *continued*
  conduct (*see also* Disorder, conduct) — *continued*
    disruptive F91.9
      hyperkinetic — *see* Disorder, attention-deficit hy-
        peractivity
    socialized F91.2
    specified NEC F91.8
    unsocialized F91.1
  coordination R27.8
  cranial nerve — *see* Disorder, nerve, cranial
  deep sensibility — *see* Disturbance, sensation
  digestive K30
    psychogenic F45.8
  electrolyte (*see also* Imbalance, electrolyte)
    newborn, transitory P74.4
      hyperammonemia P74.6
      potassium balance P74.3
      sodium balance P74.2
      specified type NEC P74.4
  emotions specific to childhood and adolescence F93.9
    with
      anxiety and fearfulness NEC F93.8
      elective mutism F94.0
      oppositional disorder F91.3
      sensitivity (withdrawal) F40.10
      shyness F40.10
      social withdrawal F40.10
    involving relationship problems F93.8
    mixed F93.8
    specified NEC F93.8
  endocrine (gland) E34.9
    neonatal, transitory P72.9
      specified NEC P72.8
  equilibrium R42
  fructose metabolism E74.10
  gait — *see* Gait
    hysterical F44.4
    psychogenic F44.4
  gastrointestinal (functional) K30
    psychogenic F45.8
  habit, child F98.9
  hearing, except deafness and tinnitus — *see* Abnormal,
    auditory perception
  heart, functional (conditions in I44-I50)
    due to presence of (cardiac) prosthesis I97.19- ☑
    postoperative I97.89
      cardiac surgery (*see also* Infarct, myocardium,
        associated with revascularization proce-
        dure) I97.19- ☑
  hormones E34.9
  innervation uterus (parasympathetic) (sympathetic)
    N85.8
  keratinization NEC
    gingiva K05.10
      nonplaque induced K05.11
      plaque induced K05.10
    lip K13.0
    oral (mucosa) (soft tissue) K13.29
    tongue K13.29
  learning (specific) — *see* Disorder, learning
  memory — *see* Amnesia
    mild, following organic brain damage F06.8
  mental F99
    associated with diseases classified elsewhere F54
  metabolism E88.9
    with
      abortion — *see* Abortion, by type with other
        specified complication
      ectopic pregnancy O08.5
      molar pregnancy O08.5
    amino-acid E72.9
      aromatic E70.9
      branched-chain E71.2
      straight-chain E72.8
      sulfur-bearing E72.10
    ammonia E72.20
    arginine E72.21
    arginosuccinic acid E72.22
    carbohydrate E74.9
    cholesterol E78.9
    citrulline E72.23
    cystathionine E72.19
    general E88.9
    glutamine E72.8
    histidine E70.40
    homocystine E72.19
    hydroxylysine E72.3
    in labor or delivery O75.89

Disturbance(s) — *continued*
  metabolism — *continued*
    iron E83.10
    lipoid E78.9
    lysine E72.3
    methionine E72.19
    neonatal, transitory P74.9
      calcium and magnesium P71.9
        specified type NEC P71.8
      carbohydrate metabolism P70.9
        specified type NEC P70.8
      specified NEC P74.8
    ornithine E72.4
    phosphate E83.39
    sodium NEC E87.8
    threonine E72.8
    tryptophan E70.5
    tyrosine E70.20
    urea cycle E72.20
  motor R29.2
  nervous, functional R45.0
  neuromuscular mechanism (eye), due to syphilis A52.15
  nutritional E63.9
    nail L60.3
  ocular motion H51.9
    psychogenic F45.8
  oculogyric H51.8
    psychogenic F45.8
  oculomotor H51.9
    psychogenic F45.8
  olfactory nerve R43.1
  optic nerve NEC — *see* Disorder, nerve, optic
  oral epithelium, including tongue NEC K13.29
  perceptual due to
    alcohol withdrawal F10.232
    amphetamine intoxication F15.922
      in
        abuse F15.122
        dependence F15.222
    anxiolytic withdrawal F13.232
    cannabis intoxication (acute) F12.922
      in
        abuse F12.122
        dependence F12.222
    cocaine intoxication (acute) F14.922
      in
        abuse F14.122
        dependence F14.222
    hypnotic withdrawal F13.232
    opioid intoxication (acute) F11.922
      in
        abuse F11.122
        dependence F11.222
    phencyclidine intoxication (acute) F16.122
    sedative withdrawal F13.232
  personality (pattern) (trait) (*see also* Disorder, personality) F60.9
  following organic brain damage F07.9
  polyglandular E31.9
    specified NEC E31.8
  potassium balance, newborn P74.3
  psychogenic F45.9
  psychomotor F44.4
  psychophysical visual H53.16
  pupillary — *see* Anomaly, pupil, function
  reflex R29.2
  rhythm, heart I49.9
  salivary secretion K11.7
  sensation (cold) (heat) (localization) (tactile discrimination) (texture) (vibratory) NEC R20.9
    hysterical F44.6
    skin R20.9
      anesthesia R20.0
      hyperesthesia R20.3
      hypoesthesia R20.1
      paresthesia R20.2
      specified type NEC R20.8
    smell R43.9
      and taste (mixed) R43.8
      anosmia R43.0
      parosmia R43.1
      specified NEC R43.8
    taste R43.9
      and smell (mixed) R43.8
      parageusia R43.2
      specified NEC R43.8
  sensory — *see* Disturbance, sensation

Disturbance(s) — *continued*
  situational (transient) (*see also* Disorder, adjustment)
    acute F43.0
  sleep G47.9
    nonorganic origin F51.9
  smell — *see* Disturbance, sensation, smell
  sociopathic F60.2
  sodium balance, newborn P74.2
  speech R47.9
    developmental F80.9
    specified NEC R47.89
  stomach (functional) K31.9
  sympathetic (nerve) G90.9
  taste — *see* Disturbance, sensation, taste
  temperature
    regulation, newborn P81.9
      specified NEC P81.8
    sense R20.8
      hysterical F44.6
  tooth
    eruption K00.6
    formation K00.4
    structure, hereditary NEC K00.5
  touch — *see* Disturbance, sensation
  vascular I99.9
    arteriosclerotic — *see* Arteriosclerosis
  vasomotor I73.9
  vasospastic I73.9
  vision, visual H53.9
    following
      cerebral infarction I69.398
      cerebrovascular disease I69.998
        specified NEC I69.898
      intracerebral hemorrhage I69.198
      nontraumatic intracranial hemorrhage NEC I69.298
      specified disease NEC I69.898
      subarachnoid hemorrhage I69.098
    psychophysical H53.16
    specified NEC H53.8
    subjective H53.10
      day blindness H53.11
      discomfort H53.14- ☑
      distortions of shape and size H53.15
      loss
        sudden H53.13- ☑
        transient H53.12- ☑
      specified type NEC H53.19
  voice R49.9
    psychogenic F44.4
    specified NEC R49.8
Diuresis R35.8
Diver's palsy, paralysis or squeeze T70.3 ☑
Diverticulitis (acute) K57.92
  bladder — *see* Cystitis
  ileum — *see* Diverticulitis, intestine, small
  intestine K57.92
    with
      abscess, perforation or peritonitis K57.80
        with bleeding K57.81
      bleeding K57.93
    congenital Q43.8
    large K57.32
      with
        abscess, perforation or peritonitis K57.20
          with bleeding K57.21
        bleeding K57.33
        small intestine K57.52
          with
            abscess, perforation or peritonitis K57.40
              with bleeding K57.41
            bleeding K57.53
    small K57.12
      with
        abscess, perforation or peritonitis K57.00
          with bleeding K57.01
        bleeding K57.13
        large intestine K57.52
          with
            abscess, perforation or peritonitis K57.40
              with bleeding K57.41
            bleeding K57.53
Diverticulosis K57.90
  with bleeding K57.91
  large intestine K57.30

Diverticulosis — *continued*
  large intestine — *continued*
    with
      bleeding K57.31
      small intestine K57.50
        with bleeding K57.51
  small intestine K57.10
    with
      bleeding K57.11
      large intestine K57.50
        with bleeding K57.51
Diverticulum, diverticula (multiple) K57.90
  appendix (noninflammatory) K38.2
  bladder (sphincter) N32.3
    congenital Q64.6
  bronchus (congenital) Q32.4
    acquired J98.09
  calyx, calyceal (kidney) N28.89
  cardia (stomach) K31.4
  cecum — *see* Diverticulosis, intestine, large
    congenital Q43.8
  colon — *see* Diverticulosis, intestine, large
    congenital Q43.8
  duodenum — *see* Diverticulosis, intestine, small
    congenital Q43.8
  epiphrenic (esophagus) K22.5
  esophagus (congenital) Q39.6
    acquired (epiphrenic) (pulsion) (traction) K22.5
  eustachian tube — *see* Disorder, eustachian tube, specified NEC
  fallopian tube N83.8
  gastric K31.4
  heart (congenital) Q24.8
  ileum — *see* Diverticulosis, intestine, small
  jejunum — *see* Diverticulosis, intestine, small
  kidney (pelvis) (calyces) N28.89
    with calculus — *see* Calculus, kidney
  Meckel's (displaced) (hypertrophic) Q43.0
    malignant — *see* Table of Neoplasms, small intestine, malignant
  midthoracic K22.5
  organ or site, congenital NEC — *see* Distortion
  pericardium (congenital) (cyst) Q24.8
    acquired I31.8
  pharyngoesophageal (congenital) Q39.6
    acquired K22.5
  pharynx (congenital) Q38.7
  rectosigmoid — *see* Diverticulosis, intestine, large
    congenital Q43.8
  rectum — *see* Diverticulosis, intestine, large
  Rokitansky's K22.5
  seminal vesicle N50.89
  sigmoid — *see* Diverticulosis, intestine, large
    congenital Q43.8
  stomach (acquired) K31.4
    congenital Q40.2
  trachea (acquired) J39.8
  ureter (acquired) N28.89
    congenital Q62.8
  ureterovesical orifice N28.89
  urethra (acquired) N36.1
    congenital Q64.79
  ventricle, left (congenital) Q24.8
  vesical N32.3
    congenital Q64.6
  Zenker's (esophagus) K22.5
Division
  cervix uteri (acquired) N88.8
  glans penis Q55.69
  labia minora (congenital) Q52.79
  ligament (partial or complete) (current) (*see also* Sprain)
    with open wound — *see* Wound, open
  muscle (partial or complete) (current) (*see also* Injury, muscle)
    with open wound — *see* Wound, open
  nerve (traumatic) — *see* Injury, nerve
  spinal cord — *see* Injury, spinal cord, by region
  vein I87.8
Divorce, causing family disruption Z63.5
Dix-Hallpike neurolabyrinthitis — *see* Neuronitis, vestibular
Dizziness R42
  hysterical F44.89
  psychogenic F45.8
DMAC (disseminated mycobacterium avium- intracellulare complex) A31.2
DNR (do not resuscitate) Z66

Index

Disturbance(s) — DNR

Doan-Wiseman syndrome (primary splenic neutropenia) — see Agranulocytosis
Doehle-Heller aortitis A52.02
Dog bite — see Bite
Dohle body panmyelopathic syndrome D72.0
Dolichocephaly Q67.2
Dolichocolon Q43.8
Dolichostenomelia — see Syndrome, Marfan's
Donohue's syndrome E34.8
Donor (organ or tissue) Z52.9
  blood (whole) Z52.000
    autologous Z52.010
    specified component (lymphocytes) (platelets) NEC Z52.008
      autologous Z52.018
      specified donor NEC Z52.098
    specified donor NEC Z52.090
    stem cells Z52.001
      autologous Z52.011
      specified donor NEC Z52.091
  bone Z52.20
    autologous Z52.21
    marrow 752.3
    specified type NEC Z52.29
  cornea Z52.5
  egg (Oocyte) Z52.819
    age 35 and over Z52.812
      anonymous recipient Z52.812
      designated recipient Z52.813
    under age 35 Z52.810
      anonymous recipient Z52.810
      designated recipient Z52.811
  kidney Z52.4
  liver Z52.6
  lung Z52.89
  lymphocyte — see Donor, blood, specified components NEC
  Oocyte — see Donor, egg
  platelets Z52.008
  potential, examination of Z00.5
  semen Z52.89
  skln Z52.10
    autologous Z52.11
    specified type NEC Z52.19
  specified organ or tissue NEC Z52.89
  sperm Z52.89
Donovanosis A58
Dorsalgia M54.9
  psychogenic F45.41
  specified NEC M54.89
Dorsopathy M53.9
  deforming M43.9
    specified NEC — see subcategory M43.8 ☑
  specified NEC M53.80
    cervical region M53.82
    cervicothoracic region M53.83
    lumbar region M53.86
    lumbosacral region M53.87
    occipito-atlanto-axial region M53.81
    sacrococcygeal region M53.88
    thoracic region M53.84
    thoracolumbar region M53.85
Double
  albumin E88.09
  aortic arch Q25.45
  auditory canal Q17.8
  auricle (heart) Q20.8
  bladder Q64.79
  cervix Q51.820
    with doubling of uterus (and vagina) Q51.10
      with obstruction Q51.11
  inlet ventricle Q20.4
  kidney with double pelvis (renal) Q63.0
  meatus urinarius Q64.75
  monster Q89.4
  outlet
    left ventricle Q20.2
    right ventricle Q20.1
  pelvis (renal) with double ureter Q62.5
  tongue Q38.3
  ureter (one or both sides) Q62.5
    with double pelvis (renal) Q62.5
  urethra Q64.74
  urinary meatus Q64.75
  uterus Q51.2
    with
      doubling of cervix (and vagina) Q51.10
        with obstruction Q51.11

Double — continued
  uterus — continued
    in pregnancy or childbirth O34.59- ☑
      causing obstructed labor O65.5
  vagina Q52.10
    with doubling of uterus (and cervix) Q51.10
      with obstruction Q51.11
  vision H53.2
  vulva Q52.79
Douglas' pouch, cul-de-sac — see condition
Down syndrome Q90.9
  meiotic nondisjunction Q90.0
  mitotic nondisjunction Q90.1
  mosaicism Q90.1
  translocation Q90.2
DPD (dihydropyrimidine dehydrogenase deficiency) E88.89
Dracontiasis B72
Dracunculiasis, dracunculosis B72
Dream state, hysterical F44.89
Drepanocytic anemia — see Disease, sickle-cell
Dresbach's syndrome (elliptocytosis) D58.1
Dreschlera (hawaiiensis) (infection) B43.8
Dressler's syndrome I24.1
Drift, ulnar — see Deformity, limb, specified type NEC, forearm
Drinking (alcohol)
  excessive, to excess NEC (without dependence) F10.10
    habitual (continual) (without remission) F10.20
      with remission F10.21
Drip, postnasal (chronic) R09.82
  due to
    allergic rhinitis — see Rhinitis, allergic
    common cold J00
    gastroesophageal reflux — see Reflux, gastroesophageal
    nasopharyngitis — see Nasopharyngitis
    other known condition — code to condition
    sinusitis — see Sinusitis
Droop
  facial R29.810
    cerebrovascular disease I69.992
      cerebral infarction I69.392
      intracerebral hemorrhage I69.192
      nontraumatic intracranial hemorrhage NEC I69.292
      specified disease NEC I69.892
      subarachnoid hemorrhage I69.092
Drop (in)
  attack NEC R55
  finger — see Deformity, finger
  foot — see Deformity, limb, foot, drop
  hematocrit (precipitous) R71.0
  hemoglobin R71.0
  toe — see Deformity, toe, specified NEC
  wrist — see Deformity, limb, wrist drop
Dropped heart beats I45.9
Dropsy, dropsical (see also Hydrops)
  abdomen R18.8
  brain — see Hydrocephalus
  cardiac, heart — see Failure, heart, congestive
  gangrenous — see Gangrene
  heart — see Failure, heart, congestive
  kidney — see Nephrosis
  lung — see Edema, lung
  newborn due to isoimmunization P56.0
  pericardium — see Pericarditis
Drowned, drowning (near) T75.1 ☑
Drowsiness R40.0
Drug
  abuse counseling and surveillance Z71.51
  addiction — see Dependence
  dependence — see Dependence
  habit — see Dependence
  harmful use — see Abuse, drug
  induced fever R50.2
  overdose — see Table of Drugs and Chemicals, by drug, poisoning
  poisoning — see Table of Drugs and Chemicals, by drug, poisoning
  resistant organism infection (see also Resistant, organism, to, drug) Z16.30
  therapy
    long term (current) (prophylactic) — see Therapy, drug long-term (current) (prophylactic)

Drug — continued
  therapy — continued
    short term — omit code
  wrong substance given or taken in error — see Table of Drugs and Chemicals, by drug, poisoning
Drunkenness (without dependence) F10.129
  acute in alcoholism F10.229
  chronic (without remission) F10.20
    with remission F10.21
  pathological (without dependence) F10.129
    with dependence F10.229
  sleep F51.9
Drusen
  macula (degenerative) (retina) — see Degeneration, macula, drusen
  optic disc H47.32- ☑
Dry, dryness (see also condition)
  larynx J38.7
  mouth R68.2
    due to dehydration E86.0
  nose J34.89
  socket (teeth) M27.3
  throat J39.2
DSAP L56.5
Duane's syndrome H50.81- ☑
Dubin-Johnson disease or syndrome E80.6
Dubois' disease (thymus gland) A50.59 [E35]
Dubowitz' syndrome Q87.1
Duchenne-Aran muscular atrophy G12.21
Duchenne-Griesinger disease G71.0
Duchenne's
  disease or syndrome
    motor neuron disease G12.22
    muscular dystrophy G71.0
  locomotor ataxia (syphilitic) A52.11
  paralysis
    birth injury P14.0
    due to or associated with
      motor neuron disease G12.22
      muscular dystrophy G71.0
Ducrey's chancre A57
Duct, ductus — see condition
Duhring's disease (dermatitis herpetiformis) L13.0
Dullness, cardiac (decreased) (increased) R01.2
Dumb ague — see Malaria
Dumbness — see Aphasia
Dumdum fever B55.0
Dumping syndrome (postgastrectomy) K91.1
Duodenitis (nonspecific) (peptic) K29.80
  with bleeding K29.81
Duodenocholangitis — see Cholangitis
Duodenum, duodenal — see condition
Duplay's bursitis or periarthritis — see Tendinitis, calcific, shoulder
Duplication, duplex (see also Accessory)
  alimentary tract Q45.8
  anus Q43.4
  appendix (and cecum) Q43.4
  biliary duct (any) Q44.5
  bladder Q64.79
  cecum (and appendix) Q43.4
  cervix Q51.820
  chromosome NEC
    with complex rearrangements NEC Q92.5
    seen only at prometaphase Q92.8
  cystic duct Q44.5
  digestive organs Q45.8
  esophagus Q39.8
  frontonasal process Q75.8
  intestine (large) (small) Q43.4
  kidney Q63.0
  liver Q44.7
  pancreas Q45.3
  penis Q55.69
  respiratory organs NEC Q34.8
  salivary duct Q38.4
  spinal cord (incomplete) Q06.2
  stomach Q40.2
Dupré's disease (meningism) R29.1
Dupuytren's contraction or disease M72.0
Durand-Nicolas-Favre disease A55
Durotomy (inadvertent) (incidental) G97.41
Duroziez's disease (congenital mitral stenosis) Q23.2
Dutton's relapsing fever (West African) A68.1
Dwarfism E34.3
  achondroplastic Q77.4
  congenital E34.3
  constitutional E34.3

Dwarfism — *continued*
  hypochondroplastic Q77.4
  hypophyseal E23.0
  infantile E34.3
  Laron-type E34.3
  Lorain (-Levi) type E23.0
  metatropic Q77.8
  nephrotic-glycosuric (with hypophosphatemic rickets) E72.09
  nutritional E45
  pancreatic K86.89
  pituitary E23.0
  renal N25.0
  thanatophoric Q77.1
Dyke-Young anemia (secondary) (symptomatic) D59.1
Dysacusis — *see* Abnormal, auditory perception
Dysadrenocortism E27.9
  hyperfunction E27.0
Dysarthria R47.1
  following
    cerebral infarction I69.322
    cerebrovascular disease I69.922
      specified disease NEC I69.822
    intracerebral hemorrhage I69.122
    nontraumatic intracranial hemorrhage NEC I69.222
    subarachnoid hemorrhage I69.022
Dysautonomia (familial) G90.1
Dysbarism T70.3 ☑
Dysbasia R26.2
  angiosclerotica intermittens I73.9
  hysterical F44.4
  lordotica (progressiva) G24.1
  nonorganic origin F44.4
  psychogenic F44.4
Dysbetalipoproteinemia (familial) E78.2
Dyscalculia R48.8
  developmental F81.2
Dyschezia K59.00
Dyschondroplasia (with hemangiomata) Q78.4
Dyschromia (skin) L81.9
Dyscollagenosis M35.9
Dyscranio-pygo-phalangy Q87.0
Dyscrasia
  blood (with) D75.9
    antepartum hemorrhage — *see* Hemorrhage, antepartum, with coagulation defect
    intrapartum hemorrhage O67.0
    newborn P61.9
      specified type NEC P61.8
    puerperal, postpartum O72.3
    polyglandular, pluriglandular E31.9
Dysendocrinism E34.9
Dysentery, dysenteric (catarrhal) (diarrhea) (epidemic) (hemorrhagic) (infectious) (sporadic) (tropical) A09
  abscess, liver A06.4
  amebic (*see also* Amebiasis) A06.0
    with abscess — *see* Abscess, amebic
    acute A06.0
    chronic A06.1
  arthritis (*see also* category M01) A09
    bacillary (*see also* category M01) A03.9
  bacillary A03.9
    arthritis (*see also* category M01) A03.9
    Boyd A03.2
    Flexner A03.1
    Schmitz (-Stutzer) A03.0
    Shiga (-Kruse) A03.0
    Shigella A03.9
      boydii A03.2
      dysenteriae A03.0
      flexneri A03.1
      group A A03.0
      group B A03.1
      group C A03.2
      group D A03.3
      sonnei A03.3
      specified type NEC A03.8
    Sonne A03.3
    specified type NEC A03.8
  balantidial A07.0
  Balantidium coli A07.0
  Boyd's A03.2
  candidal B37.82
  Chilomastix A07.8
  Chinese A03.9
  coccidial A07.3
  Dientamoeba (fragilis) A07.8
  Embadomonas A07.8

Dysentery, dysenteric — *continued*
  Entamoeba, entamebic — *see* Dysentery, amebic
  Flexner-Boyd A03.2
  Flexner's A03.1
  Giardia lamblia A07.1
  Hiss-Russell A03.1
  Lamblia A07.1
  leishmanial B55.0
  malarial — *see* Malaria
  metazoal B82.0
  monilial B37.82
  protozoal A07.9
  Salmonella A02.0
  schistosomal B65.1
  Schmitz (-Stutzer) A03.0
  Shiga (-Kruse) A03.0
  Shigella NOS — *see* Dysentery, bacillary
  Sonne A03.3
  strongyloidiasis B78.0
  trichomonal A07.8
  viral (*see also* Enteritis, viral) A08.4
Dysequilibrium R42
Dysesthesia R20.8
  hysterical F44.6
Dysfibrinogenemia (congenital) D68.2
Dysfunction
  adrenal E27.9
    hyperfunction E27.0
  autonomic
    due to alcohol G31.2
    somatoform F45.8
  bladder N31.9
    neurogenic NOS — *see* Dysfunction, bladder, neuromuscular
    neuromuscular NOS N31.9
      atonic (motor) (sensory) N31.2
      autonomous N31.2
      flaccid N31.2
      nonreflex N31.2
      reflex N31.1
      specified NEC N31.8
      uninhibited N31.0
  bleeding, uterus N93.8
  cerebral G93.89
  colon K59.9
    psychogenic F45.8
  colostomy K94.03
  cystic duct K82.8
  cystostomy (stoma) — *see* Complications, cystostomy
  ejaculatory N53.19
    anejaculatory orgasm N53.13
    painful N53.12
    premature F52.4
    retarded N53.11
  endocrine NOS E34.9
  endometrium N85.8
  enterostomy K94.13
  erectile — *see* Dysfunction, sexual, male, erectile
  gallbladder K82.8
  gastrostomy (stoma) K94.23
  gland, glandular NOS E34.9
  heart I51.89
  hemoglobin D75.89
  hepatic K76.89
  hypophysis E23.7
  hypothalamic NEC E23.3
  ileostomy (stoma) K94.13
  jejunostomy (stoma) K94.13
  kidney — *see* Disease, renal
  labyrinthine — *see* subcategory H83.2 ☑
  left ventricular, following sudden emotional stress I51.81
  liver K76.89
  male — *see* Dysfunction, sexual, male
  orgasmic (female) F52.31
    male F52.32
  ovary E28.9
    specified NEC E28.8
  papillary muscle I51.89
  parathyroid E21.4
  physiological NEC R68.89
    psychogenic F59
  pineal gland E34.8
  pituitary (gland) E23.3
  platelets D69.1
  polyglandular E31.9
    specified NEC E31.8
  psychophysiologic F59

Dysfunction — *continued*
  psychosexual F52.9
    with
      dyspareunia F52.6
      premature ejaculation F52.4
      vaginismus F52.5
  pylorus K31.9
  rectum K59.9
    psychogenic F45.8
  reflex (sympathetic) — *see* Syndrome, pain, complex regional I
  segmental — *see* Dysfunction, somatic
  senile R54
  sexual (due to) R37
    alcohol F10.981
    amphetamine F15.981
      in
        abuse F15.181
        dependence F15.281
    anxiolytic F13.981
      in
        abuse F13.181
        dependence F13.281
    cocaine F14.981
      in
        abuse F14.181
        dependence F14.281
    excessive sexual drive F52.8
    failure of genital response (male) F52.21
      female F52.22
    female N94.9
      aversion F52.1
      dyspareunia N94.10
        psychogenic F52.6
      frigidity F52.22
      nymphomania F52.8
      orgasmic F52.31
      psychogenic F52.9
        aversion F52.1
        dyspareunia F52.6
        frigidity F52.22
        nymphomania F52.8
        orgasmic F52.31
        vaginismus F52.5
      vaginismus N94.2
        psychogenic F52.5
    hypnotic F13.981
      in
        abuse F13.181
        dependence F13.281
    inhibited orgasm (female) F52.31
      male F52.32
    lack
      of sexual enjoyment F52.1
      or loss of sexual desire F52.0
    male N53.9
      anejaculatory orgasm N53.13
      ejaculatory N53.19
        painful N53.12
        premature F52.4
        retarded N53.11
      erectile N52.9
        drug induced N52.2
        due to
          disease classified elsewhere N52.1
          drug N52.2
        postoperative (postprocedural) N52.39
          following
            cryotherapy N52.37
            interstitial seed therapy N52.36
            prostate ablative therapy N52.37
            prostatectomy N52.34
              radical N52.31
            radiation therapy N52.35
            radical cystectomy N52.32
            ultrasound ablative therapy N52.37
            urethral surgery N52.33
        psychogenic F52.21
        specified cause NEC N52.8
        vasculogenic
          arterial insufficiency N52.01
            with corporo-venous occlusive N52.03
          corporo-venous occlusive N52.02
            with arterial insufficiency N52.03
      impotence — *see* Dysfunction, sexual, male, erectile
    psychogenic F52.9
      aversion F52.1

Dysfunction — continued
  sexual — continued
    male — continued
      psychogenic — continued
        erectile F52.21
        orgasmic F52.32
        premature ejaculation F52.4
        satyriasis F52.8
        specified type NEC F52.8
      specified type NEC N53.8
    nonorganic F52.9
      specified NEC F52.8
    opioid F11.981
      in
        abuse F11.181
        dependence F11.281
    orgasmic dysfunction (female) F52.31
      male F52.32
    premature ejaculation F52.4
    psychoactive substances NEC F19.981
      in
        abuse F19.181
        dependence F19.281
    psychogenic F52.9
    sedative F13.981
      in
        abuse F13.181
        dependence F13.281
    sexual aversion F52.1
    vaginismus (nonorganic) (psychogenic) F52.5
  sinoatrial node I49.5
  somatic M99.09
    abdomen M99.09
    acromioclavicular M99.07
    cervical region M99.01
    cervicothoracic M99.01
    costochondral M99.08
    costovertebral M99.08
    head region M99.00
    hip M99.05
    lower extremity M99.06
    lumbar region M99.03
    lumbosacral M99.03
    occipitocervical M99.00
    pelvic region M99.05
    pubic M99.05
    rib cage M99.08
    sacral region M99.04
    sacrococcygeal M99.04
    sacroiliac M99.04
    specified NEC M99.09
    sternochondral M99.08
    sternoclavicular M99.07
    thoracic region M99.02
    thoracolumbar M99.02
    upper extremity M99.07
  somatoform autonomic F45.8
  stomach K31.89
    psychogenic F45.8
  suprarenal E27.9
    hyperfunction E27.0
  symbolic R48.9
    specified type NEC R48.8
  temporomandibular (joint) M26.69
    joint-pain syndrome M26.62- ☑
  testicular (endocrine) E29.9
    specified NEC E29.8
  thymus E32.9
  thyroid E07.9
  ureterostomy (stoma) — see Complications, stoma, urinary tract
  urethrostomy (stoma) — see Complications, stoma, urinary tract
  uterus, complicating delivery O62.9
    hypertonic O62.4
    hypotonic O62.2
      primary O62.0
      secondary O62.1
  ventricular I51.9
    with congestive heart failure (see also Failure, heart) I50.9
    left, reversible, following sudden emotional stress I51.81
Dysgenesis
  gonadal (due to chromosomal anomaly) Q96.9
    pure Q99.1
  renal Q60.5
    bilateral Q60.4
    unilateral Q60.3

Dysgenesis — continued
  reticular D72.0
  tidal platelet D69.3
Dysgerminoma
  specified site — see Neoplasm, malignant, by site
  unspecified site
    female C56.9
    male C62.90
Dysgeusia R43.2
Dysgraphia R27.8
Dyshidrosis, dysidrosis L30.1
Dyskaryotic cervical smear R87.619
Dyskeratosis L85.8
  cervix — see Dysplasia, cervix
  congenital Q82.8
  uterus NEC N85.8
Dyskinesia G24.9
  biliary (cystic duct or gallbladder) K82.8
  drug induced
    orofacial G24.01
  esophagus K22.4
  hysterical F44.4
  intestinal K59.8
  nonorganic origin F44.4
  orofacial (idiopathic) G24.4
    drug induced G24.01
  psychogenic F44.4
  subacute, drug induced G24.01
  tardive G24.01
    neuroleptic induced G24.01
  trachea J39.8
  tracheobronchial J98.09
Dyslalia (developmental) F80.0
Dyslexia R48.0
  developmental F81.0
Dyslipidemia E78.5
  depressed HDL cholesterol E78.6
  elevated fasting triglycerides E78.1
Dysmaturity (see also Light for dates)
  pulmonary (newborn) (Wilson-Mikity) P27.0
Dysmenorrhea (essential) (exfoliative) N94.6
  congestive (syndrome) N94.6
  primary N94.4
  psychogenic F45.8
  secondary N94.5
Dysmetabolic syndrome X E88.81
Dysmetria R27.8
Dysmorphism (due to)
  alcohol Q86.0
  exogenous cause NEC Q86.8
  hydantoin Q86.1
  warfarin Q86.2
Dysmorphophobia (nondelusional) F45.22
  delusional F22
Dysnomia R47.01
Dysorexia R63.0
  psychogenic F50.89
Dysostosis
  cleidocranial, cleidocranialis Q74.0
  craniofacial Q75.1
  Fairbank's (idiopathic familial generalized osteophyto-sis) Q78.9
  mandibulofacial (incomplete) Q75.4
  multiplex E76.01
  oculomandibular Q75.5
Dyspareunia (female) N94.10
  deep N94.12
  male N53.12
  nonorganic F52.6
  psychogenic F52.6
  secondary N94.19
  specified NEC N94.19
  superficial (introital) N94.11
Dyspepsia R10.13
  atonic K30
  functional (allergic) (congenital) (gastrointestinal) (occupational) (reflex) K30
  intestinal K59.8
  nervous F45.8
  neurotic F45.8
  psychogenic F45.8
Dysphagia R13.10
  cervical R13.19
  following
    cerebral infarction I69.391
    cerebrovascular disease I69.991
      specified NEC I69.891
    intracerebral hemorrhage I69.191

Dysphagia — continued
  following — continued
    nontraumatic intracranial hemorrhage NEC I69.291
    specified disease NEC I69.891
    subarachnoid hemorrhage I69.091
  functional (hysterical) F45.8
  hysterical F45.8
  nervous (hysterical) F45.8
  neurogenic R13.19
  oral phase R13.11
  oropharyngeal phase R13.12
  pharyngeal phase R13.13
  pharyngoesophageal phase R13.14
  psychogenic F45.8
  sideropenic D50.1
  spastica K22.4
  specified NEC R13.19
Dysphagocytosis, congenital D71
Dysphasia R47.02
  developmental
    expressive type F80.1
    receptive type F80.2
  following
    cerebrovascular disease I69.921
      cerebral infarction I69.321
      intracerebral hemorrhage I69.121
      nontraumatic intracranial hemorrhage NEC I69.221
      specified disease NEC I69.821
      subarachnoid hemorrhage I69.021
Dysphonia R49.0
  functional F44.4
  hysterical F44.4
  psychogenic F44.4
  spastica J38.3
Dysphoria
  gender F64.9
    in
      adolescence and adulthood F64.0
      children F64.2
    specified NEC F64.8
  postpartal O90.6
Dyspituitarism E23.3
Dysplasia (see also Anomaly)
  acetabular, congenital Q65.89
  alveolar capillary, with vein misalignment J84.843
  anus (histologically confirmed) (mild) (moderate) K62.82
    severe D01.3
  arrhythmogenic right ventricular I42.8
  arterial, fibromuscular I77.3
  asphyxiating thoracic (congenital) Q77.2
  brain Q07.9
  bronchopulmonary, perinatal P27.1
  cervix (uteri) N87.9
    mild N87.0
    moderate N87.1
    severe D06.9
  chondroectodermal Q77.6
  colon D12.6
  craniometaphyseal Q78.8
  dentinal K00.5
  diaphyseal, progressive Q78.3
  dystrophic Q77.5
  ectodermal (anhidrotic) (congenital) (hereditary) Q82.4
    hydrotic Q82.8
  epithelial, uterine cervix — see Dysplasia, cervix
  eye (congenital) Q11.2
  fibrous
    bone NEC (monostotic) M85.00
      ankle M85.07- ☑
      foot M85.07- ☑
      forearm M85.03- ☑
      hand M85.04- ☑
      lower leg M85.06- ☑
      multiple site M85.09
      neck M85.08
      rib M85.08
      shoulder M85.01- ☑
      skull M85.08
      specified site NEC M85.08
      thigh M85.05- ☑
      toe M85.07- ☑
      upper arm M85.02- ☑
      vertebra M85.08
    diaphyseal, progressive Q78.3
    jaw M27.8
    polyostotic Q78.1

Dysplasia — continued
  florid osseous (see also Cyst, calcifying odontogenic)
  high grade, focal D12.6
  hip, congenital Q65.89
  joint, congenital Q74.8
  kidney Q61.4
    multicystic Q61.4
  leg Q74.2
  lung, congenital (not associated with short gestation)
    Q33.6
  mammary (gland) (benign) N60.9- ☑
    cyst (solitary) — see Cyst, breast
    cystic — see Mastopathy, cystic
    duct ectasia — see Ectasia, mammary duct
    fibroadenosis — see Fibroadenosis, breast
    fibrosclerosis — see Fibrosclerosis, breast
    specified type NEC N60.8- ☑
  metaphyseal Q78.5
  muscle Q79.8
  oculodentodigital Q87.0
  periapical (cemental) (cemento-osseous) — see Cyst,
    calcifying odontogenic
  periosteum — see Disorder, bone, specified type NEC
  polyostotic fibrous Q78.1
  prostate (see also Neoplasia, intraepithelial, prostate)
    N42.30
    severe D07.5
    specified NEC N42.39
  renal Q61.4
    multicystic Q61.4
  retinal, congenital Q14.1
  right ventricular, arrhythmogenic I42.8
  septo-optic Q04.4
  skin L98.8
  spinal cord Q06.1
  spondyloepiphyseal Q77.7
  thymic, with immunodeficiency D82.1
  vagina N89.3
    mild N89.0
    moderate N89.1
    severe NEC D07.2
  vulva N90.3
    mild N90.0
    moderate N90.1
    severe NEC D07.1
Dyspnea (nocturnal) (paroxysmal) R06.00
  asthmatic (bronchial) J45.909
    with
      bronchitis J45.909
        with
          exacerbation (acute) J45.901
          status asthmaticus J45.902
        chronic J44.9
      exacerbation (acute) J45.901
      status asthmaticus J45.902
    cardiac — see Failure, ventricular, left
  cardiac — see Failure, ventricular, left
  functional F45.8
  hyperventilation R06.4
  hysterical F45.8
  newborn P28.89
  orthopnea R06.01
  psychogenic F45.8
  shortness of breath R06.02
  specified type NEC R06.09
Dyspraxia R27.8
  developmental (syndrome) F82
Dysproteinemia E88.09
Dysreflexia, autonomic G90.4
Dysrhythmia
  cardiac I49.9
    newborn
      bradycardia P29.12
      occurring before birth P03.819
        before onset of labor P03.810
        during labor P03.811
      tachycardia P29.11
    postoperative I97.89
  cerebral or cortical — see Epilepsy
Dyssomnia — see Disorder, sleep
Dyssynergia
  biliary K83.8
  bladder sphincter N36.44
  cerebellaris myoclonica (Hunt's ataxia) G11.1
Dysthymia F34.1
Dysthyroidism E07.9
Dystocia O66.9
  affecting newborn P03.1

Dystocia — continued
  cervical (hypotonic) O62.2
    affecting newborn P03.6
    primary O62.0
    secondary O62.1
  contraction ring O62.4
  fetal O66.9
    abnormality NEC O66.3
    conjoined twins O66.3
    oversize O66.2
  maternal O66.9
  positional O64.9 ☑
  shoulder (girdle) O66.0
    causing obstructed labor O66.0
  uterine NEC O62.4
Dystonia G24.9
  deformans progressiva G24.1
  drug induced NEC G24.09
    acute G24.02
    specified NEC G24.09
  familial G24.1
  idiopathic G24.1
    familial G24.1
    nonfamilial G24.2
    orofacial G24.4
  lenticularis G24.8
  musculorum deformans G24.1
  neuroleptic induced (acute) G24.02
  orofacial (idiopathic) G24.4
  oromandibular G24.4
    due to drug G24.01
  specified NEC G24.8
  torsion (familial) (idiopathic) G24.1
    acquired G24.8
    genetic G24.1
    symptomatic (nonfamilial) G24.2
Dystonic movements R25.8
Dystrophy, dystrophia
  adiposogenital E23.6
  Becker's type G71.0
  cervical sympathetic G90.2
  choroid (hereditary) H31.20
    central areolar H31.22
    choroideremia H31.21
    gyrate atrophy H31.23
    specified type NEC H31.29
  cornea (hereditary) H18.50
    endothelial H18.51
    epithelial H18.52
    granular H18.53
    lattice H18.54
    macular H18.55
    specified type NEC H18.59
  Duchenne's type G71.0
  due to malnutrition E45
  Erb's G71.0
  Fuchs' H18.51
  Gower's muscular G71.0
  hair L67.8
  infantile neuraxonal G31.89
  Landouzy-Déjérine G71.0
  Leyden-Möbius G71.0
  muscular G71.0
    benign (Becker type) G71.0
    congenital (hereditary) (progressive) (with specific
      morphological abnormalities of the muscle
      fiber) G71.0
      myotonic G71.11
    distal G71.0
    Duchenne type G71.0
    Emery-Dreifuss G71.0
    Erb type G71.0
    facioscapulohumeral G71.0
    Gower's G71.0
    hereditary (progressive) G71.0
    Landouzy-Déjérine type G71.0
    limb-girdle G71.0
    myotonic G71.11
    progressive (hereditary) G71.0
      Charcot-Marie (-Tooth) type G60.0
    pseudohypertrophic (infantile) G71.0
    severe (Duchenne type) G71.0
  myocardium, myocardial — see Degeneration, myocar-
    dial
  nail L60.3
    congenital Q84.6
  nutritional E45
  ocular G71.0
  oculocerebrorenal E72.03

Dystrophy, dystrophia — continued
  oculopharyngeal G71.0
  ovarian N83.8
  polyglandular E31.8
  reflex (neuromuscular) (sympathetic) — see Syndrome,
    pain, complex regional I
  retinal (hereditary) H35.50
    in
      lipid storage disorders E75.6 [H36]
      systemic lipidoses E75.6 [H36]
    involving
      pigment epithelium H35.54
      sensory area H35.53
    pigmentary H35.52
    vitreoretinal H35.51
  Salzmann's nodular — see Degeneration, cornea,
    nodular
  scapuloperoneal G71.0
  skin NEC L98.8
  sympathetic (reflex) — see Syndrome, pain, complex
    regional I
    cervical G90.2
  tapetoretinal H35.54
  thoracic, asphyxiating Q77.2
  unguium L60.3
    congenital Q84.6
  vitreoretinal H35.51
  vulva N90.4
  yellow (liver) — see Failure, hepatic
Dysuria R30.0
  psychogenic F45.8

E

Eales' disease H35.06- ☑
Ear (see also condition)
  piercing Z41.3
  tropical NEC B36.9 [H62.40]
    in
      aspergillosis B44.89
      candidiasis B37.84
      moniliasis B37.84
  wax (impacted) H61.20
    left H61.22
      with right H61.23
    right H61.21
      with left H61.23
Earache — see subcategory H92.0 ☑
Early satiety R68.81
Eaton-Lambert syndrome — see Syndrome, Lambert-
  Eaton
Eberth's disease (typhoid fever) A01.00
Ebola virus disease A98.4
Ebstein's anomaly or syndrome (heart) Q22.5
Eccentro-osteochondrodysplasia E76.29
Ecchondroma — see Neoplasm, bone, benign
Ecchondrosis D48.0
Ecchymosis R58
  conjunctiva — see Hemorrhage, conjunctiva
  eye (traumatic) — see Contusion, eyeball
  eyelid (traumatic) — see Contusion, eyelid
  newborn P54.5
  spontaneous R23.3
  traumatic — see Contusion
Echinococciasis — see Echinococcus
Echinococcosis — see Echinococcus
Echinococcus (infection) B67.90
  granulosus B67.4
    bone B67.2
    liver B67.0
    lung B67.1
    multiple sites B67.32
    specified site NEC B67.39
    thyroid B67.31
  liver NOS B67.8
    granulosus B67.0
    multilocularis B67.5
  lung NEC B67.99
    granulosus B67.1
    multilocularis B67.69
  multilocularis B67.7
    liver B67.5
    multiple sites B67.61
    specified site NEC B67.69
  specified site NEC B67.99
    granulosus B67.39
    multilocularis B67.69
  thyroid NEC B67.99

Echinococcus — *continued*
  thyroid — *continued*
    granulosus B67.31
    multilocularis B67.69 [E35]
Echinorhynchiasis B83.8
Echinostomiasis B66.8
Echolalia R48.8
Echovirus, as cause of disease classified elsewhere
  B97.12
Eclampsia, eclamptic (coma) (convulsions) (delirium)
  (with hypertension) NEC O15.9
  complicating
    labor and delivery O15.1
    postpartum O15.2
    pregnancy O15.0- ☑
    puerperium O15.2
Economic circumstances affecting care Z59.9
Economo's disease A85.8
Ectasia, ectasis
  annuloaortic I35.8
  aorta I77.819
    with aneurysm — *see* Aneurysm, aorta
    abdominal I77.811
    thoracic I77.810
    thoracoabdominal I77.812
  breast — *see* Ectasia, mammary duct
  capillary I78.8
  cornea H18.71- ☑
  gastric antral vascular (GAVE) K31.819
    with hemorrhage K31.811
    without hemorrhage K31.819
  mammary duct N60.4- ☑
  salivary gland (duct) K11.8
  sclera — *see* Sclerectasia
Ecthyma L08.0
  contagiosum B08.02
  gangrenosum L08.0
  infectiosum B08.02
Ectocardia Q24.8
Ectodermal dysplasia (anhidrotic) Q82.4
Ectodermosis erosiva pluriorificialis L51.1
Ectoplc, ectopia (congenital)
  abdominal viscera Q45.8
    due to defect in anterior abdominal wall Q79.59
  ACTH syndrome E24.3
  adrenal gland Q89.1
  anus Q43.5
  atrial beats I49.1
  beats I49.49
    atrial I49.1
    ventricular I49.3
  bladder Q64.10
  bone and cartilage in lung Q33.5
  brain Q04.8
  breast tissue Q83.8
  cardiac Q24.8
  cerebral Q04.8
  cordis Q24.8
  endometrium — *see* Endometriosis
  gastric mucosa Q40.2
  gestation — *see* Pregnancy, by site
  heart Q24.8
  hormone secretion NEC E34.2
  kidney (crossed) (pelvis) Q63.2
  lens, lentis Q12.1
  mole — *see* Pregnancy, by site
  organ or site NEC — *see* Malposition, congenital
  pancreas Q45.3
  pregnancy — *see* Pregnancy, ectopic
  pupil — *see* Abnormality, pupillary
  renal Q63.2
  sebaceous glands of mouth Q38.6
  spleen Q89.09
  testis Q53.00
    bilateral Q53.02
    unilateral Q53.01
  thyroid Q89.2
  tissue in lung Q33.5
  ureter Q62.63
  ventricular beats I49.3
  vesicae Q64.10
Ectromelia Q73.8
  lower limb — *see* Defect, reduction, limb, lower,
    specified type NEC
  upper limb — *see* Defect, reduction, limb, upper,
    specified type NEC
Ectropion H02.109
  cervix N86

Ectropion — *continued*
  cervix — *continued*
    with cervicitis N72
  congenital Q10.1
  eyelid (paralytic) H02.109
    cicatricial H02.119
      left H02.116
        lower H02.115
        upper H02.114
      right H02.113
        lower H02.112
        upper H02.111
    congenital Q10.1
    left H02.106
      lower H02.105
      upper H02.104
    mechanical H02.129
      left H02.126
        lower H02.125
        upper H02.124
      right H02.123
        lower H02.122
        upper H02.121
    right H02.103
      lower H02.102
      upper H02.101
    senile H02.139
      left H02.136
        lower H02.135
        upper H02.134
      right H02.133
        lower H02.132
        upper H02.131
    spastic H02.149
      left H02.146
        lower H02.145
        upper H02.144
      right H02.143
        lower H02.142
        upper H02.141
  iris H21.89
  lip (acquired) K13.0
    congenital Q38.0
  urethra N36.8
  uvea H21.89
Eczema (acute) (chronic) (erythematous) (fissum)
  (rubrum) (squamous) (*see also* Dermatitis) L30.9
  contact — *see* Dermatitis, contact
  dyshydrotic L30.1
  external ear — *see* Otitis, externa, acute, eczematoid
  flexural L20.82
  herpeticum B00.0
  hypertrophicum L28.0
  hypostatic — *see* Varix, leg, with, inflammation
  impetiginous L01.1
  infantile (due to any substance) L20.83
    intertriginous L21.1
    seborrheic L21.1
  intertriginous NEC L30.4
    infantile L21.1
  intrinsic (allergic) L20.84
  lichenified NEC L28.0
  marginatum (hebrae) B35.6
  pustular L30.3
  stasis I87.2
    with varicose veins — *see* Varix, leg, with, inflam-
      mation
  vaccination, vaccinatum T88.1 ☑
  varicose — *see* Varix, leg, with, inflammation
Eczematid L30.2
Eddowes (-Spurway) **syndrome** Q78.0
Edema, edematous (infectious) (pitting) (toxic) R60.9
  with nephritis — *see* Nephrosis
  allergic T78.3 ☑
  amputation stump (surgical) (sequelae (late effect))
    T87.89
  angioneurotic (allergic) (any site) (with urticaria)
    T78.3 ☑
    hereditary D84.1
  angiospastic I73.9
  Berlin's (traumatic) S05.8X- ☑
  brain (cytotoxic) (vasogenic) G93.6
    due to birth injury P11.0
    newborn (anoxia or hypoxia) P52.4
      birth injury P11.0
    traumatic — *see* Injury, intracranial, cerebral edema
  cardiac — *see* Failure, heart, congestive
  cardiovascular — *see* Failure, heart, congestive

Edema, edematous — *continued*
  cerebral — *see* Edema, brain
  cerebrospinal — *see* Edema, brain
  cervix (uteri) (acute) N88.8
    puerperal, postpartum O90.89
  chronic hereditary Q82.0
  circumscribed, acute T78.3 ☑
    hereditary D84.1
  conjunctiva H11.42- ☑
  cornea H18.2- ☑
    idiopathic H18.22- ☑
    secondary H18.23- ☑
      due to contact lens H18.21- ☑
  due to
    lymphatic obstruction I89.0
    salt retention E87.0
  epiglottis — *see* Edema, glottis
  essential, acute T78.3 ☑
    hereditary D84.1
  extremities, lower — *see* Edema, legs
  eyelid NEC H02.849
    left H02.846
      lower H02.845
      upper H02.844
    right H02.843
      lower H02.842
      upper H02.841
  familial, hereditary Q82.0
  famine — *see* Malnutrition, severe
  generalized R60.1
  glottis, glottic, glottidis (obstructive) (passive) J38.4
    allergic T78.3 ☑
      hereditary D84.1
  heart — *see* Failure, heart, congestive
  heat T67.7 ☑
  hereditary Q82.0
  inanition — *see* Malnutrition, severe
  intracranial G93.6
  iris H21.89
  joint — *see* Effusion, joint
  larynx — *see* Edema, glottis
  legs R60.0
    due to venous obstruction I87.1
    hereditary Q82.0
  localized R60.0
    due to venous obstruction I87.1
  lower limbs — *see* Edema, legs
  lung J81.1
    with heart condition or failure — *see* Failure, ven-
      tricular, left
    acute J81.0
      chemical (acute) J68.1
        chronic J68.1
      chronic J81.1
        due to
          chemicals, gases, fumes or vapors (inhala-
            tion) J68.1
          external agent J70.9
            specified NEC J70.8
          radiation J70.1
      due to
        chemicals, fumes or vapors (inhalation) J68.1
        external agent J70.9
          specified NEC J70.8
        high altitude T70.29 ☑
        near drowning T75.1 ☑
        radiation J70.0
    meaning failure, left ventricle I50.1
  lymphatic I89.0
    due to mastectomy I97.2
  macula H35.81
    cystoid, following cataract surgery — *see* Compli-
      cations, postprocedural, following cataract
      surgery
    diabetic — *see* Diabetes, by type, with, retinopathy,
      with macular edema
  malignant — *see* Gangrene, gas
  Milroy's Q82.0
  nasopharynx J39.2
  newborn P83.30
    hydrops fetalis — *see* Hydrops, fetalis
    specified NEC P83.39
  nutritional (*see also* Malnutrition, severe)
    with dyspigmentation, skin and hair E40
  optic disc or nerve — *see* Papilledema
  orbit H05.22- ☑
  pancreas K86.89
  papilla, optic — *see* Papilledema

Index

Elephantiasis — continued
- eyelid — continued
  - right — continued
    - upper H02.851
  - filarial, filariensis — see Infestation, filarial
  - glandular I89.0
  - graecorum A30.9
  - lymphangiectatic I89.0
  - lymphatic vessel I89.0
    - due to mastectomy I97.2
  - scrotum (nonfilarial) I89.0
  - streptococcal I89.0
  - surgical I97.89
    - postmastectomy I97.2
  - telangiectodes I89.0
  - vulva (nonfilarial) N90.89

Elevated, elevation
- antibody titer R76.0
- basal metabolic rate R94.8
- blood pressure (see also Hypertension)
  - reading (incidental) (isolated) (nonspecific), no diagnosis of hypertension R03.0
- blood sugar R73.9
- body temperature (of unknown origin) R50.9
- cancer antigen 125 [CA 125] R97.1
- carcinoembryonic antigen [CEA] R97.0
- cholesterol E78.00
  - with high triglycerides E78.2
- conjugate, eye H51.0
- C-reactive protein (CRP) R79.82
- diaphragm, congenital Q79.1
- erythrocyte sedimentation rate R70.0
- fasting glucose R73.01
- fasting triglycerides E78.1
- finding on laboratory examination — see Findings, abnormal, inconclusive, without diagnosis, by type of exam
- GFR (glomerular filtration rate) — see Findings, abnormal, inconclusive, without diagnosis, by type of exam
- glucose tolerance (oral) R73.02
- immunoglobulin level R76.8
- indoleacetic acid R82.5
- lactic acid dehydrogenase (LDH) level R74.0
- leukocytes D72.829
- lipoprotein a level E78.8 ☑
- liver function
  - study R94.5
  - test R79.89
    - alkaline phosphatase R74.8
    - aminotransferase R74.0
    - bilirubin R17
    - hepatic enzyme R74.8
    - lactate dehydrogenase R74.0
- lymphocytes D72.820
- prostate specific antigen [PSA] R97.20
- Rh titer — see Complication(s), transfusion, incompatibility reaction, Rh (factor)
- scapula, congenital Q74.0
- sedimentation rate R70.0
- SGOT R74.0
- SGPT R74.0
- transaminase level R74.0
- triglycerides E78.1
  - with high cholesterol E78.2
- tumor associated antigens [TAA] NEC R97.8
- tumor specific antigens [TSA] NEC R97.8
- urine level of
  - 17-ketosteroids R82.5
  - catecholamine R82.5
  - indoleacetic acid R82.5
  - steroids R82.5
  - vanillylmandelic acid (VMA) R82.5
- venous pressure I87.8
- white blood cell count D72.829
  - specified NEC D72.828

Elliptocytosis (congenital) (hereditary) D58.1
- Hb C (disease) D58.1
- hemoglobin disease D58.1
- sickle-cell (disease) D57.8- ☑
  - trait D57.3

Ellison-Zollinger syndrome E16.4
Ellis-van Creveld syndrome (chondroectodermal dysplasia) Q77.6
Elongated, elongation (congenital) (see also Distortion)
- bone Q79.9
- cervix (uteri) Q51.828
  - acquired N88.4

Elongated, elongation — continued
- cervix — continued
  - hypertrophic N88.4
- colon Q43.8
- common bile duct Q44.5
- cystic duct Q44.5
- frenulum, penis Q55.69
- labia minora (acquired) N90.69
- ligamentum patellae Q74.1
- petiolus (epiglottidis) Q31.8
- tooth, teeth K00.2
- uvula Q38.6

Eltor cholera A00.1
Emaciation (due to malnutrition) E41
Embadomoniasis A07.8
Embedded tooth, teeth K01.0
- root only K08.3

Embolic — see condition
Embolism (multiple) (paradoxical) I74.9
- air (any site) (traumatic) T79.0 ☑
  - following
    - abortion — see Abortion by type complicated by embolism
    - ectopic pregnancy O08.2
    - infusion, therapeutic injection or transfusion T80.0 ☑
    - molar pregnancy O08.2
    - procedure NEC
      - artery T81.719 ☑
        - mesenteric T81.710 ☑
        - renal T81.711 ☑
        - specified NEC T81.718 ☑
      - vein T81.72 ☑
  - in pregnancy, childbirth or puerperium — see Embolism, obstetric
- amniotic fluid (pulmonary) (see also Embolism, obstetric)
  - following
    - abortion — see Abortion by type complicated by embolism
    - ectopic pregnancy O08.2
    - molar pregnancy O08.2
- aorta, aortic I74.10
  - abdominal I74.09
    - saddle I74.01
  - bifurcation I74.09
  - saddle I74.01
  - thoracic I74.11
- artery I74.9
  - auditory, internal I65.8
  - basilar — see Occlusion, artery, basilar
  - carotid (common) (internal) — see Occlusion, artery, carotid
  - cerebellar (anterior inferior) (posterior inferior) (superior) I66.3
  - cerebral — see Occlusion, artery, cerebral
  - choroidal (anterior) I65.8
  - communicating posterior I65.8
  - coronary (see also Infarct, myocardium)
    - not resulting in infarction I24.0
  - extremity I74.9
    - lower I74.3
    - upper I74.2
  - hypophyseal I65.8
  - iliac I74.5
  - limb I74.4
    - lower I74.3
    - upper I74.2
  - mesenteric (with gangrene) (see also Ischemia, intestine, acute) K55.059
  - ophthalmic — see Occlusion, artery, retina
  - peripheral I74.4
  - pontine I65.8
  - precerebral — see Occlusion, artery, precerebral
  - pulmonary — see Embolism, pulmonary
  - renal N28.0
  - retinal — see Occlusion, artery, retina
  - septic I76
  - specified NEC I74.8
  - vertebral — see Occlusion, artery, vertebral
- basilar (artery) I65.1
- blood clot
  - following
    - abortion — see Abortion by type complicated by embolism
    - ectopic or molar pregnancy O08.2
  - in pregnancy, childbirth or puerperium — see Embolism, obstetric

Embolism — continued
- brain (see also Occlusion, artery, cerebral)
  - following
    - abortion — see Abortion by type complicated by embolism
    - ectopic or molar pregnancy O08.2
  - puerperal, postpartum, childbirth — see Embolism, obstetric
- capillary I78.8
- cardiac (see also Infarct, myocardium)
  - not resulting in infarction I51.3
- carotid (artery) (common) (internal) — see Occlusion, artery, carotid
- cavernous sinus (venous) — see Embolism, intracranial venous sinus
- cerebral — see Occlusion, artery, cerebral
- cholesterol — see Atheroembolism
- coronary (artery or vein) (systemic) — see Occlusion, coronary
- due to device, implant or graft (see also Complications, by site and type, specified NEC)
  - arterial graft NEC T82.818 ☑
  - breast (implant) T85.818 ☑
  - catheter NEC T85.818 ☑
    - dialysis (renal) T82.818 ☑
      - intraperitoneal T85.818 ☑
    - infusion NEC T82.818 ☑
      - spinal (epidural) (subdural) T85.810 ☑
    - urinary (indwelling) T83.81 ☑
  - electronic (electrode) (pulse generator) (stimulator)
    - bone T84.81 ☑
    - cardiac T82.817 ☑
    - nervous system (brain) (peripheral nerve) (spinal) T85.810 ☑
    - urinary T83.81 ☑
  - fixation, internal (orthopedic) NEC T84.81 ☑
  - gastrointestinal (bile duct) (esophagus) T85.818 ☑
  - genital NEC T83.81 ☑
  - heart (graft) (valve) T82.817 ☑
  - joint prosthesis T84.81 ☑
  - ocular (corneal graft) (orbital implant) T85.818 ☑
  - orthopedic (bone graft) NEC T86.838
  - specified NEC T85.818 ☑
  - urinary (graft) NEC T83.81 ☑
  - vascular NEC T82.818 ☑
  - ventricular intracranial shunt T85.810 ☑
- extremities
  - lower — see Embolism, vein, lower extremity
    - arterial I74.3
  - upper I74.2
- eye H34.9
- fat (cerebral) (pulmonary) (systemic) T79.1 ☑
  - complicating delivery — see Embolism, obstetric
  - following
    - abortion — see Abortion by type complicated by embolism
    - ectopic or molar pregnancy O08.2
  - following
    - abortion — see Abortion by type complicated by embolism
    - ectopic or molar pregnancy O08.2
    - infusion, therapeutic injection or transfusion air T80.0 ☑
- heart (fatty) (see also Infarct, myocardium)
  - not resulting in infarction I51.3
- hepatic (vein) I82.0
- in pregnancy, childbirth or puerperium — see Embolism, obstetric
- intestine (artery) (vein) (with gangrene) (see also Ischemia, intestine, acute) K55.039
- intracranial (see also Occlusion, artery, cerebral)
  - venous sinus (any) G08
    - nonpyogenic I67.6
- intraspinal venous sinuses or veins G08
  - nonpyogenic G95.19
- kidney (artery) N28.0
- lateral sinus (venous) — see Embolism, intracranial, venous sinus
- leg — see Embolism, vein, lower extremity
  - arterial I74.3
- longitudinal sinus (venous) — see Embolism, intracranial, venous sinus
- lung (massive) — see Embolism, pulmonary
- meninges I66.8
- mesenteric (artery) (vein) (with gangrene) (see also Ischemia, intestine, acute) K55.059

☑ Additional Character Required — Refer to the Tabular List for Character Selection   ⬐ Subterms under main terms may continue to next column or page

Elephantiasis — Embolism

Embolism — continued
obstetric (in) (pulmonary)
childbirth O88.22
air O88.02
amniotic fluid O88.12
blood clot O88.22
fat O88.82
pyemic O88.32
septic O88.32
specified type NEC O88.82
pregnancy O88.21- ☑
air O88.01- ☑
amniotic fluid O88.11- ☑
blood clot O88.21- ☑
fat O88.81- ☑
pyemic O88.31- ☑
septic O88.31- ☑
specified type NEC O88.81- ☑
puerperal O88.23
air O88.03
amniotic fluid O88.13
blood clot O88.23
fat O88.83
pyemic O88.33
septic O88.33
specified type NEC O88.83
ophthalmic — see Occlusion, artery, retina
penis N48.81
peripheral artery NOS I74.4
pituitary E23.6
popliteal (artery) I74.3
portal (vein) I81
postoperative, postprocedural
artery T81.719 ☑
mesenteric T81.710 ☑
renal T81.711 ☑
specified NEC T81.718 ☑
vein T81.72 ☑
precerebral artery — see Occlusion, artery, precerebral
puerperal — see Embolism, obstetric
pulmonary (acute) (artery) (vein) I26.99
with acute cor pulmonale I26.09
chronic I27.82
following
abortion — see Abortion by type complicated by embolism
ectopic or molar pregnancy O08.2
healed or old Z86.711
in pregnancy, childbirth or puerperium — see Embolism, obstetric
personal history of Z86.711
saddle I26.92
with acute cor pulmonale I26.02
septic I26.90
with acute cor pulmonale I26.01
pyemic (multiple) I76
following
abortion — see Abortion by type complicated by embolism
ectopic or molar pregnancy O08.2
Hemophilus influenzae A41.3
pneumococcal A40.3
with pneumonia J13
puerperal, postpartum, childbirth (any organism) — see Embolism, obstetric
specified organism NEC A41.89
staphylococcal A41.2
streptococcal A40.9
renal (artery) N28.0
vein I82.3
retina, retinal — see Occlusion, artery, retina
saddle
abdominal aorta I74.01
pulmonary artery I26.92
with acute cor pulmonale I26.02
septic (arterial) I76
complicating abortion — see Abortion, by type, complicated by, embolism
sinus — see Embolism, intracranial, venous sinus
soap complicating abortion — see Abortion, by type, complicated by, embolism
spinal cord G95.19
pyogenic origin G06.1
spleen, splenic (artery) I74.8
upper extremity I74.2
vein (acute) I82.90
antecubital I82.61- ☑
chronic I82.71- ☑

Embolism — continued
vein — continued
axillary I82.A1- ☑ (following I82.7)
chronic I82.A2- ☑ (following I82.7)
basilic I82.61- ☑
chronic I82.71- ☑
brachial I82.62- ☑
chronic I82.72- ☑
brachiocephalic (innominate) I82.290
chronic I82.291
cephalic I82.61- ☑
chronic I82.71- ☑
chronic I82.91
deep (DVT) I82.40- ☑
calf I82.4Z- ☑
chronic I82.5Z- ☑
lower leg I82.4Z- ☑
chronic I82.5Z- ☑
thigh I82.4Y- ☑
chronic I82.5Y- ☑
upper leg I82.4Y
chronic I82.5Y-
femoral I82.41- ☑
chronic I82.51- ☑
iliac (iliofemoral) I82.42- ☑
chronic I82.52- ☑
innominate I82.290
chronic I82.291
internal jugular I82.C1- ☑ (following I82.7)
chronic I82.C2- ☑ (following I82.7)
lower extremity
deep I82.40- ☑
chronic I82.50- ☑
specified NEC I82.49- ☑
chronic NEC I82.59- ☑
distal
deep I82.4Z- ☑
proximal
deep I82.4Y- ☑
chronic I82.5Y- ☑
superficial I82.81- ☑
popliteal I82.43- ☑
chronic I82.53- ☑
radial I82.62- ☑
chronic I82.72- ☑
renal I82.3
saphenous (greater) (lesser) I82.81- ☑
specified NEC I82.890
chronic NEC I82.891
subclavian I82.B1- ☑ (following I82.7)
chronic I82.B2- ☑ (following I82.7)
thoracic NEC I82.290
chronic I82.291
tibial I82.44- ☑
chronic I82.54- ☑
ulnar I82.62- ☑
chronic I82.72- ☑
upper extremity I82.60- ☑
chronic I82.70- ☑
deep I82.62- ☑
chronic I82.72- ☑
superficial I82.61- ☑
chronic I82.71- ☑
vena cava
inferior (acute) I82.220
chronic I82.221
superior (acute) I82.210
chronic I82.211
venous sinus G08
vessels of brain — see Occlusion, artery, cerebral
Embolus — see Embolism
Embryoma (see also Neoplasm, uncertain behavior, by site)
benign — see Neoplasm, benign, by site
kidney C64.- ☑
liver C22.0
malignant (see also Neoplasm, malignant, by site)
kidney C64.- ☑
liver C22.0
testis C62.9- ☑
descended (scrotal) C62.1- ☑
undescended C62.0- ☑
testis C62.9- ☑
descended (scrotal) C62.1- ☑
undescended C62.0- ☑

Embryonic
circulation Q28.9
heart Q28.9
vas deferens Q55.4
Embryopathia NOS Q89.9
Embryotoxon Q13.4
Emesis — see Vomiting
Emotional lability R45.86
Emotionality, pathological F60.3
Emotogenic disease — see Disorder, psychogenic
Emphysema (atrophic) (bullous) (chronic) (interlobular) (lung) (obstructive) (pulmonary) (senile) (vesicular) J43.9
cellular tissue (traumatic) T79.7 ☑
surgical T81.82 ☑
centrilobular J43.2
compensatory J98.3
congenital (interstitial) P25.0
conjunctiva H11.89
connective tissue (traumatic) T79.7 ☑
surgical T81.82 ☑
due to chemicals, gases, fumes or vapors J68.4
eyelid(s) — see Disorder, eyelid, specified type NEC
surgical T81.82 ☑
traumatic T79.7 ☑
interstitial J98.2
congenital P25.0
perinatal period P25.0
laminated tissue T79.7 ☑
surgical T81.82 ☑
mediastinal J98.2
newborn P25.2
orbit, orbital — see Disorder, orbit, specified type NEC
panacinar J43.1
panlobular J43.1
specified NEC J43.8
subcutaneous (traumatic) T79.7 ☑
nontraumatic J98.2
postprocedural T81.82 ☑
surgical T81.82 ☑
surgical T81.82 ☑
thymus (gland) (congenital) E32.8
traumatic (subcutaneous) T79.7 ☑
unilateral J43.0
Empty nest syndrome Z60.0
Empyema (acute) (chest) (double) (pleura) (supradi-aphragmatic) (thorax) J86.9
with fistula J86.0
accessory sinus (chronic) — see Sinusitis
antrum (chronic) — see Sinusitis, maxillary
brain (any part) — see Abscess, brain
ethmoidal (chronic) (sinus) — see Sinusitis, ethmoidal
extradural — see Abscess, extradural
frontal (chronic) (sinus) — see Sinusitis, frontal
gallbladder K81.0
mastoid (process) (acute) — see Mastoiditis, acute
maxilla, maxillary M27.2
sinus (chronic) — see Sinusitis, maxillary
nasal sinus (chronic) — see Sinusitis
sinus (accessory) (chronic) (nasal) — see Sinusitis
sphenoidal (sinus) (chronic) — see Sinusitis, sphenoidal
subarachnoid — see Abscess, extradural
subdural — see Abscess, subdural
tuberculous A15.6
ureter — see Ureteritis
ventricular — see Abscess, brain
En coup de sabre lesion L94.1
Enamel pearls K00.2
Enameloma K00.2
Enanthema, viral B09
Encephalitis (chronic) (hemorrhagic) (idiopathic) (nonepidemic) (spurious) (subacute) G04.90
acute (see also Encephalitis, viral) A86
disseminated G04.00
infectious G04.01
noninfectious G04.81
postimmunization (postvaccination) G04.02
postinfectious G04.01
inclusion body A85.8
necrotizing hemorrhagic G04.30
postimmunization G04.32
postinfectious G04.31
specified NEC G04.39
arboviral, arbovirus NEC A85.2
arthropod-borne NEC (viral) A85.2
Australian A83.4

Encephalitis — *continued*
California (virus) A83.5
Central European (tick-borne) A84.1
Czechoslovakian A84.1
Dawson's (inclusion body) A81.1
diffuse sclerosing A81.1
disseminated, acute G04.00
due to
cat scratch disease A28.1
human immunodeficiency virus (HIV) disease
B20 [G05.3]
malaria — *see* Malaria
rickettsiosis — *see* Rickettsiosis
smallpox inoculation G04.02
typhus — *see* Typhus
Eastern equine A83.2
endemic (viral) A86
epidemic NEC (viral) A86
equine (acute) (infectious) (viral) A83.9
Eastern A83.2
Venezuelan A92.2
Western A83.1
Far Eastern (tick-borne) A84.0
following vaccination or other immunization procedure G04.02
herpes zoster B02.0
herpesviral B00.4
due to herpesvirus 6 B10.01
due to herpesvirus 7 B10.09
specified NEC B10.09
Ilheus (virus) A83.8
in (due to)
actinomycosis A42.82
adenovirus A85.1
African trypanosomiasis B56.9 [G05.3]
Chagas' disease (chronic) B57.42
cytomegalovirus B25.8
enterovirus A85.0
herpes (simplex) virus B00.4
due to herpesvirus 6 B10.01
due to herpesvirus 7 B10.09
specified NEC B10.09
Infectious disease NEC B99 ☑ [G05.3]
influenza — *see* Influenza, with, encephalopathy
listeriosis A32.12
measles B05.0
mumps B26.2
naegleriasis B60.2
parasitic disease NEC B89 [G05.3]
poliovirus A80.9 [G05.3]
rubella B06.01
syphilis
congenital A50.42
late A52.14
systemic lupus erythematosus M32.19
toxoplasmosis (acquired) B58.2
congenital P37.1
tuberculosis A17.82
zoster B02.0
inclusion body A81.1
infectious (acute) (virus) NEC A86
Japanese (B type) A83.0
La Crosse A83.5
lead — *see* Poisoning, lead
lethargica (acute) (infectious) A85.8
louping ill A84.8
lupus erythematosus, systemic M32.19
lymphatica A87.2
Mengo A85.8
meningococcal A39.81
Murray Valley A83.4
otitic NEC H66.40 [G05.3]
parasitic NOS B71.9
periaxial G37.0
periaxialis (concentrica) (diffuse) G37.5
postchickenpox B01.11
postexanthematous NEC B09
postimmunization G04.02
postinfectious NEC G04.01
postmeasles B05.0
postvaccinal G04.02
postvaricella B01.11
postviral NEC A86
Powassan A84.8
Rasmussen G04.81
Rio Bravo A85.8
Russian
autumnal A83.0
spring-summer (taiga) A84.0

Encephalitis — *continued*
saturnine — *see* Poisoning, lead
specified NEC G04.81
St. Louis A83.3
subacute sclerosing A81.1
summer A83.0
suppurative G04.81
tick-borne A84.9
Torula, torular (cryptococcal) B45.1
toxic NEC G92
trichinosis B75 [G05.3]
type
B A83.0
C A83.3
van Bogaert's A81.1
Venezuelan equine A92.2
Vienna A85.8
viral, virus A86
arthropod-borne NEC A85.2
mosquito-borne A83.9
Australian X disease A83.4
California virus A83.5
Eastern equine A83.2
Japanese (B type) A83.0
Murray Valley A83.4
specified NEC A83.8
St. Louis A83.3
type B A83.0
type C A83.3
Western equine A83.1
tick-borne A84.9
biundulant A84.1
central European A84.1
Czechoslovakian A84.1
diphasic meningoencephalitis A84.1
Far Eastern A84.0
Russian spring-summer (taiga) A84.0
specified NEC A84.8
specified type NEC A85.8
Western equine A83.1
Encephalocele Q01.9
frontal Q01.0
nasofrontal Q01.1
occipital Q01.2
specified NEC Q01.8
Encephalocystocele — *see* Encephalocele
Encephaloduroarteriomyosynangiosis (EDAMS) I67.5
Encephalomalacia (brain) (cerebellar) (cerebral) — *see*
Softening, brain
Encephalomeningitis — *see* Meningoencephalitis
Encephalomeningocele — *see* Encephalocele
Encephalomeningomyelitis — *see* Meningoencephalitis
Encephalomyelitis (*see also* Encephalitis) G04.90
acute disseminated G04.00
infectious G04.01
noninfectious G04.81
postimmunization G04.02
postinfectious G04.01
acute necrotizing hemorrhagic G04.30
postimmunization G04.32
postinfectious G04.31
specified NEC G04.39
benign myalgic G93.3
equine A83.9
Eastern A83.2
Venezuelan A92.2
Western A83.1
in diseases classified elsewhere G05.3
myalgic, benign G93.3
postchickenpox B01.11
postinfectious NEC G04.01
postmeasles B05.0
postvaccinal G04.02
postvaricella B01.11
rubella B06.01
specified NEC G04.81
Venezuelan equine A92.2
Encephalomyelocele — *see* Encephalocele
Encephalomyelomeningitis — *see* Meningoencephalitis
Encephalomyelopathy G96.9
Encephalomyeloradiculitis (acute) G61.0
Encephalomyeloradiculoneuritis (acute) (Guillain-
Barré) G61.0
Encephalomyeloradiculopathy G96.9
Encephalopathia hyperbilirubinemica, newborn
P57.9

Encephalopathia hyperbilirubinemica, newborn —
continued
due to isoimmunization (conditions in P55) P57.0
Encephalopathy (acute) G93.40
acute necrotizing hemorrhagic G04.30
postimmunization G04.32
postinfectious G04.31
specified NEC G04.39
alcoholic G31.2
anoxic — *see* Damage, brain, anoxic
arteriosclerotic I67.2
centrolobar progressive (Schilder) G37.0
congenital Q07.9
degenerative, in specified disease NEC G32.89
demyelinating callosal G37.1
due to
drugs (*see also* Table of Drugs and Chemicals) G92
hepatic — *see* Failure, hepatic
hyperbilirubinemic, newborn P57.9
due to isoimmunization (conditions in P55) P57.0
hypertensive I67.4
hypoglycemic E16.2
hypoxic — *see* Damage, brain, anoxic
hypoxic ischemic P91.60
mild P91.61
moderate P91.62
severe P91.63
in (due to) (with)
birth injury P11.1
hyperinsulinism E16.1 [G94]
influenza — *see* Influenza, with, encephalopathy
lack of vitamin (*see also* Deficiency, vitamin)
E56.9 [G32.89]
neoplastic disease (*see also* Neoplasm)
D49.9 [G13.1]
serum (*see also* Reaction, serum) T80.69 ☑
syphilis A52.17
trauma (postconcussional) F07.81
current injury — *see* Injury, intracranial
vaccination G04.02
lead — *see* Poisoning, lead
metabolic G93.41
drug induced G92
toxic G92
myoclonic, early, symptomatic — *see* Epilepsy, generalized, specified NEC
necrotizing, subacute (Leigh) G31.82
neonatal P91.819
in diseases classified elsewhere P91.811
pellagrous E52 [G32.89]
portosystemic — *see* Failure, hepatic
postcontusional F07.81
current injury — *see* Injury, intracranial, diffuse
posthypoglycemic (coma) E16.1 [G94]
postradiation G93.89
saturnine — *see* Poisoning, lead
septic G93.41
specified NEC G93.49
spongiform, subacute (viral) A81.09
toxic G92
metabolic G92
traumatic (postconcussional) F07.81
current injury — *see* Injury, intracranial
vitamin B deficiency NEC E53.9 [G32.89]
vitamin B1 E51.2
Wernicke's E51.2
Encephalorrhagia — *see* Hemorrhage, intracranial, intracerebral
Encephalosis, posttraumatic F07.81
Enchondroma (*see also* Neoplasm, bone, benign)
Enchondromatosis (cartilaginous) (multiple) Q78.4
Encopresis R15.9
functional F98.1
nonorganic origin F98.1
psychogenic F98.1
Encounter (with health service) (for) Z76.89
adjustment and management (of)
breast implant Z45.81 ☑
implanted device NEC Z45.89
myringotomy device (stent) (tube) Z45.82
administrative purpose only Z02.9
examination for
adoption Z02.82
armed forces Z02.3
disability determination Z02.71
driving license Z02.4
employment Z02.1
insurance Z02.6

☑ Additional Character Required — Refer to the Tabular List for Character Selection ▽ Subterms under main terms may continue to next column or page

Encounter — *continued*
  administrative purpose only — *continued*
    examination for — *continued*
      medical certificate NEC Z02.79
      paternity testing Z02.81
      residential institution admission Z02.2
      school admission Z02.0
      sports Z02.5
      specified reason NEC Z02.89
  aftercare — *see* Aftercare
  antenatal screening Z36.9
    cervical length Z36.86
    chromosomal anomalies Z36.0
    congenital cardiac abnormalities Z36.83
    elevated maternal serum alphafetoprotein Z36.1
    fetal growth retardation Z36.4
    fetal lung maturity Z36.84
    fetal macrosomia Z36.88
    hydrops fetalis Z36.81
    intrauterine growth restriction (IUGR) /small-for-dates Z36.4
    isoimmunization Z36.5
    large-for-dates Z36.88
    malformations Z36.3
    non-visualized anatomy on a previous scan Z36.2
    nuchal translucency Z36.82
    raised alphafetoprotein level Z36.1
    risk of pre-term labor Z36.86
    specified follow-up NEC Z36.2
    specified genetic defects NEC Z36.8A
    specified type NEC Z36.89
    Streptococcus B Z36.85
    suspected anomaly Z36.3
    uncertain dates Z36.87
  assisted reproductive fertility procedure cycle Z31.83
  blood typing Z01.83
    Rh typing Z01.83
  breast augmentation or reduction Z41.1
  breast implant exchange (different material) (different size) Z45.81 ☑
  breast reconstruction following mastectomy Z42.1
  check-up — *see* Examination
  chemotherapy for neoplasm Z51.11
  colonoscopy, screening Z12.11
  counseling — *see* Counseling
  delivery, full-term, uncomplicated O80
    cesarean, without indication O82
  desensitization to allergens Z51.6
  ear piercing Z41.3
  examination — *see* Examination
  expectant parent(s) (adoptive) pre-birth pediatrician visit Z76.81
  fertility preservation procedure (prior to cancer therapy) (prior to removal of gonads) Z31.84
  fitting (of) — *see* Fitting (and adjustment) (of)
  genetic
    counseling
      nonprocreative Z71.83
      procreative Z31.5
    testing — *see* Test, genetic
  hearing conservation and treatment Z01.12
  immunotherapy for neoplasm Z51.12
  in vitro fertilization cycle Z31.83
  instruction (in)
    child care (postpartal) (prenatal) Z32.3
    childbirth Z32.2
    natural family planning
      procreative Z31.61
      to avoid pregnancy Z30.02
  insulin pump titration Z46.81
  joint prosthesis insertion following prior explantation of joint prosthesis (staged procedure)
    hip Z47.32
    knee Z47.33
    shoulder Z47.31
  laboratory (as part of a general medical examination) Z00.00
    with abnormal findings Z00.01
  mental health services (for)
    abuse NEC
      perpetrator Z69.82
      victim Z69.81
    child abuse
      nonparental
        perpetrator Z69.021
        victim Z69.020
      parental
        perpetrator Z69.011

Encounter — *continued*
  mental health services — *continued*
    child abuse — *continued*
      parental — *continued*
        victim Z69.010
    child neglect
      nonparental
        perpetrator Z69.021
        victim Z69.020
      parental
        perpetrator Z69.011
        victim Z69.010
    child psychological abuse
      nonparental
        perpetrator Z69.021
        victim Z69.020
      parental
        perpetrator Z69.011
        victim Z69.010
    child sexual abuse
      nonparental
        perpetrator Z69.021
        victim Z69.020
      parental
        perpetrator Z69.011
        victim Z69.010
    non-spousal adult abuse (perpetrator) (victim) Z69.81
    spousal or partner
      abuse
        perpetrator Z69.12
        victim Z69.11
      neglect
        perpetrator Z69.12
        victim Z69.11
      psychological abuse
        perpetrator Z69.12
        victim Z69.11
      violence
        perpetrator (physical) (sexual) Z69.12
        victim (physical) Z69.11
          sexual Z69.81
  observation (for) (ruled out)
    exposure to (suspected)
      anthrax Z03.810
      biological agent NEC Z03.818
  pediatrician visit, by expectant parent(s) (adoptive) Z76.81
  placental sample (taken vaginally) (*see also* Encounter, antenatal screening) Z36.9
  plastic and reconstructive surgery following medical procedure or healed injury NEC Z42.8
  pregnancy
    supervision of — *see* Pregnancy, supervision of
    test Z32.00
      result negative Z32.02
      result positive Z32.01
  procreative management and counseling for gestational carrier Z31.7
  prophylactic measures Z29.9
    antivenin Z29.12
    fluoride administration Z29.3
    immunotherapy for respiratory syncytial virus (RSV) Z29.11
    rabies immune globin Z29.14
    Rho (D) immune globulin Z29.13
    specified NEC Z29.8
  radiation therapy (antineoplastic) Z51.0
  radiological (as part of a general medical examination) Z00.00
    with abnormal findings Z00.01
  reconstructive surgery following medical procedure or healed injury NEC Z42.8
  removal (of) (*see also* Removal)
    artificial
      arm Z44.00- ☑
        complete Z44.01- ☑
        partial Z44.02- ☑
      eye Z44.2- ☑
      leg Z44.10- ☑
        complete Z44.11- ☑
        partial Z44.12- ☑
    breast implant Z45.81 ☑
      tissue expander (without synchronous insertion of permanent implant) Z45.81 ☑
    device Z46.9
      specified NEC Z46.89

Encounter — *continued*
  removal (*see also* Removal) — *continued*
    external
      fixation device — *code to* fracture with seventh character D
      prosthesis, prosthetic device Z44.9
        breast Z44.3- ☑
        specified NEC Z44.8
    implanted device NEC Z45.89
    insulin pump Z46.81
    internal fixation device Z47.2
    myringotomy device (stent) (tube) Z45.82
    nervous system device NEC Z46.2
      brain neuropacemaker Z46.2
      visual substitution device Z46.2
        implanted Z45.31
    non-vascular catheter Z46.82
    orthodontic device Z46.4
    stent
      ureteral Z46.6
    urinary device Z46.6
  repeat cervical smear to confirm findings of recent normal smear following initial abnormal smear Z01.42
  respirator [ventilator] use during power failure Z99.12
  Rh typing Z01.83
  screening — *see* Screening
  specified NEC Z76.89
  sterilization Z30.2
  suspected condition, ruled out
    amniotic cavity and membrane Z03.71
    cervical shortening Z03.75
    fetal anomaly Z03.73
    fetal growth Z03.74
    maternal and fetal conditions NEC Z03.79
    oligohydramnios Z03.71
    placental problem Z03.72
    polyhydramnios Z03.71
  suspected exposure (to), ruled out
    anthrax Z03.810
    biological agents NEC Z03.818
  termination of pregnancy, elective Z33.2
  testing — *see* Test
  therapeutic drug level monitoring Z51.81
  titration, insulin pump Z46.81
  to determine fetal viability of pregnancy O36.80 ☑
  training
    insulin pump Z46.81
  X-ray of chest (as part of a general medical examination) Z00.00
    with abnormal findings Z00.01

Encystment — *see* Cyst

Endarteritis (bacterial, subacute) (infective) I77.6
  brain I67.7
  cerebral or cerebrospinal I67.7
  deformans — *see* Arteriosclerosis
  embolic — *see* Embolism
  obliterans (*see also* Arteriosclerosis)
    pulmonary I28.8
  pulmonary I28.8
  retina — *see* Vasculitis, retina
  senile — *see* Arteriosclerosis
  syphilitic A52.09
    brain or cerebral A52.04
    congenital A50.54 [I79.8]
  tuberculous A18.89

Endemic — *see* condition

Endocarditis (chronic) (marantic) (nonbacterial) (thrombotic) (valvular) I38
  with rheumatic fever (conditions in I00)
    active — *see* Endocarditis, acute, rheumatic
    inactive or quiescent (with chorea) I09.1
  acute or subacute I33.9
    infective I33.0
    rheumatic (aortic) (mitral) (pulmonary) (tricuspid) I01.1
      with chorea (acute) (rheumatic) (Sydenham's) I02.0
  aortic (heart) (nonrheumatic) (valve) I35.8
    with
      mitral disease I08.0
        with tricuspid (valve) disease I08.3
        active or acute I01.1
          with chorea (acute) (rheumatic) (Sydenham's) I02.0
      rheumatic fever (conditions in I00)
        active — *see* Endocarditis, acute, rheumatic
        inactive or quiescent (with chorea) I06.9

Endocarditis — continued
aortic — continued
  with — continued
    tricuspid (valve) disease I08.2
      with mitral (valve) disease I08.3
    acute or subacute I33.9
    arteriosclerotic I35.8
    rheumatic I06.9
      with mitral disease I08.0
        with tricuspid (valve) disease I08.3
          active or acute I01.1
            with chorea (acute) (rheumatic) (Syden-
              ham's) I02.0
      active or acute I01.1
        with chorea (acute) (rheumatic) (Syden-
          ham's) I02.0
      specified NEC I06.8
    specified cause NEC I35.8
    syphilitic A52.03
  arteriosclerotic I38
  atypical verrucous (Libman-Sacks) M32.11
  bacterial (acute) (any valve) (subacute) I33.0
  candidal B37.6
  congenital Q24.8
  constrictive I33.0
  Coxiella burnetii A78 [I39]
  Coxsackie B33.21
  due to
    prosthetic cardiac valve T82.6 ☑
    Q fever A78 [I39]
    Serratia marcescens I33.0
    typhoid (fever) A01.02
  gonococcal A54.83
  infectious or infective (acute) (any valve) (subacute)
    I33.0
  lenta (acute) (any valve) (subacute) I33.0
  Libman-Sacks M32.11
  listerial A32.82
  Löffler's I42.3
  malignant (acute) (any valve) (subacute) I33.0
  meningococcal A39.51
  mitral (chronic) (double) (fibroid) (heart) (inactive)
    (valve) (with chorea) I05.9
    with
      aortic (valve) disease I08.0
        with tricuspid (valve) disease I08.3
          active or acute I01.1
            with chorea (acute) (rheumatic) (Syden-
              ham's) I02.0
        rheumatic fever (conditions in I00)
          active — see Endocarditis, acute, rheumatic
          inactive or quiescent (with chorea) I05.9
      tricuspid (valve) disease I08.1
        with aortic (valve) disease I08.3
      active or acute I01.1
        with chorea (acute) (rheumatic) (Sydenham's)
          I02.0
      bacterial I33.0
    arteriosclerotic I34.8
    nonrheumatic I34.8
      acute or subacute I33.9
    specified NEC I05.8
  monilial B37.6
  multiple valves I08.9
    specified disorders I08.8
  mycotic (acute) (any valve) (subacute) I33.0
  pneumococcal (acute) (any valve) (subacute) I33.0
  pulmonary (chronic) (heart) (valve) I37.8
    with rheumatic fever (conditions in I00)
      active — see Endocarditis, acute, rheumatic
      inactive or quiescent (with chorea) I09.89
        with aortic, mitral or tricuspid disease I08.8
    acute or subacute I33.9
      rheumatic I01.1
        with chorea (acute) (rheumatic) (Syden-
          ham's) I02.0
    arteriosclerotic I37.8
    congenital Q22.2
    rheumatic (chronic) (inactive) (with chorea) I09.89
      active or acute I01.1
        with chorea (acute) (rheumatic) (Syden-
          ham's) I02.0
    syphilitic A52.03
  purulent (acute) (any valve) (subacute) I33.0
  Q fever A78 [I39]
  rheumatic (chronic) (inactive) (with chorea) I09.1
    active or acute (aortic) (mitral) (pulmonary) (tricus-
      pid) I01.1

Endocarditis — continued
rheumatic — continued
  active or acute — continued
    with chorea (acute) (rheumatic) (Sydenham's)
      I02.0
  rheumatoid — see Rheumatoid, carditis
  septic (acute) (any valve) (subacute) I33.0
  streptococcal (acute) (any valve) (subacute) I33.0
  subacute — see Endocarditis, acute
  suppurative (acute) (any valve) (subacute) I33.0
  syphilitic A52.03
  toxic I33.9
  tricuspid (chronic) (heart) (inactive) (rheumatic) (valve)
    (with chorea) I07.9
    with
      aortic (valve) disease I08.2
        mitral (valve) disease I08.3
      mitral (valve) disease I08.1
        aortic (valve) disease I08.3
      rheumatic fever (conditions in I00)
        active — see Endocarditis, acute, rheumatic
        inactive or quiescent (with chorea) I07.8
    active or acute I01.1
      with chorea (acute) (rheumatic) (Sydenham's)
        I02.0
    arteriosclerotic I36.8
    nonrheumatic I36.8
      acute or subacute I33.9
    specified cause, except rheumatic I36.8
  tuberculous — see Tuberculosis, endocarditis
  typhoid A01.02
  ulcerative (acute) (any valve) (subacute) I33.0
  vegetative (acute) (any valve) (subacute) I33.0
  verrucous (atypical) (nonbacterial) (nonrheumatic)
    M32.11
Endocardium, endocardial (see also condition)
  cushion defect Q21.2
Endocervicitis (see also Cervicitis)
  due to intrauterine (contraceptive) device T83.69 ☑
  hyperplastic N72
Endocrine — see condition
Endocrinopathy, pluriglandular E31.9
Endodontic
  overfill M27.52
  underfill M27.53
Endodontitis K04.01
  irreversible K04.02
  reversible K04.01
Endomastoiditis — see Mastoiditis
Endometrioma N80.9
Endometriosis N80.9
  appendix N80.5
  bladder N80.8
  bowel N80.5
  broad ligament N80.3
  cervix N80.0
  colon N80.5
  cul-de-sac (Douglas') N80.3
  exocervix N80.0
  fallopian tube N80.2
  female genital organ NEC N80.8
  gallbladder N80.8
  in scar of skin N80.6
  internal N80.0
  intestine N80.5
  lung N80.8
  myometrium N80.0
  ovary N80.1
  parametrium N80.3
  pelvic peritoneum N80.3
  peritoneal (pelvic) N80.3
  rectovaginal septum N80.4
  rectum N80.5
  round ligament N80.3
  skin (scar) N80.6
  specified site NEC N80.8
  stromal D39.0
  thorax N80.8
  umbilicus N80.8
  uterus (internal) N80.0
  vagina N80.4
  vulva N80.8
Endometritis (decidual) (nonspecific) (purulent) (senile)
  (atrophic) (suppurative) N71.9
  with ectopic pregnancy O08.0
  acute N71.0
  blenorrhagic (gonococcal) (acute) (chronic) A54.24

Endometritis — continued
  cervix, cervical (with erosion or ectropion) (see also
    Cervicitis)
    hyperplastic N72
  chlamydial A56.11
  chronic N71.1
  following
    abortion — see Abortion by type complicated by
      genital infection
    ectopic or molar pregnancy O08.0
  gonococcal, gonorrheal (acute) (chronic) A54.24
  hyperplastic (see also Hyperplasia, endometrial) N85.00
    cervix N72
  puerperal, postpartum, childbirth O86.12
  subacute N71.0
  tuberculous A18.17
Endometrium — see condition
Endomyocardiopathy, South African I42.3
Endomyocarditis — see Endocarditis
Endomyofibrosis I42.3
Endomyometritis — see Endometritis
Endopericarditis — see Endocarditis
Endoperineuritis — see Disorder, nerve
Endophlebitis — see Phlebitis
Endophthalmia — see Endophthalmitis, purulent
Endophthalmitis (acute) (infective) (metastatic) (suba-
  cute) H44.009
  bleb associated (see also Bleb, inflamed (infected),
    postprocedural H59.4 ☑
  gonorrheal A54.39
  in (due to)
    cysticercosis B69.1
    onchocerciasis B73.01
    toxocariasis B83.0
  panuveitis — see Panuveitis
  parasitic H44.12- ☑
  purulent H44.00- ☑
    panophthalmitis — see Panophthalmitis
    vitreous abscess H44.02- ☑
  specified NEC H44.19
  sympathetic — see Uveitis, sympathetic
Endosalpingioma D28.2
Endosalpingiosis N94.89
Endosteitis — see Osteomyelitis
Endothelioma, bone — see Neoplasm, bone, malignant
Endotheliosis (hemorrhagic infectional) D69.8
Endotoxemia — code to condition
Endotrachelitis — see Cervicitis
Engelmann (-Camurati) **syndrome** Q78.3
English disease — see Rickets
Engman's disease L30.3
Engorgement
  breast N64.59
    newborn P83.4
    puerperal, postpartum O92.79
  lung (passive) — see Edema, lung
  pulmonary (passive) — see Edema, lung
  stomach K31.89
  venous, retina — see Occlusion, retina, vein, engorge-
    ment
Enlargement, enlarged (see also Hypertrophy)
  adenoids J35.2
    with tonsils J35.3
  alveolar ridge K08.89
    congenital — see Anomaly, alveolar
  apertures of diaphragm (congenital) Q79.1
  gingival K06.1
  heart, cardiac — see Hypertrophy, cardiac
  labium majus, childhood asymmetric (CALME) N90.61
  lacrimal gland, chronic H04.03- ☑
  liver — see Hypertrophy, liver
  lymph gland or node R59.9
    generalized R59.1
    localized R59.0
  orbit H05.34- ☑
  organ or site, congenital NEC — see Anomaly, by site
  parathyroid (gland) E21.0
  pituitary fossa R93.0
  prostate N40.0
    with lower urinary tract symptoms (LUTS) N40.1
    without lower urinary tract symptoms (LUTS) N40.0
  sella turcica R93.0
  spleen — see Splenomegaly
  thymus (gland) (congenital) E32.0
  thyroid (gland) — see Goiter
  tongue K14.8
  tonsils J35.1

Enlargement, enlarged — *continued*
  tonsils — *continued*
    with adenoids J35.3
  uterus N85.2
  vestibular aqueduct Q16.5
Enophthalmos H05.40- ☑
  due to
    orbital tissue atrophy H05.41- ☑
    trauma or surgery H05.42- ☑
Enostosis M27.8
Entamebic, entamebiasis — *see* Amebiasis
Entanglement
  umbilical cord(s) O69.82 ☑
    with compression O69.2 ☑
    without compression O69.82 ☑
    around neck (with compression) O69.81 ☑
      with compression O69.1 ☑
      without compression O69.81 ☑
    of twins in monoamniotic sac O69.2 ☑
Enteralgia — *see* Pain, abdominal
Enteric — *see* condition
Enteritis (acute) (diarrheal) (hemorrhagic) (noninfective) K52.9
  adenovirus A08.2
  aertrycke infection A02.0
  allergic K52.29
    with
      eosinophilic gastritis or gastroenteritis K52.81
      food protein-induced enterocolitis syndrome K52.21
      food protein-induced enteropathy K52.22
  amebic (acute) A06.0
    with abscess — *see* Abscess, amebic
    chronic A06.1
      with abscess — *see* Abscess, amebic
      nondysenteric A06.2
    nondysenteric A06.2
  astrovirus A08.32
  bacillary NOS A03.9
  bacterial A04.9
    specified NEC A04.8
  calicivirus A08.31
  candidal B37.82
  Chilomastix A07.8
  choleriformis A00.1
  chronic (noninfectious) K52.9
    ulcerative — *see* Colitis, ulcerative
  cicatrizing (chronic) — *see* Enteritis, regional, small intestine
  Clostridium
    botulinum (food poisoning) A05.1
    difficile
      not specified as recurrent A04.72
      recurrent A04.71
  coccidial A07.3
  coxsackie virus A08.39
  dietetic (*see also* Enteritis, allergic) K52.29
  drug-induced K52.1
  due to
    astrovirus A08.32
    calicivirus A08.31
    coxsackie virus A08.39
    drugs K52.1
    echovirus A08.39
    enterovirus NEC A08.39
    food hypersensitivity (*see also* Enteritis, allergic) K52.29
    infectious organism (bacterial) (viral) — *see* Enteritis, infectious
    torovirus A08.39
    Yersinia enterocolitica A04.6
  echovirus A08.39
  eltor A00.1
  enterovirus NEC A08.39
  eosinophilic K52.81
  epidemic (infectious) A09
  fulminant (*see also* Ischemia, intestine, acute) K55.019
  gangrenous — *see* Enteritis, infectious
  giardial A07.1
  infectious NOS A09
    due to
      adenovirus A08.2
      Aerobacter aerogenes A04.8
      Arizona (bacillus) A02.0
      bacteria NOS A04.9
        specified NEC A04.8
      Campylobacter A04.5

Enteritis — *continued*
  infectious — *continued*
    due to — *continued*
      Clostridium difficile
        not specified as recurrent A04.72
        recurrent A04.71
      Clostridium perfringens A04.8
      Enterobacter aerogenes A04.8
      enterovirus A08.39
      Escherichia coli A04.4
        enteroaggregative A04.4
        enterohemorrhagic A04.3
        enteroinvasive A04.2
        enteropathogenic A04.0
        enterotoxigenic A04.1
        specified NEC A04.4
      specified
        bacteria NEC A04.8
        virus NEC A08.39
      Staphylococcus A04.8
      virus NEC A08.4
        specified type NEC A08.39
      Yersinia enterocolitica A04.6
      specified organism NEC A08.8
  influenzal — *see* Influenza, with, digestive manifestations
  ischemic K55.9
    acute (*see also* Ischemia, intestine, acute) K55.019
    chronic K55.1
  microsporidial A07.8
  mucomembranous, myxomembranous — *see* Syndrome, irritable bowel
  mucous — *see* Syndrome, irritable bowel
  necroticans A05.2
  necrotizing of newborn — *see* Enterocolitis, necrotizing, in newborn
  neurogenic — *see* Syndrome, irritable bowel
  newborn necrotizing — *see* Enterocolitis, necrotizing, in newborn
  noninfectious K52.9
  norovirus A08.11
  parasitic NEC B82.9
  paratyphoid (fever) — *see* Fever, paratyphoid
  protozoal A07.9
    specified NEC A07.8
  radiation K52.0
  regional (of) K50.90
    with
      complication K50.919
        abscess K50.914
        fistula K50.913
        intestinal obstruction K50.912
        rectal bleeding K50.911
        specified complication NEC K50.918
    colon — *see* Enteritis, regional, large intestine
    duodenum — *see* Enteritis, regional, small intestine
    ileum — *see* Enteritis, regional, small intestine
    jejunum — *see* Enteritis, regional, small intestine
    large bowel — *see* Enteritis, regional, large intestine
    large intestine (colon) (rectum) K50.10
      with
        complication K50.119
          abscess K50.114
          fistula K50.113
          intestinal obstruction K50.112
          rectal bleeding K50.111
          small intestine (duodenum) (ileum) (jejunum) involvement K50.80
            with
              complication K50.819
                abscess K50.814
                fistula K50.813
                intestinal obstruction K50.812
                rectal bleeding K50.811
                specified complication NEC K50.818
          specified complication NEC K50.118
    rectum — *see* Enteritis, regional, large intestine
    small intestine (duodenum) (ileum) (jejunum) K50.00
      with
        complication K50.019
          abscess K50.014
          fistula K50.013
          intestinal obstruction K50.012
          large intestine (colon) (rectum) involvement K50.80

Enteritis — *continued*
  regional — *continued*
    small intestine — *continued*
      with — *continued*
        complication — *continued*
          large intestine involvement — *continued*
            with
              complication K50.819
                abscess K50.814
                fistula K50.813
                intestinal obstruction K50.812
                rectal bleeding K50.811
                specified complication NEC K50.818
          rectal bleeding K50.011
          specified complication NEC K50.018
  rotaviral A08.0
  Salmonella, salmonellosis (arizonae) (cholerae-suis) (enteritidis) (typhimurium) A02.0
  segmental — *see* Enteritis, regional
  septic A09
  Shigella — *see* Infection, Shigella
  small round structured NEC A08.19
  spasmodic, spastic — *see* Syndrome, irritable bowel
  staphylococcal A04.8
    due to food A05.0
  torovirus A08.39
  toxic NEC K52.1
    due to Clostridium difficile
      not specified as recurrent A04.72
      recurrent A04.71
  trichomonal A07.8
  tuberculous A18.32
  typhosa A01.00
  ulcerative (chronic) — *see* Colitis, ulcerative
  viral A08.4
    adenovirus A08.2
    enterovirus A08.39
    Rotavirus A08.0
    small round structured NEC A08.19
    specified NEC A08.39
    virus specified NEC A08.39
Enterobiasis B80
Enterobius vermicularis (infection) (infestation) B80
Enterocele (*see also* Hernia, abdomen)
  pelvic, pelvis (acquired) (congenital) N81.5
  vagina, vaginal (acquired) (congenital) NEC N81.5
Enterocolitis (*see also* Enteritis) K52.9
  due to Clostridium difficile
    not specified as recurrent A04.72
    recurrent A04.71
  fulminant Ischemic (*see also* Ischemia, intestine, acute) K55.059
  granulomatous — *see* Enteritis, regional
  hemorrhagic (acute) (*see also* Ischemia, intestine, acute) K55.059
    chronic K55.1
  infectious NEC A09
  ischemic K55.9
  necrotizing K55.30
    with
      perforation K55.33
      pneumatosis K55.32
        and perforation K55.33
    without pneumatosis or perforation K55.31
    due to Clostridium difficile
      not specified as recurrent A04.72
      recurrent A04.71
    in newborn P77.9
      stage 1 (without pneumatosis, without perforation) P77.1
      stage 2 (with pneumatosis, without perforation) P77.2
      stage 3 (with pneumatosis, with perforation) P77.3
    in non-newborn K55.30
      stage 1 (without pneumatosis, without perforation) K55.31
      stage 2 (with pneumatosis, without perforation) K55.32
      stage 3 (with pneumatosis, with perforation) K55.33
  noninfectious K52.9
    newborn — *see* Enterocolitis, necrotizing, in newborn
  pseudomembranous (newborn)
    not specified as recurrent A04.72

Enterocolitis — *continued*
pseudomembranous — *continued*
recurrent A04.71
radiation K52.0
newborn — *see* Enterocolitis, necrotizing, in new-born
ulcerative (chronic) — *see* Pancolitis, ulcerative (chronic)
Enterogastritis — *see* Enteritis
Enteropathy K63.9
celiac-gluten-sensitive K90.0
non-celiac K90.41
food protein-induced enterocolitis K52.22
hemorrhagic, terminal (*see also* Ischemia, intestine, acute) K55.059
protein-losing K90.49
Enteroperitonitis — *see* Peritonitis
Enteroptosis K63.4
Enterorrhagia K92.2
Enterospasm (*see also* Syndrome, irritable, bowel)
psychogenic F45.8
Enterostenosis (*see also* Obstruction, intestine, specified NEC) K56.699
Enterostomy
complication — *see* Complication, enterostomy
status Z93.4
Enterovirus, as cause of disease classified elsewhere B97.10
coxsackievirus B97.11
echovirus B97.12
other specified B97.19
Enthesopathy (peripheral) M77.9
Achilles tendinitis — *see* Tendinitis, Achilles
ankle and tarsus M77.9
specified type NEC — *see* Enthesopathy, foot, specified type NEC
anterior tibial syndrome M76.81- ☑
calcaneal spur — *see* Spur, bone, calcaneal
elbow region M77.8
lateral epicondylitis — *see* Epicondylitis, lateral
medial epicondylitis — *see* Epicondylitis, medial
foot NEC M77.9
metatarsalgia — *see* Metatarsalgia
specified type NEC M77.5- ☑
forearm M77.9
gluteal tendinitis — *see* Tendinitis, gluteal
hand M77.9
hip — *see* Enthesopathy, lower limb, specified type NEC
iliac crest spur — *see* Spur, bone, iliac crest
iliotibial band syndrome — *see* Syndrome, iliotibial band
knee — *see* Enthesopathy, lower limb, lower leg, specified type NEC
lateral epicondylitis — *see* Epicondylitis, lateral
lower limb (excluding foot) M76.9
Achilles tendinitis — *see* Tendinitis, Achilles
anterior tibial syndrome M76.81- ☑
gluteal tendinitis — *see* Tendinitis, gluteal
iliac crest spur — *see* Spur, bone, iliac crest
iliotibial band syndrome — *see* Syndrome, iliotibial band
patellar tendinitis — *see* Tendinitis, patellar
pelvic region — *see* Enthesopathy, lower limb, specified type NEC
peroneal tendinitis — *see* Tendinitis, peroneal
posterior tibial syndrome M76.82- ☑
psoas tendinitis — *see* Tendinitis, psoas
shoulder M77.9
specified type NEC M76.89- ☑
tibial collateral bursitis — *see* Bursitis, tibial collateral
medial epicondylitis — *see* Epicondylitis, medial
metatarsalgia — *see* Metatarsalgia
multiple sites M77.9
patellar tendinitis — *see* Tendinitis, patellar
pelvis M77.9
periarthritis of wrist — *see* Periarthritis, wrist
peroneal tendinitis — *see* Tendinitis, peroneal
posterior tibial syndrome M76.82- ☑
psoas tendinitis — *see* Tendinitis, psoas
shoulder region — *see* Lesion, shoulder
specified site NEC M77.9
specified type NEC M77.8
spinal M46.00
cervical region M46.02
cervicothoracic region M46.03

Enthesopathy — *continued*
spinal — *continued*
lumbar region M46.06
lumbosacral region M46.07
multiple sites M46.09
occipito-atlanto-axial region M46.01
sacrococcygeal region M46.08
thoracic region M46.04
thoracolumbar region M46.05
tibial collateral bursitis — *see* Bursitis, tibial collateral
upper arm M77.9
wrist and carpus NEC M77.8
calcaneal spur — *see* Spur, bone, calcaneal
periarthritis of wrist — *see* Periarthritis, wrist
Entomophobia F40.218
Entomophthoromycosis B46.8
Entrance, air into vein — *see* Embolism, air
Entrapment, nerve — *see* Neuropathy, entrapment
Entropion (eyelid) (paralytic) H02.009
cicatricial H02.019
left H02.016
lower H02.015
upper H02.014
right H02.013
lower H02.012
upper H02.011
congenital Q10.2
left H02.006
lower H02.005
upper H02.004
mechanical H02.029
left H02.026
lower H02.025
upper H02.024
right H02.023
lower H02.022
upper H02.021
right H02.003
lower H02.002
upper H02.001
senile H02.039
left H02.036
lower H02.035
upper H02.034
right H02.033
lower H02.032
upper H02.031
spastic H02.049
left H02.046
lower H02.045
upper H02.044
right H02.043
lower H02.042
upper H02.041
Enucleated eye (traumatic, current) S05.7- ☑
Enuresis R32
functional F98.0
habit disturbance F98.0
nocturnal N39.44
psychogenic F98.0
nonorganic origin F98.0
psychogenic F98.0
Eosinopenia — *see* Agranulocytosis
Eosinophilia (allergic) (hereditary) (idiopathic) (secondary) D72.1
with
angiolymphoid hyperplasia (ALHE) D18.01
infiltrative J82
Löffler's J82
peritoneal — *see* Peritonitis, eosinophilic
pulmonary NEC J82
tropical (pulmonary) J82
Eosinophilia-myalgia syndrome M35.8
Ependymitis (acute) (cerebral) (chronic) (granular) — *see* Encephalomyelitis
Ependymoblastoma
specified site — *see* Neoplasm, malignant, by site
unspecified site C71.9
Ependymoma (epithelial) (malignant)
anaplastic
specified site — *see* Neoplasm, malignant, by site
unspecified site C71.9
benign
specified site — *see* Neoplasm, benign, by site
unspecified site D33.2
myxopapillary D43.2
specified site — *see* Neoplasm, uncertain behavior, by site

Ependymoma — *continued*
myxopapillary — *continued*
unspecified site D43.2
papillary D43.2
specified site — *see* Neoplasm, uncertain behavior, by site
unspecified site D43.2
specified site — *see* Neoplasm, malignant, by site
unspecified site C71.9
Ependymopathy G93.89
Ephelis, ephelides L81.2
Epiblepharon (congenital) Q10.3
Epicanthus, epicanthic fold (eyelid) (congenital) Q10.3
Epicondylitis (elbow)
lateral M77.1- ☑
medial M77.0- ☑
Epicystitis — *see* Cystitis
Epidemic — *see* condition
Epidermidalization, cervix — *see* Dysplasia, cervix
Epidermis, epidermal — *see* condition
Epidermodysplasia verruciformis B07.8
Epidermolysis
bullosa (congenital) Q81.9
acquired L12.30
drug-induced L12.31
specified cause NEC L12.35
dystrophica Q81.2
letalis Q81.1
simplex Q81.0
specified NEC Q81.8
necroticans combustiformis L51.2
due to drug — *see* Table of Drugs and Chemicals, by drug
Epidermophytid — *see* Dermatophytosis
Epidermophytosis (infected) — *see* Dermatophytosis
Epididymis — *see* condition
Epididymitis (acute) (nonvenereal) (recurrent) (residual) N45.1
with orchitis N45.3
blennorrhagic (gonococcal) A54.23
caseous (tuberculous) A18.15
chlamydial A56.19
filarial (*see also* Infestation, filarial) B74.9 [N51]
gonococcal A54.23
syphilitic A52.76
tuberculous A18.15
Epididymo-orchitis (*see also* Epididymitis) N45.3
Epidural — *see* condition
Epigastrium, epigastric — *see* condition
Epigastrocele — *see* Hernia, ventral
Epiglottis — *see* condition
Epiglottitis, epiglottiditis (acute) J05.10
with obstruction J05.11
chronic J37.0
Epignathus Q89.4
Epilepsia partialis continua (*see also* Kozhevnikof's epilepsy) G40.1- ☑
Epilepsy, epileptic, epilepsia (attack) (cerebral) (convulsion) (fit) (seizure) G40.909

> *Note: the following terms are to be considered equivalent to intractable: pharmacoresistant (pharmacologically resistant), treatment resistant, refractory (medically) and poorly controlled*

with
complex partial seizures — *see* Epilepsy, localization-related, symptomatic, with complex partial seizures
grand mal seizures on awakening — *see* Epilepsy, generalized, specified NEC
myoclonic absences — *see* Epilepsy, generalized, specified NEC
myoclonic-astatic seizures — *see* Epilepsy, generalized, specified NEC
simple partial seizures — *see* Epilepsy, localization-related, symptomatic, with simple partial seizures
akinetic — *see* Epilepsy, generalized, specified NEC
benign childhood with centrotemporal EEG spikes — *see* Epilepsy, localization-related, idiopathic
benign myoclonic in infancy G40.80- ☑
Bravais-jacksonian — *see* Epilepsy, localization-related, symptomatic, with simple partial seizures
childhood
with occipital EEG paroxysms — *see* Epilepsy, localization-related, idiopathic
absence G40.A09 (*following* G40.3)

☑ **Additional Character Required** — **Refer to the Tabular List for Character Selection** 🔽 Subterms under main terms may continue to next column or page

Epilepsy, epileptic, epilepsia — *continued*
  childhood — *continued*
    absence — *continued*
      intractable G40.A19 (*following* G40.3)
        with status epilepticus G40.A11 (*following* G40.3)
        without status epilepticus G40.A19 (*following* G40.3)
      not intractable G40.A09 (*following* G40.3)
        with status epilepticus G40.A01 (*following* G40.3)
        without status epilepticus G40.A09 (*following* G40.3)
  climacteric — *see* Epilepsy, specified NEC
  cysticercosis B69.0
  deterioration (mental) F06.8
  due to syphilis A52.19
  focal — *see* Epilepsy, localization-related, symptomatic, with simple partial seizures
  generalized
    idiopathic G40.309
      intractable G40.319
        with status epilepticus G40.311
        without status epilepticus G40.319
      not intractable G40.309
        with status epilepticus G40.301
        without status epilepticus G40.309
    specified NEC G40.409
      intractable G40.419
        with status epilepticus G40.411
        without status epilepticus G40.419
      not intractable G40.409
        with status epilepticus G40.401
        without status epilepticus G40.409
  impulsive petit mal — *see* Epilepsy, juvenile myoclonic
  intractable G40.919
    with status epilepticus G40.911
    without status epilepticus G40.919
  juvenile absence G40.A09 (*following* G40.3)
    intractable G40.A19 (*following* G40.3)
      with status epilepticus G40.A11 (*following* G40.3)
      without status epilepticus G40.A19 (*following* G40.3)
    not intractable G40.A09 (*following* G40.3)
      with status epilepticus G40.A01 (*following* G40.3)
      without status epilepticus G40.A09 (*following* G40.3)
  juvenile myoclonic G40.B09 (*following* G40.3)
    intractable G40.B19 (*following* G40.3)
      with status epilepticus G40.B11 (*following* G40.3)
      without status epilepticus G40.B19 (*following* G40.3)
    not intractable G40.B09 (*following* G40.3)
      with status epilepticus G40.B01 (*following* G40.3)
      without status epilepticus G40.B09 (*following* G40.3)
  localization-related (focal) (partial)
    idiopathic G40.009
      with seizures of localized onset G40.009
        intractable G40.019
          with status epilepticus G40.011
          without status epilepticus G40.019
        not intractable G40.009
          with status epilepticus G40.001
          without status epilepticus G40.009
    symptomatic
      with complex partial seizures G40.209
        intractable G40.219
          with status epilepticus G40.211
          without status epilepticus G40.219
        not intractable G40.209
          with status epilepticus G40.201
          without status epilepticus G40.209
      with simple partial seizures G40.109
        intractable G40.119
          with status epilepticus G40.111
          without status epilepticus G40.119
        not intractable G40.109
          with status epilepticus G40.101
          without status epilepticus G40.109
  myoclonus, myoclonic — *see* Epilepsy, generalized, specified NEC
  progressive — *see* Epilepsy, generalized, idiopathic
  not intractable G40.909
    with status epilepticus G40.901

Epilepsy, epileptic, epilepsia — *continued*
  not intractable — *continued*
    without status epilepticus G40.909
  on awakening — *see* Epilepsy, generalized, specified NEC
  parasitic NOS B71.9 [G94]
  partialis continua (*see also* Kozhevnikof's epilepsy) G40.1- ☑
  peripheral — *see* Epilepsy, specified NEC
  procursiva — *see* Epilepsy, localization-related, symptomatic, with simple partial seizures
  progressive (familial) myoclonic — *see* Epilepsy, generalized, idiopathic
  reflex — *see* Epilepsy, specified NEC
  related to
    alcohol G40.509
      not intractable G40.509
        with status epilepticus G40.501
        without status epilepticus G40.509
    drugs G40.509
      not intractable G40.509
        with status epilepticus G40.501
        without status epilepticus G40.509
    external causes G40.509
      not intractable G40.509
        with status epilepticus G40.501
        without status epilepticus G40.509
    hormonal changes G40.509
      not intractable G40.509
        with status epilepticus G40.501
        without status epilepticus G40.509
    sleep deprivation G40.509
      not intractable G40.509
        with status epilepticus G40.501
        without status epilepticus G40.509
    stress G40.509
      not intractable G40.509
        with status epilepticus G40.501
        without status epilepticus G40.509
  somatomotor — *see* Epilepsy, localization-related, symptomatic, with simple partial seizures
  somatosensory — *see* Epilepsy, localization-related, symptomatic, with simple partial seizures
  spasms G40.822
    intractable G40.824
      with status epilepticus G40.823
      without status epilepticus G40.824
    not intractable G40.822
      with status epilepticus G40.821
      without status epilepticus G40.822
  specified NEC G40.802
    intractable G40.804
      with status epilepticus G40.803
      without status epilepticus G40.804
    not intractable G40.802
      with status epilepticus G40.801
      without status epllepticus G40.802
  syndromes
    generalized
      idiopathic G40.309
        intractable G40.319
          with status epilepticus G40.311
          without status epilepticus G40.319
        not intractable G40.309
          with status epilepticus G40.301
          without status epilepticus G40.309
      specified NEC G40.409
        intractable G40.419
          with status epilepticus G40.411
          without status epilepticus G40.419
        not intractable G40.409
          with status epilepticus G40.401
          without status epilepticus G40.409
    localization-related (focal) (partial)
      idiopathic G40.009
        with seizures of localized onset G40.009
          intractable G40.019
            with status epilepticus G40.011
            without status epilepticus G40.019
          not intractable G40.009
            with status epilepticus G40.001
            without status epilepticus G40.009
      symptomatic
        with complex partial seizures G40.209
          intractable G40.219
            with status epilepticus G40.211
            without status epilepticus G40.219
          not intractable G40.209

Epilepsy, epileptic, epilepsia — *continued*
  syndromes — *continued*
    localization-related — *continued*
      symptomatic — *continued*
        with complex partial seizures — *continued*
          not intractable — *continued*
            with status epilepticus G40.201
            without status epilepticus G40.209
        with simple partial seizures G40.109
          intractable G40.119
            with status epilepticus G40.111
            without status epilepticus G40.119
          not intractable G40.109
            with status epilepticus G40.101
            without status epilepticus G40.109
      specified NEC G40.802
        intractable G40.804
          with status epilepticus G40.803
          without status epilepticus G40.804
        not intractable G40.802
          with status epilepticus G40.801
          without status epilepticus G40.802
    tonic (-clonic) — *see* Epilepsy, generalized, specified NEC
    twilight F05
    uncinate (gyrus) — *see* Epilepsy, localization-related, symptomatic, with complex partial seizures
    Unverricht (-Lundborg) (familial myoclonic) — *see* Epilepsy, generalized, idiopathic
    visceral — *see* Epilepsy, specified NEC
    visual — *see* Epilepsy, specified NEC
Epiloia Q85.1
Epimenorrhea N92.0
Epipharyngitis — *see* Nasopharyngitis
Epiphora H04.20- ☑
  due to
    excess lacrimation H04.21- ☑
    insufficient drainage H04.22- ☑
Epiphyseal arrest — *see* Arrest, epiphyseal
Epiphyseolysis, epiphysiolysis — *see* Osteochondropathy
Epiphysitis (*see also* Osteochondropathy)
  juvenile M92.9
  syphilitic (congenital) A50.02
Epiplocele — *see* Hernia, abdomen
Epiploitis — *see* Peritonitis
Epiplosarcomphalocele — *see* Hernia, umbilicus
Episcleritis (suppurative) H15.10- ☑
  in (due to)
    syphilis A52.71
    tuberculosis A18.51
  nodular H15.12- ☑
  periodica fugax H15.11- ☑
  angioneurotic — *see* Edema, angioneurotic
  syphilitic (late) A52.71
  tuberculous A18.51
Episode
  affective, mixed F39
  depersonalization (in neurotic state) F48.1
  depressive F32.9
    major F32.9
      mild F32.0
      moderate F32.1
      severe (without psychotic symptoms) F32.2
        with psychotic symptoms F32.3
    recurrent F33.9
      brief F33.8
    specified NEC F32.89
  hypomanic F30.8
  manic F30.9
    with
      psychotic symptoms F30.2
      remission (full) F30.4
        partial F30.3
    without psychotic symptoms F30.10
      mild F30.11
      moderate F30.12
      severe (without psychotic symptoms) F30.13
        with psychotic symptoms F30.2
    other specified F30.8
    recurrent F31.89
  psychotic F23
    organic F06.8
  schizophrenic (acute) NEC, brief F23
Epispadias (female) (male) Q64.0
Episplenitis D73.89
Epistaxis (multiple) R04.0

Esthesioneuroepithelioma C30.Ø
Esthiomene A55
Estivo-autumnal malaria (fever) B5Ø.9
Estrangement (marital) Z63.5
  parent-child NEC Z62.89Ø
Estriasis — *see* Myiasis
Ethanolism — *see* Alcoholism
Etherism — *see* Dependence, drug, inhalant
Ethmoid, ethmoidal — *see* condition
Ethmoiditis (chronic) (nonpurulent) (purulent) (*see also* Sinusitis, ethmoidal)
  influenzal — *see* Influenza, with, respiratory manifestations NEC
  Woakes' J33.1
Ethylism — *see* Alcoholism
Eulenburg's disease (congenital paramyotonia) G71.19
Eumycetoma B47.Ø
Eunuchoidism E29.1
  hypogonadotropic E23.Ø
European blastomycosis — *see* Cryptococcosis
Eustachian — *see* condition
Evaluation (for) (of)
  development state
    adolescent Z00.3
    period of
      delayed growth in childhood Z00.70
        with abnormal findings Z00.71
      rapid growth in childhood Z00.2
      puberty Z00.3
  growth and developmental state (period of rapid growth) Z00.2
    delayed growth Z00.70
      with abnormal findings Z00.71
  mental health (status) Z00.8
    requested by authority Z04.6
  period of
    delayed growth in childhood Z00.70
      with abnormal findings Z00.71
    rapid growth in childhood Z00.2
  suspected condition — *see* Observation
Evans syndrome D69.41
Event
  apparent life threatening in newborn and infant (ALTE) R68.13
  brief resolved unexplained event (BRUE) R68.13
Eventration (*see also* Hernia, ventral)
  colon into chest — *see* Hernia, diaphragm
  diaphragm (congenital) Q79.1
Eversion
  bladder N32.89
  cervix (uteri) N86
    with cervicitis N72
  foot NEC (*see also* Deformity, valgus, ankle)
    congenital Q66.6
  punctum lacrimale (postinfectional) (senile) H04.52- ☑
  ureter (meatus) N28.89
  urethra (meatus) N36.8
  uterus N81.4
Evidence
  cytologic
    of malignancy on anal smear R85.614
    of malignancy on cervical smear R87.614
    of malignancy on vaginal smear R87.624
Evisceration
  birth injury P15.8
  traumatic NEC
    eye — *see* Enucleated eye
Evulsion — *see* Avulsion
Ewing's sarcoma or tumor — *see* Neoplasm, bone, malignant
Examination (for) (following) (general) (of) (routine) Z00.00
  with abnormal findings Z00.01
  abuse, physical (alleged), ruled out
    adult Z04.71
    child Z04.72
  adolescent (development state) Z00.3
  alleged rape or sexual assault (victim), ruled out
    adult Z04.41
    child Z04.42
  allergy Z01.82
  annual (adult) (periodic) (physical) Z00.00
    with abnormal findings Z00.01
    gynecological Z01.419
      with abnormal findings Z01.411
  antibody response Z01.84
  blood — *see* Examination, laboratory
  blood pressure Z01.30

Examination — *continued*
  blood pressure — *continued*
    with abnormal findings Z01.31
  cancer staging — *see* Neoplasm, malignant, by site
  cervical Papanicolaou smear Z12.4
    as part of routine gynecological examination Z01.419
    with abnormal findings Z01.411
  child (over 28 days old) Z00.129
    with abnormal findings Z00.121
    under 28 days old — *see* Newborn, examination
  clinical research control or normal comparison (control) (participant) Z00.6
  contraceptive (drug) maintenance (routine) Z30.8
    device (intrauterine) Z30.431
  dental Z01.20
    with abnormal findings Z01.21
  developmental — *see* Examination, child
  donor (potential) Z00.5
  ear Z01.10
    with abnormal findings NEC Z01.118
  eye Z01.00
    with abnormal findings Z01.01
  following
    accident NEC Z04.3
      transport Z04.1
      work Z04.2
    assault, alleged, ruled out
      adult Z04.71
      child Z04.72
    motor vehicle accident Z04.1
    treatment (for) Z09
      combined NEC Z09
        fracture Z09
        malignant neoplasm Z08
      malignant neoplasm Z08
      mental disorder Z09
      specified condition NEC Z09
  follow-up (routine) (following) Z09
    chemotherapy NEC Z09
      malignant neoplasm Z08
    fracture Z09
    malignant neoplasm Z08
    postpartum Z39.2
    psychotherapy Z09
    radiotherapy NEC Z09
      malignant neoplasm Z08
    surgery NEC Z09
      malignant neoplasm Z08
  gynecological Z01.419
    with abnormal findings Z01.411
    for contraceptive maintenance Z30.8
  health — *see* Examination, medical
  hearing Z01.10
    with abnormal findings NEC Z01.118
    following failed hearing screening Z01.110
  immunity status testing Z01.84
  laboratory (as part of a general medical examination) Z00.00
    with abnormal findings Z00.01
    preprocedural Z01.812
  lactating mother Z39.1
  medical (adult) (for) (of) Z00.00
    with abnormal findings Z00.01
    administrative purpose only Z02.9
      specified NEC Z02.89
    admission to
      armed forces Z02.3
      old age home Z02.2
      prison Z02.89
      residential institution Z02.2
      school Z02.0
        following illness or medical treatment Z02.0
      summer camp Z02.89
    adoption Z02.82
    blood alcohol or drug level Z02.83
    camp (summer) Z02.89
    clinical research, normal subject (control) (participant) Z00.6
    control subject in clinical research (normal comparison) (participant) Z00.6
    donor (potential) Z00.5
    driving license Z02.4
    general (adult) Z00.00
      with abnormal findings Z00.01
    immigration Z02.89
    insurance purposes Z02.6
    marriage Z02.89
    medicolegal reasons NEC Z04.8

Examination — *continued*
  medical — *continued*
    naturalization Z02.89
    participation in sport Z02.5
    paternity testing Z02.81
    population survey Z00.8
    pre-employment Z02.1
    pre-operative — *see* Examination, pre-procedural
    pre-procedural
      cardiovascular Z01.810
      respiratory Z01.811
      specified NEC Z01.818
    preschool children
      for admission to school Z02.0
    prisoners
      for entrance into prison Z02.89
    recruitment for armed forces Z02.3
    specified NEC Z00.8
    sport competition Z02.5
  medicolegal reason NEC Z04.8
  newborn — *see* Newborn, examination
  pelvic (annual) (periodic) Z01.419
    with abnormal findings Z01.411
  period of rapid growth in childhood Z00.2
  periodic (adult) (annual) (routine) Z00.00
    with abnormal findings Z00.01
  physical (adult) (*see also* Examination, medical) Z00.00
    sports Z02.5
  postpartum
    immediately after delivery Z39.0
    routine follow-up Z39.2
  pre-chemotherapy (antineoplastic) Z01.818
  prenatal (normal pregnancy) (*see also* Pregnancy, normal) Z34.9- ☑
  pre-procedural (pre-operative)
    cardiovascular Z01.810
    laboratory Z01.812
    respiratory Z01.811
    specified NEC Z01.818
  prior to chemotherapy (antineoplastic) Z01.818
  psychiatric NEC Z00.8
    follow-up not needing further care Z09
    requested by authority Z04.6
  radiological (as part of a general medical examination) Z00.00
    with abnormal findings Z00.01
  repeat cervical smear to confirm findings of recent normal smear following initial abnormal smear Z01.42
  skin (hypersensitivity) Z01.82
  special (*see also* Examination, by type) Z01.89
    specified type NEC Z01.89
  specified type or reason NEC Z04.8
  teeth Z01.20
    with abnormal findings Z01.21
  urine — *see* Examination, laboratory
  vision Z01.00
    with abnormal findings Z01.01
Exanthem, exanthema (*see also* Rash)
  with enteroviral vesicular stomatitis B08.4
  Boston A88.0
  epidemic with meningitis A88.0 [G02]
  subitum B08.20
    due to human herpesvirus 6 B08.21
    due to human herpesvirus 7 B08.22
  viral, virus B09
    specified type NEC B08.8
Excess, excessive, excessively
  alcohol level in blood R78.0
  androgen (ovarian) E28.1
  attrition, tooth, teeth K03.0
  carotene, carotin (dietary) E67.1
  cold, effects of T69.9 ☑
    specified effect NEC T69.8 ☑
  convergence H51.12
  crying
    in child, adolescent, or adult R45.83
    in infant R68.11
  development, breast N62
  divergence H51.8
  drinking (alcohol) NEC (without dependence) F10.10
    habitual (continual) (without remission) F10.20
  eating R63.2
  estrogen E28.0
  fat (*see also* Obesity)
    in heart — *see* Degeneration, myocardial
    localized E65
  foreskin N47.8

Excess, excessive, excessively — *continued*
  gas R14.0
  glucagon E16.3
  heat — *see* Heat
  intermaxillary vertical dimension of fully erupted teeth
      M26.37
  interocclusal distance of fully erupted teeth M26.37
  kalium E87.5
  large
      colon K59.39
          congenital Q43.8
      infant P08.0
      organ or site, congenital NEC — *see* Anomaly, by
          site
  long
      organ or site, congenital NEC — *see* Anomaly, by
          site
  menstruation (with regular cycle) N92.0
      with irregular cycle N92.1
  napping Z72.821
  natrium E87.0
  number of teeth K00.1
  nutrient (dietary) NEC R63.2
  potassium (K) E87.5
  salivation K11.7
  secretion (*see also* Hypersecretion)
      milk O92.6
      sputum R09.3
      sweat R61
  sexual drive F52.8
  short
      organ or site, congenital NEC — *see* Anomaly, by
          site
      umbilical cord in labor or delivery O69.3 ☑
  skin L98.7
      and subcutaneous tissue L98.7
      eyelid (acquired) — *see* Blepharochalasis
          congenital Q10.3
  sodium (Na) E87.0
  spacing of fully erupted teeth M26.32
  sputum R09.3
  sweating R61
  thirst R63.1
      due to deprivation of water T73.1 ☑
  tuberosity of jaw M26.07
  vitamin
      A (dietary) E67.0
          administered as drug (prolonged intake) — *see*
              Table of Drugs and Chemicals, vitamins,
              adverse effect
          overdose or wrong substance given or taken
              — *see* Table of Drugs and Chemicals, vi-
              tamins, poisoning
      D (dietary) E67.3
          administered as drug (prolonged intake) — *see*
              Table of Drugs and Chemicals, vitamins,
              adverse effect
          overdose or wrong substance given or taken
              — *see* Table of Drugs and Chemicals, vi-
              tamins, poisoning
  weight
      gain R63.5
      loss R63.4
Excitability, abnormal, under minor stress (personal-
      ity disorder) F60.3
Excitation
  anomalous atrioventricular I45.6
  psychogenic F30.8
  reactive (from emotional stress, psychological trauma)
      F30.8
Excitement
  hypomanic F30.8
  manic F30.9
  mental, reactive (from emotional stress, psychological
      trauma) F30.8
  state, reactive (from emotional stress, psychological
      trauma) F30.8
Excoriation (traumatic) (*see also* Abrasion)
  neurotic L98.1
  skin picking disorder F42.4
Exfoliation
  due to erythematous conditions according to extent
      of body surface involved L49.0
      less than 10 percent of body surface L49.0
      10-19 percent of body surface L49.1
      20-29 percent of body surface L49.2
      30-39 percent of body surface L49.3
      40-49 percent of body surface L49.4

Exfoliation — *continued*
  due to erythematous conditions according to extent
      of body surface involved — *continued*
      50-59 percent of body surface L49.5
      60-69 percent of body surface L49.6
      70-79 percent of body surface L49.7
      80-89 percent of body surface L49.8
      90-99 percent of body surface L49.9
  teeth, due to systemic causes K08.0
Exfoliative — *see* condition
Exhaustion, exhaustive (physical NEC) R53.83
  battle F43.0
  cardiac — *see* Failure, heart
  delirium F43.0
  due to
      cold T69.8 ☑
      excessive exertion T73.3 ☑
      exposure T73.2 ☑
      neurasthenia F48.8
  heart — *see* Failure, heart
  heat (*see also* Heat, exhaustion) T67.5 ☑
      due to
          salt depletion T67.4 ☑
          water depletion T67.3 ☑
  maternal, complicating delivery O75.81
  mental F48.8
  myocardium, myocardial — *see* Failure, heart
  nervous F48.8
  old age R54
  psychogenic F48.8
  psychosis F43.0
  senile R54
  vital NEC Z73.0
Exhibitionism F65.2
Exocervicitis — *see* Cervicitis
Exomphalos Q79.2
  meaning hernia — *see* Hernia, umbilicus
Exophoria H50.52
  convergence, insufficiency H51.11
  divergence, excess H51.8
Exophthalmos H05.2- ☑
  congenital Q15.8
  constant NEC H05.24- ☑
  displacement, globe — *see* Displacement, globe
  due to thyrotoxicosis (hyperthyroidism) — *see* Hyper-
      thyroidism, with, goiter (diffuse)
  dysthyroid — *see* Hyperthyroidism, with, goiter (dif-
      fuse)
  goiter — *see* Hyperthyroidism, with, goiter (diffuse)
  intermittent NEC H05.25- ☑
  malignant — *see* Hyperthyroidism, with, goiter (dif-
      fuse)
  orbital
      edema — *see* Edema, orbit
      hemorrhage — *see* Hemorrhage, orbit
  pulsating NEC H05.26- ☑
  thyrotoxic, thyrotropic — *see* Hyperthyroidism, with,
      goiter (diffuse)
Exostosis (*see also* Disorder, bone)
  cartilaginous — *see* Neoplasm, bone, benign
  congenital (multiple) Q78.6
  external ear canal H61.81- ☑
  gonococcal A54.49
  jaw (bone) M27.8
  multiple, congenital Q78.6
  orbit H05.35- ☑
  osteocartilaginous — *see* Neoplasm, bone, benign
  syphilitic A52.77
Exotropia — *see* Strabismus, divergent concomitant
Explanation of
  investigation finding Z71.2
  medication Z71.89
Exposure (to) (*see also* Contact, with) T75.89 ☑
  acariasis Z20.7
  AIDS virus Z20.6
  air pollution Z77.110
  algae and algae toxins Z77.121
  algae bloom Z77.121
  anthrax Z20.810
  aromatic amines Z77.020
  aromatic (hazardous) compounds NEC Z77.028
  aromatic dyes NOS Z77.028
  arsenic Z77.010
  asbestos Z77.090
  benzene Z77.021
  blue-green algae bloom Z77.121

Exposure — *continued*
  body fluids (potentially hazardous) Z77.21
  brown tide Z77.121
  chemicals (chiefly nonmedicinal) (hazardous) NEC
      Z77.098
  cholera Z20.09
  chromium compounds Z77.018
  cold, effects of T69.9 ☑
      specified effect NEC T69.8 ☑
  communicable disease Z20.9
      bacterial NEC Z20.818
      specified NEC Z20.89
      viral NEC Z20.828
  cyanobacteria bloom Z77.121
  disaster Z65.5
  discrimination Z60.5
  dyes Z77.098
  effects of T73.9 ☑
  environmental tobacco smoke (acute) (chronic) Z77.22
  Escherichia coli (E. coli) Z20.01
  exhaustion due to T73.2 ☑
  fiberglass — *see* Table of Drugs and Chemicals, fiber-
      glass
  German measles Z20.4
  gonorrhea Z20.2
  hazardous metals NEC Z77.018
  hazardous substances NEC Z77.29
  hazards in the physical environment NEC Z77.128
  hazards to health NEC Z77.9
  human immunodeficiency virus (HIV) Z20.6
  human T-lymphotropic virus type-1 (HTLV-1) Z20.89
  implanted
      mesh — *see* Complications, mesh
      prosthetic materials NEC — *see* Complications,
          prosthetic materials NEC
  infestation (parasitic) NEC Z20.7
  intestinal infectious disease NEC Z20.09
      Escherichia coli (E. coli) Z20.01
  lead Z77.011
  meningococcus Z20.811
  mold (toxic) Z77.120
  nickel dust Z77.018
  noise Z77.122
  occupational
      air contaminants NEC Z57.39
      dust Z57.2
      environmental tobacco smoke Z57.31
      extreme temperature Z57.6
      noise Z57.0
      radiation Z57.1
      risk factors Z57.9
          specified NEC Z57.8
      toxic agents (gases) (liquids) (solids) (vapors) in
          agriculture Z57.4
      toxic agents (gases) (liquids) (solids) (vapors) in
          industry NEC Z57.5
      vibration Z57.7
  parasitic disease NEC Z20.7
  pediculosis Z20.7
  persecution Z60.5
  pfiesteria piscicida Z77.121
  poliomyelitis Z20.89
  pollution
      air Z77.110
      environmental NEC Z77.118
      soil Z77.112
      water Z77.111
  polycyclic aromatic hydrocarbons Z77.028
  prenatal (drugs) (toxic chemicals) — *see* Newborn,
      affected by, noxious substances transmitted via
      placenta or breast milk
  rabies Z20.3
  radiation, naturally occurring NEC Z77.123
  radon Z77.123
  red tide (Florida) Z77.121
  rubella Z20.4
  second hand tobacco smoke (acute) (chronic) Z77.22
      in the perinatal period P96.81
  sexually-transmitted disease Z20.2
  smallpox (laboratory) Z20.89
  syphilis Z20.2
  terrorism Z65.4
  torture Z65.4
  tuberculosis Z20.1
  uranium Z77.012
  varicella Z20.820
  venereal disease Z20.2
  viral disease NEC Z20.828

Exposure — *continued*
  war Z65.5
  water pollution Z77.111
Exsanguination — *see* Hemorrhage
Exstrophy
  abdominal contents Q45.8
  bladder Q64.10
    cloacal Q64.12
    specified type NEC Q64.19
    supravesical fissure Q64.11
Extensive — *see* condition
Extra (*see also* Accessory)
  marker chromosomes (normal individual) Q92.61
    in abnormal individual Q92.62
  rib Q76.6
    cervical Q76.5
Extrasystoles (supraventricular) I49.49
  atrial I49.1
  auricular I49.1
  junctional I49.2
  ventricular I49.3
Extrauterine gestation or pregnancy — *see* Pregnancy, by site
Extravasation
  blood R58
  chyle into mesentery I89.8
  pelvicalyceal N13.8
  pyelosinus N13.8
  urine (from ureter) R39.0
  vesicant agent
    antineoplastic chemotherapy T80.810 ☑
    other agent NEC T80.818 ☑
Extremity — *see* condition, limb
Extrophy — *see* Exstrophy
Extroversion
  bladder Q64.19
  uterus N81.4
    complicating delivery O71.2
    postpartal (old) N81.4
Extruded tooth (teeth) M26.34
Extrusion
  breast implant (prosthetic) T85.42 ☑
  eye implant (globe) (ball) T85.328 ☑
  intervertebral disc — *see* Displacement, intervertebral disc
  ocular lens implant (prosthetic) — *see* Complications, intraocular lens
  vitreous — *see* Prolapse, vitreous
Exudate
  pleural — *see* Effusion, pleura
  retina H35.89
Exudative — *see* condition
Eye, eyeball, eyelid — *see* condition
Eyestrain — *see* Disturbance, vision, subjective
Eyeworm disease of Africa B74.3

F

Faber's syndrome (achlorhydric anemia) D50.9
Fabry (-Anderson) **disease** E75.21
Faciocephalalgia, autonomic (*see also* Neuropathy, peripheral, autonomic) G90.09
Factor(s)
  psychic, associated with diseases classified elsewhere F54
  psychological
    affecting physical conditions F54
    or behavioral
      affecting general medical condition F54
      associated with disorders or diseases classified elsewhere F54
Fahr disease (of brain) G23.8
Fahr Volhard disease (of kidney) I12.- ☑
Failure, failed
  abortion — *see* Abortion, attempted
  aortic (valve) I35.8
    rheumatic I06.8
  attempted abortion — *see* Abortion, attempted
  biventricular I50.82
    due to left heart failure I50.814
  bone marrow — *see* Anemia, aplastic
  cardiac — *see* Failure, heart
  cardiorenal (chronic) (*see also* Failure, renal, and Failure, heart) I50.9
    hypertensive I13.2
  cardiorespiratory (*see also* Failure, heart) R09.2
  cardiovascular (chronic) — *see* Failure, heart

Failure, failed — *continued*
  cerebrovascular I67.9
  cervical dilatation in labor O62.0
  circulation, circulatory (peripheral) R57.9
    newborn P29.89
  compensation — *see* Disease, heart
  compliance with medical treatment or regimen — *see* Noncompliance
  congestive — *see* Failure, heart, congestive
  dental implant (endosseous) M27.69
    due to
      failure of dental prosthesis M27.63
      lack of attached gingiva M27.62
      occlusal trauma (poor prosthetic design) M27.62
      parafunctional habits M27.62
      periodontal infection (peri-implantitis) M27.62
      poor oral hygiene M27.62
      osseointegration M27.61
        due to
          complications of systemic disease M27.61
          poor bone quality M27.61
        iatrogenic M27.61
      post-osseointegration
        biological M27.62
          due to complications of systemic disease M27.62
        iatrogenic M27.62
        mechanical M27.63
      pre-integration M27.61
      pre-osseointegration M27.61
      specified NEC M27.69
  descent of head (at term) of pregnancy (mother) O32.4 ☑
  endosseous dental implant — *see* Failure, dental implant
  engagement of head (term of pregnancy) (mother) O32.4 ☑
  erection (penile) (*see also* Dysfunction, sexual, male, erectile) N52.9
    nonorganic F52.21
  examination(s), anxiety concerning Z55.2
  expansion terminal respiratory units (newborn) (primary) P28.0
  forceps NOS (with subsequent cesarean delivery) O66.5
  gain weight (child over 28 days old) R62.51
    adult R62.7
    newborn P92.6
  genital response (male) F52.21
    female F52.22
  heart (acute) (senile) (sudden) I50.9
    with
      acute pulmonary edema — *see* Failure, ventricular, left
      decompensation (*see also* Failure, heart, by type as diastolic or systolic, acute and chronic) I50.9
      dilatation — *see* Disease, heart
      normal ejection fraction — *see* Failure, heart, diastolic
      preserved ejection fraction — *see* Failure, heart, diastolic
      reduced ejection fraction — *see* Failure, heart, systolic
    arteriosclerotic I70.90
    biventricular I50.82
      due to left heart failure I50.814
      combined left-right sided I50.82
        due to left heart failure I50.814
    compensated (*see also* Failure, heart, by type as diastolic or systolic, chronic) I50.9
    complicating
      anesthesia (general) (local) or other sedation in labor and delivery O74.2
      in pregnancy O29.12- ☑
      postpartum, puerperal O89.1
      delivery (cesarean) (instrumental) O75.4
    congestive I50.9
      with rheumatic fever (conditions in I00)
        active I01.8
        inactive or quiescent (with chorea) I09.81
      newborn P29.0
      rheumatic (chronic) (inactive) (with chorea) I09.81
        active or acute I01.8
          with chorea I02.0
    decompensated (*see also* Failure, heart, by type as diastolic or systolic, acute and chronic) I50.9

Failure, failed — *continued*
  heart — *continued*
    degenerative — *see* Degeneration, myocardial
    diastolic (congestive) (left ventricular) I50.30
      acute (congestive) I50.31
        and (on) chronic (congestive) I50.33
      chronic (congestive) I50.32
        and (on) acute (congestive) I50.33
      combined with systolic (congestive) I50.40
        acute (congestive) I50.41
          and (on) chronic (congestive) I50.43
        chronic (congestive) I50.42
          and (on) acute (congestive) I50.43
    due to presence of cardiac prosthesis I97.13- ☑
    end stage (*see also* Failure, heart, by type as diastolic or systolic, chronic) I50.84
    following cardiac surgery I97.13- ☑
    high output NOS I50.83
    hypertensive — *see* Hypertension, heart
    left (ventricular) (*see also* Failure, ventricular, left)
      combined diastolic and systolic — *see* Failure, heart, diastolic, combined with systolic
      diastolic — *see* Failure, heart, diastolic
      systolic — *see* Failure, heart, systolic
    low output (syndrome) NOS I50.9
    newborn P29.0
    organic — *see* Disease, heart
    peripartum O90.3
    postprocedural I97.13- ☑
    rheumatic (chronic) (inactive) I09.9
    right (isolated) (ventricular) I50.810
      acute I50.811
        and (on) chronic I50.813
      chronic I50.812
        and acute I50.813
      secondary to left heart failure I50.814
    specified NEC I50.89

Note: heart failure stages A, B, C, and D are based on the American College of Cardiology and American Heart Association stages of heart failure, which complement and should not be confused with the New York Heart Association Classification of Heart Failure, into Class I, Class II, Class III, and Class IV

    stage A Z91.89
    stage B (*see also* Failure, heart, by type as diastolic or systolic) I50.9
    stage C (*see also* Failure, heart, by type as diastolic or systolic) I50.9
    stage D (*see also* Failure, heart, by type as diastolic or systolic, chronic) I50.84
    systolic (congestive) (left ventricular) I50.20
      acute (congestive) I50.21
        and (on) chronic (congestive) I50.23
      chronic (congestive) I50.22
        and (on) acute (congestive) I50.23
      combined with diastolic (congestive) I50.40
        acute (congestive) I50.41
          and (on) chronic (congestive) I50.43
        chronic (congestive) I50.42
          and (on) acute (congestive) I50.43
    thyrotoxic (*see also* Thyrotoxicosis) E05.90 [I43]
      with
        high output (*see also* Thyrotoxicosis) I50.83
        thyroid storm E05.91 [I43]
          high output (*see also* Thyrotoxicosis) I50.83
    valvular — *see* Endocarditis
  hepatic K72.90
    with coma K72.91
    acute or subacute K72.00
      with coma K72.01
      due to drugs K71.10
        with coma K71.11
    alcoholic (acute) (chronic) (subacute) K70.40
      with coma K70.41
    chronic K72.10
      with coma K72.11
      due to drugs (acute) (subacute) (chronic) K71.10
        with coma K71.11
    due to drugs (acute) (subacute) (chronic) K71.10
      with coma K71.11
    postprocedural K91.82
  hepatorenal K76.7
  induction (of labor) O61.9
    abortion — *see* Abortion, attempted
    by
      oxytocic drugs O61.0

Failure, failed — *continued*
  induction — *continued*
    by — *continued*
      prostaglandins O61.0
    instrumental O61.1
    mechanical O61.1
    medical O61.0
    specified NEC O61.8
    surgical O61.1
  intubation during anesthesia T88.4 ☑
    in pregnancy O29.6- ☑
    labor and delivery O74.7
    postpartum, puerperal O89.6
  involution, thymus (gland) E32.0
  kidney (*see also* Disease, kidney, chronic) N19
    acute (*see also* Failure, renal, acute) N17.9
  lactation (complete) O92.3
    partial O92.4
  Leydig's cell, adult E29.1
  liver — *see* Failure, hepatic
  menstruation at puberty N91.0
  mitral I05.8
  myocardial, myocardium (*see also* Failure, heart) I50.9
    chronic (*see also* Failure, heart, congestive) I50.9
    congestive (*see also* Failure, heart, congestive) I50.9
  orgasm (female) (psychogenic) F52.31
    male F52.32
  ovarian (primary) E28.39
    iatrogenic E89.40
      asymptomatic E89.40
      symptomatic E89.41
    postprocedural (postablative) (postirradiation) (postsurgical) E89.40
      asymptomatic E89.40
      symptomatic E89.41
  ovulation causing infertility N97.0
  polyglandular, autoimmune E31.0
  prosthetic joint implant — *see* Complications, joint prosthesis, mechanical, breakdown, by site
  renal N19
    with
      tubular necrosis (acute) N17.0
    acute N17.9
      with
        cortical necrosis N17.1
        medullary necrosis N17.2
        tubular necrosis N17.0
      specified NEC N17.8
    chronic N18.9
      hypertensive — *see* Hypertension, kidney
    congenital P96.0
    end stage (chronic) N18.6
      due to hypertension I12.0
    following
      abortion — *see* Abortion by type complicated by specified condition NEC
      crushing T79.5 ☑
      ectopic or molar pregnancy O08.4
      labor and delivery (acute) O90.4
    hypertensive — *see* Hypertension, kidney
    postprocedural N99.0
  respiration, respiratory J96.90
    with
      hypercapnia J96.92
      hypercarbia J96.02
      hypoxia J96.91
    acute J96.00
      with
        hypercapnia J96.02
        hypercarbia J96.02
        hypoxia J96.01
    acute and (on) chronic J96.20
      with
        hypercapnia J96.22
        hypercarbia J96.22
        hypoxia J96.21
    center G93.89
    chronic J96.10
      with
        hypercapnia J96.12
        hypercarbia J96.12
        hypoxia J96.11
    newborn P28.5
    postprocedural (acute) J95.821
      acute and chronic J95.822
  rotation
    cecum Q43.3
    colon Q43.3

Failure, failed — *continued*
  rotation — *continued*
    intestine Q43.3
    kidney Q63.2
  sedation (conscious) (moderate) during procedure T88.52 ☑
    history of Z92.83
  segmentation (*see also* Fusion)
    fingers — *see* Syndactylism, complex, fingers
    vertebra Q76.49
      with scoliosis Q76.3
  seminiferous tubule, adult E29.1
  senile (general) R54
  sexual arousal (male) F52.21
    female F52.22
  testicular endocrine function E29.1
  to thrive (child over 28 days old) R62.51
    adult R62.7
    newborn P92.6
  transplant T86.92
    bone T86.831
      marrow T86.02
    cornea T86.841
    heart T86.22
      with lung(s) T86.32
    intestine T86.851
    kidney T86.12
    liver T86.42
    lung(s) T86.811
      with heart T86.32
    pancreas T86.891
    skin (allograft) (autograft) T86.821
    specified organ or tissue NEC T86.891
    stem cell (peripheral blood) (umbilical cord) T86.5
  trial of labor (with subsequent cesarean delivery) O66.40
    following previous cesarean delivery O66.41
  tubal ligation N99.89
  urinary — *see* Disease, kidney, chronic
  vacuum extraction NOS (with subsequent cesarean delivery) O66.5
  vasectomy N99.89
  ventouse NOS (with subsequent cesarean delivery) O66.5
  ventricular (*see also* Failure, heart) I50.9
    left (*see also* Failure, heart, left) I50.1
      with rheumatic fever (conditions in I00)
        active I01.8
          with chorea I02.0
        inactive or quiescent (with chorea) I09.81
        rheumatic (chronic) (inactive) (with chorea) I09.81
          active or acute I01.8
            with chorea I02.0
    right — *see* Failure, heart, right
  vital centers, newborn P91.88
Fainting (fit) R55
Fallen arches — *see* Deformity, limb, flat foot
Falling, falls (repeated) R29.6
  any organ or part — *see* Prolapse
Fallopian
  insufflation Z31.41
  tube — *see* condition
Fallot's
  pentalogy Q21.8
  tetrad or tetralogy Q21.3
  triad or trilogy Q22.3
False (*see also* condition)
  croup J38.5
  joint — *see* Nonunion, fracture
  labor (pains) O47.9
    at or after 37 completed weeks of gestation O47.1
    before 37 completed weeks of gestation O47.0- ☑
  passage, urethra (prostatic) N36.5
  pregnancy F45.8
Family, familial (*see also* condition)
  disruption Z63.8
    involving divorce or separation Z63.5
  Li-Fraumeni (syndrome) Z15.01
  planning advice Z30.09
  problem Z63.9
    specified NEC Z63.8
  retinoblastoma C69.2- ☑
Famine (effects of) T73.0 ☑
  edema — *see* Malnutrition, severe
Fanconi (-de Toni)(-Debré) **syndrome** E72.09
  with cystinosis E72.04
Fanconi's anemia (congenital pancytopenia) D61.09

Farber's disease or syndrome E75.29
Farcy A24.0
Farmer's
  lung J67.0
  skin L57.8
Farsightedness — *see* Hypermetropia
Fascia — *see* condition
Fasciculation R25.3
Fasciitis M72.9
  diffuse (eosinophilic) M35.4
  infective M72.8
    necrotizing M72.6
  necrotizing M72.6
  nodular M72.4
  perirenal (with ureteral obstruction) N13.5
    with infection N13.6
  plantar M72.2
  specified NEC M72.8
  traumatic (old) M72.8
    current — *code by* site under Sprain
Fascioliasis B66.3
Fasciolopsis, fasciolopsiasis (intestinal) B66.5
Fascioscapulohumeral myopathy G71.0
Fast pulse R00.0
Fat
  embolism — *see* Embolism, fat
  excessive (*see also* Obesity)
    in heart — *see* Degeneration, myocardial
  in stool R19.5
  localized (pad) E65
    heart — *see* Degeneration, myocardial
    knee M79.4
    retropatellar M79.4
  necrosis
    breast N64.1
    mesentery K65.4
    omentum K65.4
  pad E65
    knee M79.4
Fatigue R53.83
  auditory deafness — *see* Deafness
  chronic R53.82
  combat F43.0
  general R53.83
    psychogenic F48.8
  heat (transient) T67.6 ☑
  muscle M62.89
  myocardium — *see* Failure, heart
  neoplasm-related R53.0
  nervous, neurosis F48.8
  operational F48.8
  psychogenic (general) F48.8
  senile R54
  voice R49.8
Fatness — *see* Obesity
Fatty (*see also* condition)
  apron E65
  degeneration — *see* Degeneration, fatty
  heart (enlarged) — *see* Degeneration, myocardial
  liver NEC K76.0
    alcoholic K70.0
    nonalcoholic K76.0
  necrosis — *see* Degeneration, fatty
Fauces — *see* condition
Fauchard's disease (periodontitis) — *see* Periodontitis
Faucitis J02.9
Favism (anemia) D55.0
Favus — *see* Dermatophytosis
Fazio-Londe disease or syndrome G12.1
Fear complex or reaction F40.9
Fear of — *see* Phobia
Feared complaint unfounded Z71.1
Febris, febrile (*see also* Fever)
  flava (*see also* Fever, yellow) A95.9
  melitensis A23.0
  pestis — *see* Plague
  recurrens — *see* Fever, relapsing
  rubra A38.9
Fecal
  incontinence R15.9
  smearing R15.1
  soiling R15.1
  urgency R15.2
Fecalith (impaction) K56.41
  appendix K38.1
  congenital P76.8
Fede's disease K14.0

☑ Additional Character Required — Refer to the Tabular List for Character Selection ▽ Subterms under main terms may continue to next column or page

Feeble rapid pulse due to shock following injury T79.4 ☑
Feeble-minded F70
Feeding
 difficulties R63.3
 problem R63.3
  newborn P92.9
   specified NEC P92.8
  nonorganic (adult) — see Disorder, eating
Feeling (of)
 foreign body in throat R09.89
Feer's disease — see Poisoning, mercury
Feet — see condition
Feigned illness Z76.5
Feil-Klippel syndrome (brevicollis) Q76.1
Feinmesser's (hidrotic) **ectodermal dysplasia** Q82.4
Felinophobia F40.218
Felon (see also Cellulitis, digit)
 with lymphangitis — see Lymphangitis, acute, digit
Felty's syndrome M05.00
 ankle M05.07- ☑
 elbow M05.02- ☑
 foot joint M05.07- ☑
 hand joint M05.04- ☑
 hip M05.05- ☑
 knee M05.06- ☑
 multiple site M05.09
 shoulder M05.01- ☑
 vertebra — see Spondylitis, ankylosing
 wrist M05.03- ☑
Female genital cutting status — see Female genital mutilation status (FGM)
Female genital mutilation status (FGM) N90.810
 specified NEC N90.818
 type I (clitorectomy status) N90.811
 type II (clitorectomy with excision of labia minora status) N90.812
 type III (infibulation status) N90.813
 type IV N90.818
Femur, femoral — see condition
Fenestration, fenestrated (see also Imperfect, closure)
 aortico-pulmonary Q21.4
 cusps, heart valve NEC Q24.8
  pulmonary Q22.3
 pulmonic cusps Q22.3
Fernell's disease (aortic aneurysm) I71.9
Fertile eunuch syndrome E23.0
Fetid
 breath R19.6
 sweat L75.0
Fetishism F65.0
 transvestic F65.1
Fetus, fetal (see also condition)
 alcohol syndrome (dysmorphic) Q86.0
 compressus O31.0- ☑
 hydantoin syndrome Q86.1
 lung tissue P28.0
 papyraceous O31.0- ☑
Fever (inanition) (of unknown origin) (persistent) (with chills) (with rigor) R50.9
 abortus A23.1
 Aden (dengue) A90
 African tick-borne A68.1
 American
  mountain (tick) A93.2
  spotted A77.0
 aphthous B08.8
 arbovirus, arboviral A94
  hemorrhagic A94
  specified NEC A93.8
 Argentinian hemorrhagic A96.0
 Assam B55.0
 Australian Q A78
 Bangkok hemorrhagic A91
 Barmah forest A92.8
 Bartonella A44.0
 bilious, hemoglobinuric B50.8
 blackwater B50.8
 blister B00.1
 Bolivian hemorrhagic A96.1
 Bonvale dam T73.3 ☑
 boutonneuse A77.1
 brain — see Encephalitis
 Brazilian purpuric A48.4
 breakbone A90
 Bullis A77.0
 Bunyamwera A92.8

Fever — continued
 Burdwan B55.0
 Bwamba A92.8
 Cameroon — see Malaria
 Canton A75.9
 catarrhal (acute) J00
  chronic J31.0
 cat-scratch A28.1
 Central Asian hemorrhagic A98.0
 cerebral — see Encephalitis
 cerebrospinal meningococcal A39.0
 Chagres B50.9
 Chandipura A92.8
 Changuinola A93.1
 Charcot's (biliary) (hepatic) (intermittent) — see Calculus, bile duct
 Chikungunya (viral) (hemorrhagic) A92.0
 Chitral A93.1
 Colombo — see Fever, paratyphoid
 Colorado tick (virus) A93.2
 congestive (remittent) — see Malaria
 Congo virus A98.0
 continued malarial B50.9
 Corsican — see Malaria
 Crimean-Congo hemorrhagic A98.0
 Cyprus — see Brucellosis
 dandy A90
 deer fly — see Tularemia
 dengue (virus) A90
  hemorrhagic A91
  sandfly A93.1
 desert B38.0
 drug induced R50.2
 due to
  conditions classified elsewhere R50.81
  heat T67.0 ☑
 enteric A01.00
 enteroviral exanthematous (Boston exanthem) A88.0
 ephemeral (of unknown origin) R50.9
 epidemic hemorrhagic A98.5
 erysipelatous — see Erysipelas
 estivo-autumnal (malarial) B50.9
 famine A75.0
 five day A79.0
 following delivery O86.4
 Fort Bragg A27.89
 gastroenteric A01.00
 gastromalarial — see Malaria
 Gibraltar — see Brucellosis
 glandular — see Mononucleosis, infectious
 Guama (viral) A92.8
 Haverhill A25.1
 hay (allergic) J30.1
  with asthma (bronchial) J45.909
   with
    exacerbation (acute) J45.901
    status asthmaticus J45.902
   due to
    allergen other than pollen J30.89
    pollen, any plant or tree J30.1
 heat (effects) T67.0 ☑
 hematuric, bilious B50.8
 hemoglobinuric (malarial) (bilious) B50.8
 hemorrhagic (arthropod-borne) NOS A94
  with renal syndrome A98.5
  arenaviral A96.9
   specified NEC A96.8
  Argentinian A96.0
  Bangkok A91
  Bolivian A96.1
  Central Asian A98.0
  Chikungunya A92.0
  Crimean-Congo A98.0
  dengue (virus) A91
  epidemic A98.5
  Junin (virus) A96.0
  Korean A98.5
  Kyasanur forest A98.2
  Machupo (virus) A96.1
  mite-borne A93.8
  mosquito-borne A92.8
  Omsk A98.1
  Philippine A91
  Russian A98.5
  Singapore A91
  Southeast Asia A91
  Thailand A91
  tick-borne NEC A93.8

Fever — continued
 hemorrhagic — continued
  viral A99
   specified NEC A98.8
 hepatic — see Cholecystitis
 herpetic — see Herpes
 icterohemorrhagic A27.0
 Indiana A93.8
 infective B99.9
  specified NEC B99.8
 intermittent (bilious) (see also Malaria)
  of unknown origin R50.9
  pernicious B50.9
 iodide R50.2
 Japanese river A75.3
 jungle (see also Malaria)
  yellow A95.0
 Junin (virus) hemorrhagic A96.0
 Katayama B65.2
 kedani A75.3
 Kenya (tick) A77.1
 Kew Garden A79.1
 Korean hemorrhagic A98.5
 Lassa A96.2
 Lone Star A77.0
 Machupo (virus) hemorrhagic A96.1
 malaria, malarial — see Malaria
 Malta A23.9
 Marseilles A77.1
 marsh — see Malaria
 Mayaro (viral) A92.8
 Mediterranean (see also Brucellosis) A23.9
  familial M04.1
  tick A77.1
 meningeal — see Meningitis
 Meuse A79.0
 Mexican A75.2
 mianeh A68.1
 miasmatic — see Malaria
 mosquito-borne (viral) A92.9
  hemorrhagic A92.8
 mountain (see also Brucellosis)
  meaning Rocky Mountain spotted fever A77.0
  tick (American) (Colorado) (viral) A93.2
 Mucambo (viral) A92.8
 mud A27.9
 Neapolitan — see Brucellosis
 neutropenic D70.9
 newborn P81.9
  environmental P81.0
 Nine-Mile A78
 non-exanthematous tick A93.2
 North Aslan tick-borne A77.2
 Omsk hemorrhagic A98.1
 O'nyong-nyong (viral) A92.1
 Oropouche (viral) A93.0
 Oroya A44.0
 paludal — see Malaria
 Panama (malarial) B50.9
 Pappataci A93.1
 paratyphoid A01.4
  A A01.1
  B A01.2
  C A01.3
 parrot A70
 periodic (Mediterranean) M04.1
 persistent (of unknown origin) R50.9
 petechial A39.0
 pharyngoconjunctival B30.2
 Philippine hemorrhagic A91
 phlebotomus A93.1
 Piry (virus) A93.8
 Pixuna (viral) A92.8
 Plasmodium ovale B53.0
 polioviral (nonparalytic) A80.4
 Pontiac A48.2
 postimmunization R50.83
 postoperative R50.82
  due to infection T81.4 ☑
 posttransfusion R50.84
 postvaccination R50.83
 presenting with conditions classified elsewhere R50.81
 pretibial A27.89
 puerperal O86.4
 Q A78
 quadrilateral A78
 quartan (malaria) B52.9
 Queensland (coastal) (tick) A77.3

Fever — *continued*
quintan A79.0
rabbit — *see* Tularemia
rat-bite A25.9
  due to
    Spirillum A25.0
    Streptobacillus moniliformis A25.1
recurrent — *see* Fever, relapsing
relapsing (Borrelia) A68.9
  Carter's (Asiatic) A68.1
  Dutton's (West African) A68.1
  Koch's A68.9
  louse-borne A68.0
  Novy's
    louse-borne A68.0
    tick-borne A68.1
  Obermeyer's (European) A68.0
  tick-borne A68.1
remittent (bilious) (congestive) (gastric) — *see* Malaria
rheumatic (active) (acute) (chronic) (subacute) I00
  with central nervous system involvement I02.9
  active with heart involvement — *see* category
    I01 ☑
  inactive or quiescent with
    cardiac hypertrophy I09.89
    carditis I09.9
    endocarditis I09.1
      aortic (valve) I06.9
        with mitral (valve) disease I08.0
      mitral (valve) I05.9
        with aortic (valve) disease I08.0
      pulmonary (valve) I09.89
      tricuspid (valve) I07.8
    heart disease NEC I09.89
    heart failure (congestive) (conditions in I50.)
      I09.81
    left ventricular failure (conditions in I50.1-I50.4-)
      I09.81
    myocarditis, myocardial degeneration (condi-
      tions in I51.4) I09.0
    pancarditis I09.9
    pericarditis I09.2
Rift Valley (viral) A92.4
Rocky Mountain spotted A77.0
rose J30.1
Ross River B33.1
Russian hemorrhagic A98.5
San Joaquin (Valley) B38.0
sandfly A93.1
Sao Paulo A77.0
scarlet A38.9
seven day (leptospirosis) (autumnal) (Japanese) A27.89
  dengue A90
shin-bone A79.0
Singapore hemorrhagic A91
solar A90
Songo A98.5
sore B00.1
South African tick-bite A68.1
Southeast Asia hemorrhagic A91
spinal — *see* Meningitis
spirillary A25.0
splenic — *see* Anthrax
spotted A77.9
  American A77.0
  Brazilian A77.0
  cerebrospinal meningitis A39.0
  Colombian A77.0
  due to Rickettsia
    australis A77.3
    conorii A77.1
    rickettsii A77.0
    sibirica A77.2
    specified type NEC A77.8
  Ehrlichiosis A77.40
    due to
      E. chafeensis A77.41
      specified organism NEC A77.49
  Rocky Mountain A77.0
steroid R50.2
streptobacillary A25.1
subtertian B50.9
Sumatran mite A75.3
sun A90
swamp A27.9
swine A02.8
sylvatic, yellow A95.0
Tahyna B33.8

Fever — *continued*
tertian — *see* Malaria, tertian
Thailand hemorrhagic A91
thermic T67.0 ☑
three-day A93.1
tick
  American mountain A93.2
  Colorado A93.2
  Kemerovo A93.8
  Mediterranean A77.1
  mountain A93.2
  nonxanthematous A93.2
  Quaranfil A93.8
tick-bite NEC A93.8
tick-borne (hemorrhagic) NEC A93.8
trench A79.0
tsutsugamushi A75.3
typhogastric A01.00
typhoid (abortive) (hemorrhagic) (intermittent) (malignant) A01.00
  complicated by
    arthritis A01.04
    heart involvement A01.02
    meningitis A01.01
    osteomyelitis A01.05
    pneumonia A01.03
    specified NEC A01.09
typhomalarial — *see* Malaria
typhus — *see* Typhus (fever)
undulant — *see* Brucellosis
unknown origin R50.9
uveoparotid D86.89
valley B38.0
Venezuelan equine A92.2
vesicular stomatitis A93.8
viral hemorrhagic — *see* Fever, hemorrhagic, by type
  of virus
Volhynian A79.0
Wesselsbron (viral) A92.8
West
  African B50.8
  Nile (viral) A92.30
    with
      complications NEC A92.39
      cranial nerve disorders A92.32
      encephalitis A92.31
      encephalomyelitis A92.31
      neurologic manifestation NEC A92.32
      optic neuritis A92.32
      polyradiculitis A92.32
Whitmore's — *see* Melioidosis
Wolhynian A79.0
worm B83.9
yellow A95.9
  jungle A95.0
  sylvatic A95.0
  urban A95.1
Zika virus A92.5
Fibrillation
atrial or auricular (established) I48.91
  chronic I48.2
  paroxysmal I48.0
  permanent I48.2
  persistent I48.1
cardiac I49.8
heart I49.8
muscular M62.89
ventricular I49.01
Fibrin
ball or bodies, pleural (sac) J94.1
chamber, anterior (eye) (gelatinous exudate) — *see*
  Iridocyclitis, acute
Fibrinogenolysis — *see* Fibrinolysis
Fibrinogenopenia D68.8
acquired D65
congenital D68.2
Fibrinolysis (hemorrhagic) (acquired) D65
antepartum hemorrhage — *see* Hemorrhage, antepartum, with coagulation defect
following
  abortion — *see* Abortion by type complicated by
    hemorrhage
  ectopic or molar pregnancy O08.1
intrapartum O67.0
newborn, transient P60
postpartum O72.3
Fibrinopenia (hereditary) D68.2
acquired D68.4

Fibrinopurulent — *see* condition
Fibrinous — *see* condition
Fibroadenoma
cellular intracanalicular D24- ☑
giant D24- ☑
intracanalicular
  cellular D24- ☑
  giant D24- ☑
  specified site — *see* Neoplasm, benign, by site
  unspecified site D24- ☑
juvenile D24- ☑
pericanalicular
  specified site — *see* Neoplasm, benign, by site
  unspecified site D24- ☑
phyllodes D24- ☑
prostate D29.1
specified site NEC — *see* Neoplasm, benign, by site
unspecified site D24- ☑
Fibroadenosis, breast (chronic) (cystic) (diffuse) (periodic) (segmental) N60.2- ☑
Fibroangioma (*see also* Neoplasm, benign, by site)
juvenile
  specified site — *see* Neoplasm, benign, by site
  unspecified site D10.6
Fibrochondrosarcoma — *see* Neoplasm, cartilage,
  malignant
Fibrocystic
disease (*see also* Fibrosis, cystic)
  breast — *see* Mastopathy, cystic
  jaw M27.49
  kidney (congenital) Q61.8
  liver Q44.6
  pancreas E84.9
kidney (congenital) Q61.8
Fibrodysplasia ossificans progressiva — *see* Myositis,
  ossificans, progressiva
Fibroelastosis (cordis) (endocardial) (endomyocardial)
  I42.4
Fibroid (tumor) (*see also* Neoplasm, connective tissue,
  benign)
disease, lung (chronic) — *see* Fibrosis, lung
heart (disease) — *see* Myocarditis
in pregnancy or childbirth O34.1- ☑
  causing obstructed labor O65.5
induration, lung (chronic) — *see* Fibrosis, lung
lung — *see* Fibrosis, lung
pneumonia (chronic) — *see* Fibrosis, lung
uterus (*see also* Leiomyoma, uterus) D25.9
Fibrolipoma — *see* Lipoma
Fibroliposarcoma — *see* Neoplasm, connective tissue,
  malignant
Fibroma (*see also* Neoplasm, connective tissue, benign)
ameloblastic — *see* Cyst, calcifying odontogenic
bone (nonossifying) — *see* Disorder, bone, specified
  type NEC
  ossifying — *see* Neoplasm, bone, benign
cementifying — *see* Neoplasm, bone, benign
chondromyxoid — *see* Neoplasm, bone, benign
desmoplastic — *see* Neoplasm, connective tissue,
  uncertain behavior
durum — *see* Neoplasm, connective tissue, benign
fascial — *see* Neoplasm, connective tissue, benign
invasive — *see* Neoplasm, connective tissue, uncertain
  behavior
molle — *see* Lipoma
myxoid — *see* Neoplasm, connective tissue, benign
nasopharynx, nasopharyngeal (juvenile) D10.6
nonosteogenic (nonossifying) — *see* Dysplasia, fibrous
odontogenic (central) — *see* Cyst, calcifying odontogenic
ossifying — *see* Neoplasm, bone, benign
periosteal — *see* Neoplasm, bone, benign
soft — *see* Lipoma
Fibromatosis M72.9
abdominal — *see* Neoplasm, connective tissue, uncertain behavior
aggressive — *see* Neoplasm, connective tissue, uncertain behavior
congenital generalized — *see* Neoplasm, connective
  tissue, uncertain behavior
Dupuytren's M72.0
gingival K06.1
palmar (fascial) M72.0
plantar (fascial) M72.2
pseudosarcomatous (proliferative) (subcutaneous)
  M72.4
retroperitoneal D48.3

Fibromatosis — *continued*
  specified NEC M72.8
Fibromyalgia M79.7
Fibromyoma (*see also* Neoplasm, connective tissue, benign)
  uterus (corpus) (*see also* Leiomyoma, uterus)
    in pregnancy or childbirth — *see* Fibroid, in pregnancy or childbirth
      causing obstructed labor O65.5
Fibromyositis M79.7
Fibromyxolipoma D17.9
Fibromyxoma — *see* Neoplasm, connective tissue, benign
Fibromyxosarcoma — *see* Neoplasm, connective tissue, malignant
Fibro-odontoma, ameloblastic — *see* Cyst, calcifying odontogenic
Fibro-osteoma — *see* Neoplasm, bone, benign
Fibroplasia, retrolental H35.17- ☑
Fibropurulent — *see* condition
Fibrosarcoma (*see also* Neoplasm, connective tissue, malignant)
  ameloblastic C41.1
    upper jaw (bone) C41.0
  congenital — *see* Neoplasm, connective tissue, malignant
  fascial — *see* Neoplasm, connective tissue, malignant
  infantile — *see* Neoplasm, connective tissue, malignant
  odontogenic C41.1
    upper jaw (bone) C41.0
  periosteal — *see* Neoplasm, bone, malignant
Fibrosclerosis
  breast N60.3- ☑
  multifocal M35.5
  penis (corpora cavernosa) N48.6
Fibrosis, fibrotic
  adrenal (gland) E27.8
  amnion O41.8X- ☑
  anal papillae K62.89
  arteriocapillary — *see* Arteriosclerosis
  bladder N32.89
    interstitial — *see* Cystitis, chronic, interstitial
    localized submucosal — *see* Cystitis, chronic, interstitial
    panmural — *see* Cystitis, chronic, interstitial
  breast — *see* Fibrosclerosis, breast
  capillary (*see also* Arteriosclerosis) I70.90
    lung (chronic) — *see* Fibrosis, lung
  cardiac — *see* Myocarditis
  cervix N88.8
  chorion O41.8X- ☑
  corpus cavernosum (sclerosing) N48.6
  cystic (of pancreas) E84.9
    with
      distal intestinal obstruction syndrome E84.19
      fecal impaction E84.19
      intestinal manifestations NEC E84.19
      pulmonary manifestations E84.0
      specified manifestations NEC E84.8
  due to device, implant or graft (*see also* Complications, by site and type, specified NEC) T85.828 ☑
    arterial graft NEC T82.828 ☑
    breast (implant) T85.828 ☑
    catheter NEC T85.828 ☑
      dialysis (renal) T82.828 ☑
        intraperitoneal T85.828 ☑
      infusion NEC T82.828 ☑
        spinal (epidural) (subdural) T85.820 ☑
      urinary (indwelling) T83.82 ☑
    electronic (electrode) (pulse generator) (stimulator)
      bone T84.82 ☑
      cardiac T82.827 ☑
      nervous system (brain) (peripheral nerve) (spinal) T85.820 ☑
      urinary T83.82 ☑
    fixation, internal (orthopedic) NEC T84.82 ☑
    gastrointestinal (bile duct) (esophagus) T85.828 ☑
    genital NEC T83.82 ☑
    heart NEC T82.827 ☑
    joint prosthesis T84.82 ☑
    ocular (corneal graft) (orbital implant) NEC T85.828 ☑
    orthopedic NEC T84.82 ☑
    specified NEC T85.828 ☑
    urinary NEC T83.82 ☑
    vascular NEC T82.828 ☑

Fibrosis, fibrotic — *continued*
  due to device, implant or graft (*see also* Complications, by site and type, specified) — *continued*
    ventricular intracranial shunt T85.820 ☑
  ejaculatory duct N50.89
  endocardium — *see* Endocarditis
  endomyocardial (tropical) I42.3
  epididymis N50.89
  eye muscle — *see* Strabismus, mechanical
  heart — *see* Myocarditis
  hepatic — *see* Fibrosis, liver
  hepatolienal (portal hypertension) K76.6
  hepatosplenic (portal hypertension) K76.6
  infrapatellar fat pad M79.4
  intrascrotal N50.89
  kidney N26.9
  liver K74.0
    with sclerosis K74.2
    alcoholic K70.2
  lung (atrophic) (chronic) (confluent) (massive) (perialveolar) (peribronchial) J84.10
    with
      anthracosilicosis J60
      anthracosis J60
      asbestosis J61
      bagassosis J67.1
      bauxite J63.1
      berylliosis J63.2
      byssinosis J66.0
      calcicosis J62.8
      chalicosis J62.8
      dust reticulation J64
      farmer's lung J67.0
      ganister disease J62.8
      graphite J63.3
      pneumoconiosis NOS J64
      siderosis J63.4
      silicosis J62.8
    capillary J84.10
    congenital P27.8
    diffuse (idiopathic) J84.10
      chemicals, gases, fumes or vapors (inhalation) J68.4
      interstitial J84.10
        acute J84.114
      talc J62.0
    following radiation J70.1
    idiopathic J84.112
    postinflammatory J84.10
    silicotic J62.8
    tuberculous — *see* Tuberculosis, pulmonary
  lymphatic gland I89.8
  median bar — *see* Hyperplasia, prostate
  mediastinum (idiopathic) J98.59
  meninges G96.19
  myocardium, myocardial — *see* Myocarditis
  ovary N83.8
  oviduct N83.8
  pancreas K86.89
  penis NEC N48.6
  pericardium I31.0
  perineum, in pregnancy or childbirth O34.7- ☑
    causing obstructed labor O65.5
  pleura J94.1
  popliteal fat pad M79.4
  prostate (chronic) — *see* Hyperplasia, prostate
  pulmonary (*see also* Fibrosis, lung) J84.10
    congenital P27.8
    idiopathic J84.112
  rectal sphincter K62.89
  retroperitoneal, idiopathic (with ureteral obstruction) N13.5
    with infection N13.6
  sclerosing mesenteric (idiopathic) K65.4
  scrotum N50.89
  seminal vesicle N50.89
  senile R54
  skin L90.5
  spermatic cord N50.89
  spleen D73.89
    in schistosomiasis (bilharziasis) B65.9 [D77]
  subepidermal nodular — *see* Neoplasm, skin, benign
  submucous (oral) (tongue) K13.5
  testis N44.8
    chronic, due to syphilis A52.76
  thymus (gland) E32.8
  tongue, submucous K13.5
  tunica vaginalis N50.89

Fibrosis, fibrotic — *continued*
  uterus (non-neoplastic) N85.8
  vagina N89.8
  valve, heart — *see* Endocarditis
  vas deferens N50.89
  vein I87.8
Fibrositis (periarticular) M79.7
  nodular, chronic (Jaccoud's) (rheumatoid) — *see* Arthropathy, postrheumatic, chronic
Fibrothorax J94.1
Fibrotic — *see* Fibrosis
Fibrous — *see* condition
Fibroxanthoma (*see also* Neoplasm, connective tissue, benign)
  atypical — *see* Neoplasm, connective tissue, uncertain behavior
  malignant — *see* Neoplasm, connective tissue, malignant
Fibroxanthosarcoma — *see* Neoplasm, connective tissue, malignant
Fiedler's
  disease (icterohemorrhagic leptospirosis) A27.0
  myocarditis (acute) I40.1
Fifth disease B08.3
  venereal A55
Filaria, filarial, filariasis — *see* Infestation, filarial
Filatov's disease — *see* Mononucleosis, infectious
File-cutter's disease — *see* Poisoning, lead
Filling defect
  biliary tract R93.2
  bladder R93.41
  duodenum R93.3
  gallbladder R93.2
  gastrointestinal tract R93.3
  intestine R93.3
  kidney R93.42- ☑
  stomach R93.3
  ureter R93.41
  urinary organs, specified NEC R93.49
Fimbrial cyst Q50.4
Financial problem affecting care NOS Z59.9
  bankruptcy Z59.8
  foreclosure on loan Z59.8
Findings, abnormal, inconclusive, without diagnosis
  (*see also* Abnormal)
  17-ketosteroids, elevated R82.5
  acetonuria R82.4
  alcohol in blood R78.0
  anisocytosis R71.8
  antenatal screening of mother O28.9
    biochemical O28.1
    chromosomal O28.5
    cytological O28.2
    genetic O28.5
    hematological O28.0
    radiological O28.4
    specified NEC O28.8
    ultrasonic O28.3
  antibody titer, elevated R76.0
  anticardiolipin antibody R76.0
  antiphosphatidylglycerol antibody R76.0
  antiphosphatidylinositol antibody R76.0
  antiphosphatidylserine antibody R76.0
  antiphospholipid antibody R76.0
  bacteriuria R82.71
  bicarbonate E87.8
  bile in urine R82.2
  blood sugar R73.09
    high R73.9
    low (transient) E16.2
  body fluid or substance, specified NEC R88.8
  casts, urine R82.99
  catecholamines R82.5
  cells, urine R82.99
  chloride E87.8
  cholesterol E78.9
    high E78.00
      with high triglycerides E78.2
  chyluria R82.0
  cloudy
    dialysis effluent R88.0
    urine R82.90
  creatinine clearance R94.4
  crystals, urine R82.99
  culture
    blood R78.81
    positive — *see* Positive, culture
  echocardiogram R93.1

Findings, abnormal, inconclusive, without diagnosis
— continued
electrolyte level, urinary R82.99
function study NEC R94.8
  bladder R94.8
  endocrine NEC R94.7
    thyroid R94.6
  kidney R94.4
  liver R94.5
  pancreas R94.8
  placenta R94.8
  pulmonary R94.2
  spleen R94.8
gallbladder, nonvisualization R93.2
glucose (tolerance test) (non-fasting) R73.09
glycosuria R81
heart
  shadow R93.1
  sounds R01.2
hematinuria R82.3
hematocrit drop (precipitous) R71.0
hemoglobinuria R82.3
human papillomavirus (HPV) DNA test positive
  cervix
    high risk R87.810
    low risk R87.820
  vagina
    high risk R87.811
    low risk R87.821
in blood (of substance not normally found in blood) R78.9
  addictive drug NEC R78.4
  alcohol (excessive level) R78.0
  cocaine R78.2
  hallucinogen R78.3
  heavy metals (abnormal level) R78.79
  lead R78.71
  lithium (abnormal level) R78.89
  opiate drug R78.1
  psychotropic drug R78.5
  specified substance NEC R78.89
  steroid agent R78.6
Indoleacetic acid, elevated R82.5
ketonuria R82.4
lactic acid dehydrogenase (LDH) R74.0
liver function test R79.89
mammogram NEC R92.8
  calcification (calculus) R92.1
  inconclusive result (due to dense breasts) R92.2
  microcalcification R92.0
mediastinal shift R93.8
melanin, urine R82.99
myoglobinuria R82.1
neonatal screening P09
nonvisualization of gallbladder R93.2
odor of urine NOS R82.90
Papanicolaou cervix R87.619
  non-atypical endometrial cells R87.618
pneumoencephalogram R93.0
poikilocytosis R71.8
potassium (deficiency) E87.6
  excess E87.5
PPD R76.11
radiologic (X-ray) R93.8
  abdomen R93.5
  biliary tract R93.2
  breast R92.8
  gastrointestinal tract R93.3
  genitourinary organs R93.8
  head R93.0
  inconclusive due to excess body fat of patient R93.9
  intrathoracic organs NEC R93.1
  placenta R93.8
  retroperitoneum R93.5
  skin R93.8
  skull R93.0
  subcutaneous tissue R93.8
red blood cell (count) (morphology) (sickling) (volume) R71.8
scan NEC R94.8
  bladder R94.8
  bone R94.8
  kidney R94.4
  liver R93.2
  lung R94.2
  pancreas R94.8
  placenta R94.8
  spleen R94.8
  thyroid R94.6

Findings, abnormal, inconclusive, without diagnosis
— continued
sedimentation rate, elevated R70.0
SGOT R74.0
SGPT R74.0
sodium (deficiency) E87.1
  excess E87.0
specified body fluid NEC R88.8
stress test R94.39
thyroid (function) (metabolic rate) (scan) (uptake) R94.6
transaminase (level) R74.0
triglycerides E78.9
  high E78.1
    with high cholesterol E78.2
tuberculin skin test (without active tuberculosis) R76.11
urine R82.90
  acetone R82.4
  bacteria R82.71
  bile R82.2
  casts or cells R82.99
  chyle R82.0
  culture positive R82.79
  glucose R81
  hemoglobin R82.3
  ketone R82.4
  sugar R81
vanillylmandelic acid (VMA), elevated R82.5
vectorcardiogram (VCG) R94.39
ventriculogram R93.0
white blood cell (count) (differential) (morphology) D72.9
xerography R92.8
Finger — see condition
Fire, Saint Anthony's — see Erysipelas
Fire-setting
pathological (compulsive) F63.1
Fish hook stomach K31.89
Fishmeal-worker's lung J67.8
Fissure, fissured
anus, anal K60.2
  acute K60.0
  chronic K60.1
  congenital Q43.8
ear, lobule, congenital Q17.8
epiglottis (congenital) Q31.8
larynx J38.7
  congenital Q31.8
lip K13.0
  congenital — see Cleft, lip
nipple N64.0
  associated with
    lactation O92.13
    pregnancy O92.11- ☑
    puerperium O92.12
nose Q30.2
palate (congenital) — see Cleft, palate
skin R23.4
spine (congenital) (see also Spina bifida)
  with hydrocephalus — see Spina bifida, by site, with hydrocephalus
tongue (acquired) K14.5
  congenital Q38.3
Fistula (cutaneous) L98.8
abdomen (wall) K63.2
  bladder N32.2
  intestine NEC K63.2
  ureter N28.89
  uterus N82.5
abdominorectal K63.2
abdominosigmoidal K63.2
abdominothoracic J86.0
abdominouterine N82.5
  congenital Q51.7
abdominovesical N32.2
accessory sinuses — see Sinusitis
actinomycotic — see Actinomycosis
alveolar antrum — see Sinusitis, maxillary
alveolar process K04.6
anorectal K60.5
antrobuccal — see Sinusitis, maxillary
antrum — see Sinusitis, maxillary
anus, anal (recurrent) (infectional) K60.3
  congenital Q43.6
    with absence, atresia and stenosis Q42.2
  tuberculous A18.32
aorta-duodenal I77.2

Fistula — continued
appendix, appendicular K38.3
arteriovenous (acquired) (nonruptured) I77.0
  brain I67.1
    congenital Q28.2
      ruptured I60.8
    ruptured I60.8
  cerebral — see Fistula, arteriovenous, brain
  congenital (peripheral) (see also Malformation, arteriovenous)
    brain Q28.2
      ruptured I60.8
    coronary Q24.5
    pulmonary Q25.72
  coronary I25.41
    congenital Q24.5
  pulmonary I28.0
    congenital Q25.72
  surgically created (for dialysis) Z99.2
    complication — see Complication, arteriovenous, fistula, surgically created
  traumatic — see Injury, blood vessel
artery I77.2
aural (mastoid) — see Mastoiditis, chronic
auricle (see also Disorder, pinna, specified type NEC)
  congenital Q18.1
Bartholin's gland N82.8
bile duct (common) (hepatic) K83.3
  with calculus, stones — see Calculus, bile duct
biliary (tract) — see Fistula, bile duct
bladder (sphincter) NEC (see also Fistula, vesico-) N32.2
  into seminal vesicle N32.2
bone (see also Disorder, bone, specified type NEC)
  with osteomyelitis, chronic — see Osteomyelitis, chronic, with draining sinus
brain G93.89
  arteriovenous (acquired) I67.1
    congenital Q28.2
branchial (cleft) Q18.0
branchiogenous Q18.0
breast N61.0
  puerperal, postpartum or gestational, due to mastitis (purulent) — see Mastitis, obstetric, purulent
bronchial J86.0
bronchocutaneous, bronchomediastinal, bronchopleural, bronchopleuromediastinal (infective) J86.0
  tuberculous NEC A15.5
bronchoesophageal J86.0
  congenital Q39.2
    with atresia of esophagus Q39.1
bronchovisceral J86.0
buccal cavity (infective) K12.2
cecosigmoidal K63.2
cecum K63.2
cerebrospinal (fluid) G96.0
cervical, lateral Q18.1
cervicoaural Q18.1
cervicosigmoidal N82.4
cervicovesical N82.1
cervix N82.8
chest (wall) J86.0
cholecystenteric — see Fistula, gallbladder
cholecystocolic — see Fistula, gallbladder
cholecystocolonic — see Fistula, gallbladder
cholecystoduodenal — see Fistula, gallbladder
cholecystogastric — see Fistula, gallbladder
cholecystointestinal — see Fistula, gallbladder
choledochoduodenal — see Fistula, bile duct
cholocolic K82.3
coccyx — see Sinus, pilonidal
colon K63.2
colostomy K94.09
common duct — see Fistula, bile duct
congenital, site not listed — see Anomaly, by site
coronary, arteriovenous I25.41
  congenital Q24.5
costal region J86.0
cul-de-sac, Douglas' N82.8
cystic duct (see also Fistula, gallbladder)
  congenital Q44.5
dental K04.6
diaphragm J86.0
duodenum K31.6
ear (external) (canal) — see Disorder, ear, external, specified type NEC
enterocolic K63.2
enterocutaneous K63.2

Fistula — *continued*
- enterouterine N82.4
  - congenital Q51.7
- enterovaginal N82.4
  - congenital Q52.2
  - large intestine N82.3
  - small intestine N82.2
- enterovesical N32.1
- epididymis N50.89
  - tuberculous A18.15
- esophagobronchial J86.0
  - congenital Q39.2
    - with atresia of esophagus Q39.1
- esophagocutaneous K22.8
- esophagopleural-cutaneous J86.0
- esophagotracheal J86.0
  - congenital Q39.2
    - with atresia of esophagus Q39.1
- esophagus K22.8
  - congenital Q39.2
    - with atresia of esophagus Q39.1
- ethmoid — *see* Sinusitis, ethmoidal
- eyeball (cornea) (sclera) — *see* Disorder, globe, hypotony
- eyelid H01.8
- fallopian tube, external N82.5
- fecal K63.2
  - congenital Q43.6
- from periapical abscess K04.6
- frontal sinus — *see* Sinusitis, frontal
- gallbladder K82.3
  - with calculus, cholelithiasis, stones — *see* Calculus, gallbladder
- gastric K31.6
- gastrocolic K31.6
  - congenital Q40.2
  - tuberculous A18.32
- gastroenterocolic K31.6
- gastroesophageal K31.6
- gastrojejunal K31.6
- gastrojejunocolic K31.6
- genital tract (female) N82.9
  - specified NEC N82.8
  - to intestine NEC N82.4
  - to skin N82.5
- hepatic artery-portal vein, congenital Q26.6
- hepatopleural J86.0
- hepatopulmonary J86.0
- ileorectal or ileosigmoidal K63.2
- ileovaginal N82.2
- ileovesical N32.1
- ileum K63.2
- in ano K60.3
  - tuberculous A18.32
- inner ear (labyrinth) — *see* subcategory H83.1 ☑
- intestine NEC K63.2
- intestinocolonic (abdominal) K63.2
- intestinoureteral N28.89
- intestinouterine N82.4
- intestinovaginal N82.4
  - large intestine N82.3
  - small intestine N82.2
- intestinovesical N32.1
- ischiorectal (fossa) K61.3
- jejunum K63.2
- joint M25.10
  - ankle M25.17- ☑
  - elbow M25.12- ☑
  - foot joint M25.17- ☑
  - hand joint M25.14- ☑
  - hip M25.15- ☑
  - knee M25.16- ☑
  - shoulder M25.11- ☑
  - specified joint NEC M25.18
  - tuberculous — *see* Tuberculosis, joint
  - vertebrae M25.18
  - wrist M25.13- ☑
- kidney N28.89
- labium (majus) (minus) N82.8
- labyrinth — *see* subcategory H83.1 ☑
- lacrimal (gland) (sac) H04.61- ☑
- lacrimonasal duct — *see* Fistula, lacrimal
- laryngotracheal, congenital Q34.8
- larynx J38.7
- lip K13.0
  - congenital Q38.0
- lumbar, tuberculous A18.01
- lung J86.0

Fistula — *continued*
- lymphatic I89.8
- mammary (gland) N61.0
- mastoid (process) (region) — *see* Mastoiditis, chronic
- maxillary J32.0
- medial, face and neck Q18.8
- mediastinal J86.0
- mediastinobronchial J86.0
- mediastinocutaneous J86.0
- middle ear — *see* subcategory H74.8 ☑
- mouth K12.2
- nasal J34.89
  - sinus — *see* Sinusitis
- nasopharynx J39.2
- nipple N64.0
- nose J34.89
- oral (cutaneous) K12.2
  - maxillary J32.0
  - nasal (with cleft palate) — *see* Cleft, palate
- orbit, orbital — *see* Disorder, orbit, specified type NEC
- oroantral J32.0
- oviduct, external N82.5
- palate (hard) M27.8
- pancreatic K86.89
- pancreaticoduodenal K86.89
- parotid (gland) K11.4
  - region K12.2
- penis N48.89
- perianal K60.3
- pericardium (pleura) (sac) — *see* Pericarditis
- pericecal K63.2
- perineorectal K60.4
- perineosigmoidal K63.2
- perineum, perineal (with urethral involvement) NEC N36.0
  - tuberculous A18.13
  - ureter N28.89
- perirectal K60.4
  - tuberculous A18.32
- peritoneum K65.9
- pharyngoesophageal J39.2
- pharynx J39.2
  - branchial cleft (congenital) Q18.0
- pilonidal (infected) (rectum) — *see* Sinus, pilonidal
- pleura, pleural, pleurocutaneous, pleuroperitoneal J86.0
  - tuberculous NEC A15.6
- pleuropericardial I31.8
- portal vein-hepatic artery, congenital Q26.6
- postauricular H70.81- ☑
- postoperative, persistent T81.83 ☑
  - specified site — *see* Fistula, by site
- preauricular (congenital) Q18.1
- prostate N42.89
- pulmonary J86.0
  - arteriovenous I28.0
    - congenital Q25.72
  - tuberculous — *see* Tuberculosis, pulmonary
- pulmonoperitoneal J86.0
- rectolabial N82.4
- rectosigmoid (intercommunicating) K63.2
- rectoureteral N28.89
- rectourethral N36.0
  - congenital Q64.73
- rectouterine N82.4
  - congenital Q51.7
- rectovaginal N82.3
  - congenital Q52.2
  - tuberculous A18.18
- rectovesical N32.1
  - congenital Q64.79
- rectovesicovaginal N82.3
- rectovulval N82.4
  - congenital Q52.79
- rectum (to skin) K60.4
  - congenital Q43.6
    - with absence, atresia and stenosis Q42.0
  - tuberculous A18.32
- renal N28.89
- retroauricular — *see* Fistula, postauricular
- salivary duct or gland (any) K11.4
  - congenital Q38.4
- scrotum (urinary) N50.89
  - tuberculous A18.15
- semicircular canals — *see* subcategory H83.1 ☑
- sigmoid K63.2
  - to bladder N32.1
- sinus — *see* Sinusitis

Fistula — *continued*
- skin L98.8
  - to genital tract (female) N82.5
- splenocolic D73.89
- stercoral K63.2
- stomach K31.6
- sublingual gland K11.4
- submandibular gland K11.4
- submaxillary (gland) K11.4
  - region K12.2
- thoracic J86.0
  - duct I89.8
- thoracoabdominal J86.0
- thoracogastric J86.0
- thoracointestinal J86.0
- thorax J86.0
- thyroglossal duct Q89.2
- thyroid E07.89
- trachea, congenital (external) (internal) Q32.1
- tracheoesophageal J86.0
  - congenital Q39.2
    - with atresia of esophagus Q39.1
  - following tracheostomy J95.04
- traumatic arteriovenous — *see* Injury, blood vessel, by site
- tuberculous — *code by* site under Tuberculosis
- typhoid A01.09
- umbilicourinary Q64.8
- urachus, congenital Q64.4
- ureter (persistent) N28.89
- ureteroabdominal N28.89
- ureterorectal N28.89
- ureterosigmoido-abdominal N28.89
- ureterovaginal N82.1
- ureterovesical N32.2
- urethra N36.0
  - congenital Q64.79
  - tuberculous A18.13
- urethroperineal N36.0
- urethroperineovesical N32.2
- urethrorectal N36.0
  - congenital Q64.73
- urethroscrotal N50.89
- urethrovaginal N82.1
- urethrovesical N32.2
- urinary (tract) (persistent) (recurrent) N36.0
- uteroabdominal N82.5
  - congenital Q51.7
- uteroenteric, uterointestinal N82.4
  - congenital Q51.7
- uterorectal N82.4
  - congenital Q51.7
- uteroureteric N82.1
- uterourethral Q51.7
- uterovaginal N82.8
  - congenital Q51.7
- uterovesical N82.1
  - congenital Q51.7
- uterus N82.8
- vagina (postpartal) (wall) N82.8
- vaginocutaneous (postpartal) N82.5
- vaginointestinal NEC N82.4
  - large intestine N82.3
  - small intestine N82.2
- vaginoperineal N82.5
- vasocutaneous, congenital Q55.7
- vesical NEC N32.2
- vesicoabdominal N32.2
- vesicocervicovaginal N82.1
- vesicocolic N32.1
- vesicocutaneous N32.2
- vesicoenteric N32.1
- vesicointestinal N32.1
- vesicometrorectal N82.4
- vesicoperineal N32.2
- vesicorectal N32.1
  - congenital Q64.79
- vesicosigmoidal N32.1
- vesicosigmoidovaginal N82.3
- vesicoureteral N32.2
- vesicoureterovaginal N82.1
- vesicourethral N32.2
- vesicourethrorectal N32.1
- vesicouterine N82.1
  - congenital Q51.7
- vesicovaginal N82.0
- vulvorectal N82.4
  - congenital Q52.79

Fit R56.9
- epileptic — *see* Epilepsy

Fit — *continued*
  fainting R55
  hysterical F44.5
  newborn P90
Fitting (and adjustment) (of)
  artificial
    arm — *see* Admission, adjustment, artificial, arm
    breast Z44.3 ☑
    eye Z44.2 ☑
    leg — *see* Admission, adjustment, artificial, leg
  automatic implantable cardiac defibrillator (with synchronous cardiac pacemaker) Z45.02
  brain neuropacemaker Z46.2
    implanted Z45.42
  cardiac defibrillator — *see* Fitting (and adjustment) (of), automatic implantable cardiac defibrillator
  catheter, non-vascular Z46.82
  colostomy belt Z46.89
  contact lenses Z46.0
  CRT-D (resynchronization therapy defibrillator) Z45.02
  CRT-P (cardiac resynchronization therapy pacemaker) Z45.018
    pulse generator Z45.010
  cystostomy device Z46.6
  defibrillator, cardiac — *see* Fitting (and adjustment) (of), automatic implantable cardiac defibrillator
  dentures Z46.3
  device NOS Z46.9
    abdominal Z46.89
    gastrointestinal NEC Z46.59
    implanted NEC Z45.89
    nervous system Z46.2
      implanted — *see* Admission, adjustment, device, implanted, nervous system
    orthodontic Z46.4
    orthoptic Z46.0
    orthotic Z46.89
    prosthetic (external) Z44.9
      breast Z44.3 ☑
      dental Z46.3
      eye Z44.2 ☑
      specified NEC Z44.8
    specified NEC Z46.89
    substitution
      auditory Z46.2
        implanted — *see* Admission, adjustment, device, implanted, hearing device
      nervous system Z46.2
        implanted — *see* Admission, adjustment, device, implanted, nervous system
      visual Z46.2
        implanted Z45.31
    urinary Z46.6
  gastric lap band Z46.51
  gastrointestinal appliance NEC Z46.59
  glasses (reading) Z46.0
  hearing aid Z46.1
  ileostomy device Z46.89
  insulin pump Z46.81
  intestinal appliance NEC Z46.89
  myringotomy device (stent) (tube) Z45.82
  neuropacemaker Z46.2
    implanted Z45.42
  non-vascular catheter Z46.82
  orthodontic device Z46.4
  orthopedic device (brace) (cast) (corset) (shoes) Z46.89
  pacemaker (cardiac) (cardiac resynchronization therapy (CRT-P)) Z45.018
    nervous system (brain) (peripheral nerve) (spinal cord) Z46.2
      implanted Z45.42
    pulse generator Z45.010
  portacath (port-a-cath) Z45.2
  prosthesis (external) Z44.9
    arm — *see* Admission, adjustment, artificial, arm
    breast Z44.3 ☑
    dental Z46.3
    eye Z44.2 ☑
    leg — *see* Admission, adjustment, artificial, leg
    specified NEC Z44.8
  spectacles Z46.0
  wheelchair Z46.89
Fitzhugh-Curtis syndrome
  due to
    Chlamydia trachomatis A74.81
    Neisseria gonorrhorea (gonococcal peritonitis) A54.85

Fitz's syndrome (acute hemorrhagic pancreatitis) (*see also* Pancreatitis, acute) K85.80
Fixation
  joint — *see* Ankylosis
  larynx J38.7
  stapes — *see* Ankylosis, ear ossicles
    deafness — *see* Deafness, conductive
  uterus (acquired) — *see* Malposition, uterus
  vocal cord J38.3
Flabby ridge K06.8
Flaccid (*see also* condition)
  palate, congenital Q38.5
Flail
  chest S22.5 ☑
    newborn (birth injury) P13.8
  joint (paralytic) M25.20
    ankle M25.27- ☑
    elbow M25.22- ☑
    foot joint M25.27- ☑
    hand joint M25.24- ☑
    hip M25.25- ☑
    knee M25.26- ☑
    shoulder M25.21- ☑
    specified joint NEC M25.28
    wrist M25.23- ☑
Flajani's disease — *see* Hyperthyroidism, with, goiter (diffuse)
Flap, liver K71.3
Flashbacks (residual to hallucinogen use) F16.283
Flat
  chamber (eye) — *see* Disorder, globe, hypotony, flat anterior chamber
  chest, congenital Q67.8
  foot (acquired) (fixed type) (painful) (postural) (*see also* Deformity, limb, flat foot)
    congenital (rigid) (spastic) (everted) Q66.5- ☑
    rachitic sequelae (late effect) E64.3
  organ or site, congenital NEC — *see* Anomaly, by site
  pelvis M95.5
    with disproportion (fetopelvic) O33.0
      causing obstructed labor O65.0
    congenital Q74.2
Flatau-Schilder disease G37.0
Flatback syndrome M40.30
  lumbar region M40.36
  lumbosacral region M40.37
  thoracolumbar region M40.35
Flattening
  head, femur M89.8X5
  hip — *see* Coxa, plana
  lip (congenital) Q18.8
  nose (congenital) Q67.4
    acquired M95.0
Flatulence R14.3
  psychogenic F45.8
Flatus R14.3
  vaginalis N89.8
Flax-dresser's disease J66.1
Flea bite — *see* Injury, bite, by site, superficial, insect
Flecks, glaucomatous (subcapsular) — *see* Cataract, complicated
Fleischer (-Kayser) **ring** (cornea) H18.04- ☑
Fleshy mole O02.0
Flexibilitas cerea — *see* Catalepsy
Flexion
  amputation stump (surgical) T87.89
  cervix — *see* Malposition, uterus
  contracture, joint — *see* Contraction, joint
  deformity, joint (*see also* Deformity, limb, flexion) M21.20
    hip, congenital Q65.89
  uterus (*see also* Malposition, uterus)
    lateral — *see* Lateroversion, uterus
Flexner-Boyd dysentery A03.2
Flexner's dysentery A03.1
Flexure — *see* Flexion
Flint murmur (aortic insufficiency) I35.1
Floater, vitreous — *see* Opacity, vitreous
Floating
  cartilage (joint) (*see also* Loose, body, joint)
    knee — *see* Derangement, knee, loose body
  gallbladder, congenital Q44.1
  kidney N28.89
    congenital Q63.8
  spleen D73.89
Flooding N92.0
Floor — *see* condition

Floppy
  baby syndrome (nonspecific) P94.2
  iris syndrome (intraoperative) (IFIS) H21.81
  nonrheumatic mitral valve syndrome I34.1
Flu (*see also* Influenza)
  avian (*see also* Influenza, due to, identified novel influenza A virus) J09.X2
  bird (*see also* Influenza, due to, identified novel influenza A virus) J09.X2
  intestinal NEC A08.4
  swine (viruses that normally cause infections in pigs) (*see also* Influenza, due to, identified novel influenza A virus) J09.X2
Fluctuating blood pressure I99.8
Fluid
  abdomen R18.8
  chest J94.8
  heart — *see* Failure, heart, congestive
  joint — *see* Effusion, joint
  loss (acute) E86.9
  lung — *see* Edema, lung
  overload E87.70
    specified NEC E87.79
  peritoneal cavity R18.8
  pleural cavity J94.8
  retention R60.9
Flukes NEC (*see also* Infestation, fluke)
  blood NEC — *see* Schistosomiasis
  liver B66.3
Fluor (vaginalis) N89.8
  trichomonal or due to Trichomonas (vaginalis) A59.00
Fluorosis
  dental K00.3
  skeletal M85.10
    ankle M85.17- ☑
    foot M85.17- ☑
    forearm M85.13- ☑
    hand M85.14- ☑
    lower leg M85.16- ☑
    multiple site M85.19
    neck M85.18
    rib M85.18
    shoulder M85.11- ☑
    skull M85.18
    specified site NEC M85.18
    thigh M85.15- ☑
    toe M85.17- ☑
    upper arm M85.12- ☑
    vertebra M85.18
Flush syndrome E34.0
Flushing R23.2
  menopausal N95.1
Flutter
  atrial or auricular I48.92
    atypical I48.4
    type I I48.3
    type II I48.4
    typical I48.3
  heart I49.8
    atrial or auricular I48.92
      atypical I48.4
      type I I48.3
      type II I48.4
      typical I48.3
    ventricular I49.02
  ventricular I49.02
FNHTR (febrile nonhemolytic transfusion reaction) R50.84
Fochier's abscess — *code by* site under Abscess
Focus, Assmann's — *see* Tuberculosis, pulmonary
Fogo selvagem L10.3
Foix-Alajouanine syndrome G95.19
Fold, folds (anomalous) (*see also* Anomaly, by site)
  Descemet's membrane — *see* Change, corneal membrane, Descemet's, fold
  epicanthic Q10.3
  heart Q24.8
Folie à deux F24
Follicle
  cervix (nabothian) (ruptured) N88.8
  graafian, ruptured, with hemorrhage N83.0- ☑
  nabothian N88.8
Follicular — *see* condition
Folliculitis (superficial) L73.9
  abscedens et suffodiens L66.3
  cyst N83.0- ☑
  decalvans L66.2
  deep — *see* Furuncle, by site

Foreign body — *continued*
- entering through orifice — *continued*
  - stomach T18.2 ☑
  - suffocation by — *see* Foreign body, by site
  - tear ducts or glands — *see* Foreign body, entering through orifice, eye, specified part NEC
  - throat — *see* Foreign body, pharynx
  - tongue T18.0 ☑
  - tonsil, tonsillar (fossa) — *see* Foreign body, pharynx
  - trachea — *see* Foreign body, trachea
  - ureter T19.8 ☑
  - urethra T19.0 ☑
  - uterus (any part) T19.3 ☑
  - vagina T19.2 ☑
  - vulva T19.2 ☑
- esophagus T18.108 ☑
  - causing
    - injury NEC T18.108 ☑
      - food (bone) (seed) T18.128 ☑
      - gastric contents (vomitus) T18.118 ☑
      - specified type NEC T18.198 ☑
    - tracheal compression T18.100 ☑
      - food (bone) (seed) T18.120 ☑
      - gastric contents (vomitus) T18.110 ☑
      - specified type NEC T18.190 ☑
- feeling of, in throat R09.89
- fragment — *see* Retained, foreign body fragments (type of)
- genitourinary tract T19.9 ☑
  - bladder T19.1 ☑
  - multiple parts T19.8 ☑
  - penis T19.4 ☑
  - specified site NEC T19.8 ☑
  - urethra T19.0 ☑
  - uterus T19.3 ☑
    - IUD Z97.5
  - vagina T19.2 ☑
    - contraceptive device Z97.5
  - vulva T19.2 ☑
- granuloma (old) (soft tissue) (*see also* Granuloma, foreign body)
  - skin L92.3
- in
  - laceration — *see* Laceration, by site, with foreign body
  - puncture wound — *see* Puncture, by site, with foreign body
  - soft tissue (residual) M79.5
- inadvertently left in operation wound — *see* Foreign body, accidentally left during a procedure
- ingestion, ingested NOS T18.9 ☑
- inhalation or inspiration — *see* Foreign body, by site
- internal organ, not entering through a natural orifice — code as specific injury with foreign body
- intraocular S05.5- ☑
  - old, retained (nonmagnetic) H44.70- ☑
    - anterior chamber H44.71- ☑
    - ciliary body H44.72- ☑
    - iris H44.72- ☑
    - lens H44.73- ☑
    - magnetic H44.60- ☑
      - anterior chamber H44.61- ☑
      - ciliary body H44.62- ☑
      - iris H44.62- ☑
      - lens H44.63- ☑
      - posterior wall H44.64- ☑
      - specified site NEC H44.69- ☑
      - vitreous body H44.65- ☑
    - posterior wall H44.74- ☑
    - specified site NEC H44.79- ☑
    - vitreous body H44.75- ☑
- iris — *see* Foreign body, intraocular
- lacrimal punctum — *see* Foreign body, entering through orifice, eye, specified part NEC
- larynx T17.308 ☑
  - causing
    - asphyxiation T17.300 ☑
      - food (bone) (seed) T17.320 ☑
      - gastric contents (vomitus) T17.310 ☑
      - specified type NEC T17.390 ☑
    - injury NEC T17.308 ☑
      - food (bone) (seed) T17.328 ☑
      - gastric contents (vomitus) T17.318 ☑
      - specified type NEC T17.398 ☑
- lens — *see* Foreign body, intraocular
- ocular muscle S05.4- ☑

Foreign body — *continued*
- ocular muscle — *continued*
  - old, retained — *see* Foreign body, orbit, old
- old or residual
  - soft tissue (residual) M79.5
- operation wound, left accidentally — *see* Foreign body, accidentally left during a procedure
- orbit S05.4- ☑
  - old, retained H05.5- ☑
- pharynx T17.208 ☑
  - causing
    - asphyxiation T17.200 ☑
      - food (bone) (seed) T17.220 ☑
      - gastric contents (vomitus) T17.210 ☑
      - specified type NEC T17.290 ☑
    - injury NEC T17.208 ☑
      - food (bone) (seed) T17.228 ☑
      - gastric contents (vomitus) T17.218 ☑
      - specified type NEC T17.298 ☑
- respiratory tract T17.908 ☑
  - bronchioles — *see* Foreign body, respiratory tract, specified site NEC
  - bronchus — *see* Foreign body, bronchus
  - causing
    - asphyxiation T17.900 ☑
      - food (bone) (seed) T17.920 ☑
      - gastric contents (vomitus) T17.910 ☑
      - specified type NEC T17.990 ☑
    - injury NEC T17.908 ☑
      - food (bone) (seed) T17.928 ☑
      - gastric contents (vomitus) T17.918 ☑
      - specified type NEC T17.998 ☑
  - larynx — *see* Foreign body, larynx
  - lung — *see* Foreign body, respiratory tract, specified site NEC
  - multiple parts — *see* Foreign body, respiratory tract, specified site NEC
  - nasal sinus T17.0 ☑
  - nasopharynx — *see* Foreign body, pharynx
  - nose T17.1 ☑
  - nostril T17.1 ☑
  - pharynx — *see* Foreign body, pharynx
  - specified site NEC T17.808 ☑
    - causing
      - asphyxiation T17.800 ☑
        - food (bone) (seed) T17.820 ☑
        - gastric contents (vomitus) T17.810 ☑
        - specified type NEC T17.890 ☑
      - injury NEC T17.808 ☑
        - food (bone) (seed) T17.828 ☑
        - gastric contents (vomitus) T17.818 ☑
        - specified type NEC T17.898 ☑
  - throat — *see* Foreign body, pharynx
  - trachea — *see* Foreign body, trachea
- retained (old) (nonmagnetic) (in)
  - anterior chamber (eye) — *see* Foreign body, intraocular, old, retained, anterior chamber
    - magnetic — *see* Foreign body, intraocular, old, retained, magnetic, anterior chamber
  - ciliary body — *see* Foreign body, intraocular, old, retained, ciliary body
    - magnetic — *see* Foreign body, intraocular, old, retained, magnetic, ciliary body
  - eyelid H02.819
    - left H02.816
      - lower H02.815
      - upper H02.814
    - right H02.813
      - lower H02.812
      - upper H02.811
  - fragments — *see* Retained, foreign body fragments (type of)
  - globe — *see* Foreign body, intraocular, old, retained
    - magnetic — *see* Foreign body, intraocular, old, retained, magnetic
  - intraocular — *see* Foreign body, intraocular, old, retained
    - magnetic — *see* Foreign body, intraocular, old, retained, magnetic
  - iris — *see* Foreign body, intraocular, old, retained, iris
    - magnetic — *see* Foreign body, intraocular, old, retained, magnetic, iris
  - lens — *see* Foreign body, intraocular, old, retained, lens

Foreign body — *continued*
- retained — *continued*
  - lens — *see* Foreign body, intraocular, old, retained, lens — *continued*
    - magnetic — *see* Foreign body, intraocular, old, retained, magnetic, lens
  - muscle — *see* Foreign body, retained, soft tissue
  - orbit — *see* Foreign body, orbit, old
  - posterior wall of globe — *see* Foreign body, intraocular, old, retained, posterior wall
    - magnetic — *see* Foreign body, intraocular, old, retained, magnetic, posterior wall
  - retrobulbar — *see* Foreign body, orbit, old, retrobulbar
  - soft tissue M79.5
  - vitreous — *see* Foreign body, intraocular, old, retained, vitreous body
    - magnetic — *see* Foreign body, intraocular, old, retained, magnetic, vitreous body
- retina S05.5- ☑
- superficial, without open wound
  - abdomen, abdominal (wall) S30.851 ☑
  - alveolar process S00.552 ☑
  - ankle S90.55- ☑
  - antecubital space — *see* Foreign body, superficial, forearm
  - anus S30.857 ☑
  - arm (upper) S40.85- ☑
  - auditory canal — *see* Foreign body, superficial, ear
  - auricle — *see* Foreign body, superficial, ear
  - axilla — *see* Foreign body, superficial, arm
  - back, lower S30.850 ☑
  - breast S20.15- ☑
  - brow S00.85 ☑
  - buttock S30.850 ☑
  - calf — *see* Foreign body, superficial, leg
  - canthus — *see* Foreign body, superficial, eyelid
  - cheek S00.85 ☑
    - internal S00.552 ☑
  - chest wall — *see* Foreign body, superficial, thorax
  - chin S00.85 ☑
  - clitoris S30.854 ☑
  - costal region — *see* Foreign body, superficial, thorax
  - digit(s)
    - foot — *see* Foreign body, superficial, toe
    - hand — *see* Foreign body, superficial, finger
  - ear S00.45- ☑
  - elbow S50.35- ☑
  - epididymis S30.853 ☑
  - epigastric region S30.851 ☑
  - epiglottis S10.15 ☑
  - esophagus, cervical S10.15 ☑
  - eyebrow — *see* Foreign body, superficial, eyelid
  - eyelid S00.25- ☑
  - face S00.85 ☑
  - finger(s) S60.459 ☑
    - index S60.45- ☑
    - little S60.45- ☑
    - middle S60.45- ☑
    - ring S60.45- ☑
  - flank S30.851 ☑
  - foot (except toe(s) alone) S90.85- ☑
    - toe — *see* Foreign body, superficial, toe
  - forearm S50.85- ☑
    - elbow only — *see* Foreign body, superficial, elbow
  - forehead S00.85 ☑
  - genital organs, external
    - female S30.856 ☑
    - male S30.855 ☑
  - groin S30.851 ☑
  - gum S00.552 ☑
  - hand S60.55- ☑
  - head S00.95 ☑
    - ear — *see* Foreign body, superficial, ear
    - eyelid — *see* Foreign body, superficial, eyelid
    - lip S00.551 ☑
    - nose S00.35 ☑
    - oral cavity S00.552 ☑
    - scalp S00.05 ☑
    - specified site NEC S00.85 ☑
  - heel — *see* Foreign body, superficial, foot
  - hip S70.25- ☑
  - inguinal region S30.851 ☑
  - interscapular region S20.459 ☑

☑ Additional Character Required — Refer to the Tabular List for Character Selection   ▽ Subterms under main terms may continue to next column or page

Foreign body — *continued*
  superficial, without open wound — *continued*
    jaw S00.85- ☑
    knee S80.25- ☑
    labium (majus) (minus) S30.854 ☑
    larynx S10.15 ☑
    leg (lower) S80.85- ☑
      knee — *see* Foreign body, superficial, knee
      upper — *see* Foreign body, superficial, thigh
    lip S00.551 ☑
    lower back S30.850 ☑
    lumbar region S30.850 ☑
    malar region S00.85 ☑
    mammary — *see* Foreign body, superficial, breast
    mastoid region S00.85 ☑
    mouth S00.552 ☑
    nail
      finger — *see* Foreign body, superficial, finger
      toe — *see* Foreign body, superficial, toe
    nape S10.85 ☑
    nasal S00.35 ☑
    neck S10.95 ☑
      specified site NEC S10.85 ☑
      throat S10.15 ☑
    nose S00.35 ☑
    occipital region S00.05 ☑
    oral cavity S00.552 ☑
    orbital region — *see* Foreign body, superficial, eyelid
    palate S00.552 ☑
    palm — *see* Foreign body, superficial, hand
    parietal region S00.05 ☑
    pelvis S30.850 ☑
    penis S30.852 ☑
    perineum
      female S30.854 ☑
      male S30.850 ☑
    periocular area — *see* Foreign body, superficial, eyelid
    phalanges
      finger — *see* Foreign body, superficial, finger
      toe — *see* Foreign body, superficial, toe
    pharynx S10.15 ☑
    pinna — *see* Foreign body, superficial, ear
    popliteal space — *see* Foreign body, superficial, knee
    prepuce S30.852 ☑
    pubic region S30.850 ☑
    pudendum
      female S30.856 ☑
      male S30.855 ☑
    sacral region S30.850 ☑
    scalp S00.05 ☑
    scapular region — *see* Foreign body, superficial, shoulder
    scrotum S30.853 ☑
    shin — *see* Foreign body, superficial, leg
    shoulder S40.25- ☑
    sternal region S20.359 ☑
    submaxillary region S00.85 ☑
    submental region S00.85 ☑
    subungual
      finger(s) — *see* Foreign body, superficial, finger
      toe(s) — *see* Foreign body, superficial, toe
    supraclavicular fossa S10.85 ☑
    supraorbital S00.85 ☑
    temple S00.85 ☑
    temporal region S00.85 ☑
    testis S30.853 ☑
    thigh S70.35- ☑
    thorax, thoracic (wall) S20.95 ☑
      back S20.45- ☑
      front S20.35- ☑
    throat S10.15 ☑
    thumb S60.35- ☑
    toe(s) (lesser) S90.456 ☑
      great S90.45- ☑
    tongue S00.552 ☑
    trachea S10.15 ☑
    tunica vaginalis S30.853 ☑
    tympanum, tympanic membrane — *see* Foreign body, superficial, ear
    uvula S00.552 ☑
    vagina S30.854 ☑
    vocal cords S10.15 ☑
    vulva S30.854 ☑

Foreign body — *continued*
  superficial, without open wound — *continued*
    wrist S60.85- ☑
    swallowed T18.9 ☑
    trachea T17.408 ☑
      causing
        asphyxiation T17.400 ☑
          food (bone) (seed) T17.420 ☑
          gastric contents (vomitus) T17.410 ☑
          specified type NEC T17.490 ☑
        injury NEC T17.408 ☑
          food (bone) (seed) T17.428 ☑
          gastric contents (vomitus) T17.418 ☑
          specified type NEC T17.498 ☑
    type of fragment — *see* Retained, foreign body fragments (type of)
    vitreous (humor) S05.5- ☑
Forestier's disease (rhizomelic pseudopolyarthritis) M35.3
  meaning ankylosing hyperostosis — *see* Hyperostosis, ankylosing
Formation
  hyalin in cornea — *see* Degeneration, cornea
  sequestrum in bone (due to infection) — *see* Osteomyelitis, chronic
  valve
    colon, congenital Q43.8
    ureter (congenital) Q62.39
Formication R20.2
Fort Bragg fever A27.89
Fossa (*see also* condition)
  pyriform — *see* condition
Foster-Kennedy syndrome H47.14- ☑
Fothergill's
  disease (trigeminal neuralgia) (*see also* Neuralgia, trigeminal)
    scarlatina anginosa A38.9
Foul breath R19.6
Foundling Z76.1
Fournier disease or gangrene N49.3
  female N76.89
Fourth
  cranial nerve — *see* condition
  molar K00.1
Foville's (peduncular) **disease or syndrome** G46.3
Fox (-Fordyce) disease (apocrine miliaria) L75.2
Fracture, burst — *see* Fracture, traumatic, by site
Fracture, chronic — *see* Fracture, pathological, by site
Fracture, insufficiency — *see* Fracture, pathological, by site
Fracture, nontraumatic, NEC
  atypical
    femur M84.750- ☑
      complete
        oblique M84.759 ☑
          left side M84.758 ☑
          right side M84.757 ☑
        transverse M84.756 ☑
          left side M84.755 ☑
          right side M84.754 ☑
      incomplete M84.753 ☑
        left side M84.752 ☑
        right side M84.751 ☑
Fracture, pathological (pathologic) (*see also* Fracture, traumatic) M84.40 ☑
  ankle M84.47- ☑
  carpus M84.44- ☑
  clavicle M84.41- ☑
  compression (not due to trauma) (*see also* Collapse, vertebra) M48.50- ☑
  dental implant M27.63
  dental restorative material K08.539
    with loss of material K08.531
    without loss of material K08.530
  due to
    neoplastic disease NEC (*see also* Neoplasm) M84.50
      ankle M84.57- ☑
      carpus M84.54- ☑
      clavicle M84.51- ☑
      femur M84.55- ☑
      fibula M84.56- ☑
      finger M84.54- ☑
      hip M84.559
      humerus M84.52- ☑
      ilium M84.550 ☑

Fracture, pathological — *continued*
  due to — *continued*
    neoplastic disease (*see also* Neoplasm) — *continued*
      ischium M84.550 ☑
      metacarpus M84.54- ☑
      metatarsus M84.57- ☑
      neck M84.58 ☑
      pelvis M84.550 ☑
      radius M84.53- ☑
      rib M84.58 ☑
      scapula M84.51- ☑
      skull M84.58 ☑
      specified site NEC M84.58 ☑
      tarsus M84.57- ☑
      tibia M84.56- ☑
      toe M84.57- ☑
      ulna M84.53- ☑
      vertebra M84.58 ☑
    osteoporosis M80.00 ☑
      disuse — *see* Osteoporosis, specified type NEC, with pathological fracture
      drug-induced — *see* Osteoporosis, drug-induced, with pathological fracture
      idiopathic — *see* Osteoporosis, specified type NEC, with pathological fracture
      postmenopausal — *see* Osteoporosis, postmenopausal, with pathological fracture
      postoophorectomy — *see* Osteoporosis, postoophorectomy, with pathological fracture
      postsurgical malabsorption — *see* Osteoporosis, specified type NEC, with pathological fracture
      specified cause NEC — *see* Osteoporosis, specified type NEC, with pathological fracture
    specified disease NEC M84.60 ☑
      ankle M84.67- ☑
      carpus M84.64- ☑
      clavicle M84.61- ☑
      femur M84.65- ☑
      fibula M84.66- ☑
      finger M84.64- ☑
      hip M84.65- ☑
      humerus M84.62- ☑
      ilium M84.650 ☑
      ischium M84.650 ☑
      metacarpus M84.64- ☑
      metatarsus M84.67- ☑
      neck M84.68 ☑
      radius M84.63- ☑
      rib M84.68 ☑
      scapula M84.61- ☑
      skull M84.68 ☑
      tarsus M84.67- ☑
      tibia M84.66- ☑
      toe M84.67- ☑
      ulna M84.63- ☑
      vertebra M84.68 ☑
  femur M84.45- ☑
  fibula M84.46- ☑
  finger M84.44- ☑
  hip M84.459 ☑
  humerus M84.42- ☑
  ilium M84.454 ☑
  ischium M84.454 ☑
  joint prosthesis — *see* Complications, joint prosthesis, mechanical, breakdown, by site
  periprosthetic — *see* Fracture, pathological, periprosthetic
  metacarpus M84.44- ☑
  metatarsus M84.47- ☑
  neck M84.48 ☑
  pelvis M84.454 ☑
  periprosthetic M97.9 ☑
    ankle M97.2- ☑
    elbow M97.4- ☑
    finger M97.8 ☑
    hip M97.0- ☑
    knee M97.1- ☑
    other specified joint M97.8 ☑
    shoulder M97.3- ☑
    spinal joint M97.8 ☑
    toe joint M97.8 ☑
    wrist joint M97.8 ☑
  radius M84.43- ☑

Fracture, pathological — *continued*
    restorative material (dental) K08.539
      with loss of material K08.531
      without loss of material K08.530
    rib M84.48 ☑
    scapula M84.41- ☑
    skull M84.48 ☑
    tarsus M84.47- ☑
    tibia M84.46- ☑
    toe M84.47- ☑
    ulna M84.43- ☑
    vertebra M84.48 ☑
Fracture, traumatic (abduction) (adduction) (separation)
    (*see also* Fracture, pathological) T14.8 ☑
    acetabulum S32.40- ☑
      column
        anterior (displaced) (iliopubic) S32.43- ☑
          nondisplaced S32.436 ☑
        posterior (displaced) (ilioischial) S32.443 ☑
          nondisplaced S32.44- ☑
      dome (displaced) S32.48- ☑
        nondisplaced S32.48 ☑
      specified NEC S32.49- ☑
      transverse (displaced) S32.45- ☑
        with associated posterior wall fracture (displaced) S32.46- ☑
          nondisplaced S32.46- ☑
        nondisplaced S32.45- ☑
      wall
        anterior (displaced) S32.41- ☑
          nondisplaced S32.41- ☑
        medial (displaced) S32.47- ☑
          nondisplaced S32.47- ☑
        posterior (displaced) S32.42- ☑
          with associated transverse fracture (displaced) S32.46- ☑
            nondisplaced S32.46- ☑
          nondisplaced S32.42- ☑
    acromion — *see* Fracture, scapula, acromial process
    ankle S82.899 ☑
      bimalleolar (displaced) S82.84- ☑
        nondisplaced S82.84- ☑
      lateral malleolus only (displaced) S82.6- ☑
        nondisplaced S82.6- ☑
      medial malleolus (displaced) S82.5- ☑
        associated with Maisonneuve's fracture — *see* Fracture, Maisonneuve's
        nondisplaced S82.5- ☑
      talus — *see* Fracture, tarsal, talus
      trimalleolar (displaced) S82.85- ☑
        nondisplaced S82.85- ☑
    arm (upper) (*see also* Fracture, humerus, shaft)
      humerus — *see* Fracture, humerus
      radius — *see* Fracture, radius
      ulna — *see* Fracture, ulna
    astragalus — *see* Fracture, tarsal, talus
    atlas — *see* Fracture, neck, cervical **vertebra**, first
    axis — *see* Fracture, neck, cervical **vertebra**, second
    back — *see* Fracture, vertebra
    Barton's — *see* Barton's fracture
    base of skull — *see* Fracture, skull, base
    basicervical (basal) (femoral) S72.0 ☑
    Bennett's — *see* Bennett's fracture
    bimalleolar — *see* Fracture, ankle, bimalleolar
    blow-out S02.3- ☑
    bone NEC T14.8 ☑
      birth injury P13.9
      following insertion of orthopedic implant, joint prosthesis or bone plate — *see* Fracture, following insertion of orthopedic implant, joint prosthesis or bone plate
      in (due to) neoplastic disease NEC — *see* Fracture, pathological, due to, neoplastic disease
      pathological (cause unknown) — *see* Fracture, pathological
    breast bone — *see* Fracture, sternum
    bucket handle (semilunar cartilage) — *see* Tear, meniscus
    burst — *see* Fracture, traumatic, by site
    calcaneus — *see* Fracture, tarsal, calcaneus
    carpal bone(s) S62.10- ☑
      capitate (displaced) S62.13- ☑
        nondisplaced S62.13- ☑
      cuneiform — *see* Fracture, carpal bone, triquetrum
      hamate (body) (displaced) S62.143 ☑
        hook process (displaced) S62.15- ☑

Fracture, traumatic — *continued*
    carpal bone(s) — *continued*
      hamate — *continued*
        hook process — *continued*
          nondisplaced S62.15- ☑
        nondisplaced S62.14- ☑
      larger multangular — *see* Fracture, carpal bones, trapezium
      lunate (displaced) S62.12- ☑
        nondisplaced S62.12- ☑
      navicular S62.00- ☑
        distal pole (displaced) S62.01- ☑
          nondisplaced S62.01- ☑
        middle third (displaced) S62.02- ☑
          nondisplaced S62.02- ☑
        proximal third (displaced) S62.03- ☑
          nondisplaced S62.03- ☑
        volar tuberosity — *see* Fracture, carpal bones, navicular, distal pole
      os magnum — *see* Fracture, carpal bones, capitate
      pisiform (displaced) S62.16- ☑
        nondisplaced S62.16- ☑
      semilunar — *see* Fracture, carpal bones, lunate
      smaller multangular — *see* Fracture, carpal bones, trapezoid
      trapezium (displaced) S62.17- ☑
        nondisplaced S62.17- ☑
      trapezoid (displaced) S62.18- ☑
        nondisplaced S62.18- ☑
      triquetrum (displaced) S62.11- ☑
        nondisplaced S62.11- ☑
      unciform — *see* Fracture, carpal bones, hamate
    cervical — *see* Fracture, vertebra, cervical
    clavicle S42.00- ☑
      acromial end (displaced) S42.03- ☑
        nondisplaced S42.03- ☑
      birth injury P13.4
      lateral end — *see* Fracture, clavicle, acromial end
      shaft (displaced) S42.02- ☑
        nondisplaced S42.02- ☑
      sternal end (anterior) (displaced) S42.01- ☑
        nondisplaced S42.01- ☑
        posterior S42.01- ☑
    coccyx S32.2 ☑
    collapsed — *see* Collapse, vertebra
    collar bone — *see* Fracture, clavicle
    Colles' — *see* Colles' fracture
    coronoid process — *see* Fracture, ulna, upper end, coronoid process
    corpus cavernosum penis S39.840 ☑
    costochondral cartilage S23.41 ☑
    costochondral, costosternal junction — *see* Fracture, rib
    cranium — *see* Fracture, skull
    cricoid cartilage S12.8 ☑
    cuboid (ankle) — *see* Fracture, tarsal, cuboid
    cuneiform
      foot — *see* Fracture, tarsal, cuneiform
      wrist — *see* Fracture, carpal, triquetrum
    delayed union — *see* Delay, union, fracture
    dental restorative material K08.539
      with loss of material K08.531
      without loss of material K08.530
    due to
      birth injury — *see* Birth, injury, fracture
      osteoporosis — *see* Osteoporosis, with fracture
    Dupuytren's — *see* Fracture, ankle, lateral malleolus
    elbow S42.40- ☑
    ethmoid (bone) (sinus) — *see* Fracture, skull, base
    face bone S02.92 ☑
    fatigue (*see also* Fracture, stress)
      vertebra M48.40 ☑
        cervical region M48.42 ☑
        cervicothoracic region M48.43 ☑
        lumbar region M48.46 ☑
        lumbosacral region M48.47 ☑
        occipito-atlanto-axial region M48.41 ☑
        sacrococcygeal region M48.48 ☑
        thoracic region M48.44 ☑
        thoracolumbar region M48.45 ☑
    femur, femoral S72.9- ☑
      basicervical (basal) S72.0 ☑
      birth injury P13.2
      capital epiphyseal S79.01- ☑
      condyles, epicondyles — *see* Fracture, femur, lower end

Fracture, traumatic — *continued*
    femur, femoral — *continued*
      distal end — *see* Fracture, femur, lower end
      epiphysis
        head — *see* Fracture, femur, upper end, epiphysis
        lower — *see* Fracture, femur, lower end, epiphysis
        upper — *see* Fracture, femur, upper end, epiphysis
      following insertion of implant, prosthesis or plate M96.66- ☑
      head — *see* Fracture, femur, upper end, head
      intertrochanteric — *see* Fracture, femur, trochanteric
      intratrochanteric — *see* Fracture, femur, trochanteric
      lower end S72.40- ☑
        condyle (displaced) S72.41- ☑
          lateral (displaced) S72.42- ☑
            nondisplaced S72.42- ☑
          medial (displaced) S72.43- ☑
            nondisplaced S72.43- ☑
          nondisplaced S72.41- ☑
        epiphysis (displaced) S72.44- ☑
          nondisplaced S72.44- ☑
        physeal S79.10- ☑
          Salter-Harris
            Type I S79.11- ☑
            Type II S79.12- ☑
            Type III S79.13- ☑
            Type IV S79.14- ☑
          specified NEC S79.19- ☑
        specified NEC S72.49- ☑
        supracondylar (displaced) S72.45- ☑
          with intracondylar extension (displaced) S72.46- ☑
            nondisplaced S72.46- ☑
          nondisplaced S72.45- ☑
        torus S72.47- ☑
      neck — *see* Fracture, femur, upper end, neck
      pertrochanteric — *see* Fracture, femur, trochanteric
      shaft (lower third) (middle third) (upper third) S72.30- ☑
        comminuted (displaced) S72.35- ☑
          nondisplaced S72.35- ☑
        oblique (displaced) S72.33- ☑
          nondisplaced S72.33- ☑
        segmental (displaced) S72.36- ☑
          nondisplaced S72.36- ☑
        specified NEC S72.39- ☑
        spiral (displaced) S72.34- ☑
          nondisplaced S72.34- ☑
        transverse (displaced) S72.32- ☑
          nondisplaced S72.32- ☑
      specified site NEC — *see* subcategory S72.8 ☑
      subcapital (displaced) S72.01- ☑
      subtrochanteric (region) (section) (displaced) S72.2- ☑
        nondisplaced S72.2- ☑
      transcervical — *see* Fracture, femur, upper end, neck
      transtrochanteric — *see* Fracture, femur, trochanteric
      trochanteric S72.10- ☑
        apophyseal (displaced) S72.13- ☑
          nondisplaced S72.13- ☑
        greater trochanter (displaced) S72.11- ☑
          nondisplaced S72.11- ☑
        intertrochanteric (displaced) S72.14- ☑
          nondisplaced S72.14- ☑
        lesser trochanter (displaced) S72.12- ☑
          nondisplaced S72.12- ☑
      upper end S72.00- ☑
        apophyseal (displaced) S72.13- ☑
          nondisplaced S72.13- ☑
        cervicotrochanteric — *see* Fracture, femur, upper end, neck, base
        epiphysis (displaced) S72.02- ☑
          nondisplaced S72.02- ☑
        head S72.05- ☑
          articular (displaced) S72.06- ☑
            nondisplaced S72.06- ☑
          specified NEC S72.09- ☑
        intertrochanteric (displaced) S72.14- ☑

☑ **Additional Character Required** — Refer to the Tabular List for Character Selection   ▽ **Subterms under main terms may continue to next column or page**

Fracture, traumatic — *continued*
  femur, femoral — *continued*
    upper end — *continued*
      intertrochanteric — *continued*
        nondisplaced S72.14- ☑
      intracapsular S72.01- ☑
      midcervical (displaced) S72.03- ☑
        nondisplaced S72.03- ☑
      neck S72.00- ☑
        base (displaced) S72.04- ☑
          nondisplaced S72.04- ☑
        specified NEC S72.09- ☑
      pertrochanteric — *see* Fracture, femur, upper end, trochanteric
      physeal S79.00- ☑
        Salter-Harris type I S79.01- ☑
        specified NEC S79.09- ☑
      subcapital (displaced) S72.01- ☑
      subtrochanteric (displaced) S72.2- ☑
        nondisplaced S72.2- ☑
      transcervical — *see* Fracture, femur, upper end, midcervical
      trochanteric S72.10- ☑
        greater (displaced) S72.11- ☑
          nondisplaced S72.11- ☑
        lesser (displaced) S72.12- ☑
          nondisplaced S72.12- ☑
  fibula (shaft) (styloid) S82.40- ☑
    comminuted (displaced) S82.45- ☑
      nondisplaced S82.45- ☑
    following insertion of implant, prosthesis or plate M96.67- ☑
    involving ankle or malleolus — *see* Fracture, fibula, lateral malleolus
    lateral malleolus (displaced) S82.6- ☑
      nondisplaced S82.6- ☑
    lower end
      physeal S89.30- ☑
        Salter-Harris
          Type I S89.31- ☑
          Type II S89.32- ☑
        specified NEC S89.39- ☑
      specified NEC S82.83- ☑
      torus S82.82- ☑
    oblique (displaced) S82.43- ☑
      nondisplaced S82.43- ☑
    segmental (displaced) S82.46- ☑
      nondisplaced S82.46- ☑
    specified NEC S82.49- ☑
    spiral (displaced) S82.44- ☑
      nondisplaced S82.44- ☑
    transverse (displaced) S82.42- ☑
      nondisplaced S82.42- ☑
    upper end
      physeal S89.20- ☑
        Salter-Harris
          Type I S89.21- ☑
          Type II S89.22- ☑
        specified NEC S89.29- ☑
      specified NEC S82.83- ☑
      torus S82.81- ☑
  finger (except thumb) S62.60- ☑
    distal phalanx (displaced) S62.63- ☑
      nondisplaced S62.66- ☑
    index S62.60- ☑
      distal phalanx (displaced) S62.63- ☑
        nondisplaced S62.66- ☑
      medial phalanx (displaced) S62.62- ☑
        nondisplaced S62.65- ☑
      proximal phalanx (displaced) S62.61- ☑
        nondisplaced S62.64- ☑
    little S62.60- ☑
      distal phalanx (displaced) S62.63- ☑
        nondisplaced S62.66- ☑
      medial phalanx (displaced) S62.62- ☑
        nondisplaced S62.65- ☑
      proximal phalanx (displaced) S62.61- ☑
        nondisplaced S62.64- ☑
    medial phalanx (displaced) S62.62- ☑
      nondisplaced S62.65- ☑
    middle S62.60- ☑
      distal phalanx (displaced) S62.63- ☑
        nondisplaced S62.66- ☑
      medial phalanx (displaced) S62.62- ☑
        nondisplaced S62.65- ☑
      proximal phalanx (displaced) S62.61- ☑

Fracture, traumatic — *continued*
  finger — *continued*
    middle — *continued*
      proximal phalanx — *continued*
        nondisplaced S62.64- ☑
      proximal phalanx (displaced) S62.61- ☑
        nondisplaced S62.64- ☑
    ring S62.60- ☑
      distal phalanx (displaced) S62.63- ☑
        nondisplaced S62.66- ☑
      medial phalanx (displaced) S62.62- ☑
        nondisplaced S62.65- ☑
      proximal phalanx (displaced) S62.61- ☑
        nondisplaced S62.64- ☑
    thumb — *see* Fracture, thumb
  following insertion (intraoperative) (postoperative) of orthopedic implant, joint prosthesis or bone plate M96.69
    femur M96.66- ☑
    fibula M96.67- ☑
    humerus M96.62- ☑
    pelvis M96.65
    radius M96.63- ☑
    specified bone NEC M96.69
    tibia M96.67- ☑
    ulna M96.63- ☑
  foot S92.90- ☑
    astragalus — *see* Fracture, tarsal, talus
    calcaneus — *see* Fracture, tarsal, calcaneus
    cuboid — *see* Fracture, tarsal, cuboid
    cuneiform — *see* Fracture, tarsal, cuneiform
    metatarsal — *see* Fracture, metatarsal
    navicular — *see* Fracture, tarsal, navicular
    sesamoid S92.81- ☑
    specified NEC S92.81- ☑
    talus — *see* Fracture, tarsal, talus
    tarsal — *see* Fracture, tarsal
    toe — *see* Fracture, toe
  forearm S52.9- ☑
    radius — *see* Fracture, radius
    ulna — *see* Fracture, ulna
  fossa (anterior) (middle) (posterior) S02.19 ☑
  frontal (bone) (skull) S02.0 ☑
    sinus S02.19 ☑
  glenoid (cavity) (scapula) — *see* Fracture, scapula, glenoid cavity
  greenstick — *see* Fracture, by site
  hallux — *see* Fracture, toe, great
  hand S62.9- ☑
    carpal — *see* Fracture, carpal bone
    finger (except thumb) — *see* Fracture, finger
    metacarpal — *see* Fracture, metacarpal
    navicular (scaphoid) (hand) — *see* Fracture, carpal bone, navicular
    thumb — *see* Fracture, thumb
  healed or old
    with complications — *code by* Nature of the complication
  heel bone — *see* Fracture, tarsal, calcaneus
  Hill-Sachs S42.29- ☑
  hip — *see* Fracture, femur, neck
  humerus S42.30- ☑
    anatomical neck — *see* Fracture, humerus, upper end
    articular process — *see* Fracture, humerus, lower end
    capitellum — *see* Fracture, humerus, lower end, condyle, lateral
    distal end — *see* Fracture, humerus, lower end
    epiphysis
      lower — *see* Fracture, humerus, lower end, physeal
      upper — *see* Fracture, humerus, upper end, physeal
    external condyle — *see* Fracture, humerus, lower end, condyle, lateral
    following insertion of implant, prosthesis or plate M96.62- ☑
    great tuberosity — *see* Fracture, humerus, upper end, greater tuberosity
    intercondylar — *see* Fracture, humerus, lower end
    internal epicondyle — *see* Fracture, humerus, lower end, epicondyle, medial
    lesser tuberosity — *see* Fracture, humerus, upper end, lesser tuberosity
    lower end S42.40- ☑

Fracture, traumatic — *continued*
  humerus — *continued*
    lower end — *continued*
      condyle
        lateral (displaced) S42.45- ☑
          nondisplaced S42.45- ☑
        medial (displaced) S42.46- ☑
          nondisplaced S42.46- ☑
      epicondyle
        lateral (displaced) S42.43- ☑
          nondisplaced S42.43- ☑
        medial (displaced) S42.44- ☑
          incarcerated S42.44- ☑
          nondisplaced S42.44- ☑
      physeal S49.10- ☑
        Salter-Harris
          Type I S49.11- ☑
          Type II S49.12- ☑
          Type III S49.13- ☑
          Type IV S49.14- ☑
        specified NEC S49.19- ☑
      specified NEC (displaced) S42.49- ☑
        nondisplaced S42.49- ☑
      supracondylar (simple) (displaced) S42.41- ☑
        with intercondylar fracture — *see* Fracture, humerus, lower end
        comminuted (displaced) S42.42- ☑
          nondisplaced S42.42- ☑
        nondisplaced S42.41- ☑
      torus S42.48- ☑
      transcondylar (displaced) S42.47- ☑
        nondisplaced S42.47- ☑
    proximal end — *see* Fracture, humerus, upper end
    shaft S42.30- ☑
      comminuted (displaced) S42.35- ☑
        nondisplaced S42.35- ☑
      greenstick S42.31- ☑
      oblique (displaced) S42.33- ☑
        nondisplaced S42.33- ☑
      segmental (displaced) S42.36- ☑
        nondisplaced S42.36- ☑
      specified NEC S42.39- ☑
      spiral (displaced) S42.34- ☑
        nondisplaced S42.34- ☑
      transverse (displaced) S42.32- ☑
        nondisplaced S42.32- ☑
    supracondylar — *see* Fracture, humerus, lower end
    surgical neck — *see* Fracture, humerus, upper end, surgical neck
    trochlea — *see* Fracture, humerus, lower end, condyle, medial
    tuberosity — *see* Fracture, humerus, upper end
    upper end S42.20- ☑
      anatomical neck — *see* Fracture, humerus, upper end, specified NEC
      articular head — *see* Fracture, humerus, upper end, specified NEC
      epiphysis — *see* Fracture, humerus, upper end, physeal
      greater tuberosity (displaced) S42.25- ☑
        nondisplaced S42.25- ☑
      lesser tuberosity (displaced) S42.26- ☑
        nondisplaced S42.26- ☑
      physeal S49.00- ☑
        Salter-Harris
          Type I S49.01- ☑
          Type II S49.02- ☑
          Type III S49.03- ☑
          Type IV S49.04- ☑
        specified NEC S49.09- ☑
      specified NEC (displaced) S42.29- ☑
        nondisplaced S42.29- ☑
      surgical neck (displaced) S42.21- ☑
        four-part S42.24- ☑
        nondisplaced S42.21- ☑
        three-part S42.23- ☑
        two-part (displaced) S42.22- ☑
          nondisplaced S42.22- ☑
      torus S42.27- ☑
      transepiphyseal — *see* Fracture, humerus, upper end, physeal
  hyoid bone S12.8 ☑
  ilium S32.30- ☑
    with disruption of pelvic ring — *see* Disruption, pelvic ring
    avulsion (displaced) S32.31- ☑

Fracture, traumatic — *continued*
- ilium — *continued*
  - avulsion — *continued*
    - nondisplaced S32.31- ☑
    - specified NEC S32.39- ☑
- impaction, impacted — *code as* Fracture, by site
- innominate bone — *see* Fracture, ilium
- instep — *see* Fracture, foot
- ischium S32.60- ☑
  - with disruption of pelvic ring — *see* Disruption, pelvic ring
  - avulsion (displaced) S32.61- ☑
    - nondisplaced S32.61- ☑
  - specified NEC S32.69- ☑
- jaw (bone) (lower) — *see* Fracture, mandible
  - upper — *see* Fracture, maxilla
- joint prosthesis — *see* Complications, joint prosthesis, mechanical, breakdown, by site
  - periprosthetic — *see* Fracture, traumatic, periprosthetic
- knee cap — *see* Fracture, patella
- larynx S12.8 ☑
- late effects — *see* Sequelae, fracture
- leg (lower) S82.9- ☑
  - ankle — *see* Fracture, ankle
  - femur — *see* Fracture, femur
  - fibula — *see* Fracture, fibula
  - malleolus — *see* Fracture, ankle
  - patella — *see* Fracture, patella
  - specified site NEC S82.89- ☑
  - tibia — *see* Fracture, tibia
- lumbar spine — *see* Fracture, vertebra, lumbar
- lumbosacral spine S32.9 ☑
- Maisonneuve's (displaced) S82.86- ☑
  - nondisplaced S82.86- ☑
- malar bone (*see also* Fracture, maxilla) S02.400 ☑
  - left side S02.40B ☑
  - right side S02.40A ☑
- malleolus — *see* Fracture, ankle
- malunion — *see* Fracture, by site
- mandible (lower jaw (bone)) S02.609 ☑
  - alveolus S02.67- ☑
  - angle (of jaw) S02.65- ☑
  - body, unspecified S02.600 ☑
    - left side S02.602 ☑
    - right side S02.601 ☑
  - condylar process S02.61- ☑
  - coronoid process S02.63- ☑
  - ramus, unspecified S02.64- ☑
  - specified site NEC S02.69 ☑
  - subcondylar process S02.62- ☑
  - symphysis S02.66 ☑
- manubrium (sterni) S22.21 ☑
  - dissociation from sternum S22.23 ☑
- march — *see* Fracture, traumatic, stress, by site
- maxilla, maxillary (bone) (sinus) (superior) (upper jaw) S02.401 ☑
  - alveolus S02.42 ☑
  - inferior — *see* Fracture, mandible
  - LeFort I S02.411 ☑
  - LeFort II S02.412 ☑
  - LeFort III S02.413 ☑
  - left side S02.40D ☑
  - right side S02.40C ☑
- metacarpal S62.309 ☑
  - base (displaced) S62.319 ☑
    - nondisplaced S62.349 ☑
  - fifth S62.30- ☑
    - base (displaced) S62.31- ☑
      - nondisplaced S62.34- ☑
    - neck (displaced) S62.33- ☑
      - nondisplaced S62.36- ☑
    - shaft (displaced) S62.32- ☑
      - nondisplaced S62.35- ☑
    - specified NEC S62.398 ☑
  - first S62.20- ☑
    - base NEC (displaced) S62.23- ☑
      - nondisplaced S62.23- ☑
    - Bennett's — *see* Bennett's fracture
    - neck (displaced) S62.25- ☑
      - nondisplaced S62.25- ☑
    - shaft (displaced) S62.24- ☑
      - nondisplaced S62.24- ☑
    - specified NEC S62.29- ☑
  - fourth S62.30- ☑
    - base (displaced) S62.31- ☑

Fracture, traumatic — *continued*
- metacarpal — *continued*
  - fourth — *continued*
    - base — *continued*
      - nondisplaced S62.34- ☑
    - neck (displaced) S62.33- ☑
      - nondisplaced S62.36- ☑
    - shaft (displaced) S62.32- ☑
      - nondisplaced S62.35- ☑
    - specified NEC S62.39- ☑
  - neck (displaced) S62.33- ☑
    - nondisplaced S62.36- ☑
  - Rolando's — *see* Rolando's fracture
  - second S62.30- ☑
    - base (displaced) S62.31- ☑
      - nondisplaced S62.34- ☑
    - neck (displaced) S62.33- ☑
      - nondisplaced S62.36- ☑
    - shaft (displaced) S62.32- ☑
      - nondisplaced S62.35- ☑
    - specified NEC S62.39- ☑
  - shaft (displaced) S62.32- ☑
    - nondisplaced S62.35- ☑
  - specified NEC S62.399 ☑
  - third S62.30- ☑
    - base (displaced) S62.31- ☑
      - nondisplaced S62.34- ☑
    - neck (displaced) S62.33- ☑
      - nondisplaced S62.36- ☑
    - shaft (displaced) S62.32- ☑
      - nondisplaced S62.35- ☑
    - specified NEC S62.39- ☑
- metastatic — *see* Fracture, pathological, due to, neoplastic disease (*see also* Neoplasm)
- metatarsal bone S92.30- ☑
  - fifth (displaced) S92.35- ☑
    - nondisplaced S92.35- ☑
  - first (displaced) S92.31- ☑
    - nondisplaced S92.31- ☑
  - fourth (displaced) S92.34- ☑
    - nondisplaced S92.34- ☑
  - physeal S99.10- ☑
    - Salter-Harris
      - Type I S99.11- ☑
      - Type II S99.12- ☑
      - Type III S99.13- ☑
      - Type IV S99.14- ☑
    - specified NEC S99.19- ☑
  - second (displaced) S92.32- ☑
    - nondisplaced S92.32- ☑
  - third (displaced) S92.33- ☑
    - nondisplaced S92.33- ☑
- Monteggia's — *see* Monteggia's fracture
- multiple
  - hand (and wrist) NEC — *see* Fracture, by site
  - ribs — *see* Fracture, rib, multiple
- nasal (bone(s)) S02.2 ☑
- navicular (scaphoid) (foot) (*see also* Fracture, tarsal, navicular)
  - hand — *see* Fracture, carpal, navicular
- neck S12.9 ☑
  - cervical vertebra S12.9 ☑
    - fifth (displaced) S12.400 ☑
      - nondisplaced S12.401 ☑
      - specified type NEC (displaced) S12.490 ☑
        - nondisplaced S12.491 ☑
    - first (displaced) S12.000 ☑
      - burst (stable) S12.01 ☑
        - unstable S12.02 ☑
      - lateral mass (displaced) S12.040 ☑
        - nondisplaced S12.041 ☑
      - nondisplaced S12.001 ☑
      - posterior arch (displaced) S12.030 ☑
        - nondisplaced S12.031 ☑
      - specified type NEC (displaced) S12.090 ☑
        - nondisplaced S12.091 ☑
    - fourth (displaced) S12.300 ☑
      - nondisplaced S12.301 ☑
      - specified type NEC (displaced) S12.390 ☑
        - nondisplaced S12.391 ☑
    - second (displaced) S12.100 ☑
      - dens (anterior) (displaced) (type II) S12.110 ☑
        - nondisplaced S12.112 ☑
        - posterior S12.111 ☑

Fracture, traumatic — *continued*
- neck — *continued*
  - cervical vertebra — *continued*
    - second — *continued*
      - dens — *continued*
        - specified type NEC (displaced) S12.120 ☑
        - nondisplaced S12.121 ☑
      - nondisplaced S12.101 ☑
      - specified type NEC (displaced) S12.190 ☑
        - nondisplaced S12.191 ☑
    - seventh (displaced) S12.600 ☑
      - nondisplaced S12.601 ☑
      - specified type NEC (displaced) S12.690 ☑
        - nondisplaced S12.691 ☑
    - sixth (displaced) S12.500 ☑
      - nondisplaced S12.501 ☑
      - specified type NEC (displaced) S12.590 ☑
        - nondisplaced S12.591 ☑
    - third (displaced) S12.200 ☑
      - nondisplaced S12.201 ☑
      - specified type NEC (displaced) S12.290 ☑
        - nondisplaced S12.291 ☑
  - hyoid bone S12.8 ☑
  - larynx S12.8 ☑
  - specified site NEC S12.8 ☑
  - thyroid cartilage S12.8 ☑
  - trachea S12.8 ☑
- neoplastic NEC — *see* Fracture, pathological, due to, neoplastic disease
- neural arch — *see* Fracture, vertebra
- newborn — *see* Birth, injury, fracture
- nontraumatic — *see* Fracture, pathological
- nonunion — *see* Nonunion, fracture
- nose, nasal (bone) (septum) S02.2 ☑
- occiput — *see* Fracture, skull, base, occiput
- odontoid process — *see* Fracture, neck, cervical vertebra, second
- olecranon (process) (ulna) — *see* Fracture, ulna, upper end, olecranon process
- orbit, orbital (bone) (region) S02.8- ☑
  - floor (blow-out) S02.3- ☑
  - roof S02.19 ☑
- os
  - calcis — *see* Fracture, tarsal, calcaneus
  - magnum — *see* Fracture, carpal, capitate
  - pubis — *see* Fracture, pubis
- palate S02.8- ☑
- parietal bone (skull) S02.0 ☑
- patella S82.00- ☑
  - comminuted (displaced) S82.04- ☑
    - nondisplaced S82.04- ☑
  - longitudinal (displaced) S82.02- ☑
    - nondisplaced S82.02- ☑
  - osteochondral (displaced) S82.01- ☑
    - nondisplaced S82.01- ☑
  - specified NEC S82.09- ☑
  - transverse (displaced) S82.03- ☑
    - nondisplaced S82.03- ☑
- pedicle (of vertebral arch) — *see* Fracture, vertebra
- pelvis, pelvic (bone) S32.9 ☑
  - acetabulum — *see* Fracture, acetabulum
  - circle — *see* Disruption, pelvic ring
  - following insertion of implant, prosthesis or plate M96.65
  - ilium — *see* Fracture, ilium
  - ischium — *see* Fracture, ischium
  - multiple
    - with disruption of pelvic ring (circle) — *see* Disruption, pelvic ring
    - without disruption of pelvic ring (circle) S32.82 ☑
  - pubis — *see* Fracture, pubis
  - sacrum — *see* Fracture, sacrum
  - specified site NEC S32.89 ☑
- periprosthetic, around internal prosthetic joint M97.9 ☑
  - ankle M97.2- ☑
  - elbow M97.4- ☑
  - finger M97.8 ☑
  - hip M97.0- ☑
  - knee M97.1- ☑
  - shoulder M97.3- ☑
  - specified joint NEC M97.8 ☑
  - spine M97.8 ☑
  - toe M97.8 ☑

Fracture, traumatic — *continued*
- periprosthetic, around internal prosthetic joint — *continued*
  - wrist M97.8 ☑
- phalanx
  - foot — *see* Fracture, toe
  - hand — *see* Fracture, finger
- pisiform — *see* Fracture, carpal, pisiform
- pond — *see* Fracture, skull
- prosthetic device, internal — *see* Complications, prosthetic device, by site, mechanical
- pubis S32.50- ☑
  - with disruption of pelvic ring — *see* Disruption, pelvic ring
  - specified site NEC S32.59- ☑
  - superior rim S32.51- ☑
- radius S52.9-
  - distal end — *see* Fracture, radius, lower end
  - following insertion of implant, prosthesis or plate M96.63- ☑
  - head — *see* Fracture, radius, upper end, head
  - lower end S52.50- ☑
    - Barton's — *see* Barton's fracture
    - Colles' — *see* Colles' fracture
    - extraarticular NEC S52.55- ☑
    - intraarticular NEC S52.57- ☑
    - physeal S59.20- ☑
      - Salter-Harris
        - Type I S59.21- ☑
        - Type II S59.22- ☑
        - Type III S59.23- ☑
        - Type IV S59.24- ☑
      - specified NEC S59.29- ☑
    - Smith's — *see* Smith's fracture
    - specified NEC S52.59- ☑
    - styloid process (displaced) S52.51- ☑
      - nondisplaced S52.51- ☑
    - torus S52.52- ☑
  - neck — *see* Fracture, radius, upper end
  - proximal end — *see* Fracture, radius, upper end
  - shaft S52.30- ☑
    - bent bone S52.38- ☑
    - comminuted (displaced) S52.35- ☑
      - nondisplaced S52.35- ☑
    - Galeazzi's — *see* Galeazzi's fracture
    - greenstick S52.31- ☑
    - oblique (displaced) S52.33- ☑
      - nondisplaced S52.33- ☑
    - segmental (displaced) S52.36- ☑
      - nondisplaced S52.36- ☑
    - specified NEC S52.39- ☑
    - spiral (displaced) S52.34- ☑
      - nondisplaced S52.34- ☑
    - transverse (displaced) S52.32- ☑
      - nondisplaced S52.32- ☑
  - upper end S52.10- ☑
    - head (displaced) S52.12- ☑
      - nondisplaced S52.12- ☑
    - neck (displaced) S52.13- ☑
      - nondisplaced S52.13- ☑
    - physeal S59.10- ☑
      - Salter-Harris
        - Type I S59.11- ☑
        - Type II S59.12- ☑
        - Type III S59.13- ☑
        - Type IV S59.14- ☑
      - specified NEC S59.19- ☑
    - specified NEC S52.18- ☑
    - torus S52.11- ☑
- ramus
  - inferior or superior, pubis — *see* Fracture, pubis
  - mandible — *see* Fracture, mandible
- restorative material (dental) K08.539
  - with loss of material K08.531
  - without loss of material K08.530
- rib S22.3- ☑
  - with flail chest — *see* Flail, chest
  - multiple S22.4- ☑
    - with flail chest — *see* Flail, chest
- root, tooth — *see* Fracture, tooth
- sacrum S32.10 ☑
  - specified NEC S32.19 ☑
  - Type
    - 1 S32.14 ☑
    - 2 S32.15 ☑
    - 3 S32.16 ☑

Fracture, traumatic — *continued*
- sacrum — *continued*
  - Type — *continued*
    - 4 S32.17 ☑
  - Zone
    - I S32.119 ☑
      - displaced (minimally) S32.111 ☑
        - severely S32.112 ☑
      - nondisplaced S32.110 ☑
    - II S32.129 ☑
      - displaced (minimally) S32.121 ☑
        - severely S32.122 ☑
      - nondisplaced S32.120 ☑
    - III S32.139 ☑
      - displaced (minimally) S32.131 ☑
        - severely S32.132 ☑
      - nondisplaced S32.130 ☑
- scaphoid (hand) (*see also* Fracture, carpal, navicular)
  - foot — *see* Fracture, tarsal, navicular
- scapula S42.10- ☑
  - acromial process (displaced) S42.12- ☑
    - nondisplaced S42.12- ☑
  - body (displaced) S42.11- ☑
    - nondisplaced S42.11- ☑
  - coracoid process (displaced) S42.13- ☑
    - nondisplaced S42.13- ☑
  - glenoid cavity (displaced) S42.14- ☑
    - nondisplaced S42.14- ☑
  - neck (displaced) S42.15- ☑
    - nondisplaced S42.15- ☑
  - specified NEC S42.19- ☑
- semilunar bone, wrist — *see* Fracture, carpal, lunate
- sequelae — *see* Sequelae, fracture
- sesamoid bone
  - foot S92.81- ☑
  - hand — *see* Fracture, carpal
  - other — *see* Fracture, traumatic, by site
- shepherd's — *see* Fracture, tarsal, talus
- shoulder (girdle) S42.9- ☑
  - blade — *see* Fracture, scapula
- sinus (ethmoid) (frontal) S02.19 ☑
- skull S02.91 ☑
  - base S02.10- ☑
    - occiput S02.119 ☑
      - condyle S02.113 ☑
        - specified NEC S02.118 ☑
          - left side S02.11H ☑
          - right side S02.11G ☑
        - type I S02.110 ☑
          - left side S02.11B ☑
          - right side S02.11A ☑
        - type II S02.111 ☑
          - left side S02.11D ☑
          - right side S02.11C ☑
        - type III S02.112 ☑
          - left side S02.11F ☑
          - right side S02.11E ☑
      - specified NEC S02.19 ☑
  - birth injury P13.0
  - frontal bone S02.0 ☑
  - parietal bone S02.0 ☑
  - specified site NEC S02.8- ☑
  - temporal bone S02.19 ☑
  - vault S02.0 ☑
- Smith's — *see* Smith's fracture
- sphenoid (bone) (sinus) S02.19 ☑
- spine — *see* Fracture, vertebra
- spinous process — *see* Fracture, vertebra
- spontaneous (cause unknown) — *see* Fracture, pathological
- stave (of thumb) — *see* Fracture, metacarpal, first
- sternum S22.20 ☑
  - with flail chest — *see* Flail, chest
  - body S22.22 ☑
  - manubrium S22.21 ☑
  - xiphoid (process) S22.24 ☑
- stress M84.30 ☑
  - ankle M84.37- ☑
  - carpus M84.34- ☑
  - clavicle M84.31- ☑
  - femoral neck M84.359 ☑
  - femur M84.35- ☑
  - fibula M84.36- ☑
  - finger M84.34- ☑
  - hip M84.359 ☑
  - humerus M84.32- ☑

Fracture, traumatic — *continued*
- stress — *continued*
  - ilium M84.350 ☑
  - ischium M84.350 ☑
  - metacarpus M84.34- ☑
  - metatarsus M84.37- ☑
  - neck — *see* Fracture, fatigue, vertebra
  - pelvis M84.350 ☑
  - radius M84.33- ☑
  - rib M84.38 ☑
  - scapula M84.31- ☑
  - skull M84.38 ☑
  - tarsus M84.37- ☑
  - tibia M84.36- ☑
  - toe M84.37- ☑
  - ulna M84.33- ☑
  - vertebra — *see* Fracture, fatigue, vertebra
- supracondylar, elbow — *see* Fracture, humerus, lower end, supracondylar
- symphysis pubis — *see* Fracture, pubis
- talus (ankle bone) — *see* Fracture, tarsal, talus
- tarsal bone(s) S92.20- ☑
  - astragalus — *see* Fracture, tarsal, talus
  - calcaneus S92.00- ☑
    - anterior process (displaced) S92.02- ☑
      - nondisplaced S92.02- ☑
    - body (displaced) S92.01- ☑
      - nondisplaced S92.01- ☑
    - extraarticular NEC (displaced) S92.05- ☑
      - nondisplaced S92.05- ☑
    - intraarticular (displaced) S92.06- ☑
      - nondisplaced S92.06- ☑
    - physeal S99.00- ☑
      - Salter-Harris
        - Type I S99.01- ☑
        - Type II S99.02- ☑
        - Type III S99.03- ☑
        - Type IV S99.04- ☑
      - specified NEC S99.09- ☑
    - tuberosity (displaced) S92.04- ☑
      - avulsion (displaced) S92.03- ☑
        - nondisplaced S92.03- ☑
      - nondisplaced S92.04- ☑
  - cuboid (displaced) S92.21- ☑
    - nondisplaced S92.21- ☑
  - cuneiform
    - intermediate (displaced) S92.23- ☑
      - nondisplaced S92.23- ☑
    - lateral (displaced) S92.22- ☑
      - nondisplaced S92.22- ☑
    - medial (displaced) S92.24- ☑
      - nondisplaced S92.24- ☑
  - navicular (displaced) S92.25- ☑
    - nondisplaced S92.25- ☑
  - scaphoid — *see* Fracture, tarsal, navicular
  - talus S92.10- ☑
    - avulsion (displaced) S92.15- ☑
      - nondisplaced S92.15- ☑
    - body (displaced) S92.12- ☑
      - nondisplaced S92.12- ☑
    - dome (displaced) S92.14- ☑
      - nondisplaced S92.14- ☑
    - head (displaced) S92.12- ☑
      - nondisplaced S92.12- ☑
    - lateral process (displaced) S92.14- ☑
      - nondisplaced S92.14- ☑
    - neck (displaced) S92.11- ☑
      - nondisplaced S92.11- ☑
    - posterior process (displaced) S92.13- ☑
      - nondisplaced S92.13- ☑
    - specified NEC S92.19- ☑
- temporal bone (styloid) S02.19 ☑
- thorax (bony) S22.9 ☑
  - with flail chest — *see* Flail, chest
  - rib S22.3- ☑
    - multiple S22.4- ☑
      - with flail chest — *see* Flail, chest
  - sternum S22.20 ☑
    - body S22.22 ☑
    - manubrium S22.21 ☑
    - xiphoid process S22.24 ☑
  - vertebra (displaced) S22.009 ☑
    - burst (stable) S22.001 ☑
      - unstable S22.002 ☑
    - eighth S22.069 ☑
      - burst (stable) S22.061 ☑

Fracture, traumatic — *continued*
   vertebra, vertebral — *continued*
      lumbar — *continued*
         third S32.039 ☑
            burst (stable) S32.031 ☑
               unstable S32.032 ☑
            specified type NEC S32.038 ☑
            wedge compression S32.030 ☑
            wedge compression S32.000 ☑
         metastatic — *see* Collapse, vertebra, in, specified
            disease NEC (*see also* Neoplasm)
         newborn (birth injury) P11.5
         sacrum S32.10 ☑
            specified NEC S32.19 ☑
            Type
               1 S32.14 ☑
               2 S32.15 ☑
               3 S32.16 ☑
               4 S32.17 ☑
            Zone
               I S32.119 ☑
                  displaced (minimally) S32.111 ☑
                     severely S32.112 ☑
                  nondisplaced S32.110 ☑
               II S32.129 ☑
                  displaced (minimally) S32.121 ☑
                     severely S32.122 ☑
                  nondisplaced S32.120 ☑
               III S32.139 ☑
                  displaced (minimally) S32.131 ☑
                     severely S32.132 ☑
                  nondisplaced S32.130 ☑
         thoracic — *see* Fracture, thorax, vertebra
      vertex S02.0 ☑
      vomer (bone) S02.2 ☑
      wrist S62.10- ☑
         carpal — *see* Fracture, carpal bone
         navicular (scaphoid) (hand) — *see* Fracture, carpal,
            navicular
      xiphisternum, xiphoid (process) S22.24 ☑
      zygoma S02.402 ☑
         left side S02.40F ☑
         right side S02.40E ☑
Fragile, fragility
   autosomal site Q95.5
   bone, congenital (with blue sclera) Q78.0
   capillary (hereditary) D69.8
   hair L67.8
   nails L60.3
   non-sex chromosome site Q95.5
   X chromosome Q99.2
Fragilitas
   crinium L67.8
   ossium (with blue sclerae) (hereditary) Q78.0
   unguium L60.3
      congenital Q84.6
Fragments, cataract (lens), **following cataract surgery**
   H59.02- ☑
      retained foreign body — *see* Retained, foreign body
         fragments (type of)
Frailty (frail) R54
   mental R41.81
Frambesia, frambesial (tropica) (*see also* Yaws)
   initial lesion or ulcer A66.0
   primary A66.0
Frambeside
   gummatous A66.4
   of early yaws A66.2
Frambesioma A66.1
Franceschetti-Klein (-Wildervanck) **disease or syn-**
   drome Q75.4
Francis' disease — *see* Tularemia
Franklin disease C88.2
Frank's essential thrombocytopenia D69.3
Fraser's syndrome Q87.0
Freckle(s) L81.2
   malignant melanoma in — *see* Melanoma
   melanotic (Hutchinson's) — *see* Melanoma, in situ
   retinal D49.81
Frederickson's hyperlipoproteinemia, type
   I and V E78.3
   IIA E78.00
   IIB and III E78.2
   IV E78.1
Freeman Sheldon syndrome Q87.0
Freezing (*see also* Effect, adverse, cold) T69.9 ☑

Freiberg's disease (infraction of metatarsal head or osteochondrosis) — *see* Osteochondrosis, juvenile,
   metatarsus
Frei's disease A55
Fremitus, friction, cardiac R01.2
Frenum, frenulum
   external os Q51.828
   tongue (shortening) (congenital) Q38.1
Frequency micturition (nocturnal) R35.0
   psychogenic F45.8
Frey's syndrome
   auriculotemporal G50.8
   hyperhidrosis L74.52
Friction
   burn — *see* Burn, by site
   fremitus, cardiac R01.2
   precordial R01.2
   sounds, chest R09.89
Friderichsen-Waterhouse syndrome or disease A39.1
Friedländer's B (bacillus) **NEC** (*see also* condition) A49.8
Friedreich's
   ataxia G11.1
   combined systemic disease G11.1
   facial hemihypertrophy Q67.4
   sclerosis (cerebellum) (spinal cord) G11.1
Frigidity F52.22
Fröhlich's syndrome E23.6
Frontal (*see also* condition)
   lobe syndrome F07.0
Frostbite (superficial) T33.90 ☑
   with
      partial thickness skin loss — *see* Frostbite (superfi-
         cial), by site
      tissue necrosis T34.90 ☑
   abdominal wall T33.3
      with tissue necrosis T34.3 ☑
   ankle T33.81- ☑
      with tissue necrosis T34.81- ☑
   arm T33.4-
      with tissue necrosis T34.4- ☑
      finger(s) — *see* Frostbite, finger
      hand — *see* Frostbite, hand
      wrist — *see* Frostbite, wrist
   ear T33.01- ☑
      with tissue necrosis T34.01- ☑
   face T33.09 ☑
      with tissue necrosis T34.09 ☑
   finger T33.53- ☑
      with tissue necrosis T34.53- ☑
   foot T33.82- ☑
      with tissue necrosis T34.82- ☑
   hand T33.52- ☑
      with tissue necrosis T34.52- ☑
   head T33.09 ☑
      with tissue necrosis T34.09 ☑
      ear — *see* Frostbite, ear
      nose — *see* Frostbite, nose
   hip (and thigh) T33.6- ☑
      with tissue necrosis T34.6- ☑
   knee T33.7- ☑
      with tissue necrosis T34.7- ☑
   leg T33.9- ☑
      with tissue necrosis T34.9- ☑
      ankle — *see* Frostbite, ankle
      foot — *see* Frostbite, foot
      knee — *see* Frostbite, knee
      lower T33.7- ☑
         with tissue necrosis T34.7- ☑
      thigh — *see* Frostbite, hip
      toe — *see* Frostbite, toe
   limb
      lower T33.99 ☑
         with tissue necrosis T34.99 ☑
      upper — *see* Frostbite, arm
   neck T33.1 ☑
      with tissue necrosis T34.1 ☑
   nose T33.02 ☑
      with tissue necrosis T34.02 ☑
   pelvis T33.3 ☑
      with tissue necrosis T34.3 ☑
   specified site NEC T33.99 ☑
      with tissue necrosis T34.99 ☑
   thigh — *see* Frostbite, hip
   thorax T33.2 ☑
      with tissue necrosis T34.2 ☑
   toes T33.83- ☑

Frostbite — *continued*
   toes — *continued*
      with tissue necrosis T34.83- ☑
   trunk T33.99 ☑
      with tissue necrosis T34.99 ☑
   wrist T33.51- ☑
      with tissue necrosis T34.51- ☑
Frotteurism F65.81
Frozen (*see also* Effect, adverse, cold) T69.9 ☑
   pelvis (female) N94.89
      male K66.8
   shoulder — *see* Capsulitis, adhesive
Fructokinase deficiency E74.11
Fructose 1,6 diphosphatase deficiency E74.19
Fructosemia (benign) (essential) E74.12
Fructosuria (benign) (essential) E74.11
Fuchs'
   black spot (myopic) (*see also* Myopia, degenerative)
      H44.2- ☑
   dystrophy (corneal endothelium) H18.51
   heterochromic cyclitis — *see* Cyclitis, Fuchs' hete-
      rochromic
Fucosidosis E77.1
Fugue R68.89
   dissociative F44.1
   hysterical (dissociative) F44.1
   postictal in epilepsy — *see* Epilepsy
   reaction to exceptional stress (transient) F43.0
Fulminant, fulminating — *see* condition
Functional (*see also* condition)
   bleeding (uterus) N93.8
Functioning, intellectual, borderline R41.83
Fundus — *see* condition
Fungemia NOS B49
Fungus, fungous
   cerebral G93.89
   disease NOS B49
   infection — *see* Infection, fungus
Funiculitis (acute) (chronic) (endemic) N49.1
   gonococcal (acute) (chronic) A54.23
   tuberculous A18.15
Funnel
   breast (acquired) M95.4
      congenital Q67.6
      sequelae (late effect) of rickets E64.3
   chest (acquired) M95.4
      congenital Q67.6
      sequelae (late effect) of rickets E64.3
   pelvis (acquired) M95.5
      with disproportion (fetopelvic) O33.3 ☑
         causing obstructed labor O65.3
      congenital Q74.2
FUO (fever of unknown origin) R50.9
Furfur L21.0
   microsporon B36.0
Furrier's lung J67.8
Furrowed K14.5
   nail(s) (transverse) L60.4
      congenital Q84.6
   tongue K14.5
      congenital Q38.3
Furuncle L02.92
   abdominal wall L02.221
   ankle — *see* Furuncle, lower limb
   antecubital space — *see* Furuncle, upper limb
   anus K61.0
   arm — *see* Furuncle, upper limb
   auditory canal, external — *see* Abscess, ear, external
   auricle (ear) — *see* Abscess, ear, external
   axilla (region) L02.42- ☑
   back (any part) L02.222
   breast N61.1
   buttock L02.32
   cheek (external) L02.02
   chest wall L02.223
   chin L02.02
   corpus cavernosum N48.21
   ear, external — *see* Abscess, ear, external
   external auditory canal — *see* Abscess, ear, external
   eyelid — *see* Abscess, eyelid
   face L02.02
   femoral (region) — *see* Furuncle, lower limb
   finger — *see* Furuncle, hand
   flank L02.221
   foot L02.62- ☑
   forehead L02.02
   gluteal (region) L02.32

Index

Fracture, traumatic — Furuncle

Furuncle — *continued*
  groin L02.224
  hand L02.52- ☑
  head L02.821
    face L02.02
  hip — *see* Furuncle, lower limb
  kidney — *see* Abscess, kidney
  knee — *see* Furuncle, lower limb
  labium (majus) (minus) N76.4
  lacrimal
    gland — *see* Dacryoadenitis
    passages (duct) (sac) — *see* Inflammation, lacrimal, passages, acute
  leg (any part) — *see* Furuncle, lower limb
  lower limb L02.42- ☑
  malignant A22.0
  mouth K12.2
  navel L02.226
  neck L02.12
  nose J34.0
  orbit, orbital — *see* Abscess, orbit
  palmar (space) — *see* Furuncle, hand
  partes posteriores L02.32
  pectoral region L02.223
  penis N48.21
  perineum L02.225
  pinna — *see* Abscess, ear, external
  popliteal — *see* Furuncle, lower limb
  prepatellar — *see* Furuncle, lower limb
  scalp L02.821
  seminal vesicle N49.0
  shoulder — *see* Furuncle, upper limb
  specified site NEC L02.828
  submandibular K12.2
  temple (region) L02.02
  thumb — *see* Furuncle, hand
  toe — *see* Furuncle, foot
  trunk L02.229
    abdominal wall L02.221
    back L02.222

Furuncle — *continued*
  trunk — *continued*
    chest wall L02.223
    groin L02.224
    perineum L02.225
    umbilicus L02.226
  umbilicus L02.226
  upper limb L02.42- ☑
  vulva N76.4
Furunculosis — *see* Furuncle
Fused — *see* Fusion, fused
Fusion, fused (congenital)
  astragaloscaphoid Q74.2
  atria Q21.1
  auditory canal Q16.1
  auricles, heart Q21.1
  binocular with defective stereopsis H53.32
  bone Q79.8
  cervical spine M43.22
  choanal Q30.0
  commissure, mitral valve Q23.2
  cusps, heart valve NEC Q24.8
    mitral Q23.2
    pulmonary Q22.1
    tricuspid Q22.4
  ear ossicles Q16.3
  fingers Q70.0 ☑
  hymen Q52.3
  joint (acquired) (*see also* Ankylosis)
    congenital Q74.8
  kidneys (incomplete) Q63.1
  labium (majus) (minus) Q52.5
  larynx and trachea Q34.8
  limb, congenital Q74.8
    lower Q74.2
    upper Q74.0
  lobes, lung Q33.8
  lumbosacral (acquired) M43.27
    arthrodesis status Z98.1
    congenital Q76.49

Fusion, fused — *continued*
  lumbosacral — *continued*
    postprocedural status Z98.1
  nares, nose, nasal, nostril(s) Q30.0
  organ or site not listed — *see* Anomaly, by site
  ossicles Q79.9
    auditory Q16.3
  pulmonic cusps Q22.1
  ribs Q76.6
  sacroiliac (joint) (acquired) M43.28
    arthrodesis status Z98.1
    congenital Q74.2
    postprocedural status Z98.1
  spine (acquired) NEC M43.20
    arthrodesis status Z98.1
    cervical region M43.22
    cervicothoracic region M43.23
    congenital Q76.49
    lumbar M43.26
    lumbosacral region M43.27
    occipito-atlanto-axial region M43.21
    postoperative status Z98.1
    sacrococcygeal region M43.28
    thoracic region M43.24
    thoracolumbar region M43.25
  sublingual duct with submaxillary duct at opening in mouth Q38.4
  testes Q55.1
  toes Q70.2- ☑
  tooth, teeth K00.2
  trachea and esophagus Q39.8
  twins Q89.4
  vagina Q52.4
  ventricles, heart Q21.0
  vertebra (arch) — *see* Fusion, spine
  vulva Q52.5
Fusospirillosis (mouth) (tongue) (tonsil) A69.1
Fussy baby R68.12

156

☑ **Additional Character Required** — Refer to the Tabular List for Character Selection   ▽ **Subterms under main terms may continue to next column or page**

Furuncle — Fussy baby

G

Gain in weight (abnormal) (excessive) (*see also* Weight, gain)
Gaisböck's disease (polycythemia hypertonica) D75.1
Gait abnormality R26.9
 ataxic R26.0
 falling R29.6
 hysterical (ataxic) (staggering) F44.4
 paralytic R26.1
 spastic R26.1
 specified type NEC R26.89
 staggering R26.0
 unsteadiness R26.81
 walking difficulty NEC R26.2
Galactocele (breast) N64.89
 puerperal, postpartum O92.79
Galactokinase deficiency E74.29
Galactophoritis N61.0
 gestational, puerperal, postpartum O91.2- ☑
Galactorrhea O92.6
 not associated with childbirth N64.3
Galactosemia (classic) (congenital) E74.21
Galactosuria E74.29
Galacturia R82.0
 schistosomiasis (bilharziasis) B65.0
GALD (gestational alloimmune liver disease) P78.84
Galeazzi's fracture S52.37- ☑
Galen's vein — *see* condition
Galeophobia F40.218
Gall duct — *see* condition
Gallbladder (*see also* condition)
 acute K81.0
Gallop rhythm R00.8
Gallstone (colic) (cystic duct) (gallbladder) (impacted) (multiple) (*see also* Calculus, gallbladder)
 with
  cholecystitis — *see* Calculus, gallbladder, with cholecystitis
 bile duct (common) (hepatic) — *see* Calculus, bile duct
 causing intestinal obstruction K56.3
 specified NEC K80.80
  with obstruction K80.81
Gambling Z72.6
 pathological (compulsive) F63.0
Gammopathy (of undetermined significance [MGUS]) D47.2
 associated with lymphoplasmacytic dyscrasia D47.2
 monoclonal D47.2
 polyclonal D89.0
Gamna's disease (siderotic splenomegaly) D73.1
Gamophobia F40.298
Gampsodactylia (congenital) Q66.7
Gamstorp's disease (adynamia episodica hereditaria) G72.3
Gandy-Nanta disease (siderotic splenomegaly) D73.1
Gang
 membership offenses Z72.810
Gangliocytoma D36.10
Ganglioglioma — *see* Neoplasm, uncertain behavior, by site
Ganglion (compound) (diffuse) (joint) (tendon (sheath)) M67.40
 ankle M67.47- ☑
 foot M67.47- ☑
 forearm M67.43- ☑
 hand M67.44- ☑
 lower leg M67.46- ☑
 multiple sites M67.49
 of yaws (early) (late) A66.6
 pelvic region M67.45- ☑
 periosteal — *see* Periostitis
 shoulder region M67.41- ☑
 specified site NEC M67.48
 thigh region M67.45- ☑
 tuberculous A18.09
 upper arm M67.42- ☑
 wrist M67.43- ☑
Ganglioneuroblastoma — *see* Neoplasm, nerve, malignant
Ganglioneuroma D36.10
 malignant — *see* Neoplasm, nerve, malignant
Ganglioneuromatosis D36.10
Ganglionitis
 fifth nerve — *see* Neuralgia, trigeminal
 gasserian (postherpetic) (postzoster) B02.21

Ganglionitis — *continued*
 geniculate G51.1
  newborn (birth injury) P11.3
  postherpetic, postzoster B02.21
 herpes zoster B02.21
 postherpetic geniculate B02.21
Gangliosidosis E75.10
 GM1 E75.19
 GM2 E75.00
  other specified E75.09
  Sandhoff disease E75.01
  Tay-Sachs disease E75.02
 GM3 E75.19
 mucolipidosis IV E75.11
Gangosa A66.5
Gangrene, gangrenous (connective tissue) (dropsical) (dry) (moist) (skin) (ulcer) (*see also* Necrosis) I96
 with diabetes (mellitus) — *see* Diabetes, gangrene
 abdomen (wall) I96
 alveolar M27.3
 appendix K35.80
  with
   perforation or rupture K35.2
   peritoneal abscess K35.3
   peritonitis NEC K35.3
    generalized (with perforation or rupture) K35.2
    localized (with perforation or rupture) K35.3
 arteriosclerotic (general) (senile) — *see* Arteriosclerosis, extremities, with, gangrene
 auricle I96
 Bacillus welchii A48.0
 bladder (infectious) — *see* Cystitis, specified type NEC
 bowel, cecum, or colon — *see* Gangrene, intestine
 Clostridium perfringens or welchii A48.0
 cornea H18.89- ☑
 corpora cavernosa N48.29
  noninfective N48.89
 cutaneous, spreading I96
 decubital — *see* Ulcer, pressure, by site
 diabetic (any site) — *see* Diabetes, gangrene
 emphysematous — *see* Gangrene, gas
 epidemic — *see* Poisoning, food, noxious, plant
 epididymis (infectional) N45.1
 erysipelas — *see* Erysipelas
 extremity (lower) (upper) I96
 Fournier N49.3
  female N76.89
 fusospirochetal A69.0
 gallbladder — *see* Cholecystitis, acute
 gas (bacillus) A48.0
  following
   abortion — *see* Abortion by type complicated by infection
   ectopic or molar pregnancy O08.0
 glossitis K14.0
 hernia — *see* Hernia, by site, with gangrene
 intestine, intestinal (hemorrhagic) (massive) (*see also* Infarct, intestine) K55.069
  with
   mesenteric embolism (*see also* Infarct, intestine) K55.069
   obstruction — *see* Obstruction, intestine
 laryngitis J04.0
 limb (lower) (upper) I96
 lung J85.0
  spirochetal A69.8
 lymphangitis I89.1
 Meleney's (synergistic) — *see* Ulcer, skin
 mesentery (*see also* Infarct, intestine) K55.069
  with
   embolism (*see also* Infarct, intestine) K55.069
   intestinal obstruction — *see* Obstruction, intestine
 mouth A69.0
 ovary — *see* Oophoritis
 pancreas — *see* Pancreatitis, acute
 penis N48.29
  noninfective N48.89
 perineum I96
 pharynx (*see also* Pharyngitis)
  Vincent's A69.1
 presenile I73.1
 progressive synergistic — *see* Ulcer, skin
 pulmonary J85.0
 pulpal (dental) K04.1
 quinsy J36
 Raynaud's (symmetric gangrene) I73.01

Gangrene, gangrenous — *continued*
 retropharyngeal J39.2
 scrotum N49.3
  noninfective N50.89
 senile (atherosclerotic) — *see* Arteriosclerosis, extremities, with, gangrene
 spermatic cord N49.1
  noninfective N50.89
 spine I96
 spirochetal NEC A69.8
 spreading cutaneous I96
 stomatitis A69.0
 symmetrical I73.01
 testis (infectional) N45.2
  noninfective N44.8
 throat (*see also* Pharyngitis)
  diphtheritic A36.0
  Vincent's A69.1
 thyroid (gland) E07.89
 tooth (pulp) K04.1
 tuberculous NEC — *see* Tuberculosis
 tunica vaginalis N49.1
  noninfective N50.89
 umbilicus I96
 uterus — *see* Endometritis
 uvulitis K12.2
 vas deferens N49.1
  noninfective N50.89
 vulva N76.89
Ganister disease J62.8
Ganser's syndrome (hysterical) F44.89
Gardner-Diamond syndrome (autoerythrocyte sensitization) D69.2
Gargoylism E76.01
Garré's disease, osteitis (sclerosing), osteomyelitis — *see* Osteomyelitis, specified type NEC
Garrod's pad, knuckle M72.1
Gartner's duct
 cyst Q52.4
 persistent Q50.6
Gas R14.3
 asphyxiation, inhalation, poisoning, suffocation NEC — *see* Table of Drugs and Chemicals
 excessive R14.0
 gangrene A48.0
  following
   abortion — *see* Abortion by type complicated by infection
   ectopic or molar pregnancy O08.0
 on stomach R14.0
 pains R14.1
Gastralgia (*see also* Pain, abdominal)
Gastrectasis K31.0
 psychogenic F45.8
Gastric — *see* condition
Gastrinoma
 malignant
  pancreas C25.4
  specified site NEC — *see* Neoplasm, malignant, by site
  unspecified site C25.4
 specified site — *see* Neoplasm, uncertain behavior
 unspecified site D37.9
Gastritis (simple) K29.70
 with bleeding K29.71
 acute (erosive) K29.00
  with bleeding K29.01
 alcoholic K29.20
  with bleeding K29.21
 allergic K29.60
  with bleeding K29.61
 atrophic (chronic) K29.40
  with bleeding K29.41
 chronic (antral) (fundal) K29.50
  with bleeding K29.51
  atrophic K29.40
   with bleeding K29.41
  superficial K29.30
   with bleeding K29.31
 dietary counseling and surveillance Z71.3
 due to diet deficiency E63.9
 eosinophilic K52.81
 giant hypertrophic K29.60
  with bleeding K29.61
 granulomatous K29.60
  with bleeding K29.61
 hypertrophic (mucosa) K29.60
  with bleeding K29.61

Gastritis — *continued*
nervous F54
spastic K29.60
with bleeding K29.61
specified NEC K29.60
with bleeding K29.61
superficial chronic K29.30
with bleeding K29.31
tuberculous A18.83
viral NEC A08.4
Gastrocarcinoma — *see* Neoplasm, malignant, stomach
Gastrocolic — *see* condition
Gastrodisciasis, gastrodiscoidiasis B66.8
Gastroduodenitis K29.90
with bleeding K29.91
virus, viral A08.4
specified type NEC A08.39
Gastrodynia — *see* Pain, abdominal
Gastroenteritis (acute) (chronic) (noninfectious) (*see also* Enteritis) K52.9
allergic K52.29
with
eosinophilic gastritis or gastroenteritis K52.81
food protein-induced enterocolitis syndrome K52.21
food protein-induced enteropathy K52.22
dietetic (*see also* Gastroenteritis, allergic) K52.29
drug-induced K52.1
due to
Cryptosporidium A07.2
drugs K52.1
food poisoning — *see* Intoxication, foodborne
radiation K52.0
eosinophilic K52.81
epidemic (infectious) A09
food hypersensitivity (*see also* Gastroenteritis, allergic) K52.29
infectious — *see* Enteritis, infectious
influenzal — *see* Influenza, with gastroenteritis
noninfectious K52.9
specified NEC K52.89
rotaviral A08.0
Salmonella A02.0
toxic K52.1
viral NEC A08.4
acute infectious A08.39
type Norwalk A08.11
infantile (acute) A08.39
Norwalk agent A08.11
rotaviral A08.0
severe of infants A08.39
specified type NEC A08.39
Gastroenteropathy (*see also* Gastroenteritis) K52.9
acute, due to Norovirus A08.11
acute, due to Norwalk agent A08.11
infectious A09
Gastroenteroptosis K63.4
Gastroesophageal laceration- hemorrhage syndrome K22.6
Gastrointestinal — *see* condition
Gastrojejunal — *see* condition
Gastrojejunitis (*see also* Enteritis) K52.9
Gastrojejunocolic — *see* condition
Gastroliths K31.89
Gastromalacia K31.89
Gastroparalysis K31.84
diabetic — *see* Diabetes, gastroparalysis
Gastroparesis K31.84
diabetic — *see* Diabetes, by type, with gastroparesis
Gastropathy K31.9
congestive portal K31.89
erythematous K29.70
exudative K90.89
portal hypertensive K31.89
Gastroptosis K31.89
Gastrorrhagia K92.2
psychogenic F45.8
Gastroschisis (congenital) Q79.3
Gastrospasm (neurogenic) (reflex) K31.89
neurotic F45.8
psychogenic F45.8
Gastrostaxis — *see* Gastritis, with bleeding
Gastrostenosis K31.89
Gastrostomy
attention to Z43.1
status Z93.1
Gastrosuccorrhea (continuous) (intermittent) K31.89
neurotic F45.8

Gastrosuccorrhea — *continued*
psychogenic F45.8
Gatophobia F40.218
Gaucher's disease or splenomegaly (adult) (infantile) E75.22
Gee (-Herter)(-Thaysen) **disease** (nontropical sprue) K90.0
Gélineau's syndrome G47.419
with cataplexy G47.411
Gemination, tooth, teeth K00.2
Gemistocytoma
specified site — *see* Neoplasm, malignant, by site
unspecified site C71.9
General, generalized — *see* condition
Genetic
carrier (status)
cystic fibrosis Z14.1
hemophilia A (asymptomatic) Z14.01
symptomatic Z14.02
specified NEC Z14.8
susceptibility to disease NEC Z15.89
malignant neoplasm Z15.09
breast Z15.01
endometrium Z15.04
ovary Z15.02
prostate Z15.03
specified NEC Z15.09
multiple endocrine neoplasia Z15.81
Genital — *see* condition
Genito-anorectal syndrome A55
Genitourinary system — *see* condition
Genu
congenital Q74.1
extrorsum (acquired) (*see also* Deformity, varus, knee)
congenital Q74.1
sequelae (late effect) of rickets E64.3
introrsum (acquired) (*see also* Deformity, valgus, knee)
congenital Q74.1
sequelae (late effect) of rickets E64.3
rachitic (old) E64.3
recurvatum (acquired) (*see also* Deformity, limb, specified type NEC, lower leg)
congenital Q68.2
sequelae (late effect) of rickets E64.3
valgum (acquired) (knock-knee) M21.06- ☑
congenital Q74.1
sequelae (late effect) of rickets E64.3
varum (acquired) (bowleg) M21.16- ☑
congenital Q74.1
sequelae (late effect) of rickets E64.3
Geographic tongue K14.1
Geophagia — *see* Pica
Geotrichosis B48.3
stomatitis B48.3
Gephyrophobia F40.242
Gerbode defect Q21.0
GERD (gastroesophageal reflux disease) K21.9
Gerhardt's
disease (erythromelalgia) I73.81
syndrome (vocal cord paralysis) J38.00
bilateral J38.02
unilateral J38.01
German measles (*see also* Rubella)
exposure to Z20.4
Germinoblastoma (diffuse) C85.9- ☑
follicular C82.9- ☑
Germinoma — *see* Neoplasm, malignant, by site
Gerontoxon — *see* Degeneration, cornea, senile
Gerstmann's syndrome R48.8
developmental F81.2
Gerstmann-Sträussler-Scheinker syndrome (GSS) A81.82
Gestation (period) (*see also* Pregnancy)
ectopic — *see* Pregnancy, by site
multiple O30.9- ☑
greater than quadruplets — *see* Pregnancy, multiple (gestation), specified NEC
specified NEC — *see* Pregnancy, multiple (gestation), specified NEC
Gestational
mammary abscess O91.11- ☑
purulent mastitis O91.11- ☑
subareolar abscess O91.11- ☑
Ghon tubercle, primary infection A15.7
Ghost
teeth K00.4
vessels (cornea) H16.41- ☑
Ghoul hand A66.3

Gianotti-Crosti disease L44.4
Giant
cell
epulis K06.8
peripheral granuloma K06.8
esophagus, congenital Q39.5
kidney, congenital Q63.3
urticaria T78.3 ☑
hereditary D84.1
Giardiasis A07.1
Gibert's disease or pityriasis L42
Giddiness R42
hysterical F44.89
psychogenic F45.8
Gierke's disease (glycogenosis I) E74.01
Gigantism (cerebral) (hypophyseal) (pituitary) E22.0
constitutional E34.4
Gilbert's disease or syndrome E80.4
Gilchrist's disease B40.9
Gilford-Hutchinson disease E34.8
Gilles de la Tourette's disease or syndrome (motor-verbal tic) F95.2
Gingivitis K05.10
acute (catarrhal) K05.00
necrotizing A69.1
nonplaque induced K05.01
plaque induced K05.00
chronic (desquamative) (hyperplastic) (simple marginal) (pregnancy associated) (ulcerative) K05.10
nonplaque induced K05.11
plaque induced K05.10
expulsiva — *see* Periodontitis
necrotizing ulcerative (acute) A69.1
pellagrous E52
acute necrotizing A69.1
Vincent's A69.1
Gingivoglossitis K14.0
Gingivopericementitis — *see* Periodontitis
Gingivosis — *see* Gingivitis, chronic
Gingivostomatitis K05.10
herpesviral B00.2
necrotizing ulcerative (acute) A69.1
Gland, glandular — *see* condition
Glanders A24.0
Glanzmann (-Naegeli) **disease or thrombasthenia** D69.1
Glasgow coma scale
total score
3-8 R40.243 ☑
9-12 R40.242 ☑
13-15 R40.241 ☑
Glass-blower's disease (cataract) — *see* Cataract, specified NEC
Glaucoma H40.9
with
increased episcleral venous pressure H40.81- ☑
pseudoexfoliation of lens — *see* Glaucoma, open angle, primary, capsular
absolute H44.51- ☑
angle-closure (primary) H40.20- ☑
acute (attack) (crisis) H40.21- ☑
chronic H40.22- ☑
intermittent H40.23- ☑
residual stage H40.24- ☑
borderline H40.00- ☑
capsular (with pseudoexfoliation of lens) — *see* Glaucoma, open angle, primary, capsular
childhood Q15.0
closed angle — *see* Glaucoma, angle-closure
congenital Q15.0
corticosteroid-induced — *see* Glaucoma, secondary, drugs
hypersecretion H40.82- ☑
in (due to)
amyloidosis E85.4 [H42]
aniridia Q13.1 [H42]
concussion of globe — *see* Glaucoma, secondary, trauma
dislocation of lens — *see* Glaucoma, secondary
disorder of lens NEC — *see* Glaucoma, secondary
drugs — *see* Glaucoma, secondary, drugs
endocrine disease NOS E34.9 [H42]
eye
inflammation — *see* Glaucoma, secondary, inflammation
trauma — *see* Glaucoma, secondary, trauma

Glaucoma — *continued*
  in — *continued*
    hypermature cataract — *see* Glaucoma, secondary
    iridocyclitis — *see* Glaucoma, secondary, inflammation
    lens disorder — *see* Glaucoma, secondary
    Lowe's syndrome E72.03 [H42]
    metabolic disease NOS E88.9 [H42]
    ocular disorders NEC — *see* Glaucoma, secondary
    onchocerciasis B73.02
    pupillary block — *see* Glaucoma, secondary
    retinal vein occlusion — *see* Glaucoma, secondary
    Rieger's anomaly Q13.81 [H42]
    rubeosis of iris — *see* Glaucoma, secondary
    tumor of globe — *see* Glaucoma, secondary
  infantile Q15.0
  low tension — *see* Glaucoma, open angle, primary, low-tension
  malignant H40.83- ☑
  narrow angle — *see* Glaucoma, angle-closure
  newborn Q15.0
  noncongestive (chronic) — *see* Glaucoma, open angle
  nonobstructive — *see* Glaucoma, open angle
  obstructive (*see also* Glaucoma, angle-closure)
    due to lens changes — *see* Glaucoma, secondary
  open angle H40.10- ☑
    primary H40.11- ☑
      capsular (with pseudoexfoliation of lens) H40.14- ☑
      low-tension H40.12- ☑
      pigmentary H40.13- ☑
      residual stage H40.15- ☑
  phacolytic — *see* Glaucoma, secondary
  pigmentary — *see* Glaucoma, open angle, primary, pigmentary
  postinfectious — *see* Glaucoma, secondary, inflammation
  secondary (to) H40.5- ☑
    drugs H40.6- ☑
    inflammation H40.4- ☑
    trauma H40.3- ☑
  simple (chronic) H40.11- ☑
  simplex H40.11- ☑
  specified type NEC H40.89
  suspect H40.00- ☑
  syphilitic A52.71
  traumatic (*see also* Glaucoma, secondary, trauma)
    newborn (birth injury) P15.3
  tuberculous A18.59
Glaucomatous flecks (subcapsular) — *see* Cataract, complicated
Glazed tongue K14.4
Gleet (gonococcal) A54.01
Glénard's disease K63.4
Glioblastoma (multiforme)
  with sarcomatous component
    specified site — *see* Neoplasm, malignant, by site
    unspecified site C71.9
  giant cell
    specified site — *see* Neoplasm, malignant, by site
    unspecified site C71.9
  specified site — *see* Neoplasm, malignant, by site
  unspecified site C71.9
Glioma (malignant)
  astrocytic
    specified site — *see* Neoplasm, malignant, by site
    unspecified site C71.9
  mixed
    specified site — *see* Neoplasm, malignant, by site
    unspecified site C71.9
  nose Q30.8
  specified site NEC — *see* Neoplasm, malignant, by site
  subependymal D43.2
    specified site — *see* Neoplasm, uncertain behavior, by site
    unspecified site D43.2
  unspecified site C71.9
Gliomatosis cerebri C71.0
Glioneuroma — *see* Neoplasm, uncertain behavior, by site
Gliosarcoma
  specified site — *see* Neoplasm, malignant, by site
  unspecified site C71.9
Gliosis (cerebral) G93.89
  spinal G95.89
Glisson's disease — *see* Rickets
Globinuria R82.3

Globus (hystericus) F45.8
Glomangioma D18.00
  intra-abdominal D18.03
  intracranial D18.02
  skin D18.01
  specified site NEC D18.09
Glomangiomyoma D18.00
  intra-abdominal D18.03
  intracranial D18.02
  skin D18.01
  specified site NEC D18.09
Glomangiosarcoma — *see* Neoplasm, connective tissue, malignant
Glomerular
  disease in syphilis A52.75
  nephritis — *see* Glomerulonephritis
Glomerulitis — *see* Glomerulonephritis
Glomerulonephritis (*see also* Nephritis) N05.9
  with
    edema — *see* Nephrosis
    minimal change N05.0
    minor glomerular abnormality N05.0
  acute N00.9
  chronic N03.9
  crescentic (diffuse) NEC (*see also* N00-N07 with fourth character .7) N05.7
  dense deposit (*see also* N00-N07 with fourth character .6) N05.6
  diffuse
    crescentic (*see also* N00-N07 with fourth character .7) N05.7
    endocapillary proliferative (*see also* N00-N07 with fourth character .4) N05.4
    membranous (*see also* N00-N07 with fourth character .2) N05.2
    mesangial proliferative (*see also* N00-N07 with fourth character .3) N05.3
    mesangiocapillary (*see also* N00-N07 with fourth character .5) N05.5
    sclerosing N18.9
  endocapillary proliferative (diffuse) NEC (*see also* N00-N07 with fourth character .4) N05.4
  extracapillary NEC (*see also* N00-N07 with fourth character .7) N05.7
  focal (and segmental) (*see also* N00-N07 with fourth character .1) N05.1
  hypocomplementemic — *see* Glomerulonephritis, membranoproliferative
  IgA — *see* Nephropathy, IgA
  immune complex (circulating) NEC N05.8
  in (due to)
    amyloidosis E85.4 [N08]
    bilharziasis B65.9 [N08]
    cryoglobulinemia D89.1 [N08]
    defibrination syndrome D65 [N08]
    diabetes mellitus — *see* Diabetes, glomerulosclerosis
    disseminated intravascular coagulation D65 [N08]
    Fabry (-Anderson) disease E75.21 [N08]
    Goodpasture's syndrome M31.0
    hemolytic-uremic syndrome D59.3
    Henoch (-Schönlein) purpura D69.0 [N08]
    lecithin cholesterol acyltransferase deficiency E78.6 [N08]
    microscopic polyangiitis M31.7 [N08]
    multiple myeloma C90.0- ☑ [N08]
    Plasmodium malariae B52.0
    schistosomiasis B65.9 [N08]
    sepsis A41.9 [N08]
      streptococcal A40.- ☑ [N08]
    sickle-cell disorders D57.- ☑ [N08]
    strongyloidiasis B78.9 [N08]
    subacute bacterial endocarditis I33.0 [N08]
    syphilis (late) congenital A50.59 [N08]
    systemic lupus erythematosus M32.14
    thrombotic thrombocytopenic purpura M31.1 [N08]
    typhoid fever A01.09
    Waldenström macroglobulinemia C88.0 [N08]
    Wegener's granulomatosis M31.31
  latent or quiescent N03.9
  lobular, lobulonodular — *see* Glomerulonephritis, membranoproliferative
  membranoproliferative (diffuse)(type 1 or 3) (*see also* N00-N07 with fourth character .5) N05.5
    dense deposit (type 2) NEC (*see also* N00-N07 with fourth character .6) N05.6

Glomerulonephritis — *continued*
  membranous (diffuse) NEC (*see also* N00-N07 with fourth character .2) N05.2
  mesangial
    IgA/IgG — *see* Nephropathy, IgA
    proliferative (diffuse) NEC (*see also* N00-N07 with fourth character .3) N05.3
  mesangiocapillary (diffuse) NEC (*see also* N00-N07 with fourth character .5) N05.5
  necrotic, necrotizing NEC (*see also* N00- N07 with fourth character .8) N05.8
  nodular — *see* Glomerulonephritis, membranoproliferative
  poststreptococcal NEC N05.9
    acute N00.9
    chronic N03.9
    rapidly progressive N01.9
  proliferative NEC (*see also* N00-N07 with fourth character .8) N05.8
    diffuse (lupus) M32.14
  rapidly progressive N01.9
  sclerosing, diffuse N18.9
  specified pathology NEC (*see also* N00- N07 with fourth character .8) N05.8
  subacute N01.9
Glomerulopathy — *see* Glomerulonephritis
Glomerulosclerosis (*see also* Sclerosis, renal)
  intercapillary (nodular) (with diabetes) — *see* Diabetes, glomerulosclerosis
  intracapillary — *see* Diabetes, glomerulosclerosis
Glossagra K14.6
Glossalgia K14.6
Glossitis (chronic superficial) (gangrenous) (Moeller's) K14.0
  areata exfoliativa K14.1
  atrophic K14.4
  benign migratory K14.1
  cortical superficial, sclerotic K14.0
  Hunter's D51.0
  interstitial, sclerous K14.0
  median rhomboid K14.2
  pellagrous E52
  superficial, chronic K14.0
Glossocele K14.8
Glossodynia K14.6
  exfoliativa K14.4
Glossoncus K14.8
Glossopathy K14.9
Glossophytia K14.3
Glossoplegia K14.8
Glossoptosis K14.8
Glossopyrosis K14.6
Glossotrichia K14.3
Glossy skin L90.8
Glottis — *see* condition
Glottitis (*see also* Laryngitis) J04.0
Glucagonoma
  pancreas
    benign D13.7
    malignant C25.4
    uncertain behavior D37.8
  specified site NEC
    benign — *see* Neoplasm, benign, by site
    malignant — *see* Neoplasm, malignant, by site
    uncertain behavior — *see* Neoplasm, uncertain behavior, by site
  unspecified site
    benign D13.7
    malignant C25.4
    uncertain behavior D37.8
Glucoglycinuria E72.51
Glucose-galactose malabsorption E74.39
Glue
  ear — *see* Otitis, media, nonsuppurative, chronic, mucoid
  sniffing (airplane) — *see* Abuse, drug, inhalant
    dependence — *see* Dependence, drug, inhalant
Glutaric aciduria E72.3
Glycinemia E72.51
Glycinuria (renal) (with ketosis) E72.09
Glycogen
  infiltration — *see* Disease, glycogen storage
  storage disease — *see* Disease, glycogen storage
Glycogenosis (diffuse) (generalized) (*see also* Disease, glycogen storage)
  cardiac E74.02 [I43]

Glycogenosis — continued
  diabetic, secondary — see Diabetes, glycogenosis,
    secondary
  pulmonary interstitial J84.842
Glycopenia E16.2
Glycosuria R81
  renal E74.8
Gnathostoma spinigerum (infection) (infestation),
  gnathostomiasis (wandering swelling) B83.1
Goiter (plunging) (substernal) E04.9
  with
    hyperthyroidism (recurrent) — see Hyperthy-
      roidism, with, goiter
    thyrotoxicosis — see Hyperthyroidism, with, goiter
  adenomatous — see Goiter, nodular
  cancerous C73
  congenital (nontoxic) E03.0
    diffuse E03.0
    parenchymatous E03.0
    transitory, with normal functioning P72.0
  cystic E04.2
    due to iodine-deficiency E01.1
  due to
    enzyme defect in synthesis of thyroid hormone
      E07.1
    iodine-deficiency (endemic) E01.2
  dyshormonogenetic (familial) E07.1
  endemic (iodine-deficiency) E01.2
    diffuse E01.0
    multinodular E01.1
  exophthalmic — see Hyperthyroidism, with, goiter
  iodine-deficiency (endemic) E01.2
    diffuse E01.0
    multinodular E01.1
    nodular E01.1
  lingual Q89.2
  lymphadenoid E06.3
  malignant C73
  multinodular (cystic) (nontoxic) E04.2
    toxic or with hyperthyroidism E05.20
      with thyroid storm E05.21
  neonatal NEC P72.0
  nodular (nontoxic) (due to) E04.9
    with
      hyperthyroidism E05.20
        with thyroid storm E05.21
      thyrotoxicosis E05.20
        with thyroid storm E05.21
    endemic E01.1
    iodine-deficiency E01.1
    sporadic E04.9
    toxic E05.20
      with thyroid storm E05.21
  nontoxic E04.9
    diffuse (colloid) E04.0
    multinodular E04.2
    simple E04.0
    specified NEC E04.8
    uninodular E04.1
  simple E04.0
  toxic — see Hyperthyroidism, with, goiter
  uninodular (nontoxic) E04.1
    toxic or with hyperthyroidism E05.10
      with thyroid storm E05.11
Goiter-deafness syndrome E07.1
Goldberg syndrome Q89.8
Goldberg-Maxwell syndrome E34.51
Goldblatt's hypertension or kidney I70.1
Goldenhar (-Gorlin) **syndrome** Q87.0
Goldflam-Erb disease or syndrome G70.00
  with exacerbation (acute) G70.01
  in crisis G70.01
Goldscheider's disease Q81.8
Goldstein's disease (familial hemorrhagic telangiectasia)
  I78.0
Golfer's elbow — see Epicondylitis, medial
Gonadoblastoma
  specified site — see Neoplasm, uncertain behavior,
    by site
  unspecified site
    female D39.10
    male D40.10
Gonecystitis — see Vesiculitis
Gongylonemiasis B83.8
Goniosynechiae — see Adhesions, iris, goniosynechiae
Gonococcemia A54.86
Gonococcus, gonococcal (disease) (infection) (see also
  condition) A54.9

Gonococcus, gonococcal — continued
  anus A54.6
  bursa, bursitis A54.49
  conjunctiva, conjunctivitis (neonatorum) A54.31
  endocardium A54.83
  eye A54.30
    conjunctivitis A54.31
    iridocyclitis A54.32
    keratitis A54.33
    newborn A54.31
    other specified A54.39
  fallopian tubes (acute) (chronic) A54.24
  genitourinary (organ) (system) (tract) (acute)
    lower A54.00
      with abscess (accessory gland) (periurethral)
        A54.1
    upper (see also condition) A54.29
  heart A54.83
  iridocyclitis A54.32
  joint A54.42
  lymphatic (gland) (node) A54.89
  meninges, meningitis A54.81
  musculoskeletal A54.40
    arthritis A54.42
    osteomyelitis A54.43
    other specified A54.49
    spondylopathy A54.41
  pelviperitonitis A54.24
  pelvis (acute) (chronic) A54.24
  pharynx A54.5
  proctitis A54.6
  pyosalpinx (acute) (chronic) A54.24
  rectum A54.6
  skin A54.89
  specified site NEC A54.89
  tendon sheath A54.49
  throat A54.5
  urethra (acute) (chronic) A54.01
    with abscess (accessory gland) (periurethral) A54.1
  vulva (acute) (chronic) A54.02
Gonocytoma
  specified site — see Neoplasm, uncertain behavior,
    by site
  unspecified site
    female D39.10
    male D40.10
Gonorrhea (acute) (chronic) A54.9
  Bartholin's gland (acute) (chronic) (purulent) A54.02
    with abscess (accessory gland) (periurethral) A54.1
  bladder A54.01
  cervix A54.03
  conjunctiva, conjunctivitis (neonatorum) A54.31
  contact Z20.2
  Cowper's gland (with abscess) A54.1
  exposure to Z20.2
  fallopian tube (acute) (chronic) A54.24
  kidney (acute) (chronic) A54.21
  lower genitourinary tract A54.00
    with abscess (accessory gland) (periurethral) A54.1
  ovary (acute) (chronic) A54.24
  pelvis (acute) (chronic) A54.24
    female pelvic inflammatory disease A54.24
  penis A54.09
  prostate (acute) (chronic) A54.22
  seminal vesicle (acute) (chronic) A54.23
  specified site not listed (see also Gonococcus) A54.89
  spermatic cord (acute) (chronic) A54.23
  urethra A54.01
    with abscess (accessory gland) (periurethral) A54.1
  vagina A54.02
  vas deferens (acute) (chronic) A54.23
  vulva A54.02
Goodall's disease A08.19
Goodpasture's syndrome M31.0
Gopalan's syndrome (burning feet) E53.0
Gorlin-Chaudry-Moss syndrome Q87.0
Gottron's papules L94.4
Gougerot-Blum syndrome (pigmented purpuric
  lichenoid dermatitis) L81.7
Gougerot-Carteaud disease or syndrome (confluent
  reticulate papillomatosis) L83
Gougerot's syndrome (trisymptomatic) L81.7
Gouley's syndrome (constrictive pericarditis) I31.1
Goundou A66.6
Gout, chronic (see also Gout, gouty) M1A.9 ☑ (following
  M08)
  drug-induced M1A.20 ☑ (following M08)
    ankle M1A.27- ☑ (following M08)

Gout, chronic — continued
  drug-induced — continued
    elbow M1A.22- ☑ (following M08)
    foot joint M1A.27- ☑ (following M08)
    hand joint M1A.24- ☑ (following M08)
    hip M1A.25- ☑ (following M08)
    knee M1A.26- ☑ (following M08)
    multiple site M1A.29- ☑ (following M08)
    shoulder M1A.21- ☑ (following M08)
    vertebrae M1A.28 ☑ (following M08)
    wrist M1A.23- ☑ (following M08)
  idiopathic M1A.00 ☑ (following M08)
    ankle M1A.07- ☑ (following M08)
    elbow M1A.02- ☑ (following M08)
    foot joint M1A.07- ☑ (following M08)
    hand joint M1A.04- ☑ (following M08)
    hip M1A.05- ☑ (following M08)
    knee M1A.06- ☑ (following M08)
    multiple site M1A.09 ☑ (following M08)
    shoulder M1A.01- ☑ (following M08)
    vertebrae M1A.08 ☑ (following M08)
    wrist M1A.03- ☑ (following M08)
  in (due to) renal impairment M1A.30 ☑ (following
    M08)
    ankle M1A.37- ☑ (following M08)
    elbow M1A.32- ☑ (following M08)
    foot joint M1A.37- ☑ (following M08)
    hand joint M1A.34- ☑ (following M08)
    hip M1A.35- ☑ (following M08)
    knee M1A.36- ☑ (following M08)
    multiple site M1A.39 ☑ (following M08)
    shoulder M1A.31- ☑ (following M08)
    vertebrae M1A.38 ☑ (following M08)
    wrist M1A.33- ☑ (following M08)
  lead-induced M1A.10 ☑ (following M08)
    ankle M1A.17- ☑ (following M08)
    elbow M1A.12- ☑ (following M08)
    foot joint M1A.17- ☑ (following M08)
    hand joint M1A.14- ☑ (following M08)
    hip M1A.15- ☑ (following M08)
    knee M1A.16- ☑ (following M08)
    multiple site M1A.19 ☑ (following M08)
    shoulder M1A.11- ☑ (following M08)
    vertebrae M1A.18 ☑ (following M08)
    wrist M1A.13- ☑ (following M08)
  primary — see Gout, chronic, idiopathic
  saturnine — see Gout, chronic, lead-induced
  secondary NEC M1A.40 ☑ (following M08)
    ankle M1A.47- ☑ (following M08)
    elbow M1A.42- ☑ (following M08)
    foot joint M1A.47- ☑ (following M08)
    hand joint M1A.44- ☑ (following M08)
    hip M1A.45- ☑ (following M08)
    knee M1A.46- ☑ (following M08)
    multiple site M1A.49 ☑ (following M08)
    shoulder M1A.41- ☑ (following M08)
    vertebrae M1A.48 ☑ (following M08)
    wrist M1A.43- ☑ (following M08)
  syphilitic (see also subcategory M14.8-) A52.77
  tophi M1A.9 ☑ (following M08)
Gout, gouty (acute) (attack) (flare) (see also Gout,
  chronic) M10.9
  drug-induced M10.20
    ankle M10.27- ☑
    elbow M10.22- ☑
    foot joint M10.27- ☑
    hand joint M10.24- ☑
    hip M10.25- ☑
    knee M10.26- ☑
    multiple site M10.29
    shoulder M10.21- ☑
    vertebrae M10.28
    wrist M10.23- ☑
  idiopathic M10.00
    ankle M10.07- ☑
    elbow M10.02- ☑
    foot joint M10.07- ☑
    hand joint M10.04- ☑
    hip M10.05- ☑
    knee M10.06- ☑
    multiple site M10.09
    shoulder M10.01- ☑
    vertebrae M10.08
    wrist M10.03- ☑
  in (due to) renal impairment M10.30
    ankle M10.37- ☑

☑ **Additional Character Required** — Refer to the Tabular List for Character Selection   ▽ **Subterms under main terms may continue to next column or page**

Gout, gouty — *continued*
  in renal impairment — *continued*
    elbow M10.32- ☑
    foot joint M10.37- ☑
    hand joint M10.34- ☑
    hip M10.35- ☑
    knee M10.36- ☑
    multiple site M10.39
    shoulder M10.31- ☑
    vertebrae M10.38
    wrist M10.33- ☑
  lead-induced M10.10
    ankle M10.17- ☑
    elbow M10.12- ☑
    foot joint M10.17- ☑
    hand joint M10.14- ☑
    hip M10.15- ☑
    knee M10.16- ☑
    multiple site M10.19
    shoulder M10.11- ☑
    vertebrae M10.18
    wrist M10.13- ☑
  primary — *see* Gout, idiopathic
  saturnine — *see* Gout, lead-induced
  secondary NEC M10.40
    ankle M10.47- ☑
    elbow M10.42- ☑
    foot joint M10.47- ☑
    hand joint M10.44- ☑
    hip M10.45- ☑
    knee M10.46- ☑
    multiple site M10.49
    shoulder M10.41- ☑
    vertebrae M10.48
    wrist M10.43- ☑
  syphilitic (*see also* subcategory M14.8-) A52.77
  tophi — *see* Gout, chronic
Gower's
  muscular dystrophy G71.0
  syndrome (vasovagal attack) R55
Gradenigo's syndrome — *see* Otitis, media, suppurative, acute
Graefe's disease — *see* Strabismus, paralytic, ophthalmoplegia, progressive
Graft-versus-host disease D89.813
  acute D89.810
  acute on chronic D89.812
  chronic D89.811
Grain mite (itch) B88.0
Grainhandler's disease or lung J67.8
Grand mal — *see* Epilepsy, generalized, specified NEC
Grand multipara status only (not pregnant) Z64.1
  pregnant — *see* Pregnancy, complicated by, grand multiparity
Granite worker's lung J62.8
Granular (*see also* condition)
  inflammation, pharynx J31.2
  kidney (contracting) — *see* Sclerosis, renal
  liver K74.69
Granulation tissue (abnormal) (excessive) L92.9
  postmastoidectomy cavity — *see* Complications, postmastoidectomy, granulation
Granulocytopenia (primary) (malignant) — *see* Agranulocytosis
Granuloma L92.9
  abdomen K66.8
    from residual foreign body L92.3
    pyogenicum L98.0
  actinic L57.5
  annulare (perforating) L92.0
  apical K04.5
  aural — *see* Otitis, externa, specified NEC
  beryllium (skin) L92.3
  bone
    eosinophilic C96.6
    from residual foreign body — *see* Osteomyelitis, specified type NEC
    lung C96.6
  brain (any site) G06.0
    schistosomiasis B65.9 [G07]
  canaliculus lacrimalis — *see* Granuloma, lacrimal
  candidal (cutaneous) B37.2
  cerebral (any site) G06.0
  coccidioidal (primary) (progressive) B38.7
    lung B38.1
    meninges B38.4
  colon K63.89

Granuloma — *continued*
  conjunctiva H11.22- ☑
  dental K04.5
  ear, middle — *see* Cholesteatoma
  eosinophilic C96.6
    bone C96.6
    lung C96.6
    oral mucosa K13.4
    skin L92.2
  eyelid H01.8
  facial (e) L92.2
  foreign body (in soft tissue) NEC M60.20
    ankle M60.27- ☑
    foot M60.27- ☑
    forearm M60.23- ☑
    hand M60.24- ☑
    in operation wound — *see* Foreign body, accidentally left during a procedure
    lower leg M60.26- ☑
    pelvic region M60.25- ☑
    shoulder region M60.21- ☑
    skin L92.3
    specified site NEC M60.28
    subcutaneous tissue L92.3
    thigh M60.25- ☑
    upper arm M60.22- ☑
  gangraenescens M31.2
  genito-inguinale A58
  giant cell (central) (reparative) (jaw) M27.1
    gingiva (peripheral) K06.8
  gland (lymph) I88.8
  hepatic NEC K75.3
    in (due to)
      berylliosis J63.2 [K77]
      sarcoidosis D86.89
  Hodgkin C81.9 ☑
  ileum K63.89
  infectious B99.9
    specified NEC B99.8
  inguinale (Donovan) (venereal) A58
  intestine NEC K63.89
  intracranial (any site) G06.0
  intraspinal (any part) G06.1
  iridocyclitis — *see* Iridocyclitis, chronic
  jaw (bone) (central) M27.1
    reparative giant cell M27.1
  kidney (*see also* Infection, kidney) N15.8
  lacrimal H04.81- ☑
  larynx J38.7
  lethal midline (faciale(e)) M31.2
  liver NEC — *see* Granuloma, hepatic
  lung (infectious) (*see also* Fibrosis, lung)
    coccidioidal B38.1
    eosinophilic C96.6
  Majocchi's B35.8
  malignant (facial(e)) M31.2
  mandible (central) M27.1
  midline (lethal) M31.2
  monilial (cutaneous) B37.2
  nasal sinus — *see* Sinusitis
  operation wound T81.89 ☑
    foreign body — *see* Foreign body, accidentally left during a procedure
    stitch T81.89 ☑
    talc — *see* Foreign body, accidentally left during a procedure
  oral mucosa K13.4
  orbit, orbital H05.11- ☑
  paracoccidioidal B41.8
  penis, venereal A58
  periapical K04.5
  peritoneum K66.8
    due to ova of helminths NOS (*see also* Helminthiasis) B83.9 [K67]
  postmastoidectomy cavity — *see* Complications, postmastoidectomy, recurrent cholesteatoma
  prostate N42.89
  pudendi (ulcerating) A58
  pulp, internal (tooth) K03.3
  pyogenic, pyogenicum (of) (skin) L98.0
    gingiva K06.8
    maxillary alveolar ridge K04.5
    oral mucosa K13.4
  rectum K62.89
  reticulohistiocytic D76.3
  rubrum nasi L74.8
  Schistosoma — *see* Schistosomiasis
  septic (skin) L98.0

Granuloma — *continued*
  silica (skin) L92.3
  sinus (accessory) (infective) (nasal) — *see* Sinusitis
  skin L92.9
    from residual foreign body L92.3
    pyogenicum L98.0
  spine
    syphilitic (epidural) A52.19
    tuberculous A18.01
  stitch (postoperative) T81.89 ☑
  suppurative (skin) L98.0
  swimming pool A31.1
  talc (*see also* Granuloma, foreign body)
    in operation wound — *see* Foreign body, accidentally left during a procedure
  telangiectaticum (skin) L98.0
  tracheostomy J95.09
  trichophyticum B35.8
  tropicum A66.4
  umbilical P83.81
  umbilicus P83.81
  urethra N36.8
  uveitis — *see* Iridocyclitis, chronic
  vagina A58
  venereum A58
  vocal cord J38.3
Granulomatosis L92.9
  lymphoid C83.8- ☑
  miliary (listerial) A32.89
  necrotizing, respiratory M31.30
  progressive septic D71
  specified NEC L92.8
  Wegener's M31.30
    with renal involvement M31.31
Granulomatous tissue (abnormal) (excessive) L92.9
Granulosis rubra nasi L74.8
Graphite fibrosis (of lung) J63.3
Graphospasm F48.8
  organic G25.89
Grating scapula M89.8X1
Gravel (urinary) — *see* Calculus, urinary
Graves' disease — *see* Hyperthyroidism, with, goiter
Gravis — *see* condition
Grawitz tumor C64.- ☑
Gray syndrome (newborn) P93.0
Grayness, hair (premature) L67.1
  congenital Q84.2
Green sickness D50.8
Greenfield's disease
  meaning
    concentric sclerosis (encephalitis periaxialis concentrica) G37.5
    metachromatic leukodystrophy E75.25
Greenstick fracture — *code as* Fracture, by site
Grey syndrome (newborn) P93.0
Grief F43.21
  prolonged F43.29
  reaction (*see also* Disorder, adjustment) F43.20
Griesinger's disease B76.9
Grinder's lung or pneumoconiosis J62.8
Grinding, teeth
  psychogenic F45.8
  sleep related G47.63
Grip
  Dabney's B33.0
  devil's B33.0
Grippe, grippal (*see also* Influenza)
  Balkan A78
  summer, of Italy A93.1
Grisel's disease M43.6
Groin — *see* condition
Grooved tongue K14.5
Ground itch B76.9
Grover's disease or syndrome L11.1
Growing pains, children R29.898
Growth (fungoid) (neoplastic) (new) (*see also* Neoplasm)
  adenoid (vegetative) J35.8
  benign — *see* Neoplasm, benign, by site
  malignant — *see* Neoplasm, malignant, by site
  rapid, childhood Z00.2
  secondary — *see* Neoplasm, secondary, by site
Gruby's disease B35.0
Gubler-Millard paralysis or syndrome G46.3
Guerin-Stern syndrome Q74.3
Guidance, insufficient anterior (occlusal) M26.54
Guillain-Barré disease or syndrome G61.0
  sequelae G65.0

Guinea worms (infection) (infestation) B72
Guinon's disease (motor-verbal tic) F95.2
Gull's disease E03.4
Gum — *see* condition
Gumboil K04.7
  with sinus K04.6
Gumma (syphilitic) A52.79
  artery A52.09
    cerebral A52.04
  bone A52.77
    of yaws (late) A66.6
  brain A52.19
  cauda equina A52.19
  central nervous system A52.3
  ciliary body A52.71
  congenital A50.59
  eyelid A52.71
  heart A52.06
  intracranial A52.19
  iris A52.71
  kidney A52.75
  larynx A52.73
  leptomeninges A52.19
  liver A52.74
  meninges A52.19
  myocardium A52.06
  nasopharynx A52.73
  neurosyphilitic A52.3
  nose A52.73
  orbit A52.71
  palate (soft) A52.79
  penis A52.76
  pericardium A52.06
  pharynx A52.73
  pituitary A52.79
  scrofulous (tuberculous) A18.4
  skin A52.79
  specified site NEC A52.79
  spinal cord A52.19
  tongue A52.79
  tonsil A52.73
  trachea A52.73
  tuberculous A18.4
  ulcerative due to yaws A66.4
  ureter A52.75
  yaws A66.4
    bone A66.6
Gunn's syndrome Q07.8
Gunshot wound (*see also* Wound, open)
  fracture — *code as* Fracture, by site
  internal organs — *see* Injury, by site
Gynandrism Q56.0
Gynandroblastoma
  specified site — *see* Neoplasm, uncertain behavior,
    by site
  unspecified site
    female D39.10
    male D40.10
Gynecological examination (periodic) (routine) Z01.419
  with abnormal findings Z01.411
Gynecomastia N62
Gynephobia F40.291
Gyrate scalp Q82.8

H

H (Hartnup's) **disease** E72.02
Haas' disease or osteochondrosis (juvenile) (head of
  humerus) — *see* Osteochondrosis, juvenile,
  humerus
Habit, habituation
  bad sleep Z72.821
  chorea F95.8
  disturbance, child F98.9
  drug — *see* Dependence, drug
  irregular sleep Z72.821
  laxative F55.2
  spasm — *see* Tic
  tic — *see* Tic
Haemophilus (H.) **influenzae, as cause of disease
  classified elsewhere** B96.3
Haff disease — *see* Poisoning, mercury
Hageman's factor defect, deficiency or disease D68.2
Haglund's disease or osteochondrosis (juvenile) (os
  tibiale externum) — *see* Osteochondrosis, juvenile,
  tarsus
Hailey-Hailey disease Q82.8

Hair (*see also* condition)
  plucking F63.3
    in stereotyped movement disorder F98.4
  tourniquet syndrome (*see also* Constriction, external,
    by site)
    finger S60.44- ☑
    penis S30.842 ☑
    thumb S60.34- ☑
    toe S90.44- ☑
Hairball in stomach T18.2 ☑
Hair-pulling, pathological (compulsive) F63.3
Hairy black tongue K14.3
Half vertebra Q76.49
Halitosis R19.6
Hallerman-Streiff syndrome Q87.0
Hallervorden-Spatz disease G23.0
Hallopeau's acrodermatitis or disease L40.2
Hallucination R44.3
  auditory R44.0
  gustatory R44.2
  olfactory R44.2
  specified NEC R44.2
  tactile R44.2
  visual R44.1
Hallucinosis (chronic) F28
  alcoholic (acute) F10.951
    in
      abuse F10.151
      dependence F10.251
  drug-induced F19.951
    cannabis F12.951
    cocaine F14.951
    hallucinogen F16.151
    in
      abuse F19.151
        cannabis F12.151
        cocaine F14.151
        hallucinogen F16.151
        inhalant F18.151
        opioid F11.151
        sedative, anxiolytic or hypnotic F13.151
        stimulant NEC F15.151
      dependence F19.251
        cannabis F12.251
        cocaine F14.251
        hallucinogen F16.251
        inhalant F18.251
        opioid F11.251
        sedative, anxiolytic or hypnotic F13.251
        stimulant NEC F15.251
    inhalant F18.951
    opioid F11.951
    sedative, anxiolytic or hypnotic F13.951
    stimulant NEC F15.951
  organic F06.0
Hallux
  deformity (acquired) NEC M20.5X- ☑
  limitus M20.5X- ☑
  malleus (acquired) NEC M20.3- ☑
  rigidus (acquired) M20.2- ☑
    congenital Q74.2
    sequelae (late effect) of rickets E64.3
  valgus (acquired) M20.1- ☑
    congenital Q66.6
  varus (acquired) M20.3- ☑
    congenital Q66.3
Halo, visual H53.19
Hamartoma, hamartoblastoma Q85.9
  epithelial (gingival), odontogenic, central or peripheral
    — *see* Cyst, calcifying odontogenic
Hamartosis Q85.9
Hamman-Rich syndrome J84.114
Hammer toe (acquired) NEC (*see also* Deformity, toe,
  hammer toe)
  congenital Q66.89
  sequelae (late effect) of rickets E64.3
Hand — *see* condition
Hand-foot syndrome L27.1
Handicap, handicapped
  educational Z55.9
    specified NEC Z55.8
Hand-Schüller-Christian disease or syndrome C96.5
Hanging (asphyxia) (strangulation) (suffocation) — *see*
  Asphyxia, traumatic, due to mechanical threat
Hangnail (*see also* Cellulitis, digit)
  with lymphangitis — *see* Lymphangitis, acute, digit
Hangover (alcohol) F10.129

Hanhart's syndrome Q87.0
Hanot-Chauffard (-Troisier) **syndrome** E83.19
Hanot's cirrhosis or disease K74.3
Hansen's disease — *see* Leprosy
Hantaan virus disease (Korean hemorrhagic fever) A98.5
Hantavirus disease (with renal manifestations) (Dobra-
  va) (Puumala) (Seoul) A98.5
  with pulmonary manifestations (Andes) (Bayou)
    (Bermejo) (Black Creek Canal) (Choclo) (Juquiti-
    ba) (Laguna negra) (Lechiguanas) (New York)
    (Oran) (Sin nombre) B33.4
Happy puppet syndrome Q93.5
Harada's disease or syndrome H30.81- ☑
Hardening
  artery — *see* Arteriosclerosis
  brain G93.89
Harelip (complete) (incomplete) — *see* Cleft, lip
Harlequin (newborn) Q80.4
Harley's disease D59.6
Harmful use (of)
  alcohol F10.10
  anxiolytics — *see* Abuse, drug, sedative
  cannabinoids — *see* Abuse, drug, cannabis
  cocaine — *see* Abuse, drug, cocaine
  drug — *see* Abuse, drug
  hallucinogens — *see* Abuse, drug, hallucinogen
  hypnotics — *see* Abuse, drug, sedative
  opioids — *see* Abuse, drug, opioid
  PCP (phencyclidine) — *see* Abuse, drug, hallucinogen
  sedatives — *see* Abuse, drug, sedative
  stimulants NEC — *see* Abuse, drug, stimulant
Harris' lines — *see* Arrest, epiphyseal
Hartnup's disease E72.02
Harvester's lung J67.0
Harvesting ovum for in vitro fertilization Z31.83
Hashimoto's disease or thyroiditis E06.3
Hashitoxicosis (transient) E06.3
Hassal-Henle bodies or warts (cornea) H18.49
Haut mal — *see* Epilepsy, generalized, specified NEC
Haverhill fever A25.1
Hay fever (*see also* Fever, hay) J30.1
Hayem-Widal syndrome D59.8
Haygarth's nodes M15.8
Haymaker's lung J67.0
Hb (abnormal)
  Bart's disease D56.0
  disease — *see* Disease, hemoglobin
  trait — *see* Trait
Head — *see* condition
Headache R51
  allergic NEC G44.89
  associated with sexual activity G44.82
  chronic daily R51
  cluster G44.009
    chronic G44.029
      intractable G44.021
      not intractable G44.029
    episodic G44.019
      intractable G44.011
      not intractable G44.019
    intractable G44.001
    not intractable G44.009
  cough (primary) G44.83
  daily chronic R51
  drug-induced NEC G44.40
    intractable G44.41
    not intractable G44.40
  exertional (primary) G44.84
  histamine G44.009
    intractable G44.001
    not intractable G44.009
  hypnic G44.81
  lumbar puncture G97.1
  medication overuse G44.40
    intractable G44.41
    not intractable G44.40
  menstrual — *see* Migraine, menstrual
  migraine (type) (*see also* Migraine) G43.909
  nasal septum R51
  neuralgiform, short lasting unilateral, with conjunctival
    injection and tearing (SUNCT) G44.059
    intractable G44.051
    not intractable G44.059
  new daily persistent (NDPH) G44.52
  orgasmic G44.82
  periodic syndromes in adults and children G43.C0
    (*following* G43.7)

☑ Additional Character Required — Refer to the Tabular List for Character Selection   Subterms under main terms may continue to next column or page

Headache — *continued*
  periodic syndromes in adults and children — *continued*
    with refractory migraine G43.C1 (*following* G43.7)
    without refractory migraine G43.C0 (*following* G43.7)
    intractable G43.C1 (*following* G43.7)
    not intractable G43.C0 (*following* G43.7)
  postspinal puncture G97.1
  post-traumatic G44.309
    acute G44.319
      intractable G44.311
      not intractable G44.319
    chronic G44.329
      intractable G44.321
      not intractable G44.329
    intractable G44.301
    not intractable G44.309
  pre-menstrual — *see* Migraine, menstrual
  preorgasmic G44.82
  primary
    cough G44.83
    exertional G44.84
    stabbing G44.85
    thunderclap G44.53
  rebound G44.40
    intractable G44.41
    not intractable G44.40
  short lasting unilateral neuralgiform, with conjunctival injection and tearing (SUNCT) G44.059
    intractable G44.051
    not intractable G44.059
  specified syndrome NEC G44.89
  spinal and epidural anesthesia - induced T88.59 ☑
    in labor and delivery O74.5
    in pregnancy O29.4- ☑
    postpartum, puerperal O89.4
  spinal fluid loss (from puncture) G97.1
  stabbing (primary) G44.85
  tension (-type) G44.209
    chronic G44.229
      intractable G44.221
      not intractable G44.229
    episodic G44.219
      intractable G44.211
      not intractable G44.219
    intractable G44.201
    not intractable G44.209
  thunderclap (primary) G44.53
  vascular NEC G44.1
Healthy
  infant
    accompanying sick mother Z76.3
    receiving care Z76.2
  person accompanying sick person Z76.3
Hearing examination Z01.10
  with abnormal findings NEC Z01.118
  following failed hearing screening Z01.110
  for hearing conservation and treatment Z01.12
Heart — *see* condition
Heart beat
  abnormality R00.9
    specified NEC R00.8
  awareness R00.2
  rapid R00.0
  slow R00.1
Heartburn R12
  psychogenic F45.8
Heartland virus disease A93.8
Heat (effects) T67.9 ☑
  apoplexy T67.0 ☑
  burn (*see also* Burn) L55.9
  collapse T67.1 ☑
  cramps T67.2 ☑
  dermatitis or eczema L59.0
  edema T67.7 ☑
  erythema — *code by site under* Burn, first degree
  excessive T67.9 ☑
    specified effect NEC T67.8 ☑
  exhaustion T67.5 ☑
    anhydrotic T67.3 ☑
    due to
      salt (and water) depletion T67.4 ☑
      water depletion T67.3 ☑
        with salt depletion T67.4 ☑
  fatigue (transient) T67.6 ☑
  fever T67.0 ☑
  hyperpyrexia T67.0 ☑

Heat — *continued*
  prickly L74.0
  prostration — *see* Heat, exhaustion
  pyrexia T67.0 ☑
  rash L74.0
  specified effect NEC T67.8 ☑
  stroke T67.0 ☑
  sunburn — *see* Sunburn
  syncope T67.1 ☑
Heavy-for-dates NEC (infant) (4000g to 4499g) P08.1
  exceptionally (4500g or more) P08.0
Hebephrenia, hebephrenic (schizophrenia) F20.1
Heberden's disease or nodes (with arthropathy) M15.1
Hebra's
  pityriasis L26
  prurigo L28.2
Heel — *see* condition
Heerfordt's disease D86.89
Hegglin's anomaly or syndrome D72.0
Heilmeyer-Schoner disease D45
Heine-Medin disease A80.9
Heinz body anemia, congenital D58.2
Heliophobia F40.228
Heller's disease or syndrome F84.3
HELLP syndrome (hemolysis, elevated liver enzymes and low platelet count) O14.2- ☑
  complicating
    childbirth O14.24
    puerperium O14.25
Helminthiasis (*see also* Infestation, helminth)
  Ancylostoma B76.0
  intestinal B82.0
    mixed types (types classifiable to more than one of the titles B65.0-B81.3 and B81.8) B81.4
    specified type NEC B81.8
  mixed types (intestinal) (types classifiable to more than one of the titles B65.0-B81.3 and B81.8) B81.4
  Necator (americanus) B76.1
  specified type NEC B83.8
Heloma L84
Hemangioblastoma — *see* Neoplasm, connective tissue, uncertain behavior
  malignant — *see* Neoplasm, connective tissue, malignant
Hemangioendothelioma (*see also* Neoplasm, uncertain behavior, by site)
  benign D18.00
    intra-abdominal D18.03
    intracranial D18.02
    skin D18.01
    specified site NEC D18.09
  bone (diffuse) — *see* Neoplasm, bone, malignant
  epithelioid (*see also* Neoplasm, uncertain behavior, by site)
    malignant — *see* Neoplasm, malignant, by site
  malignant — *see* Neoplasm, connective tissue, malignant
Hemangiofibroma — *see* Neoplasm, benign, by site
Hemangiolipoma — *see* Lipoma
Hemangioma D18.00
  arteriovenous D18.00
    intra-abdominal D18.03
    intracranial D18.02
    skin D18.01
    specified site NEC D18.09
  capillary D18.00
    intra-abdominal D18.03
    intracranial D18.02
    skin D18.01
    specified site NEC D18.09
  cavernous D18.00
    intra-abdominal D18.03
    intracranial D18.02
    skin D18.01
    specified site NEC D18.09
  epithelioid D18.00
    intra-abdominal D18.03
    intracranial D18.02
    skin D18.01
    specified site NEC D18.09
  histiocytoid D18.00
    intra-abdominal D18.03
    intracranial D18.02
    skin D18.01
    specified site NEC D18.09
  infantile D18.00
    intra-abdominal D18.03

Hemangioma — *continued*
  infantile — *continued*
    intracranial D18.02
    skin D18.01
    specified site NEC D18.09
  intra-abdominal D18.03
  intracranial D18.02
  intramuscular D18.00
    intra-abdominal D18.03
    intracranial D18.02
    skin D18.01
    specified site NEC D18.09
  intrathoracic structures D18.09
  juvenile D18.00
  malignant — *see* Neoplasm, connective tissue, malignant
  plexiform D18.00
    intra-abdominal D18.03
    intracranial D18.02
    skin D18.01
    specified site NEC D18.09
  racemose D18.00
    intra-abdominal D18.03
    intracranial D18.02
    skin D18.01
    specified site NEC D18.09
  sclerosing — *see* Neoplasm, skin, benign
  simplex D18.00
    intra-abdominal D18.03
    intracranial D18.02
    skin D18.01
    specified site NEC D18.09
  skin D18.01
  specified site NEC D18.09
  venous D18.00
    intra-abdominal D18.03
    intracranial D18.02
    skin D18.01
    specified site NEC D18.09
  verrucous keratotic D18.00
    intra-abdominal D18.03
    intracranial D18.02
    skin D18.01
    specified site NEC D18.09
Hemangiomatosis (systemic) I78.8
  involving single site — *see* Hemangioma
Hemangiopericytoma (*see also* Neoplasm, connective tissue, uncertain behavior)
  benign — *see* Neoplasm, connective tissue, benign
  malignant — *see* Neoplasm, connective tissue, malignant
Hemangiosarcoma — *see* Neoplasm, connective tissue, malignant
Hemarthrosis (nontraumatic) M25.00
  ankle M25.07- ☑
  elbow M25.02- ☑
  foot joint M25.07- ☑
  hand joint M25.04- ☑
  hip M25.05- ☑
  in hemophilic arthropathy — *see* Arthropathy, hemophilic
  knee M25.06- ☑
  shoulder M25.01- ☑
  specified joint NEC M25.08
  traumatic — *see* Sprain, by site
  vertebrae M25.08
  wrist M25.03- ☑
Hematemesis K92.0
  with ulcer — *code by site under* Ulcer, with hemorrhage K27.4
  newborn, neonatal P54.0
    due to swallowed maternal blood P78.2
Hematidrosis L74.8
Hematinuria (*see also* Hemoglobinuria)
  malarial B50.8
Hematobilia K83.8
Hematocele
  female NEC N94.89
    with ectopic pregnancy O00.90
      with intrauterine pregnancy O00.91
    ovary N83.8
  male N50.1
Hematochezia (*see also* Melena) K92.1
Hematochyluria (*see also* Infestation, filarial)
  schistosomiasis (bilharziasis) B65.0
Hematocolpos (with hematometra or hematosalpinx) N89.7
Hematocornea — *see* Pigmentation, cornea, stromal

▽ Subterms under main terms may continue to next column or page   ☑ Additional Character Required — Refer to the Tabular List for Character Selection   **163**

Headache — Hematocornea

Hematogenous — *see* condition
Hematoma (traumatic) (skin surface intact) (*see also* Contusion)
  with
    injury of internal organs — *see* Injury, by site
    open wound — *see* Wound, open
  amputation stump (surgical) (late) T87.89
  aorta, dissecting I71.00
    abdominal I71.02
    thoracic I71.01
    thoracoabdominal I71.03
  aortic intramural — *see* Dissection, aorta
  arterial (complicating trauma) — *see* Injury, blood vessel, by site
  auricle — *see* Contusion, ear
    nontraumatic — *see* Disorder, pinna, hematoma
  birth injury NEC P15.8
  brain (traumatic)
    with
      cerebral laceration or contusion (diffuse) — *see* Injury, intracranial, diffuse
        focal — *see* Injury, intracranial, focal
    cerebellar, traumatic S06.37- ☑
    intracerebral, traumatic — *see* Injury, intracranial, intracerebral hemorrhage
    newborn NEC P52.4
      birth injury P10.1
    nontraumatic — *see* Hemorrhage, intracranial
    subarachnoid, arachnoid, traumatic — *see* Injury, intracranial, subarachnoid hemorrhage
    subdural, traumatic — *see* Injury, intracranial, subdural hemorrhage
  breast (nontraumatic) N64.89
  broad ligament (nontraumatic) N83.7
    traumatic S37.892 ☑
  cerebellar, traumatic S06.37- ☑
  cerebral — *see* Hematoma, brain
  cerebrum S06.36- ☑
    left S06.35- ☑
    right S06.34- ☑
  cesarean delivery wound O90.2
  complicating delivery (perineal) (pelvic) (vagina) (vulva) O71.7
  corpus cavernosum (nontraumatic) N48.89
  epididymis (nontraumatic) N50.1
  epidural (traumatic) — *see* Injury, intracranial, epidural hemorrhage
    spinal — *see* Injury, spinal cord, by region
  episiotomy O90.2
  face, birth injury P15.4
  genital organ NEC (nontraumatic)
    female (nonobstetric) N94.89
      traumatic S30.202 ☑
    male N50.1
      traumatic S30.201 ☑
  internal organs — *see* Injury, by site
  intracerebral, traumatic — *see* Injury, intracranial, intracerebral hemorrhage
  intraoperative — *see* Complications, intraoperative, hemorrhage
  labia (nontraumatic) (nonobstetric) N90.89
  liver (subcapsular) (nontraumatic) K76.89
    birth injury P15.0
  mediastinum — *see* Injury, intrathoracic
  mesosalpinx (nontraumatic) N83.7
    traumatic S37.898 ☑
  muscle — code by site under Contusion
  nontraumatic
    muscle M79.81
    soft tissue M79.81
  obstetrical surgical wound O90.2
  orbit, orbital (nontraumatic) (*see also* Hemorrhage, orbit)
    traumatic — *see* Contusion, orbit
  pelvis (female) (nontraumatic) (nonobstetric) N94.89
    obstetric O71.7
    traumatic — *see* Injury, by site
  penis (nontraumatic) N48.89
    birth injury P15.5
  perianal (nontraumatic) K64.5
  perineal S30.23 ☑
    complicating delivery O71.7
  perirenal — *see* Injury, kidney
  pinna — *see* Contusion, ear
    nontraumatic — *see* Disorder, pinna, hematoma
  placenta O43.89- ☑

Hematoma — *continued*
  postoperative (postprocedural) — *see* Complication, postprocedural, hematoma
  retroperitoneal (nontraumatic) K66.1
    traumatic S36.892 ☑
  scrotum, superficial S30.22 ☑
    birth injury P15.5
  seminal vesicle (nontraumatic) N50.1
    traumatic S37.892 ☑
  spermatic cord (traumatic) S37.892 ☑
    nontraumatic N50.1
  spinal (cord) (meninges) (*see also* Injury, spinal cord, by region)
    newborn (birth injury) P11.5
  spleen D73.5
    intraoperative — *see* Complications, intraoperative, hemorrhage, spleen
    postprocedural (postoperative) — *see* Complications, postprocedural, hemorrhage, spleen
  sternocleidomastoid, birth injury P15.2
  sternomastoid, birth injury P15.2
  subarachnoid (traumatic) — *see* Injury, intracranial, subarachnoid hemorrhage
    newborn (nontraumatic) P52.5
      due to birth injury P10.3
    nontraumatic — *see* Hemorrhage, intracranial, subarachnoid
  subdural (traumatic) — *see* Injury, intracranial, subdural hemorrhage
    newborn (localized) P52.8
      birth injury P10.0
    nontraumatic — *see* Hemorrhage, intracranial, subdural
  superficial, newborn P54.5
  testis (nontraumatic) N50.1
    birth injury P15.5
  tunica vaginalis (nontraumatic) N50.1
  umbilical cord, complicating delivery O69.5 ☑
  uterine ligament (broad) (nontraumatic) N83.7
    traumatic S37.892 ☑
  vagina (ruptured) (nontraumatic) N89.8
    complicating delivery O71.7
  vas deferens (nontraumatic) N50.1
    traumatic S37.892 ☑
  vitreous — *see* Hemorrhage, vitreous
  vulva (nontraumatic) (nonobstetric) N90.89
    complicating delivery O71.7
    newborn (birth injury) P15.5
Hematometra N85.7
  with hematocolpos N89.7
Hematomyelia (central) G95.19
  newborn (birth injury) P11.5
  traumatic T14.8 ☑
Hematomyelitis G04.90
Hematoperitoneum — *see* Hemoperitoneum
Hematophobia F40.230
Hematopneumothorax (see Hemothorax)
Hematopoiesis, cyclic D70.4
Hematoporphyria — *see* Porphyria
Hematorachis, hematorrhachis G95.19
  newborn (birth injury) P11.5
Hematosalpinx N83.6
  with
    hematocolpos N89.7
    hematometra N85.7
      with hematocolpos N89.7
  infectional — *see* Salpingitis
Hematospermia R36.1
Hematothorax (see Hemothorax)
Hematuria R31.9
  benign (familial) (of childhood) (*see also* Hematuria, idiopathic)
    essential microscopic R31.1
  due to sulphonamide, sulfonamide — *see* Table of Drugs and Chemicals, by drug
  endemic (*see also* Schistosomiasis) B65.0
  gross R31.0
  idiopathic N02.9
    with glomerular lesion
      crescentic (diffuse) glomerulonephritis N02.7
      dense deposit disease N02.6
      endocapillary proliferative glomerulonephritis N02.4
      focal and segmental hyalinosis or sclerosis N02.1
      membranoproliferative (diffuse) N02.5
      membranous (diffuse) N02.2
      mesangial proliferative (diffuse) N02.3

Hematuria — *continued*
  idiopathic — *continued*
    with glomerular lesion — *continued*
      mesangiocapillary (diffuse) N02.5
      minor abnormality N02.0
      proliferative NEC N02.8
      specified pathology NEC N02.8
  intermittent — *see* Hematuria, idiopathic
  malarial B50.8
  microscopic NEC (with symptoms) R31.29
    asymptomatic R31.21
    benign essential R31.1
  paroxysmal (*see also* Hematuria, idiopathic)
    nocturnal D59.5
  persistent — *see* Hematuria, idiopathic
  recurrent — *see* Hematuria, idiopathic
  tropical (*see also* Schistosomiasis) B65.0
  tuberculous A18.13
Hemeralopia (day blindness) H53.11
  vitamin A deficiency E50.5
Hemi-akinesia R41.4
Hemianalgesia R20.0
Hemianencephaly Q00.0
Hemianesthesia R20.0
Hemianopia, hemianopsia (heteronymous) H53.47
  homonymous H53.46- ☑
  syphilitic A52.71
Hemiathetosis R25.8
Hemiatrophy R68.89
  cerebellar G31.9
  face, facial, progressive (Romberg) G51.8
  tongue K14.8
Hemiballism (us) G25.5
Hemicardia Q24.8
Hemicephalus, hemicephaly Q00.0
Hemichorea G25.5
Hemicolitis, left — *see* Colitis, left sided
Hemicrania
  congenital malformation Q00.0
  continua G44.51
  meaning migraine (*see also* Migraine) G43.909
  paroxysmal G44.039
    chronic G44.049
      intractable G44.041
      not intractable G44.049
    episodic G44.039
      intractable G44.031
      not intractable G44.039
    intractable G44.031
    not intractable G44.039
Hemidystrophy — *see* Hemiatrophy
Hemiectromelia Q73.8
Hemihypalgesia R20.8
Hemihypesthesia R20.1
Hemi-inattention R41.4
Hemimelia Q73.8
  lower limb — *see* Defect, reduction, lower limb, specified type NEC
  upper limb — *see* Defect, reduction, upper limb, specified type NEC
Hemiparalysis — *see* Hemiplegia
Hemiparesis — *see* Hemiplegia
Hemiparesthesia R20.2
Hemiparkinsonism G20
Hemiplegia G81.9- ☑
  alternans facialis G83.89
  ascending NEC G81.90
    spinal G95.89
  congenital (cerebral) G80.8
    spastic G80.2
  embolic (current episode) I63.4- ☑
  flaccid G81.0- ☑
  following
    cerebrovascular disease I69.959
      cerebral infarction I69.35- ☑
      intracerebral hemorrhage I69.15- ☑
      nontraumatic intracranial hemorrhage NEC I69.25- ☑
      specified disease NEC I69.85- ☑
      stroke NOS I69.35- ☑
      subarachnoid hemorrhage I69.05- ☑
  hysterical F44.4
  newborn NEC P91.88
    birth injury P11.9
  spastic G81.1- ☑
    congenital G80.2
  thrombotic (current episode) I63.3- ☑

☑ **Additional Character Required** — **Refer to the Tabular List for Character Selection**   ▽ Subterms under main terms may continue to next column or page

Hemisection, spinal cord — *see* Injury, spinal cord, by region
Hemispasm (facial) R25.2
Hemisporosis B48.8
Hemitremor R25.1
Hemivertebra Q76.49
  failure of segmentation with scoliosis Q76.3
  fusion with scoliosis Q76.3
Hemochromatosis E83.119
  with refractory anemia D46.1
  due to repeated red blood cell transfusion E83.111
  hereditary (primary) E83.110
  neonatal P78.84
  primary E83.110
  specified NEC E83.118
Hemoglobin (*see also* condition)
  abnormal (disease) — *see* Disease, hemoglobin
  AS genotype D57.3
  Constant Spring D58.2
  E-beta thalassemia D56.5
  fetal, hereditary persistence (HPFH) D56.4
  H Constant Spring D56.0
  low NOS D64.9
  S (Hb S), heterozygous D57.3
Hemoglobinemia D59.9
  due to blood transfusion T80.89 ☑
  paroxysmal D59.6
   nocturnal D59.5
Hemoglobinopathy (mixed) D58.2
  with thalassemia D56.8
  sickle-cell D57.1
   with thalassemia D57.40
    with crisis (vasoocclusive pain) D57.419
     with
      acute chest syndrome D57.411
      splenic sequestration D57.412
    without crisis D57.40
Hemoglobinuria R82.3
  with anemia, hemolytic, acquired (chronic) NEC D59.6
  cold (agglutinin) (paroxysmal) (with Raynaud's syndrome) D59.6
  due to exertion or hemolysis NEC D59.6
  intermittent D59.6
  malarial B50.8
  march D59.6
  nocturnal (paroxysmal) D59.5
  paroxysmal (cold) D59.6
   nocturnal D59.5
Hemolymphangioma D18.1
Hemolysis
  intravascular
   with
    abortion — *see* Abortion, by type, complicated by, hemorrhage
    ectopic or molar pregnancy O08.1
    hemorrhage
     antepartum — *see* Hemorrhage, antepartum, with coagulation defect
     intrapartum (*see also* Hemorrhage, complicating, delivery) O67.0
    postpartum O72.3
  neonatal (excessive) P58.9
   specified NEC P58.8
Hemolytic — *see* condition
Hemopericardium I31.2
  following acute myocardial infarction (current complication) I23.0
  newborn P54.8
  traumatic — *see* Injury, heart, with hemopericardium
Hemoperitoneum K66.1
  infectional K65.9
  traumatic S36.899 ☑
   with open wound — *see* Wound, open, with penetration into peritoneal cavity
Hemophilia (classical) (familial) (hereditary) D66
  A D66
  acquired D68.311
  autoimmune D68.311
  B D67
  C D68.1
  calcipriva (*see also* Defect, coagulation) D68.4
  nonfamilial (*see also* Defect, coagulation) D68.4
  secondary D68.311
  vascular D68.0
Hemophthalmos H44.81- ☑
Hemopneumothorax (*see also* Hemothorax)
  traumatic S27.2 ☑
Hemoptysis R04.2

Hemoptysis — *continued*
  newborn P26.9
  tuberculous — *see* Tuberculosis, pulmonary
Hemorrhage, hemorrhagic (concealed) R58
  abdomen R58
  accidental antepartum — *see* Hemorrhage, antepartum
  acute idiopathic pulmonary, in infants R04.81
  adenoid J35.8
  adrenal (capsule) (gland) E27.49
   medulla E27.8
   newborn P54.4
  after delivery — *see* Hemorrhage, postpartum
  alveolar
   lung, newborn P26.8
   process K08.89
  alveolus K08.89
  amputation stump (surgical) T87.89
  anemia (chronic) D50.0
   acute D62
  antepartum (with) O46.90
   with coagulation defect O46.00- ☑
    afibrinogenemia O46.01- ☑
    disseminated intravascular coagulation O46.02- ☑
    hypofibrinogenemia O46.01- ☑
    specified defect NEC O46.09- ☑
   before 20 weeks gestation O20.9
    specified type NEC O20.8
    threatened abortion O20.0
   due to
    abruptio placenta (*see also* Abruptio placentae) O45.9- ☑
    leiomyoma, uterus — *see* Hemorrhage, antepartum, specified cause NEC
    placenta previa O44.1- ☑
   specified cause NEC — *see* subcategory O46.8X- ☑
  anus (sphincter) K62.5
  apoplexy (stroke) — *see* Hemorrhage, intracranial, intracerebral
  arachnoid — *see* Hemorrhage, intracranial, subarachnoid
  artery R58
   brain — *see* Hemorrhage, intracranial, intracerebral
  basilar (ganglion) I61.0
  bladder N32.89
  bowel K92.2
   newborn P54.3
  brain (miliary) (nontraumatic) — *see* Hemorrhage, intracranial, intracerebral
   due to
    birth injury P10.1
    syphilis A52.05
   epidural or extradural (traumatic) — *see* Injury, intracranial, epidural hemorrhage
   newborn P52.4
    birth injury P10.1
   subarachnoid — *see* Hemorrhage, intracranial, subarachnoid
   subdural — *see* Hemorrhage, intracranial, subdural
  brainstem (nontraumatic) I61.3
   traumatic S06.38- ☑
  breast N64.59
  bronchial tube — *see* Hemorrhage, lung
  bronchopulmonary — *see* Hemorrhage, lung
  bronchus — *see* Hemorrhage, lung
  bulbar I61.5
  capillary I78.8
   primary D69.8
  cecum K92.2
  cerebellar, cerebellum (nontraumatic) I61.4
   newborn P52.6
   traumatic S06.37- ☑
  cerebral, cerebrum (*see also* Hemorrhage, intracranial, intracerebral)
   lobe I61.1
   newborn (anoxic) P52.4
    birth injury P10.1
  cerebromeningeal I61.8
  cerebrospinal — *see* Hemorrhage, intracranial, intracerebral
  cervix (uteri) (stump) NEC N88.8
  chamber, anterior (eye) — *see* Hyphema
  childbirth — *see* Hemorrhage, complicating, delivery
  choroid H31.30- ☑
   expulsive H31.31- ☑
  ciliary body — *see* Hyphema
  cochlea — *see* subcategory H83.8 ☑

Hemorrhage, hemorrhagic — *continued*
  colon K92.2
  complicating
   abortion — *see* Abortion, by type, complicated by, hemorrhage
   delivery O67.9
    associated with coagulation defect (afibrinogenemia) (DIC) (hyperfibrinolysis) O67.0
    specified cause NEC O67.8
   surgical procedure — *see* Hemorrhage, intraoperative
  conjunctiva H11.3- ☑
   newborn P54.8
  cord, newborn (stump) P51.9
  corpus luteum (ruptured) cyst N83.1- ☑
  cortical (brain) I61.1
  cranial — *see* Hemorrhage, intracranial
  cutaneous R23.3
   due to autosensitivity, erythrocyte D69.2
   newborn P54.5
  delayed
   following ectopic or molar pregnancy O08.1
   postpartum O72.2
  diathesis (familial) D69.9
  disease D69.9
   newborn P53
   specified type NEC D69.8
  due to or associated with
   afibrinogenemia or other coagulation defect (conditions in categories D65- D69)
    antepartum — *see* Hemorrhage, antepartum, with coagulation defect
    intrapartum O67.0
   dental implant M27.61
   device, implant or graft (*see also* Complications, by site and type, specified NEC) T85.838 ☑
    arterial graft NEC T82.838 ☑
    breast T85.838 ☑
    catheter NEC T85.838 ☑
     dialysis (renal) T82.838 ☑
      intraperitoneal T85.838 ☑
     infusion NEC T82.838 ☑
      spinal (epidural) (subdural) T85.830 ☑
     urinary (indwelling) T83.83 ☑
    electronic (electrode) (pulse generator) (stimulator)
     bone T84.83 ☑
     cardiac T82.837 ☑
     nervous system (brain) (peripheral nerve) (spinal) T85.830 ☑
     urinary T83.83 ☑
    fixation, internal (orthopedic) NEC T84.83 ☑
    gastrointestinal (bile duct) (esophagus) T85.838 ☑
    genital NEC T83.83 ☑
    heart NEC T82.837 ☑
    joint prosthesis T84.83 ☑
    ocular (corneal graft) (orbital implant) NEC T85.838 ☑
    orthopedic NEC T84.83 ☑
     bone graft T86.838 ☑
    specified NEC T85.838 ☑
    urinary NEC T83.83 ☑
    vascular NEC T82.838 ☑
    ventricular intracranial shunt T85.830 ☑
  duodenum, duodenal K92.2
   ulcer — *see* Ulcer, duodenum, with hemorrhage
  dura mater — *see* Hemorrhage, intracranial, subdural
  endotracheal — *see* Hemorrhage, lung
  epicranial subaponeurotic (massive), birth injury P12.2
  epidural (traumatic) (*see also* Injury, intracranial, epidural hemorrhage)
   nontraumatic I62.1
  esophagus K22.8
   varix I85.01
    secondary I85.11
  excessive, following ectopic gestation (subsequent episode) O08.1
  extradural (traumatic) — *see* Injury, intracranial, epidural hemorrhage
   birth injury P10.8
   newborn (anoxic) (nontraumatic) P52.8
   nontraumatic I62.1
  eye NEC H57.8
   fundus — *see* Hemorrhage, retina
   lid — *see* Disorder, eyelid, specified type NEC
  fallopian tube N83.6

Hemorrhage, hemorrhagic — *continued*
- fibrinogenolysis — *see* Fibrinolysis
- fibrinolytic (acquired) — *see* Fibrinolysis
- from
  - ear (nontraumatic) — *see* Otorrhagia
  - tracheostomy stoma J95.01
- fundus, eye — *see* Hemorrhage, retina
- funis — *see* Hemorrhage, umbilicus, cord
- gastric — *see* Hemorrhage, stomach
- gastroenteric K92.2
  - newborn P54.3
- gastrointestinal (tract) K92.2
  - newborn P54.3
- genital organ, male N50.1
- genitourinary (tract) NOS R31.9
- gingiva K06.8
- globe (eye) — *see* Hemophthalmos
- graafian follicle cyst (ruptured) N83.0- ☑
- gum K06.8
- heart I51.89
- hypopharyngeal (throat) R04.1
- intermenstrual (regular) N92.3
  - irregular N92.1
- internal (organs) NEC R58
  - capsule I61.0
  - ear — *see* subcategory H83.8 ☑
  - newborn P54.8
- intestine K92.2
  - newborn P54.3
- intra-abdominal R58
- intra-alveolar (lung), newborn P26.8
- intracerebral (nontraumatic) — *see* Hemorrhage, intracranial, intracerebral
- intracranial (nontraumatic) I62.9
  - birth injury P10.9
  - epidural, nontraumatic I62.1
  - extradural, nontraumatic I62.1
  - intracerebral (nontraumatic) (in) I61.9
    - brain stem I61.3
    - cerebellum I61.4
    - hemisphere I61.2
      - cortical (superficial) I61.1
      - subcortical (deep) I61.0
    - intraoperative
      - during a nervous system procedure G97.31
      - during other procedure G97.32
    - intraventricular I61.5
    - multiple localized I61.6
    - newborn P52.4
      - birth injury P10.1
    - postprocedural
      - following a nervous system procedure G97.51
      - following other procedure G97.52
    - specified NEC I61.8
    - superficial I61.1
    - traumatic (diffuse) — *see* Injury, intracranial, diffuse
      - focal — *see* Injury, intracranial, focal
  - newborn P52.9
    - specified NEC P52.8
  - subarachnoid (nontraumatic) (from) I60.9
    - intracranial (cerebral) artery I60.7
      - anterior communicating I60.2
      - basilar I60.4
      - carotid siphon and bifurcation I60.0- ☑
      - communicating I60.7
        - anterior I60.2
        - posterior I60.3- ☑
      - middle cerebral I60.1- ☑
      - posterior communicating I60.3- ☑
      - specified artery NEC I60.6
      - vertebral I60.5- ☑
    - newborn P52.5
      - birth injury P10.3
    - specified NEC I60.8
    - traumatic S06.6X- ☑
  - subdural (nontraumatic) I62.00
    - acute I62.01
    - birth injury P10.0
    - chronic I62.03
    - newborn (anoxic) (hypoxic) P52.8
      - birth injury P10.0
    - spinal G95.19
    - subacute I62.02
    - traumatic — *see* Injury, intracranial, subdural hemorrhage

Hemorrhage, hemorrhagic — *continued*
- intracranial — *continued*
  - traumatic — *see* Injury, intracranial, focal brain injury
- intramedullary NEC G95.19
- intraocular — *see* Hemophthalmos
- intraoperative, intraprocedural — *see* Complication, hemorrhage (hematoma), intraoperative (intraprocedural), by site
- intrapartum — *see* Hemorrhage, complicating, delivery
- intrapelvic
  - female N94.89
  - male K66.1
- intraperitoneal K66.1
- intrapontine I61.3
- intraprocedural — *see* Complication, hemorrhage (hematoma), intraoperative (intraprocedural), by site
- intrauterine N85.7
  - complicating delivery (*see also* Hemorrhage, complicating, delivery) O67.9
  - postpartum — *see* Hemorrhage, postpartum
- intraventricular I61.5
  - newborn (nontraumatic) (*see also* Newborn, affected by, hemorrhage) P52.3
    - due to birth injury P10.2
    - grade
      - 1 P52.0
      - 2 P52.1
      - 3 P52.21
      - 4 P52.22
- intravesical N32.89
- iris (postinfectional) (postinflammatory) (toxic) — *see* Hyphema
- joint (nontraumatic) — *see* Hemarthrosis
- kidney N28.89
- knee (joint) (nontraumatic) — *see* Hemarthrosis, knee
- labyrinth — *see* subcategory H83.8 ☑
- lenticular striate artery I61.0
- ligature, vessel — *see* Hemorrhage, postoperative
- liver K76.89
- lung R04.89
  - newborn P26.9
    - massive P26.1
    - specified NEC P26.8
  - tuberculous — *see* Tuberculosis, pulmonary
- massive umbilical, newborn P51.0
- mediastinum — *see* Hemorrhage, lung
- medulla I61.3
- membrane (brain) I60.8
  - spinal cord — *see* Hemorrhage, spinal cord
- meninges, meningeal (brain) (middle) I60.8
  - spinal cord — *see* Hemorrhage, spinal cord
- mesentery K66.1
- metritis — *see* Endometritis
- mouth K13.79
- mucous membrane NEC R58
  - newborn P54.8
- muscle M62.89
- nail (subungual) L60.8
- nasal turbinate R04.0
  - newborn P54.8
- navel, newborn P51.9
- newborn P54.9
  - specified NEC P54.8
- nipple N64.59
- nose R04.0
  - newborn P54.8
- omentum K66.1
- optic nerve (sheath) H47.02- ☑
- orbit, orbital H05.23- ☑
- ovary NEC N83.8
- oviduct N83.6
- pancreas K86.89
- parathyroid (gland) (spontaneous) E21.4
- parturition — *see* Hemorrhage, complicating, delivery
- penis N48.89
- pericardium, pericarditis I31.2
- peritoneum, peritoneal K66.1
- peritonsillar tissue J35.8
  - due to infection J36
- petechial R23.3
  - due to autosensitivity, erythrocyte D69.2
- pituitary (gland) E23.6
- pleura — *see* Hemorrhage, lung
- polioencephalitis, superior E51.2
- polymyositis — *see* Polymyositis

Hemorrhage, hemorrhagic — *continued*
- pons, pontine I61.3
- posterior fossa (nontraumatic) I61.8
  - newborn P52.6
- postmenopausal N95.0
- postnasal R04.0
- postoperative — *see* Complications, postprocedural, hemorrhage, by site
- postpartum NEC (following delivery of placenta) O72.1
  - delayed or secondary O72.2
    - retained placenta O72.0
  - third stage O72.0
- pregnancy — *see* Hemorrhage, antepartum
- preretinal — *see* Hemorrhage, retina
- prostate N42.1
- puerperal — *see* Hemorrhage, postpartum
  - delayed or secondary O72.2
- pulmonary R04.89
  - newborn P26.9
    - massive P26.1
    - specified NEC P26.8
  - tuberculous — *see* Tuberculosis, pulmonary
- purpura (primary) D69.3
- rectum (sphincter) K62.5
  - newborn P54.2
- recurring, following initial hemorrhage at time of injury T79.2 ☑
- renal N28.89
- respiratory passage or tract R04.9
  - specified NEC R04.89
- retina, retinal (vessels) H35.6- ☑
  - diabetic — *see* Diabetes, retinal, hemorrhage
- retroperitoneal R58
- scalp R58
- scrotum N50.1
- secondary (nontraumatic) R58
  - following initial hemorrhage at time of injury T79.2 ☑
- seminal vesicle N50.1
- skin R23.3
  - newborn P54.5
- slipped umbilical ligature P51.8
- spermatic cord N50.1
- spinal (cord) G95.19
  - newborn (birth injury) P11.5
- spleen D73.5
  - intraoperative — *see* Complications, intraoperative, hemorrhage, spleen
  - postprocedural — *see* Complications, postprocedural, hemorrhage, spleen
- stomach K92.2
  - newborn P54.3
  - ulcer — *see* Ulcer, stomach, with hemorrhage
- subarachnoid (nontraumatic) — *see* Hemorrhage, intracranial, subarachnoid
- subconjunctival (*see also* Hemorrhage, conjunctiva)
  - birth injury P15.3
- subcortical (brain) I61.0
- subcutaneous R23.3
- subdiaphragmatic R58
- subdural (acute) (nontraumatic) — *see* Hemorrhage, intracranial, subdural
- subependymal
  - newborn P52.0
    - with intraventricular extension P52.1
      - and intracerebral extension P52.22
- subgaleal P12.2
- subhyaloid — *see* Hemorrhage, retina
- subperiosteal — *see* Disorder, bone, specified type NEC
- subretinal — *see* Hemorrhage, retina
- subtentorial — *see* Hemorrhage, intracranial, subdural
- subungual L60.8
- suprarenal (capsule) (gland) E27.49
  - newborn P54.4
- tentorium (traumatic) NEC — *see* Hemorrhage, brain
  - newborn (birth injury) P10.4
- testis N50.1
- third stage (postpartum) O72.0
- thorax — *see* Hemorrhage, lung
- throat R04.1
- thymus (gland) E32.8
- thyroid (cyst) (gland) E07.89
- tongue K14.8
- tonsil J35.8
- trachea — *see* Hemorrhage, lung
- tracheobronchial R04.89
  - newborn P26.0

Hemorrhage, hemorrhagic — *continued*
　traumatic — *code to* specific injury
　　cerebellar — *see* Hemorrhage, brain
　　intracranial — *see* Hemorrhage, brain
　　recurring or secondary (following initial hemor-
　　　rhage at time of injury) T79.2 ☑
　tuberculous NEC (*see also* Tuberculosis, pulmonary)
　　A15.0
　tunica vaginalis N50.1
　ulcer — *code by* site under Ulcer, with hemorrhage
　　K27.4
　umbilicus, umbilical
　　cord
　　　after birth, newborn P51.9
　　　complicating delivery O69.5 ☑
　　newborn P51.9
　　　massive P51.0
　　　slipped ligature P51.8
　　stump P51.9
　urethra (idiopathic) N36.8
　uterus, uterine (abnormal) N93.9
　　climacteric N92.4
　　complicating delivery — *see* Hemorrhage, compli-
　　　cating, delivery
　　dysfunctional or functional N93.8
　　intermenstrual (regular) N92.3
　　　irregular N92.1
　　postmenopausal N95.0
　　postpartum — *see* Hemorrhage, postpartum
　　preclimacteric or premenopausal N92.4
　　prepubertal N93.8
　　pubertal N92.2
　vagina (abnormal) N93.9
　　newborn P54.6
　vas deferens N50.1
　vasa previa O69.4 ☑
　ventricular I61.5
　vesical N32.89
　viscera NEC R58
　　newborn P54.8
　vitreous (humor) (intraocular) H43.1- ☑
　vulva N90.89
Hemorrhoids (bleeding) (without mention of degree)
　K64.9
　1st degree (grade/stage I) (without prolapse outside
　　of anal canal) K64.0
　2nd degree (grade/stage II) (that prolapse with
　　straining but retract spontaneously) K64.1
　3rd degree (grade/stage III) (that prolapse with
　　straining and require manual replacement back
　　inside anal canal) K64.2
　4th degree (grade/stage IV) (with prolapsed tissue that
　　cannot be manually replaced) K64.3
　complicating
　　pregnancy O22.4 ☑
　　puerperium O87.2
　external K64.4
　　with
　　　thrombosis K64.5
　internal (without mention of degree) K64.8
　　prolapsed K64.8
　skin tags
　　anus K64.4
　　residual K64.4
　specified NEC K64.8
　strangulated (*see also* Hemorrhoids, by degree) K64.8
　thrombosed (*see also* Hemorrhoids, by degree) K64.5
　ulcerated (*see also* Hemorrhoids, by degree) K64.8
Hemosalpinx N83.6
　with
　　hematocolpos N89.7
　　hematometra N85.7
　　　with hematocolpos N89.7
Hemosiderosis (dietary) E83.19
　pulmonary, idiopathic E83.1- [J84.03]
　transfusion T80.89 ☑
Hemothorax (bacterial) (nontuberculous) J94.2
　newborn P54.8
　traumatic S27.1 ☑
　　with pneumothorax S27.2 ☑
　tuberculous NEC A15.6
Henoch (-Schönlein) **disease or syndrome** (purpura)
　D69.0
Henpue, henpuye A66.6
Hepar lobatum (syphilitic) A52.74
Hepatalgia K76.89
Hepatitis K75.9
　acute B17.9

Hepatitis — *continued*
　acute — *continued*
　　with coma K72.01
　　with hepatic failure — *see* Failure, hepatic
　　alcoholic — *see* Hepatitis, alcoholic
　　infectious B17.9
　　non-viral K72.0 ☑
　　viral B17.9
　alcoholic (acute) (chronic) K70.10
　　with ascites K70.11
　amebic — *see* Abscess, liver, amebic
　anicteric, (viral) — *see* Hepatitis, viral
　antigen-associated (HAA) — *see* Hepatitis, B
　Australia-antigen (positive) — *see* Hepatitis, B
　autoimmune K75.4
　B B19.10
　　with hepatic coma B19.11
　　acute B16.9
　　　with
　　　　delta-agent (coinfection) (without hepatic
　　　　　coma) B16.1
　　　　　with hepatic coma B16.0
　　　　hepatic coma (without delta-agent coinfec-
　　　　　tion) B16.2
　　chronic B18.1
　　　with delta-agent B18.0
　bacterial NEC K75.89
　C (viral) B19.20
　　with hepatic coma B19.21
　　acute B17.10
　　　with hepatic coma B17.11
　　chronic B18.2
　catarrhal (acute) B15.9
　　with hepatic coma B15.0
　cholangiolitic K75.89
　cholestatic K75.89
　chronic K73.9
　　active NEC K73.2
　　lobular NEC K73.1
　　persistent NEC K73.0
　　specified NEC K73.8
　cytomegaloviral B25.1
　due to ethanol (acute) (chronic) — *see* Hepatitis, alco-
　　holic
　epidemic B15.9
　　with hepatic coma B15.0
　fulminant NEC (viral) — *see* Hepatitis, viral
　granulomatous NEC K75.3
　herpesviral B00.81
　history of
　　B Z86.19
　　C Z86.19
　homologous serum — *see* Hepatitis, viral, type B
　in (due to)
　　mumps B26.81
　　toxoplasmosis (acquired) B58.1
　　　congenital (active) P37.1 [K77]
　infectious, infective B15.9
　　acute (subacute) B17.9
　　chronic B18.9
　inoculation — *see* Hepatitis, viral, type B
　interstitial (chronic) K74.69
　lupoid NEC K75.4
　malignant NEC (with hepatic failure) K72.90
　　with coma K72.91
　neonatal (idiopathic) (toxic) P59.29
　neonatal giant cell P59.29
　newborn P59.29
　non-viral K72.0 ☑
　postimmunization — *see* Hepatitis, viral, type B
　post-transfusion — *see* Hepatitis, viral, type B
　reactive, nonspecific K75.2
　serum — *see* Hepatitis, viral, type B
　specified type NEC
　　with hepatic failure — *see* Failure, hepatic
　syphilitic (late) A52.74
　　congenital (early) A50.08 [K77]
　　　late A50.59 [K77]
　　secondary A51.45
　toxic (*see also* Disease, liver, toxic) K71.6
　tuberculous A18.83
　viral, virus B19.9
　　with hepatic coma B19.0
　　acute B17.9
　　chronic B18.9
　　　specified NEC B18.8
　　　type
　　　　B B18.1

Hepatitis — *continued*
　viral, virus — *continued*
　　chronic — *continued*
　　　type — *continued*
　　　　B — *continued*
　　　　　with delta-agent B18.0
　　　　C B18.2
　　congenital P35.3
　　coxsackie B33.8 [K77]
　　cytomegalic inclusion B25.1
　　in remission, any type — *code to* Hepatitis, chronic,
　　　by type
　　non-A, non-B B17.8
　　specified type NEC (with or without coma) B17.8
　　type
　　　A B15.9
　　　　with hepatic coma B15.0
　　　B B19.10
　　　　with hepatic coma B19.11
　　　　acute B16.9
　　　　　with
　　　　　　delta-agent (coinfection) (without
　　　　　　　hepatic coma) B16.1
　　　　　　　with hepatic coma B16.0
　　　　　　hepatic coma (without delta-agent
　　　　　　　coinfection) B16.2
　　　　chronic B18.1
　　　　　with delta-agent B18.0
　　　C B19.20
　　　　with hepatic coma B19.21
　　　　acute B17.10
　　　　　with hepatic coma B17.11
　　　　chronic B18.2
　　　E B17.2
　　　non-A, non-B B17.8
Hepatization lung (acute) — *see* Pneumonia, lobar
Hepatoblastoma C22.2
Hepatocarcinoma C22.0
Hepatocholangiocarcinoma C22.0
Hepatocholangioma, benign D13.4
Hepatocholangitis K75.89
Hepatolenticular degeneration E83.01
Hepatoma (malignant) C22.0
　benign D13.4
　embryonal C22.0
Hepatomegaly (*see also* Hypertrophy, liver)
　with splenomegaly R16.2
　congenital Q44.7
　in mononucleosis
　　gammaherpesviral B27.09
　　infectious specified NEC B27.89
Hepatoptosis K76.89
Hepatorenal syndrome following labor and delivery
　O90.4
Hepatosis K76.89
Hepatosplenomegaly R16.2
　hyperlipemic (Bürger-Grütz type) E78.3 [K77]
Hereditary — *see* condition
Heredodegeneration, macular — *see* Dystrophy, retina
Heredopathia atactica polyneuritiformis G60.1
Heredosyphilis — *see* Syphilis, congenital
Herlitz' syndrome Q81.1
Hermansky-Pudlak syndrome E70.331
Hermaphrodite, hermaphroditism (true) Q56.0
　46,XX with streak gonads Q99.1
　46,XX/46,XY Q99.0
　46,XY with streak gonads Q99.1
　chimera 46,XX/46,XY Q99.0
Hernia, hernial (acquired) (recurrent) K46.9
　with
　　gangrene — *see* Hernia, by site, with, gangrene
　　incarceration — *see* Hernia, by site, with, obstruc-
　　　tion
　　irreducible — *see* Hernia, by site, with, obstruction
　　obstruction — *see* Hernia, by site, with, obstruction
　　strangulation — *see* Hernia, by site, with, obstruc-
　　　tion
　abdomen, abdominal K46.9
　　with
　　　gangrene (and obstruction) K46.1
　　　obstruction K46.0
　　femoral — *see* Hernia, femoral
　　incisional — *see* Hernia, incisional
　　inguinal — *see* Hernia, inguinal
　　specified site NEC K45.8
　　　with
　　　　gangrene (and obstruction) K45.1
　　　　obstruction K45.0

Hernia, hernial — *continued*
  abdomen, abdominal — *continued*
    umbilical — *see* Hernia, umbilical
    wall — *see* Hernia, ventral
  appendix — *see* Hernia, abdomen
  bladder (mucosa) (sphincter)
    congenital (female) (male) Q79.51
    female — *see* Cystocele
    male N32.89
  brain, congenital — *see* Encephalocele
  cartilage, vertebra — *see* Displacement, intervertebral disc
  cerebral, congenital (*see also* Encephalocele)
    endaural Q01.8
  ciliary body (traumatic) S05.2- ☑
  colon — *see* Hernia, abdomen
  Cooper's — *see* Hernia, abdomen, specified site NEC
  crural — *see* Hernia, femoral
  diaphragm, diaphragmatic K44.9
    with
      gangrene (and obstruction) K44.1
      obstruction K44.0
    congenital Q79.0
  direct (inguinal) — *see* Hernia, inguinal
  diverticulum, intestine — *see* Hernia, abdomen
  double (inguinal) — *see* Hernia, inguinal, bilateral
  due to adhesions (with obstruction) K56.50
  epigastric (*see also* Hernia, ventral) K43.9
  esophageal hiatus — *see* Hernia, hiatal
  external (inguinal) — *see* Hernia, inguinal
  fallopian tube N83.4- ☑
  fascia M62.89
  femoral K41.90
    with
      gangrene (and obstruction) K41.40
        not specified as recurrent K41.40
        recurrent K41.41
      obstruction K41.30
        not specified as recurrent K41.30
        recurrent K41.31
    bilateral K41.20
      with
        gangrene (and obstruction) K41.10
          not specified as recurrent K41.10
          recurrent K41.11
        obstruction K41.00
          not specified as recurrent K41.00
          recurrent K41.01
      not specified as recurrent K41.20
      recurrent K41.21
    not specified as recurrent K41.90
    recurrent K41.91
    unilateral K41.90
      with
        gangrene (and obstruction) K41.40
          not specified as recurrent K41.40
          recurrent K41.41
        obstruction K41.30
          not specified as recurrent K41.30
          recurrent K41.31
      not specified as recurrent K41.90
      recurrent K41.91
  foramen magnum G93.5
    congenital Q01.8
  funicular (umbilical) (*see also* Hernia, umbilicus)
    spermatic (cord) — *see* Hernia, inguinal
  gastrointestinal tract — *see* Hernia, abdomen
  Hesselbach's — *see* Hernia, femoral, specified site NEC
  hiatal (esophageal) (sliding) K44.9
    with
      gangrene (and obstruction) K44.1
      obstruction K44.0
    congenital Q40.1
  hypogastric — *see* Hernia, ventral
  incarcerated (*see also* Hernia, by site, with obstruction)
    with gangrene — *see* Hernia, by site, with gangrene
  incisional K43.2
    with
      gangrene (and obstruction) K43.1
      obstruction K43.0
  indirect (inguinal) — *see* Hernia, inguinal
  inguinal (direct) (external) (funicular) (indirect) (internal) (oblique) (scrotal) (sliding) K40.90
    with
      gangrene (and obstruction) K40.40
        not specified as recurrent K40.40
        recurrent K40.41

Hernia, hernial — *continued*
  inguinal — *continued*
    with — *continued*
      obstruction K40.30
        not specified as recurrent K40.30
        recurrent K40.31
    bilateral K40.20
      with
        gangrene (and obstruction) K40.10
          not specified as recurrent K40.10
          recurrent K40.11
        obstruction K40.00
          not specified as recurrent K40.00
          recurrent K40.01
      not specified as recurrent K40.20
      recurrent K40.21
    not specified as recurrent K40.90
    recurrent K40.91
    unilateral K40.90
      with
        gangrene (and obstruction) K40.40
          not specified as recurrent K40.40
          recurrent K40.41
        obstruction K40.30
          not specified as recurrent K40.30
          recurrent K40.31
      not specified as recurrent K40.90
      recurrent K40.91
  internal (*see also* Hernia, abdomen)
    inguinal — *see* Hernia, inguinal
  interstitial — *see* Hernia, abdomen
  intervertebral cartilage or disc — *see* Displacement, intervertebral disc
  intestine, intestinal — *see* Hernia, by site
  intra-abdominal — *see* Hernia, abdomen
  iris (traumatic) S05.2- ☑
  irreducible (*see also* Hernia, by site, with obstruction)
    with gangrene — *see* Hernia, by site, with gangrene
  ischiatic — *see* Hernia, abdomen, specified site NEC
  ischiorectal — *see* Hernia, abdomen, specified site NEC
  lens (traumatic) S05.2- ☑
  linea (alba) (semilunaris) — *see* Hernia, ventral
  Littre's — *see* Hernia, abdomen
  lumbar — *see* Hernia, abdomen, specified site NEC
  lung (subcutaneous) J98.4
  mediastinum J98.59
  mesenteric (internal) — *see* Hernia, abdomen
  midline — *see* Hernia, ventral
  muscle (sheath) M62.89
  nucleus pulposus — *see* Displacement, intervertebral disc
  oblique (inguinal) — *see* Hernia, inguinal
  obstructive (*see also* Hernia, by site, with obstruction)
    with gangrene — *see* Hernia, by site, with gangrene
  obturator — *see* Hernia, abdomen, specified site NEC
  omental — *see* Hernia, abdomen
  ovary N83.4- ☑
  oviduct N83.4- ☑
  paraesophageal (*see also* Hernia, diaphragm)
    congenital Q40.1
  parastomal K43.5
    with
      gangrene (and obstruction) K43.4
      obstruction K43.3
  paraumbilical — *see* Hernia, umbilicus
  perineal — *see* Hernia, abdomen, specified site NEC
  Petit's — *see* Hernia, abdomen, specified site NEC
  postoperative — *see* Hernia, incisional
  pregnant uterus — *see* Abnormal, uterus in pregnancy or childbirth
  prevesical N32.89
  properitoneal — *see* Hernia, abdomen, specified site NEC
  pudendal — *see* Hernia, abdomen, specified site NEC
  rectovaginal N81.6
  retroperitoneal — *see* Hernia, abdomen, specified site NEC
  Richter's — *see* Hernia, abdomen, with obstruction
  Rieux's, Riex's — *see* Hernia, abdomen, specified site NEC
  sac condition (adhesion) (dropsy) (inflammation) (laceration) (suppuration) — *code by site under* Hernia
  sciatic — *see* Hernia, abdomen, specified site NEC

Hernia, hernial — *continued*
  scrotum, scrotal — *see* Hernia, inguinal
  sliding (inguinal) (*see also* Hernia, inguinal)
    hiatus — *see* Hernia, hiatal
  spigelian — *see* Hernia, ventral
  spinal — *see* Spina bifida
  strangulated (*see also* Hernia, by site, with obstruction)
    with gangrene — *see* Hernia, by site, with gangrene
  subxiphoid — *see* Hernia, ventral
  supra-umbilicus — *see* Hernia, ventral
  tendon — *see* Disorder, tendon, specified type NEC
  Treitz's (fossa) — *see* Hernia, abdomen, specified site NEC
  tunica vaginalis Q55.29
  umbilicus, umbilical K42.9
    with
      gangrene (and obstruction) K42.1
      obstruction K42.0
  ureter N28.89
  urethra, congenital Q64.79
  urinary meatus, congenital Q64.79
  uterus N81.4
    pregnant — *see* Abnormal, uterus in pregnancy or childbirth
  vaginal (anterior) (wall) — *see* Cystocele
  Velpeau's — *see* Hernia, femoral
  ventral K43.9
    with
      gangrene (and obstruction) K43.7
      obstruction K43.6
    incisional K43.2
      with
        gangrene (and obstruction) K43.1
        obstruction K43.0
      recurrent — *see* Hernia, incisional
    specified NEC K43.9
      with
        gangrene (and obstruction) K43.7
        obstruction K43.6
  vesical
    congenital (female) (male) Q79.51
    female — *see* Cystocele
    male N32.89
  vitreous (into wound) S05.2- ☑
    into anterior chamber — *see* Prolapse, vitreous
Herniation (*see also* Hernia)
  brain (stem) G93.5
  cerebral G93.5
  mediastinum J98.59
  nucleus pulposus — *see* Displacement, intervertebral disc
Herpangina B08.5
Herpes, herpesvirus, herpetic B00.9
  anogenital A60.9
    perianal skin A60.1
    rectum A60.1
    urogenital tract A60.00
      cervix A60.03
      male genital organ NEC A60.02
      penis A60.01
      specified site NEC A60.09
      vagina A60.04
      vulva A60.04
  blepharitis (zoster) B02.39
    simplex B00.59
  circinatus B35.4
    bullosus L12.0
  conjunctivitis (simplex) B00.53
    zoster B02.31
  cornea B02.33
  encephalitis B00.4
    due to herpesvirus 6 B10.01
    due to herpesvirus 7 B10.09
    specified NEC B10.09
  eye (zoster) B02.30
    simplex B00.50
  eyelid (zoster) B02.39
    simplex B00.59
  facialis B00.1
  febrilis B00.1
  geniculate ganglionitis B02.21
  genital, genitalis A60.00
    female A60.09
    male A60.02
  gestational, gestationis O26.4- ☑
  gingivostomatitis B00.2
  human B00.9

Herpes, herpesvirus, herpetic — *continued*
  human — *continued*
    1 — *see* Herpes, simplex
    2 — *see* Herpes, simplex
    3 — *see* Varicella
    4 — *see* Mononucleosis, Epstein-Barr (virus)
    5 — *see* Disease, cytomegalic inclusion (general-
        ized)
    6
        encephalitis B10.01
        specified NEC B10.81
    7
        encephalitis B10.09
        specified NEC B10.82
    8 B10.89
  infection NEC B10.89
    Kaposi's sarcoma associated B10.89
  iridocyclitis (simplex) B00.51
    zoster B02.32
  iris (vesicular erythema multiforme) L51.9
  iritis (simplex) B00.51
  Kaposi's sarcoma associated B10.89
  keratitis (simplex) (dendritic) (disciform) (interstitial)
      B00.52
    zoster (interstitial) B02.33
  keratoconjunctivitis (simplex) B00.52
    zoster B02.33
  labialis B00.1
  lip B00.1
  meningitis (simplex) B00.3
    zoster B02.1
  ophthalmicus (zoster) NEC B02.30
    simplex B00.50
  penis A60.01
  perianal skin A60.1
  pharyngitis, pharyngotonsillitis B00.2
  rectum A60.1
  scrotum A60.02
  sepsis B00.7
  simplex B00.9
    complicated NEC B00.89
    congenital P35.2
    conjunctivitis B00.53
    external ear B00.1
    eyelid B00.59
    hepatitis B00.81
    keratitis (interstitial) B00.52
    myleitis B00.82
    specified complication NEC B00.89
    visceral B00.89
  stomatitis B00.2
  tonsurans B35.0
  visceral B00.89
  vulva A60.04
  whitlow B00.89
  zoster (*see also* condition) B02.9
    auricularis B02.21
    complicated NEC B02.8
    conjunctivitis B02.31
    disseminated B02.7
    encephalitis B02.0
    eye (lid) B02.39
    geniculate ganglionitis B02.21
    keratitis (interstitial) B02.33
    meningitis B02.1
    myelitis B02.24
    neuritis, neuralgia B02.29
    ophthalmicus NEC B02.30
    oticus B02.21
    polyneuropathy B02.23
    specified complication NEC B02.8
    trigeminal neuralgia B02.22
Herpesvirus (human) — *see* Herpes
Herpetophobia F40.218
Herrick's anemia — *see* Disease, sickle-cell
Hers' disease E74.09
Herter-Gee syndrome K90.0
Herxheimer's reaction R68.89
Hesitancy
  of micturition R39.11
  urinary R39.11
Hesselbach's hernia — *see* Hernia, femoral, specified
    site NEC
Heterochromia (congenital) Q13.2
  cataract — *see* Cataract, complicated
  cyclitis (Fuchs) — *see* Cyclitis, Fuchs' heterochromic
  hair L67.1
  iritis — *see* Cyclitis, Fuchs' heterochromic

Heterochromia — *continued*
  retained metallic foreign body (nonmagnetic) — *see*
      Foreign body, intraocular, old, retained
    magnetic — *see* Foreign body, intraocular, old,
        retained, magnetic
  uveitis — *see* Cyclitis, Fuchs' heterochromic
Heterophoria — *see* Strabismus, heterophoria
Heterophyes, heterophyiasis (small intestine) B66.8
Heterotopia, heterotopic (*see also* Malposition, congen-
    ital)
  cerebralis Q04.8
Heterotropia — *see* Strabismus
Heubner-Herter disease K90.0
Hexadactylism Q69.9
HGSIL (cytology finding) (high grade squamous intraep-
    ithelial lesion on cytologic smear) (Pap smear find-
    ing)
  anus R85.613
  cervix R87.613
    biopsy (histology) finding — *see* Neoplasia, intraep-
        ithelial, cervix, grade II or grade III
  vagina R87.623
    biopsy (histology) finding — *see* Neoplasia, intraep-
        ithelial, cervix, grade II or grade III
Hibernoma — *see* Lipoma
Hiccup, hiccough R06.6
  epidemic B33.0
  psychogenic F45.8
Hidden penis (congenital) Q55.64
  acquired N48.83
Hidradenitis (axillaris) (suppurative) L73.2
Hidradenoma (nodular) (*see also* Neoplasm, skin, benign)
  clear cell — *see* Neoplasm, skin, benign
  papillary — *see* Neoplasm, skin, benign
Hidrocystoma — *see* Neoplasm, skin, benign
High
  altitude effects T70.20 ☑
    anoxia T70.29 ☑
    on
      ears T70.0 ☑
      sinuses T70.1 ☑
    polycythemia D75.1
  arch
    foot Q66.7
    palate, congenital Q38.5
  arterial tension — *see* Hypertension
  basal metabolic rate R94.8
  blood pressure (*see also* Hypertension)
    borderline R03.0
    reading (incidental) (isolated) (nonspecific), with-
        out diagnosis of hypertension R03.0
  cholesterol E78.00
    with high triglycerides E78.2
  diaphragm (congenital) Q79.1
  expressed emotional level within family Z63.8
  head at term O32.4 ☑
  palate, congenital Q38.5
  risk
    infant NEC Z76.2
    sexual behavior (heterosexual) Z72.51
      bisexual Z72.53
      homosexual Z72.52
  scrotal testis, testes
    bilateral Q53.23
    unilateral Q53.13
  temperature (of unknown origin) R50.9
  thoracic rib Q76.6
  triglycerides E78.1
    with high cholesterol E78.2
Hildenbrand's disease A75.0
Hilum — *see* condition
Hip — *see* condition
Hippel's disease Q85.8
Hippophobia F40.218
Hippus H57.09
Hirschsprung's disease or megacolon Q43.1
Hirsutism, hirsuties L68.0
Hirudiniasis
  external B88.3
  internal B83.4
Hiss-Russell dysentery A03.1
Histidinemia, histidinuria E70.41
Histiocytoma (*see also* Neoplasm, skin, benign)
  fibrous (*see also* Neoplasm, skin, benign)
    atypical — *see* Neoplasm, connective tissue, uncer-
        tain behavior

Histiocytoma — *continued*
  fibrous (*see also* Neoplasm, skin, benign) — *contin-
      ued*
    malignant — *see* Neoplasm, connective tissue,
        malignant
Histiocytosis D76.3
  acute differentiated progressive C96.0
  Langerhans' cell NEC C96.6
    multifocal X
      multisystemic (disseminated) C96.0
      unisystemic C96.5
    pulmonary, adult (adult PLCH) J84.82
    unifocal (X) C96.6
  lipid, lipoid D76.3
    essential E75.29
  malignant C96.A (*following* C96.6)
  mononuclear phagocytes NEC D76.1
    Langerhans' cells C96.6
  non-Langerhans cell D76.3
  polyostotic sclerosing D76.3
  sinus, with massive lymphadenopathy D76.3
  syndrome NEC D76.3
  X NEC C96.6
    acute (progressive) C96.0
    chronic C96.6
    multifocal C96.5
    multisystemic C96.0
    unifocal C96.6
Histoplasmosis B39.9
  with pneumonia NEC B39.2
  African B39.5
  American — *see* Histoplasmosis, capsulati
  capsulati B39.4
    disseminated B39.3
    generalized B39.3
    pulmonary B39.2
      acute B39.0
      chronic B39.1
  Darling's B39.4
  duboisii B39.5
  lung NEC B39.2
History
  family (of) (*see also* History, personal (of))
    alcohol abuse Z81.1
    allergy NEC Z84.89
    anemia Z83.2
    arthritis Z82.61
    asthma Z82.5
    blindness Z82.1
    cardiac death (sudden) Z82.41
    carrier of genetic disease Z84.81
    chromosomal anomaly Z82.79
    chronic
      disabling disease NEC Z82.8
      lower respiratory disease Z82.5
    colonic polyps Z83.71
    congenital malformations and deformations Z82.79
      polycystic kidney Z82.71
    consanguinity Z84.3
    deafness Z82.2
    diabetes mellitus Z83.3
    disability NEC Z82.8
    disease or disorder (of)
      allergic NEC Z84.89
      behavioral NEC Z81.8
      blood and blood-forming organs Z83.2
      cardiovascular NEC Z82.49
      chronic disabling NEC Z82.8
      digestive Z83.79
      ear NEC Z83.52
      endocrine NEC Z83.49
      eye NEC Z83.518
        glaucoma Z83.511
      familial hypercholesterolemia Z83.42
      genitourinary NEC Z84.2
      glaucoma Z83.511
      hematological Z83.2
      immune mechanism Z83.2
      infectious NEC Z83.1
      ischemic heart Z82.49
      kidney Z84.1
      mental NEC Z81.8
      metabolic Z83.49
      musculoskeletal NEC Z82.69
      neurological NEC Z82.0
      nutritional Z83.49
      parasitic NEC Z83.1
      psychiatric NEC Z81.8
      respiratory NEC Z83.6

History — continued
  family (*see also* History, personal) — *continued*
    disease or disorder — *continued*
      skin and subcutaneous tissue NEC Z84.0
      specified NEC Z84.89
    drug abuse NEC Z81.3
    epilepsy Z82.0
    familial hypercholesterolemia Z83.42
    genetic disease carrier Z84.81
    glaucoma Z83.511
    hearing loss Z82.2
    human immunodeficiency virus (HIV) infection Z83.0
    Huntington's chorea Z82.0
    intellectual disability Z81.0
    leukemia Z80.6
    malignant neoplasm (of) NOS Z80.9
      bladder Z80.52
      breast Z80.3
      bronchus Z80.1
      digestive organ Z80.0
      gastrointestinal tract Z80.0
      genital organ Z80.49
        ovary Z80.41
        prostate Z80.42
        specified organ NEC Z80.49
        testis Z80.43
      hematopoietic NEC Z80.7
      intrathoracic organ NEC Z80.2
      kidney Z80.51
      lung Z80.1
      lymphatic NEC Z80.7
      ovary Z80.41
      prostate Z80.42
      respiratory organ NEC Z80.2
      specified site NEC Z80.8
      testis Z80.43
      trachea Z80.1
      urinary organ or tract Z80.59
        bladder Z80.52
        kidney Z80.51
    mental
      disorder NEC Z81.8
    multiple endocrine neoplasia (MEN) syndrome Z83.41
    osteoporosis Z82.62
    polycystic kidney Z82.71
    polyps (colon) Z83.71
    psychiatric disorder Z81.8
    psychoactive substance abuse NEC Z81.3
    respiratory condition NEC Z83.6
      asthma and other lower respiratory conditions Z82.5
    self-harmful behavior Z81.8
    SIDS (sudden infant death syndrome) Z84.82
    skin condition Z84.0
    specified condition NEC Z84.89
    stroke (cerebrovascular) Z82.3
    substance abuse NEC Z81.4
      alcohol Z81.1
      drug NEC Z81.3
      psychoactive NEC Z81.3
      tobacco Z81.2
    sudden
      cardiac death Z82.41
      infant death syndrome (SIDS) Z84.82
    tobacco abuse Z81.2
    violence, violent behavior Z81.8
    visual loss Z82.1
  personal (of) (*see also* History, family (of))
    abuse
      adult Z91.419
        physical and sexual Z91.410
        psychological Z91.411
      childhood Z62.819
        physical Z62.810
        psychological Z62.811
        sexual Z62.810
    alcohol dependence F10.21
    allergy (to) Z88.9
      analgesic agent NEC Z88.6
      anesthetic Z88.4
      antibiotic agent NEC Z88.1
      anti-infective agent NEC Z88.3
      contrast media Z91.041
      drugs, medicaments and biological substances Z88.9
        specified NEC Z88.8
      food Z91.018

History — continued
  personal (*see also* History, family) — *continued*
    allergy — *continued*
      food — *continued*
        additives Z91.02
        eggs Z91.012
        milk products Z91.011
        peanuts Z91.010
        seafood Z91.013
        specified food NEC Z91.018
      insect Z91.038
        bee Z91.030
      latex Z91.040
      medicinal agents Z88.9
        specified NEC Z88.8
      narcotic agent NEC Z88.5
      nonmedicinal agents Z91.048
      penicillin Z88.0
      serum Z88.7
      specified NEC Z91.09
      sulfonamides Z88.2
      vaccine Z88.7
    anaphylactic shock Z87.892
    anaphylaxis Z87.892
    behavioral disorders Z86.59
    benign carcinoid tumor Z86.012
    benign neoplasm Z86.018
      brain Z86.011
      carcinoid Z86.012
      colonic polyps Z86.010
    brain injury (traumatic) Z87.820
    breast implant removal Z98.86
    calculi, renal Z87.442
    cancer — *see* History, personal (of), malignant neoplasm (of)
    cardiac arrest (death), successfully resuscitated Z86.74
    cerebral infarction without residual deficit Z86.73
    cervical dysplasia Z87.410
    chemotherapy for neoplastic condition Z92.21
    childhood abuse — *see* History, personal (of), abuse
    cleft lip (corrected) Z87.730
    cleft palate (corrected) Z87.730
    collapsed vertebra (healed) Z87.311
      due to osteoporosis Z87.310
    combat and operational stress reaction Z86.51
    congenital malformation (corrected) Z87.798
      circulatory system (corrected) Z87.74
      digestive system (corrected) NEC Z87.738
      ear (corrected) Z87.721
      eye (corrected) Z87.720
      face and neck (corrected) Z87.790
      genitourinary system (corrected) NEC Z87.718
      heart (corrected) Z87.74
      integument (corrected) Z87.76
      limb(s) (corrected) Z87.76
      musculoskeletal system (corrected) Z87.76
      neck (corrected) Z87.790
      nervous system (corrected) NEC Z87.728
      respiratory system (corrected) Z87.75
      sense organs (corrected) NEC Z87.728
      specified NEC Z87.798
    contraception Z92.0
    deployment (military) Z91.82
    diabetic foot ulcer Z86.31
    disease or disorder (of) Z87.898
      anaphylaxis Z87.892
      blood and blood-forming organs Z86.2
      circulatory system Z86.79
        specified condition NEC Z86.79
      connective tissue Z87.39
      digestive system Z87.19
        colonic polyp Z86.010
        peptic ulcer disease Z87.11
        specified condition NEC Z87.19
      ear Z86.69
      endocrine Z86.39
        diabetic foot ulcer Z86.31
        gestational diabetes Z86.32
        specified type NEC Z86.39
      eye Z86.69
      genital (track) system NEC
        female Z87.42
        male Z87.438
      hematological Z86.2
      Hodgkin Z85.71
      immune mechanism Z86.2
      infectious Z86.19

History — continued
  personal (*see also* History, family) — *continued*
    disease or disorder — *continued*
      infectious — *continued*
        malaria Z86.13
        Methicillin resistant Staphylococcus aureus (MRSA) Z86.14
        poliomyelitis Z86.12
        specified NEC Z86.19
        tuberculosis Z86.11
      mental NEC Z86.59
      metabolic Z86.39
        diabetic foot ulcer Z86.31
        gestational diabetes Z86.32
        specified type NEC Z86.39
      musculoskeletal NEC Z87.39
      nervous system Z86.69
      nutritional Z86.39
      parasitic Z86.19
      respiratory system NEC Z87.09
      sense organs Z86.69
      skin Z87.2
      specified site or type NEC Z87.898
      subcutaneous tissue Z87.2
      trophoblastic Z87.59
      urinary system NEC Z87.448
    drug dependence — *see* Dependence, drug, by type, in remission
    drug therapy
      antineoplastic chemotherapy Z92.21
      estrogen Z92.23
      immunosupression Z92.25
      inhaled steroids Z92.240
      monoclonal drug Z92.22
      specified NEC Z92.29
      steroid Z92.241
      systemic steroids Z92.241
    dysplasia
      cervical (mild) (moderate) Z87.410
        severe (grade III) Z86.001
      prostatic Z87.430
      vaginal (mild) (moderate) Z87.411
        severe (grade III) Z86.008
      vulvar (mild) (moderate) Z87.412
        severe (grade III) Z86.008
    embolism (venous) Z86.718
      pulmonary Z86.711
    encephalitis Z86.61
    estrogen therapy Z92.23
    extracorporeal membrane oxygenation (ECMO) Z92.81
    failed conscious sedation Z92.83
    failed moderate sedation Z92.83
    fall, falling Z91.81
    fracture (healed)
      fatigue Z87.312
      fragility Z87.310
      osteoporosis Z87.310
      pathological NEC Z87.311
      stress Z87.312
      traumatic Z87.81
    gestational diabetes Z86.32
    hepatitis
      B Z86.19
      C Z86.19
    Hodgkin disease Z85.71
    hyperthermia, malignant Z88.4
    hypospadias (corrected) Z87.710
    hysterectomy Z90.710
    immunosupression therapy Z92.25
    in situ neoplasm
      breast Z86.000
      cervix uteri Z86.001
      specified NEC Z86.008
    in utero procedure during pregnancy Z98.870
    in utero procedure while a fetus Z98.871
    infection NEC Z86.19
      central nervous system Z86.61
      Methicillin resistant Staphylococcus aureus (MRSA) Z86.14
      urinary (recurrent) (tract) Z87.440
    injury NEC Z87.828
    irradiation Z92.3
    kidney stones Z87.442
    leukemia Z85.6
    lymphoma (non-Hodgkin) Z85.72
    malignant melanoma (skin) Z85.820
    malignant neoplasm (of) Z85.9
      accessory sinuses Z85.22

History — *continued*
  personal (*see also* History, family) — *continued*
    malignant neoplasm — *continued*
      anus NEC Z85.048
        carcinoid Z85.040
      bladder Z85.51
      bone Z85.830
      brain Z85.841
      breast Z85.3
      bronchus NEC Z85.118
        carcinoid Z85.110
      carcinoid — *see* History, personal (of), malignant neoplasm, by site, carcinioid
      cervix Z85.41
      colon NEC Z85.038
        carcinoid Z85.030
      digestive organ Z85.00
        specified NEC Z85.09
      endocrine gland NEC Z85.858
      epididymis Z85.48
      esophagus Z85.01
      eye Z85.840
      gastrointestinal tract — *see* History, malignant neoplasm, digestive organ
      genital organ
        female Z85.40
          specified NEC Z85.44
        male Z85.45
          specified NEC Z85.49
      hematopoietic NEC Z85.79
      intrathoracic organ Z85.20
      kidney NEC Z85.528
        carcinoid Z85.520
      large intestine NEC Z85.038
        carcinoid Z85.030
      larynx Z85.21
      liver Z85.05
      lung NEC Z85.118
        carcinoid Z85.110
      mediastinum Z85.29
      Merkel cell Z85.821
      middle ear Z85.22
      nasal cavities Z85.22
      nervous system NEC Z85.848
      oral cavity Z85.819
        specified site NEC Z85.818
      ovary Z85.43
      pancreas Z85.07
      pelvis Z85.53
      pharynx Z85.819
        specified site NEC Z85.818
      pleura Z85.29
      prostate Z85.46
      rectosigmoid junction NEC Z85.048
        carcinoid Z85.040
      rectum NEC Z85.048
        carcinoid Z85.040
      respiratory organ Z85.20
      sinuses, accessory Z85.22
      skin NEC Z85.828
        melanoma Z85.820
        Merkel cell Z85.821
      small intestine NEC Z85.068
        carcinoid Z85.060
      soft tissue Z85.831
      specified site NEC Z85.89
      stomach NEC Z85.028
        carcinoid Z85.020
      testis Z85.47
      thymus NEC Z85.238
        carcinoid Z85.230
      thyroid Z85.850
      tongue Z85.810
      trachea Z85.12
      urinary organ or tract Z85.50
        specified NEC Z85.59
      uterus Z85.42
    maltreatment Z91.89
    medical treatment NEC Z92.89
    melanoma (malignant) (skin) Z85.820
    meningitis Z86.61
    mental disorder Z86.59
    Merkel cell carcinoma (skin) Z85.821
    Methicillin resistant Staphylococcus aureus (MRSA) Z86.14
    military deployment Z91.82
    military war, peacekeeping and humanitarian deployment (current or past conflict) Z91.82
    myocardial infarction (old) I25.2

History — *continued*
  personal (*see also* History, family) — *continued*
    neglect (in)
      adult Z91.412
      childhood Z62.812
    neoplasm
      benign Z86.018
        brain Z86.011
        colon polyp Z86.010
      in situ
        breast Z86.000
        cervix uteri Z86.001
        specified NEC Z86.008
      malignant — *see* History of, malignant neoplasm
      uncertain behavior Z86.03
    nephrotic syndrome Z87.441
    nicotine dependence Z87.891
    noncompliance with medical treatment or regimen — *see* Noncompliance
    nutritional deficiency Z86.39
    obstetric complications Z87.59
      childbirth Z87.59
      pregnancy Z87.59
      pre-term labor Z87.51
      puerperium Z87.59
    osteoporosis fractures Z87.31 ☑
    parasuicide (attempt) Z91.5
    physical trauma NEC Z87.828
      self-harm or suicide attempt Z91.5
    pneumonia (recurrent) Z87.01
    poisoning NEC Z91.89
      self-harm or suicide attempt Z91.5
    poor personal hygiene Z91.89
    preterm labor Z87.51
    procedure during pregnancy Z98.870
    procedure while a fetus Z98.871
    prolonged reversible ischemic neurologic deficit (PRIND) Z86.73
    prostatic dysplasia Z87.430
    psychological
      abuse
        adult Z91.411
        child Z62.811
      trauma, specified NEC Z91.49
    radiation therapy Z92.3
    removal
      implant
        breast Z98.86
    renal calculi Z87.442
    respiratory condition NEC Z87.09
    retained foreign body fully removed Z87.821
    risk factors NEC Z91.89
    self-harm Z91.5
    self-poisoning attempt Z91.5
    sex reassignment Z87.890
    sleep-wake cycle problem Z72.821
    specified NEC Z87.898
    steroid therapy (systemic) Z92.241
      inhaled Z92.240
    stroke without residual deficits Z86.73
    substance abuse NEC F10-F19
    sudden cardiac arrest Z86.74
    sudden cardiac death successfully resuscitated Z86.74
    suicide attempt Z91.5
    surgery NEC Z98.890
      with uterine scar Z98.891
      sex reassignment Z87.890
      transplant — *see* Transplant
    thrombophlebitis Z86.72
    thrombosis (venous) Z86.718
      pulmonary Z86.711
    tobacco dependence Z87.891
    transient ischemic attack (TIA) without residual deficits Z86.73
    trauma (physical) NEC Z87.828
      psychological NEC Z91.49
      self-harm Z91.5
    traumatic brain injury Z87.820
    unhealthy sleep-wake cycle Z72.821
    unintended awareness under general anesthesia Z92.84
    urinary calculi Z87.442
    urinary (recurrent) (tract) infection(s) Z87.440
    uterine scar from previous surgery Z98.891
    vaginal dysplasia Z87.411
    venous thrombosis or embolism Z86.718
      pulmonary Z86.711

History — *continued*
  personal (*see also* History, family) — *continued*
    vulvar dysplasia Z87.412
His-Werner disease A79.0
HIV (*see also* Human, immunodeficiency virus) B20
  laboratory evidence (nonconclusive) R75
  nonconclusive test (in infants) R75
  positive, seropositive Z21
Hives (bold) — *see* Urticaria
Hoarseness R49.0
Hobo Z59.0
Hodgkin disease — *see* Lymphoma, Hodgkin
Hodgson's disease I71.2
  ruptured I71.1
Hoffa-Kastert disease E88.89
Hoffa's disease E88.89
Hoffmann-Bouveret syndrome I47.9
Hoffmann's syndrome E03.9 [G73.7]
Hole (round)
  macula H35.34- ☑
  retina (without detachment) — *see* Break, retina, round hole
    with detachment — *see* Detachment, retina, with retinal, break
Holiday relief care Z75.5
Hollenhorst's plaque — *see* Occlusion, artery, retina
Hollow foot (congenital) Q66.7
  acquired — *see* Deformity, limb, foot, specified NEC
Holoprosencephaly Q04.2
Holt-Oram syndrome Q87.2
Homelessness Z59.0
Homesickness — *see* Disorder, adjustment
Homocystinemia, homocystinuria E72.11
Homogentisate 1,2-dioxygenase deficiency E70.29
Homologous serum hepatitis (prophylactic) (therapeutic) — *see* Hepatitis, viral, type B
Honeycomb lung J98.4
  congenital Q33.0
Hooded
  clitoris Q52.6
  penis Q55.69
Hookworm (anemia) (disease) (infection) (infestation) B76.9
  specified NEC B76.8
Hordeolum (eyelid) (externum) (recurrent) H00.019
  internum H00.029
    left H00.026
      lower H00.025
      upper H00.024
    right H00.023
      lower H00.022
      upper H00.021
  left H00.016
    lower H00.015
    upper H00.014
  right H00.013
    lower H00.012
    upper H00.011
Horn
  cutaneous L85.8
  nail L60.2
    congenital Q84.6
Horner (-Claude Bernard) **syndrome** G90.2
  traumatic — *see* Injury, nerve, cervical sympathetic
Horseshoe kidney (congenital) Q63.1
Horton's headache or neuralgia G44.099
  intractable G44.091
  not intractable G44.099
Hospital hopper syndrome — *see* Disorder, factitious
Hospitalism in children — *see* Disorder, adjustment
Hostility R45.5
  towards child Z62.3
Hot flashes
  menopausal N95.1
Hourglass (contracture) (*see also* Contraction, hourglass)
  stomach K31.89
    congenital Q40.2
    stricture K31.2
Household, housing circumstance affecting care Z59.9
  specified NEC Z59.8
Housemaid's knee — *see* Bursitis, prepatellar
Hudson (-Stähli) **line** (cornea) — *see* Pigmentation, cornea, anterior
Human
  bite (open wound) (*see also* Bite)
    intact skin surface — *see* Bite, superficial

Human — *continued*
  herpesvirus — *see* Herpes
  immunodeficiency virus (HIV) disease (infection) B20
    asymptomatic status Z21
    contact Z20.6
    counseling Z71.7
    dementia B20 [F02.80]
      with behavioral disturbance B20 [F02.81]
    exposure to Z20.6
    laboratory evidence R75
    type-2 (HIV 2) as cause of disease classified else-
      where B97.35
  papillomavirus (HPV)
    DNA test positive
      high risk
        cervix R87.810
        vagina R87.811
      low risk
        cervix R87.820
        vagina R87.821
    screening for Z11.51
  T-cell lymphotropic virus
    type-1 (HTLV-I) infection B33.3
      as cause of disease classified elsewhere B97.33
      carrier Z22.6
    type-2 (HTLV-II) as cause of disease classified else-
      where B97.34
Humidifier lung or pneumonitis J67.7
Humiliation (experience) **in childhood** Z62.898
Humpback (acquired) — *see* Kyphosis
Hunchback (acquired) — *see* Kyphosis
Hunger T73.0 ☑
  air, psychogenic F45.8
Hungry bone syndrome E83.81
Hunner's ulcer — *see* Cystitis, chronic, interstitial
Hunter's
  glossitis D51.0
  syndrome E76.1
Huntington's disease or chorea G10
  with dementia G10 [F02.80]
    with behavioral disturbance G10 [F02.81]
Hunt's
  disease or syndrome (herpetic geniculate ganglionitis)
    B02.21
    dyssynergia cerebellaris myoclonica G11.1
  neuralgia B02.21
Hurler (-Scheie) **disease or syndrome** E76.02
Hurst's disease G36.1
Hurthle cell
  adenocarcinoma C73
  adenoma D34
  carcinoma C73
  tumor D34
Hutchinson-Boeck disease or syndrome — *see* Sarcoidosis
Hutchinson-Gilford disease or syndrome E34.8
Hutchinson's
  disease, meaning
    angioma serpiginosum L81.7
    pompholyx (cheiropompholyx) L30.1
    prurigo estivalis L56.4
    summer eruption or summer prurigo L56.4
  melanotic freckle — *see* Melanoma, in situ
    malignant melanoma in — *see* Melanoma
  teeth or incisors (congenital syphilis) A50.52
  triad (congenital syphilis) A50.53
Hyalin plaque, sclera, senile H15.89
Hyaline membrane (disease) (lung) (pulmonary) (newborn) P22.0
Hyalinosis
  cutis (et mucosae) E78.89
  focal and segmental (glomerular) (*see also* N00-N07
    with fourth character .1) N05.1
Hyalitis, hyalosis, asteroid (*see also* Deposit, crystalline)
  syphilitic (late) A52.71
Hydatid
  cyst or tumor — *see* Echinococcus
  mole — *see* Hydatidiform mole
  Morgagni
    female Q50.5
    male (epididymal) Q55.4
      testicular Q55.29
Hydatidiform mole (benign) (complicating pregnancy)
  (delivered) (undelivered) O01.9
  classical O01.0
  complete O01.0
  incomplete O01.1
  invasive D39.2

Hydatidiform mole — *continued*
  malignant D39.2
  partial O01.1
Hydatidosis — *see* Echinococcus
Hydradenitis (axillaris) (suppurative) L73.2
Hydradenoma — *see* Hidradenoma
Hydramnios O40.- ☑
Hydrancephaly, hydranencephaly Q04.3
  with spina bifida — *see* Spina bifida, with hydro-
    cephalus
Hydrargyrism NEC — *see* Poisoning, mercury
Hydrarthrosis (*see also* Effusion, joint)
  gonococcal A54.42
  intermittent M12.40
    ankle M12.47- ☑
    elbow M12.42- ☑
    foot joint M12.47- ☑
    hand joint M12.44- ☑
    hip M12.45- ☑
    knee M12.46- ☑
    multiple site M12.49
    shoulder M12.41- ☑
    specified joint NEC M12.48
    wrist M12.43- ☑
  of yaws (early) (late) (*see also* subcategory M14.8-)
    A66.6
  syphilitic (late) A52.77
    congenital A50.55 [M12.80]
Hydremia D64.89
Hydrencephalocele (congenital) — *see* Encephalocele
Hydrencephalomeningocele (congenital) — *see* Encephalocele
Hydroa R23.8
  aestivale L56.4
  vacciniforme L56.4
Hydroadenitis (axillaris) (suppurative) L73.2
Hydrocalycosis — *see* Hydronephrosis
Hydrocele (spermatic cord) (testis) (tunica vaginalis)
  N43.3
  canal of Nuck N94.89
  communicating N43.2
    congenital P83.5
  congenital P83.5
  encysted N43.0
  female NEC N94.89
  infected N43.1
  newborn P83.5
  round ligament N94.89
  specified NEC N43.2
  spinalis — *see* Spina bifida
  vulva N90.89
Hydrocephalus (acquired) (external) (internal) (malignant) (recurrent) G91.9
  aqueduct Sylvius stricture Q03.0
  causing disproportion O33.6 ☑
    with obstructed labor O66.3
  communicating G91.0
  congenital (external) (internal) Q03.9
    with spina bifida Q05.4
      cervical Q05.0
      dorsal Q05.1
      lumbar Q05.2
      lumbosacral Q05.2
      sacral Q05.3
      thoracic Q05.1
      thoracolumbar Q05.1
    specified NEC Q03.8
  due to toxoplasmosis (congenital) P37.1
  foramen Magendie block (acquired) G91.1
    congenital (*see also* Hydrocephalus, congenital)
      Q03.1
  in (due to)
    infectious disease NEC B89 [G91.4]
    neoplastic disease NEC (*see also* Neoplasm) G91.4
    parasitic disease B89 [G91.4]
  newborn Q03.9
    with spina bifida — *see* Spina bifida, with hydro-
      cephalus
  noncommunicating G91.1
  normal pressure G91.2
    secondary G91.2
  obstructive G91.1
  otitic G93.2
  post-traumatic NEC G91.3
  secondary G91.4
    post-traumatic G91.3
  specified NEC G91.8
  syphilitic, congenital A50.49

Hydrocolpos (congenital) N89.8
Hydrocystoma — *see* Neoplasm, skin, benign
Hydroencephalocele (congenital) — *see* Encephalocele
Hydroencephalomeningocele (congenital) — *see* En-
  cephalocele
Hydrohematopneumothorax — *see* Hemothorax
Hydromeningitis — *see* Meningitis
Hydromeningocele (spinal) (*see also* Spina bifida)
  cranial — *see* Encephalocele
Hydrometra N85.8
Hydrometrocolpos N89.8
Hydromicrocephaly Q02
Hydromyelia Q06.4
Hydromyelocele — *see* Spina bifida
Hydronephrosis (atrophic) (early) (functionless) (inter-
  mittent) (primary) (secondary) NEC N13.30
  with
    infection N13.6
    obstruction (by) (of)
      renal calculus N13.2
        with infection N13.6
      ureteral NEC N13.1
        with infection N13.6
        calculus N13.2
          with infection N13.6
      ureteropelvic junction (congenital) Q62.11
        acquired N13.0
          with infection N13.6
      ureteral stricture NEC N13.1
        with infection N13.6
  congenital Q62.0
  due to acquired occlusion of ureteropelvic junction
    N13.0
  specified type NEC N13.39
  tuberculous A18.11
Hydropericarditis — *see* Pericarditis
Hydropericardium — *see* Pericarditis
Hydroperitoneum R18.8
Hydrophobia — *see* Rabies
Hydrophthalmos Q15.0
Hydropneumohemothorax — *see* Hemothorax
Hydropneumopericarditis — *see* Pericarditis
Hydropneumopericardium — *see* Pericarditis
Hydropneumothorax J94.8
  traumatic — *see* Injury, intrathoracic, lung
  tuberculous NEC A15.6
Hydrops R60.9
  abdominis R18.8
  articulorum intermittens — *see* Hydrarthrosis, inter-
    mittent
  cardiac — *see* Failure, heart, congestive
  causing obstructed labor (mother) O66.3
  endolymphatic H81.0- ☑
  fetal — *see* Pregnancy, complicated by, hydrops, fetalis
  fetalis P83.2
    due to
      ABO isoimmunization P56.0
      alpha thalassemia D56.0
      hemolytic disease P56.90
        specified NEC P56.99
      isoimmunization (ABO) (Rh) P56.0
      other specified nonhemolytic disease NEC P83.2
      Rh incompatibility P56.0
    during pregnancy — *see* Pregnancy, complicated
      by, hydrops, fetalis
  gallbladder K82.1
  joint — *see* Effusion, joint
  labyrinth H81.0- ☑
  newborn (idiopathic) P83.2
    due to
      ABO isoimmunization P56.0
      alpha thalassemia D56.0
      hemolytic disease P56.90
        specified NEC P56.99
      isoimmunization (ABO) (Rh) P56.0
      Rh incompatibility P56.0
  nutritional — *see* Malnutrition, severe
  pericardium — *see* Pericarditis
  pleura — *see* Hydrothorax
  spermatic cord — *see* Hydrocele
Hydropyonephrosis N13.6
Hydrorachis Q06.4
Hydrorrhea (nasal) J34.89
  pregnancy — *see* Rupture, membranes, premature
Hydrosadenitis (axillaris) (suppurative) L73.2
Hydrosalpinx (fallopian tube) (follicularis) N70.11

Hydrothorax (double) (pleura) J94.8
  chylous (nonfilarial) I89.8
    filarial (*see also* Infestation, filarial) B74.9 [J91.8]
  traumatic — *see* Injury, intrathoracic
  tuberculous NEC (non primary) A15.6
Hydroureter (*see also* Hydronephrosis) N13.4
  with infection N13.6
  congenital Q62.39
Hydroureteronephrosis — *see* Hydronephrosis
Hydrourethra N36.8
Hydroxykynureninuria E70.8
Hydroxylysinemia E72.3
Hydroxyprolinemia E72.59
Hygiene, sleep
  abuse Z72.821
  inadequate Z72.821
  poor Z72.821
Hygroma (congenital) (cystic) D18.1
  praepatellare, prepatellar — *see* Bursitis, prepatellar
  subdural I62.03
Hymen — *see* condition
Hymenolepis, hymenolepiasis (diminuta) (infection)
  (infestation) (nana) B71.0
Hypalgesia R20.8
Hyperacidity (gastric) K31.89
  psychogenic F45.8
Hyperactive, hyperactivity F90.9
  basal cell, uterine cervix — *see* Dysplasia, cervix
  bowel sounds R19.12
  cervix epithelial (basal) — *see* Dysplasia, cervix
  child F90.9
    attention deficit — *see* Disorder, attention-deficit
      hyperactivity
  detrusor muscle N32.81
  gastrointestinal K31.89
    psychogenic F45.8
  nasal mucous membrane J34.3
  stomach K31.89
  thyroid (gland) — *see* Hyperthyroidism
Hyperacusis H93.23- ☑
Hyperadrenalism E27.5
Hyperadrenocorticism E24.9
  congenital E25.0
  iatrogenic E24.2
    correct substance properly administered — *see*
      Table of Drugs and Chemicals, by drug, ad-
      verse effect
    overdose or wrong substance given or taken —
      see Table of Drugs and Chemicals, by drug,
      poisoning
  not associated with Cushing's syndrome E27.0
  pituitary-dependent E24.0
Hyperaldosteronism E26.9
  familial (type I) E26.02
  glucocorticoid-remediable E26.02
  primary (due to (bilateral) adrenal hyperplasia) E26.09
  primary NEC E26.09
  secondary E26.1
  specified NEC E26.89
Hyperalgesia R20.8
Hyperalimentation R63.2
  carotene, carotin E67.1
  specified NEC E67.8
  vitamin
    A E67.0
    D E67.3
Hyperaminoaciduria
  arginine E72.21
  cystine E72.01
  lysine E72.3
  ornithine E72.4
Hyperammonemia (congenital) E72.20
Hyperazotemia — *see* Uremia
Hyperbetalipoproteinemia (familial) E78.00
  with prebetalipoproteinemia E78.2
Hyperbilirubinemia
  constitutional E80.6
  familial conjugated E80.6
  neonatal (transient) — *see* Jaundice, newborn
Hypercalcemia, hypocalciuric, familial E83.52
Hypercalciuria, idiopathic E83.52
Hypercapnia R06.89
  newborn P84
Hypercarotenemia, hypercarotinemia (dietary) E67.1
Hypercementosis K03.4
Hyperchloremia E87.8
Hyperchlorhydria K31.89

Hyperchlorhydria — *continued*
  neurotic F45.8
  psychogenic F45.8
Hypercholesterinemia — *see* Hypercholesterolemia
Hypercholesterolemia (essential) (primary) (pure)
  E78.00
  with hyperglyceridemia, endogenous E78.2
  dietary counseling and surveillance Z71.3
  familial E78.01
  hereditary E78.01
Hyperchylia gastrica, psychogenic F45.8
Hyperchylomicronemia (familial) (primary) E78.3
  with hyperbetalipoproteinemia E78.3
Hypercoagulable (state) D68.59
  activated protein C resistance D68.51
  antithrombin (III) deficiency D68.59
  factor V Leiden mutation D68.51
  primary NEC D68.59
  protein C deficiency D68.59
  protein S deficiency D68.59
  prothrombin gene mutation D68.52
  secondary D68.69
  specified NEC D68.69
Hypercoagulation (state) D68.59
Hypercorticalism, pituitary-dependent E24.0
Hypercorticosolism — *see* Cushing's, syndrome
Hypercorticosteronism E24.2
  correct substance properly administered — *see* Table
    of Drugs and Chemicals, by drug, adverse effect
  overdose or wrong substance given or taken — *see*
    Table of Drugs and Chemicals, by drug, poison-
    ing
Hypercortisonism E24.2
  correct substance properly administered — *see* Table
    of Drugs and Chemicals, by drug, adverse effect
  overdose or wrong substance given or taken — *see*
    Table of Drugs and Chemicals, by drug, poison-
    ing
Hyperekplexia Q89.8
Hyperelectrolytemia E87.8
Hyperemesis R11.10
  with nausea R11.2
  gravidarum (mild) O21.0
    with
      carbohydrate depletion O21.1
      dehydration O21.1
      electrolyte imbalance O21.1
      metabolic disturbance O21.1
    severe (with metabolic disturbance) O21.1
  projectile R11.12
  psychogenic F45.8
Hyperemia (acute) (passive) R68.89
  anal mucosa K62.89
  bladder N32.89
  cerebral I67.89
  conjunctiva H11.43- ☑
  ear internal, acute — *see* subcategory H83.0 ☑
  enteric K59.8
  eye — *see* Hyperemia, conjunctiva
  eyelid (active) (passive) — *see* Disorder, eyelid, speci-
    fied type NEC
  intestine K59.8
  iris — *see* Disorder, iris, vascular
  kidney N28.89
  labyrinth — *see* subcategory H83.0 ☑
  liver (active) K76.89
  lung (passive) — *see* Edema, lung
  pulmonary (passive) — *see* Edema, lung
  renal N28.89
  retina H35.89
  stomach K31.89
Hyperesthesia (body surface) R20.3
  larynx (reflex) J38.7
    hysterical F44.89
  pharynx (reflex) J39.2
    hysterical F44.89
Hyperestrogenism (drug-induced) (iatrogenic) E28.0
Hyperexplexia Q89.8
Hyperfibrinolysis — *see* Fibrinolysis
Hyperfructosemia E74.19
Hyperfunction
  adrenal cortex, not associated with Cushing's syn-
    drome E27.0
    medulla E27.5
      adrenomedullary E27.5
    virilism E25.9
      congenital E25.0
  ovarian E28.8

Hyperfunction — *continued*
  pancreas K86.89
  parathyroid (gland) E21.3
  pituitary (gland) (anterior) E22.9
    specified NEC E22.8
  polyglandular E31.1
  testicular E29.0
Hypergammaglobulinemia D89.2
  polyclonal D89.0
  Waldenström D89.0
Hypergastrinemia E16.4
Hyperglobulinemia R77.1
Hyperglycemia, hyperglycemic (transient) R73.9
  coma — *see* Diabetes, by type, with coma
  postpancreatectomy E89.1
Hyperglyceridemia (endogenous) (essential) (familial)
  (hereditary) (pure) E78.1
  mixed E78.3
Hyperglycinemia (non-ketotic) E72.51
Hypergonadism
  ovarian E28.8
  testicular (primary) (infantile) E29.0
Hyperheparinemia D68.32
Hyperhidrosis, hyperidrosis R61
  focal
    primary L74.519
      axilla L74.510
      face L74.511
      palms L74.512
      soles L74.513
    secondary L74.52
  generalized R61
  localized
    primary L74.519
      axilla L74.510
      face L74.511
      palms L74.512
      soles L74.513
    secondary L74.52
  psychogenic F45.8
  secondary R61
    focal L74.52
Hyperhistidinemia E70.41
Hyperhomocysteinemia E72.11
Hyperhydroxyprolinemia E72.59
Hyperinsulinism (functional) E16.1
  with
    coma (hypoglycemic) E15
    encephalopathy E16.1 [G94]
  ectopic E16.1
  therapeutic misadventure (from administration of in-
    sulin) — *see* subcategory T38.3 ☑
Hyperkalemia E87.5
Hyperkeratosis (*see also* Keratosis) L85.9
  cervix N88.0
  due to yaws (early) (late) (palmar or plantar) A66.3
  follicularis Q82.8
    penetrans (in cutem) L87.0
  palmoplantaris climacterica L85.1
  pinta A67.1
  senile (with pruritus) L57.0
  universalis congenita Q80.8
  vocal cord J38.3
  vulva N90.4
Hyperkinesia, hyperkinetic (disease) (reaction) (syndrome) (childhood) (adolescence) (*see also* Disorder,
  attention-deficit hyperactivity)
  heart I51.89
Hyperleucine-isoleucinemia E71.19
Hyperlipemia, hyperlipidemia E78.5
  combined E78.2
    familial E78.4
  group
    A E78.00
    B E78.1
    C E78.2
    D E78.3
  mixed E78.2
  specified NEC E78.4
Hyperlipidosis E75.6
  hereditary NEC E75.5
Hyperlipoproteinemia E78.5
  Fredrickson's type
    I E78.3
    IIa E78.00
    IIb E78.2
    III E78.2
    IV E78.1

Hyperlipoproteinemia — *continued*
  Fredrickson's type — *continued*
    V E78.3
    low-density-lipoprotein-type (LDL) E78.00
    very-low-density-lipoprotein-type (VLDL) E78.1
Hyperlucent lung, unilateral J43.0
Hyperlysinemia E72.3
Hypermagnesemia E83.41
  neonatal P71.8
Hypermenorrhea N92.0
Hypermethioninemia E72.19
Hypermetropia (congenital) H52.0- ☑
Hypermobility, hypermotility
  cecum — *see* Syndrome, irritable bowel
  coccyx — *see* subcategory M53.2 ☑
  colon — *see* Syndrome, irritable bowel
    psychogenic F45.8
  ileum K58.9
  intestine (*see also* Syndrome, irritable bowel) K58.9
    psychogenic F45.8
  meniscus (knee) — *see* Derangement, knee, meniscus
  scapula — *see* Instability, joint, shoulder
  stomach K31.89
    psychogenic F45.8
  syndrome M35.7
  urethra N36.41
    with intrinsic sphincter deficiency N36.43
Hypernasality R49.21
Hypernatremia E87.0
Hypernephroma C64.- ☑
Hyperopia — *see* Hypermetropia
Hyperorexia nervosa F50.2
Hyperornithinemia E72.4
Hyperosmia R43.1
Hyperosmolality E87.0
Hyperostosis (monomelic) (*see also* Disorder, bone, density and structure, specified NEC)
  ankylosing (spine) M48.10
    cervical region M48.12
    cervicothoracic region M48.13
    lumbar region M48.16
    lumbosacral region M48.17
    multiple sites M48.19
    occipito-atlanto-axial region M48.11
    sacrococcygeal region M48.18
    thoracic region M48.14
    thoracolumbar region M48.15
  cortical (skull) M85.2
    infantile M89.8X- ☑
  frontal, internal of skull M85.2
  interna frontalis M85.2
  skeletal, diffuse idiopathic — *see* Hyperostosis, ankylosing
  skull M85.2
    congenital Q75.8
  vertebral, ankylosing — *see* Hyperostosis, ankylosing
Hyperovarism E28.8
Hyperoxaluria (primary) E72.53
Hyperparathyroidism E21.3
  primary E21.0
  secondary (renal) N25.81
    non-renal E21.1
  specified NEC E21.2
  tertiary E21.2
Hyperpathia R20.8
Hyperperistalsis R19.2
  psychogenic F45.8
Hyperpermeability, capillary I78.8
Hyperphagia R63.2
Hyperphenylalaninemia NEC E70.1
Hyperphoria (alternating) H50.53
Hyperphosphatemia E83.39
Hyperpiesis, hyperpiesia — *see* Hypertension
Hyperpigmentation (*see also* Pigmentation)
  melanin NEC L81.4
  postinflammatory L81.0
Hyperpinealism E34.8
Hyperpituitarism E22.9
Hyperplasia, hyperplastic
  adenoids J35.2
  adrenal (capsule) (cortex) (gland) E27.8
    with
      sexual precocity (male) E25.9
        congenital E25.0
      virilism, adrenal E25.9
        congenital E25.0
      virilization (female) E25.9

Hyperplasia, hyperplastic — *continued*
  adrenal — *continued*
    with — *continued*
      virilization — *continued*
        congenital E25.0
    congenital E25.0
    salt-losing E25.0
  adrenomedullary E27.5
  angiolymphoid, eosinophilia (ALHE) D18.01
  appendix (lymphoid) K38.0
  artery, fibromuscular I77.3
  bone (*see also* Hypertrophy, bone)
    marrow D75.89
  breast (*see also* Hypertrophy, breast)
    ductal (atypical) N60.9- ☑
  C-cell, thyroid E07.0
  cementation (tooth) (teeth) K03.4
  cervical gland R59.0
  cervix (uteri) (basal cell) (endometrium) (polypoid) (*see also* Dysplasia, cervix)
    congenital Q51.828
  clitoris, congenital Q52.6
  denture K06.2
  endocervicitis N72
  endometrium, endometrial (adenomatous) (benign) (cystic) (glandular) (glandular-cystic) (polypoid) N85.00
    with atypia N85.02
    cervix — *see* Dysplasia, cervix
    complex (without atypia) N85.01
    simple (without atypia) N85.01
  epithelial L85.9
    focal, oral, including tongue K13.29
    nipple N62
    skin L85.9
    tongue K13.29
    vaginal wall N89.3
  erythroid D75.89
  fibromuscular of artery (carotid) (renal) I77.3
  genital
    female NEC N94.89
    male N50.89
  gingiva K06.1
  glandularis cystica uteri (interstitialis) (*see also* Hyperplasia, endometrial) N85.00
  gum K06.1
  hymen, congenital Q52.4
  irritative, edentulous (alveolar) K06.2
  jaw M26.09
    alveolar M26.79
    lower M26.03
      alveolar M26.72
    upper M26.01
      alveolar M26.71
  kidney (congenital) Q63.3
  labia N90.69
    epithelial N90.3
  liver (congenital) Q44.7
    nodular, focal K76.89
  lymph gland or node R59.9
  mandible, mandibular M26.03
    alveolar M26.72
    unilateral condylar M27.8
  maxilla, maxillary M26.01
    alveolar M26.71
  myometrium, myometrial N85.2
  neuroendocrine cell, of infancy J84.841
  nose
    lymphoid J34.89
    polypoid J33.9
  oral mucosa (irritative) K13.6
  organ or site, congenital NEC — *see* Anomaly, by site
  ovary N83.8
  palate, papillary (irritative) K13.6
  pancreatic islet cells E16.9
    alpha E16.8
      with excess
        gastrin E16.4
        glucagon E16.3
    beta E16.1
  parathyroid (gland) E21.0
  pharynx (lymphoid) J39.2
  prostate (adenofibromatous) (nodular) N40.0
    with lower urinary tract symptoms (LUTS) N40.1
    without lower urinary tract symtpoms (LUTS) N40.0
  renal artery I77.89
  reticulo-endothelial (cell) D75.89
  salivary gland (any) K11.1

Hyperplasia, hyperplastic — *continued*
  Schimmelbusch's — *see* Mastopathy, cystic
  suprarenal capsule (gland) E27.8
  thymus (gland) (persistent) E32.0
  thyroid (gland) — *see* Goiter
  tonsils (faucial) (infective) (lingual) (lymphoid) J35.1
    with adenoids J35.3
  unilateral condylar M27.8
  uterus, uterine N85.2
    endometrium (glandular) (*see also* Hyperplasia, endometrial) N85.00
  vulva N90.69
    epithelial N90.3
Hyperpnea — *see* Hyperventilation
Hyperpotassemia E87.5
Hyperprebetalipoproteinemia (familial) E78.1
Hyperprolactinemia E22.1
Hyperprolinemia (type I) (type II) E72.59
Hyperproteinemia E88.09
Hyperprothrombinemia, causing coagulation factor deficiency D68.4
Hyperpyrexia R50.9
  heat (effects) T67.0 ☑
  malignant, due to anesthetic T88.3 ☑
  rheumatic — *see* Fever, rheumatic
  unknown origin R50.9
Hyper-reflexia R29.2
Hypersalivation K11.7
Hypersecretion
  ACTH (not associated with Cushing's syndrome) E27.0
    pituitary E24.0
  adrenaline E27.5
  adrenomedullary E27.5
  androgen (testicular) E29.0
    ovarian (drug-induced) (iatrogenic) E28.1
  calcitonin E07.0
  catecholamine E27.5
  corticoadrenal E24.9
  cortisol E24.9
  epinephrine E27.5
  estrogen E28.0
  gastric K31.89
    psychogenic F45.8
  gastrin E16.4
  glucagon E16.3
  hormone(s)
    ACTH (not associated with Cushing's syndrome) E27.0
      pituitary E24.0
    antidiuretic E22.2
    growth E22.0
    intestinal NEC E34.1
    ovarian androgen E28.1
    pituitary E22.9
    testicular E29.0
    thyroid stimulating E05.80
      with thyroid storm E05.81
  insulin — *see* Hyperinsulinism
  lacrimal glands — *see* Epiphora
  medulloadrenal E27.5
  milk O92.6
  ovarian androgens E28.1
  salivary gland (any) K11.7
  thyrocalcitonin E07.0
  upper respiratory J39.8
Hypersegmentation, leukocytic, hereditary D72.0
Hypersensitive, hypersensitiveness, hypersensitivity (*see also* Allergy)
  carotid sinus G90.01
  colon — *see* Irritable, colon
  drug T88.7 ☑
  gastrointestinal K52.29
    immediate K52.29
    psychogenic F45.8
  labyrinth — *see* subcategory H83.2 ☑
  pain R20.8
  pneumonitis — *see* Pneumonitis, allergic
  reaction T78.40 ☑
  upper respiratory tract NEC J39.3
Hypersomnia (organic) G47.10
  due to
    alcohol
      abuse F10.182
      dependence F10.282
      use F10.982
    amphetamines
      abuse F15.182
      dependence F15.282

Hypersomnia — *continued*
  due to — *continued*
    amphetamines — *continued*
      use F15.982
    caffeine
      abuse F15.182
      dependence F15.282
      use F15.982
    cocaine
      abuse F14.182
      dependence F14.282
      use F14.982
    drug NEC
      abuse F19.182
      dependence F19.282
      use F19.982
    medical condition G47.14
    mental disorder F51.13
    opioid
      abuse F11.182
      dependence F11.282
      use F11.982
    psychoactive substance NEC
      abuse F19.182
      dependence F19.282
      use F19.982
    sedative, hypnotic, or anxiolytic
      abuse F13.182
      dependence F13.282
      use F13.982
    stimulant NEC
      abuse F15.182
      dependence F15.282
      use F15.982
  idiopathic G47.11
    with long sleep time G47.11
    without long sleep time G47.12
  menstrual related G47.13
  nonorganic origin F51.11
    specified NEC F51.19
  not due to a substance or known physiological condition F51.11
    specified NEC F51.19
  primary F51.11
  recurrent G47.13
  specified NEC G47.19
Hypersplenia, hypersplenism D73.1
Hyperstimulation, ovaries (associated with induced ovulation) N98.1
Hypersusceptibility — *see* Allergy
Hypertelorism (ocular) (orbital) Q75.2
Hypertension, hypertensive (accelerated) (benign) (essential) (idiopathic) (malignant) (systemic) I10
  with
    heart failure (congestive) I11.0
    heart involvement (conditions in I50.-, I51.4-I51.9 due to hypertension) — *see* Hypertension, heart
    kidney involvement — *see* Hypertension, kidney
  benign, intracranial G93.2
  borderline R03.0
  cardiorenal (disease) I13.10
    with heart failure I13.0
      with stage 1 through stage 4 chronic kidney disease I13.0
      with stage 5 or end stage renal disease I13.2
    without heart failure I13.10
      with stage 1 through stage 4 chronic kidney disease I13.10
      with stage 5 or end stage renal disease I13.11
  cardiovascular
    disease (arteriosclerotic) (sclerotic) — *see* Hypertension, heart
    renal (disease) — *see* Hypertension, cardiorenal
  chronic venous — *see* Hypertension, venous (chronic)
  complicating
    childbirth (labor) O16.4
      pre-existing O10.92
        with
          heart disease O10.12
            with renal disease O10.32
          pre-eclampsia O11.4
          renal disease O10.22
            with heart disease O10.32
          essential O10.02
      secondary O10.42
    pregnancy O16.- ☑
      with edema (*see also* Pre-eclampsia) O14.9- ☑

Hypertension, hypertensive — *continued*
  complicating — *continued*
    pregnancy — *continued*
      gestational (pregnancy induced) (without proteinuria) O13.- ☑
        with proteinuria O14.9- ☑
          mild pre-eclampsia O14.0- ☑
          moderate pre-eclampsia O14.0- ☑
          severe pre-eclampsia O14.1- ☑
            with hemolysis, elevated liver enzymes and low platelet count (HELLP) O14.2- ☑
      pre-existing O10.91-
        with
          heart disease O10.11- ☑
            with renal disease O10.31- ☑
          pre-eclampsia — *see* category O11
          renal disease O10.21- ☑
            with heart disease O10.31- ☑
        essential O10.01- ☑
        secondary O10.41- ☑
      transient O13- ☑
    puerperium, pre-existing O16.5
    pre-existing
      with
        heart disease O10.13
          with renal disease O10.33
        pre-eclampsia O11.5
        renal disease O10.23
          with heart disease O10.33
        essential O10.03
    pregnancy-induced O13.9
    secondary O10.43
  crisis I16.9
  due to
    endocrine disorders I15.2
    pheochromocytoma I15.2
    renal disorders NEC I15.1
      arterial I15.0
    renovascular disorders I15.0
    specified disease NEC I15.8
  emergency I16.1
  encephalopathy I67.4
  gestational (without significant proteinuria) (pregnancy-induced) (transient) O13.- ☑
    with significant proteinuria — *see* Pre-eclampsia
    complicating
      delivery O13.4
      puerperium O13.5
  Goldblatt's I70.1
  heart (disease) (conditions in I51.4-I51.9 due to hypertension) I11.9
    with
      heart failure (congestive) I11.0
      kidney disease (chronic) — *see* Hypertension, cardiorenal
  intracranial (benign) G93.2
  kidney I12.9
    with
      heart disease — *see* Hypertension, cardiorenal
      stage 1 through stage 4 chronic kidney disease I12.9
      stage 5 chronic kidney disease (CKD) or end stage renal disease (ESRD) I12.0
  lesser circulation I27.0
  maternal O16- ☑
  newborn P29.2
    pulmonary (persistent) P29.30
  ocular H40.05- ☑
  pancreatic duct — *code to* underlying condition
    with chronic pancreatitis K86.1
  portal (due to chronic liver disease) (idiopathic) K76.6
    gastropathy K31.89
    in (due to) schistosomiasis (bilharziasis) B65.9 [K77]
  postoperative I97.3
  psychogenic F45.8
  pulmonary I27.20
    with
      cor pulmonale (chronic) I27.29
        acute I26.09
      right heart ventricular strain/failure I27.29
        acute I26.09
      right to left shunt related to congenital heart disease I27.83
      unclear multifactorial mechanisms I27.29
    arterial (associated) (drug-induced) (toxin-induced) I27.21
    chronic thromboembolic I27.24

Hypertension, hypertensive — *continued*
  pulmonary — *continued*
    due to
      hematologic disorders I27.29
      left heart disease I27.22
      lung diseases and hypoxia I27.23
      metabolic disorders I27.29
      specified systemic disorders I27.29
    group 1 (associated) (drug-induced) (toxin-induced) I27.21
    group 2 I27.22
    group 3 I27.23
    group 4 I27.24
    group 5 I27.29
    of newborn (persistent) P29.30
    primary (idiopathic) I27.0
    secondary
      arterial I27.21
      specified NEC I27.29
  renal — *see* Hypertension, kidney
  renovascular I15.0
  secondary NEC I15.9
    due to
      endocrine disorders I15.2
      pheochromocytoma I15.2
      renal disorders NEC I15.1
        arterial I15.0
      renovascular disorders I15.0
    specified NEC I15.8
  transient, of pregnancy O13- ☑
  urgency I16.0
  venous (chronic)
    due to
      deep vein thrombosis — *see* Syndrome, post-thrombotic
      idiopathic I87.309
        with
          inflammation I87.32- ☑
            with ulcer I87.33- ☑
          specified complication NEC I87.39- ☑
          ulcer I87.31- ☑
            with inflammation I87.33- ☑
        asymptomatic I87.30- ☑
Hypertensive urgency — *see* Hypertension
Hyperthecosis ovary E28.8
Hyperthermia (of unknown origin) (*see also* Hyperpyrexia)
  malignant, due to anesthesia T88.3 ☑
  newborn P81.9
    environmental P81.0
Hyperthyroid (recurrent) — *see* Hyperthyroidism
Hyperthyroidism (latent) (pre-adult) (recurrent) E05.90
  with
    goiter (diffuse) E05.00
      with thyroid storm E05.01
      nodular (multinodular) E05.20
        with thyroid storm E05.21
        uninodular E05.10
          with thyroid storm E05.11
    storm E05.91
  due to ectopic thyroid tissue E05.30
    with thyroid storm E05.31
  neonatal, transitory P72.1
  specified NEC E05.80
    with thyroid storm E05.81
Hypertony, hypertonia, hypertonicity
  bladder N31.8
  congenital P94.1
  stomach K31.89
    psychogenic F45.8
  uterus, uterine (contractions) (complicating delivery) O62.4
Hypertrichosis L68.9
  congenital Q84.2
  eyelid H02.869
    left H02.866
      lower H02.865
      upper H02.864
    right H02.863
      lower H02.862
      upper H02.861
  lanuginosa Q84.2
    acquired L68.1
  localized L68.2
  specified NEC L68.8
Hypertriglyceridemia, essential E78.1

Hypertrophy, hypertrophic
- adenofibromatous, prostate — *see* Enlargement, enlarged, prostate
- adenoids (infective) J35.2
  - with tonsils J35.3
- adrenal cortex E27.8
- alveolar process or ridge — *see* Anomaly, alveolar
- anal papillae K62.89
- artery I77.89
  - congenital NEC Q27.8
    - digestive system Q27.8
    - lower limb Q27.8
    - specified site NEC Q27.8
    - upper limb Q27.8
- auricular — *see* Hypertrophy, cardiac
- Bartholin's gland N75.8
- bile duct (common) (hepatic) K83.8
- bladder (sphincter) (trigone) N32.89
- bone M89.30
  - carpus M89.34- ☑
  - clavicle M89.31- ☑
  - femur M89.35- ☑
  - fibula M89.36- ☑
  - finger M89.34- ☑
  - humerus M89.32- ☑
  - ilium M89.359
  - ischium M89.359
  - metacarpus M89.34- ☑
  - metatarsus M89.37- ☑
  - multiple sites M89.39
  - neck M89.38
  - radius M89.33- ☑
  - rib M89.38
  - scapula M89.31- ☑
  - skull M89.38
  - tarsus M89.37- ☑
  - tibia M89.36- ☑
  - toe M89.37- ☑
  - ulna M89.33- ☑
  - vertebra M89.38
- brain G93.89
- breast N62
  - cystic — *see* Mastopathy, cystic
  - newborn P83.4
  - pubertal, massive N62
  - puerperal, postpartum — *see* Disorder, breast, specified type NEC
  - senile (parenchymatous) N62
- cardiac (chronic) (idiopathic) I51.7
  - with rheumatic fever (conditions in I00)
    - active I01.8
    - inactive or quiescent (with chorea) I09.89
  - congenital NEC Q24.8
  - fatty — *see* Degeneration, myocardial
  - hypertensive — *see* Hypertension, heart
  - rheumatic (with chorea) I09.89
    - active or acute I01.8
      - with chorea I02.0
  - valve — *see* Endocarditis
- cartilage — *see* Disorder, cartilage, specified type NEC
- cecum — *see* Megacolon
- cervix (uteri) N88.8
  - congenital Q51.828
  - elongation N88.4
- clitoris (cirrhotic) N90.89
  - congenital Q52.6
- colon (*see also* Megacolon)
  - congenital Q43.2
- conjunctiva, lymphoid H11.89
- corpora cavernosa N48.89
- cystic duct K82.8
- duodenum K31.89
- endometrium (glandular) (*see also* Hyperplasia, endometrial) N85.00
  - cervix N88.8
- epididymis N50.89
- esophageal hiatus (congenital) Q79.1
  - with hernia — *see* Hernia, hiatal
- eyelid — *see* Disorder, eyelid, specified type NEC
- fat pad E65
  - knee (infrapatellar) (popliteal) (prepatellar) (retropatellar) M79.4
- foot (congenital) Q74.2
- frenulum, frenum (tongue) K14.8
  - lip K13.0
- gallbladder K82.8
- gastric mucosa K29.60
  - with bleeding K29.61

Hypertrophy, hypertrophic — *continued*
- gland, glandular R59.9
  - generalized R59.1
  - localized R59.0
- gum (mucous membrane) K06.1
- heart (idiopathic) (*see also* Hypertrophy, cardiac)
  - valve (*see also* Endocarditis) I38
- hemifacial Q67.4
- hepatic — *see* Hypertrophy, liver
- hiatus (esophageal) Q79.1
- hilus gland R59.0
- hymen, congenital Q52.4
- ileum K63.89
- intestine NEC K63.89
- jejunum K63.89
- kidney (compensatory) N28.81
  - congenital Q63.3
- labium (majus) (minus) N90.60
- ligament — *see* Disorder, ligament
- lingual tonsil (infective) J35.1
  - with adenoids J35.3
- lip K13.0
  - congenital Q18.6
- liver R16.0
  - acute K76.89
  - cirrhotic — *see* Cirrhosis, liver
  - congenital Q44.7
  - fatty — *see* Fatty, liver
- lymph, lymphatic gland R59.9
  - generalized R59.1
  - localized R59.0
  - tuberculous — *see* Tuberculosis, lymph gland
- mammary gland — *see* Hypertrophy, breast
- Meckel's diverticulum (congenital) Q43.0
  - malignant — *see* Table of Neoplasms, small intestine, malignant
- median bar — *see* Hyperplasia, prostate
- meibomian gland — *see* Chalazion
- meniscus, knee, congenital Q74.1
- metatarsal head — *see* Hypertrophy, bone, metatarsus
- metatarsus — *see* Hypertrophy, bone, metatarsus
- mucous membrane
  - alveolar ridge K06.2
  - gum K06.1
  - nose (turbinate) J34.3
- muscle M62.89
- muscular coat, artery I77.89
- myocardium (*see also* Hypertrophy, cardiac)
  - idiopathic I42.2
- myometrium N85.2
- nail L60.2
  - congenital Q84.5
- nasal J34.89
  - alae J34.89
  - bone J34.89
  - cartilage J34.89
  - mucous membrane (septum) J34.3
  - sinus J34.89
  - turbinate J34.3
- nasopharynx, lymphoid (infectional) (tissue) (wall) J35.2
- nipple N62
- organ or site, congenital NEC — *see* Anomaly, by site
- ovary N83.8
- palate (hard) M27.8
  - soft K13.79
- pancreas, congenital Q45.3
- parathyroid (gland) E21.0
- parotid gland K11.1
- penis N48.89
- pharyngeal tonsil J35.2
- pharynx J39.2
  - lymphoid (infectional) (tissue) (wall) J35.2
- pituitary (anterior) (fossa) (gland) E23.6
- prepuce (congenital) N47.8
  - female N90.89
- prostate — *see* Enlargement, enlarged, prostate
  - congenital Q55.4
- pseudomuscular G71.0
- pylorus (adult) (muscle) (sphincter) K31.1
  - congenital or infantile Q40.0
- rectal, rectum (sphincter) K62.89
- rhinitis (turbinate) J31.0
- salivary gland (any) K11.1
  - congenital Q38.4
- scaphoid (tarsal) — *see* Hypertrophy, bone, tarsus
- scar L91.0
- scrotum N50.89

Hypertrophy, hypertrophic — *continued*
- seminal vesicle N50.89
- sigmoid — *see* Megacolon
- skin L91.9
  - specified NEC L91.8
- spermatic cord N50.89
- spleen — *see* Splenomegaly
- spondylitis — *see* Spondylosis
- stomach K31.89
- sublingual gland K11.1
- submandibular gland K11.1
- suprarenal cortex (gland) E27.8
- synovial NEC M67.20
  - acromioclavicular M67.21- ☑
  - ankle M67.27- ☑
  - elbow M67.22- ☑
  - foot M67.27- ☑
  - hand M67.24- ☑
  - hip M67.25- ☑
  - knee M67.26- ☑
  - multiple sites M67.29
  - specified site NEC M67.28
  - wrist M67.23- ☑
- tendon — *see* Disorder, tendon, specified type NEC
- testis N44.8
  - congenital Q55.29
- thymic, thymus (gland) (congenital) E32.0
- thyroid (gland) — *see* Goiter
- toe (congenital) Q74.2
  - acquired (*see also* Deformity, toe, specified NEC)
- tongue K14.8
  - congenital Q38.2
  - papillae (foliate) K14.3
- tonsils (faucial) (infective) (lingual) (lymphoid) J35.1
  - with adenoids J35.3
- tunica vaginalis N50.89
- ureter N28.89
- urethra N36.8
- uterus N85.2
  - neck (with elongation) N88.4
  - puerperal O90.89
- uvula K13.79
- vagina N89.8
- vas deferens N50.89
- vein I87.8
- ventricle, ventricular (heart) (*see also* Hypertrophy, cardiac)
  - congenital Q24.8
  - in tetralogy of Fallot Q21.3
- verumontanum N36.8
- vocal cord J38.3
- vulva N90.60
  - stasis (nonfilarial) N90.69

Hypertropia H50.2- ☑
Hypertyrosinemia E70.21
Hyperuricemia (asymptomatic) E79.0
Hypervalinemia E71.19
Hyperventilation (tetany) R06.4
- hysterical F45.8
- psychogenic F45.8
- syndrome F45.8
Hypervitaminosis (dietary) NEC E67.8
- A E67.0
  - administered as drug (prolonged intake) — *see* Table of Drugs and Chemicals, vitamins, adverse effect
  - overdose or wrong substance given or taken — *see* Table of Drugs and Chemicals, vitamins, poisoning
- B6 E67.2
- D E67.3
  - administered as drug (prolonged intake) — *see* Table of Drugs and Chemicals, vitamins, adverse effect
  - overdose or wrong substance given or taken — *see* Table of Drugs and Chemicals, vitamins, poisoning
- K E67.8
  - administered as drug (prolonged intake) — *see* Table of Drugs and Chemicals, vitamins, adverse effect
  - overdose or wrong substance given or taken — *see* Table of Drugs and Chemicals, vitamins, poisoning
Hypervolemia E87.70
- specified NEC E87.79
Hypesthesia R20.1
- cornea — *see* Anesthesia, cornea

☑ **Additional Character Required — Refer to the Tabular List for Character Selection**   ▽ **Subterms under main terms may continue to next column or page**

Hyphema H21.0- ☑
  traumatic S05.1- ☑
Hypoacidity, gastric K31.89
  psychogenic F45.8
Hypoadrenalism, hypoadrenia E27.40
  primary E27.1
  tuberculous A18.7
Hypoadrenocorticism E27.40
  pituitary E23.0
  primary E27.1
Hypoalbuminemia E88.09
Hypoaldosteronism E27.40
Hypoalphalipoproteinemia E78.6
Hypobarism T70.29 ☑
Hypobaropathy T70.29 ☑
Hypobetalipoproteinemia (familial) E78.6
Hypocalcemia E83.51
  dietary E58
  neonatal P71.1
    due to cow's milk P71.0
  phosphate-loading (newborn) P71.1
Hypochloremia E87.8
Hypochlorhydria K31.89
  neurotic F45.8
  psychogenic F45.8
Hypochondria, hypochondriac, hypochondriasis (reaction) F45.21
  sleep F51.03
Hypochondrogenesis Q77.0
Hypochondroplasia Q77.4
Hypochromasia, blood cells D50.8
Hypodontia — *see* Anodontia
Hypoeosinophilia D72.89
Hypoesthesia R20.1
Hypofibrinogenemia D68.8
  acquired D65
  congenital (hereditary) D68.2
Hypofunction
  adrenocortical E27.40
    drug-induced E27.3
    postprocedural E89.6
    primary E27.1
  adrenomedullary, postprocedural E89.6
  cerebral R29.818
  corticoadrenal NEC E27.40
  intestinal K59.8
  labyrinth — *see* subcategory H83.2 ☑
  ovary E28.39
  pituitary (gland) (anterior) E23.0
  testicular E29.1
    postprocedural (postsurgical) (postirradiation) (iatrogenic) E89.5
Hypogalactia O92.4
Hypogammaglobulinemia (*see also* Agammaglobulinemia) D80.1
  hereditary D80.0
  nonfamilial D80.1
  transient, of infancy D80.7
Hypogenitalism (congenital) — *see* Hypogonadism
Hypoglossia Q38.3
Hypoglycemia (spontaneous) E16.2
  coma E15
    diabetic — *see* Diabetes, by type, with hypoglycemia, with coma
  diabetic — *see* Diabetes, hypoglycemia
  dietary counseling and surveillance Z71.3
  drug-induced E16.0
    with coma (nondiabetic) E15
  due to insulin E16.0
    with coma (nondiabetic) E15
    therapeutic misadventure — *see* subcategory T38.3 ☑
  functional, nonhyperinsulinemic E16.1
  iatrogenic E16.0
    with coma (nondiabetic) E15
  in infant of diabetic mother P70.1
    gestational diabetes P70.0
  infantile E16.1
  leucine-induced E71.19
  neonatal (transitory) P70.4
    iatrogenic P70.3
  reactive (not drug-induced) E16.1
  transitory neonatal P70.4
Hypogonadism
  female E28.39
  hypogonadotropic E23.0
  male E29.1
  ovarian (primary) E28.39

Hypogonadism — *continued*
  pituitary E23.0
  testicular (primary) E29.1
Hypohidrosis, hypoidrosis L74.4
Hypoinsulinemia, postprocedural E89.1
Hypokalemia E87.6
Hypoleukocytosis — *see* Agranulocytosis
Hypolipoproteinemia (alpha) (beta) E78.6
Hypomagnesemia E83.42
  neonatal P71.2
Hypomania, hypomanic reaction F30.8
Hypomenorrhea — *see* Oligomenorrhea
Hypometabolism R63.8
Hypomotility
  gastrointestinal (tract) K31.89
    psychogenic F45.8
  intestine K59.8
    psychogenic F45.8
  stomach K31.89
    psychogenic F45.8
Hyponasality R49.22
Hyponatremia E87.1
Hypo-osmolality E87.1
Hypo-ovarianism, hypo-ovarism E28.39
Hypoparathyroidism E20.9
  familial E20.8
  idiopathic E20.0
  neonatal, transitory P71.4
  postprocedural E89.2
  specified NEC E20.8
Hypoperfusion (in)
  newborn P96.89
Hypopharyngitis — *see* Laryngopharyngitis
Hypophoria H50.53
Hypophosphatemia, hypophosphatasia (acquired) (congenital) (renal) E83.39
  familial E83.31
Hypophyseal, hypophysis (*see also* condition)
  dwarfism E23.0
  gigantism E22.0
Hypopiesis — *see* Hypotension
Hypopinealism E34.8
Hypopituitarism (juvenile) E23.0
  drug-induced E23.1
  due to
    hypophysectomy E89.3
    radiotherapy E89.3
  iatrogenic NEC E23.1
  postirradiation E89.3
  postpartum O99.285
  postprocedural E89.3
Hypoplasia, hypoplastic
  adrenal (gland), congenital Q89.1
  alimentary tract, congenital Q45.8
    upper Q40.8
  anus, anal (canal) Q42.3
    with fistula Q42.2
  aorta, aortic Q25.42
    ascending, in hypoplastic left heart syndrome Q23.4
    valve Q23.1
      in hypoplastic left heart syndrome Q23.4
  areola, congenital Q83.8
  arm (congenital) — *see* Defect, reduction, upper limb
  artery (peripheral) Q27.8
    brain (congenital) Q28.3
    coronary Q24.5
    digestive system Q27.8
    lower limb Q27.8
    pulmonary Q25.79
      functional, unilateral J43.0
    retinal (congenital) Q14.1
    specified site NEC Q27.8
    umbilical Q27.0
    upper limb Q27.8
  auditory canal Q17.8
    causing impairment of hearing Q16.9
  biliary duct or passage Q44.5
  bone NOS Q79.9
    face Q75.8
    marrow D61.9
      megakaryocytic D69.49
    skull — *see* Hypoplasia, skull
  brain Q02
    gyri Q04.3
    part of Q04.3
  breast (areola) N64.82
  bronchus Q32.4

Hypoplasia, hypoplastic — *continued*
  cardiac Q24.8
  carpus — *see* Defect, reduction, upper limb, specified type NEC
  cartilage hair Q78.8
  cecum Q42.8
  cementum K00.4
  cephalic Q02
  cerebellum Q04.3
  cervix (uteri), congenital Q51.821
  clavicle (congenital) Q74.0
  coccyx Q76.49
  colon Q42.9
    specified NEC Q42.8
  corpus callosum Q04.0
  cricoid cartilage Q31.2
  digestive organ(s) or tract NEC Q45.8
    upper (congenital) Q40.8
  ear (auricle) (lobe) Q17.2
    middle Q16.4
  enamel of teeth (neonatal) (postnatal) (prenatal) K00.4
  endocrine (gland) NEC Q89.2
  endometrium N85.8
  epididymis (congenital) Q55.4
  epiglottis Q31.2
  erythroid, congenital D61.01
  esophagus (congenital) Q39.8
  eustachian tube Q17.8
  eye Q11.2
  eyelid (congenital) Q10.3
  face Q18.8
    bone(s) Q75.8
  femur (congenital) — *see* Defect, reduction, lower limb, specified type NEC
  fibula (congenital) — *see* Defect, reduction, lower limb, specified type NEC
  finger (congenital) — *see* Defect, reduction, upper limb, specified type NEC
  focal dermal Q82.8
  foot — *see* Defect, reduction, lower limb, specified type NEC
  gallbladder Q44.0
  genitalia, genital organ(s)
    female, congenital Q52.8
      external Q52.79
      internal NEC Q52.8
    in adiposogenital dystrophy E23.6
  glottis Q31.2
  hair Q84.2
  hand (congenital) — *see* Defect, reduction, upper limb, specified type NEC
  heart Q24.8
  humerus (congenital) — *see* Defect, reduction, upper limb, specified type NEC
  intestine (small) Q41.9
    large Q42.9
      specified NEC Q42.8
  jaw M26.09
    alveolar M26.79
    lower M26.04
      alveolar M26.74
    upper M26.02
      alveolar M26.73
  kidney(s) Q60.5
    bilateral Q60.4
    unilateral Q60.3
  labium (majus) (minus), congenital Q52.79
  larynx Q31.2
  left heart syndrome Q23.4
  leg (congenital) — *see* Defect, reduction, lower limb
  limb Q73.8
    lower (congenital) — *see* Defect, reduction, lower limb
    upper (congenital) — *see* Defect, reduction, upper limb
  liver Q44.7
  lung (lobe) (not associated with short gestation) Q33.6
    associated with immaturity, low birth weight, prematurity, or short gestation P28.0
  mammary (areola), congenital Q83.8
  mandible, mandibular M26.04
    alveolar M26.74
    unilateral condylar M27.8
  maxillary M26.02
    alveolar M26.73
  medullary D61.9
  megakaryocytic D69.49

Hypoplasia, hypoplastic — *continued*
    metacarpus — *see* Defect, reduction, upper limb, specified type NEC
    metatarsus — *see* Defect, reduction, lower limb, specified type NEC
    muscle Q79.8
    nail(s) Q84.6
    nose, nasal Q30.1
    optic nerve H47.03- ☑
    osseous meatus (ear) Q17.8
    ovary, congenital Q50.39
    pancreas Q45.0
    parathyroid (gland) Q89.2
    parotid gland Q38.4
    patella Q74.1
    pelvis, pelvic girdle Q74.2
    penis (congenital) Q55.62
    peripheral vascular system Q27.8
        digestive system Q27.8
        lower limb Q27.8
        specified site NEC Q27.8
        upper limb Q27.8
    pituitary (gland) (congenital) Q89.2
    pulmonary (not associated with short gestation) Q33.6
        artery, functional J43.0
        associated with short gestation P28.0
    radioulnar — *see* Defect, reduction, upper limb, specified type NEC
    radius — *see* Defect, reduction, upper limb
    rectum Q42.1
        with fistula Q42.0
    respiratory system NEC Q34.8
    rib Q76.6
    right heart syndrome Q22.6
    sacrum Q76.49
    scapula Q74.0
    scrotum Q55.1
    shoulder girdle Q74.0
    skin Q82.8
    skull (bone) Q75.8
        with
            anencephaly Q00.0
            encephalocele — *see* Encephalocele
            hydrocephalus Q03.9
                with spina bifida — *see* Spina bifida, by site, with hydrocephalus
            microcephaly Q02
    spinal (cord) (ventral horn cell) Q06.1
    spine Q76.49
    sternum Q76.7
    tarsus — *see* Defect, reduction, lower limb, specified type NEC
    testis Q55.1
    thymic, with immunodeficiency D82.1
    thymus (gland) Q89.2
        with immunodeficiency D82.1
    thyroid (gland) E03.1
        cartilage Q31.2
    tibiofibular (congenital) — *see* Defect, reduction, lower limb, specified type NEC
    toe — *see* Defect, reduction, lower limb, specified type NEC
    tongue Q38.3
    Turner's K00.4
    ulna (congenital) — *see* Defect, reduction, upper limb
    umbilical artery Q27.0
    unilateral condylar M27.8
    ureter Q62.8
    uterus, congenital Q51.811
    vagina Q52.4
    vascular NEC peripheral Q27.8
        brain Q28.3
        digestive system Q27.8
        lower limb Q27.8
        specified site NEC Q27.8
        upper limb Q27.8
    vein(s) (peripheral) Q27.8
        brain Q28.3
        digestive system Q27.8
        great Q26.8
        lower limb Q27.8
        specified site NEC Q27.8
        upper limb Q27.8
    vena cava (inferior) (superior) Q26.8
    vertebra Q76.49
    vulva, congenital Q52.79
    zonule (ciliary) Q12.8
Hypopnea, obstructive sleep apnea G47.33

Hypopotassemia E87.6
Hypoproconvertinemia, congenital (hereditary) D68.2
Hypoproteinemia E77.8
Hypoprothrombinemia (congenital) (hereditary) (idiopathic) D68.2
    acquired D68.4
    newborn, transient P61.6
Hypoptyalism K11.7
Hypopyon (eye) (anterior chamber) — *see* Iridocyclitis, acute, hypopyon
Hypopyrexia R68.0
Hyporeflexia R29.2
Hyposecretion
    ACTH E23.0
    antidiuretic hormone E23.2
    ovary E28.39
    salivary gland (any) K11.7
    vasopressin E23.2
Hyposegmentation, leukocytic, hereditary D72.0
Hyposiderinemia D50.9
Hypospadias Q54.9
    balanic Q54.0
    coronal Q54.0
    glandular Q54.0
    penile Q54.1
    penoscrotal Q54.2
    perineal Q54.3
    specified NEC Q54.8
Hypospermatogenesis — *see* Oligospermia
Hyposplenism D73.0
Hypostasis pulmonary, passive — *see* Edema, lung
Hypostatic — *see* condition
Hyposthenuria N28.89
Hypotension (arterial) (constitutional) I95.9
    chronic I95.89
    drug-induced I95.2
    due to (of) hemodialysis I95.3
    iatrogenic I95.89
    idiopathic (permanent) I95.0
    intracranial, following ventricular shunting (ventriculostomy) G97.2
    Intra-dialytic I95.3
    maternal, syndrome (following labor and delivery) O26.5- ☑
    neurogenic, orthostatic G90.3
    orthostatic (chronic) I95.1
        due to drugs I95.2
        neurogenic G90.3
    postoperative I95.81
    postural I95.1
    specified NEC I95.89
Hypothermia (accidental) T68 ☑
    due to anesthesia, anesthetic T88.51 ☑
    low environmental temperature T68 ☑
    neonatal P80.9
        environmental (mild) NEC P80.8
        mild P80.8
        severe (chronic) (cold injury syndrome) P80.0
        specified NEC P80.8
    not associated with low environmental temperature R68.0
Hypothyroidism (acquired) E03.9
    autoimmune — *see* Thyroiditis, autoimmune
    congenital (without goiter) E03.1
        with goiter (diffuse) E03.0
    due to
        exogenous substance NEC E03.2
        iodine-deficiency, acquired E01.8
            subclinical E02
        irradiation therapy E89.0
        medicament NEC E03.2
        P-aminosalicylic acid (PAS) E03.2
        phenylbutazone E03.2
        resorcinol E03.2
        sulfonamide E03.2
        surgery E89.0
        thiourea group drugs E03.2
    iatrogenic NEC E03.2
    iodine-deficiency (acquired) E01.8
        congenital — *see* Syndrome, iodine-deficiency, congenital
        subclinical E02
    neonatal, transitory P72.2
    postinfectious E03.3
    postirradiation E89.0
    postprocedural E89.0
    postsurgical E89.0
    specified NEC E03.8

Hypothyroidism — *continued*
    subclinical, iodine-deficiency related E02
Hypotonia, hypotonicity, hypotony
    bladder N31.2
    congenital (benign) P94.2
    eye — *see* Disorder, globe, hypotony
Hypotrichosis — *see* Alopecia
Hypotropia H50.2- ☑
Hypoventilation R06.89
    congenital central alveolar G47.35
    sleep related
        idiopathic nonobstructive alveolar G47.34
        in conditions classified elsewhere G47.36
Hypovitaminosis — *see* Deficiency, vitamin
Hypovolemia E86.1
    surgical shock T81.19 ☑
    traumatic (shock) T79.4 ☑
Hypoxemia R09.02
    newborn P84
    sleep related, in conditions classified elsewhere G47.36
Hypoxia (*see also* Anoxia) R09.02
    cerebral, during a procedure NEC G97.81
        postprocedural NEC G97.82
    intrauterine P84
    myocardial — *see* Insufficiency, coronary
    newborn P84
    sleep-related G47.34
Hypsarhythmia — *see* Epilepsy, generalized, specified NEC
Hysteralgia, pregnant uterus O26.89- ☑
Hysteria, hysterical (conversion) (dissociative state) F44.9
    anxiety F41.8
    convulsions F44.5
    psychosis, acute F44.9
Hysteroepilepsy F44.5

I

IBDU (colonic inflammatory bowel dissease unclassified) K52.3
Ichthyoparasitism due to Vandellia cirrhosa B88.8
Ichthyosis (congenital) Q80.9
    acquired L85.0
    fetalis Q80.4
    hystrix Q80.8
    lamellar Q80.2
    lingual K13.29
    palmaris and plantaris Q82.8
    simplex Q80.0
    vera Q80.8
    vulgaris Q80.0
    X-linked Q80.1
Ichthyotoxism — *see* Poisoning, fish
    bacterial — *see* Intoxication, foodborne
Icteroanemia, hemolytic (acquired) D59.9
    congenital — *see* Spherocytosis
Icterus (*see also* Jaundice)
    conjunctiva R17
    gravis, newborn P55.0
    hematogenous (acquired) D59.9
    hemolytic (acquired) D59.9
        congenital — *see* Spherocytosis
    hemorrhagic (acute) (leptospiral) (spirochetal) A27.0
        newborn P53
    infectious B15.9
        with hepatic coma B15.0
        leptospiral A27.0
        spirochetal A27.0
    neonatorum — *see* Jaundice, newborn
    newborn P59.9
    spirochetal A27.0
Ictus solaris, solis T67.0 ☑
Id reaction (due to bacteria) L30.2
Ideation
    homicidal R45.850
    suicidal R45.851
Identity disorder (child) F64.9
    gender role F64.2
    psychosexual F64.2
Idioglossia F80.0
Idiopathic — *see* condition
Idiot, idiocy (congenital) F73
    amaurotic (Bielschowsky(-Jansky)) (family) (infantile (late)) (juvenile (late)) (Vogt-Spielmeyer) E75.4
    microcephalic Q02
IgE asthma J45.909

IIAC (idiopathic infantile arterial calcification) Q28.8
Ileitis (chronic) (noninfectious) (see also Enteritis) K52.9
　backwash — see Pancolitis, ulcerative (chronic)
　infectious A09
　regional (ulcerative) — see Enteritis, regional, small
　　intestine
　segmental — see Enteritis, regional
　terminal (ulcerative) — see Enteritis, regional, small
　　intestine
Ileocolitis (see also Enteritis) K52.9
　infectious A09
　regional — see Enteritis, regional
　ulcerative K51.0- ☑
Ileostomy
　attention to Z43.2
　malfunctioning K94.13
　status Z93.2
　　with complication — see Complications, enteros-
　　　tomy
Ileotyphus — see Typhoid
Ileum — see condition
Ileus (bowel) (colon) (inhibitory) (intestine) K56.7
　adynamic K56.0
　due to gallstone (in intestine) K56.3
　duodenal (chronic) K31.5
　gallstone K56.3
　mechanical NEC (see also Obstruction, intestine,
　　specified NEC) K56.699
　meconium P76.0
　　in cystic fibrosis E84.11
　　meaning meconium plug (without cystic fibrosis)
　　　P76.0
　myxedema K59.8
　neurogenic K56.0
　　Hirschsprung's disease or megacolon Q43.1
　newborn
　　due to meconium P76.0
　　　in cystic fibrosis E84.11
　　　meaning meconium plug (without cystic fibro-
　　　　sis) P76.0
　　transitory P76.1
　obstructive (see also Obstruction, intestine, specified
　　NEC) K56.699
　paralytic K56.0
　postoperative K91.89
Iliac — see condition
Iliotibial band syndrome M76.3- ☑
Illiteracy Z55.0
Illness (see also Disease) R69
　manic-depressive — see Disorder, bipolar
Imbalance R26.89
　autonomic G90.8
　constituents of food intake E63.1
　electrolyte E87.8
　　with
　　　abortion — see Abortion by type, complicated
　　　　by, electrolyte imbalance
　　　molar pregnancy O08.5
　　due to hyperemesis gravidarum O21.1
　　following ectopic or molar pregnancy O08.5
　　neonatal, transitory NEC P74.4
　　　potassium P74.3
　　　sodium P74.2
　endocrine E34.9
　eye muscle NOS H50.9
　hormone E34.9
　hysterical F44.4
　labyrinth — see subcategory H83.2 ☑
　posture R29.3
　protein-energy — see Malnutrition
　sympathetic G90.8
Imbecile, imbecility (I.Q. 35-49) F71
Imbedding, intrauterine device T83.39 ☑
Imbibition, cholesterol (gallbladder) K82.4
Imbrication, teeth,, fully erupted M26.30
Imerslund (-Gräsbeck) **syndrome** D51.1
Immature (see also Immaturity)
　birth (less than 37 completed weeks) — see Preterm,
　　newborn
　extremely (less than 28 completed weeks) — see
　　Immaturity, extreme
　personality F60.89
Immaturity (less than 37 completed weeks) (see also
　Preterm, newborn)
　extreme of newborn (less than 28 completed weeks)
　　(of gestation) (less than 196 completed days of
　　gestation) (unspecified weeks of gestation)
　　P07.20

Immaturity — continued
　extreme of newborn — continued
　　gestational age
　　　less than 23 completed weeks P07.21
　　　23 completed weeks (23 weeks, 0 days through
　　　　23 weeks, 6 days) P07.22
　　　24 completed weeks (24 weeks, 0 days through
　　　　24 weeks, 6 days) P07.23
　　　25 completed weeks (25 weeks, 0 days through
　　　　25 weeks, 6 days) P07.24
　　　26 completed weeks (26 weeks, 0 days through
　　　　26 weeks, 6 days) P07.25
　　　27 completed weeks (27 weeks, 0 days through
　　　　27 weeks, 6 days) P07.26
　fetus or infant light-for-dates — see Light-for-dates
　lung, newborn P28.0
　organ or site NEC — see Hypoplasia
　pulmonary, newborn P28.0
　reaction F60.89
　sexual (female) (male), after puberty E30.0
Immersion T75.1 ☑
　foot T69.02- ☑
　hand T69.01- ☑
Immobile, immobility
　complete, due to severe physical disability or frailty
　　R53.2
　intestine K59.8
　syndrome (paraplegic) M62.3
Immune reconstitution (inflammatory) syndrome [IRIS]
　D89.3
Immunization (see also Vaccination)
　ABO — see Incompatibility, ABO
　　in newborn P55.1
　complication — see Complications, vaccination
　encounter for Z23
　not done (not carried out) Z28.9
　　because (of)
　　　acute illness of patient Z28.01
　　　allergy to vaccine (or component) Z28.04
　　　caregiver refusal Z28.82
　　　chronic illness of patient Z28.02
　　　contraindication NEC Z28.09
　　　group pressure Z28.1
　　　guardian refusal Z28.82
　　　immune compromised state of patient Z28.03
　　　parent refusal Z28.82
　　　patient had disease being vaccinated against
　　　　Z28.81
　　　patient refusal Z28.21
　　　patient's belief Z28.1
　　　religious beliefs of patient Z28.1
　　　specified reason NEC Z28.89
　　　　of patient Z28.29
　　　unspecified patient reason Z28.20
　Rh factor
　　affecting management of pregnancy NEC
　　　O36.09- ☑
　　anti-D antibody O36.01- ☑
　from transfusion — see Complication(s), transfu-
　　sion, incompatibility reaction, Rh (factor)
Immunocytoma C83.0- ☑
Immunodeficiency D84.9
　with
　　adenosine-deaminase deficiency D81.3
　　antibody defects D80.9
　　　specified type NEC D80.8
　　hyperimmunoglobulinemia D80.6
　　increased immunoglobulin M (IgM) D80.5
　　major defect D82.9
　　　specified type NEC D82.8
　　partial albinism D82.8
　　short-limbed stature D82.2
　　thrombocytopenia and eczema D82.0
　antibody with
　　hyperimmunoglobulinemia D80.6
　　near-normal immunoglobulins D80.6
　autosomal recessive, Swiss type D80.0
　combined D81.9
　　biotin-dependent carboxylase D81.819
　　　biotinidase D81.810
　　　holocarboxylase synthetase D81.818
　　　specified type NEC D81.818
　　severe (SCID) D81.9
　　　with
　　　　low or normal B-cell numbers D81.2
　　　　low T- and B-cell numbers D81.1
　　　　reticular dysgenesis D81.0
　　specified type NEC D81.89

Immunodeficiency — continued
　common variable D83.9
　　with
　　　abnormalities of B-cell numbers and function
　　　　D83.0
　　　autoantibodies to B- or T-cells D83.2
　　　immunoregulatory T-cell disorders D83.1
　　　specified type NEC D83.8
　following hereditary defective response to Epstein-
　　Barr virus (EBV) D82.3
　selective, immunoglobulin
　　A (IgA) D80.2
　　G (IgG) (subclasses) D80.3
　　M (IgM) D80.4
　severe combined (SCID) D81.9
　specified type NEC D84.8
　X-linked, with increased IgM D80.5
Immunotherapy (encounter for)
　antineoplastic Z51.12
Impaction, impacted
　bowel, colon, rectum (see also Impaction, fecal) K56.49
　　by gallstone K56.3
　calculus — see Calculus
　cerumen (ear) (external) H61.2- ☑
　cuspid — see Impaction, tooth
　dental (same or adjacent tooth) K01.1
　fecal, feces K56.41
　fracture — see Fracture, by site
　gallbladder — see Calculus, gallbladder
　gallstone(s) — see Calculus, gallbladder
　　bile duct (common) (hepatic) — see Calculus, bile
　　　duct
　　cystic duct — see Calculus, gallbladder
　　in intestine, with obstruction (any part) K56.3
　intestine (calculous) NEC (see also Impaction, fecal)
　　K56.49
　　gallstone, with ileus K56.3
　intrauterine device (IUD) T83.39 ☑
　molar — see Impaction, tooth
　shoulder, causing obstructed labor O66.0
　tooth, teeth K01.1
　turbinate J34.89
Impaired, impairment (function)
　auditory discrimination — see Abnormal, auditory
　　perception
　cognitive, mild, so stated G31.84
　dual sensory Z73.82
　fasting glucose R73.01
　glucose tolerance (oral) R73.02
　hearing — see Deafness
　heart — see Disease, heart
　kidney N28.9
　　disorder resulting from N25.9
　　　specified NEC N25.89
　liver K72.90
　　with coma K72.91
　mastication K08.89
　mild cognitive, so stated G31.84
　mobility
　　ear ossicles — see Ankylosis, ear ossicles
　　requiring care provider Z74.09
　myocardium, myocardial — see Insufficiency, myocar-
　　dial
　rectal sphincter R19.8
　renal (acute) (chronic) N28.9
　　disorder resulting from N25.9
　　　specified NEC N25.89
　vision NEC H54.7
　　both eyes H54.3
Impediment, speech R47.9
　psychogenic (childhood) F98.8
　slurring R47.81
　specified NEC R47.89
Impending
　coronary syndrome I20.0
　delirium tremens F10.239
　myocardial infarction I20.0
Imperception auditory (acquired) (see also Deafness)
　congenital H93.25
Imperfect
　aeration, lung (newborn) NEC — see Atelectasis
　closure (congenital)
　　alimentary tract NEC Q45.8
　　　lower Q43.8
　　　upper Q40.8
　　atrioventricular ostium Q21.2
　　atrium (secundum) Q21.1
　　branchial cleft NOS Q18.2

Imperfect — continued
  closure — continued
    branchial cleft — continued
      cyst Q18.0
      fistula Q18.0
      sinus Q18.0
    choroid Q14.3
    cricoid cartilage Q31.8
    cusps, heart valve NEC Q24.8
      pulmonary Q22.3
    ductus
      arteriosus Q25.0
      Botalli Q25.0
    ear drum (causing impairment of hearing) Q16.4
    esophagus with communication to bronchus or trachea Q39.1
    eyelid Q10.3
    foramen
      botalli Q21.1
      ovale Q21.1
    genitalia, genital organ(s) or system
      female Q52.8
        external Q52.79
        internal NEC Q52.8
      male Q55.8
    glottis Q31.8
    interatrial ostium or septum Q21.1
    interauricular ostium or septum Q21.1
    interventricular ostium or septum Q21.0
    larynx Q31.8
    lip — see Cleft, lip
    nasal septum Q30.3
    nose Q30.2
    omphalomesenteric duct Q43.0
    optic nerve entry Q14.2
    organ or site not listed — see Anomaly, by site
    ostium
      interatrial Q21.1
      interauricular Q21.1
      interventricular Q21.0
    palate — see Cleft, palate
    preauricular sinus Q18.1
    retina Q14.1
    roof of orbit Q75.8
    sclera Q13.5
    septum
      aorticopulmonary Q21.4
      atrial (secundum) Q21.1
      between aorta and pulmonary artery Q21.4
      heart Q21.9
      interatrial (secundum) Q21.1
      interauricular (secundum) Q21.1
      interventricular Q21.0
        in tetralogy of Fallot Q21.3
      nasal Q30.3
      ventricular Q21.0
        with pulmonary stenosis or atresia, dextraposition of aorta, and hypertrophy of right ventricle Q21.3
        in tetralogy of Fallot Q21.3
    skull Q75.0
      with
        anencephaly Q00.0
        encephalocele — see Encephalocele
        hydrocephalus Q03.9
          with spina bifida — see Spina bifida, by site, with hydrocephalus
        microcephaly Q02
    spine (with meningocele) — see Spina bifida
    trachea Q32.1
    tympanic membrane (causing impairment of hearing) Q16.4
    uterus Q51.818
    vitelline duct Q43.0
  erection — see Dysfunction, sexual, male, erectile
  fusion — see Imperfect, closure
  inflation, lung (newborn) — see Atelectasis
  posture R29.3
  rotation, intestine Q43.3
  septum, ventricular Q21.0
Imperfectly descended testis — see Cryptorchid
Imperforate (congenital) (see also Atresia)
  anus Q42.3
    with fistula Q42.2
  cervix (uteri) Q51.828
  esophagus Q39.0
    with tracheoesophageal fistula Q39.1
  hymen Q52.3

Imperforate — continued
  jejunum Q41.1
  pharynx Q38.8
  rectum Q42.1
    with fistula Q42.0
  urethra Q64.39
  vagina Q52.4
Impervious (congenital) (see also Atresia)
  anus Q42.3
    with fistula Q42.2
  bile duct Q44.2
  esophagus Q39.0
    with tracheoesophageal fistula Q39.1
  intestine (small) Q41.9
    large Q42.9
      specified NEC Q42.8
  rectum Q42.1
    with fistula Q42.0
  ureter — see Atresia, ureter
  urethra Q64.39
Impetiginization of dermatoses L01.1
Impetigo (any organism) (any site) (circinate) (contagiosa) (simplex) (vulgaris) L01.00
  Bockhart's L01.02
  bullous, bullosa L01.03
  external ear L01.00 [H62.40]
  follicularis L01.02
  furfuracea L30.5
  herpetiformis L40.1
    nonobstetrical L40.1
  neonatorum L01.03
  nonbullous L01.01
  specified type NEC L01.09
  ulcerative L01.09
Impingement (on teeth)
  soft tissue
    anterior M26.81
    posterior M26.82
Implant, endometrial N80.9
Implantation
  anomalous — see Anomaly, by site
    ureter Q62.63
  cyst
    external area or site (skin) NEC L72.0
    iris — see Cyst, iris, implantation
    vagina N89.8
    vulva N90.7
  dermoid (cyst) — see Implantation, cyst
Impotence (sexual) N52.9
  counseling Z70.1
  organic origin (see also Dysfunction, sexual, male, erectile) N52.9
  psychogenic F52.21
Impression, basilar Q75.8
Imprisonment, anxiety concerning Z65.1
Improper care (child) (newborn) — see Maltreatment
Improperly tied umbilical cord (causing hemorrhage) P51.8
Impulsiveness (impulsive) R45.87
Inability to swallow — see Aphagia
Inaccessible, inaccessibility
  health care NEC Z75.3
    due to
      waiting period Z75.2
        for admission to facility elsewhere Z75.1
    other helping agencies Z75.4
Inactive — see condition
Inadequate, inadequacy
  aesthetics of dental restoration K08.56
  biologic, constitutional, functional, or social F60.7
  development
    child R62.50
    genitalia
      after puberty NEC E30.0
      congenital
        female Q52.8
          external Q52.79
          internal Q52.8
        male Q55.8
    lungs Q33.6
      associated with short gestation P28.0
    organ or site not listed — see Anomaly, by site
  diet (causing nutritional deficiency) E63.9
  eating habits Z72.4
  environment, household Z59.1
  family support Z63.8
  food (supply) NEC Z59.4
    hunger effects T73.0 ☑

Inadequate, inadequacy — continued
  functional F60.7
  household care, due to
    family member
      handicapped or ill Z74.2
      on vacation Z75.5
      temporarily away from home Z74.2
    technical defects in home Z59.1
    temporary absence from home of person rendering care Z74.2
  housing (heating) (space) Z59.1
  income (financial) Z59.6
  intrafamilial communication Z63.8
  material resources Z59.9
  mental — see Disability, intellectual
  parental supervision or control of child Z62.0
  personality F60.7
  pulmonary
    function R06.89
      newborn P28.5
    ventilation, newborn P28.5
  sample of cytologic smear
    anus R85.615
    cervix R87.615
    vagina R87.625
  social F60.7
    insurance Z59.7
    skills NEC Z73.4
  supervision of child by parent Z62.0
  teaching affecting education Z55.8
  welfare support Z59.7
Inanition R64
  with edema — see Malnutrition, severe
  due to
    deprivation of food T73.0 ☑
    malnutrition — see Malnutrition
  fever R50.9
Inappropriate
  change in quantitative human chorionic gonadotropin (hCG) in early pregnancy O02.81
  diet or eating habits Z72.4
  level of quantitative human chorionic gonadotropin (hCG) for gestational age in early pregnancy O02.81
  secretion
    antidiuretic hormone (ADH) (excessive) E22.2
      deficiency E23.2
    pituitary (posterior) E22.2
Inattention at or after birth — see Neglect
Incarceration, incarcerated
  enterocele K46.0
    gangrenous K46.1
  epiplocele K46.0
    gangrenous K46.1
  exomphalos K42.0
    gangrenous K42.1
  hernia (see also Hernia, by site, with obstruction)
    with gangrene — see Hernia, by site, with gangrene
  iris, in wound — see Injury, eye, laceration, with prolapse
  lens, in wound — see Injury, eye, laceration, with prolapse
  omphalocele K42.0
  prison, anxiety concerning Z65.1
  rupture — see Hernia, by site
  sarcoepiplocele K46.0
    gangrenous K46.1
  sarcoepiplomphalocele K42.0
    with gangrene K42.1
  uterus N85.8
    gravid O34.51- ☑
      causing obstructed labor O65.5
Incised wound
  external — see Laceration
  internal organs — see Injury, by site
Incision, incisional
  hernia K43.2
    with
      gangrene (and obstruction) K43.1
      obstruction K43.0
    surgical, complication — see Complications, surgical procedure
    traumatic
      external — see Laceration
      internal organs — see Injury, by site
Inclusion
  azurophilic leukocytic D72.0

☑ **Additional Character Required** — Refer to the Tabular List for Character Selection   ▽ Subterms under main terms may continue to next column or page

Inclusion — *continued*
  blennorrhea (neonatal) (newborn) P39.1
  gallbladder in liver (congenital) Q44.1
Incompatibility
  ABO
    affecting management of pregnancy O36.11- ☑
      anti-A sensitization O36.11- ☑
      anti-B sensitization O36.19- ☑
      specified NEC O36.19- ☑
    infusion or transfusion reaction — *see* Complication(s), transfusion, incompatibility reaction, ABO
    newborn P55.1
  blood (group) (Duffy) (K(ell)) (Kidd) (Lewis) (M) (S) NEC
    affecting management of pregnancy O36.11- ☑
      anti-A sensitization O36.11- ☑
      anti-B sensitization O36.19- ☑
    infusion or transfusion reaction T80.89 ☑
    newborn P55.8
  divorce or estrangement Z63.5
  Rh (blood group) (factor) Z31.82
    affecting management of pregnancy NEC
      O36.09- ☑
      anti-D antibody O36.01- ☑
    infusion or transfusion reaction — *see* Complication(s), transfusion, incompatibility reaction, Rh (factor)
    newborn P55.0
  rhesus — *see* Incompatibility, Rh
Incompetency, incompetent, incompetence
  annular
    aortic (valve) — *see* Insufficiency, aortic
    mitral (valve) I34.0
    pulmonary valve (heart) I37.1
  aortic (valve) — *see* Insufficiency, aortic
  cardiac valve — *see* Endocarditis
  cervix, cervical (os) N88.3
    in pregnancy O34.3- ☑
  chronotropic I45.89
    with
      autonomic dysfunction G90.8
      ischemic heart disease I25.89
      left ventricular dysfunction I51.89
      sinus node dysfunction I49.8
  esophagogastric (junction) (sphincter) K22.0
  mitral (valve) — *see* Insufficiency, mitral
  pelvic fundus N81.89
  pubocervical tissue N81.82
  pulmonary valve (heart) I37.1
    congenital Q22.3
  rectovaginal tissue N81.83
  tricuspid (annular) (valve) — *see* Insufficiency, tricuspid
  valvular — *see* Endocarditis
    congenital Q24.8
  vein, venous (saphenous) (varicose) — *see* Varix, leg
Incomplete (*see also* condition)
  bladder, emptying R33.9
  defecation R15.0
  expansion lungs (newborn) NEC — *see* Atelectasis
  rotation, intestine Q43.3
Inconclusive
  diagnostic imaging due to excess body fat of patient R93.9
  findings on diagnostic imaging of breast NEC R92.8
  mammogram (due to dense breasts) R92.2
Incontinence R32
  anal sphincter R15.9
  coital N39.491
  feces R15.9
    nonorganic origin F98.1
  insensible (urinary) N39.42
  overflow N39.490
  postural (urinary) N39.492
  psychogenic F45.8
  rectal R15.9
  reflex N39.498
  stress (female) (male) N39.3
    and urge N39.46
  urethral sphincter R32
  urge N39.41
    and stress (female) (male) N39.46
  urine (urinary) R32
    continuous N39.45
    due to cognitive impairment, or severe physical disability or immobility R39.81
    functional R39.81
    insensible N39.42
    mixed (stress and urge) N39.46

Incontinence — *continued*
  urine — *continued*
    nocturnal N39.44
    nonorganic origin F98.0
    overflow N39.490
    post dribbling N39.43
    postural N39.492
    reflex N39.498
    specified NEC N39.498
    stress (female) (male) N39.3
      and urge N39.46
    total N39.498
    unaware N39.42
    urge N39.41
      and stress (female) (male) N39.46
Incontinentia pigmenti Q82.3
Incoordinate, incoordination
  esophageal-pharyngeal (newborn) — *see* Dysphagia
  muscular R27.8
  uterus (action) (contractions) (complicating delivery) O62.4
Increase, increased
  abnormal, in development R63.8
  androgens (ovarian) E28.1
  anticoagulants (antithrombin) (anti-VIIIa) (anti-IXa) (anti-Xa) (anti-XIa) — *see* Circulating anticoagulants
  cold sense R20.8
  estrogen E28.0
  function
    adrenal
      cortex — *see* Cushing's, syndrome
      medulla E27.5
    pituitary (gland) (anterior) (lobe) E22.9
      posterior E22.2
  heat sense R20.8
  intracranial pressure (benign) G93.2
  permeability, capillaries I78.8
  pressure, intracranial G93.2
  secretion
    gastrin E16.4
    glucagon E16.3
    pancreas, endocrine E16.9
      growth hormone-releasing hormone E16.8
      pancreatic polypeptide E16.8
      somatostatin E16.8
      vasoactive-intestinal polypeptide E16.8
  sphericity, lens Q12.4
  splenic activity D73.1
  venous pressure I87.8
    portal K76.6
Increta placenta O43.22- ☑
Incrustation, cornea, foreign body (lead)(zinc) — *see* Foreign body, cornea
Incyclophoria H50.54
Incyclotropia — *see* Cyclotropia
Indeterminate sex Q56.4
India rubber skin Q82.8
Indigestion (acid) (bilious) (functional) K30
  catarrhal K31.89
  due to decomposed food NOS A05.9
  nervous F45.8
  psychogenic F45.8
Indirect — *see* condition
Induratio penis plastica N48.6
Induration, indurated
  brain G93.89
  breast (fibrous) N64.51
    puerperal, postpartum O92.29
  broad ligament N83.8
  chancre
    anus A51.1
    congenital A50.07
    extragenital NEC A51.2
  corpora cavernosa (penis) (plastic) N48.6
  liver (chronic) K76.89
  lung (black) (chronic) (fibroid) (*see also* Fibrosis, lung) J84.10
    essential brown J84.03
  penile (plastic) N48.6
  phlebitic — *see* Phlebitis
  skin R23.4
Inebriety (without dependence) — *see* Alcohol, intoxication
Inefficiency, kidney N28.9
Inelasticity, skin R23.4
Inequality, leg (length) (acquired) (*see also* Deformity, limb, unequal length)
  congenital — *see* Defect, reduction, lower limb

Inequality, leg — *continued*
  lower leg — *see* Deformity, limb, unequal length
Inertia
  bladder (neurogenic) N31.2
  stomach K31.89
    psychogenic F45.8
  uterus, uterine during labor O62.2
    during latent phase of labor O62.0
    primary O62.0
    secondary O62.1
  vesical (neurogenic) N31.2
Infancy, infantile, infantilism (*see also* condition)
  celiac K90.0
  genitalia, genitals (after puberty) E30.0
  Herter's (nontropical sprue) K90.0
  intestinal K90.0
  Lorain E23.0
  pancreatic K86.89
  pelvis M95.5
    with disproportion (fetopelvic) O33.1
      causing obstructed labor O65.1
  pituitary E23.0
  renal N25.0
  uterus — *see* Infantile, genitalia
Infant(s) (*see also* Infancy)
  excessive crying R68.11
  irritable child R68.12
  lack of care — *see* Neglect
  liveborn (singleton) Z38.2
    born in hospital Z38.00
      by cesarean Z38.01
    born outside hospital Z38.1
    multiple NEC Z38.8
      born in hospital Z38.68
        by cesarean Z38.69
      born outside hospital Z38.7
    quadruplet Z38.8
      born in hospital Z38.63
        by cesarean Z38.64
      born outside hospital Z38.7
    quintuplet Z38.8
      born in hospital Z38.65
        by cesarean Z38.66
      born outside hospital Z38.7
    triplet Z38.8
      born in hospital Z38.61
        by cesarean Z38.62
      born outside hospital Z38.7
    twin Z38.5
      born in hospital Z38.30
        by cesarean Z38.31
      born outside hospital Z38.4
  of diabetic mother (syndrome of) P70.1
    gestational diabetes P70.0
Infantile (*see also* condition)
  genitalia, genitals E30.0
  os, uterine E30.0
  penis E30.0
  testis E29.1
  uterus E30.0
Infantilism — *see* Infancy
Infarct, infarction
  adrenal (capsule) (gland) E27.49
  appendices epiploicae (*see also* Infarct, intestine) K55.069
  bowel (*see also* Infarct, intestine) K55.069
  brain (stem) — *see* Infarct, cerebral
  breast N64.89
  brewer's (kidney) N28.0
  cardiac — *see* Infarct, myocardium
  cerebellar — *see* Infarct, cerebral
  cerebral (*see also* Occlusion, artery cerebral or precerebral, with infarction) I63.9
    aborted I63.9
    cortical I63.9
    due to
      cerebral venous thrombosis, nonpyogenic I63.6
      embolism
        cerebral arteries I63.4- ☑
        precerebral arteries I63.1- ☑
      occlusion NEC
        cerebral arteries I63.5- ☑
        precerebral arteries I63.2- ☑
      stenosis NEC
        cerebral arteries I63.5- ☑
        precerebral arteries I63.2- ☑

Infarct, infarction — *continued*
- cerebral (*see also* Occlusion, artery cerebral or precerebral, with infarction) — *continued*
  - due to — *continued*
    - thrombosis
      - cerebral artery I63.3- ☑
      - precerebral artery I63.0- ☑
    - intraoperative
      - during cardiac surgery I97.810
      - during other surgery I97.811
    - postprocedural
      - following cardiac surgery I97.820
      - following other surgery I97.821
    - specified NEC I63.8
- colon (acute) (agnogenic) (embolic) (hemorrhagic) (nonocclusive) (nonthrombotic) (occlusive) (segmental) (thrombotic) (with gangrene) (*see also* Infarct, intestine) K55.049
- coronary artery — *see* Infarct, myocardium
- embolic — *see* Embolism
- fallopian tube N83.8
- gallbladder K82.8
- heart — *see* Infarct, myocardium
- hepatic K76.3
- hypophysis (anterior lobe) E23.6
- impending (myocardium) I20.0
- intestine (acute) (agnogenic) (embolic) (hemorrhagic) (nonocclusive) (nonthrombotic) (occlusive) (thrombotic) (with gangrene) K55.069
  - diffuse K55.062
  - focal K55.061
  - large K55.049
    - diffuse K55.042
    - focal K55.041
  - small K55.029
    - diffuse K55.022
    - focal K55.021
- kidney N28.0
- liver K76.3
- lung (embolic) (thrombotic) — *see* Embolism, pulmonary
- lymph node I89.8
- mesentery, mesenteric (embolic) (thrombotic) (with gangrene) (*see also* Infarct, intestine) K55.069
- muscle (ischemic) M62.20
  - ankle M62.27- ☑
  - foot M62.27- ☑
  - forearm M62.23- ☑
  - hand M62.24- ☑
  - lower leg M62.26- ☑
  - pelvic region M62.25- ☑
  - shoulder region M62.21- ☑
  - specified site NEC M62.28
  - thigh M62.25- ☑
  - upper arm M62.22- ☑
- myocardium, myocardial (acute) (with stated duration of 4 weeks or less) I21.9
  - associated with revascularization procedure I21.A9
  - diagnosed on ECG, but presenting no symptoms I25.2
  - due to
    - demand ischemia I21.A1
    - ischemic imbalance I21.A1
  - healed or old I25.2
  - intraoperative (*see also* Infarct, myocardium, associated with revascularization procedure)
    - during cardiac surgery I97.790
    - during other surgery I97.791
  - non-Q wave I21.4
  - non-ST elevation (NSTEMI) I21.4
    - subsequent I22.2
  - nontransmural I21.4
  - past (diagnosed on ECG or other investigation, but currently presenting no symptoms) I25.2
  - postprocedural (*see also* Infarct, myocardium, associated with revascularization procedure)
    - following cardiac surgery (*see also* Infarct, myocardium, type 4 or type 5) I97.190
    - following other surgery I97.191
  - Q wave (see also, Infarct, myocardium, by site) I21.3
  - secondary to
    - demand ischemia I21.A1
    - ischemic imbalance I21.A1
  - ST elevation (STEMI) I21.3
    - anterior (anteroapical) (anterolateral) (anteroseptal) (Q wave) (wall) I21.09
      - subsequent I22.0

Infarct, infarction — *continued*
- myocardium, myocardial — *continued*
  - ST elevation — *continued*
    - inferior (diaphragmatic) (inferolateral) (inferoposterior) (wall) NEC I21.19
      - subsequent I22.1
    - inferoposterior transmural (Q wave) I21.11
    - involving
      - coronary artery of anterior wall NEC I21.09
      - coronary artery of inferior wall NEC I21.19
      - diagonal coronary artery I21.02
      - left anterior descending coronary artery I21.02
      - left circumflex coronary artery I21.21
      - left main coronary artery I21.01
      - oblique marginal coronary artery I21.21
      - right coronary artery I21.11
    - lateral (apical-lateral) (basal-lateral) (high) I21.29
      - subsequent I22.8
    - posterior (posterobasal) (posterolateral) (posteroseptal) (true) I21.29
      - subsequent I22.8
    - septal I21.29
      - subsequent I22.8
    - specified NEC I21.29
      - subsequent I22.8
    - subsequent I22.9
  - subsequent (recurrent) (reInfarction) I22.9
    - anterior (anteroapical) (anterolateral) (anteroseptal) (wall) I22.0
    - diaphragmatic (wall) I22.1
    - inferior (diaphragmatic) (inferolateral) (inferoposterior) (wall) I22.1
    - lateral (apical-lateral) (basal-lateral) (high) I22.8
    - non-ST elevation (NSTEMI) I22.2
    - posterior (posterobasal) (posterolateral) (posteroseptal) (true) I22.8
    - septal I22.8
    - specified NEC I22.8
    - ST elevation I22.9
      - anterior (anteroapical) (anterolateral) (anteroseptal) (wall) I22.0
      - inferior (diaphragmatic) (inferolateral) (inferoposterior) (wall) I22.1
      - specified NEC I22.8
    - subendocardial I22.2
    - transmural I22.9
      - anterior (anteroapical) (anterolateral) (anteroseptal) (wall) I22.0
      - diaphragmatic (wall) I22.1
      - inferior (diaphragmatic) (inferolateral) (inferoposterior) (wall) I22.1
      - lateral (apical-lateral) (basal-lateral) (high) I22.8
      - posterior (posterobasal) (posterolateral) (posteroseptal) (true) I22.8
      - specified NEC I22.8
    - type 1 (*see also* Infarction, myocardial, subsequent, by site, or by ST elevation or non-ST elevation) I22.9
    - type 2 I21.A1
    - type 3 I21.A9
    - type 4 I21.A9
    - type 5 I21.A9
  - syphilitic A52.06
  - transmural I21.9
    - anterior (anteroapical) (anterolateral) (anteroseptal) (Q wave) (wall) NEC I21.09
    - inferior (diaphragmatic) (inferolateral) (inferoposterior) (Q wave) (wall) NEC I21.19
    - inferoposterior (Q wave) I21.11
    - lateral (apical-lateral) (basal-lateral) (high) NEC I21.29
    - posterior (posterobasal) (posterolateral) (posteroseptal) (true) NEC I21.29
    - septal NEC I21.29
    - specified NEC I21.29
  - type 1 (*see also* Infarction, myocardial, by site, or by ST elevation or non-ST elevation) I21.9
  - type 2 I21.A1
  - type 3 I21.A9
  - type 4 (a) (b) (c) I21.A9
  - type 5 I21.A9
  - nontransmural I21.4
- omentum (*see also* Infarct, intestine) K55.069
- ovary N83.8
- pancreas K86.89
- papillary muscle — *see* Infarct, myocardium

Infarct, infarction — *continued*
- parathyroid gland E21.4
- pituitary (gland) E23.6
- placenta O43.81- ☑
- prostate N42.89
- pulmonary (artery) (vein) (hemorrhagic) — *see* Embolism, pulmonary
- renal (embolic) (thrombotic) N28.0
- retina, retinal (artery) — *see* Occlusion, artery, retina
- spinal (cord) (acute) (embolic) (nonembolic) G95.11
- spleen D73.5
  - embolic or thrombotic I74.8
- subendocardial (acute) (nontransmural) I21.4
- suprarenal (capsule) (gland) E27.49
- testis N50.1
- thrombotic (*see also* Thrombosis)
  - artery, arterial — *see* Embolism
- thyroid (gland) E07.89
- ventricle (heart) — *see* Infarct, myocardium

Infecting — *see* condition
Infection, infected, infective (opportunistic) B99.9
- with
  - drug resistant organism — *see* Resistance (to), drug (*see also* specific organism)
  - lymphangitis — *see* Lymphangitis
  - organ dysfunction (acute) R65.20
    - with septic shock R65.21
- abscess (skin) — *code by* site under Abscess
- Absidia — *see* Mucormycosis
- Acanthamoeba — *see* Acanthamebiasis
- Acanthocheilonema (perstans) (streptocerca) B74.4
- accessory sinus (chronic) — *see* Sinusitis
- achorion — *see* Dermatophytosis
- Acremonium falciforme B47.0
- acromioclavicular M00.9
- Actinobacillus (actinomycetem-comitans) A28.8
  - mallei A24.0
  - muris A25.1
- Actinomadura B47.1
- Actinomyces (israelii) (*see also* Actinomycosis) A42.9
- Actinomycetales — *see* Actinomycosis
- actinomycotic NOS — *see* Actinomycosis
- adenoid (and tonsil) J03.90
  - chronic J35.02
- adenovirus NEC
  - as cause of disease classified elsewhere B97.0
  - unspecified nature or site B34.0
- aerogenes capsulatus A48.0
- aertrycke — *see* Infection, salmonella
- alimentary canal NOS — *see* Enteritis, infectious
- Allescheria boydii B48.2
- Alternaria B48.8
- alveolus, alveolar (process) K04.7
- Ameba, amebic (histolytica) — *see* Amebiasis
- amniotic fluid, sac or cavity O41.10- ☑
  - chorioamnionitis O41.12- ☑
  - placentitis O41.14- ☑
- amputation stump (surgical) — *see* Complication, amputation stump, infection
- Ancylostoma (duodenalis) B76.0
- Anisakiasis, Anisakis larvae B81.0
- anthrax — *see* Anthrax
- antrum (chronic) — *see* Sinusitis, maxillary
- anus, anal (papillae) (sphincter) K62.89
- arbovirus (arbor virus) A94
  - specified type NEC A93.8
- artificial insemination N98.0
- Ascaris lumbricoides — *see* Ascariasis
- Ascomycetes B47.0
- Aspergillus (flavus) (fumigatus) (terreus) — *see* Aspergillosis
- atypical
  - acid-fast (bacilli) — *see* Mycobacterium, atypical
  - mycobacteria — *see* Mycobacterium, atypical
  - virus A81.9
    - specified type NEC A81.89
- auditory meatus (external) — *see* Otitis, externa, infective
- auricle (ear) — *see* Otitis, externa, infective
- axillary gland (lymph) L04.2
- Bacillus A49.9
  - abortus A23.1
  - anthracis — *see* Anthrax
  - Ducrey's (any location) A57
  - Flexner's A03.1
  - Friedländer's NEC A49.8
  - gas (gangrene) A48.0
  - mallei A24.0

Infection, infected, infective — *continued*
  Bacillus — *continued*
    melitensis A23.0
    paratyphoid, paratyphosus A01.4
      A A01.1
      B A01.2
      C A01.3
    Shiga (-Kruse) A03.0
    suipestifer — *see* Infection, salmonella
    swimming pool A31.1
    typhosa A01.00
    welchii — *see* Gangrene, gas
  bacterial NOS A49.9
    as cause of disease classified elsewhere B96.89
      Bacteroides fragilis [B. fragilis] B96.6
      Clostridium perfringens [C. perfringens] B96.7
      Enterobacter sakazakii B96.89
      Enterococcus B95.2
      Escherichia coli [E. coli] (*see also* Escherichia coli) B96.20
      Helicobacter pylori [H.pylori] B96.81
      Hemophilus influenzae [H. influenzae] B96.3
      Klebsiella pneumoniae [K. pneumoniae] B96.1
      Mycoplasma pneumoniae [M. pneumoniae] B96.0
      Proteus (mirabilis) (morganii) B96.4
      Pseudomonas (aeruginosa) (mallei) (pseudomallei) B96.5
      Staphylococcus B95.8
        aureus (methicillin susceptible) (MSSA) B95.61
          methicillin resistant (MRSA) B95.62
        specified NEC B95.7
      Streptococcus B95.5
        group A B95.0
        group B B95.1
        pneumoniae B95.3
        specified NEC B95.4
      Vibrio vulnificus B96.82
    specified NEC A48.8
  Bacterium
    paratyphosum A01.4
      A A01.1
      B A01.2
      C A01.3
    typhosum A01.00
  Bacteroides NEC A49.8
    fragilis, as cause of disease classified elsewhere B96.6
  Balantidium coli A07.0
  Bartholin's gland N75.8
  Basidiobolus B46.8
  bile duct (common) (hepatic) — *see* Cholangitis
  bladder — *see* Cystitis
  Blastomyces, blastomycotic (*see also* **Blastomycosis**)
    brasiliensis — *see* Paracoccidioidomycosis
    dermatitidis — *see* Blastomycosis
    European — *see* Cryptococcosis
    Loboi B48.0
    North American B40.9
    South American — *see* Paracoccidioidomycosis
  bleb, postprocedure — *see* Blebitis
  bone — *see* Osteomyelitis
  Bordetella — *see* Whooping cough
  Borrelia bergdorfi A69.20
  brain (*see also* Encephalitis) G04.90
    membranes — *see* Meningitis
    septic G06.0
      meninges — *see* Meningitis, bacterial
  branchial cyst Q18.0
  breast — *see* Mastitis
  bronchus — *see* Bronchitis
  Brucella A23.9
    abortus A23.1
    canis A23.3
    melitensis A23.0
    mixed A23.8
    specified NEC A23.8
    suis A23.2
  Brugia (malayi) B74.1
    timori B74.2
  bursa — *see* Bursitis, infective
  buttocks (skin) L08.9
  Campylobacter, intestinal A04.5
    as cause of disease classified elsewhere B96.81
  Candida (albicans) (tropicalis) — *see* Candidiasis
  candiru B88.8
  Capillaria (intestinal) B81.1

Infection, infected, infective — *continued*
  Capillaria — *continued*
    hepatica B83.8
    philippinensis B81.1
  cartilage — *see* Disorder, cartilage, specified type NEC
  cat liver fluke B66.0
  catheter-related bloodstream (CRBSI) T80.211 ☑
  cellulitis — *code by* site under Cellulitis
  central line-associated T80.219 ☑
    bloodstream (CLABSI) T80.211 ☑
    specified NEC T80.218 ☑
  Cephalosporium falciforme B47.0
  cerebrospinal — *see* Meningitis
  cervical gland (lymph) L04.0
  cervix — *see* Cervicitis
  cesarean delivery wound (puerperal) O86.0
  cestodes — *see* Infestation, cestodes
  chest J22
  Chilomastix (intestinal) A07.8
  Chlamydia, chlamydial A74.9
    anus A56.3
    genitourinary tract A56.2
      lower A56.00
      specified NEC A56.19
    lymphogranuloma A55
    pharynx A56.4
    psittaci A70
    rectum A56.3
    sexually transmitted NEC A56.8
  cholera — *see* Cholera
  Cladosporium
    bantianum (brain abscess) B43.1
    carrionii B43.0
    castellanii B36.1
    trichoides (brain abscess) B43.1
    werneckii B36.1
  Clonorchis (sinensis) (liver) B66.1
  Clostridium NEC
    bifermentans A48.0
    botulinum (food poisoning) A05.1
      infant A48.51
      wound A48.52
    difficile
      as cause of disease classified elsewhere B96.89
      foodborne (disease)
        not specified as recurrent A04.72
        recurrent A04.71
      gas gangrene A48.0
      necrotizing enterocolitis
        not specified as recurrent A04.72
        recurrent A04.71
      sepsis A41.4
    gas-forming NEC A48.0
    histolyticum A48.0
    novyi, causing gas gangrene A48.0
    oedematiens A48.0
    perfringens
      as cause of disease classified elsewhere B96.7
      due to food A05.2
      foodborne (disease) A05.2
      gas gangrene A48.0
      sepsis A41.4
    septicum, causing gas gangrene A48.0
    sordellii, causing gas gangrene A48.0
    welchii
      as cause of disease classified elsewhere B96.7
      foodborne (disease) A05.2
      gas gangrene A48.0
      necrotizing enteritis A05.2
      sepsis A41.4
  Coccidioides (immitis) — *see* Coccidioidomycosis
  colon — *see* Enteritis, infectious
  colostomy K94.02
  common duct — *see* Cholangitis
  congenital P39.9
    Candida (albicans) P37.5
    cytomegalovirus P35.1
    hepatitis, viral P35.3
    herpes simplex P35.2
    infectious or parasitic disease P37.9
      specified NEC P37.8
    listeriosis (disseminated) P37.2
    malaria NEC P37.4
      falciparum P37.3
    Plasmodium falciparum P37.3
    poliomyelitis P35.8
    rubella P35.0
    skin P39.4

Infection, infected, infective — *continued*
  congenital — *continued*
    toxoplasmosis (acute) (subacute) (chronic) P37.1
    tuberculosis P37.0
    urinary (tract) P39.3
    vaccinia P35.8
    virus P35.9
      specified type NEC P35.8
  Conidiobolus B46.8
  coronavirus NEC B34.2
    as cause of disease classified elsewhere B97.29
    severe acute respiratory syndrome (SARS associated) B97.21
  corpus luteum — *see* Salpingo-oophoritis
  Corynebacterium diphtheriae — *see* Diphtheria
  cotia virus B08.8
  Coxiella burnetii A78
  coxsackie — *see* Coxsackie
  Cryptococcus neoformans — *see* Cryptococcosis
  Cryptosporidium A07.2
  Cunninghamella — *see* Mucormycosis
  cyst — *see* Cyst
  cystic duct (*see also* Cholecystitis) K81.9
  Cysticercus cellulosae — *see* Cysticercosis
  cytomegalovirus, cytomegaloviral B25.9
    congenital P35.1
    maternal, maternal care for (suspected) damage to fetus O35.3 ☑
    mononucleosis B27.10
      with
        complication NEC B27.19
        meningitis B27.12
        polyneuropathy B27.11
  delta-agent (acute), in hepatitis B carrier B17.0
  dental (pulpal origin) K04.7
  Deuteromycetes B47.0
  Dicrocoelium dendriticum B66.2
  Dipetalonema (perstans) (streptocerca) B74.4
  diphtherial — *see* Diphtheria
  Diphyllobothrium (adult) (latum) (pacificum) B70.0
    larval B70.1
  Diplogonoporus (grandis) B71.8
  Dipylidium caninum B67.4
  Dirofilaria B74.8
  Dracunculus medinensis B72
  Drechslera (hawaiiensis) B43.8
  Ducrey Haemophilus (any location) A57
  due to or resulting from
    artificial insemination N98.0
    central venous catheter T80.219 ☑
      bloodstream T80.211 ☑
      exit or insertion site T80.212 ☑
      localized T80.212 ☑
      port or reservoir T80.212 ☑
      specified NEC T80.218 ☑
      tunnel T80.212 ☑
    device, implant or graft (*see also* Complications, by site and type, infection or inflammation) T85.79 ☑
      arterial graft NEC T82.7 ☑
      breast (implant) T85.79 ☑
      catheter NEC T85.79 ☑
        dialysis (renal) T82.7 ☑
          intraperitoneal T85.71 ☑
        infusion NEC T82.7 ☑
          cranial T85.735 ☑
          intrathecal T85.735 ☑
          spinal (epidural) (subdural) T85.735 ☑
          subarachnoid T85.735 ☑
        urinary T83.518 ☑
          cystostomy T83.510 ☑
          Hopkins T83.518 ☑
          ileostomy T83.518 ☑
          nephrostomy T83.512 ☑
          specified NEC T83.518 ☑
          urethral indwelling T83.511 ☑
          urostomy T83.518 ☑
      electronic (electrode) (pulse generator) (stimulator)
        bone T84.7 ☑
        cardiac T82.7 ☑
        nervous system T85.738 ☑
          brain T85.731 ☑
          cranial nerve T85.732 ☑
          gastric nerve T85.732 ☑
          generator pocket T85.734 ☑
          neurostimulator generator T85.734 ☑

Infection, infected, infective — *continued*
- due to or resulting from — *continued*
  - device, implant or graft (*see also* Complications, by site and type, infection or inflammation) — *continued*
    - electronic — *continued*
      - nervous system — *continued*
        - peripheral nerve T85.732 ☑
        - sacral nerve T85.732 ☑
        - spinal cord T85.733 ☑
        - vagal nerve T85.732 ☑
      - urinary (indwelling) T83.51 ☑
    - fixation, internal (orthopedic) NEC — *see* Complication, fixation device, infection
    - gastrointestinal (bile duct) (esophagus) T85.79 ☑
    - neurostimulator electrode (lead) T85.732 ☑
    - genital NEC T83.69 ☑
    - heart NEC T82.7 ☑
      - valve (prosthesis) T82.6 ☑
        - graft T82.7 ☑
    - joint prosthesis — *see* Complication, joint prosthesis, Infection
    - ocular (corneal graft) (orbital implant) NEC T85.79 ☑
    - orthopedic NEC T84.7 ☑
    - penile (cylinder) (pump) (resevoir) T83.61 ☑
    - specified NEC T85.79 ☑
    - testicular T83.62 ☑
    - urinary NEC T83.598 ☑
      - ileal conduit stent T83.593 ☑
      - implanted neurostimulation T83.590 ☑
      - implanted sphincter T83.591 ☑
      - indwelling ureteral stent T83.592 ☑
      - nephroureteral stent T83.593 ☑
      - specified stent NEC T83.593 ☑
    - vascular NEC T82.7 ☑
    - ventricular intracranial (communicating) shunt T85.730 ☑
  - Hickman catheter T80.219 ☑
    - bloodstream T80.211 ☑
    - localized T80.212 ☑
    - specified NEC T80.218 ☑
  - immunization or vaccination T88.0 ☑
  - infusion, injection or transfusion NEC T80.29 ☑
  - injury NEC — *code by* site under Wound, open
  - peripherally inserted central catheter (PICC) T80.219 ☑
    - bloodstream T80.211 ☑
    - localized T80.212 ☑
    - specified NEC T80.218 ☑
  - portacath (port-a-cath) T80.219 ☑
    - bloodstream T80.211 ☑
    - localized T80.212 ☑
    - specified NEC T80.218 ☑
  - pulmonary artery catheter — *see* Infection, due to or resulting from, central venous catheter
  - surgery T81.4 ☑
  - Swan Ganz catheter — *see* Infection, due to or resulting from, central venous catheter
  - triple lumen catheter T80.219 ☑
    - bloodstream T80.211 ☑
    - localized T80.212 ☑
    - specified NEC T80.218 ☑
  - umbilical venous catheter T80.219 ☑
    - bloodstream T80.211 ☑
    - localized T80.212 ☑
    - specified NEC T80.218 ☑
- during labor NEC O75.3
- ear (middle) (*see also* Otitis media)
  - external — *see* Otitis, externa, infective
  - inner — *see* subcategory H83.0 ☑
- Eberthella typhosa A01.00
- Echinococcus — *see* Echinococcus
- echovirus
  - as cause of disease classified elsewhere B97.12
  - unspecified nature or site B34.1
- endocardium I33.0
- endocervix — *see* Cervicitis
- Entamoeba — *see* Amebiasis
- enteric — *see* Enteritis, infectious
- Enterobacter sakazakii B96.89
- Enterobius vermicularis B80
- enterostomy K94.12
- enterovirus B34.1
  - as cause of disease classified elsewhere B97.10

- enterovirus — *continued*
  - as cause of disease classified elsewhere — *continued*
    - coxsackievirus B97.11
    - echovirus B97.12
    - specified NEC B97.19
- Entomophthora B46.8
- Epidermophyton — *see* Dermatophytosis
- epididymis — *see* Epididymitis
- episiotomy (puerperal) O86.0
- Erysipelothrix (insidiosa) (rhusiopathiae) — *see* Erysipeloid
- erythema infectiosum B08.3
- Escherichia (E.) coli NEC A49.8
  - as cause of disease classified elsewhere (*see also* Escherichia coli) B96.20
  - congenital P39.8
    - sepsis P36.4
  - generalized A41.51
  - intestinal — *see* Enteritis, infectious, due to, Escherichia coli
- ethmoidal (chronic) (sinus) — *see* Sinusitis, ethmoidal
- eustachian tube (ear) — *see* Salpingitis, eustachian
- external auditory canal (meatus) NEC — *see* Otitis, externa, infective
- eye (purulent) — *see* Endophthalmitis, purulent
- eyelid — *see* Inflammation, eyelid
- fallopian tube — *see* Salpingo-oophoritis
- Fasciola (gigantica) (hepatica) (indica) B66.3
- Fasciolopsis (buski) B66.5
- filarial — *see* Infestation, filarial
- finger (skin) L08.9
  - nail L03.01- ☑
    - fungus B35.1
- fish tapeworm B70.0
  - larval B70.1
- flagellate, intestinal A07.9
- fluke — *see* Infestation, fluke
- focal
  - teeth (pulpal origin) K04.7
  - tonsils J35.01
- Fonsecaea (compactum) (pedrosoi) B43.0
- food — *see* Intoxication, foodborne
- foot (skin) L08.9
  - dermatophytic fungus B35.3
- Francisella tularensis — *see* Tularemia
- frontal (sinus) (chronic) — *see* Sinusitis, frontal
- fungus NOS B49
  - beard B35.0
  - dermatophytic — *see* Dermatophytosis
  - foot B35.3
  - groin B35.6
  - hand B35.2
  - nail B35.1
  - pathogenic to compromised host only B48.8
  - perianal (area) B35.6
  - scalp B35.0
  - skin B36.9
    - foot B35.3
    - hand B35.2
    - toenails B35.1
- Fusarium B48.8
- gallbladder — *see* Cholecystitis
- gas bacillus — *see* Gangrene, gas
- gastrointestinal — *see* Enteritis, infectious
- generalized NEC — *see* Sepsis
- generator pocket, implanted electronic neurostimulator T85.734 ☑
- genital organ or tract
  - female — *see* Disease, pelvis, inflammatory
  - male N49.9
    - multiple sites N49.8
    - specified NEC N49.8
- Ghon tubercle, primary A15.7
- Giardia lamblia A07.1
- gingiva (chronic) K05.10
  - acute K05.00
    - nonplaque induced K05.01
    - plaque induced K05.00
  - nonplaque induced K05.11
  - plaque induced K05.10
- glanders A24.0
- glenosporopsis B48.0
- Gnathostoma (spinigerum) B83.1
- Gongylonema B83.8
- gonococcal — *see* Gonococcus
- gram-negative bacilli NOS A49.9

- guinea worm B72
- gum (chronic) K05.10
  - acute K05.00
    - nonplaque induced K05.01
    - plaque induced K05.00
  - nonplaque induced K05.11
  - plaque induced K05.10
- Haemophilus — *see* Infection, Hemophilus
- heart — *see* Carditis
- Helicobacter pylori A04.8
  - as cause of disease classified elsewhere B96.81
- helminths B83.9
  - intestinal B82.0
    - mixed (types classifiable to more than one of the titles B65.0-B81.3 and B81.8) B81.4
    - specified type NEC B81.8
  - specified type NEC B83.8
- Hemophilus
  - aegyptius, systemic A48.4
  - ducreyi (any location) A57
  - generalized A41.3
  - influenzae NEC A49.2
    - as cause of disease classified elsewhere B96.3
- herpes (simplex) (*see also* Herpes)
  - congenital P35.2
  - disseminated B00.7
  - zoster B02.9
- herpesvirus, herpesviral — *see* Herpes
- Heterophyes (heterophyes) B66.8
- hip (joint) NEC M00.9
  - due to internal joint prosthesis
    - left T84.52 ☑
    - right T84.51 ☑
  - skin NEC L08.9
- Histoplasma — *see* Histoplasmosis
  - American B39.4
  - capsulatum B39.4
- hookworm B76.9
- human
  - papilloma virus A63.0
  - T-cell lymphotropic virus type-1 (HTLV-1) B33.3
- hydrocele N43.0
- Hymenolepis B71.0
- hypopharynx — *see* Pharyngitis
- inguinal (lymph) glands L04.1
  - due to soft chancre A57
- intervertebral disc, pyogenic M46.30
  - cervical region M46.32
  - cervicothoracic region M46.33
  - lumbar region M46.36
  - lumbosacral region M46.37
  - multiple sites M46.39
  - occipito-atlanto-axial region M46.31
  - sacrococcygeal region M46.38
  - thoracic region M46.34
  - thoracolumbar region M46.35
- intestine, intestinal — *see* Enteritis, infectious
  - specified NEC A08.8
- intra-amniotic affecting newborn NEC P39.2
- Isospora belli or hominis A07.3
- Japanese B encephalitis A83.0
- jaw (bone) (lower) (upper) M27.2
- joint NEC M00.9
  - due to internal joint prosthesis T84.50 ☑
- kidney (cortex) (hematogenous) N15.9
  - with calculus N20.0
    - with hydronephrosis N13.6
  - following ectopic gestation O08.83
  - pelvis and ureter (cystic) N28.85
  - puerperal (postpartum) O86.21
  - specified NEC N15.8
- Klebsiella (K.) pneumoniae NEC A49.8
  - as cause of disease classified elsewhere B96.1
- knee (joint) NEC M00.9
  - due to internal joint prosthesis
    - left T84.54 ☑
    - right T84.53 ☑
  - joint M00.9
  - skin L08.9
- Koch's — *see* Tuberculosis
- labia (majora) (minora) (acute) — *see* Vulvitis
- lacrimal
  - gland — *see* Dacryoadenitis
  - passages (duct) (sac) — *see* Inflammation, lacrimal, passages
- lancet fluke B66.2
- larynx NEC J38.7

Infection, infected, infective — *continued*
  leg (skin) NOS L08.9
  Legionella pneumophila A48.1
    nonpneumonic A48.2
  Leishmania (*see also* Leishmaniasis)
    aethiopica B55.1
    braziliensis B55.2
    chagasi B55.0
    donovani B55.0
    infantum B55.0
    major B55.1
    mexicana B55.1
    tropica B55.1
  lentivirus, as cause of disease classified elsewhere B97.31
  Leptosphaeria senegalensis B47.0
  Leptospira interrogans A27.9
    autumnalis A27.89
    canicola A27.89
    hebdomadis A27.89
    icterohaemorrhagiae A27.0
    pomona A27.89
    specified type NEC A27.89
  leptospirochetal NEC — *see* Leptospirosis
  Listeria monocytogenes (*see also* Listeriosis)
    congenital P37.2
  Loa loa B74.3
    with conjunctival infestation B74.3
    eyelid B74.3
  Loboa loboi B48.0
  local, skin (staphylococcal) (streptococcal) L08.9
    abscess — *code by* site under Abscess
    cellulitis — *code by* site under Cellulitis
    specified NEC L08.89
    ulcer — *see* Ulcer, skin
  Loefflerella mallei A24.0
  lung (*see also* Pneumonia) J18.9
    atypical Mycobacterium A31.0
    spirochetal A69.8
    tuberculous — *see* Tuberculosis, pulmonary
    virus — *see* Pneumonia, viral
  lymph gland (*see also* Lymphadenitis, acute)
    mesenteric I88.0
  lymphoid tissue, base of tongue or posterior pharynx, NEC (chronic) J35.03
  Madurella (grisea) (mycetomii) B47.0
  major
    following ectopic or molar pregnancy O08.0
    puerperal, postpartum, childbirth O85
  Malassezia furfur B36.0
  Malleomyces
    mallei A24.0
    pseudomallei (whitmori) — *see* Melioidosis
  mammary gland N61.0
  Mansonella (ozzardi) (perstans) (streptocerca) B74.4
  mastoid — *see* Mastoiditis
  maxilla, maxillary M27.2
    sinus (chronic) — *see* Sinusitis, maxillary
  mediastinum J98.51
  Medina (worm) B72
  meibomian cyst or gland — *see* Hordeolum
  meninges — *see* Meningitis, bacterial
  meningococcal (*see also* condition) A39.9
    adrenals A39.1
    brain A39.81
    cerebrospinal A39.0
    conjunctiva A39.89
    endocardium A39.51
    heart A39.50
      endocardium A39.51
      myocardium A39.52
      pericardium A39.53
    joint A39.83
    meninges A39.0
    meningococcemia A39.4
      acute A39.2
      chronic A39.3
    myocardium A39.52
    pericardium A39.53
    retrobulbar neuritis A39.82
    specified site NEC A39.89
  mesenteric lymph nodes or glands NEC I88.0
  Metagonimus B66.8
  metatarsophalangeal M00.9
  methicillin
    resistant Staphylococcus aureus (MRSA) A49.02
    susceptible Staphylococcus aureus (MSSA) A49.01
  Microsporum, microsporic — *see* Dermatophytosis

Infection, infected, infective — *continued*
  mixed flora (bacterial) NEC A49.8
  Monilia — *see* Candidiasis
  Monosporium apiospermum B48.2
  mouth, parasitic B37.0
  Mucor — *see* Mucormycosis
  muscle NEC — *see* Myositis, infective
  mycelium NOS B49
  mycetoma B47.9
    actinomycotic NEC B47.1
    mycotic NEC B47.0
  Mycobacterium, mycobacterial — *see* Mycobacterium
  Mycoplasma NEC A49.3
    pneumoniae, as cause of disease classified elsewhere B96.0
  mycotic NOS B49
    pathogenic to compromised host only B48.8
    skin NOS B36.9
  myocardium NEC I40.0
  nail (chronic)
    with lymphangitis — *see* Lymphangitis, acute, digit
    finger L03.01- ☑
      fungus B35.1
    ingrowing L60.0
    toe L03.03- ☑
      fungus B35.1
  nasal sinus (chronic) — *see* Sinusitis
  nasopharynx — *see* Nasopharyngitis
  navel L08.82
  Necator americanus B76.1
  Neisseria — *see* Gonococcus
  Neotestudina rosatii B47.0
  newborn P39.9
    intra-amniotic NEC P39.2
    skin P39.4
    specified type NEC P39.8
  nipple N61.0
    associated with
      lactation O91.03
      pregnancy O91.01- ☑
      puerperium O91.02
  Nocardia — *see* Nocardiosis
  obstetrical surgical wound (puerperal) O86.0
  Oesophagostomum (apiostomum) B81.8
  Oestrus ovis — *see* Myiasis
  Oidium albicans B37.9
  Onchocerca (volvulus) — *see* Onchocerciasis
  oncovirus, as cause of disease classified elsewhere B97.32
  operation wound T81.4 ☑
  Opisthorchis (felineus) (viverrini) B66.0
  orbit, orbital — *see* Inflammation, orbit
  orthopoxvirus NEC B08.09
  ovary — *see* Salpingo-oophoritis
  Oxyuris vermicularis B80
  pancreas (acute) — *see* Pancreatitis, acute
    abscess — *see* Pancreatitis, acute
    specified NEC (*see also* Pancreatitis, acute) K85.80
  papillomavirus, as cause of disease classified elsewhere B97.7
  papovavirus NEC B34.4
  Paracoccidioides brasiliensis — *see* Paracoccidioidomycosis
  Paragonimus (westermani) B66.4
  parainfluenza virus B34.8
  parameningococcus NOS A39.9
  parapoxvirus B08.60
    specified NEC B08.69
  parasitic B89
  Parastrongylus
    cantonensis B83.2
    costaricensis B81.3
    paratyphoid A01.4
      Type A A01.1
      Type B A01.2
      Type C A01.3
  paraurethral ducts N34.2
  parotid gland — *see* Sialoadenitis
  parvovirus NEC B34.3
    as cause of disease classified elsewhere B97.6
  Pasteurella NEC A28.0
    multocida A28.0
    pestis — *see* Plague
    pseudotuberculosis A28.0
    septica (cat bite) (dog bite) A28.0
    tularensis — *see* Tularemia
  pelvic, female — *see* Disease, pelvis, inflammatory

Infection, infected, infective — *continued*
  Penicillium (marneffei) B48.4
  penis (glans) (retention) NEC N48.29
  periapical K04.5
  peridental, periodontal K05.20
    generalized — *see* Peridontitis, aggressive, generalized
    localized — *see* Peridontitis, aggressive, localized
  perinatal period P39.9
    specified type NEC P39.8
  perineal repair (puerperal) O86.0
  periorbital — *see* Inflammation, orbit
  perirectal K62.89
  perirenal — *see* Infection, kidney
  peritoneal — *see* Peritonitis
  periureteral N28.89
  Petriellidium boydii B48.2
  pharynx (*see also* Pharyngitis)
    coxsackievirus B08.5
    posterior, lymphoid (chronic) J35.03
  Phialophora
    gougerotii (subcutaneous abscess or cyst) B43.2
    jeanselmei (subcutaneous abscess or cyst) B43.2
    verrucosa (skin) B43.0
  Piedraia hortae B36.3
  pinta A67.9
    intermediate A67.1
    late A67.2
    mixed A67.3
    primary A67.0
  pinworm B80
  pityrosporum furfur B36.0
  pleuro-pneumonia-like organism (PPLO) NEC A49.3
    as cause of disease classified elsewhere B96.0
  pneumococcus, pneumococcal NEC A49.1
    as cause of disease classified elsewhere B95.3
    generalized (purulent) A40.3
      with pneumonia J13
  Pneumocystis carinii (pneumonia) B59
  Pneumocystis jiroveci (pneumonia) B59
  port or reservoir T80.212 ☑
  postoperative T81.4 ☑
  postoperative wound T81.4 ☑
  postprocedural T81.4 ☑
  postvaccinal T88.0 ☑
  prepuce NEC N47.7
    with penile inflammation N47.6
  prion — *see* Disease, prion, central nervous system
  prostate (capsule) — *see* Prostatitis
  Proteus (mirabilis) (morganii) (vulgaris) NEC A49.8
    as cause of disease classified elsewhere B96.4
  protozoal NEC B64
    intestinal A07.9
      specified NEC A07.8
    specified NEC B60.8
  Pseudoallescheria boydii B48.2
  Pseudomonas NEC A49.8
    as cause of disease classified elsewhere B96.5
    mallei A24.0
    pneumonia J15.1
    pseudomallei — *see* Melioidosis
  puerperal O86.4
    genitourinary tract NEC O86.89
    major or generalized O85
    minor O86.4
    specified NEC O86.89
  pulmonary — *see* Infection, lung
  purulent — *see* Abscess
  Pyrenochaeta romeroi B47.0
  Q fever A78
  rectum (sphincter) K62.89
  renal (*see also* Infection, kidney)
    pelvis and ureter (cystic) N28.85
  reovirus, as cause of disease classified elsewhere B97.5
  respiratory (tract) NEC J98.8
    acute J22
    chronic J98.8
    influenzal (upper) (acute) — *see* Influenza, with, respiratory manifestations NEC
    lower (acute) J22
      chronic — *see* Bronchitis, chronic
    rhinovirus J00
    syncytial virus, as cause of disease classified elsewhere B97.4
    upper (acute) NOS J06.9
      chronic J39.8
      streptococcal J06.9
      viral NOS J06.9

Infection, infected, infective — *continued*
  resulting from
    presence of internal prosthesis, implant, graft —
      see Complications, by site and type, infection
  retortamoniasis A07.8
  retroperitoneal NEC K68.9
  retrovirus B33.3
    as cause of disease classified elsewhere B97.30
      human
        immunodeficiency, type 2 (HIV 2) B97.35
        T-cell lymphotropic
          type I (HTLV-I) B97.33
          type II (HTLV-II) B97.34
      lentivirus B97.31
      oncovirus B97.32
      specified NEC B97.39
  Rhinosporidium (seeberi) B48.1
  rhinovirus
    as cause of disease classified elsewhere B97.89
    unspecified nature or site B34.8
  Rhizopus — *see* Mucormycosis
  rickettsial NOS A79.9
  roundworm (large) NEC B82.0
    Ascariasis (*see also* Ascariasis) B77.9
  rubella — *see* Rubella
  Saccharomyces — *see* Candidiasis
  salivary duct or gland (any) — *see* Sialoadenitis
  Salmonella (aertrycke) (arizonae) (callinarum)
    (cholerae-suis) (enteritidis) (suipestifer) (ty-
    phimurium) A02.9
    with
      (gastro)enteritis A02.0
      sepsis A02.1
      specified manifestation NEC A02.8
    due to food (poisoning) A02.9
    hirschfeldii A01.3
    localized A02.20
      arthritis A02.23
      meningitis A02.21
      osteomyelitis A02.24
      pneumonia A02.22
      pyelonephritis A02.25
      specified NEC A02.29
    paratyphi A01.4
      A A01.1
      B A01.2
      C A01.3
    schottmuelleri A01.2
    typhi, typhosa — *see* Typhoid
  Sarcocystis A07.8
  scabies B86
  Schistosoma — *see* Infestation, Schistosoma
  scrotum (acute) NEC N49.2
  seminal vesicle — *see* Vesiculitis
  septic
    localized, skin — *see* Abscess
  sheep liver fluke B66.3
  Shigella A03.9
    boydii A03.2
    dysenteriae A03.0
    flexneri A03.1
    group
      A A03.0
      B A03.1
      C A03.2
      D A03.3
    Schmitz (-Stutzer) A03.0
    schmitzii A03.0
    shigae A03.0
    sonnei A03.3
    specified NEC A03.8
  shoulder (joint) NEC M00.9
    due to internal joint prosthesis T84.59 ☑
    skin NEC L08.9
  sinus (accessory) (chronic) (nasal) (*see also* Sinusitis)
    pilonidal — *see* Sinus, pilonidal
    skin NEC L08.89
  Skene's duct or gland — *see* Urethritis
  skin (local) (staphylococcal) (streptococcal) L08.9
    abscess — *code by* site under Abscess
    cellulitis — *code by* site under Cellulitis
    due to fungus B36.9
      specified type NEC B36.8
    mycotic B36.9
      specified type NEC B36.8
    newborn P39.4
    ulcer — *see* Ulcer, skin
  slow virus A81.9

Infection, infected, infective — *continued*
  slow virus — *continued*
    specified NEC A81.89
  Sparganum (mansoni) (proliferum) (baxteri) B70.1
  specific (*see also* Syphilis)
    to perinatal period — *see* Infection, congenital
  specified NEC B99.8
  spermatic cord NEC N49.1
  sphenoidal (sinus) — *see* Sinusitis, sphenoidal
  spinal cord NOS (*see also* Myelitis) G04.91
    abscess G06.1
    meninges — *see* Meningitis
    streptococcal G04.89
  Spirillum A25.0
  spirochetal NOS A69.9
    lung A69.8
    specified NEC A69.8
  Spirometra larvae B70.1
  spleen D73.89
  Sporotrichum, Sporothrix (schenckii) — *see* Sporotri-
    chosis
  staphylococcal, unspecified site
    as cause of disease classified elsewhere B95.8
      aureus (methicillin susceptible) (MSSA) B95.61
        methicillin resistant (MRSA) B95.62
      specified NEC B95.7
    aureus (methicillin susceptible) (MSSA) A49.01
      methicillin resistant (MRSA) A49.02
    food poisoning A05.0
    generalized (purulent) A41.2
    pneumonia — *see* Pneumonia, staphylococcal
  Stellantchasmus falcatus B66.8
  streptobacillus moniliformis A25.1
  streptococcal NEC A49.1
    as cause of disease classified elsewhere B95.5
    B genitourinary complicating
      childbirth O98.82
      pregnancy O98.81- ☑
      puerperium O98.83
    congenital
      sepsis P36.10
        group B P36.0
        specified NEC P36.19
    generalized (purulent) A40.9
  Streptomyces B47.1
  Strongyloides (stercoralis) — *see* Strongyloidiasis
  stump (amputation) (surgical) — *see* Complication,
    amputation stump, infection
  subcutaneous tissue, local L08.9
  suipestifer — *see* Infection, salmonella
  swimming pool bacillus A31.1
  Taenia — *see* Infestation, Taenia
  Taeniarhynchus saginatus B68.1
  tapeworm — *see* Infestation, tapeworm
  tendon (sheath) — *see* Tenosynovitis, infective NEC
  Ternidens diminutus B81.8
  testis — *see* Orchitis
  threadworm B80
  throat — *see* Pharyngitis
  thyroglossal duct K14.8
  toe (skin) L08.9
    cellulitis L03.03- ☑
      fungus B35.1
    nail L03.03- ☑
      fungus B35.1
  tongue NEC K14.0
    parasitic B37.0
  tonsil (and adenoid) (faucial) (lingual) (pharyngeal) —
    see Tonsillitis
  tooth, teeth K04.7
    periapical K04.7
    peridental, periodontal K05.20
      generalized — *see* Peridontitis, aggressive,
        generalized
      localized — *see* Peridontitis, aggressive, local-
        ized
    pulp K04.01
      irreversible K04.02
      reversible K04.01
    socket M27.3
  TORCH — *see* Infection, congenital
    without active infection P00.2
  Torula histolytica — *see* Cryptococcosis
  Toxocara (canis) (cati) (felis) B83.0
  Toxoplasma gondii — *see* Toxoplasma
  trachea, chronic J42
  trematode NEC — *see* Infestation, fluke
  trench fever A79.0

Infection, infected, infective — *continued*
  Treponema pallidum — *see* Syphilis
  Trichinella (spiralis) B75
  Trichomonas A59.9
    cervix A59.09
    intestine A07.8
    prostate A59.02
    specified site NEC A59.8
    urethra A59.03
    urogenitalis A59.00
    vagina A59.01
    vulva A59.01
  Trichophyton, trichophytic — *see* Dermatophytosis
  Trichosporon (beigelii) cutaneum B36.2
  Trichostrongylus B81.2
  Trichuris (trichiura) B79
  Trombicula (irritans) B88.0
  Trypanosoma
    brucei
      gambiense B56.0
      rhodesiense B56.1
    cruzi — *see* Chagas' disease
  tubal — *see* Salpingo-oophoritis
  tuberculous NEC — *see* Tuberculosis
  tubo-ovarian — *see* Salpingo-oophoritis
  tunica vaginalis N49.1
  tunnel T80.212 ☑
  tympanic membrane NEC — *see* Myringitis
  typhoid (abortive) (ambulant) (bacillus) — *see* Typhoid
  typhus A75.9
    flea-borne A75.2
    mite-borne A75.3
    recrudescent A75.1
    tick-borne A77.9
      African A77.1
      North Asian A77.2
  umbilicus L08.82
  ureter N28.86
  urethra — *see* Urethritis
  urinary (tract) N39.0
    bladder — *see* Cystitis
    complicating
      pregnancy O23.4- ☑
        specified type NEC O23.3- ☑
    kidney — *see* Infection, kidney
    newborn P39.3
    puerperal (postpartum) O86.20
    tuberculous A18.13
    urethra — *see* Urethritis
  uterus, uterine — *see* Endometritis
  vaccination T88.0 ☑
  vaccinia not from vaccination B08.011
  vagina (acute) — *see* Vaginitis
  varicella B01.9
  varicose veins — *see* Varix
  vas deferens NEC N49.1
  vesical — *see* Cystitis
  Vibrio
    cholerae A00.0
      El Tor A00.1
    parahaemolyticus (food poisoning) A05.3
    vulnificus
      as cause of disease classified elsewhere B96.82
      foodborne intoxication A05.5
  Vincent's (gum) (mouth) (tonsil) A69.1
  virus, viral NOS B34.9
    adenovirus
      as cause of disease classified elsewhere B97.0
      unspecified nature or site B34.0
    arborvirus, arbovirus arthropod-borne A94
    as cause of disease classified elsewhere B97.89
      adenovirus B97.0
      coronavirus B97.29
        SARS-associated B97.21
      coxsackievirus B97.11
      echovirus B97.12
      enterovirus B97.10
        coxsackievirus B97.11
        echovirus B97.12
        specified NEC B97.19
      human
        immunodeficiency, type 2 (HIV 2) B97.35
        metapneumovirus B97.81
        T-cell lymphotropic,
          type I (HTLV-I) B97.33
          type II (HTLV-II) B97.34
      papillomavirus B97.7
      parvovirus B97.6

Infection, infected, infective — *continued*
  virus, viral — *continued*
    as cause of disease classified elsewhere — *continued*
      reovirus B97.5
      respiratory syncytial B97.4
      retrovirus B97.30
        human
          immunodeficiency, type 2 (HIV 2) B97.35
          T-cell lymphotropic,
            type I (HTLV-I) B97.33
            type II (HTLV-II) B97.34
        lentivirus B97.31
        oncovirus B97.32
        specified NEC B97.39
      specified NEC B97.89
    central nervous system A89
      atypical A81.9
        specified NEC A81.89
      enterovirus NEC A88.8
        meningitis A87.0
      slow virus A81.9
        specified NEC A81.89
      specified NEC A88.8
    chest J98.8
    cotia B08.8
    coxsackie (*see also* Infection, coxsackie) B34.1
      as cause of disease classified elsewhere B97.11
    ECHO
      as cause of disease classified elsewhere B97.12
      unspecified nature or site B34.1
    encephalitis, tick-borne A84.9
    enterovirus, as cause of disease classified elsewhere B97.10
      coxsackievirus B97.11
      echovirus B97.12
      specified NEC B97.19
    exanthem NOS B09
    human metapneumovirus as cause of disease classified elsewhere B97.81
    human papilloma as cause of disease classified elsewhere B97.7
    intestine — *see* Enteritis, viral
    respiratory syncytial
      as cause of disease classified elsewhere B97.4
      bronchopneumonia J12.1
      common cold syndrome J00
      nasopharyngitis (acute) J00
    rhinovirus
      as cause of disease classified elsewhere B97.89
      unspecified nature or site B34.8
    slow A81.9
      specified NEC A81.89
    specified type NEC B33.8
      as cause of disease classified elsewhere B97.89
      unspecified nature or site B34.8
    unspecified nature or site B34.9
    West Nile — *see* Virus, West Nile
  vulva (acute) — *see* Vulvitis
  West Nile — *see* Virus, West Nile
  whipworm B79
  worms B83.9
    specified type NEC B83.8
  Wuchereria (bancrofti) B74.0
    malayi B74.1
  yatapoxvirus B08.70
    specified NEC B08.79
  yeast (*see also* Candidiasis) B37.9
  yellow fever — *see* Fever, yellow
  Yersinia
    enterocolitica (intestinal) A04.6
    pestis — *see* Plague
    pseudotuberculosis A28.2
  Zeis' gland — *see* Hordeolum
  Zika virus A92.5
  zoonotic bacterial NOS A28.9
  Zopfia senegalensis B47.0
Infective, infectious — *see* condition
Infertility
  female N97.9
    age-related N97.8
    associated with
      anovulation N97.0
      cervical (mucus) disease or anomaly N88.3
      congenital anomaly
        cervix N88.3
        fallopian tube N97.1
        uterus N97.2

Infertility — *continued*
  female — *continued*
    associated with — *continued*
      congenital anomaly — *continued*
        vagina N97.8
      dysmucorrhea N88.3
      fallopian tube disease or anomaly N97.1
      pituitary-hypothalamic origin E23.0
      specified origin NEC N97.8
      Stein-Leventhal syndrome E28.2
      uterine disease or anomaly N97.2
      vaginal disease or anomaly N97.8
    due to
      cervical anomaly N88.3
      fallopian tube anomaly N97.1
      ovarian failure E28.39
      Stein-Leventhal syndrome E28.2
      uterine anomaly N97.2
      vaginal anomaly N97.8
    nonimplantation N97.2
    origin
      cervical N88.3
      tubal (block) (occlusion) (stenosis) N97.1
      uterine N97.2
      vaginal N97.8
  male N46.9
    azoospermia N46.01
      extratesticular cause N46.029
        drug therapy N46.021
        efferent duct obstruction N46.023
        infection N46.022
        radiation N46.024
        specified cause NEC N46.029
        systemic disease N46.025
    oligospermia N46.11
      extratesticular cause N46.129
        drug therapy N46.121
        efferent duct obstruction N46.123
        infection N46.122
        radiation N46.124
        specified cause NEC N46.129
        systemic disease N46.125
    specified type NEC N46.8
Infestation B88.9
  Acanthocheilonema (perstans) (streptocerca) B74.4
  Acariasis B88.0
    demodex folliculorum B88.0
    sarcoptes scabiei B86
    trombiculae B88.0
  Agamofilaria streptocerca B74.4
  Ancylostoma, ankylostoma (braziliense) (caninum) (ceylanicum) (duodenale) B76.0
    americanum B76.1
    new world B76.1
  Anisakis larvae, anisakiasis B81.0
  arthropod NEC B88.2
  Ascaris lumbricoides — *see* Ascariasis
  Balantidium coli A07.0
  beef tapeworm B68.1
  Bothriocephalus (latus) B70.0
    larval B70.1
  broad tapeworm B70.0
    larval B70.1
  Brugia (malayi) B74.1
    timori B74.2
  candiru B88.8
  Capillaria
    hepatica B83.8
    philippinensis B81.1
  cat liver fluke B66.0
  cestodes B71.9
    diphyllobothrium — *see* Infestation, diphyllobothrium
    dipylidiasis B71.1
    hymenolepiasis B71.0
    specified type NEC B71.8
  chigger B88.0
  chigo, chigoe B88.1
  Clonorchis (sinensis) (liver) B66.1
  coccidial A07.3
  crab-lice B85.3
  Cysticercus cellulosae — *see* Cysticercosis
  Demodex (folliculorum) B88.0
  Dermanyssus gallinae B88.0
  Dermatobia (hominis) — *see* Myiasis
  Dibothriocephalus (latus) B70.0
    larval B70.1
  Dicrocoelium dendriticum B66.2

Infestation — *continued*
  Diphyllobothrium (adult) (latum) (intestinal) (pacificum) B70.0
    larval B70.1
  Diplogonoporus (grandis) B71.8
  Dipylidium caninum B67.4
  Distoma hepaticum B66.3
  dog tapeworm B67.4
  Dracunculus medinensis B72
  dragon worm B72
  dwarf tapeworm B71.0
  Echinococcus — *see* Echinococcus
  Echinostomum ilocanum B66.8
  Entamoeba (histolytica) — *see* Infection, Ameba
  Enterobius vermicularis B80
  eyelid
    in (due to)
      leishmaniasis B55.1
      loiasis B74.3
      onchocerciasis B73.09
      phthiriasis B85.3
    parasitic NOS B89
  eyeworm B74.3
  Fasciola (gigantica) (hepatica) (indica) B66.3
  Fasciolopsis (buski) (intestine) B66.5
  filarial B74.9
    bancroftian B74.0
    conjunctiva B74.9
    due to
      Acanthocheilonema (perstans) (streptocerca) B74.4
      Brugia (malayi) B74.1
        timori B74.2
      Dracunculus medinensis B72
      guinea worm B72
      loa loa B74.3
      Mansonella (ozzardi) (perstans) (streptocerca) B74.4
      Onchocerca volvulus B73.00
        eye B73.00
        eyelid B73.09
      Wuchereria (bancrofti) B74.0
    Malayan B74.1
    ozzardi B74.4
    specified type NEC B74.8
  fish tapeworm B70.0
    larval B70.1
  fluke B66.9
    blood NOS — *see* Schistosomiasis
    cat liver B66.0
    intestinal B66.5
    lancet B66.2
    liver (sheep) B66.3
      cat B66.0
      Chinese B66.1
      due to clonorchiasis B66.1
      oriental B66.1
    lung (oriental) B66.4
    sheep liver B66.3
    specified type NEC B66.8
  fly larvae — *see* Myiasis
  Gasterophilus (intestinalis) — *see* Myiasis
  Gastrodiscoides hominis B66.8
  Giardia lamblia A07.1
  Gnathostoma (spinigerum) B83.1
  Gongylonema B83.8
  guinea worm B72
  helminth B83.9
    angiostrongyliasis B83.2
      intestinal B81.3
    gnathostomiasis B83.1
    hirudiniasis, internal B83.4
    intestinal B82.0
      angiostrongyliasis B81.3
      anisakiasis B81.0
      ascariasis — *see* Ascariasis
      capillariasis B81.1
      cysticercosis — *see* Cysticercosis
      diphyllobothriasis — *see* Infestation, diphyllobothriasis
      dracunculiasis B72
      echinococcus — *see* Echinococcosis
      enterobiasis B80
      filariasis — *see* Infestation, filarial
      fluke — *see* Infestation, fluke
      hookworm — *see* Infestation, hookworm
      mixed (types classifiable to more than one of the titles B65.0-B81.3 and B81.8) B81.4

Infestation — continued
  helminth — continued
    intestinal — continued
      onchocerciasis — see Onchocerciasis
      schistosomiasis — see Infestation, schistosoma
      specified
        cestode NEC — see Infestation, cestode
        type NEC B81.8
      strongyloidiasis — see Strongyloidiasis
      taenia — see Infestation, taenia
      trichinellosis B75
      trichostrongyliasis B81.2
      trichuriasis B79
    specified type NEC B83.8
    syngamiasis B83.3
    visceral larva migrans B83.0
  Heterophyes (heterophyes) B66.8
  hookworm B76.9
    ancylostomiasis B76.0
    necatoriasis B76.1
    specified type NEC B76.8
  Hymenolepis (diminuta) (nana) B71.0
  intestinal NEC B82.9
  leeches (aquatic) (land) — see Hirudiniasis
  Leishmania — see Leishmaniasis
  lice, louse — see Infestation, Pediculus
  Linguatula B88.8
  Liponyssoides sanguineus B88.0
  Loa loa B74.3
    conjunctival B74.3
    eyelid B74.3
  louse — see Infestation, Pediculus
  maggots — see Myiasis
  Mansonella (ozzardi) (perstans) (streptocerca) B74.4
  Medina (worm) B72
  Metagonimus (yokogawai) B66.8
  microfilaria streptocerca — see Onchocerciasis
    eye B73.00
    eyelid B73.09
  mites B88.9
    scabic B86
  Monilia (albicans) — see Candidiasis
  mouth B37.0
  Necator americanus B76.1
  nematode NEC (intestinal) B82.0
    Ancylostoma B76.0
    conjunctiva NEC B83.9
    Enterobius vermicularis B80
    Gnathostoma spinigerum B83.1
    physaloptera B80
    specified NEC B81.8
    trichostrongylus B81.2
    trichuris (trichuria) B79
  Oesophagostomum (apiostomum) B81.8
  Oestrus ovis (see also Myiasis) B87.9
  Onchocerca (volvulus) — see Onchocerciasis
  Opisthorchis (felineus) (viverrini) B66.0
  orbit, parasitic NOS B89
  Oxyuris vermicularis B80
  Paragonimus (westermani) B66.4
  parasite, parasitic B89
    eyelid B89
    intestinal NOS B82.9
    mouth B37.0
    skin B88.9
    tongue B37.0
  Parastrongylus
    cantonensis B83.2
    costaricensis B81.3
  Pediculus B85.2
    body B85.1
    capitis (humanus) (any site) B85.0
    corporis (humanus) (any site) B85.1
    head B85.0
    mixed (classifiable to more than one of the titles B85.0 - B85.3) B85.4
    pubis (any site) B85.3
  Pentastoma B88.8
  Phthirus (pubis) (any site) B85.3
    with any infestation classifiable to B85.0 - B85.2 B85.4
  pinworm B80
  pork tapeworm (adult) B68.0
  protozoal NEC B64
    intestinal A07.9
      specified NEC A07.8
    specified NEC B60.8
  pubic, louse B85.3

Infestation — continued
  rat tapeworm B71.0
  red bug B88.0
  roundworm (large) NEC B82.0
    Ascariasis (see also Ascariasis) B77.9
  sandflea B88.1
  Sarcoptes scabiei B86
  scabies B86
  Schistosoma B65.9
    bovis B65.8
    cercariae B65.3
    haematobium B65.0
    intercalatum B65.8
    japonicum B65.2
    mansoni B65.1
    mattheei B65.8
    mekongi B65.8
    specified type NEC B65.8
    spindale B65.8
  screw worms — see Myiasis
  skin NOS B88.9
  Sparganum (mansoni) (proliferum) (baxteri) B70.1
    larval B70.1
  specified type NEC B88.8
  Spirometra larvae B70.1
  Stellantchasmus falcatus B66.8
  Strongyloides stercoralis — see Strongyloidiasis
  Taenia B68.9
    diminuta B71.0
    echinococcus — see Echinococcus
    mediocanellata B68.1
    nana B71.0
    saginata B68.1
    solium (intestinal form) B68.0
      larval form — see Cysticercosis
  Taeniarhynchus saginatus B68.1
  tapeworm B71.9
    beef B68.1
    broad B70.0
      larval B70.1
    dog B67.4
    dwarf B71.0
    fish B70.0
      larval B70.1
    pork B68.0
    rat B71.0
  Ternidens diminutus B81.8
  Tetranychus molestissimus B88.0
  threadworm B80
  tongue B37.0
  Toxocara (canis) (cati) (felis) B83.0
  trematode(s) NEC — see Infestation, fluke
  Trichinella (spiralis) B75
  Trichocephalus B79
  Trichomonas — see Trichomoniasis
  Trichostrongylus B81.2
  Trichuris (trichiura) B79
  Trombicula (irritans) B88.0
  Tunga penetrans B88.1
  Uncinaria americana B76.1
  Vandellia cirrhosa B88.8
  whipworm B79
  worms B83.9
    intestinal B82.0
  Wuchereria (bancrofti) B74.0

Infiltrate, infiltration
  amyloid (generalized) (localized) — see Amyloidosis
  calcareous NEC R89.7
    localized — see Degeneration, by site
  calcium salt R89.7
  cardiac
    fatty — see Degeneration, myocardial
    glycogenic E74.02 [I43]
  corneal — see Edema, cornea
  eyelid — see Inflammation, eyelid
  glycogen, glycogenic — see Disease, glycogen storage
  heart, cardiac
    fatty — see Degeneration, myocardial
    glycogenic E74.02 [I43]
  inflammatory in vitreous H43.89
  kidney N28.89
  leukemic — see Leukemia
  liver K76.89
    fatty — see Fatty, liver NEC
    glycogen (see also Disease, glycogen storage) E74.03 [K77]
  lung R91.8
    eosinophilic J82

Infiltrate, infiltration — continued
  lymphatic (see also Leukemia, lymphatic) C91.9- ☑
    gland I88.9
  muscle, fatty M62.89
  myocardium, myocardial
    fatty — see Degeneration, myocardial
    glycogenic E74.02 [I43]
  on chest x-ray R91.8
  pulmonary R91.8
    with eosinophilia J82
  skin (lymphocytic) L98.6
  thymus (gland) (fatty) E32.8
  urine R39.0
  vesicant agent
    antineoplastic chemotherapy T80.810 ☑
    other agent NEC T80.818 ☑
  vitreous body H43.89
Infirmity R68.89
  senile R54
Inflammation, inflamed, inflammatory (with exudation)
  abducent (nerve) — see Strabismus, paralytic, sixth nerve
  accessory sinus (chronic) — see Sinusitis
  adrenal (gland) E27.8
  alveoli, teeth M27.3
    scorbutic E54
  anal canal, anus K62.89
  antrum (chronic) — see Sinusitis, maxillary
  appendix — see Appendicitis
  arachnoid — see Meningitis
  areola N61.0
    puerperal, postpartum or gestational — see Infection, nipple
  areolar tissue NOS L08.9
  artery — see Arteritis
  auditory meatus (external) — see Otitis, externa
  Bartholin's gland N75.8
  bile duct (common) (hepatic) or passage — see Cholangitis
  bladder — see Cystitis
  bone — see Osteomyelitis
  brain (see also Encephalitis)
    membrane — see Meningitis
  breast N61.0
    puerperal, postpartum, gestational — see Mastitis, obstetric
  broad ligament — see Disease, pelvis, inflammatory
  bronchi — see Bronchitis
  catarrhal J00
  cecum — see Appendicitis
  cerebral (see also Encephalitis)
    membrane — see Meningitis
  cerebrospinal
    meningococcal A39.0
  cervix (uteri) — see Cervicitis
  chest J98.8
  chorioretinal H30.9- ☑
    cyclitis — see Cyclitis
    disseminated H30.10- ☑
      generalized H30.13- ☑
      peripheral H30.12- ☑
      posterior pole H30.11- ☑
    epitheliopathy — see Epitheliopathy
    focal H30.00- ☑
      juxtapapillary H30.01- ☑
      macular H30.04- ☑
      paramacular — see Inflammation, chorioretinal, focal, macular
      peripheral H30.03- ☑
      posterior pole H30.02- ☑
    specified type NEC H30.89- ☑
  choroid — see Inflammation, chorioretinal
  chronic, postmastoidectomy cavity — see Complications, postmastoidectomy, inflammation
  colon — see Enteritis
  connective tissue (diffuse) NEC — see Disorder, soft tissue, specified type NEC
  cornea — see Keratitis
  corpora cavernosa N48.29
  cranial nerve — see Disorder, nerve, cranial
  Douglas' cul-de-sac or pouch (chronic) N73.0
  due to device, implant or graft (see also Complications, by site and type, infection or inflammation)
    arterial graft T82.7 ☑
    breast (implant) T85.79 ☑
    catheter T85.79 ☑

Inflammation, inflamed, inflammatory — *continued*
- due to device, implant or graft (*see also* Complications, by site and type, infection or inflammation) — *continued*
  - catheter — *continued*
    - dialysis (renal) T82.7 ☑
      - intraperitoneal T85.71 ☑
    - infusion T82.7 ☑
      - cranial T85.735 ☑
      - intrathecal T85.735 ☑
      - spinal (epidural) (subdural) T85.735 ☑
      - subarachnoid T85.735 ☑
    - urinary T83.518 ☑
      - cystostomy T83.510 ☑
      - Hopkins T83.518 ☑
      - ileostomy T83.518 ☑
      - nephrostomy T83.512 ☑
      - specified NEC T83.518 ☑
      - urethral indwelling T83.511 ☑
      - urostomy T83.518 ☑
  - electronic (electrode) (pulse generator) (stimulator)
    - bone T84.7 ☑
    - cardiac T82.7 ☑
    - nervous system T85.738 ☑
      - brain T85.731 ☑
      - cranial nerve T85.732 ☑
      - gastric nerve T85.732 ☑
      - neurostimulator generator T85.734 ☑
      - peripheral nerve T85.732 ☑
      - sacral nerve T85.732 ☑
      - spinal cord T85.733 ☑
      - vagal nerve T85.732 ☑
    - urinary T83.590 ☑
  - fixation, internal (orthopedic) NEC — *see* Complication, fixation device, infection
  - gastrointestinal (bile duct) (esophagus) T85.79 ☑
    - neurostimulator electrode (lead) T85.732 ☑
  - genital NEC T83.69 ☑
  - heart NEC T82.7 ☑
    - valve (prosthesis) T82.6 ☑
      - graft T82.7 ☑
  - joint prosthesis — *see* Complication, joint prosthesis, infection
  - ocular (corneal graft) (orbital implant) NEC T85.79 ☑
  - orthopedic NEC T84.7 ☑
  - penile (cylinder) (pump) (resevoir) T83.61 ☑
  - specified NEC T85.79 ☑
  - testicular T83.62 ☑
  - urinary NEC T83.598 ☑
    - ileal conduit stent T83.593 ☑
    - implanted neurostimulation T83.590 ☑
    - implanted sphincter T83.591 ☑
    - indwelling ureteral stent T83.592 ☑
    - nephroureteral stent T83.593 ☑
    - specified stent NEC T83.593 ☑
  - vascular NEC T82.7 ☑
  - ventricular intracranial (communicating) shunt T85.730 ☑
- duodenum K29.80
  - with bleeding K29.81
- dura mater — *see* Meningitis
- ear (middle) (*see also* Otitis, media)
  - external — *see* Otitis, externa
  - inner — *see* subcategory H83.0 ☑
- epididymis — *see* Epididymitis
- esophagus K20.9
- ethmoidal (sinus) (chronic) — *see* Sinusitis, ethmoidal
- eustachian tube (catarrhal) — *see* Salpingitis, eustachian
- eyelid H01.9
  - abscess — *see* Abscess, eyelid
  - blepharitis — *see* Blepharitis
  - chalazion — *see* Chalazion
  - dermatosis (noninfectious) — *see* Dermatosis, eyelid
  - hordeolum — *see* Hordeolum
  - specified NEC H01.8
- fallopian tube — *see* Salpingo-oophoritis
- fascia — *see* Myositis
- follicular, pharynx J31.2
- frontal (sinus) (chronic) — *see* Sinusitis, frontal
- gallbladder — *see* Cholecystitis
- gastric — *see* Gastritis
- gastrointestinal — *see* Enteritis

Inflammation, inflamed, inflammatory — *continued*
- genital organ (internal) (diffuse)
  - female — *see* Disease, pelvis, inflammatory
  - male N49.9
    - multiple sites N49.8
    - specified NEC N49.8
- gland (lymph) — *see* Lymphadenitis
- glottis — *see* Laryngitis
- granular, pharynx J31.2
- gum K05.10
  - nonplaque induced K05.11
  - plaque induced K05.10
- heart — *see* Carditis
- hepatic duct — *see* Cholangitis
- ileoanal (internal) pouch K91.850
- ileum (*see also* Enteritis)
  - regional or terminal — *see* Enteritis, regional
- intestinal pouch K91.850
- intestine (any part) — *see* Enteritis
- jaw (acute) (bone) (chronic) (lower) (suppurative) (upper) M27.2
- joint NEC — *see* Arthritis
  - sacroiliac M46.1
- kidney — *see* Nephritis
- knee (joint) M13.169
  - tuberculous A18.02
- labium (majus) (minus) — *see* Vulvitis
- lacrimal
  - gland — *see* Dacryoadenitis
  - passages (duct) (sac) (*see also* Dacryocystitis)
    - canaliculitis — *see* Canaliculitis, lacrimal
- larynx — *see* Laryngitis
- leg NOS L08.9
- lip K13.0
- liver (capsule) (*see also* Hepatitis)
  - chronic K73.9
  - suppurative K75.0
- lung (acute) (*see also* Pneumonia)
  - chronic J98.4
- lymph gland or node — *see* Lymphadenitis
- lymphatic vessel — *see* Lymphangitis
- maxilla, maxillary M27.2
  - sinus (chronic) — *see* Sinusitis, maxillary
- membranes of brain or spinal cord — *see* Meningitis
- meninges — *see* Meningitis
- mouth K12.1
- muscle — *see* Myositis
- myocardium — *see* Myocarditis
- nasal sinus (chronic) — *see* Sinusitis
- nasopharynx — *see* Nasopharyngitis
- navel L08.82
- nerve NEC — *see* Neuralgia
- nipple N61.0
  - puerperal, postpartum or gestational — *see* Infection, nipple
- nose — *see* Rhinitis
- oculomotor (nerve) — *see* Strabismus, paralytic, third nerve
- optic nerve — *see* Neuritis, optic
- orbit (chronic) H05.10
  - acute H05.00
    - abscess — *see* Abscess, orbit
    - cellulitis — *see* Cellulitis, orbit
    - osteomyelitis — *see* Osteomyelitis, orbit
    - periostitis — *see* Periostitis, orbital
    - tenonitis — *see* Tenonitis, eye
  - granuloma — *see* Granuloma, orbit
  - myositis — *see* Myositis, orbital
- ovary — *see* Salpingo-oophoritis
- oviduct — *see* Salpingo-oophoritis
- pancreas (acute) — *see* Pancreatitis
- parametrium N73.0
- parotid region L08.9
- pelvis, female — *see* Disease, pelvis, inflammatory
- penis (corpora cavernosa) N48.29
- perianal K62.89
- pericardium — *see* Pericarditis
- perineum (female) (male) L08.9
- perirectal K62.89
- peritoneum — *see* Peritonitis
- periuterine — *see* Disease, pelvis, inflammatory
- perivesical — *see* Cystitis
- petrous bone (acute) (chronic) — *see* Petrositis
- pharynx (acute) — *see* Pharyngitis
- pia mater — *see* Meningitis
- pleura — *see* Pleurisy

Inflammation, inflamed, inflammatory — *continued*
- polyp, colon (*see also* Polyp, colon, inflammatory) K51.40
- prostate (*see also* Prostatitis)
  - specified type NEC N41.8
- rectosigmoid — *see* Rectosigmoiditis
- rectum (*see also* Proctitis) K62.89
- respiratory, upper (*see also* Infection, respiratory, upper) J06.9
  - acute, due to radiation J70.0
  - chronic, due to external agent — *see* condition, respiratory, chronic, due to
  - due to
    - chemicals, gases, fumes or vapors (inhalation) J68.2
    - radiation J70.1
- retina — *see* Chorioretinitis
- retrocecal — *see* Appendicitis
- retroperitoneal — *see* Peritonitis
- salivary duct or gland (any) (suppurative) — *see* Sialoadenitis
- scorbutic, alveoli, teeth E54
- scrotum N49.2
- seminal vesicle — *see* Vesiculitis
- sigmoid — *see* Enteritis
- sinus — *see* Sinusitis
- Skene's duct or gland — *see* Urethritis
- skin L08.9
- spermatic cord N49.1
- sphenoidal (sinus) — *see* Sinusitis, sphenoidal
- spinal
  - cord — *see* Encephalitis
  - membrane — *see* Meningitis
  - nerve — *see* Disorder, nerve
- spine — *see* Spondylopathy, inflammatory
- spleen (capsule) D73.89
- stomach — *see* Gastritis
- subcutaneous tissue L08.9
- suprarenal (gland) E27.8
- synovial — *see* Tenosynovitis
- tendon (sheath) NEC — *see* Tenosynovitis
- testis — *see* Orchitis
- throat (acute) — *see* Pharyngitis
- thymus (gland) E32.8
- thyroid (gland) — *see* Thyroiditis
- tongue K14.0
- tonsil — *see* Tonsillitis
- trachea — *see* Tracheitis
- trochlear (nerve) — *see* Strabismus, paralytic, fourth nerve
- tubal — *see* Salpingo-oophoritis
- tuberculous NEC — *see* Tuberculosis
- tubo-ovarian — *see* Salpingo-oophoritis
- tunica vaginalis N49.1
- tympanic membrane — *see* Tympanitis
- umbilicus, umbilical L08.82
- uterine ligament — *see* Disease, pelvis, inflammatory
- uterus (catarrhal) — *see* Endometritis
- uveal tract (anterior) NOS (*see also* Iridocyclitis)
  - posterior — *see* Chorioretinitis
- vagina — *see* Vaginitis
- vas deferens N49.1
- vein (*see also* Phlebitis)
  - intracranial or intraspinal (septic) G08
  - thrombotic I80.9
    - leg — *see* Phlebitis, leg
    - lower extremity — *see* Phlebitis, leg
- vocal cord J38.3
- vulva — *see* Vulvitis
- Wharton's duct (suppurative) — *see* Sialoadenitis

Inflation, lung, imperfect (newborn) — *see* Atelectasis

Influenza (bronchial) (epidemic) (respiratory (upper)) (unidentified influenza virus) J11.1
- with
  - digestive manifestations J11.2
  - encephalopathy J11.81
  - enteritis J11.2
  - gastroenteritis J11.2
  - gastrointestinal manifestations J11.2
  - laryngitis J11.1
  - myocarditis J11.82
  - otitis media J11.83
  - pharyngitis J11.1
  - pneumonia J11.00
    - specified type J11.08
  - respiratory manifestations NEC J11.1

Influenza — *continued*
  with — *continued*
    specified manifestation NEC J11.89
  A/H5N1 (*see also* Influenza, due to, identified novel
    influenza A virus) J09.X2
  avian (*see also* Influenza, due to, identified novel in-
    fluenza A virus) J09.X2
  bird (*see also* Influenza, due to, identified novel influen-
    za A virus) J09.X2
  due to
    avian (*see also* Influenza, due to, identified novel
      influenza A virus) J09.X2
    identified influenza virus NEC J10.1
      with
        digestive manifestations J10.2
        encephalopathy J10.81
        enteritis J10.2
        gastroenteritis J10.2
        gastrointestinal manifestations J10.2
        laryngitis J10.1
        myocarditis J10.82
        otitis media J10.83
        pharyngitis J10.1
        pneumonia (unspecified type) J10.00
          with same identified influenza virus J10.01
          specified type NEC J10.08
        respiratory manifestations NEC J10.1
        specified manifestation NEC J10.89
    identified novel influenza A virus J09.X2
      with
        digestive manifestations J09.X3
        encephalopathy J09.X9
        enteritis J09.X3
        gastroenteritis J09.X3
        gastrointestinal manifestations J09.X3
        laryngitis J09.X2
        myocarditis J09.X9
        otitis media J09.X9
        pharyngitis J09.X2
        pneumonia J09.X1
        respiratory manifestations NEC J09.X2
        specified manifestation NEC J09.X9
        upper respiratory symptoms J09.X2
  novel (2009) H1N1 influenza (*see also* Influenza, due
    to, identified influenza virus NEC) J10.1
  novel influenza A/H1N1 (*see also* Influenza, due to,
    identified influenza virus NEC) J10.1
  of other animal origin, not bird or swine (*see also* In-
    fluenza, due to, identified novel influenza A
    virus) J09.X2
  swine (viruses that normally cause infections in pigs)
    (*see also* Influenza, due to, identified novel in-
    fluenza A virus) J09.X2
Influenzal — *see* Influenza
Influenza-like disease — *see* Influenza
Infraction, Freiberg's (metatarsal head) — *see* Osteochondrosis, juvenile, metatarsus
Infraeruption of tooth (teeth) M26.34
Infusion complication, misadventure, or reaction
  — *see* Complications, infusion
Ingestion
  chemical — *see* Table of Drugs and Chemicals, by
    substance, poisoning
  drug or medicament
    correct substance properly administered — *see*
      Table of Drugs and Chemicals, by drug, ad-
      verse effect
    overdose or wrong substance given or taken —
      see Table of Drugs and Chemicals, by drug,
      poisoning
  foreign body — *see* Foreign body, alimentary tract
  tularemia A21.3
Ingrowing
  hair (beard) L73.1
  nail (finger) (toe) L60.0
Inguinal (*see also* condition)
  testicle Q53.9
    bilateral Q53.212
    unilateral Q53.112
Inhalant-induced
  anxiety disorder F18.980
  depressive disorder F18.94
  major neurocognitive disorder F18.97
  mild neurocognitive disorder F18.988
  psychotic disorder F18.959
Inhalation
  anthrax A22.1

Inhalation — *continued*
  flame T27.3 ☑
  food or foreign body — *see* Foreign body, by site
  gases, fumes, or vapors NEC T59.9-
    specified agent — *see* Table of Drugs and Chemi-
      cals, by substance
  liquid or vomitus — *see* Asphyxia
  meconium (newborn) P24.00
    with
      with respiratory symptoms P24.01
      pneumonia (pneumonitis) P24.01
  mucus — *see* Asphyxia, mucus
  oil or gasoline (causing suffocation) — *see* Foreign
    body, by site
  smoke J70.5
    due to chemicals, gases, fumes and vapors J68.9
  steam — *see* Toxicity, vapors
  stomach contents or secretions — *see* Foreign body,
    by site
    due to anesthesia (general) (local) or other sedation
      T88.59 ☑
      in labor and delivery O74.0
      in pregnancy O29.01- ☑
      postpartum, puerperal O89.01
Inhibition, orgasm
  female F52.31
  male F52.32
Inhibitor, systemic lupus erythematosus (presence
  of) D68.62
Iniencephalus, iniencephaly Q00.2
Injection, traumatic jet (air) (industrial) (water) (paint
  or dye) T70.4 ☑
Injury (*see also* specified injury type) T14.90 ☑
  abdomen, abdominal S39.91 ☑
    blood vessel — *see* Injury, blood vessel, abdomen
    cavity — *see* Injury, intra-abdominal
    contusion S30.1 ☑
    internal — *see* Injury, intra-abdominal
    intra-abdominal organ — *see* Injury, intra-abdom-
      inal
    nerve — *see* Injury, nerve, abdomen
    open — *see* Wound, open, abdomen
    specified NEC S39.81 ☑
    superficial — *see* Injury, superficial, abdomen
  Achilles tendon S86.00- ☑
    laceration S86.02- ☑
    specified type NEC S86.09- ☑
    strain S86.01- ☑
  acoustic, resulting in deafness — *see* Injury, nerve,
    acoustic
  adrenal (gland) S37.819 ☑
    contusion S37.812 ☑
    laceration S37.813 ☑
    specified type NEC S37.818 ☑
  alveolar (process) S09.93 ☑
  ankle S99.91- ☑
    contusion — *see* Contusion, ankle
    dislocation — *see* Dislocation, ankle
    fracture — *see* Fracture, ankle
    nerve — *see* Injury, nerve, ankle
    open — *see* Wound, open, ankle
    specified type NEC S99.81- ☑
    sprain — *see* Sprain, ankle
    superficial — *see* Injury, superficial, ankle
  anterior chamber, eye — *see* Injury, eye, specified site
    NEC
  anus — *see* Injury, abdomen
  aorta (thoracic) S25.00 ☑
    abdominal S35.00 ☑
      laceration (minor) (superficial) S35.01 ☑
        major S35.02 ☑
      specified type NEC S35.09 ☑
    laceration (minor) (superficial) S25.01 ☑
      major S25.02 ☑
    specified type NEC S25.09 ☑
  arm (upper) S49.9- ☑
    blood vessel — *see* Injury, blood vessel, arm
    contusion — *see* Contusion, arm, upper
    fracture — *see* Fracture, humerus
    lower — *see* Injury, forearm
    muscle — *see* Injury, muscle, shoulder
    nerve — *see* Injury, nerve, arm
    open — *see* Wound, open, arm
    specified type NEC S49.8- ☑
    superficial — *see* Injury, superficial, arm

Injury — *continued*
  artery (complicating trauma) (*see also* Injury, blood
    vessel, by site)
    cerebral or meningeal — *see* Injury, intracranial
  auditory canal (external) (meatus) S09.91 ☑
  auricle, auris, ear S09.91 ☑
  axilla — *see* Injury, shoulder
  back — *see* Injury, back, lower
  bile duct S36.13 ☑
  birth (*see also* Birth, injury) P15.9
  bladder (sphincter) S37.20 ☑
    at delivery O71.5
    contusion S37.22 ☑
    laceration S37.23 ☑
    obstetrical trauma O71.5
    specified type NEC S37.29 ☑
  blast (air) (hydraulic) (immersion) (underwater) NEC
    T14.8 ☑
    acoustic nerve trauma — *see* Injury, nerve, acoustic
    bladder — *see* Injury, bladder
    brain — *see* Concussion
    colon — *see* Injury, intestine, large
    ear (primary) S09.31- ☑
      secondary S09.39- ☑
    generalized T70.8 ☑
    lung — *see* Injury, intrathoracic, lung
    multiple body organs T70.8 ☑
    peritoneum S36.81 ☑
    rectum S36.61 ☑
    retroperitoneum S36.898 ☑
    small intestine S36.419 ☑
      duodenum S36.410 ☑
      specified site NEC S36.418 ☑
    specified
      intra-abdominal organ NEC S36.898 ☑
      pelvic organ NEC S37.899 ☑
  blood vessel NEC T14.8 ☑
    abdomen S35.9 ☑
      aorta — *see* Injury, aorta, abdominal
      celiac artery — *see* Injury, blood vessel, celiac
        artery
      iliac vessel — *see* Injury, blood vessel, iliac
      laceration S35.91 ☑
      mesenteric vessel — *see* Injury, mesenteric
      portal vein — *see* Injury, blood vessel, portal
        vein
      renal vessel — *see* Injury, blood vessel, renal
      specified vessel NEC S35.8X- ☑
      splenic vessel — *see* Injury, blood vessel,
        splenic
      vena cava — *see* Injury, vena cava, inferior
    ankle — *see* Injury, blood vessel, foot
    aorta (abdominal) (thoracic) — *see* Injury, aorta
    arm (upper) NEC S45.90- ☑
      forearm — *see* Injury, blood vessel, forearm
      laceration S45.91- ☑
      specified
        site NEC S45.80- ☑
          laceration S45.81- ☑
          specified type NEC S45.89- ☑
        type NEC S45.99- ☑
      superficial vein S45.30- ☑
        laceration S45.31- ☑
        specified type NEC S45.39- ☑
    axillary
      artery S45.00- ☑
        laceration S45.01- ☑
        specified type NEC S45.09- ☑
      vein S45.20- ☑
        laceration S45.21- ☑
        specified type NEC S45.29- ☑
    azygos vein — *see* Injury, blood vessel, thoracic,
      specified site NEC
    brachial
      artery S45.10- ☑
        laceration S45.11- ☑
        specified type NEC S45.19- ☑
      vein S45.20- ☑
        laceration S45.219 ☑
        specified type NEC S45.29- ☑
    carotid artery (common) (external) (internal, ex-
      tracranial) S15.00- ☑
      internal, intracranial S06.8- ☑
      laceration (minor) (superficial) S15.01- ☑
        major S15.02- ☑
      specified type NEC S15.09- ☑

Injury — *continued*
blood vessel — *continued*
celiac artery S35.219 ☑
branch S35.299 ☑
laceration (minor) (superficial) S35.291 ☑
major S35.292 ☑
specified NEC S35.298 ☑
laceration (minor) (superficial) S35.211 ☑
major S35.212 ☑
specified type NEC S35.218 ☑
cerebral — *see* Injury, intracranial
deep plantar — *see* Injury, blood vessel, plantar
artery
digital (hand) — *see* Injury, blood vessel, finger
dorsal
artery (foot) S95.00- ☑
laceration S95.01- ☑
specified type NEC S95.09- ☑
vein (foot) S95.20- ☑
laceration S95.21- ☑
specified type NEC S95.29- ☑
due to accidental laceration during procedure —
see Laceration, accidental complicating
surgery
extremity — *see* Injury, blood vessel, limb
femoral
artery (common) (superficial) S75.00- ☑
laceration (minor) (superficial) S75.01- ☑
major S75.02- ☑
specified type NEC S75.09- ☑
vein (hip level) (thigh level) S75.10- ☑
laceration (minor) (superficial) S75.11- ☑
major S75.12- ☑
specified type NEC S75.19- ☑
finger S65.50- ☑
index S65.50- ☑
laceration S65.51- ☑
specified type NEC S65.59- ☑
laceration S65.51- ☑
little S65.50- ☑
laceration S65.51- ☑
specified type NEC S65.59- ☑
middle S65.50- ☑
laceration S65.51- ☑
specified type NEC S65.59- ☑
specified type NEC S65.59- ☑
thumb — *see* Injury, blood vessel, thumb
foot S95.90- ☑
dorsal
artery — *see* Injury, blood vessel, dorsal,
artery
vein — *see* Injury, blood vessel, dorsal, vein
laceration S95.91- ☑
plantar artery — *see* Injury, blood vessel, plantar artery
specified
site NEC S95.80- ☑
laceration S95.81- ☑
specified type NEC S95.89- ☑
specified type NEC S95.99- ☑
forearm S55.90- ☑
laceration S55.91- ☑
radial artery — *see* Injury, blood vessel, radial
artery
specified
site NEC S55.80- ☑
laceration S55.81- ☑
specified type NEC S55.89- ☑
type NEC S55.99- ☑
ulnar artery — *see* Injury, blood vessel, ulnar
artery
vein S55.20- ☑
laceration S55.21- ☑
specified type NEC S55.29- ☑
gastric
artery — *see* Injury, mesenteric, artery, branch
vein — *see* Injury, blood vessel, abdomen
gastroduodenal artery — *see* Injury, mesenteric,
artery, branch
greater saphenous vein (lower leg level) S85.30- ☑
hip (and thigh) level S75.20- ☑
laceration (minor) (superficial) S75.21- ☑
major S75.22- ☑
specified type NEC S75.29- ☑
laceration S85.31- ☑
specified type NEC S85.39- ☑

Injury — *continued*
blood vessel — *continued*
hand (level) S65.90- ☑
finger — *see* Injury, blood vessel, finger
laceration S65.91- ☑
palmar arch — *see* Injury, blood vessel, palmar
arch
radial artery — *see* Injury, blood vessel, radial
artery, hand
specified
site NEC S65.80- ☑
laceration S65.81- ☑
specified type NEC S65.89- ☑
type NEC S65.99- ☑
thumb — *see* Injury, blood vessel, thumb
ulnar artery — *see* Injury, blood vessel, ulnar
artery, hand
head S09.0 ☑
intracranial — *see* Injury, intracranial
multiple S09.0 ☑
hepatic
artery — *see* Injury, mesenteric, artery
vein — *see* Injury, vena cava, inferior
hip S75.90- ☑
femoral artery — *see* Injury, blood vessel,
femoral, artery
femoral vein — *see* Injury, blood vessel,
femoral, vein
greater saphenous vein — *see* Injury, blood
vessel, greater saphenous, hip level
laceration S75.91- ☑
specified
site NEC S75.80- ☑
laceration S75.81- ☑
specified type NEC S75.89- ☑
type NEC S75.99- ☑
hypogastric (artery) (vein) — *see* Injury, blood
vessel, iliac
iliac S35.5- ☑
artery S35.51- ☑
specified vessel NEC S35.5- ☑
uterine vessel — *see* Injury, blood vessel, uterine
vein S35.51- ☑
innominate — *see* Injury, blood vessel, thoracic,
innominate
intercostal (artery) (vein) — *see* Injury, blood vessel,
thoracic, intercostal
jugular vein (external) S15.20- ☑
internal S15.30- ☑
laceration (minor) (superficial) S15.31- ☑
major S15.32- ☑
specified type NEC S15.39- ☑
laceration (minor) (superficial) S15.21- ☑
major S15.22- ☑
specified type NEC S15.29- ☑
leg (level) (lower) S85.90- ☑
greater saphenous — *see* Injury, blood vessel,
greater saphenous
laceration S85.91- ☑
lesser saphenous — *see* Injury, blood vessel,
lesser saphenous
peroneal artery — *see* Injury, blood vessel,
peroneal artery
popliteal
artery — *see* Injury, blood vessel, popliteal,
artery
vein — *see* Injury, blood vessel, popliteal,
vein
specified
site NEC S85.80- ☑
laceration S85.81- ☑
specified type NEC S85.89- ☑
type NEC S85.99- ☑
thigh — *see* Injury, blood vessel, hip
tibial artery — *see* Injury, blood vessel, tibial
artery
lesser saphenous vein (lower leg level) S85.40- ☑
laceration S85.41- ☑
specified type NEC S85.49- ☑
limb
lower — *see* Injury, blood vessel, leg
upper — *see* Injury, blood vessel, arm
lower back — *see* Injury, blood vessel, abdomen
specified NEC — *see* Injury, blood vessel, abdomen, specified, site NEC

Injury — *continued*
blood vessel — *continued*
mammary (artery) (vein) — *see* Injury, blood vessel,
thoracic, specified site NEC
mesenteric (inferior) (superior)
artery — *see* Injury, mesenteric, artery
vein — *see* Injury, blood vessel, mesenteric,
vein
neck S15.9 ☑
specified site NEC S15.8 ☑
ovarian (artery) (vein) — *see* subcategory S35.8 ☑
palmar arch (superficial) S65.20- ☑
deep S65.30- ☑
laceration S65.31- ☑
specified type NEC S65.39- ☑
laceration S65.21- ☑
specified type NEC S65.29- ☑
pelvis — *see* Injury, blood vessel, abdomen
specified NEC — *see* Injury, blood vessel, abdomen, specified, site NEC
peroneal artery S85.20- ☑
laceration S85.21- ☑
specified type NEC S85.29- ☑
plantar artery (deep) (foot) S95.10- ☑
laceration S95.11- ☑
specified type NEC S95.19- ☑
popliteal
artery S85.00- ☑
laceration S85.01- ☑
specified type NEC S85.09- ☑
vein S85.50- ☑
laceration S85.51- ☑
specified type NEC S85.59- ☑
portal vein S35.319 ☑
laceration S35.311 ☑
specified type NEC S35.318 ☑
precerebral — *see* Injury, blood vessel, neck
pulmonary (artery) (vein) — *see* Injury, blood vessel, thoracic, pulmonary
radial artery (forearm level) S55.10- ☑
hand and wrist (level) S65.10- ☑
laceration S65.11- ☑
specified type NEC S65.19- ☑
laceration S55.11- ☑
specified type NEC S55.19- ☑
renal
artery S35.40- ☑
laceration S35.41- ☑
specified NEC S35.49- ☑
vein S35.40- ☑
laceration S35.41- ☑
specified NEC S35.49- ☑
saphenous vein (greater) (lower leg level) — *see*
Injury, blood vessel, greater saphenous
hip and thigh level — *see* Injury, blood vessel,
greater saphenous, hip level
lesser — *see* Injury, blood vessel, lesser saphenous
shoulder
specified NEC — *see* Injury, blood vessel, arm,
specified site NEC
superficial vein — *see* Injury, blood vessel, arm,
superficial vein
specified NEC T14.8 ☑
splenic
artery — *see* Injury, blood vessel, celiac artery,
branch
vein S35.329 ☑
laceration S35.321 ☑
specified NEC S35.328 ☑
subclavian — *see* Injury, blood vessel, thoracic, innominate
thigh — *see* Injury, blood vessel, hip
thoracic S25.90 ☑
aorta S25.00 ☑
laceration (minor) (superficial) S25.01 ☑
major S25.02 ☑
specified type NEC S25.09 ☑
azygos vein — *see* Injury, blood vessel, thoracic,
specified, site NEC
innominate
artery S25.10- ☑
laceration (minor) (superficial)
S25.11- ☑
major S25.12- ☑
specified type NEC S25.19- ☑

▽ Subterms under main terms may continue to next column or page   ☑ Additional Character Required — Refer to the Tabular List for Character Selection   **191**

Injury — Injury

Index

Injury — Injury

Injury — *continued*
blood vessel — *continued*
thoracic — *continued*
innominate — *continued*
vein S25.30- ☑
laceration (minor) (superficial)
S25.31- ☑
major S25.32- ☑
specified type NEC S25.39- ☑
intercostal S25.50- ☑
laceration S25.51- ☑
specified type NEC S25.59- ☑
laceration S25.91- ☑
mammary vessel — *see* Injury, blood vessel,
thoracic, specified, site NEC
pulmonary S25.40- ☑
laceration (minor) (superficial) S25.41- ☑
major S25.42- ☑
specified type NEC S25.49- ☑
specified
site NEC S25.80- ☑
laceration S25.81 ☑
specified type NEC S25.89 ☑
type NEC S25.99 ☑
subclavian — *see* Injury, blood vessel, thoracic,
innominate
vena cava (superior) S25.20 ☑
laceration (minor) (superficial) S25.21 ☑
major S25.22 ☑
specified type NEC S25.29 ☑
thumb S65.40- ☑
laceration S65.41- ☑
specified type NEC S65.49- ☑
tibial artery S85.10- ☑
anterior S85.13- ☑
laceration S85.14- ☑
specified injury NEC S85.15- ☑
laceration S85.11- ☑
posterior S85.16- ☑
laceration S85.17- ☑
specified injury NEC S85.18- ☑
specified injury NEC S85.12- ☑
ulnar artery (forearm level) S55.00- ☑
hand and wrist (level) S65.00- ☑
laceration S65.01- ☑
specified type NEC S65.09- ☑
laceration S55.01- ☑
specified type NEC S55.09- ☑
upper arm (level) — *see* Injury, blood vessel, arm
superficial vein — *see* Injury, blood vessel, arm,
superficial vein
uterine S35.5- ☑
artery S35.53- ☑
vein S35.53- ☑
vena cava — *see* Injury, vena cava
vertebral artery S15.10- ☑
laceration (minor) (superficial) S15.11- ☑
major S15.12- ☑
specified type NEC S15.19- ☑
wrist (level) — *see* Injury, blood vessel, hand
brachial plexus S14.3 ☑
newborn P14.3
brain (traumatic) S06.9- ☑
diffuse (axonal) S06.2X- ☑
focal S06.30- ☑
brainstem S06.38- ☑
breast NOS S29.9 ☑
broad ligament — *see* Injury, pelvic organ, specified
site NEC
bronchus, bronchi — *see* Injury, intrathoracic,
bronchus
brow S09.90 ☑
buttock S39.92 ☑
canthus, eye S05.90 ☑
cardiac plexus — *see* Injury, nerve, thorax, sympathetic
cauda equina S34.3 ☑
cavernous sinus — *see* Injury, intracranial
cecum — *see* Injury, colon
celiac ganglion or plexus — *see* Injury, nerve, lumbosacral, sympathetic
cerebellum — *see* Injury, intracranial
cerebral — *see* Injury, intracranial
cervix (uteri) — *see* Injury, uterus
cheek (wall) S09.93 ☑
chest — *see* Injury, thorax

Injury — *continued*
childbirth (newborn) (*see also* Birth, injury)
maternal NEC O71.9
chin S09.93 ☑
choroid (eye) — *see* Injury, eye, specified site NEC
clitoris S39.94 ☑
coccyx (*see also* Injury, back, lower)
complicating delivery O71.6
colon — *see* Injury, intestine, large
common bile duct — *see* Injury, liver
conjunctiva (superficial) — *see* Injury, eye, conjunctiva
conus medullaris — *see* Injury, spinal, sacral
cord
spermatic (pelvic region) S37.898 ☑
scrotal region S39.848 ☑
spinal — *see* Injury, spinal cord, by region
cornea — *see* Injury, eye, specified site NEC
abrasion — *see* Injury, eye, cornea, abrasion
cortex (cerebral) (*see also* Injury, intracranial)
visual — *see* Injury, nerve, optic
costal region NEC S29.9 ☑
costochondral NEC S29.9 ☑
cranial
cavity — *see* Injury, intracranial
nerve — *see* Injury, nerve, cranial
crushing — *see* Crush
cutaneous sensory nerve
cystic duct — *see* Injury, liver
deep tissue — *see* Contusion, by site
meaning pressure ulcer — *see* Ulcer, pressure, unstageable, by site
delivery (newborn) P15.9
maternal NEC O71.9
Descemet's membrane — *see* Injury, eyeball, penetrating
diaphragm — *see* Injury, intrathoracic, diaphragm
duodenum — *see* Injury, intestine, small, duodenum
ear (auricle) (external) (canal) S09.91 ☑
abrasion — *see* Abrasion, ear
bite — *see* Bite, ear
blister — *see* Blister, ear
bruise — *see* Contusion, ear
contusion — *see* Contusion, ear
external constriction — *see* Constriction, external,
ear
hematoma — *see* Hematoma, ear
inner — *see* Injury, ear, middle
laceration — *see* Laceration, ear
middle S09.30- ☑
blast — *see* Injury, blast, ear
specified NEC S09.39- ☑
puncture — *see* Puncture, ear
superficial — *see* Injury, superficial, ear
eighth cranial nerve (acoustic or auditory) — *see* Injury,
nerve, acoustic
elbow S59.90- ☑
contusion — *see* Contusion, elbow
dislocation — *see* Dislocation, elbow
fracture — *see* Fracture, ulna, upper end
open — *see* Wound, open, elbow
specified NEC S59.80- ☑
sprain — *see* Sprain, elbow
superficial — *see* Injury, superficial, elbow
eleventh cranial nerve (accessory) — *see* Injury, nerve,
accessory
epididymis S39.94 ☑
epigastric region S39.91 ☑
epiglottis NEC S19.89 ☑
esophageal plexus — *see* Injury, nerve, thorax, sympathetic
esophagus (thoracic part) (*see also* Injury, intrathoracic,
esophagus)
cervical NEC S19.85 ☑
eustachian tube S09.30 ☑
eye S05.9- ☑
avulsion S05.7- ☑
ball — *see* Injury, eyeball
conjunctiva S05.0- ☑
cornea
abrasion S05.0- ☑
laceration S05.3- ☑
with prolapse S05.2- ☑
lacrimal apparatus S05.8X- ☑
orbit penetration S05.4- ☑
specified site NEC S05.8X- ☑
eyeball S05.8X- ☑

Injury — *continued*
eyeball — *continued*
contusion S05.1- ☑
penetrating S05.6- ☑
with
foreign body S05.5- ☑
prolapse or loss of intraocular tissue
S05.2- ☑
without prolapse or loss of intraocular tissue
S05.3- ☑
specified type NEC S05.8- ☑
eyebrow S09.93 ☑
eyelid S09.93 ☑
abrasion — *see* Abrasion, eyelid
contusion — *see* Contusion, eyelid
open — *see* Wound, open, eyelid
face S09.93 ☑
fallopian tube S37.509 ☑
bilateral S37.502 ☑
blast injury S37.512 ☑
contusion S37.522 ☑
laceration S37.532 ☑
specified type NEC S37.592 ☑
blast injury (primary) S37.519 ☑
bilateral S37.512 ☑
secondary — *see* Injury, fallopian tube, specified type NEC
unilateral S37.511 ☑
contusion S37.529 ☑
bilateral S37.522 ☑
unilateral S37.521 ☑
laceration S37.539 ☑
bilateral S37.532 ☑
unilateral S37.531 ☑
specified type NEC S37.599 ☑
bilateral S37.592 ☑
unilateral S37.591 ☑
unilateral S37.501 ☑
blast injury S37.511 ☑
contusion S37.521 ☑
laceration S37.531 ☑
specified type NEC S37.591 ☑
fascia — *see* Injury, muscle
fifth cranial nerve (trigeminal) — *see* Injury, nerve,
trigeminal
finger (nail) S69.9- ☑
blood vessel — *see* Injury, blood vessel, finger
contusion — *see* Contusion, finger
dislocation — *see* Dislocation, finger
fracture — *see* Fracture, finger
muscle — *see* Injury, muscle, finger
nerve — *see* Injury, nerve, digital, finger
open — *see* Wound, open, finger
specified NEC S69.8- ☑
sprain — *see* Sprain, finger
superficial — *see* Injury, superficial, finger
first cranial nerve (olfactory) — *see* Injury, nerve, olfactory
flank — *see* Injury, abdomen
foot S99.92- ☑
blood vessel — *see* Injury, blood vessel, foot
contusion — *see* Contusion, foot
dislocation — *see* Dislocation, foot
fracture — *see* Fracture, foot
muscle — *see* Injury, muscle, foot
open — *see* Wound, open, foot
specified type NEC S99.82- ☑
sprain — *see* Sprain, foot
superficial — *see* Injury, superficial, foot
forceps NOS P15.9
forearm S59.91- ☑
blood vessel — *see* Injury, blood vessel, forearm
contusion — *see* Contusion, forearm
fracture — *see* Fracture, forearm
muscle — *see* Injury, muscle, forearm
nerve — *see* Injury, nerve, forearm
open — *see* Wound, open, forearm
specified NEC S59.81- ☑
superficial — *see* Injury, superficial, forearm
forehead S09.90 ☑
fourth cranial nerve (trochlear) — *see* Injury, nerve,
trochlear
gallbladder S36.129 ☑
contusion S36.122 ☑
laceration S36.123 ☑
specified NEC S36.128 ☑

☑ Additional Character Required — Refer to the Tabular List for Character Selection   ▽ Subterms under main terms may continue to next column or page

Injury — *continued*
  ganglion
    celiac, coeliac — *see* Injury, nerve, lumbosacral, sympathetic
    gasserian — *see* Injury, nerve, trigeminal
    stellate — *see* Injury, nerve, thorax, sympathetic
    thoracic sympathetic — *see* Injury, nerve, thorax, sympathetic
  gasserian ganglion — *see* Injury, nerve, trigeminal
  gastric artery — *see* Injury, blood vessel, celiac artery, branch
  gastroduodenal artery — *see* Injury, blood vessel, celiac artery, branch
  gastrointestinal tract — *see* Injury, intra-abdominal
    with open wound into abdominal cavity — *see* Wound, open, with penetration into peritoneal cavity
    colon — *see* Injury, intestine, large
    rectum — *see* Injury, intestine, large, rectum
      with open wound into abdominal cavity S36.61 ☑
    small intestine — *see* Injury, intestine, small
    specified site NEC — *see* Injury, intra-abdominal, specified, site NEC
    stomach — *see* Injury, stomach
  genital organ(s)
    external S39.94 ☑
      specified NEC S39.848 ☑
    internal S37.90 ☑
      fallopian tube — *see* Injury, fallopian tube
      ovary — *see* Injury, ovary
      prostate — *see* Injury, prostate
      seminal vesicle — *see* Injury, pelvis, organ, specified site NEC
      uterus — *see* Injury, uterus
      vas deferens — *see* Injury, pelvis, organ, specified site NEC
    obstetrical trauma O71.9
  gland
    lacrimal laceration — *see* Injury, eye, specified site NEC
    salivary S09.93 ☑
    thyroid NEC S19.84 ☑
  globe (eye) S05.90 ☑
    specified NEC S05.8X- ☑
  groin — *see* Injury, abdomen
  gum S09.90 ☑
  hand S69.9- ☑
    blood vessel — *see* Injury, blood vessel, hand
    contusion — *see* Contusion, hand
    fracture — *see* Fracture, hand
    muscle — *see* Injury, muscle, hand
    nerve — *see* Injury, nerve, hand
    open — *see* Wound, open, hand
    specified NEC S69.8- ☑
    sprain — *see* Sprain, hand
    superficial — *see* Injury, superficial, hand
  head S09.90 ☑
    with loss of consciousness S06.9- ☑
    specified NEC S09.8 ☑
  heart S26.90 ☑
    with hemopericardium S26.00 ☑
      contusion S26.01 ☑
      laceration (mild) S26.020 ☑
        major S26.022 ☑
        moderate S26.021 ☑
      specified type NEC S26.09 ☑
    without hemopericardium S26.10 ☑
      contusion S26.11 ☑
      laceration S26.12 ☑
      specified type NEC S26.19 ☑
    contusion S26.91 ☑
    laceration S26.92 ☑
    specified type NEC S26.99 ☑
  heel — *see* Injury, foot
  hepatic
    artery — *see* Injury, blood vessel, celiac artery, branch
    duct — *see* Injury, liver
    vein — *see* Injury, vena cava, inferior
  hip S79.91- ☑
    blood vessel — *see* Injury, blood vessel, hip
    contusion — *see* Contusion, hip
    dislocation — *see* Dislocation, hip
    fracture — *see* Fracture, femur, neck
    muscle — *see* Injury, muscle, hip

hip — *continued*
    nerve — *see* Injury, nerve, hip
    open — *see* Wound, open, hip
    specified NEC S79.81- ☑
    sprain — *see* Sprain, hip
    superficial — *see* Injury, superficial, hip
  hymen S39.94 ☑
  hypogastric
    blood vessel — *see* Injury, blood vessel, iliac
    plexus — *see* Injury, nerve, lumbosacral, sympathetic
  ileum — *see* Injury, intestine, small
  iliac region S39.91 ☑
  instrumental (during surgery) — *see* Laceration, accidental complicating surgery
    birth injury — *see* Birth, injury
    nonsurgical — *see* Injury, by site
    obstetrical O71.9
      bladder O71.5
      cervix O71.3
      high vaginal O71.4
      perineal NOS O70.9
      urethra O71.5
      uterus O71.5
        with rupture or perforation O71.1
  internal T14.8 ☑
    aorta — *see* Injury, aorta
    bladder (sphincter) — *see* Injury, bladder
      with
        ectopic or molar pregnancy O08.6
        following ectopic or molar pregnancy O08.6
        obstetrical trauma O71.5
    bronchus, bronchi — *see* Injury, intrathoracic, bronchus
    cecum — *see* Injury, intestine, large
    cervix (uteri) (*see also* Injury, uterus)
      with ectopic or molar pregnancy O08.6
      following ectopic or molar pregnancy O08.6
      obstetrical trauma O71.3
    chest — *see* Injury, intrathoracic
    gastrointestinal tract — *see* Injury, intra-abdominal
    heart — *see* Injury, heart
    intestine NEC — *see* Injury, intestine
    intrauterine — *see* Injury, uterus
    mesentery — *see* Injury, intra-abdominal, specified, site NEC
    pelvis, pelvic (organ) S37.90 ☑
      following ectopic or molar pregnancy (subsequent episode) O08.6
      obstetrical trauma NEC O71.5
        rupture or perforation O71.1
      specified NEC S39.83 ☑
    rectum — *see* Injury, intestine, large, rectum
    stomach — *see* Injury, stomach
    ureter — *see* Injury, ureter
    urethra (sphincter) following ectopic or molar pregnancy O08.6
    uterus — *see* Injury, uterus
  interscapular area — *see* Injury, thorax
  intestine
    large S36.509 ☑
      ascending (right) S36.500 ☑
        blast injury (primary) S36.510 ☑
          secondary S36.590 ☑
        contusion S36.520 ☑
        laceration S36.530 ☑
        specified type NEC S36.590 ☑
      blast injury (primary) S36.519 ☑
        ascending (right) S36.510 ☑
        descending (left) S36.512 ☑
        rectum S36.61 ☑
        sigmoid S36.513 ☑
        specified site NEC S36.518 ☑
        transverse S36.511 ☑
      contusion S36.529 ☑
        ascending (right) S36.520 ☑
        descending (left) S36.522 ☑
        rectum S36.62 ☑
        sigmoid S36.523 ☑
        specified site NEC S36.528 ☑
        transverse S36.521 ☑
      descending (left) S36.502 ☑
        blast injury (primary) S36.512 ☑
          secondary S36.592 ☑
        contusion S36.522 ☑
        laceration S36.532 ☑

Injury — *continued*
  intestine — *continued*
    large — *continued*
      descending — *continued*
        specified type NEC S36.592 ☑
      laceration S36.539 ☑
        ascending (right) S36.530 ☑
        descending (left) S36.532 ☑
        rectum S36.63 ☑
        sigmoid S36.533 ☑
        specified site NEC S36.538 ☑
        transverse S36.531 ☑
      rectum S36.60 ☑
        blast injury (primary) S36.61 ☑
          secondary S36.69 ☑
        contusion S36.62 ☑
        laceration S36.63 ☑
        specified type NEC S36.69 ☑
      sigmoid S36.503 ☑
        blast injury (primary) S36.513 ☑
          secondary S36.593 ☑
        contusion S36.523 ☑
        laceration S36.533 ☑
        specified type NEC S36.593 ☑
      specified
        site NEC S36.508 ☑
          blast injury (primary) S36.518 ☑
            secondary S36.598 ☑
          contusion S36.528 ☑
          laceration S36.538 ☑
          specified type NEC S36.598 ☑
        type NEC S36.599 ☑
          ascending (right) S36.590 ☑
          descending (left) S36.592 ☑
          rectum S36.69 ☑
          sigmoid S36.593 ☑
          specified site NEC S36.598 ☑
          transverse S36.591 ☑
      transverse S36.501 ☑
        blast injury (primary) S36.511 ☑
          secondary S36.591 ☑
        contusion S36.521 ☑
        laceration S36.531 ☑
        specified type NEC S36.591 ☑
    small S36.409 ☑
      blast injury (primary) S36.419 ☑
        duodenum S36.410 ☑
        secondary S36.499 ☑
          duodenum S36.490 ☑
          specified site NEC S36.498 ☑
        specified site NEC S36.418 ☑
      contusion S36.429 ☑
        duodenum S36.420 ☑
        specified site NEC S36.428 ☑
      duodenum S36.400 ☑
        blast injury (primary) S36.410 ☑
          secondary S36.490 ☑
        contusion S36.420 ☑
        laceration S36.430 ☑
        specified NEC S36.490 ☑
      laceration S36.439 ☑
        duodenum S36.430 ☑
        specified site NEC S36.438 ☑
      specified
        site NEC S36.408 ☑
        type NEC S36.499 ☑
          duodenum S36.490 ☑
          specified site NEC S36.498 ☑
  intra-abdominal S36.90 ☑
    adrenal gland — *see* Injury, adrenal gland
    bladder — *see* Injury, bladder
    colon — *see* Injury, intestine, large
    contusion S36.92 ☑
    fallopian tube — *see* Injury, fallopian tube
    gallbladder — *see* Injury, gallbladder
    intestine — *see* Injury, intestine
    kidney — *see* Injury, kidney
    laceration S36.93 ☑
    liver — *see* Injury, liver
    ovary — *see* Injury, ovary
    pancreas — *see* Injury, pancreas
    pelvic NOS S37.90 ☑
    peritoneum — *see* Injury, intra-abdominal, specified, site NEC
    prostate — *see* Injury, prostate
    rectum — *see* Injury, intestine, large, rectum

Injury — *continued*
  intra-abdominal — *continued*
    retroperitoneum — *see* Injury, intra-abdominal, specified, site NEC
    seminal vesicle — *see* Injury, pelvis, organ, specified site NEC
    small intestine — *see* Injury, intestine, small
    specified
      pelvic S37.90 ☑
        specified
          site NEC S37.899 ☑
            specified type NEC S37.898 ☑
          type NEC S37.99 ☑
        site NEC S36.899 ☑
          contusion S36.892 ☑
          laceration S36.893 ☑
          specified type NEC S36.898 ☑
        type NEC S36.99 ☑
    spleen — *see* Injury, spleen
    stomach — *see* Injury, stomach
    ureter — *see* Injury, ureter
    urethra — *see* Injury, urethra
    uterus — *see* Injury, uterus
    vas deferens — *see* Injury, pelvis, organ, specified site NEC
  intracranial (traumatic) S06.9- ☑
    cerebellar hemorrhage, traumatic — *see* Injury, intracranial, focal
    cerebral edema, traumatic S06.1X- ☑
      diffuse S06.1X- ☑
      focal S06.1X- ☑
    diffuse (axonal) S06.2X- ☑
    epidural hemorrhage (traumatic) S06.4X- ☑
    focal brain injury S06.30- ☑
      contusion — *see* Contusion, cerebral
      laceration — *see* Laceration, cerebral
    intracerebral hemorrhage, traumatic S06.36- ☑
      left side S06.35- ☑
      right side S06.34- ☑
    subarachnoid hemorrhage, traumatic S06.6X- ☑
    subdural hemorrhage, traumatic S06.5X- ☑
  Intraocular — *see* Injury, eyeball, penetrating
  intrathoracic S27.9 ☑
    bronchus S27.409 ☑
      bilateral S27.402 ☑
      blast injury (primary) S27.419 ☑
        bilateral S27.412 ☑
        secondary — *see* Injury, intrathoracic, bronchus, specified type NEC
        unilateral S27.411 ☑
      contusion S27.429 ☑
        bilateral S27.422 ☑
        unilateral S27.421 ☑
      laceration S27.439 ☑
        bilateral S27.432 ☑
        unilateral S27.431 ☑
      specified type NEC S27.499 ☑
        bilateral S27.492 ☑
        unilateral S27.491 ☑
      unilateral S27.401 ☑
    diaphragm S27.809 ☑
      contusion S27.802 ☑
      laceration S27.803 ☑
      specified type NEC S27.808 ☑
    esophagus (thoracic) S27.819 ☑
      contusion S27.812 ☑
      laceration S27.813 ☑
      specified type NEC S27.818 ☑
    heart — *see* Injury, heart
    hemopneumothorax S27.2 ☑
    hemothorax S27.1 ☑
    lung S27.309 ☑
      aspiration J69.0
      bilateral S27.302 ☑
      blast injury (primary) S27.319 ☑
        bilateral S27.312 ☑
        secondary — *see* Injury, intrathoracic, lung, specified type NEC
        unilateral S27.311 ☑
      contusion S27.329 ☑
        bilateral S27.322 ☑
        unilateral S27.321 ☑
      laceration S27.339 ☑
        bilateral S27.332 ☑
        unilateral S27.331 ☑
      specified type NEC S27.399 ☑

Injury — *continued*
  intrathoracic — *continued*
    lung — *continued*
      specified type — *continued*
        bilateral S27.392 ☑
        unilateral S27.391 ☑
        unilateral S27.301 ☑
      pleura S27.60 ☑
        laceration S27.63 ☑
        specified type NEC S27.69 ☑
      pneumothorax S27.0 ☑
      specified organ NEC S27.899 ☑
        contusion S27.892 ☑
        laceration S27.893 ☑
        specified type NEC S27.898 ☑
      thoracic duct — *see* Injury, intrathoracic, specified organ NEC
      thymus gland — *see* Injury, intrathoracic, specified organ NEC
      trachea, thoracic S27.50 ☑
        blast (primary) S27.51 ☑
        contusion S27.52 ☑
        laceration S27.53 ☑
        specified type NEC S27.59 ☑
    iris — *see* Injury, eye, specified site NEC
      penetrating — *see* Injury, eyeball, penetrating
    jaw S09.93 ☑
    jejunum — *see* Injury, intestine, small
    joint NOS T14.8 ☑
      old or residual — *see* Disorder, joint, specified type NEC
    kidney S37.00- ☑
      acute (nontraumatic) N17.9
      contusion — *see* Contusion, kidney
      laceration — *see* Laceration, kidney
      specified NEC S37.09- ☑
    knee S89.9- ☑
      contusion — *see* Contusion, knee
      dislocation — *see* Dislocation, knee
      meniscus (lateral) (medial) — *see* Sprain, knee, specified site NEC
        old injury or tear — *see* Derangement, knee, meniscus, due to old injury
      open — *see* Wound, open, knee
      specified NEC S89.8- ☑
      sprain — *see* Sprain, knee
      superficial — *see* Injury, superficial, knee
    labium (majus) (minus) S39.94 ☑
    labyrinth, ear S09.30- ☑
    lacrimal apparatus, duct, gland, or sac — *see* Injury, eye, specified site NEC
    larynx NEC S19.81 ☑
    leg (lower) S89.9- ☑
      blood vessel — *see* Injury, blood vessel, leg
      contusion — *see* Contusion, leg
      fracture — *see* Fracture, leg
      muscle — *see* Injury, muscle, leg
      nerve — *see* Injury, nerve, leg
      open — *see* Wound, open, leg
      specified NEC S89.8- ☑
      superficial — *see* Injury, superficial, leg
    lens, eye — *see* Injury, eye, specified site NEC
      penetrating — *see* Injury, eyeball, penetrating
    limb NEC T14.8 ☑
    lip S09.93 ☑
    liver S36.119 ☑
      contusion S36.112 ☑
      laceration S36.113 ☑
        major (stellate) S36.116 ☑
        minor S36.114 ☑
        moderate S36.115 ☑
      specified NEC S36.118 ☑
    lower back S39.92 ☑
      specified NEC S39.82 ☑
    lumbar, lumbosacral (region) S39.92 ☑
      plexus — *see* Injury, lumbosacral plexus
    lumbosacral plexus S34.4 ☑
    lung (*see also* Injury, intrathoracic, lung)
      aspiration J69.0
      transfusion-related (TRALI) J95.84
    lymphatic thoracic duct — *see* Injury, intrathoracic, specified organ NEC
    malar region S09.93 ☑
    mastoid region S09.90 ☑
    maxilla S09.93 ☑

Injury — *continued*
  mediastinum — *see* Injury, intrathoracic, specified organ NEC
  membrane, brain — *see* Injury, intracranial
  meningeal artery — *see* Injury, intracranial, subdural hemorrhage
  meninges (cerebral) — *see* Injury, intracranial
  mesenteric
    artery
      branch S35.299 ☑
        laceration (minor) (superficial) S35.291 ☑
          major S35.292 ☑
          specified NEC S35.298 ☑
      inferior S35.239 ☑
        laceration (minor) (superficial) S35.231 ☑
          major S35.232 ☑
          specified NEC S35.238 ☑
      superior S35.229 ☑
        laceration (minor) (superficial) S35.221 ☑
          major S35.222 ☑
          specified NEC S35.228 ☑
    plexus (inferior) (superior) — *see* Injury, nerve, lumbosacral, sympathetic
    vein
      inferior S35.349 ☑
        laceration S35.341 ☑
        specified NEC S35.348 ☑
      superior S35.339 ☑
        laceration S35.331 ☑
        specified NEC S35.338 ☑
  mesentery — *see* Injury, intra-abdominal, specified site NEC
  mesosalpinx — *see* Injury, pelvic organ, specified site NEC
  middle ear S09.30- ☑
  midthoracic region NOS S29.9 ☑
  mouth S09.93 ☑
  multiple NOS T07 ☑
  muscle (and fascia) (and tendon)
    abdomen S39.001 ☑
      laceration S39.021 ☑
      specified type NEC S39.091 ☑
      strain S39.011 ☑
    abductor
      thumb, forearm level — *see* Injury, muscle, thumb, abductor
    adductor
      thigh S76.20- ☑
        laceration S76.22- ☑
        specified type NEC S76.29- ☑
        strain S76.21- ☑
    ankle — *see* Injury, muscle, foot
    anterior muscle group, at leg level (lower) S86.20- ☑
      laceration S86.22- ☑
      specified type NEC S86.29- ☑
      strain S86.21- ☑
    arm (upper) — *see* Injury, muscle, shoulder
    biceps (parts NEC) S46.20- ☑
      laceration S46.22- ☑
      long head S46.10- ☑
        laceration S46.12- ☑
        specified type NEC S46.19- ☑
        strain S46.11- ☑
      specified type NEC S46.29- ☑
      strain S46.21- ☑
    extensor
      finger(s) (other than thumb) — *see* Injury, muscle, finger by site, extensor
      forearm level, specified NEC — *see* Injury, muscle, forearm, extensor
      thumb — *see* Injury, muscle, thumb, extensor
      toe (large) (ankle level) (foot level) — *see* Injury, muscle, toe, extensor
    finger
      extensor (forearm level) S56.40- ☑
        hand level S66.309 ☑
          laceration S66.329 ☑
          specified type NEC S66.399 ☑
          strain S66.319 ☑
        laceration S56.429 ☑
        specified type NEC S56.499 ☑
        strain S56.419 ☑
      flexor (forearm level) S56.10- ☑
        hand level S66.109 ☑
          laceration S66.129 ☑

☑ Additional Character Required — Refer to the Tabular List for Character Selection　　🔺 Subterms under main terms may continue to next column or page

Injury — *continued*
  muscle — *continued*
    finger — *continued*
      flexor — *continued*
        hand level — *continued*
          specified type NEC S66.199 ☑
          strain S66.119 ☑
        laceration S56.129 ☑
        specified type NEC S56.199 ☑
        strain S56.119 ☑
      index
        extensor (forearm level)
          hand level S66.308 ☑
            laceration S66.32- ☑
            specified type NEC S66.39- ☑
            strain S66.31- ☑
          specified type NEC S56.492- ☑
        flexor (forearm level)
          hand level S66.108 ☑
            laceration S66.12- ☑
            specified type NEC S66.19- ☑
            strain S66.11- ☑
          specified type NEC S56.19- ☑
          strain S56.11- ☑
        intrinsic S66.50- ☑
          laceration S66.52- ☑
          specified type NEC S66.59- ☑
          strain S66.51- ☑
      intrinsic S66.509 ☑
        laceration S66.529 ☑
        specified type NEC S66.599 ☑
        strain S66.519 ☑
      little
        extensor (forearm level)
          hand level S66.30- ☑
            laceration S66.32- ☑
            specified type NEC S66.39- ☑
            strain S66.31- ☑
          laceration S56.42- ☑
          specified type NEC S56.49- ☑
          strain S56.41- ☑
        flexor (forearm level)
          hand level S66.10- ☑
            laceration S66.12- ☑
            specified type NEC S66.19- ☑
            strain S66.11- ☑
          laceration S56.12- ☑
          specified type NEC S56.19- ☑
          strain S56.11- ☑
        intrinsic S66.50- ☑
          laceration S66.52- ☑
          specified type NEC S66.59- ☑
          strain S66.51- ☑
      middle
        extensor (forearm level)
          hand level S66.30- ☑
            laceration S66.32- ☑
            specified type NEC S66.39- ☑
            strain S66.31- ☑
          laceration S56.42- ☑
          specified type NEC S56.49- ☑
          strain S56.41- ☑
        flexor (forearm level)
          hand level S66.10- ☑
            laceration S66.12- ☑
            specified type NEC S66.19- ☑
            strain S66.11- ☑
          laceration S56.12- ☑
          specified type NEC S56.19- ☑
          strain S56.11- ☑
        intrinsic S66.50- ☑
          laceration S66.52- ☑
          specified type NEC S66.59- ☑
          strain S66.51- ☑
      ring
        extensor (forearm level)
          hand level S66.30- ☑
            laceration S66.32- ☑
            specified type NEC S66.39- ☑
            strain S66.31- ☑
          laceration S56.42- ☑
          specified type NEC S56.49- ☑
          strain S56.41- ☑
        flexor (forearm level)
          hand level S66.10- ☑
            laceration S66.12- ☑

Injury — *continued*
  muscle — *continued*
    finger — *continued*
      ring — *continued*
        flexor — *continued*
          hand level — *continued*
            specified type NEC S66.19- ☑
            strain S66.11- ☑
          laceration S56.12- ☑
          specified type NEC S56.19- ☑
          strain S56.11- ☑
        intrinsic S66.50- ☑
          laceration S66.52- ☑
          specified type NEC S66.59- ☑
          strain S66.51- ☑
    flexor
      finger(s) (other than thumb) — *see* Injury, muscle, finger
      forearm level, specified NEC — *see* Injury, muscle, forearm, flexor
      thumb — *see* Injury, muscle, thumb, flexor
      toe (long) (ankle level) (foot level) — *see* Injury, muscle, toe, flexor
    foot S96.90- ☑
      intrinsic S96.20- ☑
        laceration S96.22- ☑
        specified type NEC S96.29- ☑
        strain S96.21- ☑
      laceration S96.92- ☑
      long extensor, toe — *see* Injury, muscle, toe, extensor
      long flexor, toe — *see* Injury, muscle, toe, flexor
      specified
        site NEC S96.80- ☑
          laceration S96.82- ☑
          specified type NEC S96.89- ☑
          strain S96.81- ☑
        type S96.99- ☑
      strain S96.91- ☑
    forearm (level) S56.90- ☑
      extensor S56.50- ☑
        laceration S56.52- ☑
        specified type NEC S56.59- ☑
        strain S56.51- ☑
      flexor S56.20- ☑
        laceration S56.22- ☑
        specified type NEC S56.29- ☑
        strain S56.21- ☑
      laceration S56.92- ☑
      specified S56.99- ☑
        site NEC S56.80- ☑
          laceration S56.82- ☑
          strain S56.81- ☑
          type NEC S56.89- ☑
      strain S56.91- ☑
    hand (level) S66.90- ☑
      laceration S66.92- ☑
      specified
        site NEC S66.80- ☑
          laceration S66.82- ☑
          specified type NEC S66.89- ☑
          strain S66.81- ☑
          type NEC S66.99- ☑
      strain S66.91- ☑
    head S09.10 ☑
      laceration S09.12 ☑
      specified type NEC S09.19 ☑
      strain S09.11 ☑
    hip NEC S76.00- ☑
      laceration S76.02- ☑
      specified type NEC S76.09- ☑
      strain S76.01- ☑
    intrinsic
      ankle and foot level — *see* Injury, muscle, foot, intrinsic
      finger (other than thumb) — *see* Injury, muscle, finger by site, intrinsic
      foot (level) — *see* Injury, muscle, foot, intrinsic
      thumb — *see* Injury, muscle, thumb, intrinsic
    leg (level) (lower) S86.90- ☑
      Achilles tendon — *see* Injury, Achilles tendon
      anterior muscle group — *see* Injury, muscle, anterior muscle group
      laceration S86.92- ☑
      peroneal muscle group — *see* Injury, muscle, peroneal muscle group

Injury — *continued*
  muscle — *continued*
    leg — *continued*
      posterior muscle group — *see* Injury, muscle, posterior muscle group, leg level
      specified
        site NEC S86.80- ☑
          laceration S86.82- ☑
          specified type NEC S86.89- ☑
          strain S86.81- ☑
        type NEC S86.99- ☑
      strain S86.91- ☑
    long
      extensor toe, at ankle and foot level — *see* Injury, muscle, toe, extensor
      flexor, toe, at ankle and foot level — *see* Injury, muscle, toe, flexor
      head, biceps — *see* Injury, muscle, biceps, long head
    lower back S39.002 ☑
      laceration S39.022 ☑
      specified type NEC S39.092 ☑
      strain S39.012 ☑
    neck (level) S16.9
      laceration S16.2
      specified type NEC S16.8
      strain S16.1
    pelvis S39.003 ☑
      laceration S39.023 ☑
      specified type NEC S39.093 ☑
      strain S39.013 ☑
    peroneal muscle group, at leg level (lower) S86.30- ☑
      laceration S86.32- ☑
      specified type NEC S86.39- ☑
      strain S86.31- ☑
    posterior muscle (group)
      leg level (lower) S86.10- ☑
        laceration S86.12- ☑
        specified type NEC S86.19- ☑
        strain S86.11- ☑
      thigh level S76.30- ☑
        laceration S76.32- ☑
        specified type NEC S76.39- ☑
        strain S76.31- ☑
    quadriceps (thigh) S76.10- ☑
      laceration S76.12- ☑
      specified type NEC S76.19- ☑
      strain S76.11- ☑
    shoulder S46.90- ☑
      laceration S46.92- ☑
      rotator cuff — *see* Injury, rotator cuff
      specified site NEC S46.80- ☑
        laceration S46.82- ☑
        specified type NEC S46.89- ☑
        strain S46.81- ☑
      specified type NEC S46.99- ☑
      strain S46.91- ☑
    thigh NEC (level) S76.90- ☑
      adductor — *see* Injury, muscle, adductor, thigh
      laceration S76.92- ☑
      posterior muscle (group) — *see* Injury, muscle, posterior muscle, thigh level
      quadriceps — *see* Injury, muscle, quadriceps
      specified
        site NEC S76.80- ☑
          laceration S76.82- ☑
          specified type NEC S76.89- ☑
          strain S76.81- ☑
        type NEC S76.99- ☑
      strain S76.91- ☑
    thorax (level) S29.009 ☑
      back wall S29.002 ☑
      front wall S29.001 ☑
      laceration S29.029 ☑
        back wall S29.022 ☑
        front wall S29.021 ☑
      specified type NEC S29.099 ☑
        back wall S29.092 ☑
        front wall S29.091 ☑
      strain S29.019 ☑
        back wall S29.012 ☑
        front wall S29.011 ☑
    thumb
      abductor (forearm level) S56.30- ☑
        laceration S56.32- ☑

🔽 Subterms under main terms may continue to next column or page   ☑ Additional Character Required — Refer to the Tabular List for Character Selection   195

Injury — Injury

Injury — *continued*
muscle — *continued*
thumb — *continued*
abductor — *continued*
specified type NEC S56.39- ☑
strain S56.31- ☑
extensor (forearm level) S56.30- ☑
hand level S66.20- ☑
laceration S66.22- ☑
specified type NEC S66.29- ☑
strain S66.21- ☑
laceration S56.32- ☑
specified type NEC S56.39- ☑
strain S56.31- ☑
flexor (forearm level) S56.00- ☑
hand level S66.00- ☑
laceration S66.02- ☑
specified type NEC S66.09- ☑
strain S66.01- ☑
laceration S56.02- ☑
specified type NEC S56.09- ☑
strain S56.01- ☑
wrist level — *see* Injury, muscle, thumb, flexor, hand level
intrinsic S66.40- ☑
laceration S66.42- ☑
specified type NEC S66.49- ☑
strain S66.41- ☑
toe (*see also* Injury, muscle, foot)
extensor, long S96.10- ☑
laceration S96.12- ☑
specified type NEC S96.19- ☑
strain S96.11- ☑
flexor, long S96.00- ☑
laceration S96.02- ☑
specified type NEC S96.09- ☑
strain S96.01- ☑
triceps S46.30- ☑
laceration S46.32- ☑
specified type NEC S46.39- ☑
strain S46.31- ☑
wrist (and hand) level — *see* Injury, muscle, hand
musculocutaneous nerve — *see* Injury, nerve, musculocutaneous
myocardium — *see* Injury, heart
nape — *see* Injury, neck
nasal (septum) (sinus) S09.92 ☑
nasopharynx S09.92 ☑
neck S19.9 ☑
specified NEC S19.80 ☑
specified site NEC S19.89 ☑
nerve NEC T14.8 ☑
abdomen S34.9 ☑
peripheral S34.6 ☑
specified site NEC S34.8 ☑
abducens S04.4- ☑
contusion S04.4- ☑
laceration S04.4- ☑
specified type NEC S04.4- ☑
abducent — *see* Injury, nerve, abducens
accessory S04.7- ☑
contusion S04.7- ☑
laceration S04.7- ☑
specified type NEC S04.7- ☑
acoustic S04.6- ☑
contusion S04.6- ☑
laceration S04.6- ☑
specified type NEC S04.6- ☑
ankle S94.9- ☑
cutaneous sensory S94.3- ☑
specified site NEC — *see* subcategory S94.8 ☑
anterior crural, femoral — *see* Injury, nerve, femoral
arm (upper) S44.9- ☑
axillary — *see* Injury, nerve, axillary
cutaneous — *see* Injury, nerve, cutaneous, arm
median — *see* Injury, nerve, median, upper arm
musculocutaneous — *see* Injury, nerve, musculocutaneous
radial — *see* Injury, nerve, radial, upper arm
specified site NEC — *see* subcategory S44.8 ☑
ulnar — *see* Injury, nerve, ulnar, arm
auditory — *see* Injury, nerve, acoustic
axillary S44.3- ☑
brachial plexus — *see* Injury, brachial plexus
cervical sympathetic S14.5 ☑
cranial S04.9 ☑

Injury — *continued*
nerve — *continued*
cranial — *continued*
contusion S04.9 ☑
eighth (acoustic or auditory) — *see* Injury, nerve, acoustic
eleventh (accessory) — *see* Injury, nerve, accessory
fifth (trigeminal) — *see* Injury, nerve, trigeminal
first (olfactory) — *see* Injury, nerve, olfactory
fourth (trochlear) — *see* Injury, nerve, trochlear
laceration S04.9 ☑
ninth (glossopharyngeal) — *see* Injury, nerve, glossopharyngeal
second (optic) — *see* Injury, nerve, optic
seventh (facial) — *see* Injury, nerve, facial
sixth (abducent) — *see* Injury, nerve, abducens
specified
nerve NEC S04.89- ☑
contusion S04.89- ☑
laceration S04.89- ☑
specified type NEC S04.89- ☑
type NEC S04.9 ☑
tenth (pneumogastric or vagus) — *see* Injury, nerve, vagus
third (oculomotor) — *see* Injury, nerve, oculomotor
twelfth (hypoglossal) — *see* Injury, nerve, hypoglossal
cutaneous sensory
ankle (level) S94.3- ☑
arm (upper) (level) S44.5- ☑
foot (level) — *see* Injury, nerve, cutaneous sensory, ankle
forearm (level) S54.3- ☑
hip (level) S74.2- ☑
leg (lower level) S84.2- ☑
shoulder (level) — *see* Injury, nerve, cutaneous sensory, arm
thigh (level) — *see* Injury, nerve, cutaneous sensory, hip
deep peroneal — *see* Injury, nerve, peroneal, foot
digital
finger S64.4- ☑
index S64.49- ☑
little S64.49- ☑
middle S64.49- ☑
ring S64.49- ☑
thumb S64.3- ☑
toe — *see* Injury, nerve, ankle, specified site NEC
eighth cranial (acoustic or auditory) — *see* Injury, nerve, acoustic
eleventh cranial (accessory) — *see* Injury, nerve, accessory
facial S04.5- ☑
contusion S04.5- ☑
laceration S04.5- ☑
newborn P11.3
specified type NEC S04.5- ☑
femoral (hip level) (thigh level) S74.1- ☑
fifth cranial (trigeminal) — *see* Injury, nerve, trigeminal
finger (digital) — *see* Injury, nerve, digital, finger
first cranial (olfactory) — *see* Injury, nerve, olfactory
foot S94.9- ☑
cutaneous sensory S94.3- ☑
deep peroneal S94.2- ☑
lateral plantar S94.0- ☑
medial plantar S94.1- ☑
specified site NEC — *see* subcategory S94.8
forearm (level) S54.9- ☑
cutaneous sensory — *see* Injury, nerve, cutaneous sensory, forearm
median — *see* Injury, nerve, median
radial — *see* Injury, nerve, radial
specified site NEC — *see* subcategory S54.8 ☑
ulnar — *see* Injury, nerve, ulnar
fourth cranial (trochlear) — *see* Injury, nerve, trochlear
glossopharyngeal S04.89- ☑
specified type NEC S04.89- ☑
hand S64.9- ☑
median — *see* Injury, nerve, median, hand
radial — *see* Injury, nerve, radial, hand
specified NEC — *see* subcategory S64.8 ☑

Injury — *continued*
nerve — *continued*
hand — *continued*
ulnar — *see* Injury, nerve, ulnar, hand
hip (level) S74.9- ☑
cutaneous sensory — *see* Injury, nerve, cutaneous sensory, hip
femoral — *see* Injury, nerve, femoral
sciatic — *see* Injury, nerve, sciatic
specified site NEC — *see* subcategory S74.8 ☑
hypoglossal S04.89- ☑
specified type NEC S04.89- ☑
lateral plantar S94.0- ☑
leg (lower) S84.9- ☑
cutaneous sensory — *see* Injury, nerve, cutaneous sensory, leg
peroneal — *see* Injury, nerve, peroneal
specified site NEC — *see* subcategory S84.8 ☑
tibial — *see* Injury, nerve, tibial
upper — *see* Injury, nerve, thigh
lower
back — *see* Injury, nerve, abdomen, specified site NEC
peripheral — *see* Injury, nerve, abdomen, peripheral
limb — *see* Injury, nerve, leg
lumbar plexus — *see* Injury, nerve, lumbosacral, sympathetic
lumbar spinal — *see* Injury, nerve, spinal, lumbar
lumbosacral
plexus — *see* Injury, nerve, lumbosacral, sympathetic
sympathetic S34.5 ☑
medial plantar S94.1- ☑
median (forearm level) S54.1- ☑
hand (level) S64.1- ☑
upper arm (level) S44.1- ☑
wrist (level) — *see* Injury, nerve, median, hand
musculocutaneous S44.4- ☑
musculospiral (upper arm level) — *see* Injury, nerve, radial, upper arm
neck S14.9 ☑
peripheral S14.4 ☑
specified site NEC S14.8 ☑
sympathetic S14.5 ☑
ninth cranial (glossopharyngeal) — *see* Injury, nerve, glossopharyngeal
oculomotor S04.1- ☑
contusion S04.1- ☑
laceration S04.1- ☑
specified type NEC S04.1- ☑
olfactory S04.81- ☑
specified type NEC S04.81- ☑
optic S04.01- ☑
contusion S04.01- ☑
laceration S04.01- ☑
specified type NEC S04.01- ☑
pelvic girdle — *see* Injury, nerve, hip
pelvis — *see* Injury, nerve, abdomen, specified site NEC
peripheral — *see* Injury, nerve, abdomen, peripheral
peripheral NEC T14.8 ☑
abdomen — *see* Injury, nerve, abdomen, peripheral
lower back — *see* Injury, nerve, abdomen, peripheral
neck — *see* Injury, nerve, neck, peripheral
pelvis — *see* Injury, nerve, abdomen, peripheral
specified NEC T14.8 ☑
peroneal (lower leg level) S84.1- ☑
foot S94.2- ☑
plexus
brachial — *see* Injury, brachial plexus
celiac, coeliac — *see* Injury, nerve, lumbosacral, sympathetic
mesenteric, inferior — *see* Injury, nerve, lumbosacral, sympathetic
sacral — *see* Injury, lumbosacral plexus
spinal
brachial — *see* Injury, brachial plexus
lumbosacral — *see* Injury, lumbosacral plexus
pneumogastric — *see* Injury, nerve, vagus
radial (forearm level) S54.2- ☑
hand (level) S64.2- ☑

☑ **Additional Character Required** — Refer to the Tabular List for Character Selection   ⬇ **Subterms under main terms may continue to next column or page**

Injury — *continued*
  nerve — *continued*
    radial — *continued*
      upper arm (level) S44.2- ☑
      wrist (level) — *see* Injury, nerve, radial, hand
    root — *see* Injury, nerve, spinal, root
    sacral plexus — *see* Injury, lumbosacral plexus
    sacral spinal — *see* Injury, nerve, spinal, sacral
    sciatic (hip level) (thigh level) S74.0- ☑
    second cranial (optic) — *see* Injury, nerve, optic
    seventh cranial (facial) — *see* Injury, nerve, facial
    shoulder — *see* Injury, nerve, arm
    sixth cranial (abducent) — *see* Injury, nerve, abducens
    spinal
      plexus — *see* Injury, nerve, plexus, spinal
      root
        cervical S14.2 ☑
        dorsal S24.2 ☑
        lumbar S34.21 ☑
        sacral S34.22 ☑
        thoracic — *see* Injury, nerve, spinal, root, dorsal
    splanchnic — *see* Injury, nerve, lumbosacral, sympathetic
    sympathetic NEC — *see* Injury, nerve, lumbosacral, sympathetic
      cervical — *see* Injury, nerve, cervical sympathetic
    tenth cranial (pneumogastric or vagus) — *see* Injury, nerve, vagus
    thigh (level) — *see* Injury, nerve, hip
      cutaneous sensory — *see* Injury, nerve, cutaneous sensory, hip
      femoral — *see* Injury, nerve, femoral
      sciatic — *see* Injury, nerve, sciatic
      specified NEC — *see* Injury, nerve, hip
    third cranial (oculomotor) — *see* Injury, nerve, oculomotor
    thorax S24.9 ☑
      peripheral S24.3 ☑
      specified site NEC S24.8 ☑
      sympathetic S24.4 ☑
    thumb, digital — *see* Injury, nerve, digital, thumb
    tibial (lower leg level) (posterior) S84.0- ☑
    toe — *see* Injury, nerve, ankle
    trigeminal S04.3- ☑
      contusion S04.3- ☑
      laceration S04.3- ☑
      specified type NEC S04.3- ☑
    trochlear S04.2- ☑
      contusion S04.2- ☑
      laceration S04.2- ☑
      specified type NEC S04.2- ☑
    twelfth cranial (hypoglossal) — *see* Injury, nerve, hypoglossal
    ulnar (forearm level) S54.0- ☑
      arm (upper) (level) S44.0- ☑
      hand (level) S64.0- ☑
      wrist (level) — *see* Injury, nerve, ulnar, hand
    vagus S04.89- ☑
      specified type NEC S04.89- ☑
    wrist (level) — *see* Injury, nerve, hand
    ninth cranial nerve (glossopharyngeal) — *see* Injury, nerve, glossopharyngeal
  nose (septum) S09.92 ☑
  obstetrical O71.9
    specified NEC O71.89
  occipital (region) (scalp) S09.90 ☑
    lobe — *see* Injury, intracranial
  optic chiasm S04.02 ☑
  optic radiation S04.03- ☑
  optic tract and pathways S04.03- ☑
  orbit, orbital (region) — *see* Injury, eye
    penetrating (with foreign body) — *see* Injury, eye, orbit, penetrating
    specified NEC — *see* Injury, eye, specified site NEC
  ovary, ovarian S37.409 ☑
    bilateral S37.402 ☑
      contusion S37.422 ☑
      laceration S37.432 ☑
      specified type NEC S37.492 ☑
    blood vessel — *see* Injury, blood vessel, ovarian
    contusion S37.429 ☑
      bilateral S37.422 ☑
      unilateral S37.421 ☑

Injury — *continued*
  ovary, ovarian — *continued*
    laceration S37.439 ☑
      bilateral S37.432 ☑
      unilateral S37.431 ☑
    specified type NEC S37.499 ☑
      bilateral S37.492 ☑
      unilateral S37.491 ☑
    unilateral S37.401 ☑
      contusion S37.421 ☑
      laceration S37.431 ☑
      specified type NEC S37.491 ☑
  palate (hard) (soft) S09.93 ☑
  pancreas S36.209 ☑
    body S36.201 ☑
      contusion S36.221 ☑
      laceration S36.231 ☑
        major S36.261 ☑
        minor S36.241 ☑
        moderate S36.251 ☑
      specified type NEC S36.291 ☑
    contusion S36.229 ☑
    head S36.200 ☑
      contusion S36.220 ☑
      laceration S36.230 ☑
        major S36.260 ☑
        minor S36.240 ☑
        moderate S36.250 ☑
      specified type NEC S36.290 ☑
    laceration S36.239 ☑
      major S36.269 ☑
      minor S36.249 ☑
      moderate S36.259 ☑
    specified type NEC S36.299 ☑
    tail S36.202 ☑
      contusion S36.222 ☑
      laceration S36.232 ☑
        major S36.262 ☑
        minor S36.242 ☑
        moderate S36.252 ☑
      specified type NEC S36.292 ☑
  parietal (region) (scalp) S09.90 ☑
    lobe — *see* Injury, intracranial
  patellar ligament (tendon) S76.10- ☑
    laceration S76.12- ☑
    specified NEC S76.19- ☑
    strain S76.11- ☑
  pelvis, pelvic (floor) S39.93 ☑
    complicating delivery O70.1
    joint or ligament, complicating delivery O71.6
    organ S37.90 ☑
      with ectopic or molar pregnancy O08.6
      complication of abortion — *see* Abortion
      contusion S37.92 ☑
      following ectopic or molar pregnancy O08.6
      laceration S37.93 ☑
      obstetrical trauma NEC O71.5
      specified
        site NEC S37.899 ☑
          contusion S37.892 ☑
          laceration S37.893 ☑
          specified type NEC S37.898 ☑
        type NEC S37.99 ☑
    specified NEC S39.83 ☑
  penis S39.94 ☑
  perineum S39.94 ☑
  peritoneum S36.81 ☑
    laceration S36.893 ☑
  periurethral tissue — *see* Injury, urethra
    complicating delivery O71.82
  phalanges
    foot — *see* Injury, foot
    hand — *see* Injury, hand
  pharynx NEC S19.85 ☑
  pleura — *see* Injury, intrathoracic, pleura
  plexus
    brachial — *see* Injury, brachial plexus
    cardiac — *see* Injury, nerve, thorax, sympathetic
    celiac, coeliac — *see* Injury, nerve, lumbosacral, sympathetic
    esophageal — *see* Injury, nerve, thorax, sympathetic
    hypogastric — *see* Injury, nerve, lumbosacral, sympathetic
    lumbar, lumbosacral — *see* Injury, lumbosacral plexus

Injury — *continued*
  plexus — *continued*
    mesenteric — *see* Injury, nerve, lumbosacral, sympathetic
    pulmonary — *see* Injury, nerve, thorax, sympathetic
  postcardiac surgery (syndrome) I97.0
  prepuce S39.94 ☑
  prostate S37.829 ☑
    contusion S37.822 ☑
    laceration S37.823 ☑
    specified type NEC S37.828 ☑
  pubic region S39.94 ☑
  pudendum S39.94 ☑
  pulmonary plexus — *see* Injury, nerve, thorax, sympathetic
  rectovaginal septum NEC S39.83 ☑
  rectum — *see* Injury, intestine, large, rectum
  retina — *see* Injury, eye, specified site NEC
    penetrating — *see* Injury, eyeball, penetrating
  retroperitoneal — *see* Injury, intra-abdominal, specified site NEC
  rotator cuff (muscle(s)) (tendon(s)) S46.00- ☑
    laceration S46.02- ☑
    specified type NEC S46.09- ☑
    strain S46.01- ☑
  round ligament — *see* Injury, pelvic organ, specified site NEC
  sacral plexus — *see* Injury, lumbosacral plexus
  salivary duct or gland S09.93 ☑
  scalp S09.90 ☑
    newborn (birth injury) P12.9
      due to monitoring (electrode) (sampling incision) P12.4
      specified NEC P12.89
        caput succedaneum P12.81
  scapular region — *see* Injury, shoulder
  sclera — *see* Injury, eye, specified site NEC
    penetrating — *see* Injury, eyeball, penetrating
  scrotum S39.94 ☑
  second cranial nerve (optic) — *see* Injury, nerve, optic
  seminal vesicle — *see* Injury, pelvic organ, specified site NEC
  seventh cranial nerve (facial) — *see* Injury, nerve, facial
  shoulder S49.9- ☑
    blood vessel — *see* Injury, blood vessel, arm
    contusion — *see* Contusion, shoulder
    dislocation — *see* Dislocation, shoulder
    fracture — *see* Fracture, shoulder
    muscle — *see* Injury, muscle, shoulder
    nerve — *see* Injury, nerve, shoulder
    open — *see* Wound, open, shoulder
    specified type NEC S49.8- ☑
    sprain — *see* Sprain, shoulder girdle
    superficial — *see* Injury, superficial, shoulder
  sinus
    cavernous — *see* Injury, intracranial
    nasal S09.92 ☑
  sixth cranial nerve (abducent) — *see* Injury, nerve, abducens
  skeleton, birth injury P13.9
    specified part NEC P13.8
  skin NEC T14.8 ☑
    surface intact — *see* Injury, superficial
  skull NEC S09.90 ☑
    specified NEC T14.8 ☑
  spermatic cord (pelvic region) S37.898 ☑
    scrotal region S39.848 ☑
  spinal (cord)
    cervical (neck) S14.109 ☑
      anterior cord syndrome S14.139 ☑
        C1 level S14.131 ☑
        C2 level S14.132 ☑
        C3 level S14.133 ☑
        C4 level S14.134 ☑
        C5 level S14.135 ☑
        C6 level S14.136 ☑
        C7 level S14.137 ☑
        C8 level S14.138 ☑
      Brown-Séquard syndrome S14.149 ☑
        C1 level S14.141 ☑
        C2 level S14.142 ☑
        C3 level S14.143 ☑
        C4 level S14.144 ☑
        C5 level S14.145 ☑
        C6 level S14.146 ☑

Injury — *continued*
  spinal — *continued*
    cervical — *continued*
      Brown-Séquard syndrome — *continued*
        C7 level S14.147 ☑
        C8 level S14.148 ☑
      C1 level S14.101 ☑
      C2 level S14.102 ☑
      C3 level S14.103 ☑
      C4 level S14.104 ☑
      C5 level S14.105 ☑
      C6 level S14.106 ☑
      C7 level S14.107 ☑
      C8 level S14.108 ☑
      central cord syndrome S14.129 ☑
        C1 level S14.121 ☑
        C2 level S14.122 ☑
        C3 level S14.123 ☑
        C4 level S14.124 ☑
        C5 level S14.125 ☑
        C6 level S14.126 ☑
        C7 level S14.127 ☑
        C8 level S14.128 ☑
      complete lesion S14.119 ☑
        C1 level S14.111 ☑
        C2 level S14.112 ☑
        C3 level S14.113 ☑
        C4 level S14.114 ☑
        C5 level S14.115 ☑
        C6 level S14.116 ☑
        C7 level S14.117 ☑
        C8 level S14.118 ☑
      concussion S14.0 ☑
      edema S14.0 ☑
      incomplete lesion specified NEC S14.159 ☑
        C1 level S14.151 ☑
        C2 level S14.152 ☑
        C3 level S14.153 ☑
        C4 level S14.154 ☑
        C5 level S14.155 ☑
        C6 level S14.156 ☑
        C7 level S14.157 ☑
        C8 level S14.158 ☑
      posterior cord syndrome S14.159 ☑
        C1 level S14.151 ☑
        C2 level S14.152 ☑
        C3 level S14.153 ☑
        C4 level S14.154 ☑
        C5 level S14.155 ☑
        C6 level S14.156 ☑
        C7 level S14.157 ☑
        C8 level S14.158 ☑
    dorsal — *see* Injury, spinal, thoracic
    lumbar S34.109 ☑
      complete lesion S34.119 ☑
        L1 level S34.111 ☑
        L2 level S34.112 ☑
        L3 level S34.113 ☑
        L4 level S34.114 ☑
        L5 level S34.115 ☑
      concussion S34.01 ☑
      edema S34.01 ☑
      incomplete lesion S34.129 ☑
        L1 level S34.121 ☑
        L2 level S34.122 ☑
        L3 level S34.123 ☑
        L4 level S34.124 ☑
        L5 level S34.125 ☑
      L1 level S34.101 ☑
      L2 level S34.102 ☑
      L3 level S34.103 ☑
      L4 level S34.104 ☑
      L5 level S34.105 ☑
    nerve root NEC
      cervical — *see* Injury, nerve, spinal, root, cervical
      dorsal — *see* Injury, nerve, spinal, root, dorsal
      lumbar S34.21 ☑
      sacral S34.22 ☑
      thoracic — *see* Injury, nerve, spinal, root, dorsal
    plexus
      brachial — *see* Injury, brachial plexus
      lumbosacral — *see* Injury, lumbosacral plexus
    sacral S34.139 ☑
      complete lesion S34.131 ☑
      incomplete lesion S34.132 ☑

Injury — *continued*
  spinal — *continued*
    thoracic S24.109 ☑
      anterior cord syndrome S24.139 ☑
        T1 level S24.131 ☑
        T2-T6 level S24.132 ☑
        T7-T10 level S24.133 ☑
        T11-T12 level S24.134 ☑
      Brown-Séquard syndrome S24.149 ☑
        T1 level S24.141 ☑
        T2-T6 level S24.142 ☑
        T7-T10 level S24.143 ☑
        T11-T12 level S24.144 ☑
      complete lesion S24.119 ☑
        T1 level S24.111 ☑
        T2-T6 level S24.112 ☑
        T7-T10 level S24.113 ☑
        T11-T12 level S24.114 ☑
      concussion S24.0 ☑
      edema S24.0 ☑
      incomplete lesion specified NEC S24.159 ☑
        T1 level S24.151 ☑
        T2-T6 level S24.152 ☑
        T7-T10 level S24.153 ☑
        T11-T12 level S24.154 ☑
      posterior cord syndrome S24.159 ☑
        T1 level S24.151 ☑
        T2-T6 level S24.152 ☑
        T7-T10 level S24.153 ☑
        T11-T12 level S24.154 ☑
      T1 level S24.101 ☑
      T2-T6 level S24.102 ☑
      T7-T10 level S24.103 ☑
      T11-T12 level S24.104 ☑
  splanchnic nerve — *see* Injury, nerve, lumbosacral, sympathetic
  spleen S36.00 ☑
    contusion S36.029 ☑
      major S36.021 ☑
      minor S36.020 ☑
    laceration S36.039 ☑
      major (massive) (stellate) S36.032 ☑
      moderate S36.031 ☑
      superficial (capsular) (minor) S36.030 ☑
    specified type NEC S36.09 ☑
  splenic artery — *see* Injury, blood vessel, celiac artery, branch
  stellate ganglion — *see* Injury, nerve, thorax, sympathetic
  sternal region S29.9 ☑
  stomach S36.30 ☑
    contusion S36.32 ☑
    laceration S36.33 ☑
    specified type NEC S36.39 ☑
  subconjunctival — *see* Injury, eye, conjunctiva
  subcutaneous NEC T14.8 ☑
  submaxillary region S09.93 ☑
  submental region S09.93 ☑
  subungual
    fingers — *see* Injury, hand
    toes — *see* Injury, foot
  superficial NEC T14.8 ☑
    abdomen, abdominal (wall) S30.92 ☑
      abrasion S30.811 ☑
      bite S30.871 ☑
        insect S30.861 ☑
      contusion S30.1 ☑
      external constriction S30.841 ☑
      foreign body S30.851 ☑
    abrasion — *see* Abrasion, by site
    adnexa, eye NEC — *see* Injury, eye, specified site NEC
    alveolar process — *see* Injury, superficial, oral cavity
    ankle S90.91- ☑
      abrasion — *see* Abrasion, ankle
      bite — *see* Bite, ankle
      blister — *see* Blister, ankle
      contusion — *see* Contusion, ankle
      external constriction — *see* Constriction, external, ankle
      foreign body — *see* Foreign body, superficial, ankle
    anus S30.98 ☑
    arm (upper) S40.92- ☑
      abrasion — *see* Abrasion, arm

Injury — *continued*
  superficial — *continued*
    arm — *continued*
      bite — *see* Bite, superficial, arm
      blister — *see* Blister, arm (upper)
      contusion — *see* Contusion, arm
      external constriction — *see* Constriction, external, arm
      foreign body — *see* Foreign body, superficial, arm
    auditory canal (external) (meatus) — *see* Injury, superficial, ear
    auricle — *see* Injury, superficial, ear
    axilla — *see* Injury, superficial, arm
    back (*see also* Injury, superficial, thorax, back)
      lower S30.91 ☑
        abrasion S30.810 ☑
        contusion S30.0 ☑
        external constriction S30.840 ☑
        superficial
          bite NEC S30.870 ☑
            insect S30.860 ☑
          foreign body S30.850 ☑
    bite NEC — *see* Bite, superficial NEC, by site
    blister — *see* Blister, by site
    breast S20.10- ☑
      abrasion — *see* Abrasion, breast
      bite — *see* Bite, superficial, breast
      contusion — *see* Contusion, breast
      external constriction — *see* Constriction, external, breast
      foreign body — *see* Foreign body, superficial, breast
    brow — *see* Injury, superficial, head, specified NEC
    buttock S30.91 ☑
    calf — *see* Injury, superficial, leg
    canthus, eye — *see* Injury, superficial, periocular area
    cheek (external) — *see* Injury, superficial, head, specified NEC
      internal — *see* Injury, superficial, oral cavity
    chest wall — *see* Injury, superficial, thorax
    chin — *see* Injury, superficial, head NEC
    clitoris S30.95 ☑
    conjunctiva — *see* Injury, eye, conjunctiva
      with foreign body (in conjunctival sac) — *see* Foreign body, conjunctival sac
    contusion — *see* Contusion, by site
    costal region — *see* Injury, superficial, thorax
    digit(s)
      hand — *see* Injury, superficial, finger
    ear (auricle) (canal) (external) S00.40- ☑
      abrasion — *see* Abrasion, ear
      bite — *see* Bite, superficial, ear
      contusion — *see* Contusion, ear
      external constriction — *see* Constriction, external, ear
      foreign body — *see* Foreign body, superficial, ear
    elbow S50.90- ☑
      abrasion — *see* Abrasion, elbow
      bite — *see* Bite, superficial, elbow
      blister — *see* Blister, elbow
      contusion — *see* Contusion, elbow
      external constriction — *see* Constriction, external, elbow
      foreign body — *see* Foreign body, superficial, elbow
    epididymis S30.94 ☑
    epigastric region S30.92 ☑
    epiglottis — *see* Injury, superficial, throat
    esophagus
      cervical — *see* Injury, superficial, throat
    external constriction — *see* Constriction, external, by site
    extremity NEC T14.8 ☑
    eyeball NEC — *see* Injury, eye, specified site NEC
    eyebrow — *see* Injury, superficial, periocular area
    eyelid S00.20- ☑
      abrasion — *see* Abrasion, eyelid
      bite — *see* Bite, superficial, eyelid
      contusion — *see* Contusion, eyelid
      external constriction — *see* Constriction, external, eyelid
      foreign body — *see* Foreign body, superficial, eyelid

☑ **Additional Character Required** — Refer to the Tabular List for Character Selection   ▽ **Subterms under main terms may continue to next column or page**

Injury — *continued*
  superficial — *continued*
    face NEC — *see* Injury, superficial, head, specified NEC
    finger(s) S60.949 ☑
      abrasion — *see* Abrasion, finger
      bite — *see* Bite, superficial, finger
      blister — *see* Blister, finger
      contusion — *see* Contusion, finger
      external constriction — *see* Constriction, external, finger
      foreign body — *see* Foreign body, superficial, finger
      index S60.94- ☑
      insect bite — *see* Bite, by site, superficial, insect
      little S60.94- ☑
      middle S60.94- ☑
      ring S60.94- ☑
    flank S30.92 ☑
    foot S90.92- ☑
      abrasion — *see* Abrasion, foot
      bite — *see* Bite, foot
      blister — *see* Blister, foot
      contusion — *see* Contusion, foot
      external constriction — *see* Constriction, external, foot
      foreign body — *see* Foreign body, superficial, foot
    forearm S50.91- ☑
      abrasion — *see* Abrasion, forearm
      bite — *see* Bite, forearm, superficial
      blister — *see* Blister, forearm
      contusion — *see* Contusion, forearm
      elbow only — *see* Injury, superficial, elbow
      external constriction — *see* Constriction, external, forearm
      foreign body — *see* Foreign body, superficial, forearm
    forehead — *see* Injury, superficial, head NEC
    foreign body — *see* Foreign body, superficial
    genital organs, external
      female S30.97 ☑
      male S30.96 ☑
    globe (eye) — *see* Injury, eye, specified site NEC
    groin S30.92 ☑
    gum — *see* Injury, superficial, oral cavity
    hand S60.92- ☑
      abrasion — *see* Abrasion, hand
      bite — *see* Bite, superficial, hand
      contusion — *see* Contusion, hand
      external constriction — *see* Constriction, external, hand
      foreign body — *see* Foreign body, superficial, hand
    head S00.90 ☑
      ear — *see* Injury, superficial, ear
      eyelid — *see* Injury, superficial, eyelid
      nose S00.30 ☑
      oral cavity S00.502 ☑
      scalp S00.00 ☑
      specified site NEC S00.80 ☑
    heel — *see* Injury, superficial, foot
    hip S70.91- ☑
      abrasion — *see* Abrasion, hip
      bite — *see* Bite, superficial, hip
      blister — *see* Blister, hip
      contusion — *see* Contusion, hip
      external constriction — *see* Constriction, external, hip
      foreign body — *see* Foreign body, superficial, hip
    iliac region — *see* Injury, superficial, abdomen
    inguinal region — *see* Injury, superficial, abdomen
    insect bite — *see* Bite, by site, superficial, insect
    interscapular region — *see* Injury, superficial, thorax, back
    jaw — *see* Injury, superficial, head, specified NEC
    knee S80.91- ☑
      abrasion — *see* Abrasion, knee
      bite — *see* Bite, superficial, knee
      blister — *see* Blister, knee
      contusion — *see* Contusion, knee
      external constriction — *see* Constriction, external, knee
      foreign body — *see* Foreign body, superficial, knee

Injury — *continued*
  superficial — *continued*
    labium (majus) (minus) S30.95 ☑
    lacrimal (apparatus) (gland) (sac) — *see* Injury, eye, specified site NEC
    larynx — *see* Injury, superficial, throat
    leg (lower) S80.92- ☑
      abrasion — *see* Abrasion, leg
      bite — *see* Bite, superficial, leg
      contusion — *see* Contusion, leg
      external constriction — *see* Constriction, external, leg
      foreign body — *see* Foreign body, superficial, leg
      knee — *see* Injury, superficial, knee
    limb NEC T14.8 ☑
    lip S00.501 ☑
    lower back S30.91 ☑
    lumbar region S30.91 ☑
    malar region — *see* Injury, superficial, head, specified NEC
    mammary — *see* Injury, superficial, breast
    mastoid region — *see* Injury, superficial, head, specified NEC
    mouth — *see* Injury, superficial, oral cavity
    muscle NEC T14.8 ☑
    nail NEC T14.8 ☑
      finger — *see* Injury, superficial, finger
      toe — *see* Injury, superficial, toe
    nasal (septum) — *see* Injury, superficial, nose
    neck S10.90 ☑
      specified site NEC S10.80 ☑
    nose (septum) S00.30 ☑
    occipital region — *see* Injury, superficial, scalp
    oral cavity S00.502 ☑
    orbital region — *see* Injury, superficial, periocular area
    palate — *see* Injury, superficial, oral cavity
    palm — *see* Injury, superficial, hand
    parietal region — *see* Injury, superficial, scalp
    pelvis S30.91 ☑
      girdle — *see* Injury, superficial, hip
    penis S30.93 ☑
    perineum
      female S30.95 ☑
      male S30.91 ☑
    periocular area S00.20- ☑
      abrasion — *see* Abrasion, eyelid
      bite — *see* Bite, superficial, eyelid
      contusion — *see* Contusion, eyelid
      external constriction — *see* Constriction, external, eyelid
      foreign body — *see* Foreign body, superficial, eyelid
    phalanges
      finger — *see* Injury, superficial, finger
      toe — *see* Injury, superficial, toe
    pharynx — *see* Injury, superficial, throat
    pinna — *see* Injury, superficial, ear
    popliteal space — *see* Injury, superficial, knee
    prepuce S30.93 ☑
    pubic region S30.91 ☑
    pudendum
      female S30.97 ☑
      male S30.96 ☑
    sacral region S30.91 ☑
    scalp S00.00 ☑
    scapular region — *see* Injury, superficial, shoulder
    sclera — *see* Injury, eye, specified site NEC
    scrotum S30.94 ☑
    shin — *see* Injury, superficial, leg
    shoulder S40.91- ☑
      abrasion — *see* Abrasion, shoulder
      bite — *see* Bite, superficial, shoulder
      blister — *see* Blister, shoulder
      contusion — *see* Contusion, shoulder
      external constriction — *see* Constriction, external, shoulder
      foreign body — *see* Foreign body, superficial, shoulder
    skin NEC T14.8 ☑
    sternal region — *see* Injury, superficial, thorax, front
    subconjunctival — *see* Injury, eye, specified site NEC
    subcutaneous NEC T14.8 ☑

Injury — *continued*
  superficial — *continued*
    submaxillary region — *see* Injury, superficial, head, specified NEC
    submental region — *see* Injury, superficial, head, specified NEC
    subungual
      finger(s) — *see* Injury, superficial, finger
      toe(s) — *see* Injury, superficial, toe
    supraclavicular fossa — *see* Injury, superficial, neck
    supraorbital — *see* Injury, superficial, head, specified NEC
    temple — *see* Injury, superficial, head, specified NEC
    temporal region — *see* Injury, superficial, head, specified NEC
    testis S30.94 ☑
    thigh S70.92- ☑
      abrasion — *see* Abrasion, thigh
      bite — *see* Bite, superficial, thigh
      blister — *see* Blister, thigh
      contusion — *see* Contusion, thigh
      external constriction — *see* Constriction, external, thigh
      foreign body — *see* Foreign body, superficial, thigh
    thorax, thoracic (wall) S20.90 ☑
      abrasion — *see* Abrasion, thorax
      back S20.40- ☑
      bite — *see* Bite, thorax, superficial
      blister — *see* Blister, thorax
      contusion — *see* Contusion, thorax
      external constriction — *see* Constriction, external, thorax
      foreign body — *see* Foreign body, superficial, thorax
      front S20.30- ☑
    throat S10.10 ☑
      abrasion S10.11 ☑
      bite S10.17 ☑
        insect S10.16 ☑
      blister S10.12 ☑
      contusion S10.0 ☑
      external constriction S10.14 ☑
      foreign body S10.15 ☑
    thumb S60.93- ☑
      abrasion — *see* Abrasion, thumb
      bite — *see* Bite, superficial, thumb
      blister — *see* Blister, thumb
      contusion — *see* Contusion, thumb
      external constriction — *see* Constriction, external, thumb
      foreign body — *see* Foreign body, superficial, thumb
      insect bite — *see* Bite, by site, superficial, insect
      specified type NEC S60.39 ☑
    toe(s) S90.93- ☑
      abrasion — *see* Abrasion, toe
      bite — *see* Bite, toe
      blister — *see* Blister, toe
      contusion — *see* Contusion, toe
      external constriction — *see* Constriction, external, toe
      foreign body — *see* Foreign body, superficial, toe
      great S90.93- ☑
    tongue — *see* Injury, superficial, oral cavity
    tooth, teeth — *see* Injury, superficial, oral cavity
    trachea S10.10 ☑
    tunica vaginalis S30.94 ☑
    tympanum, tympanic membrane — *see* Injury, superficial, ear
    uvula — *see* Injury, superficial, oral cavity
    vagina S30.95 ☑
    vocal cords — *see* Injury, superficial, throat
    vulva S30.95 ☑
    wrist S60.91- ☑
  supraclavicular region — *see* Injury, neck
  supraorbital S09.93 ☑
  suprarenal gland (multiple) — *see* Injury, adrenal
  surgical complication (external or internal site) — *see* Laceration, accidental complicating surgery
  temple S09.90 ☑
  temporal region S09.90 ☑
  tendon (*see also* Injury, muscle, by site)
    abdomen — *see* Injury, muscle, abdomen

▽ Subterms under main terms may continue to next column or page   ☑ Additional Character Required — Refer to the Tabular List for Character Selection   **199**

Injury — Injury

Injury — continued

tendon (see also Injury, muscle, by site) — continued
  Achilles — see Injury, Achilles tendon
  lower back — see Injury, muscle, lower back
  pelvic organs — see Injury, muscle, pelvis
tenth cranial nerve (pneumogastric or vagus) — see Injury, nerve, vagus
testis S39.94 ☑
thigh S79.92- ☑
  blood vessel — see Injury, blood vessel, hip
  contusion — see Contusion, thigh
  fracture — see Fracture, femur
  muscle — see Injury, muscle, thigh
  nerve — see Injury, nerve, thigh
  open — see Wound, open, thigh
  specified NEC S79.82- ☑
  superficial — see Injury, superficial, thigh
third cranial nerve (oculomotor) — see Injury, nerve, oculomotor
thorax, thoracic S29.9 ☑
  blood vessel — see Injury, blood vessel, thorax
  cavity — see Injury, intrathoracic
  dislocation — see Dislocation, thorax
  external (wall) S29.9 ☑
    contusion — see Contusion, thorax
    nerve — see Injury, nerve, thorax
    open — see Wound, open, thorax
    specified NEC S29.8 ☑
    sprain — see Sprain, thorax
    superficial — see Injury, superficial, thorax
  fracture — see Fracture, thorax
  internal — see Injury, intrathoracic
  intrathoracic organ — see Injury, intrathoracic
  sympathetic ganglion — see Injury, nerve, thorax, sympathetic
throat (see also Injury, neck) S19.9 ☑
thumb S69.9- ☑
  blood vessel — see Injury, blood vessel, thumb
  contusion — see Contusion, thumb
  dislocation — see Dislocation, thumb
  fracture — see Fracture, thumb
  muscle — see Injury, muscle, thumb
  nerve — see Injury, nerve, digital, thumb
  open — see Wound, open, thumb
  specified NEC S69.8- ☑
  sprain — see Sprain, thumb
  superficial — see Injury, superficial, thumb
thymus (gland) — see Injury, intrathoracic, specified organ NEC
thyroid (gland) NEC S19.84 ☑
toe S99.92- ☑
  contusion — see Contusion, toe
  dislocation — see Dislocation, toe
  fracture — see Fracture, toe
  muscle — see Injury, muscle, toe
  open — see Wound, open, toe
  specified type NEC S99.82- ☑
  sprain — see Sprain, toe
  superficial — see Injury, superficial, toe
tongue S09.93 ☑
tonsil S09.93 ☑
tooth S09.93 ☑
trachea (cervical) NEC S19.82 ☑
  thoracic — see Injury, intrathoracic, trachea, thoracic
transfusion-related acute lung (TRALI) J95.84
tunica vaginalis S39.94 ☑
twelfth cranial nerve (hypoglossal) — see Injury, nerve, hypoglossal
ureter S37.10 ☑
  contusion S37.12 ☑
  laceration S37.13 ☑
  specified type NEC S37.19 ☑
urethra (sphincter) S37.30 ☑
  at delivery O71.5
  contusion S37.32 ☑
  laceration S37.33 ☑
  specified type NEC S37.39 ☑
urinary organ S37.90 ☑
  contusion S37.92 ☑
  laceration S37.93 ☑
  specified
    site NEC S37.899 ☑
      contusion S37.892 ☑
      laceration S37.893 ☑

Injury — continued

urinary organ — continued
  specified — continued
    site — continued
      specified type NEC S37.898 ☑
      type NEC S37.99 ☑
uterus, uterine S37.60 ☑
  with ectopic or molar pregnancy O08.6
  blood vessel — see Injury, blood vessel, iliac
  contusion S37.62 ☑
  laceration S37.63 ☑
    cervix at delivery O71.3
  rupture associated with obstetrics — see Rupture, uterus
  specified type NEC S37.69 ☑
uvula S09.93 ☑
vagina S39.93 ☑
  abrasion S30.814 ☑
  bite S31.45 ☑
    insect S30.864 ☑
    superficial NEC S30.874 ☑
  contusion S30.23 ☑
  crush S38.03 ☑
  during delivery — see Laceration, vagina, during delivery
  external constriction S30.844 ☑
  insect bite S30.864 ☑
  laceration S31.41 ☑
    with foreign body S31.42 ☑
  open wound S31.40 ☑
  puncture S31.43 ☑
    with foreign body S31.44 ☑
  superficial S30.95 ☑
    foreign body S30.854 ☑
vas deferens — see Injury, pelvic organ, specified site NEC
vascular NEC T14.8 ☑
vein — see Injury, blood vessel
vena cava (superior) S25.20 ☑
  inferior S35.10 ☑
    laceration (minor) (superficial) S35.11 ☑
      major S35.12 ☑
    specified type NEC S35.19 ☑
  laceration (minor) (superficial) S25.21 ☑
    major S25.22 ☑
  specified type NEC S25.29 ☑
vesical (sphincter) — see Injury, bladder
visual cortex S04.04- ☑
vitreous (humor) S05.90 ☑
  specified NEC S05.8X- ☑
vocal cord NEC S19.83 ☑
vulva S39.94 ☑
  abrasion S30.814 ☑
  bite S31.45 ☑
    insect S30.864 ☑
    superficial NEC S30.874 ☑
  contusion S30.23 ☑
  crush S38.03 ☑
  during delivery — see Laceration, perineum, female, during delivery
  external constriction S30.844 ☑
  insect bite S30.864 ☑
  laceration S31.41 ☑
    with foreign body S31.42 ☑
  open wound S31.40 ☑
  puncture S31.43 ☑
    with foreign body S31.44 ☑
  superficial S30.95 ☑
    foreign body S30.854 ☑
whiplash (cervical spine) S13.4 ☑
wrist S69.9- ☑
  blood vessel — see Injury, blood vessel, hand
  contusion — see Contusion, wrist
  dislocation — see Dislocation, wrist
  fracture — see Fracture, wrist
  muscle — see Injury, muscle, hand
  nerve — see Injury, nerve, hand
  open — see Wound, open, wrist
  specified NEC S69.8- ☑
  sprain — see Sprain, wrist
  superficial — see Injury, superficial, wrist
Inoculation (see also Vaccination)
complication or reaction — see Complications, vaccination
Insanity, insane (see also Psychosis)
adolescent — see Schizophrenia

Insanity, insane — continued
confusional F28
  acute or subacute F05
delusional F22
senile F03 ☑
Insect
bite — see Bite, by site, superficial, insect
venomous, poisoning NEC (by) — see Venom, arthropod
Insensitivity
adrenocorticotropin hormone (ACTH) E27.49
androgen E34.50
  complete E34.51
  partial E34.52
Insertion
cord (umbilical) lateral or velamentous O43.12- ☑
intrauterine contraceptive device (encounter for) — see Intrauterine contraceptive device
Insolation (sunstroke) T67.0 ☑
Insomnia (organic) G47.00
without objective findings F51.02
adjustment F51.02
adjustment disorder F51.02
behavioral, of childhood Z73.819
  combined type Z73.812
  limit setting type Z73.811
  sleep-onset association type Z73.810
childhood Z73.819
chronic F51.04
  somatized tension F51.04
conditioned F51.04
due to
  alcohol
    abuse F10.182
    dependence F10.282
    use F10.982
  amphetamines
    abuse F15.182
    dependence F15.282
    use F15.982
  anxiety disorder F51.05
  caffeine
    abuse F15.182
    dependence F15.282
    use F15.982
  cocaine
    abuse F14.182
    dependence F14.282
    use F14.982
  depression F51.05
  drug NEC
    abuse F19.182
    dependence F19.282
    use F19.982
  medical condition G47.01
  mental disorder NEC F51.05
  opioid
    abuse F11.182
    dependence F11.282
    use F11.982
  psychoactive substance NEC
    abuse F19.182
    dependence F19.182
    use F19.982
  sedative, hypnotic, or anxiolytic
    abuse F13.182
    dependence F13.282
    use F13.982
  stimulant NEC
    abuse F15.182
    dependence F15.282
    use F15.982
fatal familial (FFI) A81.83
idiopathic F51.01
learned F51.3
nonorganic origin F51.01
not due to a substance or known physiological condition F51.01
  specified NEC F51.09
paradoxical F51.03
primary F51.01
psychiatric F51.05
psychophysiologic F51.04
related to psychopathology F51.05
short-term F51.02
specified NEC G47.09
stress-related F51.02
transient F51.02

☑ Additional Character Required — Refer to the Tabular List for Character Selection   ▽ Subterms under main terms may continue to next column or page

Inspiration
  food or foreign body — *see* Foreign body, by site
  mucus — *see* Asphyxia, mucus
Inspissated bile syndrome (newborn) P59.1
Instability
  emotional (excessive) F60.3
  joint (post-traumatic) M25.30
    ankle M25.37- ☑
    due to old ligament injury — *see* Disorder, ligament
    elbow M25.32- ☑
    flail — *see* Flail, joint
    foot M25.37- ☑
    hand M25.34- ☑
    hip M25.35- ☑
    knee M25.36- ☑
    lumbosacral — *see* subcategory M53.2 ☑
    prosthesis — *see* Complications, joint prosthesis, mechanical, displacement, by site
    sacroiliac — *see* subcategory M53.2 ☑
    secondary to
      old ligament injury — *see* Disorder, ligament
      removal of joint prosthesis M96.89
    shoulder (region) M25.31- ☑
    spine — *see* subcategory M53.2 ☑
    wrist M25.33- ☑
  knee (chronic) M23.5- ☑
  lumbosacral — *see* subcategory M53.2 ☑
  nervous F48.8
  personality (emotional) F60.3
  spine — *see* Instability, joint, spine
  vasomotor R55
Institutional syndrome (childhood) F94.2
Institutionalization, affecting child Z62.22
  disinhibited attachment F94.2
Insufficiency, insufficient
  accommodation, old age H52.4
  adrenal (gland) E27.40
    primary E27.1
  adrenocortical E27.40
    drug-induced E27.3
    iatrogenic E27.3
    primary E27.1
  anatomic crown height K08.89
  anterior (occlusal) guidance M26.54
  anus K62.89
  aortic (valve) I35.1
    with
      mitral (valve) disease I08.0
        with tricuspid (valve) disease I08.3
      stenosis I35.2
      tricuspid (valve) disease I08.2
        with mitral (valve) disease I08.3
    congenital Q23.1
    rheumatic I06.1
      with
        mitral (valve) disease I08.0
          with tricuspid (valve) disease I08.3
        stenosis I06.2
          with mitral (valve) disease I08.0
            with tricuspid (valve) disease I08.3
        tricuspid (valve) disease I08.2
          with mitral (valve) disease I08.3
    specified cause NEC I35.1
    syphilitic A52.03
  arterial I77.1
    basilar G45.0
    carotid (hemispheric) G45.1
    cerebral I67.81
    coronary (acute or subacute) I24.8
    mesenteric K55.1
    peripheral I73.9
    precerebral (multiple) (bilateral) G45.2
    vertebral G45.0
  arteriovenous I99.8
  biliary K83.8
  cardiac (*see also* Insufficiency, myocardial)
    due to presence of (cardiac) prosthesis I97.11- ☑
    postprocedural I97.11- ☑
  cardiorenal, hypertensive I13.2
  cardiovascular — *see* Disease, cardiovascular
  cerebrovascular (acute) I67.81
    with transient focal neurological signs and symptoms G45.8
  circulatory NEC I99.8
    newborn P29.89
  clinical crown length K08.89
  convergence H51.11

Insufficiency, insufficient — *continued*
  coronary (acute or subacute) I24.8
    chronic or with a stated duration of over 4 weeks I25.89
  corticoadrenal E27.40
    primary E27.1
  dietary E63.9
  divergence H51.8
  food T73.0 ☑
  gastroesophageal K22.8
  gonadal
    ovary E28.39
    testis E29.1
  heart (*see also* Insufficiency, myocardial)
    newborn P29.0
    valve — *see* Endocarditis
  hepatic — *see* Failure, hepatic
  idiopathic autonomic G90.09
  interocclusal distance of fully erupted teeth (ridge) M26.36
  kidney N28.9
    acute N28.9
    chronic N18.9
  lacrimal (secretion) H04.12- ☑
    passages — *see* Stenosis, lacrimal
  liver — *see* Failure, hepatic
  lung — *see* Insufficiency, pulmonary
  mental (congenital) — *see* Disability, intellectual
  mesenteric K55.1
  mitral (valve) I34.0
    with
      aortic valve disease I08.0
        with tricuspid (valve) disease I08.3
      obstruction or stenosis I05.2
        with aortic valve disease I08.0
      tricuspid (valve) disease I08.1
        with aortic (valve) disease I08.3
    congenital Q23.3
    rheumatic I05.1
      with
        aortic valve disease I08.0
          with tricuspid (valve) disease I08.3
        obstruction or stenosis I05.2
          with aortic valve disease I08.0
            with tricuspid (valve) disease I08.3
        tricuspid (valve) disease I08.1
          with aortic (valve) disease I08.3
      active or acute I01.1
        with chorea, rheumatic (Sydenham's) I02.0
    specified cause, except rheumatic I34.0
  muscle (*see also* Disease, muscle)
    heart — *see* Insufficiency, myocardial
    ocular NEC H50.9
  myocardial, myocardium (with arteriosclerosis) (*see also* Failure, heart) I50.9
    with
      rheumatic fever (conditions in I00) I09.0
        active, acute or subacute I01.2
          with chorea I02.0
        inactive or quiescent (with chorea) I09.0
    congenital Q24.8
    hypertensive — *see* Hypertension, heart
    newborn P29.0
    rheumatic I09.0
      active, acute, or subacute I01.2
    syphilitic A52.06
  nourishment T73.0 ☑
  pancreatic K86.89
    exocrine K86.81
  parathyroid (gland) E20.9
  peripheral vascular (arterial) I73.9
  pituitary E23.0
  placental (mother) O36.51- ☑
  platelets D69.6
  prenatal care affecting management of pregnancy O09.3- ☑
  progressive pluriglandular E31.0
  pulmonary J98.4
    acute, following surgery (nonthoracic) J95.2
      thoracic J95.1
    chronic, following surgery J95.3
    following
      shock J98.4
      trauma J98.4
    newborn P28.5
    valve I37.1
      with stenosis I37.2
      congenital Q22.2

Insufficiency, insufficient — *continued*
  pulmonary — *continued*
    valve — *continued*
      rheumatic I09.89
        with aortic, mitral or tricuspid (valve) disease I08.8
  pyloric K31.89
  renal (acute) N28.9
    chronic N18.9
  respiratory R06.89
    newborn P28.5
  rotation — *see* Malrotation
  sleep syndrome F51.12
  social insurance Z59.7
  suprarenal E27.40
    primary E27.1
  tarso-orbital fascia, congenital Q10.3
  testis E29.1
  thyroid (gland) (acquired) E03.9
    congenital E03.1
  tricuspid (valve) (rheumatic) I07.1
    with
      aortic (valve) disease I08.2
        with mitral (valve) disease I08.3
      mitral (valve) disease I08.1
        with aortic (valve) disease I08.3
      obstruction or stenosis I07.2
        with aortic (valve) disease I08.2
          with mitral (valve) disease I08.3
    congenital Q22.8
    nonrheumatic I36.1
      with stenosis I36.2
  urethral sphincter R32
  valve, valvular (heart) I38
    aortic — *see* Insufficiency, aortic (valve)
    congenital Q24.8
    mitral — *see* Insufficiency, mitral (valve)
    pulmonary — *see* Insufficiency, pulmonary, valve
    tricuspid — *see* Insufficiency, tricuspid (valve)
  vascular I99.8
    intestine K55.9
      acute (*see also* Ischemia, intestine, acute) K55.059
    mesenteric K55.1
    peripheral I73.9
    renal — *see* Hypertension, kidney
  velopharyngeal
    acquired K13.79
    congenital Q38.8
  venous (chronic) (peripheral) I87.2
  ventricular — *see* Insufficiency, myocardial
  welfare support Z59.7
Insufflation, fallopian Z31.41
Insular — *see* condition
Insulinoma
  pancreas
    benign D13.7
    malignant C25.4
    uncertain behavior D37.8
  specified site
    benign — *see* Neoplasm, by site, benign
    malignant — *see* Neoplasm, by site, malignant
    uncertain behavior — *see* Neoplasm, by site, uncertain behavior
  unspecified site
    benign D13.7
    malignant C25.4
    uncertain behavior D37.8
Insuloma — *see* Insulinoma
Interference
  balancing side M26.56
  non-working side M26.56
Intermenstrual — *see* condition
Intermittent — *see* condition
Internal — *see* condition
Interrogation
  cardiac defibrillator (automatic) (implantable) Z45.02
  cardiac pacemaker Z45.018
  cardiac (event) (loop) recorder Z45.09
  infusion pump (implanted) (intrathecal) Z45.1
  neurostimulator Z46.2
Interruption
  aortic arch Q25.21
  bundle of His I44.30
  phase-shift, sleep cycle — *see* Disorder, sleep, circadian rhythm
  sleep phase-shift, or 24 hour sleep-wake cycle — *see* Disorder, sleep, circadian rhythm

---

▼ Subterms under main terms may continue to next column or page   ☑ Additional Character Required — Refer to the Tabular List for Character Selection

Interstitial — see condition
Intertrigo L30.4
  labialis K13.0
Intervertebral disc — see condition
Intestine, intestinal — see condition
Intolerance
  carbohydrate K90.49
  disaccharide, hereditary E73.0
  fat NEC K90.49
    pancreatic K90.3
  food K90.49
    dietary counseling and surveillance Z71.3
  fructose E74.10
    hereditary E74.12
  glucose (-galactose) E74.39
  gluten K90.41
  lactose E73.9
    specified NEC E73.8
  lysine E72.3
  milk NEC K90.49
    lactose E73.9
  protein K90.49
  starch NEC K90.49
  sucrose (-isomaltose) E74.31
Intoxicated NEC (without dependence) — see Alcohol,
    intoxication
Intoxication
  acid E87.2
  alcoholic (acute) (without dependence) — see Alcohol,
    intoxication
  alimentary canal K52.1
  amphetamine (without dependence) — see Abuse,
    drug, stimulant, with intoxication
    with dependence — see Dependence, drug, stim-
      ulant, with intoxication
  anxiolytic (acute) (without dependence) — see Abuse,
    drug, sedative, with intoxication
    with dependence — see Dependence, drug, seda-
      tive, with intoxication
  caffeine F15.929
    with dependence — see Dependence, drug, stim-
      ulant, with intoxication
  cannabinoids (acute) (without dependence) — see
    Use, cannabis, with intoxication
    with
      abuse — see Abuse, drug, cannabis, with intox-
        ication
      dependence — see Dependence, drug,
        cannabis, with intoxication
  chemical — see Table of Drugs and Chemicals
    via placenta or breast milk — see - Absorption,
      chemical, through placenta
  cocaine (acute) (without dependence) — see Abuse,
    drug, cocaine, with intoxication
    with dependence — see Dependence, drug, co-
      caine, with intoxication
  drug
    acute (without dependence) — see Abuse, drug,
      by type with intoxication
      with dependence — see Dependence, drug, by
        type with intoxication
    addictive
      via placenta or breast milk — see Absorption,
        drug, addictive, through placenta
    newborn P93.8
      gray baby syndrome P93.0
    overdose or wrong substance given or taken —
      see Table of Drugs and Chemicals, by drug,
      poisoning
  enteric K52.1
  foodborne A05.9
    bacterial A05.9
    classical (Clostridium botulinum) A05.1
    due to
      Bacillus cereus A05.4
      bacterium A05.9
        specified NEC A05.8
      Clostridium
        botulinum A05.1
        perfringens A05.2
        welchii A05.2
      Salmonella A02.9
        with
          (gastro)enteritis A02.0
          localized infection(s) A02.20
            arthritis A02.23
            meningitis A02.21
            osteomyelitis A02.24

Intoxication — continued
  foodborne — continued
    due to — continued
      Salmonella — continued
        with — continued
          localized infection(s) — continued
            pneumonia A02.22
            pyelonephritis A02.25
            specified NEC A02.29
          sepsis A02.1
          specified manifestation NEC A02.8
      Staphylococcus A05.0
      Vibrio
        parahaemolyticus A05.3
        vulnificus A05.5
    enterotoxin, staphylococcal A05.0
    noxious — see Poisoning, food, noxious
  gastrointestinal K52.1
  hallucinogenic (without dependence) — see Abuse,
    drug, hallucinogen, with intoxication
    with dependence — see Dependence, drug, hallu-
      cinogen, with intoxication
  hypnotic (acute) (without dependence) — see Abuse,
    drug, sedative, with intoxication
    with dependence — see Dependence, drug, seda-
      tive, with intoxication
  inhalant (acute) (without dependence) — see Abuse,
    drug, inhalant, with intoxication
    with dependence — see Dependence, drug, in-
      halant, with intoxication
  meaning
    inebriation — see category F10 ☑
    poisoning — see Table of Drugs and Chemicals
  methyl alcohol (acute) (without dependence) — see
    Alcohol, intoxication
  opioid (acute) (without dependence) — see Abuse,
    drug, opioid, with intoxication
    with dependence — see Dependence, drug, opioid,
      with intoxication
  pathologic NEC (without dependence) — see Alcohol,
    intoxication
  phencyclidine (without dependence) — see Abuse,
    drug, hallucinogen, with intoxication
    with dependence — see Dependence, drug, hallu-
      cinogen, with intoxication
  potassium (K) E87.5
  psychoactive substance NEC (without dependence)
    — see Abuse, drug, psychoactive NEC, with in-
    toxication
    with dependence — see Dependence, drug, psy-
      choactive NEC, with intoxication
  sedative (acute) (without dependence) — see Abuse,
    drug, sedative, with intoxication
    with dependence — see Dependence, drug, seda-
      tive, with intoxication
  serum (see also Reaction, serum) T80.69 ☑
  uremic — see Uremia
  volatile solvents (acute) (without dependence) — see
    Abuse, drug, inhalant, with intoxication
    with dependence — see Dependence, drug, in-
      halant, with intoxication
  water E87.79
Intraabdominal testis, testes
  bilateral Q53.211
  unilateral Q53.111
Intracranial — see condition
Intrahepatic gallbladder Q44.1
Intraligamentous — see condition
Intrathoracic (see also condition)
  kidney Q63.2
Intrauterine contraceptive device
  checking Z30.431
  in situ Z97.5
  insertion Z30.430
    immediately following removal Z30.433
  management Z30.431
  reinsertion Z30.433
  removal Z30.432
  replacement Z30.433
  retention in pregnancy O26.3- ☑
Intraventricular — see condition
Intrinsic deformity — see Deformity
Intumescence, lens (eye) (cataract) — see Cataract
Intussusception (bowel) (colon) (enteric) (ileocecal)
    (ileocolic) (intestine) (rectum) K56.1
  appendix K38.8
  congenital Q43.8

Intussusception — continued
  ureter (with obstruction) N13.5
Invagination (bowel, colon, intestine or rectum) K56.1
Inversion
  albumin-globulin (A-G) ratio E88.09
  bladder N32.89
  cecum — see Intussusception
  cervix N88.8
  chromosome in normal individual Q95.1
  circadian rhythm — see Disorder, sleep, circadian
    rhythm
  nipple N64.59
    congenital Q83.8
    gestational — see Retraction, nipple
    puerperal, postpartum — see Retraction, nipple
  nyctohemeral rhythm — see Disorder, sleep, circadian
    rhythm
  optic papilla Q14.2
  organ or site, congenital NEC — see Anomaly, by site
  sleep rhythm — see Disorder, sleep, circadian rhythm
  testis (congenital) Q55.29
  uterus (chronic) (postinfectional) (postpartal, old)
    N85.5
    postpartum O71.2
  vagina (posthysterectomy) N99.3
  ventricular Q20.5
Investigation (see also Examination) Z04.9
  clinical research subject (control) (normal comparison)
    (participant) Z00.6
Involuntary movement, abnormal R25.9
Involution, involutional (see also condition)
  breast, cystic — see Dysplasia, mammary, specified
    type NEC
  depression (single episode) F32.89
    recurrent episode F33.9
  melancholia (single episode) F32.89
    recurrent episode F33.8
  ovary, senile — see Atrophy, ovary
  thymus failure E32.8
I.Q.
  under 20 F73
  20-34 F72
  35-49 F71
  50-69 F70
IRDS (type I) P22.0
  type II P22.1
Irideremia Q13.1
Iridis rubeosis — see Disorder, iris, vascular
Iridochoroiditis (panuveitis) — see Panuveitis
Iridocyclitis H20.9
  acute H20.0- ☑
    hypopyon H20.05- ☑
    primary H20.01- ☑
    recurrent H20.02- ☑
    secondary (noninfectious) H20.04- ☑
      infectious H20.03- ☑
  chronic H20.1- ☑
  due to allergy — see Iridocyclitis, acute, secondary
  endogenous — see Iridocyclitis, acute, primary
  Fuchs' — see Cyclitis, Fuchs' heterochromic
  gonococcal A54.32
  granulomatous — see Iridocyclitis, chronic
  herpes, herpetic (simplex) B00.51
    zoster B02.32
  hypopyon — see Iridocyclitis, acute, hypopyon
  in (due to)
    ankylosing spondylitis M45.9
    gonococcal infection A54.32
    herpes (simplex) virus B00.51
      zoster B02.32
    infectious disease NOS B99 ☑
    parasitic disease NOS B89 [H22]
    sarcoidosis D86.83
    syphilis A51.43
    tuberculosis A18.54
    zoster B02.32
  lens-induced H20.2- ☑
  nongranulomatous — see Iridocyclitis, acute
  recurrent — see Iridocyclitis, acute, recurrent
  rheumatic — see Iridocyclitis, chronic
  subacute — see Iridocyclitis, acute
  sympathetic — see Uveitis, sympathetic
  syphilitic (secondary) A51.43
  tuberculous (chronic) A18.54
  Vogt-Koyanagi H20.82- ☑
Iridocyclochoroiditis (panuveitis) — see Panuveitis
Iridodialysis H21.53- ☑

☑ Additional Character Required — Refer to the Tabular List for Character Selection   ▽ Subterms under main terms may continue to next column or page

Iridodonesis H21.89
Iridoplegia (complete) (partial) (reflex) H57.09
Iridoschisis H21.25- ☑
Iris (see also condition)
  bombé — see Membrane, pupillary
Iritis (see also Iridocyclitis)
  chronic — see Iridocyclitis, chronic
  diabetic — see E08-E13 with .39
  due to
    herpes simplex B00.51
    leprosy A30.9 [H22]
  gonococcal A54.32
  gouty (see also Gout, by type) M10.9 [H22]
  granulomatous — see Iridocyclitis, chronic
  lens induced — see Iridocyclitis, lens-induced
  papulosa (syphilitic) A52.71
  rheumatic — see Iridocyclitis, chronic
  syphilitic (secondary) A51.43
    congenital (early) A50.01
    late A52.71
  tuberculous A18.54
Iron — see condition
Iron-miner's lung J63.4
Irradiated enamel (tooth, teeth) K03.89
Irradiation effects, adverse T66 ☑
Irreducible, irreducibility — see condition
Irregular, irregularity
  action, heart I49.9
  alveolar process K08.89
  bleeding N92.6
  breathing R06.89
  contour of cornea (acquired) — see Deformity, cornea
    congenital Q13.4
  contour, reconstructed breast N65.0
  dentin (in pulp) K04.3
  eye movements H55.89
    nystagmus — see Nystagmus
    saccadic H55.81
  labor O62.2
  menstruation (cause unknown) N92.6
  periods N92.6
  prostate N42.9
  pupil — see Abnormality, pupillary
  reconstructed breast N65.0
  respiratory R06.89
  septum (nasal) J34.2
  shape, organ or site, congenital NEC — see Distortion
  sleep-wake pattern (rhythm) G47.23
Irritable, irritability R45.4
  bladder N32.89
  bowel (syndrome) K58.9
    with
      constipation K58.1
      diarrhea K58.0
    mixed K58.2
    psychogenic F45.8
    specified NEC K58.8
  bronchial — see Bronchitis
  cerebral, in newborn P91.3
  colon (see also Irritable, bowel) K58.9
    with diarrhea K58.0
    psychogenic F45.8
  duodenum K59.8
  heart (psychogenic) F45.8
  hip — see Derangement, joint, specified type NEC, hip
  ileum K59.8
  infant R68.12
  jejunum K59.8
  rectum K59.8
  stomach K31.89
    psychogenic F45.8
  sympathetic G90.8
  urethra N36.8
Irritation
  anus K62.89
  axillary nerve G54.0
  bladder N32.89
  brachial plexus G54.0
  bronchial — see Bronchitis
  cervical plexus G54.2
  cervix — see Cervicitis
  choroid, sympathetic — see Endophthalmitis
  cranial nerve — see Disorder, nerve, cranial
  gastric K31.89
    psychogenic F45.8
  globe, sympathetic — see Uveitis, sympathetic
  labyrinth — see subcategory H83.2 ☑
  lumbosacral plexus G54.1

Irritation — continued
  meninges (traumatic) — see Injury, intracranial
    nontraumatic — see Meningismus
  nerve — see Disorder, nerve
  nervous R45.0
  penis N48.89
  perineum NEC L29.3
  peripheral autonomic nervous system G90.8
  peritoneum — see Peritonitis
  pharynx J39.2
  plantar nerve — see Lesion, nerve, plantar
  spinal (cord) (traumatic) (see also Injury, spinal cord, by region)
    nerve G58.9
      root NEC — see Radiculopathy
    nontraumatic — see Myelopathy
  stomach K31.89
    psychogenic F45.8
  sympathetic nerve NEC G90.8
  ulnar nerve — see Lesion, nerve, ulnar
  vagina N89.8
Ischemia, ischemic I99.8
  bowel (transient)
    acute (see also Ischemia, intestine, acute) K55.059
    chronic K55.1
    due to mesenteric artery insufficiency K55.1
  brain — see Ischemia, cerebral
  cardiac (see Disease, heart, ischemic)
  cardiomyopathy I25.5
  cerebral (chronic) (generalized) I67.82
    arteriosclerotic I67.2
    intermittent G45.9
    newborn P91.0
    recurrent focal G45.8
    transient G45.9
  colon chronic (due to mesenteric artery insufficiency) K55.1
  coronary — see Disease, heart, ischemic
  demand (coronary) (see also Angina) I24.8
    with myocardial infarction I21.A1
    resulting in myocardial infarction I21.A1
  heart (chronic or with a stated duration of over 4 weeks) I25.9
    acute or with a stated duration of 4 weeks or less I24.9
    subacute I24.9
  infarction, muscle — see Infarct, muscle
  intestine (large) (small) (transient) K55.9
    acute K55.059
      diffuse K55.052
      focal K55.051
      large K55.039
        diffuse K55.032
        focal K55.031
      small K55.019
        diffuse K55.012
        focal K55.011
    chronic K55.1
    due to mesenteric artery insufficiency K55.1
  kidney N28.0
  mesenteric, acute (see also Ischemia, intestine, acute) K55.059
  muscle, traumatic T79.6 ☑
  myocardium, myocardial (chronic or with a stated duration of over 4 weeks) I25.9
    acute, without myocardial infarction I51.3
    silent (asymptomatic) I25.6
    transient of newborn P29.4
  renal N28.0
  retina, retinal — see Occlusion, artery, retina
  small bowel
    acute K55.019
      diffuse K55.012
      focal K55.011
    chronic K55.1
    due to mesenteric artery insufficiency K55.1
  spinal cord G95.11
  subendocardial — see Insufficiency, coronary
  supply (coronary) (see also Angina) I25.9
    due to vasospasm I20.1
Ischial spine — see condition
Ischialgia — see Sciatica
Ischiopagus Q89.4
Ischium, ischial — see condition
Ischuria R34
Iselin's disease or osteochondrosis — see Osteochondrosis, juvenile, metatarsus

Islands of
  parotid tissue in
    lymph nodes Q38.6
    neck structures Q38.6
  submaxillary glands in
    fascia Q38.6
    lymph nodes Q38.6
    neck muscles Q38.6
Islet cell tumor, pancreas D13.7
Isoimmunization NEC (see also Incompatibility)
  affecting management of pregnancy (ABO) (with hydrops fetalis) O36.11- ☑
    anti-A sensitization O36.11- ☑
    anti-B sensitization O36.19- ☑
    anti-c sensitization O36.09- ☑
    anti-C sensitization O36.09- ☑
    anti-e sensitization O36.09- ☑
    anti-E sensitization O36.09- ☑
    Rh NEC O36.09- ☑
      anti-D antibody O36.01- ☑
    specified NEC O36.19- ☑
  newborn P55.9
    with
      hydrops fetalis P56.0
      kernicterus P57.0
    ABO (blood groups) P55.1
    Rhesus (Rh) factor P55.0
    specified type NEC P55.8
Isolation, isolated
  dwelling Z59.8
  family Z63.79
  social Z60.4
Isoleucinosis E71.19
Isomerism atrial appendages (with asplenia or polysplenia) Q20.6
Isosporiasis, isosporosis A07.3
Isovaleric acidemia E71.110
Issue of
  medical certificate Z02.79
    for disability determination Z02.71
  repeat prescription (appliance) (glasses) (medicinal substance, medicament, medicine) Z76.0
    contraception — see Contraception
Itch, itching (see also Pruritus)
  baker's L23.6
  barber's B35.0
  bricklayer's L24.5
  cheese B88.0
  clam digger's B65.3
  coolie B76.9
  copra B88.0
  dew B76.9
  dhobi B35.6
  filarial — see Infestation, filarial
  grain B88.0
  grocer's B88.0
  ground B76.9
  harvest B88.0
  jock B35.6
  Malabar B35.5
    beard B35.0
    foot B35.3
    scalp B35.0
  meaning scabies B86
  Norwegian B86
  perianal L29.0
  poultrymen's B88.0
  sarcoptic B86
  scabies B86
  scrub B88.0
  straw B88.0
  swimmer's B65.3
  water B76.9
  winter L29.8
Ivemark's syndrome (asplenia with congenital heart disease) Q89.01
Ivory bones Q78.2
Ixodiasis NEC B88.8

J

Jaccoud's syndrome — see Arthropathy, postrheumatic, chronic
Jackson's
  membrane Q43.3
  paralysis or syndrome G83.89
  veil Q43.3
Jacquet's dermatitis (diaper dermatitis) L22

Jadassohn-Pellizari's disease or anetoderma L90.2
Jadassohn's
  blue nevus — see Nevus
  intraepidermal epithelioma — see Neoplasm, skin, benign
Jaffe-Lichtenstein (-Uehlinger) **syndrome** — see Dysplasia, fibrous, bone NEC
Jakob-Creutzfeldt disease or syndrome — see Creutzfeldt-Jakob disease or syndrome
Jaksch-Luzet disease D64.89
Jamaican
  neuropathy G92
  paraplegic tropical ataxic-spastic syndrome G92
Janet's disease F48.8
Janiceps Q89.4
Jansky-Bielschowsky amaurotic idiocy E75.4
Japanese
  B-type encephalitis A83.0
  river fever A75.3
Jaundice (yellow) R17
  acholuric (familial) (splenomegalic) (see also Spherocytosis)
    acquired D59.8
  breast-milk (Inhibitor) P59.3
  catarrhal (acute) B15.9
    with hepatic coma B15.0
  cholestatic (benign) R17
  due to or associated with
    delayed conjugation P59.8
      associated with (due to) preterm delivery P59.0
    preterm delivery P59.0
  epidemic (catarrhal) B15.9
    with hepatic coma B15.0
    leptospiral A27.0
    spirochetal A27.0
  familial nonhemolytic (congenital) (Gilbert) E80.4
    Crigler-Najjar E80.5
  febrile (acute) B15.9
    with hepatic coma B15.0
    leptospiral A27.0
    spirochetal A27.0
  hematogenous D59.9
  hemolytic (acquired) D59.9
    congenital — see Spherocytosis
  hemorrhagic (acute) (leptospiral) (spirochetal) A27.0
  infectious (acute) (subacute) B15.9
    with hepatic coma B15.0
    leptospiral A27.0
    spirochetal A27.0
  leptospiral (hemorrhagic) A27.0
  malignant (without coma) K72.90
    with coma K72.91
  neonatal — see Jaundice, newborn
  newborn P59.9
    due to or associated with
      ABO
        antibodies P55.1
        incompatibility, maternal/fetal P55.1
        isoimmunization P55.1
      absence or deficiency of enzyme system for bilirubin conjugation (congenital) P59.8
      bleeding P58.1
      breast milk inhibitors to conjugation P59.3
        associated with preterm delivery P59.0
      bruising P58.0
      Crigler-Najjar syndrome E80.5
      delayed conjugation P59.8
        associated with preterm delivery P59.0
      drugs or toxins
        given to newborn P58.42
        transmitted from mother P58.41
      excessive hemolysis P58.9
        due to
          bleeding P58.1
          bruising P58.0
          drugs or toxins
            given to newborn P58.42
            transmitted from mother P58.41
          infection P58.2
          polycythemia P58.3
          swallowed maternal blood P58.5
        specified type NEC P58.8
      galactosemia E74.21
      Gilbert syndrome E80.4
      hemolytic disease P55.9
        ABO isoimmunization P55.1
        Rh isoimmunization P55.0
        specified NEC P55.8

Jaundice — continued
  newborn — continued
    due to or associated with — continued
      hepatocellular damage P59.20
        specified NEC P59.29
      hereditary hemolytic anemia P58.8
      hypothyroidism, congenital E03.1
      incompatibility, maternal/fetal NOS P55.9
      infection P58.2
      inspissated bile syndrome P59.1
      isoimmunization NOS P55.9
      mucoviscidosis E84.9
      polycythemia P58.3
      preterm delivery P59.0
      Rh
        antibodies P55.0
        incompatibility, maternal/fetal P55.0
        isoimmunization P55.0
      specified cause NEC P59.8
      swallowed maternal blood P58.5
    spherocytosis (congenital) D58.0
  nonhemolytic congenital familial (Gilbert) E80.4
  nuclear, newborn (see also Kernicterus of newborn) P57.9
  obstructive (see also Obstruction, bile duct) K83.1
  post-immunization — see Hepatitis, viral, type, B
  post-transfusion — see Hepatitis, viral, type, B
  regurgitation (see also Obstruction, bile duct) K83.1
  serum (homologous) (prophylactic) (therapeutic) — see Hepatitis, viral, type, B
  spirochetal (hemorrhagic) A27.0
  symptomatic R17
    newborn P59.9
Jaw — see condition
Jaw-winking phenomenon or syndrome Q07.8
Jealousy
  alcoholic F10.988
  childhood F93.8
  sibling F93.8
Jejunitis — see Enteritis
Jejunostomy status Z93.4
Jejunum, jejunal — see condition
Jensen's disease — see Inflammation, chorioretinal, focal, Juxtapapillary
Jerks, myoclonic G25.3
Jervell-Lange-Nielsen syndrome I45.81
Jeune's disease Q77.2
Jigger disease B88.1
Job's syndrome (chronic granulomatous disease) D71
Joint (see also condition)
  mice — see Loose, body, joint
    knee M23.4- ☑
Jordan's anomaly or syndrome D72.0
Joseph-Diamond-Blackfan anemia (congenital hypoplastic) D61.01
Jungle yellow fever A95.0
Jüngling's disease — see Sarcoidosis
Juvenile — see condition

K

Kahler's disease C90.0- ☑
Kakke E51.11
Kala-azar B55.0
Kallmann's syndrome E23.0
Kanner's syndrome (autism) — see Psychosis, childhood
Kaposi's
  dermatosis (xeroderma pigmentosum) Q82.1
  lichen ruber L44.0
    acuminatus L44.0
  sarcoma
    colon C46.4
    connective tissue C46.1
    gastrointestinal organ C46.4
    lung C46.5- ☑
    lymph node (multiple) C46.3
    palate (hard) (soft) C46.2
    rectum C46.4
    skin (multiple sites) C46.0
    specified site NEC C46.7
    stomach C46.4
    unspecified site C46.9
  varicelliform eruption B00.0
    vaccinia T88.1 ☑
Kartagener's syndrome or triad (sinusitis, bronchiectasis, situs inversus) Q89.3

Karyotype
  with abnormality except iso (Xq) Q96.2
  45,X Q96.0
  46,X
    iso (Xq) Q96.1
  46,XX Q98.3
    with streak gonads Q50.32
    hermaphrodite (true) Q99.1
    male Q98.3
  46,XY
    with streak gonads Q56.1
    female Q97.3
    hermaphrodite (true) Q99.1
  47,XXX Q97.0
  47,XXY Q98.0
  47,XYY Q98.5
Kaschin-Beck disease — see Disease, Kaschin-Beck
Katayama's disease or fever B65.2
Kawasaki's syndrome M30.3
Kayser-Fleischer ring (cornea) (pseudosclerosis) H18.04- ☑
Kaznelson's syndrome (congenital hypoplastic anemia) D61.01
Kearns-Sayre syndrome H49.81- ☑
Kedani fever A75.3
Kelis L91.0
Kelly (-Patterson) **syndrome** (sideropenic dysphagia) D50.1
Keloid, cheloid L91.0
  acne L73.0
  Addison's L94.0
  cornea — see Opacity, cornea
  Hawkin's L91.0
  scar L91.0
Keloma L91.0
Kenya fever A77.1
Keratectasia (see also Ectasia, cornea)
  congenital Q13.4
Keratinization of alveolar ridge mucosa
  excessive K13.23
  minimal K13.22
Keratinized residual ridge mucosa
  excessive K13.23
  minimal K13.22
Keratitis (nodular) (nonulcerative) (simple) (zonular) H16.9
  with ulceration (central) (marginal) (perforated) (ring) — see Ulcer, cornea
  actinic — see Photokeratitis
  arborescens (herpes simplex) B00.52
  areolar H16.11- ☑
  bullosa H16.8
  deep H16.309
    specified type NEC H16.399
  dendritic (a) (herpes simplex) B00.52
  disciform (is) (herpes simplex) B00.52
    varicella B01.81
  filamentary H16.12- ☑
  gonococcal (congenital or prenatal) A54.33
  herpes, herpetic (simplex) B00.52
    zoster B02.33
  in (due to)
    acanthamebiasis B60.13
    adenovirus B30.0
    exanthema (see also Exanthem) B09
    herpes (simplex) virus B00.52
    measles B05.81
    syphilis A50.31
    tuberculosis A18.52
    zoster B02.33
  interstitial (nonsyphilitic) H16.30- ☑
    diffuse H16.32- ☑
    herpes, herpetic (simplex) B00.52
      zoster B02.33
    sclerosing H16.33- ☑
    specified type NEC H16.39- ☑
    syphilitic (congenital) (late) A50.31
    tuberculous A18.52
  macular H16.11- ☑
  nummular H16.11- ☑
  oyster shuckers' H16.8
  parenchymatous — see Keratitis, interstitial
  petrificans H16.8
  postmeasles B05.81
  punctata
    leprosa A30.9 [H16.14-] ☑
    syphilitic (profunda) A50.31
  punctate H16.14- ☑

☑ Additional Character Required — Refer to the Tabular List for Character Selection   ⬇ Subterms under main terms may continue to next column or page

Keratitis — *continued*
  purulent H16.8
  rosacea L71.8
  sclerosing H16.33- ☑
  specified type NEC H16.8
  stellate H16.11- ☑
  striate H16.11- ☑
  superficial H16.10- ☑
    with conjunctivitis — *see* Keratoconjunctivitis
    due to light — *see* Photokeratitis
  suppurative H16.8
  syphilitic (congenital) (prenatal) A50.31
  trachomatous A71.1
    sequelae B94.0
  tuberculous A18.52
  vesicular H16.8
  xerotic (*see also* Keratomalacia) H16.8
    vitamin A deficiency E50.4
Keratoacanthoma L85.8
Keratocele — *see* Descemetocele
Keratoconjunctivitis H16.20- ☑
  Acanthamoeba B60.13
  adenoviral B30.0
  epidemic B30.0
  exposure H16.21- ☑
  herpes, herpetic (simplex) B00.52
    zoster B02.33
  in exanthema (*see also* Exanthem) B09
  infectious B30.0
  lagophthalmic — *see* Keratoconjunctivitis, specified
    type NEC
  neurotrophic H16.23- ☑
  phlyctenular H16.25- ☑
  postmeasles B05.81
  shipyard B30.0
  sicca (Sjogren's) M35.0- ☑
    not Sjogren's H16.22- ☑
  specified type NEC H16.29- ☑
  tuberculous (phlyctenular) A18.52
  vernal H16.26- ☑
Keratoconus H18.60- ☑
  congenital Q13.4
  stable H18.61- ☑
  unstable H18.62- ☑
Keratocyst (dental) (odontogenic) — *see* Cyst, calcifying
  odontogenic
Keratoderma, keratodermia (congenital) (palmaris et
  plantaris) (symmetrical) Q82.8
  acquired L85.1
    in diseases classified elsewhere L86
  climactericum L85.1
  gonococcal A54.89
  gonorrheal A54.89
  punctata L85.2
  Reiter's — *see* Reiter's disease
Keratodermatocele — *see* Descemetocele
Keratoglobus H18.79 ☑
  congenital Q15.8
    with glaucoma Q15.0
Keratohemia — *see* Pigmentation, cornea, stromal
Keratoiritis (*see also* Iridocyclitis)
  syphilitic A50.39
  tuberculous A18.54
Keratoma L57.0
  palmaris and plantaris hereditarium Q82.8
  senile L57.0
Keratomalacia H18.44- ☑
  vitamin A deficiency E50.4
Keratomegaly Q13.4
Keratomycosis B49
  nigrans, nigricans (palmaris) B36.1
Keratopathy H18.9
  band H18.42- ☑
  bullous (aphakic), following cataract surgery
    H59.01- ☑
  bullous H18.1- ☑
Keratoscleritis, tuberculous A18.52
Keratosis L57.0
  actinic L57.0
  arsenical L85.8
  congenital, specified NEC Q80.8
  female genital NEC N94.89
  follicularis Q82.8
    acquired L11.0
    congenita Q82.8
    et parafollicularis in cutem penetrans L87.0
    spinulosa (decalvans) Q82.8

Keratosis — *continued*
  follicularis — *continued*
    vitamin A deficiency E50.8
  gonococcal A54.89
  male genital (external) N50.89
  nigricans L83
  obturans, external ear (canal) — *see* Cholesteatoma,
    external ear
  palmaris et plantaris (inherited) (symmetrical) Q82.8
    acquired L85.1
  penile N48.89
  pharynx J39.2
  pilaris, acquired L85.8
  punctata (palmaris et plantaris) L85.2
  scrotal N50.89
  seborrheic L82.1
    inflamed L82.0
  senile L57.0
  solar L57.0
  tonsillaris J35.8
  vagina N89.4
  vegetans Q82.8
  vitamin A deficiency E50.8
  vocal cord J38.3
Kerato-uveitis — *see* Iridocyclitis
Kerion (celsi) B35.0
Kernicterus of newborn (not due to isoimmunization)
  P57.9
  due to isoimmunization (conditions in P55.0-P55.9)
    P57.0
  specified type NEC P57.8
Kerunoparalysis T75.09 ☑
Keshan disease E59
Ketoacidosis E87.2
  diabetic — *see* Diabetes, by type, with ketoacidosis
Ketonuria R82.4
Ketosis NEC E88.89
  diabetic — *see* Diabetes, by type, with with ketoacido-
    sis
Kew Garden fever A79.1
Kidney — *see* condition
Kienböck's disease (*see also* Osteochondrosis, juvenile,
  hand, carpal lunate)
  adult M93.1
Kimmelstiel (-Wilson) **disease** — *see* Diabetes, Kimmelstiel (-Wilson) disease
Kink, kinking
  artery I77.1
  hair (acquired) L67.8
  ileum or intestine — *see* Obstruction, intestine
  Lane's — *see* Obstruction, intestine
  organ or site, congenital NEC — *see* Anomaly, by site
  ureter (pelvic junction) N13.5
    with
      hydronephrosis N13.1
        with infection N13.6
      pyelonephritis (chronic) N11.1
    congenital Q62.39
  vein(s) I87.8
    caval I87.1
    peripheral I87.1
Kinnier Wilson's disease (hepatolenticular degeneration) E83.01
Kissing spine M48.20
  cervical region M48.22
  cervicothoracic region M48.23
  lumbar region M48.26
  lumbosacral region M48.27
  occipito-atlanto-axial region M48.21
  thoracic region M48.24
  thoracolumbar region M48.25
Klatskin's tumor C22.1
Klauder's disease A26.8
Klebs' disease (*see also* Glomerulonephritis) N05- ☑
Klebsiella (K.) **pneumoniae, as cause of disease
  classified elsewhere** B96.1
Klein (e)-**Levin syndrome** G47.13
Kleptomania F63.2
Klinefelter's syndrome Q98.4
  karyotype 47,XXY Q98.0
  male with more than two X chromosomes Q98.1
Klippel-Feil deficiency, disease, or syndrome (brevi-
  collis) Q76.1
Klippel's disease I67.2
Klippel-Trenaunay (-Weber) **syndrome** Q87.2
Klumpke (-Déjerine) **palsy, paralysis** (birth) (newborn)
  P14.1
Knee — *see* condition

Knock knee (acquired) M21.06- ☑
  congenital Q74.1
Knot(s)
  intestinal, syndrome (volvulus) K56.2
  surfer S89.8- ☑
  umbilical cord (true) O69.2 ☑
Knotting (of)
  hair L67.8
  intestine K56.2
Knuckle pad (Garrod's) M72.1
Koch's
  infection — *see* Tuberculosis
  relapsing fever A68.9
Koch-Weeks' conjunctivitis — *see* Conjunctivitis, acute,
  mucopurulent
Köebner's syndrome Q81.8
Köenig's disease (osteochondritis dissecans) — *see* Osteochondritis, dissecans
Köhler-Pellegrini-Steida disease or syndrome (calcification, knee joint) — *see* Bursitis, tibial collateral
Köhler's disease
  patellar — *see* Osteochondrosis, juvenile, patella
  tarsal navicular — *see* Osteochondrosis, juvenile, tarsus
Koilonychia L60.3
  congenital Q84.6
Kojevnikov's, epilepsy — *see* Kozhevnikof's epilepsy
Koplik's spots B05.9
Kopp's asthma E32.8
Korsakoff's (Wernicke) **disease, psychosis or syn-
  drome** (alcoholic) F10.96
  with dependence F10.26
  drug-induced
    due to drug abuse — *see* Abuse, drug, by type,
      with amnestic disorder
    due to drug dependence — *see* Dependence, drug,
      by type, with amnestic disorder
  nonalcoholic F04
Korsakov's disease, psychosis or syndrome — *see*
  Korsakoff's disease
Korsakow's disease, psychosis or syndrome — *see*
  Korsakoff's disease
Kostmann's disease or syndrome (infantile genetic
  agranulocytosis) — *see* Agranulocytosis
Kozhevnikof's epilepsy G40.109
  intractable G40.119
    with status epilepticus G40.111
    without status epilepticus G40.119
  not intractable G40.109
    with status epilepticus G40.101
    without status epilepticus G40.109
Krabbe's
  disease E75.23
  syndrome, congenital muscle hypoplasia Q79.8
Kraepelin-Morel disease — *see* Schizophrenia
Kraft-Weber-Dimitri disease Q85.8
Kraurosis
  ani K62.89
  penis N48.0
  vagina N89.8
  vulva N90.4
Kreotoxism A05.9
Krukenberg's
  spindle — *see* Pigmentation, cornea, posterior
  tumor C79.6- ☑
Kufs' disease E75.4
Kugelberg-Welander disease G12.1
Kuhnt-Junius degeneration (*see also* Degeneration,
  macula) H35.32- ☑
Kümmell's disease or spondylitis — *see* Spondylopa-
  thy, traumatic
Kupffer cell sarcoma C22.3
Kuru A81.81
Kussmaul's
  disease M30.0
  respiration E87.2
    in diabetic acidosis — *see* Diabetes, by type, with
      ketoacidosis
Kwashiorkor E40
  marasmic, marasmus type E42
Kyasanur Forest disease A98.2
Kyphoscoliosis, kyphoscoliotic (acquired) (*see also*
  Scoliosis) M41.9
  congenital Q67.5
  heart (disease) I27.1
  sequelae of rickets E64.3
  tuberculous A18.01
Kyphosis, kyphotic (acquired) M40.209

Kyphosis, kyphotic — *continued*
cervical region M40.202
cervicothoracic region M40.203
congenital Q76.419
cervical region Q76.412
cervicothoracic region Q76.413
occipito-atlanto-axial region Q76.411
thoracic region Q76.414
thoracolumbar region Q76.415
Morquio-Brailsford type (spinal) (*see also* subcategory M49.8) E76.219
postlaminectomy M96.3
postradiation therapy M96.2
postural (adolescent) M40.00
cervicothoracic region M40.03
thoracic region M40.04
thoracolumbar region M40.05
secondary NEC M40.10
cervical region M40.12
cervicothoracic region M40.13
thoracic region M40.14
thoracolumbar region M40.15
sequelae of rickets E64.3
specified type NEC M40.299
cervical region M40.292
cervicothoracic region M40.293
thoracic region M40.294
thoracolumbar region M40.295
syphilitic, congenital A50.56
thoracic region M40.204
thoracolumbar region M40.205
tuberculous A18.01
Kyrle disease L87.0

L

Labia, labium — *see* condition
Labile
blood pressure R09.89
vasomotor system I73.9
Labioglossal paralysis G12.29
Labium leporinum — *see* Cleft, lip
Labor — *see* Delivery
Labored breathing — *see* Hyperventilation
Labyrinthitis (circumscribed) (destructive) (diffuse) (inner ear) (latent) (purulent) (suppurative) (*see also* subcategory) H83.0 ☑
syphilitic A52.79
Laceration
with abortion — *see* Abortion, by type, complicated by laceration of pelvic organs
abdomen, abdominal
wall S31.119 ☑
with
foreign body S31.129 ☑
penetration into peritoneal cavity S31.619 ☑
with foreign body S31.629 ☑
epigastric region S31.112 ☑
with
foreign body S31.122 ☑
penetration into peritoneal cavity S31.612 ☑
with foreign body S31.622 ☑
left
lower quadrant S31.114 ☑
with
foreign body S31.124 ☑
penetration into peritoneal cavity S31.614 ☑
with foreign body S31.624 ☑
upper quadrant S31.111 ☑
with
foreign body S31.121 ☑
penetration into peritoneal cavity S31.611 ☑
with foreign body S31.621 ☑
periumbilic region S31.115 ☑
with
foreign body S31.125 ☑
penetration into peritoneal cavity S31.615 ☑
with foreign body S31.625 ☑
right
lower quadrant S31.113 ☑
with
foreign body S31.123 ☑

Laceration — *continued*
abdomen, abdominal — *continued*
wall — *continued*
right — *continued*
lower quadrant — *continued*
with — *continued*
penetration into peritoneal cavity S31.613 ☑
with foreign body S31.623 ☑
upper quadrant S31.110 ☑
with
foreign body S31.120 ☑
penetration into peritoneal cavity S31.610 ☑
with foreign body S31.620 ☑
accidental, complicating surgery — *see* Complications, surgical, accidental puncture or laceration
Achilles tendon S86.02- ☑
adrenal gland S37.813 ☑
alveolar (process) — *see* Laceration, oral cavity
ankle S91.01- ☑
with
foreign body S91.02- ☑
antecubital space — *see* Laceration, elbow
anus (sphincter) S31.831 ☑
with
ectopic or molar pregnancy O08.6
foreign body S31.832 ☑
complicating delivery — *see* Delivery, complicated, by, laceration, anus (sphincter)
following ectopic or molar pregnancy O08.6
nontraumatic, nonpuerperal — *see* Fissure, anus
arm (upper) S41.11- ☑
with foreign body S41.12- ☑
lower — *see* Laceration, forearm
auditory canal (external) (meatus) — *see* Laceration, ear
auricle, ear — *see* Laceration, ear
axilla — *see* Laceration, arm
back (*see also* Laceration, thorax, back)
lower S31.010 ☑
with
foreign body S31.020 ☑
with penetration into retroperitoneal space S31.021 ☑
penetration into retroperitoneal space S31.011 ☑
bile duct S36.13 ☑
bladder S37.23 ☑
with ectopic or molar pregnancy O08.6
following ectopic or molar pregnancy O08.6
obstetrical trauma O71.5
blood vessel — *see* Injury, blood vessel
bowel (*see also* Laceration, intestine)
with ectopic or molar pregnancy O08.6
complicating abortion — *see* Abortion, by type, complicated by, specified condition NEC
following ectopic or molar pregnancy O08.6
obstetrical trauma O71.5
brain (any part) (cortex) (diffuse) (membrane) (*see also* Injury, intracranial, diffuse)
during birth P10.8
with hemorrhage P10.1
focal — *see* Injury, intracranial, focal brain injury
brainstem S06.38- ☑
breast S21.01- ☑
with foreign body S21.02- ☑
broad ligament S37.893 ☑
with ectopic or molar pregnancy O08.6
following ectopic or molar pregnancy O08.6
laceration syndrome N83.8
obstetrical trauma O71.6
syndrome (laceration) N83.8
buttock S31.801 ☑
with foreign body S31.802 ☑
left S31.821 ☑
with foreign body S31.822 ☑
right S31.811 ☑
with foreign body S31.812 ☑
calf — *see* Laceration, leg
canaliculus lacrimalis — *see* Laceration, eyelid
canthus, eye — *see* Laceration, eyelid
capsule, joint — *see* Sprain
causing eversion of cervix uteri (old) N86
central (perineal), complicating delivery O70.9
cerebellum, traumatic S06.37- ☑
cerebral S06.33- ☑

Laceration — *continued*
cerebral — *continued*
during birth P10.8
with hemorrhage P10.1
left side S06.32- ☑
right side S06.31- ☑
cervix (uteri)
with ectopic or molar pregnancy O08.6
following ectopic or molar pregnancy O08.6
nonpuerperal, nontraumatic N88.1
obstetrical trauma (current) O71.3
old (postpartal) N88.1
traumatic S37.63 ☑
cheek (external) S01.41- ☑
with foreign body S01.42- ☑
internal — *see* Laceration, oral cavity
chest wall — *see* Laceration, thorax
chin — *see* Laceration, head, specified site NEC
chordae tendinae NEC I51.1
concurrent with acute myocardial infarction — *see* Infarct, myocardium
following acute myocardial infarction (current complication) I23.4
clitoris — *see* Laceration, vulva
colon — *see* Laceration, intestine, large, colon
common bile duct S36.13 ☑
cortex (cerebral) — *see* Injury, intracranial, diffuse
costal region — *see* Laceration, thorax
cystic duct S36.13 ☑
diaphragm S27.803 ☑
digit(s)
foot — *see* Laceration, toe
hand — *see* Laceration, finger
duodenum S36.430 ☑
ear (canal) (external) S01.31- ☑
with foreign body S01.32- ☑
drum S09.2- ☑
elbow S51.01- ☑
with
foreign body S51.02- ☑
epididymis — *see* Laceration, testis
epigastric region — *see* Laceration, abdomen, wall, epigastric region
esophagus K22.8
traumatic
cervical S11.21 ☑
with foreign body S11.22 ☑
thoracic S27.813 ☑
eye (ball) S05.3- ☑
with prolapse or loss of intraocular tissue S05.2- ☑
penetrating S05.6- ☑
eyebrow — *see* Laceration, eyelid
eyelid S01.11- ☑
with foreign body S01.12- ☑
face NEC — *see* Laceration, head, specified site NEC
fallopian tube S37.539 ☑
bilateral S37.532 ☑
unilateral S37.531 ☑
finger(s) S61.219 ☑
with
damage to nail S61.319 ☑
with
foreign body S61.329 ☑
foreign body S61.229 ☑
index S61.218 ☑
with
damage to nail S61.318 ☑
with
foreign body S61.328 ☑
foreign body S61.228 ☑
left S61.211 ☑
with
damage to nail S61.311 ☑
with
foreign body S61.321 ☑
foreign body S61.221 ☑
right S61.210 ☑
with
damage to nail S61.310 ☑
with
foreign body S61.320 ☑
foreign body S61.220 ☑
little S61.218 ☑
with
damage to nail S61.318 ☑
with
foreign body S61.328 ☑

☑ Additional Character Required — Refer to the Tabular List for Character Selection — Subterms under main terms may continue to next column or page

Laceration — *continued*
finger(s) — *continued*
  little — *continued*
    with — *continued*
      foreign body S61.228 ☑
    left S61.217 ☑
      with
        damage to nail S61.317 ☑
          with
            foreign body S61.327 ☑
        foreign body S61.227 ☑
    right S61.216 ☑
      with
        damage to nail S61.316 ☑
          with
            foreign body S61.326 ☑
        foreign body S61.226 ☑
  middle S61.218 ☑
    with
      damage to nail S61.318 ☑
        with
          foreign body S61.328 ☑
      foreign body S61.228 ☑
    left S61.213 ☑
      with
        damage to nail S61.313 ☑
          with
            foreign body S61.323 ☑
        foreign body S61.223 ☑
    right S61.212 ☑
      with
        damage to nail S61.312 ☑
          with
            foreign body S61.322 ☑
        foreign body S61.222 ☑
  ring S61.218 ☑
    with
      damage to nail S61.318 ☑
        with
          foreign body S61.328 ☑
      foreign body S61.228 ☑
    left S61.215 ☑
      with
        damage to nail S61.315 ☑
          with
            foreign body S61.325 ☑
        foreign body S61.225 ☑
    right S61.214 ☑
      with
        damage to nail S61.314 ☑
          with
            foreign body S61.324 ☑
        foreign body S61.224 ☑
flank S31.119 ☑
  with foreign body S31.129 ☑
foot (except toe(s) alone) S91.319 ☑
  with foreign body S91.329 ☑
  left S91.312 ☑
    with foreign body S91.322 ☑
  right S91.311 ☑
    with foreign body S91.321 ☑
  toe — *see* Laceration, toe
forearm S51.819 ☑
  with
    foreign body S51.829 ☑
  elbow only — *see* Laceration, elbow
  left S51.812 ☑
    with
      foreign body S51.822 ☑
  right S51.811 ☑
    with
      foreign body S51.821 ☑
forehead S01.81 ☑
  with foreign body S01.82 ☑
fourchette O70.0
  with ectopic or molar pregnancy O08.6
  complicating delivery O70.0
  following ectopic or molar pregnancy O08.6
gallbladder S36.123 ☑
genital organs, external
  female S31.512 ☑
    with foreign body S31.522 ☑
    vagina — *see* Laceration, vagina
    vulva — *see* Laceration, vulva
  male S31.511 ☑
    with foreign body S31.521 ☑

Laceration — *continued*
genital organs, external — *continued*
  male — *continued*
    penis — *see* Laceration, penis
    scrotum — *see* Laceration, scrotum
    testis — *see* Laceration, testis
groin — *see* Laceration, abdomen, wall
gum — *see* Laceration, oral cavity
hand S61.419 ☑
  with
    foreign body S61.429 ☑
  finger — *see* Laceration, finger
  left S61.412 ☑
    with
      foreign body S61.422 ☑
  right S61.411 ☑
    with
      foreign body S61.421 ☑
  thumb — *see* Laceration, thumb
head S01.91 ☑
  with foreign body S01.92 ☑
  cheek — *see* Laceration, cheek
  ear — *see* Laceration, ear
  eyelid — *see* Laceration, eyelid
  lip — *see* Laceration, lip
  nose — *see* Laceration, nose
  oral cavity — *see* Laceration, oral cavity
  scalp S01.01 ☑
    with foreign body S01.02 ☑
  specified site NEC S01.81 ☑
    with foreign body S01.82 ☑
  temporomandibular area — *see* Laceration, cheek
heart — *see* Injury, heart, laceration
heel — *see* Laceration, foot
hepatic duct S36.13 ☑
hip S71.019 ☑
  with foreign body S71.029 ☑
  left S71.012 ☑
    with foreign body S71.022 ☑
  right S71.011 ☑
    with foreign body S71.021 ☑
hymen — *see* Laceration, vagina
hypochondrium — *see* Laceration, abdomen, wall
hypogastric region — *see* Laceration, abdomen, wall
ileum S36.438 ☑
inguinal region — *see* Laceration, abdomen, wall
instep — *see* Laceration, foot
internal organ — *see* Injury, by site
interscapular region — *see* Laceration, thorax, back
intestine
  large
    colon S36.539 ☑
      ascending S36.530 ☑
      descending S36.532 ☑
      sigmoid S36.533 ☑
      specified site NEC S36.538 ☑
    rectum S36.63 ☑
    transverse S36.531 ☑
  small S36.439 ☑
    duodenum S36.430 ☑
    specified site NEC S36.438 ☑
intra-abdominal organ S36.93 ☑
  intestine — *see* Laceration, intestine
  liver — *see* Laceration, liver
  pancreas — *see* Laceration, pancreas
  peritoneum S36.81 ☑
  specified site NEC S36.893 ☑
  spleen — *see* Laceration, spleen
  stomach — *see* Laceration, stomach
intracranial NEC (*see also* Injury, intracranial, diffuse)
  birth injury P10.9
jaw — *see* Laceration, head, specified site NEC
jejunum S36.438 ☑
joint capsule — *see* Sprain, by site
kidney S37.03- ☑
  major (greater than 3 cm) (massive) (stellate) S37.06- ☑
  minor (less than 1 cm) S37.04- ☑
  moderate (1 to 3 cm) S37.05- ☑
    multiple S37.06- ☑
knee S81.01- ☑
  with foreign body S81.02- ☑
labium (majus) (minus) — *see* Laceration, vulva
lacrimal duct — *see* Laceration, eyelid
large intestine — *see* Laceration, intestine, large
larynx S11.011 ☑

Laceration — *continued*
larynx — *continued*
  with foreign body S11.012 ☑
leg (lower) S81.819 ☑
  with foreign body S81.829 ☑
  foot — *see* Laceration, foot
  knee — *see* Laceration, knee
  left S81.812 ☑
    with foreign body S81.822 ☑
  right S81.811 ☑
    with foreign body S81.821 ☑
  upper — *see* Laceration, thigh
ligament — *see* Sprain
lip S01.511 ☑
  with foreign body S01.521 ☑
liver S36.113 ☑
  major (stellate) S36.116 ☑
  minor S36.114 ☑
  moderate S36.115 ☑
loin — *see* Laceration, abdomen, wall
lower back — *see* Laceration, back, lower
lumbar region — *see* Laceration, back, lower
lung S27.339 ☑
  bilateral S27.332 ☑
  unilateral S27.331 ☑
malar region — *see* Laceration, head, specified site NEC
mammary — *see* Laceration, breast
mastoid region — *see* Laceration, head, specified site NEC
meninges — *see* Injury, intracranial, diffuse
meniscus — *see* Tear, meniscus
mesentery S36.893 ☑
mesosalpinx S37.893 ☑
mouth — *see* Laceration, oral cavity
muscle — *see* Injury, muscle, by site, laceration
nail
  finger — *see* Laceration, finger, with damage to nail
  toe — *see* Laceration, toe, with damage to nail
nasal (septum) (sinus) — *see* Laceration, nose
nasopharynx — *see* Laceration, head, specified site NEC
neck S11.91 ☑
  with foreign body S11.92 ☑
  involving
    cervical esophagus S11.21 ☑
      with foreign body S11.22 ☑
    larynx — *see* Laceration, larynx
    pharynx — *see* Laceration, pharynx
    thyroid gland — *see* Laceration, thyroid gland
    trachea — *see* Laceration, trachea
  specified site NEC S11.81 ☑
    with foreign body S11.82 ☑
nerve — *see* Injury, nerve
nose (septum) (sinus) S01.21 ☑
  with foreign body S01.22 ☑
ocular NOS S05.3- ☑
  adnexa NOS S01.11- ☑
oral cavity S01.512 ☑
  with foreign body S01.522 ☑
orbit (eye) — *see* Wound, open, ocular, orbit
ovary S37.439 ☑
  bilateral S37.432 ☑
  unilateral S37.431 ☑
palate — *see* Laceration, oral cavity
palm — *see* Laceration, hand
pancreas S36.239 ☑
pelvic S31.010 ☑
  with
    foreign body S31.020 ☑
      penetration into retroperitoneal cavity S31.021 ☑
    penetration into retroperitoneal cavity S31.011 ☑
  floor (*see also* Laceration, back, lower)
    with ectopic or molar pregnancy O08.6
    complicating delivery O70.1
    following ectopic or molar pregnancy O08.6
    old (postpartal) N81.89
  organ S37.93 ☑
penis S31.21 ☑
  with foreign body S31.22 ☑
perineum
  female S31.41 ☑

Laceration — *continued*
  perineum — *continued*
    female — *continued*
      with
        ectopic or molar pregnancy O08.6
        foreign body S31.42 ☑
      during delivery O70.9
        first degree O70.0
        fourth degree O70.3
        second degree O70.1
        third degree (*see also* Delivery, complicated, by, laceration, perineum, third degree) O70.20
      old (postpartal) N81.89
      postpartal N81.89
      secondary (postpartal) O90.1
    male S31.119 ☑
      with foreign body S31.129 ☑
  periocular area (with or without lacrimal passages) — *see* Laceration, eyelid
  peritoneum S36.893 ☑
  periumbilic region — *see* Laceration, abdomen, wall, periumbilic
  periurethral tissue — *see* Laceration, urethra
  phalanges
    finger — *see* Laceration, finger
    toe — *see* Laceration, toe
  pharynx S11.21 ☑
    with foreign body S11.22 ☑
  pinna — *see* Laceration, ear
  popliteal space — *see* Laceration, knee
  prepuce — *see* Laceration, penis
  prostate S37.823 ☑
  pubic region S31.119 ☑
    with foreign body S31.129 ☑
  pudendum — *see* Laceration, genital organs, external
  rectovaginal septum — *see* Laceration, vagina
  rectum S36.63 ☑
  retroperitoneum S36.893 ☑
  round ligament S37.893 ☑
  sacral region — *see* Laceration, back, lower
  sacroiliac region — *see* Laceration, back, lower
  salivary gland — *see* Laceration, oral cavity
  scalp S01.01 ☑
    with foreign body S01.02 ☑
  scapular region — *see* Laceration, shoulder
  scrotum S31.31 ☑
    with foreign body S31.32 ☑
  seminal vesicle S37.893 ☑
  shin — *see* Laceration, leg
  shoulder S41.019 ☑
    with foreign body S41.029 ☑
    left S41.012 ☑
      with foreign body S41.022 ☑
    right S41.011 ☑
      with foreign body S41.021 ☑
  small intestine — *see* Laceration, intestine, small
  spermatic cord — *see* Laceration, testis
  spinal cord (meninges) (*see also* Injury, spinal cord, by region)
    due to injury at birth P11.5
    newborn (birth injury) P11.5
  spleen S36.039 ☑
    major (massive) (stellate) S36.032 ☑
    moderate S36.031 ☑
    superficial (minor) S36.030 ☑
  sternal region — *see* Laceration, thorax, front
  stomach S36.33 ☑
  submaxillary region — *see* Laceration, head, specified site NEC
  submental region — *see* Laceration, head, specified site NEC
  subungual
    finger(s) — *see* Laceration, finger, with damage to nail
    toe(s) — *see* Laceration, toe, with damage to nail
  suprarenal gland — *see* Laceration, adrenal gland
  temple, temporal region — *see* Laceration, head, specified site NEC
  temporomandibular area — *see* Laceration, cheek
  tendon — *see* Injury, muscle, by site, laceration
    Achilles S86.02- ☑
  tentorium cerebelli — *see* Injury, intracranial, diffuse
  testis S31.31 ☑
    with foreign body S31.32 ☑
  thigh S71.11- ☑
    with foreign body S71.12- ☑

Laceration — *continued*
  thorax, thoracic (wall) S21.91 ☑
    with foreign body S21.92 ☑
      back S21.22- ☑
        with penetration into thoracic cavity S21.42- ☑
      front S21.12- ☑
        with penetration into thoracic cavity S21.32- ☑
    back S21.21- ☑
      with
        foreign body S21.22- ☑
          with penetration into thoracic cavity S21.42- ☑
        penetration into thoracic cavity S21.41- ☑
    breast — *see* Laceration, breast
    front S21.11- ☑
      with
        foreign body S21.12- ☑
          with penetration into thoracic cavity S21.32- ☑
        penetration into thoracic cavity S21.31- ☑
  thumb S61.019 ☑
    with
      damage to nail S61.119 ☑
        with
          foreign body S61.129 ☑
      foreign body S61.029 ☑
    left S61.012 ☑
      with
        damage to nail S61.112 ☑
          with
            foreign body S61.122 ☑
        foreign body S61.022 ☑
    right S61.011 ☑
      with
        damage to nail S61.111 ☑
          with
            foreign body S61.121 ☑
        foreign body S61.021 ☑
  thyroid gland S11.11 ☑
    with foreign body S11.12 ☑
  toe(s) S91.119 ☑
    with
      damage to nail S91.219 ☑
        with
          foreign body S91.229 ☑
      foreign body S91.129 ☑
    great S91.113 ☑
      with
        damage to nail S91.213 ☑
          with
            foreign body S91.223 ☑
        foreign body S91.123 ☑
      left S91.112 ☑
        with
          damage to nail S91.212 ☑
            with
              foreign body S91.222 ☑
          foreign body S91.122 ☑
      right S91.111 ☑
        with
          damage to nail S91.211 ☑
            with
              foreign body S91.221 ☑
          foreign body S91.121 ☑
    lesser S91.116 ☑
      with
        damage to nail S91.216 ☑
          with
            foreign body S91.226 ☑
        foreign body S91.126 ☑
      left S91.115 ☑
        with
          damage to nail S91.215 ☑
            with
              foreign body S91.225 ☑
          foreign body S91.125 ☑
      right S91.114 ☑
        with
          damage to nail S91.214 ☑
            with
              foreign body S91.224 ☑
          foreign body S91.124 ☑
  tongue — *see* Laceration, oral cavity
  trachea S11.021 ☑

Laceration — *continued*
  trachea — *continued*
    with foreign body S11.022 ☑
  tunica vaginalis — *see* Laceration, testis
  tympanum, tympanic membrane — *see* Laceration, ear, drum
  umbilical region S31.115 ☑
    with foreign body S31.125 ☑
  ureter S37.13 ☑
  urethra S37.33 ☑
    with or following ectopic or molar pregnancy O08.6
    obstetrical trauma O71.5
  urinary organ NEC S37.893 ☑
  uterus S37.63 ☑
    with ectopic or molar pregnancy O08.6
    following ectopic or molar pregnancy O08.6
    nonpuerperal, nontraumatic N85.8
    obstetrical trauma NEC O71.81
    old (postpartal) N85.8
  uvula — *see* Laceration, oral cavity
  vagina S31.41 ☑
    with
      ectopic or molar pregnancy O08.6
      foreign body S31.42 ☑
    during delivery O71.4
      with perineal laceration — *see* Laceration, perineum, female, during delivery
    following ectopic or molar pregnancy O08.6
    nonpuerperal, nontraumatic N89.8
    old (postpartal) N89.8
  vas deferens S37.893 ☑
  vesical — *see* Laceration, bladder
  vocal cords S11.031 ☑
    with foreign body S11.032 ☑
  vulva S31.41 ☑
    with
      ectopic or molar pregnancy O08.6
      foreign body S31.42 ☑
    complicating delivery O70.0
    following ectopic or molar pregnancy O08.6
    nonpuerperal, nontraumatic N90.89
    old (postpartal) N90.89
  wrist S61.519 ☑
    with
      foreign body S61.529 ☑
    left S61.512 ☑
      with
        foreign body S61.522 ☑
    right S61.511 ☑
      with
        foreign body S61.521 ☑

Lack of
  achievement in school Z55.3
  adequate
    food Z59.4
    intermaxillary vertical dimension of fully erupted teeth M26.36
    sleep Z72.820
  appetite (*see* Anorexia) R63.0
  awareness R41.9
  care
    in home Z74.2
    of infant (at or after birth) T76.02 ☑
      confirmed T74.02 ☑
  cognitive functions R41.9
  coordination R27.9
    ataxia R27.0
    specified type NEC R27.8
  development (physiological) R62.50
    failure to thrive (child over 28 days old) R62.51
      adult R62.7
      newborn P92.6
    short stature R62.52
    specified type NEC R62.59
  energy R53.83
  financial resources Z59.6
  food T73.0 ☑
  growth R62.52
  heating Z59.1
  housing (permanent) (temporary) Z59.0
    adequate Z59.1
  learning experiences in childhood Z62.898
  leisure time (affecting life-style) Z73.2
  material resources Z59.9
  memory (*see also* Amnesia)
    mild, following organic brain damage F06.8
  ovulation N97.0
  parental supervision or control of child Z62.0

☑ Additional Character Required — Refer to the Tabular List for Character Selection   ▽ Subterms under main terms may continue to next column or page

Lack of — continued
  person able to render necessary care Z74.2
  physical exercise Z72.3
  play experience in childhood Z62.898
  posterior occlusal support M26.57
  relaxation (affecting life-style) Z73.2
  sexual
    desire F52.0
    enjoyment F52.1
  shelter Z59.0
  sleep (adequate) Z72.820
  supervision of child by parent Z62.0
  support, posterior occlusal M26.57
  water T73.1 ☑
Lacrimal — see condition
Lacrimation, abnormal — see Epiphora
Lacrimonasal duct — see condition
Lactation, lactating (breast) (puerperal, postpartum)
  associated
    cracked nipple O92.13
    retracted nipple O92.03
  defective O92.4
  disorder NEC O92.79
  excessive O92.6
  failed (complete) O92.3
    partial O92.4
  mastitis NEC — see Mastitis, obstetric
  mother (care and/or examination) Z39.1
  nonpuerperal N64.3
Lacticemia, excessive E87.2
Lacunar skull Q75.8
Laennec's cirrhosis K70.30
  with ascites K70.31
  nonalcoholic K74.69
Lafora's disease — see Epilepsy, generalized, idiopathic
Lag, lid (nervous) — see Retraction, lid
Lagophthalmos (eyelid) (nervous) H02.209
  cicatricial H02.219
    left H02.216
      lower H02.215
      upper H02.214
    right H02.213
      lower H02.212
      upper H02.211
  keratoconjunctivitis — see Keratoconjunctivitis
  left H02.206
    lower H02.205
    upper H02.204
  mechanical H02.229
    left H02.226
      lower H02.225
      upper H02.224
    right H02.223
      lower H02.222
      upper H02.221
  paralytic H02.239
    left H02.236
      lower H02.235
      upper H02.234
    right H02.233
      lower H02.232
      upper H02.231
  right H02.203
    lower H02.202
    upper H02.201
Laki-Lorand factor deficiency — see Defect, coagulation, specified type NEC
Lalling F80.0
Lambert-Eaton syndrome — see Syndrome, Lambert-Eaton
Lambliasis, lambliosis A07.1
Landau-Kleffner syndrome — see Epilepsy, specified NEC
Landouzy-Déjérine dystrophy or facioscapulohumeral atrophy G71.0
Landouzy's disease (icterohemorrhagic leptospirosis) A27.0
Landry-Guillain-Barré, syndrome or paralysis G61.0
Landry's disease or paralysis G61.0
Lane's
  band Q43.3
  kink — see Obstruction, intestine
  syndrome K90.2
Langdon Down syndrome — see Trisomy, 21
Lapsed immunization schedule status Z28.3
Large
  baby (regardless of gestational age) (4000g to 4499g) P08.1

Large — continued
  ear, congenital Q17.1
  physiological cup Q14.2
  stature R68.89
Large-for-dates NEC (infant) (4000g to 4499g) P08.1
  affecting management of pregnancy O36.6- ☑
  exceptionally (4500g or more) P08.0
Larsen-Johansson disease orosteochondrosis — see Osteochondrosis, juvenile, patella
Larsen's syndrome (flattened facies and multiple congenital dislocations) Q74.8
Larva migrans
  cutaneous B76.9
    Ancylostoma B76.0
  visceral B83.0
Laryngeal — see condition
Laryngismus (stridulus) J38.5
  congenital P28.89
  diphtheritic A36.2
Laryngitis (acute) (edematous) (fibrinous) (infective) (infiltrative) (malignant) (membranous) (phlegmonous) (pneumococcal) (pseudomembranous) (septic) (subglottic) (suppurative) (ulcerative) J04.0
  with
    influenza, flu, or grippe — see Influenza, with, laryngitis
    tracheitis (acute) — see Laryngotracheitis
  atrophic J37.0
  catarrhal J37.0
  chronic J37.0
    with tracheitis (chronic) J37.1
  diphtheritic A36.2
  due to external agent — see Inflammation, respiratory, upper, due to
  H. influenzae J04.0
  Hemophilus influenzae J04.0
  hypertrophic J37.0
  influenzal — see Influenza, with, respiratory manifestations NEC
  obstructive J05.0
  sicca J37.0
  spasmodic J05.0
    acute J04.0
  streptococcal J04.0
  stridulous J05.0
  syphilitic (late) A52.73
    congenital A50.59 [J99]
      early A50.03 [J99]
  tuberculous A15.5
  Vincent's A69.1
Laryngocele (congenital) (ventricular) Q31.3
Laryngofissure J38.7
  congenital Q31.8
Laryngomalacia (congenital) Q31.5
Laryngopharyngitis (acute) J06.0
  chronic J37.0
  due to external agent — see Inflammation, respiratory, upper, due to
Laryngoplegia J38.00
  bilateral J38.02
  unilateral J38.01
Laryngoptosis J38.7
Laryngospasm J38.5
Laryngostenosis J38.6
Laryngotracheitis (acute) (Infectional) (infective) (viral) J04.2
  atrophic J37.1
  catarrhal J37.1
  chronic J37.1
  diphtheritic A36.2
  due to external agent — see Inflammation, respiratory, upper, due to
  Hemophilus influenzae J04.2
  hypertrophic J37.1
  influenzal — see Influenza, with, respiratory manifestations NEC
  pachydermic J38.7
  sicca J37.1
  spasmodic J38.5
    acute J05.0
  streptococcal J04.2
  stridulous J38.5
  syphilitic (late) A52.73
    congenital A50.59 [J99]
      early A50.03 [J99]
  tuberculous A15.5
  Vincent's A69.1
Laryngotracheobronchitis — see Bronchitis

Larynx, laryngeal — see condition
Lassa fever A96.2
Lassitude — see Weakness
Late
  talker R62.0
  walker R62.0
Late effect(s) — see Sequelae
Latent — see condition
Laterocession — see Lateroversion
Lateroflexion — see Lateroversion
Lateroversion
  cervix — see Lateroversion, uterus
  uterus, uterine (cervix) (postinfectional) (postpartal, old) N85.4
    congenital Q51.818
    in pregnancy or childbirth O34.59- ☑
Lathyrism — see Poisoning, food, noxious, plant
Launois' syndrome (pituitary gigantism) E22.0
Launois-Bensaude adenolipomatosis E88.89
Laurence-Moon (-Bardet)-**Biedl syndrome** Q87.89
Lax, laxity (see also Relaxation)
  ligament (ous) (see also Disorder, ligament)
    familial M35.7
    knee — see Derangement, knee
  skin (acquired) L57.4
    congenital Q82.8
Laxative habit F55.2
Lazy leukocyte syndrome D70.8
Lead miner's lung J63.6
Leak, leakage
  air NEC J93.82
    postprocedural J95.812
  amniotic fluid — see Rupture, membranes, premature
  blood (microscopic), fetal, into maternal circulation affecting management of pregnancy — see Pregnancy, complicated by
  cerebrospinal fluid G96.0
    from spinal (lumbar) puncture G97.0
  device, implant or graft (see also Complications, by site and type, mechanical)
    arterial graft NEC — see Complication, cardiovascular device, mechanical, vascular
    breast (implant) T85.43 ☑
    catheter NEC T85.638 ☑
      dialysis (renal) T82.43 ☑
        intraperitoneal T85.631 ☑
      infusion NEC T82.534 ☑
        spinal (epidural) (subdural) T85.630 ☑
      urinary T83.038 ☑
        cystostomy T83.030 ☑
        Hopkins T83.038 ☑
        ileostomy T83.038 ☑
        indwelling T83.031 ☑
        nephrostomy T83.032 ☑
        specified T83.038 ☑
        urostomy T83.038 ☑
    gastrointestinal — see Complications, prosthetic device, mechanical, gastrointestinal device
    genital NEC T83.498 ☑
      penile prosthesis (cylinder) (implanted) (pump) (reservoir) T83.490 ☑
      testicular prosthesis T83.491 ☑
    heart NEC — see Complication, cardiovascular device, mechanical
    joint prosthesis — see Complications, joint prosthesis, mechanical, specified NEC, by site
    ocular NEC — see Complications, prosthetic device, mechanical, ocular device
    orthopedic NEC — see Complication, orthopedic, device, mechanical
    persistent air J93.82
    specified NEC T85.638 ☑
    urinary NEC (see also Complication, genitourinary, device, urinary, mechanical)
      graft T83.23 ☑
    vascular NEC — see Complication, cardiovascular device, mechanical
    ventricular intracranial shunt T85.03 ☑
  urine — see Incontinence
Leaky heart — see Endocarditis
Learning defect (specific) F81.9
Leather bottle stomach C16.9
Leber's
  congenital amaurosis H35.50
  optic atrophy (hereditary) H47.22
Lederer's anemia D59.1
Leeches (external) — see Hirudiniasis

Leg — see condition
Legg (-Calvé)-Perthes disease, syndrome or osteochondrosis M91.1- ☑
Legionellosis A48.1
nonpneumonic A48.2
Legionnaires'
disease A48.1
nonpneumonic A48.2
pneumonia A48.1
Leigh's disease G31.82
Leiner's disease L21.1
Leiofibromyoma — see Leiomyoma
Leiomyoblastoma — see Neoplasm, connective tissue,
benign
Leiomyofibroma (see also Neoplasm, connective tissue,
benign)
uterus (cervix) (corpus) D25.9
Leiomyoma (see also Neoplasm, connective tissue, benign)
bizarre — see Neoplasm, connective tissue, benign
cellular — see Neoplasm, connective tissue, benign
epithelioid — see Neoplasm, connective tissue, benign
uterus (cervix) (corpus) D25.9
intramural D25.1
submucous D25.0
subserosal D25.2
vascular — see Neoplasm, connective tissue, benign
Leiomyoma, leiomyomatosis (intravascular) — see
Neoplasm, connective tissue, uncertain behavior
Leiomyosarcoma (see also Neoplasm, connective tissue,
malignant)
epithelioid — see Neoplasm, connective tissue, malignant
myxoid — see Neoplasm, connective tissue, malignant
Leishmaniasis B55.9
American (mucocutaneous) B55.2
cutaneous B55.1
Asian Desert B55.1
Brazilian B55.2
cutaneous (any type) B55.1
dermal (see also Leishmaniasis, cutaneous)
post-kala-azar B55.0
eyelid B55.1
infantile B55.0
Mediterranean B55.0
mucocutaneous (American) (New World) B55.2
naso-oral B55.2
nasopharyngeal B55.2
old world B55.1
tegumentaria diffusa B55.1
visceral B55.0
Leishmanoid, dermal (see also Leishmaniasis, cutaneous)
post-kala-azar B55.0
Lenegre's disease I44.2
Lengthening, leg — see Deformity, limb, unequal length
Lennert's lymphoma — see Lymphoma, Lennert's
Lennox-Gastaut syndrome G40.812
intractable G40.814
with status epilepticus G40.813
without status epilepticus G40.814
not intractable G40.812
with status epilepticus G40.811
without status epilepticus G40.812
Lens — see condition
Lenticonus (anterior) (posterior) (congenital) Q12.8
Lenticular degeneration, progressive E83.01
Lentiglobus (posterior) (congenital) Q12.8
Lentigo (congenital) L81.4
maligna (see also Melanoma, in situ)
melanoma — see Melanoma
Lentivirus, as cause of disease classified elsewhere
B97.31
Leontiasis
ossium M85.2
syphilitic (late) A52.78
congenital A50.59
Lepothrix A48.8
Lepra — see Leprosy
Leprechaunism E34.8
Leprosy A30.- ☑
with muscle disorder A30.9 [M63.80]
ankle A30.9 [M63.87-] ☑
foot A30.9 [M63.87-] ☑
forearm A30.9 [M63.83-] ☑
hand A30.9 [M63.84-] ☑
lower leg A30.9 [M63.86-] ☑

Leprosy — continued
with muscle disorder — continued
multiple sites A30.9 [M63.89]
pelvic region A30.9 [M63.85-] ☑
shoulder region A30.9 [M63.81-] ☑
specified site NEC A30.9 [M63.88]
thigh A30.9 [M63.85-] ☑
upper arm A30.9 [M63.82-] ☑
anesthetic A30.9
BB A30.3
BL A30.4
borderline (infiltrated) (neuritic) A30.3
lepromatous A30.4
tuberculoid A30.2
BT A30.2
dimorphous (infiltrated) (neuritic) A30.3
I A30.0
indeterminate (macular) (neuritic) A30.0
lepromatous (diffuse) (infiltrated) (macular) (neuritic)
(nodular) A30.5
LL A30.5
macular (early) (neuritic) (simple) A30.9
maculoanesthetic A30.9
mixed A30.3
neural A30.9
nodular A30.5
primary neuritic A30.3
specified type NEC A30.8
TT A30.1
tuberculoid (major) (minor) A30.1
Leptocytosis, hereditary D56.9
Leptomeningitis (chronic) (circumscribed) (hemorrhagic)
(nonsuppurative) — see Meningitis
Leptomeningopathy G96.19
Leptospiral — see condition
Leptospirochetal — see condition
Leptospirosis A27.9
canicola A27.89
due to Leptospira interrogans serovar icterohaemor-
rhagiae A27.0
icterohemorrhagica A27.0
pomona A27.89
Weil's disease A27.0
Leptus dermatitis B88.0
Leriche's syndrome (aortic bifurcation occlusion) I74.09
Leri's pleonosteosis Q78.8
Leri-Weill syndrome Q77.8
Lermoyez' syndrome — see Vertigo, peripheral NEC
Lesch-Nyhan syndrome E79.1
Leser-Trélat disease L82.1
inflamed L82.0
Lesion(s) (nontraumatic)
abducens nerve — see Strabismus, paralytic, sixth
nerve
alveolar process K08.9
angiocentric immunoproliferative D47.Z9 (following
D47.4)
anorectal K62.9
aortic (valve) I35.9
auditory nerve — see subcategory H93.3 ☑
basal ganglion G25.9
bile duct — see Disease, bile duct
biomechanical M99.9
specified type NEC M99.89
abdomen M99.89
acromioclavicular M99.87
cervical region M99.81
cervicothoracic M99.81
costochondral M99.88
costovertebral M99.88
head region M99.80
hip M99.85
lower extremity M99.86
lumbar region M99.83
lumbosacral M99.83
occipitocervical M99.80
pelvic region M99.85
pubic M99.85
rib cage M99.88
sacral region M99.84
sacrococcygeal M99.84
sacroiliac M99.84
specified NEC M99.89
sternochondral M99.88
sternoclavicular M99.87
thoracic region M99.82
thoracolumbar M99.82
upper extremity M99.87

Lesion(s) — continued
bladder N32.9
bone — see Disorder, bone
brachial plexus G54.0
brain G93.9
congenital Q04.9
vascular I67.9
degenerative I67.9
hypertensive I67.4
buccal cavity K13.79
calcified — see Calcification
canthus — see Disorder, eyelid
carate — see Pinta, lesions
cardia K31.9
cardiac (see also Disease, heart) I51.9
congenital Q24.9
valvular — see Endocarditis
cauda equina G83.4
cecum K63.9
cerebral — see Lesion, brain
cerebrovascular I67.9
degenerative I67.9
hypertensive I67.4
cervical (nerve) root NEC G54.2
chiasmal — see Disorder, optic, chiasm
chorda tympani G51.8
coin, lung R91.1
colon K63.9
combined periodontic - endodontic K05.5
congenital — see Anomaly, by site
conjunctiva H11.9
conus medullaris — see Injury, conus medullaris
coronary artery — see Ischemia, heart
cranial nerve G52.9
eighth — see Disorder, ear
eleventh G52.9
fifth G50.9
first G52.0
fourth — see Strabismus, paralytic, fourth nerve
seventh G51.9
sixth — see Strabismus, paralytic, sixth nerve
tenth G52.2
twelfth G52.3
cystic — see Cyst
degenerative — see Degeneration
duodenum K31.9
edentulous (alveolar) ridge, associated with trauma,
due to traumatic occlusion K06.2
en coup de sabre L94.1
eyelid — see Disorder, eyelid
gasserian ganglion G50.8
gastric K31.9
gastroduodenal K31.9
gastrointestinal K63.9
gingiva, associated with trauma K06.2
glomerular
focal and segmental (see also N00-N07 with fourth
character .1) N05.1
minimal change (see also N00-N07 with fourth
character .0) N05.0
heart (organic) — see Disease, heart
hyperchromic, due to pinta (carate) A67.1
hyperkeratotic — see Hyperkeratosis
hypothalamic E23.7
ileocecal K63.9
ileum K63.9
iliohypogastric nerve G57.8- ☑
inflammatory — see Inflammation
intestine K63.9
intracerebral — see Lesion, brain
intrachiasmal (optic) — see Disorder, optic, chiasm
intracranial, space-occupying R90.0
joint — see Disorder, joint
sacroiliac (old) M53.3
keratotic — see Keratosis
kidney — see Disease, renal
laryngeal nerve (recurrent) G52.2
lip K13.0
liver K76.9
lumbosacral
plexus G54.1
root (nerve) NEC G54.4
lung (coin) R91.1
maxillary sinus J32.0
mitral I05.9
Morel-Lavallée — see Hematoma, by site
motor cortex NEC G93.89
mouth K13.79

☑ Additional Character Required — Refer to the Tabular List for Character Selection   ▽ Subterms under main terms may continue to next column or page

Lesion(s) — *continued*
- nerve G58.9
  - femoral G57.2- ☑
  - median G56.1- ☑
    - carpal tunnel syndrome — *see* Syndrome, carpal tunnel
  - plantar G57.6- ☑
  - popliteal (lateral) G57.3- ☑
    - medial G57.4- ☑
  - radial G56.3- ☑
  - sciatic G57.0- ☑
  - spinal — *see* Injury, nerve, spinal
  - ulnar G56.2- ☑
- nervous system, congenital Q07.9
- nonallopathic — *see* Lesion, biomechanical
- nose (internal) J34.89
- obstructive — *see* Obstruction
- obturator nerve G57.8- ☑
- oral mucosa K13.70
- organ or site NEC — *see* Disease, by site
- osteolytic — *see* Osteolysis
- peptic K27.9
- periodontal, due to traumatic occlusion K05.5
- pharynx J39.2
- pigment, pigmented (skin) L81.9
- pinta — *see* Pinta, lesions
- polypoid — *see* Polyp
- prechiasmal (optic) — *see* Disorder, optic, chiasm
- primary (*see also* Syphilis, primary) A51.0
  - carate A67.0
  - pinta A67.0
  - yaws A66.0
- pulmonary J98.4
  - valve I37.9
- pylorus K31.9
- rectosigmoid K63.9
- retina, retinal H35.9
- sacroiliac (joint) (old) M53.3
- salivary gland K11.9
  - benign lymphoepithelial K11.8
- saphenous nerve G57.8- ☑
- sciatic nerve G57.0- ☑
- secondary — *see* Syphilis, secondary
- shoulder (region) M75.9- ☑
  - specified NEC M75.8- ☑
- sigmoid K63.9
- sinus (accessory) (nasal) J34.89
- skin L98.9
  - suppurative L08.0
- SLAP S43.43- ☑
- spinal cord G95.9
  - congenital Q06.9
- spleen D73.89
- stomach K31.9
- superior glenoid labrum S43.43- ☑
- syphilitic — *see* Syphilis
- tertiary — *see* Syphilis, tertiary
- thoracic root (nerve) NEC G54.3
- tonsillar fossa J35.9
- tooth, teeth K08.9
  - white spot
    - chewing surface K02.51
    - pit and fissure surface K02.51
    - smooth surface K02.61
- traumatic — *see* specific type of injury by site
- tricuspid (valve) I07.9
  - nonrheumatic I36.9
- trigeminal nerve G50.9
- ulcerated or ulcerative — *see* Ulcer, skin
- uterus N85.9
- vagus nerve G52.2
- valvular — *see* Endocarditis
- vascular I99.9
  - affecting central nervous system I67.9
  - following trauma NEC T14.8 ☑
  - umbilical cord, complicating delivery O69.5 ☑
- warty — *see* Verruca
- white spot (tooth)
  - chewing surface K02.51
  - pit and fissure surface K02.51
  - smooth surface K02.61

Lethargic — *see* condition
Lethargy R53.83
Letterer-Siwe's disease C96.0
Leukemia, leukemic C95.9- ☑
- acute basophilic C94.8- ☑
- acute bilineal C95.0- ☑

Leukemia, leukemic — *continued*
- acute erythroid C94.0- ☑
- acute lymphoblastic C91.0- ☑
- acute megakaryoblastic C94.2- ☑
- acute megakaryocytic C94.2- ☑
- acute mixed lineage C95.0- ☑
- acute monoblastic (monoblastic/monocytic) C93.0- ☑
- acute monocytic (monoblastic/monocytic) C93.0- ☑
- acute myeloblastic (minimal differentiation) (with maturation) C92.0- ☑
- acute myeloid
  - with
    - 11q23-abnormality C92.6- ☑
    - dysplasia of remaining hematopoesis and/or myelodysplastic disease in its history C92.A- ☑ (*following* C92.6)
    - multilineage dysplasia C92.A- ☑ (*following* C92.6)
    - variation of MLL-gene C92.6- ☑
  - M6 (a)(b) C94.0- ☑
  - M7 C94.2- ☑
- acute myelomonocytic C92.5- ☑
- acute promyelocytic C92.4- ☑
- adult T-cell (HTLV-1-associated) (acute variant) (chronic variant) (lymphomatoid variant) (smouldering variant) C91.5- ☑
- aggressive NK-cell C94.8- ☑
- AML (1/ETO) (M0) (M1) (M2) (without a FAB classification) C92.0- ☑
- AML M3 C92.4- ☑
- AML M4 (Eo with inv(16) or t(16;16)) C92.5- ☑
- AML M5 C93.0- ☑
- AML M5a C93.0- ☑
- AML M5b C93.0- ☑
- AML Me with t (15;17) and variants C92.4- ☑
- atypical chronic myeloid, BCR/ABL-negative C92.2- ☑
- biphenotypic acute C95.0- ☑
- blast cell C95.0- ☑
- Burkitt-type, mature B-cell C91.A- ☑ (*following* C91.6)
- chronic lymphocytic, of B-cell type C91.1- ☑
- chronic monocytic C93.1- ☑
- chronic myelogenous (Philadelphia chromosome (Ph1) positive) (t(9;22)) (q34;q11) (with crisis of blast cells) C92.1- ☑
- chronic myeloid, BCR/ABL-positive C92.1- ☑
  - atypical, BCR/ABL-negative C92.2- ☑
- chronic myelomonocytic C93.1- ☑
- chronic neutrophilic D47.1
- CMML (-1) (-2) (with eosinophilia) C93.1- ☑
- granulocytic (*see also* Category C92) C92.9- ☑
- hairy cell C91.4- ☑
- juvenile myelomonocytic C93.3- ☑
- lymphoid C91.9- ☑
  - specified NEC C91.Z- ☑ (*following* C91.6)
- mast cell C94.3- ☑
- mature B-cell, Burkitt-type C91.A- ☑ (*following* C91.6)
- monocytic (subacute) C93.9- ☑
  - specified NEC C93.Z- ☑ (*following* C93.3)
- myelogenous (*see also* Category C92) C92.9- ☑
- myeloid C92.9- ☑
  - specified NEC C92.Z- ☑ (*following* C92.6)
- plasma cell C90.1- ☑
- plasmacytic C90.1- ☑
- prolymphocytic
  - of B-cell type C91.3- ☑
  - of T-cell type C91.6- ☑
- specified NEC C94.8- ☑
- stem cell, of unclear lineage C95.0- ☑
- subacute lymphocytic C91.9- ☑
- T-cell large granular lymphocytic C91.Z- ☑ (*following* C91.6)
- unspecified cell type C95.9- ☑
  - acute C95.0- ☑
  - chronic C95.1- ☑

Leukemoid reaction (*see also* Reaction, leukemoid) D72.823
Leukoaraiosis (hypertensive) I67.81
Leukoariosis — *see* Leukoaraiosis
Leukocoria — *see* Disorder, globe, degenerated condition, leucocoria
Leukocytopenia D72.819
Leukocytosis D72.829
- eosinophilic D72.1
Leukoderma, leukodermia NEC L81.5
- syphilitic A51.39
  - late A52.79

Leukodystrophy E75.29
Leukoedema, oral epithelium K13.29
Leukoencephalitis G04.81
- acute (subacute) hemorrhagic G36.1
  - postimmunization or postvaccinal G04.02
- postinfectious G04.01
- subacute sclerosing A81.1
- van Bogaert's (sclerosing) A81.1
Leukoencephalopathy (*see also* Encephalopathy) G93.49
- Binswanger's I67.3
- heroin vapor G92
- metachromatic E75.25
- multifocal (progressive) A81.2
- postimmunization and postvaccinal G04.02
- progressive multifocal A81.2
- reversible, posterior G93.6
- van Bogaert's (sclerosing) A81.1
- vascular, progressive I67.3
Leukoerythroblastosis D75.9
Leukokeratosis (*see also* Leukoplakia)
- mouth K13.21
- nicotina palati K13.24
- oral mucosa K13.21
- tongue K13.21
- vocal cord J38.3
Leukokraurosis vulva (e) N90.4
Leukoma (cornea) (*see also* Opacity, cornea)
- adherent H17.0- ☑
- interfering with central vision — *see* Opacity, cornea, central
Leukomalacia, cerebral, newborn P91.2
- periventricular P91.2
Leukomelanopathy, hereditary D72.0
Leukonychia (punctata) (striata) L60.8
- congenital Q84.4
Leukopathia unguium L60.8
- congenital Q84.4
Leukopenia D72.819
- basophilic D72.818
- chemotherapy (cancer) induced D70.1
- congenital D70.0
- cyclic D70.0
- drug induced NEC D70.2
  - due to cytoreductive cancer chemotherapy D70.1
- eosinophilic D72.818
- familial D70.0
- infantile genetic D70.0
- malignant D70.9
- periodic D70.0
- transitory neonatal P61.5
Leukopenic — *see* condition
Leukoplakia
- anus K62.89
- bladder (postinfectional) N32.89
- buccal K13.21
- cervix (uteri) N88.0
- esophagus K22.8
- gingiva K13.21
- hairy (oral mucosa) (tongue) K13.3
- kidney (pelvis) N28.89
- larynx J38.7
- lip K13.21
- mouth K13.21
- oral epithelium, including tongue (mucosa) K13.21
- palate K13.21
- pelvis (kidney) N28.89
- penis (infectional) N48.0
- rectum K62.89
- syphilitic (late) A52.79
- tongue K13.21
- ureter (postinfectional) N28.89
- urethra (postinfectional) N36.8
- uterus N85.8
- vagina N89.4
- vocal cord J38.3
- vulva N90.4
Leukorrhea N89.8
- due to Trichomonas (vaginalis) A59.00
- trichomonal A59.00
Leukosarcoma C85.9- ☑
Levocardia (isolated) Q24.1
- with situs inversus Q89.3
Levotransposition Q20.5
Lev's disease or syndrome (acquired complete heart block) I44.2
Levulosuria — *see* Fructosuria
Levurid L30.2

Lewy body (ies) (dementia) (disease) G31.83
Leyden-Moebius dystrophy G71.0
Leydig cell
  carcinoma
    specified site — *see* Neoplasm, malignant, by site
    unspecified site
      female C56.9
        male C62.9- ☑
  tumor
    benign
      specified site — *see* Neoplasm, benign, by site
      unspecified site
        female D27.- ☑
        male D29.2- ☑
    malignant
      specified site — *see* Neoplasm, malignant, by site
      unspecified site
        female C56.- ☑
        male C62.9- ☑
    specified site — *see* Neoplasm, uncertain behavior, by site
    unspecified site
      female D39.1- ☑
      male D40.1- ☑
Leydig-Sertoli cell tumor
  specified site — *see* Neoplasm, benign, by site
  unspecified site
    female D27.- ☑
    male D29.2- ☑
LGSIL (Low grade squamous intraepithelial lesion on cytologic smear of)
  anus R85.612
  cervix R87.612
  vagina R87.622
Liar, pathologic F60.2
Libido
  decreased R68.82
Libman-Sacks disease M32.11
Lice (infestation) B85.2
  body (Pediculus corporis) B85.1
  crab B85.3
  head (Pediculus capitis) B85.0
  mixed (classifiable to more than one of the titles B85.0-B85.3) B85.4
  pubic (Phthirus pubis) B85.3
Lichen L28.0
  albus L90.0
    penis N48.0
    vulva N90.4
  amyloidosis E85.4 [L99]
  atrophicus L90.0
    penis N48.0
    vulva N90.4
  congenital Q82.8
  myxedematosus L98.5
  nitidus L44.1
  pilaris Q82.8
    acquired L85.8
  planopilaris L66.1
  planus (chronicus) L43.9
    annularis L43.8
    bullous L43.1
    follicular L66.1
    hypertrophic L43.0
    moniliformis L44.3
    of Wilson L43.9
    specified NEC L43.8
    subacute (active) L43.3
    tropicus L43.3
  ruber
    acuminatus L44.0
    moniliformis L44.3
    planus L43.9
  sclerosus (et atrophicus) L90.0
    penis N48.0
    vulva N90.4
  scrofulosus (primary) (tuberculous) A18.4
  simplex (chronicus) (circumscriptus) L28.0
  striatus L44.2
  urticatus L28.2
Lichenification L28.0
Lichenoides tuberculosis (primary) A18.4
Lichtheim's disease or syndrome — *see* Degeneration, combined
Lien migrans D73.89
Ligament — *see* condition

Light
  for gestational age — *see* Light for dates
  headedness R42
Light-for-dates (infant) P05.00
  with weight of
    1000-1249 grams P05.04
    1250-1499 grams P05.05
    1500-1749 grams P05.06
    1750-1999 grams P05.07
    2000-2499 grams P05.08
    2500 grams and over P05.09
    499 grams or less P05.01
    500-749 grams P05.02
    750-999 grams P05.03
  affecting management of pregnancy O36.59- ☑
  and small-for-dates — *see* Small for dates
  specified NEC P05.09
Lightning (effects) (stroke) (struck by) T75.00 ☑
  burn — *see* Burn
  foot E53.8
  shock T75.01 ☑
  specified effect NEC T75.09 ☑
Lightwood-Albright syndrome N25.89
Lightwood's disease or syndrome (renal tubular acidosis) N25.89
Lignac (-de Toni) (-Fanconi) (-Debré) **disease or syndrome** E72.09
  with cystinosis E72.04
Ligneous thyroiditis E06.5
Likoff's syndrome I20.8
Limb — *see* condition
Limbic epilepsy personality syndrome F07.0
Limitation, limited
  activities due to disability Z73.6
  cardiac reserve — *see* Disease, heart
  eye muscle duction, traumatic — *see* Strabismus, mechanical
  mandibular range of motion M26.52
Lindau (-von Hippel) **disease** Q85.8
Line(s)
  Beau's L60.4
  Harris' — *see* Arrest, epiphyseal
  Hudson's (cornea) — *see* Pigmentation, cornea, anterior
  Stähli's (cornea) — *see* Pigmentation, cornea, anterior
Linea corneae senilis — *see* Change, cornea, senile
Lingua
  geographica K14.1
  nigra (villosa) K14.3
  plicata K14.5
  tylosis K13.29
Lingual — *see* condition
Linguatulosis B88.8
Linitis (gastric) **plastica** C16.9
Lip — *see* condition
Lipedema — *see* Edema
Lipemia (*see also* Hyperlipidemia)
  retina, retinalis E78.3
Lipidosis E75.6
  cerebral (infantile) (juvenile) (late) E75.4
  cerebroretinal E75.4
  cerebroside E75.22
  cholesterol (cerebral) E75.5
  glycolipid E75.21
  hepatosplenomegalic E78.3
  sphingomyelin — *see* Niemann-Pick disease or syndrome
  sulfatide E75.29
Lipoadenoma — *see* Neoplasm, benign, by site
Lipoblastoma — *see* Lipoma
Lipoblastomatosis — *see* Lipoma
Lipochondrodystrophy E76.01
Lipochrome histiocytosis (familial) D71
Lipodermatosclerosis — *see* Varix, leg, with, inflammation
  ulcerated — *see* Varix, leg, with, ulcer, with inflammation by site
Lipodystrophia progressiva E88.1
Lipodystrophy (progressive) E88.1
  insulin E88.1
  intestinal K90.81
  mesenteric K65.4
Lipofibroma — *see* Lipoma
Lipofuscinosis, neuronal (with ceroidosis) E75.4
Lipogranuloma, sclerosing L92.8
Lipogranulomatosis E78.89
Lipoid (*see also* condition)

Lipoid — *continued*
  histiocytosis D76.3
    essential E75.29
  nephrosis N04.9
  proteinosis of Urbach E78.89
Lipoidemia — *see* Hyperlipidemia
Lipoidosis — *see* Lipidosis
Lipoma D17.9
  fetal D17.9
    fat cell D17.9
  infiltrating D17.9
  intramuscular D17.9
  pleomorphic D17.9
  site classification
    arms (skin) (subcutaneous) D17.2- ☑
    connective tissue D17.30
      intra-abdominal D17.5
      intrathoracic D17.4
      peritoneum D17.79
      retroperitoneum D17.79
      specified site NEC D17.39
      spermatic cord D17.6
    face (skin) (subcutaneous) D17.0
    genitourinary organ NEC D17.72
    head (skin) (subcutaneous) D17.0
    intra-abdominal D17.5
    intrathoracic D17.4
    kidney D17.71
    legs (skin) (subcutaneous) D17.2- ☑
    neck (skin) (subcutaneous) D17.0
    peritoneum D17.79
    retroperitoneum D17.79
    skin D17.30
      specified site NEC D17.39
    specified site NEC D17.79
    spermatic cord D17.6
    subcutaneous D17.30
      specified site NEC D17.39
    trunk (skin) (subcutaneous) D17.1
    unspecified D17.9
  spindle cell D17.9
Lipomatosis E88.2
  dolorosa (Dercum) E88.2
  fetal — *see* Lipoma
  Launois-Bensaude E88.89
Lipomyoma — *see* Lipoma
Lipomyxoma — *see* Lipoma
Lipomyxosarcoma — *see* Neoplasm, connective tissue, malignant
Lipoprotein metabolism disorder E78.9
Lipoproteinemia E78.5
  broad-beta E78.2
  floating-beta E78.2
  hyper-pre-beta E78.1
Liposarcoma (*see also* Neoplasm, connective tissue, malignant)
  dedifferentiated — *see* Neoplasm, connective tissue, malignant
  differentiated type — *see* Neoplasm, connective tissue, malignant
  embryonal — *see* Neoplasm, connective tissue, malignant
  mixed type — *see* Neoplasm, connective tissue, malignant
  myxoid — *see* Neoplasm, connective tissue, malignant
  pleomorphic — *see* Neoplasm, connective tissue, malignant
  round cell — *see* Neoplasm, connective tissue, malignant
  well differentiated type — *see* Neoplasm, connective tissue, malignant
Liposynovitis prepatellaris E88.89
Lipping, cervix N86
Lipschütz disease or ulcer N76.6
Lipuria R82.0
  schistosomiasis (bilharziasis) B65.0
Lisping F80.0
Lissauer's paralysis A52.17
Lissencephalia, lissencephaly Q04.3
Listeriosis, listerellosis A32.9
  congenital (disseminated) P37.2
  cutaneous A32.0
  neonatal, newborn (disseminated) P37.2
  oculoglandular A32.81
  specified NEC A32.89
Lithemia E79.0
Lithiasis — *see* Calculus
Lithosis J62.8

Lithuria R82.99
Litigation, anxiety concerning Z65.3
Little leaguer's elbow — see Epicondylitis, medial
Little's disease G80.9
Littre's
  gland — see condition
  hernia — see Hernia, abdomen
Littritis — see Urethrltls
Livedo (annularis) (racemosa) (reticularis) R23.1
Liver — see condition
Living alone (problems with) Z60.2
  with handicapped person Z74.2
Lloyd's syndrome — see Adenomatosis, endocrine
Loa loa, loaiasis, loasis B74.3
Lobar — see condition
Lobomycosis B48.0
Lobo's disease B48.0
Lobotomy syndrome F07.0
Lobstein (-Ekman) **disease or syndrome** Q78.0
Lobster-claw hand Q71.6- ☑
Lobulation (congenital) (see also Anomaly, by site)
  kidney, Q63.1
  liver, abnormal Q44.7
  spleen Q89.09
Lobule, lobular — see condition
Local, localized — see condition
Locked twins causing obstructed labor O66.1
Locked-in state G83.5
Locking
  joint — see Derangement, joint, specified type NEC
  knee — see Derangement, knee
Lockjaw — see Tetanus
Löffler's
  endocarditis I42.3
  eosinophilia J82
  pneumonia J82
  syndrome (eosinophilic pneumonitis) J82
Loiasis (with conjunctival infestation) (eyelid) B74.3
Lone Star fever A77.0
Long
  labor O63.9
    first stage O63.0
    second stage O63.1
  QT syndrome I45.81
Longitudinal stripes or grooves, nails L60.8
  congenital Q84.6
Long-term (current) (prophylactic) **drug therapy** (use of)
  agents affecting estrogen receptors and estrogen levels NEC Z79.818
  anastrozole (Arimidex) Z79.811
  antibiotics Z79.2
    short-term use — omit code
  anticoagulants Z79.01
  anti-inflammatory, non-steroidal (NSAID) Z79.1
  antiplatelet Z79.02
  antithrombotics Z79.02
  aromatase inhibitors Z79.811
  aspirin Z79.82
  birth control pill or patch Z79.3
  bisphosphonates Z79.83
  contraceptive, oral Z79.3
  drug, specified NEC Z79.899
  estrogen receptor downregulators Z79.818
  Evista Z79.810
  exemestane (Aromasin) Z79.811
  Fareston Z79.810
  fulvestrant (Faslodex) Z79.818
  gonadotropin-releasing hormone (GnRH) agonist Z79.818
  goserelin acetate (Zoladex) Z79.818
  hormone replacement Z79.890
  insulin Z79.4
  letrozole (Femara) Z79.811
  leuprolide acetate (leuprorelin) (Lupron) Z79.818
  megestrol acetate (Megace) Z79.818
  methadone for pain management Z79.891
  Nolvadex Z79.810
  non-steroidal anti-inflammatories (NSAID) Z79.1
  opiate analgesic Z79.891
  oral
    antidiabetic Z79.84
    contraceptive Z79.3
    hypoglycemic Z79.84
  raloxifene (Evista) Z79.810
  selective estrogen receptor modulators (SERMs) Z79.810

Long-term (current) (prophylactic) **drug therapy** — continued
  steroids
    inhaled Z79.51
    systemic Z79.52
  tamoxifen (Nolvadex) Z79.810
  toremifene (Fareston) Z79.810
Loop
  intestine — see Volvulus
  vascular on papilla (optic) Q14.2
Loose (see also condition)
  body
    joint M24.00
      ankle M24.07- ☑
      elbow M24.02- ☑
      hand M24.04- ☑
      hip M24.05- ☑
      knee M23.4- ☑
      shoulder (region) M24.01- ☑
      specified site NEC M24.08
      toe M24.07- ☑
      vertebra M24.08
      wrist M24.03- ☑
    knee M23.4- ☑
    sheath, tendon — see Disorder, tendon, specified type NEC
  cartilage — see Loose, body, joint
  skin and subcutaneous tissue (following bariatric surgery weight loss) (following dietary weight loss) L98.7
  tooth, teeth K08.89
Loosening
  aseptic
    joint prosthesis — see Complications, joint prosthesis, mechanical, loosening, by site
    epiphysis — see Osteochondropathy
  mechanical
    joint prosthesis — see Complications, joint prosthesis, mechanical, loosening, by site
Looser-Milkman (-Debray) **syndrome** M83.8
Lop ear (deformity) Q17.3
Lorain (-Levi) **short stature syndrome** E23.0
Lordosis M40.50
  acquired — see Lordosis, specified type NEC
  congenital Q76.429
    lumbar region Q76.426
    lumbosacral region Q76.427
    sacral region Q76.428
    sacrococcygeal region Q76.428
    thoracolumbar region Q76.425
  lumbar region M40.56
  lumbosacral region M40.57
  postsurgical M96.4
  postural — see Lordosis, specified type NEC
  rachitic (late effect) (sequelae) E64.3
  sequelae of rickets E64.3
  specified type NEC M40.40
    lumbar region M40.46
    lumbosacral region M40.47
    thoracolumbar region M40.45
  thoracolumbar region M40.55
  tuberculous A18.01
Loss (of)
  appetite (see also Anorexia) R63.0
    hysterical F50.89
    nonorganic origin F50.89
    psychogenic F50.89
  blood — see Hemorrhage
  bone — see Loss, substance of, bone
  consciousness, transient R55
    traumatic — see Injury, intracranial
  control, sphincter, rectum R15.9
    nonorganic origin F98.1
  elasticity, skin R23.4
  family (member) in childhood Z62.898
  fluid (acute) E86.9
  function of labyrinth — see subcategory H83.2 ☑
  hair, nonscarring — see Alopecia
  hearing (see also Deafness)
    central NOS H90.5
    conductive H90.2
      bilateral H90.0
      unilateral
        with
          restricted hearing on the contralateral side H90.A1- ☑
          unrestricted hearing on the contralateral side H90.1- ☑

Loss — continued
  hearing (see also Deafness) — continued
    mixed conductive and sensorineural hearing loss H90.8
      bilateral H90.6
      unilateral
        with
          restricted hearing on the contralateral side H90.A3- ☑
          unrestricted hearing on the contralateral side H90.7- ☑
    neural NOS H90.5
    perceptive NOS H90.5
    sensorineural NOS H90.5
      bilateral H90.3
      unilateral
        with
          restricted hearing onthe contralateral side H90.A2- ☑
          unrestricted hearing on the contralateral side H90.4- ☑
    sensory NOS H90.5
  height R29.890
  limb or member, traumatic, current — see Amputation, traumatic
  love relationship in childhood Z62.898
  memory (see also Amnesia)
    mild, following organic brain damage F06.8
  mind — see Psychosis
  occlusal vertical dimension of fully erupted teeth M26.37
  organ or part — see Absence, by site, acquired
  ossicles, ear (partial) H74.32- ☑
  parent in childhood Z63.4
  pregnancy, recurrent N96
    without current pregnancy N96
    care in current pregnancy O26.2- ☑
  recurrent pregnancy — see Loss, pregnancy, recurrent
  self-esteem, in childhood Z62.898
  sense of
    smell — see Disturbance, sensation, smell
    taste — see Disturbance, sensation, taste
    touch R20.8
  sensory R44.9
    dissociative F44.6
  sexual desire F52.0
  sight (acquired) (complete) (congenital) — see Blindness
  substance of
    bone — see Disorder, bone, density and structure, specified NEC
      horizontal alveolar K06.3
    cartilage — see Disorder, cartilage, specified type NEC
    auricle (ear) — see Disorder, pinna, specified type NEC
    vitreous (humor) H15.89
  tooth, teeth — see Absence, teeth, acquired
  vision, visual H54.7
    both eyes H54.3
    one eye H54.60
      left (normal vision on right) H54.62
      right (normal vision on left) H54.61
    specified as blindness — see Blindness
    subjective
      sudden H53.13- ☑
      transient H53.12- ☑
  vitreous — see Prolapse, vitreous
  voice — see Aphonia
  weight (abnormal) (cause unknown) R63.4
Louis-Bar syndrome (ataxia-telangiectasia) G11.3
Louping ill (encephalitis) A84.8
Louse, lousiness — see Lice
Low
  achiever, school Z55.3
  back syndrome M54.5
  basal metabolic rate R94.8
  birthweight (2499 grams or less) P07.10
    with weight of
      1000-1249 grams P07.14
      1250-1499 grams P07.15
      1500-1749 grams P07.16
      1750-1999 grams P07.17
      2000-2499 grams P07.18
    extreme (999 grams or less) P07.00
      with weight of
        499 grams or less P07.01
        500-749 grams P07.02

Low — continued
  birthweight — continued
    extreme — continued
      with weight of — continued
        750-999 grams P07.03
    for gestational age — see Light for dates
  blood pressure (see also Hypotension)
    reading (incidental) (isolated) (nonspecific) R03.1
  cardiac reserve — see Disease, heart
  function (see also Hypofunction)
    kidney N28.9
  hematocrit D64.9
  hemoglobin D64.9
  income Z59.6
  level of literacy Z55.0
  lying
    kidney N28.89
    organ or site, congenital — see Malposition, congenital
  output syndrome (cardiac) — see Failure, heart
  platelets (blood) — see Thrombocytopenia
  reserve, kidney N28.89
  salt syndrome E87.1
  self esteem R45.81
  set ears Q17.4
  vision H54.2X- ☑
    one eye (other eye normal) H54.50
      left (normal vision on right) H54.52A- ☑
      other eye blind — see Blindness
      right (normal vision on left) H54.511- ☑
Low-density-lipoprotein-type (LDL) **hyperlipoproteinemia** E78.00
Lowe's syndrome E72.03
Lown-Ganong-Levine syndrome I45.6
LSD reaction (acute) (without dependence) F16.90
  with dependence F16.20
L-shaped kidney Q63.8
Ludwig's angina or disease K12.2
Lues (venerea), **luetic** — see Syphilis
Luetscher's syndrome (dehydration) E86.0
Lumbago, lumbalgia M54.5
  with sciatica M54.4-
    due to intervertebral disc disorder M51.17
  due to displacement, intervertebral disc M51.27
    with sciatica M51.17
Lumbar — see condition
Lumbarization, vertebra, congenital Q76.49
Lumbermen's itch B88.0
Lump (see also Mass)
  breast N63.0
    axillary tail
      left N63.32
      right N63.31
    left
      lower inner quadrant N63.24
      lower outer quadrant N63.23
      unspecified quadrant N63.20
      upper inner quadrant N63.22
      upper outer quadrant N63.21
    right
      lower inner quadrant N63.14
      lower outer quadrant N63.13
      unspecified quadrant N63.10
      upper inner quadrant N63.12
      upper outer quadrant N63.11
    subareolar
      left N63.42
      right N63.41
Lunacy — see Psychosis
Lung — see condition
Lupoid (miliary) **of Boeck** D86.3
Lupus
  anticoagulant D68.62
    with
      hemorrhagic disorder D68.312
      hypercoagulable state D68.62
      finding without diagnosis R76.0
  discoid (local) L93.0
  erythematosus (discoid) (local) L93.0
    disseminated — see Lupus, erythematosus, systemic
    eyelid H01.129
      left H01.126
        lower H01.125
        upper H01.124
      right H01.123
        lower H01.122
        upper H01.121

Lupus — continued
  erythematosus — continued
    profundus L93.2
    specified NEC L93.2
    subacute cutaneous L93.1
    systemic M32.9
      with organ or system involvement M32.10
        endocarditis M32.11
        lung M32.13
        pericarditis M32.12
        renal (glomerular) M32.14
          tubulo-interstitial M32.15
        specified organ or system NEC M32.19
      drug-induced M32.0
      inhibitor (presence of) D68.62
        with
          hemorrhagic disorder D68.312
          hypercoagulable state D68.62
        finding without diagnosis R76.0
      specified NEC M32.8
  exedens A18.4
  hydralazine M32.0
    correct substance properly administered — see Table of Drugs and Chemicals, by drug, adverse effect
    overdose or wrong substance given or taken — see Table of Drugs and Chemicals, by drug, poisoning
  nephritis (chronic) M32.14
  nontuberculous, not disseminated L93.0
  panniculitis L93.2
  pernio (Besnier) D86.3
  systemic — see Lupus, erythematosus, systemic
  tuberculous A18.4
    eyelid A18.4
  vulgaris A18.4
    eyelid A18.4
Luteinoma D27.- ☑
Lutembacher's disease or syndrome (atrial septal defect with mitral stenosis) Q21.1
Luteoma D27.- ☑
Lutz (-Splendore-de Almeida) **disease** — see Paracoccidioidomycosis
Luxation (see also Dislocation)
  eyeball (nontraumatic) — see Luxation, globe
    birth injury P15.3
  globe, nontraumatic H44.82- ☑
  lacrimal gland — see Dislocation, lacrimal gland
  lens (old) (partial) (spontaneous)
    congenital Q12.1
      syphilitic A50.39
Lycanthropy F22
Lyell's syndrome L51.2
  due to drug L51.2
    correct substance properly administered — see Table of Drugs and Chemicals, by drug, adverse effect
    overdose or wrong substance given or taken — see Table of Drugs and Chemicals, by drug, poisoning
Lyme disease A69.20
Lymph
  gland or node — see condition
  scrotum — see Infestation, filarial
Lymphadenitis I88.9
  with ectopic or molar pregnancy O08.0
  acute L04.9
    axilla L04.2
    face L04.0
    head L04.0
    hip L04.3
    limb
      lower L04.3
      upper L04.2
    neck L04.0
    shoulder L04.2
    specified site NEC L04.8
    trunk L04.1
  anthracosis (occupational) J60
  any site, except mesenteric I88.9
    chronic I88.1
    subacute I88.1
  breast
    gestational — see Mastitis, obstetric
    puerperal, postpartum (nonpurulent) O91.22
  chancroidal (congenital) A57
  chronic I88.1
    mesenteric I88.0

Lymphadenitis — continued
  due to
    Brugia (malayi) B74.1
      timori B74.2
    chlamydial lymphogranuloma A55
    diphtheria (toxin) A36.89
    lymphogranuloma venereum A55
    Wuchereria bancrofti B74.0
  following ectopic or molar pregnancy O08.0
  gonorrheal A54.89
  infective — see Lymphadenitis, acute
  mesenteric (acute) (chronic) (nonspecific) (subacute) I88.0
    due to Salmonella typhi A01.09
    tuberculous A18.39
  mycobacterial A31.8
  purulent — see Lymphadenitis, acute
  pyogenic — see Lymphadenitis, acute
  regional, nonbacterial I88.8
  septic — see Lymphadenitis, acute
  subacute, unspecified site I88.1
  suppurative — see Lymphadenitis, acute
  syphilitic (early) (secondary) A51.49
    late A52.79
  tuberculous — see Tuberculosis, lymph gland
  venereal (chlamydial) A55
Lymphadenoid goiter E06.3
Lymphadenopathy (generalized) R59.1
  angioimmunoblastic, with dysproteinemia (AILD) C86.5
  due to toxoplasmosis (acquired) B58.89
    congenital (acute) (subacute) (chronic) P37.1
  localized R59.0
  syphilitic (early) (secondary) A51.49
Lymphadenosis R59.1
Lymphangiectasis I89.0
  conjunctiva H11.89
  postinfectional I89.0
  scrotum I89.0
Lymphangiectatic elephantiasis, nonfilarial I89.0
Lymphangioendothelioma D18.1
  malignant — see Neoplasm, connective tissue, malignant
Lymphangioleiomyomatosis J84.81
Lymphangioma D18.1
  capillary D18.1
  cavernous D18.1
  cystic D18.1
  malignant — see Neoplasm, connective tissue, malignant
Lymphangiomyoma D18.1
Lymphangiomyomatosis J84.81
Lymphangiosarcoma — see Neoplasm, connective tissue, malignant
Lymphangitis I89.1
  with
    abscess — code by site under Abscess
    cellulitis — code by site under Cellulitis
    ectopic or molar pregnancy O08.0
  acute L03.91
    abdominal wall L03.321
    ankle — see Lymphangitis, acute, lower limb
    arm — see Lymphangitis, acute, upper limb
    auricle (ear) — see Lymphangitis, acute, ear
    axilla L03.12- ☑
    back (any part) L03.322
    buttock L03.327
    cervical (meaning neck) L03.222
    cheek (external) L03.212
    chest wall L03.323
    digit
      finger — see Lymphangitis, acute, finger
      toe — see Lymphangitis, acute, toe
    ear (external) H60.1- ☑
    external auditory canal — see Lymphangitis, acute, ear
    eyelid — see Abscess, eyelid
    face NEC L03.212
    finger (intrathecal) (periosteal) (subcutaneous) (subcuticular) L03.02- ☑
    foot — see Lymphangitis, acute, lower limb
    gluteal (region) L03.327
    groin L03.324
    hand — see Lymphangitis, acute, upper limb
    head NEC L03.891
      face (any part, except ear, eye and nose) L03.212
    heel — see Lymphangitis, acute, lower limb

☑ **Additional Character Required** — **Refer to the Tabular List for Character Selection**

☒ **Subterms under main terms may continue to next column or page**

Lymphangitis — continued
  acute — continued
    hip — see Lymphangitis, acute, lower limb
    jaw (region) L03.212
    knee — see Lymphangitis, acute, lower limb
    leg — see Lymphangitis, acute, lower limb
    lower limb L03.12- ☑
      toe — see Lymphangitis, acute, toe
    navel L03.326
    neck (region) L03.222
    orbit, orbital — see Cellulitis, orbit
    pectoral (region) L03.323
    perineal, perineum L03.325
    scalp (any part) L03.891
    shoulder — see Lymphangitis, acute, upper limb
    specified site NEC L03.898
    thigh — see Lymphangitis, acute, lower limb
    thumb (intrathecal) (periosteal) (subcutaneous)
      (subcuticular) — see Lymphangitis, acute,
      finger
    toe (intrathecal) (periosteal) (subcutaneous) (sub-
      cuticular) L03.04- ☑
    trunk L03.329
      abdominal wall L03.321
      back (any part) L03.322
      buttock L03.327
      chest wall L03.323
      groin L03.324
      perineal, perineum L03.325
      umbilicus L03.326
    umbilicus L03.326
    upper limb L03.12- ☑
      axilla — see Lymphangitis, acute, axilla
      finger — see Lymphangitis, acute, finger
      thumb — see Lymphangitis, acute, finger
    wrist — see Lymphangitis, acute, upper limb
  breast
    gestational — see Mastitis, obstetric
  chancroidal A57
  chronic (any site) I89.1
  due to
    Brugia (malayi) B74.1
      timori B74.2
    Wuchereria bancrofti B74.0
  following ectopic or molar pregnancy O08.89
  penis
    acute N48.29
    gonococcal (acute) (chronic) A54.09
  puerperal, postpartum, childbirth O86.89
  strumous, tuberculous A18.2
  subacute (any site) I89.1
  tuberculous — see Tuberculosis, lymph gland
Lymphatic (vessel) — see condition
Lymphatism E32.8
Lymphectasia I89.0
Lymphedema (acquired) (see also Elephantiasis)
  congenital Q82.0
  hereditary (chronic) (idiopathic) Q82.0
  postmastectomy I97.2
  praecox I89.0
  secondary I89.0
  surgical NEC I97.89
    postmastectomy (syndrome) I97.2
Lymphoblastic — see condition
Lymphoblastoma (diffuse) — see Lymphoma, lymphoblastic (diffuse)
  giant follicular — see Lymphoma, lymphoblastic (dif-
    fuse)
  macrofollicular — see Lymphoma, lymphoblastic
    (diffuse)
Lymphocele I89.8
Lymphocytic
  chorioencephalitis (acute) (serous) A87.2
  choriomeningitis (acute) (serous) A87.2
  meningoencephalitis A87.2
Lymphocytoma, benign cutis L98.8
Lymphocytopenia D72.810
Lymphocytosis (symptomatic) D72.820
  infectious (acute) B33.8
Lymphoepithelioma — see Neoplasm, malignant, by
  site
Lymphogranuloma (malignant) (see also Lymphoma,
  Hodgkin)
  chlamydial A55
  inguinale A55
  venereum (any site) (chlamydial) (with stricture of
    rectum) A55

Lymphogranulomatosis (malignant) (see also Lymphoma, Hodgkin)
  benign (Boeck's sarcoid) (Schaumann's) D86.1
Lymphohistiocytosis, hemophagocytic (familial) D76.1
Lymphoid — see condition
Lymphoma (of) (malignant) C85.90
  adult T-cell (HTLV-1-associated) (acute variant)
    (chronic variant) (lymphomatoid variant)
    (smouldering variant) C91.5- ☑
  anaplastic large cell
    ALK-negative C84.7- ☑
    ALK-positive C84.6- ☑
    CD30-positive C84.6- ☑
    primary cutaneous C86.6
  angioimmunoblastic T-cell C86.5
  BALT C88.4
  B-cell C85.1- ☑
  blastic NK-cell C86.4
  blastic plasmacytoid dendritic cell neoplasm (BPDCN)
    C86.4
  B-precursor C83.5- ☑
  bronchial-associated lymphoid tissue [BALT-lym-
    phoma] C88.4
  Burkitt (atypical) C83.7- ☑
  Burkitt-like C83.7- ☑
  centrocytic C83.1- ☑
  cutaneous follicle center C82.6- ☑
  cutaneous T-cell C84.A- ☑ (following C84.7)
  diffuse follicle center C82.5- ☑
  diffuse large cell C83.3- ☑
    anaplastic C83.3- ☑
    B-cell C83.3- ☑
    CD30-positive C83.3- ☑
    centroblastic C83.3- ☑
    immunoblastic C83.3- ☑
    plasmablastic C83.3- ☑
    subtype not specified C83.3- ☑
    T-cell rich C83.3- ☑
  enteropathy-type (associated) (intestinal) T-cell C86.2
  extranodal marginal zone B-cell lymphoma of mucosa-
    associated lymphoid tissue [MALT-lymphoma]
    C88.4
  extranodal NK/T-cell, nasal type C86.0
  follicular C82.9- ☑
    grade
      I C82.0- ☑
      II C82.1- ☑
      III C82.2- ☑
      IIIa C82.3- ☑
      IIIb C82.4- ☑
    specified NEC C82.8- ☑
  hepatosplenic T-cell (alpha-beta) (gamma-delta) C86.1
  histiocytic C85.9- ☑
    true C96.A (following C96.6)
  Hodgkin C81.9 ☑
    lymphocyte depleted (classical) C81.3- ☑
    lymphocyte-rich (classical) C81.4- ☑
    mixed cellularity (classical) C81.2- ☑
    nodular
      lymphocyte predominant C81.0- ☑
      sclerosis (classical) C81.1- ☑
    nodular sclerosis (classical) C81.1- ☑
    specified NEC (classical) C81.7- ☑
  intravascular large B-cell C83.8- ☑
  Lennert's C84.4- ☑
  lymphoblastic (diffuse) C83.5- ☑
  lymphoblastic B-cell C83.5- ☑
  lymphoblastic T-cell C83.5- ☑
  lymphoepithelioid C84.4- ☑
  lymphoplasmacytic C83.0- ☑
    with IgM-production C88.0
  MALT C88.4
  mantle cell C83.1- ☑
  mature T-cell NEC C84.4- ☑
  mature T/NK-cell C84.9- ☑
    specified NEC C84.Z- ☑ (following C84.7)
  mediastinal (thymic) large B-cell C85.2- ☑
  Mediterranean C88.3
  mucosa-associated lymphoid tissue [MALT-lymphoma]
    C88.4
  NK/T cell C84.9- ☑
  nodal marginal zone C83.0- ☑
  non-follicular (diffuse) C83.9- ☑
    specified NEC C83.8- ☑
  non-Hodgkin (see also Lymphoma, by type) C85.9- ☑
    specified NEC C85.8- ☑

Lymphoma — continued
  non-leukemic variant of B-CLL C83.0- ☑
  peripheral T-cell, not classified C84.4- ☑
  primary cutaneous
    anaplastic large cell C86.6
    CD30-positive large T-cell C86.6
  primary effusion B-cell C83.8- ☑
  SALT C88.4
  skin-associated lymphoid tissue [SALT-lymphoma]
    C88.4
  small cell B-cell C83.0- ☑
  splenic marginal zone C83.0- ☑
  subcutaneous panniculitis-like T-cell C86.3
  T-precursor C83.5- ☑
  true histiocytic C96.A (following C96.6)
Lymphomatosis — see Lymphoma
Lymphopathia venereum, veneris A55
Lymphopenia D72.810
Lymphoplasmacytic leukemia — see Leukemia,
  chronic lymphocytic, B-cell type
Lymphoproliferation, X-linked disease D82.3
Lymphoreticulosis, benign (of inoculation) A28.1
Lymphorrhea I89.8
Lymphosarcoma (diffuse) (see also Lymphoma)
  C85.9- ☑
Lymphostasis I89.8
Lypemania — see Melancholia
Lysine and hydroxylysine metabolism disorder E72.3
Lyssa — see Rabies

M

Macacus ear Q17.3
Maceration, wet feet, tropical (syndrome) T69.02- ☑
MacLeod's syndrome J43.0
Macrocephalia, macrocephaly Q75.3
Macrocheilia, macrochilia (congenital) Q18.6
Macrocolon (see also Megacolon) Q43.1
Macrocornea Q15.8
  with glaucoma Q15.0
Macrocytic — see condition
Macrocytosis D75.89
Macrodactylia, macrodactylism (fingers) (thumbs)
  Q74.0
  toes Q74.2
Macrodontia K00.2
Macrogenia M26.05
Macrogenitosomia (adrenal) (male) (praecox) E25.9
  congenital E25.0
Macroglobulinemia (idiopathic) (primary) C88.0
  monoclonal (essential) D47.2
  Waldenström C88.0
Macroglossia (congenital) Q38.2
  acquired K14.8
Macrognathia, macrognathism (congenital)
  (mandibular) (maxillary) M26.09
Macrogyria (congenital) Q04.8
Macrohydrocephalus — see Hydrocephalus
Macromastia — see Hypertrophy, breast
Macrophthalmos Q11.3
  in congenital glaucoma Q15.0
Macropsia H53.15
Macrosigmoid K59.39
  congenital Q43.2
Macrospondylitis , acromegalic E22.0
Macrostomia (congenital) Q18.4
Macrotia (external ear) (congenital) Q17.1
Macula
  cornea, corneal — see Opacity, cornea
  degeneration (atrophic) (exudative) (senile) (see also
    Degeneration, macula)
    hereditary — see Dystrophy, retina
Maculae ceruleae B85.1
Maculopathy, toxic — see Degeneration, macula, toxic
Madarosis (eyelid) H02.729
  left H02.726
    lower H02.725
    upper H02.724
  right H02.723
    lower H02.722
    upper H02.721
Madelung's
  deformity (radius) Q74.0
  disease
    radial deformity Q74.0
    symmetrical lipomas, neck E88.89
Madness — see Psychosis

Madura
foot B47.9
  actinomycotic B47.1
  mycotic B47.0
Maduromycosis B47.0
Maffucci's syndrome Q78.4
Magnesium metabolism disorder — *see* Disorder, metabolism, magnesium
Main en griffe (acquired) (*see also* Deformity, limb, clawhand)
  congenital Q74.0
Maintenance (encounter for)
  antineoplastic chemotherapy Z51.11
  antineoplastic radiation therapy Z51.0
  methadone F11.20
Majocchi's
  disease L81.7
  granuloma B35.8
Major — *see* condition
Mal de los pintos — *see* Pinta
Mal de mer T75.3 ☑
Malabar itch (any site) B35.5
Malabsorption K90.9
  calcium K90.89
  carbohydrate K90.49
  disaccharide E73.9
  fat K90.49
  galactose E74.20
  glucose (-galactose) E74.39
  intestinal K90.9
   specified NEC K90.89
  isomaltose E74.31
  lactose E73.9
  methionine E72.19
  monosaccharide E74.39
  postgastrectomy K91.2
  postsurgical K91.2
  protein K90.49
  starch K90.49
  sucrose E74.39
  syndrome K90.9
   postsurgical K91.2
Malacia, bone (adult) M83.9
  juvenile — *see* Rickets
Malacoplakia
  bladder N32.89
  pelvis (kidney) N28.89
  ureter N28.89
  urethra N36.8
Malacosteon, juvenile — *see* Rickets
Maladaptation — *see* Maladjustment
Maladie de Roger Q21.0
Maladjustment
  conjugal Z63.0
   involving divorce or estrangement Z63.5
  educational Z55.4
  family Z63.9
  marital Z63.0
   involving divorce or estrangement Z63.5
  occupational NEC Z56.89
  simple, adult — *see* Disorder, adjustment
  situational — *see* Disorder, adjustment
  social Z60.9
   due to
    acculturation difficulty Z60.3
    discrimination and persecution (perceived) Z60.5
    exclusion and isolation Z60.4
    life-cycle (phase of life) transition Z60.0
    rejection Z60.4
    specified reason NEC Z60.8
Malaise R53.81
Malakoplakia — *see* Malacoplakia
Malaria, malarial (fever) B54
  with
   blackwater fever B50.8
   hemoglobinuric (bilious) B50.8
   hemoglobinuria B50.8
  accidentally induced (therapeutically) — *code by* type under Malaria
  algid B50.9
  cerebral B50.0 [G94]
  clinically diagnosed (without parasitological confirmation) B54
  congenital NEC P37.4
   falciparum P37.3
  congestion, congestive B54
  continued (fever) B50.9

Malaria, malarial — *continued*
  estivo-autumnal B50.9
  falciparum B50.9
   with complications NEC B50.8
    cerebral B50.0 [G94]
   severe B50.8
  hemorrhagic B54
  malariae B52.9
   with
    complications NEC B52.8
    glomerular disorder B52.0
  malignant (tertian) — *see* Malaria, falciparum
  mixed infections — *code to* first listed type in B50-B53
  ovale B53.0
  parasitologically confirmed NEC B53.8
  pernicious, acute — *see* Malaria, falciparum
  Plasmodium (P.)
   falciparum NEC — *see* Malaria, falciparum
   malariae NEC B52.9
    with Plasmodium
     falciparum (and or vivax) — *see* Malaria, falciparum
     vivax (*see also* Malaria, vivax)
      and falciparum — *see* Malaria, falciparum
   ovale B53.0
    with Plasmodium malariae (*see also* Malaria, malariae)
     and vivax (*see also* Malaria, vivax)
      and falciparum — *see* Malaria, falciparum
   simian B53.1
    with Plasmodium malariae (*see also* Malaria, malariae)
     and vivax (*see also* Malaria, vivax)
      and falciparum — *see* Malaria, falciparum
   vivax NEC B51.9
    with Plasmodium falciparum — *see* Malaria, falciparum
  quartan — *see* Malaria, malariae
  quotidian — *see* Malaria, falciparum
  recurrent B54
  remittent B54
  specified type NEC (parasitologically confirmed) B53.8
  spleen B54
  subtertian (fever) — *see* Malaria, falciparum
  tertian (benign) (*see also* Malaria, vivax)
   malignant B50.9
  tropical B50.9
  typhoid B54
  vivax B51.9
   with
    complications NEC B51.8
    ruptured spleen B51.0
Malassez's disease (cystic) N50.89
Malassimilation K90.9
Maldescent, testis Q53.9
  bilateral Q53.20
   abdominal Q53.211
   perineal Q53.22
  unilateral Q53.10
   abdominal Q53.111
   perineal Q53.12
Maldevelopment (*see also* Anomaly)
  brain Q07.9
  colon Q43.9
  hip Q74.2
   congenital dislocation Q65.2
    bilateral Q65.1
    unilateral Q65.0- ☑
  mastoid process Q75.8
  middle ear Q16.4
   except ossicles Q16.4
   ossicles Q16.3
  ossicles Q16.3
  spine Q76.49
  toe Q74.2
Male type pelvis Q74.2
  with disproportion (fetopelvic) O33.3 ☑
   causing obstructed labor O65.3
Malformation (congenital) (*see also* Anomaly)
  adrenal gland Q89.1
  affecting multiple systems with skeletal changes NEC Q87.5
  alimentary tract Q45.9
   specified type NEC Q45.8
   upper Q40.9

Malformation — *continued*
  alimentary tract — *continued*
   upper — *continued*
    specified type NEC Q40.8
  aorta Q25.40
   absence Q25.41
   aneurysm, congenital Q25.43
   aplasia Q25.41
   atresia Q25.29
    aortic arch Q25.21
   coarctation (preductal) (postductal) Q25.1
   dilatation, congenital Q25.44
   hypoplasia Q25.42
   patent ductus arteriosus Q25.0
   specified type NEC Q25.49
   stenosis Q25.1
    supravalvular Q25.3
  aortic valve Q23.9
   specified NEC Q23.8
  arteriovenous, aneurysmatic (congenital) Q27.30
   brain Q28.2
   cerebral Q28.2
   peripheral Q27.30
    digestive system Q27.33
    lower limb Q27.32
    other specified site Q27.39
    renal vessel Q27.34
    upper limb Q27.31
   precerebral vessels (nonruptured) Q28.0
  auricle
   ear (congenital) Q17.3
    acquired H61.119
     left H61.112
      with right H61.113
     right H61.111
      with left H61.113
  bile duct Q44.5
  bladder Q64.79
   aplasia Q64.5
   diverticulum Q64.6
   exstrophy — *see* Exstrophy, bladder
   neck obstruction Q64.31
  bone Q79.9
   face Q75.9
    specified type NEC Q75.8
   skull Q75.9
    specified type NEC Q75.8
  brain (multiple) Q04.9
   arteriovenous Q28.2
   specified type NEC Q04.8
  branchial cleft Q18.2
  breast Q83.9
   specified type NEC Q83.8
  broad ligament Q50.6
  bronchus Q32.4
  bursa Q79.9
  cardiac
   chambers Q20.9
    specified type NEC Q20.8
   septum Q21.9
    specified type NEC Q21.8
  cerebral Q04.9
   vessels Q28.3
  cervix uteri Q51.9
   specified type NEC Q51.828
  Chiari
   Type I G93.5
   Type II Q07.01
  choroid (congenital) Q14.3
   plexus Q07.8
  circulatory system Q28.9
  cochlea Q16.5
  cornea Q13.4
  coronary vessels Q24.5
  corpus callosum (congenital) Q04.0
  diaphragm Q79.1
  digestive system NEC, specified type NEC Q45.8
  dura Q07.9
   brain Q04.9
   spinal Q06.9
  ear Q17.9
   causing impairment of hearing Q16.9
   external Q17.9
    accessory auricle Q17.0
    causing impairment of hearing Q16.9
     absence of
      auditory canal Q16.1
      auricle Q16.0
    macrotia Q17.1

Malformation — *continued*
- ear — *continued*
  - external — *continued*
    - microtia Q17.2
    - misplacement Q17.4
    - misshapen NEC Q17.3
    - prominence Q17.5
    - specified type NEC Q17.8
  - inner Q16.5
  - middle Q16.4
    - absence of eustachian tube Q16.2
    - ossicles (fusion) Q16.3
  - ossicles Q16.3
  - specified type NEC Q17.8
- epididymis Q55.4
- esophagus Q39.9
  - specified type NEC Q39.8
- eye Q15.9
  - lid Q10.3
  - specified NEC Q15.8
- fallopian tube Q50.6
- genital organ — *see* Anomaly, genitalia
- great
  - artery Q25.9
    - aorta — *see* Malformation, aorta
    - pulmonary artery — *see* Malformation, pulmonary, artery
    - specified type NEC Q25.8
  - vein Q26.9
    - anomalous
      - portal venous connection Q26.5
      - pulmonary venous connection Q26.4
        - partial Q26.3
        - total Q26.2
    - persistent left superior vena cava Q26.1
    - portal vein-hepatic artery fistula Q26.6
    - specified type NEC Q26.8
    - vena cava stenosis, congenital Q26.0
- gum Q38.6
- hair Q84.2
- heart Q24.9
  - specified type NEC Q24.8
- integument Q84.9
  - specified type NEC Q84.8
- internal ear Q16.5
- intestine Q43.9
  - specified type NEC Q43.8
- iris Q13.2
- joint Q74.9
  - ankle Q74.2
  - lumbosacral Q76.49
  - sacroiliac Q74.2
  - specified type NEC Q74.8
- kidney Q63.9
  - accessory Q63.0
  - giant Q63.3
  - horseshoe Q63.1
  - hydronephrosis Q62.0
  - malposition Q63.2
  - specified type NEC Q63.8
- lacrimal apparatus Q10.6
- lingual Q38.3
- lip Q38.0
- liver Q44.7
- lung Q33.9
- meninges or membrane (congenital) Q07.9
  - cerebral Q04.8
  - spinal (cord) Q06.9
- middle ear Q16.4
  - ossicles Q16.3
- mitral valve Q23.9
  - specified NEC Q23.8
- Mondini's (congenital) (malformation, cochlea) Q16.5
- mouth (congenital) Q38.6
- multiple types NEC Q89.7
- musculoskeletal system Q79.9
- myocardium Q24.8
- nail Q84.6
- nervous system (central) Q07.9
- nose Q30.9
  - specified type NEC Q30.8
- optic disc Q14.2
- orbit Q10.7
- ovary Q50.39
- palate Q38.5
- parathyroid gland Q89.2
- pelvic organs or tissues NEC
  - in pregnancy or childbirth O34.8- ☑
    - causing obstructed labor O65.5

Malformation — *continued*
- penis Q55.69
  - aplasia Q55.5
  - curvature (lateral) Q55.61
  - hypoplasia Q55.62
- pericardium Q24.8
- peripheral vascular system Q27.9
  - specified type NEC Q27.8
- pharynx Q38.8
- precerebral vessels Q28.1
- prostate Q55.4
- pulmonary
  - arteriovenous Q25.72
  - artery Q25.9
    - atresia Q25.5
    - specified type NEC Q25.79
    - stenosis Q25.6
  - valve Q22.3
- renal artery Q27.2
- respiratory system Q34.9
- retina Q14.1
- scrotum — *see* Malformation, testis and scrotum
- seminal vesicles Q55.4
- sense organs NEC Q07.9
- skin Q82.9
- specified NEC Q89.8
- spinal
  - cord Q06.9
  - nerve root Q07.8
- spine Q76.49
  - kyphosis — *see* Kyphosis, congenital
  - lordosis — *see* Lordosis, congenital
- spleen Q89.09
- stomach Q40.3
  - specified type NEC Q40.2
- teeth, tooth K00.9
- tendon Q79.9
- testis and scrotum Q55.20
  - aplasia Q55.0
  - hypoplasia Q55.1
  - polyorchism Q55.21
  - retractile testis Q55.22
  - scrotal transposition Q55.23
  - specified NEC Q55.29
- thorax, bony Q76.9
- throat Q38.8
- thyroid gland Q89.2
- tongue (congenital) Q38.3
  - hypertrophy Q38.2
  - tie Q38.1
- trachea Q32.1
- tricuspid valve Q22.9
  - specified type NEC Q22.8
- umbilical cord NEC (complicating delivery) O69.89 ☑
- umbilicus Q89.9
- ureter Q62.8
  - agenesis Q62.4
  - duplication Q62.5
  - malposition — *see* Malposition, congenital, ureter
  - obstructive defect — *see* Defect, obstructive, ureter
  - vesico-uretero-renal reflux Q62.7
- urethra Q64.79
  - aplasia Q64.5
  - duplication Q64.74
  - posterior valves Q64.2
  - prolapse Q64.71
  - stricture Q64.32
- urinary system Q64.9
- uterus Q51.9
  - specified type NEC Q51.818
- vagina Q52.4
- vas deferens Q55.4
  - atresia Q55.3
- vascular system, peripheral Q27.9
- venous — *see* Anomaly, vein(s)
- vulva Q52.70

Malfunction (*see also* Dysfunction)
- cardiac electronic device T82.119 ☑
  - electrode T82.110 ☑
  - pulse generator T82.111 ☑
  - specified type NEC T82.118 ☑
- catheter device NEC T85.618 ☑
  - cystostomy T83.010 ☑
  - dialysis (renal) (vascular) T82.41 ☑
    - intraperitoneal T85.611 ☑
  - infusion NEC T82.514 ☑
    - cranial T85.610 ☑
    - epidural T85.610 ☑

Malfunction — *continued*
- catheter device — *continued*
  - infusion — *continued*
    - intrathecal T85.610 ☑
    - spinal T85.610 ☑
    - subarachnoid T85.610 ☑
    - subdural T85.610 ☑
  - urinary (*see also* Breakdown, device, catheter) T83.018 ☑
- colostomy K94.03
  - valve K94.03
- cystostomy (stoma) N99.512
  - catheter T83.010 ☑
- enteric stoma K94.13
- enterostomy K94.13
- esophagostomy K94.33
- gastroenteric K31.89
- gastrostomy K94.23
- ileostomy K94.13
  - valve K94.13
- intrathecal infusion pump T85.615 ☑
- jejunostomy K94.13
- nervous system device, implant or graft, specified NEC T85.615 ☑
- pacemaker — *see* Malfunction, cardiac electronic device
- prosthetic device, internal — *see* Complications, prosthetic device, by site, mechanical
- tracheostomy J95.03
- urinary device NEC — *see* Complication, genitourinary, device, urinary, mechanical
- valve
  - colostomy K94.03
  - heart T82.09 ☑
  - ileostomy K94.13
- vascular graft or shunt NEC — *see* Complication, cardiovascular device, mechanical, vascular
- ventricular (communicating shunt) T85.01 ☑

Malherbe's tumor — *see* Neoplasm, skin, benign
Malibu disease L98.8
Malignancy (*see also* Neoplasm, malignant, by site)
- unspecified site (primary) C80.1
Malignant — *see* condition
Malingerer, malingering Z76.5
Mallet finger (acquired) — *see* Deformity, finger, mallet finger
- congenital Q74.0
- sequelae of rickets E64.3
Malleus A24.0
Mallory's bodies R89.7
Mallory-Weiss syndrome K22.6
Malnutrition E46
- degree
  - first E44.1
    - mild (protein) E44.1
    - moderate (protein) E44.0
  - second E44.0
  - severe (protein-energy) E43
    - intermediate form E42
      - with
        - kwashiorkor (and marasmus) E42
        - marasmus E41
  - third E43
- following gastrointestinal surgery K91.2
- intrauterine
  - light-for-dates — *see* Light for dates
  - small-for-dates — *see* Small for dates
- lack of care, or neglect (child) (infant) T76.02 ☑
  - confirmed T74.02 ☑
- malignant E40
- protein E46
  - calorie E46
    - mild E44.1
    - moderate E44.0
    - severe E43
      - intermediate form E42
        - with
          - kwashiorkor (and marasmus) E42
          - marasmus E41
  - energy E46
    - mild E44.1
    - moderate E44.0
    - severe E43
      - intermediate form E42
        - with
          - kwashiorkor (and marasmus) E42
          - marasmus E41
- severe (protein-energy) E43

Malnutrition — *continued*
  severe — *continued*
    with
      kwashiorkor (and marasmus) E42
      marasmus E41
Malocclusion (teeth) M26.4
  Angle's M26.219
    class I M26.211
    class II M26.212
    class III M26.213
  due to
    abnormal swallowing M26.59
    mouth breathing M26.59
    tongue, lip or finger habits M26.59
  temporomandibular (joint) M26.69
Malposition
  cervix — *see* Malposition, uterus
  congenital
    adrenal (gland) Q89.1
    alimentary tract Q45.8
      lower Q43.8
      upper Q40.8
    aorta Q25.49
    appendix Q43.8
    arterial trunk Q20.0
    artery (peripheral) Q27.8
      coronary Q24.5
      digestive system Q27.8
      lower limb Q27.8
      pulmonary Q25.79
      specified site NEC Q27.8
      upper limb Q27.8
    auditory canal Q17.8
      causing impairment of hearing Q16.9
    auricle (ear) Q17.4
      causing impairment of hearing Q16.9
      cervical Q18.2
    biliary duct or passage Q44.5
    bladder (mucosa) — *see* Exstrophy, bladder
    brachial plexus Q07.8
    brain tissue Q04.8
    breast Q83.8
    bronchus Q32.4
    cecum Q43.8
    clavicle Q74.0
    colon Q43.8
    digestive organ or tract NEC Q45.8
      lower Q43.8
      upper Q40.8
    ear (auricle) (external) Q17.4
      ossicles Q16.3
    endocrine (gland) NEC Q89.2
    epiglottis Q31.8
    eustachian tube Q17.8
    eye Q15.8
    facial features Q18.8
    fallopian tube Q50.6
    finger(s) Q68.1
      supernumerary Q69.0
    foot Q66.9
    gallbladder Q44.1
    gastrointestinal tract Q45.8
    genitalia, genital organ(s) or tract
      female Q52.8
        external Q52.79
        internal NEC Q52.8
      male Q55.8
    glottis Q31.8
    hand Q68.1
    heart Q24.8
      dextrocardia Q24.0
        with complete transposition of viscera Q89.3
    hepatic duct Q44.5
    hip (joint) Q65.89
    intestine (large) (small) Q43.8
      with anomalous adhesions, fixation or malrotation Q43.3
    joint NEC Q68.8
    kidney Q63.2
    larynx Q31.8
    limb Q68.8
      lower Q68.8
      upper Q68.8
    liver Q44.7
    lung (lobe) Q33.8
    nail(s) Q84.6
    nerve Q07.8
    nervous system NEC Q07.8
    nose, nasal (septum) Q30.8

Malposition — *continued*
  congenital — *continued*
    organ or site not listed — *see* Anomaly, by site
    ovary Q50.39
    pancreas Q45.3
    parathyroid (gland) Q89.2
    patella Q74.1
    peripheral vascular system Q27.8
    pituitary (gland) Q89.2
    respiratory organ or system NEC Q34.8
    rib (cage) Q76.6
      supernumerary in cervical region Q76.5
    scapula Q74.0
    shoulder Q74.0
    spinal cord Q06.8
    spleen Q89.09
    sternum NEC Q76.7
    stomach Q40.2
    symphysis pubis Q74.2
    thymus (gland) Q89.2
    thyroid (gland) (tissue) Q89.2
      cartilage Q31.8
    toe(s) Q66.9
      supernumerary Q69.2
    tongue Q38.3
    trachea Q32.1
    ureter Q62.60
      deviation Q62.61
      displacement Q62.62
      ectopia Q62.63
      specified type NEC Q62.69
    uterus Q51.818
    vein(s) (peripheral) Q27.8
      great Q26.8
    vena cava (inferior) (superior) Q26.8
  device, implant or graft (*see also* Complications, by site and type, mechanical) T85.628 ☑
    arterial graft NEC — *see* Complication, cardiovascular device, mechanical, vascular
    breast (implant) T85.42 ☑
    catheter NEC T85.628 ☑
      cystostomy T83.020 ☑
      dialysis (renal) T82.42 ☑
        intraperitoneal T85.621 ☑
      infusion NEC T82.524 ☑
        spinal (epidural) (subdural) T85.620 ☑
      urinary (*see also* Displacement, device, catheter, urinary) T83.028 ☑
    electronic (electrode) (pulse generator) (stimulator)
      bone T84.320 ☑
      cardiac T82.129 ☑
        electrode T82.120 ☑
        pulse generator T82.121 ☑
        specified type NEC T82.128 ☑
      nervous system — *see* Complication, prosthetic device, mechanical, electronic nervous system stimulator
      urinary — *see* Complication, genitourinary, device, urinary, mechanical
    fixation, internal (orthopedic) NEC — *see* Complication, fixation device, mechanical
    gastrointestinal — *see* Complications, prosthetic device, mechanical, gastrointestinal device
    genital NEC T83.428 ☑
      intrauterine contraceptive device (string) T83.32 ☑
      penile prosthesis (cylinder) (implanted) (pump) (reservoir) T83.420 ☑
      testicular prosthesis T83.421 ☑
    heart NEC — *see* Complication, cardiovascular device, mechanical
    joint prosthesis — *see* Complication, joint prosthesis, mechanical
    ocular NEC — *see* Complications, prosthetic device, mechanical, ocular device
    orthopedic NEC — *see* Complication, orthopedic, device, mechanical
    specified NEC T85.628 ☑
    urinary NEC (*see also* Complication, genitourinary, device, urinary, mechanical)
      graft T83.22 ☑
    vascular NEC — *see* Complication, cardiovascular device, mechanical
    ventricular intracranial shunt T85.02 ☑
  fetus — *see* Pregnancy, complicated by (management affected by), presentation, fetal
  gallbladder K82.8

Malposition — *continued*
  gastrointestinal tract, congenital Q45.8
  heart, congenital NEC Q24.8
  joint prosthesis — *see* Complications, joint prosthesis, mechanical, displacement, by site
  stomach K31.89
    congenital Q40.2
  tooth, teeth, fully erupted M26.30
  uterus (acute) (acquired) (adherent) (asymptomatic) (postinfectional) (postpartal, old) N85.4
    anteflexion or anteversion N85.4
      congenital Q51.818
    flexion N85.4
      lateral — *see* Lateroversion, uterus
    inversion N85.5
    lateral (flexion) (version) — *see* Lateroversion, uterus
      in pregnancy or childbirth — *see* subcategory O34.5 ☑
    retroflexion or retroversion — *see* Retroversion, uterus
Malposture R29.3
Malrotation
  cecum Q43.3
  colon Q43.3
  intestine Q43.3
  kidney Q63.2
Malta fever — *see* Brucellosis
Maltreatment
  adult
    abandonment
      confirmed T74.01 ☑
      suspected T76.01 ☑
    confirmed T74.91 ☑
    history of Z91.419
    neglect
      confirmed T74.01 ☑
      suspected T76.01 ☑
    physical abuse
      confirmed T74.11 ☑
      suspected T76.11 ☑
    psychological abuse
      confirmed T74.31 ☑
      history of Z91.411
      suspected T76.31 ☑
    sexual abuse
      confirmed T74.21 ☑
      suspected T76.21 ☑
    suspected T76.91 ☑
  child
    abandonment
      confirmed T74.02 ☑
      suspected T76.02 ☑
    confirmed T74.92 ☑
    history of — *see* History, personal (of), abuse
    neglect
      confirmed T74.02 ☑
      history of — *see* History, personal (of), abuse
      suspected T76.02 ☑
    physical abuse
      confirmed T74.12 ☑
      history of — *see* History, personal (of), abuse
      suspected T76.12 ☑
    psychological abuse
      confirmed T74.32 ☑
      history of — *see* History, personal (of), abuse
      suspected T76.32 ☑
    sexual abuse
      confirmed T74.22 ☑
      history of — *see* History, personal (of), abuse
      suspected T76.22 ☑
    suspected T76.92 ☑
  personal history of Z91.89
Maltworker's lung J67.4
Malunion, fracture — *see* Fracture, by site
Mammillitis N61.0
  puerperal, postpartum O91.02
Mammitis — *see* Mastitis
Mammogram (examination) Z12.39
  routine Z12.31
Mammoplasia N62
Management (of)
  bone conduction hearing device (implanted) Z45.320
  cardiac pacemaker NEC Z45.018
  cerebrospinal fluid drainage device Z45.41
  cochlear device (implanted) Z45.321
  contraceptive Z30.9

Management — *continued*
  contraceptive — *continued*
    specified NEC Z30.8
    implanted device Z45.9
      specified NEC Z45.89
    infusion pump Z45.1
    procreative Z31.9
      male factor infertility in female Z31.81
      specified NEC Z31.89
    prosthesis (external) (*see also* Fitting) Z44.9
      implanted Z45.9
        specified NEC Z45.89
    renal dialysis catheter Z49.01
    vascular access device Z45.2
Mangled — *see* specified injury by site
Mania (monopolar) (*see also* Disorder, mood, manic
    episode)
  with psychotic symptoms F30.2
  without psychotic symptoms F30.10
    mild F30.11
    moderate F30.12
    severe F30.13
  Bell's F30.8
  chronic (recurrent) F31.89
  hysterical F44.89
  puerperal F30.8
  recurrent F31.89
Manic depression F31.9
Manic-depressive insanity, psychosis, or syndrome
    — *see* Disorder, bipolar
Mannosidosis E77.1
Mansonelliasis, mansonellosis B74.4
Manson's
  disease B65.1
  schistosomiasis B65.1
Manual — *see* condition
Maple-bark-stripper's lung (disease) J67.6
Maple-syrup-urine disease E71.0
Marable's syndrome (celiac artery compression) I77.4
Marasmus E41
  due to malnutrition E41
  intestinal E41
  nutritional E41
  senile R54
  tuberculous NEC — *see* Tuberculosis
Marble
  bones Q78.2
  skin R23.8
Marburg virus disease A98.3
March
  fracture — *see* Fracture, traumatic, stress, by site
  hemoglobinuria D59.6
Marchesani (-Weill) **syndrome** Q87.0
Marchiafava (-Bignami) **syndrome or disease** G37.1
Marchiafava-Micheli syndrome D59.5
Marcus Gunn's syndrome Q07.8
Marfan's syndrome — *see* Syndrome, Marfan's
Marie-Bamberger disease — *see* Osteoarthropathy,
  hypertrophic, specified NEC
Marie-Charcot-Tooth neuropathic muscular atrophy
  G60.0
Marie's
  cerebellar ataxia (late-onset) G11.2
  disease or syndrome (acromegaly) E22.0
Marie-Strümpell arthritis, disease or spondylitis —
  see Spondylitis, ankylosing
Marion's disease (bladder neck obstruction) N32.0
Marital conflict Z63.0
Mark
  port wine Q82.5
  raspberry Q82.5
  strawberry Q82.5
  stretch L90.6
  tattoo L81.8
Marker heterochromatin — *see* Extra, marker chromo-
  somes
Maroteaux-Lamy syndrome (mild) (severe) E76.29
Marrow (bone)
  arrest D61.9
  poor function D75.89
Marseilles fever A77.1
Marsh fever — *see* Malaria
Marshall's (hidrotic) **ectodermal dysplasia** Q82.4
Marsh's disease (exophthalmic goiter) E05.00
  with storm E05.01
Masculinization (female) **with adrenal hyperplasia**
  E25.9

Masculinization (female) **with adrenal hyperplasia**
  — *continued*
  congenital E25.0
Masculinovoblastoma D27.- ☑
Masochism (sexual) F65.51
Mason's lung J62.8
Mass
  abdominal R19.00
    epigastric R19.06
    generalized R19.07
    left lower quadrant R19.04
    left upper quadrant R19.02
    periumbilic R19.05
    right lower quadrant R19.03
    right upper quadrant R19.01
    specified site NEC R19.09
  breast (*see also* Lump, breast) N63.0
  chest R22.2
  cystic — *see* Cyst
  ear H93.8- ☑
  head R22.0
  intra-abdominal (diffuse) (generalized) — *see* Mass,
    abdominal
  kidney N28.89
  liver R16.0
  localized (skin) R22.9
    chest R22.2
    head R22.0
    limb
      lower R22.4- ☑
      upper R22.3- ☑
    neck R22.1
    trunk R22.2
  lung R91.8
  malignant — *see* Neoplasm, malignant, by site
  neck R22.1
  pelvic (diffuse) (generalized) — *see* Mass, abdominal
  specified organ NEC — *see* Disease, by site
  splenic R16.1
  substernal thyroid — *see* Goiter
  superficial (localized) R22.9
  umbilical (diffuse) (generalized) R19.09
Massive — *see* condition
Mast cell
  disease, systemic tissue D47.02
  leukemia C94.3- ☑
  neoplasm
    malignant C96.20
      specified type NEC C96.29
    of uncertain behavior NEC D47.09
  sarcoma C96.22
  tumor D47.09
Mastalgia N64.4
Masters-Allen syndrome N83.8
Mastitis (acute) (diffuse) (nonpuerperal) (subacute) N61.0
  with abscess N61.1
  without abscess N61.0
  chronic (cystic) — *see* Mastopathy, cystic
  cystic (Schimmelbusch's type) — *see* Mastopathy,
    cystic
  fibrocystic — *see* Mastopathy, cystic
  infective N61.0
    newborn P39.0
  interstitial, gestational or puerperal — *see* Mastitis,
    obstetric
  neonatal (noninfective) P83.4
    infective P39.0
  obstetric (interstitial) (nonpurulent)
    associated with
      lactation O91.23
      pregnancy O91.21- ☑
      puerperium O91.22
    purulent
      associated with
        lactation O91.13
        pregnancy O91.11- ☑
        puerperium O91.12
  periductal — *see* Ectasia, mammary duct
  phlegmonous — *see* Mastopathy, cystic
  plasma cell — *see* Ectasia, mammary duct
Mastocytoma (extracutaneous) D47.09
  malignant C96.29
  solitary D47.01
Mastocytosis D47.09
  aggressive systemic C96.21
  cutaneous (diffuse) (maculopapular) D47.01
    congenital Q82.2
    of neonatal onset Q82.2

Mastocytosis — *continued*
  cutaneous — *continued*
    of newborn onset Q82.2
  indolent systemic D47.02
  isolated bone marrow D47.02
  malignant C96.29
  systemic (indolent) (smoldering)
    with an associated hematological non-mast cell
      lineage disease (SM-AHNMD) D47.02
Mastodynia N64.4
Mastoid — *see* condition
Mastoidalgia — *see* subcategory H92.0 ☑
Mastoiditis (coalescent) (hemorrhagic) (suppurative)
  H70.9- ☑
  acute, subacute H70.00- ☑
    complicated NEC H70.09- ☑
    subperiosteal H70.01- ☑
  chronic (necrotic) (recurrent) H70.1- ☑
  in (due to)
    infectious disease NEC B99 ☑ [H75.0-] ☑
    parasitic disease NEC B89 [H75.0-] ☑
    tuberculosis A18.03
  petrositis — *see* Petrositis
  postauricular fistula — *see* Fistula, postauricular
  specified NEC H70.89- ☑
  tuberculous A18.03
Mastopathy, mastopathia N64.9
  chronica cystica — *see* Mastopathy, cystic
  cystic (chronic) (diffuse) N60.1- ☑
    with epithelial proliferation N60.3- ☑
  diffuse cystic — *see* Mastopathy, cystic
  estrogenic, oestrogenica N64.89
  ovarian origin N64.89
Mastoplasia, mastoplastia N62
Masturbation (excessive) F98.8
Maternal care (for) — *see* Pregnancy (complicated by)
  (management affected by)
Matheiu's disease (leptospiral jaundice) A27.0
Mauclaire's disease or osteochondrosis — *see* Osteo-
  chondrosis, juvenile, hand, metacarpal
Maxcy's disease A75.2
Maxilla, maxillary — *see* condition
May (-Hegglin) **anomaly or syndrome** D72.0
McArdle (-Schmid)(-Pearson) **disease** (glycogen storage)
  E74.04
McCune-Albright syndrome Q78.1
McQuarrie's syndrome (idiopathic familial hypo-
  glycemia) E16.2
Meadow's syndrome Q86.1
Measles (black) (hemorrhagic) (suppressed) B05.9
  with
    complications NEC B05.89
    encephalitis B05.0
    intestinal complications B05.4
    keratitis (keratoconjunctivitis) B05.81
    meningitis B05.1
    otitis media B05.3
    pneumonia B05.2
  French — *see* Rubella
  German — *see* Rubella
  Liberty — *see* Rubella
Meatitis, urethral — *see* Urethritis
Meatus, meatal — *see* condition
Meat-wrappers' asthma J68.9
Meckel-Gruber syndrome Q61.9
Meckel's diverticulitis, diverticulum (displaced) (hypertrophic) Q43.0
  malignant — *see* Table of Neoplasms, small intestine,
    malignant
Meconium
  ileus, newborn P76.0
    in cystic fibrosis E84.11
    meaning meconium plug (without cystic fibrosis)
      P76.0
  obstruction, newborn P76.0
    due to fecaliths P76.0
    in mucoviscidosis E84.11
  peritonitis P78.0
  plug syndrome (newborn) NEC P76.0
Median (*see also* condition)
  arcuate ligament syndrome I77.4
  bar (prostate) (vesical orifice) — *see* Hyperplasia,
    prostate
  rhomboid glossitis K14.2
Mediastinal shift R93.8
Mediastinitis (acute) (chronic) J98.51
  syphilitic A52.73

Mediastinitis — continued
  tuberculous A15.8
Mediastinopericarditis (see also Pericarditis)
  acute I30.9
  adhesive I31.0
  chronic I31.8
    rheumatic I09.2
Mediastinum, mediastinal — see condition
Medicine poisoning — see Table of Drugs and Chemicals, by drug, poisoning
Mediterranean
  fever — see Brucellosis
    familial M04.1
    tick A77.1
  kala-azar B55.0
  leishmaniasis B55.0
  tick fever A77.1
Medulla — see condition
Medullary cystic kidney Q61.5
Medullated fibers
  optic (nerve) Q14.8
  retina Q14.1
Medulloblastoma
  desmoplastic C71.6
  specified site — see Neoplasm, malignant, by site
  unspecified site C71.6
Medulloepithelioma (see also Neoplasm, malignant, by site)
  teratoid — see Neoplasm, malignant, by site
Medullomyoblastoma
  specified site — see Neoplasm, malignant, by site
  unspecified site C71.6
Meekeren-Ehlers-Danlos syndrome Q79.6
Megacolon (acquired) (functional) (not Hirschsprung's disease) (in) K59.39
  Chagas' disease B57.32
  congenital, congenitum (aganglionic) Q43.1
  Hirschsprung's (disease) Q43.1
  toxic NEC K59.31
    due to Clostridium difficile
      not specified as recurrent A04.72
      recurrent A04.71
Megaesophagus (functional) K22.0
  congenital Q39.5
  in (due to) Chagas' disease B57.31
Megalencephaly Q04.5
Megalerythema (epidemic) B08.3
Megaloappendix Q43.8
Megalocephalus, megalocephaly NEC Q75.3
Megalocornea Q15.8
  with glaucoma Q15.0
Megalocytic anemia D53.1
Megalodactylia (fingers) (thumbs) (congenital) Q74.0
  toes Q74.2
Megaloduodenum Q43.8
Megaloesophagus (functional) K22.0
  congenital Q39.5
Megalogastria (acquired) K31.89
  congenital Q40.2
Megalophthalmos Q11.3
Megalopsia H53.15
Megalosplenia — see Splenomegaly
Megaloureter N28.82
  congenital Q62.2
Megarectum K62.89
Megasigmoid K59.39
  congenital Q43.2
Megaureter N28.82
  congenital Q62.2
Megavitamin-B6 syndrome E67.2
Megrim — see Migraine
Meibomian
  cyst, infected — see Hordeolum
  gland — see condition
  sty, stye — see Hordeolum
Meibomitis — see Hordeolum
Meige-Milroy disease (chronic hereditary edema) Q82.0
Meige's syndrome Q82.0
Melalgia, nutritional E53.8
Melancholia F32.9
  climacteric (single episode) F32.89
    recurrent episode F33.8
  hypochondriac F45.29
  intermittent (single episode) F32.89
    recurrent episode F33.8
  involutional (single episode) F32.89
    recurrent episode F33.8

Melancholia — continued
  menopausal (single episode) F32.89
    recurrent episode F33.8
  puerperal F32.89
  reactive (emotional stress or trauma) F32.3
  recurrent F33.9
  senile F03 ☑
  stuporous (single episode) F32.89
    recurrent episode F33.8
Melanemia R79.89
Melanoameloblastoma — see Neoplasm, bone, benign
Melanoblastoma — see Melanoma
Melanocarcinoma — see Melanoma
Melanocytoma, eyeball D31.9- ☑
Melanocytosis, neurocutaneous Q82.8
Melanoderma, melanodermia L81.4
Melanodontia, infantile K03.89
Melanodontoclasia K03.89
Melanoepithelioma — see Melanoma
Melanoma (malignant) C43.9
  acral lentiginous, malignant — see Melanoma, skin, by site
  amelanotic — see Melanoma, skin, by site
  balloon cell — see Melanoma, skin, by site
  benign — see Nevus
  desmoplastic, malignant — see Melanoma, skin, by site
  epithelioid cell — see Melanoma, skin, by site
    with spindle cell, mixed — see Melanoma, skin, by site
  in
    giant pigmented nevus — see Melanoma, skin, by site
    Hutchinson's melanotic freckle — see Melanoma, skin, by site
    junctional nevus — see Melanoma, skin, by site
    precancerous melanosis — see Melanoma, skin, by site
  in situ D03.9
    abdominal wall D03.59
    ala nasi D03.39
    ankle D03.7- ☑
    anus, anal (margin) (skin) D03.51
    arm D03.6- ☑
    auditory canal D03.2- ☑
    auricle (ear) D03.2- ☑
    auricular canal (external) D03.2- ☑
    axilla, axillary fold D03.59
    back D03.59
    breast D03.52
    brow D03.39
    buttock D03.59
    canthus (eye) D03.1- ☑
    cheek (external) D03.39
    chest wall D03.59
    chin D03.39
    choroid D03.8
    conjunctiva D03.8
    ear (external) D03.2- ☑
    external meatus (ear) D03.2- ☑
    eye D03.8
    eyebrow D03.39
    eyelid (lower) (upper) D03.1- ☑
    face D03.30
      specified NEC D03.39
    female genital organ (external) NEC D03.8
    finger D03.6- ☑
    flank D03.59
    foot D03.7- ☑
    forearm D03.6- ☑
    forehead D03.39
    foreskin D03.8
    gluteal region D03.59
    groin D03.59
    hand D03.6- ☑
    heel D03.7- ☑
    helix D03.2- ☑
    hip D03.7- ☑
    interscapular region D03.59
    iris D03.8
    jaw D03.39
    knee D03.7- ☑
    labium (majus) (minus) D03.8
    lacrimal gland D03.8
    leg D03.7- ☑
    lip (lower) (upper) D03.0
    lower limb NEC D03.7- ☑

Melanoma — continued
  in situ — continued
    male genital organ (external) NEC D03.8
    nail D03.9
      finger D03.6- ☑
      toe D03.7- ☑
    neck D03.4
    nose (external) D03.39
    orbit D03.8
    penis D03.8
    perianal skin D03.51
    perineum D03.51
    pinna D03.2- ☑
    popliteal fossa or space D03.7- ☑
    prepuce D03.8
    pudendum D03.8
    retina D03.8
    retrobulbar D03.8
    scalp D03.4
    scrotum D03.8
    shoulder D03.6- ☑
    specified site NEC D03.8
    submammary fold D03.52
    temple D03.39
    thigh D03.7- ☑
    toe D03.7- ☑
    trunk NEC D03.59
    umbilicus D03.59
    upper limb NEC D03.6- ☑
    vulva D03.8
  juvenile — see Nevus
  malignant, of soft parts except skin — see Neoplasm, connective tissue, malignant
  metastatic
    breast C79.81
    genital organ C79.82
    specified site NEC C79.89
  neurotropic, malignant — see Melanoma, skin, by site
  nodular — see Melanoma, skin, by site
  regressing, malignant — see Melanoma, skin, by site
  skin C43.9
    abdominal wall C43.59
    ala nasi C43.31
    ankle C43.7- ☑
    anus, anal (skin) C43.51
    arm C43.6- ☑
    auditory canal (external) C43.2- ☑
    auricle (ear) C43.2- ☑
    auricular canal (external) C43.2- ☑
    axilla, axillary fold C43.59
    back C43.59
    breast (female) (male) C43.52
    brow C43.39
    buttock C43.59
    canthus (eye) C43.1- ☑
    cheek (external) C43.39
    chest wall C43.59
    chin C43.39
    ear (external) C43.2- ☑
    elbow C43.6- ☑
    external meatus (ear) C43.2- ☑
    eyebrow C43.39
    eyelid (lower) (upper) C43.1- ☑
    face C43.30
      specified NEC C43.39
    female genital organ (external) NEC C51.9
    finger C43.6- ☑
    flank C43.59
    foot C43.7- ☑
    forearm C43.6- ☑
    forehead C43.39
    foreskin C60.0
    glabella C43.39
    gluteal region C43.59
    groin C43.59
    hand C43.6- ☑
    heel C43.7- ☑
    helix C43.2- ☑
    hip C43.7- ☑
    interscapular region C43.59
    jaw (external) C43.39
    knee C43.7- ☑
    labium C51.9
      majus C51.0
      minus C51.1
    leg C43.7- ☑
    lip (lower) (upper) C43.0

Index

Mediastinitis — Melanoma

Melanoma — *continued*
- skin — *continued*
  - lower limb NEC C43.7- ☑
  - male genital organ (external) NEC C63.9
  - nail
    - finger C43.6- ☑
    - toe C43.7- ☑
  - nasolabial groove C43.39
  - nates C43.59
  - neck C43.4
  - nose (external) C43.31
  - overlapping site C43.8
  - palpebra C43.1- ☑
  - penis C60.9
  - perianal skin C43.51
  - perineum C43.51
  - pinna C43.2- ☑
  - popliteal fossa or space C43.7- ☑
  - prepuce C60.0
  - pudendum C51.9
  - scalp C43.4
  - scrotum C63.2
  - shoulder C43.6- ☑
  - skin NEC C43.9
  - submammary fold C43.52
  - temple C43.39
  - thigh C43.7- ☑
  - toe C43.7- ☑
  - trunk NEC C43.59
  - umbilicus C43.59
  - upper limb NEC C43.6- ☑
  - vulva C51.9
    - overlapping sites C51.8
- spindle cell
  - with epithelioid, mixed — *see* Melanoma, skin, by site
  - type A C69.4- ☑
  - type B C69.4- ☑
- superficial spreading — *see* Melanoma, skin, by site

Melanosarcoma (*see also* Melanoma)
- epithelioid cell — *see* Melanoma

Melanosis L81.4
- addisonian E27.1
  - tuberculous A18.7
- adrenal E27.1
- colon K63.89
- conjunctiva — *see* Pigmentation, conjunctiva
  - congenital Q13.89
- cornea (presenile) (senile) (*see also* Pigmentation, cornea)
  - congenital Q13.4
- eye NEC H57.8
  - congenital Q15.8
- lenticularis progressiva Q82.1
- liver K76.89
- precancerous (*see also* Melanoma, in situ)
  - malignant melanoma in — *see* Melanoma
- Riehl's L81.4
- sclera H15.89
  - congenital Q13.89
- suprarenal E27.1
- tar L81.4
- toxic L81.4

Melanuria R82.99

MELAS syndrome E88.41

Melasma L81.1
- adrenal (gland) E27.1
- suprarenal (gland) E27.1

Melena K92.1
- with ulcer — *code by* site under Ulcer, with hemorrhage K27.4
- due to swallowed maternal blood P78.2
- newborn, neonatal P54.1
  - due to swallowed maternal blood P78.2

Meleney's
- gangrene (cutaneous) — *see* Ulcer, skin
- ulcer (chronic undermining) — *see* Ulcer, skin

Melioidosis A24.9
- acute A24.1
- chronic A24.2
- fulminating A24.1
- pneumonia A24.1
- pulmonary (chronic) A24.2
  - acute A24.1
  - subacute A24.2
- sepsis A24.1
- specified NEC A24.3
- subacute A24.2

Melitensis, febris A23.0
Melkersson (-Rosenthal) **syndrome** G51.2
Mellitus, diabetes — *see* Diabetes
Melorheostosis (bone) — *see* Disorder, bone, density and structure, specified NEC
Meloschisis Q18.4
Melotia Q17.4
Membrana
- capsularis lentis posterior Q13.89
- epipapillaris Q14.2

Membranacea placenta O43.19- ☑
Membranaceous uterus N85.8
Membrane(s), membranous (*see also* condition)
- cyclitic — *see* Membrane, pupillary
- folds, congenital — *see* Web
- Jackson's Q43.3
- over face of newborn P28.9
- premature rupture — *see* Rupture, membranes, premature
- pupillary H21.4- ☑
  - persistent Q13.89
- retained (with hemorrhage) (complicating delivery) O72.2
  - without hemorrhage O73.1
- secondary cataract — *see* Cataract, secondary
- unruptured (causing asphyxia) — *see* Asphyxia, newborn
- vitreous — *see* Opacity, vitreous, membranes and strands

Membranitis — *see* Chorioamnionitis
Memory disturbance, lack or loss (*see also* Amnesia)
- mild, following organic brain damage F06.8

Menadione deficiency E56.1
Menarche
- delayed E30.0
- precocious E30.1

Mendacity, pathologic F60.2
Mendelson's syndrome (due to anesthesia) J95.4
- in labor and delivery O74.0
- in pregnancy O29.01- ☑
- obstetric O74.0
- postpartum, puerperal O89.01

Ménétrier's disease or syndrome K29.60
- with bleeding K29.61

Ménière's disease, syndrome or vertigo H81.0- ☑
Meninges, meningeal — *see* condition
Meningioma (*see also* Neoplasm, meninges, benign)
- angioblastic — *see* Neoplasm, meninges, benign
- angiomatous — *see* Neoplasm, meninges, benign
- endotheliomatous — *see* Neoplasm, meninges, benign
- fibroblastic — *see* Neoplasm, meninges, benign
- fibrous — *see* Neoplasm, meninges, benign
- hemangioblastic — *see* Neoplasm, meninges, benign
- hemangiopericytic — *see* Neoplasm, meninges, benign
- malignant — *see* Neoplasm, meninges, malignant
- meningiothelial — *see* Neoplasm, meninges, benign
- meningotheliomatous — *see* Neoplasm, meninges, benign
- mixed — *see* Neoplasm, meninges, benign
- multiple — *see* Neoplasm, meninges, uncertain behavior
- papillary — *see* Neoplasm, meninges, uncertain behavior
- psammomatous — *see* Neoplasm, meninges, benign
- syncytial — *see* Neoplasm, meninges, benign
- transitional — *see* Neoplasm, meninges, benign

Meningiomatosis (diffuse) — *see* Neoplasm, meninges, uncertain behavior
Meningism — *see* Meningismus
Meningismus (infectional) (pneumococcal) R29.1
- due to serum or vaccine R29.1
- influenzal — *see* Influenza, with, manifestations NEC

Meningitis (basal) (basic) (brain) (cerebral) (cervical) (congestive) (diffuse) (hemorrhagic) (infantile) (membranous) (metastatic) (nonspecific) (pontine) (progressive) (simple) (spinal) (subacute) (sympathetic) (toxic) G03.9
- abacterial G03.0
- actinomycotic A42.81
- adenoviral A87.1
- arbovirus A87.8
- aseptic (acute) G03.0
- bacterial G00.9
  - Escherichia coli (E. coli) G00.8
  - Friedländer (bacillus) G00.8
  - gram-negative G00.9

Meningitis — *continued*
- bacterial — *continued*
  - H. influenzae G00.0
  - Klebsiella G00.8
  - pneumococcal G00.1
  - specified organism NEC G00.8
  - staphylococcal G00.3
  - streptococcal (acute) G00.2
- benign recurrent (Mollaret) G03.2
- candidal B37.5
- caseous (tuberculous) A17.0
- cerebrospinal A39.0
- chronic NEC G03.1
- clear cerebrospinal fluid NEC G03.0
- coxsackievirus A87.0
- cryptococcal B45.1
- diplococcal (gram positive) A39.0
- echovirus A87.0
- enteroviral A87.0
- eosinophilic B83.2
- epidemic NEC A39.0
- Escherichia coli (E. coli) G00.8
- fibrinopurulent G00.9
  - specified organism NEC G00.8
- Friedländer (bacillus) G00.8
- gonococcal A54.81
- gram-negative cocci G00.9
- gram-positive cocci G00.9
- H. influenzae G00.0
- Haemophilus (influenzae) G00.0
- in (due to)
  - adenovirus A87.1
  - African trypanosomiasis B56.9 [G02]
  - anthrax A22.8
  - bacterial disease NEC A48.8 [G01]
  - Chagas' disease (chronic) B57.41
  - chickenpox B01.0
  - coccidioidomycosis B38.4
  - Diplococcus pneumoniae G00.1
  - enterovirus A87.0
  - herpes (simplex) virus B00.3
    - zoster B02.1
  - infectious mononucleosis B27.92
  - leptospirosis A27.81
  - Listeria monocytogenes A32.11
  - Lyme disease A69.21
  - measles B05.1
  - mumps (virus) B26.1
  - neurosyphilis (late) A52.13
  - parasitic disease NEC B89 [G02]
  - poliovirus A80.9 [G02]
  - preventive immunization, inoculation or vaccination G03.8
  - rubella B06.02
  - Salmonella infection A02.21
  - specified cause NEC G03.8
  - Streptococcal pneumoniae G00.1
  - typhoid fever A01.01
  - varicella B01.0
  - viral disease NEC A87.8
  - whooping cough A37.90
  - zoster B02.1
- infectious G00.9
- influenzal (H. influenzae) G00.0
- Klebsiella G00.8
- leptospiral (aseptic) A27.81
- lymphocytic (acute) (benign) (serous) A87.2
- meningococcal A39.0
- Mima polymorpha G00.8
- Mollaret (benign recurrent) G03.2
- monilial B37.5
- mycotic NEC B49 [G02]
- Neisseria A39.0
- nonbacterial G03.0
- nonpyogenic NEC G03.0
- ossificans G96.19
- pneumococcal streptococcus pneumoniae G00.1
- poliovirus A80.9 [G02]
- postmeasles B05.1
- purulent G00.9
  - specified organism NEC G00.8
- pyogenic G00.9
  - specified organism NEC G00.8
- Salmonella (arizonae) (Cholerae-Suis) (enteritidis) (typhimurium) A02.21
- septic G00.9
  - specified organism NEC G00.8
- serosa circumscripta NEC G03.0
- serous NEC G93.2

Meningitis — *continued*
specified organism NEC G00.8
sporotrichosis B42.81
staphylococcal G00.3
sterile G03.0
Streptococcal (acute) G00.2
pneumoniae G00.1
suppurative G00.9
specified organism NEC G00.8
syphilitic (late) (tertiary) A52.13
acute A51.41
congenital A50.41
secondary A51.41
Torula histolytica (cryptococcal) B45.1 ☑
traumatic (complication of injury) T79.8 ☑
tuberculous A17.0
typhoid A01.01
viral NEC A87.9
Yersinia pestis A20.3
Meningocele (spinal) (*see also* Spina bifida)
with hydrocephalus — *see* Spina bifida, by site, with hydrocephalus
acquired (traumatic) G96.19
cerebral — *see* Encephalocele
Meningocerebritis — *see* Meningoencephalitis
Meningococcemia A39.4
acute A39.2
chronic A39.3
Meningococcus, meningococcal (*see also* condition) A39.9
adrenalitis, hemorrhagic A39.1
carrier (suspected) of Z22.31
meningitis (cerebrospinal) A39.0
Meningoencephalitis (*see also* Encephalitis) G04.90
acute NEC (*see also* Encephalitis, viral) A86
bacterial NEC G04.2
California A83.5
diphasic A84.1
eosinophilic B83.2
epidemic A39.81
herpesviral, herpetic B00.4
due to herpesvirus 6 B10.01
due to herpesvirus 7 B10.09
specified NEC B10.09
in (due to)
blastomycosis NEC B40.81
diseases classified elsewhere G05.3
free-living amebae B60.2
H. influenzae G00.0
Hemophilus influenzae (H .influenzae) G00.0
herpes B00.4
due to herpesvirus 6 B10.01
due to herpesvirus 7 B10.09
specified NEC B10.09
Lyme disease A69.22
mercury — *see* subcategory T56.1 ☑
mumps B26.2
Naegleria (amebae) (organisms) (fowleri) B60.2
Parastrongylus cantonensis B83.2
toxoplasmosis (acquired) B58.2
congenital P37.1
infectious (acute) (viral) A86
influenzal (H. influenzae) G00.0
Listeria monocytogenes A32.12
lymphocytic (serous) A87.2
mumps B26.2
parasitic NEC B89 [G05.3]
pneumococcal G04.2
primary amebic B60.2
specific (syphilitic) A52.14
specified organism NEC G04.81
staphylococcal G04.2
streptococcal G04.2
syphilitic A52.14
toxic NEC G92
due to mercury — *see* subcategory T56.1 ☑
tuberculous A17.82
virus NEC A86
Meningoencephalocele (*see also* Encephalocele)
syphilitic A52.19
congenital A50.49
Meningoencephalomyelitis (*see also* Meningoencephalitis)
acute NEC (viral) A86
disseminated G04.00
postimmunization or postvaccination G04.02
postinfectious G04.01

Meningoencephalomyelitis — *continued*
due to
actinomycosis A42.82
Torula B45.1
Toxoplasma or toxoplasmosis (acquired) B58.2
congenital P37.1
postimmunization or postvaccination G04.02
Meningoencephalomyelopathy G96.9
Meningoencephalopathy G96.9
Meningomyelitis (*see also* Meningoencephalitis)
bacterial NEC G04.2
blastomycotic NEC B40.81
cryptococcal B45.1
in diseases classified elsewhere G05.4
meningococcal A39.81
syphilitic A52.14
tuberculous A17.82
Meningomyelocele (*see also* Spina bifida)
syphilitic A52.19
Meningomyeloneuritis — *see* Meningoencephalitis
Meningoradiculitis — *see* Meningitis
Meningovascular — *see* condition
Menkes' disease or syndrome E83.09
meaning maple-syrup-urine disease E71.0
Menometrorrhagia N92.1
Menopause, menopausal (asymptomatic) (state) Z78.0
arthritis (any site) NEC — *see* Arthritis, specified form NEC
bleeding N92.4
depression (single episode) F32.89
agitated (single episode) F32.2
recurrent episode F33.9
psychotic (single episode) F32.89
recurrent episode F33.9
recurrent episode F33.8
melancholia (single episode) F32.89
recurrent episode F33.8
paranoid state F22
premature E28.319
asymptomatic E28.319
postirradiation E89.40
postsurgical E89.40
symptomatic E28.310
postirradiation E89.41
postsurgical E89.41
psychosis NEC F28
symptomatic N95.1
toxic polyarthritis NEC — *see* Arthritis, specified form NEC
Menorrhagia (primary) N92.0
climacteric N92.4
menopausal N92.4
menopausal N92.4
postclimacteric N95.0
postmenopausal N95.0
preclimacteric or premenopausal N92.4
pubertal (menses retained) N92.2
Menostaxis N92.0
Menses, retention N94.89
Menstrual — *see* Menstruation
Menstruation
absent — *see* Amenorrhea
anovulatory N97.0
cycle, irregular N92.6
delayed N91.0
disorder N93.9
psychogenic F45.8
during pregnancy O20.8
excessive (with regular cycle) N92.0
with irregular cycle N92.1
at puberty N92.2
frequent N92.0
infrequent — *see* Oligomenorrhea
irregular N92.6
specified NEC N92.5
latent N92.5
membranous N92.5
painful (*see also* Dysmenorrhea) N94.6
primary N94.4
psychogenic F45.8
secondary N94.5
passage of clots N92.0
precocious E30.1
protracted N92.5
rare — *see* Oligomenorrhea
retained N94.89
retrograde N92.5
scanty — *see* Oligomenorrhea

Menstruation — *continued*
suppression N94.89
vicarious (nasal) N94.89
Mental (*see also* condition)
deficiency — *see* Disability, intellectual
deterioration — *see* Psychosis
disorder — *see* Disorder, mental
exhaustion F48.8
insufficiency (congenital) — *see* Disability, intellectual
observation without need for further medical care Z03.89
retardation — *see* Disability, intellectual
subnormality — *see* Disability, intellectuall
upset — *see* Disorder, mental
Meralgia paresthetica G57.1- ☑
Mercurial — *see* condition
Mercurialism — *see* subcategory T56.1 ☑
Merkel cell tumor — *see* Carcinoma, Merkel cell
Merocele — *see* Hernia, femoral
Meromelia
lower limb — *see* Defect, reduction, lower limb
intercalary
femur — *see* Defect, reduction, lower limb, specified type NEC
tibiofibular (complete) (incomplete) — *see* Defect, reduction, lower limb
upper limb — *see* Defect, reduction, upper limb
intercalary, humeral, radioulnar — *see* Agenesis, arm, with hand present
MERRF syndrome (myoclonic epilepsy associated with ragged-red fiber) E88.42
Merzbacher-Pelizaeus disease E75.29
Mesaortitis — *see* Aortitis
Mesarteritis — *see* Arteritis
Mesencephalitis — *see* Encephalitis
Mesenchymoma (*see also* Neoplasm, connective tissue, uncertain behavior)
benign — *see* Neoplasm, connective tissue, benign
malignant — *see* Neoplasm, connective tissue, malignant
Mesenteritis
retractile K65.4
sclerosing K65.4
Mesentery, mesenteric — *see* condition
Mesiodens, mesiodentes K00.1
Mesio-occlusion M26.213
Mesocolon — *see* condition
Mesonephroma (malignant) — *see* Neoplasm, malignant, by site
benign — *see* Neoplasm, benign, by site
Mesophlebitis — *see* Phlebitis
Mesostromal dysgenesis Q13.89
Mesothelioma (malignant) C45.9
benign
mesentery D19.1
mesocolon D19.1
omentum D19.1
peritoneum D19.1
pleura D19.0
specified site NEC D19.7
unspecified site D19.9
biphasic C45.9
benign
mesentery D19.1
mesocolon D19.1
omentum D19.1
peritoneum D19.1
pleura D19.0
specified site NEC D19.7
unspecified site D19.9
cystic D48.4
epithelioid C45.9
benign
mesentery D19.1
mesocolon D19.1
omentum D19.1
peritoneum D19.1
pleura D19.0
specified site NEC D19.7
unspecified site D19.9
fibrous C45.9
benign
mesentery D19.1
mesocolon D19.1
omentum D19.1
peritoneum D19.1
pleura D19.0
specified site NEC D19.7

Mesothelioma — *continued*
  fibrous — *continued*
    benign — *continued*
      unspecified site D19.9
  site classification
    liver C45.7
    lung C45.7
    mediastinum C45.7
    mesentery C45.1
    mesocolon C45.1
    omentum C45.1
    pericardium C45.2
    peritoneum C45.1
    pleura C45.0
      parietal C45.0
    retroperitoneum C45.7
    specified site NEC C45.7
    unspecified C45.9
Metabolic syndrome E88.81
Metagonimiasis B66.8
Metagonimus infestation (intestine) B66.8
Metal
  pigmentation L81.8
  polisher's disease J62.8
Metamorphopsia H53.15
Metaplasia
  apocrine (breast) — *see* Dysplasia, mammary, specified
    type NEC
  cervix (squamous) — *see* Dysplasia, cervix
  endometrium (squamous) (uterus) N85.8
  esophagus K22.7- ☑
  kidney (pelvis) (squamous) N28.89
  myelogenous D73.1
  myeloid (agnogenic) (megakaryocytic) D73.1
  spleen D73.1
  squamous cell, bladder N32.89
Metastasis, metastatic
  abscess — *see* Abscess
  calcification E83.59
  cancer
    from specified site — *see* Neoplasm, malignant,
      by site
    to specified site — *see* Neoplasm, secondary, by
      site
  deposits (in) — *see* Neoplasm, secondary, by site
  disease (*see also* Neoplasm, secondary, by site) C79.9
  spread (to) — *see* Neoplasm, secondary, by site
Metastrongyliasis B83.8
Metatarsalgia M77.4- ☑
  anterior G57.6- ☑
  Morton's G57.6- ☑
Metatarsus, metatarsal (*see also* condition)
  adductus, congenital Q66.22
  valgus (abductus), congenital Q66.6
  varus (congenital) Q66.22
    primus Q66.21
Methadone use — *see* Use, opioid
Methemoglobinemia D74.9
  acquired (with sulfhemoglobinemia) D74.8
  congenital D74.0
  enzymatic (congenital) D74.0
  Hb M disease D74.0
  hereditary D74.0
  toxic D74.8
Methemoglobinuria — *see* Hemoglobinuria
Methioninemia E72.19
Methylmalonic acidemia E71.120
Metritis (catarrhal) (hemorrhagic) (septic) (suppurative)
  (*see also* Endometritis)
  cervical — *see* Cervicitis
Metropathia hemorrhagica N93.8
Metroperitonitis — *see* Peritonitis, pelvic, female
Metrorrhagia N92.1
  climacteric N92.4
  menopausal N92.4
  postpartum NEC (atonic) (following delivery of placen-
    ta) O72.1
    delayed or secondary O72.2
  preclimacteric or premenopausal N92.4
  psychogenic F45.8
Metrorrhexis — *see* Rupture, uterus
Metrosalpingitis N70.91
Metrostaxis N93.8
Metrovaginitis — *see* Endometritis
Meyer-Schwickerath and Weyers syndrome Q87.0
Meynert's amentia (nonalcoholic) F04
  alcoholic F10.96

Meynert's amentia — *continued*
  alcoholic — *continued*
    with dependence F10.26
Mibelli's disease (porokeratosis) Q82.8
Mice, joint — *see* Loose, body, joint
  knee M23.4- ☑
Micrencephalon, micrencephaly Q02
Microalbuminuria R80.9
Microaneurysm, retinal (*see also* Disorder, retina, mi-
  croaneurysms)
  diabetic — *see* E08-E13 with .31
Microangiopathy (peripheral) I73.9
  thrombotic M31.1
Microcalcifications, breast R92.0
Microcephalus, microcephalic, microcephaly Q02
  due to toxoplasmosis (congenital) P37.1
Microcheilia Q18.7
Microcolon (congenital) Q43.8
Microcornea (congenital) Q13.4
Microcytic — *see* condition
Microdeletions NEC Q93.88
Microdontia K00.2
Microdrepanocytosis D57.40
  with crisis (vasoocclusive pain) D57.419
    with
      acute chest syndrome D57.411
      splenic sequestration D57.412
Microembolism
  atherothrombotic — *see* Atheroembolism
  retinal — *see* Occlusion, artery, retina
Microencephalon Q02
Microfilaria streptocerca infestation — *see* Onchocer-
  ciasis
Microgastria (congenital) Q40.2
Microgenia M26.06
Microgenitalia, congenital
  female Q52.8
  male Q55.8
Microglioma — *see* Lymphoma, non-Hodgkin, specified
  NEC
Microglossia (congenital) Q38.3
Micrognathia, micrognathism (congenital)
  (mandibular) (maxillary) M26.09
Microgyria (congenital) Q04.3
Microinfarct of heart — *see* Insufficiency, coronary
Microlentia (congenital) Q12.8
Microlithiasis, alveolar, pulmonary J84.02
Micromastia N64.82
Micromyelia (congenital) Q06.8
Micropenis Q55.62
Microphakia (congenital) Q12.8
Microphthalmos, microphthalmia (congenital) Q11.2
  due to toxoplasmosis P37.1
Micropsia H53.15
Microscopic polyangiitis (polyarteritis) M31.7
Microsporidiosis B60.8
  intestinal A07.8
Microsporon furfur infestation B36.0
Microsporosis (*see also* Dermatophytosis)
  nigra B36.1
Microstomia (congenital) Q18.5
Microtia (congenital) (external ear) Q17.2
Microtropia H50.40
Microvillus inclusion disease (MVD) (MVID) Q43.8
Micturition
  disorder NEC (*see also* Difficulty, micturition) R39.198
    psychogenic F45.8
  frequency R35.0
    psychogenic F45.8
  hesitancy R39.11
  incomplete emptying R39.14
  nocturnal R35.1
  painful R30.9
    dysuria R30.0
    psychogenic F45.8
    tenesmus R30.1
  poor stream R39.12
  position dependent R39.192
  split stream R39.13
  straining R39.16
  urgency R39.15
Mid plane — *see* condition
Middle
  ear — *see* condition
  lobe (right) syndrome J98.19
Miescher's elastoma L87.2
Mietens' syndrome Q87.2

Migraine (idiopathic) G43.909
  with aura (acute-onset) (prolonged) (typical) (without
    headache) G43.109
    with refractory migraine G43.119
      with status migrainosus G43.111
      without status migrainosus G43.119
    without mention of refractory migraine G43.109
      with status migrainosus G43.101
      without status migrainosus G43.109
    intractable G43.119
      with status migrainosus G43.111
      without status migrainosus G43.119
    not intractable G43.109
      with status migrainosus G43.101
      without status migrainosus G43.109
    persistent G43.509
      with cerebral infarction G43.609
        with refractory migraine G43.619
          with status migrainosus G43.611
          without status migrainosus G43.619
        without refractory migraine G43.609
          with status migrainosus G43.601
          without status migrainosus G43.609
        intractable G43.619
          with status migrainosus G43.611
          without status migrainosus G43.619
        not intractable G43.609
          with status migrainosus G43.601
          without status migrainosus G43.609
      without cerebral infarction G43.509
        with refractory migraine G43.519
          with status migrainosus G43.511
          without status migrainosus G43.519
        without refractory migraine G43.509
          with status migrainosus G43.501
          without status migrainosus G43.509
        intractable G43.519
          with status migrainosus G43.511
          without status migrainosus G43.519
        not intractable G43.509
          with status migrainosus G43.501
          without status migrainosus G43.509
  with refractory migraine G43.919
    with status migrainosus G43.911
    without status migrainosus G43.919
  without aura G43.009
    with refractory migraine G43.019
      with status migrainosus G43.011
      without status migrainosus G43.019
    without mention of refractory migraine G43.009
      with status migrainosus G43.001
      without status migrainosus G43.009
  chronic G43.709
    with refractory migraine G43.719
      with status migrainosus G43.711
      without status migrainosus G43.719
    without refractory migraine G43.709
      with status migrainosus G43.701
      without status migrainosus G43.709
    intractable
      with status migrainosus G43.711
      without status migrainosus G43.719
    not intractable
      with status migrainosus G43.701
      without status migrainosus G43.709
  intractable
    with status migrainosus G43.011
    without status migrainosus G43.019
  not intractable
    with status migrainosus G43.001
    without status migrainosus G43.009
  without refractory migraine G43.909
    with status migrainosus G43.901
    without status migrainosus G43.919
  abdominal G43.D0 (*following* G43.7)
    with refractory migraine G43.D1 (*following* G43.7)
    without refractory migraine G43.D0 (*following*
      G43.7)
    intractable G43.D1 (*following* G43.7)
    not intractable G43.D0 (*following* G43.7)
  basilar — *see* Migraine, with aura
  classical — *see* Migraine, with aura
  common — *see* Migraine, without aura
  complicated G43.109
  equivalents — *see* Migraine, with aura
  familiar — *see* Migraine, hemiplegic
  hemiplegic G43.409
    with refractory migraine G43.419
      with status migrainosus G43.411

Migraine — continued
  hemiplegic — continued
    with refractory migraine — continued
      without status migrainosus G43.419
    without refractory migraine G43.409
      with status migrainosus G43.401
      without status migrainosus G43.409
    intractable G43.419
      with status migrainosus G43.411
      without status migrainosus G43.419
    not intractable G43.409
      with status migrainosus G43.401
      without status migrainosus G43.409
  intractable G43.919
    with status migrainosus G43.911
    without status migrainosus G43.919
  menstrual G43.829
    with refractory migraine G43.839
      with status migrainosus G43.831
      without status migrainosus G43.839
    without refractory migraine G43.829
      with status migrainosus G43.821
      without status migrainosus G43.829
    intractable G43.839
      with status migrainosus G43.831
      without status migrainosus G43.839
    not intractable 4G43.829
      with status migrainosus G43.821
      without status migrainosus G43.829
  menstrually related — see Migraine, menstrual
  not intractable G43.909
    with status migrainosus G43.901
    without status migrainosus G43.919
  ophthalmoplegic G43.B0 (following G43.7)
    with refractory migraine G43.B1 (following G43.7)
    without refractory migraine G43.B0 (following G43.7)
    intractable G43.B1 (following G43.7)
    not intractable G43.B0 (following G43.7)
  persistent aura (with, without) cerebral infarction — see Migraine, with aura, persistent
  preceded or accompanied by transient focal neurological phenomena — see Migraine, with aura
  pre-menstrual — see Migraine, menstrual
  pure menstrual — see Migraine, menstrual
  retinal — see Migraine, with aura
  specified NEC G43.809
    intractable G43.819
      with status migrainosus G43.811
      without status migrainosus G43.819
    not intractable G43.809
      with status migrainosus G43.801
      without status migrainosus G43.809
  sporadic — see Migraine, hemiplegic
  transformed — see Migraine, without aura, chronic
  triggered seizures — see Migraine, with aura
Migrant, social Z59.0
Migration, anxiety concerning Z60.3
Migratory, migrating (see also condition)
  person Z59.0
  testis Q55.29
Mikity-Wilson disease or syndrome P27.0
Mikulicz' disease or syndrome K11.8
Miliaria L74.3
  alba L74.1
  apocrine L75.2
  crystallina L74.1
  profunda L74.2
  rubra L74.0
  tropicalis L74.2
Miliary — see condition
Milium L72.0
  colloid L57.8
Milk
  crust L21.0
  excessive secretion O92.6
  poisoning — see Poisoning, food, noxious
  retention O92.79
  sickness — see Poisoning, food, noxious
  spots I31.0
Milk-alkali disease or syndrome E83.52
Milk-leg (deep vessels) (nonpuerperal) — see Embolism, vein, lower extremity
  complicating pregnancy O22.3- ☑
  puerperal, postpartum, childbirth O87.1
Milkman's disease or syndrome M83.8
Milky urine — see Chyluria
Millard-Gubler (-Foville) **paralysis or syndrome** G46.3

Millar's asthma J38.5
Miller Fisher syndrome G61.0
Mills' disease — see Hemiplegia
Millstone maker's pneumoconiosis J62.8
Milroy's disease (chronic hereditary edema) Q82.0
Minamata disease T56.1 ☑
Miners' asthma or lung J60
Minkowski-Chauffard syndrome — see Spherocytosis
Minor — see condition
Minor's disease (hematomyelia) G95.19
Minot's disease (hemorrhagic disease), newborn P53
Minot-von Willebrand-Jurgens disease or syndrome (angiohemophilia) D68.0
Minus (and plus) **hand** (intrinsic) — see Deformity, limb, specified type NEC, forearm
Miosis (pupil) H57.03
Mirizzi's syndrome (hepatic duct stenosis) K83.1
Mirror writing F81.0
Misadventure (of) (prophylactic) (therapeutic) (see also Complications) T88.9 ☑
  administration of insulin (by accident) — see subcategory T38.3 ☑
  infusion — see Complications, infusion
  local applications (of fomentations, plasters, etc.) T88.9 ☑
    burn or scald — see Burn
    specified NEC T88.8 ☑
  medical care (early) (late) T88.9 ☑
    adverse effect of drugs or chemicals — see Table of Drugs and Chemicals
    burn or scald — see Burn
    specified NEC T88.8 ☑
  specified NEC T88.8 ☑
  surgical procedure (early) (late) — see Complications, surgical procedure
  transfusion — see Complications, transfusion
  vaccination or other immunological procedure — see Complications, vaccination
Miscarriage O03.9
Misdirection, aqueous H40.83- ☑
Misperception, sleep state F51.02
Misplaced, misplacement
  ear Q17.4
  kidney (acquired) N28.89
    congenital Q63.2
  organ or site, congenital NEC — see Malposition, congenital
Missed
  abortion O02.1
  delivery O36.4 ☑
Missing (see also Absence)
  string of intrauterine contraceptive device T83.32- ☑
Misuse of drugs F19.99
Mitchell's disease (erythromelalgia) I73.81
Mite(s) (infestation) B88.9
  diarrhea B88.0
  grain (itch) B88.0
  hair follicle (itch) B88.0
  in sputum B88.0
Mitral — see condition
Mittelschmerz N94.0
Mixed — see condition
MMN (multifocal motor neuropathy) G61.82
MNGIE (Mitochondrial Neurogastrointestinal Encephalopathy) **syndrome** E88.49
Mobile, mobility
  cecum Q43.3
  excessive — see Hypermobility
  gallbladder, congenital Q44.1
  kidney N28.89
  organ or site, congenital NEC — see Malposition, congenital
Mobitz heart block (atrioventricular) I44.1
Moebius, Möbius
  disease (ophthalmoplegic migraine) — see Migraine, ophthalmoplegic
  syndrome Q87.0
    congenital oculofacial paralysis (with other anomalies) Q87.0
    ophthalmoplegic migraine — see Migraine, ophthalmoplegic
Moeller's glossitis K14.0
Mohr's syndrome (Types I and II) Q87.0
Mola destruens D39.2
Molar pregnancy O02.0
Molarization of premolars K00.2

Molding, head (during birth) — omit code
Mole (pigmented) (see also Nevus)
  blood O02.0
  Breus' O02.0
  cancerous — see Melanoma
  carneous O02.0
  destructive D39.2
  fleshy O02.0
  hydatid, hydatidiform (benign) (complicating pregnancy) (delivered) (undelivered) O01.9
    classical O01.0
    complete O01.0
    incomplete O01.1
    invasive D39.2
    malignant D39.2
    partial O01.1
  intrauterine O02.0
  invasive (hydatidiform) D39.2
  malignant
    meaning
      malignant hydatidiform mole D39.2
      melanoma — see Melanoma
  nonhydatidiform O02.0
  nonpigmented — see Nevus
  pregnancy NEC O02.0
  skin — see Nevus
  tubal O00.10- ☑
    with intrauterine pregnancy O00.11- ☑
  vesicular — see Mole, hydatidiform
Molimen, molimina (menstrual) N94.3
Molluscum contagiosum (epitheliale) B08.1
Mönckeberg's arteriosclerosis, disease, or sclerosis — see Arteriosclerosis, extremities
Mondini's malformation (cochlea) Q16.5
Mondor's disease I80.8
Monge's disease T70.29 ☑
Monilethrix (congenital) Q84.1
Moniliasis (see also Candidiasis) B37.9
  neonatal P37.5
Monitoring (encounter for)
  therapeutic drug level Z51.81
Monkey malaria B53.1
Monkeypox B04
Monoarthritis M13.10
  ankle M13.17- ☑
  elbow M13.12- ☑
  foot joint M13.17- ☑
  hand joint M13.14- ☑
  hip M13.15- ☑
  knee M13.16- ☑
  shoulder M13.11- ☑
  wrist M13.13- ☑
Monoblastic — see condition
Monochromat (ism), monochromatopsia (acquired) (congenital) H53.51
Monocytic — see condition
Monocytopenia D72.818
Monocytosis (symptomatic) D72.821
Monomania — see Psychosis
Mononeuritis G58.9
  cranial nerve — see Disorder, nerve, cranial
  femoral nerve G57.2- ☑
  lateral
    cutaneous nerve of thigh G57.1- ☑
    popliteal nerve G57.3- ☑
  lower limb G57.9- ☑
    specified nerve NEC G57.8- ☑
  medial popliteal nerve G57.4- ☑
  median nerve G56.1- ☑
  multiplex G58.7
  plantar nerve G57.6- ☑
  posterior tibial nerve G57.5- ☑
  radial nerve G56.3- ☑
  sciatic nerve G57.0- ☑
  specified NEC G58.8
  tibial nerve G57.4- ☑
  ulnar nerve G56.2- ☑
  upper limb G56.9- ☑
    specified nerve NEC G56.8- ☑
  vestibular — see subcategory H93.3 ☑
Mononeuropathy G58.9
  carpal tunnel syndrome — see Syndrome, carpal tunnel
  diabetic NEC — see E08-E13 with .41
  femoral nerve — see Lesion, nerve, femoral
  ilioinguinal nerve G57.8- ☑
  in diseases classified elsewhere — see category G59

Mononeuropathy — continued
  intercostal G58.Ø
  lower limb G57.9- ☑
    causalgia — see Causalgia, lower limb
    femoral nerve — see Lesion, nerve, femoral
    meralgia paresthetica G57.1- ☑
    plantar nerve — see Lesion, nerve, plantar
    popliteal nerve — see Lesion, nerve, popliteal
    sciatic nerve — see Lesion, nerve, sciatic
    specified NEC G57.8- ☑
    tarsal tunnel syndrome — see Syndrome, tarsal
      tunnel
  median nerve — see Lesion, nerve, median
  multiplex G58.7
  obturator nerve G57.8- ☑
  popliteal nerve — see Lesion, nerve, popliteal
  radial nerve — see Lesion, nerve, radial
  saphenous nerve G57.8- ☑
  specified NEC G58.8
  tarsal tunnel syndrome — see Syndrome, tarsal tunnel
  tuberculous A17.83
  ulnar nerve — see Lesion, nerve, ulnar
  upper limb G56.9- ☑
    carpal tunnel syndrome — see Syndrome, carpal
      tunnel
    causalgia — see Causalgia
    median nerve — see Lesion, nerve, median
    radial nerve — see Lesion, nerve, radial
    specified site NEC G56.8- ☑
    ulnar nerve — see Lesion, nerve, ulnar
Mononucleosis, infectious B27.9Ø
  with
    complication NEC B27.99
    meningitis B27.92
    polyneuropathy B27.91
  cytomegaloviral B27.1Ø
    with
      complication NEC B27.19
      meningitis B27.12
      polyneuropathy B27.11
  Epstein-Barr (virus) B27.ØØ
    with
      complication NEC B27.Ø9
      meningitis B27.Ø2
      polyneuropathy B27.Ø1
  gammaherpesviral B27.ØØ
    with
      complication NEC B27.Ø9
      meningitis B27.Ø2
      polyneuropathy B27.Ø1
  specified NEC B27.8Ø
    with
      complication NEC B27.89
      meningitis B27.82
      polyneuropathy B27.81
Monoplegia G83.3- ☑
  congenital (cerebral) G8Ø.8
    spastic G8Ø.1
  embolic (current episode) I63.4- ☑
  following
    cerebrovascular disease
      cerebral infarction
        lower limb I69.34- ☑
        upper limb I69.33- ☑
      intracerebral hemorrhage
        lower limb I69.14- ☑
        upper limb I69.13- ☑
      lower limb I69.94- ☑
      nontraumatic intracranial hemorrhage NEC
        lower limb I69.24- ☑
        upper limb I69.23- ☑
      specified disease NEC
        lower limb I69.84- ☑
        upper limb I69.83- ☑
      stroke NOS
        lower limb I69.34- ☑
        upper limb I69.33- ☑
      subarachnoid hemorrhage
        lower limb I69.Ø4- ☑
        upper limb I69.Ø3- ☑
    upper limb I69.93- ☑
  hysterical (transient) F44.4
  lower limb G83.1- ☑
  psychogenic (conversion reaction) F44.4
  thrombotic (current episode) I63.3- ☑
  transient R29.818
  upper limb G83.2- ☑

Monorchism, monorchidism Q55.Ø
Monosomy (see also Deletion, chromosome) Q93.9
  specified NEC Q93.89
  whole chromosome
    meiotic nondisjunction Q93.Ø
    mitotic nondisjunction Q93.1
    mosaicism Q93.1
  X Q96.9
Monster, monstrosity (single) Q89.7
  acephalic QØØ.Ø
  twin Q89.4
Monteggia's fracture (-dislocation) S52.27- ☑
Mooren's ulcer (cornea) — see Ulcer, cornea, Mooren's
Moore's syndrome — see Epilepsy, specified NEC
Mooser-Neill reaction A75.2
Mooser's bodies A75.2
Morbidity not stated or unknown R69
Morbilli — see Measles
Morbus (see also Disease)
  angelicus, anglorum E55.Ø
  Beigel B36.2
  caducus — see Epilepsy
  celiacus K9Ø.Ø
  comitialis — see Epilepsy
  cordis (see also Disease, heart) I51.9
    valvulorum — see Endocarditis
  coxae senilis M16.9
    tuberculous A18.Ø2
  hemorrhagicus neonatorum P53
  maculosus neonatorum P54.5
Morel (-Stewart)(-Morgagni) **syndrome** M85.2
Morel-Kraepelin disease — see Schizophrenia
Morel-Moore syndrome M85.2
Morgagni's
  cyst, organ, hydatid, or appendage
    female Q5Ø.5
    male (epididymal) Q55.4
      testicular Q55.29
  syndrome M85.2
Morgagni-Stewart-Morel syndrome M85.2
Morgagni-Stokes-Adams syndrome I45.9
Morgagni-Turner (-Albright) **syndrome** Q96.9
Moria FØ7.Ø
Moron (I.Q. 5Ø-69) F7Ø
Morphea L94.Ø
Morphinism (without remission) F11.2Ø
  with remission F11.21
Morphinomania (without remission) F11.2Ø
  with remission F11.21
Morquio (-Ullrich)(-Brailsford) **disease or syndrome** —
  see Mucopolysaccharidosis
Mortification (dry) (moist) — see Gangrene
Morton's metatarsalgia (neuralgia)(neuroma) (syn-
  drome) G57.6- ☑
Morvan's disease or syndrome G6Ø.8
Mosaicism, mosaic (autosomal) (chromosomal)
  45,X/46,XX Q96.3
  45,X/other cell lines NEC with abnormal sex chromo-
    some Q96.4
  sex chromosome
    female Q97.8
    lines with various numbers of X chromosomes
      Q97.2
    male Q98.7
  XY Q96.3
Moschowitz' disease M31.1
Mother yaw A66.Ø
Motion sickness (from travel, any vehicle) (from round-
  abouts or swings) T75.3 ☑
Mottled, mottling, teeth (enamel) (endemic) (nonen-
  demic) KØØ.3
Mounier-Kuhn syndrome Q32.4
  with bronchiectasis J47.9
    exacerbation (acute) J47.1
    lower respiratory infection J47.Ø
  acquired J98.Ø9
    with bronchiectasis J47.9
      with
        exacerbation (acute) J47.1
        lower respiratory infection J47.Ø
Mountain
  sickness T7Ø.29 ☑
    with polycythemia , acquired (acute) D75.1
  tick fever A93.2
Mouse, joint — see Loose, body, joint
  knee M23.4- ☑
Mouth — see condition

Movable
  coccyx — see subcategory M53.2 ☑
  kidney N28.89
    congenital Q63.8
  spleen D73.89
Movements, dystonic R25.8
Moyamoya disease I67.5
MRSA (Methicillin resistant Staphylococcus aureus)
  infection A49.Ø2
    as the cause of diseases classified elsewhere B95.62
  sepsis A41.Ø2
MSSA (Methicillin susceptible Staphylococcus aureus)
  infection A49.Ø1
    as the cause of diseases classified elsewhere B95.61
  sepsis A41.Ø1
Mucha-Habermann disease L41.Ø
Mucinosis (cutaneous) (focal) (papular) (skin) L98.5
  oral K13.79
Mucocele
  appendix K38.8
  buccal cavity K13.79
  gallbladder K82.1
  lacrimal sac, chronic HØ4.43- ☑
  nasal sinus J34.1
  nose J34.1
  salivary gland (any) K11.6
  sinus (accessory) (nasal) J34.1
  turbinate (bone) (middle) (nasal) J34.1
  uterus N85.8
Mucolipidosis
  I E77.1
  II, III E77.Ø
  IV E75.11
Mucopolysaccharidosis E76.3
  beta-gluduronidase deficiency E76.29
  cardiopathy E76.3 [I52]
  Hunter's syndrome E76.1
  Hurler's syndrome E76.Ø1
  Hurler-Scheie syndrome E76.Ø2
  Maroteaux-Lamy syndrome E76.29
  Morquio syndrome E76.219
    A E76.21Ø
    B E76.211
    classic E76.21Ø
  Sanfilippo syndrome E76.22
  Scheie's syndrome E76.Ø3
  specified NEC E76.29
  type
    I
      Hurler's syndrome E76.Ø1
      Hurler-Scheie syndrome E76.Ø2
      Scheie's syndrome E76.Ø3
    II E76.1
    III E76.22
    IV E76.219
    IVA E76.21Ø
    IVB E76.211
    VI E76.29
    VII E76.29
Mucormycosis B46.5
  cutaneous B46.3
  disseminated B46.4
  gastrointestinal B46.2
  generalized B46.4
  pulmonary B46.Ø
  rhinocerebral B46.1
  skin B46.3
  subcutaneous B46.3
Mucositis (ulcerative) K12.3Ø
  due to drugs NEC K12.32
  gastrointestinal K92.81
  mouth (oral) (oropharyngeal) K12.3Ø
    due to antineoplastic therapy K12.31
    due to drugs NEC K12.32
    due to radiation K12.33
    specified NEC K12.39
    viral K12.39
  nasal J34.81
  oral cavity — see Mucositis, mouth
  oral soft tissues — see Mucositis, mouth
  vagina and vulva N76.81
Mucositis necroticans agranulocytica — see Agranulocytosis
Mucous (see also condition)
  patches (syphilitic) A51.39
    congenital A5Ø.Ø7
Mucoviscidosis E84.9
  with meconium obstruction E84.11

Mucus
asphyxia or suffocation — *see* Asphyxia, mucus
in stool R19.5
plug — *see* Asphyxia, mucus
Muguet B37.0
Mulberry molars (congenital syphilis) A50.52
Müllerian mixed tumor
specified site — *see* Neoplasm, malignant, by site
unspecified site C54.9
Multicystic kidney (development) Q61.4
Multiparity (grand) Z64.1
affecting management of pregnancy, labor and delivery (supervision only) O09.4- ☑
requiring contraceptive management — *see* Contraception
Multipartita placenta O43.19- ☑
Multiple, multiplex (*see also* condition)
digits (congenital) Q69.9
endocrine neoplasia — *see* Neoplasia, endocrine, multiple (MEN)
personality F44.81
Mumps B26.9
arthritis B26.85
complication NEC B26.89
encephalitis B26.2
hepatitis B26.81
meningitis (aseptic) B26.1
meningoencephalitis B26.2
myocarditis B26.82
oophoritis B26.89
orchitis B26.0
pancreatitis B26.3
polyneuropathy B26.84
Mumu (*see also* Infestation, filarial) B74.9 [N51]
Münchhausen's syndrome — *see* Disorder, factitious
Münchmeyer's syndrome — *see* Myositis, ossificans, progressiva
Mural — *see* condition
Murmur (cardiac) (heart) (organic) R01.1
abdominal R19.15
aortic (valve) — *see* Endocarditis, aortic
benign R01.0
diastolic — *see* Endocarditis
Flint I35.1
functional R01.0
Graham Steell I37.1
innocent R01.0
mitral (valve) — *see* Insufficiency, mitral
nonorganic R01.0
presystolic, mitral — *see* Insufficiency, mitral
pulmonic (valve) I37.8
systolic R01.1
tricuspid (valve) I07.9
valvular — *see* Endocarditis
Murri's disease (intermittent hemoglobinuria) D59.6
Muscle, muscular (*see also* condition)
carnitine (palmityltransferase) deficiency E71.314
Musculoneuralgia — *see* Neuralgia
Mushrooming hip — *see* Derangement, joint, specified NEC, hip
Mushroom-workers' (pickers') **disease or lung** J67.5
Mutation(s)
factor V Leiden D68.51
prothrombin gene D68.52
surfactant, of lung J84.83
Mutism (*see also* Aphasia)
deaf (acquired) (congenital) NEC H91.3
elective (adjustment reaction) (childhood) F94.0
hysterical F44.4
selective (childhood) F94.0
MVD (microvillus inclusion disease) Q43.8
MVID (microvillus inclusion disease) Q43.8
Myalgia M79.1
epidemic (cervical) B33.0
traumatic NEC T14.8 ☑
Myasthenia G70.9
congenital G70.2
cordis — *see* Failure, heart
developmental G70.2
gravis G70.00
with exacerbation (acute) G70.01
in crisis G70.01
neonatal, transient P94.0
pseudoparalytica G70.00
with exacerbation (acute) G70.01
in crisis G70.01
stomach, psychogenic F45.8

Myasthenia — *continued*
syndrome
in
diabetes mellitus — *see* E08-E13 with .44
neoplastic disease (*see also* Neoplasm) D49.9 [G73.3]
pernicious anemia D51.0 [G73.3]
thyrotoxicosis E05.90 [G73.3]
with thyroid storm E05.91 [G73.3]
Myasthenic M62.81
Mycelium infection B49
Mycetismus — *see* Poisoning, food, noxious, mushroom
Mycetoma B47.9
actinomycotic B47.1
bone (mycotic) B47.9 [M90.80]
eumycotic B47.0
foot B47.9
actinomycotic B47.1
mycotic B47.0
madurae NEC B47.9
mycotic B47.0
maduromycotic B47.0
mycotic B47.0
nocardial B47.1
Mycobacteriosis — *see* Mycobacterium
Mycobacterium, mycobacterial (infection) A31.9
anonymous A31.9
atypical A31.9
cutaneous A31.1
pulmonary A31.0
tuberculous — *see* Tuberculosis, pulmonary
specified site NEC A31.8
avium (intracellulare complex) A31.0
balnei A31.1
Battey A31.0
chelonei A31.8
cutaneous A31.1
extrapulmonary systemic A31.8
fortuitum A31.8
intracellulare (Battey bacillus) A31.0
kakaferifu A31.8
kansasii (yellow bacillus) A31.0
kasongo A31.8
leprae (*see also* Leprosy) A30.9
luciflavum A31.1
marinum (M. balnei) A31.1
nonspecific — *see* Mycobacterium, atypical
pulmonary (atypical) A31.0
tuberculous — *see* Tuberculosis, pulmonary
scrofulaceum A31.8
simiae A31.8
systemic, extrapulmonary A31.8
szulgai A31.8
terrae A31.8
triviale A31.8
tuberculosis (human, bovine) — *see* Tuberculosis
ulcerans A31.1
xenopi A31.8
Mycoplasma (M.) **pneumoniae, as cause of disease classified elsewhere** B96.0
Mycosis, mycotic B49
cutaneous NEC B36.9
ear B36.9
in
aspergillosis B44.89
candidiasis B37.84
moniliasis B37.84
fungoides (extranodal) (solid organ) C84.0- ☑
mouth B37.0
nails B35.1
opportunistic B48.8
skin NEC B36.9
specified NEC B48.8
stomatitis B37.0
vagina, vaginitis (candidal) B37.3
Mydriasis (pupil) H57.04
Myelatelia Q06.1
Myelinolysis, pontine, central G37.2
Myelitis (acute) (ascending) (childhood) (chronic) (descending) (diffuse) (disseminated) (idiopathic) (pressure) (progressive) (spinal cord) (subacute) (*see also* Encephalitis) G04.91
herpes simplex B00.82
herpes zoster B02.24
in diseases classified elsewhere G05.4
necrotizing, subacute G37.4
optic neuritis in G36.0
postchickenpox B01.12

Myelitis — *continued*
postherpetic B02.24
postimmunization G04.02
postinfectious NEC G04.89
postvaccinal G04.02
specified NEC G04.89
syphilitic (transverse) A52.14
toxic G92
transverse (in demyelinating diseases of central nervous system) G37.3
tuberculous A17.82
varicella B01.12
Myeloblastic — *see* condition
Myeloblastoma
granular cell (*see also* Neoplasm, connective tissue)
malignant — *see* Neoplasm, connective tissue, malignant
tongue D10.1
Myelocele — *see* Spina bifida
Myelocystocele — *see* Spina bifida
Myelocytic — *see* condition
Myelodysplasia D46.9
specified NEC D46.Z (*following* D46.4)
spinal cord (congenital) Q06.1
Myelodysplastic syndrome D46.9
with
5q deletion D46.C (*following* D46.2)
isolated del (5q) chromosomal abnormality D46.C (*following* D46.2)
specified NEC D46.Z (*following* D46.4)
Myeloencephalitis — *see* Encephalitis
Myelofibrosis D75.81
with myeloid metaplasia D47.4
acute C94.4- ☑
idiopathic (chronic) D47.4
primary D47.1
secondary D75.81
in myeloproliferative disease D47.4
Myelogenous — *see* condition
Myeloid — *see* condition
Myelokathexis D70.9
Myeloleukodystrophy E75.29
Myelolipoma — *see* Lipoma
Myeloma (multiple) C90.0- ☑
monostotic C90.3 ☑
plasma cell C90.0- ☑
plasma cell C90.0- ☑
solitary (*see also* Plasmacytoma, solitary) C90.3- ☑
Myelomalacia G95.89
Myelomatosis C90.0- ☑
Myelomeningitis — *see* Meningoencephalitis
Myelomeningocele (spinal cord) — *see* Spina bifida
Myelo-osteo-musculodysplasia hereditaria Q79.8
Myelopathic
anemia D64.89
muscle atrophy — *see* Atrophy, muscle, spinal
pain syndrome G89.0
Myelopathy (spinal cord) G95.9
drug-induced G95.89
in (due to)
degeneration or displacement, intervertebral disc NEC — *see* Disorder, disc, with, myelopathy
infection — *see* Encephalitis
intervertebral disc disorder (*see also* Disorder, disc, with, myelopathy)
mercury — *see* subcategory T56.1 ☑
neoplastic disease (*see also* Neoplasm) D49.9 [G99.2]
pernicious anemia D51.0 [G99.2]
spondylosis — *see* Spondylosis, with myelopathy NEC
necrotic (subacute) (vascular) G95.19
radiation-induced G95.89
spondylogenic NEC — *see* Spondylosis, with myelopathy NEC
toxic G95.89
transverse, acute G37.3
vascular G95.19
vitamin B12 E53.8 [G32.0]
Myelophthisis D61.82
Myeloradiculitis G04.91
Myeloradiculodysplasia (spinal) Q06.1
Myelosarcoma C92.3- ☑
Myelosclerosis D75.89
with myeloid metaplasia D47.4
disseminated, of nervous system G35
megakaryocytic D47.4

☑ **Additional Character Required** — Refer to the Tabular List for Character Selection   ▽ **Subterms under main terms may continue to next column or page**

Myelosclerosis — *continued*
  megakaryocytic — *continued*
    with myeloid metaplasia D47.4
Myelosis
  acute C92.0- ☑
  aleukemic C92.9- ☑
  chronic D47.1
  erythremic (acute) C94.0- ☑
  megakaryocytic C94.2- ☑
  nonleukemic D72.828
  subacute C92.9- ☑
Myiasis (cavernous) B87.9
  aural B87.4
  creeping B87.0
  cutaneous B87.0
  dermal B87.0
  ear (external) (middle) B87.4
  eye B87.2
  genitourinary B87.81
  intestinal B87.82
  laryngeal B87.3
  nasopharyngeal B87.3
  ocular B87.2
  orbit B87.2
  skin B87.0
  specified site NEC B87.89
  traumatic B87.1
  wound B87.1
Myoadenoma, prostate — *see* Hyperplasia, prostate
Myoblastoma
  granular cell (*see also* Neoplasm, connective tissue, benign)
    malignant — *see* Neoplasm, connective tissue, malignant
  tongue D10.1
Myocardial — *see* condition
Myocardiopathy (congestive) (constrictive) (familial) (hypertrophic nonobstructive) (idiopathic) (infiltrative) (obstructive) (primary) (restrictive) (sporadic) (*see also* Cardiomyopathy) I42.9
  alcoholic I42.6
  cobalt-beer I42.6
  glycogen storage E74.02 [I43]
  hypertrophic obstructive I42.1
  in (due to)
    beriberi E51.12
    cardiac glycogenosis E74.02 [I43]
    Friedreich's ataxia G11.1 [I43]
    myotonia atrophica G71.11 [I43]
    progressive muscular dystrophy G71.0 [I43]
  obscure (African) I42.8
  secondary I42.9
  thyrotoxic E05.90 [I43]
    with storm E05.91 [I43]
  toxic NEC I42.7
Myocarditis (with arteriosclerosis)(chronic)(fibroid) (interstitial) (old) (progressive) (senile) I51.4
  with
    rheumatic fever (conditions in I00) I09.0
      active — *see* Myocarditis, acute, rheumatic
      inactive or quiescent (with chorea) I09.0
  active I40.9
    rheumatic I01.2
      with chorea (acute) (rheumatic) (Sydenham's) I02.0
  acute or subacute (interstitial) I40.9
    due to
      streptococcus (beta-hemolytic) I01.2
    idiopathic I40.1
    rheumatic I01.2
      with chorea (acute) (rheumatic) (Sydenham's) I02.0
    specified NEC I40.8
  aseptic of newborn B33.22
  bacterial (acute) I40.0
  Coxsackie (virus) B33.22
  diphtheritic A36.81
  eosinophilic I40.1
  epidemic of newborn (Coxsackie) B33.22
  Fiedler's (acute) (isolated) I40.1
  giant cell (acute) (subacute) I40.1
  gonococcal A54.83
  granulomatous (idiopathic) (isolated) (nonspecific) I40.1
  hypertensive — *see* Hypertension, heart
  idiopathic (granulomatous) I40.1
  in (due to)
    diphtheria A36.81

Myocarditis — *continued*
  in — *continued*
    epidemic louse-borne typhus A75.0 [I41]
    Lyme disease A69.29
    sarcoidosis D86.85
    scarlet fever A38.1
    toxoplasmosis (acquired) B58.81
    typhoid A01.02
    typhus NEC A75.9 [I41]
  infective I40.0
  influenzal — *see* Influenza, with, myocarditis
  isolated (acute) I40.1
  meningococcal A39.52
  mumps B26.82
  nonrheumatic, active I40.9
  parenchymatous I40.9
  pneumococcal I40.0
  rheumatic (chronic) (inactive) (with chorea) I09.0
    active or acute I01.2
      with chorea (acute) (rheumatic) (Sydenham's) I02.0
  rheumatoid — *see* Rheumatoid, carditis
  septic I40.0
  staphylococcal I40.0
  suppurative I40.0
  syphilitic (chronic) A52.06
  toxic I40.8
    rheumatic — *see* Myocarditis, acute, rheumatic
  tuberculous A18.84
  typhoid A01.02
  valvular — *see* Endocarditis
  virus, viral I40.0
    of newborn (Coxsackie) B33.22
Myocardium, myocardial — *see* condition
Myocardosis — *see* Cardiomyopathy
Myoclonus, myoclonic, myoclonia (familial) (essential) (multifocal) (simplex) G25.3
  drug-induced G25.3
  epilepsy (*see also* Epilepsy, generalized, specified NEC) G40.4- ☑
    familial (progressive) G25.3
  epileptica G40.409
    with status epilepticus G40.401
  facial G51.3
  familial progressive G25.3
  Friedreich's G25.3
  jerks G25.3
  massive G25.3
  palatal G25.3
  pharyngeal G25.3
Myocytolysis I51.5
Myodiastasis — *see* Diastasis, muscle
Myoendocarditis — *see* Endocarditis
Myoepithelioma — *see* Neoplasm, benign, by site
Myofasciitis (acute) — *see* Myositis
Myofibroma (*see also* Neoplasm, connective tissue, benign)
  uterus (cervix) (corpus) — *see* Leiomyoma
Myofibromatosis D48.1
  infantile Q89.8
Myofibrosis M62.89
  heart — *see* Myocarditis
  scapulohumeral — *see* Lesion, shoulder, specified NEC
Myofibrositis M79.7
  scapulohumeral — *see* Lesion, shoulder, specified NEC
Myoglobulinuria, myoglobinuria (primary) R82.1
Myokymia, facial G51.4
Myolipoma — *see* Lipoma
Myoma (*see also* Neoplasm, connective tissue, benign)
  malignant — *see* Neoplasm, connective tissue, malignant
  prostate D29.1
  uterus (cervix) (corpus) — *see* Leiomyoma
Myomalacia M62.89
Myometritis — *see* Endometritis
Myometrium — *see* condition
Myonecrosis, clostridial A48.0
Myopathy G72.9
  acute
    necrotizing G72.81
      quadriplegic G72.81
  alcoholic G72.1
  benign congenital G71.2
  central core G71.2
  centronuclear G71.2
  congenital (benign) G71.2
  critical illness G72.81
  distal G71.0

Myopathy — *continued*
  drug-induced G72.0
  endocrine NEC E34.9 [G73.7]
  extraocular muscles H05.82- ☑
  facioscapulohumeral G71.0
  hereditary G71.9
    specified NEC G71.8
  immune NEC G72.49
  in (due to)
    Addison's disease E27.1 [G73.7]
    alcohol G72.1
    amyloidosis E85.0 [G73.7]
    cretinism E00.9 [G73.7]
    Cushing's syndrome E24.9 [G73.7]
    drugs G72.0
    endocrine disease NEC E34.9 [G73.7]
    giant cell arteritis M31.6 [G73.7]
    glycogen storage disease E74.00 [G73.7]
    hyperadrenocorticism E24.9 [G73.7]
    hyperparathyroidism NEC E21.3 [G73.7]
    hypoparathyroidism E20.9 [G73.7]
    hypopituitarism E23.0 [G73.7]
    hypothyroidism E03.9 [G73.7]
    infectious disease NEC B99 ☑ [G73.7]
    lipid storage disease E75.6 [G73.7]
    metabolic disease NEC E88.9 [G73.7]
    myxedema E03.9 [G73.7]
    parasitic disease NEC B89 [G73.7]
    polyarteritis nodosa M30.0 [G73.7]
    rheumatoid arthritis — *see* Rheumatoid, myopathy
    sarcoidosis D86.87
    scleroderma M34.82
    sicca syndrome M35.03
    Sjögren's syndrome M35.03
    systemic lupus erythematosus M32.19
    thyrotoxicosis (hyperthyroidism) E05.90 [G73.7]
      with thyroid storm E05.91 [G73.7]
    toxic agent NEC G72.2
  inflammatory NEC G72.49
  intensive care (ICU) G72.81
  limb-girdle G71.0
  mitochondrial NEC G71.3
  myotubular G71.2
  mytonic, proximal (PROMM) G71.11
  nemaline G71.2
  ocular G71.0
  oculopharyngeal G71.0
  of critical illness G72.81
  primary G71.9
    specified NEC G71.8
  progressive NEC G72.89
  proximal myotonic (PROMM) G71.11
  rod G71.2
  scapulohumeral G71.0
  specified NEC G72.89
  toxic G72.2
Myopericarditis (*see also* Pericarditis)
  chronic rheumatic I09.2
Myopia (axial) (congenital) H52.1- ☑
  degenerative (malignant) H44.20
    with
      choroidal neovascularization H44.2A- ☑
      foveoschisis H44.2D- ☑
      macular hole H44.2B- ☑
      retinal detachment H44.2C- ☑
      specified maculopathy NEC H44.2E- ☑
  bilateral H44.23
  left eye H44.22
  right eye H44.21
  malignant (*see also* Myopia, degenerative) H44.2- ☑
  pernicious (*see also* Myopia, degenerative) H44.2- ☑
  progressive high (degenerative) (*see also* Myopia, degenerative) H44.2- ☑
Myosarcoma — *see* Neoplasm, connective tissue, malignant
Myosis (pupil) H57.03
  stromal (endolymphatic) D39.0
Myositis M60.9
  clostridial A48.0
  due to posture — *see* Myositis, specified type NEC
  epidemic B33.0
  fibrosa or fibrous (chronic), Volkmann's T79.6
  foreign body granuloma — *see* Granuloma, foreign body
  in (due to)
    bilharziasis B65.9 [M63.8-] ☑
    cysticercosis B69.81
    leprosy A30.9 [M63.8-] ☑

Myositis — *continued*
  in — *continued*
    mycosis B49 [M63.8-] ☑
    sarcoidosis D86.87
    schistosomiasis B65.9 [M63.8-] ☑
    syphilis
      late A52.78
      secondary A51.49
    toxoplasmosis (acquired) B58.82
    trichinellosis B75 [M63.8-] ☑
    tuberculosis A18.09
  inclusion body [IBM] G72.41
  infective M60.009
    arm M60.002
      left M60.001
      right M60.000
    leg M60.005
      left M60.004
      right M60.003
    lower limb M60.005
      ankle M60.07- ☑
      foot M60.07- ☑
      lower leg M60.06- ☑
      thigh M60.05- ☑
      toe M60.07- ☑
    multiple sites M60.09
    specified site NEC M60.08
    upper limb M60.002
      finger M60.04- ☑
      forearm M60.03- ☑
      hand M60.04- ☑
      shoulder region M60.01- ☑
      upper arm M60.02- ☑
  interstitial M60.10
    ankle M60.17- ☑
    foot M60.17- ☑
    forearm M60.13- ☑
    hand M60.14- ☑
    lower leg M60.16- ☑
    multiple sites M60.19
    shoulder region M60.11- ☑
    specified site NEC M60.18
    thigh M60.15- ☑
    upper arm M60.12- ☑
  mycotic B49 [M63.8-] ☑
  orbital, chronic H05.12- ☑
  ossificans or ossifying (circumscripta) (*see also* Ossification, muscle, specified NEC)
    in (due to)
      burns M61.30
        ankle M61.37- ☑
        foot M61.37- ☑
        forearm M61.33- ☑
        hand M61.34- ☑
        lower leg M61.36- ☑
        multiple sites M61.39
        pelvic region M61.35- ☑

Myositis — *continued*
  ossificans or ossifying (*see also* Ossification, muscle, specified) — *continued*
    in — *continued*
      burns — *continued*
        shoulder region M61.31- ☑
        specified site NEC M61.38
        thigh M61.35- ☑
        upper arm M61.32- ☑
      quadriplegia or paraplegia M61.20
        ankle M61.27- ☑
        foot M61.27- ☑
        forearm M61.23- ☑
        hand M61.24- ☑
        lower leg M61.26- ☑
        multiple sites M61.29
        pelvic region M61.25- ☑
        shoulder region M61.21- ☑
        specified site NEC M61.28
        thigh M61.25- ☑
        upper arm M61.22- ☑
    progressiva M61.10
      ankle M61.17- ☑
      finger M61.14- ☑
      foot M61.17- ☑
      forearm M61.13- ☑
      hand M61.14- ☑
      lower leg M61.16- ☑
      multiple sites M61.19
      pelvic region M61.15- ☑
      shoulder region M61.11- ☑
      specified site NEC M61.18
      thigh M61.15- ☑
      toe M61.17- ☑
      upper arm M61.12- ☑
    traumatica M61.00
      ankle M61.07- ☑
      foot M61.07- ☑
      forearm M61.03- ☑
      hand M61.04- ☑
      lower leg M61.06- ☑
      multiple sites M61.09
      pelvic region M61.05- ☑
      shoulder region M61.01- ☑
      specified site NEC M61.08
      thigh M61.05- ☑
      upper arm M61.02- ☑
  purulent — *see* Myositis, infective
  specified type NEC M60.80
    ankle M60.87- ☑
    foot M60.87- ☑
    forearm M60.83- ☑
    hand M60.84- ☑
    lower leg M60.86- ☑
    multiple sites M60.89
    pelvic region M60.85- ☑
    shoulder region M60.81- ☑

Myositis — *continued*
  specified type — *continued*
    specified site NEC M60.88
    thigh M60.85- ☑
    upper arm M60.82- ☑
  suppurative — *see* Myositis, infective
  traumatic (old) — *see* Myositis, specified type NEC
Myospasia impulsiva F95.2
Myotonia (acquisita) (intermittens) M62.89
  atrophica G71.11
  chondrodystrophic G71.13
  congenita (acetazolamide responsive) (dominant) (recessive) G71.12
  drug-induced G71.14
  dystrophica G71.11
  fluctuans G71.19
  levior G71.12
  permanens G71.19
  symptomatic G71.19
Myotonic pupil — *see* Anomaly, pupil, function, tonic pupil
Myriapodiasis B88.2
Myringitis H73.2- ☑
  with otitis media — *see* Otitis, media
  acute H73.00- ☑
    bullous H73.01- ☑
    specified NEC H73.09- ☑
  bullous — *see* Myringitis, acute, bullous
  chronic H73.1- ☑
Mysophobia F40.228
Mytilotoxism — *see* Poisoning, fish
Myxadenitis labialis K13.0
Myxedema (adult) (idiocy) (infantile) (juvenile) (*see also* Hypothyroidism) E03.9
  circumscribed E05.90
    with storm E05.91
  coma E03.5
  congenital E00.1
  cutis L98.5
  localized (pretibial) E05.90
    with storm E05.91
  papular L98.5
Myxochondrosarcoma — *see* Neoplasm, cartilage, malignant
Myxofibroma — *see* Neoplasm, connective tissue, benign
  odontogenic — *see* Cyst, calcifying odontogenic
Myxofibrosarcoma — *see* Neoplasm, connective tissue, malignant
Myxolipoma D17.9
Myxoliposarcoma — *see* Neoplasm, connective tissue, malignant
Myxoma (*see also* Neoplasm, connective tissue, benign)
  nerve sheath — *see* Neoplasm, nerve, benign
  odontogenic — *see* Cyst, calcifying odontogenic
Myxosarcoma — *see* Neoplasm, connective tissue, malignant

N

Naegeli's
  disease Q82.8
  leukemia, monocytic C93.1- ☑
Naegleriasis (with meningoencephalitis) B60.2
Naffziger's syndrome G54.0
Naga sore — *see* Ulcer, skin
Nägele's pelvis M95.5
  with disproportion (fetopelvic) O33.0
    causing obstructed labor O65.0
Nail (*see also* condition)
  biting F98.8
  patella syndrome Q87.2
Nanism, nanosomia — *see* Dwarfism
Nanophyetiasis B66.8
Nanukayami A27.89
Napkin rash L22
Narcolepsy G47.419
  with cataplexy G47.411
  in conditions classified elsewhere G47.429
    with cataplexy G47.421
Narcosis R06.89
Narcotism — *see* Dependence
NARP (Neuropathy, Ataxia and Retinitis pigmentosa)
  syndrome E88.49
Narrow
  anterior chamber angle H40.03- ☑
  gingival width (of periodontal soft tissue) K05.5
  pelvis — *see* Contraction, pelvis
Narrowing (*see also* Stenosis)
  artery I77.1
    auditory, internal I65.8
    basilar — *see* Occlusion, artery, basilar
    carotid — *see* Occlusion, artery, carotid
    cerebellar — *see* Occlusion, artery, cerebellar
    cerebral — *see* Occlusion artery, cerebral
    choroidal — *see* Occlusion, artery, cerebral, specified NEC
    communicating posterior — *see* Occlusion, artery, cerebral, specified NEC
    coronary (*see also* Disease, heart, ischemic, atherosclerotic)
      congenital Q24.5
      syphilitic A50.54 [I52]
      due to syphilis NEC A52.06
    hypophyseal — *see* Occlusion, artery, cerebral, specified NEC
    pontine — *see* Occlusion, artery, cerebral, specified NEC
    precerebral — *see* Occlusion, artery, precerebral
    vertebral — *see* Occlusion, artery, vertebral
  auditory canal (external) — *see* Stenosis, external ear canal
  eustachian tube — *see* Obstruction, eustachian tube
  eyelid — *see* Disorder, eyelid function
  larynx J38.6
  mesenteric artery (*see also* Ischemia, intestine, acute) K55.059
  palate M26.89
  palpebral fissure — *see* Disorder, eyelid function
  ureter N13.5
    with infection N13.6
  urethra — *see* Stricture, urethra
Narrowness, abnormal, eyelid Q10.3
Nasal — *see* condition
Nasolachrymal, nasolacrimal — *see* condition
Nasopharyngeal (*see also* condition)
  pituitary gland Q89.2
  torticollis M43.6
Nasopharyngitis (acute) (infective) (streptococcal) (subacute) J00
  chronic (suppurative) (ulcerative) J31.1
Nasopharynx, nasopharyngeal — *see* condition
Natal tooth, teeth K00.6
Nausea (without vomiting) R11.0
  with vomiting R11.2
  gravidarum — *see* Hyperemesis, gravidarum
  marina T75.3 ☑
  navalis T75.3 ☑
Navel — *see* condition
Neapolitan fever — *see* Brucellosis
Near drowning T75.1 ☑
Nearsightedness — *see* Myopia
Near-syncope R55
Nebula, cornea — *see* Opacity, cornea

Necator americanus infestation B76.1
Necatoriasis B76.1
Neck — *see* condition
Necrobiosis R68.89
  lipoidica NEC L92.1
    with diabetes — *see* E08-E13 with .620
Necrolysis, toxic epidermal L51.2
  due to drug
    correct substance properly administered — *see* Table of Drugs and Chemicals, by drug, adverse effect
    overdose or wrong substance given or taken — *see* Table of Drugs and Chemicals, by drug, poisoning
Necrophilia F65.89
Necrosis, necrotic (ischemic) (*see also* Gangrene)
  adrenal (capsule) (gland) E27.49
  amputation stump (surgical) (late) T87.50
    arm T87.5- ☑
    leg T87.5- ☑
  antrum J32.0
  aorta (hyaline) (*see also* Aneurysm, aorta)
    cystic medial — *see* Dissection, aorta
  artery I77.5
  bladder (aseptic) (sphincter) N32.89
  bone (*see also* Osteonecrosis) M87.9
    aseptic or avascular — *see* Osteonecrosis
      idiopathic M87.00
    ethmoid J32.2
    jaw M27.2
    tuberculous — *see* Tuberculosis, bone
  brain I67.89
  breast (aseptic) (fat) (segmental) N64.1
  bronchus J98.09
  central nervous system NEC I67.89
  cerebellar I67.89
  cerebral I67.89
  colon (*see also* Infarct, intestine) K55.049
  cornea H18.89- ☑
  cortical (acute) (renal) N17.1
  cystic medial (aorta) — *see* Dissection, aorta
  dental pulp K04.1
  esophagus K22.8
  ethmoid (bone) J32.2
  eyelid — *see* Disorder, eyelid, degenerative
  fat, fatty (generalized) (*see also* Disorder, soft tissue, specified type NEC)
    abdominal wall K65.4
    breast (aseptic) (segmental) N64.1
    localized — *see* Degeneration, by site, fatty
    mesentery K65.4
    omentum K65.4
    pancreas K86.89
    peritoneum K65.4
    skin (subcutaneous), newborn P83.0
    subcutaneous, due to birth injury P15.6
  gallbladder — *see* Cholecystitis, acute
  heart — *see* Infarct, myocardium
  hip, aseptic or avascular — *see* Osteonecrosis, by type, femur
  intestine (acute) (hemorrhagic) (massive) (*see also* Infarct, intestine) K55.069
  jaw M27.2
  kidney (bilateral) N28.0
    acute N17.9
    cortical (acute) (bilateral) N17.1
      with ectopic or molar pregnancy O08.4
    medullary (bilateral) (in acute renal failure) (papillary) N17.2
    papillary (bilateral) (in acute renal failure) N17.2
    tubular N17.0
      with ectopic or molar pregnancy O08.4
      complicating
        abortion — *see* Abortion, by type, complicated by, tubular necrosis
        ectopic or molar pregnancy O08.4
        pregnancy — *see* Pregnancy, complicated by, diseases of, specified type or system NEC
      following ectopic or molar pregnancy O08.4
      traumatic T79.5 ☑
  larynx J38.7
  liver (with hepatic failure) (cell) — *see* Failure, hepatic
    hemorrhagic, central K76.2
  lung J85.0
  lymphatic gland — *see* Lymphadenitis, acute
  mammary gland (fat) (segmental) N64.1
  mastoid (chronic) — *see* Mastoiditis, chronic

Necrosis, necrotic — *continued*
  medullary (acute) (renal) N17.2
  mesentery (*see also* Infarct, intestine) K55.069
    fat K65.4
  mitral valve — *see* Insufficiency, mitral
  myocardium, myocardial — *see* Infarct, myocardium
  nose J34.0
  omentum (with mesenteric infarction) (*see also* Infarct, intestine) K55.069
    fat K65.4
  orbit, orbital — *see* Osteomyelitis, orbit
  ossicles, ear — *see* Abnormal, ear ossicles
  ovary N70.92
  pancreas (aseptic) (duct) (fat) K86.89
    acute (infective) — *see* Pancreatitis, acute
    infective — *see* Pancreatitis, acute
  papillary (acute) (renal) N17.2
  perineum N90.89
  peritoneum (with mesenteric infarction) (*see also* Infarct, intestine) K55.069
    fat K65.4
  pharynx J02.9
    in granulocytopenia — *see* Neutropenia
    Vincent's A69.1
  phosphorus — *see* subcategory T54.2 ☑
  pituitary (gland) E23.0
    postpartum O99.285
    Sheehan O99.285
  pressure — *see* Ulcer, pressure, by site
  pulmonary J85.0
  pulp (dental) K04.1
  radiation — *see* Necrosis, by site
  radium — *see* Necrosis, by site
  renal — *see* Necrosis, kidney
  sclera H15.89
  scrotum N50.89
  skin or subcutaneous tissue NEC I96
  spine, spinal (column) (*see also* Osteonecrosis, by type, vertebra)
    cord G95.19
  spleen D73.5
  stomach K31.89
  stomatitis (ulcerative) A69.0
  subcutaneous fat, newborn P83.88
  subendocardial (acute) I21.4
    chronic I25.89
  suprarenal (capsule) (gland) E27.49
  testis N50.89
  thymus (gland) E32.8
  tonsil J35.8
  trachea J39.8
  tuberculous NEC — *see* Tuberculosis
  tubular (acute) (anoxic) (renal) (toxic) N17.0
    postprocedural N99.0
  vagina N89.8
  vertebra (*see also* Osteonecrosis, by type, vertebra)
    tuberculous A18.01
  vulva N90.89
  X-ray — *see* Necrosis, by site
Necrospermia — *see* Infertility, male
Need (for)
  care provider because (of)
    assistance with personal care Z74.1
    continuous supervision required Z74.3
    impaired mobility Z74.09
    no other household member able to render care Z74.2
    specified reason NEC Z74.8
  immunization — *see* Vaccination
  vaccination — *see* Vaccination
Neglect
  adult
    confirmed T74.01 ☑
    history of Z91.412
    suspected T76.01 ☑
  child (childhood)
    confirmed T74.02 ☑
    history of Z62.812
    suspected T76.02 ☑
  emotional, in childhood Z62.898
  hemispatial R41.4
  left-sided R41.4
  sensory R41.4
  visuospatial R41.4
Neisserian infection NEC — *see* Gonococcus
Nelaton's syndrome G60.8
Nelson's syndrome E24.1
Nematodiasis (intestinal) B82.0

Nematodiasis — continued
Ancylostoma B76.0
Neonatal (see also Newborn)
acne L70.4
bradycardia P29.12
screening, abnormal findings on P09
tachycardia P29.11
tooth, teeth K00.6
Neonatorum — see condition
Neoplasia
endocrine, multiple (MEN) E31.20
type I E31.21
type IIA E31.22
type IIB E31.23
intraepithelial (histologically confirmed)
anal (AIN) (histologically confirmed) K62.82
grade I K62.82
grade II K62.82
severe D01.3
cervical glandular (histologically confirmed) D06.9
cervix (uteri) (CIN) (histologically confirmed) N87.9
glandular D06.9
grade I N87.0
grade II N87.1
grade III (severe dysplasia) (see also Carcinoma, cervix uteri, in situ) D06.9
prostate (histologically confirmed) (PIN) N42.31
grade I N42.31
grade II N42.31
grade III (severe dysplasia) D07.5
vagina (histologically confirmed) (VAIN) N89.3
grade I N89.0
grade II N89.1
grade III (severe dysplasia) D07.2
vulva (histologically confirmed) (VIN) N90.3
grade I N90.0
grade II N90.1
grade III (severe dysplasia) D07.1
Neoplasm, neoplastic (see also Table of Neoplasms)
lipomatous, benign — see Lipoma
malignant mast cell C96.20
specified type NEC C96.29
mast cell, of uncertain behavior NEC D47.09
Neovascularization
ciliary body — see Disorder, iris, vascular
cornea H16.40- ☑
deep H16.44- ☑
ghost vessels — see Ghost, vessels
localized H16.43- ☑
pannus — see Pannus
iris — see Disorder, iris, vascular
retina H35.05- ☑
Nephralgia N23
Nephritis, nephritic (albuminuric) (azotemic) (congenital) (disseminated) (epithelial) (familial) (focal) (granulomatous) (hemorrhagic) (infantile) (nonsuppurative, excretory) (uremic) N05.9
with
dense deposit disease N05.6
diffuse
crescentic glomerulonephritis N05.7
endocapillary proliferative glomerulonephritis N05.4
membranous glomerulonephritis N05.2
mesangial proliferative glomerulonephritis N05.3
mesangiocapillary glomerulonephritis N05.5
edema — see Nephrosis
focal and segmental glomerular lesions N05.1
foot process disease N04.9
glomerular lesion
diffuse sclerosing N05.8
hypocomplementemic — see Nephritis, membranoproliferative
IgA — see Nephropathy, IgA
lobular, lobulonodular — see Nephritis, membranoproliferative
nodular — see Nephritis, membranoproliferative
lesion of
glomerulonephritis, proliferative N05.8
renal necrosis N05.9
minor glomerular abnormality N05.0
specified morphological changes NEC N05.8
acute N00.9
with
dense deposit disease N00.6

Nephritis, nephritic — continued
acute — continued
with — continued
diffuse
crescentic glomerulonephritis N00.7
endocapillary proliferative glomerulonephritis N00.4
membranous glomerulonephritis N00.2
mesangial proliferative glomerulonephritis N00.3
mesangiocapillary glomerulonephritis N00.5
focal and segmental glomerular lesions N00.1
minor glomerular abnormality N00.0
specified morphological changes NEC N00.8
amyloid E85.4 [N08]
antiglomerular basement membrane (anti-GBM) antibody NEC
in Goodpasture's syndrome M31.0
antitubular basement membrane (tubulo-interstitial) NEC N12
toxic — see Nephropathy, toxic
arteriolar — see Hypertension, kidney
arteriosclerotic — see Hypertension, kidney
ascending — see Nephritis, tubulo-interstitial
atrophic N03.9
Balkan (endemic) N15.0
calculous, calculus — see Calculus, kidney
cardiac — see Hypertension, kidney
cardiovascular — see Hypertension, kidney
chronic N03.9
with
dense deposit disease N03.6
diffuse
crescentic glomerulonephritis N03.7
endocapillary proliferative glomerulonephritis N03.4
membranous glomerulonephritis N03.2
mesangial proliferative glomerulonephritis N03.3
mesangiocapillary glomerulonephritis N03.5
focal and segmental glomerular lesions N03.1
minor glomerular abnormality N03.0
specified morphological changes NEC N03.8
arteriosclerotic — see Hypertension, kidney
cirrhotic N26.9
complicating pregnancy O26.83- ☑
croupous N00.9
degenerative — see Nephrosis
diffuse sclerosing N05.8
due to
diabetes mellitus — see E08-E13 with .21
subacute bacterial endocarditis I33.0
systemic lupus erythematosus (chronic) M32.14
typhoid fever A01.09
gonococcal (acute) (chronic) A54.21
hypocomplementemic — see Nephritis, membranoproliferative
IgA — see Nephropathy, IgA
immune complex (circulating) NEC N05.8
infective — see Nephritis, tubulo-interstitial
interstitial — see Nephritis, tubulo-interstitial
lead N14.3
membranoproliferative (diffuse) (type 1 or 3) (see also N00-N07 with fourth character .5) N05.5
type 2 (see also N00-N07 with fourth character .6) N05.6
minimal change N05.0
necrotic, necrotizing NEC (see also N00-N07 with fourth character .8) N05.8
nephrotic — see Nephrosis
nodular — see Nephritis, membranoproliferative
polycystic Q61.3
adult type Q61.2
autosomal
dominant Q61.2
recessive NEC Q61.19
childhood type NEC Q61.19
infantile type NEC Q61.19
poststreptococcal N05.9
acute N00.9
chronic N03.9
rapidly progressive N01.9
proliferative NEC (see also N00-N07 with fourth character .8) N05.8
purulent — see Nephritis, tubulo-interstitial
rapidly progressive N01.9
with
dense deposit disease N01.6

Nephritis, nephritic — continued
rapidly progressive — continued
with — continued
diffuse
crescentic glomerulonephritis N01.7
endocapillary proliferative glomerulonephritis N01.4
membranous glomerulonephritis N01.2
mesangial proliferative glomerulonephritis N01.3
mesangiocapillary glomerulonephritis N01.5
focal and segmental glomerular lesions N01.1
minor glomerular abnormality N01.0
specified morphological changes NEC N01.8
salt losing or wasting N28.89
saturnine N14.3
sclerosing, diffuse N05.8
septic — see Nephritis, tubulo-interstitial
specified pathology NEC (see also N00-N07 with fourth character .8) N05.8
subacute N01.9
suppurative — see Nephritis, tubulo-interstitial
syphilitic (late) A52.75
congenital A50.59 [N08]
early (secondary) A51.44
toxic — see Nephropathy, toxic
tubal, tubular — see Nephritis, tubulo-interstitial
tuberculous A18.11
tubulo-interstitial (in) N12
acute (infectious) N10
chronic (infectious) N11.9
nonobstructive N11.8
reflux-associated N11.0
obstructive N11.1
specified NEC N11.8
due to
brucellosis A23.9 [N16]
cryoglobulinemia D89.1 [N16]
glycogen storage disease E74.00 [N16]
Sjögren's syndrome M35.04
vascular — see Hypertension, kidney
war N00.9
Nephroblastoma (epithelial) (mesenchymal) C64- ☑
Nephrocalcinosis E83.59 [N29]
Nephrocystitis, pustular — see Nephritis, tubulo-interstitial
Nephrolithiasis (congenital) (pelvis) (recurrent) (see also Calculus, kidney)
Nephroma C64- ☑
mesoblastic D41.0- ☑
Nephronephritis — see Nephrosis
Nephronophthisis Q61.5
Nephropathia epidemica A98.5
Nephropathy (see also Nephritis) N28.9
with
edema — see Nephrosis
glomerular lesion — see Glomerulonephritis
amyloid, hereditary E85.0
analgesic N14.0
with medullary necrosis, acute N17.2
Balkan (endemic) N15.0
chemical — see Nephropathy, toxic
diabetic — see E08-E13 with .21
drug-induced N14.2
specified NEC N14.1
focal and segmental hyalinosis or sclerosis N02.1
heavy metal-induced N14.3
hereditary NEC N07.9
with
dense deposit disease N07.6
diffuse
crescentic glomerulonephritis N07.7
endocapillary proliferative glomerulonephritis N07.4
membranous glomerulonephritis N07.2
mesangial proliferative glomerulonephritis N07.3
mesangiocapillary glomerulonephritis N07.5
focal and segmental glomerular lesions N07.1
minor glomerular abnormality N07.0
specified morphological changes NEC N07.8
hypercalcemic N25.89
hypertensive — see Hypertension, kidney
hypokalemic (vacuolar) N25.89
IgA N02.8
with glomerular lesion N02.9
focal and segmental hyalinosis or sclerosis N02.1

☑ **Additional Character Required** — Refer to the Tabular List for Character Selection   ▽ **Subterms under main terms may continue to next column or page**

Nephropathy — *continued*
  IgA — *continued*
    with glomerular lesion — *continued*
      membranoproliferative (diffuse) N02.5
      membranous (diffuse) N02.2
      mesangial proliferative (diffuse) N02.3
      mesangiocapillary (diffuse) N02.5
      proliferative NEC N02.8
      specified pathology NEC N02.8
  lead N14.3
  membranoproliferative (diffuse) N02.5
  membranous (diffuse) N02.2
  mesangial (IgA/IgG) — *see* Nephropathy, IgA
    proliferative (diffuse) N02.3
  mesangiocapillary (diffuse) N02.5
  obstructive N13.8
  phenacetin N17.2
  phosphate-losing N25.0
  potassium depletion N25.89
  pregnancy-related O26.83- ☑
  proliferative NEC (*see also* N00-N07 with fourth character .8) N05.8
  protein-losing N25.89
  saturnine N14.3
  sickle-cell D57.- ☑ [N08]
  toxic NEC N14.4
    due to
      drugs N14.2
        analgesic N14.0
        specified NEC N14.1
      heavy metals N14.3
  vasomotor N17.0
  water-losing N25.89
Nephroptosis N28.83
Nephropyosis — *see* Abscess, kidney
Nephrorrhagia N28.89
Nephrosclerosis (arteriolar)(arteriosclerotic) (chronic) (hyaline) (*see also* Hypertension, kidney)
  hyperplastic — *see* Hypertension, kidney
  senile N26.9
Nephrosis, nephrotic (Epstein's) (syndrome) (congenital) N04.9
  with
    foot process disease N04.9
    glomerular lesion N04.1
    hypocomplementemic N04.5
  acute N04.9
  anoxic — *see* Nephrosis, tubular
  chemical — *see* Nephrosis, tubular
  cholemic K76.7
  diabetic — *see* E08-E13 with .21
  Finnish type (congenital) Q89.8
  hemoglobin N10
  hemoglobinuric — *see* Nephrosis, tubular
  in
    amyloidosis E85.4 [N08]
    diabetes mellitus — *see* E08-E13 with .21
    epidemic hemorrhagic fever A98.5
    malaria (malariae) B52.0
  ischemic — *see* Nephrosis, tubular
  lipoid N04.9
  lower nephron — *see* Nephrosis, tubular
  malarial (malariae) B52.0
  minimal change N04.0
  myoglobin N10
  necrotizing — *see* Nephrosis, tubular
  osmotic (sucrose) N25.89
  radiation N04.9
  syphilitic (late) A52.75
  toxic — *see* Nephrosis, tubular
  tubular (acute) N17.0
    postprocedural N99.0
    radiation N04.9
Nephrosonephritis, hemorrhagic (endemic) A98.5
Nephrostomy
  attention to Z43.6
  status Z93.6
Nerve (*see also* condition)
  injury — *see* Injury, nerve, by body site
Nerves R45.0
Nervous (*see also* condition) R45.0
  heart F45.8
  stomach F45.8
  tension R45.0
Nervousness R45.0
Nesidioblastoma
  pancreas D13.7
  specified site NEC — *see* Neoplasm, benign, by site

Nesidioblastoma — *continued*
  unspecified site D13.7
Nettleship's syndrome — *see* Urticaria pigmentosa
Neumann's disease or syndrome L10.1
Neuralgia, neuralgic (acute) M79.2
  accessory (nerve) G52.8
  acoustic (nerve) — *see* subcategory H93.3 ☑
  auditory (nerve) — *see* subcategory H93.3 ☑
  ciliary G44.009
    intractable G44.001
    not intractable G44.009
  cranial
    nerve (*see also* Disorder, nerve, cranial)
      fifth or trigeminal — *see* Neuralgia, trigeminal
      postherpetic, postzoster B02.29
  ear — *see* subcategory H92.0 ☑
  facialis vera G51.1
  Fothergill's — *see* Neuralgia, trigeminal
  glossopharyngeal (nerve) G52.1
  Horton's G44.009
    intractable G44.091
    not intractable G44.099
  Hunt's B02.21
  hypoglossal (nerve) G52.3
  infraorbital — *see* Neuralgia, trigeminal
  malarial — *see* Malaria
  migrainous G44.009
    intractable G44.001
    not intractable G44.009
  Morton's G57.6- ☑
  nerve, cranial — *see* Disorder, nerve, cranial
  nose G52.0
  occipital M54.81
  olfactory G52.0
  penis N48.9
  perineum R10.2
  postherpetic NEC B02.29
    trigeminal B02.22
  pubic region R10.2
  scrotum R10.2
  Sluder's G44.89
  specified nerve NEC G58.8
  spermatic cord R10.2
  sphenopalatine (ganglion) G90.09
  trifacial — *see* Neuralgia, trigeminal
  trigeminal G50.0
    postherpetic, postzoster B02.22
  vagus (nerve) G52.2
  writer's F48.8
    organic G25.89
Neurapraxia — *see* Injury, nerve
Neurasthenia F48.8
  cardiac F45.8
  gastric F45.8
  heart F45.8
Neurilemmoma (*see also* Neoplasm, nerve, benign)
  acoustic (nerve) D33.3
  malignant (*see also* Neoplasm, nerve, malignant)
    acoustic (nerve) C72.4- ☑
Neurilemmosarcoma — *see* Neoplasm, nerve, malignant
Neurinoma — *see* Neoplasm, nerve, benign
Neurinomatosis — *see* Neoplasm, nerve, uncertain behavior
Neuritis (rheumatoid) M79.2
  abducens (nerve) — *see* Strabismus, paralytic, sixth nerve
  accessory (nerve) G52.8
  acoustic (nerve) (*see also* subcategory H93.3 ☑
    in (due to)
      infectious disease NEC B99 ☑ [H94.0-] ☑
      parasitic disease NEC B89 [H94.0-] ☑
    syphilitic A52.15
  alcoholic G62.1
    with psychosis — *see* Psychosis, alcoholic
  amyloid, any site E85.4 [G63]
  auditory (nerve) — *see* subcategory H93.3 ☑
  brachial — *see* Radiculopathy
    due to displacement, intervertebral disc — *see* Disorder, disc, cervical, with neuritis
  cranial nerve
    due to Lyme disease A69.22
    eighth or acoustic or auditory — *see* subcategory H93.3 ☑
    eleventh or accessory G52.8
    fifth or trigeminal G51.0
    first or olfactory G52.0

Neuritis — *continued*
  cranial nerve — *continued*
    fourth or trochlear — *see* Strabismus, paralytic, fourth nerve
    second or optic — *see* Neuritis, optic
    seventh or facial G51.8
      newborn (birth injury) P11.3
    sixth or abducent — *see* Strabismus, paralytic, sixth nerve
    tenth or vagus G52.2
    third or oculomotor — *see* Strabismus, paralytic, third nerve
    twelfth or hypoglossal G52.3
  Déjérine-Sottas G60.0
  diabetic (mononeuropathy) — *see* E08-E13 with .41
    polyneuropathy — *see* E08-E13 with .42
  due to
    beriberi E51.11
    displacement, prolapse or rupture, intervertebral disc — *see* Disorder, disc, with, radiculopathy
    herniation, nucleus pulposus M51.9 [G55]
  endemic E51.11
  facial G51.8
    newborn (birth injury) P11.3
  general — *see* Polyneuropathy
  geniculate ganglion G51.1
    due to herpes (zoster) B02.21
  gouty (*see also* Gout, by type) M10.9 [G63]
  hypoglossal (nerve) G52.3
  ilioinguinal (nerve) G57.9- ☑
  infectious (multiple) NEC G61.0
  interstitial hypertrophic progressive G60.0
  lumbar M54.16
  lumbosacral M54.17
  multiple (*see also* Polyneuropathy)
    endemic E51.11
    infective, acute G61.0
  multiplex endemica E51.11
  nerve root — *see* Radiculopathy
  oculomotor (nerve) — *see* Strabismus, paralytic, third nerve
  olfactory nerve G52.0
  optic (nerve) (hereditary) (sympathetic) H46.9
    with demyelination G36.0
    in myelitis G36.0
    nutritional H46.2
    papillitis — *see* Papillitis, optic
    retrobulbar H46.1- ☑
    specified type NEC H46.8
    toxic H46.3
  peripheral (nerve) G62.9
    multiple — *see* Polyneuropathy
    single — *see* Mononeuritis
  pneumogastric (nerve) G52.2
  postherpetic, postzoster B02.29
  progressive hypertrophic interstitial G60.0
  retrobulbar (*see also* Neuritis, optic, retrobulbar)
    in (due to)
      late syphilis A52.15
      meningococcal infection A39.82
    meningococcal A39.82
    syphilitic A52.15
  sciatic (nerve) (*see also* Sciatica)
    due to displacement of intervertebral disc — *see* Disorder, disc, with, radiculopathy
  serum (*see also* Reaction, serum) T80.69 ☑
  shoulder-girdle G54.5
  specified nerve NEC G58.8
  spinal (nerve) root — *see* Radiculopathy
  syphilitic A52.15
  thenar (median) G56.1- ☑
  thoracic M54.14
  toxic NEC G62.2
  trochlear (nerve) — *see* Strabismus, paralytic, fourth nerve
  vagus (nerve) G52.2
Neuroastrocytoma — *see* Neoplasm, uncertain behavior, by site
Neuroavitaminosis E56.9 [G99.8]
Neuroblastoma
  olfactory C30.0
  specified site — *see* Neoplasm, malignant, by site
  unspecified site C74.90
Neurochorioretinitis — *see* Chorioretinitis
Neurocirculatory asthenia F45.8
Neurocysticercosis B69.0
Neurocytoma — *see* Neoplasm, benign, by site

Neurodermatitis (circumscribed) (circumscripta) (local) L28.0
  atopic L20.81
  diffuse (Brocq) L20.81
  disseminated L20.81
Neuroencephalomyelopathy, optic G36.0
Neuroepithelioma (see also Neoplasm, malignant, by site)
  olfactory C30.0
Neurofibroma (see also Neoplasm, nerve, benign)
  melanotic — see Neoplasm, nerve, benign
  multiple — see Neurofibromatosis
  plexiform — see Neoplasm, nerve, benign
Neurofibromatosis (multiple) (nonmalignant) Q85.00
  acoustic Q85.02
  malignant — see Neoplasm, nerve, malignant
  specified NEC Q85.09
  type 1 (von Recklinghausen) Q85.01
  type 2 Q85.02
Neurofibrosarcoma — see Neoplasm, nerve, malignant
Neurogenic (see also condition)
  bladder (see also Dysfunction, bladder, neuromuscular) N31.9
    cauda equina syndrome G83.4
  bowel NEC K59.2
  heart F45.8
Neuroglioma — see Neoplasm, uncertain behavior, by site
Neurolabyrinthitis (of Dix and Hallpike) — see Neuronitis, vestibular
Neurolathyrism — see Poisoning, food, noxious, plant
Neuroleprosy A30.9
Neuroma (see also Neoplasm, nerve, benign)
  acoustic (nerve) D33.3
  amputation (stump) (traumatic) (surgical complication) (late) T87.3- ☑
    arm T87.3- ☑
    leg T87.3- ☑
  digital (toe) G57.6- ☑
  interdigital G58.8
    lower limb (toe) G57.8- ☑
    upper limb G56.8- ☑
  intermetatarsal G57.8- ☑
  Morton's G57.6- ☑
  nonneoplastic
    arm G56.9- ☑
    leg G57.9- ☑
    lower extremity G57.9- ☑
    upper extremity G56.9- ☑
  optic (nerve) D33.3
  plantar G57.6- ☑
  plexiform — see Neoplasm, nerve, benign
  surgical (nonneoplastic)
    arm G56.9- ☑
    leg G57.9- ☑
    lower extremity G57.9- ☑
    upper extremity G56.9- ☑
Neuromyalgia — see Neuralgia
Neuromyasthenia (epidemic) (postinfectious) G93.3
Neuromyelitis G36.9
  ascending G61.0
  optica G36.0
Neuromyopathy G70.9
  paraneoplastic D49.9 [G13.0]
Neuromyotonia (Isaacs) G71.19
Neuronevus — see Nevus
Neuronitis G58.9
  ascending (acute) G57.2- ☑
  vestibular H81.2- ☑
Neuroparalytic — see condition
Neuropathy, neuropathic G62.9
  acute motor G62.81
  alcoholic G62.1
    with psychosis — see Psychosis, alcoholic
  arm G56.9- ☑
  autonomic, peripheral — see Neuropathy, peripheral, autonomic
  axillary G56.9- ☑
  bladder N31.9
    atonic (motor) (sensory) N31.2
    autonomous N31.2
    flaccid N31.2
    nonreflex N31.2
    reflex N31.1
    uninhibited N31.0
  brachial plexus G54.0
  cervical plexus G54.2

Neuropathy, neuropathic — continued
  chronic
    progressive segmentally demyelinating G62.89
    relapsing demyelinating G62.89
  Déjérine-Sottas G60.0
  diabetic — see E08-E13 with .40
    mononeuropathy — see E08-E13 with .41
    polyneuropathy — see E08-E13 with .42
  entrapment G58.9
    iliohypogastric nerve G57.8- ☑
    ilioinguinal nerve G57.8- ☑
    lateral cutaneous nerve of thigh G57.1- ☑
    median nerve G56.0- ☑
    obturator nerve G57.8- ☑
    peroneal nerve G57.3- ☑
    posterior tibial nerve G57.5- ☑
    saphenous nerve G57.8- ☑
    ulnar nerve G56.2- ☑
  facial nerve G51.9
  hereditary G60.9
    motor and sensory (types I-IV) G60.0
    sensory G60.8
    specified NEC G60.8
  hypertrophic G60.0
    Charcot-Marie-Tooth G60.0
    Déjérine-Sottas G60.0
    interstitial progressive G60.0
    of infancy G60.0
    Refsum G60.1
  idiopathic G60.9
    progressive G60.3
    specified NEC G60.8
  in association with hereditary ataxia G60.2
  intercostal G58.0
  ischemic — see Disorder, nerve
  Jamaica (ginger) G62.2
  leg NEC G57.9- ☑
  lower extremity G57.9- ☑
  lumbar plexus G54.1
  median nerve G56.1- ☑
  motor and sensory (see also Polyneuropathy)
    hereditary (types I-IV) G60.0
  multifocal motor (MMN) G61.82
  multiple (acute) (chronic) — see Polyneuropathy
  optic (nerve) (see also Neuritis, optic)
    ischemic H47.01- ☑
  paraneoplastic (sensorial) (Denny Brown) D49.9 [G13.0]
  peripheral (nerve) (see also Polyneuropathy) G62.9
    autonomic G90.9
      idiopathic G90.09
      in (due to)
        amyloidosis E85.4 [G99.0]
        diabetes mellitus — see E08-E13 with .43
        endocrine disease NEC E34.9 [G99.0]
        gout M10.00 [G99.0]
        hyperthyroidism E05.90 [G99.0]
          with thyroid storm E05.91 [G99.0]
        metabolic disease NEC E88.9 [G99.0]
    idiopathic G60.9
      progressive G60.3
    in (due to)
      antitetanus serum G62.0
      arsenic G62.2
      drugs NEC G62.0
      lead G62.2
      organophosphate compounds G62.2
      toxic agent NEC G62.2
  plantar nerves G57.6- ☑
  progressive
    hypertrophic interstitial G60.0
    inflammatory G62.81
  radicular NEC — see Radiculopathy
  sacral plexus G54.1
  sciatic G57.0- ☑
  serum G61.1
  toxic NEC G62.2
  trigeminal sensory G50.8
  ulnar nerve G56.2- ☑
  uremic N18.9 [G63]
  vitamin B12 E53.8 [G63]
    with anemia (pernicious) D51.0 [G63]
    due to dietary deficiency D51.3 [G63]
Neurophthisis (see also Disorder, nerve)
  peripheral, diabetic — see E08-E13 with .42
Neuroretinitis — see Chorioretinitis
Neuroretinopathy, hereditary optic H47.22
Neurosarcoma — see Neoplasm, nerve, malignant
Neurosclerosis — see Disorder, nerve

Neurosis, neurotic F48.9
  anankastic F42.8
  anxiety (state) F41.1
    panic type F41.0
  asthenic F48.8
  bladder F45.8
  cardiac (reflex) F45.8
  cardiovascular F45.8
  character F60.9
  colon F45.8
  compensation F68.1 ☑
  compulsive, compulsion F42.8
  conversion F44.9
  craft F48.8
  cutaneous F45.8
  depersonalization F48.1
  depressive (reaction) (type) F34.1
  environmental F48.8
  excoriation L98.1
  fatigue F48.8
  functional — see Disorder, somatoform
  gastric F45.8
  gastrointestinal F45.8
  heart F45.8
  hypochondriacal F45.21
  hysterical F44.9
  incoordination F45.8
    larynx F45.8
    vocal cord F45.8
  intestine F45.8
  larynx (sensory) F45.8
    hysterical F44.4
  mixed NEC F48.8
  musculoskeletal F45.8
  obsessional F42.8
  obsessive-compulsive F42.8
  occupational F48.8
  ocular NEC F45.8
  organ — see Disorder, somatoform
  pharynx F45.8
  phobic F40.9
  posttraumatic (situational) F43.10
    acute F43.11
    chronic F43.12
  psychasthenic (type) F48.8
  railroad F48.8
  rectum F45.8
  respiratory F45.8
  rumination F45.8
  sexual F65.9
  situational F48.8
  social F40.10
    generalized F40.11
  specified type NEC F48.8
  state F48.9
    with depersonalization episode F48.1
  stomach F45.8
  traumatic F43.10
    acute F43.11
    chronic F43.12
  vasomotor F45.8
  visceral F45.8
  war F48.8
Neurospongioblastosis diffusa Q85.1
Neurosyphilis (arrested) (early) (gumma) (late) (latent) (recurrent) (relapse) A52.3
  with ataxia (cerebellar) (locomotor) (spastic) (spinal) A52.19
  aneurysm (cerebral) A52.05
  arachnoid (adhesive) A52.13
  arteritis (any artery) (cerebral) A52.04
  asymptomatic A52.2
  congenital A50.40
  dura (mater) A52.13
  general paresis A52.17
  hemorrhagic A52.05
  juvenile (asymptomatic) (meningeal) A50.40
  leptomeninges (aseptic) A52.13
  meningeal, meninges (adhesive) A52.13
  meningitis A52.13
  meningovascular (diffuse) A52.13
  optic atrophy A52.15
  parenchymatous (degenerative) A52.19
  paresis, paretic A52.17
    juvenile A50.45
  remission in (sustained) A52.3
  serological (without symptoms) A52.2
  specified nature or site NEC A52.19
  tabes, tabetic (dorsalis) A52.11

Neurosyphilis — *continued*
tabes, tabetic — *continued*
juvenile A50.45
taboparesis A52.17
juvenile A50.45
thrombosis (cerebral) A52.05
vascular (cerebral) NEC A52.05
Neurothekeoma — *see* Neoplasm, nerve, benign
Neurotic — *see* Neurosis
Neurotoxemia — *see* Toxemia
Neutroclusion M26.211
Neutropenia, neutropenic (chronic) (genetic) (idiopathic) (immune) (infantile) (malignant) (pernicious) (splenic) D70.9
congenital (primary) D70.0
cyclic D70.4
cytoreductive cancer chemotherapy sequela D70.1
drug-induced D70.2
due to cytoreductive cancer chemotherapy D70.1
due to infection D70.3
fever D70.9
neonatal, transitory (isoimmune) (maternal transfer) P61.5
periodic D70.4
secondary (cyclic) (periodic) (splenic) D70.4
drug-induced D70.2
due to cytoreductive cancer chemotherapy D70.1
toxic D70.8
Neutrophilia, hereditary giant D72.0
Nevocarcinoma — *see* Melanoma
Nevus D22.9
achromic — *see* Neoplasm, skin, benign
amelanotic — *see* Neoplasm, skin, benign
angiomatous D18.00
intra-abdominal D18.03
intracranial D18.02
skin D18.01
specified site NEC D18.09
araneus I78.1
balloon cell — *see* Neoplasm, skin, benign
bathing trunk D48.5
blue — *see* Neoplasm, skin, benign
cellular — *see* Neoplasm, skin, benign
giant — *see* Neoplasm, skin, benign
Jadassohn's — *see* Neoplasm, skin, benign
malignant — *see* Melanoma
capillary D18.00
intra-abdominal D18.03
intracranial D18.02
skin D18.01
specified site NEC D18.09
cavernous D18.00
intra-abdominal D18.03
intracranial D18.02
skin D18.01
specified site NEC D18.09
cellular — *see* Neoplasm, skin, benign
blue — *see* Neoplasm, skin, benign
choroid D31.3- ☑
comedonicus Q82.5
conjunctiva D31.0- ☑
dermal — *see* Neoplasm, skin, benign
with epidermal nevus — *see* Neoplasm, skin, benign
dysplastic — *see* Neoplasm, skin, benign
eye D31.9- ☑
flammeus Q82.5
hemangiomatous D18.00
intra-abdominal D18.03
intracranial D18.02
skin D18.01
specified site NEC D18.09
iris D31.4- ☑
lacrimal gland D31.5- ☑
lymphatic D18.1
magnocellular
specified site — *see* Neoplasm, benign, by site
unspecified site D31.40
malignant — *see* Melanoma
meaning hemangioma D18.00
intra-abdominal D18.03
intracranial D18.02
skin D18.01
specified site NEC D18.09
mouth (mucosa) D10.30
specified site NEC D10.39
white sponge Q38.6

Nevus — *continued*
multiplex Q85.1
non-neoplastic I78.1
oral mucosa D10.30
specified site NEC D10.39
white sponge Q38.6
orbit D31.6- ☑
pigmented
giant (*see also* Neoplasm, skin, uncertain behavior) D48.5
malignant melanoma in — *see* Melanoma
portwine Q82.5
retina D31.2- ☑
retrobulbar D31.6- ☑
sanguineous Q82.5
senile I78.1
skin D22.9
abdominal wall D22.5
ala nasi D22.39
ankle D22.7- ☑
anus, anal D22.5
arm D22.6- ☑
auditory canal (external) D22.2- ☑
auricle (ear) D22.2- ☑
auricular canal (external) D22.2- ☑
axilla, axillary fold D22.5
back D22.5
breast D22.5
brow D22.39
buttock D22.5
canthus (eye) D22.1- ☑
cheek (external) D22.39
chest wall D22.5
chin D22.39
ear (external) D22.2- ☑
external meatus (ear) D22.2- ☑
eyebrow D22.39
eyelid (lower) (upper) D22.1- ☑
face D22.30
specified NEC D22.39
female genital organ (external) NEC D28.0
finger D22.6- ☑
flank D22.5
foot D22.7- ☑
forearm D22.6- ☑
forehead D22.39
foreskin D29.0
genital organ (external) NEC
female D28.0
male D29.9
gluteal region D22.5
groin D22.5
hand D22.6- ☑
heel D22.7- ☑
helix D22.2- ☑
hip D22.7- ☑
interscapular region D22.5
jaw D22.39
knee D22.7- ☑
labium (majus) (minus) D28.0
leg D22.7- ☑
lip (lower) (upper) D22.0
lower limb D22.7- ☑
male genital organ (external) D29.9
nail D22.9
finger D22.6- ☑
toe D22.7- ☑
nasolabial groove D22.39
nates D22.5
neck D22.4
nose (external) D22.39
palpebra D22.1- ☑
penis D29.0
perianal skin D22.5
perineum D22.5
pinna D22.2- ☑
popliteal fossa or space D22.7- ☑
prepuce D29.0
pudendum D28.0
scalp D22.4
scrotum D29.4
shoulder D22.6- ☑
submammary fold D22.5
temple D22.39
thigh D22.7- ☑
toe D22.7- ☑
trunk NEC D22.5

Nevus — *continued*
skin — *continued*
umbilicus D22.5
upper limb D22.6- ☑
vulva D28.0
specified site NEC — *see* Neoplasm, by site, benign
spider I78.1
stellar I78.1
strawberry Q82.5
Sutton's benign D22.9
unius lateris Q82.5
Unna's Q82.5
vascular Q82.5
verrucous Q82.5
Newborn (infant) (liveborn) (singleton) Z38.2
abstinence syndrome P96.1
acne L70.4
affected by
abnormalities of membranes P02.9
specified NEC P02.8
abruptio placenta P02.1
amino-acid metabolic disorder, transitory P74.8
amniocentesis (while in utero) P00.6
amnionitis P02.7
apparent life threatening event (ALTE) R68.13
bleeding (into)
cerebral cortex P52.22
germinal matrix P52.0
ventricles P52.1
breech delivery P03.0
cardiac arrest P29.81
cardiomyopathy I42.8
congenital I42.4
cerebral ischemia P91.0
Cesarean delivery P03.4
chemotherapy agents P04.1
chorioamnionitis P02.7
cocaine (crack) P04.41
complications of labor and delivery P03.9
specified NEC P03.89
compression of umbilical cord NEC P02.5
contracted pelvis P03.1
delivery P03.9
Cesarean P03.4
forceps P03.2
vacuum extractor P03.3
entanglement (knot) in umbilical cord P02.5
environmental chemicals P04.6
fetal (intrauterine)
growth retardation P05.9
malnutrition not light or small for gestational age P05.2
forceps delivery P03.2
heart rate abnormalities
bradycardia P29.12
intrauterine P03.819
before onset of labor P03.810
during labor P03.811
tachycardia P29.11
hemorrhage (antepartum) P02.1
cerebellar (nontraumatic) P52.6
intracerebral (nontraumatic) P52.4
intracranial (nontraumatic) P52.9
specified NEC P52.8
intraventricular (nontraumatic) P52.3
grade 1 P52.0
grade 2 P52.1
grade 3 P52.21
grade 4 P52.22
posterior fossa (nontraumatic) P52.6
subarachnoid (nontraumatic) P52.5
subependymal P52.0
with intracerebral extension P52.22
with intraventricular extension P52.1
with enlargment of ventricles P52.21
without intraventricular extension P52.0
hypoxic ischemic encephalopathy [HIE] P91.60
mild P91.61
moderate P91.62
severe P91.63
induction of labor P03.89
intestinal perforation P78.0
intrauterine (fetal) blood loss P50.9
due to (from)
cut end of co-twin cord P50.5
hemorrhage into
co-twin P50.3
maternal circulation P50.4
placenta P50.2

Newborn — *continued*
  affected by — *continued*
    intrauterine blood loss — *continued*
      due to — *continued*
        ruptured cord blood P50.1
        vasa previa P50.0
      specified NEC P50.8
    intrauterine (fetal) hemorrhage P50.9
    intrauterine (in utero) procedure P96.5
    malpresentation (malposition) NEC P03.1
    maternal (complication of) (use of)
      alcohol P04.3
      analgesia (maternal) P04.0
      anesthesia (maternal) P04.0
      blood loss P02.1
      circulatory disease P00.3
      condition P00.9
        specified NEC P00.89
      delivery P03.9
        Cesarean P03.4
        forceps P03.2
        vacuum extractor P03.3
      diabetes mellitus (pre-existing) P70.1
      disorder P00.9
        specified NEC P00.89
      drugs (addictive) (illegal) NEC P04.49
      ectopic pregnancy P01.4
      gestational diabetes P70.0
      hemorrhage P02.1
      hypertensive disorder P00.0
      incompetent cervix P01.0
      infectious disease P00.2
      injury P00.5
      labor and delivery P03.9
      malpresentation before labor P01.7
      maternal death P01.6
      medical procedure P00.7
      medication P04.1
      multiple pregnancy P01.5
      nutritional disorder P00.4
      oligohydramnios P01.2
      parasitic disease P00.2
      periodontal disease P00.81
      placenta previa P02.0
      polyhydramnios P01.3
      precipitate delivery P03.5
      pregnancy P01.9
        specified P01.8
      premature rupture of membranes P01.1
      renal disease P00.1
      respiratory disease P00.3
      surgical procedure P00.6
      urinary tract disease P00.1
      uterine contraction (abnormal) P03.6
    meconium peritonitis P78.0
    medication (legal) (maternal use) (prescribed) P04.1
    membrane abnormalities P02.9
      specified NEC P02.8
    membranitis P02.7
    methamphetamine(s) P04.49
    mixed metabolic and respiratory acidosis P84
    neonatal abstinence syndrome P96.1
    noxious substances transmitted via placenta or
      breast milk P04.9
      specified NEC P04.8
    nutritional supplements P04.5
    placenta previa P02.0
    placental
      abnormality (functional) (morphological)
        P02.20
        specified NEC P02.29
      dysfunction P02.29
      infarction P02.29
      insufficiency P02.29
      separation NEC P02.1
      transfusion syndromes P02.3
    placentitis P02.7
    precipitate delivery P03.5
    prolapsed cord P02.4
    respiratory arrest P28.81
    slow intrauterine growth P05.9
    tobacco P04.2
    twin to twin transplacental transfusion P02.3
    umbilical cord (tightly) around neck P02.5
    umbilical cord condition P02.60
      short cord P02.69
      specified NEC P02.69
    uterine contractions (abnormal) P03.6
    vasa previa P02.69

Newborn — *continued*
  affected by — *continued*
    vasa previa — *continued*
      from intrauterine blood loss P50.0
  apnea P28.4
    obstructive P28.4
    primary P28.3
    sleep (central) (obstructive) (primary) P28.3
  born in hospital Z38.00
    by cesarean Z38.01
  born outside hospital Z38.1
  breast buds P96.89
  breast engorgement P83.4
  check-up — *see* Newborn, examination
  convulsion P90
  dehydration P74.1
  examination
    8 to 28 days old Z00.111
    under 8 days old Z00.110
  fever P81.9
    environmentally-induced P81.0
  hyperbilirubinemia P59.9
    of prematurity P59.0
  hypernatremia P74.2
  hyponatremia P74.2
  infection P39.9
    candidal P37.5
    specified NEC P39.8
    urinary tract P39.3
  jaundice P59.9
    due to
      breast milk inhibitor P59.3
      hepatocellular damage P59.20
        specified NEC P59.29
      preterm delivery P59.0
    of prematurity P59.0
    specified NEC P59.8
  late metabolic acidosis P74.0
  mastitis P39.0
    infective P39.0
    noninfective P83.4
  multiple born NEC Z38.8
    born in hospital Z38.68
      by cesarean Z38.69
    born outside hospital Z38.7
  omphalitis P38.9
    with mild hemorrhage P38.1
    without hemorrhage P38.9
  post-term P08.21
  prolonged gestation (over 42 completed weeks)
    P08.22
  quadruplet Z38.8
    born in hospital Z38.63
      by cesarean Z38.64
    born outside hospital Z38.7
  quintuplet Z38.8
    born in hospital Z38.65
      by cesarean Z38.66
    born outside hospital Z38.7
  seizure P90
  sepsis (congenital) P36.9
    due to
      anaerobes NEC P36.5
      Escherichia coli P36.4
      Staphylococcus P36.30
        aureus P36.2
        specified NEC P36.39
      Streptococcus P36.10
        group B P36.0
        specified NEC P36.19
      specified NEC P36.8
  triplet Z38.8
    born in hospital Z38.61
      by cesarean Z38.62
    born outside hospital Z38.7
  twin Z38.5
    born in hospital Z38.30
      by cesarean Z38.31
    born outside hospital Z38.4
  vomiting P92.09
    bilious P92.01
  weight check Z00.111
Newcastle conjunctivitis or disease B30.8
Nezelof's syndrome (pure alymphocytosis) D81.4
Niacin (amide) **deficiency** E52
Nicolas (-Durand)-**Favre disease** A55
Nicotine — *see* Tobacco
Nicotinic acid deficiency E52

Niemann-Pick disease or syndrome E75.249
  specified NEC E75.248
  type
    A E75.240
    B E75.241
    C E75.242
    D E75.243
Night
  blindness — *see* Blindness, night
  sweats R61
  terrors (child) F51.4
Nightmares (REM sleep type) F51.5
NIHSS (National Institutes of Health Stroke Scale) **score**
  R29.7- ☑
Nipple — *see* condition
Nisbet's chancre A57
Nishimoto (-Takeuchi) **disease** I67.5
Nitritoid crisis or reaction — *see* Crisis, nitritoid
Nitrosohemoglobinemia D74.8
Njovera A65
Nocardiosis, nocardiasis A43.9
  cutaneous A43.1
  lung A43.0
  pneumonia A43.0
  pulmonary A43.0
  specified site NEC A43.8
Nocturia R35.1
  psychogenic F45.8
Nocturnal — *see* condition
Nodal rhythm I49.8
Node(s) (*see also* Nodule)
  Bouchard's (with arthropathy) M15.2
  Haygarth's M15.8
  Heberden's (with arthropathy) M15.1
  larynx J38.7
  lymph — *see* condition
  milker's B08.03
  Osler's I33.0
  Schmorl's — *see* Schmorl's disease
  singer's J38.2
  teacher's J38.2
  tuberculous — *see* Tuberculosis, lymph gland
  vocal cord J38.2
Nodule(s), **nodular**
  actinomycotic — *see* Actinomycosis
  breast NEC (*see also* Lump, breast) N63.0
  colloid (cystic), thyroid E04.1
  cutaneous — *see* Swelling, localized
  endometrial (stromal) D26.1
  Haygarth's M15.8
  inflammatory — *see* Inflammation
  juxta-articular
    syphilitic A52.77
    yaws A66.7
  larynx J38.7
  lung, solitary (subsegmental branch of the bronchial
    tree) R91.1
    multiple R91.8
  milker's B08.03
  prostate N40.2
    with lower urinary tract symptoms (LUTS) N40.3
    without lower urinary tract symtpoms (LUTS) N40.2
  pulmonary, solitary (subsegmental branch of the
    bronchial tree) R91.1
  retrocardiac R09.89
  rheumatoid M06.30
    ankle M06.37- ☑
    elbow M06.32- ☑
    foot joint M06.37- ☑
    hand joint M06.34- ☑
    hip M06.35- ☑
    knee M06.36- ☑
    multiple site M06.39
    shoulder M06.31- ☑
    vertebra M06.38
    wrist M06.33- ☑
  scrotum (Inflammatory) N49.2
  singer's J38.2
  solitary, lung (subsegmental branch of the bronchial
    tree) R91.1
    multiple R91.8
  subcutaneous — *see* Swelling, localized
  teacher's J38.2
  thyroid (cold) (gland) (nontoxic) E04.1
    with thyrotoxicosis E05.20
      with thyroid storm E05.21
    toxic or with hyperthyroidism E05.20
      with thyroid storm E05.21

Nodule(s), nodular — *continued*
  vocal cord J38.2
Noma (gangrenous) (hospital) (infective) A69.0
  auricle I96
  mouth A69.0
  pudendi N76.89
  vulvae N76.89
Nomad, nomadism Z59.0
NOMID (neonatal onset multisystemic inflammatory disorder) M04.2
Nonadherence to medical treatment Z91.19
Nonautoimmune hemolytic anemia D59.4
  drug-induced D59.2
Nonclosure (*see also* Imperfect, closure)
  ductus arteriosus (Botallo's) Q25.0
  foramen
    botalli Q21.1
    ovale Q21.1
Noncompliance Z91.19
  with
    dialysis Z91.15
    dietary regimen Z91.11
    medical treatment Z91.19
    medication regimen NEC Z91.14
      underdosing (*see also* Table of Drugs and Chemicals, categories T36-T50, with final character 6) Z91.14
        intentional NEC Z91.128
          due to financial hardship of patient Z91.120
        unintentional NEC Z91.138
          due to patient's age related debility Z91.130
    renal dialysis Z91.15
Nondescent (congenital) (*see also* Malposition, congenital)
  cecum Q43.3
  colon Q43.3
  testicle Q53.9
    bilateral Q53.20
      abdominal Q53.211
      perineal Q53.22
    unilateral Q53.10
      abdominal Q53.111
      perineal Q53.12
Nondevelopment
  brain Q02
    part of Q04.3
  heart Q24.8
  organ or site, congenital NEC — *see* Hypoplasia
Nonengagement
  head NEC O32.4 ☑
    in labor, causing obstructed labor O64.8 ☑
Nonexanthematous tick fever A93.2
Nonexpansion, lung (newborn) P28.0
Nonfunctioning
  cystic duct (*see also* Disease, gallbladder) K82.8
  gallbladder (*see also* Disease, gallbladder) K82.8
  kidney N28.9
  labyrinth — *see* subcategory H83.2 ☑
Non-Hodgkin lymphoma NEC — *see* Lymphoma, non-Hodgkin
Nonimplantation, ovum N97.2
Noninsufflation, fallopian tube N97.1
Non-ketotic hyperglycinemia E72.51
Nonne-Milroy syndrome Q82.0
Nonovulation N97.0
Non-palpable testicle(s)
  bilateral R39.84
  unilateral R39.83
Nonpatent fallopian tube N97.1
Nonpneumatization, lung NEC P28.0
Nonrotation — *see* Malrotation
Nonsecretion, urine — *see* Anuria
Nonunion
  fracture — *see* Fracture, by site
  joint, following fusion or arthrodesis M96.0
  organ or site, congenital NEC — *see* Imperfect, closure
  symphysis pubis, congenital Q74.2
Nonvisualization, gallbladder R93.2
Nonvital, nonvitalized tooth K04.99
Non-working side interference M26.56
Noonan's syndrome Q87.1
Normocytic anemia (infectional) due to blood loss (chronic) D50.0
  acute D62
Norrie's disease (congenital) Q15.8

North American blastomycosis B40.9
Norwegian itch B86
Nose, nasal — *see* condition
Nosebleed R04.0
Nose-picking F98.8
Nosomania F45.21
Nosophobia F45.22
Nostalgia F43.20
Notch of iris Q13.2
Notching nose, congenital (tip) Q30.2
Nothnagel's
  syndrome — *see* Strabismus, paralytic, third nerve
  vasomotor acroparesthesia I73.89
Novy's relapsing fever A68.9
  louse-borne A68.0
  tick-borne A68.1
Noxious
  foodstuffs, poisoning by — *see* Poisoning, food, noxious, plant
  substances transmitted through placenta or breast milk P04.9
Nucleus pulposus — *see* condition
Numbness R20.0
Nuns' knee — *see* Bursitis, prepatellar
Nursemaid's elbow S53.03- ☑
Nutcracker esophagus K22.4
Nutmeg liver K76.1
Nutrient element deficiency E61.9
  specified NEC E61.8
Nutrition deficient or insufficient (*see also* Malnutrition) E46
  due to
    insufficient food T73.0 ☑
    lack of
      care (child) T76.02 ☑
        adult T76.01 ☑
      food T73.0 ☑
Nutritional stunting E45
Nyctalopia (night blindness) — *see* Blindness, night
Nycturia R35.1
  psychogenic F45.8
Nymphomania F52.8
Nystagmus H55.00
  benign paroxysmal — *see* Vertigo, benign paroxysmal
  central positional H81.4- ☑
  congenital H55.01
  dissociated H55.04
  latent H55.02
  miners' H55.09
  positional
    benign paroxysmal H81.4- ☑
    central H81.4- ☑
  specified form NEC H55.09
  visual deprivation H55.03

O

Obermeyer's relapsing fever (European) A68.0
Obesity E66.9
  with alveolar hypoventilation E66.2
  adrenal E27.8
  complicating
    childbirth O99.214
    pregnancy O99.21- ☑
    puerperium O99.215
  constitutional E66.8
  dietary counseling and surveillance Z71.3
  drug-induced E66.1
  due to
    drug E66.1
    excess calories E66.09
      morbid E66.01
      severe E66.01
  endocrine E66.8
  endogenous E66.8
  exogenous E66.09
  familial E66.8
  glandular E66.8
  hypothyroid — *see* Hypothyroidism
  hypoventilation syndrome (OHS) E66.2
  morbid E66.01
    with
      alveolar hypoventilation E66.2
      obesity hypoventilation syndrome (OHS) E66.2
    due to excess calories E66.01
  nutritional E66.09
  pituitary E23.6

Obesity — *continued*
  severe E66.01
  specified type NEC E66.8
Oblique — *see* condition
Obliteration
  appendix (lumen) K38.8
  artery I77.1
  bile duct (noncalculous) K83.1
  common duct (noncalculous) K83.1
  cystic duct — *see* Obstruction, gallbladder
  disease, arteriolar I77.1
  endometrium N85.8
  eye, anterior chamber — *see* Disorder, globe, hypotony
  fallopian tube N97.1
  lymphatic vessel I89.0
    due to mastectomy I97.2
  organ or site, congenital NEC — *see* Atresia, by site
  ureter N13.5
    with infection N13.6
  urethra — *see* Stricture, urethra
  vein I87.8
  vestibule (oral) K08.89
Observation (following) (for) (without need for further medical care) Z04.9
  accident NEC Z04.3
    at work Z04.2
    transport Z04.1
  adverse effect of drug Z03.6
  alleged rape or sexual assault (victim), ruled out
    adult Z04.41
    child Z04.42
  criminal assault Z04.8
  development state
    adolescent Z00.3
    period of rapid growth in childhood Z00.2
    puberty Z00.3
  disease, specified NEC Z03.89
  following work accident Z04.2
  growth and development state — *see* Observation, development state
  injuries (accidental) NEC (*see also* Observation, accident)
  newborn (for)
    suspected condition, related to exposure from the mother or birth process — *see* Newborn, affected by, maternal
    ruled out Z05.9
      cardiac Z05.0
      connective tissue Z05.73
      gastrointestinal Z05.5
      genetic Z05.41
      genitourinary Z05.6
      immunologic Z05.43
      infectious Z05.1
      metabolic Z05.42
      musculoskeletal Z05.72
      neurological Z05.2
      respiratory Z05.3
      skin and subcutaneous tissue Z05.71
      specified condition NEC Z05.8
  postpartum
    immediately after delivery Z39.0
    routine follow-up Z39.2
  pregnancy (normal) (without complication) Z34.9- ☑
    high risk O09.9- ☑
  suicide attempt, alleged NEC Z03.89
    self-poisoning Z03.6
  suspected, ruled out (*see also* Suspected condition, ruled out)
    abuse, physical
      adult Z04.71
      child Z04.72
    accident at work Z04.2
    adult battering victim Z04.71
    child battering victim Z04.72
    condition NEC Z03.89
      newborn (*see also* Observation, newborn (for), suspected condition, ruled out) Z05.9
    drug poisoning or adverse effect Z03.6
    exposure (to)
      anthrax Z03.810
      biological agent NEC Z03.818
    inflicted injury NEC Z04.8
    suicide attempt, alleged Z03.89
      self-poisoning Z03.6
    toxic effects from ingested substance (drug) (poison) Z03.6

☑ Subterms under main terms may continue to next column or page   ☑ Additional Character Required — Refer to the Tabular List for Character Selection   **235**

Nodule — Observation

Observation — *continued*
  toxic effects from ingested substance (drug) (poison) Z03.6
Obsession, obsessional state F42.8
  mixed thoughts and acts F42.2
Obsessive-compulsive neurosis or reaction F42.8
Obstetric embolism, septic — *see* Embolism, obstetric, septic
Obstetrical trauma (complicating delivery) O71.9
  with or following ectopic or molar pregnancy O08.6
  specified type NEC O71.89
Obstipation — *see* Constipation
Obstruction, obstructed, obstructive
  airway J98.8
    with
      allergic alveolitis J67.9
      asthma J45.909
        with
          exacerbation (acute) J45.901
          status asthmaticus J45.902
      bronchiectasis J47.9
        with
          exacerbation (acute) J47.1
          lower respiratory infection J47.0
      bronchitis (chronic) J44.9
      emphysema J43.9
    chronic J44.9
      with
        allergic alveolitis — *see* Pneumonitis, hypersensitivity
        bronchiectasis J47.9
          with
            exacerbation (acute) J47.1
            lower respiratory infection J47.0
    due to
      foreign body — *see* Foreign body, by site, causing asphyxia
      inhalation of fumes or vapors J68.9
      laryngospasm J38.5
  ampulla of Vater K83.1
  aortic (heart) (valve) — *see* Stenosis, aortic
  aortoiliac I74.09
  aqueduct of Sylvius G91.1
    congenital Q03.0
      with spina bifida — *see* Spina bifida, by site, with hydrocephalus
  Arnold-Chiari — *see* Arnold-Chiari disease
  artery (*see also* Atherosclerosis, artery) I70.9 ☑
    basilar (complete) (partial) — *see* Occlusion, artery, basilar
    carotid (complete) (partial) — *see* Occlusion, artery, carotid
    cerebellar — *see* Occlusion, artery, cerebellar
    cerebral (anterior) (middle) (posterior) — *see* Occlusion, artery, cerebral
    precerebral — *see* Occlusion, artery, precerebral
    renal N28.0
    retinal NEC — *see* Occlusion, artery, retina
    stent — *see* Restenosis, stent
    vertebral (complete) (partial) — *see* Occlusion, artery, vertebral
  band (intestinal) (*see also* Obstruction, intestine, specified NEC) K56.699
  bile duct or passage (common) (hepatic) (noncalculous) K83.1
    with calculus K80.51
    congenital (causing jaundice) Q44.3
  biliary (duct) (tract) K83.1
    gallbladder K82.0
  bladder-neck (acquired) N32.0
    congenital Q64.31
    due to hyperplasia (hypertrophy) of prostate — *see* Hyperplasia, prostate
  bowel — *see* Obstruction, intestine
  bronchus J98.09
  canal, ear — *see* Stenosis, external ear canal
  cardia K22.2
  caval veins (inferior) (superior) I87.1
  cecum — *see* Obstruction, intestine
  circulatory I99.8
  colon — *see* Obstruction, intestine
  common duct (noncalculous) K83.1
  coronary (artery) — *see* Occlusion, coronary
  cystic duct (*see also* Obstruction, gallbladder)
    with calculus K80.21
  device, implant or graft (*see also* Complications, by site and type, mechanical) T85.698 ☑

Obstruction, obstructed, obstructive — *continued*
  device, implant or graft (*see also* Complications, by site and type, mechanical) — *continued*
    arterial graft NEC — *see* Complication, cardiovascular device, mechanical, vascular
    catheter NEC T85.628 ☑
      cystostomy T83.090 ☑
      dialysis (renal) T82.49 ☑
        intraperitoneal T85.691 ☑
      Hopkins T83.098 ☑
      ileostomy T83.098 ☑
      infusion NEC T82.594 ☑
        spinal (epidural) (subdural) T85.690 ☑
      nephrostomy T83.092 ☑
      urethral indwelling T83.091 ☑
      urinary T83.098 ☑
      urostomy T83.098 ☑
    due to infection T85.79 ☑
    gastrointestinal — *see* Complications, prosthetic device, mechanical, gastrointestinal device
    genital NEC T83.498 ☑
      intrauterine contraceptive device T83.39 ☑
      penile prosthesis (cylinder) (implanted) (pump) (resevoir) T83.490 ☑
      testicular prosthesis T83.491 ☑
    heart NEC — *see* Complication, cardiovascular device, mechanical
    joint prosthesis — *see* Complications, joint prosthesis, mechanical, specified NEC, by site
    orthopedic NEC — *see* Complication, orthopedic, device, mechanical
    specified NEC T85.628 ☑
    urinary NEC (*see also* Complication, genitourinary, device, urinary, mechanical)
      graft T83.29 ☑
    vascular NEC — *see* Complication, cardiovascular device, mechanical
    ventricular intracranial shunt T85.09 ☑
  due to foreign body accidentally left in operative wound T81.529 ☑
  duodenum K31.5
  ejaculatory duct N50.89
  esophagus K22.2
  eustachian tube (complete) (partial) H68.10- ☑
    cartilagenous (extrinsic) H68.13- ☑
      intrinsic H68.12- ☑
    osseous H68.11- ☑
  fallopian tube (bilateral) N97.1
  fecal K56.41
    with hernia — *see* Hernia, by site, with obstruction
  foramen of Monro (congenital) Q03.8
    with spina bifida — *see* Spina bifida, by site, with hydrocephalus
  foreign body — *see* Foreign body
  gallbladder K82.0
    with calculus, stones K80.21
    congenital Q44.1
  gastric outlet K31.1
  gastrointestinal — *see* Obstruction, intestine
  hepatic K76.89
    duct (noncalculous) K83.1
  ileum — *see* Obstruction, intestine
  iliofemoral (artery) I74.5
  intestine K56.609
    with
      adhesions (intestinal) (peritoneal) K56.50
        complete K56.52
        incomplete K56.51
        partial K56.51
    adynamic K56.0
    by gallstone K56.3
    complete K56.601
    congenital (small) Q41.9
      large Q42.9
        specified part NEC Q42.8
    incomplete K56.600
    neurogenic K56.0
      Hirschsprung's disease or megacolon Q43.1
    newborn P76.9
      due to
        fecaliths P76.8
        inspissated milk P76.2
        meconium (plug) P76.0
          in mucoviscidosis E84.11
      specified NEC P76.8
    partial K56.600
    postoperative K91.30

Obstruction, obstructed, obstructive — *continued*
  intestine — *continued*
    postoperative — *continued*
      complete K91.32
      incomplete K91.31
      partial K91.31
    reflex K56.0
    specified NEC K56.699
      complete K56.691
      incomplete K56.690
      partial K56.690
    volvulus K56.2
  intracardiac ball valve prosthesis T82.09 ☑
  jejunum — *see* Obstruction, intestine
  joint prosthesis — *see* Complications, joint prosthesis, mechanical, specified NEC, by site
  kidney (calices) N28.89
  labor — *see* Delivery
  lacrimal (passages) (duct)
    by
      dacryolith — *see* Dacryolith
      stenosis — *see* Stenosis, lacrimal
    congenital Q10.5
    neonatal H04.53- ☑
  lacrimonasal duct — *see* Obstruction, lacrimal
  lacteal, with steatorrhea K90.2
  laryngitis — *see* Laryngitis
  larynx NEC J38.6
    congenital Q31.8
  lung J98.4
    disease, chronic J44.9
  lymphatic I89.0
  meconium (plug)
    newborn P76.0
      due to fecaliths P76.0
      in mucoviscidosis E84.11
  mitral — *see* Stenosis, mitral
  nasal J34.89
  nasolacrimal duct (*see also* Obstruction, lacrimal)
    congenital Q10.5
  nasopharynx J39.2
  nose J34.89
  organ or site, congenital NEC — *see* Atresia, by site
  pancreatic duct K86.89
  parotid duct or gland K11.8
  pelviureteral junction N13.5
    with hydronephrosis N13.0
    congenital Q62.39
  pharynx J39.2
  portal (circulation) (vein) I81
  prostate (*see also* Hyperplasia, prostate)
    valve (urinary) N32.0
  pulmonary valve (heart) I37.0
  pyelonephritis (chronic) N11.1
  pylorus
    adult K31.1
    congenital or infantile Q40.0
  rectosigmoid — *see* Obstruction, intestine
  rectum K62.4
  renal N28.89
    outflow N13.8
    pelvis, congenital Q62.39
  respiratory J98.8
    chronic J44.9
  retinal (vessels) H34.9
  salivary duct (any) K11.8
    with calculus K11.5
  sigmoid — *see* Obstruction, intestine
  sinus (accessory) (nasal) J34.89
  Stensen's duct K11.8
  stomach NEC K31.89
    acute K31.0
    congenital Q40.2
    due to pylorospasm K31.3
  submandibular duct K11.8
  submaxillary gland K11.8
    with calculus K11.5
  thoracic duct I89.0
  thrombotic — *see* Thrombosis
  trachea J39.8
  tracheostomy airway J95.03
  tricuspid (valve) — *see* Stenosis, tricuspid
  upper respiratory, congenital Q34.8
  ureter (functional) (pelvic junction) NEC N13.5
    with
      hydronephrosis N13.1
        with infection N13.6
      pyelonephritis (chronic) N11.1

Obstruction, obstructed, obstructive — *continued*
ureter — *continued*
congenital Q62.39
due to calculus — *see* Calculus, ureter
urethra NEC N36.8
congenital Q64.39
urinary (moderate) N13.9
due to hyperplasia (hypertrophy) of prostate —
see Hyperplasia, prostate
organ or tract (lower) N13.9
prostatic valve N32.0
specified NEC N13.8
uropathy N13.9
uterus N85.8
vagina N89.5
valvular — *see* Endocarditis
vein, venous I87.1
caval (inferior) (superior) I87.1
thrombotic — *see* Thrombosis
vena cava (inferior) (superior) I87.1
vesical NEC N32.0
vesicourethral orifice N32.0
congenital Q64.31
vessel NEC I99.8
stent — *see* Restenosis, stent
Obturator — *see* condition
Occlusal wear, teeth K03.0
Occlusio pupillae — *see* Membrane, pupillary
Occlusion, occluded
anus K62.4
congenital Q42.3
with fistula Q42.2
aortoiliac (chronic) I74.09
aqueduct of Sylvius G91.1
congenital Q03.0
with spina bifida — *see* Spina bifida, by site,
with hydrocephalus
artery (*see also* Atherosclerosis, artery) I70.9 ☑
auditory, internal I65.8
basilar I65.1
with
infarction I63.22
due to
embolism I63.12
thrombosis I63.02
brain or cerebral I66.9
with infarction (due to) I63.5- ☑
embolism I63.4- ☑
thrombosis I63.3- ☑
carotid I65.2- ☑
with
infarction I63.23- ☑
due to
embolism I63.13- ☑
thrombosis I63.03- ☑
cerebellar (anterior inferior) (posterior inferior)
(superior) I66.3
with infarction I63.54- ☑
due to
embolism I63.44- ☑
thrombosis I63.34- ☑
cerebral I66.9
with infarction I63.50
due to
embolism I63.40
specified NEC I63.49
thrombosis I63.30
specified NEC I63.39
anterior I66.1- ☑
with infarction I63.52- ☑
due to
embolism I63.42- ☑
thrombosis I63.32- ☑
middle I66.0- ☑
with infarction I63.51- ☑
due to
embolism I63.41- ☑
thrombosis I63.31- ☑
posterior I66.2- ☑
with infarction I63.53- ☑
due to
embolism I63.43- ☑
thrombosis I63.33- ☑
specified NEC I66.8
with infarction I63.59
due to
embolism I63.4- ☑

Occlusion, occluded — *continued*
artery (*see also* Atherosclerosis, artery) — *continued*
cerebral — *continued*
specified — *continued*
with infarction — *continued*
due to — *continued*
thrombosis I63.3- ☑
choroidal (anterior) — *see* Occlusion, artery, precerebral, specified NEC
communicating posterior — *see* Occlusion, artery, precerebral, specified NEC
complete
coronary I25.82
extremities I70.92
coronary (acute) (thrombotic) (without myocardial infarction) I24.0
with myocardial infarction — *see* Infarction, myocardium
chronic total I25.82
complete I25.82
healed or old I25.2
total (chronic) I25.82
hypophyseal — *see* Occlusion, artery, precerebral, specified NEC
iliac I74.5
lower extremities due to stenosis or stricture I77.1
mesenteric (embolic) (thrombotic) (*see also* Infarct, intestine) K55.069
perforating — *see* Occlusion, artery, cerebral, specified NEC
peripheral I77.9
thrombotic or embolic I74.4
pontine — *see* Occlusion, artery, precerebral, specified NEC
precerebral I65.9
with infarction I63.20
due to
embolism I63.10
specified NEC I63.19
thrombosis I63.00
specified NEC I63.09
specified NEC I63.29
basilar — *see* Occlusion, artery, basilar
carotid — *see* Occlusion, artery, carotid
puerperal O88.23
specified NEC I65.8
with infarction I63.29
due to
embolism I63.19
thrombosis I63.09
vertebral — *see* Occlusion, artery, vertebral
renal N28.0
retinal
branch H34.23- ☑
central H34.1- ☑
partial H34.21- ☑
transient H34.0- ☑
spinal — *see* Occlusion, artery, precerebral, vertebral
total (chronic)
coronary I25.82
extremities I70.92
vertebral I65.0- ☑
with
infarction I63.21- ☑
due to
embolism I63.11- ☑
thrombosis I63.01- ☑
basilar artery — *see* Occlusion, artery, basilar
bile duct (common) (hepatic) (noncalculous) K83.1
bowel — *see* Obstruction, intestine
carotid (artery) (common) (internal) — *see* Occlusion, artery, carotid
centric (of teeth) M26.59
maximum intercuspation discrepancy M26.55
cerebellar (artery) — *see* Occlusion, artery, cerebellar
cerebral (artery) — *see* Occlusion, artery, cerebral
cerebrovascular (*see also* Occlusion, artery, cerebral)
with infarction I63.5- ☑
cervical canal — *see* Stricture, cervix
cervix (uteri) — *see* Stricture, cervix
choanal Q30.0
choroidal (artery) — *see* Occlusion, artery, precerebral, specified NEC
colon — *see* Obstruction, intestine
communicating posterior artery — *see* Occlusion, artery, precerebral, specified NEC

Occlusion, occluded — *continued*
coronary (artery) (vein) (thrombotic) (*see also* Infarct, myocardium)
chronic total I25.82
healed or old I25.2
not resulting in infarction I24.0
total (chronic) I25.82
cystic duct — *see* Obstruction, gallbladder
embolic — *see* Embolism
fallopian tube N97.1
congenital Q50.6
gallbladder (*see also* Obstruction, gallbladder)
congenital (causing jaundice) Q44.1
gingiva, traumatic K06.2
hymen N89.6
congenital Q52.3
hypophyseal (artery) — *see* Occlusion, artery, precerebral, specified NEC
iliac artery I74.5
intestine — *see* Obstruction, intestine
lacrimal passages — *see* Obstruction, lacrimal
lung J98.4
lymph or lymphatic channel I89.0
mammary duct N64.89
mesenteric artery (embolic) (thrombotic) (*see also* Infarct, intestine) K55.069
nose J34.89
congenital Q30.0
organ or site, congenital NEC — *see* Atresia, by site
oviduct N97.1
congenital Q50.6
peripheral arteries
due to stricture or stenosis I77.1
upper extremity I74.2
pontine (artery) — *see* Occlusion, artery, precerebral, specified NEC
posterior lingual, of mandibular teeth M26.29
precerebral artery — *see* Occlusion, artery, precerebral
punctum lacrimale — *see* Obstruction, lacrimal
pupil — *see* Membrane, pupillary
pylorus, adult (*see also* Stricture, pylorus) K31.1
renal artery N28.0
retina, retinal
artery — *see* Occlusion, artery, retinal
vein (central) H34.81- ☑
engorgement H34.82- ☑
tributary H34.83- ☑
vessels H34.9
spinal artery — *see* Occlusion, artery, precerebral, vertebral
teeth (mandibular) (posterior lingual) M26.29
thoracic duct I89.0
thrombotic — *see* Thrombosis, artery
traumatic
edentulous (alveolar) ridge K06.2
gingiva K06.2
periodontal K05.5
tubal N97.1
ureter (complete) (partial) N13.5
congenital Q62.10
ureteropelvic junction N13.5
congenital Q62.11
ureterovesical orifice N13.5
congenital Q62.12
urethra — *see* Stricture, urethra
uterus N85.8
vagina N89.5
vascular NEC I99.8
vein — *see* Thrombosis
retinal — *see* Occlusion, retinal, vein
vena cava (inferior) (superior) — *see* Embolism, vena cava
ventricle (brain) NEC G91.1
vertebral (artery) — *see* Occlusion, artery, vertebral
vessel (blood) I99.8
vulva N90.5
Occult
blood in feces (stools) R19.5
Occupational
problems NEC Z56.89
Ochlophobia — *see* Agoraphobia
Ochronosis (endogenous) E70.29
Ocular muscle — *see* condition
Oculogyric crisis or disturbance H51.8
psychogenic F45.8
Oculomotor syndrome H51.9
Oculopathy
syphilitic NEC A52.71

Oculopathy — *continued*
  syphilitic — *continued*
    congenital
      early A50.01
      late A50.30
    early (secondary) A51.43
    late A52.71
Oddi's sphincter spasm K83.4
Odontalgia K08.89
Odontoameloblastoma — *see* Cyst, calcifying odontogenic
Odontoclasia K03.89
Odontodysplasia, regional K00.4
Odontogenesis imperfecta K00.5
Odontoma (ameloblastic) (complex) (compound) (fibroameloblastic) — *see* Cyst, calcifying odontogenic
Odontomyelitis (closed) (open) K04.01
  irreversible K04.02
  reversible K04.01
Odontorrhagia K08.89
Odontosarcoma, ameloblastic C41.1
  upper jaw (bone) C41.0
Oestriasis — *see* Myiasis
Oguchi's disease H53.63
Ohara's disease — *see* Tularemia
OHS (obesity hypoventilation syndrome) E66.2
Oidiomycosis — *see* Candidiasis
Oidium albicans infection — *see* Candidiasis
Old age (without mention of debility) R54
  dementia F03 ☑
Old (previous) **myocardial infarction** I25.2
Olfactory — *see* condition
Oligemia — *see* Anemia
Oligoastrocytoma
  specified site — *see* Neoplasm, malignant, by site
  unspecified site C71.9
Oligocythemia D64.9
Oligodendroblastoma
  specified site — *see* Neoplasm, malignant
  unspecified site C71.9
Oligodendroglioma
  anaplastic type
    specified site — *see* Neoplasm, malignant, by site
    unspecified site C71.9
  specified site — *see* Neoplasm, malignant, by site
  unspecified site C71.9
Oligodontia — *see* Anodontia
Oligoencephalon Q02
Oligohidrosis L74.4
Oligohydramnios O41.0- ☑
Oligohydrosis L74.4
Oligomenorrhea N91.5
  primary N91.3
  secondary N91.4
Oligophrenia (*see also* Disability, intellectual)
  phenylpyruvic E70.0
Oligospermia N46.11
  due to
    drug therapy N46.121
    efferent duct obstruction N46.123
    infection N46.122
    radiation N46.124
    specified cause NEC N46.129
    systemic disease N46.125
Oligotrichia — *see* Alopecia
Oliguria R34
  postprocedural N99.0
  with, complicating or following ectopic or molar pregnancy O08.4
Ollier's disease Q78.4
Omenotocele — *see* Hernia, abdomen, specified site NEC
Omentitis — *see* Peritonitis
Omentum, omental — *see* condition
Omphalitis (congenital) (newborn) P38.9
  with mild hemorrhage P38.1
  without hemorrhage P38.9
  not of newborn L08.82
  tetanus A33
Omphalocele Q79.2
Omphalomesenteric duct, persistent Q43.0
Omphalorrhagia, newborn P51.9
Omsk hemorrhagic fever A98.1
Onanism (excessive) F98.8
Onchocerciasis, onchocercosis B73.1
  with
    eye disease B73.00

Onchocerciasis, onchocercosis — *continued*
  with — *continued*
    eye disease — *continued*
      endophthalmitis B73.01
      eyelid B73.09
      glaucoma B73.02
      specified NEC B73.09
    eyelid B73.09
    eye NEC B73.00
Oncocytoma — *see* Neoplasm, benign, by site
Oncovirus, as cause of disease classified elsewhere B97.32
Ondine's curse — *see* Apnea, sleep
Oneirophrenia F23
Onychauxis L60.2
  congenital Q84.5
Onychia (*see also* Cellulitis, digit)
  with lymphangitis — *see* Lymphangitis, acute, digit
  candidal B37.2
  dermatophytic B35.1
Onychitis (*see also* Cellulitis, digit)
  with lymphangitis — *see* Lymphangitis, acute, digit
Onychocryptosis L60.0
Onychodystrophy L60.3
  congenital Q84.6
Onychogryphosis, onychogryposis L60.2
Onycholysis L60.1
Onychomadesis L60.8
Onychomalacia L60.3
Onychomycosis (finger) (toe) B35.1
Onycho-osteodysplasia Q87.2
Onychophagia F98.8
Onychophosis L60.8
Onychoptosis L60.8
Onychorrhexis L60.3
  congenital Q84.6
Onychoschizia L60.3
Onyxis (finger) (toe) L60.0
Onyxitis (*see also* Cellulitis, digit)
  with lymphangitis — *see* Lymphangitis, acute, digit
Oophoritis (cystic) (infectional) (interstitial) N70.92
  with salpingitis N70.93
  acute N70.02
    with salpingitis N70.03
  chronic N70.12
    with salpingitis N70.13
  complicating abortion — *see* Abortion, by type, complicated by, oophoritis
Oophorocele N83.4- ☑
Opacity, opacities
  cornea H17.- ☑
    central H17.1- ☑
    congenital Q13.3
    degenerative — *see* Degeneration, cornea
    hereditary — *see* Dystrophy, cornea
    inflammatory — *see* Keratitis
    minor H17.81- ☑
    peripheral H17.82- ☑
    sequelae of trachoma (healed) B94.0
    specified NEC H17.89
  enamel (teeth) (fluoride) (nonfluoride) K00.3
  lens — *see* Cataract
  snowball — *see* Deposit, crystalline
  vitreous (humor) NEC H43.39- ☑
    congenital Q14.0
    membranes and strands H43.31- ☑
Opalescent dentin (hereditary) K00.5
Open, opening
  abnormal, organ or site, congenital — *see* Imperfect, closure
  angle with
    borderline
      findings
        high risk H40.02- ☑
        low risk H40.01- ☑
      intraocular pressure H40.00- ☑
    cupping of discs H40.01- ☑
    glaucoma (primary) — *see* Glaucoma, open angle
  bite
    anterior M26.220
    posterior M26.221
  false — *see* Imperfect, closure
  margin on tooth restoration K08.51
  restoration margins of tooth K08.51
  wound — *see* Wound, open
Operational fatigue F48.8
Operative — *see* condition

Operculitis — *see* Periodontitis
Operculum — *see* Break, retina
Ophiasis L63.2
Ophthalmia (*see also* Conjunctivitis) H10.9
  actinic rays — *see* Photokeratitis
  allergic (acute) — *see* Conjunctivitis, acute, atopic
  blennorrhagic (gonococcal) (neonatorum) A54.31
  diphtheritic A36.86
  Egyptian A71.1
  electrica — *see* Photokeratitis
  gonococcal (neonatorum) A54.31
  metastatic — *see* Endophthalmitis, purulent
  migraine — *see* Migraine, ophthalmoplegic
  neonatorum, newborn P39.1
    gonococcal A54.31
  nodosa H16.24- ☑
  purulent — *see* Conjunctivitis, acute, mucopurulent
  spring — *see* Conjunctivitis, acute, atopic
  sympathetic — *see* Uveitis, sympathetic
Ophthalmitis — *see* Ophthalmia
Ophthalmocele (congenital) Q15.8
Ophthalmoneuromyelitis G36.0
Ophthalmoplegia (*see also* Strabismus, paralytic)
  anterior internuclear — *see* Ophthalmoplegia, internuclear
  ataxia-areflexia G61.0
  diabetic — *see* E08-E13 with .39
  exophthalmic E05.00
    with thyroid storm E05.01
  external H49.88- ☑
    progressive H49.4- ☑
      with pigmentary retinopathy — *see* Kearns-Sayre syndrome
    total H49.3- ☑
  internal (complete) (total) H52.51- ☑
  internuclear H51.2- ☑
  migraine — *see* Migraine, ophthalmoplegic
  Parinaud's H49.88- ☑
  progressive external — *see* Ophthalmoplegia, external, progressive
  supranuclear, progressive G23.1
  total (external) — *see* Ophthalmoplegia, external, total
Opioid(s)
  abuse — *see* Abuse, drug, opioids
  dependence — *see* Dependence, drug, opioids
  induced, without use disorder
    anxiety disorder F11.988
    delirium F11.921
    depressive disorder F11.94
    sexual dysfunction F11.981
    sleep disorder F11.982
Opisthognathism M26.09
Opisthorchiasis (felineus) (viverrini) B66.0
Opitz' disease D73.2
Opiumism — *see* Dependence, drug, opioid
Oppenheim's disease G70.2
Oppenheim-Urbach disease (necrobiosis lipoidica diabeticorum) — *see* E08-E13 with .620
Optic nerve — *see* condition
Orbit — *see* condition
Orchioblastoma C62.9- ☑
Orchitis (gangrenous) (nonspecific) (septic) (suppurative) N45.2
  blennorrhagic (gonococcal) (acute) (chronic) A54.23
  chlamydial A56.19
  filarial (*see also* Infestation, filarial) B74.9 [N51]
  gonococcal (acute) (chronic) A54.23
  mumps B26.0
  syphilitic A52.76
  tuberculous A18.15
Orf (virus disease) B08.02
Organic (*see also* condition)
  brain syndrome F09
  heart — *see* Disease, heart
  mental disorder F09
  psychosis F09
Orgasm
  anejaculatory N53.13
Oriental
  bilharziasis B65.2
  schistosomiasis B65.2
Orifice — *see* condition
Origin of both great vessels from right ventricle Q20.1
Ormond's disease (with ureteral obstruction) N13.5
  with infection N13.6
Ornithine metabolism disorder E72.4

Ornithinemia (Type I) (Type II) E72.4
Ornithosis A70
Orotaciduria, oroticaciduria (congenital) (hereditary)
    (pyrimidine deficiency) E79.8
    anemia D53.0
Orthodontics
    adjustment Z46.4
    fitting Z46.4
Orthopnea R06.01
Orthopoxvirus B08.09
    specified NEC B08.09
Os, uterus — see condition
Osgood-Schlatter disease or osteochondrosis — see
    Osteochondrosis, juvenile, tibia
Osler (-Weber)-Rendu disease I78.0
Osler's nodes I33.0
Osmidrosis L75.0
Osseous — see condition
Ossification
    artery — see Arteriosclerosis
    auricle (ear) — see Disorder, pinna, specified type NEC
    bronchial J98.09
    cardiac — see Degeneration, myocardial
    cartilage (senile) — see Disorder, cartilage, specified
        type NEC
    coronary (artery) — see Disease, heart, ischemic,
        atherosclerotic
    diaphragm J98.6
    ear, middle — see Otosclerosis
    falx cerebri G96.19
    fontanel, premature Q75.0
    heart (see also Degeneration, myocardial)
        valve — see Endocarditis
    larynx J38.7
    ligament — see Disorder, tendon, specified type NEC
        posterior longitudinal — see Spondylopathy,
            specified NEC
    meninges (cerebral) (spinal) G96.19
    multiple, eccentric centers — see Disorder, bone, de-
        velopment or growth
    muscle (see also Calcification, muscle)
        due to burns — see Myositis, ossificans, in, burns
        paralytic — see Myositis, ossificans, in, quadriplegia
        progressive — see Myositis, ossificans, progressiva
        specified NEC M61.50
            ankle M61.57- ☑
            foot M61.57- ☑
            forearm M61.53- ☑
            hand M61.54- ☑
            lower leg M61.56- ☑
            multiple sites M61.59
            pelvic region M61.55- ☑
            shoulder region M61.51- ☑
            specified site NEC M61.58
            thigh M61.55- ☑
            upper arm M61.52- ☑
        traumatic — see Myositis, ossificans, traumatica
    myocardium, myocardial — see Degeneration, myocar-
        dial
    penis N48.89
    periarticular — see Disorder, joint, specified type NEC
    pinna — see Disorder, pinna, specified type NEC
    rider's bone — see Ossification, muscle, specified NEC
    sclera H15.89
    subperiosteal, post-traumatic M89.8X- ☑
    tendon — see Disorder, tendon, specified type NEC
    trachea J39.8
    tympanic membrane — see Disorder, tympanic
        membrane, specified NEC
    vitreous (humor) — see Deposit, crystalline
Osteitis (see also Osteomyelitis)
    alveolar M27.3
    condensans M85.30
        ankle M85.37- ☑
        foot M85.37- ☑
        forearm M85.33- ☑
        hand M85.34- ☑
        lower leg M85.36- ☑
        multiple site M85.39
        neck M85.38
        rib M85.38
        shoulder M85.31- ☑
        skull M85.38
        specified site NEC M85.38
        thigh M85.35- ☑
        toe M85.37- ☑
        upper arm M85.32- ☑

Osteitis — continued
    condensans — continued
        vertebra M85.38
    deformans M88.9
        in (due to)
            malignant neoplasm of bone C41.9 [M90.60]
            neoplastic disease (see also Neoplasm)
                D49.9 [M90.60]
                carpus D49.9 [M90.64-] ☑
                clavicle D49.9 [M90.61-] ☑
                femur D49.9 [M90.65-] ☑
                fibula D49.9 [M90.66-] ☑
                finger D49.9 [M90.64-] ☑
                humerus D49.9 [M90.62-] ☑
                ilium D49.9 [M90.65-] ☑
                ischium D49.9 [M90.65-] ☑
                metacarpus D49.9 [M90.64-] ☑
                metatarsus D49.9 [M90.67-] ☑
                multiple sites D49.9 [M90.69]
                neck D49.9 [M90.68]
                radius D49.9 [M90.63-] ☑
                rib D49.9 [M90.68]
                scapula D49.9 [M90.61-] ☑
                skull D49.9 [M90.68]
                tarsus D49.9 [M90.67-] ☑
                tibia D49.9 [M90.66-] ☑
                toe D49.9 [M90.67-] ☑
                ulna D49.9 [M90.63-] ☑
                vertebra D49.9 [M90.68]
        skull M88.0
        specified NEC — see Paget's disease, bone, by site
        vertebra M88.1
    due to yaws A66.6
    fibrosa NEC — see Cyst, bone, by site
        circumscripta — see Dysplasia, fibrous, bone NEC
        cystica (generalisata) E21.0
        disseminata D78.1
        osteoplastica E21.0
    fragilitans Q78.0
    Garr's (sclerosing) — see Osteomyelitis, specified type
        NEC
    jaw (acute) (chronic) (lower) (suppurative) (upper)
        M27.2
    parathyroid E21.0
    petrous bone (acute) (chronic) — see Petrositis
    sclerotic, nonsuppurative — see Osteomyelitis, speci-
        fied type NEC
    tuberculosa A18.09
        cystica D86.89
        multiplex cystoides D86.89
Osteoarthritis M19.90
    ankle M19.07- ☑
    elbow M19.02- ☑
    foot joint M19.07- ☑
    generalized M15.9
        erosive M15.4
        primary M15.0
        specified NEC M15.8
    hand joint M19.04- ☑
        first carpometacarpal joint M18.9
    hip M16.1- ☑
        bilateral M16.0
        due to hip dysplasia (unilateral) M16.3- ☑
            bilateral M16.2
    interphalangeal
        distal (Heberden) M15.1
        proximal (Bouchard) M15.2
    knee M17.1- ☑
        bilateral M17.0
    post-traumatic NEC M19.92
        ankle M19.17- ☑
        elbow M19.12- ☑
        foot joint M19.17- ☑
        hand joint M19.14- ☑
            first carpometacarpal joint M18.3- ☑
                bilateral M18.2
        hip M16.5- ☑
            bilateral M16.4
        knee M17.3- ☑
            bilateral M17.2
        shoulder M19.11- ☑
        wrist M19.13- ☑
    primary M19.91
        ankle M19.07- ☑
        elbow M19.02- ☑
        foot joint M19.07- ☑
        hand joint M19.04- ☑

Osteoarthritis — continued
    primary — continued
        hand joint — continued
            first carpometacarpal joint M18.1- ☑
                bilateral M18.0
            hip M16.1- ☑
                bilateral M16.0
            knee M17.1- ☑
                bilateral M17.0
            shoulder M19.01- ☑
            spine — see Spondylosis
            wrist M19.03- ☑
        secondary M19.93
            ankle M19.27- ☑
            elbow M19.22- ☑
            foot joint M19.27- ☑
            hand joint M19.24- ☑
                first carpometacarpal joint M18.5- ☑
                    bilateral M18.4
            hip M16.7
                bilateral M16.6
            knee M17.5
                bilateral M17.4
            multiple M15.3
            shoulder M19.21- ☑
            spine — see Spondylosis
            wrist M19.23- ☑
    shoulder M19.01- ☑
    spine — see Spondylosis
    wrist M19.03- ☑
Osteoarthropathy (hypertrophic) M19.90
    ankle — see Osteoarthritis, primary, ankle
    elbow — see Osteoarthritis, primary, elbow
    foot joint — see Osteoarthritis, primary, foot
    hand joint — see Osteoarthritis, primary, hand joint
    knee joint — see Osteoarthritis, primary, knee
    multiple site — see Osteoarthritis, primary, multiple
        joint
    pulmonary (see also Osteoarthropathy, specified type
        NEC)
        hypertrophic — see Osteoarthropathy, hyper-
            trophic, specified type NEC
    secondary — see Osteoarthropathy, specified type
        NEC
    secondary hypertrophic — see Osteoarthropathy,
        specified type NEC
    shoulder — see Osteoarthritis, primary, shoulder
    specified joint NEC — see Osteoarthritis, primary,
        specified joint NEC
    specified type NEC M89.40
        carpus M89.44- ☑
        clavicle M89.41- ☑
        femur M89.45- ☑
        fibula M89.46- ☑
        finger M89.44- ☑
        humerus M89.42- ☑
        ilium M89.459
        ischium M89.459
        metacarpus M89.44- ☑
        metatarsus M89.47- ☑
        multiple sites M89.49
        neck M89.48
        radius M89.43- ☑
        rib M89.48
        scapula M89.41- ☑
        skull M89.48
        tarsus M89.47- ☑
        tibia M89.46- ☑
        toe M89.47- ☑
        ulna M89.43- ☑
        vertebra M89.48
    spine — see Spondylosis
    wrist — see Osteoarthritis, primary, wrist
Osteoarthrosis (degenerative) (hypertrophic) (joint) (see
    also Osteoarthritis)
    deformans alkaptonurica E70.29 [M36.8]
    erosive M15.4
    generalized M15.9
        primary M15.0
    polyarticular M15.9
    spine — see Spondylosis
Osteoblastoma — see Neoplasm, bone, benign
    aggressive — see Neoplasm, bone, uncertain behavior
Osteochondritis (see also Osteochondropathy, by site)
    Brailsford's — see Osteochondrosis, juvenile, radius
    dissecans M93.20
        ankle M93.27- ☑

Osteochondritis — *continued*
dissecans — *continued*
elbow M93.22- ☑
foot M93.27- ☑
hand M93.24- ☑
hip M93.25- ☑
knee M93.26- ☑
multiple sites M93.29
shoulder joint M93.21- ☑
specified site NEC M93.28
wrist M93.23- ☑
juvenile M92.9
patellar — *see* Osteochondrosis, juvenile, patella
syphilitic (congenital) (early) A50.02 [M90.80]
ankle A50.02 [M90.87-] ☑
elbow A50.02 [M90.82-] ☑
foot A50.02 [M90.87-] ☑
forearm A50.02 [M90.83-] ☑
hand A50.02 [M90.84-] ☑
hip A50.02 [M90.85-] ☑
knee A50.02 [M90.86-] ☑
multiple sites A50.02 [M90.89]
shoulder joint A50.02 [M90.81-] ☑
specified site NEC A50.02 [M90.88]
Osteochondroarthrosis deformans endemica — *see* Disease, Kaschin-Beck
Osteochondrodysplasia Q78.9
with defects of growth of tubular bones and spine Q77.9
specified NEC Q77.8
specified NEC Q78.8
Osteochondrodystrophy E78.9
Osteochondrolysis — *see* Osteochondritis, dissecans
Osteochondroma — *see* Neoplasm, bone, benign
Osteochondromatosis D48.0
syndrome Q78.4
Osteochondromyxosarcoma — *see* Neoplasm, bone, malignant
Osteochondropathy M93.90
ankle M93.97- ☑
elbow M93.92- ☑
foot M93.97- ☑
hand M93.94- ☑
hip M93.95- ☑
Kienböck's disease of adults M93.1
knee M93.96- ☑
multiple joints M93.99
osteochondritis dissecans — *see* Osteochondritis, dissecans
osteochondrosis — *see* Osteochondrosis
shoulder region M93.91- ☑
slipped upper femoral epiphysis — *see* Slipped, epiphysis, upper femoral
specified joint NEC M93.98
specified type NEC M93.80
ankle M93.87- ☑
elbow M93.82- ☑
foot M93.87- ☑
hand M93.84- ☑
hip M93.85- ☑
knee M93.86- ☑
multiple joints M93.89
shoulder region M93.81- ☑
specified joint NEC M93.88
wrist M93.83- ☑
syphilitic, congenital
early A50.02 [M90.80]
late A50.56 [M90.80]
wrist M93.93- ☑
Osteochondrosarcoma — *see* Neoplasm, bone, malignant
Osteochondrosis (*see also* Osteochondropathy, by site)
acetabulum (juvenile) M91.0
adult — *see* Osteochondropathy, specified type NEC, by site
astragalus (juvenile) — *see* Osteochondrosis, juvenile, tarsus
Blount's — *see* Osteochondrosis, juvenile, tibia
Buchanan's M91.0
Burns' — *see* Osteochondrosis, juvenile, ulna
calcaneus (juvenile) — *see* Osteochondrosis, juvenile, tarsus
capitular epiphysis (femur) (juvenile) — *see* Legg-Calvé-Perthes disease
carpal (juvenile) (lunate) (scaphoid) — *see* Osteochondrosis, juvenile, hand, carpal lunate
adult M93.1

Osteochondrosis — *continued*
coxae juvenilis — *see* Legg-Calvé-Perthes disease
deformans juvenilis, coxae — *see* Legg-Calvé-Perthes disease
Diaz's — *see* Osteochondrosis, juvenile, tarsus
dissecans (knee) (shoulder) — *see* Osteochondritis, dissecans
femoral capital epiphysis (juvenile) — *see* Legg-Calvé-Perthes disease
femur (head), juvenile — *see* Legg-Calvé-Perthes disease
fibula (juvenile) — *see* Osteochondrosis, juvenile, fibula
foot NEC (juvenile) M92.8
Freiberg's — *see* Osteochondrosis, juvenile, metatarsus
Haas' (juvenile) — *see* Osteochondrosis, juvenile, humerus
Haglund's — *see* Osteochondrosis, juvenile, tarsus
hip (juvenile) — *see* Legg-Calvé-Perthes disease
humerus (capitulum) (head) (juvenile) — *see* Osteochondrosis, juvenile, humerus
ilium, iliac crest (juvenile) M91.0
ischiopubic synchondrosis M91.0
Iselin's — *see* Osteochondrosis, juvenile, metatarsus
juvenile, juvenilis M92.9
after congenital dislocation of hip reduction — *see* Osteochondrosis, juvenile, hip, specified NEC
arm — *see* Osteochondrosis, juvenile, upper limb NEC
capitular epiphysis (femur) — *see* Legg-Calvé-Perthes disease
clavicle, sternal epiphysis — *see* Osteochondrosis, juvenile, upper limb NEC
coxae — *see* Legg-Calvé-Perthes disease
deformans M92.9
fibula M92.5- ☑
foot NEC M92.8
hand M92.20- ☑
carpal lunate M92.21- ☑
metacarpal head M92.22- ☑
specified site NEC M92.29- ☑
head of femur — *see* Legg-Calvé-Perthes disease
hip and pelvis M91.9- ☑
coxa plana — *see* Coxa, plana
femoral head — *see* Legg-Calvé-Perthes disease
pelvis M91.0
pseudocoxalgia — *see* Pseudocoxalgia
specified NEC M91.8- ☑
humerus M92.0- ☑
limb
lower NEC M92.8
upper NEC — *see* Osteochondrosis, juvenile, upper limb NEC
medial cuneiform bone — *see* Osteochondrosis, juvenile, tarsus
metatarsus M92.7- ☑
patella M92.4- ☑
radius M92.1- ☑
specified site NEC M92.8
spine M42.00
cervical region M42.02
cervicothoracic region M42.03
lumbar region M42.06
lumbosacral region M42.07
multiple sites M42.09
occipito-atlanto-axial region M42.01
sacrococcygeal region M42.08
thoracic region M42.04
thoracolumbar region M42.05
tarsus M92.6- ☑
tibia M92.5- ☑
ulna M92.1- ☑
upper limb NEC M92.3- ☑
vertebra (body) (epiphyseal plates) (Calvé's) (Scheuermann's) — *see* Osteochondrosis, juvenile, spine
Kienböck's — *see* Osteochondrosis, juvenile, hand, carpal lunate
adult M93.1
Köhler's
patellar — *see* Osteochondrosis, juvenile, patella
tarsal navicular — *see* Osteochondrosis, juvenile, tarsus
Legg-Perthes (-Calvé)(-Waldenström) — *see* Legg-Calvé-Perthes disease
limb
lower NEC (juvenile) M92.8

Osteochondrosis — *continued*
limb — *continued*
upper NEC (juvenile) — *see* Osteochondrosis, juvenile, upper limb NEC
lunate bone (carpal) (juvenile) (*see also* Osteochondrosis, juvenile, hand, carpal lunate)
adult M93.1
Mauclaire's — *see* Osteochondrosis, juvenile, hand, metacarpal
metacarpal (head) (juvenile) — *see* Osteochondrosis, juvenile, hand, metacarpal
metatarsus (fifth) (head) (juvenile) (second) — *see* Osteochondrosis, juvenile, metatarsus
navicular (juvenile) — *see* Osteochondrosis, juvenile, tarsus
os
calcis (juvenile) — *see* Osteochondrosis, juvenile, tarsus
tibiale externum (juvenile) — *see* Osteochondrosis, juvenile, tarsus
Osgood-Schlatter — *see* Osteochondrosis, juvenile, tibia
Panner's — *see* Osteochondrosis, juvenile, humerus
patellar center (juvenile) (primary) (secondary) — *see* Osteochondrosis, juvenile, patella
pelvis (juvenile) M91.0
Pierson's M91.0
radius (head) (juvenile) — *see* Osteochondrosis, juvenile, radius
Scheuermann's — *see* Osteochondrosis, juvenile, spine
Sever's — *see* Osteochondrosis, juvenile, tarsus
Sinding-Larsen — *see* Osteochondrosis, juvenile, patella
spine M42.9
adult M42.10
cervical region M42.12
cervicothoracic region M42.13
lumbar region M42.16
lumbosacral region M42.17
multiple sites M42.19
occipito-atlanto-axial region M42.11
sacrococcygeal region M42.18
thoracic region M42.14
thoracolumbar region M42.15
juvenile — *see* Osteochondrosis, juvenile, spine
symphysis pubis (juvenile) M91.0
syphilitic (congenital) A50.02
talus (juvenile) — *see* Osteochondrosis, juvenile, tarsus
tarsus (navicular) (juvenile) — *see* Osteochondrosis, juvenile, tarsus
tibia (proximal) (tubercle) (juvenile) — *see* Osteochondrosis, juvenile, tibia
tuberculous — *see* Tuberculosis, bone
ulna (lower) (juvenile) — *see* Osteochondrosis, juvenile, ulna
van Neck's M91.0
vertebral — *see* Osteochondrosis, spine
Osteoclastoma D48.0
malignant — *see* Neoplasm, bone, malignant
Osteodynia — *see* Disorder, bone, specified type NEC
Osteodystrophy Q78.9
azotemic N25.0
congenital Q78.9
parathyroid, secondary E21.1
renal N25.0
Osteofibroma — *see* Neoplasm, bone, benign
Osteofibrosarcoma — *see* Neoplasm, bone, malignant
Osteogenesis imperfecta Q78.0
Osteogenic — *see* condition
Osteolysis M89.50
carpus M89.54- ☑
clavicle M89.51- ☑
femur M89.55- ☑
fibula M89.56- ☑
finger M89.54- ☑
humerus M89.52- ☑
ilium M89.559
ischium M89.559
joint prosthesis (periprosthetic) — *see* Complications, joint prosthesis, mechanical, periprosthetic, osteolysis, by site
metacarpus M89.54- ☑
metatarsus M89.57- ☑
multiple sites M89.59
neck M89.58
periprosthetic — *see* Complications, joint prosthesis, mechanical, periprosthetic, osteolysis, by site

Osteolysis — *continued*
  radius M89.53- ☑
  rib M89.58
  scapula M89.51- ☑
  skull M89.58
  tarsus M89.57- ☑
  tibia M89.56- ☑
  toe M89.57- ☑
  ulna M89.53- ☑
  vertebra M89.58
Osteoma (*see also* Neoplasm, bone, benign)
  osteoid (*see also* Neoplasm, bone, benign)
    giant — *see* Neoplasm, bone, benign
Osteomalacia M83.9
  adult M83.9
    drug-induced NEC M83.5
    due to
      malabsorption (postsurgical) M83.2
      malnutrition M83.3
    specified NEC M83.8
  aluminium-induced M83.4
  infantile — *see* Rickets
  juvenile — *see* Rickets
  oncogenic E83.89
  pelvis M83.8
  puerperal M83.0
  senile M83.1
  vitamin-D-resistant in adults E83.31 [M90.8-] ☑
    carpus E83.31 [M90.84-] ☑
    clavicle E83.31 [M90.81-] ☑
    femur E83.31 [M90.85-] ☑
    fibula E83.31 [M90.86-] ☑
    finger E83.31 [M90.84-] ☑
    humerus E83.31 [M90.82-] ☑
    ilium E83.31 [M90.859]
    ischium E83.31 [M90.859]
    metacarpus E83.31 [M90.84-] ☑
    metatarsus E83.31 [M90.87-] ☑
    multiple sites E83.31 [M90.89]
    neck E83.31 [M90.88]
    radius E83.31 [M90.83-] ☑
    rib E83.31 [M90.88]
    scapula E83.31 [M90.819]
    skull E83.31 [M90.88]
    tarsus E83.31 [M90.879]
    tibia E83.31 [M90.869]
    toe E83.31 [M90.879]
    ulna E83.31 [M90.839]
    vertebra E83.31 [M90.88]
Osteomyelitis (general) (infective) (localized) (neonatal) (purulent) (septic) (staphylococcal) (streptococcal) (suppurative) (with periostitis) M86.9
  acute M86.10
    carpus M86.14- ☑
    clavicle M86.11- ☑
    femur M86.15- ☑
    fibula M86.16- ☑
    finger M86.14- ☑
    hematogenous M86.00
      carpus M86.04- ☑
      clavicle M86.01- ☑
      femur M86.05- ☑
      fibula M86.06- ☑
      finger M86.04- ☑
      humerus M86.02- ☑
      ilium M86.059
      ischium M86.059
      mandible M27.2
      metacarpus M86.04- ☑
      metatarsus M86.07- ☑
      multiple sites M86.09
      neck M86.08
      orbit H05.02- ☑
      petrous bone — *see* Petrositis
      radius M86.03- ☑
      rib M86.08
      scapula M86.01- ☑
      skull M86.08
      tarsus M86.07- ☑
      tibia M86.06- ☑
      toe M86.07- ☑
      ulna M86.03- ☑
      vertebra — *see* Osteomyelitis, vertebra
    humerus M86.12- ☑
    ilium M86.159
    ischium M86.159
    mandible M27.2

Osteomyelitis — *continued*
  acute — *continued*
    metacarpus M86.14- ☑
    metatarsus M86.17- ☑
    multiple sites M86.19
    neck M86.18
    orbit H05.02- ☑
    petrous bone — *see* Petrositis
    radius M86.13- ☑
    rib M86.18
    scapula M86.11- ☑
    skull M86.18
    tarsus M86.17- ☑
    tibia M86.16- ☑
    toe M86.17- ☑
    ulna M86.13- ☑
    vertebra — *see* Osteomyelitis, vertebra
  chronic (or old) M86.60
    with draining sinus M86.40
      carpus M86.44- ☑
      clavicle M86.41- ☑
      femur M86.45- ☑
      fibula M86.46- ☑
      finger M86.44- ☑
      humerus M86.42- ☑
      ilium M86.459
      ischium M86.459
      mandible M27.2
      metacarpus M86.44- ☑
      metatarsus M86.47- ☑
      multiple sites M86.49
      neck M86.48
      orbit H05.02- ☑
      petrous bone — *see* Petrositis
      radius M86.43- ☑
      rib M86.48
      scapula M86.41- ☑
      skull M86.48
      tarsus M86.47- ☑
      tibia M86.46- ☑
      toe M86.47- ☑
      ulna M86.43- ☑
      vertebra — *see* Osteomyelitis, vertebra
    carpus M86.64- ☑
    clavicle M86.61- ☑
    femur M86.65- ☑
    fibula M86.66- ☑
    finger M86.64- ☑
    hematogenous NEC M86.50
      carpus M86.54- ☑
      clavicle M86.51- ☑
      femur M86.55- ☑
      fibula M86.56- ☑
      finger M86.54- ☑
      humerus M86.52- ☑
      ilium M86.559
      ischium M86.559
      mandible M27.2
      metacarpus M86.54- ☑
      metatarsus M86.57- ☑
      multifocal M86.30
        carpus M86.34- ☑
        clavicle M86.31- ☑
        femur M86.35- ☑
        fibula M86.36- ☑
        finger M86.34- ☑
        humerus M86.32- ☑
        ilium M86.359
        ischium M86.359
        metacarpus M86.34- ☑
        metatarsus M86.37- ☑
        multiple sites M86.39
        neck M86.38
        radius M86.33- ☑
        rib M86.38
        scapula M86.31- ☑
        skull M86.38
        tarsus M86.37- ☑
        tibia M86.36- ☑
        toe M86.37- ☑
        ulna M86.33- ☑
        vertebra — *see* Osteomyelitis, vertebra
      multiple sites M86.59
      neck M86.58
      orbit H05.02- ☑
      petrous bone — *see* Petrositis

Osteomyelitis — *continued*
  chronic — *continued*
    hematogenous — *continued*
      radius M86.53- ☑
      rib M86.58
      scapula M86.51- ☑
      skull M86.58
      tarsus M86.57- ☑
      tibia M86.56- ☑
      toe M86.57- ☑
      ulna M86.53- ☑
      vertebra — *see* Osteomyelitis, vertebra
    humerus M86.62- ☑
    ilium M86.659
    ischium M86.659
    mandible M27.2
    metacarpus M86.64- ☑
    metatarsus M86.67- ☑
    multifocal — *see* Osteomyelitis, chronic, hematogenous, multifocal
    multiple sites M86.69
    neck M86.68
    orbit H05.02- ☑
    petrous bone — *see* Petrositis
    radius M86.63- ☑
    rib M86.68
    scapula M86.61- ☑
    skull M86.68
    tarsus M86.67- ☑
    tibia M86.66- ☑
    toe M86.67- ☑
    ulna M86.63- ☑
    vertebra — *see* Osteomyelitis, vertebra
  echinococcal B67.2
  Garr's — *see* Osteomyelitis, specified type NEC
  in diabetes mellitus — *see* E08-E13 with .69
  jaw (acute) (chronic) (lower) (neonatal) (suppurative) (upper) M27.2
  nonsuppurating — *see* Osteomyelitis, specified type NEC
  orbit H05.02- ☑
  petrous bone — *see* Petrositis
  Salmonella (arizonae) (cholerae-suis) (enteritidis) (typhimurium) A02.24
  sclerosing, nonsuppurative — *see* Osteomyelitis, specified type NEC
  specified type NEC (*see also* subcategory) M86.8X- ☑
    mandible M27.2
    orbit H05.02- ☑
    petrous bone — *see* Petrositis
    vertebra — *see* Osteomyelitis, vertebra
  subacute M86.20
    carpus M86.24- ☑
    clavicle M86.21- ☑
    femur M86.25- ☑
    fibula M86.26- ☑
    finger M86.24- ☑
    humerus M86.22- ☑
    mandible M27.2
    metacarpus M86.24- ☑
    metatarsus M86.27- ☑
    multiple sites M86.29
    neck M86.28
    orbit H05.02- ☑
    petrous bone — *see* Petrositis
    radius M86.23- ☑
    rib M86.28
    scapula M86.21- ☑
    skull M86.28
    tarsus M86.27- ☑
    tibia M86.26- ☑
    toe M86.27- ☑
    ulna M86.23- ☑
    vertebra — *see* Osteomyelitis, vertebra
  syphilitic A52.77
    congenital (early) A50.02 [M90.80]
  tuberculous — *see* Tuberculosis, bone
  typhoid A01.05
  vertebra M46.20
    cervical region M46.22
    cervicothoracic region M46.23
    lumbar region M46.26
    lumbosacral region M46.27
    occipito-atlanto-axial region M46.21
    sacrococcygeal region M46.28
    thoracic region M46.24
    thoracolumbar region M46.25

▽ Subterms under main terms may continue to next column or page   ☑ Additional Character Required — Refer to the Tabular List for Character Selection   **241**

Osteolysis — Osteomyelitis

Osteomyelofibrosis D47.4
Osteomyelosclerosis D75.89
Osteonecrosis M87.9
  due to
    drugs — see Osteonecrosis, secondary, due to, drugs
    trauma — see Osteonecrosis, secondary, due to, trauma
  idiopathic aseptic M87.00
    ankle M87.07- ☑
    carpus M87.03- ☑
    clavicle M87.01- ☑
    femur M87.05- ☑
    fibula M87.06- ☑
    finger M87.04- ☑
    humerus M87.02- ☑
    ilium M87.050
    ischium M87.050
    metacarpus M87.04- ☑
    metatarsus M87.07- ☑
    multiple sites M87.09
    neck M87.08
    pelvis M87.050
    radius M87.03- ☑
    rib M87.08
    scapula M87.01- ☑
    skull M87.08
    tarsus M87.07- ☑
    tibia M87.06- ☑
    toe M87.07- ☑
    ulna M87.03- ☑
    vertebra M87.08
  secondary NEC M87.30
    carpus M87.33- ☑
    clavicle M87.31- ☑
    due to
      drugs M87.10
        carpus M87.13- ☑
        clavicle M87.11- ☑
        femur M87.15- ☑
        fibula M87.16- ☑
        finger M87.14- ☑
        humerus M87.12- ☑
        ilium M87.159
        ischium M87.159
        jaw M87.180
        metacarpus M87.14- ☑
        metatarsus M87.17- ☑
        multiple sites M87.19
        neck M87.18 ☑
        radius M87.13- ☑
        rib M87.18 ☑
        scapula M87.11- ☑
        skull M87.18 ☑
        tarsus M87.17- ☑
        tibia M87.16- ☑
        toe M87.17- ☑
        ulna M87.13- ☑
        vertebra M87.18 ☑
      hemoglobinopathy NEC D58.2 [M90.50]
        carpus D58.2 [M90.54-] ☑
        clavicle D58.2 [M90.51-] ☑
        femur D58.2 [M90.55-] ☑
        fibula D58.2 [M90.56-] ☑
        finger D58.2 [M90.54-] ☑
        humerus D58.2 [M90.52-] ☑
        ilium D58.2 [M90.55-] ☑
        ischium D58.2 [M90.55-] ☑
        metacarpus D58.2 [M90.54-] ☑
        metatarsus D58.2 [M90.57-] ☑
        multiple sites D58.2 [M90.58]
        neck D58.2 [M90.58]
        radius D58.2 [M90.53-] ☑
        rib D58.2 [M90.58]
        scapula D58.2 [M90.51-] ☑
        skull D58.2 [M90.58]
        tarsus D58.2 [M90.57-] ☑
        tibia D58.2 [M90.56-] ☑
        toe D58.2 [M90.57-] ☑
        ulna D58.2 [M90.53-] ☑
        vertebra D58.2 [M90.58]
      trauma (previous) M87.20
        carpus M87.23- ☑
        clavicle M87.21- ☑
        femur M87.25- ☑
        fibula M87.26- ☑

Osteonecrosis — continued
  secondary — continued
    due to — continued
      trauma — continued
        finger M87.24- ☑
        humerus M87.22- ☑
        ilium M87.25- ☑
        ischium M87.25- ☑
        metacarpus M87.24- ☑
        metatarsus M87.27- ☑
        multiple sites M87.29
        neck M87.28
        radius M87.23- ☑
        rib M87.28
        scapula M87.21- ☑
        skull M87.28
        tarsus M87.27- ☑
        tibia M87.26- ☑
        toe M87.27- ☑
        ulna M87.23- ☑
        vertebra M87.28
    femur M87.35- ☑
    fibula M87.36- ☑
    finger M87.34- ☑
    humerus M87.32- ☑
    ilium M87.350
    in
      caisson disease T70.3 [M90.50]
        carpus T70.3 ☑ [M90.54-] ☑
        clavicle T70.3 ☑ [M90.51-] ☑
        femur T70.3 ☑ [M90.55-] ☑
        fibula T70.3 ☑ [M90.56-] ☑
        finger T70.3 ☑ [M90.54-] ☑
        humerus T70.3 ☑ [M90.52-] ☑
        ilium T70.3 ☑ [M90.55-] ☑
        ischium T70.3 ☑ [M90.55-] ☑
        metacarpus T70.3 ☑ [M90.54-] ☑
        metatarsus T70.3 ☑ [M90.57-] ☑
        multiple sites T70.3 ☑ [M90.59]
        neck T70.3 ☑ [M90.58]
        radius T70.3 ☑ [M90.53-] ☑
        rib T70.3 ☑ [M90.58]
        scapula T70.3 ☑ [M90.51-] ☑
        skull T70.3 ☑ [M90.58]
        tarsus T70.3 ☑ [M90.57-] ☑
        tibia T70.3 ☑ [M90.56-] ☑
        toe T70.3 ☑ [M90.57-] ☑
        ulna T70.3 ☑ [M90.53-] ☑
        vertebra T70.3 ☑ [M90.58]
    ischium M87.350
    metacarpus M87.34- ☑
    metatarsus M87.37- ☑
    multiple site M87.39
    neck M87.38
    radius M87.33- ☑
    rib M87.38
    scapula M87.319
    skull M87.38
    tarsus M87.379
    tibia M87.366
    toe M87.379
    ulna M87.33- ☑
    vertebra M87.38
  specified type NEC M87.80
    carpus M87.83- ☑
    clavicle M87.81- ☑
    femur M87.85- ☑
    fibula M87.86- ☑
    finger M87.84- ☑
    humerus M87.82- ☑
    ilium M87.85- ☑
    ischium M87.85- ☑
    metacarpus M87.84- ☑
    metatarsus M87.87- ☑
    multiple sites M87.89
    neck M87.88
    radius M87.83- ☑
    rib M87.88
    scapula M87.81- ☑
    skull M87.88
    tarsus M87.87- ☑
    tibia M87.86- ☑
    toe M87.87- ☑
    ulna M87.83- ☑
    vertebra M87.88
Osteo-onycho-arthro-dysplasia Q87.2

Osteo-onychodysplasia, hereditary Q87.2
Osteopathia condensans disseminata Q78.8
Osteopathy (see also Osteomyelitis, Osteonecrosis, Osteoporosis)
  after poliomyelitis M89.60
    carpus M89.64- ☑
    clavicle M89.61- ☑
    femur M89.65- ☑
    fibula M89.66- ☑
    finger M89.64- ☑
    humerus M89.62- ☑
    ilium M89.659
    ischium M89.659
    metacarpus M89.64- ☑
    metatarsus M89.67- ☑
    multiple sites M89.69
    neck M89.68
    radius M89.63- ☑
    rib M89.68
    scapula M89.61- ☑
    skull M89.68
    tarsus M89.67- ☑
    tibia M89.66- ☑
    toe M89.67- ☑
    ulna M89.63- ☑
    vertebra M89.68
  in (due to)
    renal osteodystrophy N25.0
    specified diseases classified elsewhere — see subcategory M90.8 ☑
Osteopenia M85.8- ☑
  borderline M85.8- ☑
Osteoperiostitis — see Osteomyelitis, specified type NEC
Osteopetrosis (familial) Q78.2
Osteophyte M25.70
  ankle M25.77- ☑
  elbow M25.72- ☑
  foot joint M25.77- ☑
  hand joint M25.74- ☑
  hip M25.75- ☑
  knee M25.76- ☑
  shoulder M25.71- ☑
  spine M25.78
  vertebrae M25.78
  wrist M25.73- ☑
Osteopoikilosis Q78.8
Osteoporosis (female) (male) M81.0
  with current pathological fracture M80.00 ☑
  age-related M81.0
    with current pathologic fracture M80.00 ☑
      carpus M80.04- ☑
      clavicle M80.01- ☑
      fibula M80.06- ☑
      finger M80.04- ☑
      humerus M80.02- ☑
      ilium M80.05- ☑
      ischium M80.05- ☑
      metacarpus M80.04- ☑
      metatarsus M80.07- ☑
      pelvis M80.05- ☑
      radius M80.03- ☑
      scapula M80.01- ☑
      tarsus M80.07- ☑
      tibia M80.06- ☑
      toe M80.07- ☑
      ulna M80.03- ☑
      vertebra M80.08 ☑
  disuse M81.8
    with current pathological fracture M80.80 ☑
      carpus M80.84- ☑
      clavicle M80.81- ☑
      fibula M80.86- ☑
      finger M80.84- ☑
      humerus M80.82- ☑
      ilium M80.85- ☑
      ischium M80.85- ☑
      metacarpus M80.84- ☑
      metatarsus M80.87- ☑
      pelvis M80.85- ☑
      radius M80.83- ☑
      scapula M80.81- ☑
      tarsus M80.87- ☑
      tibia M80.86- ☑
      toe M80.87- ☑
      ulna M80.83- ☑

☑ Additional Character Required — Refer to the Tabular List for Character Selection   ▽ Subterms under main terms may continue to next column or page

Osteoporosis — *continued*
  disuse — *continued*
    with current pathological fracture — *continued*
      vertebra M80.88 ☑
  drug-induced — *see* Osteoporosis, specified type NEC
  idiopathic — *see* Osteoporosis, specified type NEC
  involutional — *see* Osteoporosis, age-related
  Lequesne M81.6
  localized M81.6
  postmenopausal M81.0
    with pathological fracture M80.00 ☑
      carpus M80.04- ☑
      clavicle M80.01- ☑
      fibula M80.06- ☑
      finger M80.04- ☑
      humerus M80.02- ☑
      ilium M80.05- ☑
      ischium M80.05- ☑
      metacarpus M80.04- ☑
      metatarsus M80.07- ☑
      pelvis M80.05- ☑
      radius M80.03- ☑
      scapula M80.01- ☑
      tarsus M80.07- ☑
      tibia M80.06- ☑
      toe M80.07- ☑
      ulna M80.03- ☑
      vertebra M80.08 ☑
  postoophorectomy — *see* Osteoporosis, specified type NEC
  postsurgical malabsorption — *see* Osteoporosis, specified type NEC
  post-traumatic — *see* Osteoporosis, specified type NEC
  senile — *see* Osteoporosis, age-related
  specified type NEC M81.8
    with pathological fracture M80.80 ☑
      carpus M80.84- ☑
      clavicle M80.81- ☑
      fibula M80.86- ☑
      finger M80.84- ☑
      humerus M80.82- ☑
      ilium M80.85- ☑
      ischium M80.85- ☑
      metacarpus M80.84- ☑
      metatarsus M80.87- ☑
      pelvis M80.85- ☑
      radius M80.83- ☑
      scapula M80.81- ☑
      tarsus M80.87- ☑
      tibia M80.86- ☑
      toe M80.87- ☑
      ulna M80.83- ☑
      vertebra M80.88 ☑

Osteopsathyrosis (idiopathica) Q78.0
Osteoradionecrosis, jaw (acute) (chronic) (lower) (suppurative) (upper) M27.2
Osteosarcoma (any form) — *see* Neoplasm, bone, malignant
Osteosclerosis Q78.2
  acquired M85.8- ☑
  congenita Q77.4
  fragilitas (generalisata) Q78.2
  myelofibrosis D75.81
Osteosclerotic anemia D64.89
Osteosis
  cutis L94.2
  renal fibrocystic N25.0
Österreicher-Turner syndrome Q87.2
Ostium
  atrioventriculare commune Q21.2
  primum (arteriosum) (defect) (persistent) Q21.2
  secundum (arteriosum) (defect) (patent) (persistent) Q21.1
Ostrum-Furst syndrome Q75.8
Otalgia H92.0 ☑
Otitis (acute) H66.90
  with effusion (*see also* Otitis, media, nonsuppurative)
    purulent — *see* Otitis, media, suppurative
  adhesive — *see* subcategory H74.1 ☑
  chronic (*see also* Otitis, media, chronic)
    with effusion (*see also* Otitis, media, nonsuppurative, chronic)
  externa H60.9- ☑
    abscess — *see* Abscess, ear, external
    acute (noninfective) H60.50- ☑

Otitis — *continued*
  externa — *continued*
    acute — *continued*
      actinic H60.51- ☑
      chemical H60.52- ☑
      contact H60.53- ☑
      eczematoid H60.54- ☑
      infective — *see* Otitis, externa, infective
      reactive H60.55- ☑
      specified NEC H60.59- ☑
    cellulitis — *see* Cellulitis, ear
    chronic H60.6- ☑
    diffuse — *see* Otitis, externa, infective, diffuse
    hemorrhagic — *see* Otitis, externa, infective, hemorrhagic
    in (due to)
      aspergillosis B44.89
      candidiasis B37.84
      erysipelas A46 [H62.40]
      herpes (simplex) virus infection B00.1
        zoster B02.8
      impetigo L01.00 [H62.40]
      infectious disease NEC B99 ☑ [H62.4-] ☑
      mycosis NEC B36.9 [H62.40]
      parasitic disease NEC B89 [H62.40]
      viral disease NEC B34.9 [H62.40]
      zoster B02.8
    infective NEC H60.39- ☑
      abscess — *see* Abscess, ear, external
      cellulitis — *see* Cellulitis, ear
      diffuse H60.31- ☑
      hemorrhagic H60.32- ☑
      swimmer's ear — *see* Swimmer's, ear
    malignant H60.2- ☑
    mycotic NEC B36.9 [H62.40]
      in
        aspergillosis B44.89
        candidiasis B37.84
        moniliasis B37.84
    necrotizing — *see* Otitis, externa, malignant
    Pseudomonas aeruginosa — *see* Otitis, externa, malignant
    reactive — *see* Otitis, externa, acute, reactive
    specified NEC — *see* subcategory H60.8 ☑
    tropical NEC B36.9 [H62.40]
      in
        aspergillosis B44.89
        candidiasis B37.84
        moniliasis B37.84
  insidiosa — *see* Otosclerosis
  interna H83.0 ☑
  media (hemorrhagic) (staphylococcal) (streptococcal) H66.9- ☑
    with effusion (nonpurulent) — *see* Otitis, media, nonsuppurative
    acute, subacute H66.90
      allergic — *see* Otitis, media, nonsuppurative, acute, allergic
      exudative — *see* Otitis, media, suppurative, acute
      mucoid — *see* Otitis, media, nonsuppurative, acute
      necrotizing (*see also* Otitis, media, suppurative, acute)
        in
          measles B05.3
          scarlet fever A38.0
      nonsuppurative NEC — *see* Otitis, media, nonsuppurative, acute
      purulent — *see* Otitis, media, suppurative, acute
      sanguinous — *see* Otitis, media, nonsuppurative, acute
      secretory — *see* Otitis, media, nonsuppurative, acute, serous
      seromucinous — *see* Otitis, media, nonsuppurative, acute
      serous — *see* Otitis, media, nonsuppurative, acute, serous
      suppurative — *see* Otitis, media, suppurative, acute
    allergic — *see* Otitis, media, nonsuppurative
    catarrhal — *see* Otitis, media, nonsuppurative
    chronic H66.90
      with effusion (nonpurulent) — *see* Otitis, media, nonsuppurative, chronic

Otitis — *continued*
  media — *continued*
    chronic — *continued*
      allergic — *see* Otitis, media, nonsuppurative, chronic, allergic
      benign suppurative — *see* Otitis, media, suppurative, chronic, tubotympanic
      catarrhal — *see* Otitis, media, nonsuppurative, chronic, serous
      exudative — *see* Otitis, media, nonsuppurative, chronic
      mucinous — *see* Otitis, media, nonsuppurative, chronic, mucoid
      mucoid — *see* Otitis, media, nonsuppurative, chronic, mucoid
      nonsuppurative NEC — *see* Otitis, media, nonsuppurative, chronic
      purulent — *see* Otitis, media, suppurative, chronic
      secretory — *see* Otitis, media, nonsuppurative, chronic, mucoid
      seromucinous — *see* Otitis, media, nonsuppurative, chronic
      serous — *see* Otitis, media, nonsuppurative, chronic, serous
      suppurative — *see* Otitis, media, suppurative, chronic
      transudative — *see* Otitis, media, nonsuppurative, chronic, mucoid
    exudative — *see* Otitis, media, suppurative
    in (due to) (with)
      influenza — *see* Influenza, with, otitis media
      measles B05.3
      scarlet fever A38.0
      tuberculosis A18.6
      viral disease NEC B34.- ☑ [H67.-] ☑
    mucoid — *see* Otitis, media, nonsuppurative
    nonsuppurative H65.9- ☑
      acute or subacute NEC H65.19- ☑
        allergic H65.11- ☑
          recurrent H65.11- ☑
        recurrent H65.19- ☑
        secretory — *see* Otitis, media, nonsuppurative, serous
        serous H65.0- ☑
          recurrent H65.0- ☑
      chronic H65.49- ☑
        allergic H65.41- ☑
        mucoid H65.3- ☑
        serous H65.2- ☑
    postmeasles B05.3
    purulent — *see* Otitis, media, suppurative
    secretory — *see* Otitis, media, nonsuppurative
    seromucinous — *see* Otitis, media, nonsuppurative
    serous — *see* Otitis, media, nonsuppurative
    suppurative H66.4- ☑
      acute H66.00- ☑
        with rupture of ear drum H66.01- ☑
        recurrent H66.00- ☑
          with rupture of ear drum H66.01- ☑
      chronic (*see also* subcategory) H66.3 ☑
        atticoantral H66.2- ☑
        benign — *see* Otitis, media, suppurative, chronic, tubotympanic
        tubotympanic H66.1- ☑
    transudative — *see* Otitis, media, nonsuppurative
    tuberculous A18.6
Otocephaly Q18.2
Otolith syndrome — *see* subcategory H81.8 ☑
Otomycosis (diffuse) NEC B36.9 [H62.40]
  in
    aspergillosis B44.89
    candidiasis B37.84
    moniliasis B37.84
Otoporosis — *see* Otosclerosis
Otorrhagia (nontraumatic) H92.2- ☑
  traumatic — *code by* Type of injury
Otorrhea H92.1- ☑
  cerebrospinal G96.0
Otosclerosis (general) H80.9- ☑
  cochlear (endosteal) H80.2- ☑
  involving
    otic capsule — *see* Otosclerosis, cochlear
    oval window
      nonobliterative H80.0- ☑
      obliterative H80.1- ☑
    round window — *see* Otosclerosis, cochlear

Otosclerosis — *continued*
nonobliterative — *see* Otosclerosis, involving, oval window, nonobliterative
obliterative — *see* Otosclerosis, involving, oval window, obliterative
specified NEC H80.8- ☑
Otospongiosis — *see* Otosclerosis
Otto's disease or pelvis M24.7
Outcome of delivery Z37.9
multiple births Z37.9
all liveborn Z37.50
quadruplets Z37.52
quintuplets Z37.53
sextuplets Z37.54
specified number NEC Z37.59
triplets Z37.51
all stillborn Z37.7
some liveborn Z37.60
quadruplets Z37.62
quintuplets Z37.63
sextuplets Z37.64
specified number NEC Z37.69
triplets Z37.61
single NEC Z37.9
liveborn Z37.0
stillborn Z37.1
twins NEC Z37.9
both liveborn Z37.2
both stillborn Z37.4
one liveborn, one stillborn Z37.3
Outlet — *see* condition
Ovalocytosis (congenital) (hereditary) — *see* Elliptocytosis
Ovarian — *see* Condition
Ovariocele N83.4- ☑
Ovaritis (cystic) — *see* Oophoritis
Ovary, ovarian (*see also* condition)
resistant syndrome E28.39
vein syndrome N13.8
Overactive (*see also* Hyperfunction)
adrenal cortex NEC E27.0
bladder N32.81
hypothalamus E23.3
thyroid — *see* Hyperthyroidism
Overactivity R46.3
child — *see* Disorder, attention-deficit hyperactivity
Overbite (deep) (excessive) (horizontal) (vertical) M26.29
Overbreathing — *see* Hyperventilation
Overconscientious personality F60.5
Overdevelopment — *see* Hypertrophy
Overdistension — *see* Distension
Overdose, overdosage (drug) — *see* Table of Drugs and Chemicals, by drug, poisoning
Overeating R63.2
nonorganic origin F50.89
psychogenic F50.89
Overexertion (effects) (exhaustion) T73.3 ☑
Overexposure (effects) T73.9 ☑
exhaustion T73.2 ☑
Overfeeding — *see* Overeating
newborn P92.4
Overfill, endodontic M27.52
Overgrowth, bone — *see* Hypertrophy, bone
Overhanging of dental restorative material (unrepairable) K08.52
Overheated (places) (effects) — *see* Heat
Overjet (excessive horizontal) M26.23
Overlaid, overlying (suffocation) — *see* Asphyxia, traumatic, due to mechanical threat
Overlap, excessive horizontal (teeth) M26.23
Overlapping toe (acquired) (*see also* Deformity, toe, specified NEC)
congenital (fifth toe) Q66.89
Overload
circulatory, due to transfusion (blood) (blood components) (TACO) E87.71
fluid E87.70
due to transfusion (blood) (blood components) E87.71
specified NEC E87.79
iron, due to repeated red blood cell transfusions E83.111
potassium (K) E87.5
sodium (Na) E87.0
Overnutrition — *see* Hyperalimentation
Overproduction (*see also* Hypersecretion)
ACTH E27.0

Overproduction — *continued*
catecholamine E27.5
growth hormone E22.0
Overprotection, child by parent Z62.1
Overriding
aorta Q25.49
finger (acquired) — *see* Deformity, finger
congenital Q68.1
toe (acquired) (*see also* Deformity, toe, specified NEC)
congenital Q66.89
Overstrained R53.83
heart — *see* Hypertrophy, cardiac
Overuse, muscle NEC M70.8- ☑
Overweight E66.3
Overworked R53.83
Oviduct — *see* condition
Ovotestis Q56.0
Ovulation (cycle)
failure or lack of N97.0
pain N94.0
Ovum — *see* condition
Owren's disease or syndrome (parahemophilia) D68.2
Ox heart — *see* Hypertrophy, cardiac
Oxalosis E72.53
Oxaluria E72.53
Oxycephaly, oxycephalic Q75.0
syphilitic, congenital A50.02
Oxyuriasis B80
Oxyuris vermicularis (infestation) B80
Ozena J31.0

P

Pachyderma, pachydermia L85.9
larynx (verrucosa) J38.7
Pachydermatocele (congenital) Q82.8
Pachydermoperiostosis (*see also* Osteoarthropathy, hypertrophic, specified type NEC)
clubbed nail M89.40 [L62]
Pachygyria Q04.3
Pachymeningitis (adhesive) (basal) (brain) (cervical) (chronic)(circumscribed) (external) (fibrous) (hemorrhagic) (hypertrophic) (internal) (purulent) (spinal) (suppurative) — *see* Meningitis
Pachyonychia (congenital) Q84.5
Pacinian tumor — *see* Neoplasm, skin, benign
Pad, knuckle or Garrod's M72.1
Paget's disease
with infiltrating duct carcinoma — *see* Neoplasm, breast, malignant
bone M88.9
carpus M88.84- ☑
clavicle M88.81- ☑
femur M88.85- ☑
fibula M88.86- ☑
finger M88.84- ☑
humerus M88.82- ☑
ilium M88.85- ☑
in neoplastic disease — *see* Osteitis, deformans, in neoplastic disease
ischium M88.85- ☑
metacarpus M88.84- ☑
metatarsus M88.87- ☑
multiple sites M88.89
neck M88.88
radius M88.83- ☑
rib M88.88
scapula M88.81- ☑
skull M88.0
tarsus M88.87- ☑
tibia M88.86- ☑
toe M88.87- ☑
ulna M88.83- ☑
vertebra M88.88
breast (female) C50.01- ☑
male C50.02- ☑
extramammary (*see also* Neoplasm, skin, malignant)
anus C21.0
margin C44.590
skin C44.590
intraductal carcinoma — *see* Neoplasm, breast, malignant
malignant — *see* Neoplasm, skin, malignant
breast (female) C50.01- ☑
male C50.02- ☑
unspecified site (female) C50.01- ☑
male C50.02- ☑

Paget's disease — *continued*
mammary — *see* Paget's disease, breast
nipple — *see* Paget's disease, breast
osteitis deformans — *see* Paget's disease, bone
Paget-Schroetter syndrome I82.890
Pain(s) (*see also* Painful) R52
abdominal R10.9
colic R10.83
generalized R10.84
with acute abdomen R10.0
lower R10.30
left quadrant R10.32
pelvic or perineal R10.2
periumbilical R10.33
right quadrant R10.31
rebound — *see* Tenderness, abdominal, rebound
severe with abdominal rigidity R10.0
tenderness — *see* Tenderness, abdominal
upper R10.10
epigastric R10.13
left quadrant R10.12
right quadrant R10.11
acute R52
due to trauma G89.11
neoplasm related G89.3
postprocedural NEC G89.18
post-thoracotomy G89.12
specified by site — *code to* Pain, by site
adnexa (uteri) R10.2
anginoid — *see* Pain, precordial
anus K62.89
arm — *see* Pain, limb, upper
axillary (axilla) M79.62- ☑
back (postural) M54.9
bladder R39.89
associated with micturition — *see* Micturition, painful
chronic R39.82
bone — *see* Disorder, bone, specified type NEC
breast N64.4
broad ligament R10.2
cancer associated (acute) (chronic) G89.3
cecum — *see* Pain, abdominal
cervicobrachial M53.1
chest (central) R07.9
anterior wall R07.89
atypical R07.89
ischemic I20.9
musculoskeletal R07.89
non-cardiac R07.89
on breathing R07.1
pleurodynia R07.81
precordial R07.2
wall (anterior) R07.89
chronic G89.29
associated with significant psychosocial dysfunction G89.4
due to trauma G89.21
neoplasm related G89.3
postoperative NEC G89.28
postprocedural NEC G89.28
post-thoracotomy G89.22
specified NEC G89.29
coccyx M53.3
colon — *see* Pain, abdominal
coronary — *see* Angina
costochondral R07.1
diaphragm R07.1
due to cancer G89.3
due to device, implant or graft (*see also* Complications, by site and type, specified NEC) T85.848 ☑
arterial graft NEC T82.848 ☑
breast (implant) T85.848 ☑
catheter NEC T85.848 ☑
dialysis (renal) T82.848 ☑
intraperitoneal T85.848 ☑
infusion NEC T82.848 ☑
spinal (epidural) (subdural) T85.840 ☑
urinary (indwelling) T83.84 ☑
electronic (electrode) (pulse generator) (stimulator)
bone T85.840 ☑
cardiac T82.847 ☑
nervous system (brain) (peripheral nerve) (spinal) T85.84 ☑
urinary T83.84 ☑
fixation, internal (orthopedic) NEC T84.84 ☑
gastrointestinal (bile duct) (esophagus) T85.848 ☑
genital NEC T83.84 ☑

☑ **Additional Character Required** — **Refer to the Tabular List for Character Selection** ⚐ **Subterms under main terms may continue to next column or page**

Pain(s) — *continued*
  due to device, implant or graft (*see also* Complications, by site and type, specified) — *continued*
    heart NEC T82.847 ☑
    infusion NEC T85.848 ☑
    joint prosthesis T84.84 ☑
    ocular (corneal graft) (orbital implant) NEC T85.848 ☑
    orthopedic NEC T84.84 ☑
    specified NEC T85.848 ☑
    urinary NEC T83.84 ☑
    vascular NEC T82.848 ☑
    ventricular intracranial shunt T85.840 ☑
  due to malignancy (primary) (secondary) G89.3
  ear — *see* subcategory H92.0 ☑
  epigastric, epigastrium R10.13
  eye — *see* Pain, ocular
  face, facial R51
    atypical G50.1
  female genital organs NEC N94.89
  finger — *see* Pain, limb, upper
  flank — *see* Pain, abdominal
  foot — *see* Pain, limb, lower
  gallbladder K82.9
  gas (intestinal) R14.1
  gastric — *see* Pain, abdominal
  generalized NOS R52
  genital organ
    female N94.89
    male N50.89
  groin — *see* Pain, abdominal, lower
  hand — *see* Pain, limb, upper
  head — *see* Headache
  heart — *see* Pain, precordial
  infra-orbital — *see* Neuralgia, trigeminal
  intercostal R07.82
  intermenstrual N94.0
  jaw R68.84
  joint M25.50
    ankle M25.57- ☑
    elbow M25.52- ☑
    finger M25.54- ☑
    foot M25.57- ☑
    hand M25.54- ☑
    hip M25.55- ☑
    knee M25.56- ☑
    shoulder M25.51- ☑
    toe M25.57- ☑
    wrist M25.53- ☑
  kidney N23
  laryngeal R07.0
  leg — *see* Pain, limb, lower
  limb M79.609
    lower M79.60- ☑
      foot M79.67- ☑
      lower leg M79.66- ☑
      thigh M79.65- ☑
      toe M79.67- ☑
    upper M79.60- ☑
      axilla M79.62- ☑
      finger M79.64- ☑
      forearm M79.63- ☑
      hand M79.64- ☑
      upper arm M79.62- ☑
  loin M54.5
  low back M54.5
  lumbar region M54.5
  mandibular R68.84
  mastoid — *see* subcategory H92.0 ☑
  maxilla R68.84
  menstrual (*see also* Dysmenorrhea) N94.6
  metacarpophalangeal (joint) — *see* Pain, joint, hand
  metatarsophalangeal (joint) — *see* Pain, joint, foot
  mouth K13.79
  muscle — *see* Myalgia
  musculoskeletal (*see also* Pain, by site) M79.1
  myofascial M79.1
  nasal J34.89
  nasopharynx J39.2
  neck NEC M54.2
  nerve NEC — *see* Neuralgia
  neuromuscular — *see* Neuralgia
  nose J34.89
  ocular H57.1- ☑
  ophthalmic — *see* Pain, ocular
  orbital region — *see* Pain, ocular
  ovary N94.89

Pain(s) — *continued*
  over heart — *see* Pain, precordial
  ovulation N94.0
  pelvic (female) R10.2
  penis N48.89
  pericardial — *see* Pain, precordial
  perineal, perineum R10.2
  pharynx J39.2
  pleura, pleural, pleuritic R07.81
  postoperative NOS G89.18
  postprocedural NOS G89.18
  post-thoracotomy G89.12
  precordial (region) R07.2
  premenstrual N94.3
  psychogenic (persistent) (any site) F45.41
  radicular (spinal) — *see* Radiculopathy
  rectum K62.89
  respiration R07.1
  retrosternal R07.2
  rheumatoid, muscular — *see* Myalgia
  rib R07.81
  root (spinal) — *see* Radiculopathy
  round ligament (stretch) R10.2
  sacroiliac M53.3
  sciatic — *see* Sciatica
  scrotum N50.82
  seminal vesicle N50.89
  shoulder M25.51- ☑
  spermatic cord N50.89
  spinal root — *see* Radiculopathy
  spine M54.9
    cervical M54.2
    low back M54.5
      with sciatica M54.4- ☑
    thoracic M54.6
  stomach — *see* Pain, abdominal
  substernal R07.2
  temporomandibular (joint) M26.62- ☑
  testis N50.81- ☑
  thoracic spine M54.6
    with radicular and visceral pain M54.14
  throat R07.0
  tibia — *see* Pain, limb, lower
  toe — *see* Pain, limb, lower
  tongue K14.6
  tooth K08.89
  trigeminal — *see* Neuralgia, trigeminal
  tumor associated G89.3
  ureter N23
  urinary (organ) (system) N23
  uterus NEC N94.89
  vagina R10.2
  vertebrogenic (syndrome) M54.89
  vesical R39.89
    associated with micturition — *see* Micturition, painful
  vulva R10.2

Painful (*see also* Pain)
  coitus
    female N94.10
    male N53.12
    psychogenic F52.6
  ejaculation (semen) N53.12
    psychogenic F52.6
  erection — *see* Priapism
  feet syndrome E53.8
  joint replacement (hip) (knee) T84.84 ☑
  menstruation — *see* Dysmenorrhea
    psychogenic F45.8
  micturition — *see* Micturition, painful
  respiration R07.1
  scar NEC L90.5
  wire sutures T81.89 ☑
Painter's colic — *see* subcategory T56.0 ☑
Palate — *see* condition
Palatoplegia K13.79
Palatoschisis — *see* Cleft, palate
Palilalia R48.8
Palliative care Z51.5
Pallor R23.1
  optic disc, temporal — *see* Atrophy, optic
Palmar (*see also* condition)
  fascia — *see* condition
Palpable
  cecum K63.89
  kidney N28.89
  ovary N83.8
  prostate N42.9

Palpable — *continued*
  spleen — *see* Splenomegaly
Palpitations (heart) R00.2
  psychogenic F45.8
Palsy (*see also* Paralysis) G83.9
  atrophic diffuse (progressive) G12.22
  Bell's (*see also* Palsy, facial)
    newborn P11.3
  brachial plexus NEC G54.0
    newborn (birth injury) P14.3
  brain — *see* Palsy, cerebral
  bulbar (progressive) (chronic) G12.22
    of childhood (Fazio-Londe) G12.1
    pseudo NEC G12.29
    supranuclear (progressive) G23.1
  cerebral (congenital) G80.9
    ataxic G80.4
    athetoid G80.3
    choreathetoid G80.3
    diplegic G80.8
      spastic G80.1
    dyskinetic G80.3
      athetoid G80.3
      choreathetoid G80.3
      distonic G80.3
    dystonic G80.3
    hemiplegic G80.8
      spastic G80.2
    mixed G80.8
    monoplegic G80.8
      spastic G80.1
    paraplegic G80.8
      spastic G80.1
    quadriplegic G80.8
      spastic G80.0
    spastic G80.1
      diplegic G80.1
      hemiplegic G80.2
      monoplegic G80.1
      quadriplegic G80.0
      specified NEC G80.1
      tetrapelgic G80.0
    specified NEC G80.8
    syphilitic A52.12
      congenital A50.49
    tetraplegic G80.8
      spastic G80.0
  cranial nerve (*see also* Disorder, nerve, cranial)
    multiple G52.7
      in
        infectious disease B99 ☑ [G53]
        neoplastic disease (*see also* Neoplasm) D49.9 [G53]
        parasitic disease B89 [G53]
        sarcoidosis D86.82
  creeping G12.22
  diver's T70.3 ☑
  Erb's P14.0
  facial G51.0
    newborn (birth injury) P11.3
  glossopharyngeal G52.1
  Klumpke (-Déjérine) P14.1
  lead — *see* subcategory T56.0 ☑
  median nerve (tardy) G56.1- ☑
  nerve G58.9
    specified NEC G58.8
  peroneal nerve (acute) (tardy) G57.3- ☑
  progressive supranuclear G23.1
  pseudobulbar NEC G12.29
  radial nerve (acute) G56.3- ☑
  seventh nerve (*see also* Palsy, facial)
    newborn P11.3
  shaking — *see* Parkinsonism
  spastic (cerebral) (spinal) G80.1
  ulnar nerve (tardy) G56.2- ☑
  wasting G12.29
Paludism — *see* Malaria
Panangiitis M30.0
Panaris, panaritium (*see also* Cellulitis, digit)
  with lymphangitis — *see* Lymphangitis, acute, digit
Panarteritis nodosa M30.0
  brain or cerebral I67.7
Pancake heart R93.1
  with cor pulmonale (chronic) I27.81
Pancarditis (acute) (chronic) I51.89
  rheumatic I09.89
    active or acute I01.8
Pancoast's syndrome or tumor C34.1- ☑

Pancolitis, ulcerative (chronic) K51.00
  with
    abscess K51.014
    complication K51.019
    fistula K51.013
    obstruction K51.012
    rectal bleeding K51.011
    specified complication NEC K51.018
Pancreas, pancreatic — *see* condition
Pancreatitis (annular) (apoplectic) (calcareous) (edematous) (hemorrhagic) (malignant) (recurrent) (subacute) (suppurative) K85.90
  with necrosis (uninfected) K85.91
    infected K85.92
  acute (without necrosis or infection) K85.90
    with necrosis (uninfected) K85.91
      infected K85.92
    alcohol induced (without necrosis or infection) K85.20
      with necrosis (uninfected) K85.21
        infected K85.22
    biliary (without necrosis or infection) K85.10
      with necrosis (uninfected) K85.11
        infected K85.12
    drug induced (without necrosis or infection) K85.30
      with necrosis (uninfected) K85.31
        infected K85.32
    gallstone (without necrosis or infection) K85.10
      with necrosis (uninfected) K85.11
        infected K85.12
    idiopathic (without necrosis or infection) K85.00
      with necrosis (uninfected) K85.01
        infected K85.02
    specified NEC (without necrosis or infection) K85.80
      with necrosis (uninfected) K85.81
        infected K85.82
  chronic (infectious) K86.1
    alcohol-induced K86.0
    recurrent K86.1
    relapsing K86.1
  cystic (chronic) K86.1
  cytomegaloviral B25.2
  fibrous (chronic) K86.1
  gallstone (without necrosis or infection) K85.10
    with necrosis (uninfected) K85.11
      infected K85.12
  gangrenous — *see* Pancreatitis, acute
  interstitial (chronic) K86.1
    acute (*see also* Pancreatitis, acute) K85.80
  mumps B26.3
  recurrent (chronic) K86.1
  relapsing, chronic K86.1
  syphilitic A52.74
Pancreatoblastoma — *see* Neoplasm, pancreas, malignant
Pancreolithiasis K86.89
Pancytolysis D75.89
Pancytopenia (acquired) D61.818
  with
    malformations D61.09
    myelodysplastic syndrome — *see* Syndrome, myelodysplastic
  antineoplastic chemotherapy induced D61.810
  congenital D61.09
  drug-induced NEC D61.811
PANDAS (pediatric autoimmune neuropsychiatric disorders associated with streptococcal infections syndrome) D89.89
Panencephalitis, subacute, sclerosing A81.1
Panhematopenia D61.9
  congenital D61.09
  constitutional D61.09
  splenic, primary D73.1
Panhemocytopenia D61.9
  congenital D61.09
  constitutional D61.09
Panhypogonadism E29.1
Panhypopituitarism E23.0
  prepubertal E23.0
Panic (attack) (state) F41.0
  reaction to exceptional stress (transient) F43.0
Panmyelopathy, familial, constitutional D61.09
Panmyelophthisis D61.82
  congenital D61.09
Panmyelosis (acute) (with myelofibrosis) C94.4- ☑
Panner's disease — *see* Osteochondrosis, juvenile, humerus
Panneuritis endemica E51.11

Panniculitis (nodular) (nonsuppurative) M79.3
  back M54.00
    cervical region M54.02
    cervicothoracic region M54.03
    lumbar region M54.06
    lumbosacral region M54.07
    multiple sites M54.09
    occipito-atlanto-axial region M54.01
    sacrococcygeal region M54.08
    thoracic region M54.04
    thoracolumbar region M54.05
  lupus L93.2
  mesenteric K65.4
  neck M54.02
    cervicothoracic region M54.03
    occipito-atlanto-axial region M54.01
  relapsing M35.6
Panniculus adiposus (abdominal) E65
Pannus (allergic) (cornea) (degenerativus) (keratic) H16.42- ☑
  abdominal (symptomatic) E65
  trachomatosus, trachomatous (active) A71.1
Panophthalmitis H44.01- ☑
Pansinusitis (chronic) (hyperplastic) (nonpurulent) (purulent) J32.4
  acute J01.40
    recurrent J01.41
  tuberculous A15.8
Panuveitis (sympathetic) H44.11- ☑
Panvalvular disease I08.9
  specified NEC I08.8
PAPA (pyogenic arthritis, pyoderma gangrenosum, and acne syndrome) M04.8
Papanicolaou smear, cervix Z12.4
  as part of routine gynecological examination Z01.419
    with abnormal findings Z01.411
  for suspected neoplasm Z12.4
  nonspecific abnormal finding R87.619
  routine Z01.419
    with abnormal findings Z01.411
Papilledema (choked disc) H47.10
  associated with
    decreased ocular pressure H47.12
    increased intracranial pressure H47.11
    retinal disorder H47.13
  Foster-Kennedy syndrome H47.14- ☑
Papillitis H46.00
  anus K62.89
  chronic lingual K14.4
  necrotizing, kidney N17.2
  optic H46.0- ☑
  rectum K62.89
  renal, necrotizing N17.2
  tongue K14.0
Papilloma (*see also* Neoplasm, benign, by site)
  acuminatum (female) (male) (anogenital) A63.0
  basal cell L82.1
    inflamed L82.0
  benign pinta (primary) A67.0
  bladder (urinary) (transitional cell) D41.4
  choroid plexus (lateral ventricle) (third ventricle) D33.0
    anaplastic C71.5
    fourth ventricle D33.1
    malignant C71.5
  renal pelvis (transitional cell) D41.1- ☑
    benign D30.1- ☑
  Schneiderian
    specified site — *see* Neoplasm, benign, by site
    unspecified site D14.0
  serous surface
    borderline malignancy
      specified site — *see* Neoplasm, uncertain behavior, by site
      unspecified site D39.10
    specified site — *see* Neoplasm, benign, by site
    unspecified site D27.9
  transitional (cell)
    bladder (urinary) D41.4
    inverted type — *see* Neoplasm, uncertain behavior, by site
    renal pelvis D41.1- ☑
    ureter D41.2- ☑
  ureter (transitional cell) D41.2- ☑
    benign D30.2- ☑
  urothelial — *see* Neoplasm, uncertain behavior, by site
  villous — *see* Neoplasm, uncertain behavior, by site

Papilloma — *continued*
  villous — *see* Neoplasm, uncertain behavior, by site
    — *continued*
      adenocarcinoma in — *see* Neoplasm, malignant, by site
      in situ — *see* Neoplasm, in situ
  yaws, plantar or palmar A66.1
Papillomata, multiple, of yaws A66.1
Papillomatosis (*see also* Neoplasm, benign, by site)
  confluent and reticulated L83
  cystic, breast — *see* Mastopathy, cystic
  ductal, breast — *see* Mastopathy, cystic
  intraductal (diffuse) — *see* Neoplasm, benign, by site
  subareolar duct D24- ☑
Papillomavirus, as cause of disease classified elsewhere B97.7
Papillon-Léage and Psaume syndrome Q87.0
Papule(s) R23.8
  carate (primary) A67.0
  fibrous, of nose D22.39
  Gottron's L94.4
  pinta (primary) A67.0
Papulosis
  lymphomatoid C86.6
  malignant I77.89
Papyraceous fetus O31.0- ☑
Para-albuminemia E88.09
Paracephalus Q89.7
Parachute mitral valve Q23.2
Paracoccidioidomycosis B41.9
  disseminated B41.7
  generalized B41.7
  mucocutaneous-lymphangitic B41.8
  pulmonary B41.0
  specified NEC B41.8
  visceral B41.8
Paradentosis K05.4
Paraffinoma T88.8 ☑
Paraganglioma D44.7
  adrenal D35.0- ☑
    malignant C74.1- ☑
  aortic body D44.7
    malignant C75.5
  carotid body D44.6
    malignant C75.4
  chromaffin (*see also* Neoplasm, benign, by site)
    malignant — *see* Neoplasm, malignant, by site
  extra-adrenal D44.7
    malignant C75.5
      specified site — *see* Neoplasm, malignant, by site
      unspecified site C75.5
    specified site — *see* Neoplasm, uncertain behavior, by site
    unspecified site D44.7
  gangliocytic D13.2
    specified site — *see* Neoplasm, benign, by site
    unspecified site D13.2
  glomus jugulare D44.7
    malignant C75.5
  jugular D44.7
  malignant C75.5
    specified site — *see* Neoplasm, malignant, by site
    unspecified site C75.5
  nonchromaffin D44.7
    malignant C75.5
      specified site — *see* Neoplasm, malignant, by site
      unspecified site C75.5
    specified site — *see* Neoplasm, uncertain behavior, by site
    unspecified site D44.7
  parasympathetic D44.7
    specified site — *see* Neoplasm, uncertain behavior, by site
    unspecified site D44.7
  specified site — *see* Neoplasm, uncertain behavior, by site
  sympathetic D44.7
    specified site — *see* Neoplasm, uncertain behavior, by site
    unspecified site D44.7
  unspecified site D44.7
Parageusia R43.2
  psychogenic F45.8
Paragonimiasis B66.4

☑ **Additional Character Required** — Refer to the Tabular List for Character Selection   ▽ Subterms under main terms may continue to next column or page

Paragranuloma, Hodgkin — *see* Lymphoma, Hodgkin, specified NEC
Parahemophilia (*see also* Defect, coagulation) D68.2
Parakeratosis R23.4
  variegata L41.0
Paralysis, paralytic (complete) (incomplete) G83.9
  with
    syphilis A52.17
  abducens, abducent (nerve) — *see* Strabismus, paralytic, sixth nerve
  abductor, lower extremity G57.9- ☑
  accessory nerve G52.8
  accommodation (*see also* Paresis, of accommodation)
    hysterical F44.89
  acoustic nerve (except Deafness) H93.3 ☑
  agitans (*see also* Parkinsonism) G20
    arteriosclerotic G21.4
  alternating (oculomotor) G83.89
  amyotrophic G12.21
  ankle G57.9- ☑
  anus (sphincter) K62.89
  arm — *see* Monoplegia, upper limb
  ascending (spinal), acute G61.0
  association G12.29
  asthenic bulbar G70.00
    with exacerbation (acute) G70.01
    in crisis G70.01
  ataxic (hereditary) G11.9
    general (syphilitic) A52.17
  atrophic G58.9
    infantile, acute — *see* Poliomyelitis, paralytic
    progressive G12.22
    spinal (acute) — *see* Poliomyelitis, paralytic
  axillary G54.0
  Babinski-Nageotte's G83.89
  Bell's G51.0
    newborn P11.3
  Benedikt's G46.3
  birth injury P14.9
    spinal cord P11.5
  bladder (neurogenic) (sphincter) N31.2
  bowel, colon or intestine K56.0
  brachial plexus G54.0
    birth injury P14.3
    newborn (birth injury) P14.3
  brain G83.9
    diplegia G83.0
    triplegia G83.89
  bronchial J98.09
  Brown-Séquard G83.81
  bulbar (chronic) (progressive) G12.22
    infantile — *see* Poliomyelitis, paralytic
    poliomyelitic — *see* Poliomyelitis, paralytic
    pseudo G12.29
  bulbospinal G70.00
    with exacerbation (acute) G70.01
    in crisis G70.01
  cardiac (*see also* Failure, heart) I50.9
  cerebrocerebellar, diplegic G80.1
  cervical
    plexus G54.2
    sympathetic G90.09
  Céstan-Chenais G46.3
  Charcot-Marie-Tooth type G60.0
  Clark's G80.9
  colon K56.0
  compressed air T70.3 ☑
  compression
    arm G56.9- ☑
    leg G57.9- ☑
    lower extremity G57.9- ☑
    upper extremity G56.9- ☑
  congenital (cerebral) — *see* Palsy, cerebral
  conjugate movement (gaze) (of eye) H51.0
    cortical (nuclear) (supranuclear) H51.0
  cordis — *see* Failure, heart
  cranial or cerebral nerve G52.9
  creeping G12.22
  crossed leg G83.89
  crutch — *see* Injury, brachial plexus
  deglutition R13.0
    hysterical F44.4
  dementia A52.17
  descending (spinal) NEC G12.29
  diaphragm (flaccid) J98.6
    due to accidental dissection of phrenic nerve during procedure — *see* Puncture, accidental complicating surgery

Paralysis, paralytic — *continued*
  digestive organs NEC K59.8
  diplegic — *see* Diplegia
  divergence (nuclear) H51.8
  diver's T70.3 ☑
  Duchenne's
    birth injury P14.0
    due to or associated with
      motor neuron disease G12.22
      muscular dystrophy G71.0
  due to intracranial or spinal birth injury — *see* Palsy, cerebral
  embolic (current episode) I63.4- ☑
  Erb (-Duchenne) (birth) (newborn) P14.0
  Erb's syphilitic spastic spinal A52.17
  esophagus K22.8
  eye muscle (extrinsic) H49.9
    intrinsic (*see also* Paresis, of accommodation)
  facial (nerve) G51.0
    birth injury P11.3
    congenital P11.3
    following operation NEC — *see* Puncture, accidental complicating surgery
    newborn (birth injury) P11.3
  familial (recurrent) (periodic) G72.3
    spastic G11.4
  fauces J39.2
  finger G56.9- ☑
  gait R26.1
  gastric nerve (nondiabetic) G52.2
  gaze, conjugate H51.0
  general (progressive) (syphilitic) A52.17
    juvenile A50.45
  glottis J38.00
    bilateral J38.02
    unilateral J38.01
  gluteal G54.1
  Gubler (-Millard) G46.3
  hand — *see* Monoplegia, upper limb
  heart — *see* Arrest, cardiac
  hemiplegic — *see* Hemiplegia
  hyperkalemic periodic (familial) G72.3
  hypoglossal (nerve) G52.3
  hypokalemic periodic G72.3
  hysterical F44.4
  ileus K56.0
  infantile (*see also* Poliomyelitis, paralytic) A80.30
    bulbar — *see* Poliomyelitis, paralytic
    cerebral — *see* Palsy, cerebral
    spastic — *see* Palsy, cerebral, spastic
  infective — *see* Poliomyelitis, paralytic
  inferior nuclear G83.9
  internuclear — *see* Ophthalmoplegia, internuclear
  intestine K56.0
  iris H57.09
    due to diphtheria (toxin) A36.89
  ischemic, Volkmann's (complicating trauma) T79.6 ☑
  Jackson's G83.89
  jake — *see* Poisoning, food, noxious, plant
  Jamaica ginger (jake) G62.2
  juvenile general A50.45
  Klumpke (-Déjérine) (birth) (newborn) P14.1
  labioglossal (laryngeal) (pharyngeal) G12.29
  Landry's G61.0
  laryngeal nerve (recurrent) (superior) (unilateral) J38.00
    bilateral J38.02
    unilateral J38.01
  larynx J38.00
    bilateral J38.02
    due to diphtheria (toxin) A36.2
    unilateral J38.01
  lateral G12.23
  lead T56.0 ☑
  left side — *see* Hemiplegia
  leg G83.1- ☑
    both — *see* Paraplegia
    crossed G83.89
    hysterical F44.4
    psychogenic F44.4
    transient or transitory R29.818
      traumatic NEC — *see* Injury, nerve, leg
  levator palpebrae superioris — *see* Blepharoptosis, paralytic
  limb — *see* Monoplegia
  lip K13.0
  Lissauer's A52.17
  lower limb — *see* Monoplegia, lower limb
    both — *see* Paraplegia

Paralysis, paralytic — *continued*
  lung J98.4
  median nerve G56.1- ☑
  medullary (tegmental) G83.89
  mesencephalic NEC G83.89
    tegmental G83.89
  middle alternating G83.89
  Millard-Gubler-Foville G46.3
  monoplegic — *see* Monoplegia
  motor G83.9
  muscle, muscular NEC G72.89
    due to nerve lesion G58.9
    eye (extrinsic) H49.9
      intrinsic — *see* Paresis, of accommodation
      oblique — *see* Strabismus, paralytic, fourth nerve
    iris sphincter H21.9
    ischemic (Volkmann's) (complicating trauma) T79.6 ☑
    progressive G12.21
    pseudohypertrophic G71.0
  musculocutaneous nerve G56.9- ☑
  musculospiral G56.9- ☑
  nerve (*see also* Disorder, nerve)
    abducent — *see* Strabismus, paralytic, sixth nerve
    accessory G52.8
    auditory (except Deafness) H93.3 ☑
    birth injury P14.9
    cranial or cerebral G52.9
    facial G51.0
      birth injury P11.3
      congenital P11.3
      newborn (birth injury) P11.3
    fourth or trochlear — *see* Strabismus, paralytic, fourth nerve
    newborn (birth injury) P14.9
    oculomotor — *see* Strabismus, paralytic, third nerve
    phrenic (birth injury) P14.2
    radial G56.3- ☑
    seventh or facial G51.0
      newborn (birth injury) P11.3
    sixth or abducent — *see* Strabismus, paralytic, sixth nerve
    syphilitic A52.15
    third or oculomotor — *see* Strabismus, paralytic, third nerve
    trigeminal G50.9
    trochlear — *see* Strabismus, paralytic, fourth nerve
    ulnar G56.2- ☑
  normokalemic periodic G72.3
  ocular H49.9
    alternating G83.89
  oculofacial, congenital (Moebius) Q87.0
  oculomotor (external bilateral) (nerve) — *see* Strabismus, paralytic, third nerve
  palate (soft) K13.79
  paratrigeminal G50.9
  periodic (familial) (hyperkalemic) (hypokalemic) (myotonic) (normokalemic) (potassium sensitive) (secondary) G72.3
  peripheral autonomic nervous system — *see* Neuropathy, peripheral, autonomic
  peroneal (nerve) G57.3- ☑
  pharynx J39.2
  phrenic nerve G56.8- ☑
  plantar nerve(s) G57.6- ☑
  pneumogastric nerve G52.2
  poliomyelitis (current) — *see* Poliomyelitis, paralytic
  popliteal nerve G57.3- ☑
  postepileptic transitory G83.84
  progressive (atrophic) (bulbar) (spinal) G12.22
    general A52.17
    infantile acute — *see* Poliomyelitis, paralytic
    supranuclear G23.1
  pseudobulbar G12.29
  pseudohypertrophic (muscle) G71.0
  psychogenic F44.4
  quadriceps G57.9- ☑
  quadriplegic — *see* Tetraplegia
  radial nerve G56.3- ☑
  rectus muscle (eye) H49.9
  recurrent isolated sleep G47.53
  respiratory (muscle) (system) (tract) R06.81
    center NEC G93.89
    congenital P28.89
    newborn P28.89
  right side — *see* Hemiplegia

Paralysis, paralytic — *continued*
   saturnine T56.0 ☑
   sciatic nerve G57.0- ☑
   senile G83.9
   shaking — *see* Parkinsonism
   shoulder G56.9- ☑
   sleep, recurrent isolated G47.53
   spastic G83.9
      cerebral — *see* Palsy, cerebral, spastic
      congenital (cerebral) — *see* Palsy, cerebral, spastic
      familial G11.4
      hereditary G11.4
      quadriplegic G80.0
      syphilitic (spinal) A52.17
   sphincter, bladder — *see* Paralysis, bladder
   spinal (cord) G83.9
      accessory nerve G52.8
      acute — *see* Poliomyelitis, paralytic
      ascending acute G61.0
      atrophic (acute) (*see also* Poliomyelitis, paralytic)
         spastic, syphilitic A52.17
      congenital NEC — *see* Palsy, cerebral
      hereditary G95.89
      infantile — *see* Poliomyelitis, paralytic
      progressive G12.21
      sequelae NEC G83.89
   sternomastoid G52.8
   stomach K31.84
      diabetic — *see* Diabetes, by type, with gastropare-
         sis
      nerve G52.2
         diabetic — *see* Diabetes, by type, with gastro-
            paresis
   stroke — *see* Infarct, brain
   subcapsularis G56.8- ☑
   supranuclear (progressive) G23.1
   sympathetic G90.8
      cervical G90.09
      nervous system — *see* Neuropathy, peripheral,
         autonomic
   syndrome G83.9
      specified NEC G83.89
   syphilitic spastic spinal (Erb's) A52.17
   thigh G57.9- ☑
   throat J39.2
      diphtheritic A36.0
      muscle J39.2
   thrombotic (current episode) I63.3- ☑
   thumb G56.9- ☑
   tick — *see* Toxicity, venom, arthropod, specified NEC
   Todd's (postepileptic transitory paralysis) G83.84
   toe G57.6- ☑
   tongue K14.8
   transient R29.5
      arm or leg NEC R29.818
      traumatic NEC — *see* Injury, nerve
   trapezius G52.8
   traumatic, transient NEC — *see* Injury, nerve
   trembling — *see* Parkinsonism
   triceps brachii G56.9- ☑
   trigeminal nerve G50.9
   trochlear (nerve) — *see* Strabismus, paralytic, fourth
      nerve
   ulnar nerve G56.2- ☑
   upper limb — *see* Monoplegia, upper limb
   uremic N18.9 [G99.8]
   uveoparotitic D86.89
   uvula K13.79
      postdiphtheritic A36.0
   vagus nerve G52.2
   vasomotor NEC G90.8
   velum palati K13.79
   vesical — *see* Paralysis, bladder
   vestibular nerve (except Vertigo) H93.3 ☑
   vocal cords J38.00
      bilateral J38.02
      unilateral J38.01
   Volkmann's (complicating trauma) T79.6 ☑
   wasting G12.29
   Weber's G46.3
   wrist G56.9- ☑
Paramedial urethrovesical orifice Q64.79
Paramenia N92.6
Parametritis (*see also* Disease, pelvis, inflammatory)
   N73.2
   acute N73.0

Parametritis — *continued*
   complicating abortion — *see* Abortion, by type, com-
      plicated by, parametritis
Parametrium, parametric — *see* condition
Paramnesia — *see* Amnesia
Paramolar K00.1
Paramyloidosis E85.89
Paramyoclonus multiplex G25.3
Paramyotonia (congenita) G71.19
Parangi — *see* Yaws
Paranoia (querulans) F22
   senile F03 ☑
Paranoid
   dementia (senile) F03 ☑
      praecox — *see* Schizophrenia
   personality F60.0
   psychosis (climacteric) (involutional) (menopausal)
      F22
      psychogenic (acute) F23
      senile F03 ☑
   reaction (acute) F23
      chronic F22
   schizophrenia F20.0
   state (climacteric) (involutional) (menopausal) (simple)
      F22
      senile F03 ☑
   tendencies F60.0
   traits F60.0
   trends F60.0
   type, psychopathic personality F60.0
Paraparesis — *see* Paraplegia
Paraphasia R47.02
Paraphilia F65.9
Paraphimosis (congenital) N47.2
   chancroidal A57
Paraphrenia, paraphrenic (late) F22
   schizophrenia F20.0
Paraplegia (lower) G82.20
   ataxic — *see* Degeneration, combined, spinal cord
   complete G82.21
   congenital (cerebral) G80.8
      spastic G80.1
   familial spastic G11.4
   functional (hysterical) F44.4
   hereditary, spastic G11.4
   hysterical F44.4
   incomplete G82.22
   Pott's A18.01
   psychogenic F44.4
   spastic
      Erb's spinal, syphilitic A52.17
      hereditary G11.4
      tropical G04.1
   syphilitic (spastic) A52.17
   tropical spastic G04.1
Parapoxvirus B08.60
   specified NEC B08.69
Paraproteinemia D89.2
   benign (familial) D89.2
   monoclonal D47.2
   secondary to malignant disease D47.2
Parapsoriasis L41.9
   en plaques L41.4
   guttata L41.1
   large plaque L41.4
   retiform, retiformis L41.5
   small plaque L41.3
   specified NEC L41.8
   varioliformis (acuta) L41.0
Parasitic (*see also* condition)
   disease NEC B89
   stomatitis B37.0
   sycosis (beard) (scalp) B35.0
   twin Q89.4
Parasitism B89
   intestinal B82.9
   skin B88.9
   specified — *see* Infestation
Parasitophobia F40.218
Parasomnia G47.50
   due to
      alcohol
         abuse F10.182
         dependence F10.282
         use F10.982
      amphetamines
         abuse F15.182
         dependence F15.282

Parasomnia — *continued*
   due to — *continued*
      amphetamines — *continued*
         use F15.982
      caffeine
         abuse F15.182
         dependence F15.282
         use F15.982
      cocaine
         abuse F14.182
         dependence F14.282
         use F14.982
      drug NEC
         abuse F19.182
         dependence F19.282
         use F19.982
      opioid
         abuse F11.182
         dependence F11.282
         use F11.982
      psychoactive substance NEC
         abuse F19.182
         dependence F19.282
         use F19.982
      sedative, hypnotic, or anxiolytic
         abuse F13.182
         dependence F13.282
         use F13.982
      stimulant NEC
         abuse F15.182
         dependence F15.282
         use F15.982
   in conditions classified elsewhere G47.54
   nonorganic origin F51.8
   organic G47.50
   specified NEC G47.59
Paraspadias Q54.9
Paraspasmus facialis G51.8
Parasuicide (attempt)
   history of (personal) Z91.5
      in family Z81.8
Parathyroid gland — *see* condition
Parathyroid tetany E20.9
Paratrachoma A74.0
Paratyphlitis — *see* Appendicitis
Paratyphoid (fever) — *see* Fever, paratyphoid
Paratyphus — *see* Fever, paratyphoid
Paraurethral duct Q64.79
   nonorganic origin F51.5
Paraurethritis (*see also* Urethritis)
   gonococcal (acute) (chronic) (with abscess) A54.1
Paravaccinia NEC B08.04
Paravaginitis — *see* Vaginitis
Parencephalitis (*see also* Encephalitis)
   sequelae G09
Parent-child conflict — *see* Conflict, parent-child
   estrangement NEC Z62.890
Paresis (*see also* Paralysis)
   accommodation — *see* Paresis, of accommodation
   Bernhardt's G57.1- ☑
   bladder (sphincter) (*see also* Paralysis, bladder)
      tabetic A52.17
   bowel, colon or intestine K56.0
   extrinsic muscle, eye H49.9
   general (progressive) (syphilitic) A52.17
      juvenile A50.45
   heart — *see* Failure, heart
   insane (syphilitic) A52.17
   juvenile (general) A50.45
   of accommodation H52.52- ☑
   peripheral progressive (idiopathic) G60.3
   pseudohypertrophic G71.0
   senile G83.9
   syphilitic (general) A52.17
      congenital A50.45
   vesical NEC N31.2
Paresthesia (*see also* Disturbance, sensation, skin) R20.2
   Bernhardt G57.1- ☑
Paretic — *see* condition
Parinaud's
   conjunctivitis H10.89
   oculoglandular syndrome H10.89
   ophthalmoplegia H49.88- ☑
Parkinsonism (idiopathic) (primary) G20
   with neurogenic orthostatic hypotension (symptomat-
      ic) G90.3
   arteriosclerotic G21.4
   dementia G31.83 [F02.80]

248

☑ **Additional Character Required — Refer to the Tabular List for Character Selection**   ▽ Subterms under main terms may continue to next column or page

Paralysis, paralytic — Parkinsonism

Parkinsonism — *continued*
dementia — *continued*
with behavioral disturbance G31.83 [F02.81]
due to
drugs NEC G21.19
neuroleptic G21.11
medication-induced NEC G21.19
neuroleptic induced G21.11
postencephalitic G21.3
secondary G21.9
due to
arteriosclerosis G21.4
drugs NEC G21.19
neuroleptic G21.11
encephalitis G21.3
external agents NEC G21.2
syphilis A52.19
specified NEC G21.8
syphilitic A52.19
treatment-induced NEC G21.19
vascular G21.4
Parkinson's disease, syndrome or tremor — *see* Parkinsonism
Parodontitis — *see* Periodontitis
Parodontosis K05.4
Paronychia (*see also* Cellulitis, digit)
with lymphangitis — *see* Lymphangitis, acute, digit
candidal (chronic) B37.2
tuberculous (primary) A18.4
Parorexia (psychogenic) F50.89
Parosmia R43.1
psychogenic F45.8
Parotid gland — *see* condition
Parotitis, parotiditis (allergic)(nonspecific toxic) (purulent) (septic) (suppurative) (*see also* Sialoadenitis)
epidemic — *see* Mumps
infectious — *see* Mumps
postoperative K91.89
surgical K91.89
Parrot fever A70
Parrot's disease (early congenital syphilitic pseudoparalysis) A50.02
Parry-Romberg syndrome G51.8
Parry's disease or syndrome E05.00
with thyroid storm E05.01
Pars planitis — *see* Cyclitis
Parsonage (-Aldren)-**Turner syndrome** G54.5
Parson's disease (exophthalmic goiter) E05.00
with thyroid storm E05.01
Particolored infant Q82.8
Parturition — *see* Delivery
Parulis K04.7
with sinus K04.6
Parvovirus, as cause of disease classified elsewhere B97.6
Pasini and Pierini's atrophoderma L90.3
Passage
false, urethra N36.5
meconium (newborn) during delivery P03.82
of sounds or bougies — *see* Attention to, artificial, opening
Passive — *see* condition
smoking Z77.22
Pasteurella septica A28.0
Pasteurellosis — *see* Infection, Pasteurella
PAT (paroxysmal atrial tachycardia) I47.1
Patau's syndrome — *see* Trisomy, 13
Patches
mucous (syphilitic) A51.39
congenital A50.07
smokers' (mouth) K13.24
Patellar — *see* condition
Patent (*see also* Imperfect, closure)
canal of Nuck Q52.4
cervix N88.3
ductus arteriosus or Botallo's Q25.0
foramen
botalli Q21.1
ovale Q21.1
interauricular septum Q21.1
interventricular septum Q21.0
omphalomesenteric duct Q43.0
os (uteri) — *see* Patent, cervix
ostium secundum Q21.1
urachus Q64.4
vitelline duct Q43.0
Paterson (-Brown)(-Kelly) **syndrome or web** D50.1

Pathologic, pathological (*see also* condition)
asphyxia R09.01
fire-setting F63.1
gambling F63.0
ovum O02.0
resorption, tooth K03.3
stealing F63.2
Pathology (of) — *see* Disease
periradicular, associated with previous endodontic treatment NEC M27.59
Pattern, sleep-wake, irregular G47.23
Patulous (*see also* Imperfect, closure (congenital))
alimentary tract Q45.8
lower Q43.8
upper Q40.8
eustachian tube H69.0- ☑
Pause, sinoatrial I49.5
Paxton's disease B36.2
Pearl(s)
enamel K00.2
Epstein's K09.8
Pearl-worker's disease — *see* Osteomyelitis, specified type NEC
Pectenosis K62.4
Pectoral — *see* condition
Pectus
carinatum (congenital) Q67.7
acquired M95.4
rachitic sequelae (late effect) E64.3
excavatum (congenital) Q67.6
acquired M95.4
rachitic sequelae (late effect) E64.3
recurvatum (congenital) Q67.6
Pedatrophia E41
Pederosis F65.4
Pediculosis (infestation) B85.2
capitis (head-louse) (any site) B85.0
corporis (body-louse) (any site) B85.1
eyelid B85.0
mixed (classifiable to more than one of the titles B85.0-B85.3) B85.4
pubis (pubic louse) (any site) B85.3
vestimenti B85.1
vulvae B85.3
Pediculus (infestation) — *see* Pediculosis
Pedophilia F65.4
Peg-shaped teeth K00.2
Pelade — *see* Alopecia, areata
Pelger-Huët anomaly or syndrome D72.0
Peliosis (rheumatica) D69.0
hepatis K76.4
with toxic liver disease K71.8
Pelizaeus-Merzbacher disease E75.29
Pellagra (alcoholic) (with polyneuropathy) E52
Pellagra-cerebellar-ataxia-renal aminoaciduria syndrome E72.02
Pellegrini (-Stieda) **disease or syndrome** — *see* Bursitis, tibial collateral
Pellizzi's syndrome E34.8
Pel's crisis A52.11
Pelvic (*see also* condition)
examination (periodic) (routine) Z01.419
with abnormal findings Z01.411
kidney, congenital Q63.2
Pelviolithiasis — *see* Calculus, kidney
Pelviperitonitis (*see also* Peritonitis, pelvic)
gonococcal A54.24
puerperal O85
Pelvis — *see* condition or type
Pemphigoid L12.9
benign, mucous membrane L12.1
bullous L12.0
cicatricial L12.1
juvenile L12.2
ocular L12.1
specified NEC L12.8
Pemphigus L10.9
benign familial (chronic) Q82.8
Brazilian L10.3
circinatus L13.0
conjunctiva L12.1
drug-induced L10.5
erythematosus L10.4
foliaceus L10.2
gangrenous — *see* Gangrene
neonatorum L01.03
ocular L12.1
paraneoplastic L10.81

Pemphigus — *continued*
specified NEC L10.89
syphilitic (congenital) A50.06
vegetans L10.1
vulgaris L10.0
wildfire L10.3
Pendred's syndrome E07.1
Pendulous
abdomen, in pregnancy — *see* Pregnancy, complicated by, abnormal, pelvic organs or tissues NEC
breast N64.89
Penetrating wound (*see also* Puncture)
with internal injury — *see* Injury, by site
eyeball — *see* Puncture, eyeball
orbit (with or without foreign body) — *see* Puncture, orbit
uterus by instrument with or following ectopic or molar pregnancy O08.6
Penicillosis B48.4
Penis — *see* condition
Penitis N48.29
Pentalogy of Fallot Q21.8
Pentasomy X syndrome Q97.1
Pentosuria (essential) E74.8
Percreta placenta - O43.23 ☑
Peregrinating patient — *see* Disorder, factitious
Perforation, perforated (nontraumatic) (of)
accidental during procedure (blood vessel) (nerve) (organ) — *see* Complication, accidental puncture or laceration
antrum — *see* Sinusitis, maxillary
appendix K35.2
with localized peritonitis K35.3
atrial septum, multiple Q21.1
attic, ear — *see* Perforation, tympanum, attic
bile duct (common) (hepatic) K83.2
cystic K82.2
bladder (urinary)
with or following ectopic or molar pregnancy O08.6
obstetrical trauma O71.5
traumatic S37.29 ☑
at delivery O71.5
bowel K63.1
with or following ectopic or molar pregnancy O08.6
newborn P78.0
obstetrical trauma O71.5
traumatic — *see* Laceration, intestine
broad ligament N83.8
with or following ectopic or molar pregnancy O08.6
obstetrical trauma O71.6
by
device, implant or graft (*see also* Complications, by site and type, mechanical) T85.628 ☑
arterial graft NEC — *see* Complication, cardiovascular device, mechanical, vascular
breast (implant) T85.49 ☑
catheter NEC T85.698 ☑
cystostomy T83.090 ☑
dialysis (renal) T82.49 ☑
intraperitoneal T85.691 ☑
infusion NEC T82.594 ☑
spinal (epidural) (subdural) T85.690 ☑
urinary (*see also* Complications, catheter, urinary T83.098 ☑
electronic (electrode) (pulse generator) (stimulator)
bone T84.390 ☑
cardiac T82.199 ☑
electrode T82.190 ☑
pulse generator T82.191 ☑
specified type NEC T82.198 ☑
nervous system — *see* Complication, prosthetic device, mechanical, electronic nervous system stimulator
urinary — *see* Complication, genitourinary, device, urinary, mechanical
fixation, internal (orthopedic) NEC — *see* Complication, fixation device, mechanical
gastrointestinal — *see* Complications, prosthetic device, mechanical, gastrointestinal device
genital NEC T83.498 ☑
intrauterine contraceptive device T83.39 ☑
penile prosthesis T83.490 ☑
heart NEC — *see* Complication, cardiovascular device, mechanical

☝ Subterms under main terms may continue to next column or page   ☑ Additional Character Required — Refer to the Tabular List for Character Selection   249

Parkinsonism — Perforation, perforated

Perforation, perforated — *continued*
  by — *continued*
    device, implant or graft (*see also* Complications, by site and type, mechanical) — *continued*
      joint prosthesis — *see* Complications, joint prosthesis, mechanical, specified NEC, by site
      ocular NEC — *see* Complications, prosthetic device, mechanical, ocular device
      orthopedic NEC — *see* Complication, orthopedic, device, mechanical
      specified NEC T85.628 ☑
      urinary NEC (*see also* Complication, genitourinary, device, urinary, mechanical)
        graft T83.29 ☑
      vascular NEC — *see* Complication, cardiovascular device, mechanical
      ventricular intracranial shunt T85.09 ☑
    foreign body left accidentally in operative wound T81.539 ☑
    instrument (any) during a procedure, accidental — *see* Puncture, accidental complicating surgery
  cecum K35.2
    with localized peritonitis K35.3
  cervix (uteri) N88.8
    with or following ectopic or molar pregnancy O08.6
    obstetrical trauma O71.3
  colon K63.1
    newborn P78.0
    obstetrical trauma O71.5
    traumatic — *see* Laceration, intestine, large
  common duct (bile) K83.2
  cornea (due to ulceration) — *see* Ulcer, cornea, perforated
  cystic duct K82.2
  diverticulum (intestine) K57.80
    with bleeding K57.81
    large intestine K57.20
      with
        bleeding K57.21
        small intestine K57.40
          with bleeding K57.41
    small intestine K57.00
      with
        bleeding K57.01
        large intestine K57.40
          with bleeding K57.41
  ear drum — *see* Perforation, tympanum
  esophagus K22.3
  ethmoidal sinus — *see* Sinusitis, ethmoidal
  frontal sinus — *see* Sinusitis, frontal
  gallbladder K82.2
  heart valve — *see* Endocarditis
  ileum K63.1
    newborn P78.0
    obstetrical trauma O71.5
    traumatic — *see* Laceration, intestine, small
  instrumental, surgical (accidental) (blood vessel) (nerve) (organ) — *see* Puncture, accidental complicating surgery
  intestine NEC K63.1
    with ectopic or molar pregnancy O08.6
    newborn P78.0
    obstetrical trauma O71.5
    traumatic — *see* Laceration, intestine
    ulcerative NEC K63.1
      newborn P78.0
  jejunum, jejunal K63.1
    obstetrical trauma O71.5
    traumatic — *see* Laceration, intestine, small
    ulcer — *see* Ulcer, gastrojejunal, with perforation
  joint prosthesis — *see* Complications, joint prosthesis, mechanical, specified NEC, by site
  mastoid (antrum) (cell) — *see* Disorder, mastoid, specified NEC
  maxillary sinus — *see* Sinusitis, maxillary
  membrana tympani — *see* Perforation, tympanum
  nasal
    septum J34.89
      congenital Q30.3
      syphilitic A52.73
    sinus J34.89
      congenital Q30.8
      due to sinusitis — *see* Sinusitis
  palate (*see also* Cleft, palate) Q35.9
    syphilitic A52.79
  palatine vault (*see also* Cleft, palate, hard) Q35.1

Perforation, perforated — *continued*
  palatine vault (*see also* Cleft, palate, hard) — *continued*
    syphilitic A52.79
      congenital A50.59
  pars flaccida (ear drum) — *see* Perforation, tympanum, attic
  pelvic
    floor S31.030 ☑
      with
        ectopic or molar pregnancy O08.6
        penetration into retroperitoneal space S31.031 ☑
        retained foreign body S31.040 ☑
          with penetration into retroperitoneal space S31.041 ☑
      following ectopic or molar pregnancy O08.6
      obstetrical trauma O70.1
    organ S37.99 ☑
      adrenal gland S37.818 ☑
      bladder — *see* Perforation, bladder
      fallopian tube S37.599 ☑
        bilateral S37.592 ☑
        unilateral S37.591 ☑
      kidney S37.09- ☑
      obstetrical trauma O71.5
      ovary S37.499 ☑
        bilateral S37.492 ☑
        unilateral S37.491 ☑
      prostate S37.828 ☑
      specified organ NEC S37.898 ☑
      ureter — *see* Perforation, ureter
      urethra — *see* Perforation, urethra
      uterus — *see* Perforation, uterus
  perineum — *see* Laceration, perineum
  pharynx J39.2
  rectum K63.1
    newborn P78.0
    obstetrical trauma O71.5
    traumatic S36.63 ☑
  root canal space due to endodontic treatment M27.51
  sigmoid K63.1
    newborn P78.0
    obstetrical trauma O71.5
    traumatic S36.533 ☑
  sinus (accessory) (chronic) (nasal) J34.89
  sphenoidal sinus — *see* Sinusitis, sphenoidal
  surgical (accidental) (by instrument) (blood vessel) (nerve) (organ) — *see* Puncture, accidental complicating surgery
  traumatic
    external — *see* Puncture
    eye — *see* Puncture, eyeball
    internal organ — *see* Injury, by site
  tympanum, tympanic (membrane) (persistent post-traumatic) (postinflammatory) H72.9- ☑
    attic H72.1- ☑
      multiple — *see* Perforation, tympanum, multiple
      total — *see* Perforation, tympanum, total
    central H72.0- ☑
      multiple — *see* Perforation, tympanum, multiple
      total — *see* Perforation, tympanum, total
    marginal NEC — *see* subcategory H72.2 ☑
    multiple H72.81- ☑
    pars flaccida — *see* Perforation, tympanum, attic
    total H72.82- ☑
    traumatic, current episode S09.2- ☑
  typhoid, gastrointestinal — *see* Typhoid
  ulcer — *see* Ulcer, by site, with perforation
  ureter N28.89
    traumatic S37.19 ☑
  urethra N36.8
    with ectopic or molar pregnancy O08.6
    following ectopic or molar pregnancy O08.6
    obstetrical trauma O71.5
    traumatic S37.39 ☑
      at delivery O71.5
  uterus
    with ectopic or molar pregnancy O08.6
    by intrauterine contraceptive device T83.39 ☑
    following ectopic or molar pregnancy O08.6
    obstetrical trauma O71.1
    traumatic S37.69 ☑
      obstetric O71.1
  uvula K13.79

Perforation, perforated — *continued*
  uvula — *continued*
    syphilitic A52.79
  vagina O71.4
    obstetrical trauma O71.4
    other trauma — *see* Puncture, vagina
Periadenitis mucosa necrotica recurrens K12.0
Periappendicitis (acute) — *see* Appendicitis
Periarteritis nodosa (disseminated) (infectious) (necrotizing) M30.0
Periarthritis (joint) (*see also* Enthesopathy)
  Duplay's M75.0-
  gonococcal A54.42
  humeroscapularis — *see* Capsulitis, adhesive
  scapulohumeral — *see* Capsulitis, adhesive
  shoulder — *see* Capsulitis, adhesive
  wrist M77.2- ☑
Periarthrosis (angioneural) — *see* Enthesopathy
Pericapsulitis, adhesive (shoulder) — *see* Capsulitis, adhesive
Pericarditis (with decompensation) (with effusion) I31.9
  with rheumatic fever (conditions in I00)
    active — *see* Pericarditis, rheumatic
    inactive or quiescent I09.2
  acute (hemorrhagic) (nonrheumatic) (Sicca) I30.9
    with chorea (acute) (rheumatic) (Sydenham's) I02.0
    benign I30.8
    nonspecific I30.0
    rheumatic I01.0
      with chorea (acute) (Sydenham's) I02.0
  adhesive or adherent (chronic) (external) (internal) I31.0
    acute — *see* Pericarditis, acute
    rheumatic I09.2
  bacterial (acute) (subacute) (with serous or seropurulent effusion) I30.1
  calcareous I31.1
  cholesterol (chronic) I31.8
    acute I30.9
  chronic (nonrheumatic) I31.9
    rheumatic I09.2
  constrictive (chronic) I31.1
  coxsackie B33.23
  fibrinocaseous (tuberculous) A18.84
  fibrinopurulent I30.1
  fibrinous I30.8
  fibrous I31.0
  gonococcal A54.83
  idiopathic I30.0
  in systemic lupus erythematosus M32.12
  infective I30.1
  meningococcal A39.53
  neoplastic (chronic) I31.8
    acute I30.9
  obliterans, obliterating I31.0
  plastic I31.0
  pneumococcal I30.1
  postinfarction I24.1
  purulent I30.1
  rheumatic (active) (acute) (with effusion) (with pneumonia) I01.0
    with chorea (acute) (rheumatic) (Sydenham's) I02.0
    chronic or inactive (with chorea) I09.2
  rheumatoid — *see* Rheumatoid, carditis
  septic I30.1
  serofibrinous I30.8
  staphylococcal I30.1
  streptococcal I30.1
  suppurative I30.1
  syphilitic A52.06
  tuberculous A18.84
  uremic N18.9 [I32]
  viral I30.1
Pericardium, pericardial — *see* condition
Pericellulitis — *see* Cellulitis
Pericementitis (chronic) (suppurative) (*see also* Periodontitis)
  acute K05.20
    generalized — *see* Peridontitis, aggressive, generalized
    localized — *see* Peridontitis, aggressive, localized
Perichondritis
  auricle — *see* Perichondritis, ear
  bronchus J98.09
  ear (external) H61.00- ☑
    acute H61.01- ☑
    chronic H61.02- ☑
  external auditory canal — *see* Perichondritis, ear

Perichondritis — *continued*
　larynx J38.7
　　syphilitic A52.73
　　typhoid A01.09
　nose J34.89
　pinna — *see* Perichondritis, ear
　trachea J39.8
Periclasia K05.4
Pericoronitis — *see* Periodontitis
Pericystitis N30.90
　with hematuria N30.91
Peridiverticulitis (intestine) K57.92
　cecum — *see* Diverticulitis, intestine, large
　colon — *see* Diverticulitis, intestine, large
　duodenum — *see* Diverticulitis, intestine, small
　intestine — *see* Diverticulitis, intestine
　jejunum — *see* Diverticulitis, intestine, small
　rectosigmoid — *see* Diverticulitis, intestine, large
　rectum — *see* Diverticulitis, intestine, large
　sigmoid — *see* Diverticulitis, intestine, large
Periendocarditis — *see* Endocarditis
Periepididymitis N45.1
Perifolliculitis L01.02
　abscedens, caput, scalp L66.3
　capitis, abscedens (et suffodiens) L66.3
　superficial pustular L01.02
Perihepatitis K65.8
Perilabyrinthitis (acute) — *see* subcategory H83.0 ☑
Perimeningitis — *see* Meningitis
Perimetritis — *see* Endometritis
Perimetrosalpingitis — *see* Salpingo-oophoritis
Perineocele N81.81
Perinephric, perinephritic — *see* condition
Perinephritis (*see also* Infection, kidney)
　purulent — *see* Abscess, kidney
Perineum, perineal — *see* condition
Perineuritis NEC — *see* Neuralgia
Periodic — *see* condition
Periodontitis (chronic) (complex) (compound) (local)
　　(simplex) K05.30
　acute K05.20
　　generalized K05.229
　　　moderate K05.222
　　　severe K05.223
　　　slight K05.221
　　localized K05.219
　　　moderate K05.212
　　　severe K05.213
　　　slight K05.211
　apical K04.5
　　acute (pulpal origin) K04.4
　generalized K05.329
　　moderate K05.322
　　severe K05.323
　　slight K05.321
　localized K05.319
　　moderate K05.312
　　severe K05.313
　　slight K05.311
Periodontoclasia K05.4
Periodontosis (juvenile) K05.4
Periods (*see also* Menstruation)
　heavy N92.0
　irregular N92.6
　shortened intervals (irregular) N92.1
Perionychia (*see also* Cellulitis, digit)
　with lymphangitis — *see* Lymphangitis, acute, digit
Perioophoritis — *see* Salpingo-oophoritis
Periorchitis N45.2
Periosteum, periosteal — *see* condition
Periostitis (albuminosa) (circumscribed) (diffuse) (infec-
　　tive) (monomelic) (*see also* Osteomyelitis)
　alveolar M27.3
　alveolodental M27.3
　dental M27.3
　gonorrheal A54.43
　jaw (lower) (upper) M27.2
　orbit H05.03- ☑
　syphilitic A52.77
　　congenital (early) A50.02 [M90.80]
　　secondary A51.46
　tuberculous — *see* Tuberculosis, bone
　yaws (hypertrophic) (early) (late) A66.6 [M90.80]
Periostosis (hyperplastic) (*see also* Disorder, bone,
　　specified type NEC)
　with osteomyelitis — *see* Osteomyelitis, specified type
　　NEC

Peripartum
　cardiomyopathy O90.3
Periphlebitis — *see* Phlebitis
Periproctitis K62.89
Periprostatitis — *see* Prostatitis
Perirectal — *see* condition
Perirenal — *see* condition
Perisalpingitis — *see* Salpingo-oophoritis
Perisplenitis (infectional) D73.89
Peristalsis, visible or reversed R19.2
Peritendinitis — *see* Enthesopathy
Peritoneum, peritoneal — *see* condition
Peritonitis (adhesive) (bacterial) (fibrinous) (hemorrhag-
　　ic) (idiopathic) (localized) (perforative) (primary)
　　(with adhesions) (with effusion) K65.9
　with or following
　　abscess K65.1
　　appendicitis K35.3
　　　with perforation or rupture K35.2
　　　generalized K35.2
　　　localized K35.3
　　diverticular disease (intestine) K57.80
　　　with bleeding K57.81
　　　ectopic or molar pregnancy O08.0
　　　large intestine K57.20
　　　　with
　　　　　bleeding K57.21
　　　　small intestine K57.40
　　　　　with bleeding K57.41
　　　small intestine K57.00
　　　　with
　　　　　bleeding K57.01
　　　　large intestine K57.40
　　　　　with bleeding K57.41
　acute (generalized) K65.0
　aseptic T81.61 ☑
　bile, biliary K65.3
　chemical T81.61 ☑
　chlamydial A74.81
　chronic proliferative K65.8
　complicating abortion — *see* Abortion, by type, com-
　　plicated by, pelvic peritonitis
　congenital P78.1
　diaphragmatic K65.0
　diffuse K65.0
　diphtheritic A36.89
　disseminated K65.0
　due to
　　bile K65.3
　　foreign
　　　body or object accidentally left during a proce-
　　　　dure (instrument) (sponge) (swab)
　　　　T81.599 ☑
　　　substance accidentally left during a procedure
　　　　(chemical) (powder) (talc) T81.61 ☑
　　talc T81.61 ☑
　　urine K65.8
　eosinophilic K65.8
　　acute K65.0
　fibrocaseous (tuberculous) A18.31
　fibropurulent K65.0
　following ectopic or molar pregnancy O08.0
　general (ized) K65.0
　gonococcal A54.85
　meconium (newborn) P78.0
　neonatal P78.1
　　meconium P78.0
　pancreatic K65.0
　paroxysmal, familial E85.0
　　benign E85.0
　pelvic
　　female N73.5
　　　acute N73.3
　　　chronic N73.4
　　　　with adhesions N73.6
　　male K65.0
　periodic, familial E85.0
　proliferative, chronic K65.8
　puerperal, postpartum, childbirth O85
　purulent K65.0
　septic K65.0
　specified NEC K65.8
　spontaneous bacterial K65.2
　subdiaphragmatic K65.0
　subphrenic K65.0
　suppurative K65.0
　syphilitic A52.74
　　congenital (early) A50.08 [K67]

Peritonitis — *continued*
　talc T81.61 ☑
　tuberculous A18.31
　urine K65.8
Peritonsillar — *see* condition
Peritonsillitis J36
Perityphlitis K37
Periureteritis N28.89
Periurethral — *see* condition
Periurethritis (gangrenous) — *see* Urethritis
Periuterine — *see* condition
Perivaginitis — *see* Vaginitis
Perivasculitis, retinal H35.06- ☑
Perivasitis (chronic) N49.1
Perivesiculitis (seminal) — *see* Vesiculitis
Perlèche NEC K13.0
　due to
　　candidiasis B37.83
　　moniliasis B37.83
　　riboflavin deficiency E53.0
　　vitamin B2 (riboflavin) deficiency E53.0
Pernicious — *see* condition
Pernio, perniosis T69.1 ☑
Perpetrator (of abuse) — *see* Index to External Causes
　　of Injury, Perpetrator
Persecution
　delusion F22
　social Z60.5
Perseveration (tonic) R48.8
Persistence, persistent (congenital)
　anal membrane Q42.3
　　with fistula Q42.2
　arteria stapedia Q16.3
　atrioventricular canal Q21.2
　branchial cleft NOS Q18.2
　　cyst Q18.0
　　fistula Q18.0
　　sinus Q18.0
　bulbus cordis in left ventricle Q21.8
　canal of Cloquet Q14.0
　capsule (opaque) Q12.8
　cilioretinal artery or vein Q14.8
　cloaca Q43.7
　communication — *see* Fistula, congenital
　convolutions
　　aortic arch Q25.46
　　fallopian tube Q50.6
　　oviduct Q50.6
　　uterine tube Q50.6
　double aortic arch Q25.45
　ductus arteriosus (Botalli) Q25.0
　fetal
　　circulation P29.38
　　form of cervix (uteri) Q51.828
　　hemoglobin, hereditary (HPFH) D56.4
　foramen
　　Botalli Q21.1
　　ovale Q21.1
　Gartner's duct Q52.4
　hemoglobin, fetal (hereditary) (HPFH) D56.4
　hyaloid
　　artery (generally incomplete) Q14.0
　　system Q14.8
　hymen, in pregnancy or childbirth — *see* Pregnancy,
　　complicated by, abnormal, vulva
　lanugo Q84.2
　left
　　posterior cardinal vein Q26.8
　　root with right arch of aorta Q25.49
　　superior vena cava Q26.1
　Meckel's diverticulum Q43.0
　　malignant — *see* Table of Neoplasms, small intes-
　　　tine, malignant
　mucosal disease (middle ear) — *see* Otitis, media,
　　suppurative, chronic, tubotympanic
　nail(s), anomalous Q84.6
　omphalomesenteric duct Q43.0
　organ or site not listed — *see* Anomaly, by site
　ostium
　　atrioventriculare commune Q21.2
　　primum Q21.2
　　secundum Q21.1
　ovarian rests in fallopian tube Q50.6
　pancreatic tissue in intestinal tract Q43.8
　primary (deciduous)
　　teeth K00.6
　　vitreous hyperplasia Q14.0
　pupillary membrane Q13.89

Persistence, persistent — continued
    rhesus (Rh) titer — see Complication(s), transfusion, incompatibility reaction, Rh (factor)
    right aortic arch Q25.47
    sinus
      urogenitalis
        female Q52.8
        male Q55.8
      venosus with imperfect incorporation in right auricle Q26.8
    thymus (gland) (hyperplasia) E32.0
    thyroglossal duct Q89.2
    thyrolingual duct Q89.2
    truncus arteriosus or communis Q20.0
    tunica vasculosa lentis Q12.2
    umbilical sinus Q64.4
    urachus Q64.4
    vitelline duct Q43.0
Person (with)
    admitted for clinical research, as a control subject (normal comparison) (participant) Z00.6
    awaiting admission to adequate facility elsewhere Z75.1
    concern (normal) about sick person in family Z63.6
    consulting on behalf of another Z71.0
    feigning illness Z76.5
    living (in)
      without
        adequate housing (heating) (space) Z59.1
        housing (permanent) (temporary) Z59.0
        person able to render necessary care Z74.2
        shelter Z59.0
      alone Z60.2
      boarding school Z59.3
      residential institution Z59.3
    on waiting list Z75.1
    sick or handicapped in family Z63.6
Personality (disorder) F60.9
    accentuation of traits (type A pattern) Z73.1
    affective F34.0
    aggressive F60.3
    amoral F60.2
    anacastic, anankastic F60.5
    antisocial F60.2
    anxious F60.6
    asocial F60.2
    asthenic F60.7
    avoidant F60.6
    borderline F60.3
    change due to organic condition (enduring) F07.0
    compulsive F60.5
    cycloid F34.0
    cyclothymic F34.0
    dependent F60.7
    depressive F34.1
    dissocial F60.2
    dual F44.81
    eccentric F60.89
    emotionally unstable F60.3
    expansive paranoid F60.0
    explosive F60.3
    fanatic F60.0
    haltose type F60.89
    histrionic F60.4
    hyperthymic F34.0
    hypothymic F34.1
    hysterical F60.4
    immature F60.89
    inadequate F60.7
    labile (emotional) F60.3
    mixed (nonspecific) F60.89
    morally defective F60.2
    multiple F44.81
    narcissistic F60.81
    obsessional F60.5
    obsessive (-compulsive) F60.5
    organic F07.0
    overconscientious F60.5
    paranoid F60.0
    passive (-dependent) F60.7
    passive-aggressive F60.89
    pathologic F60.9
    pattern defect or disturbance F60.9
    pseudopsychopathic (organic) F07.0
    pseudoretarded (organic) F07.0
    psychoinfantile F60.4
    psychoneurotic NEC F60.89
    psychopathic F60.2
    querulant F60.0

Personality — continued
    sadistic F60.89
    schizoid F60.1
    self-defeating F60.7
    sensitive paranoid F60.0
    sociopathic (amoral) (antisocial) (asocial) (dissocial) F60.2
    specified NEC F60.89
    type A Z73.1
    unstable (emotional) F60.3
Perthes' disease — see Legg-Calvé-Perthes disease
Pertussis (see also Whooping cough) A37.90
Perversion, perverted
    appetite F50.89
      psychogenic F50.89
    function
      pituitary gland E23.2
        posterior lobe E22.2
    sense of smell and taste R43.8
      psychogenic F45.8
    sexual — see Deviation, sexual
Pervious, congenital (see also Imperfect, closure)
    ductus arteriosus Q25.0
Pes (congenital) (see also Talipes)
    acquired (see also Deformity, limb, foot, specified NEC)
      planus — see Deformity, limb, flat foot
    adductus Q66.89
    cavus Q66.7
    deformity NEC, acquired — see Deformity, limb, foot, specified NEC
    planus (acquired) (any degree) (see also Deformity, limb, flat foot)
      rachitic sequelae (late effect) E64.3
    valgus Q66.6
Pest, pestis — see Plague
Petechia, petechiae R23.3
    newborn P54.5
Petechial typhus A75.9
Peter's anomaly Q13.4
Petit mal seizure — see Epilepsy, generalized, specified NEC
Petit's hernia — see Hernia, abdomen, specified site NEC
Petrellidosis B48.2
Petrositis H70.20- ☑
    acute H70.21- ☑
    chronic H70.22- ☑
Peutz-Jeghers disease or syndrome Q85.8
Peyronie's disease N48.6
PFAPA (periodic fever, aphthous stomatitis, pharyngitis, and adenopathy syndrome) M04.8
Pfeiffer's disease — see Mononucleosis, infectious
Phagedena (dry) (moist) (sloughing) (see also Gangrene)
    geometric L88
    penis N48.29
    tropical — see Ulcer, skin
    vulva N76.6
Phagedenic — see condition
Phakoma H35.89
Phakomatosis (see also specific eponymous syndromes) Q85.9
    Bourneville's Q85.1
    specified NEC Q85.8
Phantom limb syndrome (without pain) G54.7
    with pain G54.6
Pharyngeal pouch syndrome D82.1
Pharyngitis (acute) (catarrhal)(gangrenous) (infective) (malignant) (membranous) (phlegmonous) (pseudomembranous) (simple) (subacute) (suppurative) (ulcerative) (viral) J02.9
    with influenza, flu, or grippe — see Influenza, with, pharyngitis
    aphthous B08.5
    atrophic J31.2
    chlamydial A56.4
    chronic (atrophic) (granular) (hypertrophic) J31.2
    coxsackievirus B08.5
    diphtheritic A36.0
    enteroviral vesicular B08.5
    follicular (chronic) J31.2
    fusospirochetal A69.1
    gonococcal A54.5
    granular (chronic) J31.2
    herpesviral B00.2
    hypertrophic J31.2
    infectional, chronic J31.2
    influenzal — see Influenza, with, respiratory manifestations NEC

Pharyngitis — continued
    lymphonodular, acute (enteroviral) B08.8
    pneumococcal J02.8
    purulent J02.9
    putrid J02.9
    septic J02.0
    sicca J31.2
    specified organism NEC J02.8
    staphylococcal J02.8
    streptococcal J02.0
    syphilitic, congenital (early) A50.03
    tuberculous A15.8
    vesicular, enteroviral B08.5
    viral NEC J02.8
Pharyngoconjunctivitis, viral B30.2
Pharyngolaryngitis (acute) J06.0
    chronic J37.0
Pharyngoplegia J39.2
Pharyngotonsillitis, herpesviral B00.2
Pharyngotracheitis, chronic J42
Pharynx, pharyngeal — see condition
Phencyclidine-induced
    anxiety disorder F16.980
    bipolar and related disorder F16.94
    depressive disorder F16.94
    psychotic disorder F16.959
Phenomenon
    Arthus' — see Arthus' phenomenon
    jaw-winking Q07.8
    lupus erythematosus (LE) cell M32.9
    Raynaud's (secondary) I73.00
      with gangrene I73.01
    vasomotor R55
    vasospastic I73.9
    vasovagal R55
    Wenckebach's I44.1
Phenylketonuria E70.1
    classical E70.0
    maternal E70.1
Pheochromoblastoma
    specified site — see Neoplasm, malignant, by site
    unspecified site C74.10
Pheochromocytoma
    malignant
      specified site — see Neoplasm, malignant, by site
      unspecified site C74.10
    specified site — see Neoplasm, benign, by site
    unspecified site D35.00
Pheohyphomycosis — see Chromomycosis
Pheomycosis — see Chromomycosis
Phimosis (congenital) (due to infection) N47.1
    chancroidal A57
Phlebectasia (see also Varix)
    congenital Q27.4
Phlebitis (infective) (pyemic) (septic) (suppurative) I80.9
    antepartum — see Thrombophlebitis, antepartum
    blue — see Phlebitis, leg, deep
    breast, superficial I80.8
    cavernous (venous) sinus — see Phlebitis, intracranial (venous) sinus
    cerebral (venous) sinus — see Phlebitis, intracranial (venous) sinus
    chest wall, superficial I80.8
    cranial (venous) sinus — see Phlebitis, intracranial (venous) sinus
    deep (vessels) — see Phlebitis, leg, deep
    due to implanted device — see Complications, by site and type, specified NEC
    during or resulting from a procedure T81.72 ☑
    femoral vein (superficial) I80.1- ☑
    femoropopliteal vein I80.0- ☑
    gestational — see Phlebopathy, gestational
    hepatic veins I80.8
    iliofemoral — see Phlebitis, femoral vein
    intracranial (venous) sinus (any) G08
      nonpyogenic I67.6
    intraspinal venous sinuses and veins G08
      nonpyogenic G95.19
    lateral (venous) sinus — see Phlebitis, intracranial (venous) sinus
    leg I80.3
      antepartum — see Thrombophlebitis, antepartum
      deep (vessels) NEC I80.20- ☑
        iliac I80.21- ☑
        popliteal vein I80.22- ☑
        specified vessel NEC I80.29- ☑
        tibial vein I80.23- ☑

☑ Additional Character Required — Refer to the Tabular List for Character Selection   ▽ Subterms under main terms may continue to next column or page

Phlebitis — *continued*
  leg — *continued*
    femoral vein (superficial) I80.1- ☑
    superficial (vessels) I80.0- ☑
    longitudinal sinus — *see* Phlebitis, intracranial (venous) sinus
    lower limb — *see* Phlebitis, leg
  migrans, migrating (superficial) I82.1
  pelvic
    with ectopic or molar pregnancy O08.0
    following ectopic or molar pregnancy O08.0
    puerperal, postpartum O87.1
  popliteal vein — *see* Phlebitis, leg, deep, popliteal
  portal (vein) K75.1
  postoperative T81.72 ☑
  pregnancy — *see* Thrombophlebitis, antepartum
  puerperal, postpartum, childbirth O87.0
    deep O87.1
    pelvic O87.1
    superficial O87.0
  retina — *see* Vasculitis, retina
  saphenous (accessory) (great) (long) (small) — *see* Phlebitis, leg, superficial
  sinus (meninges) — *see* Phlebitis, intracranial (venous) sinus
  specified site NEC I80.8
  syphilitic A52.09
  tibial vein — *see* Phlebitis, leg, deep, tibial
  ulcerative I80.9
    leg — *see* Phlebitis, leg
  umbilicus I80.8
  uterus (septic) — *see* Endometritis
  varicose (leg) (lower limb) — *see* Varix, leg, with, inflammation
Phlebofibrosis I87.8
Pheboliths I87.8
Phlebopathy,
  gestational O22.9- ☑
  puerperal O87.9
Phlebosclerosis I87.8
Phlebothrombosis (*see also* Thrombosis)
  antepartum — *see* Thrombophlebitis, antepartum
  pregnancy — *see* Thrombophlebitis, antepartum
  puerperal — *see* Thrombophlebitis, puerperal
Phlebotomus fever A93.1
Phlegmasia
  alba dolens O87.1
    nonpuerperal — *see* Phlebitis, femoral vein
  cerulea dolens — *see* Phlebitis, leg, deep
Phlegmon — *see* Abscess
Phlegmonous — *see* condition
Phlyctenulosis (allergic) (keratoconjunctivitis) (nontuberculous) (*see also* Keratoconjunctivitis)
  cornea — *see* Keratoconjunctivitis
  tuberculous A18.52
Phobia, phobic F40.9
  animal F40.218
    spiders F40.210
  examination F40.298
  reaction F40.9
  simple F40.298
  social F40.10
    generalized F40.11
  specific (isolated) F40.298
    animal F40.218
      spiders F40.210
    blood F40.230
    injection F40.231
    injury F40.233
    men F40.290
    natural environment F40.228
      thunderstorms F40.220
    situational F40.248
      bridges F40.242
      closed in spaces F40.240
      flying F40.243
      heights F40.241
    specified focus NEC F40.298
    transfusion F40.231
    women F40.291
  specified NEC F40.8
    medical care NEC F40.232
  state F40.9
Phocas' disease — *see* Mastopathy, cystic
Phocomelia Q73.1
  lower limb — *see* Agenesis, leg, with foot present
  upper limb — *see* Agenesis, arm, with hand present

Phoria H50.50
Phosphate-losing tubular disorder N25.0
Phosphatemia E83.39
Phosphaturia E83.39
Photodermatitis (sun) L56.8
  chronic L57.8
  due to drug L56.8
  light other than sun L59.8
Photokeratitis H16.13- ☑
Photophobia H53.14- ☑
Photophthalmia — *see* Photokeratitis
Photopsia H53.19
Photoretinitis — *see* Retinopathy, solar
Photosensitivity, photosensitization (sun) skin L56.8
  light other than sun L59.8
Phrenitis — *see* Encephalitis
Phrynoderma (vitamin A deficiency) E50.8
Phthiriasis (pubis) B85.3
  with any infestation classifiable to B85.0-B85.2 B85.4
Phthirus infestation — *see* Phthiriasis
Phthisis (*see also* Tuberculosis)
  bulbi (infectional) — *see* Disorder, globe, degenerated condition, atrophy
  eyeball (due to infection) — *see* Disorder, globe, degenerated condition, atrophy
Phycomycosis — *see* Zygomycosis
Physalopteriasis B81.8
Physical restraint status Z78.1
Phytobezoar T18.9 ☑
  intestine T18.3 ☑
  stomach T18.2 ☑
Pian — *see* Yaws
Pianoma A66.1
Pica F50.89
  in adults F50.89
  infant or child F98.3
Picking, nose F98.8
Pick-Niemann disease — *see* Niemann-Pick disease or syndrome
Pick's
  cerebral atrophy G31.01 [F02.80]
    with behavioral disturbance G31.01 [F02.81]
  disease or syndrome (brain) G31.01 [F02.80]
    with behavioral disturbance G31.01 [F02.81]
    brain G31.01 [F02.80]
      with behavioral disturbance G31.01 [F02.81]
    pericardium (pericardial pseudocirrhosis of liver) I31.1
  syndrome
    brain G31.01 [F02.80]
      with behavioral disturbance G31.01 [F02.81]
    of heart (pericardial pseudocirrhosis of liver) I31.1
Pickwickian syndrome E66.2
Piebaldism E70.39
Piedra (beard) (scalp) B36.8
  black B36.3
  white B36.2
Pierre Robin deformity or syndrome Q87.0
Pierson's disease or osteochondrosis M91.0
Pig-bel A05.2
Pigeon
  breast or chest (acquired) M95.4
    congenital Q67.7
    rachitic sequelae (late effect) E64.3
  breeder's disease or lung J67.2
  fancier's disease or lung J67.2
  toe — *see* Deformity, toe, specified NEC
Pigmentation (abnormal) (anomaly) L81.9
  conjunctiva H11.13- ☑
  cornea (anterior) H18.01- ☑
    posterior H18.05- ☑
    stromal H18.06- ☑
  diminished melanin formation NEC L81.6
  iron L81.8
  lids, congenital Q82.8
  limbus corneae — *see* Pigmentation, cornea
  metals L81.8
  optic papilla, congenital Q14.2
  retina, congenital (grouped) (nevoid) Q14.1
  scrotum, congenital Q82.8
  tattoo L81.8
Piles (*see also* Hemorrhoids) K64.9
Pili
  annulati or torti (congenital) Q84.1
  incarnati L73.1
Pill roller hand (intrinsic) — *see* Parkinsonism
Pilomatrixoma — *see* Neoplasm, skin, benign

Pilomatrixoma — *continued*
  malignant — *see* Neoplasm, skin, malignant
Pilonidal — *see* condition
Pimple R23.8
PIN — *see* Neoplasia, intraepithelial, prostate
Pinched nerve — *see* Neuropathy, entrapment
Pindborg tumor — *see* Cyst, calcifying odontogenic
Pineal body or gland — *see* condition
Pinealoblastoma C75.3
Pinealoma D44.5
  malignant C75.3
Pineoblastoma C75.3
Pineocytoma D44.5
Pinguecula H11.15- ☑
Pingueculitis H10.81- ☑
Pinhole meatus (*see also* Stricture, urethra) N35.9
Pink
  disease — *see* subcategory T56.1 ☑
  eye — *see* Conjunctivitis, acute, mucopurulent
Pinkus' disease (lichen nitidus) L44.1
Pinpoint
  meatus — *see* Stricture, urethra
  os (uteri) — *see* Stricture, cervix
Pins and needles R20.2
Pinta A67.9
  cardiovascular lesions A67.2
  chancre (primary) A67.0
  erythematous plaques A67.1
  hyperchromic lesions A67.1
  hyperkeratosis A67.1
  lesions A67.9
    cardiovascular A67.2
    hyperchromic A67.1
    intermediate A67.1
    late A67.2
    mixed A67.3
    primary A67.0
    skin (achromic) (cicatricial) (dyschromic) A67.2
      hyperchromic A67.1
      mixed (achromic and hyperchromic) A67.3
  papule (primary) A67.0
  skin lesions (achromic) (cicatricial) (dyschromic) A67.2
    hyperchromic A67.1
    mixed (achromic and hyperchromic) A67.3
  vitiligo A67.2
Pintids A67.1
Pinworm (disease) (infection) (infestation) B80
Piroplasmosis B60.0
Pistol wound — *see* Gunshot wound
Pitchers' elbow — *see* Derangement, joint, specified type NEC, elbow
Pithecoid pelvis Q74.2
  with disproportion (fetopelvic) O33.0
    causing obstructed labor O65.0
Pithiatism F48.8
Pitted — *see* Pitting
Pitting (*see also* Edema) R60.9
  lip R60.0
  nail L60.8
  teeth K00.4
Pituitary gland — *see* condition
Pituitary-snuff-taker's disease J67.8
Pityriasis (capitis) L21.0
  alba L30.5
  circinata (et maculata) L42
  furfuracea L21.0
  Hebra's L26
  lichenoides L41.0
    chronica L41.1
    et varioliformis (acuta) L41.0
  maculata (et circinata) L30.5
  nigra B36.1
  pilaris, Hebra's L44.0
  rosea L42
  rotunda L44.8
  rubra (Hebra) pilaris L44.0
  simplex L30.5
  specified type NEC L30.5
  streptogenes L30.5
  versicolor (scrotal) B36.0
Placenta, placental — *see* Pregnancy, complicated by (care of) (management affected by), specified condition
Placentitis O41.14- ☑
Plagiocephaly Q67.3
Plague A20.9
  abortive A20.8

Plague — *continued*
- ambulatory A20.8
- asymptomatic A20.8
- bubonic A20.0
- cellulocutaneous A20.1
- cutaneobubonic A20.1
- lymphatic gland A20.0
- meningitis A20.3
- pharyngeal A20.8
- pneumonic (primary) (secondary) A20.2
- pulmonary, pulmonic A20.2
- septicemic A20.7
- tonsillar A20.8
    - septicemic A20.7

Planning, family
- contraception Z30.9
- procreation Z31.69

Plaque(s)
- artery, arterial — *see* Arteriosclerosis
- calcareous — *see* Calcification
- coronary, lipid rich I25.83
- epicardial I31.8
- erythematous, of pinta A67.1
- Hollenhorst's — *see* Occlusion, artery, retina
- lipid rich, coronary I25.83
- pleural (without asbestos) J92.9
    - with asbestos J92.0
- tongue K13.29

Plasmacytoma C90.3- ☑
- extramedullary C90.2- ☑
- medullary C90.0- ☑
- solitary C90.3- ☑

Plasmacytopenia D72.818
Plasmacytosis D72.822
Plaster ulcer — *see* Ulcer, pressure, by site
Plateau iris syndrome (post-iridectomy) (postprocedural) (without glaucoma) H21.82
- with glaucoma H40.22- ☑

Platybasia Q75.8
Platyonychia (congenital) Q84.6
- acquired L60.8

Platypelloid pelvis M95.5
- with disproportion (fetopelvic) O33.0
    - causing obstructed labor O65.0
- congenital Q74.2

Platyspondylisis Q76.49
Plaut (-Vincent) **disease** (*see also* Vincent's) A69.1
Plethora R23.2
- newborn P61.1

Pleura, pleural — *see* condition
Pleuralgia R07.81
Pleurisy (acute) (adhesive) (chronic) (costal) (diaphragmatic) (double) (dry) (fibrinous) (fibrous) (interlobar) (latent) (plastic) (primary) (residual) (sicca) (sterile) (subacute) (unresolved) R09.1
- with
    - adherent pleura J86.0
    - effusion J90
        - chylous, chyliform J94.0
        - tuberculous (non primary) A15.6
            - primary (progressive) A15.7
    - tuberculosis — *see* Pleurisy, tuberculous (non primary)
- encysted — *see* Pleurisy, with effusion
- exudative — *see* Pleurisy, with effusion
- fibrinopurulent, fibropurulent — *see* Pyothorax
- hemorrhagic — *see* Hemothorax
- pneumococcal J90
- purulent — *see* Pyothorax
- septic — *see* Pyothorax
- serofibrinous — *see* Pleurisy, with effusion
- seropurulent — *see* Pyothorax
- serous — *see* Pleurisy, with effusion
- staphylococcal J86.9
- streptococcal J90
- suppurative — *see* Pyothorax
- traumatic (post) (current) — *see* Injury, intrathoracic, pleura
- tuberculous (with effusion) (non primary) A15.6
    - primary (progressive) A15.7

Pleuritis sicca — *see* Pleurisy
Pleurobronchopneumonia — *see* Pneumonia, broncho-
Pleurodynia R07.81
- epidemic B33.0
- viral B33.0

Pleuropericarditis (*see also* Pericarditis)
- acute I30.9

Pleuropneumonia (acute) (bilateral) (double) (septic) (*see also* Pneumonia) J18.8
- chronic — *see* Fibrosis, lung

Pleuro-pneumonia-like-organism (PPLO), as cause of disease classified elsewhere B96.0
Pleurorrhea — *see* Pleurisy, with effusion
Plexitis, brachial G54.0
Plica
- polonica B85.0
- syndrome, knee M67.5- ☑
- tonsil J35.8

Plicated tongue K14.5
Plug
- bronchus NEC J98.09
- meconium (newborn) NEC syndrome P76.0
- mucus — *see* Asphyxia, mucus

Plumbism — *see* subcategory T56.0 ☑
Plummer's disease E05.20
- with thyroid storm E05.21

Plummer-Vinson syndrome D50.1
Pluricarential syndrome of infancy E40
Plus (and minus) **hand** (intrinsic) — *see* Deformity, limb, specified type NEC, forearm
Pneumathemia — *see* Air, embolism
Pneumatic hammer (drill) syndrome T75.21 ☑
Pneumatocele (lung) J98.4
- intracranial G93.89
- tension J44.9

Pneumatosis
- cystoides intestinalis K63.89
- intestinalis K63.89
- peritonei K66.8

Pneumaturia R39.89
Pneumoblastoma — *see* Neoplasm, lung, malignant
Pneumocephalus G93.89
Pneumococcemia A40.3
Pneumococcus, pneumococcal — *see* condition
Pneumoconiosis (due to) (inhalation of) J64
- with tuberculosis (any type in A15) J65
- aluminum J63.0
- asbestos J61
- bagasse, bagassosis J67.1
- bauxite J63.1
- beryllium J63.2
- coal miners' (simple) J60
- coalworkers' (simple) J60
- collier's J60
- cotton dust J66.0
- diatomite (diatomaceous earth) J62.8
- dust
    - inorganic NEC J63.6
    - lime J62.8
    - marble J62.8
    - organic NEC J66.8
- fumes or vapors (from silo) J68.9
- graphite J63.3
- grinder's J62.8
- kaolin J62.8
- mica J62.8
- millstone maker's J62.8
- mineral fibers NEC J61
- miner's J60
- moldy hay J67.0
- potter's J62.8
- rheumatoid — *see* Rheumatoid, lung
- sandblaster's J62.8
- silica, silicate NEC J62.8
    - with carbon J60
- stonemason's J62.8
- talc (dust) J62.0

Pneumocystis carinii pneumonia B59
Pneumocystis jiroveci (pneumonia) B59
Pneumocystosis (with pneumonia) B59
Pneumohemopericardium I31.2
Pneumohemothorax J94.2
- traumatic S27.2 ☑

Pneumohydropericardium — *see* Pericarditis
Pneumohydrothorax — *see* Hydrothorax
Pneumomediastinum J98.2
- congenital or perinatal P25.2

Pneumomycosis B49 [J99]
Pneumonia (acute) (double) (migratory) (purulent) (septic) (unresolved) J18.9
- with
    - influenza — *see* Influenza, with, pneumonia
    - lung abscess J85.1

Pneumonia — *continued*
- with — *continued*
    - lung abscess — *continued*
        - due to specified organism — *see* Pneumonia, in (due to)
- adenoviral J12.0
- adynamic J18.2
- alba A50.04
- allergic (eosinophilic) J82
- alveolar — *see* Pneumonia, lobar
- anaerobes J15.8
- anthrax A22.1
- apex, apical — *see* Pneumonia, lobar
- Ascaris B77.81
- aspiration J69.0
    - due to
        - aspiration of microorganisms
            - bacterial J15.9
            - viral J12.9
        - food (regurgitated) J69.0
        - gastric secretions J69.0
        - milk (regurgitated) J69.0
        - oils, essences J69.1
        - solids, liquids NEC J69.8
        - vomitus J69.0
    - newborn P24.81
        - amniotic fluid (clear) P24.11
        - blood P24.21
        - food (regurgitated) P24.31
        - liquor (amnii) P24.11
        - meconium P24.01
        - milk P24.31
        - mucus P24.11
        - specified NEC P24.81
        - stomach contents P24.31
    - postprocedural J95.4
- atypical NEC J18.9
- bacillus J15.9
    - specified NEC J15.8
- bacterial J15.9
    - specified NEC J15.8
- Bacteroides (fragilis) (oralis) (melaninogenicus) J15.8
- basal, basic, basilar — *see* Pneumonia, by type
- bronchiolitis obliterans organized (BOOP) J84.89
- broncho-, bronchial (confluent) (croupous) (diffuse) (disseminated) (hemorrhagic) (involving lobes) (lobar) (terminal) J18.0
    - allergic (eosinophilic) J82
    - aspiration — *see* Pneumonia, aspiration
    - bacterial J15.9
        - specified NEC J15.8
    - chronic — *see* Fibrosis, lung
    - diplococcal J13
    - Eaton's agent J15.7
    - Escherichia coli (E. coli) J15.5
    - Friedländer's bacillus J15.0
    - Hemophilus influenzae J14
    - hypostatic J18.2
    - inhalation (*see also* Pneumonia, aspiration)
        - due to fumes or vapors (chemical) J68.0
        - of oils or essences J69.1
    - Klebsiella (pneumoniae) J15.0
    - lipid, lipoid J69.1
        - endogenous J84.89
    - Mycoplasma (pneumoniae) J15.7
    - pleuro-pneumonia-like-organisms (PPLO) J15.7
    - pneumococcal J13
    - Proteus J15.6
    - Pseudomonas J15.1
    - Serratia marcescens J15.6
    - specified organism NEC J16.8
    - staphylococcal — *see* Pneumonia, staphylococcal
    - streptococcal NEC J15.4
        - group B J15.3
        - pneumoniae J13
    - viral, virus — *see* Pneumonia, viral
- Butyrivibrio (fibriosolvens) J15.8
- Candida B37.1
- caseous — *see* Tuberculosis, pulmonary
- catarrhal — *see* Pneumonia, broncho
- chlamydial J16.0
    - congenital P23.1
- cholesterol J84.89
- cirrhotic (chronic) — *see* Fibrosis, lung
- Clostridium (haemolyticum) (novyi) J15.8
- confluent — *see* Pneumonia, broncho
- congenital (infective) P23.9

☑ **Additional Character Required** — Refer to the Tabular List for Character Selection   ▽ Subterms under main terms may continue to next column or page

Pneumonia — *continued*
  congenital — *continued*
    due to
      bacterium NEC P23.6
      Chlamydia P23.1
      Escherichia coli P23.4
      Haemophilus influenzae P23.6
      infective organism NEC P23.8
      Klebsiella pneumoniae P23.6
      Mycoplasma P23.6
      Pseudomonas P23.5
      Staphylococcus P23.2
      Streptococcus (except group B) P23.6
        group B P23.3
      viral agent P23.0
    specified NEC P23.8
  croupous — *see* Pneumonia, lobar
  cryptogenic organizing J84.116
  cytomegalic inclusion B25.0
  cytomegaloviral B25.0
  deglutition — *see* Pneumonia, aspiration
  desquamative interstitial J84.117
  diffuse — *see* Pneumonia, broncho
  diplococcal, diplococcus (broncho-) (lobar) J13
  disseminated (focal) — *see* Pneumonia, broncho
  Eaton's agent J15.7
  embolic, embolism — *see* Embolism, pulmonary
  Enterobacter J15.6
  eosinophilic J82
  Escherichia coli (E. coli) J15.5
  Eubacterium J15.8
  fibrinous — *see* Pneumonia, lobar
  fibroid, fibrous (chronic) — *see* Fibrosis, lung
  Friedländer's bacillus J15.0
  Fusobacterium (nucleatum) J15.8
  gangrenous J85.0
  giant cell (measles) B05.2
  gonococcal A54.84
  gram-negative bacteria NEC J15.6
    anaerobic J15.8
  Hemophilus influenzae (broncho) (lobar) J14
  human metapneumovirus J12.3
  hypostatic (broncho) (lobar) J18.2
  in (due to)
    actinomycosis A42.0
    adenovirus J12.0
    anthrax A22.1
    ascariasis B77.81
    aspergillosis B44.9
    Bacillus anthracis A22.1
    Bacterium anitratum J15.6
    candidiasis B37.1
    chickenpox B01.2
    Chlamydia J16.0
      neonatal P23.1
    coccidioidomycosis B38.2
      acute B38.0
      chronic B38.1
    cytomegalovirus disease B25.0
    Diplococcus (pneumoniae) J13
    Eaton's agent J15.7
    Enterobacter J15.6
    Escherichia coli (E. coli) J15.5
    Friedländer's bacillus J15.0
    fumes and vapors (chemical) (inhalation) J68.0
    gonorrhea A54.84
    Hemophilus influenzae (H. influenzae) J14
    Herellea J15.6
    histoplasmosis B39.2
      acute B39.0
      chronic B39.1
    human metapneumovirus J12.3
    Klebsiella (pneumoniae) J15.0
    measles B05.2
    Mycoplasma (pneumoniae) J15.7
    nocardiosis, nocardiasis A43.0
    ornithosis A70
    parainfluenza virus J12.2
    pleuro-pneumonia-like-organism (PPLO) J15.7
    pneumococcus J13
    pneumocystosis (Pneumocystis carinii) (Pneumocystis jiroveci) B59
    Proteus J15.6
    Pseudomonas NEC J15.1
      pseudomallei A24.1
    psittacosis A70
    Q fever A78
    respiratory syncytial virus J12.1

Pneumonia — *continued*
  in — *continued*
    rheumatic fever I00 [J17]
    rubella B06.81
    Salmonella (infection) A02.22
      typhi A01.03
    schistosomiasis B65.9 [J17]
    Serratia marcescens J15.6
    specified
      bacterium NEC J15.8
      organism NEC J16.8
    spirochetal NEC A69.8
    Staphylococcus J15.20
      aureus (methicillin susceptible) (MSSA) J15.211
        methicillin resistant (MRSA) J15.212
      specified NEC J15.29
    Streptococcus J15.4
      group B J15.3
      pneumoniae J13
      specified NEC J15.4
    toxoplasmosis B58.3
    tularemia A21.2
    typhoid (fever) A01.03
    varicella B01.2
    virus — *see* Pneumonia, viral
    whooping cough A37.91
      due to
        Bordetella parapertussis A37.11
        Bordetella pertussis A37.01
        specified NEC A37.81
    Yersinia pestis A20.2
  inhalation of food or vomit — *see* Pneumonia, aspiration
  interstitial J84.9
    chronic J84.111
    desquamative J84.117
    due to
      collagen vascular disease J84.17
      known underlying cause J84.17
    idiopathic NOS J84.111
    in disease classified elsewhere J84.17
    lymphocytic (due to collagen vascular disease) (in diseases classified elsewhere) J84.17
    lymphoid J84.2
    non-specific J84.89
      due to
        collagen vascular disease J84.17
        known underlying cause J84.17
      idiopathic J84.113
      in diseases classified elsewhere J84.17
    plasma cell B59
    pseudomonas J15.1
    usual J84.112
      due to collagen vascular disease J84.17
      idiopathic J84.112
      in diseases classified elsewhere J84.17
  Klebsiella (pneumoniae) J15.0
  lipid, lipoid (exogenous) J69.1
    endogenous J84.89
  lobar (disseminated) (double) (interstitial) J18.1
    bacterial J15.9
      specified NEC J15.8
    chronic — *see* Fibrosis, lung
    Escherichia coli (E. coli) J15.5
    Friedländer's bacillus J15.0
    Hemophilus influenzae J14
    hypostatic J18.2
    Klebsiella (pneumoniae) J15.0
    pneumococcal J13
    Proteus J15.6
    Pseudomonas J15.1
    specified organism NEC J16.8
    staphylococcal — *see* Pneumonia, staphylococcal
    streptococcal NEC J15.4
    Streptococcus pneumoniae J13
    viral, virus — *see* Pneumonia, viral
  lobular — *see* Pneumonia, broncho
  Löffler's J82
  lymphoid interstitial J84.2
  massive — *see* Pneumonia, lobar
  meconium P24.01
  MRSA (methicillin resistant Staphylococcus aureus) J15.212
  MSSA (methicillin susceptible Staphylococcus aureus) J15.211
  multilobar — *see* Pneumonia, by type
  Mycoplasma (pneumoniae) J15.7
  necrotic J85.0

Pneumonia — *continued*
  neonatal P23.9
    aspiration — *see* Aspiration, by substance, with pneumonia
  nitrogen dioxide J68.0
  organizing J84.89
    due to
      collagen vascular disease J84.17
      known underlying cause J84.17
    in diseases classified elsewhere J84.17
  orthostatic J18.2
  parainfluenza virus J12.2
  parenchymatous — *see* Fibrosis, lung
  passive J18.2
  patchy — *see* Pneumonia, broncho
  Peptococcus J15.8
  Peptostreptococcus J15.8
  plasma cell (of infants) B59
  pleurolobar — *see* Pneumonia, lobar
  pleuro-pneumonia-like organism (PPLO) J15.7
  pneumococcal (broncho) (lobar) J13
  Pneumocystis (carinii) (jiroveci) B59
  postinfectional NEC B99 ☑ [J17]
  postmeasles B05.2
  Proteus J15.6
  Pseudomonas J15.1
  psittacosis A70
  radiation J70.0
  respiratory syncytial virus J12.1
  resulting from a procedure J95.89
  rheumatic I00 [J17]
  Salmonella (arizonae) (cholerae-suis) (enteritidis) (typhimurium) A02.22
    typhi A01.03
    typhoid fever A01.03
  SARS-associated coronavirus J12.81
  segmented, segmental — *see* Pneumonia, broncho-
  Serratia marcescens J15.6
  specified NEC J18.8
    bacterium NEC J15.8
    organism NEC J16.8
    virus NEC J12.89
  spirochetal NEC A69.8
  staphylococcal (broncho) (lobar) J15.20
    aureus (methicillin susceptible) (MSSA) J15.211
      methicillin resistant (MRSA) J15.212
    specified NEC J15.29
  static, stasis J18.2
  streptococcal NEC (broncho) (lobar) J15.4
    group
      A J15.4
      B J15.3
      specified NEC J15.4
  Streptococcus pneumoniae J13
  syphilitic, congenital (early) A50.04
  traumatic (complication) (early) (secondary) T79.8 ☑
  tuberculous (any) — *see* Tuberculosis, pulmonary
  tularemic A21.2
  varicella B01.2
  Veillonella J15.8
  ventilator associated J95.851
  viral, virus (broncho) (interstitial) (lobar) J12.9
    adenoviral J12.0
    congenital P23.0
    human metapneumovirus J12.3
    parainfluenza J12.2
    respiratory syncytial J12.1
    SARS-associated coronavirus J12.81
    specified NEC J12.89
  white (congenital) A50.04
Pneumonic — *see* condition
Pneumonitis (acute) (primary) (*see also* Pneumonia)
  air-conditioner J67.7
  allergic (due to) J67.9
    organic dust NEC J67.8
    red cedar dust J67.8
    sequoiosis J67.8
    wood dust J67.8
  aspiration J69.0
    due to
      anesthesia J95.4
        during
          labor and delivery O74.0
          pregnancy O29.01- ☑
          puerperium O89.01
      fumes or gases J68.0
    obstetric O74.0

Pneumonitis — *continued*
  chemical (due to gases, fumes or vapors) (inhalation)
    J68.Ø
    due to anesthesia J95.4
  cholesterol J84.89
  chronic — *see* Fibrosis, lung
  congenital rubella P35.Ø
  crack (cocaine) J68.Ø
  due to
    beryllium J68.Ø
    cadmium J68.Ø
    crack (cocaine) J68.Ø
    detergent J69.8
    fluorocarbon-polymer J68.Ø
    food, vomit (aspiration) J69.Ø
    fumes or vapors J68.Ø
    gases, fumes or vapors (inhalation) J68.Ø
    inhalation
      blood J69.8
      essences J69.1
      food (regurgitated), milk, vomit J69.Ø
      oils, essences J69.1
      saliva J69.Ø
      solids, liquids NEC J69.8
    manganese J68.Ø
    nitrogen dioxide J68.Ø
    oils, essences J69.1
    solids, liquids NEC J69.8
    toxoplasmosis (acquired) B58.3
      congenital P37.1
    vanadium J68.Ø
    ventilator J95.851
  eosinophilic J82
  hypersensitivity J67.9
    air conditioner lung J67.7
    bagassosis J67.1
    bird fancier's lung J67.2
    farmer's lung J67.Ø
    maltworker's lung J67.4
    maple bark-stripper's lung J67.6
    mushroom worker's lung J67.5
    specified organic dust NEC J67.8
    suberosis J67.3
  interstitial (chronic) J84.89
    acute J84.114
    lymphoid J84.2
    non-specific J84.89
      idiopathic J84.113
  lymphoid, interstitial J84.2
  meconium P24.Ø1
  postanesthetic J95.4
    correct substance properly administered — *see*
      Table of Drugs and Chemicals, by drug, ad-
      verse effect
    in labor and delivery O74.Ø
    in pregnancy O29.Ø1- ☑
    obstetric O74.Ø
    overdose or wrong substance given or taken (by
      accident) — *see* Table of Drugs and Chemi-
      cals, by drug, poisoning
    postpartum, puerperal O89.Ø1
  postoperative J95.4
    obstetric O74.Ø
  radiation J7Ø.Ø
  rubella, congenital P35.Ø
  ventilation (air-conditioning) J67.7
  ventilator associated J95.851
  wood-dust J67.8
Pneumonoconiosis — *see* Pneumoconiosis
Pneumoparotid K11.8
Pneumopathy NEC J98.4
  alveolar J84.Ø9
  due to organic dust NEC J66.8
  parietoalveolar J84.Ø9
Pneumopericarditis (*see also* Pericarditis)
  acute I3Ø.9
Pneumopericardium (*see also* Pericarditis)
  congenital P25.3
  newborn P25.3
  traumatic (post) — *see* Injury, heart
Pneumophagia (psychogenic) F45.8
Pneumopleurisy, pneumopleuritis (*see also* Pneumonia) J18.8
Pneumopyopericardium I3Ø.1
Pneumopyothorax — *see* Pyopneumothorax
  with fistula J86.Ø
Pneumorrhagia (*see also* Hemorrhage, lung)
  tuberculous — *see* Tuberculosis, pulmonary

Pneumothorax NOS J93.9
  acute J93.83
  chronic J93.81
  congenital P25.1
  perinatal period P25.1
  postprocedural J95.811
  specified NEC J93.83
  spontaneous NOS J93.83
    newborn P25.1
    primary J93.11
    secondary J93.12
    tension J93.Ø
  tense valvular, infectional J93.Ø
  tension (spontaneous) J93.Ø
  traumatic S27.Ø ☑
    with hemothorax S27.2 ☑
  tuberculous — *see* Tuberculosis, pulmonary
Podagra (*see also* Gout) M1Ø.9
Podencephalus Q01.9
Poikilocytosis R71.8
Poikiloderma L81.6
  Civatte's L57.3
  congenital Q82.8
  vasculare atrophicans L94.5
Poikilodermatomyositis M33.1Ø
  with
    myopathy M33.12
    respiratory involvement M33.11
    specified organ involvement NEC M33.19
Pointed ear (congenital) Q17.3
Poison ivy, oak, sumac or other plant dermatitis
  (allergic) (contact) L23.7
Poisoning (acute) (*see also* Table of Drugs and Chemicals)
  algae and toxins T65.82- ☑
  Bacillus B (aertrycke) (cholerae (suis)) (paratyphosus)
    (suipestifer) A02.9
    botulinus A05.1
  bacterial toxins A05.9
  berries, noxious — *see* Poisoning, food, noxious,
    berries
  botulism A05.1
  ciguatera fish T61.Ø- ☑
  Clostridium botulinum A05.1
  death-cap (Amanita phalloides) (Amanita verna) —
    see Poisoning, food, noxious, mushrooms
  drug — *see* Table of Drugs and Chemicals, by drug,
    poisoning
  epidemic, fish (noxious) — *see* Poisoning, seafood
    bacterial A05.9
  fava bean D55.Ø
  fish (noxious) T61.9- ☑
    bacterial — *see* Intoxication, foodborne, by agent
    ciguatera fish — *see* Poisoning, ciguatera fish
    scombroid fish — *see* Poisoning, scombroid fish
    specified type NEC T61.77- ☑
  food (acute) (diseased) (infected) (noxious) NEC
    T62.9- ☑
    bacterial — *see* Intoxication, foodborne, by agent
    due to
      Bacillus (aertrycke) (choleraesuis) (paratypho-
        sus) (suipestifer) A02.9
        botulinus A05.1
      Clostridium (perfringens) (Welchii) A05.2
      salmonella (aertrycke) (callinarum) (choleraesu-
        is) (enteritidis) (paratyphi) (suipestifer)
        A02.9
        with
          gastroenteritis A02.Ø
          sepsis A02.1
      staphylococcus A05.Ø
      Vibrio
        parahaemolyticus A05.3
        vulnificus A05.5
    noxious or naturally toxic T62.9- ☑
      berries — *see* subcategory T62.1 ☑
      fish — *see* Poisoning, seafood
      mushrooms — *see* subcategory T62.ØX ☑
      plants NEC — *see* subcategory T62.2X ☑
      seafood — *see* Poisoning, seafood
      specified NEC — *see* subcategory T62.8X ☑
  ichthyotoxism — *see* Poisoning, seafood
  kreotoxism, food A05.9
  latex T65.81- ☑
  lead T56.Ø- ☑
  mushroom — *see* Poisoning, food, noxious, mushroom
  mussels (*see also* Poisoning, shellfish)
    bacterial — *see* Intoxication, foodborne, by agent

Poisoning — *continued*
  nicotine (tobacco) T65.2- ☑
  noxious foodstuffs — *see* Poisoning, food, noxious
  plants, noxious — *see* Poisoning, food, noxious, plants
    NEC
  ptomaine — *see* Poisoning, food
  radiation J7Ø.Ø
  Salmonella (arizonae) (cholerae-suis) (enteritidis) (ty-
    phimurium) A02.9
  scombroid fish T61.1- ☑
  seafood (noxious) T61.9- ☑
    bacterial — *see* Intoxication, foodborne, by agent
    fish — *see* Poisoning, fish
    shellfish — *see* Poisoning, shellfish
    specified NEC — *see* subcategory T61.8X ☑
  shellfish (amnesic) (azaspiracid) (diarrheic) (neurotoxic)
    (noxious) (paralytic) T61.78- ☑
    bacterial — *see* Intoxication, foodborne, by agent
    ciguatera mollusk — *see* Poisoning, ciguatera fish
  specified substance NEC T65.891 ☑
  Staphylococcus, food A05.Ø
  tobacco (nicotine) T65.2- ☑
  water E87.79
Poker spine — *see* Spondylitis, ankylosing
Poland syndrome Q79.8
Polioencephalitis (acute) (bulbar) A8Ø.9
  inferior G12.22
  influenzal — *see* Influenza, with, encephalopathy
  superior hemorrhagic (acute) (Wernicke's) E51.2
  Wernicke's E51.2
Polioencephalomyelitis (acute) (anterior) A8Ø.9
  with beriberi E51.2
Polioencephalopathy, superior hemorrhagic E51.2
  with
    beriberi E51.11
    pellagra E52
Poliomeningoencephalitis — *see* Meningoencephalitis
Poliomyelitis (acute) (anterior) (epidemic) A8Ø.9
  with paralysis (bulbar) — *see* Poliomyelitis, paralytic
  abortive A8Ø.4
  ascending (progressive) — *see* Poliomyelitis, paralytic
  bulbar (paralytic) — *see* Poliomyelitis, paralytic
  congenital P35.8
  nonepidemic A8Ø.9
  nonparalytic A8Ø.4
  paralytic A8Ø.3Ø
    specified NEC A8Ø.39
    vaccine-associated A8Ø.Ø
    wild virus
      imported A8Ø.1
      indigenous A8Ø.2
  spinal, acute A8Ø.9
Poliosis (eyebrow) (eyelashes) L67.1
  circumscripta, acquired L67.1
Pollakiuria R35.Ø
  psychogenic F45.8
Pollinosis J3Ø.1
Pollitzer's disease L73.2
Polyadenitis (*see also* Lymphadenitis)
  malignant A2Ø.Ø
Polyalgia M79.89
Polyangiitis M3Ø.Ø
  microscopic M31.7
  overlap syndrome M3Ø.8
Polyarteritis
  microscopic M31.7
  nodosa M3Ø.Ø
    with lung involvement M3Ø.1
    juvenile M3Ø.2
    related condition NEC M3Ø.8
Polyarthralgia — *see* Pain, joint
Polyarthritis, polyarthropathy (*see also* Arthritis) M13.Ø
  due to or associated with other specified conditions
    — *see* Arthritis
  epidemic (Australian) (with exanthema) B33.1
  infective — *see* Arthritis, pyogenic or pyemic
  inflammatory MØ6.4
  juvenile (chronic) (seronegative) MØ8.3
  migratory — *see* Fever, rheumatic
  rheumatic, acute — *see* Fever, rheumatic
Polyarthrosis M15.9
  post-traumatic M15.3
  primary M15.Ø
  specified NEC M15.8
Polycarential syndrome of infancy E4Ø
Polychondritis (atrophic) (chronic) (*see also* Disorder,
  cartilage, specified type NEC)
  relapsing M94.1

Polycoria Q13.2
Polycystic (disease)
  degeneration, kidney Q61.3
    autosomal dominant (adult type) Q61.2
    autosomal recessive (infantile type)
      NEC Q61.19
  kidney Q61.3
    autosomal
      dominant Q61.2
      recessive NEC Q61.19
    autosomal dominant (adult type) Q61.2
    autosomal recessive (childhood type) NEC Q61.19
    infantile type NEC Q61.19
  liver Q44.6
  lung J98.4
    congenital Q33.0
  ovary, ovaries E28.2
  spleen Q89.09
Polycythemia (secondary) D75.1
  acquired D75.1
  benign (familial) D75.0
  due to
    donor twin P61.1
    erythropoietin D75.1
    fall in plasma volume D75.1
    high altitude D75.1
    maternal-fetal transfusion P61.1
    stress D75.1
  emotional D75.1
  erythropoietin D75.1
  familial (benign) D75.0
  Gaisböck's (hypertonica) D75.1
  high altitude D75.1
  hypertonica D75.1
  hypoxemic D75.1
  neonatorum P61.1
  nephrogenous D75.1
  relative D75.1
  secondary D75.1
  spurious D75.1
  stress D75.1
  vera D45
Polycytosis cryptogenica D75.1
Polydactylism, polydactyly Q69.9
  toes Q69.2
Polydipsia R63.1
Polydystrophy, pseudo-Hurler E77.0
Polyembryoma — see Neoplasm, malignant, by site
Polyglandular
  deficiency E31.0
  dyscrasia E31.9
  dysfunction E31.9
  syndrome E31.8
Polyhydramnios O40.- ☑
Polymastia Q83.1
Polymenorrhea N92.0
Polymyalgia M35.3
  arteritica, giant cell M31.5
  rheumatica M35.3
    with giant cell arteritis M31.5
Polymyositis (acute) (chronic) (hemorrhagic) M33.20
  with
    myopathy M33.22
    respiratory involvement M33.21
    skin involvement — see Dermatopolymyositis
    specified organ involvement NEC M33.29
  ossificans (generalisata) (progressiva) — see Myositis, ossificans, progressiva
Polyneuritis, polyneuritic (see also Polyneuropathy)
  acute (post-)infective G61.0
  alcoholic G62.1
  cranialis G52.7
  demyelinating, chronic inflammatory (CIDP) G61.81
  diabetic — see Diabetes, polyneuropathy
  diphtheritic A36.83
  due to lack of vitamin NEC E56.9 [G63]
  endemic E51.11
  erythredema — see subcategory T56.1 ☑
  febrile, acute G61.0
  hereditary ataxic G60.1
  idiopathic, acute G61.0
  infective (acute) G61.0
  inflammatory, chronic demyelinating (CIDP) G61.81
  nutritional E63.9 [G63]
  postinfective (acute) G61.0
  specified NEC G62.89
Polyneuropathy (peripheral) G62.9

Polyneuropathy — continued
  alcoholic G62.1
  amyloid (Portuguese) E85.1 [G63]
    transthyretin-related (ATTR) familial E85.1
  arsenical G62.2
  critical illness G62.81
  demyelinating, chronic inflammatory (CIDP) G61.81
  diabetic — see Diabetes, polyneuropathy
  drug-induced G62.0
  hereditary G60.9
    specified NEC G60.8
  idiopathic G60.9
    progressive G60.3
  in (due to)
    alcohol G62.1
      sequelae G65.2
    amyloidosis, familial (Portuguese) E85.1 [G63]
    antitetanus serum G61.1
    arsenic G62.2
      sequelae G65.2
    avitaminosis NEC E56.9 [G63]
    beriberi E51.11
    collagen vascular disease NEC M35.9 [G63]
    deficiency (of)
      B (-complex) vitamins E53.9 [G63]
      vitamin B6 E53.1 [G63]
    diabetes — see Diabetes, polyneuropathy
    diphtheria A36.83
    drug or medicament G62.0
      correct substance properly administered — see Table of Drugs and Chemicals, by drug, adverse effect
      overdose or wrong substance given or taken — see Table of Drugs and Chemicals, by drug, poisoning
    endocrine disease NEC E34.9 [G63]
    herpes zoster B02.23
    hypoglycemia E16.2 [G63]
    infectious
      disease NEC B99 ☑ [G63]
      mononucleosis B27.91
    lack of vitamin NEC E56.9 [G63]
    lead G62.2
      sequelae G65.2
    leprosy A30.9 [G63]
    Lyme disease A69.22
    metabolic disease NEC E88.9 [G63]
    microscopic polyangiitis M31.7 [G63]
    mumps B26.84
    neoplastic disease (see also Neoplasm) D49.9 [G63]
    nutritional deficiency NEC E63.9 [G63]
    organophosphate compounds G62.2
      sequelae G65.2
    parasitic disease NEC B89 [G63]
    pellagra E52 [G63]
    polyarteritis nodosa M30.0
    porphyria E80.20 [G63]
    radiation G62.82
    rheumatoid arthritis — see Rheumatoid, polyneuropathy
    sarcoidosis D86.89
    serum G61.1
    syphilis (late) A52.15
      congenital A50.43
    systemic
      connective tissue disorder M35.9 [G63]
      lupus erythematosus M32.19
    toxic agent NEC G62.2
      sequelae G65.2
  inflammatory G61.9
    chronic demyelinating (CIDP) G61.81
    sequelae G65.1
    specified NEC G61.89
  lead G62.2
    sequelae G65.2
  nutritional NEC E63.9 [G63]
  postherpetic (zoster) B02.23
  progressive G60.3
  radiation-induced G62.82
  sensory (hereditary) (idiopathic) G60.8
  specified NEC G62.89
  syphilitic (late) A52.15
    congenital A50.43
  transthyretin-related (ATTR) familial amyloid E85.1
    triorthocresyl phosphate G62.2
      sequelae G65.2
    tuberculosis A17.89
    uremia N18.9 [G63]

Polyneuropathy — continued
  transthyretin-related familial amyloid — continued
    vitamin B12 deficiency E53.8 [G63]
      with anemia (pernicious) D51.0 [G63]
        due to dietary deficiency D51.3 [G63]
    zoster B02.23
Polyopia H53.8
Polyorchism, polyorchidism Q55.21
Polyosteoarthritis (see also Osteoarthritis, generalized) M15.9
  post-traumatic M15.3
  specified NEC M15.8
Polyostotic fibrous dysplasia Q78.1
Polyotia Q17.0
Polyp, polypus
  accessory sinus J33.8
  adenocarcinoma in — see Neoplasm, malignant, by site
  adenocarcinoma in situ in — see Neoplasm, in situ, by site
  adenoid tissue J33.0
  adenomatous (see also Neoplasm, benign, by site)
    adenocarcinoma in — see Neoplasm, malignant, by site
    adenocarcinoma in situ in — see Neoplasm, in situ, by site
    carcinoma in — see Neoplasm, malignant, by site
    carcinoma in situ in — see Neoplasm, in situ, by site
    multiple — see Neoplasm, benign
      adenocarcinoma in — see Neoplasm, malignant, by site
      adenocarcinoma in situ in — see Neoplasm, in situ, by site
  antrum J33.8
  anus, anal (canal) K62.0
  Bartholin's gland N84.3
  bladder D41.4
  carcinoma in — see Neoplasm, malignant, by site
  carcinoma in situ in — see Neoplasm, in situ, by site
  cecum D12.0
  cervix (uteri) N84.1
    in pregnancy or childbirth — see Pregnancy, complicated by, abnormal, cervix
    mucous N84.1
    nonneoplastic N84.1
  choanal J33.0
  cholesterol K82.4
  clitoris N84.3
  colon K63.5
    adenomatous D12.6
    ascending D12.2
    cecum D12.0
    descending D12.4
    inflammatory K51.40
      with
        abscess K51.414
        complication K51.419
          specified NEC K51.418
        fistula K51.413
        intestinal obstruction K51.412
        rectal bleeding K51.411
    sigmoid D12.5
    transverse D12.3
  corpus uteri N84.0
  dental K04.01
    irreversible K04.02
    reversible K04.01
  duodenum K31.7
  ear (middle) H74.4- ☑
  endometrium N84.0
  ethmoidal (sinus) J33.8
  fallopian tube N84.8
  female genital tract N84.9
    specified NEC N84.8
  frontal (sinus) J33.8
  gallbladder K82.4
  gingiva, gum K06.8
  labia, labium (majus) (minus) N84.3
  larynx (mucous) J38.1
    adenomatous D14.1
  malignant — see Neoplasm, malignant, by site
  maxillary (sinus) J33.8
  middle ear — see Polyp, ear (middle)
  myometrium N84.0
  nares
    anterior J33.9
    posterior J33.0

Polyp, polypus — *continued*
nasal (mucous) J33.9
cavity J33.0
septum J33.0
nasopharyngeal J33.0
nose (mucous) J33.9
oviduct N84.8
pharynx J39.2
placenta O90.89
prostate — *see* Enlargement, enlarged, prostate
pudenda, pudendum N84.3
pulpal (dental) K04.01
irreversible K04.02
reversible K04.01
rectum (nonadenomatous) K62.1
adenomatous — *see* Polyp, adenomatous
septum (nasal) J33.0
sinus (accessory) (ethmoidal) (frontal) (maxillary) (sphenoidal) J33.8
sphenoidal (sinus) J33.8
stomach K31.7
adenomatous D13.1
tube, fallopian N84.8
turbinate, mucous membrane J33.8
umbilical, newborn P83.6
ureter N28.89
urethra N36.2
uterus (body) (corpus) (mucous) N84.0
cervix N84.1
in pregnancy or childbirth — *see* Pregnancy, complicated by, tumor, uterus
vagina N84.2
vocal cord (mucous) J38.1
vulva N84.3
Polyphagia R63.2
Polyploidy Q92.7
Polypoid — *see* condition
Polyposis (*see also* Polyp)
coli (adenomatous) D12.6
adenocarcinoma in C18.9
adenocarcinoma in situ in — *see* Neoplasm, in situ, by site
carcinoma In C18.9
colon (adenomatous) D12.6
familial D12.6
adenocarcinoma in situ in — *see* Neoplasm, in situ, by site
intestinal (adenomatous) D12.6
malignant lymphomatous C83.1- ☑
multiple, adenomatous (*see also* Neoplasm, benign) D36.9
Polyradiculitis — *see* Polyneuropathy
Polyradiculoneuropathy (acute) (postinfective) (segmentally demyelinating) G61.0
Polyserositis
due to pericarditis I31.1
pericardial I31.1
periodic, familial E85.0
tuberculous A19.9
acute A19.1
chronic A19.8
Polysplenia syndrome Q89.09
Polysyndactyly (*see also* Syndactylism, syndactyly) Q70.4
Polytrichia L68.3
Polyunguia Q84.6
Polyuria R35.8
nocturnal R35.1
psychogenic F45.8
Pompe's disease (glycogen storage) E74.02
Pompholyx L30.1
Poncet's disease (tuberculous rheumatism) A18.09
Pond fracture — *see* Fracture, skull
Ponos B55.0
Pons, pontine — *see* condition
Poor
aesthetic of existing restoration of tooth K08.56
contractions, labor O62.2
gingival margin to tooth restoration K08.51
personal hygiene R46.0
prenatal care, affecting management of pregnancy — *see* Pregnancy, complicated by, insufficient, prenatal care
sucking reflex (newborn) R29.2
urinary stream R39.12
vision NEC H54.7
Poradenitis, nostras inguinalis or venerea A55
Porencephaly (congenital) (developmental) (true) Q04.6
acquired G93.0

Porencephaly — *continued*
nondevelopmental G93.0
traumatic (post) F07.89
Porocephaliasis B88.8
Porokeratosis Q82.8
Poroma, eccrine — *see* Neoplasm, skin, benign
Porphyria (South African) E80.20
acquired E80.20
acute intermittent (hepatic) (Swedish) E80.21
cutanea tarda (hereditary) (symptomatic) E80.1
due to drugs E80.20
correct substance properly administered — *see* Table of Drugs and Chemicals, by drug, adverse effect
overdose or wrong substance given or taken — *see* Table of Drugs and Chemicals, by drug, poisoning
erythropoietic (congenital) (hereditary) E80.0
hepatocutaneous type E80.1
secondary E80.20
toxic NEC E80.20
variegata E80.20
Porphyrinuria — *see* Porphyria
Porphyruria — *see* Porphyria
Port wine nevus, mark, or stain Q82.5
Portal — *see* condition
Posadas-Wernicke disease B38.9
Positive
culture (nonspecific)
blood R78.81
bronchial washings R84.5
cerebrospinal fluid R83.5
cervix uteri R87.5
nasal secretions R84.5
nipple discharge R89.5
nose R84.5
staphylococcus (Methicillin susceptible) Z22.321
Methicillin resistant Z22.322
peritoneal fluid R85.5
pleural fluid R84.5
prostatic secretions R86.5
saliva R85.5
seminal fluid R86.5
sputum R84.5
synovial fluid R89.5
throat scrapings R84.5
urine R82.79
vagina R87.5
vulva R87.5
wound secretions R89.5
PPD (skin test) R76.11
serology for syphilis A53.0
with signs or symptoms — *code as* Syphilis, by site and stage
false R76.8
skin test, tuberculin (without active tuberculosis) R76.11
test, human immunodeficiency virus (HIV) R75
VDRL A53.0
with signs or symptoms — *code by* site and stage under Syphilis A53.9
Wassermann reaction A53.0
Postcardiotomy syndrome I97.0
Postcaval ureter Q62.62
Postcholecystectomy syndrome K91.5
Postclimacteric bleeding N95.0
Postcommissurotomy syndrome I97.0
Postconcussional syndrome F07.81
Postcontusional syndrome F07.81
Postcricoid region — *see* condition
Post-dates (40-42 weeks) (pregnancy) (mother) O48.0
more than 42 weeks gestation O48.1
Postencephalitic syndrome F07.89
Posterior — *see* condition
Posterolateral sclerosis (spinal cord) — *see* Degeneration, combined
Postexanthematous — *see* condition
Postfebrile — *see* condition
Postgastrectomy dumping syndrome K91.1
Posthemiplegic chorea — *see* Monoplegia
Posthemorrhagic anemia (chronic) D50.0
acute D62
newborn P61.3
Postherpetic neuralgia (zoster) B02.29
trigeminal B02.22
Posthitis N47.7
Postimmunization complication or reaction — *see* Complications, vaccination

Postinfectious — *see* condition
Postlaminectomy syndrome NEC M96.1
Postleukotomy syndrome F07.0
Postmastectomy lymphedema (syndrome) I97.2
Postmaturity, postmature (over 42 weeks)
maternal (over 42 weeks gestation) O48.1
newborn P08.22
Postmeasles complication NEC (*see also* condition) B05.89
Postmenopausal
endometrium (atrophic) N95.8
suppurative (*see also* Endometritis) N71.9
osteoporosis — *see* Osteoporosis, postmenopausal
Postnasal drip R09.82
due to
allergic rhinitis — *see* Rhinitis, allergic
common cold J00
gastroesophageal reflux — *see* Reflux, gastroesophageal
nasopharyngitis — *see* Nasopharyngitis
other known condition — *code to* condition
sinusitis — *see* Sinusitis
Postnatal — *see* condition
Postoperative (postprocedural) — *see* Complication, postoperative
pneumothorax, therapeutic Z98.3
state NEC Z98.890
Postpancreatectomy hyperglycemia E89.1
Postpartum — *see* Puerperal
Postphlebitic syndrome — *see* Syndrome, postthrombotic
Postpolio (myelitic) **syndrome** G14
Postpoliomyelitic (*see also* condition)
osteopathy — *see* Osteopathy, after poliomyelitis
Postprocedural (*see also* Postoperative)
hypoinsulinemia E89.1
Postschizophrenic depression F32.89
Postsurgery status (*see also* Status (post))
pneumothorax, therapeutic Z98.3
Post-term (40-42 weeks) (pregnancy) (mother) O48.0
infant P08.21
more than 42 weeks gestation (mother) O48.1
Post-traumatic brain syndrome, nonpsychotic F07.81
Post-typhoid abscess A01.09
Postures, hysterical F44.2
Postvaccinal reaction or complication — *see* Complications, vaccination
Postvalvulotomy syndrome I97.0
Potain's
disease (pulmonary edema) — *see* Edema, lung
syndrome (gastrectasis with dyspepsia) K31.0
Potter's
asthma J62.8
facies Q60.6
lung J62.8
syndrome (with renal agenesis) Q60.6
Pott's
curvature (spinal) A18.01
disease or paraplegia A18.01
spinal curvature A18.01
tumor, puffy — *see* Osteomyelitis, specified type NEC
Pouch
bronchus Q32.4
Douglas' — *see* condition
esophagus, esophageal, congenital Q39.6
acquired K22.5
gastric K31.4
Hartmann's K82.8
pharynx, pharyngeal (congenital) Q38.7
Pouchitis K91.850
Poultrymen's itch B88.0
Poverty NEC Z59.6
extreme Z59.5
Poxvirus NEC B08.8
Prader-Willi syndrome Q87.1
Preauricular appendage or tag Q17.0
Prebetalipoproteinemia (acquired) (essential) (familial) (hereditary) (primary) (secondary) E78.1
with chylomicronemia E78.3
Precipitate labor or delivery O62.3
Preclimacteric bleeding (menorrhagia) N92.4
Precocious
adrenarche E30.1
menarche E30.1
menstruation E30.1
pubarche E30.1
puberty E30.1

Precocious — *continued*
  puberty — *continued*
    central E22.8
    sexual development NEC E30.1
    thelarche E30.8
Precocity, sexual (constitutional) (cryptogenic) (female) (idiopathic) (male) E30.1
  with adrenal hyperplasia E25.9
    congenital E25.0
Precordial pain R07.2
Predeciduous teeth K00.2
Prediabetes, prediabetic R73.03
  complicating
    pregnancy — *see* Pregnancy, complicated by, diseases of, specified type or system NEC
    puerperium O99.89
Predislocation status of hip at birth Q65.6
Pre-eclampsia O14.9- ☑
  with pre-existing hypertension — *see* Hypertension, complicating pregnancy, pre-existing, with, pre-eclampsia
  complicating
    childbirth O14.94
    puerperium O14.95
  mild O14.0- ☑
    complicating
      childbirth O14.04
      puerperium O14.05
  moderate O14.0- ☑
    complicating
      childbirth O14.04
      puerperium O14.05
  severe O14.1- ☑
    with hemolysis, elevated liver enzymes and low platelet count (HELLP) O14.2- ☑
      complicating
        childbirth O14.24
        puerperium O14.25
    complicating
      childbirth O14.14
      puerperium O14.15
Pre-eruptive color change, teeth, tooth K00.8
Pre-excitation atrioventricular conduction I45.6
Preglaucoma H40.00- ☑
Pregnancy (single) (uterine) (*see also* Delivery and Puerperal)

> *Note: The Tabular must be reviewed for assignment of appropriate seventh character for multiple gestation codes in Chapter 15*

> *Note: The Tabular must be reviewed for assignment of the appropriate character indicating the trimester of the pregnancy*

  abdominal (ectopic) O00.00
    with intrauterine pregnancy O00.01
      with viable fetus O36.7- ☑
  ampullar O00.10- ☑
    with intrauterine pregnancy O00.11- ☑
  biochemical O02.81
  broad ligament O00.80
    with intrauterine pregnancy O00.81
  cervical O00.8
    with intrauterine pregnancy O00.81
  chemical O02.81
  complicated by (care of) (management affected by)
    abnormal, abnormality
      cervix O34.4- ☑
        causing obstructed labor O65.5
      cord (umbilical) O69.9 ☑
      fetal heart rate or rhythm O36.83- ☑
      findings on antenatal screening of mother O28.9
        biochemical O28.1
        chromosomal O28.5
        cytological O28.2
        genetic O28.5
        hematological O28.0
        radiological O28.4
        specified NEC O28.8
        ultrasonic O28.3
      glucose (tolerance) NEC O99.810
      pelvic organs O34.9- ☑
        specified NEC O34.8- ☑
          causing obstructed labor O65.5
      pelvis (bony) (major) NEC O33.0
      perineum O34.7- ☑

Pregnancy — *continued*
  complicated by — *continued*
    abnormal, abnormality — *continued*
      position
        placenta O44.0- ☑
          with hemorrhage O44.1- ☑
        uterus O34.59- ☑
      uterus O34.59- ☑
        causing obstructed labor O65.5
        congenital O34.0- ☑
      vagina O34.6- ☑
        causing obstructed labor O65.5
      vulva O34.7- ☑
        causing obstructed labor O65.5
    abruptio placentae — *see* Abruptio placentae
    abscess or cellulitis
      bladder O23.1- ☑
      breast O91.11- ☑
      genital organ or tract O23.9- ☑
    abuse
      physical O9A.31 ☑ (*following* O99)
      psychological O9A.51 ☑ (*following* O99)
      sexual O9A.41 ☑ (*following* O99)
    adverse effect anesthesia O29.9- ☑
      aspiration pneumonitis O29.01- ☑
      cardiac arrest O29.11- ☑
      cardiac complication NEC O29.19- ☑
      cardiac failure O29.12- ☑
      central nervous system complication NEC O29.29- ☑
      cerebral anoxia O29.21- ☑
      failed or difficult intubation O29.6- ☑
      inhalation of stomach contents or secretions NOS O29.01- ☑
      local, toxic reaction O29.3X ☑
      Mendelson's syndrome O29.01- ☑
      pressure collapse of lung O29.02- ☑
      pulmonary complications NEC O29.09- ☑
      specified NEC O29.8X- ☑
      spinal and epidural type NEC O29.5X ☑
        induced headache O29.4- ☑
    albuminuria (*see also* Proteinuria, gestational) O12.1- ☑
    alcohol use O99.31- ☑
    amnionitis O41.12- ☑
    anaphylactoid syndrome of pregnancy O88.01- ☑
    anemia (conditions in D50-D64) (pre-existing) O99.01- ☑
      complicating the puerperium O99.03
    antepartum hemorrhage O46.9- ☑
      with coagulation defect — *see* Hemorrhage, antepartum, with coagulation defect
      specified NEC O46.8X- ☑
    appendicitis O99.61- ☑
    atrophy (yellow) (acute) liver (subacute) O26.61- ☑
    bariatric surgery status O99.84- ☑
    bicornis or bicornuate uterus O34.0- ☑
    biliary tract problems O26.61- ☑
    breech presentation O32.1 ☑
    cardiovascular diseases (conditions in I00-I09, I20-I52, I70-I99) O99.41- ☑
    cerebrovascular disorders (conditions in I60-I69) O99.41- ☑
    cervical shortening O26.87- ☑
    cervicitis O23.51- ☑
    chloasma (gravidarum) O26.89- ☑
    cholecystitis O99.61- ☑
    cholestasis (intrahepatic) O26.61- ☑
    chorioamnionitis O41.12- ☑
    circulatory system disorder (conditions in I00-I09, I20-I99, O99.41-)
    compound presentation O32.6 ☑
    conjoined twins O30.02- ☑
    connective system disorders (conditions in M00-M99) O99.89
    contracted pelvis (general) O33.1
      inlet O33.2
      outlet O33.3
    convulsions (eclamptic) (uremic) (*see also* Eclampsia) O15.9
    cracked nipple O92.11- ☑
    cystitis O23.1- ☑
    cystocele O34.8- ☑
    death of fetus (near term) O36.4 ☑
      early pregnancy O02.1

Pregnancy — *continued*
  complicated by — *continued*
    death of fetus — *continued*
      of one fetus or more in multiple gestation O31.2- ☑
    deciduitis O41.14- ☑
    decreased fetal movement O36.81- ☑
    dental problems O99.61- ☑
    diabetes (mellitus) O24.91- ☑
      gestational (pregnancy induced) — *see* Diabetes, gestational
      pre-existing O24.31- ☑
        specified NEC O24.81- ☑
        type 1 O24.01- ☑
        type 2 O24.11- ☑
    digestive system disorders (conditions in K00-K93) O99.61- ☑
    diseases of — *see* Pregnancy, complicated by, specified body system disease
      biliary tract O26.61- ☑
      blood NEC (conditions in D65-D77) O99.11- ☑
      liver O26.61- ☑
      specified NEC O99.89
    disorders of — *see* Pregnancy, complicated by, specified body system disorder
      amniotic fluid and membranes O41.9- ☑
        specified NEC O41.8X- ☑
      biliary tract O26.61- ☑
      ear and mastoid process (conditions in H60-H95) O99.89
      eye and adnexa (conditions in H00-H59) O99.89
      liver O26.61- ☑
      skin (conditions in L00-L99) O99.71- ☑
      specified NEC O99.89
    displacement, uterus NEC O34.59- ☑
      causing obstructed labor O65.5
    disproportion (due to) O33.9
      fetal (ascites) (hydrops) (meningomyelocele) (sacral teratoma) (tumor) deformities NEC O33.7
      generally contracted pelvis O33.1
      hydrocephalic fetus O33.6
      inlet contraction of pelvis O33.2
      mixed maternal and fetal origin O33.4 ☑
      specified NEC O33.8
    double uterus O34.0- ☑
      causing obstructed labor O65.5
    drug use (conditions in F11-F19) O99.32- ☑
    eclampsia, eclamptic (coma) (convulsions) (delirium) (nephritis) (uremia) (*see also* Eclampsia) O15.- ☑
    ectopic pregnancy — *see* Pregnancy, ectopic
    edema O12.0- ☑
      with
        gestational hypertension, mild (*see also* Pre-eclampsia) O14.0- ☑
        proteinuria O12.2- ☑
    effusion, amniotic fluid — *see* Pregnancy, complicated by, premature rupture of membranes
    elderly
      multigravida O09.52- ☑
      primigravida O09.51- ☑
    embolism (*see also* Embolism, obstetric, pregnancy) O88.- ☑
    endocrine diseases NEC O99.28- ☑
    endometritis O86.12
    excessive weight gain O26.0- ☑
    exhaustion O26.81- ☑
      during labor and delivery O75.81
    face presentation O32.3 ☑
    failed induction of labor O61.9
      instrumental O61.1
      mechanical O61.1
      medical O61.0
      specified NEC O61.8
      surgical O61.1
    failed or difficult intubation for anesthesia O29.6- ☑
    false labor (pains) O47.9
      at or after 37 completed weeks of pregnancy O47.1
      before 37 completed weeks of pregnancy O47.0- ☑
    fatigue O26.81- ☑
      during labor and delivery O75.81
    fatty metamorphosis of liver O26.61- ☑
    female genital mutilation O34.8- ☑ [N90.81-] ☑

⛛ Subterms under main terms may continue to next column or page   ☑ Additional Character Required — Refer to the Tabular List for Character Selection   259

Precocious — Pregnancy

Pregnancy — *continued*
  complicated by — *continued*
    fetal (maternal care for)
      abnormality or damage O35.9 ☑
        acid-base balance O68
        specified type NEC O35.8 ☑
      acidemia O68
      acidosis O68
      alkalosis O68
      anemia and thrombocytopenia O36.82- ☑
      anencephaly O35.0 ☑
      chromosomal abnormality (conditions in Q90-Q99) O35.1 ☑
      conjoined twins O30.02- ☑
      damage from
        amniocentesis O35.7 ☑
        biopsy procedures O35.7 ☑
        drug addiction O35.5 ☑
        hematological investigation O35.7 ☑
        intrauterine contraceptive device O35.7 ☑
        maternal
          alcohol addiction O35.4 ☑
          cytomegalovirus infection O35.3 ☑
          disease NEC O35.8 ☑
          drug addiction O35.5 ☑
          listeriosis O35.8 ☑
          rubella O35.3 ☑
          toxoplasmosis O35.8 ☑
          viral infection O35.3 ☑
        medical procedure NEC O35.7 ☑
        radiation O35.6 ☑
      death (near term) O36.4 ☑
        early pregnancy O02.1
      decreased movement O36.81- ☑
      disproportion due to deformity (fetal) O33.7 ☑
      excessive growth (large for dates) O36.6- ☑
      growth retardation O36.59- ☑
        light for dates O36.59- ☑
        small for dates O36.59- ☑
      heart rate irregularity (bradycardia) (decelerations) (tachycardia) O76
      hereditary disease O35.2 ☑
      hydrocephalus O35.0 ☑
      intrauterine death O36.4 ☑
      poor growth O36.59- ☑
        light for dates O36.59- ☑
        small for dates O36.59- ☑
      problem O36.9- ☑
        specified NEC O36.89- ☑
      reduction (elective) O31.3- ☑
      selective termination O31.3- ☑
      spina bifida O35.0 ☑
      thrombocytopenia O36.82- ☑
    fibroid (tumor) (uterus) O34.1- ☑
    fissure of nipple O92.11- ☑
    gallstones O99.61- ☑
    gastric banding status O99.84- ☑
    gastric bypass status O99.84- ☑
    genital herpes (asymptomatic) (history of) (inactive) O98.3- ☑
    genital tract infection O23.9- ☑
    glomerular diseases (conditions in N00-N07) O26.83- ☑
      with hypertension, pre-existing — *see* Hypertension, complicating, pregnancy, pre-existing, with, renal disease
    gonorrhea O98.21- ☑
    grand multiparity O09.4 ☑
    habitual aborter — *see* Pregnancy, complicated by, recurrent pregnancy loss
    HELLP syndrome (hemolysis, elevated liver enzymes and low platelet count) O14.2- ☑
    hemorrhage
      antepartum — *see* Hemorrhage, antepartum
      before 20 completed weeks gestation O20.9
        specified NEC O20.8
      due to premature separation, placenta (*see also* Abruptio placentae) O45.9- ☑
      early O20.9
        specified NEC O20.8
      threatened abortion O20.0
    hemorrhoids O22.4- ☑
    hepatitis (viral) O98.41- ☑
    herniation of uterus O34.59- ☑
    high
      head at term O32.4 ☑

Pregnancy — *continued*
  complicated by — *continued*
    high — *continued*
      risk — *see* Supervision (of) (for), high-risk
    history of in utero procedure during previous pregnancy O09.82- ☑
    HIV O98.71- ☑
    human immunodeficiency virus (HIV) disease O98.71- ☑
    hydatidiform mole (*see also* Mole, hydatidiform) O01.9
    hydramnios O40.- ☑
    hydrocephalic fetus (disproportion) O33.6 ☑
    hydrops
      amnii O40.- ☑
      fetalis O36.2- ☑
        associated with isoimmunization (*see also* Pregnancy, complicated by, isoimmunization) O36.11- ☑
    hydrorrhea O42.90
    hyperemesis (gravidarum) (mild) (*see also* Hyperemesis, gravidarum) O21.0
    hypertension — *see* Hypertension, complicating pregnancy
    hypertensive
      heart and renal disease, pre-existing — *see* Hypertension, complicating, pregnancy, pre-existing, with, heart disease, with renal disease
      heart disease, pre-existing — *see* Hypertension, complicating, pregnancy, pre-existing, with, heart disease
      renal disease, pre-existing — *see* Hypertension, complicating, pregnancy, pre-existing, with, renal disease
    hypotension O26.5- ☑
    immune disorders NEC (conditions in D80-D89) O99.11- ☑
    incarceration, uterus O34.51- ☑
    incompetent cervix O34.3- ☑
    inconclusive fetal viability O36.80 ☑
    infection(s) O98.91- ☑
      amniotic fluid or sac O41.10- ☑
      bladder O23.1- ☑
      carrier state NEC O99.830
        streptococcus B O99.820
      genital organ or tract O23.9- ☑
        specified NEC O23.59- ☑
      genitourinary tract O23.9- ☑
      gonorrhea O98.21- ☑
      hepatitis (viral) O98.41- ☑
      HIV O98.71- ☑
      human immunodeficiency virus (HIV) O98.71- ☑
      kidney O23.0- ☑
      nipple O91.01- ☑
      parasitic disease O98.91- ☑
        specified NEC O98.81- ☑
      protozoal disease O98.61- ☑
      sexually transmitted NEC O98.31- ☑
      specified type NEC O98.81- ☑
      syphilis O98.11- ☑
      tuberculosis O98.01- ☑
      urethra O23.2- ☑
      urinary (tract) O23.4- ☑
        specified NEC O23.3- ☑
      viral disease O98.51- ☑
    injury or poisoning (conditions in S00-T88) O9A.21- ☑ (*following* O99)
      due to abuse
        physical O9A.31- ☑ (*following* O99)
        psychological O9A.51- ☑ (*following* O99)
        sexual O9A.41- ☑ (*following* O99)
    insufficient
      prenatal care O09.3- ☑
      weight gain O26.1- ☑
    insulin resistance O26.89 ☑
    intrauterine fetal death (near term) O36.4 ☑
      early pregnancy O02.1
      multiple gestation (one fetus or more) O31.2- ☑
    isoimmunization O36.11- ☑
      anti-A sensitization O36.11- ☑
      anti-B sensitization O36.19- ☑
      Rh O36.09- ☑
        anti-D antibody O36.01- ☑

Pregnancy — *continued*
  complicated by — *continued*
    isoimmunization — *continued*
      specified NEC O36.19- ☑
    laceration of uterus NEC O71.81
    malformation
      placenta, placental (vessel) O43.10- ☑
        specified NEC O43.19- ☑
      uterus (congenital) O34.0- ☑
    malnutrition (conditions in E40-E46) O25.1- ☑
    maternal hypotension syndrome O26.5- ☑
    mental disorders (conditions in F01-F09, F20-F99) O99.34- ☑
      alcohol use O99.31- ☑
      drug use O99.32- ☑
      smoking O99.33- ☑
    mentum presentation O32.3 ☑
    metabolic disorders O99.28- ☑
    missed
      abortion O02.1
      delivery O36.4 ☑
    multiple gestations O30.9- ☑
      conjoined twins O30.02- ☑
      quadruplet — *see* Pregnancy, quadruplet
      specified complication NEC O31.8X- ☑
      specified number of multiples NEC — *see* Pregnancy, multiple (gestation), specified NEC
      triplet — *see* Pregnancy, triplet
      twin — *see* Pregnancy, twin
    musculoskeletal condition (conditions is M00-M99) O99.89
    necrosis, liver (conditions in K72) O26.61- ☑
    neoplasm
      benign
        cervix O34.4- ☑
        corpus uteri O34.1- ☑
        uterus O34.1- ☑
      malignant O9A.11- ☑ (*following* O99)
    nephropathy NEC O26.83- ☑
    nervous system condition (conditions in G00-G99) O99.35- ☑
    nutritional diseases NEC O99.28- ☑
    obesity (pre-existing) O99.21- ☑
    obesity surgery status O99.84- ☑
    oblique lie or presentation O32.2 ☑
    older mother — *see* Pregnancy, complicated by, elderly
    oligohydramnios O41.0- ☑
      with premature rupture of membranes (*see also* Pregnancy, complicated by, premature rupture of membranes) O42.- ☑
    onset (spontaneous) of labor after 37 completed weeks of gestation but before 39 completed weeks gestation, with delivery by (planned) cesarean section O75.82
    oophoritis O23.52- ☑
    overdose, drug (*see also* Table of Drugs and Chemicals, by drug, poisoning) O9A.21- ☑ (*following* O99)
    oversize fetus O33.5 ☑
    papyraceous fetus O31.0- ☑
    pelvic inflammatory disease O99.89
    periodontal disease O99.61- ☑
    peripheral neuritis O26.82- ☑
    peritoneal (pelvic) adhesions O99.89
    phlebitis O22.9- ☑
    phlebopathy O22.9- ☑
    phlebothrombosis (superficial) O22.2- ☑
      deep O22.3- ☑
    placenta accreta O43.21- ☑
    placenta increta O43.22- ☑
    placenta percreta O43.23- ☑
    placenta previa O44.0- ☑
      complete O44.0- ☑
        with hemorrhage O44.1- ☑
      marginal O44.2- ☑
        with hemorrhage O44.3- ☑
      partial O44.2- ☑
        with hemorrhage O44.3- ☑
    placental disorder O43.9- ☑
      specified NEC O43.89- ☑
    placental dysfunction O43.89- ☑
    placental infarction O43.81- ☑
    placental insufficiency O36.51- ☑

☑ **Additional Character Required** — Refer to the Tabular List for Character Selection   ▽ **Subterms under main terms may continue to next column or page**

Pregnancy — *continued*
  complicated by — *continued*
    placental transfusion syndromes
      fetomaternal O43.01- ☑
      fetus to fetus O43.02- ☑
      maternofetal O43.01- ☑
    placentitis O41.14- ☑
    pneumonia O99.51- ☑
    poisoning (*see also* Table of Drugs and Chemicals) O9A.21 ☑ (*following* O99)
    polyhydramnios O40- ☑
    polymorphic eruption of pregnancy O26.86
    poor obstetric history NEC O09.29- ☑
    postmaturity (post-term) (40 to 42 weeks) O48.0
      more than 42 completed weeks gestation (prolonged) O48.1
    pre-eclampsia O14.9- ☑
      mild O14.0- ☑
      moderate O14.0- ☑
      severe O14.1- ☑
        with hemolysis, elevated liver enzymes and low platelet count (HELLP) O14.2- ☑
    premature labor — *see* Pregnancy, complicated by, preterm labor
    premature rupture of membranes O42.90
      with onset of labor
        after 24 hours O42.10
          at or after 37 weeks gestation, onset of labor more than 24 hours following rupture O42.12
          pre-term (before 37 completed weeks of gestation) O42.11- ☑
        within 24 hours O42.00
          at or after 37 weeks gestation, onset of labor within 24 hours of rupture O42.02
          pre-term (before 37 completed weeks of gestation) O42.01- ☑
      at or after 37 weeks gestation, unspecified as to length of time between rupture and onset of labor O42.92
      full-term, unspecified as to length of time between rupture and onset of labor O42.92
      pre-term (before 37 completed weeks of gestation) O42.91- ☑
    premature separation of placenta (*see also* Abruptio placentae) O45.9- ☑
    presentation, fetal — *see* Delivery, complicated by, malposition
    preterm delivery O60.10 ☑
    preterm labor
      with delivery O60.10 ☑
        preterm O60.10 ☑
        term O60.20 ☑
      without delivery O60.00
        second trimester O60.02
        third trimester O60.03
      second trimester
        with preterm delivery
          second trimester O60.12 ☑
          third trimester O60.13 ☑
        with term delivery O60.22 ☑
        without delivery O60.02
      third trimester
        with term delivery O60.23 ☑
        with third trimester preterm delivery O60.14 ☑
        without delivery O60.03
    previous history of — *see* Pregnancy, supervision of, high-risk
    prolapse, uterus O34.52- ☑
    proteinuria (gestational) (*see also* Proteinuria, gestational) O12.1- ☑
      with edema O12.2- ☑
    pruritic urticarial papules and plaques of pregnancy (PUPPP) O26.86
    pruritus (neurogenic) O26.89- ☑
    psychosis or psychoneurosis (puerperal) F53
    ptyalism O26.89- ☑
    PUPPP (pruritic urticarial papules and plaques of pregnancy) O26.86
    pyelitis O23.0- ☑
    recurrent pregnancy loss O26.2- ☑
    renal disease or failure NEC O26.83- ☑
      with secondary hypertension, pre-existing — *see* Hypertension, complicating, pregnancy, pre-existing, secondary

Pregnancy — *continued*
  complicated by — *continued*
    renal disease or failure — *continued*
      hypertensive, pre-existing — *see* Hypertension, complicating, pregnancy, pre-existing, with, renal disease
    respiratory condition (conditions in J00-J99) O99.51- ☑
    retained, retention
      dead ovum O02.0
      intrauterine contraceptive device O26.3- ☑
    retroversion, uterus O34.53- ☑
    Rh immunization, incompatibility or sensitization NEC O36.09- ☑
      anti-D antibody O36.01- ☑
    rupture
      amnion (premature) (*see also* Pregnancy, complicated by, premature rupture of membranes) O42- ☑
      membranes (premature) (*see also* Pregnancy, complicated by, premature rupture of membranes) O42- ☑
      uterus (during labor) O71.1
        before onset of labor O71.0- ☑
    salivation (excessive) O26.89- ☑
    salpingitis O23.52- ☑
    salpingo-oophoritis O23.52- ☑
    sepsis (conditions in A40, A41) O98.81- ☑
    size date discrepancy (uterine) O26.84- ☑
    skin condition (conditions in L00-L99) O99.71- ☑
    smoking (tobacco) O99.33- ☑
    social problem O09.7- ☑
    specified condition NEC O26.89- ☑
    spotting O26.85- ☑
    streptococcus group B (GBS) carrier state O99.820
    subluxation of symphysis (pubis) O26.71- ☑
    syphilis (conditions in A50-A53) O98.11- ☑
    threatened
      abortion O20.0
      labor O47.9
        at or after 37 completed weeks of gestation O47.1
        before 37 completed weeks of gestation O47.0- ☑
    thrombophlebitis (superficial) O22.2- ☑
    thrombosis O22.9- ☑
      cerebral venous O22.5- ☑
      cerebrovenous sinus O22.5- ☑
      deep O22.3- ☑
    tobacco use disorder (smoking) O99.33- ☑
    torsion of uterus O34.59- ☑
    toxemia O14.9- ☑
    transverse lie or presentation O32.2 ☑
    tuberculosis (conditions in A15-A19) O98.01- ☑
    tumor (benign)
      cervix O34.4- ☑
      malignant O9A.11- ☑ (*following* O99)
      uterus O34.1- ☑
    unstable lie O32.0 ☑
    upper respiratory infection O99.51- ☑
    uterine size date discrepancy O26.84- ☑
    vaginitis or vulvitis O23.59- ☑
    varicose veins (lower extremities) O22.0- ☑
      genitals O22.1- ☑
      legs O22.0- ☑
      perineal O22.1- ☑
      vaginal or vulval O22.1- ☑
    venereal disease NEC (conditions in A63.8) O98.31- ☑
    venous disorders O22.9- ☑
      specified NEC O22.8X- ☑
    very young mother — *see* Pregnancy, complicated by, young mother
    viral diseases (conditions in A80-B09, B25-B34) O98.51- ☑
    vomiting O21.9
      due to diseases classified elsewhere O21.8
      hyperemesis gravidarum (mild) (*see also* Hyperemesis, gravidarum) O21.0
      late (occurring after 20 weeks of gestation) O21.2
    young mother
      multigravida O09.62- ☑
      primigravida O09.61- ☑
  complicated NOS O26.9- ☑
  concealed O09.3- ☑

Pregnancy — *continued*
  continuing following
    elective fetal reduction of one or more fetus O31.3- ☑
    intrauterine death of one or more fetus O31.2- ☑
    spontaneous abortion of one or more fetus O31.1- ☑
  cornual O00.80
    with intrauterine pregnancy O00.81
  ectopic (ruptured) O00.90
    with intrauterine pregnancy O00.91
    abdominal O00.00
      with
        intrauterine pregnancy O00.01
        viable fetus O36.7- ☑
    cervical O00.80
      with intrauterine pregnancy O00.81
    complicated (by) O08.9
      afibrinogenemia O08.1
      cardiac arrest O08.81
      chemical damage of pelvic organ(s) O08.6
      circulatory collapse O08.3
      defibrination syndrome O08.1
      electrolyte imbalance O08.5
      embolism (amniotic fluid) (blood clot) (pulmonary) (septic) O08.2
      endometritis O08.0
      genital tract and pelvic infection O08.0
      hemorrhage (delayed) (excessive) O08.1
      infection
        genital tract or pelvic O08.0
        kidney O08.83
        urinary tract O08.3
      intravascular coagulation O08.1
      laceration of pelvic organ(s) O08.6
      metabolic disorder O08.5
      oliguria O08.4
      oophoritis O08.0
      parametritis O08.0
      pelvic peritonitis O08.0
      perforation of pelvic organ(s) O08.6
      renal failure or shutdown O08.4
      salpingitis or salpingo-oophoritis O08.0
      sepsis O08.82
      shock O08.83
        septic O08.82
      specified condition NEC O08.89
      tubular necrosis (renal) O08.4
      uremia O08.4
      urinary infection O08.83
      venous complication NEC O08.7
        embolism O08.2
    cornual O00.80
      with intrauterine pregnancy O00.81
    intraligamentous O00.80
      with intrauterine pregnancy O00.81
    mural O00.80
      with intrauterine pregnancy O00.81
    ovarian O00.20- ☑
      with intrauterine pregnancy O00.21- ☑
    specified site NEC O00.80
      with intrauterine pregnancy O00.81
    tubal (ruptured) O00.10- ☑
      with intrauterine pregnancy O00.11- ☑
  examination (normal) Z34.9- ☑
    first Z34.0- ☑
    high-risk — *see* Pregnancy, supervision of, high-risk
    specified Z34.8- ☑
  extrauterine — *see* Pregnancy, ectopic
  fallopian O00.10- ☑
    with intrauterine pregnancy O00.11- ☑
  false F45.8
  gestational carrier Z33.3
  hidden O09.3- ☑
  high-risk — *see* Pregnancy, supervision of, high-risk
  incidental finding Z33.1
  interstitial O00.80
    with intrauterine pregnancy O00.81
  intraligamentous O00.80
    with intrauterine pregnancy O00.81
  intramural O00.80
    with intrauterine pregnancy O00.81
  intraperitoneal O00.00
    with intrauterine pregnancy O00.01
  isthmian O00.10- ☑
    with intrauterine pregnancy O00.11- ☑
  mesometric (mural) O00.80

▽ Subterms under main terms may continue to next column or page   ☑ Additional Character Required — Refer to the Tabular List for Character Selection   261

Pregnancy — Pregnancy

Pregnancy — *continued*
  mesometric — *continued*
    with intrauterine pregnancy O00.81
  molar NEC O02.0
    complicated (by) O08.9
      afibrinogenemia O08.1
      cardiac arrest O08.81
      chemical damage of pelvic organ(s) O08.6
      circulatory collapse O08.3
      defibrination syndrome O08.1
      electrolyte imbalance O08.5
      embolism (amniotic fluid) (blood clot) (pulmonary) (septic) O08.2
      endometritis O08.0
      genital tract and pelvic infection O08.0
      hemorrhage (delayed) (excessive) O08.1
      infection
        genital tract or pelvic O08.0
        kidney O08.83
        urinary tract O08.83
      intravascular coagulation O08.1
      laceration of pelvic organ(s) O08.6
      metabolic disorder O08.5
      oliguria O08.4
      oophoritis O08.0
      parametritis O08.0
      pelvic peritonitis O08.0
      perforation of pelvic organ(s) O08.6
      renal failure or shutdown O08.4
      salpingitis or salpingo-oophoritis O08.0
      sepsis O08.82
      shock O08.3
        septic O08.82
      specified condition NEC O08.89
      tubular necrosis (renal) O08.4
      uremia O08.4
      urinary infection O08.83
      venous complication NEC O08.7
        embolism O08.2
  hydatidiform (*see also* Mole, hydatidiform) O01.9
  multiple (gestation) O30.9- ☑
    greater than quadruplets — *see* Pregnancy, multiple (gestation), specified NEC
    specified NEC O30.80- ☑
      with
        two or more monoamniotic fetuses O30.82- ☑
        two or more monochorionic fetuses O30.81- ☑
      two or more monoamniotic fetuses O30.82- ☑
      two or more monochorionic fetuses O30.81- ☑
      unable to determine number of placenta and number of amniotic sacs O30.89- ☑
      unspecified number of placenta and unspecified number of amniotic sacs O30.80- ☑
  mural O00.80
    with intrauterine pregnancy O00.81
  normal (supervision of) Z34.9- ☑
    first Z34.0- ☑
    high-risk — *see* Pregnancy, supervision of, high-risk
    specified Z34.8- ☑
  ovarian O00.20- ☑
    with intrauterine pregnancy O00.21- ☑
  postmature (40 to 42 weeks) O48.0
    more than 42 weeks gestation O48.1
  post-term (40 to 42 weeks) O48.0
  prenatal care only Z34.9- ☑
    first Z34.0- ☑
    high-risk — *see* Pregnancy, supervision of, high-risk
    specified Z34.8- ☑
  prolonged (more than 42 weeks gestation) O48.1
  quadruplet O30.20- ☑
    with
      two or more monoamniotic fetuses O30.22- ☑
      two or more monochorionic fetuses O30.21- ☑
    two or more monoamniotic fetuses O30.22- ☑
    two or more monochorionic fetuses O30.21- ☑
    unable to determine number of placenta and number of amniotic sacs O30.29- ☑
    unspecified number of placenta and unspecified number of amniotic sacs O30.20- ☑
  quintuplet — *see* Pregnancy, multiple (gestation), specified NEC
  sextuplet — *see* Pregnancy, multiple (gestation), specified NEC

Pregnancy — *continued*
  supervision of
    concealed pregnancy O09.3- ☑
    elderly mother
      multigravida O09.52- ☑
      primigravida O09.51- ☑
    hidden pregnancy O09.3- ☑
    high-risk O09.9- ☑
      due to (history of)
        ectopic pregnancy O09.1- ☑
        elderly — *see* Pregnancy, supervision, elderly mother
        grand multiparity O09.4 ☑
        in utero procedure during previous pregnancy O09.82- ☑
        in vitro fertilization O09.81- ☑
        infertility O09.0- ☑
        insufficient prenatal care O09.3- ☑
        molar pregnancy O09.A- ☑
        multiple previous pregnancies O09.4- ☑
        older mother — *see* Pregnancy, supervision of, elderly mother
        poor reproductive or obstetric history NEC O09.29- ☑
        pre-term labor O09.21- ☑
        previous
          neonatal death O09.29- ☑
        social problems O09.7- ☑
        specified NEC O09.89- ☑
        very young mother — *see* Pregnancy, supervision, young mother
      resulting from in vitro fertilization O09.81- ☑
    normal Z34.9- ☑
      first Z34.0- ☑
      specified NEC Z34.8- ☑
    young mother
      multigravida O09.62- ☑
      primigravida O09.61- ☑
  triplet O30.10- ☑
    with
      two or more monoamniotic fetuses O30.12- ☑
      two or more monochorionic fetuses O30.11- ☑
    two or more monoamniotic fetuses O30.12- ☑
    two or more monochorionic fetuses O30.11- ☑
    unable to determine number of placenta and number of amniotic sacs O30.19- ☑
    unspecified number of placenta and unspecified number of amniotic sacs O30.10- ☑
  tubal (with abortion) (with rupture) O00.10- ☑
    with intrauterine pregnancy O00.11- ☑
  twin O30.00- ☑
    conjoined O30.02- ☑
    dichorionic/diamniotic (two placenta, two amniotic sacs) O30.04- ☑
    monochorionic/diamniotic (one placenta, two amniotic sacs) O30.03- ☑
    monochorionic/monoamniotic (one placenta, one amniotic sac) O30.01- ☑
    unable to determine number of placenta and number of amniotic sacs O30.09- ☑
    unspecified number of placenta and unspecified number of amniotic sacs O30.00- ☑
  unwanted Z64.0
  weeks of gestation
    less than 8 weeks Z3A.01 (*following* Z36)
    8 weeks Z3A.08 (*following* Z36)
    9 weeks Z3A.09 (*following* Z36)
    10 weeks Z3A.10 (*following* Z36)
    11 weeks Z3A.11 (*following* Z36)
    12 weeks Z3A.12 (*following* Z36)
    13 weeks Z3A.13 (*following* Z36)
    14 weeks Z3A.14 (*following* Z36)
    15 weeks Z3A.15 (*following* Z36)
    16 weeks Z3A.16 (*following* Z36)
    17 weeks Z3A.17 (*following* Z36)
    18 weeks Z3A.18 (*following* Z36)
    19 weeks Z3A.19 (*following* Z36)
    20 weeks Z3A.20 (*following* Z36)
    21 weeks Z3A.21 (*following* Z36)
    22 weeks Z3A.22 (*following* Z36)
    23 weeks Z3A.23 (*following* Z36)
    24 weeks Z3A.24 (*following* Z36)
    25 weeks Z3A.25 (*following* Z36)
    26 weeks Z3A.26 (*following* Z36)
    27 weeks Z3A.27 (*following* Z36)
    28 weeks Z3A.28 (*following* Z36)
    29 weeks Z3A.29 (*following* Z36)

Pregnancy — *continued*
  weeks of gestation — *continued*
    30 weeks Z3A.30 (*following* Z36)
    31 weeks Z3A.31 (*following* Z36)
    32 weeks Z3A.32 (*following* Z36)
    33 weeks Z3A.33 (*following* Z36)
    34 weeks Z3A.34 (*following* Z36)
    35 weeks Z3A.35 (*following* Z36)
    36 weeks Z3A.36 (*following* Z36)
    37 weeks Z3A.37 (*following* Z36)
    38 weeks Z3A.38 (*following* Z36)
    39 weeks Z3A.39 (*following* Z36)
    40 weeks Z3A.40 (*following* Z36)
    41 weeks Z3A.41 (*following* Z36)
    42 weeks Z3A.42 (*following* Z36)
    greater than 42 weeks Z3A.49 (*following* Z36)
    not specified Z3A.00 (*following* Z36)
Preiser's disease — *see* Osteonecrosis, secondary, due to, trauma, metacarpus
Pre-kwashiorkor — *see* Malnutrition, severe
Preleukemia (syndrome) D46.9
Preluxation, hip, congenital Q65.6
Premature (*see also* condition)
  adrenarche E27.0
  aging E34.8
  beats I49.40
    atrial I49.1
    auricular I49.1
    supraventricular I49.1
  birth NEC — *see* Preterm, newborn
  closure, foramen ovale Q21.8
  contraction
    atrial I49.1
    atrioventricular I49.2
    auricular I49.1
    auriculoventricular I49.49
    heart (extrasystole) I49.49
    junctional I49.2
    ventricular I49.3
  delivery (*see also* Pregnancy, complicated by, preterm labor) O60.10 ☑
  ejaculation F52.4
  infant NEC — *see* Preterm, newborn
    light-for-dates — *see* Light for dates
  labor — *see* Pregnancy, complicated by, preterm labor
  lungs P28.0
  menopause E28.319
    asymptomatic E28.319
    symptomatic E28.310
  newborn
    less than 37 completed weeks — *see* Preterm, newborn
    extreme (less than 28 completed weeks) — *see* Immaturity, extreme
  puberty E30.1
  rupture membranes or amnion — *see* Pregnancy, complicated by, premature rupture of membranes
  senility E34.8
  thelarche E30.8
  ventricular systole I49.3
Prematurity NEC (less than 37 completed weeks) — *see* Preterm, newborn
  extreme (less than 28 completed weeks) — *see* Immaturity, extreme
Premenstrual
  dysphoric disorder (PMDD) F32.81
  tension (syndrome) N94.3
Premolarization, cuspids K00.2
Prenatal
  care, normal pregnancy — *see* Pregnancy, normal
  screening of mother (*see also* Encounter, antenatal screening) Z36.9
  teeth K00.6
Preparatory care for subsequent treatment NEC
  for dialysis Z49.01
    peritoneal Z49.02
Prepartum — *see* condition
Preponderance, left or right ventricular I51.7
Prepuce — *see* condition
PRES (posterior reversible encephalopathy syndrome) I67.83
Presbycardia R54
Presbycusis, presbyacusia H91.1- ☑
Presbyesophagus K22.8
Presbyophrenia F03 ☑
Presbyopia H52.4
Prescription of contraceptives (initial) Z30.019

Prescription of contraceptives — *continued*
  barrier Z30.018
  diaphragm Z30.018
  emergency (postcoital) Z30.012
  implantable subdermal Z30.017
  injectable Z30.013
  intrauterine contraceptive device Z30.014
  pills Z30.011
  postcoital (emergency) Z30.012
  repeat Z30.40
    barrier Z30.49
    diaphragm Z30.49
    implantable subdermal Z30.46
    injectable Z30.42
    pills Z30.41
    specified type NEC Z30.49
    transdermal patch hormonal Z30.45
    vaginal ring hormonal Z30.44
  specified type NEC Z30.018
    transdermal patch hormonal Z30.016
    vaginal ring hormonal Z30.015
Presence (of)
  ankle-joint implant (functional) (prosthesis) Z96.66- ☑
  aortocoronary (bypass) graft Z95.1
  arterial-venous shunt (dialysis) Z99.2
  artificial
    eye (globe) Z97.0
    heart (fully implantable) (mechanical) Z95.812
      valve Z95.2
    larynx Z96.3
    lens (intraocular) Z96.1
    limb (complete) (partial) Z97.1- ☑
      arm Z97.1- ☑
        bilateral Z97.15
      leg Z97.1- ☑
        bilateral Z97.16
  audiological implant (functional) Z96.29
  bladder implant (functional) Z96.0
  bone
    conduction hearing device Z96.29
    implant (functional) NEC Z96.7
    joint (prosthesis) — *see* Presence, joint implant
  cardiac
    defibrillator (functional) (with synchronous cardiac pacemaker) Z95.810
    implant or graft Z95.9
      specified type NEC Z95.818
    pacemaker Z95.0
    resynchronization therapy
      defibrillator Z95.810
      pacemaker Z95.0
  cardioverter-defibrillator (ICD) Z95.810
  cerebrospinal fluid drainage device Z98.2
  cochlear implant (functional) Z96.21
  contact lens (es) Z97.3
  coronary artery graft or prosthesis Z95.5
  CRT-D (cardiac resynchronization therapy defibrillator) Z95.810
  CRT-P (cardiac resynchronization therapy pacemaker) Z95.0
  CSF shunt Z98.2
  dental prosthesis device Z97.2
  dentures Z97.2
  device (external) NEC Z97.8
    cardiac NEC Z95.818
    heart assist Z95.811
    implanted (functional) Z96.9
      specified NEC Z96.89
    prosthetic Z97.8
  ear implant Z96.20
    cochlear implant Z96.21
    myringotomy tube Z96.22
    specified type NEC Z96.29
  elbow-joint implant (functional) (prosthesis) Z96.62- ☑
  endocrine implant (functional) NEC Z96.49
  eustachian tube stent or device (functional) Z96.29
  external hearing-aid or device Z97.4
  finger-joint implant (functional) (prosthetic) Z96.69- ☑
  functional implant Z96.9
    specified NEC Z96.89
  graft
    cardiac NEC Z95.818
    vascular NEC Z95.828
  hearing-aid or device (external) Z97.4
    implant (bone) (cochlear) (functional) Z96.21
  heart assist device Z95.811
  heart valve implant (functional) Z95.2

Presence — *continued*
  heart valve implant — *continued*
    prosthetic Z95.2
    specified type NEC Z95.4
    xenogenic Z95.3
  hip-joint implant (functional) (prosthesis) Z96.64- ☑
  ICD (cardioverter-defibrillator) Z95.810
  implanted device (artificial) (functional) (prosthetic) Z96.9
    automatic cardiac defibrillator (with synchronous cardiac pacemaker) Z95.810
    cardiac pacemaker Z95.0
    cochlear Z96.21
    dental Z96.5
    heart Z95.812
    heart valve Z95.2
      prosthetic Z95.2
      specified NEC Z95.4
      xenogenic Z95.3
    insulin pump Z96.41
    intraocular lens Z96.1
    joint Z96.60
      ankle Z96.66- ☑
      elbow Z96.62- ☑
      finger Z96.69- ☑
      hip Z96.64- ☑
      knee Z96.65- ☑
      shoulder Z96.61- ☑
      specified NEC Z96.698
      wrist Z96.63- ☑
    larynx Z96.3
    myringotomy tube Z96.22
    otological Z96.20
      cochlear Z96.21
      eustachian stent Z96.29
      myringotomy Z96.22
      specified NEC Z96.29
      stapes Z96.29
    skin Z96.81
    skull plate Z96.7
    specified NEC Z96.89
    urogenital Z96.0
  insulin pump (functional) Z96.41
  intestinal bypass or anastomosis Z98.0
  intraocular lens (functional) Z96.1
  intrauterine contraceptive device (IUD) Z97.5
  intravascular implant (functional) (prosthetic) NEC Z95.9
    coronary artery Z95.5
    defibrillator (with synchronous cardiac pacemaker) Z95.810
    peripheral vessel (with angioplasty) Z95.820
  joint implant (prosthetic) (any) Z96.60
    ankle — *see* Presence, ankle joint implant
    elbow — *see* Presence, elbow joint implant
    finger — *see* Presence, finger joint implant
    hip — *see* Presence, hip joint implant
    knee — *see* Presence, knee joint implant
    shoulder — *see* Presence, shoulder joint implant
    specified joint NEC Z96.698
    wrist — *see* Presence, wrist joint implant
  knee-joint implant (functional) (prosthesis) Z96.65- ☑
  laryngeal implant (functional) Z96.3
  mandibular implant (dental) Z96.5
  myringotomy tube(s) Z96.22
  orthopedic-joint implant (prosthetic) (any) — *see* Presence, joint implant
  otological implant (functional) Z96.29
  shoulder-joint implant (functional) (prosthesis) Z96.61- ☑
  skull-plate implant Z96.7
  spectacles Z97.3
  stapes implant (functional) Z96.29
  systemic lupus erythematosus [SLE] inhibitor D68.62
  tendon implant (functional) (graft) Z96.7
  tooth root(s) implant Z96.5
  ureteral stent Z96.0
  urethral stent Z96.0
  urogenital implant (functional) Z96.0
  vascular implant or device Z95.9
    access port device Z95.828
    specified type NEC Z95.828
  wrist-joint implant (functional) (prosthesis) Z96.63- ☑
Presenile (*see also* condition)
  dementia F03
  premature aging E34.8
Presentation, fetal — *see* Delivery, complicated by, malposition

Prespondylolisthesis (congenital) Q76.2
Pressure
  area, skin — *see* Ulcer, pressure, by site
  brachial plexus G54.0
  brain G93.5
    injury at birth NEC P11.1
    cerebral — *see* Pressure, brain
  chest R07.89
  cone, tentorial G93.5
  hyposystolic (*see also* Hypotension)
    incidental reading, without diagnosis of hypotension R03.1
  increased
    intracranial (benign) G93.2
      injury at birth P11.0
    intraocular H40.05- ☑
  lumbosacral plexus G54.1
  mediastinum J98.59
  necrosis (chronic) — *see* Ulcer, pressure, by site
  parental, inappropriate (excessive) Z62.6
  sore (chronic) — *see* Ulcer, pressure, by site
  spinal cord G95.20
  ulcer (chronic) — *see* Ulcer, pressure, by site
  venous, increased I87.8
Pre-syncope R55
Preterm
  delivery (*see also* Pregnancy, complicated by, preterm labor) O60.10 ☑
  labor — *see* Pregnancy, complicated by, preterm labor
  newborn (infant) P07.30
    gestational age
      28 completed weeks (28 weeks, 0 days through 28 weeks, 6 days) P07.31
      29 completed weeks (29 weeks, 0 days through 29 weeks, 6 days) P07.32
      30 completed weeks (30 weeks, 0 days through 30 weeks, 6 days) P07.33
      31 completed weeks (31 weeks, 0 days through 31 weeks, 6 days) P07.34
      32 completed weeks (32 weeks, 0 days through 32 weeks, 6 days) P07.35
      33 completed weeks (33 weeks, 0 days through 33 weeks, 6 days) P07.36
      34 completed weeks (34 weeks, 0 days through 34 weeks, 6 days) P07.37
      35 completed weeks (35 weeks, 0 days through 35 weeks, 6 days) P07.38
      36 completed weeks (36 weeks, 0 days through 36 weeks, 6 days) P07.39
Previa
  placenta (total) (without hemorrhage) O44.0- ☑
    with hemorrhage O44.1- ☑
    complete O44.0- ☑
      with hemorrhage O44.1- ☑
    low (*see also* Delivery, complicated, by, placenta, low) O44.4- ☑
      with hemorrhage O44.5- ☑
    marginal O44.2- ☑
      with hemorrhage O44.3- ☑
    partial O44.2- ☑
      with hemorrhage O44.3- ☑
  vasa O69.4 ☑
Priapism N48.30
  due to
    disease classified elsewhere N48.32
    drug N48.33
    specified cause NEC N48.39
    trauma N48.31
Prickling sensation (skin) R20.2
Prickly heat L74.0
Primary — *see* condition
Primigravida
  elderly, affecting management of pregnancy, labor and delivery (supervision only) — *see* Pregnancy, complicated by, elderly, primigravida
  older, affecting management of pregnancy, labor and delivery (supervision only) — *see* Pregnancy, complicated by, elderly, primigravida
  very young, affecting management of pregnancy, labor and delivery (supervision only) — *see* Pregnancy, complicated by, young mother, primigravida
Primipara
  elderly, affecting management of pregnancy, labor and delivery (supervision only) — *see* Pregnancy, complicated by, elderly, primigravida

Primipara — continued
- older, affecting management of pregnancy, labor and delivery (supervision only) — see Pregnancy, complicated by, elderly, primigravida
- very young, affecting management of pregnancy, labor and delivery (supervision only) — see Pregnancy, complicated by, young mother, primigravida

Primus varus (bilateral) Q66.2 ☑
PRIND (Prolonged reversible ischemic neurologic deficit) I63.9
Pringle's disease (tuberous sclerosis) Q85.1
Prinzmetal angina I20.1
Prizefighter ear — see Cauliflower ear
Problem (with) (related to)
- academic Z55.8
- acculturation Z60.3
- adjustment (to)
  - change of job Z56.1
  - life-cycle transition Z60.0
  - pension Z60.0
  - retirement Z60.0
- adopted child Z62.821
- alcoholism in family Z63.72
- atypical parenting situation Z62.9
- bankruptcy Z59.8
- behavioral (adult) F69
  - drug seeking Z76.5
- birth of sibling affecting child Z62.898
- care (of)
  - provider dependency Z74.9
    - specified NEC Z74.8
  - sick or handicapped person in family or household Z63.6
- child
  - abuse (affecting the child) — see Maltreatment, child
  - custody or support proceedings Z65.3
  - in care of non-parental family member Z62.21
  - in foster care Z62.21
  - in welfare custody Z62.21
  - living in orphanage or group home Z62.22
- child-rearing Z62.9
  - specified NEC Z62.898
- communication (developmental) F80.9
- conflict or discord (with)
  - boss Z56.4
  - classmates Z55.4
  - counselor Z64.4
  - employer Z56.4
  - family Z63.9
    - specified NEC Z63.8
  - probation officer Z64.4
  - social worker Z64.4
  - teachers Z55.4
  - workmates Z56.4
- conviction in legal proceedings Z65.0
  - with imprisonment Z65.1
- counselor Z64.4
- creditors Z59.8
- digestive K92.9
- drug addict in family Z63.72
- ear — see Disorder, ear
- economic Z59.9
  - affecting care Z59.9
  - specified NEC Z59.8
- education Z55.9
  - specified NEC Z55.8
- employment Z56.9
  - change of job Z56.1
  - discord Z56.4
  - environment Z56.5
  - sexual harassment Z56.81
  - specified NEC Z56.89
  - stressful schedule Z56.3
  - stress NEC Z56.6
  - threat of job loss Z56.2
  - unemployment Z56.0
- enuresis, child F98.0
- eye H57.9
- failed examinations (school) Z55.2
- falling Z91.81
- family (see also Disruption, family) Z63.9
  - specified NEC Z63.8
- feeding (elderly) (infant) R63.3
  - newborn P92.9
    - breast P92.5
    - overfeeding P92.4
    - slow P92.2

Problem — continued
- feeding — continued
  - newborn — continued
    - specified NEC P92.8
    - underfeeding P92.3
  - nonorganic F50.89
- finance Z59.9
  - specified NEC Z59.8
- foreclosure on loan Z59.8
- foster child Z62.822
- frightening experience(s) in childhood Z62.898
- genital NEC
  - female N94.9
  - male N50.9
- health care Z75.9
  - specified NEC Z75.8
- hearing — see Deafness
- homelessness Z59.0
- housing Z59.9
  - inadequate Z59.1
  - isolated Z59.8
  - specified NEC Z59.8
- identity (of childhood) F93.8
- illegitimate pregnancy (unwanted) Z64.0
- illiteracy Z55.0
- impaired mobility Z74.09
- imprisonment or incarceration Z65.1
- inadequate teaching affecting education Z55.8
- inappropriate (excessive) parental pressure Z62.6
- influencing health status NEC Z78.9
- in-law Z63.1
- institutionalization, affecting child Z62.22
- intrafamilial communication Z63.8
- jealousy, child F93.8
- landlord Z59.2
- language (developmental) F80.9
- learning (developmental) F81.9
- legal Z65.3
  - conviction without imprisonment Z65.0
  - imprisonment Z65.1
  - release from prison Z65.2
- life-management Z73.9
  - specified NEC Z73.89
- life-style Z72.9
  - gambling Z72.6
  - high-risk sexual behavior (heterosexual) Z72.51
    - bisexual Z72.53
    - homosexual Z72.52
  - inappropriate eating habits Z72.4
  - self-damaging behavior NEC Z72.89
  - specified NEC Z72.89
  - tobacco use Z72.0
- literacy Z55.9
  - low level Z55.0
  - specified NEC Z55.8
- living alone Z60.2
- lodgers Z59.2
- loss of love relationship in childhood Z62.898
- marital Z63.0
  - involving
    - divorce Z63.5
    - estrangement Z63.5
    - gender identity F66
- mastication K08.89
- medical
  - care, within family Z63.6
  - facilities Z75.9
    - specified NEC Z75.8
- mental F48.9
- multiparity Z64.1
- negative life events in childhood Z62.9
  - altered pattern of family relationships Z62.898
  - frightening experience Z62.898
  - loss of
    - love relationship Z62.898
    - self-esteem Z62.898
  - physical abuse (alleged) — see Maltreatment, child
  - removal from home Z62.29
  - specified event NEC Z62.898
- neighbor Z59.2
- neurological NEC R29.818
- new step-parent affecting child Z62.898
- none (feared complaint unfounded) Z71.1
- occupational NEC Z56.89
- parent-child — see Conflict, parent-child
- personal hygiene Z91.89
- personality F69
- phase-of-life transition, adjustment Z60.0

Problem — continued
- presence of sick or disabled person in family or household Z63.79
  - needing care Z63.6
- primary support group (family) Z63.9
  - specified NEC Z63.8
- probation officer Z64.4
- psychiatric F99
- psychosexual (development) F66
- psychosocial Z65.9
  - religious or spiritual Z65.8
  - specified NEC Z65.8
- relationship Z63.9
  - childhood F93.8
- release from prison Z65.2
  - religious or spiritual Z65.8
- removal from home affecting child Z62.29
- seeking and accepting known hazardous and harmful behavioral or psychological interventions Z65.8
  - chemical, nutritional or physical interventions Z65.8
- sexual function (nonorganic) F52.9
- sight H54.7
- sleep disorder, child F51.9
- smell — see Disturbance, sensation, smell
- social
  - environment Z60.9
    - specified NEC Z60.8
  - exclusion and rejection Z60.4
  - worker Z64.4
- speech R47.9
  - developmental F80.9
  - specified NEC R47.89
- swallowing — see Dysphagia
- taste — see Disturbance, sensation, taste
- tic, child F95.0
- underachievement in school Z55.3
- unemployment Z56.0
  - threatened Z56.2
- unwanted pregnancy Z64.0
- upbringing Z62.9
  - specified NEC Z62.898
- urinary N39.9
- voice production R47.89
- work schedule (stressful) Z56.3

Procedure (surgical)
- converted
  - arthroscopic to open Z53.33
  - laparoscopic to open Z53.31
  - specified procedure NEC to open Z53.39
  - thoracoscopic to open Z53.32
- for purpose other than remedying health state Z41.9
  - specified NEC Z41.8
- not done Z53.9
  - because of
    - administrative reasons Z53.8
    - contraindication Z53.09
      - smoking Z53.01
    - patient's decision Z53.20
      - for reasons of belief or group pressure Z53.1
      - left against medical advice (AMA) Z53.21
      - specified reason NEC Z53.29
    - specified reason NEC Z53.8

Procidentia (uteri) N81.3
Proctalgia K62.89
- fugax K59.4
- spasmodic K59.4
Proctitis K62.89
- amebic (acute) A06.0
- chlamydial A56.3
- gonococcal A54.6
- granulomatous — see Enteritis, regional, large intestine
- herpetic A60.1
- radiation K62.7
- tuberculous A18.32
- ulcerative (chronic) K51.20
  - with
    - complication K51.219
      - abscess K51.214
      - fistula K51.213
      - obstruction K51.212
      - rectal bleeding K51.211
      - specified NEC K51.218
Proctocele
- female (without uterine prolapse) N81.6
  - with uterine prolapse N81.2
    - complete N81.3
- male K62.3

☑ Additional Character Required — Refer to the Tabular List for Character Selection   ▽ Subterms under main terms may continue to next column or page

Proctocolitis
  food protein-induced K52.82
  food-induced eosinophilic K52.82
  milk protein-induced K52.82
  mucosal — see Rectosigmoiditis, ulcerative
Proctoptosis K62.3
Proctorrhagia K62.5
Proctosigmoiditis K63.89
  ulcerative (chronic) — see Rectosigmoiditis, ulcerative
Proctospasm K59.4
  psychogenic F45.8
Profichet's disease — see Disorder, soft tissue, specified
    type NEC
Progeria E34.8
Prognathism (mandibular) (maxillary) M26.19
Progonoma (melanotic) — see Neoplasm, benign, by
    site
Progressive — see condition
Prolactinoma
  specified site — see Neoplasm, benign, by site
  unspecified site D35.2
Prolapse, prolapsed
  anus, anal (canal) (sphincter) K62.2
  arm or hand O32.2 ☑
    causing obstructed labor O64.4 ☑
  bladder (mucosa) (sphincter) (acquired)
    congenital Q79.4
    female — see Cystocele
    male N32.89
  breast implant (prosthetic) T85.49 ☑
  cecostomy K94.09
  cecum K63.4
  cervix, cervical (hypertrophied) N81.2
    anterior lip, obstructing labor O65.5
    congenital Q51.828
    postpartal, old N81.2
    stump N81.85
  ciliary body (traumatic) — see Laceration, eye(ball),
    with prolapse or loss of interocular tissue
  colon (pedunculated) K63.4
  colostomy K94.09
  disc (intervertebral) — see Displacement, interverte-
    bral disc
  eye implant (orbital) T85.398 ☑
    lens (ocular) — see Complications, intraocular lens
  fallopian tube N83.4- ☑
  gastric (mucosa) K31.89
  genital, female N81.9
    specified NEC N81.89
  globe, nontraumatic — see Luxation, globe
  ileostomy bud K94.19
  intervertebral disc — see Displacement, intervertebral
    disc
  intestine (small) K63.4
  iris (traumatic) — see Laceration, eye(ball), with pro-
    lapse or loss of interocular tissue
    nontraumatic H21.89
  kidney N28.83
    congenital Q63.2
  laryngeal muscles or ventricle J38.7
  liver K76.89
  meatus urinarius N36.8
  mitral (valve) I34.1
  ocular lens implant — see Complications, intraocular
    lens
  organ or site, congenital NEC — see Malposition,
    congenital
  ovary N83.4- ☑
  pelvic floor, female N81.89
  perineum, female N81.89
  rectum (mucosa) (sphincter) K62.3
    due to trichuris trichuria B79
  spleen D73.89
  stomach K31.89
  umbilical cord
    complicating delivery O69.0 ☑
  urachus, congenital Q64.4
  ureter N28.89
    with obstruction N13.5
      with infection N13.6
  ureterovesical orifice N28.89
  urethra (acquired) (infected) (mucosa) N36.8
    congenital Q64.71
  urinary meatus N36.8
    congenital Q64.72
  uterovaginal N81.4
    complete N81.3
    incomplete N81.2

Prolapse, prolapsed — continued
  uterus (with prolapse of vagina) N81.4
    complete N81.3
    congenital Q51.818
    first degree N81.2
    in pregnancy or childbirth — see Pregnancy,
      complicated by, abnormal, uterus
    incomplete N81.2
    postpartal (old) N81.4
    second degree N81.2
    third degree N81.3
  uveal (traumatic) — see Laceration, eye(ball), with
    prolapse or loss of interocular tissue
  vagina (anterior) (wall) — see Cystocele
    with prolapse of uterus N81.4
      complete N81.3
      incomplete N81.2
    posterior wall N81.6
    posthysterectomy N99.3
  vitreous (humor) H43.0- ☑
    in wound — see Laceration, eye(ball), with pro-
      lapse or loss of interocular tissue
  womb — see Prolapse, uterus
Prolapsus, female N81.9
  specified NEC N81.89
Proliferation(s)
  primary cutaneous CD30-positive large T-cell C86.6
  prostate, atypical small acinar N42.32
Proliferative — see condition
Prolonged, prolongation (of)
  bleeding (time) (idiopathic) R79.1
  coagulation (time) R79.1
  gestation (over 42 completed weeks)
    mother O48.1
    newborn P08.22
  interval I44.0
  labor O63.9
    first stage O63.0
    second stage O63.1
  partial thromboplastin time (PTT) R79.1
  pregnancy (more than 42 weeks gestation) O48.1
  prothrombin time R79.1
  QT interval I45.81
  uterine contractions in labor O62.4
Prominence, prominent
  auricle (congenital) (ear) Q17.5
  ischial spine or sacral promontory
    with disproportion (fetopelvic) O33.0
      causing obstructed labor O65.0
  nose (congenital) acquired M95.0
Promiscuity — see High, risk, sexual behavior
Pronation
  ankle — see Deformity, limb, foot, specified NEC
  foot (see also Deformity, limb, foot, specified NEC)
    congenital Q74.2
Prophylactic
  administration of
    antibiotics, long-term Z79.2
      short-term use — omit code
    drug (see also Long-term (current) drug therapy
      (use of)) Z79.899
  medication Z79.899
  organ removal (for neoplasia management) Z40.00
    breast Z40.01
    fallopian tube(s) Z40.03
      with ovary(s) Z40.02
    ovary(s) Z40.02
    specified site NEC Z40.09
  surgery Z40.9
    for risk factors related to malignant neoplasm —
      see Prophylactic, organ removal
    specified NEC Z40.8
  vaccination Z23
Propionic acidemia E71.121
Proptosis (ocular) (see also Exophthalmos)
  thyroid — see Hyperthyroidism, with goiter
Prosecution, anxiety concerning Z65.3
Prosopagnosia R48.3
Prostadynia N42.81
Prostate, prostatic — see condition
Prostatism — see Hyperplasia, prostate
Prostatitis (congestive) (suppurative) (with cystitis) N41.9
  acute N41.0
  cavitary N41.8
  chronic N41.1
  diverticular N41.8
  due to Trichomonas (vaginalis) A59.02
  fibrous N41.1

Prostatitis — continued
  gonococcal (acute) (chronic) A54.22
  granulomatous N41.4
  hypertrophic N41.1
  subacute N41.1
  trichomonal A59.02
  tuberculous A18.14
Prostatocystitis N41.3
Prostatorrhea N42.89
Prostatosis N42.82
Prostration R53.83
  heat (see also Heat, exhaustion)
    anhydrotic T67.3 ☑
    due to
      salt (and water) depletion T67.4 ☑
      water depletion T67.3 ☑
  nervous F48.8
  senile R54
Protanomaly (anomalous trichromat) H53.54
Protanopia (complete) (incomplete) H53.54
Protection (against) (from) — see Prophylactic
Protein
  deficiency NEC — see Malnutrition
  malnutrition — see Malnutrition
  sickness (see also Reaction, serum) T80.69 ☑
Proteinemia R77.9
Proteinosis
  alveolar (pulmonary) J84.01
  lipid or lipoid (of Urbach) E78.89
Proteinuria R80.9
  Bence Jones R80.3
  complicating pregnancy — see Proteinuria, gestational
  gestational
    complicating
      childbirth O12.14
      pregnancy O12.1- ☑
        with edema O12.2- ☑
      puerperium O12.15
  idiopathic R80.0
  isolated R80.0
    with glomerular lesion N06.9
      dense deposit disease N06.6
      diffuse
        crescentic glomerulonephritis N06.7
        endocapillary proliferative glomerulonephri-
          tis N06.4
        mesangiocapillary glomerulonephritis N06.5
      focal and segmental hyalinosis or sclerosis
        N06.1
      membranous (diffuse) N06.2
      mesangial proliferative (diffuse) N06.3
      minimal change N06.0
      specified pathology NEC N06.8
  orthostatic R80.2
    with glomerular lesion — see Proteinuria, isolated,
      with glomerular lesion
  persistent R80.1
    with glomerular lesion — see Proteinuria, isolated,
      with glomerular lesion
  postural R80.2
    with glomerular lesion — see Proteinuria, isolated,
      with glomerular lesion
  pre-eclamptic — see Pre-eclampsia
  puerperal O12.15
  specified type NEC R80.8
Proteolysis, pathologic D65
Proteus (mirabilis) (morganii), **as cause of disease
    classified elsewhere** B96.4
Prothrombin gene mutation D68.52
Protoporphyria, erythropoietic E80.0
Protozoal (see also condition)
  disease B64
    specified NEC B60.8
Protrusion, protrusio
  acetabuli M24.7
  acetabulum (into pelvis) M24.7
  device, implant or graft (see also Complications, by
    site and type, mechanical) T85.698 ☑
    arterial graft NEC — see Complication, cardiovas-
      cular device, mechanical, vascular
    breast (implant) T85.49 ☑
    catheter NEC T85.698 ☑
      cystostomy T83.090 ☑
      dialysis (renal) T82.49 ☑
        intraperitoneal T85.691 ☑
      infusion NEC T82.594 ☑
        spinal (epidural) (subdural) T85.690 ☑

Protrusion, protrusio — *continued*
 device, implant or graft (*see also* Complications, by site and type, mechanical) — *continued*
  catheter — *continued*
   urinary (*see also* Complications, catheter, urinary) T83.098 ☑
   electronic (electrode) (pulse generator) (stimulator)
    bone T84.390 ☑
    nervous system — *see* Complication, prosthetic device, mechanical, electronic nervous system stimulator
  fixation, internal (orthopedic) NEC — *see* Complication, fixation device, mechanical
  gastrointestinal — *see* Complications, prosthetic device, mechanical, gastrointestinal device
  genital NEC T83.498 ☑
   intrauterine contraceptive device T83.39 ☑
   penile prosthesis (cylinder) (implanted) (pump) (resevoir) T83.490 ☑
   testicular prosthesis T83.491 ☑
  heart NEC — *see* Complication, cardiovascular device, mechanical
  joint prosthesis — *see* Complications, joint prosthesis, mechanical, specified NEC, by site
  ocular NEC — *see* Complications, prosthetic device, mechanical, ocular device
  orthopedic NEC — *see* Complication, orthopedic, device, mechanical
  specified NEC T85.628 ☑
  urinary NEC (*see also* Complication, genitourinary, device, urinary, mechanical)
   graft T83.29 ☑
  vascular NEC — *see* Complication, cardiovascular device, mechanical
  ventricular intracranial shunt T85.09 ☑
 intervertebral disc — *see* Displacement, intervertebral disc
 joint prosthesis — *see* Complications, joint prosthesis, mechanical, specified NEC, by site
 nucleus pulposus — *see* Displacement, intervertebral disc
Prune belly (syndrome) Q79.4
Prurigo (ferox) (gravis) (Hebrae) (Hebra's) (mitis) (simplex) L28.2
 Besnier's L20.0
 estivalis L56.4
 nodularis L28.1
 psychogenic F45.8
Pruritus, pruritic (essential) L29.9
 ani, anus L29.0
  psychogenic F45.8
 anogenital L29.3
  psychogenic F45.8
 due to onchocerca volvulus B73.1
 gravidarum — *see* Pregnancy, complicated by, specified pregnancy-related condition NEC
 hiemalis L29.8
 neurogenic (any site) F45.8
 perianal L29.0
 psychogenic (any site) F45.8
 scroti, scrotum L29.1
  psychogenic F45.8
 senile, senilis L29.8
 specified NEC L29.8
  psychogenic F45.8
 Trichomonas A59.9
 vulva, vulvae L29.2
  psychogenic F45.8
Pseudarthrosis, pseudoarthrosis (bone) — *see* Nonunion, fracture
 clavicle, congenital Q74.0
 joint, following fusion or arthrodesis M96.0
Pseudoaneurysm — *see* Aneurysm
Pseudoangina (pectoris) — *see* Angina
Pseudoangioma I81
Pseudoarteriosus Q28.8
Pseudoarthrosis — *see* Pseudarthrosis
Pseudobulbar affect (PBA) F48.2
Pseudochromhidrosis L67.8
Pseudocirrhosis, liver, pericardial I31.1
Pseudocowpox B08.03
Pseudocoxalgia M91.3- ☑
Pseudocroup J38.5
Pseudo-Cushing's syndrome, alcohol-induced E24.4
Pseudocyesis F45.8
Pseudocyst
 lung J98.4

Pseudocyst — *continued*
 pancreas K86.3
 retina — *see* Cyst, retina
Pseudoelephantiasis neuroarthritica Q82.0
Pseudoexfoliation, capsule (lens) — *see* Cataract, specified NEC
Pseudofolliculitis barbae L73.1
Pseudoglioma H44.89
Pseudohemophilia (Bernuth's) (hereditary) (type B) D68.0
 Type A D69.8
 vascular D69.8
Pseudohermaphroditism Q56.3
 adrenal E25.8
 female Q56.2
  with adrenocortical disorder E25.8
  without adrenocortical disorder Q56.2
  adrenal (congenital) E25.0
  unspecified E25.9
 male Q56.1
  with
   5-alpha-reductase deficiency E29.1
   adrenocortical disorder E25.8
   androgen resistance E34.51
   cleft scrotum Q56.1
   feminizing testis E34.51
  without gonadal disorder Q56.1
  adrenal E25.8
  unspecified E25.9
Pseudo-Hurler's polydystrophy E77.0
Pseudohydrocephalus G93.2
Pseudohypertrophic muscular dystrophy (Erb's) G71.0
Pseudohypertrophy, muscle G71.0
Pseudohypoparathyroidism E20.1
Pseudoinsomnia F51.03
Pseudoleukemia, infantile D64.89
Pseudomembranous — *see* condition
Pseudomeningocele (cerebral) (infective) (post-traumatic) G96.19
 postprocedural (spinal) G97.82
Pseudomenses (newborn) P54.6
Pseudomenstruation (newborn) P54.6
Pseudomonas
 aeruginosa, as cause of disease classified elsewhere B96.5
 mallei infection A24.0
  as cause of disease classified elsewhere B96.5
 pseudomallei, as cause of disease classified elsewhere B96.5
Pseudomyotonia G71.19
Pseudomyxoma peritonei C78.6
Pseudoneuritis, optic (nerve) (disc) (papilla), **congenital** Q14.2
Pseudo-obstruction intestine (acute) (chronic) (idiopathic) (intermittent secondary) (primary) K59.8
Pseudopapilledema H47.33- ☑
 congenital Q14.2
Pseudoparalysis
 arm or leg R29.818
 atonic, congenital P94.2
Pseudopelade L66.0
Pseudophakia Z96.1
Pseudopolyarthritis, rhizomelic M35.3
Pseudopolycythemia D75.1
Pseudopseudohypoparathyroidism E20.1
Pseudopterygium H11.81- ☑
Pseudoptosis (eyelid) — *see* Blepharochalasis
Pseudopuberty, precocious
 female heterosexual E25.8
 male isosexual E25.8
Pseudorickets (renal) N25.0
Pseudorubella B08.20
Pseudosclerema, newborn P83.88
Pseudosclerosis (brain)
 Jakob's — *see* Creutzfeldt-Jakob disease or syndrome of Westphal (Strümpell) E83.01
 spastic — *see* Creutzfeldt-Jakob disease or syndrome
Pseudotetanus — *see* Convulsions
Pseudotetany R29.0
 hysterical F44.5
Pseudotruncus arteriosus Q25.49
Pseudotuberculosis A28.2
 enterocolitis A04.8
 pasteurella (infection) A28.0
Pseudotumor
 cerebri G93.2
 orbital H05.11 ☑

Pseudoxanthoma elasticum Q82.8
Psilosis (sprue) (tropical) K90.1
 nontropical K90.0
Psittacosis A70
Psoitis M60.88
Psoriasis L40.9
 arthropathic L40.50
  arthritis mutilans L40.52
  distal interphalangeal L40.51
  juvenile L40.54
  other specified L40.59
  spondylitis L40.53
 buccal K13.29
 flexural L40.8
 guttate L40.4
 mouth K13.29
 nummular L40.0
 plaque L40.0
 psychogenic F54
 pustular (generalized) L40.1
  palmaris et plantaris L40.3
 specified NEC L40.8
 vulgaris L40.0
Psychasthenia F48.8
Psychiatric disorder or problem F99
Psychogenic (*see also* condition)
 factors associated with physical conditions F54
Psychological and behavioral factors affecting medical condition F59
Psychoneurosis, psychoneurotic (*see also* Neurosis)
 anxiety (state) F41.1
 depersonalization F48.1
 hypochondriacal F45.21
 hysteria F44.9
 neurasthenic F48.8
 personality NEC F60.89
Psychopathy, psychopathic
 affectionless F94.2
 autistic F84.5
 constitution, post-traumatic F07.81
 personality — *see* Disorder, personality
 sexual — *see* Deviation, sexual
 state F60.2
Psychosexual identity disorder of childhood F64.2
Psychosis, psychotic F29
 acute (transient) F23
  hysterical F44.9
 affective — *see* Disorder, mood
 alcoholic F10.959
  with
   abuse F10.159
   anxiety disorder F10.980
    with
     abuse F10.180
     dependence F10.280
   delirium tremens F10.231
   delusions F10.950
    with
     abuse F10.150
     dependence F10.250
   dementia F10.97
    with dependence F10.27
   dependence F10.259
   hallucinosis F10.951
    with
     abuse F10.151
     dependence F10.251
   mood disorder F10.94
    with
     abuse F10.14
     dependence F10.24
   paranoia F10.950
    with
     abuse F10.150
     dependence F10.250
   persisting amnesia F10.96
    with dependence F10.26
  amnestic confabulatory F10.96
   with dependence F10.26
  delirium tremens F10.231
  Korsakoff's, Korsakov's, Korsakow's F10.26
  paranoid type F10.950
   with
    abuse F10.150
    dependence F10.250
 anergastic — *see* Psychosis, organic
 arteriosclerotic (simple type) (uncomplicated) F01.50
  with behavioral disturbance F01.51

Psychosis, psychotic — *continued*
　childhood F84.0
　　atypical F84.8
　climacteric — *see* Psychosis, involutional
　confusional F29
　　acute or subacute F05
　　reactive F23
　cycloid F23
　depressive — *see* Disorder, depressive
　disintegrative (childhood) F84.3
　drug-induced — *see* F11-F19 with .X59
　　paranoid and hallucinatory states — *see* F11-F19
　　　with .X50 or .X51
　due to or associated with
　　addiction, drug — *see* F11-F19 with .X59
　　dependence
　　　alcohol F10.259
　　　drug — *see* F11-F19 with .X59
　　epilepsy F06.8
　　Huntington's chorea F06.8
　　ischemia, cerebrovascular (generalized) F06.8
　　multiple sclerosis F06.8
　　physical disease F06.8
　　presenile dementia F03 ☑
　　senile dementia F03 ☑
　　vascular disease (arteriosclerotic) (cerebral) F01.50
　　　with behavioral disturbance F01.51
　epileptic F06.8
　episode F23
　　due to or associated with physical condition F06.8
　exhaustive F43.0
　hallucinatory, chronic F28
　hypomanic F30.8
　hysterical (acute) F44.9
　induced F24
　infantile F84.0
　　atypical F84.8
　infective (acute) (subacute) F05
　involutional F28
　　depressive — *see* Disorder, depressive
　　melancholic — *see* Disorder, depressive
　　paranoid (state) F22
　Korsakoff's, Korsakov's, Korsakow's (nonalcoholic) F04
　　alcoholic F10.96
　　　in dependence F10.26
　　induced by other psychoactive substance — *see*
　　　categories F11-F19 with .X5X
　mania, manic (single episode) F30.2
　　recurrent type F31.89
　manic-depressive — *see* Disorder, bipolar
　menopausal — *see* Psychosis, involutional
　mixed schizophrenic and affective F25.8
　multi-infarct (cerebrovascular) F01.50
　　with behavioral disturbance F01.51
　nonorganic F29
　　specified NEC F28
　organic F09
　　due to or associated with
　　　arteriosclerosis (cerebral) — *see* Psychosis, ar-
　　　　teriosclerotic
　　　cerebrovascular disease, arteriosclerotic — *see*
　　　　Psychosis, arteriosclerotic
　　　childbirth — *see* Psychosis, puerperal
　　　Creutzfeldt-Jakob disease or syndrome — *see*
　　　　Creutzfeldt-Jakob disease or syndrome
　　　dependence, alcohol F10.259
　　　disease
　　　　alcoholic liver F10.259
　　　　brain, arteriosclerotic — *see* Psychosis, arte-
　　　　　riosclerotic
　　　　cerebrovascular F01.50
　　　　　with behavioral disturbance F01.51
　　　　Creutzfeldt-Jakob — *see* Creutzfeldt-Jakob
　　　　　disease or syndrome
　　　　endocrine or metabolic F06.8
　　　　　acute or subacute F05
　　　　liver, alcoholic F10.259
　　　epilepsy transient (acute) F05
　　　infection
　　　　brain (intracranial) F06.8
　　　　　acute or subacute F05
　　　intoxication
　　　　alcoholic (acute) F10.259
　　　　drug F11-F19 with .X59
　　　ischemia, cerebrovascular (generalized) — *see*
　　　　Psychosis, arteriosclerotic
　　　puerperium — *see* Psychosis, puerperal

Psychosis, psychotic — *continued*
　organic — *continued*
　　due to or associated with — *continued*
　　　trauma, brain (birth) (from electric current)
　　　　(surgical) F06.8
　　　　acute or subacute F05
　　infective F06.8
　　　acute or subacute F05
　　post-traumatic F06.8
　　　acute or subacute F05
　paranoiac F22
　paranoid (climacteric) (involutional) (menopausal) F22
　　psychogenic (acute) F23
　　schizophrenic F20.0
　　senile F03 ☑
　postpartum F53
　presbyophrenic (type) F03 ☑
　presenile F03 ☑
　psychogenic (paranoid) F23
　　depressive F32.3
　puerperal F53
　　specified type — *see* Psychosis, by type
　reactive (brief) (transient) (emotional stress) (psycho-
　　logical trauma) F23
　　depressive F32.3
　　　recurrent F33.3
　　excitative type F30.8
　schizoaffective F25.9
　　depressive type F25.1
　　manic type F25.0
　schizophrenia, schizophrenic — *see* Schizophrenia
　schizophrenia-like, in epilepsy F06.2
　schizophreniform F20.81
　　affective type F25.9
　　brief F23
　　confusional type F23
　　mixed type F25.0
　senile NEC F03 ☑
　　depressed or paranoid type F03 ☑
　　simple deterioration F03 ☑
　　specified type — *code to* condition
　shared F24
　situational (reactive) F23
　symbiotic (childhood) F84.3
　symptomatic F09
Psychosomatic — *see* Disorder, psychosomatic
Psychosyndrome, organic F07.9
Psychotic episode due to or associated with physical
　condition F06.8
Pterygium (eye) H11.00- ☑
　amyloid H11.01- ☑
　central H11.02- ☑
　colli Q18.3
　double H11.03- ☑
　peripheral
　　progressive H11.05- ☑
　　stationary H11.04- ☑
　recurrent H11.06- ☑
Ptilosis (eyelid) — *see* Madarosis
Ptomaine (poisoning) — *see* Poisoning, food
Ptosis (*see also* Blepharoptosis)
　adiposa (false) — *see* Blepharoptosis
　breast N64.81
　cecum K63.4
　colon K63.4
　congenital (eyelid) Q10.0
　　specified site NEC — *see* Anomaly, by site
　eyelid — *see* Blepharoptosis
　　congenital Q10.0
　gastric K31.89
　intestine K63.4
　kidney N28.83
　liver K76.89
　renal N28.83
　splanchnic K63.4
　spleen D73.89
　stomach K31.89
　viscera K63.4
PTP D69.51
Ptyalism (periodic) K11.7
　hysterical F45.8
　pregnancy — *see* Pregnancy, complicated by, specified
　　pregnancy-related condition NEC
　psychogenic F45.8
Ptyalolithiasis K11.5
Pubarche, precocious E30.1
Pubertas praecox E30.1
Puberty (development state) Z00.3

Puberty — *continued*
　bleeding (excessive) N92.2
　delayed E30.0
　precocious (constitutional) (cryptogenic) (idiopathic)
　　E30.1
　　central E22.8
　　due to
　　　ovarian hyperfunction E28.1
　　　　estrogen E28.0
　　　testicular hyperfunction E29.0
　premature E30.1
　　due to
　　　adrenal cortical hyperfunction E25.8
　　　pineal tumor E34.8
　　　pituitary (anterior) hyperfunction E22.8
Puckering, macula — *see* Degeneration, macula, puck-
　ering
Pudenda, pudendum — *see* condition
Puente's disease (simple glandular cheilitis) K13.0
Puerperal, puerperium (complicated by, complications)
　abnormal glucose (tolerance test) O99.815
　abscess
　　areola O91.02
　　　associated with lactation O91.03
　　Bartholin's gland O86.19
　　breast O91.12
　　　associated with lactation O91.13
　　cervix (uteri) O86.11
　　genital organ NEC O86.19
　　kidney O86.21
　　mammary O91.12
　　　associated with lactation O91.13
　　nipple O91.02
　　　associated with lactation O91.03
　　peritoneum O85
　　subareolar O91.12
　　　associated with lactation O91.13
　　urinary tract — *see* Puerperal, infection, urinary
　　uterus O86.12
　　vagina (wall) O86.13
　　vaginorectal O86.13
　　vulvovaginal gland O86.13
　adnexitis O86.19
　afibrinogenemia, or other coagulation defect O72.3
　albuminuria (acute) (subacute) — *see* Proteinuria,
　　gestational
　alcohol use O99.315
　anemia O90.81
　　pre-existing (pre-pregnancy) O99.03
　anesthetic death O89.8
　apoplexy O99.43
　bariatric surgery status O99.845
　blood disorder NEC O99.13
　blood dyscrasia O72.3
　cardiomyopathy O90.3
　cerebrovascular disorder (conditions in I60-I69) O99.43
　cervicitis O86.11
　circulatory system disorder O99.43
　coagulopathy (any) O99.13
　　with hemorrhage O72.3
　complications O90.9
　　specified NEC O90.89
　convulsions — *see* Eclampsia
　cystitis O86.22
　cystopyelitis O86.29
　delirium NEC F05
　diabetes O24.93
　　gestational — *see* Puerperal, gestational diabetes
　　pre-existing O24.33
　　　specified NEC O24.83
　　　type 1 O24.03
　　　type 2 O24.13
　digestive system disorder O99.63
　disease O90.9
　　breast NEC O92.29
　　cerebrovascular (acute) O99.43
　　nonobstetric NEC O99.89
　　tubo-ovarian O86.19
　　Valsuani's O99.03
　disorder O90.9
　　biliary tract O26.63
　　lactation O92.70
　　liver O26.63
　　nonobstetric NEC O99.89
　disruption
　　cesarean wound O90.0
　　episiotomy wound O90.1
　　perineal laceration wound O90.1

Index

Psychosis, psychotic — Puerperal, puerperium

Puerperal, puerperium — *continued*
- drug use O99.325
- eclampsia (with pre-existing hypertension) O15.2
- embolism (pulmonary) (blood clot) — *see* Embolism, obstetric, puerperal
- endocrine, nutritional or metabolic disease NEC O99.285
- endophlebitis — *see* Puerperal, phlebitis
- endotrachelitis O86.11
- failure
  - lactation (complete) O92.3
    - partial O92.4
  - renal, acute O90.4
- fever (of unknown origin) O86.4
  - septic O85
- fissure, nipple O92.12
  - associated with lactation O92.13
- fistula
  - breast (due to mastitis) O91.12
    - associated with lactation O91.13
  - nipple O91.02
    - associated with lactation O91.03
- galactophoritis O91.22
  - associated with lactation O91.23
- galactorrhea O92.6
- gastric banding status O99.845
- gastric bypass status O99.845
- gastrointestinal disease NEC O99.63
- gestational
  - diabetes O24.439
    - diet controlled O24.430
    - insulin (and diet) controlled O24.434
    - oral drug controlled (antidiabetic) (hypo-glycemic) O24.435
  - edema O12.05
    - with proteinuria O12.25
  - proteinuria O12.15
- gonorrhea O98.23
- hematoma, subdural O99.43
- hemiplegia, cerebral O99.355
  - due to cerbrovascular disorder O99.43
- hemorrhage O72.1
  - brain O99.43
  - bulbar O99.43
  - cerebellar O99.43
  - cerebral O99.43
  - cortical O99.43
  - delayed or secondary O72.2
  - extradural O99.43
  - internal capsule O99.43
  - intracranial O99.43
  - intrapontine O99.43
  - meningeal O99.43
  - pontine O99.43
  - retained placenta O72.0
  - subarachnoid O99.43
  - subcortical O99.43
  - subdural O99.43
  - third stage O72.0
  - uterine, delayed O72.2
  - ventricular O99.43
- hemorrhoids O87.2
- hepatorenal syndrome O90.4
- hypertension — *see* Hypertension, complicating, puerperium
- hypertrophy, breast O92.29
- induration breast (fibrous) O92.29
- infection O86.4
  - cervix O86.11
  - generalized O85
  - genital tract NEC O86.19
    - obstetric surgical wound O86.0
  - kidney (bacillus coli) O86.21
  - maternal O98.93
    - carrier state NEC O99.835
    - gonorrhea O98.23
    - human immunodeficiency virus (HIV) O98.73
    - protozoal O98.63
    - sexually transmitted NEC O98.33
    - specified NEC O98.83
    - streptococcus group B (GBS) carrier state O99.825
    - syphilis O98.13
    - tuberculosis O98.03
    - viral hepatitis O98.43
    - viral NEC O98.53
  - nipple O91.02
    - associated with lactation O91.03
  - peritoneum O85

Puerperal, puerperium — *continued*
- infection — *continued*
  - renal O86.21
  - specified NEC O86.89
  - urinary (asymptomatic) (tract) NEC O86.20
    - bladder O86.22
    - kidney O86.21
    - specified site NEC O86.29
    - urethra O86.22
  - vagina O86.13
  - vein — *see* Puerperal, phlebitis
- ischemia, cerebral O99.43
- lymphangitis O86.89
  - breast O91.22
    - associated with lactation O91.23
- malignancy O9A.13 (*following* O99)
- malnutrition O25.3
- mammillitis O91.02
  - associated with lactation O91.03
- mammitis O91.22
  - associated with lactation O91.23
- mania F30.8
- mastitis O91.22
  - associated with lactation O91.23
  - purulent O91.12
    - associated with lactation O91.13
- melancholia — *see* Disorder, depressive
- mental disorder NEC O99.345
- metroperitonitis O85
- metrorrhagia — *see* Hemorrhage, postpartum
- metrosalpingitis O86.19
- metrovaginitis O86.13
- milk leg O87.1
- monoplegia, cerebral O99.43
- mood disturbance O90.6
- necrosis, liver (acute) (subacute) (conditions in subcat-egory K72.0) O26.63
  - with renal failure O90.4
- nervous system disorder O99.355
- obesity (pre-existing prior to pregnancy) O99.215
- obesity surgery status O99.845
- occlusion, precerebral artery O99.43
- paralysis
  - bladder (sphincter) O90.89
  - cerebral O99.43
- paralytic stroke O99.43
- parametritis O85
- paravaginitis O86.13
- pelviperitonitis O85
- perimetritis O86.12
- perimetrosalpingitis O86.19
- perinephritis O86.21
- periphlebitis — *see* Puerperal phlebitis
- peritoneal infection O85
- peritonitis (pelvic) O85
- perivaginitis O86.13
- phlebitis O87.0
  - deep O87.1
  - pelvic O87.1
  - superficial O87.0
- phlebothrombosis, deep O87.1
- phlegmasia alba dolens O87.1
- placental polyp O90.89
- pneumonia, embolic — *see* Embolism, obstetric, puerperal
- pre-eclampsia — *see* Pre-eclampsia
- psychosis F53
- pyelitis O86.21
- pyelocystitis O86.29
- pyelonephritis O86.21
- pyelonephrosis O86.21
- pyemia O85
- pyocystitis O86.29
- pyohemia O85
- pyometra O86.12
- pyonephritis O86.21
- pyosalpingitis O86.19
- pyrexia (of unknown origin) O86.4
- renal
  - disease NEC O90.89
  - failure O90.4
- respiratory disease NEC O99.53
- retention
  - decidua — *see* Retention, decidua
  - placenta O72.0
  - secundines — *see* Retention, secundines
- retracted nipple O92.02
- salpingo-ovaritis O86.19

Puerperal, puerperium — *continued*
- salpingoperitonitis O85
- secondary perineal tear O90.1
- sepsis (pelvic) O85
- sepsis O85
- septic thrombophlebitis O86.81
- skin disorder NEC O99.73
- specified condition NEC O99.89
- stroke O99.43
- subinvolution (uterus) O90.89
- subluxation of symphysis (pubis) O26.73
- suppuration — *see* Puerperal, abscess
- tetanus A34
- thelitis O91.02
  - associated with lactation O91.03
- thrombocytopenia O72.3
- thrombophlebitis (superficial) O87.0
  - deep O87.1
  - pelvic O87.1
  - septic O86.81
- thrombosis (venous) — *see* Thrombosis, puerperal
- thyroiditis O90.5
- toxemia (eclamptic) (pre-eclamptic) (with convulsions) O15.2
- trauma, non-obstetric O9A.23 (*following* O99)
  - caused by abuse (physical) (suspected) O9A.33 (*following* O99)
    - confirmed O9A.33 (*following* O99)
    - psychological (suspected) O9A.53 (*following* O99)
      - confirmed O9A.53 (*following* O99)
    - sexual (suspected) O9A.43 (*following* O99)
      - confirmed O9A.43 (*following* O99)
- uremia (due to renal failure) O90.4
- urethritis O86.22
- vaginitis O86.13
- varicose veins (legs) O87.4
  - vulva or perineum O87.8
- venous O87.9
- vulvitis O86.19
- vulvovaginitis O86.13
- white leg O87.1

Puerperium — *see* Puerperal
Pulmolithiasis J98.4
Pulmonary — *see* condition
Pulpitis (acute) (anachoretic) (chronic) (hyperplastic) (putrescent) (suppurative) (ulcerative) K04.01
- irreversible K04.02
- reversible K04.01

Pulpless tooth K04.99
Pulse
- alternating R00.8
- bigeminal R00.8
- fast R00.0
- feeble, rapid due to shock following injury T79.4 ☑
- rapid R00.0
- weak R09.89

Pulsus alternans or trigeminus R00.8
Punch drunk F07.81
Punctum lacrimale occlusion — *see* Obstruction, lacrimal
Puncture
- abdomen, abdominal
  - wall S31.139 ☑
    - with
      - foreign body S31.149 ☑
      - penetration into peritoneal cavity S31.639 ☑
        - with foreign body S31.649 ☑
  - epigastric region S31.132 ☑
    - with
      - foreign body S31.142 ☑
      - penetration into peritoneal cavity S31.632 ☑
        - with foreign body S31.642 ☑
  - left
    - lower quadrant S31.134 ☑
      - with
        - foreign body S31.144 ☑
        - penetration into peritoneal cavity S31.634 ☑
          - with foreign body S31.644 ☑
    - upper quadrant S31.131 ☑
      - with
        - foreign body S31.141 ☑
        - penetration into peritoneal cavity S31.631 ☑
          - with foreign body S31.641 ☑

Puncture — *continued*
  abdomen, abdominal — *continued*
    wall — *continued*
      periumbilic region S31.135 ☑
        with
          foreign body S31.145 ☑
          penetration into peritoneal cavity
            S31.635 ☑
            with foreign body S31.645 ☑
      right
        lower quadrant S31.133 ☑
          with
            foreign body S31.143 ☑
            penetration into peritoneal cavity
              S31.633 ☑
              with foreign body S31.643 ☑
        upper quadrant S31.130 ☑
          with
            foreign body S31.140 ☑
            penetration into peritoneal cavity
              S31.630 ☑
              with foreign body S31.640 ☑
  accidental, complicating surgery — *see* Complication,
    accidental puncture or laceration
  alveolar (process) — *see* Puncture, oral cavity
  ankle S91.039 ☑
    with
      foreign body S91.049 ☑
    left S91.032 ☑
      with
        foreign body S91.042 ☑
    right S91.031 ☑
      with
        foreign body S91.041 ☑
  anus S31.833 ☑
    with foreign body S31.834 ☑
  arm (upper) S41.139 ☑
    with foreign body S41.149 ☑
    left S41.132 ☑
      with foreign body S41.142 ☑
    lower — *see* Puncture, forearm
    right S41.131 ☑
      with foreign body S41.141 ☑
  auditory canal (external) (meatus) — *see* Puncture,
    ear
  auricle, ear — *see* Puncture, ear
  axilla — *see* Puncture, arm
  back (*see also* Puncture, thorax, back)
    lower S31.030 ☑
      with
        foreign body S31.040 ☑
          with penetration into retroperitoneal
            space S31.041 ☑
        penetration into retroperitoneal space
          S31.031 ☑
  bladder (traumatic) S37.29 ☑
    nontraumatic N32.89
  breast S21.039 ☑
    with foreign body S21.049 ☑
    left S21.032 ☑
      with foreign body S21.042 ☑
    right S21.031 ☑
      with foreign body S21.041 ☑
  buttock S31.803 ☑
    with foreign body S31.804 ☑
    left S31.823 ☑
      with foreign body S31.824 ☑
    right S31.813 ☑
      with foreign body S31.814 ☑
  by
    device, implant or graft — *see* Complications, by
      site and type, mechanical
    foreign body left accidentally in operative wound
      T81.539 ☑
    instrument (any) during a procedure, accidental
      — *see* Puncture, accidental complicating
      surgery
  calf — *see* Puncture, leg
  canaliculus lacrimalis — *see* Puncture, eyelid
  canthus, eye — *see* Puncture, eyelid
  cervical esophagus S11.23 ☑
    with foreign body S11.24 ☑
  cheek (external) S01.439 ☑
    with foreign body S01.449 ☑
    internal — *see* Puncture, oral cavity
    left S01.432 ☑

Puncture — *continued*
  cheek — *continued*
    left — *continued*
      with foreign body S01.442 ☑
    right S01.431 ☑
      with foreign body S01.441 ☑
  chest wall — *see* Puncture, thorax
  chin — *see* Puncture, head, specified site NEC
  clitoris — *see* Puncture, vulva
  costal region — *see* Puncture, thorax
  digit(s)
    foot — *see* Puncture, toe
    hand — *see* Puncture, finger
  ear (canal) (external) S01.339 ☑
    with foreign body S01.349 ☑
    drum S09.2- ☑
    left S01.332 ☑
      with foreign body S01.342 ☑
    right S01.331 ☑
      with foreign body S01.341 ☑
  elbow S51.039 ☑
    with
      foreign body S51.049 ☑
    left S51.032 ☑
      with
        foreign body S51.042 ☑
    right S51.031 ☑
      with
        foreign body S51.041 ☑
  epididymis — *see* Puncture, testis
  epigastric region — *see* Puncture, abdomen, wall,
    epigastric
  epiglottis S11.83 ☑
    with foreign body S11.84 ☑
  esophagus
    cervical S11.23 ☑
      with foreign body S11.24 ☑
    thoracic S27.818 ☑
  eyeball S05.6- ☑
    with foreign body S05.5- ☑
  eyebrow — *see* Puncture, eyelid
  eyelid S01.13- ☑
    with foreign body S01.14- ☑
    left S01.132 ☑
      with foreign body S01.142 ☑
    right S01.131 ☑
      with foreign body S01.141 ☑
  face NEC — *see* Puncture, head, specified site NEC
  finger(s) S61.239 ☑
    with
      damage to nail S61.339 ☑
        with
          foreign body S61.349 ☑
      foreign body S61.249 ☑
    index S61.238 ☑
      with
        damage to nail S61.338 ☑
          with
            foreign body S61.348 ☑
        foreign body S61.248 ☑
      left S61.231 ☑
        with
          damage to nail S61.331 ☑
            with
              foreign body S61.341 ☑
          foreign body S61.241 ☑
      right S61.230 ☑
        with
          damage to nail S61.330 ☑
            with
              foreign body S61.340 ☑
          foreign body S61.240 ☑
    little S61.238 ☑
      with
        damage to nail S61.338 ☑
          with
            foreign body S61.348 ☑
        foreign body S61.248 ☑
      left S61.237 ☑
        with
          damage to nail S61.337 ☑
            with
              foreign body S61.347 ☑
          foreign body S61.247 ☑
      right S61.236 ☑

Puncture — *continued*
  finger(s) — *continued*
    little — *continued*
      right — *continued*
        with
          damage to nail S61.336 ☑
            with
              foreign body S61.346 ☑
          foreign body S61.246 ☑
    middle S61.238 ☑
      with
        damage to nail S61.338 ☑
          with
            foreign body S61.348 ☑
        foreign body S61.248 ☑
      left S61.233 ☑
        with
          damage to nail S61.333 ☑
            with
              foreign body S61.343 ☑
          foreign body S61.243 ☑
      right S61.232 ☑
        with
          damage to nail S61.332 ☑
            with
              foreign body S61.342 ☑
          foreign body S61.242 ☑
    ring S61.238 ☑
      with
        damage to nail S61.338 ☑
          with
            foreign body S61.348 ☑
        foreign body S61.248 ☑
      left S61.235 ☑
        with
          damage to nail S61.335 ☑
            with
              foreign body S61.345 ☑
          foreign body S61.245 ☑
      right S61.234 ☑
        with
          damage to nail S61.334 ☑
            with
              foreign body S61.344 ☑
          foreign body S61.244 ☑
  flank S31.139 ☑
    with foreign body S31.149 ☑
  foot (except toe(s) alone) S91.339 ☑
    with foreign body S91.349 ☑
    left S91.332 ☑
      with foreign body S91.342 ☑
    right S91.331 ☑
      with foreign body S91.341 ☑
    toe — *see* Puncture, toe
  forearm S51.839 ☑
    with
      foreign body S51.849 ☑
    elbow only — *see* Puncture, elbow
    left S51.832 ☑
      with
        foreign body S51.842 ☑
    right S51.831 ☑
      with
        foreign body S51.841 ☑
  forehead — *see* Puncture, head, specified site NEC
  genital organs, external
    female S31.532 ☑
      with foreign body S31.542 ☑
      vagina — *see* Puncture, vagina
      vulva — *see* Puncture, vulva
    male S31.531 ☑
      with foreign body S31.541 ☑
      penis — *see* Puncture, penis
      scrotum — *see* Puncture, scrotum
      testis — *see* Puncture, testis
  groin — *see* Puncture, abdomen, wall
  gum — *see* Puncture, oral cavity
  hand S61.439 ☑
    with
      foreign body S61.449 ☑
    finger — *see* Puncture, finger
    left S61.432 ☑
      with
        foreign body S61.442 ☑
    right S61.431 ☑

Puncture — *continued*
  hand — *continued*
    right — *continued*
      with
        foreign body S61.441 ✓
      thumb — *see* Puncture, thumb
  head S01.93 ✓
    with foreign body S01.94 ✓
    cheek — *see* Puncture, cheek
    ear — *see* Puncture, ear
    eyelid — *see* Puncture, eyelid
    lip — *see* Puncture, oral cavity
    nose — *see* Puncture, nose
    oral cavity — *see* Puncture, oral cavity
    scalp S01.03 ✓
      with foreign body S01.04 ✓
    specified site NEC S01.83 ✓
      with foreign body S01.84 ✓
    temporomandibular area — *see* Puncture, cheek
  heart S26.99 ✓
    with hemopericardium S26.09 ✓
    without hemopericardium S26.19 ✓
  heel — *see* Puncture, foot
  hip S71.039 ✓
    with foreign body S71.049 ✓
    left S71.032 ✓
      with foreign body S71.042 ✓
    right S71.031 ✓
      with foreign body S71.041 ✓
  hymen — *see* Puncture, vagina
  hypochondrium — *see* Puncture, abdomen, wall
  hypogastric region — *see* Puncture, abdomen, wall
  inguinal region — *see* Puncture, abdomen, wall
  instep — *see* Puncture, foot
  internal organs — *see* Injury, by site
  interscapular region — *see* Puncture, thorax, back
  intestine
    large
      colon S36.599 ✓
        ascending S36.590 ✓
        descending S36.592 ✓
        sigmoid S36.593 ✓
        specified site NEC S36.598 ✓
        transverse S36.591 ✓
      rectum S36.69 ✓
    small S36.499 ✓
      duodenum S36.490 ✓
      specified site NEC S36.498 ✓
  intra-abdominal organ S36.99 ✓
    gallbladder S36.128 ✓
    intestine — *see* Puncture, intestine
    liver S36.118 ✓
    pancreas — *see* Puncture, pancreas
    peritoneum S36.81 ✓
    specified site NEC S36.898 ✓
    spleen S36.09 ✓
    stomach S36.39 ✓
  jaw — *see* Puncture, head, specified site NEC
  knee S81.039 ✓
    with foreign body S81.049 ✓
    left S81.032 ✓
      with foreign body S81.042 ✓
    right S81.031 ✓
      with foreign body S81.041 ✓
  labium (majus) (minus) — *see* Puncture, vulva
  lacrimal duct — *see* Puncture, eyelid
  larynx S11.013 ✓
    with foreign body S11.014 ✓
  leg (lower) S81.839 ✓
    with foreign body S81.849 ✓
    foot — *see* Puncture, foot
    knee — *see* Puncture, knee
    left S81.832 ✓
      with foreign body S81.842 ✓
    right S81.831 ✓
      with foreign body S81.841 ✓
    upper — *see* Puncture, thigh
  lip S01.531 ✓
    with foreign body S01.541 ✓
  loin — *see* Puncture, abdomen, wall
  lower back — *see* Puncture, back, lower
  lumbar region — *see* Puncture, back, lower
  malar region — *see* Puncture, head, specified site NEC
  mammary — *see* Puncture, breast
  mastoid region — *see* Puncture, head, specified site NEC

Puncture — *continued*
  mouth — *see* Puncture, oral cavity
  nail
    finger — *see* Puncture, finger, with damage to nail
    toe — *see* Puncture, toe, with damage to nail
  nasal (septum) (sinus) — *see* Puncture, nose
  nasopharynx — *see* Puncture, head, specified site NEC
  neck S11.93 ✓
    with foreign body S11.94 ✓
    involving
      cervical esophagus — *see* Puncture, cervical esophagus
      larynx — *see* Puncture, larynx
      pharynx — *see* Puncture, pharynx
      thyroid gland — *see* Puncture, thyroid gland
      trachea — *see* Puncture, trachea
    specified site NEC S11.83 ✓
      with foreign body S11.84 ✓
  nose (septum) (sinus) S01.23 ✓
    with foreign body S01.24 ✓
  ocular — *see* Puncture, eyeball
  oral cavity S01.532 ✓
    with foreign body S01.542 ✓
  orbit S05.4- ✓
  palate — *see* Puncture, oral cavity
  palm — *see* Puncture, hand
  pancreas S36.299 ✓
    body S36.291 ✓
    head S36.290 ✓
    tail S36.292 ✓
  pelvis — *see* Puncture, back, lower
  penis S31.23 ✓
    with foreign body S31.24 ✓
  perineum
    female S31.43 ✓
      with foreign body S31.44 ✓
    male S31.139 ✓
      with foreign body S31.149 ✓
  periocular area (with or without lacrimal passages) — *see* Puncture, eyelid
  phalanges
    finger — *see* Puncture, finger
    toe — *see* Puncture, toe
  pharynx S11.23 ✓
    with foreign body S11.24 ✓
  pinna — *see* Puncture, ear
  popliteal space — *see* Puncture, knee
  prepuce — *see* Puncture, penis
  pubic region S31.139 ✓
    with foreign body S31.149 ✓
  pudendum — *see* Puncture, genital organs, external
  rectovaginal septum — *see* Puncture, vagina
  sacral region — *see* Puncture, back, lower
  sacroiliac region — *see* Puncture, back, lower
  salivary gland — *see* Puncture, oral cavity
  scalp S01.03 ✓
    with foreign body S01.04 ✓
  scapular region — *see* Puncture, shoulder
  scrotum S31.33 ✓
    with foreign body S31.34 ✓
  shin — *see* Puncture, leg
  shoulder S41.039 ✓
    with foreign body S41.049 ✓
    left S41.032 ✓
      with foreign body S41.042 ✓
    right S41.031 ✓
      with foreign body S41.041 ✓
  spermatic cord — *see* Puncture, testis
  sternal region — *see* Puncture, thorax, front
  submaxillary region — *see* Puncture, head, specified site NEC
  submental region — *see* Puncture, head, specified site NEC
  subungual
    finger(s) — *see* Puncture, finger, with damage to nail
    toe — *see* Puncture, toe, with damage to nail
  supraclavicular fossa — *see* Puncture, neck, specified site NEC
  temple, temporal region — *see* Puncture, head, specified site NEC
  temporomandibular area — *see* Puncture, cheek
  testis S31.33 ✓
    with foreign body S31.34 ✓
  thigh S71.139 ✓
    with foreign body S71.149 ✓

Puncture — *continued*
  thigh — *continued*
    left S71.132 ✓
      with foreign body S71.142 ✓
    right S71.131 ✓
      with foreign body S71.141 ✓
  thorax, thoracic (wall) S21.93 ✓
    with foreign body S21.94 ✓
    back S21.23- ✓
      with
        foreign body S21.24- ✓
          with penetration S21.44 ✓
        penetration S21.43 ✓
    breast — *see* Puncture, breast
    front S21.13- ✓
      with
        foreign body S21.14- ✓
          with penetration S21.34 ✓
        penetration S21.33 ✓
  throat — *see* Puncture, neck
  thumb S61.039 ✓
    with
      damage to nail S61.139 ✓
        with
          foreign body S61.149 ✓
      foreign body S61.049 ✓
    left S61.032 ✓
      with
        damage to nail S61.132 ✓
          with
            foreign body S61.142 ✓
        foreign body S61.042 ✓
    right S61.031 ✓
      with
        damage to nail S61.131 ✓
          with
            foreign body S61.141 ✓
        foreign body S61.041 ✓
  thyroid gland S11.13 ✓
    with foreign body S11.14 ✓
  toe(s) S91.139 ✓
    with
      damage to nail S91.239 ✓
        with
          foreign body S91.249 ✓
      foreign body S91.149 ✓
    great S91.133 ✓
      with
        damage to nail S91.233 ✓
          with
            foreign body S91.243 ✓
        foreign body S91.143 ✓
      left S91.132 ✓
        with
          damage to nail S91.232 ✓
            with
              foreign body S91.242 ✓
          foreign body S91.142 ✓
      right S91.131 ✓
        with
          damage to nail S91.231 ✓
            with
              foreign body S91.241 ✓
          foreign body S91.141 ✓
    lesser S91.136 ✓
      with
        damage to nail S91.236 ✓
          with
            foreign body S91.246 ✓
        foreign body S91.146 ✓
      left S91.135 ✓
        with
          damage to nail S91.235 ✓
            with
              foreign body S91.245 ✓
          foreign body S91.145 ✓
      right S91.134 ✓
        with
          damage to nail S91.234 ✓
            with
              foreign body S91.244 ✓
          foreign body S91.144 ✓
  tongue — *see* Puncture, oral cavity
  trachea S11.023 ✓
    with foreign body S11.024 ✓
  tunica vaginalis — *see* Puncture, testis

Puncture — *continued*
- tympanum, tympanic membrane S09.2- ☑
- umbilical region S31.135 ☑
  - with foreign body S31.145 ☑
- uvula — *see* Puncture, oral cavity
- vagina S31.43 ☑
  - with foreign body S31.44 ☑
- vocal cords S11.033 ☑
  - with foreign body S11.034 ☑
- vulva S31.43 ☑
  - with foreign body S31.44 ☑
- wrist S61.539 ☑
  - with
    - foreign body S61.549 ☑
  - left S61.532 ☑
    - with
      - foreign body S61.542 ☑
  - right S61.531 ☑
    - with
      - foreign body S61.541 ☑

PUO (pyrexia of unknown origin) R50.9
Pupillary membrane (persistent) Q13.89
Pupillotonia — *see* Anomaly, pupil, function, tonic pupil
Purpura D69.2
- abdominal D69.2
- allergic D69.0
- anaphylactoid D69.0
- annularis telangiectodes L81.7
- arthritic D69.0
- autoerythrocyte sensitization D69.2
- autoimmune D69.0
- bacterial D69.0
- Bateman's (senile) D69.2
- capillary fragility (hereditary) (idiopathic) D69.8
- cryoglobulinemic D89.1
- Devil's pinches D69.2
- fibrinolytic — *see* Fibrinolysis
- fulminans, fulminous D65
- gangrenous D65
- hemorrhagic, hemorrhagica D69.3
  - not due to thrombocytopenia D69.0
- Henoch (-Schönlein) (allergic) D69.0
- hypergammaglobulinemic (benign) (Waldenström) D89.0
- idiopathic (thrombocytopenic) D69.3
  - nonthrombocytopenic D69.0
- immune thrombocytopenic D69.3
- infectious D69.0
- malignant D69.0
- neonatorum P54.5
- nervosa D69.0
- newborn P54.5
- nonthrombocytopenic D69.2
  - hemorrhagic D69.0
  - idiopathic D69.0
- nonthrombopenic D69.2
- peliosis rheumatica D69.0
- posttransfusion (post-transfusion) (from (fresh) whole blood or blood products) D69.51
- primary D69.49
- red cell membrane sensitivity D69.2
- rheumatica D69.0
- Schönlein (-Henoch) (allergic) D69.0
- scorbutic E54 [D77]
- senile D69.2
- simplex D69.2
- symptomatica D69.0
- telangiectasia annularis L81.7
- thrombocytopenic D69.49
  - congenital D69.42
  - hemorrhagic D69.3
  - hereditary D69.42
  - idiopathic D69.3
  - immune D69.3
  - neonatal, transitory P61.0
  - thrombotic M31.1
- thrombohemolytic — *see* Fibrinolysis
- thrombolytic — *see* Fibrinolysis
- thrombopenic D69.49
- thrombotic, thrombocytopenic M31.1
- toxic D69.0
- vascular D69.0
- visceral symptoms D69.0

Purpuric spots R23.3
Purulent — *see* condition
Pus
- in
  - stool R19.5

Pus — *continued*
- in — *continued*
  - urine N39.0
  - tube (rupture) — *see* Salpingo-oophoritis

Pustular rash L08.0
Pustule (nonmalignant) L08.9
- malignant A22.0

Pustulosis palmaris et plantaris L40.3
Putnam (-Dana) **disease or syndrome** — *see* Degeneration, combined
Putrescent pulp (dental) K04.1
Pyarthritis, pyarthrosis — *see* Arthritis, pyogenic or pyemic
- tuberculous — *see* Tuberculosis, joint

Pyelectasis — *see* Hydronephrosis
Pyelitis (congenital) (uremic) (*see also* Pyelonephritis)
- with
  - calculus — *see* category N20 ☑
    - with hydronephrosis N13.2
  - contracted kidney N11.9
- acute N10
- chronic N11.9
  - with calculus — *see* category N20 ☑
    - with hydronephrosis N13.2
- cystica N28.84
- puerperal (postpartum) O86.21
- tuberculous A18.11

Pyelocystitis — *see* Pyelonephritis
Pyelonephritis (*see also* Nephritis, tubulo-interstitial)
- with
  - calculus — *see* category N20 ☑
    - with hydronephrosis N13.2
  - contracted kidney N11.9
- acute N10
- calculus — *see* category N20 ☑
  - with hydronephrosis N13.2
- chronic N11.9
  - with calculus — *see* category N20 ☑
    - with hydronephrosis N13.2
  - associated with ureteral obstruction or stricture N11.1
  - nonobstructive N11.8
    - with reflux (vesicoureteral) N11.0
  - obstructive N11.1
  - specified NEC N11.8
- in (due to)
  - brucellosis A23.9 [N16]
  - cryoglobulinemia (mixed) D89.1 [N16]
  - cystinosis E72.04
  - diphtheria A36.84
  - glycogen storage disease E74.09 [N16]
  - leukemia NEC C95.9- ☑ [N16]
  - lymphoma NEC C85.90 [N16]
  - multiple myeloma C90.0- ☑ [N16]
  - obstruction N11.1
  - Salmonella infection A02.25
  - sarcoidosis D86.84
  - sepsis A41.9 [N16]
  - Sjögren's disease M35.04
  - toxoplasmosis B58.83
  - transplant rejection T86.91 [N16]
  - Wilson's disease E83.01 [N16]
- nonobstructive N12
  - with reflux (vesicoureteral) N11.0
  - chronic N11.8
- syphilitic A52.75

Pyelonephrosis (obstructive) N11.1
- chronic N11.9

Pyelophlebitis I80.8
Pyeloureteritis cystica N28.85
Pyemia, pyemic (fever) (infection) (purulent) (*see also* Sepsis)
- joint — *see* Arthritis, pyogenic or pyemic
- liver K75.1
- pneumococcal A40.3
- portal K75.1
- postvaccinal T88.0 ☑
- puerperal, postpartum, childbirth O85
- specified organism NEC A41.89
- tuberculous — *see* Tuberculosis, miliary

Pygopagus Q89.4
Pyknoepilepsy (idiopathic) — *see* Pyknolepsy
Pyknolepsy G40.A09 (*following* G40.3)
- intractable G40.A19 (*following* G40.3)
  - with status epilepticus G40.A11 (*following* G40.3)
  - without status epilepticus G40.A19 (*following* G40.3)
- not intractable G40.A09 (*following* G40.3)

Pyknolepsy — *continued*
- not intractable — *continued*
  - with status epilepticus G40.A01 (*following* G40.3)
  - without status epilepticus G40.A09 (*following* G40.3)

Pylephlebitis K75.1
Pyle's syndrome Q78.5
Pylethrombophlebitis K75.1
Pylethrombosis K75.1
Pyloritis K29.90
- with bleeding K29.91

Pylorospasm (reflex) **NEC** K31.3
- congenital or infantile Q40.0
- neurotic F45.8
- newborn Q40.0
- psychogenic F45.8

Pylorus, pyloric — *see* condition
Pyoarthrosis — *see* Arthritis, pyogenic or pyemic
Pyocele
- mastoid — *see* Mastoiditis, acute
- sinus (accessory) — *see* Sinusitis
- turbinate (bone) J32.9
- urethra (*see also* Urethritis) N34.0

Pyocolpos — *see* Vaginitis
Pyocystitis N30.80
- with hematuria N30.81

Pyoderma, pyodermia L08.0
- gangrenosum L88
- newborn P39.4
- phagedenic L88
- vegetans L08.81

Pyodermatitis L08.0
- vegetans L08.81

Pyogenic — *see* condition
Pyohydronephrosis N13.6
Pyometra, pyometrium, pyometritis — *see* Endometritis
Pyomyositis (tropical) — *see* Myositis, infective
Pyonephritis N12
Pyonephrosis N13.6
- tuberculous A18.11

Pyo-oophoritis — *see* Salpingo-oophoritis
Pyo-ovarium — *see* Salpingo-oophoritis
Pyopericarditis, pyopericardium I30.1
Pyophlebitis — *see* Phlebitis
Pyopneumopericardium I30.1
Pyopneumothorax (infective) J86.9
- with fistula J86.0
- tuberculous NEC A15.6

Pyosalpinx, pyosalpingitis (*see also* Salpingo-oophoritis)
Pyothorax J86.9
- with fistula J86.0
- tuberculous NEC A15.6

Pyoureter N28.89
- tuberculous A18.11

Pyramidopallidonigral syndrome G20
Pyrexia (of unknown origin) R50.9
- atmospheric T67.0 ☑
- during labor NEC O75.2
- heat T67.0 ☑
- newborn P81.9
  - environmentally-induced P81.0
- persistent R50.9
- puerperal O86.4

Pyroglobulinemia NEC E88.09
Pyromania F63.1
Pyrosis R12
Pyuria (bacterial) N39.0

Q

Q fever A78
- with pneumonia A78

Quadricuspid aortic valve Q23.8
Quadrilateral fever A78
Quadriparesis — *see* Quadriplegia
- meaning muscle weakness M62.81

Quadriplegia G82.50
- complete
  - C1-C4 level G82.51
  - C5-C7 level G82.53
- congenital (cerebral) (spinal) G80.8
  - spastic G80.0
- embolic (current episode) I63.4- ☑
- functional R53.2

Quadriplegia — *continued*
  incomplete
    C1-C4 level G82.52
    C5-C7 level G82.54
  thrombotic (current episode) I63.3- ☑
  traumatic — *code to* injury with seventh character S
    current episode — *see* Injury, spinal (cord), cervical
Quadruplet, pregnancy — *see* Pregnancy, quadruplet
Quarrelsomeness F60.3
Queensland fever A77.3
Quervain's disease M65.4
  thyroid E06.1
Queyrat's erythroplasia D07.4
  penis D07.4
  specified site — *see* Neoplasm, skin, in situ
  unspecified site D07.4
Quincke's disease or edema T78.3 ☑
  hereditary D84.1
Quinsy (gangrenous) J36
Quintan fever A79.0
Quintuplet, pregnancy — *see* Pregnancy, quintuplet

R

Rabbit fever — *see* Tularemia
Rabies A82.9
  contact Z20.3
  exposure to Z20.3
  inoculation reaction — *see* Complications, vaccination
  sylvatic A82.0
  urban A82.1
Rachischisis — *see* Spina bifida
Rachitic (*see also* condition)
  deformities of spine (late effect) (sequelae) E64.3
  pelvis (late effect) (sequelae) E64.3
    with disproportion (fetopelvic) O33.0
      causing obstructed labor O65.0
Rachitis, rachitism (acute) (tarda) (*see also* Rickets)
  renalis N25.0
  sequelae E64.3
Radial nerve — *see* condition
Radiation
  burn — *see* Burn
  effects NOS T66 ☑
  sickness NOS T66 ☑
  therapy, encounter for Z51.0
Radiculitis (pressure) (vertebrogenic) — *see* Radiculopathy
Radiculomyelitis (*see also* Encephalitis)
  toxic, due to
    Clostridium tetani A35
    Corynebacterium diphtheriae A36.82
Radiculopathy M54.10
  cervical region M54.12
  cervicothoracic region M54.13
  due to
    disc disorder
      C3 M50.11
      C4 M50.11
      C5 M50.121
      C6 M50.122
      C7 M50.123
    displacement of intervertebral disc — *see* Disorder,
      disc, with, radiculopathy
  leg M54.1- ☑
  lumbar region M54.16
  lumbosacral region M54.17
  occipito-atlanto-axial region M54.11
  postherpetic B02.29
  sacrococcygeal region M54.18
  syphilitic A52.11
  thoracic region (with visceral pain) M54.14
  thoracolumbar region M54.15
Radiodermal burns (acute, chronic, or occupational) —
  see Burn
Radiodermatitis L58.9
  acute L58.0
  chronic L58.1
Radiotherapy session Z51.0
RAEB (refractory anemia with excess blasts) D46.2- ☑
Rage, meaning rabies — *see* Rabies
Ragpicker's disease A22.1
Ragsorter's disease A22.1
Raillietiniasis B71.8
Railroad neurosis F48.8
Railway spine F48.8

Raised (*see also* Elevated)
  antibody titer R76.0
Rake teeth, tooth M26.39
Rales R09.89
Ramifying renal pelvis Q63.8
Ramsay-Hunt disease or syndrome (*see also* Hunt's
    disease) B02.21
  meaning dyssynergia cerebellaris myoclonica G11.1
Ranula K11.6
  congenital Q38.4
Rape
  adult
    confirmed T74.21 ☑
    suspected T76.21 ☑
  alleged, observation or examination, ruled out
    adult Z04.41
    child Z04.42
  child
    confirmed T74.22 ☑
    suspected T76.22 ☑
Rapid
  feeble pulse, due to shock, following injury T79.4 ☑
  heart (beat) R00.0
    psychogenic F45.8
  second stage (delivery) O62.3
  time-zone change syndrome — *see* Disorder, sleep,
    circadian rhythm, psychogenic
Rarefaction, bone — *see* Disorder, bone, density and
    structure, specified NEC
Rash (toxic) R21
  canker A38.9
  diaper L22
  drug (internal use) L27.0
    contact (*see also* Dermatitis, due to, drugs, external)
      L25.1
  following immunization T88.1 ☑
  food — *see* Dermatitis, due to, food
  heat L74.0
  napkin (psoriasiform) L22
  nettle — *see* Urticaria
  pustular L08.0
  rose R21
    epidemic B06.9
  scarlet A38.9
  serum (*see also* Reaction, serum) T80.69 ☑
  wandering tongue K14.1
Rasmussen aneurysm — *see* Tuberculosis, pulmonary
Rasmussen encephalitis G04.81
Rat-bite fever A25.9
  due to Streptobacillus moniliformis A25.1
  spirochetal (morsus muris) A25.0
Rathke's pouch tumor D44.3
Raymond (-Céstan) **syndrome** I65.8
Raynaud's disease, phenomenon or syndrome (secondary) I73.00
  with gangrene (symmetric) I73.01
RDS (newborn) (type I) P22.0
  type II P22.1
Reaction (*see also* Disorder)
  adaptation — *see* Disorder, adjustment
  adjustment (anxiety) (conduct disorder) (depressive-
    ness) (distress) — *see* Disorder, adjustment
    with
      mutism, elective (child) (adolescent) F94.0
  adverse
    food (any) (ingested) NEC T78.1 ☑
      anaphylactic — *see* Shock, anaphylactic, due
        to food
  affective — *see* Disorder, mood
  allergic — *see* Allergy
  anaphylactic — *see* Shock, anaphylactic
  anaphylactoid — *see* Shock, anaphylactic
  anesthesia — *see* Anesthesia, complication
  antitoxin (prophylactic) (therapeutic) — *see* Complications, vaccination
  anxiety F41.1
  Arthus — *see* Arthus' phenomenon
  asthenic F48.8
  combat and operational stress F43.0
  compulsive F42.8
  conversion F44.9
  crisis, acute F43.0
  deoxyribonuclease (DNA) (DNase) hypersensitivity
    D69.2
  depressive (single episode) F32.9
    affective (single episode) F31.4
      recurrent episode F33.9

Reaction — *continued*
  depressive — *continued*
    neurotic F34.1
      psychoneurotic F34.1
      psychotic F32.3
    recurrent — *see* Disorder, depressive, recurrent
  dissociative F44.9
  drug NEC T88.7 ☑
    addictive — *see* Dependence, drug
      transmitted via placenta or breast milk — *see*
        Absorption, drug, addictive, through
        placenta
    allergic — *see* Allergy, drug
    lichenoid L43.2
    newborn P93.8
      gray baby syndrome P93.0
    overdose or poisoning (by accident) — *see* Table
      of Drugs and Chemicals, by drug, poisoning
    photoallergic L56.1
    phototoxic L56.0
    withdrawal — *see* Dependence, by drug, with,
      withdrawal
      infant of dependent mother P96.1
      newborn P96.1
    wrong substance given or taken (by accident) —
      see Table of Drugs and Chemicals, by drug,
      poisoning
  fear F40.9
    child (abnormal) F93.8
  febrile nonhemolytic transfusion (FNHTR) R50.84
  fluid loss, cerebrospinal G97.1
  foreign
    body NEC — *see* Granuloma, foreign body
      in operative wound (inadvertently left) — *see*
        Foreign body, accidentally left during a
        procedure
    substance accidentally left during a procedure
      (chemical) (powder) (talc) T81.60 ☑
      aseptic peritonitis T81.61 ☑
      body or object (instrument) (sponge) (swab)
        — *see* Foreign body, accidentally left
        during a procedure
      specified reaction NEC T81.69 ☑
  grief — *see* Disorder, adjustment
  Herxheimer's R68.89
  hyperkinetic — *see* Hyperkinesia
  hypochondriacal F45.20
  hypoglycemic, due to insulin E16.0
    with coma (diabetic) — *see* Diabetes, coma
      nondiabetic E15
    therapeutic misadventure — *see* subcategory
      T38.3 ☑
  hypomanic F30.8
  hysterical F44.9
  immunization — *see* Complications, vaccination
  incompatibility
    ABO blood group (infusion) (transfusion) — *see*
      Complication(s), transfusion, incompatibility
      reaction, ABO
    delayed serologic T80.39 ☑
    minor blood group (Duffy) (E) (K(ell)) (Kidd) (Lewis)
      (M) (N) (P) (S) T80.89 ☑
    Rh (factor) (infusion) (transfusion) — *see* Complica-
      tion(s), transfusion, incompatibility reaction,
      Rh (factor)
  inflammatory — *see* Infection
  infusion — *see* Complications, infusion
  inoculation (immune serum) — *see* Complications,
    vaccination
  insulin T38.3- ☑
  involutional psychotic — *see* Disorder, depressive
  leukemoid D72.823
    basophilic D72.823
    lymphocytic D72.823
    monocytic D72.823
    myelocytic D72.823
    neutrophilic D72.823
  LSD (acute)
    due to drug abuse — *see* Abuse, drug, hallucino-
      gen
    due to drug dependence — *see* Dependence, drug,
      hallucinogen
  lumbar puncture G97.1
  manic-depressive — *see* Disorder, bipolar
  neurasthenic F48.8
  neurogenic — *see* Neurosis
  neurotic F48.9
  neurotic-depressive F34.1

Reaction — *continued*
  nitritoid — *see* Crisis, nitritoid
  nonspecific
    to
      cell mediated immunity measurement of gamma interferon antigen response without active tuberculosis R76.12
      QuantiFERON-TB test (QFT) without active tuberculosis R76.12
      tuberculin test (*see also* Reaction, tuberculin skin test) R76.11
  obsessive-compulsive F42.8
  organic, acute or subacute — *see* Delirium
  paranoid (acute) F23
    chronic F22
    senile F03 ☑
  passive dependency F60.7
  phobic F40.9
  post-traumatic stress, uncomplicated Z73.3
  psychogenic F99
  psychoneurotic (*see also* Neurosis)
    compulsive F42.8
    depersonalization F48.1
    depressive F34.1
    hypochondriacal F45.20
    neurasthenic F48.8
    obsessive F42.8
  psychophysiologic — *see* Disorder, somatoform
  psychosomatic — *see* Disorder, somatoform
  psychotic — *see* Psychosis
  scarlet fever toxin — *see* Complications, vaccination
  schizophrenic F23
    acute (brief) (undifferentiated) F23
    latent F21
    undifferentiated (acute) (brief) F23
  serological for syphilis — *see* Serology for syphilis
  serum T80.69
    anaphylactic (immediate) (*see also* Shock, anaphylactic) T80.59 ☑
    specified reaction NEC
      due to
        administration of blood and blood products T80.61 ☑
        immunization T80.62 ☑
        serum specified NEC T80.69 ☑
        vaccination T80.62 ☑
  situational — *see* Disorder, adjustment
  somatization — *see* Disorder, somatoform
  spinal puncture G97.1
  stress (severe) F43.9
    acute (agitation) ("daze") (disorientation) (disturbance of consciousness) (flight reaction) (fugue) F43.0
    specified NEC F43.8
  surgical procedure — *see* Complications, surgical procedure
  tetanus antitoxin — *see* Complications, vaccination
  toxic, to local anesthesia T88.59 ☑
    in labor and delivery O74.4
    in pregnancy O29.3X- ☑
    postpartum, puerperal O89.3
  toxin-antitoxin — *see* Complications, vaccination
  transfusion (blood) (bone marrow) (lymphocytes) (allergic) — *see* Complications, transfusion
  tuberculin skin test, abnormal R76.11
  vaccination (any) — *see* Complications, vaccination
  withdrawing, child or adolescent F93.8
Reactive airway disease — *see* Asthma
Reactive depression — *see* Reaction, depressive
Rearrangement
  chromosomal
    balanced (in) Q95.9
      abnormal individual (autosomal) Q95.2
      non-sex (autosomal) chromosomes Q95.2
      sex/non-sex chromosomes Q95.3
      specified NEC Q95.8
Recalcitrant patient — *see* Noncompliance
Recanalization, thrombus — *see* Thrombosis
Recession, receding
  chamber angle (eye) H21.55- ☑
  chin M26.09
  gingival (postinfective) (postoperative)
    generalized K06.020
      minimal K06.021
      moderate K06.022
      severe K06.023
    localized K06.010
      minimal K06.011

Recession, receding — *continued*
  gingival — *continued*
    localized — *continued*
      moderate K06.012
      severe K06.013
Recklinghausen disease Q85.01
  bones E21.0
Reclus' disease (cystic) — *see* Mastopathy, cystic
Recrudescent typhus (fever) A75.1
Recruitment, auditory H93.21- ☑
Rectalgia K62.89
Rectitis K62.89
Rectocele
  female (without uterine prolapse) N81.6
    with uterine prolapse N81.4
      incomplete N81.2
  in pregnancy — *see* Pregnancy, complicated by, abnormal, pelvic organs or tissues NEC
  male K62.3
Rectosigmoid junction — *see* condition
Rectosigmoiditis K63.89
  ulcerative (chronic) K51.30
    with
      complication K51.319
        abscess K51.314
        fistula K51.313
        obstruction K51.312
        rectal bleeding K51.311
        specified NEC K51.318
Rectourethral — *see* condition
Rectovaginal — *see* condition
Rectovesical — *see* condition
Rectum, rectal — *see* condition
Recurrent — *see* condition
  pregnancy loss — *see* Loss (of), pregnancy, recurrent
Red bugs B88.0
Red tide (*see also* Table of Drugs and Chemicals) T65.82- ☑
Red-cedar lung or pneumonitis J67.8
Reduced
  mobility Z74.09
  ventilatory or vital capacity R94.2
Redundant, redundancy
  anus (congenital) Q43.8
  clitoris N90.89
  colon (congenital) Q43.8
  foreskin (congenital) N47.8
  intestine (congenital) Q43.8
  labia N90.69
  organ or site, congenital NEC — *see* Accessory
  panniculus (abdominal) E65
  prepuce (congenital) N47.8
  pylorus K31.89
  rectum (congenital) Q43.8
  scrotum N50.89
  sigmoid (congenital) Q43.8
  skin L98.7
    and subcutaneous tissue L98.7
    of face L57.4
    eyelids — *see* Blepharochalasis
  stomach K31.89
Reduplication — *see* Duplication
Reflex R29.2
  hyperactive gag J39.2
  pupillary, abnormal — *see* Anomaly, pupil, function
  vasoconstriction I73.9
  vasovagal R55
Reflux K21.9
  acid K21.9
  esophageal K21.9
    with esophagitis K21.0
    newborn P78.83
  gastroesophageal K21.9
    with esophagitis K21.0
  mitral — *see* Insufficiency, mitral
  ureteral — *see* Reflux, vesicoureteral
  vesicoureteral (with scarring) N13.70
    with
      nephropathy N13.729
        with hydroureter N13.739
          bilateral N13.732
          unilateral N13.731
        without hydroureter N13.729
          bilateral N13.722
          unilateral N13.721
      bilateral N13.722
      unilateral N13.721
      pyelonephritis (chronic) N11.0

Reflux — *continued*
  vesicoureteral — *continued*
    without nephropathy N13.71
    congenital Q62.7
Reforming, artificial openings — *see* Attention to, artificial, opening
Refractive error — *see* Disorder, refraction
Refsum's disease or syndrome G60.1
Refusal of
  food, psychogenic F50.89
  treatment (because of) Z53.20
    left against medical advice (AMA) Z53.21
    patient's decision NEC Z53.29
    reasons of belief or group pressure Z53.1
Regional — *see* condition
Regurgitation R11.10
  aortic (valve) — *see* Insufficiency, aortic
  food (*see also* Vomiting)
    with reswallowing — *see* Rumination
    newborn P92.1
  gastric contents — *see* Vomiting
  heart — *see* Endocarditis
  mitral (valve) — *see* Insufficiency, mitral
    congenital Q23.3
  myocardial — *see* Endocarditis
  pulmonary (valve) (heart) I37.1
    congenital Q22.2
    syphilitic A52.03
  tricuspid — *see* Insufficiency, tricuspid
  valve, valvular — *see* Endocarditis
    congenital Q24.8
  vesicoureteral — *see* Reflux, vesicoureteral
Reichmann's disease or syndrome K31.89
Reifenstein syndrome E34.52
Reinsertion
  implantable subdermal contraceptive Z30.46
  intrauterine contraceptive device Z30.433
Reiter's disease, syndrome, or urethritis M02.30
  ankle M02.37- ☑
  elbow M02.32- ☑
  foot joint M02.37- ☑
  hand joint M02.34- ☑
  hip M02.35- ☑
  knee M02.36- ☑
  multiple site M02.39
  shoulder M02.31- ☑
  vertebra M02.38
  wrist M02.33- ☑
Rejection
  food, psychogenic F50.89
  transplant T86.91
    bone T86.830
      marrow T86.01
    cornea T86.840
    heart T86.21
      with lung(s) T86.31
    intestine T86.850
    kidney T86.11
    liver T86.41
    lung(s) T86.810
      with heart T86.31
    organ (immune or nonimmune cause) T86.91
    pancreas T86.890
    skin (allograft) (autograft) T86.820
    specified NEC T86.890
    stem cell (peripheral blood) (umbilical cord) T86.5
Relapsing fever A68.9
  Carter's (Asiatic) A68.1
  Dutton's (West African) A68.1
  Koch's A68.9
  louse-borne (epidemic) A68.0
  Novy's (American) A68.1
  Obermeyers's (European) A68.0
  Spirillum A68.9
  tick-borne (endemic) A68.1
Relationship
  occlusal
    open anterior M26.220
    open posterior M26.221
Relaxation
  anus (sphincter) K62.89
    psychogenic F45.8
  arch (foot) (*see also* Deformity, limb, flat foot)
  back ligaments — *see* Instability, joint, spine
  bladder (sphincter) N31.2
  cardioesophageal K21.9
  cervix — *see* Incompetency, cervix
  diaphragm J98.6

Relaxation — *continued*
- joint (capsule) (ligament) (paralytic) — *see* Flail, joint
  - congenital NEC Q74.8
- lumbosacral (joint) — *see* subcategory M53.2 ☑
- pelvic floor N81.89
- perineum N81.89
- posture R29.3
- rectum (sphincter) K62.89
- sacroiliac (joint) — *see* subcategory M53.2 ☑
- scrotum N50.89
- urethra (sphincter) N36.44
- vesical N31.2

Release from prison, anxiety concerning Z65.2

Remains
- canal of Cloquet Q14.0
- capsule (opaque) Q14.8

Remittent fever (malarial) B54

Remnant
- canal of Cloquet Q14.0
- capsule (opaque) Q14.8
- cervix, cervical stump (acquired) (postoperative) N88.8
- cystic duct, postcholecystectomy K91.5
- fingernail L60.8
  - congenital Q84.6
- meniscus, knee — *see* Derangement, knee, meniscus,
  - specified NEC
- thyroglossal duct Q89.2
- tonsil J35.8
  - infected (chronic) J35.01
- urachus Q64.4

Removal (from) (of)
- artificial
  - arm Z44.00- ☑
    - complete Z44.01- ☑
    - partial Z44.02- ☑
  - eye Z44.2- ☑
  - leg Z44.10- ☑
    - complete Z44.11- ☑
    - partial Z44.12- ☑
- breast implant Z45.81 ☑
- cardiac pulse generator (battery) (end-of-life) Z45.010
- catheter (urinary) (indwelling) Z46.6
  - from artificial opening — *see* Attention to, artificial,
    - opening
  - non-vascular Z46.82
  - vascular NEC Z45.2
- device Z46.9
  - contraceptive Z30.432
    - implantable subdermal Z30.46
  - implanted NEC Z45.89
  - specified NEC Z46.89
- drains Z48.03
- dressing (nonsurgical) Z48.00
  - surgical Z48.01
- external
  - fixation device — *code to* fracture with seventh
    - character D
  - prosthesis, prosthetic device Z44.9
    - breast Z44.3- ☑
    - specified NEC Z44.8
- home in childhood (to foster home or institution)
  - Z62.29
- ileostomy Z43.2
- insulin pump Z46.81
- myringotomy device (stent) (tube) Z45.82
- nervous system device NEC Z46.2
  - brain neuropacemaker Z46.2
  - visual substitution device Z46.2
    - implanted Z45.31
- non-vascular catheter Z46.82
- organ, prophylactic (for neoplasia management) —
  - *see* Prophylactic, organ removal
- orthodontic device Z46.4
- staples Z48.02
- stent
  - ureteral Z46.6
- suture Z48.02
- urinary device Z46.6
- vascular access device or catheter Z45.2

Ren
- arcuatus Q63.1
- mobile, mobilis N28.89
  - congenital Q63.8
- unguliformis Q63.1

Renal — *see* condition

Rendu-Osler-Weber disease or syndrome I78.0

Reninoma D41.0- ☑

Renon-Delille syndrome E23.3

Reovirus, as cause of disease classified elsewhere
B97.5

Repeated falls NEC R29.6

Replaced chromosome by dicentric ring Q93.2

Replacement by artificial or mechanical device or
prosthesis of
- bladder Z96.0
- blood vessel NEC Z95.828
- bone NEC Z96.7
- cochlea Z96.21
- coronary artery Z95.5
- eustachian tube Z96.29
- eye globe Z97.0
- heart Z95.812
  - valve Z95.2
    - prosthetic Z95.2
    - specified NEC Z95.4
    - xenogenic Z95.3
- intestine Z96.89
- joint Z96.60
  - hip — *see* Presence, hip joint implant
  - knee — *see* Presence, knee joint implant
  - specified site NEC Z96.698
- larynx Z96.3
- lens Z96.1
- limb(s) — *see* Presence, artificial, limb
- mandible NEC (for tooth root implant(s)) Z96.5
- organ NEC Z96.89
- peripheral vessel NEC Z95.828
- stapes Z96.29
- teeth Z97.2
- tendon Z96.7
- tissue NEC Z96.89
- tooth root(s) Z96.5
- vessel NEC Z95.828
  - coronary (artery) Z95.5

Request for expert evidence Z04.8

Reserve, decreased or low
- cardiac — *see* Disease, heart
- kidney N28.89

Residual (*see also* condition)
- ovary syndrome N99.83
- state, schizophrenic F20.5
- urine R39.198

Resistance, resistant (to)
- activated protein C D68.51
- complicating pregnancy O26.89 ☑
- insulin E88.81
- organism(s)
  - to
    - drug Z16.30
      - aminoglycosides Z16.29
      - amoxicillin Z16.11
      - ampicillin Z16.11
      - antibiotic(s) Z16.20
        - multiple Z16.24
        - specified NEC Z16.29
      - antifungal Z16.32
      - antimicrobial (single) Z16.30
        - multiple Z16.35
        - specified NEC Z16.39
      - antimycobacterial (single) Z16.341
        - multiple Z16.342
      - antiparasitic Z16.31
      - antiviral Z16.33
      - beta lactam antibiotics Z16.10
        - specified NEC Z16.19
      - cephalosporins Z16.19
      - extended beta lactamase (ESBL) Z16.12
      - fluoroquinolones Z16.23
      - macrolides Z16.29
      - methicillin — *see* MRSA
      - multiple drugs (MDRO)
        - antibiotics Z16.24
        - antimicrobial Z16.35
        - antimycobacterials Z16.342
      - penicillins Z16.11
      - quinine (and related compounds) Z16.31
      - quinolones Z16.23
      - sulfonamides Z16.29
      - tetracyclines Z16.29
      - tuberculostatics (single) Z16.341
        - multiple Z16.342
      - vancomycin Z16.21
        - related antibiotics Z16.22
    - thyroid hormone E07.89

Resorption
- dental (roots) K03.3

Resorption — *continued*
- dental — *continued*
  - alveoli M26.79
  - teeth (external) (internal) (pathological) (roots) K03.3

Respiration
- Cheyne-Stokes R06.3
- decreased due to shock, following injury T79.4 ☑
- disorder of, psychogenic F45.8
- insufficient, or poor R06.89
  - newborn P28.5
- painful R07.1
- sighing, psychogenic F45.8

Respiratory (*see also* condition)
- distress syndrome (newborn) (type I) P22.0
  - type II P22.1
- syncytial virus, as cause of disease classified elsewhere
  - B97.4

Respite care Z75.5

Response (drug)
- photoallergic L56.1
- phototoxic L56.0

Restenosis
- stent
  - vascular
    - end stent
      - adjacent to stent — *see* Arteriosclerosis
      - within the stent
        - coronary T82.855 ☑
        - peripheral T82.856 ☑
    - in stent
      - coronary vessel T82.855 ☑
      - peripheral vessel T82.856 ☑

Restless legs (syndrome) G25.81

Restlessness R45.1

Restoration (of)
- dental
  - aesthetically inadequate or displeasing K08.56
  - defective K08.50
    - specified NEC K08.59
  - failure of marginal integrity K08.51
  - failure of periodontal anatomical intergrity K08.54
- organ continuity from previous sterilization (tuboplas-
  - ty) (vasoplasty) Z31.0
  - aftercare Z31.42
- tooth (existing)
  - contours biologically incompatible with oral health
    - K08.54
  - open margins K08.51
  - overhanging K08.52
  - poor aesthetic K08.56
  - poor gingival margins K08.51
- unsatisfactory, of tooth K08.50
  - specified NEC K08.59

Restorative material (dental)
- allergy to K08.55
- fractured K08.539
  - with loss of material K08.531
  - without loss of material K08.530
- unrepairable overhanging of K08.52

Restriction of housing space Z59.1

Rests, ovarian, in fallopian tube Q50.6

Restzustand (schizophrenic) F20.5

Retained (*see also* Retention)
- cholelithiasis following cholecystectomy K91.86
- foreign body fragments (type of) Z18.9
  - acrylics Z18.2
  - animal quill(s) or spines Z18.31
  - cement Z18.83
  - concrete Z18.83
  - crystalline Z18.83
  - depleted isotope Z18.09
  - depleted uranium Z18.01
  - diethylhexylphthalates Z18.2
  - glass Z18.81
  - isocyanate Z18.2
  - magnetic metal Z18.11
  - metal Z18.10
  - nonmagnectic metal Z18.12
  - nontherapeutic radioactive Z18.09
  - organic NEC Z18.39
  - plastic Z18.2
  - quill(s) (animal) Z18.31
  - radioactive (nontherapeutic) NEC Z18.09
  - specified NEC Z18.89
  - spine(s) (animal) Z18.31
  - stone Z18.83
  - tooth (teeth) Z18.32
  - wood Z18.33

☑ **Additional Character Required** — **Refer to the Tabular List for Character Selection**   ⤳ **Subterms under main terms may continue to next column or page**

Retained — *continued*
- fragments (type of) Z18.9
  - acrylics Z18.2
  - animal quill(s) or spines Z18.31
  - cement Z18.83
  - concrete Z18.83
  - crystalline Z18.83
  - depleted isotope Z18.09
  - depleted uranium Z18.01
  - diethylhexylphthalates Z18.2
  - glass Z18.81
  - isocyanate Z18.2
  - magnetic metal Z18.11
  - metal Z18.10
  - nonmagnectic metal Z18.12
  - nontherapeutic radioactive Z18.09
  - organic NEC Z18.39
  - plastic Z18.2
  - quill(s) (animal) Z18.31
  - radioactive (nontherapeutic) NEC Z18.09
  - specified NEC Z18.89
  - spine(s) (animal) Z18.31
  - stone Z18.83
  - tooth (teeth) Z18.32
  - wood Z18.33
- gallstones, following cholecystectomy K91.86

Retardation
- development, developmental, specific — *see* Disorder, developmental
- endochondral bone growth — *see* Disorder, bone, development or growth
- growth R62.50
  - due to malnutrition E45
- mental — *see* Disability, intellectual
- motor function, specific F82
- physical (child) R62.52
  - due to malnutrition E45
- reading (specific) F81.0
- spelling (specific) (without reading disorder) F81.81

Retching — *see* Vomiting
Retention (*see also* Retained)
- bladder — *see* Retention, urine
- carbon dioxide E87.2
- cholelithiasis following cholecystectomy K91.86
- cyst — *see* Cyst
- dead
  - fetus (at or near term) (mother) O36.4 ☑
    - early fetal death O02.1
  - ovum O02.0
- decidua (fragments) (following delivery) (with hemorrhage) O72.2
  - without hemorrhage O73.1
- deciduous tooth K00.6
- dental root K08.3
- fecal — *see* Constipation
- fetus
  - dead O36.4 ☑
    - early O02.1
- fluid R60.9
- foreign body (*see also* Foreign body, retained)
  - current trauma — *code as* Foreign body, by site or type
- gallstones, following cholecystectomy K91.86
- gastric K31.89
- intrauterine contraceptive device, in pregnancy — *see* Pregnancy, complicated by, retention, intrauterine device
- membranes (complicating delivery) (with hemorrhage) O72.2
  - with abortion — *see* Abortion, by type
  - without hemorrhage O73.1
- meniscus — *see* Derangement, meniscus
- menses N94.89
- milk (puerperal, postpartum) O92.79
- nitrogen, extrarenal R39.2
- ovary syndrome N99.83
- placenta (total) (with hemorrhage) O72.0
  - without hemorrhage O73.0
  - portions or fragments (with hemorrhage) O72.2
    - without hemorrhage O73.1
- products of conception
  - early pregnancy (dead fetus) O02.1
  - following
    - delivery (with hemorrhage) O72.2
      - without hemorrhage O73.1
- secundines (following delivery) (with hemorrhage) O72.0
  - without hemorrhage O73.0

Retention — *continued*
- secundines — *continued*
  - complicating puerperium (delayed hemorrhage) O72.2
  - partial O72.2
    - without hemorrhage O73.1
- smegma, clitoris N90.89
- urine R33.9
  - drug-induced R33.0
  - due to hyperplasia (hypertrophy) of prostate — *see* Hyperplasia, prostate
  - organic R33.8
    - drug-induced R33.0
  - psychogenic F45.8
  - specified NEC R33.8
- water (in tissues) — *see* Edema
Reticulation, dust — *see* Pneumoconiosis
Reticulocytosis R70.1
Reticuloendotheliosis
- acute infantile C96.0
- leukemic C91.4- ☑
- nonlipid C96.0
Reticulohistiocytoma (giant-cell) D76.3
Reticuloid, actinic L57.1
Reticulosis (skin)
- acute of infancy C96.0
- hemophagocytic, familial D76.1
- histiocytic medullary C96.A (*following* C96.6)
- lipomelanotic I89.8
- malignant (midline) C86.0
- polymorphic C83.8- ☑
- Sézary — *see* Sézary disease
Retina, retinal (*see also* condition)
- dark area D49.81
Retinitis (*see also* Inflammation, chorioretinal)
- albuminurica N18.9 [H32]
- diabetic — *see* Diabetes, retinitis
- disciformis — *see* Degeneration, macula
- focal — *see* Inflammation, chorioretinal, focal
- gravidarum — *see* Pregnancy, complicated by, specified pregnancy-related condition NEC
- juxtapapillaris — *see* Inflammation, chorioretinal, focal, juxtapapillary
- luetic — *see* Retinitis, syphilitic
- pigmentosa H35.52
- proliferans — *see* Disorder, globe, degenerative, specified type NEC
- proliferating — *see* Disorder, globe, degenerative, specified type NEC
- renal N18.9 [H32]
- syphilitic (early) (secondary) A51.43
  - central, recurrent A52.71
  - congenital (early) A50.01 [H32]
  - late A52.71
- tuberculous A18.53
Retinoblastoma C69.2- ☑
- differentiated C69.2- ☑
- undifferentiated C69.2- ☑
Retinochoroiditis (*see also* Inflammation, chorioretinal)
- disseminated — *see* Inflammation, chorioretinal, disseminated
  - syphilitic A52.71
- focal — *see* Inflammation, chorioretinal
- juxtapapillaris — *see* Inflammation, chorioretinal, focal, juxtapapillary
Retinopathy (background) H35.00
- arteriosclerotic I70.8 [H35.0-] ☑
- atherosclerotic I70.8 [H35.0-] ☑
- central serous — *see* Chorioretinopathy, central serous
- Coats H35.02- ☑
- diabetic — *see* Diabetes, retinopathy
- exudative H35.02- ☑
- hypertensive H35.03- ☑
- in (due to)
  - diabetes — *see* Diabetes, retinopathy
  - sickle-cell disorders D57.- ☑ [H36]
- of prematurity H35.10- ☑
  - stage 0 H35.11- ☑
  - stage 1 H35.12- ☑
  - stage 2 H35.13- ☑
  - stage 3 H35.14- ☑
  - stage 4 H35.15- ☑
  - stage 5 H35.16- ☑
- pigmentary, congenital — *see* Dystrophy, retina
- proliferative NEC H35.2- ☑
  - diabetic — *see* Diabetes, retinopathy, proliferative
  - sickle-cell D57.- ☑ [H36]

Retinopathy — *continued*
- solar H31.02- ☑
Retinoschisis H33.10- ☑
- congenital Q14.1
- specified type NEC H33.19- ☑
Retortamoniasis A07.8
Retractile testis Q55.22
Retraction
- cervix — *see* Retroversion, uterus
- drum (membrane) — *see* Disorder, tympanic membrane, specified NEC
- finger — *see* Deformity, finger
- lid H02.539
  - left H02.536
    - lower H02.535
    - upper H02.534
  - right H02.533
    - lower H02.532
    - upper H02.531
- lung J98.4
- mediastinum J98.59
- nipple N64.53
  - associated with
    - lactation O92.03
    - pregnancy O92.01- ☑
    - puerperium O92.02
  - congenital Q83.8
- palmar fascia M72.0
- pleura — *see* Pleurisy
- ring, uterus (Bandl's) (pathological) O62.4
- sternum (congenital) Q76.7
  - acquired M95.4
- uterus — *see* Retroversion, uterus
- valve (heart) — *see* Endocarditis
Retrobulbar — *see* condition
Retrocecal — *see* condition
Retrocession — *see* Retroversion
Retrodisplacement — *see* Retroversion
Retroflection, retroflexion — *see* Retroversion
Retrognathia, retrognathism (mandibular) (maxillary) M26.19
Retrograde menstruation N92.5
Retroperineal — *see* condition
Retroperitoneal — *see* condition
Retroperitonitis K68.9
Retropharyngeal — *see* condition
Retroplacental — *see* condition
Retroposition — *see* Retroversion
Retroprosthetic membrane T85.398 ☑
Retrosternal thyroid (congenital) Q89.2
Retroversion, retroverted
- cervix — *see* Retroversion, uterus
- female NEC — *see* Retroversion, uterus
- iris H21.89
- testis (congenital) Q55.29
- uterus (acquired) (acute) (any degree) (asymptomatic) (cervix) (postinfectional) (postpartal, old) N85.4
  - congenital Q51.818
  - in pregnancy O34.53- ☑
Retrovirus, as cause of disease classified elsewhere B97.30
- human
  - immunodeficiency, type 2 (HIV 2) B97.35
  - T-cell lymphotropic
    - type I (HTLV-I) B97.33
    - type II (HTLV-II) B97.34
- lentivirus B97.31
- oncovirus B97.32
- specified NEC B97.39
Retrusion, premaxilla (developmental) M26.09
Rett's disease or syndrome F84.2
Reverse peristalsis R19.2
Reye's syndrome G93.7
Rh (factor)
- hemolytic disease (newborn) P55.0
- incompatibility, immunization or sensitization
  - affecting management of pregnancy NEC O36.09- ☑
    - anti-D antibody O36.01- ☑
  - newborn P55.0
  - transfusion reaction — *see* Complication(s), transfusion, incompatibility reaction, Rh (factor)
- negative mother affecting newborn P55.0
- titer elevated — *see* Complication(s), transfusion, incompatibility reaction, Rh (factor)
- transfusion reaction — *see* Complication(s), transfusion, incompatibility reaction, Rh (factor)

Rhabdomyolysis (idiopathic) NEC M62.82
  traumatic T79.6 ☑
Rhabdomyoma (see also Neoplasm, connective tissue, benign)
  adult — see Neoplasm, connective tissue, benign
  fetal — see Neoplasm, connective tissue, benign
  glycogenic — see Neoplasm, connective tissue, benign
Rhabdomyosarcoma (any type) — see Neoplasm, connective tissue, malignant
Rhabdosarcoma — see Rhabdomyosarcoma
Rhesus (factor) **incompatibility** — see Rh, incompatibility
Rheumatic (acute) (subacute) (chronic)
  adherent pericardium I09.2
  coronary arteritis I01.9
  degeneration, myocardium I09.0
  fever (acute) — see Fever, rheumatic
  heart — see Disease, heart, rheumatic
  myocardial degeneration — see Degeneration, myocardium
  myocarditis (chronic) (inactive) (with chorea) I09.0
    with chorea (acute) (rheumatic) (Sydenham's) I02.0
    active or acute I01.2
  pancarditis, acute I01.8
    with chorea (acute) (rheumatic) Sydenham's) I02.0
  pericarditis (active) (acute) (with effusion) (with pneumonia) I01.0
    with chorea (acute) (rheumatic) (Sydenham's) I02.0
    chronic or inactive I09.2
  pneumonia I00 [J17]
  torticollis M43.6
  typhoid fever A01.09
Rheumatism (articular) (neuralgic) (nonarticular) M79.0
  gout — see Arthritis, rheumatoid
  intercostal, meaning Tietze's disease M94.0
  palindromic (any site) M12.30
    ankle M12.37- ☑
    elbow M12.32- ☑
    foot joint M12.37- ☑
    hand joint M12.34- ☑
    hip M12.35- ☑
    knee M12.36- ☑
    multiple site M12.39
    shoulder M12.31- ☑
    specified joint NEC M12.38
    vertebrae M12.38
    wrist M12.33- ☑
  sciatic M54.4- ☑
Rheumatoid (see also condition)
  arthritis (see also Arthritis, rheumatoid)
    with involvement of organs NEC M05.60
      ankle M05.67- ☑
      elbow M05.62- ☑
      foot joint M05.67- ☑
      hand joint M05.64- ☑
      hip M05.65- ☑
      knee M05.66- ☑
      multiple site M05.69
      shoulder M05.61- ☑
      vertebra — see Spondylitis, ankylosing
      wrist M05.63- ☑
    seronegative — see Arthritis, rheumatoid, seronegative
    seropositive — see Arthritis, rheumatoid, seropositive
  carditis M05.30
    ankle M05.37- ☑
    elbow M05.32- ☑
    foot joint M05.37- ☑
    hand joint M05.34- ☑
    hip M05.35- ☑
    knee M05.36- ☑
    multiple site M05.39
    shoulder M05.31- ☑
    vertebra — see Spondylitis, ankylosing
    wrist M05.33- ☑
  endocarditis — see Rheumatoid, carditis
  lung (disease) M05.10
    ankle M05.17- ☑
    elbow M05.12- ☑
    foot joint M05.17- ☑
    hand joint M05.14- ☑
    hip M05.15- ☑
    knee M05.16- ☑
    multiple site M05.19
    shoulder M05.11- ☑
    vertebra — see Spondylitis, ankylosing

Rheumatoid — continued
  lung — continued
    wrist M05.13- ☑
  myocarditis — see Rheumatoid, carditis
  myopathy M05.40
    ankle M05.47- ☑
    elbow M05.42- ☑
    foot joint M05.47- ☑
    hand joint M05.44- ☑
    hip M05.45- ☑
    knee M05.46- ☑
    multiple site M05.49
    shoulder M05.41- ☑
    vertebra — see Spondylitis, ankylosing
    wrist M05.43- ☑
  pericarditis — see Rheumatoid, carditis
  polyarthritis — see Arthritis, rheumatoid
  polyneuropathy M05.50
    ankle M05.57- ☑
    elbow M05.52- ☑
    foot joint M05.57- ☑
    hand joint M05.54- ☑
    hip M05.55- ☑
    knee M05.56- ☑
    multiple site M05.59
    shoulder M05.51- ☑
    vertebra — see Spondylitis, ankylosing
    wrist M05.53- ☑
  vasculitis M05.20
    ankle M05.27- ☑
    elbow M05.22- ☑
    foot joint M05.27- ☑
    hand joint M05.24- ☑
    hip M05.25- ☑
    knee M05.26- ☑
    multiple site M05.29
    shoulder M05.21- ☑
    vertebra — see Spondylitis, ankylosing
    wrist M05.23- ☑
Rhinitis (atrophic) (catarrhal) (chronic) (croupous) (fibrinous) (granulomatous) (hyperplastic) (hypertrophic) (membranous) (obstructive) (purulent) (suppurative) (ulcerative) J31.0
  with
    sore throat — see Nasopharyngitis
  acute J00
  allergic J30.9
    with asthma J45.909
      with
        exacerbation (acute) J45.901
        status asthmaticus J45.902
    due to
      food J30.5
      pollen J30.1
    nonseasonal J30.89
    perennial J30.89
    seasonal NEC J30.2
    specified NEC J30.89
  infective J00
  pneumococcal J00
  syphilitic A52.73
    congenital A50.05 [J99]
  tuberculous A15.8
  vasomotor J30.0
Rhinoantritis (chronic) — see Sinusitis, maxillary
Rhinodacryolith — see Dacryolith
Rhinolith (nasal sinus) J34.89
Rhinomegaly J34.89
Rhinopharyngitis (acute) (subacute) (see also Nasopharyngitis)
  chronic J31.1
  destructive ulcerating A66.5
  mutilans A66.5
Rhinophyma L71.1
Rhinorrhea J34.89
  cerebrospinal (fluid) G96.0
  paroxysmal — see Rhinitis, allergic
  spasmodic — see Rhinitis, allergic
Rhinosalpingitis — see Salpingitis, eustachian
Rhinoscleroma A48.8
Rhinosporidiosis B48.1
Rhinovirus infection NEC B34.8
Rhizomelic chondrodysplasia punctata E71.540
Rhythm
  atrioventricular nodal I49.8
  disorder I49.9
    coronary sinus I49.8

Rhythm — continued
  disorder — continued
    ectopic I49.8
    nodal I49.8
    escape I49.9
    heart, abnormal I49.9
    idioventricular I44.2
    nodal I49.8
    sleep, inversion G47.2- ☑
      nonorganic origin — see Disorder, sleep, circadian rhythm, psychogenic
Rhytidosis facialis L98.8
Rib (see also condition)
  cervical Q76.5
Riboflavin deficiency E53.0
Rice bodies (see also Loose, body, joint)
  knee M23.4- ☑
Richter syndrome — see Leukemia, chronic lymphocytic, B-cell type
Richter's hernia — see Hernia, abdomen, with obstruction
Ricinism — see Poisoning, food, noxious, plant
Rickets (active) (acute) (adolescent) (chest wall) (congenital) (current) (infantile) (intestinal) E55.0
  adult — see Osteomalacia
  celiac K90.0
  hypophosphatemic with nephrotic-glycosuric dwarfism E72.09
  inactive E64.3
  kidney N25.0
  renal N25.0
  sequelae, any E64.3
  vitamin-D-resistant E83.31 [M90.80]
Rickettsial disease A79.9
  specified type NEC A79.89
Rickettsialpox (Rickettsia akari) A79.1
Rickettsiosis A79.9
  due to
    Ehrlichia sennetsu A79.81
    Rickettsia akari (rickettsialpox) A79.1
  specified type NEC A79.89
  tick-borne A77.9
  vesicular A79.1
Rider's bone — see Ossification, muscle, specified NEC
Ridge, alveolus (see also condition)
  flabby K06.8
Ridged ear, congenital Q17.3
Riedel's
  lobe, liver Q44.7
  struma, thyroiditis or disease E06.5
Rieger's anomaly or syndrome Q13.81
Riehl's melanosis L81.4
Rietti-Greppi-Micheli anemia D56.9
Rieux's hernia — see Hernia, abdomen, specified site NEC
Riga (-Fede) **disease** K14.0
Riggs' disease — see Periodontitis
Right aortic arch Q25.47
Right middle lobe syndrome J98.11
Rigid, rigidity (see also condition)
  abdominal R19.30
    with severe abdominal pain R10.0
    epigastric R19.36
    generalized R19.37
    left lower quadrant R19.34
    left upper quadrant R19.32
    periumbilic R19.35
    right lower quadrant R19.33
    right upper quadrant R19.31
  articular, multiple, congenital Q68.8
  cervix (uteri) in pregnancy — see Pregnancy, complicated by, abnormal, cervix
  hymen (acquired) (congenital) N89.6
  nuchal R29.1
  pelvic floor in pregnancy — see Pregnancy, complicated by, abnormal, pelvic organs or tissues NEC
  perineum or vulva in pregnancy — see Pregnancy, complicated by, abnormal, vulva
  spine — see Dorsopathy, specified NEC
  vagina in pregnancy — see Pregnancy, complicated by, abnormal, vagina
Rigors R68.89
  with fever R50.9
Riley-Day syndrome G90.1
RIND (reversible ischemic neurologic deficit) I63.9
Ring(s)
  aorta (vascular) Q25.45
  Bandl's O62.4

Ring(s) — *continued*
  contraction, complicating delivery O62.4
  esophageal, lower (muscular) K22.2
  Fleischer's (cornea) H18.04- ☑
  hymenal, tight (acquired) (congenital) N89.6
  Kayser-Fleischer (cornea) H18.04- ☑
  retraction, uterus, pathological O62.4
  Schatzki's (esophagus) (lower) K22.2
    congenital Q39.3
  Soemmerring's — *see* Cataract, secondary
  vascular (congenital) Q25.8
    aorta Q25.45
Ringed hair (congenital) Q84.1
Ringworm B35.9
  beard B35.0
  black dot B35.0
  body B35.4
  Burmese B35.5
  corporeal B35.4
  foot B35.3
  groin B35.6
  hand B35.2
  honeycomb B35.0
  nails B35.1
  perianal (area) B35.6
  scalp B35.0
  specified NEC B35.8
  Tokelau B35.5
Rise, venous pressure I87.8
Rising, PSA following treatment for malignant neoplasm of prostate R97.21
Risk
  for
    dental caries Z91.849
      high Z91.843
      low Z91.841
      moderate Z91.842
  suicidal
    meaning personal history of attempted suicide Z91.5
    meaning suicidal ideation — *see* Ideation, suicidal
Ritter's disease L00
Rivalry, sibling Z62.891
Rivalta's disease A42.2
River blindness B73.01
Robert's pelvis Q74.2
  with disproportion (fetopelvic) O33.0
    causing obstructed labor O65.0
Robin (-Pierre) **syndrome** Q87.0
Robinow-Silvermann-Smith syndrome Q87.1
Robinson's (hidrotic) **ectodermal dysplasia or syndrome** Q82.4
Robles' disease B73.01
Rocky Mountain (spotted) **fever** A77.0
Roetheln — *see* Rubella
Roger's disease Q21.0
Rokitansky-Aschoff sinuses (gallbladder) K82.8
Rolando's fracture (displaced) S62.22- ☑
  nondisplaced S62.22- ☑
Romano-Ward (prolonged QT interval) **syndrome** I45.81
Romberg's disease or syndrome G51.8
Roof, mouth — *see* condition
Rosacea L71.9
  acne L71.9
  keratitis L71.8
  specified NEC L71.8
Rosary, rachitic E55.0
Rose
  cold J30.1
  fever J30.1
  rash R21
    epidemic B06.9
Rosenbach's erysipeloid A26.0
Rosenthal's disease or syndrome D68.1
Roseola B09
  infantum B08.20
    due to human herpesvirus 6 B08.21
    due to human herpesvirus 7 B08.22
Ross River disease or fever B33.1
Rossbach's disease K31.89
  psychogenic F45.8
Rostan's asthma (cardiac) — *see* Failure, ventricular, left
Rotation
  anomalous, incomplete or insufficient, intestine Q43.3
  cecum (congenital) Q43.3
  colon (congenital) Q43.3

Rotation — *continued*
  spine, incomplete or insufficient — *see* Dorsopathy, deforming, specified NEC
  tooth, teeth, fully erupted M26.35
  vertebra, incomplete or insufficient — *see* Dorsopathy, deforming, specified NEC
Rotes Quérol disease or syndrome — *see* Hyperostosis, ankylosing
Roth (-Bernhardt) **disease or syndrome** — *see* Meralgia paraesthetica
Rothmund (-Thomson) **syndrome** Q82.8
Rotor's disease or syndrome E80.6
Round
  back (with wedging of vertebrae) — *see* Kyphosis
    sequelae (late effect) of rickets E64.3
  worms (large) (infestation) NEC B82.0
    Ascariasis (*see also* Ascariasis) B77.9
Roussy-Lévy syndrome G60.0
Rubella (German measles) B06.9
  complication NEC B06.09
    neurological B06.00
  congenital P35.0
  contact Z20.4
  exposure to Z20.4
  maternal
    care for (suspected) damage to fetus O35.3 ☑
      manifest rubella in infant P35.0
    suspected damage to fetus affecting management of pregnancy O35.3 ☑
  specified complications NEC B06.89
Rubeola (meaning measles) — *see* Measles
  meaning rubella — *see* Rubella
Rubeosis, iris — *see* Disorder, iris, vascular
Rubinstein-Taybi syndrome Q87.2
Rudimentary (congenital) (*see also* Agenesis)
  arm — *see* Defect, reduction, upper limb
  bone Q79.9
  cervix uteri Q51.828
  eye Q11.2
  lobule of ear Q17.3
  patella Q74.1
  respiratory organs in thoracopagus Q89.4
  tracheal bronchus Q32.4
  uterus Q51.818
    in male Q56.1
  vagina Q52.0
Ruled out condition — *see* Observation, suspected
Rumination R11.10
  with nausea R11.2
  disorder of infancy F98.21
  neurotic F42.8
  newborn P92.1
  obsessional F42.8
  psychogenic F42.8
Runeberg's disease D51.0
Runny nose R09.89
Rupia (syphilitic) A51.39
  congenital A50.06
  tertiary A52.79
Rupture, ruptured
  abscess (spontaneous) — *code by* site under Abscess
  aneurysm — *see* Aneurysm
  anus (sphincter) — *see* Laceration, anus
  aorta, aortic I71.8
    abdominal I71.3
    arch I71.1
    ascending I71.1
    descending I71.8
      abdominal I71.3
      thoracic I71.1
    syphilitic A52.01
    thoracoabdominal I71.5
    thorax, thoracic I71.1
    transverse I71.1
    traumatic — *see* Injury, aorta, laceration, major
    valve or cusp (*see also* Endocarditis, aortic) I35.8
  appendix (with peritonitis) K35.2
    with localized peritonitis K35.3
  arteriovenous fistula, brain I60.8
  artery I77.2
    brain — *see* Hemorrhage, intracranial, intracerebral
    coronary — *see* Infarct, myocardium
    heart — *see* Infarct, myocardium
    pulmonary I28.8
    traumatic (complication) — *see* Injury, blood vessel
  bile duct (common) (hepatic) K83.2
    cystic K82.2

Rupture, ruptured — *continued*
  bladder (sphincter) (nontraumatic) (spontaneous) N32.89
    following ectopic or molar pregnancy O08.6
    obstetrical trauma O71.5
    traumatic S37.29 ☑
  blood vessel (*see also* Hemorrhage)
    brain — *see* Hemorrhage, intracranial, intracerebral
    heart — *see* Infarct, myocardium
    traumatic (complication) — *see* Injury, blood vessel, laceration, major, by site
  bone — *see* Fracture
  bowel (nontraumatic) K63.1
  brain
    aneurysm (congenital) (*see also* Hemorrhage, intracranial, subarachnoid)
      syphilitic A52.05
    hemorrhagic — *see* Hemorrhage, intracranial, intracerebral
  capillaries I78.8
  cardiac (auricle) (ventricle) (wall) I23.3
    with hemopericardium I23.0
    infectional I40.9
    traumatic — *see* Injury, heart
  cartilage (articular) (current) (*see also* Sprain)
    knee S83.3- ☑
    semilunar — *see* Tear, meniscus
  cecum (with peritonitis) K65.0
    with peritoneal abscess K35.3
    traumatic S36.598 ☑
  celiac artery, traumatic — *see* Injury, blood vessel, celiac artery, laceration, major
  cerebral aneurysm (congenital) (*see* Hemorrhage, intracranial, subarachnoid)
  cervix (uteri)
    with ectopic or molar pregnancy O08.6
    following ectopic or molar pregnancy O08.6
    obstetrical trauma O71.3
    traumatic S37.69 ☑
  chordae tendineae NEC I51.1
    concurrent with acute myocardial infarction — *see* Infarct, myocardium
    following acute myocardial infarction (current complication) I23.4
  choroid (direct) (indirect) (traumatic) H31.32- ☑
  circle of Willis I60.6
  colon (nontraumatic) K63.1
    traumatic — *see* Injury, intestine, large
  cornea (traumatic) — *see* Injury, eye, laceration
  coronary (artery) (thrombotic) — *see* Infarct, myocardium
  corpus luteum (infected) (ovary) N83.1- ☑
  cyst — *see* Cyst
  cystic duct K82.2
  Descemet's membrane — *see* Change, corneal membrane, Descemet's, rupture
    traumatic — *see* Injury, eye, laceration
  diaphragm, traumatic — *see* Injury, intrathoracic, diaphragm
  disc — *see* Rupture, intervertebral disc
  diverticulum (intestine) K57.80
    with bleeding K57.81
    bladder N32.3
    large intestine K57.20
      with
        bleeding K57.21
        small intestine K57.40
          with bleeding K57.41
    small intestine K57.00
      with
        bleeding K57.01
        large intestine K57.40
          with bleeding K57.41
  duodenal stump K31.89
  ear drum (nontraumatic) (*see also* Perforation, tympanum)
    traumatic S09.2- ☑
      due to blast injury — *see* Injury, blast, ear
  esophagus K22.3
  eye (without prolapse or loss of intraocular tissue) — *see* Injury, eye, laceration
  fallopian tube NEC (nonobstetric) (nontraumatic) N83.8
    due to pregnancy O00.10- ☑
      with intrauterine pregnancy O00.11- ☑
  fontanel P13.1
  gallbladder K82.2
    traumatic S36.128 ☑

Rupture, ruptured — *continued*
  gastric (*see also* Rupture, stomach)
    vessel K92.2
  globe (eye) (traumatic) — *see* Injury, eye, laceration
  graafian follicle (hematoma) N83.0- ☑
  heart — *see* Rupture, cardiac
  hymen (nontraumatic) (nonintentional) N89.8
  internal organ, traumatic — *see* Injury, by site
  intervertebral disc — *see* Displacement, intervertebral
      disc
    traumatic — *see* Rupture, traumatic, intervertebral
        disc
  intestine NEC (nontraumatic) K63.1
    traumatic — *see* Injury, intestine
  iris (*see also* Abnormality, pupillary)
    traumatic — *see* Injury, eye, laceration
  joint capsule, traumatic — *see* Sprain
  kidney (traumatic) S37.06- ☑
    birth injury P15.8
    nontraumatic N28.89
  lacrimal duct (traumatic) — *see* Injury, eye, specified
      site NEC
  lens (cataract) (traumatic) — *see* Cataract, traumatic
  ligament, traumatic — *see* Rupture, traumatic, liga-
      ment, by site
  liver S36.116 ☑
    birth injury P15.0
  lymphatic vessel I89.8
  marginal sinus (placental) (with hemorrhage) — *see*
      Hemorrhage, antepartum, specified cause NEC
  membrana tympani (nontraumatic) — *see* Perforation,
      tympanum
  membranes (spontaneous)
    artificial
      delayed delivery following O75.5
    delayed delivery following — *see* Pregnancy,
        complicated by, premature rupture of
        membranes
  meningeal artery I60.8
  meniscus (knee) (*see also* Tear, meniscus)
    old — *see* Derangement, meniscus
    site other than knee — *code as* Sprain
  mesenteric artery, traumatic — *see* Injury, mesenteric,
      artery, laceration, major
  mesentery (nontraumatic) K66.8
    traumatic — *see* Injury, intra-abdominal, specified,
        site NEC
  mitral (valve) I34.8
  muscle (traumatic) (*see also* Strain)
    diastasis — *see* Diastasis, muscle
    nontraumatic M62.10
      ankle M62.17- ☑
      foot M62.17- ☑
      forearm M62.13- ☑
      hand M62.14- ☑
      lower leg M62.16- ☑
      pelvic region M62.15- ☑
      shoulder region M62.11- ☑
      specified site NEC M62.18
      thigh M62.15- ☑
      upper arm M62.12- ☑
    traumatic — *see* Strain, by site
  musculotendinous junction NEC, nontraumatic — *see*
      Rupture, tendon, spontaneous
  mycotic aneurysm causing cerebral hemorrhage —
      see Hemorrhage, intracranial, subarachnoid
  myocardium, myocardial — *see* Rupture, cardiac
    traumatic — *see* Injury, heart
  nontraumatic, meaning hernia — *see* Hernia
  obstructed — *see* Hernia, by site, obstructed
  operation wound — *see* Disruption, wound, operation
  ovary, ovarian N83.8
    corpus luteum cyst N83.1- ☑
    follicle (graafian) N83.0- ☑
  oviduct (nonobstetric) (nontraumatic) N83.8
    due to pregnancy O00.10- ☑
      with intrauterine pregnancy O00.11- ☑
  pancreas (nontraumatic) K86.89
    traumatic S36.299 ☑
  papillary muscle NEC I51.2
    following acute myocardial infarction (current
        complication) I23.5
  pelvic
    floor, complicating delivery O70.1
    organ NEC, obstetrical trauma O71.5
  perineum (nonobstetric) (nontraumatic) N90.89

Rupture, ruptured — *continued*
  perineum — *continued*
    complicating delivery — *see* Delivery, complicated,
        by, laceration, anus (sphincter)
  postoperative wound — *see* Disruption, wound, oper-
      ation
  prostate (traumatic) S37.828 ☑
  pulmonary
    artery I28.8
    valve (heart) I37.8
    vein I28.8
    vessel I28.8
  pus tube — *see* Salpingitis
  pyosalpinx — *see* Salpingitis
  rectum (nontraumatic) K63.1
    traumatic S36.69 ☑
  retina, retinal (traumatic) (without detachment) (*see
      also* Break, retina)
    with detachment — *see* Detachment, retina, with
        retinal, break
  rotator cuff (nontraumatic) M75.10- ☑
    complete M75.12- ☑
    incomplete M75.11- ☑
  sclera — *see* Injury, eye, laceration
  sigmoid (nontraumatic) K63.1
    traumatic S36.593 ☑
  spinal cord (*see also* Injury, spinal cord, by region)
    due to injury at birth P11.5
    newborn (birth injury) P11.5
  spleen (traumatic) S36.09 ☑
    birth injury P15.1
    congenital (birth injury) P15.1
    due to P. vivax malaria B51.0
    nontraumatic D73.5
    spontaneous D73.5
  splenic vein R58
    traumatic — *see* Injury, blood vessel, splenic vein
  stomach (nontraumatic) (spontaneous) K31.89
    traumatic S36.39 ☑
  supraspinatus (complete) (incomplete) (nontraumatic)
      — *see* Tear, rotator cuff
  symphysis pubis
    obstetric O71.6
    traumatic S33.4 ☑
  synovium (cyst) M66.10
    ankle M66.17- ☑
    elbow M66.12- ☑
    finger M66.14- ☑
    foot M66.17- ☑
    forearm M66.13- ☑
    hand M66.14- ☑
    pelvic region M66.15- ☑
    shoulder region M66.11- ☑
    specified site NEC M66.18
    thigh M66.15- ☑
    toe M66.17- ☑
    upper arm M66.12- ☑
    wrist M66.13- ☑
  tendon (traumatic) — *see* Strain
    nontraumatic (spontaneous) M66.9
      ankle M66.87- ☑
      extensor M66.20
        ankle M66.27- ☑
        foot M66.27- ☑
        forearm M66.23- ☑
        hand M66.24- ☑
        lower leg M66.26- ☑
        multiple sites M66.29
        pelvic region M66.25- ☑
        shoulder region M66.21- ☑
        specified site NEC M66.28
        thigh M66.25- ☑
        upper arm M66.22- ☑
      flexor M66.30
        ankle M66.37- ☑
        foot M66.37- ☑
        forearm M66.33- ☑
        hand M66.34- ☑
        lower leg M66.36- ☑
        multiple sites M66.39
        pelvic region M66.35- ☑
        shoulder region M66.31- ☑
        specified site NEC M66.38
        thigh M66.35- ☑
        upper arm M66.32- ☑
      foot M66.87- ☑
      forearm M66.83- ☑

Rupture, ruptured — *continued*
  tendon — *see* Strain — *continued*
    nontraumatic — *continued*
      hand M66.84- ☑
      lower leg M66.86- ☑
      multiple sites M66.89
      pelvic region M66.85- ☑
      shoulder region M66.81- ☑
      specified
        site NEC M66.88
        tendon M66.80
      thigh M66.85- ☑
      upper arm M66.82- ☑
  thoracic duct I89.8
  tonsil J35.8
  traumatic
    aorta — *see* Injury, aorta, laceration, major
    diaphragm — *see* Injury, intrathoracic, diaphragm
    external site — *see* Wound, open, by site
    eye — *see* Injury, eye, laceration
    internal organ — *see* Injury, by site
    intervertebral disc
      cervical S13.0 ☑
      lumbar S33.0 ☑
      thoracic S23.0 ☑
    kidney S37.06- ☑
    ligament (*see also* Sprain)
      ankle — *see* Sprain, ankle
      carpus — *see* Rupture, traumatic, ligament,
          wrist
      collateral (hand) — *see* Rupture, traumatic,
          ligament, finger, collateral
      finger (metacarpophalangeal) (interphalangeal)
          S63.40- ☑
        collateral S63.41- ☑
          index S63.41- ☑
          little S63.41- ☑
          middle S63.41- ☑
          ring S63.41- ☑
        index S63.40- ☑
        little S63.40- ☑
        middle S63.40- ☑
        palmar S63.42- ☑
          index S63.42- ☑
          little S63.42- ☑
          middle S63.42- ☑
          ring S63.42- ☑
        ring S63.40- ☑
        specified site NEC S63.499 ☑
          index S63.49- ☑
          little S63.49- ☑
          middle S63.49- ☑
          ring S63.49- ☑
        volar plate S63.43- ☑
          index S63.43- ☑
          little S63.43- ☑
          middle S63.43- ☑
          ring S63.43- ☑
      foot — *see* Sprain, foot
      radial collateral S53.2- ☑
      radiocarpal — *see* Rupture, traumatic, ligament,
          wrist, radiocarpal
      ulnar collateral S53.3- ☑
      ulnocarpal — *see* Rupture, traumatic, ligament,
          wrist, ulnocarpal
      wrist S63.30- ☑
        collateral S63.31- ☑
        radiocarpal S63.32- ☑
        specified site NEC S63.39- ☑
        ulnocarpal (palmar) S63.33- ☑
    liver S36.116 ☑
    membrana tympani — *see* Rupture, ear drum,
        traumatic
    muscle or tendon — *see* Strain
    myocardium — *see* Injury, heart
    pancreas S36.299 ☑
    rectum S36.69 ☑
    sigmoid S36.593 ☑
    spleen S36.09 ☑
    stomach S36.39 ☑
    symphysis pubis S33.4 ☑
    tympanum, tympanic (membrane) — *see* Rupture,
        ear drum, traumatic
    ureter S37.19 ☑
    uterus S37.69 ☑
    vagina — *see* Injury, vagina

Rupture, ruptured — *continued*
  traumatic — *continued*
    vena cava — *see* Injury, vena cava, laceration, major
    tricuspid (heart) (valve) I07.8
    tube, tubal (nonobstetric) (nontraumatic) N83.8
      abscess — *see* Salpingitis
      due to pregnancy O00.10- ☑
        with intrauterine pregnancy O00.11- ☑
    tympanum, tympanic (membrane) (nontraumatic)
        (*see also* Perforation, tympanic membrane)
        H72.9- ☑
      traumatic — *see* Rupture, ear drum, traumatic
    umbilical cord, complicating delivery O69.89 ☑
    ureter (traumatic) S37.19 ☑
      nontraumatic N28.89
    urethra (nontraumatic) N36.8
      with ectopic or molar pregnancy O08.6
      following ectopic or molar pregnancy O08.6
      obstetrical trauma O71.5
      traumatic S37.39 ☑
    uterosacral ligament (nonobstetric) (nontraumatic)
        N83.8
    uterus (traumatic) S37.69 ☑
      before labor O71.0- ☑
      during or after labor O71.1
      nonpuerperal, nontraumatic N85.8
      pregnant (during labor) O71.1
        before labor O71.0- ☑
    vagina — *see* Injury, vagina
    valve, valvular (heart) — *see* Endocarditis
    varicose vein — *see* Varix
    varix — *see* Varix
    vena cava R58
      traumatic — *see* Injury, vena cava, laceration, major
    vesical (urinary) N32.89
    vessel (blood) R58
      pulmonary I28.8
      traumatic — *see* Injury, blood vessel
    viscus R19.8
    vulva complicating delivery O70.0
Russell-Silver syndrome Q87.1
Russian spring-summer type encephalitis A84.0
Rust's disease (tuberculous cervical spondylitis) A18.01
Ruvalcaba-Myhre-Smith syndrome E71.440
Rytand-Lipsitch syndrome I44.2

S

Saber, sabre shin or tibia (syphilitic) A50.56 [M90.8-] ☑
Sac lacrimal — *see* condition
Saccharomyces infection B37.9
Saccharopinuria E72.3
Saccular — *see* condition
Sacculation
  aorta (nonsyphilitic) — *see* Aneurysm, aorta
  bladder N32.3
  intralaryngeal (congenital) (ventricular) Q31.3
  larynx (congenital) (ventricular) Q31.3
  organ or site, congenital — *see* Distortion
  pregnant uterus — *see* Pregnancy, complicated by, abnormal, uterus
  ureter N28.89
  urethra N36.1
  vesical N32.3
Sachs' amaurotic familial idiocy or disease E75.02
Sachs-Tay disease E75.02
Sacks-Libman disease M32.11
Sacralgia M53.3
Sacralization Q76.49
Sacrodynia M53.3
Sacroiliac joint — *see* condition
Sacroiliitis NEC M46.1
Sacrum — *see* condition
Saddle
  back — *see* Lordosis
  embolus
    abdominal aorta I74.01
    pulmonary artery I26.92
      with acute cor pulmonale I26.02
  injury — *code to* condition
  nose M95.0
    due to syphilis A50.57
Sadism (sexual) F65.52
Sadness, postpartal O90.6
Sadomasochism F65.50
Saemisch's ulcer (cornea) — *see* Ulcer, cornea, central

Sagging
  skin and subcutaneous tissue (following bariatric surgery weight loss) (following dietary weight loss) L98.7
Sahib disease B55.0
Sailors' skin L57.8
Saint
  Anthony's fire — *see* Erysipelas
  triad — *see* Hernia, diaphragm
  Vitus' dance — *see* Chorea, Sydenham's
Salaam
  attack(s) — *see* Epilepsy, spasms
  tic R25.8
Salicylism
  abuse F55.8
  overdose or wrong substance given — *see* Table of Drugs and Chemicals, by drug, poisoning
Salivary duct or gland — *see* condition
Salivation, excessive K11.7
Salmonella — *see* Infection, Salmonella
Salmonellosis A02.0
Salpingitis (catarrhal) (fallopian tube) (nodular) (pseudofollicular) (purulent) (septic) N70.91
  with oophoritis N70.93
  acute N70.01
    with oophoritis N70.03
  chlamydial A56.11
  chronic N70.11
    with oophoritis N70.13
  complicating abortion — *see* Abortion, by type, complicated by, salpingitis
  ear — *see* Salpingitis, eustachian
  eustachian (tube) H68.00- ☑
    acute H68.01- ☑
    chronic H68.02- ☑
  follicularis N70.11
    with oophoritis N70.13
  gonococcal (acute) (chronic) A54.24
  interstitial, chronic N70.11
    with oophoritis N70.13
  isthmica nodosa N70.11
    with oophoritis N70.13
  specific (gonococcal) (acute) (chronic) A54.24
  tuberculous (acute) (chronic) A18.17
  venereal (gonococcal) (acute) (chronic) A54.24
Salpingocele N83.4- ☑
Salpingo-oophoritis (catarrhal) (purulent) (ruptured) (septic) (suppurative) N70.93
  acute N70.03
    with ectopic or molar pregnancy O08.0
      following ectopic or molar pregnancy O08.0
      gonococcal A54.24
  chronic N70.13
  following ectopic or molar pregnancy O08.0
  gonococcal (acute) (chronic) A54.24
  puerperal O86.19
  specific (gonococcal) (acute) (chronic) A54.24
  subacute N70.03
  tuberculous (acute) (chronic) A18.17
  venereal (gonococcal) (acute) (chronic) A54.24
Salpingo-ovaritis — *see* Salpingo-oophoritis
Salpingoperitonitis — *see* Salpingo-oophoritis
Salzmann's nodular dystrophy — *see* Degeneration, cornea, nodular
Sampson's cyst or tumor N80.1
San Joaquin (Valley) **fever** B38.0
Sandblaster's asthma, lung or pneumoconiosis J62.8
Sander's disease (paranoia) F22
Sandfly fever A93.1
Sandhoff's disease E75.01
Sanfilippo (Type B) (Type C) (Type D) **syndrome** E76.22
Sanger-Brown ataxia G11.2
Sao Paulo fever or typhus A77.0
Saponification, mesenteric K65.8
Sarcocele (benign)
  syphilitic A52.76
    congenital A50.59
Sarcocystosis A07.8
Sarcoepiplocele — *see* Hernia
Sarcoepiplomphalocele Q79.2
Sarcoid (*see also* Sarcoidosis)
  arthropathy D86.86
  Boeck's D86.9
  Darier-Roussy D86.3
  iridocyclitis D86.83
  meningitis D86.81
  myocarditis D86.85

Sarcoid — *continued*
  myositis D86.87
  pyelonephritis D86.84
  Spiegler-Fendt L08.89
Sarcoidosis D86.9
  with
    cranial nerve palsies D86.82
    hepatic granuloma D86.89
    polyarthritis D86.86
    tubulo-interstitial nephropathy D86.84
  combined sites NEC D86.89
  lung D86.0
    and lymph nodes D86.2
  lymph nodes D86.1
    and lung D86.2
  meninges D86.81
  skin D86.3
  specified type NEC D86.89
Sarcoma (of) (*see also* Neoplasm, connective tissue, malignant)
  alveolar soft part — *see* Neoplasm, connective tissue, malignant
  ameloblastic C41.1
    upper jaw (bone) C41.0
  botryoid — *see* Neoplasm, connective tissue, malignant
  botryoides — *see* Neoplasm, connective tissue, malignant
  cerebellar C71.6
    circumscribed (arachnoidal) C71.6
  circumscribed (arachnoidal) cerebellar C71.6
  clear cell (*see also* Neoplasm, connective tissue, malignant)
    kidney C64.- ☑
  dendritic cells (accessory cells) C96.4
  embryonal — *see* Neoplasm, connective tissue, malignant
  endometrial (stromal) C54.1
    isthmus C54.0
  epithelioid (cell) — *see* Neoplasm, connective tissue, malignant
  Ewing's — *see* Neoplasm, bone, malignant
  follicular dendritic cell C96.4
  germinoblastic (diffuse) — *see* Lymphoma, diffuse large cell
    follicular — *see* Lymphoma, follicular, specified NEC
  giant cell (except of bone) (*see also* Neoplasm, connective tissue, malignant)
    bone — *see* Neoplasm, bone, malignant
  glomoid — *see* Neoplasm, connective tissue, malignant
  granulocytic C92.3- ☑
  hemangioendothelial — *see* Neoplasm, connective tissue, malignant
  hemorrhagic, multiple — *see* Sarcoma, Kaposi's
  histiocytic C96.A (*following* C96.6)
  Hodgkin — *see* Lymphoma, Hodgkin
  immunoblastic (diffuse) — *see* Lymphoma, diffuse large cell
  interdigitating dendritic cell C96.4
  Kaposi's
    colon C46.4
    connective tissue C46.1
    gastrointestinal organ C46.4
    lung C46.5- ☑
    lymph node(s) C46.3
    palate (hard) (soft) C46.2
    rectum C46.4
    skin C46.0
    specified site NEC C46.7
    stomach C46.4
    unspecified site C46.9
  Kupffer cell C22.3
  Langerhans cell C96.4
  leptomeningeal — *see* Neoplasm, meninges, malignant
  liver NEC C22.4
  lymphangioendothelial — *see* Neoplasm, connective tissue, malignant
  lymphoblastic — *see* Lymphoma, lymphoblastic (diffuse)
  lymphocytic — *see* Lymphoma, small cell B-cell
  mast cell C96.22
  melanotic — *see* Melanoma
  meningeal — *see* Neoplasm, meninges, malignant
  meningothelial — *see* Neoplasm, meninges, malignant

Sarcoma — *continued*
  mesenchymal (*see also* Neoplasm, connective tissue, malignant)
    mixed — *see* Neoplasm, connective tissue, malignant
  mesothelial — *see* Mesothelioma
  monstrocellular
    specified site — *see* Neoplasm, malignant, by site
    unspecified site C71.9
  myeloid C92.3- ☑
  neurogenic — *see* Neoplasm, nerve, malignant
  odontogenic C41.1
    upper jaw (bone) C41.Ø
  osteoblastic — *see* Neoplasm, bone, malignant
  osteogenic (*see also* Neoplasm, bone, malignant)
    juxtacortical — *see* Neoplasm, bone, malignant
    periosteal — *see* Neoplasm, bone, malignant
  periosteal (*see also* Neoplasm, bone, malignant)
    osteogenic — *see* Neoplasm, bone, malignant
  pleomorphic cell — *see* Neoplasm, connective tissue, malignant
  reticulum cell (diffuse) — *see* Lymphoma, diffuse large cell
    nodular — *see* Lymphoma, follicular
    pleomorphic cell type — *see* Lymphoma, diffuse large cell
  rhabdoid — *see* Neoplasm, malignant, by site
  round cell — *see* Neoplasm, connective tissue, malignant
  small cell — *see* Neoplasm, connective tissue, malignant
  soft tissue — *see* Neoplasm, connective tissue, malignant
  spindle cell — *see* Neoplasm, connective tissue, malignant
  stromal (endometrial) C54.1
    isthmus C54.Ø
  synovial (*see also* Neoplasm, connective tissue, malignant)
    biphasic — *see* Neoplasm, connective tissue, malignant
    epithelioid cell — *see* Neoplasm, connective tissue, malignant
    spindle cell — *see* Neoplasm, connective tissue, malignant
Sarcomatosis
  meningeal — *see* Neoplasm, meninges, malignant
  specified site NEC — *see* Neoplasm, connective tissue, malignant
  unspecified site C8Ø.1
Sarcopenia (age-related) M62.84
Sarcosinemia E72.59
Sarcosporidiosis (intestinal) AØ7.8
Satiety, early R68.81
Saturnine — *see* condition
Saturnism
  overdose or wrong substance given or taken — *see* Table of Drugs and Chemicals, by drug, poisoning
Satyriasis F52.8
Sauriasis — *see* Ichthyosis
SBE (subacute bacterial endocarditis) I33.Ø
Scabies (any site) B86
Scabs R23.4
Scaglietti-Dagnini syndrome E22.Ø
Scald — *see* Burn
Scalenus anticus (anterior) **syndrome** G54.Ø
Scales R23.4
Scaling, skin R23.4
Scalp — *see* condition
Scapegoating affecting child Z62.3
Scaphocephaly Q75.Ø
Scapulalgia M89.8X1
Scapulohumeral myopathy G71.Ø
Scar, scarring (*see also* Cicatrix) L9Ø.5
  adherent L9Ø.5
  atrophic L9Ø.5
  cervix
    in pregnancy or childbirth — *see* Pregnancy, complicated by, abnormal cervix
  cheloid L91.Ø
  chorioretinal H31.ØØ- ☑
    posterior pole macula H31.Ø1- ☑
    postsurgical H59.81- ☑
    solar retinopathy H31.Ø2- ☑
    specified type NEC H31.Ø9- ☑
  choroid — *see* Scar, chorioretinal

Scar, scarring — *continued*
  conjunctiva H11.24- ☑
  cornea H17.9
    xerophthalmic (*see also* Opacity, cornea)
      vitamin A deficiency E5Ø.6
  duodenum, obstructive K31.5
  hypertrophic L91.Ø
  keloid L91.Ø
  labia N9Ø.89
  lung (base) J98.4
  macula — *see* Scar, chorioretinal, posterior pole
  muscle M62.89
  myocardium, myocardial I25.2
  painful L9Ø.5
  posterior pole (eye) — *see* Scar, chorioretinal, posterior pole
  retina — *see* Scar, chorioretinal
  trachea J39.8
  transmural uterine, in pregnancy O34.29
  uterus N85.8
    in pregnancy O34.29
  vagina N89.8
    postoperative N99.2
  vulva N9Ø.89
Scarabiasis B88.2
Scarlatina (anginosa) (maligna) A38.9
  myocarditis (acute) A38.1
    old — *see* Myocarditis
  otitis media A38.Ø
  ulcerosa A38.8
Scarlet fever (albuminuria) (angina) A38.9
Schamberg's disease (progressive pigmentary dermatosis) L81.7
Schatzki's ring (acquired) (esophagus) (lower) K22.2
  congenital Q39.3
Schaufenster krankheit I2Ø.8
Schaumann's
  benign lymphogranulomatosis D86.1
  disease or syndrome — *see* Sarcoidosis
Scheie's syndrome E76.Ø3
Schenck's disease B42.1
Scheuermann's disease or osteochondrosis — *see* Osteochondrosis, juvenile, spine
Schilder (-Flatau) **disease** G37.Ø
Schilling-type monocytic leukemia C93.Ø- ☑
Schimmelbusch's disease, cystic mastitis, or hyperplasia — *see* Mastopathy, cystic
Schistosoma infestation — *see* Infestation, Schistosoma
Schistosomiasis B65.9
  with muscle disorder B65.9 [M63.8Ø]
    ankle B65.9 [M63.87-] ☑
    foot B65.9 [M63.87-] ☑
    forearm B65.9 [M63.83-] ☑
    hand B65.9 [M63.84-] ☑
    lower leg B65.9 [M63.86-] ☑
    multiple sites B65.9 [M63.89]
    pelvic region B65.9 [M63.85-] ☑
    shoulder region B65.9 [M63.81-] ☑
    specified site NEC B65.9 [M63.88]
    thigh B65.9 [M63.85-] ☑
    upper arm B65.9 [M63.82-] ☑
  Asiatic B65.2
  bladder B65.Ø
  chestermani B65.8
  colon B65.1
  cutaneous B65.3
  due to
    S. haematobium B65.Ø
    S. japonicum B65.2
    S. mansoni B65.1
    S. mattheii B65.8
  Eastern B65.2
  genitourinary tract B65.Ø
  intestinal B65.1
  lung NEC B65.9 [J99]
    pneumonia B65.9 [J17]
  Manson's (intestinal) B65.1
  oriental B65.2
  pulmonary NEC B65.9 [J99]
    pneumonia B65.9
  Schistosoma
    haematobium B65.Ø
    japonicum B65.2
    mansoni B65.1
  specified type NEC B65.8
  urinary B65.Ø
  vesical B65.Ø
Schizencephaly QØ4.6

Schizoaffective psychosis F25.9
Schizodontia KØØ.2
Schizoid personality F6Ø.1
Schizophrenia, schizophrenic F2Ø.9
  acute (brief) (undifferentiated) F23
  atypical (form) F2Ø.3
  borderline F21
  catalepsy F2Ø.2
  catatonic (type) (excited) (withdrawn) F2Ø.2
  cenesthopathic, cenesthesiopathic F2Ø.89
  childhood type F84.5
  chronic undifferentiated F2Ø.5
  cyclic F25.Ø
  disorganized (type) F2Ø.1
  flexibilitas cerea F2Ø.2
  hebephrenic (type) F2Ø.1
  incipient F21
  latent F21
  negative type F2Ø.5
  paranoid (type) F2Ø.Ø
  paraphrenic F2Ø.Ø
  post-psychotic depression F32.89
  prepsychotic F21
  prodromal F21
  pseudoneurotic F21
  pseudopsychopathic F21
  reaction F23
  residual (state) (type) F2Ø.5
  restzustand F2Ø.5
  schizoaffective (type) — *see* Psychosis, schizoaffective
  simple (type) F2Ø.89
  simplex F2Ø.89
  specified type NEC F2Ø.89
  spectrum and other psychotic disorder F29
    specified NEC F28
  stupor F2Ø.2
  syndrome of childhood F84.5
  undifferentiated (type) F2Ø.3
    chronic F2Ø.5
Schizothymia (persistent) F6Ø.1
Schlatter-Osgood disease or osteochondrosis — *see* Osteochondrosis, juvenile, tibia
Schlatter's tibia — *see* Osteochondrosis, juvenile, tibia
Schmidt's syndrome (polyglandular, autoimmune) E31.Ø
Schmincke's carcinoma or tumor — *see* Neoplasm, nasopharynx, malignant
Schmitz (-Stutzer) **dysentery** AØ3.Ø
Schmorl's disease or nodes
  lumbar region M51.46
  lumbosacral region M51.47
  sacrococcygeal region M53.3
  thoracic region M51.44
  thoracolumbar region M51.45
Schneiderian
  papilloma — *see* Neoplasm, nasopharynx, benign
    specified site — *see* Neoplasm, benign, by site
    unspecified site D14.Ø
  specified site — *see* Neoplasm, malignant, by site
    unspecified site C3Ø.Ø
Scholte's syndrome (malignant carcinoid) E34.Ø
Scholz (-Bielchowsky-Henneberg) **disease or syndrome** E75.25
Schönlein (-Henoch) disease or purpura (primary) (rheumatic) D69.Ø
Schottmuller's disease AØ1.4
Schroeder's syndrome (endocrine hypertensive) E27.Ø
Schüller-Christian disease or syndrome C96.5
Schultze's type acroparesthesia, simple I73.89
Schultz's disease or syndrome — *see* Agranulocytosis
Schwalbe-Ziehen-Oppenheim disease G24.1
Schwannoma (*see also* Neoplasm, nerve, benign)
  malignant (*see also* Neoplasm, nerve, malignant)
    with rhabdomyoblastic differentiation — *see* Neoplasm, nerve, malignant
  melanocytic — *see* Neoplasm, nerve, benign
  pigmented — *see* Neoplasm, nerve, benign
Schwannomatosis Q85.Ø3
Schwartz (-Jampel) **syndrome** G71.13
Schwartz-Bartter syndrome E22.2
Schweniger-Buzzi anetoderma L9Ø.1
Sciatic — *see* condition
Sciatica (infective)
  with lumbago M54.4- ☑
    due to intervertebral disc disorder — *see* Disorder, disc, with, radiculopathy
    due to displacement of intervertebral disc (with lumbago) — *see* Disorder, disc, with, radiculopathy

Sciatica — *continued*
  wallet M54.3- ☑
Scimitar syndrome Q26.8
Sclera — *see* condition
Sclerectasia H15.84- ☑
Scleredema
  adultorum — *see* Sclerosis, systemic
  Buschke's — *see* Sclerosis, systemic
  newborn P83.0
Sclerema (adiposum) (edematosum) (neonatorum)
    (newborn) P83.0
  adultorum — *see* Sclerosis, systemic
Scleriasis — *see* Scleroderma
Scleritis H15.00- ☑
  with corneal involvement H15.04- ☑
  anterior H15.01- ☑
  brawny H15.02- ☑
  in (due to) zoster B02.34
  posterior H15.03- ☑
  specified type NEC H15.09- ☑
  syphilitic A52.71
  tuberculous (nodular) A18.51
Sclerochoroiditis H31.8
Scleroconjunctivitis — *see* Scleritis
Sclerocystic ovary syndrome E28.2
Sclerodactyly, sclerodactylia L94.3
Scleroderma, sclerodermia (acrosclerotic) (diffuse)
    (generalized) (progressive) (pulmonary) (*see also*
    Sclerosis, systemic) M34.9
  circumscribed L94.0
  linear L94.1
  localized L94.0
  newborn P83.88
  systemic M34.9
Sclerokeratitis H16.8
  tuberculous A18.52
Scleroma nasi A48.8
Scleromalacia (perforans) H15.05- ☑
Scleromyxedema L98.5
Sclérose en plaques G35
Sclerosis, sclerotic
  adrenal (gland) E27.8
  Alzheimer's — *see* Disease, Alzheimer's
  amyotrophic (lateral) G12.21
  aorta, aortic I70.0
    valve — *see* Endocarditis, aortic
  artery, arterial, arteriolar, arteriovascular — *see* Arteriosclerosis
  ascending multiple G35
  brain (generalized) (lobular) G37.9
    artery, arterial I67.2
    diffuse G37.0
    disseminated G35
    insular G35
    Krabbe's E75.23
    miliary G35
    multiple G35
    presenile (Alzheimer's) — *see* Disease, Alzheimer's, early onset
    senile (arteriosclerotic) I67.2
    stem, multiple G35
    tuberous Q85.1
  bulbar, multiple G35
  bundle of His I44.39
  cardiac — *see* Disease, heart, ischemic, atherosclerotic
  cardiorenal — *see* Hypertension, cardiorenal
  cardiovascular (*see also* Disease, cardiovascular)
    renal — *see* Hypertension, cardiorenal
  cerebellar — *see* Sclerosis, brain
  cerebral — *see* Sclerosis, brain
  cerebrospinal (disseminated) (multiple) G35
  cerebrovascular I67.2
  choroid — *see* Degeneration, choroid
  combined (spinal cord) (*see also* Degeneration, combined)
    multiple G35
  concentric (Balo) G37.5
  cornea — *see* Opacity, cornea
  coronary (artery) I25.10
    with angina pectoris — *see* Arteriosclerosis, coronary (artery),
  corpus cavernosum
    female N90.89
    male N48.6
  diffuse (brain) (spinal cord) G37.0
  disseminated G35
  dorsal G35

Sclerosis, sclerotic — *continued*
  dorsolateral (spinal cord) — *see* Degeneration, combined
  endometrium N85.5
  extrapyramidal G25.9
  eye, nuclear (senile) — *see* Cataract, senile, nuclear
  focal and segmental (glomerular) (*see also* N00-N07
      with fourth character .1) N05.1
  Friedreich's (spinal cord) G11.1
  funicular (spermatic cord) N50.89
  general (vascular) — *see* Arteriosclerosis
  gland (lymphatic) I89.8
  hepatic K74.1
    alcoholic K70.2
  hereditary
    cerebellar G11.9
    spinal (Friedreich's ataxia) G11.1
  hippocampal G93.81
  insular G35
  kidney — *see* Sclerosis, renal
  larynx J38.7
  lateral (amyotrophic) (descending) (spinal) G12.21
    primary G12.23
  lens, senile nuclear — *see* Cataract, senile, nuclear
  liver K74.1
    with fibrosis K74.2
      alcoholic K70.2
    alcoholic K70.2
    cardiac K76.1
  lung — *see* Fibrosis, lung
  mastoid — *see* Mastoiditis, chronic
  mesial temporal G93.81
  mitral I05.8
  Mönckeberg's (medial) — *see* Arteriosclerosis, extremities
  multiple (brain stem) (cerebral) (generalized) (spinal cord) G35
  myocardium, myocardial — *see* Disease, heart, ischemic, atherosclerotic
  nuclear (senile), eye — *see* Cataract, senile, nuclear
  ovary N83.8
  pancreas K86.89
  penis N48.6
  peripheral arteries — *see* Arteriosclerosis, extremities
  plaques G35
  pluriglandular E31.8
  polyglandular E31.8
  posterolateral (spinal cord) — *see* Degeneration, combined
  presenile (Alzheimer's) — *see* Disease, Alzheimer's, early onset
  primary, lateral G12.23
  progressive, systemic M34.0
  pulmonary — *see* Fibrosis, lung
    artery I27.0
    valve (heart) — *see* Endocarditis, pulmonary
  renal N26.9
    with
      cystine storage disease E72.09
      hypertensive heart disease (conditions in I11) — *see* Hypertension, cardiorenal
      arteriolar (hyaline) (hyperplastic) — *see* Hypertension, kidney
  retina (senile) (vascular) H35.00
  senile (vascular) — *see* Arteriosclerosis
  spinal (cord) (progressive) G95.89
    ascending G61.0
    combined (*see also* Degeneration, combined)
      multiple G35
      syphilitic A52.11
    disseminated G35
    dorsolateral — *see* Degeneration, combined
    hereditary (Friedreich's) (mixed form) G11.1
    lateral (amyotrophic) G12.23
    multiple G35
    posterior (syphilitic) A52.11
  stomach K31.89
  subendocardial, congenital I42.4
  systemic M34.9
    with
      lung involvement M34.81
      myopathy M34.82
      polyneuropathy M34.83
    drug-induced M34.2
    due to chemicals NEC M34.2
    progressive M34.0
    specified NEC M34.89
  temporal (mesial) G93.81

Sclerosis, sclerotic — *continued*
  tricuspid (heart) (valve) I07.8
  tuberous (brain) Q85.1
  tympanic membrane — *see* Disorder, tympanic membrane, specified NEC
  valve, valvular (heart) — *see* Endocarditis
  vascular — *see* Arteriosclerosis
  vein I87.8
Scoliosis (acquired) (postural) M41.9
  adolescent (idiopathic) — *see* Scoliosis, idiopathic, adolescent
  congenital Q67.5
    due to bony malformation Q76.3
    failure of segmentation (hemivertebra) Q76.3
    hemivertebra fusion Q76.3
    postural Q67.5
  idiopathic M41.20
    adolescent M41.129
      cervical region M41.122
      cervicothoracic region M41.123
      lumbar region M41.126
      lumbosacral region M41.127
      thoracic region M41.124
      thoracolumbar region M41.125
    cervical region M41.22
    cervicothoracic region M41.23
    infantile M41.00
      cervical region M41.02
      cervicothoracic region M41.03
      lumbar region M41.06
      lumbosacral region M41.07
      sacrococcygeal region M41.08
      thoracic region M41.04
      thoracolumbar region M41.05
    juvenile M41.119
      cervical region M41.112
      cervicothoracic region M41.113
      lumbar region M41.116
      lumbosacral region M41.117
      thoracic region M41.114
      thoracolumbar region M41.115
    lumbar region M41.26
    lumbosacral region M41.27
    thoracic region M41.24
    thoracolumbar region M41.25
  infantile — *see* Scoliosis, idiopathic, infantile
  neuromuscular M41.40
    cervical region M41.42
    cervicothoracic region M41.43
    lumbar region M41.46
    lumbosacral region M41.47
    occipito-atlanto-axial region M41.41
    thoracic region M41.44
    thoracolumbar region M41.45
  paralytic — *see* Scoliosis, neuromuscular
  postradiation therapy M96.5
  rachitic (late effect or sequelae) E64.3 [M49.80]
    cervical region E64.3 [M49.82]
    cervicothoracic region E64.3 [M49.83]
    lumbar region E64.3 [M49.86]
    lumbosacral region E64.3 [M49.87]
    multiple sites E64.3 [M49.89]
    occipito-atlanto-axial region E64.3 [M49.81]
    sacrococcygeal region E64.3 [M49.88]
    thoracic region E64.3 [M49.84]
    thoracolumbar region E64.3 [M49.85]
  sciatic M54.4- ☑
  secondary (to) NEC M41.50
    cerebral palsy, Friedreich's ataxia, poliomyelitis, neuromuscular disorders — *see* Scoliosis, neuromuscular
    cervical region M41.52
    cervicothoracic region M41.53
    lumbar region M41.56
    lumbosacral region M41.57
    thoracic region M41.54
    thoracolumbar region M41.55
  specified form NEC M41.80
    cervical region M41.82
    cervicothoracic region M41.83
    lumbar region M41.86
    lumbosacral region M41.87
    thoracic region M41.84
    thoracolumbar region M41.85
  thoracogenic M41.30
    thoracic region M41.34
    thoracolumbar region M41.35
  tuberculous A18.01

Scoliotic pelvis
   with disproportion (fetopelvic) O33.0
      causing obstructed labor O65.0
Scorbutus, scorbutic (see also Scurvy)
   anemia D53.2
Score, NIHSS (National Institutes of Health Stroke Scale)
   R29.7- ☑
Scotoma (arcuate) (Bjerrum) (central) (ring) (see also
   Defect, visual field, localized, scotoma)
   scintillating H53.19
Scratch — see Abrasion
Scratchy throat R09.89
Screening (for) Z13.9
   alcoholism Z13.89
   anemia Z13.0
   anomaly, congenital Z13.89
   antenatal, of mother (see also Encounter, antenatal
      screening) Z36.9
   arterial hypertension Z13.6
   arthropod-borne viral disease NEC Z11.59
   bacteriuria, asymptomatic Z13.89
   behavioral disorder Z13.89
   brain injury, traumatic Z13.850
   bronchitis, chronic Z13.83
   brucellosis Z11.2
   cardiovascular disorder Z13.6
   cataract Z13.5
   chlamydial diseases Z11.8
   cholera Z11.0
   chromosomal abnormalities (nonprocreative) NEC
      Z13.79
   colonoscopy Z12.11
   congenital
      dislocation of hip Z13.89
      eye disorder Z13.5
      malformation or deformation Z13.89
   contamination NEC Z13.88
   cystic fibrosis Z13.228
   dengue fever Z11.59
   dental disorder Z13.84
   depression Z13.89
   developmental handicap Z13.4
      in early childhood Z13.4
      infant Z13.4
   diabetes mellitus Z13.1
   diphtheria Z11.2
   disability, intellectual Z13.4
      infant Z13.4
   disease or disorder Z13.9
      bacterial NEC Z11.2
         intestinal infectious Z11.0
         respiratory tuberculosis Z11.1
      blood or blood-forming organ Z13.0
      cardiovascular Z13.6
      Chagas' Z11.6
      chlamydial Z11.8
      dental Z13.89
      developmental Z13.4
         in child Z13.4
         infant Z13.4
      digestive tract NEC Z13.818
         lower GI Z13.811
         upper GI Z13.810
      ear Z13.5
      endocrine Z13.29
      eye Z13.5
      genitourinary Z13.89
      heart Z13.6
      human immunodeficiency virus (HIV) infection
         Z11.4
      immunity Z13.0
      infection
         intestinal Z11.0
            specified NEC Z11.6
         infectious Z11.9
      mental Z13.89
      metabolic Z13.228
      neurological Z13.89
      nutritional Z13.21
         metabolic Z13.228
            lipoid disorders Z13.220
      protozoal Z11.6
         intestinal Z11.0
      respiratory Z13.83
      rheumatic Z13.828
      rickettsial Z11.8
      sexually-transmitted NEC Z11.3
         human immunodeficiency virus (HIV) Z11.4

Screening — continued
   disease or disorder — continued
      sickle-cell (trait) Z13.0
      skin Z13.89
      specified NEC Z13.89
      spirochetal Z11.8
      thyroid Z13.29
      vascular Z13.6
      venereal Z11.3
      viral NEC Z11.59
         human immunodeficiency virus (HIV) Z11.4
         intestinal Z11.0
   elevated titer Z13.89
   emphysema Z13.83
   encephalitis, viral (mosquito- or tick-borne) Z11.59
   exposure to contaminants (toxic) Z13.88
   fever
      dengue Z11.59
      hemorrhagic Z11.59
      yellow Z11.59
   filariasis Z11.6
   galactosemia Z13.228
   gastrointestinal condition Z13.818
   genetic (nonprocreative) - for procreative manage-
      ment — see Testing, genetic, for procreative
      management
      disease carrier status (nonprocreative) Z13.71
      specified NEC (nonprocreative) Z13.79
   genitourinary condition Z13.89
   glaucoma Z13.5
   gonorrhea Z11.3
   gout Z13.89
   helminthiasis (intestinal) Z11.6
   hematopoietic malignancy Z12.89
   hemoglobinopathies NEC Z13.0
   hemorrhagic fever Z11.59
   Hodgkin disease Z12.89
   human immunodeficiency virus (HIV) Z11.4
   human papillomavirus Z11.51
   hypertension Z13.6
   immunity disorders Z13.0
   infection
      mycotic Z11.8
      parasitic Z11.8
   ingestion of radioactive substance Z13.88
   intellectual disability Z13.4
      infant Z13.4
   intestinal
      helminthiasis Z11.6
      infectious disease Z11.0
   leishmaniasis Z11.6
   leprosy Z11.2
   leptospirosis Z11.8
   leukemia Z12.89
   lymphoma Z12.89
   malaria Z11.6
   malnutrition Z13.29
      metabolic Z13.228
      nutritional Z13.21
   measles Z11.59
   mental disorder Z13.89
   metabolic errors, inborn Z13.228
   multiphasic Z13.89
   musculoskeletal disorder Z13.828
      osteoporosis Z13.820
   mycoses Z11.8
   myocardial infarction (acute) Z13.6
   neoplasm (malignant) (of) Z12.9
      bladder Z12.6
      blood Z12.89
      breast Z12.39
         routine mammogram Z12.31
      cervix Z12.4
      colon Z12.11
      genitourinary organs NEC Z12.79
         bladder Z12.6
         cervix Z12.4
         ovary Z12.73
         prostate Z12.5
         testis Z12.71
         vagina Z12.72
      hematopoietic system Z12.89
      intestinal tract Z12.10
         colon Z12.11
         rectum Z12.12
         small intestine Z12.13
      lung Z12.2
      lymph (glands) Z12.89
      nervous system Z12.82

Screening — continued
   neoplasm — continued
      oral cavity Z12.81
      prostate Z12.5
      rectum Z12.12
      respiratory organs Z12.2
      skin Z12.83
      small intestine Z12.13
      specified site NEC Z12.89
      stomach Z12.0
   nephropathy Z13.89
   nervous system disorders NEC Z13.858
   neurological condition Z13.89
   osteoporosis Z13.820
   parasitic infestation Z11.9
      specified NEC Z11.8
   phenylketonuria Z13.228
   plague Z11.2
   poisoning (chemical) (heavy metal) Z13.88
   poliomyelitis Z11.59
   postnatal, chromosomal abnormalities Z13.89
   prenatal, of mother (see also Encounter, antenatal
      screening) Z36.9
   protozoal disease Z11.6
      intestinal Z11.0
   pulmonary tuberculosis Z11.1
   radiation exposure Z13.88
   respiratory condition Z13.83
   respiratory tuberculosis Z11.1
   rheumatoid arthritis Z13.828
   rubella Z11.59
   schistosomiasis Z11.6
   sexually-transmitted disease NEC Z11.3
      human immunodeficiency virus (HIV) Z11.4
   sickle-cell disease or trait Z13.0
   skin condition Z13.89
   sleeping sickness Z11.6
   special Z13.9
      specified NEC Z13.89
   syphilis Z11.3
   tetanus Z11.2
   trachoma Z11.8
   traumatic brain injury Z13.850
   trypanosomiasis Z11.6
   tuberculosis, respiratory Z11.1
   venereal disease Z11.3
   viral encephalitis (mosquito- or tick-borne) Z11.59
   whooping cough Z11.2
   worms, intestinal Z11.6
   yaws Z11.8
   yellow fever Z11.59
Scrofula, scrofulosis (tuberculosis of cervical lymph
   glands) A18.2
Scrofulide (primary) (tuberculous) A18.4
Scrofuloderma, scrofulodermia (any site) (primary)
   A18.4
Scrofulosus lichen (primary) (tuberculous) A18.4
Scrofulous — see condition
Scrotal tongue K14.5
Scrotum — see condition
Scurvy, scorbutic E54
   anemia D53.2
   gum E54
   infantile E54
   rickets E55.0 [M90.80]
Sealpox B08.62
Seasickness T75.3 ☑
Seatworm (infection) (infestation) B80
Sebaceous (see also condition)
   cyst — see Cyst, sebaceous
Seborrhea, seborrheic L21.9
   capillitii R23.8
   capitis L21.0
   dermatitis L21.9
      infantile L21.1
   eczema L21.9
      infantile L21.1
   sicca L21.0
Seckel's syndrome Q87.1
Seclusion, pupil — see Membrane, pupillary
Second hand tobacco smoke exposure (acute)
   (chronic) Z77.22
   in the perinatal period P96.81
Secondary
   dentin (in pulp) K04.3
   neoplasm, secondaries — see Table of Neoplasms,
      secondary

☑ **Additional Character Required** — Refer to the Tabular List for Character Selection   ⩊ **Subterms under main terms may continue to next column or page**

Secretion
- antidiuretic hormone, inappropriate E22.2
- catecholamine, by pheochromocytoma E27.5
- hormone
  - antidiuretic, inappropriate (syndrome) E22.2
  - by
    - carcinoid tumor E34.0
    - pheochromocytoma E27.5
  - ectopic NEC E34.2
- urinary
  - excessive R35.8
  - suppression R34

Section
- nerve, traumatic — *see* Injury, nerve

Sedative, hypnotic, or anxiolytic-induced
- anxiety disorder F13.980
- bipolar and related disorder F13.94
- delirium F13.921
- depressive disorder F13.94
- major neurocognitive disorder F13.97
- mild neurocognitive disorder F13.988
- psychotic disorder F13.959
- sexual dysfunction F13.981
- sleep disorder F13.982

Segmentation, incomplete (congenital) (*see also* Fusion)
- bone NEC Q78.8
- lumbosacral (joint) (vertebra) Q76.49

Seitelberger's syndrome (infantile neuraxonal dystrophy) G31.89

Seizure(s) (*see also* Convulsions) R56.9
- akinetic — *see* Epilepsy, generalized, specified NEC
- atonic — *see* Epilepsy, generalized, specified NEC
- autonomic (hysterical) F44.5
- convulsive — *see* Convulsions
- cortical (focal) (motor) — *see* Epilepsy, localization-related, symptomatic, with simple partial seizures
- disorder (*see also* Epilepsy) G40.909
- due to stroke — *see* Sequelae (of), disease, cerebrovascular, by type, specified NEC
- epileptic — *see* Epilepsy
- febrile (simple) R56.00
  - with status epilepticus G40.901
  - complex (atypical) (complicated) R56.01
    - with status epilepticus G40.901
- grand mal G40.409
  - intractable G40.419
    - with status epilepticus G40.411
    - without status epilepticus G40.419
  - not intractable G40.409
    - with status epilepticus G40.401
    - without status epilepticus G40.409
- heart — *see* Disease, heart
- hysterical F44.5
- intractable G40.919
  - with status epilepticus G40.911
- Jacksonian (focal) (motor type) (sensory type) — *see* Epilepsy, localization-related, symptomatic, with simple partial seizures
- newborn P90
- nonspecific epileptic
  - atonic — *see* Epilepsy, generalized, specified NEC
  - clonic — *see* Epilepsy, generalized, specified NEC
  - myoclonic — *see* Epilepsy, generalized, specified NEC
  - tonic — *see* Epilepsy, generalized, specified NEC
  - tonic-clonic — *see* Epilepsy, generalized, specified NEC
- partial, developing into secondarily generalized seizures
  - complex — *see* Epilepsy, localization-related, symptomatic, with complex partial seizures
  - simple — *see* Epilepsy, localization-related, symptomatic, with simple partial seizures
- petit mal G40.409
  - intractable G40.419
    - with status epilepticus G40.411
    - without status epilepticus G40.419
  - not intractable G40.409
    - with status epilepticus G40.401
    - without status epilepticus G40.409
- post traumatic R56.1
- recurrent G40.909
- specified NEC G40.89
- uncinate — *see* Epilepsy, localization-related, symptomatic, with complex partial seizures

Selenium deficiency, dietary E59

Self-damaging behavior (life-style) Z72.89
Self-harm (attempted)
- history (personal) Z91.5
  - in family Z81.8
Self-mutilation (attempted)
- history (personal) Z91.5
  - in family Z81.8
Self-poisoning
- history (personal) Z91.5
  - in family Z81.8
- observation following (alleged) attempt Z03.6
Semicoma R40.1
Seminal vesiculitis N49.0
Seminoma C62.9-
- specified site — *see* Neoplasm, malignant, by site
Senear-Usher disease or syndrome L10.4
Senectus R54
Senescence (without mention of psychosis) R54
Senile, senility (*see also* condition) R41.81
- with
  - acute confusional state F05
  - mental changes NOS F03
  - psychosis NEC — *see* Psychosis, senile
- asthenia R54
- cervix (atrophic) N88.8
- debility R54
- endometrium (atrophic) N85.8
- fallopian tube (atrophic) — *see* Atrophy, fallopian tube
- heart (failure) R54
- ovary (atrophic) — *see* Atrophy, ovary
- premature E34.8
- vagina, vaginitis (atrophic) N95.2
- wart L82.1
Sensation
- burning (skin) R20.8
  - tongue K14.6
- loss of R20.8
- prickling (skin) R20.2
- tingling (skin) R20.2
Sense loss
- smell — *see* Disturbance, sensation, smell
- taste — *see* Disturbance, sensation, taste
- touch R20.8
Sensibility disturbance (cortical) (deep) (vibratory) R20.9
Sensitive, sensitivity (*see also* Allergy)
- carotid sinus G90.01
- child (excessive) F93.8
- cold, autoimmune D59.1
- dentin K03.89
- gluten (non-celiac) K90.41
- latex Z91.040
- methemoglobin D74.8
- tuberculin, without clinical or radiological symptoms R76.11
- visual
  - glare H53.71
  - impaired contrast H53.72
Sensitiver Beziehungswahn F22
Sensitization, auto-erythrocytic D69.2
Separation
- anxiety, abnormal (of childhood) F93.0
- apophysis, traumatic — *code as* Fracture, by site
- choroid — *see* Detachment, choroid
- epiphysis, epiphyseal
  - nontraumatic (*see also* Osteochondropathy, specified type NEC)
    - upper femoral — *see* Slipped, epiphysis, upper femoral
  - traumatic — *code as* Fracture, by site
- fracture — *see* Fracture
- infundibulum cardiac from right ventricle by a partition Q24.3
- joint (traumatic) (current) — *code by* site under Dislocation
- pubic bone, obstetrical trauma O71.6
- retina, retinal — *see* Detachment, retina
- symphysis pubis, obstetrical trauma O71.6
- tracheal ring, incomplete, congenital Q32.1
Sepsis (generalized) (unspecified organism) A41.9
- with
  - organ dysfunction (acute) (multiple) R65.20
    - with septic shock R65.21
- actinomycotic A42.7
- adrenal hemorrhage syndrome (meningococcal) A39.1
- anaerobic A41.4
- Bacillus anthracis A22.7
- Brucella (*see also* Brucellosis) A23.9

Sepsis — *continued*
- candidal B37.7
- cryptogenic A41.9
- due to device, implant or graft T85.79 ☑
  - arterial graft NEC T82.7 ☑
  - breast (implant) T85.79 ☑
  - catheter NEC T85.79 ☑
    - dialysis (renal) T82.7 ☑
      - intraperitoneal T85.71 ☑
    - infusion NEC T82.7 ☑
      - spinal (cranial) (epidural) (intrathecal) (spinal) (subarachnoid) (subdural) T85.735 ☑
    - urethral indwelling T83.511 ☑
    - urinary T83.518 ☑
  - ectopic or molar pregnancy O08.82
  - electronic (electrode) (pulse generator) (stimulator)
    - bone T84.7 ☑
    - cardiac T82.7 ☑
    - nervous system T85.738 ☑
      - brain T85.731 ☑
      - neurostimulator generator T85.734 ☑
      - peripheral nerve T85.732 ☑
      - spinal cord T85.733 ☑
    - urinary T83.590 ☑
  - fixation, internal (orthopedic) — *see* Complication, fixation device, infection
  - gastrointestinal (bile duct) (esophagus) T85.79 ☑
    - neurostimulator electrode (lead) T85.732 ☑
  - genital T83.69 ☑
  - heart NEC T82.7 ☑
    - valve (prosthesis) T82.6 ☑
      - graft T82.7 ☑
  - joint prosthesis — *see* Complication, joint prosthesis, infection
  - ocular (corneal graft) (orbital implant) T85.79 ☑
  - orthopedic NEC T84.7 ☑
    - fixation device, internal — *see* Complication, fixation device, infection
  - specified NEC T85.79 ☑
  - vascular T82.7 ☑
  - ventricular intracranial (communicating) shunt T85.730 ☑
- during labor O75.3
- Enterococcus A41.81
- Erysipelothrix (rhusiopathiae) (erysipeloid) A26.7
- Escherichia coli (E. coli) A41.5 ☑
- extraintestinal yersiniosis A28.2
- following
  - abortion (subsequent episode) O08.0
    - current episode — *see* Abortion
  - ectopic or molar pregnancy O08.82
  - immunization T88.0 ☑
  - infusion, therapeutic injection or transfusion NEC T80.29 ☑
- gangrenous A41.9
- gonococcal A54.86
- Gram-negative (organism) A41.5 ☑
  - anaerobic A41.4
- Haemophilus influenzae A41.3
- herpesviral B00.7
- intra-abdominal K65.1
- intraocular — *see* Endophthalmitis, purulent
- Listeria monocytogenes A32.7
- localized — *code to* specific localized infection
  - in operation wound T81.4 ☑
  - skin — *see* Abscess
- malleus A24.0
- melioidosis A24.1
- meningeal — *see* Meningitis
- meningococcal A39.4
  - acute A39.2
  - chronic A39.3
- MSSA (Methicillin susceptible Staphylococcus aureus) A41.01
- newborn P36.9
  - due to
    - anaerobes NEC P36.5
    - Escherichia coli P36.4
    - Staphylococcus P36.30
      - aureus P36.2
      - specified NEC P36.39
    - Streptococcus P36.10
      - group B P36.0
      - specified NEC P36.19
  - specified NEC P36.8
- Pasteurella multocida A28.0

Index

Secretion — Sepsis

Sepsis — *continued*
pelvic, puerperal, postpartum, childbirth O85
pneumococcal A40.3
postprocedural T81.4 ☑
puerperal, postpartum, childbirth (pelvic) O85
Salmonella (arizonae) (cholerae-suis) (enteritidis) (typhimurium) A02.1
severe R65.20
with septic shock R65.21
Shigella (*see also* Dysentery, bacillary) A03.9
skin, localized — *see* Abscess
specified organism NEC A41.89
Staphylococcus, staphylococcal A41.2
aureus (methicillin susceptible) (MSSA) A41.01
methicillin resistant (MRSA) A41.02
coagulase-negative A41.1
specified NEC A41.1
Streptococcus, streptococcal A40.9
agalactiae A40.1
group
A A40.0
B A40.1
D A41.81
neonatal P36.10
group B P36.0
specified NEC P36.19
pneumoniae A40.3
pyogenes A40.0
specified NEC A40.8
tracheostomy stoma J95.02
tularemic A21.7
umbilical, umbilical cord (newborn) — *see* Sepsis, newborn
Yersinia pestis A20.7
Septate — *see* Septum
Septic — *see* condition
arm — *see* Cellulitis, upper limb
with lymphangitis — *see* Lymphangitis, acute, upper limb
embolus — *see* Embolism
finger — *see* Cellulitis, digit
with lymphangitis — *see* Lymphangitis, acute, digit
foot — *see* Cellulitis, lower limb
with lymphangitis — *see* Lymphangitis, acute, lower limb
gallbladder (acute) K81.0
hand — *see* Cellulitis, upper limb
with lymphangitis — *see* Lymphangitis, acute, upper limb
joint — *see* Arthritis, pyogenic or pyemic
leg — *see* Cellulitis, lower limb
with lymphangitis — *see* Lymphangitis, acute, lower limb
nail (*see also* Cellulitis, digit)
with lymphangitis — *see* Lymphangitis, acute, digit
sore (*see also* Abscess)
throat J02.0
streptococcal J02.0
spleen (acute) D73.89
teeth, tooth (pulpal origin) K04.4
throat — *see* Pharyngitis
thrombus — *see* Thrombosis
toe — *see* Cellulitis, digit
with lymphangitis — *see* Lymphangitis, acute, digit
tonsils, chronic J35.01
with adenoiditis J35.03
uterus — *see* Endometritis
Septicemia A41.9
meaning sepsis — *see* Sepsis
Septum, septate (congenital) (*see also* Anomaly, by site)
anal Q42.3
with fistula Q42.2
aqueduct of Sylvius Q03.0
with spina bifida — *see* Spina bifida, by site, with hydrocephalus
uterus (complete) (partial) Q51.2
vagina Q52.10
in pregnancy — *see* Pregnancy, complicated by, abnormal vagina
causing obstructed labor O65.5
longitudinal Q52.129
microperforate
left side Q52.124
right side Q52.123
nonobstruction Q52.120

Septum, septate — *continued*
vagina — *continued*
longitudinal — *continued*
obstructing Q52.129
left side Q52.122
right side Q52.121
transverse Q52.11
Sequelae (of) (*see also* condition)
abscess, intracranial or intraspinal (conditions in G06) G09
amputation — *code to* injury with seventh character S
burn and corrosion — *code to* injury with seventh character S
calcium deficiency E64.8
cerebrovascular disease — *see* Sequelae, disease, cerebrovascular
childbirth O94
contusion — *code to* injury with seventh character S
corrosion — *see* Sequelae, burn and corrosion
crushing injury — *code to* injury with seventh character S
disease
cerebrovascular I69.90
alteration of sensation I69.998
aphasia I69.920
apraxia I69.990
ataxia I69.993
cognitive deficits I69.91 ☑
disturbance of vision I69.998
dysarthria I69.922
dysphagia I69.991
dysphasia I69.921
facial droop I69.992
facial weakness I69.992
fluency disorder I69.923
hemiplegia I69.95- ☑
hemorrhage
intracerebral — *see* Sequelae, hemorrhage, intracerebral
intracranial, nontraumatic NEC — *see* Sequelae, hemorrhage, intracranial, nontraumatic
subarachnoid — *see* Sequelae, hemorrhage, subarachnoid
language deficit I69.928
monoplegia
lower limb I69.94- ☑
upper limb I69.93- ☑
paralytic syndrome I69.96- ☑
specified effect NEC I69.998
specified type NEC I69.80
alteration of sensation I69.898
aphasia I69.820
apraxia I69.890
ataxia I69.893
cognitive deficits I69.81 ☑
disturbance of vision I69.898
dysarthria I69.822
dysphagia I69.891
dysphasia I69.821
facial droop I69.892
facial weakness I69.892
fluency disorder I69.823
hemiplegia I69.85- ☑
language deficit I69.828
monoplegia
lower limb I69.84- ☑
upper limb I69.83- ☑
paralytic syndrome I69.86- ☑
specified effect NEC I69.898
speech deficit I69.928
speech deficit I69.828
stroke NOS — *see* Sequelae, stroke NOS
dislocation — *code to* injury with seventh character S
encephalitis or encephalomyelitis (conditions in G04) G09
in infectious disease NEC B94.8
viral B94.1
external cause — *code to* injury with seventh character S
foreign body entering natural orifice — *code to* injury with seventh character S
fracture — *code to* injury with seventh character S
frostbite — *code to* injury with seventh character S
Hansen's disease B92
hemorrhage
intracerebral I69.10

Sequelae — *continued*
hemorrhage — *continued*
intracerebral — *continued*
alteration of sensation I69.198
aphasia I69.120
apraxia I69.190
ataxia I69.193
cognitive deficits I69.11 ☑
disturbance of vision I69.198
dysarthria I69.122
dysphagia I69.191
dysphasia I69.121
facial droop I69.192
facial weakness I69.192
fluency disorder I69.123
hemiplegia I69.15- ☑
language deficit NEC I69.128
monoplegia
lower limb I69.14- ☑
upper limb I69.13- ☑
paralytic syndrome I69.16- ☑
specified effect NEC I69.198
speech deficit NEC I69.128
intracranial, nontraumatic NEC I69.20
alteration of sensation I69.298
aphasia I69.220
apraxia I69.290
ataxia I69.293
cognitive deficits I69.21 ☑
disturbance of vision I69.298
dysarthria I69.222
dysphagia I69.291
dysphasia I69.221
facial droop I69.292
facial weakness I69.292
fluency disorder I69.223
hemiplegia I69.25- ☑
language deficit NEC I69.228
monoplegia
lower limb I69.24- ☑
upper limb I69.23- ☑
paralytic syndrome I69.26- ☑
specified effect NEC I69.298
speech deficit NEC I69.228
subarachnoid I69.00
alteration of sensation I69.098
aphasia I69.020
apraxia I69.090
ataxia I69.093
cognitive deficits — *see* subcategory I69.01- ☑
disturbance of vision I69.098
dysarthria I69.022
dysphagia I69.091
dysphasia I69.021
facial droop I69.092
facial weakness I69.092
fluency disorder I69.023
hemiplegia I69.05- ☑
language deficit NEC I69.028
monoplegia
lower limb I69.04- ☑
upper limb I69.03- ☑
paralytic syndrome I69.06- ☑
specified effect NEC I69.098
speech deficit NEC I69.028
hepatitis, viral B94.2
hyperalimentation E68
infarction
cerebral I69.30
alteration of sensation I69.398
aphasia I69.320
apraxia I69.390
ataxia I69.393
cognitive deficits I69.31 ☑
disturbance of vision I69.398
dysarthria I69.322
dysphagia I69.391
dysphasia I69.321
facial droop I69.392
facial weakness I69.392
fluency disorder I69.323
hemiplegia I69.35- ☑
language deficit NEC I69.328
monoplegia
lower limb I69.34- ☑
upper limb I69.33- ☑
paralytic syndrome I69.36- ☑
specified effect NEC I69.398

Sequelae — *continued*
  infarction — *continued*
    cerebral — *continued*
      speech deficit NEC I69.328
  infection, pyogenic, intracranial or intraspinal G09
  infectious disease B94.9
    specified NEC B94.8
  injury — *code to* Injury with seventh character S
  leprosy B92
  meningitis
    bacterial (conditions in G00) G09
    other or unspecified cause (conditions in G03) G09
  muscle (and tendon) injury — *code to* injury with seventh character S
  myelitis — *see* Sequelae, encephalitis
  niacin deficiency E64.8
  nutritional deficiency E64.9
    specified NEC E64.8
  obstetrical condition O94
  parasitic disease B94.9
  phlebitis or thrombophlebitis of intracranial or intraspinal venous sinuses and veins (conditions in G08) G09
  poisoning — *code to* poisoning with seventh character S
    nonmedicinal substance — *see* Sequelae, toxic effect, nonmedicinal substance
  poliomyelitis (acute) B91
  pregnancy O94
  protein-energy malnutrition E64.0
  puerperium O94
  rickets E64.3
  selenium deficiency E64.8
  sprain and strain — *code to* injury with seventh character S
  stroke NOS I69.30
    alteration in sensation I69.398
    aphasia I69.320
    apraxia I69.390
    ataxia I69.393
    cognitive deficits I69.31 ☑
    disturbance of vision I69.398
    dysarthria I69.322
    dysphagia I69.391
    dysphasia I69.321
    facial droop I69.392
    facial weakness I69.392
    hemiplegia I69.35- ☑
    language deficit NEC I69.328
    monoplegia
      lower limb I69.34- ☑
      upper limb I69.33- ☑
    paralytic syndrome I69.36- ☑
    specified effect NEC I69.398
    speech deficit NEC I69.328
  tendon and muscle injury — *code to* injury with seventh character S
  thiamine deficiency E64.8
  trachoma B94.0
  tuberculosis B90.9
    bones and joints B90.2
    central nervous system B90.0
    genitourinary B90.1
    pulmonary (respiratory) B90.9
    specified organs NEC B90.8
  viral
    encephalitis B94.1
    hepatitis B94.2
  vitamin deficiency NEC E64.8
    A E64.1
    B E64.8
    C E64.2
  wound, open — *code to* injury with seventh character S
Sequestration (*see also* Sequestrum)
  disk — *see* Displacement, intervertebral disk
  lung, congenital Q33.2
Sequestrum
  bone — *see* Osteomyelitis, chronic
  dental M27.2
  jaw bone M27.2
  orbit — *see* Osteomyelitis, orbit
  sinus (accessory) (nasal) — *see* Sinusitis
Sequoiosis lung or pneumonitis J67.8

Serology for syphilis
  doubtful
    with signs or symptoms — *code by* site and stage under Syphilis
    follow-up of latent syphilis — *see* Syphilis, latent
  negative, with signs or symptoms — *code by* site and stage under Syphilis
  positive A53.9
    with signs or symptoms — *code by* site and stage under Syphilis
  reactivated A53.0
Seroma (*see also* Hematoma)
  postprocedural — *see* Complication, postprocedural, seroma
  traumatic, secondary and recurrent T79.2 ☑
Seropurulent — *see* condition
Serositis, multiple K65.8
  pericardial I31.1
  peritoneal K65.8
Serous — *see* condition
Sertoli cell
  adenoma
    specified site — *see* Neoplasm, benign, by site
    unspecified site
      female D27.9
      male D29.20
  carcinoma
    specified site — *see* Neoplasm, malignant, by site
    unspecified site (male) C62.9- ☑
      female C56.9
  tumor
    with lipid storage
      specified site — *see* Neoplasm, benign, by site
      unspecified site
        female D27.9
        male D29.20
    specified site — *see* Neoplasm, benign, by site
    unspecified site
      female D27.9
      male D29.20
Sertoli-Leydig cell tumor — *see* Neoplasm, benign, by site
  specified site — *see* Neoplasm, benign, by site
  unspecified site
    female D27.9
    male D29.20
Serum
  allergy, allergic reaction (*see also* Reaction, serum) T80.69 ☑
    shock (*see also* Shock, anaphylactic) T80.59 ☑
  arthritis (*see also* Reaction, serum) T80.69 ☑
  complication or reaction NEC (*see also* Reaction, serum) T80.69 ☑
  disease NEC (*see also* Reaction, serum) T80.69 ☑
  hepatitis (*see also* Hepatitis, viral, type B)
    carrier (suspected) of B18.1
  intoxication (*see also* Reaction, serum) T80.69 ☑
  neuritis (*see also* Reaction, serum) T80.69 ☑
  neuropathy G61.1
  poisoning NEC (*see also* Reaction, serum) T80.69 ☑
  rash NEC (*see also* Reaction, serum) T80.69 ☑
  reaction NEC (*see also* Reaction, serum) T80.69 ☑
  sickness NEC (*see also* Reaction, serum) T80.69 ☑
  urticaria (*see also* Reaction, serum) T80.69 ☑
Sesamoiditis M25.8- ☑
Severe sepsis R65.20
  with septic shock R65.21
Sever's disease or osteochondrosis — *see* Osteochondrosis, juvenile, tarsus
Sex
  chromosome mosaics Q97.8
    lines with various numbers of X chromosomes Q97.2
  education Z70.8
  reassignment surgery status Z87.890
Sextuplet pregnancy — *see* Pregnancy, sextuplet
Sexual
  function, disorder of (psychogenic) F52.9
  immaturity (female) (male) E30.0
  impotence (psychogenic) organic origin NEC — *see* Dysfunction, sexual, male
  precocity (constitutional) (cryptogenic)(female) (idiopathic) (male) E30.1
Sexuality, pathologic — *see* Deviation, sexual
Sézary disease C84.1- ☑
Shadow, lung R91.8
Shaking palsy or paralysis — *see* Parkinsonism

Shallowness, acetabulum — *see* Derangement, joint, specified type NEC, hip
Shaver's disease J63.1
Sheath (tendon) — *see* condition
Sheathing, retinal vessels H35.01- ☑
Shedding
  nail L60.8
  premature, primary (deciduous) teeth K00.6
Sheehan's disease or syndrome E23.0
Shelf, rectal K62.89
Shell teeth K00.5
Shellshock (current) F43.0
  lasting state — *see* Disorder, post-traumatic stress
Shield kidney Q63.1
Shift
  auditory threshold (temporary) H93.24- ☑
  mediastinal R93.8
Shifting sleep-work schedule (affecting sleep) G47.26
Shiga (-Kruse) **dysentery** A03.0
Shiga's bacillus A03.0
Shigella (dysentery) — *see* Dysentery, bacillary
Shigellosis A03.9
  Group A A03.0
  Group B A03.1
  Group C A03.2
  Group D A03.3
Shin splints S86.89- ☑
Shingles — *see* Herpes, zoster
Shipyard disease or eye B30.0
Shirodkar suture, in pregnancy — *see* Pregnancy, complicated by, incompetent cervix
Shock R57.9
  with ectopic or molar pregnancy O08.3
  adrenal (cortical) (Addisonian) E27.2
  adverse food reaction (anaphylactic) — *see* Shock, anaphylactic, due to food
  allergic — *see* Shock, anaphylactic
  anaphylactic T78.2 ☑
    chemical — *see* Table of Drugs and Chemicals
    due to drug or medicinal substance
      correct substance properly administered T88.6 ☑
      overdose or wrong substance given or taken (by accident) — *see* Table of Drugs and Chemicals, by drug, poisoning
    due to food (nonpoisonous) T78.00 ☑
      additives T78.06 ☑
      dairy products T78.07 ☑
      eggs T78.08 ☑
      fish T78.03 ☑
        shellfish T78.02 ☑
      fruit T78.04 ☑
      milk T78.07 ☑
      nuts T78.05 ☑
        multiple types T78.05 ☑
        peanuts T78.01 ☑
      peanuts T78.01 ☑
      seeds T78.05 ☑
      specified type NEC T78.09 ☑
      vegetable T78.04 ☑
    following sting(s) — *see* Venom
    immunization T80.52 ☑
    serum T80.59 ☑
      blood and blood products T80.51 ☑
      immunization T80.52 ☑
      specified NEC T80.59 ☑
      vaccination T80.52 ☑
  anaphylactoid — *see* Shock, anaphylactic
  anesthetic
    correct substance properly administered T88.2 ☑
    overdose or wrong substance given or taken — *see* Table of Drugs and Chemicals, by drug, poisoning
      specified anesthetic — *see* Table of Drugs and Chemicals, by drug, poisoning
  cardiogenic R57.0
  chemical substance — *see* Table of Drugs and Chemicals
  complicating ectopic or molar pregnancy O08.3
  culture — *see* Disorder, adjustment
  drug
    due to correct substance properly administered T88.6 ☑
    overdose or wrong substance given or taken (by accident) — *see* Table of Drugs and Chemicals, by drug, poisoning
  during or after labor and delivery O75.1

⛛ Subterms under main terms may continue to next column or page   ☑ Additional Character Required — Refer to the Tabular List for Character Selection   285

Sequelae — Shock

Shock — *continued*
  electric T75.4 ☑
    (taser) T75.4 ☑
  endotoxic R65.21
    postprocedural (resulting from a procedure, not elsewhere classified) T81.12 ☑
  following
    ectopic or molar pregnancy O08.3
    injury (immediate) (delayed) T79.4 ☑
    labor and delivery O75.1
  food (anaphylactic) — *see* Shock, anaphylactic, due to food
  from electroshock gun (taser) T75.4 ☑
  gram-negative R65.21
    postprocedural (resulting from a procedure, not elsewhere classified) T81.12 ☑
  hematologic R57.8
  hemorrhagic R57.8
    surgery (intraoperative) (postoperative) T81.19 ☑
    trauma T79.4 ☑
  hypovolemic R57.1
    surgical T81.19 ☑
    traumatic T79.4 ☑
  insulin E15
    therapeutic misadventure — *see* subcategory T38.3 ☑
  kidney N17.0
    traumatic (following crushing) T79.5 ☑
  lightning T75.01 ☑
  liver K72.00
  lung J80
  obstetric O75.1
    with ectopic or molar pregnancy O08.3
    following ectopic or molar pregnancy O08.3
  pleural (surgical) T81.19 ☑
    due to trauma T79.4 ☑
  postprocedural (postoperative) T81.10 ☑
    with ectopic or molar pregnancy O08.3
    cardiogenic T81.11 ☑
    endotoxic T81.12 ☑
    following ectopic or molar pregnancy O08.3
    gram-negative T81.12 ☑
    hypovolemic T81.19 ☑
    septic T81.12 ☑
    specified type NEC T81.19 ☑
  psychic F43.0
  septic (due to severe sepsis) R65.21
  specified NEC R57.8
  surgical T81.10 ☑
  taser gun (taser) T75.4 ☑
  therapeutic misadventure NEC T81.10 ☑
  thyroxin
    overdose or wrong substance given or taken — *see* Table of Drugs and Chemicals, by drug, poisoning
  toxic, syndrome A48.3
  transfusion — *see* Complications, transfusion
  traumatic (immediate) (delayed) T79.4 ☑
Shoemaker's chest M95.4
Short, shortening, shortness
  arm (acquired) (*see also* Deformity, limb, unequal length)
    congenital Q71.81- ☑
    forearm — *see* Deformity, limb, unequal length
  bowel syndrome K91.2
  breath R06.02
  cervical (complicating pregnancy) O26.87- ☑
    non-gravid uterus N88.3
  common bile duct, congenital Q44.5
  cord (umbilical), complicating delivery O69.3 ☑
  cystic duct, congenital Q44.5
  esophagus (congenital) Q39.8
  femur (acquired) — *see* Deformity, limb, unequal length, femur
    congenital — *see* Defect, reduction, lower limb, longitudinal, femur
  frenum, frenulum, linguae (congenital) Q38.1
  hip (acquired) (*see also* Deformity, limb, unequal length)
    congenital Q65.89
  leg (acquired) (*see also* Deformity, limb, unequal length)
    congenital Q72.81- ☑
    lower leg (*see also* Deformity, limb, unequal length)
  limbed stature, with immunodeficiency D82.2
  lower limb (acquired) (*see also* Deformity, limb, unequal length)

Short, shortening, shortness — *continued*
  lower limb (*see also* Deformity, limb, unequal length) — *continued*
    congenital Q72.81- ☑
  organ or site, congenital NEC — *see* Distortion
  palate, congenital Q38.5
  radius (acquired) (*see also* Deformity, limb, unequal length)
    congenital — *see* Defect, reduction, upper limb, longitudinal, radius
  rib syndrome Q77.2
  stature (child) (hereditary) (idiopathic) NEC R62.52
    constitutional E34.3
    due to endocrine disorder E34.3
    Laron-type E34.3
  tendon (*see also* Contraction, tendon)
    with contracture of joint — *see* Contraction, joint
    Achilles (acquired) M67.0- ☑
      congenital Q66.89
    congenital Q79.8
  thigh (acquired) (*see also* Deformity, limb, unequal length, femur)
    congenital — *see* Defect, reduction, lower limb, longitudinal, femur
  tibialis anterior (tendon) — *see* Contraction, tendon
  umbilical cord
    complicating delivery O69.3 ☑
  upper limb, congenital — *see* Defect, reduction, upper limb, specified type NEC
  urethra N36.8
  uvula, congenital Q38.5
  vagina (congenital) Q52.4
Shortsightedness — *see* Myopia
Shoshin (acute fulminating beriberi) E51.11
Shoulder — *see* condition
Shovel-shaped incisors K00.2
Shower, thromboembolic — *see* Embolism
Shunt
  arterial-venous (dialysis) Z99.2
  arteriovenous, pulmonary (acquired) I28.0
    congenital Q25.72
  cerebral ventricle (communicating) in situ Z98.2
  surgical, prosthetic, with complications — *see* Complications, cardiovascular, device or implant
Shutdown, renal N28.9
Shy-Drager syndrome G90.3
Sialadenitis, sialadenosis (any gland) (chronic) (periodic) (suppurative) — *see* Sialoadenitis
Sialectasia K11.8
Sialidosis E77.1
Sialitis, silitis (any gland) (chronic) (suppurative) — *see* Sialoadenitis
Sialoadenitis (any gland) (periodic) (suppurative) K11.20
  acute K11.21
    recurrent K11.22
  chronic K11.23
Sialoadenopathy K11.9
Sialoangitis — *see* Sialoadenitis
Sialodochitis (fibrinosa) — *see* Sialoadenitis
Sialodocholithiasis K11.5
Sialolithiasis K11.5
Sialometaplasia, necrotizing K11.8
Sialorrhea (*see also* Ptyalism)
  periodic — *see* Sialoadenitis
Sialosis K11.7
Siamese twin Q89.4
Sibling rivalry Z62.891
Sicard's syndrome G52.7
Sicca syndrome M35.00
  with
    keratoconjunctivitis M35.01
    lung involvement M35.02
    myopathy M35.03
    renal tubulo-interstitial disorders M35.04
    specified organ involvement NEC M35.09
Sick R69
  or handicapped person in family Z63.79
    needing care at home Z63.6
  sinus (syndrome) I49.5
Sick-euthyroid syndrome E07.81
Sickle-cell
  anemia — *see* Disease, sickle-cell
  trait D57.3
Sicklemia (*see also* Disease, sickle-cell)
  trait D57.3
Sickness
  air (travel) T75.3 ☑

Sickness — *continued*
  airplane T75.3 ☑
  alpine T70.29 ☑
  altitude T70.20 ☑
  Andes T70.29 ☑
  aviator's T70.29 ☑
  balloon T70.29 ☑
  car T75.3 ☑
  compressed air T70.3 ☑
  decompression T70.3 ☑
  green D50.8
  milk — *see* Poisoning, food, noxious
  motion T75.3 ☑
  mountain T70.29 ☑
    acute D75.1
  protein (*see also* Reaction, serum) T80.69 ☑
  radiation T66
  roundabout (motion) T75.3 ☑
  sea T75.3 ☑
  serum NEC (*see also* Reaction, serum) T80.69 ☑
  sleeping (African) B56.9
    by Trypanosoma B56.9
      brucei
        gambiense B56.0
        rhodesiense B56.1
    East African B56.1
    Gambian B56.0
    Rhodesian B56.1
    West African B56.0
  swing (motion) T75.3 ☑
  train (railway) (travel) T75.3 ☑
  travel (any vehicle) T75.3 ☑
Sideropenia — *see* Anemia, iron deficiency
Siderosilicosis J62.8
Siderosis (lung) J63.4
  eye (globe) — *see* Disorder, globe, degenerative, siderosis
Siemens' syndrome (ectodermal dysplasia) Q82.8
Sighing R06.89
  psychogenic F45.8
Sigmoid (*see also* condition)
  flexure — *see* condition
  kidney Q63.1
Sigmoiditis (*see also* Enteritis) K52.9
  infectious A09
  noninfectious K52.9
Silfversköld's syndrome Q78.9
Silicosiderosis J62.8
Silicosis, silicotic (simple) (complicated) J62.8
  with tuberculosis J65
Silicotuberculosis J65
Silo-fillers' disease J68.8
  bronchitis J68.0
  pneumonitis J68.0
  pulmonary edema J68.1
Silver's syndrome Q87.1
Simian malaria B53.1
Simmonds' cachexia or disease E23.0
Simons' disease or syndrome (progressive lipodystrophy) E88.1
Simple, simplex — *see* condition
Simulation, conscious (of illness) Z76.5
Simultanagnosia (asimultagnosia) R48.3
Sin Nombre virus disease (Hantavirus) (cardio)-pulmonary syndrome) B33.4
Sinding-Larsen disease or osteochondrosis — *see* Osteochondrosis, juvenile, patella
Singapore hemorrhagic fever A91
Singer's node or nodule J38.2
Single
  atrium Q21.2
  coronary artery Q24.5
  umbilical artery Q27.0
  ventricle Q20.4
Singultus R06.6
  epidemicus B33.0
Sinus (*see also* Fistula)
  abdominal K63.89
  arrest I45.5
  arrhythmia I49.8
  bradycardia R00.1
  branchial cleft (internal) (external) Q18.0
  coccygeal — *see* Sinus, pilonidal
  dental K04.6
  dermal (congenital) Q06.8
    with abscess Q06.8
    coccygeal, pilonidal — *see* Sinus, coccygeal

☑ Additional Character Required — Refer to the Tabular List for Character Selection   🔻 Subterms under main terms may continue to next column or page

Sinus — *continued*
  infected, skin NEC L08.89
  marginal, ruptured or bleeding — *see* Hemorrhage, antepartum, specified cause NEC
  medial, face and neck Q18.8
  pause I45.5
  pericranii Q01.9
  pilonidal (infected) (rectum) L05.92
    with abscess L05.02
  preauricular Q18.1
  rectovaginal N82.3
  Rokitansky-Aschoff (gallbladder) K82.8
  sacrococcygeal (dermoid) (infected) — *see* Sinus, pilonidal
  tachycardia R00.0
    paroxysmal I47.1
  tarsi syndrome M25.57- ☑
  testis N50.89
  tract (postinfective) — *see* Fistula
  urachus Q64.4
Sinusitis (accessory) (chronic) (hyperplastic) (nasal) (nonpurulent) (purulent) J32.9
  acute J01.90
    ethmoidal J01.20
      recurrent J01.21
    frontal J01.10
      recurrent J01.11
    involving more than one sinus, other than pansinusitis J01.80
      recurrent J01.81
    maxillary J01.00
      recurrent J01.01
    pansinusitis J01.40
      recurrent J01.41
    recurrent J01.91
    specified NEC J01.80
      recurrent J01.81
    sphenoidal J01.30
      recurrent J01.31
  allergic — *see* Rhinitis, allergic
  due to high altitude T70.1 ☑
  ethmoidal J32.2
    acute J01.20
      recurrent J01.21
  frontal J32.1
    acute J01.10
      recurrent J01.11
  influenzal — *see* Influenza, with, respiratory manifestations NEC
  involving more than one sinus but not pansinusitis J32.8
    acute J01.80
      recurrent J01.81
  maxillary J32.0
    acute J01.00
      recurrent J01.01
  sphenoidal J32.3
    acute J01.30
      recurrent J01.31
  tuberculous, any sinus A15.8
Sinusitis-bronchiectasis-situs inversus (syndrome) (triad) Q89.3
Sipple's syndrome E31.22
Sirenomelia (syndrome) Q87.2
Siriasis T67.0 ☑
Sirkari's disease B55.0
Siti A65
Situation, psychiatric F99
Situational
  disturbance (transient) — *see* Disorder, adjustment
    acute F43.0
  maladjustment — *see* Disorder, adjustment
  reaction — *see* Disorder, adjustment
    acute F43.0
Situs inversus or transversus (abdominalis) (thoracis) Q89.3
Sixth disease B08.20
  due to human herpesvirus 6 B08.21
  due to human herpesvirus 7 B08.22
Sjögren-Larsson syndrome Q87.1
Sjögren's syndrome or disease — *see* Sicca syndrome
Skeletal — *see* condition
Skene's gland — *see* condition
Skenitis — *see* Urethritis
Skerljevo A65
Skevas-Zerfus disease — *see* Toxicity, venom, marine animal, sea anemone
Skin (*see also* condition)

Skin — *continued*
  clammy R23.1
  donor — *see* Donor, skin
  hidebound M35.9
Slate-dressers' or slate-miners' lung J62.8
Sleep
  apnea — *see* Apnea, sleep
  deprivation Z72.820
  disorder or disturbance G47.9
    child F51.9
    nonorganic origin F51.9
    specified NEC G47.8
  disturbance G47.9
    nonorganic origin F51.9
  drunkenness F51.9
  rhythm inversion G47.2- ☑
  terrors F51.4
  walking F51.3
    hysterical F44.89
Sleep hygiene
  abuse Z72.821
  inadequate Z72.821
  poor Z72.821
Sleeping sickness — *see* Sickness, sleeping
Sleeplessness — *see* Insomnia
  menopausal N95.1
Sleep-wake schedule disorder G47.20
Slim disease (in HIV infection) B20
Slipped, slipping
  epiphysis (traumatic) (*see also* Osteochondropathy, specified type NEC)
    capital femoral (traumatic)
      acute (on chronic) S79.01- ☑
      current traumatic — *code as* Fracture, by site
      upper femoral (nontraumatic) M93.00- ☑
        acute M93.01- ☑
          on chronic M93.03- ☑
        chronic M93.02- ☑
  intervertebral disc — *see* Displacement, intervertebral disc
  ligature, umbilical P51.8
  patella — *see* Disorder, patella, derangement NEC
  rib M89.8X8
  sacroiliac joint — *see* subcategory M53.2 ☑
  tendon — *see* Disorder, tendon
  ulnar nerve, nontraumatic — *see* Lesion, nerve, ulnar
  vertebra NEC — *see* Spondylolisthesis
Slocumb's syndrome E27.0
Sloughing (multiple) (phagedena) (skin) (*see also* Gangrene)
  abscess — *see* Abscess
  appendix K38.8
  fascia — *see* Disorder, soft tissue, specified type NEC
  scrotum N50.89
  tendon — *see* Disorder, tendon
  transplanted organ — *see* Rejection, transplant
  ulcer — *see* Ulcer, skin
Slow
  feeding, newborn P92.2
  flow syndrome, coronary I20.8
  heart (beat) R00.1
Slowing, urinary stream R39.198
Sluder's neuralgia (syndrome) G44.89
Slurred, slurring speech R47.81
Small (ness)
  for gestational age — *see* Small for dates
  introitus, vagina N89.6
  kidney (unknown cause) N27.9
    bilateral N27.1
    unilateral N27.0
  ovary (congenital) Q50.39
  pelvis
    with disproportion (fetopelvic) O33.1
      causing obstructed labor O65.1
  uterus N85.8
  white kidney N03.9
Small-and-light-for-dates — *see* Small for dates
Small-for-dates (infant) P05.10
  with weight of
    499 grams or less P05.11
    500-749 grams P05.12
    750-999 grams P05.13
    1000-1249 grams P05.14
    1250-1499 grams P05.15
    1500-1749 grams P05.16
    1750-1999 grams P05.17
    2000-2499 grams P05.18

Small-for-dates — *continued*
  with weight of — *continued*
    2500 grams and over P05.19
    specified NEC P05.19
Smallpox B03
Smearing, fecal R15.1
Smith-Lemli-Opitz syndrome E78.72
Smith's fracture S52.54- ☑
Smoker — *see* Dependence, drug, nicotine
Smoker's
  bronchitis J41.0
  cough J41.0
  palate K13.24
  throat J31.2
  tongue K13.24
Smoking
  passive Z77.22
Smothering spells R06.81
Snaggle teeth, tooth M26.39
Snapping
  finger — *see* Trigger finger
  hip — *see* Derangement, joint, specified type NEC, hip
    involving the iliotiblial band M76.3- ☑
  knee — *see* Derangement, knee
    involving the iliotiblial band M76.3- ☑
Sneddon-Wilkinson disease or syndrome (sub-corneal pustular dermatosis) L13.1
Sneezing (intractable) R06.7
Sniffing
  cocaine
    abuse — *see* Abuse, drug, cocaine
    dependence — *see* Dependence, drug, cocaine
  gasoline
    abuse — *see* Abuse, drug, inhalant
    dependence — *see* Dependence, drug, inhalant
  glue (airplane)
    abuse — *see* Abuse, drug, inhalant
    drug dependence — *see* Dependence, drug, inhalant
Sniffles
  newborn P28.89
Snoring R06.83
Snow blindness — *see* Photokeratitis
Snuffles (non-syphilitic) R06.5
  newborn P28.89
  syphilitic (infant) A50.05 [J99]
Social
  exclusion Z60.4
    due to discrimination or persecution (perceived) Z60.5
  migrant Z59.0
    acculturation difficulty Z60.3
  rejection Z60.4
    due to discrimination or persecution Z60.5
  role conflict NEC Z73.5
  skills inadequacy NEC Z73.4
  transplantation Z60.3
Sodoku A25.0
Soemmerring's ring — *see* Cataract, secondary
Soft (*see also* condition)
  nails L60.3
Softening
  bone — *see* Osteomalacia
  brain (necrotic) (progressive) G93.89
    congenital Q04.8
    embolic I63.4- ☑
    hemorrhagic — *see* Hemorrhage, intracranial, intracerebral
    occlusive I63.5- ☑
    thrombotic I63.3- ☑
  cartilage M94.2- ☑
    patella M22.4- ☑
  cerebellar — *see* Softening, brain
  cerebral — *see* Softening, brain
  cerebrospinal — *see* Softening, brain
  myocardial, heart — *see* Degeneration, myocardial
  spinal cord G95.89
  stomach K31.89
Soldier's
  heart F45.8
  patches I31.0
Solitary
  cyst, kidney N28.1
  kidney, congenital Q60.0
Solvent abuse — *see* Abuse, drug, inhalant
  dependence — *see* Dependence, drug, inhalant

Somatization reaction, somatic reaction — *see* Disorder, somatoform
Somnambulism F51.3
  hysterical F44.89
Somnolence R40.0
  nonorganic origin F51.11
Sonne dysentery A03.3
Soor B37.0
Sore
  bed — *see* Ulcer, pressure, by site
  chiclero B55.1
  Delhi B55.1
  desert — *see* Ulcer, skin
  eye H57.1- ☑
  Lahore B55.1
  mouth K13.79
    canker K12.0
  muscle M79.1
  Naga — *see* Ulcer, skin
  of skin — *see* Ulcer, skin
  oriental B55.1
  pressure — *see* Ulcer, pressure, by site
  skin L98.9
  soft A57
  throat (acute) (*see also* Pharyngitis)
    with influenza, flu, or grippe — *see* Influenza, with, respiratory manifestations NEC
    chronic J31.2
    coxsackie (virus) B08.5
    diphtheritic A36.0
    herpesviral B00.2
    influenzal — *see* Influenza, with, respiratory manifestations NEC
    septic J02.0
    streptococcal (ulcerative) J02.0
    viral NEC J02.8
      coxsackie B08.5
  tropical — *see* Ulcer, skin
  veldt — *see* Ulcer, skin
Soto's syndrome (cerebral gigantism) Q87.3
South African cardiomyopathy syndrome I42.8
Southeast Asian hemorrhagic fever A91
Spacing
  abnormal, tooth, teeth, fully erupted M26.30
  excessive, tooth, fully erupted M26.32
Spade-like hand (congenital) Q68.1
Spading nail L60.8
  congenital Q84.6
Spanish collar N47.1
Sparganosis B70.1
Spasm(s), spastic, spasticity (*see also* condition) R25.2
  accommodation — *see* Spasm, of accommodation
  ampulla of Vater K83.4
  anus, ani (sphincter) (reflex) K59.4
    psychogenic F45.8
  artery I73.9
    cerebral G45.9
  Bell's G51.3
  bladder (sphincter, external or internal) N32.89
    psychogenic F45.8
  bronchus, bronchiole J98.01
  cardia K22.0
  cardiac I20.1
  carpopedal — *see* Tetany
  cerebral (arteries) (vascular) G45.9
  cervix, complicating delivery O62.4
  ciliary body (of accommodation) — *see* Spasm, of accommodation
  colon (*see also* Irritable, bowel) K58.9
    with diarrhea K58.0
    psychogenic F45.8
  common duct K83.8
  compulsive — *see* Tic
  conjugate H51.8
  coronary (artery) I20.1
  diaphragm (reflex) R06.6
    epidemic B33.0
    psychogenic F45.8
  duodenum K59.8
  epidemic diaphragmatic (transient) B33.0
  esophagus (diffuse) K22.4
    psychogenic F45.8
  facial G51.3
  fallopian tube N83.8
  gastrointestinal (tract) K31.89
    psychogenic F45.8
  glottis J38.5
    hysterical F44.4

Spasm(s), spastic, spasticity — *continued*
  glottis — *continued*
    psychogenic F45.8
      conversion reaction F44.4
    reflex through recurrent laryngeal nerve J38.5
  habit — *see* Tic
  heart I20.1
  hemifacial (clonic) G51.3
  hourglass — *see* Contraction, hourglass
  hysterical F44.4
  infantile — *see* Epilepsy, spasms
  inferior oblique, eye H51.8
  intestinal (*see also* Syndrome, irritable bowel) K58.9
    psychogenic F45.8
  larynx, laryngeal J38.5
    hysterical F44.4
    psychogenic F45.8
      conversion reaction F44.4
  levator palpebrae superioris — *see* Disorder, eyelid function
  muscle NEC M62.838
    back M62.830
  nerve, trigeminal G51.0
  nervous F45.8
  nodding F98.4
  occupational F48.8
  oculogyric H51.8
    psychogenic F45.8
  of accommodation H52.53- ☑
  ophthalmic artery — *see* Occlusion, artery, retina
  perineal, female N94.89
  peroneo-extensor (*see also* Deformity, limb, flat foot)
  pharynx (reflex) J39.2
    hysterical F45.8
    psychogenic F45.8
  psychogenic F45.8
  pylorus NEC K31.3
    adult hypertrophic K31.89
    congenital or infantile Q40.0
    psychogenic F45.8
  rectum (sphincter) K59.4
    psychogenic F45.8
  retinal (artery) — *see* Occlusion, artery, retina
  sigmoid (*see also* Syndrome, irritable bowel) K58.9
    psychogenic F45.8
  sphincter of Oddi K83.4
  stomach K31.89
    neurotic F45.8
  throat J39.2
    hysterical F45.8
    psychogenic F45.8
  tic F95.9
    chronic F95.1
    transient of childhood F95.0
  tongue K14.8
  torsion (progressive) G24.1
  trigeminal nerve — *see* Neuralgia, trigeminal
  ureter N13.5
  urethra (sphincter) N35.9
  uterus N85.8
    complicating labor O62.4
  vagina N94.2
    psychogenic F52.5
  vascular I73.9
  vasomotor I73.9
  vein NEC I87.8
  viscera — *see* Pain, abdominal
Spasmodic — *see* condition
Spasmophilia — *see* Tetany
Spasmus nutans F98.4
Spastic, spasticity (*see also* Spasm)
  child (cerebral) (congenital) (paralysis) G80.1
Speaker's throat R49.8
Specific, specified — *see* condition
Speech
  defect, disorder, disturbance, impediment R47.9
    psychogenic, in childhood and adolescence F98.8
    slurring R47.81
    specified NEC R47.89
Spencer's disease A08.19
Spens' syndrome (syncope with heart block) I45.9
Sperm counts (fertility testing) Z31.41
  postvasectomy Z30.8
    reversal Z31.42
Spermatic cord — *see* condition
Spermatocele N43.40
  congenital Q55.4
  multiple N43.42

Spermatocele — *continued*
  single N43.41
Spermatocystitis N49.0
Spermatocytoma C62.9- ☑
  specified site — *see* Neoplasm, malignant, by site
Spermatorrhea N50.89
Sphacelus — *see* Gangrene
Sphenoidal — *see* condition
Sphenoiditis (chronic) — *see* Sinusitis, sphenoidal
Sphenopalatine ganglion neuralgia G90.09
Sphericity, increased, lens (congenital) Q12.4
Spherocytosis (congenital) (familial) (hereditary) D58.0
  hemoglobin disease D58.0
  sickle-cell (disease) D57.8- ☑
Spherophakia Q12.4
Sphincter — *see* condition
Sphincteritis, sphincter of Oddi — *see* Cholangitis
Sphingolipidosis E75.3
  specified NEC E75.29
Sphingomyelinosis E75.3
Spicule tooth K00.2
Spider
  bite — *see* Toxicity, venom, spider
  fingers — *see* Syndrome, Marfan's
  nevus I78.1
  toes — *see* Syndrome, Marfan's
  vascular I78.1
Spiegler-Fendt
  benign lymphocytoma L98.8
  sarcoid L08.89
Spielmeyer-Vogt disease E75.4
Spina bifida (aperta) Q05.9
  with hydrocephalus NEC Q05.4
  cervical Q05.5
    with hydrocephalus Q05.0
  dorsal Q05.6
    with hydrocephalus Q05.1
  lumbar Q05.7
    with hydrocephalus Q05.2
  lumbosacral Q05.7
    with hydrocephalus Q05.2
  occulta Q76.0
  sacral Q05.8
    with hydrocephalus Q05.3
  thoracic Q05.6
    with hydrocephalus Q05.1
  thoracolumbar Q05.6
    with hydrocephalus Q05.1
Spindle, Krukenberg's — *see* Pigmentation, cornea, posterior
Spine, spinal — *see* condition
Spiradenoma (eccrine) — *see* Neoplasm, skin, benign
Spirillosis A25.0
Spirillum
  minus A25.0
  obermeieri infection A68.0
Spirochetal — *see* condition
Spirochetosis A69.9
  arthritic, arthritica A69.9
  bronchopulmonary A69.8
  icterohemorrhagic A27.0
  lung A69.8
Spirometrosis B70.1
Spitting blood — *see* Hemoptysis
Splanchnoptosis K63.4
Spleen, splenic — *see* condition
Splenectasis — *see* Splenomegaly
Splenitis (interstitial) (malignant) (nonspecific) D73.89
  malarial (*see also* Malaria) B54 [D77]
  tuberculous A18.85
Splenocele D73.89
Splenomegaly, splenomegalia (Bengal) (cryptogenic) (idiopathic) (tropical) R16.1
  with hepatomegaly R16.2
  cirrhotic D73.2
  congenital Q89.09
  congestive, chronic D73.2
  Egyptian B65.1
  Gaucher's E75.22
  malarial (*see also* Malaria) B54 [D77]
  neutropenic D73.81
  Niemann-Pick — *see* Niemann-Pick disease or syndrome
  siderotic D73.2
  syphilitic A52.79
    congenital (early) A50.08 [D77]
Splenopathy D73.9

Splenoptosis D73.89
Splenosis D73.89
Splinter — *see* Foreign body, superficial, by site
Split, splitting
  foot Q72.7- ☑
  hand Q71.6 ☑
  heart sounds R01.2
  lip, congenital — *see* Cleft, lip
  nails L60.3
  urinary stream R39.13
Spondylarthrosis — *see* Spondylosis
Spondylitis (chronic) (*see also* Spondylopathy, inflammatory)
  ankylopoietica — *see* Spondylitis, ankylosing
  ankylosing (chronic) M45.9
    with lung involvement M45.9 [J99]
    cervical region M45.2
    cervicothoracic region M45.3
    juvenile M08.1
    lumbar region M45.6
    lumbosacral region M45.7
    multiple sites M45.0
    occipito-atlanto-axial region M45.1
    sacrococcygeal region M45.8
    thoracic region M45.4
    thoracolumbar region M45.5
  atrophic (ligamentous) — *see* Spondylitis, ankylosing
  deformans (chronic) — *see* Spondylosis
  gonococcal A54.41
  gouty (*see also* Gout, by type, vertebrae) M10.08
  in (due to)
    brucellosis A23.9 [M49.80]
      cervical region A23.9 [M49.82]
      cervicothoracic region A23.9 [M49.83]
      lumbar region A23.9 [M49.86]
      lumbosacral region A23.9 [M49.87]
      multiple sites A23.9 [M49.89]
      occipito-atlanto-axial region A23.9 [M49.81]
      sacrococcygeal region A23.9 [M49.88]
      thoracic region A23.9 [M49.84]
      thoracolumbar region A23.9 [M49.85]
    enterobacteria (*see also* subcategory M49.8) A04.9
    tuberculosis A18.01
  infectious NEC — *see* Spondylopathy, infective
  juvenile ankylosing (chronic) M08.1
  Kümmell's — *see* Spondylopathy, traumatic
  Marie-Strümpell — *see* Spondylitis, ankylosing
  muscularis — *see* Spondylopathy, specified NEC
  psoriatic L40.53
  rheumatoid — *see* Spondylitis, ankylosing
  rhizomelica — *see* Spondylitis, ankylosing
  sacroiliac NEC M46.1
  senescent, senile — *see* Spondylosis
  traumatic (chronic) or post-traumatic — *see* Spondy-
    lopathy, traumatic
  tuberculous A18.01
  typhosa A01.05
Spondylolisthesis (acquired) (degenerative) M43.10
  with disproportion (fetopelvic) O33.0
    causing obstructed labor O65.0
  cervical region M43.12
  cervicothoracic region M43.13
  congenital Q76.2
  lumbar region M43.16
  lumbosacral region M43.17
  multiple sites M43.19
  occipito-atlanto-axial region M43.11
  sacrococcygeal region M43.18
  thoracic region M43.14
  thoracolumbar region M43.15
  traumatic (old) M43.10
    acute
      fifth cervical (displaced) S12.430 ☑
        nondisplaced S12.431 ☑
        specified type NEC (displaced) S12.450 ☑
          nondisplaced S12.451 ☑
        type III S12.44 ☑
      fourth cervical (displaced) S12.330 ☑
        nondisplaced S12.331 ☑
        specified type NEC (displaced) S12.350 ☑
          nondisplaced S12.351 ☑
        type III S12.34 ☑
      second cervical (displaced) S12.130 ☑
        nondisplaced S12.131 ☑
        specified type NEC (displaced) S12.150 ☑
          nondisplaced S12.151 ☑
        type III S12.14 ☑

Spondylolisthesis — *continued*
  traumatic — *continued*
    acute — *continued*
      seventh cervical (displaced) S12.630 ☑
        nondisplaced S12.631 ☑
        specified type NEC (displaced) S12.650 ☑
          nondisplaced S12.651 ☑
        type III S12.64 ☑
      sixth cervical (displaced) S12.530 ☑
        nondisplaced S12.531 ☑
        specified type NEC (displaced) S12.550 ☑
          nondisplaced S12.551 ☑
        type III S12.54 ☑
      third cervical (displaced) S12.230 ☑
        nondisplaced S12.231 ☑
        specified type NEC (displaced) S12.250 ☑
          nondisplaced S12.251 ☑
        type III S12.24 ☑
Spondylolysis (acquired) M43.00
  cervical region M43.02
  cervicothoracic region M43.03
  congenital Q76.2
  lumbar region M43.06
  lumbosacral region M43.07
    with disproportion (fetopelvic) O33.0
      causing obstructed labor O65.8
  multiple sites M43.09
  occipito-atlanto-axial region M43.01
  sacrococcygeal region M43.08
  thoracic region M43.04
  thoracolumbar region M43.05
Spondylopathy M48.9
  infective NEC M46.50
    cervical region M46.52
    cervicothoracic region M46.53
    lumbar region M46.56
    lumbosacral region M46.57
    multiple sites M46.59
    occipito-atlanto-axial region M46.51
    sacrococcygeal region M46.58
    thoracic region M46.54
    thoracolumbar region M46.55
  inflammatory M46.90
    cervical region M46.92
    cervicothoracic region M46.93
    lumbar region M46.96
    lumbosacral region M46.97
    multiple sites M46.99
    occipito-atlanto-axial region M46.91
    sacrococcygeal region M46.98
    specified type NEC M46.80
      cervical region M46.82
      cervicothoracic region M46.83
      lumbar region M46.86
      lumbosacral region M46.87
      multiple sites M46.89
      occipito-atlanto-axial region M46.81
      sacrococcygeal region M46.88
      thoracic region M46.84
      thoracolumbar region M46.85
    thoracic region M46.94
    thoracolumbar region M46.95
  neuropathic, in
    syringomyelia and syringobulbia G95.0
    tabes dorsalis A52.11
  specified NEC — *see* subcategory M48.8 ☑
  traumatic M48.30
    cervical region M48.32
    cervicothoracic region M48.33
    lumbar region M48.36
    lumbosacral region M48.37
    occipito-atlanto-axial region M48.31
    sacrococcygeal region M48.38
    thoracic region M48.34
    thoracolumbar region M48.35
Spondylosis M47.9
  with
    disproportion (fetopelvic) O33.0
      causing obstructed labor O65.0
    myelopathy NEC M47.10
      cervical region M47.12
      cervicothoracic region M47.13
      lumbar region M47.16
      occipito-atlanto-axial region M47.11
      thoracic region M47.14
      thoracolumbar region M47.15
    radiculopathy M47.20
      cervical region M47.22

Spondylosis — *continued*
  with — *continued*
    radiculopathy — *continued*
      cervicothoracic region M47.23
      lumbar region M47.26
      lumbosacral region M47.27
      occipito-atlanto-axial region M47.21
      sacrococcygeal region M47.28
      thoracic region M47.24
      thoracolumbar region M47.25
  without myelopathy or radiculopathy M47.819
    cervical region M47.812
    cervicothoracic region M47.813
    lumbar region M47.816
    lumbosacral region M47.817
    occipito-atlanto-axial region M47.811
    sacrococcygeal region M47.818
    thoracic region M47.814
    thoracolumbar region M47.815
  specified NEC M47.899
    cervical region M47.892
    cervicothoracic region M47.893
    lumbar region M47.896
    lumbosacral region M47.897
    occipito-atlanto-axial region M47.891
    sacrococcygeal region M47.898
    thoracic region M47.894
    thoracolumbar region M47.895
  traumatic — *see* Spondylopathy, traumatic
Sponge
  inadvertently left in operation wound — *see* Foreign
    body, accidentally left during a procedure
  kidney (medullary) Q61.5
Sponge-diver's disease — *see* Toxicity, venom, marine
  animal, sea anemone
Spongioblastoma (any type) — *see* Neoplasm, malignant, by site
  specified site — *see* Neoplasm, malignant, by site
  unspecified site C71.9
Spongioneuroblastoma — *see* Neoplasm, malignant,
  by site
Spontaneous (*see also* condition)
  fracture (cause unknown) — *see* Fracture, pathological
Spoon nail L60.3
  congenital Q84.6
Sporadic — *see* condition
Sporothrix schenckii infection — *see* Sporotrichosis
Sporotrichosis B42.9
  arthritis B42.82
  disseminated B42.7
  generalized B42.7
  lymphocutaneous (fixed) (progressive) B42.1
  pulmonary B42.0
  specified NEC B42.89
Spots, spotting (in) (of)
  Bitot's (*see also* Pigmentation, conjunctiva)
    in the young child E50.1
    vitamin A deficiency E50.1
  café, au lait L81.3
  Cayenne pepper I78.1
  cotton wool, retina — *see* Occlusion, artery, retina
  de Morgan's (senile angiomas) I78.1
  Fuchs' black (myopic) (*see also* Myopia, degenerative)
    H44.2- ☑
  intermenstrual (regular) N92.0
    irregular N92.1
  Koplik's B05.9
  liver L81.4
  pregnancy O26.85- ☑
  purpuric R23.3
  ruby I78.1
Spotted fever — *see* Fever, spotted N92.3
Sprain (joint) (ligament)
  acromioclavicular joint or ligament S43.5- ☑
  ankle S93.40- ☑
    calcaneofibular ligament S93.41- ☑
    deltoid ligament S93.42- ☑
    internal collateral ligament — *see* Sprain, ankle,
      specified ligament NEC
    specified ligament NEC S93.49- ☑
    talofibular ligament — *see* Sprain, ankle, specified
      ligament NEC
    tibiofibular ligament S93.43- ☑
  anterior longitudinal, cervical S13.4 ☑
  atlas, atlanto-axial, atlanto-occipital S13.4 ☑
  breast bone — *see* Sprain, sternum
  calcaneofibular — *see* Sprain, ankle
  carpal — *see* Sprain, wrist

▽ Subterms under main terms may continue to next column or page   ☑ Additional Character Required — Refer to the Tabular List for Character Selection   289

Splenoptosis — Sprain

Sprain — *continued*
  carpometacarpal — *see* Sprain, hand, specified site NEC
  cartilage
    costal S23.41 ☑
    semilunar (knee) — *see* Sprain, knee, specified site NEC
      with current tear — *see* Tear, meniscus
    thyroid region S13.5 ☑
    xiphoid — *see* Sprain, sternum
  cervical, cervicodorsal, cervicothoracic S13.4 ☑
  chondrosternal S23.421 ☑
  coracoclavicular S43.8- ☑
  coracohumeral S43.41- ☑
  coronary, knee — *see* Sprain, knee, specified site NEC
  costal cartilage S23.41 ☑
  cricoarytenoid articulation or ligament S13.5 ☑
  cricothyroid articulation S13.5 ☑
  cruciate, knee — *see* Sprain, knee, cruciate
  deltoid, ankle — *see* Sprain, ankle
  dorsal (spine) S23.3 ☑
  elbow S53.40- ☑
    radial collateral ligament S53.43- ☑
    radiohumeral S53.41- ☑
    rupture
      radial collateral ligament — *see* Rupture, traumatic, ligament, radial collateral
      ulnar collateral ligament — *see* Rupture, traumatic, ligament, ulnar collateral
    specified type NEC S53.49- ☑
    ulnar collateral ligament S53.44- ☑
    ulnohumeral S53.42- ☑
  femur, head — *see* Sprain, hip
  fibular collateral, knee — *see* Sprain, knee, collateral
  fibulocalcaneal — *see* Sprain, ankle
  finger(s) S63.61- ☑
    index S63.61- ☑
    interphalangeal (joint) S63.63- ☑
      index S63.63- ☑
      little S63.63- ☑
      middle S63.63- ☑
      ring S63.63- ☑
    little S63.61- ☑
    metacarpophalangeal (joint) S63.65- ☑
    middle S63.61- ☑
    ring S63.61- ☑
    specified site NEC S63.69- ☑
      index S63.69- ☑
      little S63.69- ☑
      middle S63.69- ☑
      ring S63.69- ☑
  foot S93.60- ☑
    specified ligament NEC S93.69- ☑
    tarsal ligament S93.61- ☑
    tarsometatarsal ligament S93.62- ☑
    toe — *see* Sprain, toe
  hand S63.9- ☑
    finger — *see* Sprain, finger
    specified site NEC — *see* subcategory S63.8 ☑
    thumb — *see* Sprain, thumb
  head S03.9 ☑
  hip S73.10- ☑
    iliofemoral ligament S73.11- ☑
    ischiocapsular (ligament) S73.12- ☑
    specified NEC S73.19- ☑
  iliofemoral — *see* Sprain, hip
  innominate
    acetabulum — *see* Sprain, hip
    sacral junction S33.6 ☑
  internal
    collateral, ankle — *see* Sprain, ankle
    semilunar cartilage — *see* Sprain, knee, specified site NEC
  interphalangeal
    finger — *see* Sprain, finger, interphalangeal (joint)
    toe — *see* Sprain, toe, interphalangeal joint
  ischiocapsular — *see* Sprain, hip
  ischiofemoral — *see* Sprain, hip
  jaw (articular disc) (cartilage) (meniscus) S03.4- ☑
    old M26.69
  knee S83.9- ☑
    collateral ligament S83.40- ☑
      lateral (fibular) S83.42- ☑
      medial (tibial) S83.41- ☑
    cruciate ligament S83.50- ☑
      anterior S83.51- ☑

Sprain — *continued*
  knee — *continued*
    cruciate ligament — *continued*
      posterior S83.52- ☑
    lateral (fibular) collateral ligament S83.42- ☑
    medial (tibial) collateral ligament S83.41- ☑
    patellar ligament S76.11- ☑
    specified site NEC S83.8X- ☑
    superior tibiofibular joint (ligament) S83.6- ☑
  lateral collateral, knee — *see* Sprain, knee, collateral
  lumbar (spine) S33.5 ☑
  lumbosacral S33.9 ☑
  mandible (articular disc) S03.4- ☑
    old M26.69
  medial collateral, knee — *see* Sprain, knee, collateral
  meniscus
    jaw S03.4- ☑
      old M26.69
    knee — *see* Sprain, knee, specified site NEC
      with current tear — *see* Tear, meniscus
        old — *see* Derangement, knee, meniscus, due to old tear
    mandible S03.4- ☑
      old M26.69
  metacarpal (distal) (proximal) — *see* Sprain, hand, specified site NEC
  metacarpophalangeal — *see* Sprain, finger, metacarpophalangeal (joint)
  metatarsophalangeal — *see* Sprain, toe, metatarsophalangeal joint
  midcarpal — *see* Sprain, hand, specified site NEC
  midtarsal — *see* Sprain, foot, specified site NEC
  neck S13.9 ☑
    anterior longitudinal cervical ligament S13.4 ☑
    atlanto-axial joint S13.4 ☑
    atlanto-occipital joint S13.4 ☑
    cervical spine S13.4 ☑
    cricoarytenoid ligament S13.5 ☑
    cricothyroid ligament S13.5 ☑
    specified site NEC S13.8 ☑
    thyroid region (cartilage) S13.5 ☑
  nose S03.8 ☑
  orbicular, hip — *see* Sprain, hip
  patella — *see* Sprain, knee, specified site NEC
  patellar ligament S76.11- ☑
  pelvis NEC S33.8 ☑
  phalanx
    finger — *see* Sprain, finger
    toe — *see* Sprain, toe
  pubofemoral — *see* Sprain, hip
  radiocarpal — *see* Sprain, wrist
  radiohumeral — *see* Sprain, elbow
  radius, collateral — *see* Rupture, traumatic, ligament, radial collateral
  rib (cage) S23.41 ☑
  rotator cuff (capsule) S43.42- ☑
  sacroiliac (region)
    chronic or old — *see* subcategory M53.2 ☑
    joint S33.6 ☑
  scaphoid (hand) — *see* Sprain, hand, specified site NEC
  scapula (r) — *see* Sprain, shoulder girdle, specified site NEC
  semilunar cartilage (knee) — *see* Sprain, knee, specified site NEC
    with current tear — *see* Tear, meniscus
      old — *see* Derangement, knee, meniscus, due to old tear
  shoulder joint S43.40- ☑
    acromioclavicular joint (ligament) — *see* Sprain, acromioclavicular joint
    blade — *see* Sprain, shoulder, girdle, specified site NEC
    coracoclavicular joint (ligament) — *see* Sprain, coracoclavicular joint
    coracohumeral ligament — *see* Sprain, coracohumeral joint
    girdle S43.9- ☑
      specified site NEC S43.8- ☑
    rotator cuff — *see* Sprain, rotator cuff
    specified site NEC S43.49- ☑
    sternoclavicular joint (ligament) — *see* Sprain, sternoclavicular joint
  spine
    cervical S13.4 ☑
    lumbar S33.5 ☑

Sprain — *continued*
  spine — *continued*
    thoracic S23.3 ☑
  sternoclavicular joint S43.6- ☑
  sternum S23.429 ☑
    chondrosternal joint S23.421 ☑
    specified site NEC S23.428 ☑
    sternoclavicular (joint) (ligament) S23.420 ☑
  symphysis
    jaw S03.4- ☑
      old M26.69
    mandibular S03.4- ☑
      old M26.69
  talofibular — *see* Sprain, ankle
  tarsal — *see* Sprain, foot, specified site NEC
  tarsometatarsal — *see* Sprain, foot, specified site NEC
  temporomandibular S03.4- ☑
    old M26.69
  thorax S23.9 ☑
    ribs S23.41 ☑
    specified site NEC S23.8 ☑
    spine S23.3 ☑
    sternum — *see* Sprain, sternum
  thumb S63.60- ☑
    interphalangeal (joint) S63.62- ☑
    metacarpophalangeal (joint) S63.64- ☑
    specified site NEC S63.68- ☑
  thyroid cartilage or region S13.5 ☑
  tibia (proximal end) — *see* Sprain, knee, specified site NEC
  tibial collateral, knee — *see* Sprain, knee, collateral
  tibiofibular
    distal — *see* Sprain, ankle
    superior — *see* Sprain, knee, specified site NEC
  toe(s) S93.50- ☑
    great S93.50- ☑
    interphalangeal joint S93.51- ☑
      great S93.51- ☑
      lesser S93.51- ☑
    lesser S93.50- ☑
    metatarsophalangeal joint S93.52- ☑
      great S93.52- ☑
      lesser S93.52- ☑
  ulna, collateral — *see* Rupture, traumatic, ligament, ulnar collateral
  ulnohumeral — *see* Sprain, elbow
  wrist S63.50- ☑
    carpal S63.51- ☑
    radiocarpal S63.52- ☑
    specified site NEC S63.59- ☑
  xiphoid cartilage — *see* Sprain, sternum
Sprengel's deformity (congenital) Q74.0
Sprue (tropical) K90.1
  celiac K90.0
  idiopathic K90.49
  meaning thrush B37.0
  nontropical K90.0
Spur, bone (*see also* Enthesopathy)
  calcaneal M77.3- ☑
  iliac crest M76.2- ☑
  nose (septum) J34.89
Spurway's syndrome Q78.0
Sputum
  abnormal (amount) (color) (odor) (purulent) R09.3
  blood-stained R04.2
  excessive (cause unknown) R09.3
Squamous (*see also* condition)
  epithelium in
    cervical canal (congenital) Q51.828
    uterine mucosa (congenital) Q51.818
Squashed nose M95.0
  congenital Q67.4
Squeeze, diver's T70.3 ☑
Squint (*see also* Strabismus)
  accommodative — *see* Strabismus, convergent concomitant
St. Hubert's disease A82.9
Stab (*see also* Laceration)
  internal organs — *see* Injury, by site
Stafne's cyst or cavity M27.0
Staggering gait R26.0
  hysterical F44.4
Staghorn calculus — *see* Calculus, kidney
Stähli's line (cornea) (pigment) — *see* Pigmentation, cornea, anterior

Stain, staining
meconium (newborn) P96.83
port wine Q82.5
tooth, teeth (hard tissues) (extrinsic) K03.6
due to
accretions K03.6
deposits (betet) (black) (green) (materia alba) (orange) (soft) (tobacco) K03.6
metals (copper) (silver) K03.7
nicotine K03.6
pulpal bleeding K03.7
tobacco K03.6
intrinsic K00.8
Stammering (see also Disorder, fluency) F80.81
Standstill
auricular I45.5
cardiac — see Arrest, cardiac
sinoatrial I45.5
ventricular — see Arrest, cardiac
Stannosis J63.5
Stanton's disease — see Melioidosis
Staphylitis (acute) (catarrhal) (chronic) (gangrenous) (membranous) (suppurative) (ulcerative) K12.2
Staphylococcal scalded skin syndrome L00
Staphylococcemia A41.2
Staphylococcus, staphylococcal (see also condition)
as cause of disease classified elsewhere B95.8
aureus (methicillin susceptible) (MSSA) B95.61
methicillin resistant (MRSA) B95.62
specified NEC, as cause of disease classified elsewhere B95.7
Staphyloma (sclera)
cornea H18.72- ☑
equatorial H15.81- ☑
localized (anterior) H15.82- ☑
posticum H15.83- ☑
ring H15.85- ☑
Stargardt's disease — see Dystrophy, retina
Starvation (inanition) (due to lack of food) T73.0 ☑
edema — see Malnutrition, severe
Stasis
bile (noncalculous) K83.1
bronchus J98.09
with infection — see Bronchitis
cardiac — see Failure, heart, congestive
cecum K59.8
colon K59.8
dermatitis I87.2
with
varicose ulcer — see Varix, leg, with ulcer, with inflammation
varicose veins — see Varix, leg, with, inflammation
due to postthrombotic syndrome — see Syndrome, postthrombotic
duodenal K31.5
eczema — see Varix, leg, with, inflammation
edema — see Hypertension, venous (chronic), idiopathic
foot T69.0- ☑
ileocecal coil K59.8
ileum K59.8
intestinal K59.8
jejunum K59.8
kidney N19
liver (cirrhotic) K76.1
lymphatic I89.8
pneumonia J18.2
pulmonary — see Edema, lung
rectal K59.8
renal N19
tubular N17.0
ulcer — see Varix, leg, with, ulcer
without varicose veins I87.2
urine — see Retention, urine
venous I87.8
State (of)
affective and paranoid, mixed, organic psychotic F06.8
agitated R45.1
acute reaction to stress F43.0
anxiety (neurotic) F41.1
apprehension F41.1
burn-out Z73.0
climacteric, female Z78.0
symptomatic N95.1
compulsive F42.8
mixed with obsessional thoughts F42.2
confusional (psychogenic) F44.89

State — continued
confusional — continued
acute (see also Delirium)
with
arteriosclerotic dementia F01.50
with behavioral disturbance F01.51
senility or dementia F05
alcoholic F10.231
epileptic F05
reactive (from emotional stress, psychological trauma) F44.89
subacute — see Delirium
convulsive — see Convulsions
crisis F43.0
depressive F32.9
neurotic F34.1
dissociative F44.9
emotional shock (stress) R45.7
hypercoagulation — see Hypercoagulable
locked-in G83.5
menopausal Z78.0
symptomatic N95.1
neurotic F48.9
with depersonalization F48.1
obsessional F42.8
oneiroid (schizophrenia-like) F23
organic
hallucinatory (nonalcoholic) F06.0
paranoid (-hallucinatory) F06.2
panic F41.0
paranoid F22
climacteric F22
involutional F22
menopausal F22
organic F06.2
senile F03 ☑
simple F22
persistent vegetative R40.3
phobic F40.9
postleukotomy F07.0
pregnant
gestational carrier Z33.3
incidental Z33.1
psychogenic, twilight F44.89
psychopathic (constitutional) F60.2
psychotic, organic (see also Psychosis, organic)
mixed paranoid and affective F06.8
senile or presenile F03 ☑
transient NEC F06.8
with
depression F06.31
hallucinations F06.0
residual schizophrenic F20.5
restlessness R45.1
stress (emotional) R45.7
tension (mental) F48.9
specified NEC F48.8
transient organic psychotic NEC F06.8
depressive type F06.31
hallucinatory type F06.0
twilight
epileptic F05
psychogenic F44.89
vegetative, persistent R40.3
vital exhaustion Z73.0
withdrawal, — see Withdrawal, state
Status (post) (see also Presence (of))
absence, epileptic — see Epilepsy, by type, with status epilepticus
administration of tPA (rtPA) in a different facility within the last 24 hours prior to admission to current facility Z92.82
adrenalectomy (unilateral) (bilateral) E89.6
anastomosis Z98.0
anginosus I20.9
angioplasty (peripheral) Z98.62
with implant Z95.820
coronary artery Z98.61
with implant Z95.5
aortocoronary bypass Z95.1
arthrodesis Z98.1
artificial opening (of) Z93.9
gastrointestinal tract Z93.4
specified NEC Z93.8
urinary tract Z93.6
vagina Z93.8
asthmaticus — see Asthma, by type, with status asthmaticus

Status — continued
awaiting organ transplant Z76.82
bariatric surgery Z98.84
bed confinement Z74.01
bleb, filtering (vitreous), after glaucoma surgery Z98.83
breast implant Z98.82
removal Z98.86
cataract extraction Z98.4- ☑
cholecystectomy Z90.49
clitorectomy N90.811
with excision of labia minora N90.812
colectomy (complete) (partial) Z90.49
colonization — see Carrier (suspected) of
colostomy Z93.3
convulsivus idiopathicus — see Epilepsy, by type, with status epilepticus
coronary artery angioplasty — see Status, angioplasty, coronary artery
coronary artery bypass graft Z95.1
cystectomy (urinary bladder) Z90.6
cystostomy Z93.50
appendico-vesicostomy Z93.52
cutaneous Z93.51
specified NEC Z93.59
delinquent immunization Z28.3
dental Z98.818
crown Z98.811
fillings Z98.811
restoration Z98.811
sealant Z98.810
specified NEC Z98.818
deployment (current) (military) Z56.82
dialysis (hemodialysis) (peritoneal) Z99.2
do not resuscitate (DNR) Z66
donor — see Donor
embedded fragments — see Retained, foreign body fragments (type of)
embedded splinter — see Retained, foreign body fragments (type of)
enterostomy Z93.4
epileptic, epilepticus (see also Epilepsy, by type, with status epilepticus) G40.901
estrogen receptor
negative Z17.1
positive Z17.0
female genital cutting — see Female genital mutilation status
female genital mutilation — see Female genital mutilation status
filtering (vitreous) bleb after glaucoma surgery Z98.83
gastrectomy (complete) (partial) Z90.3
gastric banding Z98.84
gastric bypass for obesity Z98.84
gastrostomy Z93.1
human immunodeficiency virus (HIV) infection, asymptomatic Z21
hysterectomy (complete) (total) Z90.710
partial (with remaining cervial stump) Z90.711
ileostomy Z93.2
implant
breast Z98.82
infibulation N90.813
intestinal bypass Z98.0
jejunostomy Z93.4
lapsed immunization schedule Z28.3
laryngectomy Z90.02
lymphaticus E32.8
malignancy
castrate resistant prostate Z19.2
hormone resistant Z19.2
hormone sensitive Z19.1
marmoratus G80.3
mastectomy (unilateral) (bilateral) Z90.1- ☑
military deployment status (current) Z56.82
in theater or in support of military war, peacekeeping and humanitarian operations Z56.82
nephrectomy (unilateral) (bilateral) Z90.5
nephrostomy Z93.6
obesity surgery Z98.84
oophorectomy
bilateral Z90.722
unilateral Z90.721
organ replacement
by artificial or mechanical device or prosthesis of
artery Z95.828
bladder Z96.0
blood vessel Z95.828
breast Z97.8

▽ Subterms under main terms may continue to next column or page ☑ Additional Character Required — Refer to the Tabular List for Character Selection 291

Stain, staining — Status

Status — continued
  organ replacement — continued
    by artificial or mechanical device or prosthesis of — continued
      eye globe Z97.0
      heart Z95.812
        valve Z95.2
      intestine Z97.8
      joint Z96.60
        hip — see Presence, hip joint implant
        knee — see Presence, knee joint implant
        specified site NEC Z96.698
      kidney Z97.8
      larynx Z96.3
      lens Z96.1
      limbs — see Presence, artificial, limb
      liver Z97.8
      lung Z97.8
      pancreas Z97.8
    by organ transplant (heterologous)(homologous) — see Transplant
  pacemaker
    brain Z96.89
    cardiac Z95.0
    specified NEC Z96.89
  pancreatectomy Z90.410
    complete Z90.410
    partial Z90.411
    total Z90.410
  physical restraint Z78.1
  pneumonectomy (complete) (partial) Z90.2
  pneumothorax, therapeutic Z98.3
  postcommotio cerebri F07.81
  postoperative (postprocedural) NEC Z98.890
    breast implant Z98.82
    dental Z98.818
      crown Z98.811
      fillings Z98.811
      restoration Z98.811
      sealant Z98.810
      specified NEC Z98.818
    pneumothorax, therapeutic Z98.3
    uterine scar Z98.891
  postpartum (routine follow-up) Z39.2
    care immediately after delivery Z39.0
  postsurgical (postprocedural) NEC Z98.890
    pneumothorax, therapeutic Z98.3
  pregnancy, incidental Z33.1
  prosthesis coronary angioplasty Z95.5
  pseudophakia Z96.1
  renal dialysis (hemodialysis) (peritoneal) Z99.2
  retained foreign body — see Retained, foreign body fragments (type of)
  reversed jejunal transposition (for bypass) Z98.0
  salpingo-oophorectomy
    bilateral Z90.722
    unilateral Z90.721
  sex reassignment surgery status Z87.890
  shunt
    arteriovenous (for dialysis) Z99.2
    cerebrospinal fluid Z98.2
    ventricular (communicating) (for drainage) Z98.2
  splenectomy Z90.81
  thymicolymphaticus E32.8
  thymicus E32.8
  thymolymphaticus E32.8
  thyroidectomy (hypothyroidism) E89.0
  tooth (teeth) extraction (see also Absence, teeth, acquired) K08.409
  tPA (rtPA) administration in a different facility within the last 24 hours prior to admission to current facility Z92.82
  tracheostomy Z93.0
  transplant — see Transplant
    organ removed Z98.85
  tubal ligation Z98.51
  underimmunization Z28.3
  ureterostomy Z93.6
  urethrostomy Z93.6
  vagina, artificial Z93.8
  vasectomy Z98.52
  wheelchair confinement Z99.3
Stealing
  child problem F91.8
    in company with others Z72.810
  pathological (compulsive) F63.2
Steam burn — see Burn
Steatocystoma multiplex L72.2

Steatohepatitis (nonalcoholic) (NASH) K75.81
Steatoma L72.3
  eyelid (cystic) — see Dermatosis, eyelid
    infected — see Hordeolum
Steatorrhea (chronic) K90.9
  with lacteal obstruction K90.2
  idiopathic (adult) (infantile) K90.9
  pancreatic K90.3
  primary K90.0
  tropical K90.1
Steatosis E88.89
  heart — see Degeneration, myocardial
  kidney N28.89
  liver NEC K76.0
Steele-Richardson-Olszewski disease or syndrome G23.1
Steinbrocker's syndrome G90.8
Steinert's disease G71.11
Stein-Leventhal syndrome E28.2
Stein's syndrome E28.2
STEMI (see also Infarct, myocardium, ST elevation) I21.3
Stenocardia I20.8
Stenocephaly Q75.8
Stenosis, stenotic (cicatricial) (see also Stricture)
  ampulla of Vater K83.1
  anus, anal (canal) (sphincter) K62.4
    and rectum K62.4
    congenital Q42.3
      with fistula Q42.2
  aorta (ascending) (supraventricular) (congenital) Q25.1
    arteriosclerotic I70.0
    calcified I70.0
    supravalvular Q25.3
  aortic (valve) I35.0
    with insufficiency I35.2
    congenital Q23.0
    rheumatic I06.0
      with
        incompetency, insufficiency or regurgitation I06.2
          with mitral (valve) disease I08.0
            with tricuspid (valve) disease I08.3
        mitral (valve) disease I08.0
          with tricuspid (valve) disease I08.3
        tricuspid (valve) disease I08.2
          with mitral (valve) disease I08.3
    specified cause NEC I35.0
    syphilitic A52.03
  aqueduct of Sylvius (congenital) Q03.0
    with spina bifida — see Spina bifida, by site, with hydrocephalus
    acquired G91.1
  artery NEC (see also Arteriosclerosis) I77.1
    celiac I77.4
    cerebral — see Occlusion, artery, cerebral
    extremities — see Arteriosclerosis, extremities
    precerebral — see Occlusion, artery, precerebral
    pulmonary (congenital) Q25.6
      acquired I28.8
    renal I70.1
    stent
      coronary T82.855 ✓
      peripheral T82.856 ✓
  bile duct (common) (hepatic) K83.1
    congenital Q44.3
  bladder-neck (acquired) N32.0
    congenital Q64.31
  brain G93.89
  bronchus J98.09
    congenital Q32.3
    syphilitic A52.72
  cardia (stomach) K22.2
    congenital Q39.3
  cardiovascular — see Disease, cardiovascular
  caudal M48.08
  cervix, cervical (canal) N88.2
    congenital Q51.828
    in pregnancy or childbirth — see Pregnancy, complicated by, abnormal cervix
  colon (see also Obstruction, intestine)
    congenital Q42.9
      specified NEC Q42.8
  colostomy K94.03
  common (bile) duct K83.1
    congenital Q44.3
  coronary (artery) — see Disease, heart, ischemic, atherosclerotic
  cystic duct — see Obstruction, gallbladder

Stenosis, stenotic — continued
  due to presence of device, implant or graft (see also Complications, by site and type, specified NEC) T85.858 ✓
    arterial graft NEC T82.858 ✓
    breast (implant) T85.858 ✓
    catheter T85.858 ✓
      dialysis (renal) T82.858 ✓
        intraperitoneal T85.858 ✓
      infusion NEC T82.858 ✓
        spinal (epidural) (subdural) T85.850 ✓
      urinary (indwelling) T83.85 ✓
    fixation, internal (orthopedic) NEC T84.85 ✓
    gastrointestinal (bile duct) (esophagus) T85.858 ✓
    genital NEC T83.85 ✓
    heart NEC T82.857 ✓
    joint prosthesis T84.85 ✓
    ocular (corneal graft) (orbital implant) NEC T85.858 ✓
    orthopedic NEC T84.85 ✓
    specified NEC T85.858 ✓
    urinary NEC T83.85 ✓
    vascular NEC T82.858 ✓
    ventricular intracranial shunt T85.850 ✓
  duodenum K31.5
    congenital Q41.0
  ejaculatory duct NEC N50.89
    stent
      vascular
        end stent
          adjacent to stent — see Arteriosclerosis
          within the stent
            coronary T82.855 ✓
            peripheral T82.856 ✓
        in stent
          coronary vessel T82.855 ✓
          peripheral vessel T82.856 ✓
  endocervical os — see Stenosis, cervix
  enterostomy K94.13
  esophagus K22.2
    congenital Q39.3
    syphilitic A52.79
      congenital A50.59 [K23]
  eustachian tube — see Obstruction, eustachian tube
  external ear canal (acquired) H61.30- ✓
    congenital Q16.1
    due to
      inflammation H61.32- ✓
      trauma H61.31- ✓
    postprocedural H95.81- ✓
    specified cause NEC H61.39- ✓
  gallbladder — see Obstruction, gallbladder
  glottis J38.6
  heart valve (congenital) Q24.8
    aortic Q23.0
    mitral Q23.2
    pulmonary Q22.1
    tricuspid Q22.4
  hepatic duct K83.1
  hymen N89.6
  hypertrophic subaortic (idiopathic) I42.1
  ileum (see also Obstruction, intestine, specified NEC) K56.699
    congenital Q41.2
  infundibulum cardia Q24.3
  intervertebral foramina (see also Lesion, biomechanical, specified NEC)
    connective tissue M99.79
      abdomen M99.79
      cervical region M99.71
      cervicothoracic M99.71
      head region M99.70
      lumbar region M99.73
      lumbosacral M99.73
      occipitocervical M99.70
      sacral region M99.74
      sacrococcygeal M99.74
      sacroiliac M99.74
      specified NEC M99.79
      thoracic region M99.72
      thoracolumbar M99.72
    disc M99.79
      abdomen M99.79
      cervical region M99.71
      cervicothoracic M99.71
      head region M99.70
      lower extremity M99.76

Stenosis, stenotic — *continued*
  intervertebral foramina (*see also* Lesion, biomechanical, specified) — *continued*
    disc — *continued*
      lumbar region M99.73
      lumbosacral M99.73
      occipitocervical M99.70
      pelvic M99.75
      rib cage M99.78
      sacral region M99.74
      sacrococcygeal M99.74
      sacroiliac M99.74
      specified NEC M99.79
      thoracic region M99.72
      thoracolumbar M99.72
      upper extremity M99.77
    osseous M99.69
      abdomen M99.69
      cervical region M99.61
      cervicothoracic M99.61
      head region M99.60
      lower extremity M99.66
      lumbar region M99.63
      lumbosacral M99.63
      occipitocervical M99.60
      pelvic M99.65
      rib cage M99.68
      sacral region M99.64
      sacrococcygeal M99.64
      sacroiliac M99.64
      specified NEC M99.69
      thoracic region M99.62
      thoracolumbar M99.62
      upper extremity M99.67
    subluxation — *see* Stenosis, intervertebral foramina, osseous
  intestine (*see also* Obstruction, intestine)
    congenital (small) Q41.9
      large Q42.9
        specified NEC Q42.8
      specified NEC Q41.8
  jejunum (*see also* Obstruction, intestine, specified NEC) K56.699
    congenital Q41.1
  lacrimal (passage)
    canaliculi H04.54- ☑
    congenital Q10.5
    duct H04.55- ☑
    punctum H04.56- ☑
    sac H04.57- ☑
  lacrimonasal duct — *see* Stenosis, lacrimal, duct
    congenital Q10.5
  larynx J38.6
    congenital NEC Q31.8
      subglottic Q31.1
    syphilitic A52.73
      congenital A50.59 [J99]
  mitral (chronic) (inactive) (valve) I05.0
    with
      aortic valve disease I08.0
      incompetency, insufficiency or regurgitation I05.2
    active or acute I01.1
      with rheumatic or Sydenham's chorea I02.0
    congenital Q23.2
    specified cause, except rheumatic I34.2
    syphilitic A52.03
  myocardium, myocardial (*see also* Degeneration, myocardial)
    hypertrophic subaortic (idiopathic) I42.1
  nares (anterior) (posterior) J34.89
    congenital Q30.0
  nasal duct (*see also* Stenosis, lacrimal, duct)
    congenital Q10.5
  nasolacrimal duct (*see also* Stenosis, lacrimal, duct)
    congenital Q10.5
  neural canal (*see also* Lesion, biomechanical, specified NEC)
    connective tissue M99.49
      abdomen M99.49
      cervical region M99.41
      cervicothoracic M99.41
      head region M99.40
      lower extremity M99.46
      lumbar region M99.43
      lumbosacral M99.43
      occipitocervical M99.40
      pelvic M99.45

Stenosis, stenotic — *continued*
  neural canal (*see also* Lesion, biomechanical, specified) — *continued*
    connective tissue — *continued*
      rib cage M99.48
      sacral region M99.44
      sacrococcygeal M99.44
      sacroiliac M99.44
      specified NEC M99.49
      thoracic region M99.42
      thoracolumbar M99.42
      upper extremity M99.47
    intervertebral disc M99.59
      abdomen M99.59
      cervical region M99.51
      cervicothoracic M99.51
      head region M99.50
      lower extremity M99.56
      lumbar region M99.53
      lumbosacral M99.53
      occipitocervical M99.50
      pelvic M99.55
      rib cage M99.58
      sacral region M99.54
      sacrococcygeal M99.54
      sacroiliac M99.54
      specified NEC M99.59
      thoracic region M99.52
      thoracolumbar M99.52
      upper extremity M99.57
    osseous M99.39
      abdomen M99.39
      cervical region M99.31
      cervicothoracic M99.31
      head region M99.30
      lower extremity M99.36
      lumbar region M99.33
      lumbosacral M99.33
      occipitocervical M99.30
      pelvic M99.35
      rib cage M99.38
      sacral region M99.34
      sacrococcygeal M99.34
      sacroiliac M99.34
      specified NEC M99.39
      thoracic region M99.32
      thoracolumbar M99.32
      upper extremity M99.37
    subluxation M99.29
      cervical region M99.21
      cervicothoracic M99.21
      head region M99.20
      lower extremity M99.26
      lumbar region M99.23
      lumbosacral M99.23
      occipitocervical M99.20
      pelvic M99.25
      rib cage M99.28
      sacral region M99.24
      sacrococcygeal M99.24
      sacroiliac M99.24
      specified NEC M99.29
      thoracic region M99.22
      thoracolumbar M99.22
      upper extremity M99.27
  organ or site, congenital NEC — *see* Atresia, by site
  papilla of Vater K83.1
  pulmonary (artery) (congenital) Q25.6
    with ventricular septal defect, transposition of aorta, and hypertrophy of right ventricle Q21.3
    acquired I28.8
    in tetralogy of Fallot Q21.3
    infundibular Q24.3
    subvalvular Q24.3
    supravalvular Q25.6
    valve I37.0
      with insufficiency I37.2
      congenital Q22.1
      rheumatic I09.89
        with aortic, mitral or tricuspid (valve) disease I08.8
    vein, acquired I28.8
    vessel NEC I28.8
  pulmonic (congenital) Q22.1
    infundibular Q24.3
    subvalvular Q24.3
  pylorus (hypertrophic) (acquired) K31.1
    adult K31.1

Stenosis, stenotic — *continued*
  pylorus — *continued*
    congenital Q40.0
    infantile Q40.0
  rectum (sphincter) — *see* Stricture, rectum
  renal artery I70.1
    congenital Q27.1
  salivary duct (any) K11.8
  sphincter of Oddi K83.1
  spinal M48.00
    cervical region M48.02
    cervicothoracic region M48.03
    lumbar region (NOS) (without neurogenic claudication) M48.061
      with neurogenic claudication M48.062
    lumbosacral region M48.07
    occipito-atlanto-axial region M48.01
    sacrococcygeal region M48.08
    thoracic region M48.04
    thoracolumbar region M48.05
  stomach, hourglass K31.2
  subaortic (congenital) Q24.4
    hypertrophic (idiopathic) I42.1
  subglottic J38.6
    congenital Q31.1
    postprocedural J95.5
  trachea J39.8
    congenital Q32.1
    syphilitic A52.73
    tuberculous NEC A15.5
  tracheostomy J95.03
  tricuspid (valve) I07.0
    with
      aortic (valve) disease I08.2
      incompetency, insufficiency or regurgitation I07.2
        with aortic (valve) disease I08.2
          with mitral (valve) disease I08.3
      mitral (valve) disease I08.1
        with aortic (valve) disease I08.3
    congenital Q22.4
    nonrheumatic I36.0
      with insufficiency I36.2
  tubal N97.1
  ureter — *see* Atresia, ureter
  ureteropelvic junction, congenital Q62.11
  ureterovesical orifice, congenital Q62.12
  urethra (valve) (*see also* Stricture, urethra)
    congenital Q64.32
  urinary meatus, congenital Q64.33
  vagina N89.5
    congenital Q52.4
    in pregnancy — *see* Pregnancy, complicated by, abnormal vagina
    causing obstructed labor O65.5
  valve (cardiac) (heart) (*see also* Endocarditis) I38
    congenital Q24.8
      aortic Q23.0
      mitral Q23.2
      pulmonary Q22.1
      tricuspid Q22.4
  vena cava (inferior) (superior) I87.1
    congenital Q26.0
  vesicourethral orifice Q64.31
  vulva N90.5
Stent jail T82.897 ☑
Stercolith (impaction) K56.41
  appendix K38.1
Stercoraceous, stercoral ulcer K63.3
  anus or rectum K62.6
Stereotypies NEC F98.4
Sterility — *see* Infertility
Sterilization — *see* Encounter (for), sterilization
Sternalgia — *see* Angina
Sternopagus Q89.4
Sternum bifidum Q76.7
Steroid
  effects (adverse) (adrenocortical) (iatrogenic)
    cushingoid E24.2
      correct substance properly administered — *see* Table of Drugs and Chemicals, by drug, adverse effect
      overdose or wrong substance given or taken — *see* Table of Drugs and Chemicals, by drug, poisoning
    diabetes — *see* subcategory E09 ☑

⬇ Subterms under main terms may continue to next column or page   ☑ **Additional Character Required** — Refer to the Tabular List for Character Selection   **293**

Stenosis, stenotic — Steroid

Steroid — *continued*
  effects — *continued*
    diabetes — *see* subcategory — *continued*
      correct substance properly administered — *see* Table of Drugs and Chemicals, by drug, adverse effect
      overdose or wrong substance given or taken — *see* Table of Drugs and Chemicals, by drug, poisoning
    fever R50.2
    insufficiency E27.3
      correct substance properly administered — *see* Table of Drugs and Chemicals, by drug, adverse effect
      overdose or wrong substance given or taken — *see* Table of Drugs and Chemicals, by drug, poisoning
    responder H40.04- ☑
Stevens-Johnson disease or syndrome L51.1
  toxic epidermal necrolysis overlap L51.3
Stewart-Morel syndrome M85.2
Sticker's disease B08.3
Sticky eye — *see* Conjunctivitis, acute, mucopurulent
Stieda's disease — *see* Bursitis, tibial collateral
Stiff neck — *see* Torticollis
Stiff-man syndrome G25.82
Stiffness, joint NEC M25.60
  ankle M25.67- ☑
  ankylosis — *see* Ankylosis, joint
  contracture — *see* Contraction, joint
  elbow M25.62- ☑
  foot M25.67- ☑
  hand M25.64- ☑
  hip M25.65- ☑
  knee M25.66- ☑
  shoulder M25.61- ☑
  wrist M25.63- ☑
Stigmata congenital syphilis A50.59
Stillbirth P95
Still-Felty syndrome — *see* Felty's syndrome
Still's disease or syndrome (juvenile) M08.20
  adult-onset M06.1
  ankle M08.27- ☑
  elbow M08.22- ☑
  foot joint M08.27- ☑
  hand joint M08.24- ☑
  hip M08.25- ☑
  knee M08.26- ☑
  multiple site M08.29
  shoulder M08.21- ☑
  vertebra M08.28
  wrist M08.23- ☑
Stimulation, ovary E28.1
Sting (venomous) (with allergic or anaphylactic shock) — *see* Table of Drugs and Chemicals, by animal or substance, poisoning
Stippled epiphyses Q78.8
Stitch
  abscess T81.4 ☑
  burst (in operation wound) — *see* Disruption, wound, operation
Stokes' disease E05.00
  with thyroid storm E05.01
Stokes-Adams disease or syndrome I45.9
Stokvis (-Talma) **disease** D74.8
Stoma malfunction
  colostomy K94.03
  enterostomy K94.13
  gastrostomy K94.23
  ileostomy K94.13
  tracheostomy J95.03
Stomach — *see* condition
Stomatitis (denture) (ulcerative) K12.1
  angular K13.0
    due to dietary or vitamin deficiency E53.0
  aphthous K12.0
  bovine B08.61
  candidal B37.0
  catarrhal K12.1
  diphtheritic A36.89
  due to
    dietary deficiency E53.0
    thrush B37.0
    vitamin deficiency
      B group NEC E53.9
      B2 (riboflavin) E53.0
  epidemic B08.8

Stomatitis — *continued*
  epizootic B08.8
  follicular K12.1
  gangrenous A69.0
  Geotrichum B48.3
  herpesviral, herpetic B00.2
  herpetiformis K12.0
  malignant K12.1
  membranous acute K12.1
  monilial B37.0
  mycotic B37.0
  necrotizing ulcerative A69.0
  parasitic B37.0
  septic K12.1
  spirochetal A69.1
  suppurative (acute) K12.2
  ulceromembranous A69.1
  vesicular K12.1
    with exanthem (enteroviral) B08.4
    virus disease A93.8
  Vincent's A69.1
Stomatocytosis D58.8
Stomatomycosis B37.0
Stomatorrhagia K13.79
Stone(s) (*see also* Calculus)
  bladder (diverticulum) N21.0
  cystine E72.09
  heart syndrome I50.1
  kidney N20.0
  prostate N42.0
  pulpal (dental) K04.2
  renal N20.0
  salivary gland or duct (any) K11.5
  urethra (impacted) N21.1
  urinary (duct) (impacted) (passage) N20.9
    bladder (diverticulum) N21.0
    lower tract N21.9
    specified NEC N21.8
  xanthine E79.8 [N22]
Stonecutter's lung J62.8
Stonemason's asthma, disease, lung or pneumoconiosis J62.8
Stoppage
  heart — *see* Arrest, cardiac
  urine — *see* Retention, urine
Storm, thyroid — *see* Thyrotoxicosis
Strabismus (congenital) (nonparalytic) H50.9
  concomitant H50.40
    convergent — *see* Strabismus, convergent concomitant
    divergent — *see* Strabismus, divergent concomitant
  convergent concomitant H50.00
    accommodative component H50.43
    alternating H50.05
      with
        A pattern H50.06
        specified nonconcomitances NEC H50.08
        V pattern H50.07
    monocular H50.01- ☑
      with
        A pattern H50.02- ☑
        specified nonconcomitances NEC H50.04- ☑
        V pattern H50.03- ☑
      intermittent H50.31- ☑
        alternating H50.32
  cyclotropia H50.41 ☑
  divergent concomitant H50.10
    alternating H50.15
      with
        A pattern H50.16
        specified noncomitances NEC H50.18
        V pattern H50.17
    monocular H50.11- ☑
      with
        A pattern H50.12- ☑
        specified nonconcomitances NEC H50.14- ☑
        V pattern H50.13- ☑
      intermittent H50.33- ☑
        alternating H50.34
  Duane's syndrome H50.81- ☑
  due to adhesions, scars H50.69
  heterophoria H50.50
    alternating H50.55
    cyclophoria H50.54
    esophoria H50.51
    exophoria H50.52
    vertical H50.53

Strabismus — *continued*
  heterotropia H50.40
    intermittent H50.30
  hypertropia H50.2- ☑
  hypotropia — *see* Hypertropia
  latent H50.50
  mechanical H50.60
    Brown's sheath syndrome H50.61- ☑
    specified type NEC H50.69
  monofixation syndrome H50.42
  paralytic H49.9
    abducens nerve H49.2- ☑
    fourth nerve H49.1- ☑
    Kearns-Sayre syndrome H49.81- ☑
    ophthalmoplegia (external)
      progressive H49.4- ☑
        with pigmentary retinopathy H49.81- ☑
      total H49.3- ☑
    sixth nerve H49.2- ☑
    specified type NEC H49.88- ☑
    third nerve H49.0- ☑
    trochlear nerve H49.1- ☑
  specified type NEC H50.89
  vertical H50.2- ☑
Strain
  back S39.012 ☑
  cervical S16.1 ☑
  eye NEC — *see* Disturbance, vision, subjective
  heart — *see* Disease, heart
  low back S39.012 ☑
  mental NOS Z73.3
    work-related Z56.6
  muscle (tendon) — *see* Injury, muscle, by site, strain
  neck S16.1 ☑
  physical NOS Z73.3
    work-related Z56.6
  postural (*see also* Disorder, soft tissue, due to use)
  psychological NEC Z73.3
  tendon — *see* Injury, muscle, by site, strain
Straining, on urination R39.16
Strand, vitreous — *see* Opacity, vitreous, membranes and strands
Strangulation, strangulated (*see also* Asphyxia, traumatic)
  appendix K38.8
  bladder-neck N32.0
  bowel or colon K56.2
  food or foreign body — *see* Foreign body, by site
  hemorrhoids — *see* Hemorrhoids, with complication
  hernia (*see also* Hernia, by site, with obstruction)
    with gangrene — *see* Hernia, by site, with gangrene
  intestine (large) (small) K56.2
    with hernia (*see also* Hernia, by site, with obstruction)
      with gangrene — *see* Hernia, by site, with gangrene
  mesentery K56.2
  mucus — *see* Asphyxia, mucus
  omentum K56.2
  organ or site, congenital NEC — *see* Atresia, by site
  ovary — *see* Torsion, ovary
  penis N48.89
    foreign body T19.4 ☑
  rupture — *see* Hernia, by site, with obstruction
  stomach due to hernia (*see also* Hernia, by site, with obstruction)
    with gangrene — *see* Hernia, by site, with gangrene
  vesicourethral orifice N32.0
Strangury R30.0
Straw itch B88.0
Strawberry
  gallbladder K82.4
  mark Q82.5
  tongue (red) (white) K14.3
Streak(s)
  macula, angioid H35.33
  ovarian Q50.32
Strephosymbolia F81.0
  secondary to organic lesion R48.8
Streptobacillary fever A25.1
Streptobacillosis A25.1
Streptobacillus moniliformis A25.1
Streptococcus, streptococcal (*see also* condition)
  as cause of disease classified elsewhere B95.5

☑ **Additional Character Required** — Refer to the Tabular List for Character Selection   ▽ **Subterms under main terms may continue to next column or page**

Streptococcus, streptococcal — *continued*
group
A, as cause of disease classified elsewhere B95.Ø
B, as cause of disease classified elsewhere B95.1
D, as cause of disease classified elsewhere B95.2
pneumoniae, as cause of disease classified elsewhere B95.3
specified NEC, as cause of disease classified elsewhere B95.4
Streptomycosis B47.1
Streptotrichosis A48.8
Stress F43.9
family — *see* Disruption, family
fetal P84
complicating pregnancy O77.9
due to drug administration O77.1
mental NEC Z73.3
work-related Z56.6
physical NEC Z73.3
work-related Z56.6
polycythemia D75.1
reaction (*see also* Reaction, stress) F43.9
work schedule Z56.3
Stretching, nerve — *see* Injury, nerve
Striae albicantes, atrophicae or distensae (cutis) L9Ø.6
Stricture (*see also* Stenosis)
ampulla of Vater K83.1
anus (sphincter) K62.4
congenital Q42.3
with fistula Q42.2
infantile Q42.3
with fistula Q42.2
aorta (ascending) (congenital) Q25.1
arteriosclerotic I7Ø.Ø
calcified I7Ø.Ø
supravalvular, congenital Q25.3
aortic (valve) — *see* Stenosis, aortic
aqueduct of Sylvius (congenital) QØ3.Ø
with spina bifida — *see* Spina bifida, by site, with hydrocephalus
acquired G91.1
artery I77.1
basilar — *see* Occlusion, artery, basilar
carotid — *see* Occlusion, artery, carotid
celiac I77.4
congenital (peripheral) Q27.8
cerebral Q28.3
coronary Q24.5
digestive system Q27.8
lower limb Q27.8
retinal Q14.1
specified site NEC Q27.8
umbilical Q27.Ø
upper limb Q27.8
coronary — *see* Disease, heart, ischemic, atherosclerotic
congenital Q24.5
precerebral — *see* Occlusion, artery, precerebral
pulmonary (congenital) Q25.6
acquired I28.8
renal I7Ø.1
vertebral — *see* Occlusion, artery, vertebral
auditory canal (external) (congenital)
acquired — *see* Stenosis, external ear canal
bile duct (common) (hepatic) K83.1
congenital Q44.3
postoperative K91.89
bladder N32.89
neck N32.Ø
bowel — *see* Obstruction, intestine
brain G93.89
bronchus J98.Ø9
congenital Q32.3
syphilitic A52.72
cardia (stomach) K22.2
congenital Q39.3
cardiac (*see also* Disease, heart)
orifice (stomach) K22.2
cecum — *see* Obstruction, intestine
cervix, cervical (canal) N88.2
congenital Q51.828
in pregnancy — *see* Pregnancy, complicated by, abnormal cervix
causing obstructed labor O65.5
colon (*see also* Obstruction, intestine)
congenital Q42.9
specified NEC Q42.8
colostomy K94.Ø3

Stricture — *continued*
common (bile) duct K83.1
coronary (artery) — *see* Disease, heart, ischemic, atherosclerotic
cystic duct — *see* Obstruction, gallbladder
digestive organs NEC, congenital Q45.8
duodenum K31.5
congenital Q41.Ø
ear canal (external) (congenital) Q16.1
acquired — *see* Stricture, auditory canal, acquired
ejaculatory duct N5Ø.89
enterostomy K94.13
esophagus K22.2
congenital Q39.3
syphilitic A52.79
congenital A5Ø.59 [K23]
eustachian tube (*see also* Obstruction, eustachian tube)
congenital Q17.8
fallopian tube N97.1
gonococcal A54.24
tuberculous A18.17
gallbladder — *see* Obstruction, gallbladder
glottis J38.6
heart (*see also* Disease, heart)
valve (*see also* Endocarditis) I38
aortic Q23.Ø
mitral Q23.2
pulmonary Q22.1
tricuspid Q22.4
hepatic duct K83.1
hourglass, of stomach K31.2
hymen N89.6
hypopharynx J39.2
ileum (*see also* Obstruction, intestine, specified NEC) K56.699
congenital Q41.2
intestine (*see also* Obstruction, intestine)
congenital (small) Q41.9
large Q42.9
specified NEC Q42.8
specified NEC Q41.8
ischemic K55.1
jejunum (*see also* Obstruction, intestine, specified NEC) K56.699
congenital Q41.1
lacrimal passages (*see also* Stenosis, lacrimal)
congenital Q1Ø.5
larynx J38.6
congenital NEC Q31.8
subglottic Q31.1
syphilitic A52.73
congenital A5Ø.59 [J99]
meatus
ear (congenital) Q16.1
acquired — *see* Stricture, auditory canal, acquired
osseous (ear) (congenital) Q16.1
acquired — *see* Stricture, auditory canal, acquired
urinarius (*see also* Stricture, urethra)
congenital Q64.33
mitral (valve) — *see* Stenosis, mitral
myocardium, myocardial I51.5
hypertrophic subaortic (idiopathic) I42.1
nares (anterior) (posterior) J34.89
congenital Q3Ø.Ø
nasal duct (*see also* Stenosis, lacrimal, duct)
congenital Q1Ø.5
nasolacrimal duct (*see also* Stenosis, lacrimal, duct)
congenital Q1Ø.5
nasopharynx J39.2
syphilitic A52.73
nose J34.89
congenital Q3Ø.Ø
nostril (anterior) (posterior) J34.89
congenital Q3Ø.Ø
syphilitic A52.73
congenital A5Ø.59 [J99]
organ or site, congenital NEC — *see* Atresia, by site
os uteri — *see* Stricture, cervix
osseous meatus (ear) (congenital) Q16.1
acquired — *see* Stricture, auditory canal, acquired
oviduct — *see* Stricture, fallopian tube
pelviureteric junction (congenital) Q62.11
acquired, with hydronephrosis N13.Ø
penis, by foreign body T19.4 ☑
pharynx J39.2
prostate N42.89

Stricture — *continued*
pulmonary, pulmonic
artery (congenital) Q25.6
acquired I28.8
noncongenital I28.8
infundibulum (congenital) Q24.3
valve I37.Ø
congenital Q22.1
vein, acquired I28.8
vessel NEC I28.8
punctum lacrimale (*see also* Stenosis, lacrimal, punctum)
congenital Q1Ø.5
pylorus (hypertrophic) K31.1
adult K31.1
congenital Q4Ø.Ø
infantile Q4Ø.Ø
rectosigmoid (*see also* Obstruction, intestine, specified NEC) K56.699
rectum (sphincter) K62.4
congenital Q42.1
with fistula Q42.Ø
due to
chlamydial lymphogranuloma A55
irradiation K91.89
lymphogranuloma venereum A55
gonococcal A54.6
inflammatory (chlamydial) A55
syphilitic A52.74
tuberculous A18.32
renal artery I7Ø.1
congenital Q27.1
salivary duct or gland (any) K11.8
sigmoid (flexure) — *see* Obstruction, intestine
spermatic cord N5Ø.89
stoma (following) (of)
colostomy K94.Ø3
enterostomy K94.13
gastrostomy K94.23
ileostomy K94.13
tracheostomy J95.Ø3
stomach K31.89
congenital Q4Ø.2
hourglass K31.2
subaortic Q24.4
hypertrophic (acquired) (idiopathic) I42.1
subglottic J38.6
syphilitic NEC A52.79
trachea J39.8
congenital Q32.1
syphilitic A52.73
tuberculous NEC A15.5
tracheostomy J95.Ø3
tricuspid (valve) — *see* Stenosis, tricuspid
tunica vaginalis N5Ø.89
ureter (postoperative) N13.5
with
hydronephrosis N13.1
with infection N13.6
pyelonephritis (chronic) N11.1
congenital — *see* Atresia, ureter
tuberculous A18.11
ureteropelvic junction (congenital) Q62.11
acquired, with hydronephrosis N13.Ø
ureterovesical orifice N13.5
with infection N13.6
urethra (organic) (spasmodic) N35.9
associated with schistosomiasis B65.Ø [N37]
congenital Q64.39
valvular (posterior) Q64.2
due to
infection — *see* Stricture, urethra, postinfective
trauma — *see* Stricture, urethra, post-traumatic
gonococcal, gonorrheal A54.Ø1
infective NEC — *see* Stricture, urethra, postinfective
late effect (sequelae) of injury — *see* Stricture, urethra, post-traumatic
postcatheterization — *see* Stricture, urethra, postprocedural
postinfective NEC
female N35.12
male N35.119
anterior urethra N35.114
bulbous urethra N35.112
meatal N35.111
membranous urethra N35.113
postobstetric N35.Ø21

Stricture — continued
  urethra — continued
    postoperative — see Stricture, urethra, postproce-
      dural
    postprocedural
      female N99.12
      male N99.114
        anterior bulbous urethra N99.113
        bulbous urethra N99.111
        fossa navicularis N99.115
        meatal N99.110
        membranous urethra N99.112
    post-traumatic
      female N35.028
        due to childbirth N35.021
      male N35.014
        anterior urethra N35.013
        bulbous urethra N35.011
        meatal N35.010
        membranous urethra N35.012
    sequela (late effect) of
      childbirth N35.021
      injury — see Stricture, urethra, post-traumatic
    specified cause NEC N35.8
    syphilitic A52.76
    traumatic — see Stricture, urethra, post-traumatic
    valvular (posterior), congenital Q64.2
  urinary meatus — see Stricture, urethra
  uterus, uterine (synechiae) N85.6
    os (external) (internal) — see Stricture, cervix
  vagina (outlet) — see Stenosis, vagina
  valve (cardiac) (heart) (see also Endocarditis)
    congenital
      aortic Q23.0
      mitral Q23.2
      pulmonary Q22.1
      tricuspid Q22.4
  vas deferens N50.89
    congenital Q55.4
  vein I87.1
  vena cava (inferior) (superior) NEC I87.1
    congenital Q26.0
  vesicourethral orifice N32.0
    congenital Q64.31
  vulva (acquired) N90.5
Stridor R06.1
  congenital (larynx) P28.89
Stridulous — see condition
Stroke (apoplectic) (brain) (embolic) (ischemic) (paralytic)
    (thrombotic) I63.9
  cryptogenic (see also infarction, cerebral) I63.9
  epileptic — see Epilepsy
  heat T67.0 ☑
  in evolution I63.9
  intraoperative
    during cardiac surgery I97.810
    during other surgery I97.811
  lightning — see Lightning
  meaning
    cerebral hemorrhage — code to Hemorrhage, in-
      tracranial
    cerebral infarction — code to Infarction, cerebral
  postprocedural
    following cardiac surgery I97.820
    following other surgery I97.821
  unspecified (NOS) I63.9
Stromatosis, endometrial D39.0
Strongyloidiasis, strongyloidosis B78.9
  cutaneous B78.1
  disseminated B78.7
  intestinal B78.0
Strophulus pruriginosus L28.2
Struck by lightning — see Lightning
Struma (see also Goiter)
  Hashimoto E06.3
  lymphomatosa E06.3
  nodosa (simplex) E04.9
    endemic E01.2
      multinodular E01.1
    multinodular E04.2
      iodine-deficiency related E01.1
    toxic or with hyperthyroidism E05.20
      with thyroid storm E05.21
      multinodular E05.20
        with thyroid storm E05.21
      uninodular E05.10
        with thyroid storm E05.11
    toxicosa E05.20

Struma — continued
  nodosa — continued
    toxicosa — continued
      with thyroid storm E05.21
      multinodular E05.20
        with thyroid storm E05.21
      uninodular E05.10
        with thyroid storm E05.11
    uninodular E04.1
  ovarii D27.-☑
  Riedel's E06.5
Strumipriva cachexia E03.4
Strümpell-Marie spine — see Spondylitis, ankylosing
Strümpell-Westphal pseudosclerosis E83.01
Stuart deficiency disease (factor X) D68.2
Stuart-Prower factor deficiency (factor X) D68.2
Student's elbow — see Bursitis, elbow, olecranon
Stump — see Amputation
Stunting, nutritional E45
Stupor (catatonic) R40.1
  depressive (single episode) F32.89
    recurrent episode F33.8
  dissociative F44.2
  manic F30.2
  manic-depressive F31.89
  psychogenic (anergic) F44.2
  reaction to exceptional stress (transient) F43.0
Sturge (-Weber) (-Dimitri) (-Kalischer) **disease or syn-
    drome** Q85.8
Stuttering F80.81
  adult onset F98.5
  childhood onset F80.81
  following cerebrovascular disease — see Disorder,
    fluency. following cerebrovascular disease
  in conditions classified elsewhere R47.82
Sty, stye (external) (internal) (meibomian) (zeisian) —
    see Hordeolum
Subacidity, gastric K31.89
  psychogenic F45.8
Subacute — see condition
Subarachnoid — see condition
Subcortical — see condition
Subcostal syndrome, nerve compression — see
    Mononeuropathy, upper limb, specified site NEC
Subcutaneous, subcuticular — see condition
Subdural — see condition
Subendocardium — see condition
Subependymoma
  specified site — see Neoplasm, uncertain behavior,
    by site
  unspecified site D43.2
Suberosis J67.3
Subglossitis — see Glossitis
Subhemophilia D66
Subinvolution
  breast (postlactational) (postpuerperal) N64.89
  puerperal O90.89
  uterus (chronic) (nonpuerperal) N85.3
    puerperal O90.89
Sublingual — see condition
Sublinguitis — see Sialoadenitis
Subluxatable hip Q65.6
Subluxation (see also Dislocation)
  acromioclavicular S43.11- ☑
  ankle S93.0- ☑
  atlantoaxial, recurrent M43.4
    with myelopathy M43.3
  carpometacarpal (joint) NEC S63.05- ☑
    thumb S63.04- ☑
  complex, vertebral — see Complex, subluxation
  congenital (see also Malposition, congenital)
    hip — see Dislocation, hip, congenital, partial
    joint (excluding hip)
      lower limb Q68.8
      shoulder Q68.8
      upper limb Q68.8
  elbow (traumatic) S53.10- ☑
    anterior S53.11- ☑
    lateral S53.14- ☑
    medial S53.13- ☑
    posterior S53.12- ☑
    specified type NEC S53.19- ☑
  finger S63.20- ☑
    index S63.20- ☑
    interphalangeal S63.22- ☑
      distal S63.24- ☑
        index S63.24- ☑

Subluxation — continued
  finger — continued
    interphalangeal — continued
      distal — continued
        little S63.24- ☑
        middle S63.24- ☑
        ring S63.24- ☑
      index S63.22- ☑
      little S63.22- ☑
      middle S63.22- ☑
      proximal S63.23- ☑
        index S63.23- ☑
        little S63.23- ☑
        middle S63.23- ☑
        ring S63.23- ☑
      ring S63.22- ☑
    little S63.20- ☑
    metacarpophalangeal S63.21- ☑
      index S63.21- ☑
      little S63.21- ☑
      middle S63.21- ☑
      ring S63.21- ☑
    middle S63.20- ☑
    ring S63.20- ☑
  foot S93.30- ☑
    specified site NEC S93.33- ☑
    tarsal joint S93.31- ☑
    tarsometatarsal joint S93.32- ☑
    toe — see Subluxation, toe
  hip S73.00- ☑
    anterior S73.03- ☑
      obturator S73.02- ☑
    central S73.04- ☑
    posterior S73.01- ☑
  interphalangeal (joint)
    finger S63.22- ☑
      distal joint S63.24- ☑
        index S63.24- ☑
        little S63.24- ☑
        middle S63.24- ☑
        ring S63.24- ☑
      index S63.22- ☑
      little S63.22- ☑
      middle S63.22- ☑
      proximal joint S63.23- ☑
        index S63.23- ☑
        little S63.23- ☑
        middle S63.23- ☑
        ring S63.23- ☑
      ring S63.22- ☑
    thumb S63.12- ☑
      distal joint S63.14- ☑
      proximal joint S63.13- ☑
    toe S93.13- ☑
      great S93.13- ☑
      lesser S93.13- ☑
  joint prosthesis — see Complications, joint prosthesis,
    mechanical, displacement, by site
  knee S83.10- ☑
    cap — see Subluxation, patella
    patella — see Subluxation, patella
    proximal tibia
      anteriorly S83.11- ☑
      laterally S83.14- ☑
      medially S83.13- ☑
      posteriorly S83.12- ☑
    specified type NEC S83.19- ☑
  lens — see Dislocation, lens, partial
  ligament, traumatic — see Sprain, by site
  metacarpal (bone)
    proximal end S63.06- ☑
  metacarpophalangeal (joint)
    finger S63.21- ☑
      index S63.21- ☑
      little S63.21- ☑
      middle S63.21- ☑
      ring S63.21- ☑
    thumb S63.11- ☑
  metatarsophalangeal joint S93.14- ☑
    great toe S93.14- ☑
    lesser toe S93.14- ☑
  midcarpal (joint) S63.03- ☑
  patella S83.00- ☑
    lateral S83.01- ☑
    recurrent (nontraumatic) — see Dislocation,
      patella, recurrent, incomplete

☑ **Additional Character Required** — Refer to the Tabular List for Character Selection   ⬛ **Subterms under main terms may continue to next column or page**

Subluxation — *continued*
  patella — *continued*
    specified type NEC S83.09- ☑
  pathological — *see* Dislocation, pathological
  radial head S53.00- ☑
    anterior S53.01- ☑
    nursemaid's elbow S53.03- ☑
    posterior S53.02- ☑
    specified type NEC S53.09- ☑
  radiocarpal (joint) S63.02- ☑
  radioulnar (joint)
    distal S63.01- ☑
    proximal — *see* Subluxation, elbow
  shoulder
    congenital Q68.8
    girdle S43.30- ☑
      scapula S43.31- ☑
      specified site NEC S43.39- ☑
    traumatic S43.00- ☑
      anterior S43.01- ☑
      inferior S43.03- ☑
      posterior S43.02- ☑
      specified type NEC S43.08- ☑
  sternoclavicular (joint) S43.20- ☑
    anterior S43.21- ☑
    posterior S43.22- ☑
  symphysis (pubis)
  thumb S63.103 ☑
    interphalangeal joint — *see* Subluxation, interpha-
      langeal (joint), thumb
    metacarpophalangeal joint — *see* Subluxation,
      metacarpophalangeal (joint), thumb
  toe(s) S93.10- ☑
    great S93.10- ☑
      interphalangeal joint S93.13- ☑
      metatarsophalangeal joint S93.14- ☑
    interphalangeal joint S93.13- ☑
    lesser S93.10- ☑
      interphalangeal joint S93.13- ☑
      metatarsophalangeal joint S93.14- ☑
    metatarsophalangeal joint S93.149 ☑
  ulna
    distal end S63.07- ☑
    proximal end — *see* Subluxation, elbow
  ulnohumeral joint — *see* Subluxation, elbow
  vertebral
    recurrent NEC — *see* subcategory M43.5
    traumatic
      cervical S13.100 ☑
        atlantoaxial joint S13.120 ☑
        atlantooccipital joint S13.110 ☑
        atloidooccipital joint S13.110 ☑
        joint between
          C0 and C1 S13.110 ☑
          C1 and C2 S13.120 ☑
          C2 and C3 S13.130 ☑
          C3 and C4 S13.140 ☑
          C4 and C5 S13.150 ☑
          C5 and C6 S13.160 ☑
          C6 and C7 S13.170 ☑
          C7 and T1 S13.180 ☑
        occipitoatloid joint S13.110 ☑
      lumbar S33.100 ☑
        joint between
          L1 and L2 S33.110 ☑
          L2 and L3 S33.120 ☑
          L3 and L4 S33.130 ☑
          L4 and L5 S33.140 ☑
      thoracic S23.100 ☑
        joint between
          T1 and T2 S23.110 ☑
          T2 and T3 S23.120 ☑
          T3 and T4 S23.122 ☑
          T4 and T5 S23.130 ☑
          T5 and T6 S23.132 ☑
          T6 and T7 S23.140 ☑
          T7 and T8 S23.142 ☑
          T8 and T9 S23.150 ☑
          T9 and T10 S23.152 ☑
          T10 and T11 S23.160 ☑
          T11 and T12 S23.162 ☑
          T12 and L1 S23.170 ☑
  wrist (carpal bone) S63.00- ☑
    carpometacarpal joint — *see* Subluxation, car-
      pometacarpal (joint)

Subluxation — *continued*
  wrist — *continued*
    distal radioulnar joint — *see* Subluxation, radioul-
      nar (joint), distal
    metacarpal bone, proximal — *see* Subluxation,
      metacarpal (bone), proximal end
    midcarpal — *see* Subluxation, midcarpal (joint)
    radiocarpal joint — *see* Subluxation, radiocarpal
      (joint)
    recurrent — *see* Dislocation, recurrent, wrist
    specified site NEC S63.09- ☑
    ulna — *see* Subluxation, ulna, distal end
Submaxillary — *see* condition
Submersion (fatal) (nonfatal) T75.1 ☑
Submucous — *see* condition
Subnormal, subnormality
  accommodation (old age) H52.4
  mental — *see* Disability, intellectual
  temperature (accidental) T68 ☑
Subphrenic — *see* condition
Subscapular nerve — *see* condition
Subseptus uterus Q51.2
Subsiding appendicitis K36
Substance (other psychoactive) **-induced**
  anxiety disorder F19.980
  bipolar and related disorder F19.94
  delirium F19.921
  depressive disorder F19.94
  major neurocognitive disorder F19.97
  mild neurocognitive disorder F19.988
  obsessive-compulsive and related disorder F19.988
  psychotic disorder F19.959
  sexual dysfunction F19.981
  sleep disorder F19.982
Substernal thyroid E04.9
  congenital Q89.2
Substitution disorder F44.9
Subtentorial — *see* condition
Subthyroidism (acquired) (*see also* Hypothyroidism)
  congenital E03.1
Succenturiate placenta O43.19- ☑
Sucking thumb, child (excessive) F98.8
Sudamen, sudamina L74.1
Sudanese kala-azar B55.0
Sudden
  hearing loss — *see* Deafness, sudden
  heart failure — *see* Failure, heart
Sudeck's atrophy, disease, or syndrome — *see* Algoneurodystrophy
Suffocation — *see* Asphyxia, traumatic
Sugar
  blood
    high (transient) R73.9
    low (transient) E16.2
  in urine R81
Suicide, suicidal (attempted) T14.91 ☑
  by poisoning — *see* Table of Drugs and Chemicals
  history of (personal) Z91.5
    in family Z81.8
  ideation — *see* Ideation, suicidal
  risk
    meaning personal history of attempted suicide
      Z91.5
    meaning suicidal ideation — *see* Ideation, suicidal
  tendencies
    meaning personal history of attempted suicide
      Z91.5
    meaning suicidal ideation — *see* Ideation, suicidal
  trauma — *see* nature of injury by site
Suipestifer infection — *see* Infection, salmonella
Sulfhemoglobinemia, sulphemoglobinemia (acquired) (with methemoglobinemia) D74.8
Sumatran mite fever A75.3
Summer — *see* condition
Sunburn L55.9
  due to
    tanning bed (acute) L56.8
      chronic L57.8
    ultraviolet radiation (acute) L56.8
      chronic L57.8
  first degree L55.0
  second degree L55.1
  third degree L55.2
SUNCT (short lasting unilateral neuralgiform headache
  with conjunctival injection and tearing) G44.059
  intractable G44.051
  not intractable G44.059

Sundowning F05
Sunken acetabulum — *see* Derangement, joint, specified type NEC, hip
Sunstroke T67.0 ☑
Superfecundation — *see* Pregnancy, multiple
Superfetation — *see* Pregnancy, multiple
Superinvolution (uterus) N85.8
Supernumerary (congenital)
  aortic cusps Q23.8
  auditory ossicles Q16.3
  bone Q79.8
  breast Q83.1
  carpal bones Q74.0
  cusps, heart valve NEC Q24.8
    aortic Q23.8
    mitral Q23.2
    pulmonary Q22.3
  digit(s) Q69.9
  ear (lobule) Q17.0
  fallopian tube Q50.6
  finger Q69.0
  hymen Q52.4
  kidney Q63.0
  lacrimonasal duct Q10.6
  lobule (ear) Q17.0
  mitral cusps Q23.2
  muscle Q79.8
  nipple(s) Q83.3
  organ or site not listed — *see* Accessory
  ossicles, auditory Q16.3
  ovary Q50.31
  oviduct Q50.6
  pulmonary, pulmonic cusps Q22.3
  rib Q76.6
    cervical or first (syndrome) Q76.5
  roots (of teeth) K00.2
  spleen Q89.09
  tarsal bones Q74.2
  teeth K00.1
  testis Q55.29
  thumb Q69.1
  toe Q69.2
  uterus Q51.2
  vagina Q52.1 ☑
  vertebra Q76.49
Supervision (of)
  contraceptive — *see* Prescription, contraceptives
  dietary (for) Z71.3
    allergy (food) Z71.3
    colitis Z71.3
    diabetes mellitus Z71.3
    food allergy or intolerance Z71.3
    gastritis Z71.3
    hypercholesterolemia Z71.3
    hypoglycemia Z71.3
    intolerance (food) Z71.3
    obesity Z71.3
    specified NEC Z71.3
  healthy infant or child Z76.2
    foundling Z76.1
  high-risk pregnancy — *see* Pregnancy, complicated
    by, high, risk
  lactation Z39.1
  pregnancy — *see* Pregnancy, supervision of
Supplemental teeth K00.1
Suppression
  binocular vision H53.34
  lactation O92.5
  menstruation N94.89
  ovarian secretion E28.39
  renal N28.9
  urine, urinary secretion R34
Suppuration, suppurative (*see also* condition)
  accessory sinus (chronic) — *see* Sinusitis
  adrenal gland
  antrum (chronic) — *see* Sinusitis, maxillary
  bladder — *see* Cystitis
  brain G06.0
    sequelae G09
  breast N61.1
    puerperal, postpartum or gestational — *see* Masti-
      tis, obstetric, purulent
  dental periosteum M27.3
  ear (middle) (*see also* Otitis, media)
    external NEC — *see* Otitis, externa, infective
    internal — *see* subcategory H83.0 ☑
  ethmoidal (chronic) (sinus) — *see* Sinusitis, ethmoidal
  fallopian tube — *see* Salpingo-oophoritis

Suppuration, suppurative — *continued*
- frontal (chronic) (sinus) — *see* Sinusitis, frontal
- gallbladder (acute) K81.0
- gum K05.20
  - generalized — *see* Peridontitis, aggressive, generalized
  - localized — *see* Peridontitis, aggressive, localized
- intracranial G06.0
- joint — *see* Arthritis, pyogenic or pyemic
- labyrinthine — *see* subcategory H83.0 ☑
- lung — *see* Abscess, lung
- mammary gland N61.1
  - puerperal, postpartum O91.12
    - associated with lactation O91.13
- maxilla, maxillary M27.2
  - sinus (chronic) — *see* Sinusitis, maxillary
- muscle — *see* Myositis, infective
- nasal sinus (chronic) — *see* Sinusitis
- pancreas, acute (*see also* Pancreatitis, acute) K85.80
- parotid gland — *see* Sialoadenitis
- pelvis, pelvic
  - female — *see* Disease, pelvis, inflammatory
  - male K65.0
- pericranial — *see* Osteomyelitis
- salivary duct or gland (any) — *see* Sialoadenitis
- sinus (accessory) (chronic) (nasal) — *see* Sinusitis
- sphenoidal sinus (chronic) — *see* Sinusitis, sphenoidal
- thymus (gland) E32.1
- thyroid (gland) E06.0
- tonsil — *see* Tonsillitis
- uterus — *see* Endometritis

Supraeruption of tooth (teeth) M26.34
Supraglottitis J04.30
- with obstruction J04.31

Suprarenal (gland) — *see* condition
Suprascapular nerve — *see* condition
Suprasellar — *see* condition
Surfer's knots or nodules S89.8- ☑
Surgical
- emphysema T81.82 ☑
- procedures, complication or misadventure — *see* Complications, surgical procedures
- shock T81.10 ☑

Surveillance (of) (for) (*see also* Observation)
- alcohol abuse Z71.41
- contraceptive — *see* Prescription, contraceptives
- dietary Z71.3
- drug abuse Z71.51

Susceptibility to disease, genetic Z15.89
- malignant neoplasm Z15.09
  - breast Z15.01
  - endometrium Z15.04
  - ovary Z15.02
  - prostate Z15.03
  - specified NEC Z15.09
- multiple endocrine neoplasia Z15.81

Suspected condition, ruled out (*see also* Observation, suspected)
- amniotic cavity and membrane Z03.71
- cervical shortening Z03.75
- fetal anomaly Z03.73
- fetal growth Z03.74
- maternal and fetal conditions NEC Z03.79
- newborn (*see also* Observation, newborn, suspected condition ruled out) Z05.9
- oligohydramnios Z03.71
- placental problem Z03.72
- polyhydramnios Z03.71

Suspended uterus
- in pregnancy or childbirth — *see* Pregnancy, complicated by, abnormal uterus

Sutton's nevus D22.9
Suture
- burst (in operation wound) T81.31 ☑
  - external operation wound T81.31 ☑
  - internal operation wound T81.32 ☑
- inadvertently left in operation wound — *see* Foreign body, accidentally left during a procedure
- removal Z48.02

Swab inadvertently left in operation wound — *see* Foreign body, accidentally left during a procedure
Swallowed, swallowing
- difficulty — *see* Dysphagia
- foreign body — *see* Foreign body, alimentary tract

Swan-neck deformity (finger) — *see* Deformity, finger, swan-neck
Swearing, compulsive F42.8

Swearing, compulsive — *continued*
- in Gilles de la Tourette's syndrome F95.2

Sweat, sweats
- fetid L75.0
- night R61

Sweating, excessive R61
Sweeley-Klionsky disease E75.21
Sweet's disease or dermatosis L98.2
Swelling (of) R60.9
- abdomen, abdominal (not referable to any particular organ) — *see* Mass, abdominal
- ankle — *see* Effusion, joint, ankle
- arm M79.89
  - forearm M79.89
- breast (*see also* Lump, breast) N63.0
- Calabar B74.3
- cervical gland R59.0
- chest, localized R22.2
- ear H93.8- ☑
- extremity (lower) (upper) — *see* Disorder, soft tissue, specified type NEC
- finger M79.89
- foot M79.89
- glands R59.9
  - generalized R59.1
  - localized R59.0
- hand M79.89
- head (localized) R22.0
- inflammatory — *see* Inflammation
- intra-abdominal — *see* Mass, abdominal
- joint — *see* Effusion, joint
- leg M79.89
  - lower M79.89
- limb — *see* Disorder, soft tissue, specified type NEC
- localized (skin) R22.9
  - chest R22.2
  - head R22.0
  - limb
    - lower — *see* Mass, localized, limb, lower
    - upper — *see* Mass, localized, limb, upper
  - neck R22.1
  - trunk R22.2
- neck (localized) R22.1
- pelvic — *see* Mass, abdominal
- scrotum N50.89
- splenic — *see* Splenomegaly
- testis N50.89
- toe M79.89
- umbilical R19.09
- wandering, due to Gnathostoma (spinigerum) B83.1
- white — *see* Tuberculosis, arthritis

Swift (-Feer) **disease**
- overdose or wrong substance given or taken — *see* Table of Drugs and Chemicals, by drug, poisoning

Swimmer's
- cramp T75.1 ☑
- ear H60.33- ☑
- itch B65.3

Swimming in the head R42
Swollen — *see* Swelling
Swyer syndrome Q99.1
Sycosis L73.8
- barbae (not parasitic) L73.8
- contagiosa (mycotic) B35.0
- lupoides L73.8
- mycotic B35.0
- parasitic B35.0
- vulgaris L73.8

Sydenham's chorea — *see* Chorea, Sydenham's
Sylvatic yellow fever A95.0
Sylvest's disease B33.0
Symblepharon H11.23- ☑
- congenital Q10.3

Symond's syndrome G93.2
Sympathetic — *see* condition
Sympatheticotonia G90.8
Sympathicoblastoma
- specified site — *see* Neoplasm, malignant, by site
- unspecified site C74.90

Sympathogonioma — *see* Sympathicoblastoma
Symphalangy (fingers) (toes) Q70.9
Symptoms NEC R68.89
- breast NEC N64.59
- cold J00
- development NEC R63.8
- factitious, self-induced — *see* Disorder, factitious

Symptoms — *continued*
- genital organs, female R10.2
- involving
  - abdomen NEC R19.8
  - appearance NEC R46.89
  - awareness R41.9
    - altered mental status R41.82
    - amnesia — *see* Amnesia
    - borderline intellectual functioning R41.83
    - coma — *see* Coma
    - disorientation R41.0
    - neurologic neglect syndrome R41.4
    - senile cognitive decline R41.81
    - specified symptom NEC R41.89
  - behavior NEC R46.89
  - cardiovascular system NEC R09.89
  - chest NEC R09.89
  - circulatory system NEC R09.89
  - cognitive functions R41.9
    - altered mental status R41.82
    - amnesia — *see* Amnesia
    - borderline intellectual functioning R41.83
    - coma — *see* Coma
    - disorientation R41.0
    - neurologic neglect syndrome R41.4
    - senile cognitive decline R41.81
    - specified symptom NEC R41.89
  - development NEC R62.50
  - digestive system NEC R19.8
  - emotional state NEC R45.89
    - emotional lability R45.86
  - food and fluid intake R63.8
  - general perceptions and sensations R44.9
    - specified NEC R44.8
  - musculoskeletal system R29.91
    - specified NEC R29.898
  - nervous system R29.90
    - specified NEC R29.818
  - pelvis NEC R19.8
  - respiratory system NEC R09.89
  - skin and integument R23.9
  - urinary system R39.9
- menopausal N95.1
- metabolism NEC R63.8
- neurotic F48.8
- of infancy R68.19
- pelvis NEC, female R10.2
- skin and integument NEC R23.9
- subcutaneous tissue NEC R23.9
- viral cold J00

Sympus Q74.2
Syncephalus Q89.4
Synchondrosis
- abnormal (congenital) Q78.8
- ischiopubic M91.0

Synchysis (scintillans) (senile) (vitreous body) H43.89
Syncope (near) (pre-) R55
- anginosa I20.8
- bradycardia R00.1
- cardiac R55
- carotid sinus G90.01
- due to spinal (lumbar) puncture G97.1
- heart R55
- heat T67.1 ☑
- laryngeal R05
- psychogenic F48.8
- tussive R05
- vasoconstriction R55
- vasodepressor R55
- vasomotor R55
- vasovagal R55

Syndactylism, syndactyly Q70.9
- complex (with synostosis)
  - fingers Q70.0- ☑
  - toes Q70.2- ☑
- simple (without synostosis)
  - fingers Q70.1- ☑
  - toes Q70.3- ☑

Syndrome (*see also* Disease)
- 48,XXXX Q97.1
- 49,XXXXX Q97.1
- 5q minus NOS D46.C (*following* D46.2)
- abdominal
  - acute R10.0
  - muscle deficiency Q79.4
- abnormal innervation H02.519
  - left H02.516
    - lower H02.515

Syndrome — *continued*
- abnormal innervation — *continued*
  - left — *continued*
    - upper H02.514
  - right H02.513
    - lower H02.512
    - upper H02.511
- abstinence, neonatal P96.1
- acid pulmonary aspiration, obstetric O74.0
- acquired immunodeficiency — *see* Human, immunodeficiency virus (HIV) disease
- acute abdominal R10.0
- acute respiratory distress (adult) (child) J80
  - idiopathic J84.114
- Adair-Dighton Q78.0
- Adams-Stokes (-Morgagni) I45.9
- adiposogenital E23.6
- adrenal
  - hemorrhage (meningococcal) A39.1
  - meningococcic A39.1
- adrenocortical — *see* Cushing's, syndrome
- adrenogenital E25.9
  - congenital, associated with enzyme deficiency E25.0
- afferent loop NEC K91.89
- Alagille's Q44.7
- alcohol withdrawal (without convulsions) — *see* Dependence, alcohol, with, withdrawal
- Alder's D72.0
- Aldrich (-Wiskott) D82.0
- alien hand R41.4
- Alport Q87.81
- alveolar hypoventilation E66.2
- alveolocapillary block J84.10
- amnesic, amnestic (confabulatory) (due to) — *see* Disorder, amnesic
- amyostatic (Wilson's disease) E83.01
- androgen insensitivity E34.50
  - complete E34.51
  - partial E34.52
- androgen resistance (*see also* Syndrome, androgen insensitivity) E34.50
- Angelman Q93.5
- anginal — *see* Angina
- ankyloglossia superior Q38.1
- anterior
  - chest wall R07.89
  - cord G83.82
  - spinal artery G95.19
    - compression M47.019
      - cervical region M47.012
      - cervicothoracic region M47.013
      - lumbar region M47.016
      - occipito-atlanto-axial region M47.011
      - thoracic region M47.014
      - thoracolumbar region M47.015
  - tibial M76.81- ☑
- antibody deficiency D80.9
  - agammaglobulinemic D80.1
    - hereditary D80.0
  - congenital D80.0
  - hypogammaglobulinemic D80.1
    - hereditary D80.0
- anticardiolipin (-antibody) D68.61
- antidepressant discontinuation T43.205 ☑
- antiphospholipid (-antibody) D68.61
- aortic
  - arch M31.4
  - bifurcation I74.09
- aortomesenteric duodenum occlusion K31.5
- apical ballooning (transient left ventricular) I51.81
- arcuate ligament I77.4
- argentaffin, argentaffinoma E34.0
- Arnold-Chiari — *see* Arnold-Chiari disease
- Arrillaga-Ayerza I27.0
- arterial tortuosity Q87.82
- arteriovenous steal T82.898- ☑
- Asherman's N85.6
- aspiration, of newborn — *see* Aspiration, by substance, with pneumonia
  - meconium P24.01
- ataxia-telangiectasia G11.3
- auriculotemporal G50.8
- autoerythrocyte sensitization (Gardner-Diamond) D69.2
- autoimmune lymphoproliferative [ALPS] D89.82
- autoimmune polyglandular E31.0
- autoinflammatory M04.9

Syndrome — *continued*
- autoinflammatory — *continued*
  - specified type NEC M04.8
- autosomal — *see* Abnormal, autosomes
- Avellis' G46.8
- Ayerza (-Arrillaga) I27.0
- Babinski-Nageotte G83.89
- Bakwin-Krida Q78.5
- bare lymphocyte D81.6
- Barré-Guillain G61.0
- Barré-Liéou M53.0
- Barrett's — *see* Barrett's, esophagus
- Barsony-Polgar K22.4
- Bársony-Teschendorf K22.4
- Barth E78.71
- Bartter's E26.81
- basal cell nevus Q87.89
- Basedow's E05.00
  - with thyroid storm E05.01
- basilar artery G45.0
- Batten-Steinert G71.11
- battered
  - baby or child — *see* Maltreatment, child, physical abuse
  - spouse — *see* Maltreatment, adult, physical abuse
- Beals Q87.40
- Beau's I51.5
- Beck's I65.8
- Benedikt's G46.3
- Béquez César (-Steinbrinck-Chédiak-Higashi) E70.330
- Bernhardt-Roth — *see* Meralgia paresthetica
- Bernheim's — *see* Failure, heart, right
- big spleen D73.1
- bilateral polycystic ovarian E28.2
- Bing-Horton's — *see* Horton's headache
- Birt-Hogg-Dube syndrome Q87.89
- Björck (-Thorsen) E34.0
- black
  - lung J60
  - widow spider bite — *see* Toxicity, venom, spider, black widow
- Blackfan-Diamond D61.01
- Blau M04.8
- blind loop K90.2
  - congenital Q43.8
  - postsurgical K91.2
- blue sclera Q78.0
- blue toe I75.02- ☑
- Boder-Sedgewick G11.3
- Boerhaave's K22.3
- Borjeson Forssman Lehmann Q89.8
- Bouillaud's I01.9
- Bourneville (-Pringle) Q85.1
- Bouveret (-Hoffman) I47.9
- brachial plexus G54.0
- bradycardia-tachycardia I49.5
- brain (nonpsychotic) F09
  - with psychosis, psychotic reaction F09
  - acute or subacute — *see* Delirium
  - congenital — *see* Disability, intellectual
  - organic F09
    - post-traumatic (nonpsychotic) F07.81
      - psychotic F09
    - personality change F07.0
    - postcontusional F07.81
    - post-traumatic, nonpsychotic F07.81
    - psycho-organic F09
    - psychotic F06.8
- brain stem stroke G46.3
- Brandt's (acrodermatitis enteropathica) E83.2
- broad ligament laceration N83.8
- Brock's J98.11
- bronze baby P83.88
- Brown-Sequard G83.81
- Brugada I49.8
- bubbly lung P27.0
- Buchem's M85.2
- Budd-Chiari I82.0
- bulbar (progressive) G12.22
- Bürger-Grütz E78.3
- Burke's K86.89
- Burnett's (milk-alkali) E83.52
- burning feet E53.9
- Bywaters' T79.5 ☑
- Call-Fleming I67.841
- carbohydrate-deficient glycoprotein (CDGS) E77.8
- carcinogenic thrombophlebitis I82.1
- carcinoid E34.0

Syndrome — *continued*
- cardiac asthma I50.1
- cardiacos negros I27.0
- cardiofaciocutaneous Q87.89
- cardiopulmonary-obesity E66.2
- cardiorenal — *see* Hypertension, cardiorenal
- cardiorespiratory distress (idiopathic), newborn P22.0
- cardiovascular renal — *see* Hypertension, cardiorenal
- carotid
  - artery (hemispheric) (internal) G45.1
  - body G90.01
  - sinus G90.01
- carpal tunnel G56.0- ☑
- Cassidy (-Scholte) E34.0
- cat cry Q93.4
- cat eye Q92.8
- cauda equina G83.4
- causalgia — *see* Causalgia
- celiac K90.0
  - artery compression I77.4
  - axis I77.4
- central pain G89.0
- cerebellar
  - hereditary G11.9
  - stroke G46.4
- cerebellomedullary malformation — *see* Spina bifida
- cerebral
  - artery
    - anterior G46.1
    - middle G46.0
    - posterior G46.2
  - gigantism E22.0
- cervical M53.1
  - disc — *see* Disorder, disc, cervical, with neuritis
  - fusion Q76.1
  - posterior, sympathicus M53.0
  - rib Q76.5
  - sympathetic paralysis G90.2
- cervicobrachial (diffuse) M53.1
- cervicocranial M53.0
- cervicodorsal outlet G54.2
- cervicothoracic outlet G54.0
- Céstan (-Raymond) I65.8
- Charcot's (angina cruris) (intermittent claudication) I73.9
- Charcot-Weiss-Baker G90.09
- CHARGE Q89.8
- Chédiak-Higashi (-Steinbrinck) E70.330
- chest wall R07.1
- Chiari's (hepatic vein thrombosis) I82.0
- Chilaiditi's Q43.3
- child maltreatment — *see* Maltreatment, child
- chondrocostal junction M94.0
- chondroectodermal dysplasia Q77.6
- chromosome 4 short arm deletion Q93.3
- chromosome 5 short arm deletion Q93.4
- chronic
  - infantile neurological, cutaneous and articular (CINCA) M04.2
  - pain G89.4
    - personality F68.8
- Clarke-Hadfield K86.89
- Clerambault's automatism G93.89
- Clouston's (hidrotic ectodermal dysplasia) Q82.4
- clumsiness, clumsy child F82
- cluster headache G44.009
  - intractable G44.001
  - not intractable G44.009
- Coffin-Lowry Q89.8
- cold injury (newborn) P80.0
- combined immunity deficiency D81.9
- compartment (deep) (posterior) (traumatic) T79.A0 ☑ (*following* T79.7)
  - abdomen T79.A3 ☑ (*following* T79.7)
  - lower extremity (hip, buttock, thigh, leg, foot, toes) T79.A2 ☑ (*following* T79.7)
  - nontraumatic
    - abdomen M79.A3 (*following* M79.7)
    - lower extremity (hip, buttock, thigh, leg, foot, toes) M79.A2- ☑ (*following* M79.7)
    - specified site NEC M79.A9 (*following* M79.7)
    - upper extremity (shoulder, arm, forearm, wrist, hand, fingers) M79.A1- ☑ (*following* M79.7)
  - postprocedural — *see* Syndrome, compartment, nontraumatic
  - specified site NEC T79.A9 ☑ (*following* T79.7)

Syndrome — *continued*
compartment — *continued*
  upper extremity (shoulder, arm, forearm, wrist, hand, fingers) T79.A1 ☑ (*following* T79.7)
complex regional pain — *see* Syndrome, pain, complex regional
compression T79.5 ☑
  anterior spinal — *see* Syndrome, anterior, spinal artery, compression
  cauda equina G83.4
  celiac artery I77.4
  vertebral artery M47.029
    cervical region M47.022
    occipito-atlanto-axial region M47.021
concussion F07.81
congenital
  affecting multiple systems NEC Q87.89
  central alveolar hypoventilation G47.35
  facial diplegia Q87.0
  muscular hypertrophy-cerebral Q87.89
  oculo-auriculovertebral Q87.0
  oculofacial diplegia (Moebius) Q87.0
  rubella (manifest) P35.0
congestion-fibrosis (pelvic), female N94.89
congestive dysmenorrhea N94.6
connective tissue M35.9
  overlap NEC M35.1
Conn's E26.01
conus medullaris G95.81
cord
  anterior G83.82
  posterior G83.83
coronary
  acute NEC I24.9
  insufficiency or intermediate I20.0
  slow flow I20.8
Costen's (complex) M26.69
costochondral junction M94.0
costoclavicular G54.0
costovertebral E22.0
Cowden Q85.8
craniovertebral M53.0
Creutzfeldt-Jakob — *see* Creutzfeldt-Jakob disease or syndrome
crib death R99
cricopharyngeal — *see* Dysphagia
cri-du-chat Q93.4
croup J05.0
CRPS I — *see* Syndrome, pain, complex regional I
crush T79.5 ☑
cryopyrin-associated periodic M04.2
cryptophthalmos Q87.0
cubital tunnel — *see* Lesion, nerve, ulnar
Curschmann (-Batten) (-Steinert) G71.11
Cushing's E24.9
  alcohol-induced E24.4
  drug-induced E24.2
  due to
    alcohol
    drugs E24.2
    ectopic ACTH E24.3
    overproduction of pituitary ACTH E24.0
    overdose or wrong substance given or taken — *see* Table of Drugs and Chemicals, by drug, poisoning
  pituitary-dependent E24.0
  specified type NEC E24.8
cystic duct stump K91.5
Dana-Putnam D51.0
Danbolt (-Cross) (acrodermatitis enteropathica) E83.2
Dandy-Walker Q03.1
  with spina bifida Q07.01
Danlos' Q79.6
De Quervain E34.51
de Toni-Fanconi (-Debré) E72.09
  with cystinosis E72.04
defibrination (*see also* Fibrinolysis)
  with
    antepartum hemorrhage — *see* Hemorrhage, antepartum, with coagulation defect
    intrapartum hemorrhage — *see* Hemorrhage, complicating, delivery
  newborn P60
  postpartum O72.3
Degos' I77.89
Déjérine-Roussy G89.0
delayed sleep phase G47.21
demyelinating G37.9

Syndrome — *continued*
dependence — *see* F10-F19 with fourth character .2
depersonalization (-derealization) F48.1
di George's D82.1
diabetes mellitus in newborn infant P70.2
diabetes mellitus-hypertension-nephrosis — *see* Diabetes, nephrosis
diabetes-nephrosis — *see* Diabetes, nephrosis
diabetic amyotrophy — *see* Diabetes, amyotrophy
dialysis associated steal T82.898- ☑
Diamond-Blackfan D61.01
Diamond-Gardener D69.2
DIC (diffuse or disseminated intravascular coagulopathy) D65
Dighton's Q78.0
disequilibrium E87.8
Döhle body-panmyelopathic D72.0
dorsolateral medullary G46.4
double athetosis G80.3
Down (*see also* Down syndrome) Q90.9
Dresbach's (elliptocytosis) D58.1
Dressler's (postmyocardial infarction) I24.1
  postcardiotomy I97.0
drug withdrawal, infant of dependent mother P96.1
dry eye H04.12- ☑
due to abnormality
  chromosomal Q99.9
    sex
      female phenotype Q97.9
      male phenotype Q98.9
    specified NEC Q99.8
dumping (postgastrectomy) K91.1
  nonsurgical K31.89
Dupré's (meningism) R29.1
dysmetabolic X E88.81
dyspraxia, developmental F82
Eagle-Barrett Q79.4
Eaton-Lambert — *see* Syndrome, Lambert-Eaton
Ebstein's Q22.5
ectopic ACTH E24.3
eczema-thrombocytopenia D82.0
Eddowes' Q78.0
effort (psychogenic) F45.8
Ehlers-Danlos Q79.6
Eisenmenger's I27.83
Ekman's Q78.0
electric feet E53.8
Ellis-van Creveld Q77.6
empty nest Z60.0
endocrine-hypertensive E27.0
entrapment — *see* Neuropathy, entrapment
eosinophilia-myalgia M35.8
epileptic (*see also* Epilepsy, by type)
  absence G40.A09 (*following* G40.3)
    intractable G40.A19 (*following* G40.3)
      with status epilepticus G40.A11 (*following* G40.3)
      without status epilepticus G40.A19 (*following* G40.3)
    not intractable G40.A09 (*following* G40.3)
      with status epilepticus G40.A01 (*following* G40.3)
      without status epilepticus G40.A09 (*following* G40.3)
Erdheim-Chester (ECD) E88.89
Erdheim's E22.0
erythrocyte fragmentation D59.4
Evans D69.41
exhaustion F48.8
extrapyramidal G25.9
  specified NEC G25.89
eye retraction — *see* Strabismus
eyelid-malar-mandible Q87.0
Faber's D50.9
facial pain, paroxysmal G50.0
Fallot's Q21.3
familial cold autoinflammatory M04.2
familial eczema-thrombocytopenia (Wiskott-Aldrich) D82.0
Fanconi (-de Toni) (-Debré) E72.09
  with cystinosis E72.04
Fanconi's (anemia) (congenital pancytopenia) D61.09
fatigue
  chronic R53.82
  psychogenic F48.8
faulty bowel habit K59.39
Feil-Klippel (brevicollis) Q76.1
Felty's — *see* Felty's syndrome

Syndrome — *continued*
fertile eunuch E23.0
fetal
  alcohol (dysmorphic) Q86.0
  hydantoin Q86.1
Fiedler's I40.1
first arch Q87.0
fish odor E72.8
Fisher's G61.0
Fitzhugh-Curtis
  due to
    Chlamydia trachomatis A74.81
    Neisseria gonorrhorea (gonococcal peritonitis) A54.85
Fitz's (*see also* Pancreatitis, acute) K85.80
Flajani (-Basedow) E05.00
  with thyroid storm E05.01
flatback — *see* Flatback syndrome
floppy
  baby P94.2
  iris (intraoperative) (IFIS) H21.81
  mitral valve I34.1
flush E34.0
Foix-Alajouanine G95.19
Fong's Q87.2
food protein-induced enterocolitis K52.21
foramen magnum G93.5
Foster-Kennedy H47.14- ☑
Foville's (peduncular) G46.3
fragile X Q99.2
Franceschetti Q75.4
Frey's
  auriculotemporal G50.8
  hyperhidrosis L74.52
Friderichsen-Waterhouse A39.1
Froin's G95.89
frontal lobe F07.0
Fukuhara E88.49
functional
  bowel K59.9
  prepubertal castrate E29.1
Gaisböck's D75.1
ganglion (basal ganglia brain) G25.9
  geniculi G51.1
Gardner-Diamond D69.2
gastroesophageal
  junction K22.0
  laceration-hemorrhage K22.6
gastrojejunal loop obstruction K91.89
Gee-Herter-Heubner K90.0
Gelineau's G47.419
  with cataplexy G47.411
genito-anorectal A55
Gerstmann-Sträussler-Scheinker (GSS) A81.82
Gianotti-Crosti L44.4
giant platelet (Bernard-Soulier) D69.1
Gilles de la Tourette's F95.2
goiter-deafness E07.1
Goldberg Q89.8
Goldberg-Maxwell E34.51
Good's D83.8
Gopalan' (burning feet) E53.8
Gorlin's Q87.89
Gougerot-Blum L81.7
Gouley's I31.1
Gower's R55
gray or grey (newborn) P93.0
  platelet D69.1
Gubler-Millard G46.3
Guillain-Barré (-Strohl) G61.0
gustatory sweating G50.8
Hadfield-Clarke K86.89
hair tourniquet — *see* Constriction, external, by site
Hamman's J98.19
hand-foot L27.1
hand-shoulder G90.8
hantavirus (cardio)-pulmonary (HPS) (HCPS) B33.4
happy puppet Q93.5
Harada's H30.81- ☑
Hayem-Faber D50.9
headache NEC G44.89
  complicated NEC G44.59
Heberden's I20.8
Hedinger's E34.0
Hegglin's D72.0
HELLP (hemolysis, elevated liver enzymes and low platelet count) O14.2- ☑
  complicating
    childbirth O14.24

Syndrome — *continued*
  HELLP — *continued*
    complicating — *continued*
      puerperium O14.25
  hemolytic-uremic D59.3
  hemophagocytic, infection-associated D76.2
  Henoch-Schönlein D69.0
  hepatic flexure K59.8
  hepatopulmonary K76.81
  hepatorenal K76.7
    following delivery O90.4
    postoperative or postprocedural K91.83
    postpartum, puerperal O90.4
  hepatourologic K76.7
  Herter (-Gee) (nontropical sprue) K90.0
  Heubner-Herter K90.0
  Heyd's K76.7
  Hilger's G90.09
  histamine-like (fish poisoning) — *see* Poisoning, fish
  histiocytic D76.3
  histiocytosis NEC D76.3
  HIV infection, acute B20
  Hoffmann-Werdnig G12.0
  Hollander-Simons E88.1
  Hoppe-Goldflam G70.00
    with exacerbation (acute) G70.01
    in crisis G70.01
  Horner's G90.2
  hungry bone E83.81
  hunterian glossitis D51.0
  Hutchinson's triad A50.53
  hyperabduction G54.0
  hyperammonemia-hyperornithinemia-homocitrulline-mia E72.4
  hypereosinophilic (idiopathic) D72.1
  hyperimmunoglobulin D M04.1
  hyperimmunoglobulin E (IgE) D82.4
  hyperkalemic E87.5
  hyperkinetic — *see* Hyperkinesia
  hypermobility M35.7
  hypernatremia E87.0
  hyperosmolarity E87.0
  hyperperfusion G97.82
  hypersplenic D73.1
  hypertransfusion, newborn P61.1
  hyperventilation F45.8
  hyperviscosity (of serum)
    polycythemic D75.1
    sclerothymic D58.8
  hypoglycemic (familial) (neonatal) E16.2
  hypokalemic E87.6
  hyponatremic E87.1
  hypopituitarism E23.0
  hypoplastic left-heart Q23.4
  hypopotassemia E87.6
  hyposmolality E87.1
  hypotension, maternal O26.5- ☑
  hypothenar hammer I73.89
  hypoventilation, obesity (OHS) E66.2
  ICF (intravascular coagulation-fibrinolysis) D65
  idiopathic
    cardiorespiratory distress, newborn P22.0
    nephrotic (infantile) N04.9
  iliotibial band M76.3- ☑
  immobility, immobilization (paraplegic) M62.3
  immune reconstitution D89.3
  immune reconstitution inflammatory [IRIS] D89.3
  immunity deficiency, combined D81.9
  immunodeficiency
    acquired — *see* Human, immunodeficiency virus (HIV) disease
    combined D81.9
  impending coronary I20.0
  impingement, shoulder M75.4- ☑
  inappropriate secretion of antidiuretic hormone E22.2
  infant
    gestational diabetes P70.0
    of diabetic mother P70.1
  infantilism (pituitary) E23.0
  inferior vena cava I87.1
  inspissated bile (newborn) P59.1
  institutional (childhood) F94.2
  insufficient sleep F51.12
  intermediate coronary (artery) I20.0
  interspinous ligament — *see* Spondylopathy, specified NEC
  intestinal
    carcinoid E34.0

Syndrome — *continued*
  intestinal — *continued*
    knot K56.2
  intravascular coagulation-fibrinolysis (ICF) D65
  iodine-deficiency, congenital E00.9
    type
      mixed E00.2
      myxedematous E00.1
      neurological E00.0
  IRDS (idiopathic respiratory distress, newborn) P22.0
  irritable
    bowel K58.9
      with
        constipation K58.1
        diarrhea K58.0
      mixed K58.2
      psychogenic F45.8
      specified NEC K58.8
    heart (psychogenic) F45.8
    weakness F48.8
  ischemic
    bowel (transient) K55.9
      chronic K55.1
      due to mesenteric artery insufficiency K55.1
    steal T82.898 ☑
  IVC (intravascular coagulopathy) D65
  Ivemark's Q89.01
  Jaccoud's — *see* Arthropathy, postrheumatic, chronic
  Jackson's G83.89
  Jakob-Creutzfeldt — *see* Creutzfeldt-Jakob disease or syndrome
  jaw-winking Q07.8
  Jervell-Lange-Nielsen I45.81
  jet lag G47.25
  Job's D71
  Joseph-Diamond-Blackfan D61.01
  jugular foramen G52.7
  Kabuki Q89.8
  Kanner's (autism) F84.0
  Kartagener's Q89.3
  Kelly's D50.1
  Kimmelstiel-Wilson — *see* Diabetes, specified type, with Kimmelstiel-Wilson disease
  Klein (e)-Levine G47.13
  Klippel-Feil (brevicollis) Q76.1
  Köhler-Pellegrini-Steida — *see* Bursitis, tibial collateral
  König's K59.8
  Korsakoff (-Wernicke) (nonalcoholic) F04
    alcoholic F10.26
  Kostmann's D70.0
  Krabbe's congenital muscle hypoplasia Q79.8
  labyrinthine — *see* subcategory H83.2 ☑
  lacunar NEC G46.7
  Lambert-Eaton G70.80
    in
      neoplastic disease G73.1
      specified disease NEC G70.81
  Landau-Kleffner — *see* Epilepsy, specified NEC
  Larsen's Q74.8
  lateral
    cutaneous nerve of thigh G57.1- ☑
    medullary G46.4
  Launois' E22.0
  lazy
    leukocyte D70.8
    posture M62.3
  Lemiere I80.8
  Lennox-Gastaut G40.812
    intractable G40.814
      with status epilepticus G40.813
      without status epilepticus G40.814
    not intractable G40.812
      with status epilepticus G40.811
      without status epilepticus G40.812
  lenticular, progressive E83.01
  Leopold-Levi's E05.90
  Lev's I44.2
  Lichtheim's D51.0
  Li-Fraumeni Z15.01
  Lightwood's N25.89
  Lignac (de Toni) (-Fanconi) (-Debré) E72.09
    with cystinosis E72.04
  Likoff's I20.8
  limbic epilepsy personality F07.0
  liver-kidney K76.7
  lobotomy F07.0
  Loffler's J82
  long arm 18 or 21 deletion Q93.89

Syndrome — *continued*
  long QT I45.81
  Louis-Barré G11.3
  low
    atmospheric pressure T70.29 ☑
    back M54.5
    output (cardiac) I50.9
  lower radicular, newborn (birth injury) P14.8
  Luetscher's (dehydration) E86.0
  Lupus anticoagulant D68.62
  Lutembacher's Q21.1
  macrophage activation D76.1
    due to infection D76.2
  magnesium-deficiency R29.0
  Majeed M04.8
  Mal de Debarquement R42
  malabsorption K90.9
    postsurgical K91.2
  malformation, congenital, due to
    alcohol Q86.0
    exogenous cause NEC Q86.8
    hydantoin Q86.1
    warfarin Q86.2
  malignant
    carcinoid E34.0
    neuroleptic G21.0
  Mallory-Weiss K22.6
  mandibulofacial dysostosis Q75.4
  manic-depressive — *see* Disorder, bipolar
  maple-syrup-urine E71.0
  Marable's I77.4
  Marfan's Q87.40
    with
      cardiovascular manifestations Q87.418
        aortic dilation Q87.410
      ocular manifestations Q87.42
      skeletal manifestations Q87.43
  Marie's (acromegaly) E22.0
  mast cell activation — *see* Activation, mast cell
  maternal hypotension — *see* Syndrome, hypotension, maternal
  May (-Hegglin) D72.0
  McArdle (-Schmidt) (-Pearson) E74.04
  McQuarrie's E16.2
  meconium plug (newborn) P76.0
  median arcuate ligament I77.4
  Meekeren-Ehlers-Danlos Q79.6
  megavitamin-B6 E67.2
  Meige G24.4
  MELAS E88.41
  Mendelson's O74.0
  MERRF (myoclonic epilepsy associated with ragged-red fibers) E88.42
  mesenteric
    artery (superior) K55.1
    vascular insufficiency K55.1
  metabolic E88.81
  metastatic carcinoid E34.0
  micrognathia-glossoptosis Q87.0
  midbrain NEC G93.89
  middle lobe (lung) J98.19
  middle radicular G54.0
  migraine (*see also* Migraine) G43.909
  Mikulicz' K11.8
  milk-alkali E83.52
  Millard-Gubler G46.3
  Miller-Dieker Q93.88
  Miller-Fisher G61.0
  Minkowski-Chauffard D58.0
  Mirizzi's K83.1
  MNGIE (Mitochondrial Neurogastrointestinal En-cephalopathy) E88.49
  Möbius, ophthalmoplegic migraine — *see* Migraine, ophthalmoplegic
  monofixation H50.42
  Morel-Moore M85.2
  Morel-Morgagni M85.2
  Morgagni (-Morel) (-Stewart) M85.2
  Morgagni-Adams-Stokes I45.9
  Mounier-Kuhn Q32.4
    with bronchiectasis J47.9
      with
        exacerbation (acute) J47.1
        lower respiratory infection J47.0
    acquired J98.09
      with bronchiectasis J47.9
        with
          exacerbation (acute) J47.1
          lower respiratory infection J47.0

Syndrome — *continued*
- Muckle-Wells M04.2
- mucocutaneous lymph node (acute febrile) (MCLS) M30.3
- multiple endocrine neoplasia (MEN) — *see* Neoplasia, endocrine, multiple (MEN)
- multiple operations — *see* Disorder, factitious
- myasthenic G70.9
  - in
    - diabetes mellitus — *see* Diabetes, amyotrophy
    - endocrine disease NEC E34.9 [G73.3]
    - neoplastic disease (*see also* Neoplasm) D49.9 [G73.3]
    - thyrotoxicosis (hyperthyroidism) E05.90 [G73.3]
      - with thyroid storm E05.91 [G73.3]
- myelodysplastic D46.9
  - with
    - 5q deletion D46.C (*following* D46.2)
    - isolated del (5q) chromosomal abnormality D46.C (*following* D46.2)
    - lesions, low grade D46.20
    - specified NEC D46.Z (*following* D46.4)
- myelopathic pain G89.0
- myeloproliferative (chronic) D47.1
- myofascial pain M79.1
- Naffziger's G54.0
- nail patella Q87.2
- NARP (Neuropathy, Ataxia and Retinitis pigmentosa) E88.49
- neonatal abstinence P96.1
- nephritic (*see also* Nephritis)
  - with edema — *see* Nephrosis
  - acute N00.9
  - chronic N03.9
  - rapidly progressive N01.9
- nephrotic (congenital) (*see also* Nephrosis) N04.9
  - with
    - dense deposit disease N04.6
    - diffuse
      - crescentic glomerulonephritis N04.7
      - endocapillary proliferative glomerulonephritis N04.4
      - membranous glomerulonephritis N04.2
      - mesangial proliferative glomerulonephritis N04.3
      - mesangiocapillary glomerulonephritis N04.5
    - focal and segmental glomerular lesions N04.1
    - minor glomerular abnormality N04.0
    - specified morphological changes NEC N04.8
  - diabetic — *see* Diabetes, nephrosis
- neurologic neglect R41.4
- Nezelof's D81.4
- Nonne-Milroy-Meige Q82.0
- Nothnagel's vasomotor acroparesthesia I73.89
- obesity hypoventilation (OHS) E66.2
- oculomotor H51.9
- ophthalmoplegia-cerebellar ataxia — *see* Strabismus, paralytic, third nerve
- oral allergy T78.1 ☑
- oral-facial-digital Q87.0
- organic
  - affective F06.30
  - amnesic (not alcohol- or drug-induced) F04
  - brain F09
  - depressive F06.31
  - hallucinosis F06.0
  - personality F07.0
- Ormond's N13.5
- oro-facial-digital Q87.0
- os trigonum Q68.8
- Osler-Weber-Rendu I78.0
- osteoporosis-osteomalacia M83.8
- Osterreicher-Turner Q87.2
- otolith — *see* subcategory H81.8 ☑
- oto-palatal-digital Q87.0
- outlet (thoracic) G54.0
- ovary
  - polycystic E28.2
  - resistant E28.39
  - sclerocystic E28.2
- Owren's D68.2
- Paget-Schroetter I82.890
- pain (*see also* Pain)
  - complex regional I G90.50
    - lower limb G90.52- ☑
    - specified site NEC G90.59
    - upper limb G90.51- ☑
  - complex regional II — *see* Causalgia

Syndrome — *continued*
- painful
  - bruising D69.2
  - feet E53.8
  - prostate N42.81
- paralysis agitans — *see* Parkinsonism
- paralytic G83.9
  - specified NEC G83.89
- Parinaud's H51.0
- parkinsonian — *see* Parkinsonism
- Parkinson's — *see* Parkinsonism
- paroxysmal facial pain G50.0
- Parry's E05.00
  - with thyroid storm E05.01
- Parsonage (-Aldren)-Turner G54.5
- patella clunk M25.86- ☑
- Paterson (-Brown) (-Kelly) D50.1
- pectoral girdle I77.89
- pectoralis minor I77.89
- pediatric autoimmune neuropsychiatric disorders associated with streptococcal infections (PANDAS) D89.89
- Pelger-Huet D72.0
- pellagra-cerebellar ataxia-renal aminoaciduria E72.02
- pellagroid E52
- Pellegrini-Stieda — *see* Bursitis, tibial collateral
- pelvic congestion-fibrosis, female N94.89
- penta X Q97.1
- peptic ulcer — *see* Ulcer, peptic
- perabduction I77.89
- periodic fever M04.1
- periodic fever, aphthous stomatitis, pharyngitis, and adenopathy [PFAPA] M04.8
- periodic headache, in adults and children — *see* Headache, periodic syndromes in adults and children
- periurethral fibrosis N13.5
- phantom limb (without pain) G54.7
  - with pain G54.6
- pharyngeal pouch D82.1
- Pick's — *see* Disease, Pick's
- Pickwickian E66.2
- PIE (pulmonary infiltration with eosinophilia) J82
- pigmentary pallidal degeneration (progressive) G23.0
- pineal E34.8
- pituitary E22.0
- placental transfusion — *see* Pregnancy, complicated by, placental transfusion syndromes
- plantar fascia M72.2
- plateau iris (post-iridectomy) (postprocedural) H21.82
- Plummer-Vinson D50.1
- pluricarential of infancy E40
- plurideficiency E40
- pluriglandular (compensatory) E31.8
  - autoimmune E31.0
- pneumatic hammer T75.21 ☑
- polyangiitis overlap M30.8
- polycarential of infancy E40
- polyglandular E31.8
  - autoimmune E31.0
- polysplenia Q89.09
- pontine NEC G93.89
- popliteal
  - artery entrapment I77.89
  - web Q87.89
- post chemoembolization — *code to* associated conditions
- postcardiac injury
  - postcardiotomy I97.0
  - postmyocardial infarction I24.1
- postcardiotomy I97.0
- postcholecystectomy K91.5
- postcommissurotomy I97.0
- postconcussional F07.81
- postcontusional F07.81
- postencephalitic F07.89
- posterior
  - cervical sympathetic M53.0
  - cord G83.83
  - fossa compression G93.5
  - reversible encephalopathy (PRES) I67.83
- postgastrectomy (dumping) K91.1
- postgastric surgery K91.1
- postinfarction I24.1
- postlaminectomy NEC M96.1
- postleukotomy F07.0
- postmastectomy lymphedema I97.2
- postmyocardial infarction I24.1

Syndrome — *continued*
- postoperative NEC T81.9 ☑
  - blind loop K90.2
- postpartum panhypopituitary (Sheehan) E23.0
- postpolio (myelitic) G14
- postthrombotic I87.009
  - with
    - inflammation I87.02- ☑
      - with ulcer I87.03- ☑
    - specified complication NEC I87.09- ☑
    - ulcer I87.01- ☑
      - with inflammation I87.03- ☑
  - asymptomatic I87.00- ☑
- postvagotomy K91.1
- postvalvulotomy I97.0
- postviral NEC G93.3
  - fatigue G93.3
- Potain's K31.0
- potassium intoxication E87.5
- precerebral artery (multiple) (bilateral) G45.2
- preinfarction I20.0
- preleukemic D46.9
- premature senility E34.8
- premenstrual dysphoric F32.89
- premenstrual tension N94.3
- Prinzmetal-Massumi R07.1
- prune belly Q79.4
- pseudo -Turner's Q87.1
- pseudocarpal tunnel (sublimis) — *see* Syndrome, carpal tunnel
- pseudoparalytica G70.00
  - with exacerbation (acute) G70.01
  - in crisis G70.01
- psycho-organic (nonpsychotic severity) F07.9
  - acute or subacute F05
  - depressive type F06.31
  - hallucinatory type F06.0
  - nonpsychotic severity F07.0
  - specified NEC F07.89
- pulmonary
  - arteriosclerosis I27.0
  - dysmaturity (Wilson-Mikity) P27.0
  - hypoperfusion (idiopathic) P22.0
  - renal (hemorrhagic) (Goodpasture's) M31.0
- pure
  - motor lacunar G46.5
  - sensory lacunar G46.6
- Putnam-Dana D51.0
- pyogenic arthritis, pyoderma gangrenosum, and acne [PAPA] M04.8
- pyramidopallidonigral G20
- pyriformis — *see* Lesion, nerve, sciatic
- QT interval prolongation I45.81
- radicular NEC — *see* Radiculopathy
  - upper limbs, newborn (birth injury) P14.3
- rapid time-zone change G47.25
- Rasmussen G04.81
- Raymond (-Céstan) I65.8
- Raynaud's I73.00
  - with gangrene I73.01
- RDS (respiratory distress syndrome, newborn) P22.0
- reactive airways dysfunction J68.3
- Refsum's G60.1
- Reifenstein E34.52
- renal glomerulohyalinosis-diabetic — *see* Diabetes, nephrosis
- Rendu-Osler-Weber I78.0
- residual ovary N99.83
- resistant ovary E28.39
- respiratory
  - distress
    - acute J80
      - adult J80
      - child J80
      - idiopathic J84.114
    - newborn (idiopathic) (type I) P22.0
      - type II P22.1
- restless legs G25.81
- retinoblastoma (familial) C69.2 ☑
- retroperitoneal fibrosis N13.5
- retroviral seroconversion (acute) Z21
- Reye's G93.7
- Richter — *see* Leukemia, chronic lymphocytic, B-cell type
- Ridley's I50.1
- right
  - heart, hypoplastic Q22.6

☑ **Additional Character Required** — Refer to the Tabular List for Character Selection   ▽ **Subterms under main terms may continue to next column or page**

Syndrome — *continued*
    right — *continued*
        ventricular obstruction — *see* Failure, heart, congestive
    Romano-Ward (prolonged QT interval) I45.81
    rotator cuff, shoulder (*see also* Tear, rotator cuff) M75.10- ☑
    Rotes Quérol — *see* Hyperostosis, ankylosing
    Roth — *see* Meralgia paresthetica
    rubella (congenital) P35.0
    Ruvalcaba-Myhre-Smith E71.440
    Rytand-Lipsitch I44.2
    salt
        depletion E87.1
            due to heat NEC T67.8 ☑
                causing heat exhaustion or prostration T67.4 ☑
        low E87.1
    salt-losing N28.89
    Scaglietti-Dagnini E22.0
    scalenus anticus (anterior) G54.0
    scapulocostal — *see* Mononeuropathy, upper limb, specified site NEC
    scapuloperoneal G71.0
    schizophrenic, of childhood NEC F84.5
    Schnitzler D47.2
    Scholte's E34.0
    Schroeder's E27.0
    Schüller-Christian C96.5
    Schwachman's — *see* Syndrome, Shwachman's
    Schwartz (-Jampel) G71.13
    Schwartz-Bartter E22.2
    scimitar Q26.8
    sclerocystic ovary E28.2
    Seitelberger's G31.89
    septicemic adrenal hemorrhage A39.1
    seroconversion, retroviral (acute) Z21
    serous meningitis G93.2
    severe acute respiratory (SARS) J12.81
    shaken infant T74.4 ☑
    shock (traumatic) T79.4 ☑
        kidney N17.0
            following crush injury T79.5 ☑
        toxic A48.3
    shock-lung J80
    Shone's — *code to* specific anomalies
    short
        bowel K91.2
        rib Q77.2
    shoulder-hand — *see* Algoneurodystrophy
    Shwachman's D70.4
    sicca — *see* Sicca syndrome
    sick
        cell E87.1
        sinus I49.5
    sick-euthyroid E07.81
    sideropenic D50.1
    Siemens' ectodermal dysplasia Q82.4
    Silfversköld's Q78.9
    Simons' E88.1
    sinus tarsi M25.57- ☑
    sinusitis-bronchiectasis-situs inversus Q89.3
    Sipple's E31.22
    sirenomelia Q87.2
    Slocumb's E27.0
    slow flow, coronary I20.8
    Sluder's G44.89
    Smith-Magenis Q93.88
    Sneddon-Wilkinson L13.1
    Sotos' Q87.3
    South African cardiomyopathy I42.8
    spasmodic
        upward movement, eyes H51.8
        winking F95.8
    Spen's I45.9
    splenic
        agenesis Q89.01
        flexure K59.8
        neutropenia D73.81
    Spurway's Q78.0
    staphylococcal scalded skin L00
    steal
        arteriovenous T82.898- ☑
        ischemic T82.898- ☑
        subclavian G45.8
    Stein-Leventhal E28.2
    Stein's E28.2
    Stevens-Johnson syndrome L51.1

Syndrome — *continued*
    Stevens-Johnson syndrome — *continued*
        toxic epidermal necrolysis overlap L51.3
    Stewart-Morel M85.2
    Stickler Q89.8
    stiff baby Q89.8
    stiff man G25.82
    Still-Felty — *see* Felty's syndrome
    Stokes (-Adams) I45.9
    stone heart I50.1
    straight back, congenital Q76.49
    subclavian steal G45.8
    subcoracoid-pectoralis minor G54.0
    subcostal nerve compression I77.89
    subphrenic interposition Q43.3
    superior
        cerebellar artery I63.8
        mesenteric artery K55.1
        semi-circular canal dehiscence H83.8X- ☑
        vena cava I87.1
    supine hypotensive (maternal) — *see* Syndrome, hypotension, maternal
    suprarenal cortical E27.0
    supraspinatus (*see also* Tear, rotator cuff) M75.10- ☑
    Susac G93.49
    swallowed blood P78.2
    sweat retention L74.0
    Swyer Q99.1
    Symond's G93.2
    sympathetic
        cervical paralysis G90.2
        pelvic, female N94.89
    systemic inflammatory response (SIRS), of non-infectious origin (without organ dysfunction) R65.10
        with acute organ dysfunction R65.11
    tachycardia-bradycardia I49.5
    takotsubo I51.81
    TAR (thrombocytopenia with absent radius) Q87.2
    tarsal tunnel G57.5- ☑
    teething K00.7
    tegmental G93.89
    telangiectasic-pigmentation-cataract Q82.8
    temporal pyramidal apex — *see* Otitis, media, suppurative, acute
    temporomandibular joint-pain-dysfunction M26.62- ☑
    Terry's (*see also* Myopia, degenerative) H44.2- ☑
    testicular feminization (*see also* Syndrome, androgen insensitivity) E34.51
    thalamic pain (hyperesthetic) G89.0
    thoracic outlet (compression) G54.0
    Thorson-Björck E34.0
    thrombocytopenia with absent radius (TAR) Q87.2
    thyroid-adrenocortical insufficiency E31.0
    tibial
        anterior M76.81- ☑
        posterior M76.82- ☑
    Tietze's M94.0
    time-zone (rapid) G47.25
    Toni-Fanconi E72.09
        with cystinosis E72.04
    Touraine's Q79.8
    tourniquet — *see* Constriction, external, by site
    toxic shock A48.3
    transient left ventricular apical ballooning I51.81
    traumatic vasospastic T75.22 ☑
    Treacher Collins Q75.4
    triple X, female Q97.0
    trisomy Q92.9
        13 Q91.7
            meiotic nondisjunction Q91.4
            mitotic nondisjunction Q91.5
            mosaicism Q91.5
            translocation Q91.6
        18 Q91.3
            meiotic nondisjunction Q91.0
            mitotic nondisjunction Q91.1
            mosaicism Q91.1
            translocation Q91.2
        20 (q)(p) Q92.8
        21 Q90.9
            meiotic nondisjunction Q90.0
            mitotic nondisjunction Q90.1
            mosaicism Q90.1
            translocation Q90.2
        22 Q92.8
    tropical wet feet T69.0- ☑
    Trousseau's I82.1

Syndrome — *continued*
    tumor lysis (following antineoplastic chemotherapy) (spontaneous) NEC E88.3
    tumor necrosis factor receptor associated periodic (TRAPS) M04.1
    Twiddler's (due to)
        automatic implantable defibrillator T82.198 ☑
        cardiac pacemaker T82.198 ☑
    Unverricht (-Lundborg) — *see* Epilepsy, generalized, idiopathic
    upward gaze H51.8
    uremia, chronic (*see also* Disease, kidney, chronic) N18.9
    urethral N34.3
    urethro-oculo-articular — *see* Reiter's disease
    urohepatic K76.7
    vago-hypoglossal G52.7
    van Buchem's M85.2
    van der Hoeve's Q78.0
    vascular NEC in cerebrovascular disease G46.8
    vasoconstriction, reversible cerebrovascular I67.841
    vasomotor I73.9
    vasospastic (traumatic) T75.22 ☑
    vasovagal R55
    VATER Q87.2
    velo-cardio-facial Q93.81
    vena cava (inferior) (superior) (obstruction) I87.1
    vertebral
        artery G45.0
            compression — *see* Syndrome, anterior, spinal artery, compression
        steal G45.0
    vertebro-basilar artery G45.0
    vertebrogenic (pain) M54.89
    vertiginous — *see* Disorder, vestibular function
    Vinson-Plummer D50.1
    virus B34.9
    visceral larva migrans B83.0
    visual disorientation H53.8
    vitamin B6 deficiency E53.1
    vitreal corneal H59.01- ☑
    vitreous (touch) H59.01- ☑
    Vogt-Koyanagi H20.82- ☑
    Volkmann's T79.6 ☑
    von Schroetter's I82.890
    von Willebrand (-Jürgen) D68.0
    Waldenström-Kjellberg D50.1
    Wallenberg's G46.3
    water retention E87.79
    Waterhouse (-Friderichsen) A39.1
    Weber-Gubler G46.3
    Weber-Leyden G46.3
    Weber's G46.3
    Wegener's M31.30
        with
            kidney involvement M31.31
            lung involvement M31.30
                with kidney involvement M31.31
    Weingarten's (tropical eosinophilia) J82
    Weiss-Baker G90.09
    Werdnig-Hoffman G12.0
    Wermer's E31.21
    Werner's E34.8
    Wernicke-Korsakoff (nonalcoholic) F04
        alcoholic F10.26
    Westphal-Strümpell E83.01
    West's — *see* Epilepsy, spasms
    wet
        feet (maceration) (tropical) T69.0- ☑
        lung, newborn P22.1
    whiplash S13.4 ☑
    whistling face Q87.0
    Wilkie's K55.1
    Wilkinson-Sneddon L13.1
    Willebrand (-Jürgens) D68.0
    Wilson's (hepatolenticular degeneration) E83.01
    Wiskott-Aldrich D82.0
    withdrawal — *see* Withdrawal, state
        drug
            infant of dependent mother P96.1
            therapeutic use, newborn P96.2
    Woakes' (ethmoiditis) J33.1
    Wright's (hyperabduction) G54.0
    X I20.9
    XXXX Q97.1
    XXXXX Q97.1
    XXXXY Q98.1
    XXY Q98.0

Syndrome — *continued*
  yellow nail L60.5
  Zahorsky's B08.5
  Zellweger syndrome E71.510
  Zellweger-like syndrome E71.541
Synechia (anterior) (iris) (posterior) (pupil) (*see also* Adhesions, iris)
  intra-uterine (traumatic) N85.6
Synesthesia R20.8
Syngamiasis, syngamosis B83.3
Synodontia K00.2
Synorchidism, synorchism Q55.1
Synostosis (congenital) Q78.8
  astragalo-scaphoid Q74.2
  radioulnar Q74.0
Synovial sarcoma — *see* Neoplasm, connective tissue, malignant
Synovioma (malignant) (*see also* Neoplasm, connective tissue, malignant)
  benign — *see* Neoplasm, connective tissue, benign
Synoviosarcoma — *see* Neoplasm, connective tissue, malignant
Synovitis (*see also* Tenosynovitis) M65.9
  crepitant
    hand M70.0- ☑
    wrist M70.03- ☑
  gonococcal A54.49
  gouty — *see* Gout
  in (due to)
    crystals M65.8- ☑
    gonorrhea A54.49
    syphilis (late) A52.78
    use, overuse, pressure — *see* Disorder, soft tissue, due to use
  infective NEC — *see* Tenosynovitis, infective NEC
  specified NEC — *see* Tenosynovitis, specified type NEC
  syphilitic A52.78
    congenital (early) A50.02
  toxic — *see* Synovitis, transient
  transient M67.3- ☑
    ankle M67.37- ☑
    elbow M67.32- ☑
    foot joint M67.37- ☑
    hand joint M67.34- ☑
    hip M67.35- ☑
    knee M67.36- ☑
    multiple site M67.39
    pelvic region M67.35- ☑
    shoulder M67.31- ☑
    specified joint NEC M67.38
    wrist M67.33- ☑
  traumatic, current — *see* Sprain
  tuberculous — *see* Tuberculosis, synovitis
  villonodular (pigmented) M12.2- ☑
    ankle M12.27- ☑
    elbow M12.22- ☑
    foot joint M12.27- ☑
    hand joint M12.24- ☑
    hip M12.25- ☑
    knee M12.26- ☑
    multiple site M12.29
    pelvic region M12.25- ☑
    shoulder M12.21- ☑
    specified joint NEC M12.28
    vertebrae M12.28
    wrist M12.23- ☑
Syphilid A51.39
  congenital A50.06
  newborn A50.06
  tubercular (late) A52.79
Syphilis, syphilitic (acquired) A53.9
  abdomen (late) A52.79
  acoustic nerve A52.15
  adenopathy (secondary) A51.49
  adrenal (gland) (with cortical hypofunction) A52.79
  age under 2 years NOS (*see also* Syphilis, congenital, early)
    acquired A51.9
  alopecia (secondary) A51.32
  anemia (late) A52.79 [D63.8]
  aneurysm (aorta) (ruptured) A52.01
    central nervous system A52.05
    congenital A50.54 [I79.0]
  anus (late) A52.74
    primary A51.1
    secondary A51.39
  aorta (arch) (abdominal) (thoracic) A52.02

Syphilis, syphilitic — *continued*
  aorta — *continued*
    aneurysm A52.01
  aortic (insufficiency) (regurgitation) (stenosis) A52.03
    aneurysm A52.01
  arachnoid (adhesive) (cerebral) (spinal) A52.13
  asymptomatic — *see* Syphilis, latent
  ataxia (locomotor) A52.11
  atrophoderma maculatum A51.39
  auricular fibrillation A52.06
  bladder (late) A52.76
  bone A52.77
    secondary A51.46
  brain A52.17
  breast (late) A52.79
  bronchus (late) A52.72
  bubo (primary) A51.0
  bulbar palsy A52.19
  bursa (late) A52.78
  cardiac decompensation A52.06
  cardiovascular A52.00
  central nervous system (late) (recurrent) (relapse) (tertiary) A52.3
    with
      ataxia A52.11
      general paralysis A52.17
        juvenile A50.45
      paresis (general) A52.17
        juvenile A50.45
      tabes (dorsalis) A52.11
        juvenile A50.45
      taboparesis A52.17
        juvenile A50.45
    aneurysm A52.05
    congenital A50.40
    juvenile A50.40
    remission in (sustained) A52.3
    serology doubtful, negative, or positive A52.3
    specified nature or site NEC A52.19
    vascular A52.05
  cerebral A52.17
    meningovascular A52.13
    nerves (multiple palsies) A52.15
    sclerosis A52.17
    thrombosis A52.05
  cerebrospinal (tabetic type) A52.12
  cerebrovascular A52.05
  cervix (late) A52.76
  chancre (multiple) A51.0
    extragenital A51.2
    Rollet's A51.0
  Charcot's joint A52.16
  chorioretinitis A51.43
    congenital A50.01
    late A52.71
    prenatal A50.01
  choroiditis — *see* Syphilitic chorioretinitis
  choroidoretinitis — *see* Syphilitic chorioretinitis
  ciliary body (secondary) A51.43
    late A52.71
  colon (late) A52.74
  combined spinal sclerosis A52.11
  condyloma (latum) A51.31
  congenital A50.9
    with
      paresis (general) A50.45
      tabes (dorsalis) A50.45
      taboparesis A50.45
    early, or less than 2 years after birth NEC A50.2
      with manifestations — *see* Syphilis, congenital, early, symptomatic
      latent (without manifestations) A50.1
        negative spinal fluid test A50.1
        serology positive A50.1
      symptomatic A50.09
        cutaneous A50.06
        mucocutaneous A50.07
        oculopathy A50.01
        osteochondropathy A50.02
        pharyngitis A50.03
        pneumonia A50.04
        rhinitis A50.05
        visceral A50.08
    chorioretinitis, choroiditis A50.01 [H32]
    interstitial keratitis A50.31
    juvenile neurosyphilis A50.45
    late, or 2 years or more after birth NEC A50.7
      chorioretinitis, choroiditis A50.32
      interstitial keratitis A50.31

Syphilis, syphilitic — *continued*
  congenital — *continued*
    late, or 2 years or more after birth — *continued*
      juvenile neurosyphilis A50.45
      latent (without manifestations) A50.6
        negative spinal fluid test A50.6
        serology positive A50.6
      symptomatic or with manifestations NEC A50.59
        arthropathy A50.55
        cardiovascular A50.54
        Clutton's joints A50.51
        Hutchinson's teeth A50.52
        Hutchinson's triad A50.53
        osteochondropathy A50.56
        saddle nose A50.57
  conjugal A53.9
    tabes A52.11
  conjunctiva (late) A52.71
  contact Z20.2
  cord bladder A52.19
  cornea, late A52.71
  coronary (artery) (sclerosis) A52.06
  coryza, congenital A50.05
  cranial nerve A52.15
    multiple palsies A52.15
  cutaneous — *see* Syphilis, skin
  dacryocystitis (late) A52.71
  degeneration, spinal cord A52.12
  dementia paralytica A52.17
    juvenilis A50.45
  destruction of bone A52.77
  dilatation, aorta A52.01
  due to blood transfusion A53.9
  dura mater A52.13
  ear A52.79
    inner A52.79
      nerve (eighth) A52.15
      neurorecurrence A52.15
  early A51.9
    cardiovascular A52.00
    central nervous system A52.3
    latent (without manifestations) (less than 2 years after Infection) A51.5
      negative spinal fluid test A51.5
      serological relapse after treatment A51.5
      serology positive A51.5
    relapse (treated, untreated) A51.9
    skin A51.39
    symptomatic A51.9
      extragenital chancre A51.2
      primary, except extragenital chancre A51.0
      secondary (*see also* Syphilis, secondary) A51.39
        relapse (treated, untreated) A51.49
    ulcer A51.39
  eighth nerve (neuritis) A52.15
  endemic A65
  endocarditis A52.03
    aortic A52.03
    pulmonary A52.03
  epididymis (late) A52.76
  epiglottis (late) A52.73
  epiphysitis (congenital) (early) A50.02
  episcleritis (late) A52.71
  esophagus A52.79
  eustachian tube A52.73
  exposure to Z20.2
  eye A52.71
  eyelid (late) (with gumma) A52.71
  fallopian tube (late) A52.76
  fracture A52.77
  gallbladder (late) A52.74
  gastric (polyposis) (late) A52.74
  general A53.9
    paralysis A52.17
      juvenile A50.45
  genital (primary) A51.0
  glaucoma A52.71
  gumma NEC A52.79
    cardiovascular system A52.00
    central nervous system A52.3
    congenital A50.59
  heart (block) (decompensation) (disease) (failure) A52.06 [I52]
    valve NEC A52.03
  hemianesthesia A52.19
  hemianopsia A52.71
  hemiparesis A52.17
  hemiplegia A52.17

☑ **Additional Character Required** — Refer to the Tabular List for Character Selection   ▽ **Subterms under main terms may continue to next column or page**

Syphilis, syphilitic — *continued*
hepatic artery A52.09
hepatis A52.74
hepatomegaly, congenital A50.08
hereditaria tarda — *see* Syphilis, congenital, late
hereditary — *see* Syphilis, congenital
Hutchinson's teeth A50.52
hyalitis A52.71
inactive — *see* Syphilis, latent
infantum — *see* Syphilis, congenital
inherited — *see* Syphilis, congenital
internal ear A52.79
intestine (late) A52.74
iris, iritis (secondary) A51.43
    late A52.71
joint (late) A52.77
keratitis (congenital) (interstitial) (late) A50.31
kidney (late) A52.75
lacrimal passages (late) A52.71
larynx (late) A52.73
late A52.9
    cardiovascular A52.00
    central nervous system A52.3
    kidney A52.75
    latent or 2 years or more after infection (without
        manifestations) A52.8
        negative spinal fluid test A52.8
        serology positive A52.8
    paresis A52.17
    specified site NEC A52.79
    symptomatic or with manifestations A52.79
    tabes A52.11
latent A53.0
    with signs or symptoms — *code by* site and stage
        under Syphilis
    early, or less than 2 years after infection A51.5
    central nervous system A52.2
    date of infection unspecified A53.0
    follow-up of latent syphilis A53.0
        date of infection unspecified A53.0
        late, or 2 years or more after infection A52.8
    late, or 2 years or more after infection A52.8
    positive serology (only finding) A53.0
        early, or less than 2 years after infection A51.5
        date of infection unspecified A53.0
        late, or 2 years or more after infection A52.8
lens (late) A52.71
leukoderma A51.39
    late A52.79
lienitis A52.79
lip A51.39
    chancre (primary) A51.2
    late A52.79
Lissauer's paralysis A52.17
liver A52.74
locomotor ataxia A52.11
lung A52.72
lymph gland (early) (secondary) A51.49
    late A52.79
lymphadenitis (secondary) A51.49
macular atrophy of skin A51.39
    striated A52.79
mediastinum (late) A52.73
meninges (adhesive) (brain) (spinal cord) A52.13
meningitis A52.13
    acute (secondary) A51.41
    congenital A50.41
meningoencephalitis A52.14
meningovascular A52.13
    congenital A50.41
mesarteritis A52.09
    brain A52.04
middle ear A52.77
mitral stenosis A52.03
monoplegia A52.17
mouth (secondary) A51.39
    late A52.79
mucocutaneous (secondary) A51.39
    late A52.79
mucous
    membrane (secondary) A51.39
        late A52.79
    patches A51.39
        congenital A50.07
mulberry molars A50.52
muscle A52.78
myocardium A52.06
nasal sinus (late) A52.73

Syphilis, syphilitic — *continued*
neonatorum — *see* Syphilis, congenital
nephrotic syndrome (secondary) A51.44
nerve palsy (any cranial nerve) A52.15
    multiple A52.15
nervous system, central A52.3
neuritis A52.15
    acoustic A52.15
neurorecidive of retina A52.19
neuroretinitis A52.19
newborn — *see* Syphilis, congenital
nodular superficial (late) A52.79
nonvenereal A65
nose (late) A52.73
    saddle back deformity A50.57
occlusive arterial disease A52.09
oculopathy A52.71
ophthalmic (late) A52.71
optic nerve (atrophy) (neuritis) (papilla) A52.15
orbit (late) A52.71
organic A53.9
osseous (late) A52.77
osteochondritis (congenital) (early) A50.02 [M90.80]
osteoporosis A52.77
ovary (late) A52.76
oviduct (late) A52.76
palate (late) A52.79
pancreas (late) A52.74
paralysis A52.17
    general A52.17
        juvenile A50.45
paresis (general) A52.17
    juvenile A50.45
paresthesia A52.19
Parkinson's disease or syndrome A52.19
paroxysmal tachycardia A52.06
pemphigus (congenital) A50.06
penis (chancre) A51.0
    late A52.76
pericardium A52.06
perichondritis, larynx (late) A52.73
periosteum (late) A52.77
    congenital (early) A50.02 [M90.80]
    early (secondary) A51.46
peripheral nerve A52.79
petrous bone (late) A52.77
pharynx (late) A52.73
    secondary A51.39
pituitary (gland) A52.79
pleura (late) A52.73
pneumonia, white A50.04
pontine lesion A52.17
portal vein A52.09
primary A51.0
    anal A51.1
    and secondary — *see* Syphilis, secondary
    central nervous system A52.3
    extragenital chancre NEC A51.2
    fingers A51.2
    genital A51.0
    lip A51.2
    specified site NEC A51.2
    tonsils A51.2
prostate (late) A52.76
ptosis (eyelid) A52.71
pulmonary (late) A52.72
    artery A52.09
pyelonephritis (late) A52.75
recently acquired, symptomatic A51.9
rectum (late) A52.74
respiratory tract (late) A52.73
retina, late A52.71
retrobulbar neuritis A52.15
salpingitis A52.76
sclera (late) A52.71
sclerosis
    cerebral A52.17
    coronary A52.06
    multiple A52.11
scotoma (central) A52.71
scrotum (late) A52.76
secondary (and primary) A51.49
    adenopathy A51.49
    anus A51.39
    bone A51.46
    chorioretinitis, choroiditis A51.43
    hepatitis A51.45
    liver A51.45
    lymphadenitis A51.49

Syphilis, syphilitic — *continued*
secondary — *continued*
    meningitis (acute) A51.41
    mouth A51.39
    mucous membranes A51.39
    periosteum, periostitis A51.46
    pharynx A51.39
    relapse (treated, untreated) A51.49
    skin A51.39
    specified form NEC A51.49
    tonsil A51.39
    ulcer A51.39
    viscera NEC A51.49
    vulva A51.39
seminal vesicle (late) A52.76
seronegative with signs or symptoms — *code by* site
    and stage under Syphilis
seropositive
    with signs or symptoms — *code by* site and stage
        under Syphilis
    follow-up of latent syphilis — *see* Syphilis, latent
    only finding — *see* Syphilis, latent
seventh nerve (paralysis) A52.15
sinus, sinusitis (late) A52.73
skeletal system A52.77
skin (with ulceration) (early) (secondary) A51.39
    late or tertiary A52.79
small intestine A52.74
spastic spinal paralysis A52.17
spermatic cord (late) A52.76
spinal (cord) A52.12
spleen A52.79
splenomegaly A52.79
spondylitis A52.77
staphyloma A52.71
stigmata (congenital) A50.59
stomach A52.74
synovium A52.78
tabes dorsalis (late) A52.11
    juvenile A50.45
tabetic type A52.11
    juvenile A50.45
taboparesis A52.17
    juvenile A50.45
tachycardia A52.06
tendon (late) A52.78
tertiary A52.9
    with symptoms NEC A52.79
    cardiovascular A52.00
    central nervous system A52.3
    multiple NEC A52.79
    specified site NEC A52.79
testis A52.76
thorax A52.73
throat A52.73
thymus (gland) (late) A52.79
thyroid (late) A52.79
tongue (late) A52.79
tonsil (lingual) (late) A52.73
    primary A51.2
    secondary A51.39
trachea (late) A52.73
tunica vaginalis (late) A52.76
ulcer (any site) (early) (secondary) A51.39
    late A52.79
    perforating A52.79
        foot A52.11
urethra (late) A52.76
urogenital (late) A52.76
uterus (late) A52.76
uveal tract (secondary) A51.43
    late A52.71
uveitis (secondary) A51.43
    late A52.71
uvula (late) (perforated) A52.79
vagina A51.0
    late A52.76
valvulitis NEC A52.03
vascular A52.00
    brain (cerebral) A52.05
ventriculi A52.74
vesicae urinariae (late) A52.76
viscera (abdominal) (late) A52.74
    secondary A51.49
vitreous (opacities) (late) A52.71
    hemorrhage A52.71
vulva A51.0
    late A52.76
    secondary A51.39

Syphiloma A52.79
   cardiovascular system A52.00
   central nervous system A52.3
   circulatory system A52.00
   congenital A50.59
Syphilophobia F45.29
Syringadenoma (*see also* Neoplasm, skin, benign)
   papillary — *see* Neoplasm, skin, benign

Syringobulbia G95.0
Syringocystadenoma — *see* Neoplasm, skin, benign
   papillary — *see* Neoplasm, skin, benign
Syringoma (*see also* Neoplasm, skin, benign)
   chondroid — *see* Neoplasm, skin, benign
Syringomyelia G95.0
Syringomyelitis — *see* Encephalitis
Syringomyelocele — *see* Spina bifida

Syringopontia G95.0
System, systemic (*see also* condition)
   disease, combined — *see* Degeneration, combined
   inflammatory response syndrome (SIRS) of non-infectious origin (without organ dysfunction) R65.10
     with acute organ dysfunction R65.11
   lupus erythematosus M32.9
     inhibitor present D68.62

☑ **Additional Character Required** — Refer to the Tabular List for Character Selection   ▽ **Subterms under main terms may continue to next column or page**

T

Tabacism, tabacosis, tabagism (*see also* Poisoning, tobacco)
  meaning dependence (without remission) F17.200
    with
      disorder F17.299
        in remission F17.211
        specified disorder NEC F17.298
        withdrawal F17.203
Tabardillo A75.9
  flea-borne A75.2
  louse-borne A75.0
Tabes, tabetic A52.10
  with
    central nervous system syphilis A52.10
    Charcot's joint A52.16
    cord bladder A52.19
    crisis, viscera (any) A52.19
    paralysis, general A52.17
    paresis (general) A52.17
    perforating ulcer (foot) A52.19
  arthropathy (Charcot) A52.16
  bladder A52.19
  bone A52.11
  cerebrospinal A52.12
  congenital A50.45
  conjugal A52.10
  dorsalis A52.11
    juvenile A50.49
  juvenile A50.49
  latent A52.19
  mesenterica A18.39
  paralysis, insane, general A52.17
  spasmodic A52.17
  syphilis (cerebrospinal) A52.12
Taboparalysis A52.17
Taboparesis (remission) A52.17
  juvenile A50.45
TAC (trigeminal autonomic cephalgia) **NEC** G44.099
  intractable G44.091
  not intractable G44.099
Tache noir S60.22- ☑
Tachyalimentation K91.2
Tachyarrhythmia, tachyrhythmia — *see* Tachycardia
Tachycardia R00.0
  atrial (paroxysmal) I47.1
  auricular I47.1
  AV nodal re-entry (re-entrant) I47.1
  junctional (paroxysmal) I47.1
  newborn P29.11
  nodal (paroxysmal) I47.1
  non-paroxysmal AV nodal I45.89
  paroxysmal (sustained) (nonsustained) I47.9
    with sinus bradycardia I49.5
    atrial (PAT) I47.1
    atrioventricular (AV) (re-entrant) I47.1
      psychogenic F54
    junctional I47.1
      ectopic I47.1
    nodal I47.1
    psychogenic (atrial) (supraventricular) (ventricular) F54
    supraventricular (sustained) I47.1
      psychogenic F54
    ventricular I47.2
      psychogenic F54
  psychogenic F45.8
  sick sinus I49.5
  sinoauricular NOS R00.0
    paroxysmal I47.1
  sinus [sinusal] NOS R00.0
    paroxysmal I47.1
  supraventricular I47.1
  ventricular (paroxysmal) (sustained) I47.2
    psychogenic F54
Tachygastria K31.89
Tachypnea R06.82
  hysterical F45.8
  newborn (idiopathic) (transitory) P22.1
  psychogenic F45.8
  transitory, of newborn P22.1
TACO (transfusion associated circulatory overload) E87.71
Taenia (infection) (infestation) B68.9
  diminuta B71.0
  echinococcal infestation B67.90
  mediocanellata B68.1

Taenia — *continued*
  nana B71.0
  saginata B68.1
  solium (intestinal form) B68.0
    larval form — *see* Cysticercosis
Taeniasis (intestine) — *see* Taenia
Tag (hypertrophied skin) (infected) L91.8
  adenoid J35.8
  anus K64.4
  hemorrhoidal K64.4
  hymen N89.8
  perineal N90.89
  preauricular Q17.0
  sentinel K64.4
  skin L91.8
    accessory (congenital) Q82.8
    anus K64.4
    congenital Q82.8
    preauricular Q17.0
  tonsil J35.8
  urethra, urethral N36.8
  vulva N90.89
Tahyna fever B33.8
Takahara's disease E80.3
Takayasu's disease or syndrome M31.4
Talcosis (pulmonary) J62.0
Talipes (congenital) Q66.89
  acquired, planus — *see* Deformity, limb, flat foot
  asymmetric Q66.89
  calcaneovalgus Q66.4
  calcaneovarus Q66.1
  calcaneus Q66.89
  cavus Q66.7
  equinovalgus Q66.6
  equinovarus Q66.0
  equinus Q66.89
  percavus Q66.7
  planovalgus Q66.6
  planus (acquired) (any degree) (*see also* Deformity, limb, flat foot)
    congenital Q66.5- ☑
    due to rickets (sequelae) E64.3
  valgus Q66.6
  varus Q66.3
Tall stature, constitutional E34.4
Talma's disease M62.89
Talon noir S90.3- ☑
  hand S60.22- ☑
  heel S90.3- ☑
  toe S90.1- ☑
Tamponade, heart I31.4
Tanapox (virus disease) B08.71
Tangier disease E78.6
Tantrum, child problem F91.8
Tapeworm (infection) (infestation) — *see* Infestation, tapeworm
Tapia's syndrome G52.7
TAR (thrombocytopenia with absent radius) **syndrome** Q87.2
Tarral-Besnier disease L44.0
Tarsal tunnel syndrome — *see* Syndrome, tarsal tunnel
Tarsalgia — *see* Pain, limb, lower
Tarsitis (eyelid) H01.8
  syphilitic A52.71
  tuberculous A18.4
Tartar (teeth) (dental calculus) K03.6
Tattoo (mark) L81.8
Tauri's disease E74.09
Taurodontism K00.2
Taussig-Bing syndrome Q20.1
Taybi's syndrome Q87.2
Tay-Sachs amaurotic familial idiocy or disease E75.02
TBI (traumatic brain injury) S06.9 ☑
Teacher's node or nodule J38.2
Tear, torn (traumatic) (*see also* Laceration)
  with abortion — *see* Abortion
  annular fibrosis M51.35
  anus, anal (sphincter) S31.831 ☑
    complicating delivery
      with third degree perineal laceration (*see also* Delivery, complicated, by, laceration, perineum, third degree) O70.20
        with mucosa O70.3
      without third degree perineal laceration O70.4
    nontraumatic (healed) (old) K62.81
  articular cartilage, old — *see* Derangement, joint, articular cartilage, by site

Tear, torn — *continued*
  bladder
    with ectopic or molar pregnancy O08.6
    following ectopic or molar pregnancy O08.6
    obstetrical O71.5
    traumatic — *see* Injury, bladder
  bowel
    with ectopic or molar pregnancy O08.6
    following ectopic or molar pregnancy O08.6
    obstetrical trauma O71.5
  broad ligament
    with ectopic or molar pregnancy O08.6
    following ectopic or molar pregnancy O08.6
    obstetrical trauma O71.6
  bucket handle (knee) (meniscus) — *see* Tear, meniscus
  capsule, joint — *see* Sprain
  cartilage (*see also* Sprain)
    articular, old — *see* Derangement, joint, articular cartilage, by site
  cervix
    with ectopic or molar pregnancy O08.6
    following ectopic or molar pregnancy O08.6
    obstetrical trauma (current) O71.3
    old N88.1
    traumatic — *see* Injury, uterus
  dural G97.41
    nontraumatic G96.11
  internal organ — *see* Injury, by site
  knee cartilage
    articular (current) S83.3- ☑
    old — *see* Derangement, knee, meniscus, due to old tear
  ligament — *see* Sprain
  meniscus (knee) (current injury) S83.209 ☑
    bucket-handle S83.20- ☑
    lateral
      bucket-handle S83.25- ☑
      complex S83.27- ☑
      peripheral S83.26- ☑
      specified type NEC S83.28- ☑
    medial
      bucket-handle S83.21- ☑
      complex S83.23- ☑
      peripheral S83.22- ☑
      specified type NEC S83.24- ☑
    old — *see* Derangement, knee, meniscus, due to old tear
    site other than knee — *code as* Sprain
    specified type NEC S83.20- ☑
  muscle — *see* Strain
  pelvic
    floor, complicating delivery O70.1
    organ NEC, obstetrical trauma O71.5
      with ectopic or molar pregnancy O08.6
      following ectopic or molar pregnancy O08.6
  perineal, secondary O90.1
  periurethral tissue, obstetrical trauma O71.82
    with ectopic or molar pregnancy O08.6
    following ectopic or molar pregnancy O08.6
  rectovaginal septum — *see* Laceration, vagina
  retina, retinal (without detachment) (horseshoe) (*see also* Break, retina, horseshoe)
    with detachment — *see* Detachment, retina, with retinal, break
  rotator cuff (nontraumatic) M75.10- ☑
    complete M75.12- ☑
    incomplete M75.11- ☑
    traumatic S46.01- ☑
      capsule S43.42- ☑
  semilunar cartilage, knee — *see* Tear, meniscus
  supraspinatus (complete) (incomplete) (nontraumatic) (*see also* Tear, rotator cuff) M75.10- ☑
  tendon — *see* Strain
  tentorial, at birth P10.4
  umbilical cord
    complicating delivery O69.89 ☑
  urethra
    with ectopic or molar pregnancy O08.6
    following ectopic or molar pregnancy O08.6
    obstetrical trauma O71.5
  uterus — *see* Injury, uterus
  vagina — *see* Laceration, vagina
  vessel, from catheter — *see* Puncture, accidental complicating surgery
  vulva, complicating delivery O70.0
Tear-stone — *see* Dacryolith

Teeth (*see also* condition)
  grinding
    psychogenic F45.8
    sleep related G47.63
Teething (syndrome) K00.7
Telangiectasia, telangiectasis (verrucous) I78.1
  ataxic (cerebellar) (Louis-Bar) G11.3
  familial I78.0
  hemorrhagic, hereditary (congenital) (senile) I78.0
  hereditary, hemorrhagic (congenital) (senile) I78.0
  juxtafoveal H35.07- ☑
  macular H35.07- ☑
  macularis eruptiva perstans D47.01
  parafoveal H35.07- ☑
  retinal (idiopathic) (juxtafoveal) (macular) (parafoveal) H35.07- ☑
  spider I78.1
Telephone scatologia F65.89
Telescoped bowel or intestine K56.1
  congenital Q43.8
Temperature
  body, high (of unknown origin) R50.9
  cold, trauma from T69.9 ☑
    newborn P80.0
    specified effect NEC T69.8 ☑
Temple — *see* condition
Temporal — *see* condition
Temporomandibular joint pain-dysfunction syndrome M26.62- ☑
Temporosphenoidal — *see* condition
Tendency
  bleeding — *see* Defect, coagulation
  suicide
    meaning personal history of attempted suicide Z91.5
    meaning suicidal ideation — *see* Ideation, suicidal
  to fall R29.6
Tenderness, abdominal R10.819
  epigastric R10.816
  generalized R10.817
  left lower quadrant R10.814
  left upper quadrant R10.812
  periumbilic R10.815
  rebound R10.829
    epigastric R10.826
    generalized R10.827
    left lower quadrant R10.824
    left upper quadrant R10.822
    periumbilic R10.825
    right lower quadrant R10.823
    right upper quadrant R10.821
  right lower quadrant R10.813
  right upper quadrant R10.811
Tendinitis, tendonitis (*see also* Enthesopathy)
  Achilles M76.6- ☑
  adhesive — *see* Tenosynovitis, specified type NEC
    shoulder — *see* Capsulitis, adhesive
  bicipital M75.2- ☑
  calcific M65.2- ☑
    ankle M65.27- ☑
    foot M65.27- ☑
    forearm M65.23- ☑
    hand M65.24- ☑
    lower leg M65.26- ☑
    multiple sites M65.29
    pelvic region M65.25- ☑
    shoulder M75.3- ☑
    specified site NEC M65.28
    thigh M65.25- ☑
    upper arm M65.22- ☑
  due to use, overuse, pressure (*see also* Disorder, soft tissue, due to use)
    specified NEC — *see* Disorder, soft tissue, due to use, specified NEC
  gluteal M76.0- ☑
  patellar M76.5- ☑
  peroneal M76.7- ☑
  psoas M76.1- ☑
  tibial (posterior) M76.82- ☑
    anterior M76.81- ☑
  trochanteric — *see* Bursitis, hip, trochanteric
Tendon — *see* condition
Tendosynovitis — *see* Tenosynovitis
Tenesmus (rectal) R19.8
  vesical R30.1
Tennis elbow — *see* Epicondylitis, lateral

Tenonitis (*see also* Tenosynovitis)
  eye (capsule) H05.04- ☑
Tenontosynovitis — *see* Tenosynovitis
Tenontothecitis — *see* Tenosynovitis
Tenophyte — *see* Disorder, synovium, specified type NEC
Tenosynovitis (*see also* Synovitis) M65.9
  adhesive — *see* Tenosynovitis, specified type NEC
    shoulder — *see* Capsulitis, adhesive
  bicipital (calcifying) — *see* Tendinitis, bicipital
  gonococcal A54.49
  in (due to)
    crystals M65.8- ☑
    gonorrhea A54.49
    syphilis (late) A52.78
    use, overuse, pressure (*see also* Disorder, soft tissue, due to use)
      specified NEC — *see* Disorder, soft tissue, due to use, specified NEC
  infective NEC M65.1- ☑
    ankle M65.17- ☑
    foot M65.17- ☑
    forearm M65.13- ☑
    hand M65.14- ☑
    lower leg M65.16- ☑
    multiple sites M65.19
    pelvic region M65.15- ☑
    shoulder region M65.11- ☑
    specified site NEC M65.18
    thigh M65.15- ☑
    upper arm M65.12- ☑
  radial styloid M65.4
  shoulder region M65.81- ☑
    adhesive — *see* Capsulitis, adhesive
  specified type NEC M65.88
    ankle M65.87- ☑
    foot M65.87- ☑
    forearm M65.83- ☑
    hand M65.84- ☑
    lower leg M65.86- ☑
    multiple sites M65.89
    pelvic region M65.85- ☑
    shoulder region M65.81- ☑
    specified site NEC M65.88
    thigh M65.85- ☑
    upper arm M65.82- ☑
  tuberculous — *see* Tuberculosis, tenosynovitis
Tenovaginitis — *see* Tenosynovitis
Tension
  arterial, high (*see also* Hypertension)
    without diagnosis of hypertension R03.0
  headache G44.209
    intractable G44.201
    not intractable G44.209
  nervous R45.0
  pneumothorax J93.0
  premenstrual N94.3
  state (mental) F48.9
Tentorium — *see* condition
Teratencephalus Q89.8
Teratism Q89.7
Teratoblastoma (malignant) — *see* Neoplasm, malignant, by site
Teratocarcinoma (*see also* Neoplasm, malignant, by site)
  liver C22.7
Teratoma (solid) (*see also* Neoplasm, uncertain behavior, by site)
  with embryonal carcinoma, mixed — *see* Neoplasm, malignant, by site
  with malignant transformation — *see* Neoplasm, malignant, by site
  adult (cystic) — *see* Neoplasm, benign, by site
  benign — *see* Neoplasm, benign, by site
  combined with choriocarcinoma — *see* Neoplasm, malignant, by site
  cystic (adult) — *see* Neoplasm, benign, by site
  differentiated — *see* Neoplasm, benign, by site
  embryonal (*see also* Neoplasm, malignant, by site)
    liver C22.7
  immature — *see* Neoplasm, malignant, by site
  liver C22.7
    adult, benign, cystic, differentiated type or mature D13.4
  malignant (*see also* Neoplasm, malignant, by site)
    anaplastic — *see* Neoplasm, malignant, by site
    intermediate — *see* Neoplasm, malignant, by site

Teratoma — *continued*
  malignant (*see also* Neoplasm, malignant, by site) — *continued*
    intermediate — *see* Neoplasm, malignant, by site — *continued*
      specified site — *see* Neoplasm, malignant, by site
    unspecified site C62.90
    undifferentiated — *see* Neoplasm, malignant, by site
  mature — *see* Neoplasm, uncertain behavior, by site
    malignant — *see* Neoplasm, by site, malignant, by site
  ovary D27.- ☑
    embryonal, immature or malignant C56- ☑
  solid — *see* Neoplasm, uncertain behavior, by site
  testis C62.9- ☑
    adult, benign, cystic, differentiated type or mature D29.2- ☑
    scrotal C62.1- ☑
    undescended C62.0- ☑
Termination
  anomalous (*see also* Malposition, congenital)
    right pulmonary vein Q26.3
  pregnancy, elective Z33.2
Ternidens diminutus infestation B81.8
Ternidensiasis B81.8
Terror(s) night (child) F51.4
Terrorism, victim of Z65.4
Terry's syndrome (*see also* Myopia, degenerative) H44.2- ☑
Tertiary — *see* condition
Test, tests, testing (for)
  adequacy (for dialysis)
    hemodialysis Z49.31
    peritoneal Z49.32
  blood pressure Z01.30
    abnormal reading — *see* Blood, pressure
  blood typing Z01.83
    Rh typing Z01.83
  blood-alcohol Z04.8
    positive — *see* Findings, abnormal, in blood
  blood-drug Z04.8
    positive — *see* Findings, abnormal, in blood
  cardiac pulse generator (battery) Z45.010
  fertility Z31.41
  genetic
    disease carrier status for procreative management
      female Z31.430
      male Z31.440
    male partner of patient with recurrent pregnancy loss Z31.441
    procreative management NEC
      female Z31.438
      male Z31.448
  hearing Z01.10
    with abnormal findings NEC Z01.118
  HIV (human immunodeficiency virus)
    nonconclusive (in infants) R75
    positive Z21
    seropositive Z21
  immunity status Z01.84
  intelligence NEC Z01.89
  laboratory (as part of a general medical examination) Z00.00
    with abnormal finding Z00.01
    for medicolegal reason NEC Z04.8
  male partner of patient with recurrent pregnancy loss Z31.441
  Mantoux (for tuberculosis) Z11.1
    abnormal result R76.11
  pregnancy, positive first pregnancy — *see* Pregnancy, normal, first
  procreative Z31.49
    fertility Z31.41
  skin, diagnostic
    allergy Z01.82
      special screening examination — *see* Screening, by name of disease
    Mantoux Z11.1
    tuberculin Z11.1
  specified NEC Z01.89
  tuberculin Z11.1
    abnormal result R76.11
  vision Z01.00
    with abnormal findings Z01.01
  Wassermann Z11.3
    positive — *see* Serology for syphilis, positive

☑ Additional Character Required — Refer to the Tabular List for Character Selection   ▽ Subterms under main terms may continue to next column or page

Testicle, testicular, testis (see also condition)
  feminization syndrome (see also Syndrome, androgen insensitivity) E34.51
  migrans Q55.29
Tetanus, tetanic (cephalic) (convulsions) A35
  with
    abortion A34
    ectopic or molar pregnancy O08.0
  following ectopic or molar pregnancy O08.0
  inoculation reaction (due to serum) — see Complications, vaccination
  neonatorum A33
  obstetrical A34
  puerperal, postpartum, childbirth A34
Tetany (due to) R29.0
  alkalosis E87.3
  associated with rickets E55.0
  convulsions R29.0
    hysterical F44.5
  functional (hysterical) F44.5
  hyperkinetic R29.0
    hysterical F44.5
  hyperpnea R06.4
    hysterical F44.5
    psychogenic F45.8
  hyperventilation (see also Hyperventilation) R06.4
    hysterical F44.5
  neonatal (without calcium or magnesium deficiency) P71.3
  parathyroid (gland) E20.9
  parathyroprival E89.2
  post- (para)thyroidectomy E89.2
  postoperative E89.2
  pseudotetany R29.0
  psychogenic (conversion reaction) F44.5
Tetralogy of Fallot Q21.3
Tetraplegia (chronic) (see also Quadriplegia) G82.50
Thailand hemorrhagic fever A91
Thalassanemia — see Thalassemia
Thalassemia (anemia) (disease) D56.9
  with other hemoglobinopathy D56.8
  alpha (major) (severe) (triple gene defect) D56.0
    minor D56.3
    silent carrier D56.3
    trait D56.3
  beta (severe) D56.1
    homozygous D56.1
    major D56.1
    minor D56.3
    trait D56.3
  delta-beta (homozygous) D56.2
    minor D56.3
    trait D56.3
  dominant D56.8
  hemoglobin
    C D56.8
    E-beta D56.5
  intermedia D56.1
  major D56.1
  minor D56.3
  mixed D56.8
  sickle-cell — see Disease, sickle-cell, thalassemia
  specified type NEC D56.8
  trait D56.3
  variants D56.8
Thanatophoric dwarfism or short stature Q77.1
Thaysen-Gee disease (nontropical sprue) K90.0
Thaysen's disease K90.0
Thecoma D27- ☑
  luteinized D27- ☑
  malignant C56- ☑
Thelarche, premature E30.8
Thelaziasis B83.8
Thelitis N61.0
  puerperal, postpartum or gestational — see Infection, nipple
Therapeutic — see condition
Therapy
  drug, long-term (current) (prophylactic)
    agents affecting estrogen receptors and estrogen levels NEC Z79.818
    anastrozole (Arimidex) Z79.811
    antibiotics Z79.2
      short-term use — omit code
    anticoagulants Z79.01
    anti-inflammatory Z79.1
    antiplatelet Z79.02
    antithrombotics Z79.02

Therapy — continued
  drug, long-term — continued
    aromatase inhibitors Z79.811
    aspirin Z79.82
    birth control pill or patch Z79.3
    bisphosphonates Z79.83
    contraceptive, oral Z79.3
    drug, specified NEC Z79.899
    estrogen receptor downregulators Z79.818
    Evista Z79.810
    exemestane (Aromasin) Z79.811
    Fareston Z79.810
    fulvestrant (Faslodex) Z79.818
    gonadotropin-releasing hormone (GnRH) agonist Z79.818
    goserelin acetate (Zoladex) Z79.818
    hormone replacement Z79.890
    insulin Z79.4
    letrozole (Femara) Z79.811
    leuprolide acetate (leuprorelin) (Lupron) Z79.818
    megestrol acetate (Megace) Z79.818
    methadone
      for pain management Z79.891
      maintenance therapy F11.20
    Nolvadex Z79.810
    opiate analgesic Z79.891
    oral contraceptive Z79.3
    raloxifene (Evista) Z79.810
    selective estrogen receptor modulators (SERMs) Z79.810
    short term — omit code
    steroids
      inhaled Z79.51
      systemic Z79.52
    tamoxifen (Nolvadex) Z79.810
    toremifene (Fareston) Z79.810
Thermic — see condition
Thermography (abnormal) (see also Abnormal, diagnostic imaging) R93.8
  breast R92.8
Thermoplegia T67.0 ☑
Thesaurismosis, glycogen — see Disease, glycogen storage
Thiamin deficiency E51.9
  specified NEC E51.8
Thiaminic deficiency with beriberi E51.11
Thibierge-Weissenbach syndrome — see Sclerosis, systemic
Thickening
  bone — see Hypertrophy, bone
  breast N64.59
  endometrium R93.8
  epidermal L85.9
    specified NEC L85.8
  hymen N89.6
  larynx J38.7
  nail L60.2
    congenital Q84.5
  periosteal — see Hypertrophy, bone
  pleura J92.9
    with asbestos J92.0
  skin R23.4
  subepiglottic J38.7
  tongue K14.8
  valve, heart — see Endocarditis
Thigh — see condition
Thinning vertebra — see Spondylopathy, specified NEC
Thirst, excessive R63.1
  due to deprivation of water T73.1 ☑
Thomsen disease G71.12
Thoracic (see also condition)
  kidney Q63.2
  outlet syndrome G54.0
Thoracogastroschisis (congenital) Q79.8
Thoracopagus Q89.4
Thorax — see condition
Thorn's syndrome N28.89
Thorson-Björck syndrome E34.0
Threadworm (infection) (infestation) B80
Threatened
  abortion O20.0
    with subsequent abortion O03.9
  job loss, anxiety concerning Z56.2
  labor (without delivery) O47.9
    at or after 37 completed weeks of gestation O47.1
    before 37 completed weeks of gestation O47.0- ☑
  loss of job, anxiety concerning Z56.2
  miscarriage O20.0

Threatened — continued
  unemployment, anxiety concerning Z56.2
Three-day fever A93.1
Threshers' lung J67.0
Thrix annulata (congenital) Q84.1
Throat — see condition
Thrombasthenia (Glanzmann) (hemorrhagic) (hereditary) D69.1
Thromboangiitis I73.1
  obliterans (general) I73.1
    cerebral I67.89
    vessels
      brain I67.89
      spinal cord I67.89
Thromboarteritis — see Arteritis
Thromboasthenia (Glanzmann) (hemorrhagic) (hereditary) D69.1
Thrombocytasthenia (Glanzmann) D69.1
Thrombocythemia (essential) (hemorrhagic) (idiopathic) (primary) D47.3
Thrombocytopathy (dystrophic) (granulopenic) D69.1
Thrombocytopenia, thrombocytopenic D69.6
  with absent radius (TAR) Q87.2
  congenital D69.42
  dilutional D69.59
  due to
    (massive) blood transfusion D69.59
    drugs D69.59
    extracorporeal circulation of blood D69.59
    platelet alloimmunization D69.59
  essential D69.3
  heparin induced (HIT) D75.82
  hereditary D69.42
  idiopathic D69.3
  neonatal, transitory P61.0
    due to
      exchange transfusion P61.0
      idiopathic maternal thrombocytopenia P61.0
      isoimmunization P61.0
  primary NEC D69.49
    idiopathic D69.3
  puerperal, postpartum O72.3
  secondary D69.59
  transient neonatal P61.0
Thrombocytosis, essential D47.3
  primary D47.3
Thromboembolism — see Embolism
Thrombopathy (Bernard-Soulier) D69.1
  constitutional D68.0
  Willebrand-Jurgens D68.0
Thrombopenia — see Thrombocytopenia
Thrombophilia D68.59
  primary NEC D68.59
  secondary NEC D68.69
  specified NEC D68.69
Thrombophlebitis I80.9
  antepartum O22.2- ☑
    deep O22.3- ☑
    superficial O22.2- ☑
  cavernous (venous) sinus G08
    complicating pregnancy O22.5- ☑
    nonpyogenic I67.6
  cerebral (sinus) (vein) G08
    nonpyogenic I67.6
    sequelae G09
  due to implanted device — see Complications, by site and type, specified NEC
  during or resulting from a procedure NEC T81.72 ☑
  femoral vein (superficial) I80.1- ☑
  femoropopliteal vein I80.0- ☑
  hepatic (vein) I80.8
  idiopathic, recurrent I82.1
  iliofemoral I80.1- ☑
  intracranial venous sinus (any) G08
    nonpyogenic I67.6
    sequelae G09
  intraspinal venous sinuses and veins G08
    nonpyogenic G95.19
  lateral (venous) sinus G08
    nonpyogenic I67.6
  leg I80.3
    superficial I80.0- ☑
  longitudinal (venous) sinus G08
    nonpyogenic I67.6
  lower extremity I80.299
  migrans, migrating I82.1
  pelvic
    with ectopic or molar pregnancy O08.0

Thrombophlebitis — continued
- pelvic — continued
  - following ectopic or molar pregnancy O08.0
  - puerperal O87.1
- popliteal vein — see Phlebitis, leg, deep, popliteal
- portal (vein) K75.1
- postoperative T81.72 ☑
- pregnancy — see Thrombophlebitis, antepartum
- puerperal, postpartum, childbirth O87.0
  - deep O87.1
  - pelvic O87.1
  - septic O86.81
  - superficial O87.0
- saphenous (greater) (lesser) I80.0- ☑
- sinus (intracranial) G08
  - nonpyogenic I67.6
- specified site NEC I80.8
- tibial vein I80.23- ☑

Thrombosis, thrombotic (bland) (multiple) (progressive) (silent) (vessel) I82.90
- anal K64.5
- antepartum — see Thrombophlebitis, antepartum
- aorta, aortic I74.10
  - abdominal I74.09
    - saddle I74.01
  - bifurcation I74.09
  - saddle I74.01
  - specified site NEC I74.19
  - terminal I74.09
  - thoracic I74.11
  - valve — see Endocarditis, aortic
- apoplexy I63.3- ☑
- artery, arteries (postinfectional) I74.9
  - auditory, internal — see Occlusion, artery, precerebral, specified NEC
  - basilar — see Occlusion, artery, basilar
  - carotid (common) (internal) — see Occlusion, artery, carotid
  - cerebellar (anterior inferior) (posterior inferior) (superior) — see Occlusion, artery, cerebellar
  - cerebral — see Occlusion, artery, cerebral
  - choroidal (anterior) — see Occlusion, artery, precerebral, specified NEC
  - communicating, posterior — see Occlusion, artery, precerebral, specified NEC
  - coronary (see also Infarct, myocardium)
    - not resulting in infarction I24.0
  - hepatic I74.8
  - hypophyseal — see Occlusion, artery, precerebral, specified NEC
  - iliac I74.5
  - limb I74.4
    - lower I74.3
    - upper I74.2
  - meningeal, anterior or posterior — see Occlusion, artery, cerebral, specified NEC
  - mesenteric (with gangrene) (see also Infarct, intestine) K55.069
  - ophthalmic — see Occlusion, artery, retina
  - pontine — see Occlusion, artery, precerebral, specified NEC
  - precerebral — see Occlusion, artery, precerebral
  - pulmonary (iatrogenic) — see Embolism, pulmonary
  - renal N28.0
  - retinal — see Occlusion, artery, retina
  - spinal, anterior or posterior G95.11
  - traumatic NEC T14.8 ☑
  - vertebral — see Occlusion, artery, vertebral
- atrium, auricular (see also Infarct, myocardium)
  - following acute myocardial infarction (current complication) I23.6
  - not resulting in infarction I51.3
  - old I51.3
- basilar (artery) — see Occlusion, artery, basilar
- brain (artery) (stem) (see also Occlusion, artery, cerebral)
  - due to syphilis A52.05
  - puerperal O99.43
  - sinus — see Thrombosis, intracranial venous sinus
- capillary I78.8
- cardiac (see also Infarct, myocardium)
  - not resulting in infarction I51.3
  - old I51.3
  - valve — see Endocarditis
- carotid (artery) (common) (internal) — see Occlusion, artery, carotid

Thrombosis, thrombotic — continued
- cavernous (venous) sinus — see Thrombosis, intracranial venous sinus
- cerebellar artery (anterior inferior) (posterior inferior) (superior) I66.3
- cerebral (artery) — see Occlusion, artery, cerebral
- cerebrovenous sinus (see also Thrombosis, intracranial venous sinus)
  - puerperium O87.3
- chronic I82.91
- coronary (artery) (vein) (see also Infarct, myocardium)
  - not resulting in infarction I24.0
- corpus cavernosum N48.89
- cortical I66.9
- deep — see Embolism, vein, lower extremity
- due to device, implant or graft (see also Complications, by site and type, specified NEC) T85.868 ☑
  - arterial graft NEC T82.868 ☑
  - breast (implant) T85.868 ☑
  - catheter NEC T85.868 ☑
    - dialysis (renal) T82.868 ☑
      - intraperitoneal T85.868 ☑
    - infusion NEC T82.868 ☑
      - spinal (epidural) (subdural) T85.860 ☑
    - urinary (indwelling) T83.86 ☑
  - electronic (electrode) (pulse generator) (stimulator)
    - bone T84.86 ☑
    - cardiac T82.867 ☑
    - nervous system (brain) (peripheral nerve) (spinal) T85.860 ☑
    - urinary T83.86 ☑
  - fixation, internal (orthopedic) NEC T84.86 ☑
  - gastrointestinal (bile duct) (esophagus) T85.868 ☑
  - genital NEC T83.86 ☑
  - heart T82.867 ☑
  - joint prosthesis T84.86 ☑
  - ocular (corneal graft) (orbital implant) NEC T85.868 ☑
  - orthopedic NEC T84.86 ☑
  - specified NEC T85.868 ☑
  - urinary NEC T83.86 ☑
  - vascular NEC T82.868 ☑
  - ventricular intracranial shunt T85.860 ☑
- during the puerperium — see Thrombosis, puerperal
- endocardial (see also Infarct, myocardium)
  - not resulting in infarction I51.3
- eye — see Occlusion, retina
- genital organ
  - female NEC N94.89
    - pregnancy — see Thrombophlebitis, antepartum
  - male N50.1
- gestational — see Phlebopathy, gestational
- heart (chamber) (see also Infarct, myocardium)
  - not resulting in infarction I51.3
  - old I51.3
- hepatic (vein) I82.0
  - artery I74.8
- history (of) Z86.718
- intestine (with gangrene) (see also Infarct, intestine) K55.069
- intracardiac NEC (apical) (atrial) (auricular) (ventricular) (old) I51.3
- intracranial (arterial) I66.9
  - venous sinus (any) G08
    - nonpyogenic origin I67.6
    - puerperium O87.3
- intramural (see also Infarct, myocardium)
  - not resulting in infarction I51.3
  - old I51.3
- intraspinal venous sinuses and veins G08
  - nonpyogenic G95.19
- kidney (artery) N28.0
- lateral (venous) sinus — see Thrombosis, intracranial venous sinus
- leg — see Thrombosis, vein, lower extremity
  - arterial I74.3
- liver (venous) I82.0
  - artery I74.8
  - portal vein I81
- longitudinal (venous) sinus — see Thrombosis, intracranial venous sinus
- lower limb — see Thrombosis, vein, lower extremity
- lung (iatrogenic) (postoperative) — see Embolism, pulmonary
- meninges (brain) (arterial) I66.8

Thrombosis, thrombotic — continued
- mesenteric (artery) (with gangrene) (see also Infarct, intestine) K55.069
  - vein (inferior) (superior) I81
- mitral I34.8
- mural (see also Infarct, myocardium)
  - due to syphilis A52.06
  - not resulting in infarction I51.3
  - old I51.3
- omentum (with gangrene) (see also Infarct, intestine) K55.069
- ophthalmic — see Occlusion, retina
- pampiniform plexus (male) N50.1
- parietal (see also Infarct, myocardium)
  - not resulting in infarction I24.0
- penis, superficial vein N48.81
- perianal venous K64.5
- peripheral arteries I74.4
  - upper I74.2
- personal history (of) Z86.718
- portal I81
  - due to syphilis A52.09
- precerebral artery — see Occlusion, artery, precerebral
- puerperal, postpartum O87.0
  - brain (artery) O99.43
    - venous (sinus) O87.3
  - cardiac O99.43
  - cerebral (artery) O99.43
    - venous (sinus) O87.3
  - superficial O87.0
- pulmonary (artery) (iatrogenic) (postoperative) (vein) — see Embolism, pulmonary
- renal (artery) N28.0
  - vein I82.3
- resulting from presence of device, implant or graft — see Complications, by site and type, specified NEC
- retina, retinal — see Occlusion, retina
- scrotum N50.1
- seminal vesicle N50.1
- sigmoid (venous) sinus — see Thrombosis, intracranial venous sinus
- sinus, intracranial (any) — see Thrombosis, intracranial venous sinus
- specified site NEC I82.890
  - chronic I82.891
- spermatic cord N50.1
- spinal cord (arterial) G95.11
  - due to syphilis A52.09
  - pyogenic origin G06.1
- spleen, splenic D73.5
  - artery I74.8
- testis N50.1
- traumatic NEC T14.8 ☑
- tricuspid I07.8
- tumor — see Neoplasm, unspecified behavior, by site
- tunica vaginalis N50.1
- umbilical cord (vessels), complicating delivery O69.5 ☑
- vas deferens N50.1
- vein (acute) I82.90
  - antecubital I82.61- ☑
    - chronic I82.71- ☑
  - axillary I82.A1- ☑ (following I82.7)
    - chronic I82.A2- ☑ (following I82.7)
  - basilic I82.61- ☑
    - chronic I82.71- ☑
  - brachial I82.62- ☑
    - chronic I82.72- ☑
  - brachiocephalic (innominate) I82.290
    - chronic I82.291
  - cephalic I82.61- ☑
    - chronic I82.71- ☑
  - cerebral, nonpyogenic I67.6
  - chronic I82.91
  - deep (DVT) I82.40- ☑
    - calf I82.4Z- ☑
      - chronic I82.5Z- ☑
    - lower leg I82.4Z- ☑
      - chronic I82.5Z- ☑
    - thigh I82.4Y- ☑
      - chronic I82.5Y- ☑
    - upper leg I82.4Y ☑
      - chronic I82.5Y- ☑
  - femoral I82.41- ☑
    - chronic I82.51- ☑
  - iliac (iliofemoral) I82.42- ☑
    - chronic I82.52- ☑

Thrombosis, thrombotic — *continued*
  vein — *continued*
    innominate I82.290
      chronic I82.291
    internal jugular I82.C1- ☑ (*following* I82.7)
      chronic I82.C2- ☑ (*following* I82.7)
    lower extremity
      deep I82.40- ☑
        chronic I82.50- ☑
        specified NEC I82.49- ☑
          chronic NEC I82.59- ☑
      distal
        deep I82.4Z- ☑
      proximal
        deep I82.4Y- ☑
        chronic I82.5Y- ☑
      superficial I82.81- ☑
    perianal K64.5
    popliteal I82.43- ☑
      chronic I82.53- ☑
    radial I82.62- ☑
      chronic I82.72- ☑
    renal I82.3
    saphenous (greater) (lesser) I82.81- ☑
    specified NEC I82.890
      chronic NEC I82.891
    subclavian I82.B1- ☑ (*following* I82.7)
      chronic I82.B2- ☑ (*following* I82.7)
    thoracic NEC I82.290
      chronic I82.291
    tibial I82.44- ☑
      chronic I82.54- ☑
    ulnar I82.62- ☑
      chronic I82.72- ☑
    upper extremity I82.60- ☑
      chronic I82.70- ☑
      deep I82.62- ☑
        chronic I82.72- ☑
      superficial I82.61- ☑
        chronic I82.71- ☑
  vena cava
    inferior I82.220
      chronic I82.221
    superior I82.210
      chronic I82.211
  venous, perianal K64.5
  ventricle (*see also* Infarct, myocardium)
    following acute myocardial infarction (current complication) I23.6
    not resulting in infarction I24.0
    old I51.3
Thrombus — *see* Thrombosis
Thrush (*see also* Candidiasis)
  newborn P37.5
  oral B37.0
  vaginal B37.3
Thumb (*see also* condition)
  sucking (child problem) F98.8
Thymitis E32.8
Thymoma (benign) D15.0
  malignant C37
Thymus, thymic (gland) — *see* condition
Thyrocele — *see* Goiter
Thyroglossal (*see also* condition)
  cyst Q89.2
  duct, persistent Q89.2
Thyroid (gland) (body) (*see also* condition)
  hormone resistance E07.89
  lingual Q89.2
  nodule (cystic) (nontoxic) (single) E04.1
Thyroiditis E06.9
  acute (nonsuppurative) (pyogenic) (suppurative) E06.0
  autoimmune E06.3
  chronic (nonspecific) (sclerosing) E06.5
    with thyrotoxicosis, transient E06.2
    fibrous E06.5
    lymphadenoid E06.3
    lymphocytic E06.3
    lymphoid E06.3
  de Quervain's E06.1
  drug-induced E06.4
  fibrous (chronic) E06.5
  giant-cell (follicular) E06.1
  granulomatous (de Quervain) (subacute) E06.1
  Hashimoto's (struma lymphomatosa) E06.3
  iatrogenic E06.4
  ligneous E06.5

Thyroiditis — *continued*
  lymphocytic (chronic) E06.3
  lymphoid E06.3
  lymphomatous E06.3
  nonsuppurative E06.1
  postpartum, puerperal O90.5
  pseudotuberculous E06.1
  pyogenic E06.0
  radiation E06.4
  Riedel's E06.5
  subacute (granulomatous) E06.1
  suppurative E06.0
  tuberculous A18.81
  viral E06.1
  woody E06.5
Thyrolingual duct, persistent Q89.2
Thyromegaly E01.0
Thyrotoxic
  crisis — *see* Thyrotoxicosis
  heart disease or failure (*see also* Thyrotoxicosis) E05.90 [I43]
    with thyroid storm E05.91 [I43]
  storm — *see* Thyrotoxicosis
Thyrotoxicosis (recurrent) E05.90
  with
    goiter (diffuse) E05.00
      with thyroid storm E05.01
      adenomatous uninodular E05.10
        with thyroid storm E05.11
      multinodular E05.20
        with thyroid storm E05.21
      nodular E05.20
        with thyroid storm E05.21
      uninodular E05.10
        with thyroid storm E05.11
    infiltrative
      dermopathy E05.00
        with thyroid storm E05.01
      ophthalmopathy E05.00
        with thyroid storm E05.01
    single thyroid nodule E05.10
      with thyroid storm E05.11
    thyroid storm E05.91
  due to
    ectopic thyroid nodule or tissue E05.30
      with thyroid storm E05.31
    ingestion of (excessive) thyroid material E05.40
      with thyroid storm E05.41
    overproduction of thyroid-stimulating hormone E05.80
      with thyroid storm E05.81
    specified cause NEC E05.80
      with thyroid storm E05.81
  factitia E05.40
    with thyroid storm E05.41
  heart (*see also* Failure, heart, high-output) E05.90 [I43]
    with thyroid storm (*see also* Failure, heart, high-output) E05.91 [I43]
    failure (*see also* Failure, heart, high-output) E05.90 [I43]
  neonatal (transient) P72.1
  transient with chronic thyroiditis E06.2
Tibia vara — *see* Osteochondrosis, juvenile, tibia
Tic (disorder) F95.9
  breathing F95.8
  child problem F95.0
  compulsive F95.1
  de la Tourette F95.2
  degenerative (generalized) (localized) G25.69
    facial G25.69
  disorder
    chronic
      motor F95.1
      vocal F95.1
    combined vocal and multiple motor F95.2
    transient F95.0
  douloureux G50.0
    atypical G50.1
    postherpetic, postzoster B02.22
  drug-induced G25.61
  eyelid F95.8
  habit F95.9
    chronic F95.1
    transient of childhood F95.0
  lid, transient of childhood F95.0
  motor-verbal F95.2
  occupational F48.8
  orbicularis F95.8

Tic — *continued*
  orbicularis — *continued*
    transient of childhood F95.0
  organic origin G25.69
  postchoreic G25.69
  provisional F95.0
  psychogenic, compulsive F95.1
  salaam R25.8
  spasm (motor or vocal) F95.9
    chronic F95.1
    transient of childhood F95.0
  specified NEC F95.8
Tick-borne — *see* condition
Tietze's disease or syndrome M94.0
Tight, tightness
  anus K62.89
  chest R07.89
  fascia (lata) M62.89
  foreskin (congenital) N47.1
  hymen, hymenal ring N89.6
  introitus (acquired) (congenital) N89.6
  rectal sphincter K62.89
  tendon — *see* Short, tendon
  urethral sphincter N35.9
Tilting vertebra — *see* Dorsopathy, deforming, specified NEC
Timidity, child F93.8
Tinea (intersecta) (tarsi) B35.9
  amiantacea L44.8
  asbestina B35.0
  barbae B35.0
  beard B35.0
  black dot B35.0
  blanca B36.2
  capitis B35.0
  corporis B35.4
  cruris B35.6
  flava B36.0
  foot B35.3
  furfuracea B36.0
  imbricata (Tokelau) B35.5
  kerion B35.0
  manuum B35.2
  microsporic — *see* Dermatophytosis
  nigra B36.1
  nodosa — *see* Piedra
  pedis B35.3
  scalp B35.0
  specified NEC B35.8
  sycosis B35.0
  tonsurans B35.0
  trichophytic — *see* Dermatophytosis
  ungulum B35.1
  versicolor B36.0
Tingling sensation (skin) R20.2
Tin-miner's lung J63.5
Tinnitus NOS H93.1- ☑
  audible H93.1- ☑
  aurium H93.1- ☑
  pulsatile H93.A- ☑
  subjective H93.1- ☑
Tipped tooth (teeth) M26.33
Tipping
  pelvis M95.5
    with disproportion (fetopelvic) O33.0
      causing obstructed labor O65.0
  tooth (teeth), fully erupted M26.33
Tiredness R53.83
Tissue — *see* condition
Tobacco (nicotine)
  abuse — *see* Tobacco, use
  dependence — *see* Dependence, drug, nicotine
  harmful use Z72.0
  heart — *see* Tobacco, toxic effect
  maternal use, affecting newborn P04.2
  toxic effect — *see* Table of Drugs and Chemicals, by substance, poisoning
    chewing tobacco — *see* Table of Drugs and Chemicals, by substance, poisoning
    cigarettes — *see* Table of Drugs and Chemicals, by substance, poisoning
  use Z72.0
    complicating
      childbirth O99.334
      pregnancy O99.33- ☑
      puerperium O99.335
    counseling and surveillance Z71.6
    history Z87.891

Tobacco — *continued*
  withdrawal state (*see also* Dependence, drug, nicotine) F17.203
Tocopherol deficiency E56.0
Todd's
  cirrhosis K74.3
  paralysis (postepileptic) (transitory) G83.84
Toe — *see* condition
Toilet, artificial opening — *see* Attention to, artificial, opening
Tokelau (ringworm) B35.5
Tollwut — *see* Rabies
Tommaselli's disease R31.9
  correct substance properly administered — *see* Table of Drugs and Chemicals, by drug, adverse effect
  overdose or wrong substance given or taken — *see* Table of Drugs and Chemicals, by drug, poisoning
Tongue (*see also* condition)
  tie Q38.1
Tonic pupil — *see* Anomaly, pupil, function, tonic pupil
Toni-Fanconi syndrome (cystinosis) E72.09
  with cystinosis E72.04
Tonsil — *see* condition
Tonsillitis (acute) (catarrhal) (croupous) (follicular) (gangrenous) (infective) (lacunar) (lingual) (malignant) (membranous) (parenchymatous) (phlegmonous) (pseudomembranous) (purulent) (septic) (subacute) (suppurative) (toxic) (ulcerative) (vesicular) (viral) J03.90
  chronic J35.01
    with adenoiditis J35.03
  diphtheritic A36.0
  hypertrophic J35.01
    with adenoiditis J35.03
  recurrent J03.91
  specified organism NEC J03.80
    recurrent J03.81
  staphylococcal J03.80
    recurrent J03.81
  streptococcal J03.00
    recurrent J03.01
  tuberculous A15.8
  Vincent's A69.1
Tooth, teeth — *see* condition
Toothache K08.89
Topagnosis R20.8
Tophi — *see* Gout, chronic
TORCH infection — *see* Infection, congenital
  without active infection P00.2
Torn — *see* Tear
Tornwaldt's cyst or disease J39.2
Torsion
  accessory tube — *see* Torsion, fallopian tube
  adnexa (female) — *see* Torsion, fallopian tube
  aorta, acquired I77.1
  appendix epididymis N44.04
  appendix testis N44.03
  bile duct (common) (hepatic) K83.8
    congenital Q44.5
  bowel, colon or intestine K56.2
  cervix — *see* Malposition, uterus
  cystic duct K82.8
  dystonia — *see* Dystonia, torsion
  epididymis (appendix) N44.04
  fallopian tube N83.52- ☑
    with ovary N83.53
  gallbladder K82.8
    congenital Q44.1
  hydatid of Morgagni
    female N83.52- ☑
    male N44.03
  kidney (pedicle) (leading to infarction) N28.0
  Meckel's diverticulum (congenital) Q43.0
    malignant — *see* Table of Neoplasms, small intestine, malignant
  mesentery K56.2
  omentum K56.2
  organ or site, congenital NEC — *see* Anomaly, by site
  ovary (pedicle) N83.51- ☑
    with fallopian tube N83.53
    congenital Q50.2
  oviduct — *see* Torsion, fallopian tube
  penis (acquired) N48.82
    congenital Q55.63
  spasm — *see* Dystonia, torsion
  spermatic cord N44.02
    extravaginal N44.01

Torsion — *continued*
  spermatic cord — *continued*
    intravaginal N44.02
  spleen D73.5
  testis, testicle N44.00
    appendix N44.03
  tibia — *see* Deformity, limb, specified type NEC, lower leg
  uterus — *see* Malposition, uterus
Torticollis (intermittent) (spastic) M43.6
  congenital (sternomastoid) Q68.0
  due to birth injury P15.8
  hysterical F44.4
  ocular R29.891
  psychogenic F45.8
    conversion reaction F44.4
  rheumatic M43.6
  rheumatoid M06.88
  spasmodic G24.3
  traumatic, current S13.4 ☑
Tortipelvis G24.1
Tortuous
  aortic arch Q25.46
  artery I77.1
  organ or site, congenital NEC — *see* Distortion
  retinal vessel, congenital Q14.1
  ureter N13.8
  urethra N36.8
  vein — *see* Varix
Torture, victim of Z65.4
Torula, torular (histolytica) (infection) — *see* Cryptococcosis
Torulosis — *see* Cryptococcosis
Torus (mandibularis) (palatinus) M27.0
  fracture — *see* Fracture, by site, torus
Touraine's syndrome Q79.8
Tourette's syndrome F95.2
Tourniquet syndrome — *see* Constriction, external, by site
Tower skull Q75.0
  with exophthalmos Q87.0
Toxemia R68.89
  bacterial — *see* Sepsis
  burn — *see* Burn
  eclamptic (with pre-existing hypertension) — *see* Eclampsia
  erysipelatous — *see* Erysipelas
  fatigue R68.89
  food — *see* Poisoning, food
  gastrointestinal K52.1
  intestinal K52.1
  kidney — *see* Uremia
  malarial — *see* Malaria
  myocardial — *see* Myocarditis, toxic
  of pregnancy — *see* Pre-eclampsia
  pre-eclamptic — *see* Pre-eclampsia
  small intestine K52.1
  staphylococcal, due to food A05.0
  stasis R68.89
  uremic — *see* Uremia
  urinary — *see* Uremia
Toxemica cerebropathia psychica (nonalcoholic) F04
  alcoholic — *see* Alcohol, amnestic disorder
Toxic (poisoning) (*see also* condition) T65.91 ☑
  effect — *see* Table of Drugs and Chemicals, by substance, poisoning
  shock syndrome A48.3
  thyroid (gland) — *see* Thyrotoxicosis
Toxicemia — *see* Toxemia
Toxicity — *see* Table of Drugs and Chemicals, by substance, poisoning
  fava bean D55.0
  food, noxious — *see* Poisoning, food
  from drug or nonmedicinal substance — *see* Table of Drugs and Chemicals, by drug
Toxicosis (*see also* Toxemia)
  capillary, hemorrhagic D69.0
Toxinfection, gastrointestinal K52.1
Toxocariasis B83.0
Toxoplasma, toxoplasmosis (acquired) B58.9
  with
    hepatitis B58.1
    meningoencephalitis B58.2
    ocular involvement B58.00
    other organ involvement B58.89
    pneumonia, pneumonitis B58.3
  congenital (acute) (subacute) (chronic) P37.1

Toxoplasma, toxoplasmosis — *continued*
  maternal, manifest toxoplasmosis in infant (acute) (subacute) (chronic) P37.1
tPA (rtPA) administration in a different facility within the last 24 hours prior to admission to current facility Z92.82
Trabeculation, bladder N32.89
Trachea — *see* condition
Tracheitis (catarrhal) (infantile) (membranous) (plastic) (septal) (suppurative) (viral) J04.10
  with
    bronchitis (15 years of age and above) J40
      acute or subacute — *see* Bronchitis, acute
      chronic J42
      tuberculous NEC A15.5
      under 15 years of age J20.9
    laryngitis (acute) J04.2
      chronic J37.1
      tuberculous NEC A15.5
  acute J04.10
    with obstruction J04.11
  chronic J42
    with
      bronchitis (chronic) J42
      laryngitis (chronic) J37.1
  diphtheritic (membranous) A36.89
  due to external agent — *see* Inflammation, respiratory, upper, due to
  syphilitic A52.73
  tuberculous A15.5
Trachelitis (nonvenereal) — *see* Cervicitis
Tracheobronchial — *see* condition
Tracheobronchitis (15 years of age and above) (*see also* Bronchitis)
  due to
    Bordetella bronchiseptica A37.80
      with pneumonia A37.81
    Francisella tularensis A21.8
Tracheobronchomegaly Q32.4
  with bronchiectasis J47.9
    with
      exacerbation (acute) J47.1
      lower respiratory infection J47.0
  acquired J98.09
    with bronchiectasis J47.9
      with
        exacerbation (acute) J47.1
        lower respiratory infection J47.0
Tracheobronchopneumonitis — *see* Pneumonia, broncho-
Tracheocele (external) (internal) J39.8
  congenital Q32.1
Tracheomalacia J39.8
  congenital Q32.0
Tracheopharyngitis (acute) J06.9
  chronic J42
  due to external agent — *see* Inflammation, respiratory, upper, due to
Tracheostenosis J39.8
Tracheostomy
  complication — *see* Complication, tracheostomy
  status Z93.0
    attention to Z43.0
    malfunctioning J95.03
Trachoma, trachomatous A71.9
  active (stage) A71.1
  contraction of conjunctiva A71.1
  dubium A71.0
  healed or sequelae B94.0
  initial (stage) A71.0
  pannus A71.1
  Türck's J37.0
Traction, vitreomacular H43.82- ☑
Train sickness T75.3 ☑
Trait(s)
  Hb-S D57.3
  hemoglobin
    abnormal NEC D58.2
      with thalassemia D56.3
    C — *see* Disease, hemoglobin C
    S (Hb-S) D57.3
  Lepore D56.3
  personality, accentuated Z73.1
  sickle-cell D57.3
    with elliptocytosis or spherocytosis D57.3
  type A personality Z73.1
Tramp Z59.0
Trance R41.89

☑ **Additional Character Required** — Refer to the Tabular List for Character Selection   ▽ **Subterms under main terms may continue to next column or page**

Trance — *continued*
  hysterical F44.89
Transaminasemia R74.0
Transection
  abdomen (partial) S38.3 ☑
  aorta (incomplete) (*see also* Injury, aorta)
    complete — *see* Injury, aorta, laceration, major
  carotid artery (incomplete) (*see also* Injury, blood vessel, carotid, laceration)
    complete — *see* Injury, blood vessel, carotid, laceration, major
  celiac artery (incomplete) S35.211 ☑
    branch (incomplete) S35.291 ☑
      complete S35.292 ☑
    complete S35.212 ☑
  innominate
    artery (incomplete) (*see also* Injury, blood vessel, thoracic, innominate, artery, laceration)
      complete — *see* Injury, blood vessel, thoracic, innominate, artery, laceration, major
    vein (incomplete) (*see also* Injury, blood vessel, thoracic, innominate, vein, laceration)
      complete — *see* Injury, blood vessel, thoracic, innominate, vein, laceration, major
  jugular vein (external) (incomplete) (*see also* Injury, blood vessel, jugular vein, laceration)
    complete — *see* Injury, blood vessel, jugular vein, laceration, major
    internal (incomplete) (*see also* Injury, blood vessel, jugular vein, internal, laceration)
      complete — *see* Injury, blood vessel, jugular vein, internal, laceration, major
  mesenteric artery (incomplete) (*see also* Injury, mesenteric, artery, laceration)
    complete — *see* Injury, mesenteric artery, laceration, major
  pulmonary vessel (incomplete) (*see also* Injury, blood vessel, thoracic, pulmonary, laceration)
    complete — *see* Injury, blood vessel, thoracic, pulmonary, laceration, major
  subclavian — *see* Transection, innominate
  vena cava (incomplete) (*see also* Injury, vena cava)
    complete — *see* Injury, vena cava, laceration, major
  vertebral artery (incomplete) (*see also* Injury, blood vessel, vertebral, laceration)
    complete — *see* Injury, blood vessel, vertebral, laceration, major
Transfusion
  associated (red blood cell) hemochromatosis E83.111
  blood
    ABO incompatible — *see* Complication(s), transfusion, incompatibility reaction, ABO
    minor blood group (Duffy) (E) (K(ell)) (Kidd) (Lewis) (M) (N) (P) (S) T80.89 ☑
    reaction or complication — *see* Complications, transfusion
  fetomaternal (mother) — *see* Pregnancy, complicated by, placenta, transfusion syndrome
  maternofetal (mother) — *see* Pregnancy, complicated by, placenta, transfusion syndrome
  placental (syndrome) (mother) — *see* Pregnancy, complicated by, placenta, transfusion syndrome
  reaction (adverse) — *see* Complications, transfusion
  related acute lung injury (TRALI) J95.84
  twin-to-twin — *see* Pregnancy, complicated by, placenta, transfusion syndrome, fetus to fetus
Transient (meaning homeless) (*see also* condition) Z59.0
Translocation
  balanced autosomal Q95.9
    in normal individual Q95.0
  chromosomes NEC Q99.8
    balanced and insertion in normal individual Q95.0
  Down syndrome Q90.2
  trisomy
    13 Q91.6
    18 Q91.2
    21 Q90.2
Translucency, iris — *see* Degeneration, iris
Transmission of chemical substances through the placenta — *see* Absorption, chemical, through placenta
Transparency, lung, unilateral J43.0
Transplant (ed) (status) Z94.9
  awaiting organ Z76.82
  bone Z94.6
    marrow Z94.81
  candidate Z76.82

Transplant — *continued*
  complication — *see* Complication, transplant
  cornea Z94.7
  heart Z94.1
    and lung(s) Z94.3
    valve Z95.2
      prosthetic Z95.2
      specified NEC Z95.4
      xenogenic Z95.3
  intestine Z94.82
  kidney Z94.0
  liver Z94.4
  lung(s) Z94.2
    and heart Z94.3
  organ (failure) (infection) (rejection) Z94.9
    removal status Z98.85
  pancreas Z94.83
  skin Z94.5
  social Z60.3
  specified organ or tissue NEC Z94.89
  stem cells Z94.84
  tissue Z94.9
Transplants, ovarian, endometrial N80.1
Transposed — *see* Transposition
Transposition (congenital) (*see also* Malposition, congenital)
  abdominal viscera Q89.3
  aorta (dextra) Q20.3
  appendix Q43.8
  colon Q43.8
  corrected Q20.5
  great vessels (complete) (partial) Q20.3
  heart Q24.0
    with complete transposition of viscera Q89.3
  intestine (large) (small) Q43.8
  reversed jejunal (for bypass) (status) Z98.0
  scrotum Q55.23
  stomach Q40.2
    with general transposition of viscera Q89.3
  tooth, teeth, fully erupted M26.30
  vessels, great (complete) (partial) Q20.3
  viscera (abdominal) (thoracic) Q89.3
Transsexualism F64.0
Transverse (*see also* condition)
  arrest (deep), in labor O64.0 ☑
  lie (mother) O32.2 ☑
    causing obstructed labor O64.8 ☑
Transvestism, transvestitism (dual-role) F64.1
  fetishistic F65.1
Trapped placenta (with hemorrhage) O72.0
  without hemorrhage O73.0
TRAPS (tumor necrosis factor receptor associated periodic syndrome) M04.1
Trauma, traumatism (*see also* Injury)
  acoustic — *see* subcategory H83.3 ☑
  birth — *see* Birth, injury
  complicating ectopic or molar pregnancy O08.6
  during delivery O71.9
  following ectopic or molar pregnancy O08.6
  obstetric O71.9
    specified NEC O71.89
  occusal
    primary K08.81
    secondary K08.82
Traumatic (*see also* condition)
  brain injury S06.9 ☑
Treacher Collins syndrome Q75.4
Treitz's hernia — *see* Hernia, abdomen, specified site NEC
Trematode infestation — *see* Infestation, fluke
Trematodiasis — *see* Infestation, fluke
Trembling paralysis — *see* Parkinsonism
Tremor(s) R25.1
  drug induced G25.1
  essential (benign) G25.0
  familial G25.0
  hereditary G25.0
  hysterical F44.4
  intention G25.2
  medication induced postural G25.1
  mercurial — *see* subcategory T56.1 ☑
  Parkinson's — *see* Parkinsonism
  psychogenic (conversion reaction) F44.4
  senilis R54
  specified type NEC G25.2
Trench
  fever A79.0
  foot — *see* Immersion, foot

Trench — *continued*
  mouth A69.1
Treponema pallidum infection — *see* Syphilis
Treponematosis
  due to
    T. pallidum — *see* Syphilis
    T. pertenue — *see* Yaws
Triad
  Hutchinson's (congenital syphilis) A50.53
  Kartagener's Q89.3
  Saint's — *see* Hernia, diaphragm
Trichiasis (eyelid) H02.059
  with entropion — *see* Entropion
  left H02.056
    lower H02.055
    upper H02.054
  right H02.053
    lower H02.052
    upper H02.051
Trichinella spiralis (infection) (infestation) B75
Trichinellosis, trichiniasis, trichinelliasis, trichinosis B75
  with muscle disorder B75 [M63.80]
    ankle B75 [M63.87-] ☑
    foot B75 [M63.87-] ☑
    forearm B75 [M63.83-] ☑
    hand B75 [M63.84-] ☑
    lower leg B75 [M63.86-] ☑
    multiple sites B75 [M63.89]
    pelvic region B75 [M63.85-] ☑
    shoulder region B75 [M63.81-] ☑
    specified site NEC B75 [M63.88]
    thigh B75 [M63.85-] ☑
    upper arm B75 [M63.82-] ☑
Trichobezoar T18.9 ☑
  intestine T18.3 ☑
  stomach T18.2 ☑
Trichocephaliasis, trichocephalosis B79
Trichocephalus infestation B79
Trichoclasis L67.8
Trichoepithelioma (*see also* Neoplasm, skin, benign)
  malignant — *see* Neoplasm, skin, malignant
Trichofolliculoma — *see* Neoplasm, skin, benign
Tricholemmoma — *see* Neoplasm, skin, benign
Trichomoniasis A59.9
  bladder A59.03
  cervix A59.09
  intestinal A07.8
  prostate A59.02
  seminal vesicles A59.09
  specified site NEC A59.8
  urethra A59.03
  urogenitalis A59.00
  vagina A59.01
  vulva A59.01
Trichomycosis
  axillaris A48.8
  nodosa, nodularis B36.8
Trichonodosis L67.8
Trichophytid, trichophyton infection — *see* Dermatophytosis
Trichophytobezoar T18.9 ☑
  intestine T18.3 ☑
  stomach T18.2 ☑
Trichophytosis — *see* Dermatophytosis
Trichoptilosis L67.8
Trichorrhexis (nodosa) (invaginata) L67.0
Trichosis axillaris A48.8
Trichosporosis nodosa B36.2
Trichostasis spinulosa (congenital) Q84.1
Trichostrongyliasis, trichostrongylosis (small intestine) B81.2
Trichostrongylus infection B81.2
Trichotillomania F63.3
Trichromat, trichromatopsia, anomalous (congenital) H53.55
Trichuriasis B79
Trichuris trichiura (infection) (infestation) (any site) B79
Tricuspid (valve) — *see* condition
Trifid (*see also* Accessory)
  kidney (pelvis) Q63.8
  tongue Q38.3
Trigeminal neuralgia — *see* Neuralgia, trigeminal
Trigeminy R00.8
Trigger finger (acquired) M65.30
  congenital Q74.0
  index finger M65.32- ☑

▽ **Subterms under main terms may continue to next column or page**   ☑ **Additional Character Required — Refer to the Tabular List for Character Selection**   313

Trance — Trigger finger

Trigger finger — *continued*
  little finger M65.35- ☑
  middle finger M65.33- ☑
  ring finger M65.34- ☑
  thumb M65.31- ☑
Trigonitis (bladder) (chronic) (pseudomembranous) N30.30
  with hematuria N30.31
Trigonocephaly Q75.0
Trilocular heart — *see* Cor triloculare
Trimethylaminuria E72.52
Tripartite placenta O43.19- ☑
Triphalangeal thumb Q74.0
Triple (*see also* Accessory)
  kidneys Q63.0
  uteri Q51.818
  X, female Q97.0
Triplegia G83.89
  congenital G80.8
Triplet (newborn) (*see also* Newborn, triplet)
  complicating pregnancy — *see* Pregnancy, triplet
Triplication — *see* Accessory
Triploidy Q92.7
Trismus R25.2
  neonatorum A33
  newborn A33
Trisomy (syndrome) Q92.9
  13 (partial) Q91.7
    meiotic nondisjunction Q91.4
    mitotic nondisjunction Q91.5
    mosaicism Q91.5
    translocation Q91.6
  18 (partial) Q91.3
    meiotic nondisjunction Q91.0
    mitotic nondisjunction Q91.1
    mosaicism Q91.1
    translocation Q91.2
  20 Q92.8
  21 (partial) Q90.9
    meiotic nondisjunction Q90.0
    mitotic nondisjunction Q90.1
    mosaiclsm Q90.1
    translocation Q90.2
  22 Q92.8
  autosomes Q92.9
  chromosome specified NEC Q92.8
    partial Q92.2
      due to unbalanced translocation Q92.5
    specified NEC Q92.8
    whole (nonsex chromosome)
      meiotic nondisjunction Q92.0
      mitotic nondisjunction Q92.1
      mosaicism Q92.1
  due to
    dicentrics — *see* Extra, marker chromosomes
    extra rings — *see* Extra, marker chromosomes
    isochromosomes — *see* Extra, marker chromosomes
  specified NEC Q92.8
  whole chromosome Q92.9
    meiotic nondisjunction Q92.0
    mitotic nondisjunction Q92.1
    mosaicism Q92.1
    partial Q92.9
    specified NEC Q92.8
Tritanomaly, tritanopia H53.55
Trombiculosis, trombiculiasis, trombidiosis B88.0
Trophedema (congenital) (hereditary) Q82.0
Trophoblastic disease (*see also* Mole, hydatidiform) O01.9
Tropholymphedema Q82.0
Trophoneurosis NEC G96.8
  disseminated M34.9
Tropical — *see* condition
Trouble (*see also* Disease)
  heart — *see* Disease, heart
  kidney — *see* Disease, renal
  nervous R45.0
  sinus — *see* Sinusitis
Trousseau's syndrome (thrombophlebitis migrans) I82.1
Truancy, childhood
  from school Z72.810
Truncus
  arteriosus (persistent) Q20.0
  communis Q20.0
Trunk — *see* condition

Trypanosomiasis
  African B56.9
    by Trypanosoma brucei
      gambiense B56.0
      rhodesiense B56.1
  American — *see* Chagas' disease
  Brazilian — *see* Chagas' disease
  by Trypanosoma
    brucei gambiense B56.0
    brucei rhodesiense B56.1
    cruzi — *see* Chagas' disease
  gambiense, Gambian B56.0
  rhodesiensis, Rhodesian B56.1
  South American — *see* Chagas' disease
  where
    African trypanosomiasis is prevalent B56.9
    Chagas' disease is prevalent B57.2
T-shaped incisors K00.2
Tsutsugamushi (disease) (fever) A75.3
Tube, tubal, tubular — *see* condition
Tubercle (*see also* Tuberculosis)
  brain, solitary A17.81
  Darwin's Q17.8
  Ghon, primary infection A15.7
Tuberculid, tuberculide (indurating, subcutaneous) (lichenoid) (miliary) (papulonecrotic) (primary) (skin) A18.4
Tuberculoma (*see also* Tuberculosis)
  brain A17.81
  meninges (cerebral) (spinal) A17.1
  spinal cord A17.81
Tuberculosis, tubercular, tuberculous (calcification) (calcified) (caseous) (chromogenic acid-fast bacilli) (degeneration) (fibrocaseous) (fistula) (interstitial) (isolated circumscribed lesions) (necrosis) (parenchymatous) (ulcerative) A15.9
  with pneumoconiosis (any condition in J60-J64) J65
  abdomen (lymph gland) A18.39
  abscess (respiratory) A15.9
    bone A18.03
      hip A18.02
      knee A18.02
      sacrum A18.01
      specified site NEC A18.03
      spinal A18.01
      vertebra A18.01
    brain A17.81
    breast A18.89
    Cowper's gland A18.15
    dura (mater) (cerebral) (spinal) A17.81
    epidural (cerebral) (spinal) A17.81
    female pelvis A18.17
    frontal sinus A15.8
    genital organs NEC A18.10
    genitourinary A18.10
    gland (lymphatic) — *see* Tuberculosis, lymph gland
    hip A18.02
    intestine A18.32
    ischiorectal A18.32
    joint NEC A18.02
      hip A18.02
      knee A18.02
      specified NEC A18.02
      vertebral A18.01
    kidney A18.11
    knee A18.02
    latent R76.11
    lumbar (spine) A18.01
    lung — *see* Tuberculosis, pulmonary
    meninges (cerebral) (spinal) A17.0
    muscle A18.09
    perianal (fistula) A18.32
    perinephritic A18.11
    perirectal A18.32
    rectum A18.32
    retropharyngeal A15.8
    sacrum A18.01
    scrofulous A18.2
    scrotum A18.15
    skin (primary) A18.4
    spinal cord A17.81
    spine or vertebra (column) A18.01
    subdiaphragmatic A18.31
    testis A18.15
    urinary A18.13
    uterus A18.17
  accessory sinus — *see* Tuberculosis, sinus
  Addison's disease A18.7

Tuberculosis, tubercular, tuberculous — *continued*
  adenitis — *see* Tuberculosis, lymph gland
  adenoids A15.8
  adenopathy — *see* Tuberculosis, lymph gland
  adherent pericardium A18.84
  adnexa (uteri) A18.17
  adrenal (capsule) (gland) A18.7
  alimentary canal A18.32
  anemia A18.89
  ankle (joint) (bone) A18.02
  anus A18.32
  apex, apical — *see* Tuberculosis, pulmonary
  appendicitis, appendix A18.32
  arachnoid A17.0
  artery, arteritis A18.89
    cerebral A18.89
  arthritis (chronic) (synovial) A18.02
    spine or vertebra (column) A18.01
  articular — *see* Tuberculosis, joint
  ascites A18.31
  asthma — *see* Tuberculosis, pulmonary
  axilla, axillary (gland) A18.2
  bladder A18.12
  bone A18.03
    hip A18.02
    knee A18.02
    limb NEC A18.03
    sacrum A18.01
    spine or vertebral column A18.01
  bowel (miliary) A18.32
  brain A17.81
  breast A18.89
  broad ligament A18.17
  bronchi, bronchial, bronchus A15.5
    ectasia, ectasis (bronchiectasis) — *see* Tuberculosis, pulmonary
    fistula A15.5
      primary (progressive) A15.7
    gland or node A15.4
      primary (progressive) A15.7
    lymph gland or node A15.4
      primary (progressive) A15.7
  bronchiectasis — *see* Tuberculosis, pulmonary
  bronchitis A15.5
  bronchopleural A15.6
  bronchopneumonia, bronchopneumonic — *see* Tuberculosis, pulmonary
  bronchorrhagia A15.5
  bronchotracheal A15.5
  bronze disease A18.7
  buccal cavity A18.83
  bulbourethral gland A18.15
  bursa A18.09
  cachexia A15.9
  cardiomyopathy A18.84
  caries — *see* Tuberculosis, bone
  cartilage A18.02
    intervertebral A18.01
  catarrhal — *see* Tuberculosis, respiratory
  cecum A18.32
  cellulitis (primary) A18.4
  cerebellum A17.81
  cerebral, cerebrum A17.81
  cerebrospinal A17.81
    meninges A17.0
  cervical (lymph gland or node) A18.2
  cervicitis, cervix (uteri) A18.16
  chest — *see* Tuberculosis, respiratory
  chorioretinitis A18.53
  choroid, choroiditis A18.53
  ciliary body A18.54
  colitis A18.32
  collier's J65
  colliquativa (primary) A18.4
  colon A18.32
  complex, primary A15.7
  congenital P37.0
  conjunctiva A18.59
  connective tissue (systemic) A18.89
  contact Z20.1
  cornea (ulcer) A18.52
  Cowper's gland A18.15
  coxae A18.02
  coxalgia A18.02
  cul-de-sac of Douglas A18.17
  curvature, spine A18.01
  cutis (colliquativa) (primary) A18.4
  cyst, ovary A18.18

☑ **Additional Character Required** — Refer to the Tabular List for Character Selection   ▽ **Subterms under main terms may continue to next column or page**

Tuberculosis, tubercular, tuberculous — *continued*
- cystitis A18.12
- dactylitis A18.03
- diarrhea A18.32
- diffuse — *see* Tuberculosis, miliary
- digestive tract A18.32
- disseminated — *see* Tuberculosis, miliary
- duodenum A18.32
- dura (mater) (cerebral) (spinal) A17.0
  - abscess (cerebral) (spinal) A17.81
- dysentery A18.32
- ear (inner) (middle) A18.6
  - bone A18.03
  - external (primary) A18.4
  - skin (primary) A18.4
- elbow A18.02
- emphysema — *see* Tuberculosis, pulmonary
- empyema A15.6
- encephalitis A17.82
- endarteritis A18.89
- endocarditis A18.84
  - aortic A18.84
  - mitral A18.84
  - pulmonary A18.84
  - tricuspid A18.84
- endocrine glands NEC A18.82
- endometrium A18.17
- enteric, enterica, enteritis A18.32
- enterocolitis A18.32
- epididymis, epididymitis A18.15
- epidural abscess (cerebral) (spinal) A17.81
- epiglottis A15.5
- episcleritis A18.51
- erythema (induratum) (nodosum) (primary) A18.4
- esophagus A18.83
- eustachian tube A18.6
- exposure (to) Z20.1
- exudative — *see* Tuberculosis, pulmonary
- eye A18.50
- eyelid (primary) (lupus) A18.4
- fallopian tube (acute) (chronic) A18.17
- fascia A18.09
- fauces A15.8
- female pelvic inflammatory disease A18.17
- finger A18.03
- first infection A15.7
- gallbladder A18.83
- ganglion A18.09
- gastritis A18.83
- gastrocolic fistula A18.32
- gastroenteritis A18.32
- gastrointestinal tract A18.32
- general, generalized — *see* Tuberculosis, miliary
- genital organs A18.10
- genitourinary A18.10
- genu A18.02
- glandula suprarenalis A18.7
- glandular, general A18.2
- glottis A15.5
- grinder's J65
- gum A18.83
- hand A18.03
- heart A18.84
- hematogenous — *see* Tuberculosis, miliary
- hemoptysis — *see* Tuberculosis, pulmonary
- hemorrhage NEC — *see* Tuberculosis, pulmonary
- hemothorax A15.6
- hepatitis A18.83
- hilar lymph nodes A15.4
  - primary (progressive) A15.7
- hip (joint) (disease) (bone) A18.02
- hydropneumothorax A15.6
- hydrothorax A15.6
- hypoadrenalism A18.7
- hypopharynx A15.8
- ileocecal (hyperplastic) A18.32
- ileocolitis A18.32
- ileum A18.32
- iliac spine (superior) A18.03
- immunological findings only A15.7
- indurativa (primary) A18.4
- infantile A15.7
- infection A15.9
  - without clinical manifestations A15.7
- infraclavicular gland A18.2
- inguinal gland A18.2
- inguinalis A18.2
- intestine (any part) A18.32

Tuberculosis, tubercular, tuberculous — *continued*
- iridocyclitis A18.54
- iris, iritis A18.54
- ischiorectal A18.32
- jaw A18.03
- jejunum A18.32
- joint A18.02
  - vertebral A18.01
- keratitis (interstitial) A18.52
- keratoconjunctivitis A18.52
- kidney A18.11
- knee (joint) A18.02
- kyphosis, kyphoscoliosis A18.01
- laryngitis A15.5
- larynx A15.5
- latent R76.11
- leptomeninges, leptomeningitis (cerebral) (spinal) A17.0
- lichenoides (primary) A18.4
- linguae A18.83
- lip A18.83
- liver A18.83
- lordosis A18.01
- lung — *see* Tuberculosis, pulmonary
- lupus vulgaris A18.4
- lymph gland or node (peripheral) A18.2
  - abdomen A18.39
  - bronchial A15.4
    - primary (progressive) A15.7
  - cervical A18.2
  - hilar A15.4
    - primary (progressive) A15.7
  - intrathoracic A15.4
    - primary (progressive) A15.7
  - mediastinal A15.4
    - primary (progressive) A15.7
  - mesenteric A18.39
  - retroperitoneal A18.39
  - tracheobronchial A15.4
    - primary (progressive) A15.7
- lymphadenitis — *see* Tuberculosis, lymph gland
- lymphangitis — *see* Tuberculosis, lymph gland
- lymphatic (gland) (vessel) — *see* Tuberculosis, lymph gland
- mammary gland A18.89
- marasmus A15.9
- mastoiditis A18.03
- mediastinal lymph gland or node A15.4
  - primary (progressive) A15.7
- mediastinitis A15.8
  - primary (progressive) A15.7
- mediastinum A15.8
  - primary (progressive) A15.7
- medulla A17.81
- melanosis, Addisonian A18.7
- meninges, meningitis (basilar) (cerebral) (cerebrospinal) (spinal) A17.0
- meningoencephalitis A17.82
- mesentery, mesenteric (gland or node) A18.39
- miliary A19.9
  - acute A19.2
    - multiple sites A19.1
    - single specified site A19.0
  - chronic A19.8
  - specified NEC A19.8
- millstone makers' J65
- miner's J65
- molder's J65
- mouth A18.83
- multiple A19.9
  - acute A19.1
  - chronic A19.8
- muscle A18.09
- myelitis A17.82
- myocardium, myocarditis A18.84
- nasal (passage) (sinus) A15.8
- nasopharynx A15.8
- neck gland A18.2
- nephritis A18.11
- nerve (mononeuropathy) A17.83
- nervous system A17.9
- nose (septum) A15.8
- ocular A18.50
- omentum A18.31
- oophoritis (acute) (chronic) A18.17
- optic (nerve trunk) (papilla) A18.59
- orbit A18.59
- orchitis A18.15
- organ, specified NEC A18.89

Tuberculosis, tubercular, tuberculous — *continued*
- osseous — *see* Tuberculosis, bone
- osteitis — *see* Tuberculosis, bone
- osteomyelitis — *see* Tuberculosis, bone
- otitis media A18.6
- ovary, ovaritis (acute) (chronic) A18.17
- oviduct (acute) (chronic) A18.17
- pachymeningitis A17.0
- palate (soft) A18.83
- pancreas A18.83
- papulonecrotic (a) (primary) A18.4
- parathyroid glands A18.82
- paronychia (primary) A18.4
- parotid gland or region A18.83
- pelvis (bony) A18.03
- penis A18.15
- peribronchitis A15.5
- pericardium, pericarditis A18.84
- perichondritis, larynx A15.5
- periostitis — *see* Tuberculosis, bone
- perirectal fistula A18.32
- peritoneum NEC A18.31
- peritonitis A18.31
- pharynx, pharyngitis A15.8
- phlyctenulosis (keratoconjunctivitis) A18.52
- phthisis NEC — *see* Tuberculosis, pulmonary
- pituitary gland A18.82
- pleura, pleural, pleurisy, pleuritis (fibrinous) (obliterative) (purulent) (simple plastic) (with effusion) A15.6
  - primary (progressive) A15.7
- pneumonia, pneumonic — *see* Tuberculosis, pulmonary
- pneumothorax (spontaneous) (tense valvular) — *see* Tuberculosis, pulmonary
- polyneuropathy A17.89
- polyserositis A19.9
  - acute A19.1
  - chronic A19.8
- potter's J65
- prepuce A18.15
- primary (complex) A15.7
- proctitis A18.32
- prostate, prostatitis A18.14
- pulmonalis — *see* Tuberculosis, pulmonary
- pulmonary (cavitated) (fibrotic) (infiltrative) (nodular) A15.0
  - childhood type or first infection A15.7
  - primary (complex) A15.7
- pyelitis A18.11
- pyelonephritis A18.11
- pyemia — *see* Tuberculosis, miliary
- pyonephrosis A18.11
- pyopneumothorax A15.6
- pyothorax A15.6
- rectum (fistula) (with abscess) A18.32
- reinfection stage — *see* Tuberculosis, pulmonary
- renal A18.11
- renis A18.11
- respiratory A15.9
  - primary A15.7
  - specified site NEC A15.8
- retina, retinitis A18.53
- retroperitoneal (lymph gland or node) A18.39
- rheumatism NEC A18.09
- rhinitis A15.8
- sacroiliac (joint) A18.01
- sacrum A18.01
- salivary gland A18.83
- salpingitis (acute) (chronic) A18.17
- sandblaster's J65
- sclera A18.51
- scoliosis A18.01
- scrofulous A18.2
- scrotum A18.15
- seminal tract or vesicle A18.15
- senile A15.9
- septic — *see* Tuberculosis, miliary
- shoulder (joint) A18.02
  - blade A18.03
- sigmoid A18.32
- sinus (any nasal) A15.8
  - bone A18.03
  - epididymis A18.15
- skeletal NEC A18.03
- skin (any site) (primary) A18.4
- small intestine A18.32
- soft palate A18.83

Tuberculosis, tubercular, tuberculous — continued
- spermatic cord A18.15
- spine, spinal (column) A18.01
  - cord A17.81
  - medulla A17.81
  - membrane A17.0
  - meninges A17.0
- spleen, splenitis A18.85
- spondylitis A18.01
- sternoclavicular joint A18.02
- stomach A18.83
- stonemason's J65
- subcutaneous tissue (cellular) (primary) A18.4
- subcutis (primary) A18.4
- subdeltoid bursa A18.83
- submaxillary (region) A18.83
- supraclavicular gland A18.2
- suprarenal (capsule) (gland) A18.7
- swelling, joint (see also category M01) (see also Tuberculosis, joint) A18.02
- symphysis pubis A18.02
- synovitis A18.09
  - articular A18.02
  - spine or vertebra A18.01
- systemic — see Tuberculosis, miliary
- tarsitis A18.4
- tendon (sheath) — see Tuberculosis, tenosynovitis
- tenosynovitis A18.09
  - spine or vertebra A18.01
- testis A18.15
- throat A15.8
- thymus gland A18.82
- thyroid gland A18.81
- tongue A18.83
- tonsil, tonsillitis A15.8
- trachea, tracheal A15.5
  - lymph gland or node A15.4
    - primary (progressive) A15.7
- tracheobronchial A15.5
  - lymph gland or node A15.4
    - primary (progressive) A15.7
- tubal (acute) (chronic) A18.17
- tunica vaginalis A18.15
- ulcer (skin) (primary) A18.4
  - bowel or intestine A18.32
  - specified NEC — see Tuberculosis, by site
- unspecified site A15.9
- ureter A18.11
- urethra, urethral (gland) A18.13
- urinary organ or tract A18.13
- uterus A18.17
- uveal tract A18.54
- uvula A18.83
- vagina A18.18
- vas deferens A18.15
- verruca, verrucosa (cutis) (primary) A18.4
- vertebra (column) A18.01
- vesiculitis A18.15
- vulva A18.18
- wrist (joint) A18.02

Tuberculum
- Carabelli — see Excludes Note at K00.2
- occlusal — see Excludes Note at K00.2
- paramolare K00.2

Tuberosity, enitre maxillary M26.07

Tuberous sclerosis (brain) Q85.1

Tubo-ovarian — see condition

Tuboplasty, after previous sterilization Z31.0
- aftercare Z31.42

Tubotympanitis, catarrhal (chronic) — see Otitis, media, nonsuppurative, chronic, serous

Tularemia A21.9
- with
  - conjunctivitis A21.1
  - pneumonia A21.2
- abdominal A21.3
- bronchopneumonic A21.2
- conjunctivitis A21.1
- cryptogenic A21.3
- enteric A21.3
- gastrointestinal A21.3
- generalized A21.7
- ingestion A21.3
- intestinal A21.3
- oculoglandular A21.1
- ophthalmic A21.1
- pneumonia (any), pneumonic A21.2
- pulmonary A21.2

Tularemia — continued
- sepsis A21.7
- specified NEC A21.8
- typhoidal A21.7
- ulceroglandular A21.0

Tularensis conjunctivitis A21.1

Tumefaction (see also Swelling)
- liver — see Hypertrophy, liver

Tumor (see also Neoplasm, unspecified behavior, by site)
- acinar cell — see Neoplasm, uncertain behavior, by site
- acinic cell — see Neoplasm, uncertain behavior, by site
- adenocarcinoid — see Neoplasm, malignant, by site
- adenomatoid (see also Neoplasm, benign, by site)
  - odontogenic — see Cyst, calcifying odontogenic
- adnexal (skin) — see Neoplasm, skin, benign, by site
- adrenal
  - cortical (benign) D35.0- ☑
    - malignant C74.0- ☑
  - rest — see Neoplasm, benign, by site
- alpha-cell
  - malignant
    - pancreas C25.4
    - specified site NEC — see Neoplasm, malignant, by site
    - unspecified site C25.4
  - pancreas D13.7
  - specified site NEC — see Neoplasm, benign, by slte
  - unspecified site D13.7
- aneurysmal — see Aneurysm
- aortic body D44.7
  - malignant C75.5
- Askin's — see Neoplasm, connective tissue, malignant
- basal cell (see also Neoplasm, skin, uncertain behavior) D48.5
- Bednar — see Neoplasm, skin, malignant
- benign (unclassified) — see Neoplasm, benign, by site
- beta-cell
  - malignant
    - pancreas C25.4
    - specified site NEC — see Neoplasm, malignant, by site
    - unspecified site C25.4
  - pancreas D13.7
  - specified site NEC — see Neoplasm, benign, by site
  - unspecified site D13.7
- Brenner D27.9
  - borderline malignancy D39.1- ☑
  - malignant C56- ☑
  - proliferating D39.1- ☑
- bronchial alveolar, intravascular D38.1
- Brooke's — see Neoplasm, skin, benign
- brown fat — see Lipoma
- Burkitt — see Lymphoma, Burkitt
- calcifying epithelial odontogenic — see Cyst, calcifying odontogenic
- carcinoid
  - benign D3A.00 (following D36)
    - appendix D3A.020 (following D36)
    - ascending colon D3A.022 (following D36)
    - bronchus (lung) D3A.090 (following D36)
    - cecum D3A.021 (following D36)
    - colon D3A.029 (following D36)
    - descending colon D3A.024 (following D36)
    - duodenum D3A.010 (following D36)
    - foregut NOS D3A.094 (following D36)
    - hindgut NOS D3A.096 (following D36)
    - ileum D3A.012 (following D36)
    - jejunum D3A.011 (following D36)
    - kidney D3A.093 (following D36)
    - large intestine D3A.029 (following D36)
    - lung (bronchus) D3A.090 (following D36)
    - midgut NOS D3A.095 (following D36)
    - rectum D3A.026 (following D36)
    - sigmoid colon D3A.025 (following D36)
    - small intestine D3A.019 (following D36)
    - specified NEC D3A.098 (following D36)
    - stomach D3A.092 (following D36)
    - thymus D3A.091 (following D36)
    - transverse colon D3A.023 (following D36)
  - malignant C7A.00 (following C75)
    - appendix C7A.020 (following C75)
    - ascending colon C7A.022 (following C75)
    - bronchus (lung) C7A.090 (following C75)
    - cecum C7A.021 (following C75)
    - colon C7A.029 (following C75)
    - descending colon C7A.024 (following C75)

Tumor — continued
- carcinoid — continued
  - malignant — continued
    - duodenum C7A.010 (following C75)
    - foregut NOS C7A.094 (following C75)
    - hindgut NOS C7A.096 (following C75)
    - ileum C7A.012 (following C75)
    - jejunum C7A.011 (following C75)
    - kidney C7A.093 (following C75)
    - large intestine C7A.029 (following C75)
    - lung (bronchus) C7A.090 (following C75)
    - midgut NOS C7A.095 (following C75)
    - rectum C7A.026 (following C75)
    - sigmoid colon C7A.025 (following C75)
    - small intestine C7A.019 (following C75)
    - specified NEC C7A.098 (following C75)
    - stomach C7A.092 (following C75)
    - thymus C7A.091 (following C75)
    - transverse colon C7A.023 (following C75)
  - mesentary metastasis C7B.04 (following C75)
  - secondary C7B.00 (following C75)
    - bone C7B.03 (following C75)
    - distant lymph nodes C7B.01 (following C75)
    - liver C7B.02 (following C75)
    - peritoneum C7B.04 (following C75)
    - specified NEC C7B.09 (following C75)
- carotid body D44.6
  - malignant C75.4
- cells (see also Neoplasm, unspecified behavior, by site)
  - benign — see Neoplasm, benign, by site
  - malignant — see Neoplasm, malignant, by site
  - uncertain whether benign or malignant — see Neoplasm, uncertain behavior, by site
- cervix, in pregnancy or childbirth — see Pregnancy, complicated by, tumor, cervix
- chondromatous giant cell — see Neoplasm, bone, benign
- chromaffin (see also Neoplasm, benign, by site)
  - malignant — see Neoplasm, malignant, by site
- Cock's peculiar L72.3
- Codman's — see Neoplasm, bone, benign
- dentigerous, mixed — see Cyst, calcifying odontogenic
- dermoid — see Neoplasm, benign, by site
  - with malignant transformatlon C56- ☑
- desmoid (extra-abdominal) (see also Neoplasm, connective tissue, uncertain behavior)
  - abdominal — see Neoplasm, connective tissue, uncertain behavior
- embolus — see Neoplasm, secondary, by site
- embryonal (mixed) (see also Neoplasm, uncertain behavior, by site)
  - liver C22.7
- endodermal sinus
  - specified site — see Neoplasm, malignant, by site
  - unspecified site
    - female C56.- ☑
    - male C62.90
- epithelial
  - benign — see Neoplasm, benign, by site
  - malignant — see Neoplasm, malignant, by site
- Ewing's — see Neoplasm, bone, malignant, by site
- fatty — see Lipoma
- fibroid — see Leiomyoma
- G cell
  - malignant
    - pancreas C25.4
    - specified site NEC — see Neoplasm, malignant, by site
    - unspecified site C25.4
  - specified site — see Neoplasm, uncertain behavior, by site
  - unspecified site D37.8
- germ cell (see also Neoplasm, malignant, by site)
  - mixed — see Neoplasm, malignant, by site
- ghost cell, odontogenic — see Cyst, calcifying odontogenic
- giant cell (see also Neoplasm, uncertain behavior, by site)
  - bone D48.0
    - malignant — see Neoplasm, bone, malignant
    - chondromatous — see Neoplasm, bone, benign
    - malignant — see Neoplasm, malignant, by site
  - soft parts — see Neoplasm, connective tissue, uncertain behavior
    - malignant — see Neoplasm, connective tissue, malignant
- glomus D18.00
  - intra-abdominal D18.03

Tumor — *continued*
- glomus — *continued*
  - intracranial D18.Ø2
  - jugulare D44.7
    - malignant C75.5
  - skin D18.Ø1
  - specified site NEC D18.Ø9
- gonadal stromal — *see* Neoplasm, uncertain behavior, by site
- granular cell (*see also* Neoplasm, connective tissue, benign)
  - malignant — *see* Neoplasm, connective tissue, malignant
- granulosa cell D39.1- ☑
  - juvenile D39.1-
  - malignant C56- ☑
- granulosa cell-theca cell D39.1- ☑
  - malignant C56- ☑
- Grawitz's C64- ☑
- hemorrhoidal — *see* Hemorrhoids
- hilar cell D27- ☑
- hilus cell D27- ☑
- Hurthle cell (benign) D34
  - malignant C73
- hydatid — *see* Echinococcus
- hypernephroid (*see also* Neoplasm, uncertain behavior, by site)
- interstitial cell (*see also* Neoplasm, uncertain behavior, by site)
  - benign — *see* Neoplasm, benign, by site
  - malignant — *see* Neoplasm, malignant, by site
- intravascular bronchial alveolar D38.1
- islet cell — *see* Neoplasm, benign, by site
  - malignant — *see* Neoplasm, malignant, by site
    - pancreas C25.4
    - specified site NEC — *see* Neoplasm, malignant, by site
    - unspecified site C25.4
  - pancreas D13.7
  - specified site NEC — *see* Neoplasm, benign, by site
  - unspecified site D13.7
- juxtaglomerular D41.Ø- ☑
- Klatskin's C22.1
- Krukenberg's C79.6- ☑
- Leydig cell — *see* Neoplasm, uncertain behavior, by site
  - benign — *see* Neoplasm, benign, by site
    - specified site — *see* Neoplasm, benign, by site
    - unspecified site
      - female D27.9
      - male D29.2Ø
  - malignant — *see* Neoplasm, malignant, by site
    - specified site — *see* Neoplasm, malignant, by site
    - unspecified site
      - female C56.9
      - male C62.9Ø
  - specified site — *see* Neoplasm, uncertain behavior, by site
  - unspecified site
    - female D39.1Ø
    - male D4Ø.1Ø
- lipid cell, ovary D27- ☑
- lipoid cell, ovary D27- ☑
- malignant (*see also* Neoplasm, malignant, by site) C8Ø.1
  - fusiform cell (type) C8Ø.1
  - giant cell (type) C8Ø.1
  - localized, plasma cell — *see* Plasmacytoma, solitary
  - mixed NEC C8Ø.1
  - small cell (type) C8Ø.1
  - spindle cell (type) C8Ø.1
  - unclassified C8Ø.1
- mast cell D47.Ø9
- melanotic, neuroectodermal — *see* Neoplasm, benign, by site
- Merkel cell — *see* Carcinoma, Merkel cell
- mesenchymal
  - malignant — *see* Neoplasm, connective tissue, malignant
  - mixed — *see* Neoplasm, connective tissue, uncertain behavior
- mesodermal, mixed (*see also* Neoplasm, malignant, by site)
  - liver C22.4

Tumor — *continued*
- mesonephric (*see also* Neoplasm, uncertain behavior, by site)
  - malignant — *see* Neoplasm, malignant, by site
- metastatic
  - from specified site — *see* Neoplasm, malignant, by site
  - of specified site — *see* Neoplasm, malignant, by site
  - to specified site — *see* Neoplasm, secondary, by site
- mixed NEC (*see also* Neoplasm, benign, by site)
  - malignant — *see* Neoplasm, malignant, by site
- mucinous of low malignant potential
  - specified site — *see* Neoplasm, malignant, by site
  - unspecified site C56.9
- mucocarcinoid
  - specified site — *see* Neoplasm, malignant, by site
  - unspecified site C18.1
- mucoepidermoid — *see* Neoplasm, uncertain behavior, by site
- Müllerian, mixed
  - specified site — *see* Neoplasm, malignant, by site
  - unspecified site C54.9
- myoepithelial — *see* Neoplasm, benign, by site
- neuroectodermal (peripheral) — *see* Neoplasm, malignant, by site
  - primitive
    - specified site — *see* Neoplasm, malignant, by site
    - unspecified site C71.9
- neuroendocrine D3A.8 (*following* D36)
  - malignant poorly differentiated C7A.1 (*following* C75)
  - secondary NEC C7B.8 (*following* C75)
  - specified NEC C7A.8 (*following* C75)
- neurogenic olfactory C3Ø.Ø
- nonencapsulated sclerosing C73
- odontogenic (adenomatoid) (benign) (calcifying epithelial) (keratocystic) (squamous) — *see* Cyst, calcifying odontogenic
  - malignant C41.1
    - upper jaw (bone) C41.Ø
- ovarian stromal D39.1- ☑
- ovary, in pregnancy — *see* Pregnancy, complicated by
- pacinian — *see* Neoplasm, skin, benign
- Pancoast's — *see* Pancoast's syndrome
- papillary (*see also* Papilloma)
  - cystic D37.9
  - mucinous of low malignant potential C56- ☑
    - specified site — *see* Neoplasm, malignant, by site
    - unspecified site C56.9
  - serous of low malignant potential
    - specified site — *see* Neoplasm, malignant, by site
    - unspecified site C56.9
- pelvic, in pregnancy or childbirth — *see* Pregnancy, complicated by
- phantom F45.8
- phyllodes D48.6- ☑
  - benign D24- ☑
  - malignant — *see* Neoplasm, breast, malignant
- Pindborg — *see* Cyst, calcifying odontogenic
- placental site trophoblastic D39.2
- plasma cell (malignant) (localized) — *see* Plasmacytoma, solitary
- polyvesicular vitelline
  - specified site — *see* Neoplasm, malignant, by site
  - unspecified site
    - female C56.9
    - male C62.9Ø
- Pott's puffy — *see* Osteomyelitis, specified NEC
- Rathke's pouch D44.3
- retinal anlage — *see* Neoplasm, benign, by site
- salivary gland type, mixed — *see* Neoplasm, salivary gland, benign
  - malignant — *see* Neoplasm, salivary gland, malignant
- Sampson's N8Ø.1
- Schmincke's — *see* Neoplasm, nasopharynx, malignant
- sclerosing stromal D27- ☑
- sebaceous — *see* Cyst, sebaceous
- secondary — *see* Neoplasm, secondary, by site
  - carcinoid C7B.ØØ (*following* C75)
    - bone C7B.Ø3 (*following* C75)
    - distant lymph nodes C7B.Ø1 (*following* C75)

Tumor — *continued*
- secondary — *see* Neoplasm, secondary, by site — *continued*
  - carcinoid — *continued*
    - liver C7B.Ø2 (*following* C75)
    - peritoneum C7B.Ø4 (*following* C75)
    - specified NEC C7B.Ø9 (*following* C75)
  - neuroendocrine NEC C7B.8 (*following* C75)
- serous of low malignant potential
  - specified site — *see* Neoplasm, malignant, by site
  - unspecified site C56.9
- Sertoli cell — *see* Neoplasm, benign, by site
  - with lipid storage
    - specified site — *see* Neoplasm, benign, by site
    - unspecified site
      - female D27.9
      - male D29.2Ø
  - specified site — *see* Neoplasm, benign, by site
  - unspecified site
    - female D27.9
    - male D29.2Ø
- Sertoli-Leydig cell — *see* Neoplasm, benign, by site
  - specified site — *see* Neoplasm, benign, by site
  - unspecified site
    - female D27.9
    - male D29.2Ø
- sex cord (-stromal) — *see* Neoplasm, uncertain behavior, by site
  - with annular tubules D39.1- ☑
- skin appendage — *see* Neoplasm, skin, benign
- smooth muscle — *see* Neoplasm, connective tissue, uncertain behavior
- soft tissue
  - benign — *see* Neoplasm, connective tissue, benign
  - malignant — *see* Neoplasm, connective tissue, malignant
- sternomastoid (congenital) Q68.Ø
- stromal
  - endometrial D39.Ø
  - gastric D48.1
    - benign D21.4
    - malignant C16.9
    - uncertain behavior D48.1
  - gastrointestinal C49.A- ☑
    - benign D21.4
    - esophagus C49.A1
    - malignant C49.AØ
      - colon C49.A4
      - duodenum C49.A3
      - esophagus C49.A1
      - ileum C49.A3
      - jejunum C49.A3
      - large intestine C49.A4
      - Meckel diverticulum C49.A3
      - omentum C49.A9
      - peritoneum C49.A9
      - rectum C49.A5
      - small intestine C49.A3
      - specified site NEC C49.A9
      - stomach C49.A2
    - rectum C49.A5
    - small intestine C49.A3
    - specified site NEC C49.A9
    - stomach C49.A2
    - uncertain behavior D48.1
  - intestine
    - benign D21.4
    - malignant
      - large C49.A4
      - small C49.A3
    - uncertain behavior D48.1
  - ovarian D39.1- ☑
  - stomach C49.A2
    - benign D21.4
    - malignant C49.A2
    - uncertain behavior D48.1
- sweat gland (*see also* Neoplasm, skin, uncertain behavior)
  - benign — *see* Neoplasm, skin, benign
  - malignant — *see* Neoplasm, skin, malignant
- syphilitic, brain A52.17
- testicular D4Ø.1Ø
- testicular stromal D4Ø.1- ☑
- theca cell D27.- ☑
- theca cell-granulosa cell D39.1- ☑
- Triton, malignant — *see* Neoplasm, nerve, malignant
- trophoblastic, placental site D39.2
- turban D23.4

Tumor — *continued*
 uterus (body), in pregnancy or childbirth — *see* Pregnancy, complicated by, tumor, uterus
 vagina, in pregnancy or childbirth — *see* Pregnancy, complicated by
 varicose — *see* Varix
 von Recklinghausen's — *see* Neurofibromatosis
 vulva or perineum, in pregnancy or childbirth — *see* Pregnancy, complicated by
  causing obstructed labor O65.5
 Warthin's — *see* Neoplasm, salivary gland, benign
 Wilms' C64- ☑
 yolk sac — *see* Neoplasm, malignant, by site
  specified site — *see* Neoplasm, malignant, by site
  unspecified site
   female C56.9
   male C62.90
Tumor lysis syndrome (following antineoplastic chemotherapy) (spontaneous) NEC E88.3
Tumorlet — *see* Neoplasm, uncertain behavior, by site
Tungiasis B88.1
Tunica vasculosa lentis Q12.2
Turban tumor D23.4
Türck's trachoma J37.0
Turner-Kieser syndrome Q87.2
Turner-like syndrome Q87.1
Turner's
 hypoplasia (tooth) K00.4
 syndrome Q96.9
  specified NEC Q96.8
 tooth K00.4
Turner-Ullrich syndrome Q96.9
Tussis convulsiva — *see* Whooping cough
Twiddler's syndrome (due to)
 automatic implantable defibrillator T82.198
 cardiac pacemaker T82.198 ☑
Twilight state
 epileptic F05
 psychogenic F44.89
Twin (newborn) (*see also* Newborn, twin)
 conjoined Q89.4
 pregnancy — *see* Pregnancy, twin
Twinning, teeth K00.2
Twist, twisted
 bowel, colon or intestine K56.2
 hair (congenital) Q84.1
 mesentery K56.2
 omentum K56.2
 organ or site, congenital NEC — *see* Anomaly, by site
 ovarian pedicle — *see* Torsion, ovary
Twitching R25.3
Tylosis (acquired) L84
 buccalis K13.29
 linguae K13.29
 palmaris et plantaris (congenital) (inherited) Q82.8
  acquired L85.1
Tympanism R14.0
Tympanites (abdominal) (intestinal) R14.0
Tympanitis — *see* Myringitis
Tympanosclerosis H74.0 ☑
Tympanum — *see* condition
Tympany
 abdomen R14.0
 chest R09.89
Type A behavior pattern Z73.1
Typhlitis — *see* Appendicitis
Typhoenteritis — *see* Typhoid
Typhoid (abortive) (ambulant) (any site) (clinical) (fever) (hemorrhagic) (infection) (intermittent) (malignant) (rheumatic) (Widal negative) A01.00
 with pneumonia A01.03
 abdominal A01.09
 arthritis A01.04
 carrier (suspected) of Z22.0
 cholecystitis (current) A01.09
 endocarditis A01.02
 heart involvement A01.02
 inoculation reaction — *see* Complications, vaccination
 meningitis A01.01
 mesenteric lymph nodes A01.09
 myocarditis A01.02
 osteomyelitis A01.05
 perichondritis, larynx A01.09
 pneumonia A01.03
 specified NEC A01.09
 spine A01.05
 ulcer (perforating) A01.09

Typhomalaria (fever) — *see* Malaria
Typhomania A01.00
Typhoperitonitis A01.09
Typhus (fever) A75.9
 abdominal, abdominalis — *see* Typhoid
 African tick A77.1
 amarillic A95.9
 brain A75.9 [G94]
 cerebral A75.9 [G94]
 classical A75.0
 due to Rickettsia
  prowazekii A75.0
   recrudescent A75.1
  tsutsugamushi A75.3
  typhi A75.2
 endemic (flea-borne) A75.2
 epidemic (louse-borne) A75.0
 exanthematicus SAI A75.0
  brillii SAI A75.1
  mexicanus SAI A75.2
  typhus murinus A75.2
 exanthematic NEC A75.0
 flea-borne A75.2
 India tick A77.1
 Kenya (tick) A77.1
 louse-borne A75.0
 Mexican A75.2
 mite-borne A75.3
 murine A75.2
 North Asian tick-borne A77.2
 petechial A75.9
 Queensland tick A77.3
 rat A75.2
 recrudescent A75.1
 recurrens — *see* Fever, relapsing
 Sao Paulo A77.0
 scrub (China) (India) (Malaysia) (New Guinea) A75.3
 shop (of Malaysia) A75.2
 Siberian tick A77.2
 tick-borne A77.9
 tropical (mite-borne) A75.3
Tyrosinemia E70.21
 newborn, transitory P74.5
Tyrosinosis E70.21
Tyrosinuria E70.29

U

Uhl's anomaly or disease Q24.8
Ulcer, ulcerated, ulcerating, ulceration, ulcerative
 alveolar process M27.3
 amebic (intestine) A06.1
  skin A06.7
 anastomotic — *see* Ulcer, gastrojejunal
 anorectal K62.6
 antral — *see* Ulcer, stomach
 anus (sphincter) (solitary) K62.6
 aorta — *see* Aneurysm
 aphthous (oral) (recurrent) K12.0
  genital organ(s)
   female N76.6
   male N50.89
 artery I77.2
 atrophic — *see* Ulcer, skin
  decubitus — *see* Ulcer, pressure, by site
 back L98.429
  with
   bone involvement without evidence of necrosis L98.426
   bone necrosis L98.424
   exposed fat layer L98.422
   muscle involvement without evidence of necrosis L98.425
   muscle necrosis L98.423
   skin breakdown only L98.421
   specified severity NEC L98.428
 Barrett's (esophagus) K22.10
  with bleeding K22.11
 bile duct (common) (hepatic) K83.8
 bladder (solitary) (sphincter) NEC N32.89
  bilharzial B65.9 [N33]
  in schistosomiasis (bilharzial) B65.9 [N33]
  submucosal — *see* Cystitis, interstitial
  tuberculous A18.12
 bleeding K27.4
 bone — *see* Osteomyelitis, specified type NEC
 bowel — *see* Ulcer, intestine
 breast N61.1

Ulcer, ulcerated, ulcerating, ulceration, ulcerative
 — *continued*
 bronchus J98.09
 buccal (cavity) (traumatic) K12.1
 Buruli A31.1
 buttock L98.419
  with
   bone involvement without evidence of necrosis L98.416
   bone necrosis L98.414
   exposed fat layer L98.412
   muscle involvement without evidence of necrosis L98.415
   muscle necrosis L98.413
   skin breakdown only L98.411
   specified severity NEC L98.418
 cancerous — *see* Neoplasm, malignant, by site
 cardia K22.10
  with bleeding K22.11
 cardioesophageal (peptic) K22.10
  with bleeding K22.11
 cecum — *see* Ulcer, intestine
 cervix (uteri) (decubitus) (trophic) N86
  with cervicitis N72
 chancroidal A57
 chiclero B55.1
 chronic (cause unknown) — *see* Ulcer, skin
 Cochin-China B55.1
 colon — *see* Ulcer, intestine
 conjunctiva H10.89
 cornea H16.00- ☑
  with hypopyon H16.03- ☑
  central H16.01- ☑
  dendritic (herpes simplex) B00.52
  marginal H16.04- ☑
  Mooren's H16.05- ☑
  mycotic H16.06- ☑
  perforated H16.07- ☑
  ring H16.02- ☑
  tuberculous (phlyctenular) A18.52
 corpus cavernosum (chronic) N48.5
 crural — *see* Ulcer, lower limb
 Curling's — *see* Ulcer, peptic, acute
 Cushing's — *see* Ulcer, peptic, acute
 cystic duct K82.8
 cystitis (interstitial) — *see* Cystitis, interstitial
 decubitus — *see* Ulcer, pressure, by site
 dendritic, cornea (herpes simplex) B00.52
 diabetes, diabetic — *see* Diabetes, ulcer
 Dieulafoy's K25.0
 due to
  infection NEC — *see* Ulcer, skin
  radiation NEC L59.8
  trophic disturbance (any region) — *see* Ulcer, skin
  X-ray L58.1
 duodenum, duodenal (eroded) (peptic) K26.9
  with
   hemorrhage K26.4
    and perforation K26.6
   perforation K26.5
  acute K26.3
   with
    hemorrhage K26.0
     and perforation K26.2
    perforation K26.1
  chronic K26.7
   with
    hemorrhage K26.4
     and perforation K26.6
    perforation K26.5
 dysenteric A09
 elusive — *see* Cystitis, interstitial
 endocarditis (acute) (chronic) (subacute) I28.8
 epiglottis J38.7
 esophagus (peptic) K22.10
  with bleeding K22.11
  due to
   aspirin K22.10
    with bleeding K22.11
   gastrointestinal reflux disease K21.0
   ingestion of chemical or medicament K22.10
    with bleeding K22.11
  fungal K22.10
   with bleeding K22.11
  infective K22.10
   with bleeding K22.11
  varicose — *see* Varix, esophagus
 eyelid (region) H01.8

☑ **Additional Character Required** — **Refer to the Tabular List for Character Selection** ▽ **Subterms under main terms may continue to next column or page**

Ulcer, ulcerated, ulcerating, ulceration, ulcerative
— continued
- fauces J39.2
- Fenwick (-Hunner) (solitary) — see Cystitis, interstitial
- fistulous — see Ulcer, skin
- foot (indolent) (trophic) — see Ulcer, lower limb
- frambesial, initial A66.0
- frenum (tongue) K14.0
- gallbladder or duct K82.8
- gangrenous — see Gangrene
- gastric — see Ulcer, stomach
- gastrocolic — see Ulcer, gastrojejunal
- gastroduodenal — see Ulcer, peptic
- gastroesophageal — see Ulcer, stomach
- gastrointestinal — see Ulcer, gastrojejunal
- gastrojejunal (peptic) K28.9
  - with
    - hemorrhage K28.4
      - and perforation K28.6
    - perforation K28.5
  - acute K28.3
    - with
      - hemorrhage K28.0
        - and perforation K28.2
      - perforation K28.1
  - chronic K28.7
    - with
      - hemorrhage K28.4
        - and perforation K28.6
      - perforation K28.5
- gastrojejunocolic — see Ulcer, gastrojejunal
- gingiva K06.8
- gingivitis K05.10
  - nonplaque induced K05.11
  - plaque induced K05.10
- glottis J38.7
- granuloma of pudenda A58
- gum K06.8
- gumma, due to yaws A66.4
- heel — see Ulcer, lower limb
- hemorrhoid (see also Hemorrhoids, by degree) K64.8
- Hunner's — see Cystitis, interstitial
- hypopharynx J39.2
- hypopyon (chronic) (subacute) — see Ulcer, cornea, with hypopyon
- hypostaticum — see Ulcer, varicose
- ileum — see Ulcer, intestine
- intestine, intestinal K63.3
  - with perforation K63.1
  - amebic A06.1
  - duodenal — see Ulcer, duodenum
  - granulocytopenic (with hemorrhage) — see Neutropenia
  - marginal — see Ulcer, gastrojejunal
  - perforating K63.1
    - newborn P78.0
  - primary, small intestine K63.3
  - rectum K62.6
  - stercoraceous, stercoral K63.3
  - tuberculous A18.32
  - typhoid (fever) — see Typhoid
  - varicose I86.8
- jejunum, jejunal — see Ulcer, gastrojejunal
- keratitis — see Ulcer, cornea
- knee — see Ulcer, lower limb
- labium (majus) (minus) N76.6
- laryngitis — see Laryngitis
- larynx (aphthous) (contact) J38.7
  - diphtheritic A36.2
- leg — see Ulcer, lower limb
- lip K13.0
- Lipschütz's N76.6
- lower limb (atrophic) (chronic) (neurogenic) (perforating) (pyogenic) (trophic) (tropical) L97.909
  - with
    - bone involvement without evidence of necrosis L97.906
    - bone necrosis L97.904
    - exposed fat layer L97.902
    - muscle involvement without evidence of necrosis L97.905
    - muscle necrosis L97.903
    - skin breakdown only L97.901
    - specified severity NEC L97.908
  - ankle L97.309
    - with
      - bone involvement without evidence of necrosis L97.306

Ulcer, ulcerated, ulcerating, ulceration, ulcerative
— continued
- lower limb — continued
  - ankle — continued
    - with — continued
      - bone necrosis L97.304
      - exposed fat layer L97.302
      - muscle involvement without evidence of necrosis L97.305
      - muscle necrosis L97.303
      - skin breakdown only L97.301
      - specified severity NEC L97.308
    - left L97.329
      - with
        - bone involvement without evidence of necrosis L97.326
        - bone necrosis L97.324
        - exposed fat layer L97.322
        - muscle involvement without evidence of necrosis L97.325
        - muscle necrosis L97.323
        - skin breakdown only L97.321
        - specified severity NEC L97.328
    - right L97.319
      - with
        - bone involvement without evidence of necrosis L97.316
        - bone necrosis L97.314
        - exposed fat layer L97.312
        - muscle involvement without evidence of necrosis L97.315
        - muscle necrosis L97.313
        - skin breakdown only L97.311
        - specified severity NEC L97.318
  - calf L97.209
    - with
      - bone involvement without evidence of necrosis L97.206
      - bone necrosis L97.204
      - exposed fat layer L97.202
      - muscle involvement without evidence of necrosis L97.205
      - muscle necrosis L97.203
      - skin breakdown only L97.201
      - specified severity NEC L97.208
    - left L97.229
      - with
        - bone involvement without evidence of necrosis L97.226
        - bone necrosis L97.224
        - exposed fat layer L97.222
        - muscle involvement without evidence of necrosis L97.225
        - muscle necrosis L97.223
        - skin breakdown only L97.221
        - specified severity NEC L97.228
    - right L97.219
      - with
        - bone involvement without evidence of necrosis L97.216
        - bone necrosis L97.214
        - exposed fat layer L97.212
        - muscle involvement without evidence of necrosis L97.215
        - muscle necrosis L97.213
        - skin breakdown only L97.211
        - specified severity NEC L97.218
  - decubitus — see Ulcer, pressure, by site
  - foot specified NEC L97.509
    - with
      - bone involvement without evidence of necrosis L97.506
      - bone necrosis L97.504
      - exposed fat layer L97.502
      - muscle involvement without evidence of necrosis L97.505
      - muscle necrosis L97.503
      - skin breakdown only L97.501
      - specified severity NEC L97.508
    - left L97.529
      - with
        - bone involvement without evidence of necrosis L97.526
        - bone necrosis L97.524
        - exposed fat layer L97.522
        - muscle involvement without evidence of necrosis L97.525
        - muscle necrosis L97.523
        - skin breakdown only L97.521

Ulcer, ulcerated, ulcerating, ulceration, ulcerative
— continued
- lower limb — continued
  - foot specified — continued
    - left — continued
      - with — continued
        - specified severity NEC L97.528
    - right L97.519
      - with
        - bone involvement without evidence of necrosis L97.516
        - bone necrosis L97.514
        - exposed fat layer L97.512
        - muscle involvement without evidence of necrosis L97.515
        - muscle necrosis L97.513
        - skin breakdown only L97.511
        - specified severity NEC L97.518
  - heel L97.409
    - with
      - bone involvement without evidence of necrosis L97.406
      - bone necrosis L97.404
      - exposed fat layer L97.402
      - muscle involvement without evidence of necrosis L97.405
      - muscle necrosis L97.403
      - skin breakdown only L97.401
      - specified severity NEC L97.408
    - left L97.429
      - with
        - bone involvement without evidence of necrosis L97.426
        - bone necrosis L97.424
        - exposed fat layer L97.422
        - muscle involvement without evidence of necrosis L97.425
        - muscle necrosis L97.423
        - skin breakdown only L97.421
        - specified severity NEC L97.428
    - right L97.419
      - with
        - bone involvement without evidence of necrosis L97.416
        - bone necrosis L97.414
        - exposed fat layer L97.412
        - muscle involvement without evidence of necrosis L97.415
        - muscle necrosis L97.413
        - skin breakdown only L97.411
        - specified severity NEC L97.418
  - left L97.929
    - with
      - bone involvement without evidence of necrosis L97.926
      - bone necrosis L97.924
      - exposed fat layer L97.922
      - muscle involvement without evidence of necrosis L97.925
      - muscle necrosis L97.923
      - skin breakdown only L97.921
      - specified severity NEC L97.928
  - leprous A30.1
  - lower leg NOS L97.909
    - with
      - bone involvement without evidence of necrosis L97.906
      - bone necrosis L97.904
      - exposed fat layer L97.902
      - muscle involvement without evidence of necrosis L97.905
      - muscle necrosis L97.903
      - skin breakdown only L97.901
      - specified severity NEC L97.908
    - left L97.929
      - with
        - bone involvement without evidence of necrosis L97.926
        - bone necrosis L97.924
        - exposed fat layer L97.922
        - muscle involvement without evidence of necrosis L97.925
        - muscle necrosis L97.923
        - skin breakdown only L97.921
        - specified severity NEC L97.928
    - right L97.919
      - with
        - bone involvement without evidence of necrosis L97.916

Ulcer, ulcerated, ulcerating, ulceration, ulcerative
— continued
lower limb — continued
  lower leg — continued
    right — continued
      with — continued
        bone necrosis L97.914
        exposed fat layer L97.912
        muscle involvement without evidence of necrosis L97.915
        muscle necrosis L97.913
        skin breakdown only L97.911
        specified severity NEC L97.918
  specified site NEC L97.809
    with
      bone involvement without evidence of necrosis L97.806
      bone necrosis L97.804
      exposed fat layer L97.802
      muscle involvement without evidence of necrosis L97.805
      muscle necrosis L97.803
      skin breakdown only L97.801
      specified severity NEC L97.808
    left L97.829
      with
        bone involvement without evidence of necrosis L97.826
        bone necrosis L97.824
        exposed fat layer L97.822
        muscle involvement without evidence of necrosis L97.825
        muscle necrosis L97.823
        skin breakdown only L97.821
        specified severity NEC L97.828
    right L97.819
      with
        bone involvement without evidence of necrosis L97.816
        bone necrosis L97.814
        exposed fat layer L97.812
        muscle involvement without evidence of necrosis L97.815
        muscle necrosis L97.813
        skin breakdown only L97.811
        specified severity NEC L97.818
  midfoot L97.409
    with
      bone involvement without evidence of necrosis L97.406
      bone necrosis L97.404
      exposed fat layer L97.402
      muscle involvement without evidence of necrosis L97.405
      muscle necrosis L97.403
      skin breakdown only L97.401
      specified severity NEC L97.408
    left L97.429
      with
        bone involvement without evidence of necrosis L97.426
        bone necrosis L97.424
        exposed fat layer L97.422
        muscle involvement without evidence of necrosis L97.425
        muscle necrosis L97.423
        skin breakdown only L97.421
        specified severity NEC L97.428
    right L97.419
      with
        bone involvement without evidence of necrosis L97.416
        bone necrosis L97.414
        exposed fat layer L97.412
        muscle involvement without evidence of necrosis L97.415
        muscle necrosis L97.413
        skin breakdown only L97.411
        specified severity NEC L97.418
  right L97.919
    with
      bone involvement without evidence of necrosis L97.916
      bone necrosis L97.914
      exposed fat layer L97.912
      muscle involvement without evidence of necrosis L97.915
      muscle necrosis L97.913
      skin breakdown only L97.911

Ulcer, ulcerated, ulcerating, ulceration, ulcerative
— continued
lower limb — continued
  right — continued
    with — continued
      specified severity NEC L97.918
  syphilitic A52.19
  thigh L97.109
    with
      bone involvement without evidence of necrosis L97.106
      bone necrosis L97.104
      exposed fat layer L97.102
      muscle involvement without evidence of necrosis L97.105
      muscle necrosis L97.103
      skin breakdown only L97.101
      specified severity NEC L97.108
    left L97.129
      with
        bone involvement without evidence of necrosis L97.126
        bone necrosis L97.124
        exposed fat layer L97.122
        muscle involvement without evidence of necrosis L97.125
        muscle necrosis L97.123
        skin breakdown only L97.121
        specified severity NEC L97.128
    right L97.119
      with
        bone involvement without evidence of necrosis L97.116
        bone necrosis L97.114
        exposed fat layer L97.112
        muscle involvement without evidence of necrosis L97.115
        muscle necrosis L97.113
        skin breakdown only L97.111
        specified severity NEC L97.118
  toe L97.509
    with
      bone involvement without evidence of necrosis L97.506
      bone necrosis L97.504
      exposed fat layer L97.502
      muscle involvement without evidence of necrosis L97.505
      muscle necrosis L97.503
      skin breakdown only L97.501
      specified severity NEC L97.508
    left L97.529
      with
        bone involvement without evidence of necrosis L97.526
        bone necrosis L97.524
        exposed fat layer L97.522
        muscle involvement without evidence of necrosis L97.525
        muscle necrosis L97.523
        skin breakdown only L97.521
        specified severity NEC L97.528
    right L97.519
      with
        bone involvement without evidence of necrosis L97.516
        bone necrosis L97.514
        exposed fat layer L97.512
        muscle involvement without evidence of necrosis L97.515
        muscle necrosis L97.513
        skin breakdown only L97.511
        specified severity NEC L97.518
  varicose — see Varix, leg, with, ulcer
  luetic — see Ulcer, syphilitic
  lung J98.4
    tuberculous — see Tuberculosis, pulmonary
  malignant — see Neoplasm, malignant, by site
  marginal NEC — see Ulcer, gastrojejunal
  meatus (urinarius) N34.2
  Meckel's diverticulum Q43.0
    malignant — see Table of Neoplasms, small intestine, malignant
  Meleney's (chronic undermining) — see Ulcer, skin
  Mooren's (cornea) — see Ulcer, cornea, Mooren's
  mycobacterial (skin) A31.1
  nasopharynx J39.2
  neck, uterus N86

Ulcer, ulcerated, ulcerating, ulceration, ulcerative
— continued
neurogenic NEC — see Ulcer, skin
nose, nasal (passage) (infective) (septum) J34.0
  skin — see Ulcer, skin
  spirochetal A69.8
  varicose (bleeding) I86.8
oral mucosa (traumatic) K12.1
palate (soft) K12.1
penis (chronic) N48.5
peptic (site unspecified) K27.9
  with
    hemorrhage K27.4
      and perforation K27.6
    perforation K27.5
  acute K27.3
    with
      hemorrhage K27.0
        and perforation K27.2
      perforation K27.1
  chronic K27.7
    with
      hemorrhage K27.4
        and perforation K27.6
      perforation K27.5
  esophagus K22.10
    with bleeding K22.11
  newborn P78.82
perforating K27.5
  skin — see Ulcer, skin
peritonsillar J35.8
phagedenic (tropical) — see Ulcer, skin
pharynx J39.2
phlebitis — see Phlebitis
plaster — see Ulcer, pressure, by site
popliteal space — see Ulcer, lower limb
postpyloric — see Ulcer, duodenum
prepuce N47.7
prepyloric — see Ulcer, stomach
pressure (pressure area) L89.9- ☑
  ankle L89.5- ☑
  back L89.1- ☑
  buttock L89.3- ☑
  coccyx L89.15- ☑
  contiguous site of back, buttock, hip L89.4- ☑
  elbow L89.0- ☑
  face L89.81- ☑
  head L89.81- ☑
  heel L89.6- ☑
  hip L89.2- ☑
  sacral region (tailbone) L89.15- ☑
  specified site NEC L89.89- ☑
  stage 1 (healing) (pre-ulcer skin changes limited to persistent focal edema)
    ankle L89.5- ☑
    back L89.1- ☑
    buttock L89.3- ☑
    coccyx L89.15- ☑
    contiguous site of back, buttock, hip L89.4- ☑
    elbow L89.0- ☑
    face L89.81- ☑
    head L89.81- ☑
    heel L89.6- ☑
    hip L89.2- ☑
    sacral region (tailbone) L89.15- ☑
    specified site NEC L89.89- ☑
  stage 2 (healing) (abrasion, blister, partial thickness skin loss involving epidermis and/or dermis)
    ankle L89.5- ☑
    back L89.1- ☑
    buttock L89.3- ☑
    coccyx L89.15- ☑
    contiguous site of back, buttock, hip L89.4- ☑
    elbow L89.0- ☑
    face L89.81- ☑
    head L89.81- ☑
    heel L89.6- ☑
    hip L89.2- ☑
    sacral region (tailbone) L89.15- ☑
    specified site NEC L89.89- ☑
  stage 3 (healing) (full thickness skin loss involving damage or necrosis of subcutaneous tissue)
    ankle L89.5- ☑
    back L89.1- ☑
    buttock L89.3- ☑
    coccyx L89.15- ☑
    contiguous site of back, buttock, hip L89.4- ☑

Ulcer, ulcerated, ulcerating, ulceration, ulcerative
— *continued*
pressure — *continued*
  stage 3 — *continued*
    elbow L89.0- ☑
    face L89.81- ☑
    head L89.81- ☑
    heel L89.6- ☑
    hip L89.2- ☑
    sacral region (tailbone) L89.15- ☑
    specified site NEC L89.89- ☑
  stage 4 (healing) (necrosis of soft tissues through
    to underlying muscle, tendon, or bone)
    ankle L89.5- ☑
    back L89.1- ☑
    buttock L89.3- ☑
    coccyx L89.15- ☑
    contiguous site of back, buttock, hip L89.4- ☑
    elbow L89.0- ☑
    face L89.81- ☑
    head L89.81- ☑
    heel L89.6- ☑
    hip L89.2- ☑
    sacral region (tailbone) L89.15- ☑
    specified site NEC L89.89- ☑
  unspecified stage
    ankle L89.5- ☑
    back L89.1- ☑
    buttock L89.3- ☑
    coccyx L89.15- ☑
    contiguous site of back, buttock, hip L89.4- ☑
    elbow L89.0- ☑
    face L89.81- ☑
    head L89.81- ☑
    heel L89.6- ☑
    hip L89.2- ☑
    sacral region (tailbone) L89.15- ☑
    specified site NEC L89.89- ☑
  unstageable
    ankle L89.5- ☑
    back L89.1- ☑
    buttock L89.3- ☑
    coccyx L89.15- ☑
    contiguous site of back, buttock, hip L89.4- ☑
    elbow L89.0- ☑
    face L89.81- ☑
    head L89.81- ☑
    heel L89.6- ☑
    hip L89.2- ☑
    sacral region (tailbone) L89.15- ☑
    specified site NEC L89.89- ☑
primary of intestine K63.3
  with perforation K63.1
prostate N41.9
pyloric — *see* Ulcer, stomach
rectosigmoid K63.3
  with perforation K63.1
rectum (sphincter) (solitary) K62.6
  stercoraceous, stercoral K62.6
retina — *see* Inflammation, chorioretinal
rodent (*see also* Neoplasm, skin, malignant)
sclera — *see* Scleritis
scrofulous (tuberculous) A18.2
scrotum N50.89
  tuberculous A18.15
  varicose I86.1
seminal vesicle N50.89
sigmoid — *see* Ulcer, intestine
skin (atrophic) (chronic) (neurogenic) (non-healing)
  (perforating) (pyogenic) (trophic) (tropical)
  L98.499
  with gangrene — *see* Gangrene
  amebic A06.7
  back — *see* Ulcer, back
  buttock — *see* Ulcer, buttock
  decubitus — *see* Ulcer, pressure
  lower limb — *see* Ulcer, lower limb
  mycobacterial A31.1
  specified site NEC L98.499
    with
      bone involvement without evidence of
        necrosis L98.496
      bone necrosis L98.494
      exposed fat layer L98.492
      muscle involvement without evidence of
        necrosis L98.495
      muscle necrosis L98.493

Ulcer, ulcerated, ulcerating, ulceration, ulcerative
— *continued*
skin — *continued*
  specified site — *continued*
    with — *continued*
      skin breakdown only L98.491
      specified severity NEC L98.498
  tuberculous (primary) A18.4
  varicose — *see* Ulcer, varicose
sloughing — *see* Ulcer, skin
solitary, anus or rectum (sphincter) K62.6
sore throat J02.9
  streptococcal J02.0
spermatic cord N50.89
spine (tuberculous) A18.01
stasis (venous) — *see* Varix, leg, with, ulcer
  without varicose veins I87.2
stercoraceous, stercoral K63.3
  with perforation K63.1
  anus or rectum K62.6
stoma, stomal — *see* Ulcer, gastrojejunal
stomach (eroded) (peptic) (round) K25.9
  with
    hemorrhage K25.4
      and perforation K25.6
    perforation K25.5
  acute K25.3
    with
      hemorrhage K25.0
        and perforation K25.2
      perforation K25.1
  chronic K25.7
    with
      hemorrhage K25.4
        and perforation K25.6
      perforation K25.5
stomal — *see* Ulcer, gastrojejunal
stomatitis K12.1
stress — *see* Ulcer, peptic
strumous (tuberculous) A18.2
submucosal, bladder — *see* Cystitis, interstitial
syphilitic (any site) (early) (secondary) A51.39
  late A52.79
  perforating A52.79
    foot A52.11
testis N50.89
thigh — *see* Ulcer, lower limb
throat J39.2
  diphtheritic A36.0
toe — *see* Ulcer, lower limb
tongue (traumatic) K14.0
tonsil J35.8
  diphtheritic A36.0
trachea J39.8
trophic — *see* Ulcer, skin
tropical — *see* Ulcer, skin
tuberculous — *see* Tuberculosis, ulcer
tunica vaginalis N50.89
turbinate J34.89
typhoid (perforating) — *see* Typhoid
unspecified site — *see* Ulcer, skin
urethra (meatus) — *see* Urethritis
uterus N85.8
  cervix N86
    with cervicitis N72
  neck N86
    with cervicitis N72
vagina N76.5
  in Behçet's disease M35.2 [N77.0]
  pessary N89.8
valve, heart I33.0
varicose (lower limb, any part) (*see also* Varix, leg, with,
  ulcer)
  broad ligament I86.2
  esophagus — *see* Varix, esophagus
  inflamed or infected — *see* Varix, leg, with ulcer,
    with inflammation
  nasal septum I86.8
  perineum I86.3
  scrotum I86.1
  specified site NEC I86.8
  sublingual I86.0
  vulva I86.3
vas deferens N50.89
vulva (acute) (infectional) N76.6
  in (due to)
    Behçet's disease M35.2 [N77.0]
    herpesviral (herpes simplex) infection A60.04

Ulcer, ulcerated, ulcerating, ulceration, ulcerative
— *continued*
vulva — *continued*
  in — *continued*
    tuberculosis A18.18
vulvobuccal, recurring N76.6
X-ray L58.1
yaws A66.4
Ulcerosa scarlatina A38.8
Ulcus (*see also* Ulcer)
cutis tuberculosum A18.4
duodeni — *see* Ulcer, duodenum
durum (syphilitic) A51.0
  extragenital A51.2
gastrojejunale — *see* Ulcer, gastrojejunal
hypostaticum — *see* Ulcer, varicose
molle (cutis) (skin) A57
serpens corneae — *see* Ulcer, cornea, central
ventriculi — *see* Ulcer, stomach
Ulegyria Q04.8
Ulerythema
ophryogenes, congenital Q84.2
sycosiforme L73.8
Ullrich (-Bonnevie)(-Turner) **syndrome** (*see also* Turner's
  syndrome) Q87.1
Ullrich-Feichtiger syndrome Q87.0
Ulnar — *see* condition
Ulorrhagia, ulorrhea K06.8
Umbilicus, umbilical — *see* condition
Unacceptable
contours of tooth K08.54
morphology of tooth K08.54
Unavailability (of)
bed at medical facility Z75.1
health service-related agencies Z75.4
medical facilities (at) Z75.3
  due to
    investigation by social service agency Z75.2
    lack of services at home Z75.0
    remoteness from facility Z75.3
    waiting list Z75.1
  home Z75.0
  outpatient clinic Z75.3
schooling Z55.1
social service agencies Z75.4
Uncinaria americana infestation B76.1
Uncinariasis B76.9
Uncongenial work Z56.5
Unconscious (ness) — *see* Coma
Under observation — *see* Observation
Underachievement in school Z55.3
Underdevelopment (*see also* Undeveloped)
nose Q30.1
sexual E30.0
Underdosing (*see also* Table of Drugs and Chemicals,
  categories T36-T50, with final character 6) Z91.14
intentional NEC Z91.128
  due to financial hardship of patient Z91.120
unintentional NEC Z91.138
  due to patient's age related debility Z91.130
Underfeeding, newborn P92.3
Underfill, endodontic M27.53
Underimmunization status Z28.3
Undernourishment — *see* Malnutrition
Undernutrition — *see* Malnutrition
Underweight R63.6
for gestational age — *see* Light for dates
Underwood's disease P83.0
Undescended (*see also* Malposition, congenital)
cecum Q43.3
colon Q43.3
testicle — *see* Cryptorchid
Undeveloped, undevelopment (*see also* Hypoplasia)
brain (congenital) Q02
cerebral (congenital) Q02
heart Q24.8
lung Q33.6
testis E29.1
uterus E30.0
Undiagnosed (disease) R69
Undulant fever — *see* Brucellosis
Unemployment, anxiety concerning Z56.0
threatened Z56.2
Unequal length (acquired) (limb) (*see also* Deformity,
  limb, unequal length)
leg (*see also* Deformity, limb, unequal length)
  congenital Q72.9- ☑

Unextracted dental root K08.3
Unguis incarnatus L60.0
Unhappiness R45.2
Unicornate uterus Q51.4
  in pregnancy or childbirth O34.00
Unilateral (*see also* condition)
  development, breast N64.89
  organ or site, congenital NEC — *see* Agenesis, by site
Unilocular heart Q20.8
Union, abnormal (*see also* Fusion)
  larynx and trachea Q34.8
Universal mesentery Q43.3
Unrepairable overhanging of dental restorative materials K08.52
Unsatisfactory
  restoration of tooth K08.50
    specified NEC K08.59
  sample of cytologic smear
    anus R85.615
    cervix R87.615
    vagina R87.625
  surroundings Z59.1
    work Z56.5
Unsoundness of mind — *see* Psychosis
Unstable
  back NEC — *see* Instability, joint, spine
  hip (congenital) Q65.6
    acquired — *see* Derangement, joint, specified type NEC, hip
  joint — *see* Instability, joint
    secondary to removal of joint prosthesis M96.89
  lie (mother) O32.0 ☑
  lumbosacral joint (congenital)
    acquired — *see* subcategory M53.2 ☑
  sacroiliac — *see* subcategory M53.2 ☑
  spine NEC — *see* Instability, joint, spine
Unsteadiness on feet R26.81
Untruthfulness, child problem F91.8
Unverricht (-Lundborg) **disease or epilepsy** — *see* Epilepsy, generalized, idiopathic
Unwanted pregnancy Z64.0
Upbringing, institutional Z62.22
  away from parents NEC Z62.29
  in care of non-parental family member Z62.21
  in foster care Z62.21
  in orphanage or group home Z62.22
  in welfare custody Z62.21
Upper respiratory — *see* condition
Upset
  gastric K30
  gastrointestinal K30
    psychogenic F45.8
  intestinal (large) (small) K59.9
    psychogenic F45.8
  menstruation N93.9
  mental F48.9
  stomach K30
    psychogenic F45.8
Urachus (*see also* condition)
  patent or persistent Q64.4
Urbach-Oppenheim disease (necrobiosis lipoidica diabeticorum) — *see* E08-E13 with .620
Urbach's lipoid proteinosis E78.89
Urbach-Wiethe disease E78.89
Urban yellow fever A95.1
Urea
  blood, high — *see* Uremia
  cycle metabolism disorder — *see* Disorder, urea cycle metabolism
Uremia, uremic N19
  with
    ectopic or molar pregnancy O08.4
    polyneuropathy N18.9 [G63]
  chronic NOS (*see also* Disease, kidney, chronic) N18.9
    due to hypertension — *see* Hypertensive, kidney
  complicating
    ectopic or molar pregnancy O08.4
  congenital P96.0
  extrarenal R39.2
  following ectopic or molar pregnancy O08.4
  newborn P96.0
  prerenal R39.2
Ureter, ureteral — *see* condition
Ureteralgia N23
Ureterectasis — *see* Hydroureter
Ureteritis N28.89
  cystica N28.86

Ureteritis — *continued*
  due to calculus N20.1
    with calculus, kidney N20.2
      with hydronephrosis N13.2
  gonococcal (acute) (chronic) A54.21
  nonspecific N28.89
Ureterocele N28.89
  congenital (orthotopic) Q62.31
    ectopic Q62.32
Ureterolith, ureterolithiasis — *see* Calculus, ureter
Ureterostomy
  attention to Z43.6
  status Z93.6
Urethra, urethral — *see* condition
Urethralgia R39.89
Urethritis (anterior) (posterior) N34.2
  calculous N21.1
  candidal B37.41
  chlamydial A56.01
  diplococcal (gonococcal) A54.01
    with abscess (accessory gland) (periurethral) A54.1
  gonococcal A54.01
    with abscess (accessory gland) (periurethral) A54.1
  nongonococcal N34.1
    Reiter's — *see* Reiter's disease
  nonspecific N34.1
  nonvenereal N34.1
  postmenopausal N34.2
  puerperal O86.22
  Reiter's — *see* Reiter's disease
  specified NEC N34.2
  trichomonal or due to Trichomonas (vaginalis) A59.03
Urethrocele N81.0
  with
    cystocele — *see* Cystocele
    prolapse of uterus — *see* Prolapse, uterus
Urethrolithiasis (with colic or infection) N21.1
Urethrorectal — *see* condition
Urethrorrhagia N36.8
Urethrorrhea R36.9
Urethrostomy
  attention to Z43.6
  status Z93.6
Urethrotrigonitis — *see* Trigonitis
Urethrovaginal — *see* condition
Urgency
  fecal R15.2
  hypertensive — *see* Hypertension
  urinary R39.15
Urhidrosis, uridrosis L74.8
Uric acid in blood (increased) E79.0
Uricacidemia (asymptomatic) E79.0
Uricemia (asymptomatic) E79.0
Uricosuria R82.99
Urinary — *see* condition
Urination
  frequent R35.0
  painful R30.9
Urine
  blood in — *see* Hematuria
  discharge, excessive R35.8
  enuresis, nonorganic origin F98.0
  extravasation R39.0
  frequency R35.0
  incontinence R32
    nonorganic origin F98.0
  intermittent stream R39.198
  pus in N39.0
  retention or stasis R33.9
    organic R33.8
      drug-induced R33.0
    psychogenic F45.8
  secretion
    deficient R34
    excessive R35.8
    frequency R35.0
  stream
    intermittent R39.198
    slowing R39.198
    splitting R39.13
    weak R39.12
Urinemia — *see* Uremia
Urinoma, urethra N36.8
Uroarthritis, infectious (Reiter's) — *see* Reiter's disease
Urodialysis R34
Urolithiasis — *see* Calculus, urinary
Uronephrosis — *see* Hydronephrosis
Uropathy N39.9

Uropathy — *continued*
  obstructive N13.9
    specified NEC N13.8
  reflux N13.9
    specified NEC N13.8
  vesicoureteral reflux-associated — *see* Reflux, vesicoureteral
Urosepsis — *code to* condition
Urticaria L50.9
  with angioneurotic edema T78.3 ☑
    hereditary D84.1
  allergic L50.0
  cholinergic L50.5
  chronic L50.8
  cold, familial L50.2
  contact L50.6
  dermatographic L50.3
  due to
    cold or heat L50.2
    drugs L50.0
    food L50.0
    inhalants L50.0
    plants L50.6
    serum (*see also* Reaction, serum) T80.69 ☑
  factitial L50.3
  familial cold M04.2
  giant T78.3 ☑
    hereditary D84.1
  gigantea T78.3 ☑
  idiopathic L50.1
  larynx T78.3 ☑
    hereditary D84.1
  neonatorum P83.88
  nonallergic L50.1
  papulosa (Hebra) L28.2
  pigmentosa D47.01
    congenital Q82.2
    of neonatal onset Q82.2
    of newborn onset Q82.2
  recurrent periodic L50.8
  serum (*see also* Reaction, serum) T80.69 ☑
  solar L56.3
  specified type NEC L50.8
  thermal (cold) (heat) L50.2
  vibratory L50.4
  xanthelasmoidea — *see* Urticaria pigmentosa
Use (of)
  alcohol Z72.89
    with
      intoxication F10.929
      sleep disorder F10.982
    harmful — *see* Abuse, alcohol
  amphetamines — *see* Use, stimulant NEC
  caffeine — *see* Use, stimulant NEC
  cannabis F12.90
    with
      anxiety disorder F12.980
      intoxication F12.929
        with
          delirium F12.921
          perceptual disturbance F12.922
        uncomplicated F12.920
      other specified disorder F12.988
      psychosis F12.959
        delusions F12.950
        hallucinations F12.951
      unspecified disorder F12.99
  cocaine F14.90
    with
      anxiety disorder F14.980
      intoxication F14.929
        with
          delirium F14.921
          perceptual disturbance F14.922
        uncomplicated F14.920
      other specified disorder F14.988
      psychosis F14.959
        delusions F14.950
        hallucinations F14.951
      sexual dysfunction F14.981
      sleep disorder F14.982
      unspecified disorder F14.99
    harmful — *see* Abuse, drug, cocaine
  drug(s) NEC F19.90
    with sleep disorder F19.982
    harmful — *see* Abuse, drug, by type
  hallucinogen NEC F16.90

☑ **Additional Character Required** — Refer to the Tabular List for Character Selection   ▽ **Subterms under main terms may continue to next column or page**

Use — *continued*
hallucinogen — *continued*
  with
    anxiety disorder F16.980
    intoxication F16.929
      with
        delirium F16.921
      uncomplicated F16.920
    mood disorder F16.94
    other specified disorder F16.988
    perception disorder (flashbacks) F16.983
    psychosis F16.959
      delusions F16.950
      hallucinations F16.951
    unspecified disorder F16.99
  harmful — *see* Abuse, drug, hallucinogen NEC
inhalants F18.90
  with
    anxiety disorder F18.980
    intoxication F18.929
      with delirium F18.921
      uncomplicated F18.920
    mood disorder F18.94
    other specified disorder F18.988
    persisting dementia F18.97
    psychosis F18.959
      delusions F18.950
      hallucinations F18.951
    unspecified disorder F18.99
  harmful — *see* Abuse, drug, inhalant
methadone — *see* Use, opioid
nonprescribed drugs F19.90
  harmful — *see* Abuse, non-psychoactive substance
opioid F11.90
  with
    disorder F11.99
      mood F11.94
      sleep F11.982
      specified type NEC F11.988
    intoxication F11.929
      with
        delirium F11.921
        perceptual disturbance F11.922
      uncomplicated F11.920
    withdrawal F11.93
  harmful — *see* Abuse, drug, opioid
patent medicines F19.90
  harmful — *see* Abuse, non-psychoactive substance
psychoactive drug NEC F19.90
  with
    anxiety disorder F19.980
    intoxication F19.929
      with
        delirium F19.921
        perceptual disturbance F19.922
      uncomplicated F19.920
    mood disorder F19.94
    other specified disorder F19.988
    persisting
      amnestic disorder F19.96
      dementia F19.97
    psychosis F19.959
      delusions F19.950
      hallucinations F19.951
    sexual dysfunction F19.981
    sleep disorder F19.982
    unspecified disorder F19.99
    withdrawal F19.939
      with
        delirium F19.931
        perceptual disturbance F19.932
      uncomplicated F19.930
  harmful — *see* Abuse, drug NEC, psychoactive NEC
sedative, hypnotic, or anxiolytic F13.90
  with
    anxiety disorder F13.980
    intoxication F13.929
      with
        delirium F13.921
      uncomplicated F13.920
    other specified disorder F13.988
    persisting
      amnestic disorder F13.96
      dementia F13.97
    psychosis F13.959
      delusions F13.950
      hallucinations F13.951
    sexual dysfunction F13.981

Use — *continued*
sedative, hypnotic, or anxiolytic — *continued*
  with — *continued*
    sleep disorder F13.982
    unspecified disorder F13.99
  harmful — *see* Abuse, drug, sedative, hypnotic, or anxiolytic
stimulant NEC F15.90
  with
    anxiety disorder F15.980
    intoxication F15.929
      with
        delirium F15.921
        perceptual disturbance F15.922
      uncomplicated F15.920
    mood disorder F15.94
    other specified disorder F15.988
    psychosis F15.959
      delusions F15.950
      hallucinations F15.951
    sexual dysfunction F15.981
    sleep disorder F15.982
    unspecified disorder F15.99
    withdrawal F15.93
  harmful — *see* Abuse, drug, stimulant NEC
tobacco Z72.0
  with dependence — *see* Dependence, drug, nicotine
volatile solvents (*see also* Use, inhalant) F18.90
  harmful — *see* Abuse, drug, inhalant
Usher-Senear disease or syndrome L10.4
Uta B55.1
Uteromegaly N85.2
Uterovaginal — *see* condition
Uterovesical — *see* condition
Uveal — *see* condition
Uveitis (anterior) (*see also* Iridocyclitis)
  acute — *see* Iridocyclitis, acute
  chronic — *see* Iridocyclitis, chronic
  due to toxoplasmosis (acquired) B58.09
    congenital P37.1
  granulomatous — *see* Iridocyclitis, chronic
  heterochromic — *see* Cyclitis, Fuchs' heterochromic
  lens-induced — *see* Iridocyclitis, lens-induced
  posterior — *see* Chorioretinitis
  sympathetic H44.13- ☑
  syphilitic (secondary) A51.43
    congenital (early) A50.01
    late A52.71
  tuberculous A18.54
Uveoencephalitis — *see* Inflammation, chorioretinal
Uveokeratitis — *see* Iridocyclitis
Uveoparotitis D86.89
Uvula — *see* condition
Uvulitis (acute) (catarrhal) (chronic) (membranous) (suppurative) (ulcerative) K12.2

V

Vaccination (prophylactic)
  complication or reaction — *see* Complications, vaccination
  delayed Z28.9
  encounter for Z23
  not done — *see* Immunization, not done, because of)
Vaccinia (generalized) (localized) T88.1 ☑
  without vaccination B08.011
  congenital P35.8
Vacuum, in sinus (accessory) (nasal) J34.89
Vagabond, vagabondage Z59.0
Vagabond's disease B85.1
Vagina, vaginal — *see* condition
Vaginalitis (tunica) (testis) N49.1
Vaginismus (reflex) N94.2
  functional F52.5
  nonorganic F52.5
  psychogenic F52.5
  secondary N94.2
Vaginitis (acute) (circumscribed) (diffuse) (emphysematous) (nonvenereal) (ulcerative) N76.0
  with ectopic or molar pregnancy O08.0
  amebic A06.82
  atrophic, postmenopausal N95.2
  bacterial N76.0
  blennorrhagic (gonococcal) A54.02
  candidal B37.3
  chlamydial A56.02

Vaginitis — *continued*
  chronic N76.1
  due to Trichomonas (vaginalis) A59.01
  following ectopic or molar pregnancy O08.0
  gonococcal A54.02
    with abscess (accessory gland) (periurethral) A54.1
  granuloma A58
  in (due to)
    candidiasis B37.3
    herpesviral (herpes simplex) infection A60.04
    pinworm infection B80 [N77.1]
  monilial B37.3
  mycotic (candidal) B37.3
  postmenopausal atrophic N95.2
  puerperal (postpartum) O86.13
  senile (atrophic) N95.2
  subacute or chronic N76.1
  syphilitic (early) A51.0
    late A52.76
  trichomonal A59.01
  tuberculous A18.18
Vaginosis — *see* Vaginitis
Vagotonia G52.2
Vagrancy Z59.0
VAIN — *see* Neoplasia, intraepithelial, vagina
Vallecula — *see* condition
Valley fever B38.0
Valsuani's disease — *see* Anemia, obstetric
Valve, valvular (formation) (*see also* condition)
  cerebral ventricle (communicating) in situ Z98.2
  cervix, internal os Q51.828
  congenital NEC — *see* Atresia, by site
  ureter (pelvic junction) (vesical orifice) Q62.39
  urethra (congenital) (posterior) Q64.2
Valvulitis (chronic) — *see* Endocarditis
Valvulopathy — *see* Endocarditis
Van Bogaert's leukoencephalopathy (sclerosing) (subacute) A81.1
Van Bogaert-Scherer-Epstein disease or syndrome E75.5
Van Buchem's syndrome M85.2
Van Creveld-von Gierke disease E74.01
Van der Hoeve (-de Kleyn) **syndrome** Q78.0
Van der Woude's syndrome Q38.0
Van Neck's disease or osteochondrosis M91.0
Vanishing lung J44.9
Vapor asphyxia or suffocation T59.9 ☑
  specified agent — *see* Table of Drugs and Chemicals
Variance, lethal ball, prosthetic heart valve T82.09 ☑
Variants, thalassemic D56.8
Variations in hair color L67.1
Varicella B01.9
  with
    complications NEC B01.89
    encephalitis B01.11
    encephalomyelitis B01.11
    meningitis B01.0
    myelitis B01.12
    pneumonia B01.2
  congenital P35.8
Varices — *see* Varix
Varicocele (scrotum) (thrombosed) I86.1
  ovary I86.2
  perineum I86.3
  spermatic cord (ulcerated) I86.1
Varicose
  aneurysm (ruptured) I77.0
  dermatitis — *see* Varix, leg, with, inflammation
  eczema — *see* Varix, leg, with, inflammation
  phlebitis — *see* Varix, with, inflammation
  tumor — *see* Varix
  ulcer (lower limb, any part) (*see also* Varix, leg, with, ulcer)
    anus (*see also* Hemorrhoids) K64.8
    esophagus — *see* Varix, esophagus
    inflamed or infected — *see* Varix, leg, with ulcer, with inflammation
    nasal septum I86.8
    perineum I86.3
    scrotum I86.1
    specified site NEC I86.8
  vein — *see* Varix
  vessel — *see* Varix, leg
Varicosis, varicosities, varicosity — *see* Varix
Variola (major) (minor) B03
Varioloid B03
Varix (lower limb) (ruptured) I83.90

Varix — continued
  with
    edema I83.899
    inflammation I83.10
      with ulcer (venous) I83.209
    pain I83.819
    specified complication NEC I83.899
    stasis dermatitis I83.10
      with ulcer (venous) I83.209
    swelling I83.899
    ulcer I83.009
      with inflammation I83.209
  aneurysmal I77.0
  asymptomatic I83.9- ☑
  bladder I86.2
  broad ligament I86.2
  complicating
    childbirth (lower extremity) O87.4
      anus or rectum O87.2
      genital (vagina, vulva or perineum) O87.8
    pregnancy (lower extremity) O22.0- ☑
      anus or rectum O22.4- ☑
      genital (vagina, vulva or perineum) O22.1- ☑
    puerperium (lower extremity) O87.4
      anus or rectum O87.2
      genital (vagina, vulva, perineum) O87.8
  congenital (any site) Q27.8
  esophagus (idiopathic) (primary) (ulcerated) I85.00
    bleeding I85.01
    congenital Q27.8
    in (due to)
      alcoholic liver disease I85.10
        bleeding I85.11
      cirrhosis of liver I85.10
        bleeding I85.11
      portal hypertension I85.10
        bleeding I85.11
      schistosomiasis I85.10
        bleeding I85.11
      toxic liver disease I85.10
        bleeding I85.11
    secondary I85.10
      bleeding I85.11
  gastric I86.4
  inflamed or infected I83.10
    ulcerated I83.209
  labia (majora) I86.3
  leg (asymptomatic) I83.90
    with
      edema I83.899
      inflammation I83.10
        with ulcer — see Varix, leg, with, ulcer, with inflammation by site
      pain I83.819
      specified complication NEC I83.899
      swelling I83.899
      ulcer I83.009
        with inflammation I83.209
        ankle I83.003
          with inflammation I83.203
        calf I83.002
          with inflammation I83.202
        foot NEC I83.005
          with inflammation I83.205
        heel I83.004
          with inflammation I83.204
        lower leg NEC I83.008
          with inflammation I83.208
        midfoot I83.004
          with inflammation I83.204
        thigh I83.001
          with inflammation I83.201
    bilateral (asymptomatic) I83.93
      with
        edema I83.893
        pain I83.813
        specified complication NEC I83.893
        swelling I83.893
        ulcer I83.0- ☑
          with inflammation I83.209
    left (asymptomatic) I83.92
      with
        edema I83.892
        inflammation I83.12
          with ulcer — see Varix, leg, with, ulcer, with inflammation by site
        pain I83.812
        specified complication NEC I83.892

Varix — continued
  leg — continued
    left — continued
      with — continued
        swelling I83.892
        ulcer I83.029
          with inflammation I83.229
          ankle I83.023
            with inflammation I83.223
          calf I83.022
            with inflammation I83.222
          foot NEC I83.025
            with inflammation I83.225
          heel I83.024
            with inflammation I83.224
          lower leg NEC I83.028
            with inflammation I83.228
          midfoot I83.024
            with inflammation I83.224
          thigh I83.021
            with inflammation I83.221
    right (asymptomatic) I83.91
      with
        edema I83.891
        inflammation I83.11
          with ulcer — see Varix, leg, with, ulcer, with inflammation by site
        pain I83.811
        specified complication NEC I83.891
        swelling I83.891
        ulcer I83.019
          with inflammation I83.219
          ankle I83.013
            with inflammation I83.213
          calf I83.012
            with inflammation I83.212
          foot NEC I83.015
            with inflammation I83.215
          heel I83.014
            with inflammation I83.214
          lower leg NEC I83.018
            with inflammation I83.218
          midfoot I83.014
            with inflammation I83.214
          thigh I83.011
            with inflammation I83.211
  nasal septum I86.8
  orbit I86.8
    congenital Q27.8
  ovary I86.2
  papillary I78.1
  pelvis I86.2
  perineum I86.3
  pharynx I86.8
  placenta O43.89- ☑
  renal papilla I86.8
  retina H35.09
  scrotum (ulcerated) I86.1
  sigmoid colon I86.8
  specified site NEC I86.8
  spinal (cord) (vessels) I86.8
  spleen, splenic (vein) (with phlebolith) I86.8
  stomach I86.4
  sublingual I86.0
  ulcerated I83.009
    inflamed or infected I83.209
  uterine ligament I86.2
  vagina I86.8
  vocal cord I86.8
  vulva I86.3
Vas deferens — see condition
Vas deferentitis N49.1
Vasa previa O69.4 ☑
  hemorrhage from, affecting newborn P50.0
Vascular (see also condition)
  loop on optic papilla Q14.2
  spasm I73.9
  spider I78.1
Vascularization, cornea — see Neovascularization, cornea
Vasculitis I77.6
  allergic D69.0
  cryoglobulinemic D89.1
  disseminated I77.6
  hypocomplementemic M31.8
  kidney I77.89
  livedoid L95.0
  nodular L95.8

Vasculitis — continued
  retina H35.06- ☑
  rheumatic — see Fever, rheumatic
  rheumatoid — see Rheumatoid, vasculitis
  skin (limited to) L95.9
    specified NEC L95.8
  systemic M31.8
Vasculopathy, necrotizing M31.9
  cardiac allograft T86.290
  specified NEC M31.8
Vasitis (nodosa) N49.1
  tuberculous A18.15
Vasodilation I73.9
Vasomotor — see condition
Vasoplasty, after previous sterilization Z31.0
  aftercare Z31.42
Vasospasm (vasoconstriction) I73.9
  cerebral (cerebrovascular) (artery) I67.848
    reversible I67.841
  coronary I20.1
  nerve
    arm — see Mononeuropathy, upper limb
    brachial plexus G54.0
    cervical plexus G54.2
    leg — see Mononeuropathy, lower limb
  peripheral NOS I73.9
  retina (artery) — see Occlusion, artery, retina
Vasospastic — see condition
Vasovagal attack (paroxysmal) R55
  psychogenic F45.8
VATER syndrome Q87.2
Vater's ampulla — see condition
Vegetation, vegetative
  adenoid (nasal fossa) J35.8
  endocarditis (acute) (any valve) (subacute) I33.0
  heart (mycotic) (valve) I33.0
Veil
  Jackson's Q43.3
Vein, venous — see condition
Veldt sore — see Ulcer, skin
Velpeau's hernia — see Hernia, femoral
Venereal
  bubo A55
  disease A64
  granuloma inguinale A58
  lymphogranuloma (Durand-Nicolas-Favre) A55
Venofibrosis I87.8
Venom, venomous — see Table of Drugs and Chemicals, by animal or substance, poisoning
Venous — see condition
Ventilator lung, newborn P27.8
Ventral — see condition
Ventricle, ventricular (see also condition)
  escape I49.3
  inversion Q20.5
Ventriculitis (cerebral) (see also Encephalitis) G04.90
Ventriculostomy status Z98.2
Vernet's syndrome G52.7
Verneuil's disease (syphilitic bursitis) A52.78
Verruca (due to HPV) (filiformis) (simplex) (viral) (vulgaris) B07.9
  acuminata A63.0
  necrogenica (primary) (tuberculosa) A18.4
  plana B07.8
  plantaris B07.0
  seborrheica L82.1
    inflamed L82.0
  senile (seborrheic) L82.1
    inflamed L82.0
  tuberculosa (primary) A18.4
  venereal A63.0
Verrucosities — see Verruca
Verruga peruana, peruviana A44.1
Version
  with extraction
  cervix — see Malposition, uterus
  uterus (postinfectional) (postpartal, old) — see Malposition, uterus
Vertebra, vertebral — see condition
Vertical talus (congenital) Q66.80
  left foot Q66.82
  right foot Q66.81
Vertigo R42
  auditory — see Vertigo, aural
  aural H81.31- ☑
  benign paroxysmal (positional) H81.1- ☑
  central (origin) H81.4- ☑

Vertigo — *continued*
  cerebral H81.4- ☑
  Dix and Hallpike (epidemic) — *see* Neuronitis,
    vestibular
  due to infrasound T75.23 ☑
  epidemic A88.1
    Dix and Hallpike — *see* Neuronitis, vestibular
    Pedersen's — *see* Neuronitis, vestibular
    vestibular neuronitis — *see* Neuronitis, vestibular
  hysterical F44.89
  infrasound T75.23 ☑
  labyrinthine — *see* subcategory H81.0 ☑
  laryngeal R05
  malignant positional H81.4- ☑
  Ménière's — *see* subcategory H81.0 ☑
  menopausal N95.1
  otogenic — *see* Vertigo, aural
  paroxysmal positional, benign — *see* Vertigo, benign
    paroxysmal
  Pedersen's (epidemic) — *see* Neuronitis, vestibular
  peripheral NEC H81.39- ☑
  positional
    benign paroxysmal — *see* Vertigo, benign parox-
      ysmal
    malignant H81.4- ☑
Very-low-density-lipoprotein-type (VLDL) **hyperlipoproteinemia** E78.1
Vesania — *see* Psychosis
Vesical — *see* condition
Vesicle
  cutaneous R23.8
  seminal — *see* condition
  skin R23.8
Vesicocolic — *see* condition
Vesicoperineal — *see* condition
Vesicorectal — *see* condition
Vesicourethrorectal — *see* condition
Vesicovaginal — *see* condition
Vesicular — *see* condition
Vesiculitis (seminal) N49.0
  amebic A06.82
  gonorrheal (acute) (chronic) A54.23
  trichomonal A59.09
  tuberculous A18.15
Vestibulitis (ear) (*see also* subcategory) H83.0 ☑
  nose (external) J34.89
  vulvar N94.810
Vestibulopathy , acute peripheral (recurrent) — *see*
  Neuronitis, vestibular
Vestige, vestigial (*see also* Persistence)
  branchial Q18.0
  structures in vitreous Q14.0
Vibration
  adverse effects T75.20 ☑
    pneumatic hammer syndrome T75.21 ☑
    specified effect NEC T75.29 ☑
    vasospastic syndrome T75.22 ☑
    vertigo from infrasound T75.23 ☑
  exposure (occupational) Z57.7
  vertigo T75.23 ☑
Vibriosis A28.9
Victim (of)
  crime Z65.4
  disaster Z65.5
  terrorism Z65.4
  torture Z65.4
  war Z65.5
Vidal's disease L28.0
Villaret's syndrome G52.7
Villous — *see* condition
VIN — *see* Neoplasia, intraepithelial, vulva
Vincent's infection (angina) (gingivitis) A69.1
  stomatitis NEC A69.1
Vinson-Plummer syndrome D50.1
Violence, physical R45.6
Viosterol deficiency — *see* Deficiency, calciferol
Vipoma — *see* Neoplasm, malignant, by site
Viremia B34.9
Virilism (adrenal) E25.9
  congenital E25.0
Virilization (female) (suprarenal) E25.9
  congenital E25.0
  isosexual E28.2
Virulent bubo A57
Virus, viral (*see also* condition)
  as cause of disease classified elsewhere B97.89
  cytomegalovirus B25.9

Virus, viral — *continued*
  human immunodeficiency (HIV) — *see* Human, immun-
    odeficiency virus (HIV) disease
  infection — *see* Infection, virus
  specified NEC B34.8
  swine influenza (viruses that normally cause infections
    in pigs) (*see also* Influenza, due to, identified
    novel influenza A virus) J09.X2
  West Nile (fever) A92.30
    with
      complications NEC A92.39
      cranial nerve disorders A92.32
      encephalitis A92.31
      encephalomyelitis A92.31
      neurologic manifestation NEC A92.32
      optic neuritis A92.32
      polyradiculitis A92.32
Viscera, visceral — *see* condition
Visceroptosis K63.4
Visible peristalsis R19.2
Vision, visual
  binocular, suppression H53.34
  blurred, blurring H53.8
    hysterical F44.6
  defect, defective NEC H54.7
  disorientation (syndrome) H53.8
  disturbance H53.9
    hysterical F44.6
  double H53.2
  examination Z01.00
    with abnormal findings Z01.01
  field, limitation (defect) — *see* Defect, visual field
  hallucinations R44.1
  halos H53.19
  loss — *see* Loss, vision
    sudden — *see* Disturbance, vision, subjective, loss,
      sudden
  low (both eyes) — *see* Low, vision
  perception, simultaneous without fusion H53.33
Vitality, lack or want of R53.83
  newborn P96.89
Vitamin deficiency — *see* Deficiency, vitamin
Vitelline duct, persistent Q43.0
Vitiligo L80
  eyelid H02.739
    left H02.736
      lower H02.735
      upper H02.734
    right H02.733
      lower H02.732
      upper H02.731
  pinta A67.2
  vulva N90.89
Vitreal corneal syndrome H59.01- ☑
Vitreoretinopathy, proliferative (*see also* Retinopathy,
  proliferative)
  with retinal detachment — *see* Detachment, retina,
    traction
Vitreous (*see also* condition)
  touch syndrome — *see* Complication, postprocedural,
    following cataract surgery
Vocal cord — *see* condition
Vogt-Koyanagi syndrome H20.82- ☑
Vogt's disease or syndrome G80.3
Vogt-Spielmeyer amaurotic idiocy or disease E75.4
Voice
  change R49.9
    specified NEC R49.8
  loss — *see* Aphonia
Volhynian fever A79.0
Volkmann's ischemic contracture or paralysis (complicating trauma) T79.6 ☑
Volvulus (bowel) (colon) (intestine) K56.2
  with perforation K56.2
  congenital Q43.8
  duodenum K31.5
  fallopian tube — *see* Torsion, fallopian tube
  oviduct — *see* Torsion, fallopian tube
  stomach (due to absence of gastrocolic ligament)
    K31.89
Vomiting R11.10
  with nausea R11.2
  without nausea R11.11
  asphyxia — *see* Foreign body, by site, causing asphyx-
    ia, gastric contents
  bilious (cause unknown) R11.14
    following gastro-intestinal surgery K91.0
    in newborn P92.01

Vomiting — *continued*
  blood — *see* Hematemesis
  causing asphyxia, choking, or suffocation — *see* For-
    eign body, by site
  cyclical G43.A0 (*following* G43.7)
    with refractory migraine G43.A1 (*following* G43.7)
    without refractory migraine G43.A0 (*following*
      G43.7)
    intractable G43.A1 (*following* G43.7)
    not intractable G43.A0 (*following* G43.7)
    psychogenic F50.89
  fecal mater R11.13
  following gastrointestinal surgery K91.0
    psychogenic F50.89
  functional K31.89
  hysterical F50.89
  nervous F50.89
  neurotic F50.89
  newborn NEC P92.09
    bilious P92.01
  periodic R11.10
    psychogenic F50.89
  projectile R11.12
  psychogenic F50.89
  uremic — *see* Uremia
Vomito negro — *see* Fever, yellow
Von Bezold's abscess — *see* Mastoiditis, acute
Von Economo-Cruchet disease A85.8
Von Eulenburg's disease G71.19
Von Gierke's disease E74.01
Von Hippel (-Lindau) **disease or syndrome** Q85.8
Von Jaksch's anemia or disease D64.89
Von Recklinghausen
  disease (neurofibromatosis) Q85.01
    bones E21.0
Von Schroetter's syndrome I82.890
Von Willebrand (-Jurgens)(-Minot) **disease or syn-
  drome** D68.0
Von Zumbusch's disease L40.1
Voyeurism F65.3
Vrolik's disease Q78.0
Vulva — *see* condition
Vulvismus N94.2
Vulvitis (acute) (allergic) (atrophic) (hypertrophic) (intertriginous) (senile) N76.2
  with ectopic or molar pregnancy O08.0
  adhesive, congenital Q52.79
  blennorrhagic (gonococcal) A54.02
  candidal B37.3
  chlamydial A56.02
  due to Haemophilus ducreyi A57
  following ectopic or molar pregnancy O08.0
  gonococcal A54.02
    with abscess (accessory gland) (periurethral) A54.1
  herpesviral A60.04
  leukoplakic N90.4
  monilial B37.3
  puerperal (postpartum) O86.19
  subacute or chronic N76.3
  syphilitic (early) A51.0
    late A52.76
  trichomonal A59.01
  tuberculous A18.18
Vulvodynia N94.819
  specified NEC N94.818
Vulvorectal — *see* condition
Vulvovaginitis (acute) — *see* Vaginitis

W

Waiting list, person on Z75.1
  for organ transplant Z76.82
  undergoing social agency investigation Z75.2
Waldenström
  hypergammaglobulinemia D89.0
  syndrome or macroglobulinemia C88.0
Waldenström-Kjellberg syndrome D50.1
Walking
  difficulty R26.2
    psychogenic F44.4
  sleep F51.3
    hysterical F44.89
Wall, abdominal — *see* condition
Wallenberg's disease or syndrome G46.3
Wallgren's disease I87.8
Wandering
  gallbladder, congenital Q44.1
  in diseases classified elsewhere Z91.83

▽ **Subterms under main terms may continue to next column or page**   ☑ **Additional Character Required — Refer to the Tabular List for Character Selection**   **325**

Vertigo — Wandering

Wandering — *continued*
- kidney, congenital Q63.8
- organ or site, congenital NEC — *see* Malposition, congenital, by site
- pacemaker (heart) I49.8
- spleen D73.89

War neurosis F48.8

Wart (due to HPV) (filiform) (infectious) (viral) B07.9
- anogenital region (venereal) A63.0
- common B07.8
- external genital organs (venereal) A63.0
- flat B07.8
- Hassal-Henle's (of cornea) H18.49
- Peruvian A44.1
- plantar B07.0
- prosector (tuberculous) A18.4
- seborrheic L82.1
    - inflamed L82.0
- senile (seborrheic) L82.1
    - inflamed L82.0
- tuberculous A18.4
- venereal A63.0

Warthin's tumor — *see* Neoplasm, salivary gland, benign

Wassilieff's disease A27.0

Wasting
- disease R64
    - due to malnutrition E41
- extreme (due to malnutrition) E41
- muscle NEC — *see* Atrophy, muscle

Water
- clefts (senile cataract) — *see* Cataract, senile, incipient
- deprivation of T73.1 ☑
- intoxication E87.79
- itch B76.9
- lack of T73.1 ☑
- loading E87.70
- on
    - brain — *see* Hydrocephalus
    - chest J94.8
- poisoning E87.79

Waterbrash R12

Waterhouse (-Friderichsen) **syndrome or disease** (meningococcal) A39.1

Water-losing nephritis N25.89

Watermelon stomach K31.819
- with hemorrhage K31.811
- without hemorrhage K31.819

Watsoniasis B66.8

Wax in ear — *see* Impaction, cerumen

Weak, weakening, weakness (generalized) R53.1
- arches (acquired) (*see also* Deformity, limb, flat foot)
- bladder (sphincter) R32
- facial R29.810
    - following
        - cerebrovascular disease I69.992
            - cerebral infarction I69.392
            - intracerebral hemorrhage I69.192
            - nontraumatic intracranial hemorrhage NEC I69.292
            - specified disease NEC I69.892
            - stroke I69.392
            - subarachnoid hemorrhage I69.092
- foot (double) — *see* Weak, arches
- heart, cardiac — *see* Failure, heart
- mind F70
- muscle M62.81
- myocardium — *see* Failure, heart
- newborn P96.89
- pelvic fundus N81.89
- pubocervical tissue N81.82
- rectovaginal tissue N81.83
- senile R54
- urinary stream R39.12
- valvular — *see* Endocarditis

Wear, worn (with normal or routine use)
- articular bearing surface of internal joint prosthesis — *see* Complications, joint prosthesis, mechanical, wear of articular bearing surfaces, by site
- device, implant or graft — *see* Complications, by site, mechanical complication
- tooth, teeth (approximal) (hard tissues) (interproximal) (occlusal) K03.0

Weather, weathered
- effects of
    - cold T69.9 ☑
        - specified effect NEC T69.8 ☑
    - hot — *see* Heat
- skin L57.8

Weaver's syndrome Q87.3

Web, webbed (congenital)
- duodenal Q43.8
- esophagus Q39.4
- fingers Q70.1- ☑
- larynx (glottic) (subglottic) Q31.0
- neck (pterygium colli) Q18.3
- Paterson-Kelly D50.1
- popliteal syndrome Q87.89
- toes Q70.3- ☑

Weber-Christian disease M35.6

Weber-Cockayne syndrome (epidermolysis bullosa) Q81.8

Weber-Gubler syndrome G46.3

Weber-Leyden syndrome G46.3

Weber-Osler syndrome I78.0

Weber's paralysis or syndrome G46.3

Wedge-shaped or wedging vertebra — *see* Collapse, vertebra NEC

Wegener's granulomatosis or syndrome M31.30
- with
    - kidney involvement M31.31
    - lung involvement M31.30
        - with kidney involvement M31.31

Wegner's disease A50.02

Weight
- 1000-2499 grams at birth (low) — *see* Low, birthweight
- 999 grams or less at birth (extremely low) — *see* Low, birthweight, extreme
- and length below 10th percentile for gestational age P05.1- ☑
- below but length above 10th percentile for gestational age P05.0- ☑
- gain (abnormal) (excessive) R63.5
    - in pregnancy — *see* Pregnancy, complicated by, excessive weight gain
    - low — *see* Pregnancy, complicated by, insufficient, weight gain
- loss (abnormal) (cause unknown) R63.4

Weightlessness (effect of) T75.82 ☑

Weil (I)-**Marchesani syndrome** Q87.1

Weil's disease A27.0

Weingarten's syndrome J82

Weir Mitchell's disease I73.81

Weiss-Baker syndrome G90.09

Wells' disease L98.3

Wen — *see* Cyst, sebaceous

Wenckebach's block or phenomenon I44.1

Werdnig-Hoffmann syndrome (muscular atrophy) G12.0

Werlhof's disease D69.3

Wermer's disease or syndrome E31.21

Werner-His disease A79.0

Werner's disease or syndrome E34.8

Wernicke-Korsakoff's syndrome or psychosis (alcoholic) F10.96
- with dependence F10.26
- drug-induced
    - due to drug abuse — *see* Abuse, drug, by type, with amnestic disorder
    - due to drug dependence — *see* Dependence, drug, by type, with amnestic disorder
- nonalcoholic F04

Wernicke-Posadas disease B38.9

Wernicke's
- developmental aphasia F80.2
- disease or syndrome E51.2
- encephalopathy E51.2
- polioencephalitis, superior E51.2

West African fever B50.8

Westphal-Strümpell syndrome E83.01

West's syndrome — *see* Epilepsy, spasms

Wet
- feet, tropical (maceration) (syndrome) — *see* Immersion, foot
- lung (syndrome), newborn P22.1

Wharton's duct — *see* condition

Wheal — *see* Urticaria

Wheezing R06.2

Whiplash injury S13.4 ☑

Whipple's disease (*see also* subcategory M14.8-) K90.81

Whipworm (disease) (infection) (infestation) B79

Whistling face Q87.0

White (*see also* condition)
- kidney, small N03.9
- leg, puerperal, postpartum, childbirth O87.1

White — *continued*
- mouth B37.0
- patches of mouth K13.29
- spot lesions, teeth
    - chewing surface K02.51
    - pit and fissure surface K02.51
    - smooth surface K02.61

Whitehead L70.0

Whitlow (*see also* Cellulitis, digit)
- with lymphangitis — *see* Lymphangitis, acute, digit
- herpesviral B00.89

Whitmore's disease or fever — *see* Melioidosis

Whooping cough A37.90
- with pneumonia A37.91
    - due to Bordetella
        - bronchiseptica A37.81
        - parapertussis A37.11
        - pertussis A37.01
    - specified organism NEC A37.81
- due to
    - Bordetella
        - bronchiseptica A37.80
            - with pneumonia A37.81
        - parapertussis A37.10
            - with pneumonia A37.11
        - pertussis A37.00
            - with pneumonia A37.01
    - specified NEC A37.80
        - with pneumonia A37.81

Wichman's asthma J38.5

Wide cranial sutures, newborn P96.3

Widening aorta — *see* Ectasia, aorta
- with aneurysm — *see* Aneurysm, aorta

Wilkie's disease or syndrome K55.1

Wilkinson-Sneddon disease or syndrome L13.1

Willebrand (-Jürgens) **thrombopathy** D68.0

Willige-Hunt disease or syndrome G23.1

Wilms' tumor C64- ☑

Wilson-Mikity syndrome P27.0

Wilson's
- disease or syndrome E83.01
- hepatolenticular degeneration E83.01
- lichen ruber L43.9

Window (*see also* Imperfect, closure)
- aorticopulmonary Q21.4

Winter — *see* condition

Wiskott-Aldrich syndrome D82.0

Withdrawal state (*see also* Dependence, drug by type, with withdrawal)
- alcohol
    - with perceptual disturbances F10.232
    - without perceptual disturbances F10.239
- caffeine F15.93
- cannabis F12.288
- newborn
    - correct therapeutic substance properly administered P96.2
    - infant of dependent mother P96.1
- therapeutic substance, neonatal P96.2

Witts' anemia D50.8

Witzelsucht F07.0

Woakes' ethmoiditis or syndrome J33.1

Wolff-Hirschorn syndrome Q93.3

Wolff-Parkinson-White syndrome I45.6

Wolhynian fever A79.0

Wolman's disease E75.5

Wood lung or pneumonitis J67.8

Woolly, wooly hair (congenital) (nevus) Q84.1

Woolsorter's disease A22.1

Word
- blindness (congenital) (developmental) F81.0
- deafness (congenital) (developmental) H93.25

Worm(s) (infection) (infestation) (*see also* Infestation, helminth)
- guinea B72
- in intestine NEC B82.0

Worm-eaten soles A66.3

Worn out — *see* Exhaustion
- cardiac
    - defibrillator (with synchronous cardiace pacemaker) Z45.02
    - pacemaker
        - battery Z45.010
        - lead Z45.018
    - device, implant or graft — *see* Complications, by site, mechanical

Worried well Z71.1

Worries R45.82

Wound check Z48.0- ☑
    due to injury — *code to* Injury, by site, using appropriate seventh character for subsequent encounter
Wound, open T14.8- ☑
    abdomen, abdominal
        wall S31.109 ☑
            with penetration into peritoneal cavity S31.609 ☑
            bite — *see* Bite, abdomen, wall
            epigastric region S31.102 ☑
                with penetration into peritoneal cavity S31.602 ☑
                bite — *see* Bite, abdomen, wall, epigastric region
                laceration — *see* Laceration, abdomen, wall, epigastric region
                puncture — *see* Puncture, abdomen, wall, epigastric region
            laceration — *see* Laceration, abdomen, wall
            left
                lower quadrant S31.104 ☑
                    with penetration into peritoneal cavity S31.604 ☑
                    bite — *see* Bite, abdomen, wall, left, lower quadrant
                    laceration — *see* Laceration, abdomen, wall, left, lower quadrant
                    puncture — *see* Puncture, abdomen, wall, left, lower quadrant
                upper quadrant S31.101 ☑
                    with penetration into peritoneal cavity S31.601 ☑
                    bite — *see* Bite, abdomen, wall, left, upper quadrant
                    laceration — *see* Laceration, abdomen, wall, left, upper quadrant
                    puncture — *see* Puncture, abdomen, wall, left, upper quadrant
            periumbilic region S31.105 ☑
                with penetration into peritoneal cavity S31.605 ☑
                bite — *see* Bite, abdomen, wall, periumbilic region
                laceration — *see* Laceration, abdomen, wall, periumbilic region
                puncture — *see* Puncture, abdomen, wall, periumbilic region
            puncture — *see* Puncture, abdomen, wall
            right
                lower quadrant S31.103 ☑
                    with penetration into peritoneal cavity S31.603 ☑
                    bite — *see* Bite, abdomen, wall, right, lower quadrant
                    laceration — *see* Laceration, abdomen, wall, right, lower quadrant
                    puncture — *see* Puncture, abdomen, wall, right, lower quadrant
                upper quadrant S31.100 ☑
                    with penetration into peritoneal cavity S31.600 ☑
                    bite — *see* Bite, abdomen, wall, right, upper quadrant
                    laceration — *see* Laceration, abdomen, wall, right, upper quadrant
                    puncture — *see* Puncture, abdomen, wall, right, upper quadrant
    alveolar (process) — *see* Wound, open, oral cavity
    ankle S91.00- ☑
        bite — *see* Bite, ankle
        laceration — *see* Laceration, ankle
        puncture — *see* Puncture, ankle
    antecubital space — *see* Wound, open, elbow
    anterior chamber, eye — *see* Wound, open, ocular
    anus S31.839 ☑
        bite S31.835 ☑
        laceration — *see* Laceration, anus
        puncture — *see* Puncture, anus
    arm (upper) S41.10- ☑
        with amputation — *see* Amputation, traumatic, arm
        bite — *see* Bite, arm
        forearm — *see* Wound, open, forearm
        laceration — *see* Laceration, arm
        puncture — *see* Puncture, arm
    auditory canal (external) (meatus) — *see* Wound, open, ear

Wound, open — *continued*
    auricle, ear — *see* Wound, open, ear
    axilla — *see* Wound, open, arm
    back (*see also* Wound, open, thorax, back)
        lower S31.000 ☑
            with penetration into retroperitoneal space S31.001 ☑
            bite — *see* Bite, back, lower
            laceration — *see* Laceration, back, lower
            puncture — *see* Puncture, back, lower
    bite — *see* Bite
    blood vessel — *see* Injury, blood vessel
    breast S21.00- ☑
        with amputation — *see* Amputation, traumatic, breast
        bite — *see* Bite, breast
        laceration — *see* Laceration, breast
        puncture — *see* Puncture, breast
    buttock S31.809 ☑
        bite — *see* Bite, buttock
        laceration — *see* Laceration, buttock
        left S31.829 ☑
        puncture — *see* Puncture, buttock
        right S31.819 ☑
    calf — *see* Wound, open, leg
    canaliculus lacrimalis — *see* Wound, open, eyelid
    canthus, eye — *see* Wound, open, eyelid
    cervical esophagus S11.20 ☑
        bite S11.25 ☑
        laceration — *see* Laceration, esophagus, traumatic, cervical
        puncture — *see* Puncture, cervical esophagus
    cheek (external) S01.40- ☑
        bite — *see* Bite, cheek
        internal — *see* Wound, open, oral cavity
        laceration — *see* Laceration, cheek
        puncture — *see* Puncture, cheek
    chest wall — *see* Wound, open, thorax
    chin — *see* Wound, open, head, specified site NEC
    choroid — *see* Wound, open, ocular
    ciliary body (eye) — *see* Wound, open, ocular
    clitoris S31.40 ☑
        with amputation — *see* Amputation, traumatic, clitoris
        bite S31.45 ☑
        laceration — *see* Laceration, vulva
        puncture — *see* Puncture, vulva
    conjunctiva — *see* Wound, open, ocular
    cornea — *see* Wound, open, ocular
    costal region — *see* Wound, open, thorax
    Descemet's membrane — *see* Wound, open, ocular
    digit(s)
        foot — *see* Wound, open, toe
        hand — *see* Wound, open, finger
    ear (canal) (external) S01.30- ☑
        with amputation — *see* Amputation, traumatic, ear
        bite — *see* Bite, ear
        drum S09.2- ☑
        laceration — *see* Laceration, ear
        puncture — *see* Puncture, ear
    elbow S51.00- ☑
        bite — *see* Bite, elbow
        laceration — *see* Laceration, elbow
        puncture — *see* Puncture, elbow
    epididymis — *see* Wound, open, testis
    epigastric region S31.102 ☑
        with penetration into peritoneal cavity S31.602 ☑
        bite — *see* Bite, abdomen, wall, epigastric region
        laceration — *see* Laceration, abdomen, wall, epigastric region
        puncture — *see* Puncture, abdomen, wall, epigastric region
    epiglottis — *see* Wound, open, neck, specified site NEC
    esophagus (thoracic) S27.819 ☑
        cervical — *see* Wound, open, cervical esophagus
        laceration S27.813 ☑
        specified type NEC S27.818 ☑
    eye — *see* Wound, open, ocular
    eyeball — *see* Wound, open, ocular
    eyebrow — *see* Wound, open, eyelid
    eyelid S01.10- ☑
        bite — *see* Bite, eyelid
        laceration — *see* Laceration, eyelid
        puncture — *see* Puncture, eyelid

Wound, open — *continued*
    face NEC — *see* Wound, open, head, specified site NEC
    finger(s) S61.209 ☑
        with
            amputation — *see* Amputation, traumatic, finger
            damage to nail S61.309 ☑
        bite — *see* Bite, finger
        index S61.208 ☑
            with
                damage to nail S61.308 ☑
            left S61.201 ☑
                with
                    damage to nail S61.301 ☑
            right S61.200 ☑
                with
                    damage to nail S61.300 ☑
        laceration — *see* Laceration, finger
        little S61.208 ☑
            with
                damage to nail S61.308 ☑
            left S61.207 ☑
                with damage to nail S61.307 ☑
            right S61.206 ☑
                with damage to nail S61.306 ☑
        middle S61.208 ☑
            with
                damage to nail S61.308 ☑
            left S61.203 ☑
                with damage to nail S61.303 ☑
            right S61.202 ☑
                with damage to nail S61.302 ☑
        puncture — *see* Puncture, finger
        ring S61.208 ☑
            with
                damage to nail S61.308 ☑
            left S61.205 ☑
                with damage to nail S61.305 ☑
            right S61.204 ☑
                with damage to nail S61.304 ☑
    flank — *see* Wound, open, abdomen, wall
    foot (except toe(s) alone) S91.30- ☑
        with amputation — *see* Amputation, traumatic, foot
        bite — *see* Bite, foot
        laceration — *see* Laceration, foot
        puncture — *see* Puncture, foot
        toe — *see* Wound, open, toe
    forearm S51.80- ☑
        with
            amputation — *see* Amputation, traumatic, forearm
        bite — *see* Bite, forearm
        elbow only — *see* Wound, open, elbow
        laceration — *see* Laceration, forearm
        puncture — *see* Puncture, forearm
    forehead — *see* Wound, open, head, specified site NEC
    genital organs, external
        with amputation — *see* Amputation, traumatic, genital organs
        bite — *see* Bite, genital organ
        female S31.502 ☑
            vagina S31.40 ☑
            vulva S31.40 ☑
        laceration — *see* Laceration, genital organ
        male S31.501 ☑
            penis S31.20 ☑
            scrotum S31.30 ☑
            testes S31.30 ☑
        puncture — *see* Puncture, genital organ
    globe (eye) — *see* Wound, open, ocular
    groin — *see* Wound, open, abdomen, wall
    gum — *see* Wound, open, oral cavity
    hand S61.40- ☑
        with
            amputation — *see* Amputation, traumatic, hand
        bite — *see* Bite, hand
        finger(s) — *see* Wound, open, finger
        laceration — *see* Laceration, hand
        puncture — *see* Puncture, hand
        thumb — *see* Wound, open, thumb
    head S01.90 ☑
        bite — *see* Bite, head
        cheek — *see* Wound, open, cheek
        ear — *see* Wound, open, ear

☑ Additional Character Required — Refer to the Tabular List for Character Selection   ▽ Subterms under main terms may continue to next column or page

Wound, open — *continued*
thorax, thoracic — *continued*
back — *continued*
with penetration S21.40 ☑
bite — *see* Bite, thorax
breast — *see* Wound, open, breast
front S21.10- ☑
with penetration S21.30 ☑
laceration — *see* Laceration, thorax
puncture — *see* Puncture, thorax
throat — *see* Wound, open, neck
thumb S61.009 ☑
with
amputation — *see* Amputation, traumatic, thumb
damage to nail S61.109 ☑
bite — *see* Bite, thumb
laceration — *see* Laceration, thumb
left S61.002 ☑
with
damage to nail S61.102 ☑
puncture — *see* Puncture, thumb
right S61.001 ☑
with
damage to nail S61.101 ☑
thyroid (gland) — *see* Wound, open, neck, thyroid
toe(s) S91.109 ☑
with
amputation — *see* Amputation, traumatic, toe
damage to nail S91.209 ☑
bite — *see* Bite, toe
great S91.103 ☑
with
damage to nail S91.203 ☑
left S91.102 ☑
with
damage to nail S91.202 ☑
right S91.101 ☑
with
damage to nail S91.201 ☑
laceration — *see* Laceration, toe
lesser S91.106 ☑
with
damage to nail S91.206 ☑
left S91.105 ☑
with
damage to nail S91.205 ☑
right S91.104 ☑
with
damage to nail S91.204 ☑
puncture — *see* Puncture, toe
tongue — *see* Wound, open, oral cavity
trachea (cervical region) — *see* Wound, open, neck, trachea
tunica vaginalis — *see* Wound, open, testis
tympanum, tympanic membrane S09.2- ☑
laceration — *see* Laceration, ear, drum
puncture — *see* Puncture, tympanum
umbilical region — *see* Wound, open, abdomen, wall, periumbilic region
uvula — *see* Wound, open, oral cavity
vagina S31.40 ☑
bite S31.45 ☑
laceration — *see* Laceration, vagina
puncture — *see* Puncture, vagina
vitreous (humor) — *see* Wound, open, ocular
vocal cord S11.039 ☑
bite — *see* Bite, vocal cord
laceration S11.031 ☑
with foreign body S11.032 ☑
puncture S11.033 ☑
with foreign body S11.034 ☑
vulva S31.40 ☑
with amputation — *see* Amputation, traumatic, vulva
bite S31.45 ☑
laceration — *see* Laceration, vulva
puncture — *see* Puncture, vulva
wrist S61.50- ☑
bite — *see* Bite, wrist
laceration — *see* Laceration, wrist
puncture — *see* Puncture, wrist
Wound, superficial — *see* Injury (*see also* specified injury type)

Wright's syndrome G54.0
Wrist — *see* condition
Wrong drug (by accident) (given in error) — *see* Table of Drugs and Chemicals, by drug, poisoning
Wry neck — *see* Torticollis
Wuchereria (bancrofti) **infestation** B74.0
Wuchereriasis B74.0
Wuchernde Struma Langhans C73

X

Xanthelasma (eyelid) (palpebrarum) H02.60
left H02.66
lower H02.65
upper H02.64
right H02.63
lower H02.62
upper H02.61
Xanthelasmatosis (essential) E78.2
Xanthinuria, hereditary E79.8
Xanthoastrocytoma
specified site — *see* Neoplasm, malignant, by site
unspecified site C71.9
Xanthofibroma — *see* Neoplasm, connective tissue, benign
Xanthogranuloma D76.3
Xanthoma(s), xanthomatosis (primary) (familial) (hereditary) E75.5
with
hyperlipoproteinemia
Type I E78.3
Type III E78.2
Type IV E78.1
Type V E78.3
bone (generalisata) C96.5
cerebrotendinous E75.5
cutaneotendinous E75.5
disseminatum (skin) E78.2
eruptive E78.2
hypercholesterinemic E78.00
hypercholesterolemic E78.00
hyperlipidemic E78.5
joint E75.5
multiple (skin) E78.2
tendon (sheath) E75.5
tuberosum E78.2
tuberous E78.2
tubo-eruptive E78.2
verrucous, oral mucosa K13.4
Xanthosis R23.8
Xenophobia F40.10
Xeroderma (*see also* Ichthyosis)
acquired L85.0
eyelid H01.149
left H01.146
lower H01.145
upper H01.144
right H01.143
lower H01.142
upper H01.141
pigmentosum Q82.1
vitamin A deficiency E50.8
Xerophthalmia (vitamin A deficiency) E50.7
unrelated to vitamin A deficiency — *see* Keratoconjunctivitis
Xerosis
conjunctiva H11.14- ☑
with Bitot's spots (*see also* Pigmentation, conjunctiva)
vitamin A deficiency E50.1
vitamin A deficiency E50.0
cornea H18.89- ☑
with ulceration — *see* Ulcer, cornea
vitamin A deficiency E50.3
vitamin A deficiency E50.2
cutis L85.3
skin L85.3
Xerostomia K11.7
Xiphopagus Q89.4
XO syndrome Q96.9
X-ray (of)
abnormal findings — *see* Abnormal, diagnostic imaging
breast (mammogram) (routine) Z12.31

X-ray — *continued*
chest
routine (as part of a general medical examination) Z00.00
with abnormal findings Z00.01
routine (as part of a general medical examination) Z00.00
with abnormal findings Z00.01
XXXXY syndrome Q98.1
XXY syndrome Q98.0

Y

Yaba pox (virus disease) B08.72
Yatapoxvirus B08.70
specified NEC B08.79
Yawning R06.89
psychogenic F45.8
Yaws A66.9
cutaneous, less than five years after infection A66.2
bone lesions A66.6
butter A66.1
chancre A66.0
early (cutaneous) (macular) (maculopapular) (micropapular) (papular) A66.2
frambeside A66.2
skin lesions NEC A66.2
eyelid A66.2
ganglion A66.6
gangosis, gangosa A66.5
gumma, gummata A66.4
bone A66.6
gummatous
frambeside A66.4
osteitis A66.6
periostitis A66.6
hydrarthrosis (*see also* subcategory M14.8-) A66.6
hyperkeratosis (early) (late) A66.3
initial lesions A66.0
joint lesions (*see also* subcategory M14.8-) A66.6
juxta-articular nodules A66.7
late nodular (ulcerated) A66.4
latent (without clinical manifestations) (with positive serology) A66.8
mother A66.0
mucosal A66.7
multiple papillomata A66.1
nodular, late (ulcerated) A66.4
osteitis A66.6
papilloma, plantar or palmar A66.1
periostitis (hypertrophic) A66.6
specified NEC A66.7
ulcers A66.4
wet crab A66.1
Yeast infection (*see also* Candidiasis) B37.9
Yellow
atrophy (liver) — *see* Failure, hepatic
fever — *see* Fever, yellow
jack — *see* Fever, yellow
jaundice — *see* Jaundice
nail syndrome L60.5
Yersiniosis (*see also* Infection, Yersinia)
extraintestinal A28.2
intestinal A04.6

Z

Zahorsky's syndrome (herpangina) B08.5
Zellweger's syndrome Q87.89
Zenker's diverticulum (esophagus) K22.5
Ziehen-Oppenheim disease G24.1
Zieve's syndrome K70.0
Zika NOS A92.5
Zinc
deficiency, dietary E60
metabolism disorder E83.2
Zollinger-Ellison syndrome E16.4
Zona — *see* Herpes, zoster
Zoophobia F40.218
Zoster (herpes) — *see* Herpes, zoster
Zygomycosis B46.9
specified NEC B46.8
Zymotic — *see* condition

Wound, open — Zymotic

☟ Subterms under main terms may continue to next column or page   ☑ Additional Character Required — Refer to the Tabular List for Character Selection   329

	Malignant Primary	Malignant Secondary	Ca in situ	Benign	Uncertain	Unspecified Behavior

Note: The list below gives the code number for neoplasms by anatomical site. For each site there are six possible code numbers according to whether the neoplasm in question is malignant, benign, in situ, of uncertain behavior, or of unspecified nature. The description of the neoplasm will often indicate which of the six columns is appropriate; e.g., malignant melanoma of skin, benign fibroadenoma of breast, carcinoma in situ of cervix uteri. Where such descriptors are not present, the remainder of the Index should be consulted where guidance is given to the appropriate column for each morphological (histological) variety listed; e.g., Mesonephroma – see Neoplasm, malignant; Embryoma (see also Neoplasm, uncertain behavior); Disease, Bowen's – see Neoplasm, skin, in situ. However, the guidance in the Index can be overridden if one of the descriptors mentioned above is present; e.g., malignant adenoma of colon is coded to C18.9 and not to D12.6 as the adjective "malignant" overrides the Index entry "Adenoma (see also Neoplasm, benign, by site)." Codes listed with a dash -, following the code have a required additional character for laterality. The tabular list must be reviewed for the complete code.

	Malignant Primary	Malignant Secondary	Ca in situ	Benign	Uncertain	Unspecified Behavior
Neoplasm, neoplastic	C80.1	C79.9	D09.9	D36.9	D48.9	D49.9
abdomen, abdominal	C76.2	C79.8-☑	D09.8	D36.7	D48.7	D49.89
cavity	C76.2	C79.8-☑	D09.8	D36.7	D48.7	D49.89
organ	C76.2	C79.8-☑	D09.8	D36.7	D48.7	D49.89
viscera	C76.2	C79.8-☑	D09.8	D36.7	D48.7	D49.89
wall — *see also* Neoplasm, abdomen, wall, skin	C44.509	C79.2	D04.5	D23.5	D48.5	D49.2
connective tissue	C49.4	C79.8-☑	—	D21.4	D48.1	D49.2
skin	C44.509	—	—	—	—	—
basal cell carcinoma	C44.519	—	—	—	—	—
specified type NEC	C44.599	—	—	—	—	—
squamous cell carcinoma	C44.529	—	—	—	—	—
abdominopelvic	C76.8	C79.8-☑	—	D36.7	D48.7	D49.89
accessory sinus — *see* Neoplasm, sinus						
acoustic nerve	C72.4-☑	C79.49	—	D33.3	D43.3	D49.7
adenoid (pharynx) (tissue)	C11.1	C79.89	D00.08	D10.6	D37.05	D49.0
adipose tissue — *see also* Neoplasm, connective tissue	C49.4	C79.89	—	D21.9	D48.1	D49.2
adnexa (uterine)	C57.4	C79.89	D07.39	D28.7	D39.8	D49.59
adrenal	C74.9-☑	C79.7-☑	D09.3	D35.0-☑	D44.1-☑	D49.7
capsule	C74.9-☑	C79.7-☑	D09.3	D35.0-☑	D44.1-☑	D49.7
cortex	C74.0-☑	C79.7-☑	D09.3	D35.0-☑	D44.1-☑	D49.7
gland	C74.9-☑	C79.7-☑	D09.3	D35.0-☑	D44.1-☑	D49.7
medulla	C74.1-☑	C79.7-☑	D09.3	D35.0-☑	D44.1-☑	D49.7
ala nasi (external) — *see also* Neoplasm, skin, nose	C44.301	C79.2	D04.39	D23.39	D48.5	D49.2
alimentary canal or tract NEC	C26.9	C78.80	D01.9	D13.9	D37.9	D49.0
alveolar	C03.9	C79.89	D00.03	D10.39	D37.09	D49.0
mucosa	C03.9	C79.89	D00.03	D10.39	D37.09	D49.0
lower	C03.1	C79.89	D00.03	D10.39	D37.09	D49.0
upper	C03.0	C79.89	D00.03	D10.39	D37.09	D49.0
ridge or process	C41.1	C79.51	—	D16.5	D48.0	D49.2
carcinoma	C03.9	C79.8-☑	—	—	—	—
lower	C03.1	C79.8-☑	—	—	—	—
upper	C03.0	C79.8-☑	—	—	—	—
lower	C41.1	C79.51	—	D16.5	D48.0	D49.2
mucosa	C03.9	C79.89	D00.03	D10.39	D37.09	D49.0
lower	C03.1	C79.89	D00.03	D10.39	D37.09	D49.0
upper	C03.0	C79.89	D00.03	D10.39	D37.09	D49.0
upper	C41.0	C79.51	—	D16.4	D48.0	D49.2
sulcus	C06.1	C79.89	D00.02	D10.39	D37.09	D49.0
alveolus	C03.9	C79.89	D00.03	D10.39	D37.09	D49.0
lower	C03.1	C79.89	D00.03	D10.39	D37.09	D49.0
upper	C03.0	C79.89	D00.03	D10.39	D37.09	D49.0
ampulla of Vater	C24.1	C78.89	D01.5	D13.5	D37.6	D49.0
ankle NEC	C76.5-☑	C79.89	D04.7-☑	D36.7	D48.7	D49.89
anorectum, anorectal (junction)	C21.8	C78.5	D01.3	D12.9	D37.8	D49.0
antecubital fossa or space	C76.4-☑	C79.89	D04.6-☑	D36.7	D48.7	D49.89

	Malignant Primary	Malignant Secondary	Ca in situ	Benign	Uncertain	Unspecified Behavior
Neoplasm, neoplastic — *continued*						
antrum (Highmore) (maxillary)	C31.0	C78.39	D02.3	D14.0	D38.5	D49.1
pyloric	C16.3	C78.89	D00.2	D13.1	D37.1	D49.0
tympanicum	C30.1	C78.39	D02.3	D14.0	D38.5	D49.1
anus, anal	C21.0	C78.5	D01.3	D12.9	D37.8	D49.0
canal	C21.1	C78.5	D01.3	D12.9	D37.8	D49.0
cloacogenic zone	C21.2	C78.5	D01.3	D12.9	D37.8	D49.0
margin — *see also* Neoplasm, anus, skin	C44.500	C79.2	D04.5	D23.5	D48.5	D49.2
overlapping lesion with rectosigmoid junction or rectum	C21.8	—	—	—	—	—
skin	C44.500	C79.2	D04.5	D23.5	D48.5	D49.2
basal cell carcinoma	C44.510	—	—	—	—	—
specified type NEC	C44.590	—	—	—	—	—
squamous cell carcinoma	C44.520	—	—	—	—	—
sphincter	C21.1	C78.5	D01.3	D12.9	D37.8	D49.0
aorta (thoracic)	C49.3	C79.89	—	D21.3	D48.1	D49.2
abdominal	C49.4	C79.89	—	D21.4	D48.1	D49.2
aortic body	C75.5	C79.89	—	D35.6	D44.7	D49.7
aponeurosis	C49.9	C79.89	—	D21.9	D48.1	D49.2
palmar	C49.1-☑	C79.89	—	D21.1-☑	D48.1	D49.2
plantar	C49.2-☑	C79.89	—	D21.2-☑	D48.1	D49.2
appendix	C18.1	C78.5	D01.0	D12.1	D37.3	D49.0
arachnoid	C70.9	C79.49	—	D32.9	D42.9	D49.7
cerebral	C70.0	C79.32	—	D32.0	D42.0	D49.7
spinal	C70.1	C79.49	—	D32.1	D42.1	D49.7
areola	C50.0-☑	C79.81	D05-☑	D24-☑	D48.6-☑	D49.3
arm NEC	C76.4-☑	C79.89	D04.6-☑	D36.7	D48.7	D49.89
artery — *see* Neoplasm, connective tissue						
aryepiglottic fold	C13.1	C79.89	D00.08	D10.7	D37.05	D49.0
hypopharyngeal aspect	C13.1	C79.89	D00.08	D10.7	D37.05	D49.0
laryngeal aspect	C32.1	C78.39	D02.0	D14.1	D38.0	D49.1
marginal zone	C13.1	C79.89	D00.08	D10.7	D37.05	D49.0
arytenoid (cartilage)	C32.3	C78.39	D02.0	D14.1	D38.0	D49.1
fold — *see* Neoplasm, aryepiglottic						
associated with transplanted organ	C80.2	—	—	—	—	—
atlas	C41.2	C79.51	—	D16.6	D48.0	D49.2
atrium, cardiac	C38.0	C79.89	—	D15.1	D48.7	D49.89
auditory						
canal (external) (skin)	C44.20-☑	C79.2	D04.2-☑	D23.2-☑	D48.5	D49.2
internal	C30.1	C78.39	D02.3	D14.0	D38.5	D49.1
nerve	C72.4-☑	C79.49	—	D33.3	D43.3	D49.7
tube	C30.1	C78.39	D02.3	D14.0	D38.5	D49.1
opening	C11.2	C79.89	D00.08	D10.6	D37.05	D49.0
auricle, ear — *see also* Neoplasm, skin, ear	C44.20-☑	C79.2	D04.2-☑	D23.2-☑	D48.5	D49.2
auricular canal (external) — *see also* Neoplasm, skin, ear	C44.20-☑	C79.2	D04.2-☑	D23.2-☑	D48.5	D49.2
internal	C30.1	C78.39	D02.3	D14.0	D38.5	D49.2
autonomic nerve or nervous system NEC (see Neoplasm, nerve, peripheral)						
axilla, axillary	C76.1	C79.89	D09.8	D36.7	D48.7	D49.89
fold — *see also* Neoplasm, skin, trunk	C44.509	C79.2	D04.5	D23.5	D48.5	D49.2
back NEC	C76.8	C79.89	D04.5	D36.7	D48.7	D49.89
Bartholin's gland	C51.0	C79.82	D07.1	D28.0	D39.8	D49.59
basal ganglia	C71.0	C79.31	—	D33.0	D43.0	D49.6
basis pedunculi	C71.7	C79.31	—	D33.1	D43.1	D49.6
bile or biliary (tract)	C24.9	C78.89	D01.5	D13.5	D37.6	D49.0
canaliculi (biliferi) (intrahepatic)	C22.1	C78.7	D01.5	D13.4	D37.6	D49.0
canals, interlobular	C22.1	C78.89	D01.5	D13.4	D37.6	D49.0

Neoplasm Table
Neoplasm, bile or biliary — Neoplasm, brain NEC

Neoplasm, neoplastic — continued	Malignant Primary	Malignant Secondary	Ca in situ	Benign	Uncertain	Unspecified Behavior
bile or biliary — continued						
duct or passage (common) (cystic) (extrahepatic)	C24.0	C78.89	D01.5	D13.5	D37.6	D49.0
interlobular	C22.1	C78.89	D01.5	D13.4	D37.6	D49.0
intrahepatic	C22.1	C78.7	D01.5	D13.4	D37.6	D49.0
and extrahepatic	C24.8	C78.89	D01.5	D13.5	D37.6	D49.0
bladder (urinary)	C67.9	C79.11	D09.0	D30.3	D41.4	D49.4
dome	C67.1	C79.11	D09.0	D30.3	D41.4	D49.4
neck	C67.5	C79.11	D09.0	D30.3	D41.4	D49.4
orifice	C67.9	C79.11	D09.0	D30.3	D41.4	D49.4
ureteric	C67.6	C79.11	D09.0	D30.3	D41.4	D49.4
urethral	C67.5	C79.11	D09.0	D30.3	D41.4	D49.4
overlapping lesion	C67.8	—	—	—	—	—
sphincter	C67.8	C79.11	D09.0	D30.3	D41.4	D49.4
trigone	C67.0	C79.11	D09.0	D30.3	D41.4	D49.4
urachus	C67.7	C79.11	D09.0	D30.3	D41.4	D49.4
wall	C67.9	C79.11	D09.0	D30.3	D41.4	D49.4
anterior	C67.3	C79.11	D09.0	D30.3	D41.4	D49.4
lateral	C67.2	C79.11	D09.0	D30.3	D41.4	D49.4
posterior	C67.4	C79.11	D09.0	D30.3	D41.4	D49.4
blood vessel — see Neoplasm, connective tissue						
bone (periosteum)	C41.9	C79.51	—	D16.9	D48.0	D49.2
acetabulum	C41.4	C79.51	—	D16.8	D48.0	D49.2
ankle	C40.3-✓	C79.51	—	D16.3-✓	—	—
arm NEC	C40.0-✓	C79.51	—	D16.0-✓	—	—
astragalus	C40.3-✓	C79.51	—	D16.3-✓	—	—
atlas	C41.2	C79.51	—	D16.6	D48.0	D49.2
axis	C41.2	C79.51	—	D16.6	D48.0	D49.2
back NEC	C41.2	C79.51	—	D16.6	D48.0	D49.2
calcaneus	C40.3-✓	C79.51	—	D16.3-✓	—	—
calvarium	C41.0	C79.51	—	D16.4	D48.0	D49.2
carpus (any)	C40.1-✓	C79.51	—	D16.1-✓	—	—
cartilage NEC	C41.9	C79.51	—	D16.9	D48.0	D49.2
clavicle	C41.3	C79.51	—	D16.7	D48.0	D49.2
clivus	C41.0	C79.51	—	D16.4	D48.0	D49.2
coccygeal vertebra	C41.4	C79.51	—	D16.8	D48.0	D49.2
coccyx	C41.4	C79.51	—	D16.8	D48.0	D49.2
costal cartilage	C41.3	C79.51	—	D16.7	D48.0	D49.2
costovertebral joint	C41.3	C79.51	—	D16.7	D48.0	D49.2
cranial	C41.0	C79.51	—	D16.4	D48.0	D49.2
cuboid	C40.3-✓	C79.51	—	D16.3-✓	—	—
cuneiform	C41.9	C79.51	—	D16.9	D48.0	D49.2
elbow	C40.0-✓	C79.51	—	D16.0-✓	—	—
ethmoid (labyrinth)	C41.0	C79.51	—	D16.4	D48.0	D49.2
face	C41.0	C79.51	—	D16.4	D48.0	D49.2
femur (any part)	C40.2-✓	C79.51	—	D16.2-✓	—	—
fibula (any part)	C40.2-✓	C79.51	—	D16.2-✓	—	—
finger (any)	C40.1-✓	C79.51	—	D16.1-✓	—	—
foot	C40.3-✓	C79.51	—	D16.3-✓	—	—
forearm	C40.0-✓	C79.51	—	D16.0-✓	—	—
frontal	C41.0	C79.51	—	D16.4	D48.0	D49.2
hand	C40.1-✓	C79.51	—	D16.1-✓	—	—
heel	C40.3-✓	C79.51	—	D16.3-✓	—	—
hip	C41.4	C79.51	—	D16.8	D48.0	D49.2
humerus (any part)	C40.0-✓	C79.51	—	D16.0-✓	—	—
hyoid	C41.0	C79.51	—	D16.4	D48.0	D49.2
ilium	C41.4	C79.51	—	D16.8	D48.0	D49.2
innominate	C41.4	C79.51	—	D16.8	D48.0	D49.2
intervertebral cartilage or disc	C41.2	C79.51	—	D16.6	D48.0	D49.2
ischium	C41.4	C79.51	—	D16.8	D48.0	D49.2
jaw (lower)	C41.1	C79.51	—	D16.5	D48.0	D49.2
knee	C40.2-✓	C79.51	—	D16.2-✓	—	—
leg NEC	C40.2-✓	C79.51	—	D16.2-✓	—	—
limb NEC	C40.9-✓	C79.51	—	D16.9	—	—
lower (long bones)	C40.2-✓	C79.51	—	D16.2-✓	—	—
short bones	C40.3-✓	C79.51	—	D16.3-✓	—	—
upper (long bones)	C40.0-✓	C79.51	—	D16.0-✓	—	—
short bones	C40.1-✓	C79.51	—	D16.1-✓	—	—
malar	C41.0	C79.51	—	D16.4	D48.0	D49.2

Neoplasm, neoplastic — continued	Malignant Primary	Malignant Secondary	Ca in situ	Benign	Uncertain	Unspecified Behavior
bone — continued						
mandible	C41.1	C79.51	—	D16.5	D48.0	D49.2
marrow NEC (any bone)	C96.9	C79.52	—	—	D47.9	D49.89
mastoid	C41.0	C79.51	—	D16.4	D48.0	D49.2
maxilla, maxillary (superior)	C41.0	C79.51	—	D16.4	D48.0	D49.2
inferior	C41.1	C79.51	—	D16.5	D48.0	D49.2
metacarpus (any)	C40.1-✓	C79.51	—	D16.1-✓	—	—
metatarsus (any)	C40.3-✓	C79.51	—	D16.3-✓	—	—
navicular						
ankle	C40.3-✓	C79.51	—	—	—	—
hand	C40.1-✓	C79.51	—	—	—	—
nose, nasal	C41.0	C79.51	—	D16.4	D48.0	D49.2
occipital	C41.0	C79.51	—	D16.4	D48.0	D49.2
orbit	C41.0	C79.51	—	D16.4	D48.0	D49.2
overlapping sites	C40.8-✓	—	—	—	—	—
parietal	C41.0	C79.51	—	D16.4	D48.0	D49.2
patella	C40.2-✓	C79.51	—	—	—	—
pelvic	C41.4	C79.51	—	D16.8	D48.0	D49.2
phalanges						
foot	C40.3-✓	C79.51	—	—	—	—
hand	C40.1-✓	C79.51	—	—	—	—
pubic	C41.4	C79.51	—	D16.8	D48.0	D49.2
radius (any part)	C40.0-✓	C79.51	—	D16.0-✓	—	—
rib	C41.3	C79.51	—	D16.7	D48.0	D49.2
sacral vertebra	C41.4	C79.51	—	D16.8	D48.0	D49.2
sacrum	C41.4	C79.51	—	D16.8	D48.0	D49.2
scaphoid						
of ankle	C40.3-✓	C79.51	—	—	—	—
of hand	C40.1-✓	C79.51	—	—	—	—
scapula (any part)	C40.0-✓	C79.51	—	D16.0-✓	—	—
sella turcica	C41.0	C79.51	—	D16.4	D48.0	D49.2
shoulder	C40.0-✓	C79.51	—	D16.0-✓	—	—
skull	C41.0	C79.51	—	D16.4	D48.0	D49.2
sphenoid	C41.0	C79.51	—	D16.4	D48.0	D49.2
spine, spinal (column)	C41.2	C79.51	—	D16.6	D48.0	D49.2
coccyx	C41.4	C79.51	—	D16.8	D48.0	D49.2
sacrum	C41.4	C79.51	—	D16.8	D48.0	D49.2
sternum	C41.3	C79.51	—	D16.7	D48.0	D49.2
tarsus (any)	C40.3-✓	C79.51	—	—	—	—
temporal	C41.0	C79.51	—	D16.4	D48.0	D49.2
thumb	C40.1-✓	C79.51	—	—	—	—
tibia (any part)	C40.2-✓	C79.51	—	—	—	—
toe (any)	C40.3-✓	C79.51	—	—	—	—
trapezium	C40.1-✓	C79.51	—	—	—	—
trapezoid	C40.1-✓	C79.51	—	—	—	—
turbinate	C41.0	C79.51	—	D16.4	D48.0	D49.2
ulna (any part)	C40.0-✓	C79.51	—	D16.0-✓	—	—
unciform	C40.1-✓	C79.51	—	—	—	—
vertebra (column)	C41.2	C79.51	—	D16.6	D48.0	D49.2
coccyx	C41.4	C79.51	—	D16.8	D48.0	D49.2
sacrum	C41.4	C79.51	—	D16.8	D48.0	D49.2
vomer	C41.0	C79.51	—	D16.4	D48.0	D49.2
wrist	C40.1-✓	C79.51	—	—	—	—
xiphoid process	C41.3	C79.51	—	D16.7	D48.0	D49.2
zygomatic	C41.0	C79.51	—	D16.4	D48.0	D49.2
book-leaf (mouth) — ventral surface of tongue and floor of mouth	C06.89	C79.89	D00.00	D10.39	D37.09	D49.0
bowel — see Neoplasm, intestine						
brachial plexus	C47.1-✓	C79.89	—	D36.12	D48.2	D49.2
brain NEC	C71.9	C79.31	—	D33.2	D43.2	D49.6
basal ganglia	C71.0	C79.31	—	D33.0	D43.0	D49.6
cerebellopontine angle	C71.6	C79.31	—	D33.1	D43.1	D49.6
cerebellum NOS	C71.6	C79.31	—	D33.1	D43.1	D49.6
cerebrum	C71.0	C79.31	—	D33.0	D43.0	D49.6
choroid plexus	C71.7	C79.31	—	D33.1	D43.1	D49.6
corpus callosum	C71.8	C79.31	—	D33.2	D43.2	D49.6
corpus striatum	C71.0	C79.31	—	D33.0	D43.0	D49.6
cortex (cerebral)	C71.0	C79.31	—	D33.0	D43.0	D49.6
frontal lobe	C71.1	C79.31	—	D33.0	D43.0	D49.6
globus pallidus	C71.0	C79.31	—	D33.0	D43.0	D49.6
hippocampus	C71.2	C79.31	—	D33.0	D43.0	D49.6
hypothalamus	C71.0	C79.31	—	D33.0	D43.0	D49.6
internal capsule	C71.0	C79.31	—	D33.0	D43.0	D49.6

✓ Additional Character Required — Refer to the Tabular List for Character Selection   ▽ Subterms under main terms may continue to next column or page

Neoplasm, neoplastic — continued	Malignant Primary	Malignant Secondary	Ca in situ	Benign	Uncertain	Unspecified Behavior
brain — continued						
medulla						
oblongata	C71.7	C79.31	—	D33.1	D43.1	D49.6
meninges	C70.0	C79.32	—	D32.0	D42.0	D49.7
midbrain	C71.7	C79.31	—	D33.1	D43.1	D49.6
occipital lobe	C71.4	C79.31	—	D33.0	D43.0	D49.6
overlapping lesion	C71.8	C79.31	—	—	—	—
parietal lobe	C71.3	C79.31	—	D33.0	D43.0	D49.6
peduncle	C71.7	C79.31	—	D33.1	D43.1	D49.6
pons	C71.7	C79.31	—	D33.1	D43.1	D49.6
stem	C71.7	C79.31	—	D33.1	D43.1	D49.6
tapetum	C71.8	C79.31	—	D33.2	D43.2	D49.6
temporal lobe	C71.2	C79.31	—	D33.0	D43.0	D49.6
thalamus	C71.0	C79.31	—	D33.0	D43.0	D49.6
uncus	C71.2	C79.31	—	D33.0	D43.0	D49.6
ventricle (floor)	C71.5	C79.31	—	D33.0	D43.0	D49.6
fourth	C71.7	C79.31	—	D33.1	D43.1	D49.6
branchial (cleft) (cyst) (vestiges)	C10.4	C79.89	D00.08	D10.5	D37.05	D49.0
breast (connective tissue) (glandular tissue) (soft parts)	C50.9-☑	C79.81	D05.-☑	D24.-☑	D48.6-☑	D49.3
areola	C50.0-☑	C79.81	D05.-☑	D24.-☑	D48.6-☑	D49.3
axillary tail	C50.6-☑	C79.81	D05.-☑	D24.-☑	D48.6-☑	D49.3
central portion	C50.1-☑	C79.81	D05.-☑	D24.-☑	D48.6-☑	D49.3
inner	C50.8-☑	C79.81	D05.-☑	D24.-☑	D48.6-☑	D49.3
lower	C50.8-☑	C79.81	D05.-☑	D24.-☑	D48.6-☑	D49.3
lower-inner quadrant	C50.3-☑	C79.81	D05.-☑	D24.-☑	D48.6-☑	D49.3
lower-outer quadrant	C50.5-☑	C79.81	D05.-☑	D24.-☑	D48.6-☑	D49.3
mastectomy site (skin) — see also Neoplasm, breast, skin	C44.501	C79.2	—	—	—	—
specified as breast tissue	C50.8-☑	C79.81	—	—	—	—
midline	C50.8-☑	C79.81	D05.-☑	D24.-☑	D48.6-☑	D49.3
nipple	C50.0-☑	C79.81	D05.-☑	D24.-☑	D48.6-☑	D49.3
outer	C50.8-☑	C79.81	D05.-☑	D24.-☑	D48.6-☑	D49.3
overlapping lesion	C50.8-☑					
skin	C44.501	C79.2	D04.5	D23.5	D48.5	D49.2
basal cell carcinoma	C44.511	—	—	—	—	—
specified type NEC	C44.591	—	—	—	—	—
squamous cell carcinoma	C44.521	—	—	—	—	—
tail (axillary)	C50.6-☑	C79.81	D05.-☑	D24.-☑	D48.6-☑	D49.3
upper	C50.8-☑	C79.81	D05.-☑	D24.-☑	D48.6-☑	D49.3
upper-inner quadrant	C50.2-☑	C79.81	D05.-☑	D24.-☑	D48.6-☑	D49.3
upper-outer quadrant	C50.4-☑	C79.81	D05.-☑	D24.-☑	D48.6-☑	D49.3
broad ligament	C57.1-☑	C79.82	D07.39	D28.2	D39.8	D49.59
bronchiogenic, bronchogenic (lung)	C34.9-☑	C78.0-☑	D02.2-☑	D14.3-☑	D38.1	D49.1
bronchiole	C34.9-☑	C78.0-☑	D02.2-☑	D14.3-☑	D38.1	D49.1
bronchus	C34.9-☑	C78.0-☑	D02.2-☑	D14.3-☑	D38.1	D49.1
carina	C34.0-☑	C78.0-☑	D02.2-☑	D14.3-☑	D38.1	D49.1
lower lobe of lung	C34.3-☑	C78.0-☑	D02.2-☑	D14.3-☑	D38.1	D49.1
main	C34.0-☑	C78.0-☑	D02.2-☑	D14.3-☑	D38.1	D49.1
middle lobe of lung	C34.2	C78.0-☑	D02.21	D14.31	D38.1	D49.1
overlapping lesion	C34.8-☑	—	—	—	—	—
upper lobe of lung	C34.1-☑	C78.0-☑	D02.2-☑	D14.3-☑	D38.1	D49.1
brow	C44.309	C79.2	D04.39	D23.39	D48.5	D49.2
basal cell carcinoma	C44.319	—	—	—	—	—
specified type NEC	C44.399	—	—	—	—	—
squamous cell carcinoma	C44.329	—	—	—	—	—
buccal (cavity)	C06.9	C79.89	D00.00	D10.39	D37.09	D49.0
commissure	C06.0	C79.89	D00.02	D10.39	D37.09	D49.0
groove (lower) (upper)	C06.1	C79.89	D00.02	D10.39	D37.09	D49.0
mucosa	C06.0	C79.89	D00.02	D10.39	D37.09	D49.0
sulcus (lower) (upper)	C06.1	C79.89	D00.02	D10.39	D37.09	D49.0

Neoplasm, neoplastic — continued	Malignant Primary	Malignant Secondary	Ca in situ	Benign	Uncertain	Unspecified Behavior
bulbourethral gland	C68.0	C79.19	D09.19	D30.4	D41.3	D49.59
bursa — see Neoplasm, connective tissue						
buttock NEC	C76.3	C79.89	D04.5	D36.7	D48.7	D49.89
calf	C76.5-☑	C79.89	D04.7-☑	D36.7	D48.7	D49.89
calvarium	C41.0	C79.51	—	D16.4	D48.0	D49.2
calyx, renal	C65-☑	C79.0-☑	D09.19	D30.1-☑	D41.1-☑	D49.51-☑
canal						
anal	C21.1	C78.5	D01.3	D12.9	D37.8	D49.0
auditory (external) — see also Neoplasm, skin, ear	C44.20-☑	C79.2	D04.2-☑	D23.2-☑	D48.5	D49.2
auricular (external) — see also Neoplasm, skin, ear	C44.20-☑	C79.2	D04.2-☑	D23.2-☑	D48.5	D49.2
canaliculi, biliary (biliferi) (intrahepatic)	C22.1	C78.7	D01.5	D13.4	D37.6	D49.0
canthus (eye) (inner) (outer)	C44.10-☑	C79.2	D04.1-☑	D23.1-☑	D48.5	D49.2
basal cell carcinoma	C44.11-☑	—	—	—	—	—
specified type NEC	C44.19-☑	—	—	—	—	—
squamous cell carcinoma	C44.12-☑	—	—	—	—	—
capillary — see Neoplasm, connective tissue						
caput coli	C18.0	C78.5	D01.0	D12.0	D37.4	D49.0
carcinoid — see Tumor, carcinoid						
cardia (gastric)	C16.0	C78.89	D00.2	D13.1	D37.1	D49.0
cardiac orifice (stomach)	C16.0	C78.89	D00.2	D13.1	D37.1	D49.0
cardio-esophageal junction	C16.0	C78.89	D00.2	D13.1	D37.1	D49.0
cardio-esophagus	C16.0	C78.89	D00.2	D13.1	D37.1	D49.0
carina (bronchus)	C34.0-☑	C78.0-☑	D02.2-☑	D14.3-☑	D38.1	D49.1
carotid (artery)	C49.0	C79.89	—	D21.0	D48.1	D49.2
body	C75.4	C79.89	—	D35.5	D44.6	D49.7
carpus (any bone)	C40.1-☑	C79.51	—	D16.1-☑	—	—
cartilage (articular) (joint) NEC — see also Neoplasm, bone	C41.9	C79.51	—	D16.9	D48.0	D49.2
arytenoid	C32.3	C78.39	D02.0	D14.1	D38.0	D49.1
auricular	C49.0	C79.89	—	D21.0	D48.1	D49.2
bronchi	C34.0-☑	C78.39	—	D14.3-☑	D38.1	D49.1
costal	C41.3	C79.51	—	D16.7	D48.0	D49.2
cricoid	C32.3	C78.39	D02.0	D14.1	D38.0	D49.1
cuneiform	C32.3	C78.39	D02.0	D14.1	D38.0	D49.1
ear (external)	C49.0	C79.89	—	D21.0	D48.1	D49.2
ensiform	C41.3	C79.51	—	D16.7	D48.0	D49.2
epiglottis	C32.1	C78.39	D02.0	D14.1	D38.0	D49.1
anterior surface	C10.1	C79.89	D00.08	D10.5	D37.05	D49.0
eyelid	C49.0	C79.89	—	D21.0	D48.1	D49.2
intervertebral	C41.2	C79.51	—	D16.6	D48.0	D49.2
larynx, laryngeal	C32.3	C78.39	D02.0	D14.1	D38.0	D49.1
nose, nasal	C30.0	C78.39	D02.3	D14.0	D38.5	D49.1
pinna	C49.0	C79.89	—	D21.0	D48.1	D49.2
rib	C41.3	C79.51	—	D16.7	D48.0	D49.2
semilunar (knee)	C40.2-☑	C79.51	—	D16.2-☑	D48.0	D49.2
thyroid	C32.3	C78.39	D02.0	D14.1	D38.0	D49.1
trachea	C33	C78.39	D02.1	D14.2	D38.1	D49.1
cauda equina	C72.1	C79.49	—	D33.4	D43.4	D49.7
cavity						
buccal	C06.9	C79.89	D00.00	D10.30	D37.09	D49.0
nasal	C30.0	C78.39	D02.3	D14.0	D38.5	D49.1
oral	C06.9	C79.89	D00.00	D10.30	D37.09	D49.0
peritoneal	C48.2	C78.6	—	D20.1	D48.4	D49.0
tympanic	C30.1	C78.39	D02.3	D14.0	D38.5	D49.1
cecum	C18.0	C78.5	D01.0	D12.0	D37.4	D49.0
central nervous system	C72.9	C79.40	—	—	—	—
cerebellopontine (angle)	C71.6	C79.31	—	D33.1	D43.1	D49.6
cerebellum, cerebellar	C71.6	C79.31	—	D33.1	D43.1	D49.6
cerebrum, cerebral (cortex) (hemisphere) (white matter)	C71.0	C79.31	—	D33.0	D43.0	D49.6
meninges	C70.0	C79.32	—	D32.0	D42.0	D49.7
peduncle	C71.7	C79.31	—	D33.1	D43.1	D49.6

Neoplasm Table

	Malignant Primary	Malignant Secondary	Ca in situ	Benign	Uncertain	Unspecified Behavior
Neoplasm, neoplastic — *continued*						
cerebrum, cerebral — *continued*						
ventricle	C71.5	C79.31	—	D33.0	D43.0	D49.6
fourth	C71.7	C79.31	—	D33.1	D43.1	D49.6
cervical region	C76.0	C79.89	D09.8	D36.7	D48.7	D49.89
cervix (cervical) (uteri) (uterus)	C53.9	C79.82	D06.9	D26.0	D39.0	D49.59
canal	C53.0	C79.82	D06.0	D26.0	D39.0	D49.59
endocervix (canal) (gland)	C53.0	C79.82	D06.0	D26.0	D39.0	D49.59
exocervix	C53.1	C79.82	D06.1	D26.0	D39.0	D49.59
external os	C53.1	C79.82	D06.1	D26.0	D39.0	D49.59
internal os	C53.0	C79.82	D06.0	D26.0	D39.0	D49.59
nabothian gland	C53.0	C79.82	D06.0	D26.0	D39.0	D49.59
overlapping lesion	C53.8	—	—	—	—	—
squamocolumnar junction	C53.8	C79.82	D06.7	D26.0	D39.0	D49.59
stump	C53.8	C79.82	D06.7	D26.0	D39.0	D49.59
cheek	C76.0	C79.89	D09.8	D36.7	D48.7	D49.89
external	C44.309	C79.2	D04.39	D23.39	D48.5	D49.2
basal cell carcinoma	C44.319	—	—	—	—	—
specified type NEC	C44.399	—	—	—	—	—
squamous cell carcinoma	C44.329	—	—	—	—	—
inner aspect	C06.0	C79.89	D00.02	D10.39	D37.09	D49.0
internal	C06.0	C79.89	D00.02	D10.39	D37.09	D49.0
mucosa	C06.0	C79.89	D00.02	D10.39	D37.09	D49.0
chest (wall) NEC	C76.1	C79.89	D09.8	D36.7	D48.7	D49.89
chiasma opticum	C72.3-☑	C79.49	—	D33.3	D43.3	D49.7
chin	C44.309	C79.2	D04.39	D23.39	D48.5	D49.2
basal cell carcinoma	C44.319	—	—	—	—	—
specified type NEC	C44.399	—	—	—	—	—
squamous cell carcinoma	C44.329	—	—	—	—	—
choana	C11.3	C79.89	D00.08	D10.6	D37.05	D49.0
cholangiole	C22.1	C78.89	D01.5	D13.4	D37.6	D49.0
choledochal duct	C24.0	C78.89	D01.5	D13.5	D37.6	D49.0
choroid	C69.3-☑	C79.49	D09.2-☑	D31.3-☑	D48.7	D49.81
plexus	C71.5	C79.31	—	D33.0	D43.0	D49.6
ciliary body	C69.4-☑	C79.49	D09.2-☑	D31.4-☑	D48.7	D49.89
clavicle	C41.3	C79.51	—	D16.7	D48.0	D49.2
clitoris	C51.2	C79.82	D07.1	D28.0	D39.8	D49.59
clivus	C41.0	C79.51	—	D16.4	D48.0	D49.2
cloacogenic zone	C21.2	C78.5	D01.3	D12.9	D37.8	D49.0
coccygeal						
body or glomus	C49.5	C79.89	—	D21.5	D48.1	D49.2
vertebra	C41.4	C79.51	—	D16.8	D48.0	D49.2
coccyx	C41.4	C79.51	—	D16.8	D48.0	D49.2
colon — *see also* Neoplasm, intestine, large	C18.9	C78.5	—	—	—	—
with rectum	C19	C78.5	D01.1	D12.7	D37.5	D49.0
columnella — *see also* Neoplasm, skin, face	C44.390	C79.2	D04.39	D23.39	D48.5	D49.2
column, spinal — *see* Neoplasm, spine						
commissure						
labial, lip	C00.6	C79.89	D00.01	D10.39	D37.01	D49.0
laryngeal	C32.0	C78.39	D02.0	D14.1	D38.0	D49.1
common (bile) duct	C24.0	C78.89	D01.5	D13.5	D37.6	D49.0
concha — *see also* Neoplasm, skin, ear	C44.20-☑	C79.2	D04.2-☑	D23.2-☑	D48.5	D49.2
nose	C30.0	C78.39	D02.3	D14.0	D38.5	D49.1
conjunctiva	C69.0-☑	C79.49	D09.2-☑	D31.0-☑	D48.7	D49.89

	Malignant Primary	Malignant Secondary	Ca in situ	Benign	Uncertain	Unspecified Behavior
Neoplasm, neoplastic — *continued*						
connective tissue NEC	C49.9	C79.89	—	D21.9	D48.1	D49.2

> Note: For neoplasms of connective tissue (blood vessel, bursa, fascia, ligament, muscle, peripheral nerves, sympathetic and parasympathetic nerves and ganglia, synovia, tendon, etc.) or of morphological types that indicate connective tissue, code according to the list under "Neoplasm, connective tissue". For sites that do not appear in this list, code to neoplasm of that site; e.g., fibrosarcoma, pancreas (C25.9)

> Note: Morphological types that indicate connective tissue appear in their proper place in the alphabetic index with the instruction "see Neoplasm, connective tissue ...."

	Malignant Primary	Malignant Secondary	Ca in situ	Benign	Uncertain	Unspecified Behavior
abdomen	C49.4	C79.89	—	D21.4	D48.1	D49.2
abdominal wall	C49.4	C79.89	—	D21.4	D48.1	D49.2
ankle	C49.2-☑	C79.89	—	D21.2-☑	D48.1	D49.2
antecubital fossa or space	C49.1-☑	C79.89	—	D21.1-☑	D48.1	D49.2
arm	C49.1-☑	C79.89	—	D21.1-☑	D48.1	D49.2
auricle (ear)	C49.0	C79.89	—	D21.0	D48.1	D49.2
axilla	C49.3	C79.89	—	D21.3	D48.1	D49.2
back	C49.6	C79.89	—	D21.6	D48.1	D49.2
breast — *see* Neoplasm, breast						
buttock	C49.5	C79.89	—	D21.5	D48.1	D49.2
calf	C49.2-☑	C79.89	—	D21.2-☑	D48.1	D49.2
cervical region	C49.0	C79.89	—	D21.0	D48.1	D49.2
cheek	C49.0	C79.89	—	D21.0	D48.1	D49.2
chest (wall)	C49.3	C79.89	—	D21.3	D48.1	D49.2
chin	C49.0	C79.89	—	D21.0	D48.1	D49.2
diaphragm	C49.3	C79.89	—	D21.3	D48.1	D49.2
ear (external)	C49.0	C79.89	—	D21.0	D48.1	D49.2
elbow	C49.1-☑	C79.89	—	D21.1-☑	D48.1	D49.2
extrarectal	C49.5	C79.89	—	D21.5	D48.1	D49.2
extremity	C49.9	C79.89	—	D21.9	D48.1	D49.2
lower	C49.2-☑	C79.89	—	D21.2-☑	D48.1	D49.2
upper	C49.1-☑	C79.89	—	D21.1-☑	D48.1	D49.2
eyelid	C49.0	C79.89	—	D21.0	D48.1	D49.2
face	C49.0	C79.89	—	D21.0	D48.1	D49.2
finger	C49.1-☑	C79.89	—	D21.1-☑	D48.1	D49.2
flank	C49.6	C79.89	—	D21.6	D48.1	D49.2
foot	C49.2-☑	C79.89	—	D21.2-☑	D48.1	D49.2
forearm	C49.1-☑	C79.89	—	D21.1-☑	D48.1	D49.2
forehead	C49.0	C79.89	—	D21.0	D48.1	D49.2
gastric	C49.4	C79.89	—	D21.4	D48.1	D49.2
gastrointestinal	C49.4	C79.89	—	D21.4	D48.1	D49.2
gluteal region	C49.5	C79.89	—	D21.5	D48.1	D49.2
great vessels NEC	C49.3	C79.89	—	D21.3	D48.1	D49.2
groin	C49.5	C79.89	—	D21.5	D48.1	D49.2
hand	C49.1-☑	C79.89	—	D21.1-☑	D48.1	D49.2
head	C49.0	C79.89	—	D21.0	D48.1	D49.2
heel	C49.2-☑	C79.89	—	D21.2-☑	D48.1	D49.2
hip	C49.2-☑	C79.89	—	D21.2-☑	D48.1	D49.2
hypochondrium	C49.4	C79.89	—	D21.4	D48.1	D49.2
iliopsoas muscle	C49.5	C79.89	—	D21.5	D48.1	D49.2
infraclavicular region	C49.3	C79.89	—	D21.3	D48.1	D49.2
inguinal (canal) (region)	C49.5	C79.89	—	D21.5	D48.1	D49.2
intestinal	C49.4	C79.89	—	D21.4	D48.1	D49.2
intrathoracic	C49.3	C79.89	—	D21.3	D48.1	D49.2
ischiorectal fossa	C49.5	C79.89	—	D21.5	D48.1	D49.2
jaw	C03.9	C79.89	D00.03	D10.39	D48.1	D49.0
knee	C49.2-☑	C79.89	—	D21.2-☑	D48.1	D49.2
leg	C49.2-☑	C79.89	—	D21.2-☑	D48.1	D49.2
limb NEC	C49.9	C79.89	—	D21.9	D48.1	D49.2
lower	C49.2-☑	C79.89	—	D21.2-☑	D48.1	D49.2
upper	C49.1-☑	C79.89	—	D21.1-☑	D48.1	D49.2
nates	C49.5	C79.89	—	D21.5	D48.1	D49.2
neck	C49.0	C79.89	—	D21.0	D48.1	D49.2
orbit	C69.6-☑	C79.49	D09.2-☑	D31.6-☑	D48.1	D49.89
overlapping lesion	C49.8	—	—	—	—	—
pararectal	C49.5	C79.89	—	D21.5	D48.1	D49.2
para-urethral	C49.5	C79.89	—	D21.5	D48.1	D49.2
paravaginal	C49.5	C79.89	—	D21.5	D48.1	D49.2
pelvis (floor)	C49.5	C79.89	—	D21.5	D48.1	D49.2
pelvo-abdominal	C49.8	C79.89	—	D21.6	D48.1	D49.2
perineum	C49.5	C79.89	—	D21.5	D48.1	D49.2
perirectal (tissue)	C49.5	C79.89	—	D21.5	D48.1	D49.2

(Side tab: Neoplasm Table — Neoplasm, cerebrum, cerebral — Neoplasm, connective tissue NEC)

Neoplasm, neoplastic — continued	Malignant Primary	Malignant Secondary	Ca in situ	Benign	Uncertain	Unspecified Behavior
connective tissue — continued						
periurethral (tissue)	C49.5	C79.89	—	D21.5	D48.1	D49.2
popliteal fossa or space	C49.2-☑	C79.89	—	D21.2-☑	D48.1	D49.2
presacral	C49.5	C79.89	—	D21.5	D48.1	D49.2
psoas muscle	C49.4	C79.89	—	D21.4	D48.1	D49.2
pterygoid fossa	C49.0	C79.89	—	D21.0	D48.1	D49.2
rectovaginal septum or wall	C49.5	C79.89	—	D21.5	D48.1	D49.2
rectovesical	C49.5	C79.89	—	D21.5	D48.1	D49.2
retroperitoneum	C48.0	C78.6		D20.0	D48.3	D49.0
sacrococcygeal region	C49.5	C79.89	—	D21.5	D48.1	D49.2
scalp	C49.0	C79.89	—	D21.0	D48.1	D49.2
scapular region	C49.3	C79.89	—	D21.3	D48.1	D49.2
shoulder	C49.1-☑	C79.89	—	D21.1-☑	D48.1	D49.2
skin (dermis) NEC — see also Neoplasm, skin, by site	C44.90	C79.2	D04.9	D23.9	D48.5	D49.2
stomach	C49.4	C79.89	—	D21.4	D48.1	D49.2
submental	C49.0	C79.89	—	D21.0	D48.1	D49.2
supraclavicular region	C49.0	C79.89	—	D21.0	D48.1	D49.2
temple	C49.0	C79.89	—	D21.0	D48.1	D49.2
temporal region	C49.0	C79.89	—	D21.0	D48.1	D49.2
thigh	C49.2-☑	C79.89	—	D21.2-☑	D48.1	D49.2
thoracic (duct) (wall)	C49.3	C79.89	—	D21.3	D48.1	D49.2
thorax	C49.3	C79.89	—	D21.3	D48.1	D49.2
thumb	C49.1-☑	C79.89	—	D21.1-☑	D48.1	D49.2
toe	C49.2-☑	C79.89	—	D21.2-☑	D48.1	D49.2
trunk	C49.6	C79.89	—	D21.6	D48.1	D49.2
umbilicus	C49.4	C79.89	—	D21.4	D48.1	D49.2
vesicorectal	C49.5	C79.89	—	D21.5	D48.1	D49.2
wrist	C49.1-☑	C79.89	—	D21.1-☑	D48.1	D49.2
conus medullaris	C72.0	C79.49	—	D33.4	D43.4	D49.7
cord (true) (vocal)	C32.0	C78.39	D02.0	D14.1	D38.0	D49.1
false	C32.1	C78.39	D02.0	D14.1	D38.0	D49.1
spermatic	C63.1-☑	C79.82	D07.69	D29.8	D40.8	D49.59
spinal (cervical) (lumbar) (thoracic)	C72.0	C79.49	—	D33.4	D43.4	D49.7
cornea (limbus)	C69.1-☑	C79.49	D09.2-☑	D31.1-☑	D48.7	D49.89
corpus						
albicans	C56.-☑	C79.6-☑	D07.39	D27.-☑	D39.1-☑	D49.59
callosum, brain	C71.0	C79.31	—	D33.2	D43.2	D49.6
cavernosum	C60.2	C79.82	D07.4	D29.0	D40.8	D49.59
gastric	C16.2	C78.89	D00.2	D13.1	D37.1	D49.0
overlapping sites	C54.8	—	—	—	—	—
penis	C60.2	C79.82	D07.4	D29.0	D40.8	D49.59
striatum, cerebrum	C71.0	C79.31	—	D33.0	D43.0	D49.6
uteri	C54.9	C79.82	D07.0	D26.1	D39.0	D49.59
isthmus	C54.0	C79.82	D07.0	D26.1	D39.0	D49.59
cortex						
adrenal	C74.0-☑	C79.7-☑	D09.3	D35.0-☑	D44.1-☑	D49.7
cerebral	C71.0	C79.31	—	D33.0	D43.0	D49.6
costal cartilage	C41.3	C79.51	—	D16.7	D48.0	D49.2
costovertebral joint	C41.3	C79.51	—	D16.7	D48.0	D49.2
Cowper's gland	C68.0	C79.19	D09.19	D30.4	D41.3	D49.59
cranial (fossa, any)	C71.9	C79.31	—	D33.2	D43.2	D49.6
meninges	C70.0	C79.32	—	D32.0	D42.0	D49.7
nerve	C72.50	C79.49	—	D33.3	D43.3	D49.7
specified NEC	C72.59	C79.49	—	D33.3	D43.3	D49.7
craniobuccal pouch	C75.2	C79.89	D09.3	D35.2	D44.3	D49.7
craniopharyngeal (duct) (pouch)	C75.2	C79.89	D09.3	D35.3	D44.4	D49.7
cricoid	C13.0	C79.89	D00.08	D10.7	D37.05	D49.0
cartilage	C32.3	C78.39	D02.0	D14.1	D38.0	D49.1
cricopharynx	C13.0	C79.89	D00.08	D10.7	D37.05	D49.0
crypt of Morgagni	C21.8	C78.5	D01.3	D12.9	D37.8	D49.0
crystalline lens	C69.4-☑	C79.49	D09.2-☑	D31.4-☑	D48.7	D49.89
cul-de-sac (Douglas')	C48.1	C78.6	—	D20.1	D48.4	D49.0
cuneiform cartilage	C32.3	C78.39	D02.0	D14.1	D38.0	D49.1
cutaneous — see Neoplasm, skin						
cutis — see Neoplasm, skin						

Neoplasm, neoplastic — continued	Malignant Primary	Malignant Secondary	Ca in situ	Benign	Uncertain	Unspecified Behavior
cystic (bile) duct (common)	C24.0	C78.89	D01.5	D13.5	D37.6	D49.0
dermis — see Neoplasm, skin						
diaphragm	C49.3	C79.89	—	D21.3	D48.1	D49.2
digestive organs, system, tube, or tract						
NEC	C26.9	C78.89	D01.9	D13.9	D37.9	D49.0
disc, intervertebral	C41.2	C79.51	—	D16.6	D48.0	D49.2
disease, generalized	C80.0	—	—	—	—	—
disseminated	C80.0	—	—	—	—	—
Douglas' cul-de-sac or pouch	C48.1	C78.6	—	D20.1	D48.4	D49.0
duodenojejunal junction	C17.8	C78.4	D01.49	D13.39	D37.2	D49.0
duodenum	C17.0	C78.4	D01.49	D13.2	D37.2	D49.0
dura (cranial) (mater)	C70.9	C79.49	—	D32.9	D42.9	D49.7
cerebral	C70.0	C79.32	—	D32.0	D42.0	D49.7
spinal	C70.1	C79.49	—	D32.1	D42.1	D49.7
ear (external) — see also Neoplasm, skin, ear	C44.20-☑	C79.2	D04.2-☑	D23.2-☑	D48.5	D49.2
auricle or auris — see also Neoplasm, skin, ear	C44.20-☑	C79.2	D04.2-☑	D23.2-☑	D48.5	D49.2
canal, external — see also Neoplasm, skin, ear	C44.20-☑	C79.2	D04.2-☑	D23.2-☑	D48.5	D49.2
cartilage	C49.0	C79.89	—	D21.0	D48.1	D49.2
external meatus — see also Neoplasm, skin, ear	C44.20-☑	C79.2	D04.2-☑	D23.2-☑	D48.5	D49.2
inner	C30.1	C78.39	D02.3	D14.0	D38.5	D49.1
lobule — see also Neoplasm, skin, ear	C44.20-☑	C79.2	D04.2-☑	D23.2-☑	D48.5	D49.2
middle	C30.1	C78.39	D02.3	D14.0	D38.5	D49.1
overlapping lesion with accessory sinuses	C31.8	—	—	—	—	—
skin	C44.20-☑	C79.2	D04.2-☑	D23.2-☑	D48.5	D49.2
basal cell carcinoma	C44.21-☑	—	—	—	—	—
specified type NEC	C44.29-☑	—	—	—	—	—
squamous cell carcinoma	C44.22-☑	—	—	—	—	—
earlobe	C44.20-☑	C79.2	D04.2-☑	D23.2-☑	D48.5	D49.2
basal cell carcinoma	C44.21-☑	—	—	—	—	—
specified type NEC	C44.29-☑	—	—	—	—	—
squamous cell carcinoma	C44.22-☑	—	—	—	—	—
ejaculatory duct	C63.7	C79.82	D07.69	D29.8	D40.8	D49.59
elbow NEC	C76.4-☑	C79.89	D04.6-☑	D36.7	D48.7	D49.89
endocardium	C38.0	C79.89		D15.1	D48.7	D49.89
endocervix (canal) (gland)	C53.0	C79.82	D06.0	D26.0	D39.0	D49.59
endocrine gland NEC	C75.9	C79.89	D09.3	D35.9	D44.9	D49.7
pluriglandular	C75.8	C79.89	D09.3	D35.7	D44.9	D49.7
endometrium (gland) (stroma)	C54.1	C79.82	D07.0	D26.1	D39.0	D49.59
ensiform cartilage	C41.3	C79.51	—	D16.7	D48.0	D49.2
enteric — see Neoplasm, intestine						
ependyma (brain)	C71.5	C79.31	—	D33.0	D43.0	D49.6
fourth ventricle	C71.7	C79.31	—	D33.1	D43.1	D49.6
epicardium	C38.0	C79.89	—	D15.1	D48.7	D49.89
epididymis	C63.0-☑	C79.82	D07.69	D29.3-☑	D40.8	D49.59
epidural	C72.9	C79.49	—	D33.9	D43.9	D49.7
epiglottis	C32.1	C78.39	D02.0	D14.1	D38.0	D49.1
anterior aspect or surface	C10.1	C79.89	D00.08	D10.5	D37.05	D49.0
cartilage	C32.3	C78.39	D02.0	D14.1	D38.0	D49.1
free border (margin)	C10.1	C79.89	D00.08	D10.5	D37.05	D49.0
junctional region	C10.8	C79.89	D00.08	D10.5	D37.05	D49.0
posterior (laryngeal) surface	C32.1	C78.39	D02.0	D14.1	D38.0	D49.1

Neoplasm Table

Neoplasm, epiglottis — Neoplasm, gland, glandular

	Malignant Primary	Malignant Secondary	Ca in situ	Benign	Uncertain	Unspecified Behavior
Neoplasm, neoplastic — *continued*						
epiglottis — *continued*						
suprahyoid portion	C32.1	C78.39	D02.0	D14.1	D38.0	D49.1
esophagogastric junction	C16.0	C78.89	D00.2	D13.1	D37.1	D49.0
esophagus	C15.9	C78.89	D00.1	D13.0	D37.8	D49.0
abdominal	C15.5	C78.89	D00.1	D13.0	D37.8	D49.0
cervical	C15.3	C78.89	D00.1	D13.0	D37.8	D49.0
distal (third)	C15.5	C78.89	D00.1	D13.0	D37.8	D49.0
lower (third)	C15.5	C78.89	D00.1	D13.0	D37.8	D49.0
middle (third)	C15.4	C78.89	D00.1	D13.0	D37.8	D49.0
overlapping lesion	C15.8	—	—	—	—	—
proximal (third)	C15.3	C78.89	D00.1	D13.0	D37.8	D49.0
thoracic	C15.4	C78.89	D00.1	D13.0	D37.8	D49.0
upper (third)	C15.3	C78.89	D00.1	D13.0	D37.8	D49.0
ethmoid (sinus)	C31.1	C78.39	D02.3	D14.0	D38.5	D49.1
bone or labyrinth	C41.0	C79.51	—	D16.4	D48.0	D49.2
eustachian tube	C30.1	C78.39	D02.3	D14.0	D38.5	D49.1
exocervix	C53.1	C79.82	D06.1	D26.0	D39.0	D49.59
external						
meatus (ear) — *see also* Neoplasm, skin, ear	C44.20-☑	C79.2	D04.2-☑	D23.2-☑	D48.5	D49.2
os, cervix uteri	C53.1	C79.82	D06.1	D26.0	D39.0	D49.59
extradural	C72.9	C79.49	—	D33.9	D43.9	D49.7
extrahepatic (bile) duct	C24.0	C78.89	D01.5	D13.5	D37.6	D49.0
overlapping lesion with gallbladder	C24.8	—	—	—	—	—
extraocular muscle	C69.6-☑	C79.49	D09.2-☑	D31.6-☑	D48.7	D49.89
extrarectal	C76.3	C79.89	D09.8	D36.7	D48.7	D49.89
extremity	C76.8	C79.89	D04.8	D36.7	D48.7	D49.8
lower	C76.5-☑	C79.89	D04.7-☑	D36.7	D48.7	D49.89
upper	C76.4-☑	C79.89	D04.6-☑	D36.7	D48.7	D49.89
eyeball	C69.9-☑	C79.49	D09.2-☑	D31.9-☑	D48.7	D49.89
eyebrow	C44.309	C79.2	D04.39	D23.39	D48.5	D49.2
basal cell carcinoma	C44.319	—	—	—	—	—
specified type NEC	C44.399	—	—	—	—	—
squamous cell carcinoma	C44.329	—	—	—	—	—
eyelid (lower) (skin) (upper)	C44.10-☑	—	—	—	—	—
basal cell carcinoma	C44.11-☑	—	—	—	—	—
cartilage	C49.0	C79.89	—	D21.0	D48.1	D49.2
specified type NEC	C44.19-☑	—	—	—	—	—
squamous cell carcinoma	C44.12-☑	—	—	—	—	—
eye NEC	C69.9-☑	C79.49	D09.2-☑	D31.9-☑	D48.7	D49.89
overlapping sites	C69.8-☑	—	—	—	—	—
face NEC	C76.0	C79.89	D04.39	D36.7	D48.7	D49.89
fallopian tube (accessory)	C57.0-☑	C79.82	D07.39	D28.2	D39.8	D49.59
falx (cerebella) (cerebri)	C70.0	C79.32	—	D32.0	D42.0	D49.7
fascia — *see also* Neoplasm, connective tissue						
palmar	C49.1-☑	C79.89	—	D21.1-☑	D48.1	D49.2
plantar	C49.2-☑	C79.89	—	D21.2-☑	D48.1	D49.2
fatty tissue — *see* Neoplasm, connective tissue						
fauces, faucial NEC	C10.9	C79.89	D00.08	D10.5	D37.05	D49.0
pillars	C09.1	C79.89	D00.08	D10.5	D37.05	D49.0
tonsil	C09.9	C79.89	D00.08	D10.4	D37.05	D49.0
femur (any part)	C40.2-☑	—	—	D16.2-☑	—	—
fetal membrane	C58	C79.82	D07.0	D26.7	D39.2	D49.59
fibrous tissue — *see* Neoplasm, connective tissue						
fibula (any part)	C40.2-☑	C79.51	—	D16.2-☑	—	—
filum terminale	C72.0	C79.49	—	D33.4	D43.4	D49.7
finger NEC	C76.4-☑	C79.89	D04.6-☑	D36.7	D48.7	D49.89
flank NEC	C76.8	C79.89	D04.5	D36.7	D48.7	D49.89
follicle, nabothian	C53.0	C79.82	D06.0	D26.0	D39.0	D49.59
foot NEC	C76.5-☑	C79.89	D04.7-☑	D36.7	D48.7	D49.89
forearm NEC	C76.4-☑	C79.89	D04.6-☑	D36.7	D48.7	D49.89
forehead (skin)	C44.309	C79.2	D04.39	D23.39	D48.5	D49.2

	Malignant Primary	Malignant Secondary	Ca in situ	Benign	Uncertain	Unspecified Behavior
Neoplasm, neoplastic — *continued*						
forehead — *continued*						
basal cell carcinoma	C44.319	—	—	—	—	—
specified type NEC	C44.399	—	—	—	—	—
squamous cell carcinoma	C44.329	—	—	—	—	—
foreskin	C60.0	C79.82	D07.4	D29.0	D40.8	D49.59
fornix						
pharyngeal	C11.3	C79.89	D00.08	D10.6	D37.05	D49.0
vagina	C52	C79.82	D07.2	D28.1	D39.8	D49.59
fossa (of)						
anterior (cranial)	C71.9	C79.31	—	D33.2	D43.2	D49.6
cranial	C71.9	C79.31	—	D33.2	D43.2	D49.6
ischiorectal	C76.3	C79.89	D09.8	D36.7	D48.7	D49.89
middle (cranial)	C71.9	C79.31	—	D33.2	D43.2	D49.6
piriform	C12	C79.89	D00.08	D10.7	D37.05	D49.0
pituitary	C75.1	C79.89	D09.3	D35.2	D44.3	D49.7
posterior (cranial)	C71.9	C79.31	—	D33.2	D43.2	D49.6
pterygoid	C49.0	C79.89	—	D21.0	D48.1	D49.2
pyriform	C12	C79.89	D00.08	D10.7	D37.05	D49.0
Rosenmuller	C11.2	C79.89	D00.08	D10.6	D37.05	D49.0
tonsillar	C09.0	C79.89	D00.08	D10.5	D37.05	D49.0
fourchette	C51.9	C79.82	D07.1	D28.0	D39.8	D49.59
frenulum						
labii — *see* Neoplasm, lip, internal						
linguae	C02.2	C79.89	D00.07	D10.1	D37.02	D49.0
frontal						
bone	C41.0	C79.51	—	D16.4	D48.0	D49.2
lobe, brain	C71.1	C79.31	—	D33.0	D43.0	D49.6
pole	C71.1	C79.31	—	D33.0	D43.0	D49.6
sinus	C31.2	C78.39	D02.3	D14.0	D38.5	D49.1
fundus						
stomach	C16.1	C78.89	D00.2	D13.1	D37.1	D49.0
uterus	C54.3	C79.82	D07.0	D26.1	D39.0	D49.59
gallbladder	C23	C78.89	D01.5	D13.5	D37.6	D49.0
overlapping lesion with extrahepatic bile ducts	C24.8	—	—	—	—	—
gall duct (extrahepatic)	C24.0	C78.89	D01.5	D13.5	D37.6	D49.0
intrahepatic	C22.1	C78.7	D01.5	D13.4	D37.6	D49.0
ganglia — *see also* Neoplasm, nerve, peripheral	C47.9	C79.89	—	D36.10	D48.2	D49.2
basal	C71.0	C79.31	—	D33.0	D43.0	D49.6
cranial nerve	C72.50	C79.49	—	D33.3	D43.3	D49.7
Gartner's duct	C52	C79.82	D07.2	D28.1	D39.8	D49.59
gastric — *see* Neoplasm, stomach						
gastrocolic	C26.9	C78.89	D01.9	D13.9	D37.9	D49.0
gastroesophageal junction	C16.0	C78.89	D00.2	D13.1	D37.1	D49.0
gastrointestinal (tract) NEC	C26.9	C78.89	D01.9	D13.9	D37.9	D49.0
generalized	C80.0	—	—	—	—	—
genital organ or tract						
female NEC	C57.9	C79.82	D07.30	D28.9	D39.9	D49.59
overlapping lesion	C57.8	—	—	—	—	—
specified site NEC	C57.7	C79.82	D07.39	D28.7	D39.8	D49.59
male NEC	C63.9	C79.82	D07.60	D29.9	D40.9	D49.59
overlapping lesion	C63.8	—	—	—	—	—
specified site NEC	C63.7	C79.82	D07.69	D29.8	D40.8	D49.59
genitourinary tract						
female	C57.9	C79.82	D07.30	D28.9	D39.9	D49.59
male	C63.9	C79.82	D07.60	D29.9	D40.9	D49.59
gingiva (alveolar) (marginal)	C03.9	C79.89	D00.03	D10.39	D37.09	D49.0
lower	C03.1	C79.89	D00.03	D10.39	D37.09	D49.0
mandibular	C03.1	C79.89	D00.03	D10.39	D37.09	D49.0
maxillary	C03.0	C79.89	D00.03	D10.39	D37.09	D49.0
upper	C03.0	C79.89	D00.03	D10.39	D37.09	D49.0
gland, glandular (lymphatic) (system) — *see also* Neoplasm, lymph gland						
endocrine NEC	C75.9	C79.89	D09.3	D35.9	D44.9	D49.7

☑ **Additional Character Required — Refer to the Tabular List for Character Selection**   ▽ Subterms under main terms may continue to next column or page

	Malignant Primary	Malignant Secondary	Ca in situ	Benign	Uncertain	Unspecified Behavior
Neoplasm, neoplastic —						
continued						
gland, glandular — *see*						
also Neoplasm, lymph						
gland — *continued*						
salivary — *see*						
Neoplasm, salivary						
gland						
glans penis	C60.1	C79.82	D07.4	D29.0	D40.8	D49.59
globus pallidus	C71.0	C79.31	—	D33.0	D43.0	D49.6
glomus						
coccygeal	C49.5	C79.89	—	D21.5	D48.1	D49.2
jugularis	C75.5	C79.89	—	D35.6	D44.7	D49.7
glosso-epiglottic						
fold(s)	C10.1	C79.89	D00.08	D10.5	D37.05	D49.0
glossopalatine fold	C09.1	C79.89	D00.08	D10.5	D37.05	D49.0
glossopharyngeal						
sulcus	C09.0	C79.89	D00.08	D10.5	D37.05	D49.0
glottis	C32.0	C78.39	D02.0	D14.1	D38.0	D49.1
gluteal region	C76.3	C79.89	D04.5	D36.7	D48.7	D49.89
great vessels NEC	C49.3	C79.89	—	D21.3	D48.1	D49.2
groin NEC	C76.3	C79.89	D04.5	D36.7	D48.7	D49.89
gum	C03.9	C79.89	D00.03	D10.39	D37.09	D49.0
lower	C03.1	C79.89	D00.03	D10.39	D37.09	D49.0
upper	C03.0	C79.89	D00.03	D10.39	D37.09	D49.0
hand NEC	C76.4-☑	C79.89	D04.6-☑	D36.7	D48.7	D49.89
head NEC	C76.0	C79.89	D04.4	D36.7	D48.7	D49.89
heart	C38.0	C79.89	—	D15.1	D48.7	D49.89
heel NEC	C76.5-☑	C79.89	D04.7-☑	D36.7	D48.7	D49.89
helix — *see also*						
Neoplasm, skin,						
ear	C44.20-☑	C79.2	D04.2-☑	D23.2-☑	D48.5	D49.2
hematopoietic,						
hemopoietic tissue						
NEC	C96.9	—	—	—	—	—
specified NEC	C96.Z	—	—	—	—	—
hemisphere,						
cerebral	C71.0	C79.31	—	D33.0	D43.0	D49.6
hemorrhoidal zone	C21.1	C78.5	D01.3	D12.9	D37.8	D49.0
hepatic — *see also* Index						
to disease, by						
histology	C22.9	C78.7	D01.5	D13.4	D37.6	D49.0
duct (bile)	C24.0	C78.89	D01.5	D13.5	D37.6	D49.0
flexure (colon)	C18.3	C78.5	D01.0	D12.3	D37.4	D49.0
primary	C22.8	C78.7	D01.5	D13.4	D37.6	D49.0
hepatobiliary	C24.9	C78.89	D01.5	D13.5	D37.6	D49.0
hepatoblastoma	C22.2	C78.7	D01.5	D13.4	D37.6	D49.0
hepatoma	C22.0	C78.7	D01.5	D13.4	D37.6	D49.0
hilus of lung	C34.0-☑	C78.0-☑	D02.2-☑	D14.3-☑	D38.1	D49.1
hippocampus, brain	C71.2	C79.31	—	D33.0	D43.0	D49.6
hip NEC	C76.5-☑	C79.89	D04.7-☑	D36.7	D48.7	D49.89
humerus (any part)	C40.0-☑	C79.51	—	D16.0-☑	—	—
hymen	C52	C79.82	D07.2	D28.1	D39.8	D49.59
hypopharynx,						
hypopharyngeal						
NEC	C13.9	C79.89	D00.08	D10.7	D37.05	D49.0
overlapping lesion	C13.8	—	—	—	—	—
postcricoid region	C13.0	C79.89	D00.08	D10.7	D37.05	D49.0
posterior wall	C13.2	C79.89	D00.08	D10.7	D37.05	D49.0
pyriform fossa						
(sinus)	C12	C79.89	D00.08	D10.7	D37.05	D49.0
hypophysis	C75.1	C79.89	D09.3	D35.2	D44.3	D49.7
hypothalamus	C71.0	C79.31	—	D33.0	D43.0	D49.6
ileocecum, ileocecal (coil)						
(junction)						
(valve)	C18.0	C78.5	D01.0	D12.0	D37.4	D49.0
ileum	C17.2	C78.4	D01.49	D13.39	D37.2	D49.0
ilium	C41.4	C79.51	—	D16.8	D48.0	D49.2
immunoproliferative						
NEC	C88.9	—	—	—	—	—
infraclavicular						
(region)	C76.1	C79.89	D04.5	D36.7	D48.7	D49.89
inguinal (region)	C76.3	C79.89	D04.5	D36.7	D48.7	D49.89
insula	C71.0	C79.31	—	D33.0	D43.0	D49.6
insular tissue						
(pancreas)	C25.4	C78.89	D01.7	D13.7	D37.8	D49.0
brain	C71.0	C79.31	—	D33.0	D43.0	D49.6
interarytenoid fold	C13.1	C78.39	D00.08	D10.7	D37.05	D49.0
hypopharyngeal						
aspect	C13.1	C79.89	D00.08	D10.7	D37.05	D49.0
laryngeal aspect	C32.1	C78.39	D02.0	D14.1	D38.0	D49.1
marginal zone	C13.1	C79.89	D00.08	D10.7	D37.05	D49.0
interdental papillae	C03.9	C79.89	D00.03	D10.39	D37.09	D49.0

	Malignant Primary	Malignant Secondary	Ca in situ	Benign	Uncertain	Unspecified Behavior
Neoplasm, neoplastic —						
continued						
interdental papillae —						
continued						
lower	C03.1	C79.89	D00.03	D10.39	D37.09	D49.0
upper	C03.0	C79.89	D00.03	D10.39	D37.09	D49.0
internal						
capsule	C71.0	C79.31	—	D33.0	D43.0	D49.6
os (cervix)	C53.0	C79.82	D06.0	D26.0	D39.0	D49.59
intervertebral cartilage or						
disc	C41.2	C79.51	—	D16.6	D48.0	D49.2
intestine, intestinal	C26.0	C78.80	D01.40	D13.9	D37.8	D49.0
large	C18.9	C78.5	D01.0	D12.6	D37.4	D49.0
appendix	C18.1	C78.5	D01.0	D12.1	D37.3	D49.0
caput coli	C18.0	C78.5	D01.0	D12.0	D37.4	D49.0
cecum	C18.0	C78.5	D01.0	D12.0	D37.4	D49.0
colon	C18.9	C78.5	D01.0	D12.6	D37.4	D49.0
and rectum	C19	C78.5	D01.1	D12.7	D37.5	D49.0
ascending	C18.2	C78.5	D01.0	D12.2	D37.4	D49.0
caput	C18.0	C78.5	D01.0	D12.0	D37.4	D49.0
descending	C18.6	C78.5	D01.0	D12.4	D37.4	D49.0
distal	C18.6	C78.5	D01.0	D12.4	D37.4	D49.0
left	C18.6	C78.5	D01.0	D12.4	D37.4	D49.0
overlapping						
lesion	C18.8	—	—	—	—	—
pelvic	C18.7	C78.5	D01.0	D12.5	D37.4	D49.0
right	C18.2	C78.5	D01.0	D12.2	D37.4	D49.0
sigmoid						
(flexure)	C18.7	C78.5	D01.0	D12.5	D37.4	D49.0
transverse	C18.4	C78.5	D01.0	D12.3	D37.4	D49.0
hepatic flexure	C18.3	C78.5	D01.0	D12.3	D37.4	D49.0
ileocecum, ileocecal						
(coil) (valve)	C18.0	C78.5	D01.0	D12.0	D37.4	D49.0
overlapping						
lesion	C18.8	—	—	—	—	—
sigmoid flexure						
(lower)						
(upper)	C18.7	C78.5	D01.0	D12.5	D37.4	D49.0
splenic flexure	C18.5	C78.5	D01.0	D12.3	D37.4	D49.0
small	C17.9	C78.4	D01.40	D13.30	D37.2	D49.0
duodenum	C17.0	C78.4	D01.49	D13.2	D37.2	D49.0
ileum	C17.2	C78.4	D01.49	D13.39	D37.2	D49.0
jejunum	C17.1	C78.4	D01.49	D13.39	D37.2	D49.0
overlapping						
lesion	C17.8	—	—	—	—	—
tract NEC	C26.0	C78.89	D01.40	D13.9	D37.8	D49.0
intra-abdominal	C76.2	C79.89	D09.8	D36.7	D48.7	D49.89
intracranial NEC	C71.9	C79.31	—	D33.2	D43.2	D49.6
intrahepatic (bile)						
duct	C22.1	C78.7	D01.5	D13.4	D37.6	D49.0
intraocular	C69.9-☑	C79.49	D09.2-☑	D31.9-☑	D48.7	D49.89
intraorbital	C69.6-☑	C79.49	D09.2-☑	D31.6-☑	D48.7	D49.89
intrasellar	C75.1	C79.89	D09.3	D35.2	D44.3	D49.7
intrathoracic (cavity)						
(organs)	C76.1	C79.89	D09.8	D15.9	D48.7	D49.89
specified NEC	C76.1	C79.89	D09.8	D15.7	—	—
iris	C69.4-☑	C79.49	D09.2-☑	D31.4-☑	D48.7	D49.89
ischiorectal (fossa)	C76.3	C79.89	D09.8	D36.7	D48.7	D49.89
ischium	C41.4	C79.51	—	D16.8	D48.0	D49.2
island of Reil	C71.0	C79.31	—	D33.0	D43.0	D49.6
islands or islets of						
Langerhans	C25.4	C78.89	D01.7	D13.7	D37.8	D49.0
isthmus uteri	C54.0	C79.82	D07.0	D26.1	D39.0	D49.59
jaw	C76.0	C79.89	D09.8	D36.7	D48.7	D49.89
bone	C41.1	C79.51	—	D16.5	D48.0	D49.2
lower	C41.1	C79.51	—	D16.5	—	—
upper	C41.0	C79.51	—	D16.4	—	—
carcinoma (any type)						
(lower)						
(upper)	C76.0	C79.89	—	—	—	—
skin — *see also*						
Neoplasm, skin,						
face	C44.309	C79.2	D04.39	D23.39	D48.5	D49.2
soft tissues	C03.9	C79.89	D00.03	D10.39	D37.09	D49.0
lower	C03.1	C79.89	D00.03	D10.39	D37.09	D49.0
upper	C03.0	C79.89	D00.03	D10.39	D37.09	D49.0
jejunum	C17.1	C78.4	D01.49	D13.39	D37.2	D49.0
joint NEC — *see also*						
Neoplasm, bone	C41.9	C79.51	—	D16.9	D48.0	D49.2
acromioclavicular	C40.0-☑	C79.51	—	D16.0-☑	—	—

Neoplasm Table

Neoplasm, joint NEC — Neoplasm, lung

Neoplasm, neoplastic — continued	Malignant Primary	Malignant Secondary	Ca in situ	Benign	Uncertain	Unspecified Behavior
joint — see also Neoplasm, bone — continued						
bursa or synovial membrane — see Neoplasm, connective tissue						
costovertebral	C41.3	C79.51	—	D16.7	D48.0	D49.2
sternocostal	C41.3	C79.51	—	D16.7	D48.0	D49.2
temporomandibular	C41.1	C79.51	—	D16.5	D48.0	D49.2
junction						
anorectal	C21.8	C78.5	D01.3	D12.9	D37.8	D49.0
cardioesophageal	C16.0	C78.89	D00.2	D13.1	D37.1	D49.0
esophagogastric	C16.0	C78.89	D00.2	D13.1	D37.1	D49.0
gastroesophageal	C16.0	C78.89	D00.2	D13.1	D37.1	D49.0
hard and soft palate	C05.9	C79.89	D00.00	D10.39	D37.09	D49.0
ileocecal	C18.0	C78.5	D01.0	D12.0	D37.4	D49.0
pelvirectal	C19	C78.5	D01.1	D12.7	D37.5	D49.0
pelviureteric	C65.-☑	C79.0-☑	D09.19	D30.1-☑	D41.1-☑	D49.59
rectosigmoid	C19	C78.5	D01.1	D12.7	D37.5	D49.0
squamocolumnar, of cervix	C53.8	C79.82	D06.7	D26.0	D39.0	D49.59
Kaposi's sarcoma — see Kaposi's, sarcoma						
kidney (parenchymal)	C64.-☑	C79.0-☑	D09.19	D30.0-☑	D41.0-☑	D49.51-☑
calyx	C65.-☑	C79.0-☑	D09.19	D30.1-☑	D41.1-☑	D49.51-☑
hilus	C65.-☑	C79.0-☑	D09.19	D30.1-☑	D41.1-☑	D49.51-☑
pelvis	C65.-☑	C79.0-☑	D09.19	D30.1-☑	D41.1-☑	D49.51-☑
knee NEC	C76.5-☑	C79.89	D04.7-☑	D36.7	D48.7	D49.89
labia (skin)	C51.9	C79.82	D07.1	D28.0	D39.8	D49.59
majora	C51.0	C79.82	D07.1	D28.0	D39.8	D49.59
minora	C51.1	C79.82	D07.1	D28.0	D39.8	D49.59
labial — see also Neoplasm, lip	C00.9	C79.89	D00.01	D10.0	D37.01	D49.0
sulcus (lower) (upper)	C06.1	C79.89	D00.02	D10.39	D37.09	D49.0
labium (skin)	C51.9	C79.82	D07.1	D28.0	D39.8	D49.59
majus	C51.0	C79.82	D07.1	D28.0	D39.8	D49.59
minus	C51.1	C79.82	D07.1	D28.0	D39.8	D49.59
lacrimal						
canaliculi	C69.5-☑	C79.49	D09.2-☑	D31.5-☑	D48.7	D49.89
duct (nasal)	C69.5-☑	C79.49	D09.2-☑	D31.5-☑	D48.7	D49.89
gland	C69.5-☑	C79.49	D09.2-☑	D31.5-☑	D48.7	D49.89
punctum	C69.5-☑	C79.49	D09.2-☑	D31.5-☑	D48.7	D49.89
sac	C69.5-☑	C79.49	D09.2-☑	D31.5-☑	D48.7	D49.89
Langerhans, islands or islets	C25.4	C78.89	D01.7	D13.7	D37.8	D49.0
laryngopharynx	C13.9	C79.89	D00.08	D10.7	D37.05	D49.0
larynx, laryngeal NEC	C32.9	C78.39	D02.0	D14.1	D38.0	D49.1
aryepiglottic fold	C32.1	C78.39	D02.0	D14.1	D38.0	D49.1
cartilage (arytenoid) (cricoid) (cuneiform) (thyroid)	C32.3	C78.39	D02.0	D14.1	D38.0	D49.1
commissure (anterior) (posterior)	C32.0	C78.39	D02.0	D14.1	D38.0	D49.1
extrinsic NEC	C32.1	C78.39	D02.0	D14.1	D38.0	D49.1
meaning hypopharynx	C13.9	C79.89	D00.08	D10.7	D37.05	D49.0
interarytenoid fold	C32.1	C78.39	D02.0	D14.1	D38.0	D49.1
intrinsic	C32.0	C78.39	D02.0	D14.1	D38.0	D49.1
overlapping lesion	C32.8	—	—	—	—	—
ventricular band	C32.1	C78.39	D02.0	D14.1	D38.0	D49.1
leg NEC	C76.5-☑	C79.89	D04.7-☑	D36.7	D48.7	D49.89
lens, crystalline	C69.4-☑	C79.49	D09.2-☑	D31.4-☑	D48.7	D49.89
lid (lower) (upper)	C44.10-☑	C79.2	D04.1-☑	D23.1-☑	D48.5	D49.2
basal cell carcinoma	C44.11-☑	—	—	—	—	—
specified type NEC	C44.19-☑	—	—	—	—	—
squamous cell carcinoma	C44.12-☑	—	—	—	—	—

Neoplasm, neoplastic — continued	Malignant Primary	Malignant Secondary	Ca in situ	Benign	Uncertain	Unspecified Behavior
ligament — see also Neoplasm, connective tissue						
broad	C57.1-☑	C79.82	D07.39	D28.2	D39.8	D49.59
Mackenrodt's	C57.7	C79.82	D07.39	D28.7	D39.8	D49.59
non-uterine — see Neoplasm, connective tissue						
round	C57.2-☑	C79.82	—	D28.2	D39.8	D49.59
sacro-uterine	C57.3	C79.82	—	D28.2	D39.8	D49.59
uterine	C57.3	C79.82	—	D28.2	D39.8	D49.59
utero-ovarian	C57.7	C79.82	D07.39	D28.2	D39.8	D49.59
uterosacral	C57.3	C79.82	—	D28.2	D39.8	D49.59
limb	C76.8	C79.89	D04.8	D36.7	D48.7	D49.89
lower	C76.5-☑	C79.89	D04.7-☑	D36.7	D48.7	D49.89
upper	C76.4-☑	C79.89	D04.6-☑	D36.7	D48.7	D49.89
limbus of cornea	C69.1-☑	C79.49	D09.2-☑	D31.1-☑	D48.7	D49.89
lingual NEC — see also Neoplasm, tongue	C02.9	C79.89	D00.07	D10.1	D37.02	D49.0
lingula, lung	C34.1-☑	C78.0-☑	D02.2-☑	D14.3-☑	D38.1	D49.1
lip	C00.9	C79.89	D00.01	D10.0	D37.01	D49.0
buccal aspect — see Neoplasm, lip, internal						
commissure	C00.6	C79.89	D00.01	D10.0	D37.01	D49.0
external	C00.2	C79.89	D00.01	D10.0	D37.01	D49.0
lower	C00.1	C79.89	D00.01	D10.0	D37.01	D49.0
upper	C00.0	C79.89	D00.01	D10.0	D37.01	D49.0
frenulum — see Neoplasm, lip, internal						
inner aspect — see Neoplasm, lip, internal						
internal	C00.5	C79.89	D00.01	D10.0	D37.01	D49.0
lower	C00.4	C79.89	D00.01	D10.0	D37.01	D49.0
upper	C00.3	C79.89	D00.01	D10.0	D37.01	D49.0
lipstick area	C00.2	C79.89	D00.01	D10.0	D37.01	D49.0
lower	C00.1	C79.89	D00.01	D10.0	D37.01	D49.0
upper	C00.0	C79.89	D00.01	D10.0	D37.01	D49.0
lower	C00.1	C79.89	D00.01	D10.0	D37.01	D49.0
internal	C00.4	C79.89	D00.01	D10.0	D37.01	D49.0
mucosa — see Neoplasm, lip, internal						
oral aspect — see Neoplasm, lip, internal						
overlapping lesion	C00.8	—	—	—	—	—
with oral cavity or pharynx	C14.8	—	—	—	—	—
skin (commissure) (lower) (upper)	C44.00	C79.2	D04.0	D23.0	D48.5	D49.2
basal cell carcinoma	C44.01	—	—	—	—	—
specified type NEC	C44.09	—	—	—	—	—
squamous cell carcinoma	C44.02	—	—	—	—	—
upper	C00.0	C79.89	D00.01	D10.0	D37.01	D49.0
internal	C00.3	C79.89	D00.01	D10.0	D37.01	D49.0
vermilion border	C00.2	C79.89	D00.01	D10.0	D37.01	D49.0
lower	C00.1	C79.89	D00.01	D10.0	D37.01	D49.0
upper	C00.0	C79.89	D00.01	D10.0	D37.01	D49.0
lipomatous — see Lipoma, by site						
liver — see also Index to disease, by histology	C22.9	C78.7	D01.5	D13.4	D37.6	D49.0
primary	C22.8	C78.7	D01.5	D13.4	D37.6	D49.0
lumbosacral plexus	C47.5	C79.89	—	D36.16	D48.2	D49.2
lung	C34.9-☑	C78.0-☑	D02.2-☑	D14.3-☑	D38.1	D49.1
azygos lobe	C34.1-☑	C78.0-☑	D02.2-☑	D14.3-☑	D38.1	D49.1
carina	C34.0-☑	C78.0-☑	D02.2-☑	D14.3-☑	D38.1	D49.1
hilus	C34.0-☑	C78.0-☑	D02.2-☑	D14.3-☑	D38.1	D49.1
lingula	C34.1-☑	C78.0-☑	D02.2-☑	D14.3-☑	D38.1	D49.1
lobe NEC	C34.9-☑	C78.0-☑	D02.2-☑	D14.3-☑	D38.1	D49.1
lower lobe	C34.3-☑	C78.0-☑	D02.2-☑	D14.3-☑	D38.1	D49.1

☑ Additional Character Required — Refer to the Tabular List for Character Selection   ▽ Subterms under main terms may continue to next column or page

Neoplasm, neoplastic — continued	Malignant Primary	Malignant Secondary	Ca in situ	Benign	Uncertain	Unspecified Behavior
lung — continued						
main bronchus	C34.0-☑	C78.0-☑	D02.2-☑	D14.3-☑	D38.1	D49.1
mesothelioma — see Mesothelioma						
middle lobe	C34.2	C78.0-☑	D02.21	D14.31	D38.1	D49.1
overlapping lesion	C34.8-☑	—				
upper lobe	C34.1-☑	C78.0-☑	D02.2-☑	D14.3-☑	D38.1	D49.1
lymph, lymphatic channel						
NEC	C49.9	C79.89	—	D21.9	D48.1	D49.2
gland (secondary)	—	C77.9	—	D36.0	D48.7	D49.89
abdominal	—	C77.2	—	D36.0	D48.7	D49.89
aortic	—	C77.2	—	D36.0	D48.7	D49.89
arm	—	C77.3	—	D36.0	D48.7	D49.89
auricular (anterior)						
(posterior)	—	C77.0	—	D36.0	D48.7	D49.89
axilla, axillary	—	C77.3	—	D36.0	D48.7	D49.89
brachial	—	C77.3	—	D36.0	D48.7	D49.89
bronchial	—	C77.1	—	D36.0	D48.7	D49.89
bronchopulmonary	—	C77.1	—	D36.0	D48.7	D49.89
celiac	—	C77.2	—	D36.0	D48.7	D49.89
cervical	—	C77.0	—	D36.0	D48.7	D49.89
cervicofacial	—	C77.0	—	D36.0	D48.7	D49.89
Cloquet	—	C77.4	—	D36.0	D48.7	D49.89
colic	—	C77.2	—	D36.0	D48.7	D49.89
common duct	—	C77.2	—	D36.0	D48.7	D49.89
cubital	—	C77.3	—	D36.0	D48.7	D49.89
diaphragmatic	—	C77.1	—	D36.0	D48.7	D49.89
epigastric, inferior	—	C77.1	—	D36.0	D48.7	D49.89
epitrochlear	—	C77.3	—	D36.0	D48.7	D49.89
esophageal	—	C77.1	—	D36.0	D48.7	D49.89
face	—	C77.0	—	D36.0	D48.7	D49.89
femoral	—	C77.4	—	D36.0	D48.7	D49.89
gastric	—	C77.2	—	D36.0	D48.7	D49.89
groin	—	C77.4	—	D36.0	D48.7	D49.89
head	—	C77.0	—	D36.0	D48.7	D49.89
hepatic	—	C77.2	—	D36.0	D48.7	D49.89
hilar (pulmonary)	—	C77.1	—	D36.0	D48.7	D49.89
splenic	—	C77.2	—	D36.0	D48.7	D49.89
hypogastric	—	C77.5	—	D36.0	D48.7	D49.89
ileocolic	—	C77.2	—	D36.0	D48.7	D49.89
iliac	—	C77.5	—	D36.0	D48.7	D49.89
infraclavicular	—	C77.3	—	D36.0	D48.7	D49.89
inguina, inguinal	—	C77.4	—	D36.0	D48.7	D49.89
innominate	—	C77.1	—	D36.0	D48.7	D49.89
intercostal	—	C77.1	—	D36.0	D48.7	D49.89
intestinal	—	C77.2	—	D36.0	D48.7	D49.89
intrabdominal	—	C77.2	—	D36.0	D48.7	D49.89
intrapelvic	—	C77.5	—	D36.0	D48.7	D49.89
intrathoracic	—	C77.1	—	D36.0	D48.7	D49.89
jugular	—	C77.0	—	D36.0	D48.7	D49.89
leg	—	C77.4	—	D36.0	D48.7	D49.89
limb						
lower	—	C77.4	—	D36.0	D48.7	D49.89
upper	—	C77.3	—	D36.0	D48.7	D49.89
lower limb	—	C77.4	—	D36.0	D48.7	D49.89
lumbar	—	C77.2	—	D36.0	D48.7	D49.89
mandibular	—	C77.0	—	D36.0	D48.7	D49.89
mediastinal	—	C77.1	—	D36.0	D48.7	D49.89
mesenteric (inferior) (superior)	—	C77.2	—	D36.0	D48.7	D49.89
midcolic	—	C77.2	—	D36.0	D48.7	D49.89
multiple sites in categories C77.0 - C77.5	—	C77.8	—	D36.0	D48.7	D49.89
neck	—	C77.0	—	D36.0	D48.7	D49.89
obturator	—	C77.5	—	D36.0	D48.7	D49.89
occipital	—	C77.0	—	D36.0	D48.7	D49.89
pancreatic	—	C77.2	—	D36.0	D48.7	D49.89
para-aortic	—	C77.2	—	D36.0	D48.7	D49.89
paracervical	—	C77.5	—	D36.0	D48.7	D49.89
parametrial	—	C77.5	—	D36.0	D48.7	D49.89
parasternal	—	C77.1	—	D36.0	D48.7	D49.89
parotid	—	C77.0	—	D36.0	D48.7	D49.89
pectoral	—	C77.3	—	D36.0	D48.7	D49.89
pelvic	—	C77.5	—	D36.0	D48.7	D49.89
peri-aortic	—	C77.2	—	D36.0	D48.7	D49.89
peripancreatic	—	C77.2	—	D36.0	D48.7	D49.89
popliteal	—	C77.4	—	D36.0	D48.7	D49.89
porta hepatis	—	C77.2	—	D36.0	D48.7	D49.89

Right table

Neoplasm, neoplastic — continued	Malignant Primary	Malignant Secondary	Ca in situ	Benign	Uncertain	Unspecified Behavior
lymph, lymphatic channel — continued						
gland — continued						
portal	—	C77.2	—	D36.0	D48.7	D49.89
preauricular	—	C77.0	—	D36.0	D48.7	D49.89
prelaryngeal	—	C77.0	—	D36.0	D48.7	D49.89
presymphysial	—	C77.5	—	D36.0	D48.7	D49.89
pretracheal	—	C77.0	—	D36.0	D48.7	D49.89
primary (any site) NEC	C96.9	—	—	—	—	—
pulmonary (hiler)	—	C77.1	—	D36.0	D48.7	D49.89
pyloric	—	C77.2	—	D36.0	D48.7	D49.89
retroperitoneal	—	C77.2	—	D36.0	D48.7	D49.89
retropharyngeal	—	C77.0	—	D36.0	D48.7	D49.89
Rosenmuller's	—	C77.4	—	D36.0	D48.7	D49.89
sacral	—	C77.5	—	D36.0	D48.7	D49.89
scalene	—	C77.0	—	D36.0	D48.7	D49.89
site NEC	—	C77.9	—	D36.0	D48.7	D49.89
splenic (hilar)	—	C77.2	—	D36.0	D48.7	D49.89
subclavicular	—	C77.3	—	D36.0	D48.7	D49.89
subinguinal	—	C77.4	—	D36.0	D48.7	D49.89
sublingual	—	C77.0	—	D36.0	D48.7	D49.89
submandibular	—	C77.0	—	D36.0	D48.7	D49.89
submaxillary	—	C77.0	—	D36.0	D48.7	D49.89
submental	—	C77.0	—	D36.0	D48.7	D49.89
subscapular	—	C77.3	—	D36.0	D48.7	D49.89
supraclavicular	—	C77.0	—	D36.0	D48.7	D49.89
thoracic	—	C77.1	—	D36.0	D48.7	D49.89
tibial	—	C77.4	—	D36.0	D48.7	D49.89
tracheal	—	C77.1	—	D36.0	D48.7	D49.89
tracheobronchial	—	C77.1	—	D36.0	D48.7	D49.89
upper limb	—	C77.3	—	D36.0	D48.7	D49.89
Virchow's	—	C77.0	—	D36.0	D48.7	D49.89
node — see also Neoplasm, lymph gland						
primary NEC	C96.9	—	—	—	—	—
vessel — see also Neoplasm, connective tissue	C49.9	C79.89	—	D21.9	D48.1	D49.2
Mackenrodt's ligament	C57.7	C79.82	D07.39	D28.7	D39.8	D49.59
malar	C41.0	C79.51		D16.4	D48.0	D49.2
region — see Neoplasm, cheek						
mammary gland — see Neoplasm, breast						
mandible	C41.1	C79.51	—	D16.5	D48.0	D49.2
alveolar						
mucosa (carcinoma)	C03.1	C79.89	D00.03	D10.39	D37.09	D49.0
ridge or process	C41.1	C79.51	—	D16.5	D48.0	D49.2
marrow (bone) NEC	C96.9	C79.52	—	—	D47.9	D49.89
mastectomy site (skin) — see also Neoplasm, breast, skin	C44.501	C79.2	—			
specified as breast tissue	C50.8-☑	C79.81	—			
mastoid (air cells) (antrum) (cavity)	C30.1	C78.39	D02.3	D14.0	D38.5	D49.1
bone or process	C41.0	C79.51	—	D16.4	D48.0	D49.2
maxilla, maxillary (superior)	C41.0	C79.51	—	D16.4	D48.0	D49.2
alveolar						
mucosa	C03.0	C79.89	D00.03	D10.39	D37.09	D49.0
ridge or process (carcinoma)	C41.0	C79.51	—	D16.4	D48.0	D49.2
antrum	C31.0	C78.39	D02.3	D14.0	D38.5	D49.1
carcinoma	C03.0	C79.51	—	—	—	—
inferior — see Neoplasm, mandible						
sinus	C31.0	C78.39	D02.3	D14.0	D38.5	D49.1
meatus external (ear) — see also Neoplasm, skin, ear	C44.20-☑	C79.2	D04.2-☑	D23.2-☑	D48.5	D49.2
Meckel diverticulum, malignant	C17.3	C78.4	D01.49	D13.39	D37.2	D49.0
mediastinum, mediastinal	C38.3	C78.1		D15.2	D38.3	D49.89

Neoplasm, neoplastic — *continued*
mediastinum, mediastinal — *continued*

	Malignant Primary	Malignant Secondary	Ca in situ	Benign	Uncertain	Unspecified Behavior
anterior	C38.1	C78.1	—	D15.2	D38.3	D49.89
posterior	C38.2	C78.1	—	D15.2	D38.3	D49.89
medulla						
adrenal	C74.1-☑	C79.7-☑	D09.3	D35.0-☑	D44.1-☑	D49.7
oblongata	C71.7	C79.31	—	D33.1	D43.1	D49.6
meibomian gland	C44.10-☑	C79.2	D04.1-☑	D23.1-☑	D48.5	D49.2
basal cell carcinoma	C44.11-☑	—	—	—	—	—
specified type NEC	C44.19-☑	—	—	—	—	—
squamous cell carcinoma	C44.12-☑	—	—	—	—	—
melanoma — *see* Melanoma						
meninges	C70.9	C79.49	—	D32.9	D42.9	D49.7
brain	C70.0	C79.32	—	D32.0	D42.0	D49.7
cerebral	C70.0	C79.32	—	D32.0	D42.0	D49.7
crainial	C70.0	C79.32	—	D32.0	D42.0	D49.7
intracranial	C70.0	C79.32	—	D32.0	D42.0	D49.7
spinal (cord)	C70.1	C79.49	—	D32.1	D42.1	D49.7
meniscus, knee joint (lateral) (medial)	C40.2-☑	C79.51	—	D16.2-☑	D48.0	D49.2
Merkel cell — *see* Carcinoma, Merkel cell						
mesentery, mesenteric	C48.1	C78.6	—	D20.1	D48.4	D49.0
mesoappendix	C48.1	C78.6	—	D20.1	D48.4	D49.0
mesocolon	C48.1	C78.6	—	D20.1	D48.4	D49.0
mesopharynx — *see* Neoplasm, oropharynx						
mesosalpinx	C57.1-☑	C79.82	D07.39	D28.2	D39.8	D49.59
mesothelial tissue — *see* Mesothelioma						
mesothelioma — *see* Mesothelioma						
mesovarium	C57.1-☑	C79.82	D07.39	D28.2	D39.8	D49.59
metacarpus (any bone)	C40.1-☑	C79.51	—	D16.1-☑	—	—
metastatic NEC — *see also* Neoplasm, by site, secondary	—	C79.9	—	—	—	—
metatarsus (any bone)	C40.3-☑	C79.51	—	D16.3-☑	—	—
midbrain	C71.7	C79.31	—	D33.1	D43.1	D49.6
milk duct — *see* Neoplasm, breast						
mons						
pubis	C51.9	C79.82	D07.1	D28.0	D39.8	D49.59
veneris	C51.9	C79.82	D07.1	D28.0	D39.8	D49.59
motor tract	C72.9	C79.49	—	D33.9	D43.9	D49.7
brain	C71.9	C79.31	—	D33.2	D43.2	D49.6
cauda equina	C72.1	C79.49	—	D33.4	D43.4	D49.7
spinal	C72.0	C79.49	—	D33.4	D43.4	D49.7
mouth	C06.9	C79.89	D00.00	D10.30	D37.09	D49.0
book-leaf	C06.89	C79.89	—	—	—	—
floor	C04.9	C79.89	D00.06	D10.2	D37.09	D49.0
anterior portion	C04.0	C79.89	D00.06	D10.2	D37.09	D49.0
lateral portion	C04.1	C79.89	D00.06	D10.2	D37.09	D49.0
overlapping lesion	C04.8	—	—	—	—	—
overlapping NEC	C06.80	—	—	—	—	—
roof	C05.9	C79.89	D00.00	D10.39	D37.09	D49.0
specified part NEC	C06.89	C79.89	D00.00	D10.39	D37.09	D49.0
vestibule	C06.1	C79.89	D00.00	D10.39	D37.09	D49.0
mucosa						
alveolar (ridge or process)	C03.9	C79.89	D00.03	D10.39	D37.09	D49.0
lower	C03.1	C79.89	D00.03	D10.39	D37.09	D49.0
upper	C03.0	C79.89	D00.03	D10.39	D37.09	D49.0
buccal	C06.0	C79.89	D00.02	D10.39	D37.09	D49.0
cheek	C06.0	C79.89	D00.02	D10.39	D37.09	D49.0
lip — *see* Neoplasm, lip, internal						
nasal	C30.0	C78.39	D02.3	D14.0	D38.5	D49.1
oral	C06.0	C79.89	D00.02	D10.39	D37.09	D49.0
Mullerian duct						
female	C57.7	C79.82	D07.39	D28.7	D39.8	D49.59
male	C63.7	C79.82	D07.69	D29.8	D40.8	D49.59

Neoplasm, neoplastic — *continued*
muscle — *see also* Neoplasm, connective tissue

	Malignant Primary	Malignant Secondary	Ca in situ	Benign	Uncertain	Unspecified Behavior
extraocular	C69.6-☑	C79.49	D09.2-☑	D31.6-☑	D48.7	D49.89
myocardium	C38.0	C79.89	—	D15.1	D48.7	D49.89
myometrium	C54.2	C79.82	D07.0	D26.1	D39.0	D49.59
myopericardium	C38.0	C79.89	—	D15.1	D48.7	D49.89
nabothian gland (follicle)	C53.0	C79.82	D06.0	D26.0	D39.0	D49.59
nail — *see also* Neoplasm, skin, limb	C44.90	C79.2	D04.9	D23.9	D48.5	D49.2
finger — *see also* Neoplasm, skin, limb, upper	C44.60-☑	C79.2	D04.6-☑	D23.6-☑	D48.5	D49.2
toe — *see also* Neoplasm, skin, limb, lower	C44.70-☑	C79.2	D04.7-☑	D23.7-☑	D48.5	D49.2
nares, naris (anterior) (posterior)	C30.0	C78.39	D02.3	D14.0	D38.5	D49.1
nasal — *see* Neoplasm, nose						
nasolabial groove — *see also* Neoplasm, skin, face	C44.309	C79.2	D04.39	D23.39	D48.5	D49.2
nasolacrimal duct	C69.5-☑	C79.49	D09.2-☑	D31.5-☑	D48.7	D49.89
nasopharynx, nasopharyngeal	C11.9	C79.89	D00.08	D10.6	D37.05	D49.0
floor	C11.3	C79.89	D00.08	D10.6	D37.05	D49.0
overlapping lesion	C11.8	—	—	—	—	—
roof	C11.0	C79.89	D00.08	D10.6	D37.05	D49.0
wall	C11.9	C79.89	D00.08	D10.6	D37.05	D49.0
anterior	C11.3	C79.89	D00.08	D10.6	D37.05	D49.0
lateral	C11.2	C79.89	D00.08	D10.6	D37.05	D49.0
posterior	C11.1	C79.89	D00.08	D10.6	D37.05	D49.0
superior	C11.0	C79.89	D00.08	D10.6	D37.05	D49.0
nates — *see also* Neoplasm, skin, trunk	C44.509	C79.2	D04.5	D23.5	D48.5	D49.2
neck NEC	C76.0	C79.89	D09.8	D36.7	D48.7	D49.89
skin	C44.40	—	—	—	—	—
basal cell carcinoma	C44.41	—	—	—	—	—
specified type NEC	C44.49	—	—	—	—	—
squamous cell carcinoma	C44.42	—	—	—	—	—
nerve (ganglion)	C47.9	C79.89	—	D36.10	D48.2	D49.2
abducens	C72.59	C79.49	—	D33.3	D43.3	D49.7
accessory (spinal)	C72.59	C79.49	—	D33.3	D43.3	D49.7
acoustic	C72.4-☑	C79.49	—	D33.3	D43.3	D49.7
auditory	C72.4-☑	C79.49	—	D33.3	D43.3	D49.7
autonomic NEC — *see also* Neoplasm, nerve, peripheral	C47.9	C79.89	—	D36.10	D48.2	D49.2
brachial	C47.1-☑	C79.89	—	D36.12	D48.2	D49.2
cranial	C72.50	C79.49	—	D33.3	D43.3	D49.7
specified NEC	C72.59	C79.49	—	D33.3	D43.3	D49.7
facial	C72.59	C79.49	—	D33.3	D43.3	D49.7
femoral	C47.2-☑	C79.89	—	D36.13	D48.2	D49.2
ganglion NEC — *see also* Neoplasm, nerve, peripheral	C47.9	C79.89	—	D36.10	D48.2	D49.2
glossopharyngeal	C72.59	C79.49	—	D33.3	D43.3	D49.7
hypoglossal	C72.59	C79.49	—	D33.3	D43.3	D49.7
intercostal	C47.3	C79.89	—	D36.14	D48.2	D49.2
lumbar	C47.6	C79.89	—	D36.17	D48.2	D49.2
median	C47.1-☑	C79.89	—	D36.12	D48.2	D49.2
obturator	C47.2-☑	C79.89	—	D36.13	D48.2	D49.2
oculomotor	C72.59	C79.49	—	D33.3	D43.3	D49.7
olfactory	C47.2-☑	C79.49	—	D33.3	D43.3	D49.7
optic	C72.3-☑	C79.49	—	D33.3	D43.3	D49.7
parasympathetic NEC	C47.9	C79.89	—	D36.10	D48.2	D49.2
peripheral NEC	C47.9	C79.89	—	D36.10	D48.2	D49.2
abdomen	C47.4	C79.89	—	D36.15	D48.2	D49.2
abdominal wall	C47.4	C79.89	—	D36.15	D48.2	D49.2
ankle	C47.2-☑	C79.89	—	D36.13	D48.2	D49.2
antecubital fossa or space	C47.1-☑	C79.89	—	D36.12	D48.2	D49.2

☑ Additional Character Required — Refer to the Tabular List for Character Selection   ▽ Subterms under main terms may continue to next column or page

Neoplasm, neoplastic — continued

	Malignant Primary	Malignant Secondary	Ca in situ	Benign	Uncertain	Unspecified Behavior
nerve — continued						
peripheral — continued						
arm	C47.1-☑	C79.89	—	D36.12	D48.2	D49.2
auricle (ear)	C47.0	C79.89	—	D36.11	D48.2	D49.2
axilla	C47.3	C79.89	—	D36.12	D48.2	D49.2
back	C47.6	C79.89	—	D36.17	D48.2	D49.2
buttock	C47.5	C79.89	—	D36.16	D48.2	D49.2
calf	C47.2-☑	C79.89	—	D36.13	D48.2	D49.2
cervical region	C47.0	C79.89	—	D36.11	D48.2	D49.2
cheek	C47.0	C79.89	—	D36.11	D48.2	D49.2
chest (wall)	C47.3	C79.89	—	D36.14	D48.2	D49.2
chin	C47.0	C79.89	—	D36.11	D48.2	D49.2
ear (external)	C47.0	C79.89	—	D36.11	D48.2	D49.2
elbow	C47.1-☑	C79.89	—	D36.12	D48.2	D49.2
extrarectal	C47.5	C79.89	—	D36.16	D48.2	D49.2
extremity	C47.9	C79.89	—	D36.10	D48.2	D49.2
lower	C47.2-☑	C79.89	—	D36.13	D48.2	D49.2
upper	C47.1-☑	C79.89	—	D36.12	D48.2	D49.2
eyelid	C47.0	C79.89	—	D36.11	D48.2	D49.2
face	C47.0	C79.89	—	D36.11	D48.2	D49.2
finger	C47.1-☑	C79.89	—	D36.12	D48.2	D49.2
flank	C47.6	C79.89	—	D36.17	D48.2	D49.2
foot	C47.2-☑	C79.89	—	D36.13	D48.2	D49.2
forearm	C47.1-☑	C79.89	—	D36.12	D48.2	D49.2
forehead	C47.0	C79.89	—	D36.11	D48.2	D49.2
gluteal region	C47.5	C79.89	—	D36.16	D48.2	D49.2
groin	C47.5	C79.89	—	D36.16	D48.2	D49.2
hand	C47.1-☑	C79.89	—	D36.12	D48.2	D49.2
head	C47.0	C79.89	—	D36.11	D48.2	D49.2
heel	C47.2-☑	C79.89	—	D36.13	D48.2	D49.2
hip	C47.2-☑	C79.89	—	D36.13	D48.2	D49.2
infraclavicular region	C47.3	C79.89	—	D36.14	D48.2	D49.2
inguinal (canal) (region)	C47.5	C79.89	—	D36.16	D48.2	D49.2
intrathoracic	C47.3	C79.89	—	D36.14	D48.2	D49.2
ischiorectal fossa	C47.5	C79.89	—	D36.16	D48.2	D49.2
knee	C47.2-☑	C79.89	—	D36.13	D48.2	D49.2
leg	C47.2-☑	C79.89	—	D36.13	D48.2	D49.2
limb NEC	C47.9	C79.89	—	D36.10	D48.2	D49.2
lower	C47.2-☑	C79.89	—	D36.13	D48.2	D49.2
upper	C47.1-☑	C79.89	—	D36.12	D48.2	D49.2
nates	C47.5	C79.89	—	D36.16	D48.2	D49.2
neck	C47.0	C79.89	—	D36.11	D48.2	D49.2
orbit	C69.6-☑	C79.49	—	D31.6-☑	D48.7	D49.2
pararectal	C47.5	C79.89	—	D36.16	D48.2	D49.2
paraurethral	C47.5	C79.89	—	D36.16	D48.2	D49.2
paravaginal	C47.5	C79.89	—	D36.16	D48.2	D49.2
pelvis (floor)	C47.5	C79.89	—	D36.16	D48.2	D49.2
pelvoabdominal	C47.8	C79.89	—	D36.17	D48.2	D49.2
perineum	C47.5	C79.89	—	D36.16	D48.2	D49.2
perirectal (tissue)	C47.5	C79.89	—	D36.16	D48.2	D49.2
periurethral (tissue)	C47.5	C79.89	—	D36.16	D48.2	D49.2
popliteal fossa or space	C47.2-☑	C79.89	—	D36.13	D48.2	D49.2
presacral	C47.5	C79.89	—	D36.16	D48.2	D49.2
pterygoid fossa	C47.0	C79.89	—	D36.11	D48.2	D49.2
rectovaginal septum or wall	C47.5	C79.89	—	D36.16	D48.2	D49.2
rectovesical	C47.5	C79.89	—	D36.16	D48.2	D49.2
sacrococcygeal region	C47.5	C79.89	—	D36.16	D48.2	D49.2
scalp	C47.0	C79.89	—	D36.11	D48.2	D49.2
scapular region	C47.3	C79.89	—	D36.14	D48.2	D49.2
shoulder	C47.1-☑	C79.89	—	D36.12	D48.2	D49.2
submental	C47.0	C79.89	—	D36.11	D48.2	D49.2
supraclavicular region	C47.0	C79.89	—	D36.11	D48.2	D49.2
temple	C47.0	C79.89	—	D36.11	D48.2	D49.2
temporal region	C47.0	C79.89	—	D36.11	D48.2	D49.2
thigh	C47.2-☑	C79.89	—	D36.13	D48.2	D49.2
thoracic (duct) (wall)	C47.3	C79.89	—	D36.14	D48.2	D49.2
thorax	C47.3	C79.89	—	D36.14	D48.2	D49.2
thumb	C47.1-☑	C79.89	—	D36.12	D48.2	D49.2
toe	C47.2-☑	C79.89	—	D36.13	D48.2	D49.2
trunk	C47.6	C79.89	—	D36.17	D48.2	D49.2

Neoplasm, neoplastic — continued

	Malignant Primary	Malignant Secondary	Ca in situ	Benign	Uncertain	Unspecified Behavior
nerve — continued						
peripheral — continued						
umbilicus	C47.4	C79.89	—	D36.15	D48.2	D49.2
vesicorectal	C47.5	C79.89	—	D36.16	D48.2	D49.2
wrist	C47.1-☑	C79.89	—	D36.12	D48.2	D49.2
radial	C47.1-☑	C79.89	—	D36.12	D48.2	D49.2
sacral	C47.5	C79.89	—	D36.16	D48.2	D49.2
sciatic	C47.2-☑	C79.89	—	D36.13	D48.2	D49.2
spinal NEC	C47.9	C79.89	—	D36.10	D48.2	D49.2
accessory	C72.59	C79.49	—	D33.3	D43.3	D49.7
sympathetic NEC — see also Neoplasm, nerve, peripheral	C47.9	C79.89	—	D36.10	D48.2	D49.2
trigeminal	C72.59	C79.49	—	D33.3	D43.3	D49.7
trochlear	C72.59	C79.49	—	D33.3	D43.3	D49.7
ulnar	C47.1-☑	C79.89	—	D36.12	D48.2	D49.2
vagus	C72.59	C79.49	—	D33.3	D43.3	D49.7
nervous system (central)	C72.9	C79.40	—	D33.9	D43.9	D49.7
autonomic — see Neoplasm, nerve, peripheral						
parasympathetic — see Neoplasm, nerve, peripheral						
specified site NEC	—	C79.49	—	D33.7	D43.8	—
sympathetic — see Neoplasm, nerve, peripheral						
nevus — see Nevus						
nipple	C50.0-☑	C79.81	D05.-☑	D24.-☑	—	—
nose, nasal	C76.0	C79.89	D09.8	D36.7	D48.7	D49.89
ala (external) (nasi) — see also Neoplasm, nose, skin	C44.301	C79.2	D04.39	D23.39	D48.5	D49.2
bone	C41.0	C79.51	—	D16.4	D48.0	D49.2
cartilage	C30.0	C78.39	D02.3	D14.0	D38.5	D49.1
cavity	C30.0	C78.39	D02.3	D14.0	D38.5	D49.1
choana	C11.3	C79.89	D00.08	D10.6	D37.05	D49.0
external (skin) — see also Neoplasm, nose, skin	C44.301	C79.2	D04.39	D23.39	D48.5	D49.2
fossa	C30.0	C78.39	D02.3	D14.0	D38.5	D49.1
internal	C30.0	C78.39	D02.3	D14.0	D38.5	D49.1
mucosa	C30.0	C78.39	D02.3	D14.0	D38.5	D49.1
septum	C30.0	C78.39	D02.3	D14.0	D38.5	D49.1
posterior margin	C11.3	C79.89	D00.08	D10.6	D37.05	D49.0
sinus — see Neoplasm, sinus						
skin	C44.301	C79.2	D04.39	D23.39	D48.5	D49.2
basal cell carcinoma	C44.311	—	—	—	—	—
specified type NEC	C44.391	—	—	—	—	—
squamous cell carcinoma	C44.321	—	—	—	—	—
turbinate (mucosa)	C30.0	C78.39	D02.3	D14.0	D38.5	D49.1
bone	C41.0	C79.51	—	D16.4	D48.0	D49.2
vestibule	C30.0	C78.39	D02.3	D14.0	D38.5	D49.1
nostril	C30.0	C78.39	D02.3	D14.0	D38.5	D49.1
nucleus pulposus	C41.2	C79.51	—	D16.6	D48.0	D49.2
occipital						
bone	C41.0	C79.51	—	D16.4	D48.0	D49.2
lobe or pole, brain	C71.4	C79.31	—	D33.0	D43.0	D49.6
odontogenic — see Neoplasm, jaw bone						
olfactory nerve or bulb	C72.2-☑	C79.49	—	D33.3	D43.3	D49.7
olive (brain)	C71.7	C79.31	—	D33.1	D43.1	D49.6
omentum	C48.1	C78.6	—	D20.1	D48.4	D49.0
operculum (brain)	C71.0	C79.31	—	D33.0	D43.0	D49.6
optic nerve, chiasm, or tract	C72.3-☑	C79.49	—	D33.3	D43.3	D49.7
oral (cavity)	C06.9	C79.89	D00.00	D10.30	D37.09	D49.0
ill-defined	C14.8	C79.89	D00.00	D10.30	D37.09	D49.0
mucosa	C06.0	C79.89	D00.02	D10.39	D37.09	D49.0
orbit	C69.6-☑	C79.49	D09.2-☑	D31.6-☑	D48.7	D49.89
autonomic nerve	C69.6-☑	C79.49	—	D31.6-☑	D48.7	D49.2
bone	C41.0	C79.51	—	D16.4	D48.0	D49.2

Neoplasm, neoplastic — *continued*

orbit — *continued*	Malignant Primary	Malignant Secondary	Ca in situ	Benign	Uncertain	Unspecified Behavior
eye	C69.6-✓	C79.49	D09.2-✓	D31.6-✓	D48.7	D49.89
peripheral nerves	C69.6-✓	C79.49	—	D31.6-✓	D48.7	D49.2
soft parts	C69.6-✓	C79.49	D09.2-✓	D31.6-✓	D48.7	D49.89
organ of Zuckerkandl	C75.5	C79.89	—	D35.6	D44.7	D49.7
oropharynx	C10.9	C79.89	D00.08	D10.5	D37.05	D49.0
branchial cleft (vestige)	C10.4	C79.89	D00.08	D10.5	D37.05	D49.0
junctional region	C10.8	C79.89	D00.08	D10.5	D37.05	D49.0
lateral wall	C10.2	C79.89	D00.08	D10.5	D37.05	D49.0
overlapping lesion	C10.8	—	—	—	—	—
pillars or fauces	C09.1	C79.89	D00.08	D10.5	D37.05	D49.0
posterior wall	C10.3	C79.89	D00.08	D10.5	D37.05	D49.0
vallecula	C10.0	C79.89	D00.08	D10.5	D37.05	D49.0
os						
external	C53.1	C79.82	D06.1	D26.0	D39.0	D49.59
internal	C53.0	C79.82	D06.0	D26.0	D39.0	D49.59
ovary	C56.-✓	C79.6-✓	D07.39	D27.-✓	D39.1-✓	D49.59
oviduct	C57.0-✓	C79.82	D07.39	D28.2	D39.8	D49.59
palate	C05.9	C79.89	D00.00	D10.39	D37.09	D49.0
hard	C05.0	C79.89	D00.05	D10.39	D37.09	D49.0
junction of hard and soft palate	C05.9	C79.89	D00.00	D10.39	D37.09	D49.0
overlapping lesions	C05.8	—	—	—	—	—
soft	C05.1	C79.89	D00.04	D10.39	D37.09	D49.0
nasopharyngeal surface	C11.3	C79.89	D00.08	D10.6	D37.05	D49.0
posterior surface	C11.3	C79.89	D00.08	D10.6	D37.05	D49.0
superior surface	C11.3	C79.89	D00.08	D10.6	D37.05	D49.0
palatoglossal arch	C09.1	C79.89	D00.00	D10.5	D37.09	D49.0
palatopharyngeal arch	C09.1	C79.89	D00.00	D10.5	D37.09	D49.0
pallium	C71.0	C79.31	—	D33.0	D43.0	D49.6
palpebra	C44.10-✓	C79.2	D04.1-✓	D23.1-✓	D48.5	D49.2
basal cell carcinoma	C44.11-✓	—	—	—	—	—
specified type NEC	C44.19-✓	—	—	—	—	—
squamous cell carcinoma	C44.12-✓	—	—	—	—	—
pancreas	C25.9	C78.89	D01.7	D13.6	D37.8	D49.0
body	C25.1	C78.89	D01.7	D13.6	D37.8	D49.0
duct (of Santorini) (of Wirsung)	C25.3	C78.89	D01.7	D13.6	D37.8	D49.0
ectopic tissue	C25.7	C78.89	—	D13.6	D37.8	D49.0
head	C25.0	C78.89	D01.7	D13.6	D37.8	D49.0
islet cells	C25.4	C78.89	D01.7	D13.7	D37.8	D49.0
neck	C25.7	C78.89	D01.7	D13.6	D37.8	D49.0
overlapping lesion	C25.8	—	—	—	—	—
tail	C25.2	C78.89	D01.7	D13.6	D37.8	D49.0
para-aortic body	C75.5	C79.89	—	D35.6	D44.7	D49.7
paraganglion NEC	C75.5	C79.89	—	D35.6	D44.7	D49.7
parametrium	C57.3	C79.82	—	D28.2	D39.8	D49.59
paranephric	C48.0	C78.6	—	D20.0	D48.3	D49.0
pararectal	C76.3	C79.89	—	D36.7	D48.7	D49.89
parasagittal (region)	C76.0	C79.89	D09.8	D36.7	D48.7	D49.89
parasellar	C72.9	C79.49	—	D33.9	D43.8	D49.7
parathyroid (gland)	C75.0	C79.89	D09.3	D35.1	D44.2	D49.7
paraurethral	C76.3	C79.89	—	D36.7	D48.7	D49.89
gland	C68.1	C79.19	D09.19	D30.8	D41.8	D49.59
paravaginal	C76.3	C79.89	—	D36.7	D48.7	D49.89
parenchyma, kidney	C64.-✓	C79.0-✓	D09.19	D30.0-✓	D41.0-✓	D49.51-✓
parietal						
bone	C41.0	C79.51	—	D16.4	D48.0	D49.2
lobe, brain	C71.3	C79.31	—	D33.0	D43.0	D49.6
paroophoron	C57.1-✓	C79.82	D07.39	D28.2	D39.8	D49.59
parotid (duct) (gland)	C07	C79.89	D00.00	D11.0	D37.030	D49.0
parovarium	C57.1-✓	C79.82	D07.39	D28.2	D39.8	D49.59
patella	C40.20	C79.51				
peduncle, cerebral	C71.7	C79.31	—	D33.1	D43.1	D49.6
pelvirectal junction	C19	C78.5	D01.1	D12.7	D37.5	D49.0
pelvis, pelvic	C76.3	C79.89	D09.8	D36.7	D48.7	D49.89
bone	C41.4	C79.51	—	D16.8	D48.0	D49.2
floor	C76.3	C79.89	D09.8	D36.7	D48.7	D49.89
renal	C65.-✓	C79.0-✓	D09.19	D30.1-✓	D41.1-✓	D49.51-✓
viscera	C76.3	C79.89	D09.8	D36.7	D48.7	D49.89
wall	C76.3	C79.89	D09.8	D36.7	D48.7	D49.89
pelvo-abdominal	C76.8	C79.89	D09.8	D36.7	D48.7	D49.89
penis	C60.9	C79.82	D07.4	D29.0	D40.8	D49.59

Neoplasm, neoplastic — *continued*

penis — *continued*	Malignant Primary	Malignant Secondary	Ca in situ	Benign	Uncertain	Unspecified Behavior
body	C60.2	C79.82	D07.4	D29.0	D40.8	D49.59
corpus (cavernosum)	C60.2	C79.82	D07.4	D29.0	D40.8	D49.59
glans	C60.1	C79.82	D07.4	D29.0	D40.8	D49.59
overlapping sites	C60.8	—	—	—	—	—
skin NEC	C60.9	C79.82	D07.4	D29.0	D40.8	D49.59
periadrenal (tissue)	C48.0	C78.6	—	D20.0	D48.3	D49.0
perianal (skin) — *see also* Neoplasm, anus, skin	C44.500	C79.2	D04.5	D23.5	D48.5	D49.2
pericardium	C38.0	C79.89	—	D15.1	D48.7	D49.89
perinephric	C48.0	C78.6	—	D20.0	D48.3	D49.0
perineum	C76.3	C79.89	D09.8	D36.7	D48.7	D49.89
periodontal tissue NEC	C03.9	C79.89	D00.03	D10.39	D37.09	D49.0
periosteum — *see* Neoplasm, bone						
peripancreatic	C48.0	C78.6	—	D20.0	D48.3	D49.0
peripheral nerve NEC	C47.9	C79.89	—	D36.10	D48.2	D49.2
perirectal (tissue)	C76.3	C79.89	—	D36.7	D48.7	D49.89
perirenal (tissue)	C48.0	C78.6	—	D20.0	D48.3	D49.0
peritoneum, peritoneal (cavity)	C48.2	C78.6	—	D20.1	D48.4	D49.0
benign mesothelial tissue — *see* Mesothelioma, benign						
overlapping lesion with digestive organs	C48.8	—	—	—	—	—
parietal	C48.1	C78.6	—	D20.1	D48.4	D49.0
pelvic	C48.1	C78.6	—	D20.1	D48.4	D49.0
specified part NEC	C48.1	C78.6	—	D20.1	D48.4	D49.0
peritonsillar (tissue)	C76.0	C79.89	D09.8	D36.7	D48.7	D49.89
periurethral tissue	C76.3	C79.89	—	D36.7	D48.7	D49.89
phalanges						
foot	C40.3-✓	C79.51	—	D16.3-✓	—	—
hand	C40.1-✓	C79.51	—	D16.1-✓	—	—
pharynx, pharyngeal	C14.0	C79.89	D00.08	D10.9	D37.05	D49.0
bursa	C11.1	C79.89	D00.08	D10.6	D37.05	D49.0
fornix	C11.3	C79.89	D00.08	D10.6	D37.05	D49.0
recess	C11.2	C79.89	D00.08	D10.6	D37.05	D49.0
region	C14.0	C79.89	D00.08	D10.9	D37.05	D49.0
tonsil	C11.1	C79.89	D00.08	D10.6	D37.05	D49.0
wall (lateral) (posterior)	C14.0	C79.89	D00.08	D10.9	D37.05	D49.0
pia mater	C70.9	C79.40	—	D32.9	D42.9	D49.7
cerebral	C70.0	C79.32	—	D32.0	D42.0	D49.7
cranial	C70.0	C79.32	—	D32.0	D42.0	D49.7
spinal	C70.1	C79.49	—	D32.1	D42.1	D49.7
pillars of fauces	C09.1	C79.89	D00.08	D10.5	D37.05	D49.0
pineal (body) (gland)	C75.3	C79.89	D09.3	D35.4	D44.5	D49.7
pinna (ear) NEC — *see also* Neoplasm, skin, ear	C44.20-✓	C79.2	D04.2-✓	D23.2-✓	D48.5	D49.2
piriform fossa or sinus	C12	C79.89	D00.08	D10.7	D37.05	D49.0
pituitary (body) (fossa) (gland) (lobe)	C75.1	C79.89	D09.3	D35.2	D44.3	D49.7
placenta	C58	C79.82	D07.0	D26.7	D39.2	D49.59
pleura, pleural (cavity)	C38.4	C78.2	—	D19.0	D38.2	D49.1
overlapping lesion with heart or mediastinum	C38.8	—	—	—	—	—
parietal	C38.4	C78.2	—	D19.0	D38.2	D49.1
visceral	C38.4	C78.2	—	D19.0	D38.2	D49.1
plexus						
brachial	C47.1-✓	C79.89	—	D36.12	D48.2	D49.2
cervical	C47.0	C79.89	—	D36.11	D48.2	D49.2
choroid	C71.5	C79.31	—	D33.0	D43.0	D49.6
lumbosacral	C47.5	C79.89	—	D36.16	D48.2	D49.2
sacral	C47.5	C79.89	—	D36.16	D48.2	D49.2
pluriendocrine	C75.8	C79.89	D09.3	D35.7	D44.9	D49.7
pole						
frontal	C71.1	C79.31	—	D33.0	D43.0	D49.6
occipital	C71.4	C79.31	—	D33.0	D43.0	D49.6
pons (varolii)	C71.7	C79.31	—	D33.1	D43.1	D49.6

✓ **Additional Character Required — Refer to the Tabular List for Character Selection**　　　▽ **Subterms under main terms may continue to next column or page**

(left margin: Neoplasm Table — Neoplasm, orbit — Neoplasm, pons)

Neoplasm, neoplastic — *continued*	Malignant Primary	Malignant Secondary	Ca in situ	Benign	Uncertain	Unspecified Behavior
popliteal fossa or space	C76.5-☑	C79.89	D04.7-☑	D36.7	D48.7	D49.89
postcricoid (region)	C13.0	C79.89	D00.08	D10.7	D37.05	D49.0
posterior fossa (cranial)	C71.9	C79.31	—	D33.2	D43.2	D49.6
postnasal space	C11.9	C79.89	D00.08	D10.6	D37.05	D49.0
prepuce	C60.0	C79.82	D07.4	D29.0	D40.8	D49.59
prepylorus	C16.4	C78.89	D00.2	D13.1	D37.1	D49.0
presacral (region)	C76.3	C79.89	—	D36.7	D48.7	D49.89
prostate (gland)	C61	C79.82	D07.5	D29.1	D40.0	D49.59
utricle	C68.0	C79.19	D09.19	D30.4	D41.3	D49.59
pterygoid fossa	C49.0	C79.89	—	D21.0	D48.1	D49.2
pubic bone	C41.4	C79.51	—	D16.8	D48.0	D49.2
pudenda, pudendum (femaie)	C51.9	C79.82	D07.1	D28.0	D39.8	D49.59
pulmonary — *see also* Neoplasm, lung	C34.9-☑	C78.0-☑	D02.2-☑	D14.3-☑	D38.1	D49.1
putamen	C71.0	C79.31	—	D33.0	D43.0	D49.6
pyloric						
antrum	C16.3	C78.89	D00.2	D13.1	D37.1	D49.0
canal	C16.4	C78.89	D00.2	D13.1	D37.1	D49.0
pylorus	C16.4	C78.89	D00.2	D13.1	D37.1	D49.0
pyramid (brain)	C71.7	C79.31	—	D33.1	D43.1	D49.6
pyriform fossa or sinus	C12	C79.89	D00.08	D10.7	D37.05	D49.0
radius (any part)	C40.0-☑	C79.51	—	D16.0-☑	—	—
Rathke's pouch	C75.1	C79.89	D09.3	D35.2	D44.3	D49.7
rectosigmoid (junction)	C19	C78.5	D01.1	D12.7	D37.5	D49.0
overlapping lesion with anus or rectum	C21.8	—	—	—	—	—
rectouterine pouch	C48.1	C78.6	—	D20.1	D48.4	D49.0
rectovaginal septum or wall	C76.3	C79.89	D09.8	D36.7	D48.7	D49.89
rectovesical septum	C76.3	C79.89	D09.8	D36.7	D48.7	D49.89
rectum (ampulla)	C20	C78.5	D01.2	D12.8	D37.5	D49.0
and colon	C19	C78.5	D01.1	D12.7	D37.5	D49.0
overlapping lesion with anus or rectosigmoid junction	C21.8	—	—	—	—	—
renal	C64.-☑	C79.0-☑	D09.19	D30.0-☑	D41.0-☑	D49.51-☑
calyx	C65.-☑	C79.0-☑	D09.19	D30.1-☑	D41.1-☑	D49.51-☑
hilus	C65.-☑	C79.0-☑	D09.19	D30.1-☑	D41.1-☑	D49.51-☑
parenchyma	C64.-☑	C79.0-☑	D09.19	D30.0-☑	D41.0-☑	D49.51-☑
pelvis	C65.-☑	C79.0-☑	D09.19	D30.1-☑	D41.1-☑	D49.51-☑
respiratory						
organs or system NEC	C39.9	C78.30	D02.4	D14.4	D38.6	D49.1
tract NEC	C39.9	C78.30	D02.4	D14.4	D38.5	D49.1
upper	C39.0	C78.30	D02.4	D14.4	D38.5	D49.1
retina	C69.2-☑	C79.49	D09.2-☑	D31.2-☑	D48.7	D49.81
retrobulbar	C69.6-☑	C79.49	—	D31.6-☑	D48.7	D49.89
retrocecal	C48.0	C78.6	—	D20.0	D48.3	D49.0
retromolar (area) (triangle) (trigone)	C06.2	C79.89	D00.00	D10.39	D37.09	D49.0
retro-orbital	C76.0	C79.89	D09.8	D36.7	D48.7	D49.89
retroperitoneal (space) (tissue)	C48.0	C78.6	—	D20.0	D48.3	D49.0
retroperitoneum	C48.0	C78.6	—	D20.0	D48.3	D49.0
retropharyngeal	C14.0	C79.89	D00.08	D10.9	D37.05	D49.0
retrovesical (septum)	C76.3	C79.89	D09.8	D36.7	D48.7	D49.89
rhinencephalon	C71.0	C79.31	—	D33.0	D43.0	D49.6
rib	C41.3	C79.51	—	D16.7	D48.0	D49.2
Rosenmuller's fossa	C11.2	C79.89	D00.08	D10.6	D37.05	D49.0
round ligament	C57.2-☑	C79.82	—	D28.2	D39.8	D49.59
sacrococcyx, sacrococcygeal	C41.4	C79.51	—	D16.8	D48.0	D49.2
region	C76.3	C79.89	D09.8	D36.7	D48.7	D49.89
sacrouterine ligament	C57.3	C79.82	—	D28.2	D39.8	D49.59
sacrum, sacral (vertebra)	C41.4	C79.51	—	D16.8	D48.0	D49.2
salivary gland or duct (major)	C08.9	C79.89	D00.00	D11.9	D37.039	D49.0
minor NEC	C06.9	C79.89	D00.00	D10.39	D37.04	D49.0
overlapping lesion	C08.9	—	—	D11.9	—	D49.0
parotid	C07	C79.89	D00.00	D11.0	D37.030	D49.0

Neoplasm, neoplastic — *continued*	Malignant Primary	Malignant Secondary	Ca in situ	Benign	Uncertain	Unspecified Behavior
sallvary gland or duct — *continued*						
pluriglandular	C08.9	C79.89	D00.00	D11.9	D37.039	D49.0
sublingual	C08.1	C79.89	D00.00	D11.7	D37.031	D49.0
submandibular	C08.0	C79.89	D00.00	D11.7	D37.032	D49.0
submaxillary	C08.0	C79.89	D00.00	D11.7	D37.032	D49.0
salpinx (uterine)	C57.0-☑	C79.82	D07.39	D28.2	D39.8	D49.59
Santorini's duct	C25.3	C78.89	D01.7	D13.6	D37.8	D49.0
scalp	C44.40	C79.2	D04.4	D23.4	D48.5	D49.2
basal cell carcinoma	C44.41	—	—	—	—	—
specified type NEC	C44.49	—	—	—	—	—
squamous cell carcinoma	C44.42	—	—	—	—	—
scapula (any part)	C40.0-☑	C79.51	—	D16.0-☑	—	—
scapular region	C76.1	C79.89	D09.8	D36.7	D48.7	D49.89
scar NEC — *see also* Neoplasm, skin, by site	C44.90	C79.2	D04.9	D23.9	D48.5	D49.2
sciatic nerve	C47.2-☑	C79.89	—	D36.13	D48.2	D49.2
sclera	C69.4-☑	C79.49	D09.2-☑	D31.4-☑	D48.7	D49.89
scrotum (skin)	C63.2	C79.82	D07.61	D29.4	D40.8	D49.59
sebaceous gland — *see* Neoplasm, skin						
sella turcica	C75.1	C79.89	D09.3	D35.2	D44.3	D49.7
bone	C41.0	C79.51	—	D16.4	D48.0	D49.2
semilunar cartilage (knee)	C40.2-☑	C79.51	—	D16.2-☑	D48.0	D49.2
seminal vesicle	C63.7	C79.82	D07.69	D29.8	D40.8	D49.59
septum						
nasal	C30.0	C78.39	D02.3	D14.0	D38.5	D49.1
posterior margin	C11.3	C79.89	D00.08	D10.6	D37.05	D49.0
rectovaginal	C76.3	C79.89	D09.8	D36.7	D48.7	D49.89
rectovesical	C76.3	C79.89	D09.8	D36.7	D48.7	D49.89
urethrovaginal	C57.9	C79.82	D07.30	D28.9	D39.9	D49.59
vesicovaginal	C57.9	C79.82	D07.30	D28.9	D39.9	D49.59
shoulder NEC	C76.4-☑	C79.89	D04.6-☑	D36.7	D48.7	D49.89
sigmoid flexure (lower) (upper)	C18.7	C78.5	D01.0	D12.5	D37.4	D49.0
sinus (accessory)	C31.9	C78.39	D02.3	D14.0	D38.5	D49.1
bone (any)	C41.0	C79.51	—	D16.4	D48.0	D49.2
ethmoidal	C31.1	C78.39	D02.3	D14.0	D38.5	D49.1
frontal	C31.2	C78.39	D02.3	D14.0	D38.5	D49.1
maxillary	C31.0	C78.39	D02.3	D14.0	D38.5	D49.1
nasal, paranasal NEC	C31.9	C78.39	D02.3	D14.0	D38.5	D49.1
overlapping lesion	C31.8	—	—	—	—	—
pyriform	C12	C79.89	D00.08	D10.7	D37.05	D49.0
sphenoid	C31.3	C78.39	D02.3	D14.0	D38.5	D49.1
skeleton, skeletal NEC	C41.9	C79.51	—	D16.9	D48.0	D49.2
Skene's gland	C68.1	C79.19	D09.19	D30.8	D41.8	D49.59
skin NOS	C44.90	C79.2	D04.9	D23.9	D48.5	D49.2
abdominal wall	C44.509	C79.2	D04.5	D23.5	D48.5	D49.2
basal cell carcinoma specified type	C44.519	—	—	—	—	—
NEC	C44.599	—	—	—	—	—
squamous cell carcinoma	C44.529	—	—	—	—	—
ala nasi — *see also* Neoplasm, nose, skin	C44.301	C79.2	D04.39	D23.39	D48.5	D49.2
ankle — *see also* Neoplasm, skin, limb, lower	C44.70-☑	C79.2	D04.7-☑	D23.7-☑	D48.5	D49.2
antecubital space — *see also* Neoplasm, skin, limb, upper	C44.60-☑	C79.2	D04.6-☑	D23.6-☑	D48.5	D49.2
anus	C44.500	C79.2	D04.5	D23.5	D48.5	D49.2
basal cell carcinoma	C44.510	—	—	—	—	—
specified type NEC	C44.590	—	—	—	—	—
squamous cell carcinoma	C44.520	—	—	—	—	—
arm — *see also* Neoplasm, skin, limb, upper	C44.60-☑	C79.2	D04.6-☑	D23.6-☑	D48.5	D49.2

☑ **Subterms under main terms may continue to next column or page**   ☑ **Additional Character Required — Refer to the Tabular List for Character Selection**

Neoplasm Table

Neoplasm, skin NOS — Neoplasm, skin NOS

Neoplasm, neoplastic — *continued*	Malignant Primary	Malignant Secondary	Ca in situ	Benign	Uncertain	Unspecified Behavior
skin — *continued*						
auditory canal (external) — *see also* Neoplasm, skin, ear	C44.20-☑	C79.2	D04.2-☑	D23.2-☑	D48.5	D49.2
auricle (ear) — *see also* Neoplasm, skin, ear	C44.20-☑	C79.2	D04.2-☑	D23.2-☑	D48.5	D49.2
auricular canal (external) — *see also* Neoplasm, skin, ear	C44.20-☑	C79.2	D04.2-☑	D23.2-☑	D48.5	D49.2
axilla, axillary fold — *see also* Neoplasm, skin, trunk	C44.509	C79.2	D04.5	D23.5	D48.5	D49.2
back — *see also* Neoplasm, skin, trunk	C44.509	C79.2	D04.5	D23.5	D48.5	D49.2
basal cell carcinoma	C44.91	—	—	—	—	—
breast	C44.501	C79.2	D04.5	D23.5	D48.5	D49.2
basal cell carcinoma	C44.511	—	—	—	—	—
specified type NEC	C44.591	—	—	—	—	—
squamous cell carcinoma	C44.521	—	—	—	—	—
brow — *see also* Neoplasm, skin, face	C44.309	C79.2	D04.39	D23.39	D48.5	D49.2
buttock — *see also* Neoplasm, skin, trunk	C44.509	C79.2	D04.5	D23.5	D48.5	D49.2
calf — *see also* Neoplasm, skin, limb, lower	C44.70-☑	C79.2	D04.7-☑	D23.7-☑	D48.5	D49.2
canthus (eye) (inner) (outer)	C44.10-☑	C79.2	D04.1-☑	D23.1-☑	D48.5	D49.2
basal cell carcinoma	C44.11-☑	—	—	—	—	—
specified type NEC	C44.19-☑	—	—	—	—	—
squamous cell carcinoma	C44.12-☑	—	—	—	—	—
cervical region — *see also* Neoplasm, skin, neck	C44.40	C79.2	D04.4	D23.4	D48.5	D49.2
cheek (external) — *see also* Neoplasm, skin, face	C44.309	C79.2	D04.39	D23.39	D48.5	D49.2
chest (wall) — *see also* Neoplasm, skin, trunk	C44.509	C79.2	D04.5	D23.5	D48.5	D49.2
chin — *see also* Neoplasm, skin, face	C44.309	C79.2	D04.39	D23.39	D48.5	D49.2
clavicular area — *see also* Neoplasm, skin, trunk	C44.509	C79.2	D04.5	D23.5	D48.5	D49.2
clitoris	C51.2	C79.82	D07.1	D28.0	D39.8	D49.59
columnella — *see also* Neoplasm, skin, face	C44.309	C79.2	D04.39	D23.39	D48.5	D49.2
concha — *see also* Neoplasm, skin, ear	C44.20-☑	C79.2	D04.2-☑	D23.2-☑	D48.5	D49.2
ear (external)	C44.20-☑	C79.2	D04.2-☑	D23.2-☑	D48.5	D49.2
basal cell carcinoma	C44.21-☑	—	—	—	—	—
specified type NEC	C44.29-☑	—	—	—	—	—
squamous cell carcinoma	C44.22-☑	—	—	—	—	—
elbow — *see also* Neoplasm, skin, limb, upper	C44.60-☑	C79.2	D04.6-☑	D23.6-☑	D48.5	D49.2
eyebrow — *see also* Neoplasm, skin, face	C44.309	C79.2	D04.39	D23.39	D48.5	D49.2
eyelid	C44.10-☑	C79.2	D04.1-☑	D23.1-☑	D48.5	D49.2

Neoplasm, neoplastic — *continued*	Malignant Primary	Malignant Secondary	Ca in situ	Benign	Uncertain	Unspecified Behavior
skin — *continued*						
eyelid — *continued*						
basal cell carcinoma	C44.11-☑	—	—	—	—	—
specified type NEC	C44.19-☑	—	—	—	—	—
squamous cell carcinoma	C44.12-☑	—	—	—	—	—
face NOS	C44.300	C79.2	D04.30	D23.30	D48.5	D49.2
basal cell carcinoma	C44.310	—	—	—	—	—
specified type NEC	C44.390	—	—	—	—	—
squamous cell carcinoma	C44.320	—	—	—	—	—
female genital organs (external)	C51.9	C79.82	D07.1	D28.0	D39.8	D49.59
clitoris	C51.2	C79.82	D07.1	D28.0	D39.8	D49.59
labium NEC	C51.9	C79.82	D07.1	D28.0	D39.8	D49.59
majus	C51.0	C79.82	D07.1	D28.0	D39.8	D49.59
minus	C51.1	C79.82	D07.1	D28.0	D39.8	D49.59
pudendum	C51.9	C79.82	D07.1	D28.0	D39.8	D49.59
vulva	C51.9	C79.82	D07.1	D28.0	D39.8	D49.59
finger — *see also* Neoplasm, skin, limb, upper	C44.60-☑	C79.2	D04.6-☑	D23.6-☑	D48.5	D49.2
flank — *see also* Neoplasm, skin, trunk	C44.509	C79.2	D04.5	D23.5	D48.5	D49.2
foot — *see also* Neoplasm, skin, limb, lower	C44.70-☑	C79.2	D04.7-☑	D23.7-☑	D48.5	D49.2
forearm — *see also* Neoplasm, skin, limb, upper	C44.60-☑	C79.2	D04.6-☑	D23.6-☑	D48.5	D49.2
forehead — *see also* Neoplasm, skin, face	C44.309	C79.2	D04.39	D23.39	D48.5	D49.2
glabella — *see also* Neoplasm, skin, face	C44.309	C79.2	D04.39	D23.39	D48.5	D49.2
gluteal region — *see also* Neoplasm, skin, trunk	C44.509	C79.2	D04.5	D23.5	D48.5	D49.2
groin — *see also* Neoplasm, skin, trunk	C44.509	C79.2	D04.5	D23.5	D48.5	D49.2
hand — *see also* Neoplasm, skin, limb, upper	C44.60-☑	C79.2	D04.6-☑	D23.6-☑	D48.5	D49.2
head NEC — *see also* Neoplasm, skin, scalp	C44.40	C79.2	D04.4	D23.4	D48.5	D49.2
heel — *see also* Neoplasm, skin, limb, lower	C44.70-☑	C79.2	D04.7-☑	D23.7-☑	D48.5	D49.2
helix — *see also* Neoplasm, skin, ear	C44.20-☑	C79.2	D04.2-☑	D23.2-☑	D48.5	D49.2
hip — *see also* Neoplasm, skin, limb, lower	C44.70-☑	C79.2	D04.7-☑	D23.7-☑	D48.5	D49.2
infraclavicular region — *see also* Neoplasm, skin, trunk	C44.509	C79.2	D04.5	D23.5	D48.5	D49.2
inguinal region — *see also* Neoplasm, skin, trunk	C44.509	C79.2	D04.5	D23.5	D48.5	D49.2
jaw — *see also* Neoplasm, skin, face	C44.309	C79.2	D04.39	D23.39	D48.5	D49.2
Kaposi's sarcoma — *see* Kaposi's, sarcoma, skin						
knee — *see also* Neoplasm, skin, limb, lower	C44.70-☑	C79.2	D04.7-☑	D23.7-☑	D48.5	D49.2
labia						
majora	C51.0	C79.82	D07.1	D28.0	D39.8	D49.59
minora	C51.1	C79.82	D07.1	D28.0	D39.8	D49.59

☑ Additional Character Required — Refer to the Tabular List for Character Selection   ▽ Subterms under main terms may continue to next column or page

Neoplasm, neoplastic —	Malignant Primary	Malignant Secondary	Ca in situ	Benign	Uncertain	Unspecified Behavior
continued						
skin — *continued*						
leg — *see also*						
Neoplasm, skin, limb, lower	C44.70-✓	C79.2	D04.7-✓	D23.7-✓	D48.5	D49.2
lid (lower) (upper)	C44.10-✓	C79.2	D04.1-✓	D23.1-✓	D48.5	D49.2
basal cell carcinoma	C44.11-✓	—	—	—	—	—
specified type NEC	C44.19-✓	—	—	—	—	—
squamous cell carcinoma	C44.12-✓	—	—	—	—	—
limb NEC	C44.90	C79.2	D04.9	D23.9	D48.5	D49.2
basal cell carcinoma	C44.91	—	—	—	—	—
lower	C44.70-✓	C79.2	D04.7-✓	D23.7-✓	D48.5	D49.2
basal cell carcinoma	C44.71-✓	—	—	—	—	—
specified type NEC	C44.79-✓	—	—	—	—	—
squamous cell carcinoma	C44.72-✓	—	—	—	—	—
upper	C44.60-✓	C79.2	D04.6-✓	D23.6-✓	D48.5	D49.2
basal cell carcinoma	C44.61-✓	—	—	—	—	—
specified type NEC	C44.69-✓	—	—	—	—	—
squamous cell carcinoma	C44.62-✓	—	—	—	—	—
lip (lower) (upper)	C44.00	C79.2	D04.0	D23.0	D48.5	D49.2
basal cell carcinoma	C44.01	—	—	—	—	—
specified type NEC	C44.09	—	—	—	—	—
squamous cell carcinoma	C44.02	—	—	—	—	—
male genital organs	C63.9	C79.82	D07.60	D29.9	D40.8	D49.59
penis	C60.9	C79.82	D07.4	D29.0	D40.8	D49.59
prepuce	C60.0	C79.82	D07.4	D29.0	D40.8	D49.59
scrotum	C63.2	C79.82	D07.61	D29.4	D40.8	D49.59
mastectomy site (skin) — *see also* Neoplasm, skin, breast	C44.501	C79.2	—	—	—	—
specified as breast tissue	C50.8-✓	C79.81	—	—	—	—
meatus, acoustic (external) — *see also* Neoplasm, skin, ear	C44.20-✓	C79.2	D04.2-✓	D23.2-✓	D48.5	D49.2
melanotic — *see* Melanoma						
Merkel cell — *see* Carcinoma, Merkel cell						
nates — *see also* Neoplasm, skin, trunk	C44.509	C79.2	D04.5	D23.5	D48.5	D49.2
neck	C44.40	C79.2	D04.4	D23.4	D48.5	D49.2
basal cell carcinoma	C44.41	—	—	—	—	—
specified type NEC	C44.49	—	—	—	—	—
squamous cell carcinoma	C44.42	—	—	—	—	—
nevus — *see* Nevus, skin						
nose (external) — *see also* Neoplasm, nose, skin	C44.301	C79.2	D04.39	D23.39	D48.5	D49.2
overlapping lesion	C44.80	—	—	—	—	—
basal cell carcinoma	C44.81	—	—	—	—	—
specified type NEC	C44.89	—	—	—	—	—
squamous cell carcinoma	C44.82	—	—	—	—	—
palm — *see also* Neoplasm, skin, limb, upper	C44.60-✓	C79.2	D04.6-✓	D23.6-✓	D48.5	D49.2
palpebra	C44.10-✓	C79.2	D04.1-✓	D23.1-✓	D48.5	D49.2

Neoplasm, neoplastic —	Malignant Primary	Malignant Secondary	Ca in situ	Benign	Uncertain	Unspecified Behavior
continued						
skin — *continued*						
palpebra — *continued*						
basal cell carcinoma	C44.11-✓	—	—	—	—	—
specified type NEC	C44.19-✓	—	—	—	—	—
squamous cell carcinoma	C44.12-✓	—	—	—	—	—
penis NEC	C60.9	C79.82	D07.4	D29.0	D40.8	D49.59
perianal — *see also* Neoplasm, skin, anus	C44.500	C79.2	D04.5	D23.5	D48.5	D49.2
perineum — *see also* Neoplasm, skin, anus	C44.500	C79.2	D04.5	D23.5	D48.5	D49.2
pinna — *see also* Neoplasm, skin, ear	C44.20-✓	C79.2	D04.2-✓	D23.2-✓	D48.5	D49.2
plantar — *see also* Neoplasm, skin, limb, lower	C44.70-✓	C79.2	D04.7-✓	D23.7-✓	D48.5	D49.2
popliteal fossa or space — *see also* Neoplasm, skin, limb, lower	C44.70-✓	C79.2	D04.7-✓	D23.7-✓	D48.5	D49.2
prepuce	C60.0	C79.82	D07.4	D29.0	D40.8	D49.59
pubes — *see also* Neoplasm, skin, trunk	C44.509	C79.2	D04.5	D23.5	D48.5	D49.2
sacrococcygeal region — *see also* Neoplasm, skin, trunk	C44.509	C79.2	D04.5	D23.5	D48.5	D49.2
scalp	C44.40	C79.2	D04.4	D23.4	D48.5	D49.2
basal cell carcinoma	C44.41	—	—	—	—	—
specified type NEC	C44.49	—	—	—	—	—
squamous cell carcinoma	C44.42	—	—	—	—	—
scapular region — *see also* Neoplasm, skin, trunk	C44.509	C79.2	D04.5	D23.5	D48.5	D49.2
scrotum	C63.2	C79.82	D07.61	D29.4	D40.8	D49.59
shoulder — *see also* Neoplasm, skin, limb, upper	C44.60-✓	C79.2	D04.6-✓	D23.6-✓	D48.5	D49.2
sole (foot) — *see also* Neoplasm, skin, limb, lower	C44.70-✓	C79.2	D04.7-✓	D23.7-✓	D48.5	D49.2
specified sites NEC	C44.80	C79.2	D04.8	D23.9	D48.5	D49.2
basal cell carcinoma	C44.81	—	—	—	—	—
specified type NEC	C44.89	—	—	—	—	—
squamous cell carcinoma	C44.82	—	—	—	—	—
specified type NEC	C44.99	—	—	—	—	—
squamous cell carcinoma	C44.92	—	—	—	—	—
submammary fold — *see also* Neoplasm, skin, trunk	C44.509	C79.2	D04.5	D23.5	D48.5	D49.2
supraclavicular region — *see also* Neoplasm, skin, neck	C44.40	C79.2	D04.4	D23.4	D48.5	D49.2
temple — *see also* Neoplasm, skin, face	C44.309	C79.2	D04.39	D23.39	D48.5	D49.2
thigh — *see also* Neoplasm, skin, limb, lower	C44.70-✓	C79.2	D04.7-✓	D23.7-✓	D48.5	D49.2
thoracic wall — *see also* Neoplasm, skin, trunk	C44.509	C79.2	D04.5	D23.5	D48.5	D49.2
thumb — *see also* Neoplasm, skin, limb, upper	C44.60-✓	C79.2	D04.6-✓	D23.6-✓	D48.5	D49.2
toe — *see also* Neoplasm, skin, limb, lower	C44.70-✓	C79.2	D04.7-✓	D23.7-✓	D48.5	D49.2

▽ **Subterms under main terms may continue to next column or page**   ☑ **Additional Character Required — Refer to the Tabular List for Character Selection**

Neoplasm, neoplastic — continued	Malignant Primary	Malignant Secondary	Ca in situ	Benign	Uncertain	Unspecified Behavior
skin — continued						
tragus — *see also Neoplasm, skin, ear*	C44.20-☑	C79.2	D04.2-☑	D23.2-☑	D48.5	D49.2
trunk	C44.509	C79.2	D04.5	D23.5	D48.5	D49.2
basal cell carcinoma	C44.519	—	—	—	—	—
specified type NEC	C44.599	—	—	—	—	—
squamous cell carcinoma	C44.529	—	—	—	—	—
umbilicus — *see also Neoplasm, skin, trunk*	C44.509	C79.2	D04.5	D23.5	D48.5	D49.2
vulva	C51.9	C79.82	D07.1	D28.0	D39.8	D49.59
overlapping lesion	C51.8	—	—	—	—	—
wrist — *see also Neoplasm, skin, limb, upper*	C44.60-☑	C79.2	D04.6-☑	D23.6-☑	D48.5	D49.2
skull	C41.0	C79.51		D16.4	D48.0	D49.2
soft parts or tissues — *see Neoplasm, connective tissue*						
specified site NEC	C76.8	C79.89	D09.8	D36.7	D48.7	D49.89
spermatic cord	C63.1-☑	C79.82	D07.69	D29.8	D40.8	D49.59
sphenoid	C31.3	C78.39	D02.3	D14.0	D38.5	D49.1
bone	C41.0	C79.51	—	D16.4	D48.0	D49.2
sinus	C31.3	C78.39	D02.3	D14.0	D38.5	D49.1
sphincter						
anal	C21.1	C78.5	D01.3	D12.9	D37.8	D49.0
of Oddi	C24.0	C78.89	D01.5	D13.5	D37.6	D49.0
spine, spinal						
(column)	C41.2	C79.51	—	D16.6	D48.0	D49.2
bulb	C71.7	C79.31	—	D33.1	D43.1	D49.6
coccyx	C41.4	C79.51	—	D16.8	D48.0	D49.2
cord (cervical) (lumbar) (sacral) (thoracic)	C72.0	C79.49	—	D33.4	D43.4	D49.7
dura mater	C70.1	C79.49	—	D32.1	D42.1	D49.7
lumbosacral	C41.2	C79.51	—	D16.6	D48.0	D49.2
marrow NEC	C96.9	C79.52	—	—	D47.9	D49.89
membrane	C70.1	C79.49	—	D32.1	D42.1	D49.7
meninges	C70.1	C79.49	—	D32.1	D42.1	D49.7
nerve (root)	C47.9	C79.89	—	D36.10	D48.2	D49.2
pia mater	C70.1	C79.49	—	D32.1	D42.1	D49.7
root	C47.9	C79.89	—	D36.10	D48.2	D49.2
sacrum	C41.4	C79.51	—	D16.8	D48.0	D49.2
spleen, splenic NEC	C26.1	C78.89	D01.7	D13.9	D37.8	D49.0
flexure (colon)	C18.5	C78.5	D01.0	D12.3	D37.4	D49.0
stem, brain	C71.7	C79.31	—	D33.1	D43.1	D49.6
Stensen's duct	C07	C79.89	D00.00	D11.0	D37.030	D49.0
sternum	C41.3	C79.51	—	D16.7	D48.0	D49.2
stomach	C16.9	C78.89	D00.2	D13.1	D37.1	D49.0
antrum (pyloric)	C16.3	C78.89	D00.2	D13.1	D37.1	D49.0
body	C16.2	C78.89	D00.2	D13.1	D37.1	D49.0
cardia	C16.0	C78.89	D00.2	D13.1	D37.1	D49.0
cardiac orifice	C16.0	C78.89	D00.2	D13.1	D37.1	D49.0
corpus	C16.2	C78.89	D00.2	D13.1	D37.1	D49.0
fundus	C16.1	C78.89	D00.2	D13.1	D37.1	D49.0
greater curvature NEC	C16.6	C78.89	D00.2	D13.1	D37.1	D49.0
lesser curvature NEC	C16.5	C78.89	D00.2	D13.1	D37.1	D49.0
overlapping lesion	C16.8	—	—	—	—	—
prepylorus	C16.4	C78.89	D00.2	D13.1	D37.1	D49.0
pylorus	C16.4	C78.89	D00.2	D13.1	D37.1	D49.0
wall NEC	C16.9	C78.89	D00.2	D13.1	D37.1	D49.0
anterior NEC	C16.8	C78.89	D00.2	D13.1	D37.1	D49.0
posterior NEC	C16.8	C78.89	D00.2	D13.1	D37.1	D49.0
stroma, endometrial	C54.1	C79.82	D07.0	D26.1	D39.0	D49.59
stump, cervical	C53.8	C79.82	D06.7	D26.0	D39.0	D49.59
subcutaneous (nodule) (tissue) NEC — *see Neoplasm, connective tissue*						
subdural	C70.9	C79.32	—	D32.9	D42.9	D49.7
subglottis, subglottic	C32.2	C78.39	D02.0	D14.1	D38.0	D49.1
sublingual	C04.9	C79.89	D00.06	D10.2	D37.09	D49.0
gland or duct	C08.1	C79.89	D00.00	D11.7	D37.031	D49.0

Neoplasm, neoplastic — continued	Malignant Primary	Malignant Secondary	Ca in situ	Benign	Uncertain	Unspecified Behavior
submandibular gland	C08.0	C79.89	D00.00	D11.7	D37.032	D49.0
submaxillary gland or duct	C08.0	C79.89	D00.00	D11.7	D37.032	D49.0
submental	C76.0	C79.89	D09.8	D36.7	D48.7	D49.89
subpleural	C34.9-☑	C78.0-☑	D02.2-☑	D14.3-☑	D38.1	D49.1
substernal	C38.1	C78.1	—	D15.2	D38.3	D49.89
sudoriferous, sudoriparous gland, site unspecified	C44.90	C79.2	D04.9	D23.9	D48.5	D49.2
specified site — *see Neoplasm, skin*						
supraclavicular region	C76.0	C79.89	D09.8	D36.7	D48.7	D49.89
supraglottis	C32.1	C78.39	D02.0	D14.1	D38.0	D49.1
suprarenal	C74.9-☑	C79.7-☑	D09.3	D35.0-☑	D44.1-☑	D49.7
capsule	C74.9-☑	C79.7-☑	D09.3	D35.0-☑	D44.1-☑	D49.7
cortex	C74.0-☑	C79.7-☑	D09.3	D35.0-☑	D44.1-☑	D49.7
gland	C74.9-☑	C79.7-☑	D09.3	D35.0-☑	D44.1-☑	D49.7
medulla	C74.1-☑	C79.7-☑	D09.3	D35.0-☑	D44.1-☑	D49.7
suprasellar (region)	C71.9	C79.31	—	D33.2	D43.2	D49.6
supratentorial (brain) NEC	C71.0	C79.31	—	D33.0	D43.0	D49.6
sweat gland (apocrine) (eccrine), site unspecified	C44.90	C79.2	D04.9	D23.9	D48.5	D49.2
specified site — *see Neoplasm, skin*						
sympathetic nerve or nervous system NEC	C47.9	C79.89	—	D36.10	D48.2	D49.2
symphysis pubis	C41.4	C79.51	—	D16.8	D48.0	D49.2
synovial membrane — *see Neoplasm, connective tissue*						
tapetum, brain	C71.8	C79.31	—	D33.2	D43.2	D49.6
tarsus (any bone)	C40.3-☑	C79.51	—	D16.3-☑	—	—
temple (skin) — *see also Neoplasm, skin, face*	C44.309	C79.2	D04.39	D23.39	D48.5	D49.2
temporal						
bone	C41.0	C79.51	—	D16.4	D48.0	D49.2
lobe or pole	C71.2	C79.31	—	D33.0	D43.0	D49.6
region	C76.0	C79.89	D09.8	D36.7	D48.7	D49.89
skin — *see also Neoplasm, skin, face*	C44.309	C79.2	D04.39	D23.39	D48.5	D49.2
tendon (sheath) — *see Neoplasm, connective tissue*						
tentorium (cerebelli)	C70.0	C79.32	—	D32.0	D42.0	D49.7
testis, testes	C62.9-☑	C79.82	D07.69	D29.2-☑	D40.1-☑	D49.59
descended	C62.1-☑	C79.82	D07.69	D29.2-☑	D40.1-☑	D49.59
ectopic	C62.0-☑	C79.82	D07.69	D29.2-☑	D40.1-☑	D49.59
retained	C62.0-☑	C79.82	D07.69	D29.2-☑	D40.1-☑	D49.59
scrotal	C62.1-☑	C79.82	D07.69	D29.2-☑	D40.1-☑	D49.59
undescended	C62.0-☑	C79.82	D07.69	D29.2-☑	D40.1-☑	D49.59
unspecified whether descended or undescended	C62.9-☑	C79.82	D07.69	D29.2-☑	D40.1-☑	D49.59
thalamus	C71.0	C79.31	—	D33.0	D43.0	D49.6
thigh NEC	C76.5-☑	C79.89	D04.7-☑	D36.7	D48.7	D49.89
thorax, thoracic (cavity) (organs NEC)	C76.1	C79.89	D09.8	D36.7	D48.7	D49.89
duct	C49.3	C79.89	—	D21.3	D48.1	D49.2
wall NEC	C76.1	C79.89	D09.8	D36.7	D48.7	D49.89
throat	C14.0	C79.89	D00.08	D10.9	D37.05	D49.0
thumb NEC	C76.4-☑	C79.89	D04.6-☑	D36.7	D48.7	D49.89
thymus (gland)	C37	C79.89	D09.3	D15.0	D38.4	D49.89
thyroglossal duct	C73	C79.89	D09.3	D34	D44.0	D49.7
thyroid (gland)	C73	C79.89	D09.3	D34	D44.0	D49.7
cartilage	C32.3	C78.39	D02.0	D14.1	D38.0	D49.1
tibia (any part)	C40.2-☑	C79.51	—	D16.2-☑	—	—
toe NEC	C76.5-☑	C79.89	D04.7-☑	D36.7	D48.7	D49.89
tongue	C02.9	C79.89	D00.07	D10.1	D37.02	D49.0
anterior (two-thirds) NEC	C02.3	C79.89	D00.07	D10.1	D37.02	D49.0
dorsal surface	C02.0	C79.89	D00.07	D10.1	D37.02	D49.0
ventral surface	C02.2	C79.89	D00.07	D10.1	D37.02	D49.0

☑ Additional Character Required — Refer to the Tabular List for Character Selection   ▽ Subterms under main terms may continue to next column or page

Neoplasm, neoplastic —	Malignant Primary	Malignant Secondary	Ca in situ	Benign	Uncertain	Unspecified Behavior
continued						
tongue — *continued*						
base (dorsal surface)	C01	C79.89	D00.07	D10.1	D37.02	D49.0
border (lateral)	C02.1	C79.89	D00.07	D10.1	D37.02	D49.0
dorsal surface NEC	C02.0	C79.89	D00.07	D10.1	D37.02	D49.0
fixed part NEC	C01	C79.89	D00.07	D10.1	D37.02	D49.0
foreamen cecum	C02.0	C79.89	D00.07	D10.1	D37.02	D49.0
frenulum linguae	C02.2	C79.89	D00.07	D10.1	D37.02	D49.0
junctional zone	C02.8	C79.89	D00.07	D10.1	D37.02	D49.0
margin (lateral)	C02.1	C79.89	D00.07	D10.1	D37.02	D49.0
midline NEC	C02.0	C79.89	D00.07	D10.1	D37.02	D49.0
mobile part NEC	C02.3	C79.89	D00.07	D10.1	D37.02	D49.0
overlapping lesion	C02.8	—	—	—	—	—
posterior (third)	C01	C79.89	D00.07	D10.1	D37.02	D49.0
root	C01	C79.89	D00.07	D10.1	D37.02	D49.0
surface (dorsal)	C02.0	C79.89	D00.07	D10.1	D37.02	D49.0
base	C01	C79.89	D00.07	D10.1	D37.02	D49.0
ventral	C02.2	C79.89	D00.07	D10.1	D37.02	D49.0
tip	C02.1	C79.89	D00.07	D10.1	D37.02	D49.0
tonsil	C02.4	C79.89	D00.07	D10.1	D37.02	D49.0
tonsil	C09.9	C79.89	D00.08	D10.4	D37.05	D49.0
fauces, faucial	C09.9	C79.89	D00.08	D10.4	D37.05	D49.0
lingual	C02.4	C79.89	D00.07	D10.1	D37.02	D49.0
overlapping sites	C09.8	—	—	—	—	—
palatine	C09.9	C79.89	D00.08	D10.4	D37.05	D49.0
pharyngeal	C11.1	C79.89	D00.08	D10.6	D37.05	D49.0
pillar (anterior) (posterior)	C09.1	C79.89	D00.08	D10.5	D37.05	D49.0
tonsillar fossa	C09.0	C79.89	D00.08	D10.5	D37.05	D49.0
tooth socket NEC	C03.9	C79.89	D00.03	D10.39	D37.09	D49.0
trachea (cartilage) (mucosa)	C33	C78.39	D02.1	D14.2	D38.1	D49.1
overlapping lesion with bronchus or lung	C34.8-☑	—	—	—	—	—
tracheobronchial	C34.8-☑	C78.39	D02.1	D14.2	D38.1	D49.1
overlapping lesion with lung	C34.8-☑	—	—	—	—	—
tragus — *see also* Neoplasm, skin, ear	C44.20-☑	C79.2	D04.2-☑	D23.2-☑	D48.5	D49.2
trunk NEC	C76.8	C79.89	D04.5	D36.7	D48.7	D49.89
tubo-ovarian	C57.8	C79.82	D07.39	D28.7	D39.8	D49.59
tunica vaginalis	C63.7	C79.82	D07.69	D29.8	D40.8	D49.59
turbinate (bone)	C41.0	C79.51	—	D16.4	D48.0	D49.2
nasal	C30.0	C78.39	D02.3	D14.0	D38.5	D49.1
tympanic cavity	C30.1	C78.39	D02.3	D14.0	D38.5	D49.1
ulna (any part)	C40.0-☑	C79.51	—	D16.0-☑	—	—
umbilicus, umbilical — *see also* Neoplasm, skin, trunk	C44.509	C79.2	D04.5	D23.5	D48.5	D49.2
uncus, brain	C71.2	C79.31		D33.0	D43.0	D49.6
unknown site or unspecified	C80.1	C79.9	D09.9	D36.9	D48.9	D49.9
urachus	C67.7	C79.11	D09.0	D30.3	D41.4	D49.4
ureter-bladder (junction)	C67.6	C79.11	D09.0	D30.3	D41.4	D49.4
ureter, ureteral	C66.-☑	C79.19	D09.19	D30.2-☑	D41.2-☑	D49.59
orifice (bladder)	C67.6	C79.11	D09.0	D30.3	D41.4	D49.4
urethra, urethral (gland)	C68.0	C79.19	D09.19	D30.4	D41.3	D49.59
orifice, internal	C67.5	C79.11	D09.0	D30.3	D41.4	D49.4
urethrovaginal (septum)	C57.9	C79.82	D07.30	D28.9	D39.8	D49.59
urinary organ or system	C68.9	C79.10	D09.10	D30.9	D41.9	D49.59
bladder — *see* Neoplasm, bladder						
overlapping lesion	C68.8	—	—	—	—	—
specified sites NEC	C68.8	C79.19	D09.19	D30.8	D41.8	D49.59
utero-ovarian	C57.8	C79.82	D07.39	D28.7	D39.8	D49.59
ligament	C57.1-☑	C79.82	D07.39	D28.2	D39.8	D49.59
uterosacral ligament	C57.3	C79.82	—	D28.2	D39.8	D49.59
uterus, uteri, uterine	C55	C79.82	D07.0	D26.9	D39.0	D49.59
adnexa NEC	C57.4	C79.82	D07.39	D28.7	D39.8	D49.59
body	C54.9	C79.82	D07.0	D26.1	D39.0	D49.59
cervix	C53.9	C79.82	D06.9	D26.0	D39.0	D49.59
cornu	C54.9	C79.82	D07.0	D26.1	D39.0	D49.59
corpus	C54.9	C79.82	D07.0	D26.1	D39.0	D49.59
endocervix (canal) (gland)	C53.0	C79.82	D06.0	D26.0	D39.0	D49.59

Neoplasm, neoplastic —	Malignant Primary	Malignant Secondary	Ca in situ	Benign	Uncertain	Unspecified Behavior
continued						
uterus, uteri, uterine — *continued*						
endometrium	C54.1	C79.82	D07.0	D26.1	D39.0	D49.59
exocervix	C53.1	C79.82	D06.1	D26.0	D39.0	D49.59
external os	C53.1	C79.82	D06.1	D26.0	D39.0	D49.59
fundus	C54.3	C79.82	D07.0	D26.1	D39.0	D49.59
internal os	C53.0	C79.82	D06.0	D26.0	D39.0	D49.59
isthmus	C54.0	C79.82	D07.0	D26.1	D39.0	D49.59
ligament	C57.3	C79.82	—	D28.2	D39.8	D49.59
broad	C57.1-☑	C79.82	D07.39	D28.2	D39.8	D49.59
round	C57.2-☑	C79.82	—	D28.2	D39.8	D49.59
lower segment	C54.0	C79.82	D07.0	D26.1	D39.0	D49.59
myometrium	C54.2	C79.82	D07.0	D26.1	D39.0	D49.59
overlapping sites	C54.8	—	—	—	—	—
squamocolumnar junction	C53.8	C79.82	D06.7	D26.0	D39.0	D49.59
tube	C57.0-☑	C79.82	D07.39	D28.2	D39.8	D49.59
utricle, prostatic	C68.0	C79.19	D09.19	D30.4	D41.3	D49.59
uveal tract	C69.4-☑	C79.49	D09.2-☑	D31.4-☑	D48.7	D49.89
uvula	C05.2	C79.89	D00.04	D10.39	D37.09	D49.0
vagina, vaginal (fornix) (vault) (wall)	C52	C79.82	D07.2	D28.1	D39.8	D49.59
vaginovesical	C57.9	C79.82	D07.30	D28.9	D39.9	D49.59
septum	C57.9	C79.82	D07.30	D28.9	D39.9	D49.59
vallecula (epiglottis)	C10.0	C79.89	D00.08	D10.5	D37.05	D49.0
vascular — *see* Neoplasm, connective tissue						
vas deferens	C63.1-☑	C79.82	D07.69	D29.8	D40.8	D49.59
Vater's ampulla	C24.1	C78.89	D01.5	D13.5	D37.6	D49.0
vein, venous — *see* Neoplasm, connective tissue						
vena cava (abdominal) (inferior)	C49.4	C79.89	—	D21.4	D48.1	D49.2
superior	C49.3	C79.89	—	D21.3	D48.1	D49.2
ventricle (cerebral) (floor) (lateral) (third)	C71.5	C79.31	—	D33.0	D43.0	D49.6
cardiac (left) (right)	C38.0	C79.89	—	D15.1	D48.7	D49.89
fourth	C71.7	C79.31	—	D33.1	D43.1	D49.6
ventricular band of larynx	C32.1	C78.39	D02.0	D14.1	D38.0	D49.1
ventriculus — *see* Neoplasm, stomach						
vermillion border — *see* Neoplasm, lip						
vermis, cerebellum	C71.6	C79.31	—	D33.1	D43.1	D49.6
vertebra (column)	C41.2	C79.51	—	D16.6	D48.0	D49.2
coccyx	C41.4	C79.51	—	D16.8	D48.0	D49.2
marrow NEC	C96.9	C79.52	—	—	D47.9	D49.89
sacrum	C41.4	C79.51	—	D16.8	D48.0	D49.2
vesical — *see* Neoplasm, bladder						
vesicle, seminal	C63.7	C79.82	D07.69	D29.8	D40.8	D49.59
vesicocervical tissue	C57.9	C79.82	D07.30	D28.9	D39.9	D49.59
vesicorectal	C76.3	C79.89	D09.8	D36.7	D48.7	D49.89
vesicovaginal	C57.9	C79.82	D07.30	D28.9	D39.9	D49.59
septum	C57.9	C79.82	D07.30	D28.9	D39.8	D49.59
vessel (blood) — *see* Neoplasm, connective tissue						
vestibular gland, greater	C51.0	C79.82	D07.1	D28.0	D39.8	D49.59
vestibule						
mouth	C06.1	C79.89	D00.00	D10.39	D37.09	D49.0
nose	C30.0	C78.39	D02.3	D14.0	D38.5	D49.1
Virchow's gland	C77.0	C77.0	—	D36.0	D48.7	D49.89
viscera NEC	C76.8	C79.89	D09.8	D36.7	D48.7	D49.89
vocal cords (true)	C32.0	C78.39	D02.0	D14.1	D38.0	D49.1
false	C32.1	C78.39	D02.0	D14.1	D38.0	D49.1
vomer	C41.0	C79.51	—	D16.4	D48.0	D49.2
vulva	C51.9	C79.82	D07.1	D28.0	D39.8	D49.59
vulvovaginal gland	C51.0	C79.82	D07.1	D28.0	D39.8	D49.59
Waldeyer's ring	C14.2	C79.89	D00.08	D10.9	D37.05	D49.0
Wharton's duct	C08.0	C79.89	D00.00	D11.7	D37.032	D49.0
white matter (central) (cerebral)	C71.0	C79.31	—	D33.0	D43.0	D49.6
windpipe	C33	C78.39	D02.1	D14.2	D38.1	D49.1
Wirsung's duct	C25.3	C78.89	D01.7	D13.6	D37.8	D49.0
wolffian (body) (duct) female	C57.7	C79.82	D07.39	D28.7	D39.8	D49.59

☒ **Subterms under main terms may continue to next column or page**   ☑ **Additional Character Required — Refer to the Tabular List for Character Selection**   **347**

Neoplasm Table

	Malignant Primary	Malignant Secondary	Ca in situ	Benign	Uncertain	Unspecified Behavior
Neoplasm, neoplastic — *continued*						
wolffian — *continued*						
male	C63.7	C79.82	DØ7.69	D29.8	D4Ø.8	D49.59
womb — *see* Neoplasm, uterus						
wrist NEC	C76.4-☑	C79.89	DØ4.6-☑	D36.7	D48.7	D49.89
xiphoid process	C41.3	C79.51	—	D16.7	D48.Ø	D49.2
Zuckerkandl organ	C75.5	C79.89	—	D35.6	D44.7	D49.7

Substance	Poisoning, Accidental (unintentional)	Poisoning, Intentional Self-harm	Poisoning, Assault	Poisoning, Undetermined	Adverse Effect	Under-dosing
14-Hydroxydihydromorphinone	T40.2X1	T40.2X2	T40.2X3	T40.2X4	T40.2X5	T40.2X6
1-Propanol	T51.3X1	T51.3X2	T51.3X3	T51.3X4	—	—
2,3,7,8-Tetrachlorodibenzo-p-dioxin	T53.7X1	T53.7X2	T53.7X3	T53.7X4	—	—
2,4,5-T (trichlorophenoxyacetic acid)	T60.1X1	T60.1X2	T60.1X3	T60.1X4	—	—
2,4,5-Trichlorophenoxyacetic acid	T60.3X1	T60.3X2	T60.3X3	T60.3X4	—	—
2,4-D (dichlorophenoxyacetic acid)	T60.3X1	T60.3X2	T60.3X3	T60.3X4	—	—
2,4-Toluene diisocyanate	T65.0X1	T65.0X2	T65.0X3	T65.0X4		
2-Deoxy-5-fluorouridine	T45.1X1	T45.1X2	T45.1X3	T45.1X4	T45.1X5	T45.1X6
2-Ethoxyethanol	T52.3X1	T52.3X2	T52.3X3	T52.3X4		
2-Methoxyethanol	T52.3X1	T52.3X2	T52.3X3	T52.3X4		
2-Propanol	T51.2X1	T51.2X2	T51.2X3	T51.2X4		
4-Aminobutyric acid	T43.8X1	T43.8X2	T43.8X3	T43.8X4	T43.8X5	T43.8X6
4-Aminophenol derivatives	T39.1X1	T39.1X2	T39.1X3	T39.1X4	T39.1X5	T39.1X6
5-Deoxy-5-fluorouridine	T45.1X1	T45.1X2	T45.1X3	T45.1X4	T45.1X5	T45.1X6
5-Methoxypsoralen (5-MOP)	T50.991	T50.992	T50.993	T50.994	T50.995	T50.996
8-Aminoquinoline drugs	T37.2X1	T37.2X2	T37.2X3	T37.2X4	T37.2X5	T37.2X6
8-Methoxypsoralen (8-MOP)	T50.991	T50.992	T50.993	T50.994	T50.995	T50.996
ABOB	T37.5X1	T37.5X2	T37.5X3	T37.5X4	T37.5X5	T37.5X6
Abrine	T62.2X1	T62.2X2	T62.2X3	T62.2X4	—	—
Abrus (seed)	T62.2X1	T62.2X2	T62.2X3	T62.2X4	—	—
Absinthe	T51.0X1	T51.0X2	T51.0X3	T51.0X4	—	—
beverage	T51.0X1	T51.0X2	T51.0X3	T51.0X4	—	—
Acaricide	T60.8X1	T60.8X2	T60.8X3	T60.8X4	—	—
Acebutolol	T44.7X1	T44.7X2	T44.7X3	T44.7X4	T44.7X5	T44.7X6
Acecarbromal	T42.6X1	T42.6X2	T42.6X3	T42.6X4	T42.6X5	T42.6X6
Aceclidine	T44.1X1	T44.1X2	T44.1X3	T44.1X4	T44.1X5	T44.1X6
Acedapsone	T37.0X1	T37.0X2	T37.0X3	T37.0X4	T37.0X5	T37.0X6
Acefylline piperazine	T48.6X1	T48.6X2	T48.6X3	T48.6X4	T48.6X5	T48.6X6
Acemorphan	T40.2X1	T40.2X2	T40.2X3	T40.2X4	T40.2X5	T40.2X6
Acenocoumarin	T45.511	T45.512	T45.513	T45.514	T45.515	T45.516
Acenocoumarol	T45.511	T45.512	T45.513	T45.514	T45.515	T45.516
Acepifylline	T48.6X1	T48.6X2	T48.6X3	T48.6X4	T48.6X5	T48.6X6
Acepromazine	T43.3X1	T43.3X2	T43.3X3	T43.3X4	T43.3X5	T43.3X6
Acesulfamethoxypyridazine	T37.0X1	T37.0X2	T37.0X3	T37.0X4	T37.0X5	T37.0X6
Acetal	T52.8X1	T52.8X2	T52.8X3	T52.8X4	—	—
Acetaldehyde (vapor)	T52.8X1	T52.8X2	T52.8X3	T52.8X4	—	—
liquid	T65.891	T65.892	T65.893	T65.894	—	—
Acetaminophen	T39.1X1	T39.1X2	T39.1X3	T39.1X4	T39.1X5	T39.1X6
Acetaminosalol	T39.1X1	T39.1X2	T39.1X3	T39.1X4	T39.1X5	T39.1X6
Acetanilide	T39.1X1	T39.1X2	T39.1X3	T39.1X4	T39.1X5	T39.1X6
Acetarsol	T37.3X1	T37.3X2	T37.3X3	T37.3X4	T37.3X5	T37.3X6
Acetazolamide	T50.2X1	T50.2X2	T50.2X3	T50.2X4	T50.2X5	T50.2X6
Acetiamine	T45.2X1	T45.2X2	T45.2X3	T45.2X4	T45.2X5	T45.2X6
Acetic						
acid	T54.2X1	T54.2X2	T54.2X3	T54.2X4	—	—
with sodium acetate (ointment)	T49.3X1	T49.3X2	T49.3X3	T49.3X4	T49.3X5	T49.3X6
ester (solvent)(vapor)	T52.8X1	T52.8X2	T52.8X3	T52.8X4	—	—
irrigating solution	T50.3X1	T50.3X2	T50.3X3	T50.3X4	T50.3X5	T50.3X6
medicinal (lotion)	T49.2X1	T49.2X2	T49.2X3	T49.2X4	T49.2X5	T49.2X6
anhydride	T65.891	T65.892	T65.893	T65.894	—	—
ether (vapor)	T52.8X1	T52.8X2	T52.8X3	T52.8X4	—	—
Acetohexamide	T38.3X1	T38.3X2	T38.3X3	T38.3X4	T38.3X5	T38.3X6
Acetohydroxamic acid	T50.991	T50.992	T50.993	T50.994	T50.995	T50.996
Acetomenaphthone	T45.7X1	T45.7X2	T45.7X3	T45.7X4	T45.7X5	T45.7X6
Acetomorphine	T40.1X1	T40.1X2	T40.1X3	T40.1X4	—	—
Acetone (oils)	T52.4X1	T52.4X2	T52.4X3	T52.4X4	—	—
chlorinated	T52.4X1	T52.4X2	T52.4X3	T52.4X4	—	—
vapor	T52.4X1	T52.4X2	T52.4X3	T52.4X4	—	—
Acetonitrile	T52.8X1	T52.8X2	T52.8X3	T52.8X4	—	—
Acetophenazine	T43.3X1	T43.3X2	T43.3X3	T43.3X4	T43.3X5	T43.3X6
Acetophenetedin	T39.1X1	T39.1X2	T39.1X3	T39.1X4	T39.1X5	T39.1X6
Acetophenone	T52.4X1	T52.4X2	T52.4X3	T52.4X4	—	—
Acetorphine	T40.2X1	T40.2X2	T40.2X3	T40.2X4	—	—
Acetosulfone (sodium)	T37.1X1	T37.1X2	T37.1X3	T37.1X4	T37.1X5	T37.1X6
Acetrizoate (sodium)	T50.8X1	T50.8X2	T50.8X3	T50.8X4	T50.8X5	T50.8X6
Acetrizoic acid	T50.8X1	T50.8X2	T50.8X3	T50.8X4	T50.8X5	T50.8X6
Acetyl						
bromide	T53.6X1	T53.6X2	T53.6X3	T53.6X4	—	—
chloride	T53.6X1	T53.6X2	T53.6X3	T53.6X4	—	—
Acetylcarbromal	T42.6X1	T42.6X2	T42.6X3	T42.6X4	T42.6X5	T42.6X6
Acetylcholine						
chloride	T44.1X1	T44.1X2	T44.1X3	T44.1X4	T44.1X5	T44.1X6
derivative	T44.1X1	T44.1X2	T44.1X3	T44.1X4	T44.1X5	T44.1X6
Acetylcysteine	T48.4X1	T48.4X2	T48.4X3	T48.4X4	T48.4X5	T48.4X6
Acetyldigitoxin	T46.0X1	T46.0X2	T46.0X3	T46.0X4	T46.0X5	T46.0X6
Acetyldigoxin	T46.0X1	T46.0X2	T46.0X3	T46.0X4	T46.0X5	T46.0X6

Substance	Poisoning, Accidental (unintentional)	Poisoning, Intentional Self-harm	Poisoning, Assault	Poisoning, Undetermined	Adverse Effect	Under-dosing
Acetyldihydrocodeine	T40.2X1	T40.2X2	T40.2X3	T40.2X4	—	—
Acetyldihydrocodeinone	T40.2X1	T40.2X2	T40.2X3	T40.2X4	—	—
Acetylene (gas)	T59.891	T59.892	T59.893	T59.894	—	—
dichloride	T53.6X1	T53.6X2	T53.6X3	T53.6X4	—	—
incomplete combustion of	T58.11	T58.12	T58.13	T58.14	—	—
industrial	T59.891	T59.892	T59.893	T59.894	—	—
tetrachloride	T53.6X1	T53.6X2	T53.6X3	T53.6X4	—	—
vapor	T53.6X1	T53.6X2	T53.6X3	T53.6X4	—	—
Acetylpheneturide	T42.6X1	T42.6X2	T42.6X3	T42.6X4	T42.6X5	T42.6X6
Acetylphenylhydrazine	T39.8X1	T39.8X2	T39.8X3	T39.8X4	T39.8X5	T39.8X6
Acetylsalicylic acid (salts)	T39.011	T39.012	T39.013	T39.014	T39.015	T39.016
enteric coated	T39.011	T39.012	T39.013	T39.014	T39.015	T39.016
Acetylsulfamethoxypyridazine	T37.0X1	T37.0X2	T37.0X3	T37.0X4	T37.0X5	T37.0X6
Achromycin	T36.4X1	T36.4X2	T36.4X3	T36.4X4	T36.4X5	T36.4X6
ophthalmic preparation	T49.5X1	T49.5X2	T49.5X3	T49.5X4	T49.5X5	T49.5X6
topical NEC	T49.0X1	T49.0X2	T49.0X3	T49.0X4	T49.0X5	T49.0X6
Aciclovir	T37.5X1	T37.5X2	T37.5X3	T37.5X4	T37.5X5	T37.5X6
Acidifying agent NEC	T50.901	T50.902	T50.903	T50.904	T50.905	T50.906
Acid (corrosive) NEC	T54.2X1	T54.2X2	T54.2X3	T54.2X4	—	—
Acipimox	T46.6X1	T46.6X2	T46.6X3	T46.6X4	T46.6X5	T46.6X6
Acitretin	T50.991	T50.992	T50.993	T50.994	T50.995	T50.996
Aclarubicin	T45.1X1	T45.1X2	T45.1X3	T45.1X4	T45.1X5	T45.1X6
Aclatonium napadisilate	T48.1X1	T48.1X2	T48.1X3	T48.1X4	T48.1X5	T48.1X6
Aconite (wild)	T46.991	T46.992	T46.993	T46.994	T46.995	T46.996
Aconitine	T46.991	T46.992	T46.993	T46.994	T46.995	T46.996
Aconitum ferox	T46.991	T46.992	T46.993	T46.994	T46.995	T46.996
Acridine	T65.6X1	T65.6X2	T65.6X3	T65.6X4	—	—
vapor	T59.891	T59.892	T59.893	T59.894	—	—
Acriflavine	T37.91	T37.92	T37.93	T37.94	T37.95	T37.96
Acriflavinium chloride	T49.0X1	T49.0X2	T49.0X3	T49.0X4	T49.0X5	T49.0X6
Acrinol	T49.0X1	T49.0X2	T49.0X3	T49.0X4	T49.0X5	T49.0X6
Acrisorcin	T49.0X1	T49.0X2	T49.0X3	T49.0X4	T49.0X5	T49.0X6
Acrivastine	T45.0X1	T45.0X2	T45.0X3	T45.0X4	T45.0X5	T45.0X6
Acrolein (gas)	T59.891	T59.892	T59.893	T59.894	—	—
liquid	T54.1X1	T54.1X2	T54.1X3	T54.1X4	—	—
Acrylamide	T65.891	T65.892	T65.893	T65.894	—	—
Acrylic resin	T49.3X1	T49.3X2	T49.3X3	T49.3X4	T49.3X5	T49.3X6
Acrylonitrile	T65.891	T65.892	T65.893	T65.894	—	—
Actaea spicata	T62.2X1	T62.2X2	T62.2X3	T62.2X4	—	—
berry	T62.1X1	T62.1X2	T62.1X3	T62.1X4	—	—
Acterol	T37.3X1	T37.3X2	T37.3X3	T37.3X4	T37.3X5	T37.3X6
ACTH	T38.811	T38.812	T38.813	T38.814	T38.815	T38.816
Actinomycin C	T45.1X1	T45.1X2	T45.1X3	T45.1X4	T45.1X5	T45.1X6
Actinomycin D	T45.1X1	T45.1X2	T45.1X3	T45.1X4	T45.1X5	T45.1X6
Activated charcoal — see also Charcoal, medicinal	T47.6X1	T47.6X2	T47.6X3	T47.6X4	T47.6X5	T47.6X6
Acyclovir	T37.5X1	T37.5X2	T37.5X3	T37.5X4	T37.5X5	T37.5X6
Adenine	T45.2X1	T45.2X2	T45.2X3	T45.2X4	T45.2X5	T45.2X6
arabinoside	T37.5X1	T37.5X2	T37.5X3	T37.5X4	T37.5X5	T37.5X6
Adenosine (phosphate)	T46.2X1	T46.2X2	T46.2X3	T46.2X4	T46.2X5	T46.2X6
ADH	T38.891	T38.892	T38.893	T38.894	T38.895	T38.896
Adhesive NEC	T65.891	T65.892	T65.893	T65.894	—	—
Adicillin	T36.0X1	T36.0X2	T36.0X3	T36.0X4	T36.0X5	T36.0X6
Adiphenine	T44.3X1	T44.3X2	T44.3X3	T44.3X4	T44.3X5	T44.3X6
Adipiodone	T50.8X1	T50.8X2	T50.8X3	T50.8X4	T50.8X5	T50.8X6
Adjunct, pharmaceutical	T50.901	T50.902	T50.903	T50.904	T50.905	T50.906
Adrenal (extract, cortex or medulla) (glucocorticoids) (hormones) (mineralocorticoids)	T38.0X1	T38.0X2	T38.0X3	T38.0X4	T38.0X5	T38.0X6
ENT agent	T49.6X1	T49.6X2	T49.6X3	T49.6X4	T49.6X5	T49.6X6
ophthalmic preparation	T49.5X1	T49.5X2	T49.5X3	T49.5X4	T49.5X5	T49.5X6
topical NEC	T49.0X1	T49.0X2	T49.0X3	T49.0X4	T49.0X5	T49.0X6
Adrenalin — see Adrenaline						
Adrenaline	T44.5X1	T44.5X2	T44.5X3	T44.5X4	T44.5X5	T44.5X6
Adrenergic NEC	T44.901	T44.902	T44.903	T44.904	T44.905	T44.906
blocking agent NEC	T44.8X1	T44.8X2	T44.8X3	T44.8X4	T44.8X5	T44.8X6
beta, heart	T44.7X1	T44.7X2	T44.7X3	T44.7X4	T44.7X5	T44.7X6
specified NEC	T44.991	T44.992	T44.993	T44.994	T44.995	T44.996
Adrenochrome						
derivative	T46.991	T46.992	T46.993	T46.994	T46.995	T46.996
(mono) semicarbazone	T46.991	T46.992	T46.993	T46.994	T46.995	T46.996
Adrenocorticotrophic hormone	T38.811	T38.812	T38.813	T38.814	T38.815	T38.816
Adrenocorticotrophin	T38.811	T38.812	T38.813	T38.814	T38.815	T38.816
Adriamycin	T45.1X1	T45.1X2	T45.1X3	T45.1X4	T45.1X5	T45.1X6
Aerosol spray NEC	T65.91	T65.92	T65.93	T65.94	—	—
Aerosporin	T36.8X1	T36.8X2	T36.8X3	T36.8X4	T36.8X5	T36.8X6
ENT agent	T49.6X1	T49.6X2	T49.6X3	T49.6X4	T49.6X5	T49.6X6
ophthalmic preparation	T49.5X1	T49.5X2	T49.5X3	T49.5X4	T49.5X5	T49.5X6
topical NEC	T49.0X1	T49.0X2	T49.0X3	T49.0X4	T49.0X5	T49.0X6
Aethusa cynapium	T62.2X1	T62.2X2	T62.2X3	T62.2X4	—	—
Afghanistan black	T40.7X1	T40.7X2	T40.7X3	T40.7X4	T40.7X5	T40.7X6

Table of Drugs and Chemicals

Aflatoxin — Amanita phalloides

Substance	Poisoning, Accidental (unintentional)	Poisoning, Intentional Self-harm	Poisoning, Assault	Poisoning, Undetermined	Adverse Effect	Under-dosing
Aflatoxin	T64.Ø1	T64.Ø2	T64.Ø3	T64.Ø4	—	—
Afloqualone	T42.8X1	T42.8X2	T42.8X3	T42.8X4	T42.8X5	T42.8X6
African boxwood	T62.2X1	T62.2X2	T62.2X3	T62.2X4		
Agar	T47.4X1	T47.4X2	T47.4X3	T47.4X4	T47.4X5	T47.4X6
Agonist						
predominantly						
alpha-adrenoreceptor	T44.4X1	T44.4X2	T44.4X3	T44.4X4	T44.4X5	T44.4X6
beta-adrenoreceptor	T44.5X1	T44.5X2	T44.5X3	T44.5X4	T44.5X5	T44.5X6
Agricultural agent NEC	T65.91	T65.92	T65.93	T65.94	—	—
Agrypnal	T42.3X1	T42.3X2	T42.3X3	T42.3X4	T42.3X5	T42.3X6
AHLG	T50.Z11	T50.Z12	T50.Z13	T50.Z14	T50.Z15	T50.Z16
Air contaminant(s), source/type NOS	T65.91	T65.92	T65.93	T65.94		
Ajmaline	T46.2X1	T46.2X2	T46.2X3	T46.2X4	T46.2X5	T46.2X6
Akee	T62.1X1	T62.1X2	T62.1X3	T62.1X4		
Akrinol	T49.ØX1	T49.ØX2	T49.ØX3	T49.ØX4	T49.ØX5	T49.ØX6
Akritoin	T37.8X1	T37.8X2	T37.8X3	T37.8X4	T37.8X5	T37.8X6
Alacepril	T46.4X1	T46.4X2	T46.4X3	T46.4X4	T46.4X5	T46.4X6
Alantolactone	T37.4X1	T37.4X2	T37.4X3	T37.4X4	T37.4X5	T37.4X6
Albamycin	T36.8X1	T36.8X2	T36.8X3	T36.8X4	T36.8X5	T36.8X6
Albendazole	T37.4X1	T37.4X2	T37.4X3	T37.4X4	T37.4X5	T37.4X6
Albumin						
bovine	T45.8X1	T45.8X2	T45.8X3	T45.8X4	T45.8X5	T45.8X6
human serum	T45.8X1	T45.8X2	T45.8X3	T45.8X4	T45.8X5	T45.8X6
salt-poor	T45.8X1	T45.8X2	T45.8X3	T45.8X4	T45.8X5	T45.8X6
normal human serum	T45.8X1	T45.8X2	T45.8X3	T45.8X4	T45.8X5	T45.8X6
Albuterol	T48.6X1	T48.6X2	T48.6X3	T48.6X4	T48.6X5	T48.6X6
Albutoin	T42.ØX1	T42.ØX2	T42.ØX3	T42.ØX4	T42.ØX5	T42.ØX6
Alclometasone	T49.ØX1	T49.ØX2	T49.ØX3	T49.ØX4	T49.ØX5	T49.ØX6
Alcohol	T51.91	T51.92	T51.93	T51.94	—	—
absolute	T51.ØX1	T51.ØX2	T51.ØX3	T51.ØX4	—	—
beverage	T51.ØX1	T51.ØX2	T51.ØX3	T51.ØX4	—	—
allyl	T51.8X1	T51.8X2	T51.8X3	T51.8X4		
amyl	T51.3X1	T51.3X2	T51.3X3	T51.3X4		
antifreeze	T51.1X1	T51.1X2	T51.1X3	T51.1X4		
beverage	T51.ØX1	T51.ØX2	T51.ØX3	T51.ØX4	—	—
butyl	T51.3X1	T51.3X2	T51.3X3	T51.3X4		
dehydrated	T51.ØX1	T51.ØX2	T51.ØX3	T51.ØX4	—	—
beverage	T51.ØX1	T51.ØX2	T51.ØX3	T51.ØX4	—	—
denatured	T51.ØX1	T51.ØX2	T51.ØX3	T51.ØX4	—	
deterrent NEC	T50.6X1	T50.6X2	T50.6X3	T50.6X4	T50.6X5	T50.6X6
diagnostic (gastric function)	T50.8X1	T50.8X2	T50.8X3	T50.8X4	T50.8X5	T50.8X6
ethyl	T51.ØX1	T51.ØX2	T51.ØX3	T51.ØX4	—	—
beverage	T51.ØX1	T51.ØX2	T51.ØX3	T51.ØX4	—	—
grain	T51.ØX1	T51.ØX2	T51.ØX3	T51.ØX4	—	—
beverage	T51.ØX1	T51.ØX2	T51.ØX3	T51.ØX4	—	—
industrial	T51.ØX1	T51.ØX2	T51.ØX3	T51.ØX4	—	—
isopropyl	T51.2X1	T51.2X2	T51.2X3	T51.2X4		
methyl	T51.1X1	T51.1X2	T51.1X3	T51.1X4		
preparation for consumption	T51.ØX1	T51.ØX2	T51.ØX3	T51.ØX4	—	—
propyl	T51.3X1	T51.3X2	T51.3X3	T51.3X4		
secondary	T51.2X1	T51.2X2	T51.2X3	T51.2X4	—	—
radiator	T51.1X1	T51.1X2	T51.1X3	T51.1X4		
rubbing	T51.2X1	T51.2X2	T51.2X3	T51.2X4	—	—
specified type NEC	T51.8X1	T51.8X2	T51.8X3	T51.8X4	—	—
surgical	T51.ØX1	T51.ØX2	T51.ØX3	T51.ØX4	—	—
vapor (from any type of Alcohol)	T59.891	T59.892	T59.893	T59.894		
wood	T51.1X1	T51.1X2	T51.1X3	T51.1X4	—	—
Alcuronium (chloride)	T48.1X1	T48.1X2	T48.1X3	T48.1X4	T48.1X5	T48.1X6
Aldactone	T50.ØX1	T50.ØX2	T50.ØX3	T50.ØX4	T50.ØX5	T50.ØX6
Aldesulfone sodium	T37.1X1	T37.1X2	T37.1X3	T37.1X4	T37.1X5	T37.1X6
Aldicarb	T60.ØX1	T60.ØX2	T60.ØX3	T60.ØX4	—	—
Aldomet	T46.5X1	T46.5X2	T46.5X3	T46.5X4	T46.5X5	T46.5X6
Aldosterone	T50.ØX1	T50.ØX2	T50.ØX3	T50.ØX4	T50.ØX5	T50.ØX6
Aldrin (dust)	T60.1X1	T60.1X2	T60.1X3	T60.1X4		
Aleve — see Naproxen						
Alexitol sodium	T47.1X1	T47.1X2	T47.1X3	T47.1X4	T47.1X5	T47.1X6
Alfacalcidol	T45.2X1	T45.2X2	T45.2X3	T45.2X4	T45.2X5	T45.2X6
Alfadolone	T41.1X1	T41.1X2	T41.1X3	T41.1X4	T41.1X5	T41.1X6
Alfaxalone	T41.1X1	T41.1X2	T41.1X3	T41.1X4	T41.1X5	T41.1X6
Alfentanil	T40.4X1	T40.4X2	T40.4X3	T40.4X4	T40.4X5	T40.4X6
Alfuzosin (hydrochloride)	T44.8X1	T44.8X2	T44.8X3	T44.8X4	T44.8X5	T44.8X6
Algae (harmful) (toxin)	T65.821	T65.822	T65.823	T65.824		
Algeldrate	T47.1X1	T47.1X2	T47.1X3	T47.1X4	T47.1X5	T47.1X6
Algin	T47.8X1	T47.8X2	T47.8X3	T47.8X4	T47.8X5	T47.8X6
Alglucerase	T45.3X1	T45.3X2	T45.3X3	T45.3X4	T45.3X5	T45.3X6
Alidase	T45.3X1	T45.3X2	T45.3X3	T45.3X4	T45.3X5	T45.3X6
Alimemazine	T43.3X1	T43.3X2	T43.3X3	T43.3X4	T43.3X5	T43.3X6
Aliphatic thiocyanates	T65.ØX1	T65.ØX2	T65.ØX3	T65.ØX4	—	—
Alizapride	T45.ØX1	T45.ØX2	T45.ØX3	T45.ØX4	T45.ØX5	T45.ØX6
Alkali (caustic)	T54.3X1	T54.3X2	T54.3X3	T54.3X4	—	—
Alkaline antiseptic solution (aromatic)	T49.6X1	T49.6X2	T49.6X3	T49.6X4	T49.6X5	T49.6X6
Alkalinizing agents (medicinal)	T50.9Ø1	T50.9Ø2	T50.9Ø3	T50.9Ø4	T50.9Ø5	T50.9Ø6
Alkalizing agent NEC	T50.9Ø1	T50.9Ø2	T50.9Ø3	T50.9Ø4	T50.9Ø5	T50.9Ø6
Alka-seltzer	T39.Ø11	T39.Ø12	T39.Ø13	T39.Ø14	T39.Ø15	T39.Ø16
Alkavervir	T46.5X1	T46.5X2	T46.5X3	T46.5X4	T46.5X5	T46.5X6
Alkonium (bromide)	T49.ØX1	T49.ØX2	T49.ØX3	T49.ØX4	T49.ØX5	T49.ØX6
Alkylating drug NEC	T45.1X1	T45.1X2	T45.1X3	T45.1X4	T45.1X5	T45.1X6
antimyeloproliferative	T45.1X1	T45.1X2	T45.1X3	T45.1X4	T45.1X5	T45.1X6
lymphatic	T45.1X1	T45.1X2	T45.1X3	T45.1X4	T45.1X5	T45.1X6
Alkylisocyanate	T65.ØX1	T65.ØX2	T65.ØX3	T65.ØX4	—	—
Allantoin	T49.4X1	T49.4X2	T49.4X3	T49.4X4	T49.4X5	T49.4X6
Allegron	T43.Ø11	T43.Ø12	T43.Ø13	T43.Ø14	T43.Ø15	T43.Ø16
Allethrin	T49.ØX1	T49.ØX2	T49.ØX3	T49.ØX4	T49.ØX5	T49.ØX6
Allobarbital	T42.3X1	T42.3X2	T42.3X3	T42.3X4	T42.3X5	T42.3X6
Allopurinol	T50.4X1	T50.4X2	T50.4X3	T50.4X4	T50.4X5	T50.4X6
Allyl						
alcohol	T51.8X1	T51.8X2	T51.8X3	T51.8X4	—	—
disulfide	T46.6X1	T46.6X2	T46.6X3	T46.6X4	T46.6X5	T46.6X6
Allylestrenol	T38.5X1	T38.5X2	T38.5X3	T38.5X4	T38.5X5	T38.5X6
Allylisopropylacetylurea	T42.6X1	T42.6X2	T42.6X3	T42.6X4	T42.6X5	T42.6X6
Allylisopropylmalonylurea	T42.3X1	T42.3X2	T42.3X3	T42.3X4	T42.3X5	T42.3X6
Allylthiourea	T49.3X1	T49.3X2	T49.3X3	T49.3X4	T49.3X5	T49.3X6
Allyltribromide	T42.6X1	T42.6X2	T42.6X3	T42.6X4	T42.6X5	T42.6X6
Allypropymal	T42.3X1	T42.3X2	T42.3X3	T42.3X4	T42.3X5	T42.3X6
Almagate	T47.1X1	T47.1X2	T47.1X3	T47.1X4	T47.1X5	T47.1X6
Almasilate	T47.1X1	T47.1X2	T47.1X3	T47.1X4	T47.1X5	T47.1X6
Almitrine	T50.7X1	T50.7X2	T50.7X3	T50.7X4	T50.7X5	T50.7X6
Aloes	T47.2X1	T47.2X2	T47.2X3	T47.2X4	T47.2X5	T47.2X6
Aloglutamol	T47.1X1	T47.1X2	T47.1X3	T47.1X4	T47.1X5	T47.1X6
Aloin	T47.2X1	T47.2X2	T47.2X3	T47.2X4	T47.2X5	T47.2X6
Aloxidone	T42.2X1	T42.2X2	T42.2X3	T42.2X4	T42.2X5	T42.2X6
Alpha						
acetyldigoxin	T46.ØX1	T46.ØX2	T46.ØX3	T46.ØX4	T46.ØX5	T46.ØX6
adrenergic blocking drug	T44.6X1	T44.6X2	T44.6X3	T44.6X4	T44.6X5	T44.6X6
amylase	T45.3X1	T45.3X2	T45.3X3	T45.3X4	T45.3X5	T45.3X6
tocoferol (acetate)	T45.2X1	T45.2X2	T45.2X3	T45.2X4	T45.2X5	T45.2X6
tocopherol	T45.2X1	T45.2X2	T45.2X3	T45.2X4	T45.2X5	T45.2X6
Alphadolone	T41.1X1	T41.1X2	T41.1X3	T41.1X4	T41.1X5	T41.1X6
Alphaprodine	T40.4X1	T40.4X2	T40.4X3	T40.4X4	T40.4X5	T40.4X6
Alphaxalone	T41.1X1	T41.1X2	T41.1X3	T41.1X4	T41.1X5	T41.1X6
Alprazolam	T42.4X1	T42.4X2	T42.4X3	T42.4X4	T42.4X5	T42.4X6
Alprenolol	T44.7X1	T44.7X2	T44.7X3	T44.7X4	T44.7X5	T44.7X6
Alprostadil	T46.7X1	T46.7X2	T46.7X3	T46.7X4	T46.7X5	T46.7X6
Alsactide	T38.811	T38.812	T38.813	T38.814	T38.815	T38.816
Alseroxylon	T46.5X1	T46.5X2	T46.5X3	T46.5X4	T46.5X5	T46.5X6
Alteplase	T45.611	T45.612	T45.613	T45.614	T45.615	T45.616
Altizide	T50.2X1	T50.2X2	T50.2X3	T50.2X4	T50.2X5	T50.2X6
Altretamine	T45.1X1	T45.1X2	T45.1X3	T45.1X4	T45.1X5	T45.1X6
Alum (medicinal)	T49.4X1	T49.4X2	T49.4X3	T49.4X4	T49.4X5	T49.4X6
nonmedicinal (ammonium) (potassium)	T56.891	T56.892	T56.893	T56.894	—	—
Aluminium, aluminum						
acetate	T49.2X1	T49.2X2	T49.2X3	T49.2X4	T49.2X5	T49.2X6
solution	T49.ØX1	T49.ØX2	T49.ØX3	T49.ØX4	T49.ØX5	T49.ØX6
aspirin	T39.Ø11	T39.Ø12	T39.Ø13	T39.Ø14	T39.Ø15	T39.Ø16
bis (acetylsalicylate)	T39.Ø11	T39.Ø12	T39.Ø13	T39.Ø14	T39.Ø15	T39.Ø16
carbonate (gel, basic)	T47.1X1	T47.1X2	T47.1X3	T47.1X4	T47.1X5	T47.1X6
chlorhydroxide-complex	T47.1X1	T47.1X2	T47.1X3	T47.1X4	T47.1X5	T47.1X6
chloride	T49.2X1	T49.2X2	T49.2X3	T49.2X4	T49.2X5	T49.2X6
clofibrate	T46.6X1	T46.6X2	T46.6X3	T46.6X4	T46.6X5	T46.6X6
diacetate	T49.2X1	T49.2X2	T49.2X3	T49.2X4	T49.2X5	T49.2X6
glycinate	T47.1X1	T47.1X2	T47.1X3	T47.1X4	T47.1X5	T47.1X6
hydroxide (gel)	T47.1X1	T47.1X2	T47.1X3	T47.1X4	T47.1X5	T47.1X6
hydroxide-magnesium carb. gel	T47.1X1	T47.1X2	T47.1X3	T47.1X4	T47.1X5	T47.1X6
magnesium silicate	T47.1X1	T47.1X2	T47.1X3	T47.1X4	T47.1X5	T47.1X6
nicotinate	T46.7X1	T46.7X2	T46.7X3	T46.7X4	T46.7X5	T46.7X6
ointment (surgical) (topical)	T49.3X1	T49.3X2	T49.3X3	T49.3X4	T49.3X5	T49.3X6
phosphate	T47.1X1	T47.1X2	T47.1X3	T47.1X4	T47.1X5	T47.1X6
salicylate	T39.Ø91	T39.Ø92	T39.Ø93	T39.Ø94	T39.Ø95	T39.Ø96
silicate	T47.1X1	T47.1X2	T47.1X3	T47.1X4	T47.1X5	T47.1X6
sodium silicate	T47.1X1	T47.1X2	T47.1X3	T47.1X4	T47.1X5	T47.1X6
subacetate	T49.2X1	T49.2X2	T49.2X3	T49.2X4	T49.2X5	T49.2X6
sulfate	T49.ØX1	T49.ØX2	T49.ØX3	T49.ØX4	T49.ØX5	T49.ØX6
tannate	T47.6X1	T47.6X2	T47.6X3	T47.6X4	T47.6X5	T47.6X6
topical NEC	T49.3X1	T49.3X2	T49.3X3	T49.3X4	T49.3X5	T49.3X6
Alurate	T42.3X1	T42.3X2	T42.3X3	T42.3X4	T42.3X5	T42.3X6
Alverine	T44.3X1	T44.3X2	T44.3X3	T44.3X4	T44.3X5	T44.3X6
Alvodine	T40.2X1	T40.2X2	T40.2X3	T40.2X4	T40.2X5	T40.2X6
Amanita phalloides	T62.ØX1	T62.ØX2	T62.ØX3	T62.ØX4	—	—

Substance	Poisoning, Accidental (unintentional)	Poisoning, Intentional Self-harm	Poisoning, Assault	Poisoning, Undetermined	Adverse Effect	Under-dosing
Amanitine	T62.0X1	T62.0X2	T62.0X3	T62.0X4	—	—
Amantadine	T42.8X1	T42.8X2	T42.8X3	T42.8X4	T42.8X5	T42.8X6
Ambazone	T49.6X1	T49.6X2	T49.6X3	T49.6X4	T49.6X5	T49.6X6
Ambenonium (chloride)	T44.0X1	T44.0X2	T44.0X3	T44.0X4	T44.0X5	T44.0X6
Ambroxol	T48.4X1	T48.4X2	T48.4X3	T48.4X4	T48.4X5	T48.4X6
Ambuphylline	T48.6X1	T48.6X2	T48.6X3	T48.6X4	T48.6X5	T48.6X6
Ambutonium bromide	T44.3X1	T44.3X2	T44.3X3	T44.3X4	T44.3X5	T44.3X6
Amcinonide	T49.0X1	T49.0X2	T49.0X3	T49.0X4	T49.0X5	T49.0X6
Amdinocilline	T36.0X1	T36.0X2	T36.0X3	T36.0X4	T36.0X5	T36.0X6
Ametazole	T50.8X1	T50.8X2	T50.8X3	T50.8X4	T50.8X5	T50.8X6
Amethocaine	T41.3X1	T41.3X2	T41.3X3	T41.3X4	T41.3X5	T41.3X6
regional	T41.3X1	T41.3X2	T41.3X3	T41.3X4	T41.3X5	T41.3X6
spinal	T41.3X1	T41.3X2	T41.3X3	T41.3X4	T41.3X5	T41.3X6
Amethopterin	T45.1X1	T45.1X2	T45.1X3	T45.1X4	T45.1X5	T45.1X6
Amezinium metilsulfate	T44.992	T44.992	T44.993	T44.994	T44.995	T44.996
Amfebutamone	T43.291	T43.292	T43.293	T43.294	T43.295	T43.296
Amfepramone	T50.5X1	T50.5X2	T50.5X3	T50.5X4	T50.5X5	T50.5X6
Amfetamine	T43.621	T43.622	T43.623	T43.624	T43.625	T43.626
Amfetaminil	T43.621	T43.622	T43.623	T43.624	T43.625	T43.626
Amfomycin	T36.8X1	T36.8X2	T36.8X3	T36.8X4	T36.8X5	T36.8X6
Amidefrine mesilate	T48.5X1	T48.5X2	T48.5X3	T48.5X4	T48.5X5	T48.5X6
Amidone	T40.3X1	T40.3X2	T40.3X3	T40.3X4	T40.3X5	T40.3X6
Amidopyrine	T39.2X1	T39.2X2	T39.2X3	T39.2X4	T39.2X5	T39.2X6
Amidotrizoate	T50.8X1	T50.8X2	T50.8X3	T50.8X4	T50.8X5	T50.8X6
Amiflamine	T43.1X1	T43.1X2	T43.1X3	T43.1X4	T43.1X5	T43.1X6
Amikacin	T36.5X1	T36.5X2	T36.5X3	T36.5X4	T36.5X5	T36.5X6
Amikhelline	T46.3X1	T46.3X2	T46.3X3	T46.3X4	T46.3X5	T46.3X6
Amiloride	T50.2X1	T50.2X2	T50.2X3	T50.2X4	T50.2X5	T50.2X6
Aminacrine	T49.0X1	T49.0X2	T49.0X3	T49.0X4	T49.0X5	T49.0X6
Amineptine	T43.011	T43.012	T43.013	T43.014	T43.015	T43.016
Aminitrozole	T37.3X1	T37.3X2	T37.3X3	T37.3X4	T37.3X5	T37.3X6
Aminoacetic acid (derivatives)	T50.3X1	T50.3X2	T50.3X3	T50.3X4	T50.3X5	T50.3X6
Amino acids	T50.3X1	T50.3X2	T50.3X3	T50.3X4	T50.3X5	T50.3X6
Aminoacridine	T49.0X1	T49.0X2	T49.0X3	T49.0X4	T49.0X5	T49.0X6
Aminobenzoic acid (-p)	T49.3X1	T49.3X2	T49.3X3	T49.3X4	T49.3X5	T49.3X6
Aminocaproic acid	T45.621	T45.622	T45.623	T45.624	T45.625	T45.626
Aminoethylisothiourium	T45.8X1	T45.8X2	T45.8X3	T45.8X4	T45.8X5	T45.8X6
Aminofenazone	T39.2X1	T39.2X2	T39.2X3	T39.2X4	T39.2X5	T39.2X6
Aminoglutethimide	T45.1X1	T45.1X2	T45.1X3	T45.1X4	T45.1X5	T45.1X6
Aminohippuric acid	T50.8X1	T50.8X2	T50.8X3	T50.8X4	T50.8X5	T50.8X6
Aminomethylbenzoic acid	T45.691	T45.692	T45.693	T45.694	T45.695	T45.696
Aminometradine	T50.2X1	T50.2X2	T50.2X3	T50.2X4	T50.2X5	T50.2X6
Aminopentamide	T44.3X1	T44.3X2	T44.3X3	T44.3X4	T44.3X5	T44.3X6
Aminophenazone	T39.2X1	T39.2X2	T39.2X3	T39.2X4	T39.2X5	T39.2X6
Aminophenol	T54.0X1	T54.0X2	T54.0X3	T54.0X4	—	—
Aminophenylpyridone	T43.591	T43.592	T43.593	T43.594	T43.595	T43.596
Aminophylline	T48.6X1	T48.6X2	T48.6X3	T48.6X4	T48.6X5	T48.6X6
Aminopterin sodium	T45.1X1	T45.1X2	T45.1X3	T45.1X4	T45.1X5	T45.1X6
Aminopyrine	T39.2X1	T39.2X2	T39.2X3	T39.2X4	T39.2X5	T39.2X6
Aminorex	T50.5X1	T50.5X2	T50.5X3	T50.5X4	T50.5X5	T50.5X6
Aminosalicylic acid	T37.1X1	T37.1X2	T37.1X3	T37.1X4	T37.1X5	T37.1X6
Aminosalylum	T37.1X1	T37.1X2	T37.1X3	T37.1X4	T37.1X5	T37.1X6
Amiodarone	T46.2X1	T46.2X2	T46.2X3	T46.2X4	T46.2X5	T46.2X6
Amiphenazole	T50.7X1	T50.7X2	T50.7X3	T50.7X4	T50.7X5	T50.7X6
Amiquinsin	T46.5X1	T46.5X2	T46.5X3	T46.5X4	T46.5X5	T46.5X6
Amisometradine	T50.2X1	T50.2X2	T50.2X3	T50.2X4	T50.2X5	T50.2X6
Amisulpride	T43.591	T43.592	T43.593	T43.594	T43.595	T43.596
Amitriptyline	T43.011	T43.012	T43.013	T43.014	T43.015	T43.016
Amitriptylinoxide	T43.011	T43.012	T43.013	T43.014	T43.015	T43.016
Amlexanox	T48.6X1	T48.6X2	T48.6X3	T48.6X4	T48.6X5	T48.6X6
Ammonia (fumes) (gas) (vapor)	T59.891	T59.892	T59.893	T59.894	—	—
aromatic spirit	T48.991	T48.992	T48.993	T48.994	T48.995	T48.996
liquid (household)	T54.3X1	T54.3X2	T54.3X3	T54.3X4	—	—
Ammoniated mercury	T49.0X1	T49.0X2	T49.0X3	T49.0X4	T49.0X5	T49.0X6
Ammonium						
acid tartrate	T49.5X1	T49.5X2	T49.5X3	T49.5X4	T49.5X5	T49.5X6
bromide	T42.6X1	T42.6X2	T42.6X3	T42.6X4	T42.6X5	T42.6X6
carbonate	T54.3X1	T54.3X2	T54.3X3	T54.3X4	—	—
chloride	T50.991	T50.992	T50.993	T50.994	T50.995	T50.996
expectorant	T48.4X1	T48.4X2	T48.4X3	T48.4X4	T48.4X5	T48.4X6
compounds (household) NEC	T54.3X1	T54.3X2	T54.3X3	T54.3X4	—	—
fumes (any usage)	T59.891	T59.892	T59.893	T59.894	—	—
industrial	T54.3X1	T54.3X2	T54.3X3	T54.3X4	—	—
ichthyosulronate	T49.4X1	T49.4X2	T49.4X3	T49.4X4	T49.4X5	T49.4X6
mandelate	T37.91	T37.92	T37.93	T37.94	T37.95	T37.96
sulfamate	T60.3X1	T60.3X2	T60.3X3	T60.3X4	—	—
sulfonate resin	T47.8X1	T47.8X2	T47.8X3	T47.8X4	T47.8X5	T47.8X6
Amobarbital (sodium)	T42.3X1	T42.3X2	T42.3X3	T42.3X4	T42.3X5	T42.3X6
Amodiaquine	T37.2X1	T37.2X2	T37.2X3	T37.2X4	T37.2X5	T37.2X6
Amopyroquin (e)	T37.2X1	T37.2X2	T37.2X3	T37.2X4	T37.2X5	T37.2X6
Amoxapine	T43.011	T43.012	T43.013	T43.014	T43.015	T43.016
Amoxicillin	T36.0X1	T36.0X2	T36.0X3	T36.0X4	T36.0X5	T36.0X6
Amperozide	T43.591	T43.592	T43.593	T43.594	T43.595	T43.596
Amphenidone	T43.591	T43.592	T43.593	T43.594	T43.595	T43.596
Amphetamine NEC	T43.621	T43.622	T43.623	T43.624	T43.625	T43.626
Amphomycin	T36.8X1	T36.8X2	T36.8X3	T36.8X4	T36.8X5	T36.8X6
Amphotalide	T37.4X1	T37.4X2	T37.4X3	T37.4X4	T37.4X5	T37.4X6
Amphotericin B	T36.7X1	T36.7X2	T36.7X3	T36.7X4	T36.7X5	T36.7X6
topical	T49.0X1	T49.0X2	T49.0X3	T49.0X4	T49.0X5	T49.0X6
Ampicillin	T36.0X1	T36.0X2	T36.0X3	T36.0X4	T36.0X5	T36.0X6
Amprotropine	T44.3X1	T44.3X2	T44.3X3	T44.3X4	T44.3X5	T44.3X6
Amsacrine	T45.1X1	T45.1X2	T45.1X3	T45.1X4	T45.1X5	T45.1X6
Amygdaline	T62.2X1	T62.2X2	T62.2X3	T62.2X4	—	—
Amyl						
acetate	T52.8X1	T52.8X2	T52.8X3	T52.8X4	—	—
vapor	T59.891	T59.892	T59.893	T59.894	—	—
alcohol	T51.3X1	T51.3X2	T51.3X3	T51.3X4	—	—
chloride	T53.6X1	T53.6X2	T53.6X3	T53.6X4	—	—
formate	T52.8X1	T52.8X2	T52.8X3	T52.8X4	—	—
nitrite	T46.3X1	T46.3X2	T46.3X3	T46.3X4	T46.3X5	T46.3X6
propionate	T65.891	T65.892	T65.893	T65.894	—	—
Amylase	T47.5X1	T47.5X2	T47.5X3	T47.5X4	T47.5X5	T47.5X6
Amyleine, regional	T41.3X1	T41.3X2	T41.3X3	T41.3X4	T41.3X5	T41.3X6
Amylene						
dichloride	T53.6X1	T53.6X2	T53.6X3	T53.6X4	—	—
hydrate	T51.3X1	T51.3X2	T51.3X3	T51.3X4	—	—
Amylmetacresol	T49.6X1	T49.6X2	T49.6X3	T49.6X4	T49.6X5	T49.6X6
Amylobarbitone	T42.3X1	T42.3X2	T42.3X3	T42.3X4	T42.3X5	T42.3X6
Amylocaine, regional	T41.3X1	T41.3X2	T41.3X3	T41.3X4	T41.3X5	T41.3X6
infiltration (subcutaneous)	T41.3X1	T41.3X2	T41.3X3	T41.3X4	T41.3X5	T41.3X6
nerve block (peripheral) (plexus)	T41.3X1	T41.3X2	T41.3X3	T41.3X4	T41.3X5	T41.3X6
spinal				T41.3X4	T41.3X5	T41.3X6
topical (surface)	T41.3X1	T41.3X2	T41.3X3	T41.3X4	T41.3X5	T41.3X6
Amylopectin	T47.6X1	T47.6X2	T47.6X3	T47.6X4	T47.6X5	T47.6X6
Amytal (sodium)	T42.3X1	T42.3X2	T42.3X3	T42.3X4	T42.3X5	T42.3X6
Anabolic steroid	T38.7X1	T38.7X2	T38.7X3	T38.7X4	T38.7X5	T38.7X6
Analeptic NEC	T50.7X1	T50.7X2	T50.7X3	T50.7X4	T50.7X5	T50.7X6
Analgesic	T39.91	T39.92	T39.93	T39.94	T39.95	T39.96
anti-inflammatory NEC	T39.91	T39.92	T39.93	T39.94	T39.95	T39.96
propionic acid derivative	T39.311	T39.312	T39.313	T39.314	T39.315	T39.316
antirheumatic NEC	T39.4X1	T39.4X2	T39.4X3	T39.4X4	T39.4X5	T39.4X6
aromatic NEC	T39.1X1	T39.1X2	T39.1X3	T39.1X4	T39.1X5	T39.1X6
narcotic NEC	T40.601	T40.602	T40.603	T40.604	T40.605	T40.606
combination	T40.601	T40.602	T40.603	T40.604	T40.605	T40.606
obstetric	T40.601	T40.602	T40.603	T40.604	T40.605	T40.606
non-narcotic NEC	T39.91	T39.92	T39.93	T39.94	T39.95	T39.96
combination	T39.91	T39.92	T39.93	T39.94	T39.95	T39.96
pyrazole	T39.2X1	T39.2X2	T39.2X3	T39.2X4	T39.2X5	T39.2X6
specified NEC	T39.8X1	T39.8X2	T39.8X3	T39.8X4	T39.8X5	T39.8X6
Analgin	T39.2X1	T39.2X2	T39.2X3	T39.2X4	T39.2X5	T39.2X6
Anamirta cocculus	T62.1X1	T62.1X2	T62.1X3	T62.1X4	—	—
Ancillin	T36.0X1	T36.0X2	T36.0X3	T36.0X4	T36.0X5	T36.0X6
Ancrod	T45.691	T45.692	T45.693	T45.694	T45.695	T45.696
Androgen	T38.7X1	T38.7X2	T38.7X3	T38.7X4	T38.7X5	T38.7X6
Androgen-estrogen mixture	T38.7X1	T38.7X2	T38.7X3	T38.7X4	T38.7X5	T38.7X6
Androstalone	T38.7X1	T38.7X2	T38.7X3	T38.7X4	T38.7X5	T38.7X6
Androstanolone	T38.7X1	T38.7X2	T38.7X3	T38.7X4	T38.7X5	T38.7X6
Androsterone	T38.7X1	T38.7X2	T38.7X3	T38.7X4	T38.7X5	T38.7X6
Anemone pulsatilla	T62.2X1	T62.2X2	T62.2X3	T62.2X4	—	—
Anesthesia						
caudal	T41.3X1	T41.3X2	T41.3X3	T41.3X4	T41.3X5	T41.3X6
endotracheal	T41.0X1	T41.0X2	T41.0X3	T41.0X4	T41.0X5	T41.0X6
epidural	T41.3X1	T41.3X2	T41.3X3	T41.3X4	T41.3X5	T41.3X6
inhalation	T41.0X1	T41.0X2	T41.0X3	T41.0X4	T41.0X5	T41.0X6
local	T41.3X1	T41.3X2	T41.3X3	T41.3X4	T41.3X5	T41.3X6
mucosal	T41.3X1	T41.3X2	T41.3X3	T41.3X4	T41.3X5	T41.3X6
muscle relaxation	T48.1X1	T48.1X2	T48.1X3	T48.1X4	T48.1X5	T48.1X6
nerve blocking	T41.3X1	T41.3X2	T41.3X3	T41.3X4	T41.3X5	T41.3X6
plexus blocking	T41.3X1	T41.3X2	T41.3X3	T41.3X4	T41.3X5	T41.3X6
potentiated	T41.201	T41.202	T41.203	T41.204	T41.205	T41.206
rectal	T41.201	T41.202	T41.203	T41.204	T41.205	T41.206
general	T41.201	T41.202	T41.203	T41.204	T41.205	T41.206
local	T41.3X1	T41.3X2	T41.3X3	T41.3X4	T41.3X5	T41.3X6
regional	T41.3X1	T41.3X2	T41.3X3	T41.3X4	T41.3X5	T41.3X6
surface	T41.3X1	T41.3X2	T41.3X3	T41.3X4	T41.3X5	T41.3X6
Anesthetic NEC — see also Anesthesia	T41.41	T41.42	T41.43	T41.44	T41.45	T41.46
with muscle relaxant	T41.201	T41.202	T41.203	T41.204	T41.205	T41.206
general	T41.201	T41.202	T41.203	T41.204	T41.205	T41.206
local	T41.3X1	T41.3X2	T41.3X3	T41.3X4	T41.3X5	T41.3X6
gaseous NEC	T41.0X1	T41.0X2	T41.0X3	T41.0X4	T41.0X5	T41.0X6

Table of Drugs and Chemicals

Substance	Poisoning, Accidental (unintentional)	Poisoning, Intentional Self-harm	Poisoning, Assault	Poisoning, Undetermined	Adverse Effect	Under-dosing
Anesthetic — *see also* Anesthesia — continued						
general NEC	T41.201	T41.202	T41.203	T41.204	T41.205	T41.206
halogenated hydrocarbon derivatives NEC	T41.0X1	T41.0X2	T41.0X3	T41.0X4	T41.0X5	T41.0X6
infiltration NEC	T41.3X1	T41.3X2	T41.3X3	T41.3X4	T41.3X5	T41.3X6
intravenous NEC	T41.1X1	T41.1X2	T41.1X3	T41.1X4	T41.1X5	T41.1X6
local NEC	T41.3X1	T41.3X2	T41.3X3	T41.3X4	T41.3X5	T41.3X6
rectal	T41.201	T41.202	T41.203	T41.204	T41.205	T41.206
general	T41.201	T41.202	T41.203	T41.204	T41.205	T41.206
local	T41.3X1	T41.3X2	T41.3X3	T41.3X4	T41.3X5	T41.3X6
regional NEC	T41.3X1	T41.3X2	T41.3X3	T41.3X4	T41.3X5	T41.3X6
spinal NEC	T41.3X1	T41.3X2	T41.3X3	T41.3X4	T41.3X5	T41.3X6
thiobarbiturate	T41.1X1	T41.1X2	T41.1X3	T41.1X4	T41.1X5	T41.1X6
topical	T41.3X1	T41.3X2	T41.3X3	T41.3X4	T41.3X5	T41.3X6
Aneurine	T45.2X1	T45.2X2	T45.2X3	T45.2X4	T45.2X5	T45.2X6
Angio-Conray	T50.8X1	T50.8X2	T50.8X3	T50.8X4	T50.8X5	T50.8X6
Angiotensin	T44.5X1	T44.5X2	T44.5X3	T44.5X4	T44.5X5	T44.5X6
Angiotensinamide	T44.991	T44.992	T44.993	T44.994	T44.995	T44.996
Anhydrohydroxy-progesterone	T38.5X1	T38.5X2	T38.5X3	T38.5X4	T38.5X5	T38.5X6
Anhydron	T50.2X1	T50.2X2	T50.2X3	T50.2X4	T50.2X5	T50.2X6
Anileridine	T40.4X1	T40.4X2	T40.4X3	T40.4X4	T40.4X5	T40.4X6
Aniline (dye) (liquid)	T65.3X1	T65.3X2	T65.3X3	T65.3X4	—	—
analgesic	T39.1X1	T39.1X2	T39.1X3	T39.1X4	T39.1X5	T39.1X6
derivatives, therapeutic NEC	T39.1X1	T39.1X2	T39.1X3	T39.1X4	T39.1X5	T39.1X6
vapor	T65.3X1	T65.3X2	T65.3X3	T65.3X4	—	—
Aniscoropine	T44.3X1	T44.3X2	T44.3X3	T44.3X4	T44.3X5	T44.3X6
Anise oil	T47.5X1	T47.5X2	T47.5X3	T47.5X4	T47.5X5	T47.5X6
Anisidine	T65.3X1	T65.3X2	T65.3X3	T65.3X4	—	—
Anisindione	T45.511	T45.512	T45.513	T45.514	T45.515	T45.516
Anisotropine methyl-bromide	T44.3X1	T44.3X2	T44.3X3	T44.3X4	T44.3X5	T44.3X6
Anistreplase	T45.611	T45.612	T45.613	T45.614	T45.615	T45.616
Anorexiant (central)	T50.5X1	T50.5X2	T50.5X3	T50.5X4	T50.5X5	T50.5X6
Anorexic agents	T50.5X1	T50.5X2	T50.5X3	T50.5X4	T50.5X5	T50.5X6
Ansamycin	T36.6X1	T36.6X2	T36.6X3	T36.6X4	T36.6X5	T36.6X6
Ant (bite) (sting)	T63.421	T63.422	T63.423	T63.424	—	—
Antabuse	T50.6X1	T50.6X2	T50.6X3	T50.6X4	T50.6X5	T50.6X6
Antacid NEC	T47.1X1	T47.1X2	T47.1X3	T47.1X4	T47.1X5	T47.1X6
Antagonist						
Aldosterone	T50.0X1	T50.0X2	T50.0X3	T50.0X4	T50.0X5	T50.0X6
alpha-adrenoreceptor	T44.6X1	T44.6X2	T44.6X3	T44.6X4	T44.6X5	T44.6X6
anticoagulant	T45.7X1	T45.7X2	T45.7X3	T45.7X4	T45.7X5	T45.7X6
beta-adrenoreceptor	T44.7X1	T44.7X2	T44.7X3	T44.7X4	T44.7X5	T44.7X6
extrapyramidal NEC	T44.3X1	T44.3X2	T44.3X3	T44.3X4	T44.3X5	T44.3X6
folic acid	T45.1X1	T45.1X2	T45.1X3	T45.1X4	T45.1X5	T45.1X6
H2 receptor	T47.0X1	T47.0X2	T47.0X3	T47.0X4	T47.0X5	T47.0X6
heavy metal	T45.8X1	T45.8X2	T45.8X3	T45.8X4	T45.8X5	T45.8X6
narcotic analgesic	T50.7X1	T50.7X2	T50.7X3	T50.7X4	T50.7X5	T50.7X6
opiate	T50.7X1	T50.7X2	T50.7X3	T50.7X4	T50.7X5	T50.7X6
pyrimidine	T45.1X1	T45.1X2	T45.1X3	T45.1X4	T45.1X5	T45.1X6
serotonin	T46.5X1	T46.5X2	T46.5X3	T46.5X4	T46.5X5	T46.5X6
Antazolin(e)	T45.0X1	T45.0X2	T45.0X3	T45.0X4	T45.0X5	T45.0X6
Anterior pituitary hormone NEC	T38.811	T38.812	T38.813	T38.814	T38.815	T38.816
Anthelmintic NEC	T37.4X1	T37.4X2	T37.4X3	T37.4X4	T37.4X5	T37.4X6
Anthiolimine	T37.4X1	T37.4X2	T37.4X3	T37.4X4	T37.4X5	T37.4X6
Anthralin	T49.4X1	T49.4X2	T49.4X3	T49.4X4	T49.4X5	T49.4X6
Anthramycin	T45.1X1	T45.1X2	T45.1X3	T45.1X4	T45.1X5	T45.1X6
Antiadrenergic NEC	T44.8X1	T44.8X2	T44.8X3	T44.8X4	T44.8X5	T44.8X6
Antiallergic NEC	T45.0X1	T45.0X2	T45.0X3	T45.0X4	T45.0X5	T45.0X6
Antiandrogen NEC	T38.6X1	T38.6X2	T38.6X3	T38.6X4	T38.6X5	T38.6X6
Anti-anemic (drug) (preparation)	T45.8X1	T45.8X2	T45.8X3	T45.8X4	T45.8X5	T45.8X6
Antianxiety drug NEC	T43.501	T43.502	T43.503	T43.504	T43.505	T43.506
Antiaris toxicaria	T65.891	T65.892	T65.893	T65.894	—	—
Antiarteriosclerotic drug	T46.6X1	T46.6X2	T46.6X3	T46.6X4	T46.6X5	T46.6X6
Antiasthmatic drug NEC	T48.6X1	T48.6X2	T48.6X3	T48.6X4	T48.6X5	T48.6X6
Antibiotic NEC	T36.91	T36.92	T36.93	T36.94	T36.95	T36.96
aminoglycoside	T36.5X1	T36.5X2	T36.5X3	T36.5X4	T36.5X5	T36.5X6
anticancer	T45.1X1	T45.1X2	T45.1X3	T45.1X4	T45.1X5	T45.1X6
antifungal	T36.7X1	T36.7X2	T36.7X3	T36.7X4	T36.7X5	T36.7X6
antimycobacterial	T36.5X1	T36.5X2	T36.5X3	T36.5X4	T36.5X5	T36.5X6
antineoplastic	T45.1X1	T45.1X2	T45.1X3	T45.1X4	T45.1X5	T45.1X6
b-lactam NEC	T36.1X1	T36.1X2	T36.1X3	T36.1X4	T36.1X5	T36.1X6
cephalosporin (group)	T36.1X1	T36.1X2	T36.1X3	T36.1X4	T36.1X5	T36.1X6
chloramphenicol (group)	T36.2X1	T36.2X2	T36.2X3	T36.2X4	T36.2X5	T36.2X6
ENT	T49.6X1	T49.6X2	T49.6X3	T49.6X4	T49.6X5	T49.6X6
eye	T49.5X1	T49.5X2	T49.5X3	T49.5X4	T49.5X5	T49.5X6
fungicidal (local)	T49.0X1	T49.0X2	T49.0X3	T49.0X4	T49.0X5	T49.0X6
intestinal	T36.8X1	T36.8X2	T36.8X3	T36.8X4	T36.8X5	T36.8X6
local	T49.0X1	T49.0X2	T49.0X3	T49.0X4	T49.0X5	T49.0X6
Antibiotic — *continued*						
macrolides	T36.3X1	T36.3X2	T36.3X3	T36.3X4	T36.3X5	T36.3X6
polypeptide	T36.8X1	T36.8X2	T36.8X3	T36.8X4	T36.8X5	T36.8X6
specified NEC	T36.8X1	T36.8X2	T36.8X3	T36.8X4	T36.8X5	T36.8X6
tetracycline (group)	T36.4X1	T36.4X2	T36.4X3	T36.4X4	T36.4X5	T36.4X6
throat	T49.6X1	T49.6X2	T49.6X3	T49.6X4	T49.6X5	T49.6X6
Anticancer agents NEC	T45.1X1	T45.1X2	T45.1X3	T45.1X4	T45.1X5	T45.1X6
Anticholesterolemic drug NEC	T46.6X1	T46.6X2	T46.6X3	T46.6X4	T46.6X5	T46.6X6
Anticholinergic NEC	T44.3X1	T44.3X2	T44.3X3	T44.3X4	T44.3X5	T44.3X6
Anticholinesterase	T44.0X1	T44.0X2	T44.0X3	T44.0X4	T44.0X5	T44.0X6
organophosphorus	T44.0X1	T44.0X2	T44.0X3	T44.0X4	T44.0X5	T44.0X6
insecticide	T60.0X1	T60.0X2	T60.0X3	T60.0X4	—	—
nerve gas	T59.891	T59.892	T59.893	T59.894	—	—
reversible	T44.0X1	T44.0X2	T44.0X3	T44.0X4	T44.0X5	T44.0X6
ophthalmological	T49.5X1	T49.5X2	T49.5X3	T49.5X4	T49.5X5	T49.5X6
Anticoagulant NEC	T45.511	T45.512	T45.513	T45.514	T45.515	T45.516
Antagonist	T45.7X1	T45.7X2	T45.7X3	T45.7X4	T45.7X5	T45.7X6
Anti-common-cold drug NEC	T48.5X1	T48.5X2	T48.5X3	T48.5X4	T48.5X5	T48.5X6
Anticonvulsant	T42.71	T42.72	T42.73	T42.74	T42.75	T42.76
barbiturate	T42.3X1	T42.3X2	T42.3X3	T42.3X4	T42.3X5	T42.3X6
combination (with barbiturate)	T42.3X1	T42.3X2	T42.3X3	T42.3X4	T42.3X5	T42.3X6
hydantoin	T42.0X1	T42.0X2	T42.0X3	T42.0X4	T42.0X5	T42.0X6
hypnotic NEC	T42.6X1	T42.6X2	T42.6X3	T42.6X4	T42.6X5	T42.6X6
oxazolidinedione	T42.2X1	T42.2X2	T42.2X3	T42.2X4	T42.2X5	T42.2X6
pyrimidinedione	T42.6X1	T42.6X2	T42.6X3	T42.6X4	T42.6X5	T42.6X6
specified NEC	T42.6X1	T42.6X2	T42.6X3	T42.6X4	T42.6X5	T42.6X6
succinimide	T42.2X1	T42.2X2	T42.2X3	T42.2X4	T42.2X5	T42.2X6
Antidepressant	T43.201	T43.202	T43.203	T43.204	T43.205	T43.206
monoamine oxidase inhibitor	T43.1X1	T43.1X2	T43.1X3	T43.1X4	T43.1X5	T43.1X6
selective serotonin norepinephrine reuptake inhibitor	T43.211	T43.212	T43.213	T43.214	T43.215	T43.216
selective serotonin reuptake inhibitor	T43.221	T43.222	T43.223	T43.224	T43.225	T43.226
specified NEC	T43.291	T43.292	T43.293	T43.294	T43.295	T43.296
tetracyclic	T43.021	T43.022	T43.023	T43.024	T43.025	T43.026
triazolopyridine	T43.211	T43.212	T43.213	T43.214	T43.215	T43.216
tricyclic	T43.011	T43.012	T43.013	T43.014	T43.015	T43.016
Antidiabetic NEC	T38.3X1	T38.3X2	T38.3X3	T38.3X4	T38.3X5	T38.3X6
biguanide	T38.3X1	T38.3X2	T38.3X3	T38.3X4	T38.3X5	T38.3X6
and sulfonyl combined	T38.3X1	T38.3X2	T38.3X3	T38.3X4	T38.3X5	T38.3X6
combined	T38.3X1	T38.3X2	T38.3X3	T38.3X4	T38.3X5	T38.3X6
sulfonylurea	T38.3X1	T38.3X2	T38.3X3	T38.3X4	T38.3X5	T38.3X6
Antidiarrheal drug NEC	T47.6X1	T47.6X2	T47.6X3	T47.6X4	T47.6X5	T47.6X6
absorbent	T47.6X1	T47.6X2	T47.6X3	T47.6X4	T47.6X5	T47.6X6
Anti-D immunoglobulin (human)	T50.Z11	T50.Z12	T50.Z13	T50.Z14	T50.Z15	T50.Z16
Antidiphtheria serum	T50.Z11	T50.Z12	T50.Z13	T50.Z14	T50.Z15	T50.Z16
Antidiuretic hormone	T38.891	T38.892	T38.893	T38.894	T38.895	T38.896
Antidote NEC	T50.6X1	T50.6X2	T50.6X3	T50.6X4	T50.6X5	T50.6X6
heavy metal	T45.8X1	T45.8X2	T45.8X3	T45.8X4	T45.8X5	T45.8X6
Antidysrhythmic NEC	T46.2X1	T46.2X2	T46.2X3	T46.2X4	T46.2X5	T46.2X6
Antiemetic drug	T45.0X1	T45.0X2	T45.0X3	T45.0X4	T45.0X5	T45.0X6
Antiepilepsy agent	T42.71	T42.72	T42.73	T42.74	T42.75	T42.76
combination	T42.5X1	T42.5X2	T42.5X3	T42.5X4	T42.5X5	T42.5X6
mixed	T42.5X1	T42.5X2	T42.5X3	T42.5X4	T42.5X5	T42.5X6
specified, NEC	T42.6X1	T42.6X2	T42.6X3	T42.6X4	T42.6X5	T42.6X6
Antiestrogen NEC	T38.6X1	T38.6X2	T38.6X3	T38.6X4	T38.6X5	T38.6X6
Antifertility pill	T38.4X1	T38.4X2	T38.4X3	T38.4X4	T38.4X5	T38.4X6
Antifibrinolytic drug	T45.621	T45.622	T45.623	T45.624	T45.625	T45.626
Antifilarial drug	T37.4X1	T37.4X2	T37.4X3	T37.4X4	T37.4X5	T37.4X6
Antiflatulent	T47.5X1	T47.5X2	T47.5X3	T47.5X4	T47.5X5	T47.5X6
Antifreeze	T65.91	T65.92	T65.93	T65.94	—	—
alcohol	T51.1X1	T51.1X2	T51.1X3	T51.1X4	—	—
ethylene glycol	T51.8X1	T51.8X2	T51.8X3	T51.8X4	—	—
Antifungal						
antibiotic (systemic)	T36.7X1	T36.7X2	T36.7X3	T36.7X4	T36.7X5	T36.7X6
anti-infective NEC	T37.91	T37.92	T37.93	T37.94	T37.95	T37.96
disinfectant, local	T49.0X1	T49.0X2	T49.0X3	T49.0X4	T49.0X5	T49.0X6
nonmedicinal (spray)	T60.3X1	T60.3X2	T60.3X3	T60.3X4	—	—
topical	T49.0X1	T49.0X2	T49.0X3	T49.0X4	T49.0X5	T49.0X6
Anti-gastric-secretion drug NEC	T47.1X1	T47.1X2	T47.1X3	T47.1X4	T47.1X5	T47.1X6
Antigonadotrophin NEC	T38.6X1	T38.6X2	T38.6X3	T38.6X4	T38.6X5	T38.6X6
Antihallucinogen	T43.501	T43.502	T43.503	T43.504	T43.505	T43.506
Antihelmintics	T37.4X1	T37.4X2	T37.4X3	T37.4X4	T37.4X5	T37.4X6
Antihemophilic						
factor	T45.8X1	T45.8X2	T45.8X3	T45.8X4	T45.8X5	T45.8X6
fraction	T45.8X1	T45.8X2	T45.8X3	T45.8X4	T45.8X5	T45.8X6

Additional Character May Be Required — Refer to the Tabular List for Character Selection   Subterms under main terms may continue to next column or page

Substance	Poisoning, Accidental (unintentional)	Poisoning, Intentional Self-harm	Poisoning, Assault	Poisoning, Undetermined	Adverse Effect	Under-dosing
Antihemophilic — *continued*						
globulin concentrate	T45.7X1	T45.7X2	T45.7X3	T45.7X4	T45.7X5	T45.7X6
human plasma	T45.8X1	T45.8X2	T45.8X3	T45.8X4	T45.8X5	T45.8X6
plasma, dried	T45.7X1	T45.7X2	T45.7X3	T45.7X4	T45.7X5	T45.7X6
Antihemorrhoidal preparation	T49.2X1	T49.2X2	T49.2X3	T49.2X4	T49.2X5	T49.2X6
Antiheparin drug	T45.7X1	T45.7X2	T45.7X3	T45.7X4	T45.7X5	T45.7X6
Antihistamine	T45.0X1	T45.0X2	T45.0X3	T45.0X4	T45.0X5	T45.0X6
Antihookworm drug	T37.4X1	T37.4X2	T37.4X3	T37.4X4	T37.4X5	T37.4X6
Anti-human lymphocytic globulin	T50.Z11	T50.Z12	T50.Z13	T50.Z14	T50.Z15	T50.Z16
Antihyperlipidemic drug	T46.6X1	T46.6X2	T46.6X3	T46.6X4	T46.6X5	T46.6X6
Antihypertensive drug NEC	T46.5X1	T46.5X2	T46.5X3	T46.5X4	T46.5X5	T46.5X6
Anti-infective NEC	T37.91	T37.92	T37.93	T37.94	T37.95	T37.96
anthelmintic	T37.4X1	T37.4X2	T37.4X3	T37.4X4	T37.4X5	T37.4X6
antibiotics	T36.91	T36.92	T36.93	T36.94	T36.95	T36.96
specified NEC	T36.8X1	T36.8X2	T36.8X3	T36.8X4	T36.8X5	T36.8X6
antimalarial	T37.2X1	T37.2X2	T37.2X3	T37.2X4	T37.2X5	T37.2X6
antimycobacterial NEC	T37.1X1	T37.1X2	T37.1X3	T37.1X4	T37.1X5	T37.1X6
antibiotics	T36.5X1	T36.5X2	T36.5X3	T36.5X4	T36.5X5	T36.5X6
antiprotozoal NEC	T37.3X1	T37.3X2	T37.3X3	T37.3X4	T37.3X5	T37.3X6
blood	T37.2X1	T37.2X2	T37.2X3	T37.2X4	T37.2X5	T37.2X6
antiviral	T37.5X1	T37.5X2	T37.5X3	T37.5X4	T37.5X5	T37.5X6
arsenical	T37.8X1	T37.8X2	T37.8X3	T37.8X4	T37.8X5	T37.8X6
bismuth, local	T49.0X1	T49.0X2	T49.0X3	T49.0X4	T49.0X5	T49.0X6
ENT	T49.6X1	T49.6X2	T49.6X3	T49.6X4	T49.6X5	T49.6X6
eye NEC	T49.5X1	T49.5X2	T49.5X3	T49.5X4	T49.5X5	T49.5X6
heavy metals NEC	T37.8X1	T37.8X2	T37.8X3	T37.8X4	T37.8X5	T37.8X6
local NEC	T49.0X1	T49.0X2	T49.0X3	T49.0X4	T49.0X5	T49.0X6
specified NEC	T49.0X1	T49.0X2	T49.0X3	T49.0X4	T49.0X5	T49.0X6
mixed	T37.91	T37.92	T37.93	T37.94	T37.95	T37.96
ophthalmic preparation	T49.5X1	T49.5X2	T49.5X3	T49.5X4	T49.5X5	T49.5X6
topical NEC	T49.0X1	T49.0X2	T49.0X3	T49.0X4	T49.0X5	T49.0X6
Anti-inflammatory drug NEC	T39.391	T39.392	T39.393	T39.394	T39.395	T39.396
local	T49.0X1	T49.0X2	T49.0X3	T49.0X4	T49.0X5	T49.0X6
nonsteroidal NEC	T39.391	T39.392	T39.393	T39.394	T39.395	T39.396
propionic acid derivative	T39.311	T39.312	T39.313	T39.314	T39.315	T39.316
specified NEC	T39.391	T39.392	T39.393	T39.394	T39.395	T39.396
Antikaluretic	T50.3X1	T50.3X2	T50.3X3	T50.3X4	T50.3X5	T50.3X6
Antiknock (tetraethyl lead)	T56.0X1	T56.0X2	T56.0X3	T56.0X4	—	—
Antilipemic drug NEC	T46.6X1	T46.6X2	T46.6X3	T46.6X4	T46.6X5	T46.6X6
Antimalarial	T37.2X1	T37.2X2	T37.2X3	T37.2X4	T37.2X5	T37.2X6
prophylactic NEC	T37.2X1	T37.2X2	T37.2X3	T37.2X4	T37.2X5	T37.2X6
pyrimidine derivative	T37.2X1	T37.2X2	T37.2X3	T37.2X4	T37.2X5	T37.2X6
Antimetabolite	T45.1X1	T45.1X2	T45.1X3	T45.1X4	T45.1X5	T45.1X6
Antimitotic agent	T45.1X1	T45.1X2	T45.1X3	T45.1X4	T45.1X5	T45.1X6
Antimony (compounds) (vapor) NEC	T56.891	T56.892	T56.893	T56.894	—	—
anti-infectives	T37.8X1	T37.8X2	T37.8X3	T37.8X4	T37.8X5	T37.8X6
dimercaptosuccinate	T37.3X1	T37.3X2	T37.3X3	T37.3X4	T37.3X5	T37.3X6
hydride	T56.891	T56.892	T56.893	T56.894	—	—
pesticide (vapor)	T60.8X1	T60.8X2	T60.8X3	T60.8X4	—	—
potassium (sodium) tartrate	T37.8X1	T37.8X2	T37.8X3	T37.8X4	T37.8X5	T37.8X6
sodium	T37.3X1	T37.3X2	T37.3X3	T37.3X4	T37.3X5	T37.3X6
dimercaptosuccinate						
tartrated	T37.8X1	T37.8X2	T37.8X3	T37.8X4	T37.8X5	T37.8X6
Antimuscarinic NEC	T44.3X1	T44.3X2	T44.3X3	T44.3X4	T44.3X5	T44.3X6
Antimycobacterial drug NEC	T37.1X1	T37.1X2	T37.1X3	T37.1X4	T37.1X5	T37.1X6
antibiotics	T36.5X1	T36.5X2	T36.5X3	T36.5X4	T36.5X5	T36.5X6
combination	T37.1X1	T37.1X2	T37.1X3	T37.1X4	T37.1X5	T37.1X6
Antinausea drug	T45.0X1	T45.0X2	T45.0X3	T45.0X4	T45.0X5	T45.0X6
Antinematode drug	T37.4X1	T37.4X2	T37.4X3	T37.4X4	T37.4X5	T37.4X6
Antineoplastic NEC	T45.1X1	T45.1X2	T45.1X3	T45.1X4	T45.1X5	T45.1X6
alkaloidal	T45.1X1	T45.1X2	T45.1X3	T45.1X4	T45.1X5	T45.1X6
antibiotics	T45.1X1	T45.1X2	T45.1X3	T45.1X4	T45.1X5	T45.1X6
combination	T45.1X1	T45.1X2	T45.1X3	T45.1X4	T45.1X5	T45.1X6
estrogen	T38.5X1	T38.5X2	T38.5X3	T38.5X4	T38.5X5	T38.5X6
steroid	T38.7X1	T38.7X2	T38.7X3	T38.7X4	T38.7X5	T38.7X6
Antiparasitic drug (systemic)	T37.91	T37.92	T37.93	T37.94	T37.95	T37.96
local	T49.0X1	T49.0X2	T49.0X3	T49.0X4	T49.0X5	T49.0X6
specified NEC	T37.8X1	T37.8X2	T37.8X3	T37.8X4	T37.8X5	T37.8X6
Antiparkinsonism drug NEC	T42.8X1	T42.8X2	T42.8X3	T42.8X4	T42.8X5	T42.8X6
Antiperspirant NEC	T49.2X1	T49.2X2	T49.2X3	T49.2X4	T49.2X5	T49.2X6
Antiphlogistic NEC	T39.4X1	T39.4X2	T39.4X3	T39.4X4	T39.4X5	T39.4X6
Antiplatyhelmintic drug	T37.4X1	T37.4X2	T37.4X3	T37.4X4	T37.4X5	T37.4X6
Antiprotozoal drug NEC	T37.3X1	T37.3X2	T37.3X3	T37.3X4	T37.3X5	T37.3X6
blood	T37.2X1	T37.2X2	T37.2X3	T37.2X4	T37.2X5	T37.2X6
local	T49.0X1	T49.0X2	T49.0X3	T49.0X4	T49.0X5	T49.0X6

Substance	Poisoning, Accidental (unintentional)	Poisoning, Intentional Self-harm	Poisoning, Assault	Poisoning, Undetermined	Adverse Effect	Under-dosing
Antipruritic drug NEC	T49.1X1	T49.1X2	T49.1X3	T49.1X4	T49.1X5	T49.1X6
Antipsychotic drug	T43.501	T43.502	T43.503	T43.504	T43.505	T43.506
specified NEC	T43.591	T43.592	T43.593	T43.594	T43.595	T43.596
Antipyretic	T39.91	T39.92	T39.93	T39.94	T39.95	T39.96
specified NEC	T39.8X1	T39.8X2	T39.8X3	T39.8X4	T39.8X5	T39.8X6
Antipyrine	T39.2X1	T39.2X2	T39.2X3	T39.2X4	T39.2X5	T39.2X6
Antirabies hyperimmune serum	T50.Z11	T50.Z12	T50.Z13	T50.Z14	T50.Z15	T50.Z16
Antirheumatic NEC	T39.4X1	T39.4X2	T39.4X3	T39.4X4	T39.4X5	T39.4X6
Antirigidity drug NEC	T42.8X1	T42.8X2	T42.8X3	T42.8X4	T42.8X5	T42.8X6
Antischistosomal drug	T37.4X1	T37.4X2	T37.4X3	T37.4X4	T37.4X5	T37.4X6
Antiscorpion sera	T50.Z11	T50.Z12	T50.Z13	T50.Z14	T50.Z15	T50.Z16
Antiseborrheics	T49.4X1	T49.4X2	T49.4X3	T49.4X4	T49.4X5	T49.4X6
Antiseptics (external) (medicinal)	T49.0X1	T49.0X2	T49.0X3	T49.0X4	T49.0X5	T49.0X6
Antistine	T45.0X1	T45.0X2	T45.0X3	T45.0X4	T45.0X5	T45.0X6
Antitapeworm drug	T37.4X1	T37.4X2	T37.4X3	T37.4X4	T37.4X5	T37.4X6
Antitetanus immunoglobulin	T50.Z11	T50.Z12	T50.Z13	T50.Z14	T50.Z15	T50.Z16
Antithrombotic	T45.521	T45.522	T45.523	T45.524	T45.525	T45.526
Antithyroid drug NEC	T38.2X1	T38.2X2	T38.2X3	T38.2X4	T38.2X5	T38.2X6
Antitoxin	T50.Z11	T50.Z12	T50.Z13	T50.Z14	T50.Z15	T50.Z16
diphtheria	T50.Z11	T50.Z12	T50.Z13	T50.Z14	T50.Z15	T50.Z16
gas gangrene	T50.Z11	T50.Z12	T50.Z13	T50.Z14	T50.Z15	T50.Z16
tetanus	T50.Z11	T50.Z12	T50.Z13	T50.Z14	T50.Z15	T50.Z16
Antitrichomonal drug	T37.3X1	T37.3X2	T37.3X3	T37.3X4	T37.3X5	T37.3X6
Antituberculars	T37.1X1	T37.1X2	T37.1X3	T37.1X4	T37.1X5	T37.1X6
antibiotics	T36.5X1	T36.5X2	T36.5X3	T36.5X4	T36.5X5	T36.5X6
Antitussive NEC	T48.3X1	T48.3X2	T48.3X3	T48.3X4	T48.3X5	T48.3X6
codeine mixture	T40.2X1	T40.2X2	T40.2X3	T40.2X4	T40.2X5	T40.2X6
opiate	T40.2X1	T40.2X2	T40.2X3	T40.2X4	T40.2X5	T40.2X6
Antivaricose drug	T46.8X1	T46.8X2	T46.8X3	T46.8X4	T46.8X5	T46.8X6
Antivenin, antivenom (sera)	T50.Z11	T50.Z12	T50.Z13	T50.Z14	T50.Z15	T50.Z16
crotaline	T50.Z11	T50.Z12	T50.Z13	T50.Z14	T50.Z15	T50.Z16
spider bite	T50.Z11	T50.Z12	T50.Z13	T50.Z14	T50.Z15	T50.Z16
Antivertigo drug	T45.0X1	T45.0X2	T45.0X3	T45.0X4	T45.0X5	T45.0X6
Antiviral drug NEC	T37.5X1	T37.5X2	T37.5X3	T37.5X4	T37.5X5	T37.5X6
eye	T49.5X1	T49.5X2	T49.5X3	T49.5X4	T49.5X5	T49.5X6
Antiwhipworm drug	T37.4X1	T37.4X2	T37.4X3	T37.4X4	T37.4X5	T37.4X6
Ant poison — *see also* by specific chemical substance	T60.91	T60.92	T60.93	T60.94	—	—
Antrol — *see also* by specific chemical substance	T60.91	T60.92	T60.93	T60.94	—	—
fungicide	T60.91	T60.92	T60.93	T60.94	—	—
ANTU (alpha naphthylthiourea)	T60.4X1	T60.4X2	T60.4X3	T60.4X4	—	—
Apalcillin	T36.0X1	T36.0X2	T36.0X3	T36.0X4	T36.0X5	T36.0X6
APC	T48.5X1	T48.5X2	T48.5X3	T48.5X4	T48.5X5	T48.5X6
Aplonidine	T44.4X1	T44.4X2	T44.4X3	T44.4X4	T44.4X5	T44.4X6
Apomorphine	T47.7X1	T47.7X2	T47.7X3	T47.7X4	T47.7X5	T47.7X6
Appetite depressants, central	T50.5X1	T50.5X2	T50.5X3	T50.5X4	T50.5X5	T50.5X6
Apraclonidine (hydrochloride)	T44.4X1	T44.4X2	T44.4X3	T44.4X4	T44.4X5	T44.4X6
Apresoline	T46.5X1	T46.5X2	T46.5X3	T46.5X4	T46.5X5	T46.5X6
Aprindine	T46.2X1	T46.2X2	T46.2X3	T46.2X4	T46.2X5	T46.2X6
Aprobarbital	T42.3X1	T42.3X2	T42.3X3	T42.3X4	T42.3X5	T42.3X6
Apronalide	T42.6X1	T42.6X2	T42.6X3	T42.6X4	T42.6X5	T42.6X6
Aprotinin	T45.621	T45.622	T45.623	T45.624	T45.625	T45.626
Aptocaine	T41.3X1	T41.3X2	T41.3X3	T41.3X4	T41.3X5	T41.3X6
Aqua fortis	T54.2X1	T54.2X2	T54.2X3	T54.2X4	—	—
Ara-A	T37.5X1	T37.5X2	T37.5X3	T37.5X4	T37.5X5	T37.5X6
Ara-C	T45.1X1	T45.1X2	T45.1X3	T45.1X4	T45.1X5	T45.1X6
Arachis oil	T49.3X1	T49.3X2	T49.3X3	T49.3X4	T49.3X5	T49.3X6
cathartic	T47.4X1	T47.4X2	T47.4X3	T47.4X4	T47.4X5	T47.4X6
Aralen	T37.2X1	T37.2X2	T37.2X3	T37.2X4	T37.2X5	T37.2X6
Arecoline	T44.1X1	T44.1X2	T44.1X3	T44.1X4	T44.1X5	T44.1X6
Arginine	T50.991	T50.992	T50.993	T50.994	T50.995	T50.996
glutamate	T50.991	T50.992	T50.993	T50.994	T50.995	T50.996
Argyrol	T49.0X1	T49.0X2	T49.0X3	T49.0X4	T49.0X5	T49.0X6
ENT agent	T49.6X1	T49.6X2	T49.6X3	T49.6X4	T49.6X5	T49.6X6
ophthalmic preparation	T49.5X1	T49.5X2	T49.5X3	T49.5X4	T49.5X5	T49.5X6
Aristocort	T38.0X1	T38.0X2	T38.0X3	T38.0X4	T38.0X5	T38.0X6
ENT agent	T49.6X1	T49.6X2	T49.6X3	T49.6X4	T49.6X5	T49.6X6
ophthalmic preparation	T49.5X1	T49.5X2	T49.5X3	T49.5X4	T49.5X5	T49.5X6
topical NEC	T49.0X1	T49.0X2	T49.0X3	T49.0X4	T49.0X5	T49.0X6
Aromatics, corrosive	T54.1X1	T54.1X2	T54.1X3	T54.1X4	—	—
disinfectants	T54.1X1	T54.1X2	T54.1X3	T54.1X4	—	—
Arsenate of lead	T57.0X1	T57.0X2	T57.0X3	T57.0X4	—	—
herbicide	T57.0X1	T57.0X2	T57.0X3	T57.0X4	—	—
Arsenic, arsenicals (compounds) (dust) (vapor) NEC	T57.0X1	T57.0X2	T57.0X3	T57.0X4	—	—
anti-infectives	T37.8X1	T37.8X2	T37.8X3	T37.8X4	T37.8X5	T37.8X6
pesticide (dust) (fumes)	T57.0X1	T57.0X2	T57.0X3	T57.0X4	—	—

Table of Drugs and Chemicals

Substance	Poisoning, Accidental (unintentional)	Poisoning, Intentional Self-harm	Poisoning, Assault	Poisoning, Undetermined	Adverse Effect	Under-dosing
Arsine (gas)	T57.0X1	T57.0X2	T57.0X3	T57.0X4	—	—
Arsphenamine (silver)	T37.8X1	T37.8X2	T37.8X3	T37.8X4	T37.8X5	T37.8X6
Arsthinol	T37.3X1	T37.3X2	T37.3X3	T37.3X4	T37.3X5	T37.3X6
Artane	T44.3X1	T44.3X2	T44.3X3	T44.3X4	T44.3X5	T44.3X6
Arthropod (venomous) **NEC**	T63.481	T63.482	T63.483	T63.484	—	—
Articaine	T41.3X1	T41.3X2	T41.3X3	T41.3X4	T41.3X5	T41.3X6
Asbestos	T57.8X1	T57.8X2	T57.8X3	T57.8X4	—	—
Ascaridole	T37.4X1	T37.4X2	T37.4X3	T37.4X4	T37.4X5	T37.4X6
Ascorbic acid	T45.2X1	T45.2X2	T45.2X3	T45.2X4	T45.2X5	T45.2X6
Asiaticoside	T49.0X1	T49.0X2	T49.0X3	T49.0X4	T49.0X5	T49.0X6
Asparaginase	T45.1X1	T45.1X2	T45.1X3	T45.1X4	T45.1X5	T45.1X6
Aspidium (oleoresin)	T37.4X1	T37.4X2	T37.4X3	T37.4X4	T37.4X5	T37.4X6
Aspirin (aluminum) (soluble)	T39.011	T39.012	T39.013	T39.014	T39.015	T39.016
Aspoxicillin	T36.0X1	T36.0X2	T36.0X3	T36.0X4	T36.0X5	T36.0X6
Astemizole	T45.0X1	T45.0X2	T45.0X3	T45.0X4	T45.0X5	T45.0X6
Astringent (local)	T49.2X1	T49.2X2	T49.2X3	T49.2X4	T49.2X5	T49.2X6
specified NEC	T49.2X1	T49.2X2	T49.2X3	T49.2X4	T49.2X5	T49.2X6
Astromicin	T36.5X1	T36.5X2	T36.5X3	T36.5X4	T36.5X5	T36.5X6
Ataractic drug NEC	T43.501	T43.502	T43.503	T43.504	T43.505	T43.506
Atenolol	T44.7X1	T44.7X2	T44.7X3	T44.7X4	T44.7X5	T44.7X6
Atonia drug, intestinal	T47.4X1	T47.4X2	T47.4X3	T47.4X4	T47.4X5	T47.4X6
Atophan	T50.4X1	T50.4X2	T50.4X3	T50.4X4	T50.4X5	T50.4X6
Atracurium besilate	T48.1X1	T48.1X2	T48.1X3	T48.1X4	T48.1X5	T48.1X6
Atropine	T44.3X1	T44.3X2	T44.3X3	T44.3X4	T44.3X5	T44.3X6
derivative	T44.3X1	T44.3X2	T44.3X3	T44.3X4	T44.3X5	T44.3X6
methonitrate	T44.3X1	T44.3X2	T44.3X3	T44.3X4	T44.3X5	T44.3X6
Attapulgite	T47.6X1	T47.6X2	T47.6X3	T47.6X4	T47.6X5	T47.6X6
Auramine	T65.891	T65.892	T65.893	T65.894	—	—
dye	T65.6X1	T65.6X2	T65.6X3	T65.6X4	—	—
fungicide	T60.3X1	T60.3X2	T60.3X3	T60.3X4	—	—
Auranofin	T39.4X1	T39.4X2	T39.4X3	T39.4X4	T39.4X5	T39.4X6
Aurantiin	T46.991	T46.992	T46.993	T46.994	T46.995	T46.996
Aureomycin	T36.4X1	T36.4X2	T36.4X3	T36.4X4	T36.4X5	T36.4X6
ophthalmic preparation	T49.5X1	T49.5X2	T49.5X3	T49.5X4	T49.5X5	T49.5X6
topical NEC	T49.0X1	T49.0X2	T49.0X3	T49.0X4	T49.0X5	T49.0X6
Aurothioglucose	T39.4X1	T39.4X2	T39.4X3	T39.4X4	T39.4X5	T39.4X6
Aurothioglycanide	T39.4X1	T39.4X2	T39.4X3	T39.4X4	T39.4X5	T39.4X6
Aurothiomalate sodium	T39.4X1	T39.4X2	T39.4X3	T39.4X4	T39.4X5	T39.4X6
Aurotioprol	T39.4X1	T39.4X2	T39.4X3	T39.4X4	T39.4X5	T39.4X6
Automobile fuel	T52.0X1	T52.0X2	T52.0X3	T52.0X4	—	—
Autonomic nervous system agent NEC	T44.901	T44.902	T44.903	T44.904	T44.905	T44.906
Avlosulfon	T37.1X1	T37.1X2	T37.1X3	T37.1X4	T37.1X5	T37.1X6
Avomine	T42.6X1	T42.6X2	T42.6X3	T42.6X4	T42.6X5	T42.6X6
Axerophthol	T45.2X1	T45.2X2	T45.2X3	T45.2X4	T45.2X5	T45.2X6
Azacitidine	T45.1X1	T45.1X2	T45.1X3	T45.1X4	T45.1X5	T45.1X6
Azacyclonol	T43.591	T43.592	T43.593	T43.594	T43.595	T43.596
Azadirachta	T60.2X1	T60.2X2	T60.2X3	T60.2X4	—	—
Azanidazole	T37.3X1	T37.3X2	T37.3X3	T37.3X4	T37.3X5	T37.3X6
Azapetine	T46.7X1	T46.7X2	T46.7X3	T46.7X4	T46.7X5	T46.7X6
Azapropazone	T39.2X1	T39.2X2	T39.2X3	T39.2X4	T39.2X5	T39.2X6
Azaribine	T45.1X1	T45.1X2	T45.1X3	T45.1X4	T45.1X5	T45.1X6
Azaserine	T45.1X1	T45.1X2	T45.1X3	T45.1X4	T45.1X5	T45.1X6
Azatadine	T45.0X1	T45.0X2	T45.0X3	T45.0X4	T45.0X5	T45.0X6
Azatepa	T45.1X1	T45.1X2	T45.1X3	T45.1X4	T45.1X5	T45.1X6
Azathioprine	T45.1X1	T45.1X2	T45.1X3	T45.1X4	T45.1X5	T45.1X6
Azelaic acid	T49.0X1	T49.0X2	T49.0X3	T49.0X4	T49.0X5	T49.0X6
Azelastine	T45.0X1	T45.0X2	T45.0X3	T45.0X4	T45.0X5	T45.0X6
Azidocillin	T36.0X1	T36.0X2	T36.0X3	T36.0X4	T36.0X5	T36.0X6
Azidothymidine	T37.5X1	T37.5X2	T37.5X3	T37.5X4	T37.5X5	T37.5X6
Azinphos (ethyl) (methyl)	T60.0X1	T60.0X2	T60.0X3	T60.0X4	—	—
Aziridine (chelating)	T54.1X1	T54.1X2	T54.1X3	T54.1X4	—	—
Azithromycin	T36.3X1	T36.3X2	T36.3X3	T36.3X4	T36.3X5	T36.3X6
Azlocillin	T36.0X1	T36.0X2	T36.0X3	T36.0X4	T36.0X5	T36.0X6
Azobenzene smoke	T65.3X1	T65.3X2	T65.3X3	T65.3X4	—	—
acaricide	T60.8X1	T60.8X2	T60.8X3	T60.8X4	—	—
Azosulfamide	T37.0X1	T37.0X2	T37.0X3	T37.0X4	T37.0X5	T37.0X6
AZT	T37.5X1	T37.5X2	T37.5X3	T37.5X4	T37.5X5	T37.5X6
Aztreonam	T36.1X1	T36.1X2	T36.1X3	T36.1X4	T36.1X5	T36.1X6
Azulfidine	T37.0X1	T37.0X2	T37.0X3	T37.0X4	T37.0X5	T37.0X6
Azuresin	T50.8X1	T50.8X2	T50.8X3	T50.8X4	T50.8X5	T50.8X6
b-acetyldigoxin	T46.0X1	T46.0X2	T46.0X3	T46.0X4	T46.0X5	T46.0X6
P-Acetamidophenol	T39.1X1	T39.1X2	T39.1X3	T39.1X4	T39.1X5	T39.1X6
Bacampicillin	T36.0X1	T36.0X2	T36.0X3	T36.0X4	T36.0X5	T36.0X6
Bacillus						
lactobacillus	T47.8X1	T47.8X2	T47.8X3	T47.8X4	T47.8X5	T47.8X6
subtilis	T47.6X1	T47.6X2	T47.6X3	T47.6X4	T47.6X5	T47.6X6
Bacimycin	T49.0X1	T49.0X2	T49.0X3	T49.0X4	T49.0X5	T49.0X6
ophthalmic preparation	T49.5X1	T49.5X2	T49.5X3	T49.5X4	T49.5X5	T49.5X6
Bacitracin zinc	T49.0X1	T49.0X2	T49.0X3	T49.0X4	T49.0X5	T49.0X6
with neomycin	T49.0X1	T49.0X2	T49.0X3	T49.0X4	T49.0X5	T49.0X6
ENT agent	T49.6X1	T49.6X2	T49.6X3	T49.6X4	T49.6X5	T49.6X6
ophthalmic preparation	T49.5X1	T49.5X2	T49.5X3	T49.5X4	T49.5X5	T49.5X6

Substance	Poisoning, Accidental (unintentional)	Poisoning, Intentional Self-harm	Poisoning, Assault	Poisoning, Undetermined	Adverse Effect	Under-dosing
Bacitracin zinc — continued						
topical NEC	T49.0X1	T49.0X2	T49.0X3	T49.0X4	T49.0X5	T49.0X6
Baclofen	T42.8X1	T42.8X2	T42.8X3	T42.8X4	T42.8X5	T42.8X6
Baking soda	T50.991	T50.992	T50.993	T50.994	T50.995	T50.996
BAL	T45.8X1	T45.8X2	T45.8X3	T45.8X4	T45.8X5	T45.8X6
Bambuterol	T48.6X1	T48.6X2	T48.6X3	T48.6X4	T48.6X5	T48.6X6
Bamethan (sulfate)	T46.7X1	T46.7X2	T46.7X3	T46.7X4	T46.7X5	T46.7X6
Bamifylline	T48.6X1	T48.6X2	T48.6X3	T48.6X4	T48.6X5	T48.6X6
Bamipine	T45.0X1	T45.0X2	T45.0X3	T45.0X4	T45.0X5	T45.0X6
Baneberry — see Actaea spicata						
Banewort — see Belladonna						
Barbenyl	T42.3X1	T42.3X2	T42.3X3	T42.3X4	T42.3X5	T42.3X6
Barbexaclone	T42.6X1	T42.6X2	T42.6X3	T42.6X4	T42.6X5	T42.6X6
Barbital	T42.3X1	T42.3X2	T42.3X3	T42.3X4	T42.3X5	T42.3X6
sodium	T42.3X1	T42.3X2	T42.3X3	T42.3X4	T42.3X5	T42.3X6
Barbitone	T42.3X1	T42.3X2	T42.3X3	T42.3X4	T42.3X5	T42.3X6
Barbiturate NEC	T42.3X1	T42.3X2	T42.3X3	T42.3X4	T42.3X5	T42.3X6
with tranquilizer	T42.3X1	T42.3X2	T42.3X3	T42.3X4	T42.3X5	T42.3X6
anesthetic (intravenous)	T41.1X1	T41.1X2	T41.1X3	T41.1X4	T41.1X5	T41.1X6
Barium (carbonate) (chloride)	T57.8X1	T57.8X2	T57.8X3	T57.8X4	—	—
(sulfite)						
diagnostic agent	T50.8X1	T50.8X2	T50.8X3	T50.8X4	T50.8X5	T50.8X6
pesticide	T60.4X1	T60.4X2	T60.4X3	T60.4X4	—	—
rodenticide	T60.4X1	T60.4X2	T60.4X3	T60.4X4	—	—
sulfate (medicinal)	T50.8X1	T50.8X2	T50.8X3	T50.8X4	T50.8X5	T50.8X6
Barrier cream	T49.3X1	T49.3X2	T49.3X3	T49.3X4	T49.3X5	T49.3X6
Basic fuchsin	T49.0X1	T49.0X2	T49.0X3	T49.0X4	T49.0X5	T49.0X6
Battery acid or fluid	T54.2X1	T54.2X2	T54.2X3	T54.2X4	—	—
Bay rum	T51.8X1	T51.8X2	T51.8X3	T51.8X4	—	—
b-benzalbutyramide	T46.6X1	T46.6X2	T46.6X3	T46.6X4	T46.6X5	T46.6X6
BCG (vaccine)	T50.A91	T50.A92	T50.A93	T50.A94	T50.A95	T50.A96
BCNU	T45.1X1	T45.1X2	T45.1X3	T45.1X4	T45.1X5	T45.1X6
Bearsfoot	T62.2X1	T62.2X2	T62.2X3	T62.2X4	—	—
Beclamide	T42.6X1	T42.6X2	T42.6X3	T42.6X4	T42.6X5	T42.6X6
Beclomethasone	T44.5X1	T44.5X2	T44.5X3	T44.5X4	T44.5X5	T44.5X6
Bee (sting) (venom)	T63.441	T63.442	T63.443	T63.444	—	—
Befunolol	T49.5X1	T49.5X2	T49.5X3	T49.5X4	T49.5X5	T49.5X6
Bekanamycin	T36.5X1	T36.5X2	T36.5X3	T36.5X4	T36.5X5	T36.5X6
Belladonna — see also						
Nightshade						
alkaloids	T44.3X1	T44.3X2	T44.3X3	T44.3X4	T44.3X5	T44.3X6
extract	T44.3X1	T44.3X2	T44.3X3	T44.3X4	T44.3X5	T44.3X6
herb	T44.3X1	T44.3X2	T44.3X3	T44.3X4	T44.3X5	T44.3X6
Bemegride	T50.7X1	T50.7X2	T50.7X3	T50.7X4	T50.7X5	T50.7X6
Benactyzine	T44.3X1	T44.3X2	T44.3X3	T44.3X4	T44.3X5	T44.3X6
Benadryl	T45.0X1	T45.0X2	T45.0X3	T45.0X4	T45.0X5	T45.0X6
Benaprizine	T44.3X1	T44.3X2	T44.3X3	T44.3X4	T44.3X5	T44.3X6
Benazepril	T46.4X1	T46.4X2	T46.4X3	T46.4X4	T46.4X5	T46.4X6
Bencyclane	T46.7X1	T46.7X2	T46.7X3	T46.7X4	T46.7X5	T46.7X6
Bendazol	T46.3X1	T46.3X2	T46.3X3	T46.3X4	T46.3X5	T46.3X6
Bendrofluazide	T50.2X1	T50.2X2	T50.2X3	T50.2X4	T50.2X5	T50.2X6
Bendroflumethiazide	T50.2X1	T50.2X2	T50.2X3	T50.2X4	T50.2X5	T50.2X6
Benemid	T50.4X1	T50.4X2	T50.4X3	T50.4X4	T50.4X5	T50.4X6
Benethamine penicillin	T36.0X1	T36.0X2	T36.0X3	T36.0X4	T36.0X5	T36.0X6
Benexate	T47.1X1	T47.1X2	T47.1X3	T47.1X4	T47.1X5	T47.1X6
Benfluorex	T46.6X1	T46.6X2	T46.6X3	T46.6X4	T46.6X5	T46.6X6
Benfotiamine	T45.2X1	T45.2X2	T45.2X3	T45.2X4	T45.2X5	T45.2X6
Benisone	T49.0X1	T49.0X2	T49.0X3	T49.0X4	T49.0X5	T49.0X6
Benomyl	T60.0X1	T60.0X2	T60.0X3	T60.0X4	—	—
Benoquin	T49.8X1	T49.8X2	T49.8X3	T49.8X4	T49.8X5	T49.8X6
Benoxinate	T41.3X1	T41.3X2	T41.3X3	T41.3X4	T41.3X5	T41.3X6
Benperidol	T43.4X1	T43.4X2	T43.4X3	T43.4X4	T43.4X5	T43.4X6
Benproperine	T48.3X1	T48.3X2	T48.3X3	T48.3X4	T48.3X5	T48.3X6
Benserazide	T42.8X1	T42.8X2	T42.8X3	T42.8X4	T42.8X5	T42.8X6
Bentazepam	T42.4X1	T42.4X2	T42.4X3	T42.4X4	T42.4X5	T42.4X6
Bentiromide	T50.8X1	T50.8X2	T50.8X3	T50.8X4	T50.8X5	T50.8X6
Bentonite	T49.3X1	T49.3X2	T49.3X3	T49.3X4	T49.3X5	T49.3X6
Benzalbutyramide	T46.6X1	T46.6X2	T46.6X3	T46.6X4	T46.6X5	T46.6X6
Benzalkonium (chloride)	T49.0X1	T49.0X2	T49.0X3	T49.0X4	T49.0X5	T49.0X6
ophthalmic preparation	T49.5X1	T49.5X2	T49.5X3	T49.5X4	T49.5X5	T49.5X6
Benzamidosalicylate (calcium)	T37.1X1	T37.1X2	T37.1X3	T37.1X4	T37.1X5	T37.1X6
Benzamine	T41.3X1	T41.3X2	T41.3X3	T41.3X4	T41.3X5	T41.3X6
lactate	T49.1X1	T49.1X2	T49.1X3	T49.1X4	T49.1X5	T49.1X6
Benzamphetamine	T50.5X1	T50.5X2	T50.5X3	T50.5X4	T50.5X5	T50.5X6
Benzapril hydrochloride	T46.5X1	T46.5X2	T46.5X3	T46.5X4	T46.5X5	T46.5X6
Benzathine	T36.0X1	T36.0X2	T36.0X3	T36.0X4	T36.0X5	T36.0X6
benzylpenicillin						
Benzathine penicillin	T36.0X1	T36.0X2	T36.0X3	T36.0X4	T36.0X5	T36.0X6
Benzatropine	T42.8X1	T42.8X2	T42.8X3	T42.8X4	T42.8X5	T42.8X6
Benzbromarone	T50.4X1	T50.4X2	T50.4X3	T50.4X4	T50.4X5	T50.4X6
Benzcarbimine	T45.1X1	T45.1X2	T45.1X3	T45.1X4	T45.1X5	T45.1X6
Benzedrex	T44.991	T44.992	T44.993	T44.994	T44.995	T44.996

Additional Character May Be Required — Refer to the Tabular List for Character Selection ▽ **Subterms under main terms may continue to next column or page**

Substance	Poisoning, Accidental (unintentional)	Poisoning, Intentional Self-harm	Poisoning, Assault	Poisoning, Undetermined	Adverse Effect	Under-dosing
Benzedrine (amphetamine)	T43.621	T43.622	T43.623	T43.624	T43.625	T43.626
Benzenamine	T65.3X1	T65.3X2	T65.3X3	T65.3X4	—	—
Benzene	T52.1X1	T52.1X2	T52.1X3	T52.1X4	—	—
homologues (acetyl) (dimethyl) (methyl) (solvent)	T52.2X1	T52.2X2	T52.2X3	T52.2X4	—	—
Benzethonium (chloride)	T49.0X1	T49.0X2	T49.0X3	T49.0X4	T49.0X5	T49.0X6
Benzfetamine	T50.5X1	T50.5X2	T50.5X3	T50.5X4	T50.5X5	T50.5X6
Benzhexol	T44.3X1	T44.3X2	T44.3X3	T44.3X4	T44.3X5	T44.3X6
Benzhydramine (chloride)	T45.0X1	T45.0X2	T45.0X3	T45.0X4	T45.0X5	T45.0X6
Benzidine	T65.891	T65.892	T65.893	T65.894		
Benzilonium bromide	T44.3X1	T44.3X2	T44.3X3	T44.3X4	T44.3X5	T44.3X6
Benzimidazole	T60.3X1	T60.3X2	T60.3X3	T60.3X4		
Benzin (e) — see Ligroin						
Benziodarone	T46.3X1	T46.3X2	T46.3X3	T46.3X4	T46.3X5	T46.3X6
Benznidazole	T37.3X1	T37.3X2	T37.3X3	T37.3X4	T37.3X5	T37.3X6
Benzocaine	T41.3X1	T41.3X2	T41.3X3	T41.3X4	T41.3X5	T41.3X6
Benzodiapin	T42.4X1	T42.4X2	T42.4X3	T42.4X4	T42.4X5	T42.4X6
Benzodiazepine NEC	T42.4X1	T42.4X2	T42.4X3	T42.4X4	T42.4X5	T42.4X6
Benzoic acid	T49.0X1	T49.0X2	T49.0X3	T49.0X4	T49.0X5	T49.0X6
with salicylic acid	T49.0X1	T49.0X2	T49.0X3	T49.0X4	T49.0X5	T49.0X6
Benzoin (tincture)	T48.5X1	T48.5X2	T48.5X3	T48.5X4	T48.5X5	T48.5X6
Benzol (benzene)	T52.1X1	T52.1X2	T52.1X3	T52.1X4	—	—
vapor	T52.0X1	T52.0X2	T52.0X3	T52.0X4	—	—
Benzomorphan	T40.2X1	T40.2X2	T40.2X3	T40.2X4	T40.2X5	T40.2X6
Benzonatate	T48.3X1	T48.3X2	T48.3X3	T48.3X4	T48.3X5	T48.3X6
Benzophenones	T49.3X1	T49.3X2	T49.3X3	T49.3X4	T49.3X5	T49.3X6
Benzopyrone	T46.991	T46.992	T46.993	T46.994	T46.995	T46.996
Benzothiadiazides	T50.2X1	T50.2X2	T50.2X3	T50.2X4	T50.2X5	T50.2X6
Benzoxonium chloride	T49.0X1	T49.0X2	T49.0X3	T49.0X4	T49.0X5	T49.0X6
Benzoylpas calcium	T37.1X1	T37.1X2	T37.1X3	T37.1X4	T37.1X5	T37.1X6
Benzoyl peroxide	T49.0X1	T49.0X2	T49.0X3	T49.0X4	T49.0X5	T49.0X6
Benzperidin	T43.591	T43.592	T43.593	T43.594	T43.595	T43.596
Benzperidol	T43.591	T43.592	T43.593	T43.594	T43.595	T43.596
Benzphetamine	T50.5X1	T50.5X2	T50.5X3	T50.5X4	T50.5X5	T50.5X6
Benzpyrinium bromide	T44.1X1	T44.1X2	T44.1X3	T44.1X4	T44.1X5	T44.1X6
Benzquinamide	T45.0X1	T45.0X2	T45.0X3	T45.0X4	T45.0X5	T45.0X6
Benzthiazide	T50.2X1	T50.2X2	T50.2X3	T50.2X4	T50.2X5	T50.2X6
Benztropine						
anticholinergic	T44.3X1	T44.3X2	T44.3X3	T44.3X4	T44.3X5	T44.3X6
antiparkinson	T42.8X1	T42.8X2	T42.8X3	T42.8X4	T42.8X5	T42.8X6
Benzydamine	T49.0X1	T49.0X2	T49.0X3	T49.0X4	T49.0X5	T49.0X6
Benzyl						
acetate	T52.8X1	T52.8X2	T52.8X3	T52.8X4	—	—
alcohol	T49.0X1	T49.0X2	T49.0X3	T49.0X4	T49.0X5	T49.0X6
benzoate	T49.0X1	T49.0X2	T49.0X3	T49.0X4	T49.0X5	T49.0X6
Benzoic acid	T49.0X1	T49.0X2	T49.0X3	T49.0X4	T49.0X5	T49.0X6
morphine	T40.2X1	T40.2X2	T40.2X3	T40.2X4	—	—
nicotinate	T46.6X1	T46.6X2	T46.6X3	T46.6X4	T46.6X5	T46.6X6
penicillin	T36.0X1	T36.0X2	T36.0X3	T36.0X4	T36.0X5	T36.0X6
BenzylhydrochlorthiazIde	T50.2X1	T50.2X2	T50.2X3	T50.2X4	T50.2X5	T50.2X6
Benzylpenicillin	T36.0X1	T36.0X2	T36.0X3	T36.0X4	T36.0X5	T36.0X6
Benzylthiouracil	T38.2X1	T38.2X2	T38.2X3	T38.2X4	T38.2X5	T38.2X6
Bephenium hydroxynaphthoate	T37.4X1	T37.4X2	T37.4X3	T37.4X4	T37.4X5	T37.4X6
Bepridil	T46.1X1	T46.1X2	T46.1X3	T46.1X4	T46.1X5	T46.1X6
Bergamot oil	T65.891	T65.892	T65.893	T65.894	—	—
Bergapten	T50.991	T50.992	T50.993	T50.994	T50.995	T50.996
Berries, poisonous	T62.1X1	T62.1X2	T62.1X3	T62.1X4	—	—
Beryllium (compounds)	T56.7X1	T56.7X2	T56.7X3	T56.7X4	—	—
beta adrenergic blocking agent, heart	T44.7X1	T44.7X2	T44.7X3	T44.7X4	T44.7X5	T44.7X6
Betacarotene	T45.2X1	T45.2X2	T45.2X3	T45.2X4	T45.2X5	T45.2X6
Beta-Chlor	T42.6X1	T42.6X2	T42.6X3	T42.6X4	T42.6X5	T42.6X6
Betahistine	T46.7X1	T46.7X2	T46.7X3	T46.7X4	T46.7X5	T46.7X6
Betaine	T47.5X1	T47.5X2	T47.5X3	T47.5X4	T47.5X5	T47.5X6
Betamethasone	T49.0X1	T49.0X2	T49.0X3	T49.0X4	T49.0X5	T49.0X6
topical	T49.0X1	T49.0X2	T49.0X3	T49.0X4	T49.0X5	T49.0X6
Betamicin	T36.8X1	T36.8X2	T36.8X3	T36.8X4	T36.8X5	T36.8X6
Betanidine	T46.5X1	T46.5X2	T46.5X3	T46.5X4	T46.5X5	T46.5X6
Betaxolol	T44.7X1	T44.7X2	T44.7X3	T44.7X4	T44.7X5	T44.7X6
Betazole	T50.8X1	T50.8X2	T50.8X3	T50.8X4	T50.8X5	T50.8X6
Bethanechol	T44.1X1	T44.1X2	T44.1X3	T44.1X4	T44.1X5	T44.1X6
chloride	T44.1X1	T44.1X2	T44.1X3	T44.1X4	T44.1X5	T44.1X6
Bethanidine	T46.5X1	T46.5X2	T46.5X3	T46.5X4	T46.5X5	T46.5X6
Betoxycaine	T41.3X1	T41.3X2	T41.3X3	T41.3X4	T41.3X5	T41.3X6
Betula oil	T49.3X1	T49.3X2	T49.3X3	T49.3X4	T49.3X5	T49.3X6
Bevantolol	T44.7X1	T44.7X2	T44.7X3	T44.7X4	T44.7X5	T44.7X6
Bevonium metilsulfate	T44.3X1	T44.3X2	T44.3X3	T44.3X4	T44.3X5	T44.3X6
Bezafibrate	T46.6X1	T46.6X2	T46.6X3	T46.6X4	T46.6X5	T46.6X6
Bezitramide	T40.4X1	T40.4X2	T40.4X3	T40.4X4	T40.4X5	T40.4X6
BHA	T50.991	T50.992	T50.993	T50.994	T50.995	T50.996
Bhang	T40.7X1	T40.7X2	T40.7X3	T40.7X4	T40.7X5	T40.7X6
BHC (medicinal)	T49.0X1	T49.0X2	T49.0X3	T49.0X4	T49.0X5	T49.0X6
BHC — continued						
nonmedicinal (vapor)	T53.6X1	T53.6X2	T53.6X3	T53.6X4	—	—
Bialamicol	T37.3X1	T37.3X2	T37.3X3	T37.3X4	T37.3X5	T37.3X6
Bibenzonium bromide	T48.3X1	T48.3X2	T48.3X3	T48.3X4	T48.3X5	T48.3X6
Bibrocathol	T49.5X1	T49.5X2	T49.5X3	T49.5X4	T49.5X5	T49.5X6
Bichloride of mercury — see Mercury, chloride						
Bichromates (calcium) (potassium)(sodium) (crystals)	T57.8X1	T57.8X2	T57.8X3	T57.8X4		
fumes	T56.2X1	T56.2X2	T56.2X3	T56.2X4	—	
Biclotymol	T49.6X1	T49.6X2	T49.6X3	T49.6X4	T49.6X5	T49.6X6
Bicucculine	T50.7X1	T50.7X2	T50.7X3	T50.7X4	T50.7X5	T50.7X6
Bifemelane	T43.291	T43.292	T43.293	T43.294	T43.295	T43.296
Biguanide derivatives, oral	T38.3X1	T38.3X2	T38.3X3	T38.3X4	T38.3X5	T38.3X6
Bile salts	T47.5X1	T47.5X2	T47.5X3	T47.5X4	T47.5X5	T47.5X6
Biligrafin	T50.8X1	T50.8X2	T50.8X3	T50.8X4	T50.8X5	T50.8X6
Bilopaque	T50.8X1	T50.8X2	T50.8X3	T50.8X4	T50.8X5	T50.8X6
Binifibrate	T46.6X1	T46.6X2	T46.6X3	T46.6X4	T46.6X5	T46.6X6
Binitrobenzol	T65.3X1	T65.3X2	T65.3X3	T65.3X4		
Bioflavonoid(s)	T46.991	T46.992	T46.993	T46.994	T46.995	T46.996
Biological substance NEC	T50.901	T50.902	T50.903	T50.904	T50.905	T50.906
Biotin	T45.2X1	T45.2X2	T45.2X3	T45.2X4	T45.2X5	T45.2X6
Biperiden	T44.3X1	T44.3X2	T44.3X3	T44.3X4	T44.3X5	T44.3X6
Bisacodyl	T47.2X1	T47.2X2	T47.2X3	T47.2X4	T47.2X5	T47.2X6
Bisbentiamine	T45.2X1	T45.2X2	T45.2X3	T45.2X4	T45.2X5	T45.2X6
Bisbutiamine	T45.2X1	T45.2X2	T45.2X3	T45.2X4	T45.2X5	T45.2X6
Bisdequalinium (salts) (diacetate)	T49.6X1	T49.6X2	T49.6X3	T49.6X4	T49.6X5	T49.6X6
Bishydroxycoumarin	T45.511	T45.512	T45.513	T45.514	T45.515	T45.516
Bismarsen	T37.8X1	T37.8X2	T37.8X3	T37.8X4	T37.8X5	T37.8X6
Bismuth salts	T47.6X1	T47.6X2	T47.6X3	T47.6X4	T47.6X5	T47.6X6
aluminate	T47.1X1	T47.1X2	T47.1X3	T47.1X4	T47.1X5	T47.1X6
anti-infectives	T37.8X1	T37.8X2	T37.8X3	T37.8X4	T37.8X5	T37.8X6
formic iodide	T49.0X1	T49.0X2	T49.0X3	T49.0X4	T49.0X5	T49.0X6
glycolylarsenate	T49.0X1	T49.0X2	T49.0X3	T49.0X4	T49.0X5	T49.0X6
nonmedicinal (compounds) NEC	T65.91	T65.92	T65.93	T65.94	—	—
subcarbonate	T47.6X1	T47.6X2	T47.6X3	T47.6X4	T47.6X5	T47.6X6
subsalicylate	T37.8X1	T37.8X2	T37.8X3	T37.8X4	T37.8X5	T37.8X6
sulfarsphenamine	T37.8X1	T37.8X2	T37.8X3	T37.8X4	T37.8X5	T37.8X6
Bisoprolol	T44.7X1	T44.7X2	T44.7X3	T44.7X4	T44.7X5	T44.7X6
Bisoxatin	T47.2X1	T47.2X2	T47.2X3	T47.2X4	T47.2X5	T47.2X6
Bisulepin (hydrochloride)	T45.0X1	T45.0X2	T45.0X3	T45.0X4	T45.0X5	T45.0X6
Bithionol	T37.8X1	T37.8X2	T37.8X3	T37.8X4	T37.8X5	T37.8X6
anthelminthic	T37.4X1	T37.4X2	T37.4X3	T37.4X4	T37.4X5	T37.4X6
Bitolterol	T48.6X1	T48.6X2	T48.6X3	T48.6X4	T48.6X5	T48.6X6
Bitoscanate	T37.4X1	T37.4X2	T37.4X3	T37.4X4	T37.4X5	T37.4X6
Bitter almond oil	T62.8X1	T62.8X2	T62.8X3	T62.8X4	—	—
Bittersweet	T62.2X1	T62.2X2	T62.2X3	T62.2X4	—	—
Black						
flag	T60.91	T60.92	T60.93	T60.94	—	—
henbane	T62.2X1	T62.2X2	T62.2X3	T62.2X4	—	—
leaf (40)	T60.91	T60.92	T60.93	T60.94	—	—
widow spider (bite)	T63.311	T63.312	T63.313	T63.314		
antivenin	T50.Z11	T50.Z12	T50.Z13	T50.Z14	T50.Z15	T50.Z16
Blast furnace gas (carbon monoxide from)	T58.8X1	T58.8X2	T58.8X3	T58.8X4		
Bleach	T54.91	T54.92	T54.93	T54.94		
Bleaching agent (medicinal)	T49.4X1	T49.4X2	T49.4X3	T49.4X4	T49.4X5	T49.4X6
Bleomycin	T45.1X1	T45.1X2	T45.1X3	T45.1X4	T45.1X5	T45.1X6
Blockain	T41.3X1	T41.3X2	T41.3X3	T41.3X4	T41.3X5	T41.3X6
infiltration (subcutaneous)	T41.3X1	T41.3X2	T41.3X3	T41.3X4	T41.3X5	T41.3X6
nerve block (peripheral) (plexus)	T41.3X1	T41.3X2	T41.3X3	T41.3X4	T41.3X5	T41.3X6
topical (surface)	T41.3X1	T41.3X2	T41.3X3	T41.3X4	T41.3X5	T41.3X6
Blockers, calcium channel	T46.1X1	T46.1X2	T46.1X3	T46.1X4	T46.1X5	T46.1X6
Blood (derivatives) (natural) (plasma) (whole)	T45.8X1	T45.8X2	T45.8X3	T45.8X4	T45.8X5	T45.8X6
dried	T45.8X1	T45.8X2	T45.8X3	T45.8X4	T45.8X5	T45.8X6
drug affecting NEC	T45.91	T45.92	T45.93	T45.94	T45.95	T45.96
expander NEC	T45.8X1	T45.8X2	T45.8X3	T45.8X4	T45.8X5	T45.8X6
fraction NEC	T45.8X1	T45.8X2	T45.8X3	T45.8X4	T45.8X5	T45.8X6
substitute (macromolecular)	T45.8X1	T45.8X2	T45.8X3	T45.8X4	T45.8X5	T45.8X6
Blue velvet	T40.2X1	T40.2X2	T40.2X3	T40.2X4	—	—
Bone meal	T62.8X1	T62.8X2	T62.8X3	T62.8X4	—	—
Bonine	T45.0X1	T45.0X2	T45.0X3	T45.0X4	T45.0X5	T45.0X6
Bopindolol	T44.7X1	T44.7X2	T44.7X3	T44.7X4	T44.7X5	T44.7X6
Boracic acid	T49.0X1	T49.0X2	T49.0X3	T49.0X4	T49.0X5	T49.0X6
ENT agent	T49.6X1	T49.6X2	T49.6X3	T49.6X4	T49.6X5	T49.6X6
ophthalmic preparation	T49.5X1	T49.5X2	T49.5X3	T49.5X4	T49.5X5	T49.5X6
Borane complex	T57.8X1	T57.8X2	T57.8X3	T57.8X4	—	—

Table of Drugs and Chemicals

Substance	Poisoning, Accidental (unintentional)	Poisoning, Intentional Self-harm	Poisoning, Assault	Poisoning, Undetermined	Adverse Effect	Underdosing
Borate(s)	T57.8X1	T57.8X2	T57.8X3	T57.8X4	—	—
buffer	T50.991	T50.992	T50.993	T50.994	T50.995	T50.996
cleanser	T54.91	T54.92	T54.93	T54.94	—	—
sodium	T57.8X1	T57.8X2	T57.8X3	T57.8X4	—	—
Borax (cleanser)	T54.91	T54.92	T54.93	T54.94	—	—
Bordeaux mixture	T60.3X1	T60.3X2	T60.3X3	T60.3X4	—	—
Boric acid	T49.0X1	T49.0X2	T49.0X3	T49.0X4	T49.0X5	T49.0X6
ENT agent	T49.6X1	T49.6X2	T49.6X3	T49.6X4	T49.6X5	T49.6X6
ophthalmic preparation	T49.5X1	T49.5X2	T49.5X3	T49.5X4	T49.5X5	T49.5X6
Bornaprine	T44.3X1	T44.3X2	T44.3X3	T44.3X4	T44.3X5	T44.3X6
Boron	T57.8X1	T57.8X2	T57.8X3	T57.8X4	—	—
hydride NEC	T57.8X1	T57.8X2	T57.8X3	T57.8X4	—	—
fumes or gas	T57.8X1	T57.8X2	T57.8X3	T57.8X4	—	—
trifluoride	T59.891	T59.892	T59.893	T59.894	—	—
Botox	T48.291	T48.292	T48.293	T48.294	T48.295	T48.296
Botulinus anti-toxin (type A, B)	T50.Z11	T50.Z12	T50.Z13	T50.Z14	T50.Z15	T50.Z16
Brake fluid vapor	T59.891	T59.892	T59.893	T59.894	—	—
Brallobarbital	T42.3X1	T42.3X2	T42.3X3	T42.3X4	T42.3X5	T42.3X6
Bran (wheat)	T47.4X1	T47.4X2	T47.4X3	T47.4X4	T47.4X5	T47.4X6
Brass (fumes)	T56.891	T56.892	T56.893	T56.894	—	—
Brasso	T52.0X1	T52.0X2	T52.0X3	T52.0X4	—	—
Bretylium tosilate	T46.2X1	T46.2X2	T46.2X3	T46.2X4	T46.2X5	T46.2X6
Brevital (sodium)	T41.1X1	T41.1X2	T41.1X3	T41.1X4	T41.1X5	T41.1X6
Brinase	T45.3X1	T45.3X2	T45.3X3	T45.3X4	T45.3X5	T45.3X6
British antilewisite	T45.8X1	T45.8X2	T45.8X3	T45.8X4	T45.8X5	T45.8X6
Brodifacoum	T60.4X1	T60.4X2	T60.4X3	T60.4X4	—	—
Bromal (hydrate)	T42.6X1	T42.6X2	T42.6X3	T42.6X4	T42.6X5	T42.6X6
Bromazepam	T42.4X1	T42.4X2	T42.4X3	T42.4X4	T42.4X5	T42.4X6
Bromazine	T45.0X1	T45.0X2	T45.0X3	T45.0X4	T45.0X5	T45.0X6
Brombenzylcyanide	T59.3X1	T59.3X2	T59.3X3	T59.3X4	—	—
Bromelains	T45.3X1	T45.3X2	T45.3X3	T45.3X4	T45.3X5	T45.3X6
Bromethalin	T60.4X1	T60.4X2	T60.4X3	T60.4X4	—	—
Bromhexine	T48.4X1	T48.4X2	T48.4X3	T48.4X4	T48.4X5	T48.4X6
Bromide salts	T42.6X1	T42.6X2	T42.6X3	T42.6X4	T42.6X5	T42.6X6
Bromindione	T45.511	T45.512	T45.513	T45.514	T45.515	T45.516
Bromine						
compounds (medicinal)	T42.6X1	T42.6X2	T42.6X3	T42.6X4	T42.6X5	T42.6X6
sedative	T42.6X1	T42.6X2	T42.6X3	T42.6X4	T42.6X5	T42.6X6
vapor	T59.891	T59.892	T59.893	T59.894	—	—
Bromisoval	T42.6X1	T42.6X2	T42.6X3	T42.6X4	T42.6X5	T42.6X6
Bromisovalum	T42.6X1	T42.6X2	T42.6X3	T42.6X4	T42.6X5	T42.6X6
Bromobenzylcyanide	T59.3X1	T59.3X2	T59.3X3	T59.3X4	—	—
Bromochlorosalicylani-lide	T49.0X1	T49.0X2	T49.0X3	T49.0X4	T49.0X5	T49.0X6
Bromocriptine	T42.8X1	T42.8X2	T42.8X3	T42.8X4	T42.8X5	T42.8X6
Bromodiphenhydramine	T45.0X1	T45.0X2	T45.0X3	T45.0X4	T45.0X5	T45.0X6
Bromoform	T42.6X1	T42.6X2	T42.6X3	T42.6X4	T42.6X5	T42.6X6
Bromophenol blue reagent	T50.991	T50.992	T50.993	T50.994	T50.995	T50.996
Bromopride	T47.8X1	T47.8X2	T47.8X3	T47.8X4	T47.8X5	T47.8X6
Bromosalicylchloranitide	T49.0X1	T49.0X2	T49.0X3	T49.0X4	T49.0X5	T49.0X6
Bromosalicylhydroxamic acid	T37.1X1	T37.1X2	T37.1X3	T37.1X4	T37.1X5	T37.1X6
Bromo-seltzer	T39.1X1	T39.1X2	T39.1X3	T39.1X4	T39.1X5	T39.1X6
Bromoxynil	T60.3X1	T60.3X2	T60.3X3	T60.3X4	—	—
Bromperidol	T43.4X1	T43.4X2	T43.4X3	T43.4X4	T43.4X5	T43.4X6
Brompheniramine	T45.0X1	T45.0X2	T45.0X3	T45.0X4	T45.0X5	T45.0X6
Bromsulfophthalein	T50.8X1	T50.8X2	T50.8X3	T50.8X4	T50.8X5	T50.8X6
Bromural	T42.6X1	T42.6X2	T42.6X3	T42.6X4	T42.6X5	T42.6X6
Bromvaletone	T42.6X1	T42.6X2	T42.6X3	T42.6X4	T42.6X5	T42.6X6
Bronchodilator NEC	T48.6X1	T48.6X2	T48.6X3	T48.6X4	T48.6X5	T48.6X6
Brotizolam	T42.4X1	T42.4X2	T42.4X3	T42.4X4	T42.4X5	T42.4X6
Brovincamine	T46.7X1	T46.7X2	T46.7X3	T46.7X4	T46.7X5	T46.7X6
Brown recluse spider (bite) (venom)	T63.331	T63.332	T63.333	T63.334	—	—
Brown spider (bite) (venom)	T63.391	T63.392	T63.393	T63.394	—	—
Broxaterol	T48.6X1	T48.6X2	T48.6X3	T48.6X4	T48.6X5	T48.6X6
Broxuridine	T45.1X1	T45.1X2	T45.1X3	T45.1X4	T45.1X5	T45.1X6
Broxyquinoline	T37.8X1	T37.8X2	T37.8X3	T37.8X4	T37.8X5	T37.8X6
Bruceine	T48.291	T48.292	T48.293	T48.294	T48.295	T48.296
Brucia	T62.2X1	T62.2X2	T62.2X3	T62.2X4	—	—
Brucine	T65.1X1	T65.1X2	T65.1X3	T65.1X4	—	—
Brunswick green — see Copper						
Bruten — see Ibuprofen						
Bryonia	T47.2X1	T47.2X2	T47.2X3	T47.2X4	T47.2X5	T47.2X6
Buclizine	T45.0X1	T45.0X2	T45.0X3	T45.0X4	T45.0X5	T45.0X6
Buclosamide	T49.0X1	T49.0X2	T49.0X3	T49.0X4	T49.0X5	T49.0X6
Budesonide	T44.5X1	T44.5X2	T44.5X3	T44.5X4	T44.5X5	T44.5X6
Budralazine	T46.5X1	T46.5X2	T46.5X3	T46.5X4	T46.5X5	T46.5X6
Bufferin	T39.011	T39.012	T39.013	T39.014	T39.015	T39.016
Buflomedil	T46.7X1	T46.7X2	T46.7X3	T46.7X4	T46.7X5	T46.7X6
Buformin	T38.3X1	T38.3X2	T38.3X3	T38.3X4	T38.3X5	T38.3X6
Bufotenine	T40.991	T40.992	T40.993	T40.994		
Bufrolin	T48.6X1	T48.6X2	T48.6X3	T48.6X4	T48.6X5	T48.6X6

Substance	Poisoning, Accidental (unintentional)	Poisoning, Intentional Self-harm	Poisoning, Assault	Poisoning, Undetermined	Adverse Effect	Underdosing
Bufylline	T48.6X1	T48.6X2	T48.6X3	T48.6X4	T48.6X5	T48.6X6
Bulk filler	T50.5X1	T50.5X2	T50.5X3	T50.5X4	T50.5X5	T50.5X6
cathartic	T47.4X1	T47.4X2	T47.4X3	T47.4X4	T47.4X5	T47.4X6
Bumetanide	T50.1X1	T50.1X2	T50.1X3	T50.1X4	T50.1X5	T50.1X6
Bunaftine	T46.2X1	T46.2X2	T46.2X3	T46.2X4	T46.2X5	T46.2X6
Bunamiodyl	T50.8X1	T50.8X2	T50.8X3	T50.8X4	T50.8X5	T50.8X6
Bunazosin	T44.6X1	T44.6X2	T44.6X3	T44.6X4	T44.6X5	T44.6X6
Bunitrolol	T44.7X1	T44.7X2	T44.7X3	T44.7X4	T44.7X5	T44.7X6
Buphenine	T46.7X1	T46.7X2	T46.7X3	T46.7X4	T46.7X5	T46.7X6
Bupivacaine	T41.3X1	T41.3X2	T41.3X3	T41.3X4	T41.3X5	T41.3X6
infiltration (subcutaneous)	T41.3X1	T41.3X2	T41.3X3	T41.3X4	T41.3X5	T41.3X6
nerve block (peripheral) (plexus)	T41.3X1	T41.3X2	T41.3X3	T41.3X4	T41.3X5	T41.3X6
spinal	T41.3X1	T41.3X2	T41.3X3	T41.3X4	T41.3X5	T41.3X6
Bupranolol	T44.7X1	T44.7X2	T44.7X3	T44.7X4	T44.7X5	T44.7X6
Buprenorphine	T40.4X1	T40.4X2	T40.4X3	T40.4X4	T40.4X5	T40.4X6
Bupropion	T43.291	T43.292	T43.293	T43.294	T43.295	T43.296
Burimamide	T47.1X1	T47.1X2	T47.1X3	T47.1X4	T47.1X5	T47.1X6
Buserelin	T38.891	T38.892	T38.893	T38.894	T38.895	T38.896
Buspirone	T43.591	T43.592	T43.593	T43.594	T43.595	T43.596
Busulfan, busulphan	T45.1X1	T45.1X2	T45.1X3	T45.1X4	T45.1X5	T45.1X6
Butabarbital (sodium)	T42.3X1	T42.3X2	T42.3X3	T42.3X4	T42.3X5	T42.3X6
Butabarbitone	T42.3X1	T42.3X2	T42.3X3	T42.3X4	T42.3X5	T42.3X6
Butabarpal	T42.3X1	T42.3X2	T42.3X3	T42.3X4	T42.3X5	T42.3X6
Butacaine	T41.3X1	T41.3X2	T41.3X3	T41.3X4	T41.3X5	T41.3X6
Butalamine	T46.7X1	T46.7X2	T46.7X3	T46.7X4	T46.7X5	T46.7X6
Butalbital	T42.3X1	T42.3X2	T42.3X3	T42.3X4	T42.3X5	T42.3X6
Butallylonal	T42.3X1	T42.3X2	T42.3X3	T42.3X4	T42.3X5	T42.3X6
Butamben	T41.3X1	T41.3X2	T41.3X3	T41.3X4	T41.3X5	T41.3X6
Butamirate	T48.3X1	T48.3X2	T48.3X3	T48.3X4	T48.3X5	T48.3X6
Butane (distributed in mobile container)	T59.891	T59.892	T59.893	T59.894		
distributed through pipes	T59.891	T59.892	T59.893	T59.894	—	—
incomplete combustion	T58.11	T58.12	T58.13	T58.14	—	—
Butanilicaine	T41.3X1	T41.3X2	T41.3X3	T41.3X4	T41.3X5	T41.3X6
Butanol	T51.3X1	T51.3X2	T51.3X3	T51.3X4		
Butanone, 2-butanone	T52.4X1	T52.4X2	T52.4X3	T52.4X4	—	
Butantrone	T49.4X1	T49.4X2	T49.4X3	T49.4X4	T49.4X5	T49.4X6
Butaperazine	T43.3X1	T43.3X2	T43.3X3	T43.3X4	T43.3X5	T43.3X6
Butazolidin	T39.2X1	T39.2X2	T39.2X3	T39.2X4	T39.2X5	T39.2X6
Butetamate	T48.6X1	T48.6X2	T48.6X3	T48.6X4	T48.6X5	T48.6X6
Butethal	T42.3X1	T42.3X2	T42.3X3	T42.3X4	T42.3X5	T42.3X6
Butethamate	T44.3X1	T44.3X2	T44.3X3	T44.3X4	T44.3X5	T44.3X6
Buthalitone (sodium)	T41.1X1	T41.1X2	T41.1X3	T41.1X4	T41.1X5	T41.1X6
Butisol (sodium)	T42.3X1	T42.3X2	T42.3X3	T42.3X4	T42.3X5	T42.3X6
Butizide	T50.2X1	T50.2X2	T50.2X3	T50.2X4	T50.2X5	T50.2X6
Butobarbital	T42.3X1	T42.3X2	T42.3X3	T42.3X4	T42.3X5	T42.3X6
sodium	T42.3X1	T42.3X2	T42.3X3	T42.3X4	T42.3X5	T42.3X6
Butobarbitone	T42.3X1	T42.3X2	T42.3X3	T42.3X4	T42.3X5	T42.3X6
Butoconazole (nitrate)	T49.0X1	T49.0X2	T49.0X3	T49.0X4	T49.0X5	T49.0X6
Butorphanol	T40.4X1	T40.4X2	T40.4X3	T40.4X4	T40.4X5	T40.4X6
Butriptyline	T43.011	T43.012	T43.013	T43.014	T43.015	T43.016
Butropium bromide	T44.3X1	T44.3X2	T44.3X3	T44.3X4	T44.3X5	T44.3X6
Buttercups	T62.2X1	T62.2X2	T62.2X3	T62.2X4	—	—
Butter of antimony — see Antimony						
Butyl						
acetate (secondary)	T52.8X1	T52.8X2	T52.8X3	T52.8X4	—	—
alcohol	T51.3X1	T51.3X2	T51.3X3	T51.3X4	—	—
aminobenzoate	T41.3X1	T41.3X2	T41.3X3	T41.3X4	T41.3X5	T41.3X6
butyrate	T52.8X1	T52.8X2	T52.8X3	T52.8X4	—	—
carbinol	T51.3X1	T51.3X2	T51.3X3	T51.3X4	—	—
carbitol	T52.3X1	T52.3X2	T52.3X3	T52.3X4	—	—
cellosolve	T52.3X1	T52.3X2	T52.3X3	T52.3X4	—	—
chloral (hydrate)	T42.6X1	T42.6X2	T42.6X3	T42.6X4	T42.6X5	T42.6X6
formate	T52.8X1	T52.8X2	T52.8X3	T52.8X4	—	—
lactate	T52.8X1	T52.8X2	T52.8X3	T52.8X4	—	—
propionate	T52.8X1	T52.8X2	T52.8X3	T52.8X4	—	—
scopolamine bromide	T44.3X1	T44.3X2	T44.3X3	T44.3X4	T44.3X5	T44.3X6
thiobarbital sodium	T41.1X1	T41.1X2	T41.1X3	T41.1X4	T41.1X5	T41.1X6
Butylated hydroxyanisole	T50.991	T50.992	T50.993	T50.994	T50.995	T50.996
Butylchloral hydrate	T42.6X1	T42.6X2	T42.6X3	T42.6X4	T42.6X5	T42.6X6
Butyltoluene	T52.2X1	T52.2X2	T52.2X3	T52.2X4	—	—
Butyn	T41.3X1	T41.3X2	T41.3X3	T41.3X4	T41.3X5	T41.3X6
Butyrophenone (-based tranquilizers)	T43.4X1	T43.4X2	T43.4X3	T43.4X4	T43.4X5	T43.4X6
Cabergoline	T42.8X1	T42.8X2	T42.8X3	T42.8X4	T42.8X5	T42.8X6
Cacodyl, cacodylic acid	T57.0X1	T57.0X2	T57.0X3	T57.0X4	—	—
Cactinomycin	T45.1X1	T45.1X2	T45.1X3	T45.1X4	T45.1X5	T45.1X6
Cade oil	T49.4X1	T49.4X2	T49.4X3	T49.4X4	T49.4X5	T49.4X6
Cadexomer iodine	T49.0X1	T49.0X2	T49.0X3	T49.0X4	T49.0X5	T49.0X6
Cadmium (chloride) (fumes) (oxide)	T56.3X1	T56.3X2	T56.3X3	T56.3X4		

Borate — Cadmium

Substance	Poisoning, Accidental (unintentional)	Poisoning, Intentional Self-harm	Poisoning, Assault	Poisoning, Undetermined	Adverse Effect	Under-dosing
Cadmium — *continued*						
sulfide (medicinal) NEC	T49.4X1	T49.4X2	T49.4X3	T49.4X4	T49.4X5	T49.4X6
Cadralazine	T46.5X1	T46.5X2	T46.5X3	T46.5X4	T46.5X5	T46.5X6
Caffeine	T43.611	T43.612	T43.613	T43.614	T43.615	T43.616
Calabar bean	T62.2X1	T62.2X2	T62.2X3	T62.2X4	—	—
Caladium seguinum	T62.2X1	T62.2X2	T62.2X3	T62.2X4	—	—
Calamine (lotion)	T49.3X1	T49.3X2	T49.3X3	T49.3X4	T49.3X5	T49.3X6
Calcifediol	T45.2X1	T45.2X2	T45.2X3	T45.2X4	T45.2X5	T45.2X6
Calciferol	T45.2X1	T45.2X2	T45.2X3	T45.2X4	T45.2X5	T45.2X6
Calcitonin	T50.991	T50.992	T50.993	T50.994	T50.995	T50.996
Calcitriol	T45.2X1	T45.2X2	T45.2X3	T45.2X4	T45.2X5	T45.2X6
Calcium	T50.3X1	T50.3X2	T50.3X3	T50.3X4	T50.3X5	T50.3X6
actylsalicylate	T39.011	T39.012	T39.013	T39.014	T39.015	T39.016
benzamidosalicylate	T37.1X1	T37.1X2	T37.1X3	T37.1X4	T37.1X5	T37.1X6
bromide	T42.6X1	T42.6X2	T42.6X3	T42.6X4	T42.6X5	T42.6X6
bromolactobionate	T42.6X1	T42.6X2	T42.6X3	T42.6X4	T42.6X5	T42.6X6
carbaspirin	T39.011	T39.012	T39.013	T39.014	T39.015	T39.016
carbimide	T50.6X1	T50.6X2	T50.6X3	T50.6X4	T50.6X5	T50.6X6
carbonate	T47.1X1	T47.1X2	T47.1X3	T47.1X4	T47.1X5	T47.1X6
chloride	T50.991	T50.992	T50.993	T50.994	T50.995	T50.996
anhydrous	T50.991	T50.992	T50.993	T50.994	T50.995	T50.996
cyanide	T57.8X1	T57.8X2	T57.8X3	T57.8X4	—	—
dioctyl sulfosuccinate	T47.4X1	T47.4X2	T47.4X3	T47.4X4	T47.4X5	T47.4X6
disodium edathamil	T45.8X1	T45.8X2	T45.8X3	T45.8X4	T45.8X5	T45.8X6
disodium edetate	T45.8X1	T45.8X2	T45.8X3	T45.8X4	T45.8X5	T45.8X6
dobesilate	T46.991	T46.992	T46.993	T46.994	T46.995	T46.996
EDTA	T45.8X1	T45.8X2	T45.8X3	T45.8X4	T45.8X5	T45.8X6
ferrous citrate	T45.4X1	T45.4X2	T45.4X3	T45.4X4	T45.4X5	T45.4X6
folinate	T45.8X1	T45.8X2	T45.8X3	T45.8X4	T45.8X5	T45.8X6
glubionate	T50.3X1	T50.3X2	T50.3X3	T50.3X4	T50.3X5	T50.3X6
gluconate	T50.3X1	T50.3X2	T50.3X3	T50.3X4	T50.3X5	T50.3X6
gluconogalactogluconate	T50.3X1	T50.3X2	T50.3X3	T50.3X4	T50.3X5	T50.3X6
hydrate, hydroxide	T54.3X1	T54.3X2	T54.3X3	T54.3X4	—	—
hypochlorite	T54.3X1	T54.3X2	T54.3X3	T54.3X4	—	—
iodide	T48.4X1	T48.4X2	T48.4X3	T48.4X4	T48.4X5	T48.4X6
ipodate	T50.8X1	T50.8X2	T50.8X3	T50.8X4	T50.8X5	T50.8X6
lactate	T50.3X1	T50.3X2	T50.3X3	T50.3X4	T50.3X5	T50.3X6
leucovorin	T45.8X1	T45.8X2	T45.8X3	T45.8X4	T45.8X5	T45.8X6
mandelate	T37.91	T37.92	T37.93	T37.94	T37.95	T37.96
oxide	T54.3X1	T54.3X2	T54.3X3	T54.3X4	—	—
pantothenate	T45.2X1	T45.2X2	T45.2X3	T45.2X4	T45.2X5	T45.2X6
phosphate	T50.3X1	T50.3X2	T50.3X3	T50.3X4	T50.3X5	T50.3X6
salicylate	T39.091	T39.092	T39.093	T39.094	T39.095	T39.096
salts	T50.3X1	T50.3X2	T50.3X3	T50.3X4	T50.3X5	T50.3X6
Calculus-dissolving drug	T50.991	T50.992	T50.993	T50.994	T50.995	T50.996
Calomel	T49.0X1	T49.0X2	T49.0X3	T49.0X4	T49.0X5	T49.0X6
Caloric agent	T50.3X1	T50.3X2	T50.3X3	T50.3X4	T50.3X5	T50.3X6
Calusterone	T38.7X1	T38.7X2	T38.7X3	T38.7X4	T38.7X5	T38.7X6
Camazepam	T42.4X1	T42.4X2	T42.4X3	T42.4X4	T42.4X5	T42.4X6
Camomile	T49.0X1	T49.0X2	T49.0X3	T49.0X4	T49.0X5	T49.0X6
Camoquin	T37.2X1	T37.2X2	T37.2X3	T37.2X4	T37.2X5	T37.2X6
Camphor						
Insecticide	T60.2X1	T60.2X2	T60.2X3	T60.2X4	—	—
medicinal	T49.8X1	T49.8X2	T49.8X3	T49.8X4	T49.8X5	T49.8X6
Camylofin	T44.3X1	T44.3X2	T44.3X3	T44.3X4	T44.3X5	T44.3X6
Cancer chemotherapy drug regimen	T45.1X1	T45.1X2	T45.1X3	T45.1X4	T45.1X5	T45.1X6
Candeptin	T49.0X1	T49.0X2	T49.0X3	T49.0X4	T49.0X5	T49.0X6
Candicidin	T49.0X1	T49.0X2	T49.0X3	T49.0X4	T49.0X5	T49.0X6
Cannabinol	T40.7X1	T40.7X2	T40.7X3	T40.7X4	T40.7X5	T40.7X6
Cannabis (derivatives)	T40.7X1	T40.7X2	T40.7X3	T40.7X4	T40.7X5	T40.7X6
Canned heat	T51.1X1	T51.1X2	T51.1X3	T51.1X4	—	—
Canrenoic acid	T50.0X1	T50.0X2	T50.0X3	T50.0X4	T50.0X5	T50.0X6
Canrenone	T50.0X1	T50.0X2	T50.0X3	T50.0X4	T50.0X5	T50.0X6
Cantharides, cantharidin, cantharis	T49.8X1	T49.8X2	T49.8X3	T49.8X4	T49.8X5	T49.8X6
Canthaxanthin	T50.991	T50.992	T50.993	T50.994	T50.995	T50.996
Capillary-active drug NEC	T46.901	T46.902	T46.903	T46.904	T46.905	T46.906
Capreomycin	T36.8X1	T36.8X2	T36.8X3	T36.8X4	T36.8X5	T36.8X6
Capsicum	T49.4X1	T49.4X2	T49.4X3	T49.4X4	T49.4X5	T49.4X6
Captafol	T60.3X1	T60.3X2	T60.3X3	T60.3X4	—	—
Captan	T60.3X1	T60.3X2	T60.3X3	T60.3X4	—	—
Captodiame, captodiamine	T43.591	T43.592	T43.593	T43.594	T43.595	T43.596
Captopril	T46.4X1	T46.4X2	T46.4X3	T46.4X4	T46.4X5	T46.4X6
Caramiphen	T44.3X1	T44.3X2	T44.3X3	T44.3X4	T44.3X5	T44.3X6
Carazolol	T44.7X1	T44.7X2	T44.7X3	T44.7X4	T44.7X5	T44.7X6
Carbachol	T44.1X1	T44.1X2	T44.1X3	T44.1X4	T44.1X5	T44.1X6
Carbacrylamine (resin)	T50.3X1	T50.3X2	T50.3X3	T50.3X4	T50.3X5	T50.3X6
Carbamate (insecticide)	T60.0X1	T60.0X2	T60.0X3	T60.0X4	—	—
Carbamate (sedative)	T42.6X1	T42.6X2	T42.6X3	T42.6X4	T42.6X5	T42.6X6
herbicide	T60.0X1	T60.0X2	T60.0X3	T60.0X4	—	—
insecticide	T60.0X1	T60.0X2	T60.0X3	T60.0X4	—	—
Carbamazepine	T42.1X1	T42.1X2	T42.1X3	T42.1X4	T42.1X5	T42.1X6

Substance	Poisoning, Accidental (unintentional)	Poisoning, Intentional Self-harm	Poisoning, Assault	Poisoning, Undetermined	Adverse Effect	Under-dosing
Carbamide	T47.3X1	T47.3X2	T47.3X3	T47.3X4	T47.3X5	T47.3X6
peroxide	T49.0X1	T49.0X2	T49.0X3	T49.0X4	T49.0X5	T49.0X6
topical	T49.8X1	T49.8X2	T49.8X3	T49.8X4	T49.8X5	T49.8X6
Carbamylcholine chloride	T44.1X1	T44.1X2	T44.1X3	T44.1X4	T44.1X5	T44.1X6
Carbaril	T60.0X1	T60.0X2	T60.0X3	T60.0X4	—	—
Carbarsone	T37.3X1	T37.3X2	T37.3X3	T37.3X4	T37.3X5	T37.3X6
Carbaryl	T60.0X1	T60.0X2	T60.0X3	T60.0X4	—	—
Carbaspirin	T39.011	T39.012	T39.013	T39.014	T39.015	T39.016
Carbazochrome (salicylate) (sodium sulfonate)	T49.4X1	T49.4X2	T49.4X3	T49.4X4	T49.4X5	T49.4X6
Carbenicillin	T36.0X1	T36.0X2	T36.0X3	T36.0X4	T36.0X5	T36.0X6
Carbenoxolone	T47.1X1	T47.1X2	T47.1X3	T47.1X4	T47.1X5	T47.1X6
Carbetapentane	T48.3X1	T48.3X2	T48.3X3	T48.3X4	T48.3X5	T48.3X6
Carbethyl salicylate	T39.091	T39.092	T39.093	T39.094	T39.095	T39.096
Carbidopa (with levodopa)	T42.8X1	T42.8X2	T42.8X3	T42.8X4	T42.8X5	T42.8X6
Carbimazole	T38.2X1	T38.2X2	T38.2X3	T38.2X4	T38.2X5	T38.2X6
Carbinol	T51.1X1	T51.1X2	T51.1X3	T51.1X4	—	—
Carbinoxamine	T45.0X1	T45.0X2	T45.0X3	T45.0X4	T45.0X5	T45.0X6
Carbiphene	T39.8X1	T39.8X2	T39.8X3	T39.8X4	T39.8X5	T39.8X6
Carbitol	T52.3X1	T52.3X2	T52.3X3	T52.3X4	—	—
Carbocaine	T41.3X1	T41.3X2	T41.3X3	T41.3X4	T41.3X5	T41.3X6
infiltration (subcutaneous)	T41.3X1	T41.3X2	T41.3X3	T41.3X4	T41.3X5	T41.3X6
nerve block (peripheral) (plexus)	T41.3X1	T41.3X2	T41.3X3	T41.3X4	T41.3X5	T41.3X6
topical (surface)	T41.3X1	T41.3X2	T41.3X3	T41.3X4	T41.3X5	T41.3X6
Carbocisteine	T48.4X1	T48.4X2	T48.4X3	T48.4X4	T48.4X5	T48.4X6
Carbocromen	T46.3X1	T46.3X2	T46.3X3	T46.3X4	T46.3X5	T46.3X6
Carbol fuchsin	T49.0X1	T49.0X2	T49.0X3	T49.0X4	T49.0X5	T49.0X6
Carbolic acid — *see also* Phenol	T54.0X1	T54.0X2	T54.0X3	T54.0X4	—	—
Carbolonium (bromide)	T48.1X1	T48.1X2	T48.1X3	T48.1X4	T48.1X5	T48.1X6
Carbo medicinalis	T47.6X1	T47.6X2	T47.6X3	T47.6X4	T47.6X5	T47.6X6
Carbomycin	T36.8X1	T36.8X2	T36.8X3	T36.8X4	T36.8X5	T36.8X6
Carbon						
bisulfide (liquid)	T65.4X1	T65.4X2	T65.4X3	T65.4X4	—	—
vapor	T65.4X1	T65.4X2	T65.4X3	T65.4X4	—	—
dioxide (gas)	T59.7X1	T59.7X2	T59.7X3	T59.7X4	—	—
medicinal	T41.5X1	T41.5X2	T41.5X3	T41.5X4	T41.5X5	T41.5X6
nonmedicinal	T59.7X1	T59.7X2	T59.7X3	T59.7X4	—	—
snow	T49.4X1	T49.4X2	T49.4X3	T49.4X4	T49.4X5	T49.4X6
disulfide (liquid)	T65.4X1	T65.4X2	T65.4X3	T65.4X4	—	—
vapor	T65.4X1	T65.4X2	T65.4X3	T65.4X4	—	—
monoxide (from incomplete combustion)	T58.91	T58.92	T58.93	T58.94	—	—
blast furnace gas	T58.8X1	T58.8X2	T58.8X3	T58.8X4	—	—
butane (distributed in mobile container)	T58.11	T58.12	T58.13	T58.14	—	—
distributed through pipes	T58.11	T58.12	T58.13	T58.14	—	—
charcoal fumes	T58.2X1	T58.2X2	T58.2X3	T58.2X4	—	—
coal	T58.2X1	T58.2X2	T58.2X3	T58.2X4	—	—
coke (in domestic stoves, fireplaces)	T58.2X1	T58.2X2	T58.2X3	T58.2X4	—	—
exhaust gas (motor) not in transit	T58.01	T58.02	T58.03	T58.04	—	—
combustion engine, any not in watercraft	T58.01	T58.02	T58.03	T58.04	—	—
farm tractor, not in transit	T58.01	T58.02	T58.03	T58.04	—	—
gas engine	T58.01	T58.02	T58.03	T58.04	—	—
motor pump	T58.01	T58.02	T58.03	T58.04	—	—
motor vehicle, not in transit	T58.01	T58.02	T58.03	T58.04	—	—
fuel (in domestic use)	T58.2X1	T58.2X2	T58.2X3	T58.2X4	—	—
gas (piped)	T58.11	T58.12	T58.13	T58.14	—	—
in mobile container	T58.11	T58.12	T58.13	T58.14	—	—
piped (natural)	T58.11	T58.12	T58.13	T58.14	—	—
utility	T58.11	T58.12	T58.13	T58.14	—	—
in mobile container	T58.11	T58.12	T58.13	T58.14	—	—
gas (piped)	T58.11	T58.12	T58.13	T58.14	—	—
illuminating gas	T58.11	T58.12	T58.13	T58.14	—	—
industrial fuels or gases, any	T58.8X1	T58.8X2	T58.8X3	T58.8X4	—	—
kerosene (in domestic stoves, fireplaces)	T58.2X1	T58.2X2	T58.2X3	T58.2X4	—	—
kiln gas or vapor	T58.8X1	T58.8X2	T58.8X3	T58.8X4	—	—
motor exhaust gas, not in transit	T58.01	T58.02	T58.03	T58.04	—	—
piped gas (manufactured) (natural)	T58.11	T58.12	T58.13	T58.14	—	—
producer gas	T58.8X1	T58.8X2	T58.8X3	T58.8X4	—	—
propane (distributed in mobile container)	T58.11	T58.12	T58.13	T58.14	—	—

Substance	Poisoning, Accidental (unintentional)	Poisoning, Intentional Self-harm	Poisoning, Assault	Poisoning, Undetermined	Adverse Effect	Under-dosing
Carbon — *continued*						
monoxide — *continued*						
propane — *continued*						
distributed through pipes	T58.11	T58.12	T58.13	T58.14	—	—
solid (in domestic stoves, fireplaces)	T58.2X1	T58.2X2	T58.2X3	T58.2X4	—	—
specified source NEC	T58.8X1	T58.8X2	T58.8X3	T58.8X4	—	—
stove gas	T58.11	T58.12	T58.13	T58.14	—	—
piped	T58.11	T58.12	T58.13	T58.14	—	—
utility gas	T58.11	T58.12	T58.13	T58.14	—	—
piped	T58.11	T58.12	T58.13	T58.14	—	—
water gas	T58.11	T58.12	T58.13	T58.14	—	—
wood (in domestic stoves, fireplaces)	T58.2X1	T58.2X2	T58.2X3	T58.2X4	—	—
tetrachloride (vapor) NEC	T53.0X1	T53.0X2	T53.0X3	T53.0X4	—	—
liquid (cleansing agent) NEC	T53.0X1	T53.0X2	T53.0X3	T53.0X4	—	—
solvent	T53.0X1	T53.0X2	T53.0X3	T53.0X4	—	—
Carbonic acid gas	T59.7X1	T59.7X2	T59.7X3	T59.7X4	—	—
anhydrase inhibitor NEC	T50.2X1	T50.2X2	T50.2X3	T50.2X4	T50.2X5	T50.2X6
Carbophenothion	T60.0X1	T60.0X2	T60.0X3	T60.0X4	—	—
Carboplatin	T45.1X1	T45.1X2	T45.1X3	T45.1X4	T45.1X5	T45.1X6
Carboprost	T48.0X1	T48.0X2	T48.0X3	T48.0X4	T48.0X5	T48.0X6
Carboquone	T45.1X1	T45.1X2	T45.1X3	T45.1X4	T45.1X5	T45.1X6
Carbowax	T49.3X1	T49.3X2	T49.3X3	T49.3X4	T49.3X5	T49.3X6
Carboxymethylcellulose	T47.4X1	T47.4X2	T47.4X3	T47.4X4	T47.4X5	T47.4X6
Carbrital	T42.3X1	T42.3X2	T42.3X3	T42.3X4	T42.3X5	T42.3X6
Carbromal	T42.6X1	T42.6X2	T42.6X3	T42.6X4	T42.6X5	T42.6X6
Carbutamide	T38.3X1	T38.3X2	T38.3X3	T38.3X4	T38.3X5	T38.3X6
Carbuterol	T48.6X1	T48.6X2	T48.6X3	T48.6X4	T48.6X5	T48.6X6
Cardiac						
depressants	T46.2X1	T46.2X2	T46.2X3	T46.2X4	T46.2X5	T46.2X6
rhythm regulator	T46.2X1	T46.2X2	T46.2X3	T46.2X4	T46.2X5	T46.2X6
specified NEC	T46.2X1	T46.2X2	T46.2X3	T46.2X4	T46.2X5	T46.2X6
Cardiografin	T50.8X1	T50.8X2	T50.8X3	T50.8X4	T50.8X5	T50.8X6
Cardiogreen	T50.8X1	T50.8X2	T50.8X3	T50.8X4	T50.8X5	T50.8X6
Cardiotonic (glycoside) **NEC**	T46.0X1	T46.0X2	T46.0X3	T46.0X4	T46.0X5	T46.0X6
Cardiovascular drug NEC	T46.901	T46.902	T46.903	T46.904	T46.905	T46.906
Cardrase	T50.2X1	T50.2X2	T50.2X3	T50.2X4	T50.2X5	T50.2X6
Carfecillin	T36.0X1	T36.0X2	T36.0X3	T36.0X4	T36.0X5	T36.0X6
Carfenazine	T43.3X1	T43.3X2	T43.3X3	T43.3X4	T43.3X5	T43.3X6
Carfusin	T49.0X1	T49.0X2	T49.0X3	T49.0X4	T49.0X5	T49.0X6
Carindacillin	T36.0X1	T36.0X2	T36.0X3	T36.0X4	T36.0X5	T36.0X6
Carisoprodol	T42.8X1	T42.8X2	T42.8X3	T42.8X4	T42.8X5	T42.8X6
Carmellose	T47.4X1	T47.4X2	T47.4X3	T47.4X4	T47.4X5	T47.4X6
Carminative	T47.5X1	T47.5X2	T47.5X3	T47.5X4	T47.5X5	T47.5X6
Carmofur	T45.1X1	T45.1X2	T45.1X3	T45.1X4	T45.1X5	T45.1X6
Carmustine	T45.1X1	T45.1X2	T45.1X3	T45.1X4	T45.1X5	T45.1X6
Carotene	T45.2X1	T45.2X2	T45.2X3	T45.2X4	T45.2X5	T45.2X6
Carphenazine	T43.3X1	T43.3X2	T43.3X3	T43.3X4	T43.3X5	T43.3X6
Carpipramine	T42.4X1	T42.4X2	T42.4X3	T42.4X4	T42.4X5	T42.4X6
Carprofen	T39.311	T39.312	T39.313	T39.314	T39.315	T39.316
Carpronium chloride	T44.3X1	T44.3X2	T44.3X3	T44.3X4	T44.3X5	T44.3X6
Carrageenan	T47.8X1	T47.8X2	T47.8X3	T47.8X4	T47.8X5	T47.8X6
Carteolol	T44.7X1	T44.7X2	T44.7X3	T44.7X4	T44.7X5	T44.7X6
Carter's Little Pills	T47.2X1	T47.2X2	T47.2X3	T47.2X4	T47.2X5	T47.2X6
Cascara (sagrada)	T47.2X1	T47.2X2	T47.2X3	T47.2X4	T47.2X5	T47.2X6
Cassava	T62.2X1	T62.2X2	T62.2X3	T62.2X4	—	—
Castellani's paint	T49.0X1	T49.0X2	T49.0X3	T49.0X4	T49.0X5	T49.0X6
Castor						
bean	T62.2X1	T62.2X2	T62.2X3	T62.2X4	—	—
oil	T47.2X1	T47.2X2	T47.2X3	T47.2X4	T47.2X5	T47.2X6
Catalase	T45.3X1	T45.3X2	T45.3X3	T45.3X4	T45.3X5	T45.3X6
Caterpillar (sting)	T63.431	T63.432	T63.433	T63.434	—	—
Catha (edulis) (tea)	T43.691	T43.692	T43.693	T43.694	—	—
Cathartic NEC	T47.4X1	T47.4X2	T47.4X3	T47.4X4	T47.4X5	T47.4X6
anthacene derivative	T47.2X1	T47.2X2	T47.2X3	T47.2X4	T47.2X5	T47.2X6
bulk	T47.4X1	T47.4X2	T47.4X3	T47.4X4	T47.4X5	T47.4X6
contact	T47.2X1	T47.2X2	T47.2X3	T47.2X4	T47.2X5	T47.2X6
emollient NEC	T47.4X1	T47.4X2	T47.4X3	T47.4X4	T47.4X5	T47.4X6
irritant NEC	T47.2X1	T47.2X2	T47.2X3	T47.2X4	T47.2X5	T47.2X6
mucilage	T47.4X1	T47.4X2	T47.4X3	T47.4X4	T47.4X5	T47.4X6
saline	T47.3X1	T47.3X2	T47.3X3	T47.3X4	T47.3X5	T47.3X6
vegetable	T47.2X1	T47.2X2	T47.2X3	T47.2X4	T47.2X5	T47.2X6
Cathine	T50.5X1	T50.5X2	T50.5X3	T50.5X4	T50.5X5	T50.5X6
Cathomycin	T36.8X1	T36.8X2	T36.8X3	T36.8X4	T36.8X5	T36.8X6
Cation exchange resin	T50.3X1	T50.3X2	T50.3X3	T50.3X4	T50.3X5	T50.3X6
Caustic(s) **NEC**	T54.91	T54.92	T54.93	T54.94	—	—
alkali	T54.3X1	T54.3X2	T54.3X3	T54.3X4	—	—
hydroxide	T54.3X1	T54.3X2	T54.3X3	T54.3X4	—	—
potash	T54.3X1	T54.3X2	T54.3X3	T54.3X4	—	—
soda	T54.3X1	T54.3X2	T54.3X3	T54.3X4	—	—

Substance	Poisoning, Accidental (unintentional)	Poisoning, Intentional Self-harm	Poisoning, Assault	Poisoning, Undetermined	Adverse Effect	Under-dosing
Caustic(s) **NEC** — *continued*						
specified NEC	T54.91	T54.92	T54.93	T54.94	—	—
Ceepryn	T49.0X1	T49.0X2	T49.0X3	T49.0X4	T49.0X5	T49.0X6
ENT agent	T49.6X1	T49.6X2	T49.6X3	T49.6X4	T49.6X5	T49.6X6
lozenges	T49.6X1	T49.6X2	T49.6X3	T49.6X4	T49.6X5	T49.6X6
Cefacetrile	T36.1X1	T36.1X2	T36.1X3	T36.1X4	T36.1X5	T36.1X6
Cefaclor	T36.1X1	T36.1X2	T36.1X3	T36.1X4	T36.1X5	T36.1X6
Cefadroxil	T36.1X1	T36.1X2	T36.1X3	T36.1X4	T36.1X5	T36.1X6
Cefalexin	T36.1X1	T36.1X2	T36.1X3	T36.1X4	T36.1X5	T36.1X6
Cefaloglycin	T36.1X1	T36.1X2	T36.1X3	T36.1X4	T36.1X5	T36.1X6
Cefaloridine	T36.1X1	T36.1X2	T36.1X3	T36.1X4	T36.1X5	T36.1X6
Cefalosporins	T36.1X1	T36.1X2	T36.1X3	T36.1X4	T36.1X5	T36.1X6
Cefalotin	T36.1X1	T36.1X2	T36.1X3	T36.1X4	T36.1X5	T36.1X6
Cefamandole	T36.1X1	T36.1X2	T36.1X3	T36.1X4	T36.1X5	T36.1X6
Cefamycin antibiotic	T36.1X1	T36.1X2	T36.1X3	T36.1X4	T36.1X5	T36.1X6
Cefapirin	T36.1X1	T36.1X2	T36.1X3	T36.1X4	T36.1X5	T36.1X6
Cefatrizine	T36.1X1	T36.1X2	T36.1X3	T36.1X4	T36.1X5	T36.1X6
Cefazedone	T36.1X1	T36.1X2	T36.1X3	T36.1X4	T36.1X5	T36.1X6
Cefazolin	T36.1X1	T36.1X2	T36.1X3	T36.1X4	T36.1X5	T36.1X6
Cefbuperazone	T36.1X1	T36.1X2	T36.1X3	T36.1X4	T36.1X5	T36.1X6
Cefetamet	T36.1X1	T36.1X2	T36.1X3	T36.1X4	T36.1X5	T36.1X6
Cefixime	T36.1X1	T36.1X2	T36.1X3	T36.1X4	T36.1X5	T36.1X6
Cefmenoxime	T36.1X1	T36.1X2	T36.1X3	T36.1X4	T36.1X5	T36.1X6
Cefmetazole	T36.1X1	T36.1X2	T36.1X3	T36.1X4	T36.1X5	T36.1X6
Cefminox	T36.1X1	T36.1X2	T36.1X3	T36.1X4	T36.1X5	T36.1X6
Cefonicid	T36.1X1	T36.1X2	T36.1X3	T36.1X4	T36.1X5	T36.1X6
Cefoperazone	T36.1X1	T36.1X2	T36.1X3	T36.1X4	T36.1X5	T36.1X6
Ceforanide	T36.1X1	T36.1X2	T36.1X3	T36.1X4	T36.1X5	T36.1X6
Cefotaxime	T36.1X1	T36.1X2	T36.1X3	T36.1X4	T36.1X5	T36.1X6
Cefotetan	T36.1X1	T36.1X2	T36.1X3	T36.1X4	T36.1X5	T36.1X6
Cefotiam	T36.1X1	T36.1X2	T36.1X3	T36.1X4	T36.1X5	T36.1X6
Cefoxitin	T36.1X1	T36.1X2	T36.1X3	T36.1X4	T36.1X5	T36.1X6
Cefpimizole	T36.1X1	T36.1X2	T36.1X3	T36.1X4	T36.1X5	T36.1X6
Cefpiramide	T36.1X1	T36.1X2	T36.1X3	T36.1X4	T36.1X5	T36.1X6
Cefradine	T36.1X1	T36.1X2	T36.1X3	T36.1X4	T36.1X5	T36.1X6
Cefroxadine	T36.1X1	T36.1X2	T36.1X3	T36.1X4	T36.1X5	T36.1X6
Cefsulodin	T36.1X1	T36.1X2	T36.1X3	T36.1X4	T36.1X5	T36.1X6
Ceftazidime	T36.1X1	T36.1X2	T36.1X3	T36.1X4	T36.1X5	T36.1X6
Cefteram	T36.1X1	T36.1X2	T36.1X3	T36.1X4	T36.1X5	T36.1X6
Ceftezole	T36.1X1	T36.1X2	T36.1X3	T36.1X4	T36.1X5	T36.1X6
Ceftizoxime	T36.1X1	T36.1X2	T36.1X3	T36.1X4	T36.1X5	T36.1X6
Ceftriaxone	T36.1X1	T36.1X2	T36.1X3	T36.1X4	T36.1X5	T36.1X6
Cefuroxime	T36.1X1	T36.1X2	T36.1X3	T36.1X4	T36.1X5	T36.1X6
Cefuzonam	T36.1X1	T36.1X2	T36.1X3	T36.1X4	T36.1X5	T36.1X6
Celestone	T38.0X1	T38.0X2	T38.0X3	T38.0X4	T38.0X5	T38.0X6
topical	T49.0X1	T49.0X2	T49.0X3	T49.0X4	T49.0X5	T49.0X6
Celiprolol	T44.7X1	T44.7X2	T44.7X3	T44.7X4	T44.7X5	T44.7X6
Cellosolve	T52.91	T52.92	T52.93	T52.94	—	—
Cell stimulants and proliferants	T49.8X1	T49.8X2	T49.8X3	T49.8X4	T49.8X5	T49.8X6
Cellulose						
cathartic	T47.4X1	T47.4X2	T47.4X3	T47.4X4	T47.4X5	T47.4X6
hydroxyethyl	T47.4X1	T47.4X2	T47.4X3	T47.4X4	T47.4X5	T47.4X6
nitrates (topical)	T49.3X1	T49.3X2	T49.3X3	T49.3X4	T49.3X5	T49.3X6
oxidized	T49.4X1	T49.4X2	T49.4X3	T49.4X4	T49.4X5	T49.4X6
Centipede (bite)	T63.411	T63.412	T63.413	T63.414	—	—
Central nervous system						
depressants	T42.71	T42.72	T42.73	T42.74	T42.75	T42.76
anesthetic (general) NEC	T41.201	T41.202	T41.203	T41.204	T41.205	T41.206
gases NEC	T41.0X1	T41.0X2	T41.0X3	T41.0X4	T41.0X5	T41.0X6
intravenous	T41.1X1	T41.1X2	T41.1X3	T41.1X4	T41.1X5	T41.1X6
barbiturates	T42.3X1	T42.3X2	T42.3X3	T42.3X4	T42.3X5	T42.3X6
benzodiazepines	T42.4X1	T42.4X2	T42.4X3	T42.4X4	T42.4X5	T42.4X6
bromides	T42.6X1	T42.6X2	T42.6X3	T42.6X4	T42.6X5	T42.6X6
cannabis sativa	T40.7X1	T40.7X2	T40.7X3	T40.7X4	T40.7X5	T40.7X6
chloral hydrate	T42.6X1	T42.6X2	T42.6X3	T42.6X4	T42.6X5	T42.6X6
ethanol	T51.0X1	T51.0X2	T51.0X3	T51.0X4	—	—
hallucinogenics	T40.901	T40.902	T40.903	T40.904	T40.905	T40.906
hypnotics	T42.71	T42.72	T42.73	T42.74	T42.75	T42.76
specified NEC	T42.6X1	T42.6X2	T42.6X3	T42.6X4	T42.6X5	T42.6X6
muscle relaxants	T42.8X1	T42.8X2	T42.8X3	T42.8X4	T42.8X5	T42.8X6
paraldehyde	T42.6X1	T42.6X2	T42.6X3	T42.6X4	T42.6X5	T42.6X6
sedatives; sedative-hypnotics	T42.71	T42.72	T42.73	T42.74	T42.75	T42.76
mixed NEC	T42.6X1	T42.6X2	T42.6X3	T42.6X4	T42.6X5	T42.6X6
specified NEC	T42.6X1	T42.6X2	T42.6X3	T42.6X4	T42.6X5	T42.6X6
muscle-tone depressants	T42.8X1	T42.8X2	T42.8X3	T42.8X4	T42.8X5	T42.8X6
stimulants	T43.601	T43.602	T43.603	T43.604	T43.605	T43.606
amphetamines	T43.621	T43.622	T43.623	T43.624	T43.625	T43.626
analeptics	T50.7X1	T50.7X2	T50.7X3	T50.7X4	T50.7X5	T50.7X6
antidepressants	T43.201	T43.202	T43.203	T43.204	T43.205	T43.206
opiate antagonists	T50.7X1	T50.7X2	T50.7X3	T50.7X4	T50.7X5	T50.7X6
specified NEC	T43.691	T43.692	T43.693	T43.694	T43.695	T43.696

358

Additional Character May Be Required — Refer to the Tabular List for Character Selection ▽ Subterms under main terms may continue to next column or page

Substance	Poisoning, Accidental (unintentional)	Poisoning, Intentional Self-harm	Poisoning, Assault	Poisoning, Undetermined	Adverse Effect	Under-dosing
Cephalexin	T36.1X1	T36.1X2	T36.1X3	T36.1X4	T36.1X5	T36.1X6
Cephaloglycin	T36.1X1	T36.1X2	T36.1X3	T36.1X4	T36.1X5	T36.1X6
Cephaloridine	T36.1X1	T36.1X2	T36.1X3	T36.1X4	T36.1X5	T36.1X6
Cephalosporins	T36.1X1	T36.1X2	T36.1X3	T36.1X4	T36.1X5	T36.1X6
N (adicillin)	T36.0X1	T36.0X2	T36.0X3	T36.0X4	T36.0X5	T36.0X6
Cephalothin	T36.1X1	T36.1X2	T36.1X3	T36.1X4	T36.1X5	T36.1X6
Cephalotin	T36.1X1	T36.1X2	T36.1X3	T36.1X4	T36.1X5	T36.1X6
Cephradine	T36.1X1	T36.1X2	T36.1X3	T36.1X4	T36.1X5	T36.1X6
Cerbera (odallam)	T62.2X1	T62.2X2	T62.2X3	T62.2X4	—	—
Cerberin	T46.0X1	T46.0X2	T46.0X3	T46.0X4	T46.0X5	T46.0X6
Cerebral stimulants	T43.601	T43.602	T43.603	T43.604	T43.605	T43.606
psychotherapeutic	T43.601	T43.602	T43.603	T43.604	T43.605	T43.606
specified NEC	T43.691	T43.692	T43.693	T43.694	T43.695	T43.696
Cerium oxalate	T45.0X1	T45.0X2	T45.0X3	T45.0X4	T45.0X5	T45.0X6
Cerous oxalate	T45.0X1	T45.0X2	T45.0X3	T45.0X4	T45.0X5	T45.0X6
Ceruletide	T50.8X1	T50.8X2	T50.8X3	T50.8X4	T50.8X5	T50.8X6
Cetalkonium (chloride)	T49.0X1	T49.0X2	T49.0X3	T49.0X4	T49.0X5	T49.0X6
Cethexonium chloride	T49.0X1	T49.0X2	T49.0X3	T49.0X4	T49.0X5	T49.0X6
Cetiedil	T46.7X1	T46.7X2	T46.7X3	T46.7X4	T46.7X5	T46.7X6
Cetirizine	T45.0X1	T45.0X2	T45.0X3	T45.0X4	T45.0X5	T45.0X6
Cetomacrogol	T50.991	T50.992	T50.993	T50.994	T50.995	T50.996
Cetotiamine	T45.2X1	T45.2X2	T45.2X3	T45.2X4	T45.2X5	T45.2X6
Cetoxime	T45.0X1	T45.0X2	T45.0X3	T45.0X4	T45.0X5	T45.0X6
Cetraxate	T47.1X1	T47.1X2	T47.1X3	T47.1X4	T47.1X5	T47.1X6
Cetrimide	T49.0X1	T49.0X2	T49.0X3	T49.0X4	T49.0X5	T49.0X6
Cetrimonium (bromide)	T49.0X1	T49.0X2	T49.0X3	T49.0X4	T49.0X5	T49.0X6
Cetylpyridinium chloride	T49.0X1	T49.0X2	T49.0X3	T49.0X4	T49.0X5	T49.0X6
ENT agent	T49.6X1	T49.6X2	T49.6X3	T49.6X4	T49.6X5	T49.6X6
lozenges	T49.6X1	T49.6X2	T49.6X3	T49.6X4	T49.6X5	T49.6X6
Cevadilla — see Sabadilla						
Cevitamic acid	T45.2X1	T45.2X2	T45.2X3	T45.2X4	T45.2X5	T45.2X6
Chalk, precipitated	T47.1X1	T47.1X2	T47.1X3	T47.1X4	T47.1X5	T47.1X6
Chamomile	T49.0X1	T49.0X2	T49.0X3	T49.0X4	T49.0X5	T49.0X6
Ch'an su	T46.0X1	T46.0X2	T46.0X3	T46.0X4	T46.0X5	T46.0X6
Charcoal	T47.6X1	T47.6X2	T47.6X3	T47.6X4	T47.6X5	T47.6X6
activated — see also Charcoal, medicinal	T47.6X1	T47.6X2	T47.6X3	T47.6X4	T47.6X5	T47.6X6
fumes (Carbon monoxide)	T58.2X1	T58.2X2	T58.2X3	T58.2X4	—	—
industrial	T58.8X1	T58.8X2	T58.8X3	T58.8X4	—	—
medicinal (activated)	T47.6X1	T47.6X2	T47.6X3	T47.6X4	T47.6X5	T47.6X6
antidiarrheal	T47.6X1	T47.6X2	T47.6X3	T47.6X4	T47.6X5	T47.6X6
poison control	T47.8X1	T47.8X2	T47.8X3	T47.8X4	T47.8X5	T47.8X6
specified use other than for diarrhea	T47.8X1	T47.8X2	T47.8X3	T47.8X4	T47.8X5	T47.8X6
topical	T49.8X1	T49.8X2	T49.8X3	T49.8X4	T49.8X5	T49.8X6
Chaulmosulfone	T37.1X1	T37.1X2	T37.1X3	T37.1X4	T37.1X5	T37.1X6
Chelating agent NEC	T50.6X1	T50.6X2	T50.6X3	T50.6X4	T50.6X5	T50.6X6
Chelidonium majus	T62.2X1	T62.2X2	T62.2X3	T62.2X4	—	—
Chemical substance NEC	T65.91	T65.92	T65.93	T65.94	—	—
Chenodeoxycholic acid	T47.5X1	T47.5X2	T47.5X3	T47.5X4	T47.5X5	T47.5X6
Chenodiol	T47.5X1	T47.5X2	T47.5X3	T47.5X4	T47.5X5	T47.5X6
Chenopodium	T37.4X1	T37.4X2	T37.4X3	T37.4X4	T37.4X5	T37.4X6
Cherry laurel	T62.2X1	T62.2X2	T62.2X3	T62.2X4	—	—
Chinidin (e)	T46.2X1	T46.2X2	T46.2X3	T46.2X4	T46.2X5	T46.2X6
Chiniofon	T37.8X1	T37.8X2	T37.8X3	T37.8X4	T37.8X5	T37.8X6
Chlophedianol	T48.3X1	T48.3X2	T48.3X3	T48.3X4	T48.3X5	T48.3X6
Chloral	T42.6X1	T42.6X2	T42.6X3	T42.6X4	T42.6X5	T42.6X6
derivative	T42.6X1	T42.6X2	T42.6X3	T42.6X4	T42.6X5	T42.6X6
hydrate	T42.6X1	T42.6X2	T42.6X3	T42.6X4	T42.6X5	T42.6X6
Chloralamide	T42.6X1	T42.6X2	T42.6X3	T42.6X4	T42.6X5	T42.6X6
Chloralodol	T42.6X1	T42.6X2	T42.6X3	T42.6X4	T42.6X5	T42.6X6
Chloralose	T60.4X1	T60.4X2	T60.4X3	T60.4X4	—	—
Chlorambucil	T45.1X1	T45.1X2	T45.1X3	T45.1X4	T45.1X5	T45.1X6
Chloramine	T57.8X1	T57.8X2	T57.8X3	T57.8X4	—	—
T	T49.0X1	T49.0X2	T49.0X3	T49.0X4	T49.0X5	T49.0X6
topical	T49.0X1	T49.0X2	T49.0X3	T49.0X4	T49.0X5	T49.0X6
Chloramphenicol	T36.2X1	T36.2X2	T36.2X3	T36.2X4	T36.2X5	T36.2X6
ENT agent	T49.6X1	T49.6X2	T49.6X3	T49.6X4	T49.6X5	T49.6X6
ophthalmic preparation	T49.5X1	T49.5X2	T49.5X3	T49.5X4	T49.5X5	T49.5X6
topical NEC	T49.0X1	T49.0X2	T49.0X3	T49.0X4	T49.0X5	T49.0X6
Chlorate (potassium) (sodium) NEC	T60.3X1	T60.3X2	T60.3X3	T60.3X4	—	—
herbicide	T60.3X1	T60.3X2	T60.3X3	T60.3X4	—	—
Chlorazanil	T50.2X1	T50.2X2	T50.2X3	T50.2X4	T50.2X5	T50.2X6
Chlorbenzene, chlorbenzol	T53.7X1	T53.7X2	T53.7X3	T53.7X4	—	—
Chlorbenzoxamine	T44.3X1	T44.3X2	T44.3X3	T44.3X4	T44.3X5	T44.3X6
Chlorbutol	T42.6X1	T42.6X2	T42.6X3	T42.6X4	T42.6X5	T42.6X6
Chlorcyclizine	T45.0X1	T45.0X2	T45.0X3	T45.0X4	T45.0X5	T45.0X6
Chlordan (e) (dust)	T60.1X1	T60.1X2	T60.1X3	T60.1X4	—	—
Chlordantoin	T49.0X1	T49.0X2	T49.0X3	T49.0X4	T49.0X5	T49.0X6
Chlordiazepoxide	T42.4X1	T42.4X2	T42.4X3	T42.4X4	T42.4X5	T42.4X6
Chlordiethyl benzamide	T49.3X1	T49.3X2	T49.3X3	T49.3X4	T49.3X5	T49.3X6
Chloresium	T49.8X1	T49.8X2	T49.8X3	T49.8X4	T49.8X5	T49.8X6

Substance	Poisoning, Accidental (unintentional)	Poisoning, Intentional Self-harm	Poisoning, Assault	Poisoning, Undetermined	Adverse Effect	Under-dosing
Chlorethiazol	T42.6X1	T42.6X2	T42.6X3	T42.6X4	T42.6X5	T42.6X6
Chlorethyl — see Ethyl chloride						
Chloretone	T42.6X1	T42.6X2	T42.6X3	T42.6X4	T42.6X5	T42.6X6
Chlorex	T53.6X1	T53.6X2	T53.6X3	T53.6X4	—	—
insecticide	T60.1X1	T60.1X2	T60.1X3	T60.1X4	—	—
Chlorfenvinphos	T60.0X1	T60.0X2	T60.0X3	T60.0X4	—	—
Chlorhexadol	T42.6X1	T42.6X2	T42.6X3	T42.6X4	T42.6X5	T42.6X6
Chlorhexamide	T45.1X1	T45.1X2	T45.1X3	T45.1X4	T45.1X5	T45.1X6
Chlorhexidine	T49.0X1	T49.0X2	T49.0X3	T49.0X4	T49.0X5	T49.0X6
Chlorhydroxyquinolin	T49.0X1	T49.0X2	T49.0X3	T49.0X4	T49.0X5	T49.0X6
Chloride of lime (bleach)	T54.3X1	T54.3X2	T54.3X3	T54.3X4	—	—
Chlorimipramine	T43.011	T43.012	T43.013	T43.014	T43.015	T43.016
Chlorinated						
camphene	T53.6X1	T53.6X2	T53.6X3	T53.6X4	—	—
diphenyl	T53.7X1	T53.7X2	T53.7X3	T53.7X4	—	—
hydrocarbons NEC	T53.91	T53.92	T53.93	T53.94	—	—
solvents	T53.91	T53.92	T53.93	T53.94	—	—
lime (bleach)	T54.3X1	T54.3X2	T54.3X3	T54.3X4	—	—
and boric acid solution	T49.0X1	T49.0X2	T49.0X3	T49.0X4	T49.0X5	T49.0X6
naphthalene (insecticide)	T60.1X1	T60.1X2	T60.1X3	T60.1X4	—	—
industrial (non-pesticide)	T53.7X1	T53.7X2	T53.7X3	T53.7X4	—	—
pesticide NEC	T60.8X1	T60.8X2	T60.8X3	T60.8X4	—	—
soda — see also sodium hypochlorite						
solution	T49.0X1	T49.0X2	T49.0X3	T49.0X4	T49.0X5	T49.0X6
Chlorine (fumes) (gas)	T59.4X1	T59.4X2	T59.4X3	T59.4X4	—	—
bleach	T54.3X1	T54.3X2	T54.3X3	T54.3X4	—	—
compound gas NEC	T59.4X1	T59.4X2	T59.4X3	T59.4X4	—	—
disinfectant	T59.4X1	T59.4X2	T59.4X3	T59.4X4	—	—
releasing agents NEC	T59.4X1	T59.4X2	T59.4X3	T59.4X4	—	—
Chlorisondamine chloride	T46.991	T46.992	T46.993	T46.994	T46.995	T46.996
Chlormadinone	T38.5X1	T38.5X2	T38.5X3	T38.5X4	T38.5X5	T38.5X6
Chlormephos	T60.0X1	T60.0X2	T60.0X3	T60.0X4	—	—
Chlormerodrin	T50.2X1	T50.2X2	T50.2X3	T50.2X4	T50.2X5	T50.2X6
Chlormethiazole	T42.6X1	T42.6X2	T42.6X3	T42.6X4	T42.6X5	T42.6X6
Chlormethine	T45.1X1	T45.1X2	T45.1X3	T45.1X4	T45.1X5	T45.1X6
Chlormethylenecycline	T36.4X1	T36.4X2	T36.4X3	T36.4X4	T36.4X5	T36.4X6
Chlormezanone	T42.6X1	T42.6X2	T42.6X3	T42.6X4	T42.6X5	T42.6X6
Chloroacetic acid	T60.3X1	T60.3X2	T60.3X3	T60.3X4	—	—
Chloroacetone	T59.3X1	T59.3X2	T59.3X3	T59.3X4	—	—
Chloroacetophenone	T59.3X1	T59.3X2	T59.3X3	T59.3X4	—	—
Chloroaniline	T53.7X1	T53.7X2	T53.7X3	T53.7X4	—	—
Chlorobenzene, chlorobenzol	T53.7X1	T53.7X2	T53.7X3	T53.7X4	—	—
Chlorobromomethane (fire extinguisher)	T53.6X1	T53.6X2	T53.6X3	T53.6X4	—	—
Chlorobutanol	T49.0X1	T49.0X2	T49.0X3	T49.0X4	T49.0X5	T49.0X6
Chlorocresol	T49.0X1	T49.0X2	T49.0X3	T49.0X4	T49.0X5	T49.0X6
Chlorodehydromethyltestosterone	T38.7X1	T38.7X2	T38.7X3	T38.7X4	T38.7X5	T38.7X6
Chlorodinitrobenzene	T53.7X1	T53.7X2	T53.7X3	T53.7X4	—	—
dust or vapor	T53.7X1	T53.7X2	T53.7X3	T53.7X4	—	—
Chlorodiphenyl	T53.7X1	T53.7X2	T53.7X3	T53.7X4	—	—
Chloroethane — see Ethyl chloride						
Chloroethylene	T53.6X1	T53.6X2	T53.6X3	T53.6X4	—	—
Chlorofluorocarbons	T53.5X1	T53.5X2	T53.5X3	T53.5X4	—	—
Chloroform (fumes) (vapor)	T53.1X1	T53.1X2	T53.1X3	T53.1X4	—	—
anesthetic	T41.0X1	T41.0X2	T41.0X3	T41.0X4	T41.0X5	T41.0X6
solvent	T53.1X1	T53.1X2	T53.1X3	T53.1X4	—	—
water, concentrated	T41.0X1	T41.0X2	T41.0X3	T41.0X4	T41.0X5	T41.0X6
Chloroguanide	T37.2X1	T37.2X2	T37.2X3	T37.2X4	T37.2X5	T37.2X6
Chloromycetin	T36.2X1	T36.2X2	T36.2X3	T36.2X4	T36.2X5	T36.2X6
ENT agent	T49.6X1	T49.6X2	T49.6X3	T49.6X4	T49.6X5	T49.6X6
ophthalmic preparation	T49.5X1	T49.5X2	T49.5X3	T49.5X4	T49.5X5	T49.5X6
otic solution	T49.6X1	T49.6X2	T49.6X3	T49.6X4	T49.6X5	T49.6X6
topical NEC	T49.0X1	T49.0X2	T49.0X3	T49.0X4	T49.0X5	T49.0X6
Chloronitrobenzene	T53.7X1	T53.7X2	T53.7X3	T53.7X4	—	—
dust or vapor	T53.7X1	T53.7X2	T53.7X3	T53.7X4	—	—
Chlorophacinone	T60.4X1	T60.4X2	T60.4X3	T60.4X4	—	—
Chlorophenol	T53.7X1	T53.7X2	T53.7X3	T53.7X4	—	—
Chlorophenothane	T60.1X1	T60.1X2	T60.1X3	T60.1X4	—	—
Chlorophyll	T50.991	T50.992	T50.993	T50.994	T50.995	T50.996
Chloropicrin (fumes)	T53.6X1	T53.6X2	T53.6X3	T53.6X4	—	—
fumigant	T60.8X1	T60.8X2	T60.8X3	T60.8X4	—	—
fungicide	T60.3X1	T60.3X2	T60.3X3	T60.3X4	—	—
pesticide	T60.8X1	T60.8X2	T60.8X3	T60.8X4	—	—
Chloroprocaine	T41.3X1	T41.3X2	T41.3X3	T41.3X4	T41.3X5	T41.3X6
infiltration (subcutaneous)	T41.3X1	T41.3X2	T41.3X3	T41.3X4	T41.3X5	T41.3X6
nerve block (peripheral) (plexus)	T41.3X1	T41.3X2	T41.3X3	T41.3X4	T41.3X5	T41.3X6
spinal	T41.3X1	T41.3X2	T41.3X3	T41.3X4	T41.3X5	T41.3X6
Chloroptic	T49.5X1	T49.5X2	T49.5X3	T49.5X4	T49.5X5	T49.5X6
Chloropurine	T45.1X1	T45.1X2	T45.1X3	T45.1X4	T45.1X5	T45.1X6

Table of Drugs and Chemicals

Chloropyramine — Cloponone

Substance	Poisoning, Accidental (unintentional)	Poisoning, Intentional Self-harm	Poisoning, Assault	Poisoning, Undetermined	Adverse Effect	Under-dosing
Chloropyramine	T45.0X1	T45.0X2	T45.0X3	T45.0X4	T45.0X5	T45.0X6
Chloropyrifos	T60.0X1	T60.0X2	T60.0X3	T60.0X4	—	—
Chloropyrilene	T45.0X1	T45.0X2	T45.0X3	T45.0X4	T45.0X5	T45.0X6
Chloroquine	T37.2X1	T37.2X2	T37.2X3	T37.2X4	T37.2X5	T37.2X6
Chlorothalonil	T60.3X1	T60.3X2	T60.3X3	T60.3X4	—	—
Chlorothen	T45.0X1	T45.0X2	T45.0X3	T45.0X4	T45.0X5	T45.0X6
Chlorothiazide	T50.2X1	T50.2X2	T50.2X3	T50.2X4	T50.2X5	T50.2X6
Chlorothymol	T49.4X1	T49.4X2	T49.4X3	T49.4X4	T49.4X5	T49.4X6
Chlorotrianisene	T38.5X1	T38.5X2	T38.5X3	T38.5X4	T38.5X5	T38.5X6
Chlorovinyldichloroarsine, not in war	T57.0X1	T57.0X2	T57.0X3	T57.0X4	—	—
Chloroxine	T49.4X1	T49.4X2	T49.4X3	T49.4X4	T49.4X5	T49.4X6
Chloroxylenol	T49.0X1	T49.0X2	T49.0X3	T49.0X4	T49.0X5	T49.0X6
Chlorphenamine	T45.0X1	T45.0X2	T45.0X3	T45.0X4	T45.0X5	T45.0X6
Chlorphenesin	T42.8X1	T42.8X2	T42.8X3	T42.8X4	T42.8X5	T42.8X6
topical (antifungal)	T49.0X1	T49.0X2	T49.0X3	T49.0X4	T49.0X5	T49.0X6
Chlorpheniramine	T45.0X1	T45.0X2	T45.0X3	T45.0X4	T45.0X5	T45.0X6
Chlorphenoxamine	T45.0X1	T45.0X2	T45.0X3	T45.0X4	T45.0X5	T45.0X6
Chlorphentermine	T50.5X1	T50.5X2	T50.5X3	T50.5X4	T50.5X5	T50.5X6
Chlorprocaine — see Chloroprocaine						
Chlorproguanil	T37.2X1	T37.2X2	T37.2X3	T37.2X4	T37.2X5	T37.2X6
Chlorpromazine	T43.3X1	T43.3X2	T43.3X3	T43.3X4	T43.3X5	T43.3X6
Chlorpropamide	T38.3X1	T38.3X2	T38.3X3	T38.3X4	T38.3X5	T38.3X6
Chlorprothixene	T43.4X1	T43.4X2	T43.4X3	T43.4X4	T43.4X5	T43.4X6
Chlorquinaldol	T49.0X1	T49.0X2	T49.0X3	T49.0X4	T49.0X5	T49.0X6
Chlorquinol	T49.0X1	T49.0X2	T49.0X3	T49.0X4	T49.0X5	T49.0X6
Chlortalidone	T50.2X1	T50.2X2	T50.2X3	T50.2X4	T50.2X5	T50.2X6
Chlortetracycline	T36.4X1	T36.4X2	T36.4X3	T36.4X4	T36.4X5	T36.4X6
Chlorthalidone	T50.2X1	T50.2X2	T50.2X3	T50.2X4	T50.2X5	T50.2X6
Chlorthion	T60.0X1	T60.0X2	T60.0X3	T60.0X4	—	—
Chlorthiophos	T60.0X1	T60.0X2	T60.0X3	T60.0X4	—	—
Chlortrianisene	T38.5X1	T38.5X2	T38.5X3	T38.5X4	T38.5X5	T38.5X6
Chlor-Trimeton	T45.0X1	T45.0X2	T45.0X3	T45.0X4	T45.0X5	T45.0X6
Chlorzoxazone	T42.8X1	T42.8X2	T42.8X3	T42.8X4	T42.8X5	T42.8X6
Choke damp	T59.7X1	T59.7X2	T59.7X3	T59.7X4	—	—
Cholagogues	T47.5X1	T47.5X2	T47.5X3	T47.5X4	T47.5X5	T47.5X6
Cholebrine	T50.8X1	T50.8X2	T50.8X3	T50.8X4	T50.8X5	T50.8X6
Cholecalciferol	T45.2X1	T45.2X2	T45.2X3	T45.2X4	T45.2X5	T45.2X6
Cholecystokinin	T50.8X1	T50.8X2	T50.8X3	T50.8X4	T50.8X5	T50.8X6
Cholera vaccine	T50.A91	T50.A92	T50.A93	T50.A94	T50.A95	T50.A96
Choleretic	T47.5X1	T47.5X2	T47.5X3	T47.5X4	T47.5X5	T47.5X6
Cholesterol-lowering agents	T46.6X1	T46.6X2	T46.6X3	T46.6X4	T46.6X5	T46.6X6
Cholestyramine (resin)	T46.6X1	T46.6X2	T46.6X3	T46.6X4	T46.6X5	T46.6X6
Cholic acid	T47.5X1	T47.5X2	T47.5X3	T47.5X4	T47.5X5	T47.5X6
Choline	T48.6X1	T48.6X2	T48.6X3	T48.6X4	T48.6X5	T48.6X6
chloride	T50.991	T50.992	T50.993	T50.994	T50.995	T50.996
dihydrogen citrate	T50.991	T50.992	T50.993	T50.994	T50.995	T50.996
salicylate	T39.091	T39.092	T39.093	T39.094	T39.095	T39.096
theophyllinate	T48.6X1	T48.6X2	T48.6X3	T48.6X4	T48.6X5	T48.6X6
Cholinergic (drug) NEC	T44.1X1	T44.1X2	T44.1X3	T44.1X4	T44.1X5	T44.1X6
muscle tone enhancer	T44.1X1	T44.1X2	T44.1X3	T44.1X4	T44.1X5	T44.1X6
organophosphorus	T44.0X1	T44.0X2	T44.0X3	T44.0X4	T44.0X5	T44.0X6
insecticide	T60.0X1	T60.0X2	T60.0X3	T60.0X4	—	—
nerve gas	T59.891	T59.892	T59.893	T59.894	—	—
trimethyl ammonium propanediol	T44.1X1	T44.1X2	T44.1X3	T44.1X4	T44.1X5	T44.1X6
Cholinesterase reactivator	T50.6X1	T50.6X2	T50.6X3	T50.6X4	T50.6X5	T50.6X6
Cholografin	T50.8X1	T50.8X2	T50.8X3	T50.8X4	T50.8X5	T50.8X6
Chorionic gonadotropin	T38.891	T38.892	T38.893	T38.894	T38.895	T38.896
Chromate	T56.2X1	T56.2X2	T56.2X3	T56.2X4	—	—
dust or mist	T56.2X1	T56.2X2	T56.2X3	T56.2X4	—	—
lead — see also lead	T56.0X1	T56.0X2	T56.0X3	T56.0X4	—	—
paint	T56.0X1	T56.0X2	T56.0X3	T56.0X4	—	—
Chromic						
acid	T56.2X1	T56.2X2	T56.2X3	T56.2X4	—	—
dust or mist	T56.2X1	T56.2X2	T56.2X3	T56.2X4	—	—
phosphate 32P	T45.1X1	T45.1X2	T45.1X3	T45.1X4	T45.1X5	T45.1X6
Chromium	T56.2X1	T56.2X2	T56.2X3	T56.2X4	—	—
compounds — see Chromate						
sesquioxide	T50.8X1	T50.8X2	T50.8X3	T50.8X4	T50.8X5	T50.8X6
Chromomycin A3	T45.1X1	T45.1X2	T45.1X3	T45.1X4	T45.1X5	T45.1X6
Chromonar	T46.3X1	T46.3X2	T46.3X3	T46.3X4	T46.3X5	T46.3X6
Chromyl chloride	T56.2X1	T56.2X2	T56.2X3	T56.2X4	—	—
Chrysarobin	T49.4X1	T49.4X2	T49.4X3	T49.4X4	T49.4X5	T49.4X6
Chrysazin	T47.2X1	T47.2X2	T47.2X3	T47.2X4	T47.2X5	T47.2X6
Chymar	T45.3X1	T45.3X2	T45.3X3	T45.3X4	T45.3X5	T45.3X6
ophthalmic preparation	T49.5X1	T49.5X2	T49.5X3	T49.5X4	T49.5X5	T49.5X6
Chymopapain	T45.3X1	T45.3X2	T45.3X3	T45.3X4	T45.3X5	T45.3X6
Chymotrypsin	T45.3X1	T45.3X2	T45.3X3	T45.3X4	T45.3X5	T45.3X6
ophthalmic preparation	T49.5X1	T49.5X2	T49.5X3	T49.5X4	T49.5X5	T49.5X6
Cianidanol	T50.991	T50.992	T50.993	T50.994	T50.995	T50.996
Cianopramine	T43.011	T43.012	T43.013	T43.014	T43.015	T43.016
Cibenzoline	T46.2X1	T46.2X2	T46.2X3	T46.2X4	T46.2X5	T46.2X6
Ciclacillin	T36.0X1	T36.0X2	T36.0X3	T36.0X4	T36.0X5	T36.0X6
Ciclobarbital — see Hexobarbital						
Ciclonicate	T46.7X1	T46.7X2	T46.7X3	T46.7X4	T46.7X5	T46.7X6
Ciclopirox (olamine)	T49.0X1	T49.0X2	T49.0X3	T49.0X4	T49.0X5	T49.0X6
Ciclosporin	T45.1X1	T45.1X2	T45.1X3	T45.1X4	T45.1X5	T45.1X6
Cicuta maculata or virosa	T62.2X1	T62.2X2	T62.2X3	T62.2X4	—	—
Cicutoxin	T62.2X1	T62.2X2	T62.2X3	T62.2X4	—	—
Cigarette lighter fluid	T52.0X1	T52.0X2	T52.0X3	T52.0X4	—	—
Cigarettes (tobacco)	T65.221	T65.222	T65.223	T65.224	—	—
Ciguatoxin	T61.01	T61.02	T61.03	T61.04	—	—
Cilazapril	T46.4X1	T46.4X2	T46.4X3	T46.4X4	T46.4X5	T46.4X6
Cimetidine	T47.0X1	T47.0X2	T47.0X3	T47.0X4	T47.0X5	T47.0X6
Cimetropium bromide	T44.3X1	T44.3X2	T44.3X3	T44.3X4	T44.3X5	T44.3X6
Cinchocaine	T41.3X1	T41.3X2	T41.3X3	T41.3X4	T41.3X5	T41.3X6
topical (surface)	T41.3X1	T41.3X2	T41.3X3	T41.3X4	T41.3X5	T41.3X6
Cinchona	T37.2X1	T37.2X2	T37.2X3	T37.2X4	T37.2X5	T37.2X6
Cinchonine alkaloids	T37.2X1	T37.2X2	T37.2X3	T37.2X4	T37.2X5	T37.2X6
Cinchophen	T50.4X1	T50.4X2	T50.4X3	T50.4X4	T50.4X5	T50.4X6
Cinepazide	T46.7X1	T46.7X2	T46.7X3	T46.7X4	T46.7X5	T46.7X6
Cinnamedrine	T48.5X1	T48.5X2	T48.5X3	T48.5X4	T48.5X5	T48.5X6
Cinnarizine	T45.0X1	T45.0X2	T45.0X3	T45.0X4	T45.0X5	T45.0X6
Cinoxacin	T37.8X1	T37.8X2	T37.8X3	T37.8X4	T37.8X5	T37.8X6
Ciprofibrate	T46.6X1	T46.6X2	T46.6X3	T46.6X4	T46.6X5	T46.6X6
Ciprofloxacin	T36.8X1	T36.8X2	T36.8X3	T36.8X4	T36.8X5	T36.8X6
Cisapride	T47.8X1	T47.8X2	T47.8X3	T47.8X4	T47.8X5	T47.8X6
Cisplatin	T45.1X1	T45.1X2	T45.1X3	T45.1X4	T45.1X5	T45.1X6
Citalopram	T43.221	T43.222	T43.223	T43.224	T43.225	T43.226
Citanest	T41.3X1	T41.3X2	T41.3X3	T41.3X4	T41.3X5	T41.3X6
infiltration (subcutaneous)	T41.3X1	T41.3X2	T41.3X3	T41.3X4	T41.3X5	T41.3X6
nerve block (peripheral) (plexus)	T41.3X1	T41.3X2	T41.3X3	T41.3X4	T41.3X5	T41.3X6
Citric acid	T47.5X1	T47.5X2	T47.5X3	T47.5X4	T47.5X5	T47.5X6
Citrovorum (factor)	T45.8X1	T45.8X2	T45.8X3	T45.8X4	T45.8X5	T45.8X6
Claviceps purpurea	T62.2X1	T62.2X2	T62.2X3	T62.2X4	—	—
Clavulanic acid	T36.1X1	T36.1X2	T36.1X3	T36.1X4	T36.1X5	T36.1X6
Cleaner, cleansing agent, type not specified	T65.891	T65.892	T65.893	T65.894	—	—
of paint or varnish	T52.91	T52.92	T52.93	T52.94	—	—
specified type NEC	T65.891	T65.892	T65.893	T65.894	—	—
Clebopride	T47.8X1	T47.8X2	T47.8X3	T47.8X4	T47.8X5	T47.8X6
Clefamide	T37.3X1	T37.3X2	T37.3X3	T37.3X4	T37.3X5	T37.3X6
Clemastine	T45.0X1	T45.0X2	T45.0X3	T45.0X4	T45.0X5	T45.0X6
Clematis vitalba	T62.2X1	T62.2X2	T62.2X3	T62.2X4	—	—
Clemizole	T45.0X1	T45.0X2	T45.0X3	T45.0X4	T45.0X5	T45.0X6
penicillin	T36.0X1	T36.0X2	T36.0X3	T36.0X4	T36.0X5	T36.0X6
Clenbuterol	T48.6X1	T48.6X2	T48.6X3	T48.6X4	T48.6X5	T48.6X6
Clidinium bromide	T44.3X1	T44.3X2	T44.3X3	T44.3X4	T44.3X5	T44.3X6
Clindamycin	T36.8X1	T36.8X2	T36.8X3	T36.8X4	T36.8X5	T36.8X6
Clinofibrate	T46.6X1	T46.6X2	T46.6X3	T46.6X4	T46.6X5	T46.6X6
Clioquinol	T37.8X1	T37.8X2	T37.8X3	T37.8X4	T37.8X5	T37.8X6
Cliradon	T40.2X1	T40.2X2	T40.2X3	T40.2X4	—	—
Clobazam	T42.4X1	T42.4X2	T42.4X3	T42.4X4	T42.4X5	T42.4X6
Clobenzorex	T50.5X1	T50.5X2	T50.5X3	T50.5X4	T50.5X5	T50.5X6
Clobetasol	T49.0X1	T49.0X2	T49.0X3	T49.0X4	T49.0X5	T49.0X6
Clobetasone	T49.0X1	T49.0X2	T49.0X3	T49.0X4	T49.0X5	T49.0X6
Clobutinol	T48.3X1	T48.3X2	T48.3X3	T48.3X4	T48.3X5	T48.3X6
Clocortolone	T38.0X1	T38.0X2	T38.0X3	T38.0X4	T38.0X5	T38.0X6
Clodantoin	T49.0X1	T49.0X2	T49.0X3	T49.0X4	T49.0X5	T49.0X6
Clodronic acid	T50.991	T50.992	T50.993	T50.994	T50.995	T50.996
Clofazimine	T37.1X1	T37.1X2	T37.1X3	T37.1X4	T37.1X5	T37.1X6
Clofedanol	T48.3X1	T48.3X2	T48.3X3	T48.3X4	T48.3X5	T48.3X6
Clofenamide	T50.2X1	T50.2X2	T50.2X3	T50.2X4	T50.2X5	T50.2X6
Clofenotane	T49.0X1	T49.0X2	T49.0X3	T49.0X4	T49.0X5	T49.0X6
Clofezone	T39.2X1	T39.2X2	T39.2X3	T39.2X4	T39.2X5	T39.2X6
Clofibrate	T46.6X1	T46.6X2	T46.6X3	T46.6X4	T46.6X5	T46.6X6
Clofibride	T46.6X1	T46.6X2	T46.6X3	T46.6X4	T46.6X5	T46.6X6
Cloforex	T50.5X1	T50.5X2	T50.5X3	T50.5X4	T50.5X5	T50.5X6
Clomethiazole	T42.6X1	T42.6X2	T42.6X3	T42.6X4	T42.6X5	T42.6X6
Clometocillin	T36.0X1	T36.0X2	T36.0X3	T36.0X4	T36.0X5	T36.0X6
Clomifene	T38.5X1	T38.5X2	T38.5X3	T38.5X4	T38.5X5	T38.5X6
Clomiphene	T38.5X1	T38.5X2	T38.5X3	T38.5X4	T38.5X5	T38.5X6
Clomipramine	T43.011	T43.012	T43.013	T43.014	T43.015	T43.016
Clomocycline	T36.4X1	T36.4X2	T36.4X3	T36.4X4	T36.4X5	T36.4X6
Clonazepam	T42.4X1	T42.4X2	T42.4X3	T42.4X4	T42.4X5	T42.4X6
Clonidine	T46.5X1	T46.5X2	T46.5X3	T46.5X4	T46.5X5	T46.5X6
Clonixin	T39.8X1	T39.8X2	T39.8X3	T39.8X4	T39.8X5	T39.8X6
Clopamide	T50.2X1	T50.2X2	T50.2X3	T50.2X4	T50.2X5	T50.2X6
Clopenthixol	T43.4X1	T43.4X2	T43.4X3	T43.4X4	T43.4X5	T43.4X6
Cloperastine	T48.3X1	T48.3X2	T48.3X3	T48.3X4	T48.3X5	T48.3X6
Clophedianol	T48.3X1	T48.3X2	T48.3X3	T48.3X4	T48.3X5	T48.3X6
Cloponone	T36.2X1	T36.2X2	T36.2X3	T36.2X4	T36.2X5	T36.2X6

Additional Character May Be Required — Refer to the Tabular List for Character Selection

▽ Subterms under main terms may continue to next column or page

Substance	Poisoning, Accidental (unintentional)	Poisoning, Intentional Self-harm	Poisoning, Assault	Poisoning, Undetermined	Adverse Effect	Under-dosing
Cloprednol	T38.0X1	T38.0X2	T38.0X3	T38.0X4	T38.0X5	T38.0X6
Cloral betaine	T42.6X1	T42.6X2	T42.6X3	T42.6X4	T42.6X5	T42.6X6
Cloramfenicol	T36.2X1	T36.2X2	T36.2X3	T36.2X4	T36.2X5	T36.2X6
Clorazepate (dipotassium)	T42.4X1	T42.4X2	T42.4X3	T42.4X4	T42.4X5	T42.4X6
Clorexolone	T50.2X1	T50.2X2	T50.2X3	T50.2X4	T50.2X5	T50.2X6
Clorfenamine	T45.0X1	T45.0X2	T45.0X3	T45.0X4	T45.0X5	T45.0X6
Clorgiline	T43.1X1	T43.1X2	T43.1X3	T43.1X4	T43.1X5	T43.1X6
Clorotepine	T44.3X1	T44.3X2	T44.3X3	T44.3X4	T44.3X5	T44.3X6
Clorox (bleach)	T54.91	T54.92	T54.93	T54.94	—	—
Clorprenaline	T48.6X1	T48.6X2	T48.6X3	T48.6X4	T48.6X5	T48.6X6
Clortermine	T50.5X1	T50.5X2	T50.5X3	T50.5X4	T50.5X5	T50.5X6
Clotiapine	T43.591	T43.592	T43.593	T43.594	T43.595	T43.596
Clotiazepam	T42.4X1	T42.4X2	T42.4X3	T42.4X4	T42.4X5	T42.4X6
Clotibric acid	T46.6X1	T46.6X2	T46.6X3	T46.6X4	T46.6X5	T46.6X6
Clotrimazole	T49.0X1	T49.0X2	T49.0X3	T49.0X4	T49.0X5	T49.0X6
Cloxacillin	T36.0X1	T36.0X2	T36.0X3	T36.0X4	T36.0X5	T36.0X6
Cloxazolam	T42.4X1	T42.4X2	T42.4X3	T42.4X4	T42.4X5	T42.4X6
Cloxiquine	T49.0X1	T49.0X2	T49.0X3	T49.0X4	T49.0X5	T49.0X6
Clozapine	T42.4X1	T42.4X2	T42.4X3	T42.4X4	T42.4X5	T42.4X6
Coagulant NEC	T45.7X1	T45.7X2	T45.7X3	T45.7X4	T45.7X5	T45.7X6
Coal (carbon monoxide from) —	T58.2X1	T58.2X2	T58.2X3	T58.2X4	—	—
see also Carbon, monoxide,						
coal						
oil — *see* Kerosene						
tar	T49.1X1	T49.1X2	T49.1X3	T49.1X4	T49.1X5	T49.1X6
fumes	T59.891	T59.892	T59.893	T59.894	—	—
medicinal (ointment)	T49.4X1	T49.4X2	T49.4X3	T49.4X4	T49.4X5	T49.4X6
analgesics NEC	T39.2X1	T39.2X2	T39.2X3	T39.2X4	T39.2X5	T39.2X6
naphtha (solvent)	T52.0X1	T52.0X2	T52.0X3	T52.0X4	—	—
Cobalamine	T45.2X1	T45.2X2	T45.2X3	T45.2X4	T45.2X5	T45.2X6
Cobalt (nonmedicinal) (fumes)	T56.891	T56.892	T56.893	T56.894	—	—
(industrial)						
medicinal (trace) (chloride)	T45.8X1	T45.8X2	T45.8X3	T45.8X4	T45.8X5	T45.8X6
Cobra (venom)	T63.041	T63.042	T63.043	T63.044	—	—
Coca (leaf)	T40.5X1	T40.5X2	T40.5X3	T40.5X4	T40.5X5	T40.5X6
Cocaine	T40.5X1	T40.5X2	T40.5X3	T40.5X4	T40.5X5	T40.5X6
topical anesthetic	T41.3X1	T41.3X2	T41.3X3	T41.3X4	T41.3X5	T41.3X6
Cocarboxylase	T45.3X1	T45.3X2	T45.3X3	T45.3X4	T45.3X5	T45.3X6
Coccidioidin	T50.8X1	T50.8X2	T50.8X3	T50.8X4	T50.8X5	T50.8X6
Cocculus indicus	T62.1X1	T62.1X2	T62.1X3	T62.1X4	—	—
Cochineal	T65.6X1	T65.6X2	T65.6X3	T65.6X4	—	—
medicinal products	T50.991	T50.992	T50.993	T50.994	T50.995	T50.996
Codeine	T40.2X1	T40.2X2	T40.2X3	T40.2X4	T40.2X5	T40.2X6
Cod-liver oil	T45.2X1	T45.2X2	T45.2X3	T45.2X4	T45.2X5	T45.2X6
Coenzyme A	T50.991	T50.992	T50.993	T50.994	T50.995	T50.996
Coffee	T62.8X1	T62.8X2	T62.8X3	T62.8X4	—	—
Cogalactoisomerase	T50.991	T50.992	T50.993	T50.994	T50.995	T50.996
Cogentin	T44.3X1	T44.3X2	T44.3X3	T44.3X4	T44.3X5	T44.3X6
Coke fumes or gas (carbon	T58.2X1	T58.2X2	T58.2X3	T58.2X4	—	—
monoxide)						
industrial use	T58.8X1	T58.8X2	T58.8X3	T58.8X4	—	—
Colace	T47.4X1	T47.4X2	T47.4X3	T47.4X4	T47.4X5	T47.4X6
Colaspase	T45.1X1	T45.1X2	T45.1X3	T45.1X4	T45.1X5	T45.1X6
Colchicine	T50.4X1	T50.4X2	T50.4X3	T50.4X4	T50.4X5	T50.4X6
Colchicum	T62.2X1	T62.2X2	T62.2X3	T62.2X4	—	—
Cold cream	T49.3X1	T49.3X2	T49.3X3	T49.3X4	T49.3X5	T49.3X6
Colecalciferol	T45.2X1	T45.2X2	T45.2X3	T45.2X4	T45.2X5	T45.2X6
Colestipol	T46.6X1	T46.6X2	T46.6X3	T46.6X4	T46.6X5	T46.6X6
Colestyramine	T46.6X1	T46.6X2	T46.6X3	T46.6X4	T46.6X5	T46.6X6
Colimycin	T36.8X1	T36.8X2	T36.8X3	T36.8X4	T36.8X5	T36.8X6
Colistimethate	T36.8X1	T36.8X2	T36.8X3	T36.8X4	T36.8X5	T36.8X6
Colistin	T36.8X1	T36.8X2	T36.8X3	T36.8X4	T36.8X5	T36.8X6
sulfate (eye preparation)	T49.5X1	T49.5X2	T49.5X3	T49.5X4	T49.5X5	T49.5X6
Collagen	T50.991	T50.992	T50.993	T50.994	T50.995	T50.996
Collagenase	T49.4X1	T49.4X2	T49.4X3	T49.4X4	T49.4X5	T49.4X6
Collodion	T49.3X1	T49.3X2	T49.3X3	T49.3X4	T49.3X5	T49.3X6
Colocynth	T47.2X1	T47.2X2	T47.2X3	T47.2X4	T47.2X5	T47.2X6
Colophony adhesive	T49.3X1	T49.3X2	T49.3X3	T49.3X4	T49.3X5	T49.3X6
Colorant — *see also* Dye	T50.991	T50.992	T50.993	T50.994	T50.995	T50.996
Coloring matter — *see* Dye(s)						
Combustion gas (after						
combustion) — *see* Carbon,						
monoxide						
prior to combustion	T59.891	T59.892	T59.893	T59.894	—	—
Compazine	T43.3X1	T43.3X2	T43.3X3	T43.3X4	T43.3X5	T43.3X6
Compound						
42 (warfarin)	T60.4X1	T60.4X2	T60.4X3	T60.4X4	—	—
269 (endrin)	T60.1X1	T60.1X2	T60.1X3	T60.1X4	—	—
497 (dieldrin)	T60.1X1	T60.1X2	T60.1X3	T60.1X4	—	—
1080 (sodium	T60.4X1	T60.4X2	T60.4X3	T60.4X4	—	—
fluoroacetate)						
3422 (parathion)	T60.0X1	T60.0X2	T60.0X3	T60.0X4	—	—
3911 (phorate)	T60.0X1	T60.0X2	T60.0X3	T60.0X4	—	—
Compound — *continued*						
3956 (toxaphene)	T60.1X1	T60.1X2	T60.1X3	T60.1X4	—	—
4049 (malathion)	T60.0X1	T60.0X2	T60.0X3	T60.0X4	—	—
4069 (malathion)	T60.0X1	T60.0X2	T60.0X3	T60.0X4	—	—
4124 (dicapthon)	T60.0X1	T60.0X2	T60.0X3	T60.0X4	—	—
E (cortisone)	T38.0X1	T38.0X2	T38.0X3	T38.0X4	T38.0X5	T38.0X6
F (hydrocortisone)	T38.0X1	T38.0X2	T38.0X3	T38.0X4	T38.0X5	T38.0X6
Congener, anabolic	T38.7X1	T38.7X2	T38.7X3	T38.7X4	T38.7X5	T38.7X6
Congo red	T50.8X1	T50.8X2	T50.8X3	T50.8X4	T50.8X5	T50.8X6
Coniine, conine	T62.2X1	T62.2X2	T62.2X3	T62.2X4	—	—
Conium (maculatum)	T62.2X1	T62.2X2	T62.2X3	T62.2X4	—	—
Conjugated estrogenic	T38.5X1	T38.5X2	T38.5X3	T38.5X4	T38.5X5	T38.5X6
substances						
Contac	T48.5X1	T48.5X2	T48.5X3	T48.5X4	T48.5X5	T48.5X6
Contact lens solution	T49.5X1	T49.5X2	T49.5X3	T49.5X4	T49.5X5	T49.5X6
Contraceptive (oral)	T38.4X1	T38.4X2	T38.4X3	T38.4X4	T38.4X5	T38.4X6
vaginal	T49.8X1	T49.8X2	T49.8X3	T49.8X4	T49.8X5	T49.8X6
Contrast medium,	T50.8X1	T50.8X2	T50.8X3	T50.8X4	T50.8X5	T50.8X6
radiography						
Convallaria glycosides	T46.0X1	T46.0X2	T46.0X3	T46.0X4	T46.0X5	T46.0X6
Convallaria majalis	T62.2X1	T62.2X2	T62.2X3	T62.2X4	—	—
berry	T62.1X1	T62.1X2	T62.1X3	T62.1X4	—	—
Copperhead snake (bite)	T63.061	T63.062	T63.063	T63.064	—	—
(venom)						
Copper (dust) (fumes)	T56.4X1	T56.4X2	T56.4X3	T56.4X4	—	—
(nonmedicinal) NEC						
arsenate, arsenite	T57.0X1	T57.0X2	T57.0X3	T57.0X4	—	—
insecticide	T60.2X1	T60.2X2	T60.2X3	T60.2X4	—	—
emetic	T47.7X1	T47.7X2	T47.7X3	T47.7X4	T47.7X5	T47.7X6
fungicide	T60.3X1	T60.3X2	T60.3X3	T60.3X4	—	—
gluconate	T49.0X1	T49.0X2	T49.0X3	T49.0X4	T49.0X5	T49.0X6
insecticide	T60.2X1	T60.2X2	T60.2X3	T60.2X4	—	—
medicinal (trace)	T45.8X1	T45.8X2	T45.8X3	T45.8X4	T45.8X5	T45.8X6
oleate	T49.0X1	T49.0X2	T49.0X3	T49.0X4	T49.0X5	T49.0X6
sulfate	T56.4X1	T56.4X2	T56.4X3	T56.4X4	—	—
cupric	T56.4X1	T56.4X2	T56.4X3	T56.4X4	—	—
fungicide	T60.3X1	T60.3X2	T60.3X3	T60.3X4	—	—
medicinal						
ear	T49.6X1	T49.6X2	T49.6X3	T49.6X4	T49.6X5	T49.6X6
emetic	T47.7X1	T47.7X2	T47.7X3	T47.7X4	T47.7X5	T47.7X6
eye	T49.5X1	T49.5X2	T49.5X3	T49.5X4	T49.5X5	T49.5X6
cuprous	T56.4X1	T56.4X2	T56.4X3	T56.4X4	—	—
fungicide	T60.3X1	T60.3X2	T60.3X3	T60.3X4	—	—
medicinal						
ear	T49.6X1	T49.6X2	T49.6X3	T49.6X4	T49.6X5	T49.6X6
emetic	T47.7X1	T47.7X2	T47.7X3	T47.7X4	T47.7X5	T47.7X6
eye	T49.5X1	T49.5X2	T49.5X3	T49.5X4	T49.5X5	T49.5X6
Coral (sting)	T63.691	T63.692	T63.693	T63.694	—	—
snake (bite) (venom)	T63.021	T63.022	T63.023	T63.024	—	—
Corbadrine	T49.6X1	T49.6X2	T49.6X3	T49.6X4	T49.6X5	T49.6X6
Cordite	T65.891	T65.892	T65.893	T65.894	—	—
vapor	T59.891	T59.892	T59.893	T59.894	—	—
Cordran	T49.0X1	T49.0X2	T49.0X3	T49.0X4	T49.0X5	T49.0X6
Corn cures	T49.4X1	T49.4X2	T49.4X3	T49.4X4	T49.4X5	T49.4X6
Cornhusker's lotion	T49.3X1	T49.3X2	T49.3X3	T49.3X4	T49.3X5	T49.3X6
Corn starch	T49.3X1	T49.3X2	T49.3X3	T49.3X4	T49.3X5	T49.3X6
Coronary vasodilator NEC	T46.3X1	T46.3X2	T46.3X3	T46.3X4	T46.3X5	T46.3X6
Corrosive NEC	T54.91	T54.92	T54.93	T54.94	—	—
acid NEC	T54.2X1	T54.2X2	T54.2X3	T54.2X4	—	—
aromatics	T54.1X1	T54.1X2	T54.1X3	T54.1X4	—	—
disinfectant	T54.1X1	T54.1X2	T54.1X3	T54.1X4	—	—
fumes NEC	T54.91	T54.92	T54.93	T54.94	—	—
specified NEC	T54.91	T54.92	T54.93	T54.94	—	—
sublimate	T56.1X1	T56.1X2	T56.1X3	T56.1X4	—	—
Cortate	T38.0X1	T38.0X2	T38.0X3	T38.0X4	T38.0X5	T38.0X6
Cort-Dome	T38.0X1	T38.0X2	T38.0X3	T38.0X4	T38.0X5	T38.0X6
ENT agent	T49.6X1	T49.6X2	T49.6X3	T49.6X4	T49.6X5	T49.6X6
ophthalmic preparation	T49.5X1	T49.5X2	T49.5X3	T49.5X4	T49.5X5	T49.5X6
topical NEC	T49.0X1	T49.0X2	T49.0X3	T49.0X4	T49.0X5	T49.0X6
Cortef	T38.0X1	T38.0X2	T38.0X3	T38.0X4	T38.0X5	T38.0X6
ENT agent	T49.6X1	T49.6X2	T49.6X3	T49.6X4	T49.6X5	T49.6X6
ophthalmic preparation	T49.5X1	T49.5X2	T49.5X3	T49.5X4	T49.5X5	T49.5X6
topical NEC	T49.0X1	T49.0X2	T49.0X3	T49.0X4	T49.0X5	T49.0X6
Corticosteroid	T38.0X1	T38.0X2	T38.0X3	T38.0X4	T38.0X5	T38.0X6
ENT agent	T49.6X1	T49.6X2	T49.6X3	T49.6X4	T49.6X5	T49.6X6
mineral	T50.0X1	T50.0X2	T50.0X3	T50.0X4	T50.0X5	T50.0X6
ophthalmic	T49.5X1	T49.5X2	T49.5X3	T49.5X4	T49.5X5	T49.5X6
topical NEC	T49.0X1	T49.0X2	T49.0X3	T49.0X4	T49.0X5	T49.0X6
Corticotropin	T38.811	T38.812	T38.813	T38.814	T38.815	T38.816
Cortisol	T49.0X1	T49.0X2	T49.0X3	T49.0X4	T49.0X5	T49.0X6
ENT agent	T49.6X1	T49.6X2	T49.6X3	T49.6X4	T49.6X5	T49.6X6
ophthalmic preparation	T49.5X1	T49.5X2	T49.5X3	T49.5X4	T49.5X5	T49.5X6
topical NEC	T49.0X1	T49.0X2	T49.0X3	T49.0X4	T49.0X5	T49.0X6

Substance	Poisoning, Accidental (unintentional)	Poisoning, Intentional Self-harm	Poisoning, Assault	Poisoning, Undetermined	Adverse Effect	Underdosing
Cortisone (acetate)	T38.0X1	T38.0X2	T38.0X3	T38.0X4	T38.0X5	T38.0X6
ENT agent	T49.6X1	T49.6X2	T49.6X3	T49.6X4	T49.6X5	T49.6X6
ophthalmic preparation	T49.5X1	T49.5X2	T49.5X3	T49.5X4	T49.5X5	T49.5X6
topical NEC	T49.0X1	T49.0X2	T49.0X3	T49.0X4	T49.0X5	T49.0X6
Cortivazol	T38.0X1	T38.0X2	T38.0X3	T38.0X4	T38.0X5	T38.0X6
Cortogen	T38.0X1	T38.0X2	T38.0X3	T38.0X4	T38.0X5	T38.0X6
ENT agent	T49.6X1	T49.6X2	T49.6X3	T49.6X4	T49.6X5	T49.6X6
ophthalmic preparation	T49.5X1	T49.5X2	T49.5X3	T49.5X4	T49.5X5	T49.5X6
Cortone	T38.0X1	T38.0X2	T38.0X3	T38.0X4	T38.0X5	T38.0X6
ENT agent	T49.6X1	T49.6X2	T49.6X3	T49.6X4	T49.6X5	T49.6X6
ophthalmic preparation	T49.5X1	T49.5X2	T49.5X3	T49.5X4	T49.5X5	T49.5X6
Cortril	T38.0X1	T38.0X2	T38.0X3	T38.0X4	T38.0X5	T38.0X6
ENT agent	T49.6X1	T49.6X2	T49.6X3	T49.6X4	T49.6X5	T49.6X6
ophthalmic preparation	T49.5X1	T49.5X2	T49.5X3	T49.5X4	T49.5X5	T49.5X6
topical NEC	T49.0X1	T49.0X2	T49.0X3	T49.0X4	T49.0X5	T49.0X6
Corynebacterium parvum	T45.1X1	T45.1X2	T45.1X3	T45.1X4	T45.1X5	T45.1X6
Cosmetic preparation	T49.8X1	T49.8X2	T49.8X3	T49.8X4	T49.8X5	T49.8X6
Cosmetics	T49.8X1	T49.8X2	T49.8X3	T49.8X4	T49.8X5	T49.8X6
Cosyntropin	T38.811	T38.812	T38.813	T38.814	T38.815	T38.816
Cotarnine	T45.7X1	T45.7X2	T45.7X3	T45.7X4	T45.7X5	T45.7X6
Co-trimoxazole	T36.8X1	T36.8X2	T36.8X3	T36.8X4	T36.8X5	T36.8X6
Cottonseed oil	T49.3X1	T49.3X2	T49.3X3	T49.3X4	T49.3X5	T49.3X6
Cough mixture (syrup)	T48.4X1	T48.4X2	T48.4X3	T48.4X4	T48.4X5	T48.4X6
containing opiates	T40.2X1	T40.2X2	T40.2X3	T40.2X4	T40.2X5	T40.2X6
expectorants	T48.4X1	T48.4X2	T48.4X3	T48.4X4	T48.4X5	T48.4X6
Coumadin	T45.511	T45.512	T45.513	T45.514	T45.515	T45.516
rodenticide	T60.4X1	T60.4X2	T60.4X3	T60.4X4	—	—
Coumaphos	T60.0X1	T60.0X2	T60.0X3	T60.0X4	—	—
Coumarin	T45.511	T45.512	T45.513	T45.514	T45.515	T45.516
Coumetarol	T45.511	T45.512	T45.513	T45.514	T45.515	T45.516
Cowbane	T62.2X1	T62.2X2	T62.2X3	T62.2X4	—	—
Cozyme	T45.2X1	T45.2X2	T45.2X3	T45.2X4	T45.2X5	T45.2X6
Crack	T40.5X1	T40.5X2	T40.5X3	T40.5X4	—	—
Crataegus extract	T46.0X1	T46.0X2	T46.0X3	T46.0X4	T46.0X5	T46.0X6
Creolin	T54.1X1	T54.1X2	T54.1X3	T54.1X4	—	—
disinfectant	T54.1X1	T54.1X2	T54.1X3	T54.1X4	—	—
Creosol (compound)	T49.0X1	T49.0X2	T49.0X3	T49.0X4	T49.0X5	T49.0X6
Creosote (coal tar)	T49.0X1	T49.0X2	T49.0X3	T49.0X4	T49.0X5	T49.0X6
(beechwood)						
medicinal (expectorant)	T48.4X1	T48.4X2	T48.4X3	T48.4X4	T48.4X5	T48.4X6
syrup	T48.4X1	T48.4X2	T48.4X3	T48.4X4	T48.4X5	T48.4X6
Cresol(s)	T49.0X1	T49.0X2	T49.0X3	T49.0X4	T49.0X5	T49.0X6
and soap solution	T49.0X1	T49.0X2	T49.0X3	T49.0X4	T49.0X5	T49.0X6
Cresyl acetate	T49.0X1	T49.0X2	T49.0X3	T49.0X4	T49.0X5	T49.0X6
Cresylic acid	T49.0X1	T49.0X2	T49.0X3	T49.0X4	T49.0X5	T49.0X6
Crimidine	T60.4X1	T60.4X2	T60.4X3	T60.4X4	—	—
Croconazole	T37.8X1	T37.8X2	T37.8X3	T37.8X4	T37.8X5	T37.8X6
Cromoglicic acid	T48.6X1	T48.6X2	T48.6X3	T48.6X4	T48.6X5	T48.6X6
Cromolyn	T48.6X1	T48.6X2	T48.6X3	T48.6X4	T48.6X5	T48.6X6
Cromonar	T46.3X1	T46.3X2	T46.3X3	T46.3X4	T46.3X5	T46.3X6
Cropropamide	T39.8X1	T39.8X2	T39.8X3	T39.8X4	T39.8X5	T39.8X6
with crotethamide	T50.7X1	T50.7X2	T50.7X3	T50.7X4	T50.7X5	T50.7X6
Crotamiton	T49.0X1	T49.0X2	T49.0X3	T49.0X4	T49.0X5	T49.0X6
Crotethamide	T39.8X1	T39.8X2	T39.8X3	T39.8X4	T39.8X5	T39.8X6
with cropropamide	T50.7X1	T50.7X2	T50.7X3	T50.7X4	T50.7X5	T50.7X6
Croton (oil)	T47.2X1	T47.2X2	T47.2X3	T47.2X4	T47.2X5	T47.2X6
chloral	T42.6X1	T42.6X2	T42.6X3	T42.6X4	T42.6X5	T42.6X6
Crude oil	T52.0X1	T52.0X2	T52.0X3	T52.0X4	—	—
Cryogenine	T39.8X1	T39.8X2	T39.8X3	T39.8X4	T39.8X5	T39.8X6
Cryolite (vapor)	T60.1X1	T60.1X2	T60.1X3	T60.1X4	—	—
insecticide	T60.1X1	T60.1X2	T60.1X3	T60.1X4	—	—
Cryptenamine (tannates)	T46.5X1	T46.5X2	T46.5X3	T46.5X4	T46.5X5	T46.5X6
Crystal violet	T49.0X1	T49.0X2	T49.0X3	T49.0X4	T49.0X5	T49.0X6
Cuckoopint	T62.2X1	T62.2X2	T62.2X3	T62.2X4	—	—
Cumetharol	T45.511	T45.512	T45.513	T45.514	T45.515	T45.516
Cupric						
acetate	T60.3X1	T60.3X2	T60.3X3	T60.3X4	—	—
acetoarsenite	T57.0X1	T57.0X2	T57.0X3	T57.0X4	—	—
arsenate	T57.0X1	T57.0X2	T57.0X3	T57.0X4	—	—
gluconate	T49.0X1	T49.0X2	T49.0X3	T49.0X4	T49.0X5	T49.0X6
oleate	T49.0X1	T49.0X2	T49.0X3	T49.0X4	T49.0X5	T49.0X6
sulfate	T56.4X1	T56.4X2	T56.4X3	T56.4X4	—	—
Cuprous sulfate — *see also*	T56.4X1	T56.4X2	T56.4X3	T56.4X4	—	—
Copper sulfate						
Curare, curarine	T48.1X1	T48.1X2	T48.1X3	T48.1X4	T48.1X5	T48.1X6
Cyamemazine	T43.3X1	T43.3X2	T43.3X3	T43.3X4	T43.3X5	T43.3X6
Cyamopsis tetragonoloba	T46.6X1	T46.6X2	T46.6X3	T46.6X4	T46.6X5	T46.6X6
Cyanacetyl hydrazide	T37.1X1	T37.1X2	T37.1X3	T37.1X4	T37.1X5	T37.1X6
Cyanic acid (gas)	T59.891	T59.892	T59.893	T59.894	—	—
Cyanide(s) (compounds)	T65.0X1	T65.0X2	T65.0X3	T65.0X4	—	—
(potassium) (sodium)						
NEC						
dust or gas (inhalation) NEC	T57.3X1	T57.3X2	T57.3X3	T57.3X4	—	—

Substance	Poisoning, Accidental (unintentional)	Poisoning, Intentional Self-harm	Poisoning, Assault	Poisoning, Undetermined	Adverse Effect	Underdosing
Cyanide(s) (compounds) (potassium) (sodium) NEC — *continued*						
fumigant	T65.0X1	T65.0X2	T65.0X3	T65.0X4	—	—
hydrogen	T57.3X1	T57.3X2	T57.3X3	T57.3X4	—	—
mercuric — *see* Mercury						
pesticide (dust) (fumes)	T65.0X1	T65.0X2	T65.0X3	T65.0X4	—	—
Cyanoacrylate adhesive	T49.3X1	T49.3X2	T49.3X3	T49.3X4	T49.3X5	T49.3X6
Cyanocobalamin	T45.8X1	T45.8X2	T45.8X3	T45.8X4	T45.8X5	T45.8X6
Cyanogen (chloride) (gas) NEC	T59.891	T59.892	T59.893	T59.894	—	—
Cyclacillin	T36.0X1	T36.0X2	T36.0X3	T36.0X4	T36.0X5	T36.0X6
Cyclaine	T41.3X1	T41.3X2	T41.3X3	T41.3X4	T41.3X5	T41.3X6
Cyclamate	T50.991	T50.992	T50.993	T50.994	T50.995	T50.996
Cyclamen europaeum	T62.2X1	T62.2X2	T62.2X3	T62.2X4	—	—
Cyclandelate	T46.7X1	T46.7X2	T46.7X3	T46.7X4	T46.7X5	T46.7X6
Cyclazocine	T50.7X1	T50.7X2	T50.7X3	T50.7X4	T50.7X5	T50.7X6
Cyclizine	T45.0X1	T45.0X2	T45.0X3	T45.0X4	T45.0X5	T45.0X6
Cyclobarbital	T42.3X1	T42.3X2	T42.3X3	T42.3X4	T42.3X5	T42.3X6
Cyclobarbitone	T42.3X1	T42.3X2	T42.3X3	T42.3X4	T42.3X5	T42.3X6
Cyclobenzaprine	T48.1X1	T48.1X2	T48.1X3	T48.1X4	T48.1X5	T48.1X6
Cyclodrine	T44.3X1	T44.3X2	T44.3X3	T44.3X4	T44.3X5	T44.3X6
Cycloguanil embonate	T37.2X1	T37.2X2	T37.2X3	T37.2X4	T37.2X5	T37.2X6
Cyclohexane	T52.8X1	T52.8X2	T52.8X3	T52.8X4	—	—
Cyclohexanol	T51.8X1	T51.8X2	T51.8X3	T51.8X4	—	—
Cyclohexanone	T52.4X1	T52.4X2	T52.4X3	T52.4X4	—	—
Cycloheximide	T60.3X1	T60.3X2	T60.3X3	T60.3X4	—	—
Cyclohexyl acetate	T52.8X1	T52.8X2	T52.8X3	T52.8X4	—	—
Cycloleucin	T45.1X1	T45.1X2	T45.1X3	T45.1X4	T45.1X5	T45.1X6
Cyclomethycaine	T41.3X1	T41.3X2	T41.3X3	T41.3X4	T41.3X5	T41.3X6
Cyclopentamine	T44.4X1	T44.4X2	T44.4X3	T44.4X4	T44.4X5	T44.4X6
Cyclopenthiazide	T50.2X1	T50.2X2	T50.2X3	T50.2X4	T50.2X5	T50.2X6
Cyclopentolate	T44.3X1	T44.3X2	T44.3X3	T44.3X4	T44.3X5	T44.3X6
Cyclophosphamide	T45.1X1	T45.1X2	T45.1X3	T45.1X4	T45.1X5	T45.1X6
Cycloplegic drug	T49.5X1	T49.5X2	T49.5X3	T49.5X4	T49.5X5	T49.5X6
Cyclopropane	T41.291	T41.292	T41.293	T41.294	T41.295	T41.296
Cyclopyrabital	T39.8X1	T39.8X2	T39.8X3	T39.8X4	T39.8X5	T39.8X6
Cycloserine	T37.1X1	T37.1X2	T37.1X3	T37.1X4	T37.1X5	T37.1X6
Cyclosporin	T45.1X1	T45.1X2	T45.1X3	T45.1X4	T45.1X5	T45.1X6
Cyclothiazide	T50.2X1	T50.2X2	T50.2X3	T50.2X4	T50.2X5	T50.2X6
Cycrimine	T44.3X1	T44.3X2	T44.3X3	T44.3X4	T44.3X5	T44.3X6
Cyhalothrin	T60.1X1	T60.1X2	T60.1X3	T60.1X4	—	—
Cymarin	T46.0X1	T46.0X2	T46.0X3	T46.0X4	T46.0X5	T46.0X6
Cypermethrin	T60.1X1	T60.1X2	T60.1X3	T60.1X4	—	—
Cyphenothrin	T60.2X1	T60.2X2	T60.2X3	T60.2X4	—	—
Cyproheptadine	T45.0X1	T45.0X2	T45.0X3	T45.0X4	T45.0X5	T45.0X6
Cyproterone	T38.6X1	T38.6X2	T38.6X3	T38.6X4	T38.6X5	T38.6X6
Cysteamine	T50.6X1	T50.6X2	T50.6X3	T50.6X4	T50.6X5	T50.6X6
Cytarabine	T45.1X1	T45.1X2	T45.1X3	T45.1X4	T45.1X5	T45.1X6
Cytisus						
laburnum	T62.2X1	T62.2X2	T62.2X3	T62.2X4	—	—
scoparius	T62.2X1	T62.2X2	T62.2X3	T62.2X4	—	—
Cytochrome C	T47.5X1	T47.5X2	T47.5X3	T47.5X4	T47.5X5	T47.5X6
Cytomel	T38.1X1	T38.1X2	T38.1X3	T38.1X4	T38.1X5	T38.1X6
Cytosine arabinoside	T45.1X1	T45.1X2	T45.1X3	T45.1X4	T45.1X5	T45.1X6
Cytoxan	T45.1X1	T45.1X2	T45.1X3	T45.1X4	T45.1X5	T45.1X6
Cytozyme	T45.7X1	T45.7X2	T45.7X3	T45.7X4	T45.7X5	T45.7X6
S-Carboxymethylcysteine	T48.4X1	T48.4X2	T48.4X3	T48.4X4	T48.4X5	T48.4X6
Dacarbazine	T45.1X1	T45.1X2	T45.1X3	T45.1X4	T45.1X5	T45.1X6
Dactinomycin	T45.1X1	T45.1X2	T45.1X3	T45.1X4	T45.1X5	T45.1X6
DADPS	T37.1X1	T37.1X2	T37.1X3	T37.1X4	T37.1X5	T37.1X6
Dakin's solution	T49.0X1	T49.0X2	T49.0X3	T49.0X4	T49.0X5	T49.0X6
Dalapon (sodium)	T60.3X1	T60.3X2	T60.3X3	T60.3X4	—	—
Dalmane	T42.4X1	T42.4X2	T42.4X3	T42.4X4	T42.4X5	T42.4X6
Danazol	T38.6X1	T38.6X2	T38.6X3	T38.6X4	T38.6X5	T38.6X6
Danilone	T45.511	T45.512	T45.513	T45.514	T45.515	T45.516
Danthron	T47.2X1	T47.2X2	T47.2X3	T47.2X4	T47.2X5	T47.2X6
Dantrolene	T42.8X1	T42.8X2	T42.8X3	T42.8X4	T42.8X5	T42.8X6
Dantron	T47.2X1	T47.2X2	T47.2X3	T47.2X4	T47.2X5	T47.2X6
Daphne (gnidium) (mezereum)	T62.2X1	T62.2X2	T62.2X3	T62.2X4	—	—
berry	T62.1X1	T62.1X2	T62.1X3	T62.1X4	—	—
Dapsone	T37.1X1	T37.1X2	T37.1X3	T37.1X4	T37.1X5	T37.1X6
Daraprim	T37.2X1	T37.2X2	T37.2X3	T37.2X4	T37.2X5	T37.2X6
Darnel	T62.2X1	T62.2X2	T62.2X3	T62.2X4	—	—
Darvon	T39.8X1	T39.8X2	T39.8X3	T39.8X4	T39.8X5	T39.8X6
Daunomycin	T45.1X1	T45.1X2	T45.1X3	T45.1X4	T45.1X5	T45.1X6
Daunorubicin	T45.1X1	T45.1X2	T45.1X3	T45.1X4	T45.1X5	T45.1X6
DBI	T38.3X1	T38.3X2	T38.3X3	T38.3X4	T38.3X5	T38.3X6
D-Con	T60.91	T60.92	T60.93	T60.94	—	—
insecticide	T60.2X1	T60.2X2	T60.2X3	T60.2X4	—	—
rodenticide	T60.4X1	T60.4X2	T60.4X3	T60.4X4	—	—
DDAVP	T38.891	T38.892	T38.893	T38.894	T38.895	T38.896

Substance	Poisoning, Accidental (unintentional)	Poisoning, Intentional Self-harm	Poisoning, Assault	Poisoning, Undetermined	Adverse Effect	Under-dosing
DDE (bis(chlorophenyl)-dichloroethylene)	T60.2X1	T60.2X2	T60.2X3	T60.2X4	—	—
DDS	T37.1X1	T37.1X2	T37.1X4	T37.1X4	T37.1X5	T37.1X6
DDT (dust)	T60.1X1	T60.1X2	T60.1X3	T60.1X4	—	—
Deadly nightshade — see also Belladonna	T62.2X1	T62.2X2	T62.2X3	T62.2X4	—	—
berry	T62.1X1	T62.1X2	T62.1X3	T62.1X4	—	—
Deamino-D-arginine vasopressin	T38.891	T38.892	T38.893	T38.894	T38.895	T38.896
Deanol (aceglumate)	T50.991	T50.992	T50.993	T50.994	T50.995	T50.996
Debrisoquine	T46.5X1	T46.5X2	T46.5X3	T46.5X4	T46.5X5	T46.5X6
Decaborane	T57.8X1	T57.8X2	T57.8X3	T57.8X4	—	—
fumes	T59.891	T59.892	T59.893	T59.894	—	—
Decadron	T38.0X1	T38.0X2	T38.0X3	T38.0X4	T38.0X5	T38.0X6
ENT agent	T49.6X1	T49.6X2	T49.6X3	T49.6X4	T49.6X5	T49.6X6
ophthalmic preparation	T49.5X1	T49.5X2	T49.5X3	T49.5X4	T49.5X5	T49.5X6
topical NEC	T49.0X1	T49.0X2	T49.0X3	T49.0X4	T49.0X5	T49.0X6
Decahydronaphthalene	T52.8X1	T52.8X2	T52.8X3	T52.8X4	—	—
Decalin	T52.8X1	T52.8X2	T52.8X3	T52.8X4	—	—
Decamethonium (bromide)	T48.1X1	T48.1X2	T48.1X3	T48.1X4	T48.1X5	T48.1X6
Decholin	T47.5X1	T47.5X2	T47.5X3	T47.5X4	T47.5X5	T47.5X6
Declomycin	T36.4X1	T36.4X2	T36.4X3	T36.4X4	T36.4X5	T36.4X6
Decongestant, nasal (mucosa)	T48.5X1	T48.5X2	T48.5X3	T48.5X4	T48.5X5	T48.5X6
combination	T48.5X1	T48.5X2	T48.5X3	T48.5X4	T48.5X5	T48.5X6
Deet	T60.8X1	T60.8X2	T60.8X3	T60.8X4	—	—
Deferoxamine	T45.8X1	T45.8X2	T45.8X3	T45.8X4	T45.8X5	T45.8X6
Deflazacort	T38.0X1	T38.0X2	T38.0X3	T38.0X4	T38.0X5	T38.0X6
Deglycyrrhizinized extract of licorice	T48.4X1	T48.4X2	T48.4X3	T48.4X4	T48.4X5	T48.4X6
Dehydrocholic acid	T47.5X1	T47.5X2	T47.5X3	T47.5X4	T47.5X5	T47.5X6
Dehydroemetine	T37.3X1	T37.3X2	T37.3X3	T37.3X4	T37.3X5	T37.3X6
Dekalin	T52.8X1	T52.8X2	T52.8X3	T52.8X4	—	—
Delalutin	T38.5X1	T38.5X2	T38.5X3	T38.5X4	T38.5X5	T38.5X6
Delorazepam	T42.4X1	T42.4X2	T42.4X3	T42.4X4	T42.4X5	T42.4X6
Delphinium	T62.2X1	T62.2X2	T62.2X3	T62.2X4	—	—
Deltamethrin	T60.1X1	T60.1X2	T60.1X3	T60.1X4	—	—
Deltasone	T38.0X1	T38.0X2	T38.0X3	T38.0X4	T38.0X5	T38.0X6
Deltra	T38.0X1	T38.0X2	T38.0X3	T38.0X4	T38.0X5	T38.0X6
Delvinal	T42.3X1	T42.3X2	T42.3X3	T42.3X4	T42.3X5	T42.3X6
Demecarium (bromide)	T49.5X1	T49.5X2	T49.5X3	T49.5X4	T49.5X5	T49.5X6
Demeclocycline	T36.4X1	T36.4X2	T36.4X3	T36.4X4	T36.4X5	T36.4X6
Demecolcine	T45.1X1	T45.1X2	T45.1X3	T45.1X4	T45.1X5	T45.1X6
Demegestone	T38.5X1	T38.5X2	T38.5X3	T38.5X4	T38.5X5	T38.5X6
Demelanizing agents	T49.8X1	T49.8X2	T49.8X3	T49.8X4	T49.8X5	T49.8X6
Demephion -O and -S	T60.0X1	T60.0X2	T60.0X3	T60.0X4	—	—
Demerol	T40.2X1	T40.2X2	T40.2X3	T40.2X4	T40.2X5	T40.2X6
Demethylchlortetracycline	T36.4X1	T36.4X2	T36.4X3	T36.4X4	T36.4X5	T36.4X6
Demethyltetracycline	T36.4X1	T36.4X2	T36.4X3	T36.4X4	T36.4X5	T36.4X6
Demeton -O and -S	T60.0X1	T60.0X2	T60.0X3	T60.0X4	—	—
Demulcent (external)	T49.3X1	T49.3X2	T49.3X3	T49.3X4	T49.3X5	T49.3X6
specified NEC	T49.3X1	T49.3X2	T49.3X3	T49.3X4	T49.3X5	T49.3X6
Demulen	T38.4X1	T38.4X2	T38.4X3	T38.4X4	T38.4X5	T38.4X6
Denatured alcohol	T51.0X1	T51.0X2	T51.0X3	T51.0X4	—	—
Dendrid	T49.5X1	T49.5X2	T49.5X3	T49.5X4	T49.5X5	T49.5X6
Dental drug, topical application NEC	T49.7X1	T49.7X2	T49.7X3	T49.7X4	T49.7X5	T49.7X6
Dentifrice	T49.7X1	T49.7X2	T49.7X3	T49.7X4	T49.7X5	T49.7X6
Deodorant spray (feminine hygiene)	T49.8X1	T49.8X2	T49.8X3	T49.8X4	T49.8X5	T49.8X6
Deoxycortone	T50.0X1	T50.0X2	T50.0X3	T50.0X4	T50.0X5	T50.0X6
Deoxyribonuclease (pancreatic)	T45.3X1	T45.3X2	T45.3X3	T45.3X4	T45.3X5	T45.3X6
Depilatory	T49.4X1	T49.4X2	T49.4X3	T49.4X4	T49.4X5	T49.4X6
Deprenalin	T42.8X1	T42.8X2	T42.8X3	T42.8X4	T42.8X5	T42.8X6
Deprenyl	T42.8X1	T42.8X2	T42.8X3	T42.8X4	T42.8X5	T42.8X6
Depressant						
appetite (central)	T50.5X1	T50.5X2	T50.5X3	T50.5X4	T50.5X5	T50.5X6
cardiac	T46.2X1	T46.2X2	T46.2X3	T46.2X4	T46.2X5	T46.2X6
central nervous system (anesthetic) — see also Central nervous system, depressants	T42.71	T42.72	T42.73	T42.74	T42.75	T42.76
general anesthetic	T41.201	T41.202	T41.203	T41.204	T41.205	T41.206
muscle tone	T42.8X1	T42.8X2	T42.8X3	T42.8X4	T42.8X5	T42.8X6
muscle tone, central	T42.8X1	T42.8X2	T42.8X3	T42.8X4	T42.8X5	T42.8X6
psychotherapeutic	T43.501	T43.502	T43.503	T43.504	T43.505	T43.506
Depressant, appetite	T50.5X1	T50.5X2	T50.5X3	T50.5X4	T50.5X5	T50.5X6
Deptropine	T45.0X1	T45.0X2	T45.0X3	T45.0X4	T45.0X5	T45.0X6
Dequalinium (chloride)	T49.0X1	T49.0X2	T49.0X3	T49.0X4	T49.0X5	T49.0X6
Derris root	T60.2X1	T60.2X2	T60.2X3	T60.2X4	—	—
Deserpidine	T46.5X1	T46.5X2	T46.5X3	T46.5X4	T46.5X5	T46.5X6
Desferrioxamine	T45.8X1	T45.8X2	T45.8X3	T45.8X4	T45.8X5	T45.8X6

Substance	Poisoning, Accidental (unintentional)	Poisoning, Intentional Self-harm	Poisoning, Assault	Poisoning, Undetermined	Adverse Effect	Under-dosing
Desipramine	T43.011	T43.012	T43.013	T43.014	T43.015	T43.016
Deslanoside	T46.0X1	T46.0X2	T46.0X3	T46.0X4	T46.0X5	T46.0X6
Desloughing agent	T49.4X1	T49.4X2	T49.4X3	T49.4X4	T49.4X5	T49.4X6
Desmethylimipramine	T43.011	T43.012	T43.013	T43.014	T43.015	T43.016
Desmopressin	T38.891	T38.892	T38.893	T38.894	T38.895	T38.896
Desocodeine	T40.2X1	T40.2X2	T40.2X3	T40.2X4	T40.2X5	T40.2X6
Desogestrel	T38.5X1	T38.5X2	T38.5X3	T38.5X4	T38.5X5	T38.5X6
Desomorphine	T40.2X1	T40.2X2	T40.2X3	T40.2X4	—	—
Desonide	T49.0X1	T49.0X2	T49.0X3	T49.0X4	T49.0X5	T49.0X6
Desoximetasone	T49.0X1	T49.0X2	T49.0X3	T49.0X4	T49.0X5	T49.0X6
Desoxycorticosteroid	T50.0X1	T50.0X2	T50.0X3	T50.0X4	T50.0X5	T50.0X6
Desoxycortone	T50.0X1	T50.0X2	T50.0X3	T50.0X4	T50.0X5	T50.0X6
Desoxyephedrine	T43.621	T43.622	T43.623	T43.624	T43.625	T43.626
Detaxtran	T46.6X1	T46.6X2	T46.6X3	T46.6X4	T46.6X5	T46.6X6
Detergent	T49.2X1	T49.2X2	T49.2X3	T49.2X4	T49.2X5	T49.2X6
external medication	T49.2X1	T49.2X2	T49.2X3	T49.2X4	T49.2X5	T49.2X6
local	T49.2X1	T49.2X2	T49.2X3	T49.2X4	T49.2X5	T49.2X6
medicinal	T49.2X1	T49.2X2	T49.2X3	T49.2X4	T49.2X5	T49.2X6
nonmedicinal	T55.1X1	T55.1X2	T55.1X3	T55.1X4	—	—
specified NEC	T55.1X1	T55.1X2	T55.1X3	T55.1X4	—	—
Deterrent, alcohol	T50.6X1	T50.6X2	T50.6X3	T50.6X4	T50.6X5	T50.6X6
Detoxifying agent	T50.6X1	T50.6X2	T50.6X3	T50.6X4	T50.6X5	T50.6X6
Detrothyronine	T38.1X1	T38.1X2	T38.1X3	T38.1X4	T38.1X5	T38.1X6
Dettol (external medication)	T49.0X1	T49.0X2	T49.0X3	T49.0X4	T49.0X5	T49.0X6
Dexamethasone	T38.0X1	T38.0X2	T38.0X3	T38.0X4	T38.0X5	T38.0X6
ENT agent	T49.6X1	T49.6X2	T49.6X3	T49.6X4	T49.6X5	T49.6X6
ophthalmic preparation	T49.5X1	T49.5X2	T49.5X3	T49.5X4	T49.5X5	T49.5X6
topical NEC	T49.0X1	T49.0X2	T49.0X3	T49.0X4	T49.0X5	T49.0X6
Dexamfetamine	T43.621	T43.622	T43.623	T43.624	T43.625	T43.626
Dexamphetamine	T43.621	T43.622	T43.623	T43.624	T43.625	T43.626
Dexbrompheniramine	T45.0X1	T45.0X2	T45.0X3	T45.0X4	T45.0X5	T45.0X6
Dexchlorpheniramine	T45.0X1	T45.0X2	T45.0X3	T45.0X4	T45.0X5	T45.0X6
Dexedrine	T43.621	T43.622	T43.623	T43.624	T43.625	T43.626
Dexetimide	T44.3X1	T44.3X2	T44.3X3	T44.3X4	T44.3X5	T44.3X6
Dexfenfluramine	T50.5X1	T50.5X2	T50.5X3	T50.5X4	T50.5X5	T50.5X6
Dexpanthenol	T45.2X1	T45.2X2	T45.2X3	T45.2X4	T45.2X5	T45.2X6
Dextran (40) (70) (150)	T45.8X1	T45.8X2	T45.8X3	T45.8X4	T45.8X5	T45.8X6
Dextriferron	T45.4X1	T45.4X2	T45.4X3	T45.4X4	T45.4X5	T45.4X6
Dextroamphetamine	T43.621	T43.622	T43.623	T43.624	T43.625	T43.626
Dextro calcium pantothenate	T45.2X1	T45.2X2	T45.2X3	T45.2X4	T45.2X5	T45.2X6
Dextromethorphan	T48.3X1	T48.3X2	T48.3X3	T48.3X4	T48.3X5	T48.3X6
Dextromoramide	T40.4X1	T40.4X2	T40.4X3	T40.4X4	—	—
topical	T49.8X1	T49.8X2	T49.8X3	T49.8X4	T49.8X5	T49.8X6
Dextro pantothenyl alcohol	T45.2X1	T45.2X2	T45.2X3	T45.2X4	T45.2X5	T45.2X6
Dextropropoxyphene	T40.4X1	T40.4X2	T40.4X3	T40.4X4	T40.4X5	T40.4X6
Dextrorphan	T40.2X1	T40.2X2	T40.2X3	T40.2X4	T40.2X5	T40.2X6
Dextrose	T50.3X1	T50.3X2	T50.3X3	T50.3X4	T50.3X5	T50.3X6
concentrated solution, intravenous	T46.8X1	T46.8X2	T46.8X3	T46.8X4	T46.8X5	T46.8X6
Dextrothyroxin	T38.1X1	T38.1X2	T38.1X3	T38.1X4	T38.1X5	T38.1X6
Dextrothyroxine sodium	T38.1X1	T38.1X2	T38.1X3	T38.1X4	T38.1X5	T38.1X6
DFP	T44.0X1	T44.0X2	T44.0X3	T44.0X4	T44.0X5	T44.0X6
DHE	T37.3X1	T37.3X2	T37.3X3	T37.3X4	T37.3X5	T37.3X6
45	T46.5X1	T46.5X2	T46.5X3	T46.5X4	T46.5X5	T46.5X6
Diabinese	T38.3X1	T38.3X2	T38.3X3	T38.3X4	T38.3X5	T38.3X6
Diacetone alcohol	T52.4X1	T52.4X2	T52.4X3	T52.4X4	—	—
Diacetyl monoxime	T50.991	T50.992	T50.993	T50.994	—	—
Diacetylmorphine	T40.1X1	T40.1X2	T40.1X3	T40.1X4	—	—
Diachylon plaster	T49.4X1	T49.4X2	T49.4X3	T49.4X4	T49.4X5	T49.4X6
Diaethylstilboestrolum	T38.5X1	T38.5X2	T38.5X3	T38.5X4	T38.5X5	T38.5X6
Diagnostic agent NEC	T50.8X1	T50.8X2	T50.8X3	T50.8X4	T50.8X5	T50.8X6
Dial (soap)	T49.2X1	T49.2X2	T49.2X3	T49.2X4	T49.2X5	T49.2X6
sedative	T42.3X1	T42.3X2	T42.3X3	T42.3X4	T42.3X5	T42.3X6
Dialkyl carbonate	T52.91	T52.92	T52.93	T52.94	—	—
Diallylbarbituric acid	T42.3X1	T42.3X2	T42.3X3	T42.3X4	T42.3X5	T42.3X6
Diallymal	T42.3X1	T42.3X2	T42.3X3	T42.3X4	T42.3X5	T42.3X6
Dialysis solution (intraperitoneal)	T50.3X1	T50.3X2	T50.3X3	T50.3X4	T50.3X5	T50.3X6
Diaminodiphenylsulfone	T37.1X1	T37.1X2	T37.1X3	T37.1X4	T37.1X5	T37.1X6
Diamorphine	T40.1X1	T40.1X2	T40.1X3	T40.1X4	—	—
Diamox	T50.2X1	T50.2X2	T50.2X3	T50.2X4	T50.2X5	T50.2X6
Diamthazole	T49.0X1	T49.0X2	T49.0X3	T49.0X4	T49.0X5	T49.0X6
Dianthone	T47.2X1	T47.2X2	T47.2X3	T47.2X4	T47.2X5	T47.2X6
Diaphenylsulfone	T37.0X1	T37.0X2	T37.0X3	T37.0X4	T37.0X5	T37.0X6
Diasone (sodium)	T37.1X1	T37.1X2	T37.1X3	T37.1X4	T37.1X5	T37.1X6
Diastase	T47.5X1	T47.5X2	T47.5X3	T47.5X4	T47.5X5	T47.5X6
Diatrizoate	T50.8X1	T50.8X2	T50.8X3	T50.8X4	T50.8X5	T50.8X6
Diazepam	T42.4X1	T42.4X2	T42.4X3	T42.4X4	T42.4X5	T42.4X6
Diazinon	T60.0X1	T60.0X2	T60.0X3	T60.0X4	—	—
Diazomethane (gas)	T59.891	T59.892	T59.893	T59.894	—	—
Diazoxide	T46.5X1	T46.5X2	T46.5X3	T46.5X4	T46.5X5	T46.5X6
Dibekacin	T36.5X1	T36.5X2	T36.5X3	T36.5X4	T36.5X5	T36.5X6

Substance	Poisoning, Accidental (unintentional)	Poisoning, Intentional Self-harm	Poisoning, Assault	Poisoning, Undetermined	Adverse Effect	Under-dosing
Dibenamine	T44.6X1	T44.6X2	T44.6X3	T44.6X4	T44.6X5	T44.6X6
Dibenzepin	T43.011	T43.012	T43.013	T43.014	T43.015	T43.016
Dibenzheptropine	T45.0X1	T45.0X2	T45.0X3	T45.0X4	T45.0X5	T45.0X6
Dibenzyline	T44.6X1	T44.6X2	T44.6X3	T44.6X4	T44.6X5	T44.6X6
Diborane (gas)	T59.891	T59.892	T59.893	T59.894	—	—
Dibromochloropropane	T60.8X1	T60.8X2	T60.8X3	T60.8X4	—	—
Dibromodulcitol	T45.1X1	T45.1X2	T45.1X3	T45.1X4	T45.1X5	T45.1X6
Dibromoethane	T53.6X1	T53.6X2	T53.6X3	T53.6X4	—	—
Dibromomannitol	T45.1X1	T45.1X2	T45.1X3	T45.1X4	T45.1X5	T45.1X6
Dibromopropamidine isethionate	T49.0X1	T49.0X2	T49.0X3	T49.0X4	T49.0X5	T49.0X6
Dibrompropamidine	T49.0X1	T49.0X2	T49.0X3	T49.0X4	T49.0X5	T49.0X6
Dibucaine	T41.3X1	T41.3X2	T41.3X3	T41.3X4	T41.3X5	T41.3X6
topical (surface)	T41.3X1	T41.3X2	T41.3X3	T41.3X4	T41.3X5	T41.3X6
Dibunate sodium	T48.3X1	T48.3X2	T48.3X3	T48.3X4	T48.3X5	T48.3X6
Dibutoline sulfate	T44.3X1	T44.3X2	T44.3X3	T44.3X4	T44.3X5	T44.3X6
Dicamba	T60.3X1	T60.3X2	T60.3X3	T60.3X4	—	—
Dicapthon	T60.0X1	T60.0X2	T60.0X3	T60.0X4	—	—
Dichlobenil	T60.3X1	T60.3X2	T60.3X3	T60.3X4	—	—
Dichlone	T60.3X1	T60.3X2	T60.3X3	T60.3X4	—	—
Dichloralphenozone	T42.6X1	T42.6X2	T42.6X3	T42.6X4	T42.6X5	T42.6X6
Dichlorbenzidine	T65.3X1	T65.3X2	T65.3X3	T65.3X4	—	—
Dichlorhydrin	T52.8X1	T52.8X2	T52.8X3	T52.8X4	—	—
Dichlorhydroxyquinoline	T37.8X1	T37.8X2	T37.8X3	T37.8X4	T37.8X5	T37.8X6
Dichlorobenzene	T53.7X1	T53.7X2	T53.7X3	T53.7X4	—	—
Dichlorobenzyl alcohol	T49.6X1	T49.6X2	T49.6X3	T49.6X4	T49.6X5	T49.6X6
Dichlorodifluoromethane	T53.5X1	T53.5X2	T53.5X3	T53.5X4	—	—
Dichloroethane	T52.8X1	T52.8X2	T52.8X3	T52.8X4	—	—
Dichloroethylene	T53.6X1	T53.6X2	T53.6X3	T53.6X4	—	—
Dichloroethyl sulfide, not in war	T59.891	T59.892	T59.893	T59.894	—	—
Dichloroformoxine, not in war	T59.891	T59.892	T59.893	T59.894	—	—
Dichlorohydrin, alpha-dichlorohydrin	T52.8X1	T52.8X2	T52.8X3	T52.8X4	—	—
Dichloromethane (solvent)	T53.4X1	T53.4X2	T53.4X3	T53.4X4	—	—
vapor	T53.4X1	T53.4X2	T53.4X3	T53.4X4	—	—
Dichloronaphthoquinone	T60.3X1	T60.3X2	T60.3X3	T60.3X4	—	—
Dichlorophen	T37.4X1	T37.4X2	T37.4X3	T37.4X4	T37.4X5	T37.4X6
Dichloropropene	T60.3X1	T60.3X2	T60.3X3	T60.3X4	—	—
Dichloropropionic acid	T60.3X1	T60.3X2	T60.3X3	T60.3X4	—	—
Dichlorphenamide	T50.2X1	T50.2X2	T50.2X3	T50.2X4	T50.2X5	T50.2X6
Dichlorvos	T60.0X1	T60.0X2	T60.0X3	T60.0X4	—	—
Diclofenac	T39.391	T39.392	T39.393	T39.394	T39.395	T39.396
Diclofenamide	T50.2X1	T50.2X2	T50.2X3	T50.2X4	T50.2X5	T50.2X6
Diclofensine	T43.291	T43.292	T43.293	T43.294	T43.295	T43.296
Diclonixine	T39.8X1	T39.8X2	T39.8X3	T39.8X4	T39.8X5	T39.8X6
Dicloxacillin	T36.0X1	T36.0X2	T36.0X3	T36.0X4	T36.0X5	T36.0X6
Dicophane	T49.0X1	T49.0X2	T49.0X3	T49.0X4	T49.0X5	T49.0X6
Dicoumarol, dicoumarin, dicumarol	T45.511	T45.512	T45.513	T45.514	T45.515	T45.516
Dicrotophos	T60.0X1	T60.0X2	T60.0X3	T60.0X4	—	—
Dicyanogen (gas)	T65.0X1	T65.0X2	T65.0X3	T65.0X4	—	—
Dicyclomine	T44.3X1	T44.3X2	T44.3X3	T44.3X4	T44.3X5	T44.3X6
Dicycloverine	T44.3X1	T44.3X2	T44.3X3	T44.3X4	T44.3X5	T44.3X6
Dideoxycytidine	T37.5X1	T37.5X2	T37.5X3	T37.5X4	T37.5X5	T37.5X6
Dideoxyinosine	T37.5X1	T37.5X2	T37.5X3	T37.5X4	T37.5X5	T37.5X6
Dieldrin (vapor)	T60.1X1	T60.1X2	T60.1X3	T60.1X4	—	—
Diemal	T42.3X1	T42.3X2	T42.3X3	T42.3X4	T42.3X5	T42.3X6
Dienestrol	T38.5X1	T38.5X2	T38.5X3	T38.5X4	T38.5X5	T38.5X6
Dienoestrol	T38.5X1	T38.5X2	T38.5X3	T38.5X4	T38.5X5	T38.5X6
Dietetic drug NEC	T50.901	T50.902	T50.903	T50.904	T50.905	T50.906
Diethazine	T42.8X1	T42.8X2	T42.8X3	T42.8X4	T42.8X5	T42.8X6
Diethyl						
barbituric acid	T42.3X1	T42.3X2	T42.3X3	T42.3X4	T42.3X5	T42.3X6
carbamazine	T37.4X1	T37.4X2	T37.4X3	T37.4X4	T37.4X5	T37.4X6
carbinol	T51.3X1	T51.3X2	T51.3X3	T51.3X4	—	—
carbonate	T52.8X1	T52.8X2	T52.8X3	T52.8X4	—	—
ether (vapor) — see also ether	T41.0X1	T41.0X2	T41.0X3	T41.0X4	T41.0X5	T41.0X6
oxide	T52.8X1	T52.8X2	T52.8X3	T52.8X4	—	—
propion	T50.5X1	T50.5X2	T50.5X3	T50.5X4	T50.5X5	T50.5X6
stilbestrol	T38.5X1	T38.5X2	T38.5X3	T38.5X4	T38.5X5	T38.5X6
toluamide (nonmedicinal)	T60.8X1	T60.8X2	T60.8X3	T60.8X4	—	—
medicinal	T49.3X1	T49.3X2	T49.3X3	T49.3X4	T49.3X5	T49.3X6
Diethylcarbamazine	T37.4X1	T37.4X2	T37.4X3	T37.4X4	T37.4X5	T37.4X6
Diethylene						
dioxide	T52.8X1	T52.8X2	T52.8X3	T52.8X4	—	—
glycol (monoacetate) (monobutyl ether) (monoethyl ether)	T52.3X1	T52.3X2	T52.3X3	T52.3X4	—	—
Diethylhexylphthalate	T65.891	T65.892	T65.893	T65.894	—	—
Diethylpropion	T50.5X1	T50.5X2	T50.5X3	T50.5X4	T50.5X5	T50.5X6

Substance	Poisoning, Accidental (unintentional)	Poisoning, Intentional Self-harm	Poisoning, Assault	Poisoning, Undetermined	Adverse Effect	Under-dosing
Diethylstilbestrol	T38.5X1	T38.5X2	T38.5X3	T38.5X4	T38.5X5	T38.5X6
Diethylstilboestrol	T38.5X1	T38.5X2	T38.5X3	T38.5X4	T38.5X5	T38.5X6
Diethylsulfone-diethylmethane	T42.6X1	T42.6X2	T42.6X3	T42.6X4	T42.6X5	T42.6X6
Diethyltoluamide	T49.0X1	T49.0X2	T49.0X3	T49.0X4	T49.0X5	T49.0X6
Diethyltryptamine (DET)	T40.991	T40.992	T40.993	T40.994		
Difebarbamate	T42.3X1	T42.3X2	T42.3X3	T42.3X4	T42.3X5	T42.3X6
Difencloxazine	T40.2X1	T40.2X2	T40.2X3	T40.2X4	T40.2X5	T40.2X6
Difenidol	T45.0X1	T45.0X2	T45.0X3	T45.0X4	T45.0X5	T45.0X6
Difenoxin	T47.6X1	T47.6X2	T47.6X3	T47.6X4	T47.6X5	T47.6X6
Difetarsone	T37.3X1	T37.3X2	T37.3X3	T37.3X4	T37.3X5	T37.3X6
Diffusin	T45.3X1	T45.3X2	T45.3X3	T45.3X4	T45.3X5	T45.3X6
Diflorasone	T49.0X1	T49.0X2	T49.0X3	T49.0X4	T49.0X5	T49.0X6
Diflos	T44.0X1	T44.0X2	T44.0X3	T44.0X4	T44.0X5	T44.0X6
Diflubenzuron	T60.1X1	T60.1X2	T60.1X3	T60.1X4	—	—
Diflucortolone	T49.0X1	T49.0X2	T49.0X3	T49.0X4	T49.0X5	T49.0X6
Diflunisal	T39.091	T39.092	T39.093	T39.094	T39.095	T39.096
Difluoromethyldopa	T42.8X1	T42.8X2	T42.8X3	T42.8X4	T42.8X5	T42.8X6
Difluorophate	T44.0X1	T44.0X2	T44.0X3	T44.0X4	T44.0X5	T44.0X6
Digestant NEC	T47.5X1	T47.5X2	T47.5X3	T47.5X4	T47.5X5	T47.5X6
Digitalin (e)	T46.0X1	T46.0X2	T46.0X3	T46.0X4	T46.0X5	T46.0X6
Digitalis (leaf)(glycoside)	T46.0X1	T46.0X2	T46.0X3	T46.0X4	T46.0X5	T46.0X6
lanata	T46.0X1	T46.0X2	T46.0X3	T46.0X4	T46.0X5	T46.0X6
purpurea	T46.0X1	T46.0X2	T46.0X3	T46.0X4	T46.0X5	T46.0X6
Digitoxin	T46.0X1	T46.0X2	T46.0X3	T46.0X4	T46.0X5	T46.0X6
Digitoxose	T46.0X1	T46.0X2	T46.0X3	T46.0X4	T46.0X5	T46.0X6
Digoxin	T46.0X1	T46.0X2	T46.0X3	T46.0X4	T46.0X5	T46.0X6
Digoxine	T46.0X1	T46.0X2	T46.0X3	T46.0X4	T46.0X5	T46.0X6
Dihydralazine	T46.5X1	T46.5X2	T46.5X3	T46.5X4	T46.5X5	T46.5X6
Dihydrazine	T46.5X1	T46.5X2	T46.5X3	T46.5X4	T46.5X5	T46.5X6
Dihydrocodeine	T40.2X1	T40.2X2	T40.2X3	T40.2X4	T40.2X5	T40.2X6
Dihydrocodeinone	T40.2X1	T40.2X2	T40.2X3	T40.2X4	T40.2X5	T40.2X6
Dihydroergocornine	T46.7X1	T46.7X2	T46.7X3	T46.7X4	T46.7X5	T46.7X6
Dihydroergocristine (mesilate)	T46.7X1	T46.7X2	T46.7X3	T46.7X4	T46.7X5	T46.7X6
Dihydroergokryptine	T46.7X1	T46.7X2	T46.7X3	T46.7X4	T46.7X5	T46.7X6
Dihydroergotamine	T46.5X1	T46.5X2	T46.5X3	T46.5X4	T46.5X5	T46.5X6
Dihydroergotoxine	T46.7X1	T46.7X2	T46.7X3	T46.7X4	T46.7X5	T46.7X6
mesilate	T46.7X1	T46.7X2	T46.7X3	T46.7X4	T46.7X5	T46.7X6
Dihydrohydroxycodeinone	T40.2X1	T40.2X2	T40.2X3	T40.2X4	T40.2X5	T40.2X6
Dihydrohydroxymorphinone	T40.2X1	T40.2X2	T40.2X3	T40.2X4	T40.2X5	T40.2X6
Dihydroisocodeine	T40.2X1	T40.2X2	T40.2X3	T40.2X4	T40.2X5	T40.2X6
Dihydromorphine	T40.2X1	T40.2X2	T40.2X3	T40.2X4	—	—
Dihydromorphinone	T40.2X1	T40.2X2	T40.2X3	T40.2X4	T40.2X5	T40.2X6
Dihydrostreptomycin	T36.5X1	T36.5X2	T36.5X3	T36.5X4	T36.5X5	T36.5X6
Dihydrotachysterol	T45.2X1	T45.2X2	T45.2X3	T45.2X4	T45.2X5	T45.2X6
Dihydroxyaluminum aminoacetate	T47.1X1	T47.1X2	T47.1X3	T47.1X4	T47.1X5	T47.1X6
Dihydroxyaluminum sodium carbonate	T47.1X1	T47.1X2	T47.1X3	T47.1X4	T47.1X5	T47.1X6
Dihydroxyanthraquinone	T47.2X1	T47.2X2	T47.2X3	T47.2X4	T47.2X5	T47.2X6
Dihydroxycodeinone	T40.2X1	T40.2X2	T40.2X3	T40.2X4	T40.2X5	T40.2X6
Dihydroxypropyl theophylline	T50.2X1	T50.2X2	T50.2X3	T50.2X4	T50.2X5	T50.2X6
Diiodohydroxyquin	T37.8X1	T37.8X2	T37.8X3	T37.8X4	T37.8X5	T37.8X6
topical	T49.0X1	T49.0X2	T49.0X3	T49.0X4	T49.0X5	T49.0X6
Diiodohydroxyquinoline	T37.8X1	T37.8X2	T37.8X3	T37.8X4	T37.8X5	T37.8X6
Diiodotyrosine	T38.2X1	T38.2X2	T38.2X3	T38.2X4	T38.2X5	T38.2X6
Diisopromine	T44.3X1	T44.3X2	T44.3X3	T44.3X4	T44.3X5	T44.3X6
Diisopropylamine	T46.3X1	T46.3X2	T46.3X3	T46.3X4	T46.3X5	T46.3X6
Diisopropylfluorophosphonate	T44.0X1	T44.0X2	T44.0X3	T44.0X4	T44.0X5	T44.0X6
Dilantin	T42.0X1	T42.0X2	T42.0X3	T42.0X4	T42.0X5	T42.0X6
Dilaudid	T40.2X1	T40.2X2	T40.2X3	T40.2X4	T40.2X5	T40.2X6
Dilazep	T46.3X1	T46.3X2	T46.3X3	T46.3X4	T46.3X5	T46.3X6
Dill	T47.5X1	T47.5X2	T47.5X3	T47.5X4	T47.5X5	T47.5X6
Diloxanide	T37.3X1	T37.3X2	T37.3X3	T37.3X4	T37.3X5	T37.3X6
Diltiazem	T46.1X1	T46.1X2	T46.1X3	T46.1X4	T46.1X5	T46.1X6
Dimazole	T49.0X1	T49.0X2	T49.0X3	T49.0X4	T49.0X5	T49.0X6
Dimefline	T50.7X1	T50.7X2	T50.7X3	T50.7X4	T50.7X5	T50.7X6
Dimefox	T60.0X1	T60.0X2	T60.0X3	T60.0X4	—	—
Dimemorfan	T48.3X1	T48.3X2	T48.3X3	T48.3X4	T48.3X5	T48.3X6
Dimenhydrinate	T45.0X1	T45.0X2	T45.0X3	T45.0X4	T45.0X5	T45.0X6
Dimercaprol (British anti-lewisite)	T45.8X1	T45.8X2	T45.8X3	T45.8X4	T45.8X5	T45.8X6
Dimercaptopropanol	T45.8X1	T45.8X2	T45.8X3	T45.8X4	T45.8X5	T45.8X6
Dimestrol	T38.5X1	T38.5X2	T38.5X3	T38.5X4	T38.5X5	T38.5X6
Dimetane	T45.0X1	T45.0X2	T45.0X3	T45.0X4	T45.0X5	T45.0X6
Dimethicone	T47.1X1	T47.1X2	T47.1X3	T47.1X4	T47.1X5	T47.1X6
Dimethindene	T45.0X1	T45.0X2	T45.0X3	T45.0X4	T45.0X5	T45.0X6
Dimethisoquin	T49.1X1	T49.1X2	T49.1X3	T49.1X4	T49.1X5	T49.1X6
Dimethisterone	T38.5X1	T38.5X2	T38.5X3	T38.5X4	T38.5X5	T38.5X6
Dimethoate	T60.0X1	T60.0X2	T60.0X3	T60.0X4	—	—
Dimethocaine	T41.3X1	T41.3X2	T41.3X3	T41.3X4	T41.3X5	T41.3X6
Dimethoxanate	T48.3X1	T48.3X2	T48.3X3	T48.3X4	T48.3X5	T48.3X6

Additional Character May Be Required — Refer to the Tabular List for Character Selection ▽ Subterms under main terms may continue to next column or page

Substance	Poisoning, Accidental (unintentional)	Poisoning, Intentional Self-harm	Poisoning, Assault	Poisoning, Undetermined	Adverse Effect	Under-dosing
Dimethyl						
arsine, arsinic acid	T57.0X1	T57.0X2	T57.0X3	T57.0X4	—	—
carbinol	T51.2X1	T51.2X2	T51.2X3	T51.2X4	—	—
carbonate	T52.8X1	T52.8X2	T52.8X3	T52.8X4	—	—
diguanide	T38.3X1	T38.3X2	T38.3X3	T38.3X4	T38.3X5	T38.3X6
ketone	T52.4X1	T52.4X2	T52.4X3	T52.4X4	—	—
vapor	T52.4X1	T52.4X2	T52.4X3	T52.4X4	—	—
meperidine	T40.2X1	T40.2X2	T40.2X3	T40.2X4	T40.2X5	T40.2X6
parathion	T60.0X1	T60.0X2	T60.0X3	T60.0X4	—	—
phthlate	T49.3X1	T49.3X2	T49.3X3	T49.3X4	T49.3X5	T49.3X6
polysiloxane	T47.8X1	T47.8X2	T47.8X3	T47.8X4	T47.8X5	T47.8X6
sulfate (fumes)	T59.891	T59.892	T59.893	T59.894	—	—
liquid	T65.891	T65.892	T65.893	T65.894	—	—
sulfoxide (nonmedicinal)	T52.8X1	T52.8X2	T52.8X3	T52.8X4	—	—
medicinal	T49.4X1	T49.4X2	T49.4X3	T49.4X4	T49.4X5	T49.4X6
tryptamine	T40.991	T40.992	T40.993	T40.994	—	—
tubocurarine	T48.1X1	T48.1X2	T48.1X3	T48.1X4	T48.1X5	T48.1X6
Dimethylamine sulfate	T49.4X1	T49.4X2	T49.4X3	T49.4X4	T49.4X5	T49.4X6
Dimethylformamide	T52.8X1	T52.8X2	T52.8X3	T52.8X4	—	—
Dimethyltubocurarinium chloride	T48.1X1	T48.1X2	T48.1X3	T48.1X4	T48.1X5	T48.1X6
Dimeticone	T47.1X1	T47.1X2	T47.1X3	T47.1X4	T47.1X5	T47.1X6
Dimetilan	T60.0X1	T60.0X2	T60.0X3	T60.0X4	—	—
Dimetindene	T45.0X1	T45.0X2	T45.0X3	T45.0X4	T45.0X5	T45.0X6
Dimetotiazine	T43.3X1	T43.3X2	T43.3X3	T43.3X4	T43.3X5	T43.3X6
Dimorpholamine	T50.7X1	T50.7X2	T50.7X3	T50.7X4	T50.7X5	T50.7X6
Dimoxyline	T46.3X1	T46.3X2	T46.3X3	T46.3X4	T46.3X5	T46.3X6
Dinitrobenzene	T65.3X1	T65.3X2	T65.3X3	T65.3X4	—	—
vapor	T59.891	T59.892	T59.893	T59.894	—	—
Dinitrobenzol	T65.3X1	T65.3X2	T65.3X3	T65.3X4	—	—
vapor	T59.891	T59.892	T59.893	T59.894	—	—
Dinitrobutylphenol	T65.3X1	T65.3X2	T65.3X3	T65.3X4	—	—
Dinitro (-ortho-)cresol (pesticide) (spray)	T65.3X1	T65.3X2	T65.3X3	T65.3X4	—	—
Dinitrocyclohexylphenol	T65.3X1	T65.3X2	T65.3X3	T65.3X4	—	—
Dinitrophenol	T65.3X1	T65.3X2	T65.3X3	T65.3X4	—	—
Dinoprost	T48.0X1	T48.0X2	T48.0X3	T48.0X4	T48.0X5	T48.0X6
Dinoprostone	T48.0X1	T48.0X2	T48.0X3	T48.0X4	T48.0X5	T48.0X6
Dinoseb	T60.3X1	T60.3X2	T60.3X3	T60.3X4	—	—
Dioctyl sulfosuccinate (calcium) (sodium)	T47.4X1	T47.4X2	T47.4X3	T47.4X4	T47.4X5	T47.4X6
Diodone	T50.8X1	T50.8X2	T50.8X3	T50.8X4	T50.8X5	T50.8X6
Diodoquin	T37.8X1	T37.8X2	T37.8X3	T37.8X4	T37.8X5	T37.8X6
Dionin	T40.2X1	T40.2X2	T40.2X3	T40.2X4	T40.2X5	T40.2X6
Diosmin	T46.991	T46.992	T46.993	T46.994	T46.995	T46.996
Dioxane	T52.8X1	T52.8X2	T52.8X3	T52.8X4	—	—
Dioxathion	T60.0X1	T60.0X2	T60.0X3	T60.0X4	—	—
Dioxin	T53.7X1	T53.7X2	T53.7X3	T53.7X4	—	—
Dioxopromethazine	T43.3X1	T43.3X2	T43.3X3	T43.3X4	T43.3X5	T43.3X6
Dioxyline	T46.3X1	T46.3X2	T46.3X3	T46.3X4	T46.3X5	T46.3X6
Dipentene	T52.8X1	T52.8X2	T52.8X3	T52.8X4	—	—
Diperodon	T41.3X1	T41.3X2	T41.3X3	T41.3X4	T41.3X5	T41.3X6
Diphacinone	T60.4X1	T60.4X2	T60.4X3	T60.4X4	—	—
Diphemanil	T44.3X1	T44.3X2	T44.3X3	T44.3X4	T44.3X5	T44.3X6
metilsulfate	T44.3X1	T44.3X2	T44.3X3	T44.3X4	T44.3X5	T44.3X6
Diphenadione	T45.511	T45.512	T45.513	T45.514	T45.515	T45.516
rodenticide	T60.4X1	T60.4X2	T60.4X3	T60.4X4	—	—
Diphenhydramine	T45.0X1	T45.0X2	T45.0X3	T45.0X4	T45.0X5	T45.0X6
Diphenidol	T45.0X1	T45.0X2	T45.0X3	T45.0X4	T45.0X5	T45.0X6
Diphenoxylate	T47.6X1	T47.6X2	T47.6X3	T47.6X4	T47.6X5	T47.6X6
Diphenylamine	T65.3X1	T65.3X2	T65.3X3	T65.3X4	—	—
Diphenylbutazone	T39.2X1	T39.2X2	T39.2X3	T39.2X4	T39.2X5	T39.2X6
Diphenylchloroarsine, not in war	T57.0X1	T57.0X2	T57.0X3	T57.0X4	—	—
Diphenylhydantoin	T42.0X1	T42.0X2	T42.0X3	T42.0X4	T42.0X5	T42.0X6
Diphenylmethane dye	T52.1X1	T52.1X2	T52.1X3	T52.1X4	—	—
Diphenylpyraline	T45.0X1	T45.0X2	T45.0X3	T45.0X4	T45.0X5	T45.0X6
Diphtheria						
antitoxin	T50.Z11	T50.Z12	T50.Z13	T50.Z14	T50.Z15	T50.Z16
toxoid	T50.A91	T50.A92	T50.A93	T50.A94	T50.A95	T50.A96
with tetanus toxoid	T50.A21	T50.A22	T50.A23	T50.A24	T50.A25	T50.A26
with pertussis component	T50.A11	T50.A12	T50.A13	T50.A14	T50.A15	T50.A16
vaccine	T50.A91	T50.A92	T50.A93	T50.A94	T50.A95	T50.A96
combination						
without pertussis	T50.A21	T50.A22	T50.A23	T50.A24	T50.A25	T50.A26
including pertussis	T50.A11	T50.A12	T50.A13	T50.A14	T50.A15	T50.A16
Diphylline	T50.2X1	T50.2X2	T50.2X3	T50.2X4	T50.2X5	T50.2X6
Dipipanone	T40.4X1	T40.4X2	T40.4X3	T40.4X4	—	—
Dipivefrine	T49.5X1	T49.5X2	T49.5X3	T49.5X4	T49.5X5	T49.5X6
Diplovax	T50.B91	T50.B92	T50.B93	T50.B94	T50.B95	T50.B96
Diprophylline	T50.2X1	T50.2X2	T50.2X3	T50.2X4	T50.2X5	T50.2X6
Dipropyline	T48.291	T48.292	T48.293	T48.294	T48.295	T48.296

Substance	Poisoning, Accidental (unintentional)	Poisoning, Intentional Self-harm	Poisoning, Assault	Poisoning, Undetermined	Adverse Effect	Under-dosing
Dipyridamole	T46.3X1	T46.3X2	T46.3X3	T46.3X4	T46.3X5	T46.3X6
Dipyrone	T39.2X1	T39.2X2	T39.2X3	T39.2X4	T39.2X5	T39.2X6
Diquat (dibromide)	T60.3X1	T60.3X2	T60.3X3	T60.3X4	—	—
Disinfectant	T65.891	T65.892	T65.893	T65.894	—	—
alkaline	T54.3X1	T54.3X2	T54.3X3	T54.3X4	—	—
aromatic	T54.1X1	T54.1X2	T54.1X3	T54.1X4	—	—
intestinal	T37.8X1	T37.8X2	T37.8X3	T37.8X4	T37.8X5	T37.8X6
Disipal	T42.8X1	T42.8X2	T42.8X3	T42.8X4	T42.8X5	T42.8X6
Disodium edetate	T50.6X1	T50.6X2	T50.6X3	T50.6X4	T50.6X5	T50.6X6
Disoprofol	T41.291	T41.292	T41.293	T41.294	T41.295	T41.296
Disopyramide	T46.2X1	T46.2X2	T46.2X3	T46.2X4	T46.2X5	T46.2X6
Distigmine (bromide)	T44.0X1	T44.0X2	T44.0X3	T44.0X4	T44.0X5	T44.0X6
Disulfamide	T50.2X1	T50.2X2	T50.2X3	T50.2X4	T50.2X5	T50.2X6
Disulfanilamide	T37.0X1	T37.0X2	T37.0X3	T37.0X4	T37.0X5	T37.0X6
Disulfiram	T50.6X1	T50.6X2	T50.6X3	T50.6X4	T50.6X5	T50.6X6
Disulfoton	T60.0X1	T60.0X2	T60.0X3	T60.0X4	—	—
Dithiazanine iodide	T37.4X1	T37.4X2	T37.4X3	T37.4X4	T37.4X5	T37.4X6
Dithiocarbamate	T60.0X1	T60.0X2	T60.0X3	T60.0X4	—	—
Dithranol	T49.4X1	T49.4X2	T49.4X3	T49.4X4	T49.4X5	T49.4X6
Diucardin	T50.2X1	T50.2X2	T50.2X3	T50.2X4	T50.2X5	T50.2X6
Diupres	T50.2X1	T50.2X2	T50.2X3	T50.2X4	T50.2X5	T50.2X6
Diuretic NEC	T50.2X1	T50.2X2	T50.2X3	T50.2X4	T50.2X5	T50.2X6
benzothiadiazine	T50.2X1	T50.2X2	T50.2X3	T50.2X4	T50.2X5	T50.2X6
carbonic acid anhydrase inhibitors	T50.2X1	T50.2X2	T50.2X3	T50.2X4	T50.2X5	T50.2X6
furfuryl NEC	T50.2X1	T50.2X2	T50.2X3	T50.2X4	T50.2X5	T50.2X6
loop (high-ceiling)	T50.1X1	T50.1X2	T50.1X3	T50.1X4	T50.1X5	T50.1X6
mercurial NEC	T50.2X1	T50.2X2	T50.2X3	T50.2X4	T50.2X5	T50.2X6
osmotic	T50.2X1	T50.2X2	T50.2X3	T50.2X4	T50.2X5	T50.2X6
purine NEC	T50.2X1	T50.2X2	T50.2X3	T50.2X4	T50.2X5	T50.2X6
saluretic NEC	T50.2X1	T50.2X2	T50.2X3	T50.2X4	T50.2X5	T50.2X6
sulfonamide	T50.2X1	T50.2X2	T50.2X3	T50.2X4	T50.2X5	T50.2X6
thiazide NEC	T50.2X1	T50.2X2	T50.2X3	T50.2X4	T50.2X5	T50.2X6
xanthine	T50.2X1	T50.2X2	T50.2X3	T50.2X4	T50.2X5	T50.2X6
Diurgin	T50.2X1	T50.2X2	T50.2X3	T50.2X4	T50.2X5	T50.2X6
Diuril	T50.2X1	T50.2X2	T50.2X3	T50.2X4	T50.2X5	T50.2X6
Diuron	T60.3X1	T60.3X2	T60.3X3	T60.3X4	—	—
Divalproex	T42.6X1	T42.6X2	T42.6X3	T42.6X4	T42.6X5	T42.6X6
Divinyl ether	T41.0X1	T41.0X2	T41.0X3	T41.0X4	T41.0X5	T41.0X6
Dixanthogen	T49.0X1	T49.0X2	T49.0X3	T49.0X4	T49.0X5	T49.0X6
Dixyrazine	T43.3X1	T43.3X2	T43.3X3	T43.3X4	T43.3X5	T43.3X6
D-lysergic acid diethylamide	T40.8X1	T40.8X2	T40.8X3	T40.8X4	—	—
DMCT	T36.4X1	T36.4X2	T36.4X3	T36.4X4	T36.4X5	T36.4X6
DMSO — see Dimethyl sulfoxide						
DNBP	T60.3X1	T60.3X2	T60.3X3	T60.3X4	—	—
DNOC	T65.3X1	T65.3X2	T65.3X3	T65.3X4	—	—
Dobutamine	T44.5X1	T44.5X2	T44.5X3	T44.5X4	T44.5X5	T44.5X6
DOCA	T38.0X1	T38.0X2	T38.0X3	T38.0X4	T38.0X5	T38.0X6
Docusate sodium	T47.4X1	T47.4X2	T47.4X3	T47.4X4	T47.4X5	T47.4X6
Dodicin	T49.0X1	T49.0X2	T49.0X3	T49.0X4	T49.0X5	T49.0X6
Dofamium chloride	T49.0X1	T49.0X2	T49.0X3	T49.0X4	T49.0X5	T49.0X6
Dolophine	T40.3X1	T40.3X2	T40.3X3	T40.3X4	T40.3X5	T40.3X6
Doloxene	T39.8X1	T39.8X2	T39.8X3	T39.8X4	T39.8X5	T39.8X6
Domestic gas (after combustion) — see Gas, utility						
prior to combustion	T59.891	T59.892	T59.893	T59.894	—	—
Domiodol	T48.4X1	T48.4X2	T48.4X3	T48.4X4	T48.4X5	T48.4X6
Domiphen (bromide)	T49.0X1	T49.0X2	T49.0X3	T49.0X4	T49.0X5	T49.0X6
Domperidone	T45.0X1	T45.0X2	T45.0X3	T45.0X4	T45.0X5	T45.0X6
Dopa	T42.8X1	T42.8X2	T42.8X3	T42.8X4	T42.8X5	T42.8X6
Dopamine	T44.991	T44.992	T44.993	T44.994	T44.995	T44.996
Doriden	T42.6X1	T42.6X2	T42.6X3	T42.6X4	T42.6X5	T42.6X6
Dormiral	T42.3X1	T42.3X2	T42.3X3	T42.3X4	T42.3X5	T42.3X6
Dormison	T42.6X1	T42.6X2	T42.6X3	T42.6X4	T42.6X5	T42.6X6
Dornase	T48.4X1	T48.4X2	T48.4X3	T48.4X4	T48.4X5	T48.4X6
Dorsacaine	T41.3X1	T41.3X2	T41.3X3	T41.3X4	T41.3X5	T41.3X6
Dosulepin	T43.011	T43.012	T43.013	T43.014	T43.015	T43.016
Dothiepin	T43.011	T43.012	T43.013	T43.014	T43.015	T43.016
Doxantrazole	T48.6X1	T48.6X2	T48.6X3	T48.6X4	T48.6X5	T48.6X6
Doxapram	T50.7X1	T50.7X2	T50.7X3	T50.7X4	T50.7X5	T50.7X6
Doxazosin	T44.6X1	T44.6X2	T44.6X3	T44.6X4	T44.6X5	T44.6X6
Doxepin	T43.011	T43.012	T43.013	T43.014	T43.015	T43.016
Doxifluridine	T45.1X1	T45.1X2	T45.1X3	T45.1X4	T45.1X5	T45.1X6
Doxorubicin	T45.1X1	T45.1X2	T45.1X3	T45.1X4	T45.1X5	T45.1X6
Doxycycline	T36.4X1	T36.4X2	T36.4X3	T36.4X4	T36.4X5	T36.4X6
Doxylamine	T45.0X1	T45.0X2	T45.0X3	T45.0X4	T45.0X5	T45.0X6
Dramamine	T45.0X1	T45.0X2	T45.0X3	T45.0X4	T45.0X5	T45.0X6
Drano (drain cleaner)	T54.3X1	T54.3X2	T54.3X3	T54.3X4	—	—
Dressing, live pulp	T49.7X1	T49.7X2	T49.7X3	T49.7X4	T49.7X5	T49.7X6
Drocode	T40.2X1	T40.2X2	T40.2X3	T40.2X4	T40.2X5	T40.2X6
Dromoran	T40.2X1	T40.2X2	T40.2X3	T40.2X4	T40.2X5	T40.2X6
Dromostanolone	T38.7X1	T38.7X2	T38.7X3	T38.7X4	T38.7X5	T38.7X6

▽ Subterms under main terms may continue to next column or page　　　Additional Character May Be Required — Refer to the Tabular List for Character Selection　　　365

Dimethyl — Dromostanolone

Substance	Poisoning, Accidental (unintentional)	Poisoning, Intentional Self-harm	Poisoning, Assault	Poisoning, Undetermined	Adverse Effect	Under-dosing
Dronabinol	T40.7X1	T40.7X2	T40.7X3	T40.7X4	T40.7X5	T40.7X6
Droperidol	T43.591	T43.592	T43.593	T43.594	T43.595	T43.596
Dropropizine	T48.3X1	T48.3X2	T48.3X3	T48.3X4	T48.3X5	T48.3X6
Drostanolone	T38.7X1	T38.7X2	T38.7X3	T38.7X4	T38.7X5	T38.7X6
Drotaverine	T44.3X1	T44.3X2	T44.3X3	T44.3X4	T44.3X5	T44.3X6
Drotrecogin alfa	T45.511	T45.512	T45.513	T45.514	T45.515	T45.516
Drug NEC	T50.901	T50.902	T50.903	T50.904	T50.905	T50.906
specified NEC	T50.991	T50.992	T50.993	T50.994	T50.995	T50.996
DTIC	T45.1X1	T45.1X2	T45.1X3	T45.1X4	T45.1X5	T45.1X6
Duboisine	T44.3X1	T44.3X2	T44.3X3	T44.3X4	T44.3X5	T44.3X6
Dulcolax	T47.2X1	T47.2X2	T47.2X3	T47.2X4	T47.2X5	T47.2X6
Duponol (C) (EP)	T49.2X1	T49.2X2	T49.2X3	T49.2X4	T49.2X5	T49.2X6
Durabolin	T38.7X1	T38.7X2	T38.7X3	T38.7X4	T38.7X5	T38.7X6
Dyclone	T41.3X1	T41.3X2	T41.3X3	T41.3X4	T41.3X5	T41.3X6
Dyclonine	T41.3X1	T41.3X2	T41.3X3	T41.3X4	T41.3X5	T41.3X6
Dydrogesterone	T38.5X1	T38.5X2	T38.5X3	T38.5X4	T38.5X5	T38.5X6
Dye NEC	T65.6X1	T65.6X2	T65.6X3	T65.6X4		
antiseptic	T49.0X1	T49.0X2	T49.0X3	T49.0X4	T49.0X5	T49.0X6
diagnostic agents	T50.8X1	T50.8X2	T50.8X3	T50.8X4	T50.8X5	T50.8X6
pharmaceutical NEC	T50.901	T50.902	T50.903	T50.904	T50.905	T50.906
Dyflos	T44.0X1	T44.0X2	T44.0X3	T44.0X4	T44.0X5	T44.0X6
Dymelor	T38.3X1	T38.3X2	T38.3X3	T38.3X4	T38.3X5	T38.3X6
Dynamite	T65.3X1	T65.3X2	T65.3X3	T65.3X4	—	—
fumes	T59.891	T59.892	T59.893	T59.894		
Dyphylline	T44.3X1	T44.3X2	T44.3X3	T44.3X4	T44.3X5	T44.3X6
b-eucaine	T49.1X1	T49.1X2	T49.1X3	T49.1X4	T49.1X5	T49.1X6
Ear drug NEC	T49.6X1	T49.6X2	T49.6X3	T49.6X4	T49.6X5	T49.6X6
Ear preparations	T49.6X1	T49.6X2	T49.6X3	T49.6X4	T49.6X5	T49.6X6
Echothiophate, echothiopate, ecothiopate	T49.5X1	T49.5X2	T49.5X3	T49.5X4	T49.5X5	T49.5X6
Econazole	T49.0X1	T49.0X2	T49.0X3	T49.0X4	T49.0X5	T49.0X6
Ecothiopate iodide	T49.5X1	T49.5X2	T49.5X3	T49.5X4	T49.5X5	T49.5X6
Ecstasy	T43.621	T43.622	T43.623	T43.624	T43.625	T43.626
Ectylurea	T42.6X1	T42.6X2	T42.6X3	T42.6X4	T42.6X5	T42.6X6
Edathamil disodium	T45.8X1	T45.8X2	T45.8X3	T45.8X4	T45.8X5	T45.8X6
Edecrin	T50.1X1	T50.1X2	T50.1X3	T50.1X4	T50.1X5	T50.1X6
Edetate, disodium (calcium)	T45.8X1	T45.8X2	T45.8X3	T45.8X4	T45.8X5	T45.8X6
Edoxudine	T49.5X1	T49.5X2	T49.5X3	T49.5X4	T49.5X5	T49.5X6
Edrophonium	T44.0X1	T44.0X2	T44.0X3	T44.0X4	T44.0X5	T44.0X6
chloride	T44.0X1	T44.0X2	T44.0X3	T44.0X4	T44.0X5	T44.0X6
EDTA	T50.6X1	T50.6X2	T50.6X3	T50.6X4	T50.6X5	T50.6X6
Eflornithine	T37.2X1	T37.2X2	T37.2X3	T37.2X4	T37.2X5	T37.2X6
Efloxate	T46.3X1	T46.3X2	T46.3X3	T46.3X4	T46.3X5	T46.3X6
Elase	T49.8X1	T49.8X2	T49.8X3	T49.8X4	T49.8X5	T49.8X6
Elastase	T47.5X1	T47.5X2	T47.5X3	T47.5X4	T47.5X5	T47.5X6
Elaterium	T47.2X1	T47.2X2	T47.2X3	T47.2X4	T47.2X5	T47.2X6
Elcatonin	T50.991	T50.992	T50.993	T50.994	T50.995	T50.996
Elder	T62.2X1	T62.2X2	T62.2X3	T62.2X4	—	—
berry, (unripe)	T62.1X1	T62.1X2	T62.1X3	T62.1X4	—	—
Electrolyte balance drug	T50.3X1	T50.3X2	T50.3X3	T50.3X4	T50.3X5	T50.3X6
Electrolytes NEC	T50.3X1	T50.3X2	T50.3X3	T50.3X4	T50.3X5	T50.3X6
Electrolytic agent NEC	T50.3X1	T50.3X2	T50.3X3	T50.3X4	T50.3X5	T50.3X6
Elemental diet	T50.901	T50.902	T50.903	T50.904	T50.905	T50.906
Elliptinium acetate	T45.1X1	T45.1X2	T45.1X3	T45.1X4	T45.1X5	T45.1X6
Embramine	T45.0X1	T45.0X2	T45.0X3	T45.0X4	T45.0X5	T45.0X6
Emepronium (salts)	T44.3X1	T44.3X2	T44.3X3	T44.3X4	T44.3X5	T44.3X6
bromide	T44.3X1	T44.3X2	T44.3X3	T44.3X4	T44.3X5	T44.3X6
Emetic NEC	T47.7X1	T47.7X2	T47.7X3	T47.7X4	T47.7X5	T47.7X6
Emetine	T37.3X1	T37.3X2	T37.3X3	T37.3X4	T37.3X5	T37.3X6
Emollient NEC	T49.3X1	T49.3X2	T49.3X3	T49.3X4	T49.3X5	T49.3X6
Emorfazone	T39.8X1	T39.8X2	T39.8X3	T39.8X4	T39.8X5	T39.8X6
Emylcamate	T43.591	T43.592	T43.593	T43.594	T43.595	T43.596
Enalapril	T46.4X1	T46.4X2	T46.4X3	T46.4X4	T46.4X5	T46.4X6
Enalaprilat	T46.4X1	T46.4X2	T46.4X3	T46.4X4	T46.4X5	T46.4X6
Encainide	T46.2X1	T46.2X2	T46.2X3	T46.2X4	T46.2X5	T46.2X6
Endocaine	T41.3X1	T41.3X2	T41.3X3	T41.3X4	T41.3X5	T41.3X6
Endosulfan	T60.2X1	T60.2X2	T60.2X3	T60.2X4	—	—
Endothall	T60.3X1	T60.3X2	T60.3X3	T60.3X4	—	—
Endralazine	T46.5X1	T46.5X2	T46.5X3	T46.5X4	T46.5X5	T46.5X6
Endrin	T60.1X1	T60.1X2	T60.1X3	T60.1X4	—	—
Enflurane	T41.0X1	T41.0X2	T41.0X3	T41.0X4	T41.0X5	T41.0X6
Enhexymal	T42.3X1	T42.3X2	T42.3X3	T42.3X4	T42.3X5	T42.3X6
Enocitabine	T45.1X1	T45.1X2	T45.1X3	T45.1X4	T45.1X5	T45.1X6
Enovid	T38.4X1	T38.4X2	T38.4X3	T38.4X4	T38.4X5	T38.4X6
Enoxacin	T36.8X1	T36.8X2	T36.8X3	T36.8X4	T36.8X5	T36.8X6
Enoxaparin (sodium)	T45.511	T45.512	T45.513	T45.514	T45.515	T45.516
Enpiprazole	T43.591	T43.592	T43.593	T43.594	T43.595	T43.596
Enprofylline	T48.6X1	T48.6X2	T48.6X3	T48.6X4	T48.6X5	T48.6X6
Enprostil	T47.1X1	T47.1X2	T47.1X3	T47.1X4	T47.1X5	T47.1X6
Enterogastrone	T38.891	T38.892	T38.893	T38.894	T38.895	T38.896
ENT preparations (anti-infectives)	T49.6X1	T49.6X2	T49.6X3	T49.6X4	T49.6X5	T49.6X6
Enviomycin	T36.8X1	T36.8X2	T36.8X3	T36.8X4	T36.8X5	T36.8X6

Substance	Poisoning, Accidental (unintentional)	Poisoning, Intentional Self-harm	Poisoning, Assault	Poisoning, Undetermined	Adverse Effect	Under-dosing
Enzodase	T45.3X1	T45.3X2	T45.3X3	T45.3X4	T45.3X5	T45.3X6
Enzyme NEC	T45.3X1	T45.3X2	T45.3X3	T45.3X4	T45.3X5	T45.3X6
depolymerizing	T49.8X1	T49.8X2	T49.8X3	T49.8X4	T49.8X5	T49.8X6
fibrolytic	T45.3X1	T45.3X2	T45.3X3	T45.3X4	T45.3X5	T45.3X6
gastric	T47.5X1	T47.5X2	T47.5X3	T47.5X4	T47.5X5	T47.5X6
intestinal	T47.5X1	T47.5X2	T47.5X3	T47.5X4	T47.5X5	T47.5X6
local action	T49.4X1	T49.4X2	T49.4X3	T49.4X4	T49.4X5	T49.4X6
proteolytic	T49.4X1	T49.4X2	T49.4X3	T49.4X4	T49.4X5	T49.4X6
thrombolytic	T45.3X1	T45.3X2	T45.3X3	T45.3X4	T45.3X5	T45.3X6
EPAB	T41.3X1	T41.3X2	T41.3X3	T41.3X4	T41.3X5	T41.3X6
Epanutin	T42.0X1	T42.0X2	T42.0X3	T42.0X4	T42.0X5	T42.0X6
Ephedra	T44.991	T44.992	T44.993	T44.994	T44.995	T44.996
Ephedrine	T44.991	T44.992	T44.993	T44.994	T44.995	T44.996
Epichlorhydrin, epichlorohydrin	T52.8X1	T52.8X2	T52.8X3	T52.8X4		
Epicillin	T36.0X1	T36.0X2	T36.0X3	T36.0X4	T36.0X5	T36.0X6
Epiestriol	T38.5X1	T38.5X2	T38.5X3	T38.5X4	T38.5X5	T38.5X6
Epilim — see Sodium valproate						
Epimestrol	T38.5X1	T38.5X2	T38.5X3	T38.5X4	T38.5X5	T38.5X6
Epinephrine	T44.5X1	T44.5X2	T44.5X3	T44.5X4	T44.5X5	T44.5X6
Epirubicin	T45.1X1	T45.1X2	T45.1X3	T45.1X4	T45.1X5	T45.1X6
Epitiostanol	T38.7X1	T38.7X2	T38.7X3	T38.7X4	T38.7X5	T38.7X6
Epitizide	T50.2X1	T50.2X2	T50.2X3	T50.2X4	T50.2X5	T50.2X6
EPN	T60.0X1	T60.0X2	T60.0X3	T60.0X4	—	—
EPO	T45.8X1	T45.8X2	T45.8X3	T45.8X4	T45.8X5	T45.8X6
Epoetin alpha	T45.8X1	T45.8X2	T45.8X3	T45.8X4	T45.8X5	T45.8X6
Epomediol	T50.991	T50.992	T50.993	T50.994	T50.995	T50.996
Epoprostenol	T45.521	T45.522	T45.523	T45.524	T45.525	T45.526
Epoxy resin	T65.891	T65.892	T65.893	T65.894		
Eprazinone	T48.4X1	T48.4X2	T48.4X3	T48.4X4	T48.4X5	T48.4X6
Epsilon aminocaproic acid	T45.621	T45.622	T45.623	T45.624	T45.625	T45.626
Epsom salt	T47.3X1	T47.3X2	T47.3X3	T47.3X4	T47.3X5	T47.3X6
Eptazocine	T40.4X1	T40.4X2	T40.4X3	T40.4X4	T40.4X5	T40.4X6
Equanil	T43.591	T43.592	T43.593	T43.594	T43.595	T43.596
Equisetum	T62.2X1	T62.2X2	T62.2X3	T62.2X4	—	—
diuretic	T50.2X1	T50.2X2	T50.2X3	T50.2X4	T50.2X5	T50.2X6
Ergobasine	T48.0X1	T48.0X2	T48.0X3	T48.0X4	T48.0X5	T48.0X6
Ergocalciferol	T45.2X1	T45.2X2	T45.2X3	T45.2X4	T45.2X5	T45.2X6
Ergoloid mesylates	T46.7X1	T46.7X2	T46.7X3	T46.7X4	T46.7X5	T46.7X6
Ergometrine	T48.0X1	T48.0X2	T48.0X3	T48.0X4	T48.0X5	T48.0X6
Ergonovine	T48.0X1	T48.0X2	T48.0X3	T48.0X4	T48.0X5	T48.0X6
Ergotamine	T46.5X1	T46.5X2	T46.5X3	T46.5X4	T46.5X5	T46.5X6
Ergotocine	T48.0X1	T48.0X2	T48.0X3	T48.0X4	T48.0X5	T48.0X6
Ergotrate	T48.0X1	T48.0X2	T48.0X3	T48.0X4	T48.0X5	T48.0X6
Ergot NEC	T64.81	T64.82	T64.83	T64.84	—	—
derivative	T48.0X1	T48.0X2	T48.0X3	T48.0X4	T48.0X5	T48.0X6
medicinal (alkaloids)	T48.0X1	T48.0X2	T48.0X3	T48.0X4	T48.0X5	T48.0X6
prepared	T48.0X1	T48.0X2	T48.0X3	T48.0X4	T48.0X5	T48.0X6
Eritrityl tetranitrate	T46.3X1	T46.3X2	T46.3X3	T46.3X4	T46.3X5	T46.3X6
Erythrityl tetranitrate	T46.3X1	T46.3X2	T46.3X3	T46.3X4	T46.3X5	T46.3X6
Erythrol tetranitrate	T46.3X1	T46.3X2	T46.3X3	T46.3X4	T46.3X5	T46.3X6
Erythromycin (salts)	T36.3X1	T36.3X2	T36.3X3	T36.3X4	T36.3X5	T36.3X6
ophthalmic preparation	T49.5X1	T49.5X2	T49.5X3	T49.5X4	T49.5X5	T49.5X6
topical NEC	T49.0X1	T49.0X2	T49.0X3	T49.0X4	T49.0X5	T49.0X6
Erythropoietin	T45.8X1	T45.8X2	T45.8X3	T45.8X4	T45.8X5	T45.8X6
human	T45.8X1	T45.8X2	T45.8X3	T45.8X4	T45.8X5	T45.8X6
Escin	T46.991	T46.992	T46.993	T46.994	T46.995	T46.996
Esculin	T45.2X1	T45.2X2	T45.2X3	T45.2X4	T45.2X5	T45.2X6
Esculoside	T45.2X1	T45.2X2	T45.2X3	T45.2X4	T45.2X5	T45.2X6
ESDT (ether-soluble tar distillate)	T49.1X1	T49.1X2	T49.1X3	T49.1X4	T49.1X5	T49.1X6
Eserine	T49.5X1	T49.5X2	T49.5X3	T49.5X4	T49.5X5	T49.5X6
Esflurbiprofen	T39.311	T39.312	T39.313	T39.314	T39.315	T39.316
Eskabarb	T42.3X1	T42.3X2	T42.3X3	T42.3X4	T42.3X5	T42.3X6
Eskalith	T43.8X1	T43.8X2	T43.8X3	T43.8X4	T43.8X5	T43.8X6
Esmolol	T44.7X1	T44.7X2	T44.7X3	T44.7X4	T44.7X5	T44.7X6
Estanozolol	T38.7X1	T38.7X2	T38.7X3	T38.7X4	T38.7X5	T38.7X6
Estazolam	T42.4X1	T42.4X2	T42.4X3	T42.4X4	T42.4X5	T42.4X6
Estradiol	T38.5X1	T38.5X2	T38.5X3	T38.5X4	T38.5X5	T38.5X6
with testosterone	T38.7X1	T38.7X2	T38.7X3	T38.7X4	T38.7X5	T38.7X6
benzoate	T38.5X1	T38.5X2	T38.5X3	T38.5X4	T38.5X5	T38.5X6
Estramustine	T45.1X1	T45.1X2	T45.1X3	T45.1X4	T45.1X5	T45.1X6
Estriol	T38.5X1	T38.5X2	T38.5X3	T38.5X4	T38.5X5	T38.5X6
Estrogen	T38.5X1	T38.5X2	T38.5X3	T38.5X4	T38.5X5	T38.5X6
with progesterone	T38.5X1	T38.5X2	T38.5X3	T38.5X4	T38.5X5	T38.5X6
conjugated	T38.5X1	T38.5X2	T38.5X3	T38.5X4	T38.5X5	T38.5X6
Estrone	T38.5X1	T38.5X2	T38.5X3	T38.5X4	T38.5X5	T38.5X6
Estropipate	T38.5X1	T38.5X2	T38.5X3	T38.5X4	T38.5X5	T38.5X6
Etacrynate sodium	T50.1X1	T50.1X2	T50.1X3	T50.1X4	T50.1X5	T50.1X6
Etacrynic acid	T50.1X1	T50.1X2	T50.1X3	T50.1X4	T50.1X5	T50.1X6
Etafedrine	T48.6X1	T48.6X2	T48.6X3	T48.6X4	T48.6X5	T48.6X6
Etafenone	T46.3X1	T46.3X2	T46.3X3	T46.3X4	T46.3X5	T46.3X6
Etambutol	T37.1X1	T37.1X2	T37.1X3	T37.1X4	T37.1X5	T37.1X6

Additional Character May Be Required — Refer to the Tabular List for Character Selection   ▽ Subterms under main terms may continue to next column or page

Substance	Poisoning, Accidental (unintentional)	Poisoning, Intentional Self-harm	Poisoning, Assault	Poisoning, Undetermined	Adverse Effect	Under-dosing
Etamiphyllin	T48.6X1	T48.6X2	T48.6X3	T48.6X4	T48.6X5	T48.6X6
Etamivan	T50.7X1	T50.7X2	T50.7X3	T50.7X4	T50.7X5	T50.7X6
Etamsylate	T45.7X1	T45.7X2	T45.7X3	T45.7X4	T45.7X5	T45.7X6
Etebenecid	T50.4X1	T50.4X2	T50.4X3	T50.4X4	T50.4X5	T50.4X6
Ethacridine	T49.0X1	T49.0X2	T49.0X3	T49.0X4	T49.0X5	T49.0X6
Ethacrynic acid	T50.1X1	T50.1X2	T50.1X3	T50.1X4	T50.1X5	T50.1X6
Ethadione	T42.2X1	T42.2X2	T42.2X3	T42.2X4	T42.2X5	T42.2X6
Ethambutol	T37.1X1	T37.1X2	T37.1X3	T37.1X4	T37.1X5	T37.1X6
Ethamide	T50.2X1	T50.2X2	T50.2X3	T50.2X4	T50.2X5	T50.2X6
Ethamivan	T50.7X1	T50.7X2	T50.7X3	T50.7X4	T50.7X5	T50.7X6
Ethamsylate	T45.7X1	T45.7X2	T45.7X3	T45.7X4	T45.7X5	T45.7X6
Ethanol	T51.0X1	T51.0X2	T51.0X3	T51.0X4	—	—
beverage	T51.0X1	T51.0X2	T51.0X3	T51.0X4	—	—
Ethanolamine oleate	T46.8X1	T46.8X2	T46.8X3	T46.8X4	T46.8X5	T46.8X6
Ethaverine	T44.3X1	T44.3X2	T44.3X3	T44.3X4	T44.3X5	T44.3X6
Ethchlorvynol	T42.6X1	T42.6X2	T42.6X3	T42.6X4	T42.6X5	T42.6X6
Ethebenecid	T50.4X1	T50.4X2	T50.4X3	T50.4X4	T50.4X5	T50.4X6
Ether (vapor)	T41.0X1	T41.0X2	T41.0X3	T41.0X4	T41.0X5	T41.0X6
anesthetic	T41.0X1	T41.0X2	T41.0X3	T41.0X4	T41.0X5	T41.0X6
divinyl	T41.0X1	T41.0X2	T41.0X3	T41.0X4	T41.0X5	T41.0X6
ethyl (medicinal)	T41.0X1	T41.0X2	T41.0X3	T41.0X4	T41.0X5	T41.0X6
nonmedicinal	T52.8X1	T52.8X2	T52.8X3	T52.8X4	—	—
petroleum — see Ligroin						
solvent	T52.8X1	T52.8X2	T52.8X3	T52.8X4	—	—
Ethiazide	T50.2X1	T50.2X2	T50.2X3	T50.2X4	T50.2X5	T50.2X6
Ethidium chloride (vapor)	T59.891	T59.892	T59.893	T59.894		
Ethinamate	T42.6X1	T42.6X2	T42.6X3	T42.6X4	T42.6X5	T42.6X6
Ethinylestradiol, ethinyloestradiol	T38.5X1	T38.5X2	T38.5X3	T38.5X4	T38.5X5	T38.5X6
with						
levonorgestrel	T38.4X1	T38.4X2	T38.4X3	T38.4X4	T38.4X5	T38.4X6
norethisterone	T38.4X1	T38.4X2	T38.4X3	T38.4X4	T38.4X5	T38.4X6
Ethiodized oil (131 I)	T50.8X1	T50.8X2	T50.8X3	T50.8X4	T50.8X5	T50.8X6
Ethion	T60.0X1	T60.0X2	T60.0X3	T60.0X4		
Ethionamide	T37.1X1	T37.1X2	T37.1X3	T37.1X4	T37.1X5	T37.1X6
Ethioniamide	T37.1X1	T37.1X2	T37.1X3	T37.1X4	T37.1X5	T37.1X6
Ethisterone	T38.5X1	T38.5X2	T38.5X3	T38.5X4	T38.5X5	T38.5X6
Ethobral	T42.3X1	T42.3X2	T42.3X3	T42.3X4	T42.3X5	T42.3X6
Ethocaine (infiltration)	T41.3X1	T41.3X2	T41.3X3	T41.3X4	T41.3X5	T41.3X6
(topical)	T41.3X1	T41.3X2	T41.3X3	T41.3X4	T41.3X5	T41.3X6
nerve block (peripheral) (plexus)	T41.3X1	T41.3X2	T41.3X3	T41.3X4	T41.3X5	T41.3X6
spinal	T41.3X1	T41.3X2	T41.3X3	T41.3X4	T41.3X5	T41.3X6
Ethoheptazine	T40.4X1	T40.4X2	T40.4X3	T40.4X4	T40.4X5	T40.4X6
Ethopropazine	T44.3X1	T44.3X2	T44.3X3	T44.3X4	T44.3X5	T44.3X6
Ethosuximide	T42.2X1	T42.2X2	T42.2X3	T42.2X4	T42.2X5	T42.2X6
Ethotoin	T42.0X1	T42.0X2	T42.0X3	T42.0X4	T42.0X5	T42.0X6
Ethoxazene	T37.91	T37.92	T37.93	T37.94	T37.95	T37.96
Ethoxazorutoside	T46.991	T46.992	T46.993	T46.994	T46.995	T46.996
Ethoxzolamide	T50.2X1	T50.2X2	T50.2X3	T50.2X4	T50.2X5	T50.2X6
Ethyl						
acetate	T52.8X1	T52.8X2	T52.8X3	T52.8X4	—	—
alcohol	T51.0X1	T51.0X2	T51.0X3	T51.0X4	—	—
beverage	T51.0X1	T51.0X2	T51.0X3	T51.0X4	—	—
aldehyde (vapor)	T59.891	T59.892	T59.893	T59.894	—	—
liquid	T52.8X1	T52.8X2	T52.8X3	T52.8X4	—	—
aminobenzoate	T41.3X1	T41.3X2	T41.3X3	T41.3X4	T41.3X5	T41.3X6
aminophenothiazine	T43.3X1	T43.3X2	T43.3X3	T43.3X4	T43.3X5	T43.3X6
benzoate	T52.8X1	T52.8X2	T52.8X3	T52.8X4	—	—
biscoumacetate	T45.511	T45.512	T45.513	T45.514	T45.515	T45.516
bromide (anesthetic)	T41.0X1	T41.0X2	T41.0X3	T41.0X4	T41.0X5	T41.0X6
carbamate	T45.1X1	T45.1X2	T45.1X3	T45.1X4	T45.1X5	T45.1X6
carbinol	T51.3X1	T51.3X2	T51.3X3	T51.3X4	—	—
carbonate	T52.8X1	T52.8X2	T52.8X3	T52.8X4	—	—
chaulmoograte	T37.1X1	T37.1X2	T37.1X3	T37.1X4	T37.1X5	T37.1X6
chloride (anesthetic)	T41.0X1	T41.0X2	T41.0X3	T41.0X4	T41.0X5	T41.0X6
anesthetic (local)	T41.3X1	T41.3X2	T41.3X3	T41.3X4	T41.3X5	T41.3X6
inhaled	T41.0X1	T41.0X2	T41.0X3	T41.0X4	T41.0X5	T41.0X6
local	T49.4X1	T49.4X2	T49.4X3	T49.4X4	T49.4X5	T49.4X6
solvent	T53.6X1	T53.6X2	T53.6X3	T53.6X4	—	—
dibunate	T48.3X1	T48.3X2	T48.3X3	T48.3X4	T48.3X5	T48.3X6
dichloroarsine (vapor)	T57.0X1	T57.0X2	T57.0X3	T57.0X4	—	—
estranol	T38.7X1	T38.7X2	T38.7X3	T38.7X4	T38.7X5	T38.7X6
ether — see also ether	T52.8X1	T52.8X2	T52.8X3	T52.8X4	—	—
formate NEC (solvent)	T52.0X1	T52.0X2	T52.0X3	T52.0X4	—	—
fumarate	T49.4X1	T49.4X2	T49.4X3	T49.4X4	T49.4X5	T49.4X6
hydroxyisobutyrate NEC (solvent)	T52.8X1	T52.8X2	T52.8X3	T52.8X4	—	—
iodoacetate	T59.3X1	T59.3X2	T59.3X3	T59.3X4	—	—
lactate NEC (solvent)	T52.8X1	T52.8X2	T52.8X3	T52.8X4	—	—
loflazepate	T42.4X1	T42.4X2	T42.4X3	T42.4X4	T42.4X5	T42.4X6
mercuric chloride	T56.1X1	T56.1X2	T56.1X3	T56.1X4	—	—
methylcarbinol	T51.8X1	T51.8X2	T51.8X3	T51.8X4	—	—
Ethyl — continued						
morphine	T40.2X1	T40.2X2	T40.2X3	T40.2X4	T40.2X5	T40.2X6
noradrenaline	T48.6X1	T48.6X2	T48.6X3	T48.6X4	T48.6X5	T48.6X6
oxybutyrate NEC (solvent)	T52.8X1	T52.8X2	T52.8X3	T52.8X4		
Ethylene (gas)	T59.891	T59.892	T59.893	T59.894	—	—
anesthetic (general)	T41.0X1	T41.0X2	T41.0X3	T41.0X4	T41.0X5	T41.0X6
chlorohydrin	T52.8X1	T52.8X2	T52.8X3	T52.8X4	—	—
vapor	T53.6X1	T53.6X2	T53.6X3	T53.6X4	—	—
dichloride	T52.8X1	T52.8X2	T52.8X3	T52.8X4	—	—
vapor	T53.6X1	T53.6X2	T53.6X3	T53.6X4	—	—
dinitrate	T52.3X1	T52.3X2	T52.3X3	T52.3X4	—	—
glycol(s)	T52.8X1	T52.8X2	T52.8X3	T52.8X4	—	—
dinitrate	T52.3X1	T52.3X2	T52.3X3	T52.3X4	—	—
monobutyl ether	T52.3X1	T52.3X2	T52.3X3	T52.3X4	—	—
imine	T54.1X1	T54.1X2	T54.1X3	T54.1X4	—	—
oxide (fumigant) (nonmedicinal)	T59.891	T59.892	T59.893	T59.894	—	—
medicinal	T49.0X1	T49.0X2	T49.0X3	T49.0X4	T49.0X5	T49.0X6
Ethylenediaminetetra-acetic acid	T50.6X1	T50.6X2	T50.6X3	T50.6X4	T50.6X5	T50.6X6
Ethylenediamine theophylline	T48.6X1	T48.6X2	T48.6X3	T48.6X4	T48.6X5	T48.6X6
Ethylenedinitrilotetra-acetate	T50.6X1	T50.6X2	T50.6X3	T50.6X4	T50.6X5	T50.6X6
Ethylestrenol	T38.7X1	T38.7X2	T38.7X3	T38.7X4	T38.7X5	T38.7X6
Ethylhydroxycellulose	T47.4X1	T47.4X2	T47.4X3	T47.4X4	T47.4X5	T47.4X6
Ethylidene						
chloride NEC	T53.6X1	T53.6X2	T53.6X3	T53.6X4	—	—
diacetate	T60.3X1	T60.3X2	T60.3X3	T60.3X4	—	—
dicoumarin	T45.511	T45.512	T45.513	T45.514	T45.515	T45.516
dicoumarol	T45.511	T45.512	T45.513	T45.514	T45.515	T45.516
diethyl ether	T52.0X1	T52.0X2	T52.0X3	T52.0X4	—	—
Ethylmorphine	T40.2X1	T40.2X2	T40.2X3	T40.2X4	T40.2X5	T40.2X6
Ethylnorepinephrine	T48.6X1	T48.6X2	T48.6X3	T48.6X4	T48.6X5	T48.6X6
Ethylparachlorophen-oxyisobutyrate	T46.6X1	T46.6X2	T46.6X3	T46.6X4	T46.6X5	T46.6X6
Ethynodiol	T38.4X1	T38.4X2	T38.4X3	T38.4X4	T38.4X5	T38.4X6
with mestranol diacetate	T38.4X1	T38.4X2	T38.4X3	T38.4X4	T38.4X5	T38.4X6
Etidocaine	T41.3X1	T41.3X2	T41.3X3	T41.3X4	T41.3X5	T41.3X6
infiltration (subcutaneous)	T41.3X1	T41.3X2	T41.3X3	T41.3X4	T41.3X5	T41.3X6
nerve (peripheral) (plexus)	T41.3X1	T41.3X2	T41.3X3	T41.3X4	T41.3X5	T41.3X6
Etidronate	T50.991	T50.992	T50.993	T50.994	T50.995	T50.996
Etidronic acid (disodium salt)	T50.991	T50.992	T50.993	T50.994	T50.995	T50.996
Etifoxine	T42.6X1	T42.6X2	T42.6X3	T42.6X4	T42.6X5	T42.6X6
Etilefrine	T44.4X1	T44.4X2	T44.4X3	T44.4X4	T44.4X5	T44.4X6
Etilfen	T42.3X1	T42.3X2	T42.3X3	T42.3X4	T42.3X5	T42.3X6
Etinodiol	T38.4X1	T38.4X2	T38.4X3	T38.4X4	T38.4X5	T38.4X6
Etiroxate	T46.6X1	T46.6X2	T46.6X3	T46.6X4	T46.6X5	T46.6X6
Etizolam	T42.4X1	T42.4X2	T42.4X3	T42.4X4	T42.4X5	T42.4X6
Etodolac	T39.391	T39.392	T39.393	T39.394	T39.395	T39.396
Etofamide	T37.3X1	T37.3X2	T37.3X3	T37.3X4	T37.3X5	T37.3X6
Etofibrate	T46.6X1	T46.6X2	T46.6X3	T46.6X4	T46.6X5	T46.6X6
Etofylline	T46.7X1	T46.7X2	T46.7X3	T46.7X4	T46.7X5	T46.7X6
clofibrate	T46.6X1	T46.6X2	T46.6X3	T46.6X4	T46.6X5	T46.6X6
Etoglucid	T45.1X1	T45.1X2	T45.1X3	T45.1X4	T45.1X5	T45.1X6
Etomidate	T41.1X1	T41.1X2	T41.1X3	T41.1X4	T41.1X5	T41.1X6
Etomide	T39.8X1	T39.8X2	T39.8X3	T39.8X4	T39.8X5	T39.8X6
Etomidoline	T44.3X1	T44.3X2	T44.3X3	T44.3X4	T44.3X5	T44.3X6
Etoposide	T45.1X1	T45.1X2	T45.1X3	T45.1X4	T45.1X5	T45.1X6
Etorphine	T40.2X1	T40.2X2	T40.2X3	T40.2X4	T40.2X5	T40.2X6
Etoval	T42.3X1	T42.3X2	T42.3X3	T42.3X4	T42.3X5	T42.3X6
Etozolin	T50.1X1	T50.1X2	T50.1X3	T50.1X4	T50.1X5	T50.1X6
Etretinate	T50.991	T50.992	T50.993	T50.994	T50.995	T50.996
Etryptamine	T43.691	T43.692	T43.693	T43.694	T43.695	T43.696
Etybenzatropine	T44.3X1	T44.3X2	T44.3X3	T44.3X4	T44.3X5	T44.3X6
Etynodiol	T38.4X1	T38.4X2	T38.4X3	T38.4X4	T38.4X5	T38.4X6
Eucaine	T41.3X1	T41.3X2	T41.3X3	T41.3X4	T41.3X5	T41.3X6
Eucalyptus oil	T49.7X1	T49.7X2	T49.7X3	T49.7X4	T49.7X5	T49.7X6
Eucatropine	T49.5X1	T49.5X2	T49.5X3	T49.5X4	T49.5X5	T49.5X6
Eucodal	T40.2X1	T40.2X2	T40.2X3	T40.2X4	T40.2X5	T40.2X6
Euneryl	T42.3X1	T42.3X2	T42.3X3	T42.3X4	T42.3X5	T42.3X6
Euphthalmine	T44.3X1	T44.3X2	T44.3X3	T44.3X4	T44.3X5	T44.3X6
Eurax	T49.0X1	T49.0X2	T49.0X3	T49.0X4	T49.0X5	T49.0X6
Euresol	T49.4X1	T49.4X2	T49.4X3	T49.4X4	T49.4X5	T49.4X6
Euthroid	T38.1X1	T38.1X2	T38.1X3	T38.1X4	T38.1X5	T38.1X6
Evans blue	T50.8X1	T50.8X2	T50.8X3	T50.8X4	T50.8X5	T50.8X6
Evipal	T42.3X1	T42.3X2	T42.3X3	T42.3X4	T42.3X5	T42.3X6
sodium	T41.1X1	T41.1X2	T41.1X3	T41.1X4	T41.1X5	T41.1X6
Evipan	T42.3X1	T42.3X2	T42.3X3	T42.3X4	T42.3X5	T42.3X6
sodium	T41.1X1	T41.1X2	T41.1X3	T41.1X4	T41.1X5	T41.1X6
Exalamide	T49.0X1	T49.0X2	T49.0X3	T49.0X4	T49.0X5	T49.0X6
Exalgin	T39.1X1	T39.1X2	T39.1X3	T39.1X4	T39.1X5	T39.1X6
Excipients, pharmaceutical	T50.901	T50.902	T50.903	T50.904	T50.905	T50.906

Substance	Poisoning, Accidental (unintentional)	Poisoning, Intentional Self-harm	Poisoning, Assault	Poisoning, Undetermined	Adverse Effect	Under-dosing
Exhaust gas (engine) (motor vehicle)	T58.01	T58.02	T58.03	T58.04	—	—
Ex-Lax (phenolphthalein)	T47.2X1	T47.2X2	T47.2X3	T47.2X4	T47.2X5	T47.2X6
Expectorant NEC	T48.4X1	T48.4X2	T48.4X3	T48.4X4	T48.4X5	T48.4X6
Extended insulin zinc suspension	T38.3X1	T38.3X2	T38.3X3	T38.3X4	T38.3X5	T38.3X6
External medications (skin) (mucous membrane)	T49.91	T49.92	T49.93	T49.94	T49.95	T49.96
dental agent	T49.7X1	T49.7X2	T49.7X3	T49.7X4	T49.7X5	T49.7X6
ENT agent	T49.6X1	T49.6X2	T49.6X3	T49.6X4	T49.6X5	T49.6X6
ophthalmic preparation	T49.5X1	T49.5X2	T49.5X3	T49.5X4	T49.5X5	T49.5X6
specified NEC	T49.8X1	T49.8X2	T49.8X3	T49.8X4	T49.8X5	T49.8X6
Extrapyramidal antagonist NEC	T44.3X1	T44.3X2	T44.3X3	T44.3X4	T44.3X5	T44.3X6
Eye agents (anti-infective)	T49.5X1	T49.5X2	T49.5X3	T49.5X4	T49.5X5	T49.5X6
Eye drug NEC	T49.5X1	T49.5X2	T49.5X3	T49.5X4	T49.5X5	T49.5X6
FAC (fluorouracil + doxorubicin + cyclophosphamide)	T45.1X1	T45.1X2	T45.1X3	T45.1X4	T45.1X5	T45.1X6
Factor						
I (fibrinogen)	T45.8X1	T45.8X2	T45.8X3	T45.8X4	T45.8X5	T45.8X6
III (thromboplastin)	T45.8X1	T45.8X2	T45.8X3	T45.8X4	T45.8X5	T45.8X6
VIII (antihemophilic Factor) (concentrate)	T45.8X1	T45.8X2	T45.8X3	T45.8X4	T45.8X5	T45.8X6
IX complex	T45.7X1	T45.7X2	T45.7X3	T45.7X4	T45.7X5	T45.7X6
human	T45.8X1	T45.8X2	T45.8X3	T45.8X4	T45.8X5	T45.8X6
Famotidine	T47.0X1	T47.0X2	T47.0X3	T47.0X4	T47.0X5	T47.0X6
Fat suspension, intravenous	T50.991	T50.992	T50.993	T50.994	T50.995	T50.996
Fazadinium bromide	T48.1X1	T48.1X2	T48.1X3	T48.1X4	T48.1X5	T48.1X6
Febarbamate	T42.3X1	T42.3X2	T42.3X3	T42.3X4	T42.3X5	T42.3X6
Fecal softener	T47.4X1	T47.4X2	T47.4X3	T47.4X4	T47.4X5	T47.4X6
Fedrilate	T48.3X1	T48.3X2	T48.3X3	T48.3X4	T48.3X5	T48.3X6
Felodipine	T46.1X1	T46.1X2	T46.1X3	T46.1X4	T46.1X5	T46.1X6
Felypressin	T38.891	T38.892	T38.893	T38.894	T38.895	T38.896
Femoxetine	T43.221	T43.222	T43.223	T43.224	T43.225	T43.226
Fenalcomine	T46.3X1	T46.3X2	T46.3X3	T46.3X4	T46.3X5	T46.3X6
Fenamisal	T37.1X1	T37.1X2	T37.1X3	T37.1X4	T37.1X5	T37.1X6
Fenazone	T39.2X1	T39.2X2	T39.2X3	T39.2X4	T39.2X5	T39.2X6
Fenbendazole	T37.4X1	T37.4X2	T37.4X3	T37.4X4	T37.4X5	T37.4X6
Fenbutrazate	T50.5X1	T50.5X2	T50.5X3	T50.5X4	T50.5X5	T50.5X6
Fencamfamine	T43.691	T43.692	T43.693	T43.694	T43.695	T43.696
Fendiline	T46.1X1	T46.1X2	T46.1X3	T46.1X4	T46.1X5	T46.1X6
Fenetylline	T43.691	T43.692	T43.693	T43.694	T43.695	T43.696
Fenflumizole	T39.391	T39.392	T39.393	T39.394	T39.395	T39.396
Fenfluramine	T50.5X1	T50.5X2	T50.5X3	T50.5X4	T50.5X5	T50.5X6
Fenobarbital	T42.3X1	T42.3X2	T42.3X3	T42.3X4	T42.3X5	T42.3X6
Fenofibrate	T46.6X1	T46.6X2	T46.6X3	T46.6X4	T46.6X5	T46.6X6
Fenoprofen	T39.311	T39.312	T39.313	T39.314	T39.315	T39.316
Fenoterol	T48.6X1	T48.6X2	T48.6X3	T48.6X4	T48.6X5	T48.6X6
Fenoverine	T44.3X1	T44.3X2	T44.3X3	T44.3X4	T44.3X5	T44.3X6
Fenoxazoline	T48.5X1	T48.5X2	T48.5X3	T48.5X4	T48.5X5	T48.5X6
Fenproporex	T50.5X1	T50.5X2	T50.5X3	T50.5X4	T50.5X5	T50.5X6
Fenquizone	T50.2X1	T50.2X2	T50.2X3	T50.2X4	T50.2X5	T50.2X6
Fentanyl	T40.4X1	T40.4X2	T40.4X3	T40.4X4	T40.4X5	T40.4X6
Fentazin	T43.3X1	T43.3X2	T43.3X3	T43.3X4	T43.3X5	T43.3X6
Fenthion	T60.0X1	T60.0X2	T60.0X3	T60.0X4	—	—
Fenticlor	T49.0X1	T49.0X2	T49.0X3	T49.0X4	T49.0X5	T49.0X6
Fenylbutazone	T39.2X1	T39.2X2	T39.2X3	T39.2X4	T39.2X5	T39.2X6
Feprazone	T39.2X1	T39.2X2	T39.2X3	T39.2X4	T39.2X5	T39.2X6
Fer de lance (bite) (venom)	T63.061	T63.062	T63.063	T63.064	—	—
Ferric — see also Iron						
chloride	T45.4X1	T45.4X2	T45.4X3	T45.4X4	T45.4X5	T45.4X6
citrate	T45.4X1	T45.4X2	T45.4X3	T45.4X4	T45.4X5	T45.4X6
hydroxide						
colloidal	T45.4X1	T45.4X2	T45.4X3	T45.4X4	T45.4X5	T45.4X6
polymaltose	T45.4X1	T45.4X2	T45.4X3	T45.4X4	T45.4X5	T45.4X6
pyrophosphate	T45.4X1	T45.4X2	T45.4X3	T45.4X4	T45.4X5	T45.4X6
Ferritin	T45.4X1	T45.4X2	T45.4X3	T45.4X4	T45.4X5	T45.4X6
Ferrocholinate	T45.4X1	T45.4X2	T45.4X3	T45.4X4	T45.4X5	T45.4X6
Ferrodextrane	T45.4X1	T45.4X2	T45.4X3	T45.4X4	T45.4X5	T45.4X6
Ferropolimaler	T45.4X1	T45.4X2	T45.4X3	T45.4X4	T45.4X5	T45.4X6
Ferrous — see also Iron						
phosphate	T45.4X1	T45.4X2	T45.4X3	T45.4X4	T45.4X5	T45.4X6
salt	T45.4X1	T45.4X2	T45.4X3	T45.4X4	T45.4X5	T45.4X6
with folic acid	T45.4X1	T45.4X2	T45.4X3	T45.4X4	T45.4X5	T45.4X6
Ferrous fumarate, gluconate, lactate, salt NEC, sulfate (medicinal)	T45.4X1	T45.4X2	T45.4X3	T45.4X4	T45.4X5	T45.4X6
Ferrovanadium (fumes)	T59.891	T59.892	T59.893	T59.894	—	—
Ferrum — see Iron						
Fertilizers NEC	T65.891	T65.892	T65.893	T65.894	—	—
with herbicide mixture	T60.3X1	T60.3X2	T60.3X3	T60.3X4	—	—
Fetoxilate	T47.6X1	T47.6X2	T47.6X3	T47.6X4	T47.6X5	T47.6X6
Fiber, dietary	T47.4X1	T47.4X2	T47.4X3	T47.4X4	T47.4X5	T47.4X6
Fiberglass	T65.831	T65.832	T65.833	T65.834	—	—
Fibrinogen (human)	T45.8X1	T45.8X2	T45.8X3	T45.8X4	T45.8X5	T45.8X6
Fibrinolysin (human)	T45.691	T45.692	T45.693	T45.694	T45.695	T45.696
Fibrinolysis						
affecting drug	T45.601	T45.602	T45.603	T45.604	T45.605	T45.606
inhibitor NEC	T45.621	T45.622	T45.623	T45.624	T45.625	T45.626
Fibrinolytic drug	T45.611	T45.612	T45.613	T45.614	T45.615	T45.616
Filix mas	T37.4X1	T37.4X2	T37.4X3	T37.4X4	T37.4X5	T37.4X6
Filtering cream	T49.3X1	T49.3X2	T49.3X3	T49.3X4	T49.3X5	T49.3X6
Fiorinal	T39.011	T39.012	T39.013	T39.014	T39.015	T39.016
Firedamp	T59.891	T59.892	T59.893	T59.894	—	—
Fish, noxious, nonbacterial	T61.91	T61.92	T61.93	T61.94	—	—
ciguatera	T61.01	T61.02	T61.03	T61.04	—	—
scombroid	T61.11	T61.12	T61.13	T61.14	—	—
shell	T61.781	T61.782	T61.783	T61.784	—	—
specified NEC	T61.771	T61.772	T61.773	T61.774	—	—
Flagyl	T37.3X1	T37.3X2	T37.3X3	T37.3X4	T37.3X5	T37.3X6
Flavine adenine dinucleotide	T45.2X1	T45.2X2	T45.2X3	T45.2X4	T45.2X5	T45.2X6
Flavodic acid	T46.991	T46.992	T46.993	T46.994	T46.995	T46.996
Flavoxate	T44.3X1	T44.3X2	T44.3X3	T44.3X4	T44.3X5	T44.3X6
Flaxedil	T48.1X1	T48.1X2	T48.1X3	T48.1X4	T48.1X5	T48.1X6
Flaxseed (medicinal)	T49.3X1	T49.3X2	T49.3X3	T49.3X4	T49.3X5	T49.3X6
Flecainide	T46.2X1	T46.2X2	T46.2X3	T46.2X4	T46.2X5	T46.2X6
Fleroxacin	T36.8X1	T36.8X2	T36.8X3	T36.8X4	T36.8X5	T36.8X6
Floctafenine	T39.8X1	T39.8X2	T39.8X3	T39.8X4	T39.8X5	T39.8X6
Flomax	T44.6X1	T44.6X2	T44.6X3	T44.6X4	T44.6X5	T44.6X6
Flomoxef	T36.1X1	T36.1X2	T36.1X3	T36.1X4	T36.1X5	T36.1X6
Flopropione	T44.3X1	T44.3X2	T44.3X3	T44.3X4	T44.3X5	T44.3X6
Florantyrone	T47.5X1	T47.5X2	T47.5X3	T47.5X4	T47.5X5	T47.5X6
Floraquin	T37.8X1	T37.8X2	T37.8X3	T37.8X4	T37.8X5	T37.8X6
Florinef	T38.0X1	T38.0X2	T38.0X3	T38.0X4	T38.0X5	T38.0X6
ENT agent	T49.6X1	T49.6X2	T49.6X3	T49.6X4	T49.6X5	T49.6X6
ophthalmic preparation	T49.5X1	T49.5X2	T49.5X3	T49.5X4	T49.5X5	T49.5X6
topical NEC	T49.0X1	T49.0X2	T49.0X3	T49.0X4	T49.0X5	T49.0X6
Flowers of sulfur	T49.4X1	T49.4X2	T49.4X3	T49.4X4	T49.4X5	T49.4X6
Floxuridine	T45.1X1	T45.1X2	T45.1X3	T45.1X4	T45.1X5	T45.1X6
Fluanlsone	T43.4X1	T43.4X2	T43.4X3	T43.4X4	T43.4X5	T43.4X6
Flubendazole	T37.4X1	T37.4X2	T37.4X3	T37.4X4	T37.4X5	T37.4X6
Fluclorolone acetonide	T49.0X1	T49.0X2	T49.0X3	T49.0X4	T49.0X5	T49.0X6
Flucloxacillin	T36.0X1	T36.0X2	T36.0X3	T36.0X4	T36.0X5	T36.0X6
Fluconazole	T37.8X1	T37.8X2	T37.8X3	T37.8X4	T37.8X5	T37.8X6
Flucytosine	T37.8X1	T37.8X2	T37.8X3	T37.8X4	T37.8X5	T37.8X6
Fludeoxyglucose (18F)	T50.8X1	T50.8X2	T50.8X3	T50.8X4	T50.8X5	T50.8X6
Fludiazepam	T42.4X1	T42.4X2	T42.4X3	T42.4X4	T42.4X5	T42.4X6
Fludrocortisone	T50.0X1	T50.0X2	T50.0X3	T50.0X4	T50.0X5	T50.0X6
ENT agent	T49.6X1	T49.6X2	T49.6X3	T49.6X4	T49.6X5	T49.6X6
ophthalmic preparation	T49.5X1	T49.5X2	T49.5X3	T49.5X4	T49.5X5	T49.5X6
topical NEC	T49.0X1	T49.0X2	T49.0X3	T49.0X4	T49.0X5	T49.0X6
Fludroxycortide	T49.0X1	T49.0X2	T49.0X3	T49.0X4	T49.0X5	T49.0X6
Flufenamic acid	T39.391	T39.392	T39.393	T39.394	T39.395	T39.396
Fluindione	T45.511	T45.512	T45.513	T45.514	T45.515	T45.516
Flumequine	T37.8X1	T37.8X2	T37.8X3	T37.8X4	T37.8X5	T37.8X6
Flumethasone	T49.0X1	T49.0X2	T49.0X3	T49.0X4	T49.0X5	T49.0X6
Flumethiazide	T50.2X1	T50.2X2	T50.2X3	T50.2X4	T50.2X5	T50.2X6
Flumidin	T37.5X1	T37.5X2	T37.5X3	T37.5X4	T37.5X5	T37.5X6
Flunarizine	T46.7X1	T46.7X2	T46.7X3	T46.7X4	T46.7X5	T46.7X6
Flunidazole	T37.8X1	T37.8X2	T37.8X3	T37.8X4	T37.8X5	T37.8X6
Flunisolide	T48.6X1	T48.6X2	T48.6X3	T48.6X4	T48.6X5	T48.6X6
Flunitrazepam	T42.4X1	T42.4X2	T42.4X3	T42.4X4	T42.4X5	T42.4X6
Fluocinolone (acetonide)	T49.0X1	T49.0X2	T49.0X3	T49.0X4	T49.0X5	T49.0X6
Fluocinonide	T49.0X1	T49.0X2	T49.0X3	T49.0X4	T49.0X5	T49.0X6
Fluocortin (butyl)	T49.0X1	T49.0X2	T49.0X3	T49.0X4	T49.0X5	T49.0X6
Fluocortolone	T49.0X1	T49.0X2	T49.0X3	T49.0X4	T49.0X5	T49.0X6
Fluohydrocortisone	T38.0X1	T38.0X2	T38.0X3	T38.0X4	T38.0X5	T38.0X6
ENT agent	T49.6X1	T49.6X2	T49.6X3	T49.6X4	T49.6X5	T49.6X6
ophthalmic preparation	T49.5X1	T49.5X2	T49.5X3	T49.5X4	T49.5X5	T49.5X6
topical NEC	T49.0X1	T49.0X2	T49.0X3	T49.0X4	T49.0X5	T49.0X6
Fluonid	T49.0X1	T49.0X2	T49.0X3	T49.0X4	T49.0X5	T49.0X6
Fluopromazine	T43.3X1	T43.3X2	T43.3X3	T43.3X4	T43.3X5	T43.3X6
Fluoracetate	T60.8X1	T60.8X2	T60.8X3	T60.8X4	—	—
Fluorescein	T50.8X1	T50.8X2	T50.8X3	T50.8X4	T50.8X5	T50.8X6
Fluorhydrocortisone	T50.0X1	T50.0X2	T50.0X3	T50.0X4	T50.0X5	T50.0X6
Fluoride (nonmedicinal) (pesticide) (sodium) **NEC**	T60.8X1	T60.8X2	T60.8X3	T60.8X4	—	—
hydrogen — see Hydrofluoric acid						
medicinal NEC	T50.991	T50.992	T50.993	T50.994	T50.995	T50.996
dental use	T49.7X1	T49.7X2	T49.7X3	T49.7X4	T49.7X5	T49.7X6
not pesticide NEC	T54.91	T54.92	T54.93	T54.94	—	—
stannous	T49.7X1	T49.7X2	T49.7X3	T49.7X4	T49.7X5	T49.7X6
Fluorinated corticosteroids	T38.0X1	T38.0X2	T38.0X3	T38.0X4	T38.0X5	T38.0X6

Substance	Poisoning, Accidental (unintentional)	Poisoning, Intentional Self-harm	Poisoning, Assault	Poisoning, Undetermined	Adverse Effect	Under-dosing
Fluorine (gas)	T59.5X1	T59.5X2	T59.5X3	T59.5X4	—	—
salt — see Fluoride(s)						
Fluoristan	T49.7X1	T49.7X2	T49.7X3	T49.7X4	T49.7X5	T49.7X6
Fluormetholone	T49.0X1	T49.0X2	T49.0X3	T49.0X4	T49.0X5	T49.0X6
Fluoroacetate	T60.8X1	T60.8X2	T60.8X3	T60.8X4	—	—
Fluorocarbon monomer	T53.6X1	T53.6X2	T53.6X3	T53.6X4	—	—
Fluorocytosine	T37.8X1	T37.8X2	T37.8X3	T37.8X4	T37.8X5	T37.8X6
Fluorodeoxyuridine	T45.1X1	T45.1X2	T45.1X3	T45.1X4	T45.1X5	T45.1X6
Fluorometholone	T49.0X1	T49.0X2	T49.0X3	T49.0X4	T49.0X5	T49.0X6
ophthalmic preparation	T49.5X1	T49.5X2	T49.5X3	T49.5X4	T49.5X5	T49.5X6
Fluorophosphate insecticide	T60.0X1	T60.0X2	T60.0X3	T60.0X4	—	—
Fluorosol	T46.3X1	T46.3X2	T46.3X3	T46.3X4	T46.3X5	T46.3X6
Fluorouracil	T45.1X1	T45.1X2	T45.1X3	T45.1X4	T45.1X5	T45.1X6
Fluorphenylalanine	T49.5X1	T49.5X2	T49.5X3	T49.5X4	T49.5X5	T49.5X6
Fluothane	T41.0X1	T41.0X2	T41.0X3	T41.0X4	T41.0X5	T41.0X6
Fluoxetine	T43.221	T43.222	T43.223	T43.224	T43.225	T43.226
Fluoxymesterone	T38.7X1	T38.7X2	T38.7X3	T38.7X4	T38.7X5	T38.7X6
Flupenthixol	T43.4X1	T43.4X2	T43.4X3	T43.4X4	T43.4X5	T43.4X6
Flupentixol	T43.4X1	T43.4X2	T43.4X3	T43.4X4	T43.4X5	T43.4X6
Fluphenazine	T43.3X1	T43.3X2	T43.3X3	T43.3X4	T43.3X5	T43.3X6
Fluprednidene	T49.0X1	T49.0X2	T49.0X3	T49.0X4	T49.0X5	T49.0X6
Fluprednisolone	T38.0X1	T38.0X2	T38.0X3	T38.0X4	T38.0X5	T38.0X6
Fluradoline	T39.8X1	T39.8X2	T39.8X3	T39.8X4	T39.8X5	T39.8X6
Flurandrenolide	T49.0X1	T49.0X2	T49.0X3	T49.0X4	T49.0X5	T49.0X6
Flurandrenolone	T49.0X1	T49.0X2	T49.0X3	T49.0X4	T49.0X5	T49.0X6
Flurazepam	T42.4X1	T42.4X2	T42.4X3	T42.4X4	T42.4X5	T42.4X6
Flurbiprofen	T39.311	T39.312	T39.313	T39.314	T39.315	T39.316
Flurobate	T49.0X1	T49.0X2	T49.0X3	T49.0X4	T49.0X5	T49.0X6
Fluroxene	T41.0X1	T41.0X2	T41.0X3	T41.0X4	T41.0X5	T41.0X6
Fluspirilene	T43.591	T43.592	T43.593	T43.594	T43.595	T43.596
Flutamide	T38.6X1	T38.6X2	T38.6X3	T38.6X4	T38.6X5	T38.6X6
Flutazolam	T38.0X1	T38.0X2	T38.0X3	T38.0X4	T38.0X5	T38.0X6
Fluticasone propionate	T38.0X1	T38.0X2	T38.0X3	T38.0X4	T38.0X5	T38.0X6
Flutoprazepam	T42.4X1	T42.4X2	T42.4X3	T42.4X4	T42.4X5	T42.4X6
Flutropium bromide	T48.6X1	T48.6X2	T48.6X3	T48.6X4	T48.6X5	T48.6X6
Fluvoxamine	T43.221	T43.222	T43.223	T43.224	T43.225	T43.226
Folacin	T45.8X1	T45.8X2	T45.8X3	T45.8X4	T45.8X5	T45.8X6
Folic acid	T45.8X1	T45.8X2	T45.8X3	T45.8X4	T45.8X5	T45.8X6
with ferrous salt	T45.2X1	T45.2X2	T45.2X3	T45.2X4	T45.2X5	T45.2X6
antagonist	T45.1X1	T45.1X2	T45.1X3	T45.1X4	T45.1X5	T45.1X6
Folinic acid	T45.8X1	T45.8X2	T45.8X3	T45.8X4	T45.8X5	T45.8X6
Folium stramoniae	T48.6X1	T48.6X2	T48.6X3	T48.6X4	T48.6X5	T48.6X6
Follicle-stimulating hormone, human	T38.811	T38.812	T38.813	T38.814	T38.815	T38.816
Folpet	T60.3X1	T60.3X2	T60.3X3	T60.3X4	—	—
Fominoben	T48.3X1	T48.3X2	T48.3X3	T48.3X4	T48.3X5	T48.3X6
Food, foodstuffs, noxious, nonbacterial, NEC	T62.91	T62.92	T62.93	T62.94	—	—
berries	T62.1X1	T62.1X2	T62.1X3	T62.1X4	—	—
fish — see also Fish	T61.91	T61.92	T61.93	T61.94	—	—
mushrooms	T62.0X1	T62.0X2	T62.0X3	T62.0X4	—	—
plants	T62.2X1	T62.2X2	T62.2X3	T62.2X4	—	—
seafood	T61.91	T61.92	T61.93	T61.94	—	—
specified NEC	T61.8X1	T61.8X2	T61.8X3	T61.8X4	—	—
seeds	T62.2X1	T62.2X2	T62.2X3	T62.2X4	—	—
shellfish	T61.781	T61.782	T61.783	T61.784	—	—
specified NEC	T62.8X1	T62.8X2	T62.8X3	T62.8X4	—	—
Fool's parsley	T62.2X1	T62.2X2	T62.2X3	T62.2X4	—	—
Formaldehyde (solution), gas or vapor	T59.2X1	T59.2X2	T59.2X3	T59.2X4	—	—
fungicide	T60.3X1	T60.3X2	T60.3X3	T60.3X4	—	—
Formalin	T59.2X1	T59.2X2	T59.2X3	T59.2X4	—	—
fungicide	T60.3X1	T60.3X2	T60.3X3	T60.3X4	—	—
vapor	T59.2X1	T59.2X2	T59.2X3	T59.2X4	—	—
Formic acid	T54.2X1	T54.2X2	T54.2X3	T54.2X4	—	—
vapor	T59.891	T59.892	T59.893	T59.894	—	—
Foscarnet sodium	T37.5X1	T37.5X2	T37.5X3	T37.5X4	T37.5X5	T37.5X6
Fosfestrol	T38.5X1	T38.5X2	T38.5X3	T38.5X4	T38.5X5	T38.5X6
Fosfomycin	T36.8X1	T36.8X2	T36.8X3	T36.8X4	T36.8X5	T36.8X6
Fosfonet sodium	T37.5X1	T37.5X2	T37.5X3	T37.5X4	T37.5X5	T37.5X6
Fosinopril	T46.4X1	T46.4X2	T46.4X3	T46.4X4	T46.4X5	T46.4X6
sodium	T46.4X1	T46.4X2	T46.4X3	T46.4X4	T46.4X5	T46.4X6
Fowler's solution	T57.0X1	T57.0X2	T57.0X3	T57.0X4	—	—
Foxglove	T62.2X1	T62.2X2	T62.2X3	T62.2X4	—	—
Framycetin	T36.5X1	T36.5X2	T36.5X3	T36.5X4	T36.5X5	T36.5X6
Frangula	T47.2X1	T47.2X2	T47.2X3	T47.2X4	T47.2X5	T47.2X6
extract	T47.2X1	T47.2X2	T47.2X3	T47.2X4	T47.2X5	T47.2X6
Frei antigen	T50.8X1	T50.8X2	T50.8X3	T50.8X4	T50.8X5	T50.8X6
Freon	T53.5X1	T53.5X2	T53.5X3	T53.5X4	—	—
Fructose	T50.3X1	T50.3X2	T50.3X3	T50.3X4	T50.3X5	T50.3X6
Frusemide	T50.1X1	T50.1X2	T50.1X3	T50.1X4	T50.1X5	T50.1X6
FSH	T38.811	T38.812	T38.813	T38.814	T38.815	T38.816

Substance	Poisoning, Accidental (unintentional)	Poisoning, Intentional Self-harm	Poisoning, Assault	Poisoning, Undetermined	Adverse Effect	Under-dosing
Ftorafur	T45.1X1	T45.1X2	T45.1X3	T45.1X4	T45.1X5	T45.1X6
Fuel						
automobile	T52.0X1	T52.0X2	T52.0X3	T52.0X4	—	—
exhaust gas, not in transit	T58.01	T58.02	T58.03	T58.04	—	—
vapor NEC	T52.0X1	T52.0X2	T52.0X3	T52.0X4	—	—
gas (domestic use) — see also Carbon, monoxide, fuel, utility	T59.891	T59.892	T59.893	T59.894	—	—
utility	T59.891	T59.892	T59.893	T59.894	—	—
incomplete combustion of — see Carbon, monoxide, fuel, utility						
in mobile container	T59.891	T59.892	T59.893	T59.894	—	—
piped (natural)	T59.891	T59.892	T59.893	T59.894	—	—
industrial, incomplete combustion	T58.8X1	T58.8X2	T58.8X3	T58.8X4	—	—
Fugillin	T36.8X1	T36.8X2	T36.8X3	T36.8X4	T36.8X5	T36.8X6
Fulminate of mercury	T56.1X1	T56.1X2	T56.1X3	T56.1X4	—	—
Fulvicin	T36.7X1	T36.7X2	T36.7X3	T36.7X4	T36.7X5	T36.7X6
Fumadil	T36.8X1	T36.8X2	T36.8X3	T36.8X4	T36.8X5	T36.8X6
Fumagillin	T36.8X1	T36.8X2	T36.8X3	T36.8X4	T36.8X5	T36.8X6
Fumaric acid	T49.4X1	T49.4X2	T49.4X3	T49.4X4	T49.4X5	T49.4X6
Fumes (from)	T59.91	T59.92	T59.93	T59.94	—	—
carbon monoxide — see Carbon, monoxide						
charcoal (domestic use) — see Charcoal, fumes						
chloroform — see Chloroform						
coke (in domestic stoves, fireplaces) — see Coke fumes						
corrosive NEC	T54.91	T54.92	T54.93	T54.94	—	—
ether — see ether						
freons	T53.5X1	T53.5X2	T53.5X3	T53.5X4	—	—
hydrocarbons	T59.891	T59.892	T59.893	T59.894	—	—
petroleum (liquefied)	T59.891	T59.892	T59.893	T59.894	—	—
distributed through pipes (pure or mixed with air)	T59.891	T59.892	T59.893	T59.894	—	—
lead — see lead						
metal — see Metals, or the specified metal						
nitrogen dioxide	T59.0X1	T59.0X2	T59.0X3	T59.0X4	—	—
pesticides — see Pesticides						
petroleum (liquefied)	T59.891	T59.892	T59.893	T59.894	—	—
distributed through pipes (pure or mixed with air)	T59.891	T59.892	T59.893	T59.894	—	—
polyester	T59.891	T59.892	T59.893	T59.894	—	—
specified source NEC — see also substance specified	T59.891	T59.892	T59.893	T59.894	—	—
sulfur dioxide	T59.1X1	T59.1X2	T59.1X3	T59.1X4	—	—
Fumigant NEC	T60.91	T60.92	T60.93	T60.94	—	—
Fungicide NEC (nonmedicinal)	T60.3X1	T60.3X2	T60.3X3	T60.3X4	—	—
Fungi, noxious, used as food	T62.0X1	T62.0X2	T62.0X3	T62.0X4	—	—
Fungizone	T36.7X1	T36.7X2	T36.7X3	T36.7X4	T36.7X5	T36.7X6
topical	T49.0X1	T49.0X2	T49.0X3	T49.0X4	T49.0X5	T49.0X6
Furacin	T49.0X1	T49.0X2	T49.0X3	T49.0X4	T49.0X5	T49.0X6
Furadantin	T37.91	T37.92	T37.93	T37.94	T37.95	T37.96
Furazolidone	T37.8X1	T37.8X2	T37.8X3	T37.8X4	T37.8X5	T37.8X6
Furazolium chloride	T49.0X1	T49.0X2	T49.0X3	T49.0X4	T49.0X5	T49.0X6
Furfural	T52.8X1	T52.8X2	T52.8X3	T52.8X4	—	—
Furnace (coal burning) (domestic), gas from	T58.2X1	T58.2X2	T58.2X3	T58.2X4	—	—
industrial	T58.8X1	T58.8X2	T58.8X3	T58.8X4	—	—
Furniture polish	T65.891	T65.892	T65.893	T65.894	—	—
Furosemide	T50.1X1	T50.1X2	T50.1X3	T50.1X4	T50.1X5	T50.1X6
Furoxone	T37.91	T37.92	T37.93	T37.94	T37.95	T37.96
Fursultiamine	T45.2X1	T45.2X2	T45.2X3	T45.2X4	T45.2X5	T45.2X6
Fusafungine	T36.8X1	T36.8X2	T36.8X3	T36.8X4	T36.8X5	T36.8X6
Fusel oil (any) (amyl) (butyl) (propyl), vapor	T51.3X1	T51.3X2	T51.3X3	T51.3X4	—	—
Fusidate (ethanolamine) (sodium)	T36.8X1	T36.8X2	T36.8X3	T36.8X4	T36.8X5	T36.8X6
Fusidic acid	T36.8X1	T36.8X2	T36.8X3	T36.8X4	T36.8X5	T36.8X6
Fytic acid, nonasodium	T50.6X1	T50.6X2	T50.6X3	T50.6X4	T50.6X5	T50.6X6
b-Galactosidase	T47.5X1	T47.5X2	T47.5X3	T47.5X4	T47.5X5	T47.5X6
GABA	T43.8X1	T43.8X2	T43.8X3	T43.8X4	T43.8X5	T43.8X6
Gadopentetic acid	T50.8X1	T50.8X2	T50.8X3	T50.8X4	T50.8X5	T50.8X6
Galactose	T50.3X1	T50.3X2	T50.3X3	T50.3X4	T50.3X5	T50.3X6
Galantamine	T44.0X1	T44.0X2	T44.0X3	T44.0X4	T44.0X5	T44.0X6

Table of Drugs and Chemicals

Substance	Poisoning, Accidental (unintentional)	Poisoning, Intentional Self-harm	Poisoning, Assault	Poisoning, Undetermined	Adverse Effect	Under-dosing
Gallamine (triethiodide)	T48.1X1	T48.1X2	T48.1X3	T48.1X4	T48.1X5	T48.1X6
Gallium citrate	T50.991	T50.992	T50.993	T50.994	T50.995	T50.996
Gallopamil	T46.1X1	T46.1X2	T46.1X3	T46.1X4	T46.1X5	T46.1X6
Gamboge	T47.2X1	T47.2X2	T47.2X3	T47.2X4	T47.2X5	T47.2X6
Gamimune	T50.Z11	T50.Z12	T50.Z13	T50.Z14	T50.Z15	T50.Z16
Gamma-aminobutyric acid	T43.8X1	T43.8X2	T43.8X3	T43.8X4	T43.8X5	T43.8X6
Gamma-benzene hexachloride (medicinal)	T49.0X1	T49.0X2	T49.0X3	T49.0X4	T49.0X5	T49.0X6
nonmedicinal, vapor	T53.6X1	T53.6X2	T53.6X3	T53.6X4	—	—
Gamma-BHC (medicinal) — *see also* Gamma-benzene hexachloride	T49.0X1	T49.0X2	T49.0X3	T49.0X4	T49.0X5	T49.0X6
Gamma globulin	T50.Z11	T50.Z12	T50.Z13	T50.Z14	T50.Z15	T50.Z16
Gamulin	T50.Z11	T50.Z12	T50.Z13	T50.Z14	T50.Z15	T50.Z16
Ganciclovir (sodium)	T37.5X1	T37.5X2	T37.5X3	T37.5X4	T37.5X5	T37.5X6
Ganglionic blocking drug NEC	T44.2X1	T44.2X2	T44.2X3	T44.2X4	T44.2X5	T44.2X6
specified NEC	T44.2X1	T44.2X2	T44.2X3	T44.2X4	T44.2X5	T44.2X6
Ganja	T40.7X1	T40.7X2	T40.7X3	T40.7X4	T40.7X5	T40.7X6
Garamycin	T36.5X1	T36.5X2	T36.5X3	T36.5X4	T36.5X5	T36.5X6
ophthalmic preparation	T49.5X1	T49.5X2	T49.5X3	T49.5X4	T49.5X5	T49.5X6
topical NEC	T49.0X1	T49.0X2	T49.0X3	T49.0X4	T49.0X5	T49.0X6
Gardenal	T42.3X1	T42.3X2	T42.3X3	T42.3X4	T42.3X5	T42.3X6
Gardepanyl	T42.3X1	T42.3X2	T42.3X3	T42.3X4	T42.3X5	T42.3X6
Gaseous substance — *see* Gas						
Gasoline	T52.0X1	T52.0X2	T52.0X3	T52.0X4	—	—
vapor	T52.0X1	T52.0X2	T52.0X3	T52.0X4	—	—
Gastric enzymes	T47.5X1	T47.5X2	T47.5X3	T47.5X4	T47.5X5	T47.5X6
Gastrografin	T50.8X1	T50.8X2	T50.8X3	T50.8X4	T50.8X5	T50.8X6
Gastrointestinal drug	T47.91	T47.92	T47.93	T47.94	T47.95	T47.96
biological	T47.8X1	T47.8X2	T47.8X3	T47.8X4	T47.8X5	T47.8X6
specified NEC	T47.8X1	T47.8X2	T47.8X3	T47.8X4	T47.8X5	T47.8X6
Gas NEC	T59.91	T59.92	T59.93	T59.94	—	—
acetylene	T59.891	T59.892	T59.893	T59.894	—	—
incomplete combustion of	T58.11	T58.12	T58.13	T58.14	—	—
air contaminants, source or type not specified	T59.91	T59.92	T59.93	T59.94	—	—
anesthetic	T41.0X1	T41.0X2	T41.0X3	T41.0X4	T41.0X5	T41.0X6
blast furnace	T58.8X1	T58.8X2	T58.8X3	T58.8X4	—	—
butane — *see* butane						
carbon monoxide — *see* Carbon, monoxide						
chlorine	T59.4X1	T59.4X2	T59.4X3	T59.4X4	—	—
coal	T58.2X1	T58.2X2	T58.2X3	T58.2X4	—	—
cyanide	T57.3X1	T57.3X2	T57.3X3	T57.3X4	—	—
dicyanogen	T65.0X1	T65.0X2	T65.0X3	T65.0X4	—	—
domestic — *see* Domestic gas						
exhaust	T58.01	T58.02	T58.03	T58.04	—	—
from utility (for cooking, heating, or lighting) (after combustion) — *see* Carbon, monoxide, fuel, utility						
prior to combustion	T59.891	T59.892	T59.893	T59.894	—	—
from wood- or coal-burning stove or fireplace	T58.2X1	T58.2X2	T58.2X3	T58.2X4	—	—
fuel (domestic use) (after combustion) — *see also* Carbon, monoxide, fuel						
industrial use	T58.8X1	T58.8X2	T58.8X3	T58.8X4	—	—
prior to combustion	T59.891	T59.892	T59.893	T59.894	—	—
utility	T59.891	T59.892	T59.893	T59.894	—	—
incomplete combustion of — *see* Carbon, monoxide, fuel, utility						
in mobile container	T59.891	T59.892	T59.893	T59.894	—	—
piped (natural)	T59.891	T59.892	T59.893	T59.894	—	—
garage	T58.01	T58.02	T58.03	T58.04	—	—
hydrocarbon NEC	T59.891	T59.892	T59.893	T59.894	—	—
incomplete combustion of — *see* Carbon, monoxide, fuel, utility						
liquefied — *see* butane						
piped	T59.891	T59.892	T59.893	T59.894	—	—
hydrocyanic acid	T65.0X1	T65.0X2	T65.0X3	T65.0X4	—	—
illuminating (after combustion)	T58.11	T58.12	T58.13	T58.14	—	—
prior to combustion	T59.891	T59.892	T59.893	T59.894	—	—
incomplete combustion, any — *see* Carbon, monoxide						
kiln	T58.8X1	T58.8X2	T58.8X3	T58.8X4	—	—
lacrimogenic	T59.3X1	T59.3X2	T59.3X3	T59.3X4	—	—
Gas — *continued*						
liquefied petroleum — *see* butane						
marsh	T59.891	T59.892	T59.893	T59.894	—	—
motor exhaust, not in transit	T58.01	T58.02	T58.03	T58.04	—	—
mustard, not in war	T59.891	T59.892	T59.893	T59.894	—	—
natural	T59.891	T59.892	T59.893	T59.894	—	—
nerve, not in war	T59.91	T59.92	T59.93	T59.94	—	—
oil	T52.0X1	T52.0X2	T52.0X3	T52.0X4	—	—
petroleum (liquefied) (distributed in mobile containers)	T59.891	T59.892	T59.893	T59.894	—	—
piped (pure or mixed with air)	T59.891	T59.892	T59.893	T59.894	—	—
piped (manufactured) (natural) NEC	T59.891	T59.892	T59.893	T59.894	—	—
producer	T58.8X1	T58.8X2	T58.8X3	T58.8X4	—	—
propane — *see* propane						
refrigerant (chlorofluoro-carbon)	T53.5X1	T53.5X2	T53.5X3	T53.5X4	—	—
not chlorofluoro-carbon	T59.891	T59.892	T59.893	T59.894	—	—
sewer	T59.91	T59.92	T59.93	T59.94	—	—
specified source NEC	T59.91	T59.92	T59.93	T59.94	—	—
stove (after combustion)	T58.11	T58.12	T58.13	T58.14	—	—
prior to combustion	T59.891	T59.892	T59.893	T59.894	—	—
tear	T59.3X1	T59.3X2	T59.3X3	T59.3X4	—	—
therapeutic	T41.5X1	T41.5X2	T41.5X3	T41.5X4	T41.5X5	T41.5X6
utility (for cooking, heating, or lighting) (piped) NEC	T59.891	T59.892	T59.893	T59.894	—	—
incomplete combustion of — *see* Carbon, monoxide, fuel, utilty						
in mobile container	T59.891	T59.892	T59.893	T59.894	—	—
piped (natural)	T59.891	T59.892	T59.893	T59.894	—	—
water	T58.11	T58.12	T58.13	T58.14	—	—
incomplete combustion of — *see* Carbon, monoxide, fuel, utility						
Gaultheria procumbens	T62.2X1	T62.2X2	T62.2X3	T62.2X4	—	—
Gefarnate	T44.3X1	T44.3X2	T44.3X3	T44.3X4	T44.3X5	T44.3X6
Gelatin (intravenous)	T45.8X1	T45.8X2	T45.8X3	T45.8X4	T45.8X5	T45.8X6
absorbable (sponge)	T45.7X1	T45.7X2	T45.7X3	T45.7X4	T45.7X5	T45.7X6
Gelfilm	T49.8X1	T49.8X2	T49.8X3	T49.8X4	T49.8X5	T49.8X6
Gelfoam	T45.7X1	T45.7X2	T45.7X3	T45.7X4	T45.7X5	T45.7X6
Gelsemine	T50.991	T50.992	T50.993	T50.994	T50.995	T50.996
Gelsemium (sempervirens)	T62.2X1	T62.2X2	T62.2X3	T62.2X4	—	—
Gemeprost	T48.0X1	T48.0X2	T48.0X3	T48.0X4	T48.0X5	T48.0X6
Gemfibrozil	T46.6X1	T46.6X2	T46.6X3	T46.6X4	T46.6X5	T46.6X6
Gemonil	T42.3X1	T42.3X2	T42.3X3	T42.3X4	T42.3X5	T42.3X6
Gentamicin	T36.5X1	T36.5X2	T36.5X3	T36.5X4	T36.5X5	T36.5X6
ophthalmic preparation	T49.5X1	T49.5X2	T49.5X3	T49.5X4	T49.5X5	T49.5X6
topical NEC	T49.0X1	T49.0X2	T49.0X3	T49.0X4	T49.0X5	T49.0X6
Gentian	T47.5X1	T47.5X2	T47.5X3	T47.5X4	T47.5X5	T47.5X6
violet	T49.0X1	T49.0X2	T49.0X3	T49.0X4	T49.0X5	T49.0X6
Gepefrine	T44.4X1	T44.4X2	T44.4X3	T44.4X4	T44.4X5	T44.4X6
Gestonorone caproate	T38.5X1	T38.5X2	T38.5X3	T38.5X4	T38.5X5	T38.5X6
Gexane	T49.0X1	T49.0X2	T49.0X3	T49.0X4	T49.0X5	T49.0X6
Gila monster (venom)	T63.111	T63.112	T63.113	T63.114	—	—
Ginger	T47.5X1	T47.5X2	T47.5X3	T47.5X4	T47.5X5	T47.5X6
Jamaica — *see* Jamaica, ginger						
Gitalin	T46.0X1	T46.0X2	T46.0X3	T46.0X4	T46.0X5	T46.0X6
amorphous	T46.0X1	T46.0X2	T46.0X3	T46.0X4	T46.0X5	T46.0X6
Gitaloxin	T46.0X1	T46.0X2	T46.0X3	T46.0X4	T46.0X5	T46.0X6
Gitoxin	T46.0X1	T46.0X2	T46.0X3	T46.0X4	T46.0X5	T46.0X6
Glafenine	T39.8X1	T39.8X2	T39.8X3	T39.8X4	T39.8X5	T39.8X6
Glandular extract (medicinal) NEC	T50.Z91	T50.Z92	T50.Z93	T50.Z94	T50.Z95	T50.Z96
Glaucarubin	T37.3X1	T37.3X2	T37.3X3	T37.3X4	T37.3X5	T37.3X6
Glibenclamide	T38.3X1	T38.3X2	T38.3X3	T38.3X4	T38.3X5	T38.3X6
Glibornuride	T38.3X1	T38.3X2	T38.3X3	T38.3X4	T38.3X5	T38.3X6
Gliclazide	T38.3X1	T38.3X2	T38.3X3	T38.3X4	T38.3X5	T38.3X6
Glimidine	T38.3X1	T38.3X2	T38.3X3	T38.3X4	T38.3X5	T38.3X6
Glipizide	T38.3X1	T38.3X2	T38.3X3	T38.3X4	T38.3X5	T38.3X6
Gliquidone	T38.3X1	T38.3X2	T38.3X3	T38.3X4	T38.3X5	T38.3X6
Glisolamide	T38.3X1	T38.3X2	T38.3X3	T38.3X4	T38.3X5	T38.3X6
Glisoxepide	T38.3X1	T38.3X2	T38.3X3	T38.3X4	T38.3X5	T38.3X6
Globin zinc insulin	T38.3X1	T38.3X2	T38.3X3	T38.3X4	T38.3X5	T38.3X6
Globulin						
antilymphocytic	T50.Z11	T50.Z12	T50.Z13	T50.Z14	T50.Z15	T50.Z16
antirhesus	T50.Z11	T50.Z12	T50.Z13	T50.Z14	T50.Z15	T50.Z16
antivenin	T50.Z11	T50.Z12	T50.Z13	T50.Z14	T50.Z15	T50.Z16
antiviral	T50.Z11	T50.Z12	T50.Z13	T50.Z14	T50.Z15	T50.Z16

Gallamine — Globulin

Substance	Poisoning, Accidental (unintentional)	Poisoning, Intentional Self-harm	Poisoning, Assault	Poisoning, Undetermined	Adverse Effect	Under-dosing
Glucagon	T38.3X1	T38.3X2	T38.3X3	T38.3X4	T38.3X5	T38.3X6
Glucocorticoids	T38.0X1	T38.0X2	T38.0X3	T38.0X4	T38.0X5	T38.0X6
Glucocorticosteroid	T38.0X1	T38.0X2	T38.0X3	T38.0X4	T38.0X5	T38.0X6
Gluconic acid	T50.991	T50.992	T50.993	T50.994	T50.995	T50.996
Glucosamine sulfate	T39.4X1	T39.4X2	T39.4X3	T39.4X4	T39.4X5	T39.4X6
Glucose	T50.3X1	T50.3X2	T50.3X3	T50.3X4	T50.3X5	T50.3X6
with sodium chloride	T50.3X1	T50.3X2	T50.3X3	T50.3X4	T50.3X5	T50.3X6
Glucosulfone sodium	T37.1X1	T37.1X2	T37.1X3	T37.1X4	T37.1X5	T37.1X6
Glucurolactone	T47.8X1	T47.8X2	T47.8X3	T47.8X4	T47.8X5	T47.8X6
Glue NEC	T52.8X1	T52.8X2	T52.8X3	T52.8X4	—	—
Glutamic acid	T47.5X1	T47.5X2	T47.5X3	T47.5X4	T47.5X5	T47.5X6
Glutaral (medicinal)	T49.0X1	T49.0X2	T49.0X3	T49.0X4	T49.0X5	T49.0X6
nonmedicinal	T65.891	T65.892	T65.893	T65.894	—	—
Glutaraldehyde (nonmedicinal)	T65.891	T65.892	T65.893	T65.894	—	—
medicinal	T49.0X1	T49.0X2	T49.0X3	T49.0X4	T49.0X5	T49.0X6
Glutathione	T50.6X1	T50.6X2	T50.6X3	T50.6X4	T50.6X5	T50.6X6
Glutethimide	T42.6X1	T42.6X2	T42.6X3	T42.6X4	T42.6X5	T42.6X6
Glyburide	T38.3X1	T38.3X2	T38.3X3	T38.3X4	T38.3X5	T38.3X6
Glycerin	T47.4X1	T47.4X2	T47.4X3	T47.4X4	T47.4X5	T47.4X6
Glycerol	T47.4X1	T47.4X2	T47.4X3	T47.4X4	T47.4X5	T47.4X6
borax	T49.6X1	T49.6X2	T49.6X3	T49.6X4	T49.6X5	T49.6X6
intravenous	T50.3X1	T50.3X2	T50.3X3	T50.3X4	T50.3X5	T50.3X6
iodinated	T48.4X1	T48.4X2	T48.4X3	T48.4X4	T48.4X5	T48.4X6
Glycerophosphate	T50.991	T50.992	T50.993	T50.994	T50.995	T50.996
Glyceryl						
gualacolate	T48.4X1	T48.4X2	T48.4X3	T48.4X4	T48.4X5	T48.4X6
nitrate	T46.3X1	T46.3X2	T46.3X3	T46.3X4	T46.3X5	T46.3X6
triacetate (topical)	T49.0X1	T49.0X2	T49.0X3	T49.0X4	T49.0X5	T49.0X6
trinitrate	T46.3X1	T46.3X2	T46.3X3	T46.3X4	T46.3X5	T46.3X6
Glycine	T50.3X1	T50.3X2	T50.3X3	T50.3X4	T50.3X5	T50.3X6
Glyclopyramide	T38.3X1	T38.3X2	T38.3X3	T38.3X4	T38.3X5	T38.3X6
Glycobiarsol	T37.3X1	T37.3X2	T37.3X3	T37.3X4	T37.3X5	T37.3X6
Glycols (ether)	T52.3X1	T52.3X2	T52.3X3	T52.3X4	—	—
Glyconiazide	T37.1X1	T37.1X2	T37.1X3	T37.1X4	T37.1X5	T37.1X6
Glycopyrrolate	T44.3X1	T44.3X2	T44.3X3	T44.3X4	T44.3X5	T44.3X6
Glycopyrronium	T44.3X1	T44.3X2	T44.3X3	T44.3X4	T44.3X5	T44.3X6
bromide	T44.3X1	T44.3X2	T44.3X3	T44.3X4	T44.3X5	T44.3X6
Glycoside, cardiac (stimulant)	T46.0X1	T46.0X2	T46.0X3	T46.0X4	T46.0X5	T46.0X6
Glycyclamide	T38.3X1	T38.3X2	T38.3X3	T38.3X4	T38.3X5	T38.3X6
Glycyrrhiza extract	T48.4X1	T48.4X2	T48.4X3	T48.4X4	T48.4X5	T48.4X6
Glycyrrhizic acid	T48.4X1	T48.4X2	T48.4X3	T48.4X4	T48.4X5	T48.4X6
Glycyrrhizinate potassium	T48.4X1	T48.4X2	T48.4X3	T48.4X4	T48.4X5	T48.4X6
Glymidine sodium	T38.3X1	T38.3X2	T38.3X3	T38.3X4	T38.3X5	T38.3X6
Glyphosate	T60.3X1	T60.3X2	T60.3X3	T60.3X4	—	—
Glyphylline	T48.6X1	T48.6X2	T48.6X3	T48.6X4	T48.6X5	T48.6X6
Gold						
colloidal (I98Au)	T45.1X1	T45.1X2	T45.1X3	T45.1X4	T45.1X5	T45.1X6
salts	T39.4X1	T39.4X2	T39.4X3	T39.4X4	T39.4X5	T39.4X6
Golden sulfide of antimony	T56.891	T56.892	T56.893	T56.894	—	—
Goldylocks	T62.2X1	T62.2X2	T62.2X3	T62.2X4	—	—
Gonadal tissue extract	T38.901	T38.902	T38.903	T38.904	T38.905	T38.906
female	T38.5X1	T38.5X2	T38.5X3	T38.5X4	T38.5X5	T38.5X6
male	T38.7X1	T38.7X2	T38.7X3	T38.7X4	T38.7X5	T38.7X6
Gonadorelin	T38.891	T38.892	T38.893	T38.894	T38.895	T38.896
Gonadotropin	T38.891	T38.892	T38.893	T38.894	T38.895	T38.896
chorionic	T38.891	T38.892	T38.893	T38.894	T38.895	T38.896
pituitary	T38.811	T38.812	T38.813	T38.814	T38.815	T38.816
Goserelin	T45.1X1	T45.1X2	T45.1X3	T45.1X4	T45.1X5	T45.1X6
Grain alcohol	T51.0X1	T51.0X2	T51.0X3	T51.0X4	—	—
Gramicidin	T49.0X1	T49.0X2	T49.0X3	T49.0X4	T49.0X5	T49.0X6
Granisetron	T45.0X1	T45.0X2	T45.0X3	T45.0X4	T45.0X5	T45.0X6
Gratiola officinalis	T62.2X1	T62.2X2	T62.2X3	T62.2X4	—	—
Grease	T65.891	T65.892	T65.893	T65.894	—	—
Green hellebore	T62.2X1	T62.2X2	T62.2X3	T62.2X4	—	—
Green soap	T49.2X1	T49.2X2	T49.2X3	T49.2X4	T49.2X5	T49.2X6
Grifulvin	T36.7X1	T36.7X2	T36.7X3	T36.7X4	T36.7X5	T36.7X6
Griseofulvin	T36.7X1	T36.7X2	T36.7X3	T36.7X4	T36.7X5	T36.7X6
Growth hormone	T38.811	T38.812	T38.813	T38.814	T38.815	T38.816
Guaiacol derivatives	T48.4X1	T48.4X2	T48.4X3	T48.4X4	T48.4X5	T48.4X6
Guaiac reagent	T50.991	T50.992	T50.993	T50.994	T50.995	T50.996
Guaifenesin	T48.4X1	T48.4X2	T48.4X3	T48.4X4	T48.4X5	T48.4X6
Guaimesal	T48.4X1	T48.4X2	T48.4X3	T48.4X4	T48.4X5	T48.4X6
Guaiphenesin	T48.4X1	T48.4X2	T48.4X3	T48.4X4	T48.4X5	T48.4X6
Guamecycline	T36.4X1	T36.4X2	T36.4X3	T36.4X4	T36.4X5	T36.4X6
Guanabenz	T46.5X1	T46.5X2	T46.5X3	T46.5X4	T46.5X5	T46.5X6
Guanacline	T46.5X1	T46.5X2	T46.5X3	T46.5X4	T46.5X5	T46.5X6
Guanadrel	T46.5X1	T46.5X2	T46.5X3	T46.5X4	T46.5X5	T46.5X6
Guanatol	T37.2X1	T37.2X2	T37.2X3	T37.2X4	T37.2X5	T37.2X6
Guanethidine	T46.5X1	T46.5X2	T46.5X3	T46.5X4	T46.5X5	T46.5X6
Guanfacine	T46.5X1	T46.5X2	T46.5X3	T46.5X4	T46.5X5	T46.5X6
Guano	T65.891	T65.892	T65.893	T65.894	—	—
Guanochlor	T46.5X1	T46.5X2	T46.5X3	T46.5X4	T46.5X5	T46.5X6
Guanoclor	T46.5X1	T46.5X2	T46.5X3	T46.5X4	T46.5X5	T46.5X6
Guanoctine	T46.5X1	T46.5X2	T46.5X3	T46.5X4	T46.5X5	T46.5X6
Guanoxabenz	T46.5X1	T46.5X2	T46.5X3	T46.5X4	T46.5X5	T46.5X6
Guanoxan	T46.5X1	T46.5X2	T46.5X3	T46.5X4	T46.5X5	T46.5X6
Guar gum (medicinal)	T46.6X1	T46.6X2	T46.6X3	T46.6X4	T46.6X5	T46.6X6
Hachimycin	T36.7X1	T36.7X2	T36.7X3	T36.7X4	T36.7X5	T36.7X6
Hair						
dye	T49.4X1	T49.4X2	T49.4X3	T49.4X4	T49.4X5	T49.4X6
preparation NEC	T49.4X1	T49.4X2	T49.4X3	T49.4X4	T49.4X5	T49.4X6
Halazepam	T42.4X1	T42.4X2	T42.4X3	T42.4X4	T42.4X5	T42.4X6
Halcinolone	T49.0X1	T49.0X2	T49.0X3	T49.0X4	T49.0X5	T49.0X6
Halcinonide	T49.0X1	T49.0X2	T49.0X3	T49.0X4	T49.0X5	T49.0X6
Halethazole	T49.0X1	T49.0X2	T49.0X3	T49.0X4	T49.0X5	T49.0X6
Hallucinogen NEC	T40.901	T40.902	T40.903	T40.904	T40.905	T40.906
Halofantrine	T37.2X1	T37.2X2	T37.2X3	T37.2X4	T37.2X5	T37.2X6
Halofenate	T46.6X1	T46.6X2	T46.6X3	T46.6X4	T46.6X5	T46.6X6
Halometasone	T49.0X1	T49.0X2	T49.0X3	T49.0X4	T49.0X5	T49.0X6
Haloperidol	T43.4X1	T43.4X2	T43.4X3	T43.4X4	T43.4X5	T43.4X6
Haloprogin	T49.0X1	T49.0X2	T49.0X3	T49.0X4	T49.0X5	T49.0X6
Halotex	T49.0X1	T49.0X2	T49.0X3	T49.0X4	T49.0X5	T49.0X6
Halothane	T41.0X1	T41.0X2	T41.0X3	T41.0X4	T41.0X5	T41.0X6
Haloxazolam	T42.4X1	T42.4X2	T42.4X3	T42.4X4	T42.4X5	T42.4X6
Halquinols	T49.0X1	T49.0X2	T49.0X3	T49.0X4	T49.0X5	T49.0X6
Hamamelis	T49.2X1	T49.2X2	T49.2X3	T49.2X4	T49.2X5	T49.2X6
Haptendextran	T45.8X1	T45.8X2	T45.8X3	T45.8X4	T45.8X5	T45.8X6
Harmonyl	T46.5X1	T46.5X2	T46.5X3	T46.5X4	T46.5X5	T46.5X6
Hartmann's solution	T50.3X1	T50.3X2	T50.3X3	T50.3X4	T50.3X5	T50.3X6
Hashish	T40.7X1	T40.7X2	T40.7X3	T40.7X4	T40.7X5	T40.7X6
Hawaiian Woodrose seeds	T40.991	T40.992	T40.993	T40.994	—	—
HCB	T60.3X1	T60.3X2	T60.3X3	T60.3X4	—	—
HCH	T53.6X1	T53.6X2	T53.6X3	T53.6X4	—	—
medicinal	T49.0X1	T49.0X2	T49.0X3	T49.0X4	T49.0X5	T49.0X6
HCN	T57.3X1	T57.3X2	T57.3X3	T57.3X4	—	—
Headache cures, drugs, powders NEC	T50.901	T50.902	T50.903	T50.904	T50.905	T50.906
Heavenly Blue (morning glory)	T40.991	T40.992	T40.993	T40.994	—	—
Heavy metal antidote	T45.8X1	T45.8X2	T45.8X3	T45.8X4	T45.8X5	T45.8X6
Hedaquinium	T49.0X1	T49.0X2	T49.0X3	T49.0X4	T49.0X5	T49.0X6
Hedge hyssop	T62.2X1	T62.2X2	T62.2X3	T62.2X4	—	—
Heet	T49.8X1	T49.8X2	T49.8X3	T49.8X4	T49.8X5	T49.8X6
Helenin	T37.4X1	T37.4X2	T37.4X3	T37.4X4	T37.4X5	T37.4X6
Helium (nonmedicinal) NEC	T59.891	T59.892	T59.893	T59.894	—	—
medicinal	T48.991	T48.992	T48.993	T48.994	T48.995	T48.996
Hellebore (black) (green) (white)	T62.2X1	T62.2X2	T62.2X3	T62.2X4	—	—
Hematin	T45.8X1	T45.8X2	T45.8X3	T45.8X4	T45.8X5	T45.8X6
Hematinic preparation	T45.8X1	T45.8X2	T45.8X3	T45.8X4	T45.8X5	T45.8X6
Hematological agent	T45.91	T45.92	T45.93	T45.94	T45.95	T45.96
specified NEC	T45.8X1	T45.8X2	T45.8X3	T45.8X4	T45.8X5	T45.8X6
Hemlock	T62.2X1	T62.2X2	T62.2X3	T62.2X4	—	—
Hemostatic	T45.621	T45.622	T45.623	T45.624	T45.625	T45.626
drug, systemic	T45.621	T45.622	T45.623	T45.624	T45.625	T45.626
Hemostyptic	T49.4X1	T49.4X2	T49.4X3	T49.4X4	T49.4X5	T49.4X6
Henbane	T62.2X1	T62.2X2	T62.2X3	T62.2X4	—	—
Heparin (sodium)	T45.511	T45.512	T45.513	T45.514	T45.515	T45.516
action reverser	T45.7X1	T45.7X2	T45.7X3	T45.7X4	T45.7X5	T45.7X6
Heparin-fraction	T45.511	T45.512	T45.513	T45.514	T45.515	T45.516
Heparinoid (systemic)	T45.511	T45.512	T45.513	T45.514	T45.515	T45.516
Hepatic secretion stimulant	T47.8X1	T47.8X2	T47.8X3	T47.8X4	T47.8X5	T47.8X6
Hepatitis B						
immune globulin	T50.Z11	T50.Z12	T50.Z13	T50.Z14	T50.Z15	T50.Z16
vaccine	T50.B91	T50.B92	T50.B93	T50.B94	T50.B95	T50.B96
Hepronicate	T46.7X1	T46.7X2	T46.7X3	T46.7X4	T46.7X5	T46.7X6
Heptabarbital	T42.3X1	T42.3X2	T42.3X3	T42.3X4	T42.3X5	T42.3X6
Heptabarbitone	T42.3X1	T42.3X2	T42.3X3	T42.3X4	T42.3X5	T42.3X6
Heptachlor	T60.1X1	T60.1X2	T60.1X3	T60.1X4	—	—
Heptalgin	T40.2X1	T40.2X2	T40.2X3	T40.2X4	T40.2X5	T40.2X6
Heptaminol	T46.3X1	T46.3X2	T46.3X3	T46.3X4	T46.3X5	T46.3X6
Herbicide NEC	T60.3X1	T60.3X2	T60.3X3	T60.3X4	—	—
Heroin	T40.1X1	T40.1X2	T40.1X3	T40.1X4	—	—
Herplex	T49.5X1	T49.5X2	T49.5X3	T49.5X4	T49.5X5	T49.5X6
HES	T45.8X1	T45.8X2	T45.8X3	T45.8X4	T45.8X5	T45.8X6
Hesperidin	T46.991	T46.992	T46.993	T46.994	T46.995	T46.996
Hetacillin	T36.0X1	T36.0X2	T36.0X3	T36.0X4	T36.0X5	T36.0X6
Hetastarch	T45.8X1	T45.8X2	T45.8X3	T45.8X4	T45.8X5	T45.8X6
HETP	T60.0X1	T60.0X2	T60.0X3	T60.0X4	—	—
Hexachlorobenzene (vapor)	T60.3X1	T60.3X2	T60.3X3	T60.3X4	—	—
Hexachlorocyclohexane	T53.6X1	T53.6X2	T53.6X3	T53.6X4	—	—
Hexachlorophene	T49.0X1	T49.0X2	T49.0X3	T49.0X4	T49.0X5	T49.0X6

Table of Drugs and Chemicals

Glucagon — Hexachlorophene

Substance	Poisoning, Accidental (unintentional)	Poisoning, Intentional Self-harm	Poisoning, Assault	Poisoning, Undetermined	Adverse Effect	Under- dosing
Hexadiline	T46.3X1	T46.3X2	T46.3X3	T46.3X4	T46.3X5	T46.3X6
Hexadimethrine (bromide)	T45.7X1	T45.7X2	T45.7X3	T45.7X4	T45.7X5	T45.7X6
Hexadylamine	T46.3X1	T46.3X2	T46.3X3	T46.3X4	T46.3X5	T46.3X6
Hexaethyl tetraphosphate	T60.0X1	T60.0X2	T60.0X3	T60.0X4	—	—
Hexafluorenium bromide	T48.1X1	T48.1X2	T48.1X3	T48.1X4	T48.1X5	T48.1X6
Hexafluronium (bromide)	T48.1X1	T48.1X2	T48.1X3	T48.1X4	T48.1X5	T48.1X6
Hexa-germ	T49.2X1	T49.2X2	T49.2X3	T49.2X4	T49.2X5	T49.2X6
Hexahydrobenzol	T52.8X1	T52.8X2	T52.8X3	T52.8X4	—	—
Hexahydrocresol(s)	T51.8X1	T51.8X2	T51.8X3	T51.8X4	—	—
arsenide	T57.0X1	T57.0X2	T57.0X3	T57.0X4	—	—
arseniurated	T57.0X1	T57.0X2	T57.0X3	T57.0X4	—	—
cyanide	T57.3X1	T57.3X2	T57.3X3	T57.3X4	—	—
gas	T59.891	T59.892	T59.893	T59.894	—	—
Fluoride (liquid)	T57.8X1	T57.8X2	T57.8X3	T57.8X4	—	—
vapor	T59.891	T59.892	T59.893	T59.894	—	—
phophorated	T60.0X1	T60.0X2	T60.0X3	T60.0X4	—	—
sulfate	T57.8X1	T57.8X2	T57.8X3	T57.8X4	—	—
sulfide (gas)	T59.6X1	T59.6X2	T59.6X3	T59.6X4	—	—
arseniurated	T57.0X1	T57.0X2	T57.0X3	T57.0X4	—	—
sulfurated	T57.8X1	T57.8X2	T57.8X3	T57.8X4	—	—
Hexahydrophenol	T51.8X1	T51.8X2	T51.8X3	T51.8X4	—	—
Hexalen	T51.8X1	T51.8X2	T51.8X3	T51.8X4	—	—
Hexamethonium bromide	T44.2X1	T44.2X2	T44.2X3	T44.2X4	T44.2X5	T44.2X6
Hexamethylene	T52.8X1	T52.8X2	T52.8X3	T52.8X4	—	—
Hexamethylmelamine	T45.1X1	T45.1X2	T45.1X3	T45.1X4	T45.1X5	T45.1X6
Hexamidine	T49.0X1	T49.0X2	T49.0X3	T49.0X4	T49.0X5	T49.0X6
Hexamine (mandelate)	T37.8X1	T37.8X2	T37.8X3	T37.8X4	T37.8X5	T37.8X6
Hexanone, 2-hexanone	T52.4X1	T52.4X2	T52.4X3	T52.4X4	—	—
Hexanuorenium	T48.1X1	T48.1X2	T48.1X3	T48.1X4	T48.1X5	T48.1X6
Hexapropymate	T42.6X1	T42.6X2	T42.6X3	T42.6X4	T42.6X5	T42.6X6
Hexasonium iodide	T44.3X1	T44.3X2	T44.3X3	T44.3X4	T44.3X5	T44.3X6
Hexcarbacholine bromide	T48.1X1	T48.1X2	T48.1X3	T48.1X4	T48.1X5	T48.1X6
Hexemal	T42.3X1	T42.3X2	T42.3X3	T42.3X4	T42.3X5	T42.3X6
Hexestrol	T38.5X1	T38.5X2	T38.5X3	T38.5X4	T38.5X5	T38.5X6
Hexethal (sodium)	T42.3X1	T42.3X2	T42.3X3	T42.3X4	T42.3X5	T42.3X6
Hexetidine	T37.8X1	T37.8X2	T37.8X3	T37.8X4	T37.8X5	T37.8X6
Hexobarbital	T42.3X1	T42.3X2	T42.3X3	T42.3X4	T42.3X5	T42.3X6
rectal	T41.291	T41.292	T41.293	T41.294	T41.295	T41.296
sodium	T41.1X1	T41.1X2	T41.1X3	T41.1X4	T41.1X5	T41.1X6
Hexobendine	T46.3X1	T46.3X2	T46.3X3	T46.3X4	T46.3X5	T46.3X6
Hexocyclium	T44.3X1	T44.3X2	T44.3X3	T44.3X4	T44.3X5	T44.3X6
metilsulfate	T44.3X1	T44.3X2	T44.3X3	T44.3X4	T44.3X5	T44.3X6
Hexoestrol	T38.5X1	T38.5X2	T38.5X3	T38.5X4	T38.5X5	T38.5X6
Hexone	T52.4X1	T52.4X2	T52.4X3	T52.4X4	—	—
Hexoprenaline	T48.6X1	T48.6X2	T48.6X3	T48.6X4	T48.6X5	T48.6X6
Hexylcaine	T41.3X1	T41.3X2	T41.3X3	T41.3X4	T41.3X5	T41.3X6
Hexylresorcinol	T52.2X1	T52.2X2	T52.2X3	T52.2X4	—	—
HGH (human growth hormone)	T38.811	T38.812	T38.813	T38.814	T38.815	T38.816
Hinkle's pills	T47.2X1	T47.2X2	T47.2X3	T47.2X4	T47.2X5	T47.2X6
Histalog	T50.8X1	T50.8X2	T50.8X3	T50.8X4	T50.8X5	T50.8X6
Histamine (phosphate)	T50.8X1	T50.8X2	T50.8X3	T50.8X4	T50.8X5	T50.8X6
Histoplasmin	T50.8X1	T50.8X2	T50.8X3	T50.8X4	T50.8X5	T50.8X6
Holly berries	T62.2X1	T62.2X2	T62.2X3	T62.2X4	—	—
Homatropine	T44.3X1	T44.3X2	T44.3X3	T44.3X4	T44.3X5	T44.3X6
methylbromide	T44.3X1	T44.3X2	T44.3X3	T44.3X4	T44.3X5	T44.3X6
Homochlorcyclizine	T45.0X1	T45.0X2	T45.0X3	T45.0X4	T45.0X5	T45.0X6
Homosalate	T49.3X1	T49.3X2	T49.3X3	T49.3X4	T49.3X5	T49.3X6
Homo-tet	T50.Z11	T50.Z12	T50.Z13	T50.Z14	T50.Z15	T50.Z16
Hormone	T38.801	T38.802	T38.803	T38.804	T38.805	T38.806
adrenal cortical steroids	T38.0X1	T38.0X2	T38.0X3	T38.0X4	T38.0X5	T38.0X6
androgenic	T38.7X1	T38.7X2	T38.7X3	T38.7X4	T38.7X5	T38.7X6
anterior pituitary NEC	T38.811	T38.812	T38.813	T38.814	T38.815	T38.816
antidiabetic agents	T38.3X1	T38.3X2	T38.3X3	T38.3X4	T38.3X5	T38.3X6
antidiuretic	T38.891	T38.892	T38.893	T38.894	T38.895	T38.896
cancer therapy	T45.1X1	T45.1X2	T45.1X3	T45.1X4	T45.1X5	T45.1X6
follicle stimulating	T38.811	T38.812	T38.813	T38.814	T38.815	T38.816
gonadotropic	T38.891	T38.892	T38.893	T38.894	T38.895	T38.896
pituitary	T38.811	T38.812	T38.813	T38.814	T38.815	T38.816
growth	T38.811	T38.812	T38.813	T38.814	T38.815	T38.816
luteinizing	T38.811	T38.812	T38.813	T38.814	T38.815	T38.816
ovarian	T38.5X1	T38.5X2	T38.5X3	T38.5X4	T38.5X5	T38.5X6
oxytocic	T48.0X1	T48.0X2	T48.0X3	T48.0X4	T48.0X5	T48.0X6
parathyroid (derivatives)	T50.991	T50.992	T50.993	T50.994	T50.995	T50.996
pituitary (posterior) NEC	T38.891	T38.892	T38.893	T38.894	T38.895	T38.896
anterior	T38.811	T38.812	T38.813	T38.814	T38.815	T38.816
specified, NEC	T38.891	T38.892	T38.893	T38.894	T38.895	T38.896
thyroid	T38.1X1	T38.1X2	T38.1X3	T38.1X4	T38.1X5	T38.1X6
Hornet (sting)	T63.451	T63.452	T63.453	T63.454	—	—
Horse anti-human lymphocytic serum	T50.Z11	T50.Z12	T50.Z13	T50.Z14	T50.Z15	T50.Z16
Horticulture agent NEC	T65.91	T65.92	T65.93	T65.94	—	—
with pesticide	T60.91	T60.92	T60.93	T60.94	—	—

Substance	Poisoning, Accidental (unintentional)	Poisoning, Intentional Self-harm	Poisoning, Assault	Poisoning, Undetermined	Adverse Effect	Under- dosing
Human						
albumin	T45.8X1	T45.8X2	T45.8X3	T45.8X4	T45.8X5	T45.8X6
growth hormone (HGH)	T38.811	T38.812	T38.813	T38.814	T38.815	T38.816
immune serum	T50.Z11	T50.Z12	T50.Z13	T50.Z14	T50.Z15	T50.Z16
Hyaluronidase	T45.3X1	T45.3X2	T45.3X3	T45.3X4	T45.3X5	T45.3X6
Hyazyme	T45.3X1	T45.3X2	T45.3X3	T45.3X4	T45.3X5	T45.3X6
Hycodan	T40.2X1	T40.2X2	T40.2X3	T40.2X4	T40.2X5	T40.2X6
Hydantoin derivative NEC	T42.0X1	T42.0X2	T42.0X3	T42.0X4	T42.0X5	T42.0X6
Hydeltra	T38.0X1	T38.0X2	T38.0X3	T38.0X4	T38.0X5	T38.0X6
Hydergine	T44.6X1	T44.6X2	T44.6X3	T44.6X4	T44.6X5	T44.6X6
Hydrabamine penicillin	T36.0X1	T36.0X2	T36.0X3	T36.0X4	T36.0X5	T36.0X6
Hydralazine	T46.5X1	T46.5X2	T46.5X3	T46.5X4	T46.5X5	T46.5X6
Hydrargaphen	T49.0X1	T49.0X2	T49.0X3	T49.0X4	T49.0X5	T49.0X6
Hydrargyri aminochloridum	T49.0X1	T49.0X2	T49.0X3	T49.0X4	T49.0X5	T49.0X6
Hydrastine	T48.291	T48.292	T48.293	T48.294	T48.295	T48.296
Hydrazine	T54.1X1	T54.1X2	T54.1X3	T54.1X4	—	—
monoamine oxidase inhibitors	T43.1X1	T43.1X2	T43.1X3	T43.1X4	T43.1X5	T43.1X6
Hydrazoic acid, azides	T54.2X1	T54.2X2	T54.2X3	T54.2X4	—	—
Hydriodic acid	T48.4X1	T48.4X2	T48.4X3	T48.4X4	T48.4X5	T48.4X6
Hydrocarbon gas	T59.891	T59.892	T59.893	T59.894	—	—
incomplete combustion of — see Carbon, monoxide, fuel, utility						
liquefied (mobile container)	T59.891	T59.892	T59.893	T59.894	—	—
piped (natural)	T59.891	T59.892	T59.893	T59.894	—	—
Hydrochloric acid (liquid)	T54.2X1	T54.2X2	T54.2X3	T54.2X4	—	—
medicinal (digestant)	T47.5X1	T47.5X2	T47.5X3	T47.5X4	T47.5X5	T47.5X6
vapor	T59.891	T59.892	T59.893	T59.894	—	—
Hydrochlorothiazide	T50.2X1	T50.2X2	T50.2X3	T50.2X4	T50.2X5	T50.2X6
Hydrocodone	T40.2X1	T40.2X2	T40.2X3	T40.2X4	T40.2X5	T40.2X6
Hydrocortisone (derivatives)	T38.0X1	T38.0X2	T38.0X3	T38.0X4	T38.0X5	T38.0X6
aceponate	T49.0X1	T49.0X2	T49.0X3	T49.0X4	T49.0X5	T49.0X6
ENT agent	T49.6X1	T49.6X2	T49.6X3	T49.6X4	T49.6X5	T49.6X6
ophthalmic preparation	T49.5X1	T49.5X2	T49.5X3	T49.5X4	T49.5X5	T49.5X6
topical NEC	T49.0X1	T49.0X2	T49.0X3	T49.0X4	T49.0X5	T49.0X6
Hydrocortone	T38.0X1	T38.0X2	T38.0X3	T38.0X4	T38.0X5	T38.0X6
ENT agent	T49.6X1	T49.6X2	T49.6X3	T49.6X4	T49.6X5	T49.6X6
ophthalmic preparation	T49.5X1	T49.5X2	T49.5X3	T49.5X4	T49.5X5	T49.5X6
topical NEC	T49.0X1	T49.0X2	T49.0X3	T49.0X4	T49.0X5	T49.0X6
Hydrocyanic acid (liquid)	T57.3X1	T57.3X2	T57.3X3	T57.3X4	—	—
gas	T65.0X1	T65.0X2	T65.0X3	T65.0X4	—	—
Hydroflumethiazide	T50.2X1	T50.2X2	T50.2X3	T50.2X4	T50.2X5	T50.2X6
Hydrofluoric acid (liquid)	T54.2X1	T54.2X2	T54.2X3	T54.2X4	—	—
vapor	T59.891	T59.892	T59.893	T59.894	—	—
Hydrogen	T59.891	T59.892	T59.893	T59.894	—	—
arsenide	T57.0X1	T57.0X2	T57.0X3	T57.0X4	—	—
arseniureted	T57.0X1	T57.0X2	T57.0X3	T57.0X4	—	—
chloride	T57.8X1	T57.8X2	T57.8X3	T57.8X4	—	—
cyanide (salts)	T57.3X1	T57.3X2	T57.3X3	T57.3X4	—	—
gas	T57.3X1	T57.3X2	T57.3X3	T57.3X4	—	—
Fluoride	T59.5X1	T59.5X2	T59.5X3	T59.5X4	—	—
vapor	T59.5X1	T59.5X2	T59.5X3	T59.5X4	—	—
peroxide	T49.0X1	T49.0X2	T49.0X3	T49.0X4	T49.0X5	T49.0X6
phosphureted	T57.1X1	T57.1X2	T57.1X3	T57.1X4	—	—
sulfide	T59.6X1	T59.6X2	T59.6X3	T59.6X4	—	—
arseniureted	T57.0X1	T57.0X2	T57.0X3	T57.0X4	—	—
sulfureted	T59.6X1	T59.6X2	T59.6X3	T59.6X4	—	—
Hydromethylpyridine	T46.7X1	T46.7X2	T46.7X3	T46.7X4	T46.7X5	T46.7X6
Hydromorphinol	T40.2X1	T40.2X2	T40.2X3	T40.2X4	—	—
Hydromorphinone	T40.2X1	T40.2X2	T40.2X3	T40.2X4	T40.2X5	T40.2X6
Hydromorphone	T40.2X1	T40.2X2	T40.2X3	T40.2X4	T40.2X5	T40.2X6
Hydromox	T50.2X1	T50.2X2	T50.2X3	T50.2X4	T50.2X5	T50.2X6
Hydrophilic lotion	T49.3X1	T49.3X2	T49.3X3	T49.3X4	T49.3X5	T49.3X6
Hydroquinidine	T46.2X1	T46.2X2	T46.2X3	T46.2X4	T46.2X5	T46.2X6
Hydroquinone	T52.2X1	T52.2X2	T52.2X3	T52.2X4	—	—
vapor	T59.891	T59.892	T59.893	T59.894	—	—
Hydrosulfuric acid (gas)	T59.6X1	T59.6X2	T59.6X3	T59.6X4	—	—
Hydrotalcite	T47.1X1	T47.1X2	T47.1X3	T47.1X4	T47.1X5	T47.1X6
Hydrous wool fat	T49.3X1	T49.3X2	T49.3X3	T49.3X4	T49.3X5	T49.3X6
Hydroxide, caustic	T54.3X1	T54.3X2	T54.3X3	T54.3X4	—	—
Hydroxocobalamin	T45.8X1	T45.8X2	T45.8X3	T45.8X4	T45.8X5	T45.8X6
Hydroxyamphetamine	T49.5X1	T49.5X2	T49.5X3	T49.5X4	T49.5X5	T49.5X6
Hydroxycarbamide	T45.1X1	T45.1X2	T45.1X3	T45.1X4	T45.1X5	T45.1X6
Hydroxychloroquine	T37.8X1	T37.8X2	T37.8X3	T37.8X4	T37.8X5	T37.8X6
Hydroxydihydrocodeinone	T40.2X1	T40.2X2	T40.2X3	T40.2X4	T40.2X5	T40.2X6
Hydroxyestrone	T38.5X1	T38.5X2	T38.5X3	T38.5X4	T38.5X5	T38.5X6
Hydroxyethyl starch	T45.8X1	T45.8X2	T45.8X3	T45.8X4	T45.8X5	T45.8X6
Hydroxymethylpentanone	T52.4X1	T52.4X2	T52.4X3	T52.4X4	—	—
Hydroxyphenamate	T43.591	T43.592	T43.593	T43.594	T43.595	T43.596
Hydroxyphenylbutazone	T39.2X1	T39.2X2	T39.2X3	T39.2X4	T39.2X5	T39.2X6
Hydroxyprogesterone	T38.5X1	T38.5X2	T38.5X3	T38.5X4	T38.5X5	T38.5X6

Substance	Poisoning, Accidental (unintentional)	Poisoning, Intentional Self-harm	Poisoning, Assault	Poisoning, Undetermined	Adverse Effect	Underdosing
Hydroxyprogesterone — *continued*						
caproate	T38.5X1	T38.5X2	T38.5X3	T38.5X4	T38.5X5	T38.5X6
Hydroxyquinoline (derivatives) **NEC**	T37.8X1	T37.8X2	T37.8X3	T37.8X4	T37.8X5	T37.8X6
Hydroxystilbamidine	T37.3X1	T37.3X2	T37.3X3	T37.3X4	T37.3X5	T37.3X6
Hydroxytoluene (nonmedicinal)	T54.0X1	T54.0X2	T54.0X3	T54.0X4	—	—
medicinal	T49.0X1	T49.0X2	T49.0X3	T49.0X4	T49.0X5	T49.0X6
Hydroxyurea	T45.1X1	T45.1X2	T45.1X3	T45.1X4	T45.1X5	T45.1X6
Hydroxyzine	T43.591	T43.592	T43.593	T43.594	T43.595	T43.596
Hyoscine	T44.3X1	T44.3X2	T44.3X3	T44.3X4	T44.3X5	T44.3X6
Hyoscyamine	T44.3X1	T44.3X2	T44.3X3	T44.3X4	T44.3X5	T44.3X6
Hyoscyamus	T44.3X1	T44.3X2	T44.3X3	T44.3X4	T44.3X5	T44.3X6
dry extract	T44.3X1	T44.3X2	T44.3X3	T44.3X4	T44.3X5	T44.3X6
Hypaque	T50.8X1	T50.8X2	T50.8X3	T50.8X4	T50.8X5	T50.8X6
Hypertussis	T50.Z11	T50.Z12	T50.Z13	T50.Z14	T50.Z15	T50.Z16
Hypnotic	T42.71	T42.72	T42.73	T42.74	T42.75	T42.76
anticonvulsant	T42.71	T42.72	T42.73	T42.74	T42.75	T42.76
specified NEC	T42.6X1	T42.6X2	T42.6X3	T42.6X4	T42.6X5	T42.6X6
Hypochlorite	T49.0X1	T49.0X2	T49.0X3	T49.0X4	T49.0X5	T49.0X6
Hypophysis, posterior	T38.891	T38.892	T38.893	T38.894	T38.895	T38.896
Hypotensive NEC	T46.5X1	T46.5X2	T46.5X3	T46.5X4	T46.5X5	T46.5X6
Hypromellose	T49.5X1	T49.5X2	T49.5X3	T49.5X4	T49.5X5	T49.5X6
Ibacitabine	T37.5X1	T37.5X2	T37.5X3	T37.5X4	T37.5X5	T37.5X6
Ibopamine	T44.991	T44.992	T44.993	T44.994	T44.995	T44.996
Ibufenac	T39.311	T39.312	T39.313	T39.314	T39.315	T39.316
Ibuprofen	T39.311	T39.312	T39.313	T39.314	T39.315	T39.316
Ibuproxam	T39.311	T39.312	T39.313	T39.314	T39.315	T39.316
Ibuterol	T48.6X1	T48.6X2	T48.6X3	T48.6X4	T48.6X5	T48.6X6
Ichthammol	T49.0X1	T49.0X2	T49.0X3	T49.0X4	T49.0X5	T49.0X6
Ichthyol	T49.4X1	T49.4X2	T49.4X3	T49.4X4	T49.4X5	T49.4X6
Idarubicin	T45.1X1	T45.1X2	T45.1X3	T45.1X4	T45.1X5	T45.1X6
Idrocilamide	T42.8X1	T42.8X2	T42.8X3	T42.8X4	T42.8X5	T42.8X6
Ifenprodil	T46.7X1	T46.7X2	T46.7X3	T46.7X4	T46.7X5	T46.7X6
Ifosfamide	T45.1X1	T45.1X2	T45.1X3	T45.1X4	T45.1X5	T45.1X6
Iletin	T38.3X1	T38.3X2	T38.3X3	T38.3X4	T38.3X5	T38.3X6
Ilex	T62.2X1	T62.2X2	T62.2X3	T62.2X4	—	—
Illuminating gas (after combustion)	T58.11	T58.12	T58.13	T58.14	—	—
prior to combustion	T59.891	T59.892	T59.893	T59.894	—	—
Ilopan	T45.2X1	T45.2X2	T45.2X3	T45.2X4	T45.2X5	T45.2X6
Iloprost	T46.7X1	T46.7X2	T46.7X3	T46.7X4	T46.7X5	T46.7X6
Ilotycin	T36.3X1	T36.3X2	T36.3X3	T36.3X4	T36.3X5	T36.3X6
ophthalmic preparation	T49.5X1	T49.5X2	T49.5X3	T49.5X4	T49.5X5	T49.5X6
topical NEC	T49.0X1	T49.0X2	T49.0X3	T49.0X4	T49.0X5	T49.0X6
Imidazole-4-carboxamide	T45.1X1	T45.1X2	T45.1X3	T45.1X4	T45.1X5	T45.1X6
Iminostilbene	T42.1X1	T42.1X2	T42.1X3	T42.1X4	T42.1X5	T42.1X6
Imipenem	T36.0X1	T36.0X2	T36.0X3	T36.0X4	T36.0X5	T36.0X6
Imipramine	T43.011	T43.012	T43.013	T43.014	T43.015	T43.016
Immu-G	T50.Z11	T50.Z12	T50.Z13	T50.Z14	T50.Z15	T50.Z16
Immuglobin	T50.Z11	T50.Z12	T50.Z13	T50.Z14	T50.Z15	T50.Z16
Immune						
globulin	T50.Z11	T50.Z12	T50.Z13	T50.Z14	T50.Z15	T50.Z16
serum globulin	T50.Z11	T50.Z12	T50.Z13	T50.Z14	T50.Z15	T50.Z16
Immunoglobin human (intravenous) (normal)	T50.Z11	T50.Z12	T50.Z13	T50.Z14	T50.Z15	T50.Z16
unmodified	T50.Z11	T50.Z12	T50.Z13	T50.Z14	T50.Z15	T50.Z16
Immunosuppressive drug	T45.1X1	T45.1X2	T45.1X3	T45.1X4	T45.1X5	T45.1X6
Immu-tetanus	T50.Z11	T50.Z12	T50.Z13	T50.Z14	T50.Z15	T50.Z16
Indalpine	T43.221	T43.222	T43.223	T43.224	T43.225	T43.226
Indanazoline	T48.5X1	T48.5X2	T48.5X3	T48.5X4	T48.5X5	T48.5X6
Indandione (derivatives)	T45.511	T45.512	T45.513	T45.514	T45.515	T45.516
Indapamide	T46.5X1	T46.5X2	T46.5X3	T46.5X4	T46.5X5	T46.5X6
Indendione (derivatives)	T45.511	T45.512	T45.513	T45.514	T45.515	T45.516
Indenolol	T44.7X1	T44.7X2	T44.7X3	T44.7X4	T44.7X5	T44.7X6
Inderal	T44.7X1	T44.7X2	T44.7X3	T44.7X4	T44.7X5	T44.7X6
Indian						
hemp	T40.7X1	T40.7X2	T40.7X3	T40.7X4	T40.7X5	T40.7X6
tobacco	T62.2X1	T62.2X2	T62.2X3	T62.2X4	—	—
Indigo carmine	T50.8X1	T50.8X2	T50.8X3	T50.8X4	T50.8X5	T50.8X6
Indobufen	T45.521	T45.522	T45.523	T45.524	T45.525	T45.526
Indocin	T39.2X1	T39.2X2	T39.2X3	T39.2X4	T39.2X5	T39.2X6
Indocyanine green	T50.8X1	T50.8X2	T50.8X3	T50.8X4	T50.8X5	T50.8X6
Indometacin	T39.391	T39.392	T39.393	T39.394	T39.395	T39.396
Indomethacin	T39.391	T39.392	T39.393	T39.394	T39.395	T39.396
farnesil	T39.4X1	T39.4X2	T39.4X3	T39.4X4	T39.4X5	T39.4X6
Indoramin	T44.6X1	T44.6X2	T44.6X3	T44.6X4	T44.6X5	T44.6X6
Industrial						
alcohol	T51.0X1	T51.0X2	T51.0X3	T51.0X4	—	—
fumes	T59.891	T59.892	T59.893	T59.894	—	—
solvents (fumes) (vapors)	T52.91	T52.92	T52.93	T52.94	—	—
Influenza vaccine	T50.B91	T50.B92	T50.B93	T50.B94	T50.B95	T50.B96
Ingested substance NEC	T65.91	T65.92	T65.93	T65.94	—	—
INH	T37.1X1	T37.1X2	T37.1X3	T37.1X4	T37.1X5	T37.1X6
Inhalation, gas (noxious) — *see* Gas						
Inhibitor						
angiotensin-converting enzyme	T46.4X1	T46.4X2	T46.4X3	T46.4X4	T46.4X5	T46.4X6
carbonic anhydrase	T50.2X1	T50.2X2	T50.2X3	T50.2X4	T50.2X5	T50.2X6
fibrinolysis	T45.621	T45.622	T45.623	T45.624	T45.625	T45.626
monoamine oxidase NEC	T43.1X1	T43.1X2	T43.1X3	T43.1X4	T43.1X5	T43.1X6
hydrazine	T43.1X1	T43.1X2	T43.1X3	T43.1X4	T43.1X5	T43.1X6
postsynaptic	T43.8X1	T43.8X2	T43.8X3	T43.8X4	T43.8X5	T43.8X6
prothrombin synthesis	T45.511	T45.512	T45.513	T45.514	T45.515	T45.516
Ink	T65.891	T65.892	T65.893	T65.894	—	—
Inorganic substance NEC	T57.91	T57.92	T57.93	T57.94	—	—
Inosine pranobex	T37.5X1	T37.5X2	T37.5X3	T37.5X4	T37.5X5	T37.5X6
Inositol	T50.991	T50.992	T50.993	T50.994	T50.995	T50.996
nicotinate	T46.7X1	T46.7X2	T46.7X3	T46.7X4	T46.7X5	T46.7X6
Inproquone	T45.1X1	T45.1X2	T45.1X3	T45.1X4	T45.1X5	T45.1X6
Insecticide NEC	T60.91	T60.92	T60.93	T60.94	—	—
carbamate	T60.0X1	T60.0X2	T60.0X3	T60.0X4	—	—
chlorinated	T60.1X1	T60.1X2	T60.1X3	T60.1X4	—	—
mixed	T60.91	T60.92	T60.93	T60.94	—	—
organochlorine	T60.1X1	T60.1X2	T60.1X3	T60.1X4	—	—
organophosphorus	T60.0X1	T60.0X2	T60.0X3	T60.0X4	—	—
Insect (sting), venomous	T63.481	T63.482	T63.483	T63.484	—	—
ant	T63.421	T63.422	T63.423	T63.424	—	—
bee	T63.441	T63.442	T63.443	T63.444	—	—
caterpillar	T63.431	T63.432	T63.433	T63.434	—	—
hornet	T63.451	T63.452	T63.453	T63.454	—	—
wasp	T63.461	T63.462	T63.463	T63.464	—	—
Insular tissue extract	T38.3X1	T38.3X2	T38.3X3	T38.3X4	T38.3X5	T38.3X6
Insulin (amorphous) (globin) (isophane) (Lente) (NPH) (Semilente) (Ultralente)	T38.3X1	T38.3X2	T38.3X3	T38.3X4	T38.3X5	T38.3X6
defalan	T38.3X1	T38.3X2	T38.3X3	T38.3X4	T38.3X5	T38.3X6
human	T38.3X1	T38.3X2	T38.3X3	T38.3X4	T38.3X5	T38.3X6
injection, soluble	T38.3X1	T38.3X2	T38.3X3	T38.3X4	T38.3X5	T38.3X6
biphasic	T38.3X1	T38.3X2	T38.3X3	T38.3X4	T38.3X5	T38.3X6
intermediate acting	T38.3X1	T38.3X2	T38.3X3	T38.3X4	T38.3X5	T38.3X6
protamine zinc	T38.3X1	T38.3X2	T38.3X3	T38.3X4	T38.3X5	T38.3X6
slow acting	T38.3X1	T38.3X2	T38.3X3	T38.3X4	T38.3X5	T38.3X6
zinc						
protamine injection	T38.3X1	T38.3X2	T38.3X3	T38.3X4	T38.3X5	T38.3X6
suspension (amorphous) (crystalline)	T38.3X1	T38.3X2	T38.3X3	T38.3X4	T38.3X5	T38.3X6
Interferon (alpha) (beta) (gamma)	T37.5X1	T37.5X2	T37.5X3	T37.5X4	T37.5X5	T37.5X6
Intestinal motility control drug	T47.6X1	T47.6X2	T47.6X3	T47.6X4	T47.6X5	T47.6X6
biological	T47.8X1	T47.8X2	T47.8X3	T47.8X4	T47.8X5	T47.8X6
Intranarcon	T41.1X1	T41.1X2	T41.1X3	T41.1X4	T41.1X5	T41.1X6
Intravenous						
amino acids	T50.991	T50.992	T50.993	T50.994	T50.995	T50.996
fat suspension	T50.991	T50.992	T50.993	T50.994	T50.995	T50.996
Inulin	T50.8X1	T50.8X2	T50.8X3	T50.8X4	T50.8X5	T50.8X6
Invert sugar	T50.3X1	T50.3X2	T50.3X3	T50.3X4	T50.3X5	T50.3X6
Inza — *see* Naproxen						
Iobenzamic acid	T50.8X1	T50.8X2	T50.8X3	T50.8X4	T50.8X5	T50.8X6
Iocarmic acid	T50.8X1	T50.8X2	T50.8X3	T50.8X4	T50.8X5	T50.8X6
Iocetamic acid	T50.8X1	T50.8X2	T50.8X3	T50.8X4	T50.8X5	T50.8X6
Iodamide	T50.8X1	T50.8X2	T50.8X3	T50.8X4	T50.8X5	T50.8X6
Iodide NEC — *see also* Iodine	T49.0X1	T49.0X2	T49.0X3	T49.0X4	T49.0X5	T49.0X6
mercury (ointment)	T49.0X1	T49.0X2	T49.0X3	T49.0X4	T49.0X5	T49.0X6
methylate	T49.0X1	T49.0X2	T49.0X3	T49.0X4	T49.0X5	T49.0X6
potassium (expectorant) NEC	T48.4X1	T48.4X2	T48.4X3	T48.4X4	T48.4X5	T48.4X6
Iodinated						
contrast medium	T50.8X1	T50.8X2	T50.8X3	T50.8X4	T50.8X5	T50.8X6
glycerol	T48.4X1	T48.4X2	T48.4X3	T48.4X4	T48.4X5	T48.4X6
human serum albumin (131I)	T50.8X1	T50.8X2	T50.8X3	T50.8X4	T50.8X5	T50.8X6
Iodine (antiseptic, external) (tincture) **NEC**	T49.0X1	T49.0X2	T49.0X3	T49.0X4	T49.0X5	T49.0X6
125 — *see also* Radiation sickness, and Exposure to radioactivce isotopes	T50.8X1	T50.8X2	T50.8X3	T50.8X4	T50.8X5	T50.8X6
therapeutic	T50.991	T50.992	T50.993	T50.994	T50.995	T50.996
131 — *see also* Radiation sickness, and Exposure to radioactivce isotopes	T50.8X1	T50.8X2	T50.8X3	T50.8X4	T50.8X5	T50.8X6
therapeutic	T38.2X1	T38.2X2	T38.2X3	T38.2X4	T38.2X5	T38.2X6
diagnostic	T50.8X1	T50.8X2	T50.8X3	T50.8X4	T50.8X5	T50.8X6

Substance	Poisoning, Accidental (unintentional)	Poisoning, Intentional Self-harm	Poisoning, Assault	Poisoning, Undetermined	Adverse Effect	Underdosing
Iodine (antiseptic, external) (tincture) NEC — continued						
for thyroid conditions (antithyroid)	T38.2X1	T38.2X2	T38.2X3	T38.2X4	T38.2X5	T38.2X6
solution	T49.0X1	T49.0X2	T49.0X3	T49.0X4	T49.0X5	T49.0X6
vapor	T59.891	T59.892	T59.893	T59.894	—	—
Iodipamide	T50.8X1	T50.8X2	T50.8X3	T50.8X4	T50.8X5	T50.8X6
Iodized (poppy seed) oil	T50.8X1	T50.8X2	T50.8X3	T50.8X4	T50.8X5	T50.8X6
Iodobismitol	T37.8X1	T37.8X2	T37.8X3	T37.8X4	T37.8X5	T37.8X6
Iodochlorhydroxyquin	T37.8X1	T37.8X2	T37.8X3	T37.8X4	T37.8X5	T37.8X6
topical	T49.0X1	T49.0X2	T49.0X3	T49.0X4	T49.0X5	T49.0X6
Iodochlorhydroxyquinoline	T37.8X1	T37.8X2	T37.8X3	T37.8X4	T37.8X5	T37.8X6
Iodocholesterol (131I)	T50.8X1	T50.8X2	T50.8X3	T50.8X4	T50.8X5	T50.8X6
Iodoform	T49.0X1	T49.0X2	T49.0X3	T49.0X4	T49.0X5	T49.0X6
Iodohippuric acid	T50.8X1	T50.8X2	T50.8X3	T50.8X4	T50.8X5	T50.8X6
Iodopanoic acid	T50.8X1	T50.8X2	T50.8X3	T50.8X4	T50.8X5	T50.8X6
Iodophthalein (sodium)	T50.8X1	T50.8X2	T50.8X3	T50.8X4	T50.8X5	T50.8X6
Iodopyracet	T50.8X1	T50.8X2	T50.8X3	T50.8X4	T50.8X5	T50.8X6
Iodoquinol	T37.8X1	T37.8X2	T37.8X3	T37.8X4	T37.8X5	T37.8X6
Iodoxamic acid	T50.8X1	T50.8X2	T50.8X3	T50.8X4	T50.8X5	T50.8X6
Iofendylate	T50.8X1	T50.8X2	T50.8X3	T50.8X4	T50.8X5	T50.8X6
Ioglycamic acid	T50.8X1	T50.8X2	T50.8X3	T50.8X4	T50.8X5	T50.8X6
Iohexol	T50.8X1	T50.8X2	T50.8X3	T50.8X4	T50.8X5	T50.8X6
Ion exchange resin						
anion	T47.8X1	T47.8X2	T47.8X3	T47.8X4	T47.8X5	T47.8X6
cation	T50.3X1	T50.3X2	T50.3X3	T50.3X4	T50.3X5	T50.3X6
cholestyramine	T46.6X1	T46.6X2	T46.6X3	T46.6X4	T46.6X5	T46.6X6
intestinal	T47.8X1	T47.8X2	T47.8X3	T47.8X4	T47.8X5	T47.8X6
Iopamidol	T50.8X1	T50.8X2	T50.8X3	T50.8X4	T50.8X5	T50.8X6
Iopanoic acid	T50.8X1	T50.8X2	T50.8X3	T50.8X4	T50.8X5	T50.8X6
Iophenoic acid	T50.8X1	T50.8X2	T50.8X3	T50.8X4	T50.8X5	T50.8X6
Iopodate, sodium	T50.8X1	T50.8X2	T50.8X3	T50.8X4	T50.8X5	T50.8X6
Iopodic acid	T50.8X1	T50.8X2	T50.8X3	T50.8X4	T50.8X5	T50.8X6
Iopromide	T50.8X1	T50.8X2	T50.8X3	T50.8X4	T50.8X5	T50.8X6
Iopydol	T50.8X1	T50.8X2	T50.8X3	T50.8X4	T50.8X5	T50.8X6
Iotalamic acid	T50.8X1	T50.8X2	T50.8X3	T50.8X4	T50.8X5	T50.8X6
Iothalamate	T50.8X1	T50.8X2	T50.8X3	T50.8X4	T50.8X5	T50.8X6
Iothiouracil	T38.2X1	T38.2X2	T38.2X3	T38.2X4	T38.2X5	T38.2X6
Iotrol	T50.8X1	T50.8X2	T50.8X3	T50.8X4	T50.8X5	T50.8X6
Iotrolan	T50.8X1	T50.8X2	T50.8X3	T50.8X4	T50.8X5	T50.8X6
Iotroxate	T50.8X1	T50.8X2	T50.8X3	T50.8X4	T50.8X5	T50.8X6
Iotroxic acid	T50.8X1	T50.8X2	T50.8X3	T50.8X4	T50.8X5	T50.8X6
Ioversol	T50.8X1	T50.8X2	T50.8X3	T50.8X4	T50.8X5	T50.8X6
Ioxaglate	T50.8X1	T50.8X2	T50.8X3	T50.8X4	T50.8X5	T50.8X6
Ioxaglic acid	T50.8X1	T50.8X2	T50.8X3	T50.8X4	T50.8X5	T50.8X6
Ioxitalamic acid	T50.8X1	T50.8X2	T50.8X3	T50.8X4	T50.8X5	T50.8X6
Ipecac	T47.7X1	T47.7X2	T47.7X3	T47.7X4	T47.7X5	T47.7X6
Ipecacuanha	T48.4X1	T48.4X2	T48.4X3	T48.4X4	T48.4X5	T48.4X6
Ipodate, calcium	T50.8X1	T50.8X2	T50.8X3	T50.8X4	T50.8X5	T50.8X6
Ipral	T42.3X1	T42.3X2	T42.3X3	T42.3X4	T42.3X5	T42.3X6
Ipratropium (bromide)	T48.6X1	T48.6X2	T48.6X3	T48.6X4	T48.6X5	T48.6X6
Ipriflavone	T46.3X1	T46.3X2	T46.3X3	T46.3X4	T46.3X5	T46.3X6
Iprindole	T43.011	T43.012	T43.013	T43.014	T43.015	T43.016
Iproclozide	T43.1X1	T43.1X2	T43.1X3	T43.1X4	T43.1X5	T43.1X6
Iprofenin	T50.8X1	T50.8X2	T50.8X3	T50.8X4	T50.8X5	T50.8X6
Iproheptine	T49.2X1	T49.2X2	T49.2X3	T49.2X4	T49.2X5	T49.2X6
Iproniazid	T43.1X1	T43.1X2	T43.1X3	T43.1X4	T43.1X5	T43.1X6
Iproplatin	T45.1X1	T45.1X2	T45.1X3	T45.1X4	T45.1X5	T45.1X6
Iproveratril	T46.1X1	T46.1X2	T46.1X3	T46.1X4	T46.1X5	T46.1X6
Iron (compounds) (medicinal) NEC	T45.4X1	T45.4X2	T45.4X3	T45.4X4	T45.4X5	T45.4X6
ammonium	T45.4X1	T45.4X2	T45.4X3	T45.4X4	T45.4X5	T45.4X6
dextran injection	T45.4X1	T45.4X2	T45.4X3	T45.4X4	T45.4X5	T45.4X6
nonmedicinal	T56.891	T56.892	T56.893	T56.894	—	—
salts	T45.4X1	T45.4X2	T45.4X3	T45.4X4	T45.4X5	T45.4X6
sorbitex	T45.4X1	T45.4X2	T45.4X3	T45.4X4	T45.4X5	T45.4X6
sorbitol citric acid complex	T45.4X1	T45.4X2	T45.4X3	T45.4X4	T45.4X5	T45.4X6
Irrigating fluid (vaginal)	T49.8X1	T49.8X2	T49.8X3	T49.8X4	T49.8X5	T49.8X6
eye	T49.5X1	T49.5X2	T49.5X3	T49.5X4	T49.5X5	T49.5X6
Isepamicin	T36.5X1	T36.5X2	T36.5X3	T36.5X4	T36.5X5	T36.5X6
Isoaminile (citrate)	T48.3X1	T48.3X2	T48.3X3	T48.3X4	T48.3X5	T48.3X6
Isoamyl nitrite	T46.3X1	T46.3X2	T46.3X3	T46.3X4	T46.3X5	T46.3X6
Isobenzan	T60.1X1	T60.1X2	T60.1X3	T60.1X4	—	—
Isobutyl acetate	T52.8X1	T52.8X2	T52.8X3	T52.8X4	—	—
Isocarboxazid	T43.1X1	T43.1X2	T43.1X3	T43.1X4	T43.1X5	T43.1X6
Isoconazole	T49.0X1	T49.0X2	T49.0X3	T49.0X4	T49.0X5	T49.0X6
Isocyanate	T65.0X1	T65.0X2	T65.0X3	T65.0X4	—	—
Isoephedrine	T44.991	T44.992	T44.993	T44.994	T44.995	T44.996
Isoetarine	T48.6X1	T48.6X2	T48.6X3	T48.6X4	T48.6X5	T48.6X6
Isoethadione	T42.2X1	T42.2X2	T42.2X3	T42.2X4	T42.2X5	T42.2X6
Isoetharine	T44.5X1	T44.5X2	T44.5X3	T44.5X4	T44.5X5	T44.5X6
Isoflurane	T41.0X1	T41.0X2	T41.0X3	T41.0X4	T41.0X5	T41.0X6
Isoflurophate	T44.0X1	T44.0X2	T44.0X3	T44.0X4	T44.0X5	T44.0X6
Isomaltose, ferric complex	T45.4X1	T45.4X2	T45.4X3	T45.4X4	T45.4X5	T45.4X6
Isometheptene	T44.3X1	T44.3X2	T44.3X3	T44.3X4	T44.3X5	T44.3X6
Isoniazid	T37.1X1	T37.1X2	T37.1X3	T37.1X4	T37.1X5	T37.1X6
with						
rifampicin	T36.6X1	T36.6X2	T36.6X3	T36.6X4	T36.6X5	T36.6X6
thioacetazone	T37.1X1	T37.1X2	T37.1X3	T37.1X4	T37.1X5	T37.1X6
Isonicotinic acid hydrazide	T37.1X1	T37.1X2	T37.1X3	T37.1X4	T37.1X5	T37.1X6
Isonipecaine	T40.4X1	T40.4X2	T40.4X3	T40.4X4	T40.4X5	T40.4X6
Isopentaquine	T37.2X1	T37.2X2	T37.2X3	T37.2X4	T37.2X5	T37.2X6
Isophane insulin	T38.3X1	T38.3X2	T38.3X3	T38.3X4	T38.3X5	T38.3X6
Isophorone	T65.891	T65.892	T65.893	T65.894	—	—
Isophosphamide	T45.1X1	T45.1X2	T45.1X3	T45.1X4	T45.1X5	T45.1X6
Isopregnenone	T38.5X1	T38.5X2	T38.5X3	T38.5X4	T38.5X5	T38.5X6
Isoprenaline	T48.6X1	T48.6X2	T48.6X3	T48.6X4	T48.6X5	T48.6X6
Isopromethazine	T43.3X1	T43.3X2	T43.3X3	T43.3X4	T43.3X5	T43.3X6
Isopropamide	T44.3X1	T44.3X2	T44.3X3	T44.3X4	T44.3X5	T44.3X6
iodide	T44.3X1	T44.3X2	T44.3X3	T44.3X4	T44.3X5	T44.3X6
Isopropanol	T51.2X1	T51.2X2	T51.2X3	T51.2X4	—	—
Isopropyl						
acetate	T52.8X1	T52.8X2	T52.8X3	T52.8X4	—	—
alcohol	T51.2X1	T51.2X2	T51.2X3	T51.2X4	—	—
medicinal	T49.4X1	T49.4X2	T49.4X3	T49.4X4	T49.4X5	T49.4X6
ether	T52.8X1	T52.8X2	T52.8X3	T52.8X4	—	—
Isopropylaminophenazone	T39.2X1	T39.2X2	T39.2X3	T39.2X4	T39.2X5	T39.2X6
Isoproterenol	T48.6X1	T48.6X2	T48.6X3	T48.6X4	T48.6X5	T48.6X6
Isosorbide dinitrate	T46.3X1	T46.3X2	T46.3X3	T46.3X4	T46.3X5	T46.3X6
Isothipendyl	T45.0X1	T45.0X2	T45.0X3	T45.0X4	T45.0X5	T45.0X6
Isotretinoin	T50.991	T50.992	T50.993	T50.994	T50.995	T50.996
Isoxazolyl penicillin	T36.0X1	T36.0X2	T36.0X3	T36.0X4	T36.0X5	T36.0X6
Isoxicam	T39.391	T39.392	T39.393	T39.394	T39.395	T39.396
Isoxsuprine	T46.7X1	T46.7X2	T46.7X3	T46.7X4	T46.7X5	T46.7X6
Ispagula	T47.4X1	T47.4X2	T47.4X3	T47.4X4	T47.4X5	T47.4X6
husk	T47.4X1	T47.4X2	T47.4X3	T47.4X4	T47.4X5	T47.4X6
Isradipine	T46.1X1	T46.1X2	T46.1X3	T46.1X4	T46.1X5	T46.1X6
I-thyroxine sodium	T38.1X1	T38.1X2	T38.1X3	T38.1X4	T38.1X5	T38.1X6
Itraconazole	T37.8X1	T37.8X2	T37.8X3	T37.8X4	T37.8X5	T37.8X6
Itramin tosilate	T46.3X1	T46.3X2	T46.3X3	T46.3X4	T46.3X5	T46.3X6
Ivermectin	T37.4X1	T37.4X2	T37.4X3	T37.4X4	T37.4X5	T37.4X6
Izoniazid	T37.1X1	T37.1X2	T37.1X3	T37.1X4	T37.1X5	T37.1X6
with thioacetazone	T37.1X1	T37.1X2	T37.1X3	T37.1X4	T37.1X5	T37.1X6
Jalap	T47.2X1	T47.2X2	T47.2X3	T47.2X4	T47.2X5	T47.2X6
Jamaica						
dogwood (bark)	T39.8X1	T39.8X2	T39.8X3	T39.8X4	T39.8X5	T39.8X6
ginger	T65.891	T65.892	T65.893	T65.894	—	—
root	T62.2X1	T62.2X2	T62.2X3	T62.2X4	—	—
Jatropha	T62.2X1	T62.2X2	T62.2X3	T62.2X4	—	—
curcas	T62.2X1	T62.2X2	T62.2X3	T62.2X4	—	—
Jectofer	T45.4X1	T45.4X2	T45.4X3	T45.4X4	T45.4X5	T45.4X6
Jellyfish (sting)	T63.621	T63.622	T63.623	T63.624	—	—
Jequirity (bean)	T62.2X1	T62.2X2	T62.2X3	T62.2X4	—	—
Jimson weed (stramonium)	T62.2X1	T62.2X2	T62.2X3	T62.2X4	—	—
seeds	T62.2X1	T62.2X2	T62.2X3	T62.2X4	—	—
Josamycin	T36.3X1	T36.3X2	T36.3X3	T36.3X4	T36.3X5	T36.3X6
Juniper tar	T49.1X1	T49.1X2	T49.1X3	T49.1X4	T49.1X5	T49.1X6
Kallidinogenase	T46.7X1	T46.7X2	T46.7X3	T46.7X4	T46.7X5	T46.7X6
Kallikrein	T46.7X1	T46.7X2	T46.7X3	T46.7X4	T46.7X5	T46.7X6
Kanamycin	T36.5X1	T36.5X2	T36.5X3	T36.5X4	T36.5X5	T36.5X6
Kantrex	T36.5X1	T36.5X2	T36.5X3	T36.5X4	T36.5X5	T36.5X6
Kaolin	T47.6X1	T47.6X2	T47.6X3	T47.6X4	T47.6X5	T47.6X6
light	T47.6X1	T47.6X2	T47.6X3	T47.6X4	T47.6X5	T47.6X6
Karaya (gum)	T47.4X1	T47.4X2	T47.4X3	T47.4X4	T47.4X5	T47.4X6
Kebuzone	T39.2X1	T39.2X2	T39.2X3	T39.2X4	T39.2X5	T39.2X6
Kelevan	T60.1X1	T60.1X2	T60.1X3	T60.1X4	—	—
Kemithal	T41.1X1	T41.1X2	T41.1X3	T41.1X4	T41.1X5	T41.1X6
Kenacort	T38.0X1	T38.0X2	T38.0X3	T38.0X4	T38.0X5	T38.0X6
Keratolytic drug NEC	T49.4X1	T49.4X2	T49.4X3	T49.4X4	T49.4X5	T49.4X6
anthracene	T49.4X1	T49.4X2	T49.4X3	T49.4X4	T49.4X5	T49.4X6
Keratoplastic NEC	T49.4X1	T49.4X2	T49.4X3	T49.4X4	T49.4X5	T49.4X6
Kerosene, kerosine (fuel) (solvent) NEC	T52.0X1	T52.0X2	T52.0X3	T52.0X4	—	—
insecticide	T52.0X1	T52.0X2	T52.0X3	T52.0X4	—	—
vapor	T52.0X1	T52.0X2	T52.0X3	T52.0X4	—	—
Ketamine	T41.291	T41.292	T41.293	T41.294	T41.295	T41.296
Ketazolam	T42.4X1	T42.4X2	T42.4X3	T42.4X4	T42.4X5	T42.4X6
Ketazon	T39.2X1	T39.2X2	T39.2X3	T39.2X4	T39.2X5	T39.2X6
Ketobemidone	T40.4X1	T40.4X2	T40.4X3	T40.4X4	—	—
Ketoconazole	T49.0X1	T49.0X2	T49.0X3	T49.0X4	T49.0X5	T49.0X6
Ketols	T52.4X1	T52.4X2	T52.4X3	T52.4X4	—	—
Ketone oils	T52.4X1	T52.4X2	T52.4X3	T52.4X4	—	—
Ketoprofen	T39.311	T39.312	T39.313	T39.314	T39.315	T39.316
Ketorolac	T39.8X1	T39.8X2	T39.8X3	T39.8X4	T39.8X5	T39.8X6
Ketotifen	T45.0X1	T45.0X2	T45.0X3	T45.0X4	T45.0X5	T45.0X6
Khat	T43.691	T43.692	T43.693	T43.694	—	—

Substance	Poisoning, Accidental (unintentional)	Poisoning, Intentional Self-harm	Poisoning, Assault	Poisoning, Undetermined	Adverse Effect	Under-dosing
Khellin	T46.3X1	T46.3X2	T46.3X3	T46.3X4	T46.3X5	T46.3X6
Khelloside	T46.3X1	T46.3X2	T46.3X3	T46.3X4	T46.3X5	T46.3X6
Kiln gas or vapor (carbon monoxide)	T58.8X1	T58.8X2	T58.8X3	T58.8X4	—	—
Kitasamycin	T36.3X1	T36.3X2	T36.3X3	T36.3X4	T36.3X5	T36.3X6
Konsyl	T47.4X1	T47.4X2	T47.4X3	T47.4X4	T47.4X5	T47.4X6
Kosam seed	T62.2X1	T62.2X2	T62.2X3	T62.2X4	—	—
Krait (venom)	T63.091	T63.092	T63.093	T63.094	—	—
Kwell (insecticide)	T60.1X1	T60.1X2	T60.1X3	T60.1X4	—	—
anti-infective (topical)	T49.0X1	T49.0X2	T49.0X3	T49.0X4	T49.0X5	T49.0X6
Labetalol	T44.8X1	T44.8X2	T44.8X3	T44.8X4	T44.8X5	T44.8X6
Laburnum (seeds)	T62.2X1	T62.2X2	T62.2X3	T62.2X4	—	—
leaves	T62.2X1	T62.2X2	T62.2X3	T62.2X4	—	—
Lachesine	T49.5X1	T49.5X2	T49.5X3	T49.5X4	T49.5X5	T49.5X6
Lacidipine	T46.5X1	T46.5X2	T46.5X3	T46.5X4	T46.5X5	T46.5X6
Lacquer	T65.6X1	T65.6X2	T65.6X3	T65.6X4	—	—
Lacrimogenic gas	T59.3X1	T59.3X2	T59.3X3	T59.3X4	—	—
Lactated potassic saline	T50.3X1	T50.3X2	T50.3X3	T50.3X4	T50.3X5	T50.3X6
Lactic acid	T49.8X1	T49.8X2	T49.8X3	T49.8X4	T49.8X5	T49.8X6
Lactobacillus						
acidophilus	T47.6X1	T47.6X2	T47.6X3	T47.6X4	T47.6X5	T47.6X6
compound	T47.6X1	T47.6X2	T47.6X3	T47.6X4	T47.6X5	T47.6X6
bifidus, lyophilized	T47.6X1	T47.6X2	T47.6X3	T47.6X4	T47.6X5	T47.6X6
bulgaricus	T47.6X1	T47.6X2	T47.6X3	T47.6X4	T47.6X5	T47.6X6
sporogenes	T47.6X1	T47.6X2	T47.6X3	T47.6X4	T47.6X5	T47.6X6
Lactoflavin	T45.2X1	T45.2X2	T45.2X3	T45.2X4	T45.2X5	T45.2X6
Lactose (as excipient)	T50.901	T50.902	T50.903	T50.904	T50.905	T50.906
Lactuca (virosa) (extract)	T42.6X1	T42.6X2	T42.6X3	T42.6X4	T42.6X5	T42.6X6
Lactucarium	T42.6X1	T42.6X2	T42.6X3	T42.6X4	T42.6X5	T42.6X6
Lactulose	T47.3X1	T47.3X2	T47.3X3	T47.3X4	T47.3X5	T47.3X6
Laevo — see Levo-						
Lanatosides	T46.0X1	T46.0X2	T46.0X3	T46.0X4	T46.0X5	T46.0X6
Lanolin	T49.3X1	T49.3X2	T49.3X3	T49.3X4	T49.3X5	T49.3X6
Largactil	T43.3X1	T43.3X2	T43.3X3	T43.3X4	T43.3X5	T43.3X6
Larkspur	T62.2X1	T62.2X2	T62.2X3	T62.2X4	—	—
Laroxyl	T43.011	T43.012	T43.013	T43.014	T43.015	T43.016
Lasix	T50.1X1	T50.1X2	T50.1X3	T50.1X4	T50.1X5	T50.1X6
Lassar's paste	T49.4X1	T49.4X2	T49.4X3	T49.4X4	T49.4X5	T49.4X6
Latamoxef	T36.1X1	T36.1X2	T36.1X3	T36.1X4	T36.1X5	T36.1X6
Latex	T65.811	T65.812	T65.813	T65.814	—	—
Lathyrus (seed)	T62.2X1	T62.2X2	T62.2X3	T62.2X4	—	—
Laudanum	T40.0X1	T40.0X2	T40.0X3	T40.0X4	T40.0X5	T40.0X6
Laudexium	T48.1X1	T48.1X2	T48.1X3	T48.1X4	T48.1X5	T48.1X6
Laughing gas	T41.0X1	T41.0X2	T41.0X3	T41.0X4	T41.0X5	T41.0X6
Laurel, black or cherry	T62.2X1	T62.2X2	T62.2X3	T62.2X4	—	—
Laurolinium	T49.0X1	T49.0X2	T49.0X3	T49.0X4	T49.0X5	T49.0X6
Lauryl sulfoacetate	T49.2X1	T49.2X2	T49.2X3	T49.2X4	T49.2X5	T49.2X6
Laxative NEC	T47.4X1	T47.4X2	T47.4X3	T47.4X4	T47.4X5	T47.4X6
osmotic	T47.3X1	T47.3X2	T47.3X3	T47.3X4	T47.3X5	T47.3X6
saline	T47.3X1	T47.3X2	T47.3X3	T47.3X4	T47.3X5	T47.3X6
stimulant	T47.2X1	T47.2X2	T47.2X3	T47.2X4	T47.2X5	T47.2X6
L-dopa	T42.8X1	T42.8X2	T42.8X3	T42.8X4	T42.8X5	T42.8X6
Lead (dust) (fumes) (vapor)	T56.0X1	T56.0X2	T56.0X3	T56.0X4	—	—
NEC						
acetate	T49.2X1	T49.2X2	T49.2X3	T49.2X4	T49.2X5	T49.2X6
alkyl (fuel additive)	T56.0X1	T56.0X2	T56.0X3	T56.0X4	—	—
anti-infectives	T37.8X1	T37.8X2	T37.8X3	T37.8X4	T37.8X5	T37.8X6
antiknock compound (tetraethyl)	T56.0X1	T56.0X2	T56.0X3	T56.0X4	—	—
arsenate, arsenite (dust)(herbicide) (insecticide) (vapor)	T57.0X1	T57.0X2	T57.0X3	T57.0X4		—
carbonate	T56.0X1	T56.0X2	T56.0X3	T56.0X4	—	—
paint	T56.0X1	T56.0X2	T56.0X3	T56.0X4	—	—
chromate	T56.0X1	T56.0X2	T56.0X3	T56.0X4	—	—
paint	T56.0X1	T56.0X2	T56.0X3	T56.0X4	—	—
dioxide	T56.0X1	T56.0X2	T56.0X3	T56.0X4	—	—
inorganic	T56.0X1	T56.0X2	T56.0X3	T56.0X4	—	—
iodide	T56.0X1	T56.0X2	T56.0X3	T56.0X4	—	—
pigment (paint)	T56.0X1	T56.0X2	T56.0X3	T56.0X4	—	—
monoxide (dust)	T56.0X1	T56.0X2	T56.0X3	T56.0X4	—	—
paint	T56.0X1	T56.0X2	T56.0X3	T56.0X4	—	—
organic	T56.0X1	T56.0X2	T56.0X3	T56.0X4	—	—
oxide	T56.0X1	T56.0X2	T56.0X3	T56.0X4	—	—
paint	T56.0X1	T56.0X2	T56.0X3	T56.0X4	—	—
paint	T56.0X1	T56.0X2	T56.0X3	T56.0X4	—	—
salts	T56.0X1	T56.0X2	T56.0X3	T56.0X4	—	—
specified compound NEC	T56.0X1	T56.0X2	T56.0X3	T56.0X4	—	—
tetra-ethyl	T56.0X1	T56.0X2	T56.0X3	T56.0X4	—	—
Lebanese red	T40.7X1	T40.7X2	T40.7X3	T40.7X4	T40.7X5	T40.7X6
Lefetamine	T39.8X1	T39.8X2	T39.8X3	T39.8X4	T39.8X5	T39.8X6
Lenperone	T43.4X1	T43.4X2	T43.4X3	T43.4X4	T43.4X5	T43.4X6
Lente lietin (insulin)	T38.3X1	T38.3X2	T38.3X3	T38.3X4	T38.3X5	T38.3X6

Substance	Poisoning, Accidental (unintentional)	Poisoning, Intentional Self-harm	Poisoning, Assault	Poisoning, Undetermined	Adverse Effect	Under-dosing
Leptazol	T50.7X1	T50.7X2	T50.7X3	T50.7X4	T50.7X5	T50.7X6
Leptophos	T60.0X1	T60.0X2	T60.0X3	T60.0X4	—	—
Leritine	T40.2X1	T40.2X2	T40.2X3	T40.2X4	T40.2X5	T40.2X6
Letosteine	T48.4X1	T48.4X2	T48.4X3	T48.4X4	T48.4X5	T48.4X6
Letter	T38.1X1	T38.1X2	T38.1X3	T38.1X4	T38.1X5	T38.1X6
Lettuce opium	T42.6X1	T42.6X2	T42.6X3	T42.6X4	T42.6X5	T42.6X6
Leucinocaine	T41.3X1	T41.3X2	T41.3X3	T41.3X4	T41.3X5	T41.3X6
Leucocianidol	T46.991	T46.992	T46.993	T46.994	T46.995	T46.996
Leucovorin (factor)	T45.8X1	T45.8X2	T45.8X3	T45.8X4	T45.8X5	T45.8X6
Leukeran	T45.1X1	T45.1X2	T45.1X3	T45.1X4	T45.1X5	T45.1X6
Leuprolide	T38.891	T38.892	T38.893	T38.894	T38.895	T38.896
Levalbuterol	T48.6X1	T48.6X2	T48.6X3	T48.6X4	T48.6X5	T48.6X6
Levallorphan	T50.7X1	T50.7X2	T50.7X3	T50.7X4	T50.7X5	T50.7X6
Levamisole	T37.4X1	T37.4X2	T37.4X3	T37.4X4	T37.4X5	T37.4X6
Levanil	T42.6X1	T42.6X2	T42.6X3	T42.6X4	T42.6X5	T42.6X6
Levarterenol	T44.4X1	T44.4X2	T44.4X3	T44.4X4	T44.4X5	T44.4X6
Levdropropizine	T48.3X1	T48.3X2	T48.3X3	T48.3X4	T48.3X5	T48.3X6
Levobunolol	T49.5X1	T49.5X2	T49.5X3	T49.5X4	T49.5X5	T49.5X6
Levocabastine (hydrochloride)	T45.0X1	T45.0X2	T45.0X3	T45.0X4	T45.0X5	T45.0X6
Levocarnitine	T50.991	T50.992	T50.993	T50.994	T50.995	T50.996
Levodopa	T42.8X1	T42.8X2	T42.8X3	T42.8X4	T42.8X5	T42.8X6
with carbidopa	T42.8X1	T42.8X2	T42.8X3	T42.8X4	T42.8X5	T42.8X6
Levo-dromoran	T40.2X1	T40.2X2	T40.2X3	T40.2X4	T40.2X5	T40.2X6
Levoglutamide	T50.991	T50.992	T50.993	T50.994	T50.995	T50.996
Levoid	T38.1X1	T38.1X2	T38.1X3	T38.1X4	T38.1X5	T38.1X6
Levo-isomethadone	T40.3X1	T40.3X2	T40.3X3	T40.3X4	T40.3X5	T40.3X6
Levomepromazine	T43.3X1	T43.3X2	T43.3X3	T43.3X4	T43.3X5	T43.3X6
Levonordefrin	T49.6X1	T49.6X2	T49.6X3	T49.6X4	T49.6X5	T49.6X6
Levonorgestrel	T38.4X1	T38.4X2	T38.4X3	T38.4X4	T38.4X5	T38.4X6
with ethinylestradiol	T38.5X1	T38.5X2	T38.5X3	T38.5X4	T38.5X5	T38.5X6
Levopromazine	T43.3X1	T43.3X2	T43.3X3	T43.3X4	T43.3X5	T43.3X6
Levoprome	T42.6X1	T42.6X2	T42.6X3	T42.6X4	T42.6X5	T42.6X6
Levopropoxyphene	T40.4X1	T40.4X2	T40.4X3	T40.4X4	T40.4X5	T40.4X6
Levopropylhexedrine	T50.5X1	T50.5X2	T50.5X3	T50.5X4	T50.5X5	T50.5X6
Levoproxyphylline	T48.6X1	T48.6X2	T48.6X3	T48.6X4	T48.6X5	T48.6X6
Levorphanol	T40.4X1	T40.4X2	T40.4X3	T40.4X4	T40.4X5	T40.4X6
Levothyroxine	T38.1X1	T38.1X2	T38.1X3	T38.1X4	T38.1X5	T38.1X6
sodium	T38.1X1	T38.1X2	T38.1X3	T38.1X4	T38.1X5	T38.1X6
Levsin	T44.3X1	T44.3X2	T44.3X3	T44.3X4	T44.3X5	T44.3X6
Levulose	T50.3X1	T50.3X2	T50.3X3	T50.3X4	T50.3X5	T50.3X6
Lewisite (gas), not in war	T57.0X1	T57.0X2	T57.0X3	T57.0X4		
Librium	T42.4X1	T42.4X2	T42.4X3	T42.4X4	T42.4X5	T42.4X6
Lidex	T49.0X1	T49.0X2	T49.0X3	T49.0X4	T49.0X5	T49.0X6
Lidocaine	T41.3X1	T41.3X2	T41.3X3	T41.3X4	T41.3X5	T41.3X6
regional	T41.3X1	T41.3X2	T41.3X3	T41.3X4	T41.3X5	T41.3X6
spinal	T41.3X1	T41.3X2	T41.3X3	T41.3X4	T41.3X5	T41.3X6
Lidofenin	T50.8X1	T50.8X2	T50.8X3	T50.8X4	T50.8X5	T50.8X6
Lidoflazine	T46.1X1	T46.1X2	T46.1X3	T46.1X4	T46.1X5	T46.1X6
Lighter fluid	T52.0X1	T52.0X2	T52.0X3	T52.0X4	—	—
Lignin hemicellulose	T47.6X1	T47.6X2	T47.6X3	T47.6X4	T47.6X5	T47.6X6
Lignocaine	T41.3X1	T41.3X2	T41.3X3	T41.3X4	T41.3X5	T41.3X6
regional	T41.3X1	T41.3X2	T41.3X3	T41.3X4	T41.3X5	T41.3X6
spinal	T41.3X1	T41.3X2	T41.3X3	T41.3X4	T41.3X5	T41.3X6
Ligroin (e) (solvent)	T52.0X1	T52.0X2	T52.0X3	T52.0X4	—	—
vapor	T59.891	T59.892	T59.893	T59.894	—	—
Ligustrum vulgare	T62.2X1	T62.2X2	T62.2X3	T62.2X4	—	—
Lily of the valley	T62.2X1	T62.2X2	T62.2X3	T62.2X4	—	—
Lime (chloride)	T54.3X1	T54.3X2	T54.3X3	T54.3X4	—	—
Limonene	T52.8X1	T52.8X2	T52.8X3	T52.8X4	—	—
Lincomycin	T36.8X1	T36.8X2	T36.8X3	T36.8X4	T36.8X5	T36.8X6
Lindane (insecticide) (nonmedicinal) (vapor)	T53.6X1	T53.6X2	T53.6X3	T53.6X4	—	—
medicinal	T49.0X1	T49.0X2	T49.0X3	T49.0X4	T49.0X5	T49.0X6
Liniments NEC	T49.91	T49.92	T49.93	T49.94	T49.95	T49.96
Linoleic acid	T46.6X1	T46.6X2	T46.6X3	T46.6X4	T46.6X5	T46.6X6
Linolenic acid	T46.6X1	T46.6X2	T46.6X3	T46.6X4	T46.6X5	T46.6X6
Linseed	T47.4X1	T47.4X2	T47.4X3	T47.4X4	T47.4X5	T47.4X6
Liothyronine	T38.1X1	T38.1X2	T38.1X3	T38.1X4	T38.1X5	T38.1X6
Liotrix	T38.1X1	T38.1X2	T38.1X3	T38.1X4	T38.1X5	T38.1X6
Lipancreatin	T47.5X1	T47.5X2	T47.5X3	T47.5X4	T47.5X5	T47.5X6
Lipo-alprostadil	T46.7X1	T46.7X2	T46.7X3	T46.7X4	T46.7X5	T46.7X6
Lipo-Lutin	T38.5X1	T38.5X2	T38.5X3	T38.5X4	T38.5X5	T38.5X6
Lipotropic drug NEC	T50.901	T50.902	T50.903	T50.904	T50.905	T50.906
Liquefied petroleum gases	T59.891	T59.892	T59.893	T59.894	—	—
piped (pure or mixed with air)	T59.891	T59.892	T59.893	T59.894	—	—
Liquid						
paraffin	T47.4X1	T47.4X2	T47.4X3	T47.4X4	T47.4X5	T47.4X6
petrolatum	T47.4X1	T47.4X2	T47.4X3	T47.4X4	T47.4X5	T47.4X6
topical	T49.3X1	T49.3X2	T49.3X3	T49.3X4	T49.3X5	T49.3X6
specified NEC	T65.891	T65.892	T65.893	T65.894	—	—
substance	T65.91	T65.92	T65.93	T65.94	—	—

Table of Drugs and Chemicals

Substance	Poisoning, Accidental (unintentional)	Poisoning, Intentional Self-harm	Poisoning, Assault	Poisoning, Undetermined	Adverse Effect	Under-dosing
Liquor creosolis compositus	T65.891	T65.892	T65.893	T65.894	—	—
Liquorice	T48.4X1	T48.4X2	T48.4X3	T48.4X4	T48.4X5	T48.4X6
extract	T47.8X1	T47.8X2	T47.8X3	T47.8X4	T47.8X5	T47.8X6
Lisinopril	T46.4X1	T46.4X2	T46.4X3	T46.4X4	T46.4X5	T46.4X6
Lisuride	T42.8X1	T42.8X2	T42.8X3	T42.8X4	T42.8X5	T42.8X6
Lithane	T43.8X1	T43.8X2	T43.8X3	T43.8X4	T43.8X5	T43.8X6
Lithium	T56.891	T56.892	T56.893	T56.894		
gluconate	T43.591	T43.592	T43.593	T43.594	T43.595	T43.596
salts (carbonate)	T43.591	T43.592	T43.593	T43.594	T43.595	T43.596
Lithonate	T43.8X1	T43.8X2	T43.8X3	T43.8X4	T43.8X5	T43.8X6
Liver						
extract	T45.8X1	T45.8X2	T45.8X3	T45.8X4	T45.8X5	T45.8X6
for parenteral use	T45.8X1	T45.8X2	T45.8X3	T45.8X4	T45.8X5	T45.8X6
fraction 1	T45.8X1	T45.8X2	T45.8X3	T45.8X4	T45.8X5	T45.8X6
hydrolysate	T45.8X1	T45.8X2	T45.8X3	T45.8X4	T45.8X5	T45.8X6
Lizard (bite) (venom)	T63.121	T63.122	T63.123	T63.124	—	—
LMD	T45.8X1	T45.8X2	T45.8X3	T45.8X4	T45.8X5	T45.8X6
Lobelia	T62.2X1	T62.2X2	T62.2X3	T62.2X4	—	—
Lobeline	T50.7X1	T50.7X2	T50.7X3	T50.7X4	T50.7X5	T50.7X6
Local action drug NEC	T49.8X1	T49.8X2	T49.8X3	T49.8X4	T49.8X5	T49.8X6
Locorten	T49.0X1	T49.0X2	T49.0X3	T49.0X4	T49.0X5	T49.0X6
Lofepramine	T43.011	T43.012	T43.013	T43.014	T43.015	T43.016
Lolium temulentum	T62.2X1	T62.2X2	T62.2X3	T62.2X4	—	—
Lomotil	T47.6X1	T47.6X2	T47.6X3	T47.6X4	T47.6X5	T47.6X6
Lomustine	T45.1X1	T45.1X2	T45.1X3	T45.1X4	T45.1X5	T45.1X6
Lonidamine	T45.1X1	T45.1X2	T45.1X3	T45.1X4	T45.1X5	T45.1X6
Loperamide	T47.6X1	T47.6X2	T47.6X3	T47.6X4	T47.6X5	T47.6X6
Loprazolam	T42.4X1	T42.4X2	T42.4X3	T42.4X4	T42.4X5	T42.4X6
Lorajmine	T46.2X1	T46.2X2	T46.2X3	T46.2X4	T46.2X5	T46.2X6
Loratidine	T45.0X1	T45.0X2	T45.0X3	T45.0X4	T45.0X5	T45.0X6
Lorazepam	T42.4X1	T42.4X2	T42.4X3	T42.4X4	T42.4X5	T42.4X6
Lorcainide	T46.2X1	T46.2X2	T46.2X3	T46.2X4	T46.2X5	T46.2X6
Lormetazepam	T42.4X1	T42.4X2	T42.4X3	T42.4X4	T42.4X5	T42.4X6
Lotions NEC	T49.91	T49.92	T49.93	T49.94	T49.95	T49.96
Lotusate	T42.3X1	T42.3X2	T42.3X3	T42.3X4	T42.3X5	T42.3X6
Lovastatin	T46.6X1	T46.6X2	T46.6X3	T46.6X4	T46.6X5	T46.6X6
Lowila	T49.2X1	T49.2X2	T49.2X3	T49.2X4	T49.2X5	T49.2X6
Loxapine	T43.591	T43.592	T43.593	T43.594	T43.595	T43.596
Lozenges (throat)	T49.6X1	T49.6X2	T49.6X3	T49.6X4	T49.6X5	T49.6X6
LSD	T40.8X1	T40.8X2	T40.8X3	T40.8X4	—	—
L-Tryptophan — see amino acid						
Lubricant, eye	T49.5X1	T49.5X2	T49.5X3	T49.5X4	T49.5X5	T49.5X6
Lubricating oil NEC	T52.0X1	T52.0X2	T52.0X3	T52.0X4	—	—
Lucanthone	T37.4X1	T37.4X2	T37.4X3	T37.4X4	T37.4X5	T37.4X6
Luminal	T42.3X1	T42.3X2	T42.3X3	T42.3X4	T42.3X5	T42.3X6
Lung irritant (gas) NEC	T59.91	T59.92	T59.93	T59.94	—	—
Luteinizing hormone	T38.811	T38.812	T38.813	T38.814	T38.815	T38.816
Lutocylol	T38.5X1	T38.5X2	T38.5X3	T38.5X4	T38.5X5	T38.5X6
Lutromone	T38.5X1	T38.5X2	T38.5X3	T38.5X4	T38.5X5	T38.5X6
Lututrin	T48.291	T48.292	T48.293	T48.294	T48.295	T48.296
Lye (concentrated)	T54.3X1	T54.3X2	T54.3X3	T54.3X4	—	—
Lygranum (skin test)	T50.8X1	T50.8X2	T50.8X3	T50.8X4	T50.8X5	T50.8X6
Lymecycline	T36.4X1	T36.4X2	T36.4X3	T36.4X4	T36.4X5	T36.4X6
Lymphogranuloma venereum antigen	T50.8X1	T50.8X2	T50.8X3	T50.8X4	T50.8X5	T50.8X6
Lynestrenol	T38.4X1	T38.4X2	T38.4X3	T38.4X4	T38.4X5	T38.4X6
Lyovac Sodium Edecrin	T50.1X1	T50.1X2	T50.1X3	T50.1X4	T50.1X5	T50.1X6
Lypressin	T38.891	T38.892	T38.893	T38.894	T38.895	T38.896
Lysergic acid diethylamide	T40.8X1	T40.8X2	T40.8X3	T40.8X4	—	—
Lysergide	T40.8X1	T40.8X2	T40.8X3	T40.8X4	—	—
Lysine vasopressin	T38.891	T38.892	T38.893	T38.894	T38.895	T38.896
Lysol	T54.1X1	T54.1X2	T54.1X3	T54.1X4	—	—
Lysozyme	T49.0X1	T49.0X2	T49.0X3	T49.0X4	T49.0X5	T49.0X6
Lytta (vitatta)	T49.8X1	T49.8X2	T49.8X3	T49.8X4	T49.8X5	T49.8X6
Mace	T59.3X1	T59.3X2	T59.3X3	T59.3X4	—	—
Macrogol	T50.991	T50.992	T50.993	T50.994	T50.995	T50.996
Macrolide						
anabolic drug	T38.7X1	T38.7X2	T38.7X3	T38.7X4	T38.7X5	T38.7X6
antibiotic	T36.3X1	T36.3X2	T36.3X3	T36.3X4	T36.3X5	T36.3X6
Mafenide	T49.0X1	T49.0X2	T49.0X3	T49.0X4	T49.0X5	T49.0X6
Magaldrate	T47.1X1	T47.1X2	T47.1X3	T47.1X4	T47.1X5	T47.1X6
Magic mushroom	T40.991	T40.992	T40.993	T40.994	—	—
Magnamycin	T36.8X1	T36.8X2	T36.8X3	T36.8X4	T36.8X5	T36.8X6
Magnesia magma	T47.1X1	T47.1X2	T47.1X3	T47.1X4	T47.1X5	T47.1X6
Magnesium NEC	T56.891	T56.892	T56.893	T56.894		
carbonate	T47.1X1	T47.1X2	T47.1X3	T47.1X4	T47.1X5	T47.1X6
citrate	T47.4X1	T47.4X2	T47.4X3	T47.4X4	T47.4X5	T47.4X6
hydroxide	T47.1X1	T47.1X2	T47.1X3	T47.1X4	T47.1X5	T47.1X6
oxide	T47.1X1	T47.1X2	T47.1X3	T47.1X4	T47.1X5	T47.1X6
peroxide	T49.0X1	T49.0X2	T49.0X3	T49.0X4	T49.0X5	T49.0X6
salicylate	T39.091	T39.092	T39.093	T39.094	T39.095	T39.096
silicofluoride	T50.3X1	T50.3X2	T50.3X3	T50.3X4	T50.3X5	T50.3X6

Substance	Poisoning, Accidental (unintentional)	Poisoning, Intentional Self-harm	Poisoning, Assault	Poisoning, Undetermined	Adverse Effect	Under-dosing
Magnesium — continued						
sulfate	T47.4X1	T47.4X2	T47.4X3	T47.4X4	T47.4X5	T47.4X6
thiosulfate	T45.0X1	T45.0X2	T45.0X3	T45.0X4	T45.0X5	T45.0X6
trisilicate	T47.1X1	T47.1X2	T47.1X3	T47.1X4	T47.1X5	T47.1X6
Malathion (medicinal)	T49.0X1	T49.0X2	T49.0X3	T49.0X4	T49.0X5	T49.0X6
insecticide	T60.0X1	T60.0X2	T60.0X3	T60.0X4	—	—
Male fern extract	T37.4X1	T37.4X2	T37.4X3	T37.4X4	T37.4X5	T37.4X6
M-AMSA	T45.1X1	T45.1X2	T45.1X3	T45.1X4	T45.1X5	T45.1X6
Mandelic acid	T37.8X1	T37.8X2	T37.8X3	T37.8X4	T37.8X5	T37.8X6
Manganese (dioxide) (salts)	T57.2X1	T57.2X2	T57.2X3	T57.2X4	—	—
medicinal	T50.991	T50.992	T50.993	T50.994	T50.995	T50.996
Mannitol	T47.3X1	T47.3X2	T47.3X3	T47.3X4	T47.3X5	T47.3X6
hexanitrate	T46.3X1	T46.3X2	T46.3X3	T46.3X4	T46.3X5	T46.3X6
Mannomustine	T45.1X1	T45.1X2	T45.1X3	T45.1X4	T45.1X5	T45.1X6
MAO inhibitors	T43.1X1	T43.1X2	T43.1X3	T43.1X4	T43.1X5	T43.1X6
Mapharsen	T37.8X1	T37.8X2	T37.8X3	T37.8X4	T37.8X5	T37.8X6
Maphenide	T49.0X1	T49.0X2	T49.0X3	T49.0X4	T49.0X5	T49.0X6
Maprotiline	T43.021	T43.022	T43.023	T43.024	T43.025	T43.026
Marcaine	T41.3X1	T41.3X2	T41.3X3	T41.3X4	T41.3X5	T41.3X6
infiltration (subcutaneous)	T41.3X1	T41.3X2	T41.3X3	T41.3X4	T41.3X5	T41.3X6
nerve block (peripheral) (plexus)	T41.3X1	T41.3X2	T41.3X3	T41.3X4	T41.3X5	T41.3X6
Marezine	T45.0X1	T45.0X2	T45.0X3	T45.0X4	T45.0X5	T45.0X6
Marihuana	T40.7X1	T40.7X2	T40.7X3	T40.7X4	T40.7X5	T40.7X6
Marijuana	T40.7X1	T40.7X2	T40.7X3	T40.7X4	T40.7X5	T40.7X6
Marine (sting)	T63.691	T63.692	T63.693	T63.694	—	—
animals (sting)	T63.691	T63.692	T63.693	T63.694	—	—
plants (sting)	T63.711	T63.712	T63.713	T63.714	—	—
Marplan	T43.1X1	T43.1X2	T43.1X3	T43.1X4	T43.1X5	T43.1X6
Marsh gas	T59.891	T59.892	T59.893	T59.894	—	—
Marsilid	T43.1X1	T43.1X2	T43.1X3	T43.1X4	T43.1X5	T43.1X6
Matulane	T45.1X1	T45.1X2	T45.1X3	T45.1X4	T45.1X5	T45.1X6
Mazindol	T50.5X1	T50.5X2	T50.5X3	T50.5X4	T50.5X5	T50.5X6
MCPA	T60.3X1	T60.3X2	T60.3X3	T60.3X4	—	—
MDMA	T43.621	T43.622	T43.623	T43.624	T43.625	T43.626
Meadow saffron	T62.2X1	T62.2X2	T62.2X3	T62.2X4	—	—
Measles virus vaccine (attenuated)	T50.B91	T50.B92	T50.B93	T50.B94	T50.B95	T50.B96
Meat, noxious	T62.8X1	T62.8X2	T62.8X3	T62.8X4	—	—
Meballymal	T42.3X1	T42.3X2	T42.3X3	T42.3X4	T42.3X5	T42.3X6
Mebanazine	T43.1X1	T43.1X2	T43.1X3	T43.1X4	T43.1X5	T43.1X6
Mebaral	T42.3X1	T42.3X2	T42.3X3	T42.3X4	T42.3X5	T42.3X6
Mebendazole	T37.4X1	T37.4X2	T37.4X3	T37.4X4	T37.4X5	T37.4X6
Mebeverine	T44.3X1	T44.3X2	T44.3X3	T44.3X4	T44.3X5	T44.3X6
Mebhydrolin	T45.0X1	T45.0X2	T45.0X3	T45.0X4	T45.0X5	T45.0X6
Mebumal	T42.3X1	T42.3X2	T42.3X3	T42.3X4	T42.3X5	T42.3X6
Mebutamate	T43.591	T43.592	T43.593	T43.594	T43.595	T43.596
Mecamylamine	T44.2X1	T44.2X2	T44.2X3	T44.2X4	T44.2X5	T44.2X6
Mechlorethamine	T45.1X1	T45.1X2	T45.1X3	T45.1X4	T45.1X5	T45.1X6
Mecillinam	T36.0X1	T36.0X2	T36.0X3	T36.0X4	T36.0X5	T36.0X6
Meclizine (hydrochloride)	T45.0X1	T45.0X2	T45.0X3	T45.0X4	T45.0X5	T45.0X6
Meclocycline	T36.4X1	T36.4X2	T36.4X3	T36.4X4	T36.4X5	T36.4X6
Meclofenamate	T39.391	T39.392	T39.393	T39.394	T39.395	T39.396
Meclofenamic acid	T39.391	T39.392	T39.393	T39.394	T39.395	T39.396
Meclofenoxate	T43.691	T43.692	T43.693	T43.694	T43.695	T43.696
Meclozine	T45.0X1	T45.0X2	T45.0X3	T45.0X4	T45.0X5	T45.0X6
Mecobalamin	T45.8X1	T45.8X2	T45.8X3	T45.8X4	T45.8X5	T45.8X6
Mecoprop	T60.3X1	T60.3X2	T60.3X3	T60.3X4	—	—
Mecrilate	T49.3X1	T49.3X2	T49.3X3	T49.3X4	T49.3X5	T49.3X6
Mecysteine	T48.4X1	T48.4X2	T48.4X3	T48.4X4	T48.4X5	T48.4X6
Medazepam	T42.4X1	T42.4X2	T42.4X3	T42.4X4	T42.4X5	T42.4X6
Medicament NEC	T50.901	T50.902	T50.903	T50.904	T50.905	T50.906
Medinal	T42.3X1	T42.3X2	T42.3X3	T42.3X4	T42.3X5	T42.3X6
Medomin	T42.3X1	T42.3X2	T42.3X3	T42.3X4	T42.3X5	T42.3X6
Medrogestone	T38.5X1	T38.5X2	T38.5X3	T38.5X4	T38.5X5	T38.5X6
Medroxalol	T44.8X1	T44.8X2	T44.8X3	T44.8X4	T44.8X5	T44.8X6
Medroxyprogesterone acetate (depot)	T38.5X1	T38.5X2	T38.5X3	T38.5X4	T38.5X5	T38.5X6
Medrysone	T49.0X1	T49.0X2	T49.0X3	T49.0X4	T49.0X5	T49.0X6
Mefenamic acid	T39.391	T39.392	T39.393	T39.394	T39.395	T39.396
Mefenorex	T50.5X1	T50.5X2	T50.5X3	T50.5X4	T50.5X5	T50.5X6
Mefloquine	T37.2X1	T37.2X2	T37.2X3	T37.2X4	T37.2X5	T37.2X6
Mefruside	T50.2X1	T50.2X2	T50.2X3	T50.2X4	T50.2X5	T50.2X6
Megahallucinogen	T40.901	T40.902	T40.903	T40.904	T40.905	T40.906
Megestrol	T38.5X1	T38.5X2	T38.5X3	T38.5X4	T38.5X5	T38.5X6
Meglumine						
antimoniate	T37.8X1	T37.8X2	T37.8X3	T37.8X4	T37.8X5	T37.8X6
diatrizoate	T50.8X1	T50.8X2	T50.8X3	T50.8X4	T50.8X5	T50.8X6
iodipamide	T50.8X1	T50.8X2	T50.8X3	T50.8X4	T50.8X5	T50.8X6
iotroxate	T50.8X1	T50.8X2	T50.8X3	T50.8X4	T50.8X5	T50.8X6
MEK (methyl ethyl ketone)	T52.4X1	T52.4X2	T52.4X3	T52.4X4	—	—
Meladinin	T49.3X1	T49.3X2	T49.3X3	T49.3X4	T49.3X5	T49.3X6
Meladrazine	T44.3X1	T44.3X2	T44.3X3	T44.3X4	T44.3X5	T44.3X6

Substance	Poisoning, Accidental (unintentional)	Poisoning, Intentional Self-harm	Poisoning, Assault	Poisoning, Undetermined	Adverse Effect	Under-dosing
Melaleuca alternifolia oil	T49.0X1	T49.0X2	T49.0X3	T49.0X4	T49.0X5	T49.0X6
Melanizing agents	T49.3X1	T49.3X2	T49.3X3	T49.3X4	T49.3X5	T49.3X6
Melanocyte-stimulating hormone	T38.891	T38.892	T38.893	T38.894	T38.895	T38.896
Melarsonyl potassium	T37.3X1	T37.3X2	T37.3X3	T37.3X4	T37.3X5	T37.3X6
Melarsoprol	T37.3X1	T37.3X2	T37.3X3	T37.3X4	T37.3X5	T37.3X6
Melia azedarach	T62.2X1	T62.2X2	T62.2X3	T62.2X4	—	—
Melitracen	T43.011	T43.012	T43.013	T43.014	T43.015	T43.016
Mellaril	T43.3X1	T43.3X2	T43.3X3	T43.3X4	T43.3X5	T43.3X6
Meloxine	T49.3X1	T49.3X2	T49.3X3	T49.3X4	T49.3X5	T49.3X6
Melperone	T43.4X1	T43.4X2	T43.4X3	T43.4X4	T43.4X5	T43.4X6
Melphalan	T45.1X1	T45.1X2	T45.1X3	T45.1X4	T45.1X5	T45.1X6
Memantine	T43.8X1	T43.8X2	T43.8X3	T43.8X4	T43.8X5	T43.8X6
Menadiol	T45.7X1	T45.7X2	T45.7X3	T45.7X4	T45.7X5	T45.7X6
sodium sulfate	T45.7X1	T45.7X2	T45.7X3	T45.7X4	T45.7X5	T45.7X6
Menadione	T45.7X1	T45.7X2	T45.7X3	T45.7X4	T45.7X5	T45.7X6
sodium bisulfite	T45.7X1	T45.7X2	T45.7X3	T45.7X4	T45.7X5	T45.7X6
Menaphthone	T45.7X1	T45.7X2	T45.7X3	T45.7X4	T45.7X5	T45.7X6
Menaquinone	T45.7X1	T45.7X2	T45.7X3	T45.7X4	T45.7X5	T45.7X6
Menatetrenone	T45.7X1	T45.7X2	T45.7X3	T45.7X4	T45.7X5	T45.7X6
Meningococcal vaccine	T50.A91	T50.A92	T50.A93	T50.A94	T50.A95	T50.A96
Menningovax (-AC) (-C)	T50.A91	T50.A92	T50.A93	T50.A94	T50.A95	T50.A96
Menotropins	T38.811	T38.812	T38.813	T38.814	T38.815	T38.816
Menthol	T48.5X1	T48.5X2	T48.5X3	T48.5X4	T48.5X5	T48.5X6
Mepacrine	T37.2X1	T37.2X2	T37.2X3	T37.2X4	T37.2X5	T37.2X6
Meparfynol	T42.6X1	T42.6X2	T42.6X3	T42.6X4	T42.6X5	T42.6X6
Mepartricin	T36.7X1	T36.7X2	T36.7X3	T36.7X4	T36.7X5	T36.7X6
Mepazine	T43.3X1	T43.3X2	T43.3X3	T43.3X4	T43.3X5	T43.3X6
Mepenzolate	T44.3X1	T44.3X2	T44.3X3	T44.3X4	T44.3X5	T44.3X6
bromide	T44.3X1	T44.3X2	T44.3X3	T44.3X4	T44.3X5	T44.3X6
Meperidine	T40.4X1	T40.4X2	T40.4X3	T40.4X4	T40.4X5	T40.4X6
Mephebarbital	T42.3X1	T42.3X2	T42.3X3	T42.3X4	T42.3X5	T42.3X6
Mephenamin (e)	T42.8X1	T42.8X2	T42.8X3	T42.8X4	T42.8X5	T42.8X6
Mephenesin	T42.8X1	T42.8X2	T42.8X3	T42.8X4	T42.8X5	T42.8X6
Mephenhydramine	T45.0X1	T45.0X2	T45.0X3	T45.0X4	T45.0X5	T45.0X6
Mephenoxalone	T42.8X1	T42.8X2	T42.8X3	T42.8X4	T42.8X5	T42.8X6
Mephentermine	T44.991	T44.992	T44.993	T44.994	T44.995	T44.996
Mephenytoin	T42.0X1	T42.0X2	T42.0X3	T42.0X4	T42.0X5	T42.0X6
with phenobarbital	T42.3X1	T42.3X2	T42.3X3	T42.3X4	T42.3X5	T42.3X6
Mephobarbital	T42.3X1	T42.3X2	T42.3X3	T42.3X4	T42.3X5	T42.3X6
Mephosfolan	T60.0X1	T60.0X2	T60.0X3	T60.0X4	—	—
Mepindolol	T44.7X1	T44.7X2	T44.7X3	T44.7X4	T44.7X5	T44.7X6
Mepiperphenidol	T44.3X1	T44.3X2	T44.3X3	T44.3X4	T44.3X5	T44.3X6
Mepitiostane	T38.7X1	T38.7X2	T38.7X3	T38.7X4	T38.7X5	T38.7X6
Mepivacaine	T41.3X1	T41.3X2	T41.3X3	T41.3X4	T41.3X5	T41.3X6
epidural	T41.3X1	T41.3X2	T41.3X3	T41.3X4	T41.3X5	T41.3X6
Meprednisone	T38.0X1	T38.0X2	T38.0X3	T38.0X4	T38.0X5	T38.0X6
Meprobam	T43.591	T43.592	T43.593	T43.594	T43.595	T43.596
Meprobamate	T43.591	T43.592	T43.593	T43.594	T43.595	T43.596
Meproscillarin	T46.0X1	T46.0X2	T46.0X3	T46.0X4	T46.0X5	T46.0X6
Meprylcalne	T41.3X1	T41.3X2	T41.3X3	T41.3X4	T41.3X5	T41.3X6
Meptazinol	T39.8X1	T39.8X2	T39.8X3	T39.8X4	T39.8X5	T39.8X6
Mepyramine	T45.0X1	T45.0X2	T45.0X3	T45.0X4	T45.0X5	T45.0X6
Mequitazine	T43.3X1	T43.3X2	T43.3X3	T43.3X4	T43.3X5	T43.3X6
Meralluride	T50.2X1	T50.2X2	T50.2X3	T50.2X4	T50.2X5	T50.2X6
Merbaphen	T50.2X1	T50.2X2	T50.2X3	T50.2X4	T50.2X5	T50.2X6
Merbromin	T49.0X1	T49.0X2	T49.0X3	T49.0X4	T49.0X5	T49.0X6
Mercaptobenzothiazole salts	T49.0X1	T49.0X2	T49.0X3	T49.0X4	T49.0X5	T49.0X6
Mercaptomerin	T50.2X1	T50.2X2	T50.2X3	T50.2X4	T50.2X5	T50.2X6
Mercaptopurine	T45.1X1	T45.1X2	T45.1X3	T45.1X4	T45.1X5	T45.1X6
Mercumatilin	T50.2X1	T50.2X2	T50.2X3	T50.2X4	T50.2X5	T50.2X6
Mercuramide	T50.2X1	T50.2X2	T50.2X3	T50.2X4	T50.2X5	T50.2X6
Mercurochrome	T49.0X1	T49.0X2	T49.0X3	T49.0X4	T49.0X5	T49.0X6
Mercurophylline	T50.2X1	T50.2X2	T50.2X3	T50.2X4	T50.2X5	T50.2X6
Mercury, mercurial, mercuric, mercurous (compounds)	T56.1X1	T56.1X2	T56.1X3	T56.1X4	—	—
(cyanide) (fumes)						
(nonmedicinal) (vapor)						
NEC						
ammoniated	T49.0X1	T49.0X2	T49.0X3	T49.0X4	T49.0X5	T49.0X6
anti-infective						
local	T49.0X1	T49.0X2	T49.0X3	T49.0X4	T49.0X5	T49.0X6
systemic	T37.8X1	T37.8X2	T37.8X3	T37.8X4	T37.8X5	T37.8X6
topical	T49.0X1	T49.0X2	T49.0X3	T49.0X4	T49.0X5	T49.0X6
chloride (ammoniated)	T49.0X1	T49.0X2	T49.0X3	T49.0X4	T49.0X5	T49.0X6
fungicide	T56.1X1	T56.1X2	T56.1X3	T56.1X4	—	—
diuretic NEC	T50.2X1	T50.2X2	T50.2X3	T50.2X4	T50.2X5	T50.2X6
fungicide	T56.1X1	T56.1X2	T56.1X3	T56.1X4	—	—
organic (fungicide)	T56.1X1	T56.1X2	T56.1X3	T56.1X4	—	—
oxide, yellow	T49.0X1	T49.0X2	T49.0X3	T49.0X4	T49.0X5	T49.0X6
Mersalyl	T50.2X1	T50.2X2	T50.2X3	T50.2X4	T50.2X5	T50.2X6
Merthiolate	T49.0X1	T49.0X2	T49.0X3	T49.0X4	T49.0X5	T49.0X6

Substance	Poisoning, Accidental (unintentional)	Poisoning, Intentional Self-harm	Poisoning, Assault	Poisoning, Undetermined	Adverse Effect	Under-dosing
Merthiolate — continued						
ophthalmic preparation	T49.5X1	T49.5X2	T49.5X3	T49.5X4	T49.5X5	T49.5X6
Meruvax	T50.B91	T50.B92	T50.B93	T50.B94	T50.B95	T50.B96
Mesalazine	T47.8X1	T47.8X2	T47.8X3	T47.8X4	T47.8X5	T47.8X6
Mescal buttons	T40.991	T40.992	T40.993	T40.994	—	—
Mescaline	T40.991	T40.992	T40.993	T40.994	—	—
Mesna	T48.4X1	T48.4X2	T48.4X3	T48.4X4	T48.4X5	T48.4X6
Mesoglycan	T46.6X1	T46.6X2	T46.6X3	T46.6X4	T46.6X5	T46.6X6
Mesoridazine	T43.3X1	T43.3X2	T43.3X3	T43.3X4	T43.3X5	T43.3X6
Mestanolone	T38.7X1	T38.7X2	T38.7X3	T38.7X4	T38.7X5	T38.7X6
Mesterolone	T38.7X1	T38.7X2	T38.7X3	T38.7X4	T38.7X5	T38.7X6
Mestranol	T38.5X1	T38.5X2	T38.5X3	T38.5X4	T38.5X5	T38.5X6
Mesulergine	T42.8X1	T42.8X2	T42.8X3	T42.8X4	T42.8X5	T42.8X6
Mesulfen	T49.0X1	T49.0X2	T49.0X3	T49.0X4	T49.0X5	T49.0X6
Mesuximide	T42.2X1	T42.2X2	T42.2X3	T42.2X4	T42.2X5	T42.2X6
Metabutethamine	T41.3X1	T41.3X2	T41.3X3	T41.3X4	T41.3X5	T41.3X6
Metactesylacetate	T49.0X1	T49.0X2	T49.0X3	T49.0X4	T49.0X5	T49.0X6
Metacycline	T36.4X1	T36.4X2	T36.4X3	T36.4X4	T36.4X5	T36.4X6
Metaldehyde (snail killer) NEC	T60.8X1	T60.8X2	T60.8X3	T60.8X4	—	—
Metals (heavy) (nonmedicinal)	T56.91	T56.92	T56.93	T56.94	—	—
dust, fumes, or vapor NEC	T56.91	T56.92	T56.93	T56.94	—	—
light NEC	T56.91	T56.92	T56.93	T56.94	—	—
dust, fumes, or vapor NEC	T56.91	T56.92	T56.93	T56.94	—	—
specified NEC	T56.891	T56.892	T56.893	T56.894	—	—
thallium	T56.811	T56.812	T56.813	T56.814	—	—
Metamfetamine	T43.621	T43.622	T43.623	T43.624	T43.625	T43.626
Metamizole sodium	T39.2X1	T39.2X2	T39.2X3	T39.2X4	T39.2X5	T39.2X6
Metampicillin	T36.0X1	T36.0X2	T36.0X3	T36.0X4	T36.0X5	T36.0X6
Metamucil	T47.4X1	T47.4X2	T47.4X3	T47.4X4	T47.4X5	T47.4X6
Metandienone	T38.7X1	T38.7X2	T38.7X3	T38.7X4	T38.7X5	T38.7X6
Metandrostenolone	T38.7X1	T38.7X2	T38.7X3	T38.7X4	T38.7X5	T38.7X6
Metaphen	T49.0X1	T49.0X2	T49.0X3	T49.0X4	T49.0X5	T49.0X6
Metaphos	T60.0X1	T60.0X2	T60.0X3	T60.0X4	—	—
Metapramine	T43.011	T43.012	T43.013	T43.014	T43.015	T43.016
Metaproterenol	T48.291	T48.292	T48.293	T48.294	T48.295	T48.296
Metaraminol	T44.4X1	T44.4X2	T44.4X3	T44.4X4	T44.4X5	T44.4X6
Metaxalone	T42.8X1	T42.8X2	T42.8X3	T42.8X4	T42.8X5	T42.8X6
Metenolone	T38.7X1	T38.7X2	T38.7X3	T38.7X4	T38.7X5	T38.7X6
Metergoline	T42.8X1	T42.8X2	T42.8X3	T42.8X4	T42.8X5	T42.8X6
Metescufylline	T46.991	T46.992	T46.993	T46.994	T46.995	T46.996
Metetoin	T42.0X1	T42.0X2	T42.0X3	T42.0X4	T42.0X5	T42.0X6
Metformin	T38.3X1	T38.3X2	T38.3X3	T38.3X4	T38.3X5	T38.3X6
Methacholine	T44.1X1	T44.1X2	T44.1X3	T44.1X4	T44.1X5	T44.1X6
Methacycline	T36.4X1	T36.4X2	T36.4X3	T36.4X4	T36.4X5	T36.4X6
Methadone	T40.3X1	T40.3X2	T40.3X3	T40.3X4	T40.3X5	T40.3X6
Methallenestril	T38.5X1	T38.5X2	T38.5X3	T38.5X4	T38.5X5	T38.5X6
Methallenoestril	T38.5X1	T38.5X2	T38.5X3	T38.5X4	T38.5X5	T38.5X6
Methamphetamine	T43.621	T43.622	T43.623	T43.624	T43.625	T43.626
Methampyrone	T39.2X1	T39.2X2	T39.2X3	T39.2X4	T39.2X5	T39.2X6
Methandienone	T38.7X1	T38.7X2	T38.7X3	T38.7X4	T38.7X5	T38.7X6
Methandriol	T38.7X1	T38.7X2	T38.7X3	T38.7X4	T38.7X5	T38.7X6
Methandrostenolone	T38.7X1	T38.7X2	T38.7X3	T38.7X4	T38.7X5	T38.7X6
Methane	T59.891	T59.892	T59.893	T59.894	—	—
Methanethiol	T59.891	T59.892	T59.893	T59.894	—	—
Methaniazide	T37.1X1	T37.1X2	T37.1X3	T37.1X4	T37.1X5	T37.1X6
Methanol (vapor)	T51.1X1	T51.1X2	T51.1X3	T51.1X4	—	—
Methantheline	T44.3X1	T44.3X2	T44.3X3	T44.3X4	T44.3X5	T44.3X6
Methanthelinium bromide	T44.3X1	T44.3X2	T44.3X3	T44.3X4	T44.3X5	T44.3X6
Methaphenilene	T45.0X1	T45.0X2	T45.0X3	T45.0X4	T45.0X5	T45.0X6
Methapyrilene	T45.0X1	T45.0X2	T45.0X3	T45.0X4	T45.0X5	T45.0X6
Methaqualone (compound)	T42.6X1	T42.6X2	T42.6X3	T42.6X4	T42.6X5	T42.6X6
Metharbital	T42.3X1	T42.3X2	T42.3X3	T42.3X4	T42.3X5	T42.3X6
Methazolamide	T50.2X1	T50.2X2	T50.2X3	T50.2X4	T50.2X5	T50.2X6
Methdilazine	T43.3X1	T43.3X2	T43.3X3	T43.3X4	T43.3X5	T43.3X6
Methedrine	T43.621	T43.622	T43.623	T43.624	T43.625	T43.626
Methenamine (mandelate)	T37.8X1	T37.8X2	T37.8X3	T37.8X4	T37.8X5	T37.8X6
Methenolone	T38.7X1	T38.7X2	T38.7X3	T38.7X4	T38.7X5	T38.7X6
Methergine	T48.0X1	T48.0X2	T48.0X3	T48.0X4	T48.0X5	T48.0X6
Methetoin	T42.0X1	T42.0X2	T42.0X3	T42.0X4	T42.0X5	T42.0X6
Methiacil	T38.2X1	T38.2X2	T38.2X3	T38.2X4	T38.2X5	T38.2X6
Methicillin	T36.0X1	T36.0X2	T36.0X3	T36.0X4	T36.0X5	T36.0X6
Methimazole	T38.2X1	T38.2X2	T38.2X3	T38.2X4	T38.2X5	T38.2X6
Methiodal sodium	T50.8X1	T50.8X2	T50.8X3	T50.8X4	T50.8X5	T50.8X6
Methionine	T50.991	T50.992	T50.993	T50.994	T50.995	T50.996
Methisazone	T37.5X1	T37.5X2	T37.5X3	T37.5X4	T37.5X5	T37.5X6
Methisoprinol	T37.5X1	T37.5X2	T37.5X3	T37.5X4	T37.5X5	T37.5X6
Methitural	T42.3X1	T42.3X2	T42.3X3	T42.3X4	T42.3X5	T42.3X6
Methixene	T44.3X1	T44.3X2	T44.3X3	T44.3X4	T44.3X5	T44.3X6
Methobarbital, methobarbitone	T42.3X1	T42.3X2	T42.3X3	T42.3X4	T42.3X5	T42.3X6
Methocarbamol	T42.8X1	T42.8X2	T42.8X3	T42.8X4	T42.8X5	T42.8X6

Substance	Poisoning, Accidental (unintentional)	Poisoning, Intentional Self-harm	Poisoning, Assault	Poisoning, Undetermined	Adverse Effect	Under-dosing
Methocarbamol — *continued*						
skeletal muscle relaxant	T48.1X1	T48.1X2	T48.1X3	T48.1X4	T48.1X5	T48.1X6
Methohexital	T41.1X1	T41.1X2	T41.1X3	T41.1X4	T41.1X5	T41.1X6
Methohexitone	T41.1X1	T41.1X2	T41.1X3	T41.1X4	T41.1X5	T41.1X6
Methoin	T42.0X1	T42.0X2	T42.0X3	T42.0X4	T42.0X5	T42.0X6
Methopholine	T39.8X1	T39.8X2	T39.8X3	T39.8X4	T39.8X5	T39.8X6
Methopromazine	T43.3X1	T43.3X2	T43.3X3	T43.3X4	T43.3X5	T43.3X6
Methorate	T48.3X1	T48.3X2	T48.3X3	T48.3X4	T48.3X5	T48.3X6
Methoserpidine	T46.5X1	T46.5X2	T46.5X3	T46.5X4	T46.5X5	T46.5X6
Methotrexate	T45.1X1	T45.1X2	T45.1X3	T45.1X4	T45.1X5	T45.1X6
Methotrimeprazine	T43.3X1	T43.3X2	T43.3X3	T43.3X4	T43.3X5	T43.3X6
Methoxa-Dome	T49.3X1	T49.3X2	T49.3X3	T49.3X4	T49.3X5	T49.3X6
Methoxamine	T44.4X1	T44.4X2	T44.4X3	T44.4X4	T44.4X5	T44.4X6
Methoxsalen	T50.991	T50.992	T50.993	T50.994	T50.995	T50.996
Methoxyaniline	T65.3X1	T65.3X2	T65.3X3	T65.3X4	—	—
Methoxybenzyl penicillin	T36.0X1	T36.0X2	T36.0X3	T36.0X4	T36.0X5	T36.0X6
Methoxychlor	T53.7X1	T53.7X2	T53.7X3	T53.7X4	—	—
Methoxy-DDT	T53.7X1	T53.7X2	T53.7X3	T53.7X4	—	—
Methoxyflurane	T41.0X1	T41.0X2	I41.0X3	T41.0X4	T41.0X5	T41.0X6
Methoxyphenamine	T48.6X1	T48.6X2	T48.6X3	T48.6X4	T48.6X5	T48.6X6
Methoxypromazine	T43.3X1	T43.3X2	T43.3X3	T43.3X4	T43.3X5	T43.3X6
Methscopolamine bromide	T44.3X1	T44.3X2	T44.3X3	T44.3X4	T44.3X5	T44.3X6
Methsuximide	T42.2X1	T42.2X2	T42.2X3	T42.2X4	T42.2X5	T42.2X6
Methyclothiazide	T50.2X1	T50.2X2	T50.2X3	T50.2X4	T50.2X5	T50.2X6
Methyl						
acetate	T52.4X1	T52.4X2	T52.4X3	T52.4X4	—	—
acetone	T52.4X1	T52.4X2	T52.4X3	T52.4X4	—	—
acrylate	T65.891	T65.892	T65.893	T65.894	—	—
alcohol	T51.1X1	T51.1X2	T51.1X3	T51.1X4	—	—
aminophenol	T65.3X1	T65.3X2	T65.3X3	T65.3X4	—	—
amphetamine	T43.621	T43.622	T43.623	T43.624	T43.625	T43.626
androstanolone	T38.7X1	T38.7X2	T38.7X3	T38.7X4	T38.7X5	T38.7X6
atropine	T44.3X1	T44.3X2	T44.3X3	T44.3X4	T44.3X5	T44.3X6
benzene	T52.2X1	T52.2X2	T52.2X3	T52.2X4	—	—
benzoate	T52.8X1	T52.8X2	T52.8X3	T52.8X4	—	—
benzol	T52.2X1	T52.2X2	T52.2X3	T52.2X4	—	—
bromide (gas)	T59.891	T59.892	T59.893	T59.894	—	—
fumigant	T60.8X1	T60.8X2	T60.8X3	T60.8X4	—	—
butanol	T51.3X1	T51.3X2	T51.3X3	T51.3X4	—	—
carbinol	T51.1X1	T51.1X2	T51.1X3	T51.1X4	—	—
carbonate	T52.8X1	T52.8X2	T52.8X3	T52.8X4	—	—
CCNU	T45.1X1	T45.1X2	T45.1X3	T45.1X4	T45.1X5	T45.1X6
cellosolve	T52.91	T52.92	T52.93	T52.94	—	—
cellulose	T47.4X1	T47.4X2	T47.4X3	T47.4X4	T47.4X5	T47.4X6
chloride (gas)	T59.891	T59.892	T59.893	T59.894	—	—
chloroformate	T59.3X1	T59.3X2	T59.3X3	T59.3X4	—	—
cyclohexane	T52.8X1	T52.8X2	T52.8X3	T52.8X4	—	—
cyclohexanol	T51.8X1	T51.8X2	T51.8X3	T51.8X4	—	—
cyclohexanone	T52.8X1	T52.8X2	T52.8X3	T52.8X4	—	—
cyclohexyl acetate	T52.8X1	T52.8X2	T52.8X3	T52.8X4	—	—
demeton	T60.0X1	T60.0X2	T60.0X3	T60.0X4	—	—
dihydromorphinone	T40.2X1	T40.2X2	T40.2X3	T40.2X4	T40.2X5	T40.2X6
ergometrine	T48.0X1	T48.0X2	T48.0X3	T48.0X4	T48.0X5	T48.0X6
ergonovine	T48.0X1	T48.0X2	T48.0X3	T48.0X4	T48.0X5	T48.0X6
ethyl ketone	T52.4X1	T52.4X2	T52.4X3	T52.4X4	—	—
glucamine antimonate	T37.8X1	T37.8X2	T37.8X3	T37.8X4	T37.8X5	T37.8X6
hydrazine	T65.891	T65.892	T65.893	T65.894	—	—
iodide	T65.891	T65.892	T65.893	T65.894	—	—
isobutyl ketone	T52.4X1	T52.4X2	T52.4X3	T52.4X4	—	—
isothiocyanate	T60.3X1	T60.3X2	T60.3X3	T60.3X4	—	—
mercaptan	T59.891	T59.892	T59.893	T59.894	—	—
morphine NEC	T40.2X1	T40.2X2	T40.2X3	T40.2X4	T40.2X5	T40.2X6
nicotinate	T49.4X1	T49.4X2	T49.4X3	T49.4X4	T49.4X5	T49.4X6
paraben	T49.0X1	T49.0X2	T49.0X3	T49.0X4	T49.0X5	T49.0X6
parafynol	T42.6X1	T42.6X2	T42.6X3	T42.6X4	T42.6X5	T42.6X6
parathion	T60.0X1	T60.0X2	T60.0X3	T60.0X4	—	—
peridol	T43.4X1	T43.4X2	T43.4X3	T43.4X4	T43.4X5	T43.4X6
phenidate	T43.631	T43.632	T43.633	T43.634	T43.635	T43.636
prednisolone	T38.0X1	T38.0X2	T38.0X3	T38.0X4	T38.0X5	T38.0X6
ENT agent	T49.6X1	T49.6X2	T49.6X3	T49.6X4	T49.6X5	T49.6X6
ophthalmic preparation	T49.5X1	T49.5X2	T49.5X3	T49.5X4	T49.5X5	T49.5X6
topical NEC	T49.0X1	T49.0X2	T49.0X3	T49.0X4	T49.0X5	T49.0X6
propylcarbinol	T51.3X1	T51.3X2	T51.3X3	T51.3X4	—	—
rosaniline NEC	T49.0X1	T49.0X2	T49.0X3	T49.0X4	T49.0X5	T49.0X6
salicylate	T49.2X1	T49.2X2	T49.2X3	T49.2X4	T49.2X5	T49.2X6
sulfate (fumes)	T59.891	T59.892	T59.893	T59.894	—	—
liquid	T52.8X1	T52.8X2	T52.8X3	T52.8X4	—	—
sulfonal	T42.6X1	T42.6X2	T42.6X3	T42.6X4	T42.6X5	T42.6X6
testosterone	T38.7X1	T38.7X2	T38.7X3	T38.7X4	T38.7X5	T38.7X6
thiouracil	T38.2X1	T38.2X2	T38.2X3	T38.2X4	T38.2X5	T38.2X6
Methylamphetamine	T43.621	T43.622	T43.623	T43.624	T43.625	T43.626
Methylated spirit	T51.1X1	T51.1X2	T51.1X3	T51.1X4	—	—
Methylatropine nitrate	T44.3X1	T44.3X2	T44.3X3	T44.3X4	T44.3X5	T44.3X6

Substance	Poisoning, Accidental (unintentional)	Poisoning, Intentional Self-harm	Poisoning, Assault	Poisoning, Undetermined	Adverse Effect	Under-dosing
Methylbenactyzium bromide	T44.3X1	T44.3X2	T44.3X3	T44.3X4	T44.3X5	T44.3X6
Methylbenzethonium chloride	T49.0X1	T49.0X2	T49.0X3	T49.0X4	T49.0X5	T49.0X6
Methylcellulose	T47.4X1	T47.4X2	T47.4X3	T47.4X4	T47.4X5	T47.4X6
laxative	T47.4X1	T47.4X2	T47.4X3	T47.4X4	T47.4X5	T47.4X6
Methylchlorophenoxyacetic acid	T60.3X1	T60.3X2	T60.3X3	T60.3X4	—	—
Methyldopa	T46.5X1	T46.5X2	T46.5X3	T46.5X4	T46.5X5	T46.5X6
Methyldopate	T46.5X1	T46.5X2	T46.5X3	T46.5X4	T46.5X5	T46.5X6
Methylene						
blue	T50.6X1	T50.6X2	T50.6X3	T50.6X4	T50.6X5	T50.6X6
chloride or dichloride (solvent) NEC	T53.4X1	T53.4X2	T53.4X3	T53.4X4	—	—
Methylenedioxyamphetamine	T43.621	T43.622	T43.623	T43.624	T43.625	T43.626
Methylenedioxymethamphetamine	T43.621	T43.622	T43.623	T43.624	T43.625	T43.626
Methylergometrine	T48.0X1	T48.0X2	T48.0X3	T48.0X4	T48.0X5	T48.0X6
Methylergonovine	T48.0X1	T48.0X2	T48.0X3	T48.0X4	T48.0X5	T48.0X6
Methylestrenolone	T38.5X1	T38.5X2	T38.5X3	T38.5X4	T38.5X5	T38.5X6
Methylethyl cellulose	T50.991	T50.992	T50.993	T50.994	T50.995	T50.996
Methylhexabital	T42.3X1	T42.3X2	T42.3X3	T42.3X4	T42.3X5	T42.3X6
Methylmorphine	T40.2X1	T40.2X2	T40.2X3	T40.2X4	T40.2X5	T40.2X6
Methylparaben (ophthalmic)	T49.5X1	T49.5X2	T49.5X3	T49.5X4	T49.5X5	T49.5X6
Methylparafynol	T42.6X1	T42.6X2	T42.6X3	T42.6X4	T42.6X5	T42.6X6
Methylpentynol, methylpenthynol	T42.6X1	T42.6X2	T42.6X3	T42.6X4	T42.6X5	T42.6X6
Methylphenidate	T43.631	T43.632	T43.633	T43.634	T43.635	T43.636
Methylphenobarbital	T42.3X1	T42.3X2	T42.3X3	T42.3X4	T42.3X5	T42.3X6
Methylpolysiloxane	T47.1X1	T47.1X2	T47.1X3	T47.1X4	T47.1X5	T47.1X6
Methylprednisolone — *see* Methyl, prednisolone						
Methylrosaniline	T49.0X1	T49.0X2	T49.0X3	T49.0X4	T49.0X5	T49.0X6
Methylrosanilinium chloride	T49.0X1	T49.0X2	T49.0X3	T49.0X4	T49.0X5	T49.0X6
Methyltestosterone	T38.7X1	T38.7X2	T38.7X3	T38.7X4	T38.7X5	T38.7X6
Methylthionine chloride	T50.6X1	T50.6X2	T50.6X3	T50.6X4	T50.6X5	T50.6X6
Methylthioninium chloride	T50.6X1	T50.6X2	T50.6X3	T50.6X4	T50.6X5	T50.6X6
Methylthiouracil	T38.2X1	T38.2X2	T38.2X3	T38.2X4	T38.2X5	T38.2X6
Methyprylon	T42.6X1	T42.6X2	T42.6X3	T42.6X4	T42.6X5	T42.6X6
Methysergide	T46.5X1	T46.5X2	T46.5X3	T46.5X4	T46.5X5	T46.5X6
Metiamide	T47.1X1	T47.1X2	T47.1X3	T47.1X4	T47.1X5	T47.1X6
Meticillin	T36.0X1	T36.0X2	T36.0X3	T36.0X4	T36.0X5	T36.0X6
Meticrane	T50.2X1	T50.2X2	T50.2X3	T50.2X4	T50.2X5	T50.2X6
Metildigoxin	T46.0X1	T46.0X2	T46.0X3	T46.0X4	T46.0X5	T46.0X6
Metipranolol	T49.5X1	T49.5X2	T49.5X3	T49.5X4	T49.5X5	T49.5X6
Metirosine	T46.5X1	T46.5X2	T46.5X3	T46.5X4	T46.5X5	T46.5X6
Metisazone	T37.5X1	T37.5X2	T37.5X3	T37.5X4	T37.5X5	T37.5X6
Metixene	T44.3X1	T44.3X2	T44.3X3	T44.3X4	T44.3X5	T44.3X6
Metizoline	T48.5X1	T48.5X2	T48.5X3	T48.5X4	T48.5X5	T48.5X6
Metoclopramide	T45.0X1	T45.0X2	T45.0X3	T45.0X4	T45.0X5	T45.0X6
Metofenazate	T43.3X1	T43.3X2	T43.3X3	T43.3X4	T43.3X5	T43.3X6
Metofoline	T39.8X1	T39.8X2	T39.8X3	T39.8X4	T39.8X5	T39.8X6
Metolazone	T50.2X1	T50.2X2	T50.2X3	T50.2X4	T50.2X5	T50.2X6
Metopon	T40.2X1	T40.2X2	T40.2X3	T40.2X4	T40.2X5	T40.2X6
Metoprine	T45.1X1	T45.1X2	T45.1X3	T45.1X4	T45.1X5	T45.1X6
Metoprolol	T44.7X1	T44.7X2	T44.7X3	T44.7X4	T44.7X5	T44.7X6
Metrifonate	T60.0X1	T60.0X2	T60.0X3	T60.0X4	—	—
Metrizamide	T50.8X1	T50.8X2	T50.8X3	T50.8X4	—	T50.8X6
Metrizoic acid	T50.8X1	T50.8X2	T50.8X3	T50.8X4	T50.8X5	T50.8X6
Metronidazole	T37.8X1	T37.8X2	T37.8X3	T37.8X4	T37.8X5	T37.8X6
Metycaine	T41.3X1	T41.3X2	T41.3X3	T41.3X4	T41.3X5	T41.3X6
infiltration (subcutaneous)	T41.3X1	T41.3X2	T41.3X3	T41.3X4	T41.3X5	T41.3X6
nerve block (peripheral) (plexus)	T41.3X1	T41.3X2	T41.3X3	T41.3X4	T41.3X5	T41.3X6
topical (surface)	T41.3X1	T41.3X2	T41.3X3	T41.3X4	T41.3X5	T41.3X6
Metyrapone	T50.8X1	T50.8X2	T50.8X3	T50.8X4	T50.8X5	T50.8X6
Mevinphos	T60.0X1	T60.0X2	T60.0X3	T60.0X4	—	—
Mexazolam	T42.4X1	T42.4X2	T42.4X3	T42.4X4	T42.4X5	T42.4X6
Mexenone	T49.3X1	T49.3X2	T49.3X3	T49.3X4	T49.3X5	T49.3X6
Mexiletine	T46.2X1	T46.2X2	T46.2X3	T46.2X4	T46.2X5	T46.2X6
Mezereon	T62.2X1	T62.2X2	T62.2X3	T62.2X4	—	—
berries	T62.1X1	T62.1X2	T62.1X3	T62.1X4	—	—
Mezlocillin	T36.0X1	T36.0X2	T36.0X3	T36.0X4	T36.0X5	T36.0X6
Mianserin	T43.021	T43.022	T43.023	T43.024	T43.025	T43.026
Micatin	T49.0X1	T49.0X2	T49.0X3	T49.0X4	T49.0X5	T49.0X6
Miconazole	T49.0X1	T49.0X2	T49.0X3	T49.0X4	T49.0X5	T49.0X6
Micronomicin	T36.5X1	T36.5X2	T36.5X3	T36.5X4	T36.5X5	T36.5X6
Midazolam	T42.4X1	T42.4X2	T42.4X3	T42.4X4	T42.4X5	T42.4X6
Midecamycin	T36.3X1	T36.3X2	T36.3X3	T36.3X4	T36.3X5	T36.3X6
Mifepristone	T38.6X1	T38.6X2	T38.6X3	T38.6X4	T38.6X5	T38.6X6
Milk of magnesia	T47.1X1	T47.1X2	T47.1X3	T47.1X4	T47.1X5	T47.1X6

Additional Character May Be Required — Refer to the Tabular List for Character Selection ▽ Subterms under main terms may continue to next column or page

Substance	Poisoning, Accidental (unintentional)	Poisoning, Intentional Self-harm	Poisoning, Assault	Poisoning, Undetermined	Adverse Effect	Under-dosing
Millipede (tropical)	T63.411	T63.412	T63.413	T63.414	—	—
(venomous)						
Miltown	T43.591	T43.592	T43.593	T43.594	T43.595	T43.596
Milverine	T44.3X1	T44.3X2	T44.3X3	T44.3X4	T44.3X5	T44.3X6
Minaprine	T43.291	T43.292	T43.293	T43.294	T43.295	T43.296
Minaxolone	T41.291	T41.292	T41.293	T41.294	T41.295	T41.296
Mineral						
acids	T54.2X1	T54.2X2	T54.2X3	T54.2X4	—	—
oil (laxative)(medicinal)	T47.4X1	T47.4X2	T47.4X3	T47.4X4	T47.4X5	T47.4X6
emulsion	T47.2X1	T47.2X2	T47.2X3	T47.2X4	T47.2X5	T47.2X6
nonmedicinal	T52.0X1	T52.0X2	T52.0X3	T52.0X4	—	—
topical	T49.3X1	T49.3X2	T49.3X3	T49.3X4	T49.3X5	T49.3X6
salt NEC	T50.3X1	T50.3X2	T50.3X3	T50.3X4	T50.3X5	T50.3X6
spirits	T52.0X1	T52.0X2	T52.0X3	T52.0X4	—	—
Mineralocorticosteroid	T50.0X1	T50.0X2	T50.0X3	T50.0X4	T50.0X5	T50.0X6
Minocycline	T36.4X1	T36.4X2	T36.4X3	T36.4X4	T36.4X5	T36.4X6
Minoxidil	T46.7X1	T46.7X2	T46.7X3	T46.7X4	T46.7X5	T46.7X6
Miokamycin	T36.3X1	T36.3X2	T36.3X3	T36.3X4	T36.3X5	T36.3X6
Miotic drug	T49.5X1	T49.5X2	T49.5X3	T49.5X4	T49.5X5	T49.5X6
Mipafox	T60.0X1	T60.0X2	T60.0X3	T60.0X4	—	—
Mirex	T60.1X1	T60.1X2	T60.1X3	T60.1X4	—	—
Mirtazapine	T43.021	T43.022	T43.023	T43.024	T43.025	T43.026
Misonidazole	T37.3X1	T37.3X2	T37.3X3	T37.3X4	T37.3X5	T37.3X6
Misoprostol	T47.1X1	T47.1X2	T47.1X3	T47.1X4	T47.1X5	T47.1X6
Mithramycin	T45.1X1	T45.1X2	T45.1X3	T45.1X4	T45.1X5	T45.1X6
Mitobronitol	T45.1X1	T45.1X2	T45.1X3	T45.1X4	T45.1X5	T45.1X6
Mitoguazone	T45.1X1	T45.1X2	T45.1X3	T45.1X4	T45.1X5	T45.1X6
Mitolactol	T45.1X1	T45.1X2	T45.1X3	T45.1X4	T45.1X5	T45.1X6
Mitomycin	T45.1X1	T45.1X2	T45.1X3	T45.1X4	T45.1X5	T45.1X6
Mitopodozide	T45.1X1	T45.1X2	T45.1X3	T45.1X4	T45.1X5	T45.1X6
Mitotane	T45.1X1	T45.1X2	T45.1X3	T45.1X4	T45.1X5	T45.1X6
Mitoxantrone	T45.1X1	T45.1X2	T45.1X3	T45.1X4	T45.1X5	T45.1X6
Mivacurium chloride	T48.1X1	T48.1X2	T48.1X3	T48.1X4	T48.1X5	T48.1X6
Miyari bacteria	T47.6X1	T47.6X2	T47.6X3	T47.6X4	T47.6X5	T47.6X6
Moclobemide	T43.1X1	T43.1X2	T43.1X3	T43.1X4	T43.1X5	T43.1X6
Moderil	T46.5X1	T46.5X2	T46.5X3	T46.5X4	T46.5X5	T46.5X6
Mofebutazone	T39.2X1	T39.2X2	T39.2X3	T39.2X4	T39.2X5	T39.2X6
Mogadon — see Nitrazepam						
Molindone	T43.591	T43.592	T43.593	T43.594	T43.595	T43.596
Molsidomine	T46.3X1	T46.3X2	T46.3X3	T46.3X4	T46.3X5	T46.3X6
Mometasone	T49.0X1	T49.0X2	T49.0X3	T49.0X4	T49.0X5	T49.0X6
Monistat	T49.0X1	T49.0X2	T49.0X3	T49.0X4	T49.0X5	T49.0X6
Monkshood	T62.2X1	T62.2X2	T62.2X3	T62.2X4	—	—
Monoamine oxidase inhibitor NEC	T43.1X1	T43.1X2	T43.1X3	T43.1X4	T43.1X5	T43.1X6
hydrazine	T43.1X1	T43.1X2	T43.1X3	T43.1X4	T43.1X5	T43.1X6
Monobenzone	T49.4X1	T49.4X2	T49.4X3	T49.4X4	T49.4X5	T49.4X6
Monochloroacetic acid	T60.3X1	T60.3X2	T60.3X3	T60.3X4	—	—
Monochlorobenzene	T53.7X1	T53.7X2	T53.7X3	T53.7X4	—	—
Monoethanolamine	T46.8X1	T46.8X2	T46.8X3	T46.8X4	T46.8X5	T46.8X6
oleate	T46.8X1	T46.8X2	T46.8X3	T46.8X4	T46.8X5	T46.8X6
Monooctanoin	T50.991	T50.992	T50.993	T50.994	T50.995	T50.996
Monophenylbutazone	T39.2X1	T39.2X2	T39.2X3	T39.2X4	T39.2X5	T39.2X6
Monosodium glutamate	T65.891	T65.892	T65.893	T65.894	—	—
Monosulfiram	T49.0X1	T49.0X2	T49.0X3	T49.0X4	T49.0X5	T49.0X6
Monoxide, carbon — see Carbon,						
monoxide						
Monoxidine hydrochloride	T46.1X1	T46.1X2	T46.1X3	T46.1X4	T46.1X5	T46.1X6
Monuron	T60.3X1	T60.3X2	T60.3X3	T60.3X4	—	—
Moperone	T43.4X1	T43.4X2	T43.4X3	T43.4X4	T43.4X5	T43.4X6
Mopidamol	T45.1X1	T45.1X2	T45.1X3	T45.1X4	T45.1X5	T45.1X6
MOPP (mechloreth-amine + vincristine + prednisone + procarba-zine)	T45.1X1	T45.1X2	T45.1X3	T45.1X4	T45.1X5	T45.1X6
Morfin	T40.2X1	T40.2X2	T40.2X3	T40.2X4	T40.2X5	T40.2X6
Morinamide	T37.1X1	T37.1X2	T37.1X3	T37.1X4	T37.1X5	T37.1X6
Morning glory seeds	T40.991	T40.992	T40.993	T40.994	—	—
Moroxydine	T37.5X1	T37.5X2	T37.5X3	T37.5X4	T37.5X5	T37.5X6
Morphazinamide	T37.1X1	T37.1X2	T37.1X3	T37.1X4	T37.1X5	T37.1X6
Morphine	T40.2X1	T40.2X2	T40.2X3	T40.2X4	T40.2X5	T40.2X6
antagonist	T50.7X1	T50.7X2	T50.7X3	T50.7X4	T50.7X5	T50.7X6
Morpholinylethylmorphine	T40.2X1	T40.2X2	T40.2X3	T40.2X4	—	—
Morsuximide	T42.2X1	T42.2X2	T42.2X3	T42.2X4	T42.2X5	T42.2X6
Mosapramine	T43.591	T43.592	T43.593	T43.594	T43.595	T43.596
Moth balls — see also Pesticides	T60.2X1	T60.2X2	T60.2X3	T60.2X4	—	—
naphthalene	T60.2X1	T60.2X2	T60.2X3	T60.2X4	—	—
paradichlorobenzene	T60.1X1	T60.1X2	T60.1X3	T60.1X4	—	—
Motor exhaust gas	T58.01	T58.02	T58.03	T58.04		
Mouthwash (antiseptic) (zinc chloride)	T49.6X1	T49.6X2	T49.6X3	T49.6X4	T49.6X5	T49.6X6
Moxastine	T45.0X1	T45.0X2	T45.0X3	T45.0X4	T45.0X5	T45.0X6
Moxaverine	T44.3X1	T44.3X2	T44.3X3	T44.3X4	T44.3X5	T44.3X6
Moxisylyte	T46.7X1	T46.7X2	T46.7X3	T46.7X4	T46.7X5	T46.7X6
Mucilage, plant	T47.4X1	T47.4X2	T47.4X3	T47.4X4	T47.4X5	T47.4X6
Mucolytic drug	T48.4X1	T48.4X2	T48.4X3	T48.4X4	T48.4X5	T48.4X6
Mucomyst	T48.4X1	T48.4X2	T48.4X3	T48.4X4	T48.4X5	T48.4X6
Mucous membrane agents (external)	T49.91	T49.92	T49.93	T49.94	T49.95	T49.96
specified NEC	T49.8X1	T49.8X2	T49.8X3	T49.8X4	T49.8X5	T49.8X6
Mumps						
immune globulin (human)	T50.Z11	T50.Z12	T50.Z13	T50.Z14	T50.Z15	T50.Z16
skin test antigen	T50.8X1	T50.8X2	T50.8X3	T50.8X4	T50.8X5	T50.8X6
vaccine	T50.B91	T50.B92	T50.B93	T50.B94	T50.B95	T50.B96
Mumpsvax	T50.B91	T50.B92	T50.B93	T50.B94	T50.B95	T50.B96
Mupirocin	T49.0X1	T49.0X2	T49.0X3	T49.0X4	T49.0X5	T49.0X6
Muriatic acid — see Hydrochloric acid						
Muromonab-CD3	T45.1X1	T45.1X2	T45.1X3	T45.1X4	T45.1X5	T45.1X6
Muscle-action drug NEC	T48.201	T48.202	T48.203	T48.204	T48.205	T48.206
Muscle affecting agents NEC	T48.201	T48.202	T48.203	T48.204	T48.205	T48.206
oxytocic	T48.0X1	T48.0X2	T48.0X3	T48.0X4	T48.0X5	T48.0X6
relaxants	T48.201	T48.202	T48.203	T48.204	T48.205	T48.206
central nervous system	T42.8X1	T42.8X2	T42.8X3	T42.8X4	T42.8X5	T42.8X6
skeletal	T48.1X1	T48.1X2	T48.1X3	T48.1X4	T48.1X5	T48.1X6
smooth	T44.3X1	T44.3X2	T44.3X3	T44.3X4	T44.3X5	T44.3X6
Muscle relaxant — see Relaxant, muscle						
Muscle-tone depressant, central NEC	T42.8X1	T42.8X2	T42.8X3	T42.8X4	T42.8X5	T42.8X6
specified NEC	T42.8X1	T42.8X2	T42.8X3	T42.8X4	T42.8X5	T42.8X6
Mushroom, noxious	T62.0X1	T62.0X2	T62.0X3	T62.0X4	—	—
Mussel, noxious	T61.781	T61.782	T61.783	T61.784	—	—
Mustard (emetic)	T47.7X1	T47.7X2	T47.7X3	T47.7X4	T47.7X5	T47.7X6
black	T47.7X1	T47.7X2	T47.7X3	T47.7X4	T47.7X5	T47.7X6
gas, not in war	T59.91	T59.92	T59.93	T59.94		
nitrogen	T45.1X1	T45.1X2	T45.1X3	T45.1X4	T45.1X5	T45.1X6
Mustine	T45.1X1	T45.1X2	T45.1X3	T45.1X4	T45.1X5	T45.1X6
M-vac	T45.1X1	T45.1X2	T45.1X3	T45.1X4	T45.1X5	T45.1X6
Mycifradin	T36.5X1	T36.5X2	T36.5X3	T36.5X4	T36.5X5	T36.5X6
topical	T49.0X1	T49.0X2	T49.0X3	T49.0X4	T49.0X5	T49.0X6
Mycitracin	T36.8X1	T36.8X2	T36.8X3	T36.8X4	T36.8X5	T36.8X6
ophthalmic preparation	T49.5X1	T49.5X2	T49.5X3	T49.5X4	T49.5X5	T49.5X6
Mycostatin	T36.7X1	T36.7X2	T36.7X3	T36.7X4	T36.7X5	T36.7X6
topical	T49.0X1	T49.0X2	T49.0X3	T49.0X4	T49.0X5	T49.0X6
Mycotoxins	T64.81	T64.82	T64.83	T64.84	—	—
aflatoxin	T64.01	T64.02	T64.03	T64.04	—	—
specified NEC	T64.81	T64.82	T64.83	T64.84	—	—
Mydriacyl	T44.3X1	T44.3X2	T44.3X3	T44.3X4	T44.3X5	T44.3X6
Mydriatic drug	T49.5X1	T49.5X2	T49.5X3	T49.5X4	T49.5X5	T49.5X6
Myelobromal	T45.1X1	T45.1X2	T45.1X3	T45.1X4	T45.1X5	T45.1X6
Myleran	T45.1X1	T45.1X2	T45.1X3	T45.1X4	T45.1X5	T45.1X6
Myochrysin (e)	T39.2X1	T39.2X2	T39.2X3	T39.2X4	T39.2X5	T39.2X6
Myoneural blocking agents	T48.1X1	T48.1X2	T48.1X3	T48.1X4	T48.1X5	T48.1X6
Myralact	T49.0X1	T49.0X2	T49.0X3	T49.0X4	T49.0X5	T49.0X6
Myristica fragrans	T62.2X1	T62.2X2	T62.2X3	T62.2X4	—	—
Myristicin	T65.891	T65.892	T65.893	T65.894	—	—
Mysoline	T42.3X1	T42.3X2	T42.3X3	T42.3X4	T42.3X5	T42.3X6
Nabilone	T40.7X1	T40.7X2	T40.7X3	T40.7X4	T40.7X5	T40.7X6
Nabumetone	T39.391	T39.392	T39.393	T39.394	T39.395	T39.396
Nadolol	T44.7X1	T44.7X2	T44.7X3	T44.7X4	T44.7X5	T44.7X6
Nafcillin	T36.0X1	T36.0X2	T36.0X3	T36.0X4	T36.0X5	T36.0X6
Nafoxidine	T38.6X1	T38.6X2	T38.6X3	T38.6X4	T38.6X5	T38.6X6
Naftazone	T46.991	T46.992	T46.993	T46.994	T46.995	T46.996
Naftidrofuryl (oxalate)	T46.7X1	T46.7X2	T46.7X3	T46.7X4	T46.7X5	T46.7X6
Naftifine	T49.0X1	T49.0X2	T49.0X3	T49.0X4	T49.0X5	T49.0X6
Nail polish remover	T52.91	T52.92	T52.93	T52.94		
Nalbuphine	T40.4X1	T40.4X2	T40.4X3	T40.4X4	T40.4X5	T40.4X6
Naled	T60.0X1	T60.0X2	T60.0X3	T60.0X4	—	—
Nalidixic acid	T37.8X1	T37.8X2	T37.8X3	T37.8X4	T37.8X5	T37.8X6
Nalorphine	T50.7X1	T50.7X2	T50.7X3	T50.7X4	T50.7X5	T50.7X6
Naloxone	T50.7X1	T50.7X2	T50.7X3	T50.7X4	T50.7X5	T50.7X6
Naltrexone	T50.7X1	T50.7X2	T50.7X3	T50.7X4	T50.7X5	T50.7X6
Namenda	T43.8X1	T43.8X2	T43.8X3	T43.8X4	T43.8X5	T43.8X6
Nandrolone	T38.7X1	T38.7X2	T38.7X3	T38.7X4	T38.7X5	T38.7X6
Naphazoline	T48.5X1	T48.5X2	T48.5X3	T48.5X4	T48.5X5	T48.5X6
Naphtha (painters') (petroleum)	T52.0X1	T52.0X2	T52.0X3	T52.0X4	—	—
solvent	T52.0X1	T52.0X2	T52.0X3	T52.0X4	—	—
vapor	T52.0X1	T52.0X2	T52.0X3	T52.0X4	—	—
Naphthalene (non-chlorinated)	T60.2X1	T60.2X2	T60.2X3	T60.2X4	—	—
chlorinated	T60.1X1	T60.1X2	T60.1X3	T60.1X4	—	—
vapor	T60.1X1	T60.1X2	T60.1X3	T60.1X4	—	—

▽ Subterms under main terms may continue to next column or page   Additional Character May Be Required — Refer to the Tabular List for Character Selection   379

Millipede — Naphthalene

Substance	Poisoning, Accidental (unintentional)	Poisoning, Intentional Self-harm	Poisoning, Assault	Poisoning, Undetermined	Adverse Effect	Under-dosing
Naphthalene — *continued*						
insecticide or moth repellent	T60.2X1	T60.2X2	T60.2X3	T60.2X4	—	—
chlorinated	T60.1X1	T60.1X2	T60.1X3	T60.1X4	—	—
vapor	T60.2X1	T60.2X2	T60.2X3	T60.2X4	—	—
chlorinated	T60.1X1	T60.1X2	T60.1X3	T60.1X4	—	—
Naphthol	T65.891	T65.892	T65.893	T65.894	—	—
Naphthylamine	T65.891	T65.892	T65.893	T65.894	—	—
Naphthylthiourea (ANTU)	T60.4X1	T60.4X2	T60.4X3	T60.4X4	—	—
Naprosyn — *see* Naproxen						
Naproxen	T39.311	T39.312	T39.313	T39.314	T39.315	T39.316
Narcotic (drug)	T40.601	T40.602	T40.603	T40.604	T40.605	T40.606
analgesic NEC	T40.601	T40.602	T40.603	T40.604	T40.605	T40.606
antagonist	T50.7X1	T50.7X2	T50.7X3	T50.7X4	T50.7X5	T50.7X6
specified NEC	T40.691	T40.692	T40.693	T40.694	T40.695	T40.696
synthetic	T40.4X1	T40.4X2	T40.4X3	T40.4X4	T40.4X5	T40.4X6
Narcotine	T48.3X1	T48.3X2	T48.3X3	T48.3X4	T48.3X5	T48.3X6
Nardil	T43.1X1	T43.1X2	T43.1X3	T43.1X4	T43.1X5	T43.1X6
Nasal drug NEC	T49.6X1	T49.6X2	T49.6X3	T49.6X4	T49.6X5	T49.6X6
Natamycin	T49.0X1	T49.0X2	T49.0X3	T49.0X4	T49.0X5	T49.0X6
Natrium cyanide — *see* Cyanide(s)						
Natural						
blood (product)	T45.8X1	T45.8X2	T45.8X3	T45.8X4	T45.8X5	T45.8X6
gas (piped)	T59.891	T59.892	T59.893	T59.894	—	—
incomplete combustion	T58.11	T58.12	T58.13	T58.14	—	—
Nealbarbital	T42.3X1	T42.3X2	T42.3X3	T42.3X4	T42.3X5	T42.3X6
Nectadon	T48.3X1	T48.3X2	T48.3X3	T48.3X4	T48.3X5	T48.3X6
Nedocromil	T48.6X1	T48.6X2	T48.6X3	T48.6X4	T48.6X5	T48.6X6
Nefopam	T39.8X1	T39.8X2	T39.8X3	T39.8X4	T39.8X5	T39.8X6
Nematocyst (sting)	T63.691	T63.692	T63.693	T63.694	—	—
Nembutal	T42.3X1	T42.3X2	T42.3X3	T42.3X4	T42.3X5	T42.3X6
Nemonapride	T43.591	T43.592	T43.593	T43.594	T43.595	T43.596
Neoarsphenamine	T37.8X1	T37.8X2	T37.8X3	T37.8X4	T37.8X5	T37.8X6
Neocinchophen	T50.4X1	T50.4X2	T50.4X3	T50.4X4	T50.4X5	T50.4X6
Neomycin (derivatives)	T36.5X1	T36.5X2	T36.5X3	T36.5X4	T36.5X5	T36.5X6
with						
bacitracin	T49.0X1	T49.0X2	T49.0X3	T49.0X4	T49.0X5	T49.0X6
neostigmine	T44.0X1	T44.0X2	T44.0X3	T44.0X4	T44.0X5	T44.0X6
ENT agent	T49.6X1	T49.6X2	T49.6X3	T49.6X4	T49.6X5	T49.6X6
ophthalmic preparation	T49.5X1	T49.5X2	T49.5X3	T49.5X4	T49.5X5	T49.5X6
topical NEC	T49.0X1	T49.0X2	T49.0X3	T49.0X4	T49.0X5	T49.0X6
Neonal	T42.3X1	T42.3X2	T42.3X3	T42.3X4	T42.3X5	T42.3X6
Neoprontosil	T37.0X1	T37.0X2	T37.0X3	T37.0X4	T37.0X5	T37.0X6
Neosalvarsan	T37.8X1	T37.8X2	T37.8X3	T37.8X4	T37.8X5	T37.8X6
Neosilversalvarsan	T37.8X1	T37.8X2	T37.8X3	T37.8X4	T37.8X5	T37.8X6
Neosporin	T36.8X1	T36.8X2	T36.8X3	T36.8X4	T36.8X5	T36.8X6
ENT agent	T49.6X1	T49.6X2	T49.6X3	T49.6X4	T49.6X5	T49.6X6
opthalmic preparation	T49.5X1	T49.5X2	T49.5X3	T49.5X4	T49.5X5	T49.5X6
topical NEC	T49.0X1	T49.0X2	T49.0X3	T49.0X4	T49.0X5	T49.0X6
Neostigmine bromide	T44.0X1	T44.0X2	T44.0X3	T44.0X4	T44.0X5	T44.0X6
Neraval	T42.3X1	T42.3X2	T42.3X3	T42.3X4	T42.3X5	T42.3X6
Neravan	T42.3X1	T42.3X2	T42.3X3	T42.3X4	T42.3X5	T42.3X6
Nerium oleander	T62.2X1	T62.2X2	T62.2X3	T62.2X4	—	—
Nerve gas, not in war	T59.91	T59.92	T59.93	T59.94	—	—
Nesacaine	T41.3X1	T41.3X2	T41.3X3	T41.3X4	T41.3X5	T41.3X6
infiltration (subcutaneous)	T41.3X1	T41.3X2	T41.3X3	T41.3X4	T41.3X5	T41.3X6
nerve block (peripheral) (plexus)	T41.3X1	T41.3X2	T41.3X3	T41.3X4	T41.3X5	T41.3X6
Netilmicin	T36.5X1	T36.5X2	T36.5X3	T36.5X4	T36.5X5	T36.5X6
Neurobarb	T42.3X1	T42.3X2	T42.3X3	T42.3X4	T42.3X5	T42.3X6
Neuroleptic drug NEC	T43.501	T43.502	T43.503	T43.504	T43.505	T43.506
Neuromuscular blocking drug	T48.1X1	T48.1X2	T48.1X3	T48.1X4	T48.1X5	T48.1X6
Neutral insulin injection	T38.3X1	T38.3X2	T38.3X3	T38.3X4	T38.3X5	T38.3X6
Neutral spirits	T51.0X1	T51.0X2	T51.0X3	T51.0X4	—	—
beverage	T51.0X1	T51.0X2	T51.0X3	T51.0X4	—	—
Niacin	T46.7X1	T46.7X2	T46.7X3	T46.7X4	T46.7X5	T46.7X6
Niacinamide	T45.2X1	T45.2X2	T45.2X3	T45.2X4	T45.2X5	T45.2X6
Nialamide	T43.1X1	T43.1X2	T43.1X3	T43.1X4	T43.1X5	T43.1X6
Niaprazine	T42.6X1	T42.6X2	T42.6X3	T42.6X4	T42.6X5	T42.6X6
Nicametate	T46.7X1	T46.7X2	T46.7X3	T46.7X4	T46.7X5	T46.7X6
Nicardipine	T46.1X1	T46.1X2	T46.1X3	T46.1X4	T46.1X5	T46.1X6
Nicergoline	T46.7X1	T46.7X2	T46.7X3	T46.7X4	T46.7X5	T46.7X6
Nickel (carbonyl) (tetra-carbonyl) (fumes) (vapor)	T56.891	T56.892	T56.893	T56.894	—	—
Nickelocene	T56.891	T56.892	T56.893	T56.894	—	—
Niclosamide	T37.4X1	T37.4X2	T37.4X3	T37.4X4	T37.4X5	T37.4X6
Nicofuranose	T46.7X1	T46.7X2	T46.7X3	T46.7X4	T46.7X5	T46.7X6
Nicomorphine	T40.2X1	T40.2X2	T40.2X3	T40.2X4	—	—
Nicorandil	T46.3X1	T46.3X2	T46.3X3	T46.3X4	T46.3X5	T46.3X6
Nicotiana (plant)	T62.2X1	T62.2X2	T62.2X3	T62.2X4	—	—
Nicotinamide	T45.2X1	T45.2X2	T45.2X3	T45.2X4	T45.2X5	T45.2X6

Substance	Poisoning, Accidental (unintentional)	Poisoning, Intentional Self-harm	Poisoning, Assault	Poisoning, Undetermined	Adverse Effect	Under-dosing
Nicotine (insecticide) (spray) (sulfate) **NEC**	T60.2X1	T60.2X2	T60.2X3	T60.2X4	—	—
from tobacco	T65.291	T65.292	T65.293	T65.294	—	—
cigarettes	T65.221	T65.222	T65.223	T65.224	—	—
not insecticide	T65.291	T65.292	T65.293	T65.294	—	—
Nicotinic acid	T46.7X1	T46.7X2	T46.7X3	T46.7X4	T46.7X5	T46.7X6
Nicotinyl alcohol	T46.7X1	T46.7X2	T46.7X3	T46.7X4	T46.7X5	T46.7X6
Nicoumalone	T45.511	T45.512	T45.513	T45.514	T45.515	T45.516
Nifedipine	T46.1X1	T46.1X2	T46.1X3	T46.1X4	T46.1X5	T46.1X6
Nifenazone	T39.2X1	T39.2X2	T39.2X3	T39.2X4	T39.2X5	T39.2X6
Nifuraldezone	T37.91	T37.92	T37.93	T37.94	T37.95	T37.96
Nifuratel	T37.8X1	T37.8X2	T37.8X3	T37.8X4	T37.8X5	T37.8X6
Nifurtimox	T37.3X1	T37.3X2	T37.3X3	T37.3X4	T37.3X5	T37.3X6
Nifurtoinol	T37.8X1	T37.8X2	T37.8X3	T37.8X4	T37.8X5	T37.8X6
Nightshade, deadly (solanum) — *see also* Belladonna	T62.2X1	T62.2X2	T62.2X3	T62.2X4	—	—
berry	T62.1X1	T62.1X2	T62.1X3	T62.1X4	—	—
Nikethamide	T50.7X1	T50.7X2	T50.7X3	T50.7X4	T50.7X5	T50.7X6
Nilstat	T36.7X1	T36.7X2	T36.7X3	T36.7X4	T36.7X5	T36.7X6
topical	T49.0X1	T49.0X2	T49.0X3	T49.0X4	T49.0X5	T49.0X6
Nilutamide	T38.6X1	T38.6X2	T38.6X3	T38.6X4	T38.6X5	T38.6X6
Nimesulide	T39.391	T39.392	T39.393	T39.394	T39.395	T39.396
Nimetazepam	T42.4X1	T42.4X2	T42.4X3	T42.4X4	T42.4X5	T42.4X6
Nimodipine	T46.1X1	T46.1X2	T46.1X3	T46.1X4	T46.1X5	T46.1X6
Nimorazole	T37.3X1	T37.3X2	T37.3X3	T37.3X4	T37.3X5	T37.3X6
Nimustine	T45.1X1	T45.1X2	T45.1X3	T45.1X4	T45.1X5	T45.1X6
Niridazole	T37.4X1	T37.4X2	T37.4X3	T37.4X4	T37.4X5	T37.4X6
Nisentil	T40.2X1	T40.2X2	T40.2X3	T40.2X4	T40.2X5	T40.2X6
Nisoldipine	T46.1X1	T46.1X2	T46.1X3	T46.1X4	T46.1X5	T46.1X6
Nitramine	T65.3X1	T65.3X2	T65.3X3	T65.3X4	—	—
Nitrate, organic	T46.3X1	T46.3X2	T46.3X3	T46.3X4	T46.3X5	T46.3X6
Nitrazepam	T42.4X1	T42.4X2	T42.4X3	T42.4X4	T42.4X5	T42.4X6
Nitrefazole	T50.6X1	T50.6X2	T50.6X3	T50.6X4	T50.6X5	T50.6X6
Nitrendipine	T46.1X1	T46.1X2	T46.1X3	T46.1X4	T46.1X5	T46.1X6
Nitric						
acid (liquid)	T54.2X1	T54.2X2	T54.2X3	T54.2X4	—	—
vapor	T59.891	T59.892	T59.893	T59.894	—	—
oxide (gas)	T59.0X1	T59.0X2	T59.0X3	T59.0X4	—	—
Nitrimidazine	T37.3X1	T37.3X2	T37.3X3	T37.3X4	T37.3X5	T37.3X6
Nitrite, amyl (medicinal) (vapor)	T46.3X1	T46.3X2	T46.3X3	T46.3X4	T46.3X5	T46.3X6
Nitroaniline	T65.3X1	T65.3X2	T65.3X3	T65.3X4	—	—
vapor	T59.891	T59.892	T59.893	T59.894	—	—
Nitrobenzene, nitrobenzol	T65.3X1	T65.3X2	T65.3X3	T65.3X4	—	—
vapor	T65.3X1	T65.3X2	T65.3X3	T65.3X4	—	—
Nitrocellulose	T65.891	T65.892	T65.893	T65.894	—	—
lacquer	T65.891	T65.892	T65.893	T65.894	—	—
Nitrodiphenyl	T65.3X1	T65.3X2	T65.3X3	T65.3X4	—	—
Nitrofural	T49.0X1	T49.0X2	T49.0X3	T49.0X4	T49.0X5	T49.0X6
Nitrofurantoin	T37.8X1	T37.8X2	T37.8X3	T37.8X4	T37.8X5	T37.8X6
Nitrofurazone	T49.0X1	T49.0X2	T49.0X3	T49.0X4	T49.0X5	T49.0X6
Nitrogen	T59.0X1	T59.0X2	T59.0X3	T59.0X4	—	—
mustard	T45.1X1	T45.1X2	T45.1X3	T45.1X4	T45.1X5	T45.1X6
Nitroglycerin, nitroglycerol (medicinal)	T46.3X1	T46.3X2	T46.3X3	T46.3X4	T46.3X5	T46.3X6
nonmedicinal	T65.5X1	T65.5X2	T65.5X3	T65.5X4	—	—
fumes	T65.5X1	T65.5X2	T65.5X3	T65.5X4	—	—
Nitroglycol	T52.3X1	T52.3X2	T52.3X3	T52.3X4	—	—
Nitrohydrochloric acid	T54.2X1	T54.2X2	T54.2X3	T54.2X4	—	—
Nitromersol	T49.0X1	T49.0X2	T49.0X3	T49.0X4	T49.0X5	T49.0X6
Nitronaphthalene	T65.891	T65.892	T65.893	T65.894	—	—
Nitrophenol	T54.0X1	T54.0X2	T54.0X3	T54.0X4	—	—
Nitropropane	T52.8X1	T52.8X2	T52.8X3	T52.8X4	—	—
Nitroprusside	T46.5X1	T46.5X2	T46.5X3	T46.5X4	T46.5X5	T46.5X6
Nitrosodimethylamine	T65.3X1	T65.3X2	T65.3X3	T65.3X4	—	—
Nitrothiazol	T37.4X1	T37.4X2	T37.4X3	T37.4X4	T37.4X5	T37.4X6
Nitrotoluene, nitrotoluol	T65.3X1	T65.3X2	T65.3X3	T65.3X4	—	—
vapor	T65.3X1	T65.3X2	T65.3X3	T65.3X4	—	—
Nitrous						
acid (liquid)	T54.2X1	T54.2X2	T54.2X3	T54.2X4	—	—
fumes	T59.891	T59.892	T59.893	T59.894	—	—
ether spirit	T46.3X1	T46.3X2	T46.3X3	T46.3X4	T46.3X5	T46.3X6
oxide	T41.0X1	T41.0X2	T41.0X3	T41.0X4	T41.0X5	T41.0X6
Nitroxoline	T37.8X1	T37.8X2	T37.8X3	T37.8X4	T37.8X5	T37.8X6
Nitrozone	T49.0X1	T49.0X2	T49.0X3	T49.0X4	T49.0X5	T49.0X6
Nizatidine	T47.0X1	T47.0X2	T47.0X3	T47.0X4	T47.0X5	T47.0X6
Nizofenone	T43.8X1	T43.8X2	T43.8X3	T43.8X4	T43.8X5	T43.8X6
Noctec	T42.6X1	T42.6X2	T42.6X3	T42.6X4	T42.6X5	T42.6X6
Noludar	T42.6X1	T42.6X2	T42.6X3	T42.6X4	T42.6X5	T42.6X6
Nomegestrol	T38.5X1	T38.5X2	T38.5X3	T38.5X4	T38.5X5	T38.5X6
Nomifensine	T43.291	T43.292	T43.293	T43.294	T43.295	T43.296
Nonoxinol	T49.8X1	T49.8X2	T49.8X3	T49.8X4	T49.8X5	T49.8X6

Substance	Poisoning, Accidental (unintentional)	Poisoning, Intentional Self-harm	Poisoning, Assault	Poisoning, Undetermined	Adverse Effect	Under-dosing
Nonylphenoxy	T49.8X1	T49.8X2	T49.8X3	T49.8X4	T49.8X5	T49.8X6
(polyethoxyethanol)						
Noptil	T42.3X1	T42.3X2	T42.3X3	T42.3X4	T42.3X5	T42.3X6
Noradrenaline	T44.4X1	T44.4X2	T44.4X3	T44.4X4	T44.4X5	T44.4X6
Noramidopyrine	T39.2X1	T39.2X2	T39.2X3	T39.2X4	T39.2X5	T39.2X6
methanesulfonate sodium	T39.2X1	T39.2X2	T39.2X3	T39.2X4	T39.2X5	T39.2X6
Norbormide	T60.4X1	T60.4X2	T60.4X3	T60.4X4		
Nordazepam	T42.4X1	T42.4X2	T42.4X3	T42.4X4	T42.4X5	T42.4X6
Norepinephrine	T44.4X1	T44.4X2	T44.4X3	T44.4X4	T44.4X5	T44.4X6
Norethandrolone	T38.7X1	T38.7X2	T38.7X3	T38.7X4	T38.7X5	T38.7X6
Norethindrone	T38.4X1	T38.4X2	T38.4X3	T38.4X4	T38.4X5	T38.4X6
Norethisterone (acetate)	T38.4X1	T38.4X2	T38.4X3	T38.4X4	T38.4X5	T38.4X6
(enantate)						
with ethinylestradiol	T38.5X1	T38.5X2	T38.5X3	T38.5X4	T38.5X5	T38.5X6
Noretynodrel	T38.5X1	T38.5X2	T38.5X3	T38.5X4	T38.5X5	T38.5X6
Norfenefrine	T44.4X1	T44.4X2	T44.4X3	T44.4X4	T44.4X5	T44.4X6
Norfloxacin	T36.8X1	T36.8X2	T36.8X3	T36.8X4	T36.8X5	T36.8X6
Norgestrel	T38.4X1	T38.4X2	T38.4X3	T38.4X4	T38.4X5	T38.4X6
Norgestrienone	T38.4X1	T38.4X2	T38.4X3	T38.4X4	T38.4X5	T38.4X6
Norlestrin	T38.4X1	T38.4X2	T38.4X3	T38.4X4	T38.4X5	T38.4X6
Norlutin	T38.4X1	T38.4X2	T38.4X3	T38.4X4	T38.4X5	T38.4X6
Normal serum albumin (human),	T45.8X1	T45.8X2	T45.8X3	T45.8X4	T45.8X5	T45.8X6
salt-poor						
Normethandrone	T38.5X1	T38.5X2	T38.5X3	T38.5X4	T38.5X5	T38.5X6
Normison — see Benzodiazepines						
Normorphine	T40.2X1	T40.2X2	T40.2X3	T40.2X4	—	—
Norpseudoephedrine	T50.5X1	T50.5X2	T50.5X3	T50.5X4	T50.5X5	T50.5X6
Nortestosterone	T38.7X1	T38.7X2	T38.7X3	T38.7X4	T38.7X5	T38.7X6
(furanpropionate)						
Nortriptyline	T43.011	T43.012	T43.013	T43.014	T43.015	T43.016
Noscapine	T48.3X1	T48.3X2	T48.3X3	T48.3X4	T48.3X5	T48.3X6
Nose preparations	T49.6X1	T49.6X2	T49.6X3	T49.6X4	T49.6X5	T49.6X6
Novobiocin	T36.5X1	T36.5X2	T36.5X3	T36.5X4	T36.5X5	T36.5X6
Novocain (infiltration)	T41.3X1	T41.3X2	T41.3X3	T41.3X4	T41.3X5	T41.3X6
(topical)						
nerve block (peripheral)	T41.3X1	T41.3X2	T41.3X3	T41.3X4	T41.3X5	T41.3X6
(plexus)						
spinal	T41.3X1	T41.3X2	T41.3X3	T41.3X4	T41.3X5	T41.3X6
Noxious foodstuff	T62.91	T62.92	T62.93	T62.94	—	—
specified NEC	T62.8X1	T62.8X2	T62.8X3	T62.8X4	—	—
Noxiptiline	T43.011	T43.012	T43.013	T43.014	T43.015	T43.016
Noxytiolin	T49.0X1	T49.0X2	T49.0X3	T49.0X4	T49.0X5	T49.0X6
NPH Iletin (insulin)	T38.3X1	T38.3X2	T38.3X3	T38.3X4	T38.3X5	T38.3X6
Numorphan	T40.2X1	T40.2X2	T40.2X3	T40.2X4	T40.2X5	T40.2X6
Nunol	T42.3X1	T42.3X2	T42.3X3	T42.3X4	T42.3X5	T42.3X6
Nupercaine (spinal anesthetic)	T41.3X1	T41.3X2	T41.3X3	T41.3X4	T41.3X5	T41.3X6
topical (surface)	T41.3X1	T41.3X2	T41.3X3	T41.3X4	T41.3X5	T41.3X6
Nutmeg oil (liniment)	T49.3X1	T49.3X2	T49.3X3	T49.3X4	T49.3X5	T49.3X6
Nutritional supplement	T50.901	T50.902	T50.903	T50.904	T50.905	T50.906
Nux vomica	T65.1X1	T65.1X2	T65.1X3	T65.1X4	—	—
Nydrazid	T37.1X1	T37.1X2	T37.1X3	T37.1X4	T37.1X5	T37.1X6
Nylidrin	T46.7X1	T46.7X2	T46.7X3	T46.7X4	T46.7X5	T46.7X6
Nystatin	T36.7X1	T36.7X2	T36.7X3	T36.7X4	T36.7X5	T36.7X6
topical	T49.0X1	T49.0X2	T49.0X3	T49.0X4	T49.0X5	T49.0X6
Nytol	T45.0X1	T45.0X2	T45.0X3	T45.0X4	T45.0X5	T45.0X6
Obidoxime chloride	T50.6X1	T50.6X2	T50.6X3	T50.6X4	T50.6X5	T50.6X6
Octafonium (chloride)	T49.3X1	T49.3X2	T49.3X3	T49.3X4	T49.3X5	T49.3X6
Octamethyl pyrophosphoramide	T60.0X1	T60.0X2	T60.0X3	T60.0X4	—	—
Octanoin	T50.991	T50.992	T50.993	T50.994	T50.995	T50.996
Octatropine methylbromide	T44.3X1	T44.3X2	T44.3X3	T44.3X4	T44.3X5	T44.3X6
Octotiamine	T45.2X1	T45.2X2	T45.2X3	T45.2X4	T45.2X5	T45.2X6
Octoxinol (9)	T49.8X1	T49.8X2	T49.8X3	T49.8X4	T49.8X5	T49.8X6
Octreotide	T38.991	T38.992	T38.993	T38.994	T38.995	T38.996
Octyl nitrite	T46.3X1	T46.3X2	T46.3X3	T46.3X4	T46.3X5	T46.3X6
Oestradiol	T38.5X1	T38.5X2	T38.5X3	T38.5X4	T38.5X5	T38.5X6
Oestriol	T38.5X1	T38.5X2	T38.5X3	T38.5X4	T38.5X5	T38.5X6
Oestrogen	T38.5X1	T38.5X2	T38.5X3	T38.5X4	T38.5X5	T38.5X6
Oestrone	T38.5X1	T38.5X2	T38.5X3	T38.5X4	T38.5X5	T38.5X6
Ofloxacin	T36.8X1	T36.8X2	T36.8X3	T36.8X4	T36.8X5	T36.8X6
Oil (of)	T65.891	T65.892	T65.893	T65.894	—	—
bitter almond	T62.8X1	T62.8X2	T62.8X3	T62.8X4	—	—
cloves	T49.7X1	T49.7X2	T49.7X3	T49.7X4	T49.7X5	T49.7X6
colors	T65.6X1	T65.6X2	T65.6X3	T65.6X4	—	—
fumes	T59.891	T59.892	T59.893	T59.894	—	—
lubricating	T52.0X1	T52.0X2	T52.0X3	T52.0X4	—	—
Niobe	T52.8X1	T52.8X2	T52.8X3	T52.8X4	—	—
vitriol (liquid)	T54.2X1	T54.2X2	T54.2X3	T54.2X4	—	—
fumes	T54.2X1	T54.2X2	T54.2X3	T54.2X4	—	—
wintergreen (bitter) NEC	T49.3X1	T49.3X2	T49.3X3	T49.3X4	T49.3X5	T49.3X6
Oily preparation (for skin)	T49.3X1	T49.3X2	T49.3X3	T49.3X4	T49.3X5	T49.3X6
Ointment NEC	T49.3X1	T49.3X2	T49.3X3	T49.3X4	T49.3X5	T49.3X6
Olanzapine	T43.591	T43.592	T43.593	T43.594	T43.595	T43.596
Oleander	T62.2X1	T62.2X2	T62.2X3	T62.2X4	—	—
Oleandomycin	T36.3X1	T36.3X2	T36.3X3	T36.3X4	T36.3X5	T36.3X6
Oleandrin	T46.0X1	T46.0X2	T46.0X3	T46.0X4	T46.0X5	T46.0X6
Oleic acid	T46.6X1	T46.6X2	T46.6X3	T46.6X4	T46.6X5	T46.6X6
Oleovitamin A	T45.2X1	T45.2X2	T45.2X3	T45.2X4	T45.2X5	T45.2X6
Oleum ricini	T47.2X1	T47.2X2	T47.2X3	T47.2X4	T47.2X5	T47.2X6
Olive oil (medicinal) NEC	T47.4X1	T47.4X2	T47.4X3	T47.4X4	T47.4X5	T47.4X6
Olivomycin	T45.1X1	T45.1X2	T45.1X3	T45.1X4	T45.1X5	T45.1X6
Olsalazine	T47.8X1	T47.8X2	T47.8X3	T47.8X4	T47.8X5	T47.8X6
Omeprazole	T47.1X1	T47.1X2	T47.1X3	T47.1X4	T47.1X5	T47.1X6
OMPA	T60.0X1	T60.0X2	T60.0X3	T60.0X4	—	—
Oncovin	T45.1X1	T45.1X2	T45.1X3	T45.1X4	T45.1X5	T45.1X6
Ondansetron	T45.0X1	T45.0X2	T45.0X3	T45.0X4	T45.0X5	T45.0X6
Ophthaine	T41.3X1	T41.3X2	T41.3X3	T41.3X4	T41.3X5	T41.3X6
Ophthetic	T41.3X1	T41.3X2	T41.3X3	T41.3X4	T41.3X5	T41.3X6
Opiate NEC	T40.601	T40.602	T40.603	T40.604	T40.605	T40.606
antagonists	T50.7X1	T50.7X2	T50.7X3	T50.7X4	T50.7X5	T50.7X6
Opioid NEC	T40.2X1	T40.2X2	T40.2X3	T40.2X4	T40.2X5	T40.2X6
Opipramol	T43.011	T43.012	T43.013	T43.014	T43.015	T43.016
Opium alkaloids (total)	T40.0X1	T40.0X2	T40.0X3	T40.0X4	T40.0X5	T40.0X6
standardized powdered	T40.0X1	T40.0X2	T40.0X3	T40.0X4	T40.0X5	T40.0X6
tincture (camphorated)	T40.0X1	T40.0X2	T40.0X3	T40.0X4	T40.0X5	T40.0X6
Oracon	T38.4X1	T38.4X2	T38.4X3	T38.4X4	T38.4X5	T38.4X6
Oragrafin	T50.8X1	T50.8X2	T50.8X3	T50.8X4	T50.8X5	T50.8X6
Oral contraceptives	T38.4X1	T38.4X2	T38.4X3	T38.4X4	T38.4X5	T38.4X6
Oral rehydration salts	T50.3X1	T50.3X2	T50.3X3	T50.3X4	T50.3X5	T50.3X6
Orazamide	T50.991	T50.992	T50.993	T50.994	T50.995	T50.996
Orciprenaline	T48.291	T48.292	T48.293	T48.294	T48.295	T48.296
Organidin	T48.4X1	T48.4X2	T48.4X3	T48.4X4	T48.4X5	T48.4X6
Organonitrate NEC	T46.3X1	T46.3X2	T46.3X3	T46.3X4	T46.3X5	T46.3X6
Organophosphates	T60.0X1	T60.0X2	T60.0X3	T60.0X4	—	—
Orimune	T50.B91	T50.B92	T50.B93	T50.B94	T50.B95	T50.B96
Orinase	T38.3X1	T38.3X2	T38.3X3	T38.3X4	T38.3X5	T38.3X6
Ormeloxifene	T38.6X1	T38.6X2	T38.6X3	T38.6X4	T38.6X5	T38.6X6
Ornidazole	T37.3X1	T37.3X2	T37.3X3	T37.3X4	T37.3X5	T37.3X6
Ornithine aspartate	T50.991	T50.992	T50.993	T50.994	T50.995	T50.996
Ornoprostil	T47.1X1	T47.1X2	T47.1X3	T47.1X4	T47.1X5	T47.1X6
Orphenadrine (hydrochloride)	T42.8X1	T42.8X2	T42.8X3	T42.8X4	T42.8X5	T42.8X6
Ortal (sodium)	T42.3X1	T42.3X2	T42.3X3	T42.3X4	T42.3X5	T42.3X6
Orthoboric acid	T49.0X1	T49.0X2	T49.0X3	T49.0X4	T49.0X5	T49.0X6
ENT agent	T49.6X1	T49.6X2	T49.6X3	T49.6X4	T49.6X5	T49.6X6
ophthalmic preparation	T49.5X1	T49.5X2	T49.5X3	T49.5X4	T49.5X5	T49.5X6
Orthocaine	T41.3X1	T41.3X2	T41.3X3	T41.3X4	T41.3X5	T41.3X6
Orthodichlorobenzene	T53.7X1	T53.7X2	T53.7X3	T53.7X4	—	—
Ortho-Novum	T38.4X1	T38.4X2	T38.4X3	T38.4X4	T38.4X5	T38.4X6
Orthotolidine (reagent)	T54.2X1	T54.2X2	T54.2X3	T54.2X4	—	—
Osmic acid (liquid)	T54.2X1	T54.2X2	T54.2X3	T54.2X4	—	—
fumes	T54.2X1	T54.2X2	T54.2X3	T54.2X4	—	—
Osmotic diuretics	T50.2X1	T50.2X2	T50.2X3	T50.2X4	T50.2X5	T50.2X6
Otilonium bromide	T44.3X1	T44.3X2	T44.3X3	T44.3X4	T44.3X5	T44.3X6
Otorhinolaryngological drug NEC	T49.6X1	T49.6X2	T49.6X3	T49.6X4	T49.6X5	T49.6X6
Ouabain (e)	T46.0X1	T46.0X2	T46.0X3	T46.0X4	T46.0X5	T46.0X6
Ovarian						
hormone	T38.5X1	T38.5X2	T38.5X3	T38.5X4	T38.5X5	T38.5X6
stimulant	T38.5X1	T38.5X2	T38.5X3	T38.5X4	T38.5X5	T38.5X6
Ovral	T38.4X1	T38.4X2	T38.4X3	T38.4X4	T38.4X5	T38.4X6
Ovulen	T38.4X1	T38.4X2	T38.4X3	T38.4X4	T38.4X5	T38.4X6
Oxacillin	T36.0X1	T36.0X2	T36.0X3	T36.0X4	T36.0X5	T36.0X6
Oxalic acid	T54.2X1	T54.2X2	T54.2X3	T54.2X4	—	—
ammonium salt	T50.991	T50.992	T50.993	T50.994	T50.995	T50.996
Oxamniquine	T37.4X1	T37.4X2	T37.4X3	T37.4X4	T37.4X5	T37.4X6
Oxanamide	T43.591	T43.592	T43.593	T43.594	T43.595	T43.596
Oxandrolone	T38.7X1	T38.7X2	T38.7X3	T38.7X4	T38.7X5	T38.7X6
Oxantel	T37.4X1	T37.4X2	T37.4X3	T37.4X4	T37.4X5	T37.4X6
Oxapium iodide	T44.3X1	T44.3X2	T44.3X3	T44.3X4	T44.3X5	T44.3X6
Oxaprotiline	T43.021	T43.022	T43.023	T43.024	T43.025	T43.026
Oxaprozin	T39.311	T39.312	T39.313	T39.314	T39.315	T39.316
Oxatomide	T45.0X1	T45.0X2	T45.0X3	T45.0X4	T45.0X5	T45.0X6
Oxazepam	T42.4X1	T42.4X2	T42.4X3	T42.4X4	T42.4X5	T42.4X6
Oxazimedrine	T50.5X1	T50.5X2	T50.5X3	T50.5X4	T50.5X5	T50.5X6
Oxazolam	T42.4X1	T42.4X2	T42.4X3	T42.4X4	T42.4X5	T42.4X6
Oxazolidine derivatives	T42.2X1	T42.2X2	T42.2X3	T42.2X4	T42.2X5	T42.2X6
Oxazolidinedione (derivative)	T42.2X1	T42.2X2	T42.2X3	T42.2X4	T42.2X5	T42.2X6
Ox bile extract	T47.5X1	T47.5X2	T47.5X3	T47.5X4	T47.5X5	T47.5X6
Oxcarbazepine	T42.1X1	T42.1X2	T42.1X3	T42.1X4	T42.1X5	T42.1X6
Oxedrine	T44.4X1	T44.4X2	T44.4X3	T44.4X4	T44.4X5	T44.4X6
Oxeladin (citrate)	T48.3X1	T48.3X2	T48.3X3	T48.3X4	T48.3X5	T48.3X6

Subterms under main terms may continue to next column or page   Additional Character May Be Required — Refer to the Tabular List for Character Selection   381

Nonylphenoxy — Oxeladin

Substance	Poisoning, Accidental (unintentional)	Poisoning, Intentional Self-harm	Poisoning, Assault	Poisoning, Undetermined	Adverse Effect	Under-dosing
Oxendolone	T38.5X1	T38.5X2	T38.5X3	T38.5X4	T38.5X5	T38.5X6
Oxetacaine	T41.3X1	T41.3X2	T41.3X3	T41.3X4	T41.3X5	T41.3X6
Oxethazine	T41.3X1	T41.3X2	T41.3X3	T41.3X4	T41.3X5	T41.3X6
Oxetorone	T39.8X1	T39.8X2	T39.8X3	T39.8X4	T39.8X5	T39.8X6
Oxiconazole	T49.0X1	T49.0X2	T49.0X3	T49.0X4	T49.0X5	T49.0X6
Oxidizing agent NEC	T54.91	T54.92	T54.93	T54.94	—	—
Oxipurinol	T50.4X1	T50.4X2	T50.4X3	T50.4X4	T50.4X5	T50.4X6
Oxitriptan	T43.291	T43.292	T43.293	T43.294	T43.295	T43.296
Oxitropium bromide	T48.6X1	T48.6X2	T48.6X3	T48.6X4	T48.6X5	T48.6X6
Oxodipine	T46.1X1	T46.1X2	T46.1X3	T46.1X4	T46.1X5	T46.1X6
Oxolamine	T48.3X1	T48.3X2	T48.3X3	T48.3X4	T48.3X5	T48.3X6
Oxolinic acid	T37.8X1	T37.8X2	T37.8X3	T37.8X4	T37.8X5	T37.8X6
Oxomemazine	T43.3X1	T43.3X2	T43.3X3	T43.3X4	T43.3X5	T43.3X6
Oxophenarsine	T37.3X1	T37.3X2	T37.3X3	T37.3X4	T37.3X5	T37.3X6
Oxprenolol	T44.7X1	T44.7X2	T44.7X3	T44.7X4	T44.7X5	T44.7X6
Oxsoralen	T49.3X1	T49.3X2	T49.3X3	T49.3X4	T49.3X5	T49.3X6
Oxtriphylline	T48.6X1	T48.6X2	T48.6X3	T48.6X4	T48.6X5	T48.6X6
Oxybate sodium	T41.291	T41.292	T41.293	T41.294	T41.295	T41.296
Oxybuprocaine	T41.3X1	T41.3X2	T41.3X3	T41.3X4	T41.3X5	T41.3X6
Oxybutynin	T44.3X1	T44.3X2	T44.3X3	T44.3X4	T44.3X5	T44.3X6
Oxychlorosene	T49.0X1	T49.0X2	T49.0X3	T49.0X4	T49.0X5	T49.0X6
Oxycodone	T40.2X1	T40.2X2	T40.2X3	T40.2X4	T40.2X5	T40.2X6
Oxyfedrine	T46.3X1	T46.3X2	T46.3X3	T46.3X4	T46.3X5	T46.3X6
Oxygen	T41.5X1	T41.5X2	T41.5X3	T41.5X4	T41.5X5	T41.5X6
Oxylone	T49.0X1	T49.0X2	T49.0X3	T49.0X4	T49.0X5	T49.0X6
ophthalmic preparation	T49.5X1	T49.5X2	T49.5X3	T49.5X4	T49.5X5	T49.5X6
Oxymesterone	T38.7X1	T38.7X2	T38.7X3	T38.7X4	T38.7X5	T38.7X6
Oxymetazoline	T48.5X1	T48.5X2	T48.5X3	T48.5X4	T48.5X5	T48.5X6
Oxymetholone	T38.7X1	T38.7X2	T38.7X3	T38.7X4	T38.7X5	T38.7X6
Oxymorphone	T40.2X1	T40.2X2	T40.2X3	T40.2X4	T40.2X5	T40.2X6
Oxypertine	T43.591	T43.592	T43.593	T43.594	T43.595	T43.596
Oxyphenbutazone	T39.2X1	T39.2X2	T39.2X3	T39.2X4	T39.2X5	T39.2X6
Oxyphencyclimine	T44.3X1	T44.3X2	T44.3X3	T44.3X4	T44.3X5	T44.3X6
Oxyphenisatine	T47.2X1	T47.2X2	T47.2X3	T47.2X4	T47.2X5	T47.2X6
Oxyphenonium bromide	T44.3X1	T44.3X2	T44.3X3	T44.3X4	T44.3X5	T44.3X6
Oxypolygelatin	T45.8X1	T45.8X2	T45.8X3	T45.8X4	T45.8X5	T45.8X6
Oxyquinoline (derivatives)	T37.8X1	T37.8X2	T37.8X3	T37.8X4	T37.8X5	T37.8X6
Oxytetracycline	T36.4X1	T36.4X2	T36.4X3	T36.4X4	T36.4X5	T36.4X6
Oxytocic drug NEC	T48.0X1	T48.0X2	T48.0X3	T48.0X4	T48.0X5	T48.0X6
Oxytocin (synthetic)	T48.0X1	T48.0X2	T48.0X3	T48.0X4	T48.0X5	T48.0X6
Ozone	T59.891	T59.892	T59.893	T59.894	—	—
PABA	T49.3X1	T49.3X2	T49.3X3	T49.3X4	T49.3X5	T49.3X6
Packed red cells	T45.8X1	T45.8X2	T45.8X3	T45.8X4	T45.8X5	T45.8X6
Padimate	T49.3X1	T49.3X2	T49.3X3	T49.3X4	T49.3X5	T49.3X6
Paint NEC	T65.6X1	T65.6X2	T65.6X3	T65.6X4	—	—
cleaner	T52.91	T52.92	T52.93	T52.94	—	—
fumes NEC	T59.891	T59.892	T59.893	T59.894	—	—
lead (fumes)	T56.0X1	T56.0X2	T56.0X3	T56.0X4	—	—
solvent NEC	T52.8X1	T52.8X2	T52.8X3	T52.8X4	—	—
stripper	T52.8X1	T52.8X2	T52.8X3	T52.8X4	—	—
Palfium	T40.2X1	T40.2X2	T40.2X3	T40.2X4	—	—
Palm kernel oil	T50.991	T50.992	T50.993	T50.994	T50.995	T50.996
Paludrine	T37.2X1	T37.2X2	T37.2X3	T37.2X4	T37.2X5	T37.2X6
PAM (pralidoxime)	T50.6X1	T50.6X2	T50.6X3	T50.6X4	T50.6X5	T50.6X6
Pamaquine (naphthoute)	T37.2X1	T37.2X2	T37.2X3	T37.2X4	T37.2X5	T37.2X6
Panadol	T39.1X1	T39.1X2	T39.1X3	T39.1X4	T39.1X5	T39.1X6
Pancreatic						
digestive secretion stimulant	T47.8X1	T47.8X2	T47.8X3	T47.8X4	T47.8X5	T47.8X6
dornase	T45.3X1	T45.3X2	T45.3X3	T45.3X4	T45.3X5	T45.3X6
Pancreatin	T47.5X1	T47.5X2	T47.5X3	T47.5X4	T47.5X5	T47.5X6
Pancrelipase	T47.5X1	T47.5X2	T47.5X3	T47.5X4	T47.5X5	T47.5X6
Pancuronium (bromide)	T48.1X1	T48.1X2	T48.1X3	T48.1X4	T48.1X5	T48.1X6
Pangamic acid	T45.2X1	T45.2X2	T45.2X3	T45.2X4	T45.2X5	T45.2X6
Panthenol	T45.2X1	T45.2X2	T45.2X3	T45.2X4	T45.2X5	T45.2X6
topical	T49.8X1	T49.8X2	T49.8X3	T49.8X4	T49.8X5	T49.8X6
Pantopon	T40.0X1	T40.0X2	T40.0X3	T40.0X4	T40.0X5	T40.0X6
Pantothenic acid	T45.2X1	T45.2X2	T45.2X3	T45.2X4	T45.2X5	T45.2X6
Panwarfin	T45.511	T45.512	T45.513	T45.514	T45.515	T45.516
Papain	T47.5X1	T47.5X2	T47.5X3	T47.5X4	T47.5X5	T47.5X6
digestant	T47.5X1	T47.5X2	T47.5X3	T47.5X4	T47.5X5	T47.5X6
Papaveretum	T40.0X1	T40.0X2	T40.0X3	T40.0X4	T40.0X5	T40.0X6
Papaverine	T44.3X1	T44.3X2	T44.3X3	T44.3X4	T44.3X5	T44.3X6
Para-acetamidophenol	T39.1X1	T39.1X2	T39.1X3	T39.1X4	T39.1X5	T39.1X6
Para-aminobenzoic acid	T49.3X1	T49.3X2	T49.3X3	T49.3X4	T49.3X5	T49.3X6
Para-aminophenol derivatives	T39.1X1	T39.1X2	T39.1X3	T39.1X4	T39.1X5	T39.1X6
Para-aminosalicylic acid	T37.1X1	T37.1X2	T37.1X3	T37.1X4	T37.1X5	T37.1X6
Paracetaldehyde	T42.6X1	T42.6X2	T42.6X3	T42.6X4	T42.6X5	T42.6X6
Paracetamol	T39.1X1	T39.1X2	T39.1X3	T39.1X4	T39.1X5	T39.1X6
Parachlorophenol (camphorated)	T49.0X1	T49.0X2	T49.0X3	T49.0X4	T49.0X5	T49.0X6
Paracodin	T40.2X1	T40.2X2	T40.2X3	T40.2X4	T40.2X5	T40.2X6

Substance	Poisoning, Accidental (unintentional)	Poisoning, Intentional Self-harm	Poisoning, Assault	Poisoning, Undetermined	Adverse Effect	Under-dosing
Paradione	T42.2X1	T42.2X2	T42.2X3	T42.2X4	T42.2X5	T42.2X6
Paraffin(s) (wax)	T52.0X1	T52.0X2	T52.0X3	T52.0X4	—	—
liquid (medicinal)	T47.4X1	T47.4X2	T47.4X3	T47.4X4	T47.4X5	T47.4X6
nonmedicinal	T52.0X1	T52.0X2	T52.0X3	T52.0X4	—	—
Paraformaldehyde	T60.3X1	T60.3X2	T60.3X3	T60.3X4	—	—
Paraldehyde	T42.6X1	T42.6X2	T42.6X3	T42.6X4	T42.6X5	T42.6X6
Paramethadione	T42.2X1	T42.2X2	T42.2X3	T42.2X4	T42.2X5	T42.2X6
Paramethasone	T38.0X1	T38.0X2	T38.0X3	T38.0X4	T38.0X5	T38.0X6
acetate	T49.0X1	T49.0X2	T49.0X3	T49.0X4	T49.0X5	T49.0X6
Paraoxon	T60.0X1	T60.0X2	T60.0X3	T60.0X4	—	—
Paraquat	T60.3X1	T60.3X2	T60.3X3	T60.3X4	—	—
Parasympatholytic NEC	T44.3X1	T44.3X2	T44.3X3	T44.3X4	T44.3X5	T44.3X6
Parasympathomimetic drug NEC	T44.1X1	T44.1X2	T44.1X3	T44.1X4	T44.1X5	T44.1X6
Parathion	T60.0X1	T60.0X2	T60.0X3	T60.0X4	—	—
Parathormone	T50.991	T50.992	T50.993	T50.994	T50.995	T50.996
Parathyroid extract	T50.991	T50.992	T50.993	T50.994	T50.995	T50.996
Paratyphoid vaccine	T50.A91	T50.A92	T50.A93	T50.A94	T50.A95	T50.A96
Paredrine	T44.4X1	T44.4X2	T44.4X3	T44.4X4	T44.4X5	T44.4X6
Paregoric	T40.0X1	T40.0X2	T40.0X3	T40.0X4	T40.0X5	T40.0X6
Pargyline	T46.5X1	T46.5X2	T46.5X3	T46.5X4	T46.5X5	T46.5X6
Paris green	T57.0X1	T57.0X2	T57.0X3	T57.0X4	—	—
insecticide	T57.0X1	T57.0X2	T57.0X3	T57.0X4	—	—
Parnate	T43.1X1	T43.1X2	T43.1X3	T43.1X4	T43.1X5	T43.1X6
Paromomycin	T36.5X1	T36.5X2	T36.5X3	T36.5X4	T36.5X5	T36.5X6
Paroxypropione	T45.1X1	T45.1X2	T45.1X3	T45.1X4	T45.1X5	T45.1X6
Parzone	T40.2X1	T40.2X2	T40.2X3	T40.2X4	T40.2X5	T40.2X6
PAS	T37.1X1	T37.1X2	T37.1X3	T37.1X4	T37.1X5	T37.1X6
Pasiniazid	T37.1X1	T37.1X2	T37.1X3	T37.1X4	T37.1X5	T37.1X6
PBB (polybrominated biphenyls)	T65.891	T65.892	T65.893	T65.894	—	—
PCB	T65.891	T65.892	T65.893	T65.894	—	—
PCP						
meaning pentachlorophenol	T60.1X1	T60.1X2	T60.1X3	T60.1X4	—	—
fungicide	T60.3X1	T60.3X2	T60.3X3	T60.3X4	—	—
herbicide	T60.3X1	T60.3X2	T60.3X3	T60.3X4	—	—
insecticide	T60.1X1	T60.1X2	T60.1X3	T60.1X4	—	—
meaning phencyclidine	T40.991	T40.992	T40.993	T40.994	—	—
Peach kernel oil (emulsion)	T47.4X1	T47.4X2	T47.4X3	T47.4X4	T47.4X5	T47.4X6
Peanut oil (emulsion) NEC	T47.4X1	T47.4X2	T47.4X3	T47.4X4	T47.4X5	T47.4X6
topical	T49.3X1	T49.3X2	T49.3X3	T49.3X4	T49.3X5	T49.3X6
Pearly Gates (morning glory seeds)	T40.991	T40.992	T40.993	T40.994	—	—
Pecazine	T43.3X1	T43.3X2	T43.3X3	T43.3X4	T43.3X5	T43.3X6
Pectin	T47.6X1	T47.6X2	T47.6X3	T47.6X4	T47.6X5	T47.6X6
Pefloxacin	T37.8X1	T37.8X2	T37.8X3	T37.8X4	T37.8X5	T37.8X6
Pegademase, bovine	T50.Z91	T50.Z92	T50.Z93	T50.Z94	T50.Z95	T50.Z96
Pelletierine tannate	T37.4X1	T37.4X2	T37.4X3	T37.4X4	T37.4X5	T37.4X6
Pemirolast (potassium)	T48.6X1	T48.6X2	T48.6X3	T48.6X4	T48.6X5	T48.6X6
Pemoline	T50.7X1	T50.7X2	T50.7X3	T50.7X4	T50.7X5	T50.7X6
Pempidine	T44.2X1	T44.2X2	T44.2X3	T44.2X4	T44.2X5	T44.2X6
Penamecillin	T36.0X1	T36.0X2	T36.0X3	T36.0X4	T36.0X5	T36.0X6
Penbutolol	T44.7X1	T44.7X2	T44.7X3	T44.7X4	T44.7X5	T44.7X6
Penethamate	T36.0X1	T36.0X2	T36.0X3	T36.0X4	T36.0X5	T36.0X6
Penfluridol	T43.591	T43.592	T43.593	T43.594	T43.595	T43.596
Penflutizide	T50.2X1	T50.2X2	T50.2X3	T50.2X4	T50.2X5	T50.2X6
Pengitoxin	T46.0X1	T46.0X2	T46.0X3	T46.0X4	T46.0X5	T46.0X6
Penicillamine	T50.6X1	T50.6X2	T50.6X3	T50.6X4	T50.6X5	T50.6X6
Penicillin (any)	T36.0X1	T36.0X2	T36.0X3	T36.0X4	T36.0X5	T36.0X6
Penicillinase	T45.3X1	T45.3X2	T45.3X3	T45.3X4	T45.3X5	T45.3X6
Penicilloyl polylysine	T50.8X1	T50.8X2	T50.8X3	T50.8X4	T50.8X5	T50.8X6
Penimepicycline	T36.4X1	T36.4X2	T36.4X3	T36.4X4	T36.4X5	T36.4X6
Pentachloroethane	T53.6X1	T53.6X2	T53.6X3	T53.6X4	—	—
Pentachloronaphthalene	T53.7X1	T53.7X2	T53.7X3	T53.7X4	—	—
Pentachlorophenol (pesticide)	T60.1X1	T60.1X2	T60.1X3	T60.1X4	—	—
fungicide	T60.3X1	T60.3X2	T60.3X3	T60.3X4	—	—
herbicide	T60.3X1	T60.3X2	T60.3X3	T60.3X4	—	—
insecticide	T60.1X1	T60.1X2	T60.1X3	T60.1X4	—	—
Pentaerythritol	T46.3X1	T46.3X2	T46.3X3	T46.3X4	T46.3X5	T46.3X6
chloral	T42.6X1	T42.6X2	T42.6X3	T42.6X4	T42.6X5	T42.6X6
tetranitrate NEC	T46.3X1	T46.3X2	T46.3X3	T46.3X4	T46.3X5	T46.3X6
Pentaerythrityl tetranitrate	T46.3X1	T46.3X2	T46.3X3	T46.3X4	T46.3X5	T46.3X6
Pentagastrin	T50.8X1	T50.8X2	T50.8X3	T50.8X4	T50.8X5	T50.8X6
Pentalin	T53.6X1	T53.6X2	T53.6X3	T53.6X4	—	—
Pentamethonium bromide	T44.2X1	T44.2X2	T44.2X3	T44.2X4	T44.2X5	T44.2X6
Pentamidine	T37.3X1	T37.3X2	T37.3X3	T37.3X4	T37.3X5	T37.3X6
Pentanol	T51.3X1	T51.3X2	T51.3X3	T51.3X4	—	—
Pentapyrrolinium (bitartrate)	T44.2X1	T44.2X2	T44.2X3	T44.2X4	T44.2X5	T44.2X6
Pentaquine	T37.2X1	T37.2X2	T37.2X3	T37.2X4	T37.2X5	T37.2X6

Additional Character May Be Required — Refer to the Tabular List for Character Selection   Subterms under main terms may continue to next column or page

Substance	Poisoning, Accidental (unintentional)	Poisoning, Intentional Self-harm	Poisoning, Assault	Poisoning, Undetermined	Adverse Effect	Under-dosing
Pentazocine	T40.4X1	T40.4X2	T40.4X3	T40.4X4	T40.4X5	T40.4X6
Pentetrazole	T50.7X1	T50.7X2	T50.7X3	T50.7X4	T50.7X5	T50.7X6
Penthienate bromide	T44.3X1	T44.3X2	T44.3X3	T44.3X4	T44.3X5	T44.3X6
Pentifylline	T46.7X1	T46.7X2	T46.7X3	T46.7X4	T46.7X5	T46.7X6
Pentobarbital	T42.3X1	T42.3X2	T42.3X3	T42.3X4	T42.3X5	T42.3X6
sodium	T42.3X1	T42.3X2	T42.3X3	T42.3X4	T42.3X5	T42.3X6
Pentobarbitone	T42.3X1	T42.3X2	T42.3X3	T42.3X4	T42.3X5	T42.3X6
Pentolonium tartrate	T44.2X1	T44.2X2	T44.2X3	T44.2X4	T44.2X5	T44.2X6
Pentosan polysulfate	T39.8X1	T39.8X2	T39.8X3	T39.8X4	T39.8X5	T39.8X6
(sodium)						
Pentostatin	T45.1X1	T45.1X2	T45.1X3	T45.1X4	T45.1X5	T45.1X6
Pentothal	T41.1X1	T41.1X2	T41.1X3	T41.1X4	T41.1X5	T41.1X6
Pentoxifylline	T46.7X1	T46.7X2	T46.7X3	T46.7X4	T46.7X5	T46.7X6
Pentoxyverine	T48.3X1	T48.3X2	T48.3X3	T48.3X4	T48.3X5	T48.3X6
Pentrinat	T46.3X1	T46.3X2	T46.3X3	T46.3X4	T46.3X5	T46.3X6
Pentylenetetrazole	T50.7X1	T50.7X2	T50.7X3	T50.7X4	T50.7X5	T50.7X6
Pentylsalicylamide	T37.1X1	T37.1X2	T37.1X3	T37.1X4	T37.1X5	T37.1X6
Pentymal	T42.3X1	T42.3X2	T42.3X3	T42.3X4	T42.3X5	T42.3X6
Peplomycin	T45.1X1	T45.1X2	T45.1X3	T45.1X4	T45.1X5	T45.1X6
Peppermint (oil)	T47.5X1	T47.5X2	T47.5X3	T47.5X4	T47.5X5	T47.5X6
Pepsin	T47.5X1	T47.5X2	T47.5X3	T47.5X4	T47.5X5	T47.5X6
digestant	T47.5X1	T47.5X2	T47.5X3	T47.5X4	T47.5X5	T47.5X6
Pepstatin	T47.1X1	T47.1X2	T47.1X3	T47.1X4	T47.1X5	T47.1X6
Peptavlon	T50.8X1	T50.8X2	T50.8X3	T50.8X4	T50.8X5	T50.8X6
Perazine	T43.3X1	T43.3X2	T43.3X3	T43.3X4	T43.3X5	T43.3X6
Percaine (spinal)	T41.3X1	T41.3X2	T41.3X3	T41.3X4	T41.3X5	T41.3X6
topical (surface)	T41.3X1	T41.3X2	T41.3X3	T41.3X4	T41.3X5	T41.3X6
Perchloroethylene	T53.3X1	T53.3X2	T53.3X3	T53.3X4	—	—
medicinal	T37.4X1	T37.4X2	T37.4X3	T37.4X4	T37.4X5	T37.4X6
vapor	T53.3X1	T53.3X2	T53.3X3	T53.3X4	—	—
Percodan	T40.2X1	T40.2X2	T40.2X3	T40.2X4	T40.2X5	T40.2X6
Percogesic — see also acetaminophen	T45.0X1	T45.0X2	T45.0X3	T45.0X4	T45.0X5	T45.0X6
Percorten	T38.0X1	T38.0X2	T38.0X3	T38.0X4	T38.0X5	T38.0X6
Pergolide	T42.8X1	T42.8X2	T42.8X3	T42.8X4	T42.8X5	T42.8X6
Pergonal	T38.811	T38.812	T38.813	T38.814	T38.815	T38.816
Perhexilene	T46.3X1	T46.3X2	T46.3X3	T46.3X4	T46.3X5	T46.3X6
Perhexiline (maleate)	T46.3X1	T46.3X2	T46.3X3	T46.3X4	T46.3X5	T46.3X6
Periactin	T45.0X1	T45.0X2	T45.0X3	T45.0X4	T45.0X5	T45.0X6
Periciazine	T43.3X1	T43.3X2	T43.3X3	T43.3X4	T43.3X5	T43.3X6
Periclor	T42.6X1	T42.6X2	T42.6X3	T42.6X4	T42.6X5	T42.6X6
Perindopril	T46.4X1	T46.4X2	T46.4X3	T46.4X4	T46.4X5	T46.4X6
Perisoxal	T39.8X1	T39.8X2	T39.8X3	T39.8X4	T39.8X5	T39.8X6
Peritoneal dialysis solution	T50.3X1	T50.3X2	T50.3X3	T50.3X4	T50.3X5	T50.3X6
Peritrate	T46.3X1	T46.3X2	T46.3X3	T46.3X4	T46.3X5	T46.3X6
Perlapine	T42.4X1	T42.4X2	T42.4X3	T42.4X4	T42.4X5	T42.4X6
Permanganate	T65.891	T65.892	T65.893	T65.894		
Permethrin	T60.1X1	T60.1X2	T60.1X3	T60.1X4	—	—
Pernocton	T42.3X1	T42.3X2	T42.3X3	T42.3X4	T42.3X5	T42.3X6
Pernoston	T42.3X1	T42.3X2	T42.3X3	T42.3X4	T42.3X5	T42.3X6
Peronine	T40.2X1	T40.2X2	T40.2X3	T40.2X4	—	—
Perphenazine	T43.3X1	T43.3X2	T43.3X3	T43.3X4	T43.3X5	T43.3X6
Pertofrane	T43.011	T43.012	T43.013	T43.014	T43.015	T43.016
Pertussis						
immune serum (human)	T50.Z11	T50.Z12	T50.Z13	T50.Z14	T50.Z15	T50.Z16
vaccine (with diphtheria toxoid)	T50.A11	T50.A12	T50.A13	T50.A14	T50.A15	T50.A16
(with tetanus toxoid)						
Peruvian balsam	T49.0X1	T49.0X2	T49.0X3	T49.0X4	T49.0X5	T49.0X6
Peruvoside	T46.0X1	T46.0X2	T46.0X3	T46.0X4	T46.0X5	T46.0X6
Pesticide (dust) (fumes) (vapor) NEC	T60.91	T60.92	T60.93	T60.94	—	—
arsenic	T57.0X1	T57.0X2	T57.0X3	T57.0X4	—	—
chlorinated	T60.1X1	T60.1X2	T60.1X3	T60.1X4	—	—
cyanide	T65.0X1	T65.0X2	T65.0X3	T65.0X4	—	—
kerosene	T52.0X1	T52.0X2	T52.0X3	T52.0X4	—	—
mixture (of compounds)	T60.91	T60.92	T60.93	T60.94	—	—
naphthalene	T60.2X1	T60.2X2	T60.2X3	T60.2X4	—	—
organochlorine (compounds)	T60.1X1	T60.1X2	T60.1X3	T60.1X4	—	—
petroleum (distillate) (products) NEC	T60.8X1	T60.8X2	T60.8X3	T60.8X4	—	—
specified ingredient NEC	T60.8X1	T60.8X2	T60.8X3	T60.8X4	—	—
strychnine	T65.1X1	T65.1X2	T65.1X3	T65.1X4	—	—
thallium	T60.4X1	T60.4X2	T60.4X3	T60.4X4	—	—
Pethidine	T40.4X1	T40.4X2	T40.4X3	T40.4X4	T40.4X5	T40.4X6
Petrichloral	T42.6X1	T42.6X2	T42.6X3	T42.6X4	T42.6X5	T42.6X6
Petrol	T52.0X1	T52.0X2	T52.0X3	T52.0X4	—	—
vapor	T52.0X1	T52.0X2	T52.0X3	T52.0X4	—	—
Petrolatum	T49.3X1	T49.3X2	T49.3X3	T49.3X4	T49.3X5	T49.3X6
hydrophilic	T49.3X1	T49.3X2	T49.3X3	T49.3X4	T49.3X5	T49.3X6
liquid	T47.4X1	T47.4X2	T47.4X3	T47.4X4	T47.4X5	T47.4X6
topical	T49.3X1	T49.3X2	T49.3X3	T49.3X4	T49.3X5	T49.3X6
nonmedicinal	T52.0X1	T52.0X2	T52.0X3	T52.0X4	—	—

Substance	Poisoning, Accidental (unintentional)	Poisoning, Intentional Self-harm	Poisoning, Assault	Poisoning, Undetermined	Adverse Effect	Under-dosing
Petrolatum — continued						
red veterinary	T49.3X1	T49.3X2	T49.3X3	T49.3X4	T49.3X5	T49.3X6
white	T49.3X1	T49.3X2	T49.3X3	T49.3X4	T49.3X5	T49.3X6
Petroleum (products) NEC	T52.0X1	T52.0X2	T52.0X3	T52.0X4	—	—
benzine(s) — see Ligroin						
ether — see Ligroin						
jelly — see Petrolatum						
naphtha — see Ligroin						
pesticide	T60.8X1	T60.8X2	T60.8X3	T60.8X4	—	—
solids	T52.0X1	T52.0X2	T52.0X3	T52.0X4	—	—
solvents	T52.0X1	T52.0X2	T52.0X3	T52.0X4	—	—
vapor	T52.0X1	T52.0X2	T52.0X3	T52.0X4	—	—
Peyote	T40.991	T40.992	T40.993	T40.994	—	—
Phanodorm, phanodorn	T42.3X1	T42.3X2	T42.3X3	T42.3X4	T42.3X5	T42.3X6
Phanquinone	T37.3X1	T37.3X2	T37.3X3	T37.3X4	T37.3X5	T37.3X6
Phanquone	T37.3X1	T37.3X2	T37.3X3	T37.3X4	T37.3X5	T37.3X6
Pharmaceutical						
adjunct NEC	T50.901	T50.902	T50.903	T50.904	T50.905	T50.906
excipient NEC	T50.901	T50.902	T50.903	T50.904	T50.905	T50.906
sweetener	T50.901	T50.902	T50.903	T50.904	T50.905	T50.906
viscous agent	T50.901	T50.902	T50.903	T50.904	T50.905	T50.906
Phemitone	T42.3X1	T42.3X2	T42.3X3	T42.3X4	T42.3X5	T42.3X6
Phenacaine	T41.3X1	T41.3X2	T41.3X3	T41.3X4	T41.3X5	T41.3X6
Phenacemide	T42.6X1	T42.6X2	T42.6X3	T42.6X4	T42.6X5	T42.6X6
Phenacetin	T39.1X1	T39.1X2	T39.1X3	T39.1X4	T39.1X5	T39.1X6
Phenadoxone	T40.2X1	T40.2X2	T40.2X3	T40.2X4	—	—
Phenaglycodol	T43.591	T43.592	T43.593	T43.594	T43.595	T43.596
Phenantoin	T42.0X1	T42.0X2	T42.0X3	T42.0X4	T42.0X5	T42.0X6
Phenaphthazine reagent	T50.991	T50.992	T50.993	T50.994	T50.995	T50.996
Phenazocine	T40.4X1	T40.4X2	T40.4X3	T40.4X4	T40.4X5	T40.4X6
Phenazone	T39.2X1	T39.2X2	T39.2X3	T39.2X4	T39.2X5	T39.2X6
Phenazopyridine	T39.8X1	T39.8X2	T39.8X3	T39.8X4	T39.8X5	T39.8X6
Phenbenicillin	T36.0X1	T36.0X2	T36.0X3	T36.0X4	T36.0X5	T36.0X6
Phenbutrazate	T50.5X1	T50.5X2	T50.5X3	T50.5X4	T50.5X5	T50.5X6
Phencyclidine	T40.991	T40.992	T40.993	T40.994	T40.995	T40.996
Phendimetrazine	T50.5X1	T50.5X2	T50.5X3	T50.5X4	T50.5X5	T50.5X6
Phenelzine	T43.1X1	T43.1X2	T43.1X3	T43.1X4	T43.1X5	T43.1X6
Phenemal	T42.3X1	T42.3X2	T42.3X3	T42.3X4	T42.3X5	T42.3X6
Phenergan	T42.6X1	T42.6X2	T42.6X3	T42.6X4	T42.6X5	T42.6X6
Pheneticillin	T36.0X1	T36.0X2	T36.0X3	T36.0X4	T36.0X5	T36.0X6
Pheneturide	T42.6X1	T42.6X2	T42.6X3	T42.6X4	T42.6X5	T42.6X6
Phenformin	T38.3X1	T38.3X2	T38.3X3	T38.3X4	T38.3X5	T38.3X6
Phenglutarimide	T44.3X1	T44.3X2	T44.3X3	T44.3X4	T44.3X5	T44.3X6
Phenicarbazide	T39.8X1	T39.8X2	T39.8X3	T39.8X4	T39.8X5	T39.8X6
Phenindamine	T45.0X1	T45.0X2	T45.0X3	T45.0X4	T45.0X5	T45.0X6
Phenindione	T45.511	T45.512	T45.513	T45.514	T45.515	T45.516
Pheniprazine	T43.1X1	T43.1X2	T43.1X3	T43.1X4	T43.1X5	T43.1X6
Pheniramine	T45.0X1	T45.0X2	T45.0X3	T45.0X4	T45.0X5	T45.0X6
Phenisatin	T47.2X1	T47.2X2	T47.2X3	T47.2X4	T47.2X5	T47.2X6
Phenmetrazine	T50.5X1	T50.5X2	T50.5X3	T50.5X4	T50.5X5	T50.5X6
Phenobal	T42.3X1	T42.3X2	T42.3X3	T42.3X4	T42.3X5	T42.3X6
Phenobarbital	T42.3X1	T42.3X2	T42.3X3	T42.3X4	T42.3X5	T42.3X6
with						
mephenytoin	T42.3X1	T42.3X2	T42.3X3	T42.3X4	T42.3X5	T42.3X6
phenytoin	T42.3X1	T42.3X2	T42.3X3	T42.3X4	T42.3X5	T42.3X6
sodium	T42.3X1	T42.3X2	T42.3X3	T42.3X4	T42.3X5	T42.3X6
Phenobarbitone	T42.3X1	T42.3X2	T42.3X3	T42.3X4	T42.3X5	T42.3X6
Phenobutiodil	T50.8X1	T50.8X2	T50.8X3	T50.8X4	T50.8X5	T50.8X6
Phenoctide	T49.0X1	T49.0X2	T49.0X3	T49.0X4	T49.0X5	T49.0X6
Phenol	T49.0X1	T49.0X2	T49.0X3	T49.0X4	T49.0X5	T49.0X6
disinfectant	T54.0X1	T54.0X2	T54.0X3	T54.0X4	—	—
in oil injection	T46.8X1	T46.8X2	T46.8X3	T46.8X4	T46.8X5	T46.8X6
medicinal	T49.1X1	T49.1X2	T49.1X3	T49.1X4	T49.1X5	T49.1X6
nonmedicinal NEC	T54.0X1	T54.0X2	T54.0X3	T54.0X4	—	—
pesticide	T60.8X1	T60.8X2	T60.8X3	T60.8X4	—	—
red	T50.8X1	T50.8X2	T50.8X3	T50.8X4	T50.8X5	T50.8X6
Phenolic preparation	T49.1X1	T49.1X2	T49.1X3	T49.1X4	T49.1X5	T49.1X6
Phenolphthalein	T47.2X1	T47.2X2	T47.2X3	T47.2X4	T47.2X5	T47.2X6
Phenolsulfonphthalein	T50.8X1	T50.8X2	T50.8X3	T50.8X4	T50.8X5	T50.8X6
Phenomorphan	T40.2X1	T40.2X2	T40.2X3	T40.2X4	—	—
Phenonyl	T42.3X1	T42.3X2	T42.3X3	T42.3X4	T42.3X5	T42.3X6
Phenoperidine	T40.4X1	T40.4X2	T40.4X3	T40.4X4	—	—
Phenopyrazone	T46.991	T46.992	T46.993	T46.994	T46.995	T46.996
Phenoquin	T50.4X1	T50.4X2	T50.4X3	T50.4X4	T50.4X5	T50.4X6
Phenothiazine (psychotropic) NEC	T43.3X1	T43.3X2	T43.3X3	T43.3X4	T43.3X5	T43.3X6
insecticide	T60.2X1	T60.2X2	T60.2X3	T60.2X4	—	—
Phenothrin	T49.0X1	T49.0X2	T49.0X3	T49.0X4	T49.0X5	T49.0X6
Phenoxybenzamine	T46.7X1	T46.7X2	T46.7X3	T46.7X4	T46.7X5	T46.7X6
Phenoxyethanol	T49.0X1	T49.0X2	T49.0X3	T49.0X4	T49.0X5	T49.0X6
Phenoxymethyl penicillin	T36.0X1	T36.0X2	T36.0X3	T36.0X4	T36.0X5	T36.0X6
Phenprobamate	T42.8X1	T42.8X2	T42.8X3	T42.8X4	T42.8X5	T42.8X6
Phenprocoumon	T45.511	T45.512	T45.513	T45.514	T45.515	T45.516

Substance	Poisoning, Accidental (unintentional)	Poisoning, Intentional Self-harm	Poisoning, Assault	Poisoning, Undetermined	Adverse Effect	Under-dosing
Phensuximide	T42.2X1	T42.2X2	T42.2X3	T42.2X4	T42.2X5	T42.2X6
Phentermine	T50.5X1	T50.5X2	T50.5X3	T50.5X4	T50.5X5	T50.5X6
Phenthicillin	T36.0X1	T36.0X2	T36.0X3	T36.0X4	T36.0X5	T36.0X6
Phentolamine	T46.7X1	T46.7X2	T46.7X3	T46.7X4	T46.7X5	T46.7X6
Phenyl						
butazone	T39.2X1	T39.2X2	T39.2X3	T39.2X4	T39.2X5	T39.2X6
enediamine	T65.3X1	T65.3X2	T65.3X3	T65.3X4	—	—
hydrazine	T65.3X1	T65.3X2	T65.3X3	T65.3X4	—	—
antineoplastic	T45.1X1	T45.1X2	T45.1X3	T45.1X4	T45.1X5	T45.1X6
mercuric compounds — see Mercury						
salicylate	T49.3X1	T49.3X2	T49.3X3	T49.3X4	T49.3X5	T49.3X6
Phenylalanine mustard	T45.1X1	T45.1X2	T45.1X3	T45.1X4	T45.1X5	T45.1X6
Phenylbutazone	T39.2X1	T39.2X2	T39.2X3	T39.2X4	T39.2X5	T39.2X6
Phenylenediamine	T65.3X1	T65.3X2	T65.3X3	T65.3X4	—	—
Phenylephrine	T44.4X1	T44.4X2	T44.4X3	T44.4X4	T44.4X5	T44.4X6
Phenylethylbiguanide	T38.3X1	T38.3X2	T38.3X3	T38.3X4	T38.3X5	T38.3X6
Phenylmercuric						
acetate	T49.0X1	T49.0X2	T49.0X3	T49.0X4	T49.0X5	T49.0X6
borate	T49.0X1	T49.0X2	T49.0X3	T49.0X4	T49.0X5	T49.0X6
nitrate	T49.0X1	T49.0X2	T49.0X3	T49.0X4	T49.0X5	T49.0X6
Phenylmethylbarbitone	T42.3X1	T42.3X2	T42.3X3	T42.3X4	T42.3X5	T42.3X6
Phenylpropanol	T47.5X1	T47.5X2	T47.5X3	T47.5X4	T47.5X5	T47.5X6
Phenylpropanolamine	T44.991	T44.992	T44.993	T44.994	T44.995	T44.996
Phenylsulfthion	T60.0X1	T60.0X2	T60.0X3	T60.0X4	—	—
Phenyltoloxamine	T45.0X1	T45.0X2	T45.0X3	T45.0X4	T45.0X5	T45.0X6
Phenyramidol, phenyramidon	T39.8X1	T39.8X2	T39.8X3	T39.8X4	T39.8X5	T39.8X6
Phenytoin	T42.0X1	T42.0X2	T42.0X3	T42.0X4	T42.0X5	T42.0X6
with Phenobarbital	T42.3X1	T42.3X2	T42.3X3	T42.3X4	T42.3X5	T42.3X6
pHisoHex	T49.2X1	T49.2X2	T49.2X3	T49.2X4	T49.2X5	T49.2X6
Pholcodine	T48.3X1	T48.3X2	T48.3X3	T48.3X4	T48.3X5	T48.3X6
Pholedrine	T46.991	T46.992	T46.993	T46.994	T46.995	T46.996
Phorate	T60.0X1	T60.0X2	T60.0X3	T60.0X4	—	—
Phosdrin	T60.0X1	T60.0X2	T60.0X3	T60.0X4	—	—
Phosfolan	T60.0X1	T60.0X2	T60.0X3	T60.0X4	—	—
Phosgene (gas)	T59.891	T59.892	T59.893	T59.894	—	—
Phosphamidon	T60.0X1	T60.0X2	T60.0X3	T60.0X4	—	—
Phosphate	T65.891	T65.892	T65.893	T65.894	—	—
laxative	T47.4X1	T47.4X2	T47.4X3	T47.4X4	T47.4X5	T47.4X6
organic	T60.0X1	T60.0X2	T60.0X3	T60.0X4	—	—
solvent	T52.91	T52.92	T52.93	T52.94	—	—
tricresyl	T65.891	T65.892	T65.893	T65.894	—	—
Phosphine	T57.1X1	T57.1X2	T57.1X3	T57.1X4	—	—
fumigant	T57.1X1	T57.1X2	T57.1X3	T57.1X4	—	—
Phospholine	T49.5X1	T49.5X2	T49.5X3	T49.5X4	T49.5X5	T49.5X6
Phosphoric acid	T54.2X1	T54.2X2	T54.2X3	T54.2X4	—	—
Phosphorus (compound) NEC	T57.1X1	T57.1X2	T57.1X3	T57.1X4	—	—
pesticide	T60.0X1	T60.0X2	T60.0X3	T60.0X4	—	—
Phthalates	T65.891	T65.892	T65.893	T65.894	—	—
Phthalic anhydride	T65.891	T65.892	T65.893	T65.894	—	—
Phthalimidoglutarimide	T42.6X1	T42.6X2	T42.6X3	T42.6X4	T42.6X5	T42.6X6
Phthalylsulfathiazole	T37.0X1	T37.0X2	T37.0X3	T37.0X4	T37.0X5	T37.0X6
Phylloquinone	T45.7X1	T45.7X2	T45.7X3	T45.7X4	T45.7X5	T45.7X6
Physeptone	T40.3X1	T40.3X2	T40.3X3	T40.3X4	T40.3X5	T40.3X6
Physostigma venenosum	T62.2X1	T62.2X2	T62.2X3	T62.2X4	—	—
Physostigmine	T49.5X1	T49.5X2	T49.5X3	T49.5X4	T49.5X5	T49.5X6
Phytolacca decandra	T62.2X1	T62.2X2	T62.2X3	T62.2X4	—	—
berries	T62.1X1	T62.1X2	T62.1X3	T62.1X4	—	—
Phytomenadione	T45.7X1	T45.7X2	T45.7X3	T45.7X4	T45.7X5	T45.7X6
Phytonadione	T45.7X1	T45.7X2	T45.7X3	T45.7X4	T45.7X5	T45.7X6
Picoperine	T48.3X1	T48.3X2	T48.3X3	T48.3X4	T48.3X5	T48.3X6
Picosulfate (sodium)	T47.2X1	T47.2X2	T47.2X3	T47.2X4	T47.2X5	T47.2X6
Picric (acid)	T54.2X1	T54.2X2	T54.2X3	T54.2X4	—	—
Picrotoxin	T50.7X1	T50.7X2	T50.7X3	T50.7X4	T50.7X5	T50.7X6
Piketoprofen	T49.0X1	T49.0X2	T49.0X3	T49.0X4	T49.0X5	T49.0X6
Pilocarpine	T44.1X1	T44.1X2	T44.1X3	T44.1X4	T44.1X5	T44.1X6
Pilocarpus (jaborandi) extract	T44.1X1	T44.1X2	T44.1X3	T44.1X4	T44.1X5	T44.1X6
Pilsicainide (hydrochloride)	T46.2X1	T46.2X2	T46.2X3	T46.2X4	T46.2X5	T46.2X6
Pimaricin	T36.7X1	T36.7X2	T36.7X3	T36.7X4	T36.7X5	T36.7X6
Pimeclone	T50.7X1	T50.7X2	T50.7X3	T50.7X4	T50.7X5	T50.7X6
Pimelic ketone	T52.8X1	T52.8X2	T52.8X3	T52.8X4	—	—
Pimethixene	T45.0X1	T45.0X2	T45.0X3	T45.0X4	T45.0X5	T45.0X6
Piminodine	T40.2X1	T40.2X2	T40.2X3	T40.2X4	T40.2X5	T40.2X6
Pimozide	T43.591	T43.592	T43.593	T43.594	T43.595	T43.596
Pinacidil	T46.5X1	T46.5X2	T46.5X3	T46.5X4	T46.5X5	T46.5X6
Pinaverium bromide	T44.3X1	T44.3X2	T44.3X3	T44.3X4	T44.3X5	T44.3X6
Pinazepam	T42.4X1	T42.4X2	T42.4X3	T42.4X4	T42.4X5	T42.4X6
Pindolol	T44.7X1	T44.7X2	T44.7X3	T44.7X4	T44.7X5	T44.7X6
Pindone	T60.4X1	T60.4X2	T60.4X3	T60.4X4	—	—
Pine oil (disinfectant)	T65.891	T65.892	T65.893	T65.894	—	—

Substance	Poisoning, Accidental (unintentional)	Poisoning, Intentional Self-harm	Poisoning, Assault	Poisoning, Undetermined	Adverse Effect	Under-dosing
Pinkroot	T37.4X1	T37.4X2	T37.4X3	T37.4X4	T37.4X5	T37.4X6
Pipadone	T40.2X1	T40.2X2	T40.2X3	T40.2X4	—	—
Pipamazine	T45.0X1	T45.0X2	T45.0X3	T45.0X4	T45.0X5	T45.0X6
Pipamperone	T43.4X1	T43.4X2	T43.4X3	T43.4X4	T43.4X5	T43.4X6
Pipazetate	T48.3X1	T48.3X2	T48.3X3	T48.3X4	T48.3X5	T48.3X6
Pipemidic acid	T37.8X1	T37.8X2	T37.8X3	T37.8X4	T37.8X5	T37.8X6
Pipenzolate bromide	T44.3X1	T44.3X2	T44.3X3	T44.3X4	T44.3X5	T44.3X6
Piperacetazine	T43.3X1	T43.3X2	T43.3X3	T43.3X4	T43.3X5	T43.3X6
Piperacillin	T36.0X1	T36.0X2	T36.0X3	T36.0X4	T36.0X5	T36.0X6
Piperazine	T37.4X1	T37.4X2	T37.4X3	T37.4X4	T37.4X5	T37.4X6
estrone sulfate	T38.5X1	T38.5X2	T38.5X3	T38.5X4	T38.5X5	T38.5X6
Piper cubeba	T62.2X1	T62.2X2	T62.2X3	T62.2X4	—	—
Piperidione	T48.3X1	T48.3X2	T48.3X3	T48.3X4	T48.3X5	T48.3X6
Piperidolate	T44.3X1	T44.3X2	T44.3X3	T44.3X4	T44.3X5	T44.3X6
Piperocaine	T41.3X1	T41.3X2	T41.3X3	T41.3X4	T41.3X5	T41.3X6
infiltration (subcutaneous)	T41.3X1	T41.3X2	T41.3X3	T41.3X4	T41.3X5	T41.3X6
nerve block (peripheral) (plexus)	T41.3X1	T41.3X2	T41.3X3	T41.3X4	T41.3X5	T41.3X6
topical (surface)	T41.3X1	T41.3X2	T41.3X3	T41.3X4	T41.3X5	T41.3X6
Piperonyl butoxide	T60.8X1	T60.8X2	T60.8X3	T60.8X4	—	—
Pipethanate	T44.3X1	T44.3X2	T44.3X3	T44.3X4	T44.3X5	T44.3X6
Pipobroman	T45.1X1	T45.1X2	T45.1X3	T45.1X4	T45.1X5	T45.1X6
Pipotiazine	T43.3X1	T43.3X2	T43.3X3	T43.3X4	T43.3X5	T43.3X6
Pipoxizine	T45.0X1	T45.0X2	T45.0X3	T45.0X4	T45.0X5	T45.0X6
Pipradrol	T43.691	T43.692	T43.693	T43.694	T43.695	T43.696
Piprinhydrinate	T45.0X1	T45.0X2	T45.0X3	T45.0X4	T45.0X5	T45.0X6
Pirarubicin	T45.1X1	T45.1X2	T45.1X3	T45.1X4	T45.1X5	T45.1X6
Pirazinamide	T37.1X1	T37.1X2	T37.1X3	T37.1X4	T37.1X5	T37.1X6
Pirbuterol	T48.6X1	T48.6X2	T48.6X3	T48.6X4	T48.6X5	T48.6X6
Pirenzepine	T47.1X1	T47.1X2	T47.1X3	T47.1X4	T47.1X5	T47.1X6
Piretanide	T50.1X1	T50.1X2	T50.1X3	T50.1X4	T50.1X5	T50.1X6
Piribedil	T42.8X1	T42.8X2	T42.8X3	T42.8X4	T42.8X5	T42.8X6
Piridoxilate	T46.3X1	T46.3X2	T46.3X3	T46.3X4	T46.3X5	T46.3X6
Piritramide	T40.4X1	T40.4X2	T40.4X3	T40.4X4	—	—
Piromidic acid	T37.8X1	T37.8X2	T37.8X3	T37.8X4	T37.8X5	T37.8X6
Piroxicam	T39.391	T39.392	T39.393	T39.394	T39.395	T39.396
beta-cyclodextrin complex	T39.8X1	T39.8X2	T39.8X3	T39.8X4	T39.8X5	T39.8X6
Pirozadil	T46.6X1	T46.6X2	T46.6X3	T46.6X4	T46.6X5	T46.6X6
Piscidia (bark) (erythrina)	T39.8X1	T39.8X2	T39.8X3	T39.8X4	T39.8X5	T39.8X6
Pitch	T65.891	T65.892	T65.893	T65.894	—	—
Pitkin's solution	T41.3X1	T41.3X2	T41.3X3	T41.3X4	T41.3X5	T41.3X6
Pitocin	T48.0X1	T48.0X2	T48.0X3	T48.0X4	T48.0X5	T48.0X6
Pitressin (tannate)	T38.891	T38.892	T38.893	T38.894	T38.895	T38.896
Pituitary extracts (posterior)	T38.891	T38.892	T38.893	T38.894	T38.895	T38.896
anterior	T38.811	T38.812	T38.813	T38.814	T38.815	T38.816
Pituitrin	T38.891	T38.892	T38.893	T38.894	T38.895	T38.896
Pivampicillin	T36.0X1	T36.0X2	T36.0X3	T36.0X4	T36.0X5	T36.0X6
Pivmecillinam	T36.0X1	T36.0X2	T36.0X3	T36.0X4	T36.0X5	T36.0X6
Placental hormone	T38.891	T38.892	T38.893	T38.894	T38.895	T38.896
Placidyl	T42.6X1	T42.6X2	T42.6X3	T42.6X4	T42.6X5	T42.6X6
Plague vaccine	T50.A91	T50.A92	T50.A93	T50.A94	T50.A95	T50.A96
Plant						
food or fertilizer NEC	T65.891	T65.892	T65.893	T65.894	—	—
containing herbicide	T60.3X1	T60.3X2	T60.3X3	T60.3X4	—	—
noxious, used as food	T62.2X1	T62.2X2	T62.2X3	T62.2X4	—	—
berries	T62.1X1	T62.1X2	T62.1X3	T62.1X4	—	—
seeds	T62.2X1	T62.2X2	T62.2X3	T62.2X4	—	—
specified type NEC	T62.2X1	T62.2X2	T62.2X3	T62.2X4	—	—
Plasma	T45.8X1	T45.8X2	T45.8X3	T45.8X4	T45.8X5	T45.8X6
expander NEC	T45.8X1	T45.8X2	T45.8X3	T45.8X4	T45.8X5	T45.8X6
protein fraction (human)	T45.8X1	T45.8X2	T45.8X3	T45.8X4	T45.8X5	T45.8X6
Plasmanate	T45.8X1	T45.8X2	T45.8X3	T45.8X4	T45.8X5	T45.8X6
Plasminogen (tissue) activator	T45.611	T45.612	T45.613	T45.614	T45.615	T45.616
Plaster dressing	T49.3X1	T49.3X2	T49.3X3	T49.3X4	T49.3X5	T49.3X6
Plastic dressing	T49.3X1	T49.3X2	T49.3X3	T49.3X4	T49.3X5	T49.3X6
Plegicil	T43.3X1	T43.3X2	T43.3X3	T43.3X4	T43.3X5	T43.3X6
Plicamycin	T45.1X1	T45.1X2	T45.1X3	T45.1X4	T45.1X5	T45.1X6
Podophyllotoxin	T49.8X1	T49.8X2	T49.8X3	T49.8X4	T49.8X5	T49.8X6
Podophyllum (resin)	T49.4X1	T49.4X2	T49.4X3	T49.4X4	T49.4X5	T49.4X6
Poisonous berries	T62.1X1	T62.1X2	T62.1X3	T62.1X4	—	—
Poison NEC	T65.91	T65.92	T65.93	T65.94	—	—
Pokeweed (any part)	T62.2X1	T62.2X2	T62.2X3	T62.2X4	—	—
Poldine metilsulfate	T44.3X1	T44.3X2	T44.3X3	T44.3X4	T44.3X5	T44.3X6
Polidexide (sulfate)	T46.6X1	T46.6X2	T46.6X3	T46.6X4	T46.6X5	T46.6X6
Polidocanol	T46.8X1	T46.8X2	T46.8X3	T46.8X4	T46.8X5	T46.8X6
Poliomyelitis vaccine	T50.B91	T50.B92	T50.B93	T50.B94	T50.B95	T50.B96
Polish (car) (floor) (furniture) (metal) (porcelain) (silver)	T65.891	T65.892	T65.893	T65.894	—	—
abrasive	T65.891	T65.892	T65.893	T65.894	—	—
porcelain	T65.891	T65.892	T65.893	T65.894	—	—
Poloxalkol	T47.4X1	T47.4X2	T47.4X3	T47.4X4	T47.4X5	T47.4X6
Poloxamer	T47.4X1	T47.4X2	T47.4X3	T47.4X4	T47.4X5	T47.4X6

Additional Character May Be Required — Refer to the Tabular List for Character Selection   ▽ Subterms under main terms may continue to next column or page

Substance	Poisoning, Accidental (unintentional)	Poisoning, Intentional Self-harm	Poisoning, Assault	Poisoning, Undetermined	Adverse Effect	Underdosing
Polyaminostyrene resins	T50.3X1	T50.3X2	T50.3X3	T50.3X4	T50.3X5	T50.3X6
Polycarbophil	T47.4X1	T47.4X2	T47.4X3	T47.4X4	T47.4X5	T47.4X6
Polychlorinated biphenyl	T65.891	T65.892	T65.893	T65.894	—	—
Polycycline	T36.4X1	T36.4X2	T36.4X3	T36.4X4	T36.4X5	T36.4X6
Polyester fumes	T59.891	T59.892	T59.893	T59.894	—	—
Polyester resin hardener	T52.91	T52.92	T52.93	T52.94	—	—
fumes	T59.891	T59.892	T59.893	T59.894	—	—
Polyestradiol phosphate	T38.5X1	T38.5X2	T38.5X3	T38.5X4	T38.5X5	T38.5X6
Polyethanolamine alkyl sulfate	T49.2X1	T49.2X2	T49.2X3	T49.2X4	T49.2X5	T49.2X6
Polyethylene adhesive	T49.3X1	T49.3X2	T49.3X3	T49.3X4	T49.3X5	T49.3X6
Polyferose	T45.4X1	T45.4X2	T45.4X3	T45.4X4	T45.4X5	T45.4X6
Polygeline	T45.8X1	T45.8X2	T45.8X3	T45.8X4	T45.8X5	T45.8X6
Polymyxin	T36.8X1	T36.8X2	T36.8X3	T36.8X4	T36.8X5	T36.8X6
B	T36.8X1	T36.8X2	T36.8X3	T36.8X4	T36.8X5	T36.8X6
ENT agent	T49.6X1	T49.6X2	T49.6X3	T49.6X4	T49.6X5	T49.6X6
ophthalmic preparation	T49.5X1	T49.5X2	T49.5X3	T49.5X4	T49.5X5	T49.5X6
topical NEC	T49.0X1	T49.0X2	T49.0X3	T49.0X4	T49.0X5	T49.0X6
E sulfate (eye preparation)	T49.5X1	T49.5X2	T49.5X3	T49.5X4	T49.5X5	T49.5X6
Polynoxylin	T49.0X1	T49.0X2	T49.0X3	T49.0X4	T49.0X5	T49.0X6
Polyoestradiol phosphate	T38.5X1	T38.5X2	T38.5X3	T38.5X4	T38.5X5	T38.5X6
Polyoxymethyleneurea	T49.0X1	T49.0X2	T49.0X3	T49.0X4	T49.0X5	T49.0X6
Polysilane	T47.8X1	T47.8X2	T47.8X3	T47.8X4	T47.8X5	T47.8X6
Polytetrafluoroethylene (inhaled)	T59.891	T59.892	T59.893	T59.894	—	—
Polythiazide	T50.2X1	T50.2X2	T50.2X3	T50.2X4	T50.2X5	T50.2X6
Polyvidone	T45.8X1	T45.8X2	T45.8X3	T45.8X4	T45.8X5	T45.8X6
Polyvinylpyrrolidone	T45.8X1	T45.8X2	T45.8X3	T45.8X4	T45.8X5	T45.8X6
Pontocaine (hydrochloride) (infiltration) (topical)	T41.3X1	T41.3X2	T41.3X3	T41.3X4	T41.3X5	T41.3X6
nerve block (peripheral) (plexus)	T41.3X1	T41.3X2	T41.3X3	T41.3X4	T41.3X5	T41.3X6
spinal	T41.3X1	T41.3X2	T41.3X3	T41.3X4	T41.3X5	T41.3X6
Porfiromycin	T45.1X1	T45.1X2	T45.1X3	T45.1X4	T45.1X5	T45.1X6
Posterior pituitary hormone NEC	T38.891	T38.892	T38.893	T38.894	T38.895	T38.896
Pot	T40.7X1	T40.7X2	T40.7X3	T40.7X4	T40.7X5	T40.7X6
Potash (caustic)	T54.3X1	T54.3X2	T54.3X3	T54.3X4	—	—
Potassic saline injection (lactated)	T50.3X1	T50.3X2	T50.3X3	T50.3X4	T50.3X5	T50.3X6
Potassium-removing resin	T50.3X1	T50.3X2	T50.3X3	T50.3X4	T50.3X5	T50.3X6
Potassium-retaining drug	T50.3X1	T50.3X2	T50.3X3	T50.3X4	T50.3X5	T50.3X6
Potassium (salts) NEC	T50.3X1	T50.3X2	T50.3X3	T50.3X4	T50.3X5	T50.3X6
aminobenzoate	T45.8X1	T45.8X2	T45.8X3	T45.8X4	T45.8X5	T45.8X6
aminosalicylate	T37.1X1	T37.1X2	T37.1X3	T37.1X4	T37.1X5	T37.1X6
antimony ' tartrate'	T37.8X1	T37.8X2	T37.8X3	T37.8X4	T37.8X5	T37.8X6
arsenite (solution)	T57.0X1	T57.0X2	T57.0X3	T57.0X4	—	—
bichromate	T56.2X1	T56.2X2	T56.2X3	T56.2X4	—	—
bisulfate	T47.3X1	T47.3X2	T47.3X3	T47.3X4	T47.3X5	T47.3X6
bromide	T42.6X1	T42.6X2	T42.6X3	T42.6X4	T42.6X5	T42.6X6
canrenoate	T50.0X1	T50.0X2	T50.0X3	T50.0X4	T50.0X5	T50.0X6
carbonate	T54.3X1	T54.3X2	T54.3X3	T54.3X4	—	—
chlorate NEC	T65.891	T65.892	T65.893	T65.894	—	—
chloride	T50.3X1	T50.3X2	T50.3X3	T50.3X4	T50.3X5	T50.3X6
citrate	T50.991	T50.992	T50.993	T50.994	T50.995	T50.996
cyanide	T65.0X1	T65.0X2	T65.0X3	T65.0X4	—	—
ferric hexacyanoferrate (medicinal)	T50.6X1	T50.6X2	T50.6X3	T50.6X4	T50.6X5	T50.6X6
nonmedicinal	T65.891	T65.892	T65.893	T65.894	—	—
Fluoride	T57.8X1	T57.8X2	T57.8X3	T57.8X4	—	—
glucaldrate	T47.1X1	T47.1X2	T47.1X3	T47.1X4	T47.1X5	T47.1X6
hydroxide	T54.3X1	T54.3X2	T54.3X3	T54.3X4	—	—
iodate	T49.0X1	T49.0X2	T49.0X3	T49.0X4	T49.0X5	T49.0X6
iodide	T48.4X1	T48.4X2	T48.4X3	T48.4X4	T48.4X5	T48.4X6
nitrate	T57.8X1	T57.8X2	T57.8X3	T57.8X4	—	—
oxalate	T65.891	T65.892	T65.893	T65.894	—	—
perchlorate (nonmedicinal) NEC	T65.891	T65.892	T65.893	T65.894	—	—
antithyroid	T38.2X1	T38.2X2	T38.2X3	T38.2X4	T38.2X5	T38.2X6
medicinal	T38.2X1	T38.2X2	T38.2X3	T38.2X4	T38.2X5	T38.2X6
Permanganate (nonmedicinal)	T65.891	T65.892	T65.893	T65.894	—	—
medicinal	T49.0X1	T49.0X2	T49.0X3	T49.0X4	T49.0X5	T49.0X6
sulfate	T47.2X1	T47.2X2	T47.2X3	T47.2X4	T47.2X5	T47.2X6
Povidone	T45.8X1	T45.8X2	T45.8X3	T45.8X4	T45.8X5	T45.8X6
iodine	T49.0X1	T49.0X2	T49.0X3	T49.0X4	T49.0X5	T49.0X6
Practolol	T44.7X1	T44.7X2	T44.7X3	T44.7X4	T44.7X5	T44.7X6
Prajmalium bitartrate	T46.2X1	T46.2X2	T46.2X3	T46.2X4	T46.2X5	T46.2X6
Pralidoxime (iodide)	T50.6X1	T50.6X2	T50.6X3	T50.6X4	T50.6X5	T50.6X6
chloride	T50.6X1	T50.6X2	T50.6X3	T50.6X4	T50.6X5	T50.6X6
Pramiverine	T44.3X1	T44.3X2	T44.3X3	T44.3X4	T44.3X5	T44.3X6
Pramocaine	T49.1X1	T49.1X2	T49.1X3	T49.1X4	T49.1X5	T49.1X6
Pramoxine	T49.1X1	T49.1X2	T49.1X3	T49.1X4	T49.1X5	T49.1X6

Substance	Poisoning, Accidental (unintentional)	Poisoning, Intentional Self-harm	Poisoning, Assault	Poisoning, Undetermined	Adverse Effect	Underdosing
Prasterone	T38.7X1	T38.7X2	T38.7X3	T38.7X4	T38.7X5	T38.7X6
Pravastatin	T46.6X1	T46.6X2	T46.6X3	T46.6X4	T46.6X5	T46.6X6
Prazepam	T42.4X1	T42.4X2	T42.4X3	T42.4X4	T42.4X5	T42.4X6
Praziquantel	T37.4X1	T37.4X2	T37.4X3	T37.4X4	T37.4X5	T37.4X6
Prazitone	T43.291	T43.292	T43.293	T43.294	T43.295	T43.296
Prazosin	T44.6X1	T44.6X2	T44.6X3	T44.6X4	T44.6X5	T44.6X6
Prednicarbate	T49.0X1	T49.0X2	T49.0X3	T49.0X4	T49.0X5	T49.0X6
Prednimustine	T45.1X1	T45.1X2	T45.1X3	T45.1X4	T45.1X5	T45.1X6
Prednisolone	T38.0X1	T38.0X2	T38.0X3	T38.0X4	T38.0X5	T38.0X6
ENT agent	T49.6X1	T49.6X2	T49.6X3	T49.6X4	T49.6X5	T49.6X6
ophthalmic preparation	T49.5X1	T49.5X2	T49.5X3	T49.5X4	T49.5X5	T49.5X6
steaglate	T49.0X1	T49.0X2	T49.0X3	T49.0X4	T49.0X5	T49.0X6
topical NEC	T49.0X1	T49.0X2	T49.0X3	T49.0X4	T49.0X5	T49.0X6
Prednisone	T38.0X1	T38.0X2	T38.0X3	T38.0X4	T38.0X5	T38.0X6
Prednylidene	T38.0X1	T38.0X2	T38.0X3	T38.0X4	T38.0X5	T38.0X6
Pregnandiol	T38.5X1	T38.5X2	T38.5X3	T38.5X4	T38.5X5	T38.5X6
Pregneninolone	T38.5X1	T38.5X2	T38.5X3	T38.5X4	T38.5X5	T38.5X6
Preludin	T43.691	T43.692	T43.693	T43.694	T43.695	T43.696
Premarin	T38.5X1	T38.5X2	T38.5X3	T38.5X4	T38.5X5	T38.5X6
Premedication anesthetic	T41.201	T41.202	T41.203	T41.204	T41.205	T41.206
Prenalterol	T44.5X1	T44.5X2	T44.5X3	T44.5X4	T44.5X5	T44.5X6
Prenoxdiazine	T48.3X1	T48.3X2	T48.3X3	T48.3X4	T48.3X5	T48.3X6
Prenylamine	T46.3X1	T46.3X2	T46.3X3	T46.3X4	T46.3X5	T46.3X6
Preparation H	T49.8X1	T49.8X2	T49.8X3	T49.8X4	T49.8X5	T49.8X6
Preparation, local	T49.4X1	T49.4X2	T49.4X3	T49.4X4	T49.4X5	T49.4X6
Preservative (nonmedicinal)	T65.891	T65.892	T65.893	T65.894	—	—
medicinal	T50.901	T50.902	T50.903	T50.904	T50.905	T50.906
wood	T60.91	T60.92	T60.93	T60.94	—	—
Prethcamide	T50.7X1	T50.7X2	T50.7X3	T50.7X4	T50.7X5	T50.7X6
Pride of China	T62.2X1	T62.2X2	T62.2X3	T62.2X4	—	—
Pridinol	T44.3X1	T44.3X2	T44.3X3	T44.3X4	T44.3X5	T44.3X6
Prifinium bromide	T44.3X1	T44.3X2	T44.3X3	T44.3X4	T44.3X5	T44.3X6
Prilocaine	T41.3X1	T41.3X2	T41.3X3	T41.3X4	T41.3X5	T41.3X6
infiltration (subcutaneous)	T41.3X1	T41.3X2	T41.3X3	T41.3X4	T41.3X5	T41.3X6
nerve block (peripheral) (plexus)	T41.3X1	T41.3X2	T41.3X3	T41.3X4	T41.3X5	T41.3X6
regional	T41.3X1	T41.3X2	T41.3X3	T41.3X4	T41.3X5	T41.3X6
Primaquine	T37.2X1	T37.2X2	T37.2X3	T37.2X4	T37.2X5	T37.2X6
Primidone	T42.6X1	T42.6X2	T42.6X3	T42.6X4	T42.6X5	T42.6X6
Primula (veris)	T62.2X1	T62.2X2	T62.2X3	T62.2X4	—	—
Prinadol	T40.2X1	T40.2X2	T40.2X3	T40.2X4	T40.2X5	T40.2X6
Priscol, Priscoline	T46.6X1	T46.6X2	T46.6X3	T46.6X4	T46.6X5	T46.6X6
Pristinamycin	T36.3X1	T36.3X2	T36.3X3	T36.3X4	T36.3X5	T36.3X6
Privet	T62.2X1	T62.2X2	T62.2X3	T62.2X4	—	—
berries	T62.1X1	T62.1X2	T62.1X3	T62.1X4	—	—
Privine	T44.4X1	T44.4X2	T44.4X3	T44.4X4	T44.4X5	T44.4X6
Pro-Banthine	T44.3X1	T44.3X2	T44.3X3	T44.3X4	T44.3X5	T44.3X6
Probarbital	T42.3X1	T42.3X2	T42.3X3	T42.3X4	T42.3X5	T42.3X6
Probenecid	T50.4X1	T50.4X2	T50.4X3	T50.4X4	T50.4X5	T50.4X6
Probucol	T46.6X1	T46.6X2	T46.6X3	T46.6X4	T46.6X5	T46.6X6
Procainamide	T46.2X1	T46.2X2	T46.2X3	T46.2X4	T46.2X5	T46.2X6
Procaine	T41.3X1	T41.3X2	T41.3X3	T41.3X4	T41.3X5	T41.3X6
benzylpenicillin	T36.0X1	T36.0X2	T36.0X3	T36.0X4	T36.0X5	T36.0X6
nerve block (peripheral) (plexus)	T41.3X1	T41.3X2	T41.3X3	T41.3X4	T41.3X5	T41.3X6
penicillin G	T36.0X1	T36.0X2	T36.0X3	T36.0X4	T36.0X5	T36.0X6
regional	T41.3X1	T41.3X2	T41.3X3	T41.3X4	T41.3X5	T41.3X6
spinal	T41.3X1	T41.3X2	T41.3X3	T41.3X4	T41.3X5	T41.3X6
Procalmidol	T43.591	T43.592	T43.593	T43.594	T43.595	T43.596
Procarbazine	T45.1X1	T45.1X2	T45.1X3	T45.1X4	T45.1X5	T45.1X6
Procaterol	T44.5X1	T44.5X2	T44.5X3	T44.5X4	T44.5X5	T44.5X6
Prochlorperazine	T43.3X1	T43.3X2	T43.3X3	T43.3X4	T43.3X5	T43.3X6
Procyclidine	T44.3X1	T44.3X2	T44.3X3	T44.3X4	T44.3X5	T44.3X6
Producer gas	T58.8X1	T58.8X2	T58.8X3	T58.8X4	—	—
Profadol	T40.4X1	T40.4X2	T40.4X3	T40.4X4	T40.4X5	T40.4X6
Profenamine	T44.3X1	T44.3X2	T44.3X3	T44.3X4	T44.3X5	T44.3X6
Profenil	T44.3X1	T44.3X2	T44.3X3	T44.3X4	T44.3X5	T44.3X6
Proflavine	T49.0X1	T49.0X2	T49.0X3	T49.0X4	T49.0X5	T49.0X6
Progabide	T42.6X1	T42.6X2	T42.6X3	T42.6X4	T42.6X5	T42.6X6
Progesterone	T38.5X1	T38.5X2	T38.5X3	T38.5X4	T38.5X5	T38.5X6
Progestin	T38.5X1	T38.5X2	T38.5X3	T38.5X4	T38.5X5	T38.5X6
oral contraceptive	T38.4X1	T38.4X2	T38.4X3	T38.4X4	T38.4X5	T38.4X6
Progestogen NEC	T38.5X1	T38.5X2	T38.5X3	T38.5X4	T38.5X5	T38.5X6
Progestone	T38.5X1	T38.5X2	T38.5X3	T38.5X4	T38.5X5	T38.5X6
Proglumide	T47.1X1	T47.1X2	T47.1X3	T47.1X4	T47.1X5	T47.1X6
Proguanil	T37.2X1	T37.2X2	T37.2X3	T37.2X4	T37.2X5	T37.2X6
Prolactin	T38.811	T38.812	T38.813	T38.814	T38.815	T38.816
Prolintane	T43.691	T43.692	T43.693	T43.694	T43.695	T43.696
Proloid	T38.1X1	T38.1X2	T38.1X3	T38.1X4	T38.1X5	T38.1X6
Proluton	T38.5X1	T38.5X2	T38.5X3	T38.5X4	T38.5X5	T38.5X6
Promacetin	T37.1X1	T37.1X2	T37.1X3	T37.1X4	T37.1X5	T37.1X6
Promazine	T43.3X1	T43.3X2	T43.3X3	T43.3X4	T43.3X5	T43.3X6
Promedol	T40.2X1	T40.2X2	T40.2X3	T40.2X4	—	—

Table of Drugs and Chemicals

Substance	Poisoning, Accidental (unintentional)	Poisoning, Intentional Self-harm	Poisoning, Assault	Poisoning, Undetermined	Adverse Effect	Under-dosing
Promegestone	T38.5X1	T38.5X2	T38.5X3	T38.5X4	T38.5X5	T38.5X6
Promethazine (teoclate)	T43.3X1	T43.3X2	T43.3X3	T43.3X4	T43.3X5	T43.3X6
Promin	T37.1X1	T37.1X2	T37.1X3	T37.1X4	T37.1X5	T37.1X6
Pronase	T45.3X1	T45.3X2	T45.3X3	T45.3X4	T45.3X5	T45.3X6
Pronestyl (hydrochloride)	T46.2X1	T46.2X2	T46.2X3	T46.2X4	T46.2X5	T46.2X6
Pronetalol	T44.7X1	T44.7X2	T44.7X3	T44.7X4	T44.7X5	T44.7X6
Prontosil	T37.0X1	T37.0X2	T37.0X3	T37.0X4	T37.0X5	T37.0X6
Propachlor	T60.3X1	T60.3X2	T60.3X3	T60.3X4	—	—
Propafenone	T46.2X1	T46.2X2	T46.2X3	T46.2X4	—	T46.2X6
Propallylonal	T42.3X1	T42.3X2	T42.3X3	T42.3X4	T42.3X5	T42.3X6
Propamidine	T49.0X1	T49.0X2	T49.0X3	T49.0X4	T49.0X5	T49.0X6
Propane (distributed in mobile container)	T59.891	T59.892	T59.893	T59.894	—	—
distributed through pipes	T59.891	T59.892	T59.893	T59.894	—	—
incomplete combustion	T58.11	T58.12	T58.13	T58.14	—	—
Propanidid	T41.291	T41.292	T41.293	T41.294	T41.295	T41.296
Propanil	T60.3X1	T60.3X2	T60.3X3	T60.3X4	—	—
Propantheline	T44.3X1	T44.3X2	T44.3X3	T44.3X4	T44.3X5	T44.3X6
bromide	T44.3X1	T44.3X2	T44.3X3	T44.3X4	T44.3X5	T44.3X6
Proparacaine	T41.3X1	T41.3X2	T41.3X3	T41.3X4	T41.3X5	T41.3X6
Propatylnitrate	T46.3X1	T46.3X2	T46.3X3	T46.3X4	T46.3X5	T46.3X6
Propicillin	T36.0X1	T36.0X2	T36.0X3	T36.0X4	T36.0X5	T36.0X6
Propiolactone	T49.0X1	T49.0X2	T49.0X3	T49.0X4	T49.0X5	T49.0X6
Propiomazine	T45.0X1	T45.0X2	T45.0X3	T45.0X4	T45.0X5	T45.0X6
Propionaldehyde (medicinal)	T42.6X1	T42.6X2	T42.6X3	T42.6X4	T42.6X5	T42.6X6
Propionate (calcium) (sodium)	T49.0X1	T49.0X2	T49.0X3	T49.0X4	T49.0X5	T49.0X6
Propion gel	T49.0X1	T49.0X2	T49.0X3	T49.0X4	T49.0X5	T49.0X6
Propitocaine	T41.3X1	T41.3X2	T41.3X3	T41.3X4	T41.3X5	T41.3X6
infiltration (subcutaneous)	T41.3X1	T41.3X2	T41.3X3	T41.3X4	T41.3X5	T41.3X6
nerve block (peripheral) (plexus)	T41.3X1	T41.3X2	T41.3X3	T41.3X4	T41.3X5	T41.3X6
Propofol	T41.291	T41.292	T41.293	T41.294	T41.295	T41.296
Propoxur	T60.0X1	T60.0X2	T60.0X3	T60.0X4	—	—
Propoxycaine	T41.3X1	T41.3X2	T41.3X3	T41.3X4	T41.3X5	T41.3X6
infiltration (subcutaneous)	T41.3X1	T41.3X2	T41.3X3	T41.3X4	T41.3X5	T41.3X6
nerve block (peripheral) (plexus)	T41.3X1	T41.3X2	T41.3X3	T41.3X4	T41.3X5	T41.3X6
topical (surface)	T41.3X1	T41.3X2	T41.3X3	T41.3X4	T41.3X5	T41.3X6
Propoxyphene	T40.4X1	T40.4X2	T40.4X3	T40.4X4	T40.4X5	T40.4X6
Propranolol	T44.7X1	T44.7X2	T44.7X3	T44.7X4	T44.7X5	T44.7X6
Propyl						
alcohol	T51.3X1	T51.3X2	T51.3X3	T51.3X4	—	—
carbinol	T51.3X1	T51.3X2	T51.3X3	T51.3X4	—	—
hexadrine	T44.4X1	T44.4X2	T44.4X3	T44.4X4	T44.4X5	T44.4X6
iodone	T50.8X1	T50.8X2	T50.8X3	T50.8X4	T50.8X5	T50.8X6
thiouracil	T38.2X1	T38.2X2	T38.2X3	T38.2X4	T38.2X5	T38.2X6
Propylaminophenothiazine	T43.3X1	T43.3X2	T43.3X3	T43.3X4	T43.3X5	T43.3X6
Propylene	T59.891	T59.892	T59.893	T59.894	—	—
Propylhexedrine	T48.5X1	T48.5X2	T48.5X3	T48.5X4	T48.5X5	T48.5X6
Propyliodone	T50.8X1	T50.8X2	T50.8X3	T50.8X4	T50.8X5	T50.8X6
Propylparaben (ophthalmic)	T49.5X1	T49.5X2	T49.5X3	T49.5X4	T49.5X5	T49.5X6
Propylthiouracil	T38.2X1	T38.2X2	T38.2X3	T38.2X4	T38.2X5	T38.2X6
Propyphenazone	T39.2X1	T39.2X2	T39.2X3	T39.2X4	T39.2X5	T39.2X6
Proquazone	T39.391	T39.392	T39.393	T39.394	T39.395	T39.396
Proscillaridin	T46.0X1	T46.0X2	T46.0X3	T46.0X4	T46.0X5	T46.0X6
Prostacyclin	T45.521	T45.522	T45.523	T45.524	T45.525	T45.526
Prostaglandin (I2)	T45.521	T45.522	T45.523	T45.524	T45.525	T45.526
E1	T46.7X1	T46.7X2	T46.7X3	T46.7X4	T46.7X5	T46.7X6
E2	T48.0X1	T48.0X2	T48.0X3	T48.0X4	T48.0X5	T48.0X6
F2 alpha	T48.0X1	T48.0X2	T48.0X3	T48.0X4	T48.0X5	T48.0X6
Prostigmin	T44.0X1	T44.0X2	T44.0X3	T44.0X4	T44.0X5	T44.0X6
Prosultiamine	T45.2X1	T45.2X2	T45.2X3	T45.2X4	T45.2X5	T45.2X6
Protamine sulfate	T45.7X1	T45.7X2	T45.7X3	T45.7X4	T45.7X5	T45.7X6
zinc insulin	T38.3X1	T38.3X2	T38.3X3	T38.3X4	T38.3X5	T38.3X6
Protease	T47.5X1	T47.5X2	T47.5X3	T47.5X4	T47.5X5	T47.5X6
Protectant, skin NEC	T49.3X1	T49.3X2	T49.3X3	T49.3X4	T49.3X5	T49.3X6
Protein hydrolysate	T50.991	T50.992	T50.993	T50.994	T50.995	T50.996
Prothiaden — see Dothiepin hydrochloride						
Prothionamide	T37.1X1	T37.1X2	T37.1X3	T37.1X4	T37.1X5	T37.1X6
Prothipendyl	T43.591	T43.592	T43.593	T43.594	T43.595	T43.596
Prothoate	T60.0X1	T60.0X2	T60.0X3	T60.0X4	—	—
Prothrombin						
activator	T45.7X1	T45.7X2	T45.7X3	T45.7X4	T45.7X5	T45.7X6
synthesis inhibitor	T45.511	T45.512	T45.513	T45.514	T45.515	T45.516
Protionamide	T37.1X1	T37.1X2	T37.1X3	T37.1X4	T37.1X5	T37.1X6
Protirelin	T38.891	T38.892	T38.893	T38.894	T38.895	T38.896
Protokylol	T48.6X1	T48.6X2	T48.6X3	T48.6X4	T48.6X5	T48.6X6
Protopam	T50.6X1	T50.6X2	T50.6X3	T50.6X4	T50.6X5	T50.6X6
Protoveratrine(s) (A) (B)	T46.5X1	T46.5X2	T46.5X3	T46.5X4	T46.5X5	T46.5X6
Protriptyline	T43.011	T43.012	T43.013	T43.014	T43.015	T43.016
Provera	T38.5X1	T38.5X2	T38.5X3	T38.5X4	T38.5X5	T38.5X6
Provitamin A	T45.2X1	T45.2X2	T45.2X3	T45.2X4	T45.2X5	T45.2X6
Proxibarbal	T42.3X1	T42.3X2	T42.3X3	T42.3X4	T42.3X5	T42.3X6
Proxymetacaine	T41.3X1	T41.3X2	T41.3X3	T41.3X4	T41.3X5	T41.3X6
Proxyphylline	T48.6X1	T48.6X2	T48.6X3	T48.6X4	T48.6X5	T48.6X6
Prozac — see Fluoxetine hydrochloride						
Prunus						
laurocerasus	T62.2X1	T62.2X2	T62.2X3	T62.2X4	—	—
virginiana	T62.2X1	T62.2X2	T62.2X3	T62.2X4	—	—
Prussian blue						
commercial	T65.891	T65.892	T65.893	T65.894	—	—
therapeutic	T50.6X1	T50.6X2	T50.6X3	T50.6X4	T50.6X5	T50.6X6
Prussic acid	T65.0X1	T65.0X2	T65.0X3	T65.0X4	—	—
vapor	T57.3X1	T57.3X2	T57.3X3	T57.3X4	—	—
Pseudoephedrine	T44.991	T44.992	T44.993	T44.994	T44.995	T44.996
Psilocin	T40.991	T40.992	T40.993	T40.994	—	—
Psilocybin	T40.991	T40.992	T40.993	T40.994	—	—
Psilocybine	T40.991	T40.992	T40.993	T40.994	—	—
Psoralene (nonmedicinal)	T65.891	T65.892	T65.893	T65.894	—	—
Psoralens (medicinal)	T50.991	T50.992	T50.993	T50.994	T50.995	T50.996
PSP (phenolsulfonphthalein)	T50.8X1	T50.8X2	T50.8X3	T50.8X4	T50.8X5	T50.8X6
Psychodysleptic drug NEC	T40.901	T40.902	T40.903	T40.904	T40.905	T40.906
Psychostimulant	T43.601	T43.602	T43.603	T43.604	T43.605	T43.606
amphetamine	T43.621	T43.622	T43.623	T43.624	T43.625	T43.626
caffeine	T43.611	T43.612	T43.613	T43.614	T43.615	T43.616
methylphenidate	T43.631	T43.632	T43.633	T43.634	T43.635	T43.636
specified NEC	T43.691	T43.692	T43.693	T43.694	T43.695	T43.696
Psychotherapeutic drug NEC	T43.91	T43.92	T43.93	T43.94	T43.95	T43.96
antidepressants — see also Antidepressant	T43.201	T43.202	T43.203	T43.204	T43.205	T43.206
specified NEC	T43.8X1	T43.8X2	T43.8X3	T43.8X4	T43.8X5	T43.8X6
tranquilizers NEC	T43.501	T43.502	T43.503	T43.504	T43.505	T43.506
Psychotomimetic agents	T40.901	T40.902	T40.903	T40.904	T40.905	T40.906
Psychotropic drug NEC	T43.91	T43.92	T43.93	T43.94	T43.95	T43.96
specified NEC	T43.8X1	T43.8X2	T43.8X3	T43.8X4	T43.8X5	T43.8X6
Psyllium hydrophilic mucilloid	T47.4X1	T47.4X2	T47.4X3	T47.4X4	T47.4X5	T47.4X6
Pteroylglutamic acid	T45.8X1	T45.8X2	T45.8X3	T45.8X4	T45.8X5	T45.8X6
Pteroyltriglutamate	T45.1X1	T45.1X2	T45.1X3	T45.1X4	T45.1X5	T45.1X6
PTFE — see Polytetrafluoroethylene						
Pulp						
devitalizing paste	T49.7X1	T49.7X2	T49.7X3	T49.7X4	T49.7X5	T49.7X6
dressing	T49.7X1	T49.7X2	T49.7X3	T49.7X4	T49.7X5	T49.7X6
Pulsatilla	T62.2X1	T62.2X2	T62.2X3	T62.2X4	—	—
Pumpkin seed extract	T37.4X1	T37.4X2	T37.4X3	T37.4X4	T37.4X5	T37.4X6
Purex (bleach)	T54.91	T54.92	T54.93	T54.94	—	—
Purgative NEC — see also Cathartic	T47.4X1	T47.4X2	T47.4X3	T47.4X4	T47.4X5	T47.4X6
Purine analogue (antineoplastic)	T45.1X1	T45.1X2	T45.1X3	T45.1X4	T45.1X5	T45.1X6
Purine diuretics	T50.2X1	T50.2X2	T50.2X3	T50.2X4	T50.2X5	T50.2X6
Purinethol	T45.1X1	T45.1X2	T45.1X3	T45.1X4	T45.1X5	T45.1X6
PVP	T45.8X1	T45.8X2	T45.8X3	T45.8X4	T45.8X5	T45.8X6
Pyrabital	T39.8X1	T39.8X2	T39.8X3	T39.8X4	T39.8X5	T39.8X6
Pyramidon	T39.2X1	T39.2X2	T39.2X3	T39.2X4	T39.2X5	T39.2X6
Pyrantel	T37.4X1	T37.4X2	T37.4X3	T37.4X4	T37.4X5	T37.4X6
Pyrathiazine	T45.0X1	T45.0X2	T45.0X3	T45.0X4	T45.0X5	T45.0X6
Pyrazinamide	T37.1X1	T37.1X2	T37.1X3	T37.1X4	T37.1X5	T37.1X6
Pyrazinoic acid (amide)	T37.1X1	T37.1X2	T37.1X3	T37.1X4	T37.1X5	T37.1X6
Pyrazole (derivatives)	T39.2X1	T39.2X2	T39.2X3	T39.2X4	T39.2X5	T39.2X6
Pyrazolone analgesic NEC	T39.2X1	T39.2X2	T39.2X3	T39.2X4	T39.2X5	T39.2X6
Pyrethrin, pyrethrum (nonmedicinal)	T60.2X1	T60.2X2	T60.2X3	T60.2X4	—	—
Pyrethrum extract	T49.0X1	T49.0X2	T49.0X3	T49.0X4	T49.0X5	T49.0X6
Pyribenzamine	T45.0X1	T45.0X2	T45.0X3	T45.0X4	T45.0X5	T45.0X6
Pyridine	T52.8X1	T52.8X2	T52.8X3	T52.8X4	—	—
aldoxime methiodide	T50.6X1	T50.6X2	T50.6X3	T50.6X4	T50.6X5	T50.6X6
aldoxime methyl chloride	T50.6X1	T50.6X2	T50.6X3	T50.6X4	T50.6X5	T50.6X6
vapor	T59.891	T59.892	T59.893	T59.894	—	—
Pyridium	T39.8X1	T39.8X2	T39.8X3	T39.8X4	T39.8X5	T39.8X6
Pyridostigmine bromide	T44.0X1	T44.0X2	T44.0X3	T44.0X4	T44.0X5	T44.0X6
Pyridoxal phosphate	T45.2X1	T45.2X2	T45.2X3	T45.2X4	T45.2X5	T45.2X6
Pyridoxine	T45.2X1	T45.2X2	T45.2X3	T45.2X4	T45.2X5	T45.2X6
Pyrilamine	T45.0X1	T45.0X2	T45.0X3	T45.0X4	T45.0X5	T45.0X6
Pyrimethamine	T37.2X1	T37.2X2	T37.2X3	T37.2X4	T37.2X5	T37.2X6
with sulfadoxine	T37.2X1	T37.2X2	T37.2X3	T37.2X4	T37.2X5	T37.2X6
Pyrimidine antagonist	T45.1X1	T45.1X2	T45.1X3	T45.1X4	T45.1X5	T45.1X6
Pyriminil	T60.4X1	T60.4X2	T60.4X3	T60.4X4	—	—
Pyrithione zinc	T49.4X1	T49.4X2	T49.4X3	T49.4X4	T49.4X5	T49.4X6
Pyrithyldione	T42.6X1	T42.6X2	T42.6X3	T42.6X4	T42.6X5	T42.6X6

Promegestone — Pyrithyldione

Substance	Poisoning, Accidental (unintentional)	Poisoning, Intentional Self-harm	Poisoning, Assault	Poisoning, Undetermined	Adverse Effect	Under-dosing
Pyrogallic acid	T49.0X1	T49.0X2	T49.0X3	T49.0X4	T49.0X5	T49.0X6
Pyrogallol	T49.0X1	T49.0X2	T49.0X3	T49.0X4	T49.0X5	T49.0X6
Pyroxylin	T49.3X1	T49.3X2	T49.3X3	T49.3X4	T49.3X5	T49.3X6
Pyrrobutamine	T45.0X1	T45.0X2	T45.0X3	T45.0X4	T45.0X5	T45.0X6
Pyrrolizidine alkaloids	T62.8X1	T62.8X2	T62.8X3	T62.8X4	—	—
Pyrvinium chloride	T37.4X1	T37.4X2	T37.4X3	T37.4X4	T37.4X5	T37.4X6
PZI	T38.3X1	T38.3X2	T38.3X3	T38.3X4	T38.3X5	T38.3X6
Quaalude	T42.6X1	T42.6X2	T42.6X3	T42.6X4	T42.6X5	T42.6X6
Quarternary ammonium						
anti-infective	T49.0X1	T49.0X2	T49.0X3	T49.0X4	T49.0X5	T49.0X6
ganglion blocking	T44.2X1	T44.2X2	T44.2X3	T44.2X4	T44.2X5	T44.2X6
parasympatholytic	T44.3X1	T44.3X2	T44.3X3	T44.3X4	T44.3X5	T44.3X6
Quazepam	T42.4X1	T42.4X2	T42.4X3	T42.4X4	T42.4X5	T42.4X6
Quicklime	T54.3X1	T54.3X2	T54.3X3	T54.3X4	—	—
Quillaja extract	T48.4X1	T48.4X2	T48.4X3	T48.4X4	T48.4X5	T48.4X6
Quinacrine	T37.2X1	T37.2X2	T37.2X3	T37.2X4	T37.2X5	T37.2X6
Quinaglute	T46.2X1	T46.2X2	T46.2X3	T46.2X4	T46.2X5	T46.2X6
Quinalbarbital	T42.3X1	T42.3X2	T42.3X3	T42.3X4	T42.3X5	T42.3X6
Quinalbarbitone sodium	T42.3X1	T42.3X2	T42.3X3	T42.3X4	T42.3X5	T42.3X6
Quinalphos	T60.0X1	T60.0X2	T60.0X3	T60.0X4	—	—
Quinapril	T46.4X1	T46.4X2	T46.4X3	T46.4X4	T46.4X5	T46.4X6
Quinestradiol	T38.5X1	T38.5X2	T38.5X3	T38.5X4	T38.5X5	T38.5X6
Quinestradol	T38.5X1	T38.5X2	T38.5X3	T38.5X4	T38.5X5	T38.5X6
Quinestrol	T38.5X1	T38.5X2	T38.5X3	T38.5X4	T38.5X5	T38.5X6
Quinethazone	T50.2X1	T50.2X2	T50.2X3	T50.2X4	T50.2X5	T50.2X6
Quingestanol	T38.4X1	T38.4X2	T38.4X3	T38.4X4	T38.4X5	T38.4X6
Quinidine	T46.2X1	T46.2X2	T46.2X3	T46.2X4	T46.2X5	T46.2X6
Quinine	T37.2X1	T37.2X2	T37.2X3	T37.2X4	T37.2X5	T37.2X6
Quiniobine	T37.8X1	T37.8X2	T37.8X3	T37.8X4	T37.8X5	T37.8X6
Quinisocaine	T49.1X1	T49.1X2	T49.1X3	T49.1X4	T49.1X5	T49.1X6
Quinocide	T37.2X1	T37.2X2	T37.2X3	T37.2X4	T37.2X5	T37.2X6
Quinoline (derivatives) NEC	T37.8X1	T37.8X2	T37.8X3	T37.8X4	T37.8X5	T37.8X6
Quinupramine	T43.011	T43.012	T43.013	T43.014	T43.015	T43.016
Quotane	T41.3X1	T41.3X2	T41.3X3	T41.3X4	T41.3X5	T41.3X6
Rabies						
immune globulin (human)	T50.Z11	T50.Z12	T50.Z13	T50.Z14	T50.Z15	T50.Z16
vaccine	T50.B91	T50.B92	T50.B93	T50.B94	T50.B95	T50.B96
Racemoramide	T40.2X1	T40.2X2	T40.2X3	T40.2X4		
Racemorphan	T40.2X1	T40.2X2	T40.2X3	T40.2X4	T40.2X5	T40.2X6
Racepinefrin	T44.5X1	T44.5X2	T44.5X3	T44.5X4	T44.5X5	T44.5X6
Raclopride	T43.591	T43.592	T43.593	T43.594	T43.595	T43.596
Radiator alcohol	T51.1X1	T51.1X2	T51.1X3	T51.1X4		
Radioactive drug NEC	T50.8X1	T50.8X2	T50.8X3	T50.8X4	T50.8X5	T50.8X6
Radio-opaque (drugs) (materials)	T50.8X1	T50.8X2	T50.8X3	T50.8X4	T50.8X5	T50.8X6
Ramifenazone	T39.2X1	T39.2X2	T39.2X3	T39.2X4	T39.2X5	T39.2X6
Ramipril	T46.4X1	T46.4X2	T46.4X3	T46.4X4	T46.4X5	T46.4X6
Ranitidine	T47.0X1	T47.0X2	T47.0X3	T47.0X4	T47.0X5	T47.0X6
Ranunculus	T62.2X1	T62.2X2	T62.2X3	T62.2X4	—	—
Rat poison NEC	T60.4X1	T60.4X2	T60.4X3	T60.4X4	—	—
Rattlesnake (venom)	T63.011	T63.012	T63.013	T63.014	—	—
Raubasine	T46.7X1	T46.7X2	T46.7X3	T46.7X4	T46.7X5	T46.7X6
Raudixin	T46.5X1	T46.5X2	T46.5X3	T46.5X4	T46.5X5	T46.5X6
Rautensin	T46.5X1	T46.5X2	T46.5X3	T46.5X4	T46.5X5	T46.5X6
Rautina	T46.5X1	T46.5X2	T46.5X3	T46.5X4	T46.5X5	T46.5X6
Rautotal	T46.5X1	T46.5X2	T46.5X3	T46.5X4	T46.5X5	T46.5X6
Rauwiloid	T46.5X1	T46.5X2	T46.5X3	T46.5X4	T46.5X5	T46.5X6
Rauwoldin	T46.5X1	T46.5X2	T46.5X3	T46.5X4	T46.5X5	T46.5X6
Rauwolfia (alkaloids)	T46.5X1	T46.5X2	T46.5X3	T46.5X4	T46.5X5	T46.5X6
Razoxane	T45.1X1	T45.1X2	T45.1X3	T45.1X4	T45.1X5	T45.1X6
Realgar	T57.0X1	T57.0X2	T57.0X3	T57.0X4	—	—
Recombinant (R) — see specific protein						
Red blood cells, packed	T45.8X1	T45.8X2	T45.8X3	T45.8X4	T45.8X5	T45.8X6
Red squill (scilliroside)	T60.4X1	T60.4X2	T60.4X3	T60.4X4	—	—
Reducing agent, industrial NEC	T65.891	T65.892	T65.893	T65.894		
Refrigerant gas (chlorofluorocarbon)	T53.5X1	T53.5X2	T53.5X3	T53.5X4		
not chlorofluorocarbon	T59.891	T59.892	T59.893	T59.894		
Regroton	T50.2X1	T50.2X2	T50.2X3	T50.2X4	T50.2X5	T50.2X6
Rehydration salts (oral)	T50.3X1	T50.3X2	T50.3X3	T50.3X4	T50.3X5	T50.3X6
Rela	T42.8X1	T42.8X2	T42.8X3	T42.8X4	T42.8X5	T42.8X6
Relaxant, muscle						
anesthetic	T48.1X1	T48.1X2	T48.1X3	T48.1X4	T48.1X5	T48.1X6
central nervous system	T42.8X1	T42.8X2	T42.8X3	T42.8X4	T42.8X5	T42.8X6
skeletal NEC	T48.1X1	T48.1X2	T48.1X3	T48.1X4	T48.1X5	T48.1X6
smooth NEC	T44.3X1	T44.3X2	T44.3X3	T44.3X4	T44.3X5	T44.3X6
Remoxipride	T43.591	T43.592	T43.593	T43.594	T43.595	T43.596
Renese	T50.2X1	T50.2X2	T50.2X3	T50.2X4	T50.2X5	T50.2X6
Renografin	T50.8X1	T50.8X2	T50.8X3	T50.8X4	T50.8X5	T50.8X6
Replacement solution	T50.3X1	T50.3X2	T50.3X3	T50.3X4	T50.3X5	T50.3X6
Reproterol	T48.6X1	T48.6X2	T48.6X3	T48.6X4	T48.6X5	T48.6X6
Rescinnamine	T46.5X1	T46.5X2	T46.5X3	T46.5X4	T46.5X5	T46.5X6
Reserpin (e)	T46.5X1	T46.5X2	T46.5X3	T46.5X4	T46.5X5	T46.5X6
Resorcin, resorcinol (nonmedicinal)	T65.891	T65.892	T65.893	T65.894	—	—
medicinal	T49.4X1	T49.4X2	T49.4X3	T49.4X4	T49.4X5	T49.4X6
Respaire	T48.4X1	T48.4X2	T48.4X3	T48.4X4	T48.4X5	T48.4X6
Respiratory drug NEC	T48.901	T48.902	T48.903	T48.904	T48.905	T48.906
antiasthmatic NEC	T48.6X1	T48.6X2	T48.6X3	T48.6X4	T48.6X5	T48.6X6
anti-common-cold NEC	T48.5X1	T48.5X2	T48.5X3	T48.5X4	T48.5X5	T48.5X6
expectorant NEC	T48.4X1	T48.4X2	T48.4X3	T48.4X4	T48.4X5	T48.4X6
stimulant	T48.901	T48.902	T48.903	T48.904	T48.905	T48.906
Retinoic acid	T49.0X1	T49.0X2	T49.0X3	T49.0X4	T49.0X5	T49.0X6
Retinol	T45.2X1	T45.2X2	T45.2X3	T45.2X4	T45.2X5	T45.2X6
Rh (D) immune globulin (human)	T50.Z11	T50.Z12	T50.Z13	T50.Z14	T50.Z15	T50.Z16
Rhodine	T39.011	T39.012	T39.013	T39.014	T39.015	T39.016
RhoGAM	T50.Z11	T50.Z12	T50.Z13	T50.Z14	T50.Z15	T50.Z16
Rhubarb						
dry extract	T47.2X1	T47.2X2	T47.2X3	T47.2X4	T47.2X5	T47.2X6
tincture, compound	T47.2X1	T47.2X2	T47.2X3	T47.2X4	T47.2X5	T47.2X6
Ribavirin	T37.5X1	T37.5X2	T37.5X3	T37.5X4	T37.5X5	T37.5X6
Riboflavin	T45.2X1	T45.2X2	T45.2X3	T45.2X4	T45.2X5	T45.2X6
Ribostamycin	T36.5X1	T36.5X2	T36.5X3	T36.5X4	T36.5X5	T36.5X6
Ricin	T62.2X1	T62.2X2	T62.2X3	T62.2X4	—	—
Ricinus communis	T62.2X1	T62.2X2	T62.2X3	T62.2X4	—	—
Rickettsial vaccine NEC	T50.A91	T50.A92	T50.A93	T50.A94	T50.A95	T50.A96
Rifabutin	T36.6X1	T36.6X2	T36.6X3	T36.6X4	T36.6X5	T36.6X6
Rifamide	T36.6X1	T36.6X2	T36.6X3	T36.6X4	T36.6X5	T36.6X6
Rifampicin	T36.6X1	T36.6X2	T36.6X3	T36.6X4	T36.6X5	T36.6X6
with isoniazid	T37.1X1	T37.1X2	T37.1X3	T37.1X4	T37.1X5	T37.1X6
Rifampin	T36.6X1	T36.6X2	T36.6X3	T36.6X4	T36.6X5	T36.6X6
Rifamycin	T36.6X1	T36.6X2	T36.6X3	T36.6X4	T36.6X5	T36.6X6
Rifaximin	T36.6X1	T36.6X2	T36.6X3	T36.6X4	T36.6X5	T36.6X6
Rimantadine	T37.5X1	T37.5X2	T37.5X3	T37.5X4	T37.5X5	T37.5X6
Rimazolium metilsulfate	T39.8X1	T39.8X2	T39.8X3	T39.8X4	T39.8X5	T39.8X6
Rimifon	T37.1X1	T37.1X2	T37.1X3	T37.1X4	T37.1X5	T37.1X6
Rimiterol	T48.6X1	T48.6X2	T48.6X3	T48.6X4	T48.6X5	T48.6X6
Ringer (lactate) solution	T50.3X1	T50.3X2	T50.3X3	T50.3X4	T50.3X5	T50.3X6
Ristocetin	T36.8X1	T36.8X2	T36.8X3	T36.8X4	T36.8X5	T36.8X6
Ritalin	T43.631	T43.632	T43.633	T43.634	T43.635	T43.636
Ritodrine	T44.5X1	T44.5X2	T44.5X3	T44.5X4	T44.5X5	T44.5X6
Roach killer — see Insecticide						
Rociverine	T44.3X1	T44.3X2	T44.3X3	T44.3X4	T44.3X5	T44.3X6
Rocky Mountain spotted fever vaccine	T50.A91	T50.A92	T50.A93	T50.A94	T50.A95	T50.A96
Rodenticide NEC	T60.4X1	T60.4X2	T60.4X3	T60.4X4	—	—
Rohypnol	T42.4X1	T42.4X2	T42.4X3	T42.4X4	T42.4X5	T42.4X6
Rokitamycin	T36.3X1	T36.3X2	T36.3X3	T36.3X4	T36.3X5	T36.3X6
Rolaids	T47.1X1	T47.1X2	T47.1X3	T47.1X4	T47.1X5	T47.1X6
Rolitetracycline	T36.4X1	T36.4X2	T36.4X3	T36.4X4	T36.4X5	T36.4X6
Romilar	T48.3X1	T48.3X2	T48.3X3	T48.3X4	T48.3X5	T48.3X6
Ronifibrate	T46.6X1	T46.6X2	T46.6X3	T46.6X4	T46.6X5	T46.6X6
Rosaprostol	T47.1X1	T47.1X2	T47.1X3	T47.1X4	T47.1X5	T47.1X6
Rose bengal sodium (131I)	T50.8X1	T50.8X2	T50.8X3	T50.8X4	T50.8X5	T50.8X6
Rose water ointment	T49.3X1	T49.3X2	T49.3X3	T49.3X4	T49.3X5	T49.3X6
Rosoxacin	T37.8X1	T37.8X2	T37.8X3	T37.8X4	T37.8X5	T37.8X6
Rotenone	T60.2X1	T60.2X2	T60.2X3	T60.2X4	—	—
Rotoxamine	T45.0X1	T45.0X2	T45.0X3	T45.0X4	T45.0X5	T45.0X6
Rough-on-rats	T60.4X1	T60.4X2	T60.4X3	T60.4X4	—	—
Roxatidine	T47.0X1	T47.0X2	T47.0X3	T47.0X4	T47.0X5	T47.0X6
Roxithromycin	T36.3X1	T36.3X2	T36.3X3	T36.3X4	T36.3X5	T36.3X6
Rt-PA	T45.611	T45.612	T45.613	T45.614	T45.615	T45.616
Rubbing alcohol	T51.2X1	T51.2X2	T51.2X3	T51.2X4		
Rubefacient	T49.4X1	T49.4X2	T49.4X3	T49.4X4	T49.4X5	T49.4X6
Rubella vaccine	T50.B91	T50.B92	T50.B93	T50.B94	T50.B95	T50.B96
Rubeola vaccine	T50.B91	T50.B92	T50.B93	T50.B94	T50.B95	T50.B96
Rubidium chloride Rb82	T50.8X1	T50.8X2	T50.8X3	T50.8X4	T50.8X5	T50.8X6
Rubidomycin	T45.1X1	T45.1X2	T45.1X3	T45.1X4	T45.1X5	T45.1X6
Rue	T62.2X1	T62.2X2	T62.2X3	T62.2X4	—	—
Rufocromomycin	T45.1X1	T45.1X2	T45.1X3	T45.1X4	T45.1X5	T45.1X6
Russel's viper venin	T45.7X1	T45.7X2	T45.7X3	T45.7X4	T45.7X5	T45.7X6
Ruta (graveolens)	T62.2X1	T62.2X2	T62.2X3	T62.2X4	—	—
Rutinum	T46.991	T46.992	T46.993	T46.994	T46.995	T46.996
Rutoside	T46.991	T46.992	T46.993	T46.994	T46.995	T46.996
b-sitosterol(s)	T46.6X1	T46.6X2	T46.6X3	T46.6X4	T46.6X5	T46.6X6
Sabadilla (plant)	T62.2X1	T62.2X2	T62.2X3	T62.2X4	—	—
pesticide	T60.2X1	T60.2X2	T60.2X3	T60.2X4	—	—
Saccharated iron oxide	T45.8X1	T45.8X2	T45.8X3	T45.8X4	T45.8X5	T45.8X6
Saccharin	T50.901	T50.902	T50.903	T50.904	T50.905	T50.906
Saccharomyces boulardii	T47.6X1	T47.6X2	T47.6X3	T47.6X4	T47.6X5	T47.6X6
Safflower oil	T46.6X1	T46.6X2	T46.6X3	T46.6X4	T46.6X5	T46.6X6
Safrazine	T43.1X1	T43.1X2	T43.1X3	T43.1X4	T43.1X5	T43.1X6
Salazosulfapyridine	T37.0X1	T37.0X2	T37.0X3	T37.0X4	T37.0X5	T37.0X6

▽ Subterms under main terms may continue to next column or page   Additional Character May Be Required — Refer to the Tabular List for Character Selection

Table of Drugs and Chemicals

Salbutamol — Soda

Substance	Poisoning, Accidental (unintentional)	Poisoning, Intentional Self-harm	Poisoning, Assault	Poisoning, Undetermined	Adverse Effect	Under-dosing
Salbutamol	T48.6X1	T48.6X2	T48.6X3	T48.6X4	T48.6X5	T48.6X6
Salicylamide	T39.091	T39.092	T39.093	T39.094	T39.095	T39.096
Salicylate NEC	T39.091	T39.092	T39.093	T39.094	T39.095	T39.096
methyl	T49.3X1	T49.3X2	T49.3X3	T49.3X4	T49.3X5	T49.3X6
theobromine calcium	T50.2X1	T50.2X2	T50.2X3	T50.2X4	T50.2X5	T50.2X6
Salicylazosulfapyridine	T37.0X1	T37.0X2	T37.0X3	T37.0X4	T37.0X5	T37.0X6
Salicylhydroxamic acid	T49.0X1	T49.0X2	T49.0X3	T49.0X4	T49.0X5	T49.0X6
Salicylic acid	T49.4X1	T49.4X2	T49.4X3	T49.4X4	T49.4X5	T49.4X6
with benzoic acid	T49.4X1	T49.4X2	T49.4X3	T49.4X4	T49.4X5	T49.4X6
congeners	T39.091	T39.092	T39.093	T39.094	T39.095	T39.096
derivative	T39.091	T39.092	T39.093	T39.094	T39.095	T39.096
salts	T39.091	T39.092	T39.093	T39.094	T39.095	T39.096
Salinazid	T37.1X1	T37.1X2	T37.1X3	T37.1X4	T37.1X5	T37.1X6
Salmeterol	T48.6X1	T48.6X2	T48.6X3	T48.6X4	T48.6X5	T48.6X6
Salol	T49.3X1	T49.3X2	T49.3X3	T49.3X4	T49.3X5	T49.3X6
Salsalate	T39.091	T39.092	T39.093	T39.094	T39.095	T39.096
Salt-replacing drug	T50.901	T50.902	T50.903	T50.904	T50.905	T50.906
Salt-retaining mineralocorticoid	T50.0X1	T50.0X2	T50.0X3	T50.0X4	T50.0X5	T50.0X6
Salt substitute	T50.901	T50.902	T50.903	T50.904	T50.905	T50.906
Saluretic NEC	T50.2X1	T50.2X2	T50.2X3	T50.2X4	T50.2X5	T50.2X6
Saluron	T50.2X1	T50.2X2	T50.2X3	T50.2X4	T50.2X5	T50.2X6
Salvarsan 606 (neosilver) (silver)	T37.8X1	T37.8X2	T37.8X3	T37.8X4	T37.8X5	T37.8X6
Sambucus canadensis	T62.2X1	T62.2X2	T62.2X3	T62.2X4	—	—
berry	T62.1X1	T62.1X2	T62.1X3	T62.1X4	—	—
Sandril	T46.5X1	T46.5X2	T46.5X3	T46.5X4	T46.5X5	T46.5X6
Sanguinaria canadensis	T62.2X1	T62.2X2	T62.2X3	T62.2X4	—	—
Saniflush (cleaner)	T54.2X1	T54.2X2	T54.2X3	T54.2X4	—	—
Santonin	T37.4X1	T37.4X2	T37.4X3	T37.4X4	T37.4X5	T37.4X6
Santyl	T49.8X1	T49.8X2	T49.8X3	T49.8X4	T49.8X5	T49.8X6
Saralasin	T46.5X1	T46.5X2	T46.5X3	T46.5X4	T46.5X5	T46.5X6
Sarcolysin	T45.1X1	T45.1X2	T45.1X3	T45.1X4	T45.1X5	T45.1X6
Sarkomycin	T45.1X1	T45.1X2	T45.1X3	T45.1X4	T45.1X5	T45.1X6
Saroten	T43.011	T43.012	T43.013	T43.014	T43.015	T43.016
Saturnine — see Lead						
Savin (oil)	T49.4X1	T49.4X2	T49.4X3	T49.4X4	T49.4X5	T49.4X6
Scammony	T47.2X1	T47.2X2	T47.2X3	T47.2X4	T47.2X5	T47.2X6
Scarlet red	T49.8X1	T49.8X2	T49.8X3	T49.8X4	T49.8X5	T49.8X6
Scheele's green	T57.0X1	T57.0X2	T57.0X3	T57.0X4	—	—
insecticide	T57.0X1	T57.0X2	T57.0X3	T57.0X4	—	—
Schizontozide (blood) (tissue)	T37.2X1	T37.2X2	T37.2X3	T37.2X4	T37.2X5	T37.2X6
Schradan	T60.0X1	T60.0X2	T60.0X3	T60.0X4	—	—
Schweinfurth green	T57.0X1	T57.0X2	T57.0X3	T57.0X4	—	—
insecticide	T57.0X1	T57.0X2	T57.0X3	T57.0X4	—	—
Scilla, rat poison	T60.4X1	T60.4X2	T60.4X3	T60.4X4	—	—
Scillaren	T60.4X1	T60.4X2	T60.4X3	T60.4X4	—	—
Sclerosing agent	T46.8X1	T46.8X2	T46.8X3	T46.8X4	T46.8X5	T46.8X6
Scombrotoxin	T61.11	T61.12	T61.13	T61.14	—	—
Scopolamine	T44.3X1	T44.3X2	T44.3X3	T44.3X4	T44.3X5	T44.3X6
Scopolia extract	T44.3X1	T44.3X2	T44.3X3	T44.3X4	T44.3X5	T44.3X6
Scouring powder	T65.891	T65.892	T65.893	T65.894	—	—
Sea						
anemone (sting)	T63.631	T63.632	T63.633	T63.634	—	—
cucumber (sting)	T63.691	T63.692	T63.693	T63.694	—	—
snake (bite) (venom)	T63.091	T63.092	T63.093	T63.094	—	—
urchin spine (puncture)	T63.691	T63.692	T63.693	T63.694	—	—
Seafood	T61.91	T61.92	T61.93	T61.94	—	—
specified NEC	T61.8X1	T61.8X2	T61.8X3	T61.8X4	—	—
Secbutabarbital	T42.3X1	T42.3X2	T42.3X3	T42.3X4	T42.3X5	T42.3X6
Secbutabarbitone	T42.3X1	T42.3X2	T42.3X3	T42.3X4	T42.3X5	T42.3X6
Secnidazole	T37.3X1	T37.3X2	T37.3X3	T37.3X4	T37.3X5	T37.3X6
Secobarbital	T42.3X1	T42.3X2	T42.3X3	T42.3X4	T42.3X5	T42.3X6
Seconal	T42.3X1	T42.3X2	T42.3X3	T42.3X4	T42.3X5	T42.3X6
Secretin	T50.8X1	T50.8X2	T50.8X3	T50.8X4	T50.8X5	T50.8X6
Sedative NEC	T42.71	T42.72	T42.73	T42.74	T42.75	T42.76
mixed NEC	T42.6X1	T42.6X2	T42.6X3	T42.6X4	T42.6X5	T42.6X6
Sedormid	T42.6X1	T42.6X2	T42.6X3	T42.6X4	T42.6X5	T42.6X6
Seed disinfectant or dressing	T60.8X1	T60.8X2	T60.8X3	T60.8X4	—	—
Seeds (poisonous)	T62.2X1	T62.2X2	T62.2X3	T62.2X4	—	—
Selegiline	T42.8X1	T42.8X2	T42.8X3	T42.8X4	T42.8X5	T42.8X6
Selenium NEC	T56.891	T56.892	T56.893	T56.894	—	—
disulfide or sulfide	T49.4X1	T49.4X2	T49.4X3	T49.4X4	T49.4X5	T49.4X6
fumes	T59.891	T59.892	T59.893	T59.894	—	—
sulfide	T49.4X1	T49.4X2	T49.4X3	T49.4X4	T49.4X5	T49.4X6
Selenomethionine (75Se)	T50.8X1	T50.8X2	T50.8X3	T50.8X4	T50.8X5	T50.8X6
Selsun	T49.4X1	T49.4X2	T49.4X3	T49.4X4	T49.4X5	T49.4X6
Semustine	T45.1X1	T45.1X2	T45.1X3	T45.1X4	T45.1X5	T45.1X6
Senega syrup	T48.4X1	T48.4X2	T48.4X3	T48.4X4	T48.4X5	T48.4X6
Senna	T47.2X1	T47.2X2	T47.2X3	T47.2X4	T47.2X5	T47.2X6
Sennoside A+B	T47.2X1	T47.2X2	T47.2X3	T47.2X4	T47.2X5	T47.2X6
Septisol	T49.2X1	T49.2X2	T49.2X3	T49.2X4	T49.2X5	T49.2X6
Seractide	T38.811	T38.812	T38.813	T38.814	T38.815	T38.816
Serax	T42.4X1	T42.4X2	T42.4X3	T42.4X4	T42.4X5	T42.4X6
Serenesil	T42.6X1	T42.6X2	T42.6X3	T42.6X4	T42.6X5	T42.6X6
Serenium (hydrochloride)	T37.91	T37.92	T37.93	T37.94	T37.95	T37.96
Serepax — see Oxazepam						
Sermorelin	T38.891	T38.892	T38.893	T38.894	T38.895	T38.896
Sernyl	T41.1X1	T41.1X2	T41.1X3	T41.1X4	T41.1X5	T41.1X6
Serotonin	T50.991	T50.992	T50.993	T50.994	T50.995	T50.996
Serpasil	T46.5X1	T46.5X2	T46.5X3	T46.5X4	T46.5X5	T46.5X6
Serrapeptase	T45.3X1	T45.3X2	T45.3X3	T45.3X4	T45.3X5	T45.3X6
Serum						
antibotulinus	T50.Z11	T50.Z12	T50.Z13	T50.Z14	T50.Z15	T50.Z16
anticytotoxic	T50.Z11	T50.Z12	T50.Z13	T50.Z14	T50.Z15	T50.Z16
antidiphtheria	T50.Z11	T50.Z12	T50.Z13	T50.Z14	T50.Z15	T50.Z16
antimeningococcus	T50.Z11	T50.Z12	T50.Z13	T50.Z14	T50.Z15	T50.Z16
anti-Rh	T50.Z11	T50.Z12	T50.Z13	T50.Z14	T50.Z15	T50.Z16
anti-snake-bite	T50.Z11	T50.Z12	T50.Z13	T50.Z14	T50.Z15	T50.Z16
antitetanic	T50.Z11	T50.Z12	T50.Z13	T50.Z14	T50.Z15	T50.Z16
antitoxic	T50.Z11	T50.Z12	T50.Z13	T50.Z14	T50.Z15	T50.Z16
complement (inhibitor)	T45.8X1	T45.8X2	T45.8X3	T45.8X4	T45.8X5	T45.8X6
convalescent	T50.Z11	T50.Z12	T50.Z13	T50.Z14	T50.Z15	T50.Z16
hemolytic complement	T45.8X1	T45.8X2	T45.8X3	T45.8X4	T45.8X5	T45.8X6
immune (human)	T50.Z11	T50.Z12	T50.Z13	T50.Z14	T50.Z15	T50.Z16
protective NEC	T50.Z11	T50.Z12	T50.Z13	T50.Z14	T50.Z15	T50.Z16
Setastine	T45.0X1	T45.0X2	T45.0X3	T45.0X4	T45.0X5	T45.0X6
Setoperone	T43.591	T43.592	T43.593	T43.594	T43.595	T43.596
Sewer gas	T59.91	T59.92	T59.93	T59.94	—	—
Shampoo	T55.0X1	T55.0X2	T55.0X3	T55.0X4	—	—
Shellfish, noxious, nonbacterial	T61.781	T61.782	T61.783	T61.784	—	—
Sildenafil	T46.7X1	T46.7X2	T46.7X3	T46.7X4	T46.7X5	T46.7X6
Silibinin	T50.991	T50.992	T50.993	T50.994	T50.995	T50.996
Silicone NEC	T65.891	T65.892	T65.893	T65.894	—	—
medicinal	T49.3X1	T49.3X2	T49.3X3	T49.3X4	T49.3X5	T49.3X6
Silvadene	T49.0X1	T49.0X2	T49.0X3	T49.0X4	T49.0X5	T49.0X6
Silver	T49.0X1	T49.0X2	T49.0X3	T49.0X4	T49.0X5	T49.0X6
anti-infectives	T49.0X1	T49.0X2	T49.0X3	T49.0X4	T49.0X5	T49.0X6
arsphenamine	T37.8X1	T37.8X2	T37.8X3	T37.8X4	T37.8X5	T37.8X6
colloidal	T49.0X1	T49.0X2	T49.0X3	T49.0X4	T49.0X5	T49.0X6
nitrate	T49.0X1	T49.0X2	T49.0X3	T49.0X4	T49.0X5	T49.0X6
ophthalmic preparation	T49.5X1	T49.5X2	T49.5X3	T49.5X4	T49.5X5	T49.5X6
toughened (keratolytic)	T49.4X1	T49.4X2	T49.4X3	T49.4X4	T49.4X5	T49.4X6
nonmedicinal (dust)	T56.891	T56.892	T56.893	T56.894	—	—
protein	T49.5X1	T49.5X2	T49.5X3	T49.5X4	T49.5X5	T49.5X6
salvarsan	T37.8X1	T37.8X2	T37.8X3	T37.8X4	T37.8X5	T37.8X6
sulfadiazine	T49.4X1	T49.4X2	T49.4X3	T49.4X4	T49.4X5	T49.4X6
Silymarin	T50.991	T50.992	T50.993	T50.994	T50.995	T50.996
Simaldrate	T47.1X1	T47.1X2	T47.1X3	T47.1X4	T47.1X5	T47.1X6
Simazine	T60.3X1	T60.3X2	T60.3X3	T60.3X4	—	—
Simethicone	T47.1X1	T47.1X2	T47.1X3	T47.1X4	T47.1X5	T47.1X6
Simfibrate	T46.6X1	T46.6X2	T46.6X3	T46.6X4	T46.6X5	T46.6X6
Simvastatin	T46.6X1	T46.6X2	T46.6X3	T46.6X4	T46.6X5	T46.6X6
Sincalide	T50.8X1	T50.8X2	T50.8X3	T50.8X4	T50.8X5	T50.8X6
Sinequan	T43.011	T43.012	T43.013	T43.014	T43.015	T43.016
Singoserp	T46.5X1	T46.5X2	T46.5X3	T46.5X4	T46.5X5	T46.5X6
Sintrom	T45.511	T45.512	T45.513	T45.514	T45.515	T45.516
Sisomicin	T36.5X1	T36.5X2	T36.5X3	T36.5X4	T36.5X5	T36.5X6
Sitosterols	T46.6X1	T46.6X2	T46.6X3	T46.6X4	T46.6X5	T46.6X6
Skeletal muscle relaxants	T48.1X1	T48.1X2	T48.1X3	T48.1X4	T48.1X5	T48.1X6
Skin						
agents (external)	T49.91	T49.92	T49.93	T49.94	T49.95	T49.96
specified NEC	T49.8X1	T49.8X2	T49.8X3	T49.8X4	T49.8X5	T49.8X6
test antigen	T50.8X1	T50.8X2	T50.8X3	T50.8X4	T50.8X5	T50.8X6
Sleep-eze	T45.0X1	T45.0X2	T45.0X3	T45.0X4	T45.0X5	T45.0X6
Sleeping draught, pill	T42.71	T42.72	T42.73	T42.74	T42.75	T42.76
Smallpox vaccine	T50.B11	T50.B12	T50.B13	T50.B14	T50.B15	T50.B16
Smelter fumes NEC	T56.91	T56.92	T56.93	T56.94	—	—
Smog	T59.1X1	T59.1X2	T59.1X3	T59.1X4	—	—
Smoke NEC	T59.811	T59.812	T59.813	T59.814	—	—
Smooth muscle relaxant	T44.3X1	T44.3X2	T44.3X3	T44.3X4	T44.3X5	T44.3X6
Snail killer NEC	T60.8X1	T60.8X2	T60.8X3	T60.8X4	—	—
Snake venom or bite	T63.001	T63.002	T63.003	T63.004	—	—
hemocoagulase	T45.7X1	T45.7X2	T45.7X3	T45.7X4	T45.7X5	T45.7X6
Snuff	T65.211	T65.212	T65.213	T65.214	—	—
Soap (powder) (product)	T55.0X1	T55.0X2	T55.0X3	T55.0X4	—	—
enema	T47.4X1	T47.4X2	T47.4X3	T47.4X4	T47.4X5	T47.4X6
medicinal, soft	T49.2X1	T49.2X2	T49.2X3	T49.2X4	T49.2X5	T49.2X6
superfatted	T49.2X1	T49.2X2	T49.2X3	T49.2X4	T49.2X5	T49.2X6
Sobrerol	T48.4X1	T48.4X2	T48.4X3	T48.4X4	T48.4X5	T48.4X6
Soda (caustic)	T54.3X1	T54.3X2	T54.3X3	T54.3X4	—	—
bicarb	T47.1X1	T47.1X2	T47.1X3	T47.1X4	T47.1X5	T47.1X6

Substance	Poisoning, Accidental (unintentional)	Poisoning, Intentional Self-harm	Poisoning, Assault	Poisoning, Undetermined	Adverse Effect	Under- dosing
Soda — *continued*						
chlorinated — *see* Sodium, hypochlorite						
Sodium						
acetosulfone	T37.1X1	T37.1X2	T37.1X3	T37.1X4	T37.1X5	T37.1X6
acetrizoate	T50.8X1	T50.8X2	T50.8X3	T50.8X4	T50.8X5	T50.8X6
acid phosphate	T50.3X1	T50.3X2	T50.3X3	T50.3X4	T50.3X5	T50.3X6
alginate	T47.8X1	T47.8X2	T47.8X3	T47.8X4	T47.8X5	T47.8X6
amidotrizoate	T50.8X1	T50.8X2	T50.8X3	T50.8X4	T50.8X5	T50.8X6
aminopterin	T45.1X1	T45.1X2	T45.1X3	T45.1X4	T45.1X5	T45.1X6
amylosulfate	T47.8X1	T47.8X2	T47.8X3	T47.8X4	T47.8X5	T47.8X6
amytal	T42.3X1	T42.3X2	T42.3X3	T42.3X4	T42.3X5	T42.3X6
antimony gluconate	T37.3X1	T37.3X2	T37.3X3	T37.3X4	T37.3X5	T37.3X6
arsenate	T57.0X1	T57.0X2	T57.0X3	T57.0X4	—	—
aurothiomalate	T39.4X1	T39.4X2	T39.4X3	T39.4X4	T39.4X5	T39.4X6
aurothiosulfate	T39.4X1	T39.4X2	T39.4X3	T39.4X4	T39.4X5	T39.4X6
barbiturate	T42.3X1	T42.3X2	T42.3X3	T42.3X4	T42.3X5	T42.3X6
basic phosphate	T47.4X1	T47.4X2	T47.4X3	T47.4X4	T47.4X5	T47.4X6
bicarbonate	T47.1X1	T47.1X2	T47.1X3	T47.1X4	T47.1X5	T47.1X6
bichromate	T57.8X1	T57.8X2	T57.8X3	T57.8X4	—	—
biphosphate	T50.3X1	T50.3X2	T50.3X3	T50.3X4	T50.3X5	T50.3X6
bisulfate	T65.891	T65.892	T65.893	T65.894	—	—
borate						
cleanser	T57.8X1	T57.8X2	T57.8X3	T57.8X4	—	—
eye	T49.5X1	T49.5X2	T49.5X3	T49.5X4	T49.5X5	T49.5X6
therapeutic	T49.8X1	T49.8X2	T49.8X3	T49.8X4	T49.8X5	T49.8X6
bromide	T42.6X1	T42.6X2	T42.6X3	T42.6X4	T42.6X5	T42.6X6
cacodylate (nonmedicinal) NEC	T50.8X1	T50.8X2	T50.8X3	T50.8X4	T50.8X5	T50.8X6
anti-infective	T37.8X1	T37.8X2	T37.8X3	T37.8X4	T37.8X5	T37.8X6
herbicide	T60.3X1	T60.3X2	T60.3X3	T60.3X4	—	—
calcium edetate	T45.8X1	T45.8X2	T45.8X3	T45.8X4	T45.8X5	T45.8X6
carbonate NEC	T54.3X1	T54.3X2	T54.3X3	T54.3X4	—	—
chlorate NEC	T65.891	T65.892	T65.893	T65.894	—	—
herbicide	T54.91	T54.92	T54.93	T54.94	—	—
chloride	T50.3X1	T50.3X2	T50.3X3	T50.3X4	T50.3X5	T50.3X6
with glucose	T50.3X1	T50.3X2	T50.3X3	T50.3X4	T50.3X5	T50.3X6
chromate	T65.891	T65.892	T65.893	T65.894	—	—
citrate	T50.991	T50.992	T50.993	T50.994	T50.995	T50.996
cromoglicate	T48.6X1	T48.6X2	T48.6X3	T48.6X4	T48.6X5	T48.6X6
cyanide	T65.0X1	T65.0X2	T65.0X3	T65.0X4	—	—
cyclamate	T50.3X1	T50.3X2	T50.3X3	T50.3X4	T50.3X5	T50.3X6
dehydrocholate	T45.8X1	T45.8X2	T45.8X3	T45.8X4	T45.8X5	T45.8X6
diatrizoate	T50.8X1	T50.8X2	T50.8X3	T50.8X4	T50.8X5	T50.8X6
dibunate	T48.4X1	T48.4X2	T48.4X3	T48.4X4	T48.4X5	T48.4X6
dioctyl sulfosuccinate	T47.4X1	T47.4X2	T47.4X3	T47.4X4	T47.4X5	T47.4X6
dipantoyl ferrate	T45.8X1	T45.8X2	T45.8X3	T45.8X4	T45.8X5	T45.8X6
edetate	T45.8X1	T45.8X2	T45.8X3	T45.8X4	T45.8X5	T45.8X6
ethacrynate	T50.1X1	T50.1X2	T50.1X3	T50.1X4	T50.1X5	T50.1X6
feredetate	T45.8X1	T45.8X2	T45.8X3	T45.8X4	T45.8X5	T45.8X6
Fluoride — *see* Fluoride						
fluoroacetate (dust) (pesticide)	T60.4X1	T60.4X2	T60.4X3	T60.4X4	—	—
free salt	T50.3X1	T50.3X2	T50.3X3	T50.3X4	T50.3X5	T50.3X6
fusidate	T36.8X1	T36.8X2	T36.8X3	T36.8X4	T36.8X5	T36.8X6
glucaldrate	T47.1X1	T47.1X2	T47.1X3	T47.1X4	T47.1X5	T47.1X6
glucosulfone	T37.1X1	T37.1X2	T37.1X3	T37.1X4	T37.1X5	T37.1X6
glutamate	T45.8X1	T45.8X2	T45.8X3	T45.8X4	T45.8X5	T45.8X6
hydrogen carbonate	T50.3X1	T50.3X2	T50.3X3	T50.3X4	T50.3X5	T50.3X6
hydroxide	T54.3X1	T54.3X2	T54.3X3	T54.3X4	—	—
hypochlorite (bleach) NEC	T54.3X1	T54.3X2	T54.3X3	T54.3X4	—	—
disinfectant	T54.3X1	T54.3X2	T54.3X3	T54.3X4	—	—
medicinal (anti-infective) (external)	T49.0X1	T49.0X2	T49.0X3	T49.0X4	T49.0X5	T49.0X6
vapor	T54.3X1	T54.3X2	T54.3X3	T54.3X4	—	—
hyposulfite	T49.0X1	T49.0X2	T49.0X3	T49.0X4	T49.0X5	T49.0X6
indigotin disulfonate	T50.8X1	T50.8X2	T50.8X3	T50.8X4	T50.8X5	T50.8X6
iodide	T50.991	T50.992	T50.993	T50.994	T50.995	T50.996
I-131	T50.8X1	T50.8X2	T50.8X3	T50.8X4	T50.8X5	T50.8X6
therapeutic	T38.2X1	T38.2X2	T38.2X3	T38.2X4	T38.2X5	T38.2X6
iodohippurate (131I)	T50.8X1	T50.8X2	T50.8X3	T50.8X4	T50.8X5	T50.8X6
iopodate	T50.8X1	T50.8X2	T50.8X3	T50.8X4	T50.8X5	T50.8X6
iothalamate	T50.8X1	T50.8X2	T50.8X3	T50.8X4	T50.8X5	T50.8X6
iron edetate	T45.4X1	T45.4X2	T45.4X3	T45.4X4	T45.4X5	T45.4X6
lactate (compound solution)	T45.8X1	T45.8X2	T45.8X3	T45.8X4	T45.8X5	T45.8X6
lauryl (sulfate)	T49.2X1	T49.2X2	T49.2X3	T49.2X4	T49.2X5	T49.2X6
L-triiodothyronine	T38.1X1	T38.1X2	T38.1X3	T38.1X4	T38.1X5	T38.1X6
magnesium citrate	T50.991	T50.992	T50.993	T50.994	T50.995	T50.996
mersalate	T50.2X1	T50.2X2	T50.2X3	T50.2X4	T50.2X5	T50.2X6
metasilicate	T65.891	T65.892	T65.893	T65.894	—	—
metrizoate	T50.8X1	T50.8X2	T50.8X3	T50.8X4	T50.8X5	T50.8X6

Substance	Poisoning, Accidental (unintentional)	Poisoning, Intentional Self-harm	Poisoning, Assault	Poisoning, Undetermined	Adverse Effect	Under- dosing
Sodium — *continued*						
monofluoroacetate (pesticide)	T60.1X1	T60.1X2	T60.1X3	T60.1X4	—	—
morrhuate	T46.8X1	T46.8X2	T46.8X3	T46.8X4	T46.8X5	T46.8X6
nafcillin	T36.0X1	T36.0X2	T36.0X3	T36.0X4	T36.0X5	T36.0X6
nitrate (oxidizing agent)	T65.891	T65.892	T65.893	T65.894	—	—
nitrite	T50.6X1	T50.6X2	T50.6X3	T50.6X4	T50.6X5	T50.6X6
nitroferricyanide	T46.5X1	T46.5X2	T46.5X3	T46.5X4	T46.5X5	T46.5X6
nitroprusside	T46.5X1	T46.5X2	T46.5X3	T46.5X4	T46.5X5	T46.5X6
oxalate	T65.891	T65.892	T65.893	T65.894	—	—
oxide/peroxide	T65.891	T65.892	T65.893	T65.894	—	—
oxybate	T41.291	T41.292	T41.293	T41.294	T41.295	T41.296
para-aminohippurate	T50.8X1	T50.8X2	T50.8X3	T50.8X4	T50.8X5	T50.8X6
perborate (nonmedicinal) NEC	T65.891	T65.892	T65.893	T65.894	—	—
medicinal	T49.0X1	T49.0X2	T49.0X3	T49.0X4	T49.0X5	T49.0X6
soap	T55.0X1	T55.0X2	T55.0X3	T55.0X4	—	—
percarbonate — *see* Sodium, perborate						
pertechnetate Tc99m	T50.8X1	T50.8X2	T50.8X3	T50.8X4	T50.8X5	T50.8X6
phosphate						
cellulose	T45.8X1	T45.8X2	T45.8X3	T45.8X4	T45.8X5	T45.8X6
dibasic	T47.2X1	T47.2X2	T47.2X3	T47.2X4	T47.2X5	T47.2X6
monobasic	T47.2X1	T47.2X2	T47.2X3	T47.2X4	T47.2X5	T47.2X6
phytate	T50.6X1	T50.6X2	T50.6X3	T50.6X4	T50.6X5	T50.6X6
picosulfate	T47.2X1	T47.2X2	T47.2X3	T47.2X4	T47.2X5	T47.2X6
polyhydroxyaluminium monocarbonate	T47.1X1	T47.1X2	T47.1X3	T47.1X4	T47.1X5	T47.1X6
polystyrene sulfonate	T50.3X1	T50.3X2	T50.3X3	T50.3X4	T50.3X5	T50.3X6
propionate	T49.0X1	T49.0X2	T49.0X3	T49.0X4	T49.0X5	T49.0X6
propyl hydroxybenzoate	T50.991	T50.992	T50.993	T50.994	T50.995	T50.996
psylliate	T46.8X1	T46.8X2	T46.8X3	T46.8X4	T46.8X5	T46.8X6
removing resins	T50.3X1	T50.3X2	T50.3X3	T50.3X4	T50.3X5	T50.3X6
salicylate	T39.091	T39.092	T39.093	T39.094	T39.095	T39.096
salt NEC	T50.3X1	T50.3X2	T50.3X3	T50.3X4	T50.3X5	T50.3X6
selenate	T60.2X1	T60.2X2	T60.2X3	T60.2X4	—	—
stibogluconate	T37.3X1	T37.3X2	T37.3X3	T37.3X4	T37.3X5	T37.3X6
sulfate	T47.4X1	T47.4X2	T47.4X3	T47.4X4	T47.4X5	T47.4X6
sulfoxone	T37.1X1	T37.1X2	T37.1X3	T37.1X4	T37.1X5	T37.1X6
tetradecyl sulfate	T46.8X1	T46.8X2	T46.8X3	T46.8X4	T46.8X5	T46.8X6
thiopental	T41.1X1	T41.1X2	T41.1X3	T41.1X4	T41.1X5	T41.1X6
thiosalicylate	T39.091	T39.092	T39.093	T39.094	T39.095	T39.096
thiosulfate	T50.6X1	T50.6X2	T50.6X3	T50.6X4	T50.6X5	T50.6X6
tolbutamide	T38.3X1	T38.3X2	T38.3X3	T38.3X4	T38.3X5	T38.3X6
(L)-triiodothyronine	T38.1X1	T38.1X2	T38.1X3	T38.1X4	T38.1X5	T38.1X6
tyropanoate	T50.8X1	T50.8X2	T50.8X3	T50.8X4	T50.8X5	T50.8X6
valproate	T42.6X1	T42.6X2	T42.6X3	T42.6X4	T42.6X5	T42.6X6
versenate	T50.6X1	T50.6X2	T50.6X3	T50.6X4	T50.6X5	T50.6X6
Sodium-free salt	T50.901	T50.902	T50.903	T50.904	T50.905	T50.906
Sodium-removing resin	T50.3X1	T50.3X2	T50.3X3	T50.3X4	T50.3X5	T50.3X6
Soft soap	T55.0X1	T55.0X2	T55.0X3	T55.0X4	—	—
Solanine	T62.2X1	T62.2X2	T62.2X3	T62.2X4	—	—
berries	T62.1X1	T62.1X2	T62.1X3	T62.1X4	—	—
Solanum dulcamara	T62.2X1	T62.2X2	T62.2X3	T62.2X4	—	—
berries	T62.1X1	T62.1X2	T62.1X3	T62.1X4	—	—
Solapsone	T37.1X1	T37.1X2	T37.1X3	T37.1X4	T37.1X5	T37.1X6
Solar lotion	T49.3X1	T49.3X2	T49.3X3	T49.3X4	T49.3X5	T49.3X6
Solasulfone	T37.1X1	T37.1X2	T37.1X3	T37.1X4	T37.1X5	T37.1X6
Soldering fluid	T65.891	T65.892	T65.893	T65.894	—	—
Solid substance	T65.91	T65.92	T65.93	T65.94	—	—
specified NEC	T65.891	T65.892	T65.893	T65.894	—	—
Solvent, industrial NEC	T52.91	T52.92	T52.93	T52.94	—	—
naphtha	T52.0X1	T52.0X2	T52.0X3	T52.0X4	—	—
petroleum	T52.0X1	T52.0X2	T52.0X3	T52.0X4	—	—
specified NEC	T52.8X1	T52.8X2	T52.8X3	T52.8X4	—	—
Soma	T42.8X1	T42.8X2	T42.8X3	T42.8X4	T42.8X5	T42.8X6
Somatorelin	T38.891	T38.892	T38.893	T38.894	T38.895	T38.896
Somatostatin	T38.991	T38.992	T38.993	T38.994	T38.995	T38.996
Somatotropin	T38.811	T38.812	T38.813	T38.814	T38.815	T38.816
Somatrem	T38.811	T38.812	T38.813	T38.814	T38.815	T38.816
Somatropin	T38.811	T38.812	T38.813	T38.814	T38.815	T38.816
Sominex	T45.0X1	T45.0X2	T45.0X3	T45.0X4	T45.0X5	T45.0X6
Somnos	T42.6X1	T42.6X2	T42.6X3	T42.6X4	T42.6X5	T42.6X6
Somonal	T42.3X1	T42.3X2	T42.3X3	T42.3X4	T42.3X5	T42.3X6
Soneryl	T42.3X1	T42.3X2	T42.3X3	T42.3X4	T42.3X5	T42.3X6
Soothing syrup	T50.901	T50.902	T50.903	T50.904	T50.905	T50.906
Sopor	T42.6X1	T42.6X2	T42.6X3	T42.6X4	T42.6X5	T42.6X6
Soporific	T42.71	T42.72	T42.73	T42.74	T42.75	T42.76
Soporific drug	T42.71	T42.72	T42.73	T42.74	T42.75	T42.76
specified type NEC	T42.6X1	T42.6X2	T42.6X3	T42.6X4	T42.6X5	T42.6X6
Sorbide nitrate	T46.3X1	T46.3X2	T46.3X3	T46.3X4	T46.3X5	T46.3X6
Sorbitol	T47.4X1	T47.4X2	T47.4X3	T47.4X4	T47.4X5	T47.4X6
Sotalol	T44.7X1	T44.7X2	T44.7X3	T44.7X4	T44.7X5	T44.7X6

Substance	Poisoning, Accidental (unintentional)	Poisoning, Intentional Self-harm	Poisoning, Assault	Poisoning, Undetermined	Adverse Effect	Under-dosing
Sotradecol	T46.8X1	T46.8X2	T46.8X3	T46.8X4	T46.8X5	T46.8X6
Soysterol	T46.6X1	T46.6X2	T46.6X3	T46.6X4	T46.6X5	T46.6X6
Spacoline	T44.3X1	T44.3X2	T44.3X3	T44.3X4	T44.3X5	T44.3X6
Spanish fly	T49.8X1	T49.8X2	T49.8X3	T49.8X4	T49.8X5	T49.8X6
Sparine	T43.3X1	T43.3X2	T43.3X3	T43.3X4	T43.3X5	T43.3X6
Sparteine	T48.0X1	T48.0X2	T48.0X3	T48.0X4	T48.0X5	T48.0X6
Spasmolytic						
anticholinergics	T44.3X1	T44.3X2	T44.3X3	T44.3X4	T44.3X5	T44.3X6
autonomic	T44.3X1	T44.3X2	T44.3X3	T44.3X4	T44.3X5	T44.3X6
bronchial NEC	T48.6X1	T48.6X2	T48.6X3	T48.6X4	T48.6X5	T48.6X6
quaternary ammonium	T44.3X1	T44.3X2	T44.3X3	T44.3X4	T44.3X5	T44.3X6
skeletal muscle NEC	T48.1X1	T48.1X2	T48.1X3	T48.1X4	T48.1X5	T48.1X6
Spectinomycin	T36.5X1	T36.5X2	T36.5X3	T36.5X4	T36.5X5	T36.5X6
Speed	T43.621	T43.622	T43.623	T43.624	T43.625	T43.626
Spermicide	T49.8X1	T49.8X2	T49.8X3	T49.8X4	T49.8X5	T49.8X6
Spider (bite) (venom)	T63.391	T63.392	T63.393	T63.394	—	—
antivenin	T50.Z11	T50.Z12	T50.Z13	T50.Z14	T50.Z15	T50.Z16
Spigelia (root)	T37.4X1	T37.4X2	T37.4X3	T37.4X4	T37.4X5	T37.4X6
Spindle inactivator	T50.4X1	T50.4X2	T50.4X3	T50.4X4	T50.4X5	T50.4X6
Spiperone	T43.4X1	T43.4X2	T43.4X3	T43.4X4	T43.4X5	T43.4X6
Spiramycin	T36.3X1	T36.3X2	T36.3X3	T36.3X4	T36.3X5	T36.3X6
Spirapril	T46.4X1	T46.4X2	T46.4X3	T46.4X4	T46.4X5	T46.4X6
Spirilene	T43.591	T43.592	T43.593	T43.594	T43.595	T43.596
Spirit(s) (neutral) **NEC**	T51.0X1	T51.0X2	T51.0X3	T51.0X4	—	—
beverage	T51.0X1	T51.0X2	T51.0X3	T51.0X4	—	—
industrial	T51.0X1	T51.0X2	T51.0X3	T51.0X4	—	—
mineral	T52.0X1	T52.0X2	T52.0X3	T52.0X4	—	—
of salt — *see* Hydrochloric acid						
surgical	T51.0X1	T51.0X2	T51.0X3	T51.0X4	—	—
Spironolactone	T50.0X1	T50.0X2	T50.0X3	T50.0X4	T50.0X5	T50.0X6
Spiroperidol	T43.4X1	T43.4X2	T43.4X3	T43.4X4	T43.4X5	T43.4X6
Sponge, absorbable	T45.7X1	T45.7X2	T45.7X3	T45.7X4	T45.7X5	T45.7X6
(gelatin)						
Sporostacin	T49.0X1	T49.0X2	T49.0X3	T49.0X4	T49.0X5	T49.0X6
Spray (aerosol)	T65.91	T65.92	T65.93	T65.94	—	—
cosmetic	T65.891	T65.892	T65.893	T65.894	—	—
medicinal NEC	T50.901	T50.902	T50.903	T50.904	T50.905	T50.906
pesticides — *see* Pesticides						
specified content — *see* specific substance						
Spurge flax	T62.2X1	T62.2X2	T62.2X3	T62.2X4	—	—
Spurges	T62.2X1	T62.2X2	T62.2X3	T62.2X4	—	—
Sputum viscosity-lowering drug	T48.4X1	T48.4X2	T48.4X3	T48.4X4	T48.4X5	T48.4X6
Squill	T46.0X1	T46.0X2	T46.0X3	T46.0X4	T46.0X5	T46.0X6
rat poison	T60.4X1	T60.4X2	T60.4X3	T60.4X4	—	—
Squirting cucumber (cathartic)	T47.2X1	T47.2X2	T47.2X3	T47.2X4	T47.2X5	T47.2X6
Stains	T65.6X1	T65.6X2	T65.6X3	T65.6X4	—	—
Stannous fluoride	T49.7X1	T49.7X2	T49.7X3	T49.7X4	T49.7X5	T49.7X6
Stanolone	T38.7X1	T38.7X2	T38.7X3	T38.7X4	T38.7X5	T38.7X6
Stanozolol	T38.7X1	T38.7X2	T38.7X3	T38.7X4	T38.7X5	T38.7X6
Staphisagria or stavesacre (pediculicide)	T49.0X1	T49.0X2	T49.0X3	T49.0X4	T49.0X5	T49.0X6
Starch	T50.901	T50.902	T50.903	T50.904	T50.905	T50.906
Stelazine	T43.3X1	T43.3X2	T43.3X3	T43.3X4	T43.3X5	T43.3X6
Stemetil	T43.3X1	T43.3X2	T43.3X3	T43.3X4	T43.3X5	T43.3X6
Stepronin	T48.4X1	T48.4X2	T48.4X3	T48.4X4	T48.4X5	T48.4X6
Sterculia	T47.4X1	T47.4X2	T47.4X3	T47.4X4	T47.4X5	T47.4X6
Sternutator gas	T59.891	T59.892	T59.893	T59.894	—	—
Steroid	T38.0X1	T38.0X2	T38.0X3	T38.0X4	T38.0X5	T38.0X6
anabolic	T38.7X1	T38.7X2	T38.7X3	T38.7X4	T38.7X5	T38.7X6
androgenic	T38.7X1	T38.7X2	T38.7X3	T38.7X4	T38.7X5	T38.7X6
antineoplastic, hormone	T38.7X1	T38.7X2	T38.7X3	T38.7X4	T38.7X5	T38.7X6
estrogen	T38.5X1	T38.5X2	T38.5X3	T38.5X4	T38.5X5	T38.5X6
ENT agent	T49.6X1	T49.6X2	T49.6X3	T49.6X4	T49.6X5	T49.6X6
ophthalmic preparation	T49.5X1	T49.5X2	T49.5X3	T49.5X4	T49.5X5	T49.5X6
topical NEC	T49.0X1	T49.0X2	T49.0X3	T49.0X4	T49.0X5	T49.0X6
Stibine	T56.891	T56.892	T56.893	T56.894	—	—
Stibogluconate	T37.3X1	T37.3X2	T37.3X3	T37.3X4	T37.3X5	T37.3X6
Stibophen	T37.4X1	T37.4X2	T37.4X3	T37.4X4	T37.4X5	T37.4X6
Stilbamidine (isetionate)	T37.3X1	T37.3X2	T37.3X3	T37.3X4	T37.3X5	T37.3X6
Stilbestrol	T38.5X1	T38.5X2	T38.5X3	T38.5X4	T38.5X5	T38.5X6
Stilboestrol	T38.5X1	T38.5X2	T38.5X3	T38.5X4	T38.5X5	T38.5X6
Stimulant						
central nervous system — *see also* Psychostimulant	T43.601	T43.602	T43.603	T43.604	T43.605	T43.606
analeptics	T50.7X1	T50.7X2	T50.7X3	T50.7X4	T50.7X5	T50.7X6
opiate antagonist	T50.7X1	T50.7X2	T50.7X3	T50.7X4	T50.7X5	T50.7X6
psychotherapeutic NEC — *see also* Psychotherapeutic drug	T43.601	T43.602	T43.603	T43.604	T43.605	T43.606
specified NEC	T43.691	T43.692	T43.693	T43.694	T43.695	T43.696

Substance	Poisoning, Accidental (unintentional)	Poisoning, Intentional Self-harm	Poisoning, Assault	Poisoning, Undetermined	Adverse Effect	Under-dosing
Stimulant — *continued*						
respiratory	T48.901	T48.902	T48.903	T48.904	T48.905	T48.906
Stone-dissolving drug	T50.901	T50.902	T50.903	T50.904	T50.905	T50.906
Storage battery (cells) (acid)	T54.2X1	T54.2X2	T54.2X3	T54.2X4	—	—
Stovaine	T41.3X1	T41.3X2	T41.3X3	T41.3X4	T41.3X5	T41.3X6
infiltration (subcutaneous)	T41.3X1	T41.3X2	T41.3X3	T41.3X4	T41.3X5	T41.3X6
nerve block (peripheral) (plexus)	T41.3X1	T41.3X2	T41.3X3	T41.3X4	T41.3X5	T41.3X6
spinal	T41.3X1	T41.3X2	T41.3X3	T41.3X4	T41.3X5	T41.3X6
topical (surface)	T41.3X1	T41.3X2	T41.3X3	T41.3X4	T41.3X5	T41.3X6
Stovarsal	T37.8X1	T37.8X2	T37.8X3	T37.8X4	T37.8X5	T37.8X6
Stove gas — *see* Gas, stove						
Stoxil	T49.5X1	T49.5X2	T49.5X3	T49.5X4	T49.5X5	T49.5X6
Stramonium	T48.6X1	T48.6X2	T48.6X3	T48.6X4	T48.6X5	T48.6X6
natural state	T62.2X1	T62.2X2	T62.2X3	T62.2X4	—	—
Streptodornase	T45.3X1	T45.3X2	T45.3X3	T45.3X4	T45.3X5	T45.3X6
Streptoduocin	T36.5X1	T36.5X2	T36.5X3	T36.5X4	T36.5X5	T36.5X6
Streptokinase	T45.611	T45.612	T45.613	T45.614	T45.615	T45.616
Streptomycin (derivative)	T36.5X1	T36.5X2	T36.5X3	T36.5X4	T36.5X5	T36.5X6
Streptonivicin	T36.5X1	T36.5X2	T36.5X3	T36.5X4	T36.5X5	T36.5X6
Streptovarycin	T36.5X1	T36.5X2	T36.5X3	T36.5X4	T36.5X5	T36.5X6
Streptozocin	T45.1X1	T45.1X2	T45.1X3	T45.1X4	T45.1X5	T45.1X6
Streptozotocin	T45.1X1	T45.1X2	T45.1X3	T45.1X4	T45.1X5	T45.1X6
Stripper (paint) (solvent)	T52.8X1	T52.8X2	T52.8X3	T52.8X4	—	—
Strobane	T60.1X1	T60.1X2	T60.1X3	T60.1X4	—	—
Strofantina	T46.0X1	T46.0X2	T46.0X3	T46.0X4	T46.0X5	T46.0X6
Strophanthin (g) (k)	T46.0X1	T46.0X2	T46.0X3	T46.0X4	T46.0X5	T46.0X6
Strophanthus	T46.0X1	T46.0X2	T46.0X3	T46.0X4	T46.0X5	T46.0X6
Strophantin	T46.0X1	T46.0X2	T46.0X3	T46.0X4	T46.0X5	T46.0X6
Strophantin-g	T46.0X1	T46.0X2	T46.0X3	T46.0X4	T46.0X5	T46.0X6
Strychnine (nonmedicinal) (pesticide) (salts)	T65.1X1	T65.1X2	T65.1X3	T65.1X4	—	—
medicinal	T48.291	T48.292	T48.293	T48.294	T48.295	T48.296
Strychnos (ignatii) — *see* Strychnine						
Styramate	T42.8X1	T42.8X2	T42.8X3	T42.8X4	T42.8X5	T42.8X6
Styrene	T65.891	T65.892	T65.893	T65.894	—	—
Succinimide, antiepileptic or anticonvulsant	T42.2X1	T42.2X2	T42.2X3	T42.2X4	T42.2X5	T42.2X6
mercuric — *see* Mercury						
Succinylcholine	T48.1X1	T48.1X2	T48.1X3	T48.1X4	T48.1X5	T48.1X6
Succinylsulfathiazole	T37.0X1	T37.0X2	T37.0X3	T37.0X4	T37.0X5	T37.0X6
Sucralfate	T47.1X1	T47.1X2	T47.1X3	T47.1X4	T47.1X5	T47.1X6
Sucrose	T50.3X1	T50.3X2	T50.3X3	T50.3X4	T50.3X5	T50.3X6
Sufentanil	T40.4X1	T40.4X2	T40.4X3	T40.4X4	T40.4X5	T40.4X6
Sulbactam	T36.0X1	T36.0X2	T36.0X3	T36.0X4	T36.0X5	T36.0X6
Sulbenicillin	T36.0X1	T36.0X2	T36.0X3	T36.0X4	T36.0X5	T36.0X6
Sulbentine	T49.0X1	T49.0X2	T49.0X3	T49.0X4	T49.0X5	T49.0X6
Sulfacetamide	T49.0X1	T49.0X2	T49.0X3	T49.0X4	T49.0X5	T49.0X6
ophthalmic preparation	T49.5X1	T49.5X2	T49.5X3	T49.5X4	T49.5X5	T49.5X6
Sulfachlorpyridazine	T37.0X1	T37.0X2	T37.0X3	T37.0X4	T37.0X5	T37.0X6
Sulfacitine	T37.0X1	T37.0X2	T37.0X3	T37.0X4	T37.0X5	T37.0X6
Sulfadiasulfone sodium	T37.0X1	T37.0X2	T37.0X3	T37.0X4	T37.0X5	T37.0X6
Sulfadiazine	T37.0X1	T37.0X2	T37.0X3	T37.0X4	T37.0X5	T37.0X6
silver (topical)	T49.0X1	T49.0X2	T49.0X3	T49.0X4	T49.0X5	T49.0X6
Sulfadimethoxine	T37.0X1	T37.0X2	T37.0X3	T37.0X4	T37.0X5	T37.0X6
Sulfadimidine	T37.0X1	T37.0X2	T37.0X3	T37.0X4	T37.0X5	T37.0X6
Sulfadoxine	T37.0X1	T37.0X2	T37.0X3	T37.0X4	T37.0X5	T37.0X6
with pyrimethamine	T37.2X1	T37.2X2	T37.2X3	T37.2X4	T37.2X5	T37.2X6
Sulfaethidole	T37.0X1	T37.0X2	T37.0X3	T37.0X4	T37.0X5	T37.0X6
Sulfafurazole	T37.0X1	T37.0X2	T37.0X3	T37.0X4	T37.0X5	T37.0X6
Sulfaguanidine	T37.0X1	T37.0X2	T37.0X3	T37.0X4	T37.0X5	T37.0X6
Sulfalene	T37.0X1	T37.0X2	T37.0X3	T37.0X4	T37.0X5	T37.0X6
Sulfaloxate	T37.0X1	T37.0X2	T37.0X3	T37.0X4	T37.0X5	T37.0X6
Sulfaloxic acid	T37.0X1	T37.0X2	T37.0X3	T37.0X4	T37.0X5	T37.0X6
Sulfamazone	T39.2X1	T39.2X2	T39.2X3	T39.2X4	T39.2X5	T39.2X6
Sulfamerazine	T37.0X1	T37.0X2	T37.0X3	T37.0X4	T37.0X5	T37.0X6
Sulfameter	T37.0X1	T37.0X2	T37.0X3	T37.0X4	T37.0X5	T37.0X6
Sulfamethazine	T37.0X1	T37.0X2	T37.0X3	T37.0X4	T37.0X5	T37.0X6
Sulfamethizole	T37.0X1	T37.0X2	T37.0X3	T37.0X4	T37.0X5	T37.0X6
Sulfamethoxazole	T37.0X1	T37.0X2	T37.0X3	T37.0X4	T37.0X5	T37.0X6
with trimethoprim	T36.8X1	T36.8X2	T36.8X3	T36.8X4	T36.8X5	T36.8X6
Sulfamethoxydiazine	T37.0X1	T37.0X2	T37.0X3	T37.0X4	T37.0X5	T37.0X6
Sulfamethoxypyridazine	T37.0X1	T37.0X2	T37.0X3	T37.0X4	T37.0X5	T37.0X6
Sulfamethylthiazole	T37.0X1	T37.0X2	T37.0X3	T37.0X4	T37.0X5	T37.0X6
Sulfametoxydiazine	T37.0X1	T37.0X2	T37.0X3	T37.0X4	T37.0X5	T37.0X6
Sulfamidopyrine	T39.2X1	T39.2X2	T39.2X3	T39.2X4	T39.2X5	T39.2X6
Sulfamonomethoxine	T37.0X1	T37.0X2	T37.0X3	T37.0X4	T37.0X5	T37.0X6
Sulfamoxole	T37.0X1	T37.0X2	T37.0X3	T37.0X4	T37.0X5	T37.0X6
Sulfamylon	T49.0X1	T49.0X2	T49.0X3	T49.0X4	T49.0X5	T49.0X6
Sulfan blue (diagnostic dye)	T50.8X1	T50.8X2	T50.8X3	T50.8X4	T50.8X5	T50.8X6
Sulfanilamide	T37.0X1	T37.0X2	T37.0X3	T37.0X4	T37.0X5	T37.0X6
Sulfanilylguanidine	T37.0X1	T37.0X2	T37.0X3	T37.0X4	T37.0X5	T37.0X6

390

Additional Character May Be Required — Refer to the Tabular List for Character Selection ▽ Subterms under main terms may continue to next column or page

Substance	Poisoning, Accidental (unintentional)	Poisoning, Intentional Self-harm	Poisoning, Assault	Poisoning, Undetermined	Adverse Effect	Under-dosing
Sulfaperin	T37.0X1	T37.0X2	T37.0X3	T37.0X4	T37.0X5	T37.0X6
Sulfaphenazole	T37.0X1	T37.0X2	T37.0X3	T37.0X4	T37.0X5	T37.0X6
Sulfaphenylthiazole	T37.0X1	T37.0X2	T37.0X3	T37.0X4	T37.0X5	T37.0X6
Sulfaproxyline	T37.0X1	T37.0X2	T37.0X3	T37.0X4	T37.0X5	T37.0X6
Sulfapyridine	T37.0X1	T37.0X2	T37.0X3	T37.0X4	T37.0X5	T37.0X6
Sulfapyrimidine	T37.0X1	T37.0X2	T37.0X3	T37.0X4	T37.0X5	T37.0X6
Sulfarsphenamine	T37.8X1	T37.8X2	T37.8X3	T37.8X4	T37.8X5	T37.8X6
Sulfasalazine	T37.0X1	T37.0X2	T37.0X3	T37.0X4	T37.0X5	T37.0X6
Sulfasuxidine	T37.0X1	T37.0X2	T37.0X3	T37.0X4	T37.0X5	T37.0X6
Sulfasymazine	T37.0X1	T37.0X2	T37.0X3	T37.0X4	T37.0X5	T37.0X6
Sulfated amylopectin	T47.8X1	T47.8X2	T47.8X3	T47.8X4	T47.8X5	T47.8X6
Sulfathiazole	T37.0X1	T37.0X2	T37.0X3	T37.0X4	T37.0X5	T37.0X6
Sulfatostearate	T49.2X1	T49.2X2	T49.2X3	T49.2X4	T49.2X5	T49.2X6
Sulfinpyrazone	T50.4X1	T50.4X2	T50.4X3	T50.4X4	T50.4X5	T50.4X6
Sulfiram	T49.0X1	T49.0X2	T49.0X3	T49.0X4	T49.0X5	T49.0X6
Sulfisomidine	T37.0X1	T37.0X2	T37.0X3	T37.0X4	T37.0X5	T37.0X6
Sulfisoxazole	T37.0X1	T37.0X2	T37.0X3	T37.0X4	T37.0X5	T37.0X6
ophthalmic preparation	T49.5X1	T49.5X2	T49.5X3	T49.5X4	T49.5X5	T49.5X6
Sulfobromophthalein (sodium)	T50.8X1	T50.8X2	T50.8X3	T50.8X4	T50.8X5	T50.8X6
Sulfobromphthalein	T50.8X1	T50.8X2	T50.8X3	T50.8X4	T50.8X5	T50.8X6
Sulfogaiacol	T48.4X1	T48.4X2	T48.4X3	T48.4X4	T48.4X5	T48.4X6
Sulfomyxin	T36.8X1	T36.8X2	T36.8X3	T36.8X4	T36.8X5	T36.8X6
Sulfonal	T42.6X1	T42.6X2	T42.6X3	T42.6X4	T42.6X5	T42.6X6
Sulfonamide NEC	T37.0X1	T37.0X2	T37.0X3	T37.0X4	T37.0X5	T37.0X6
eye	T49.5X1	T49.5X2	T49.5X3	T49.5X4	T49.5X5	T49.5X6
Sulfonazide	T37.1X1	T37.1X2	T37.1X3	T37.1X4	T37.1X5	T37.1X6
Sulfones	T37.1X1	T37.1X2	T37.1X3	T37.1X4	T37.1X5	T37.1X6
Sulfonethylmethane	T42.6X1	T42.6X2	T42.6X3	T42.6X4	T42.6X5	T42.6X6
Sulfonmethane	T42.6X1	T42.6X2	T42.6X3	T42.6X4	T42.6X5	T42.6X6
Sulfonphthal, sulfonphthol	T50.8X1	T50.8X2	T50.8X3	T50.8X4	T50.8X5	T50.8X6
Sulfonylurea derivatives, oral	T38.3X1	T38.3X2	T38.3X3	T38.3X4	T38.3X5	T38.3X6
Sulforidazine	T43.3X1	T43.3X2	T43.3X3	T43.3X4	T43.3X5	T43.3X6
Sulfoxone	T37.1X1	T37.1X2	T37.1X3	T37.1X4	T37.1X5	T37.1X6
Sulfuric acid	T54.2X1	T54.2X2	T54.2X3	T54.2X4	—	—
Sulfur, sulfurated, sulfuric, sulfurous, sulfuryl (compounds NEC) (medicinal)	T49.4X1	T49.4X2	T49.4X3	T49.4X4	T49.4X5	T49.4X6
acid	T54.2X1	T54.2X2	T54.2X3	T54.2X4	—	—
dioxide (gas)	T59.1X1	T59.1X2	T59.1X3	T59.1X4	—	—
ether — see Ether(s)						
hydrogen	T59.6X1	T59.6X2	T59.6X3	T59.6X4	—	—
medicinal (keratolytic) (ointment) NEC	T49.4X1	T49.4X2	T49.4X3	T49.4X4	T49.4X5	T49.4X6
ointment	T49.0X1	T49.0X2	T49.0X3	T49.0X4	T49.0X5	T49.0X6
pesticide (vapor)	T60.91	T60.92	T60.93	T60.94	—	—
vapor NEC	T59.891	T59.892	T59.893	T59.894	—	—
Sulglicotide	T47.1X1	T47.1X2	T47.1X3	T47.1X4	T47.1X5	T47.1X6
Sulindac	T39.391	T39.392	T39.393	T39.394	T39.395	T39.396
Sulisatin	T47.2X1	T47.2X2	T47.2X3	T47.2X4	T47.2X5	T47.2X6
Sulisobenzone	T49.3X1	T49.3X2	T49.3X3	T49.3X4	T49.3X5	T49.3X6
Sulkowitch's reagent	T50.8X1	T50.8X2	T50.8X3	T50.8X4	T50.8X5	T50.8X6
Sulmetozine	T44.3X1	T44.3X2	T44.3X3	T44.3X4	T44.3X5	T44.3X6
Suloctidil	T46.7X1	T46.7X2	T46.7X3	T46.7X4	T46.7X5	T46.7X6
Sulph- — see also Sulf-						
Sulphadiazine	T37.0X1	T37.0X2	T37.0X3	T37.0X4	T37.0X5	T37.0X6
Sulphadimethoxine	T37.0X1	T37.0X2	T37.0X3	T37.0X4	T37.0X5	T37.0X6
Sulphadimidine	T37.0X1	T37.0X2	T37.0X3	T37.0X4	T37.0X5	T37.0X6
Sulphadione	T37.1X1	T37.1X2	T37.1X3	T37.1X4	T37.1X5	T37.1X6
Sulphafurazole	T37.0X1	T37.0X2	T37.0X3	T37.0X4	T37.0X5	T37.0X6
Sulphamethizole	T37.0X1	T37.0X2	T37.0X3	T37.0X4	T37.0X5	T37.0X6
Sulphamethoxazole	T37.0X1	T37.0X2	T37.0X3	T37.0X4	T37.0X5	T37.0X6
Sulphan blue	T50.8X1	T50.8X2	T50.8X3	T50.8X4	T50.8X5	T50.8X6
Sulphaphenazole	T37.0X1	T37.0X2	T37.0X3	T37.0X4	T37.0X5	T37.0X6
Sulphapyridine	T37.0X1	T37.0X2	T37.0X3	T37.0X4	T37.0X5	T37.0X6
Sulphasalazine	T37.0X1	T37.0X2	T37.0X3	T37.0X4	T37.0X5	T37.0X6
Sulphinpyrazone	T50.4X1	T50.4X2	T50.4X3	T50.4X4	T50.4X5	T50.4X6
Sulpiride	T43.591	T43.592	T43.593	T43.594	T43.595	T43.596
Sulprostone	T48.0X1	T48.0X2	T48.0X3	T48.0X4	T48.0X5	T48.0X6
Sulpyrine	T39.2X1	T39.2X2	T39.2X3	T39.2X4	T39.2X5	T39.2X6
Sultamicillin	T36.0X1	T36.0X2	T36.0X3	T36.0X4	T36.0X5	T36.0X6
Sulthiame	T42.6X1	T42.6X2	T42.6X3	T42.6X4	T42.6X5	T42.6X6
Sultiame	T42.6X1	T42.6X2	T42.6X3	T42.6X4	T42.6X5	T42.6X6
Sultopride	T43.591	T43.592	T43.593	T43.594	T43.595	T43.596
Sumatriptan	T39.8X1	T39.8X2	T39.8X3	T39.8X4	T39.8X5	T39.8X6
Sunflower seed oil	T46.6X1	T46.6X2	T46.6X3	T46.6X4	T46.6X5	T46.6X6
Superinone	T48.4X1	T48.4X2	T48.4X3	T48.4X4	T48.4X5	T48.4X6
Suprofen	T39.311	T39.312	T39.313	T39.314	T39.315	T39.316
Suramin (sodium)	T37.4X1	T37.4X2	T37.4X3	T37.4X4	T37.4X5	T37.4X6
Surfacaine	T41.3X1	T41.3X2	T41.3X3	T41.3X4	T41.3X5	T41.3X6
Surital	T41.1X1	T41.1X2	T41.1X3	T41.1X4	T41.1X5	T41.1X6
Sutilains	T45.3X1	T45.3X2	T45.3X3	T45.3X4	T45.3X5	T45.3X6
Suxamethonium (chloride)	T48.1X1	T48.1X2	T48.1X3	T48.1X4	T48.1X5	T48.1X6
Suxethonium (chloride)	T48.1X1	T48.1X2	T48.1X3	T48.1X4	T48.1X5	T48.1X6
Suxibuzone	T39.2X1	T39.2X2	T39.2X3	T39.2X4	T39.2X5	T39.2X6
Sweetener	T50.901	T50.902	T50.903	T50.904	T50.905	T50.906
Sweet niter spirit	T46.3X1	T46.3X2	T46.3X3	T46.3X4	T46.3X5	T46.3X6
Sweet oil (birch)	T49.3X1	T49.3X2	T49.3X3	T49.3X4	T49.3X5	T49.3X6
Sym-dichloroethyl ether	T53.6X1	T53.6X2	T53.6X3	T53.6X4	—	—
Sympatholytic NEC	T44.8X1	T44.8X2	T44.8X3	T44.8X4	T44.8X5	T44.8X6
haloalkylamine	T44.8X1	T44.8X2	T44.8X3	T44.8X4	T44.8X5	T44.8X6
Sympathomimetic NEC	T44.901	T44.902	T44.903	T44.904	T44.905	T44.906
anti-common-cold	T48.5X1	T48.5X2	T48.5X3	T48.5X4	T48.5X5	T48.5X6
bronchodilator	T48.6X1	T48.6X2	T48.6X3	T48.6X4	T48.6X5	T48.6X6
specified NEC	T44.991	T44.992	T44.993	T44.994	T44.995	T44.996
Synagis	T50.B91	T50.B92	T50.B93	T50.B94	T50.B95	T50.B96
Synalar	T49.0X1	T49.0X2	T49.0X3	T49.0X4	T49.0X5	T49.0X6
Synthroid	T38.1X1	T38.1X2	T38.1X3	T38.1X4	T38.1X5	T38.1X6
Syntocinon	T48.0X1	T48.0X2	T48.0X3	T48.0X4	T48.0X5	T48.0X6
Syrosingopine	T46.5X1	T46.5X2	T46.5X3	T46.5X4	T46.5X5	T46.5X6
Systemic drug	T45.91	T45.92	T45.93	T45.94	T45.95	T45.96
specified NEC	T45.8X1	T45.8X2	T45.8X3	T45.8X4	T45.8X5	T45.8X6
Tablets — see also specified substance	T50.901	T50.902	T50.903	T50.904	T50.905	T50.906
Tace	T38.5X1	T38.5X2	T38.5X3	T38.5X4	T38.5X5	T38.5X6
Tacrine	T44.0X1	T44.0X2	T44.0X3	T44.0X4	T44.0X5	T44.0X6
Tadalafil	T46.7X1	T46.7X2	T46.7X3	T46.7X4	T46.7X5	T46.7X6
Talampicillin	T36.0X1	T36.0X2	T36.0X3	T36.0X4	T36.0X5	T36.0X6
Talbutal	T42.3X1	T42.3X2	T42.3X3	T42.3X4	T42.3X5	T42.3X6
Talc powder	T49.3X1	T49.3X2	T49.3X3	T49.3X4	T49.3X5	T49.3X6
Talcum	T49.3X1	T49.3X2	T49.3X3	T49.3X4	T49.3X5	T49.3X6
Taleranol	T38.6X1	T38.6X2	T38.6X3	T38.6X4	T38.6X5	T38.6X6
Tamoxifen	T38.6X1	T38.6X2	T38.6X3	T38.6X4	T38.6X5	T38.6X6
Tamsulosin	T44.6X1	T44.6X2	T44.6X3	T44.6X4	T44.6X5	T44.6X6
Tandearil, tanderil	T39.2X1	T39.2X2	T39.2X3	T39.2X4	T39.2X5	T39.2X6
Tannic acid	T49.2X1	T49.2X2	T49.2X3	T49.2X4	T49.2X5	T49.2X6
medicinal (astringent)	T49.2X1	T49.2X2	T49.2X3	T49.2X4	T49.2X5	T49.2X6
Tannin — see Tannic acid						
Tansy	T62.2X1	T62.2X2	T62.2X3	T62.2X4	—	—
TAO	T36.3X1	T36.3X2	T36.3X3	T36.3X4	T36.3X5	T36.3X6
Tapazole	T38.2X1	T38.2X2	T38.2X3	T38.2X4	T38.2X5	T38.2X6
Taractan	T43.591	T43.592	T43.593	T43.594	T43.595	T43.596
Tarantula (venomous)	T63.321	T63.322	T63.323	T63.324	—	—
Tartar emetic	T37.8X1	T37.8X2	T37.8X3	T37.8X4	T37.8X5	T37.8X6
Tartaric acid	T65.891	T65.892	T65.893	T65.894	—	—
Tartrated antimony (anti-infective)	T37.8X1	T37.8X2	T37.8X3	T37.8X4	T37.8X5	T37.8X6
Tartrate, laxative	T47.4X1	T47.4X2	T47.4X3	T47.4X4	T47.4X5	T47.4X6
Tar NEC	T52.0X1	T52.0X2	T52.0X3	T52.0X4	—	—
camphor	T60.1X1	T60.1X2	T60.1X3	T60.1X4	—	—
distillate	T49.1X1	T49.1X2	T49.1X3	T49.1X4	T49.1X5	T49.1X6
fumes	T59.891	T59.892	T59.893	T59.894	—	—
medicinal	T49.1X1	T49.1X2	T49.1X3	T49.1X4	T49.1X5	T49.1X6
ointment	T49.1X1	T49.1X2	T49.1X3	T49.1X4	T49.1X5	T49.1X6
Tauromustine	T45.1X1	T45.1X2	T45.1X3	T45.1X4	T45.1X5	T45.1X6
TCA — see Trichloroacetic acid						
TCDD	T53.7X1	T53.7X2	T53.7X3	T53.7X4	—	—
TDI (vapor)	T65.0X1	T65.0X2	T65.0X3	T65.0X4	—	—
Tear						
gas	T59.3X1	T59.3X2	T59.3X3	T59.3X4	—	—
solution	T49.5X1	T49.5X2	T49.5X3	T49.5X4	T49.5X5	T49.5X6
Teclothiazide	T50.2X1	T50.2X2	T50.2X3	T50.2X4	T50.2X5	T50.2X6
Teclozan	T37.3X1	T37.3X2	T37.3X3	T37.3X4	T37.3X5	T37.3X6
Tegafur	T45.1X1	T45.1X2	T45.1X3	T45.1X4	T45.1X5	T45.1X6
Tegretol	T42.1X1	T42.1X2	T42.1X3	T42.1X4	T42.1X5	T42.1X6
Teicoplanin	T36.8X1	T36.8X2	T36.8X3	T36.8X4	T36.8X5	T36.8X6
Telepaque	T50.8X1	T50.8X2	T50.8X3	T50.8X4	T50.8X5	T50.8X6
Tellurium	T56.891	T56.892	T56.893	T56.894	—	—
fumes	T56.891	T56.892	T56.893	T56.894	—	—
TEM	T45.1X1	T45.1X2	T45.1X3	T45.1X4	T45.1X5	T45.1X6
Temazepam	T42.4X1	T42.4X2	T42.4X3	T42.4X4	T42.4X5	T42.4X6
Temocillin	T36.0X1	T36.0X2	T36.0X3	T36.0X4	T36.0X5	T36.0X6
Tenamfetamine	T43.621	T43.622	T43.623	T43.624	T43.625	T43.626
Teniposide	T45.1X1	T45.1X2	T45.1X3	T45.1X4	T45.1X5	T45.1X6
Tenitramine	T46.3X1	T46.3X2	T46.3X3	T46.3X4	T46.3X5	T46.3X6
Tenoglicin	T48.4X1	T48.4X2	T48.4X3	T48.4X4	T48.4X5	T48.4X6
Tenonitrozole	T37.3X1	T37.3X2	T37.3X3	T37.3X4	T37.3X5	T37.3X6
Tenoxicam	T39.391	T39.392	T39.393	T39.394	T39.395	T39.396
TEPA	T45.1X1	T45.1X2	T45.1X3	T45.1X4	T45.1X5	T45.1X6
TEPP	T60.0X1	T60.0X2	T60.0X3	T60.0X4	—	—
Teprotide	T46.5X1	T46.5X2	T46.5X3	T46.5X4	T46.5X5	T46.5X6
Terazosin	T44.6X1	T44.6X2	T44.6X3	T44.6X4	T44.6X5	T44.6X6
Terbufos	T60.0X1	T60.0X2	T60.0X3	T60.0X4	—	—
Terbutaline	T48.6X1	T48.6X2	T48.6X3	T48.6X4	T48.6X5	T48.6X6

Subterms under main terms may continue to next column or page — Additional Character May Be Required — Refer to the Tabular List for Character Selection — 391

Sulfaperin — Terbutaline

Substance	Poisoning, Accidental (unintentional)	Poisoning, Intentional Self-harm	Poisoning, Assault	Poisoning, Undetermined	Adverse Effect	Under-dosing
Terconazole	T49.0X1	T49.0X2	T49.0X3	T49.0X4	T49.0X5	T49.0X6
Terfenadine	T45.0X1	T45.0X2	T45.0X3	T45.0X4	T45.0X5	T45.0X6
Teriparatide (acetate)	T50.991	T50.992	T50.993	T50.994	T50.995	T50.996
Terizidone	T37.1X1	T37.1X2	T37.1X3	T37.1X4	T37.1X5	T37.1X6
Terlipressin	T38.891	T38.892	T38.893	T38.894	T38.895	T38.896
Terodiline	T46.3X1	T46.3X2	T46.3X3	T46.3X4	T46.3X5	T46.3X6
Teroxalene	T37.4X1	T37.4X2	T37.4X3	T37.4X4	T37.4X5	T37.4X6
Terpin (cis) hydrate	T48.4X1	T48.4X2	T48.4X3	T48.4X4	T48.4X5	T48.4X6
Terramycin	T36.4X1	T36.4X2	T36.4X3	T36.4X4	T36.4X5	T36.4X6
Tertatolol	T44.7X1	T44.7X2	T44.7X3	T44.7X4	T44.7X5	T44.7X6
Tessalon	T48.3X1	T48.3X2	T48.3X3	T48.3X4	T48.3X5	T48.3X6
Testolactone	T38.7X1	T38.7X2	T38.7X3	T38.7X4	T38.7X5	T38.7X6
Testosterone	T38.7X1	T38.7X2	T38.7X3	T38.7X4	T38.7X5	T38.7X6
Tetanus toxoid or vaccine	T50.A91	T50.A92	T50.A93	T50.A94	T50.A95	T50.A96
antitoxin	T50.Z11	T50.Z12	T50.Z13	T50.Z14	T50.Z15	T50.Z16
immune globulin (human)	T50.Z11	T50.Z12	T50.Z13	T50.Z14	T50.Z15	T50.Z16
toxoid	T50.A91	T50.A92	T50.A93	T50.A94	T50.A95	T50.A96
with diphtheria toxoid	T50.A21	T50.A22	T50.A23	T50.A24	T50.A25	T50.A26
with pertussis	T50.A11	T50.A12	T50.A13	T50.A14	T50.A15	T50.A16
Tetrabenazine	T43.591	T43.592	T43.593	143.594	T43.595	T43.596
Tetracaine	T41.3X1	T41.3X2	T41.3X3	T41.3X4	T41.3X5	T41.3X6
nerve block (peripheral) (plexus)	T41.3X1	T41.3X2	T41.3X3	T41.3X4	T41.3X5	T41.3X6
regional	T41.3X1	T41.3X2	T41.3X3	T41.3X4	T41.3X5	T41.3X6
spinal	T41.3X1	T41.3X2	T41.3X3	T41.3X4	T41.3X5	T41.3X6
Tetrachlorethylene — see Tetrachloroethylene						
Tetrachlormethiazide	T50.2X1	T50.2X2	T50.2X3	T50.2X4	T50.2X5	T50.2X6
Tetrachloroethane	T53.6X1	T53.6X2	T53.6X3	T53.6X4	—	—
vapor	T53.6X1	T53.6X2	T53.6X3	T53.6X4	—	—
paint or varnish	T53.6X1	T53.6X2	T53.6X3	T53.6X4	—	—
Tetrachloroethylene (liquid)	T53.3X1	T53.3X2	T53.3X3	T53.3X4	—	—
medicinal	T37.4X1	T37.4X2	T37.4X3	T37.4X4	T37.4X5	T37.4X6
vapor	T53.3X1	T53.3X2	T53.3X3	T53.3X4	—	—
Tetrachloromethane — see Carbon tetrachloride						
Tetracosactide	T38.811	T38.812	T38.813	T38.814	T38.815	T38.816
Tetracosactrin	T38.811	T38.812	T38.813	T38.814	T38.815	T38.816
Tetracycline	T36.4X1	T36.4X2	T36.4X3	T36.4X4	T36.4X5	T36.4X6
ophthalmic preparation	T49.5X1	T49.5X2	T49.5X3	T49.5X4	T49.5X5	T49.5X6
topical NEC	T49.0X1	T49.0X2	T49.0X3	T49.0X4	T49.0X5	T49.0X6
Tetradifon	T60.8X1	T60.8X2	T60.8X3	T60.8X4	—	—
Tetradotoxin	T61.771	T61.772	T61.773	T61.774	—	—
Tetraethyl						
lead	T56.0X1	T56.0X2	T56.0X3	T56.0X4	—	—
pyrophosphate	T60.0X1	T60.0X2	T60.0X3	T60.0X4	—	—
Tetraethylammonium chloride	T44.2X1	T44.2X2	T44.2X3	T44.2X4	T44.2X5	T44.2X6
Tetraethylthiuram disulfide	T50.6X1	T50.6X2	T50.6X3	T50.6X4	T50.6X5	T50.6X6
Tetrahydroaminoacridine	T44.0X1	T44.0X2	T44.0X3	T44.0X4	T44.0X5	T44.0X6
Tetrahydrocannabinol	T40.7X1	T40.7X2	T40.7X3	T40.7X4	T40.7X5	T40.7X6
Tetrahydrofuran	T52.8X1	T52.8X2	T52.8X3	T52.8X4	—	—
Tetrahydronaphthalene	T52.8X1	T52.8X2	T52.8X3	T52.8X4	—	—
Tetrahydrozoline	T49.5X1	T49.5X2	T49.5X3	T49.5X4	T49.5X5	T49.5X6
Tetralin	T52.8X1	T52.8X2	T52.8X3	T52.8X4	—	—
Tetramethrin	T60.2X1	T60.2X2	T60.2X3	T60.2X4	—	—
Tetramethylthiuram (disulfide) NEC	T60.3X1	T60.3X2	T60.3X3	T60.3X4	—	—
medicinal	T49.0X1	T49.0X2	T49.0X3	T49.0X4	T49.0X5	T49.0X6
Tetramisole	T37.4X1	T37.4X2	T37.4X3	T37.4X4	T37.4X5	T37.4X6
Tetranicotinoyl fructose	T46.7X1	T46.7X2	T46.7X3	T46.7X4	T46.7X5	T46.7X6
Tetrazepam	T42.4X1	T42.4X2	T42.4X3	T42.4X4	T42.4X5	T42.4X6
Tetronal	T42.6X1	T42.6X2	T42.6X3	T42.6X4	T42.6X5	T42.6X6
Tetryl	T65.3X1	T65.3X2	T65.3X3	T65.3X4	—	—
Tetrylammonium chloride	T44.2X1	T44.2X2	T44.2X3	T44.2X4	T44.2X5	T44.2X6
Tetryzoline	T49.5X1	T49.5X2	T49.5X3	T49.5X4	T49.5X5	T49.5X6
Thalidomide	T45.1X1	T45.1X2	T45.1X3	T45.1X4	T45.1X5	T45.1X6
Thallium (compounds) (dust)	T56.811	T56.812	T56.813	T56.814	—	—
NEC						
pesticide	T60.4X1	T60.4X2	T60.4X3	T60.4X4	—	—
THC	T40.7X1	T40.7X2	T40.7X3	T40.7X4	T40.7X5	T40.7X6
Thebacon	T48.3X1	T48.3X2	T48.3X3	T48.3X4	T48.3X5	T48.3X6
Thebaine	T40.2X1	T40.2X2	T40.2X3	T40.2X4	T40.2X5	T40.2X6
Thenoic acid	T49.6X1	T49.6X2	T49.6X3	T49.6X4	T49.6X5	T49.6X6
Thenyldiamine	T45.0X1	T45.0X2	T45.0X3	T45.0X4	T45.0X5	T45.0X6
Theobromine (calcium salicylate)	T48.6X1	T48.6X2	T48.6X3	T48.6X4	T48.6X5	T48.6X6
sodium salicylate	T48.6X1	T48.6X2	T48.6X3	T48.6X4	T48.6X5	T48.6X6
Theophylline	T48.6X1	T48.6X2	T48.6X3	T48.6X4	T48.6X5	T48.6X6
Theophylline	T48.6X1	T48.6X2	T48.6X3	T48.6X4	T48.6X5	T48.6X6
aminobenzoic acid	T48.6X1	T48.6X2	T48.6X3	T48.6X4	T48.6X5	T48.6X6

Substance	Poisoning, Accidental (unintentional)	Poisoning, Intentional Self-harm	Poisoning, Assault	Poisoning, Undetermined	Adverse Effect	Under-dosing
Theophylline — continued						
ethylenediamine	T48.6X1	T48.6X2	T48.6X3	T48.6X4	T48.6X5	T48.6X6
piperazine	T48.6X1	T48.6X2	T48.6X3	T48.6X4	T48.6X5	T48.6X6
p-amino-benzoate						
Thiabendazole	T37.4X1	T37.4X2	T37.4X3	T37.4X4	T37.4X5	T37.4X6
Thialbarbital	T41.1X1	T41.1X2	T41.1X3	T41.1X4	T41.1X5	T41.1X6
Thiamazole	T38.2X1	T38.2X2	T38.2X3	T38.2X4	T38.2X5	T38.2X6
Thiambutosine	T37.1X1	T37.1X2	T37.1X3	T37.1X4	T37.1X5	T37.1X6
Thiamine	T45.2X1	T45.2X2	T45.2X3	T45.2X4	T45.2X5	T45.2X6
Thiamphenicol	T36.2X1	T36.2X2	T36.2X3	T36.2X4	T36.2X5	T36.2X6
Thiamylal	T41.1X1	T41.1X2	T41.1X3	T41.1X4	T41.1X5	T41.1X6
sodium	T41.1X1	T41.1X2	T41.1X3	T41.1X4	T41.1X5	T41.1X6
Thiazesim	T43.291	T43.292	T43.293	T43.294	T43.295	T43.296
Thiazides (diuretics)	T50.2X1	T50.2X2	T50.2X3	T50.2X4	T50.2X5	T50.2X6
Thiazinamium metilsulfate	T43.3X1	T43.3X2	T43.3X3	T43.3X4	T43.3X5	T43.3X6
Thiethylperazine	T43.3X1	T43.3X2	T43.3X3	T43.3X4	T43.3X5	T43.3X6
Thimerosal	T49.0X1	T49.0X2	T49.0X3	T49.0X4	T49.0X5	T49.0X6
ophthalmic preparation	T49.5X1	T49.5X2	T49.5X3	T49.5X4	T49.5X5	T49.5X6
Thioacetazone	T37.1X1	T37.1X2	T37.1X3	T37.1X4	T37.1X5	T37.1X6
with isoniazid	T37.1X1	T37.1X2	T37.1X3	T37.1X4	T37.1X5	T37.1X6
Thiobarbital sodium	T41.1X1	T41.1X2	T41.1X3	T41.1X4	T41.1X5	T41.1X6
Thiobarbiturate anesthetic	T41.1X1	T41.1X2	T41.1X3	T41.1X4	T41.1X5	T41.1X6
Thiobismol	T37.8X1	T37.8X2	T37.8X3	T37.8X4	T37.8X5	T37.8X6
Thiobutabarbital sodium	T41.1X1	T41.1X2	T41.1X3	T41.1X4	T41.1X5	T41.1X6
Thiocarbamate (insecticide)	T60.0X1	T60.0X2	T60.0X3	T60.0X4	—	—
Thiocarbamide	T38.2X1	T38.2X2	T38.2X3	T38.2X4	T38.2X5	T38.2X6
Thiocarbarsone	T37.8X1	T37.8X2	T37.8X3	T37.8X4	T37.8X5	T37.8X6
Thiocarlide	T37.1X1	T37.1X2	T37.1X3	T37.1X4	T37.1X5	T37.1X6
Thioctamide	T50.991	T50.992	T50.993	T50.994	T50.995	T50.996
Thioctic acid	T50.991	T50.992	T50.993	T50.994	T50.995	T50.996
Thiofos	T60.0X1	T60.0X2	T60.0X3	T60.0X4	—	—
Thioglycolate	T49.4X1	T49.4X2	T49.4X3	T49.4X4	T49.4X5	T49.4X6
Thioglycolic acid	T65.891	T65.892	T65.893	T65.894	—	—
Thioguanine	T45.1X1	T45.1X2	T45.1X3	T45.1X4	T45.1X5	T45.1X6
Thiomercaptomerin	T50.2X1	T50.2X2	T50.2X3	T50.2X4	T50.2X5	T50.2X6
Thiomerin	T50.2X1	T50.2X2	T50.2X3	T50.2X4	T50.2X5	T50.2X6
Thiomersal	T49.0X1	T49.0X2	T49.0X3	T49.0X4	T49.0X5	T49.0X6
Thionazin	T60.0X1	T60.0X2	T60.0X3	T60.0X4	—	—
Thiopental (sodium)	T41.1X1	T41.1X2	T41.1X3	T41.1X4	T41.1X5	T41.1X6
Thiopentone (sodium)	T41.1X1	T41.1X2	T41.1X3	T41.1X4	T41.1X5	T41.1X6
Thiopropazate	T43.3X1	T43.3X2	T43.3X3	T43.3X4	T43.3X5	T43.3X6
Thioproperazine	T43.3X1	T43.3X2	T43.3X3	T43.3X4	T43.3X5	T43.3X6
Thioridazine	T43.3X1	T43.3X2	T43.3X3	T43.3X4	T43.3X5	T43.3X6
Thiosinamine	T49.3X1	T49.3X2	T49.3X3	T49.3X4	T49.3X5	T49.3X6
Thiotepa	T45.1X1	T45.1X2	T45.1X3	T45.1X4	T45.1X5	T45.1X6
Thiothixene	T43.4X1	T43.4X2	T43.4X3	T43.4X4	T43.4X5	T43.4X6
Thiouracil (benzyl) (methyl) (propyl)	T38.2X1	T38.2X2	T38.2X3	T38.2X4	T38.2X5	T38.2X6
Thiourea	T38.2X1	T38.2X2	T38.2X3	T38.2X4	T38.2X5	T38.2X6
Thiphenamil	T44.3X1	T44.3X2	T44.3X3	T44.3X4	T44.3X5	T44.3X6
Thiram	T60.3X1	T60.3X2	T60.3X3	T60.3X4	—	—
medicinal	T49.2X1	T49.2X2	T49.2X3	T49.2X4	T49.2X5	T49.2X6
Thonzylamine (systemic)	T45.0X1	T45.0X2	T45.0X3	T45.0X4	T45.0X5	T45.0X6
mucosal decongestant	T48.5X1	T48.5X2	T48.5X3	T48.5X4	T48.5X5	T48.5X6
Thorazine	T43.3X1	T43.3X2	T43.3X3	T43.3X4	T43.3X5	T43.3X6
Thorium dioxide suspension	T50.8X1	T50.8X2	T50.8X3	T50.8X4	T50.8X5	T50.8X6
Thornapple	T62.2X1	T62.2X2	T62.2X3	T62.2X4	—	—
Throat drug NEC	T49.6X1	T49.6X2	T49.6X3	T49.6X4	T49.6X5	T49.6X6
Thrombin	T45.7X1	T45.7X2	T45.7X3	T45.7X4	T45.7X5	T45.7X6
Thrombolysin	T45.611	T45.612	T45.613	T45.614	T45.615	T45.616
Thromboplastin	T45.7X1	T45.7X2	T45.7X3	T45.7X4	T45.7X5	T45.7X6
Thurfyl nicotinate	T46.7X1	T46.7X2	T46.7X3	T46.7X4	T46.7X5	T46.7X6
Thymol	T49.0X1	T49.0X2	T49.0X3	T49.0X4	T49.0X5	T49.0X6
Thymopentin	T37.5X1	T37.5X2	T37.5X3	T37.5X4	T37.5X5	T37.5X6
Thymoxamine	T46.7X1	T46.7X2	T46.7X3	T46.7X4	T46.7X5	T46.7X6
Thymus extract	T38.891	T38.892	T38.893	T38.894	T38.895	T38.896
Thyreotrophic hormone	T38.811	T38.812	T38.813	T38.814	T38.815	T38.816
Thyroglobulin	T38.1X1	T38.1X2	T38.1X3	T38.1X4	T38.1X5	T38.1X6
Thyroid (hormone)	T38.1X1	T38.1X2	T38.1X3	T38.1X4	T38.1X5	T38.1X6
Thyrolar	T38.1X1	T38.1X2	T38.1X3	T38.1X4	T38.1X5	T38.1X6
Thyrotrophin	T38.811	T38.812	T38.813	T38.814	T38.815	T38.816
Thyrotropic hormone	T38.811	T38.812	T38.813	T38.814	T38.815	T38.816
Thyroxine	T38.1X1	T38.1X2	T38.1X3	T38.1X4	T38.1X5	T38.1X6
Tiabendazole	T37.4X1	T37.4X2	T37.4X3	T37.4X4	T37.4X5	T37.4X6
Tiamizide	T50.2X1	T50.2X2	T50.2X3	T50.2X4	T50.2X5	T50.2X6
Tianeptine	T43.291	T43.292	T43.293	T43.294	T43.295	T43.296
Tiapamil	T46.1X1	T46.1X2	T46.1X3	T46.1X4	T46.1X5	T46.1X6
Tiapride	T43.591	T43.592	T43.593	T43.594	T43.595	T43.596
Tiaprofenic acid	T39.311	T39.312	T39.313	T39.314	T39.315	T39.316
Tiaramide	T39.8X1	T39.8X2	T39.8X3	T39.8X4	T39.8X5	T39.8X6
Ticarcillin	T36.0X1	T36.0X2	T36.0X3	T36.0X4	T36.0X5	T36.0X6
Ticlatone	T49.0X1	T49.0X2	T49.0X3	T49.0X4	T49.0X5	T49.0X6

Additional Character May Be Required — Refer to the Tabular List for Character Selection

▽ **Subterms under main terms may continue to next column or page**

Substance	Poisoning, Accidental (unintentional)	Poisoning, Intentional Self-harm	Poisoning, Assault	Poisoning, Undetermined	Adverse Effect	Under-dosing
Ticlopidine	T45.521	T45.522	T45.523	T45.524	T45.525	T45.526
Ticrynafen	T50.1X1	T50.1X2	T50.1X3	T50.1X4	T50.1X5	T50.1X6
Tidiacic	T50.991	T50.992	T50.993	T50.994	T50.995	T50.996
Tiemonium	T44.3X1	T44.3X2	T44.3X3	T44.3X4	T44.3X5	T44.3X6
iodide	T44.3X1	T44.3X2	T44.3X3	T44.3X4	T44.3X5	T44.3X6
Tienilic acid	T50.1X1	T50.1X2	T50.1X3	T50.1X4	T50.1X5	T50.1X6
Tifenamil	T44.3X1	T44.3X2	T44.3X3	T44.3X4	T44.3X5	T44.3X6
Tigan	T45.0X1	T45.0X2	T45.0X3	T45.0X4	T45.0X5	T45.0X6
Tigloidine	T44.3X1	T44.3X2	T44.3X3	T44.3X4	T44.3X5	T44.3X6
Tilactase	T47.5X1	T47.5X2	T47.5X3	T47.5X4	T47.5X5	T47.5X6
Tiletamine	T41.291	T41.292	T41.293	T41.294	T41.295	T41.296
Tilidine	T40.4X1	T40.4X2	T40.4X3	T40.4X4		
Timepidium bromide	T44.3X1	T44.3X2	T44.3X3	T44.3X4	T44.3X5	T44.3X6
Timiperone	T43.4X1	T43.4X2	T43.4X3	T43.4X4	T43.4X5	T43.4X6
Timolol	T44.7X1	T44.7X2	T44.7X3	T44.7X4	T44.7X5	T44.7X6
Tincture, iodine — see Iodine						
Tindal	T43.3X1	T43.3X2	T43.3X3	T43.3X4	T43.3X5	T43.3X6
Tinidazole	T37.3X1	T37.3X2	T37.3X3	T37.3X4	T37.3X5	T37.3X6
Tinoridine	T39.8X1	T39.8X2	T39.8X3	T39.8X4	T39.8X5	T39.8X6
Tin (chloride) (dust) (oxide)	T56.6X1	T56.6X2	T56.6X3	T56.6X4	—	—
NEC						
anti-infectives	T37.8X1	T37.8X2	T37.8X3	T37.8X4	T37.8X5	T37.8X6
Tiocarlide	T37.1X1	T37.1X2	T37.1X3	T37.1X4	T37.1X5	T37.1X6
Tioclomarol	T45.511	T45.512	T45.513	T45.514	T45.515	T45.516
Tioconazole	T49.0X1	T49.0X2	T49.0X3	T49.0X4	T49.0X5	T49.0X6
Tioguanine	T45.1X1	T45.1X2	T45.1X3	T45.1X4	T45.1X5	T45.1X6
Tiopronin	T50.991	T50.992	T50.993	T50.994	T50.995	T50.996
Tiotixene	T43.4X1	T43.4X2	T43.4X3	T43.4X4	T43.4X5	T43.4X6
Tioxolone	T49.4X1	T49.4X2	T49.4X3	T49.4X4	T49.4X5	T49.4X6
Tipepidine	T48.3X1	T48.3X2	T48.3X3	T48.3X4	T48.3X5	T48.3X6
Tiquizium bromide	T44.3X1	T44.3X2	T44.3X3	T44.3X4	T44.3X5	T44.3X6
Tiratricol	T38.1X1	T38.1X2	T38.1X3	T38.1X4	T38.1X5	T38.1X6
Tisopurine	T50.4X1	T50.4X2	T50.4X3	T50.4X4	T50.4X5	T50.4X6
Titanium (compounds)	T56.891	T56.892	T56.893	T56.894	—	—
(vapor)						
dioxide	T49.3X1	T49.3X2	T49.3X3	T49.3X4	T49.3X5	T49.3X6
ointment	T49.3X1	T49.3X2	T49.3X3	T49.3X4	T49.3X5	T49.3X6
oxide	T49.3X1	T49.3X2	T49.3X3	T49.3X4	T49.3X5	T49.3X6
tetrachloride	T56.891	T56.892	T56.893	T56.894	—	—
Titanocene	T56.891	T56.892	T56.893	T56.894	—	—
Titroid	T38.1X1	T38.1X2	T38.1X3	T38.1X4	T38.1X5	T38.1X6
Tizanidine	T42.8X1	T42.8X2	T42.8X3	T42.8X4	T42.8X5	T42.8X6
TMTD	T60.3X1	T60.3X2	T60.3X3	T60.3X4	—	—
TNT (fumes)	T65.3X1	T65.3X2	T65.3X3	T65.3X4	—	—
Toadstool	T62.0X1	T62.0X2	T62.0X3	T62.0X4	—	—
Tobacco NEC	T65.291	T65.292	T65.293	T65.294	—	—
cigarettes	T65.221	T65.222	T65.223	T65.224	—	—
Indian	T62.2X1	T62.2X2	T62.2X3	T62.2X4	—	—
smoke, second-hand	T65.221	T65.222	T65.223	T65.224	—	—
Tobramycin	T36.5X1	T36.5X2	T36.5X3	T36.5X4	T36.5X5	T36.5X6
Tocainide	T46.2X1	T46.2X2	T46.2X3	T46.2X4	T46.2X5	T46.2X6
Tocoferol	T45.2X1	T45.2X2	T45.2X3	T45.2X4	T45.2X5	T45.2X6
Tocopherol	T45.2X1	T45.2X2	T45.2X3	T45.2X4	T45.2X5	T45.2X6
acetate	T45.2X1	T45.2X2	T45.2X3	T45.2X4	T45.2X5	T45.2X6
Tocosamine	T48.0X1	T48.0X2	T48.0X3	T48.0X4	T48.0X5	T48.0X6
Todralazine	T46.5X1	T46.5X2	T46.5X3	T46.5X4	T46.5X5	T46.5X6
Tofisopam	T42.4X1	T42.4X2	T42.4X3	T42.4X4	T42.4X5	T42.4X6
Tofranil	T43.012	T43.012	T43.013	T43.014	T43.015	T43.016
Toilet deodorizer	T65.891	T65.892	T65.893	T65.894	—	—
Tolamolol	T44.7X1	T44.7X2	T44.7X3	T44.7X4	T44.7X5	T44.7X6
Tolazamide	T38.3X1	T38.3X2	T38.3X3	T38.3X4	T38.3X5	T38.3X6
Tolazoline	T46.7X1	T46.7X2	T46.7X3	T46.7X4	T46.7X5	T46.7X6
Tolbutamide (sodium)	T38.3X1	T38.3X2	T38.3X3	T38.3X4	T38.3X5	T38.3X6
Tolciclate	T49.0X1	T49.0X2	T49.0X3	T49.0X4	T49.0X5	T49.0X6
Tolmetin	T39.391	T39.392	T39.393	T39.394	T39.395	T39.396
Tolnaftate	T49.0X1	T49.0X2	T49.0X3	T49.0X4	T49.0X5	T49.0X6
Tolonidine	T46.5X1	T46.5X2	T46.5X3	T46.5X4	T46.5X5	T46.5X6
Toloxatone	T42.6X1	T42.6X2	T42.6X3	T42.6X4	T42.6X5	T42.6X6
Tolperisone	T44.3X1	T44.3X2	T44.3X3	T44.3X4	T44.3X5	T44.3X6
Tolserol	T42.8X1	T42.8X2	T42.8X3	T42.8X4	T42.8X5	T42.8X6
Toluene (liquid)	T52.2X1	T52.2X2	T52.2X3	T52.2X4	—	—
diisocyanate	T65.0X1	T65.0X2	T65.0X3	T65.0X4	—	—
Toluidine	T65.891	T65.892	T65.893	T65.894	—	—
vapor	T59.891	T59.892	T59.893	T59.894	—	—
Toluol (liquid)	T52.2X1	T52.2X2	T52.2X3	T52.2X4	—	—
vapor	T52.2X1	T52.2X2	T52.2X3	T52.2X4	—	—
Toluylenediamine	T65.3X1	T65.3X2	T65.3X3	T65.3X4	—	—
Tolylene-2,4-diisocyanate	T65.0X1	T65.0X2	T65.0X3	T65.0X4	—	—
Tonic NEC	T50.901	T50.902	T50.903	T50.904	T50.905	T50.906
Topical action drug NEC	T49.91	T49.92	T49.93	T49.94	T49.95	T49.96
ear, nose or throat	T49.6X1	T49.6X2	T49.6X3	T49.6X4	T49.6X5	T49.6X6
eye	T49.5X1	T49.5X2	T49.5X3	T49.5X4	T49.5X5	T49.5X6
skin	T49.91	T49.92	T49.93	T49.94	T49.95	T49.96

Substance	Poisoning, Accidental (unintentional)	Poisoning, Intentional Self-harm	Poisoning, Assault	Poisoning, Undetermined	Adverse Effect	Under-dosing
Topical action drug — continued						
specified NEC	T49.8X1	T49.8X2	T49.8X3	T49.8X4	T49.8X5	T49.8X6
Toquizine	T44.3X1	T44.3X2	T44.3X3	T44.3X4	T44.3X5	T44.3X6
Toremifene	T38.6X1	T38.6X2	T38.6X3	T38.6X4	T38.6X5	T38.6X6
Tosylchloramide sodium	T49.8X1	T49.8X2	T49.8X3	T49.8X4	T49.8X5	T49.8X6
Toxaphene (dust) (spray)	T60.1X1	T60.1X2	T60.1X3	T60.1X4	—	—
Toxin, diphtheria (Schick Test)	T50.8X1	T50.8X2	T50.8X3	T50.8X4	T50.8X5	T50.8X6
Toxoid						
combined	T50.A21	T50.A22	T50.A23	T50.A24	T50.A25	T50.A26
diphtheria	T50.A91	T50.A92	T50.A93	T50.A94	T50.A95	T50.A96
tetanus	T50.A91	T50.A92	T50.A93	T50.A94	T50.A95	T50.A96
Trace element NEC	T45.8X1	T45.8X2	T45.8X3	T45.8X4	T45.8X5	T45.8X6
Tractor fuel NEC	T52.0X1	T52.0X2	T52.0X3	T52.0X4	—	—
Tragacanth	T50.991	T50.992	T50.993	T50.994	T50.995	T50.996
Tramadol	T40.4X1	T40.4X2	T40.4X3	T40.4X4	T40.4X5	T40.4X6
Tramazoline	T48.5X1	T48.5X2	T48.5X3	T48.5X4	T48.5X5	T48.5X6
Tranexamic acid	T45.621	T45.622	T45.623	T45.624	T45.625	T45.626
Tranilast	T45.0X1	T45.0X2	T45.0X3	T45.0X4	T45.0X5	T45.0X6
Tranquilizer NEC	T43.501	T43.502	T43.503	T43.504	T43.505	T43.506
with hypnotic or sedative	T42.6X1	T42.6X2	T42.6X3	T42.6X4	T42.6X5	T42.6X6
benzodiazepine NEC	T42.4X1	T42.4X2	T42.4X3	T42.4X4	T42.4X5	T42.4X6
butyrophenone NEC	T43.4X1	T43.4X2	T43.4X3	T43.4X4	T43.4X5	T43.4X6
carbamate	T43.591	T43.592	T43.593	T43.594	T43.595	T43.596
dimethylamine	T43.3X1	T43.3X2	T43.3X3	T43.3X4	T43.3X5	T43.3X6
ethylamine	T43.3X1	T43.3X2	T43.3X3	T43.3X4	T43.3X5	T43.3X6
hydroxyzine	T43.591	T43.592	T43.593	T43.594	T43.595	T43.596
major NEC	T43.501	T43.502	T43.503	T43.504	T43.505	T43.506
penothiazine NEC	T43.3X1	T43.3X2	T43.3X3	T43.3X4	T43.3X5	T43.3X6
phenothiazine-based	T43.3X1	T43.3X2	T43.3X3	T43.3X4	T43.3X5	T43.3X6
piperazine NEC	T43.3X1	T43.3X2	T43.3X3	T43.3X4	T43.3X5	T43.3X6
piperidine	T43.3X1	T43.3X2	T43.3X3	T43.3X4	T43.3X5	T43.3X6
propylamine	T43.3X1	T43.3X2	T43.3X3	T43.3X4	T43.3X5	T43.3X6
specified NEC	T43.591	T43.592	T43.593	T43.594	T43.595	T43.596
thioxanthene NEC	T43.591	T43.592	T43.593	T43.594	T43.595	T43.596
Tranxene	T42.4X1	T42.4X2	T42.4X3	T42.4X4	T42.4X5	T42.4X6
Tranylcypromine	T43.1X1	T43.1X2	T43.1X3	T43.1X4	T43.1X5	T43.1X6
Trapidil	T46.3X1	T46.3X2	T46.3X3	T46.3X4	T46.3X5	T46.3X6
Trasentine	T44.3X1	T44.3X2	T44.3X3	T44.3X4	T44.3X5	T44.3X6
Travert	T50.3X1	T50.3X2	T50.3X3	T50.3X4	T50.3X5	T50.3X6
Trazodone	T43.211	T43.212	T43.213	T43.214	T43.215	T43.216
Trecator	T37.1X1	T37.1X2	T37.1X3	T37.1X4	T37.1X5	T37.1X6
Treosulfan	T45.1X1	T45.1X2	T45.1X3	T45.1X4	T45.1X5	T45.1X6
Tretamine	T45.1X1	T45.1X2	T45.1X3	T45.1X4	T45.1X5	T45.1X6
Tretinoin	T49.0X1	T49.0X2	T49.0X3	T49.0X4	T49.0X5	T49.0X6
Tretoquinol	T48.6X1	T48.6X2	T48.6X3	T48.6X4	T48.6X5	T48.6X6
Triacetin	T49.0X1	T49.0X2	T49.0X3	T49.0X4	T49.0X5	T49.0X6
Triacetoxyanthracene	T49.4X1	T49.4X2	T49.4X3	T49.4X4	T49.4X5	T49.4X6
Triacetyloleandomycin	T36.3X1	T36.3X2	T36.3X3	T36.3X4	T36.3X5	T36.3X6
Triamcinolone	T38.0X1	T38.0X2	T38.0X3	T38.0X4	T38.0X5	T38.0X6
ENT agent	T49.6X1	T49.6X2	T49.6X3	T49.6X4	T49.6X5	T49.6X6
hexacetonide	T49.0X1	T49.0X2	T49.0X3	T49.0X4	T49.0X5	T49.0X6
ophthalmic preparation	T49.5X1	T49.5X2	T49.5X3	T49.5X4	T49.5X5	T49.5X6
topical NEC	T49.0X1	T49.0X2	T49.0X3	T49.0X4	T49.0X5	T49.0X6
Triampyzine	T44.3X1	T44.3X2	T44.3X3	T44.3X4	T44.3X5	T44.3X6
Triamterene	T50.2X1	T50.2X2	T50.2X3	T50.2X4	T50.2X5	T50.2X6
Triazine (herbicide)	T60.3X1	T60.3X2	T60.3X3	T60.3X4	—	—
Triaziquone	T45.1X1	T45.1X2	T45.1X3	T45.1X4	T45.1X5	T45.1X6
Triazolam	T42.4X1	T42.4X2	T42.4X3	T42.4X4	T42.4X5	T42.4X6
Triazole (herbicide)	T60.3X1	T60.3X2	T60.3X3	T60.3X4	—	—
Tribenoside	T46.991	T46.992	T46.993	T46.994	T46.995	T46.996
Tribromacetaldehyde	T42.6X1	T42.6X2	T42.6X3	T42.6X4	T42.6X5	T42.6X6
Tribromoethanol, rectal	T41.291	T41.292	T41.293	T41.294	T41.295	T41.296
Tribromomethane	T42.6X1	T42.6X2	T42.6X3	T42.6X4	T42.6X5	T42.6X6
Trichlorethane	T53.2X1	T53.2X2	T53.2X3	T53.2X4	—	—
Trichlorethylene	T53.2X1	T53.2X2	T53.2X3	T53.2X4	—	—
Trichlorfon	T60.0X1	T60.0X2	T60.0X3	T60.0X4	—	—
Trichlormethiazide	T50.2X1	T50.2X2	T50.2X3	T50.2X4	T50.2X5	T50.2X6
Trichlormethine	T45.1X1	T45.1X2	T45.1X3	T45.1X4	T45.1X5	T45.1X6
Trichloroacetic acid, Trichloracetic acid	T54.2X1	T54.2X2	T54.2X3	T54.2X4		
medicinal	T49.4X1	T49.4X2	T49.4X3	T49.4X4	T49.4X5	T49.4X6
Trichloroethane	T53.2X1	T53.2X2	T53.2X3	T53.2X4	—	—
Trichloroethanol	T42.6X1	T42.6X2	T42.6X3	T42.6X4	T42.6X5	T42.6X6
Trichloroethylene (liquid) (vapor)	T53.2X1	T53.2X2	T53.2X3	T53.2X4	—	—
anesthetic (gas)	T41.0X1	T41.0X2	T41.0X3	T41.0X4	T41.0X5	T41.0X6
vapor NEC	T53.2X1	T53.2X2	T53.2X3	T53.2X4	—	—
Trichloroethyl phosphate	T42.6X1	T42.6X2	T42.6X3	T42.6X4	T42.6X5	T42.6X6
Trichlorofluoromethane NEC	T53.5X1	T53.5X2	T53.5X3	T53.5X4	—	—
Trichloronate	T60.0X1	T60.0X2	T60.0X3	T60.0X4	—	—
Trichloropropane	T53.6X1	T53.6X2	T53.6X3	T53.6X4		

Subterms under main terms may continue to next column or page   Additional Character May Be Required — Refer to the Tabular List for Character Selection   393

Ticlopidine — Trichloropropane

Substance	Poisoning, Accidental (unintentional)	Poisoning, Intentional Self-harm	Poisoning, Assault	Poisoning, Undetermined	Adverse Effect	Under-dosing
Trichlorotriethylamine	T45.1X1	T45.1X2	T45.1X3	T45.1X4	T45.1X5	T45.1X6
Trichomonacides NEC	T37.3X1	T37.3X2	T37.3X3	T37.3X4	T37.3X5	T37.3X6
Trichomycin	T36.7X1	T36.7X2	T36.7X3	T36.7X4	T36.7X5	T36.7X6
Triclobisonium chloride	T49.0X1	T49.0X2	T49.0X3	T49.0X4	T49.0X5	T49.0X6
Triclocarban	T49.0X1	T49.0X2	T49.0X3	T49.0X4	T49.0X5	T49.0X6
Triclofos	T42.6X1	T42.6X2	T42.6X3	T42.6X4	T42.6X5	T42.6X6
Triclosan	T49.0X1	T49.0X2	T49.0X3	T49.0X4	T49.0X5	T49.0X6
Tricresyl phosphate	T65.891	T65.892	T65.893	T65.894	—	—
solvent	T52.91	T52.92	T52.93	T52.94	—	—
Tricyclamol chloride	T44.3X1	T44.3X2	T44.3X3	T44.3X4	T44.3X5	T44.3X6
Tridesilon	T49.0X1	T49.0X2	T49.0X3	T49.0X4	T49.0X5	T49.0X6
Tridihexethyl iodide	T44.3X1	T44.3X2	T44.3X3	T44.3X4	T44.3X5	T44.3X6
Tridione	T42.2X1	T42.2X2	T42.2X3	T42.2X4	T42.2X5	T42.2X6
Trientine	T45.8X1	T45.8X2	T45.8X3	T45.8X4	T45.8X5	T45.8X6
Triethanolamine NEC	T54.3X1	T54.3X2	T54.3X3	T54.3X4	—	—
detergent	T54.3X1	T54.3X2	T54.3X3	T54.3X4	—	—
trinitrate (biphosphate)	T46.3X1	T46.3X2	T46.3X3	T46.3X4	T46.3X5	T46.3X6
Triethanomelamine	T45.1X1	T45.1X2	T45.1X3	T45.1X4	T45.1X5	T45.1X6
Triethylenemelamine	T45.1X1	T45.1X2	T45.1X3	T45.1X4	T45.1X5	T45.1X6
Triethylenephosphoramide	T45.1X1	T45.1X2	T45.1X3	T45.1X4	T45.1X5	T45.1X6
Triethylenethiophosphoramide	T45.1X1	T45.1X2	T45.1X3	T45.1X4	T45.1X5	T45.1X6
Trifluoperazine	T43.3X1	T43.3X2	T43.3X3	T43.3X4	T43.3X5	T43.3X6
Trifluoroethyl vinyl ether	T41.0X1	T41.0X2	T41.0X3	T41.0X4	T41.0X5	T41.0X6
Trifluperidol	T43.4X1	T43.4X2	T43.4X3	T43.4X4	T43.4X5	T43.4X6
Triflupromazine	T43.3X1	T43.3X2	T43.3X3	T43.3X4	T43.3X5	T43.3X6
Trifluridine	T37.5X1	T37.5X2	T37.5X3	T37.5X4	T37.5X5	T37.5X6
Triflusal	T45.521	T45.522	T45.523	T45.524	T45.525	T45.526
Trihexyphenidyl	T44.3X1	T44.3X2	T44.3X3	T44.3X4	T44.3X5	T44.3X6
Triiodothyronine	T38.1X1	T38.1X2	T38.1X3	T38.1X4	T38.1X5	T38.1X6
Trilene	T41.0X1	T41.0X2	T41.0X3	T41.0X4	T41.0X5	T41.0X6
Trilostane	T38.991	T38.992	T38.993	T38.994	T38.995	T38.996
Trimebutine	T44.3X1	T44.3X2	T44.3X3	T44.3X4	T44.3X5	T44.3X6
Trimecaine	T41.3X1	T41.3X2	T41.3X3	T41.3X4	T41.3X5	T41.3X6
Trimeprazine (tartrate)	T44.3X1	T44.3X2	T44.3X3	T44.3X4	T44.3X5	T44.3X6
Trimetaphan camsilate	T44.2X1	T44.2X2	T44.2X3	T44.2X4	T44.2X5	T44.2X6
Trimetazidine	T46.7X1	T46.7X2	T46.7X3	T46.7X4	T46.7X5	T46.7X6
Trimethadione	T42.2X1	T42.2X2	T42.2X3	T42.2X4	T42.2X5	T42.2X6
Trimethaphan	T44.2X1	T44.2X2	T44.2X3	T44.2X4	T44.2X5	T44.2X6
Trimethidinium	T44.2X1	T44.2X2	T44.2X3	T44.2X4	T44.2X5	T44.2X6
Trimethobenzamide	T45.0X1	T45.0X2	T45.0X3	T45.0X4	T45.0X5	T45.0X6
Trimethoprim	T37.8X1	T37.8X2	T37.8X3	T37.8X4	T37.8X5	T37.8X6
with sulfamethoxazole	T36.8X1	T36.8X2	T36.8X3	T36.8X4	T36.8X5	T36.8X6
Trimethylcarbinol	T51.3X1	T51.3X2	T51.3X3	T51.3X4	—	—
Trimethylpsoralen	T49.3X1	T49.3X2	T49.3X3	T49.3X4	T49.3X5	T49.3X6
Trimeton	T45.0X1	T45.0X2	T45.0X3	T45.0X4	T45.0X5	T45.0X6
Trimetrexate	T45.1X1	T45.1X2	T45.1X3	T45.1X4	T45.1X5	T45.1X6
Trimipramine	T43.011	T43.012	T43.013	T43.014	T43.015	T43.016
Trimustine	T45.1X1	T45.1X2	T45.1X3	T45.1X4	T45.1X5	T45.1X6
Trinitrine	T46.3X1	T46.3X2	T46.3X3	T46.3X4	T46.3X5	T46.3X6
Trinitrobenzol	T65.3X1	T65.3X2	T65.3X3	T65.3X4	—	—
Trinitrophenol	T65.3X1	T65.3X2	T65.3X3	T65.3X4	—	—
Trinitrotoluene (fumes)	T65.3X1	T65.3X2	T65.3X3	T65.3X4	—	—
Trional	T42.6X1	T42.6X2	T42.6X3	T42.6X4	T42.6X5	T42.6X6
Triorthocresyl phosphate	T65.891	T65.892	T65.893	T65.894	—	—
Trioxide of arsenic	T57.0X1	T57.0X2	T57.0X3	T57.0X4	—	—
Trioxysalen	T49.4X1	T49.4X2	T49.4X3	T49.4X4	T49.4X5	T49.4X6
Tripamide	T50.2X1	T50.2X2	T50.2X3	T50.2X4	T50.2X5	T50.2X6
Triparanol	T46.6X1	T46.6X2	T46.6X3	T46.6X4	T46.6X5	T46.6X6
Tripelennamine	T45.0X1	T45.0X2	T45.0X3	T45.0X4	T45.0X5	T45.0X6
Triperiden	T44.3X1	T44.3X2	T44.3X3	T44.3X4	T44.3X5	T44.3X6
Triperidol	T43.4X1	T43.4X2	T43.4X3	T43.4X4	T43.4X5	T43.4X6
Triphenylphosphate	T65.891	T65.892	T65.893	T65.894	—	—
Triple						
bromides	T42.6X1	T42.6X2	T42.6X3	T42.6X4	T42.6X5	T42.6X6
carbonate	T47.1X1	T47.1X2	T47.1X3	T47.1X4	T47.1X5	T47.1X6
vaccine						
DPT	T50.A11	T50.A12	T50.A13	T50.A14	T50.A15	T50.A16
including pertussis	T50.A11	T50.A12	T50.A13	T50.A14	T50.A15	T50.A16
MMR	T50.B91	T50.B92	T50.B93	T50.B94	T50.B95	T50.B96
Triprolidine	T45.0X1	T45.0X2	T45.0X3	T45.0X4	T45.0X5	T45.0X6
Trisodium hydrogen edetate	T50.6X1	T50.6X2	T50.6X3	T50.6X4	T50.6X5	T50.6X6
Trisoralen	T49.3X1	T49.3X2	T49.3X3	T49.3X4	T49.3X5	T49.3X6
Trisulfapyrimidines	T37.0X1	T37.0X2	T37.0X3	T37.0X4	T37.0X5	T37.0X6
Trithiozine	T44.3X1	T44.3X2	T44.3X3	T44.3X4	T44.3X5	T44.3X6
Tritiozine	T44.3X1	T44.3X2	T44.3X3	T44.3X4	T44.3X5	T44.3X6
Tritoqualine	T45.0X1	T45.0X2	T45.0X3	T45.0X4	T45.0X5	T45.0X6
Trofosfamide	T45.1X1	T45.1X2	T45.1X3	T45.1X4	T45.1X5	T45.1X6
Troleandomycin	T36.3X1	T36.3X2	T36.3X3	T36.3X4	T36.3X5	T36.3X6
Trolnitrate (phosphate)	T46.3X1	T46.3X2	T46.3X3	T46.3X4	T46.3X5	T46.3X6
Tromantadine	T37.5X1	T37.5X2	T37.5X3	T37.5X4	T37.5X5	T37.5X6
Trometamol	T50.2X1	T50.2X2	T50.2X3	T50.2X4	T50.2X5	T50.2X6
Tromethamine	T50.2X1	T50.2X2	T50.2X3	T50.2X4	T50.2X5	T50.2X6
Tronothane	T41.3X1	T41.3X2	T41.3X3	T41.3X4	T41.3X5	T41.3X6
Tropacine	T44.3X1	T44.3X2	T44.3X3	T44.3X4	T44.3X5	T44.3X6
Tropatepine	T44.3X1	T44.3X2	T44.3X3	T44.3X4	T44.3X5	T44.3X6
Tropicamide	T44.3X1	T44.3X2	T44.3X3	T44.3X4	T44.3X5	T44.3X6
Trospium chloride	T44.3X1	T44.3X2	T44.3X3	T44.3X4	T44.3X5	T44.3X6
Troxerutin	T46.991	T46.992	T46.993	T46.994	T46.995	T46.996
Troxidone	T42.2X1	T42.2X2	T42.2X3	T42.2X4	T42.2X5	T42.2X6
Tryparsamide	T37.3X1	T37.3X2	T37.3X3	T37.3X4	T37.3X5	T37.3X6
Trypsin	T45.3X1	T45.3X2	T45.3X3	T45.3X4	T45.3X5	T45.3X6
Tryptizol	T43.011	T43.012	T43.013	T43.014	T43.015	T43.016
TSH	T38.811	T38.812	T38.813	T38.814	T38.815	T38.816
Tuaminoheptane	T48.5X1	T48.5X2	T48.5X3	T48.5X4	T48.5X5	T48.5X6
Tuberculin, purified protein derivative (PPD)	T50.8X1	T50.8X2	T50.8X4	T50.8X4	T50.8X5	T50.8X6
Tubocurare	T48.1X1	T48.1X2	T48.1X3	T48.1X4	T48.1X5	T48.1X6
Tubocurarine (chloride)	T48.1X1	T48.1X2	T48.1X3	T48.1X4	T48.1X5	T48.1X6
Tulobuterol	T48.6X1	T48.6X2	T48.6X3	T48.6X4	T48.6X5	T48.6X6
Turpentine (spirits of)	T52.8X1	T52.8X2	T52.8X3	T52.8X4	—	—
vapor	T52.8X1	T52.8X2	T52.8X3	T52.8X4	—	—
Tybamate	T43.591	T43.592	T43.593	T43.594	T43.595	T43.596
Tyloxapol	T48.4X1	T48.4X2	T48.4X3	T48.4X4	T48.4X5	T48.4X6
Tymazoline	T48.5X1	T48.5X2	T48.5X3	T48.5X4	T48.5X5	T48.5X6
Typhoid-paratyphoid vaccine	T50.A91	T50.A92	T50.A93	T50.A94	T50.A95	T50.A96
Typhus vaccine	T50.A91	T50.A92	T50.A93	T50.A94	T50.A95	T50.A96
Tyropanoate	T50.8X1	T50.8X2	T50.8X3	T50.8X4	T50.8X5	T50.8X6
Tyrothricin	T49.6X1	T49.6X2	T49.6X3	T49.6X4	T49.6X5	T49.6X6
ENT agent	T49.6X1	T49.6X2	T49.6X3	T49.6X4	T49.6X5	T49.6X6
ophthalmic preparation	T49.5X1	T49.5X2	T49.5X3	T49.5X4	T49.5X5	T49.5X6
Ufenamate	T39.391	T39.392	T39.393	T39.394	T39.395	T39.396
Ultraviolet light protectant	T49.3X1	T49.3X2	T49.3X3	T49.3X4	T49.3X5	T49.3X6
Undecenoic acid	T49.0X1	T49.0X2	T49.0X3	T49.0X4	T49.0X5	T49.0X6
Undecoylium	T49.0X1	T49.0X2	T49.0X3	T49.0X4	T49.0X5	T49.0X6
Undecylenic acid (derivatives)	T49.0X1	T49.0X2	T49.0X3	T49.0X4	T49.0X5	T49.0X6
Unna's boot	T49.3X1	T49.3X2	T49.3X3	T49.3X4	T49.3X5	T49.3X6
Unsaturated fatty acid	T46.6X1	T46.6X2	T46.6X3	T46.6X4	T46.6X5	T46.6X6
Uracil mustard	T45.1X1	T45.1X2	T45.1X3	T45.1X4	T45.1X5	T45.1X6
Uramustine	T45.1X1	T45.1X2	T45.1X3	T45.1X4	T45.1X5	T45.1X6
Urapidil	T46.5X1	T46.5X2	T46.5X3	T46.5X4	T46.5X5	T46.5X6
Urari	T48.1X1	T48.1X2	T48.1X3	T48.1X4	T48.1X5	T48.1X6
Urate oxidase	T50.4X1	T50.4X2	T50.4X3	T50.4X4	T50.4X5	T50.4X6
Urea	T47.3X1	T47.3X2	T47.3X3	T47.3X4	T47.3X5	T47.3X6
peroxide	T49.0X1	T49.0X2	T49.0X3	T49.0X4	T49.0X5	T49.0X6
stibamine	T37.4X1	T37.4X2	T37.4X3	T37.4X4	T37.4X5	T37.4X6
topical	T49.8X1	T49.8X2	T49.8X3	T49.8X4	T49.8X5	T49.8X6
Urethane	T45.1X1	T45.1X2	T45.1X3	T45.1X4	T45.1X5	T45.1X6
Urginea (maritima) (scilla) — see Squill						
Uric acid metabolism drug NEC	T50.4X1	T50.4X2	T50.4X3	T50.4X4	T50.4X5	T50.4X6
Uricosuric agent	T50.4X1	T50.4X2	T50.4X3	T50.4X4	T50.4X5	T50.4X6
Urinary anti-infective	T37.8X1	T37.8X2	T37.8X3	T37.8X4	T37.8X5	T37.8X6
Urofollitropin	T38.811	T38.812	T38.813	T38.814	T38.815	T38.816
Urokinase	T45.611	T45.612	T45.613	T45.614	T45.615	T45.616
Urokon	T50.8X1	T50.8X2	T50.8X3	T50.8X4	T50.8X5	T50.8X6
Ursodeoxycholic acid	T50.991	T50.992	T50.993	T50.994	T50.995	T50.996
Ursodiol	T50.991	T50.992	T50.993	T50.994	T50.995	T50.996
Urtica	T62.2X1	T62.2X2	T62.2X3	T62.2X4	—	—
Utility gas — see Gas, utility						
Vaccine NEC	T50.Z91	T50.Z92	T50.Z93	T50.Z94	T50.Z95	T50.Z96
antineoplastic	T50.Z91	T50.Z92	T50.Z93	T50.Z94	T50.Z95	T50.Z96
bacterial NEC	T50.A91	T50.A92	T50.A93	T50.A94	T50.A95	T50.A96
with						
other bacterial component	T50.A21	T50.A22	T50.A23	T50.A24	T50.A25	T50.A26
pertussis component	T50.A11	T50.A12	T50.A13	T50.A14	T50.A15	T50.A16
viral-rickettsial component	T50.A21	T50.A22	T50.A23	T50.A24	T50.A25	T50.A26
mixed NEC	T50.A21	T50.A22	T50.A23	T50.A24	T50.A25	T50.A26
BCG	T50.A91	T50.A92	T50.A93	T50.A94	T50.A95	T50.A96
cholera	T50.A91	T50.A92	T50.A93	T50.A94	T50.A95	T50.A96
diphtheria	T50.A91	T50.A92	T50.A93	T50.A94	T50.A95	T50.A96
with tetanus	T50.A21	T50.A22	T50.A23	T50.A24	T50.A25	T50.A26
and pertussis	T50.A11	T50.A12	T50.A13	T50.A14	T50.A15	T50.A16
influenza	T50.B91	T50.B92	T50.B93	T50.B94	T50.B95	T50.B96
measles	T50.B91	T50.B92	T50.B93	T50.B94	T50.B95	T50.B96
with mumps and rubella	T50.B91	T50.B92	T50.B93	T50.B94	T50.B95	T50.B96
meningococcal	T50.A91	T50.A92	T50.A93	T50.A94	T50.A95	T50.A96
mumps	T50.B91	T50.B92	T50.B93	T50.B94	T50.B95	T50.B96
paratyphoid	T50.A91	T50.A92	T50.A93	T50.A94	T50.A95	T50.A96
pertussis	T50.A11	T50.A12	T50.A13	T50.A14	T50.A15	T50.A16
with diphtheria	T50.A11	T50.A12	T50.A13	T50.A14	T50.A15	T50.A16

Table of Drugs and Chemicals

Substance	Poisoning, Accidental (unintentional)	Poisoning, Intentional Self-harm	Poisoning, Assault	Poisoning, Undetermined	Adverse Effect	Under-dosing
Vaccine — *continued*						
pertussis — *continued*						
with diphtheria — *continued*						
and tetanus	T50.A11	T50.A12	T50.A13	T50.A14	T50.A15	T50.A16
with other component	T50.A11	T50.A12	T50.A13	T50.A14	T50.A15	T50.A16
plague	T50.A91	T50.A92	T50.A93	T50.A94	T50.A95	T50.A96
poliomyelitis	T50.B91	T50.B92	T50.B93	T50.B94	T50.B95	T50.B96
poliovirus	T50.B91	T50.B92	T50.B93	T50.B94	T50.B95	T50.B96
rabies	T50.B91	T50.B92	T50.B93	T50.B94	T50.B95	T50.B96
respiratory syncytial virus	T50.B91	T50.B92	T50.B93	T50.B94	T50.B95	T50.B96
rickettsial NEC	T50.A91	T50.A92	T50.A93	T50.A94	T50.A95	T50.A96
with						
bacterial component	T50.A21	T50.A22	T50.A23	T50.A24	T50.A25	T50.A26
Rocky Mountain spotted fever	T50.A91	T50.A92	T50.A93	T50.A94	T50.A95	T50.A96
rubella	T50.B91	T50.B92	T50.B93	T50.B94	T50.B95	T50.B96
sabin oral	T50.B91	T50.B92	T50.B93	T50.B94	T50.B95	T50.B96
smallpox	T50.B11	T50.B12	T50.B13	T50.B14	T50.B15	T50.B16
TAB	T50.A91	T50.A92	T50.A93	T50.A94	T50.A95	T50.A96
tetanus	T50.A91	T50.A92	T50.A93	T50.A94	T50.A95	T50.A96
typhoid	T50.A91	T50.A92	T50.A93	T50.A94	T50.A95	T50.A96
typhus	T50.A91	T50.A92	T50.A93	T50.A94	T50.A95	T50.A96
viral NEC	T50.B91	T50.B92	T50.B93	T50.B94	T50.B95	T50.B96
yellow fever	T50.B91	T50.B92	T50.B93	T50.B94	T50.B95	T50.B96
Vaccinia immune globulin	T50.Z11	T50.Z12	T50.Z13	T50.Z14	T50.Z15	T50.Z16
Vaginal contraceptives	T49.8X1	T49.8X2	T49.8X3	T49.8X4	T49.8X5	T49.8X6
Valerian						
root	T42.6X1	T42.6X2	T42.6X3	T42.6X4	T42.6X5	T42.6X6
tincture	T42.6X1	T42.6X2	T42.6X3	T42.6X4	T42.6X5	T42.6X6
Valethamate bromide	T44.3X1	T44.3X2	T44.3X3	T44.3X4	T44.3X5	T44.3X6
Valisone	T49.0X1	T49.0X2	T49.0X3	T49.0X4	T49.0X5	T49.0X6
Valium	T42.4X1	T42.4X2	T42.4X3	T42.4X4	T42.4X5	T42.4X6
Valmid	T42.6X1	T42.6X2	T42.6X3	T42.6X4	T42.6X5	T42.6X6
Valnoctamide	T42.6X1	T42.6X2	T42.6X3	T42.6X4	T42.6X5	T42.6X6
Valproate (sodium)	T42.6X1	T42.6X2	T42.6X3	T42.6X4	T42.6X5	T42.6X6
Valproic acid	T42.6X1	T42.6X2	T42.6X3	T42.6X4	T42.6X5	T42.6X6
Valpromide	T42.6X1	T42.6X2	T42.6X3	T42.6X4	T42.6X5	T42.6X6
Vanadium	T56.891	T56.892	T56.893	T56.894	—	—
Vancomycin	T36.8X1	T36.8X2	T36.8X3	T36.8X4	T36.8X5	T36.8X6
Vapor — *see also* Gas	T59.91	T59.92	T59.93	T59.94	—	—
kiln (carbon monoxide)	T58.8X1	T58.8X2	T58.8X3	T58.8X4	—	—
lead — *see* lead						
specified source NEC	T59.891	T59.892	T59.893	T59.894	—	—
Vardenafil	T46.7X1	T46.7X2	T46.7X3	T46.7X4	T46.7X5	T46.7X6
Varicose reduction drug	T46.8X1	T46.8X2	T46.8X3	T46.8X4	T46.8X5	T46.8X6
Varnish	T65.4X1	T65.4X2	T65.4X3	T65.4X4	—	—
cleaner	T52.91	T52.92	T52.93	T52.94	—	—
Vaseline	T49.3X1	T49.3X2	T49.3X3	T49.3X4	T49.3X5	T49.3X6
Vasodilan	T46.7X1	T46.7X2	T46.7X3	T46.7X4	T46.7X5	T46.7X6
Vasodilator						
coronary NEC	T46.3X1	T46.3X2	T46.3X3	T46.3X4	T46.3X5	T46.3X6
peripheral NEC	T46.7X1	T46.7X2	T46.7X3	T46.7X4	T46.7X5	T46.7X6
Vasopressin	T38.891	T38.892	T38.893	T38.894	T38.895	T38.896
Vasopressor drugs	T38.891	T38.892	T38.893	T38.894	T38.895	T38.896
Vecuronium bromide	T48.1X1	T48.1X2	T48.1X3	T48.1X4	T48.1X5	T48.1X6
Vegetable extract, astringent	T49.2X1	T49.2X2	T49.2X3	T49.2X4	T49.2X5	T49.2X6
Venlafaxine	T43.211	T43.212	T43.213	T43.214	T43.215	T43.216
Venom, venomous (bite) (sting)	T63.91	T63.92	T63.93	T63.94	—	—
amphibian NEC	T63.831	T63.832	T63.833	T63.834	—	—
animal NEC	T63.891	T63.892	T63.893	T63.894	—	—
ant	T63.421	T63.422	T63.423	T63.424	—	—
arthropod NEC	T63.481	T63.482	T63.483	T63.484	—	—
bee	T63.441	T63.442	T63.443	T63.444	—	—
centipede	T63.411	T63.412	T63.413	T63.414	—	—
fish	T63.591	T63.592	T63.593	T63.594	—	—
frog	T63.811	T63.812	T63.813	T63.814	—	—
hornet	T63.451	T63.452	T63.453	T63.454	—	—
insect NEC	T63.481	T63.482	T63.483	T63.484	—	—
lizard	T63.121	T63.122	T63.123	T63.124	—	—
marine						
animals	T63.691	T63.692	T63.693	T63.694	—	—
bluebottle	T63.611	T63.612	T63.613	T63.614	—	—
jellyfish NEC	T63.621	T63.622	T63.623	T63.624	—	—
Portugese Man-o-war	T63.611	T63.612	T63.613	T63.614	—	—
sea anemone	T63.631	T63.632	T63.633	T63.634	—	—
specified NEC	T63.691	T63.692	T63.693	T63.694	—	—
fish	T63.591	T63.592	T63.593	T63.594	—	—
plants	T63.711	T63.712	T63.713	T63.714	—	—
sting ray	T63.511	T63.512	T63.513	T63.514	—	—
millipede (tropical)	T63.411	T63.412	T63.413	T63.414	—	—
plant NEC	T63.791	T63.792	T63.793	T63.794	—	—

Substance	Poisoning, Accidental (unintentional)	Poisoning, Intentional Self-harm	Poisoning, Assault	Poisoning, Undetermined	Adverse Effect	Under-dosing
Venom, venomous — *continued*						
plant — *continued*						
marine	T63.711	T63.712	T63.713	T63.714	—	—
reptile	T63.191	T63.192	T63.193	T63.194	—	—
gila monster	T63.111	T63.112	T63.113	T63.114	—	—
lizard NEC	T63.121	T63.122	T63.123	T63.124	—	—
scorpion	T63.2X1	T63.2X2	T63.2X3	T63.2X4	—	—
snake	T63.001	T63.002	T63.003	T63.004	—	—
African NEC	T63.081	T63.082	T63.083	T63.084	—	—
American (North) (South) NEC	T63.061	T63.062	T63.063	T63.064	—	—
Asian	T63.081	T63.082	T63.083	T63.084	—	—
Australian	T63.071	T63.072	T63.073	T63.074	—	—
cobra	T63.041	T63.042	T63.043	T63.044	—	—
coral snake	T63.021	T63.022	T63.023	T63.024	—	—
rattlesnake	T63.011	T63.012	T63.013	T63.014	—	—
specified NEC	T63.091	T63.092	T63.093	T63.094	—	—
taipan	T63.031	T63.032	T63.033	T63.034	—	—
specified NEC	T63.891	T63.892	T63.893	T63.894	—	—
spider	T63.301	T63.302	T63.303	T63.304	—	—
black widow	T63.311	T63.312	T63.313	T63.314	—	—
brown recluse	T63.331	T63.332	T63.333	T63.334	—	—
specified NEC	T63.391	T63.392	T63.393	T63.394	—	—
tarantula	T63.321	T63.322	T63.323	T63.324	—	—
sting ray	T63.511	T63.512	T63.513	T63.514	—	—
toad	T63.821	T63.822	T63.823	T63.824	—	—
wasp	T63.461	T63.462	T63.463	T63.464	—	—
Venous sclerosing drug NEC	T46.8X1	T46.8X2	T46.8X3	T46.8X4	T46.8X5	T46.8X6
Ventolin — *see* Albuterol						
Veramon	T42.3X1	T42.3X2	T42.3X3	T42.3X4	T42.3X5	T42.3X6
Verapamil	T46.1X1	T46.1X2	T46.1X3	T46.1X4	T46.1X5	T46.1X6
Veratrine	T46.5X1	T46.5X2	T46.5X3	T46.5X4	T46.5X5	T46.5X6
Veratrum						
album	T62.2X1	T62.2X2	T62.2X3	T62.2X4	—	—
alkaloids	T46.5X1	T46.5X2	T46.5X3	T46.5X4	T46.5X5	T46.5X6
viride	T62.2X1	T62.2X2	T62.2X3	T62.2X4	—	—
Verdigris	T60.3X1	T60.3X2	T60.3X3	T60.3X4	—	—
Veronal	T42.3X1	T42.3X2	T42.3X3	T42.3X4	T42.3X5	T42.3X6
Veroxil	T37.4X1	T37.4X2	T37.4X3	T37.4X4	T37.4X5	T37.4X6
Versenate	T50.6X1	T50.6X2	T50.6X3	T50.6X4	T50.6X5	T50.6X6
Versidyne	T39.8X1	T39.8X2	T39.8X3	T39.8X4	T39.8X5	T39.8X6
Vetrabutine	T48.0X1	T48.0X2	T48.0X3	T48.0X4	T48.0X5	T48.0X6
Vidarabine	T37.5X1	T37.5X2	T37.5X3	T37.5X4	T37.5X5	T37.5X6
Vienna						
green	T57.0X1	T57.0X2	T57.0X3	T57.0X4	—	—
insecticide	T60.2X1	T60.2X2	T60.2X3	T60.2X4	—	—
red	T57.0X1	T57.0X2	T57.0X3	T57.0X4	—	—
pharmaceutical dye	T50.991	T50.992	T50.993	T50.994	T50.995	T50.996
Vigabatrin	T42.6X1	T42.6X2	T42.6X3	T42.6X4	T42.6X5	T42.6X6
Viloxazine	T43.291	T43.292	T43.293	T43.294	T43.295	T43.296
Viminol	T39.8X1	T39.8X2	T39.8X3	T39.8X4	T39.8X5	T39.8X6
Vinbarbital, vinbarbitone	T42.3X1	T42.3X2	T42.3X3	T42.3X4	T42.3X5	T42.3X6
Vinblastine	T45.1X1	T45.1X2	T45.1X3	T45.1X4	T45.1X5	T45.1X6
Vinburnine	T46.7X1	T46.7X2	T46.7X3	T46.7X4	T46.7X5	T46.7X6
Vincamine	T46.7X1	T46.7X2	T46.7X3	T46.7X4	T46.7X5	T46.7X6
Vincristine	T45.1X1	T45.1X2	T45.1X3	T45.1X4	T45.1X5	T45.1X6
Vindesine	T45.1X1	T45.1X2	T45.1X3	T45.1X4	T45.1X5	T45.1X6
Vinesthene, vinethene	T41.0X1	T41.0X2	T41.0X3	T41.0X4	T41.0X5	T41.0X6
Vinorelbine tartrate	T45.1X1	T45.1X2	T45.1X3	T45.1X4	T45.1X5	T45.1X6
Vinpocetine	T46.7X1	T46.7X2	T46.7X3	T46.7X4	T46.7X5	T46.7X6
Vinyl						
acetate	T65.891	T65.892	T65.893	T65.894	—	—
bital	T42.3X1	T42.3X2	T42.3X3	T42.3X4	T42.3X5	T42.3X6
bromide	T65.891	T65.892	T65.893	T65.894	—	—
chloride	T59.891	T59.892	T59.893	T59.894	—	—
ether	T41.0X1	T41.0X2	T41.0X3	T41.0X4	T41.0X5	T41.0X6
Vinylbital	T42.3X1	T42.3X2	T42.3X3	T42.3X4	T42.3X5	T42.3X6
Vinylidene chloride	T65.891	T65.892	T65.893	T65.894	—	—
Vioform	T37.8X1	T37.8X2	T37.8X3	T37.8X4	T37.8X5	T37.8X6
topical	T49.0X1	T49.0X2	T49.0X3	T49.0X4	T49.0X5	T49.0X6
Viomycin	T36.8X1	T36.8X2	T36.8X3	T36.8X4	T36.8X5	T36.8X6
Viosterol	T45.2X1	T45.2X2	T45.2X3	T45.2X4	T45.2X5	T45.2X6
Viper (venom)	T63.091	T63.092	T63.093	T63.094	—	—
Viprynium	T37.4X1	T37.4X2	T37.4X3	T37.4X4	T37.4X5	T37.4X6
Viquidil	T46.7X1	T46.7X2	T46.7X3	T46.7X4	T46.7X5	T46.7X6
Viral vaccine NEC	T50.B91	T50.B92	T50.B93	T50.B94	T50.B95	T50.B96
Virginiamycin	T36.8X1	T36.8X2	T36.8X3	T36.8X4	T36.8X5	T36.8X6
Virugon	T37.5X1	T37.5X2	T37.5X3	T37.5X4	T37.5X5	T37.5X6
Viscous agent	T50.901	T50.902	T50.903	T50.904	T50.905	T50.906
Visine	T49.5X1	T49.5X2	T49.5X3	T49.5X4	T49.5X5	T49.5X6
Visnadine	T46.3X1	T46.3X2	T46.3X3	T46.3X4	T46.3X5	T46.3X6
Vitamin NEC	T45.2X1	T45.2X2	T45.2X3	T45.2X4	T45.2X5	T45.2X6

Vaccine NEC — Vitamin NEC

Substance	Poisoning, Accidental (unintentional)	Poisoning, Intentional Self-harm	Poisoning, Assault	Poisoning, Undetermined	Adverse Effect	Under-dosing
Vitamin — *continued*						
A	T45.2X1	T45.2X2	T45.2X3	T45.2X4	T45.2X5	T45.2X6
B1	T45.2X1	T45.2X2	T45.2X3	T45.2X4	T45.2X5	T45.2X6
B2	T45.2X1	T45.2X2	T45.2X3	T45.2X4	T45.2X5	T45.2X6
B6	T45.2X1	T45.2X2	T45.2X3	T45.2X4	T45.2X5	T45.2X6
B12	T45.2X1	T45.2X2	T45.2X3	T45.2X4	T45.2X5	T45.2X6
B15	T45.2X1	T45.2X2	T45.2X3	T45.2X4	T45.2X5	T45.2X6
B NEC	T45.2X1	T45.2X2	T45.2X3	T45.2X4	T45.2X5	T45.2X6
nicotinic acid	T46.7X1	T46.7X2	T46.7X3	T46.7X4	T46.7X5	T46.7X6
C	T45.2X1	T45.2X2	T45.2X3	T45.2X4	T45.2X5	T45.2X6
D	T45.2X1	T45.2X2	T45.2X3	T45.2X4	T45.2X5	T45.2X6
D2	T45.2X1	T45.2X2	T45.2X3	T45.2X4	T45.2X5	T45.2X6
D3	T45.2X1	T45.2X2	T45.2X3	T45.2X4	T45.2X5	T45.2X6
E	T45.2X1	T45.2X2	T45.2X3	T45.2X4	T45.2X5	T45.2X6
E acetate	T45.2X1	T45.2X2	T45.2X3	T45.2X4	T45.2X5	T45.2X6
hematopoietic	T45.8X1	T45.8X2	T45.8X3	T45.8X4	T45.8X5	T45.8X6
K1	T45.7X1	T45.7X2	T45.7X3	T45.7X4	T45.7X5	T45.7X6
K2	T45.7X1	T45.7X2	T45.7X3	T45.7X4	T45.7X5	T45.7X6
K NEC	T45.7X1	T45.7X2	T45.7X3	T45.7X4	T45.7X5	T45.7X6
PP	T45.2X1	T45.2X2	T45.2X3	T45.2X4	T45.2X5	T45.2X6
ulceroprotectant	T47.1X1	T47.1X2	T47.1X3	T47.1X4	T47.1X5	T47.1X6
Vleminckx's solution	T49.4X1	T49.4X2	T49.4X3	T49.4X4	T49.4X5	T49.4X6
Voltaren — *see* Diclofenac						
sodium						
Warfarin	T45.511	T45.512	T45.513	T45.514	T45.515	T45.516
rodenticide	T45.511	T45.512	T45.513	T45.514	T45.515	T45.516
sodium	T45.511	T45.512	T45.513	T45.514	T45.515	T45.516
Wasp (sting)	T63.461	T63.462	T63.463	T63.464	—	—
Water						
balance drug	T50.3X1	T50.3X2	T50.3X3	T50.3X4	T50.3X5	T50.3X6
distilled	T50.3X1	T50.3X2	T50.3X3	T50.3X4	T50.3X5	T50.3X6
gas — *see* Gas, water						
incomplete combustion of —						
see Carbon, monoxide,						
fuel, utility						
hemlock	T62.2X1	T62.2X2	T62.2X3	T62.2X4	—	—
moccasin (venom)	T63.061	T63.062	T63.063	T63.064	—	—
purified	T50.3X1	T50.3X2	T50.3X3	T50.3X4	T50.3X5	T50.3X6
Wax (paraffin) (petroleum)	T52.0X1	T52.0X2	T52.0X3	T52.0X4	—	—
automobile	T65.891	T65.892	T65.893	T65.894	—	—
floor	T52.0X1	T52.0X2	T52.0X3	T52.0X4	—	—
Weed killers NEC	T60.3X1	T60.3X2	T60.3X3	T60.3X4	—	—
Welldorm	T42.6X1	T42.6X2	T42.6X3	T42.6X4	T42.6X5	T42.6X6
White						
arsenic	T57.0X1	T57.0X2	T57.0X3	T57.0X4	—	—
hellebore	T62.2X1	T62.2X2	T62.2X3	T62.2X4	—	—
lotion (keratolytic)	T49.4X1	T49.4X2	T49.4X3	T49.4X4	T49.4X5	T49.4X6
spirit	T52.0X1	T52.0X2	T52.0X3	T52.0X4	—	—
Whitewash	T65.891	T65.892	T65.893	T65.894	—	—
Whole blood (human)	T45.8X1	T45.8X2	T45.8X3	T45.8X4	T45.8X5	T45.8X6
Wild						
black cherry	T62.2X1	T62.2X2	T62.2X3	T62.2X4	—	—
poisonous plants NEC	T62.2X1	T62.2X2	T62.2X3	T62.2X4	—	—
Window cleaning fluid	T65.891	T65.892	T65.893	T65.894	—	—
Wintergreen (oil)	T49.3X1	T49.3X2	T49.3X3	T49.3X4	T49.3X5	T49.3X6
Wisterine	T62.2X1	T62.2X2	T62.2X3	T62.2X4	—	—
Witch hazel	T49.2X1	T49.2X2	T49.2X3	T49.2X4	T49.2X5	T49.2X6
Wood alcohol or spirit	T51.1X1	T51.1X2	T51.1X3	T51.1X4	—	—
Wool fat (hydrous)	T49.3X1	T49.3X2	T49.3X3	T49.3X4	T49.3X5	T49.3X6
Woorali	T48.1X1	T48.1X2	T48.1X3	T48.1X4	T48.1X5	T48.1X6
Wormseed, American	T37.4X1	T37.4X2	T37.4X3	T37.4X4	T37.4X5	T37.4X6
Xamoterol	T44.5X1	T44.5X2	T44.5X3	T44.5X4	T44.5X5	T44.5X6
Xanthine diuretics	T50.2X1	T50.2X2	T50.2X3	T50.2X4	T50.2X5	T50.2X6
Xanthinol nicotinate	T46.7X1	T46.7X2	T46.7X3	T46.7X4	T46.7X5	T46.7X6
Xanthotoxin	T49.3X1	T49.3X2	T49.3X3	T49.3X4	T49.3X5	T49.3X6
Xantinol nicotinate	T46.7X1	T46.7X2	T46.7X3	T46.7X4	T46.7X5	T46.7X6
Xantocillin	T36.0X1	T36.0X2	T36.0X3	T36.0X4	T36.0X5	T36.0X6
Xenon (127Xe) (133Xe)	T50.8X1	T50.8X2	T50.8X3	T50.8X4	T50.8X5	T50.8X6
Xenysalate	T49.4X1	T49.4X2	T49.4X3	T49.4X4	T49.4X5	T49.4X6
Xibornol	T37.8X1	T37.8X2	T37.8X3	T37.8X4	T37.8X5	T37.8X6
Xigris	T45.511	T45.512	T45.513	T45.514	T45.515	T45.516
Xipamide	T50.2X1	T50.2X2	T50.2X3	T50.2X4	T50.2X5	T50.2X6
Xylene (vapor)	T52.2X1	T52.2X2	T52.2X3	T52.2X4	—	—
Xylocaine (infiltration)	T41.3X1	T41.3X2	T41.3X3	T41.3X4	T41.3X5	T41.3X6
(topical)						
nerve block (peripheral)	T41.3X1	T41.3X2	T41.3X3	T41.3X4	T41.3X5	T41.3X6
(plexus)						
spinal	T41.3X1	T41.3X2	T41.3X3	T41.3X4	T41.3X5	T41.3X6
Xylol (vapor)	T52.2X1	T52.2X2	T52.2X3	T52.2X4	—	—
Xylometazoline	T48.5X1	T48.5X2	T48.5X3	T48.5X4	T48.5X5	T48.5X6
Yeast	T45.2X1	T45.2X2	T45.2X3	T45.2X4	T45.2X5	T45.2X6
dried	T45.2X1	T45.2X2	T45.2X3	T45.2X4	T45.2X5	T45.2X6

Substance	Poisoning, Accidental (unintentional)	Poisoning, Intentional Self-harm	Poisoning, Assault	Poisoning, Undetermined	Adverse Effect	Under-dosing
Yellow						
fever vaccine	T50.B91	T50.B92	T50.B93	T50.B94	T50.B95	T50.B96
jasmine	T62.2X1	T62.2X2	T62.2X3	T62.2X4	—	—
phenolphthalein	T47.2X1	T47.2X2	T47.2X3	T47.2X4	T47.2X5	T47.2X6
Yew	T62.2X1	T62.2X2	T62.2X3	T62.2X4	—	—
Yohimbic acid	T40.991	T40.992	T40.993	T40.994	T40.995	T40.996
Zactane	T39.8X1	T39.8X2	T39.8X3	T39.8X4	T39.8X5	T39.8X6
Zalcitabine	T37.5X1	T37.5X2	T37.5X3	T37.5X4	T37.5X5	T37.5X6
Zaroxolyn	T50.2X1	T50.2X2	T50.2X3	T50.2X4	T50.2X5	T50.2X6
Zephiran (topical)	T49.0X1	T49.0X2	T49.0X3	T49.0X4	T49.0X5	T49.0X6
ophthalmic preparation	T49.5X1	T49.5X2	T49.5X3	T49.5X4	T49.5X5	T49.5X6
Zeranol	T38.7X1	T38.7X2	T38.7X3	T38.7X4	T38.7X5	T38.7X6
Zerone	T51.1X1	T51.1X2	T51.1X3	T51.1X4	—	—
Zidovudine	T37.5X1	T37.5X2	T37.5X3	T37.5X4	T37.5X5	T37.5X6
Zimeldine	T43.221	T43.222	T43.223	T43.224	T43.225	T43.226
Zinc (compounds) (fumes) (vapor)	T56.5X1	T56.5X2	T56.5X3	T56.5X4	—	—
NEC						
anti-infectives	T49.0X1	T49.0X2	T49.0X3	T49.0X4	T49.0X5	T49.0X6
antivaricose	T46.8X1	T46.8X2	T46.8X3	T46.8X4	T46.8X5	T46.8X6
bacitracin	T49.0X1	T49.0X2	T49.0X3	T49.0X4	T49.0X5	T49.0X6
chloride (mouthwash)	T49.6X1	T49.6X2	T49.6X3	T49.6X4	T49.6X5	T49.6X6
chromate	T56.5X1	T56.5X2	T56.5X3	T56.5X4	—	—
gelatin	T49.3X1	T49.3X2	T49.3X3	T49.3X4	T49.3X5	T49.3X6
oxide	T49.3X1	T49.3X2	T49.3X3	T49.3X4	T49.3X5	T49.3X6
plaster	T49.3X1	T49.3X2	T49.3X3	T49.3X4	T49.3X5	T49.3X6
peroxide	T49.0X1	T49.0X2	T49.0X3	T49.0X4	T49.0X5	T49.0X6
pesticides	T56.5X1	T56.5X2	T56.5X3	T56.5X4	—	—
phosphide	T60.4X1	T60.4X2	T60.4X3	T60.4X4	—	—
pyrithionate	T49.4X1	T49.4X2	T49.4X3	T49.4X4	T49.4X5	T49.4X6
stearate	T49.3X1	T49.3X2	T49.3X3	T49.3X4	T49.3X5	T49.3X6
sulfate	T49.5X1	T49.5X2	T49.5X3	T49.5X4	T49.5X5	T49.5X6
ENT agent	T49.6X1	T49.6X2	T49.6X3	T49.6X4	T49.6X5	T49.6X6
ophthalmic solution	T49.5X1	T49.5X2	T49.5X3	T49.5X4	T49.5X5	T49.5X6
topical NEC	T49.0X1	T49.0X2	T49.0X3	T49.0X4	T49.0X5	T49.0X6
undecylenate	T49.0X1	T49.0X2	T49.0X3	T49.0X4	T49.0X5	T49.0X6
Zineb	T60.0X1	T60.0X2	T60.0X3	T60.0X4	—	—
Zinostatin	T45.1X1	T45.1X2	T45.1X3	T45.1X4	T45.1X5	T45.1X6
Zipeprol	T48.3X1	T48.3X2	T48.3X3	T48.3X4	T48.3X5	T48.3X6
Zofenopril	T46.4X1	T46.4X2	T46.4X3	T46.4X4	T46.4X5	T46.4X6
Zolpidem	T42.6X1	T42.6X2	T42.6X3	T42.6X4	T42.6X5	T42.6X6
Zomepirac	T39.391	T39.392	T39.393	T39.394	T39.395	T39.396
Zopiclone	T42.6X1	T42.6X2	T42.6X3	T42.6X4	T42.6X5	T42.6X6
Zorubicin	T45.1X1	T45.1X2	T45.1X3	T45.1X4	T45.1X5	T45.1X6
Zotepine	T43.591	T43.592	T43.593	T43.594	T43.595	T43.596
Zovant	T45.511	T45.512	T45.513	T45.514	T45.515	T45.516
Zoxazolamine	T42.8X1	T42.8X2	T42.8X3	T42.8X4	T42.8X5	T42.8X6
Zuclopenthixol	T43.4X1	T43.4X2	T43.4X3	T43.4X4	T43.4X5	T43.4X6
Zygadenus (venenosus)	T62.2X1	T62.2X2	T62.2X3	T62.2X4	—	—
Zyprexa	T43.591	T43.592	T43.593	T43.594	T43.595	T43.596

A

Abandonment (causing exposure to weather conditions) (with intent to injure or kill) NEC X58 ☑
Abuse (adult) (child) (mental) (physical) (sexual) X58 ☑
Accident (to) X58 ☑
  aircraft (in transit) (powered) (*see also* Accident, transport, aircraft)
    due to, caused by cataclysm — *see* Forces of nature, by type
  animal-drawn vehicle — *see* Accident, transport, animal-drawn vehicle occupant
  animal-rider — *see* Accident, transport, animal-rider
  automobile — *see* Accident, transport, car occupant
  bare foot water skier V94.4 ☑
  boat, boating (*see also* Accident, watercraft)
    striking swimmer
      powered V94.11 ☑
      unpowered V94.12 ☑
  bus — *see* Accident, transport, bus occupant
  cable car, not on rails V98.0 ☑
    on rails — *see* Accident, transport, streetcar occupant
  car — *see* Accident, transport, car occupant
  caused by, due to
    animal NEC W64 ☑
    chain hoist W24.0 ☑
    cold (excessive) — *see* Exposure, cold
    corrosive liquid, substance — *see* Table of Drugs and Chemicals
    cutting or piercing instrument — *see* Contact, with, by type of instrument
    drive belt W24.0 ☑
    electric
      current — *see* Exposure, electric current
      motor (*see also* Contact, with, by type of machine) W31.3 ☑
      current (of) W86.8 ☑
    environmental factor NEC X58 ☑
    explosive material — *see* Explosion
    fire, flames — *see* Exposure, fire
    firearm missile — *see* Discharge, firearm by type
    heat (excessive) — *see* Heat
    hot — *see* Contact, with, hot
    ignition — *see* Ignition
    lifting device W24.0 ☑
    lightning — *see* subcategory T75.0 ☑
      causing fire — *see* Exposure, fire
    machine, machinery — *see* Contact, with, by type of machine
    natural factor NEC X58 ☑
    pulley (block) W24.0 ☑
    radiation — *see* Radiation
    steam X13.1 ☑
      inhalation X13.0 ☑
      pipe X16 ☑
    thunderbolt — *see* subcategory T75.0 ☑
      causing fire — *see* Exposure, fire
    transmission device W24.1 ☑
  coach — *see* Accident, transport, bus occupant
  coal car — *see* Accident, transport, industrial vehicle occupant
  diving (*see also* Fall, into, water)
    with
      drowning or submersion — *see* Drowning
  forklift — *see* Accident, transport, industrial vehicle occupant
  heavy transport vehicle NOS — *see* Accident, transport, truck occupant
  ice yacht V98.2 ☑
  in
    medical, surgical procedure
      as, or due to misadventure — *see* Misadventure
      causing an abnormal reaction or later complication without mention of misadventure (*see also* Complication of or following, by type of procedure) Y84.9
  land yacht V98.1 ☑
  late effect of — *see* W00-X58 with 7th character S
  logging car — *see* Accident, transport, industrial vehicle occupant
  machine, machinery (*see also* Contact, with, by type of machine)
    on board watercraft V93.69 ☑
      explosion — *see* Explosion, in, watercraft

Accident — *continued*
  machine, machinery (*see also* Contact, with, by type of machine) — *continued*
    on board watercraft — *continued*
      fire — *see* Burn, on board watercraft
      powered craft V93.63 ☑
        ferry boat V93.61 ☑
        fishing boat V93.62 ☑
        jetskis V93.63 ☑
        liner V93.61 ☑
        merchant ship V93.60 ☑
        passenger ship V93.61 ☑
        sailboat V93.64 ☑
  mine tram — *see* Accident, transport, industrial vehicle occupant
  mobility scooter (motorized) — *see* Accident, transport, pedestrian, conveyance, specified type NEC
  motor scooter — *see* Accident, transport, motorcyclist
  motor vehicle NOS (traffic) (*see also* Accident, transport) V89.2 ☑
    nontraffic V89.0 ☑
    three-wheeled NOS — *see* Accident, transport, three-wheeled motor vehicle occupant
  motorcycle NOS — *see* Accident, transport, motorcyclist
  nonmotor vehicle NOS (nontraffic) (*see also* Accident, transport) V89.1 ☑
    traffic NOS V89.3 ☑
  nontraffic (victim's mode of transport NOS) V88.9 ☑
    collision (between) V88.7 ☑
      bus and truck V88.5 ☑
      car and:
        bus V88.3 ☑
        pickup V88.2 ☑
        three-wheeled motor vehicle V88.0 ☑
        train V88.6 ☑
        truck V88.4 ☑
        two-wheeled motor vehicle V88.0 ☑
        van V88.2 ☑
      specified vehicle NEC and:
        three-wheeled motor vehicle V88.1 ☑
        two-wheeled motor vehicle V88.1 ☑
    known mode of transport — *see* Accident, transport, by type of vehicle
    noncollision V88.8 ☑
  on board watercraft V93.89 ☑
    powered craft V93.83 ☑
      ferry boat V93.81 ☑
      fishing boat V93.82 ☑
      jetskis V93.83 ☑
      liner V93.81 ☑
      merchant ship V93.80 ☑
      passenger ship V93.81 ☑
    unpowered craft V93.88 ☑
      canoe V93.85 ☑
      inflatable V93.86 ☑
        in tow
          recreational V94.31 ☑
          specified NEC V94.32 ☑
      kayak V93.85 ☑
      sailboat V93.84 ☑
      surf-board V93.88 ☑
      water skis V93.87 ☑
      windsurfer V93.88 ☑
  parachutist V97.29 ☑
    entangled in object V97.21 ☑
    injured on landing V97.22 ☑
  pedal cycle — *see* Accident, transport, pedal cyclist
  pedestrian (on foot)
    with
      another pedestrian W51 ☑
        with fall W03 ☑
          due to ice or snow W00.0 ☑
      on pedestrian conveyance NEC V00.09 ☑
      roller skater (in-line) V00.01 ☑
      skate boarder V00.02 ☑
      transport vehicle — *see* Accident, transport
    on pedestrian conveyance — *see* Accident, transport, pedestrian, conveyance
  pick-up truck or van — *see* Accident, transport, pickup truck occupant
  quarry truck — *see* Accident, transport, industrial vehicle occupant
  railway vehicle (any) (in motion) — *see* Accident, transport, railway vehicle occupant
    due to cataclysm — *see* Forces of nature, by type

Accident — *continued*
  scooter (non-motorized) — *see* Accident, transport, pedestrian, conveyance, scooter
  sequelae of — *see* categories W00-X58 with 7th character S
  skateboard — *see* Accident, transport, pedestrian, conveyance, skateboard
  ski(ing) — *see* Accident, transport, pedestrian, conveyance
    lift V98.3 ☑
  specified cause NEC X58 ☑
  streetcar — *see* Accident, transport, streetcar occupant
  traffic (victim's mode of transport NOS) V87.9 ☑
    collision (between) V87.7 ☑
      bus and truck V87.5 ☑
      car and:
        bus V87.3 ☑
        pickup V87.2 ☑
        three-wheeled motor vehicle V87.0 ☑
        train V87.6 ☑
        truck V87.4 ☑
        two-wheeled motor vehicle V87.0 ☑
        van V87.2 ☑
      specified vehicle NEC and:
        three-wheeled motor vehicle V87.1 ☑
        two-wheeled motor vehicle V87.1 ☑
    known mode of transport — *see* Accident, transport, by type of vehicle
    noncollision V87.8 ☑
  transport (involving injury to) V99 ☑
    18 wheeler — *see* Accident, transport, truck occupant
    agricultural vehicle occupant (nontraffic) V84.9 ☑
      driver V84.5 ☑
      hanger-on V84.7 ☑
      passenger V84.6 ☑
      traffic V84.3 ☑
        driver V84.0 ☑
        hanger-on V84.2 ☑
        passenger V84.1 ☑
      while boarding or alighting V84.4 ☑
    aircraft NEC V97.89 ☑
      military NEC V97.818 ☑
        with civilan aircraft V97.810 ☑
        civilian injured by V97.811 ☑
      occupant injured (in)
        nonpowered craft accident V96.9 ☑
          balloon V96.00 ☑
            collision V96.03 ☑
            crash V96.01 ☑
            explosion V96.05 ☑
            fire V96.04 ☑
            forced landing V96.02 ☑
            specified type NEC V96.09 ☑
          glider V96.20 ☑
            collision V96.23 ☑
            crash V96.21 ☑
            explosion V96.25 ☑
            fire V96.24 ☑
            forced landing V96.22 ☑
            specified type NEC V96.29 ☑
          hang glider V96.10 ☑
            collision V96.13 ☑
            crash V96.11 ☑
            explosion V96.15 ☑
            fire V96.14 ☑
            forced landing V96.12 ☑
            specified type NEC V96.19 ☑
          specified craft NEC V96.8 ☑
        powered craft accident V95.9 ☑
          fixed wing NEC
            commercial V95.30 ☑
              collision V95.33 ☑
              crash V95.31 ☑
              explosion V95.35 ☑
              fire V95.34 ☑
              forced landing V95.32 ☑
              specified type NEC V95.39 ☑
            private V95.20 ☑
              collision V95.23 ☑
              crash V95.21 ☑
              explosion V95.25 ☑
              fire V95.24 ☑
              forced landing V95.22 ☑
              specified type NEC V95.29 ☑
          glider V95.10 ☑

☑ Subterms under main terms may continue to next column or page   ☑ Additional Character Required — Refer to the Tabular List for Character Selection   397

Abandonment — Accident

Accident — *continued*
  transport — *continued*
    aircraft — *continued*
      occupant injured — *continued*
        powered craft accident — *continued*
          glider — *continued*
            collision V95.13 ☑
            crash V95.11 ☑
            explosion V95.15 ☑
            fire V95.14 ☑
            forced landing V95.12 ☑
            specified type NEC V95.19 ☑
          helicopter V95.00 ☑
            collision V95.03 ☑
            crash V95.01 ☑
            explosion V95.05 ☑
            fire V95.04 ☑
            forced landing V95.02 ☑
            specified type NEC V95.09 ☑
          spacecraft V95.40 ☑
            collision V95.43 ☑
            crash V95.41 ☑
            explosion V95.45 ☑
            fire V95.44 ☑
            forced landing V95.42 ☑
            specified type NEC V95.49 ☑
          specified craft NEC V95.8 ☑
          ultralight V95.10 ☑
            collision V95.13 ☑
            crash V95.11 ☑
            explosion V95.15 ☑
            fire V95.14 ☑
            forced landing V95.12 ☑
            specified type NEC V95.19 ☑
        specified accident NEC V97.0 ☑
        while boarding or alighting V97.1 ☑
      person (injured by)
        falling from, in or on aircraft V97.0 ☑
        machinery on aircraft V97.89 ☑
        on ground with aircraft involvement V97.39 ☑
        rotating propeller V97.32 ☑
        struck by object falling from aircraft V97.31 ☑
        sucked into aircraft jet V97.33 ☑
        while boarding or alighting aircraft V97.1 ☑
    airport (battery-powered) passenger vehicle — *see* Accident, transport, industrial vehicle occupant
    all-terrain vehicle occupant (nontraffic) V86.95 ☑
      driver V86.55 ☑
      dune buggy — *see* Accident, transport, dune buggy occupant
      hanger-on V86.75 ☑
      passenger V86.65 ☑
      snowmobile — *see* Accident, transport, snowmobile occupant
      specified type NEC V86.99 ☑
      traffic V86.35 ☑
        driver V86.05 ☑
        hanger-on V86.25 ☑
        passenger V86.15 ☑
      while boarding or alighting V86.45 ☑
    ambulance occupant (traffic) V86.31 ☑
      driver V86.01 ☑
      hanger-on V86.21 ☑
      nontraffic V86.91 ☑
        driver V86.51 ☑
        hanger-on V86.71 ☑
        passenger V86.61 ☑
      passenger V86.11 ☑
      while boarding or alighting V86.41 ☑
    animal-drawn vehicle occupant (in) V80.929 ☑
      collision (with)
        animal V80.12 ☑
          being ridden V80.711 ☑
        animal-drawn vehicle V80.721 ☑
        bus V80.42 ☑
        car V80.42 ☑
        fixed or stationary object V80.82 ☑
        military vehicle V80.920 ☑
        nonmotor vehicle V80.791 ☑
        pedal cycle V80.22 ☑
        pedestrian V80.12 ☑
        pickup V80.42 ☑
        railway train or vehicle V80.62 ☑

Accident — *continued*
  transport — *continued*
    animal-drawn vehicle occupant — *continued*
      collision — *continued*
        specified motor vehicle NEC V80.52 ☑
        streetcar V80.731 ☑
        truck V80.42 ☑
        two- or three-wheeled motor vehicle V80.32 ☑
        van V80.42 ☑
      noncollision V80.02 ☑
      specified circumstance NEC V80.928 ☑
    animal-rider V80.919 ☑
      collision (with)
        animal V80.11 ☑
          being ridden V80.710 ☑
        animal-drawn vehicle V80.720 ☑
        bus V80.41 ☑
        car V80.41 ☑
        fixed or stationary object V80.81 ☑
        military vehicle V80.910 ☑
        nonmotor vehicle V80.790 ☑
        pedal cycle V80.21 ☑
        pedestrian V80.11 ☑
        pickup V80.41 ☑
        railway train or vehicle V80.61 ☑
        specified motor vehicle NEC V80.51 ☑
        streetcar V80.730 ☑
        truck V80.41 ☑
        two- or three-wheeled motor vehicle V80.31 ☑
        van V80.31 ☑
      noncollision V80.018 ☑
        specified as horse rider V80.010 ☑
      specified circumstance NEC V80.918 ☑
    armored car — *see* Accident, transport, truck occupant
    battery-powered truck (baggage) (mail) — *see* Accident, transport, industrial vehicle occupant
    bus occupant V79.9 ☑
      collision (with)
        animal (traffic) V70.9 ☑
          being ridden (traffic) V76.9 ☑
            nontraffic V76.3 ☑
            while boarding or alighting V76.4 ☑
          nontraffic V70.3 ☑
          while boarding or alighting V70.4 ☑
        animal-drawn vehicle (traffic) V76.9 ☑
          nontraffic V76.3 ☑
          while boarding or alighting V76.4 ☑
        bus (traffic) V74.9 ☑
          nontraffic V74.3 ☑
          while boarding or alighting V74.4 ☑
        car (traffic) V73.9 ☑
          nontraffic V73.3 ☑
          while boarding or alighting V73.4 ☑
        motor vehicle NOS (traffic) V79.60 ☑
          nontraffic V79.20 ☑
          specified type NEC (traffic) V79.69 ☑
            nontraffic V79.29 ☑
        pedal cycle (traffic) V71.9 ☑
          nontraffic V71.3 ☑
          while boarding or alighting V71.4 ☑
        pickup truck (traffic) V73.9 ☑
          nontraffic V73.3 ☑
          while boarding or alighting V73.4 ☑
        railway vehicle (traffic) V75.9 ☑
          nontraffic V75.3 ☑
          while boarding or alighting V75.4 ☑
        specified vehicle NEC (traffic) V76.9 ☑
          nontraffic V76.3 ☑
          while boarding or alighting V76.4 ☑
        stationary object (traffic) V77.9 ☑
          nontraffic V77.3 ☑
          while boarding or alighting V77.4 ☑
        streetcar (traffic) V76.9 ☑
          nontraffic V76.3 ☑
          while boarding or alighting V76.4 ☑
        three wheeled motor vehicle (traffic) V72.9 ☑
          nontraffic V72.3 ☑
          while boarding or alighting V72.4 ☑
        truck (traffic) V74.9 ☑
          nontraffic V74.3 ☑
          while boarding or alighting V74.4 ☑

Accident — *continued*
  transport — *continued*
    bus occupant — *continued*
      collision — *continued*
        two wheeled motor vehicle (traffic) V72.9 ☑
          nontraffic V72.3 ☑
          while boarding or alighting V72.4 ☑
        van (traffic) V73.9 ☑
          nontraffic V73.3 ☑
          while boarding or alighting V73.4 ☑
      driver
        collision (with)
          animal (traffic) V70.5 ☑
            being ridden (traffic) V76.5 ☑
              nontraffic V76.0 ☑
            nontraffic V70.0 ☑
          animal-drawn vehicle (traffic) V76.5 ☑
            nontraffic V76.0 ☑
          bus (traffic) V74.5 ☑
            nontraffic V74.0 ☑
          car (traffic) V73.5 ☑
            nontraffic V73.0 ☑
          motor vehicle NOS (traffic) V79.40 ☑
            nontraffic V79.00 ☑
            specified type NEC (traffic) V79.49 ☑
              nontraffic V79.09 ☑
          pedal cycle (traffic) V71.5 ☑
            nontraffic V71.0 ☑
          pickup truck (traffic) V73.5 ☑
            nontraffic V73.0 ☑
          railway vehicle (traffic) V75.5 ☑
            nontraffic V75.0 ☑
          specified vehicle NEC (traffic) V76.5 ☑
            nontraffic V76.0 ☑
          stationary object (traffic) V77.5 ☑
            nontraffic V77.0 ☑
          streetcar (traffic) V76.5 ☑
            nontraffic V76.0 ☑
          three wheeled motor vehicle (traffic) V72.5 ☑
            nontraffic V72.0 ☑
          truck (traffic) V74.5 ☑
            nontraffic V74.0 ☑
          two wheeled motor vehicle (traffic) V72.5 ☑
            nontraffic V72.0 ☑
          van (traffic) V73.5 ☑
            nontraffic V73.0 ☑
        noncollision accident (traffic) V78.5 ☑
          nontraffic V78.0 ☑
      hanger-on
        collision (with)
          animal (traffic) V70.7 ☑
            being ridden (traffic) V76.7 ☑
              nontraffic V76.2 ☑
            nontraffic V70.2 ☑
          animal-drawn vehicle (traffic) V76.7 ☑
            nontraffic V76.2 ☑
          bus (traffic) V74.7 ☑
            nontraffic V74.2 ☑
          car (traffic) V73.7 ☑
            nontraffic V73.2 ☑
          pedal cycle (traffic) V71.7 ☑
            nontraffic V71.2 ☑
          pickup truck (traffic) V73.7 ☑
            nontraffic V73.2 ☑
          railway vehicle (traffic) V75.7 ☑
            nontraffic V75.2 ☑
          specified vehicle NEC (traffic) V76.7 ☑
            nontraffic V76.2 ☑
          stationary object (traffic) V77.7 ☑
            nontraffic V77.2 ☑
          streetcar (traffic) V76.7 ☑
            nontraffic V76.2 ☑
          three wheeled motor vehicle (traffic) V72.7 ☑
            nontraffic V72.2 ☑
          truck (traffic) V74.7 ☑
            nontraffic V74.2 ☑
          two wheeled motor vehicle (traffic) V72.7 ☑
            nontraffic V72.2 ☑
          van (traffic) V73.7 ☑
            nontraffic V73.2 ☑
        noncollision accident (traffic) V78.7 ☑
          nontraffic V78.2 ☑

☑ Additional Character Required — Refer to the Tabular List for Character Selection   ▽ Subterms under main terms may continue to next column or page

Accident — *continued*
  transport — *continued*
    bus occupant — *continued*
      noncollision accident (traffic) V78.9 ☑
        nontraffic V78.3 ☑
        while boarding or alighting V78.4 ☑
      nontraffic V79.3 ☑
      passenger
        collision (with)
          animal (traffic) V70.6 ☑
            being ridden (traffic) V76.6 ☑
              nontraffic V76.1 ☑
            nontraffic V70.1 ☑
          animal-drawn vehicle (traffic) V76.6 ☑
            nontraffic V76.1 ☑
          bus (traffic) V74.6 ☑
            nontraffic V74.1 ☑
          car (traffic) V73.6 ☑
            nontraffic V73.1 ☑
          motor vehicle NOS (traffic) V79.50 ☑
            nontraffic V79.10 ☑
            specified type NEC (traffic) V79.59 ☑
              nontraffic V79.19 ☑
          pedal cycle (traffic) V71.6 ☑
            nontraffic V71.1 ☑
          pickup truck (traffic) V73.6 ☑
            nontraffic V73.1 ☑
          railway vehicle (traffic) V75.6 ☑
            nontraffic V75.1 ☑
          specified vehicle NEC (traffic) V76.6 ☑
            nontraffic V76.1 ☑
          stationary object (traffic) V77.6 ☑
            nontraffic V77.1 ☑
          streetcar (traffic) V76.6 ☑
            nontraffic V76.1 ☑
          three wheeled motor vehicle (traffic)
            V72.6 ☑
            nontraffic V72.1 ☑
          truck (traffic) V74.6 ☑
            nontraffic V74.1 ☑
          two wheeled motor vehicle (traffic)
            V72.6 ☑
            nontraffic V72.1 ☑
          van (traffic) V73.6 ☑
            nontraffic V73.1 ☑
        noncollision accident (traffic) V78.6 ☑
          nontraffic V78.1 ☑
        specified type NEC V79.88 ☑
        military vehicle V79.81 ☑
    cable car, not on rails V98.0 ☑
      on rails — *see* Accident, transport, streetcar
        occupant
    car occupant V49.9 ☑
      ambulance occupant — *see* Accident, transport,
        ambulance occupant
      collision (with)
        animal (traffic) V40.9 ☑
          being ridden (traffic) V46.9 ☑
            nontraffic V46.3 ☑
            while boarding or alighting V46.4 ☑
          nontraffic V40.3 ☑
          while boarding or alighting V40.4 ☑
        animal-drawn vehicle (traffic) V46.9 ☑
          nontraffic V46.3 ☑
          while boarding or alighting V46.4 ☑
        bus (traffic) V44.9 ☑
          nontraffic V44.3 ☑
          while boarding or alighting V44.4 ☑
        car (traffic) V43.92 ☑
          nontraffic V43.32 ☑
          while boarding or alighting V43.42 ☑
        motor vehicle NOS (traffic) V49.60 ☑
          nontraffic V49.20 ☑
          specified type NEC (traffic) V49.69 ☑
            nontraffic V49.29 ☑
        pedal cycle (traffic) V41.9 ☑
          nontraffic V41.3 ☑
          while boarding or alighting V41.4 ☑
        pickup truck (traffic) V43.93 ☑
          nontraffic V43.33 ☑
          while boarding or alighting V43.43 ☑
        railway vehicle (traffic) V45.9 ☑
          nontraffic V45.3 ☑
          while boarding or alighting V45.4 ☑
        specified vehicle NEC (traffic) V46.9 ☑
          nontraffic V46.3 ☑

Accident — *continued*
  transport — *continued*
    car occupant — *continued*
      collision — *continued*
        specified vehicle — *continued*
          while boarding or alighting V46.4 ☑
        sport utility vehicle (traffic) V43.91 ☑
          nontraffic V43.31 ☑
          while boarding or alighting V43.41 ☑
        stationary object (traffic) V47.9 ☑
          nontraffic V47.3 ☑
          while boarding or alighting V47.4 ☑
        streetcar (traffic) V46.9 ☑
          nontraffic V46.3 ☑
          while boarding or alighting V46.4 ☑
        three wheeled motor vehicle (traffic)
          V42.9 ☑
          nontraffic V42.3 ☑
          while boarding or alighting V42.4 ☑
        truck (traffic) V44.9 ☑
          nontraffic V44.3 ☑
          while boarding or alighting V44.4 ☑
        two wheeled motor vehicle (traffic) V42.9 ☑
          nontraffic V42.3 ☑
          while boarding or alighting V42.4 ☑
        van (traffic) V43.94 ☑
          nontraffic V43.34 ☑
          while boarding or alighting V43.44 ☑
      driver
        collision (with)
          animal (traffic) V40.5 ☑
            being ridden (traffic) V46.5 ☑
              nontraffic V46.0 ☑
            nontraffic V40.0 ☑
          animal-drawn vehicle (traffic) V46.5 ☑
            nontraffic V46.0 ☑
          bus (traffic) V44.5 ☑
            nontraffic V44.0 ☑
          car (traffic) V43.52 ☑
            nontraffic V43.02 ☑
          motor vehicle NOS (traffic) V49.40 ☑
            nontraffic V49.00 ☑
            specified type NEC (traffic) V49.49 ☑
              nontraffic V49.09 ☑
          pedal cycle (traffic) V41.5 ☑
            nontraffic V41.0 ☑
          pickup truck (traffic) V43.53 ☑
            nontraffic V43.03 ☑
          railway vehicle (traffic) V45.5 ☑
            nontraffic V45.0 ☑
          specified vehicle NEC (traffic) V46.5 ☑
            nontraffic V46.0 ☑
          sport utility vehicle (traffic) V43.51 ☑
            nontraffic V43.01 ☑
          stationary object (traffic) V47.5 ☑
            nontraffic V47.0 ☑
          streetcar (traffic) V46.5 ☑
            nontraffic V46.0 ☑
          three wheeled motor vehicle (traffic)
            V42.5 ☑
            nontraffic V42.0 ☑
          truck (traffic) V44.5 ☑
            nontraffic V44.0 ☑
          two wheeled motor vehicle (traffic)
            V42.5 ☑
            nontraffic V42.0 ☑
          van (traffic) V43.54 ☑
            nontraffic V43.04 ☑
        noncollision accident (traffic) V48.5 ☑
          nontraffic V48.0 ☑
      hanger-on
        collision (with)
          animal (traffic) V40.7 ☑
            being ridden (traffic) V46.7 ☑
              nontraffic V46.2 ☑
            nontraffic V40.2 ☑
          animal-drawn vehicle (traffic) V46.7 ☑
            nontraffic V46.2 ☑
          bus (traffic) V44.7 ☑
            nontraffic V44.2 ☑
          car (traffic) V43.72 ☑
            nontraffic V43.22 ☑
          pedal cycle (traffic) V41.7 ☑
            nontraffic V41.2 ☑
          pickup truck (traffic) V43.73 ☑
            nontraffic V43.23 ☑

Accident — *continued*
  transport — *continued*
    car occupant — *continued*
      hanger-on — *continued*
        collision — *continued*
          railway vehicle (traffic) V45.7 ☑
            nontraffic V45.2 ☑
          specified vehicle NEC (traffic) V46.7 ☑
            nontraffic V46.2 ☑
          sport utility vehicle (traffic) V43.71 ☑
            nontraffic V43.21 ☑
          stationary object (traffic) V47.7 ☑
            nontraffic V47.2 ☑
          streetcar (traffic) V46.7 ☑
            nontraffic V46.2 ☑
          three wheeled motor vehicle (traffic)
            V42.7 ☑
            nontraffic V42.2 ☑
          truck (traffic) V44.7 ☑
            nontraffic V44.2 ☑
          two wheeled motor vehicle (traffic)
            V42.7 ☑
            nontraffic V42.2 ☑
          van (traffic) V43.74 ☑
            nontraffic V43.24 ☑
        noncollision accident (traffic) V48.7 ☑
          nontraffic V48.2 ☑
      noncollision accident (traffic) V48.9 ☑
        nontraffic V48.3 ☑
        while boarding or alighting V48.4 ☑
      nontraffic V49.3 ☑
      passenger
        collision (with)
          animal (traffic) V40.6 ☑
            being ridden (traffic) V46.6 ☑
              nontraffic V46.1 ☑
            nontraffic V40.1 ☑
          animal-drawn vehicle (traffic) V46.6 ☑
            nontraffic V46.1 ☑
          bus (traffic) V44.6 ☑
            nontraffic V44.1 ☑
          car (traffic) V43.62 ☑
            nontraffic V43.12 ☑
          motor vehicle NOS (traffic) V49.50 ☑
            nontraffic V49.10 ☑
            specified type NEC (traffic) V49.59 ☑
              nontraffic V49.19 ☑
          pedal cycle (traffic) V41.6 ☑
            nontraffic V41.1 ☑
          pickup truck (traffic) V43.63 ☑
            nontraffic V43.13 ☑
          railway vehicle (traffic) V45.6 ☑
            nontraffic V45.1 ☑
          specified vehicle NEC (traffic) V46.6 ☑
            nontraffic V46.1 ☑
          sport utility vehicle (traffic) V43.61 ☑
            nontraffic V43.11 ☑
          stationary object (traffic) V47.6 ☑
            nontraffic V47.1 ☑
          streetcar (traffic) V46.6 ☑
            nontraffic V46.1 ☑
          three wheeled motor vehicle (traffic)
            V42.6 ☑
            nontraffic V42.1 ☑
          truck (traffic) V44.6 ☑
            nontraffic V44.1 ☑
          two wheeled motor vehicle (traffic)
            V42.6 ☑
            nontraffic V42.1 ☑
          van (traffic) V43.64 ☑
            nontraffic V43.14 ☑
        noncollision accident (traffic) V48.6 ☑
          nontraffic V48.1 ☑
      specified type NEC V49.88 ☑
        military vehicle V49.81 ☑
    coal car — *see* Accident, transport, industrial vehi-
      cle occupant
    construction vehicle occupant (nontraffic) V85.9 ☑
      driver V85.5 ☑
      hanger-on V85.7 ☑
      passenger V85.6 ☑
      traffic V85.3 ☑
        driver V85.0 ☑
        hanger-on V85.2 ☑
        passenger V85.1 ☑
      while boarding or alighting V85.4 ☑

Accident — *continued*
  transport — *continued*
    dirt bike rider (nontraffic) V86.96 ☑
      driver V86.56 ☑
      hanger-on V86.76 ☑
      passenger V86.66 ☑
      traffic V86.36 ☑
        driver V86.06 ☑
        hanger-on V86.26 ☑
        passenger V86.16 ☑
      while boarding or alighting V86.46 ☑
    due to cataclysm — *see* Forces of nature, by type
    dune buggy occupant (nontraffic) V86.93 ☑
      driver V86.53 ☑
      hanger-on V86.73 ☑
      passenger V86.63 ☑
      traffic V86.33 ☑
        driver V86.03 ☑
        hanger-on V86.23 ☑
        passenger V86.13 ☑
      while boarding or alighting V86.43 ☑
    forklift — *see* Accident, transport, industrial vehicle occupant
    go cart — *see* Accident, transport, all-terrain vehicle occupant
    golf cart — *see* Accident, transport, all-terrain vehicle occupant
    heavy transport vehicle occupant — *see* Accident, transport, truck occupant
    ice yacht V98.2 ☑
    industrial vehicle occupant (nontraffic) V83.9 ☑
      driver V83.5 ☑
      hanger-on V83.7 ☑
      passenger V83.6 ☑
      traffic V83.3 ☑
        driver V83.0 ☑
        hanger-on V83.2 ☑
        passenger V83.1 ☑
      while boarding or alighting V83.4 ☑
    interurban electric car — *see* Accident, transport, streetcar
    land yacht V98.1 ☑
    logging car — *see* Accident, transport, industrial vehicle occupant
    military vehicle occupant (traffic) V86.34 ☑
      driver V86.04 ☑
      hanger-on V86.24 ☑
      nontraffic V86.94 ☑
        driver V86.54 ☑
        hanger-on V86.74 ☑
        passenger V86.64 ☑
      passenger V86.14 ☑
      while boarding or alighting V86.44 ☑
    mine tram — *see* Accident, transport, industrial vehicle occupant
    motor vehicle NEC occupant (traffic) V89.2 ☑
    motorcoach — *see* Accident, transport, bus occupant
    motor/cross bike rider (*see also* Accident, transport, dirt bike rider) V86.96 ☑
    motorcyclist V29.9 ☑
      collision (with)
        animal (traffic) V20.9 ☑
          being ridden (traffic) V26.9 ☑
            nontraffic V26.2 ☑
            while boarding or alighting V26.3 ☑
          nontraffic V20.2 ☑
          while boarding or alighting V20.3 ☑
        animal-drawn vehicle (traffic) V26.9 ☑
          nontraffic V26.2 ☑
          while boarding or alighting V26.3 ☑
        bus (traffic) V24.9 ☑
          nontraffic V24.2 ☑
          while boarding or alighting V24.3 ☑
        car (traffic) V23.9 ☑
          nontraffic V23.2 ☑
          while boarding or alighting V23.3 ☑
        motor vehicle NOS (traffic) V29.60 ☑
          nontraffic V29.20 ☑
          specified type NEC (traffic) V29.69 ☑
            nontraffic V29.29 ☑
        pedal cycle (traffic) V21.9 ☑
          nontraffic V21.2 ☑
          while boarding or alighting V21.3 ☑
        pickup truck (traffic) V23.9 ☑
          nontraffic V23.2 ☑

Accident — *continued*
  transport — *continued*
    motorcyclist — *continued*
      collision — *continued*
        pickup truck — *continued*
          while boarding or alighting V23.3 ☑
        railway vehicle (traffic) V25.9 ☑
          nontraffic V25.2 ☑
          while boarding or alighting V25.3 ☑
        specified vehicle NEC (traffic) V26.9 ☑
          nontraffic V26.2 ☑
          while boarding or alighting V26.3 ☑
        stationary object (traffic) V27.9 ☑
          nontraffic V27.2 ☑
          while boarding or alighting V27.3 ☑
        streetcar (traffic) V26.9 ☑
          nontraffic V26.2 ☑
          while boarding or alighting V26.3 ☑
        three wheeled motor vehicle (traffic) V22.9 ☑
          nontraffic V22.2 ☑
          while boarding or alighting V22.3 ☑
        truck (traffic) V24.9 ☑
          nontraffic V24.2 ☑
          while boarding or alighting V24.3 ☑
        two wheeled motor vehicle (traffic) V22.9 ☑
          nontraffic V22.2 ☑
          while boarding or alighting V22.3 ☑
        van (traffic) V23.9 ☑
          nontraffic V23.2 ☑
          while boarding or alighting V23.3 ☑
      driver
        collision (with)
          animal (traffic) V20.4 ☑
            being ridden (traffic) V26.4 ☑
              nontraffic V26.0 ☑
            nontraffic V20.0 ☑
          animal-drawn vehicle (traffic) V26.4 ☑
            nontraffic V26.0 ☑
          bus (traffic) V24.4 ☑
            nontraffic V24.0 ☑
          car (traffic) V23.4 ☑
            nontraffic V23.0 ☑
          motor vehicle NOS (traffic) V29.40 ☑
            nontraffic V29.00 ☑
            specified type NEC (traffic) V29.49 ☑
              nontraffic V29.09 ☑
          pedal cycle (traffic) V21.4 ☑
            nontraffic V21.0 ☑
          pickup truck (traffic) V23.4 ☑
            nontraffic V23.0 ☑
          railway vehicle (traffic) V25.4 ☑
            nontraffic V25.0 ☑
          specified vehicle NEC (traffic) V26.4 ☑
            nontraffic V26.0 ☑
          stationary object (traffic) V27.4 ☑
            nontraffic V27.0 ☑
          streetcar (traffic) V26.4 ☑
            nontraffic V26.0 ☑
          three wheeled motor vehicle (traffic) V22.4 ☑
            nontraffic V22.0 ☑
          truck (traffic) V24.4 ☑
            nontraffic V24.0 ☑
          two wheeled motor vehicle (traffic) V22.4 ☑
            nontraffic V22.0 ☑
          van (traffic) V23.4 ☑
            nontraffic V23.0 ☑
        noncollision accident (traffic) V28.4 ☑
          nontraffic V28.0 ☑
      noncollision accident (traffic) V28.9 ☑
        nontraffic V28.2 ☑
        while boarding or alighting V28.3 ☑
      nontraffic V29.3 ☑
      passenger
        collision (with)
          animal (traffic) V20.5 ☑
            being ridden (traffic) V26.5 ☑
              nontraffic V26.1 ☑
            nontraffic V20.1 ☑
          animal-drawn vehicle (traffic) V26.5 ☑
            nontraffic V26.1 ☑
          bus (traffic) V24.5 ☑
            nontraffic V24.1 ☑
          car (traffic) V23.5 ☑

Accident — *continued*
  transport — *continued*
    motorcyclist — *continued*
      passenger — *continued*
        collision — *continued*
          car — *continued*
            nontraffic V23.1 ☑
          motor vehicle NOS (traffic) V29.50 ☑
            nontraffic V29.10 ☑
            specified type NEC (traffic) V29.59 ☑
              nontraffic V29.19 ☑
          pedal cycle (traffic) V21.5 ☑
            nontraffic V21.1 ☑
          pickup truck (traffic) V23.5 ☑
            nontraffic V23.1 ☑
          railway vehicle (traffic) V25.5 ☑
            nontraffic V25.1 ☑
          specified vehicle NEC (traffic) V26.5 ☑
            nontraffic V26.1 ☑
          stationary object (traffic) V27.5 ☑
            nontraffic V27.1 ☑
          streetcar (traffic) V26.5 ☑
            nontraffic V26.1 ☑
          three wheeled motor vehicle (traffic) V22.5 ☑
            nontraffic V22.1 ☑
          truck (traffic) V24.5 ☑
            nontraffic V24.1 ☑
          two wheeled motor vehicle (traffic) V22.5 ☑
            nontraffic V22.1 ☑
          van (traffic) V23.5 ☑
            nontraffic V23.1 ☑
        noncollision accident (traffic) V28.5 ☑
          nontraffic V28.1 ☑
      specified type NEC V29.88 ☑
      military vehicle V29.81 ☑
    occupant (of)
      aircraft (powered) V95.9 ☑
        fixed wing
          commercial — *see* Accident, transport, aircraft, occupant, powered, fixed wing, commercial
          private — *see* Accident, transport, aircraft, occupant, powered, fixed wing, private
        nonpowered V96.9 ☑
        specified NEC V95.8 ☑
      airport battery-powered vehicle — *see* Accident, transport, industrial vehicle occupant
      all-terrain vehicle (ATV) — *see* Accident, transport, all-terrain vehicle occupant
      animal-drawn vehicle — *see* Accident, transport, animal-drawn vehicle occupant
      automobile — *see* Accident, transport, car occupant
      balloon V96.00 ☑
      battery-powered vehicle — *see* Accident, transport, industrial vehicle occupant
      bicycle — *see* Accident, transport, pedal cyclist
        motorized — *see* Accident, transport, motorcycle rider
      boat NEC — *see* Accident, watercraft
      bulldozer — *see* Accident, transport, construction vehicle occupant
      bus — *see* Accident, transport, bus occupant
      cable car (on rails) (*see also* Accident, transport, streetcar occupant)
        not on rails V98.0 ☑
      car (*see also* Accident, transport, car occupant)
        cable (on rails) (*see also* Accident, transport, streetcar occupant)
        not on rails V98.0 ☑
      coach — *see* Accident, transport, bus occupant
      coal-car — *see* Accident, transport, industrial vehicle occupant
      digger — *see* Accident, transport, construction vehicle occupant
      dump truck — *see* Accident, transport, construction vehicle occupant
      earth-leveler — *see* Accident, transport, construction vehicle occupant
      farm machinery (self-propelled) — *see* Accident, transport, agricultural vehicle occupant

☑ Additional Character Required — Refer to the Tabular List for Character Selection   Subterms under main terms may continue to next column or page

Accident — *continued*
  transport — *continued*
    occupant — *continued*
      forklift — *see* Accident, transport, industrial vehicle occupant
      glider (unpowered) V96.20 ☑
        hang V96.10 ☑
        powered (microlight) (ultralight) — *see* Accident, transport, aircraft, occupant, powered, glider
      glider (unpowered) NEC V96.20 ☑
      hang-glider V96.10 ☑
      harvester — *see* Accident, transport, agricultural vehicle occupant
      heavy (transport) vehicle — *see* Accident, transport, truck occupant
      helicopter — *see* Accident, transport, aircraft, occupant, helicopter
      ice-yacht V98.2 ☑
      kite (carrying person) V96.8 ☑
      land-yacht V98.1 ☑
      logging car — *see* Accident, transport, industrial vehicle occupant
      mechanical shovel — *see* Accident, transport, construction vehicle occupant
      microlight — *see* Accident, transport, aircraft, occupant, powered, glider
      minibus — *see* Accident, transport, pickup truck occupant
      minivan — *see* Accident, transport, pickup truck occupant
      moped — *see* Accident, transport, motorcycle
      motor scooter — *see* Accident, transport, motorcycle
      motorcycle (with sidecar) — *see* Accident, transport, motorcycle
      off-road motor-vehicle (*see also* Accident, transport, all-terrain vehicle occupant) V86.99 ☑
      pedal cycle (*see also* Accident, transport, pedal cyclist)
      pick-up (truck) — *see* Accident, transport, pickup truck occupant
      railway (train) (vehicle) (subterranean) (elevated) — *see* Accident, transport, railway vehicle occupant
      rickshaw — *see* Accident, transport, pedal cycle
        motorized — *see* Accident, transport, three-wheeled motor vehicle
        pedal driven — *see* Accident, transport, pedal cyclist
      road-roller — *see* Accident, transport, construction vehicle occupant
      ship NOS V94.9 ☑
      ski-lift (chair) (gondola) V98.3 ☑
      snowmobile — *see* Accident, transport, snowmobile occupant
      spacecraft, spaceship — *see* Accident, transport, aircraft, occupant, spacecraft
      sport utility vehicle — *see* Accident, transport, pickup truck occupant
      streetcar (interurban) (operating on public street or highway) — *see* Accident, transport, streetcar occupant
      SUV — *see* Accident, transport, pickup truck occupant
      téléférique V98.0 ☑
      three-wheeled vehicle (motorized) (*see also* Accident, transport, three-wheeled motor vehicle occupant)
        nonmotorized — *see* Accident, transport, pedal cycle
      tractor (farm) (and trailer) — *see* Accident, transport, agricultural vehicle occupant
      train — *see* Accident, transport, railway vehicle occupant
      tram — *see* Accident, transport, streetcar occupant
        in mine or quarry — *see* Accident, transport, industrial vehicle occupant
      tricycle — *see* Accident, transport, pedal cycle
        motorized — *see* Accident, transport, three-wheeled motor vehicle
      trolley — *see* Accident, transport, streetcar occupant
        in mine or quarry — *see* Accident, transport, industrial vehicle occupant

Accident — *continued*
  transport — *continued*
    occupant — *continued*
      tub, in mine or quarry — *see* Accident, transport, industrial vehicle occupant
      ultralight — *see* Accident, transport, aircraft, occupant, powered, glider
      van — *see* Accident, transport, van occupant
      vehicle NEC V89.9 ☑
        heavy transport — *see* Accident, transport, truck occupant
        motor (traffic) NEC V89.2 ☑
        nontraffic NEC V89.0 ☑
      watercraft NOS V94.9 ☑
        causing drowning — *see* Drowning, resulting from accident to boat
    off-road motor-vehicle (*see also* Accident, transport, all-terrain vehicle occupant) V86.99 ☑
    parachutist V97.29 ☑
      after accident to aircraft — *see* Accident, transport, aircraft
      entangled in object V97.21 ☑
      injured on landing V97.22 ☑
    pedal cyclist V19.9 ☑
      collision (with)
        animal (traffic) V10.9 ☑
          being ridden (traffic) V16.9 ☑
            nontraffic V16.2 ☑
            while boarding or alighting V16.3 ☑
          nontraffic V10.2 ☑
          while boarding or alighting V10.3 ☑
        animal-drawn vehicle (traffic) V16.9 ☑
          nontraffic V16.2 ☑
          while boarding or alighting V16.3 ☑
        bus (traffic) V14.9 ☑
          nontraffic V14.2 ☑
          while boarding or alighting V14.3 ☑
        car (traffic) V13.9 ☑
          nontraffic V13.2 ☑
          while boarding or alighting V13.3 ☑
        motor vehicle NOS (traffic) V19.60 ☑
          nontraffic V19.20 ☑
          specified type NEC (traffic) V19.69 ☑
            nontraffic V19.29 ☑
        pedal cycle (traffic) V11.9 ☑
          nontraffic V11.2 ☑
          while boarding or alighting V11.3 ☑
        pickup truck (traffic) V13.9 ☑
          nontraffic V13.2 ☑
          while boarding or alighting V13.3 ☑
        railway vehicle (traffic) V15.9 ☑
          nontraffic V15.2 ☑
          while boarding or alighting V15.3 ☑
        specified vehicle NEC (traffic) V16.9 ☑
          nontraffic V16.2 ☑
          while boarding or alighting V16.3 ☑
        stationary object (traffic) V17.9 ☑
          nontraffic V17.2 ☑
          while boarding or alighting V17.3 ☑
        streetcar (traffic) V16.9 ☑
          nontraffic V16.2 ☑
          while boarding or alighting V16.3 ☑
        three wheeled motor vehicle (traffic) V12.9 ☑
          nontraffic V12.2 ☑
          while boarding or alighting V12.3 ☑
        truck (traffic) V14.9 ☑
          nontraffic V14.2 ☑
          while boarding or alighting V14.3 ☑
        two wheeled motor vehicle (traffic) V12.9 ☑
          nontraffic V12.2 ☑
          while boarding or alighting V12.3 ☑
        van (traffic) V13.9 ☑
          nontraffic V13.2 ☑
          while boarding or alighting V13.3 ☑
      driver
        collision (with)
          animal (traffic) V10.4 ☑
            being ridden (traffic) V16.4 ☑
              nontraffic V16.0 ☑
            nontraffic V10.0 ☑
          animal-drawn vehicle (traffic) V16.4 ☑
            nontraffic V16.0 ☑
          bus (traffic) V14.4 ☑
            nontraffic V14.0 ☑
          car (traffic) V13.4 ☑

Accident — *continued*
  transport — *continued*
    pedal cyclist — *continued*
      driver — *continued*
        collision — *continued*
          car — *continued*
            nontraffic V13.0 ☑
            motor vehicle NOS (traffic) V19.40 ☑
              nontraffic V19.00 ☑
              specified type NEC (traffic) V19.49 ☑
                nontraffic V19.09 ☑
            pedal cycle (traffic) V11.4 ☑
              nontraffic V11.0 ☑
            pickup truck (traffic) V13.4 ☑
              nontraffic V13.0 ☑
            railway vehicle (traffic) V15.4 ☑
              nontraffic V15.0 ☑
            specified vehicle NEC (traffic) V16.4 ☑
              nontraffic V16.0 ☑
            stationary object (traffic) V17.4 ☑
              nontraffic V17.0 ☑
            streetcar (traffic) V16.4 ☑
              nontraffic V16.0 ☑
            three wheeled motor vehicle (traffic) V12.4 ☑
              nontraffic V12.0 ☑
            truck (traffic) V14.4 ☑
              nontraffic V14.0 ☑
            two wheeled motor vehicle (traffic) V12.4 ☑
              nontraffic V12.0 ☑
            van (traffic) V13.4 ☑
              nontraffic V13.0 ☑
          noncollision accident (traffic) V18.4 ☑
            nontraffic V18.0 ☑
        noncollision accident (traffic) V18.9 ☑
          nontraffic V18.2 ☑
          while boarding or alighting V18.3 ☑
      nontraffic V19.3 ☑
      passenger
        collision (with)
          animal (traffic) V10.5 ☑
            being ridden (traffic) V16.5 ☑
              nontraffic V16.1 ☑
            nontraffic V10.1 ☑
          animal-drawn vehicle (traffic) V16.5 ☑
            nontraffic V16.1 ☑
          bus (traffic) V14.5 ☑
            nontraffic V14.1 ☑
          car (traffic) V13.5 ☑
            nontraffic V13.1 ☑
          motor vehicle NOS (traffic) V19.50 ☑
            nontraffic V19.10 ☑
            specified type NEC (traffic) V19.59 ☑
              nontraffic V19.19 ☑
          pedal cycle (traffic) V11.5 ☑
            nontraffic V11.1 ☑
          pickup truck (traffic) V13.5 ☑
            nontraffic V13.1 ☑
          railway vehicle (traffic) V15.5 ☑
            nontraffic V15.1 ☑
          specified vehicle NEC (traffic) V16.5 ☑
            nontraffic V16.1 ☑
          stationary object (traffic) V17.5 ☑
            nontraffic V17.1 ☑
          streetcar (traffic) V16.5 ☑
            nontraffic V16.1 ☑
          three wheeled motor vehicle (traffic) V12.5 ☑
            nontraffic V12.1 ☑
          truck (traffic) V14.5 ☑
            nontraffic V14.1 ☑
          two wheeled motor vehicle (traffic) V12.5 ☑
            nontraffic V12.1 ☑
          van (traffic) V13.5 ☑
            nontraffic V13.1 ☑
        noncollision accident (traffic) V18.5 ☑
          nontraffic V18.1 ☑
      specified type NEC V19.88 ☑
        military vehicle V19.81 ☑
    pedestrian
      conveyance (occupant) V09.9 ☑
        babystroller V00.828 ☑
          collision (with) V09.9 ☑

⏷ **Subterms under main terms may continue to next column or page**   ☑ **Additional Character Required — Refer to the Tabular List for Character Selection**   **401**

Accident — Accident

Accident — *continued*
  transport — *continued*
    pedestrian — *continued*
      conveyance — *continued*
        babystroller — *continued*
          collision — *continued*
            animal being ridden or animal drawn
              vehicle V06.99 ☑
              nontraffic V06.09 ☑
              traffic V06.19 ☑
            bus or heavy transport V04.99 ☑
              nontraffic V04.09 ☑
              traffic V04.19 ☑
            car V03.99 ☑
              nontraffic V03.09 ☑
              traffic V03.19 ☑
            pedal cycle V01.99 ☑
              nontraffic V01.09 ☑
              traffic V01.19 ☑
            pick-up truck or van V03.99 ☑
              nontraffic V03.09 ☑
              traffic V03.19 ☑
            railway (train) (vehicle) V05.99 ☑
              nontraffic V05.09 ☑
              traffic V05.19 ☑
            stationary object V00.822 ☑
            streetcar V06.99 ☑
              nontraffic V06.09 ☑
              traffic V06.19 ☑
            two- or three-wheeled motor vehicle
              V02.99 ☑
              nontraffic V02.09 ☑
              traffic V02.19 ☑
            vehicle V09.9 ☑
              animal-drawn V06.99 ☑
                nontraffic V06.09 ☑
                traffic V06.19 ☑
              motor
                nontraffic V09.00 ☑
                traffic V09.20 ☑
          fall V00.821 ☑
          nontraffic V09.1 ☑
            involving motor vehicle NEC
              V09.00 ☑
          traffic V09.3 ☑
            involving motor vehicle NEC
              V09.20 ☑
        flat-bottomed NEC V00.388 ☑
          collision (with) V09.9 ☑
            animal being ridden or animal drawn
              vehicle V06.99 ☑
              nontraffic V06.09 ☑
              traffic V06.19 ☑
            bus or heavy transport V04.99 ☑
              nontraffic V04.09 ☑
              traffic V04.19 ☑
            car V03.99 ☑
              nontraffic V03.09 ☑
              traffic V03.19 ☑
            pedal cycle V01.99 ☑
              nontraffic V01.09 ☑
              traffic V01.19 ☑
            pick-up truck or van V03.99 ☑
              nontraffic V03.09 ☑
              traffic V03.19 ☑
            railway (train) (vehicle) V05.99 ☑
              nontraffic V05.09 ☑
              traffic V05.19 ☑
            stationary object V00.382 ☑
            streetcar V06.99 ☑
              nontraffic V06.09 ☑
              traffic V06.19 ☑
            two- or three-wheeled motor vehicle
              V02.99 ☑
              nontraffic V02.09 ☑
              traffic V02.19 ☑
            vehicle V09.9 ☑
              animal-drawn V06.99 ☑
                nontraffic V06.09 ☑
                traffic V06.19 ☑
              motor
                nontraffic V09.00 ☑
                traffic V09.20 ☑
          fall V00.381 ☑
          nontraffic V09.1 ☑

Accident — *continued*
  transport — *continued*
    pedestrian — *continued*
      conveyance — *continued*
        flat-bottomed — *continued*
          nontraffic — *continued*
            involving motor vehicle NEC
              V09.00 ☑
          snow
            board — *see* Accident, transport,
              pedestrian, conveyance, snow
              board
            ski — *see* Accident, transport,
              pedestrian, conveyance, skis
              (snow)
          traffic V09.3 ☑
            involving motor vehicle NEC
              V09.20 ☑
        gliding type NEC V00.288 ☑
          collision (with) V09.9 ☑
            animal being ridden or animal drawn
              vehicle V06.99 ☑
              nontraffic V06.09 ☑
              traffic V06.19 ☑
            bus or heavy transport V04.99 ☑
              nontraffic V04.09 ☑
              traffic V04.19 ☑
            car V03.99 ☑
              nontraffic V03.09 ☑
              traffic V03.19 ☑
            pedal cycle V01.99 ☑
              nontraffic V01.09 ☑
              traffic V01.19 ☑
            pick-up truck or van V03.99 ☑
              nontraffic V03.09 ☑
              traffic V03.19 ☑
            railway (train) (vehicle) V05.99 ☑
              nontraffic V05.09 ☑
              traffic V05.19 ☑
            stationary object V00.282 ☑
            streetcar V06.99 ☑
              nontraffic V06.09 ☑
              traffic V02.19 ☑
            two- or three-wheeled motor vehicle
              V02.99 ☑
              nontraffic V02.09 ☑
              traffic V02.19 ☑
            vehicle V09.9 ☑
              animal-drawn V06.99 ☑
                nontraffic V06.09 ☑
                traffic V06.19 ☑
              motor
                nontraffic V09.00 ☑
                traffic V09.20 ☑
          fall V00.281 ☑
          heelies — *see* Accident, transport,
            pedestrian, conveyance, heelies
          ice skate — *see* Accident, transport,
            pedestrian, conveyance, ice skate
          nontraffic V09.1 ☑
            involving motor vehicle NEC
              V09.00 ☑
          sled — *see* Accident, transport, pedestri-
            an, conveyance, sled
          traffic V09.3 ☑
            involving motor vehicle NEC
              V09.20 ☑
            wheelies — *see* Accident, transport,
              pedestrian, conveyance, heel-
              ies
        heelies V00.158 ☑
          colliding with stationary object
            V00.152 ☑
          fall V00.151 ☑
        ice skates V00.218 ☑
          collision (with) V09.9 ☑
            animal being ridden or animal drawn
              vehicle V06.99 ☑
              nontraffic V06.09 ☑
              traffic V06.19 ☑
            bus or heavy transport V04.99 ☑
              nontraffic V04.09 ☑
              traffic V04.19 ☑
            car V03.99 ☑
              nontraffic V03.09 ☑
              traffic V03.19 ☑

Accident — *continued*
  transport — *continued*
    pedestrian — *continued*
      conveyance — *continued*
        ice skates — *continued*
          collision — *continued*
            pedal cycle V01.99 ☑
              nontraffic V01.09 ☑
              traffic V01.19 ☑
            pick-up truck or van V03.99 ☑
              nontraffic V03.09 ☑
              traffic V03.19 ☑
            railway (train) (vehicle) V05.99 ☑
              nontraffic V05.09 ☑
              traffic V05.19 ☑
            stationary object V00.212 ☑
            streetcar V06.99 ☑
              nontraffic V06.09 ☑
              traffic V06.19 ☑
            two- or three-wheeled motor vehicle
              V02.99 ☑
              nontraffic V02.09 ☑
              traffic V02.19 ☑
            vehicle V09.9 ☑
              animal-drawn V06.99 ☑
                nontraffic V06.09 ☑
                traffic V06.19 ☑
              motor
                nontraffic V09.00 ☑
                traffic V09.20 ☑
          fall V00.211 ☑
          nontraffic V09.1 ☑
            involving motor vehicle NEC
              V09.00 ☑
          traffic V09.3 ☑
            involving motor vehicle NEC
              V09.20 ☑
        motorized mobility scooter V00.838 ☑
          collision with stationary object
            V00.832 ☑
          fall from V00.831 ☑
        nontraffic V09.1 ☑
          involving motor vehicle V09.00 ☑
            military V09.01 ☑
            specified type NEC V09.09 ☑
        roller skates (non in-line) V00.128 ☑
          collision (with) V09.9 ☑
            animal being ridden or animal drawn
              vehicle V06.91 ☑
              nontraffic V06.01 ☑
              traffic V06.11 ☑
            bus or heavy transport V04.91 ☑
              nontraffic V04.01 ☑
              traffic V04.11 ☑
            car V03.91 ☑
              nontraffic V03.01 ☑
              traffic V03.11 ☑
            pedal cycle V01.91 ☑
              nontraffic V01.01 ☑
              traffic V01.11 ☑
            pick-up truck or van V03.91 ☑
              nontraffic V03.01 ☑
              traffic V03.11 ☑
            railway (train) (vehicle) V05.91 ☑
              nontraffic V05.01 ☑
              traffic V05.11 ☑
            stationary object V00.122 ☑
            streetcar V06.91 ☑
              nontraffic V06.01 ☑
              traffic V06.11 ☑
            two- or three-wheeled motor vehicle
              V02.91 ☑
              nontraffic V02.01 ☑
              traffic V02.11 ☑
            vehicle V09.9 ☑
              animal-drawn V06.91 ☑
                nontraffic V06.01 ☑
                traffic V06.11 ☑
              motor
                nontraffic V09.00 ☑
                traffic V09.20 ☑
          fall V00.121 ☑
          in-line V00.118 ☑

Accident — *continued*
  transport — *continued*
    pedestrian — *continued*
      conveyance — *continued*
        roller skates — *continued*
          in-line — *continued*
            collision — *see also* Accident, transport, pedestrian, conveyance occupant, roller skates, collision
              with stationary object V00.112 ☑
            fall V00.111 ☑
            nontraffic V09.1 ☑
              involving motor vehicle NEC V09.00 ☑
            traffic V09.3 ☑
              involving motor vehicle NEC V09.20 ☑
        rolling shoes V00.158 ☑
          colliding with stationary object V00.152 ☑
          fall V00.151 ☑
        rolling type NEC V00.188 ☑
          collision (with) V09.9 ☑
            animal being ridden or animal drawn vehicle V06.99 ☑
              nontraffic V06.09 ☑
              traffic V06.19 ☑
            bus or heavy transport V04.99 ☑
              nontraffic V04.09 ☑
              traffic V04.19 ☑
            car V03.99 ☑
              nontraffic V03.09 ☑
              traffic V03.19 ☑
            pedal cycle V01.99 ☑
              nontraffic V01.09 ☑
              traffic V01.19 ☑
            pick-up truck or van V03.99 ☑
              nontraffic V03.09 ☑
              traffic V03.19 ☑
            railway (train) (vehicle) V05.99 ☑
              nontraffic V05.09 ☑
              traffic V05.19 ☑
            stationary object V00.182 ☑
            streetcar V06.99 ☑
              nontraffic V06.09 ☑
              traffic V06.19 ☑
            two- or three-wheeled motor vehicle V02.99 ☑
              nontraffic V02.09 ☑
              traffic V02.19 ☑
            vehicle V09.9 ☑
              animal-drawn V06.99 ☑
                nontraffic V06.09 ☑
                traffic V06.19 ☑
              motor
                nontraffic V09.00 ☑
                traffic V09.20 ☑
          fall V00.181 ☑
        in-line roller skate — *see* Accident, transport, pedestrian, conveyance, roller skate, in-line
        nontraffic V09.1 ☑
          involving motor vehicle NEC V09.00 ☑
        roller skate — *see* Accident, transport, pedestrian, conveyance, roller skate
        scooter (non-motorized) — *see* Accident, transport, pedestrian, conveyance, scooter
        skateboard — *see* Accident, transport, pedestrian, conveyance, skateboard
        traffic V09.3 ☑
          involving motor vehicle NEC V09.20 ☑
      scooter (non-motorized) V00.148 ☑
        collision (with) V09.9 ☑
          animal being ridden or animal drawn vehicle V06.99 ☑
            nontraffic V06.09 ☑
            traffic V06.19 ☑
          bus or heavy transport V04.99 ☑
            nontraffic V04.09 ☑
            traffic V04.19 ☑

Accident — *continued*
  transport — *continued*
    pedestrian — *continued*
      conveyance — *continued*
        scooter — *continued*
          collision — *continued*
            car V03.99 ☑
              nontraffic V03.09 ☑
              traffic V03.19 ☑
            pedal cycle V01.99 ☑
              nontraffic V01.09 ☑
              traffic V01.19 ☑
            pick-up truck or van V03.99 ☑
              nontraffic V03.09 ☑
              traffic V03.19 ☑
            railway (train) (vehicle) V05.99 ☑
              nontraffic V05.09 ☑
              traffic V05.19 ☑
            stationary object V00.142 ☑
            streetcar V06.99 ☑
              nontraffic V06.09 ☑
              traffic V06.19 ☑
            two- or three-wheeled motor vehicle V02.99 ☑
              nontraffic V02.09 ☑
              traffic V02.19 ☑
            vehicle V09.9 ☑
              animal-drawn V06.99 ☑
                nontraffic V06.09 ☑
                traffic V06.19 ☑
              motor
                nontraffic V09.00 ☑
                traffic V09.20 ☑
          fall V00.141 ☑
          nontraffic V09.1 ☑
            involving motor vehicle NEC V09.00 ☑
          traffic V09.3 ☑
            involving motor vehicle NEC V09.20 ☑
        skate board V00.138 ☑
          collision (with) V09.9 ☑
            animal being ridden or animal drawn vehicle V06.92 ☑
              nontraffic V06.02 ☑
              traffic V06.12 ☑
            bus or heavy transport V04.92 ☑
              nontraffic V04.02 ☑
              traffic V04.12 ☑
            car V03.92 ☑
              nontraffic V03.02 ☑
              traffic V03.12 ☑
            pedal cycle V01.92 ☑
              nontraffic V01.02 ☑
              traffic V01.12 ☑
            pick-up truck or van V03.92 ☑
              nontraffic V03.02 ☑
              traffic V03.12 ☑
            railway (train) (vehicle) V05.92 ☑
              nontraffic V05.02 ☑
              traffic V05.12 ☑
            stationary object V00.132 ☑
            streetcar V06.92 ☑
              nontraffic V06.02 ☑
              traffic V06.12 ☑
            two- or three-wheeled motor vehicle V02.92 ☑
              nontraffic V02.02 ☑
              traffic V02.12 ☑
            vehicle V09.9 ☑
              animal-drawn V06.92 ☑
                nontraffic V06.02 ☑
                traffic V06.12 ☑
              motor
                nontraffic V09.00 ☑
                traffic V09.20 ☑
          fall V00.131 ☑
          nontraffic V09.1 ☑
            involving motor vehicle NEC V09.00 ☑
          traffic V09.3 ☑
            involving motor vehicle NEC V09.20 ☑
        skis (snow) V00.328 ☑
          collision (with) V09.9 ☑

Accident — *continued*
  transport — *continued*
    pedestrian — *continued*
      conveyance — *continued*
        skis — *continued*
          collision — *continued*
            animal being ridden or animal drawn vehicle V06.99 ☑
              nontraffic V06.09 ☑
              traffic V06.19 ☑
            bus or heavy transport V04.99 ☑
              nontraffic V04.09 ☑
              traffic V04.19 ☑
            car V03.99 ☑
              nontraffic V03.09 ☑
              traffic V03.19 ☑
            pedal cycle V01.99 ☑
              nontraffic V01.09 ☑
              traffic V01.19 ☑
            pick-up truck or van V03.99 ☑
              nontraffic V03.09 ☑
              traffic V03.19 ☑
            railway (train) (vehicle) V05.99 ☑
              nontraffic V05.09 ☑
              traffic V05.19 ☑
            stationary object V00.322 ☑
            streetcar V06.99 ☑
              nontraffic V06.09 ☑
              traffic V06.19 ☑
            two- or three-wheeled motor vehicle V02.99 ☑
              nontraffic V02.09 ☑
              traffic V02.19 ☑
            vehicle V09.9 ☑
              animal-drawn V06.99 ☑
                nontraffic V06.09 ☑
                traffic V06.19 ☑
              motor
                nontraffic V09.00 ☑
                traffic V09.20 ☑
          fall V00.321 ☑
          nontraffic V09.1 ☑
            involving motor vehicle NEC V09.00 ☑
          traffic V09.3 ☑
            involving motor vehicle NEC V09.20 ☑
        sled V00.228 ☑
          collision (with) V09.9 ☑
            animal being ridden or animal drawn vehicle V06.99 ☑
              nontraffic V06.09 ☑
              traffic V06.19 ☑
            bus or heavy transport V04.99 ☑
              nontraffic V04.09 ☑
              traffic V04.19 ☑
            car V03.99 ☑
              nontraffic V03.09 ☑
              traffic V03.19 ☑
            pedal cycle V01.99 ☑
              nontraffic V01.09 ☑
              traffic V01.19 ☑
            pick-up truck or van V03.99 ☑
              nontraffic V03.09 ☑
              traffic V03.19 ☑
            railway (train) (vehicle) V05.99 ☑
              nontraffic V05.09 ☑
              traffic V05.19 ☑
            stationary object V00.222 ☑
            streetcar V06.99 ☑
              nontraffic V06.09 ☑
              traffic V06.19 ☑
            two- or three-wheeled motor vehicle V02.99 ☑
              nontraffic V02.09 ☑
              traffic V02.19 ☑
            vehicle V09.9 ☑
              animal-drawn V06.99 ☑
                nontraffic V06.09 ☑
                traffic V06.19 ☑
              motor
                nontraffic V09.00 ☑
                traffic V09.20 ☑
          fall V00.221 ☑
          nontraffic V09.1 ☑

☷ Subterms under main terms may continue to next column or page   ☑ Additional Character Required — Refer to the Tabular List for Character Selection   403

Accident — Accident

Accident — *continued*
  transport — *continued*
    pedestrian — *continued*
      conveyance — *continued*
        sled — *continued*
          nontraffic — *continued*
            involving motor vehicle NEC
              V09.00 ☑
          traffic V09.3 ☑
            involving motor vehicle NEC
              V09.20 ☑
        snow board V00.318 ☑
          collision (with) V09.9 ☑
            animal being ridden or animal drawn
              vehicle V06.99 ☑
              nontraffic V06.09 ☑
              traffic V06.19 ☑
            bus or heavy transport V04.99 ☑
              nontraffic V04.09 ☑
              traffic V04.19 ☑
            car V03.99 ☑
              nontraffic V03.09 ☑
              traffic V03.19 ☑
            pedal cycle V01.99 ☑
              nontraffic V01.09 ☑
              traffic V01.19 ☑
            pick-up truck or van V03.99 ☑
              nontrafflc V03.09 ☑
              traffic V03.19 ☑
            railway (train) (vehicle) V05.99 ☑
              nontraffic V05.09 ☑
              traffic V05.19 ☑
            stationary object V00.312 ☑
            streetcar V06.99 ☑
              nontraffic V06.09 ☑
              traffic V06.19 ☑
            two- or three-wheeled motor vehicle
              V02.99 ☑
              nontraffic V02.09 ☑
              traffic V02.19 ☑
            vehicle V09.9 ☑
              animal-drawn V06.99 ☑
                nontraffic V06.09 ☑
                traffic V06.19 ☑
              motor
                nontraffic V09.00 ☑
                traffic V09.20 ☑
        fall V00.311 ☑
        nontraffic V09.1 ☑
          involving motor vehicle NEC
            V09.00 ☑
        traffic V09.3 ☑
          involving motor vehicle NEC
            V09.20 ☑
        specified type NEC V00.898 ☑
          collision (with) V09.9 ☑
            animal being ridden or animal drawn
              vehicle V06.99 ☑
              nontraffic V06.09 ☑
              traffic V06.19 ☑
            bus or heavy transport V04.99 ☑
              nontraffic V04.09 ☑
              traffic V04.19 ☑
            car V03.99 ☑
              nontraffic V03.09 ☑
              traffic V03.19 ☑
            pedal cycle V01.99 ☑
              nontraffic V01.09 ☑
              traffic V01.19 ☑
            pick-up truck or van V03.99 ☑
              nontraffic V03.09 ☑
              traffic V03.19 ☑
            railway (train) (vehicle) V05.99 ☑
              nontraffic V05.09 ☑
              traffic V05.19 ☑
            stationary object V00.892 ☑
            streetcar V06.99 ☑
              nontraffic V06.09 ☑
              traffic V06.19 ☑
            two- or three-wheeled motor vehicle
              V02.99 ☑
              nontraffic V02.09 ☑
              traffic V02.19 ☑
            vehicle V09.9 ☑
              animal-drawn V06.99 ☑
                nontraffic V06.09 ☑

Accident — *continued*
  transport — *continued*
    pedestrian — *continued*
      conveyance — *continued*
        specified type — *continued*
          collision — *continued*
            vehicle — *continued*
              animal-drawn — *continued*
                traffic V06.19 ☑
              motor
                nontraffic V09.00 ☑
                traffic V09.20 ☑
        fall V00.891 ☑
        nontraffic V09.1 ☑
          involving motor vehicle NEC
            V09.00 ☑
        traffic V09.3 ☑
          involving motor vehicle NEC
            V09.20 ☑
      traffic V09.3 ☑
        involving motor vehicle V09.20 ☑
          military V09.21 ☑
          specified type NEC V09.29 ☑
      wheelchair (powered) V00.818 ☑
        collision (with) V09.9 ☑
          animal being ridden or animal drawn
            vehicle V06.99 ☑
            nontraffic V06.09 ☑
            traffic V06.19 ☑
          bus or heavy transport V04.99 ☑
            nontraffic V04.09 ☑
            traffic V04.19 ☑
          car V03.99 ☑
            nontraffic V03.09 ☑
            traffic V03.19 ☑
          pedal cycle V01.99 ☑
            nontraffic V01.09 ☑
            traffic V01.19 ☑
          pick-up truck or van V03.99 ☑
            nontraffic V03.09 ☑
            traffic V03.19 ☑
          railway (train) (vehicle) V05.99 ☑
            nontraffic V05.09 ☑
            traffic V05.19 ☑
          stationary object V00.812 ☑
          streetcar V06.99 ☑
            nontraffic V06.09 ☑
            traffic V06.19 ☑
          two- or three-wheeled motor vehicle
            V02.99 ☑
            nontraffic V02.09 ☑
            traffic V02.19 ☑
          vehicle V09.9 ☑
            animal-drawn V06.99 ☑
              nontraffic V06.09 ☑
              traffic V06.19 ☑
            motor
              nontraffic V09.00 ☑
              traffic V09.20 ☑
        fall V00.811 ☑
        nontraffic V09.1 ☑
          involving motor vehicle NEC
            V09.00 ☑
        traffic V09.3 ☑
          involving motor vehicle NEC
            V09.20 ☑
      wheeled shoe V00.158 ☑
        colliding with stationary object
          V00.152 ☑
        fall V00.151 ☑
    on foot (*see also* Accident, pedestrian)
      collision (with)
        animal being ridden or animal drawn
          vehicle V06.90 ☑
           nontraffic V06.00 ☑
           traffic V06.10 ☑
        bus or heavy transport V04.90 ☑
          nontraffic V04.00 ☑
          traffic V04.10 ☑
        car V03.90 ☑
          nontraffic V03.00 ☑
          traffic V03.10 ☑
        pedal cycle V01.90 ☑
          nontraffic V01.00 ☑
          traffic V01.10 ☑
        pick-up truck or van V03.90 ☑

Accident — *continued*
  transport — *continued*
    pedestrian — *continued*
      on foot (*see also* Accident, pedestrian) — *continued*
        collision — *continued*
          pick-up truck or van — *continued*
           nontraffic V03.00 ☑
           traffic V03.10 ☑
          railway (train) (vehicle) V05.90 ☑
           nontraffic V05.00 ☑
           traffic V05.10 ☑
          streetcar V06.90 ☑
           nontraffic V06.00 ☑
           traffic V06.10 ☑
          two- or three-wheeled motor vehicle
           V02.90 ☑
           nontraffic V02.00 ☑
           traffic V02.10 ☑
          vehicle V09.9 ☑
           animal-drawn V06.90 ☑
            nontraffic V06.00 ☑
            traffic V06.10 ☑
           motor
        nontraffic V09.1 ☑
          involving motor vehicle V09.00 ☑
           military V09.01 ☑
           specified type NEC V09.09 ☑
        traffic V09.3 ☑
          involving motor vehicle V09.20 ☑
           military V09.21 ☑
           specified type NEC V09.29 ☑
    person NEC (unknown way or transportation)
      V99 ☑
    collision (between)
      bus (with)
        heavy transport vehicle (traffic) V87.5 ☑
          nontraffic V88.5 ☑
      car (with)
        bus (traffic) V87.3 ☑
          nontraffic V88.3 ☑
        heavy transport vehicle (traffic) V87.4 ☑
          nontraffic V88.4 ☑
        nontraffic V88.5 ☑
        pick-up truck or van (traffic) V87,2 ☑
          nontraffic V88.2 ☑
        train or railway vehicle (traffic) V87.6 ☑
          nontraffic V88.6 ☑
        two-or three-wheeled motor vehicle
          (traffic) V87.0 ☑
          nontraffic V88.0 ☑
      motor vehicle (traffic) NEC V87.7 ☑
        nontraffic V88.7 ☑
      two-or three-wheeled vehicle (with) (traffic)
        motor vehicle NEC V87.1 ☑
          nontraffic V88.1 ☑
      nonmotor vehicle (collision) (noncollision)
        (traffic) V87.9 ☑
        nontraffic V88.9 ☑
    pickup truck occupant V59.9 ☑
      collision (with)
        animal (traffic) V50.9 ☑
          being ridden (traffic) V56.9 ☑
           nontraffic V56.3 ☑
           while boarding or alighting V56.4 ☑
          nontraffic V50.3 ☑
          while boarding or alighting V50.4 ☑
        animal-drawn vehicle (traffic) V56.9 ☑
          nontraffic V56.3 ☑
          while boarding or alighting V56.4 ☑
        bus (traffic) V54.9 ☑
          nontraffic V54.3 ☑
          while boarding or alighting V54.4 ☑
        car (traffic) V53.9 ☑
          nontraffic V53.3 ☑
          while boarding or alighting V53.4 ☑
        motor vehicle NOS (traffic) V59.60 ☑
          nontraffic V59.20 ☑
          specified type NEC (traffic) V59.69 ☑
           nontraffic V59.29 ☑
        pedal cycle (traffic) V51.9 ☑
          nontraffic V51.3 ☑
          while boarding or alighting V51.4 ☑
        pickup truck (traffic) V53.9 ☑
          nontraffic V53.3 ☑
          while boarding or alighting V53.4 ☑

Accident — *continued*
  transport — *continued*
    pickup truck occupant — *continued*
      collision — *continued*
        railway vehicle (traffic) V55.9 ☑
          nontraffic V55.3 ☑
          while boarding or alighting V55.4 ☑
        specified vehicle NEC (traffic) V56.9 ☑
          nontraffic V56.3 ☑
          while boarding or alighting V56.4 ☑
        stationary object (traffic) V57.9 ☑
          nontraffic V57.3 ☑
          while boarding or alighting V57.4 ☑
        streetcar (traffic) V56.9 ☑
          nontraffic V56.3 ☑
          while boarding or alighting V56.4 ☑
        three wheeled motor vehicle (traffic)
          V52.9 ☑
          nontraffic V52.3 ☑
          while boarding or alighting V52.4 ☑
         truck (traffic) V54.9 ☑
          nontraffic V54.3 ☑
          while boarding or alighting V54.4 ☑
        two wheeled motor vehicle (traffic) V52.9 ☑
          nontraffic V52.3 ☑
          while boarding or alighting V52.4 ☑
        van (traffic) V53.9 ☑
          nontraffic V53.3 ☑
          while boarding or alighting V53.4 ☑
      driver
        collision (with)
          animal (traffic) V50.5 ☑
            being ridden (traffic) V56.5 ☑
              nontraffic V56.0 ☑
            nontraffic V50.0 ☑
          animal-drawn vehicle (traffic) V56.5 ☑
            nontraffic V56.0 ☑
          bus (traffic) V54.5 ☑
            nontraffic V54.0 ☑
          car (traffic) V53.5 ☑
            nontraffic V53.0 ☑
          motor vehicle NOS (traffic) V59.40 ☑
            nontraffic V59.00 ☑
            specified type NEC (traffic) V59.49 ☑
              nontraffic V59.09 ☑
          pedal cycle (traffic) V51.5 ☑
            nontraffic V51.0 ☑
          pickup truck (traffic) V53.5 ☑
            nontraffic V53.0 ☑
          railway vehicle (traffic) V55.5 ☑
            nontraffic V55.0 ☑
          specified vehicle NEC (traffic) V56.5 ☑
            nontraffic V56.0 ☑
          stationary object (traffic) V57.5 ☑
            nontraffic V57.0 ☑
          streetcar (traffic) V56.5 ☑
            nontraffic V56.0 ☑
          three wheeled motor vehicle (traffic)
            V52.5 ☑
            nontraffic V52.0 ☑
          truck (traffic) V54.5 ☑
            nontraffic V54.0 ☑
          two wheeled motor vehicle (traffic)
            V52.5 ☑
            nontraffic V52.0 ☑
          van (traffic) V53.5 ☑
            nontraffic V53.0 ☑
        noncollision accident (traffic) V58.5 ☑
          nontraffic V58.0 ☑
      hanger-on
        collision (with)
          animal (traffic) V50.7 ☑
            being ridden (traffic) V56.7 ☑
              nontraffic V56.2 ☑
            nontraffic V50.2 ☑
          animal-drawn vehicle (traffic) V56.7 ☑
            nontraffic V56.2 ☑
          bus (traffic) V54.7 ☑
            nontraffic V54.2 ☑
          car (traffic) V53.7 ☑
            nontraffic V53.2 ☑
          pedal cycle (traffic) V51.7 ☑
            nontraffic V51.2 ☑
          pickup truck (traffic) V53.7 ☑
            nontraffic V53.2 ☑
          railway vehicle (traffic) V55.7 ☑

Accident — *continued*
  transport — *continued*
    pickup truck occupant — *continued*
      hanger-on — *continued*
        collision — *continued*
          railway vehicle — *continued*
            nontraffic V55.2 ☑
          specified vehicle NEC (traffic) V56.7 ☑
            nontraffic V56.2 ☑
          stationary object (traffic) V57.7 ☑
            nontraffic V57.2 ☑
          streetcar (traffic) V56.7 ☑
            nontraffic V56.2 ☑
          three wheeled motor vehicle (traffic)
            V52.7 ☑
            nontraffic V52.2 ☑
          truck (traffic) V54.7 ☑
            nontraffic V54.2 ☑
          two wheeled motor vehicle (traffic)
            V52.7 ☑
            nontraffic V52.2 ☑
          van (traffic) V53.7 ☑
            nontraffic V53.2 ☑
        noncollision accident (traffic) V58.7 ☑
          nontraffic V58.2 ☑
      noncollision accident (traffic) V58.9 ☑
        nontraffic V58.3 ☑
        while boarding or alighting V58.4 ☑
      nontraffic V59.3 ☑
      passenger
        collision (with)
          animal (traffic) V50.6 ☑
            being ridden (traffic) V56.6 ☑
              nontraffic V56.1 ☑
            nontraffic V50.1 ☑
          animal-drawn vehicle (traffic) V56.6 ☑
            nontraffic V56.1 ☑
          bus (traffic) V54.6 ☑
            nontraffic V54.1 ☑
          car (traffic) V53.6 ☑
            nontraffic V53.1 ☑
          motor vehicle NOS (traffic) V59.50 ☑
            nontraffic V59.10 ☑
            specified type NEC (traffic) V59.59 ☑
              nontraffic V59.19 ☑
          pedal cycle (traffic) V51.6 ☑
            nontraffic V51.1 ☑
          pickup truck (traffic) V53.6 ☑
            nontraffic V53.1 ☑
          railway vehicle (traffic) V55.6 ☑
            nontraffic V55.1 ☑
          specified vehicle NEC (traffic) V56.6 ☑
            nontraffic V56.1 ☑
          stationary object (traffic) V57.6 ☑
            nontraffic V57.1 ☑
          streetcar (traffic) V56.6 ☑
            nontraffic V56.1 ☑
          three wheeled motor vehicle (traffic)
            V52.6 ☑
            nontraffic V52.1 ☑
          truck (traffic) V54.6 ☑
            nontraffic V54.1 ☑
          two wheeled motor vehicle (traffic)
            V52.6 ☑
            nontraffic V52.1 ☑
          van (traffic) V53.6 ☑
            nontraffic V53.1 ☑
        noncollision accident (traffic) V58.6 ☑
          nontraffic V58.1
      specified type NEC V59.88 ☑
        military vehicle V59.81 ☑
      quarry truck — *see* Accident, transport, industrial
        vehicle occupant
    race car — *see* Accident, transport, motor vehicle
      NEC occupant
    railway vehicle occupant V81.9 ☑
      collision (with) V81.3 ☑
        motor vehicle (non-military) (traffic)
          V81.1 ☑
          military V81.83 ☑
          nontraffic V81.0 ☑
        rolling stock V81.2 ☑
        specified object NEC V81.3 ☑
      during derailment V81.7 ☑

Accident — *continued*
  transport — *continued*
    railway vehicle occupant — *continued*
      during derailment — *continued*
        with antecedent collision — *see* Accident,
          transport, railway vehicle occupant,
          collision
      explosion V81.81 ☑
      fall (in railway vehicle) V81.5 ☑
        during derailment V81.7 ☑
          with antecedent collision — *see* Acci-
            dent, transport, railway vehicle
            occupant, collision
        from railway vehicle V81.6 ☑
          during derailment V81.7 ☑
            with antecedent collision — *see* Ac-
              cident, transport, railway vehi-
              cle occupant, collision
        while boarding or alighting V81.4 ☑
      fire V81.81 ☑
      object falling onto train V81.82 ☑
      specified type NEC V81.89 ☑
      while boarding or alighting V81.4 ☑
    ski lift V98.3 ☑
    snowmobile occupant (nontraffic) V86.92 ☑
      driver V86.52 ☑
      hanger-on V86.72 ☑
      passenger V86.62 ☑
      traffic V86.32 ☑
        driver V86.02 ☑
        hanger-on V86.22 ☑
        passenger V86.12 ☑
      while boarding or alighting V86.42 ☑
    specified NEC V98.8 ☑
    sport utility vehicle occupant (*see also* Accident,
      transport, pickup truck occupant)
    streetcar occupant V82.9 ☑
      collision (with) V82.3 ☑
        motor vehicle (traffic) V82.1 ☑
          nontraffic V82.0 ☑
        rolling stock V82.2 ☑
      during derailment V82.7 ☑
        with antecedent collision — *see* Accident,
          transport, streetcar occupant, collision
      fall (in streetcar) V82.5 ☑
        during derailment V82.7 ☑
          with antecedent collision — *see* Acci-
            dent, transport, streetcar occu-
            pant, collision
        from streetcar V82.6 ☑
          during derailment V82.7 ☑
            with antecedent collision — *see* Ac-
              cident, transport, streetcar oc-
              cupant, collision
        while boarding or alighting V82.4 ☑
      while boarding or alighting V82.4 ☑
      specified type NEC V82.8 ☑
      while boarding or alighting V82.4 ☑
    three-wheeled motor vehicle occupant V39.9 ☑
      collision (with)
        animal (traffic) V30.9 ☑
          being ridden (traffic) V36.9 ☑
            nontraffic V36.3 ☑
            while boarding or alighting V36.4 ☑
          nontraffic V30.3 ☑
          while boarding or alighting V30.4 ☑
        animal-drawn vehicle (traffic) V36.9 ☑
          nontraffic V36.3 ☑
          while boarding or alighting V36.4 ☑
        bus (traffic) V34.9 ☑
          nontraffic V34.3 ☑
          while boarding or alighting V34.4 ☑
        car (traffic) V33.9 ☑
          nontraffic V33.3 ☑
          while boarding or alighting V33.4 ☑
        motor vehicle NOS (traffic) V39.60 ☑
          nontraffic V39.20 ☑
          specified type NEC (traffic) V39.69 ☑
            nontraffic V39.29 ☑
        pedal cycle (traffic) V31.9 ☑
          nontraffic V31.3 ☑
          while boarding or alighting V31.4 ☑
        pickup truck (traffic) V33.9 ☑
          nontraffic V33.3 ☑
          while boarding or alighting V33.4 ☑
        railway vehicle (traffic) V35.9 ☑

▽ Subterms under main terms may continue to next column or page   ☑ Additional Character Required — Refer to the Tabular List for Character Selection   405

Accident — Accident

Accident — *continued*
  transport — *continued*
    three-wheeled motor vehicle occupant — *continued*
      collision — *continued*
        railway vehicle — *continued*
          nontraffic V35.3 ☑
          while boarding or alighting V35.4 ☑
        specified vehicle NEC (traffic) V36.9 ☑
          nontraffic V36.3 ☑
          while boarding or alighting V36.4 ☑
        stationary object (traffic) V37.9 ☑
          nontraffic V37.3 ☑
          while boarding or alighting V37.4 ☑
        streetcar (traffic) V36.9 ☑
          nontraffic V36.3 ☑
          while boarding or alighting V36.4 ☑
        three wheeled motor vehicle (traffic) V32.9 ☑
          nontraffic V32.3 ☑
          while boarding or alighting V32.4 ☑
         truck (traffic) V34.9 ☑
          nontraffic V34.3 ☑
          while boarding or alighting V34.4 ☑
         two wheeled motor vehicle (traffic) V32.9 ☑
          nontraffic V32.3 ☑
          while boarding or alighting V32.4 ☑
         van (traffic) V33.9 ☑
          nontraffic V33.3 ☑
          while boarding or alighting V33.4 ☑
      driver
        collision (with)
          animal (traffic) V30.5 ☑
            being ridden (traffic) V36.5 ☑
              nontraffic V36.0 ☑
            nontraffic V30.0 ☑
          animal-drawn vehicle (traffic) V36.5 ☑
            nontraffic V36.0 ☑
          bus (traffic) V34.5 ☑
            nontraffic V34.0 ☑
          car (traffic) V33.5 ☑
            nontraffic V33.0 ☑
          motor vehicle NOS (traffic) V39.40 ☑
            nontraffic V39.00 ☑
            specified type NEC (traffic) V39.49 ☑
              nontraffic V39.09 ☑
          pedal cycle (traffic) V31.5 ☑
            nontraffic V31.0 ☑
          pickup truck (traffic) V33.5 ☑
            nontraffic V33.0 ☑
          railway vehicle (traffic) V35.5 ☑
            nontraffic V35.0 ☑
          specified vehicle NEC (traffic) V36.5 ☑
            nontraffic V36.0 ☑
          stationary object (traffic) V37.5 ☑
            nontraffic V37.0 ☑
          streetcar (traffic) V36.5 ☑
            nontraffic V36.0 ☑
          three wheeled motor vehicle (traffic) V32.5 ☑
            nontraffic V32.0 ☑
          truck (traffic) V34.5 ☑
            nontraffic V34.0 ☑
          two wheeled motor vehicle (traffic) V32.5 ☑
            nontraffic V32.0 ☑
          van (traffic) V33.5 ☑
            nontraffic V33.0 ☑
        noncollision accident (traffic) V38.5 ☑
          nontraffic V38.0 ☑
      hanger-on
        collision (with)
          animal (traffic) V30.7 ☑
            being ridden (traffic) V36.7 ☑
              nontraffic V36.2 ☑
            nontraffic V30.2 ☑
          animal-drawn vehicle (traffic) V36.7 ☑
            nontraffic V36.2 ☑
          bus (traffic) V34.7 ☑
            nontraffic V34.2 ☑
          car (traffic) V33.7 ☑
            nontraffic V33.2 ☑
          pedal cycle (traffic) V31.7 ☑
            nontraffic V31.2 ☑
          pickup truck (traffic) V33.7 ☑
            nontraffic V33.2 ☑

Accident — *continued*
  transport — *continued*
    three-wheeled motor vehicle occupant — *continued*
      hanger-on — *continued*
        collision — *continued*
          railway vehicle (traffic) V35.7 ☑
            nontraffic V35.2 ☑
          specified vehicle NEC (traffic) V36.7 ☑
            nontraffic V36.2 ☑
          stationary object (traffic) V37.7 ☑
            nontraffic V37.2 ☑
          streetcar (traffic) V36.7 ☑
            nontraffic V36.2 ☑
          three wheeled motor vehicle (traffic) V32.7 ☑
            nontraffic V32.2 ☑
          truck (traffic) V34.7 ☑
            nontraffic V34.2 ☑
          two wheeled motor vehicle (traffic) V32.7 ☑
            nontraffic V32.2 ☑
          van (traffic) V33.7 ☑
            nontraffic V33.2 ☑
        noncollision accident (traffic) V38.7 ☑
          nontraffic V38.2 ☑
      noncollision accident (traffic) V38.9 ☑
        nontraffic V38.3 ☑
        while boarding or alighting V38.4 ☑
      nontraffic V39.3 ☑
      passenger
        collision (with)
          animal (traffic) V30.6 ☑
            being ridden (traffic) V36.6 ☑
              nontraffic V36.1 ☑
            nontraffic V30.1 ☑
          animal-drawn vehicle (traffic) V36.6 ☑
            nontraffic V36.1 ☑
          bus (traffic) V34.6 ☑
            nontraffic V34.1 ☑
          car (traffic) V33.6 ☑
            nontraffic V33.1 ☑
          motor vehlcle NOS (traffic) V39.50 ☑
            nontraffic V39.10 ☑
            specified type NEC (traffic) V39.59 ☑
              nontraffic V39.19 ☑
          pedal cycle (traffic) V31.6 ☑
            nontraffic V31.1 ☑
          pickup truck (traffic) V33.6 ☑
            nontraffic V33.1 ☑
          railway vehicle (traffic) V35.6 ☑
            nontraffic V35.1 ☑
          specified vehicle NEC (traffic) V36.6 ☑
            nontraffic V36.1 ☑
          stationary object (traffic) V37.6 ☑
            nontraffic V37.1 ☑
          streetcar (traffic) V36.6 ☑
            nontraffic V36.1 ☑
          three wheeled motor vehicle (traffic) V32.6 ☑
            nontraffic V32.1 ☑
          truck (traffic) V34.6 ☑
            nontraffic V34.1 ☑
          two wheeled motor vehicle (traffic) V32.6 ☑
            nontraffic V32.1 ☑
          van (traffic) V33.6 ☑
            nontraffic V33.1 ☑
        noncollision accident (traffic) V38.6 ☑
          nontraffic V38.1 ☑
      specified type NEC V39.89 ☑
        military vehicle V39.81 ☑
      tractor (farm) (and trailer) — *see* Accident, transport, agricultural vehicle occupant
      tram — *see* Accident, transport, streetcar
        in mine or quarry — *see* Accident, transport, industrial vehicle occupant
      trolley — *see* Accident, transport, streetcar
        in mine or quarry — *see* Accident, transport, industrial vehicle occupant
      truck (heavy) occupant V69.9 ☑
        collision (with)
          animal (traffic) V60.9 ☑
            being ridden (traffic) V66.9 ☑
              nontraffic V66.3 ☑
              while boarding or alighting V66.4 ☑

Accident — *continued*
  transport — *continued*
    truck occupant — *continued*
      collision — *continued*
        animal — *continued*
          nontraffic V60.3 ☑
          while boarding or alighting V60.4 ☑
        animal-drawn vehicle (traffic) V66.9 ☑
          nontraffic V66.3 ☑
          while boarding or alighting V66.4 ☑
        bus (traffic) V64.9 ☑
          nontraffic V64.3 ☑
          while boarding or alighting V64.4 ☑
        car (traffic) V63.9 ☑
          nontraffic V63.3 ☑
          while boarding or alighting V63.4 ☑
        motor vehicle NOS (traffic) V69.60 ☑
          nontraffic V69.20 ☑
          specified type NEC (traffic) V69.69 ☑
           nontraffic V69.29 ☑
        pedal cycle (traffic) V61.9 ☑
          nontraffic V61.3 ☑
          while boarding or alighting V61.4 ☑
        pickup truck (traffic) V63.9 ☑
          nontraffic V63.3 ☑
          while boarding or alighting V63.4 ☑
        railway vehicle (traffic) V65.9 ☑
          nontraffic V65.3 ☑
          while boarding or alighting V65.4 ☑
        specified vehicle NEC (traffic) V66.9 ☑
          nontraffic V66.3 ☑
          while boarding or alighting V66.4 ☑
        stationary object (traffic) V67.9 ☑
          nontraffic V67.3 ☑
          while boarding or alighting V67.4 ☑
        streetcar (traffic) V66.9 ☑
          nontraffic V66.3 ☑
          while boarding or alighting V66.4 ☑
        three wheeled motor vehicle (traffic) V62.9 ☑
          nontraffic V62.3 ☑
          while boarding or alighting V62.4 ☑
        truck (traffic) V64.9 ☑
          nontraffic V64.3 ☑
          while boarding or alighting V64.4 ☑
        two wheeled motor vehicle (traffic) V62.9 ☑
          nontraffic V62.3 ☑
          while boarding or alighting V62.4 ☑
        van (traffic) V63.9 ☑
          nontraffic V63.3 ☑
          while boarding or alighting V63.4 ☑
      driver
        collision (with)
          animal (traffic) V60.5 ☑
            being ridden (traffic) V66.5 ☑
              nontraffic V66.0 ☑
            nontraffic V60.0 ☑
          animal-drawn vehicle (traffic) V66.5 ☑
            nontraffic V66.0 ☑
          bus (traffic) V64.5 ☑
            nontraffic V64.0 ☑
          car (traffic) V63.5 ☑
            nontraffic V63.0 ☑
          motor vehicle NOS (traffic) V69.40 ☑
            nontraffic V69.00 ☑
            specified type NEC (traffic) V69.49 ☑
              nontraffic V69.09 ☑
          pedal cycle (traffic) V61.5 ☑
            nontraffic V61.0 ☑
          pickup truck (traffic) V63.5 ☑
            nontraffic V63.0 ☑
          railway vehicle (traffic) V65.5 ☑
            nontraffic V65.0 ☑
          specified vehicle NEC (traffic) V66.5 ☑
            nontraffic V66.0 ☑
          stationary object (traffic) V67.5 ☑
            nontraffic V67.0 ☑
          streetcar (traffic) V66.5 ☑
            nontraffic V66.0 ☑
          three wheeled motor vehicle (traffic) V62.5 ☑
            nontraffic V62.0 ☑
          truck (traffic) V64.5 ☑
            nontraffic V64.0 ☑
          two wheeled motor vehicle (traffic) V62.5 ☑

☑ **Additional Character Required** — Refer to the Tabular List for Character Selection   ▽ **Subterms under main terms may continue to next column or page**

Accident — *continued*
  transport — *continued*
    truck occupant — *continued*
      driver — *continued*
        collision — *continued*
          two wheeled motor vehicle — *continued*
            nontraffic V62.0 ☑
            van (traffic) V63.5 ☑
              nontraffic V63.0 ☑
          noncollision accident (traffic) V68.5 ☑
            nontraffic V68.0 ☑
      dump — *see* Accident, transport, construction vehicle occupant
      hanger-on
        collision (with)
          animal (traffic) V60.7 ☑
            being ridden (traffic) V66.7 ☑
              nontraffic V66.2 ☑
            nontraffic V60.2 ☑
          animal-drawn vehicle (traffic) V66.7 ☑
            nontraffic V66.2 ☑
          bus (traffic) V64.7 ☑
            nontraffic V64.2 ☑
          car (traffic) V63.7 ☑
            nontraffic V63.2 ☑
          pedal cycle (traffic) V61.7 ☑
            nontraffic V61.2 ☑
          pickup truck (traffic) V63.7 ☑
            nontraffic V63.2 ☑
          railway vehicle (traffic) V65.7 ☑
            nontraffic V65.2 ☑
          specified vehicle NEC (traffic) V66.7 ☑
            nontraffic V66.2 ☑
          stationary object (traffic) V67.7 ☑
            nontraffic V67.2 ☑
          streetcar (traffic) V66.7 ☑
            nontraffic V66.2 ☑
          three wheeled motor vehicle (traffic) V62.7 ☑
            nontraffic V62.2 ☑
          truck (traffic) V64.7 ☑
            nontraffic V64.2 ☑
          two wheeled motor vehicle (traffic) V62.7 ☑
            nontraffic V62.2 ☑
          van (traffic) V63.7 ☑
            nontraffic V63.2 ☑
        noncollision accident (traffic) V68.7 ☑
          nontraffic V68.2 ☑
      noncollision accident (traffic) V68.9 ☑
        nontraffic V68.3 ☑
        while boarding or alighting V68.4 ☑
      nontraffic V69.3 ☑
      passenger
        collision (with)
          animal (traffic) V60.6 ☑
            being ridden (traffic) V66.6 ☑
              nontraffic V66.1- ☑
            nontraffic V60.1 ☑
          animal-drawn vehicle (traffic) V66.6 ☑
            nontraffic V66.1 ☑
          bus (traffic) V64.6 ☑
            nontraffic V64.1 ☑
          car (traffic) V63.6 ☑
            nontraffic V63.1 ☑
          motor vehicle NOS (traffic) V69.50 ☑
            nontraffic V69.10 ☑
            specified type NEC (traffic) V69.59 ☑
              nontraffic V69.19 ☑
          pedal cycle (traffic) V61.6 ☑
            nontraffic V61.1 ☑
          pickup truck (traffic) V63.6 ☑
            nontraffic V63.1 ☑
          railway vehicle (traffic) V65.6 ☑
            nontraffic V65.1 ☑
          specified vehicle NEC (traffic) V66.6 ☑
            nontraffic V66.1 ☑
          stationary object (traffic) V67.6 ☑
            nontraffic V67.1 ☑
          streetcar (traffic) V66.6 ☑
            nontraffic V66.1 ☑
          three wheeled motor vehicle (traffic) V62.6 ☑
            nontraffic V62.1 ☑
          truck (traffic) V64.6 ☑

Accident — *continued*
  transport — *continued*
    truck occupant — *continued*
      passenger — *continued*
        collision — *continued*
          truck — *continued*
            nontraffic V64.1 ☑
          two wheeled motor vehicle (traffic) V62.6 ☑
            nontraffic V62.1 ☑
          van (traffic) V63.6 ☑
            nontraffic V63.1 ☑
        noncollision accident (traffic) V68.6 ☑
          nontraffic V68.1 ☑
      pickup — *see* Accident, transport, pickup truck occupant
      specified type NEC V69.88 ☑
      military vehicle V69.81 ☑
    van occupant V59.9 ☑
      collision (with)
        animal (traffic) V50.9 ☑
          being ridden (traffic) V56.9 ☑
            nontraffic V56.3 ☑
            while boarding or alighting V56.4 ☑
          nontraffic V50.3 ☑
          while boarding or alighting V50.4 ☑
        animal-drawn vehicle (traffic) V56.9 ☑
          nontraffic V56.3 ☑
          while boarding or alighting V56.4 ☑
        bus (traffic) V54.9 ☑
          nontraffic V54.3 ☑
          while boarding or alighting V54.4 ☑
        car (traffic) V53.9 ☑
          nontraffic V53.3 ☑
          while boarding or alighting V53.4 ☑
        motor vehicle NOS (traffic) V59.60 ☑
          nontraffic V59.20 ☑
          specified type NEC (traffic) V59.69 ☑
            nontraffic V59.29 ☑
        pedal cycle (traffic) V51.9 ☑
          nontraffic V51.3 ☑
          while boarding or alighting V51.4 ☑
        pickup truck (traffic) V53.9 ☑
          nontraffic V53.3 ☑
          while boarding or alighting V53.4 ☑
        railway vehicle (traffic) V55.9 ☑
          nontraffic V55.3 ☑
          while boarding or alighting V55.4 ☑
        specified vehicle NEC (traffic) V56.9 ☑
          nontraffic V56.3 ☑
          while boarding or alighting V56.4 ☑
        stationary object (traffic) V57.9 ☑
          nontraffic V57.3 ☑
          while boarding or alighting V57.4 ☑
        streetcar (traffic) V56.9 ☑
          nontraffic V56.3 ☑
          while boarding or alighting V56.4 ☑
        three wheeled motor vehicle (traffic) V52.9 ☑
          nontraffic V52.3 ☑
          while boarding or alighting V52.4 ☑
        truck (traffic) V54.9 ☑
          nontraffic V54.3 ☑
          while boarding or alighting V54.4 ☑
        two wheeled motor vehicle (traffic) V52.9 ☑
          nontraffic V52.3 ☑
          while boarding or alighting V52.4 ☑
        van (traffic) V53.9 ☑
          nontraffic V53.3 ☑
          while boarding or alighting V53.4 ☑
      driver
        collision (with)
          animal (traffic) V50.5 ☑
            being ridden (traffic) V56.5 ☑
              nontraffic V56.0 ☑
            nontraffic V50.0 ☑
          animal-drawn vehicle (traffic) V56.5 ☑
            nontraffic V56.0 ☑
          bus (traffic) V54.5 ☑
            nontraffic V54.0 ☑
          car (traffic) V53.5 ☑
            nontraffic V53.0 ☑
          motor vehicle NOS (traffic) V59.40 ☑
            nontraffic V59.00 ☑
            specified type NEC (traffic) V59.49 ☑
              nontraffic V59.09 ☑

Accident — *continued*
  transport — *continued*
    van occupant — *continued*
      driver — *continued*
        collision — *continued*
          pedal cycle (traffic) V51.5 ☑
            nontraffic V51.0 ☑
          pickup truck (traffic) V53.5 ☑
            nontraffic V53.0 ☑
          railway vehicle (traffic) V55.5 ☑
            nontraffic V55.0 ☑
          specified vehicle NEC (traffic) V56.5 ☑
            nontraffic V56.0 ☑
          stationary object (traffic) V57.5 ☑
            nontraffic V57.0 ☑
          streetcar (traffic) V56.5 ☑
            nontraffic V56.0 ☑
          three wheeled motor vehicle (traffic) V52.5 ☑
            nontraffic V52.0 ☑
          truck (traffic) V54.5 ☑
            nontraffic V54.0 ☑
          two wheeled motor vehicle (traffic) V52.5 ☑
            nontraffic V52.0 ☑
          van (traffic) V53.5 ☑
            nontraffic V53.0 ☑
        noncollision accident (traffic) V58.5 ☑
          nontraffic V58.0 ☑
      hanger-on
        collision (with)
          animal (traffic) V50.7 ☑
            being ridden (traffic) V56.7 ☑
              nontraffic V56.2 ☑
            nontraffic V50.2 ☑
          animal-drawn vehicle (traffic) V56.7 ☑
            nontraffic V56.2 ☑
          bus (traffic) V54.7 ☑
            nontraffic V54.2 ☑
          car (traffic) V53.7 ☑
            nontraffic V53.2 ☑
          pedal cycle (traffic) V51.7 ☑
            nontraffic V51.2 ☑
          pickup truck (traffic) V53.7 ☑
            nontraffic V53.2 ☑
          railway vehicle (traffic) V55.7 ☑
            nontraffic V55.2 ☑
          specified vehicle NEC (traffic) V56.7 ☑
            nontraffic V56.2 ☑
          stationary object (traffic) V57.7 ☑
            nontraffic V57.2 ☑
          streetcar (traffic) V56.7 ☑
            nontraffic V56.2 ☑
          three wheeled motor vehicle (traffic) V52.7 ☑
            nontraffic V52.2 ☑
          truck (traffic) V54.7 ☑
            nontraffic V54.2 ☑
          two wheeled motor vehicle (traffic) V52.7 ☑
            nontraffic V52.2 ☑
          van (traffic) V53.7 ☑
            nontraffic V53.2 ☑
        noncollision accident (traffic) V58.7 ☑
          nontraffic V58.2 ☑
      noncollision accident (traffic) V58.9 ☑
        nontraffic V58.3 ☑
        while boarding or alighting V58.4 ☑
      nontraffic V59.3 ☑
      passenger
        collision (with)
          animal (traffic) V50.6 ☑
            being ridden (traffic) V56.6 ☑
              nontraffic V56.1 ☑
            nontraffic V50.1 ☑
          animal-drawn vehicle (traffic) V56.6 ☑
            nontraffic V56.1 ☑
          bus (traffic) V54.6 ☑
            nontraffic V54.1 ☑
          car (traffic) V53.6 ☑
            nontraffic V53.1 ☑
          motor vehicle NOS (traffic) V59.50 ☑
            nontraffic V59.10 ☑
            specified type NEC (traffic) V59.59 ☑
              nontraffic V59.19 ☑
          pedal cycle (traffic) V51.6 ☑

▽ Subterms under main terms may continue to next column or page   ☑ Additional Character Required — Refer to the Tabular List for Character Selection   **407**

Accident — Accident

Accident — *continued*
  transport — *continued*
    van occupant — *continued*
      passenger — *continued*
        collision — *continued*
          pedal cycle — *continued*
            nontraffic V51.1
          pickup truck (traffic) V53.6 ☑
            nontraffic V53.1 ☑
          railway vehicle (traffic) V55.6 ☑
            nontraffic V55.1 ☑
          specified vehicle NEC (traffic) V56.6 ☑
            nontraffic V56.1 ☑
          stationary object (traffic) V57.6 ☑
            nontraffic V57.1 ☑
          streetcar (traffic) V56.6 ☑
            nontraffic V56.1 ☑
          three wheeled motor vehicle (traffic) V52.6 ☑
            nontraffic V52.1 ☑
          truck (traffic) V54.6 ☑
            nontraffic V54.1 ☑
          two wheeled motor vehicle (traffic) V52.6 ☑
            nontraffic V52.1 ☑
          van (traffic) V53.6 ☑
            nontraffic V53.1 ☑
        noncollision accident (traffic) V58.6 ☑
          nontraffic V58.1 ☑
        specified type NEC V59.88 ☑
        military vehicle V59.81 ☑
  watercraft occupant — *see* Accident, watercraft
  vehicle NEC V89.9 ☑
    animal-drawn NEC — *see* Accident, transport, animal-drawn vehicle occupant
    special
      agricultural — *see* Accident, transport, agricultural vehicle occupant
      construction — *see* Accident, transport, construction vehicle occupant
      industrial — *see* Accident, transport, industrial vehicle occupant
      three-wheeled NEC (motorized) — *see* Accident, transport, three-wheeled motor vehicle occupant
  watercraft V94.9 ☑
    causing
      drowning — *see* Drowning, due to, accident to, watercraft
      injury NEC V91.89 ☑
        crushed between craft and object V91.19 ☑
          powered craft V91.13 ☑
            ferry boat V91.11 ☑
            fishing boat V91.12 ☑
            jetskis V91.13 ☑
            liner V91.11 ☑
            merchant ship V91.10 ☑
            passenger ship V91.11 ☑
          unpowered craft V91.18 ☑
            canoe V91.15 ☑
            inflatable V91.16 ☑
            kayak V91.15 ☑
            sailboat V91.14 ☑
            surf-board V91.18 ☑
            windsurfer V91.18 ☑
        fall on board V91.29 ☑
          powered craft V91.23 ☑
            ferry boat V91.21 ☑
            fishing boat V91.22 ☑
            jetskis V91.23 ☑
            liner V91.21 ☑
            merchant ship V91.20 ☑
            passenger ship V91.21 ☑
          unpowered craft
            canoe V91.25 ☑
            inflatable V91.26 ☑
            kayak V91.25 ☑
            sailboat V91.24 ☑
        fire on board causing burn V91.09 ☑
          powered craft V91.03 ☑
            ferry boat V91.01 ☑
            fishing boat V91.02 ☑
            jetskis V91.03 ☑
            liner V91.01 ☑
            merchant ship V91.00 ☑
            passenger ship V91.01 ☑

Accident — *continued*
  watercraft — *continued*
    causing — *continued*
      injury — *continued*
        fire on board causing burn — *continued*
          unpowered craft V91.08 ☑
            canoe V91.05 ☑
            inflatable V91.06 ☑
            kayak V91.05 ☑
            sailboat V91.04 ☑
            surf-board V91.08 ☑
            water skis V91.07 ☑
            windsurfer V91.08 ☑
        hit by falling object V91.39 ☑
          powered craft V91.33 ☑
            ferry boat V91.31 ☑
            fishing boat V91.32 ☑
            jetskis V91.33 ☑
            liner V91.31 ☑
            merchant ship V91.30 ☑
            passenger ship V91.31 ☑
          unpowered craft V91.38 ☑
            canoe V91.35 ☑
            inflatable V91.36 ☑
            kayak V91.35 ☑
            sailboat V91.34 ☑
            surf-board V91.38 ☑
            water skis V91.37 ☑
            windsurfer V91.38 ☑
        specified type NEC V91.89 ☑
          powered craft V91.83 ☑
            ferry boat V91.81 ☑
            fishing boat V91.82 ☑
            jetskis V91.83 ☑
            liner V91.81 ☑
            merchant ship V91.80 ☑
            passenger ship V91.81 ☑
          unpowered craft V91.88 ☑
            canoe V91.85 ☑
            inflatable V91.86 ☑
            kayak V91.85 ☑
            sailboat V91.84 ☑
            surf-board V91.88 ☑
            water skis V91.87 ☑
            windsurfer V91.88 ☑
      due to, caused by cataclysm — *see* Forces of nature, by type
      military NEC V94.818 ☑
        with civilian watercraft V94.810 ☑
        civilian in water injured by V94.811 ☑
      nonpowered, struck by
        nonpowered vessel V94.22 ☑
        powered vessel V94.21 ☑
      specified type NEC V94.89 ☑
      striking swimmer
        powered V94.11 ☑
        unpowered V94.12 ☑

Acid throwing (assault) Y08.89 ☑

Activity (involving) (of victim at time of event) Y93.9
  aerobic and step exercise (class) Y93.A3 (*following* Y93.7)
  alpine skiing Y93.23
  animal care NEC Y93.K9 (*following* Y93.7)
  arts and handcrafts NEC Y93.D9 (*following* Y93.7)
  athletics played as a team or group NEC Y93.69
  athletics played individually NEC Y93.59
  athletics NEC Y93.79
  baking Y93.G3 (*following* Y93.7)
  ballet Y93.41
  barbells Y93.B3 (*following* Y93.7)
  BASE (Building, Antenna, Span, Earth) jumping Y93.33
  baseball Y93.64
  basketball Y93.67
  bathing (personal) Y93.E1 (*following* Y93.7)
  beach volleyball Y93.68
  bike riding Y93.55
  blackout game Y93.85
  boogie boarding Y93.18
  bowling Y93.54
  boxing Y93.71
  brass instrument playing Y93.J4 (*following* Y93.7)
  building construction Y93.H3 (*following* Y93.7)
  bungee jumping Y93.34
  calisthenics Y93.A2 (*following* Y93.7)
  canoeing (in calm and turbulent water) Y93.16
  capture the flag Y93.6A
  cardiorespiratory exercise NEC Y93.A9 (*following* Y93.7)

Activity — *continued*
  caregiving (providing) NEC Y93.F9 (*following* Y93.7)
    bathing Y93.F1 (*following* Y93.7)
    lifting Y93.F2 (*following* Y93.7)
  cellular
    communication device Y93.C2 (*following* Y93.7)
    telephone Y93.C2 (*following* Y93.7)
  challenge course Y93.A5 (*following* Y93.7)
  cheerleading Y93.45
  choking game Y93.85
  circuit training Y93.A4 (*following* Y93.7)
  cleaning
    floor Y93.E5 (*following* Y93.7)
  climbing NEC Y93.39
    mountain Y93.31
    rock Y93.31
    wall Y93.31
  clothing care and maintenance NEC Y93.E9 (*following* Y93.7)
  combatives Y93.75
  computer
    keyboarding Y93.C1 (*following* Y93.7)
    technology NEC Y93.C9 (*following* Y93.7)
  confidence course Y93.A5 (*following* Y93.7)
  construction (building) Y93.H3 (*following* Y93.7)
  cooking and baking Y93.G3 (*following* Y93.7)
  cool down exercises Y93.A2 (*following* Y93.7)
  cricket Y93.69
  crocheting Y93.D1 (*following* Y93.7)
  cross country skiing Y93.24
  dancing (all types) Y93.41
  digging
    dirt Y93.H1 (*following* Y93.7)
  dirt digging Y93.H1 (*following* Y93.7)
  dishwashing Y93.G1 (*following* Y93.7)
  diving (platform) (springboard) Y93.12
    underwater Y93.15
  dodge ball Y93.6A
  downhill skiing Y93.23
  drum playing Y93.J2 (*following* Y93.7)
  dumbbells Y93.B3 (*following* Y93.7)
  electronic
    devices NEC Y93.C9 (*following* Y93.7)
      hand held interactive Y93.C2 (*following* Y93.7)
    game playing (using) (with)
      interactive device Y93.C2 (*following* Y93.7)
      keyboard or other stationary device Y93.C1 (*following* Y93.7)
  elliptical machine Y93.A1 (*following* Y93.7)
  exercise(s)
    machines ((primarily) for)
      cardiorespiratory conditioning Y93.A1 (*following* Y93.7)
      muscle strengthening Y93.B1 (*following* Y93.7)
    muscle strengthening (non-machine) NEC Y93.B9 (*following* Y93.7)
  external motion NEC Y93.I9 (*following* Y93.7)
    rollercoaster Y93.I1 (*following* Y93.7)
  fainting game Y93.85
  field hockey Y93.65
  figure skating (pairs) (singles) Y93.21
  flag football Y93.62
  floor mopping and cleaning Y93.E5 (*following* Y93.7)
  food preparation and clean up Y93.G1 (*following* Y93.7)
  football (American) NOS Y93.61
    flag Y93.62
    tackle Y93.61
    touch Y93.62
  four square Y93.6A
  free weights Y93.B3 (*following* Y93.7)
  frisbee (ultimate) Y93.74
  furniture
    building Y93.D3 (*following* Y93.7)
    finishing Y93.D3 (*following* Y93.7)
    repair Y93.D3 (*following* Y93.7)
  game playing (electronic)
    using interactive device Y93.C2 (*following* Y93.7)
    using keyboard or other stationary device Y93.C1 (*following* Y93.7)
  gardening Y93.H2 (*following* Y93.7)
  golf Y93.53
  grass drills Y93.A6 (*following* Y93.7)
  grilling and smoking food Y93.G2 (*following* Y93.7)
  grooming and shearing an animal Y93.K3 (*following* Y93.7)
  guerilla drills Y93.A6 (*following* Y93.7)
  gymnastics (rhythmic) Y93.43
  hand held interactive electronic device Y93.C2 (*following* Y93.7)

Activity — *continued*
  handball Y93.73
  handcrafts NEC Y93.D9 (*following* Y93.7)
  hang gliding Y93.35
  hiking (on level or elevated terrain) Y93.Ø1
  hockey (ice) Y93.22
    field Y93.65
  horseback riding Y93.52
  household (interior) maintenance NEC Y93.E9 (*following* Y93.7)
  ice NEC Y93.29
    dancing Y93.21
    hockey Y93.22
    skating Y93.21
  inline roller skating Y93.51
  ironing Y93.E4 (*following* Y93.7)
  judo Y93.75
  jumping jacks Y93.A2 (*following* Y93.7)
  jumping rope Y93.56
  jumping (off) NEC Y93.39
    BASE (Building, Antenna, Span, Earth) Y93.33
    bungee Y93.34
    jacks Y93.A2 (*following* Y93.7)
    rope Y93.56
  karate Y93.75
  kayaking (in calm and turbulent water) Y93.16
  keyboarding (computer) Y93.C1 (*following* Y93.7)
  kickball Y93.6A
  knitting Y93.D1 (*following* Y93.7)
  lacrosse Y93.65
  land maintenance NEC Y93.H9 (*following* Y93.7)
  landscaping Y93.H2 (*following* Y93.7)
  laundry Y93.E2 (*following* Y93.7)
  machines (exercise)
    primarily for cardiorespiratory conditioning Y93.A1 (*following* Y93.7)
    primarily for muscle strengthening Y93.B1 (*following* Y93.7)
  maintenance
    exterior building NEC Y93.H9 (*following* Y93.7)
    household (interior) NEC Y93.E9 (*following* Y93.7)
    land Y93.H9 (*following* Y93.7)
    property Y93.H9 (*following* Y93.7)
  marching (on level or elevated terrain) Y93.Ø1
  martial arts Y93.75
  microwave oven Y93.G3 (*following* Y93.7)
  milking an animal Y93.K2 (*following* Y93.7)
  mopping (floor) Y93.E5 (*following* Y93.7)
  mountain climbing Y93.31
  muscle strengthening
    exercises (non-machine) NEC Y93.B9 (*following* Y93.7)
    machines Y93.B1 (*following* Y93.7)
  musical keyboard (electronic) playing Y93.J1 (*following* Y93.7)
  nordic skiing Y93.24
  obstacle course Y93.A5 (*following* Y93.7)
  oven (microwave) Y93.G3 (*following* Y93.7)
  packing up and unpacking in moving to a new residence Y93.E6 (*following* Y93.7)
  parasailing Y93.19
  pass out game Y93.85
  percussion instrument playing NEC Y93.J2 (*following* Y93.7)
  personal
    bathing and showering Y93.E1 (*following* Y93.7)
    hygiene NEC Y93.E8 (*following* Y93.7)
    showering Y93.E1 (*following* Y93.7)
  physical games generally associated with school recess, summer camp and children Y93.6A
  physical training NEC Y93.A9 (*following* Y93.7)
  piano playing Y93.J1 (*following* Y93.7)
  pilates Y93.B4 (*following* Y93.7)
  platform diving Y93.12
  playing musical instrument
    brass instrument Y93.J4 (*following* Y93.7)
    drum Y93.J2 (*following* Y93.7)
    musical keyboard (electronic) Y93.J1 (*following* Y93.7)
    percussion instrument NEC Y93.J2 (*following* Y93.7)
    piano Y93.J1 (*following* Y93.7)
    string instrument Y93.J3 (*following* Y93.7)
    winds instrument Y93.J4 (*following* Y93.7)
  property maintenance
    exterior NEC Y93.H9 (*following* Y93.7)
    interior NEC Y93.E9 (*following* Y93.7)
  pruning (garden and lawn) Y93.H2 (*following* Y93.7)
  pull-ups Y93.B2 (*following* Y93.7)
  push-ups Y93.B2 (*following* Y93.7)

Activity — *continued*
  racquetball Y93.73
  rafting (in calm and turbulent water) Y93.16
  raking (leaves) Y93.H1 (*following* Y93.7)
  rappelling Y93.32
  refereeing a sports activity Y93.81
  residential relocation Y93.E6 (*following* Y93.7)
  rhythmic gymnastics Y93.43
  rhythmic movement NEC Y93.49
  riding
    horseback Y93.52
    rollercoaster Y93.I1 (*following* Y93.7)
  rock climbing Y93.31
  roller skating (inline) Y93.51
  rollercoaster riding Y93.I1 (*following* Y93.7)
  rough housing and horseplay Y93.83
  rowing (in calm and turbulent water) Y93.16
  rugby Y93.63
  running Y93.Ø2
  SCUBA diving Y93.15
  sewing Y93.D2 (*following* Y93.7)
  shoveling Y93.H1 (*following* Y93.7)
    dirt Y93.H1 (*following* Y93.7)
    snow Y93.H1 (*following* Y93.7)
  showering (personal) Y93.E1 (*following* Y93.7)
  sit-ups Y93.B2 (*following* Y93.7)
  skateboarding Y93.51
  skating (ice) Y93.21
    roller Y93.51
  skiing (alpine) (downhill) Y93.23
    cross country Y93.24
    nordic Y93.24
    water Y93.17
  sledding (snow) Y93.23
  sleeping (sleep) Y93.84
  smoking and grilling food Y93.G2 (*following* Y93.7)
  snorkeling Y93.15
  snow NEC Y93.29
    boarding Y93.23
    shoveling Y93.H1 (*following* Y93.7)
    sledding Y93.23
    tubing Y93.23
  soccer Y93.66
  softball Y93.64
  specified NEC Y93.89
  spectator at an event Y93.82
  sports NEC Y93.79
    sports played as a team or group NEC Y93.69
    sports played individually NEC Y93.59
  springboard diving Y93.12
  squash Y93.73
  stationary bike Y93.A1 (*following* Y93.7)
  step (stepping) exercise (class) Y93.A3 (*following* Y93.7)
  stepper machine Y93.A1 (*following* Y93.7)
  stove Y93.G3 (*following* Y93.7)
  string instrument playing Y93.J3 (*following* Y93.7)
  surfing Y93.18
    wind Y93.18
  swimming Y93.11
  tackle football Y93.61
  tap dancing Y93.41
  tennis Y93.73
  tobogganing Y93.23
  touch football Y93.62
  track and field events (non-running) Y93.57
    running Y93.Ø2
  trampoline Y93.44
  treadmill Y93.A1 (*following* Y93.7)
  trimming shrubs Y93.H2 (*following* Y93.7)
  tubing (in calm and turbulent water) Y93.16
    snow Y93.23
  ultimate frisbee Y93.74
  underwater diving Y93.15
  unpacking in moving to a new residence Y93.E6 (*following* Y93.7)
  use of stove, oven and microwave oven Y93.G3 (*following* Y93.7)
  vacuuming Y93.E3 (*following* Y93.7)
  volleyball (beach) (court) Y93.68
  wake boarding Y93.17
  walking (on level or elevated terrain) Y93.Ø1
    an animal Y93.K1 (*following* Y93.7)
  walking an animal Y93.K1 (*following* Y93.7)
  wall climbing Y93.31
  warm up and cool down exercises Y93.A2 (*following* Y93.7)
  water NEC Y93.19
    aerobics Y93.14
    craft NEC Y93.19

Activity — *continued*
  water — *continued*
    exercise Y93.14
    polo Y93.13
    skiing Y93.17
    sliding Y93.18
    survival training and testing Y93.19
  weeding (garden and lawn) Y93.H2 (*following* Y93.7)
  wind instrument playing Y93.J4 (*following* Y93.7)
  windsurfing Y93.18
  wrestling Y93.72
  yoga Y93.42
Adverse effect of drugs — *see* Table of Drugs and Chemicals
Aerosinusitis — *see* Air, pressure
After-effect, late — *see* Sequelae
Air
  blast in war operations — *see* War operations, air blast
  pressure
    change, rapid
      during
        ascent W94.29 ☑
          while (in) (surfacing from)
            aircraft W94.23 ☑
            deep water diving W94.21 ☑
            underground W94.22 ☑
        descent W94.39 ☑
          in
            aircraft W94.31 ☑
            water W94.32 ☑
    high, prolonged W94.Ø ☑
    low, prolonged W94.12 ☑
      due to residence or long visit at high altitude W94.11 ☑
Alpine sickness W94.11 ☑
Altitude sickness W94.11 ☑
Anaphylactic shock, anaphylaxis — *see* Table of Drugs and Chemicals
Andes disease W94.11 ☑
Arachnidism, arachnoidism X58 ☑
Arson (with intent to injure or kill) X97 ☑
Asphyxia, asphyxiation
  by
    food (bone) (seed) — *see* categories T17 and T18 ☑
    gas (*see also* Table of Drugs and Chemicals)
      legal
        execution — *see* Legal, intervention, gas
        intervention — *see* Legal, intervention, gas
  from
    fire (*see also* Exposure, fire)
      in war operations — *see* War operations, fire
    ignition — *see* Ignition
    vomitus T17.81 ☑
  in war operations — *see* War operations, restriction of airway
Aspiration
  food (any type) (into respiratory tract) (with asphyxia, obstruction respiratory tract, suffocation) — *see* categories T17 and T18 ☑
  foreign body — *see* Foreign body, aspiration
  vomitus (with asphyxia, obstruction respiratory tract, suffocation) T17.81 ☑
Assassination (attempt) — *see* Assault
Assault (homicidal) (by) (in) YØ9
  arson X97 ☑
  bite (of human being) YØ4.1 ☑
  bodily force YØ4.8 ☑
    bite YØ4.1 ☑
    bumping into YØ4.2 ☑
    sexual — *see* subcategories T74.Ø, T76.Ø ☑
    unarmed fight YØ4.Ø ☑
  bomb X96.9 ☑
    antipersonnel X96.Ø ☑
    fertilizer X96.3 ☑
    gasoline X96.1 ☑
    letter X96.2 ☑
    petrol X96.1 ☑
    pipe X96.3 ☑
    specified NEC X96.8 ☑
  brawl (hand) (fists) (foot) (unarmed) YØ4.Ø ☑
  burning, burns (by fire) NEC X97 ☑
    acid YØ8.89 ☑
    caustic, corrosive substance YØ8.89 ☑
    chemical from swallowing caustic, corrosive substance — *see* Table of Drugs and Chemicals

External Causes Index

Assault — Burn, burned, burning

Assault — *continued*
burning, burns — *continued*
cigarette(s) X97 ☑
hot object X98.9 ☑
fluid NEC X98.2 ☑
household appliance X98.3 ☑
specified NEC X98.8 ☑
steam X98.0 ☑
tap water X98.1 ☑
vapors X98.0 ☑
scalding — *see* Assault, burning
steam X98.0 ☑
vitriol Y08.89 ☑
caustic, corrosive substance (gas) Y08.89 ☑
crashing of
aircraft Y08.81 ☑
motor vehicle Y03.8 ☑
pushed in front of Y02.0 ☑
run over Y03.0 ☑
specified NEC Y03.8 ☑
cutting or piercing instrument X99.9 ☑
dagger X99.2 ☑
glass X99.0 ☑
knife X99.1 ☑
specified NEC X99.8 ☑
sword X99.2 ☑
dagger X99.2 ☑
drowning (in) X92.9 ☑
bathtub X92.0 ☑
natural water X92.3 ☑
specified NEC X92.8 ☑
swimming pool X92.1 ☑
following fall X92.2 ☑
dynamite X96.8 ☑
explosive(s) (material) X96.9 ☑
fight (hand) (fists) (foot) (unarmed) Y04.0 ☑
with weapon — *see* Assault, by type of weapon
fire X97 ☑
firearm X95.9 ☑
airgun X95.01 ☑
handgun X93 ☑
hunting rifle X94.1 ☑
larger X94.9 ☑
specified NEC X94.8 ☑
machine gun X94.2 ☑
shotgun X94.0 ☑
specified NEC X95.8 ☑
from high place Y01 ☑
gunshot (wound) NEC — *see* Assault, firearm, by type
incendiary device X97 ☑
injury Y09
to child due to criminal abortion attempt NEC Y08.89 ☑
knife X99.1 ☑
late effect of — *see* categories X92-Y08 with 7th character S
placing before moving object NEC Y02.8 ☑
motor vehicle Y02.0 ☑
poisoning — *see* categories T36-T65 with 7th character S
puncture, any part of body — *see* Assault, cutting or piercing instrument
pushing
before moving object NEC Y02.8 ☑
motor vehicle Y02.0 ☑
subway train Y02.1 ☑
train Y02.1 ☑
from high place Y01 ☑
rape T74.2- ☑
scalding — *see* Assault, burning
sequelae of — *see* categories X92-Y08 with 7th character S
sexual (by bodily force) T74.2- ☑
shooting — *see* Assault, firearm
specified means NEC Y08.89 ☑
stab, any part of body — *see* Assault, cutting or piercing instrument
steam X98.0 ☑
striking against
other person Y04.2 ☑
sports equipment Y08.09 ☑
baseball bat Y08.02 ☑
hockey stick Y08.01 ☑
struck by
sports equipment Y08.09 ☑
baseball bat Y08.02 ☑

Assault — *continued*
struck by — *continued*
sports equipment — *continued*
hockey stick Y08.01 ☑
submersion — *see* Assault, drowning
violence Y09
weapon Y09
blunt Y00 ☑
cutting or piercing — *see* Assault, cutting or piercing instrument
firearm — *see* Assault, firearm
wound Y09
cutting — *see* Assault, cutting or piercing instrument
gunshot — *see* Assault, firearm
knife X99.1 ☑
piercing — *see* Assault, cutting or piercing instrument
puncture — *see* Assault, cutting or piercing instrument
stab — *see* Assault, cutting or piercing instrument
Attack by mammals NEC W55.89 ☑
Avalanche — *see* Landslide
Aviator's disease — *see* Air, pressure

B

Barotitis, barodontalgia, barosinusitis, barotrauma (otitic) (sinus) — *see* Air, pressure
Battered (baby) (child) (person) (syndrome) X58 ☑
Bayonet wound W26.1 ☑
in
legal intervention — *see* Legal, intervention, sharp object, bayonet
war operations — *see* War operations, combat
stated as undetermined whether accidental or intentional Y28.8 ☑
suicide (attempt) X78.2 ☑
Bean in nose — *see* categories T17 and T18
Bed set on fire NEC — *see* Exposure, fire, uncontrolled, building, bed
Beheading (by guillotine)
homicide X99.9 ☑
legal execution — *see* Legal, intervention
Bending, injury in (prolonged) (static) X50.1 ☑
Bends — *see* Air, pressure, change
Bite, bitten by
alligator W58.01 ☑
arthropod (nonvenomous) NEC W57 ☑
bull W55.21 ☑
cat W55.01 ☑
cow W55.21 ☑
crocodile W58.11 ☑
dog W54.0 ☑
goat W55.31 ☑
hoof stock NEC W55.31 ☑
horse W55.11 ☑
human being (accidentally) W50.3 ☑
with intent to injure or kill Y04.1 ☑
as, or caused by, a crowd or human stampede (with fall) W52 ☑
assault Y04.1 ☑
homicide (attempt) Y04.1 ☑
in
fight Y04.1 ☑
insect (nonvenomous) W57 ☑
lizard (nonvenomous) W59.01 ☑
mammal NEC W55.81 ☑
marine W56.31 ☑
marine animal (nonvenomous) W56.81 ☑
millipede W57 ☑
moray eel W56.51 ☑
mouse W53.01 ☑
person(s) (accidentally) W50.3 ☑
with intent to injure or kill Y04.1 ☑
as, or caused by, a crowd or human stampede (with fall) W52 ☑
assault Y04.1 ☑
homicide (attempt) Y04.1 ☑
in
fight Y04.1 ☑
pig W55.41 ☑
raccoon W55.51 ☑
rat W53.11 ☑
reptile W59.81 ☑
lizard W59.01 ☑

Bite, bitten by — *continued*
reptile — *continued*
snake W59.11 ☑
turtle W59.21 ☑
terrestrial W59.81 ☑
rodent W53.81 ☑
mouse W53.01 ☑
rat W53.11 ☑
specified NEC W53.81 ☑
squirrel W53.21 ☑
shark W56.41 ☑
sheep W55.31 ☑
snake (nonvenomous) W59.11 ☑
spider (nonvenomous) W57 ☑
squirrel W53.21 ☑
Blast (air) in war operations — *see* War operations, blast
Blizzard X37.2 ☑
Blood alcohol level Y90.9
less than 20mg/100ml Y90.0
20-39mg/100ml Y90.1
40-59mg/100ml Y90.2
60-79mg/100ml Y90.3
80-99mg/100ml Y90.4
100-119mg/100ml Y90.5
120-199mg/100ml Y90.6
200-239mg/100ml Y90.7
presence in blood, level not specified Y90.9
Blow X58 ☑
by law-enforcing agent, police (on duty) — *see* Legal, intervention, manhandling
blunt object — *see* Legal, intervention, blunt object
Blowing up — *see* Explosion
Brawl (hand) (fists) (foot) Y04.0 ☑
Breakage (accidental) (part of)
ladder (causing fall) W11 ☑
scaffolding (causing fall) W12 ☑
Broken
glass, contact with — *see* Contact, with, glass
power line (causing electric shock) W85 ☑
Bumping against, into (accidentally)
object NEC W22.8 ☑
with fall — *see* Fall, due to, bumping against, object
caused by crowd or human stampede (with fall) W52 ☑
sports equipment W21.9 ☑
person(s) W51 ☑
with fall W03 ☑
due to ice or snow W00.0 ☑
assault Y04.2 ☑
caused by, a crowd or human stampede (with fall) W52 ☑
homicide (attempt) Y04.2 ☑
sports equipment W21.9 ☑
Burn, burned, burning (accidental) (by) (from) (on)
acid NEC — *see* Table of Drugs and Chemicals
bed linen — *see* Exposure, fire, uncontrolled, in building, bed
blowtorch X08.8 ☑
with ignition of clothing NEC X06.2 ☑
nightwear X05 ☑
bonfire, campfire (controlled) (*see also* Exposure, fire, controlled, not in building)
uncontrolled — *see* Exposure, fire, uncontrolled, not in building
candle X08.8 ☑
with ignition of clothing NEC X06.2 ☑
nightwear X05 ☑
caustic liquid, substance (external) (internal) NEC — *see* Table of Drugs and Chemicals
chemical (external) (internal) (*see also* Table of Drugs and Chemicals)
in war operations — *see* War operations, fire
cigar(s) or cigarette(s) X08.8 ☑
with ignition of clothing NEC X06.2 ☑
nightwear X05 ☑
clothes, clothing NEC (from controlled fire) X06.2 ☑
with conflagration — *see* Exposure, fire, uncontrolled, building
not in building or structure — *see* Exposure, fire, uncontrolled, not in building
cooker (hot) X15.8 ☑
stated as undetermined whether accidental or intentional Y27.3 ☑
suicide (attempt) X77.3 ☑
electric blanket X16 ☑

Burn, burned, burning — *continued*
- engine (hot) X17 ☑
- fire, flames — *see* Exposure, fire
- flare, Very pistol — *see* Discharge, firearm NEC
- heat
  - from appliance (electrical) (household) X15.8 ☑
    - cooker X15.8 ☑
    - hotplate X15.2 ☑
    - kettle X15.8 ☑
    - light bulb X15.8 ☑
    - saucepan X15.3 ☑
    - skillet X15.3 ☑
    - stated as undetermined whether accidental or intentional Y27.3 ☑
    - stove X15.0 ☑
    - suicide (attempt) X77.3 ☑
    - toaster X15.1 ☑
  - in local application or packing during medical or surgical procedure Y63.5
- heating
  - appliance, radiator or pipe X16 ☑
- homicide (attempt) — *see* Assault, burning
- hot
  - air X14.1 ☑
  - cooker X15.8 ☑
  - drink X10.0 ☑
  - engine X17 ☑
  - fat X10.2 ☑
  - fluid NEC X12 ☑
  - food X10.1 ☑
  - gases X14.1 ☑
  - heating appliance X16 ☑
  - household appliance NEC X15.8 ☑
  - kettle X15.8 ☑
  - liquid NEC X12 ☑
  - machinery X17 ☑
  - metal (molten) (liquid) NEC X18 ☑
  - object (not producing fire or flames) NEC X19 ☑
  - oil (cooking) X10.2 ☑
  - pipe(s) X16 ☑
  - radiator X16 ☑
  - saucepan (glass) (metal) X15.3 ☑
  - stove (kitchen) X15.0 ☑
  - substance NEC X19 ☑
    - caustic or corrosive NEC — *see* Table of Drugs and Chemicals
  - toaster X15.1 ☑
  - tool X17 ☑
  - vapor X13.1 ☑
  - water (tap) — *see* Contact, with, hot, tap water
- hotplate X15.2 ☑
  - suicide (attempt) X77.3 ☑
- ignition — *see* Ignition
- in war operations — *see* War operations, fire
- inflicted by other person X97 ☑
  - by hot objects, hot vapor, and steam — *see* Assault, burning, hot object
- internal, from swallowed caustic, corrosive liquid, substance — *see* Table of Drugs and Chemicals
- iron (hot) X15.8 ☑
  - stated as undetermined whether accidental or intentional Y27.3 ☑
  - suicide (attempt) X77.3 ☑
- kettle (hot) X15.8 ☑
  - stated as undetermined whether accidental or intentional Y27.3 ☑
  - suicide (attempt) X77.3 ☑
- lamp (flame) X08.8 ☑
  - with ignition of clothing NEC X06.2 ☑
    - nightwear X05 ☑
- lighter (cigar) (cigarette) X08.8 ☑
  - with ignition of clothing NEC X06.2 ☑
    - nightwear X05 ☑
- lightning — *see* subcategory T75.0 ☑
  - causing fire — *see* Exposure, fire
- liquid (boiling) (hot) NEC X12 ☑
  - stated as undetermined whether accidental or intentional Y27.2 ☑
  - suicide (attempt) X77.2 ☑
- local application of externally applied substance in medical or surgical care Y63.5
- machinery (hot) X17 ☑
- matches X08.8 ☑
  - with ignition of clothing NEC X06.2 ☑
    - nightwear X05 ☑

Burn, burned, burning — *continued*
- mattress — *see* Exposure, fire, uncontrolled, building, bed
- medicament, externally applied Y63.5
- metal (hot) (liquid) (molten) NEC X18 ☑
- nightwear (nightclothes, nightdress, gown, pajamas, robe) X05 ☑
- object (hot) NEC X19 ☑
- on board watercraft
  - due to
    - accident to watercraft V91.09 ☑
      - powered craft V91.03 ☑
        - ferry boat V91.01 ☑
        - fishing boat V91.02 ☑
        - jetskis V91.03 ☑
        - liner V91.01 ☑
        - merchant ship V91.00 ☑
        - passenger ship V91.01 ☑
      - unpowered craft V91.08 ☑
        - canoe V91.05 ☑
        - inflatable V91.06 ☑
        - kayak V91.05 ☑
        - sailboat V91.04 ☑
        - surf-board V91.08 ☑
        - water skis V91.07 ☑
        - windsurfer V91.08 ☑
    - fire on board V93.09 ☑
      - ferry boat V93.01 ☑
      - fishing boat V93.02 ☑
      - jetskis V93.03 ☑
      - liner V93.01 ☑
      - merchant ship V93.00 ☑
      - passenger ship V93.01 ☑
      - powered craft NEC V93.03 ☑
      - sailboat V93.04 ☑
    - specified heat source NEC on board V93.19 ☑
      - ferry boat V93.11 ☑
      - fishing boat V93.12 ☑
      - jetskis V93.13 ☑
      - liner V93.11 ☑
      - merchant ship V93.10 ☑
      - passenger ship V93.11 ☑
      - powered craft NEC V93.13 ☑
      - sailboat V93.14 ☑
- pipe (hot) X16 ☑
  - smoking X08.8 ☑
    - with ignition of clothing NEC X06.2 ☑
      - nightwear X05 ☑
- powder — *see* Powder burn
- radiator (hot) X16 ☑
- saucepan (hot) (glass) (metal) X15.3 ☑
  - stated as undetermined whether accidental or intentional Y27.3 ☑
  - suicide (attempt) X77.3 ☑
- self-inflicted X76 ☑
  - stated as undetermined whether accidental or intentional Y26 ☑
- stated as undetermined whether accidental or intentional Y27.0 ☑
- steam X13.1 ☑
  - pipe X16 ☑
    - stated as undetermined whether accidental or intentional Y27.8 ☑
  - stated as undetermined whether accidental or intentional Y27.0 ☑
  - suicide (attempt) X77.0 ☑
- stove (hot) (kitchen) X15.0 ☑
  - stated as undetermined whether accidental or intentional Y27.3 ☑
  - suicide (attempt) X77.3 ☑
- substance (hot) NEC X19 ☑
  - boiling X12 ☑
    - stated as undetermined whether accidental or intentional Y27.2 ☑
    - suicide (attempt) X77.2 ☑
  - molten (metal) X18 ☑
- suicide (attempt) NEC X76 ☑
  - hot
    - household appliance X77.3 ☑
    - object X77.9 ☑
- therapeutic misadventure
  - heat in local application or packing during medical or surgical procedure Y63.5
  - overdose of radiation Y63.2
- toaster (hot) X15.1 ☑

Burn, burned, burning — *continued*
- toaster — *continued*
  - stated as undetermined whether accidental or intentional Y27.3 ☑
  - suicide (attempt) X77.3 ☑
- tool (hot) X17 ☑
- torch, welding X08.8 ☑
  - with ignition of clothing NEC X06.2 ☑
    - nightwear X05 ☑
- trash fire (controlled) — *see* Exposure, fire, controlled, not in building
  - uncontrolled — *see* Exposure, fire, uncontrolled, not in building
- vapor (hot) X13.1 ☑
  - stated as undetermined whether accidental or intentional Y27.0 ☑
  - suicide (attempt) X77.0 ☑
- Very pistol — *see* Discharge, firearm NEC
Butted by animal W55.82 ☑
- bull W55.22 ☑
- cow W55.22 ☑
- goat W55.32 ☑
- horse W55.12 ☑
- pig W55.42 ☑
- sheep W55.32 ☑

C

Caisson disease — *see* Air, pressure, change
Campfire (exposure to) (controlled) (*see also* Exposure, fire, controlled, not in building)
- uncontrolled — *see* Exposure, fire, uncontrolled, not in building
Capital punishment (any means) — *see* Legal, intervention
Car sickness T75.3 ☑
Casualty (not due to war) NEC X58 ☑
- war — *see* War operations
Cat
- bite W55.01 ☑
- scratch W55.03 ☑
Cataclysm, cataclysmic (any injury) NEC — *see* Forces of nature
Catching fire — *see* Exposure, fire
Caught
- between
  - folding object W23.0 ☑
  - objects (moving) (stationary and moving) W23.0 ☑
    - and machinery — *see* Contact, with, by type of machine
    - stationary W23.1 ☑
  - sliding door and door frame W23.0 ☑
- by, in
  - machinery (moving parts of) — *see* Contact, with, by type of machine
  - washing-machine wringer W23.0 ☑
- under packing crate (due to losing grip) W23.1 ☑
Cave-in caused by cataclysmic earth surface movement or eruption — *see* Landslide
Change(s) in air pressure — *see* Air, pressure, change
Choked, choking (on) (any object except food or vomitus)
- food (bone) (seed) — *see* categories T17 and T18 ☑
- vomitus T17.81- ☑
Civil insurrection — *see* War operations
Cloudburst (any injury) X37.8 ☑
Cold, exposure to (accidental) (excessive) (extreme) (natural) (place) NEC — *see* Exposure, cold
Collapse
- building W20.1 ☑
  - burning (uncontrolled fire) X00.2 ☑
- dam or man-made structure (causing earth movement) X36.0 ☑
- machinery — *see* Contact, with, by type of machine
- structure W20.1 ☑
  - burning (uncontrolled fire) X00.2 ☑
Collision (accidental) NEC (*see also* Accident, transport) V89.9 ☑
- pedestrian W51 ☑
  - with fall W03 ☑
    - due to ice or snow W00.0 ☑
    - involving pedestrian conveyance — *see* Accident, transport, pedestrian, conveyance
  - and
    - crowd or human stampede (with fall) W52 ☑
    - object W22.8 ☑

Collision — *continued*
 pedestrian — *continued*
  and — *continued*
   object — *continued*
    with fall — *see* Fall, due to, bumping
      against, object
 person(s) — *see* Collision, pedestrian
 transport vehicle NEC V89.9 ☑
  and
    avalanche, fallen or not moving — *see* Accident,
      transport
     falling or moving — *see* Landslide
    landslide, fallen or not moving — *see* Accident,
      transport
     falling or moving — *see* Landslide
  due to cataclysm — *see* Forces of nature, by type
  intentional, purposeful suicide (attempt) — *see*
    Suicide, collision
Combustion, spontaneous — *see* Ignition
Complication (delayed) **of or following** (medical or
  surgical procedure) Y84.9
 with misadventure — *see* Misadventure
 amputation of limb(s) Y83.5
 anastomosis (arteriovenous) (blood vessel) (gastrojejunal) (tendon) (natural or artificial material)
   Y83.2
 aspiration (of fluid) Y84.4
  tissue Y84.8
 biopsy Y84.8
 blood
  sampling Y84.7
  transfusion
   procedure Y84.8
 bypass Y83.2
 catheterization (urinary) Y84.6
  cardiac Y84.0
 colostomy Y83.3
 cystostomy Y83.3
 dialysis (kidney) Y84.1
 drug — *see* Table of Drugs and Chemicals
 due to misadventure — *see* Misadventure
 duodenostomy Y83.3
 electroshock therapy Y84.3
 external stoma, creation of Y83.3
 formation of external stoma Y83.3
 gastrostomy Y83.3
 graft Y83.2
 hypothermia (medically-induced) Y84.8
 implant, implantation (of)
  artificial
   internal device (cardiac pacemaker) (electrodes
     in brain) (heart valve prosthesis) (ortho-
     pedic) Y83.1
   material or tissue (for anastomosis or bypass)
     Y83.2
    with creation of external stoma Y83.3
  natural tissues (for anastomosis or bypass) Y83.2
   with creation of external stoma Y83.3
 infusion
  procedure Y84.8
 injection — *see* Table of Drugs and Chemicals
  procedure Y84.8
 insertion of gastric or duodenal sound Y84.5
 insulin-shock therapy Y84.3
 paracentesis (abdominal) (thoracic) (aspirative) Y84.4
 procedures other than surgical operation — *see*
   Complication of or following, by type of procedure
 radiological procedure or therapy Y84.2
 removal of organ (partial) (total) NEC Y83.6
 sampling
  blood Y84.7
  fluid NEC Y84.4
  tissue Y84.8
 shock therapy Y84.3
 surgical operation NEC (*see also* Complication of or
   following, by type of operation) Y83.9
  reconstructive NEC Y83.4
   with
    anastomosis, bypass or graft Y83.2
    formation of external stoma Y83.3
  specified NEC Y83.8
 transfusion (*see also* Table of Drugs and Chemicals)
  procedure Y84.8
 transplant, transplantation (heart) (kidney) (liver)
   (whole organ, any) Y83.0
  partial organ Y83.4
 ureterostomy Y83.3

Complication (delayed) **of or following** —
  continued
 vaccination (*see also* Table of Drugs and Chemicals)
  procedure Y84.8
Compression
 divers' squeeze — *see* Air, pressure, change
 trachea by
  food (lodged in esophagus) — *see* categories T17
    and T18 ☑
  vomitus (lodged in esophagus) T17.81- ☑
Conflagration — *see* Exposure, fire, uncontrolled
Constriction (external)
 hair W49.01 ☑
 jewelry W49.04 ☑
 ring W49.04 ☑
 rubber band W49.03 ☑
 specified item NEC W49.09 ☑
 string W49.02 ☑
 thread W49.02 ☑
Contact (accidental)
 with
  abrasive wheel (metalworking) W31.1 ☑
  alligator W58.09 ☑
   bite W58.01 ☑
   crushing W58.03 ☑
   strike W58.02 ☑
  amphibian W62.9 ☑
   frog W62.0 ☑
   toad W62.1 ☑
  animal (nonvenomous) NEC W64 ☑
   marine W56.89 ☑
    bite W56.81 ☑
    dolphin — *see* Contact, with, dolphin
    fish NEC — *see* Contact, with, fish
    mammal — *see* Contact, with, mammal,
      marine
    orca — *see* Contact, with, orca
    sea lion — *see* Contact, with, sea lion
    shark — *see* Contact, with, shark
    strike W56.82 ☑
  animate mechanical force NEC W64 ☑
  arrow W21.89 ☑
   not thrown, projected or falling W45.8 ☑
  arthropods (nonvenomous) W57 ☑
  axe W27.0 ☑
  band-saw (industrial) W31.2 ☑
  bayonet — *see* Bayonet wound
  bee(s) X58 ☑
  bench-saw (industrial) W31.2 ☑
  bird W61.99 ☑
   bite W61.91 ☑
   chicken — *see* Contact, with, chicken
   duck — *see* Contact, with, duck
   goose — *see* Contact, with, goose
   macaw — *see* Contact, with, macaw
   parrot — *see* Contact, with, parrot
   psittacine — *see* Contact, with, psittacine
   strike W61.92 ☑
   turkey — *see* Contact, with, turkey
  blender W29.0 ☑
  boiling water X12 ☑
   stated as undetermined whether accidental or
     intentional Y27.2 ☑
   suicide (attempt) X77.2 ☑
  bore, earth-drilling or mining (land) (seabed)
    W31.0 ☑
  buffalo — *see* Contact, with, hoof stock NEC
  bull W55.29 ☑
   bite W55.21 ☑
   gored W55.22 ☑
   strike W55.22 ☑
  bumper cars W31.81 ☑
  camel — *see* Contact, with, hoof stock NEC
  can
   lid W26.8 ☑
   opener W27.4 ☑
    powered W29.0 ☑
  cat W55.09 ☑
   bite W55.01 ☑
   scratch W55.03 ☑
  caterpillar (venomous) X58 ☑
  centipede (venomous) X58 ☑
  chain
   hoist W24.0 ☑
    agricultural operations W30.89 ☑
   saw W29.3 ☑

Contact — *continued*
 with — *continued*
  chicken W61.39 ☑
   peck W61.33 ☑
   strike W61.32 ☑
  chisel W27.0 ☑
  circular saw W31.2 ☑
  cobra X58 ☑
  combine (harvester) W30.0 ☑
  conveyer belt W24.1 ☑
  cooker (hot) X15.8 ☑
   stated as undetermined whether accidental or
     intentional Y27.3 ☑
   suicide (attempt) X77.3 ☑
  coral X58 ☑
  cotton gin W31.82 ☑
  cow W55.29 ☑
   bite W55.21 ☑
   strike W55.22 ☑
  crane W24.0 ☑
   agricultural operations W30.89 ☑
  crocodile W58.19 ☑
   bite W58.11 ☑
   crushing W58.13 ☑
   strike W58.12 ☑
  dagger W26.1 ☑
   stated as undetermined whether accidental or
     intentional Y28.2 ☑
   suicide (attempt) X78.2 ☑
  dairy equipment W31.82 ☑
  dart W21.89 ☑
   not thrown, projected or falling W45.8 ☑
  deer — *see* Contact, with, hoof stock NEC
  derrick W24.0 ☑
   agricultural operations W30.89 ☑
   hay W30.2 ☑
  dog W54.8 ☑
   bite W54.0 ☑
   strike W54.1 ☑
  dolphin W56.09 ☑
   bite W56.01 ☑
   strike W56.02 ☑
  donkey — *see* Contact, with, hoof stock NEC
  drill (powered) W29.8 ☑
   earth (land) (seabed) W31.0 ☑
   nonpowered W27.8 ☑
  drive belt W24.0 ☑
   agricultural operations W30.89 ☑
  dry ice — *see* Exposure, cold, man-made
  dryer (clothes) (powered) (spin) W29.2 ☑
  duck W61.69 ☑
   bite W61.61 ☑
   strike W61.62 ☑
  earth (-)
   drilling machine (industrial) W31.0 ☑
   scraping machine in stationary use W31.83 ☑
  edge of stiff paper W26.2 ☑
  electric
   beater W29.0 ☑
   blanket X16 ☑
   fan W29.2 ☑
    commercial W31.82 ☑
   knife W29.1 ☑
   mixer W29.0 ☑
  elevator (building) W24.0 ☑
   agricultural operations W30.89 ☑
    grain W30.3 ☑
  engine(s), hot NEC X17 ☑
  excavating machine W31.0 ☑
  farm machine W30.9 ☑
  feces — *see* Contact, with, by type of animal
  fer de lance X58 ☑
  fish W56.59 ☑
   bite W56.51 ☑
   shark — *see* Contact, with, shark
   strike W56.52 ☑
  flying horses W31.81 ☑
  forging (metalworking) machine W31.1 ☑
  fork W27.4 ☑
  forklift (truck) W24.0 ☑
   agricultural operations W30.89 ☑
  frog W62.0 ☑
  garden
   cultivator (powered) W29.3 ☑
    riding W30.89 ☑
   fork W27.1 ☑

Contact — *continued*
  with — *continued*
    gas turbine W31.3 ☑
    Gila monster X58 ☑
    giraffe — *see* Contact, with, hoof stock NEC
    glass (sharp) (broken) W25 ☑
      with subsequent fall W18.02 ☑
      assault X99.0 ☑
      due to fall — *see* Fall, by type
      stated as undetermined whether accidental or
        intentional Y28.0 ☑
      suicide (attempt) X78.0 ☑
    goat W55.39 ☑
      bite W55.31 ☑
      strike W55.32 ☑
    goose W61.59 ☑
      bite W61.51 ☑
      strike W61.52 ☑
    hand
      saw W27.0 ☑
      tool (not powered) NEC W27.8 ☑
        powered W29.8 ☑
    harvester W30.0 ☑
    hay-derrick W30.2 ☑
    heating
      appliance (hot) X16 ☑
      pad (electric) X16 ☑
    heat NEC X19 ☑
      from appliance (electrical) (household) — *see*
        Contact, with, hot, household appliance
      heating appliance X16 ☑
    hedge-trimmer (powered) W29.3 ☑
    hoe W27.1 ☑
    hoist (chain) (shaft) NEC W24.0 ☑
      agricultural W30.89 ☑
    hoof stock NEC W55.39 ☑
      bite W55.31 ☑
      strike W55.32 ☑
    hornet(s) X58 ☑
    horse W55.19 ☑
      bite W55.11 ☑
      strike W55.12 ☑
    hot
      air X14.1 ☑
        inhalation X14.0 ☑
      cooker X15.8 ☑
      drinks X10.0 ☑
      engine X17 ☑
      fats X10.2 ☑
      fluids NEC X12 ☑
        assault X98.2 ☑
        suicide (attempt) X77.2 ☑
        undetermined whether accidental or Inten-
          tional Y27.2 ☑
      food X10.1 ☑
      gases X14.1 ☑
        inhalation X14.0 ☑
      heating appliance X16 ☑
      household appliance X15.8 ☑
        assault X98.3 ☑
        cooker X15.8 ☑
        hotplate X15.2 ☑
        kettle X15.8 ☑
        light bulb X15.8 ☑
        object NEC X19 ☑
          assault X98.8 ☑
          stated as undetermined whether acciden-
            tal or intentional Y27.9 ☑
          suicide (attempt) X77.8 ☑
        saucepan X15.3 ☑
        skillet X15.3 ☑
        stated as undetermined whether accidental
          or intentional Y27.3 ☑
        stove X15.0 ☑
        suicide (attempt) X77.3 ☑
        toaster X15.1 ☑
      kettle X15.8 ☑
      light bulb X15.8 ☑
      liquid NEC (*see also* Burn) X12 ☑
        drinks X10.0 ☑
        stated as undetermined whether accidental
          or intentional Y27.2 ☑
        suicide (attempt) X77.2 ☑
        tap water X11.8 ☑
          stated as undetermined whether acciden-
            tal or intentional Y27.1 ☑

Contact — *continued*
  with — *continued*
    hot — *continued*
      liquid (*see also* Burn) — *continued*
        tap water — *continued*
          suicide (attempt) X77.1 ☑
      machinery X17 ☑
      metal (molten) (liquid) NEC X18 ☑
      object (not producing fire or flames) NEC X19 ☑
      oil (cooking) X10.2 ☑
      pipe X16 ☑
      plate X15.2 ☑
      radiator X16 ☑
      saucepan (glass) (metal) X15.3 ☑
      skillet X15.3 ☑
      stove (kitchen) X15.0 ☑
      substance NEC X19 ☑
      tap-water X11.8 ☑
        assault X98.1 ☑
        heated on stove X12 ☑
          stated as undetermined whether acciden-
            tal or intentional Y27.2 ☑
          suicide (attempt) X77.2 ☑
        in bathtub X11.0 ☑
        running X11.1 ☑
        stated as undetermined whether accidental
          or intentional Y27.1 ☑
        suicide (attempt) X77.1 ☑
      toaster X15.1 ☑
      tool X17 ☑
      vapors X13.1 ☑
        inhalation X13.0 ☑
      water (tap) X11.8 ☑
        boiling X12 ☑
          stated as undetermined whether acciden-
            tal or intentional Y27.2 ☑
          suicide (attempt) X77.2 ☑
        heated on stove X12 ☑
          stated as undetermined whether acciden-
            tal or intentional Y27.2 ☑
          suicide (attempt) X77.2 ☑
        in bathtub X11.0 ☑
        running X11.1 ☑
        stated as undetermined whether accidental
          or intentional Y27.1 ☑
        suicide (attempt) X77.1 ☑
    hotplate X15.2 ☑
    ice-pick W27.4 ☑
    insect (nonvenomous) NEC W57 ☑
    kettle (hot) X15.8 ☑
    knife W26.0 ☑
      assault X99.1 ☑
      electric W29.1 ☑
      stated as undetermined whether accidental or
        intentional Y28.1 ☑
      suicide (attempt) X78.1 ☑
    lathe (metalworking) W31.1 ☑
      turnings W45.8 ☑
      woodworking W31.2 ☑
    lawnmower (powered) (ridden) W28 ☑
      causing electrocution W86.8 ☑
      suicide (attempt) X83.1 ☑
      unpowered W27.1 ☑
    lift, lifting (devices) W24.0 ☑
      agricultural operations W30.89 ☑
      shaft W24.0 ☑
    liquefied gas — *see* Exposure, cold, man-made
    liquid air, hydrogen, nitrogen — *see* Exposure, cold,
      man-made
    lizard (nonvenomous) W59.09 ☑
      bite W59.01 ☑
      strike W59.02 ☑
    llama — *see* Contact, with, hoof stock NEC
    macaw W61.19 ☑
      bite W61.11 ☑
      strike W61.12 ☑
    machine, machinery W31.9 ☑
      abrasive wheel W31.1 ☑
      agricultural including animal-powered
        W30.9 ☑
        combine harvester W30.0 ☑
        grain storage elevator W30.3 ☑
        hay derrick W30.2 ☑
        power take-off device W30.1 ☑
        reaper W30.0 ☑
        specified NEC W30.89 ☑

Contact — *continued*
  with — *continued*
    machine, machinery — *continued*
      agricultural including animal-powered — *con-*
        tinued
        thresher W30.0 ☑
        transport vehicle, stationary W30.81 ☑
      band saw W31.2 ☑
      bench saw W31.2 ☑
      circular saw W31.2 ☑
      commercial NEC W31.82 ☑
      drilling, metal (industrial) W31.1 ☑
      earth-drilling W31.0 ☑
      earthmoving or scraping W31.89 ☑
      excavating W31.89 ☑
      forging machine W31.1 ☑
      gas turbine W31.3 ☑
      hot X17 ☑
      internal combustion engine W31.3 ☑
      land drill W31.0 ☑
      lathe W31.1 ☑
      lifting (devices) W24.0 ☑
      metal drill W31.1 ☑
      metalworking (industrial) W31.1 ☑
      milling, metal W31.1 ☑
      mining W31.0 ☑
      molding W31.2 ☑
      overhead plane W31.2 ☑
      power press, metal W31.1 ☑
      prime mover W31.3 ☑
      printing W31.89 ☑
      radial saw W31.2 ☑
      recreational W31.81 ☑
      roller-coaster W31.81 ☑
      rolling mill, metal W31.1 ☑
      sander W31.2 ☑
      seabed drill W31.0 ☑
      shaft
        hoist W31.0 ☑
        lift W31.0 ☑
      specified NEC W31.89 ☑
      spinning W31.89 ☑
      steam engine W31.3 ☑
      transmission W24.1 ☑
      undercutter W31.0 ☑
      water driven turbine W31.3 ☑
      weaving W31.89 ☑
      woodworking or forming (industrial) W31.2 ☑
    mammal (feces) (urine) W55.89 ☑
      bull — *see* Contact, with, bull
      cat — *see* Contact, with, cat
      cow — *see* Contact, with, cow
      goat — *see* Contact, with, goat
      hoof stock — *see* Contact, with, hoof stock
      horse — *see* Contact, with, horse
      marine W56.39 ☑
        dolphin — *see* Contact, with, dolphin
        orca — *see* Contact, with, orca
        sea lion — *see* Contact, with, sea lion
        specified NEC W56.39 ☑
          bite W56.31 ☑
          strike W56.32 ☑
      pig — *see* Contact, with, pig
      raccoon — *see* Contact, with, raccoon
      rodent — *see* Contact, with, rodent
      sheep — *see* Contact, with, sheep
      specified NEC W55.89 ☑
        bite W55.81 ☑
        strike W55.82 ☑
    marine
      animal W56.89 ☑
        bite W56.81 ☑
        dolphin — *see* Contact, with, dolphin
        fish NEC — *see* Contact, with, fish
        mammal — *see* Contact, with, mammal,
          marine
        orca — *see* Contact, with, orca
        sea lion — *see* Contact, with, sea lion
        shark — *see* Contact, with, shark
        strike W56.82 ☑
    meat
      grinder (domestic) W29.0 ☑
        industrial W31.82 ☑
        nonpowered W27.4 ☑
      slicer (domestic) W29.0 ☑
        industrial W31.82 ☑

Contact — *continued*
  with — *continued*
    merry go round W31.81 ☑
    metal, hot (liquid) (molten) NEC X18 ☑
    millipede W57 ☑
    nail W45.0 ☑
      gun W29.4 ☑
    needle (sewing) W27.3 ☑
      hypodermic W46.0 ☑
        contaminated W46.1 ☑
    object (blunt) NEC
      hot NEC X19 ☑
      legal intervention — *see* Legal, intervention, blunt object
      sharp NEC W45.8 ☑
        inflicted by other person NEC W45.8 ☑
          stated as
            intentional homicide (attempt) — *see* Assault, cutting or piercing instrument
        legal intervention — *see* Legal, intervention, sharp object
        self-inflicted X78.9 ☑
    orca W56.29 ☑
      bite W56.21 ☑
      strike W56.22 ☑
    overhead plane W31.2 ☑
    paper (as sharp object) W26.2 ☑
    paper-cutter W27.5 ☑
    parrot W61.09 ☑
      bite W61.01 ☑
      strike W61.02 ☑
    pig W55.49 ☑
      bite W55.41 ☑
      strike W55.42 ☑
    pipe, hot X16 ☑
    pitchfork W27.1 ☑
    plane (metal) (wood) W27.0 ☑
      overhead W31.2 ☑
    plant thorns, spines, sharp leaves or other mechanisms W60 ☑
    powered
      garden cultivator W29.3 ☑
      household appliance, implement, or machine W29.8 ☑
      saw (industrial) W31.2 ☑
        hand W29.8 ☑
    printing machine W31.89 ☑
    psittacine bird W61.29 ☑
      bite W61.21 ☑
      macaw — *see* Contact, with, macaw
      parrot — *see* Contact, with, parrot
      strike W61.22 ☑
    pulley (block) (transmission) W24.0 ☑
      agricultural operations W30.89 ☑
    raccoon W55.59 ☑
      bite W55.51 ☑
      strike W55.52 ☑
    radial-saw (industrial) W31.2 ☑
    radiator (hot) X16 ☑
    rake W27.1 ☑
    rattlesnake X58 ☑
    reaper W30.0 ☑
    reptile W59.89 ☑
      lizard — *see* Contact, with, lizard
      snake — *see* Contact, with, snake
      specified NEC W59.89 ☑
        bite W59.81 ☑
        crushing W59.83 ☑
        strike W59.82 ☑
      turtle — *see* Contact, with, turtle
    rivet gun (powered) W29.4 ☑
    road scraper — *see* Accident, transport, construction vehicle
    rodent (feces) (urine) W53.89 ☑
      bite W53.81 ☑
      mouse W53.09 ☑
        bite W53.01 ☑
      rat W53.19 ☑
        bite W53.11 ☑
      specified NEC W53.89 ☑
        bite W53.81 ☑
      squirrel W53.29 ☑
        bite W53.21 ☑
    roller coaster W31.81 ☑
    rope NEC W24.0 ☑

Contact — *continued*
  with — *continued*
    rope — *continued*
      agricultural operations W30.89 ☑
    saliva — *see* Contact, with, by type of animal
    sander W29.8 ☑
      industrial W31.2 ☑
    saucepan (hot) (glass) (metal) X15.3 ☑
    saw W27.0 ☑
      band (industrial) W31.2 ☑
      bench (industrial) W31.2 ☑
      chain W29.3 ☑
      hand W27.0 ☑
    sawing machine, metal W31.1 ☑
    scissors W27.2 ☑
    scorpion X58 ☑
    screwdriver W27.0 ☑
      powered W29.8 ☑
    sea
      anemone, cucumber or urchin (spine) X58 ☑
      lion W56.19 ☑
        bite W56.11 ☑
        strike W56.12 ☑
    serpent — *see* Contact, with, snake, by type
    sewing-machine (electric) (powered) W29.2 ☑
      not powered W27.8 ☑
    shaft (hoist) (lift) (transmission) NEC W24.0 ☑
      agricultural W30.89 ☑
    shark W56.49 ☑
      bite W56.41 ☑
      strike W56.42 ☑
    sharp object(s) W26.9 ☑
      specified NEC W26.8 ☑
    shears (hand) W27.2 ☑
      powered (industrial) W31.1 ☑
        domestic W29.2 ☑
    sheep W55.39 ☑
      bite W55.31 ☑
      strike W55.32 ☑
    shovel W27.8 ☑
      steam — *see* Accident, transport, construction vehicle
    snake (nonvenomous) W59.19 ☑
      bite W59.11 ☑
      crushing W59.13 ☑
      strike W59.12 ☑
    spade W27.1 ☑
    spider (venomous) X58 ☑
    spin-drier W29.2 ☑
    spinning machine W31.89 ☑
    splinter W45.8 ☑
    sports equipment W21.9 ☑
    staple gun (powered) W29.8 ☑
    steam X13.1 ☑
      engine W31.3 ☑
      inhalation X13.0 ☑
      pipe X16 ☑
      shovel W31.89 ☑
    stove (hot) (kitchen) X15.0 ☑
    substance, hot NEC X19 ☑
      molten (metal) X18 ☑
    sword W26.1 ☑
      assault X99.2 ☑
      stated as undetermined whether accidental or intentional Y28.2 ☑
      suicide (attempt) X78.2 ☑
    tarantula X58 ☑
    thresher W30.0 ☑
    tin can lid W26.8 ☑
    toad W62.1 ☑
    toaster (hot) X15.1 ☑
    tool W27.8 ☑
      hand (not powered) W27.8 ☑
        auger W27.0 ☑
        axe W27.0 ☑
        can opener W27.4 ☑
        chisel W27.0 ☑
        fork W27.4 ☑
        garden W27.1 ☑
        handsaw W27.0 ☑
        hoe W27.1 ☑
        ice-pick W27.4 ☑
        kitchen utensil W27.4 ☑
        manual
          lawn mower W27.1 ☑
            sewing machine W27.8 ☑

Contact — *continued*
  with — *continued*
    tool — *continued*
      hand — *continued*
        meat grinder W27.4 ☑
        needle (sewing) W27.3 ☑
          hypodermic W46.0 ☑
            contaminated W46.1 ☑
        paper cutter W27.5 ☑
        pitchfork W27.1 ☑
        rake W27.1 ☑
        scissors W27.2 ☑
        screwdriver W27.0 ☑
        specified NEC W27.8 ☑
        workbench W27.0 ☑
      hot X17 ☑
      powered W29.8 ☑
        blender W29.0 ☑
          commercial W31.82 ☑
        can opener W29.0 ☑
          commercial W31.82 ☑
        chainsaw W29.3 ☑
        clothes dryer W29.2 ☑
          commercial W31.82 ☑
        dishwasher W29.2 ☑
          commercial W31.82 ☑
        edger W29.3 ☑
        electric fan W29.2 ☑
          commercial W31.82 ☑
        electric knife W29.1 ☑
        food processor W29.0 ☑
          commercial W31.82 ☑
        garbage disposal W29.0 ☑
          commercial W31.82 ☑
        garden tool W29.3 ☑
        hedge trimmer W29.3 ☑
        ice maker W29.0 ☑
          commercial W31.82 ☑
        kitchen appliance W29.0 ☑
          commercial W31.82 ☑
        lawn mower W28 ☑
        meat grinder W29.0 ☑
          commercial W31.82 ☑
        mixer W29.0 ☑
          commercial W31.82 ☑
        rototiller W29.3 ☑
        sewing machine W29.2 ☑
          commercial W31.82 ☑
        washing machine W29.2 ☑
          commercial W31.82 ☑
    transmission device (belt, cable, chain, gear, pinion, shaft) W24.1 ☑
      agricultural operations W30.89 ☑
    turbine (gas) (water-driven) W31.3 ☑
    turkey W61.49 ☑
      peck W61.43 ☑
      strike W61.42 ☑
    turtle (nonvenomous) W59.29 ☑
      bite W59.21 ☑
      strike W59.22 ☑
      terrestrial W59.89 ☑
        bite W59.81 ☑
        crushing W59.83 ☑
        strike W59.82 ☑
    under-cutter W31.0 ☑
    urine — *see* Contact, with, by type of animal
    vehicle
      agricultural use (transport) — *see* Accident, transport, agricultural vehicle
        not on public highway W30.81 ☑
      industrial use (transport) — *see* Accident, transport, industrial vehicle
        not on public highway W31.83 ☑
      off-road use (transport) — *see* Accident, transport, all-terrain or off-road vehicle
        not on public highway W31.83 ☑
      special construction use (transport) — *see* Accident, transport, construction vehicle
        not on public highway W31.83 ☑
    venomous
      animal X58 ☑
      arthropods X58 ☑
      lizard X58 ☑
      marine animal NEC X58 ☑
      marine plant NEC X58 ☑
      millipedes (tropical) X58 ☑

☑ Additional Character Required — Refer to the Tabular List for Character Selection   ▽ Subterms under main terms may continue to next column or page

Contact — *continued*
  with — *continued*
    venomous — *continued*
      plant(s) X58 ☑
      snake X58 ☑
      spider X58 ☑
      viper X58 ☑
      washing-machine (powered) W29.2 ☑
      wasp X58 ☑
      weaving-machine W31.89 ☑
      winch W24.0 ☑
        agricultural operations W30.89 ☑
      wire NEC W24.0 ☑
        agricultural operations W30.89 ☑
      wood slivers W45.8 ☑
      yellow jacket X58 ☑
      zebra — *see* Contact, with, hoof stock NEC
    pressure X50.9 ☑
    stress X50.9 ☑
Coup de soleil X32 ☑
Crash
  aircraft (in transit) (powered) V95.9 ☑
    balloon V96.01 ☑
    fixed wing NEC (private) V95.21 ☑
      commercial V95.31 ☑
    glider V96.21 ☑
      hang V96.11 ☑
      powered V95.11 ☑
    helicopter V95.01 ☑
    in war operations — *see* War operations, destruction of aircraft
    microlight V95.11 ☑
    nonpowered V96.9 ☑
      specified NEC V96.8 ☑
    powered NEC V95.8 ☑
    stated as
      homicide (attempt) Y08.81 ☑
      suicide (attempt) X83.0 ☑
    ultralight V95.11 ☑
  spacecraft V95.41 ☑
  transport vehicle NEC (*see also* Accident, transport) V89.9 ☑
    homicide (attempt) Y03.8 ☑
    motor NEC (traffic) V89.2 ☑
      homicide (attempt) Y03.8 ☑
    suicide (attempt) — *see* Suicide, collision
Cruelty (mental) (physical) (sexual) X58 ☑
Crushed (accidentally) X58 ☑
  between objects (moving) (stationary and moving) W23.0 ☑
    stationary W23.1 ☑
  by
    alligator W58.03 ☑
    avalanche NEC — *see* Landslide
    cave-in W20.0 ☑
      caused by cataclysmic earth surface movement — *see* Landslide
    crocodile W58.13 ☑
    crowd or human stampede W52 ☑
    falling
      aircraft V97.39 ☑
        in war operations — *see* War operations, destruction of aircraft
      earth, material W20.0 ☑
        caused by cataclysmic earth surface movement — *see* Landslide
      object NEC W20.8 ☑
    landslide NEC — *see* Landslide
    lizard (nonvenomous) W59.09 ☑
    machinery — *see* Contact, with, by type of machine
    reptile NEC W59.89 ☑
    snake (nonvenomous) W59.13 ☑
  in
    machinery — *see* Contact, with, by type of machine
Cut, cutting (any part of body) (accidental) (*see also* Contact, with, by object or machine)
  during medical or surgical treatment as misadventure — *see* Index to Diseases and Injuries, Complications
  homicide (attempt) — *see* Assault, cutting or piercing instrument
  inflicted by other person — *see* Assault, cutting or piercing instrument
  legal
    execution — *see* Legal, intervention

Cut, cutting — *continued*
  legal — *continued*
    intervention — *see* Legal, intervention, sharp object
  machine NEC (*see also* Contact, with, by type of machine) W31.9 ☑
  self-inflicted — *see* Suicide, cutting or piercing instrument
  suicide (attempt) — *see* Suicide, cutting or piercing instrument
Cyclone (any injury) X37.1 ☑

D

Decapitation (accidental circumstances) NEC X58 ☑
  homicide X99.9 ☑
  legal execution — *see* Legal, intervention
Dehydration from lack of water X58 ☑
Deprivation X58 ☑
Derailment (accidental)
  railway (rolling stock) (train) (vehicle) (without antecedent collision) V81.7 ☑
    with antecedent collision — *see* Accident, transport, railway vehicle occupant
  streetcar (without antecedent collision) V82.7 ☑
    with antecedent collision — *see* Accident, transport, streetcar occupant
Descent
  parachute (voluntary) (without accident to aircraft) V97.29 ☑
    due to accident to aircraft — *see* Accident, transport, aircraft
Desertion X58 ☑
Destitution X58 ☑
Disability, late effect or sequela of injury — *see* Sequelae
Discharge (accidental)
  airgun W34.010 ☑
    assault X95.01 ☑
    homicide (attempt) X95.01 ☑
    stated as undetermined whether accidental or intentional Y24.0 ☑
    suicide (attempt) X74.01 ☑
  BB gun — *see* Discharge, airgun
  firearm (accidental) W34.00 ☑
    assault X95.9 ☑
    handgun (pistol) (revolver) W32.0 ☑
      assault X93 ☑
      homicide (attempt) X93 ☑
      legal intervention — *see* Legal, intervention, firearm, handgun
      stated as undetermined whether accidental or intentional Y22 ☑
      suicide (attempt) X72 ☑
    homicide (attempt) X95.9 ☑
    hunting rifle W33.02 ☑
      assault X94.1 ☑
      homicide (attempt) X94.1 ☑
      legal intervention
        injuring
          bystander Y35.032 ☑
          law enforcement personnel Y35.031 ☑
          suspect Y35.033 ☑
      stated as undetermined whether accidental or intentional Y23.1 ☑
      suicide (attempt) X73.1 ☑
    larger W33.00 ☑
      assault X94.9 ☑
      homicide (attempt) X94.9 ☑
      hunting rifle — *see* Discharge, firearm, hunting rifle
      legal intervention — *see* Legal, intervention, firearm by type of firearm
      machine gun — *see* Discharge, firearm, machine gun
      shotgun — *see* Discharge, firearm, shotgun
      specified NEC W33.09 ☑
        assault X94.8 ☑
        homicide (attempt) X94.8 ☑
        legal intervention
          injuring
            bystander Y35.092 ☑
            law enforcement personnel Y35.091 ☑
            suspect Y35.093 ☑

Discharge — *continued*
  firearm — *continued*
    larger — *continued*
      specified — *continued*
        stated as undetermined whether accidental or intentional Y23.8 ☑
        suicide (attempt) X73.8 ☑
      stated as undetermined whether accidental or intentional Y23.9 ☑
      suicide (attempt) X73.9 ☑
    legal intervention
      injuring
        bystander Y35.002 ☑
        law enforcement personnel Y35.001 ☑
        suspect Y35.03 ☑
      using rubber bullet
        injuring
          bystander Y35.042 ☑
          law enforcement personnel Y35.041 ☑
          suspect Y35.043 ☑
    machine gun W33.03 ☑
      assault X94.2 ☑
      homicide (attempt) X94.2 ☑
      legal intervention — *see* Legal, intervention, firearm, machine gun
      stated as undetermined whether accidental or intentional Y23.3 ☑
      suicide (attempt) X73.2 ☑
    pellet gun — *see* Discharge, airgun
    shotgun W33.01 ☑
      assault X94.0 ☑
      homicide (attempt) X94.0 ☑
      legal intervention — *see* Legal, intervention, firearm, specified NEC
      stated as undetermined whether accidental or intentional Y23.0 ☑
      suicide (attempt) X73.0 ☑
    specified NEC W34.09 ☑
      assault X95.8 ☑
      homicide (attempt) X95.8 ☑
      legal intervention — *see* Legal, intervention, firearm, specified NEC
      stated as undetermined whether accidental or intentional Y24.8 ☑
      suicide (attempt) X74.8 ☑
    stated as undetermined whether accidental or intentional Y24.9 ☑
    suicide (attempt) X74.9 ☑
    Very pistol W34.09 ☑
      assault X95.8 ☑
      homicide (attempt) X95.8 ☑
      stated as undetermined whether accidental or intentional Y24.8 ☑
      suicide (attempt) X74.8 ☑
  firework(s) W39 ☑
    stated as undetermined whether accidental or intentional Y25 ☑
  gas-operated gun NEC W34.018 ☑
    airgun — *see* Discharge, airgun
    assault X95.09 ☑
    homicide (attempt) X95.09 ☑
    paintball gun — *see* Discharge, paintball gun
    stated as undetermined whether accidental or intentional Y24.8 ☑
    suicide (attempt) X74.09 ☑
  gun NEC (*see also* Discharge, firearm NEC)
    air — *see* Discharge, airgun
    BB — *see* Discharge, airgun
    for single hand use — *see* Discharge, firearm, handgun
    hand — *see* Discharge, firearm, handgun
    machine — *see* Discharge, firearm, machine gun
    other specified — *see* Discharge, firearm NEC
    paintball — *see* Discharge, paintball gun
    pellet — *see* Discharge, airgun
  handgun — *see* Discharge, firearm, handgun
  machine gun — *see* Discharge, firearm, machine gun
  paintball gun W34.011 ☑
    assault X95.02 ☑
    homicide (attempt) X95.02 ☑
    stated as undetermined whether accidental or intentional Y24.8 ☑
    suicide (attempt) X74.02 ☑
  pistol — *see* Discharge, firearm, handgun
    flare — *see* Discharge, firearm, Very pistol
    pellet — *see* Discharge, airgun

Discharge — *continued*
  pistol — *see* Discharge, firearm, handgun — *contin-ued*
    Very — *see* Discharge, firearm, Very pistol
  revolver — *see* Discharge, firearm, handgun
  rifle (hunting) — *see* Discharge, firearm, hunting rifle
  shotgun — *see* Discharge, firearm, shotgun
  spring-operated gun NEC W34.018 ☑
    assault X95.09 ☑
    homicide (attempt) X95.09 ☑
    stated as undetermined whether accidental or intentional Y24.8 ☑
    suicide (attempt) X74.09 ☑
Disease
  Andes W94.11 ☑
  aviator's — *see* Air, pressure
  range W94.11 ☑
Diver's disease, palsy, paralysis, squeeze — *see* Air, pressure
Diving (into water) — *see* Accident, diving
Dog bite W54.0 ☑
Dragged by transport vehicle NEC (*see also* Accident, transport) V09.9 ☑
Drinking poison (accidental) — *see* Table of Drugs and Chemicals
Dropped (accidentally) **while being carried or supported by other person** W04 ☑
Drowning (accidental) W74 ☑
  assault X92.9 ☑
  due to
    accident (to)
      machinery — *see* Contact, with, by type of machine
      watercraft V90.89 ☑
        burning V90.29 ☑
          powered V90.23 ☑
            fishing boat V90.22 ☑
            jetskis V90.23 ☑
            merchant ship V90.20 ☑
            passenger ship V90.21 ☑
          unpowered V90.28 ☑
            canoe V90.25 ☑
            inflatable V90.26 ☑
            kayak V90.25 ☑
            sailboat V90.24 ☑
            water skis V90.27 ☑
        crushed V90.39 ☑
          powered V90.33 ☑
            fishing boat V90.32 ☑
            jetskis V90.33 ☑
            merchant ship V90.30 ☑
            passenger ship V90.31 ☑
          unpowered V90.38 ☑
            canoe V90.35 ☑
            inflatable V90.36 ☑
            kayak V90.35 ☑
            sailboat V90.34 ☑
            water skis V90.37 ☑
        overturning V90.09 ☑
          powered V90.03 ☑
            fishing boat V90.02 ☑
            jetskis V90.03 ☑
            merchant ship V90.00 ☑
            passenger ship V90.01 ☑
          unpowered V90.08 ☑
            canoe V90.05 ☑
            inflatable V90.06 ☑
            kayak V90.05 ☑
            sailboat V90.04 ☑
        sinking V90.19 ☑
          powered V90.13 ☑
            fishing boat V90.12 ☑
            jetskis V90.13 ☑
            merchant ship V90.10 ☑
            passenger ship V90.11 ☑
          unpowered V90.18 ☑
            canoe V90.15 ☑
            inflatable V90.16 ☑
            kayak V90.15 ☑
            sailboat V90.14 ☑
        specified type NEC V90.89 ☑
          powered V90.83 ☑
            fishing boat V90.82 ☑
            jetskis V90.83 ☑
            merchant ship V90.80 ☑
            passenger ship V90.81 ☑

Drowning — *continued*
  due to — *continued*
    accident — *continued*
      watercraft — *continued*
        specified type — *continued*
          unpowered V90.88 ☑
            canoe V90.85 ☑
            inflatable V90.86 ☑
            kayak V90.85 ☑
            sailboat V90.84 ☑
            water skis V90.87 ☑
  avalanche — *see* Landslide
  cataclysmic
    earth surface movement NEC — *see* Forces of nature, earth movement
    storm — *see* Forces of nature, cataclysmic storm
  cloudburst X37.8 ☑
  cyclone X37.1 ☑
  fall overboard (from) V92.09 ☑
    powered craft V92.03 ☑
      ferry boat V92.01 ☑
      fishing boat V92.02 ☑
      jetskis V92.03 ☑
      liner V92.01 ☑
      merchant ship V92.00 ☑
      passenger ship V92.01 ☑
    resulting from
      accident to watercraft — *see* Drowning, due to, accident to, watercraft
      being washed overboard (from) V92.29 ☑
        powered craft V92.23 ☑
          ferry boat V92.21 ☑
          fishing boat V92.22 ☑
          jetskis V92.23 ☑
          liner V92.21 ☑
          merchant ship V92.20 ☑
          passenger ship V92.21 ☑
        unpowered craft V92.28 ☑
          canoe V92.25 ☑
          inflatable V92.26 ☑
          kayak V92.25 ☑
          sailboat V92.24 ☑
          surf-board V92.28 ☑
          water skis V92.27 ☑
          windsurfer V92.28 ☑
      motion of watercraft V92.19 ☑
        powered craft V92.13 ☑
          ferry boat V92.11 ☑
          fishing boat V92.12 ☑
          jetskis V92.13 ☑
          liner V92.11 ☑
          merchant ship V92.10 ☑
          passenger ship V92.11 ☑
        unpowered craft
          canoe V92.15 ☑
          inflatable V92.16 ☑
          kayak V92.15 ☑
          sailboat V92.14 ☑
    unpowered craft V92.08 ☑
      canoe V92.05 ☑
      inflatable V92.06 ☑
      kayak V92.05 ☑
      sailboat V92.04 ☑
      surf-board V92.08 ☑
      water skis V92.07 ☑
      windsurfer V92.08 ☑
  hurricane X37.0 ☑
  jumping into water from watercraft (involved in accident) (*see also* Drowning, due to, accident to, watercraft)
    without accident to or on watercraft W16.711 ☑
  tidal wave NEC — *see* Forces of nature, tidal wave
  torrential rain X37.8 ☑
  following
    fall
      into
        bathtub W16.211 ☑
        bucket W16.221 ☑
        fountain — *see* Drowning, following, fall, into, water, specified NEC
        quarry — *see* Drowning, following, fall, into, water, specified NEC
        reservoir — *see* Drowning, following, fall, into, water, specified NEC

Drowning — *continued*
  following — *continued*
    fall — *continued*
      into — *continued*
        swimming-pool W16.011 ☑
          stated as undetermined whether accidental or intentional Y21.3 ☑
          striking
            bottom W16.021 ☑
            wall W16.031 ☑
          suicide (attempt) X71.2 ☑
        water NOS W16.41 ☑
          natural (lake) (open sea) (river) (stream) (pond) W16.111 ☑
            striking
              bottom W16.121 ☑
              side W16.131 ☑
          specified NEC W16.311 ☑
            striking
              bottom W16.321 ☑
              wall W16.331 ☑
      overboard NEC — *see* Drowning, due to, fall overboard
    jump or dive
      from boat W16.711 ☑
        striking bottom W16.721 ☑
      into
        fountain — *see* Drowning, following, jump or dive, into, water, specified NEC
        quarry — *see* Drowning, following, jump or dive, into, water, specified NEC
        reservoir — *see* Drowning, following, jump or dive, into, water, specified NEC
        swimming-pool W16.511 ☑
          striking
            bottom W16.521 ☑
            wall W16.531 ☑
          suicide (attempt) X71.2 ☑
        water NOS W16.91 ☑
          natural (lake) (open sea) (river) (stream) (pond) W16.611 ☑
          specified NEC W16.811 ☑
            bottom W16.821 ☑
            striking
              bottom W16.821 ☑
              wall W16.831 ☑
          striking
            bottom W16.821 ☑
            wall W16.831 ☑
          striking bottom W16.621 ☑
  homicide (attempt) X92.9 ☑
  in
    bathtub (accidental) W65 ☑
      assault X92.0 ☑
      following fall W16.211 ☑
        stated as undetermined whether accidental or intentional Y21.1 ☑
      stated as undetermined whether accidental or intentional Y21.0 ☑
      suicide (attempt) X71.0 ☑
    lake — *see* Drowning, in, natural water
    natural water (lake) (open sea) (river) (stream) (pond) W69 ☑
      assault X92.3 ☑
      following
        dive or jump W16.611 ☑
          striking bottom W16.621 ☑
        fall W16.111 ☑
          striking
            bottom W16.121 ☑
            side W16.131 ☑
      stated as undetermined whether accidental or intentional Y21.4 ☑
      suicide (attempt) X71.3 ☑
    quarry — *see* Drowning, in, specified place NEC
    quenching tank — *see* Drowning, in, specified place NEC
    reservoir — *see* Drowning, in, specified place NEC
    river — *see* Drowning, in, natural water
    sea — *see* Drowning, in, natural water
    specified place NEC W73 ☑
      assault X92.8 ☑
      following
        dive or jump W16.811 ☑
          striking
            bottom W16.821 ☑
            wall W16.831 ☑

Drowning — *continued*
  in — *continued*
    specified place — *continued*
      following — *continued*
        fall W16.311 ☑
          striking
            bottom W16.321 ☑
            wall W16.331 ☑
      stated as undetermined whether accidental or
        intentional Y21.8 ☑
      suicide (attempt) X71.8 ☑
  stream — *see* Drowning, in, natural water
  swimming-pool W67 ☑
    assault X92.1 ☑
      following fall X92.2 ☑
    following
      dive or jump W16.511 ☑
        striking
          bottom W16.521 ☑
          wall W16.531 ☑
      fall W16.011 ☑
        striking
          bottom W16.021 ☑
          wall W16.031 ☑
    stated as undetermined whether accidental or
      intentional Y21.2 ☑
      following fall Y21.3 ☑
    suicide (attempt) X71.1 ☑
      following fall X71.2 ☑
  war operations — *see* War operations, restriction
    of airway
  resulting from accident to watercraft — *see* Drowning,
    due to, accident, watercraft
  self-inflicted X71.9 ☑
  stated as undetermined whether accidental or inten-
    tional Y21.9 ☑
  suicide (attempt) X71.9 ☑

E

Earth falling (on) W20.0 ☑
  caused by cataclysmic earth surface movement or
    eruption — *see* Landslide
Earth (surface) **movement NEC** — *see* Forces of nature,
  earth movement
Earthquake (any injury) X34 ☑
Effect(s) (adverse) **of**
  air pressure (any) — *see* Air, pressure
  cold, excessive (exposure to) — *see* Exposure, cold
  heat (excessive) — *see* Heat
  hot place (weather) — *see* Heat
  insolation X30 ☑
  late — *see* Sequelae
  motion — *see* Motion
  nuclear explosion or weapon in war operations — *see*
    War operations, nuclear weapon
  radiation — *see* Radiation
  travel — *see* Travel
Electric shock (accidental) (by) (in) — *see* Exposure,
  electric current
Electrocution (accidental) — *see* Exposure, electric current
Endotracheal tube wrongly placed during anesthetic
  procedure
Entanglement
  in
    bed linen, causing suffocation T71 ☑
    wheel of pedal cycle V19.88 ☑
Entry of foreign body or material — *see* Foreign body
Environmental pollution related condition — *see*
  category Z57 ☑
Execution, legal (any method) — *see* Legal, intervention
Exhaustion
  cold — *see* Exposure, cold
  due to excessive exertion (*see also* Overexertion)
    X50.9 ☑
  heat — *see* Heat
Explosion (accidental) (of) (with secondary fire) W40.9 ☑
  acetylene W40.1 ☑
  aerosol can W36.1 ☑
  air tank (compressed) (in machinery) W36.2 ☑
  aircraft (in transit) (powered) NEC V95.9 ☑
    balloon V96.05 ☑
    fixed wing NEC (private) V95.25 ☑
      commercial V95.35 ☑
    glider V96.25 ☑

Explosion — *continued*
  aircraft — *continued*
    glider — *continued*
      hang V96.15 ☑
      powered V95.15 ☑
    helicopter V95.05 ☑
    in war operations — *see* War operations, destruc-
      tion of aircraft
    microlight V95.15 ☑
    nonpowered V96.9 ☑
      specified NEC V96.8 ☑
    powered NEC V95.8 ☑
    stated as
      homicide (attempt) Y03.8 ☑
      suicide (attempt) X83.0 ☑
    ultralight V95.15 ☑
  anesthetic gas in operating room W40.1 ☑
  antipersonnel bomb W40.8 ☑
    assault X96.0 ☑
    homicide (attempt) X96.0 ☑
    suicide (attempt) X75 ☑
  assault X96.9 ☑
  bicycle tire W37.0 ☑
  blasting (cap) (materials) W40.0 ☑
  boiler (machinery), not on transport vehicle W35 ☑
    on watercraft — *see* Explosion, in, watercraft
  butane W40.1 ☑
  caused by other person X96.9 ☑
  coal gas W40.1 ☑
  detonator W40.0 ☑
  dump (munitions) W40.8 ☑
  dynamite W40.0 ☑
    in
      assault X96.8 ☑
      homicide (attempt) X96.8 ☑
      legal intervention
        injuring
          bystander Y35.112 ☑
          law enforcement personnel Y35.111 ☑
          suspect Y35.113 ☑
      suicide (attempt) X75 ☑
  explosive (material) W40.9 ☑
    gas W40.1 ☑
    in blasting operation W40.0 ☑
    specified NEC W40.8 ☑
      in
        assault X96.8 ☑
        homicide (attempt) X96.8 ☑
        legal intervention
          injuring
            bystander Y35.192 ☑
            law enforcement personnel
              Y35.191 ☑
            suspect Y35.193 ☑
        suicide (attempt) X75 ☑
  factory (munitions) W40.8 ☑
  fertilizer bomb W40.8 ☑
    assault X96.3 ☑
    homicide (attempt) X96.3 ☑
    suicide (attempt) X75 ☑
  firearm (parts) NEC W34.19 ☑
    airgun W34.110 ☑
    BB gun W34.110 ☑
    gas, air or spring-operated gun NEC W34.118 ☑
    hangun W32.1 ☑
    hunting rifle W33.12 ☑
    larger firearm W33.10 ☑
      specified NEC W33.19 ☑
    machine gun W33.13 ☑
    paintball gun W34.111 ☑
    pellet gun W34.110 ☑
    shotgun W33.11 ☑
    Very pistol [flare] W34.19 ☑
  fire-damp W40.1 ☑
  fireworks W39 ☑
  gas (coal) (explosive) W40.1 ☑
    cylinder W36.9 ☑
      aerosol can W36.1 ☑
      air tank W36.2 ☑
      pressurized W36.3 ☑
      specified NEC W36.8 ☑
  gasoline (fumes) (tank) not in moving motor vehicle
    W40.1 ☑
    bomb W40.8 ☑
      assault X96.1 ☑
      homicide (attempt) X96.1 ☑

Explosion — *continued*
  gasoline not in moving motor vehicle — *continued*
    bomb — *continued*
      suicide (attempt) X75 ☑
    in motor vehicle — *see* Accident, transport, by type
      of vehicle
  grain store W40.8 ☑
  grenade W40.8 ☑
    in
      assault X96.8 ☑
      homicide (attempt) X96.8 ☑
      legal intervention
        injuring
          bystander Y35.192 ☑
          law enforcement personnel Y35.191 ☑
          suspect Y35.193 ☑
      suicide (attempt) X75 ☑
  handgun (parts) — *see* Explosion, firearm, hangun
    (parts)
  homicide (attempt) X96.9 ☑
    antipersonnel bomb — *see* Explosion, antiperson-
      nel bomb
    fertilizer bomb — *see* Explosion, fertilizer bomb
    gasoline bomb — *see* Explosion, gasoline bomb
    letter bomb — *see* Explosion, letter bomb
    pipe bomb — *see* Explosion, pipe bomb
    specified NEC X96.8 ☑
  hose, pressurized W37.8 ☑
  hot water heater, tank (in machinery) W35 ☑
    on watercraft — *see* Explosion, in, watercraft
  in, on
    dump W40.8 ☑
    factory W40.8 ☑
    mine (of explosive gases) NEC W40.1 ☑
    watercraft V93.59 ☑
      powered craft V93.53 ☑
        ferry boat V93.51 ☑
        fishing boat V93.52 ☑
        jetskis V93.53 ☑
        liner V93.51 ☑
        merchant ship V93.50 ☑
        passenger ship V93.51 ☑
        sailboat V93.54 ☑
  letter bomb W40.8 ☑
    assault X96.2 ☑
    homicide (attempt) X96.2 ☑
    suicide (attempt) X75 ☑
  machinery (*see also* Contact, with, by type of machine)
    on board watercraft — *see* Explosion, in, watercraft
    pressure vessel — *see* Explosion, by type of vessel
  methane W40.1 ☑
  mine W40.1 ☑
  missile NEC W40.8 ☑
  mortar bomb W40.8 ☑
    in
      assault X96.8 ☑
      homicide (attempt) X96.8 ☑
      legal intervention
        injuring
          bystander Y35.192 ☑
          law enforcement personnel Y35.191 ☑
          suspect Y35.193 ☑
      suicide (attempt) X75 ☑
  munitions (dump) (factory) W40.8 ☑
  pipe, pressurized W37.8 ☑
    bomb W40.8 ☑
      assault X96.4 ☑
      homicide (attempt) X96.4 ☑
      suicide (attempt) X75 ☑
  pressure, pressurized
    cooker W38 ☑
    gas tank (in machinery) W36.3 ☑
    hose W37.8 ☑
    pipe W37.8 ☑
    specified device NEC W38 ☑
    tire W37.8 ☑
      bicycle W37.0 ☑
    vessel (in machinery) W38 ☑
  propane W40.1 ☑
  self-inflicted X75 ☑
  shell (artillery) NEC W40.8 ☑
    during war operations — *see* War operations, ex-
      plosion

Explosion — continued
- shell — continued
  - in
    - legal intervention
      - injuring
        - bystander Y35.122 ☑
        - law enforcement personnel Y35.121 ☑
        - suspect Y35.123 ☑
    - war — see War operations, explosion
- spacecraft V95.45 ☑
- stated as undetermined whether accidental or intentional Y25 ☑
- steam or water lines (in machinery) W37.8 ☑
- stove W40.9 ☑
- suicide (attempt) X75 ☑
- tire, pressurized W37.8 ☑
  - bicycle W37.0 ☑
- undetermined whether accidental or intentional Y25 ☑
- vehicle tire NEC W37.8 ☑
  - bicycle W37.0 ☑
- war operations — see War operations, explosion

Exposure (to) X58 ☑
- air pressure change — see Air, pressure
- cold (accidental) (excessive) (extreme) (natural) (place) X31 ☑
  - assault Y08.89 ☑
  - due to
    - man-made conditions W93.8 ☑
      - dry ice (contact) W93.01 ☑
        - inhalation W93.02 ☑
      - liquid air (contact) (hydrogen) (nitrogen) W93.11 ☑
        - inhalation W93.12 ☑
      - refrigeration unit (deep freeze) W93.2 ☑
    - suicide (attempt) X83.2 ☑
    - weather (conditions) X31 ☑
  - homicide (attempt) Y08.89 ☑
  - self-inflicted X83.2 ☑
- due to abandonment or neglect X58 ☑
- electric current W86.8 ☑
  - appliance (faulty) W86.8 ☑
    - domestic W86.0 ☑
  - caused by other person Y08.89 ☑
  - conductor (faulty) W86.1 ☑
  - control apparatus (faulty) W86.1 ☑
  - electric power generating plant, distribution station W86.1 ☑
  - electroshock gun — see Exposure, electric current, taser
  - high-voltage cable W85 ☑
  - homicide (attempt) Y08.89 ☑
  - legal execution — see Legal, intervention, specified means NEC
  - lightning — see subcategory T75.0 ☑
  - live rail W86.8 ☑
  - misadventure in medical or surgical procedure in electroshock therapy Y63.4
  - motor (electric) (faulty) W86.8 ☑
    - domestic W86.0 ☑
  - self-inflicted X83.1 ☑
  - specified NEC W86.8 ☑
    - domestic W86.0 ☑
  - stun gun — see Exposure, electric current, taser
  - suicide (attempt) X83.1 ☑
  - taser W86.8 ☑
    - assault Y08.89 ☑
    - legal intervention — see category Y35 ☑
    - self-harm (intentional) X83.8 ☑
    - undetermined intent Y33 ☑
  - third rail W86.8 ☑
  - transformer (faulty) W86.1 ☑
  - transmission lines W85 ☑
- environmental tobacco smoke X58 ☑
- excessive
  - cold — see Exposure, cold
  - heat (natural) NEC X30 ☑
    - man-made W92 ☑
- factor(s) NOS X58 ☑
  - environmental NEC X58 ☑
  - man-made NEC W99 ☑
  - natural NEC — see Forces of nature
  - specified NEC X58 ☑
- fire, flames (accidental) X08.8 ☑
  - assault X97 ☑

Exposure — continued
- fire, flames — continued
  - campfire — see Exposure, fire, controlled, not in building
  - controlled (in)
    - with ignition (of) clothing (see also Ignition, clothes) X06.2 ☑
      - nightwear X05 ☑
    - bonfire — see Exposure, fire, controlled, not in building
    - brazier (in building or structure) (see also Exposure, fire, controlled, building)
      - not in building or structure — see Exposure, fire, controlled, not in building
    - building or structure X02.0 ☑
      - with
        - fall from building X02.3 ☑
        - from building X02.5 ☑
        - injury due to building collapse X02.2 ☑
        - smoke inhalation X02.1 ☑
      - hit by object from building X02.4 ☑
      - specified mode of injury NEC X02.8 ☑
    - fireplace, furnace or stove — see Exposure, fire, controlled, building
    - not in building or structure X03.0 ☑
      - with
        - fall X03.3 ☑
        - smoke inhalation X03.1 ☑
      - hit by object X03.4 ☑
      - specified mode of injury NEC X03.8 ☑
    - trash — see Exposure, fire, controlled, not in building
  - fireplace — see Exposure, fire, controlled, building
  - fittings or furniture (in building or structure) (uncontrolled) — see Exposure, fire, uncontrolled, building
  - forest (uncontrolled) — see Exposure, fire, uncontrolled, not in building
  - grass (uncontrolled) — see Exposure, fire, uncontrolled, not in building
  - hay (uncontrolled) — see Exposure, fire, uncontrolled, not in building
  - homicide (attempt) X97 ☑
  - ignition of highly flammable material X04 ☑
  - in, of, on, starting in
    - machinery — see Contact, with, by type of machine
    - motor vehicle (in motion) (see also Accident, transport, occupant by type of vehicle) V87.8 ☑
      - with collision — see Collision
    - railway rolling stock, train, vehicle V81.81 ☑
      - with collision — see Accident, transport, railway vehicle occupant
    - street car (in motion) V82.8 ☑
      - with collision — see Accident, transport, streetcar occupant
    - transport vehicle NEC (see also Accident, transport)
      - with collision — see Collision
    - war operations (see also War operations, fire)
      - from nuclear explosion — see War operations, nuclear weapons
    - watercraft (in transit) (not in transit) V91.09 ☑
      - localized — see Burn, on board watercraft, due to, fire on board
      - powered craft V91.03 ☑
        - ferry boat V91.01 ☑
        - fishing boat V91.02 ☑
        - jet skis V91.03 ☑
        - liner V91.01 ☑
        - merchant ship V91.00 ☑
        - passenger ship V91.01 ☑
      - unpowered craft V91.08 ☑
        - canoe V91.05 ☑
        - inflatable V91.06 ☑
        - kayak V91.05 ☑
        - sailboat V91.04 ☑
        - surf-board V91.08 ☑
        - waterskis V91.07 ☑
        - windsurfer V91.08 ☑
  - lumber (uncontrolled) — see Exposure, fire, uncontrolled, not in building
  - mine (uncontrolled) — see Exposure, fire, uncontrolled, not in building
  - prairie (uncontrolled) — see Exposure, fire, uncontrolled, not in building

Exposure — continued
- fire, flames — continued
  - resulting from
    - explosion — see Explosion
    - lightning X08.8 ☑
  - self-inflicted X76 ☑
  - specified NEC X08.8 ☑
  - started by other person X97 ☑
  - stated as undetermined whether accidental or intentional Y26 ☑
  - stove — see Exposure, fire, controlled, building
  - suicide (attempt) X76 ☑
  - tunnel (uncontrolled) — see Exposure, fire, uncontrolled, not in building
  - uncontrolled
    - in building or structure X00.0 ☑
      - with
        - fall from building X00.3 ☑
        - injury due to building collapse X00.2 ☑
        - jump from building X00.5 ☑
        - smoke inhalation X00.1 ☑
      - bed X08.00 ☑
        - due to
          - cigarette X08.01 ☑
          - specified material NEC X08.09 ☑
      - furniture NEC X08.20 ☑
        - due to
          - cigarette X08.21 ☑
          - specified material NEC X08.29 ☑
      - hit by object from building X00.4 ☑
      - sofa X08.10 ☑
        - due to
          - cigarette X08.11 ☑
          - specified material NEC X08.19 ☑
      - specified mode of injury NEC X00.8 ☑
    - not in building or structure (any) X01.0 ☑
      - with
        - fall X01.3 ☑
        - smoke inhalation X01.1 ☑
      - hit by object X01.4 ☑
      - specified mode of injury NEC X01.8 ☑
  - undetermined whether accidental or intentional Y26 ☑
- forces of nature NEC — see Forces of nature
- G-forces (abnormal) W49.9 ☑
- gravitational forces (abnormal) W49.9 ☑
- heat (natural) NEC — see Heat
- high-pressure jet (hydraulic) (pneumatic) W49.9 ☑
- hydraulic jet W49.9 ☑
- inanimate mechanical force W49.9 ☑
- jet, high-pressure (hydraulic) (pneumatic) W49.9 ☑
- lightning — see subcategory T75.0 ☑
  - causing fire — see Exposure, fire
- mechanical forces NEC W49.9 ☑
  - animate NEC W64
  - inanimate NEC W49.9 ☑
- noise W42.9 ☑
  - supersonic W42.0 ☑
- noxious substance — see Table of Drugs and Chemicals
- pneumatic jet W49.9 ☑
- prolonged in deep-freeze unit or refrigerator W93.2 ☑
- radiation — see Radiation
- smoke (see also Exposure, fire)
  - tobacco, second hand Z77.22
- specified factors NEC X58 ☑
- sunlight X32 ☑
  - man-made (sun lamp) W89.8 ☑
    - tanning bed W89.1 ☑
- supersonic waves W42.0 ☑
- transmission line(s), electric W85 ☑
- vibration W49.9 ☑
- waves
  - infrasound W49.9 ☑
  - sound W42.9 ☑
  - supersonic W42.0 ☑
- weather NEC — see Forces of nature

External cause status Y99.9
- child assisting in compensated work for family Y99.8
- civilian activity done for financial or other compensation Y99.0
- civilian activity done for income or pay Y99.0
- family member assisting in compensated work for other family member Y99.8
- hobby not done for income Y99.8
- leisure activity Y99.8

☑ Additional Character Required — Refer to the Tabular List for Character Selection   ▽ Subterms under main terms may continue to next column or page

External cause status — *continued*
  military activity Y99.1
  off-duty activity of military personnel Y99.8
  recreation or sport not for income or while a student
    Y99.8
  specified NEC Y99.8
  student activity Y99.8
  volunteer activity Y99.2

F

Factors, supplemental
  alcohol
    blood level
      less than 20mg/100ml Y90.0
      20-39mg/100ml Y90.1
      40-59mg/100ml Y90.2
      60-79mg/100ml Y90.3
      80-99mg/100ml Y90.4
      100-119mg/100ml Y90.5
      120-199mg/100ml Y90.6
      200-239mg/100ml Y90.7
      240mg/100ml or more Y90.8
      presence in blood, level not specified Y90.9
    presence in blood, but level not specified Y90.9
  environmental-pollution-related condition- see Z57 ☑
  nosocomial condition Y95
  work-related condition Y99.0
Failure
  in suture or ligature during surgical procedure Y65.2
  mechanical, of instrument or apparatus (any) (during
    any medical or surgical procedure) Y65.8
  sterile precautions (during medical and surgical care)
    — *see* Misadventure, failure, sterile precautions,
    by type of procedure
  to
    introduce tube or instrument Y65.4
      endotracheal tube during anesthesia Y65.3
    make curve (transport vehicle) NEC — *see* Accident,
      transport
    remove tube or instrument Y65.4
Fall, falling (accidental) W19 ☑
  building W20.1 ☑
    burning (uncontrolled fire) X00.3 ☑
  down
    embankment W17.81 ☑
    escalator W10.0 ☑
    hill W17.81 ☑
    ladder W11 ☑
    ramp W10.2 ☑
    stairs, steps W10.9 ☑
  due to
    bumping against
      object W18.00 ☑
        sharp glass W18.02 ☑
        specified NEC W18.09 ☑
        sports equipment W18.01 ☑
      person W03 ☑
        due to ice or snow W00.0 ☑
        on pedestrian conveyance — *see* Accident,
          transport, pedestrian, conveyance
    collision with another person W03 ☑
      due to ice or snow W00.0 ☑
      involving pedestrian conveyance — *see* Acci-
        dent, transport, pedestrian, conveyance
    grocery cart tipping over W17.82 ☑
    ice or snow W00.9 ☑
      from one level to another W00.2 ☑
      on stairs or steps W00.1 ☑
      involving pedestrian conveyance — *see* Acci-
        dent, transport, pedestrian, conveyance
      on same level W00.0 ☑
    slipping (on moving sidewalk) W01.0 ☑
      with subsequent striking against object
        W01.10 ☑
        furniture W01.190 ☑
        sharp object W01.119 ☑
          glass W01.110 ☑
          power tool or machine W01.111 ☑
          specified NEC W01.118 ☑
        specified NEC W01.198 ☑
    striking against
      object W18.00 ☑
        sharp glass W18.02 ☑
        specified NEC W18.09 ☑
        sports equipment W18.01 ☑
      person W03 ☑

Fall, falling — *continued*
  due to — *continued*
    striking against — *continued*
      person — *continued*
        due to ice or snow W00.0 ☑
        on pedestrian conveyance — *see* Accident,
          transport, pedestrian, conveyance
  earth (with asphyxia or suffocation (by pressure)) —
    see Earth, falling
  from, off, out of
    aircraft NEC (with accident to aircraft NEC) V97.0 ☑
      while boarding or alighting V97.1 ☑
    balcony W13.0 ☑
    bed W06 ☑
    boat, ship, watercraft NEC (with drowning or sub-
      mersion) — *see* Drowning, due to, fall over-
      board
      with hitting bottom or object V94.0 ☑
    bridge W13.1 ☑
    building W13.9 ☑
      burning (uncontrolled fire) X00.3 ☑
    cavity W17.2 ☑
    chair W07 ☑
    cherry picker W17.89 ☑
    cliff W15 ☑
    dock W17.4 ☑
    embankment W17.81 ☑
    escalator W10.0 ☑
    flagpole W13.8 ☑
    furniture NEC W08 ☑
    grocery cart W17.82 ☑
    haystack W17.89 ☑
    high place NEC W17.89 ☑
      stated as undetermined whether accidental or
        intentional Y30 ☑
    hole W17.2 ☑
    incline W10.2 ☑
    ladder W11 ☑
    lifting device W17.89 ☑
    machine, machinery (*see also* Contact, with, by
      type of machine)
      not in operation W17.89 ☑
    manhole W17.1 ☑
    mobile elevated work platform [MEWP] W17.89 ☑
    motorized mobility scooter W05.2 ☑
    one level to another NEC W17.89 ☑
      intentional, purposeful, suicide (attempt)
        X80 ☑
      stated as undetermined whether accidental or
        intentional Y30 ☑
    pit W17.2 ☑
    playground equipment W09.8 ☑
      jungle gym W09.2 ☑
      slide W09.0 ☑
      swing W09.1 ☑
    quarry W17.89 ☑
    railing W13.9 ☑
    ramp W10.2 ☑
    roof W13.2 ☑
    scaffolding W12 ☑
    scooter (nonmotorized) W05.1 ☑
      motorized mobility W05.2 ☑
    sky lift W17.89 ☑
    stairs, steps W10.9 ☑
      curb W10.1 ☑
      due to ice or snow W00.1 ☑
      escalator W10.0 ☑
      incline W10.2 ☑
      ramp W10.2 ☑
      sidewalk curb W10.1 ☑
      specified NEC W10.8 ☑
    stepladder W11 ☑
    storm drain W17.1 ☑
    streetcar W82.6 ☑
      with antecedent collision — *see* Accident,
        transport, streetcar occupant
      while boarding or alighting V82.4 ☑
    structure NEC W13.8 ☑
      burning (uncontrolled fire) X00.3 ☑
    table W08 ☑
    toilet W18.11 ☑
      with subsequent striking against object
        W18.12 ☑
    train NEC V81.6 ☑
      during derailment (without antecedent colli-
        sion) V81.7 ☑

Fall, falling — *continued*
  from, off, out of — *continued*
    train — *continued*
      during derailment — *continued*
        with antecedent collision — *see* Accident,
          transport, railway vehicle occupant
      while boarding or alighting V81.4 ☑
    transport vehicle after collision — *see* Accident,
      transport, by type of vehicle, collision
    tree W14 ☑
    vehicle (in motion) NEC (*see also* Accident, trans-
      port) V89.9 ☑
      motor NEC (*see also* Accident, transport, occu-
        pant, by type of vehicle) V87.8 ☑
      stationary W17.89 ☑
        while boarding or alighting — *see* Accident,
          transport, by type of vehicle, while
          boarding or alighting
    viaduct W13.8 ☑
    wall W13.8 ☑
    watercraft (*see also* Drowning, due to, fall over-
      board)
      with hitting bottom or object V94.0 ☑
    well W17.0 ☑
    wheelchair, non-moving W05.0 ☑
      powered — *see* Accident, transport, pedestrian,
        conveyance occupant, specified type NEC
    window W13.4 ☑
  in, on
    aircraft NEC V97.0 ☑
      with accident to aircraft V97.0 ☑
      while boarding or alighting V97.1 ☑
    bathtub (empty) W18.2 ☑
      filled W16.212 ☑
        causing drowning W16.211 ☑
    escalator W10.0 ☑
    incline W10.2 ☑
    ladder W11 ☑
    machine, machinery — *see* Contact, with, by type
      of machine
    object, edged, pointed or sharp (with cut) — *see*
      Fall, by type
    playground equipment W09.8 ☑
      jungle gym W09.2 ☑
      slide W09.0 ☑
      swing W09.1 ☑
    ramp W10.2 ☑
    scaffolding W12 ☑
    shower W18.2 ☑
      causing drowning W16.211 ☑
    staircase, stairs, steps W10.9 ☑
      curb W10.1 ☑
      due to ice or snow W00.1 ☑
      escalator W10.0 ☑
      incline W10.2 ☑
      specified NEC W10.8 ☑
    streetcar (without antecedent collision) V82.5 ☑
      with antecedent collision — *see* Accident,
        transport, streetcar occupant
      while boarding or alighting V82.4 ☑
    train (without antecedent collision) V81.5 ☑
      with antecedent collision — *see* Accident,
        transport, railway vehicle occupant
      during derailment (without antecedent colli-
        sion) V81.7 ☑
        with antecedent collision — *see* Accident,
          transport, railway vehicle occupant
      while boarding or alighting V81.4 ☑
    transport vehicle after collision — *see* Accident,
      transport, by type of vehicle, collision
    watercraft V93.39 ☑
      due to
        accident to craft V91.29 ☑
          powered craft V91.23 ☑
            ferry boat V91.21 ☑
            fishing boat V91.22 ☑
            jetskis V91.23 ☑
            liner V91.21 ☑
            merchant ship V91.20 ☑
            passenger ship V91.21 ☑
          unpowered craft
            canoe V91.25 ☑
            inflatable V91.26 ☑
            kayak V91.25 ☑
            sailboat V91.24 ☑
      powered craft V93.33 ☑

Fall, falling — *continued*
in, on — *continued*
watercraft — *continued*
powered craft — *continued*
ferry boat V93.31 ☑
fishing boat V93.32 ☑
jetskis V93.33 ☑
liner V93.31 ☑
merchant ship V93.30 ☑
passenger ship V93.31 ☑
unpowered craft V93.38 ☑
canoe V93.35 ☑
inflatable V93.36 ☑
kayak V93.35 ☑
sailboat V93.34 ☑
surf-board V93.38 ☑
windsurfer V93.38 ☑
into
cavity W17.2 ☑
dock W17.4 ☑
fire — *see* Exposure, fire, by type
haystack W17.89 ☑
hole W17.2 ☑
lake — *see* Fall, into, water
manhole W17.1 ☑
moving part of machinery — *see* Contact, with, by
type of machine
ocean — *see* Fall, into, water
opening in surface NEC W17.89 ☑
pit W17.2 ☑
pond — *see* Fall, into, water
quarry W17.89 ☑
river — *see* Fall, into, water
shaft W17.89 ☑
storm drain W17.1 ☑
stream — *see* Fall, into, water
swimming pool (*see also* Fall, into, water, in,
swimming pool)
empty W17.3 ☑
tank W17.89 ☑
water W16.42 ☑
causing drowning W16.41 ☑
from watercraft — *see* Drowning, due to, fall
overboard
hitting diving board W21.4 ☑
in
bathtub W16.212 ☑
causing drowning W16.211 ☑
bucket W16.222 ☑
causing drowning W16.221 ☑
natural body of water W16.112 ☑
causing drowning W16.111 ☑
striking
bottom W16.122 ☑
causing drowning W16.121 ☑
side W16.132 ☑
causing drowning W16.131 ☑
specified water NEC W16.312 ☑
causing drowning W16.311 ☑
striking
bottom W16.322 ☑
causing drowning W16.321 ☑
wall W16.332 ☑
causing drowning W16.331 ☑
swimming pool W16.012 ☑
causing drowning W16.011 ☑
striking
bottom W16.022 ☑
causing drowning W16.031 ☑
wall W16.032 ☑
causing drowning W16.021 ☑
utility bucket W16.222 ☑
causing drowning W16.221 ☑
well W17.0 ☑
involving
bed W06 ☑
chair W07 ☑
furniture NEC W08 ☑
glass — *see* Fall, by type
playground equipment W09.8 ☑
jungle gym W09.2 ☑
slide W09.0 ☑
swing W09.1 ☑
roller blades — *see* Accident, transport, pedestrian,
conveyance

Fall, falling — *continued*
involving — *continued*
skateboard(s) — *see* Accident, transport, pedestrian, conveyance
skates (ice) (in line) (roller) — *see* Accident, transport, pedestrian, conveyance
skis — *see* Accident, transport, pedestrian, conveyance
table W08 ☑
wheelchair, non-moving W05.0 ☑
powered — *see* Accident, transport, pedestrian, conveyance, specified type NEC
object — *see* Struck by, object, falling
off
toilet W18.11 ☑
with subsequent striking against object W18.12 ☑
on same level W18.30 ☑
due to
specified NEC W18.39 ☑
stepping on an object W18.31 ☑
out of
bed W06 ☑
building NEC W13.8 ☑
chair W07 ☑
furniture NEC W08 ☑
wheelchair, non-moving W05.0 ☑
powered — *see* Accident, transport, pedestrian, conveyance, specified type NEC
window W13.4 ☑
over
animal W01.0 ☑
cliff W15 ☑
embankment W17.81 ☑
small object W01.0 ☑
rock W20.8 ☑
same level W18.30 ☑
from
being crushed, pushed, or stepped on by a crowd or human stampede W52 ☑
collision, pushing, shoving, by or with other person W03 ☑
slipping, stumbling, tripping W01.0 ☑
involving ice or snow W00.0 ☑
involving skates (ice) (roller), skateboard, skis — *see* Accident, transport, pedestrian, conveyance
snowslide (avalanche) — *see* Landslide
stone W20.8 ☑
structure W20.1 ☑
burning (uncontrolled fire) X00.3 ☑
through
bridge W13.1 ☑
floor W13.3 ☑
roof W13.2 ☑
wall W13.8 ☑
window W13.4 ☑
timber W20.8 ☑
tree (caused by lightning) W20.8 ☑
while being carried or supported by other person(s) W04 ☑
Fallen on by
animal (not being ridden) NEC W55.89 ☑
Felo-de-se — *see* Suicide
Fight (hand) (fists) (foot) — *see* Assault, fight
Fire (accidental) — *see* Exposure, fire
Firearm discharge — *see* Discharge, firearm
Fireball effects from nuclear explosion in war operations — *see* War operations, nuclear weapons
Fireworks (explosion) W39 ☑
Flash burns from explosion — *see* Explosion
Flood (any injury) (caused by) X38 ☑
collapse of man-made structure causing earth movement X36.0 ☑
tidal wave — *see* Forces of nature, tidal wave
Food (any type) **in**
air passages (with asphyxia, obstruction, or suffocation) — *see* categories T17 and T18 ☑
alimentary tract causing asphyxia (due to compression of trachea) — *see* categories T17 and T18 ☑
Forces of nature X39.8 ☑
avalanche X36.1 ☑
causing transport accident — *see* Accident, transport, by type of vehicle
blizzard X37.2 ☑
cataclysmic storm X37.9 ☑

Forces of nature — *continued*
cataclysmic storm — *continued*
with flood X38 ☑
blizzard X37.2 ☑
cloudburst X37.8 ☑
cyclone X37.1 ☑
dust storm X37.3 ☑
hurricane X37.0 ☑
specified storm NEC X37.8 ☑
storm surge X37.0 ☑
tornado X37.1 ☑
twister X37.1 ☑
typhoon X37.0 ☑
cloudburst X37.8 ☑
cold (natural) X31 ☑
cyclone X37.1 ☑
dam collapse causing earth movement X36.0 ☑
dust storm X37.3 ☑
earth movement X36.1 ☑
caused by dam or structure collapse X36.0 ☑
earthquake X34 ☑
earthquake X34 ☑
flood (caused by) X38 ☑
dam collapse X36.0 ☑
tidal wave — *see* Forces of nature, tidal wave
heat (natural) X30 ☑
hurricane X37.0 ☑
landslide X36.1 ☑
causing transport accident — *see* Accident, transport, by type of vehicle
lightning — *see* subcategory T75.0 ☑
causing fire — *see* Exposure, fire
mudslide X36.1 ☑
causing transport accident — *see* Accident, transport, by type of vehicle
radiation (natural) X39.08 ☑
radon X39.01 ☑
radon X39.01 ☑
specified force NEC X39.8 ☑
storm surge X37.0 ☑
structure collapse causing earth movement X36.0 ☑
sunlight X32 ☑
tidal wave X37.41 ☑
due to
earthquake X37.41 ☑
landslide X37.43 ☑
storm X37.42 ☑
volcanic eruption X37.41 ☑
tornado X37.1 ☑
tsunami X37.41 ☑
twister X37.1 ☑
typhoon X37.0 ☑
volcanic eruption X35 ☑
Foreign body
aspiration — *see* Index to Diseases and Injuries, Foreign body, respiratory tract
embedded in skin W45 ☑
entering through skin W45.8 ☑
can lid W26.8 ☑
nail W45.0 ☑
paper W26.2 ☑
specified NEC W45.8 ☑
splinter W45.8 ☑
Forest fire (exposure to) — *see* Exposure, fire, uncontrolled, not in building
Found injured X58 ☑
from exposure (to) — *see* Exposure
on
highway, road(way), street V89.9 ☑
railway right of way V81.9 ☑
Fracture (circumstances unknown or unspecified) X58 ☑
due to specified cause NEC X58 ☑
Freezing — *see* Exposure, cold
Frostbite X31 ☑
due to man-made conditions — *see* Exposure, cold, man-made
Frozen — *see* Exposure, cold

G

Gored by bull W55.22 ☑
Gunshot wound W34.00 ☑

H

Hailstones, injured by X39.8 ☑

Hanged herself or himself — *see* Hanging, self-inflicted
Hanging (accidental) (*see also* category) T71 ☑
   legal execution — *see* Legal, intervention, specified
      means NEC
Heat (effects of) (excessive) X30 ☑
   due to
      man-made conditions W92 ☑
         on board watercraft V93.29 ☑
            fishing boat V93.22 ☑
            merchant ship V93.20 ☑
            passenger ship V93.21 ☑
            sailboat V93.24 ☑
            specified powered craft NEC V93.23 ☑
      weather (conditions) X30 ☑
   from
      electric heating apparatus causing burning X16 ☑
      nuclear explosion in war operations — *see* War
         operations, nuclear weapons
   inappropriate in local application or packing in medical
      or surgical procedure Y63.5
Hemorrhage
   delayed following medical or surgical treatment
      without mention of misadventure — *see* Index
      to Diseases and Injuries, Complication(s)
   during medical or surgical treatment as misadventure
      — *see* Index to Diseases and Injuries, Complica-
      tion(s)
High
   altitude (effects) — *see* Air, pressure, low
   level of radioactivity, effects — *see* Radiation
   pressure (effects) — *see* Air, pressure, high
   temperature, effects — *see* Heat
Hit, hitting (accidental) by — *see* Struck by
Hitting against — *see* Striking against
Homicide (attempt) (justifiable) — *see* Assault
Hot
   place, effects (*see also* Heat)
   weather, effects X30 ☑
House fire (uncontrolled) — *see* Exposure, fire, uncon-
   trolled, building
Humidity, causing problem X39.8 ☑
Hunger X58 ☑
Hurricane (any injury) X37.0 ☑
Hypobarism, hypobaropathy — *see* Air, pressure, low

I

Ictus
   caloris (*see also* Heat)
   solaris X30 ☑
Ignition (accidental) (*see also* Exposure, fire) X08.8 ☑
   anesthetic gas in operating room W40.1 ☑
   apparel X06.2 ☑
      from highly flammable material X04 ☑
      nightwear X05 ☑
   bed linen (sheets) (spreads) (pillows) (mattress) — *see*
      Exposure, fire, uncontrolled, building, bed
   benzine X04 ☑
   clothes, clothing NEC (from controlled fire) X06.2 ☑
      from
         highly flammable material X04 ☑
   ether X04 ☑
      in operating room W40.1 ☑
   explosive material — *see* Explosion
   gasoline X04 ☑
   jewelry (plastic) (any) X06.0 ☑
   kerosene X04 ☑
   material
      explosive — *see* Explosion
      highly flammable with secondary explosion X04 ☑
   nightwear X05 ☑
   paraffin X04 ☑
   petrol X04 ☑
Immersion (accidental) (*see also* Drowning)
   hand or foot due to cold (excessive) X31 ☑
Implantation of quills of porcupine W55.89 ☑
Inanition (from) (hunger) X58 ☑
   thirst X58 ☑
Inappropriate operation performed
   correct operation on wrong side or body part (wrong
      side) (wrong site) Y65.53
   operation intended for another patient done on wrong
      patient Y65.52
   wrong operation performed on correct patient Y65.51
Inattention after, at birth (homicidal intent) (infantici-
   dal intent) X58 ☑

Incident, adverse
   device
      anesthesiology Y70.8
         accessory Y70.2
         diagnostic Y70.0
         miscellaneous Y70.8
         monitoring Y70.0
         prosthetic Y70.2
         rehabilitative Y70.1
         surgical Y70.3
         therapeutic Y70.1
      cardiovascular Y71.8
         accessory Y71.2
         diagnostic Y71.0
         miscellaneous Y71.8
         monitoring Y71.0
         prosthetic Y71.2
         rehabilitative Y71.1
         surgical Y71.3
         therapeutic Y71.1
      gastroenterology Y73.8
         accessory Y73.2
         diagnostic Y73.0
         miscellaneous Y73.8
         monitoring Y73.0
         prosthetic Y73.2
         rehabilitative Y73.1
         surgical Y73.3
         therapeutic Y73.1
      general
         hospital Y74.8
            accessory Y74.2
            diagnostic Y74.0
            miscellaneous Y74.8
            monitoring Y74.0
            prosthetic Y74.2
            rehabilitative Y74.1
            surgical Y74.3
            therapeutic Y74.1
         surgical Y81.8
            accessory Y81.2
            diagnostic Y81.0
            miscellaneous Y81.8
            monitoring Y81.0
            prosthetic Y81.2
            rehabilitative Y81.1
            surgical Y81.3
            therapeutic Y81.1
      gynecological Y76.8
         accessory Y76.2
         diagnostic Y76.0
         miscellaneous Y76.8
         monitoring Y76.0
         prosthetic Y76.2
         rehabilitative Y76.1
         surgical Y76.3
         therapeutic Y76.1
      medical Y82.9
         specified type NEC Y82.8
      neurological Y75.8
         accessory Y75.2
         diagnostic Y75.0
         miscellaneous Y75.8
         monitoring Y75.0
         prosthetic Y75.2
         rehabilitative Y75.1
         surgical Y75.3
         therapeutic Y75.1
      obstetrical Y76.8
         accessory Y76.2
         diagnostic Y76.0
         miscellaneous Y76.8
         monitoring Y76.0
         prosthetic Y76.2
         rehabilitative Y76.1
         surgical Y76.3
         therapeutic Y76.1
      ophthalmic Y77.8
         accessory Y77.2
         diagnostic Y77.0
         miscellaneous Y77.8
         monitoring Y77.0
         prosthetic Y77.2
         rehabilitative Y77.1
         surgical Y77.3
         therapeutic Y77.1
      orthopedic Y79.8
         accessory Y79.2
         diagnostic Y79.0

Incident, adverse — *continued*
   device — *continued*
      orthopedic — *continued*
         miscellaneous Y79.8
         monitoring Y79.0
         prosthetic Y79.2
         rehabilitative Y79.1
         surgical Y79.3
         therapeutic Y79.1
      otorhinolaryngological Y72.8
         accessory Y72.2
         diagnostic Y72.0
         miscellaneous Y72.8
         monitoring Y72.0
         prosthetic Y72.2
         rehabilitative Y72.1
         surgical Y72.3
         therapeutic Y72.1
      personal use Y74.8
         accessory Y74.2
         diagnostic Y74.0
         miscellaneous Y74.8
         monitoring Y74.0
         prosthetic Y74.2
         rehabilitative Y74.1
         surgical Y74.3
         therapeutic Y74.1
      physical medicine Y80.8
         accessory Y80.2
         diagnostic Y80.0
         miscellaneous Y80.8
         monitoring Y80.0
         prosthetic Y80.2
         rehabilitative Y80.1
         surgical Y80.3
         therapeutic Y80.1
      plastic surgical Y81.8
         accessory Y81.2
         diagnostic Y81.0
         miscellaneous Y81.8
         monitoring Y81.0
         prosthetic Y81.2
         rehabilitative Y81.1
         surgical Y81.3
         therapeutic Y81.1
      radiological Y78.8
         accessory Y78.2
         diagnostic Y78.0
         miscellaneous Y78.8
         monitoring Y78.0
         prosthetic Y78.2
         rehabilitative Y78.1
         surgical Y78.3
         therapeutic Y78.1
      urology Y73.8
         accessory Y73.2
         diagnostic Y73.0
         miscellaneous Y73.8
         monitoring Y73.0
         prosthetic Y73.2
         rehabilitative Y73.1
         surgical Y73.3
         therapeutic Y73.1
Incineration (accidental) — *see* Exposure, fire
Infanticide — *see* Assault
Infrasound waves (causing injury) W49.9 ☑
Ingestion
   foreign body (causing injury) (with obstruction) — *see*
      Foreign body, alimentary canal
   poisonous
      plant(s) X58 ☑
      substance NEC — *see* Table of Drugs and Chemicals
Inhalation
   excessively cold substance, man-made — *see* Expo-
      sure, cold, man-made
   food (any type) (into respiratory tract) (with asphyxia,
      obstruction respiratory tract, suffocation) — *see*
      categories T17 and T18 ☑
   foreign body — *see* Foreign body, aspiration
   gastric contents (with asphyxia, obstruction respiratory
      passage, suffocation) T17.81- ☑
   hot air or gases X14.0 ☑
   liquid air, hydrogen, nitrogen W93.12 ☑
      suicide (attempt) X83.2 ☑
   steam X13.0 ☑
      assault X98.0 ☑
      stated as undetermined whether accidental or in-
         tentional Y27.0 ☑

Inhalation — *continued*
  steam — *continued*
    suicide (attempt) X77.0 ☑
  toxic gas — *see* Table of Drugs and Chemicals
  vomitus (with asphyxia, obstruction respiratory passage, suffocation) T17.81- ☑
Injury, injured (accidental(ly)) NOS X58 ☑
  by, caused by, from
    assault — *see* Assault
    law-enforcing agent, police, in course of legal intervention — *see* Legal intervention
    suicide (attempt) X83.8 ☑
  due to, in
    civil insurrection — *see* War operations
    fight (*see also* Assault, fight) Y04.0 ☑
    war operations — *see* War operations
  homicide (*see also* Assault) Y09
  inflicted (by)
    in course of arrest (attempted), suppression of disturbance, maintenance of order, by law-enforcing agents — *see* Legal intervention
    other person
      stated as
        accidental X58 ☑
        intentional, homicide (attempt) — *see* Assault
        undetermined whether accidental or intentional Y33 ☑
    purposely (inflicted) by other person(s) — *see* Assault
  self-inflicted X83.8 ☑
    stated as accidental X58 ☑
  specified cause NEC X58 ☑
  undetermined whether accidental or intentional Y33 ☑
Insolation, effects X30 ☑
Insufficient nourishment X58 ☑
Interruption of respiration (by)
  food (lodged in esophagus) — *see* categories T17 and T18 ☑
  vomitus (lodged in esophagus) T17.81- ☑
Intervention, legal — *see* Legal intervention
Intoxication
  drug — *see* Table of Drugs and Chemicals
  poison — *see* Table of Drugs and Chemicals

J

Jammed (accidentally)
  between objects (moving) (stationary and moving) W23.0 ☑
    stationary W23.1 ☑
Jumped, jumping
  before moving object NEC X81.8 ☑
    motor vehicle X81.0 ☑
    subway train X81.1 ☑
    train X81.1 ☑
    undetermined whether accidental or intentional Y31 ☑
  from
    boat (into water) voluntarily, without accident (to or on boat) W16.712 ☑
      with
        accident to or on boat — *see* Accident, watercraft
        drowning or submersion W16.711 ☑
          suicide (attempt) X71.3 ☑
      striking bottom W16.722 ☑
        causing drowning W16.721 ☑
    building (*see also* Jumped, from, high place) W13.9 ☑
      burning (uncontrolled fire) X00.5 ☑
    high place NEC W17.89 ☑
      suicide (attempt) X80 ☑
      undetermined whether accidental or intentional Y30 ☑
    structure (*see also* Jumped, from, high place) W13.9 ☑
      burning (uncontrolled fire) X00.5 ☑
  into water W16.92 ☑
    causing drowning W16.91 ☑
    from, off watercraft — *see* Jumped, from, boat
    in
      natural body W16.612 ☑
        causing drowning W16.611 ☑
        striking bottom W16.622 ☑
          causing drowning W16.621 ☑

Jumped, jumping — *continued*
  into water — *continued*
    in — *continued*
      specified place NEC W16.812 ☑
        causing drowning W16.811 ☑
        striking
          bottom W16.822 ☑
            causing drowning W16.821 ☑
          wall W16.832 ☑
            causing drowning W16.831 ☑
      swimming pool W16.512 ☑
        causing drowning W16.511 ☑
        striking
          bottom W16.522 ☑
            causing drowning W16.521 ☑
          wall W16.532 ☑
            causing drowning W16.531 ☑
  suicide (attempt) X71.3 ☑

K

Kicked by
  animal NEC W55.82 ☑
  person(s) (accidentally) W50.1 ☑
    with intent to injure or kill Y04.0 ☑
    as, or caused by, a crowd or human stampede (with fall) W52 ☑
    assault Y04.0 ☑
    homicide (attempt) Y04.0 ☑
    in
      fight Y04.0 ☑
      legal intervention
        injuring
          bystander Y35.812 ☑
          law enforcement personnel Y35.811 ☑
          suspect Y35.813 ☑
Kicking
  against
    object W22.8 ☑
      sports equipment W21.9 ☑
      stationary W22.09 ☑
        sports equipment W21.89 ☑
    person — *see* Striking against, person
    sports equipment W21.9 ☑
  carpet stretcher with knee X50.3 ☑
Killed, killing (accidentally) NOS (*see also* Injury) X58 ☑
  in
    action — *see* War operations
    brawl, fight (hand) (fists) (foot) Y04.0 ☑
      by weapon (*see also* Assault)
        cutting, piercing — *see* Assault, cutting or piercing instrument
        firearm — *see* Discharge, firearm, by type, homicide
  self
    stated as
      accident NOS X58 ☑
      suicide — *see* Suicide
      undetermined whether accidental or intentional Y33 ☑
Kneeling (prolonged (static) X50.1 ☑
Knocked down (accidentally) (by) NOS X58 ☑
  animal (not being ridden) NEC (*see also* Struck by, by type of animal)
  crowd or human stampede W52 ☑
  person W51 ☑
    in brawl, fight Y04.0 ☑
  transport vehicle NEC (*see also* Accident, transport) V09.9 ☑

L

Laceration NEC — *see* Injury
Lack of
  care (helpless person) (infant) (newborn) X58 ☑
  food except as result of abandonment or neglect X58 ☑
    due to abandonment or neglect X58 ☑
  water except as result of transport accident X58 ☑
    due to transport accident — *see* Accident, transport, by type
  helpless person, infant, newborn X58 ☑
Landslide (falling on transport vehicle) X36.1 ☑
  caused by collapse of man-made structure X36.0 ☑
Late effect — *see* Sequelae

Legal
  execution (any method) — *see* Legal, intervention
  intervention (by)
    baton — *see* Legal, intervention, blunt object, baton
    bayonet — *see* Legal, intervention, sharp object, bayonet
    blow — *see* Legal, intervention, manhandling
    blunt object
      baton
        injuring
          bystander Y35.312 ☑
          law enforcement personnel Y35.311 ☑
          suspect Y35.313 ☑
      injuring
        bystander Y35.302 ☑
        law enforcement personnel Y35.301 ☑
        suspect Y35.303 ☑
      specified NEC
        injuring
          bystander Y35.392 ☑
          law enforcement personnel Y35.391 ☑
          suspect Y35.393 ☑
      stave
        injuring
          bystander Y35.392 ☑
          law enforcement personnel Y35.391 ☑
          suspect Y35.393 ☑
    bomb — *see* Legal, intervention, explosive
    cutting or piercing instrument — *see* Legal, intervention, sharp object
    dynamite — *see* Legal, intervention, explosive, dynamite
    explosive(s)
      dynamite
        injuring
          bystander Y35.112 ☑
          law enforcement personnel Y35.111 ☑
          suspect Y35.113 ☑
      grenade
        injuring
          bystander Y35.192 ☑
          law enforcement personnel Y35.191 ☑
          suspect Y35.193 ☑
      injuring
        bystander Y35.102 ☑
        law enforcement personnel Y35.101 ☑
        suspect Y35.103 ☑
      mortar bomb
        injuring
          bystander Y35.192 ☑
          law enforcement personnel Y35.191 ☑
          suspect Y35.193 ☑
      shell
        injuring
          bystander Y35.122 ☑
          law enforcement personnel Y35.121 ☑
          suspect Y35.123 ☑
      specified NEC
        injuring
          bystander Y35.192 ☑
          law enforcement personnel Y35.191 ☑
          suspect Y35.193 ☑
    firearm(s) (discharge)
      handgun
        injuring
          bystander Y35.022 ☑
          law enforcement personnel Y35.021 ☑
          suspect Y35.023 ☑
      injuring
        bystander Y35.002 ☑
        law enforcement personnel Y35.001 ☑
        suspect Y35.003 ☑
      machine gun
        injuring
          bystander Y35.012 ☑
          law enforcement personnel Y35.011 ☑
          suspect Y35.013 ☑
      rifle pellet
        injuring
          bystander Y35.032 ☑
          law enforcement personnel Y35.031 ☑
          suspect Y35.033 ☑
      rubber bullet
        injuring
          bystander Y35.042 ☑
          law enforcement personnel Y35.041 ☑

☑ **Additional Character Required** — Refer to the Tabular List for Character Selection   ▽ **Subterms under main terms may continue to next column or page**

Legal — *continued*
intervention — *continued*
firearm(s) — *continued*
rubber bullet — *continued*
injuring — *continued*
suspect Y35.043 ☑
shotgun — *see* Legal, intervention, firearm, specified NEC
specified NEC
injuring
bystander Y35.092 ☑
law enforcement personnel Y35.091 ☑
suspect Y35.093 ☑
gas (asphyxiation) (poisoning)
injuring
bystander Y35.202 ☑
law enforcement personnel Y35.201 ☑
suspect Y35.203 ☑
specified NEC
injuring
bystander Y35.292 ☑
law enforcement personnel Y35.291 ☑
suspect Y35.293 ☑
tear gas
injuring
bystander Y35.212 ☑
law enforcement personnel Y35.211 ☑
suspect Y35.213 ☑
grenade — *see* Legal, intervention, explosive, grenade
injuring
bystander Y35.92 ☑
law enforcement personnel Y35.91 ☑
suspect Y35.93 ☑
late effect (of) — *see* with 7th character S Y35 ☑
manhandling
injuring
bystander Y35.812 ☑
law enforcement personnel Y35.811 ☑
suspect Y35.813 ☑
sequelae (of) — *see* with 7th character S Y35 ☑
sharp objects
bayonet
injuring
bystander Y35.412 ☑
law enforcement personnel Y35.411 ☑
suspect Y35.413 ☑
injuring
bystander Y35.402 ☑
law enforcement personnel Y35.401 ☑
suspect Y35.403 ☑
specified NEC
injuring
bystander Y35.492 ☑
law enforcement personnel Y35.491 ☑
suspect Y35.493 ☑
specified means NEC
injuring
bystander Y35.892 ☑
law enforcement personnel Y35.891 ☑
suspect Y35.893 ☑
stabbing — *see* Legal, intervention, sharp object
stave — *see* Legal, intervention, blunt object, stave
tear gas — *see* Legal, intervention, gas, tear gas
truncheon — *see* Legal, intervention, blunt object, stave

Lifting — *see also* Overexertion
heavy objects X50.0 ☑
weights X50.0 ☑

Lightning (shock) (stroke) (struck by) — *see* subcategory T75.0 ☑
causing fire — *see* Exposure, fire

Loss of control (transport vehicle) NEC — *see* Accident, transport

Lost at sea NOS — *see* Drowning, due to, fall overboard

Low
pressure (effects) — *see* Air, pressure, low
temperature (effects) — *see* Exposure, cold

Lying before train, vehicle or other moving object X81.8 ☑
subway train X81.1 ☑
train X81.1 ☑
undetermined whether accidental or intentional Y31 ☑

Lynching — *see* Assault

M

Malfunction (mechanism or component) (of)
firearm W34.10 ☑
airgun W34.110 ☑
BB gun W34.110 ☑
gas, air or spring-operated gun NEC W34.118 ☑
handgun W32.1 ☑
hunting rifle W33.12 ☑
larger firearm W33.10 ☑
specified NEC W33.19 ☑
machine gun W33.13 ☑
paintball gun W34.111 ☑
pellet gun W34.110 ☑
shotgun W33.11 ☑
specified NEC W34.19 ☑
Very pistol [flare] W34.19 ☑
handgun — *see* Malfunction, firearm, handgun

Maltreatment — *see* Perpetrator
Mangled (accidentally) NOS X58 ☑
Manhandling (in brawl, fight) Y04.0 ☑
legal intervention — *see* Legal, intervention, manhandling
Manslaughter (nonaccidental) — *see* Assault
Mauled by animal NEC W55.89 ☑
Medical procedure, complication of (delayed or as an abnormal reaction without mention of misadventure) — *see* Complication of or following, by specified type of procedure
due to or as a result of misadventure — *see* Misadventure
Melting (due to fire) (*see also* Exposure, fire)
apparel NEC X06.3 ☑
clothes, clothing NEC X06.3 ☑
nightwear X05 ☑
fittings or furniture (burning building) (uncontrolled fire) X00.8 ☑
nightwear X05 ☑
plastic jewelry X06.1 ☑
Mental cruelty X58 ☑
Military operations (injuries to military and civilians occuring during peacetime on military property and during routine military exercises and operations) (by) (from) (involving) Y37.90- ☑
air blast Y37.20- ☑
aircraft
destruction — *see* Military operations, destruction of aircraft
airway restriction — *see* Military operations, restriction of airways
asphyxiation — *see* Military operations, restriction of airways
biological weapons Y37.6X- ☑
blast Y37.20- ☑
blast fragments Y37.20- ☑
blast wave Y37.20- ☑
blast wind Y37.20- ☑
bomb Y37.20- ☑
dirty Y37.50- ☑
gasoline Y37.31- ☑
incendiary Y37.31- ☑
petrol Y37.31- ☑
bullet Y37.43- ☑
incendiary Y37.32- ☑
rubber Y37.41- ☑
chemical weapons Y37.7X- ☑
combat
hand to hand (unarmed) combat Y37.44- ☑
using blunt or piercing object Y37.45- ☑
conflagration — *see* Military operations, fire
conventional warfare NEC Y37.49- ☑
depth-charge Y37.01- ☑
destruction of aircraft Y37.10- ☑
due to
air to air missile Y37.11- ☑
collision with other aircraft Y37.12- ☑
detonation (accidental) of onboard munitions and explosives Y37.14- ☑
enemy fire or explosives Y37.11- ☑
explosive placed on aircraft Y37.11- ☑
onboard fire Y37.13- ☑
rocket propelled grenade [RPG] Y37.11- ☑
small arms fire Y37.11- ☑
surface to air missile Y37.11- ☑
specified NEC Y37.19- ☑

Military operations — *continued*
detonation (accidental) of
onboard marine weapons Y37.05- ☑
own munitions or munitions launch device Y37.24- ☑
dirty bomb Y37.50- ☑
explosion (of) Y37.20- ☑
aerial bomb Y37.21- ☑
bomb NOS (*see also* Military operations, bomb(s)) Y37.20- ☑
fragments Y37.29- ☑
grenade Y37.29- ☑
guided missile Y37.22- ☑
improvised explosive device [IED] (person-borne) (roadside) (vehicle-borne) Y37.23- ☑
land mine Y37.29- ☑
marine mine (at sea) (in harbor) Y37.02- ☑
marine weapon Y37.00- ☑
specified NEC Y37.09- ☑
own munitions or munitions launch device (accidental) Y37.24- ☑
sea-based artillery shell Y37.03- ☑
specified NEC Y37.29- ☑
torpedo Y37.04- ☑
fire Y37.30- ☑
specified NEC Y37.39- ☑
firearms
discharge Y37.43- ☑
pellets Y37.42- ☑
flamethrower Y37.33- ☑
fragments (from) (of)
improvised explosive device [IED] (person-borne) (roadside) (vehicle-borne) Y37.26- ☑
munitions Y37.25- ☑
specified NEC Y37.29- ☑
weapons Y37.27- ☑
friendly fire Y37.92- ☑
hand to hand (unarmed) combat Y37.44- ☑
hot substances — *see* Military operations, fire
incendiary bullet Y37.32- ☑
nuclear weapon (effects of) Y37.50- ☑
acute radiation exposure Y37.54- ☑
blast pressure Y37.51- ☑
direct blast Y37.51- ☑
direct heat Y37.53- ☑
fallout exposure Y37.54- ☑
fireball Y37.53- ☑
indirect blast (struck or crushed by blast debris) (being thrown by blast) Y37.52- ☑
ionizing radiation (immediate exposure) Y37.54- ☑
nuclear radiation Y37.54- ☑
radiation
ionizing (immediate exposure) Y37.54- ☑
nuclear Y37.54- ☑
thermal Y37.53- ☑
secondary effects Y37.54- ☑
specified NEC Y37.59- ☑
thermal radiation Y37.53- ☑
restriction of air (airway)
intentional Y37.46- ☑
unintentional Y37.47- ☑
rubber bullets Y37.41- ☑
shrapnel NOS Y37.29- ☑
suffocation — *see* Military operations, restriction of airways
unconventional warfare NEC Y37.7X- ☑
underwater blast NOS Y37.00- ☑
warfare
conventional NEC Y37.49- ☑
unconventional NEC Y37.7X- ☑
weapon of mass destruction [WMD] Y37.91- ☑
weapons
biological weapons Y37.6X- ☑
chemical Y37.7X- ☑
nuclear (effects of) Y37.50- ☑
acute radiation exposure Y37.54- ☑
blast pressure Y37.51- ☑
direct blast Y37.51- ☑
direct heat Y37.53- ☑
fallout exposure Y37.54- ☑
fireball Y37.53- ☑
radiation
ionizing (immediate exposure) Y37.54- ☑
nuclear Y37.54- ☑
thermal Y37.53- ☑
secondary effects Y37.54- ☑

Military operations — continued
  weapons — continued
    nuclear — continued
      specified NEC Y37.59- ☑
      of mass destruction [WMD] Y37.91- ☑
Misadventure(s) to patient(s) during surgical or medical care Y69
  contaminated medical or biological substance (blood, drug, fluid) Y64.9
    administered (by) NEC Y64.9
      immunization Y64.1
      infusion Y64.0
      injection Y64.1
      specified means NEC Y64.8
      transfusion Y64.0
      vaccination Y64.1
  excessive amount of blood or other fluid during transfusion or infusion Y63.0
  failure
    in dosage Y63.9
      electroshock therapy Y63.4
      inappropriate temperature (too hot or too cold) in local application and packing Y63.5
      infusion
        excessive amount of fluid Y63.0
        incorrect dilution of fluid Y63.1
      insulin-shock therapy Y63.4
      nonadministration of necessary drug or biological substance Y63.6
      overdose — see Table of Drugs and Chemicals
      radiation, in therapy Y63.2
      radiation
        overdose Y63.2
      specified procedure NEC Y63.8
      transfusion
        excessive amount of blood Y63.0
  mechanical, of instrument or apparatus (any) (during any procedure) Y65.8
  sterile precautions (during procedure) Y62.9
    aspiration of fluid or tissue (by puncture or catheterization, except heart) Y62.6
    biopsy (except needle aspiration) Y62.8
      needle (aspirating) Y62.6
    blood sampling Y62.6
    catheterization Y62.6
      heart Y62.5
    dialysis (kidney) Y62.2
    endoscopic examination Y62.4
    enema Y62.8
    immunization Y62.3
    infusion Y62.1
    injection Y62.3
    needle biopsy Y62.6
    paracentesis (abdominal) (thoracic) Y62.6
    perfusion Y62.2
    puncture (lumbar) Y62.6
    removal of catheter or packing Y62.8
    specified procedure NEC Y62.8
    surgical operation Y62.0
    transfusion Y62.1
    vaccination Y62.3
  suture or ligature during surgical procedure Y65.2
  to introduce or to remove tube or instrument — see Failure, to
  hemorrhage — see Index to Diseases and Injuries, Complication(s)
  inadvertent exposure of patient to radiation Y63.3
  inappropriate
    operation performed — see Inappropriate operation performed
    temperature (too hot or too cold) in local application or packing Y63.5
  infusion (see also Misadventure, by type, infusion) Y69
    excessive amount of fluid Y63.0
    incorrect dilution of fluid Y63.1
    wrong fluid Y65.1
  mismatched blood in transfusion Y65.0
  nonadministration of necessary drug or biological substance Y63.6
  overdose — see Table of Drugs and Chemicals
  radiation (in therapy) Y63.2
  perforation — see Index to Diseases and Injuries, Complication(s)
  performance of inappropriate operation — see Inappropriate operation performed
  puncture — see Index to Diseases and Injuries, Complication(s)
  specified type NEC Y65.8

Misadventure(s) to patient(s) during surgical or medical care — continued
  specified type — continued
    failure
      suture or ligature during surgical operation Y65.2
      to introduce or to remove tube or instrument — see Failure, to
    infusion of wrong fluid Y65.1
    performance of inappropriate operation — see Inappropriate operation performed
    transfusion of mismatched blood Y65.0
    wrong
      fluid in infusion Y65.1
      placement of endotracheal tube during anesthetic procedure Y65.3
  transfusion — see Misadventure, by type, transfusion
    excessive amount of blood Y63.0
    mismatched blood Y65.0
  wrong
    drug given in error — see Table of Drugs and Chemicals
    fluid in infusion Y65.1
    placement of endotracheal tube during anesthetic procedure Y65.3
Mismatched blood in transfusion Y65.0
Motion sickness T75.3 ☑
Mountain sickness W94.11 ☑
Mudslide (of cataclysmic nature) — see Landslide
Murder (attempt) — see Assault

N

Nail
  contact with W45.0 ☑
    gun W29.4 ☑
  embedded in skin W45.0 ☑
Neglect (criminal) (homicidal intent) X58 ☑
Noise (causing injury) (pollution) W42.9 ☑
  supersonic W42.0 ☑
Nonadministration (of)
  drug or biological substance (necessary) Y63.6
  surgical and medical care Y66
Nosocomial condition Y95

O

Object
  falling
    from, in, on, hitting
      machinery — see Contact, with, by type of machine
    set in motion by
      accidental explosion or rupture of pressure vessel W38 ☑
      firearm — see Discharge, firearm, by type
      machine(ry) — see Contact, with, by type of machine
Overdose (drug) — see Table of Drugs and Chemicals
  radiation Y63.2
Overexertion X50.9 ☑
  from
    prolonged static or awkward postures X50.1 ☑
    repetitive movements X50.3 ☑
    specified strenuous movements or postures NEC X50.9 ☑
    strenuous movement or load X50.0 ☑
Overexposure (accidental) (to)
  cold (see also Exposure, cold) X31 ☑
    due to man-made conditions — see Exposure, cold, man-made
  heat (see also Heat) X30 ☑
  radiation — see Radiation
  radioactivity W88.0 ☑
  sun (sunburn) X32 ☑
  weather NEC — see Forces of nature
  wind NEC — see Forces of nature
Overheated — see Heat
Overturning (accidental)
  machinery — see Contact, with, by type of machine
  transport vehicle NEC (see also Accident, transport) V89.9 ☑
  watercraft (causing drowning, submersion) (see also Drowning, due to, accident to, watercraft, overturning)
    causing injury except drowning or submersion — see Accident, watercraft, causing, injury NEC

P

Parachute descent (voluntary) (without accident to aircraft) V97.29 ☑
  due to accident to aircraft — see Accident, transport, aircraft
Pecked by bird W61.99 ☑
Perforation during medical or surgical treatment as misadventure — see Index to Diseases and Injuries, Complication(s)
Perpetrator, perpetration, of assault, maltreatment and neglect (by) Y07.9
  boyfriend Y07.03
  brother Y07.410
    stepbrother Y07.435
  coach Y07.53
  cousin
    female Y07.491
    male Y07.490
  daycare provider Y07.519
    at-home
      adult care Y07.512
      childcare Y07.510
    care center
      adult care Y07.513
      childcare Y07.511
  family member NEC Y07.499
  father Y07.11
    adoptive Y07.13
    foster Y07.420
    stepfather Y07.430
  foster father Y07.420
  foster mother Y07.421
  girl friend Y07.04
  healthcare provider Y07.529
    mental health Y07.521
    specified NEC Y07.528
  husband Y07.01
  instructor Y07.53
  mother Y07.12
    adoptive Y07.14
    foster Y07.421
    stepmother Y07.433
  nonfamily member Y07.50
    specified NEC Y07.59
  nurse Y07.528
  occupational therapist Y07.528
  partner of parent
    female Y07.434
    male Y07.432
  physical therapist Y07.528
  sister Y07.411
  speech therapist Y07.528
  stepbrother Y07.435
  stepfather Y07.430
  stepmother Y07.433
  stepsister Y07.436
  teacher Y07.53
  wife Y07.02
Piercing — see Contact, with, by type of object or machine
Pinched
  between objects (moving) (stationary and moving) W23.0 ☑
  stationary W23.1 ☑
Pinned under machine(ry) — see Contact, with, by type of machine
Place of occurrence Y92.9
  abandoned house Y92.89
  airplane Y92.813
  airport Y92.520
  ambulatory health services establishment NEC Y92.538
  ambulatory surgery center Y92.530
  amusement park Y92.831
  apartment (co-op) — see Place of occurrence, residence, apartment
  assembly hall Y92.29
  bank Y92.510
  barn Y92.71
  baseball field Y92.320
  basketball court Y92.310
  beach Y92.832
  boarding house — see Place of occurrence, residence, boarding house
  boat Y92.814
  bowling alley Y92.39
  bridge Y92.89

☑ **Additional Character Required** — Refer to the Tabular List for Character Selection   ⬇ Subterms under main terms may continue to next column or page

Place of occurrence — *continued*

building under construction Y92.61
bus Y92.811
    station Y92.521
cafe Y92.511
campsite Y92.833
campus — *see* Place of occurrence, school
canal Y92.89
car Y92.810
casino Y92.59
children's home — *see* Place of occurrence, residence, institutional, orphanage
church Y92.22
cinema Y92.26
clubhouse Y92.29
coal pit Y92.64
college (community) Y92.214
condominium — *see* Place of occurrence, residence, apartment
construction area — *see* Place of occurrence, industrial and construction area
convalescent home — *see* Place of occurrence, residence, institutional, nursing home
court-house Y92.240
cricket ground Y92.328
cultural building Y92.258
    art gallery Y92.250
    museum Y92.251
    music hall Y92.252
    opera house Y92.253
    specified NEC Y92.258
    theater Y92.254
dancehall Y92.252
day nursery Y92.210
dentist office Y92.531
derelict house Y92.89
desert Y92.820
dockyard Y92.62
dock NOS Y92.89
doctor's office Y92.531
dormitory — *see* Place of occurrence, residence, institutional, school dormitory
dry dock Y92.62
factory (building) (premises) Y92.63
farm (land under cultivation) (outbuildings) Y92.79
    barn Y92.71
    chicken coop Y92.72
    field Y92.73
    hen house Y92.72
    house — *see* Place of occurrence, residence, house
    orchard Y92.74
    specified NEC Y92.79
football field Y92.321
forest Y92.821
freeway Y92.411
gallery Y92.250
garage (commercial) Y92.59
    boarding house Y92.044
    military base Y92.135
    mobile home Y92.025
    nursing home Y92.124
    orphanage Y92.114
    private house Y92.015
    reform school Y92.155
gas station Y92.524
gasworks Y92.69
golf course Y92.39
gravel pit Y92.64
grocery Y92.512
gymnasium Y92.39
handball court Y92.318
harbor Y92.89
harness racing course Y92.39
healthcare provider office Y92.531
highway (interstate) Y92.411
hill Y92.828
hockey rink Y92.330
home — *see* Place of occurrence, residence
hospice — *see* Place of occurrence, residence, institutional, nursing home
hospital Y92.239
    cafeteria Y92.233
    corridor Y92.232
    operating room Y92.234
    patient
        bathroom Y92.231
        room Y92.230
    specified NEC Y92.238

Place of occurrence — *continued*

hotel Y92.59
house (*see also* Place of occurrence, residence)
    abandoned Y92.89
    under construction Y92.61
industrial and construction area (yard) Y92.69
    building under construction Y92.61
    dock Y92.62
    dry dock Y92.62
    factory Y92.63
    gasworks Y92.69
    mine Y92.64
    oil rig Y92.65
    pit Y92.64
    power station Y92.69
    shipyard Y92.62
    specified NEC Y92.69
    tunnel under construction Y92.69
    workshop Y92.69
kindergarten Y92.211
lacrosse field Y92.328
lake Y92.828
library Y92.241
mall Y92.59
market Y92.512
marsh Y92.828
military
    base — *see* Place of occurrence, residence, institutional, military base
    training ground Y92.84
mine Y92.64
mosque Y92.22
motel Y92.59
motorway (interstate) Y92.411
mountain Y92.828
movie-house Y92.26
museum Y92.251
music-hall Y92.252
not applicable Y92.9
nuclear power station Y92.69
nursing home — *see* Place of occurrence, residence, institutional, nursing home
office building Y92.59
offshore installation Y92.65
oil rig Y92.65
old people's home — *see* Place of occurrence, residence, institutional, specified NEC
opera-house Y92.253
orphanage — *see* Place of occurrence, residence, institutional, orphanage
outpatient surgery center Y92.530
park (public) Y92.830
    amusement Y92.831
parking garage Y92.89
    lot Y92.481
pavement Y92.480
physician office Y92.531
polo field Y92.328
pond Y92.828
post office Y92.242
power station Y92.69
prairie Y92.828
prison — *see* Place of occurrence, residence, institutional, prison
public
    administration building Y92.248
        city hall Y92.243
        courthouse Y92.240
        library Y92.241
        post office Y92.242
        specified NEC Y92.248
    building NEC Y92.29
    hall Y92.29
    place NOS Y92.89
race course Y92.39
radio station Y92.59
railway line (bridge) Y92.85
ranch (outbuildings) — *see* Place of occurrence, farm
recreation area Y92.838
    amusement park Y92.831
    beach Y92.832
    campsite Y92.833
    park (public) Y92.830
    seashore Y92.832
    specified NEC Y92.838
reform school - — *see* Place of occurrence, residence, institutional, reform school
religious institution Y92.22

Place of occurrence — *continued*

residence (non-institutional) (private) Y92.009
    apartment Y92.039
        bathroom Y92.031
        bedroom Y92.032
        kitchen Y92.030
        specified NEC Y92.038
    bathroom Y92.002
    bedroom Y92.003
    boarding house Y92.049
        bathroom Y92.041
        bedroom Y92.042
        driveway Y92.043
        garage Y92.044
        garden Y92.046
        kitchen Y92.040
        specified NEC Y92.048
        swimming pool Y92.045
        yard Y92.046
    dining room Y92.001
    garden Y92.007
    home Y92.009
    house, single family Y92.019
        bathroom Y92.012
        bedroom Y92.013
        dining room Y92.011
        driveway Y92.014
        garage Y92.015
        garden Y92.017
        kitchen Y92.010
        specified NEC Y92.018
        swimming pool Y92.016
        yard Y92.017
    institutional Y92.10
        children's home — *see* Place of occurrence, residence, institutional, orphanage
        hospice — *see* Place of occurrence, residence, institutional, nursing home
        military base Y92.139
            barracks Y92.133
            garage Y92.135
            garden Y92.137
            kitchen Y92.130
            mess hall Y92.131
            specified NEC Y92.138
            swimming pool Y92.136
            yard Y92.137
        nursing home Y92.129
            bathroom Y92.121
            bedroom Y92.122
            driveway Y92.123
            garage Y92.124
            garden Y92.126
            kitchen Y92.120
            specified NEC Y92.128
            swimming pool Y92.125
            yard Y92.126
        orphanage Y92.119
            bathroom Y92.111
            bedroom Y92.112
            driveway Y92.113
            garage Y92.114
            garden Y92.116
            kitchen Y92.110
            specified NEC Y92.118
            swimming pool Y92.115
            yard Y92.116
        prison Y92.149
            bathroom Y92.142
            cell Y92.143
            courtyard Y92.147
            dining room Y92.141
            kitchen Y92.140
            specified NEC Y92.148
            swimming pool Y92.146
        reform school Y92.159
            bathroom Y92.152
            bedroom Y92.153
            dining room Y92.151
            driveway Y92.154
            garage Y92.155
            garden Y92.157
            kitchen Y92.150
            specified NEC Y92.158
            swimming pool Y92.156
            yard Y92.157
        school dormitory Y92.169
            bathroom Y92.162
            bedroom Y92.163

External Causes Index

Place of occurrence — *continued*
  residence — *continued*
    institutional — *continued*
      school dormitory — *continued*
        dining room Y92.161
        kitchen Y92.160
        specified NEC Y92.168
      specified NEC Y92.199
        bathroom Y92.192
        bedroom Y92.193
        dining room Y92.191
        driveway Y92.194
        garage Y92.195
        garden Y92.197
        kitchen Y92.190
        specified NEC Y92.198
        swimming pool Y92.196
        yard Y92.197
    kitchen Y92.000
    mobile home Y92.029
      bathroom Y92.022
      bedroom Y92.023
      dining room Y92.021
      driveway Y92.024
      garage Y92.025
      garden Y92.027
      kitchen Y92.020
      specified NEC Y92.028
      swimming pool Y92.026
      yard Y92.027
    specified place in residence NEC Y92.008
    specified residence type NEC Y92.099
      bathroom Y92.091
      bedroom Y92.092
      driveway Y92.093
      garage Y92.094
      garden Y92.096
      kitchen Y92.090
      specified NEC Y92.098
      swimming pool Y92.095
      yard Y92.096
  restaurant Y92.511
  riding school Y92.39
  river Y92.828
  road Y92.488
  rodeo ring Y92.39
  rugby field Y92.328
  same day surgery center Y92.530
  sand pit Y92.64
  school (private) (public) (state) Y92.219
    college Y92.214
    daycare center Y92.210
    elementary school Y92.211
    high school Y92.213
    kindergarten Y92.211
    middle school Y92.212
    specified NEC Y92.218
    trace school Y92.215
    university Y92.214
    vocational school Y92.215
  sea (shore) Y92.832
  senior citizen center Y92.29
  service area
    airport Y92.520
    bus station Y92.521
    gas station Y92.524
    highway rest stop Y92.523
    railway station Y92.522
  shipyard Y92.62
  shop (commercial) Y92.513
  sidewalk Y92.480
  silo Y92.79
  skating rink (roller) Y92.331
    ice Y92.330
  slaughter house Y92.86
  soccer field Y92.322
  specified place NEC Y92.89
  sports area Y92.39
    athletic
      court Y92.318
        basketball Y92.310
        specified NEC Y92.318
        squash Y92.311
        tennis Y92.312
      field Y92.328
        baseball Y92.320
        cricket ground Y92.328
        football Y92.321
        hockey Y92.328

Place of occurrence — *continued*
  sports area — *continued*
    athletic — *continued*
      field — *continued*
        soccer Y92.322
        specified NEC Y92.328
    golf course Y92.39
    gymnasium Y92.39
    riding school Y92.39
    skating rink (roller) Y92.331
      ice Y92.330
    stadium Y92.39
    swimming pool Y92.34
  squash court Y92.311
  stadium Y92.39
  steeplechasing course Y92.39
  store Y92.512
  stream Y92.828
  street and highway Y92.410
    bike path Y92.482
    freeway Y92.411
    highway ramp Y92.415
    interstate highway Y92.411
    local residential or business street Y92.414
    motorway Y92.411
    parking lot Y92.481
    parkway Y92.412
    sidewalk Y92.480
    specified NEC Y92.488
    state road Y92.413
  subway car Y92.816
  supermarket Y92.512
  swamp Y92.828
  swimming pool (public) Y92.34
    private (at) Y92.095
      boarding house Y92.045
      military base Y92.136
      mobile home Y92.026
      nursing home Y92.125
      orphanage Y92.115
      prison Y92.146
      reform school Y92.156
      single family residence Y92.016
  synagogue Y92.22
  television station Y92.59
  tennis court Y92.312
  theater Y92.254
  trade area Y92.59
    bank Y92.510
    cafe Y92.511
    casino Y92.59
    garage Y92.59
    hotel Y92.59
    market Y92.512
    office building Y92.59
    radio station Y92.59
    restaurant Y92.511
    shop Y92.513
    shopping mall Y92.59
    store Y92.512
    supermarket Y92.512
    television station Y92.59
    warehouse Y92.59
  trailer park, residential — *see* Place of occurrence, residence, mobile home
  trailer site NOS Y92.89
  train Y92.815
    station Y92.522
  truck Y92.812
  tunnel under construction Y92.69
  university Y92.214
  urgent (health) care center Y92.532
  vehicle (transport) Y92.818
    airplane Y92.813
    boat Y92.814
    bus Y92.811
    car Y92.810
    specified NEC Y92.818
    subway car Y92.816
    train Y92.815
    truck Y92.812
  warehouse Y92.59
  water reservoir Y92.89
  wilderness area Y92.828
    desert Y92.820
    forest Y92.821
    marsh Y92.828
    mountain Y92.828
    prairie Y92.828

Place of occurrence — *continued*
  wilderness area — *continued*
    specified NEC Y92.828
    swamp Y92.828
  workshop Y92.69
  yard, private Y92.096
    boarding house Y92.046
    mobile home Y92.027
    single family house Y92.017
  youth center Y92.29
  zoo (zoological garden) Y92.834
Plumbism — *see* Table of Drugs and Chemicals, lead
Poisoning (accidental) (by) (*see also* Table of Drugs and Chemicals)
  by plant, thorns, spines, sharp leaves or other mechanisms NEC X58 ☑
  carbon monoxide
    generated by
      motor vehicle — *see* Accident, transport
      watercraft (in transit) (not in transit) V93.89 ☑
        ferry boat V93.81 ☑
        fishing boat V93.82 ☑
        jet skis V93.83 ☑
        liner V93.81 ☑
        merchant ship V93.80 ☑
        passenger ship V93.81 ☑
        powered craft NEC V93.83 ☑
  caused by injection of poisons into skin by plant
    thorns, spines, sharp leaves X58 ☑
    marine or sea plants (venomous) X58 ☑
  execution — *see* Legal, intervention, gas
  intervention
    by gas — *see* Legal, intervention, gas
    other specified means — *see* Legal, intervention, specified means NEC
  exhaust gas
    generated by
      motor vehicle — *see* Accident, transport
      watercraft (in transit) (not in transit) V93.89 ☑
        ferry boat V93.81 ☑
        fishing boat V93.82 ☑
        jet skis V93.83 ☑
        liner V93.81 ☑
        merchant ship V93.80 ☑
        passenger ship V93.81 ☑
        powered craft NEC V93.83 ☑
  fumes or smoke due to
    explosion (*see also* Explosion) W40.9 ☑
    fire — *see* Exposure, fire
    ignition — *see* Ignition
  gas
    in legal intervention — *see* Legal, intervention, gas
    legal execution — *see* Legal, intervention, gas
  in war operations — *see* War operations
  legal
Powder burn (by) (from)
  airgun W34.110 ☑
  BB gun W34.110 ☑
  firearm NEC W34.19 ☑
  gas, air or spring-operated gun NEC W34.118 ☑
  handgun W32.1 ☑
  hunting rifle W33.12 ☑
  larger firearm W33.10 ☑
    specified NEC W33.19 ☑
  machine gun W33.13 ☑
  paintball gun W34.111 ☑
  pellet gun W34.110 ☑
  shotgun W33.11 ☑
  Very pistol [flare] W34.19 ☑
Premature cessation (of) **surgical and medical care** Y66
Privation (food) (water) X58 ☑
Procedure (operation)
  correct, on wrong side or body part (wrong side) (wrong site) Y65.53
  intended for another patient done on wrong patient Y65.52
  performed on patient not scheduled for surgery Y65.52
  performed on wrong patient Y65.52
  wrong, performed on correct patient Y65.51
Prolonged
  sitting in transport vehicle — *see* Travel, by type of vehicle
  stay in
    high altitude as cause of anoxia, barodontalgia, barotitis or hypoxia W94.11 ☑
    weightless environment X52 ☑

Place of occurrence — Prolonged

Pulling, excessive (see also Overexertion) X50.9- ☑
Puncture, puncturing (see also Contact, with, by type of object or machine)
  by
    plant thorns, spines, sharp leaves or other mechanisms NEC W60 ☑
    during medical or surgical treatment as misadventure — see Index to Diseases and Injuries, Complication(s)
Pushed, pushing (accidental) (injury in)
  by other person(s) (accidental) W51 ☑
    with fall W03 ☑
      due to ice or snow W00.0 ☑
    as, or caused by, a crowd or human stampede (with fall) W52 ☑
    before moving object NEC Y02.8 ☑
      motor vehicle Y02.0 ☑
      subway train Y02.1 ☑
      train Y02.1 ☑
    from
      high place NEC
        in accidental circumstances W17.89 ☑
        stated as
          intentional, homicide (attempt) Y01 ☑
          undetermined whether accidental or intentional Y30 ☑
      transport vehicle NEC (see also Accident, transport) V89.9 ☑
        stated as
          intentional, homicide (attempt) Y08.89
  overexertion X50.9 ☑

R

Radiation (exposure to)
  arc lamps W89.0 ☑
  atomic power plant (malfunction) NEC W88.1 ☑
  complication of or abnormal reaction to medical radiotherapy Y84.2
  electromagnetic, ionizing W88.0 ☑
  gamma rays W88.1 ☑
  in
    war operations (from or following nuclear explosion) — see War operations
  inadvertent exposure of patient (receiving test or therapy) Y63.3
  infrared (heaters and lamps) W90.1 ☑
    excessive heat from W92 ☑
  ionized, ionizing (particles, artificially accelerated)
    radioisotopes W88.1 ☑
    specified NEC W88.8 ☑
    x-rays W88.0 ☑
  isotopes, radioactive — see Radiation, radioactive isotopes
  laser(s) W90.2 ☑
    in war operations — see War operations
    misadventure in medical care Y63.2
  light sources (man-made visible and ultraviolet) W89.9 ☑
    natural X32 ☑
    specified NEC W89.8 ☑
    tanning bed W89.1 ☑
    welding light W89.0 ☑
  man-made visible light W89.9 ☑
    specified NEC W89.8 ☑
    tanning bed W89.1 ☑
    welding light W89.0 ☑
  microwave W90.8 ☑
  misadventure in medical or surgical procedure Y63.2
  natural NEC X39.08 ☑
    radon X39.01 ☑
  overdose (in medical or surgical procedure) Y63.2
  radar W90.0 ☑
  radioactive isotopes (any) W88.1 ☑
    atomic power plant malfunction W88.1 ☑
    misadventure in medical or surgical treatment Y63.2
  radiofrequency W90.0 ☑
  radium NEC W88.1 ☑
  sun X32 ☑
  ultraviolet (light) (man-made) W89.9 ☑
    natural X32 ☑
    specified NEC W89.8 ☑
    tanning bed W89.1 ☑
    welding light W89.0 ☑

Radiation — continued
  welding arc, torch, or light W89.0 ☑
    excessive heat from W92 ☑
  x-rays (hard) (soft) W88.0 ☑
Range disease W94.11 ☑
Rape (attempted) T74.2- ☑
Rat bite W53.11 ☑
Reaching (prolonged) (static) X50.1 ☑
Reaction, abnormal to medical procedure (see also Complication of or following, by type of procedure) Y84.9
  with misadventure — see Misadventure
  biologicals — see Table of Drugs and Chemicals
  drugs — see Table of Drugs and Chemicals
  vaccine — see Table of Drugs and Chemicals
Recoil
  airgun W34.110 ☑
  BB gun W34.110 ☑
  firearm NEC W34.19 ☑
  gas, air or spring-operated gun NEC W34.118 ☑
  handgun W32.1 ☑
  hunting rifle W33.12 ☑
  larger firearm W33.10 ☑
    specified NEC W33.19 ☑
  machine gun W33.13 ☑
  paintball gun W34.111 ☑
  pellet W34.110 ☑
  shotgun W33.11 ☑
  Very pistol [flare] W34.19 ☑
Reduction in
  atmospheric pressure — see Air, pressure, change
Rock falling on or hitting (accidentally) (person) W20.8 ☑
  in cave-in W20.0 ☑
Run over (accidentally) (by)
  animal (not being ridden) NEC W55.89 ☑
  machinery — see Contact, with, by specified type of machine
  transport vehicle NEC (see also Accident, transport) V09.9 ☑
    intentional homicide (attempt) Y03.0 ☑
    motor NEC V09.20 ☑
      intentional homicide (attempt) Y03.0 ☑
Running
  before moving object X81.8 ☑
  motor vehicle X81.0 ☑
Running off, away
  animal (being ridden) (see also Accident, transport) V80.918 ☑
    not being ridden W55.89 ☑
  animal-drawn vehicle NEC (see also Accident, transport) V80.928 ☑
  highway, road(way), street
    transport vehicle NEC (see also Accident, transport) V89.9 ☑
Rupture pressurized devices — see Explosion, by type of device

S

Saturnism — see Table of Drugs and Chemicals, lead
Scald, scalding (accidental) (by) (from) (in) X19 ☑
  air (hot) X14.1 ☑
  gases (hot) X14.1 ☑
  homicide (attempt) — see Assault, burning, hot object
  inflicted by other person
    stated as intentional, homicide (attempt) — see Assault, burning, hot object
  liquid (boiling) (hot) NEC X12 ☑
    stated as undetermined whether accidental or intentional Y27.2 ☑
    suicide (attempt) X77.2 ☑
  local application of externally applied substance in medical or surgical care Y63.5
  metal (molten) (liquid) (hot) NEC X18 ☑
  self-inflicted X77.9 ☑
  stated as undetermined whether accidental or intentional Y27.8 ☑
  steam X13.1 ☑
    assault X98.0 ☑
    stated as undetermined whether accidental or intentional Y27.0 ☑
    suicide (attempt) X77.0 ☑
  suicide (attempt) X77.9 ☑
  vapor (hot) X13.1 ☑
    assault X98.0 ☑

Scald, scalding — continued
  vapor — continued
    stated as undetermined whether accidental or intentional Y27.0 ☑
    suicide (attempt) X77.0 ☑
Scratched by
  cat W55.03 ☑
  person(s) (accidentally) W50.4 ☑
    with intent to injure or kill Y04.0 ☑
    as, or caused by, a crowd or human stampede (with fall) W52 ☑
    assault Y04.0 ☑
    homicide (attempt) Y04.0 ☑
    in
      fight Y04.0 ☑
      legal intervention
        injuring
          bystander Y35.892 ☑
          law enforcement personnel Y35.891 ☑
          suspect Y35.893 ☑
Seasickness T75.3 ☑
Self-harm NEC (see also External cause by type, undetermined whether accidental or intentional)
  intentional — see Suicide
  poisoning NEC — see Table of Drugs and Chemicals, poisoning, accidental
Self-inflicted (injury) **NEC** (see also External cause by type, undetermined whether accidental or intentional)
  intentional — see Suicide
  poisoning NEC — see Table of Drugs and Chemicals, poisoning, accidental
Sequelae (of)
  accident NEC — see W00-X58 with 7th character S
  assault (homicidal) (any means) — see X92-Y08 with 7th character S
  homicide, attempt (any means) — see X92-Y08 with 7th character S
  injury undetermined whether accidentally or purposely inflicted — see Y21-Y33 with 7th character S
  intentional self-harm (classifiable to X71-X83) — see X71-X83 with 7th character S
  legal intervention — see with 7th character S Y35 ☑
  motor vehicle accident — see V00-V99 with 7th character S
  suicide, attempt (any means) — see X71-X83 with 7th character S
  transport accident — see V00-V99 with 7th character S
  war operations — see War operations
Shock
  electric — see Exposure, electric current
  from electric appliance (any) (faulty) W86.8 ☑
    domestic W86.0 ☑
    suicide (attempt) X83.1 ☑
Shooting, shot (accidental(ly)) (see also Discharge, firearm, by type)
  herself or himself — see Discharge, firearm by type, self-inflicted
  homicide (attempt) — see Discharge, firearm by type, homicide
  in war operations — see War operations
  inflicted by other person — see Discharge, firearm by type, homicide
    accidental — see Discharge, firearm, by type of firearm
  legal
    execution — see Legal, intervention, firearm
    intervention — see Legal, intervention, firearm
  self-inflicted — see Discharge, firearm by type, suicide
    accidental — see Discharge, firearm, by type of firearm
  suicide (attempt) — see Discharge, firearm by type, suicide
Shoving (accidentally) **by other person** — see Pushed, by other person
Sickness
  alpine W94.11 ☑
  motion — see Motion
  mountain W94.11 ☑
Sinking (accidental)
  watercraft (causing drowning, submersion) (see also Drowning, due to, accident to, watercraft, sinking)
    causing injury except drowning or submersion — see Accident, watercraft, causing, injury NEC
Siriasis X32 ☑

Sitting (prolonged) (static) X50.1 ☑
Slashed wrists — see Cut, self-inflicted
Slipping (accidental) (on same level) (with fall) W01.0 ☑
  without fall W18.40 ☑
    due to
      specified NEC W18.49 ☑
      stepping from one level to another W18.43 ☑
      stepping into hole or opening W18.42 ☑
      stepping on object W18.41 ☑
  on
    ice W00.0 ☑
      with skates — see Accident, transport, pedestrian, conveyance
    mud W01.0 ☑
    oil W01.0 ☑
    snow W00.0 ☑
      with skis — see Accident, transport, pedestrian, conveyance
    surface (slippery) (wet) NEC W01.0 ☑
Sliver, wood, contact with W45.8 ☑
Smoldering (due to fire) — see Exposure, fire
Sodomy (attempted) **by force** T74.2 ☑
Sound waves (causing injury) W42.9 ☑
  supersonic W42.0 ☑
Splinter, contact with W45.8 ☑
Stab, stabbing — see Cut
Standing (prolonged) (static) X50.1 ☑
Starvation X58 ☑
Status of external cause Y99.9
  child assisting in compensated work for family Y99.8
  civilian activity done for financial or other compensation Y99.0
  civilian activity done for income or pay Y99.0
  family member assisting in compensated work for other family member Y99.8
  hobby not done for income Y99.8
  leisure activity Y99.8
  military activity Y99.1
  off-duty activity of military personnel Y99.8
  recreation or sport not for income or while a student Y99.8
  specified NEC Y99.8
  student activity Y99.8
  volunteer activity Y99.2
Stepped on
  by
    animal (not being ridden) NEC W55.89 ☑
    crowd or human stampede W52 ☑
    person W50.0 ☑
Stepping on
  object W22.8 ☑
    with fall W18.31 ☑
    sports equipment W21.9 ☑
    stationary W22.09 ☑
      sports equipment W21.89 ☑
  person W51 ☑
    by crowd or human stampede W52 ☑
  sports equipment W21.9 ☑
Sting
  arthropod, nonvenomous W57 ☑
  insect, nonvenomous W57 ☑
Storm (cataclysmic) — see Forces of nature, cataclysmic storm
Straining, excessive (see also Overexertion) X50.9 ☑
Strangling — see Strangulation
Strangulation (accidental) T71 ☑
Strenuous movements (see also Overexertion) X50.9 ☑
Striking against
  airbag (automobile) W22.10 ☑
    driver side W22.11 ☑
    front passenger side W22.12 ☑
    specified NEC W22.19 ☑
  bottom when
    diving or jumping into water (in) W16.822 ☑
      causing drowning W16.821 ☑
      from boat W16.722 ☑
        causing drowning W16.721 ☑
      natural body W16.622 ☑
        causing drowning W16.821 ☑
      swimming pool W16.522 ☑
        causing drowning W16.521 ☑
    falling into water (in) W16.322 ☑
      causing drowning W16.321 ☑
      fountain — see Striking against, bottom when, falling into water, specified NEC
      natural body W16.122 ☑

Striking against — continued
  bottom when — continued
    falling into water — continued
      natural body — continued
        causing drowning W16.121 ☑
      reservoir — see Striking against, bottom when, falling into water, specified NEC
      specified NEC W16.322 ☑
        causing drowning W16.321 ☑
      swimming pool W16.022 ☑
        causing drowning W16.021 ☑
  diving board (swimming-pool) W21.4 ☑
  object W22.8 ☑
    with
      drowning or submersion — see Drowning
      fall — see Fall, due to, bumping against, object
    caused by crowd or human stampede (with fall) W52 ☑
    furniture W22.03 ☑
    lamppost W22.02 ☑
    sports equipment W21.9 ☑
    stationary W22.09 ☑
      sports equipment W21.89 ☑
    wall W22.01 ☑
  person(s) W51 ☑
    with fall W03 ☑
      due to ice or snow W00.0 ☑
    as, or caused by, a crowd or human stampede (with fall) W52 ☑
    assault Y04.2 ☑
    homicide (attempt) Y04.2 ☑
  sports equipment W21.9 ☑
  wall (when) W22.01 ☑
    diving or jumping into water (in) W16.832 ☑
      causing drowning W16.831 ☑
      swimming pool W16.532 ☑
        causing drowning W16.531 ☑
    falling into water (in) W16.332 ☑
      causing drowning W16.331 ☑
      fountain — see Striking against, wall when, falling into water, specified NEC
      natural body W16.132 ☑
        causing drowning W16.131 ☑
      reservoir — see Striking against, wall when, falling into water, specified NEC
      specified NEC W16.332 ☑
        causing drowning W16.331 ☑
      swimming pool W16.032 ☑
        causing drowning W16.031 ☑
    swimming pool (when) W22.042 ☑
      causing drowning W22.041 ☑
      diving or jumping into water W16.532 ☑
        causing drowning W16.531 ☑
      falling into water W16.032 ☑
        causing drowning W16.031 ☑
Struck (accidentally) **by**
  airbag (automobile) W22.10 ☑
    driver side W22.11 ☑
    front passenger side W22.12 ☑
    specified NEC W22.19 ☑
  alligator W58.02 ☑
  animal (not being ridden) NEC W55.89 ☑
  avalanche — see Landslide
  ball (hit) (thrown) W21.00 ☑
    assault Y08.09 ☑
    baseball W21.03 ☑
    basketball W21.05 ☑
    football W21.01 ☑
    golf ball W21.04 ☑
    soccer W21.02 ☑
    softball W21.07 ☑
    specified NEC W21.09 ☑
    volleyball W21.06 ☑
  bat or racquet
    baseball bat W21.11 ☑
      assault Y08.02 ☑
    golf club W21.13 ☑
      assault Y08.09 ☑
    specified NEC W21.19 ☑
      assault Y08.09 ☑
    tennis racquet W21.12 ☑
      assault Y08.09 ☑
  bullet (see also Discharge, firearm by type)
    in war operations — see War operations
  crocodile W58.12 ☑
  dog W54.1 ☑

Struck (accidentally) **by** — continued
  flare, Very pistol — see Discharge, firearm NEC
  hailstones X39.8 ☑
  hockey (ice)
    field
      puck W21.221 ☑
      stick W21.211 ☑
    puck W21.220 ☑
    stick W21.210 ☑
      assault Y08.01 ☑
  landslide — see Landslide
  law-enforcement agent (on duty) — see Legal, intervention, manhandling
    with blunt object — see Legal, intervention, blunt object
  lightning T75.0 ☑
    causing fire — see Exposure, fire
  machine — see Contact, with, by type of machine
  mammal NEC W55.89 ☑
    marine W56.32 ☑
  marine animal W56.82 ☑
  missile
    firearm — see Discharge, firearm by type
    in war operations — see War operations, missile
  object W22.8 ☑
    blunt W22.8 ☑
      assault Y00 ☑
      suicide (attempt) X79 ☑
      undetermined whether accidental or intentional Y29 ☑
    falling W20.8 ☑
      from, in, on
        building W20.1 ☑
          burning (uncontrolled fire) X00.4 ☑
        cataclysmic
          earth surface movement NEC — see Landslide
          storm — see Forces of nature, cataclysmic storm
        cave-in W20.0 ☑
        earthquake X34 ☑
        machine (in operation) — see Contact, with, by type of machine
        structure W20.1 ☑
          burning X00.4 ☑
        transport vehicle (in motion) — see Accident, transport, by type of vehicle
        watercraft V93.49 ☑
          due to
            accident to craft V91.39 ☑
              powered craft V91.33 ☑
                ferry boat V91.31 ☑
                fishing boat V91.32 ☑
                jetskis V91.33 ☑
                liner V91.31 ☑
                merchant ship V91.30 ☑
                passenger ship V91.31 ☑
              unpowered craft V91.38 ☑
                canoe V91.35 ☑
                inflatable V91.36 ☑
                kayak V91.35 ☑
                sailboat V91.34 ☑
                surf-board V91.38 ☑
                windsurfer V91.38 ☑
            powered craft V93.43 ☑
              ferry boat V93.41 ☑
              fishing boat V93.42 ☑
              jetskis V93.43 ☑
              liner V93.41 ☑
              merchant ship V93.40 ☑
              passenger ship V93.41 ☑
            unpowered craft V93.48 ☑
              sailboat V93.44 ☑
              surf-board V93.48 ☑
              windsurfer V93.48 ☑
    moving NEC W20.8 ☑
    projected W20.8 ☑
      assault Y00 ☑
      in sports W21.9 ☑
        assault Y08.09 ☑
        ball W21.00 ☑
          baseball W21.03 ☑
          basketball W21.05 ☑
          football W21.01 ☑
          golf ball W21.04 ☑
          soccer W21.02 ☑

428 ☑ Additional Character Required — Refer to the Tabular List for Character Selection ▽ Subterms under main terms may continue to next column or page

Sitting — Struck

Struck (accidentally) **by** — *continued*
  object — *continued*
    projected — *continued*
      in sports — *continued*
        ball — *continued*
          softball W21.07 ☑
          specified NEC W21.09 ☑
          volleyball W21.06 ☑
        bat or racquet
          baseball bat W21.11 ☑
            assault Y08.02 ☑
          golf club W21.13 ☑
            assault Y08.09 ☑
          specified NEC W21.19 ☑
            assault Y08.09 ☑
          tennis racquet W21.12 ☑
            assault Y08.09 ☑
        hockey (ice)
          field
            puck W21.221 ☑
            stick W21.211 ☑
          puck W21.220 ☑
          stick W21.210 ☑
            assault Y08.01 ☑
        specified NEC W21.89 ☑
    set in motion by explosion — *see* Explosion
    thrown W20.8 ☑
      assault Y00 ☑
      in sports W21.9 ☑
        assault Y08.09 ☑
        ball W21.00 ☑
          baseball W21.03 ☑
          basketball W21.05 ☑
          football W21.01 ☑
          golf ball W21.04 ☑
          soccer W21.02 ☑
          soft ball W21.07 ☑
          specified NEC W21.09 ☑
          volleyball W21.06 ☑
        bat or racquet
          baseball bat W21.11 ☑
            assault Y08.02 ☑
          golf club W21.13 ☑
            assault Y08.09 ☑
          specified NEC W21.19 ☑
            assault Y08.09 ☑
          tennis racquet W21.12 ☑
            assault Y08.09 ☑
        hockey (ice)
          field
            puck W21.221 ☑
            stick W21.211 ☑
          puck W21.220 ☑
          stick W21.210 ☑
            assault Y08.01 ☑
        specified NEC W21.89 ☑
  other person(s) W50.0 ☑
    with
      blunt object W22.8 ☑
      intentional, homicide (attempt) Y00 ☑
      sports equipment W21.9 ☑
      undetermined whether accidental or intentional Y29 ☑
    fall W03 ☑
      due to ice or snow W00.0 ☑
    as, or caused by, a crowd or human stampede (with fall) W52 ☑
    assault Y04.2 ☑
    homicide (attempt) Y04.2 ☑
    in legal intervention
      injuring
        bystander Y35.812 ☑
        law enforcement personnel Y35.811 ☑
        suspect Y35.813 ☑
    sports equipment W21.9 ☑
  police (on duty) — *see* Legal, intervention, manhandling
    with blunt object — *see* Legal, intervention, blunt object
  sports equipment W21.9 ☑
    assault Y08.09 ☑
    ball W21.00 ☑
      baseball W21.03 ☑
      basketball W21.05 ☑
      football W21.01 ☑
      golf ball W21.04 ☑

Struck (accidentally) **by** — *continued*
  sports equipment — *continued*
    ball — *continued*
      soccer W21.02 ☑
      soft ball W21.07 ☑
      specified NEC W21.09 ☑
      volleyball W21.06 ☑
    bat or racquet
      baseball bat W21.11 ☑
        assault Y08.02 ☑
      golf club W21.13 ☑
        assault Y08.09 ☑
      specified NEC W21.19 ☑
      tennis racquet W21.12 ☑
        assault Y08.09 ☑
    cleats (shoe) W21.31 ☑
    foot wear NEC W21.39 ☑
    football helmet W21.81 ☑
    hockey (ice)
      field
        puck W21.221 ☑
        stick W21.211 ☑
      puck W21.220 ☑
      stick W21.210 ☑
        assault Y08.01 ☑
    skate blades W21.32 ☑
    specified NEC W21.89 ☑
      assault Y08.09 ☑
  thunderbolt — *see* subcategory T75.0 ☑
    causing fire — *see* Exposure, fire
  transport vehicle NEC (*see also* Accident, transport) V09.9 ☑
    intentional, homicide (attempt) Y03.0 ☑
    motor NEC (*see also* Accident, transport) V09.20 ☑
      homicide Y03.0 ☑
  vehicle (transport) NEC — *see* Accident, transport, by type of vehicle
    stationary (falling from jack, hydraulic lift, ramp) W20.8 ☑
Stumbling
  without fall W18.40 ☑
    due to
      specified NEC W18.49 ☑
      stepping from one level to another W18.43 ☑
      stepping into hole or opening W18.42 ☑
      stepping on object W18.41 ☑
    over
      animal NEC W01.0 ☑
        with fall W18.09 ☑
      carpet, rug or (small) object W22.8 ☑
        with fall W18.09 ☑
      person W51 ☑
        with fall W03 ☑
          due to ice or snow W00.0 ☑
Submersion (accidental) — *see* Drowning
Suffocation (accidental) (by external means) (by pressure) (mechanical) (*see also* category) T71 ☑
  due to, by
    avalanche — *see* Landslide
    explosion — *see* Explosion
    fire — *see* Exposure, fire
    food, any type (aspiration) (ingestion) (inhalation) — *see* categories T17 and T18 ☑
    ignition — *see* Ignition
    landslide — *see* Landslide
    machine(ry) — *see* Contact, with, by type of machine
    vomitus (aspiration) (inhalation) T17.81- ☑
  in
    burning building X00.8 ☑
Suicide, suicidal (attempted) (by) X83.8 ☑
  blunt object X79 ☑
  burning, burns X76 ☑
    hot object X77.9 ☑
      fluid NEC X77.2 ☑
      household appliance X77.3 ☑
      specified NEC X77.8 ☑
      steam X77.0 ☑
      tap water X77.1 ☑
      vapors X77.0 ☑
  caustic substance — *see* Table of Drugs and Chemicals
  cold, extreme X83.2 ☑
  collision of motor vehicle with
    motor vehicle X82.0 ☑
    specified NEC X82.8 ☑
    train X82.1 ☑

Suicide, suicidal — *continued*
  collision of motor vehicle with — *continued*
    tree X82.2 ☑
  crashing of aircraft X83.0 ☑
  cut (any part of body) X78.9 ☑
  cutting or piercing instrument X78.9 ☑
    dagger X78.2 ☑
    glass X78.0 ☑
    knife X78.1 ☑
    specified NEC X78.8 ☑
    sword X78.2 ☑
  drowning (in) X71.9 ☑
    bathtub X71.0 ☑
    natural water X71.3 ☑
    specified NEC X71.8 ☑
    swimming pool X71.1 ☑
      following fall X71.2 ☑
  electrocution X83.1 ☑
  explosive(s) (material) X75 ☑
  fire, flames X76 ☑
  firearm X74.9 ☑
    airgun X74.01 ☑
    handgun X72 ☑
    hunting rifle X73.1 ☑
    larger X73.9 ☑
      specified NEC X73.8 ☑
    machine gun X73.2 ☑
    shotgun X73.0 ☑
    specified NEC X74.8 ☑
  hanging X83.8 ☑
  hot object — *see* Suicide, burning, hot object
  jumping
    before moving object X81.8 ☑
      motor vehicle X81.0 ☑
      subway train X81.1 ☑
      train X81.1 ☑
    from high place X80 ☑
  late effect of attempt — *see* X71-X83 with 7th character S
  lying before moving object, train, vehicle X81.8 ☑
  poisoning — *see* Table of Drugs and Chemicals
  puncture (any part of body) — *see* Suicide, cutting or piercing instrument
  scald — *see* Suicide, burning, hot object
  sequelae of attempt — *see* X71-X83 with 7th character S
  sharp object (any) — *see* Suicide, cutting or piercing instrument
  shooting — *see* Suicide, firearm
  specified means NEC X83.8 ☑
  stab (any part of body) — *see* Suicide, cutting or piercing instrument
  steam, hot vapors X77.0 ☑
  strangulation X83.8 ☑
  submersion — *see* Suicide, drowning
  suffocation X83.8 ☑
  wound NEC X83.8 ☑
Sunstroke X32 ☑
Supersonic waves (causing injury) W42.0 ☑
Surgical procedure, complication of (delayed or as an abnormal reaction without mention of misadventure) (*see also* Complication of or following, by type of procedure)
  due to or as a result of misadventure — *see* Misadventure
Swallowed, swallowing
  foreign body — *see* Foreign body, alimentary canal
  poison — *see* Table of Drugs and Chemicals
  substance
    caustic or corrosive — *see* Table of Drugs and Chemicals
    poisonous — *see* Table of Drugs and Chemicals

T

Tackle in sport W03 ☑
Terrorism (involving) Y38.80 ☑
  biological weapons Y38.6X- ☑
  chemical weapons Y38.7X- ☑
  conflagration Y38.3X- ☑
  drowning and submersion Y38.89- ☑
  explosion Y38.2X- ☑
    destruction of aircraft Y38.1X- ☑
    marine weapons Y38.0X- ☑
  fire Y38.3X- ☑
  firearms Y38.4X- ☑

▽ Subterms under main terms may continue to next column or page   ☑ Additional Character Required — Refer to the Tabular List for Character Selection   **429**

Struck — Terrorism

Terrorism — *continued*
  hot substances Y38.3X- ☑
  lasers Y38.89- ☑
  nuclear weapons Y38.5X- ☑
  piercing or stabbing instruments Y38.89- ☑
  secondary effects Y38.9X- ☑
  specified method NEC Y38.89- ☑
  suicide bomber Y38.81- ☑
Thirst X58 ☑
Threat to breathing
  aspiration — *see* Aspiration
  due to cave-in, falling earth or substance NEC T71 ☑
Thrown (accidentally)
  against part (any) of or object in transport vehicle (in motion) NEC (*see also* Accident, transport)
  from
    high place, homicide (attempt) Y01 ☑
    machinery — *see* Contact, with, by type of machine
    transport vehicle NEC (*see also* Accident, transport) V89.9 ☑
  off — *see* Thrown, from
Thunderbolt — *see* subcategory T75.0 ☑
  causing fire — *see* Exposure, fire
Tidal wave (any injury) **NEC** — *see* Forces of nature, tidal wave
Took
  overdose (drug) — *see* Table of Drugs and Chemicals
  poison — *see* Table of Drugs and Chemicals
Tornado (any injury) X37.1 ☑
Torrential rain (any injury) X37.8 ☑
Torture X58 ☑
Trampled by animal NEC W55.89 ☑
Trapped (accidentally)
  between objects (moving) (stationary and moving) — *see* Caught
  by part (any) of
    motorcycle V29.88 ☑
    pedal cycle V19.88 ☑
    transport vehicle NEC (*see also* Accident, transport) V89.9 ☑
Travel (effects) (sickness) T75.3 ☑
Tree falling on or hitting (accidentally) (person) W20.8 ☑
Tripping
  without fall W18.40 ☑
    due to
      specified NEC W18.49 ☑
      stepping from one level to another W18.43 ☑
      stepping into hole or opening W18.42 ☑
      stepping on object W18.41 ☑
    over
      animal W01.0 ☑
        with fall W01.0 ☑
      carpet, rug or (small) object W22.8 ☑
        with fall W18.09 ☑
      person W51 ☑
        with fall W03 ☑
          due to ice or snow W00.0 ☑
Twisted by person(s) (accidentally) W50.2 ☑
  with intent to injure or kill Y04.0 ☑
  as, or caused by, a crowd or human stampede (with fall) W52 ☑
  assault Y04.0 ☑
  homicide (attempt) Y04.0 ☑
  in
    fight Y04.0 ☑
    legal intervention — *see* Legal, intervention, manhandling
Twisting (prolonged) (static) X50.1- ☑

U

Underdosing of necessary drugs, medicaments or biological substances Y63.6
Undetermined intent (contact) (exposure)
  automobile collision Y32 ☑
  blunt object Y29 ☑
  drowning (submersion) (in) Y21.9 ☑
    bathtub Y21.0 ☑
      after fall Y21.1 ☑
    natural water (lake) (ocean) (pond) (river) (stream) Y21.4 ☑
    specified place NEC Y21.8 ☑
    swimming pool Y21.2 ☑
      after fall Y21.3 ☑
  explosive material Y25 ☑

Undetermined intent — *continued*
  fall, jump or push from high place Y30 ☑
  falling, lying or running before moving object Y31 ☑
  fire Y26 ☑
  firearm discharge Y24.9 ☑
    airgun (BB) (pellet) Y24.0 ☑
    handgun (pistol) (revolver) Y22 ☑
    hunting rifle Y23.1 ☑
    larger Y23.9 ☑
      hunting rifle Y23.1 ☑
      machine gun Y23.3 ☑
      military Y23.2 ☑
      shotgun Y23.0 ☑
      specified type NEC Y23.8 ☑
    machine gun Y23.3 ☑
    military Y23.2 ☑
    shotgun Y23.0 ☑
    specified type NEC Y24.8 ☑
    Very pistol Y24.8 ☑
  hot object Y27.9 ☑
    fluid NEC Y27.2 ☑
    household appliance Y27.3 ☑
    specified object NEC Y27.8 ☑
    steam Y27.0 ☑
    tap water Y27.1 ☑
    vapor Y27.0 ☑
  jump, fall or push from high place Y30 ☑
  lying, falling or running before moving object Y31 ☑
  motor vehicle crash Y32 ☑
  push, fall or jump from high place Y30 ☑
  running, falling or lying before moving object Y31 ☑
  sharp object Y28.9 ☑
    dagger Y28.2 ☑
    glass Y28.0 ☑
    knife Y28.1 ☑
    specified object NEC Y28.8 ☑
    sword Y28.2 ☑
  smoke Y26 ☑
  specified event NEC Y33 ☑
Use of hand as hammer X50.3 ☑

V

Vibration (causing injury) W49.9 ☑
Victim (of)
  avalanche — *see* Landslide
  earth movements NEC — *see* Forces of nature, earth movement
  earthquake X34 ☑
  flood — *see* Flood
  landslide — *see* Landslide
  lightning — *see* subcategory T75.0 ☑
    causing fire — *see* Exposure, fire
  storm (cataclysmic) NEC — *see* Forces of nature, cataclysmic storm
  volcanic eruption X35 ☑
Volcanic eruption (any injury) X35 ☑
Vomitus, gastric contents in air passages (with asphyxia, obstruction or suffocation) T17.81- ☑

W

Walked into stationary object (any) W22.09 ☑
  furniture W22.03 ☑
  lamppost W22.02 ☑
  wall W22.01 ☑
War operations (injuries to military personnel and civilians during war, civil insurrection and peacekeeping missions) (by) (from) (involving) Y36.90 ☑
  after cessation of hostilities Y36.89- ☑
    explosion (of)
      bomb placed during war operations Y36.82- ☑
      mine placed during war operations Y36.81- ☑
      specified NEC Y36.88- ☑
  air blast Y36.20- ☑
  aircraft
    destruction — *see* War operations, destruction of aircraft
    airway restriction — *see* War operations, restriction of airways
    asphyxiation — *see* War operations, restriction of airways
  biological weapons Y36.6X- ☑
  blast Y36.20- ☑
  blast fragments Y36.20- ☑
  blast wave Y36.20- ☑

War operations — *continued*
  blast wind Y36.20- ☑
  bomb Y36.20- ☑
    dirty Y36.50- ☑
    gasoline Y36.31- ☑
    incendiary Y36.31- ☑
    petrol Y36.31- ☑
  bullet Y36.43- ☑
    incendiary Y36.32- ☑
    rubber Y36.41- ☑
  chemical weapons Y36.7X- ☑
  combat
    hand to hand (unarmed) combat Y36.44- ☑
    using blunt or piercing object Y36.45- ☑
  conflagration — *see* War operations, fire
  conventional warfare NEC Y36.49- ☑
  depth-charge Y36.01- ☑
  destruction of aircraft Y36.10- ☑
    due to
      air to air missile Y36.11- ☑
      collision with other aircraft Y36.12- ☑
      detonation (accidental) of onboard munitions and explosives Y36.14- ☑
      enemy fire or explosives Y36.11- ☑
      explosive placed on aircraft Y36.11- ☑
      onboard fire Y36.13- ☑
      rocket propelled grenade [RPG] Y36.11- ☑
      small arms fire Y36.11- ☑
      surface to air missile Y36.11- ☑
      specified NEC Y36.19- ☑
  detonation (accidental) of
    onboard marine weapons Y36.05- ☑
    own munitions or munitions launch device Y36.24- ☑
  dirty bomb Y36.50- ☑
  explosion (of) Y36.20- ☑
    aerial bomb Y36.21- ☑
    after cessation of hostilities
      bomb placed during war operations Y36.82- ☑
      mine placed during war operations Y36.81- ☑
    bomb NOS (*see also* War operations, bomb(s)) Y36.20- ☑
    fragments Y36.20- ☑
    grenade Y36.29- ☑
    guided missile Y36.22- ☑
    improvised explosive device [IED] (person-borne) (roadside) (vehicle-borne) Y36.23- ☑
    land mine Y36.29- ☑
    marine mine (at sea) (in harbor) Y36.02- ☑
    marine weapon Y36.00- ☑
      specified NEC Y36.09- ☑
    own munitions or munitions launch device (accidental) Y36.24- ☑
    sea-based artillery shell Y36.03- ☑
    specified NEC Y36.29- ☑
    torpedo Y36.04- ☑
  fire Y36.30- ☑
    specified NEC Y36.39- ☑
  firearms
    discharge Y36.43- ☑
    pellets Y36.42- ☑
  flamethrower Y36.33- ☑
  fragments (from) (of)
    improvised explosive device [IED] (person-borne) (roadside) (vehicle-borne) Y36.26- ☑
    munitions Y36.25- ☑
    specified NEC Y36.29- ☑
    weapons Y36.27- ☑
  friendly fire Y36.92 ☑
  hand to hand (unarmed) combat Y36.44- ☑
  hot substances — *see* War operations, fire
  incendiary bullet Y36.32- ☑
  nuclear weapon (effects of) Y36.50- ☑
    acute radiation exposure Y36.54- ☑
    blast pressure Y36.51- ☑
    direct blast Y36.51- ☑
    direct heat Y36.53- ☑
    fallout exposure Y36.54- ☑
    fireball Y36.53- ☑
    indirect blast (struck or crushed by blast debris) (being thrown by blast) Y36.52- ☑
    ionizing radiation (immediate exposure) Y36.54- ☑
    nuclear radiation Y36.54- ☑
    radiation
      ionizing (immediate exposure) Y36.54- ☑
      nuclear Y36.54- ☑

☑ **Additional Character Required** — Refer to the Tabular List for Character Selection   ▽ **Subterms under main terms may continue to next column or page**

War operations — *continued*
  nuclear weapon — *continued*
    radiation — *continued*
      thermal Y36.53- ☑
    secondary effects Y36.54- ☑
    specified NEC Y36.59- ☑
    thermal radiation Y36.53- ☑
  restriction of air (airway)
    intentional Y36.46- ☑
    unintentional Y36.47- ☑
  rubber bullets Y36.41- ☑
  shrapnel NOS Y36.29- ☑
  suffocation — *see* War operations, restriction of airways
  unconventional warfare NEC Y36.7X- ☑
  underwater blast NOS Y36.00- ☑
  warfare
    conventional NEC Y36.49- ☑
    unconventional NEC Y36.7X- ☑

War operations — *continued*
  weapon of mass destruction [WMD] Y36.91 ☑
  weapons
    biological weapons Y36.6X- ☑
    chemical Y36.7X- ☑
    nuclear (effects of) Y36.50- ☑
      acute radiation exposure Y36.54- ☑
      blast pressure Y36.51- ☑
      direct blast Y36.51- ☑
      direct heat Y36.53- ☑
      fallout exposure Y36.54- ☑
      fireball Y36.53- ☑
      radiation
        ionizing (immediate exposure) Y36.54- ☑
        nuclear Y36.54- ☑
        thermal Y36.53- ☑
      secondary effects Y36.54- ☑
      specified NEC Y36.59- ☑
  of mass destruction [WMD] Y36.91 ☑

Washed
  away by flood — *see* Flood
  off road by storm (transport vehicle) — *see* Forces of nature, cataclysmic storm
Weather exposure NEC — *see* Forces of nature
Weightlessness (causing injury) (effects of) (in spacecraft, real or simulated) X52 ☑
Work related condition Y99.0
Wound (accidental) NEC (*see also* Injury) X58 ☑
  battle (*see also* War operations) Y36.90 ☑
  gunshot — *see* Discharge, firearm by type
Wreck transport vehicle NEC (*see also* Accident, transport) V89.9 ☑
Wrong
  device implanted into correct surgical site Y65.51
  fluid in infusion Y65.1
  patient, procedure performed on Y65.52
  procedure (operation) on correct patient Y65.51

ICD-10-CM Tabular List of Diseases and Injuries

Chapter 1. Certain Infectious and Parasitic Diseases (A00–B99)

Chapter Specific Guidelines with Coding Examples

The chapter specific guidelines from the ICD-10-CM Official Guidelines for Coding and Reporting have been provided below. Along with these guidelines are coding examples, contained in the shaded boxes, that have been developed to help illustrate the coding and/or sequencing guidance found in these guidelines.

a. Human immunodeficiency virus (HIV) infections

1) Code only confirmed cases

Code only confirmed cases of HIV infection/illness. This is an exception to the hospital inpatient guideline Section II, H.

In this context, "confirmation" does not require documentation of positive serology or culture for HIV; the provider's diagnostic statement that the patient is HIV positive, or has an HIV-related illness is sufficient.

> Patient being seen for hypothyroidism with possible HIV infection
>
> **E03.9**   **Hypothyroidism, unspecified**
>
> *Explanation:* Only the hypothyroidism is coded in this scenario because it has not been confirmed that an HIV infection is present.

2) Selection and sequencing of HIV codes

(a) Patient admitted for HIV-related condition

If a patient is admitted for an HIV-related condition, the principal diagnosis should be B20, Human immunodeficiency virus [HIV] disease followed by additional diagnosis codes for all reported HIV-related conditions.

> HIV with CMV
>
> **B20**   **Human immunodeficiency virus [HIV] disease**
>
> **B25.9**   **Cytomegaloviral disease, unspecified**
>
> *Explanation:* Cytomegaloviral infection is an HIV related condition, so the HIV diagnosis code is reported first, followed by the code for the CMV.

(b) Patient with HIV disease admitted for unrelated condition

If a patient with HIV disease is admitted for an unrelated condition (such as a traumatic injury), the code for the unrelated condition (e.g., the nature of injury code) should be the principal diagnosis. Other diagnoses would be B20 followed by additional diagnosis codes for all reported HIV-related conditions.

> Sprain of the internal collateral ligament, right ankle; HIV
>
> **S93.491A**   **Sprain of other ligament of right ankle, initial encounter**
>
> **B20**   **Human immunodeficiency virus [HIV] disease**
>
> *Explanation:* The ankle sprain is not related to HIV, so it is the first-listed diagnosis code, and HIV is reported secondarily.

(c) Whether the patient is newly diagnosed

Whether the patient is newly diagnosed or has had previous admissions/encounters for HIV conditions is irrelevant to the sequencing decision.

> Newly diagnosed multiple cutaneous Kaposi's sarcoma lesions in previously diagnosed HIV disease
>
> **B20**   **Human immunodeficiency virus [HIV] disease**
>
> **C46.0**   **Kaposi's sarcoma of skin**
>
> *Explanation:* Even though the HIV was diagnosed on a previous encounter, it is still sequenced first when coded with an HIV related condition. Kaposi's sarcoma is an HIV-related condition.

(d) Asymptomatic human immunodeficiency virus

Z21, Asymptomatic human immunodeficiency virus [HIV] infection status, is to be applied when the patient without any documentation of symptoms is listed as being "HIV positive," "known HIV," "HIV test positive," or similar terminology. Do not use this code if the term "AIDS" is used or if the patient is treated for any HIV-related illness or is described as having any condition(s) resulting from his/her HIV positive status; use B20 in these cases.

> Patient is being seen for iron deficiency anemia. Status positive HIV test on Atripla, with no prior symptoms
>
> **D50.9**   **Iron deficiency anemia, unspecified**
>
> **Z21**   **Asymptomatic human immunodeficiency virus [HIV] infection status**
>
> *Explanation:* Code Z21 is sequenced second since documentation indicates that the patient has had a positive HIV test but has been asymptomatic. Being on medication for HIV is not an indication that code B20 is used instead of Z21. Unless there has been documentation that the patient has had current or prior symptoms or HIV-related complications, code B20 is not used. The anemia is not an AIDS-related complication and is sequenced first.

(e) Patients with inconclusive HIV serology

Patients with inconclusive HIV serology, but no definitive diagnosis or manifestations of the illness, may be assigned code R75, Inconclusive laboratory evidence of human immunodeficiency virus [HIV].

(f) Previously diagnosed HIV-related illness

Patients with any known prior diagnosis of an HIV-related illness should be coded to B20. Once a patient has developed an HIV-related illness, the patient should always be assigned code B20 on every subsequent admission/encounter. Patients previously diagnosed with any HIV illness (B20) should never be assigned to R75 or Z21, Asymptomatic human immunodeficiency virus [HIV] infection status.

(g) HIV infection in pregnancy, childbirth and the puerperium

During pregnancy, childbirth or the puerperium, a patient admitted (or presenting for a health care encounter) because of an HIV-related illness should receive a principal diagnosis code of O98.7-, Human immunodeficiency [HIV] disease complicating pregnancy, childbirth and the puerperium, followed by B20 and the code(s) for the HIV-related illness(es). Codes from Chapter 15 always take sequencing priority.

Patients with asymptomatic HIV infection status admitted (or presenting for a health care encounter) during pregnancy, childbirth, or the puerperium should receive codes of O98.7- and Z21.

(h) Encounters for testing for HIV

If a patient is being seen to determine his/her HIV status, use code Z11.4, Encounter for screening for human immunodeficiency virus [HIV]. Use additional codes for any associated high risk behavior.

If a patient with signs or symptoms is being seen for HIV testing, code the signs and symptoms. An additional counseling code Z71.7, Human immunodeficiency virus [HIV] counseling, may be used if counseling is provided during the encounter for the test.

When a patient returns to be informed of his/her HIV test results and the test result is negative, use code Z71.7, Human immunodeficiency virus [HIV] counseling.

If the results are positive, see previous guidelines and assign codes as appropriate.

b. Infectious agents as the cause of diseases classified to other chapters

Certain infections are classified in chapters other than Chapter 1 and no organism is identified as part of the infection code. In these instances, it is necessary to use an additional code from Chapter 1 to identify the organism. A code from category B95, Streptococcus, Staphylococcus, and Enterococcus as the cause of diseases classified to other chapters, B96, Other bacterial agents as the cause of diseases classified to other chapters, or B97, Viral agents as the cause of diseases classified to other chapters, is to be used as an additional code to identify the organism. An instructional note will be found at the infection code advising that an additional organism code is required.

Acute *E. coli* cystitis

N30.00	**Acute cystitis without hematuria**
B96.20	**Unspecified Escherichia coli [E.coli] as the cause of diseases classified elsewhere**

Explanation: An instructional note under the category for the cystitis indicates to code also the specific organism.

c. Infections resistant to antibiotics

Many bacterial infections are resistant to current antibiotics. It is necessary to identify all infections documented as antibiotic resistant. Assign a code from category Z16, Resistance to antimicrobial drugs, following the infection code only if the infection code does not identify drug resistance.

Penicillin-resistant *Streptococcus pneumoniae* pneumonia

J13	**Pneumonia due to Streptococcus pneumoniae**
Z16.11	**Resistance to penicillins**

Explanation: Code Z16.11 is assigned as a secondary code to represent the penicillin resistance. This code includes resistance to amoxicillin and ampicillin.

d. Sepsis, severe sepsis, and septic shock

1) Coding of Sepsis and Severe Sepsis

(a) Sepsis

For a diagnosis of sepsis, assign the appropriate code for the underlying systemic infection. If the type of infection or causal organism is not further specified, assign code A41.9, Sepsis, unspecified organism.

A code from subcategory R65.2, Severe sepsis, should not be assigned unless severe sepsis or an associated acute organ dysfunction is documented.

Gram-negative sepsis

A41.50	**Gram-negative sepsis, unspecified**

Staphylococcal sepsis

A41.2	**Sepsis due to unspecified staphylococcus**

Explanation: In both examples above the organism causing the sepsis is identified, therefore A41.9 Sepsis, unspecified organism, would not be appropriate as this code would not capture the highest degree of specificity found in the documentation. Do not use an additional code for severe sepsis unless an acute organ dysfunction was also documented as "associated with" or "due to" the sepsis or the sepsis was documented as "severe."

(i) Negative or inconclusive blood cultures and sepsis

Negative or inconclusive blood cultures do not preclude a diagnosis of sepsis in patients with clinical evidence of the condition; however, the provider should be queried.

(ii) Urosepsis

The term urosepsis is a nonspecific term. It is not to be considered synonymous with sepsis. It has no default code in the Alphabetic Index. Should a provider use this term, he/she must be queried for clarification.

(iii) Sepsis with organ dysfunction

If a patient has sepsis and associated acute organ dysfunction or multiple organ dysfunction (MOD), follow the instructions for coding severe sepsis.

(iv) Acute organ dysfunction that is not clearly associated with the sepsis

If a patient has sepsis and an acute organ dysfunction, but the medical record documentation indicates that the acute organ dysfunction is related to a medical condition other than the sepsis, do not assign a code from subcategory R65.2, Severe sepsis. An acute organ dysfunction must be associated with the sepsis in order to assign the severe sepsis code. If the documentation is not clear as to whether an acute organ dysfunction is related to the sepsis or another medical condition, query the provider.

Sepsis and acute respiratory failure due to COPD exacerbation

A41.9	**Sepsis, unspecified organism**
J44.1	**Chronic obstructive pulmonary disease with (acute) exacerbation**
J96.00	**Acute respiratory failure, unspecified whether with hypoxia or hypercapnia**

Explanation: Although acute organ dysfunction is present in the form of acute respiratory failure, severe sepsis (R65.2) is not coded in this example, as the acute respiratory failure is attributed to the COPD exacerbation rather than the sepsis. Sequencing of these codes would be determined by the reason for the encounter.

(b) Severe sepsis

The coding of severe sepsis requires a minimum of 2 codes: first a code for the underlying systemic infection, followed by a code from subcategory R65.2, Severe sepsis. If the causal organism is not documented, assign code A41.9, Sepsis, unspecified organism, for the infection. Additional code(s) for the associated acute organ dysfunction are also required.

Due to the complex nature of severe sepsis, some cases may require querying the provider prior to assignment of the codes.

2) Septic shock

(a) Septic shock generally refers to circulatory failure associated with severe sepsis, and therefore, it represents a type of acute organ dysfunction.

For cases of septic shock, the code for the systemic infection should be sequenced first, followed by code R65.21, Severe sepsis with septic shock or code T81.12, Postprocedural septic shock. Any additional codes for the other acute organ dysfunctions should also be assigned. As noted in the sequencing instructions in the Tabular List, the code for septic shock cannot be assigned as a principal diagnosis.

Sepsis with septic shock

A41.9	**Sepsis, unspecified organism**
R65.21	**Severe sepsis with septic shock**

Explanation: Documentation of septic shock automatically implies severe sepsis as it is a form of acute organ dysfunction. Septic shock is not coded as the first-listed diagnosis; it is always preceded by the code for the systemic infection.

3) Sequencing of severe sepsis

If severe sepsis is present on admission, and meets the definition of principal diagnosis, the underlying systemic infection should be assigned as principal diagnosis followed by the appropriate code from subcategory R65.2 as required by the sequencing rules in the Tabular List. A code from subcategory R65.2 can never be assigned as a principal diagnosis.

When severe sepsis develops during an encounter (it was not present on admission), the underlying systemic infection and the appropriate code from subcategory R65.2 should be assigned as secondary diagnoses.

Severe sepsis may be present on admission, but the diagnosis may not be confirmed until sometime after admission. If the documentation is not clear whether severe sepsis was present on admission, the provider should be queried.

4) Sepsis and severe sepsis with a localized infection

If the reason for admission is both sepsis or severe sepsis and a localized infection, such as pneumonia or cellulitis, a code(s) for the underlying systemic infection should be assigned first and the code for the localized infection should be assigned as a secondary diagnosis. If the patient has severe sepsis, a code from subcategory R65.2 should also be assigned as a secondary diagnosis. If the patient is admitted with a localized infection, such as pneumonia, and sepsis/severe sepsis doesn't develop until after admission, the localized infection should be assigned first, followed by the appropriate sepsis/severe sepsis codes.

Patient presents with acute renal failure due to severe sepsis from *Pseudomonas pneumonia*

A41.52	Sepsis, due to Pseudomonas
J15.1	Pneumonia due to Pseudomonas
R65.20	Severe sepsis without septic shock
N17.9	Acute kidney failure, unspecified

Explanation: If all conditions are present, the systemic infection (sepsis) is sequenced first followed by the codes for the localized infection (pneumonia), severe sepsis and any organ dysfunction.

5) Sepsis due to a postprocedural infection

(a) Documentation of causal relationship

As with all postprocedural complications, code assignment is based on the provider's documentation of the relationship between the infection and the procedure.

(b) Sepsis due to a postprocedural infection

For such cases, the postprocedural infection code, such as T80.2, Infections following infusion, transfusion, and therapeutic injection, T81.4, Infection following a procedure, T88.0, Infection following immunization, or O86.0, Infection of obstetric surgical wound, should be coded first, followed by the code for the specific infection. If the patient has severe sepsis, the appropriate code from subcategory R65.2 should also be assigned with the additional code(s) for any acute organ dysfunction.

(c) Postprocedural infection and postprocedural septic shock

In cases where a postprocedural infection has occurred and has resulted in severe sepsis the code for the precipitating complication such as code T81.4, Infection following a procedure, or O86.0, Infection of obstetrical surgical wound should be coded first followed by code R65.20, Severe sepsis without septic shock. A code for the systemic infection should also be assigned.

If a postprocedural infection has resulted in postprocedural septic shock, the code for the precipitating complication such as code T81.4, Infection following a procedure, or O86.0, Infection of obstetrical surgical wound should be coded first followed by code T81.12-, Postprocedural septic shock. A code for the systemic infection should also be assigned.

6) Sepsis and severe sepsis associated with a noninfectious process (condition)

In some cases a noninfectious process (condition), such as trauma, may lead to an infection which can result in sepsis or severe sepsis. If sepsis or severe sepsis is documented as associated with a noninfectious condition, such as a burn or serious injury, and this condition meets the definition for principal diagnosis, the code for the noninfectious condition should be sequenced first, followed by the code for the resulting infection. If severe sepsis is present, a code from subcategory R65.2 should also be assigned with any associated organ dysfunction(s) codes. It is not necessary to assign a code from subcategory R65.1, Systemic inflammatory response syndrome (SIRS) of non-infectious origin, for these cases.

If the infection meets the definition of principal diagnosis, it should be sequenced before the non-infectious condition. When both the associated non-infectious condition and the infection meet the definition of principal diagnosis, either may be assigned as principal diagnosis.

Only one code from category R65, Symptoms and signs specifically associated with systemic inflammation and infection, should be assigned. Therefore, when a non-infectious condition leads to an infection resulting in severe sepsis, assign the appropriate code from subcategory R65.2, Severe sepsis. Do not additionally assign a code from subcategory R65.1, Systemic inflammatory response syndrome (SIRS) of non-infectious origin.

See Section I.C.18. SIRS due to non-infectious process

7) Sepsis and septic shock complicating abortion, pregnancy, childbirth, and the puerperium

See Section I.C.15. Sepsis and septic shock complicating abortion, pregnancy, childbirth and the puerperium

8) Newborn sepsis

See Section I.C.16. f. Bacterial sepsis of Newborn

e. Methicillin resistant *Staphylococcus aureus* (MRSA) conditions

1) Selection and sequencing of MRSA codes

(a) Combination codes for MRSA infection

When a patient is diagnosed with an infection that is due to methicillin resistant *Staphylococcus aureus* (MRSA), and that infection has a combination code that includes the causal organism (e.g., sepsis, pneumonia) assign the appropriate combination code for the condition (e.g., code A41.02, Sepsis due to Methicillin resistant Staphylococcus aureus or code J15.212, Pneumonia due to Methicillin resistant Staphylococcus aureus). Do not assign code B95.62, Methicillin resistant Staphylococcus aureus infection as the cause of diseases classified elsewhere, as an additional code, because the combination code includes the type of infection and the MRSA organism. Do not assign a code from subcategory Z16.11, Resistance to penicillins, as an additional diagnosis.

See Section C.1. for instructions on coding and sequencing of sepsis and severe sepsis.

(b) Other codes for MRSA infection

When there is documentation of a current infection (e.g., wound infection, stitch abscess, urinary tract infection) due to MRSA, and that infection does not have a combination code that includes the causal organism, assign the appropriate code to identify the condition along with code B95.62, Methicillin resistant Staphylococcus aureus infection as the cause of diseases classified elsewhere for the MRSA infection. Do not assign a code from subcategory Z16.11, Resistance to penicillins.

(c) Methicillin susceptible Staphylococcus aureus (MSSA) and MRSA colonization

The condition or state of being colonized or carrying MSSA or MRSA is called colonization or carriage, while an individual person is described as being colonized or being a carrier. Colonization means that MSSA or MSRA is present on or in the body without necessarily causing illness. A positive MRSA colonization test might be documented by the provider as "MRSA screen positive" or "MRSA nasal swab positive".

Assign code Z22.322, Carrier or suspected carrier of Methicillin resistant Staphylococcus aureus, for patients documented as having MRSA colonization. Assign code Z22.321, Carrier or suspected carrier of Methicillin susceptible Staphylococcus aureus, for patient documented as having MSSA colonization. Colonization is not necessarily indicative of a disease process or as the cause of a specific condition the patient may have unless documented as such by the provider.

(d) MRSA colonization and infection

If a patient is documented as having both MRSA colonization and infection during a hospital admission, code Z22.322, Carrier or suspected carrier of Methicillin resistant Staphylococcus aureus, and a code for the MRSA Infection may both be assigned.

f. Zika virus infections

1) Code only confirmed cases

Code only a confirmed diagnosis of Zika virus (A92.5, Zika virus disease) as documented by the provider. This is an exception to the hospital inpatient guideline Section II, H.

In this context, "confirmation" does not require documentation of the type of test performed; the physician's diagnostic statement that the condition is confirmed is sufficient. This code should be assigned regardless of the stated mode of transmission.

If the provider documents "suspected", "possible" or "probable" Zika, do not assign code A92.5. Assign a code(s) explaining the reason for encounter (such as fever, rash, or joint pain) or Z20.828, Contact with and (suspected) exposure to other viral communicable diseases.

Chapter 1. Certain Infectious and Parasitic Diseases (A00-B99)

INCLUDES   diseases generally recognized as communicable or transmissible

Use additional code to identify resistance to antimicrobial drugs (Z16.-)

EXCLUDES 1   *certain localized infections—see body system-related chapters*

EXCLUDES 2   *carrier or suspected carrier of infectious disease (Z22.-)*
infectious and parasitic diseases specific to the perinatal period (P35-P39)
infectious and parasitic diseases complicating pregnancy, childbirth and the puerperium (O98.-)
influenza and other acute respiratory infections (J00-J22)

This chapter contains the following blocks:

A00-A09   Intestinal infectious diseases
A15-A19   Tuberculosis
A20-A28   Certain zoonotic bacterial diseases
A30-A49   Other bacterial diseases
A50-A64   Infections with a predominantly sexual mode of transmission
A65-A69   Other spirochetal diseases
A70-A74   Other diseases caused by chlamydiae
A75-A79   Rickettsioses
A80-A89   Viral infections of the central nervous system
A90-A99   Arthropod-borne viral fevers and viral hemorrhagic fevers
B00-B09   Viral infections characterized by skin and mucous membrane lesions
B10   Other human herpesviruses
B15-B19   Viral hepatitis
B20   Human immunodeficiency virus [HIV] disease
B25-B34   Other viral diseases
B35-B49   Mycoses
B50-B64   Protozoal diseases
B65-B83   Helminthiases
B85-B89   Pediculosis, acariasis and other infestations
B90-B94   Sequelae of infectious and parasitic diseases
B95-B97   Bacterial and viral infectious agents
B99   Other infectious diseases

Intestinal Infectious Diseases (A00-A09)

✓4ᵗʰ **A00 Cholera**

     A00.0 Cholera due to Vibrio cholerae 01, biovar cholerae
         Classical cholera

     A00.1 Cholera due to Vibrio cholerae 01, biovar eltor
         Cholera eltor

     A00.9 Cholera, unspecified   ▽

✓4ᵗʰ **A01 Typhoid and paratyphoid fevers**

     DEF: Typhoid fever: An acute generalized illness caused by *Salmonella typhi*; clinical features are fever, headache, abdominal pain, cough, toxemia, leukopenia, abnormal pulse, rose spots on the skin, bacteremia, hyperplasia of intestinal lymph nodes, mesenteric lymphadenopathy, and Peyer's patches in the intestines.
     DEF: Paratyphoid fever: A prolonged febrile illness, caused by *Salmonella* serotypes other than *S. typhi*, especially *S. enterica* serotypes paratyphi A, B, and C.

     ✓5ᵗʰ **A01.0 Typhoid fever**
         Infection due to Salmonella typhi

         A01.00 Typhoid fever, unspecified   ▽

         A01.01 Typhoid meningitis

         A01.02 Typhoid fever with heart involvement
            Typhoid endocarditis
            Typhoid myocarditis

         A01.03 Typhoid pneumonia   HCC

         A01.04 Typhoid arthritis   HCC

         A01.05 Typhoid osteomyelitis   HCC

         A01.09 Typhoid fever with other complications

     A01.1 Paratyphoid fever A

     A01.2 Paratyphoid fever B

     A01.3 Paratyphoid fever C

     A01.4 Paratyphoid fever, unspecified   ▽
         Infection due to Salmonella paratyphi NOS

✓4ᵗʰ **A02 Other salmonella infections**
     INCLUDES   infection or foodborne intoxication due to any Salmonella species other than S. typhi and S. paratyphi

     A02.0 Salmonella enteritis
         Salmonellosis

     A02.1 Salmonella sepsis   HCC

     ✓5ᵗʰ **A02.2 Localized salmonella infections**

         A02.20 Localized salmonella infection, unspecified   ▽

         A02.21 Salmonella meningitis

         A02.22 Salmonella pneumonia   HCC

         A02.23 Salmonella arthritis   HCC

         A02.24 Salmonella osteomyelitis   HCC

         A02.25 Salmonella pyelonephritis
            Salmonella tubulo-interstitial nephropathy

         A02.29 Salmonella with other localized infection

     A02.8 Other specified salmonella infections

     A02.9 Salmonella infection, unspecified   ▽

✓4ᵗʰ **A03 Shigellosis**
     DEF: Infection caused by the genus *Shigella*, of the family *Enterobacteriaceae*; known to cause an acute dysenteric infection of the bowel with fever, drowsiness, anorexia, nausea, vomiting, bloody diarrhea, abdominal cramps, and distention.

     A03.0 Shigellosis due to Shigella dysenteriae
         Group A shigellosis [Shiga-Kruse dysentery]

     A03.1 Shigellosis due to Shigella flexneri
         Group B shigellosis

     A03.2 Shigellosis due to Shigella boydii
         Group C shigellosis

     A03.3 Shigellosis due to Shigella sonnei
         Group D shigellosis

     A03.8 Other shigellosis

     A03.9 Shigellosis, unspecified   ▽
         Bacillary dysentery NOS

✓4ᵗʰ **A04 Other bacterial intestinal infections**
     EXCLUDES 1   *bacterial foodborne intoxications, NEC (A05.-)*
                tuberculous enteritis (A18.32)

     A04.0 Enteropathogenic Escherichia coli infection

     A04.1 Enterotoxigenic Escherichia coli infection

     A04.2 Enteroinvasive Escherichia coli infection

     A04.3 Enterohemorrhagic Escherichia coli infection
         DEF: *E. coli* infection penetrating the intestinal mucosa, producing microscopic ulceration and bleeding.

     A04.4 Other intestinal Escherichia coli infections
         Escherichia coli enteritis NOS

     A04.5 Campylobacter enteritis

     A04.6 Enteritis due to Yersinia enterocolitica
         EXCLUDES 1   *extraintestinal yersiniosis (A28.2)*

     ✓5ᵗʰ **A04.7 Enterocolitis due to Clostridium difficile**
         Foodborne intoxication by Clostridium difficile
         Pseudomembraneous colitis

●   **A04.71 Enterocolitis due to Clostridium difficile, recurrent**

●   **A04.72 Enterocolitis due to Clostridium difficile, not specified as recurrent**

     A04.8 Other specified bacterial intestinal infections

     A04.9 Bacterial intestinal infection, unspecified   ▽
         Bacterial enteritis NOS

✓4ᵗʰ **A05 Other bacterial foodborne intoxications, not elsewhere classified**
     EXCLUDES 1   *Clostridium difficile foodborne intoxication and infection* ▶*(A04.7-)*◀
                Escherichia coli infection (A04.0-A04.4)
                listeriosis (A32.-)
                salmonella foodborne intoxication and infection (A02.-)
                toxic effect of noxious foodstuffs (T61-T62)

     A05.0 Foodborne staphylococcal intoxication

     A05.1 Botulism food poisoning
         Botulism NOS
         Classical foodborne intoxication due to Clostridium botulinum
         EXCLUDES 1   *infant botulism (A48.51)*
                    wound botulism (A48.52)

     A05.2 Foodborne Clostridium perfringens [Clostridium welchii] intoxication
         Enteritis necroticans
         Pig-bel

     A05.3 Foodborne Vibrio parahaemolyticus intoxication

     A05.4 Foodborne Bacillus cereus intoxication

     A05.5 Foodborne Vibrio vulnificus intoxication

     A05.8 Other specified bacterial foodborne intoxications

     A05.9 Bacterial foodborne intoxication, unspecified   ▽

☑️⁴ᵗʰ **A06 Amebiasis**
  INCLUDES infection due to Entamoeba histolytica
  EXCLUDES 1 *other protozoal intestinal diseases (A07.-)*
  EXCLUDES 2 *acanthamebiasis (B60.1-)*
           Naegleriasis (B60.2)

  A06.0 Acute amebic dysentery
       Acute amebiasis
       Intestinal amebiasis NOS

  A06.1 Chronic intestinal amebiasis

  A06.2 Amebic nondysenteric colitis

  A06.3 Ameboma of intestine
       Ameboma NOS

  A06.4 Amebic liver abscess
       Hepatic amebiasis

  A06.5 Amebic lung abscess   HCC
       Amebic abscess of lung (and liver)

  A06.6 Amebic brain abscess
       Amebic abscess of brain (and liver) (and lung)

  A06.7 Cutaneous amebiasis

☑️⁵ᵗʰ **A06.8 Amebic infection of other sites**
       A06.81 Amebic cystitis
       A06.82 Other amebic genitourinary infections
            Amebic balanitis
            Amebic vesiculitis
            Amebic vulvovaginitis
       A06.89 Other amebic infections
            Amebic appendicitis
            Amebic splenic abscess

  A06.9 Amebiasis, unspecified   ▽

☑️⁴ᵗʰ **A07 Other protozoal intestinal diseases**
  A07.0 Balantidiasis
       Balantidial dysentery

  A07.1 Giardiasis [lambliasis]

  A07.2 Cryptosporidiosis   HCC

  A07.3 Isosporiasis
       Infection due to Isospora belli and Isospora hominis
       Intestinal coccidiosis
       Isosporosis

  A07.4 Cyclosporiasis

  A07.8 Other specified protozoal intestinal diseases
       Intestinal microsporidiosis
       Intestinal trichomoniasis
       Sarcocystosis
       Sarcosporidiosis

  A07.9 Protozoal intestinal disease, unspecified   ▽
       Flagellate diarrhea
       Protozoal colitis
       Protozoal diarrhea
       Protozoal dysentery

☑️⁴ᵗʰ **A08 Viral and other specified intestinal infections**
  EXCLUDES 1 *influenza with involvement of gastrointestinal tract (J09.X3, J10.2, J11.2)*

  A08.0 Rotaviral enteritis

☑️⁵ᵗʰ **A08.1 Acute gastroenteropathy due to Norwalk agent and other small round viruses**
       A08.11 Acute gastroenteropathy due to Norwalk agent
            Acute gastroenteropathy due to Norovirus
            Acute gastroenteropathy due to Norwalk-like agent
       A08.19 Acute gastroenteropathy due to other small round viruses
            Acute gastroenteropathy due to small round virus [SRV] NOS

  A08.2 Adenoviral enteritis

☑️⁵ᵗʰ **A08.3 Other viral enteritis**
       A08.31 Calicivirus enteritis
       A08.32 Astrovirus enteritis
       A08.39 Other viral enteritis
            Coxsackie virus enteritis
            Echovirus enteritis
            Enterovirus enteritis NEC
            Torovirus enteritis

  A08.4 Viral intestinal infection, unspecified   ▽
       Viral enteritis NOS
       Viral gastroenteritis NOS
       Viral gastroenteropathy NOS
       AHA: 2016, 3Q, 12

  A08.8 Other specified intestinal infections

A09 Infectious gastroenteritis and colitis, unspecified   ▽
     Infectious colitis NOS
     Infectious enteritis NOS
     Infectious gastroenteritis NOS
     EXCLUDES 1 *colitis NOS (K52.9)*
              diarrhea NOS (R19.7)
              enteritis NOS (K52.9)
              gastroenteritis NOS (K52.9)
              noninfective gastroenteritis and colitis, unspecified (K52.9)
     DEF: Colitis: An inflammation of mucous membranes of the colon.
     DEF: Enteritis: An inflammation of mucous membranes of the small intestine.
     DEF: Gastroenteritis: An inflammation of mucous membranes of stomach and intestines.

Tuberculosis (A15-A19)

  INCLUDES infections due to Mycobacterium tuberculosis and Mycobacterium bovis
  EXCLUDES 1 *congenital tuberculosis (P37.0)*
           nonspecific reaction to test for tuberculosis without active tuberculosis (R76.1-)
           pneumoconiosis associated with tuberculosis, any type in A15 (J65)
           positive PPD (R76.11)
           positive tuberculin skin test without active tuberculosis (R76.11)
           sequelae of tuberculosis (B90.-)
           silicotuberculosis (J65)

☑️⁴ᵗʰ **A15 Respiratory tuberculosis**
  A15.0 Tuberculosis of lung
       Tuberculous bronchiectasis
       Tuberculous fibrosis of lung
       Tuberculous pneumonia
       Tuberculous pneumothorax

  A15.4 Tuberculosis of intrathoracic lymph nodes
       Tuberculosis of hilar lymph nodes
       Tuberculosis of mediastinal lymph nodes
       Tuberculosis of tracheobronchial lymph nodes
       EXCLUDES 1 *tuberculosis specified as primary (A15.7)*

  A15.5 Tuberculosis of larynx, trachea and bronchus
       Tuberculosis of bronchus   Tuberculosis of larynx
       Tuberculosis of glottis   Tuberculosis of trachea

  A15.6 Tuberculous pleurisy
       Tuberculosis of pleura Tuberculous empyema
       EXCLUDES 1 *primary respiratory tuberculosis (A15.7)*

  A15.7 Primary respiratory tuberculosis

  A15.8 Other respiratory tuberculosis
       Mediastinal tuberculosis
       Nasopharyngeal tuberculosis
       Tuberculosis of nose
       Tuberculosis of sinus [any nasal]

  A15.9 Respiratory tuberculosis unspecified   ▽

☑️⁴ᵗʰ **A17 Tuberculosis of nervous system**
  A17.0 Tuberculous meningitis
       Tuberculosis of meninges (cerebral) (spinal)
       Tuberculous leptomeningitis
       EXCLUDES 1 *tuberculous meningoencephalitis (A17.82)*

  A17.1 Meningeal tuberculoma
       Tuberculoma of meninges (cerebral) (spinal)
       EXCLUDES 2 *tuberculoma of brain and spinal cord (A17.81)*

Tuberculosis of Lung

Granulomas from Mycobacterium tuberculosis

☑️ Additional Character Req   ✕ˣ⁷ᵗʰ Placeholder Alert   Manifestation   HCC CMS-HCC Condition   ▽ Unspecified Code   ►◄ Revised Text   ● New Code   ▲ Revised Code Title

ICD-10-CM 2018   437

Chapter 1. Certain Infectious and Parasitic Diseases

A17.8 Other tuberculosis of nervous system
- **A17.81 Tuberculoma of brain and spinal cord**
  Tuberculous abscess of brain and spinal cord
- **A17.82 Tuberculous meningoencephalitis**
  Tuberculous myelitis
- **A17.83 Tuberculous neuritis**
  Tuberculous mononeuropathy
- **A17.89 Other tuberculosis of nervous system**
  Tuberculous polyneuropathy

A17.9 Tuberculosis of nervous system, unspecified ▽

A18 Tuberculosis of other organs

A18.0 Tuberculosis of bones and joints
- **A18.01 Tuberculosis of spine**
  Pott's disease or curvature of spine
  Tuberculous arthritis
  Tuberculous osteomyelitis of spine
  Tuberculous spondylitis
- **A18.02 Tuberculous arthritis of other joints**
  Tuberculosis of hip (joint)
  Tuberculosis of knee (joint)
- **A18.03 Tuberculosis of other bones**
  Tuberculous mastoiditis
  Tuberculous osteomyelitis
- **A18.09 Other musculoskeletal tuberculosis**
  Tuberculous myositis
  Tuberculous synovitis
  Tuberculous tenosynovitis

A18.1 Tuberculosis of genitourinary system
- **A18.10 Tuberculosis of genitourinary system, unspecified** ▽
- **A18.11 Tuberculosis of kidney and ureter**
- **A18.12 Tuberculosis of bladder**
- **A18.13 Tuberculosis of other urinary organs**
  Tuberculous urethritis
- **A18.14 Tuberculosis of prostate** A♂
- **A18.15 Tuberculosis of other male genital organs** ♂
- **A18.16 Tuberculosis of cervix** ♀
- **A18.17 Tuberculous female pelvic inflammatory disease** ♀
  Tuberculous endometritis
  Tuberculous oophoritis and salpingitis
- **A18.18 Tuberculosis of other female genital organs** ♀
  Tuberculous ulceration of vulva

A18.2 Tuberculous peripheral lymphadenopathy
  Tuberculous adenitis
  EXCLUDES 2 *tuberculosis of bronchial and mediastinal lymph nodes (A15.4)*
  tuberculosis of mesenteric and retroperitoneal lymph nodes (A18.39)
  tuberculous tracheobronchial adenopathy (A15.4)

A18.3 Tuberculosis of intestines, peritoneum and mesenteric glands
- **A18.31 Tuberculous peritonitis**
  Tuberculous ascites
  DEF: Tuberculous inflammation of the membrane lining the abdomen.
- **A18.32 Tuberculous enteritis**
  Tuberculosis of anus and rectum
  Tuberculosis of intestine (large) (small)
- **A18.39 Retroperitoneal tuberculosis**
  Tuberculosis of mesenteric glands
  Tuberculosis of retroperitoneal (lymph glands)

A18.4 Tuberculosis of skin and subcutaneous tissue
  Erythema induratum, tuberculous
  Lupus excedens
  Lupus vulgaris NOS
  Lupus vulgaris of eyelid
  Scrofuloderma
  Tuberculosis of external ear
  EXCLUDES 2 *lupus erythematosus (L93.-)*
  lupus NOS (M32.9)
  systemic (M32.-)

A18.5 Tuberculosis of eye
  EXCLUDES 2 *lupus vulgaris of eyelid (A18.4)*
- **A18.50 Tuberculosis of eye, unspecified** ▽
- **A18.51 Tuberculous episcleritis**
- **A18.52 Tuberculous keratitis**
  Tuberculous interstitial keratitis
  Tuberculous keratoconjunctivitis (interstitial) (phlyctenular)

- **A18.53 Tuberculous chorioretinitis**
- **A18.54 Tuberculous iridocyclitis**
- **A18.59 Other tuberculosis of eye**
  Tuberculous conjunctivitis

A18.6 Tuberculosis of (inner) (middle) ear
  Tuberculous otitis media
  EXCLUDES 2 *tuberculosis of external ear (A18.4)*
  tuberculous mastoiditis (A18.03)

A18.7 Tuberculosis of adrenal glands
  Tuberculous Addison's disease

A18.8 Tuberculosis of other specified organs
- **A18.81 Tuberculosis of thyroid gland**
- **A18.82 Tuberculosis of other endocrine glands**
  Tuberculosis of pituitary gland
  Tuberculosis of thymus gland
- **A18.83 Tuberculosis of digestive tract organs, not elsewhere classified**
  EXCLUDES 1 *tuberculosis of intestine (A18.32)*
- **A18.84 Tuberculosis of heart**
  Tuberculous cardiomyopathy
  Tuberculous endocarditis
  Tuberculous myocarditis
  Tuberculous pericarditis
- **A18.85 Tuberculosis of spleen**
- **A18.89 Tuberculosis of other sites**
  Tuberculosis of muscle
  Tuberculous cerebral arteritis

A19 Miliary tuberculosis
  INCLUDES disseminated tuberculosis
  generalized tuberculosis
  tuberculous polyserositis
- **A19.0 Acute miliary tuberculosis of a single specified site**
- **A19.1 Acute miliary tuberculosis of multiple sites**
- **A19.2 Acute miliary tuberculosis, unspecified** ▽
- **A19.8 Other miliary tuberculosis**
- **A19.9 Miliary tuberculosis, unspecified** ▽

Certain zoonotic bacterial diseases (A20-A28)

A20 Plague
  INCLUDES infection due to Yersinia pestis
- **A20.0 Bubonic plague**
- **A20.1 Cellulocutaneous plague**
- **A20.2 Pneumonic plague** HCC
- **A20.3 Plague meningitis**
- **A20.7 Septicemic plague** HCC
- **A20.8 Other forms of plague**
  Abortive plague
  Asymptomatic plague
  Pestis minor
- **A20.9 Plague, unspecified** ▽

A21 Tularemia
  INCLUDES deer-fly fever
  infection due to Francisella tularensis
  rabbit fever
  DEF: A febrile disease transmitted to humans by the bites of deer flies, fleas, and ticks; by inhaling aerosolized *F. tularensis*; or by ingesting contaminated food or water. Patients quickly develop fever, chills, weakness, headache, backache, and malaise.
- **A21.0 Ulceroglandular tularemia**
- **A21.1 Oculoglandular tularemia**
  Ophthalmic tularemia
- **A21.2 Pulmonary tularemia** HCC
- **A21.3 Gastrointestinal tularemia**
  Abdominal tularemia
- **A21.7 Generalized tularemia**
- **A21.8 Other forms of tularemia**
- **A21.9 Tularemia, unspecified** ▽

A22 Anthrax
  INCLUDES infection due to Bacillus anthracis
- **A22.0 Cutaneous anthrax**
  Malignant carbuncle
  Malignant pustule
- **A22.1 Pulmonary anthrax** HCC
  Inhalation anthrax
  Ragpicker's disease
  Woolsorter's disease

EXCLUDES 1 Not coded here   EXCLUDES 2 Not included here   N Newborn Age: 0   P Pediatric Age: 0-17   M Maternity Age: 12-55   A Adult Age: 15-124

438   ICD-10-CM 2018

A22.2 **Gastrointestinal anthrax**

A22.7 **Anthrax sepsis** `HCC`

A22.8 **Other forms of anthrax**
Anthrax meningitis

A22.9 **Anthrax, unspecified** ▽

`√4th` **A23 Brucellosis**
`INCLUDES`   Malta fever
Mediterranean fever
undulant fever

A23.0 **Brucellosis due to Brucella melitensis**

A23.1 **Brucellosis due to Brucella abortus**

A23.2 **Brucellosis due to Brucella suis**

A23.3 **Brucellosis due to Brucella canis**

A23.8 **Other brucellosis**

A23.9 **Brucellosis, unspecified** ▽

`√4th` **A24 Glanders and melioidosis**
A24.0 **Glanders**
Infection due to Pseudomonas mallei
Malleus

A24.1 **Acute and fulminating melioidosis**
Melioidosis pneumonia
Melioidosis sepsis

A24.2 **Subacute and chronic melioidosis**

A24.3 **Other melioidosis**

A24.9 **Melioidosis, unspecified** ▽
Infection due to Pseudomonas pseudomallei NOS
Whitmore's disease

`√4th` **A25 Rat-bite fevers**
A25.0 **Spirillosis**
Sodoku

A25.1 **Streptobacillosis**
Epidemic arthritic erythema
Haverhill fever
Streptobacillary rat-bite fever

A25.9 **Rat-bite fever, unspecified** ▽

`√4th` **A26 Erysipeloid**
A26.0 **Cutaneous erysipeloid**
Erythema migrans

A26.7 **Erysipelothrix sepsis** `HCC`

A26.8 **Other forms of erysipeloid**

A26.9 **Erysipeloid, unspecified** ▽

`√4th` **A27 Leptospirosis**
A27.0 **Leptospirosis icterohemorrhagica**
Leptospiral or spirochetal jaundice (hemorrhagic)
Weil's disease

`√5th` A27.8 **Other forms of leptospirosis**
A27.81 **Aseptic meningitis in leptospirosis**
A27.89 **Other forms of leptospirosis**

A27.9 **Leptospirosis, unspecified** ▽

`√4th` **A28 Other zoonotic bacterial diseases, not elsewhere classified**
A28.0 **Pasteurellosis**

A28.1 **Cat-scratch disease**
Cat-scratch fever

A28.2 **Extraintestinal yersiniosis**
`EXCLUDES 1`   enteritis due to Yersinia enterocolitica (A04.6)
plague (A20.-)

A28.8 **Other specified zoonotic bacterial diseases, not elsewhere classified**

A28.9 **Zoonotic bacterial disease, unspecified** ▽

Other bacterial diseases (A30-A49)
AHA: 2016, 3Q, 8-14

`√4th` **A30 Leprosy [Hansen's disease]**
`INCLUDES`   infection due to Mycobacterium leprae
`EXCLUDES 1`   sequelae of leprosy (B92)

A30.0 **Indeterminate leprosy**
I leprosy

A30.1 **Tuberculoid leprosy**
TT leprosy

A30.2 **Borderline tuberculoid leprosy**
BT leprosy

A30.3 **Borderline leprosy**
BB leprosy

A30.4 **Borderline lepromatous leprosy**
BL leprosy

A30.5 **Lepromatous leprosy**
LL leprosy

A30.8 **Other forms of leprosy**

A30.9 **Leprosy, unspecified** ▽

`√4th` **A31 Infection due to other mycobacteria**
`EXCLUDES 2`   leprosy (A30.-)
tuberculosis (A15-A19)

A31.0 **Pulmonary mycobacterial infection** `HCC`
Infection due to Mycobacterium avium
Infection due to Mycobacterium intracellulare [Battey bacillus]
Infection due to Mycobacterium kansasii

A31.1 **Cutaneous mycobacterial infection**
Buruli ulcer
Infection due to Mycobacterium marinum
Infection due to Mycobacterium ulcerans

A31.2 **Disseminated mycobacterium avium-intracellulare complex (DMAC)** `HCC`
MAC sepsis

A31.8 **Other mycobacterial infections**

A31.9 **Mycobacterial infection, unspecified** ▽
Atypical mycobacterial infection NOS
Mycobacteriosis NOS

`√4th` **A32 Listeriosis**
`INCLUDES`   listerial foodborne infection
`EXCLUDES 1`   neonatal (disseminated) listeriosis (P37.2)

A32.0 **Cutaneous listeriosis**

`√5th` A32.1 **Listerial meningitis and meningoencephalitis**
A32.11 **Listerial meningitis**
A32.12 **Listerial meningoencephalitis**

A32.7 **Listerial sepsis** `HCC`

`√5th` A32.8 **Other forms of listeriosis**
A32.81 **Oculoglandular listeriosis**
A32.82 **Listerial endocarditis**
A32.89 **Other forms of listeriosis**
Listerial cerebral arteritis

A32.9 **Listeriosis, unspecified** ▽

A33 Tetanus neonatorum `N`

A34 Obstetrical tetanus `M`♀

A35 Other tetanus
Tetanus NOS
`EXCLUDES 1`   obstetrical tetanus (A34)
tetanus neonatorum (A33)

`√4th` **A36 Diphtheria**
A36.0 **Pharyngeal diphtheria**
Diphtheritic membranous angina
Tonsillar diphtheria

A36.1 **Nasopharyngeal diphtheria**

A36.2 **Laryngeal diphtheria**
Diphtheritic laryngotracheitis

A36.3 **Cutaneous diphtheria**
`EXCLUDES 2`   erythrasma (L08.1)

`√5th` A36.8 **Other diphtheria**
A36.81 **Diphtheritic cardiomyopathy** `HCC`
Diphtheritic myocarditis
A36.82 **Diphtheritic radiculomyelitis**
A36.83 **Diphtheritic polyneuritis**
A36.84 **Diphtheritic tubulo-interstitial nephropathy**
A36.85 **Diphtheritic cystitis**
A36.86 **Diphtheritic conjunctivitis**
A36.89 **Other diphtheritic complications**
Diphtheritic peritonitis

A36.9 **Diphtheria, unspecified** ▽

`√4th` **A37 Whooping cough**
`√5th` A37.0 **Whooping cough due to Bordetella pertussis**
A37.00 **Whooping cough due to Bordetella pertussis without pneumonia**
A37.01 **Whooping cough due to Bordetella pertussis with pneumonia**

`√5th` A37.1 **Whooping cough due to Bordetella parapertussis**
A37.10 **Whooping cough due to Bordetella parapertussis without pneumonia**

A37.11 **Whooping cough due to Bordetella parapertussis with pneumonia**

✓5th **A37.8** **Whooping cough due to other Bordetella species**

A37.80 **Whooping cough due to other Bordetella species without pneumonia**

A37.81 **Whooping cough due to other Bordetella species with pneumonia**

✓5th **A37.9** **Whooping cough, unspecified species**

A37.90 **Whooping cough, unspecified species without pneumonia** ▽

A37.91 **Whooping cough, unspecified species with pneumonia** ▽

✓4th **A38** **Scarlet fever**
INCLUDES scarlatina
EXCLUDES 2 streptococcal sore throat (J02.0)

A38.0 **Scarlet fever with otitis media**

A38.1 **Scarlet fever with myocarditis**

A38.8 **Scarlet fever with other complications**

A38.9 **Scarlet fever, uncomplicated** ▽
Scarlet fever, NOS

✓4th **A39** **Meningococcal infection**

A39.0 **Meningococcal meningitis**

A39.1 **Waterhouse-Friderichsen syndrome** HCC
Meningococcal hemorrhagic adrenalitis
Meningococcic adrenal syndrome

A39.2 **Acute meningococcemia** HCC

A39.3 **Chronic meningococcemia** HCC

A39.4 **Meningococcemia, unspecified** HCC ▽

✓5th **A39.5** **Meningococcal heart disease**

A39.50 **Meningococcal carditis, unspecified** ▽

A39.51 **Meningococcal endocarditis**

A39.52 **Meningococcal myocarditis**

A39.53 **Meningococcal pericarditis**

✓5th **A39.8** **Other meningococcal infections**

A39.81 **Meningococcal encephalitis**

A39.82 **Meningococcal retrobulbar neuritis**

A39.83 **Meningococcal arthritis** HCC

A39.84 **Postmeningococcal arthritis** HCC

A39.89 **Other meningococcal infections**
Meningococcal conjunctivitis

A39.9 **Meningococcal infection, unspecified** ▽
Meningococcal disease NOS

✓4th **A40** **Streptococcal sepsis**
Code first: postprocedural streptococcal sepsis (T81.4-)
streptococcal sepsis during labor (O75.3)
streptococcal sepsis following abortion or ectopic or molar pregnancy (O03-O07, O08.0)
streptococcal sepsis following immunization (T88.0)
streptococcal sepsis following infusion, transfusion or therapeutic injection (T80.2-)
EXCLUDES 1 neonatal (P36.0-P36.1)
puerperal sepsis (O85)
sepsis due to Streptococcus, group D (A41.81)
AHA: 2016, 1Q, 32

A40.0 **Sepsis due to streptococcus, group A** HCC

A40.1 **Sepsis due to streptococcus, group B** HCC

A40.3 **Sepsis due to Streptococcus pneumoniae** HCC
Pneumococcal sepsis

A40.8 **Other streptococcal sepsis** HCC

A40.9 **Streptococcal sepsis, unspecified** HCC ▽

✓4th **A41** **Other sepsis**
Code first: postprocedural sepsis (T81.4-)
sepsis during labor (O75.3)
sepsis following abortion, ectopic or molar pregnancy (O03-O07, O08.0)
sepsis following immunization (T88.0)
sepsis following infusion, transfusion or therapeutic injection (T80.2-)
EXCLUDES 1 bacteremia NOS (R78.81)
neonatal (P36.-)
puerperal sepsis (O85)
streptococcal sepsis (A40.-)
EXCLUDES 2 sepsis (due to) (in) actinomycotic (A42.7)
sepsis (due to) (in) anthrax (A22.7)
sepsis (due to) (in) candidal (B37.7)
sepsis (due to) (in) Erysipelothrix (A26.7)
sepsis (due to) (in) extraintestinal yersiniosis (A28.2)
sepsis (due to) (in) gonococcal (A54.86)
sepsis (due to) (in) herpesviral (B00.7)
sepsis (due to) (in) listerial (A32.7)
sepsis (due to) (in) melioidosis (A24.1)
sepsis (due to) (in) meningococcal (A39.2-A39.4)
sepsis (due to) (in) plague (A20.7)
sepsis (due to) (in) tularemia (A21.7)
toxic shock syndrome (A48.3)
AHA: 2016, 1Q, 32; 2014, 2Q, 13

✓5th **A41.0** **Sepsis due to Staphylococcus aureus**

A41.01 **Sepsis due to Methicillin susceptible Staphylococcus aureus** HCC
MSSA sepsis
Staphylococcus aureus sepsis NOS

A41.02 **Sepsis due to Methicillin resistant Staphylococcus aureus** HCC

A41.1 **Sepsis due to other specified staphylococcus** HCC
Coagulase negative staphylococcus sepsis

A41.2 **Sepsis due to unspecified staphylococcus** HCC ▽

A41.3 **Sepsis due to Hemophilus influenzae** HCC

A41.4 **Sepsis due to anaerobes** HCC
EXCLUDES 1 gas gangrene (A48.0)

✓5th **A41.5** **Sepsis due to other Gram-negative organisms**

A41.50 **Gram-negative sepsis, unspecified** HCC ▽
Gram-negative sepsis NOS

A41.51 **Sepsis due to Escherichia coli [E. coli]** HCC

A41.52 **Sepsis due to Pseudomonas** HCC
Pseudomonas aeroginosa

A41.53 **Sepsis due to Serratia** HCC

A41.59 **Other Gram-negative sepsis** HCC

✓5th **A41.8** **Other specified sepsis**

A41.81 **Sepsis due to Enterococcus** HCC

A41.89 **Other specified sepsis** HCC
AHA: 2017, 1Q, 51; 2016, 3Q, 8-14

A41.9 **Sepsis, unspecified organism** HCC ▽
Septicemia NOS

✓4th **A42** **Actinomycosis**
EXCLUDES 1 actinomycetoma (B47.1)

A42.0 **Pulmonary actinomycosis** HCC

A42.1 **Abdominal actinomycosis**

A42.2 **Cervicofacial actinomycosis**

A42.7 **Actinomycotic sepsis** HCC

✓5th **A42.8** **Other forms of actinomycosis**

A42.81 **Actinomycotic meningitis**

A42.82 **Actinomycotic encephalitis**

A42.89 **Other forms of actinomycosis**

A42.9 **Actinomycosis, unspecified** ▽

✓4th **A43** **Nocardiosis**

A43.0 **Pulmonary nocardiosis** HCC

A43.1 **Cutaneous nocardiosis**

A43.8 **Other forms of nocardiosis**

A43.9 **Nocardiosis, unspecified** ▽

✓4th **A44** **Bartonellosis**

A44.0 **Systemic bartonellosis**
Oroya fever

A44.1 **Cutaneous and mucocutaneous bartonellosis**
Verruga peruana

A44.8 **Other forms of bartonellosis**

A44.9   Bartonellosis, unspecified ▽

A46   Erysipelas
EXCLUDES 1   postpartum or puerperal erysipelas (O86.89)
DEF: A skin infection affecting the upper dermis and superficial dermal lymphatics; lesion edges are well-demarcated with distinct raised borders; it is often caused by group A *Streptococci*.

✓4ᵗʰ A48   Other bacterial diseases, not elsewhere classified
EXCLUDES 1   actinomycetoma (B47.1)

A48.0   Gas gangrene   HCC
Clostridial cellulitis
Clostridial myonecrosis

A48.1   Legionnaires' disease   HCC
DEF: Severe and often fatal infection by *Legionella pneumophila*; symptoms include high fever, gastrointestinal pain, headache, myalgia, dry cough, and pneumonia; usually transmitted through airborne water droplets via air conditioning systems or hot tubs.

A48.2   Nonpneumonic Legionnaires' disease [Pontiac fever]

A48.3   Toxic shock syndrome   HCC
Use additional code to identify the organism (B95, B96)
EXCLUDES 1   endotoxic shock NOS (R57.8)
        sepsis NOS (A41.9)

A48.4   Brazilian purpuric fever
Systemic Hemophilus aegyptius infection

✓5ᵗʰ A48.5   Other specified botulism
Non-foodborne intoxication due to toxins of Clostridium botulinum [C. botulinum]
EXCLUDES 1   food poisoning due to toxins of Clostridium botulinum (A05.1)

    A48.51   Infant botulism   P

    A48.52   Wound botulism
       Non-foodborne botulism NOS
       Use additional code for associated wound

A48.8   Other specified bacterial diseases

✓4ᵗʰ A49   Bacterial infection of unspecified site
EXCLUDES 1   bacterial agents as the cause of diseases classified elsewhere (B95-B96)
       chlamydial infection NOS (A74.9)
       meningococcal infection NOS (A39.9)
       rickettsial infection NOS (A79.9)
       spirochetal infection NOS (A69.9)

✓5ᵗʰ A49.0   Staphylococcal infection, unspecified site

    A49.01   Methicillin susceptible Staphylococcus aureus infection, unspecified site
       Methicillin susceptible Staphylococcus aureus (MSSA) infection
       Staphylococcus aureus infection NOS

    A49.02   Methicillin resistant Staphylococcus aureus infection, unspecified site
       Methicillin resistant Staphylococcus aureus (MRSA) infection

A49.1   Streptococcal infection, unspecified site

A49.2   Hemophilus influenzae infection, unspecified site

A49.3   Mycoplasma infection, unspecified site

A49.8   Other bacterial infections of unspecified site

A49.9   Bacterial infection, unspecified ▽
EXCLUDES 1   bacteremia NOS (R78.81)

Infections with a predominantly sexual mode of transmission (A50-A64)
EXCLUDES 1   human immunodeficiency virus [HIV] disease (B20)
       nonspecific and nongonococcal urethritis (N34.1)
       Reiter's disease (M02.3-)

✓4ᵗʰ A50   Congenital syphilis

✓5ᵗʰ A50.0   Early congenital syphilis, symptomatic
Any congenital syphilitic condition specified as early or manifest less than two years after birth.

    A50.01   Early congenital syphilitic oculopathy
    A50.02   Early congenital syphilitic osteochondropathy
    A50.03   Early congenital syphilitic pharyngitis
       Early congenital syphilitic laryngitis
    A50.04   Early congenital syphilitic pneumonia
    A50.05   Early congenital syphilitic rhinitis
    A50.06   Early cutaneous congenital syphilis
    A50.07   Early mucocutaneous congenital syphilis
    A50.08   Early visceral congenital syphilis
    A50.09   Other early congenital syphilis, symptomatic

A50.1   Early congenital syphilis, latent
Congenital syphilis without clinical manifestations, with positive serological reaction and negative spinal fluid test, less than two years after birth.

A50.2   Early congenital syphilis, unspecified ▽
Congenital syphilis NOS less than two years after birth.

✓5ᵗʰ A50.3   Late congenital syphilitic oculopathy
EXCLUDES 1   Hutchinson's triad (A50.53)

    A50.30   Late congenital syphilitic oculopathy, unspecified ▽
    A50.31   Late congenital syphilitic interstitial keratitis
    A50.32   Late congenital syphilitic chorioretinitis
    A50.39   Other late congenital syphilitic oculopathy

✓5ᵗʰ A50.4   Late congenital neurosyphilis [juvenile neurosyphilis]
Use additional code to identify any associated mental disorder
EXCLUDES 1   Hutchinson's triad (A50.53)

    A50.40   Late congenital neurosyphilis, unspecified ▽
       Juvenile neurosyphilis NOS
    A50.41   Late congenital syphilitic meningitis
    A50.42   Late congenital syphilitic encephalitis
    A50.43   Late congenital syphilitic polyneuropathy
    A50.44   Late congenital syphilitic optic nerve atrophy
    A50.45   Juvenile general paresis
       Dementia paralytica juvenilis
       Juvenile tabetoparetic neurosyphilis
    A50.49   Other late congenital neurosyphilis
       Juvenile tabes dorsalis

✓5ᵗʰ A50.5   Other late congenital syphilis, symptomatic
Any congenital syphilitic condition specified as late or manifest two years or more after birth.

    A50.51   Clutton's joints
    A50.52   Hutchinson's teeth
    A50.53   Hutchinson's triad
    A50.54   Late congenital cardiovascular syphilis
    A50.55   Late congenital syphilitic arthropathy   HCC
    A50.56   Late congenital syphilitic osteochondropathy
    A50.57   Syphilitic saddle nose
    A50.59   Other late congenital syphilis, symptomatic

A50.6   Late congenital syphilis, latent
Congenital syphilis without clinical manifestations, with positive serological reaction and negative spinal fluid test, two years or more after birth.

A50.7   Late congenital syphilis, unspecified ▽
Congenital syphilis NOS two years or more after birth.

A50.9   Congenital syphilis, unspecified ▽

✓4ᵗʰ A51   Early syphilis

A51.0   Primary genital syphilis
Syphilitic chancre NOS

A51.1   Primary anal syphilis

A51.2   Primary syphilis of other sites

✓5ᵗʰ A51.3   Secondary syphilis of skin and mucous membranes
DEF: Transitory or chronic cutaneous eruptions that present within two to 10 weeks following initial syphilis infection that may include nontender lymphadenopathy along with alopecia and condylomata lata.

    A51.31   Condyloma latum
    A51.32   Syphilitic alopecia
    A51.39   Other secondary syphilis of skin
       Syphilitic leukoderma
       Syphilitic mucous patch
       EXCLUDES 1   late syphilitic leukoderma (A52.79)

✓5ᵗʰ A51.4   Other secondary syphilis

    A51.41   Secondary syphilitic meningitis
    A51.42   Secondary syphilitic female pelvic disease   ♀
    A51.43   Secondary syphilitic oculopathy
       Secondary syphilitic chorioretinitis
       Secondary syphilitic iridocyclitis, iritis
       Secondary syphilitic uveitis
    A51.44   Secondary syphilitic nephritis
    A51.45   Secondary syphilitic hepatitis
    A51.46   Secondary syphilitic osteopathy
    A51.49   Other secondary syphilitic conditions
       Secondary syphilitic lymphadenopathy
       Secondary syphilitic myositis

✓ Additional Character Req   ✓ˣ⁷ᵗʰ Placeholder Alert   Manifestation   HCC CMS-HCC Condition   ▽ Unspecified Code   ▶◀ Revised Text   ● New Code   ▲ Revised Code Title

ICD-10-CM 2018   441

A44.9-A51.49

A51.5 Early syphilis, latent
Syphilis (acquired) without clinical manifestations, with positive serological reaction and negative spinal fluid test, less than two years after infection.

A51.9 Early syphilis, unspecified ▽

✓4ᵗʰ A52 Late syphilis

✓5ᵗʰ A52.0 Cardiovascular and cerebrovascular syphilis

    A52.00 Cardiovascular syphilis, unspecified ▽

    A52.01 Syphilitic aneurysm of aorta

    A52.02 Syphilitic aortitis

    A52.03 Syphilitic endocarditis
        Syphilitic aortic valve incompetence or stenosis
        Syphilitic mitral valve stenosis
        Syphilitic pulmonary valve regurgitation

    A52.04 Syphilitic cerebral arteritis

    A52.05 Other cerebrovascular syphilis
        Syphilitic cerebral aneurysm (ruptured) (non-ruptured)
        Syphilitic cerebral thrombosis

    A52.06 Other syphilitic heart involvement
        Syphilitic coronary artery disease
        Syphilitic myocarditis
        Syphilitic pericarditis

    A52.09 Other cardiovascular syphilis

✓5ᵗʰ A52.1 Symptomatic neurosyphilis

    A52.10 Symptomatic neurosyphilis, unspecified ▽

    A52.11 Tabes dorsalis
        Locomotor ataxia (progressive)
        Tabetic neurosyphilis

    A52.12 Other cerebrospinal syphilis

    A52.13 Late syphilitic meningitis

    A52.14 Late syphilitic encephalitis

    A52.15 Late syphilitic neuropathy
        Late syphilitic acoustic neuritis
        Late syphilitic optic (nerve) atrophy
        Late syphilitic polyneuropathy
        Late syphilitic retrobulbar neuritis

    A52.16 Charcôt's arthropathy (tabetic)

    A52.17 General paresis
        Dementia paralytica

    A52.19 Other symptomatic neurosyphilis
        Syphilitic parkinsonism

A52.2 Asymptomatic neurosyphilis

A52.3 Neurosyphilis, unspecified ▽
    Gumma (syphilitic)
    Syphilis (late)
    Syphiloma

✓5ᵗʰ A52.7 Other symptomatic late syphilis

    A52.71 Late syphilitic oculopathy
        Late syphilitic chorioretinitis
        Late syphilitic episcleritis

    A52.72 Syphilis of lung and bronchus

    A52.73 Symptomatic late syphilis of other respiratory organs

    A52.74 Syphilis of liver and other viscera
        Late syphilitic peritonitis

    A52.75 Syphilis of kidney and ureter
        Syphilitic glomerular disease

    A52.76 Other genitourinary symptomatic late syphilis
        Late syphilitic female pelvic inflammatory disease

    A52.77 Syphilis of bone and joint

    A52.78 Syphilis of other musculoskeletal tissue
        Late syphilitic bursitis
        Syphilis [stage unspecified] of bursa
        Syphilis [stage unspecified] of muscle
        Syphilis [stage unspecified] of synovium
        Syphilis [stage unspecified] of tendon

    A52.79 Other symptomatic late syphilis
        Late syphilitic leukoderma
        Syphilis of adrenal gland
        Syphilis of pituitary gland
        Syphilis of thyroid gland
        Syphilitic splenomegaly
        EXCLUDES 1   *syphilitic leukoderma (secondary) (A51.39)*

A52.8 Late syphilis, latent
Syphilis (acquired) without clinical manifestations, with positive serological reaction and negative spinal fluid test, two years or more after infection.

A52.9 Late syphilis, unspecified ▽

✓4ᵗʰ A53 Other and unspecified syphilis

    A53.0 Latent syphilis, unspecified as early or late
        Latent syphilis NOS
        Positive serological reaction for syphilis

    A53.9 Syphilis, unspecified ▽
        Infection due to Treponema pallidum NOS
        Syphilis (acquired) NOS
        EXCLUDES 1   *syphilis NOS under two years of age (A50.2)*

✓4ᵗʰ A54 Gonococcal infection

✓5ᵗʰ A54.0 Gonococcal infection of lower genitourinary tract without periurethral or accessory gland abscess
        EXCLUDES 1   *gonococcal infection with genitourinary gland abscess (A54.1)*
                       gonococcal infection with periurethral abscess (A54.1)

    A54.00 Gonococcal infection of lower genitourinary tract, unspecified ▽

    A54.01 Gonococcal cystitis and urethritis, unspecified ▽

    A54.02 Gonococcal vulvovaginitis, unspecified ♀▽

    A54.03 Gonococcal cervicitis, unspecified ♀▽

    A54.09 Other gonococcal infection of lower genitourinary tract

    A54.1 Gonococcal infection of lower genitourinary tract with periurethral and accessory gland abscess
        Gonococcal Bartholin's gland abscess

✓5ᵗʰ A54.2 Gonococcal pelviperitonitis and other gonococcal genitourinary infection

    A54.21 Gonococcal infection of kidney and ureter

    A54.22 Gonococcal prostatitis ♂

    A54.23 Gonococcal infection of other male genital organs ♂
        Gonococcal epididymitis
        Gonococcal orchitis

    A54.24 Gonococcal female pelvic inflammatory disease ♀
        Gonococcal pelviperitonitis
        EXCLUDES 1   *gonococcal peritonitis (A54.85)*

    A54.29 Other gonococcal genitourinary infections

✓5ᵗʰ A54.3 Gonococcal infection of eye

    A54.30 Gonococcal infection of eye, unspecified ▽

    A54.31 Gonococcal conjunctivitis
        Ophthalmia neonatorum due to gonococcus

    A54.32 Gonococcal iridocyclitis

    A54.33 Gonococcal keratitis

    A54.39 Other gonococcal eye infection
        Gonococcal endophthalmia

✓5ᵗʰ A54.4 Gonococcal infection of musculoskeletal system

    A54.40 Gonococcal infection of musculoskeletal system, unspecified HCC ▽

    A54.41 Gonococcal spondylopathy HCC

    A54.42 Gonococcal arthritis HCC
        EXCLUDES 2   *gonococcal infection of spine (A54.41)*

    A54.43 Gonococcal osteomyelitis HCC
        EXCLUDES 2   *gonococcal infection of spine (A54.41)*

    A54.49 Gonococcal infection of other musculoskeletal tissue HCC
        Gonococcal bursitis
        Gonococcal myositis
        Gonococcal synovitis
        Gonococcal tenosynovitis

    A54.5 Gonococcal pharyngitis

    A54.6 Gonococcal infection of anus and rectum

✓5ᵗʰ A54.8 Other gonococcal infections

    A54.81 Gonococcal meningitis

    A54.82 Gonococcal brain abscess

    A54.83 Gonococcal heart infection
        Gonococcal endocarditis
        Gonococcal myocarditis
        Gonococcal pericarditis

    A54.84 Gonococcal pneumonia HCC

    A54.85 Gonococcal peritonitis HCC
        EXCLUDES 1   *gonococcal pelviperitonitis (A54.24)*

    A54.86 Gonococcal sepsis HCC

    A54.89 Other gonococcal infections
        Gonococcal keratoderma
        Gonococcal lymphadenitis

    A54.9 Gonococcal infection, unspecified ▽

EXCLUDES 1 Not coded here   **EXCLUDES 2** Not included here   **N** Newborn Age: 0   **P** Pediatric Age: 0-17   **M** Maternity Age: 12-55   **A** Adult Age: 15-124

A55 Chlamydial lymphogranuloma (venereum)
Climatic or tropical bubo
Durand-Nicolas-Favre disease
Esthiomene
Lymphogranuloma inguinale

✓4ᵗʰ **A56 Other sexually transmitted chlamydial diseases**
INCLUDES sexually transmitted diseases due to Chlamydia trachomatis
EXCLUDES 1 neonatal chlamydial conjunctivitis (P39.1)
neonatal chlamydial pneumonia (P23.1)
EXCLUDES 2 chlamydial lymphogranuloma (A55)
conditions classified to A74-

✓5ᵗʰ **A56.0 Chlamydial infection of lower genitourinary tract**
     A56.00 Chlamydial infection of lower genitourinary tract, unspecified ▽
     A56.01 Chlamydial cystitis and urethritis
     A56.02 Chlamydial vulvovaginitis ♀
     A56.09 Other chlamydial infection of lower genitourinary tract
        Chlamydial cervicitis

✓5ᵗʰ **A56.1 Chlamydial infection of pelviperitoneum and other genitourinary organs**
     A56.11 Chlamydial female pelvic inflammatory disease ♀
     A56.19 Other chlamydial genitourinary infection
        Chlamydial epididymitis
        Chlamydial orchitis

A56.2 Chlamydial infection of genitourinary tract, unspecified ▽
A56.3 Chlamydial infection of anus and rectum
A56.4 Chlamydial infection of pharynx
A56.8 Sexually transmitted chlamydial infection of other sites

A57 Chancroid
Ulcus molle

A58 Granuloma inguinale
Donovanosis

✓4ᵗʰ **A59 Trichomoniasis**
EXCLUDES 2 intestinal trichomoniasis (A07.8)

✓5ᵗʰ **A59.0 Urogenital trichomoniasis**
     A59.00 Urogenital trichomoniasis, unspecified ▽
        Fluor (vaginalis) due to Trichomonas
        Leukorrhea (vaginalis) due to Trichomonas
     A59.01 Trichomonal vulvovaginitis ♀
     A59.02 Trichomonal prostatitis ♂
     A59.03 Trichomonal cystitis and urethritis
     A59.09 Other urogenital trichomoniasis
        Trichomonas cervicitis

A59.8 Trichomoniasis of other sites
A59.9 Trichomoniasis, unspecified ▽

✓4ᵗʰ **A60 Anogenital herpesviral [herpes simplex] infections**
✓5ᵗʰ **A60.0 Herpesviral infection of genitalia and urogenital tract**
     A60.00 Herpesviral infection of urogenital system, unspecified ▽
     A60.01 Herpesviral infection of penis ♂
     A60.02 Herpesviral infection of other male genital organs ♂
     A60.03 Herpesviral cervicitis ♀
     A60.04 Herpesviral vulvovaginitis ♀
        Herpesviral [herpes simplex] ulceration
        Herpesviral [herpes simplex] vaginitis
        Herpesviral [herpes simplex] vulvitis
     A60.09 Herpesviral infection of other urogenital tract

A60.1 Herpesviral infection of perianal skin and rectum
A60.9 Anogenital herpesviral infection, unspecified ▽

✓4ᵗʰ **A63 Other predominantly sexually transmitted diseases, not elsewhere classified**
EXCLUDES 2 molluscum contagiosum (B08.1)
papilloma of cervix (D26.0)

A63.0 Anogenital (venereal) warts
Anogenital warts due to (human) papillomavirus [HPV]
Condyloma acuminatum
A63.8 Other specified predominantly sexually transmitted diseases

A64 Unspecified sexually transmitted disease ▽

Other spirochetal diseases (A65-A69)

EXCLUDES 2 leptospirosis (A27.-)
syphilis (A50-A53)

A65 Nonvenereal syphilis
Bejel   Njovera
Endemic syphilis

✓4ᵗʰ **A66 Yaws**
INCLUDES bouba
frambesia (tropica)
pian

A66.0 Initial lesions of yaws
Chancre of yaws
Frambesia, initial or primary
Initial frambesial ulcer
Mother yaw
A66.1 Multiple papillomata and wet crab yaws
Frambesioma
Pianoma
Plantar or palmar papilloma of yaws
A66.2 Other early skin lesions of yaws
Cutaneous yaws, less than five years after infection
Early yaws (cutaneous) (macular) (maculopapular) (micropapular) (papular)
Frambeside of early yaws
A66.3 Hyperkeratosis of yaws
Ghoul hand
Hyperkeratosis, palmar or plantar (early) (late) due to yaws
Worm-eaten soles
A66.4 Gummata and ulcers of yaws
Gummatous frambeside
Nodular late yaws (ulcerated)
A66.5 Gangosa
Rhinopharyngitis mutilans
A66.6 Bone and joint lesions of yaws HCC
Yaws ganglion   Yaws hydrarthrosis
Yaws goundou   Yaws osteitis
Yaws gumma, bone   Yaws periostitis (hypertrophic)
Yaws gummatous osteitis or periostitis
A66.7 Other manifestations of yaws
Juxta-articular nodules of yaws
Mucosal yaws
A66.8 Latent yaws
Yaws without clinical manifestations, with positive serology
A66.9 Yaws, unspecified ▽

✓4ᵗʰ **A67 Pinta [carate]**
A67.0 Primary lesions of pinta
Chancre (primary) of pinta
Papule (primary) of pinta
A67.1 Intermediate lesions of pinta
Erythematous plaques of pinta
Hyperchromic lesions of pinta
Hyperkeratosis of pinta
Pintids
A67.2 Late lesions of pinta
Achromic skin lesions of pinta
Cicatricial skin lesions of pinta
Dyschromic skin lesions of pinta
A67.3 Mixed lesions of pinta
Achromic with hyperchromic skin lesions of pinta [carate]
A67.9 Pinta, unspecified ▽

✓4ᵗʰ **A68 Relapsing fevers**
INCLUDES recurrent fever
EXCLUDES 2 Lyme disease (A69.2-)

A68.0 Louse-borne relapsing fever
Relapsing fever due to Borrelia recurrentis
A68.1 Tick-borne relapsing fever
Relapsing fever due to any Borrelia species other than Borrelia recurrentis
A68.9 Relapsing fever, unspecified ▽

✓4ᵗʰ **A69 Other spirochetal infections**
A69.0 Necrotizing ulcerative stomatitis
Cancrum oris
Fusospirochetal gangrene
Noma
Stomatitis gangrenosa

☑ Additional Character Req   ✓x7ᵗʰ Placeholder Alert   Manifestation   HCC CMS-HCC Condition   ▽ Unspecified Code   ►◄ Revised Text   ● New Code   ▲ Revised Code Title

A69.1 Other Vincent's infections
Fusospirochetal pharyngitis
Necrotizing ulcerative (acute) gingivitis
Necrotizing ulcerative (acute) gingivostomatitis
Spirochetal stomatitis
Trench mouth
Vincent's angina
Vincent's gingivitis

✓5th **A69.2 Lyme disease**
Erythema chronicum migrans due to Borrelia burgdorferi
DEF: A recurrent multisystem disorder through tick bites; begins with lesions of erythema chronicum migrans; followed by arthritis of the large joints, myalgia, malaise, and neurological and cardiac manifestations.

     A69.20 Lyme disease, unspecified ▽

     A69.21 Meningitis due to Lyme disease

     A69.22 Other neurologic disorders in Lyme disease
Cranial neuritis
Meningoencephalitis
Polyneuropathy

     A69.23 Arthritis due to Lyme disease   HCC

     A69.29 Other conditions associated with Lyme disease
Myopericarditis due to Lyme disease
AHA: 2016, 3Q, 12

A69.8 Other specified spirochetal infections

A69.9 Spirochetal infection, unspecified ▽

Other diseases caused by chlamydiae (A70-A74)

EXCLUDES 1   *sexually transmitted chlamydial diseases (A55-A56)*

A70 Chlamydia psittaci infections
Ornithosis
Parrot fever
Psittacosis

✓4th **A71 Trachoma**
EXCLUDES 1   *sequelae of trachoma (B94.0)*

     A71.0 Initial stage of trachoma
Trachoma dubium

     A71.1 Active stage of trachoma
Granular conjunctivitis (trachomatous)
Trachomatous follicular conjunctivitis
Trachomatous pannus

     A71.9 Trachoma, unspecified ▽

✓4th **A74 Other diseases caused by chlamydiae**
EXCLUDES 1   *neonatal chlamydial conjunctivitis (P39.1)*
neonatal chlamydial pneumonia (P23.1)
Reiter's disease (M02.3-)
sexually transmitted chlamydial diseases (A55-A56)
EXCLUDES 2   *chlamydial pneumonia (J16.0)*

     A74.0 Chlamydial conjunctivitis
Paratrachoma

✓5th   **A74.8 Other chlamydial diseases**

     A74.81 Chlamydial peritonitis

     A74.89 Other chlamydial diseases

     A74.9 Chlamydial infection, unspecified ▽
Chlamydiosis NOS

Rickettsioses (A75-A79)

✓4th **A75 Typhus fever**
EXCLUDES 1   *rickettsiosis due to Ehrlichia sennetsu (A79.81)*

     A75.0 Epidemic louse-borne typhus fever due to Rickettsia prowazekii
Classical typhus (fever)
Epidemic (louse-borne) typhus

     A75.1 Recrudescent typhus [Brill's disease]
Brill-Zinsser disease

     A75.2 Typhus fever due to Rickettsia typhi
Murine (flea-borne) typhus

     A75.3 Typhus fever due to Rickettsia tsutsugamushi
Scrub (mite-borne) typhus
Tsutsugamushi fever

     A75.9 Typhus fever, unspecified ▽
Typhus (fever) NOS

✓4th **A77 Spotted fever [tick-borne rickettsioses]**

     A77.0 Spotted fever due to Rickettsia rickettsii
Rocky Mountain spotted fever
Sao Paulo fever

     A77.1 Spotted fever due to Rickettsia conorii
African tick typhus
Boutonneuse fever
India tick typhus
Kenya tick typhus
Marseilles fever
Mediterranean tick fever

     A77.2 Spotted fever due to Rickettsia siberica
North Asian tick fever
Siberian tick typhus

     A77.3 Spotted fever due to Rickettsia australis
Queensland tick typhus

✓5th   **A77.4 Ehrlichiosis**
EXCLUDES 1   *Rickettsiosis due to Ehrlichia sennetsu (A79.81)*

     A77.40 Ehrlichiosis, unspecified ▽

     A77.41 Ehrlichiosis chafeensis [E. chafeensis]

     A77.49 Other ehrlichiosis

     A77.8 Other spotted fevers

     A77.9 Spotted fever, unspecified ▽
Tick-borne typhus NOS

A78 Q fever
Infection due to Coxiella burnetii
Nine Mile fever
Quadrilateral fever

✓4th **A79 Other rickettsioses**

     A79.0 Trench fever
Quintan fever
Wolhynian fever

     A79.1 Rickettsialpox due to Rickettsia akari
Kew Garden fever
Vesicular rickettsiosis

✓5th   **A79.8 Other specified rickettsioses**

     A79.81 Rickettsiosis due to Ehrlichia sennetsu

     A79.89 Other specified rickettsioses

     A79.9 Rickettsiosis, unspecified ▽
Rickettsial infection NOS

Viral and prion infections of the central nervous system (A80-A89)

EXCLUDES 1   *postpolio syndrome (G14)*
sequelae of poliomyelitis (B91)
sequelae of viral encephalitis (B94.1)

✓4th **A80 Acute poliomyelitis**

     A80.0 Acute paralytic poliomyelitis, vaccine-associated

     A80.1 Acute paralytic poliomyelitis, wild virus, imported

     A80.2 Acute paralytic poliomyelitis, wild virus, indigenous

✓5th   **A80.3 Acute paralytic poliomyelitis, other and unspecified**

     A80.30 Acute paralytic poliomyelitis, unspecified ▽

     A80.39 Other acute paralytic poliomyelitis

     A80.4 Acute nonparalytic poliomyelitis

     A80.9 Acute poliomyelitis, unspecified ▽

✓4th **A81 Atypical virus infections of central nervous system**
INCLUDES   diseases of the central nervous system caused by prions
Use additional code to identify:
dementia with behavioral disturbance (F02.81)
dementia without behavioral disturbance (F02.80)

✓5th   **A81.0 Creutzfeldt-Jakob disease**

     A81.00 Creutzfeldt-Jakob disease, unspecified ▽
Jakob-Creutzfeldt disease, unspecified

     A81.01 Variant Creutzfeldt-Jakob disease
vCJD

     A81.09 Other Creutzfeldt-Jakob disease
CJD
Familial Creutzfeldt-Jakob disease
Iatrogenic Creutzfeldt-Jakob disease
Sporadic Creutzfeldt-Jakob disease
Subacute spongiform encephalopathy (with dementia)

     A81.1 Subacute sclerosing panencephalitis
Dawson's inclusion body encephalitis
Van Bogaert's sclerosing leukoencephalopathy

     A81.2 Progressive multifocal leukoencephalopathy
Multifocal leukoencephalopathy NOS

EXCLUDES 1   Not coded here   EXCLUDES 2   Not included here   N Newborn Age: 0   P Pediatric Age: 0-17   M Maternity Age: 12-55   A Adult Age: 15-124

444   ICD-10-CM 2018

✓5ᵗʰ **A81.8 Other atypical virus infections of central nervous system**
     A81.81 Kuru
     A81.82 Gerstmann-Sträussler-Scheinker syndrome
         GSS syndrome
     A81.83 Fatal familial insomnia
         FFI
     A81.89 Other atypical virus infections of central nervous system

A81.9 Atypical virus infection of central nervous system, unspecified ▽
     Prion diseases of the central nervous system NOS

✓4ᵗʰ **A82 Rabies**
     A82.0 Sylvatic rabies
     A82.1 Urban rabies
     A82.9 Rabies, unspecified ▽

✓4ᵗʰ **A83 Mosquito-borne viral encephalitis**
     INCLUDES mosquito-borne viral meningoencephalitis
     EXCLUDES 2 *Venezuelan equine encephalitis (A92.2)*
                 West Nile fever (A92.3-)
                 West Nile virus (A92.3-)
     A83.0 Japanese encephalitis
     A83.1 Western equine encephalitis
     A83.2 Eastern equine encephalitis
     A83.3 St Louis encephalitis
     A83.4 Australian encephalitis
         Kunjin virus disease
     A83.5 California encephalitis
         California meningoencephalitis
         La Crosse encephalitis
     A83.6 Rocio virus disease
     A83.8 Other mosquito-borne viral encephalitis
     A83.9 Mosquito-borne viral encephalitis, unspecified ▽

✓4ᵗʰ **A84 Tick-borne viral encephalitis**
     INCLUDES tick-borne viral meningoencephalitis
     A84.0 Far Eastern tick-borne encephalitis [Russian spring-summer encephalitis]
     A84.1 Central European tick-borne encephalitis
     A84.8 Other tick-borne viral encephalitis
         Louping ill
         Powassan virus disease
     A84.9 Tick-borne viral encephalitis, unspecified ▽

✓4ᵗʰ **A85 Other viral encephalitis, not elsewhere classified**
     INCLUDES specified viral encephalomyelitis NEC
                 specified viral meningoencephalitis NEC
     EXCLUDES 1 *benign myalgic encephalomyelitis (G93.3)*
                 encephalitis due to cytomegalovirus (B25.8)
                 encephalitis due to herpesvirus NEC (B10.0-)
                 encephalitis due to herpesvirus [herpes simplex] (B00.4)
                 encephalitis due to measles virus (B05.0)
                 encephalitis due to mumps virus (B26.2)
                 encephalitis due to poliomyelitis virus (A80.-)
                 encephalitis due to zoster (B02.0
                 lymphocytic choriomeningitis (A87.2)
     A85.0 Enteroviral encephalitis
         Enteroviral encephalomyelitis
     A85.1 Adenoviral encephalitis
         Adenoviral meningoencephalitis
     A85.2 Arthropod-borne viral encephalitis, unspecified ▽
         EXCLUDES 1 *West nile virus with encephalitis (A92.31)*
     A85.8 Other specified viral encephalitis
         Encephalitis lethargica
         Von Economo-Cruchet disease

A86 Unspecified viral encephalitis ▽
     Viral encephalomyelitis NOS
     Viral meningoencephalitis NOS

✓4ᵗʰ **A87 Viral meningitis**
     EXCLUDES 1 *meningitis due to herpesvirus [herpes simplex] (B00.3)*
                 meningitis due to measles virus (B05.1)
                 meningitis due to mumps virus (B26.1)
                 meningitis due to poliomyelitis virus (A80.-)
                 meningitis due to zoster (B02.1)
     A87.0 Enteroviral meningitis
         Coxsackievirus meningitis
         Echovirus meningitis
     A87.1 Adenoviral meningitis

     A87.2 Lymphocytic choriomeningitis
         Lymphocytic meningoencephalitis
     A87.8 Other viral meningitis
     A87.9 Viral meningitis, unspecified ▽

✓4ᵗʰ **A88 Other viral infections of central nervous system, not elsewhere classified**
     EXCLUDES 1 *viral encephalitis NOS (A86)*
                 viral meningitis NOS (A87.9)
     A88.0 Enteroviral exanthematous fever [Boston exanthem]
     A88.1 Epidemic vertigo
     A88.8 Other specified viral infections of central nervous system

A89 Unspecified viral infection of central nervous system ▽

Arthropod-borne viral fevers and viral hemorrhagic fevers (A90-A99)

A90 Dengue fever [classical dengue]
     EXCLUDES 1 *dengue hemorrhagic fever (A91)*
     AHA: 2016, 3Q, 13

A91 Dengue hemorrhagic fever

✓4ᵗʰ **A92 Other mosquito-borne viral fevers**
     EXCLUDES 1 *Ross River disease (B33.1)*
     A92.0 Chikungunya virus disease
         Chikungunya (hemorrhagic) fever
     A92.1 O'nyong-nyong fever
     A92.2 Venezuelan equine fever
         Venezuelan equine encephalitis
         Venezuelan equine encephalomyelitis virus disease
     ✓5ᵗʰ **A92.3 West Nile virus infection**
         West Nile fever
         AHA: 2016, 3Q, 12
         A92.30 West Nile virus infection, unspecified ▽
             West Nile fever NOS
             West Nile fever without complications
             West Nile virus NOS
         A92.31 West Nile virus infection with encephalitis
             West Nile encephalitis
             West Nile encephalomyelitis
         A92.32 West Nile virus infection with other neurologic manifestation
             Use additional code to specify the neurologic manifestation
         A92.39 West Nile virus infection with other complications
             Use additional code to specify the other conditions
     A92.4 Rift Valley fever
     A92.5 Zika virus disease
         Zika virus fever
         Zika virus infection
         Zika NOS
     A92.8 Other specified mosquito-borne viral fevers
     A92.9 Mosquito-borne viral fever, unspecified ▽

✓4ᵗʰ **A93 Other arthropod-borne viral fevers, not elsewhere classified**
     A93.0 Oropouche virus disease
         Oropouche fever
     A93.1 Sandfly fever
         Pappataci fever
         Phlebotomus fever
     A93.2 Colorado tick fever
     A93.8 Other specified arthropod-borne viral fevers
         Piry virus disease
         Vesicular stomatitis virus disease [Indiana fever]

A94 Unspecified arthropod-borne viral fever ▽
     Arboviral fever NOS
     Arbovirus infection NOS

✓4ᵗʰ **A95 Yellow fever**
     A95.0 Sylvatic yellow fever
         Jungle yellow fever
     A95.1 Urban yellow fever
     A95.9 Yellow fever, unspecified ▽

✓4ᵗʰ **A96 Arenaviral hemorrhagic fever**
     A96.0 Junin hemorrhagic fever
         Argentinian hemorrhagic fever
     A96.1 Machupo hemorrhagic fever
         Bolivian hemorrhagic fever
     A96.2 Lassa fever

A96.8   **Other arenaviral hemorrhagic fevers**

A96.9   **Arenaviral hemorrhagic fever, unspecified**   ▽

√4ᵗʰ **A98   Other viral hemorrhagic fevers, not elsewhere classified**
  EXCLUDES 1   *chikungunya hemorrhagic fever (A92.0)*
               dengue hemorrhagic fever (A91)

A98.0   **Crimean-Congo hemorrhagic fever**
           Central Asian hemorrhagic fever

A98.1   **Omsk hemorrhagic fever**

A98.2   **Kyasanur Forest disease**

A98.3   **Marburg virus disease**

A98.4   **Ebola virus disease**

A98.5   **Hemorrhagic fever with renal syndrome**
           Epidemic hemorrhagic fever
           Korean hemorrhagic fever
           Russian hemorrhagic fever
           Hantaan virus disease
           Hantavirus disease with renal manifestations
           Nephropathia epidemica
           Songo fever
             EXCLUDES 1   *hantavirus (cardio)-pulmonary syndrome (B33.4)*

A98.8   **Other specified viral hemorrhagic fevers**

A99   **Unspecified viral hemorrhagic fever**   ▽

Viral infections characterized by skin and mucous membrane lesions (B00-B09)

√4ᵗʰ **B00   Herpesviral [herpes simplex] infections**
  EXCLUDES 1   *congenital herpesviral infections (P35.2)*
  EXCLUDES 2   *anogenital herpesviral infection (A60.-)*
               gammaherpesviral mononucleosis (B27.0-)
               herpangina (B08.5)

B00.0   **Eczema herpeticum**
           Kaposi's varicelliform eruption

B00.1   **Herpesviral vesicular dermatitis**
           Herpes simplex facialis
           Herpes simplex labialis
           Herpes simplex otitis externa
           Vesicular dermatitis of ear
           Vesicular dermatitis of lip

B00.2   **Herpesviral gingivostomatitis and pharyngotonsillitis**
           Herpesviral pharyngitis

B00.3   **Herpesviral meningitis**

B00.4   **Herpesviral encephalitis**
           Herpesviral meningoencephalitis
           Simian B disease
             EXCLUDES 1   *herpesviral encephalitis due to herpesvirus 6 and 7*
                          (B10.01, B10.09)
                          non-simplex herpesviral encephalitis (B10.0-)

√5ᵗʰ B00.5   **Herpesviral ocular disease**
           B00.50   **Herpesviral ocular disease, unspecified**   ▽
           B00.51   **Herpesviral iridocyclitis**
                       Herpesviral iritis
                       Herpesviral uveitis, anterior
           B00.52   **Herpesviral keratitis**
                       Herpesviral keratoconjunctivitis
           B00.53   **Herpesviral conjunctivitis**
           B00.59   **Other herpesviral disease of eye**
                       Herpesviral dermatitis of eyelid

B00.7   **Disseminated herpesviral disease**   HCC
           Herpesviral sepsis

√5ᵗʰ B00.8   **Other forms of herpesviral infections**
           B00.81   **Herpesviral hepatitis**
           B00.82   **Herpes simplex myelitis**   HCC
           B00.89   **Other herpesviral infection**
                       Herpesviral whitlow

B00.9   **Herpesviral infection, unspecified**   ▽
           Herpes simplex infection NOS

√4ᵗʰ **B01   Varicella [chickenpox]**
B01.0   **Varicella meningitis**

√5ᵗʰ B01.1   **Varicella encephalitis, myelitis and encephalomyelitis**
           Postchickenpox encephalitis, myelitis and encephalomyelitis
           B01.11   **Varicella encephalitis and encephalomyelitis**
                       Postchickenpox encephalitis and encephalomyelitis
           B01.12   **Varicella myelitis**   HCC
                       Postchickenpox myelitis

B01.2   **Varicella pneumonia**

√5ᵗʰ B01.8   **Varicella with other complications**
           B01.81   **Varicella keratitis**
           B01.89   **Other varicella complications**

B01.9   **Varicella without complication**   ▽
           Varicella NOS

√4ᵗʰ **B02   Zoster [herpes zoster]**
  INCLUDES   shingles
             zona

B02.0   **Zoster encephalitis**
           Zoster meningoencephalitis

B02.1   **Zoster meningitis**

√5ᵗʰ B02.2   **Zoster with other nervous system involvement**
           B02.21   **Postherpetic geniculate ganglionitis**
           B02.22   **Postherpetic trigeminal neuralgia**
           B02.23   **Postherpetic polyneuropathy**
           B02.24   **Postherpetic myelitis**   HCC
                       Herpes zoster myelitis
           B02.29   **Other postherpetic nervous system involvement**
                       Postherpetic radiculopathy

√5ᵗʰ B02.3   **Zoster ocular disease**
           B02.30   **Zoster ocular disease, unspecified**   ▽
           B02.31   **Zoster conjunctivitis**
           B02.32   **Zoster iridocyclitis**
           B02.33   **Zoster keratitis**
                       Herpes zoster keratoconjunctivitis
           B02.34   **Zoster scleritis**
           B02.39   **Other herpes zoster eye disease**
                       Zoster blepharitis

B02.7   **Disseminated zoster**

B02.8   **Zoster with other complications**
           Herpes zoster otitis externa

B02.9   **Zoster without complications**   ▽
           Zoster NOS

B03   Smallpox
  NOTE   In 1980 the 33rd World Health Assembly declared that smallpox had been eradicated.
          The classification is maintained for surveillance purposes.

B04   Monkeypox

√4ᵗʰ **B05   Measles**
  INCLUDES   morbilli
  EXCLUDES 1   *subacute sclerosing panencephalitis (A81.1)*

B05.0   **Measles complicated by encephalitis**
           Postmeasles encephalitis

B05.1   **Measles complicated by meningitis**
           Postmeasles meningitis

B05.2   **Measles complicated by pneumonia**
           Postmeasles pneumonia

B05.3   **Measles complicated by otitis media**
           Postmeasles otitis media

B05.4   **Measles with intestinal complications**

√5ᵗʰ B05.8   **Measles with other complications**
           B05.81   **Measles keratitis and keratoconjunctivitis**
           B05.89   **Other measles complications**

B05.9   **Measles without complication**   ▽
           Measles NOS

√4ᵗʰ **B06   Rubella [German measles]**
  EXCLUDES 1   *congenital rubella (P35.0)*

√5ᵗʰ B06.0   **Rubella with neurological complications**
           B06.00   **Rubella with neurological complication, unspecified**   ▽
           B06.01   **Rubella encephalitis**
                       Rubella meningoencephalitis
           B06.02   **Rubella meningitis**
           B06.09   **Other neurological complications of rubella**

√5ᵗʰ B06.8   **Rubella with other complications**
           B06.81   **Rubella pneumonia**
           B06.82   **Rubella arthritis**   HCC
           B06.89   **Other rubella complications**

B06.9   **Rubella without complication**   ▽
           Rubella NOS

EXCLUDES 1 Not coded here   EXCLUDES 2 Not included here   N Newborn Age: 0   P Pediatric Age: 0-17   M Maternity Age: 12-55   A Adult Age: 15-124

446   ICD-10-CM 2018

☑️4ᵗʰ **B07 Viral warts**
    INCLUDES   verruca simplex
              verruca vulgaris
              viral warts due to human papillomavirus
    EXCLUDES 2   *anogenital (venereal) warts (A63.0)*
              papilloma of bladder (D41.4)
              papilloma of cervix (D26.0)
              papilloma larynx (D14.1)

    B07.0 Plantar wart
         Verruca plantaris

    B07.8 Other viral warts
         Common wart
         Flat wart
         Verruca plana

    B07.9 Viral wart, unspecified ▽

☑️4ᵗʰ **B08 Other viral infections characterized by skin and mucous membrane lesions, not elsewhere classified**
    EXCLUDES 1   *vesicular stomatitis virus disease (A93.8)*

    ☑️5ᵗʰ **B08.0 Other orthopoxvirus infections**
        EXCLUDES 2   *monkeypox (B04)*

      ☑️6ᵗʰ **B08.01 Cowpox and vaccinia not from vaccine**
          B08.010 Cowpox
              DEF: A disease contracted by milking infected cows; vesicles usually appear on the fingers, hands, and adjacent areas and usually disappear without scarring; other symptoms: local edema, lymphangitis, and regional lymphadenitis with or without fever.

          B08.011 Vaccinia not from vaccine
              EXCLUDES 1   *vaccinia (from vaccination) (generalized) (T88.1)*

      B08.02 Orf virus disease
          Contagious pustular dermatitis
          Ecthyma contagiosum

      B08.03 Pseudocowpox [milker's node]

      B08.04 Paravaccinia, unspecified ▽

      B08.09 Other orthopoxvirus infections
          Orthopoxvirus infection NOS

    B08.1 Molluscum contagiosum
        DEF: Benign poxvirus infection causing small bumps on the skin or conjunctiva; transmitted by close contact.

    ☑️5ᵗʰ **B08.2 Exanthema subitum [sixth disease]**
        Roseola infantum

      B08.20 Exanthema subitum [sixth disease], unspecified P ▽
          Roseola infantum, unspecified

      B08.21 Exanthema subitum [sixth disease] due to human herpesvirus 6 P
          Roseola infantum due to human herpesvirus 6

      B08.22 Exanthema subitum [sixth disease] due to human herpesvirus 7 P
          Roseola infantum due to human herpesvirus 7

    B08.3 Erythema infectiosum [fifth disease]

    B08.4 Enteroviral vesicular stomatitis with exanthem
        Hand, foot and mouth disease

    B08.5 Enteroviral vesicular pharyngitis
        Herpangina
        DEF: Acute infectious Coxsackie virus infection causing throat lesions, fever, and vomiting; generally affects children in summer.

    ☑️5ᵗʰ **B08.6 Parapoxvirus infections**
      B08.60 Parapoxvirus infection, unspecified ▽
      B08.61 Bovine stomatitis
      B08.62 Sealpox
      B08.69 Other parapoxvirus infections

    ☑️5ᵗʰ **B08.7 Yatapoxvirus infections**
      B08.70 Yatapoxvirus infection, unspecified ▽
      B08.71 Tanapox virus disease
      B08.72 Yaba pox virus disease
          Yaba monkey tumor disease
      B08.79 Other yatapoxvirus infections

    B08.8 Other specified viral infections characterized by skin and mucous membrane lesions
        Enteroviral lymphonodular pharyngitis
        Foot-and-mouth disease
        Poxvirus NEC

B09 Unspecified viral infection characterized by skin and mucous membrane lesions ▽
        Viral enanthema NOS
        Viral exanthema NOS

Other human herpesviruses (B10)

☑️4ᵗʰ **B10 Other human herpesviruses**
    EXCLUDES 2   *cytomegalovirus (B25.9)*
              Epstein-Barr virus (B27.0-)
              herpes NOS (B00.9)
              herpes simplex (B00.-)
              herpes zoster (B02.-)
              human herpesvirus NOS (B00.-)
              human herpesvirus 1 and 2 (B00.-)
              human herpesvirus 3 (B01.-, B02.-)
              human herpesvirus 4 (B27.0-)
              human herpesvirus (B25.-)
              varicella (B01.-)
              zoster (B02.-)

    ☑️5ᵗʰ **B10.0 Other human herpesvirus encephalitis**
        EXCLUDES 2   *herpes encephalitis NOS (B00.4)*
                 herpes simplex encephalitis (B00.4)
                 human herpesvirus encephalitis (B00.4)
                 simian B herpes virus encephalitis (B00.4)

      B10.01 Human herpesvirus 6 encephalitis
      B10.09 Other human herpesvirus encephalitis
          Human herpesvirus 7 encephalitis

    ☑️5ᵗʰ **B10.8 Other human herpesvirus infection**
      B10.81 Human herpesvirus 6 infection
      B10.82 Human herpesvirus 7 infection
      B10.89 Other human herpesvirus infection
          Human herpesvirus 8 infection
          Kaposi's sarcoma-associated herpesvirus infection

Viral hepatitis (B15-B19)

    EXCLUDES 1   *sequelae of viral hepatitis (B94.2)*
    EXCLUDES 2   *cytomegaloviral hepatitis (B25.1)*
              herpesviral [herpes simplex] hepatitis (B00.81)
DEF: Hepatitis A: HAV infection is self-limiting with flulike symptoms; transmission, fecal-oral.
DEF: Hepatitis B: HBV infection can be chronic and systemic; transmission, bodily fluids.
DEF: Hepatitis C: HCV infection can be chronic and systemic; transmission, blood transfusion and unidentified agents.
DEF: Hepatitis D (delta): HDV occurs only in the presence of hepatitis B virus; transmission, contaminated blood in contact with mucous membranes.
DEF: Hepatitis E: HEV is epidemic form; transmission, fecal-oral, most often from contaminated water.

☑️4ᵗʰ **B15 Acute hepatitis A**
    B15.0 Hepatitis A with hepatic coma
    B15.9 Hepatitis A without hepatic coma
        Hepatitis A (acute)(viral) NOS

☑️4ᵗʰ **B16 Acute hepatitis B**
    AHA: 2016, 3Q, 13
    B16.0 Acute hepatitis B with delta-agent with hepatic coma
    B16.1 Acute hepatitis B with delta-agent without hepatic coma
    B16.2 Acute hepatitis B without delta-agent with hepatic coma
    B16.9 Acute hepatitis B without delta-agent and without hepatic coma
        Hepatitis B (acute) (viral) NOS

☑️4ᵗʰ **B17 Other acute viral hepatitis**
    B17.0 Acute delta-(super) infection of hepatitis B carrier
    ☑️5ᵗʰ **B17.1 Acute hepatitis C**
      B17.10 Acute hepatitis C without hepatic coma
          Acute hepatitis C NOS
      B17.11 Acute hepatitis C with hepatic coma
    B17.2 Acute hepatitis E
    B17.8 Other specified acute viral hepatitis
        Hepatitis non-A non-B (acute) (viral) NEC
    B17.9 Acute viral hepatitis, unspecified ▽
        Acute hepatitis NOS
        Acute infectious hepatitis NOS

☑️4ᵗʰ **B18 Chronic viral hepatitis**
    INCLUDES   carrier of viral hepatitis
    AHA: 2017, 1Q, 41
    B18.0 Chronic viral hepatitis B with delta-agent HCC

☑️ Additional Character Req   ✓x7ᵗʰ Placeholder Alert   Manifestation   HCC CMS-HCC Condition   ▽ Unspecified Code   ▶◀ Revised Text   ● New Code   ▲ Revised Code Title

ICD-10-CM 2018   **447**

B18.1 Chronic viral hepatitis B without delta-agent HCC
Carrier of viral hepatitis B
Chronic (viral) hepatitis B

B18.2 Chronic viral hepatitis C HCC
Carrier of viral hepatitis C

B18.8 Other chronic viral hepatitis HCC
Carrier of other viral hepatitis

B18.9 Chronic viral hepatitis, unspecified HCC ▽
Carrier of unspecified viral hepatitis

✓4th **B19 Unspecified viral hepatitis**

B19.0 Unspecified viral hepatitis with hepatic coma ▽

✓5th **B19.1 Unspecified viral hepatitis B**

B19.10 Unspecified viral hepatitis B without hepatic coma ▽
Unspecified viral hepatitis B NOS

B19.11 Unspecified viral hepatitis B with hepatic coma ▽

✓5th **B19.2 Unspecified viral hepatitis C**

B19.20 Unspecified viral hepatitis C without hepatic coma ▽
Viral hepatitis C NOS

B19.21 Unspecified viral hepatitis C with hepatic coma ▽

B19.9 Unspecified viral hepatitis without hepatic coma ▽
Viral hepatitis NOS

Human immunodeficiency virus [HIV] disease (B20)

B20 Human immunodeficiency virus [HIV] disease HCC
INCLUDES acquired immune deficiency syndrome [AIDS]
AIDS-related complex [ARC]
HIV infection, symptomatic
Code first human immunodeficiency virus [HIV] disease complicating pregnancy, childbirth and the puerperium, if applicable (O98.7-)
Use additional code(s) to identify all manifestations of HIV infection
EXCLUDES 1 asymptomatic human immunodeficiency virus [HIV] infection status (Z21)
exposure to HIV virus (Z20.6)
inconclusive serologic evidence of HIV (R75)

Other viral diseases (B25-B34)

✓4th **B25 Cytomegaloviral disease**
EXCLUDES 1 congenital cytomegalovirus infection (P35.1)
cytomegaloviral mononucleosis (B27.1-)

B25.0 Cytomegaloviral pneumonitis HCC

B25.1 Cytomegaloviral hepatitis HCC

B25.2 Cytomegaloviral pancreatitis HCC

B25.8 Other cytomegaloviral diseases HCC
Cytomegaloviral encephalitis

B25.9 Cytomegaloviral disease, unspecified HCC ▽

✓4th **B26 Mumps**
INCLUDES epidemic parotitis
infectious parotitis

B26.0 Mumps orchitis ♂

B26.1 Mumps meningitis

B26.2 Mumps encephalitis

B26.3 Mumps pancreatitis

✓5th **B26.8 Mumps with other complications**

B26.81 Mumps hepatitis

B26.82 Mumps myocarditis

B26.83 Mumps nephritis

B26.84 Mumps polyneuropathy

B26.85 Mumps arthritis HCC

B26.89 Other mumps complications

B26.9 Mumps without complication ▽
Mumps NOS
Mumps parotitis NOS

✓4th **B27 Infectious mononucleosis**
INCLUDES glandular fever
monocytic angina
Pfeiffer's disease

✓5th **B27.0 Gammaherpesviral mononucleosis**
Mononucleosis due to Epstein-Barr virus

B27.00 Gammaherpesviral mononucleosis without complication

B27.01 Gammaherpesviral mononucleosis with polyneuropathy

B27.02 Gammaherpesviral mononucleosis with meningitis

B27.09 Gammaherpesviral mononucleosis with other complications
Hepatomegaly in gammaherpesviral mononucleosis

✓5th **B27.1 Cytomegaloviral mononucleosis**

B27.10 Cytomegaloviral mononucleosis without complications

B27.11 Cytomegaloviral mononucleosis with polyneuropathy

B27.12 Cytomegaloviral mononucleosis with meningitis

B27.19 Cytomegaloviral mononucleosis with other complication
Hepatomegaly in cytomegaloviral mononucleosis

✓5th **B27.8 Other infectious mononucleosis**

B27.80 Other infectious mononucleosis without complication

B27.81 Other infectious mononucleosis with polyneuropathy

B27.82 Other infectious mononucleosis with meningitis

B27.89 Other infectious mononucleosis with other complication
Hepatomegaly in other infectious mononucleosis

✓5th **B27.9 Infectious mononucleosis, unspecified**

B27.90 Infectious mononucleosis, unspecified without complication ▽

B27.91 Infectious mononucleosis, unspecified with polyneuropathy ▽

B27.92 Infectious mononucleosis, unspecified with meningitis ▽

B27.99 Infectious mononucleosis, unspecified with other complication ▽
Hepatomegaly in unspecified infectious mononucleosis

✓4th **B30 Viral conjunctivitis**
EXCLUDES 1 herpesviral [herpes simplex] ocular disease (B00.5)
ocular zoster (B02.3)

B30.0 Keratoconjunctivitis due to adenovirus
Epidemic keratoconjunctivitis
Shipyard eye

B30.1 Conjunctivitis due to adenovirus
Acute adenoviral follicular conjunctivitis
Swimming-pool conjunctivitis

B30.2 Viral pharyngoconjunctivitis

B30.3 Acute epidemic hemorrhagic conjunctivitis (enteroviral)
Conjunctivitis due to coxsackievirus 24
Conjunctivitis due to enterovirus 70
Hemorrhagic conjunctivitis (acute)(epidemic)

B30.8 Other viral conjunctivitis
Newcastle conjunctivitis

B30.9 Viral conjunctivitis, unspecified ▽

✓4th **B33 Other viral diseases, not elsewhere classified**

B33.0 Epidemic myalgia
Bornholm disease

B33.1 Ross River disease
Epidemic polyarthritis and exanthema
Ross River fever

Viral Conjunctivitis

Normal conjunctiva

Inflamed conjunctiva

✓5ᵗʰ **B33.2 Viral carditis**
Coxsackie (virus) carditis

    B33.20 Viral carditis, unspecified ▽

    B33.21 Viral endocarditis

    B33.22 Viral myocarditis

    B33.23 Viral pericarditis

    B33.24 Viral cardiomyopathy HCC

B33.3 Retrovirus infections, not elsewhere classified
Retrovirus infection NOS

B33.4 Hantavirus (cardio)-pulmonary syndrome [HPS] [HCPS]
Hantavirus disease with pulmonary manifestations
Sin nombre virus disease
Use additional code to identify any associated acute kidney failure (N17.9)
    EXCLUDES 1   *hantavirus disease with renal manifestations (A98.5)*
                   hemorrhagic fever with renal manifestations (A98.5)

B33.8 Other specified viral diseases
    EXCLUDES 1   *anogenital human papillomavirus infection (A63.0)*
                   viral warts due to human papillomavirus infection (B07)

✓4ᵗʰ **B34 Viral infection of unspecified site**
    EXCLUDES 1   *anogenital human papillomavirus infection (A63.0)*
                   cytomegaloviral disease NOS (B25.9)
                   herpesvirus [herpes simplex] infection NOS (B00.9)
                   retrovirus infection NOS (B33.3)
                   viral agents as the cause of diseases classified elsewhere (B97.-)
                   viral warts due to human papillomavirus infection (B07)

B34.0 Adenovirus infection, unspecified ▽

B34.1 Enterovirus infection, unspecified ▽
Coxsackievirus infection NOS
Echovirus infection NOS

B34.2 Coronavirus infection, unspecified ▽
    EXCLUDES 1   *pneumonia due to SARS-associated coronavirus (J12.81)*

B34.3 Parvovirus infection, unspecified ▽

B34.4 Papovavirus infection, unspecified ▽

B34.8 Other viral infections of unspecified site ▽

B34.9 Viral infection, unspecified ▽
Viremia NOS
AHA: 2016, 3Q, 10

Mycoses (B35-B49)

EXCLUDES 2   *hypersensitivity pneumonitis due to organic dust (J67.-)*
                 mycosis fungoides (C84.0-)

✓4ᵗʰ **B35 Dermatophytosis**
    INCLUDES   favus
               infections due to species of Epidermophyton, Micro-sporum and Trichophyton
               tinea, any type except those in B36-
    DEF: Contagious superficial fungal infection of the skin that invades and grows in dead keratin.

B35.0 Tinea barbae and tinea capitis
Beard ringworm
Kerion
Scalp ringworm
Sycosis, mycotic

B35.1 Tinea unguium
Dermatophytic onychia
Dermatophytosis of nail
Onychomycosis
Ringworm of nails

B35.2 Tinea manuum
Dermatophytosis of hand
Hand ringworm

B35.3 Tinea pedis
Athlete's foot
Dermatophytosis of foot
Foot ringworm

B35.4 Tinea corporis
Ringworm of the body

B35.5 Tinea imbricata
Tokelau

B35.6 Tinea cruris
Dhobi itch
Groin ringworm
Jock itch

B35.8 Other dermatophytoses
Disseminated dermatophytosis
Granulomatous dermatophytosis

B35.9 Dermatophytosis, unspecified ▽
Ringworm NOS

✓4ᵗʰ **B36 Other superficial mycoses**
B36.0 Pityriasis versicolor
Tinea flava
Tinea versicolor

B36.1 Tinea nigra
Keratomycosis nigricans palmaris
Microsporosis nigra
Pityriasis nigra

B36.2 White piedra
Tinea blanca

B36.3 Black piedra

B36.8 Other specified superficial mycoses

B36.9 Superficial mycosis, unspecified ▽

✓4ᵗʰ **B37 Candidiasis**
    INCLUDES   candidosis
               moniliasis
    EXCLUDES 1   *neonatal candidiasis (P37.5)*

B37.0 Candidal stomatitis
Oral thrush

B37.1 Pulmonary candidiasis HCC
Candidal bronchitis
Candidal pneumonia

B37.2 Candidiasis of skin and nail
Candidal onychia
Candidal paronychia
    EXCLUDES 2   *diaper dermatitis (L22)*

B37.3 Candidiasis of vulva and vagina ♀
Candidal vulvovaginitis
Monilial vulvovaginitis
Vaginal thrush

✓5ᵗʰ **B37.4 Candidiasis of other urogenital sites**
    B37.41 Candidal cystitis and urethritis
    B37.42 Candidal balanitis
    B37.49 Other urogenital candidiasis
               Candidal pyelonephritis

B37.5 Candidal meningitis

B37.6 Candidal endocarditis

B37.7 Candidal sepsis HCC
Disseminated candidiasis
Systemic candidiasis
AHA: 2014, 4Q, 46

✓5ᵗʰ **B37.8 Candidiasis of other sites**
    B37.81 Candidal esophagitis HCC
    B37.82 Candidal enteritis
               Candidal proctitis
    B37.83 Candidal cheilitis
    B37.84 Candidal otitis externa
    B37.89 Other sites of candidiasis
               Candidal osteomyelitis

B37.9 Candidiasis, unspecified ▽
Thrush NOS

✓4ᵗʰ **B38 Coccidioidomycosis**
B38.0 Acute pulmonary coccidioidomycosis HCC
B38.1 Chronic pulmonary coccidioidomycosis HCC
B38.2 Pulmonary coccidioidomycosis, unspecified HCC ▽
B38.3 Cutaneous coccidioidomycosis
B38.4 Coccidioidomycosis meningitis
    DEF: *Coccidioides immitis* infection of the lining of the brain and/or spinal cord.
B38.7 Disseminated coccidioidomycosis
Generalized coccidioidomycosis

✓5ᵗʰ **B38.8 Other forms of coccidioidomycosis**
    B38.81 Prostatic coccidioidomycosis ♂
    B38.89 Other forms of coccidioidomycosis
B38.9 Coccidioidomycosis, unspecified ▽

✓ Additional Character Req   ✓x7ᵗʰ Placeholder Alert   Manifestation   HCC CMS-HCC Condition   ▽ Unspecified Code   ►◄ Revised Text   ● New Code   ▲ Revised Code Title

ICD-10-CM 2018   **449**

Chapter 1. Certain Infectious and Parasitic Diseases

Histoplasmosis

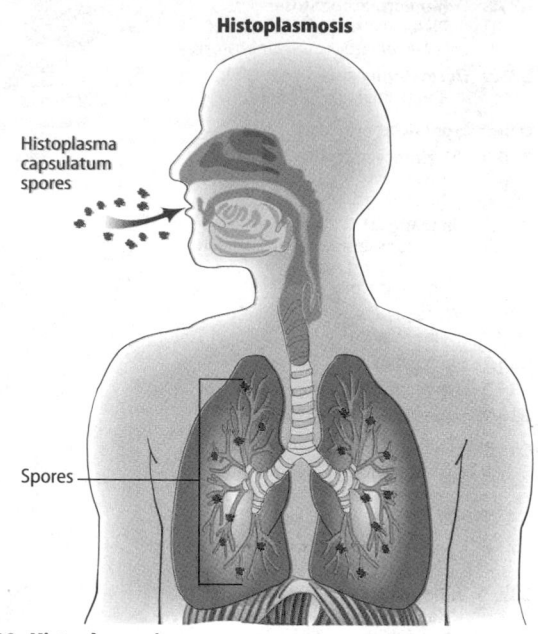

Histoplasma capsulatum spores

Spores

✓4ᵗʰ B39 Histoplasmosis

Code first associated AIDS (B2Ø)

Use additional code for any associated manifestations, such as:
  endocarditis (I39)
  meningitis (GØ2)
  pericarditis (I32)
  retinitits (H32)

DEF: Type of lung infection caused by breathing in fungal spores often found in the droppings of bats and birds or soil contaminated by their droppings.

- B39.Ø   **Acute pulmonary histoplasmosis capsulati**   HCC
- B39.1   **Chronic pulmonary histoplasmosis capsulati**   HCC
- B39.2   **Pulmonary histoplasmosis capsulati, unspecified**   HCC ▽
- B39.3   **Disseminated histoplasmosis capsulati**
  Generalized histoplasmosis capsulati
- B39.4   **Histoplasmosis capsulati, unspecified**   ▽
  American histoplasmosis
- B39.5   **Histoplasmosis duboisii**
  African histoplasmosis
- B39.9   **Histoplasmosis, unspecified**   ▽

✓4ᵗʰ B40 Blastomycosis

EXCLUDES 1   Brazilian blastomycosis (B41.-)
     keloidal blastomycosis (B48.Ø)

- B4Ø.Ø   **Acute pulmonary blastomycosis**   HCC
- B4Ø.1   **Chronic pulmonary blastomycosis**   HCC
- B4Ø.2   **Pulmonary blastomycosis, unspecified**   HCC ▽
- B4Ø.3   **Cutaneous blastomycosis**
- B4Ø.7   **Disseminated blastomycosis**
  Generalized blastomycosis
- ✓5ᵗʰ B4Ø.8   **Other forms of blastomycosis**
  - B4Ø.81   **Blastomycotic meningoencephalitis**
    Meningomyelitis due to blastomycosis
  - B4Ø.89   **Other forms of blastomycosis**
- B4Ø.9   **Blastomycosis, unspecified**   ▽

✓4ᵗʰ B41 Paracoccidioidomycosis

INCLUDES   Brazilian blastomycosis
     Lutz' disease

- B41.Ø   **Pulmonary paracoccidioidomycosis**   HCC
- B41.7   **Disseminated paracoccidioidomycosis**
  Generalized paracoccidioidomycosis
- B41.8   **Other forms of paracoccidioidomycosis**
- B41.9   **Paracoccidioidomycosis, unspecified**   ▽

✓4ᵗʰ B42 Sporotrichosis

- B42.Ø   **Pulmonary sporotrichosis**
- B42.1   **Lymphocutaneous sporotrichosis**
- B42.7   **Disseminated sporotrichosis**
  Generalized sporotrichosis

- ✓5ᵗʰ B42.8   **Other forms of sporotrichosis**
  - B42.81   **Cerebral sporotrichosis**
    Meningitis due to sporotrichosis
  - B42.82   **Sporotrichosis arthritis**   HCC
  - B42.89   **Other forms of sporotrichosis**
- B42.9   **Sporotrichosis, unspecified**   ▽

✓4ᵗʰ B43 Chromomycosis and pheomycotic abscess

- B43.Ø   **Cutaneous chromomycosis**
  Dermatitis verrucosa
- B43.1   **Pheomycotic brain abscess**
  Cerebral chromomycosis
- B43.2   **Subcutaneous pheomycotic abscess and cyst**
- B43.8   **Other forms of chromomycosis**
- B43.9   **Chromomycosis, unspecified**   ▽

✓4ᵗʰ B44 Aspergillosis

INCLUDES   aspergilloma

- B44.Ø   **Invasive pulmonary aspergillosis**   HCC
- B44.1   **Other pulmonary aspergillosis**   HCC
- B44.2   **Tonsillar aspergillosis**   HCC
- B44.7   **Disseminated aspergillosis**   HCC
  Generalized aspergillosis
- ✓5ᵗʰ B44.8   **Other forms of aspergillosis**
  - B44.81   **Allergic bronchopulmonary aspergillosis**   HCC
  - B44.89   **Other forms of aspergillosis**   HCC
- B44.9   **Aspergillosis, unspecified**   HCC ▽

✓4ᵗʰ B45 Cryptococcosis

- B45.Ø   **Pulmonary cryptococcosis**   HCC
- B45.1   **Cerebral cryptococcosis**   HCC
  Cryptococcal meningitis
  Cryptococcosis meningocerebralis
- B45.2   **Cutaneous cryptococcosis**   HCC
- B45.3   **Osseous cryptococcosis**   HCC
- B45.7   **Disseminated cryptococcosis**   HCC
  Generalized cryptococcosis
- B45.8   **Other forms of cryptococcosis**   HCC
- B45.9   **Cryptococcosis, unspecified**   HCC ▽

✓4ᵗʰ B46 Zygomycosis

- B46.Ø   **Pulmonary mucormycosis**   HCC
- B46.1   **Rhinocerebral mucormycosis**   HCC
- B46.2   **Gastrointestinal mucormycosis**   HCC
- B46.3   **Cutaneous mucormycosis**   HCC
  Subcutaneous mucormycosis
- B46.4   **Disseminated mucormycosis**   HCC
  Generalized mucormycosis
- B46.5   **Mucormycosis, unspecified**   HCC ▽
- B46.8   **Other zygomycoses**   HCC
  Entomophthoromycosis
- B46.9   **Zygomycosis, unspecified**   HCC ▽
  Phycomycosis NOS

✓4ᵗʰ B47 Mycetoma

- B47.Ø   **Eumycetoma**
  Madura foot, mycotic
  Maduromycosis
- B47.1   **Actinomycetoma**
- B47.9   **Mycetoma, unspecified**   ▽
  Madura foot NOS

✓4ᵗʰ B48 Other mycoses, not elsewhere classified

- B48.Ø   **Lobomycosis**
  Keloidal blastomycosis
  Lobo's disease
- B48.1   **Rhinosporidiosis**
- B48.2   **Allescheriasis**
  Infection due to Pseudallescheria boydii
  EXCLUDES 1   eumycetoma (B47.Ø)
- B48.3   **Geotrichosis**
  Geotrichum stomatitis
- B48.4   **Penicillosis**   HCC

EXCLUDES 1 Not coded here   EXCLUDES 2 Not included here   N Newborn Age: 0   P Pediatric Age: 0-17   M Maternity Age: 12-55   A Adult Age: 15-124

450   ICD-10-CM 2018

B48.8 Other specified mycoses   `HCC`
Adiaspiromycosis
Infection of tissue and organs by Alternaria
Infection of tissue and organs by Drechslera
Infection of tissue and organs by Fusarium
Infection of tissue and organs by saprophytic fungi NEC
AHA: 2014, 4Q, 46; 2014, 2Q, 13

B49 Unspecified mycosis   ▽
Fungemia NOS

Protozoal diseases (B50-B64)

`EXCLUDES 1`   *amebiasis (A06.-)*
other protozoal intestinal diseases (A07.-)

☑4ᵗʰ **B50 Plasmodium falciparum malaria**
`INCLUDES`   mixed infections of Plasmodium falciparum with any other Plasmodium species

B50.0 Plasmodium falciparum malaria with cerebral complications
Cerebral malaria NOS

B50.8 Other severe and complicated Plasmodium falciparum malaria
Severe or complicated Plasmodium falciparum malaria NOS

B50.9 Plasmodium falciparum malaria, unspecified   ▽

☑4ᵗʰ **B51 Plasmodium vivax malaria**
`INCLUDES`   mixed infections of Plasmodium vivax with other Plasmodium species, except Plasmodium falciparum
`EXCLUDES 1`   *plasmodium vivax with Plasmodium falciparum (B50.-)*

B51.0 Plasmodium vivax malaria with rupture of spleen

B51.8 Plasmodium vivax malaria with other complications

B51.9 Plasmodium vivax malaria without complication   ▽
Plasmodium vivax malaria NOS

☑4ᵗʰ **B52 Plasmodium malariae malaria**
`INCLUDES`   mixed infections of Plasmodium malariae with other Plasmodium species, except Plasmodium falciparum and Plasmodium vivax
`EXCLUDES 1`   *Plasmodium falciparum (B50.-)*
Plasmodium vivax (B51.-)

B52.0 Plasmodium malariae malaria with nephropathy

B52.8 Plasmodium malariae malaria with other complications

B52.9 Plasmodium malariae malaria without complication   ▽
Plasmodium malariae malaria NOS

☑4ᵗʰ **B53 Other specified malaria**

B53.0 Plasmodium ovale malaria
`EXCLUDES 1`   *Plasmodium ovale with Plasmodium falciparum (B50.-)*
Plasmodium ovale with Plasmodium malariae (B52.-)
Plasmodium ovale with Plasmodium vivax (B51.-)

B53.1 Malaria due to simian plasmodia
`EXCLUDES 1`   *Malaria due to simian plasmodia with Plasmodium falciparum (B50.-)*
Malaria due to simian plasmodia with Plasmodium malariae (B52.-)
Malaria due to simian plasmodia with Plasmodium ovale (B53.0)
Malaria due to simian plasmodia with Plasmodium vivax (B51.-)

B53.8 Other malaria, not elsewhere classified

B54 Unspecified malaria   ▽

☑4ᵗʰ **B55 Leishmaniasis**

B55.0 Visceral leishmaniasis
Kala-azar
Post-kala-azar dermal leishmaniasis

B55.1 Cutaneous leishmaniasis

B55.2 Mucocutaneous leishmaniasis

B55.9 Leishmaniasis, unspecified   ▽

☑4ᵗʰ **B56 African trypanosomiasis**

B56.0 Gambiense trypanosomiasis
Infection due to Trypanosoma brucei gambiense
West African sleeping sickness

B56.1 Rhodesiense trypanosomiasis
East African sleeping sickness
Infection due to Trypanosoma brucei rhodesiense

B56.9 African trypanosomiasis, unspecified   ▽
Sleeping sickness NOS

☑4ᵗʰ **B57 Chagas' disease**
`INCLUDES`   American trypanosomiasis
infection due to Trypanosoma cruzi

B57.0 Acute Chagas' disease with heart involvement
Acute Chagas' disease with myocarditis

B57.1 Acute Chagas' disease without heart involvement
Acute Chagas' disease NOS

B57.2 Chagas' disease (chronic) with heart involvement
American trypanosomiasis NOS
Chagas' disease (chronic) NOS
Chagas' disease (chronic) with myocarditis
Trypanosomiasis NOS

☑5ᵗʰ **B57.3 Chagas' disease (chronic) with digestive system involvement**

B57.30 Chagas' disease with digestive system involvement, unspecified   ▽

B57.31 Megaesophagus in Chagas' disease

B57.32 Megacolon in Chagas' disease

B57.39 Other digestive system involvement in Chagas' disease

☑5ᵗʰ **B57.4 Chagas' disease (chronic) with nervous system involvement**

B57.40 Chagas' disease with nervous system involvement, unspecified   ▽

B57.41 Meningitis in Chagas' disease

B57.42 Meningoencephalitis in Chagas' disease

B57.49 Other nervous system involvement in Chagas' disease

B57.5 Chagas' disease (chronic) with other organ involvement

☑4ᵗʰ **B58 Toxoplasmosis**
`INCLUDES`   infection due to Toxoplasma gondii
`EXCLUDES 1`   *congenital toxoplasmosis (P37.1)*

☑5ᵗʰ **B58.0 Toxoplasma oculopathy**

B58.00 Toxoplasma oculopathy, unspecified   ▽

B58.01 Toxoplasma chorioretinitis

B58.09 Other toxoplasma oculopathy
Toxoplasma uveitis

B58.1 Toxoplasma hepatitis

B58.2 Toxoplasma meningoencephalitis   `HCC`

B58.3 Pulmonary toxoplasmosis   `HCC`

☑5ᵗʰ **B58.8 Toxoplasmosis with other organ involvement**

B58.81 Toxoplasma myocarditis

B58.82 Toxoplasma myositis

B58.83 Toxoplasma tubulo-interstitial nephropathy
Toxoplasma pyelonephritis

B58.89 Toxoplasmosis with other organ involvement

B58.9 Toxoplasmosis, unspecified   ▽

B59 Pneumocystosis   `HCC`
Pneumonia due to Pneumocystis carinii
Pneumonia due to Pneumocystis jiroveci

☑4ᵗʰ **B60 Other protozoal diseases, not elsewhere classified**
`EXCLUDES 1`   *cryptosporidiosis (A07.2)*
intestinal microsporidiosis (A07.8)
isosporiasis (A07.3)

B60.0 Babesiosis
Piroplasmosis

☑5ᵗʰ **B60.1 Acanthamebiasis**

B60.10 Acanthamebiasis, unspecified   ▽

B60.11 Meningoencephalitis due to Acanthamoeba (culbertsoni)

B60.12 Conjunctivitis due to Acanthamoeba

B60.13 Keratoconjunctivitis due to Acanthamoeba

B60.19 Other acanthamebic disease

B60.2 Naegleriasis
Primary amebic meningoencephalitis

B60.8 Other specified protozoal diseases
Microsporidiosis

B64 Unspecified protozoal disease   ▽

☑ Additional Character Req   ᵥₓ₇ᵗʰ Placeholder Alert   Manifestation   `HCC` CMS-HCC Condition   ▽ Unspecified Code   ▶◀ Revised Text   ● New Code   ▲ Revised Code Title

ICD-10-CM 2018   451

Helminthiases (B65-B83)

✓4ᵗʰ B65   Schistosomiasis [bilharziasis]
> INCLUDES   snail fever

B65.0   Schistosomiasis due to Schistosoma haematobium [urinary schistosomiasis]

B65.1   Schistosomiasis due to Schistosoma mansoni [intestinal schistosomiasis]

B65.2   Schistosomiasis due to Schistosoma japonicum
> Asiatic schistosomiasis

B65.3   Cercarial dermatitis
> Swimmer's itch

B65.8   Other schistosomiasis
> Infection due to Schistosoma intercalatum
> Infection due to Schistosoma mattheei
> Infection due to Schistosoma mekongi

B65.9   Schistosomiasis, unspecified   ▽

✓4ᵗʰ B66   Other fluke infections

B66.0   Opisthorchiasis
> Infection due to cat liver fluke
> Infection due to Opisthorchis (felineus)(viverrini)

B66.1   Clonorchiasis
> Chinese liver fluke disease
> Infection due to Clonorchis sinensis
> Oriental liver fluke disease

B66.2   Dicroceliasis
> Infection due to Dicrocoelium dendriticum
> Lancet fluke infection

B66.3   Fascioliasis
> Infection due to Fasciola gigantica
> Infection due to Fasciola hepatica
> Infection due to Fasciola indica
> Sheep liver fluke disease

B66.4   Paragonimiasis   HCC
> Infection due to Paragonimus species
> Lung fluke disease
> Pulmonary distomiasis

B66.5   Fasciolopsiasis
> Infection due to Fasciolopsis buski
> Intestinal distomiasis

B66.8   Other specified fluke infections
> Echinostomiasis
> Heterophyiasis
> Metagonimiasis
> Nanophyetiasis
> Watsoniasis

B66.9   Fluke infection, unspecified   ▽

✓4ᵗʰ B67   Echinococcosis
> INCLUDES   hydatidosis

B67.0   Echinococcus granulosus infection of liver

B67.1   Echinococcus granulosus infection of lung   HCC

B67.2   Echinococcus granulosus infection of bone

✓5ᵗʰ B67.3   Echinococcus granulosus infection, other and multiple sites

B67.31   Echinococcus granulosus infection, thyroid gland

B67.32   Echinococcus granulosus infection, multiple sites

B67.39   Echinococcus granulosus infection, other sites

B67.4   Echinococcus granulosus infection, unspecified   ▽
> Dog tapeworm (infection)

B67.5   Echinococcus multilocularis infection of liver

✓5ᵗʰ B67.6   Echinococcus multilocularis infection, other and multiple sites

B67.61   Echinococcus multilocularis infection, multiple sites

B67.69   Echinococcus multilocularis infection, other sites

B67.7   Echinococcus multilocularis infection, unspecified   ▽

B67.8   Echinococcosis, unspecified, of liver   ▽

✓5ᵗʰ B67.9   Echinococcosis, other and unspecified

B67.90   Echinococcosis, unspecified   ▽
> Echinococcosis NOS

B67.99   Other echinococcosis

✓4ᵗʰ B68   Taeniasis
> EXCLUDES 1   cysticercosis (B69.-)

B68.0   Taenia solium taeniasis
> Pork tapeworm (infection)

B68.1   Taenia saginata taeniasis
> Beef tapeworm (infection)
> Infection due to adult tapeworm Taenia saginata

B68.9   Taeniasis, unspecified   ▽

✓4ᵗʰ B69   Cysticercosis
> INCLUDES   cysticerciasis infection due to larval form of Taenia solium

B69.0   Cysticercosis of central nervous system

B69.1   Cysticercosis of eye

✓5ᵗʰ B69.8   Cysticercosis of other sites

B69.81   Myositis in cysticercosis

B69.89   Cysticercosis of other sites

B69.9   Cysticercosis, unspecified   ▽

✓4ᵗʰ B70   Diphyllobothriasis and sparganosis

B70.0   Diphyllobothriasis
> Diphyllobothrium (adult) (latum) (pacificum) infection
> Fish tapeworm (infection)
> EXCLUDES 2   larval diphyllobothriasis (B70.1)

B70.1   Sparganosis
> Infection due to Sparganum (mansoni) (proliferum)
> Infection due to Spirometra larva
> Larval diphyllobothriasis
> Spirometrosis

✓4ᵗʰ B71   Other cestode infections

B71.0   Hymenolepiasis
> Dwarf tapeworm infection
> Rat tapeworm (infection)

B71.1   Dipylidiasis

B71.8   Other specified cestode infections
> Coenurosis

B71.9   Cestode infection, unspecified   ▽
> Tapeworm (infection) NOS

B72   Dracunculiasis
> INCLUDES   guinea worm infection
> infection due to Dracunculus medinensis

✓4ᵗʰ B73   Onchocerciasis
> INCLUDES   onchocerca volvulus infection
> onchocercosis
> river blindness

✓5ᵗʰ B73.0   Onchocerciasis with eye disease

B73.00   Onchocerciasis with eye involvement, unspecified   ▽

B73.01   Onchocerciasis with endophthalmitis

B73.02   Onchocerciasis with glaucoma

B73.09   Onchocerciasis with other eye involvement
> Infestation of eyelid due to onchocerciasis

B73.1   Onchocerciasis without eye disease

✓4ᵗʰ B74   Filariasis
> EXCLUDES 2   onchocerciasis (B73)
> tropical (pulmonary) eosinophilia NOS (J82)

B74.0   Filariasis due to Wuchereria bancrofti
> Bancroftian elephantiasis
> Bancroftian filariasis

B74.1   Filariasis due to Brugia malayi

B74.2   Filariasis due to Brugia timori

B74.3   Loiasis
> Calabar swelling
> Eyeworm disease of Africa
> Loa loa infection

B74.4   Mansonelliasis
> Infection due to Mansonella ozzardi
> Infection due to Mansonella perstans
> Infection due to Mansonella streptocerca

B74.8   Other filariases
> Dirofilariasis

B74.9   Filariasis, unspecified   ▽

B75   Trichinellosis
> INCLUDES   infection due to Trichinella species
> trichiniasis

✓4ᵗʰ B76   Hookworm diseases
> INCLUDES   uncinariasis

B76.0   Ancylostomiasis
> Infection due to Ancylostoma species

B76.1   Necatoriasis
> Infection due to Necator americanus

B76.8   Other hookworm diseases

B76.9   Hookworm disease, unspecified   ▽
> Cutaneous larva migrans NOS

EXCLUDES 1 Not coded here   EXCLUDES 2 Not included here   N Newborn Age: 0   P Pediatric Age: 0-17   M Maternity Age: 12-55   A Adult Age: 15-124

☑️4ᵗʰ **B77** **Ascariasis**
     INCLUDES   ascaridiasis
            roundworm infection
     B77.0 **Ascariasis with intestinal complications**
     ☑️5ᵗʰ **B77.8** **Ascariasis with other complications**
           B77.81 **Ascariasis pneumonia**
           B77.89 **Ascariasis with other complications**
     B77.9 **Ascariasls, unspecified** ▽

☑️4ᵗʰ **B78** **Strongyloidiasis**
     EXCLUDES 1   trichostrongyliasis (B81.2)
     B78.0 **Intestinal strongyloidiasis**
     B78.1 **Cutaneous strongyloidiasis**
     B78.7 **Disseminated strongyloidiasis**
     B78.9 **Strongyloidiasis, unspecified** ▽

B79 **Trichuriasis**
     INCLUDES   trichocephaliasis
            whipworm (disease)(infection)

B80 **Enterobiasis**
     INCLUDES   oxyuriasis
            pinworm infection
            threadworm infection

☑️4ᵗʰ **B81** **Other intestinal helminthiases, not elsewhere classified**
     EXCLUDES 1 ▶angiostrongyliasis due to:
           angiostrongylus cantonensis (B83.2)
           parastrongylus cantonensis (B83.2) ◀
     B81.0 **Anisakiasis**
           Infection due to Anisakis larva
     B81.1 **Intestinal capillariasis**
           Capillariasis NOS
           Infection due to Capillaria philippinensis
           EXCLUDES 2   hepatic capillariasis (B83.8)
     B81.2 **Trichostrongyliasis**
     B81.3 **Intestinal angiostrongyliasis**
           ▶Angiostrongyliasis due to:
           angiostrongylus costaricensis
           parastrongylus costaricensis◀
     B81.4 **Mixed intestinal helminthiases**
           Infection due to intestinal helminths classified to more than one
              of the categories B65.0-B81.3 and B81.8
           Mixed helminthiasis NOS
     B81.8 **Other specified intestinal helminthiases**
           Infection due to Oesophagostomum species
              [esophagostomiasis]
           Infection due to Ternidens diminutus [ternidensiasis]

☑️4ᵗʰ **B82** **Unspecified intestinal parasitism**
     B82.0 **Intestinal helminthiasis, unspecified** ▽
     B82.9 **Intestinal parasitism, unspecified** ▽

☑️4ᵗʰ **B83** **Other helminthiases**
     EXCLUDES 1   capillariasis NOS (B81.1)
     EXCLUDES 2   intestinal capillariasis (B81.1)
     B83.0 **Visceral larva migrans**
           Toxocariasis
     B83.1 **Gnathostomiasis**
           Wandering swelling
     B83.2 **Angiostrongyliasis due to Parastrongylus cantonensis**
           Eosinophilic meningoencephalitis due to Parastrongylus
              cantonensis
           EXCLUDES 2   intestinal angiostrongyliasis (B81.3)
     B83.3 **Syngamiasis**
           Syngamosis
     B83.4 **Internal hirudiniasis**
           EXCLUDES 2   external hirudiniasis (B88.3)
     B83.8 **Other specified helminthiases**
           Acanthocephaliasis
           Gongylonemiasis
           Hepatic capillariasis
           Metastrongyliasis
           Thelaziasis
     B83.9 **Helminthiasis, unspecified** ▽
           Worms NOS
           EXCLUDES 1   intestinal helminthiasis NOS (B82.0)

Pediculosis, acariasis and other infestations (B85-B89)

☑️4ᵗʰ **B85** **Pediculosis and phthiriasis**
     B85.0 **Pediculosis due to Pediculus humanus capitis**
           Head-louse infestation
     B85.1 **Pediculosis due to Pediculus humanus corporis**
           Body-louse infestation
     B85.2 **Pediculosis, unspecified** ▽
     B85.3 **Phthiriasis**
           Infestation by crab-louse
           Infestation by Phthirus pubis
     B85.4 **Mixed pediculosis and phthiriasis**
           Infestation classifiable to more than one of the categories
              B85.0- B85.3

B86 **Scabies**
     Sarcoptic itch

☑️4ᵗʰ **B87** **Myiasis**
     INCLUDES   infestation by larva of flies
     B87.0 **Cutaneous myiasis**
           Creeping myiasis
     B87.1 **Wound myiasis**
           Traumatic myiasis
     B87.2 **Ocular myiasis**
     B87.3 **Nasopharyngeal myiasis**
           Laryngeal myiasis
     B87.4 **Aural myiasis**
     ☑️5ᵗʰ **B87.8** **Myiasis of other sites**
           B87.81 **Genitourinary myiasis**
           B87.82 **Intestinal myiasis**
           B87.89 **Myiasis of other sites**
     B87.9 **Myiasis, unspecified** ▽

☑️4ᵗʰ **B88** **Other infestations**
     B88.0 **Other acariasis**
           Acarine dermatitis
           Dermatitis due to Demodex species
           Dermatitis due to Dermanyssus gallinae
           Dermatitis due to Liponyssoides sanguineus
           Trombiculosis
           EXCLUDES 2   scabies (B86)
     B88.1 **Tungiasis [sandflea infestation]**
     B88.2 **Other arthropod infestations**
           Scarabiasis
     B88.3 **External hirudiniasis**
           Leech infestation NOS
           EXCLUDES 2   internal hirudiniasis (B83.4)
     B88.8 **Other specified infestations**
           Ichthyoparasitism due to Vandellia cirrhosa
           Linguatulosis
           Porocephaliasis
     B88.9 **Infestation, unspecified** ▽
           Infestation (skin) NOS
           Infestation by mites NOS
           Skin parasites NOS

B89 **Unspecified parasitic disease** ▽

Sequelae of infectious and parasitic diseases (B90-B94)

     NOTE   Categories B90-B94 are to be used to indicate conditions in
           categories A00-B89 as the cause of sequelae, which are themselves
           classified elsewhere. The "sequelae" include conditions specified as
           such; they also include residuals of diseases classifiable to the above
           categories if there is evidence that the disease itself is no longer
           present. Codes from these categories are not to be used for chronic
           infections. Code chronic current infections to active infectious
           disease as appropriate.
     Code first condition resulting from (sequela) the infectious or parasitic disease

☑️4ᵗʰ **B90** **Sequelae of tuberculosis**
     B90.0 **Sequelae of central nervous system tuberculosis**
     B90.1 **Sequelae of genitourinary tuberculosis**
     B90.2 **Sequelae of tuberculosis of bones and joints**
     B90.8 **Sequelae of tuberculosis of other organs**
           EXCLUDES 2   sequelae of respiratory tuberculosis (B90.9)
     B90.9 **Sequelae of respiratory and unspecified tuberculosis** ▽
           Sequelae of tuberculosis NOS

☑️ Additional Character Req   ☑️x7ᵗʰ Placeholder Alert   Manifestation   HCC CMS-HCC Condition   ▽ Unspecified Code   ▶◀ Revised Text   ● New Code   ▲ Revised Code Title

ICD-10-CM 2018   453

B91 Sequelae of poliomyelitis
> EXCLUDES 1 postpolio syndrome (G14)

B92 Sequelae of leprosy

✓4ᵗʰ B94 Sequelae of other and unspecified infectious and parasitic diseases

   B94.0 Sequelae of trachoma

   B94.1 Sequelae of viral encephalitis

   B94.2 Sequelae of viral hepatitis

   B94.8 Sequelae of other specified infectious and parasitic diseases

   B94.9 Sequelae of unspecified infectious and parasitic disease ▽

Bacterial and viral infectious agents (B95-B97)

> NOTE These categories are provided for use as supplementary or additional codes to identify the infectious agent(s) in diseases classified elsewhere.

✓4ᵗʰ B95 Streptococcus, Staphylococcus, and Enterococcus as the cause of diseases classified elsewhere

   B95.0 Streptococcus, group A, as the cause of diseases classified elsewhere

   B95.1 Streptococcus, group B, as the cause of diseases classified elsewhere

   B95.2 Enterococcus as the cause of diseases classified elsewhere

   B95.3 Streptococcus pneumoniae as the cause of diseases classified elsewhere

   B95.4 Other streptococcus as the cause of diseases classified elsewhere

   B95.5 Unspecified streptococcus as the cause of diseases classified elsewhere ▽

   ✓5ᵗʰ B95.6 Staphylococcus aureus as the cause of diseases classified elsewhere

      B95.61 Methicillin susceptible Staphylococcus aureus infection as the cause of diseases classified elsewhere
        Methicillin susceptible Staphylococcus aureus (MSSA) infection as the cause of diseases classified elsewhere
        Staphylococcus aureus infection NOS as the cause of diseases classified elsewhere

      B95.62 Methicillin resistant Staphylococcus aureus infection as the cause of diseases classified elsewhere
        Methicillin resistant Staphylococcus aureus (MRSA) infection as the cause of diseases classified elsewhere
        AHA: 2016, 1Q, 12

   B95.7 Other staphylococcus as the cause of diseases classified elsewhere

   B95.8 Unspecified staphylococcus as the cause of diseases classified elsewhere ▽

✓4ᵗʰ B96 Other bacterial agents as the cause of diseases classified elsewhere

   B96.0 Mycoplasma pneumoniae [M. pneumoniae] as the cause of diseases classified elsewhere
      Pleuro-pneumonia-like-organism [PPLO]

   B96.1 Klebsiella pneumoniae [K. pneumoniae] as the cause of diseases classified elsewhere

   ✓5ᵗʰ B96.2 Escherichia coli [E. coli] as the cause of diseases classified elsewhere

      B96.20 Unspecified Escherichia coli [E. coli] as the cause of diseases classified elsewhere ▽
        Escherichia coli [E. coli] NOS

      B96.21 Shiga toxin-producing Escherichia coli [E. coli] (STEC) O157 as the cause of diseases classified elsewhere
        E. coli O157:H- (nonmotile) with confirmation of Shiga toxin
        E. coli O157 with confirmation of Shiga toxin when H antigen is unknown, or is not H7
        O157:H7 Escherichia coli [E.coli] with or without confirmation of Shiga toxin-production
        Shiga toxin-producing Escherichia coli [E.coli] O157:H7 with or without confirmation of Shiga toxin-production
        STEC O157:H7 with or without confirmation of Shiga toxin-production

      B96.22 Other specified Shiga toxin-producing Escherichia coli [E. coli] (STEC) as the cause of diseases classified elsewhere
        Non-O157 Shiga toxin-producing Escherichia coli [E.coli]
        Non-O157 Shiga toxin-producing Escherichia coli [E.coli] with known O group

      B96.23 Unspecified Shiga toxin-producing Escherichia coli [E. coli] (STEC) as the cause of diseases classified elsewhere ▽
        Shiga toxin-producing Escherichia coli [E. coli] with unspecified O group
        STEC NOS

      B96.29 Other Escherichia coli [E. coli] as the cause of diseases classified elsewhere
        Non-Shiga toxin-producing E. coli

   B96.3 Hemophilus influenzae [H. influenzae] as the cause of diseases classified elsewhere

   B96.4 Proteus (mirabilis) (morganii) as the cause of diseases classified elsewhere

   B96.5 Pseudomonas (aeruginosa) (mallei) (pseudomallei) as the cause of diseases classified elsewhere
      AHA: 2015, 1Q, 18

   B96.6 Bacteroides fragilis [B. fragilis] as the cause of diseases classified elsewhere

   B96.7 Clostridium perfringens [C. perfringens] as the cause of diseases classified elsewhere

   ✓5ᵗʰ B96.8 Other specified bacterial agents as the cause of diseases classified elsewhere

      B96.81 Helicobacter pylori [H. pylori] as the cause of diseases classified elsewhere

      B96.82 Vibrio vulnificus as the cause of diseases classified elsewhere

      B96.89 Other specified bacterial agents as the cause of diseases classified elsewhere

✓4ᵗʰ B97 Viral agents as the cause of diseases classified elsewhere
   AHA: 2016, 3Q, 8-10, 14

   B97.0 Adenovirus as the cause of diseases classified elsewhere

   ✓5ᵗʰ B97.1 Enterovirus as the cause of diseases classified elsewhere

      B97.10 Unspecified enterovirus as the cause of diseases classified elsewhere ▽

      B97.11 Coxsackievirus as the cause of diseases classified elsewhere

      B97.12 Echovirus as the cause of diseases classified elsewhere

      B97.19 Other enterovirus as the cause of diseases classified elsewhere

   ✓5ᵗʰ B97.2 Coronavirus as the cause of diseases classified elsewhere

      B97.21 SARS-associated coronavirus as the cause of diseases classified elsewhere
        > EXCLUDES 1 pneumonia due to SARS-associated coronavirus (J12.81)

      B97.29 Other coronavirus as the cause of diseases classified elsewhere

   ✓5ᵗʰ B97.3 Retrovirus as the cause of diseases classified elsewhere
      > EXCLUDES 1 human immunodeficiency virus [HIV] disease (B20)

      B97.30 Unspecified retrovirus as the cause of diseases classified elsewhere ▽

      B97.31 Lentivirus as the cause of diseases classified elsewhere

      B97.32 Oncovirus as the cause of diseases classified elsewhere

      B97.33 Human T-cell lymphotrophic virus, type I [HTLV-I] as the cause of diseases classified elsewhere

      B97.34 Human T-cell lymphotrophic virus, type II [HTLV-II] as the cause of diseases classified elsewhere

      B97.35 Human immunodeficiency virus, type 2 [HIV 2] HCC as the cause of diseases classified elsewhere

      B97.39 Other retrovirus as the cause of diseases classified elsewhere

   B97.4 Respiratory syncytial virus as the cause of diseases classified elsewhere

   B97.5 Reovirus as the cause of diseases classified elsewhere

   B97.6 Parvovirus as the cause of diseases classified elsewhere

   B97.7 Papillomavirus as the cause of diseases classified elsewhere

---

EXCLUDES 1 Not coded here   EXCLUDES 2 Not included here   N Newborn Age: 0   P Pediatric Age: 0-17   M Maternity Age: 12-55   A Adult Age: 15-124

454   ICD-10-CM 2018

☑5ᵗʰ **B97.8** Other viral agents as the cause of diseases classified elsewhere

     B97.81 Human metapneumovirus as the cause of diseases classified elsewhere

     B97.89 Other viral agents as the cause of diseases classified elsewhere

Other infectious diseases (B99)

☑4ᵗʰ **B99** **Other and unspecified infectious diseases**

     B99.8 Other infectious disease

     B99.9 Unspecified infectious disease   ▽

☑ Additional Character Req   ✓ₓ7ᵗʰ Placeholder Alert   Manifestation   HCC CMS-HCC Condition   ▽ Unspecified Code   ►◄ Revised Text   ● New Code   ▲ Revised Code Title

ICD-10-CM 2018   455

Chapter 2. Neoplasms (C00–D49)

Chapter Specific Guidelines with Coding Examples

The chapter specific guidelines from the ICD-10-CM Official Guidelines for Coding and Reporting have been provided below. Along with these guidelines are coding examples, contained in the shaded boxes, that have been developed to help illustrate the coding and/or sequencing guidance found in these guidelines.

General guidelines

Chapter 2 of the ICD-10-CM contains the codes for most benign and all malignant neoplasms. Certain benign neoplasms, such as prostatic adenomas, may be found in the specific body system chapters. To properly code a neoplasm it is necessary to determine from the record if the neoplasm is benign, in-situ, malignant, or of uncertain histologic behavior. If malignant, any secondary (metastatic) sites should also be determined.

Primary malignant neoplasms overlapping site boundaries

A primary malignant neoplasm that overlaps two or more contiguous (next to each other) sites should be classified to the subcategory/code .8 ('overlapping lesion'), unless the combination is specifically indexed elsewhere. For multiple neoplasms of the same site that are not contiguous such as tumors in different quadrants of the same breast, codes for each site should be assigned.

> A 62-year-old female with a malignant lesion of the upper lip that extends from the lipstick area to the labial frenulum
>
> **C00.8**   **Malignant neoplasm of overlapping sites of lip**
>
> *Explanation*: Because this is a single lesion that overlaps two contiguous sites, a single code for overlapping sites is assigned.

> A 74-year-old male is treated for two distinct malignant lesions, one in the mucosa of the upper lip and a second in the mucosa of the lower lip.
>
> **C00.3**   **Malignant neoplasm of upper lip, inner aspect**
>
> **C00.4**   **Malignant neoplasm of lower lip, inner aspect**
>
> *Explanation*: This patient has two distinct malignant lesions of the upper and lower lips. Because the lesions are not contiguous, two codes are reported.

Malignant neoplasm of ectopic tissue

Malignant neoplasms of ectopic tissue are to be coded to the site of origin mentioned, e.g., ectopic pancreatic malignant neoplasms involving the stomach are coded to pancreas, unspecified (C25.9).

The neoplasm table in the Alphabetic Index should be referenced first. However, if the histological term is documented, that term should be referenced first, rather than going immediately to the Neoplasm Table, in order to determine which column in the Neoplasm Table is appropriate. For example, if the documentation indicates "adenoma," refer to the term in the Alphabetic Index to review the entries under this term and the instructional note to "see also neoplasm, by site, benign." The table provides the proper code based on the type of neoplasm and the site. It is important to select the proper column in the table that corresponds to the type of neoplasm. The Tabular List should then be referenced to verify that the correct code has been selected from the table and that a more specific site code does not exist.

See Section I.C.21. Factors influencing health status and contact with health services, Status, for information regarding Z15.0, codes for genetic susceptibility to cancer.

a. Treatment directed at the malignancy

If the treatment is directed at the malignancy, designate the malignancy as the principal diagnosis.

The only exception to this guideline is if a patient admission/encounter is solely for the administration of chemotherapy, immunotherapy or radiation therapy, assign the appropriate Z51.-- code as the first-listed or principal diagnosis, and the diagnosis or problem for which the service is being performed as a secondary diagnosis.

b. Treatment of secondary site

When a patient is admitted because of a primary neoplasm with metastasis and treatment is directed toward the secondary site only, the secondary neoplasm is designated as the principal diagnosis even though the primary malignancy is still present.

> Patient with primary prostate cancer with metastasis to lungs presents for wedge resection of mass in right lung
>
> **C78.01**   **Secondary malignant neoplasm of right lung**
>
> **C61**   **Malignant neoplasm of prostate**
>
> *Explanation*: Since the encounter is for treatment of the lung metastasis, the secondary lung metastasis is sequenced before the primary prostate cancer.

c. Coding and sequencing of complications

Coding and sequencing of complications associated with the malignancies or with the therapy thereof are subject to the following guidelines:

1) Anemia associated with malignancy

When admission/encounter is for management of an anemia associated with the malignancy, and the treatment is only for anemia, the appropriate code for the malignancy is sequenced as the principal or first-listed diagnosis followed by the appropriate code for the anemia (such as code D63.0, Anemia in neoplastic disease).

> Patient is seen for treatment of anemia in advanced primary liver cancer
>
> **C22.8**   **Malignant neoplasm of liver, primary, unspecified as to type**
>
> **D63.0**   **Anemia in neoplastic disease**
>
> *Explanation*: Even though the admission was solely to treat the anemia, this guideline indicates that the code for the malignancy is sequenced first.

2) Anemia associated with chemotherapy, immunotherapy and radiation therapy

When the admission/encounter is for management of an anemia associated with an adverse effect of the administration of chemotherapy or immunotherapy and the only treatment is for the anemia, the anemia code is sequenced first followed by the appropriate codes for the neoplasm and the adverse effect (T45.1X5, Adverse effect of antineoplastic and immunosuppressive drugs).

> A 56-year-old Hispanic male with grade II follicular lymphoma involving multiple lymph node sites referred for blood transfusion to treat anemia due to chemotherapy
>
> **D64.81**   **Anemia due to antineoplastic chemotherapy**
>
> **C82.18**   **Follicular lymphoma grade II, lymph nodes of multiple sites**
>
> **T45.1X5A**   **Adverse effect of antineoplastic and immunosuppressive drugs, initial encounter**
>
> *Explanation*: The code for the anemia is sequenced first followed by the code for the malignant neoplasm and lastly the code for the adverse effect.

When the admission/encounter is for management of an anemia associated with an adverse effect of radiotherapy, the anemia code should be sequenced first, followed by the appropriate neoplasm code and code Y84.2, Radiological procedure and radiotherapy as the cause of abnormal reaction of the patient, or of later complication, without mention of misadventure at the time of the procedure.

A 55-year-old male with a large malignant rectal tumor has been receiving external radiation therapy to shrink the tumor prior to planned surgery. He is referred today for a blood transfusion to treat anemia related to radiation therapy.

D64.89	Other specified anemias
C20	Malignant neoplasm of rectum
Y84.2	Radiological procedure and radiotherapy as the cause of abnormal reaction of the patient, or of later complication, without mention of misadventure at the time of the procedure

Explanation: The code for the anemia is sequenced first, followed by the code for the malignancy, and lastly the code for the abnormal reaction due to radiotherapy.

3) Management of dehydration due to the malignancy

When the admission/encounter is for management of dehydration due to the malignancy and only the dehydration is being treated (intravenous rehydration), the dehydration is sequenced first, followed by the code(s) for the malignancy.

4) Treatment of a complication resulting from a surgical procedure

When the admission/encounter is for treatment of a complication resulting from a surgical procedure, designate the complication as the principal or first-listed diagnosis if treatment is directed at resolving the complication.

d. Primary malignancy previously excised

When a primary malignancy has been previously excised or eradicated from its site and there is no further treatment directed to that site and there is no evidence of any existing primary malignancy, a code from category Z85, Personal history of malignant neoplasm, should be used to indicate the former site of the malignancy. Any mention of extension, invasion, or metastasis to another site is coded as a secondary malignant neoplasm to that site. The secondary site may be the principal or first-listed with the Z85 code used as a secondary code.

History of lung cancer, left upper lobectomy 18 months ago with no current treatment; MRI of the brain shows metastatic disease in the brain

C79.31	Secondary malignant neoplasm of brain
Z85.118	Personal history of other other malignant neoplasm of bronchifus and bronchfuls and lung

Explanation: The patient has undergone a diagnostic procedure that revealed metastatic lung cancer in the brain. The code for the secondary (metastatic) site is sequenced first, followed by a personal history code to identify the former site of the primary malignancy.

e. Admissions/encounters involving chemotherapy, immunotherapy and radiation therapy

1) Episode of care involves surgical removal of neoplasm

When an episode of care involves the surgical removal of a neoplasm, primary or secondary site, followed by adjunct chemotherapy or radiation treatment during the same episode of care, the code for the neoplasm should be assigned as principal or first-listed diagnosis.

2) Patient admission/encounter solely for administration of chemotherapy, immunotherapy and radiation therapy

If a patient admission/encounter is solely for the administration of chemotherapy, immunotherapy or radiation therapy assign code Z51.0, Encounter for antineoplastic radiation therapy, or Z51.11, Encounter for antineoplastic chemotherapy, or Z51.12, Encounter for antineoplastic immunotherapy as the first-listed or principal diagnosis. If a patient receives more than one of these therapies during the same admission more than one of these codes may be assigned, in any sequence.

The malignancy for which the therapy is being administered should be assigned as a secondary diagnosis.

Patient presents for second round of rituximab and fludarabine for his chronic B cell lymphocytic leukemia

Z51.11	Encounter for antineoplastic chemotherapy
Z51.12	Encounter for antineoplastic immunotherapy
C91.10	Chronic lymphocytic leukemia of B-cell type not having achieved remission

Explanation: Rituximab is an antineoplastic immunotherapy while fludarabine is an antineoplastic chemotherapy. The two treatments are often used together. The encounter was solely for the purpose of administering this treatment and either can be sequenced first, before the neoplastic condition.

3) Patient admitted for radiation therapy, chemotherapy or immunotherapy and develops complications

When a patient is admitted for the purpose of radiotherapy, immunotherapy or chemotherapy and develops complications such as uncontrolled nausea and vomiting or dehydration, the principal or first-listed diagnosis is Z51.0, Encounter for antineoplastic radiation therapy, or Z51.11, Encounter for antineoplastic chemotherapy, or Z51.12, Encounter for antineoplastic immunotherapy followed by any codes for the complications.

f. Admission/encounter to determine extent of malignancy

When the reason for admission/encounter is to determine the extent of the malignancy, or for a procedure such as paracentesis or thoracentesis, the primary malignancy or appropriate metastatic site is designated as the principal or first-listed diagnosis, even though chemotherapy or radiotherapy is administered.

Patient with left lung cancer with malignant pleural effusion being seen for paracentesis and initiation/administration of chemotherapy

C34.92	Malignant neoplasm of unspecified part of left bronchus or lung
J91.0	Malignant pleural effusion
Z51.11	Encounter for antineoplastic chemotherapy

Explanation: The lung cancer is sequenced before the chemotherapy in this instance because the paracentesis for the malignant effusion is also being performed. An instructional note under the malignant effusion instructs that the lung cancer be sequenced first.

g. Symptoms, signs, and abnormal findings listed in Chapter 18 associated with neoplasms

Symptoms, signs, and ill-defined conditions listed in Chapter 18 characteristic of, or associated with, an existing primary or secondary site malignancy cannot be used to replace the malignancy as principal or first-listed diagnosis, regardless of the number of admissions or encounters for treatment and care of the neoplasm.

See Section I.C.21. Factors influencing health status and contact with health services, Encounter for prophylactic organ removal.

h. Admission/encounter for pain control/management

See Section I.C.6. for information on coding admission/encounter for pain control/management.

i. Malignancy in two or more noncontiguous sites

A patient may have more than one malignant tumor in the same organ. These tumors may represent different primaries or metastatic disease, depending on the site. Should the documentation be unclear, the provider should be queried as to the status of each tumor so that the correct codes can be assigned.

j. Disseminated malignant neoplasm, unspecified

Code C80.0, Disseminated malignant neoplasm, unspecified, is for use only in those cases where the patient has advanced metastatic disease and no known primary or secondary sites are specified. It should not be used in place of assigning codes for the primary site and all known secondary sites.

Patient who has had no medical care for many years is seen today and diagnosed with carcinomatosis

C80.0	Disseminated malignant neoplasm, unspecified

Explanation: Carcinomatosis NOS is an "includes" note under this code. Should seldom be used but is available for use in cases such as this.

k. Malignant neoplasm without specification of site

Code C80.1, Malignant (primary) neoplasm, unspecified, equates to Cancer, unspecified. This code should only be used when no determination can be made as to the primary site of a malignancy. This code should rarely be used in the inpatient setting.

> Evaluation of painful hip leads to diagnosis of a metastatic bone lesion from an unknown primary neoplasm source
>
> | C79.51 | Secondary malignant neoplasm of bone |
> |---|---|
> | C80.1 | Malignant (primary) neoplasm, unspecified |
>
> *Explanation*: If only the secondary site is known, use code C80.1 for the unknown primary site.

l. Sequencing of neoplasm codes

1) Encounter for treatment of primary malignancy

If the reason for the encounter is for treatment of a primary malignancy, assign the malignancy as the principal/first-listed diagnosis. The primary site is to be sequenced first, followed by any metastatic sites.

2) Encounter for treatment of secondary malignancy

When an encounter is for a primary malignancy with metastasis and treatment is directed toward the metastatic (secondary) site(s) only, the metastatic site(s) is designated as the principal/first-listed diagnosis. The primary malignancy is coded as an additional code.

> Patient has primary colon cancer with metastasis to rib and is evaluated for possible excision of portion of rib bone
>
> | C79.51 | Secondary malignant neoplasm of bone |
> |---|---|
> | C18.9 | Malignant neoplasm of colon, unspecified |
>
> *Explanation*: The treatment for this encounter is focused on the metastasis to the rib bone rather than the primary colon cancer, thus indicating that the bone metastasis is sequenced as the first-listed code.

3) Malignant neoplasm in a pregnant patient

When a pregnant woman has a malignant neoplasm, a code from subcategory O9A.1-, Malignant neoplasm complicating pregnancy, childbirth, and the puerperium, should be sequenced first, followed by the appropriate code from Chapter 2 to indicate the type of neoplasm.

> A 30-year-old pregnant female in first trimester evaluated for pituitary gland malignancy
>
> | O9A.111 | Malignant neoplasm complicating pregnancy, first trimester |
> |---|---|
> | C75.1 | Malignant neoplasm of pituitary gland |
>
> *Explanation*: Codes from chapter 15 describing complications of pregnancy are sequenced as first-listed codes, further specified by codes from other chapters such as neoplastic, unless the pregnancy is documented as incidental to the condition. See also guideline 1.C.15.a.1.

4) Encounter for complication associated with a neoplasm

When an encounter is for management of a complication associated with a neoplasm, such as dehydration, and the treatment is only for the complication, the complication is coded first, followed by the appropriate code(s) for the neoplasm.

The exception to this guideline is anemia. When the admission/encounter is for management of an anemia associated with the malignancy, and the treatment is only for anemia, the appropriate code for the malignancy is sequenced as the principal or first-listed diagnosis followed by code D63.0, Anemia in neoplastic disease.

> Patient with pancreatic cancer is seen for initiation of TPN for cancer-related moderate protein-calorie malnutrition
>
> | E44.0 | Moderate protein-calorie malnutrition |
> |---|---|
> | C25.9 | Malignant neoplasm of pancreas, unspecified |
>
> *Explanation*: The encounter is to initiate treatment for malnutrition, a common complication of many types of neoplasms, and is sequenced first.

5) Complication from surgical procedure for treatment of a neoplasm

When an encounter is for treatment of a complication resulting from a surgical procedure performed for the treatment of the neoplasm, designate the complication as the principal/first-listed diagnosis. See guideline regarding the coding of a current malignancy versus personal history to determine if the code for the neoplasm should also be assigned.

6) Pathologic fracture due to a neoplasm

When an encounter is for a pathological fracture due to a neoplasm, and the focus of treatment is the fracture, a code from subcategory M84.5, Pathological fracture in neoplastic disease, should be sequenced first, followed by the code for the neoplasm.

If the focus of treatment is the neoplasm with an associated pathological fracture, the neoplasm code should be sequenced first, followed by a code from M84.5 for the pathological fracture.

m. Current malignancy versus personal history of malignancy

When a primary malignancy has been excised but further treatment, such as an additional surgery for the malignancy, radiation therapy or chemotherapy is directed to that site, the primary malignancy code should be used until treatment is completed.

When a primary malignancy has been previously excised or eradicated from its site, there is no further treatment (of the malignancy) directed to that site, and there is no evidence of any existing primary malignancy, a code from category Z85, Personal history of malignant neoplasm, should be used to indicate the former site of the malignancy.

See Section I.C.21. Factors influencing health status and contact with health services, History (of)

> Female patient with ongoing chemotherapy after right mastectomy for breast cancer
>
> | C50.911 | Malignant neoplasm of unspecified site of right female breast |
> |---|---|
> | Z90.11 | Acquired absence of right breast and nipple |
>
> *Explanation*: Even though the breast has been removed, the breast cancer is still being treated with chemotherapy and therefore is still coded as a current condition rather than personal history.

n. Leukemia, multiple myeloma, and malignant plasma cell neoplasms in remission versus personal history

The categories for leukemia, and category C90, Multiple myeloma and malignant plasma cell neoplasms, have codes indicating whether or not the leukemia has achieved remission. There are also codes Z85.6, Personal history of leukemia, and Z85.79, Personal history of other malignant neoplasms of lymphoid, hematopoietic and related tissues. If the documentation is unclear as to whether the leukemia has achieved remission, the provider should be queried.

See Section I.C.21. Factors influencing health status and contact with health services, History (of)

o. Aftercare following surgery for neoplasm

See Section I.C.21. Factors influencing health status and contact with health services, Aftercare

p. Follow-up care for completed treatment of a malignancy

See Section I.C.21. Factors influencing health status and contact with health services, Follow-up

q. Prophylactic organ removal for prevention of malignancy

See Section I.C. 21, Factors influencing health status and contact with health services, Prophylactic organ removal

r. Malignant neoplasm associated with transplant organ

A malignant neoplasm of a transplanted organ should be coded as a transplant complication. Assign first the appropriate code from category T86.-, Complications of transplanted organs and tissue, followed by code C80.2, Malignant neoplasm associated with transplanted organ. Use an additional code for the specific malignancy.

Chapter 2. Neoplasms (C00-D49)

NOTE

Functional activity

All neoplasms are classified in this chapter, whether they are functionally active or not. An additional code from Chapter 4 may be used, to identify functional activity associated with any neoplasm.

Morphology [Histology]

Chapter 2 classifies neoplasms primarily by site (topography), with broad groupings for behavior, malignant, in situ, benign, etc. The Table of Neoplasms should be used to identify the correct topography code. In a few cases, such as for malignant melanoma and certain neuroendocrine tumors, the morphology (histologic type) is included in the category and codes.

Primary malignant neoplasms overlapping site boundaries

A primary malignant neoplasm that overlaps two or more contiguous (next to each other) sites should be classified to the subcategory/code .8 ("overlapping lesion"), unless the combination is specifically indexed elsewhere. For multiple neoplasms of the same site that are not contiguous, such as tumors in different quadrants of the same breast, codes for each site should be assigned.

Malignant neoplasm of ectopic tissue

Malignant neoplasms of ectopic tissue are to be coded to the site mentioned, e.g., ectopic pancreatic malignant neoplasms are coded to pancreas, unspecified (C25.9).

AHA: 2017, 1Q, 4, 5-6, 8

This chapter contains the following blocks:

C00-C14	Malignant neoplasms of lip, oral cavity and pharynx
C15-C26	Malignant neoplasms of digestive organs
C30-C39	Malignant neoplasms of respiratory and intrathoracic organs
C40-C41	Malignant neoplasms of bone and articular cartilage
C43-C44	Melanoma and other malignant neoplasms of skin
C45-C49	Malignant neoplasms of mesothelial and soft tissue
C50	Malignant neoplasms of breast
C51-C58	Malignant neoplasms of female genital organs
C60-C63	Malignant neoplasms of male genital organs
C64-C68	Malignant neoplasms of urinary tract
C69-C72	Malignant neoplasms of eye, brain and other parts of central nervous system
C73-C75	Malignant neoplasms of thyroid and other endocrine glands
C7A	Malignant neuroendocrine tumors
C7B	Secondary neuroendocrine tumors
C76-C80	Malignant neoplasms of ill-defined, other secondary and unspecified sites
C81-C96	Malignant neoplasms of lymphoid, hematopoietic and related tissue
D00-D09	In situ neoplasms
D10-D36	Benign neoplasms, except benign neuroendocrine tumors
D3A	Benign neuroendocrine tumors
D37-D48	Neoplasms of uncertain behavior, polycythemia vera and myelodysplastic syndromes
D49	Neoplasms of unspecified behavior

MALIGNANT NEOPLASMS (C00-C96)

Malignant neoplasms, stated or presumed to be primary (of specified sites), and certain specified histologies, except neuroendocrine, and of lymphoid, hematopoietic and related tissue (C00-C75)

Malignant neoplasms of lip, oral cavity and pharynx (C00-C14)

☑4ᵗʰ C00 Malignant neoplasm of lip

Use additional code to identify:
alcohol abuse and dependence (F10.-)
history of tobacco dependence (Z87.891)
tobacco dependence (F17.-)
tobacco use (Z72.0)

   EXCLUDES 1   *malignant melanoma of lip (C43.0)*
Merkel cell carcinoma of lip (C4A.0)
other and unspecified malignant neoplasm of skin of lip (C44.0-)

C00.0 Malignant neoplasm of external upper lip
Malignant neoplasm of lipstick area of upper lip
Malignant neoplasm of upper lip NOS
Malignant neoplasm of vermilion border of upper lip

C00.1 Malignant neoplasm of external lower lip
Malignant neoplasm of lower lip NOS
Malignant neoplasm of lipstick area of lower lip
Malignant neoplasm of vermilion border of lower lip

C00.2 Malignant neoplasm of external lip, unspecified ▽
Malignant neoplasm of vermilion border of lip NOS

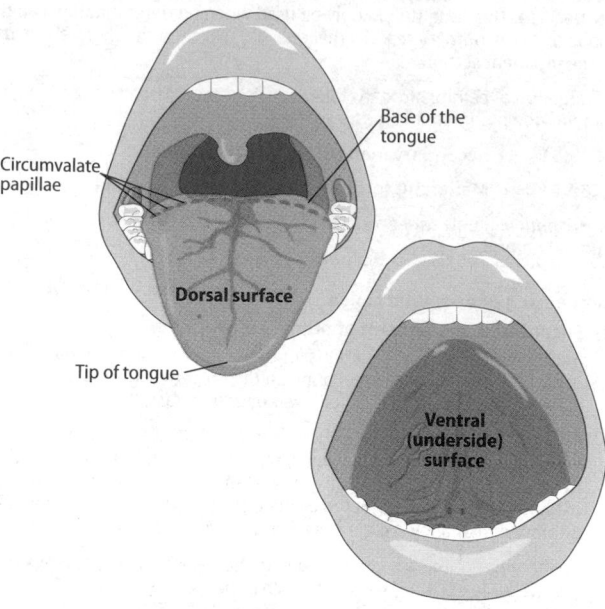

Malignant Neoplasm of Tongue

Base of the tongue
Circumvallate papillae
Dorsal surface
Tip of tongue
Ventral (underside) surface

C00.3 Malignant neoplasm of upper lip, inner aspect
Malignant neoplasm of buccal aspect of upper lip
Malignant neoplasm of frenulum of upper lip
Malignant neoplasm of mucosa of upper lip
Malignant neoplasm of oral aspect of upper lip

C00.4 Malignant neoplasm of lower lip, inner aspect
Malignant neoplasm of buccal aspect of lower lip
Malignant neoplasm of frenulum of lower lip
Malignant neoplasm of mucosa of lower lip
Malignant neoplasm of oral aspect of lower lip

C00.5 Malignant neoplasm of lip, unspecified, inner aspect ▽
Malignant neoplasm of buccal aspect of lip, unspecified
Malignant neoplasm of frenulum of lip, unspecified
Malignant neoplasm of mucosa of lip, unspecified
Malignant neoplasm of oral aspect of lip, unspecified

C00.6 Malignant neoplasm of commissure of lip, unspecified ▽

C00.8 Malignant neoplasm of overlapping sites of lip

C00.9 Malignant neoplasm of lip, unspecified ▽

C01 Malignant neoplasm of base of tongue   **HCC**
Malignant neoplasm of dorsal surface of base of tongue
Malignant neoplasm of fixed part of tongue NOS
Malignant neoplasm of posterior third of tongue
Use additional code to identify:
alcohol abuse and dependence (F10.-)
history of tobacco dependence (Z87.891)
tobacco dependence (F17.-)
tobacco use (Z72.0)

☑4ᵗʰ C02 Malignant neoplasm of other and unspecified parts of tongue
Use additional code to identify:
alcohol abuse and dependence (F10.-)
history of tobacco dependence (Z87.891)
tobacco dependence (F17.-)
tobacco use (Z72.0)

C02.0 Malignant neoplasm of dorsal surface of tongue   **HCC**
Malignant neoplasm of anterior two-thirds of tongue, dorsal surface
   EXCLUDES 2   *malignant neoplasm of dorsal surface of base of tongue (C01)*

C02.1 Malignant neoplasm of border of tongue   **HCC**
Malignant neoplasm of tip of tongue

C02.2 Malignant neoplasm of ventral surface of tongue   **HCC**
Malignant neoplasm of anterior two-thirds of tongue, ventral surface
Malignant neoplasm of frenulum linguae

C02.3 Malignant neoplasm of anterior two-thirds of tongue, part unspecified   **HCC**
Malignant neoplasm of middle third of tongue NOS
Malignant neoplasm of mobile part of tongue NOS

C02.4 Malignant neoplasm of lingual tonsil   **HCC**
   EXCLUDES 2   *malignant neoplasm of tonsil NOS (C09.9)*

C02.8 Malignant neoplasm of overlapping sites of tongue   **HCC**
Malignant neoplasm of two or more contiguous sites of tongue

EXCLUDES 1 Not coded here   **EXCLUDES 2** Not included here   **N** Newborn Age: 0   **P** Pediatric Age: 0-17   **M** Maternity Age: 12-55   **A** Adult Age: 15-124

460   ICD-10-CM 2018

C02.9   Malignant neoplasm of tongue, unspecified   HCC ▽

✓4th C03   Malignant neoplasm of gum
> INCLUDES   malignant neoplasm of alveolar (ridge) mucosa
> malignant neoplasm of gingiva
>
> Use additional code to identify:
> alcohol abuse and dependence (F10.-)
> history of tobacco dependence (Z87.891)
> tobacco dependence (F17.-)
> tobacco use (Z72.0)
> EXCLUDES 2   *malignant odontogenic neoplasms (C41.0-C41.1)*

C03.0   Malignant neoplasm of upper gum   HCC

C03.1   Malignant neoplasm of lower gum   HCC

C03.9   Malignant neoplasm of gum, unspecified   HCC ▽

✓4th C04   Malignant neoplasm of floor of mouth
> Use additional code to identify:
> alcohol abuse and dependence (F10.-)
> history of tobacco dependence (Z87.891)
> tobacco dependence (F17.-)
> tobacco use (Z72.0)

C04.0   Malignant neoplasm of anterior floor of mouth   HCC
> Malignant neoplasm of anterior to the premolar-canine junction

C04.1   Malignant neoplasm of lateral floor of mouth   HCC

C04.8   Malignant neoplasm of overlapping sites of floor of mouth   HCC

C04.9   Malignant neoplasm of floor of mouth, unspecified   HCC ▽

✓4th C05   Malignant neoplasm of palate
> Use additional code to identify:
> alcohol abuse and dependence (F10.-)
> history of tobacco dependence (Z87.891)
> tobacco dependence (F17.-)
> tobacco use (Z72.0)
> EXCLUDES 1   *Kaposi's sarcoma of palate (C46.2)*

C05.0   Malignant neoplasm of hard palate   HCC

C05.1   Malignant neoplasm of soft palate   HCC
> EXCLUDES 2   *malignant neoplasm of nasopharyngeal surface of soft palate (C11.3)*

C05.2   Malignant neoplasm of uvula   HCC

C05.8   Malignant neoplasm of overlapping sites of palate   HCC

C05.9   Malignant neoplasm of palate, unspecified   HCC ▽
> Malignant neoplasm of roof of mouth

✓4th C06   Malignant neoplasm of other and unspecified parts of mouth
> Use additional code to identify:
> alcohol abuse and dependence (F10.-)
> history of tobacco dependence (Z87.891)
> tobacco dependence (F17.-)
> tobacco use (Z72.0)

C06.0   Malignant neoplasm of cheek mucosa   HCC
> Malignant neoplasm of buccal mucosa NOS
> Malignant neoplasm of internal cheek

C06.1   Malignant neoplasm of vestibule of mouth   HCC
> Malignant neoplasm of buccal sulcus (upper) (lower)
> Malignant neoplasm of labial sulcus (upper) (lower)

C06.2   Malignant neoplasm of retromolar area   HCC

✓5th C06.8   Malignant neoplasm of overlapping sites of other and unspecified parts of mouth

> **C06.80   Malignant neoplasm of overlapping sites of unspecified parts of mouth**   HCC ▽

> **C06.89   Malignant neoplasm of overlapping sites of other parts of mouth**   HCC
> > "book leaf" neoplasm [ventral surface of tongue and floor of mouth]

C06.9   Malignant neoplasm of mouth, unspecified   HCC ▽
> Malignant neoplasm of minor salivary gland, unspecified site
> Malignant neoplasm of oral cavity NOS

C07   Malignant neoplasm of parotid gland   HCC
> Use additional code to identify:
> alcohol abuse and dependence (F10.-)
> exposure to environmental tobacco smoke (Z77.22)
> exposure to tobacco smoke in the perinatal period (P96.81)
> history of tobacco dependence (Z87.891)
> occupational exposure to environmental tobacco smoke (Z57.31)
> tobacco dependence (F17.-)
> tobacco use (Z72.0)

✓4th C08   Malignant neoplasm of other and unspecified major salivary glands
> INCLUDES   malignant neoplasm of salivary ducts
>
> Use additional code to identify:
> alcohol abuse and dependence (F10.-)
> exposure to environmental tobacco smoke (Z77.22)
> exposure to tobacco smoke in the perinatal period (P96.81)
> history of tobacco dependence (Z87.891)
> occupational exposure to environmental tobacco smoke (Z57.31)
> tobacco dependence (F17.-)
> tobacco use (Z72.0)
> EXCLUDES 1   *malignant neoplasms of specified minor salivary glands which are classified according to their anatomical location*
> EXCLUDES 2   *malignant neoplasms of minor salivary glands NOS (C06.9)*
> *malignant neoplasm of parotid gland (C07)*

C08.0   Malignant neoplasm of submandibular gland   HCC
> Malignant neoplasm of submaxillary gland

C08.1   Malignant neoplasm of sublingual gland   HCC

C08.9   Malignant neoplasm of major salivary gland, unspecified   HCC ▽
> Malignant neoplasm of salivary gland (major) NOS

✓4th C09   Malignant neoplasm of tonsil
> Use additional code to identify:
> alcohol abuse and dependence (F10.-)
> exposure to environmental tobacco smoke (Z77.22)
> exposure to tobacco smoke in the perinatal period (P96.81)
> history of tobacco dependence (Z87.891)
> occupational exposure to environmental tobacco smoke (Z57.31)
> tobacco dependence (F17.-)
> tobacco use (Z72.0)
> EXCLUDES 2   *malignant neoplasm of lingual tonsil (C02.4)*
> *malignant neoplasm of pharyngeal tonsil (C11.1)*

C09.0   Malignant neoplasm of tonsillar fossa   HCC

C09.1   Malignant neoplasm of tonsillar pillar (anterior) (posterior)   HCC

C09.8   Malignant neoplasm of overlapping sites of tonsil   HCC

C09.9   Malignant neoplasm of tonsil, unspecified   HCC ▽
> Malignant neoplasm of tonsil NOS
> Malignant neoplasm of faucial tonsils
> Malignant neoplasm of palatine tonsils

✓4th C10   Malignant neoplasm of oropharynx
> Use additional code to identify:
> alcohol abuse and dependence (F10.-)
> exposure to environmental tobacco smoke (Z77.22)
> exposure to tobacco smoke in the perinatal period (P96.81)
> history of tobacco dependence (Z87.891)
> occupational exposure to environmental tobacco smoke (Z57.31)
> tobacco dependence (F17.-)
> tobacco use (Z72.0)
> EXCLUDES 2   *malignant neoplasm of tonsil (C09.-)*

C10.0   Malignant neoplasm of vallecula   HCC

C10.1   Malignant neoplasm of anterior surface of epiglottis   HCC
> Malignant neoplasm of epiglottis, free border [margin]
> Malignant neoplasm of glossoepiglottic fold(s)
> EXCLUDES 2   *malignant neoplasm of epiglottis (suprahyoid portion) NOS (C32.1)*

C10.2   Malignant neoplasm of lateral wall of oropharynx   HCC

C10.3   Malignant neoplasm of posterior wall of oropharynx   HCC

C10.4   Malignant neoplasm of branchial cleft   HCC
> Malignant neoplasm of branchial cyst [site of neoplasm]

C10.8   Malignant neoplasm of overlapping sites of oropharynx   HCC
> Malignant neoplasm of junctional region of oropharynx

C10.9   Malignant neoplasm of oropharynx, unspecified   HCC ▽

✓4th C11   Malignant neoplasm of nasopharynx
> Use additional code to identify:
> exposure to environmental tobacco smoke (Z77.22)
> exposure to tobacco smoke in the perinatal period (P96.81)
> history of tobacco dependence (Z87.891)
> occupational exposure to environmental tobacco smoke (Z57.31)
> tobacco dependence (F17.-)
> tobacco use (Z72.0)

C11.0   Malignant neoplasm of superior wall of nasopharynx   HCC
> Malignant neoplasm of roof of nasopharynx

C11.1   Malignant neoplasm of posterior wall of nasopharynx   HCC
> Malignant neoplasm of adenoid
> Malignant neoplasm of pharyngeal tonsil

☑ Additional Character Req   ✓x7th Placeholder Alert   Manifestation   HCC CMS-HCC Condition   ▽ Unspecified Code   ►◄ Revised Text   ● New Code   ▲ Revised Code Title

C11.2 Malignant neoplasm of lateral wall of nasopharynx `HCC`
Malignant neoplasm of fossa of Rosenmüller
Malignant neoplasm of opening of auditory tube
Malignant neoplasm of pharyngeal recess

C11.3 Malignant neoplasm of anterior wall of nasopharynx `HCC`
Malignant neoplasm of floor of nasopharynx
Malignant neoplasm of nasopharyngeal (anterior) (posterior) surface of soft palate
Malignant neoplasm of posterior margin of nasal choana
Malignant neoplasm of posterior margin of nasal septum

C11.8 Malignant neoplasm of overlapping sites of nasopharynx `HCC`

C11.9 Malignant neoplasm of nasopharynx, unspecified `HCC` ▽
Malignant neoplasm of nasopharyngeal wall NOS

C12 Malignant neoplasm of pyriform sinus `HCC`
Malignant neoplasm of pyriform fossa
Use additional code to identify:
exposure to environmental tobacco smoke (Z77.22)
exposure to tobacco smoke in the perinatal period (P96.81)
history of tobacco dependence (Z87.891)
occupational exposure to environmental tobacco smoke (Z57.31)
tobacco dependence (F17.-)
tobacco use (Z72.0)

✓4ᵗʰ **C13 Malignant neoplasm of hypopharynx**
Use additional code to identify:
exposure to environmental tobacco smoke (Z77.22)
exposure to tobacco smoke in the perinatal period (P96.81)
history of tobacco dependence (Z87.891)
occupational exposure to environmental tobacco smoke (Z57.31)
tobacco dependence (F17.-)
tobacco use (Z72.0)
EXCLUDES 2   *malignant neoplasm of pyriform sinus (C12)*

C13.0 Malignant neoplasm of postcricoid region `HCC`

C13.1 Malignant neoplasm of aryepiglottic fold, hypopharyngeal aspect `HCC`
Malignant neoplasm of aryepiglottic fold, marginal zone
Malignant neoplasm of aryepiglottic fold NOS
Malignant neoplasm of interarytenoid fold, marginal zone
Malignant neoplasm of interarytenoid fold NOS
EXCLUDES 2   *malignant neoplasm of aryepiglottic fold or interarytenoid fold, laryngeal aspect (C32.1)*

C13.2 Malignant neoplasm of posterior wall of hypopharynx `HCC`

C13.8 Malignant neoplasm of overlapping sites of hypopharynx `HCC`

C13.9 Malignant neoplasm of hypopharynx, unspecified `HCC` ▽
Malignant neoplasm of hypopharyngeal wall NOS

✓4ᵗʰ **C14 Malignant neoplasm of other and ill-defined sites in the lip, oral cavity and pharynx**
Use additional code to identify:
alcohol abuse and dependence (F10.-)
exposure to environmental tobacco smoke (Z77.22)
exposure to tobacco smoke in the perinatal period (P96.81)
history of tobacco dependence (Z87.891)
occupational exposure to environmental tobacco smoke (Z57.31)
tobacco dependence (F17.-)
tobacco use (Z72.0)
EXCLUDES 1   *malignant neoplasm of oral cavity NOS (C06.9)*

C14.0 Malignant neoplasm of pharynx, unspecified `HCC` ▽

C14.2 Malignant neoplasm of Waldeyer's ring `HCC`

C14.8 Malignant neoplasm of overlapping sites of lip, oral cavity and pharynx `HCC`
Primary malignant neoplasm of two or more contiguous sites of lip, oral cavity and pharynx
EXCLUDES 1   *"book leaf" neoplasm [ventral surface of tongue and floor of mouth] (C06.89)*

Malignant neoplasms of digestive organs (C15-C26)

EXCLUDES 1   *Kaposi's sarcoma of gastrointestinal sites (C46.4)*
EXCLUDES 2   *gastrointestinal stromal tumors (C49.A-)*

✓4ᵗʰ **C15 Malignant neoplasm of esophagus**
Use additional code to identify:
alcohol abuse and dependence (F10.-)

C15.3 Malignant neoplasm of upper third of esophagus `HCC`

C15.4 Malignant neoplasm of middle third of esophagus `HCC`

C15.5 Malignant neoplasm of lower third of esophagus `HCC`
EXCLUDES 1   *malignant neoplasm of cardio-esophageal junction (C16.0)*

C15.8 Malignant neoplasm of overlapping sites of esophagus `HCC`

C15.9 Malignant neoplasm of esophagus, unspecified `HCC` ▽

✓4ᵗʰ **C16 Malignant neoplasm of stomach**
Use additional code to identify:
alcohol abuse and dependence (F10.-)
EXCLUDES 2   *malignant carcinoid tumor of the stomach (C7A.092)*

C16.0 Malignant neoplasm of cardia `HCC`
Malignant neoplasm of cardiac orifice
Malignant neoplasm of cardio-esophageal junction
Malignant neoplasm of esophagus and stomach
Malignant neoplasm of gastro-esophageal junction

C16.1 Malignant neoplasm of fundus of stomach `HCC`

C16.2 Malignant neoplasm of body of stomach `HCC`

C16.3 Malignant neoplasm of pyloric antrum `HCC`
Malignant neoplasm of gastric antrum

C16.4 Malignant neoplasm of pylorus `HCC`
Malignant neoplasm of prepylorus
Malignant neoplasm of pyloric canal

C16.5 Malignant neoplasm of lesser curvature of stomach, unspecified `HCC` ▽
Malignant neoplasm of lesser curvature of stomach, not classifiable to C16.1-C16.4

C16.6 Malignant neoplasm of greater curvature of stomach, unspecified `HCC` ▽
Malignant neoplasm of greater curvature of stomach, not classifiable to C16.0-C16.4

C16.8 Malignant neoplasm of overlapping sites of stomach `HCC`

C16.9 Malignant neoplasm of stomach, unspecified `HCC` ▽
Gastric cancer NOS

✓4ᵗʰ **C17 Malignant neoplasm of small intestine**
EXCLUDES 1   *malignant carcinoid tumors of the small intestine (C7A.01)*
AHA: 2016, 1Q, 19

C17.0 Malignant neoplasm of duodenum `HCC`

C17.1 Malignant neoplasm of jejunum `HCC`

C17.2 Malignant neoplasm of ileum `HCC`
EXCLUDES 1   *malignant neoplasm of ileocecal valve (C18.0)*

C17.3 Meckel's diverticulum, malignant `HCC`
EXCLUDES 1   *Meckel's diverticulum, congenital (Q43.0)*

C17.8 Malignant neoplasm of overlapping sites of small intestine `HCC`

C17.9 Malignant neoplasm of small intestine, unspecified `HCC` ▽

✓4ᵗʰ **C18 Malignant neoplasm of colon**
EXCLUDES 1   *malignant carcinoid tumors of the colon (C7A.02-)*

C18.0 Malignant neoplasm of cecum `HCC`
Malignant neoplasm of ileocecal valve

C18.1 Malignant neoplasm of appendix `HCC`

C18.2 Malignant neoplasm of ascending colon `HCC`

C18.3 Malignant neoplasm of hepatic flexure `HCC`

C18.4 Malignant neoplasm of transverse colon `HCC`

C18.5 Malignant neoplasm of splenic flexure `HCC`

C18.6 Malignant neoplasm of descending colon `HCC`

C18.7 Malignant neoplasm of sigmoid colon `HCC`
Malignant neoplasm of sigmoid (flexure)
EXCLUDES 1   *malignant neoplasm of rectosigmoid junction (C19)*

C18.8 Malignant neoplasm of overlapping sites of colon `HCC`

C18.9 Malignant neoplasm of colon, unspecified `HCC` ▽
Malignant neoplasm of large intestine NOS

C19 Malignant neoplasm of rectosigmoid junction `HCC`
Malignant neoplasm of colon with rectum
Malignant neoplasm of rectosigmoid (colon)
EXCLUDES 1   *malignant carcinoid tumors of the colon (C7A.02-)*

C20 Malignant neoplasm of rectum `HCC`
Malignant neoplasm of rectal ampulla
EXCLUDES 1   *malignant carcinoid tumor of the rectum (C7A.026)*

✓4ᵗʰ **C21 Malignant neoplasm of anus and anal canal**
EXCLUDES 2   *malignant carcinoid tumors of the colon (C7A.02-)*
     malignant melanoma of anal margin (C43.51)
     malignant melanoma of anal skin (C43.51)
     malignant melanoma of perianal skin (C43.51)
     other and unspecified malignant neoplasm of anal margin (C44.500, C44.510, C44.520, C44.590)
     other and unspecified malignant neoplasm of anal skin (C44.500, C44.510, C44.520, C44.590)
     other and unspecified malignant neoplasm of perianal skin (C44.500, C44.510, C44.520, C44.590)

C21.0 Malignant neoplasm of anus, unspecified `HCC` ▽

EXCLUDES 1 Not coded here   *EXCLUDES 2* Not included here   **N** Newborn Age: 0   **P** Pediatric Age: 0-17   **M** Maternity Age: 12-55   **A** Adult Age: 15-124

462   ICD-10-CM 2018

Colon

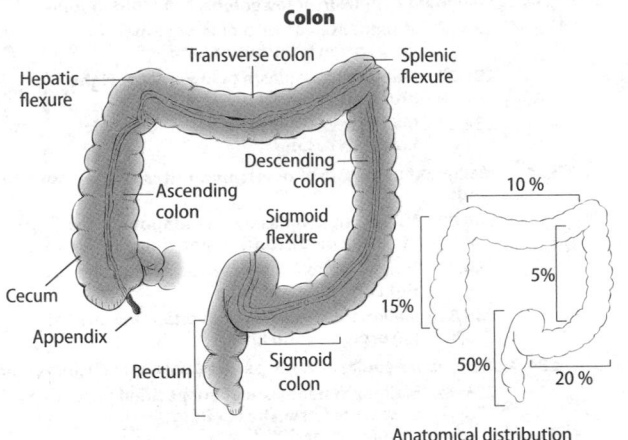

Anatomical distribution of large bowel cancers

Pancreas

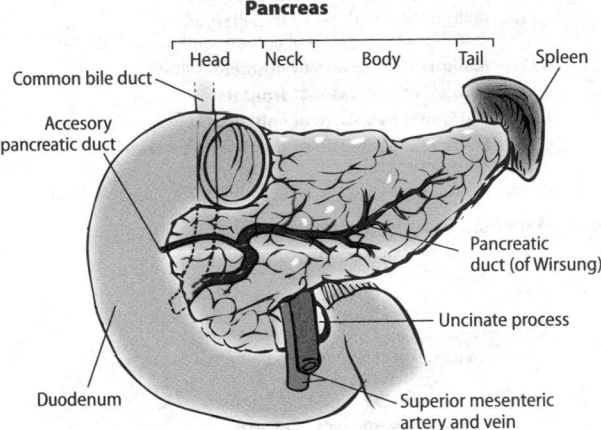

C21.1 Malignant neoplasm of anal canal `HCC`
Malignant neoplasm of anal sphincter

C21.2 Malignant neoplasm of cloacogenic zone `HCC`

C21.8 Malignant neoplasm of overlapping sites of rectum, anus and anal canal `HCC`
Malignant neoplasm of anorectal junction
Malignant neoplasm of anorectum
Primary malignant neoplasm of two or more contiguous sites of rectum, anus and anal canal

✓4ᵗʰ **C22 Malignant neoplasm of liver and intrahepatic bile ducts**
Use additional code to identify:
  alcohol abuse and dependence (F10.-)
  hepatitis B (B16.-, B18.0-B18.1)
  hepatitis C (B17.1-, B18.2)
  EXCLUDES 1   malignant neoplasm of biliary tract NOS (C24.9)
       secondary malignant neoplasm of liver and intrahepatic bile duct (C78.7)

C22.0 Liver cell carcinoma `HCC`
Hepatocellular carcinoma   Hepatoma
AHA: 2016, 1Q, 18

C22.1 Intrahepatic bile duct carcinoma `HCC`
Cholangiocarcinoma
  EXCLUDES 1   malignant neoplasm of hepatic duct (C24.0)

C22.2 Hepatoblastoma `HCC`

C22.3 Angiosarcoma of liver `HCC`
Kupffer cell sarcoma

C22.4 Other sarcomas of liver `HCC`

C22.7 Other specified carcinomas of liver `HCC`

C22.8 Malignant neoplasm of liver, primary, unspecified as to type `HCC` ▽

C22.9 Malignant neoplasm of liver, not specified as primary or secondary `HCC` ▽

C23 Malignant neoplasm of gallbladder `HCC`

✓4ᵗʰ **C24 Malignant neoplasm of other and unspecified parts of biliary tract**
  EXCLUDES 1   malignant neoplasm of intrahepatic bile duct (C22.1)

C24.0 Malignant neoplasm of extrahepatic bile duct `HCC`
Malignant neoplasm of biliary duct or passage NOS
Malignant neoplasm of common bile duct
Malignant neoplasm of cystic duct
Malignant neoplasm of hepatic duct

C24.1 Malignant neoplasm of ampulla of Vater `HCC`
DEF: Malignant neoplasm in the area of dilation at the juncture of the common bile and pancreatic ducts near the opening into the lumen of the duodenum.

C24.8 Malignant neoplasm of overlapping sites of biliary tract `HCC`
Malignant neoplasm involving both intrahepatic and extrahepatic bile ducts
Primary malignant neoplasm of two or more contiguous sites of biliary tract

C24.9 Malignant neoplasm of biliary tract, unspecified `HCC` ▽

✓4ᵗʰ **C25 Malignant neoplasm of pancreas**
Code also exocrine pancreatic insufficiency (K86.81)
Use additional code to identify:
  alcohol abuse and dependence (F10.-)

C25.0 Malignant neoplasm of head of pancreas `HCC`

C25.1 Malignant neoplasm of body of pancreas `HCC`

C25.2 Malignant neoplasm of tail of pancreas `HCC`

C25.3 Malignant neoplasm of pancreatic duct `HCC`

C25.4 Malignant neoplasm of endocrine pancreas `HCC`
Malignant neoplasm of islets of Langerhans
Use additional code to identify any functional activity

C25.7 Malignant neoplasm of other parts of pancreas `HCC`
Malignant neoplasm of neck of pancreas

C25.8 Malignant neoplasm of overlapping sites of pancreas `HCC`

C25.9 Malignant neoplasm of pancreas, unspecified `HCC` ▽

✓4ᵗʰ **C26 Malignant neoplasm of other and ill-defined digestive organs**
  EXCLUDES 1   malignant neoplasm of peritoneum and retroperitoneum (C48.-)

C26.0 Malignant neoplasm of intestinal tract, part unspecified `HCC` ▽
Malignant neoplasm of intestine NOS

C26.1 Malignant neoplasm of spleen `HCC`
  EXCLUDES 1   Hodgkin lymphoma (C81.-)
       non-Hodgkin lymphoma (C82-C85)

C26.9 Malignant neoplasm of ill-defined sites within the digestive system `HCC` ▽
Malignant neoplasm of alimentary canal or tract NOS
Malignant neoplasm of gastrointestinal tract NOS
  EXCLUDES 1   malignant neoplasm of abdominal NOS (C76.2)
       malignant neoplasm of intra-abdominal NOS (C76.2)

Malignant neoplasms of respiratory and intrathoracic organs (C30-C39)

  `INCLUDES`   malignant neoplasm of middle ear
  EXCLUDES 1   mesothelioma (C45.-)

✓4ᵗʰ **C30 Malignant neoplasm of nasal cavity and middle ear**

C30.0 Malignant neoplasm of nasal cavity `HCC`
Malignant neoplasm of cartilage of nose
Malignant neoplasm of nasal concha
Malignant neoplasm of internal nose
Malignant neoplasm of septum of nose
Malignant neoplasm of vestibule of nose
  EXCLUDES 1   malignant melanoma of skin of nose (C43.31)
       malignant neoplasm of nasal bone (C41.0)
       malignant neoplasm of nose NOS (C76.0)
       malignant neoplasm of olfactory bulb (C72.2-)
       malignant neoplasm of posterior margin of nasal septum and choana (C11.3)
       malignant neoplasm of turbinates (C41.0)
       other and unspecified malignant neoplasm of skin of nose (C44.301, C44.311, C44.321, C44.391)

C30.1 Malignant neoplasm of middle ear `HCC`
Malignant neoplasm of antrum tympanicum
Malignant neoplasm of auditory tube
Malignant neoplasm of eustachian tube
Malignant neoplasm of inner ear
Malignant neoplasm of mastoid air cells
Malignant neoplasm of tympanic cavity
  EXCLUDES 1   malignant melanoma of skin of (external) ear (C43.2-)
       malignant neoplasm of auricular canal (external) (C43.2-,C44.2-)
       malignant neoplasm of bone of ear (meatus) (C41.0)
       malignant neoplasm of cartilage of ear (C49.0)
       other and unspecified malignant neoplasm of skin of (external) ear (C44.2-)

✓ Additional Character Req   ✓x7ᵗʰ Placeholder Alert   Manifestation   `HCC` CMS-HCC Condition   ▽ Unspecified Code   ►◄ Revised Text   ● New Code   ▲ Revised Code Title

ICD-10-CM 2018   463

C21.1–C30.1

✓4th **C31** **Malignant neoplasm of accessory sinuses**

     C31.0 **Malignant neoplasm of maxillary sinus** `HCC`
         Malignant neoplasm of antrum (Highmore) (maxillary)

     C31.1 **Malignant neoplasm of ethmoidal sinus** `HCC`

     C31.2 **Malignant neoplasm of frontal sinus** `HCC`

     C31.3 **Malignant neoplasm of sphenoid sinus** `HCC`

     C31.8 **Malignant neoplasm of overlapping sites of accessory sinuses** `HCC`

     C31.9 **Malignant neoplasm of accessory sinus, unspecified** `HCC` ▽

✓4th **C32** **Malignant neoplasm of larynx**
     Use additional code to identify:
         alcohol abuse and dependence (F10.-)
         exposure to environmental tobacco smoke (Z77.22)
         exposure to tobacco smoke in the perinatal period (P96.81)
         history of tobacco dependence (Z87.891)
         occupational exposure to environmental tobacco smoke (Z57.31)
         tobacco dependence (F17.-)
         tobacco use (Z72.0)

     C32.0 **Malignant neoplasm of glottis** `HCC`
         Malignant neoplasm of intrinsic larynx
         Malignant neoplasm of laryngeal commissure (anterior)(posterior)
         Malignant neoplasm of vocal cord (true) NOS

     C32.1 **Malignant neoplasm of supraglottis** `HCC`
         Malignant neoplasm of aryepiglottic fold or interarytenoid fold, laryngeal aspect
         Malignant neoplasm of epiglottis (suprahyoid portion) NOS
         Malignant neoplasm of extrinsic larynx
         Malignant neoplasm of false vocal cord
         Malignant neoplasm of posterior (laryngeal) surface of epiglottis
         Malignant neoplasm of ventricular bands
         `EXCLUDES 2` malignant neoplasm of anterior surface of epiglottis (C10.1)
                 malignant neoplasm of aryepiglottic fold or interarytenoid fold, hypopharyngeal aspect (C13.1)
                 malignant neoplasm of aryepiglottic fold or interarytenoid fold, marginal zone (C13.1)
                 malignant neoplasm of aryepiglottic fold or interarytenoid fold NOS (C13.1)

     C32.2 **Malignant neoplasm of subglottis** `HCC`

     C32.3 **Malignant neoplasm of laryngeal cartilage** `HCC`

     C32.8 **Malignant neoplasm of overlapping sites of larynx** `HCC`

     C32.9 **Malignant neoplasm of larynx, unspecified** `HCC` ▽

C33 **Malignant neoplasm of trachea** `HCC`
     Use additional code to identify:
         exposure to environmental tobacco smoke (Z77.22)
         exposure to tobacco smoke in the perinatal period (P96.81)
         history of tobacco dependence (Z87.891)
         occupational exposure to environmental tobacco smoke (Z57.31)
         tobacco dependence (F17.-)
         tobacco use (Z72.0)

✓4th **C34** **Malignant neoplasm of bronchus and lung**
     Use additional code to identify:
         exposure to environmental tobacco smoke (Z77.22)
         exposure to tobacco smoke in the perinatal period (P96.81)
         history of tobacco dependence (Z87.891)
         occupational exposure to environmental tobacco smoke (Z57.31)
         tobacco dependence (F17.-)
         tobacco use (Z72.0)
     `EXCLUDES 1` Kaposi's sarcoma of lung (C46.5-)
             malignant carcinoid tumor of the bronchus and lung (C7A.090)

     ✓5th **C34.0** **Malignant neoplasm of main bronchus**
         Malignant neoplasm of carina
         Malignant neoplasm of hilus (of lung)

         C34.00 **Malignant neoplasm of unspecified main bronchus** `HCC` ▽

         C34.01 **Malignant neoplasm of right main bronchus** `HCC`

         C34.02 **Malignant neoplasm of left main bronchus** `HCC`

     ✓5th **C34.1** **Malignant neoplasm of upper lobe, bronchus or lung**

         C34.10 **Malignant neoplasm of upper lobe, unspecified bronchus or lung** `HCC` ▽

         C34.11 **Malignant neoplasm of upper lobe, right bronchus or lung** `HCC`

         C34.12 **Malignant neoplasm of upper lobe, left bronchus or lung** `HCC`

     C34.2 **Malignant neoplasm of middle lobe, bronchus or lung** `HCC`

     ✓5th **C34.3** **Malignant neoplasm of lower lobe, bronchus or lung**

         C34.30 **Malignant neoplasm of lower lobe, unspecified bronchus or lung** `HCC` ▽

         C34.31 **Malignant neoplasm of lower lobe, right bronchus or lung** `HCC`

         C34.32 **Malignant neoplasm of lower lobe, left bronchus or lung** `HCC`

     ✓5th **C34.8** **Malignant neoplasm of overlapping sites of bronchus and lung**

         C34.80 **Malignant neoplasm of overlapping sites of unspecified bronchus and lung** `HCC` ▽

         C34.81 **Malignant neoplasm of overlapping sites of right bronchus and lung** `HCC`

         C34.82 **Malignant neoplasm of overlapping sites of left bronchus and lung** `HCC`

     ✓5th **C34.9** **Malignant neoplasm of unspecified part of bronchus or lung**

         C34.90 **Malignant neoplasm of unspecified part of unspecified bronchus or lung** `HCC` ▽
             Lung cancer NOS

         C34.91 **Malignant neoplasm of unspecified part of right bronchus or lung** `HCC` ▽

         C34.92 **Malignant neoplasm of unspecified part of left bronchus or lung** `HCC` ▽

C37 **Malignant neoplasm of thymus** `HCC`
     `EXCLUDES 1` malignant carcinoid tumor of the thymus (C7A.091)

✓4th **C38** **Malignant neoplasm of heart, mediastinum and pleura**
     `EXCLUDES 1` mesothelioma (C45.-)

     C38.0 **Malignant neoplasm of heart** `HCC`
         Malignant neoplasm of pericardium
         `EXCLUDES 1` malignant neoplasm of great vessels (C49.3)

     C38.1 **Malignant neoplasm of anterior mediastinum** `HCC`

     C38.2 **Malignant neoplasm of posterior mediastinum** `HCC`

     C38.3 **Malignant neoplasm of mediastinum, part unspecified** `HCC` ▽

     C38.4 **Malignant neoplasm of pleura** `HCC`

     C38.8 **Malignant neoplasm of overlapping sites of heart, mediastinum and pleura** `HCC`

✓4th **C39** **Malignant neoplasm of other and ill-defined sites in the respiratory system and intrathoracic organs**
     Use additional code to identify:
         exposure to environmental tobacco smoke (Z77.22)
         exposure to tobacco smoke in the perinatal period (P96.81)
         history of tobacco dependence (Z87.891)
         occupational exposure to environmental tobacco smoke (Z57.31)
         tobacco dependence (F17.-)
         tobacco use (Z72.0)
     `EXCLUDES 1` intrathoracic malignant neoplasm NOS (C76.1)
             thoracic malignant neoplasm NOS (C76.1)

     C39.0 **Malignant neoplasm of upper respiratory tract, part unspecified** `HCC` ▽

     C39.9 **Malignant neoplasm of lower respiratory tract, part unspecified** `HCC` ▽
         Malignant neoplasm of respiratory tract NOS

Malignant neoplasms of bone and articular cartilage (C40-C41)

     `INCLUDES` malignant neoplasm of cartilage (articular) (joint)
               malignant neoplasm of periosteum
     `EXCLUDES 1` malignant neoplasm of bone marrow NOS (C96.9)
             malignant neoplasm of synovia (C49.-)

✓4th **C40** **Malignant neoplasm of bone and articular cartilage of limbs**
     Use additional code to identify major osseous defect, if applicable (M89.7-)

     ✓5th **C40.0** **Malignant neoplasm of scapula and long bones of upper limb**

         C40.00 **Malignant neoplasm of scapula and long bones of unspecified upper limb** `HCC` ▽

         C40.01 **Malignant neoplasm of scapula and long bones of right upper limb** `HCC`

         C40.02 **Malignant neoplasm of scapula and long bones of left upper limb** `HCC`

     ✓5th **C40.1** **Malignant neoplasm of short bones of upper limb**

         C40.10 **Malignant neoplasm of short bones of unspecified upper limb** `HCC` ▽

         C40.11 **Malignant neoplasm of short bones of right upper limb** `HCC`

         C40.12 **Malignant neoplasm of short bones of left upper limb** `HCC`

✓5ᵗʰ **C40.2** **Malignant neoplasm of long bones of lower limb**

     C40.20 Malignant neoplasm of long bones of unspecified lower limb   HCC ▽

     C40.21 Malignant neoplasm of long bones of right lower limb   HCC

     C40.22 Malignant neoplasm of long bones of left lower limb   HCC

✓5ᵗʰ **C40.3** **Malignant neoplasm of short bones of lower limb**

     C40.30 Malignant neoplasm of short bones of unspecified lower limb   HCC ▽

     C40.31 Malignant neoplasm of short bones of right lower limb   HCC

     C40.32 Malignant neoplasm of short bones of left lower limb   HCC

✓5ᵗʰ **C40.8** **Malignant neoplasm of overlapping sites of bone and articular cartilage of limb**

     C40.80 Malignant neoplasm of overlapping sites of bone and articular cartilage of unspecified limb   HCC ▽

     C40.81 Malignant neoplasm of overlapping sites of bone and articular cartilage of right limb   HCC

     C40.82 Malignant neoplasm of overlapping sites of bone and articular cartilage of left limb   HCC

✓5ᵗʰ **C40.9** **Malignant neoplasm of unspecified bones and articular cartilage of limb**

     C40.90 Malignant neoplasm of unspecified bones and articular cartilage of unspecified limb   HCC ▽

     C40.91 Malignant neoplasm of unspecified bones and articular cartilage of right limb   HCC ▽

     C40.92 Malignant neoplasm of unspecified bones and articular cartilage of left limb   HCC ▽

✓4ᵗʰ **C41** **Malignant neoplasm of bone and articular cartilage of other and unspecified sites**

     EXCLUDES 1   *malignant neoplasm of bones of limbs (C40.-)*
              malignant neoplasm of cartilage of ear (C49.0)
              malignant neoplasm of cartilage of eyelid (C49.0)
              malignant neoplasm of cartilage of larynx (C32.3)
              malignant neoplasm of cartilage of limbs (C40.-)
              malignant neoplasm of cartilage of nose (C30.0)

     C41.0 **Malignant neoplasm of bones of skull and face**   HCC
         Malignant neoplasm of maxilla (superior)
         Malignant neoplasm of orbital bone
         EXCLUDES 2   *carcinoma, any type except intraosseous or*
                     odontogenic of:
                         maxillary sinus (C31.0)
                         upper jaw (C03.0)
                     malignant neoplasm of jaw bone (lower) (C41.1)

     C41.1 **Malignant neoplasm of mandible**   HCC
         Malignant neoplasm of inferior maxilla
         Malignant neoplasm of lower jaw bone
         EXCLUDES 2   *carcinoma, any type except intraosseous or*
                     odontogenic of:
                         jaw NOS (C03.9)
                         lower (C03.1)
                     malignant neoplasm of upper jaw bone (C41.0)

     C41.2 **Malignant neoplasm of vertebral column**   HCC
         EXCLUDES 1   *malignant neoplasm of sacrum and coccyx (C41.4)*

     C41.3 **Malignant neoplasm of ribs, sternum and clavicle**   HCC

     C41.4 **Malignant neoplasm of pelvic bones, sacrum and coccyx**   HCC

     C41.9 **Malignant neoplasm of bone and articular cartilage, unspecified**   HCC ▽

Melanoma and other malignant neoplasms of skin (C43-C44)

✓4ᵗʰ **C43** **Malignant melanoma of skin**
     EXCLUDES 1   *melanoma in situ (D03.-)*
     EXCLUDES 2   *malignant melanoma of skin of genital organs (C51-C52, C60.-, C63.-)*
                     Merkel cell carcinoma (C4A.-)
                     sites other than skin—code to malignant neoplasm of the site

     C43.0 **Malignant melanoma of lip**   HCC
         EXCLUDES 1   *malignant neoplasm of vermilion border of lip (C00.0-C00.2)*

✓5ᵗʰ **C43.1** **Malignant melanoma of eyelid, including canthus**

     C43.10 Malignant melanoma of unspecified eyelid, including canthus   HCC ▽

     C43.11 Malignant melanoma of right eyelid, including canthus   HCC

     C43.12 Malignant melanoma of left eyelid, including canthus   HCC

✓5ᵗʰ **C43.2** **Malignant melanoma of ear and external auricular canal**

     C43.20 Malignant melanoma of unspecified ear and external auricular canal   HCC ▽

     C43.21 Malignant melanoma of right ear and external auricular canal   HCC

     C43.22 Malignant melanoma of left ear and external auricular canal   HCC

✓5ᵗʰ **C43.3** **Malignant melanoma of other and unspecified parts of face**

     C43.30 Malignant melanoma of unspecified part of face   HCC ▽

     C43.31 Malignant melanoma of nose   HCC

     C43.39 Malignant melanoma of other parts of face   HCC

     C43.4 **Malignant melanoma of scalp and neck**   HCC

✓5ᵗʰ **C43.5** **Malignant melanoma of trunk**
     EXCLUDES 2   *malignant neoplasm of anus NOS (C21.0)*
                     malignant neoplasm of scrotum (C63.2)

     C43.51 **Malignant melanoma of anal skin**   HCC
         Malignant melanoma of anal margin
         Malignant melanoma of perianal skin

     C43.52 **Malignant melanoma of skin of breast**   HCC

     C43.59 **Malignant melanoma of other part of trunk**   HCC

✓5ᵗʰ **C43.6** **Malignant melanoma of upper limb, including shoulder**

     C43.60 Malignant melanoma of unspecified upper limb, including shoulder   HCC ▽

     C43.61 Malignant melanoma of right upper limb, including shoulder   HCC

     C43.62 Malignant melanoma of left upper limb, including shoulder   HCC

✓5ᵗʰ **C43.7** **Malignant melanoma of lower limb, including hip**

     C43.70 Malignant melanoma of unspecified lower limb, including hip   HCC ▽

     C43.71 Malignant melanoma of right lower limb, including hip   HCC

     C43.72 Malignant melanoma of left lower limb, including hip   HCC

     C43.8 **Malignant melanoma of overlapping sites of skin**   HCC

     C43.9 **Malignant melanoma of skin, unspecified**   HCC ▽
         Malignant melanoma of unspecified site of skin
         Melanoma (malignant) NOS

✓4ᵗʰ **C4A** **Merkel cell carcinoma**
     DEF: Malignant cutaneous cancer predominantly found in elderly patients with sun exposure that usually presents as a flesh-colored or bluish-red lump typically seen on the neck, head and face.

     C4A.0 **Merkel cell carcinoma of lip**   HCC
         EXCLUDES 1   *malignant neoplasm of vermilion border of lip (C00.0-C00.2)*

✓5ᵗʰ **C4A.1** **Merkel cell carcinoma of eyelid, including canthus**

     C4A.10 Merkel cell carcinoma of unspecified eyelid, including canthus   HCC ▽

     C4A.11 Merkel cell carcinoma of right eyelid, including canthus   HCC

     C4A.12 Merkel cell carcinoma of left eyelid, including canthus   HCC

✓5ᵗʰ **C4A.2** **Merkel cell carcinoma of ear and external auricular canal**

     C4A.20 Merkel cell carcinoma of unspecified ear and external auricular canal   HCC ▽

     C4A.21 Merkel cell carcinoma of right ear and external auricular canal   HCC

     C4A.22 Merkel cell carcinoma of left ear and external auricular canal   HCC

✓5ᵗʰ **C4A.3** **Merkel cell carcinoma of other and unspecified parts of face**

     C4A.30 Merkel cell carcinoma of unspecified part of face   HCC ▽

     C4A.31 Merkel cell carcinoma of nose   HCC

     C4A.39 Merkel cell carcinoma of other parts of face   HCC

     C4A.4 **Merkel cell carcinoma of scalp and neck**   HCC

✓5ᵗʰ **C4A.5** **Merkel cell carcinoma of trunk**
     EXCLUDES 2   *malignant neoplasm of anus NOS (C21.0)*
                     malignant neoplasm of scrotum (C63.2)

     C4A.51 **Merkel cell carcinoma of anal skin**   HCC
         Merkel cell carcinoma of anal margin
         Merkel cell carcinoma of perianal skin

✓ Additional Character Req   ✓x7ᵗʰ Placeholder Alert   Manifestation   HCC CMS-HCC Condition   ▽ Unspecified Code   ►◄ Revised Text   ● New Code   ▲ Revised Code Title

ICD-10-CM 2018   465

Chapter 2. Neoplasms

C4A.52–C44.40

    C4A.52   Merkel cell carcinoma of **skin of breast**   HCC
    C4A.59   Merkel cell carcinoma of other part of trunk   HCC

✓5ᵗʰ **C4A.6   Merkel cell carcinoma of upper limb, including shoulder**
    C4A.60   Merkel cell carcinoma of unspecified upper limb, including shoulder   HCC ▽
    C4A.61   Merkel cell carcinoma of **right** upper limb, including shoulder   HCC
    C4A.62   Merkel cell carcinoma of **left** upper limb, including shoulder   HCC

✓5ᵗʰ **C4A.7   Merkel cell carcinoma of lower limb, including hip**
    C4A.70   Merkel cell carcinoma of unspecified lower limb, including hip   HCC ▽
    C4A.71   Merkel cell carcinoma of **right** lower limb, including hip   HCC
    C4A.72   Merkel cell carcinoma of **left** lower limb, including hip   HCC

C4A.8   Merkel cell carcinoma of overlapping sites   HCC

C4A.9   Merkel cell carcinoma, unspecified   HCC ▽
     Merkel cell carcinoma of unspecified site

✓4ᵗʰ **C44   Other and unspecified malignant neoplasm of skin**
    INCLUDES   malignant neoplasm of sebaceous glands
                malignant neoplasm of sweat glands
    EXCLUDES 1   *Kaposi's sarcoma of skin (C46.0)*
              malignant melanoma of skin (C43.-)
              malignant neoplasm of skin of genital organs (C51-C52, C60-, C63.2)
              Merkel cell carcinoma (C4A.-)

DEF: Basal cell carcinoma: An abnormal growth of skin cells that arises from the deepest layer of the epidermis and may present as an open sore, red patches, pink growth, or scar. One of the most common forms of skin cancer, typically caused by sun exposure.

DEF: Squamous cell carcinoma: An uncontrolled growth of abnormal skin cells that arises from the skin's outer layers (epidermis) and may present as an open sore; firm, red nodule; elevated growth with a central depression; or flat sore with a scaly crust.

✓5ᵗʰ **C44.0   Other and unspecified malignant neoplasm of skin of lip**
    EXCLUDES 1   *malignant neoplasm of lip (C00.-)*
    C44.00   Unspecified malignant neoplasm of skin of lip   ▽
    C44.01   **Basal cell carcinoma** of skin of lip
    C44.02   **Squamous cell carcinoma** of skin of lip
    C44.09   Other specified malignant neoplasm of skin of lip

✓5ᵗʰ **C44.1   Other and unspecified malignant neoplasm of skin of eyelid, including canthus**
    EXCLUDES 1   *connective tissue of eyelid (C49.0)*

  ✓6ᵗʰ **C44.10   Unspecified malignant neoplasm of skin of eyelid, including canthus**
    C44.101   Unspecified malignant neoplasm of skin of unspecified eyelid, including canthus   ▽
    C44.102   Unspecified malignant neoplasm of skin of **right** eyelid, including canthus   ▽
    C44.109   Unspecified malignant neoplasm of skin of **left** eyelid, including canthus   ▽

  ✓6ᵗʰ **C44.11   Basal cell carcinoma of skin of eyelid, including canthus**
    C44.111   Basal cell carcinoma of skin of unspecified eyelid, including canthus   ▽
    C44.112   Basal cell carcinoma of skin of **right** eyelid, including canthus
    C44.119   Basal cell carcinoma of skin of **left** eyelid, including canthus

  ✓6ᵗʰ **C44.12   Squamous cell carcinoma of skin of eyelid, including canthus**
    C44.121   Squamous cell carcinoma of skin of unspecified eyelid, including canthus   ▽
    C44.122   Squamous cell carcinoma of skin of **right** eyelid, including canthus
    C44.129   Squamous cell carcinoma of skin of **left** eyelid, including canthus

  ✓6ᵗʰ **C44.19   Other specified malignant neoplasm of skin of eyelid, including canthus**
    C44.191   Other specified malignant neoplasm of skin of unspecified eyelid, including canthus   ▽
    C44.192   Other specified malignant neoplasm of skin of **right** eyelid, including canthus
    C44.199   Other specified malignant neoplasm of skin of **left** eyelid, including canthus

✓5ᵗʰ **C44.2   Other and unspecified malignant neoplasm of skin of ear and external auricular canal**
    EXCLUDES 1   *connective tissue of ear (C49.0)*

  ✓6ᵗʰ **C44.20   Unspecified malignant neoplasm of skin of ear and external auricular canal**
    C44.201   Unspecified malignant neoplasm of skin of unspecified ear and external auricular canal   ▽
    C44.202   Unspecified malignant neoplasm of skin of **right** ear and external auricular canal   ▽
    C44.209   Unspecified malignant neoplasm of skin of **left** ear and external auricular canal   ▽

  ✓6ᵗʰ **C44.21   Basal cell carcinoma of skin of ear and external auricular canal**
    C44.211   Basal cell carcinoma of skin of unspecified ear and external auricular canal   ▽
    C44.212   Basal cell carcinoma of skin of **right** ear and external auricular canal
    C44.219   Basal cell carcinoma of skin of **left** ear and external auricular canal

  ✓6ᵗʰ **C44.22   Squamous cell carcinoma of skin of ear and external auricular canal**
    C44.221   Squamous cell carcinoma of skin of unspecified ear and external auricular canal   ▽
    C44.222   Squamous cell carcinoma of skin of **right** ear and external auricular canal
    C44.229   Squamous cell carcinoma of skin of **left** ear and external auricular canal

  ✓6ᵗʰ **C44.29   Other specified malignant neoplasm of skin of ear and external auricular canal**
    C44.291   Other specified malignant neoplasm of skin of unspecified ear and external auricular canal   ▽
    C44.292   Other specified malignant neoplasm of skin of **right** ear and external auricular canal
    C44.299   Other specified malignant neoplasm of skin of **left** ear and external auricular canal

✓5ᵗʰ **C44.3   Other and unspecified malignant neoplasm of skin of other and unspecified parts of face**

  ✓6ᵗʰ **C44.30   Unspecified malignant neoplasm of skin of other and unspecified parts of face**
    C44.300   Unspecified malignant neoplasm of skin of unspecified part of face   ▽
    C44.301   Unspecified malignant neoplasm of skin of **nose**   ▽
    C44.309   Unspecified malignant neoplasm of skin of other parts of face   ▽

  ✓6ᵗʰ **C44.31   Basal cell carcinoma of skin of other and unspecified parts of face**
    C44.310   Basal cell carcinoma of skin of unspecified parts of face   ▽
    C44.311   Basal cell carcinoma of skin of **nose**
    C44.319   Basal cell carcinoma of skin of other parts of face

  ✓6ᵗʰ **C44.32   Squamous cell carcinoma of skin of other and unspecified parts of face**
    C44.320   Squamous cell carcinoma of skin of unspecified parts of face   ▽
    C44.321   Squamous cell carcinoma of skin of **nose**
    C44.329   Squamous cell carcinoma of skin of other parts of face

  ✓6ᵗʰ **C44.39   Other specified malignant neoplasm of skin of other and unspecified parts of face**
    C44.390   Other specified malignant neoplasm of skin of unspecified parts of face   ▽
    C44.391   Other specified malignant neoplasm of skin of **nose**
    C44.399   Other specified malignant neoplasm of skin of other parts of face

✓5ᵗʰ **C44.4   Other and unspecified malignant neoplasm of skin of scalp and neck**
    C44.40   Unspecified malignant neoplasm of skin of scalp and neck   ▽

EXCLUDES 1 Not coded here   EXCLUDES 2 Not included here   N Newborn Age: 0   P Pediatric Age: 0-17   M Maternity Age: 12-55   A Adult Age: 15-124

C44.41   **Basal cell carcinoma of skin of scalp and neck**

C44.42   **Squamous cell carcinoma of skin of scalp and neck**

C44.49   **Other specified malignant neoplasm of skin of scalp and neck**

√5th **C44.5**   **Other and unspecified malignant neoplasm of skin of trunk**
> EXCLUDES 1   *anus NOS (C21.0)*
> *scrotum (C63.2)*

√6th **C44.50**   **Unspecified malignant neoplasm of skin of trunk**

C44.500   **Unspecified malignant neoplasm of anal skin** ▽
> Unspecified malignant neoplasm of anal margin
> Unspecified malignant neoplasm of perianal skin

C44.501   **Unspecified malignant neoplasm of skin of breast** ▽

C44.509   **Unspecified malignant neoplasm of skin of other part of trunk** ▽

√6th **C44.51**   **Basal cell carcinoma of skin of trunk**

C44.510   **Basal cell carcinoma of anal skin**
> Basal cell carcinoma of anal margin
> Basal cell carcinoma of perianal skin

C44.511   **Basal cell carcinoma of skin of breast**

C44.519   **Basal cell carcinoma of skin of other part of trunk**

√6th **C44.52**   **Squamous cell carcinoma of skin of trunk**

C44.520   **Squamous cell carcinoma of anal skin**
> Squamous cell carcinoma of anal margin
> Squamous cell carcinoma of perianal skin

C44.521   **Squamous cell carcinoma of skin of breast**

C44.529   **Squamous cell carcinoma of skin of other part of trunk**

√6th **C44.59**   **Other specified malignant neoplasm of skin of trunk**

C44.590   **Other specified malignant neoplasm of anal skin**
> Other specified malignant neoplasm of anal margin
> Other specified malignant neoplasm of perianal skin

C44.591   **Other specified malignant neoplasm of skin of breast**

C44.599   **Other specified malignant neoplasm of skin of other part of trunk**

√5th **C44.6**   **Other and unspecified malignant neoplasm of skin of upper limb, including shoulder**

√6th **C44.60**   **Unspecified malignant neoplasm of skin of upper limb, including shoulder**

C44.601   **Unspecified malignant neoplasm of skin of unspecified upper limb, including shoulder** ▽

C44.602   **Unspecified malignant neoplasm of skin of right upper limb, including shoulder** ▽

C44.609   **Unspecified malignant neoplasm of skin of left upper limb, including shoulder** ▽

√6th **C44.61**   **Basal cell carcinoma of skin of upper limb, including shoulder**

C44.611   **Basal cell carcinoma of skin of unspecified upper limb, including shoulder** ▽

C44.612   **Basal cell carcinoma of skin of right upper limb, including shoulder**

C44.619   **Basal cell carcinoma of skin of left upper limb, including shoulder**

√6th **C44.62**   **Squamous cell carcinoma of skin of upper limb, including shoulder**

C44.621   **Squamous cell carcinoma of skin of unspecified upper limb, including shoulder** ▽

C44.622   **Squamous cell carcinoma of skin of right upper limb, including shoulder**

C44.629   **Squamous cell carcinoma of skin of left upper limb, including shoulder**

√6th **C44.69**   **Other specified malignant neoplasm of skin of upper limb, including shoulder**

C44.691   **Other specified malignant neoplasm of skin of unspecified upper limb, including shoulder** ▽

C44.692   **Other specified malignant neoplasm of skin of right upper limb, including shoulder**

C44.699   **Other specified malignant neoplasm of skin of left upper limb, including shoulder**

√5th **C44.7**   **Other and unspecified malignant neoplasm of skin of lower limb, including hip**

√6th **C44.70**   **Unspecified malignant neoplasm of skin of lower limb, including hip**

C44.701   **Unspecified malignant neoplasm of skin of unspecified lower limb, including hip** ▽

C44.702   **Unspecified malignant neoplasm of skin of right lower limb, including hip** ▽

C44.709   **Unspecified malignant neoplasm of skin of left lower limb, including hip** ▽

√6th **C44.71**   **Basal cell carcinoma of skin of lower limb, including hip**

C44.711   **Basal cell carcinoma of skin of unspecified lower limb, including hip** ▽

C44.712   **Basal cell carcinoma of skin of right lower limb, including hip**

C44.719   **Basal cell carcinoma of skin of left lower limb, including hip**

√6th **C44.72**   **Squamous cell carcinoma of skin of lower limb, including hip**

C44.721   **Squamous cell carcinoma of skin of unspecified lower limb, including hip** ▽

C44.722   **Squamous cell carcinoma of skin of right lower limb, including hip**

C44.729   **Squamous cell carcinoma of skin of left lower limb, including hip**

√6th **C44.79**   **Other specified malignant neoplasm of skin of lower limb, including hip**

C44.791   **Other specified malignant neoplasm of skin of unspecified lower limb, including hip** ▽

C44.792   **Other specified malignant neoplasm of skin of right lower limb, including hip**

C44.799   **Other specified malignant neoplasm of skin of left lower limb, including hip**

√5th **C44.8**   **Other and unspecified malignant neoplasm of overlapping sites of skin**

C44.80   **Unspecified malignant neoplasm of overlapping sites of skin** ▽

C44.81   **Basal cell carcinoma of overlapping sites of skin**

C44.82   **Squamous cell carcinoma of overlapping sites of skin**

C44.89   **Other specified malignant neoplasm of overlapping sites of skin**

√5th **C44.9**   **Other and unspecified malignant neoplasm of skin, unspecified**

C44.90   **Unspecified malignant neoplasm of skin, unspecified** ▽
> Malignant neoplasm of unspecified site of skin

C44.91   **Basal cell carcinoma of skin, unspecified** ▽

C44.92   **Squamous cell carcinoma of skin, unspecified** ▽

C44.99   **Other specified malignant neoplasm of skin, unspecified** ▽

Malignant neoplasms of mesothelial and soft tissue (C45-C49)

√4th **C45**   **Mesothelioma**
> **DEF:** Rare type of cancer that forms in the thin layer of protective tissue that covers the majority of internal organs (mesothelium).

C45.0   **Mesothelioma of pleura**   HCC
> EXCLUDES 1   *other malignant neoplasm of pleura (C38.4)*
> **AHA:** 2017, 2Q, 11

C45.1   **Mesothelioma of peritoneum**   HCC
> Mesothelioma of cul-de-sac   Mesothelioma of omentum
> Mesothelioma of mesentery   Mesothelioma of peritoneum
> Mesothelioma of mesocolon   (parietal) (pelvic)
> EXCLUDES 1   *other malignant neoplasm of soft tissue of peritoneum (C48.-)*

C45.2   **Mesothelioma of pericardium**   HCC
> EXCLUDES 1   *other malignant neoplasm of pericardium (C38.0)*

C45.7   **Mesothelioma of other sites**   HCC

C45.9   **Mesothelioma, unspecified**   HCC ▽

✔ Additional Character Req   √x7th Placeholder Alert   Manifestation   HCC CMS-HCC Condition   ▽ Unspecified Code   ►◄ Revised Text   ● New Code   ▲ Revised Code Title

ICD-10-CM 2018   467

☑4ᵗʰ **C46 Kaposi's sarcoma**

Code first any human immunodeficiency virus [HIV] disease (B20)
DEF: Malignant neoplasm that causes patches of abnormal tissue to grow under the skin, in the lining of the mouth, nose, and throat, in lymph nodes, or in other visceral organs. Kaposi's sarcoma is caused by human herpesvirus8 (HHV8).

C46.0 Kaposi's sarcoma of skin `HCC`

C46.1 Kaposi's sarcoma of soft tissue `HCC`
Kaposi's sarcoma of blood vessel
Kaposi's sarcoma of connective tissue
Kaposi's sarcoma of fascia
Kaposi's sarcoma of ligament
Kaposi's sarcoma of lymphatic(s) NEC
Kaposi's sarcoma of muscle
EXCLUDES 2 Kaposi's sarcoma of lymph glands and nodes (C46.3)

C46.2 Kaposi's sarcoma of palate `HCC`

C46.3 Kaposi's sarcoma of lymph nodes `HCC`

C46.4 Kaposi's sarcoma of gastrointestinal sites `HCC`

☑5ᵗʰ **C46.5 Kaposi's sarcoma of lung**

C46.50 Kaposi's sarcoma of unspecified lung `HCC` ▽

C46.51 Kaposi's sarcoma of right lung `HCC`

C46.52 Kaposi's sarcoma of left lung `HCC`

C46.7 Kaposi's sarcoma of other sites `HCC`

C46.9 Kaposi's sarcoma, unspecified `HCC` ▽
Kaposi's sarcoma of unspecified site

☑4ᵗʰ **C47 Malignant neoplasm of peripheral nerves and autonomic nervous system**

`INCLUDES` malignant neoplasm of sympathetic and parasympathetic nerves and ganglia

EXCLUDES 1 Kaposi's sarcoma of soft tissue (C46.1)

C47.0 Malignant neoplasm of peripheral nerves of head, face and neck `HCC`
EXCLUDES 1 malignant neoplasm of peripheral nerves of orbit (C69.6-)

☑5ᵗʰ **C47.1 Malignant neoplasm of peripheral nerves of upper limb, including shoulder**

C47.10 Malignant neoplasm of peripheral nerves of unspecified upper limb, including shoulder `HCC` ▽

C47.11 Malignant neoplasm of peripheral nerves of right upper limb, including shoulder `HCC`

C47.12 Malignant neoplasm of peripheral nerves of left upper limb, including shoulder `HCC`

☑5ᵗʰ **C47.2 Malignant neoplasm of peripheral nerves of lower limb, including hip**

C47.20 Malignant neoplasm of peripheral nerves of unspecified lower limb, including hip `HCC` ▽

C47.21 Malignant neoplasm of peripheral nerves of right lower limb, including hip `HCC`

C47.22 Malignant neoplasm of peripheral nerves of left lower limb, including hip `HCC`

C47.3 Malignant neoplasm of peripheral nerves of thorax `HCC`

C47.4 Malignant neoplasm of peripheral nerves of abdomen `HCC`

C47.5 Malignant neoplasm of peripheral nerves of pelvis `HCC`

C47.6 Malignant neoplasm of peripheral nerves of trunk, unspecified `HCC` ▽
Malignant neoplasm of peripheral nerves of unspecified part of trunk

C47.8 Malignant neoplasm of overlapping sites of peripheral nerves and autonomic nervous system `HCC`

C47.9 Malignant neoplasm of peripheral nerves and autonomic nervous system, unspecified `HCC` ▽
Malignant neoplasm of unspecified site of peripheral nerves and autonomic nervous system

☑4ᵗʰ **C48 Malignant neoplasm of retroperitoneum and peritoneum**
EXCLUDES 1 Kaposi's sarcoma of connective tissue (C46.1)
mesothelioma (C45.-)

C48.0 Malignant neoplasm of retroperitoneum `HCC`

C48.1 Malignant neoplasm of specified parts of peritoneum `HCC`
Malignant neoplasm of cul-de-sac
Malignant neoplasm of mesentery
Malignant neoplasm of mesocolon
Malignant neoplasm of omentum
Malignant neoplasm of parietal peritoneum
Malignant neoplasm of pelvic peritoneum

C48.2 Malignant neoplasm of peritoneum, unspecified `HCC` ▽

C48.8 Malignant neoplasm of overlapping sites of retroperitoneum and peritoneum `HCC`

☑4ᵗʰ **C49 Malignant neoplasm of other connective and soft tissue**

`INCLUDES` malignant neoplasm of blood vessel
malignant neoplasm of bursa
malignant neoplasm of cartilage
malignant neoplasm of fascia
malignant neoplasm of fat
malignant neoplasm of ligament, except uterine
malignant neoplasm of lymphatic vessel
malignant neoplasm of muscle
malignant neoplasm of synovia
malignant neoplasm of tendon (sheath)

EXCLUDES 1 malignant neoplasm of cartilage (of):
articular (C40-C41)
larynx (C32.3)
nose (C30.0)
malignant neoplasm of connective tissue of breast (C50.-)

EXCLUDES 2 Kaposi's sarcoma of soft tissue (C46.1)
malignant neoplasm of heart (C38.0)
malignant neoplasm of peripheral nerves and autonomic nervous system (C47.-)
malignant neoplasm of peritoneum (C48.2)
malignant neoplasm of retroperitoneum (C48.0)
malignant neoplasm of uterine ligament (C57.3)
mesothelioma (C45.-)

C49.0 Malignant neoplasm of connective and soft tissue of head, face and neck `HCC`
Malignant neoplasm of connective tissue of ear
Malignant neoplasm of connective tissue of eyelid
EXCLUDES 1 connective tissue of orbit (C69.6-)

☑5ᵗʰ **C49.1 Malignant neoplasm of connective and soft tissue of upper limb, including shoulder**

C49.10 Malignant neoplasm of connective and soft tissue of unspecified upper limb, including shoulder `HCC` ▽

C49.11 Malignant neoplasm of connective and soft tissue of right upper limb, including shoulder `HCC`

C49.12 Malignant neoplasm of connective and soft tissue of left upper limb, including shoulder `HCC`

☑5ᵗʰ **C49.2 Malignant neoplasm of connective and soft tissue of lower limb, including hip**

C49.20 Malignant neoplasm of connective and soft tissue of unspecified lower limb, including hip `HCC` ▽

C49.21 Malignant neoplasm of connective and soft tissue of right lower limb, including hip `HCC`

C49.22 Malignant neoplasm of connective and soft tissue of left lower limb, including hip `HCC`

C49.3 Malignant neoplasm of connective and soft tissue of thorax `HCC`
Malignant neoplasm of axilla
Malignant neoplasm of diaphragm
Malignant neoplasm of great vessels
EXCLUDES 1 malignant neoplasm of breast (C50.-)
malignant neoplasm of heart (C38.0)
malignant neoplasm of mediastinum (C38.1-C38.3)
malignant neoplasm of thymus (C37)
AHA: 2015, 3Q, 19

C49.4 Malignant neoplasm of connective and soft tissue of abdomen `HCC`
Malignant neoplasm of abdominal wall
Malignant neoplasm of hypochondrium

C49.5 Malignant neoplasm of connective and soft tissue of pelvis `HCC`
Malignant neoplasm of buttock
Malignant neoplasm of groin
Malignant neoplasm of perineum

C49.6 Malignant neoplasm of connective and soft tissue of trunk, unspecified `HCC` ▽
Malignant neoplasm of back NOS

C49.8 Malignant neoplasm of overlapping sites of connective and soft tissue `HCC`
Primary malignant neoplasm of two or more contiguous sites of connective and soft tissue

C49.9 Malignant neoplasm of connective and soft tissue, unspecified `HCC` ▽

☑5ᵗʰ **C49.A Gastrointestinal stromal tumor**

C49.A0 Gastrointestinal stromal tumor, unspecified site `HCC` ▽

C49.A1 Gastrointestinal stromal tumor of esophagus `HCC`

C49.A2 Gastrointestinal stromal tumor of stomach `HCC`

C49.A3 Gastrointestinal stromal tumor of small intestine `HCC`

EXCLUDES 1 Not coded here   *EXCLUDES 2* Not included here   N Newborn Age: 0   P Pediatric Age: 0-17   M Maternity Age: 12-55   A Adult Age: 15-124

468

ICD-10-CM 2018

C49.A4   Gastrointestinal stromal tumor of **large intestine** ᴴᶜᶜ

C49.A5   Gastrointestinal stromal tumor of **rectum**   ᴴᶜᶜ

C49.A9   Gastrointestinal stromal tumor of other sites   ᴴᶜᶜ

Malignant neoplasms of breast (C50)

✓⁴ᵗʰ **C50** **Malignant neoplasm of breast**

INCLUDES   connective tissue of breast
Paget's disease of breast
Paget's disease of nipple

Use additional code to identify estrogen receptor status (Z17.0, Z17.1)

EXCLUDES 1   *skin of breast (C44.501, C44.511, C44.521, C44.591)*

✓⁵ᵗʰ **C50.0**   Malignant neoplasm of **nipple and areola**

✓⁶ᵗʰ **C50.01**   Malignant neoplasm of nipple and areola, **female**

    C50.011   Malignant neoplasm of nipple and areola, **right** female breast   ᴴᶜᶜ ♀

    C50.012   Malignant neoplasm of nipple and areola, **left** female breast   ᴴᶜᶜ ♀

    C50.019   Malignant neoplasm of nipple and areola, unspecified female breast   ᴴᶜᶜ ♀▽

✓⁶ᵗʰ **C50.02**   Malignant neoplasm of nipple and areola, **male**

    C50.021   Malignant neoplasm of nipple and areola, **right** male breast   ᴴᶜᶜ ♂

    C50.022   Malignant neoplasm of nipple and areola, **left** male breast   ᴴᶜᶜ ♂

    C50.029   Malignant neoplasm of nipple and areola, unspecified male breast   ᴴᶜᶜ ♂▽

✓⁵ᵗʰ **C50.1**   Malignant neoplasm of **central portion** of breast

✓⁶ᵗʰ **C50.11**   Malignant neoplasm of central portion of breast, **female**

    C50.111   Malignant neoplasm of central portion of **right** female breast   ᴴᶜᶜ ♀

    C50.112   Malignant neoplasm of central portion of **left** female breast   ᴴᶜᶜ ♀

    C50.119   Malignant neoplasm of central portion of unspecified female breast   ᴴᶜᶜ ♀▽

✓⁶ᵗʰ **C50.12**   Malignant neoplasm of central portion of breast, **male**

    C50.121   Malignant neoplasm of central portion of **right** male breast   ᴴᶜᶜ ♂

    C50.122   Malignant neoplasm of central portion of **left** male breast   ᴴᶜᶜ ♂

    C50.129   Malignant neoplasm of central portion of unspecified male breast   ᴴᶜᶜ ♂▽

✓⁵ᵗʰ **C50.2**   Malignant neoplasm of **upper-inner quadrant** of breast

✓⁶ᵗʰ **C50.21**   Malignant neoplasm of upper-inner quadrant of breast, **female**

    C50.211   Malignant neoplasm of upper-inner quadrant of **right** female breast   ᴴᶜᶜ ♀

    C50.212   Malignant neoplasm of upper-inner quadrant of **left** female breast   ᴴᶜᶜ ♀

    C50.219   Malignant neoplasm of upper-inner quadrant of unspecified female breast   ᴴᶜᶜ ♀▽

✓⁶ᵗʰ **C50.22**   Malignant neoplasm of upper-inner quadrant of breast, **male**

    C50.221   Malignant neoplasm of upper-inner quadrant of **right** male breast   ᴴᶜᶜ ♂

    C50.222   Malignant neoplasm of upper-inner quadrant of **left** male breast   ᴴᶜᶜ ♂

    C50.229   Malignant neoplasm of upper-inner quadrant of unspecified male breast   ᴴᶜᶜ ♂▽

✓⁵ᵗʰ **C50.3**   Malignant neoplasm of **lower-inner quadrant** of breast

✓⁶ᵗʰ **C50.31**   Malignant neoplasm of lower-inner quadrant of breast, **female**

    C50.311   Malignant neoplasm of lower-inner quadrant of **right** female breast   ᴴᶜᶜ ♀

    C50.312   Malignant neoplasm of lower-inner quadrant of **left** female breast   ᴴᶜᶜ ♀

    C50.319   Malignant neoplasm of lower-inner quadrant of unspecified female breast   ᴴᶜᶜ ♀▽

✓⁶ᵗʰ **C50.32**   Malignant neoplasm of lower-inner quadrant of breast, **male**

    C50.321   Malignant neoplasm of lower-inner quadrant of **right** male breast   ᴴᶜᶜ ♂

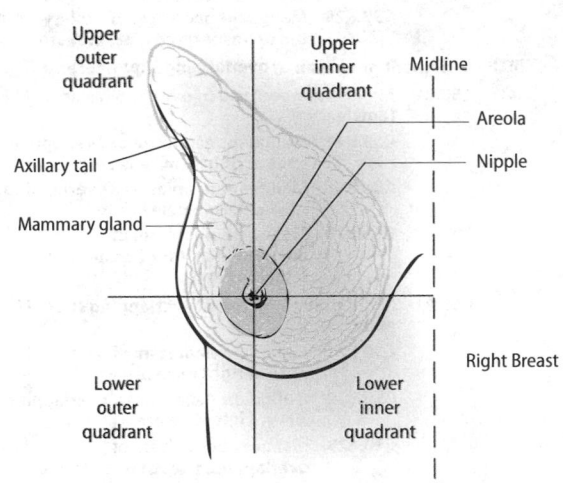

Female Breast

Upper outer quadrant · Upper inner quadrant · Midline · Areola · Nipple · Axillary tail · Mammary gland · Lower outer quadrant · Lower inner quadrant · Right Breast

    C50.322   Malignant neoplasm of lower-inner quadrant of **left** male breast   ᴴᶜᶜ ♂

    C50.329   Malignant neoplasm of lower-inner quadrant of unspecified male breast   ᴴᶜᶜ ♂▽

✓⁵ᵗʰ **C50.4**   Malignant neoplasm of **upper-outer quadrant** of breast

✓⁶ᵗʰ **C50.41**   Malignant neoplasm of upper-outer quadrant of breast, **female**

    C50.411   Malignant neoplasm of upper-outer quadrant of **right** female breast   ᴴᶜᶜ ♀

    C50.412   Malignant neoplasm of upper-outer quadrant of **left** female breast   ᴴᶜᶜ ♀

    C50.419   Malignant neoplasm of upper-outer quadrant of unspecified female breast   ᴴᶜᶜ ♀▽

✓⁶ᵗʰ **C50.42**   Malignant neoplasm of upper-outer quadrant of breast, **male**

    C50.421   Malignant neoplasm of upper-outer quadrant of **right** male breast   ᴴᶜᶜ ♂

    C50.422   Malignant neoplasm of upper-outer quadrant of **left** male breast   ᴴᶜᶜ ♂

    C50.429   Malignant neoplasm of upper-outer quadrant of unspecified male breast   ᴴᶜᶜ ♂▽

✓⁵ᵗʰ **C50.5**   Malignant neoplasm of **lower-outer quadrant** of breast

✓⁶ᵗʰ **C50.51**   Malignant neoplasm of lower-outer quadrant of breast, **female**

    C50.511   Malignant neoplasm of lower-outer quadrant of **right** female breast   ᴴᶜᶜ ♀

    C50.512   Malignant neoplasm of lower-outer quadrant of **left** female breast   ᴴᶜᶜ ♀

    C50.519   Malignant neoplasm of lower-outer quadrant of unspecified female breast   ᴴᶜᶜ ♀▽

✓⁶ᵗʰ **C50.52**   Malignant neoplasm of lower-outer quadrant of breast, **male**

    C50.521   Malignant neoplasm of lower-outer quadrant of **right** male breast   ᴴᶜᶜ ♂

    C50.522   Malignant neoplasm of lower-outer quadrant of **left** male breast   ᴴᶜᶜ ♂

    C50.529   Malignant neoplasm of lower-outer quadrant of unspecified male breast   ᴴᶜᶜ ♂▽

✓⁵ᵗʰ **C50.6**   Malignant neoplasm of **axillary tail** of breast

✓⁶ᵗʰ **C50.61**   Malignant neoplasm of axillary tail of breast, **female**

    C50.611   Malignant neoplasm of axillary tail of **right** female breast   ᴴᶜᶜ ♀

    C50.612   Malignant neoplasm of axillary tail of **left** female breast   ᴴᶜᶜ ♀

    C50.619   Malignant neoplasm of axillary tail of unspecified female breast   ᴴᶜᶜ ♀▽

✓⁶ᵗʰ **C50.62**   Malignant neoplasm of axillary tail of breast, **male**

    C50.621   Malignant neoplasm of axillary tail of **right** male breast   ᴴᶜᶜ

☑ Additional Character Req   ✗x7ᵗʰ Placeholder Alert   Manifestation   ᴴᶜᶜ CMS-HCC Condition   ▽ Unspecified Code   ►◄ Revised Text   ● New Code   ▲ Revised Code Title

ICD-10-CM 2018   469

Chapter 2. Neoplasms

C50.622   Malignant neoplasm of axillary tail of left male breast   HCC ♂

C50.629   Malignant neoplasm of axillary tail of unspecified male breast   HCC ♂ ▽

✓5ᵗʰ **C50.8   Malignant neoplasm of overlapping sites of breast**

   ✓6ᵗʰ **C50.81   Malignant neoplasm of overlapping sites of breast, female**

     C50.811   Malignant neoplasm of overlapping sites of right female breast   HCC ♀

     C50.812   Malignant neoplasm of overlapping sites of left female breast   HCC ♀

     C50.819   Malignant neoplasm of overlapping sites of unspecified female breast   HCC ♀ ▽

   ✓6ᵗʰ **C50.82   Malignant neoplasm of overlapping sites of breast, male**

     C50.821   Malignant neoplasm of overlapping sites of right male breast   HCC ♂

     C50.822   Malignant neoplasm of overlapping sites of left male breast   HCC ♂

     C50.829   Malignant neoplasm of overlapping sites of unspecified male breast   HCC ♂ ▽

✓5ᵗʰ **C50.9   Malignant neoplasm of breast of unspecified site**

   ✓6ᵗʰ **C50.91   Malignant neoplasm of breast of unspecified site, female**

     C50.911   Malignant neoplasm of unspecified site of right female breast   HCC ♀

     C50.912   Malignant neoplasm of unspecified site of left female breast   HCC ♀

     C50.919   Malignant neoplasm of unspecified site of unspecified female breast   HCC ♀ ▽

   ✓6ᵗʰ **C50.92   Malignant neoplasm of breast of unspecified site, male**

     C50.921   Malignant neoplasm of unspecified site of right male breast   HCC ♂

     C50.922   Malignant neoplasm of unspecified site of left male breast   HCC ♂

     C50.929   Malignant neoplasm of unspecified site of unspecified male breast   HCC ♂ ▽

Malignant neoplasms of female genital organs (C51-C58)

INCLUDES   malignant neoplasm of skin of female genital organs

✓4ᵗʰ **C51   Malignant neoplasm of vulva**

   EXCLUDES 1   *carcinoma in situ of vulva (D07.1)*

   C51.0   Malignant neoplasm of labium majus   HCC ♀
     Malignant neoplasm of Bartholin's [greater vestibular] gland

   C51.1   Malignant neoplasm of labium minus   HCC ♀

   C51.2   Malignant neoplasm of clitoris   HCC ♀

   C51.8   Malignant neoplasm of overlapping sites of vulva   HCC ♀

   C51.9   Malignant neoplasm of vulva, unspecified   HCC ♀ ▽
     Malignant neoplasm of external female genitalia NOS
     Malignant neoplasm of pudendum

C52   Malignant neoplasm of vagina   HCC ♀
   EXCLUDES 1   *carcinoma in situ of vagina (D07.2)*

✓4ᵗʰ **C53   Malignant neoplasm of cervix uteri**
   EXCLUDES 1   *carcinoma in situ of cervix uteri (D06.-)*

   C53.0   Malignant neoplasm of endocervix   HCC ♀

   C53.1   Malignant neoplasm of exocervix   HCC ♀

   C53.8   Malignant neoplasm of overlapping sites of cervix uteri   HCC ♀

   C53.9   Malignant neoplasm of cervix uteri, unspecified   HCC ♀ ▽

✓4ᵗʰ **C54   Malignant neoplasm of corpus uteri**

   C54.0   Malignant neoplasm of isthmus uteri   HCC ♀
     Malignant neoplasm of lower uterine segment

   C54.1   Malignant neoplasm of endometrium   HCC ♀

   C54.2   Malignant neoplasm of myometrium   HCC ♀

   C54.3   Malignant neoplasm of fundus uteri   HCC ♀

   C54.8   Malignant neoplasm of overlapping sites of corpus uteri   HCC ♀

   C54.9   Malignant neoplasm of corpus uteri, unspecified   HCC ♀ ▽

C55   Malignant neoplasm of uterus, part unspecified   HCC ♀ ▽

✓4ᵗʰ **C56   Malignant neoplasm of ovary**
   Use additional code to identify any functional activity

   C56.1   Malignant neoplasm of right ovary   HCC ♀

   C56.2   Malignant neoplasm of left ovary   HCC ♀

   C56.9   Malignant neoplasm of unspecified ovary   HCC ♀ ▽

✓4ᵗʰ **C57   Malignant neoplasm of other and unspecified female genital organs**

   ✓5ᵗʰ **C57.0   Malignant neoplasm of fallopian tube**
     Malignant neoplasm of oviduct
     Malignant neoplasm of uterine tube

     C57.00   Malignant neoplasm of unspecified fallopian tube   HCC ♀ ▽

     C57.01   Malignant neoplasm of right fallopian tube   HCC ♀

     C57.02   Malignant neoplasm of left fallopian tube   HCC ♀

   ✓5ᵗʰ **C57.1   Malignant neoplasm of broad ligament**

     C57.10   Malignant neoplasm of unspecified broad ligament   HCC ♀ ▽

     C57.11   Malignant neoplasm of right broad ligament   HCC ♀

     C57.12   Malignant neoplasm of left broad ligament   HCC ♀

   ✓5ᵗʰ **C57.2   Malignant neoplasm of round ligament**

     C57.20   Malignant neoplasm of unspecified round ligament   HCC ♀ ▽

     C57.21   Malignant neoplasm of right round ligament   HCC ♀

     C57.22   Malignant neoplasm of left round ligament   HCC ♀

   C57.3   Malignant neoplasm of parametrium   HCC ♀
     Malignant neoplasm of uterine ligament NOS

   C57.4   Malignant neoplasm of uterine adnexa, unspecified   HCC ♀ ▽

   C57.7   Malignant neoplasm of other specified female genital organs   HCC ♀
     Malignant neoplasm of wolffian body or duct

   C57.8   Malignant neoplasm of overlapping sites of female genital organs   HCC ♀
     Primary malignant neoplasm of two or more contiguous sites of the female genital organs whose point of origin cannot be determined
     Primary tubo-ovarian malignant neoplasm whose point of origin cannot be determined
     Primary utero-ovarian malignant neoplasm whose point of origin cannot be determined

   C57.9   Malignant neoplasm of female genital organ, unspecified   HCC ♀ ▽
     Malignant neoplasm of female genitourinary tract NOS

C58   Malignant neoplasm of placenta   HCC M ♀
   INCLUDES   choriocarcinoma NOS
     chorionepithelioma NOS
   EXCLUDES 1   *chorioadenoma (destruens) (D39.2)*
     hydatidiform mole NOS (O01.9)
     invasive hydatidiform mole (D39.2)
     male choriocarcinoma NOS (C62.9-)
     malignant hydatidiform mole (D39.2)

Malignant neoplasms of male genital organs (C60-C63)

INCLUDES   malignant neoplasm of skin of male genital organs

✓4ᵗʰ **C60   Malignant neoplasm of penis**

   C60.0   Malignant neoplasm of prepuce   HCC ♂
     Malignant neoplasm of foreskin

   C60.1   Malignant neoplasm of glans penis   HCC ♂

   C60.2   Malignant neoplasm of body of penis   HCC ♂
     Malignant neoplasm of corpus cavernosum

   C60.8   Malignant neoplasm of overlapping sites of penis   HCC ♂

   C60.9   Malignant neoplasm of penis, unspecified   HCC ♂ ▽
     Malignant neoplasm of skin of penis NOS

C61   Malignant neoplasm of prostate   HCC ♂
   Use additional code to identify:
     hormone sensitivity status (Z19.1-Z19.2)
     rising PSA following treatment for malignant neoplasm of prostate (R97.21)
   EXCLUDES 1   *malignant neoplasm of seminal vesicle (C63.7)*
   AHA: 2017, 1Q, 17

EXCLUDES 1 Not coded here   EXCLUDES 2 Not included here   N Newborn Age: 0   P Pediatric Age: 0-17   M Maternity Age: 12-55   A Adult Age: 15-124

✓4ᵗʰ C62 Malignant neoplasm of testis
Use additional code to identify any functional activity

     ✓5ᵗʰ C62.0 Malignant neoplasm of undescended testis
         Malignant neoplasm of ectopic testis
         Malignant neoplasm of retained testis

         C62.00 Malignant neoplasm of unspecified undescended testis   HCC ♂ ▽

         C62.01 Malignant neoplasm of undescended right testis   HCC ♂

         C62.02 Malignant neoplasm of undescended left testis   HCC ♂

     ✓5ᵗʰ C62.1 Malignant neoplasm of descended testis
         Malignant neoplasm of scrotal testis

         C62.10 Malignant neoplasm of unspecified descended testis   HCC ♂ ▽

         C62.11 Malignant neoplasm of descended right testis   HCC ♂

         C62.12 Malignant neoplasm of descended left testis   HCC ♂

     ✓5ᵗʰ C62.9 Malignant neoplasm of testis, unspecified whether descended or undescended

         C62.90 Malignant neoplasm of unspecified testis, unspecified whether descended or undescended   HCC ♂ ▽
           Malignant neoplasm of testis NOS

         C62.91 Malignant neoplasm of right testis, unspecified whether descended or undescended   HCC ♂ ▽

         C62.92 Malignant neoplasm of left testis, unspecified whether descended or undescended   HCC ♂ ▽

✓4ᵗʰ C63 Malignant neoplasm of other and unspecified male genital organs

     ✓5ᵗʰ C63.0 Malignant neoplasm of epididymis

         C63.00 Malignant neoplasm of unspecified epididymis   HCC ♂ ▽

         C63.01 Malignant neoplasm of right epididymis   HCC ♂

         C63.02 Malignant neoplasm of left epididymis   HCC ♂

     ✓5ᵗʰ C63.1 Malignant neoplasm of spermatic cord

         C63.10 Malignant neoplasm of unspecified spermatic cord   HCC ♂ ▽

         C63.11 Malignant neoplasm of right spermatic cord   HCC ♂

         C63.12 Malignant neoplasm of left spermatic cord   HCC ♂

     C63.2 Malignant neoplasm of scrotum   HCC ♂
         Malignant neoplasm of skin of scrotum

     C63.7 Malignant neoplasm of other specified male genital organs   HCC ♂
         Malignant neoplasm of seminal vesicle
         Malignant neoplasm of tunica vaginalis

     C63.8 Malignant neoplasm of overlapping sites of male genital organs   HCC ♂
         Primary malignant neoplasm of two or more contiguous sites of male genital organs whose point of origin cannot be determined

     C63.9 Malignant neoplasm of male genital organ, unspecified   HCC ♂ ▽
         Malignant neoplasm of male genitourinary tract NOS

Malignant neoplasms of urinary tract (C64-C68)

✓4ᵗʰ C64 Malignant neoplasm of kidney, except renal pelvis
     EXCLUDES 1   *malignant carcinoid tumor of the kidney (C7A.093)*
         malignant neoplasm of renal calyces (C65.-)
         malignant neoplasm of renal pelvis (C65.-)

     C64.1 Malignant neoplasm of right kidney, except renal pelvis   HCC

     C64.2 Malignant neoplasm of left kidney, except renal pelvis   HCC

     C64.9 Malignant neoplasm of unspecified kidney, except renal pelvis   HCC ▽

✓4ᵗʰ C65 Malignant neoplasm of renal pelvis
     INCLUDES   malignant neoplasm of pelviureteric junction
         malignant neoplasm of renal calyces

     C65.1 Malignant neoplasm of right renal pelvis   HCC

     C65.2 Malignant neoplasm of left renal pelvis   HCC

     C65.9 Malignant neoplasm of unspecified renal pelvis   HCC ▽

✓4ᵗʰ C66 Malignant neoplasm of ureter
     EXCLUDES 1   *malignant neoplasm of ureteric orifice of bladder (C67.6)*

     C66.1 Malignant neoplasm of right ureter   HCC

     C66.2 Malignant neoplasm of left ureter   HCC

     C66.9 Malignant neoplasm of unspecified ureter   HCC ▽

✓4ᵗʰ C67 Malignant neoplasm of bladder

     C67.0 Malignant neoplasm of trigone of bladder   HCC

     C67.1 Malignant neoplasm of dome of bladder   HCC

     C67.2 Malignant neoplasm of lateral wall of bladder   HCC

     C67.3 Malignant neoplasm of anterior wall of bladder   HCC

     C67.4 Malignant neoplasm of posterior wall of bladder   HCC

     C67.5 Malignant neoplasm of bladder neck   HCC
         Malignant neoplasm of internal urethral orifice

     C67.6 Malignant neoplasm of ureteric orifice   HCC

     C67.7 Malignant neoplasm of urachus   HCC

     C67.8 Malignant neoplasm of overlapping sites of bladder   HCC

     C67.9 Malignant neoplasm of bladder, unspecified   HCC ▽
         AHA: 2016, 1Q, 19

✓4ᵗʰ C68 Malignant neoplasm of other and unspecified urinary organs
     EXCLUDES 1   *malignant neoplasm of female genitourinary tract NOS (C57.9)*
         malignant neoplasm of male genitourinary tract NOS (C63.9)

     C68.0 Malignant neoplasm of urethra
         EXCLUDES 1   *malignant neoplasm of urethral orifice of bladder (C67.5)*

     C68.1 Malignant neoplasm of paraurethral glands   HCC

     C68.8 Malignant neoplasm of overlapping sites of urinary organs   HCC
         Primary malignant neoplasm of two or more contiguous sites of urinary organs whose point of origin cannot be determined

     C68.9 Malignant neoplasm of urinary organ, unspecified   HCC ▽
         Malignant neoplasm of urinary system NOS

Malignant neoplasms of eye, brain and other parts of central nervous system (C69-C72)

✓4ᵗʰ C69 Malignant neoplasm of eye and adnexa
     EXCLUDES 1   *malignant neoplasm of connective tissue of eyelid (C49.0)*
         malignant neoplasm of eyelid (skin) (C43.1-, C44.1-)
         malignant neoplasm of optic nerve (C72.3-)

     ✓5ᵗʰ C69.0 Malignant neoplasm of conjunctiva

         C69.00 Malignant neoplasm of unspecified conjunctiva   HCC ▽

         C69.01 Malignant neoplasm of right conjunctiva   HCC

         C69.02 Malignant neoplasm of left conjunctiva   HCC

     ✓5ᵗʰ C69.1 Malignant neoplasm of cornea

         C69.10 Malignant neoplasm of unspecified cornea   HCC ▽

         C69.11 Malignant neoplasm of right cornea   HCC

         C69.12 Malignant neoplasm of left cornea   HCC

     ✓5ᵗʰ C69.2 Malignant neoplasm of retina
         EXCLUDES 1   *dark area on retina (D49.81)*
           neoplasm of unspecified behavior of retina and choroid (D49.81)
           retinal freckle (D49.81)

         C69.20 Malignant neoplasm of unspecified retina   HCC ▽

         C69.21 Malignant neoplasm of right retina   HCC

         C69.22 Malignant neoplasm of left retina   HCC

     ✓5ᵗʰ C69.3 Malignant neoplasm of choroid

         C69.30 Malignant neoplasm of unspecified choroid   HCC ▽

         C69.31 Malignant neoplasm of right choroid   HCC

         C69.32 Malignant neoplasm of left choroid   HCC

     ✓5ᵗʰ C69.4 Malignant neoplasm of ciliary body

         C69.40 Malignant neoplasm of unspecified ciliary body   HCC ▽

         C69.41 Malignant neoplasm of right ciliary body   HCC

         C69.42 Malignant neoplasm of left ciliary body   HCC

     ✓5ᵗʰ C69.5 Malignant neoplasm of lacrimal gland and duct
         Malignant neoplasm of lacrimal sac
         Malignant neoplasm of nasolacrimal duct

         C69.50 Malignant neoplasm of unspecified lacrimal gland and duct   HCC ▽

         C69.51 Malignant neoplasm of right lacrimal gland and duct   HCC

         C69.52 Malignant neoplasm of left lacrimal gland and duct   HCC

☑ Additional Character Req   ✓ˣ7ᵗʰ Placeholder Alert   Manifestation   HCC CMS-HCC Condition   ▽ Unspecified Code   ►◄ Revised Text   ● New Code   ▲ Revised Code Title

ICD-10-CM 2018   471

Chapter 2. Neoplasms

C69.6–C75.4

✓5th **C69.6 Malignant neoplasm of orbit**
Malignant neoplasm of connective tissue of orbit
Malignant neoplasm of extraocular muscle
Malignant neoplasm of peripheral nerves of orbit
Malignant neoplasm of retrobulbar tissue
Malignant neoplasm of retro-ocular tissue
EXCLUDES 1   *malignant neoplasm of orbital bone (C41.0)*

    C69.60 Malignant neoplasm of unspecified orbit HCC ▽
    C69.61 Malignant neoplasm of right orbit HCC
    C69.62 Malignant neoplasm of left orbit HCC

✓5th **C69.8 Malignant neoplasm of overlapping sites of eye and adnexa**

    C69.80 Malignant neoplasm of overlapping sites of unspecified eye and adnexa HCC ▽
    C69.81 Malignant neoplasm of overlapping sites of right eye and adnexa HCC
    C69.82 Malignant neoplasm of overlapping sites of left eye and adnexa HCC

✓5th **C69.9 Malignant neoplasm of unspecified site of eye**
Malignant neoplasm of eyeball

    C69.90 Malignant neoplasm of unspecified site of unspecified eye HCC ▽
    C69.91 Malignant neoplasm of unspecified site of right eye HCC ▽
    C69.92 Malignant neoplasm of unspecified site of left eye HCC ▽

✓4th **C70 Malignant neoplasm of meninges**
    C70.0 Malignant neoplasm of cerebral meninges HCC
    C70.1 Malignant neoplasm of spinal meninges HCC
    C70.9 Malignant neoplasm of meninges, unspecified HCC ▽

✓4th **C71 Malignant neoplasm of brain**
EXCLUDES 1   *malignant neoplasm of cranial nerves (C72.2-C72.5)*
retrobulbar malignant neoplasm (C69.6-)

    C71.0 Malignant neoplasm of cerebrum, except lobes and ventricles HCC
Malignant neoplasm of supratentorial NOS
    C71.1 Malignant neoplasm of frontal lobe HCC
    C71.2 Malignant neoplasm of temporal lobe HCC
    C71.3 Malignant neoplasm of parietal lobe HCC
    C71.4 Malignant neoplasm of occipital lobe HCC
    C71.5 Malignant neoplasm of cerebral ventricle HCC
        EXCLUDES 1   *malignant neoplasm of fourth cerebral ventricle (C71.7)*
    C71.6 Malignant neoplasm of cerebellum HCC
    C71.7 Malignant neoplasm of brain stem HCC
Malignant neoplasm of fourth cerebral ventricle
Infratentorial malignant neoplasm NOS
    C71.8 Malignant neoplasm of overlapping sites of brain HCC
    C71.9 Malignant neoplasm of brain, unspecified HCC ▽
    AHA: 2014, 3Q, 3

✓4th **C72 Malignant neoplasm of spinal cord, cranial nerves and other parts of central nervous system**
EXCLUDES 1   *malignant neoplasm of meninges (C70.-)*
malignant neoplasm of peripheral nerves and autonomic nervous system (C47.-)

    C72.0 Malignant neoplasm of spinal cord HCC
    C72.1 Malignant neoplasm of cauda equina HCC
✓5th **C72.2 Malignant neoplasm of olfactory nerve**
Malignant neoplasm of olfactory bulb
    C72.20 Malignant neoplasm of unspecified olfactory nerve HCC ▽
    C72.21 Malignant neoplasm of right olfactory nerve HCC
    C72.22 Malignant neoplasm of left olfactory nerve HCC
✓5th **C72.3 Malignant neoplasm of optic nerve**
    C72.30 Malignant neoplasm of unspecified optic nerve HCC ▽
    C72.31 Malignant neoplasm of right optic nerve HCC
    C72.32 Malignant neoplasm of left optic nerve HCC
✓5th **C72.4 Malignant neoplasm of acoustic nerve**
    C72.40 Malignant neoplasm of unspecified acoustic nerve HCC ▽
    C72.41 Malignant neoplasm of right acoustic nerve HCC
    C72.42 Malignant neoplasm of left acoustic nerve HCC

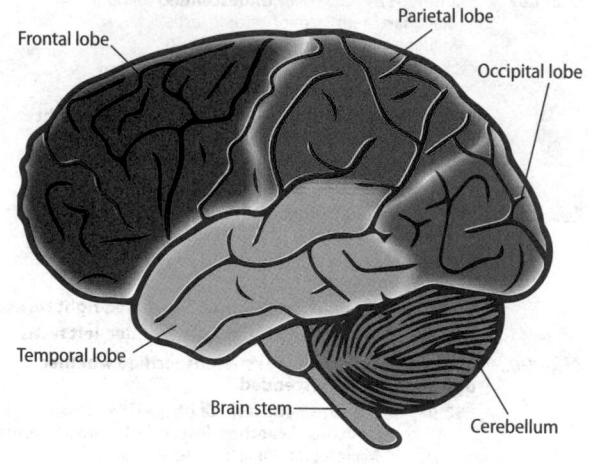

Lobes of the Brain

Frontal lobe — Parietal lobe — Occipital lobe — Temporal lobe — Brain stem — Cerebellum

✓5th **C72.5 Malignant neoplasm of other and unspecified cranial nerves**
    C72.50 Malignant neoplasm of unspecified cranial nerve HCC ▽
Malignant neoplasm of cranial nerve NOS
    C72.59 Malignant neoplasm of other cranial nerves HCC
    C72.9 Malignant neoplasm of central nervous system, unspecified HCC ▽
Malignant neoplasm of unspecified site of central nervous system
Malignant neoplasm of nervous system NOS

Malignant neoplasms of thyroid and other endocrine glands (C73-C75)

C73 Malignant neoplasm of thyroid gland HCC
Use additional code to identify any functional activity

✓4th **C74 Malignant neoplasm of adrenal gland**
✓5th **C74.0 Malignant neoplasm of cortex of adrenal gland**
    C74.00 Malignant neoplasm of cortex of unspecified adrenal gland HCC ▽
    C74.01 Malignant neoplasm of cortex of right adrenal gland HCC
    C74.02 Malignant neoplasm of cortex of left adrenal gland HCC
✓5th **C74.1 Malignant neoplasm of medulla of adrenal gland**
    C74.10 Malignant neoplasm of medulla of unspecified adrenal gland HCC ▽
    C74.11 Malignant neoplasm of medulla of right adrenal gland HCC
    C74.12 Malignant neoplasm of medulla of left adrenal gland HCC
✓5th **C74.9 Malignant neoplasm of unspecified part of adrenal gland**
    C74.90 Malignant neoplasm of unspecified part of unspecified adrenal gland HCC ▽
    C74.91 Malignant neoplasm of unspecified part of right adrenal gland HCC ▽
    C74.92 Malignant neoplasm of unspecified part of left adrenal gland HCC ▽

✓4th **C75 Malignant neoplasm of other endocrine glands and related structures**
EXCLUDES 1   *malignant carcinoid tumors (C7A.0-)*
malignant neoplasm of adrenal gland (C74.-)
malignant neoplasm of endocrine pancreas (C25.4)
malignant neoplasm of islets of Langerhans (C25.4)
malignant neoplasm of ovary (C56.-)
malignant neoplasm of testis (C62.-)
malignant neoplasm of thymus (C37)
malignant neoplasm of thyroid gland (C73)
malignant neuroendocrine tumors (C7A.-)

    C75.0 Malignant neoplasm of parathyroid gland HCC
    C75.1 Malignant neoplasm of pituitary gland HCC
    C75.2 Malignant neoplasm of craniopharyngeal duct HCC
    C75.3 Malignant neoplasm of pineal gland HCC
    C75.4 Malignant neoplasm of carotid body HCC

EXCLUDES 1 Not coded here   *EXCLUDES 2* Not included here   N Newborn Age: 0   P Pediatric Age: 0-17   M Maternity Age: 12-55   A Adult Age: 15-124

472   ICD-10-CM 2018

C75.5 Malignant neoplasm of **aortic body** and other **paraganglia**   HCC

C75.8 Malignant neoplasm with **pluriglandular involvement,** unspecified   HCC ▽

C75.9 Malignant neoplasm of endocrine gland, unspecified   HCC ▽

Malignant neuroendocrine tumors (C7A)

✓4ᵗʰ **C7A** Malignant **neuroendocrine tumors**

Code also any associated multiple endocrine neoplasia [MEN] syndromes (E31.2-)

Use additional code to identify any associated endocrine syndrome, such as:

carcinoid syndrome (E34.0)

EXCLUDES 2   malignant pancreatic islet cell tumors (C25.4)
Merkel cell carcinoma (C4A.-)

✓5ᵗʰ **C7A.0** Malignant **carcinoid tumors**

C7A.00 Malignant carcinoid tumor of unspecified site   HCC ▽

✓6ᵗʰ **C7A.01** Malignant carcinoid tumors of the **small intestine**

C7A.010 Malignant carcinoid tumor of the **duodenum**   HCC

C7A.011 Malignant carcinoid tumor of the **jejunum**   HCC

C7A.012 Malignant carcinoid tumor of the **ileum**   HCC

C7A.019 Malignant carcinoid tumor of the small intestine, unspecified portion   HCC ▽

✓6ᵗʰ **C7A.02** Malignant carcinoid tumors of the **appendix, large intestine, and rectum**

C7A.020 Malignant carcinoid tumor of the **appendix**   HCC

C7A.021 Malignant carcinoid tumor of the **cecum**   HCC

C7A.022 Malignant carcinoid tumor of the **ascending colon**   HCC

C7A.023 Malignant carcinoid tumor of the **transverse colon**   HCC

C7A.024 Malignant carcinoid tumor of the **descending colon**   HCC

C7A.025 Malignant carcinoid tumor of the **sigmoid colon**   HCC

C7A.026 Malignant carcinoid tumor of the **rectum**   HCC

C7A.029 Malignant carcinoid tumor of the large intestine, unspecified portion   HCC ▽
Malignant carcinoid tumor of the colon NOS

✓6ᵗʰ **C7A.09** Malignant carcinoid tumors of other sites

C7A.090 Malignant carcinoid tumor of the **bronchus and lung**   HCC

C7A.091 Malignant carcinoid tumor of the **thymus**   HCC

C7A.092 Malignant carcinoid tumor of the **stomach**   HCC

C7A.093 Malignant carcinoid tumor of the **kidney**   HCC

C7A.094 Malignant carcinoid tumor of the **foregut** unspecified   HCC ▽

C7A.095 Malignant carcinoid tumor of the **midgut** unspecified   HCC ▽

C7A.096 Malignant carcinoid tumor of the **hindgut** unspecified   HCC ▽

C7A.098 Malignant carcinoid tumors of other sites   HCC

C7A.1 Malignant **poorly differentiated** neuroendocrine tumors   HCC
High grade neuroendocrine carcinoma, any site
Malignant poorly differentiated neuroendocrine tumor NOS
Malignant poorly differentiated neuroendocrine carcinoma, any site

C7A.8 Other malignant neuroendocrine tumors   HCC

Secondary neuroendocrine tumors (C7B)

✓4ᵗʰ **C7B** Secondary neuroendocrine tumors
Use additional code to identify any functional activity

✓5ᵗʰ **C7B.0** Secondary **carcinoid tumors**

C7B.00 Secondary carcinoid tumors, unspecified site   HCC ▽

C7B.01 Secondary carcinoid tumors of **distant lymph nodes**   HCC

C7B.02 Secondary carcinoid tumors of **liver**   HCC

C7B.03 Secondary carcinoid tumors of **bone**   HCC

C7B.04 Secondary carcinoid tumors of **peritoneum**   HCC
Mesentery metastasis of carcinoid tumor

C7B.09 Secondary carcinoid tumors of other sites   HCC

C7B.1 Secondary **Merkel cell carcinoma**   HCC
Merkel cell carcinoma nodal presentation
Merkel cell carcinoma visceral metastatic presentation

C7B.8 Other secondary neuroendocrine tumors   HCC

Malignant neoplasms of ill-defined, other secondary and unspecified sites (C76-C80)

✓4ᵗʰ **C76** Malignant neoplasm of other and ill-defined sites

EXCLUDES 1   malignant neoplasm of female genitourinary tract NOS (C57.9)
malignant neoplasm of male genitourinary tract NOS (C63.9)
malignant neoplasm of lymphoid, hematopoietic and related tissue (C81-C96)
malignant neoplasm of skin (C44.-)
malignant neoplasm of unspecified site NOS (C80.1)

C76.0 Malignant neoplasm of **head, face and neck**   HCC
Malignant neoplasm of cheek NOS
Malignant neoplasm of nose NOS

C76.1 Malignant neoplasm of **thorax**   HCC
Intrathoracic malignant neoplasm NOS
Malignant neoplasm of axilla NOS
Thoracic malignant neoplasm NOS

C76.2 Malignant neoplasm of **abdomen**   HCC

C76.3 Malignant neoplasm of **pelvis**   HCC
Malignant neoplasm of groin NOS
Malignant neoplasm of sites overlapping systems within the pelvis
Rectovaginal (septum) malignant neoplasm
Rectovesical (septum) malignant neoplasm

✓5ᵗʰ **C76.4** Malignant neoplasm of **upper limb**

C76.40 Malignant neoplasm of unspecified upper limb   HCC ▽

C76.41 Malignant neoplasm of **right** upper limb   HCC

C76.42 Malignant neoplasm of **left** upper limb   HCC

✓5ᵗʰ **C76.5** Malignant neoplasm of **lower limb**

C76.50 Malignant neoplasm of unspecified lower limb   HCC ▽

C76.51 Malignant neoplasm of **right** lower limb   HCC

C76.52 Malignant neoplasm of **left** lower limb   HCC

C76.8 Malignant neoplasm of other **specified ill-defined sites**   HCC
Malignant neoplasm of overlapping ill-defined sites

✓4ᵗʰ **C77** Secondary and unspecified malignant neoplasm of **lymph nodes**

EXCLUDES 1   malignant neoplasm of lymph nodes, specified as primary (C81-C86, C88, C96.-)
mesentery metastasis of carcinoid tumor (C7B.04)
secondary carcinoid tumors of distant lymph nodes (C7B.01)

C77.0 Secondary and unspecified malignant neoplasm of lymph nodes of **head, face and neck**   HCC
Secondary and unspecified malignant neoplasm of supraclavicular lymph nodes

C77.1 Secondary and unspecified malignant neoplasm of **intrathoracic** lymph nodes   HCC

C77.2 Secondary and unspecified malignant neoplasm of **intra-abdominal** lymph nodes   HCC

C77.3 Secondary and unspecified malignant neoplasm of **axilla and upper limb** lymph nodes   HCC
Secondary and unspecified malignant neoplasm of pectoral lymph nodes

C77.4 Secondary and unspecified malignant neoplasm of **inguinal and lower limb** lymph nodes   HCC

C77.5 Secondary and unspecified malignant neoplasm of **intrapelvic** lymph nodes   HCC

C77.8 Secondary and unspecified malignant neoplasm of lymph nodes of **multiple regions**   HCC

C77.9 Secondary and unspecified malignant neoplasm of lymph node, unspecified   HCC ▽

☑ Additional Character Req   ✔7ᵗʰ Placeholder Alert   Manifestation   HCC CMS-HCC Condition   ▽ Unspecified Code   ►◄ Revised Text   ● New Code   ▲ Revised Code Title

✓4th C78 Secondary malignant neoplasm of respiratory and digestive organs

> EXCLUDES 1 secondary carcinoid tumors of liver (C7B.02)
> secondary carcinoid tumors of peritoneum (C7B.04)
> EXCLUDES 2 lymph node metastases (C77.0)

✓5th C78.0 Secondary malignant neoplasm of lung

- **C78.00 Secondary malignant neoplasm of unspecified lung** HCC ▽
- **C78.01 Secondary malignant neoplasm of right lung** HCC
- **C78.02 Secondary malignant neoplasm of left lung** HCC

C78.1 Secondary malignant neoplasm of mediastinum HCC

C78.2 Secondary malignant neoplasm of pleura HCC

✓5th C78.3 Secondary malignant neoplasm of other and unspecified respiratory organs

- **C78.30 Secondary malignant neoplasm of unspecified respiratory organ** HCC ▽
- **C78.39 Secondary malignant neoplasm of other respiratory organs** HCC

C78.4 Secondary malignant neoplasm of small intestine HCC

C78.5 Secondary malignant neoplasm of large intestine and rectum HCC

C78.6 Secondary malignant neoplasm of retroperitoneum and peritoneum HCC
> AHA: 2017, 2Q, 12

C78.7 Secondary malignant neoplasm of liver and intrahepatic bile duct HCC

✓5th C78.8 Secondary malignant neoplasm of other and unspecified digestive organs

- **C78.80 Secondary malignant neoplasm of unspecified digestive organ** HCC ▽
- **C78.89 Secondary malignant neoplasm of other digestive organs** HCC
  > Code also exocrine pancreatic insufficiency (K86.81)

✓4th C79 Secondary malignant neoplasm of other and unspecified sites

> EXCLUDES 1 secondary carcinoid tumors (C7B.-)
> secondary neuroendocrine tumors (C7B.-)
> EXCLUDES 2 ~~lymph node metastases (C77.0)~~

✓5th C79.0 Secondary malignant neoplasm of kidney and renal pelvis

- **C79.00 Secondary malignant neoplasm of unspecified kidney and renal pelvis** HCC ▽
- **C79.01 Secondary malignant neoplasm of right kidney and renal pelvis** HCC
- **C79.02 Secondary malignant neoplasm of left kidney and renal pelvis** HCC

✓5th C79.1 Secondary malignant neoplasm of bladder and other and unspecified urinary organs

- **C79.10 Secondary malignant neoplasm of unspecified urinary organs** HCC ▽
- **C79.11 Secondary malignant neoplasm of bladder** HCC
  > EXCLUDES 2 ►lymph node metastases (C77.0)◄
- **C79.19 Secondary malignant neoplasm of other urinary organs** HCC

C79.2 Secondary malignant neoplasm of skin HCC
> EXCLUDES 1 secondary Merkel cell carcinoma (C7B.1)

✓5th C79.3 Secondary malignant neoplasm of brain and cerebral meninges

- **C79.31 Secondary malignant neoplasm of brain** HCC
- **C79.32 Secondary malignant neoplasm of cerebral meninges** HCC

✓5th C79.4 Secondary malignant neoplasm of other and unspecified parts of nervous system

- **C79.40 Secondary malignant neoplasm of unspecified part of nervous system** HCC ▽
- **C79.49 Secondary malignant neoplasm of other parts of nervous system** HCC

✓5th C79.5 Secondary malignant neoplasm of bone and bone marrow

> EXCLUDES 1 secondary carcinoid tumors of bone (C7B.03)

- **C79.51 Secondary malignant neoplasm of bone** HCC
- **C79.52 Secondary malignant neoplasm of bone marrow** HCC

✓5th C79.6 Secondary malignant neoplasm of ovary

- **C79.60 Secondary malignant neoplasm of unspecified ovary** HCC ♀ ▽
- **C79.61 Secondary malignant neoplasm of right ovary** HCC ♀
- **C79.62 Secondary malignant neoplasm of left ovary** HCC ♀

✓5th C79.7 Secondary malignant neoplasm of adrenal gland

- **C79.70 Secondary malignant neoplasm of unspecified adrenal gland** HCC ▽
- **C79.71 Secondary malignant neoplasm of right adrenal gland** HCC
- **C79.72 Secondary malignant neoplasm of left adrenal gland** HCC

✓5th C79.8 Secondary malignant neoplasm of other specified sites

- **C79.81 Secondary malignant neoplasm of breast** HCC
- **C79.82 Secondary malignant neoplasm of genital organs** HCC
- **C79.89 Secondary malignant neoplasm of other specified sites**
  > AHA: 2017, 2Q, 11

C79.9 Secondary malignant neoplasm of unspecified site HCC ▽
> Metastatic cancer NOS
> Metastatic disease NOS
> EXCLUDES 1 carcinomatosis NOS (C80.0)
> generalized cancer NOS (C80.0)
> malignant (primary) neoplasm of unspecified site (C80.1)

✓4th C80 Malignant neoplasm without specification of site

> EXCLUDES 1 malignant carcinoid tumor of unspecified site (C7A.00)
> malignant neoplasm of specified multiple sites—code to each site

C80.0 Disseminated malignant neoplasm, unspecified HCC ▽
> Carcinomatosis NOS
> Generalized cancer, unspecified site (primary) (secondary)
> Generalized malignancy, unspecified site (primary) (secondary)

C80.1 Malignant (primary) neoplasm, unspecified HCC ▽
> Cancer NOS
> Cancer unspecified site (primary)
> Carcinoma unspecified site (primary)
> Malignancy unspecified site (primary)
> EXCLUDES 1 secondary malignant neoplasm of unspecified site (C79.9)

C80.2 Malignant neoplasm associated with transplanted organ HCC
> Code first complication of transplanted organ (T86.-)
> Use additional code to identify the specific malignancy

Malignant neoplasms of lymphoid, hematopoietic and related tissue (C81-C96)

> EXCLUDES 2 Kaposi's sarcoma of lymph nodes (C46.3)
> secondary and unspecified neoplasm of lymph nodes (C77.-)
> secondary neoplasm of bone marrow (C79.52)
> secondary neoplasm of spleen (C78.89)

✓4th C81 Hodgkin lymphoma

> EXCLUDES 1 personal history of Hodgkin lymphoma (Z85.71)

✓5th C81.0 Nodular lymphocyte predominant Hodgkin lymphoma

- **C81.00 Nodular lymphocyte predominant Hodgkin lymphoma, unspecified site** HCC ▽
- **C81.01 Nodular lymphocyte predominant Hodgkin lymphoma, lymph nodes of head, face, and neck** HCC
- **C81.02 Nodular lymphocyte predominant Hodgkin lymphoma, intrathoracic lymph nodes** HCC
- **C81.03 Nodular lymphocyte predominant Hodgkin lymphoma, intra-abdominal lymph nodes** HCC
- **C81.04 Nodular lymphocyte predominant Hodgkin lymphoma, lymph nodes of axilla and upper limb** HCC
- **C81.05 Nodular lymphocyte predominant Hodgkin lymphoma, lymph nodes of inguinal region and lower limb** HCC
- **C81.06 Nodular lymphocyte predominant Hodgkin lymphoma, intrapelvic lymph nodes** HCC
- **C81.07 Nodular lymphocyte predominant Hodgkin lymphoma, spleen** HCC
- **C81.08 Nodular lymphocyte predominant Hodgkin lymphoma, lymph nodes of multiple sites** HCC
- **C81.09 Nodular lymphocyte predominant Hodgkin lymphoma, extranodal and solid organ sites** HCC

✓5th C81.1 Nodular sclerosis Hodgkin lymphoma
> Nodular sclerosis classical Hodgkin lymphoma

- **C81.10 Nodular sclerosis Hodgkin lymphoma, unspecified site** HCC ▽
- **C81.11 Nodular sclerosis Hodgkin lymphoma, lymph nodes of head, face, and neck** HCC

EXCLUDES 1 Not coded here   EXCLUDES 2 Not included here   N Newborn Age: 0   P Pediatric Age: 0-17   M Maternity Age: 12-55   A Adult Age: 15-124

474   ICD-10-CM 2018

Chapter 2. Neoplasms

C81.12   **Nodular sclerosis Hodgkin lymphoma, intrathoracic** lymph nodes   `HCC`

C81.13   **Nodular sclerosis Hodgkin lymphoma, intra-abdominal** lymph nodes   `HCC`

C81.14   **Nodular sclerosis Hodgkin lymphoma, lymph nodes of axilla and upper limb**   `HCC`

C81.15   **Nodular sclerosis Hodgkin lymphoma, lymph nodes of inguinal region and lower limb**   `HCC`

C81.16   **Nodular sclerosis Hodgkin lymphoma, intrapelvic** lymph nodes   `HCC`

C81.17   **Nodular sclerosis Hodgkin lymphoma, spleen**   `HCC`

C81.18   **Nodular sclerosis Hodgkin lymphoma, lymph nodes of multiple sites**   `HCC`

C81.19   **Nodular sclerosis Hodgkin lymphoma, extranodal and solid organ sites**   `HCC`

✓5ᵗʰ **C81.2 Mixed cellularity Hodgkin lymphoma**
Mixed cellularity classical Hodgkin lymphoma

C81.20   **Mixed cellularity Hodgkin lymphoma, unspecified site**   `HCC` ▽

C81.21   **Mixed cellularity Hodgkin lymphoma, lymph nodes of head, face, and neck**   `HCC`

C81.22   **Mixed cellularity Hodgkin lymphoma, intrathoracic** lymph nodes   `HCC`

C81.23   **Mixed cellularity Hodgkin lymphoma, intra-abdominal** lymph nodes   `HCC`

C81.24   **Mixed cellularity Hodgkin lymphoma, lymph nodes of axilla and upper limb**   `HCC`

C81.25   **Mixed cellularity Hodgkin lymphoma, lymph nodes of inguinal region and lower limb**   `HCC`

C81.26   **Mixed cellularity Hodgkin lymphoma, intrapelvic** lymph nodes   `HCC`

C81.27   **Mixed cellularity Hodgkin lymphoma, spleen**   `HCC`

C81.28   **Mixed cellularity Hodgkin lymphoma, lymph nodes of multiple sites**   `HCC`

C81.29   **Mixed cellularity Hodgkin lymphoma, extranodal and solid organ sites**   `HCC`

✓5ᵗʰ **C81.3 Lymphocyte depleted Hodgkin lymphoma**
Lymphocyte depleted classical Hodgkin lymphoma

C81.30   **Lymphocyte depleted Hodgkin lymphoma, unspecified site**   `HCC` ▽

C81.31   **Lymphocyte depleted Hodgkin lymphoma, lymph nodes of head, face, and neck**   `HCC`

C81.32   **Lymphocyte depleted Hodgkin lymphoma, intrathoracic** lymph nodes   `HCC`

C81.33   **Lymphocyte depleted Hodgkin lymphoma, intra-abdominal** lymph nodes   `HCC`

C81.34   **Lymphocyte depleted Hodgkin lymphoma, lymph nodes of axilla and upper limb**   `HCC`

C81.35   **Lymphocyte depleted Hodgkin lymphoma, lymph nodes of inguinal region and lower limb**   `HCC`

C81.36   **Lymphocyte depleted Hodgkin lymphoma, intrapelvic** lymph nodes   `HCC`

C81.37   **Lymphocyte depleted Hodgkin lymphoma, spleen**   `HCC`

C81.38   **Lymphocyte depleted Hodgkin lymphoma, lymph nodes of multiple sites**   `HCC`

C81.39   **Lymphocyte depleted Hodgkin lymphoma, extranodal and solid organ sites**   `HCC`

✓5ᵗʰ **C81.4 Lymphocyte-rich Hodgkin lymphoma**
Lymphocyte-rich classical Hodgkin lymphoma
EXCLUDES 1   nodular lymphocyte predominant Hodgkin lymphoma (C81.0-)

C81.40   **Lymphocyte-rich Hodgkin lymphoma, unspecified site**   `HCC` ▽

C81.41   **Lymphocyte-rich Hodgkin lymphoma, lymph nodes of head, face, and neck**   `HCC`

C81.42   **Lymphocyte-rich Hodgkin lymphoma, intrathoracic** lymph nodes   `HCC`

C81.43   **Lymphocyte-rich Hodgkin lymphoma, intra-abdominal** lymph nodes   `HCC`

C81.44   **Lymphocyte-rich Hodgkin lymphoma, lymph nodes of axilla and upper limb**   `HCC`

C81.45   **Lymphocyte-rich Hodgkin lymphoma, lymph nodes of inguinal region and lower limb**   `HCC`

C81.46   **Lymphocyte-rich Hodgkin lymphoma, intrapelvic** lymph nodes   `HCC`

C81.47   **Lymphocyte-rich Hodgkin lymphoma, spleen**   `HCC`

C81.48   **Lymphocyte-rich Hodgkin lymphoma, lymph nodes of multiple sites**   `HCC`

C81.49   **Lymphocyte-rich Hodgkin lymphoma, extranodal and solid organ sites**   `HCC`

✓5ᵗʰ **C81.7 Other Hodgkin lymphoma**
Classical Hodgkin lymphoma NOS
Other classical Hodgkin lymphoma

C81.70   **Other Hodgkin lymphoma, unspecified site**   `HCC` ▽

C81.71   **Other Hodgkin lymphoma, lymph nodes of head, face, and neck**   `HCC`

C81.72   **Other Hodgkin lymphoma, intrathoracic lymph nodes**   `HCC`

C81.73   **Other Hodgkin lymphoma, intra-abdominal lymph nodes**   `HCC`

C81.74   **Other Hodgkin lymphoma, lymph nodes of axilla and upper limb**   `HCC`

C81.75   **Other Hodgkin lymphoma, lymph nodes of inguinal region and lower limb**   `HCC`

C81.76   **Other Hodgkin lymphoma, intrapelvic lymph nodes**   `HCC`

C81.77   **Other Hodgkin lymphoma, spleen**   `HCC`

C81.78   **Other Hodgkin lymphoma, lymph nodes of multiple sites**   `HCC`

C81.79   **Other Hodgkin lymphoma, extranodal and solid organ sites**   `HCC`

✓5ᵗʰ **C81.9 Hodgkin lymphoma, unspecified**

C81.90   **Hodgkin lymphoma, unspecified, unspecified site**   `HCC` ▽

C81.91   **Hodgkin lymphoma, unspecified, lymph nodes of head, face, and neck**   `HCC` ▽

C81.92   **Hodgkin lymphoma, unspecified, intrathoracic lymph nodes**   `HCC` ▽

C81.93   **Hodgkin lymphoma, unspecified, intra-abdominal lymph nodes**   `HCC` ▽

C81.94   **Hodgkin lymphoma, unspecified, lymph nodes of axilla and upper limb**   `HCC` ▽

C81.95   **Hodgkin lymphoma, unspecified, lymph nodes of inguinal region and lower limb**   `HCC` ▽

C81.96   **Hodgkin lymphoma, unspecified, intrapelvic lymph nodes**   `HCC` ▽

C81.97   **Hodgkin lymphoma, unspecified, spleen**   `HCC` ▽

C81.98   **Hodgkin lymphoma, unspecified, lymph nodes of multiple sites**   `HCC` ▽

C81.99   **Hodgkin lymphoma, unspecified, extranodal and solid organ sites**   `HCC` ▽

✓4ᵗʰ **C82 Follicular lymphoma**
INCLUDES   follicular lymphoma with or without diffuse areas
EXCLUDES 1   mature T/NK-cell lymphomas (C84.-)
      personal history of non-Hodgkin lymphoma (Z85.72)

✓5ᵗʰ **C82.0 Follicular lymphoma grade I**

C82.00   **Follicular lymphoma grade I, unspecified site**   `HCC` ▽

C82.01   **Follicular lymphoma grade I, lymph nodes of head, face, and neck**   `HCC`

C82.02   **Follicular lymphoma grade I, intrathoracic lymph nodes**   `HCC`

C82.03   **Follicular lymphoma grade I, intra-abdominal lymph nodes**   `HCC`

C82.04   **Follicular lymphoma grade I, lymph nodes of axilla and upper limb**   `HCC`

C82.05   **Follicular lymphoma grade I, lymph nodes of inguinal region and lower limb**   `HCC`

C82.06   **Follicular lymphoma grade I, intrapelvic lymph nodes**   `HCC`

C82.07   **Follicular lymphoma grade I, spleen**   `HCC`

C82.08   **Follicular lymphoma grade I, lymph nodes of multiple sites**   `HCC`

C82.09   **Follicular lymphoma grade I, extranodal and solid organ sites**   `HCC`

✓5ᵗʰ **C82.1 Follicular lymphoma grade II**

C82.10   **Follicular lymphoma grade II, unspecified site**   `HCC` ▽

C82.11   **Follicular lymphoma grade II, lymph nodes of head, face, and neck**   `HCC`

C82.12   **Follicular lymphoma grade II, intrathoracic lymph nodes**   `HCC`

C82.13   **Follicular lymphoma grade II, intra-abdominal lymph nodes**   `HCC`

☑ Additional Character Req   ✓7ᵗʰ Placeholder Alert   Manifestation   `HCC` CMS-HCC Condition   ▽ Unspecified Code   ►◄ Revised Text   ● New Code   ▲ Revised Code Title

ICD-10-CM 2018   475

C82.14 Follicular lymphoma grade II, lymph nodes of axilla and upper limb `HCC`

C82.15 Follicular lymphoma grade II, lymph nodes of inguinal region and lower limb `HCC`

C82.16 Follicular lymphoma grade II, intrapelvic lymph nodes `HCC`

C82.17 Follicular lymphoma grade II, spleen `HCC`

C82.18 Follicular lymphoma grade II, lymph nodes of multiple sites `HCC`

C82.19 Follicular lymphoma grade II, extranodal and solid organ sites `HCC`

✓5th **C82.2 Follicular lymphoma grade III, unspecified**

C82.20 Follicular lymphoma grade III, unspecified, unspecified site `HCC` ▽

C82.21 Follicular lymphoma grade III, unspecified, lymph nodes of head, face, and neck `HCC` ▽

C82.22 Follicular lymphoma grade III, unspecified, intrathoracic lymph nodes `HCC` ▽

C82.23 Follicular lymphoma grade III, unspecified, intra-abdominal lymph nodes `HCC` ▽

C82.24 Follicular lymphoma grade III, unspecified, lymph nodes of axilla and upper limb `HCC` ▽

C82.25 Follicular lymphoma grade III, unspecified, lymph nodes of inguinal region and lower limb `HCC` ▽

C82.26 Follicular lymphoma grade III, unspecified, intrapelvic lymph nodes `HCC` ▽

C82.27 Follicular lymphoma grade III, unspecified, spleen `HCC` ▽

C82.28 Follicular lymphoma grade III, unspecified, lymph nodes of multiple sites `HCC` ▽

C82.29 Follicular lymphoma grade III, unspecified, extranodal and solid organ sites `HCC` ▽

✓5th **C82.3 Follicular lymphoma grade IIIa**

C82.30 Follicular lymphoma grade IIIa, unspecified site `HCC` ▽

C82.31 Follicular lymphoma grade IIIa, lymph nodes of head, face, and neck `HCC`

C82.32 Follicular lymphoma grade IIIa, intrathoracic lymph nodes `HCC`

C82.33 Follicular lymphoma grade IIIa, intra-abdominal lymph nodes `HCC`

C82.34 Follicular lymphoma grade IIIa, lymph nodes of axilla and upper limb `HCC`

C82.35 Follicular lymphoma grade IIIa, lymph nodes of inguinal region and lower limb `HCC`

C82.36 Follicular lymphoma grade IIIa, intrapelvic lymph nodes `HCC`

C82.37 Follicular lymphoma grade IIIa, spleen `HCC`

C82.38 Follicular lymphoma grade IIIa, lymph nodes of multiple sites `HCC`

C82.39 Follicular lymphoma grade IIIa, extranodal and solid organ sites `HCC`

✓5th **C82.4 Follicular lymphoma grade IIIb**

C82.40 Follicular lymphoma grade IIIb, unspecified site `HCC` ▽

C82.41 Follicular lymphoma grade IIIb, lymph nodes of head, face, and neck `HCC`

C82.42 Follicular lymphoma grade IIIb, intrathoracic lymph nodes `HCC`

C82.43 Follicular lymphoma grade IIIb, intra-abdominal lymph nodes `HCC`

C82.44 Follicular lymphoma grade IIIb, lymph nodes of axilla and upper limb `HCC`

C82.45 Follicular lymphoma grade IIIb, lymph nodes of inguinal region and lower limb `HCC`

C82.46 Follicular lymphoma grade IIIb, intrapelvic lymph nodes `HCC`

C82.47 Follicular lymphoma grade IIIb, spleen `HCC`

C82.48 Follicular lymphoma grade IIIb, lymph nodes of multiple sites `HCC`

C82.49 Follicular lymphoma grade IIIb, extranodal and solid organ sites `HCC`

✓5th **C82.5 Diffuse follicle center lymphoma**

C82.50 Diffuse follicle center lymphoma, unspecified site `HCC` ▽

C82.51 Diffuse follicle center lymphoma, lymph nodes of head, face, and neck `HCC`

C82.52 Diffuse follicle center lymphoma, intrathoracic lymph nodes `HCC`

C82.53 Diffuse follicle center lymphoma, intra-abdominal lymph nodes `HCC`

C82.54 Diffuse follicle center lymphoma, lymph nodes of axilla and upper limb `HCC`

C82.55 Diffuse follicle center lymphoma, lymph nodes of inguinal region and lower limb `HCC`

C82.56 Diffuse follicle center lymphoma, intrapelvic lymph nodes `HCC`

C82.57 Diffuse follicle center lymphoma, spleen `HCC`

C82.58 Diffuse follicle center lymphoma, lymph nodes of multiple sites `HCC`

C82.59 Diffuse follicle center lymphoma, extranodal and solid organ sites `HCC`

✓5th **C82.6 Cutaneous follicle center lymphoma**

C82.60 Cutaneous follicle center lymphoma, unspecified site `HCC` ▽

C82.61 Cutaneous follicle center lymphoma, lymph nodes of head, face, and neck `HCC`

C82.62 Cutaneous follicle center lymphoma, intrathoracic lymph nodes `HCC`

C82.63 Cutaneous follicle center lymphoma, intra-abdominal lymph nodes `HCC`

C82.64 Cutaneous follicle center lymphoma, lymph nodes of axilla and upper limb `HCC`

C82.65 Cutaneous follicle center lymphoma, lymph nodes of inguinal region and lower limb `HCC`

C82.66 Cutaneous follicle center lymphoma, intrapelvic lymph nodes `HCC`

C82.67 Cutaneous follicle center lymphoma, spleen `HCC`

C82.68 Cutaneous follicle center lymphoma, lymph nodes of multiple sites `HCC`

C82.69 Cutaneous follicle center lymphoma, extranodal and solid organ sites `HCC`

✓5th **C82.8 Other types of follicular lymphoma**

C82.80 Other types of follicular lymphoma, unspecified site `HCC` ▽

C82.81 Other types of follicular lymphoma, lymph nodes of head, face, and neck `HCC`

C82.82 Other types of follicular lymphoma, intrathoracic lymph nodes `HCC`

C82.83 Other types of follicular lymphoma, intra-abdominal lymph nodes `HCC`

C82.84 Other types of follicular lymphoma, lymph nodes of axilla and upper limb `HCC`

C82.85 Other types of follicular lymphoma, lymph nodes of inguinal region and lower limb `HCC`

C82.86 Other types of follicular lymphoma, intrapelvic lymph nodes `HCC`

C82.87 Other types of follicular lymphoma, spleen `HCC`

C82.88 Other types of follicular lymphoma, lymph nodes of multiple sites `HCC`

C82.89 Other types of follicular lymphoma, extranodal and solid organ sites `HCC`

✓5th **C82.9 Follicular lymphoma, unspecified**

C82.90 Follicular lymphoma, unspecified, unspecified site `HCC` ▽

C82.91 Follicular lymphoma, unspecified, lymph nodes of head, face, and neck `HCC` ▽

C82.92 Follicular lymphoma, unspecified, intrathoracic lymph nodes `HCC` ▽

C82.93 Follicular lymphoma, unspecified, intra-abdominal lymph nodes `HCC` ▽

C82.94 Follicular lymphoma, unspecified, lymph nodes of axilla and upper limb `HCC` ▽

C82.95 Follicular lymphoma, unspecified, lymph nodes of inguinal region and lower limb `HCC` ▽

C82.96 Follicular lymphoma, unspecified, intrapelvic lymph nodes `HCC` ▽

C82.97 Follicular lymphoma, unspecified, spleen `HCC` ▽

EXCLUDES 1 Not coded here   *EXCLUDES 2* Not included here   N Newborn Age: 0   P Pediatric Age: 0-17   M Maternity Age: 12-55   A Adult Age: 15-124

476   ICD-10-CM 2018

C82.98   **Follicular lymphoma, unspecified, lymph nodes of multiple sites**   HCC ▽

C82.99   **Follicular lymphoma, unspecified, extranodal and solid organ sites**   HCC ▽

✓4th **C83**   **Non-follicular lymphoma**
> EXCLUDES 1   *personal history of non-Hodgkin lymphoma (Z85.72)*

✓5th   **C83.0**   **Small cell B-cell lymphoma**
> Lymphoplasmacytic lymphoma
> Nodal marginal zone lymphoma
> Non-leukemic variant of B-CLL
> Splenic marginal zone lymphoma
> EXCLUDES 1   *chronic lymphocytic leukemia (C91.1)*
>   *mature T/NK-cell lymphomas (C84.-)*
>   *Waldenström macroglobulinemia (C88.0)*

C83.00   **Small cell B-cell lymphoma, unspecified site**   HCC ▽

C83.01   **Small cell B-cell lymphoma, lymph nodes of head, face, and neck**   HCC

C83.02   **Small cell B-cell lymphoma, intrathoracic lymph nodes**   HCC

C83.03   **Small cell B-cell lymphoma, intra-abdominal lymph nodes**   HCC

C83.04   **Small cell B-cell lymphoma, lymph nodes of axilla and upper limb**   HCC

C83.05   **Small cell B-cell lymphoma, lymph nodes of inguinal region and lower limb**   HCC

C83.06   **Small cell B-cell lymphoma, intrapelvic lymph nodes**   HCC

C83.07   **Small cell B-cell lymphoma, spleen**   HCC

C83.08   **Small cell B-cell lymphoma, lymph nodes of multiple sites**   HCC

C83.09   **Small cell B-cell lymphoma, extranodal and solid organ sites**   HCC

✓5th   **C83.1**   **Mantle cell lymphoma**
> Centrocytic lymphoma
> Malignant lymphomatous polyposis
> **DEF:** Rare form of B-cell non-Hodgkin lymphoma named for the location of tumor cell production, the mantle zone of the lymph nodes.

C83.10   **Mantle cell lymphoma, unspecified site**   HCC ▽

C83.11   **Mantle cell lymphoma, lymph nodes of head, face, and neck**   HCC

C83.12   **Mantle cell lymphoma, intrathoracic lymph nodes**   HCC

C83.13   **Mantle cell lymphoma, intra-abdominal lymph nodes**   HCC

C83.14   **Mantle cell lymphoma, lymph nodes of axilla and upper limb**   HCC

C83.15   **Mantle cell lymphoma, lymph nodes of inguinal region and lower limb**   HCC

C83.16   **Mantle cell lymphoma, intrapelvic lymph nodes**   HCC

C83.17   **Mantle cell lymphoma, spleen**   HCC

C83.18   **Mantle cell lymphoma, lymph nodes of multiple sites**   HCC

C83.19   **Mantle cell lymphoma, extranodal and solid organ sites**   HCC

✓5th   **C83.3**   **Diffuse large B-cell lymphoma**
> Anaplastic diffuse large B-cell lymphoma
> CD30-positive diffuse large B-cell lymphoma
> Centroblastic diffuse large B-cell lymphoma
> Diffuse large B-cell lymphoma, subtype not specified
> Immunoblastic diffuse large B-cell lymphoma
> Plasmablastic diffuse large B-cell lymphoma
> T-cell rich diffuse large B-cell lymphoma
> EXCLUDES 1   *mature T/NK-cell lymphomas (C84.-)*
>   *mediastinal (thymic) large B-cell lymphoma (C85.2-)*

C83.30   **Diffuse large B-cell lymphoma, unspecified site**   HCC ▽

C83.31   **Diffuse large B-cell lymphoma, lymph nodes of head, face, and neck**   HCC

C83.32   **Diffuse large B-cell lymphoma, intrathoracic lymph nodes**   HCC

C83.33   **Diffuse large B-cell lymphoma, intra-abdominal lymph nodes**   HCC

C83.34   **Diffuse large B-cell lymphoma, lymph nodes of axilla and upper limb**   HCC

C83.35   **Diffuse large B-cell lymphoma, lymph nodes of inguinal region and lower limb**   HCC

C83.36   **Diffuse large B-cell lymphoma, intrapelvic lymph nodes**   HCC

C83.37   **Diffuse large B-cell lymphoma, spleen**   HCC

C83.38   **Diffuse large B-cell lymphoma, lymph nodes of multiple sites**   HCC

C83.39   **Diffuse large B-cell lymphoma, extranodal and solid organ sites**   HCC

✓5th   **C83.5**   **Lymphoblastic (diffuse) lymphoma**
> B-precursor lymphoma
> Lymphoblastic B-cell lymphoma
> Lymphoblastic lymphoma NOS
> Lymphoblastic T-cell lymphoma
> T-precursor lymphoma

C83.50   **Lymphoblastic (diffuse) lymphoma, unspecified site**   HCC ▽

C83.51   **Lymphoblastic (diffuse) lymphoma, lymph nodes of head, face, and neck**   HCC

C83.52   **Lymphoblastic (diffuse) lymphoma, intrathoracic lymph nodes**   HCC

C83.53   **Lymphoblastic (diffuse) lymphoma, intra-abdominal lymph nodes**   HCC

C83.54   **Lymphoblastic (diffuse) lymphoma, lymph nodes of axilla and upper limb**   HCC

C83.55   **Lymphoblastic (diffuse) lymphoma, lymph nodes of inguinal region and lower limb**   HCC

C83.56   **Lymphoblastic (diffuse) lymphoma, intrapelvic lymph nodes**   HCC

C83.57   **Lymphoblastic (diffuse) lymphoma, spleen**   HCC

C83.58   **Lymphoblastic (diffuse) lymphoma, lymph nodes of multiple sites**   HCC

C83.59   **Lymphoblastic (diffuse) lymphoma, extranodal and solid organ sites**   HCC

✓5th   **C83.7**   **Burkitt lymphoma**
> Atypical Burkitt lymphoma
> Burkitt-like lymphoma
> EXCLUDES 1   *mature B-cell leukemia Burkitt type (C91.A-)*
> **DEF:** Malignancy of the lymphatic system, most often seen as a large bone-deteriorating lesion within the jaw or as an abdominal mass. It is a form of non-Hodgkin's lymphoma and is recognized as the fastest growing human tumor.

C83.70   **Burkitt lymphoma, unspecified site**   HCC ▽

C83.71   **Burkitt lymphoma, lymph nodes of head, face, and neck**   HCC

C83.72   **Burkitt lymphoma, intrathoracic lymph nodes**   HCC

C83.73   **Burkitt lymphoma, intra-abdominal lymph nodes**   HCC

C83.74   **Burkitt lymphoma, lymph nodes of axilla and upper limb**   HCC

C83.75   **Burkitt lymphoma, lymph nodes of inguinal region and lower limb**   HCC

C83.76   **Burkitt lymphoma, intrapelvic lymph nodes**   HCC

C83.77   **Burkitt lymphoma, spleen**   HCC

C83.78   **Burkitt lymphoma, lymph nodes of multiple sites**   HCC

C83.79   **Burkitt lymphoma, extranodal and solid organ sites**   HCC

✓5th   **C83.8**   **Other non-follicular lymphoma**
> Intravascular large B-cell lymphoma
> Lymphoid granulomatosis
> Primary effusion B-cell lymphoma
> EXCLUDES 1   *mediastinal (thymic) large B-cell lymphoma (C85.2-)*
>   *T-cell rich B-cell lymphoma (C83.3-)*

C83.80   **Other non-follicular lymphoma, unspecified site**   HCC ▽

C83.81   **Other non-follicular lymphoma, lymph nodes of head, face, and neck**   HCC

C83.82   **Other non-follicular lymphoma, intrathoracic lymph nodes**   HCC

C83.83   **Other non-follicular lymphoma, intra-abdominal lymph nodes**   HCC

C83.84   **Other non-follicular lymphoma, lymph nodes of axilla and upper limb**   HCC

C83.85   **Other non-follicular lymphoma, lymph nodes of inguinal region and lower limb**   HCC

✓ Additional Character Req   ✓x7th Placeholder Alert   Manifestation   HCC CMS-HCC Condition   ▽ Unspecified Code   ►◄ Revised Text   ● New Code   ▲ Revised Code Title

C83.86 Other non-follicular lymphoma, intrapelvic lymph nodes `HCC`

C83.87 Other non-follicular lymphoma, spleen `HCC`

C83.88 Other non-follicular lymphoma, lymph nodes of multiple sites `HCC`

C83.89 Other non-follicular lymphoma, extranodal and solid organ sites `HCC`

☑5ᵗʰ **C83.9** Non-follicular (diffuse) lymphoma, unspecified

C83.90 Non-follicular (diffuse) lymphoma, unspecified, unspecified site `HCC` ▽

C83.91 Non-follicular (diffuse) lymphoma, unspecified, lymph nodes of head, face, and neck `HCC` ▽

C83.92 Non-follicular (diffuse) lymphoma, unspecified, intrathoracic lymph nodes `HCC` ▽

C83.93 Non-follicular (diffuse) lymphoma, unspecified, intra-abdominal lymph nodes `HCC` ▽

C83.94 Non-follicular (diffuse) lymphoma, unspecified, lymph nodes of axilla and upper limb `HCC` ▽

C83.95 Non-follicular (diffuse) lymphoma, unspecified, lymph nodes of inguinal region and lower limb `HCC` ▽

C83.96 Non-follicular (diffuse) lymphoma, unspecified, intrapelvic lymph nodes `HCC` ▽

C83.97 Non-follicular (diffuse) lymphoma, unspecified, spleen `HCC` ▽

C83.98 Non-follicular (diffuse) lymphoma, unspecified, lymph nodes of multiple sites `HCC` ▽

C83.99 Non-follicular (diffuse) lymphoma, unspecified, extranodal and solid organ sites `HCC` ▽

☑4ᵗʰ **C84 Mature T/NK-cell lymphomas**

EXCLUDES 1 personal history of non-Hodgkin lymphoma (Z85.72)

☑5ᵗʰ **C84.0** Mycosis fungoides

EXCLUDES 1 peripheral T-cell lymphoma, not classified (C84.4-)

DEF: Most common form of cutaneous T-cell lymphoma, also known as Alibert-Bazin syndrome. A type of non-Hodgkin lymphoma in which white blood cells become cancerous and affect the skin and sometimes internal organs.

C84.00 Mycosis fungoides, unspecified site `HCC` ▽

C84.01 Mycosis fungoides, lymph nodes of head, face, and neck `HCC`

C84.02 Mycosis fungoides, intrathoracic lymph nodes `HCC`

C84.03 Mycosis fungoides, intra-abdominal lymph nodes `HCC`

C84.04 Mycosis fungoides, lymph nodes of axilla and upper limb `HCC`

C84.05 Mycosis fungoides, lymph nodes of inguinal region and lower limb `HCC`

C84.06 Mycosis fungoides, intrapelvic lymph nodes `HCC`

C84.07 Mycosis fungoides, spleen `HCC`

C84.08 Mycosis fungoides, lymph nodes of multiple sites `HCC`

C84.09 Mycosis fungoides, extranodal and solid organ sites `HCC`

☑5ᵗʰ **C84.1** Sézary disease

C84.10 Sézary disease, unspecified site `HCC` ▽

C84.11 Sézary disease, lymph nodes of head, face, and neck `HCC`

C84.12 Sézary disease, intrathoracic lymph nodes `HCC`

C84.13 Sézary disease, intra-abdominal lymph nodes `HCC`

C84.14 Sézary disease, lymph nodes of axilla and upper limb `HCC`

C84.15 Sézary disease, lymph nodes of inguinal region and lower limb `HCC`

C84.16 Sézary disease, intrapelvic lymph nodes `HCC`

C84.17 Sézary disease, spleen `HCC`

C84.18 Sézary disease, lymph nodes of multiple sites `HCC`

C84.19 Sézary disease, extranodal and solid organ sites `HCC`

☑5ᵗʰ **C84.4** Peripheral T-cell lymphoma, not classified

Lennert's lymphoma
Lymphoepithelioid lymphoma
Mature T-cell lymphoma, not elsewhere classified

C84.40 Peripheral T-cell lymphoma, not classified, unspecified site `HCC` ▽

C84.41 Peripheral T-cell lymphoma, not classified, lymph nodes of head, face, and neck `HCC`

C84.42 Peripheral T-cell lymphoma, not classified, intrathoracic lymph nodes `HCC`

C84.43 Peripheral T-cell lymphoma, not classified, intra-abdominal lymph nodes `HCC`

C84.44 Peripheral T-cell lymphoma, not classified, lymph nodes of axilla and upper limb `HCC`

C84.45 Peripheral T-cell lymphoma, not classified, lymph nodes of inguinal region and lower limb `HCC`

C84.46 Peripheral T-cell lymphoma, not classified, intrapelvic lymph nodes `HCC`

C84.47 Peripheral T-cell lymphoma, not classified, spleen `HCC`

C84.48 Peripheral T-cell lymphoma, not classified, lymph nodes of multiple sites `HCC`

C84.49 Peripheral T-cell lymphoma, not classified, extranodal and solid organ sites `HCC`

☑5ᵗʰ **C84.6** Anaplastic large cell lymphoma, ALK-positive

Anaplastic large cell lymphoma, CD30-positive

C84.60 Anaplastic large cell lymphoma, ALK-positive, unspecified site `HCC` ▽

C84.61 Anaplastic large cell lymphoma, ALK-positive, lymph nodes of head, face, and neck `HCC`

C84.62 Anaplastic large cell lymphoma, ALK-positive, intrathoracic lymph nodes `HCC`

C84.63 Anaplastic large cell lymphoma, ALK-positive, intra-abdominal lymph nodes `HCC`

C84.64 Anaplastic large cell lymphoma, ALK-positive, lymph nodes of axilla and upper limb `HCC`

C84.65 Anaplastic large cell lymphoma, ALK-positive, lymph nodes of inguinal region and lower limb `HCC`

C84.66 Anaplastic large cell lymphoma, ALK-positive, intrapelvic lymph nodes `HCC`

C84.67 Anaplastic large cell lymphoma, ALK-positive, spleen `HCC`

C84.68 Anaplastic large cell lymphoma, ALK-positive, lymph nodes of multiple sites `HCC`

C84.69 Anaplastic large cell lymphoma, ALK-positive, extranodal and solid organ sites `HCC`

☑5ᵗʰ **C84.7** Anaplastic large cell lymphoma, ALK-negative

EXCLUDES 1 primary cutaneous CD30-positive T-cell proliferations (C86.6-)

C84.70 Anaplastic large cell lymphoma, ALK-negative, unspecified site `HCC` ▽

C84.71 Anaplastic large cell lymphoma, ALK-negative, lymph nodes of head, face, and neck `HCC`

C84.72 Anaplastic large cell lymphoma, ALK-negative, intrathoracic lymph nodes `HCC`

C84.73 Anaplastic large cell lymphoma, ALK-negative, intra-abdominal lymph nodes `HCC`

C84.74 Anaplastic large cell lymphoma, ALK-negative, lymph nodes of axilla and upper limb `HCC`

C84.75 Anaplastic large cell lymphoma, ALK-negative, lymph nodes of inguinal region and lower limb `HCC`

C84.76 Anaplastic large cell lymphoma, ALK-negative, intrapelvic lymph nodes `HCC`

C84.77 Anaplastic large cell lymphoma, ALK-negative, spleen `HCC`

C84.78 Anaplastic large cell lymphoma, ALK-negative, lymph nodes of multiple sites `HCC`

C84.79 Anaplastic large cell lymphoma, ALK-negative, extranodal and solid organ sites `HCC`

☑5ᵗʰ **C84.A** Cutaneous T-cell lymphoma, unspecified

C84.A0 Cutaneous T-cell lymphoma, unspecified, unspecified site `HCC` ▽

C84.A1 Cutaneous T-cell lymphoma, unspecified, lymph nodes of head, face, and neck `HCC` ▽

C84.A2 Cutaneous T-cell lymphoma, unspecified, intrathoracic lymph nodes `HCC` ▽

C84.A3 Cutaneous T-cell lymphoma, unspecified, intra-abdominal lymph nodes `HCC` ▽

C84.A4 Cutaneous T-cell lymphoma, unspecified, lymph nodes of axilla and upper limb `HCC` ▽

C84.A5 Cutaneous T-cell lymphoma, unspecified, lymph nodes of inguinal region and lower limb `HCC` ▽

C84.A6 Cutaneous T-cell lymphoma, unspecified, intrapelvic lymph nodes `HCC` ▽

EXCLUDES 1 Not coded here   EXCLUDES 2 Not included here   N Newborn Age: 0   P Pediatric Age: 0-17   M Maternity Age: 12-55   A Adult Age: 15-124

478   ICD-10-CM 2018

C84.A7   **Cutaneous T-cell lymphoma, unspecified, spleen**   HCC ▽

C84.A8   **Cutaneous T-cell lymphoma, unspecified, lymph nodes of multiple sites**   HCC ▽

C84.A9   **Cutaneous T-cell lymphoma, unspecified, extranodal and solid organ sites**   HCC ▽

✓5ᵗʰ **C84.Z**   **Other mature T/NK-cell lymphomas**

> NOTE   If T-cell lineage or involvement is mentioned in conjunction with a specific lymphoma, code to the more specific description.
>
> EXCLUDES 1   *angioimmunoblastic T-cell lymphoma (C86.5)*
> *blastic NK-cell lymphoma (C86.4)*
> *enteropathy-type T-cell lymphoma (C86.2)*
> *extranodal NK-cell lymphoma, nasal type (C86.0)*
> *hepatosplenic T-cell lymphoma (C86.1)*
> *primary cutaneous CD30-positive T-cell proliferations (C86.6)*
> *subcutaneous panniculitis-like T-cell lymphoma (C86.3)*
> *T-cell leukemia (C91.1-)*

C84.Z0   **Other mature T/NK-cell lymphomas, unspecified site**   HCC ▽

C84.Z1   **Other mature T/NK-cell lymphomas, lymph nodes of head, face, and neck**   HCC

C84.Z2   **Other mature T/NK-cell lymphomas, intrathoracic lymph nodes**   HCC

C84.Z3   **Other mature T/NK-cell lymphomas, intra-abdominal lymph nodes**   HCC

C84.Z4   **Other mature T/NK-cell lymphomas, lymph nodes of axilla and upper limb**   HCC

C84.Z5   **Other mature T/NK-cell lymphomas, lymph nodes of inguinal region and lower limb**   HCC

C84.Z6   **Other mature T/NK-cell lymphomas, intrapelvic lymph nodes**   HCC

C84.Z7   **Other mature T/NK-cell lymphomas, spleen**   HCC

C84.Z8   **Other mature T/NK-cell lymphomas, lymph nodes of multiple sites**   HCC

C84.Z9   **Other mature T/NK-cell lymphomas, extranodal and solid organ sites**   HCC

✓5ᵗʰ **C84.9**   **Mature T/NK-cell lymphomas, unspecified**

NK/T cell lymphoma NOS

> EXCLUDES 1   *mature T-cell lymphoma, not elsewhere classified (C84.4-)*

C84.90   **Mature T/NK-cell lymphomas, unspecified, unspecified site**   HCC ▽

C84.91   **Mature T/NK-cell lymphomas, unspecified, lymph nodes of head, face, and neck**   HCC ▽

C84.92   **Mature T/NK-cell lymphomas, unspecified, intrathoracic lymph nodes**   HCC ▽

C84.93   **Mature T/NK-cell lymphomas, unspecified, intra-abdominal lymph nodes**   HCC ▽

C84.94   **Mature T/NK-cell lymphomas, unspecified, lymph nodes of axilla and upper limb**   HCC ▽

C84.95   **Mature T/NK-cell lymphomas, unspecified, lymph nodes of inguinal region and lower limb**   HCC ▽

C84.96   **Mature T/NK-cell lymphomas, unspecified, intrapelvic lymph nodes**   HCC ▽

C84.97   **Mature T/NK-cell lymphomas, unspecified, spleen**   HCC ▽

C84.98   **Mature T/NK-cell lymphomas, unspecified, lymph nodes of multiple sites**   HCC ▽

C84.99   **Mature T/NK-cell lymphomas, unspecified, extranodal and solid organ sites**   HCC ▽

✓4ᵗʰ **C85**   **Other specified and unspecified types of non-Hodgkin lymphoma**

> EXCLUDES 1   *other specified types of T/NK-cell lymphoma (C86.-)*
> *personal history of non-Hodgkin lymphoma (Z85.72)*

✓5ᵗʰ **C85.1**   **Unspecified B-cell lymphoma**

> NOTE   If B-cell lineage or involvement is mentioned in conjunction with a specific lymphoma, code to the more specific description.

C85.10   **Unspecified B-cell lymphoma, unspecified site**   HCC ▽

C85.11   **Unspecified B-cell lymphoma, lymph nodes of head, face, and neck**   HCC ▽

C85.12   **Unspecified B-cell lymphoma, intrathoracic lymph nodes**   HCC ▽

C85.13   **Unspecified B-cell lymphoma, intra-abdominal lymph nodes**   HCC ▽

C85.14   **Unspecified B-cell lymphoma, lymph nodes of axilla and upper limb**   HCC ▽

C85.15   **Unspecified B-cell lymphoma, lymph nodes of inguinal region and lower limb**   HCC ▽

C85.16   **Unspecified B-cell lymphoma, intrapelvic lymph nodes**   HCC ▽

C85.17   **Unspecified B-cell lymphoma, spleen**   HCC ▽

C85.18   **Unspecified B-cell lymphoma, lymph nodes of multiple sites**   HCC ▽

C85.19   **Unspecified B-cell lymphoma, extranodal and solid organ sites**   HCC ▽

✓5ᵗʰ **C85.2**   **Mediastinal (thymic) large B-cell lymphoma**

C85.20   **Mediastinal (thymic) large B-cell lymphoma, unspecified site**   HCC ▽

C85.21   **Mediastinal (thymic) large B-cell lymphoma, lymph nodes of head, face, and neck**   HCC

C85.22   **Mediastinal (thymic) large B-cell lymphoma, intrathoracic lymph nodes**   HCC

C85.23   **Mediastinal (thymic) large B-cell lymphoma, intra-abdominal lymph nodes**   HCC

C85.24   **Mediastinal (thymic) large B-cell lymphoma, lymph nodes of axilla and upper limb**   HCC

C85.25   **Mediastinal (thymic) large B-cell lymphoma, lymph nodes of inguinal region and lower limb**   HCC

C85.26   **Mediastinal (thymic) large B-cell lymphoma, intrapelvic lymph nodes**   HCC

C85.27   **Mediastinal (thymic) large B-cell lymphoma, spleen**   HCC

C85.28   **Mediastinal (thymic) large B-cell lymphoma, lymph nodes of multiple sites**   HCC

C85.29   **Mediastinal (thymic) large B-cell lymphoma, extranodal and solid organ sites**   HCC

✓5ᵗʰ **C85.8**   **Other specified types of non-Hodgkin lymphoma**

C85.80   **Other specified types of non-Hodgkin lymphoma, unspecified site**   HCC ▽

C85.81   **Other specified types of non-Hodgkin lymphoma, lymph nodes of head, face, and neck**   HCC

C85.82   **Other specified types of non-Hodgkin lymphoma, intrathoracic lymph nodes**   HCC

C85.83   **Other specified types of non-Hodgkin lymphoma, intra-abdominal lymph nodes**   HCC

C85.84   **Other specified types of non-Hodgkin lymphoma, lymph nodes of axilla and upper limb**   HCC

C85.85   **Other specified types of non-Hodgkin lymphoma, lymph nodes of inguinal region and lower limb**   HCC

C85.86   **Other specified types of non-Hodgkin lymphoma, intrapelvic lymph nodes**   HCC

C85.87   **Other specified types of non-Hodgkin lymphoma, spleen**   HCC

C85.88   **Other specified types of non-Hodgkin lymphoma, lymph nodes of multiple sites**   HCC

C85.89   **Other specified types of non-Hodgkin lymphoma, extranodal and solid organ sites**   HCC

✓5ᵗʰ **C85.9**   **Non-Hodgkin lymphoma, unspecified**

Lymphoma NOS
Malignant lymphoma NOS
Non-Hodgkin lymphoma NOS

C85.90   **Non-Hodgkin lymphoma, unspecified, unspecified site**   HCC ▽

C85.91   **Non-Hodgkin lymphoma, unspecified, lymph nodes of head, face, and neck**   HCC ▽

C85.92   **Non-Hodgkin lymphoma, unspecified, intrathoracic lymph nodes**   HCC ▽

C85.93   **Non-Hodgkin lymphoma, unspecified, intra-abdominal lymph nodes**   HCC ▽

C85.94   **Non-Hodgkin lymphoma, unspecified, lymph nodes of axilla and upper limb**   HCC ▽

C85.95   **Non-Hodgkin lymphoma, unspecified, lymph nodes of inguinal region and lower limb**   HCC ▽

C85.96   **Non-Hodgkin lymphoma, unspecified, intrapelvic lymph nodes**   HCC ▽

C85.97   **Non-Hodgkin lymphoma, unspecified, spleen**   HCC ▽

C85.98   **Non-Hodgkin lymphoma, unspecified, lymph nodes of multiple sites**   HCC ▽

C85.99   **Non-Hodgkin lymphoma, unspecified, extranodal and solid organ sites**   HCC ▽

☑ Additional Character Req   ✓ⁿ Placeholder Alert   Manifestation   HCC CMS-HCC Condition   ▽ Unspecified Code   ►◄ Revised Text   ● New Code   ▲ Revised Code Title

ICD-10-CM 2018   479

✓4th **C86 Other specified types of T/NK-cell lymphoma**
> EXCLUDES 1   *anaplastic large cell lymphoma, ALK negative (C84.7-)*
> *anaplastic large cell lymphoma, ALK positive (C84.6-)*
> *mature T/NK-cell lymphomas (C84.-)*
> *other specified types of non-Hodgkin lymphoma (C85.8-)*

C86.0 Extranodal NK/T-cell lymphoma, nasal type   HCC

C86.1 Hepatosplenic T-cell lymphoma   HCC
Alpha-beta and gamma delta types

C86.2 Enteropathy-type (intestinal) T-cell lymphoma   HCC
Enteropathy associated T-cell lymphoma

C86.3 Subcutaneous panniculitis-like T-cell lymphoma   HCC

C86.4 Blastic NK-cell lymphoma   HCC
▶Blastic plasmacytoid dendritic cell neoplasm (BPDCN)◀

C86.5 Angioimmunoblastic T-cell lymphoma   HCC
Angioimmunoblastic lymphadenopathy with dysproteinemia [AILD]

C86.6 Primary cutaneous CD30-positive T-cell proliferations   HCC
Lymphomatoid papulosis
Primary cutaneous anaplastic large cell lymphoma
Primary cutaneous CD30-positive large T-cell lymphoma

✓4th **C88 Malignant immunoproliferative diseases and certain other B-cell lymphomas**
> EXCLUDES 1   *B-cell lymphoma, unspecified (C85.1-)*
> *personal history of other malignant neoplasms of lymphoid, hematopoietic and related tissues (Z85.79)*

C88.0 Waldenström macroglobulinemia   HCC
Lymphoplasmacytic lymphoma with IgM-production
Macroglobulinemia (idiopathic) (primary)
> EXCLUDES 1   *small cell B-cell lymphoma (C83.0)*

C88.2 Heavy chain disease   HCC
Franklin disease
Gamma heavy chain disease
Mu heavy chain disease

C88.3 Immunoproliferative small intestinal disease   HCC
Alpha heavy chain disease
Mediterranean lymphoma

C88.4 Extranodal marginal zone B-cell lymphoma of mucosa-associated lymphoid tissue [MALT-lymphoma]   HCC
Lymphoma of skin-associated lymphoid tissue [SALT-lymphoma]
Lymphoma of bronchial-associated lymphoid tissue [BALT-lymphoma]
> EXCLUDES 1   *high malignant (diffuse large B-cell) lymphoma (C83.3-)*

C88.8 Other malignant immunoproliferative diseases   HCC

C88.9 Malignant immunoproliferative disease, unspecified   HCC ▽
Immunoproliferative disease NOS

✓4th **C90 Multiple myeloma and malignant plasma cell neoplasms**
> EXCLUDES 1   *personal history of other malignant neoplasms of lymphoid, hematopoietic and related tissues (Z85.79)*

✓5th **C90.0 Multiple myeloma**
Kahler's disease   Myelomatosis
Medullary plasmacytoma   Plasma cell myeloma
> EXCLUDES 1   *solitary myeloma (C90.3-)*
> *solitary plasmactyoma (C90.3-)*

C90.00 Multiple myeloma not having achieved remission   HCC
Multiple myeloma with failed remission
Multiple myeloma NOS

C90.01 Multiple myeloma in remission   HCC

C90.02 Multiple myeloma in relapse   HCC

✓5th **C90.1 Plasma cell leukemia**
Plasmacytic leukemia

C90.10 Plasma cell leukemia not having achieved remission   HCC
Plasma cell leukemia with failed remission
Plasma cell leukemia NOS

C90.11 Plasma cell leukemia in remission   HCC

C90.12 Plasma cell leukemia in relapse   HCC

✓5th **C90.2 Extramedullary plasmacytoma**

C90.20 Extramedullary plasmacytoma not having achieved remission   HCC
Extramedullary plasmacytoma with failed remission
Extramedullary plasmacytoma NOS

C90.21 Extramedullary plasmacytoma in remission   HCC

C90.22 Extramedullary plasmacytoma in relapse   HCC

✓5th **C90.3 Solitary plasmacytoma**
Localized malignant plasma cell tumor NOS
Plasmacytoma NOS
Solitary myeloma

C90.30 Solitary plasmacytoma not having achieved remission   HCC
Solitary plasmacytoma with failed remission
Solitary plasmacytoma NOS

C90.31 Solitary plasmacytoma in remission   HCC

C90.32 Solitary plasmacytoma in relapse   HCC

✓4th **C91 Lymphoid leukemia**
> EXCLUDES 1   *personal history of leukemia (Z85.6)*

✓5th **C91.0 Acute lymphoblastic leukemia [ALL]**
> NOTE   Code C91.0 should only be used for T-cell and B-cell precursor leukemia.

C91.00 Acute lymphoblastic leukemia not having achieved remission
Acute lymphoblastic leukemia with failed remission
Acute lymphoblastic leukemia NOS

C91.01 Acute lymphoblastic leukemia, in remission   HCC

C91.02 Acute lymphoblastic leukemia, in relapse   HCC

✓5th **C91.1 Chronic lymphocytic leukemia of B-cell type**
Lymphoplasmacytic leukemia
Richter syndrome
> EXCLUDES 1   *lymphoplasmacytic lymphoma (C83.0-)*

C91.10 Chronic lymphocytic leukemia of B-cell type not having achieved remission   HCC
Chronic lymphocytic leukemia of B-cell type with failed remission
Chronic lymphocytic leukemia of B-cell type NOS

C91.11 Chronic lymphocytic leukemia of B-cell type in remission   HCC

C91.12 Chronic lymphocytic leukemia of B-cell type in relapse   HCC

✓5th **C91.3 Prolymphocytic leukemia of B-cell type**

C91.30 Prolymphocytic leukemia of B-cell type not having achieved remission   HCC
Prolymphocytic leukemia of B-cell type with failed remission
Prolymphocytic leukemia of B-cell type NOS

C91.31 Prolymphocytic leukemia of B-cell type, in remission   HCC

C91.32 Prolymphocytic leukemia of B-cell type, in relapse   HCC

✓5th **C91.4 Hairy cell leukemia**
Leukemic reticuloendotheliosis

C91.40 Hairy cell leukemia not having achieved remission   HCC
Hairy cell leukemia with failed remission
Hairy cell leukemia NOS

C91.41 Hairy cell leukemia, in remission   HCC

C91.42 Hairy cell leukemia, in relapse   HCC

✓5th **C91.5 Adult T-cell lymphoma/leukemia (HTLV-1-associated)**
Acute variant of adult T-cell lymphoma/leukemia (HTLV-1-associated)
Chronic variant of adult T-cell lymphoma/leukemia (HTLV-1-associated)
Lymphomatoid variant of adult T-cell lymphoma/leukemia (HTLV-1-associated)
Smouldering variant of adult T-cell lymphoma/leukemia (HTLV-1-associated)

C91.50 Adult T-cell lymphoma/leukemia (HTLV-1-associated) not having achieved remission   HCC A
Adult T-cell lymphoma/leukemia (HTLV-1-associated) with failed remission
Adult T-cell lymphoma/leukemia (HTLV-1-associated) NOS

C91.51 Adult T-cell lymphoma/leukemia (HTLV-1-associated), in remission   HCC A

C91.52 Adult T-cell lymphoma/leukemia (HTLV-1-associated), in relapse   HCC A

✓5th **C91.6 Prolymphocytic leukemia of T-cell type**

C91.60 Prolymphocytic leukemia of T-cell type not having achieved remission   HCC
Prolymphocytic leukemia of T-cell type with failed remission
Prolymphocytic leukemia of T-cell type NOS

C91.61   Prolymphocytic leukemia of T-cell type, in remission   HCC

C91.62   Prolymphocytic leukemia of T-cell type, in relapse   HCC

✓5th **C91.A**   **Mature B-cell leukemia Burkitt-type**
     EXCLUDES 1   *Burkitt lymphoma (C83.7-)*

     C91.A0   **Mature B-cell leukemia Burkitt-type not having achieved remission**   HCC
        Mature B-cell leukemia Burkitt-type with failed remission
        Mature B-cell leukemia Burkitt-type NOS

     C91.A1   **Mature B-cell leukemia Burkitt-type, in remission**   HCC

     C91.A2   **Mature B-cell leukemia Burkitt-type, in relapse**   HCC

✓5th **C91.Z**   **Other lymphoid leukemia**
     T-cell large granular lymphocytic leukemia (associated with rheumatoid arthritis)

     C91.Z0   **Other lymphoid leukemia not having achieved remission**   HCC
        Other lymphoid leukemia with failed remission
        Other lymphoid leukemia NOS

     C91.Z1   **Other lymphoid leukemia, in remission**   HCC

     C91.Z2   **Other lymphoid leukemia, in relapse**   HCC

✓5th **C91.9**   **Lymphoid leukemia, unspecified**

     C91.90   **Lymphoid leukemia, unspecified not having achieved remission**   HCC ▽
        Lymphoid leukemia with failed remission
        Lymphoid leukemia NOS

     C91.91   **Lymphoid leukemia, unspecified, in remission**   HCC ▽

     C91.92   **Lymphoid leukemia, unspecified, in relapse**   HCC ▽

✓4th **C92**   **Myeloid leukemia**
     INCLUDES   granulocytic leukemia
                myelogenous leukemia
     EXCLUDES 1   *personal history of leukemia (Z85.6)*

✓5th **C92.0**   **Acute myeloblastic leukemia**
     Acute myeloblastic leukemia, minimal differentiation
     Acute myeloblastic leukemia (with maturation)
     Acute myeloblastic leukemia 1/ETO
     Acute myeloblastic leukemia M0
     Acute myeloblastic leukemia M1
     Acute myeloblastic leukemia M2
     Acute myeloblastic leukemia with t(8;21)
     Acute myeloblastic leukemia (without a FAB classification) NOS
     Refractory anemia with excess blasts in transformation [RAEB T]
     EXCLUDES 1   *acute exacerbation of chronic myeloid leukemia (C92.10)*
                 refractory anemia with excess of blasts not in transformation (D46.2-)

     C92.00   **Acute myeloblastic leukemia, not having achieved remission**   HCC
        Acute myeloblastic leukemia with failed remission
        Acute myeloblastic leukemia NOS

     C92.01   **Acute myeloblastic leukemia, in remission**   HCC

     C92.02   **Acute myeloblastic leukemia, in relapse**   HCC

✓5th **C92.1**   **Chronic myeloid leukemia, BCR/ABL-positive**
     Chronic myelogenous leukemia, Philadelphia chromosome (Ph1) positive
     Chronic myelogenous leukemia, t(9;22) (q34;q11)
     Chronic myelogenous leukemia with crisis of blast cells
     EXCLUDES 1   *atypical chronic myeloid leukemia BCR/ABL-negative (C92.2-)*
                 chronic myelomonocytic leukemia (C93.1-)
                 chronic myeloproliferative disease (D47.1)

     C92.10   **Chronic myeloid leukemia, BCR/ABL-positive, not having achieved remission**   HCC
        Chronic myeloid leukemia, BCR/ABL-positive with failed remission
        Chronic myeloid leukemia, BCR/ABL-positive NOS

     C92.11   **Chronic myeloid leukemia, BCR/ABL-positive, in remission**   HCC

     C92.12   **Chronic myeloid leukemia, BCR/ABL-positive, in relapse**   HCC

✓5th **C92.2**   **Atypical chronic myeloid leukemia, BCR/ABL-negative**

     C92.20   **Atypical chronic myeloid leukemia, BCR/ABL-negative, not having achieved remission**   HCC
        Atypical chronic myeloid leukemia, BCR/ABL-negative with failed remission
        Atypical chronic myeloid leukemia, BCR/ABL-negative NOS

     C92.21   **Atypical chronic myeloid leukemia, BCR/ABL-negative, in remission**   HCC

     C92.22   **Atypical chronic myeloid leukemia, BCR/ABL-negative, in relapse**   HCC

✓5th **C92.3**   **Myeloid sarcoma**
     A malignant tumor of immature myeloid cells
     Chloroma
     Granulocytic sarcoma

     C92.30   **Myeloid sarcoma, not having achieved remission**   HCC
        Myeloid sarcoma with failed remission
        Myeloid sarcoma NOS

     C92.31   **Myeloid sarcoma, in remission**   HCC

     C92.32   **Myeloid sarcoma, in relapse**   HCC

✓5th **C92.4**   **Acute promyelocytic leukemia**
     AML M3
     AML Me with t(15;17) and variants

     C92.40   **Acute promyelocytic leukemia, not having achieved remission**   HCC
        Acute promyelocytic leukemia with failed remission
        Acute promyelocytic leukemia NOS

     C92.41   **Acute promyelocytic leukemia, in remission**   HCC

     C92.42   **Acute promyelocytic leukemia, in relapse**   HCC

✓5th **C92.5**   **Acute myelomonocytic leukemia**
     AML M4
     AML M4 Eo with inv(16) or t(16;16)

     C92.50   **Acute myelomonocytic leukemia, not having achieved remission**   HCC
        Acute myelomonocytic leukemia with failed remission
        Acute myelomonocytic leukemia NOS

     C92.51   **Acute myelomonocytic leukemia, in remission**   HCC

     C92.52   **Acute myelomonocytic leukemia, in relapse**   HCC

✓5th **C92.6**   **Acute myeloid leukemia with 11q23-abnormality**
     Acute myeloid leukemia with variation of MLL-gene

     C92.60   **Acute myeloid leukemia with 11q23-abnormality not having achieved remission**   HCC
        Acute myeloid leukemia with 11q23-abnormality with failed remission
        Acute myeloid leukemia with 11q23-abnormality NOS

     C92.61   **Acute myeloid leukemia with 11q23-abnormality in remission**   HCC

     C92.62   **Acute myeloid leukemia with 11q23-abnormality in relapse**   HCC

✓5th **C92.A**   **Acute myeloid leukemia with multilineage dysplasia**
     Acute myeloid leukemia with dysplasia of remaining hematopoesis and/or myelodysplastic disease in its history

     C92.A0   **Acute myeloid leukemia with multilineage dysplasia, not having achieved remission**   HCC
        Acute myeloid leukemia with multilineage dysplasia with failed remission
        Acute myeloid leukemia with multilineage dysplasia NOS

     C92.A1   **Acute myeloid leukemia with multilineage dysplasia, in remission**   HCC

     C92.A2   **Acute myeloid leukemia with multilineage dysplasia, in relapse**   HCC

✓5th **C92.Z**   **Other myeloid leukemia**

     C92.Z0   **Other myeloid leukemia not having achieved remission**   HCC
        Myeloid leukemia NEC with failed remission
        Myeloid leukemia NEC

     C92.Z1   **Other myeloid leukemia, in remission**   HCC

     C92.Z2   **Other myeloid leukemia, in relapse**   HCC

✓5th **C92.9**   **Myeloid leukemia, unspecified**

     C92.90   **Myeloid leukemia, unspecified, not having achieved remission**   HCC ▽
        Myeloid leukemia, unspecified with failed remission
        Myeloid leukemia, unspecified NOS

     C92.91   **Myeloid leukemia, unspecified in remission**   HCC ▽

     C92.92   **Myeloid leukemia, unspecified in relapse**   HCC ▽

✓ Additional Character Req   ✓x7th Placeholder Alert   Manifestation   HCC CMS-HCC Condition   ▽ Unspecified Code   ►◄ Revised Text   ● New Code   ▲ Revised Code Title

✓4ᵗʰ **C93 Monocytic leukemia**
INCLUDES monocytoid leukemia
EXCLUDES 1 *personal history of leukemia (Z85.6)*

✓5ᵗʰ **C93.0 Acute monoblastic/monocytic leukemia**
AML M5   AML M5b
AML M5a

   C93.00 Acute monoblastic/monocytic leukemia, HCC
not having achieved remission
Acute monoblastic/monocytic leukemia with failed remission
Acute monoblastic/monocytic leukemia NOS

   C93.01 Acute monoblastic/monocytic leukemia, HCC
in remission

   C93.02 Acute monoblastic/monocytic leukemia, HCC
in relapse

✓5ᵗʰ **C93.1 Chronic myelomonocytic leukemia**
Chronic monocytic leukemia
CMML-1
CMML-2
CMML with eosinophilia

   C93.10 Chronic myelomonocytic leukemia not having HCC
achieved remission
Chronic myelomonocytic leukemia with failed remission
Chronic myelomonocytic leukemia NOS

   C93.11 Chronic myelomonocytic leukemia, in remission HCC
   C93.12 Chronic myelomonocytic leukemia, in relapse HCC

✓5ᵗʰ **C93.3 Juvenile myelomonocytic leukemia**

   C93.30 Juvenile myelomonocytic leukemia, HCC P
not having achieved remission
Juvenile myelomonocytic leukemia with failed remission
Juvenile myelomonocytic leukemia NOS

   C93.31 Juvenile myelomonocytic leukemia, HCC P
in remission

   C93.32 Juvenile myelomonocytic leukemia, HCC P
in relapse

✓5ᵗʰ **C93.Z Other monocytic leukemia**

   C93.Z0 Other monocytic leukemia, not having HCC
achieved remission
Other monocytic leukemia NOS

   C93.Z1 Other monocytic leukemia, in remission HCC
   C93.Z2 Other monocytic leukemia, in relapse HCC

✓5ᵗʰ **C93.9 Monocytic leukemia, unspecified**

   C93.90 Monocytic leukemia, unspecified, not having HCC ▽
achieved remission
Monocytic leukemia, unspecified with failed remission
Monocytic leukemia, unspecified NOS

   C93.91 Monocytic leukemia, unspecified in remission HCC ▽
   C93.92 Monocytic leukemia, unspecified in relapse HCC ▽

✓4ᵗʰ **C94 Other leukemias of specified cell type**
EXCLUDES 1 *leukemic reticuloendotheliosis (C91.4-)*
myelodysplastic syndromes (D46.-)
personal history of leukemia (Z85.6)
plasma cell leukemia (C90.1-)

✓5ᵗʰ **C94.0 Acute erythroid leukemia**
Acute myeloid leukemia M6(a)(b)
Erythroleukemia
DEF: Erythroleukemia: A malignant blood dyscrasia (a myeloproliferative disorder).

   C94.00 Acute erythroid leukemia, not having achieved HCC
remission
Acute erythroid leukemia with failed remission
Acute erythroid leukemia NOS

   C94.01 Acute erythroid leukemia, in remission HCC
   C94.02 Acute erythroid leukemia, in relapse HCC

✓5ᵗʰ **C94.2 Acute megakaryoblastic leukemia**
Acute myeloid leukemia M7
Acute megakaryocytic leukemia

   C94.20 Acute megakaryoblastic leukemia not having HCC
achieved remission
Acute megakaryoblastic leukemia with failed remission
Acute megakaryoblastic leukemia NOS

   C94.21 Acute megakaryoblastic leukemia, in remission HCC
   C94.22 Acute megakaryoblastic leukemia, in relapse HCC

✓5ᵗʰ **C94.3 Mast cell leukemia**

   C94.30 Mast cell leukemia not having achieved HCC
remission
Mast cell leukemia with failed remission
Mast cell leukemia NOS

   C94.31 Mast cell leukemia, in remission HCC
   C94.32 Mast cell leukemia, in relapse HCC

✓5ᵗʰ **C94.4 Acute panmyelosis with myelofibrosis**
Acute myelofibrosis
EXCLUDES 1 *myelofibrosis NOS (D75.81)*
secondary myelofibrosis NOS (D75.81)

   C94.40 Acute panmyelosis with myelofibrosis not HCC
having achieved remission
Acute myelofibrosis NOS
Acute panmyelosis with myelofibrosis with failed remission
Acute panmyelosis NOS

   C94.41 Acute panmyelosis with myelofibrosis, HCC
in remission

   C94.42 Acute panmyelosis with myelofibrosis, HCC
in relapse

C94.6 Myelodysplastic disease, not classified HCC
Myeloproliferative disease, not classified

✓5ᵗʰ **C94.8 Other specified leukemias**
Aggressive NK-cell leukemia
Acute basophilic leukemia

   C94.80 Other specified leukemias not having HCC
achieved remission
Other specified leukemia with failed remission
Other specified leukemias NOS

   C94.81 Other specified leukemias, in remission HCC
   C94.82 Other specified leukemias, in relapse HCC

✓4ᵗʰ **C95 Leukemia of unspecified cell type**
EXCLUDES 1 *personal history of leukemia (Z85.6)*

✓5ᵗʰ **C95.0 Acute leukemia of unspecified cell type**
Acute bilineal leukemia
Acute mixed lineage leukemia
Biphenotypic acute leukemia
Stem cell leukemia of unclear lineage
EXCLUDES 1 *acute exacerbation of unspecified chronic leukemia (C95.10)*

   C95.00 Acute leukemia of unspecified cell type HCC
not having achieved remission
Acute leukemia of unspecified cell type with failed remission
Acute leukemia NOS

   C95.01 Acute leukemia of unspecified cell type, HCC
in remission

   C95.02 Acute leukemia of unspecified cell type, HCC
in relapse

✓5ᵗʰ **C95.1 Chronic leukemia of unspecified cell type**

   C95.10 Chronic leukemia of unspecified cell type HCC
not having achieved remission
Chronic leukemia of unspecified cell type with failed remission
Chronic leukemia NOS

   C95.11 Chronic leukemia of unspecified cell type, HCC
in remission

   C95.12 Chronic leukemia of unspecified cell type, HCC
in relapse

✓5ᵗʰ **C95.9 Leukemia, unspecified**

   C95.90 Leukemia, unspecified not having achieved HCC ▽
remission
Leukemia, unspecified with failed remission
Leukemia NOS

   C95.91 Leukemia, unspecified, in remission HCC ▽
   C95.92 Leukemia, unspecified, in relapse HCC ▽

Chapter 2. Neoplasms

✓4th **C96** **Other and unspecified malignant neoplasms of lymphoid, hematopoietic and related tissue**

    EXCLUDES 1   *personal history of other malignant neoplasms of lymphoid, hematopoietic and related tissues (Z85.79)*

    C96.0 **Multifocal and multisystemic (disseminated)**   HCC
    Langerhans-cell histiocytosis
         Histiocytosis X, multisystemic
         Letterer-Siwe disease
         EXCLUDES 1   *adult pulmonary Langerhans cell histiocytosis (J84.82)*
                multifocal and unisystemic Langerhans-cell histiocytosis (C96.5)
                unifocal Langerhans-cell histiocytosis (C96.6)

▲ ✓5th **C96.2** **Malignant mast cell neoplasm**
         ~~Aggressive systemic mastocytosis~~
         ~~Mast cell sarcoma~~
         EXCLUDES 1   *indolent mastocytosis ▶(D47.02)◀*
                mast cell leukemia (C94.30)
                mastocytosis (congenital) (cutaneous) (Q82.2)

●   **C96.20** **Malignant mast cell neoplasm, unspecified**   ▽
●   **C96.21** **Aggressive systemic mastocytosis**
●   **C96.22** **Mast cell sarcoma**
●   **C96.29** **Other malignant mast cell neoplasm**

    C96.4 **Sarcoma of dendritic cells (accessory cells)**   HCC
         Follicular dendritic cell sarcoma
         Interdigitating dendritic cell sarcoma
         Langerhans cell sarcoma

    C96.5 **Multifocal and unisystemic Langerhans-cell histiocytosis**   HCC
         Hand-Schüller-Christian disease
         Histiocytosis X, multifocal
         EXCLUDES 1   *multifocal and multisystemic (disseminated) Langerhans-cell histiocytosis (C96.0)*
                unifocal Langerhans-cell histiocytosis (C96.6)

    C96.6 **Unifocal Langerhans-cell histiocytosis**   HCC
         Eosinophilic granuloma
         Histiocytosis X, unifocal
         Histiocytosis X NOS
         Langerhans-cell histiocytosis NOS
         EXCLUDES 1   *multifocal and multisysemic (disseminated) Langerhans-cell histiocytosis (C96.0)*
                multifocal and unisystemic Langerhans-cell histiocytosis (C96.5)

    C96.A **Histiocytic sarcoma**   HCC
         Malignant histiocytosis

    C96.Z **Other specified malignant neoplasms of lymphoid, hematopoietic and related tissue**   HCC

    C96.9 **Malignant neoplasm of lymphoid, hematopoietic and related tissue, unspecified**   HCC ▽

In situ neoplasms (D00-D09)

    INCLUDES   Bowen's disease
                erythroplasia
                grade III intraepithelial neoplasia
                Queyrat's erythroplasia

✓4th **D00** **Carcinoma in situ of oral cavity, esophagus and stomach**
    EXCLUDES 1   *melanoma in situ (D03.-)*

    ✓5th **D00.0** **Carcinoma in situ of lip, oral cavity and pharynx**
         Use additional code to identify:
            exposure to environmental tobacco smoke (Z77.22)
            exposure to tobacco smoke in the perinatal period (P96.81)
            history of tobacco dependence (Z87.891)
            occupational exposure to environmental tobacco smoke (Z57.31)
            tobacco dependence (F17.-)
            tobacco use (Z72.0)
         EXCLUDES 1   *carcinoma in situ of aryepiglottic fold or interarytenoid fold, laryngeal aspect (D02.0)*
                carcinoma in situ of epiglottis NOS (D02.0)
                carcinoma in situ of epiglottis suprahyoid portion (D02.0)
                carcinoma in situ of skin of lip (D03.0, D04.0)

         D00.00 **Carcinoma in situ of oral cavity, unspecified site**   ▽
         D00.01 **Carcinoma in situ of labial mucosa and vermilion border**
         D00.02 **Carcinoma in situ of buccal mucosa**
         D00.03 **Carcinoma in situ of gingiva and edentulous alveolar ridge**
         D00.04 **Carcinoma in situ of soft palate**
         D00.05 **Carcinoma in situ of hard palate**
         D00.06 **Carcinoma in situ of floor of mouth**

         D00.07 **Carcinoma in situ of tongue**
         D00.08 **Carcinoma in situ of pharynx**
            Carcinoma in situ of aryepiglottic fold NOS
            Carcinoma in situ of hypopharyngeal aspect of aryepiglottic fold
            Carcinoma in situ of marginal zone of aryepiglottic fold

    D00.1 **Carcinoma in situ of esophagus**
    D00.2 **Carcinoma in situ of stomach**

✓4th **D01** **Carcinoma in situ of other and unspecified digestive organs**
    EXCLUDES 1   *melanoma in situ (D03.-)*

    D01.0 **Carcinoma in situ of colon**
         EXCLUDES 1   *carcinoma in situ of rectosigmoid junction (D01.1)*

    D01.1 **Carcinoma in situ of rectosigmoid junction**
    D01.2 **Carcinoma in situ of rectum**
    D01.3 **Carcinoma in situ of anus and anal canal**
         Anal intraepithelial neoplasia III [AIN III]
         Severe dysplasia of anus
         EXCLUDES 1   *anal intraepithelial neoplasia I and II [AIN I and AIN II] (K62.82)*
                carcinoma in situ of anal margin (D04.5)
                carcinoma in situ of anal skin (D04.5)
                carcinoma in situ of perianal skin (D04.5)

    ✓5th **D01.4** **Carcinoma in situ of other and unspecified parts of intestine**
         EXCLUDES 1   *carcinoma in situ of ampulla of Vater (D01.5)*

         D01.40 **Carcinoma in situ of unspecified part of intestine** ▽
         D01.49 **Carcinoma in situ of other parts of intestine**

    D01.5 **Carcinoma in situ of liver, gallbladder and bile ducts**
         Carcinoma in situ of ampulla of Vater

    D01.7 **Carcinoma in situ of other specified digestive organs**
         Carcinoma in situ of pancreas

    D01.9 **Carcinoma in situ of digestive organ, unspecified**   ▽

✓4th **D02** **Carcinoma in situ of middle ear and respiratory system**
     Use additional code to identify:
         exposure to environmental tobacco smoke (Z77.22)
         exposure to tobacco smoke in the perinatal period (P96.81)
         history of tobacco dependence (Z87.891)
         occupational exposure to environmental tobacco smoke (Z57.31)
         tobacco dependence (F17.-)
         tobacco use (Z72.0)
     EXCLUDES 1   *melanoma in situ (D03.-)*

    D02.0 **Carcinoma in situ of larynx**
         Carcinoma in situ of aryepiglottic fold or interarytenoid fold, laryngeal aspect
         Carcinoma in situ of epiglottis (suprahyoid portion)
         EXCLUDES 1   *carcinoma in situ of aryepiglottic fold or interarytenoid fold NOS (D00.08)*
                carcinoma in situ of hypopharyngeal aspect (D00.08)
                carcinoma in situ of marginal zone (D00.08)

    D02.1 **Carcinoma in situ of trachea**

    ✓5th **D02.2** **Carcinoma in situ of bronchus and lung**
         D02.20 **Carcinoma in situ of unspecified bronchus and lung**   ▽
         D02.21 **Carcinoma in situ of right bronchus and lung**
         D02.22 **Carcinoma in situ of left bronchus and lung**

    D02.3 **Carcinoma in situ of other parts of respiratory system**
         Carcinoma in situ of accessory sinuses
         Carcinoma in situ of middle ear
         Carcinoma in situ of nasal cavities
         EXCLUDES 1   *carcinoma in situ of ear (external) (skin) (D04.2-)*
                carcinoma in situ of nose NOS (D09.8)
                carcinoma in situ of skin of nose (D04.3)

    D02.4 **Carcinoma in situ of respiratory system, unspecified**   ▽

✓4th **D03** **Melanoma in situ**
    D03.0 **Melanoma in situ of lip**   HCC

    ✓5th **D03.1** **Melanoma in situ of eyelid, including canthus**
         D03.10 **Melanoma in situ of unspecified eyelid, including canthus**   HCC ▽
         D03.11 **Melanoma in situ of right eyelid, including canthus**   HCC
         D03.12 **Melanoma in situ of left eyelid, including canthus**   HCC

    ✓5th **D03.2** **Melanoma in situ of ear and external auricular canal**
         D03.20 **Melanoma in situ of unspecified ear and external auricular canal**   HCC ▽

☑ Additional Character Req   ☑x7th Placeholder Alert   Manifestation   HCC CMS-HCC Condition   ▽ Unspecified Code   ▶◀ Revised Text   ● New Code   ▲ Revised Code Title

Chapter 2. Neoplasms

D03.21   Melanoma in situ of **right** ear and external auricular canal   `HCC`

D03.22   Melanoma in situ of **left** ear and external auricular canal   `HCC`

✓5ᵗʰ **D03.3**   Melanoma in situ of other and unspecified **parts of face**

D03.30   Melanoma in situ of unspecified part of face   `HCC` ▽

D03.39   Melanoma in situ of other parts of face   `HCC`

D03.4   Melanoma in situ of **scalp and neck**

✓5ᵗʰ **D03.5**   Melanoma in situ of **trunk**

D03.51   Melanoma in situ of **anal skin**   `HCC`
    Melanoma in situ of anal margin
    Melanoma in situ of perianal skin

D03.52   Melanoma in situ of **breast (skin) (soft tissue)**   `HCC`

D03.59   Melanoma in situ of other part of trunk   `HCC`

✓5ᵗʰ **D03.6**   Melanoma in situ of **upper limb, including shoulder**

D03.60   Melanoma in situ of unspecified upper limb, including shoulder   `HCC` ▽

D03.61   Melanoma in situ of **right** upper limb, including shoulder   `HCC`

D03.62   Melanoma in situ of **left** upper limb, including shoulder   `HCC`

✓5ᵗʰ **D03.7**   Melanoma in situ of **lower limb, including hip**

D03.70   Melanoma in situ of unspecified lower limb, including hip   `HCC` ▽

D03.71   Melanoma in situ of **right** lower limb, including hip   `HCC`

D03.72   Melanoma in situ of **left** lower limb, including hip   `HCC`

D03.8   Melanoma in situ of other sites   `HCC`
    Melanoma in situ of scrotum
    EXCLUDES 1   carcinoma in situ of scrotum (D07.61)

D03.9   Melanoma in situ, unspecified   `HCC` ▽

✓4ᵗʰ **D04**   **Carcinoma in situ of skin**
    EXCLUDES 1   erythroplasia of Queyrat (penis) NOS (D07.4)
                  melanoma in situ (D03.-)

D04.0   Carcinoma in situ of skin of **lip**
    EXCLUDES 1   carcinoma in situ of vermilion border of lip (D00.01)

✓5ᵗʰ **D04.1**   Carcinoma in situ of skin of **eyelid, including canthus**

D04.10   Carcinoma in situ of skin of unspecified eyelid, including canthus   ▽

D04.11   Carcinoma in situ of skin of **right** eyelid, including canthus

D04.12   Carcinoma in situ of skin of **left** eyelid, including canthus

✓5ᵗʰ **D04.2**   Carcinoma in situ of skin of **ear and external auricular canal**

D04.20   Carcinoma in situ of skin of unspecified ear and external auricular canal   ▽

D04.21   Carcinoma in situ of skin of **right** ear and external auricular canal

D04.22   Carcinoma in situ of skin of **left** ear and external auricular canal

✓5ᵗʰ **D04.3**   Carcinoma in situ of skin of other and unspecified **parts of face**

D04.30   Carcinoma in situ of skin of unspecified part of face   ▽

D04.39   Carcinoma in situ of skin of other parts of face

D04.4   Carcinoma in situ of skin of **scalp and neck**

D04.5   Carcinoma in situ of skin of **trunk**
    Carcinoma in situ of anal margin
    Carcinoma in situ of anal skin
    Carcinoma in situ of perianal skin
    Carcinoma in situ of skin of breast
    EXCLUDES 1   carcinoma in situ of anus NOS (D01.3)
                  carcinoma in situ of scrotum (D07.61)
                  carcinoma in situ of skin of genital organs (D07.-)

✓5ᵗʰ **D04.6**   Carcinoma in situ of skin of **upper limb, including shoulder**

D04.60   Carcinoma in situ of skin of unspecified upper limb, including shoulder   ▽

D04.61   Carcinoma in situ of skin of **right** upper limb, including shoulder

D04.62   Carcinoma in situ of skin of **left** upper limb, including shoulder

✓5ᵗʰ **D04.7**   Carcinoma in situ of skin of **lower limb, including hip**

D04.70   Carcinoma in situ of skin of unspecified lower limb, including hip   ▽

D04.71   Carcinoma in situ of skin of **right** lower limb, including hip

D04.72   Carcinoma in situ of skin of **left** lower limb, including hip

D04.8   Carcinoma in situ of skin of other sites

D04.9   Carcinoma in situ of skin, unspecified   ▽

✓4ᵗʰ **D05**   **Carcinoma in situ of breast**
    EXCLUDES 1   carcinoma in situ of skin of breast (D04.5)
                  melanoma in situ of breast (skin) (D03.5)
                  Paget's disease of breast or nipple (C50.-)

✓5ᵗʰ **D05.0**   **Lobular** carcinoma in situ of breast

D05.00   Lobular carcinoma in situ of unspecified breast   ▽

D05.01   Lobular carcinoma in situ of **right** breast

D05.02   Lobular carcinoma in situ of **left** breast

✓5ᵗʰ **D05.1**   **Intraductal** carcinoma in situ of breast

D05.10   Intraductal carcinoma in situ of unspecified breast   ▽

D05.11   Intraductal carcinoma in situ of **right** breast

D05.12   Intraductal carcinoma in situ of **left** breast

✓5ᵗʰ **D05.8**   Other specified type of carcinoma in situ of breast

D05.80   Other specified type of carcinoma in situ of unspecified breast   ▽

D05.81   Other specified type of carcinoma in situ of **right** breast

D05.82   Other specified type of carcinoma in situ of **left** breast

✓5ᵗʰ **D05.9**   Unspecified type of carcinoma in situ of breast

D05.90   Unspecified type of carcinoma in situ of unspecified breast   ▽

D05.91   Unspecified type of carcinoma in situ of **right** breast   ▽

D05.92   Unspecified type of carcinoma in situ of **left** breast   ▽

✓4ᵗʰ **D06**   **Carcinoma in situ of cervix uteri**
    INCLUDES   cervical adenocarcinoma in situ
                cervical intraepithelial glandular neoplasia
                cervical intraepithelial neoplasia III [CIN III]
                severe dysplasia of cervix uteri
    EXCLUDES 1   cervical intraepithelial neoplasia II [CIN II] (N87.1)
                  cytologic evidence of malignancy of cervix without histologic
                      confirmation (R87.614)
                  high grade squamous intraepithelial lesion (HGSIL) of cervix
                      (R87.613)
                  melanoma in situ of cervix (D03.5)
                  moderate cervical dysplasia (N87.1)

D06.0   Carcinoma in situ of **endocervix**   ♀

D06.1   Carcinoma in situ of **exocervix**   ♀

D06.7   Carcinoma in situ of other **parts** of cervix   ♀

D06.9   Carcinoma in situ of cervix, unspecified   ♀ ▽

✓4ᵗʰ **D07**   **Carcinoma in situ of other and unspecified genital organs**
    EXCLUDES 1   melanoma in situ of trunk (D03.5)

D07.0   Carcinoma in situ of **endometrium**   ♀

D07.1   Carcinoma in situ of **vulva**   ♀
    Severe dysplasia of vulva
    Vulvar intraepithelial neoplasia III [VIN III]
    EXCLUDES 1   moderate dysplasia of vulva (N90.1)
                  vulvar intraepithelial neoplasia II [VIN II] (N90.1)

D07.2   Carcinoma in situ of **vagina**   ♀
    Severe dysplasia of vagina
    Vaginal intraepithelial neoplasia III [VAIN III]
    EXCLUDES 1   moderate dysplasia of vagina (N89.1)
                  vaginal intraepithelial neoplasia II [VIN II] (N89.1)

✓5ᵗʰ **D07.3**   Carcinoma in situ of other and unspecified **female genital organs**

D07.30   Carcinoma in situ of unspecified female genital organs   ♀ ▽

D07.39   Carcinoma in situ of other female genital organs   ♀

D07.4   Carcinoma in situ of **penis**   ♂
    Erythroplasia of Queyrat NOS

D07.5   Carcinoma in situ of **prostate**   ♂
    Prostatic intraepithelial neoplasia III (PIN III)
    Severe dysplasia of prostate
    EXCLUDES 1   dysplasia (mild) (moderate) of prostate (N42.3-)
                  prostatic intraepithelial neoplasia II [PIN II] (N42.3-)

✓5ᵗʰ **D07.6 Carcinoma in situ of other and unspecified male genital organs**

    D07.60 Carcinoma in situ of unspecified male genital ♂▽
         organs

    D07.61 Carcinoma in situ of scrotum   ♂

    D07.69 Carcinoma in situ of other male genital organs   ♂

✓4ᵗʰ **D09 Carcinoma in situ of other and unspecified sites**

    EXCLUDES 1   *melanoma in situ (D03.-)*

    D09.0 Carcinoma in situ of bladder

✓5ᵗʰ **D09.1 Carcinoma in situ of other and unspecified urinary organs**

    D09.10 Carcinoma in situ of unspecified urinary organ   ▽

    D09.19 Carcinoma in situ of other urinary organs

✓5ᵗʰ **D09.2 Carcinoma in situ of eye**

    EXCLUDES 1   *carcinoma in situ of skin of eyelid (D04.1-)*

    D09.20 Carcinoma in situ of unspecified eye   ▽

    D09.21 Carcinoma in situ of right eye

    D09.22 Carcinoma in situ of left eye

    D09.3 Carcinoma in situ of thyroid and other endocrine glands

    EXCLUDES 1   *carcinoma in situ of endocrine pancreas (D01.7)*
                 carcinoma in situ of ovary (D07.39)
                 carcinoma in situ of testis (D07.69)

    D09.8 Carcinoma in situ of other specified sites

    D09.9 Carcinoma in situ, unspecified   ▽

Benign neoplasms, except benign neuroendocrine tumors (D10-D36)

✓4ᵗʰ **D10 Benign neoplasm of mouth and pharynx**

    D10.0 Benign neoplasm of lip
         Benign neoplasm of lip (frenulum) (inner aspect) (mucosa)
            (vermilion border)
        EXCLUDES 1   *benign neoplasm of skin of lip (D22.0, D23.0)*

    D10.1 Benign neoplasm of tongue
         Benign neoplasm of lingual tonsil

    D10.2 Benign neoplasm of floor of mouth

✓5ᵗʰ **D10.3 Benign neoplasm of other and unspecified parts of mouth**

    D10.30 Benign neoplasm of unspecified part of mouth   ▽

    D10.39 Benign neoplasm of other parts of mouth
          Benign neoplasm of minor salivary gland NOS
         EXCLUDES 1   *benign odontogenic neoplasms*
                    (D16.4-D16.5)
                 benign neoplasm of mucosa of lip (D10.0)
                 benign neoplasm of nasopharyngeal surface
                    of soft palate (D10.6)

    D10.4 Benign neoplasm of tonsil
         Benign neoplasm of tonsil (faucial) (palatine)
        EXCLUDES 1   *benign neoplasm of lingual tonsil (D10.1)*
               benign neoplasm of pharyngeal tonsil (D10.6)
               benign neoplasm of tonsillar fossa (D10.5)
               benign neoplasm of tonsillar pillars (D10.5)

    D10.5 Benign neoplasm of other parts of oropharynx
         Benign neoplasm of epiglottis, anterior aspect
         Benign neoplasm of tonsillar fossa
         Benign neoplasm of tonsillar pillars
         Benign neoplasm of vallecula
        EXCLUDES 1   *benign neoplasm of epiglottis NOS (D14.1)*
               benign neoplasm of epiglottis, suprahyoid portion
                    (D14.1)

    D10.6 Benign neoplasm of nasopharynx
         Benign neoplasm of pharyngeal tonsil
         Benign neoplasm of posterior margin of septum and choanae

    D10.7 Benign neoplasm of hypopharynx

    D10.9 Benign neoplasm of pharynx, unspecified   ▽

✓4ᵗʰ **D11 Benign neoplasm of major salivary glands**

    EXCLUDES 1   *benign neoplasms of minor salivary glands NOS (D10.39)*
               benign neoplasms of specified minor salivary glands which are
                 classified according to their anatomical location

    D11.0 Benign neoplasm of parotid gland

    D11.7 Benign neoplasm of other major salivary glands
         Benign neoplasm of sublingual salivary gland
         Benign neoplasm of submandibular salivary gland

    D11.9 Benign neoplasm of major salivary gland, unspecified ▽

✓4ᵗʰ **D12 Benign neoplasm of colon, rectum, anus and anal canal**

    EXCLUDES 1   *benign carcinoid tumors of the large intestine, and rectum*
               (D3A.02-)

    AHA: 2017, 1Q, 15; 2015, 2Q, 14

    D12.0 Benign neoplasm of cecum
         Benign neoplasm of ileocecal valve

    D12.1 Benign neoplasm of appendix
        EXCLUDES 1   *benign carcinoid tumor of the appendix (D3A.020)*

    D12.2 Benign neoplasm of ascending colon

    D12.3 Benign neoplasm of transverse colon
         Benign neoplasm of hepatic flexure
         Benign neoplasm of splenic flexure
        AHA: 2017, 1Q, 16

    D12.4 Benign neoplasm of descending colon

    D12.5 Benign neoplasm of sigmoid colon

    D12.6 Benign neoplasm of colon, unspecified   ▽
         Adenomatosis of colon
         Benign neoplasm of large intestine NOS
         Polyposis (hereditary) of colon
        EXCLUDES 1   *inflammatory polyp of colon (K51.4-)*
               polyp of colon NOS (K63.5)

    D12.7 Benign neoplasm of rectosigmoid junction

    D12.8 Benign neoplasm of rectum
        EXCLUDES 1   *benign carcinoid tumor of the rectum (D3A.026)*

    D12.9 Benign neoplasm of anus and anal canal
         Benign neoplasm of anus NOS
        EXCLUDES 1   *benign neoplasm of anal margin (D22.5, D23.5)*
               benign neoplasm of anal skin (D22.5, D23.5)
               benign neoplasm of perianal skin (D22.5, D23.5)

✓4ᵗʰ **D13 Benign neoplasm of other and ill-defined parts of digestive system**

    EXCLUDES 1   *benign stromal tumors of digestive system (D21.4)*

    D13.0 Benign neoplasm of esophagus

    D13.1 Benign neoplasm of stomach
        EXCLUDES 1   *benign carcinoid tumor of the stomach (D3A.092)*

    D13.2 Benign neoplasm of duodenum
        EXCLUDES 1   *benign carcinoid tumor of the duodenum (D3A.010)*

✓5ᵗʰ **D13.3 Benign neoplasm of other and unspecified parts of small intestine**

    EXCLUDES 1   *benign carcinoid tumors of the small intestine*
               (D3A.01-)
               benign neoplasm of ileocecal valve (D12.0)

    D13.30 Benign neoplasm of unspecified part of small   ▽
           intestine

    D13.39 Benign neoplasm of other parts of small intestine

    D13.4 Benign neoplasm of liver
         Benign neoplasm of intrahepatic bile ducts

    D13.5 Benign neoplasm of extrahepatic bile ducts

    D13.6 Benign neoplasm of pancreas
        EXCLUDES 1   *benign neoplasm of endocrine pancreas (D13.7)*

    D13.7 Benign neoplasm of endocrine pancreas
         Islet cell tumor
         Benign neoplasm of islets of Langerhans
         Use additional code to identify any functional activity

    D13.9 Benign neoplasm of ill-defined sites within the digestive system
         Benign neoplasm of digestive system NOS
         Benign neoplasm of intestine NOS
         Benign neoplasm of spleen

✓4ᵗʰ **D14 Benign neoplasm of middle ear and respiratory system**

    D14.0 Benign neoplasm of middle ear, nasal cavity and accessory sinuses
         Benign neoplasm of cartilage of nose
        EXCLUDES 1   *benign neoplasm of auricular canal (external) (D22.2-,*
                    D23.2-)
               benign neoplasm of bone of ear (D16.4)
               benign neoplasm of bone of nose (D16.4)
               benign neoplasm of cartilage of ear (D21.0)
               benign neoplasm of ear (external)(skin) (D22.2-,
                    D23.2-)
               benign neoplasm of nose NOS (D36.7)
               benign neoplasm of skin of nose (D22.39, D23.39)
               benign neoplasm of olfactory bulb (D33.3)
               benign neoplasm of posterior margin of septum and
                    choanae (D10.6)
               polyp of accessory sinus (J33.8)
               polyp of ear (middle) (H74.4)
               polyp of nasal (cavity) (J33.-)

D14.1 Benign neoplasm of larynx
Adenomatous polyp of larynx
Benign neoplasm of epiglottis (suprahyoid portion)
> EXCLUDES 1   benign neoplasm of epiglottis, anterior aspect (D10.5)
> polyp (nonadenomatous) of vocal cord or larynx (J38.1)

D14.2 Benign neoplasm of trachea

✓5th D14.3 Benign neoplasm of bronchus and lung
> EXCLUDES 1   benign carcinoid tumor of the bronchus and lung (D3A.090)

D14.30   Benign neoplasm of unspecified bronchus and lung   ▽

D14.31   Benign neoplasm of right bronchus and lung

D14.32   Benign neoplasm of left bronchus and lung

D14.4 Benign neoplasm of respiratory system, unspecified   ▽

✓4th D15 Benign neoplasm of other and unspecified intrathoracic organs
> EXCLUDES 1   benign neoplasm of mesothelial tissue (D19.-)

D15.0   Benign neoplasm of thymus
> EXCLUDES 1   benign carcinoid tumor of the thymus (D3A.091)

D15.1   Benign neoplasm of heart
> EXCLUDES 1   benign neoplasm of great vessels (D21.3)

D15.2   Benign neoplasm of mediastinum

D15.7   Benign neoplasm of other specified intrathoracic organs

D15.9   Benign neoplasm of intrathoracic organ, unspecified   ▽

✓4th D16 Benign neoplasm of bone and articular cartilage
> EXCLUDES 1   benign neoplasm of connective tissue of ear (D21.0)
> benign neoplasm of connective tissue of eyelid (D21.0)
> benign neoplasm of connective tissue of larynx (D14.1)
> benign neoplasm of connective tissue of nose (D14.0)
> benign neoplasm of synovia (D21.-)

✓5th D16.0   Benign neoplasm of scapula and long bones of upper limb
D16.00   Benign neoplasm of scapula and long bones of unspecified upper limb   ▽
D16.01   Benign neoplasm of scapula and long bones of right upper limb
D16.02   Benign neoplasm of scapula and long bones of left upper limb

✓5th D16.1   Benign neoplasm of short bones of upper limb
D16.10   Benign neoplasm of short bones of unspecified upper limb   ▽
D16.11   Benign neoplasm of short bones of right upper limb
D16.12   Benign neoplasm of short bones of left upper limb

✓5th D16.2   Benign neoplasm of long bones of lower limb
D16.20   Benign neoplasm of long bones of unspecified lower limb   ▽
D16.21   Benign neoplasm of long bones of right lower limb
D16.22   Benign neoplasm of long bones of left lower limb

✓5th D16.3   Benign neoplasm of short bones of lower limb
D16.30   Benign neoplasm of short bones of unspecified lower limb   ▽
D16.31   Benign neoplasm of short bones of right lower limb
D16.32   Benign neoplasm of short bones of left lower limb

D16.4   Benign neoplasm of bones of skull and face
Benign neoplasm of maxilla (superior)
Benign neoplasm of orbital bone
Keratocyst of maxilla
Keratocystic odontogenic tumor of maxilla
> EXCLUDES 2   benign neoplasm of lower jaw bone (D16.5)

D16.5   Benign neoplasm of lower jaw bone
Keratocyst of mandible
Keratocystic odontogenic tumor of mandible

D16.6   Benign neoplasm of vertebral column
> EXCLUDES 1   benign neoplasm of sacrum and coccyx (D16.8)

D16.7   Benign neoplasm of ribs, sternum and clavicle

D16.8   Benign neoplasm of pelvic bones, sacrum and coccyx

D16.9   Benign neoplasm of bone and articular cartilage, unspecified   ▽

✓4th D17 Benign lipomatous neoplasm

D17.0   Benign lipomatous neoplasm of skin and subcutaneous tissue of head, face and neck

D17.1   Benign lipomatous neoplasm of skin and subcutaneous tissue of trunk

✓5th D17.2   Benign lipomatous neoplasm of skin and subcutaneous tissue of limb
D17.20   Benign lipomatous neoplasm of skin and subcutaneous tissue of unspecified limb   ▽
D17.21   Benign lipomatous neoplasm of skin and subcutaneous tissue of right arm
D17.22   Benign lipomatous neoplasm of skin and subcutaneous tissue of left arm
D17.23   Benign lipomatous neoplasm of skin and subcutaneous tissue of right leg
D17.24   Benign lipomatous neoplasm of skin and subcutaneous tissue of left leg

✓5th D17.3   Benign lipomatous neoplasm of skin and subcutaneous tissue of other and unspecified sites
D17.30   Benign lipomatous neoplasm of skin and subcutaneous tissue of unspecified sites   ▽
D17.39   Benign lipomatous neoplasm of skin and subcutaneous tissue of other sites

D17.4   Benign lipomatous neoplasm of intrathoracic organs

D17.5   Benign lipomatous neoplasm of intra-abdominal organs
> EXCLUDES 1   benign lipomatous neoplasm of peritoneum and retroperitoneum (D17.79)

D17.6   Benign lipomatous neoplasm of spermatic cord   ♂

✓5th D17.7   Benign lipomatous neoplasm of other sites
D17.71   Benign lipomatous neoplasm of kidney
D17.72   Benign lipomatous neoplasm of other genitourinary organ
D17.79   Benign lipomatous neoplasm of other sites
Benign lipomatous neoplasm of peritoneum
Benign lipomatous neoplasm of retroperitoneum

D17.9   Benign lipomatous neoplasm, unspecified   ▽
Lipoma NOS

✓4th D18 Hemangioma and lymphangioma, any site
> EXCLUDES 1   benign neoplasm of glomus jugulare (D35.6)
> blue or pigmented nevus (D22.-)
> nevus NOS (D22.-)
> vascular nevus (Q82.5)

✓5th D18.0   Hemangioma
Angioma NOS
Cavernous nevus
DEF: A common benign tumor usually occurring in infancy; composed of newly formed blood vessels due to malformation of angioblastic tissue.
D18.00   Hemangioma unspecified site   ▽
D18.01   Hemangioma of skin and subcutaneous tissue
D18.02   Hemangioma of intracranial structures   HCC
D18.03   Hemangioma of intra-abdominal structures
D18.09   Hemangioma of other sites

D18.1   Lymphangioma, any site

✓4th D19 Benign neoplasm of mesothelial tissue

D19.0   Benign neoplasm of mesothelial tissue of pleura

D19.1   Benign neoplasm of mesothelial tissue of peritoneum

D19.7   Benign neoplasm of mesothelial tissue of other sites

D19.9   Benign neoplasm of mesothelial tissue, unspecified   ▽
Benign mesothelioma NOS

✓4th D20 Benign neoplasm of soft tissue of retroperitoneum and peritoneum
> EXCLUDES 1   benign lipomatous neoplasm of peritoneum and retroperitoneum (D17.79)
> benign neoplasm of mesothelial tissue (D19.-)

D20.0   Benign neoplasm of soft tissue of retroperitoneum

D20.1   Benign neoplasm of soft tissue of peritoneum

EXCLUDES 1 Not coded here   EXCLUDES 2 Not included here   N Newborn Age: 0   P Pediatric Age: 0-17   M Maternity Age: 12-55   A Adult Age: 15-124

486   ICD-10-CM 2018

✓4th **D21** **Other benign neoplasms of connective and other soft tissue**
    INCLUDES benign neoplasm of blood vessel
                benign neoplasm of bursa
                benign neoplasm of cartilage
                benign neoplasm of fascia
                benign neoplasm of fat
                benign neoplasm of ligament, except uterine
                benign neoplasm of lymphatic channel
                benign neoplasm of muscle
                benign neoplasm of synovia
                benign neoplasm of tendon (sheath)
                benign stromal tumors
    EXCLUDES 1 *benign neoplasm of articular cartilage (D16.-)*
                benign neoplasm of cartilage of larynx (D14.1)
                benign neoplasm of cartilage of nose (D14.0)
                benign neoplasm of connective tissue of breast (D24.-)
                benign neoplasm of peripheral nerves and autonomic nervous system (D36.1-)
                benign neoplasm of peritoneum (D20.1)
                benign neoplasm of retroperitoneum (D20.0)
                benign neoplasm of uterine ligament, any (D28.2)
                benign neoplasm of vascular tissue (D18.-)
                hemangioma (D18.0-)
                lipomatous neoplasm (D17.-)
                lymphangioma (D18.1)
                uterine leiomyoma (D25.-)

D21.0 **Benign neoplasm of connective and other soft tissue of head, face and neck**
    Benign neoplasm of connective tissue of ear
    Benign neoplasm of connective tissue of eyelid
    EXCLUDES 1 *benign neoplasm of connective tissue of orbit (D31.6-)*

✓5th **D21.1** **Benign neoplasm of connective and other soft tissue of upper limb, including shoulder**
    D21.10 **Benign neoplasm of connective and other soft tissue of unspecified upper limb, including shoulder** ▽
    D21.11 **Benign neoplasm of connective and other soft tissue of right upper limb, including shoulder**
    D21.12 **Benign neoplasm of connective and other soft tissue of left upper limb, including shoulder**

✓5th **D21.2** **Benign neoplasm of connective and other soft tissue of lower limb, including hip**
    D21.20 **Benign neoplasm of connective and other soft tissue of unspecified lower limb, including hip** ▽
    D21.21 **Benign neoplasm of connective and other soft tissue of right lower limb, including hip**
    D21.22 **Benign neoplasm of connective and other soft tissue of left lower limb, including hip**

D21.3 **Benign neoplasm of connective and other soft tissue of thorax**
    Benign neoplasm of axilla
    Benign neoplasm of diaphragm
    Benign neoplasm of great vessels
    EXCLUDES 1 *benign neoplasm of heart (D15.1)*
                benign neoplasm of mediastinum (D15.2)
                benign neoplasm of thymus (D15.0)

D21.4 **Benign neoplasm of connective and other soft tissue of abdomen**
    Benign stromal tumors of abdomen

D21.5 **Benign neoplasm of connective and other soft tissue of pelvis**
    EXCLUDES 1 *benign neoplasm of any uterine ligament (D28.2)*
                uterine leiomyoma (D25.-)

D21.6 **Benign neoplasm of connective and other soft tissue of trunk, unspecified** ▽
    Benign neoplasm of back NOS

D21.9 **Benign neoplasm of connective and other soft tissue, unspecified** ▽

✓4th **D22** **Melanocytic nevi**
    INCLUDES atypical nevus
                blue hairy pigmented nevus
                nevus NOS

D22.0 **Melanocytic nevi of lip**

✓5th **D22.1** **Melanocytic nevi of eyelid, including canthus**
    D22.10 **Melanocytic nevi of unspecified eyelid, including canthus** ▽
    D22.11 **Melanocytic nevi of right eyelid, including canthus**
    D22.12 **Melanocytic nevi of left eyelid, including canthus**

✓5th **D22.2** **Melanocytic nevi of ear and external auricular canal**
    D22.20 **Melanocytic nevi of unspecified ear and external auricular canal** ▽

D22.21 **Melanocytic nevi of right ear and external auricular canal**

D22.22 **Melanocytic nevi of left ear and external auricular canal**

✓5th **D22.3** **Melanocytic nevi of other and unspecified parts of face**
    D22.30 **Melanocytic nevi of unspecified part of face** ▽
    D22.39 **Melanocytic nevi of other parts of face**

D22.4 **Melanocytic nevi of scalp and neck**

D22.5 **Melanocytic nevi of trunk**
    Melanocytic nevi of anal margin
    Melanocytic nevi of anal skin
    Melanocytic nevi of perianal skin
    Melanocytic nevi of skin of breast

✓5th **D22.6** **Melanocytic nevi of upper limb, including shoulder**
    D22.60 **Melanocytic nevi of unspecified upper limb, including shoulder** ▽
    D22.61 **Melanocytic nevi of right upper limb, including shoulder**
    D22.62 **Melanocytic nevi of left upper limb, including shoulder**

✓5th **D22.7** **Melanocytic nevi of lower limb, including hip**
    D22.70 **Melanocytic nevi of unspecified lower limb, including hip** ▽
    D22.71 **Melanocytic nevi of right lower limb, including hip**
    D22.72 **Melanocytic nevi of left lower limb, including hip**

D22.9 **Melanocytic nevi, unspecified** ▽

✓4th **D23** **Other benign neoplasms of skin**
    INCLUDES benign neoplasm of hair follicles
                benign neoplasm of sebaceous glands
                benign neoplasm of sweat glands
    EXCLUDES 1 *benign lipomatous neoplasms of skin (D17.0-D17.3)*
                melanocytic nevi (D22.-)

D23.0 **Other benign neoplasm of skin of lip**
    EXCLUDES 1 *benign neoplasm of vermilion border of lip (D10.0)*

✓5th **D23.1** **Other benign neoplasm of skin of eyelid, including canthus**
    D23.10 **Other benign neoplasm of skin of unspecified eyelid, including canthus** ▽
    D23.11 **Other benign neoplasm of skin of right eyelid, including canthus**
    D23.12 **Other benign neoplasm of skin of left eyelid, including canthus**

✓5th **D23.2** **Other benign neoplasm of skin of ear and external auricular canal**
    D23.20 **Other benign neoplasm of skin of unspecified ear and external auricular canal** ▽
    D23.21 **Other benign neoplasm of skin of right ear and external auricular canal**
    D23.22 **Other benign neoplasm of skin of left ear and external auricular canal**

✓5th **D23.3** **Other benign neoplasm of skin of other and unspecified parts of face**
    D23.30 **Other benign neoplasm of skin of unspecified part of face** ▽
    D23.39 **Other benign neoplasm of skin of other parts of face**

D23.4 **Other benign neoplasm of skin of scalp and neck**

D23.5 **Other benign neoplasm of skin of trunk**
    Other benign neoplasm of anal margin
    Other benign neoplasm of anal skin
    Other benign neoplasm of perianal skin
    Other benign neoplasm of skin of breast
    EXCLUDES 1 *benign neoplasm of anus NOS (D12.9)*

✓5th **D23.6** **Other benign neoplasm of skin of upper limb, including shoulder**
    D23.60 **Other benign neoplasm of skin of unspecified upper limb, including shoulder** ▽
    D23.61 **Other benign neoplasm of skin of right upper limb, including shoulder**
    D23.62 **Other benign neoplasm of skin of left upper limb, including shoulder**

✓5th **D23.7** **Other benign neoplasm of skin of lower limb, including hip**
    D23.70 **Other benign neoplasm of skin of unspecified lower limb, including hip** ▽
    D23.71 **Other benign neoplasm of skin of right lower limb, including hip**
    D23.72 **Other benign neoplasm of skin of left lower limb, including hip**

✓ Additional Character Req   ✓x7th Placeholder Alert   Manifestation   HCC CMS-HCC Condition   ▽ Unspecified Code   ►◄ Revised Text   ● New Code   ▲ Revised Code Title

ICD-10-CM 2018   487

D23.9   Other benign neoplasm of skin, unspecified   ▽

✓4ᵗʰ D24 Benign neoplasm of breast
    INCLUDES   benign neoplasm of connective tissue of breast
        benign neoplasm of soft parts of breast
        fibroadenoma of breast
    EXCLUDES 2 *adenofibrosis of breast (N60.2)*
        benign cyst of breast (N60.-)
        benign mammary dysplasia (N60.-)
        benign neoplasm of skin of breast (D22.5, D23.5)
        fibrocystic disease of breast (N60.-)

  D24.1 Benign neoplasm of right breast
  D24.2 Benign neoplasm of left breast
  D24.9 Benign neoplasm of unspecified breast   ▽

✓4ᵗʰ D25 Leiomyoma of uterus
    INCLUDES   uterine fibroid
        uterine fibromyoma
        uterine myoma

  D25.0 Submucous leiomyoma of uterus   ♀
  D25.1 Intramural leiomyoma of uterus   ♀
      Interstitial leiomyoma of uterus
  D25.2 Subserosal leiomyoma of uterus   ♀
      Subperitoneal leiomyoma of uterus
  D25.9 Leiomyoma of uterus, unspecified   ♀▽

✓4ᵗʰ D26 Other benign neoplasms of uterus
  D26.0 Other benign neoplasm of cervix uteri   ♀
  D26.1 Other benign neoplasm of corpus uteri   ♀
  D26.7 Other benign neoplasm of other parts of uterus   ♀
  D26.9 Other benign neoplasm of uterus, unspecified   ♀▽

✓4ᵗʰ D27 Benign neoplasm of ovary
    Use additional code to identify any functional activity
    EXCLUDES 2 *corpus albicans cyst (N83.2-)*
        corpus luteum cyst (N83.1-)
        endometrial cyst (N80.1)
        follicular (atretic) cyst (N83.0-)
        graafian follicle cyst (N83.0-)
        ovarian cyst NEC (N83.2-)
        ovarian retention cyst (N83.2-)

  D27.0 Benign neoplasm of right ovary   ♀
  D27.1 Benign neoplasm of left ovary   ♀
  D27.9 Benign neoplasm of unspecified ovary   ♀▽

✓4ᵗʰ D28 Benign neoplasm of other and unspecified female genital organs
    INCLUDES   adenomatous polyp
        benign neoplasm of skin of female genital organs
        benign teratoma
    EXCLUDES 1 *epoophoron cyst (Q50.5)*
        fimbrial cyst (Q50.4)
        Gartner's duct cyst (Q52.4)
        parovarian cyst (Q50.5)

  D28.0 Benign neoplasm of vulva   ♀
  D28.1 Benign neoplasm of vagina   ♀
  D28.2 Benign neoplasm of uterine tubes and ligaments   ♀
      Benign neoplasm of fallopian tube
      Benign neoplasm of uterine ligament (broad) (round)
  D28.7 Benign neoplasm of other specified female genital organs   ♀
  D28.9 Benign neoplasm of female genital organ, unspecified   ♀▽

Uterine Leiomyomas (Fibroids)

✓4ᵗʰ D29 Benign neoplasm of male genital organs
    INCLUDES   benign neoplasm of skin of male genital organs
  D29.0 Benign neoplasm of penis   ♂
  D29.1 Benign neoplasm of prostate   ♂
      EXCLUDES 1 *enlarged prostate (N40.-)*
  ✓5ᵗʰ **D29.2** Benign neoplasm of testis
      Use additional code to identify any functional activity
    D29.20 Benign neoplasm of unspecified testis   ♂▽
    D29.21 Benign neoplasm of right testis   ♂
    D29.22 Benign neoplasm of left testis   ♂
  ✓5ᵗʰ **D29.3** Benign neoplasm of epididymis
    D29.30 Benign neoplasm of unspecified epididymis   ♂▽
    D29.31 Benign neoplasm of right epididymis   ♂
    D29.32 Benign neoplasm of left epididymis   ♂
  D29.4 Benign neoplasm of scrotum   ♂
      Benign neoplasm of skin of scrotum
  D29.8 Benign neoplasm of other specified male genital organs   ♂
      Benign neoplasm of seminal vesicle
      Benign neoplasm of spermatic cord
      Benign neoplasm of tunica vaginalis
  D29.9 Benign neoplasm of male genital organ, unspecified   ♂▽

✓4ᵗʰ D30 Benign neoplasm of urinary organs
  ✓5ᵗʰ **D30.0** Benign neoplasm of kidney
      EXCLUDES 1 *benign carcinoid tumor of the kidney (D3A.093)*
        benign neoplasm of renal calyces (D30.1-)
        benign neoplasm of renal pelvis (D30.1-)
    D30.00 Benign neoplasm of unspecified kidney   ▽
    D30.01 Benign neoplasm of right kidney
    D30.02 Benign neoplasm of left kidney
  ✓5ᵗʰ **D30.1** Benign neoplasm of renal pelvis
    D30.10 Benign neoplasm of unspecified renal pelvis   ▽
    D30.11 Benign neoplasm of right renal pelvis
    D30.12 Benign neoplasm of left renal pelvis
  ✓5ᵗʰ **D30.2** Benign neoplasm of ureter
      EXCLUDES 1 *benign neoplasm of ureteric orifice of bladder (D30.3)*
    D30.20 Benign neoplasm of unspecified ureter   ▽
    D30.21 Benign neoplasm of right ureter
    D30.22 Benign neoplasm of left ureter
  D30.3 Benign neoplasm of bladder
      Benign neoplasm of ureteric orifice of bladder
      Benign neoplasm of urethral orifice of bladder
  D30.4 Benign neoplasm of urethra
      EXCLUDES 1 *benign neoplasm of urethral orifice of bladder (D30.3)*
  D30.8 Benign neoplasm of other specified urinary organs
      Benign neoplasm of paraurethral glands
  D30.9 Benign neoplasm of urinary organ, unspecified   ▽
      Benign neoplasm of urinary system NOS

✓4ᵗʰ D31 Benign neoplasm of eye and adnexa
    EXCLUDES 1 *benign neoplasm of connective tissue of eyelid (D21.0)*
        benign neoplasm of optic nerve (D33.3)
        benign neoplasm of skin of eyelid (D22.1-, D23.1-)
  ✓5ᵗʰ **D31.0** Benign neoplasm of conjunctiva
    D31.00 Benign neoplasm of unspecified conjunctiva   ▽
    D31.01 Benign neoplasm of right conjunctiva
    D31.02 Benign neoplasm of left conjunctiva
  ✓5ᵗʰ **D31.1** Benign neoplasm of cornea
    D31.10 Benign neoplasm of unspecified cornea   ▽
    D31.11 Benign neoplasm of right cornea
    D31.12 Benign neoplasm of left cornea
  ✓5ᵗʰ **D31.2** Benign neoplasm of retina
      EXCLUDES 1 *dark area on retina (D49.81)*
        hemangioma of retina (D49.81)
        neoplasm of unspecified behavior of retina and choroid (D49.81)
        retinal freckle (D49.81)
    D31.20 Benign neoplasm of unspecified retina   ▽
    D31.21 Benign neoplasm of right retina
    D31.22 Benign neoplasm of left retina
  ✓5ᵗʰ **D31.3** Benign neoplasm of choroid
    D31.30 Benign neoplasm of unspecified choroid   ▽
    D31.31 Benign neoplasm of right choroid
    D31.32 Benign neoplasm of left choroid

EXCLUDES 1 Not coded here   EXCLUDES 2 Not included here   N Newborn Age: 0   P Pediatric Age: 0-17   M Maternity Age: 12-55   A Adult Age: 15-124

488   ICD-10-CM 2018

✓5th **D31.4 Benign neoplasm of ciliary body**
     D31.40 Benign neoplasm of unspecified ciliary body ▽
     D31.41 Benign neoplasm of right ciliary body
     D31.42 Benign neoplasm of left ciliary body

✓5th **D31.5 Benign neoplasm of lacrimal gland and duct**
     Benign neoplasm of lacrimal sac
     Benign neoplasm of nasolacrimal duct
     D31.50 Benign neoplasm of unspecified lacrimal gland ▽
        and duct
     D31.51 Benign neoplasm of right lacrimal gland and duct
     D31.52 Benign neoplasm of left lacrimal gland and duct

✓5th **D31.6 Benign neoplasm of unspecified site of orbit**
     Benign neoplasm of connective tissue of orbit
     Benign neoplasm of extraocular muscle
     Benign neoplasm of peripheral nerves of orbit
     Benign neoplasm of retrobulbar tissue
     Benign neoplasm of retro-ocular tissue
     EXCLUDES 1   *benign neoplasm of orbital bone (D16.4)*
     D31.60 Benign neoplasm of unspecified site of ▽
        unspecified orbit
     D31.61 Benign neoplasm of unspecified site of right orbit
     D31.62 Benign neoplasm of unspecified site of left orbit

✓5th **D31.9 Benign neoplasm of unspecified part of eye**
     Benign neoplasm of eyeball
     D31.90 Benign neoplasm of unspecified part of ▽
        unspecified eye
     D31.91 Benign neoplasm of unspecified part of right eye
     D31.92 Benign neoplasm of unspecified part of left eye

✓4th **D32 Benign neoplasm of meninges**
     D32.0 Benign neoplasm of cerebral meninges   HCC
     D32.1 Benign neoplasm of spinal meninges   HCC
     D32.9 Benign neoplasm of meninges, unspecified   HCC ▽
        Meningioma NOS

✓4th **D33 Benign neoplasm of brain and other parts of central nervous system**
     EXCLUDES 1   *angioma (D18.0-)*
        benign neoplasm of meninges (D32.-)
        benign neoplasm of peripheral nerves and autonomic nervous
          system (D36.1-)
        hemangioma (D18.0-)
        neurofibromatosis (Q85.0-)
        retro-ocular benign neoplasm (D31.6-)
     D33.0 Benign neoplasm of brain, supratentorial   HCC
     Benign neoplasm of cerebral ventricle
     Benign neoplasm of cerebrum
     Benign neoplasm of frontal lobe
     Benign neoplasm of occipital lobe
     Benign neoplasm of parietal lobe
     Benign neoplasm of temporal lobe
     EXCLUDES 1   *benign neoplasm of fourth ventricle (D33.1)*
     D33.1 Benign neoplasm of brain, infratentorial   HCC
     Benign neoplasm of brain stem
     Benign neoplasm of cerebellum
     Benign neoplasm of fourth ventricle
     D33.2 Benign neoplasm of brain, unspecified   HCC ▽
     D33.3 Benign neoplasm of cranial nerves   HCC
     Benign neoplasm of olfactory bulb
     D33.4 Benign neoplasm of spinal cord   HCC
     D33.7 Benign neoplasm of other specified parts of   HCC
        central nervous system
     D33.9 Benign neoplasm of central nervous system,   HCC ▽
        unspecified
        Benign neoplasm of nervous system (central) NOS

D34 Benign neoplasm of thyroid gland
     Use additional code to identify any functional activity

✓4th **D35 Benign neoplasm of other and unspecified endocrine glands**
     Use additional code to identify any functional activity
     EXCLUDES 1   *benign neoplasm of endocrine pancreas (D13.7)*
        benign neoplasm of ovary (D27.-)
        benign neoplasm of testis (D29.2-)
        benign neoplasm of thymus (D15.0)
     ✓5th **D35.0 Benign neoplasm of adrenal gland**
     D35.00 Benign neoplasm of unspecified adrenal gland ▽
     D35.01 Benign neoplasm of right adrenal gland
     D35.02 Benign neoplasm of left adrenal gland
     D35.1 Benign neoplasm of parathyroid gland

     D35.2 Benign neoplasm of pituitary gland   HCC
        AHA: 2014, 3Q, 22
     D35.3 Benign neoplasm of craniopharyngeal duct   HCC
     D35.4 Benign neoplasm of pineal gland   HCC
     D35.5 Benign neoplasm of carotid body
     D35.6 Benign neoplasm of aortic body and other paraganglia
        Benign tumor of glomus jugulare
     D35.7 Benign neoplasm of other specified endocrine glands
     D35.9 Benign neoplasm of endocrine gland, unspecified ▽
        Benign neoplasm of unspecified endocrine gland

✓4th **D36 Benign neoplasm of other and unspecified sites**
     D36.0 Benign neoplasm of lymph nodes
        EXCLUDES 1   *lymphangioma (D18.1)*
     ✓5th **D36.1 Benign neoplasm of peripheral nerves and autonomic nervous system**
        EXCLUDES 1   *benign neoplasm of peripheral nerves of orbit (D31.6-)*
          neurofibromatosis (Q85.0-)
     D36.10 Benign neoplasm of peripheral nerves and ▽
        autonomic nervous system, unspecified
     D36.11 Benign neoplasm of peripheral nerves and
        autonomic nervous system of face, head, and neck
     D36.12 Benign neoplasm of peripheral nerves and
        autonomic nervous system, upper limb, including
        shoulder
     D36.13 Benign neoplasm of peripheral nerves and
        autonomic nervous system of lower limb, including
        hip
     D36.14 Benign neoplasm of peripheral nerves and
        autonomic nervous system of thorax
     D36.15 Benign neoplasm of peripheral nerves and
        autonomic nervous system of abdomen
     D36.16 Benign neoplasm of peripheral nerves and
        autonomic nervous system of pelvis
     D36.17 Benign neoplasm of peripheral nerves and ▽
        autonomic nervous system of trunk, unspecified
     D36.7 Benign neoplasm of other specified sites
        Benign neoplasm of nose NOS
     D36.9 Benign neoplasm, unspecified site ▽

Benign neuroendocrine tumors (D3A)

✓4th **D3A Benign neuroendocrine tumors**
     Code also any associated multiple endocrine neoplasia [MEN]
        syndromes (E31.2-)
     Use additional code to identify any associated endocrine syndrome,
        such as:
        carcinoid syndrome (E34.0)
     EXCLUDES 2   *benign pancreatic islet cell tumors (D13.7)*
     ✓5th **D3A.0 Benign carcinoid tumors**
     D3A.00 Benign carcinoid tumor of unspecified site ▽
        Carcinoid tumor NOS
     ✓6th **D3A.01 Benign carcinoid tumors of the small intestine**
        D3A.010 Benign carcinoid tumor of the duodenum
        D3A.011 Benign carcinoid tumor of the jejunum
        D3A.012 Benign carcinoid tumor of the ileum
        D3A.019 Benign carcinoid tumor of the small ▽
          intestine, unspecified portion
     ✓6th **D3A.02 Benign carcinoid tumors of the appendix, large intestine, and rectum**
        D3A.020 Benign carcinoid tumor of the appendix
        D3A.021 Benign carcinoid tumor of the cecum
        D3A.022 Benign carcinoid tumor of the ascending colon
        D3A.023 Benign carcinoid tumor of the transverse colon
        D3A.024 Benign carcinoid tumor of the descending colon
        D3A.025 Benign carcinoid tumor of the sigmoid colon
        D3A.026 Benign carcinoid tumor of the rectum
        D3A.029 Benign carcinoid tumor of the large ▽
          intestine, unspecified portion
          Benign carcinoid tumor of the colon NOS
     ✓6th **D3A.09 Benign carcinoid tumors of other sites**
        D3A.090 Benign carcinoid tumor of the bronchus and lung
        D3A.091 Benign carcinoid tumor of the thymus

✓ Additional Character Req   ✓x7th Placeholder Alert   Manifestation   HCC CMS-HCC Condition   ▽ Unspecified Code   ▶◀ Revised Text   ● New Code   ▲ Revised Code Title

D3A.092 Benign carcinoid tumor of the **stomach**
D3A.093 Benign carcinoid tumor of the **kidney**
D3A.094 Benign carcinoid tumor of the **foregut**, ▽ unspecified
D3A.095 Benign carcinoid tumor of the **midgut**, ▽ unspecified
D3A.096 Benign carcinoid tumor of the **hindgut**, ▽ unspecified
D3A.098 Benign carcinoid tumors of other sites

D3A.8 Other benign neuroendocrine tumors
Neuroendocrine tumor NOS

Neoplasms of uncertain behavior, polycythemia vera and myelodysplastic syndromes (D37-D48)

NOTE Categories D37-D44, and D48 classify by site neoplasms of uncertain behavior, i.e., histologic confirmation whether the neoplasm is malignant or benign cannot be made.
EXCLUDES 1 neoplasms of unspecified behavior (D49.-)

D37 Neoplasm of uncertain behavior of oral cavity and digestive organs
EXCLUDES 1 stromal tumors of uncertain behavior of digestive system (D48.1)

D37.0 Neoplasm of uncertain behavior of lip, oral cavity and pharynx
EXCLUDES 1 neoplasm of uncertain behavior of aryepiglottic fold or interarytenoid fold, laryngeal aspect (D38.0)
neoplasm of uncertain behavior of epiglottis NOS (D38.0)
neoplasm of uncertain behavior of skin of lip (D48.5)
neoplasm of uncertain behavior of suprahyoid portion of epiglottis (D38.0)

D37.01 Neoplasm of uncertain behavior of **lip**
Neoplasm of uncertain behavior of vermilion border of lip
D37.02 Neoplasm of uncertain behavior of **tongue**
D37.03 Neoplasm of uncertain behavior of the **major salivary glands**
D37.030 Neoplasm of uncertain behavior of the **parotid** salivary glands
D37.031 Neoplasm of uncertain behavior of the **sublingual** salivary glands
D37.032 Neoplasm of uncertain behavior of the **submandibular** salivary glands
D37.039 Neoplasm of uncertain behavior of ▽ the major salivary glands, unspecified
D37.04 Neoplasm of uncertain behavior of the **minor salivary glands**
Neoplasm of uncertain behavior of submucosal salivary glands of lip
Neoplasm of uncertain behavior of submucosal salivary glands of cheek
Neoplasm of uncertain behavior of submucosal salivary glands of hard palate
Neoplasm of uncertain behavior of submucosal salivary glands of soft palate
D37.05 Neoplasm of uncertain behavior of **pharynx**
Neoplasm of uncertain behavior of aryepiglottic fold of pharynx NOS
Neoplasm of uncertain behavior of hypopharyngeal aspect of aryepiglottic fold of pharynx
Neoplasm of uncertain behavior of marginal zone of aryepiglottic fold of pharynx
D37.09 Neoplasm of uncertain behavior of other specified sites of the oral cavity

D37.1 Neoplasm of uncertain behavior of stomach
D37.2 Neoplasm of uncertain behavior of small intestine
D37.3 Neoplasm of uncertain behavior of appendix
D37.4 Neoplasm of uncertain behavior of colon
D37.5 Neoplasm of uncertain behavior of rectum
Neoplasm of uncertain behavior of rectosigmoid junction
D37.6 Neoplasm of uncertain behavior of liver, gallbladder and bile ducts
Neoplasm of uncertain behavior of ampulla of Vater

D37.8 Neoplasm of uncertain behavior of other specified digestive organs
Neoplasm of uncertain behavior of anal canal
Neoplasm of uncertain behavior of anal sphincter
Neoplasm of uncertain behavior of anus NOS
Neoplasm of uncertain behavior of esophagus
Neoplasm of uncertain behavior of intestine NOS
Neoplasm of uncertain behavior of pancreas
EXCLUDES 1 neoplasm of uncertain behavior of anal margin (D48.5)
neoplasm of uncertain behavior of anal skin (D48.5)
neoplasm of uncertain behavior of perianal skin (D48.5)
D37.9 Neoplasm of uncertain behavior of digestive organ, ▽ unspecified

D38 Neoplasm of uncertain behavior of middle ear and respiratory and intrathoracic organs
EXCLUDES 1 neoplasm of uncertain behavior of heart (D48.7)

D38.0 Neoplasm of uncertain behavior of larynx
Neoplasm of uncertain behavior of aryepiglottic fold or interarytenoid fold, laryngeal aspect
Neoplasm of uncertain behavior of epiglottis (suprahyoid portion)
EXCLUDES 1 neoplasm of uncertain behavior of aryepiglottic fold or interarytenoid fold NOS (D37.05)
neoplasm of uncertain behavior of hypopharyngeal aspect of aryepiglottic fold (D37.05)
neoplasm of uncertain behavior of marginal zone of aryepiglottic fold (D37.05)
D38.1 Neoplasm of uncertain behavior of trachea, bronchus and lung
D38.2 Neoplasm of uncertain behavior of pleura
D38.3 Neoplasm of uncertain behavior of mediastinum
D38.4 Neoplasm of uncertain behavior of thymus
D38.5 Neoplasm of uncertain behavior of other respiratory organs
Neoplasm of uncertain behavior of accessory sinuses
Neoplasm of uncertain behavior of cartilage of nose
Neoplasm of uncertain behavior of middle ear
Neoplasm of uncertain behavior of nasal cavities
EXCLUDES 1 neoplasm of uncertain behavior of ear (external) (skin) (D48.5)
neoplasm of uncertain behavior of nose NOS (D48.7)
neoplasm of uncertain behavior of skin of nose (D48.5)
D38.6 Neoplasm of uncertain behavior of respiratory organ, ▽ unspecified

D39 Neoplasm of uncertain behavior of female genital organs
D39.0 Neoplasm of uncertain behavior of uterus ♀
D39.1 Neoplasm of uncertain behavior of ovary
Use additional code to identify any functional activity
D39.10 Neoplasm of uncertain behavior of unspecified ♀▽ ovary
D39.11 Neoplasm of uncertain behavior of **right** ovary ♀
D39.12 Neoplasm of uncertain behavior of **left** ovary ♀
D39.2 Neoplasm of uncertain behavior of placenta Ⓜ♀
Chorioadenoma destruens
Invasive hydatidiform mole
Malignant hydatidiform mole
EXCLUDES 1 hydatidiform mole NOS (O01.9)
D39.8 Neoplasm of uncertain behavior of other specified female genital organs ♀
Neoplasm of uncertain behavior of skin of female genital organs
D39.9 Neoplasm of uncertain behavior of female genital organ, ♀▽ unspecified

D40 Neoplasm of uncertain behavior of male genital organs
D40.0 Neoplasm of uncertain behavior of prostate ♂
D40.1 Neoplasm of uncertain behavior of testis
D40.10 Neoplasm of uncertain behavior of unspecified ♂▽ testis
D40.11 Neoplasm of uncertain behavior of **right** testis ♂
D40.12 Neoplasm of uncertain behavior of **left** testis ♂
D40.8 Neoplasm of uncertain behavior of other specified male ♂ **genital organs**
Neoplasm of uncertain behavior of skin of male genital organs
D40.9 Neoplasm of uncertain behavior of male genital organ, ♂▽ unspecified

Chapter 2. Neoplasms

✓4ᵗʰ **D41 Neoplasm of uncertain behavior of urinary organs**

  ✓5ᵗʰ **D41.0 Neoplasm of uncertain behavior of kidney**
       EXCLUDES 1   *neoplasm of uncertain behavior of renal pelvis (D41.1-)*

     D41.00 Neoplasm of uncertain behavior of unspecified ▽
         kidney

     D41.01 Neoplasm of uncertain behavior of right kidney

     D41.02 Neoplasm of uncertain behavior of left kidney

  ✓5ᵗʰ **D41.1 Neoplasm of uncertain behavior of renal pelvis**

     D41.10 Neoplasm of uncertain behavior of unspecified ▽
         renal pelvis

     D41.11 Neoplasm of uncertain behavior of right renal pelvis

     D41.12 Neoplasm of uncertain behavior of left renal pelvis

  ✓5ᵗʰ **D41.2 Neoplasm of uncertain behavior of ureter**

     D41.20 Neoplasm of uncertain behavior of unspecified ▽
         ureter

     D41.21 Neoplasm of uncertain behavior of right ureter

     D41.22 Neoplasm of uncertain behavior of left ureter

  D41.3 Neoplasm of uncertain behavior of urethra

  D41.4 Neoplasm of uncertain behavior of bladder

  D41.8 Neoplasm of uncertain behavior of other specified urinary organs

  D41.9 Neoplasm of uncertain behavior of unspecified urinary ▽
  organ

✓4ᵗʰ **D42 Neoplasm of uncertain behavior of meninges**

  D42.0 Neoplasm of uncertain behavior of cerebral meninges `HCC`

  D42.1 Neoplasm of uncertain behavior of spinal meninges `HCC`

  D42.9 Neoplasm of uncertain behavior of meninges, `HCC` ▽
  unspecified

✓4ᵗʰ **D43 Neoplasm of uncertain behavior of brain and central nervous system**

       EXCLUDES 1   *neoplasm of uncertain behavior of peripheral nerves and autonomic nervous system (D48.2)*

  D43.0 Neoplasm of uncertain behavior of brain, supratentorial `HCC`
     Neoplasm of uncertain behavior of cerebral ventricle
     Neoplasm of uncertain behavior of cerebrum
     Neoplasm of uncertain behavior of frontal lobe
     Neoplasm of uncertain behavior of occipital lobe
     Neoplasm of uncertain behavior of parietal lobe
     Neoplasm of uncertain behavior of temporal lobe
     EXCLUDES 1   *neoplasm of uncertain behavior of fourth ventricle (D43.1)*

  D43.1 Neoplasm of uncertain behavior of brain, infratentorial `HCC`
     Neoplasm of uncertain behavior of brain stem
     Neoplasm of uncertain behavior of cerebellum
     Neoplasm of uncertain behavior of fourth ventricle

  D43.2 Neoplasm of uncertain behavior of brain, unspecified `HCC` ▽

  D43.3 Neoplasm of uncertain behavior of cranial nerves `HCC`

  D43.4 Neoplasm of uncertain behavior of spinal cord `HCC`

  D43.8 Neoplasm of uncertain behavior of other specified `HCC`
  parts of central nervous system

  D43.9 Neoplasm of uncertain behavior of central nervous `HCC` ▽
  system, unspecified
     Neoplasm of uncertain behavior of nervous system (central)
     NOS

✓4ᵗʰ **D44 Neoplasm of uncertain behavior of endocrine glands**

       EXCLUDES 1   *multiple endocrine adenomatosis (E31.2-)*
             multiple endocrine neoplasia (E31.2-)
             neoplasm of uncertain behavior of endocrine pancreas (D37.8)
             neoplasm of uncertain behavior of ovary (D39.1-)
             neoplasm of uncertain behavior of testis (D40.1-)
             neoplasm of uncertain behavior of thymus (D38.4)

  D44.0 Neoplasm of uncertain behavior of thyroid gland

  ✓5ᵗʰ **D44.1 Neoplasm of uncertain behavior of adrenal gland**
     Use additional code to identify any functional activity

     D44.10 Neoplasm of uncertain behavior of unspecified ▽
         adrenal gland

     D44.11 Neoplasm of uncertain behavior of right adrenal
         gland

     D44.12 Neoplasm of uncertain behavior of left adrenal
         gland

  D44.2 Neoplasm of uncertain behavior of parathyroid gland

  D44.3 Neoplasm of uncertain behavior of pituitary gland `HCC`
     Use additional code to identify any functional activity

  D44.4 Neoplasm of uncertain behavior of craniopharyngeal `HCC`
  duct

  D44.5 Neoplasm of uncertain behavior of pineal gland `HCC`

  D44.6 Neoplasm of uncertain behavior of carotid body `HCC`

  D44.7 Neoplasm of uncertain behavior of aortic body and `HCC`
  other paraganglia

  D44.9 Neoplasm of uncertain behavior of unspecified ▽
  endocrine gland

D45 Polycythemia vera `HCC`
       EXCLUDES 1   *familial polycythemia (D75.0)*
             secondary polycythemia (D75.1)
  DEF: Abnormal proliferation of all bone marrow elements, increased red cell mass, and total blood volume; unknown etiology, frequently associated with splenomegaly, leukocytosis, and thrombocythemia.

✓4ᵗʰ **D46 Myelodysplastic syndromes**
   Use additional code for adverse effect, if applicable, to identify drug (T36-T50 with fifth or sixth character 5)
       EXCLUDES 2   *drug-induced aplastic anemia (D61.1)*

  D46.0 Refractory anemia without ring sideroblasts, so stated `HCC`
     Refractory anemia without sideroblasts, without excess of blasts

  D46.1 Refractory anemia with ring sideroblasts `HCC`
     RARS

  ✓5ᵗʰ **D46.2 Refractory anemia with excess of blasts [RAEB]**

     D46.20 Refractory anemia with excess of blasts, `HCC` ▽
         unspecified
         RAEB NOS

     D46.21 Refractory anemia with excess of blasts 1 `HCC`
         RAEB 1

     D46.22 Refractory anemia with excess of blasts 2 `HCC`
         RAEB 2

  D46.A Refractory cytopenia with multilineage dysplasia `HCC`

  D46.B Refractory cytopenia with multilineage dysplasia `HCC`
  and ring sideroblasts
     RCMD RS

  D46.C Myelodysplastic syndrome with isolated del(5q) `HCC`
  chromosomal abnormality
     Myelodysplastic syndrome with 5q deletion
     5q minus syndrome NOS

  D46.4 Refractory anemia, unspecified `HCC` ▽

  D46.Z Other myelodysplastic syndromes `HCC`
       EXCLUDES 1   *chronic myelomonocytic leukemia (C93.1-)*

  D46.9 Myelodysplastic syndrome, unspecified `HCC` ▽
     Myelodysplasia NOS

✓4ᵗʰ **D47 Other neoplasms of uncertain behavior of lymphoid, hematopoietic and related tissue**

▲   ✓5ᵗʰ **D47.0 Mast cell neoplasms of uncertain behavior**
     ~~Indolent systemic mastocytosis~~
     ~~Mast cell tumor NOS~~
     ~~Mastocytoma NOS~~
       EXCLUDES 1 ▶*congenital cutaneous mastocytosis (Q82.2-)*
             histiocytic neoplasms of uncertain behavior (D47.Z9)
             malignant mast cell neoplasm (C96.2-)◀
             ~~*mastocytosis (congenital) (cutaneous) (Q82.2)*~~

●   **D47.01 Cutaneous mastocytosis**
         Diffuse cutaneous mastocytosis
         Maculopapular cutaneous mastocytosis
         Solitary mastocytoma
         Telangiectasia macularis eruptiva perstans
         Urticaria pigmentosa
           EXCLUDES 1   *congenital (diffuse) (maculopapular) cutaneous mastocytosis (Q82.2)*
                 congenital urticaria pigmentosa (Q82.2)
                 extracutaneous mastocytoma (D47.09)

✓ Additional Character Req   ✓ˣ⁷ᵗʰ Placeholder Alert   Manifestation   `HCC` CMS-HCC Condition   ▽ Unspecified Code   ▶◀ Revised Text   ● New Code   ▲ Revised Code Title

Chapter 2. Neoplasms *(side tab)*

●   **D47.02**   **Systemic mastocytosis**
Indolent systemic mastocytosis
Isolated bone marrow mastocytosis
Smoldering systemic mastocytosis
Systemic mastocytosis, with an associated
    hematological non-mast cell lineage disease
    (SM-AHNMD)
Code also, if applicable, any associated hematological
    non-mast cell lineage disease, such as:
    acute myeloid leukemia (C92.6-, C92.A-)
    chronic myelomonocytic leukemia (C93.1-)
    essential thrombocytosis (D47.3)
    hypereosinophilic syndrome (D72.1)
    myelodysplastic syndrome (D46.9)
    myeloproliferative syndrome (D47.1)
    non-Hodgkin lymphoma (C82-C85)
    plasma cell myeloma (C90.0-)
    polycythemia vera (D45)
    EXCLUDES 1   *aggressive systemic mastocytosis (C96.21)*
         mast cell leukemia (C94.3-)

●   **D47.09**   **Other mast cell neoplasms of uncertain behavior**
Extracutaneous mastocytoma
Mast cell tumor NOS
Mastocytoma NOS
Mastocytosis NOS

D47.1   **Chronic myeloproliferative disease**   `HCC`
Chronic neutrophilic leukemia
Myeloproliferative disease, unspecified
    EXCLUDES 1   *atypical chronic myeloid leukemia BCR/ABL-negative*
         (C92.2-)
         chronic myeloid leukemia BCR/ABL-positive (C92.1-)
         myelofibrosis NOS (D75.81)
         myelophthisic anemia (D61.82)
         myelophthisis (D61.82)
         secondary myelofibrosis NOS (D75.81)

D47.2   **Monoclonal gammopathy**
Monoclonal gammopathy of undetermined significance [MGUS]

D47.3   **Essential (hemorrhagic) thrombocythemia**   `HCC`
Essential thrombocytosis
Idiopathic hemorrhagic thrombocythemia

D47.4   **Osteomyelofibrosis**   `HCC`
Chronic idiopathic myelofibrosis
Myelofibrosis (idiopathic) (with myeloid metaplasia)
Myelosclerosis (megakaryocytic) with myeloid metaplasia
Secondary myelofibrosis in myeloproliferative disease
    EXCLUDES 1   *acute myelofibrosis (C94.4-)*

✓5th   **D47.Z**   **Other specified neoplasms of uncertain behavior of lymphoid, hematopoietic and related tissue**

D47.Z1   **Post-transplant lymphoproliferative**   `HCC`
disorder (PTLD)
Code first complications of transplanted organs and
    tissue (T86.-)
DEF: Excessive proliferation of B-cell lymphocytes
following Epstein-Barr virus infection in organ
transplant patients; may progress to non-Hodgkin
lymphoma.

D47.Z2   **Castleman disease**   `HCC`
Code also if applicable human herpesvirus 8 infection
    (B10.89)
    EXCLUDES 2   *Kaposi's sarcoma (C46-)*

D47.Z9   **Other specified neoplasms of uncertain**   `HCC`
behavior of lymphoid, hematopoietic and related tissue
Histiocytic tumors of uncertain behavior

D47.9   **Neoplasm of uncertain behavior of lymphoid,**   `HCC` ▽
hematopoietic and related tissue, unspecified
Lymphoproliferative disease NOS

✓4th   **D48**   **Neoplasm of uncertain behavior of other and unspecified sites**
    EXCLUDES 1   *neurofibromatosis (nonmalignant) (Q85.0-)*

D48.0   **Neoplasm of uncertain behavior of bone and articular cartilage**
    EXCLUDES 1   *neoplasm of uncertain behavior of cartilage of ear*
         (D48.1)
         neoplasm of uncertain behavior of cartilage of larynx
         (D38.0)
         neoplasm of uncertain behavior of cartilage of nose
         (D38.5)
         neoplasm of uncertain behavior of connective tissue of
         eyelid (D48.1)
         neoplasm of uncertain behavior of synovia (D48.1)

D48.1   **Neoplasm of uncertain behavior of connective and other soft tissue**
Neoplasm of uncertain behavior of connective tissue of ear
Neoplasm of uncertain behavior of connective tissue of eyelid
Stromal tumors of uncertain behavior of digestive system
    EXCLUDES 1   *neoplasm of uncertain behavior of articular cartilage*
         (D48.0)
         neoplasm of uncertain behavior of cartilage of larynx
         (D38.0)
         neoplasm of uncertain behavior of cartilage of nose
         (D38.5)
         neoplasm of uncertain behavior of connective tissue of
         breast (D48.6-)

D48.2   **Neoplasm of uncertain behavior of peripheral nerves and autonomic nervous system**
    EXCLUDES 1   *neoplasm of uncertain behavior of peripheral nerves of*
         orbit (D48.7)

D48.3   **Neoplasm of uncertain behavior of retroperitoneum**

D48.4   **Neoplasm of uncertain behavior of peritoneum**

D48.5   **Neoplasm of uncertain behavior of skin**
Neoplasm of uncertain behavior of anal margin
Neoplasm of uncertain behavior of anal skin
Neoplasm of uncertain behavior of perianal skin
Neoplasm of uncertain behavior of skin of breast
    EXCLUDES 1   *neoplasm of uncertain behavior of anus NOS (D37.8)*
         neoplasm of uncertain behavior of skin of genital
         organs (D39.8, D40.8)
         neoplasm of uncertain behavior of vermilion border of
         lip (D37.0)

✓5th   **D48.6**   **Neoplasm of uncertain behavior of breast**
Neoplasm of uncertain behavior of connective tissue of breast
Cystosarcoma phyllodes
    EXCLUDES 1   *neoplasm of uncertain behavior of skin of breast*
         (D48.5)

D48.60   **Neoplasm of uncertain behavior of unspecified**   ▽
breast

D48.61   **Neoplasm of uncertain behavior of right breast**

D48.62   **Neoplasm of uncertain behavior of left breast**

D48.7   **Neoplasm of uncertain behavior of other specified sites**
Neoplasm of uncertain behavior of eye
Neoplasm of uncertain behavior of heart
Neoplasm of uncertain behavior of peripheral nerves of orbit
    EXCLUDES 1   *neoplasm of uncertain behavior of connective tissue*
         (D48.1)
         neoplasm of uncertain behavior of skin of eyelid
         (D48.5)

D48.9   **Neoplasm of uncertain behavior, unspecified**   ▽

Neoplasms of unspecified behavior (D49)

✓4th   **D49**   **Neoplasms of unspecified behavior**
    `NOTE`   Category D49 classifies by site neoplasms of unspecified
         morphology and behavior. The term "mass", unless
         otherwise stated, is not to be regarded as a neoplastic
         growth.
    `INCLUDES`   "growth" NOS
         neoplasm NOS
         new growth NOS
         tumor NOS
    EXCLUDES 1   *neoplasms of uncertain behavior (D37-D44, D48)*

D49.0   **Neoplasm of unspecified behavior of digestive system**
    EXCLUDES 1   *neoplasm of unspecified behavior of margin of anus*
         (D49.2)
         neoplasm of unspecified behavior of perianal skin
         (D49.2)
         neoplasm of unspecified behavior of skin of anus
         (D49.2)

D49.1   **Neoplasm of unspecified behavior of respiratory system**

EXCLUDES 1 Not coded here   *EXCLUDES 2* Not included here   `N` Newborn Age: 0   `P` Pediatric Age: 0-17   `M` Maternity Age: 12-55   `A` Adult Age: 15-124

492   ICD-10-CM 2018

D47.02–D49.1 *(side tab)*

D49.2 **Neoplasm of unspecified behavior of bone, soft tissue, and skin**

> EXCLUDES 1   *neoplasm of unspecified behavior of anal canal (D49.0)*
> *neoplasm of unspecified behavior of anus NOS (D49.0)*
> *neoplasm of unspecified behavior of bone marrow (D49.89)*
> *neoplasm of unspecified behavior of cartilage of larynx (D49.1)*
> *neoplasm of unspecified behavior of cartilage of nose (D49.1)*
> *neoplasm of unspecified behavior of connective tissue of breast (D49.3)*
> *neoplasm of unspecified behavior of skin of genital organs (D49.59)*
> *neoplasm of unspecified behavior of vermilion border of lip (D49.0)*

D49.3 **Neoplasm of unspecified behavior of breast**

> EXCLUDES 1   *neoplasm of unspecified behavior of skin of breast (D49.2)*

D49.4 **Neoplasm of unspecified behavior of bladder**

✓5ᵗʰ D49.5 **Neoplasm of unspecified behavior of other genitourinary organs**

     ✓6ᵗʰ D49.51 **Neoplasm of unspecified behavior of kidney**

        D49.511 **Neoplasm of unspecified behavior of right kidney**

        D49.512 **Neoplasm of unspecified behavior of left kidney**

        D49.519 **Neoplasm of unspecified behavior of unspecified kidney** ▽

     D49.59 **Neoplasm of unspecified behavior of other genitourinary organ**

D49.6 **Neoplasm of unspecified behavior of brain**   HCC

> EXCLUDES 1   *neoplasm of unspecified behavior of cerebral meninges (D49.7)*
> *neoplasm of unspecified behavior of cranial nerves (D49.7)*

D49.7 **Neoplasm of unspecified behavior of endocrine glands and other parts of nervous system**

> EXCLUDES 1   *neoplasm of unspecified behavior of peripheral, sympathetic, and parasympathetic nerves and ganglia (D49.2)*

✓5ᵗʰ D49.8 **Neoplasm of unspecified behavior of other specified sites**

> EXCLUDES 1   *neoplasm of unspecified behavior of eyelid (skin) (D49.2)*
> *neoplasm of unspecified behavior of eyelid cartilage (D49.2)*
> *neoplasm of unspecified behavior of great vessels (D49.2)*
> *neoplasm of unspecified behavior of optic nerve (D49.7)*

     D49.81 **Neoplasm of unspecified behavior of retina and choroid**
        Dark area on retina
        Retinal freckle

     D49.89 **Neoplasm of unspecified behavior of other specified sites**

D49.9 **Neoplasm of unspecified behavior of unspecified site** ▽

☑ Additional Character Req   ✓x7ᵗʰ Placeholder Alert   Manifestation   HCC CMS-HCC Condition   ▽ Unspecified Code   ►◄ Revised Text   ● New Code   ▲ Revised Code Title

ICD-10-CM 2018   493

Chapter 3. Disease of the Blood and Blood-Forming Organs and Certain Disorders Involving the Immune Mechanism (D50–D89)

Chapter Specific Coding Guidelines and Examples
Reserved for future guideline expansion.

Chapter 3. Disease of the Blood and Blood-Forming Organs *(left margin)*

D50–D56.1 *(left margin)*

Chapter 3. Diseases of the Blood and Blood-forming Organs and Certain Disorders Involving the Immune Mechanism (D50-D89)

EXCLUDES 2   *autoimmune disease (systemic) NOS (M35.9)*
certain conditions originating in the perinatal period (P00-P96)
complications of pregnancy, childbirth and the puerperium (O00-O9A)
congenital malformations, deformations and chromosomal abnormalities (Q00-Q99)
endocrine, nutritional and metabolic diseases (E00-E88)
human immunodeficiency virus [HIV] disease (B20)
injury, poisoning and certain other consequences of external causes (S00-T88)
neoplasms (C00-D49)
symptoms, signs and abnormal clinical and laboratory findings, not elsewhere classified (R00-R94)

This chapter contains the following blocks:

D50-D53   Nutritional anemias
D55-D59   Hemolytic anemias
D60-D64   Aplastic and other anemias and other bone marrow failure syndromes
D65-D69   Coagulation defects, purpura and other hemorrhagic conditions
D70-D77   Other disorders of blood and blood-forming organs
D78   Intraoperative and postprocedural complications of the spleen
D80-D89   Certain disorders involving the immune mechanism

Nutritional anemias (D50-D53)

✓4th D50   Iron deficiency anemia
INCLUDES   asiderotic anemia
      hypochromic anemia

D50.0   Iron deficiency anemia secondary to blood loss (chronic)
Posthemorrhagic anemia (chronic)
EXCLUDES 1   *acute posthemorrhagic anemia (D62)*
      congenital anemia from fetal blood loss (P61.3)

D50.1   Sideropenic dysphagia
Kelly-Paterson syndrome
Plummer-Vinson syndrome

D50.8   Other iron deficiency anemias
Iron deficiency anemia due to inadequate dietary iron intake

D50.9   Iron deficiency anemia, unspecified   ▽

✓4th D51   Vitamin B12 deficiency anemia
EXCLUDES 1   *vitamin B12 deficiency (E53.8)*

D51.0   Vitamin B12 deficiency anemia due to intrinsic factor deficiency
Addison anemia
Biermer anemia
Pernicious (congenital) anemia
Congenital intrinsic factor deficiency
DEF: Chronic progressive anemia due to vitamin B12 malabsorption; caused by lack of secretion of intrinsic factor, which is produced by the gastric mucosa of the stomach.

D51.1   Vitamin B12 deficiency anemia due to selective vitamin B12 malabsorption with proteinuria
Imerslund (Gräsbeck) syndrome
Megaloblastic hereditary anemia

D51.2   Transcobalamin II deficiency

D51.3   Other dietary vitamin B12 deficiency anemia
Vegan anemia

D51.8   Other vitamin B12 deficiency anemias

D51.9   Vitamin B12 deficiency anemia, unspecified   ▽

✓4th D52   Folate deficiency anemia
EXCLUDES 1   *folate deficiency without anemia (E53.8)*

D52.0   Dietary folate deficiency anemia
Nutritional megaloblastic anemia
DEF: The result of a poor diet with inadequate intake of folate, which is needed to produce healthy red blood cells.

D52.1   Drug-induced folate deficiency anemia
Use additional code for adverse effect, if applicable, to identify drug (T36-T50 with fifth or sixth character 5)

D52.8   Other folate deficiency anemias

D52.9   Folate deficiency anemia, unspecified   ▽
Folic acid deficiency anemia NOS

✓4th D53   Other nutritional anemias
INCLUDES   megaloblastic anemia unresponsive to vitamin B12 or folate therapy

D53.0   Protein deficiency anemia
Amino-acid deficiency anemia
Orotaciduric anemia
EXCLUDES 1   *Lesch-Nyhan syndrome (E79.1)*

D53.1   Other megaloblastic anemias, not elsewhere classified
Megaloblastic anemia NOS
EXCLUDES 1   *Di Guglielmo's disease (C94.0)*

D53.2   Scorbutic anemia
EXCLUDES 1   *scurvy (E54)*

D53.8   Other specified nutritional anemias
Anemia associated with deficiency of copper
Anemia associated with deficiency of molybdenum
Anemia associated with deficiency of zinc
EXCLUDES 1   *nutritional deficiencies without anemia, such as:*
      copper deficiency NOS (E61.0)
      molybdenum deficiency NOS (E61.5)
      zinc deficiency NOS (E60)

D53.9   Nutritional anemia, unspecified   ▽
Simple chronic anemia
EXCLUDES 1   *anemia NOS (D64.9)*

Hemolytic anemias (D55-D59)

✓4th D55   Anemia due to enzyme disorders
EXCLUDES 1   *drug-induced enzyme deficiency anemia (D59.2)*

D55.0   Anemia due to glucose-6-phosphate dehydrogenase [G6PD] deficiency   HCC
Favism
G6PD deficiency anemia

D55.1   Anemia due to other disorders of glutathione metabolism   HCC
Anemia (due to) enzyme deficiencies, except G6PD, related to the hexose monophosphate [HMP] shunt pathway
Anemia (due to) hemolytic nonspherocytic (hereditary), type I

D55.2   Anemia due to disorders of glycolytic enzymes   HCC
Hemolytic nonspherocytic (hereditary) anemia, type II
Hexokinase deficiency anemia
Pyruvate kinase [PK] deficiency anemia
Triose-phosphate isomerase deficiency anemia
EXCLUDES 1   *disorders of glycolysis not associated with anemia (E74.8)*

D55.3   Anemia due to disorders of nucleotide metabolism   HCC

D55.8   Other anemias due to enzyme disorders   HCC

D55.9   Anemia due to enzyme disorder, unspecified   HCC ▽

✓4th D56   Thalassemia
EXCLUDES 1   *sickle-cell thalassemia (D57.4-)*

D56.0   Alpha thalassemia   HCC
Alpha thalassemia major
Hemoglobin H Constant Spring
Hemoglobin H disease
Hydrops fetalis due to alpha thalassemia
Severe alpha thalassemia
Triple gene defect alpha thalassemia
Use additional code, if applicable, for hydrops fetalis due to alpha thalassemia (P56.99)
EXCLUDES 1   *alpha thalassemia trait or minor (D56.3)*
      asymptomatic alpha thalassemia (D56.3)
      hydrops fetalis due to isoimmunization (P56.0)
      hydrops fetalis not due to immune hemolysis (P83.2)
DEF: HBA1 and HBA2 genetic variant of chromosome 16 prevalent among those of African and Southeast Asian descent; associated with a wide spectrum of anemic presentation; includes hemoglobin H disease subtypes.

D56.1   Beta thalassemia   HCC
Beta thalassemia major
Cooley's anemia
Homozygous beta thalassemia
Severe beta thalassemia
Thalassemia intermedia
Thalassemia major
EXCLUDES 1   *beta thalassemia minor (D56.3)*
      beta thalassemia trait (D56.3)
      delta-beta thalassemia (D56.2)
      hemoglobin E-beta thalassemia (D56.5)
      sickle-cell beta thalassemia (D57.4-)

EXCLUDES 1   Not coded here   EXCLUDES 2   Not included here   N Newborn Age: 0   P Pediatric Age: 0-17   M Maternity Age: 12-55   A Adult Age: 15-124

496   ICD-10-CM 2018

Thalassemia

Misshapen RBC

Misshapen RBC

Healthy RBC

Sickle cell

Sickle cells

Normal RBCs

D56.2 Delta-beta thalassemia   HCC
     Homozygous delta-beta thalassemia
     EXCLUDES 1   *delta-beta thalassemia minor (D56.3)*
                 delta-beta thalassemia trait (D56.3)

D56.3 Thalassemia minor
     Alpha thalassemia minor
     Alpha thalassemia silent carrier
     Alpha thalassemia trait
     Beta thalassemia minor
     Beta thalassemia trait
     Delta-beta thalassemia minor
     Delta-beta thalassemia trait
     Thalassemia trait NOS
     EXCLUDES 1   *alpha thalassemia (D56.Ø)*
                 beta thalassemia (D56.1)
                 delta-beta thalassemia (D56.2)
                 hemoglobin E-beta thalassemia (D56.5)
                 sickle-cell trait (D57.3)
     DEF: Solitary abnormal gene that identifies a carrier of the disease, yet with an absence of symptoms or a clinically mild anemic presentation.

D56.4 Hereditary persistence of fetal hemoglobin [HPFH]   HCC

D56.5 Hemoglobin E-beta thalassemia   HCC
     EXCLUDES 1   *beta thalassemia (D56.1)*
                 beta thalassemia minor (D56.3)
                 beta thalassemia trait (D56.3)
                 delta-beta thalassemia (D56.2)
                 delta-beta thalassemia trait (D56.3)
                 hemoglobin E disease (D58.2)
                 other hemoglobinopathies (D58.2)
                 sickle-cell beta thalassemia (D57.4-)

D56.8 Other thalassemias   HCC
     Dominant thalassemia
     Hemoglobin C thalassemia
     Mixed thalassemia
     Thalassemia with other hemoglobinopathy
     EXCLUDES 1   *hemoglobin C disease (D58.2)*
                 hemoglobin E disease (D58.2)
                 other hemoglobinopathies (D58.2)
                 sickle-cell anemia (D57.-)
                 sickle-cell thalassemia (D57.4)

D56.9 Thalassemia, unspecified   ▽
     Mediterranean anemia (with other hemoglobinopathy)

✓4ᵗʰ **D57 Sickle-cell disorders**
     Use additional code for any associated fever (R5Ø.81)
     EXCLUDES 1   *other hemoglobinopathies (D58.-)*

✓5ᵗʰ **D57.Ø Hb-SS disease with crisis**
     Sickle-cell disease NOS with crisis
     Hb-SS disease with vasoocclusive pain
     D57.ØØ Hb-SS disease with crisis, unspecified   HCC ▽
     D57.Ø1 Hb-SS disease with acute chest syndrome   HCC
     D57.Ø2 Hb-SS disease with splenic sequestration   HCC
     D57.1 Sickle-cell disease without crisis   HCC ▽
         Hb-SS disease without crisis
         Sickle-cell anemia NOS
         Sickle-cell disease NOS
         Sickle-cell disorder NOS

✓5ᵗʰ **D57.2 Sickle-cell/Hb-C disease**
     Hb-SC disease
     Hb-S/Hb-C disease
     D57.2Ø Sickle-cell/Hb-C disease without crisis   HCC ▽
   ✓6ᵗʰ **D57.21 Sickle-cell/Hb-C disease with crisis**
         D57.211 Sickle-cell/Hb-C disease with acute chest syndrome   HCC
         D57.212 Sickle-cell/Hb-C disease with splenic sequestration   HCC
         D57.219 Sickle-cell/Hb-C disease with crisis, unspecified   HCC ▽
             Sickle-cell/Hb-C disease with crisis NOS

D57.3 Sickle-cell trait   HCC
     Hb-S trait
     Heterozygous hemoglobin S
     DEF: Heterozygous genetic makeup characterized by one gene for normal hemoglobin and one for sickle-cell hemoglobin; clinical disease rarely present.

✓5ᵗʰ **D57.4 Sickle-cell thalassemia**
     Sickle-cell beta thalassemia
     Thalassemia Hb-S disease
     D57.4Ø Sickle-cell thalassemia without crisis   HCC ▽
         Microdrepanocytosis
         Sickle-cell thalassemia NOS
   ✓6ᵗʰ **D57.41 Sickle-cell thalassemia with crisis**
         Sickle-cell thalassemia with vasoocclusive pain
         D57.411 Sickle-cell thalassemia with acute chest syndrome   HCC
         D57.412 Sickle-cell thalassemia with splenic sequestration   HCC
         D57.419 Sickle-cell thalassemia with crisis, unspecified   HCC ▽
             Sickle-cell thalassemia with crisis NOS

✓5ᵗʰ **D57.8 Other sickle-cell disorders**
     Hb-SD disease
     Hb-SE disease
     D57.8Ø Other sickle-cell disorders without crisis   HCC ▽
   ✓6ᵗʰ **D57.81 Other sickle-cell disorders with crisis**
         D57.811 Other sickle-cell disorders with acute chest syndrome   HCC
         D57.812 Other sickle-cell disorders with splenic sequestration   HCC
         D57.819 Other sickle-cell disorders with crisis, unspecified   HCC ▽
             Other sickle-cell disorders with crisis NOS

✓4ᵗʰ **D58 Other hereditary hemolytic anemias**
     EXCLUDES 1   *hemolytic anemia of the newborn (P55.-)*

D58.Ø Hereditary spherocytosis   HCC
     Acholuric (familial) jaundice
     Congenital (spherocytic) hemolytic icterus
     Minkowski-Chauffard syndrome

D58.1 Hereditary elliptocytosis   HCC
     Elliptocytosis (congenital)
     Ovalocytosis (congenital) (hereditary)

☑ Additional Character Req   ☑7ᵗʰ Placeholder Alert   Manifestation   HCC CMS-HCC Condition   ▽ Unspecified Code   ▶◀ Revised Text   ● New Code   ▲ Revised Code Title

ICD-10-CM 2018   497

D58.2 Other hemoglobinopathies `HCC`
Abnormal hemoglobin NOS
Congenital Heinz body anemia
Hb-C disease
Hb-D disease
Hb-E disease
Hemoglobinopathy NOS
Unstable hemoglobin hemolytic disease
> `EXCLUDES 1` *familial polycythemia (D75.0)*
> *Hb-M disease (D74.0)*
> *hemoglobin E-beta thalassemia (D56.5)*
> *hereditary persistence of fetal hemoglobin [HPFH]*
> *(D56.4)*
> *high-altitude polycythemia (D75.1)*
> *methemoglobinemia (D74.-)*
> *other hemoglobinopathies with thalassemia (D56.8)*

D58.8 Other specified hereditary hemolytic anemias `HCC`
Stomatocytosis

D58.9 Hereditary hemolytic anemia, unspecified `HCC` ▽

✓4ᵗʰ **D59 Acquired hemolytic anemia**
> **DEF:** Non-hereditary anemia characterized by premature destruction of
> red blood cells; caused by infectious organisms, poisons, and physical
> agents.

D59.0 Drug-induced autoimmune hemolytic anemia `HCC`
Use additional code for adverse effect, if applicable, to identify
drug (T36-T50 with fifth or sixth character 5)

D59.1 Other autoimmune hemolytic anemias `HCC`
Autoimmune hemolytic disease (cold type) (warm type)
Chronic cold hemagglutinin disease
Cold agglutinin disease
Cold agglutinin hemoglobinuria
Cold type (secondary) (symptomatic) hemolytic anemia
Warm type (secondary) (symptomatic) hemolytic anemia
> `EXCLUDES 1` *Evans syndrome (D69.41)*
> *hemolytic disease of newborn (P55.-)*
> *paroxysmal cold hemoglobinuria (D59.6)*

D59.2 Drug-induced nonautoimmune hemolytic anemia `HCC`
Drug-induced enzyme deficiency anemia
Use additional code for adverse effect, if applicable, to identify
drug (T36-T50 with fifth or sixth character 5)

D59.3 Hemolytic-uremic syndrome `HCC`
Use additional code to identify associated:
E. coli infection (B96.2-)
Pneumococcal pneumonia (J13)
Shigella dysenteriae (A03.9)

D59.4 Other nonautoimmune hemolytic anemias `HCC`
Mechanical hemolytic anemia
Microangiopathic hemolytic anemia
Toxic hemolytic anemia

D59.5 Paroxysmal nocturnal hemoglobinuria `HCC`
[Marchiafava-Micheli]
> `EXCLUDES 1` *hemoglobinuria NOS (R82.3)*

D59.6 Hemoglobinuria due to hemolysis from other `HCC`
external causes
Hemoglobinuria from exertion
March hemoglobinuria
Paroxysmal cold hemoglobinuria
Use additional code (Chapter 20) to identify external cause
> `EXCLUDES 1` *hemoglobinuria NOS (R82.3)*

D59.8 Other acquired hemolytic anemias `HCC`

D59.9 Acquired hemolytic anemia, unspecified `HCC` ▽
Idiopathic hemolytic anemia, chronic

Aplastic and other anemias and other bone marrow failure syndromes (D60-D64)

✓4ᵗʰ **D60 Acquired pure red cell aplasia [erythroblastopenia]**
> `INCLUDES` red cell aplasia (acquired) (adult) (with thymoma)
> `EXCLUDES 1` *congenital red cell aplasia (D61.01)*

D60.0 Chronic acquired pure red cell aplasia `HCC`

D60.1 Transient acquired pure red cell aplasia `HCC`

D60.8 Other acquired pure red cell aplasias `HCC`

D60.9 Acquired pure red cell aplasia, unspecified `HCC` ▽

✓4ᵗʰ **D61 Other aplastic anemias and other bone marrow failure**
syndromes
> `EXCLUDES 1` *neutropenia (D70.-)*
> **AHA:** 2014, 4Q, 22

✓5ᵗʰ **D61.0 Constitutional aplastic anemia**
D61.01 Constitutional (pure) red blood cell aplasia `HCC`
Blackfan-Diamond syndrome
Congenital (pure) red cell aplasia
Familial hypoplastic anemia
Primary (pure) red cell aplasia
Red cell (pure) aplasia of infants
> `EXCLUDES 1` *acquired red cell aplasia (D60.9)*

D61.09 Other constitutional aplastic anemia `HCC`
Fanconi's anemia
Pancytopenia with malformations

D61.1 Drug-induced aplastic anemia `HCC`
Use additional code for adverse effect, if applicable, to identify
drug (T36-T50 with fifth or sixth character 5)

D61.2 Aplastic anemia due to other external agents `HCC`
Code first, if applicable, toxic effects of substances chiefly
nonmedicinal as to source (T51-T65)

D61.3 Idiopathic aplastic anemia `HCC`

✓5ᵗʰ **D61.8 Other specified aplastic anemias and other bone marrow**
failure syndromes

✓6ᵗʰ **D61.81 Pancytopenia**
> `EXCLUDES 1` *pancytopenia (due to) (with) aplastic anemia*
> *(D61.9)*
> *pancytopenia (due to) (with) bone marrow*
> *infiltration (D61.82)*
> *pancytopenia (due to) (with) congenital*
> *(pure) red cell aplasia (D61.01)*
> *pancytopenia (due to) (with) hairy cell*
> *leukemia (C91.4-)*
> *pancytopenia (due to) (with) human*
> *immunodeficiency virus disease (B20)*
> *pancytopenia (due to) (with)*
> *leukoerythroblastic anemia (D61.82)*
> *pancytopenia (due to) (with)*
> *myeloproliferative disease (D47.1)*
> `EXCLUDES 2` *pancytopenia (due to) (with) myelodysplastic*
> *syndromes (D46.-)*
> **DEF:** Occurs when a person has a shortage of all three
> blood cells: white, red, and platelets.

D61.810 Antineoplastic chemotherapy `HCC`
induced pancytopenia
> `EXCLUDES 2` *aplastic anemia due to*
> *antineoplastic*
> *chemotherapy (D61.1)*

D61.811 Other drug-induced pancytopenia `HCC`
> `EXCLUDES 2` *aplastic anemia due to drugs*
> *(D61.1)*

D61.818 Other pancytopenia `HCC`

D61.82 Myelophthisis `HCC`
Leukoerythroblastic anemia
Myelophthisic anemia
Panmyelophthisis
Code also the underlying disorder, such as:
malignant neoplasm of breast (C50.-)
tuberculosis (A15.-)
> `EXCLUDES 1` *idiopathic myelofibrosis (D47.1)*
> *myelofibrosis NOS (D75.81)*
> *myelofibrosis with myeloid metaplasia*
> *(D47.4)*
> *primary myelofibrosis (D47.1)*
> *secondary myelofibrosis (D75.81)*

D61.89 Other specified aplastic anemias and other `HCC`
bone marrow failure syndromes

D61.9 Aplastic anemia, unspecified `HCC` ▽
Hypoplastic anemia NOS
Medullary hypoplasia

D62 Acute posthemorrhagic anemia
> `EXCLUDES 1` *anemia due to chronic blood loss (D50.0)*
> *blood loss anemia NOS (D50.0)*
> *congenital anemia from fetal blood loss (P61.3)*

`EXCLUDES 1` Not coded here   `EXCLUDES 2` Not included here   **N** Newborn Age: 0   **P** Pediatric Age: 0-17   **M** Maternity Age: 12-55   **A** Adult Age: 15-124

498   ICD-10-CM 2018

✓4ᵗʰ **D63 Anemia in chronic diseases classified elsewhere**

  D63.0 *Anemia in neoplastic disease*
    Code first neoplasm (C00-D49)
    EXCLUDES 1 ~~anemia due to antineoplastic chemotherapy (D64.81)~~
        aplastic anemia due to antineoplastic chemotherapy
        (D61.1)
    EXCLUDES 2 ▶anemia due to antineoplastic chemotherapy
        (D64.81)◀

  D63.1 *Anemia in chronic kidney disease*
    Erythropoietin resistant anemia (EPO resistant anemia)
    Code first underlying chronic kidney disease (CKD) (N18.-)

  D63.8 *Anemia in other chronic diseases classified elsewhere*
    Code first underlying disease, such as:
      diphyllobothriasis (B70.0)
      hookworm disease (B76.0-B76.9)
      hypothyroidism (E00.0-E03.9)
      malaria (B50.0-B54)
      symptomatic late syphilis (A52.79)
      tuberculosis (A18.89)

✓4ᵗʰ **D64 Other anemias**

  EXCLUDES 1 refractory anemia (D46.-)
        refractory anemia with excess blasts in transformation
        [RAEB T] (C92.0-)

  D64.0 Hereditary sideroblastic anemia   HCC
    Sex-linked hypochromic sideroblastic anemia

  D64.1 *Secondary sideroblastic anemia due to disease*   HCC
    Code first underlying disease

  D64.2 Secondary sideroblastic anemia due to drugs and toxins   HCC
    Code first poisoning due to drug or toxin, if applicable (T36-T65
    with fifth or sixth character 1-4 or 6)
    Use additional code for adverse effect, if applicable, to identify
    drug (T36-T50 with fifth or sixth character 5)

  D64.3 Other sideroblastic anemias   HCC
    Sideroblastic anemia NOS
    Pyridoxine-responsive sideroblastic anemia NEC

  D64.4 Congenital dyserythropoietic anemia
    Dyshematopoietic anemia (congenital)
    EXCLUDES 1 Blackfan-Diamond syndrome (D61.01)
        Di Guglielmo's disease (C94.0)

✓5ᵗʰ **D64.8 Other specified anemias**

    D64.81 Anemia due to antineoplastic chemotherapy
      Antineoplastic chemotherapy induced anemia
      EXCLUDES 1 aplastic anemia due to antineoplastic
        chemotherapy (D61.1)
      EXCLUDES 2 anemia in neoplastic disease (D63.0)
      AHA: 2014, 4Q, 22
      DEF: Reversible adverse effect of chemotherapy,
      causing inhibition of bone marrow production; decrease
      in red blood cell production prevents adequate
      oxygenation of the tissues and organs causing fatigue,
      SOB, and exacerbation of other medical conditions.

    D64.89 Other specified anemias
      Infantile pseudoleukemia

  D64.9 Anemia, unspecified   ▽
    AHA: 2017, 1Q, 7

Coagulation defects, purpura and other hemorrhagic conditions (D65-D69)

D65 Disseminated intravascular coagulation [defibrination syndrome]   HCC
    Afibrinogenemia, acquired
    Consumption coagulopathy
    Diffuse or disseminated intravascular coagulation [DIC]
    Fibrinolytic hemorrhage, acquired
    Fibrinolytic purpura
    Purpura fulminans
    EXCLUDES 1 disseminated intravascular coagulation (complicating):
        abortion or ectopic or molar pregnancy (O00-O07, O08.1)
        in newborn (P60)
        pregnancy, childbirth and the puerperium (O45.0, O46.0,
        O67.0, O72.3)

Coagulation

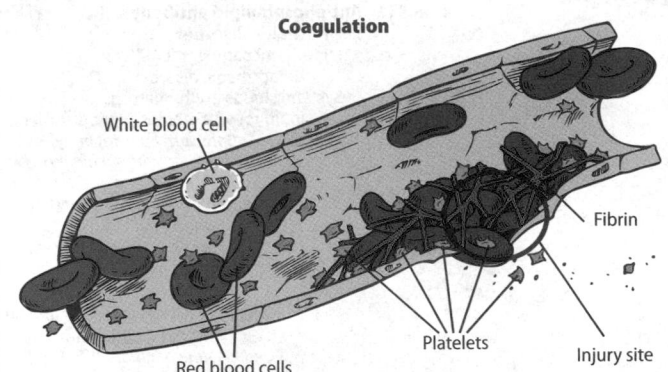

White blood cell   Fibrin   Platelets   Injury site   Red blood cells

D66 Hereditary factor VIII deficiency   HCC
    Classical hemophilia
    Deficiency factor VIII (with functional defect)
    Hemophilia A
    Hemophilia NOS
    EXCLUDES 1 factor VIII deficiency with vascular defect (D68.0)
    DEF: Hereditary, sex-linked lack of antihemophilic globulin (AHG) (factor
    VIII); causes abnormal coagulation characterized by increased bleeding,
    large bruises of skin, bleeding in mouth, nose, gastrointestinal tract;
    hemorrhages into joints, resulting in swelling and impaired function.

D67 Hereditary factor IX deficiency   HCC
    Christmas disease
    Factor IX deficiency (with functional defect)
    Hemophilia B
    Plasma thromboplastin component [PTC] deficiency

✓4ᵗʰ **D68 Other coagulation defects**

  EXCLUDES 1 abnormal coagulation profile (R79.1)
        coagulation defects complicating abortion or ectopic or molar
        pregnancy (O00-O07, O08.1)
        coagulation defects complicating pregnancy, childbirth and the
        puerperium (O45.0, O46.0, O67.0, O72.3)
  AHA: 2016, 1Q, 14

  D68.0 Von Willebrand's disease   HCC
    Angiohemophilia
    Factor VIII deficiency with vascular defect
    Vascular hemophilia
    EXCLUDES 1 capillary fragility (hereditary) (D69.8)
        factor VIII deficiency NOS (D66)
        factor VIII deficiency with functional defect (D66)
    DEF: Abnormal blood coagulation caused by deficient blood
    factor VII; congenital; symptoms include excess or prolonged
    bleeding.

  D68.1 Hereditary factor XI deficiency   HCC
    Hemophilia C
    Plasma thromboplastin antecedent [PTA] deficiency
    Rosenthal's disease

  D68.2 Hereditary deficiency of other clotting factors   HCC
    AC globulin deficiency
    Congenital afibrinogenemia
    Deficiency of factor I [fibrinogen]
    Deficiency of factor II [prothrombin]
    Deficiency of factor V [labile]
    Deficiency of factor VII [stable]
    Deficiency of factor X [Stuart-Prower]
    Deficiency of factor XII [Hageman]
    Deficiency of factor XIII [fibrin stabilizing]
    Dysfibrinogenemia (congenital)
    Hypoproconvertinemia
    Owren's disease
    Proaccelerin deficiency

✓5ᵗʰ **D68.3 Hemorrhagic disorder due to circulating anticoagulants**

    ✓6ᵗʰ **D68.31 Hemorrhagic disorder due to intrinsic circulating anticoagulants, antibodies, or inhibitors**

      D68.311 Acquired hemophilia   HCC
        Autoimmune hemophilia
        Autoimmune inhibitors to clotting factors
        Secondary hemophilia

✓ Additional Character Req   ✓x7ᵗʰ Placeholder Alert   Manifestation   HCC CMS-HCC Condition   ▽ Unspecified Code   ▶◀ Revised Text   ● New Code   ▲ Revised Code Title

ICD-10-CM 2018   **499**

Chapter 3. Disease of the Blood and Blood-Forming Organs (side margin)

D68.312 **Antiphospholipid antibody with hemorrhagic disorder** `HCC`
  Lupus anticoagulant (LAC) with hemorrhagic disorder
  Systemic lupus erythematosus [SLE] inhibitor with hemorrhagic disorder
  EXCLUDES 1   *antiphospholipid antibody, finding without diagnosis (R76.0)*
    antiphospholipid antibody syndrome (D68.61)
    antiphospholipid antibody with hypercoagulable state (D68.61)
    lupus anticoagulant (LAC) finding without diagnosis (R76.0)
    lupus anticoagulant (LAC) with hypercoagulable state (D68.62)
    systemic lupus erythematosus [SLE] inhibitor finding without diagnosis (R76.0)
    systemic lupus erythematosus [SLE] inhibitor with hypercoagulable state (D68.62)

D68.318 **Other hemorrhagic disorder due to intrinsic circulating anticoagulants, antibodies, or inhibitors** `HCC`
  Antithromboplastinemia
  Antithromboplastinogenemia
  Hemorrhagic disorder due to intrinsic increase in antithrombin
  Hemorrhagic disorder due to intrinsic increase in anti-VIIIa
  Hemorrhagic disorder due to intrinsic increase in anti-IXa
  Hemorrhagic disorder due to intrinsic increase in anti-XIa

D68.32 **Hemorrhagic disorder due to extrinsic circulating anticoagulants** `HCC`
  Drug-induced hemorrhagic disorder
  Hemorrhagic disorder due to increase in anti-IIa
  Hemorrhagic disorder due to increase in anti-Xa
  Hyperheparinemia
  Use additional code for adverse effect, if applicable, to identify drug (T45.515, T45.525)
  AHA: 2016, 1Q, 14-15

D68.4 **Acquired coagulation factor deficiency** `HCC`
  Deficiency of coagulation factor due to liver disease
  Deficiency of coagulation factor due to vitamin K deficiency
  EXCLUDES 1   *vitamin K deficiency of newborn (P53)*

✓5th **D68.5** **Primary thrombophilia**
  Primary hypercoagulable states
  EXCLUDES 1   *antiphospholipid syndrome (D68.61)*
    lupus anticoagulant (D68.62)
    secondary activated protein C resistance (D68.69)
    secondary antiphospholipid antibody syndrome (D68.69)
    secondary lupus anticoagulant with hypercoagulable state (D68.69)
    secondary systemic lupus erythematosus [SLE] inhibitor with hypercoagulable state (D68.69)
    systemic lupus erythematosus [SLE] inhibitor finding without diagnosis (R76.0)
    systemic lupus erythematosus [SLE] inhibitor with hemorrhagic disorder (D68.312)
    thrombotic thrombocytopenic purpura (M31.1)

D68.51 **Activated protein C resistance** `HCC`
  Factor V Leiden mutation

D68.52 **Prothrombin gene mutation** `HCC`

D68.59 **Other primary thrombophilia** `HCC`
  Antithrombin III deficiency
  Hypercoagulable state NOS
  Primary hypercoagulable state NEC
  Primary thrombophilia NEC
  Protein C deficiency
  Protein S deficiency
  Thrombophilia NOS

✓5th **D68.6** **Other thrombophilia**
  Other hypercoagulable states
  EXCLUDES 1   *diffuse or disseminated intravascular coagulation [DIC] (D65)*
    heparin induced thrombocytopenia (HIT) (D75.82)
    hyperhomocysteinemia (E72.11)

D68.61 **Antiphospholipid syndrome** `HCC`
  Anticardiolipin syndrome
  Antiphospholipid antibody syndrome
  EXCLUDES 1   *antiphospholipid antibody, finding without diagnosis (R76.0)*
    antiphospholipid antibody with hemorrhagic disorder (D68.312)
    lupus anticoagulant syndrome (D68.62)

D68.62 **Lupus anticoagulant syndrome** `HCC`
  Lupus anticoagulant
  Presence of systemic lupus erythematosus [SLE] inhibitor
  EXCLUDES 1   *anticardiolipin syndrome (D68.61)*
    antiphospholipid syndrome (D68.61)
    lupus anticoagulant (LAC) finding without diagnosis (R76.0)
    lupus anticoagulant (LAC) with hemorrhagic disorder (D68.312)

D68.69 **Other thrombophilia** `HCC`
  Hypercoagulable states NEC
  Secondary hypercoagulable state NOS

D68.8 **Other specified coagulation defects** `HCC`
  EXCLUDES 1   *hemorrhagic disease of newborn (P53)*

D68.9 **Coagulation defect, unspecified** `HCC` ▽

✓4th **D69** **Purpura and other hemorrhagic conditions**
  EXCLUDES 1   *benign hypergammaglobulinemic purpura (D89.0)*
    cryoglobulinemic purpura (D89.1)
    essential (hemorrhagic) thrombocythemia (D47.3)
    hemorrhagic thrombocythemia (D47.3)
    purpura fulminans (D65)
    thrombotic thrombocytopenic purpura (M31.1)
    Waldenström hypergammaglobulinemic purpura (D89.0)

D69.0 **Allergic purpura** `HCC`
  Allergic vasculitis
  Nonthrombocytopenic hemorrhagic purpura
  Nonthrombocytopenic idiopathic purpura
  Purpura anaphylactoid
  Purpura Henoch(-Schönlein)
  Purpura rheumatica
  Vascular purpura
  EXCLUDES 1   *thrombocytopenic hemorrhagic purpura (D69.3)*
  DEF: Any hemorrhagic condition, thrombocytic or nonthrombocytopenic in origin, caused by a presumed allergic reaction.

D69.1 **Qualitative platelet defects** `HCC`
  Bernard-Soulier [giant platelet] syndrome
  Glanzmann's disease
  Grey platelet syndrome
  Thromboasthenia (hemorrhagic) (hereditary)
  Thrombocytopathy
  EXCLUDES 1   *von Willebrand's disease (D68.0)*

D69.2 **Other nonthrombocytopenic purpura** `HCC`
  Purpura NOS
  Purpura simplex
  Senile purpura

D69.3 **Immune thrombocytopenic purpura** `HCC`
  Hemorrhagic (thrombocytopenic) purpura
  Idiopathic thrombocytopenic purpura
  Tidal platelet dysgenesis
  DEF: Tidal platelet dysgenesis: Platelet counts fluctuate from normal to very low within periods of 20 to 40 days and may involve autoimmune platelet destruction.

✓5th **D69.4** **Other primary thrombocytopenia**
  EXCLUDES 1   *transient neonatal thrombocytopenia (P61.0)*
    Wiskott-Aldrich syndrome (D82.0)

D69.41 **Evans syndrome** `HCC`

D69.42 **Congenital and hereditary thrombocytopenia purpura** `HCC`
  Congenital thrombocytopenia
  Hereditary thrombocytopenia
  Code first congenital or hereditary disorder, such as: thrombocytopenia with absent radius (TAR syndrome) (Q87.2)

D69.49 **Other primary thrombocytopenia** `HCC`
  Megakaryocytic hypoplasia
  Primary thrombocytopenia NOS

EXCLUDES 1 Not coded here   *EXCLUDES 2* Not included here   **N** Newborn Age: 0   **P** Pediatric Age: 0-17   **M** Maternity Age: 12-55   **A** Adult Age: 15-124

500
ICD-10-CM 2018

√5th **D69.5 Secondary thrombocytopenia**
   EXCLUDES 1   *heparin induced thrombocytopenia (HIT) (D75.82)*
           transient thrombocytopenia of newborn (P61.0)

   D69.51 Posttransfusion purpura
       Posttransfusion purpura from whole blood (fresh) or
           blood products
       PTP

   D69.59 Other secondary thrombocytopenia
       AHA: 2014, 4Q, 22

D69.6 Thrombocytopenia, unspecified   HCC ▽

D69.8 Other specified hemorrhagic conditions   HCC
     Capillary fragility (hereditary)
     Vascular pseudohemophilia

D69.9 Hemorrhagic condition, unspecified   HCC ▽

Other disorders of blood and blood-forming organs (D70-D77)

√4th **D70 Neutropenia**
   INCLUDES   agranulocytosis
          decreased absolute neurophile count (ANC)
   Use additional code for any associated:
     fever (R50.81)
     mucositis (J34.81, K12.3-, K92.81, N76.81)
   EXCLUDES 1   *neutropenic splenomegaly (D73.81)*
          transient neonatal neutropenia (P61.5)

   D70.0 Congenital agranulocytosis   HCC
     Congenital neutropenia   Kostmann's disease
     Infantile genetic agranulocytosis

   D70.1 Agranulocytosis secondary to cancer chemotherapy   HCC
     Code also underlying neoplasm
     Use additional code for adverse effect, if applicable, to identify
         drug (T45.1X5)
     AHA: 2014, 4Q, 22

   D70.2 Other drug-induced agranulocytosis   HCC
     Use additional code for adverse effect, if applicable, to identify
         drug (T36-T50 with fifth or sixth character 5)

   D70.3 Neutropenia due to infection   HCC

   D70.4 Cyclic neutropenia   HCC
     Cyclic hematopoiesis
     Periodic neutropenia

   D70.8 Other neutropenia   HCC

   D70.9 Neutropenia, unspecified   HCC ▽

D71 Functional disorders of polymorphonuclear neutrophils   HCC
     Cell membrane receptor complex [CR3] defect
     Chronic (childhood) granulomatous disease
     Congenital dysphagocytosis
     Progressive septic granulomatosis

√4th **D72 Other disorders of white blood cells**
   EXCLUDES 1   *basophilia (D72.824)*
          immunity disorders (D80-D89)
          neutropenia (D70)
          preleukemia (syndrome) (D46.9)

   D72.0 Genetic anomalies of leukocytes   HCC
     Alder (granulation) (granulocyte) anomaly
     Alder syndrome
     Hereditary leukocytic hypersegmentation
     Hereditary leukocytic hyposegmentation
     Hereditary leukomelanopathy
     May-Hegglin (granulation) (granulocyte) anomaly
     May-Hegglin syndrome
     Pelger-Huët (granulation) (granulocyte) anomaly
     Pelger-Huët syndrome
     EXCLUDES 1   *Chédiak (-Steinbrinck)-Higashi syndrome (E70.330)*

   D72.1 Eosinophilia
     Allergic eosinophilia   Hereditary eosinophilia
     EXCLUDES 1   *Löffler's syndrome (J82)*
          pulmonary eosinophilia (J82)

√5th **D72.8 Other specified disorders of white blood cells**
     EXCLUDES 1   *leukemia (C91-C95)*

   √6th **D72.81 Decreased white blood cell count**
       EXCLUDES 1   *neutropenia (D70.-)*

     D72.810 Lymphocytopenia
         Decreased lymphocytes

     D72.818 Other decreased white blood cell count
         Basophilic leukopenia
         Eosinophilic leukopenia
         Monocytopenia
         Other decreased leukocytes
         Plasmacytopenia

     D72.819 Decreased white blood cell count, unspecified ▽
         Decreased leukocytes, unspecified
         Leukocytopenia, unspecified
         Leukopenia
         EXCLUDES 1   *malignant leukopenia (D70.9)*

   √6th **D72.82 Elevated white blood cell count**
       EXCLUDES 1   *eosinophilia (D72.1)*

     D72.820 Lymphocytosis (symptomatic)
         Elevated lymphocytes

     D72.821 Monocytosis (symptomatic)
         EXCLUDES 1   *infectious mononucleosis (B27.-)*

     D72.822 Plasmacytosis

     D72.823 Leukemoid reaction
         Basophilic leukemoid reaction
         Leukemoid reaction NOS
         Lymphocytic leukemoid reaction
         Monocytic leukemoid reaction
         Myelocytic leukemoid reaction
         Neutrophilic leukemoid reaction

     D72.824 Basophilia

     D72.825 Bandemia
         Bandemia without diagnosis of specific
            infection
         EXCLUDES 1   *confirmed infection—code to*
            infection
            leukemia (C91.-, C92.-, C93.-,
              C94.-, C95.-)
         DEF: Increase in early neutrophil cells, called
            band cells; may indicate infection.

     D72.828 Other elevated white blood cell count

     D72.829 Elevated white blood cell count, unspecified ▽
         Elevated leukocytes, unspecified
         Leukocytosis, unspecified

   D72.89 Other specified disorders of white blood cells
     Abnormality of white blood cells NEC

   D72.9 Disorder of white blood cells, unspecified ▽
     Abnormal leukocyte differential NOS

√4th **D73 Diseases of spleen**
   D73.0 Hyposplenism
     Atrophy of spleen
     EXCLUDES 1   *asplenia (congenital) (Q89.01)*
          postsurgical absence of spleen (Z90.81)

   D73.1 Hypersplenism
     EXCLUDES 1   *neutropenic splenomegaly (D73.81)*
          primary splenic neutropenia (D73.81)
          splenitis, splenomegaly in late syphilis (A52.79)
          splenitis, splenomegaly in tuberculosis (A18.85)
          splenomegaly NOS (R16.1)
          splenomegaly congenital (Q89.0)

   D73.2 Chronic congestive splenomegaly

   D73.3 Abscess of spleen

   D73.4 Cyst of spleen

   D73.5 Infarction of spleen
     Splenic rupture, nontraumatic
     Torsion of spleen
     EXCLUDES 1   *rupture of spleen due to Plasmodium vivax malaria*
          (B51.0)
          traumatic rupture of spleen (S36.03-)

   √5th **D73.8 Other diseases of spleen**
     D73.81 Neutropenic splenomegaly
         Werner-Schultz disease

     D73.89 Other diseases of spleen
         Fibrosis of spleen NOS
         Perisplenitis
         Splenitis NOS

   D73.9 Disease of spleen, unspecified ▽

√4th **D74 Methemoglobinemia**
   D74.0 Congenital methemoglobinemia
     Congenital NADH-methemoglobin reductase deficiency
     Hemoglobin-M [Hb-M] disease
     Methemoglobinemia, hereditary

   D74.8 Other methemoglobinemias
     Acquired methemoglobinemia (with sulfhemoglobinemia)
     Toxic methemoglobinemia

   D74.9 Methemoglobinemia, unspecified ▽

☑ Additional Character Req   √x7th Placeholder Alert   Manifestation   HCC CMS-HCC Condition   ▽ Unspecified Code   ►◄ Revised Text   ● New Code   ▲ Revised Code Title

ICD-10-CM 2018   501

✓4th **D75** **Other and unspecified diseases of blood and blood-forming organs**

> EXCLUDES 2 *acute lymphadenitis (L04.-)*
> *chronic lymphadenitis (I88.1)*
> *enlarged lymph nodes (R59.-)*
> *hypergammaglobulinemia NOS (D89.2)*
> *lymphadenitis NOS (I88.9)*
> *mesenteric lymphadenitis (acute) (chronic) (I88.0)*

D75.0 **Familial erythrocytosis**
Benign polycythemia
Familial polycythemia
> EXCLUDES 1 *hereditary ovalocytosis (D58.1)*

D75.1 **Secondary polycythemia**
Acquired polycythemia
Emotional polycythemia
Erythrocytosis NOS
Hypoxemic polycythemia
Nephrogenous polycythemia
Polycythemia due to erythropoietin
Polycythemia due to fall in plasma volume
Polycythemia due to high altitude
Polycythemia due to stress
Polycythemia NOS
Relative polycythemia
> EXCLUDES 1 *polycythemia neonatorum (P61.1)*
> *polycythemia vera (D45)*

DEF: Elevated number of red blood cells in circulating blood as a result of reduced oxygen supply to the tissues.

✓5th **D75.8** **Other specified diseases of blood and blood-forming organs**

D75.81 **Myelofibrosis**   HCC
Myelofibrosis NOS
Secondary myelofibrosis NOS
Code first the underlying disorder, such as:
  malignant neoplasm of breast (C50.-)
Use additional code, if applicable, for associated therapy-related myelodysplastic syndrome (D46.-)
Use additional code for adverse effect, if applicable, to identify drug (T45.1X5)
> EXCLUDES 1 *acute myelofibrosis (C94.4-)*
> *idiopathic myelofibrosis (D47.1)*
> *leukoerythroblastic anemia (D61.82)*
> *myelofibrosis with myeloid metaplasia (D47.4)*
> *myelophthisic anemia (D61.82)*
> *myelophthisis (D61.82)*
> *primary myelofibrosis (D47.1)*

D75.82 **Heparin induced thrombocytopenia (HIT)**   HCC
DEF: Immune-mediated reaction to heparin therapy causing an abrupt fall in platelet count and serious complications such as pulmonary embolism, stroke, AMI, or DVT.

D75.89 **Other specified diseases of blood and blood-forming organs**

D75.9 **Disease of blood and blood-forming organs, unspecified**   ▽

✓4th **D76** **Other specified diseases with participation of lymphoreticular and reticulohistiocytic tissue**

> EXCLUDES 1 *(Abt-) Letterer-Siwe disease (C96.0)*
> *eosinophilic granuloma (C96.6)*
> *Hand-Schüller-Christian disease (C96.5)*
> *histiocytic medullary reticulosis (C96.9)*
> *histiocytic sarcoma (C96.A)*
> *histiocytosis X, multifocal (C96.5)*
> *histiocytosis X, unifocal (C96.6)*
> *Langerhans-cell histiocytosis, multifocal (C96.5)*
> *Langerhans-cell histiocytosis NOS (C96.6)*
> *Langerhans-cell histiocytosis, unifocal (C96.6)*
> *leukemic reticuloendotheliosis (C91.4-)*
> *lipomelanotic reticulosis (I89.8)*
> *malignant histiocytosis (C96.A)*
> *malignant reticulosis (C86.0)*
> *nonlipid reticuloendotheliosis (C96.0)*

D76.1 **Hemophagocytic lymphohistiocytosis**   HCC
Familial hemophagocytic reticulosis
Histiocytoses of mononuclear phagocytes

D76.2 **Hemophagocytic syndrome, infection-associated**   HCC
Use additional code to identify infectious agent or disease

D76.3 **Other histiocytosis syndromes**   HCC
Reticulohistiocytoma (giant-cell)
Sinus histiocytosis with massive lymphadenopathy
Xanthogranuloma

✓4th **D77** **Other disorders of blood and blood-forming organs in diseases classified elsewhere**
Code first underlying disease, such as:
  amyloidosis (E85.-)
  congenital early syphilis (A50.0)
  echinococcosis (B67.0-B67.9)
  malaria (B50.0-B54)
  schistosomiasis [bilharziasis] (B65.0-B65.9)
  vitamin C deficiency (E54)
> EXCLUDES 1 *rupture of spleen due to Plasmodium vivax malaria (B51.0)*
> *splenitis, splenomegaly in late syphilis (A52.79)*
> *splenitis, splenomegaly in tuberculosis (A18.85)*

Intraoperative and postprocedural complications of the spleen (D78)

✓4th **D78** **Intraoperative and postprocedural complications of the spleen**

✓5th **D78.0** **Intraoperative hemorrhage and hematoma of the spleen complicating a procedure**
> EXCLUDES 1 *intraoperative hemorrhage and hematoma of the spleen due to accidental puncture or laceration during a procedure (D78.1-)*

D78.01 **Intraoperative hemorrhage and hematoma of the spleen complicating a procedure on the spleen**

D78.02 **Intraoperative hemorrhage and hematoma of the spleen complicating other procedure**

✓5th **D78.1** **Accidental puncture and laceration of the spleen during a procedure**

D78.11 **Accidental puncture and laceration of the spleen during a procedure on the spleen**

D78.12 **Accidental puncture and laceration of the spleen during other procedure**

✓5th **D78.2** **Postprocedural hemorrhage of the spleen following a procedure**

D78.21 **Postprocedural hemorrhage of the spleen following a procedure on the spleen**

D78.22 **Postprocedural hemorrhage of the spleen following other procedure**

✓5th **D78.3** **Postprocedural hematoma and seroma of the spleen following a procedure**

D78.31 **Postprocedural hematoma of the spleen following a procedure on the spleen**

D78.32 **Postprocedural hematoma of the spleen following other procedure**

D78.33 **Postprocedural seroma of the spleen following a procedure on the spleen**

D78.34 **Postprocedural seroma of the spleen following other procedure**

✓5th **D78.8** **Other intraoperative and postprocedural complications of the spleen**
Use additional code, if applicable, to further specify disorder

D78.81 **Other intraoperative complications of the spleen**

D78.89 **Other postprocedural complications of the spleen**

Certain disorders involving the immune mechanism (D80-D89)

> INCLUDES defects in the complement system
> immunodeficiency disorders, except human immunodeficiency virus [HIV] disease
> sarcoidosis

> EXCLUDES 1 *autoimmune disease (systemic) NOS (M35.9)*
> *functional disorders of polymorphonuclear neutrophils (D71)*
> *human immunodeficiency virus [HIV] disease (B20)*

✓4th **D80** **Immunodeficiency with predominantly antibody defects**

D80.0 **Hereditary hypogammaglobulinemia**   HCC
Autosomal recessive agammaglobulinemia (Swiss type)
X-linked agammaglobulinemia [Bruton] (with growth hormone deficiency)

D80.1 **Nonfamilial hypogammaglobulinemia**   HCC
Agammaglobulinemia with immunoglobulin-bearing B-lymphocytes
Common variable agammaglobulinemia [CVAgamma]
Hypogammaglobulinemia NOS

D80.2 **Selective deficiency of immunoglobulin A [IgA]**   HCC

D80.3 **Selective deficiency of immunoglobulin G [IgG] subclasses**   HCC

D80.4 **Selective deficiency of immunoglobulin M [IgM]**   HCC

D80.5 **Immunodeficiency with increased immunoglobulin M [IgM]**   HCC

EXCLUDES 1 Not coded here   EXCLUDES 2 Not included here   N Newborn Age: 0   P Pediatric Age: 0-17   M Maternity Age: 12-55   A Adult Age: 15-124

502   ICD-10-CM 2018

D80.6 Antibody deficiency with near-normal immunoglobulins or with hyperimmunoglobulinemia `HCC`

D80.7 Transient hypogammaglobulinemia of infancy `HCC`

D80.8 Other immunodeficiencies with predominantly antibody defects `HCC`
Kappa light chain deficiency

D80.9 Immunodeficiency with predominantly antibody defects, unspecified `HCC` ▽

✓4ᵗʰ **D81 Combined immunodeficiencies**
EXCLUDES 1   *autosomal recessive agammaglobulinemia (Swiss type) (D80.0)*

D81.0 Severe combined immunodeficiency [SCID] with reticular dysgenesis `HCC`

D81.1 Severe combined immunodeficiency [SCID] with low T- and B-cell numbers `HCC`

D81.2 Severe combined immunodeficiency [SCID] with low or normal B-cell numbers `HCC`

D81.3 Adenosine deaminase [ADA] deficiency `HCC`

D81.4 Nezelof's syndrome `HCC`

D81.5 Purine nucleoside phosphorylase [PNP] deficiency `HCC`

D81.6 Major histocompatibility complex class I deficiency `HCC`
Bare lymphocyte syndrome

D81.7 Major histocompatibility complex class II deficiency `HCC`

✓5ᵗʰ **D81.8 Other combined immunodeficiencies**

    ✓6ᵗʰ **D81.81 Biotin-dependent carboxylase deficiency**
Multiple carboxylase deficiency
EXCLUDES 1   *biotin-dependent carboxylase deficiency due to dietary deficiency of biotin (E53.8)*

       D81.810 Biotinidase deficiency

       D81.818 Other biotin-dependent carboxylase deficiency
Holocarboxylase synthetase deficiency
Other multiple carboxylase deficiency

       D81.819 Biotin-dependent carboxylase deficiency, unspecified ▽
Multiple carboxylase deficiency, unspecified

    D81.89 Other combined immunodeficiencies `HCC`

D81.9 Combined immunodeficiency, unspecified `HCC` ▽
Severe combined immunodeficiency disorder [SCID] NOS

✓4ᵗʰ **D82 Immunodeficiency associated with other major defects**
EXCLUDES 1   *ataxia telangiectasia [Louis-Bar] (G11.3)*

D82.0 Wiskott-Aldrich syndrome `HCC`
Immunodeficiency with thrombocytopenia and eczema

D82.1 Di George's syndrome `HCC`
Pharyngeal pouch syndrome
Thymic alymphoplasia
Thymic aplasia or hypoplasia with immunodeficiency

D82.2 Immunodeficiency with short-limbed stature `HCC`

D82.3 Immunodeficiency following hereditary defective response to Epstein-Barr virus `HCC`
X-linked lymphoproliferative disease

D82.4 Hyperimmunoglobulin E [IgE] syndrome `HCC`

D82.8 Immunodeficiency associated with other specified major defects `HCC`

D82.9 Immunodeficiency associated with major defect, unspecified `HCC` ▽

✓4ᵗʰ **D83 Common variable immunodeficiency**

D83.0 Common variable immunodeficiency with predominant abnormalities of B-cell numbers and function `HCC`

D83.1 Common variable immunodeficiency with predominant immunoregulatory T-cell disorders `HCC`

D83.2 Common variable immunodeficiency with autoantibodies to B- or T-cells `HCC`

D83.8 Other common variable immunodeficiencies `HCC`

D83.9 Common variable immunodeficiency, unspecified `HCC` ▽

✓4ᵗʰ **D84 Other immunodeficiencies**

D84.0 Lymphocyte function antigen-1 [LFA-1] defect `HCC`

D84.1 Defects in the complement system `HCC`
C1 esterase inhibitor [C1-INH] deficiency

D84.8 Other specified immunodeficiencies `HCC`

D84.9 Immunodeficiency, unspecified `HCC` ▽

✓4ᵗʰ **D86 Sarcoidosis**

D86.0 Sarcoidosis of lung `HCC`

D86.1 Sarcoidosis of lymph nodes

D86.2 Sarcoidosis of lung with sarcoidosis of lymph nodes `HCC`

D86.3 Sarcoidosis of skin

✓5ᵗʰ **D86.8 Sarcoidosis of other sites**

    D86.81 Sarcoid meningitis

    D86.82 Multiple cranial nerve palsies in sarcoidosis `HCC`

    D86.83 Sarcoid iridocyclitis

    D86.84 Sarcoid pyelonephritis
Tubulo-interstitial nephropathy in sarcoidosis

    D86.85 Sarcoid myocarditis

    D86.86 Sarcoid arthropathy
Polyarthritis in sarcoidosis

    D86.87 Sarcoid myositis

    D86.89 Sarcoidosis of other sites
Hepatic granuloma
Uveoparotid fever [Heerfordt]

D86.9 Sarcoidosis, unspecified ▽

✓4ᵗʰ **D89 Other disorders involving the immune mechanism, not elsewhere classified**
EXCLUDES 1   *hyperglobulinemia NOS (R77.1)*
monoclonal gammopathy (of undetermined significance) (D47.2)
EXCLUDES 2   *transplant failure and rejection (T86.-)*

D89.0 Polyclonal hypergammaglobulinemia
Benign hypergammaglobulinemic purpura
Polyclonal gammopathy NOS

D89.1 Cryoglobulinemia `HCC`
Cryoglobulinemic purpura   Mixed cryoglobulinemia
Cryoglobulinemic vasculitis   Primary cryoglobulinemia
Essential cryoglobulinemia   Secondary cryoglobulinemia
Idiopathic cryoglobulinemia

D89.2 Hypergammaglobulinemia, unspecified ▽

D89.3 Immune reconstitution syndrome `HCC`
Immune reconstitution inflammatory syndrome [IRIS]
Use additional code for adverse effect, if applicable, to identify drug (T36-T50 with fifth or sixth character 5)

✓5ᵗʰ **D89.4 Mast cell activation syndrome and related disorders**
EXCLUDES 1   *aggressive systemic mastocytosis ►(C96.21)◄*
    ►congenital cutaneous mastocytosis◄ (Q82.2)
    ►(non-congenital) cutaneous mastocytosis (D47.01)
    (indolent) systemic mastocytosis (D47.02)
    malignant mast cell neoplasm (C96.2-)◄
    malignant mastocytoma ►(C96.29)◄
    mast cell leukemia (C94.3-)
    ►mast cell sarcoma (C96.22)
    mastocytoma NOS (D47.09)
    other mast cell neoplasms of uncertain behavior (D47.09)◄
    systemic mastocytosis associated with a clonal hematologic non-mast cell lineage disease (SM-AHNMD)►(D47.02)◄

    D89.40 Mast cell activation, unspecified `HCC` ▽
Mast cell activation disorder, unspecified
Mast cell activation syndrome, NOS

    D89.41 Monoclonal mast cell activation syndrome `HCC`

    D89.42 Idiopathic mast cell activation syndrome `HCC`

    D89.43 Secondary mast cell activation `HCC`
Secondary mast cell activation syndrome
Code also underlying etiology, if known

    D89.49 Other mast cell activation disorder `HCC`
Other mast cell activation syndrome

✓5ᵗʰ **D89.8 Other specified disorders involving the immune mechanism, not elsewhere classified**

    ✓6ᵗʰ **D89.81 Graft-versus-host disease**
Code first underlying cause, such as:
    complications of transplanted organs and tissue (T86.-)
    complications of blood transfusion (T80.89)
Use additional code to identify associated manifestations, such as:
    desquamative dermatitis (L30.8)
    diarrhea (R19.7)
    elevated bilirubin (R17)
    hair loss (L65.9)

       D89.810 Acute graft-versus-host disease `HCC`

       D89.811 Chronic graft-versus-host disease `HCC`

       D89.812 Acute on chronic graft-versus-host disease `HCC`

       D89.813 Graft-versus-host disease, unspecified `HCC` ▽

☑ Additional Character Req   ✓x7ᵗʰ Placeholder Alert   Manifestation   `HCC` CMS-HCC Condition   ▽ Unspecified Code   ►◄ Revised Text   ● New Code   ▲ Revised Code Title

D89.82   Autoimmune lymphoproliferative syndrome   `HCC`
        [ALPS]
        DEF: Rare genetic alteration of the Fas protein; impairs
        normal cellular apoptosis (normal cell death), causing
        abnormal accumulation of lymphocytes in the lymph
        glands, liver, and spleen; symptoms include
        neutropenia, anemia, and thrombocytopenia.

D89.89   Other specified disorders involving the immune   `HCC`
        mechanism, not elsewhere classified
            EXCLUDES 1   *human immunodeficiency virus disease (B2Ø)*

D89.9   Disorder involving the immune mechanism,   `HCC` ▽
        unspecified
        Immune disease NOS
        AHA: 2015, 3Q, 22

Chapter 4. Endocrine, Nutritional, and Metabolic Diseases (E00–E89)

Chapter Specific Guidelines with Coding Examples

The chapter specific guidelines from the ICD-10-CM Official Guidelines for Coding and Reporting have been provided below. Along with these guidelines are coding examples, contained in the shaded boxes, that have been developed to help illustrate the coding and/or sequencing guidance found in these guidelines.

a. Diabetes mellitus

The diabetes mellitus codes are combination codes that include the type of diabetes mellitus, the body system affected, and the complications affecting that body system. As many codes within a particular category as are necessary to describe all of the complications of the disease may be used. They should be sequenced based on the reason for a particular encounter. Assign as many codes from categories E08–E13 as needed to identify all of the associated conditions that the patient has.

> Patient is seen for uncontrolled diabetes, type 2, with diabetic nephropathy and diabetic gastroparesis.
>
> | | |
> |---|---|
> | E11.65 | Type 2 diabetes mellitus with hyperglycemia |
> | E11.21 | Type 2 diabetes mellitus with diabetic nephropathy |
> | E11.43 | Type 2 diabetes mellitus with diabetic automomic (poly)neuropathy |
>
> *Explanation*: Use as many codes to describe the diabetic complications as needed. Many are combination codes that describe more than one condition. Code first the reason for the encounter. "Uncontrolled" is described as "with hyperglycemia."

1) Type of diabetes

The age of a patient is not the sole determining factor, though most type 1 diabetics develop the condition before reaching puberty. For this reason type 1 diabetes mellitus is also referred to as juvenile diabetes.

> A 45-year-old patient is diagnosed with type 1 diabetes
>
> | | |
> |---|---|
> | E10.9 | Type 1 diabetes mellitus without complications |
>
> *Explanation*: Although most type 1 diabetics are diagnosed in childhood or adolescence, it can also begin in adults.

2) Type of diabetes mellitus not documented

If the type of diabetes mellitus is not documented in the medical record the default is E11.-, Type 2 diabetes mellitus.

> Office visit lists diabetic retinopathy with macular edema and hypertension on patient problem list
>
> | | |
> |---|---|
> | E11.311 | Type 2 diabetes mellitus with unspecified diabetic retinopathy with macular edema |
> | I10 | Essential (primary) hypertension |
>
> *Explanation*: Since the type of diabetes was not documented, default to category E11.

3) Diabetes mellitus and the use of insulin and oral hypoglycemics

If the documentation in a medical record does not indicate the type of diabetes but does indicate that the patient uses insulin, code E11, Type 2 diabetes mellitus, should be assigned. Code Z79.4, Long-term (current) use of insulin, or Z79.84, Long term (current) use of oral hypoglycemic drugs, should also be assigned to indicate that the patient uses insulin or hypoglycemic drugs. Code Z79.4 should not be assigned if insulin is given temporarily to bring a type 2 patient's blood sugar under control during an encounter.

> Office visit lists chronic diabetes with daily insulin use on patient problem list
>
> | | |
> |---|---|
> | E11.9 | Type 2 diabetes mellitus without complications |
> | Z79.4 | Long term (current) use of insulin |
>
> *Explanation*: Do not assume that a patient on insulin must have type 1 diabetes. The default for diabetes without further specification defaults to type 2. Add the code for long term use of insulin.

4) Diabetes mellitus in pregnancy and gestational diabetes

See Section I.C.15. Diabetes mellitus in pregnancy.

See Section I.C.15. Gestational (pregnancy induced) diabetes

5) Complications due to insulin pump malfunction

(a) Underdose of insulin due to insulin pump failure

An underdose of insulin due to an insulin pump failure should be assigned to a code from subcategory T85.6, Mechanical complication of other specified internal and external prosthetic devices, implants and grafts, that specifies the type of pump malfunction, as the principal or first-listed code, followed by code T38.3X6-, Underdosing of insulin and oral hypoglycemic [antidiabetic] drugs. Additional codes for the type of diabetes mellitus and any associated complications due to the underdosing should also be assigned.

> A 24-year-old type 1 diabetic male treated in for hyperglycemia; insulin pump found to be malfunctioning and underdosing
>
> | | |
> |---|---|
> | T85.614A | Breakdown (mechanical) of insulin pump, initial encounter |
> | T38.3X6A | Underdosing of insulin and oral hypoglycemic [antidiabetic] drugs, initial encounter |
> | E10.65 | Type 1 diabetes mellitus with hyperglycemia |
>
> *Explanation*: The complication code for the mechanical breakdown of the pump is sequenced first, followed by the underdosing code and type of diabetes with complication. Code all other diabetic complication codes necessary to describe the patient's condition.

(b) Overdose of insulin due to insulin pump failure

The principal or first-listed code for an encounter due to an insulin pump malfunction resulting in an overdose of insulin, should also be T85.6-, Mechanical complication of other specified internal and external prosthetic devices, implants and grafts, followed by code T38.3X1-, Poisoning by insulin and oral hypoglycemic [antidiabetic] drugs, accidental (unintentional).

> A 24-year-old type 1 diabetic male found down with diabetic coma, brought into ED and treated for hypoglycemia; insulin pump found to be malfunctioning and overdosing
>
> | | |
> |---|---|
> | T85.614A | Breakdown (mechanical) of insulin pump, initial encounter |
> | T38.3X1A | Poisoning by insulin and oral hypoglycemic [antidiabetic] drugs, accidental (unintentional), initial encounter |
> | E10.641 | Type 1 diabetes mellitus with hypoglycemia with coma |
>
> *Explanation*: The complication code for the mechanical breakdown of the pump is sequenced first, followed by the poisoning code and type of diabetes with complication. All the characters in the combination code must be used to form a valid code and to fully describe the type of diabetes, the hypoglycemia, and the coma.

6) Secondary diabetes mellitus

Codes under categories E08, Diabetes mellitus due to underlying condition, E09, Drug or chemical induced diabetes mellitus, and E13, Other specified diabetes mellitus, identify complications/manifestations associated with secondary diabetes mellitus. Secondary diabetes is always caused by another condition or event (e.g., cystic fibrosis, malignant neoplasm of pancreas, pancreatectomy, adverse effect of drug, or poisoning).

(a) Secondary diabetes mellitus and the use of insulin or hypoglycemic drugs

For patients who routinely use insulin or hypoglycemic drugs, code Z79.4, Long-term (current) use of insulin, or Z79.84, Long term (current) use of oral hypoglycemic drugs should also be assigned. Code Z79.4 should not be assigned if insulin is given temporarily to bring a patient's blood sugar under control during an encounter.

Type 2 diabetic with no complications, normally only on oral metformin, is given insulin for three days to maintain glucose control while in the hospital recovering from surgery

E11.9   Type 2 diabetes mellitus without complications

Z79.84   Long term (current) use of oral hypoglycemic drugs

Explanation: Although the patient was given insulin for a short time during his hospital stay, the intent was only to maintain the patient's glucose levels while off his regular oral hypoglycemic medication, not for long term use. No code is needed for long term use of insulin, but a Z code for long term use of an oral hypoglycemic should be added to identify the chronic use of this drug.

Type 2 diabetic with diabetic polyneuropathy on insulin

E11.42   Type 2 diabetes mellitus with diabetic polyneuropathy

Z79.4   Long term (current) use of insulin

Explanation: Add the Z code for the long term use of insulin because the insulin is taken chronically.

(b) Assigning and sequencing secondary diabetes codes and its causes

The sequencing of the secondary diabetes codes in relationship to codes for the cause of the diabetes is based on the Tabular List instructions for categories E08, E09 and E13.

(i) Secondary diabetes mellitus due to pancreatectomy

For postpancreatectomy diabetes mellitus (lack of insulin due to the surgical removal of all or part of the pancreas), assign code E89.1, Postprocedural hypoinsulinemia. Assign a code from category E13 and a code from subcategory Z90.41-, Acquired absence of pancreas, as additional codes.

Patient with newly diagnosed diabetes after surgical removal of part of pancreas

E89.1   Postprocedural hypoinsulinemia

E13.9   Other specified diabetes mellitus without complications

Z90.411   Acquired partial absence of pancreas

Explanation: Sequence the postprocedural complication of the hypoinsulinemia due to the partial removal of the pancreas as the first-listed code, followed by the other specified diabetes (NEC) with or without complications and the partial or total acquired absence of the pancreas.

(ii) Secondary diabetes due to drugs

Secondary diabetes may be caused by an adverse effect of correctly administered medications, poisoning or sequela of poisoning.

See section I.C.19.e for coding of adverse effects and poisoning, and section I.C.20 for external cause code reporting.

Initial encounter for corticosteroid-induced diabetes mellitus

E09.9   Drug or chemical induced diabetes mellitus without complications

T38.0X5A   Adverse effect of glucocorticoids and synthetic analogues, initial encounter

Explanation: If the diabetes is caused by an adverse effect of a drug, the diabetic condition is coded first. If it occurs from a poisoning or overdose, the poisoning code causing the diabetes is sequenced first.

Chapter 4. Endocrine, Nutritional and Metabolic Diseases (E00-E89)

NOTE All neoplasms, whether functionally active or not, are classified in Chapter 2. Appropriate codes in this chapter (i.e. E05.8, E07.0, E16-E31, E34-) may be used as additional codes to indicate either functional activity by neoplasms and ectopic endocrine tissue or hyperfunction and hypofunction of endocrine glands associated with neoplasms and other conditions classified elsewhere.

EXCLUDES 1   transitory endocrine and metabolic disorders specific to newborn (P70-P74)

This chapter contains the following blocks:

E00-E07   Disorders of thyroid gland
E08-E13   Diabetes mellitus
E15-E16   Other disorders of glucose regulation and pancreatic internal secretion
E20-E35   Disorders of other endocrine glands
E36   Intraoperative complications of endocrine system
E40-E46   Malnutrition
E50-E64   Other nutritional deficiencies
E65-E68   Overweight, obesity and other hyperalimentation
E70-E88   Metabolic disorders
E89   Postprocedural endocrine and metabolic complications and disorders, not elsewhere classified

Disorders of thyroid gland (E00-E07)

✓4ᵗʰ E00   Congenital iodine-deficiency syndrome
Use additional code (F70-F79) to identify associated intellectual disabilities
EXCLUDES 1   subclinical iodine-deficiency hypothyroidism (E02)

E00.0   Congenital iodine-deficiency syndrome, neurological type
Endemic cretinism, neurological type

E00.1   Congenital iodine-deficiency syndrome, myxedematous type
Endemic hypothyroid cretinism
Endemic cretinism, myxedematous type

E00.2   Congenital iodine-deficiency syndrome, mixed type
Endemic cretinism, mixed type

E00.9   Congenital iodine-deficiency syndrome, unspecified ▽
Congenital iodine-deficiency hypothyroidism NOS
Endemic cretinism NOS

✓4ᵗʰ E01   Iodine-deficiency related thyroid disorders and allied conditions
EXCLUDES 1   congenital iodine-deficiency syndrome (E00.-)
subclinical iodine-deficiency hypothyroidism (E02)

E01.0   Iodine-deficiency related diffuse (endemic) goiter

E01.1   Iodine-deficiency related multinodular (endemic) goiter
Iodine-deficiency related nodular goiter

E01.2   Iodine-deficiency related (endemic) goiter, unspecified ▽
Endemic goiter NOS

E01.8   Other iodine-deficiency related thyroid disorders and allied conditions
Acquired iodine-deficiency hypothyroidism NOS

E02   Subclinical iodine-deficiency hypothyroidism

✓4ᵗʰ E03   Other hypothyroidism
EXCLUDES 1   iodine-deficiency related hypothyroidism (E00-E02)
postprocedural hypothyroidism (E89.0)

E03.0   Congenital hypothyroidism with diffuse goiter
Congenital parenchymatous goiter (nontoxic)
Congenital goiter (nontoxic) NOS
EXCLUDES 1   transitory congenital goiter with normal function (P72.0)

E03.1   Congenital hypothyroidism without goiter
Aplasia of thyroid (with myxedema)
Congenital atrophy of thyroid
Congenital hypothyroidism NOS

E03.2   Hypothyroidism due to medicaments and other exogenous substances
Code first poisoning due to drug or toxin, if applicable (T36-T65 with fifth or sixth character 1-4 or 6)
Use additional code for adverse effect, if applicable, to identify drug (T36-T50 with fifth or sixth character 5)

E03.3   Postinfectious hypothyroidism

E03.4   Atrophy of thyroid (acquired)
EXCLUDES 1   congenital atrophy of thyroid (E03.1)

E03.5   Myxedema coma   `HCC`

E03.8   Other specified hypothyroidism

E03.9   Hypothyroidism, unspecified ▽
Myxedema NOS

Goiter

Pyramidal lobe
Thyroid cartilage
Healthy thyroid
Goiter (hyperfunctioning thyroid)

✓4ᵗʰ E04   Other nontoxic goiter
EXCLUDES 1   congenital goiter (NOS) (diffuse) (parenchymatous) (E03.0)
iodine-deficiency related goiter (E00-E02)

E04.0   Nontoxic diffuse goiter
Diffuse (colloid) nontoxic goiter
Simple nontoxic goiter

E04.1   Nontoxic single thyroid nodule
Colloid nodule (cystic) (thyroid)
Nontoxic uninodular goiter
Thyroid (cystic) nodule NOS
DEF: Enlarged thyroid, commonly due to decreased thyroid production, with single nodule; no clinical hypothyroidism.

E04.2   Nontoxic multinodular goiter
Cystic goiter NOS
Multinodular (cystic) goiter NOS
DEF: Enlarged thyroid, commonly due to decreased thyroid production with multiple nodules; no clinical hypothyroidism.

E04.8   Other specified nontoxic goiter

E04.9   Nontoxic goiter, unspecified ▽
Goiter NOS
Nodular goiter (nontoxic) NOS

✓4ᵗʰ E05   Thyrotoxicosis [hyperthyroidism]
EXCLUDES 1   chronic thyroiditis with transient thyrotoxicosis (E06.2)
neonatal thyrotoxicosis (P72.1)c

✓5ᵗʰ E05.0   Thyrotoxicosis with diffuse goiter
Exophthalmic or toxic goiter NOS   Graves' disease
                Toxic diffuse goiter
DEF: Diffuse thyroid enlargement accompanied by hyperthyroidism, bulging eyes, and dermopathy.

E05.00   Thyrotoxicosis with diffuse goiter without thyrotoxic crisis or storm

E05.01   Thyrotoxicosis with diffuse goiter with thyrotoxic crisis or storm

✓5ᵗʰ E05.1   Thyrotoxicosis with toxic single thyroid nodule
Thyrotoxicosis with toxic uninodular goiter
DEF: Symptomatic hyperthyroidism with a single nodule on the enlarged thyroid gland. Abrupt onset of symptoms include extreme nervousness, insomnia, weight loss, tremors, and psychosis or coma.

E05.10   Thyrotoxicosis with toxic single thyroid nodule without thyrotoxic crisis or storm

E05.11   Thyrotoxicosis with toxic single thyroid nodule with thyrotoxic crisis or storm

✓5ᵗʰ E05.2   Thyrotoxicosis with toxic multinodular goiter
Toxic nodular goiter NOS

E05.20   Thyrotoxicosis with toxic multinodular goiter without thyrotoxic crisis or storm

E05.21   Thyrotoxicosis with toxic multinodular goiter with thyrotoxic crisis or storm

✓5ᵗʰ E05.3   Thyrotoxicosis from ectopic thyroid tissue

E05.30   Thyrotoxicosis from ectopic thyroid tissue without thyrotoxic crisis or storm

E05.31   Thyrotoxicosis from ectopic thyroid tissue with thyrotoxic crisis or storm

✓5ᵗʰ E05.4   Thyrotoxicosis factitia

E05.40   Thyrotoxicosis factitia without thyrotoxic crisis or storm

E05.41   Thyrotoxicosis factitia with thyrotoxic crisis or storm

---

☑ Additional Character Req   ✓x7ᵗʰ Placeholder Alert   Manifestation   `HCC` CMS-HCC Condition   ▽ Unspecified Code   ▶◀ Revised Text   ● New Code   ▲ Revised Code Title

✓5ᵗʰ E05.8   Other thyrotoxicosis
Overproduction of thyroid-stimulating hormone

E05.80   Other thyrotoxicosis without thyrotoxic crisis or storm

E05.81   Other thyrotoxicosis with thyrotoxic crisis or storm

✓5ᵗʰ E05.9   Thyrotoxicosis, unspecified
Hyperthyroidism NOS

E05.90   Thyrotoxicosis, unspecified without thyrotoxic crisis or storm   ▽

E05.91   Thyrotoxicosis, unspecified with thyrotoxic crisis or storm   ▽

✓4ᵗʰ E06   Thyroiditis
EXCLUDES 1 *postpartum thyroiditis (O90.5)*

E06.0   Acute thyroiditis
Abscess of thyroid
Pyogenic thyroiditis
Suppurative thyroiditis
Use additional code (B95-B97) to identify infectious agent

E06.1   Subacute thyroiditis
de Quervain thyroiditis
Giant-cell thyroiditis
Granulomatous thyroiditis
Nonsuppurative thyroiditis
Viral thyroiditis
EXCLUDES 1 *autoimmune thyroiditis (E06.3)*

E06.2   Chronic thyroiditis with transient thyrotoxicosis
EXCLUDES 1 *autoimmune thyroiditis (E06.3)*

E06.3   Autoimmune thyroiditis
Hashimoto's thyroiditis
Hashitoxicosis (transient)
Lymphadenoid goiter
Lymphocytic thyroiditis
Struma lymphomatosa

E06.4   Drug-induced thyroiditis
Use additional code for adverse effect, if applicable, to identify drug (T36-T50 with fifth or sixth character 5)

E06.5   Other chronic thyroiditis
Chronic fibrous thyroiditis
Chronic thyroiditis NOS
Ligneous thyroiditis
Riedel thyroiditis

E06.9   Thyroiditis, unspecified   ▽

✓4ᵗʰ E07   Other disorders of thyroid

E07.0   Hypersecretion of calcitonin
C-cell hyperplasia of thyroid
Hypersecretion of thyrocalcitonin

E07.1   Dyshormogenetic goiter
Familial dyshormogenetic goiter
Pendred's syndrome
EXCLUDES 1 *transitory congenital goiter with normal function (P72.0)*

✓5ᵗʰ E07.8   Other specified disorders of thyroid

E07.81   Sick-euthyroid syndrome
Euthyroid sick-syndrome

E07.89   Other specified disorders of thyroid
Abnormality of thyroid-binding globulin
Hemorrhage of thyroid
Infarction of thyroid

E07.9   Disorder of thyroid, unspecified   ▽

Diabetes mellitus (E08-E13)
AHA: 2017, 1Q, 42; 2016, 2Q, 36; 2016, 1Q, 11-13

✓4ᵗʰ E08   Diabetes mellitus due to underlying condition
Code first the underlying condition, such as:
congenital rubella (P35.0)
Cushing's syndrome (E24.-)
cystic fibrosis (E84.-)
malignant neoplasm (C00-C96)
malnutrition (E40-E46)
pancreatitis and other diseases of the pancreas (K85.-, K86.-)
Use additional code to identify control using:
insulin (Z79.4)
oral antidiabetic drugs (Z79.84)
oral hypoglycemic drugs (Z79.84)
EXCLUDES 1 *drug or chemical induced diabetes mellitus (E09.-)*
gestational diabetes (O24.4-)
neonatal diabetes mellitus (P70.2)
postpancreatectomy diabetes mellitus (E13.-)
postprocedural diabetes mellitus (E13.-)
secondary diabetes mellitus NEC (E13.-)
type 1 diabetes mellitus (E10.-)
type 2 diabetes mellitus (E11.-)
AHA: 2013, 4Q, 114; 2013, 3Q, 20

✓5ᵗʰ E08.0   Diabetes mellitus due to underlying condition with hyperosmolarity

E08.00   *Diabetes mellitus due to underlying condition with hyperosmolarity without nonketotic hyperglycemic-hyperosmolar coma (NKHHC)*   HCC

E08.01   *Diabetes mellitus due to underlying condition with hyperosmolarity with coma*   HCC

✓5ᵗʰ E08.1   Diabetes mellitus due to underlying condition with ketoacidosis

E08.10   *Diabetes mellitus due to underlying condition with ketoacidosis without coma*   HCC

E08.11   *Diabetes mellitus due to underlying condition with ketoacidosis with coma*   HCC

✓5ᵗʰ E08.2   Diabetes mellitus due to underlying condition with kidney complications

E08.21   *Diabetes mellitus due to underlying condition with diabetic nephropathy*   HCC
Diabetes mellitus due to underlying condition with intercapillary glomerulosclerosis
Diabetes mellitus due to underlying condition with intracapillary glomerulonephrosis
Diabetes mellitus due to underlying condition with Kimmelstiel-Wilson disease

E08.22   *Diabetes mellitus due to underlying condition with diabetic chronic kidney disease*   HCC
Use additional code to identify stage of chronic kidney disease (N18.1-N18.6)

E08.29   *Diabetes mellitus due to underlying condition with other diabetic kidney complication*   HCC
Renal tubular degeneration in diabetes mellitus due to underlying condition

✓5ᵗʰ E08.3   Diabetes mellitus due to underlying condition with ophthalmic complications

One of the following 7th characters is to be assigned to codes in subcategories E08.32, E08.33, E08.34, E08.35, and E08.37 to designate laterality of the disease:
1   right eye
2   left eye
3   bilateral
9   unspecified eye

✓6ᵗʰ E08.31   Diabetes mellitus due to underlying condition with unspecified diabetic retinopathy

E08.311   *Diabetes mellitus due to underlying condition with unspecified diabetic retinopathy with macular edema*   HCC ▽

E08.319   *Diabetes mellitus due to underlying condition with unspecified diabetic retinopathy without macular edema*   HCC ▽

✓6ᵗʰ E08.32   Diabetes mellitus due to underlying condition with mild nonproliferative diabetic retinopathy
Diabetes mellitus due to underlying condition with nonproliferative diabetic retinopathy NOS

✓7ᵗʰ E08.321   *Diabetes mellitus due to underlying condition with mild nonproliferative diabetic retinopathy with macular edema*   HCC

☑7th **E08.329** *Diabetes mellitus due to underlying condition with mild nonproliferative diabetic retinopathy without macular edema* HCC

☑6th **E08.33** Diabetes mellitus due to underlying condition with moderate nonproliferative diabetic retinopathy

  ☑7th **E08.331** *Diabetes mellitus due to underlying condition with moderate nonproliferative diabetic retinopathy with macular edema* HCC

  ☑7th **E08.339** *Diabetes mellitus due to underlying condition with moderate nonproliferative diabetic retinopathy without macular edema* HCC

☑6th **E08.34** Diabetes mellitus due to underlying condition with severe nonproliferative diabetic retinopathy

  ☑7th **E08.341** *Diabetes mellitus due to underlying condition with severe nonproliferative diabetic retinopathy with macular edema* HCC

  ☑7th **E08.349** *Diabetes mellitus due to underlying condition with severe nonproliferative diabetic retinopathy without macular edema* HCC

☑6th **E08.35** Diabetes mellitus due to underlying condition with proliferative diabetic retinopathy

  ☑7th **E08.351** *Diabetes mellitus due to underlying condition with proliferative diabetic retinopathy with macular edema* HCC

  ☑7th **E08.352** *Diabetes mellitus due to underlying condition with proliferative diabetic retinopathy with traction retinal detachment involving the macula* HCC

  ☑7th **E08.353** *Diabetes mellitus due to underlying condition with proliferative diabetic retinopathy with traction retinal detachment not involving the macula* HCC

  ☑7th **E08.354** *Diabetes mellitus due to underlying condition with proliferative diabetic retinopathy with combined traction retinal detachment and rhegmatogenous retinal detachment* HCC

  ☑7th **E08.355** *Diabetes mellitus due to underlying condition with stable proliferative diabetic retinopathy* HCC

  ☑7th **E08.359** *Diabetes mellitus due to underlying condition with proliferative diabetic retinopathy without macular edema* HCC

E08.36 *Diabetes mellitus due to underlying condition with diabetic cataract* HCC
  AHA: 2016, 4Q, 142

☑x7th **E08.37** *Diabetes mellitus due to underlying condition with diabetic macular edema, resolved following treatment* HCC

E08.39 *Diabetes mellitus due to underlying condition with other diabetic ophthalmic complication* HCC
  Use additional code to identify manifestation, such as: diabetic glaucoma (H40-H42)

☑5th **E08.4** Diabetes mellitus due to underlying condition with neurological complications

E08.40 *Diabetes mellitus due to underlying condition with diabetic neuropathy, unspecified* HCC ▽

E08.41 *Diabetes mellitus due to underlying condition with diabetic mononeuropathy* HCC

E08.42 *Diabetes mellitus due to underlying condition with diabetic polyneuropathy* HCC
  Diabetes mellitus due to underlying condition with diabetic neuralgia

E08.43 *Diabetes mellitus due to underlying condition with diabetic autonomic (poly)neuropathy* HCC
  Diabetes mellitus due to underlying condition with diabetic gastroparesis
  AHA: 2013, 4Q, 114

E08.44 *Diabetes mellitus due to underlying condition with diabetic amyotrophy* HCC

E08.49 *Diabetes mellitus due to underlying condition with other diabetic neurological complication* HCC

☑5th **E08.5** Diabetes mellitus due to underlying condition with circulatory complications

E08.51 *Diabetes mellitus due to underlying condition with diabetic peripheral angiopathy without gangrene* HCC

E08.52 *Diabetes mellitus due to underlying condition with diabetic peripheral angiopathy with gangrene* HCC
  Diabetes mellitus due to underlying condition with diabetic gangrene

E08.59 *Diabetes mellitus due to underlying condition with other circulatory complications* HCC

☑5th **E08.6** Diabetes mellitus due to underlying condition with other specified complications

☑6th **E08.61** Diabetes mellitus due to underlying condition with diabetic arthropathy

E08.610 *Diabetes mellitus due to underlying condition with diabetic neuropathic arthropathy* HCC
  Diabetes mellitus due to underlying condition with Charcôt's joints

E08.618 *Diabetes mellitus due to underlying condition with other diabetic arthropathy* HCC

☑6th **E08.62** Diabetes mellitus due to underlying condition with skin complications

E08.620 *Diabetes mellitus due to underlying condition with diabetic dermatitis* HCC
  Diabetes mellitus due to underlying condition with diabetic necrobiosis lipoidica

E08.621 *Diabetes mellitus due to underlying condition with foot ulcer* HCC
  Use additional code to identify site of ulcer (L97.4-, L97.5-)

E08.622 *Diabetes mellitus due to underlying condition with other skin ulcer* HCC
  Use additional code to identify site of ulcer (L97.1-L97.9, L98.41-L98.49)

E08.628 *Diabetes mellitus due to underlying condition with other skin complications* HCC

☑6th **E08.63** Diabetes mellitus due to underlying condition with oral complications

E08.630 *Diabetes mellitus due to underlying condition with periodontal disease* HCC

E08.638 *Diabetes mellitus due to underlying condition with other oral complications* HCC

☑6th **E08.64** Diabetes mellitus due to underlying condition with hypoglycemia

E08.641 *Diabetes mellitus due to underlying condition with hypoglycemia with coma* HCC

E08.649 *Diabetes mellitus due to underlying condition with hypoglycemia without coma* HCC
  AHA: 2016, 3Q, 42; 2015, 3Q, 21

E08.65 *Diabetes mellitus due to underlying condition with hyperglycemia* HCC

E08.69 *Diabetes mellitus due to underlying condition with other specified complication* HCC
  Use additional code to identify complication
  AHA: 2016, 4Q, 141; 2016, 1Q, 13

E08.8 *Diabetes mellitus due to underlying condition with unspecified complications* HCC ▽

E08.9 *Diabetes mellitus due to underlying condition without complications* HCC

☑4th **E09** Drug or chemical induced diabetes mellitus
  Code first poisoning due to drug or toxin, if applicable (T36-T65 with fifth or sixth character 1-4 or 6)
  Use additional code for adverse effect, if applicable, to identify drug (T36-T50 with fifth or sixth character 5)
  Use additional code to identify control using:
    insulin (Z79.4)
    oral antidiabetic drugs (Z79.84)
    oral hypoglycemic drugs (Z79.84)
  EXCLUDES 1   diabetes mellitus due to underlying condition (E08.-)
    gestational diabetes (O24.4-)
    neonatal diabetes mellitus (P70.2)
    postpancreatectomy diabetes mellitus (E13.-)
    postprocedural diabetes mellitus (E13.-)
    secondary diabetes mellitus NEC (E13.-)
    type 1 diabetes mellitus (E10.-)
    type 2 diabetes mellitus (E11.-)
  AHA: 2013, 4Q, 114; 2013, 3Q, 20

☑5th **E09.0** Drug or chemical induced diabetes mellitus with hyperosmolarity

E09.00 Drug or chemical induced diabetes mellitus with hyperosmolarity without nonketotic hyperglycemic-hyperosmolar coma (NKHHC) HCC

☑ Additional Character Req   ☑x7th Placeholder Alert   Manifestation   HCC CMS-HCC Condition   ▽ Unspecified Code   ▶◀ Revised Text   ● New Code   ▲ Revised Code Title

E09.01   **Drug or chemical induced diabetes mellitus with hyperosmolarity with coma**   HCC

√5ᵗʰ **E09.1**   **Drug or chemical induced diabetes mellitus with ketoacidosis**

   E09.10   **Drug or chemical induced diabetes mellitus with ketoacidosis without coma**   HCC

   E09.11   **Drug or chemical induced diabetes mellitus with ketoacidosis with coma**   HCC

√5ᵗʰ **E09.2**   **Drug or chemical induced diabetes mellitus with kidney complications**

   E09.21   **Drug or chemical induced diabetes mellitus with diabetic nephropathy**   HCC

     Drug or chemical induced diabetes mellitus with intercapillary glomerulosclerosis

     Drug or chemical induced diabetes mellitus with intracapillary glomerulonephrosis

     Drug or chemical induced diabetes mellitus with Kimmelstiel-Wilson disease

   E09.22   **Drug or chemical induced diabetes mellitus with diabetic chronic kidney disease**   HCC

     Use additional code to identify stage of chronic kidney disease (N18.1-N18.6)

   E09.29   **Drug or chemical induced diabetes mellitus with other diabetic kidney complication**   HCC

     Drug or chemical induced diabetes mellitus with renal tubular degeneration

√5ᵗʰ **E09.3**   **Drug or chemical induced diabetes mellitus with ophthalmic complications**

> One of the following 7th characters is to be assigned to codes in subcategories E09.32, E09.33, E09.34, E09.35, and E09.37 to designate laterality of the disease:
> 1   right eye
> 2   left eye
> 3   bilateral
> 9   unspecified eye

√6ᵗʰ **E09.31**   **Drug or chemical induced diabetes mellitus with unspecified diabetic retinopathy**

   E09.311   **Drug or chemical induced diabetes mellitus with unspecified diabetic retinopathy with macular edema**   HCC ▽

   E09.319   **Drug or chemical induced diabetes mellitus with unspecified diabetic retinopathy without macular edema**   HCC ▽

√6ᵗʰ **E09.32**   **Drug or chemical induced diabetes mellitus with mild nonproliferative diabetic retinopathy**

     Drug or chemical induced diabetes mellitus with nonproliferative diabetic retinopathy NOS

   √7ᵗʰ **E09.321**   **Drug or chemical induced diabetes mellitus with mild nonproliferative diabetic retinopathy with macular edema**   HCC

   √7ᵗʰ **E09.329**   **Drug or chemical induced diabetes mellitus with mild nonproliferative diabetic retinopathy without macular edema**   HCC

√6ᵗʰ **E09.33**   **Drug or chemical induced diabetes mellitus with moderate nonproliferative diabetic retinopathy**

   √7ᵗʰ **E09.331**   **Drug or chemical induced diabetes mellitus with moderate nonproliferative diabetic retinopathy with macular edema**   HCC

   √7ᵗʰ **E09.339**   **Drug or chemical induced diabetes mellitus with moderate nonproliferative diabetic retinopathy without macular edema**   HCC

√6ᵗʰ **E09.34**   **Drug or chemical induced diabetes mellitus with severe nonproliferative diabetic retinopathy**

   √7ᵗʰ **E09.341**   **Drug or chemical induced diabetes mellitus with severe nonproliferative diabetic retinopathy with macular edema**   HCC

   √7ᵗʰ **E09.349**   **Drug or chemical induced diabetes mellitus with severe nonproliferative diabetic retinopathy without macular edema**   HCC

√6ᵗʰ **E09.35**   **Drug or chemical induced diabetes mellitus with proliferative diabetic retinopathy**

   √7ᵗʰ **E09.351**   **Drug or chemical induced diabetes mellitus with proliferative diabetic retinopathy with macular edema**   HCC

   √7ᵗʰ **E09.352**   **Drug or chemical induced diabetes mellitus with proliferative diabetic retinopathy with traction retinal detachment involving the macula**   HCC

   √7ᵗʰ **E09.353**   **Drug or chemical induced diabetes mellitus with proliferative diabetic retinopathy with traction retinal detachment not involving the macula**   HCC

   √7ᵗʰ **E09.354**   **Drug or chemical induced diabetes mellitus with proliferative diabetic retinopathy with combined traction retinal detachment and rhegmatogenous retinal detachment**   HCC

   √7ᵗʰ **E09.355**   **Drug or chemical induced diabetes mellitus with stable proliferative diabetic retinopathy**   HCC

   √7ᵗʰ **E09.359**   **Drug or chemical induced diabetes mellitus with proliferative diabetic retinopathy without macular edema**   HCC

   E09.36   **Drug or chemical induced diabetes mellitus with diabetic cataract**   HCC

     AHA: 2016, 4Q, 142

√x7ᵗʰ **E09.37**   **Drug or chemical induced diabetes mellitus with diabetic macular edema, resolved following treatment**   HCC

   E09.39   **Drug or chemical induced diabetes mellitus with other diabetic ophthalmic complication**   HCC

     Use additional code to identify manifestation, such as: diabetic glaucoma (H40-H42)

√5ᵗʰ **E09.4**   **Drug or chemical induced diabetes mellitus with neurological complications**

   E09.40   **Drug or chemical induced diabetes mellitus with neurological complications with diabetic neuropathy, unspecified**   HCC ▽

   E09.41   **Drug or chemical induced diabetes mellitus with neurological complications with diabetic mononeuropathy**   HCC

   E09.42   **Drug or chemical induced diabetes mellitus with neurological complications with diabetic polyneuropathy**   HCC

     Drug or chemical induced diabetes mellitus with diabetic neuralgia

   E09.43   **Drug or chemical induced diabetes mellitus with neurological complications with diabetic autonomic (poly)neuropathy**   HCC

     Drug or chemical induced diabetes mellitus with diabetic gastroparesis

     AHA: 2013, 4Q, 114

   E09.44   **Drug or chemical induced diabetes mellitus with neurological complications with diabetic amyotrophy**   HCC

   E09.49   **Drug or chemical induced diabetes mellitus with neurological complications with other diabetic neurological complication**   HCC

√5ᵗʰ **E09.5**   **Drug or chemical induced diabetes mellitus with circulatory complications**

   E09.51   **Drug or chemical induced diabetes mellitus with diabetic peripheral angiopathy without gangrene**   HCC

   E09.52   **Drug or chemical induced diabetes mellitus with diabetic peripheral angiopathy with gangrene**   HCC

     Drug or chemical induced diabetes mellitus with diabetic gangrene

   E09.59   **Drug or chemical induced diabetes mellitus with other circulatory complications**   HCC

√5ᵗʰ **E09.6**   **Drug or chemical induced diabetes mellitus with other specified complications**

√6ᵗʰ **E09.61**   **Drug or chemical induced diabetes mellitus with diabetic arthropathy**

   E09.610   **Drug or chemical induced diabetes mellitus with diabetic neuropathic arthropathy**   HCC

     Drug or chemical induced diabetes mellitus with Charcôt's joints

   E09.618   **Drug or chemical induced diabetes mellitus with other diabetic arthropathy**   HCC

EXCLUDES 1 Not coded here   EXCLUDES 2 Not included here   N Newborn Age: 0   P Pediatric Age: 0-17   M Maternity Age: 12-55   A Adult Age: 15-124

510   ICD-10-CM 2018

☑6th **E09.62 Drug or chemical induced diabetes mellitus with skin complications**

    E09.620 Drug or chemical induced diabetes HCC
    mellitus with diabetic dermatitis
        Drug or chemical induced diabetes mellitus
        with diabetic necrobiosis lipoidica

    E09.621 Drug or chemical induced diabetes HCC
    mellitus with foot ulcer
        Use additional code to identify site of ulcer
        (L97.4-, L97.5-)

    E09.622 Drug or chemical induced diabetes HCC
    mellitus with other skin ulcer
        Use additional code to identify site of ulcer
        (L97.1-L97.9, L98.41-L98.49)

    E09.628 Drug or chemical induced diabetes HCC
    mellitus with other skin complications

☑6th **E09.63 Drug or chemical induced diabetes mellitus with oral complications**

    E09.630 Drug or chemical induced diabetes HCC
    mellitus with periodontal disease

    E09.638 Drug or chemical induced diabetes HCC
    mellitus with other oral complications

☑6th **E09.64 Drug or chemical induced diabetes mellitus with hypoglycemia**

    E09.641 Drug or chemical induced diabetes HCC
    mellitus with hypoglycemia with coma

    E09.649 Drug or chemical induced diabetes HCC
    mellitus with hypoglycemia without coma
        AHA: 2016, 3Q, 42; 2015, 3Q, 21

    E09.65 Drug or chemical induced diabetes mellitus HCC
    with hyperglycemia

    E09.69 Drug or chemical induced diabetes mellitus HCC
    with other specified complication
        Use additional code to identify complication
        AHA: 2016, 4Q, 141; 2016, 1Q, 13

  E09.8 Drug or chemical induced diabetes mellitus with HCC ▽
  unspecified complications

  E09.9 Drug or chemical induced diabetes mellitus without HCC
  complications

☑4th **E10 Type 1 diabetes mellitus**

  INCLUDES   brittle diabetes (mellitus)
        diabetes (mellitus) due to autoimmune process
        diabetes (mellitus) due to immune mediated pancreatic islet
          beta-cell destruction
        idiopathic diabetes (mellitus)
        juvenile onset diabetes (mellitus)
        ketosis-prone diabetes (mellitus)

  EXCLUDES 1   *diabetes mellitus due to underlying condition (E08.-)*
        drug or chemical induced diabetes mellitus (E09.-)
        gestational diabetes (O24.4-)
        hyperglycemia NOS (R73.9)
        neonatal diabetes mellitus (P70.2)
        postpancreatectomy diabetes mellitus (E13.-)
        postprocedural diabetes mellitus (E13.-)
        secondary diabetes mellitus NEC (E13.-)
        type 2 diabetes mellitus (E11.-)
  AHA: 2013, 4Q, 114; 2013, 3Q, 20

☑5th **E10.1 Type 1 diabetes mellitus with ketoacidosis**
    AHA: 2013, 3Q, 20

    E10.10 Type 1 diabetes mellitus with ketoacidosis HCC
    without coma

    E10.11 Type 1 diabetes mellitus with ketoacidosis HCC
    with coma

☑5th **E10.2 Type 1 diabetes mellitus with kidney complications**

    E10.21 Type 1 diabetes mellitus with diabetic HCC
    nephropathy
        Type 1 diabetes mellitus with intercapillary
          glomerulosclerosis
        Type 1 diabetes mellitus with intracapillary
          glomerulonephrosis
        Type 1 diabetes mellitus with Kimmelstiel-Wilson
          disease

    E10.22 Type 1 diabetes mellitus with diabetic chronic HCC
    kidney disease
        Use additional code to identify stage of chronic kidney
          disease (N18.1-N18.6)

    E10.29 Type 1 diabetes mellitus with other diabetic HCC
    kidney complication
        Type 1 diabetes mellitus with renal tubular
          degeneration
        AHA: 2016, 1Q, 13

☑5th **E10.3 Type 1 diabetes mellitus with ophthalmic complications**

  One of the following 7th characters is to be assigned to codes
  in subcategories E10.32, E10.33, E10.34, E10.35, and E10.37 to
  designate laterality of the disease:
  1   right eye
  2   left eye
  3   bilateral
  9   unspecified eye

☑6th **E10.31 Type 1 diabetes mellitus with unspecified diabetic retinopathy**

    E10.311 Type 1 diabetes mellitus with HCC ▽
    unspecified diabetic retinopathy
    with macular edema

    E10.319 Type 1 diabetes mellitus with HCC ▽
    unspecified diabetic retinopathy
    without macular edema

☑6th **E10.32 Type 1 diabetes mellitus with mild nonproliferative diabetic retinopathy**
    Type 1 diabetes mellitus with nonproliferative diabetic
    retinopathy NOS

    ☑7th **E10.321 Type 1 diabetes mellitus with mild** HCC
    nonproliferative diabetic retinopathy
    with macular edema

    ☑7th **E10.329 Type 1 diabetes mellitus with mild** HCC
    nonproliferative diabetic retinopathy
    without macular edema

☑6th **E10.33 Type 1 diabetes mellitus with moderate nonproliferative diabetic retinopathy**

    ☑7th **E10.331 Type 1 diabetes mellitus with** HCC
    moderate nonproliferative diabetic
    retinopathy with macular edema

    ☑7th **E10.339 Type 1 diabetes mellitus with** HCC
    moderate nonproliferative diabetic
    retinopathy without macular edema

☑6th **E10.34 Type 1 diabetes mellitus with severe nonproliferative diabetic retinopathy**

    ☑7th **E10.341 Type 1 diabetes mellitus with severe** HCC
    nonproliferative diabetic retinopathy
    with macular edema

    ☑7th **E10.349 Type 1 diabetes mellitus with severe** HCC
    nonproliferative diabetic retinopathy
    without macular edema

☑6th **E10.35 Type 1 diabetes mellitus with proliferative diabetic retinopathy**

    ☑7th **E10.351 Type 1 diabetes mellitus with** HCC
    proliferative diabetic retinopathy
    with macular edema

    ☑7th **E10.352 Type 1 diabetes mellitus with** HCC
    proliferative diabetic retinopathy
    with traction retinal detachment
    involving the macula

    ☑7th **E10.353 Type 1 diabetes mellitus with** HCC
    proliferative diabetic retinopathy
    with traction retinal detachment not
    involving the macula

    ☑7th **E10.354 Type 1 diabetes mellitus with** HCC
    proliferative diabetic retinopathy with
    combined traction retinal detachment and
    rhegmatogenous retinal detachment

    ☑7th **E10.355 Type 1 diabetes mellitus with stable** HCC
    proliferative diabetic retinopathy

    ☑7th **E10.359 Type 1 diabetes mellitus with** HCC
    proliferative diabetic retinopathy
    without macular edema

    E10.36 Type 1 diabetes mellitus with diabetic cataract HCC
        AHA: 2016, 4Q, 142

  ☑x7th **E10.37 Type 1 diabetes mellitus with diabetic macular** HCC
  edema, resolved following treatment

    E10.39 Type 1 diabetes mellitus with other diabetic HCC
    ophthalmic complication
        Use additional code to identify manifestation, such as:
          diabetic glaucoma (H40-H42)

☑5th **E10.4 Type 1 diabetes mellitus with neurological complications**

    E10.40 Type 1 diabetes mellitus with diabetic HCC ▽
    neuropathy, unspecified

    E10.41 Type 1 diabetes mellitus with diabetic HCC
    mononeuropathy

☑ Additional Character Req   ✓x7th Placeholder Alert   Manifestation   HCC CMS-HCC Condition   ▽ Unspecified Code   ▶◀ Revised Text   ● New Code   ▲ Revised Code Title

ICD-10-CM 2018   511

E10.42 **Type 1 diabetes mellitus with diabetic polyneuropathy** `HCC`
Type 1 diabetes mellitus with diabetic neuralgia

E10.43 **Type 1 diabetes mellitus with diabetic autonomic (poly)neuropathy** `HCC`
Type 1 diabetes mellitus with diabetic gastroparesis
AHA: 2013, 4Q, 114

E10.44 **Type 1 diabetes mellitus with diabetic amyotrophy** `HCC`

E10.49 **Type 1 diabetes mellitus with other diabetic neurological complication** `HCC`

✓5th **E10.5** **Type 1 diabetes mellitus with circulatory complications**

E10.51 **Type 1 diabetes mellitus with diabetic peripheral angiopathy without gangrene** `HCC`

E10.52 **Type 1 diabetes mellitus with diabetic peripheral angiopathy with gangrene** `HCC`
Type 1 diabetes mellitus with diabetic gangrene

E10.59 **Type 1 diabetes mellitus with other circulatory complications** `HCC`

✓5th **E10.6** **Type 1 diabetes mellitus with other specified complications**

✓6th **E10.61** **Type 1 diabetes mellitus with diabetic arthropathy**

     E10.610 **Type 1 diabetes mellitus with diabetic neuropathic arthropathy** `HCC`
Type 1 diabetes mellitus with Charcôt's joints

     E10.618 **Type 1 diabetes mellitus with other diabetic arthropathy** `HCC`

✓6th **E10.62** **Type 1 diabetes mellitus with skin complications**

     E10.620 **Type 1 diabetes mellitus with diabetic dermatitis** `HCC`
Type 1 diabetes mellitus with diabetic necrobiosis lipoidica

     E10.621 **Type 1 diabetes mellitus with foot ulcer** `HCC`
Use additional code to identify site of ulcer (L97.4-, L97.5-)

     E10.622 **Type 1 diabetes mellitus with other skin ulcer** `HCC`
Use additional code to identify site of ulcer (L97.1-L97.9, L98.41-L98.49)

     E10.628 **Type 1 diabetes mellitus with other skin complications** `HCC`

✓6th **E10.63** **Type 1 diabetes mellitus with oral complications**

     E10.630 **Type 1 diabetes mellitus with periodontal disease** `HCC`

     E10.638 **Type 1 diabetes mellitus with other oral complications** `HCC`

✓6th **E10.64** **Type 1 diabetes mellitus with hypoglycemia**

     E10.641 **Type 1 diabetes mellitus with hypoglycemia with coma** `HCC`

     E10.649 **Type 1 diabetes mellitus with hypoglycemia without coma** `HCC`
AHA: 2016, 3Q, 42; 2016, 1Q, 13; 2015, 3Q, 21

E10.65 **Type 1 diabetes mellitus with hyperglycemia** `HCC`
AHA: 2013, 3Q, 20

E10.69 **Type 1 diabetes mellitus with other specified complication** `HCC`
Use additional code to identify complication
AHA: 2016, 4Q, 141; 2016, 1Q, 13

E10.8 **Type 1 diabetes mellitus with unspecified complications** `HCC` ▽

E10.9 **Type 1 diabetes mellitus without complications** `HCC`

✓4th **E11** **Type 2 diabetes mellitus**
`INCLUDES` diabetes (mellitus) due to insulin secretory defect
diabetes NOS
insulin resistant diabetes (mellitus)
Use additional code to identify control using:
insulin (Z79.4)
oral antidiabetic drugs (Z79.84)
oral hypoglycemic drugs (Z79.84)
`EXCLUDES 1` *diabetes mellitus due to underlying condition (E08.-)*
drug or chemical induced diabetes mellitus (E09.-)
gestational diabetes (O24.4-)
neonatal diabetes mellitus (P70.2)
postpancreatectomy diabetes mellitus (E13.-)
postprocedural diabetes mellitus (E13.-)
secondary diabetes mellitus NEC (E13.-)
type 1 diabetes mellitus (E10.-)
AHA: 2016, 2Q, 10; 2013, 4Q, 114; 2013, 3Q, 20; 2013, 1Q, 26

✓5th **E11.0** **Type 2 diabetes mellitus with hyperosmolarity**

     E11.00 **Type 2 diabetes mellitus with hyperosmolarity without nonketotic hyperglycemic-hyperosmolar coma (NKHHC)** `HCC`

     E11.01 **Type 2 diabetes mellitus with hyperosmolarity with coma** `HCC`

● ✓5th **E11.1** **Type 2 diabetes mellitus with ketoacidosis**

●   **E11.10** **Type 2 diabetes mellitus with ketoacidosis without coma**

●   **E11.11** **Type 2 diabetes mellitus with ketoacidosis with coma**

✓5th **E11.2** **Type 2 diabetes mellitus with kidney complications**

     E11.21 **Type 2 diabetes mellitus with diabetic nephropathy** `HCC`
Type 2 diabetes mellitus with intercapillary glomerulosclerosis
Type 2 diabetes mellitus with intracapillary glomerulonephrosis
Type 2 diabetes mellitus with Kimmelstiel-Wilson disease

     E11.22 **Type 2 diabetes mellitus with diabetic chronic kidney disease** `HCC`
Use additional code to identify stage of chronic kidney disease (N18.1-N18.6)
AHA: 2016, 1Q, 12

     E11.29 **Type 2 diabetes mellitus with other diabetic kidney complication** `HCC`
Type 2 diabetes mellitus with renal tubular degeneration

✓5th **E11.3** **Type 2 diabetes mellitus with ophthalmic complications**

One of the following 7th characters is to be assigned to codes in subcategories E11.32, E11.33, E11.34, E11.35, and E11.37 to designate laterality of the disease:
1   right eye
2   left eye
3   bilateral
9   unspecified eye

✓6th **E11.31** **Type 2 diabetes mellitus with unspecified diabetic retinopathy**

     E11.311 **Type 2 diabetes mellitus with unspecified diabetic retinopathy with macular edema** `HCC` ▽

     E11.319 **Type 2 diabetes mellitus with unspecified diabetic retinopathy without macular edema** `HCC` ▽

✓6th **E11.32** **Type 2 diabetes mellitus with mild nonproliferative diabetic retinopathy**
Type 2 diabetes mellitus with nonproliferative diabetic retinopathy NOS

     ✓7th **E11.321** **Type 2 diabetes mellitus with mild nonproliferative diabetic retinopathy with macular edema** `HCC`

     ✓7th **E11.329** **Type 2 diabetes mellitus with mild nonproliferative diabetic retinopathy without macular edema** `HCC`

✓6th **E11.33** **Type 2 diabetes mellitus with moderate nonproliferative diabetic retinopathy**

     ✓7th **E11.331** **Type 2 diabetes mellitus with moderate nonproliferative diabetic retinopathy with macular edema** `HCC`

     ✓7th **E11.339** **Type 2 diabetes mellitus with moderate nonproliferative diabetic retinopathy without macular edema** `HCC`

✓6ᵗʰ **E11.34**　**Type 2 diabetes mellitus with severe nonproliferative diabetic retinopathy**

　　✓7ᵗʰ **E11.341**　**Type 2 diabetes mellitus with severe nonproliferative diabetic retinopathy with macular edema** ᴴᶜᶜ

　　✓7ᵗʰ **E11.349**　**Type 2 diabetes mellitus with severe nonproliferative diabetic retinopathy without macular edema** ᴴᶜᶜ

✓6ᵗʰ **E11.35**　**Type 2 diabetes mellitus with proliferative diabetic retinopathy**

　　✓7ᵗʰ **E11.351**　**Type 2 diabetes mellitus with proliferative diabetic retinopathy with macular edema** ᴴᶜᶜ

　　✓7ᵗʰ **E11.352**　**Type 2 diabetes mellitus with proliferative diabetic retinopathy with traction retinal detachment involving the macula** ᴴᶜᶜ

　　✓7ᵗʰ **E11.353**　**Type 2 diabetes mellitus with proliferative diabetic retinopathy with traction retinal detachment not involving the macula** ᴴᶜᶜ

　　✓7ᵗʰ **E11.354**　**Type 2 diabetes mellitus with proliferative diabetic retinopathy with combined traction retinal detachment and rhegmatogenous retinal detachment** ᴴᶜᶜ

　　✓7ᵗʰ **E11.355**　**Type 2 diabetes mellitus with stable proliferative diabetic retinopathy** ᴴᶜᶜ

　　✓7ᵗʰ **E11.359**　**Type 2 diabetes mellitus with proliferative diabetic retinopathy without macular edema** ᴴᶜᶜ

E11.36　**Type 2 diabetes mellitus with diabetic cataract** ᴴᶜᶜ
　　　　AHA: 2016, 4Q, 142

✓x7ᵗʰ **E11.37**　**Type 2 diabetes mellitus with diabetic macular edema, resolved following treatment** ᴴᶜᶜ

E11.39　**Type 2 diabetes mellitus with other diabetic ophthalmic complication** ᴴᶜᶜ
　　　　Use additional code to identify manifestation, such as: diabetic glaucoma (H40-H42)

✓5ᵗʰ **E11.4**　**Type 2 diabetes mellitus with neurological complications**

E11.40　**Type 2 diabetes mellitus with diabetic neuropathy, unspecified** ᴴᶜᶜ ▽
　　　　AHA: 2013, 4Q, 129

E11.41　**Type 2 diabetes mellitus with diabetic mononeuropathy** ᴴᶜᶜ

E11.42　**Type 2 diabetes mellitus with diabetic polyneuropathy** ᴴᶜᶜ
　　　　Type 2 diabetes mellitus with diabetic neuralgia
　　　　AHA: 2016, 1Q, 12

E11.43　**Type 2 diabetes mellitus with diabetic autonomic (poly)neuropathy** ᴴᶜᶜ
　　　　Type 2 diabetes mellitus with diabetic gastroparesis
　　　　AHA: 2013, 4Q, 114

E11.44　**Type 2 diabetes mellitus with diabetic amyotrophy** ᴴᶜᶜ

E11.49　**Type 2 diabetes mellitus with other diabetic neurological complication** ᴴᶜᶜ

✓5ᵗʰ **E11.5**　**Type 2 diabetes mellitus with circulatory complications**

E11.51　**Type 2 diabetes mellitus with diabetic peripheral angiopathy without gangrene** ᴴᶜᶜ

E11.52　**Type 2 diabetes mellitus with diabetic peripheral angiopathy with gangrene** ᴴᶜᶜ
　　　　Type 2 diabetes mellitus with diabetic gangrene

E11.59　**Type 2 diabetes mellitus with other circulatory complications** ᴴᶜᶜ

✓5ᵗʰ **E11.6**　**Type 2 diabetes mellitus with other specified complications**

✓6ᵗʰ **E11.61**　**Type 2 diabetes mellitus with diabetic arthropathy**

　　E11.610　**Type 2 diabetes mellitus with diabetic neuropathic arthropathy** ᴴᶜᶜ
　　　　　Type 2 diabetes mellitus with Charcôt's joints

　　E11.618　**Type 2 diabetes mellitus with other diabetic arthropathy** ᴴᶜᶜ

✓6ᵗʰ **E11.62**　**Type 2 diabetes mellitus with skin complications**

　　E11.620　**Type 2 diabetes mellitus with diabetic dermatitis** ᴴᶜᶜ
　　　　　Type 2 diabetes mellitus with diabetic necrobiosis lipoidica

E11.621　**Type 2 diabetes mellitus with foot ulcer** ᴴᶜᶜ
　　　　Use additional code to identify site of ulcer (L97.4-, L97.5-)
　　　　AHA: 2016, 1Q, 12

E11.622　**Type 2 diabetes mellitus with other skin ulcer** ᴴᶜᶜ
　　　　Use additional code to identify site of ulcer (L97.1-L97.9, L98.41-L98.49)

E11.628　**Type 2 diabetes mellitus with other skin complications** ᴴᶜᶜ

✓6ᵗʰ **E11.63**　**Type 2 diabetes mellitus with oral complications**

E11.630　**Type 2 diabetes mellitus with periodontal disease** ᴴᶜᶜ

E11.638　**Type 2 diabetes mellitus with other oral complications** ᴴᶜᶜ

✓6ᵗʰ **E11.64**　**Type 2 diabetes mellitus with hypoglycemia**

E11.641　**Type 2 diabetes mellitus with hypoglycemia with coma** ᴴᶜᶜ

E11.649　**Type 2 diabetes mellitus with hypoglycemia without coma** ᴴᶜᶜ
　　　　AHA: 2016, 3Q, 42; 2015, 3Q, 21

E11.65　**Type 2 diabetes mellitus with hyperglycemia** ᴴᶜᶜ
　　　　AHA: 2013, 3Q, 20

E11.69　**Type 2 diabetes mellitus with other specified complication** ᴴᶜᶜ
　　　　Use additional code to identify complication
　　　　AHA: 2016, 4Q, 141; 2016, 1Q, 13

E11.8　**Type 2 diabetes mellitus with unspecified complications** ᴴᶜᶜ ▽

E11.9　**Type 2 diabetes mellitus without complications** ᴴᶜᶜ

✓4ᵗʰ **E13**　**Other specified diabetes mellitus**
　　INCLUDES　diabetes mellitus due to genetic defects of beta-cell function
　　　　diabetes mellitus due to genetic defects in insulin action
　　　　postpancreatectomy diabetes mellitus
　　　　postprocedural diabetes mellitus
　　　　secondary diabetes mellitus NEC
　　Use additional code to identify control using:
　　　　insulin (Z79.4)
　　　　oral antidiabetic drugs (Z79.84)
　　　　oral hypoglycemic drugs (Z79.84)
　　EXCLUDES 1　*diabetes (mellitus) due to autoimmune process (E10.-)*
　　　　diabetes (mellitus) due to immune mediated pancreatic islet beta-cell destruction (E10.-)
　　　　diabetes mellitus due to underlying condition (E08.-)
　　　　drug or chemical induced diabetes mellitus (E09.-)
　　　　gestational diabetes (O24.4-)
　　　　neonatal diabetes mellitus (P70.2)
　　　　type 1 diabetes mellitus (E10.-)
　　　　~~*type 2 diabetes mellitus (E11.-)*~~
　　AHA: 2013, 4Q, 114; 2013, 3Q, 20

✓5ᵗʰ **E13.0**　**Other specified diabetes mellitus with hyperosmolarity**

E13.00　**Other specified diabetes mellitus with hyperosmolarity without nonketotic hyperglycemic-hyperosmolar coma (NKHHC)** ᴴᶜᶜ
　　　　EXCLUDES 2 ▶*type 2 diabetes mellitus (E11.-)*◀

E13.01　**Other specified diabetes mellitus with hyperosmolarity with coma** ᴴᶜᶜ

✓5ᵗʰ **E13.1**　**Other specified diabetes mellitus with ketoacidosis**
　　　　AHA: 2016, 2Q, 10; 2013, 1Q, 26

E13.10　**Other specified diabetes mellitus with ketoacidosis without coma** ᴴᶜᶜ

E13.11　**Other specified diabetes mellitus with ketoacidosis with coma** ᴴᶜᶜ

✓5ᵗʰ **E13.2**　**Other specified diabetes mellitus with kidney complications**

E13.21　**Other specified diabetes mellitus with diabetic nephropathy** ᴴᶜᶜ
　　　　Other specified diabetes mellitus with intercapillary glomerulosclerosis
　　　　Other specified diabetes mellitus with intracapillary glomerulonephrosis
　　　　Other specified diabetes mellitus with Kimmelstiel-Wilson disease

E13.22　**Other specified diabetes mellitus with diabetic chronic kidney disease** ᴴᶜᶜ
　　　　Use additional code to identify stage of chronic kidney disease (N18.1-N18.6)

☑ Additional Character Req　　✓x7ᵗʰ Placeholder Alert　　Manifestation　　ᴴᶜᶜ CMS-HCC Condition　　▽ Unspecified Code　　▶◀ Revised Text　　● New Code　　▲ Revised Code Title

ICD-10-CM 2018　　　　　　　　　　　　　　　　　　　　　　　　　　　　　　　　　**513**

E13.29   **Other specified diabetes mellitus with other diabetic kidney complication**   HCC
Other specified diabetes mellitus with renal tubular degeneration

✓5th **E13.3**   **Other specified diabetes mellitus with ophthalmic complications**

> One of the following 7th characters is to be assigned to codes in subcategories E13.32, E13.33, E13.34, E13.35, and E13.37 to designate laterality of the disease:
> 1   right eye
> 2   left eye
> 3   bilateral
> 9   unspecified eye

✓6th **E13.31**   **Other specified diabetes mellitus with unspecified diabetic retinopathy**

     E13.311   **Other specified diabetes mellitus with unspecified diabetic retinopathy with macular edema**   HCC ▽

     E13.319   **Other specified diabetes mellitus with unspecified diabetic retinopathy without macular edema**   HCC ▽

✓6th **E13.32**   **Other specified diabetes mellitus with mild nonproliferative diabetic retinopathy**
Other specified diabetes mellitus with nonproliferative diabetic retinopathy NOS

     ✓7th **E13.321**   **Other specified diabetes mellitus with mild nonproliferative diabetic retinopathy with macular edema**   HCC

     ✓7th **E13.329**   **Other specified diabetes mellitus with mild nonproliferative diabetic retinopathy without macular edema**   HCC

✓6th **E13.33**   **Other specified diabetes mellitus with moderate nonproliferative diabetic retinopathy**

     ✓7th **E13.331**   **Other specified diabetes mellitus with moderate nonproliferative diabetic retinopathy with macular edema**   HCC

     ✓7th **E13.339**   **Other specified diabetes mellitus with moderate nonproliferative diabetic retinopathy without macular edema**   HCC

✓6th **E13.34**   **Other specified diabetes mellitus with severe nonproliferative diabetic retinopathy**

     ✓7th **E13.341**   **Other specified diabetes mellitus with severe nonproliferative diabetic retinopathy with macular edema**   HCC

     ✓7th **E13.349**   **Other specified diabetes mellitus with severe nonproliferative diabetic retinopathy without macular edema**   HCC

✓6th **E13.35**   **Other specified diabetes mellitus with proliferative diabetic retinopathy**

     ✓7th **E13.351**   **Other specified diabetes mellitus with proliferative diabetic retinopathy with macular edema**   HCC

     ✓7th **E13.352**   **Other specified diabetes mellitus with proliferative diabetic retinopathy with traction retinal detachment involving the macula**   HCC

     ✓7th **E13.353**   **Other specified diabetes mellitus with proliferative diabetic retinopathy with traction retinal detachment not involving the macula**   HCC

     ✓7th **E13.354**   **Other specified diabetes mellitus with proliferative diabetic retinopathy with combined traction retinal detachment and rhegmatogenous retinal detachment**   HCC

     ✓7th **E13.355**   **Other specified diabetes mellitus with stable proliferative diabetic retinopathy**   HCC

     ✓7th **E13.359**   **Other specified diabetes mellitus with proliferative diabetic retinopathy without macular edema**   HCC

     E13.36   **Other specified diabetes mellitus with diabetic cataract**   HCC
AHA: 2016, 4Q, 142

✓x7th **E13.37**   **Other specified diabetes mellitus with diabetic macular edema, resolved following treatment**   HCC

     E13.39   **Other specified diabetes mellitus with other diabetic ophthalmic complication**   HCC
Use additional code to identify manifestation, such as:
diabetic glaucoma (H40-H42)

✓5th **E13.4**   **Other specified diabetes mellitus with neurological complications**

     E13.40   **Other specified diabetes mellitus with diabetic neuropathy, unspecified**   HCC ▽

     E13.41   **Other specified diabetes mellitus with diabetic mononeuropathy**   HCC

     E13.42   **Other specified diabetes mellitus with diabetic polyneuropathy**   HCC
Other specified diabetes mellitus with diabetic neuralgia

     E13.43   **Other specified diabetes mellitus with diabetic autonomic (poly)neuropathy**   HCC
Other specified diabetes mellitus with diabetic gastroparesis
AHA: 2013, 4Q, 114

     E13.44   **Other specified diabetes mellitus with diabetic amyotrophy**   HCC

     E13.49   **Other specified diabetes mellitus with other diabetic neurological complication**   HCC

✓5th **E13.5**   **Other specified diabetes mellitus with circulatory complications**

     E13.51   **Other specified diabetes mellitus with diabetic peripheral angiopathy without gangrene**   HCC

     E13.52   **Other specified diabetes mellitus with diabetic peripheral angiopathy with gangrene**   HCC
Other specified diabetes mellitus with diabetic gangrene

     E13.59   **Other specified diabetes mellitus with other circulatory complications**   HCC

✓5th **E13.6**   **Other specified diabetes mellitus with other specified complications**

✓6th **E13.61**   **Other specified diabetes mellitus with diabetic arthropathy**

     E13.610   **Other specified diabetes mellitus with diabetic neuropathic arthropathy**   HCC
Other specified diabetes mellitus with Charcôt's joints

     E13.618   **Other specified diabetes mellitus with other diabetic arthropathy**   HCC

✓6th **E13.62**   **Other specified diabetes mellitus with skin complications**

     E13.620   **Other specified diabetes mellitus with diabetic dermatitis**   HCC
Other specified diabetes mellitus with diabetic necrobiosis lipoidica

     E13.621   **Other specified diabetes mellitus with foot ulcer**   HCC
Use additional code to identify site of ulcer (L97.4-, L97.5-)

     E13.622   **Other specified diabetes mellitus with other skin ulcer**   HCC
Use additional code to identify site of ulcer (L97.1-L97.9, L98.41-L98.49)

     E13.628   **Other specified diabetes mellitus with other skin complications**   HCC

✓6th **E13.63**   **Other specified diabetes mellitus with oral complications**

     E13.630   **Other specified diabetes mellitus with periodontal disease**   HCC

     E13.638   **Other specified diabetes mellitus with other oral complications**   HCC

✓6th **E13.64**   **Other specified diabetes mellitus with hypoglycemia**

     E13.641   **Other specified diabetes mellitus with hypoglycemia with coma**   HCC

     E13.649   **Other specified diabetes mellitus with hypoglycemia without coma**   HCC
AHA: 2016, 3Q, 42; 2015, 3Q, 21

     E13.65   **Other specified diabetes mellitus with hyperglycemia**   HCC

     E13.69   **Other specified diabetes mellitus with other specified complication**   HCC
Use additional code to identify complication
AHA: 2016, 4Q, 141; 2016, 1Q, 13

E13.8   **Other specified diabetes mellitus with unspecified complications**   HCC ▽

E13.9   **Other specified diabetes mellitus without complications**   HCC

EXCLUDES 1 Not coded here   EXCLUDES 2 Not included here   N Newborn Age: 0   P Pediatric Age: 0-17   M Maternity Age: 12-55   A Adult Age: 15-124

514   ICD-10-CM 2018

Other disorders of glucose regulation and pancreatic internal secretion (E15-E16)

E15   **Nondiabetic hypoglycemic coma**   HCC
     INCLUDES   drug-induced insulin coma in nondiabetic
              hyperinsulinism with hypoglycemic coma
              hypoglycemic coma NOS

✓4th **E16**   **Other disorders of pancreatic internal secretion**

E16.0   **Drug-induced hypoglycemia without coma**
     Use additional code for adverse effect, if applicable, to identify
     drug (T36-T50 with fifth or sixth character 5)
     EXCLUDES 1   *diabetes with hypoglycemia without coma*
           ▶*(E09.649)*◀

E16.1   **Other hypoglycemia**
     Functional hyperinsulinism
     Functional nonhyperinsulinemic hypoglycemia
     Hyperinsulinism NOS
     Hyperplasia of pancreatic islet beta cells NOS
     EXCLUDES 1   *diabetes with hypoglycemia (E08.649, E10.649,*
           E11.649, E13.649)
           hypoglycemia in infant of diabetic mother (P70.1)
           neonatal hypoglycemia (P70.4)

E16.2   **Hypoglycemia, unspecified**   ▽
     EXCLUDES 1   *diabetes with hypoglycemia (E08.649, E10.649,*
           E11.649, E13.649)
     AHA: 2016, 3Q, 42

E16.3   **Increased secretion of glucagon**
     Hyperplasia of pancreatic endocrine cells with glucagon excess

E16.4   **Increased secretion of gastrin**
     Hypergastrinemia
     Hyperplasia of pancreatic endocrine cells with gastrin excess
     Zollinger-Ellison syndrome

E16.8   **Other specified disorders of pancreatic internal secretion**
     Increased secretion from endocrine pancreas of growth
         hormone-releasing hormone
     Increased secretion from endocrine pancreas of pancreatic
         polypeptide
     Increased secretion from endocrine pancreas of somatostatin
     Increased secretion from endocrine pancreas of
         vasoactive-intestinal polypeptide

E16.9   **Disorder of pancreatic internal secretion, unspecified**   ▽
     Islet-cell hyperplasia NOS
     Pancreatic endocrine cell hyperplasia NOS

Disorders of other endocrine glands (E20-E35)

     EXCLUDES 1   *galactorrhea (N64.3)*
           gynecomastia (N62)

✓4th **E20**   **Hypoparathyroidism**
     EXCLUDES 1   *Di George's syndrome (D82.1)*
           postprocedural hypoparathyroidism (E89.2)
           tetany NOS (R29.0)
           transitory neonatal hypoparathyroidism (P71.4)

E20.0   **Idiopathic hypoparathyroidism**   HCC
     DEF: Abnormally low secretion of parathyroid hormones, with
     unknown cause, which causes decreased calcium and increased
     phosphorus in the blood, resulting in muscle cramps, tetany,
     tingling, or burning in lips, fingers, and toes, and cataracts.

E20.1   **Pseudohypoparathyroidism**

E20.8   **Other hypoparathyroidism**   HCC

E20.9   **Hypoparathyroidism, unspecified**   HCC ▽
     Parathyroid tetany

✓4th **E21**   **Hyperparathyroidism and other disorders of parathyroid gland**
     EXCLUDES 1   *adult osteomalacia (M83.-)*
           ectopic hyperparathyroidism (E34.2)
           familial hypocalciuric hypercalcemia (E83.52)
           hungry bone syndrome (E83.81)
           infantile and juvenile osteomalacia (E55.0)

E21.0   **Primary hyperparathyroidism**   HCC
     Hyperplasia of parathyroid
     Osteitis fibrosa cystica generalisata [von Recklinghausen's
         disease of bone]
     DEF: Parathyroid dysfunction commonly caused by hyperplasia of
     two or more glands; characteristic hypercalcemia and increased
     parathyroid hormone levels.

E21.1   **Secondary hyperparathyroidism, not elsewhere classified** HCC
     EXCLUDES 1   *secondary hyperparathyroidism of renal origin*
           (N25.81)

E21.2   **Other hyperparathyroidism**   HCC
     Tertiary hyperparathyroidism
     EXCLUDES 1   *familial hypocalciuric hypercalcemia (E83.52)*

E21.3   **Hyperparathyroidism, unspecified**   HCC ▽

E21.4   **Other specified disorders of parathyroid gland**   HCC

E21.5   **Disorder of parathyroid gland, unspecified**   HCC ▽

✓4th **E22**   **Hyperfunction of pituitary gland**
     EXCLUDES 1   *Cushing's syndrome (E24.-)*
           Nelson's syndrome (E24.1)
           overproduction of ACTH not associated with Cushing's disease
           (E27.0)
           overproduction of pituitary ACTH (E24.0)
           overproduction of thyroid-stimulating hormone (E05.8-)

E22.0   **Acromegaly and pituitary gigantism**   HCC
     Overproduction of growth hormone
     EXCLUDES 1   *constitutional gigantism (E34.4)*
           constitutional tall stature (E34.4)
           increased secretion from endocrine pancreas of growth
           hormone-releasing hormone (E16.8)

E22.1   **Hyperprolactinemia**   HCC
     Use additional code for adverse effect, if applicable, to identify
     drug (T36-T50 with fifth or sixth character 5)

E22.2   **Syndrome of inappropriate secretion of antidiuretic hormone**   HCC

E22.8   **Other hyperfunction of pituitary gland**   HCC
     Central precocious puberty

E22.9   **Hyperfunction of pituitary gland, unspecified**   HCC ▽

✓4th **E23**   **Hypofunction and other disorders of the pituitary gland**
     INCLUDES   the listed conditions whether the disorder is in the pituitary
              or the hypothalamus
     EXCLUDES 1   *postprocedural hypopituitarism (E89.3)*

E23.0   **Hypopituitarism**   HCC
     Fertile eunuch syndrome
     Hypogonadotropic hypogonadism
     Idiopathic growth hormone deficiency
     Isolated deficiency of gonadotropin
     Isolated deficiency of growth hormone
     Isolated deficiency of pituitary hormone
     Kallmann's syndrome
     Lorain-Levi short stature
     Necrosis of pituitary gland (postpartum)
     Panhypopituitarism
     Pituitary cachexia
     Pituitary insufficiency NOS
     Pituitary short stature
     Sheehan's syndrome
     Simmonds' disease

E23.1   **Drug-induced hypopituitarism**   HCC
     Use additional code for adverse effect, if applicable, to identify
     drug (T36-T50 with fifth or sixth character 5)

E23.2   **Diabetes insipidus**   HCC
     EXCLUDES 1   *nephrogenic diabetes insipidus (N25.1)*

E23.3   **Hypothalamic dysfunction, not elsewhere classified**   HCC
     EXCLUDES 1   *Prader-Willi syndrome (Q87.1)*
           Russell-Silver syndrome (Q87.1)

E23.6   **Other disorders of pituitary gland**   HCC
     Abscess of pituitary   Adiposogenital dystrophy

E23.7   **Disorder of pituitary gland, unspecified**   HCC ▽

✓4th **E24**   **Cushing's syndrome**
     EXCLUDES 1   *congenital adrenal hyperplasia (E25.0)*

E24.0   **Pituitary-dependent Cushing's disease**   HCC
     Overproduction of pituitary ACTH
     Pituitary-dependent hypercorticalism

E24.1   **Nelson's syndrome**   HCC

E24.2   **Drug-induced Cushing's syndrome**   HCC
     Use additional code for adverse effect, if applicable, to identify
     drug (T36-T50 with fifth or sixth character 5)

E24.3   **Ectopic ACTH syndrome**   HCC

E24.4   **Alcohol-induced pseudo-Cushing's syndrome**   HCC

E24.8   **Other Cushing's syndrome**   HCC

E24.9   **Cushing's syndrome, unspecified**   HCC ▽

✓ Additional Character Req   ✗7th Placeholder Alert   Manifestation   HCC CMS-HCC Condition   ▽ Unspecified Code   ▶◀ Revised Text   ● New Code   ▲ Revised Code Title

Chapter 4. Endocrine, Nutritional, and Metabolic Diseases

✓4ᵗʰ E25 Adrenogenital disorders

INCLUDES   adrenogenital syndromes, virilizing or feminizing, whether acquired or due to adrenal hyperplasia
consequent on inborn enzyme defects in hormone synthesis
female adrenal pseudohermaphroditism
female heterosexual precocious pseudopuberty
male isosexual precocious pseudopuberty
male macrogenitosomia praecox
male sexual precocity with adrenal hyperplasia
male virilization (female)

EXCLUDES 1   *indeterminate sex and pseudohermaphroditism (Q56)*
chromosomal abnormalities (Q90-Q99)

E25.0   Congenital adrenogenital disorders associated with enzyme deficiency   HCC
Congenital adrenal hyperplasia
21-Hydroxylase deficiency
Salt-losing congenital adrenal hyperplasia

E25.8   Other adrenogenital disorders   HCC
Idiopathic adrenogenital disorder
Use additional code for adverse effect, if applicable, to identify drug (T36-T50 with fifth or sixth character 5)

E25.9   Adrenogenital disorder, unspecified   HCC ▽
Adrenogenital syndrome NOS

✓4ᵗʰ E26 Hyperaldosteronism

✓5ᵗʰ E26.0   Primary hyperaldosteronism

E26.01   Conn's syndrome   HCC
Code also adrenal adenoma (D35.0-)

E26.02   Glucocorticoid-remediable aldosteronism   HCC
Familial aldosteronism type I
DEF: Rare autosomal dominant familial form of primary aldosteronism in which the secretion of aldosterone is under the influence of adrenocorticotrophic hormone (ACTH) rather than the renin-angiotensin mechanism; moderate hypersecretion of aldosterone and suppressed plasma renin activity that are rapidly reversed by administration of glucosteroids; symptoms include hypertension and mild hypokalemia.

E26.09   Other primary hyperaldosteronism   HCC
Primary aldosteronism due to adrenal hyperplasia (bilateral)

E26.1   Secondary hyperaldosteronism   HCC

✓5ᵗʰ E26.8   Other hyperaldosteronism

E26.81   Bartter's syndrome   HCC

E26.89   Other hyperaldosteronism   HCC

E26.9   Hyperaldosteronism, unspecified   HCC ▽
Aldosteronism NOS
Hyperaldosteronism NOS

✓4ᵗʰ E27 Other disorders of adrenal gland

E27.0   Other adrenocortical overactivity   HCC
Overproduction of ACTH, not associated with Cushing's disease
Premature adrenarche
EXCLUDES 1   *Cushing's syndrome (E24.-)*

E27.1   Primary adrenocortical insufficiency   HCC
Addison's disease
Autoimmune adrenalitis
EXCLUDES 1   *Addison only phenotype adrenoleukodystrophy (E71.528)*
amyloidosis (E85.-)
tuberculous Addison's disease (A18.7)
Waterhouse-Friderichsen syndrome (A39.1)

E27.2   Addisonian crisis   HCC
Adrenal crisis
Adrenocortical crisis

E27.3   Drug-induced adrenocortical insufficiency   HCC
Use additional code for adverse effect, if applicable, to identify drug (T36-T50 with fifth or sixth character 5)

✓5ᵗʰ E27.4   Other and unspecified adrenocortical insufficiency
EXCLUDES 1   *adrenoleukodystrophy [Addison-Schilder] (E71.528)*
Waterhouse-Friderichsen syndrome (A39.1)

E27.40   Unspecified adrenocortical insufficiency   HCC ▽
Adrenocortical insufficiency NOS
Hypoaldosteronism

E27.49   Other adrenocortical insufficiency   HCC
Adrenal hemorrhage
Adrenal infarction

E27.5   Adrenomedullary hyperfunction   HCC
Adrenomedullary hyperplasia
Catecholamine hypersecretion

E27.8   Other specified disorders of adrenal gland   HCC
Abnormality of cortisol-binding globulin

E27.9   Disorder of adrenal gland, unspecified   HCC ▽

✓4ᵗʰ E28 Ovarian dysfunction

EXCLUDES 1   *isolated gonadotropin deficiency (E23.0)*
postprocedural ovarian failure (E89.4-)

E28.0   Estrogen excess   ♀
Use additional code for adverse effect, if applicable, to identify drug (T36-T50 with fifth or sixth character 5)

E28.1   Androgen excess   ♀
Hypersecretion of ovarian androgens
Use additional code for adverse effect, if applicable, to identify drug (T36-T50 with fifth or sixth character 5)

E28.2   Polycystic ovarian syndrome   ♀
Sclerocystic ovary syndrome
Stein-Leventhal syndrome

✓5ᵗʰ E28.3   Primary ovarian failure
EXCLUDES 1   *pure gonadal dysgenesis (Q99.1)*
Turner's syndrome (Q96.-)

✓6ᵗʰ E28.31   Premature menopause

E28.310   Symptomatic premature menopause   A ♀
Symptoms such as flushing, sleeplessness, headache, lack of concentration, associated with premature menopause

E28.319   Asymptomatic premature menopause   A ♀
Premature menopause NOS

E28.39   Other primary ovarian failure   ♀
Decreased estrogen
Resistant ovary syndrome

E28.8   Other ovarian dysfunction   ♀
Ovarian hyperfunction NOS
EXCLUDES 1   *postprocedural ovarian failure (E89.4-)*

E28.9   Ovarian dysfunction, unspecified   ♀ ▽

✓4ᵗʰ E29 Testicular dysfunction

EXCLUDES 1   *androgen insensitivity syndrome (E34.5-)*
azoospermia or oligospermia NOS (N46.0-N46.1)
isolated gonadotropin deficiency (E23.0)
Klinefelter's syndrome (Q98.0-Q98.1, Q98.4)

E29.0   Testicular hyperfunction   ♂
Hypersecretion of testicular hormones

E29.1   Testicular hypofunction   ♂
Defective biosynthesis of testicular androgen NOS
5-delta-Reductase deficiency (with male pseudohermaphroditism)
Testicular hypogonadism NOS
Use additional code for adverse effect, if applicable, to identify drug (T36-T50 with fifth or sixth character 5)
EXCLUDES 1   *postprocedural testicular hypofunction (E89.5)*

E29.8   Other testicular dysfunction   ♂

E29.9   Testicular dysfunction, unspecified   ♂ ▽

✓4ᵗʰ E30 Disorders of puberty, not elsewhere classified

E30.0   Delayed puberty
Constitutional delay of puberty
Delayed sexual development

E30.1   Precocious puberty   P
Precocious menstruation
EXCLUDES 1   *Albright (-McCune) (-Sternberg) syndrome (Q78.1)*
central precocious puberty (E22.8)
congenital adrenal hyperplasia (E25.0)
female heterosexual precocious pseudopuberty (E25.-)
male isosexual precocious pseudopuberty (E25.-)

E30.8   Other disorders of puberty   P
Premature thelarche

E30.9   Disorder of puberty, unspecified   ▽

✓4ᵗʰ E31 Polyglandular dysfunction

EXCLUDES 1   *ataxia telangiectasia [Louis-Bar] (G11.3)*
dystrophia myotonica [Steinert] (G71.11)
pseudohypoparathyroidism (E20.1)

E31.0   Autoimmune polyglandular failure   HCC
Schmidt's syndrome

E31.1   Polyglandular hyperfunction   HCC
EXCLUDES 1   *multiple endocrine adenomatosis (E31.2-)*
multiple endocrine neoplasia (E31.2-)

EXCLUDES 1 Not coded here   EXCLUDES 2 Not included here   N Newborn Age: 0   P Pediatric Age: 0-17   M Maternity Age: 12-55   A Adult Age: 15-124

516   ICD-10-CM 2018

☑5ᵗʰ **E31.2 Multiple endocrine neoplasia [MEN] syndromes**
Multiple endocrine adenomatosis
Code also any associated malignancies and other conditions associated with the syndromes

     E31.20 Multiple endocrine neoplasia [MEN]   HCC ▽
     syndrome, unspecified
       Multiple endocrine adenomatosis NOS
       Multiple endocrine neoplasia [MEN] syndrome NOS

     E31.21 Multiple endocrine neoplasia [MEN] type I   HCC
       Wermer's syndrome

     E31.22 Multiple endocrine neoplasia [MEN] type IIA   HCC
       Sipple's syndrome

     E31.23 Multiple endocrine neoplasia [MEN] type IIB   HCC

E31.8 Other polyglandular dysfunction   HCC

E31.9 Polyglandular dysfunction, unspecified   HCC ▽

☑4ᵗʰ **E32 Diseases of thymus**
    EXCLUDES 1   aplasia or hypoplasia of thymus with immunodeficiency (D82.1)
            myasthenia gravis (G70.0)

E32.0 Persistent hyperplasia of thymus   HCC
Hypertrophy of thymus

E32.1 Abscess of thymus   HCC

E32.8 Other diseases of thymus   HCC
    EXCLUDES 1   aplasia or hypoplasia with immunodeficiency (D82.1)
            thymoma (D15.0)

E32.9 Disease of thymus, unspecified   HCC ▽

☑4ᵗʰ **E34 Other endocrine disorders**
    EXCLUDES 1   pseudohypoparathyroidism (E20.1)

E34.0 Carcinoid syndrome   HCC
    NOTE   May be used as an additional code to identify functional activity associated with a carcinoid tumor.

E34.1 Other hypersecretion of intestinal hormones

E34.2 Ectopic hormone secretion, not elsewhere classified
    EXCLUDES 1   ectopic ACTH syndrome (E24.3)

E34.3 Short stature due to endocrine disorder
Constitutional short stature
Laron-type short stature
    EXCLUDES 1   achondroplastic short stature (Q77.4)
            hypochondroplastic short stature (Q77.4)
            nutritional short stature (E45)
            pituitary short stature (E23.0)
            progeria (E34.8)
            renal short stature (N25.0)
            Russell-Silver syndrome (Q87.1)
            short-limbed stature with immunodeficiency (D82.2)
            short stature in specific dysmorphic syndromes— code
            to syndrome—see Alphabetical Index
            short stature NOS (R62.52)

E34.4 Constitutional tall stature   HCC
Constitutional gigantism

☑5ᵗʰ **E34.5 Androgen insensitivity syndrome**
     E34.50 Androgen insensitivity syndrome, unspecified   ▽
       Androgen insensitivity NOS

     E34.51 Complete androgen insensitivity syndrome
       Complete androgen insensitivity
       de Quervain syndrome
       Goldberg-Maxwell syndrome

     E34.52 Partial androgen insensitivity syndrome
       Partial androgen insensitivity
       Reifenstein syndrome

E34.8 Other specified endocrine disorders
Pineal gland dysfunction
Progeria
    EXCLUDES 2   pseudohypoparathyroidism (E20.1)

E34.9 Endocrine disorder, unspecified   ▽
Endocrine disturbance NOS
Hormone disturbance NOS

E35   ***Disorders of endocrine glands in diseases classified elsewhere***
Code first underlying disease, such as:
    late congenital syphilis of thymus gland [Dubois disease] (A50.5)
Use additional code, if applicable, to identify:
    sequelae of tuberculosis of other organs (B90.8)
    EXCLUDES 1   Echinococcus granulosus infection of thyroid gland (B67.3)
            meningococcal hemorrhagic adrenalitis (A39.1)
            syphilis of endocrine gland (A52.79)
            tuberculosis of adrenal gland, except calcification (A18.7)
            tuberculosis of endocrine gland NEC (A18.82)
            tuberculosis of thyroid gland (A18.81)
            Waterhouse-Friderichsen syndrome (A39.1)

Intraoperative complications of endocrine system (E36)

☑4ᵗʰ **E36 Intraoperative complications of endocrine system**
    EXCLUDES 2   postprocedural endocrine and metabolic complications and
            disorders, not elsewhere classified (E89.-)

☑5ᵗʰ **E36.0 Intraoperative hemorrhage and hematoma of an endocrine system organ or structure complicating a procedure**
     EXCLUDES 1   intraoperative hemorrhage and hematoma of an
              endocrine system organ or structure due to
              accidental puncture or laceration during a
              procedure (E36.1-)

     E36.01 Intraoperative hemorrhage and hematoma of an endocrine system organ or structure complicating an endocrine system procedure

     E36.02 Intraoperative hemorrhage and hematoma of an endocrine system organ or structure complicating other procedure

☑5ᵗʰ **E36.1 Accidental puncture and laceration of an endocrine system organ or structure during a procedure**

     E36.11 Accidental puncture and laceration of an endocrine system organ or structure during an endocrine system procedure

     E36.12 Accidental puncture and laceration of an endocrine system organ or structure during other procedure

E36.8 Other intraoperative complications of endocrine system
Use additional code, if applicable, to further specify disorder

Malnutrition (E40-E46)

    EXCLUDES 1   intestinal malabsorption (K90.-)
            sequelae of protein-calorie malnutrition (E64.0)
    EXCLUDES 2   nutritional anemias (D50-D53)
            starvation (T73.0)

E40 Kwashiorkor   HCC
Severe malnutrition with nutritional edema with dyspigmentation of skin and hair
    EXCLUDES 1   marasmic kwashiorkor (E42)

E41 Nutritional marasmus   HCC
Severe malnutrition with marasmus
    EXCLUDES 1   marasmic kwashiorkor (E42)
DEF: Protein-calorie malabsorption or malnutrition in children; characterized by tissue wasting, dehydration, and subcutaneous fat depletion; may occur with infectious disease; also called infantile atrophy.

E42 Marasmic kwashiorkor   HCC
Intermediate form severe protein-calorie malnutrition
Severe protein-calorie malnutrition with signs of both kwashiorkor and marasmus

E43 Unspecified severe protein-calorie malnutrition   HCC ▽
Starvation edema

☑4ᵗʰ **E44 Protein-calorie malnutrition of moderate and mild degree**
     E44.0 Moderate protein-calorie malnutrition   HCC
     E44.1 Mild protein-calorie malnutrition   HCC

E45 Retarded development following protein-calorie   HCC
malnutrition
Nutritional short stature
Nutritional stunting
Physical retardation due to malnutrition

E46 Unspecified protein-calorie malnutrition   HCC ▽
Malnutrition NOS
Protein-calorie imbalance NOS
    EXCLUDES 1   nutritional deficiency NOS (E63.9)

Other nutritional deficiencies (E50-E64)

    EXCLUDES 2   nutritional anemias (D50-D53)

☑4ᵗʰ **E50 Vitamin A deficiency**
    EXCLUDES 1   sequelae of vitamin A deficiency (E64.1)

E50.0 Vitamin A deficiency with conjunctival xerosis

E50.1 Vitamin A deficiency with Bitot's spot and conjunctival xerosis
Bitot's spot in the young child
DEF: Vitamin A deficiency with conjunctival dryness, superficial spots of keratinized epithelium.

E50.2 Vitamin A deficiency with corneal xerosis

E50.3 Vitamin A deficiency with corneal ulceration and xerosis

E50.4 Vitamin A deficiency with keratomalacia
DEF: Vitamin A deficiency creating corneal dryness; progresses to corneal insensitivity, softness, and necrosis; usually bilateral.

☑ Additional Character Req   ☑x7ᵗʰ Placeholder Alert   Manifestation   HCC CMS-HCC Condition   ▽ Unspecified Code   ►◄ Revised Text   ● New Code   ▲ Revised Code Title

Chapter 4. Endocrine, Nutritional, and Metabolic Diseases

E50.5   **Vitamin A deficiency with night blindness**

E50.6   **Vitamin A deficiency with xerophthalmic scars of cornea**

E50.7   **Other ocular manifestations of vitamin A deficiency**
Xerophthalmia NOS

E50.8   **Other manifestations of vitamin A deficiency**
Follicular keratosis
Xeroderma

E50.9   **Vitamin A deficiency, unspecified**   ▽
Hypovitaminosis A NOS

✓4th **E51**   **Thiamine deficiency**
EXCLUDES 1   *sequelae of thiamine deficiency (E64.8)*

   ✓5th **E51.1**   **Beriberi**

     E51.11   **Dry beriberi**
Beriberi NOS
Beriberi with polyneuropathy

     E51.12   **Wet beriberi**
Beriberi with cardiovascular manifestations
Cardiovascular beriberi
Shoshin disease

   E51.2   **Wernicke's encephalopathy**

   E51.8   **Other manifestations of thiamine deficiency**

   E51.9   **Thiamine deficiency, unspecified**   ▽

E52   **Niacin deficiency [pellagra]**
Niacin (-tryptophan) deficiency
Nicotinamide deficiency
Pellagra (alcoholic)
EXCLUDES 1   *sequelae of niacin deficiency (E64.8)*

✓4th **E53**   **Deficiency of other B group vitamins**
EXCLUDES 1   *sequelae of vitamin B deficiency (E64.8)*

   E53.0   **Riboflavin deficiency**
Ariboflavinosis
Vitamin B2 deficiency

   E53.1   **Pyridoxine deficiency**
Vitamin B6 deficiency
EXCLUDES 1   *pyridoxine-responsive sideroblastic anemia (D64.3)*

   E53.8   **Deficiency of other specified B group vitamins**
Biotin deficiency
Cyanocobalamin deficiency
Folate deficiency
Folic acid deficiency
Pantothenic acid deficiency
Vitamin B12 deficiency
EXCLUDES 1   *folate deficiency anemia (D52.-)*
vitamin B12 deficiency anemia (D51.-)

   E53.9   **Vitamin B deficiency, unspecified**   ▽

E54   **Ascorbic acid deficiency**
Deficiency of vitamin C
Scurvy
EXCLUDES 1   *scorbutic anemia (D53.2)*
sequelae of vitamin C deficiency (E64.2)
DEF: Vitamin C deficiency causing swollen gums, myalgia, weight loss, and weakness.

✓4th **E55**   **Vitamin D deficiency**
EXCLUDES 1   *adult osteomalacia (M83.-)*
osteoporosis (M80.-)
sequelae of rickets (E64.3)

   E55.0   **Rickets, active**
Infantile osteomalacia
Juvenile osteomalacia
EXCLUDES 1   *celiac rickets (K90.0)*
Crohn's rickets (K50.-)
hereditary vitamin D-dependent rickets (E83.32)
inactive rickets (E64.3)
renal rickets (N25.0)
sequelae of rickets (E64.3)
vitamin D-resistant rickets (E83.31)

   E55.9   **Vitamin D deficiency, unspecified**   ▽
Avitaminosis D

✓4th **E56**   **Other vitamin deficiencies**
EXCLUDES 1   *sequelae of other vitamin deficiencies (E64.8)*

   E56.0   **Deficiency of vitamin E**

   E56.1   **Deficiency of vitamin K**
EXCLUDES 1   *deficiency of coagulation factor due to vitamin K deficiency (D68.4)*
vitamin K deficiency of newborn (P53)

   E56.8   **Deficiency of other vitamins**

   E56.9   **Vitamin deficiency, unspecified**   ▽

E58   **Dietary calcium deficiency**
EXCLUDES 1   *disorders of calcium metabolism (E83.5-)*
sequelae of calcium deficiency (E64.8)

E59   **Dietary selenium deficiency**
Keshan disease
EXCLUDES 1   *sequelae of selenium deficiency (E64.8)*

E60   **Dietary zinc deficiency**

✓4th **E61**   **Deficiency of other nutrient elements**
Use additional code for adverse effect, if applicable, to identify drug (T36-T50 with fifth or sixth character 5)
EXCLUDES 1   *disorders of mineral metabolism (E83.-)*
iodine deficiency related thyroid disorders (E00-E02)
sequelae of malnutrition and other nutritional deficiencies (E64.-)

   E61.0   **Copper deficiency**

   E61.1   **Iron deficiency**
EXCLUDES 1   *iron deficiency anemia (D50.-)*

   E61.2   **Magnesium deficiency**

   E61.3   **Manganese deficiency**

   E61.4   **Chromium deficiency**

   E61.5   **Molybdenum deficiency**

   E61.6   **Vanadium deficiency**

   E61.7   **Deficiency of multiple nutrient elements**

   E61.8   **Deficiency of other specified nutrient elements**

   E61.9   **Deficiency of nutrient element, unspecified**   ▽

✓4th **E63**   **Other nutritional deficiencies**
EXCLUDES 1   *dehydration (E86.0)*
failure to thrive, adult (R62.7)
failure to thrive, child (R62.51)
feeding problems in newborn (P92.-)
sequelae of malnutrition and other nutritional deficiencies (E64.-)

   E63.0   **Essential fatty acid [EFA] deficiency**

   E63.1   **Imbalance of constituents of food intake**

   E63.8   **Other specified nutritional deficiencies**

   E63.9   **Nutritional deficiency, unspecified**   ▽

✓4th **E64**   **Sequelae of malnutrition and other nutritional deficiencies**
NOTE   This category is to be used to indicate conditions in categories E43, E44, E46, E50-E63 as the cause of sequelae, which are themselves classified elsewhere. The 'sequelae' include conditions specified as such; they also include the late effects of diseases classifiable to the above categories if the disease itself is no longer present.
Code first condition resulting from (sequela) of malnutrition and other nutritional deficiencies

   E64.0   **Sequelae of protein-calorie malnutrition**   HCC
EXCLUDES 2   *retarded development following protein-calorie malnutrition (E45)*

   E64.1   **Sequelae of vitamin A deficiency**

   E64.2   **Sequelae of vitamin C deficiency**

   E64.3   **Sequelae of rickets**

   E64.8   **Sequelae of other nutritional deficiencies**

   E64.9   **Sequelae of unspecified nutritional deficiency**   ▽

Overweight, obesity and other hyperalimentation (E65-E68)

E65   **Localized adiposity**
Fat pad

✓4th **E66**   **Overweight and obesity**
Code first obesity complicating pregnancy, childbirth and the puerperium, if applicable (O99.21-)
Use additional code to identify body mass index (BMI), if known (Z68.-)
EXCLUDES 1   *adiposogenital dystrophy (E23.6)*
lipomatosis NOS (E88.2)
lipomatosis dolorosa [Dercum] (E88.2)
Prader-Willi syndrome (Q87.1)

   ✓5th **E66.0**   **Obesity due to excess calories**

     E66.01   **Morbid (severe) obesity due to excess calories**   HCC
EXCLUDES 1   *morbid (severe) obesity with alveolar hypoventilation (E66.2)*

     E66.09   **Other obesity due to excess calories**

   E66.1   **Drug-induced obesity**
Use additional code for adverse effect, if applicable, to identify drug (T36-T50 with fifth or sixth character 5)

EXCLUDES 1 Not coded here   EXCLUDES 2 Not included here   N Newborn Age: 0   P Pediatric Age: 0-17   M Maternity Age: 12-55   A Adult Age: 15-124

518   ICD-10-CM 2018

E66.2   **Morbid (severe) obesity with alveolar hypoventilation**   `HCC`
     Obesity hypoventilation syndrome (OHS)
     Pickwickian syndrome

E66.3   **Overweight**

E66.8   **Other obesity**

E66.9   **Obesity, unspecified**   ▽
     Obesity NOS

✓4th **E67**   **Other hyperalimentation**
     EXCLUDES 1   *hyperalimentation NOS (R63.2)*
             sequelae of hyperalimentation (E68)

E67.0   **Hypervitaminosis A**

E67.1   **Hypercarotinemia**

E67.2   **Megavitamin-B6 syndrome**

E67.3   **Hypervitaminosis D**

E67.8   **Other specified hyperalimentation**

E68   **Sequelae of hyperalimentation**
     Code first condition resulting from (sequela) of hyperalimentation

Metabolic disorders (E70-E88)

EXCLUDES 1   *androgen insensitivity syndrome (E34.5-)*
            congenital adrenal hyperplasia (E25.0)
            Ehlers-Danlos syndrome (Q79.6)
            hemolytic anemias attributable to enzyme disorders (D55.-)
            Marfan's syndrome (Q87.4)
            5-alpha-reductase deficiency (E29.1)

✓4th **E70**   **Disorders of aromatic amino-acid metabolism**

E70.0   **Classical phenylketonuria**   `HCC`

E70.1   **Other hyperphenylalaninemias**   `HCC`

✓5th **E70.2**   **Disorders of tyrosine metabolism**
       EXCLUDES 1   *transitory tyrosinemia of newborn (P74.5)*

     E70.20   **Disorder of tyrosine metabolism, unspecified**   `HCC` ▽

     E70.21   **Tyrosinemia**   `HCC`
         Hypertyrosinemia

     E70.29   **Other disorders of tyrosine metabolism**   `HCC`
         Alkaptonuria
         Ochronosis

✓5th **E70.3**   **Albinism**

     E70.30   **Albinism, unspecified**   `HCC` ▽

     ✓6th **E70.31**   **Ocular albinism**

         E70.310   **X-linked ocular albinism**   `HCC`

         E70.311   **Autosomal recessive ocular albinism**   `HCC`

         E70.318   **Other ocular albinism**   `HCC`

         E70.319   **Ocular albinism, unspecified**   `HCC` ▽

     ✓6th **E70.32**   **Oculocutaneous albinism**
         EXCLUDES 1   *Chediak-Higashi syndrome (E70.330)*
              Hermansky-Pudlak syndrome (E70.331)

         E70.320   **Tyrosinase negative oculocutaneous albinism**   `HCC`
            Albinism I
            Oculocutaneous albinism ty-neg

         E70.321   **Tyrosinase positive oculocutaneous albinism**   `HCC`
            Albinism II
            Oculocutaneous albinism ty-pos

         E70.328   **Other oculocutaneous albinism**   `HCC`
            Cross syndrome

         E70.329   **Oculocutaneous albinism, unspecified**   `HCC` ▽

     ✓6th **E70.33**   **Albinism with hematologic abnormality**

         E70.330   **Chediak-Higashi syndrome**   `HCC`

         E70.331   **Hermansky-Pudlak syndrome**   `HCC`

         E70.338   **Other albinism with hematologic abnormality**   `HCC`

         E70.339   **Albinism with hematologic abnormality, unspecified**   `HCC` ▽

     E70.39   **Other specified albinism**   `HCC`
         Piebaldism

✓5th **E70.4**   **Disorders of histidine metabolism**

     E70.40   **Disorders of histidine metabolism, unspecified**   `HCC` ▽

     E70.41   **Histidinemia**   `HCC`

     E70.49   **Other disorders of histidine metabolism**   `HCC`

E70.5   **Disorders of tryptophan metabolism**   `HCC`

E70.8   **Other disorders of aromatic amino-acid metabolism**   `HCC`

E70.9   **Disorder of aromatic amino-acid metabolism, unspecified**   `HCC` ▽

✓4th **E71**   **Disorders of branched-chain amino-acid metabolism and fatty-acid metabolism**

E71.0   **Maple-syrup-urine disease**   `HCC`

✓5th **E71.1**   **Other disorders of branched-chain amino-acid metabolism**

     ✓6th **E71.11**   **Branched-chain organic acidurias**

         E71.110   **Isovaleric acidemia**   `HCC`

         E71.111   **3-methylglutaconic aciduria**   `HCC`

         E71.118   **Other branched-chain organic acidurias**   `HCC`

     ✓6th **E71.12**   **Disorders of propionate metabolism**

         E71.120   **Methylmalonic acidemia**   `HCC`

         E71.121   **Propionic acidemia**   `HCC`

         E71.128   **Other disorders of propionate metabolism**   `HCC`

     E71.19   **Other disorders of branched-chain amino-acid metabolism**   `HCC`
         Hyperleucine-isoleucinemia
         Hypervalinemia

E71.2   **Disorder of branched-chain amino-acid metabolism, unspecified**   `HCC` ▽

✓5th **E71.3**   **Disorders of fatty-acid metabolism**
       EXCLUDES 1   *peroxisomal disorders (E71.5)*
              Refsum's disease (G60.1)
              Schilder's disease (G37.0)
       EXCLUDES 2   *carnitine deficiency due to inborn error of metabolism (E71.42)*

     E71.30   **Disorder of fatty-acid metabolism, unspecified**   ▽

     ✓6th **E71.31**   **Disorders of fatty-acid oxidation**

         E71.310   **Long chain/very long chain acyl CoA dehydrogenase deficiency**   `HCC`
            LCAD   VLCAD

         E71.311   **Medium chain acyl CoA dehydrogenase deficiency**   `HCC`
            MCAD

         E71.312   **Short chain acyl CoA dehydrogenase deficiency**
            SCAD

         E71.313   **Glutaric aciduria type II**   `HCC`
            Glutaric aciduria type II A
            Glutaric aciduria type II B
            Glutaric aciduria type II C
            EXCLUDES 1   *glutaric aciduria (type 1) NOS (E72.3)*

         E71.314   **Muscle carnitine palmitoyltransferase deficiency**   `HCC`

         E71.318   **Other disorders of fatty-acid oxidation**   `HCC`

     E71.32   **Disorders of ketone metabolism**   `HCC`

     E71.39   **Other disorders of fatty-acid metabolism**   `HCC`

✓5th **E71.4**   **Disorders of carnitine metabolism**
       EXCLUDES 1   *muscle carnitine palmitoyltransferase deficiency (E71.314)*

     E71.40   **Disorder of carnitine metabolism, unspecified**   `HCC` ▽

     E71.41   **Primary carnitine deficiency**   `HCC`

     E71.42   **Carnitine deficiency due to inborn errors of metabolism**   `HCC`
         Code also associated inborn error or metabolism

     E71.43   **Iatrogenic carnitine deficiency**   `HCC`
         Carnitine deficiency due to hemodialysis
         Carnitine deficiency due to Valproic acid therapy

     ✓6th **E71.44**   **Other secondary carnitine deficiency**

         E71.440   **Ruvalcaba-Myhre-Smith syndrome**   `HCC`

         E71.448   **Other secondary carnitine deficiency**   `HCC`

✓5th **E71.5**   **Peroxisomal disorders**
       EXCLUDES 1   *Schilder's disease (G37.0)*

     E71.50   **Peroxisomal disorder, unspecified**   `HCC` ▽

     ✓6th **E71.51**   **Disorders of peroxisome biogenesis**
         Group 1 peroxisomal disorders
         EXCLUDES 1   *Refsum's disease (G60.1)*

         E71.510   **Zellweger syndrome**   `HCC`

         E71.511   **Neonatal adrenoleukodystrophy**   `HCC`
            EXCLUDES 1   *X-linked adrenoleuko- dystrophy (E71.52-)*

         E71.518   **Other disorders of peroxisome biogenesis**   `HCC`

✓ Additional Character Req   ✓x7th Placeholder Alert   Manifestation   `HCC` CMS-HCC Condition   ▽ Unspecified Code   ►◄ Revised Text   ● New Code   ▲ Revised Code Title

✓6ᵗʰ **E71.52 X-linked adrenoleukodystrophy**
    E71.520 Childhood cerebral X-linked adrenoleukodystrophy `HCC`
    E71.521 Adolescent X-linked adrenoleukodystrophy `HCC`
    E71.522 Adrenomyeloneuropathy `HCC`
    E71.528 Other X-linked adrenoleukodystrophy `HCC`
        Addison only phenotype adrenoleukodystrophy
        Addison-Schilder adrenoleukodystrophy
    E71.529 X-linked adrenoleukodystrophy, unspecified type `HCC` ▽

  E71.53 Other group 2 peroxisomal disorders `HCC`

✓6ᵗʰ **E71.54 Other peroxisomal disorders**
    E71.540 Rhizomelic chondrodysplasia punctata `HCC`
        EXCLUDES 1   *chondrodysplasia punctata NOS (Q77.3)*
    E71.541 Zellweger-like syndrome `HCC`
    E71.542 Other group 3 peroxisomal disorders `HCC`
    E71.548 Other peroxisomal disorders `HCC`

✓4ᵗʰ **E72 Other disorders of amino-acid metabolism**
    EXCLUDES 1   *disorders of:*
        aromatic amino-acid metabolism (E70.-)
        branched-chain amino-acid metabolism (E71.0-E71.2)
        fatty-acid metabolism (E71.3)
        purine and pyrimidine metabolism (E79.-)
        gout (M1A.-, M10.-)

✓5ᵗʰ **E72.0 Disorders of amino-acid transport**
    EXCLUDES 1   *disorders of tryptophan metabolism (E70.5)*
    E72.00 Disorders of amino-acid transport, unspecified `HCC` ▽
    E72.01 Cystinuria `HCC`
    E72.02 Hartnup's disease `HCC`
    E72.03 Lowe's syndrome `HCC`
        Use additional code for associated glaucoma (H42)
    E72.04 Cystinosis `HCC`
        Fanconi (-de Toni) (-Debré) syndrome with cystinosis
        EXCLUDES 1   *Fanconi (-de Toni) (-Debré) syndrome without cystinosis (E72.09)*
    E72.09 Other disorders of amino-acid transport `HCC`
        Fanconi (-de Toni) (-Debré) syndrome, unspecified

✓5ᵗʰ **E72.1 Disorders of sulfur-bearing amino-acid metabolism**
    EXCLUDES 1   *cystinosis (E72.04)*
        cystinuria (E72.01)
        transcobalamin II deficiency (D51.2)
    E72.10 Disorders of sulfur-bearing amino-acid metabolism, unspecified `HCC` ▽
    E72.11 Homocystinuria `HCC`
        Cystathionine synthase deficiency
    E72.12 Methylenetetrahydrofolate reductase deficiency `HCC`
    E72.19 Other disorders of sulfur-bearing amino-acid metabolism `HCC`
        Cystathioninuria
        Methioninemia
        Sulfite oxidase deficiency

✓5ᵗʰ **E72.2 Disorders of urea cycle metabolism**
    EXCLUDES 1   *disorders of ornithine metabolism (E72.4)*
    E72.20 Disorder of urea cycle metabolism, unspecified `HCC` ▽
        Hyperammonemia
        EXCLUDES 1   *hyperammonemia- hyperornithinemia-homocitrullinemia syndrome (E72.4)*
            transient hyperammonemia of newborn (P74.6)
    E72.21 Argininemia `HCC`
    E72.22 Arginosuccinic aciduria `HCC`
    E72.23 Citrullinemia `HCC`
    E72.29 Other disorders of urea cycle metabolism `HCC`

  E72.3 Disorders of lysine and hydroxylysine metabolism `HCC`
    Glutaric aciduria NOS   Hydroxylysinemia
    Glutaric aciduria (type I)   Hyperlysinemia
    EXCLUDES 1   *glutaric aciduria type II (E71.313)*
        Refsum's disease (G60.1)
        Zellweger syndrome (E71.510)

  E72.4 Disorders of ornithine metabolism `HCC`
    Hyperammonemia-hyperornithinemia-homocitrullinemia syndrome
    Ornithinemia (types I, II)
    Ornithine transcarbamylase deficiency
    EXCLUDES 1   *hereditary choroidal dystrophy (H31.2-)*

✓5ᵗʰ **E72.5 Disorders of glycine metabolism**
    E72.50 Disorder of glycine metabolism, unspecified `HCC` ▽
    E72.51 Non-ketotic hyperglycinemia `HCC`
    E72.52 Trimethylaminuria `HCC`
    E72.53 Hyperoxaluria `HCC`
        Oxalosis
        Oxaluria
    E72.59 Other disorders of glycine metabolism `HCC`
        D-glycericacidemia
        Hyperhydroxyprolinemia
        Hyperprolinemia (types I, II)
        Sarcosinemia

  E72.8 Other specified disorders of amino-acid metabolism `HCC`
    Disorders of beta-amino-acid metabolism
    Disorders of gamma-glutamyl cycle

  E72.9 Disorder of amino-acid metabolism, unspecified `HCC` ▽

✓4ᵗʰ **E73 Lactose intolerance**
  E73.0 Congenital lactase deficiency
  E73.1 Secondary lactase deficiency
  E73.8 Other lactose intolerance
  E73.9 Lactose intolerance, unspecified ▽

✓4ᵗʰ **E74 Other disorders of carbohydrate metabolism**
    EXCLUDES 1   *diabetes mellitus (E08-E13)*
        hypoglycemia NOS (E16.2)
        increased secretion of glucagon (E16.3)
        mucopolysaccharidosis (E76.0-E76.3)

✓5ᵗʰ **E74.0 Glycogen storage disease**
    E74.00 Glycogen storage disease, unspecified `HCC` ▽
    E74.01 von Gierke disease `HCC`
        Type I glycogen storage disease
    E74.02 Pompe disease `HCC`
        Cardiac glycogenosis
        Type II glycogen storage disease
    E74.03 Cori disease `HCC`
        Forbes disease
        Type III glycogen storage disease
    E74.04 McArdle disease `HCC`
        Type V glycogen storage disease
    E74.09 Other glycogen storage disease `HCC`
        Andersen disease
        Hers disease
        Tauri disease
        Glycogen storage disease, types 0, IV, VI-XI
        Liver phosphorylase deficiency
        Muscle phosphofructokinase deficiency

✓5ᵗʰ **E74.1 Disorders of fructose metabolism**
    EXCLUDES 1   *muscle phosphofructokinase deficiency (E74.09)*
    E74.10 Disorder of fructose metabolism, unspecified ▽
    E74.11 Essential fructosuria
        Fructokinase deficiency
    E74.12 Hereditary fructose intolerance
        Fructosemia
    E74.19 Other disorders of fructose metabolism
        Fructose-1, 6-diphosphatase deficiency

✓5ᵗʰ **E74.2 Disorders of galactose metabolism**
    E74.20 Disorders of galactose metabolism, unspecified `HCC` ▽
    E74.21 Galactosemia `HCC`
        DEF: Any of three genetic disorders due to defective galactose metabolism; symptoms include failure to thrive in infancy, jaundice, liver and spleen damage, cataracts, and mental retardation.
    E74.29 Other disorders of galactose metabolism `HCC`
        Galactokinase deficiency

✓5ᵗʰ **E74.3 Other disorders of intestinal carbohydrate absorption**
    EXCLUDES 2   *lactose intolerance (E73.-)*
    E74.31 Sucrase-isomaltase deficiency

EXCLUDES 1 Not coded here   *EXCLUDES 2* Not included here   **N** Newborn Age: 0   **P** Pediatric Age: 0-17   **M** Maternity Age: 12-55   **A** Adult Age: 15-124

520   ICD-10-CM 2018

Tay-Sachs Disease

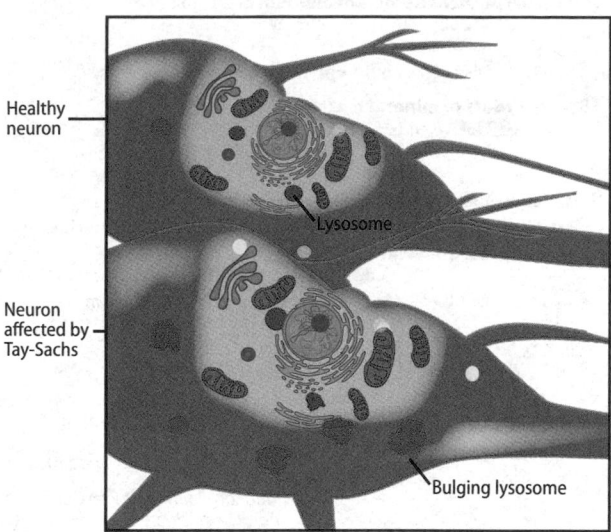

Healthy neuron

Lysosome

Neuron affected by Tay-Sachs

Bulging lysosome

E74.39   **Other disorders of intestinal carbohydrate absorption**
Disorder of intestinal carbohydrate absorption NOS
Glucose-galactose malabsorption
Sucrase deficiency

E74.4   **Disorders of pyruvate metabolism and gluconeogenesis** `HCC`
Deficiency of phosphoenolpyruvate carboxykinase
Deficiency of pyruvate carboxylase
Deficiency of pyruvate dehydrogenase
EXCLUDES 1   *disorders of pyruvate metabolism and gluconeogenesis with anemia (D55.-)*
Leigh's syndrome (G31.82)

E74.8   **Other specified disorders of carbohydrate metabolism** `HCC`
Essential pentosuria
Renal glycosuria

E74.9   **Disorder of carbohydrate metabolism, unspecified** `HCC` ▽

✓4th **E75**   **Disorders of sphingolipid metabolism and other lipid storage disorders**
EXCLUDES 1   *mucolipidosis, types I-III (E77.0-E77.1)*
Refsum's disease (G60.1)

✓5th **E75.0**   **GM2 gangliosidosis**

    E75.00   **GM2 gangliosidosis, unspecified** ▽

    E75.01   **Sandhoff disease**

    E75.02   **Tay-Sachs disease**
DEF: Genetic mutation of the HEXA gene that inhibits the breakdown of a toxic substance called ganglioside. The accumulation of ganglioside results in destruction of the neurons in the brain and spinal cord.

    E75.09   **Other GM2 gangliosidosis**
Adult GM2 gangliosidosis
Juvenile GM2 gangliosidosis

✓5th **E75.1**   **Other and unspecified gangliosidosis**

    E75.10   **Unspecified gangliosidosis** ▽
Gangliosidosis NOS

    E75.11   **Mucolipidosis IV**

    E75.19   **Other gangliosidosis**
GM1 gangliosidosis
GM3 gangliosidosis

✓5th **E75.2**   **Other sphingolipidosis**
EXCLUDES 1   *adrenoleukodystrophy [Addison-Schilder] (E71.528)*

    E75.21   **Fabry (-Anderson) disease** `HCC`

    E75.22   **Gaucher disease** `HCC`

    E75.23   **Krabbe disease**

✓6th **E75.24**   **Niemann-Pick disease**

      E75.240   **Niemann-Pick disease type A** `HCC`

      E75.241   **Niemann-Pick disease type B** `HCC`

      E75.242   **Niemann-Pick disease type C** `HCC`

      E75.243   **Niemann-Pick disease type D** `HCC`

      E75.248   **Other Niemann-Pick disease** `HCC`

      E75.249   **Niemann-Pick disease, unspecified** `HCC` ▽

    E75.25   **Metachromatic leukodystrophy**

    E75.29   **Other sphingolipidosis**
Farber's syndrome
Sulfatase deficiency
Sulfatide lipidosis

E75.3   **Sphingolipidosis, unspecified** `HCC` ▽

E75.4   **Neuronal ceroid lipofuscinosis**
Batten disease   Kufs disease
Bielschowsky-Jansky disease   Spielmeyer-Vogt disease

E75.5   **Other lipid storage disorders**
Cerebrotendinous cholesterosis [van Bogaert-Scherer-Epstein]
Wolman's disease

E75.6   **Lipid storage disorder, unspecified** ▽

✓4th **E76**   **Disorders of glycosaminoglycan metabolism**

✓5th **E76.0**   **Mucopolysaccharidosis, type I**

    E76.01   **Hurler's syndrome** `HCC`

    E76.02   **Hurler-Scheie syndrome** `HCC`

    E76.03   **Scheie's syndrome** `HCC`

    E76.1   **Mucopolysaccharidosis, type II** `HCC`
Hunter's syndrome

✓5th **E76.2**   **Other mucopolysaccharidoses**

✓6th **E76.21**   **Morquio mucopolysaccharidoses**

      E76.210   **Morquio A mucopolysaccharidoses** `HCC`
Classic Morquio syndrome
Morquio syndrome A
Mucopolysaccharidosis, type IVA

      E76.211   **Morquio B mucopolysaccharidoses** `HCC`
Morquio-like mucopolysaccharidoses
Morquio-like syndrome
Morquio syndrome B
Mucopolysaccharidosis, type IVB

      E76.219   **Morquio mucopolysaccharidoses, unspecified** `HCC` ▽
Morquio syndrome
Mucopolysaccharidosis, type IV

    E76.22   **Sanfilippo mucopolysaccharidoses** `HCC`
Mucopolysaccharidosis, type III (A) (B) (C) (D)
Sanfilippo A syndrome
Sanfilippo B syndrome
Sanfilippo C syndrome
Sanfilippo D syndrome

    E76.29   **Other mucopolysaccharidoses** `HCC`
beta-Glucuronidase deficiency
Maroteaux-Lamy (mild) (severe) syndrome
Mucopolysaccharidosis, types VI, VII

E76.3   **Mucopolysaccharidosis, unspecified** `HCC` ▽

E76.8   **Other disorders of glucosaminoglycan metabolism** `HCC`

E76.9   **Glucosaminoglycan metabolism disorder, unspecified** `HCC` ▽

✓4th **E77**   **Disorders of glycoprotein metabolism**

E77.0   **Defects in post-translational modification of lysosomal enzymes** `HCC`
Mucolipidosis II [I-cell disease]
Mucolipidosis III [pseudo-Hurler polydystrophy]

E77.1   **Defects in glycoprotein degradation** `HCC`
Aspartylglucosaminuria
Fucosidosis
Mannosidosis
Sialidosis [mucolipidosis I]

E77.8   **Other disorders of glycoprotein metabolism** `HCC`

E77.9   **Disorder of glycoprotein metabolism, unspecified** `HCC` ▽

✓4th **E78**   **Disorders of lipoprotein metabolism and other lipidemias**
EXCLUDES 1   *sphingolipidosis (E75.0-E75.3)*

✓5th **E78.0**   **Pure hypercholesterolemia**

    E78.00   **Pure hypercholesterolemia, unspecified** ▽
Fredrickson's hyperlipoproteinemia, type IIa
Hyperbetalipoproteinemia
Low-density-lipoprotein-type [LDL] hyperlipoproteinemia
▶(Pure) hypercholesterolemia NOS◀

    E78.01   **Familial hypercholesterolemia**

E78.1   **Pure hyperglyceridemia**
Elevated fasting triglycerides
Endogenous hyperglyceridemia
Fredrickson's hyperlipoproteinemia, type IV
Hyperlipidemia, group B
Hyperprebetalipoproteinemia
Very-low-density-lipoprotein-type [VLDL] hyperlipoproteinemia

E78.2   Mixed hyperlipidemia
Broad- or floating-betalipoproteinemia
Combined hyperlipidemia NOS
Elevated cholesterol with elevated triglycerides NEC
Fredrickson's hyperlipoproteinemia, type IIb or III
Hyperbetalipoproteinemia with prebetalipoproteinemia
Hypercholesteremia with endogenous hyperglyceridemia
Hyperlipidemia, group C
Tubo-eruptive xanthoma
Xanthoma tuberosum
EXCLUDES 1   *cerebrotendinous cholesterosis [van Bogaert-Scherer-Epstein] (E75.5)*
                familial combined hyperlipidemia (E78.4)

E78.3   Hyperchylomicronemia
Chylomicron retention disease
Fredrickson's hyperlipoproteinemia, type I or V
Hyperlipidemia, group D
Mixed hyperglyceridemia

E78.4   Other hyperlipidemia
Familial combined hyperlipidemia

E78.5   Hyperlipidemia, unspecified ▽

E78.6   Lipoprotein deficiency
Abetalipoproteinemia
Depressed HDL cholesterol
High-density lipoprotein deficiency
Hypoalphalipoproteinemia
Hypobetalipoproteinemia (familial)
Lecithin cholesterol acyltransferase deficiency
Tangier disease

✓5th **E78.7   Disorders of bile acid and cholesterol metabolism**
EXCLUDES 1   *Niemann-Pick disease type C (E75.242)*

　　　E78.70   Disorder of bile acid and cholesterol metabolism, ▽
　　　　　　　unspecified

　　　E78.71   Barth syndrome

　　　E78.72   Smith-Lemli-Opitz syndrome

　　　E78.79   Other disorders of bile acid and cholesterol
　　　　　　　metabolism

✓5th **E78.8   Other disorders of lipoprotein metabolism**
　　　E78.81   Lipoid dermatoarthritis
　　　E78.89   Other lipoprotein metabolism disorders

E78.9   Disorder of lipoprotein metabolism, unspecified ▽

✓4th **E79   Disorders of purine and pyrimidine metabolism**
EXCLUDES 1   *Ataxia-telangiectasia (Q87.1)*
　　　　　　 Bloom's syndrome (Q82.8)
　　　　　　 Cockayne's syndrome (Q87.1)
　　　　　　 calculus of kidney (N20.0)
　　　　　　 combined immunodeficiency disorders (D81.-)
　　　　　　 Fanconi's anemia (D61.09)
　　　　　　 gout (M1A.-, M10.-)
　　　　　　 orotaciduric anemia (D53.0)
　　　　　　 progeria (E34.8)
　　　　　　 Werner's syndrome (E34.8)
　　　　　　 xeroderma pigmentosum (Q82.1)

E79.0   Hyperuricemia without signs of inflammatory arthritis and
　　　　　tophaceous disease
Asymptomatic hyperuricemia

E79.1   Lesch-Nyhan syndrome   HCC
HGPRT deficiency

E79.2   Myoadenylate deaminase deficiency   HCC

E79.8   Other disorders of purine and pyrimidine metabolism   HCC
Hereditary xanthinuria

E79.9   Disorder of purine and pyrimidine metabolism,   HCC ▽
　　　　　unspecified

✓4th **E80   Disorders of porphyrin and bilirubin metabolism**
INCLUDES   defects of catalase and peroxidase

E80.0   Hereditary erythropoietic porphyria   HCC
Congenital erythropoietic porphyria
Erythropoietic protoporphyria

E80.1   Porphyria cutanea tarda   HCC

✓5th **E80.2   Other and unspecified porphyria**
　　　E80.20   Unspecified porphyria   HCC ▽
　　　　　　　Porphyria NOS
　　　E80.21   Acute intermittent (hepatic) porphyria   HCC
　　　E80.29   Other porphyria   HCC
　　　　　　　Hereditary coproporphyria

E80.3   Defects of catalase and peroxidase   HCC
Acatalasia [Takahara]

E80.4   Gilbert syndrome

E80.5   Crigler-Najjar syndrome

E80.6   Other disorders of bilirubin metabolism
Dubin-Johnson syndrome
Rotor's syndrome

E80.7   Disorder of bilirubin metabolism, unspecified ▽

✓4th **E83   Disorders of mineral metabolism**
EXCLUDES 1   *dietary mineral deficiency (E58-E61)*
　　　　　　 parathyroid disorders (E20-E21)
　　　　　　 vitamin D deficiency (E55.-)

✓5th **E83.0   Disorders of copper metabolism**
　　　E83.00   Disorder of copper metabolism, unspecified ▽
　　　E83.01   Wilson's disease
　　　　　　　Code also associated Kayser Fleischer ring (H18.04-)
　　　E83.09   Other disorders of copper metabolism
　　　　　　　Menkes' (kinky hair) (steely hair) disease

✓5th **E83.1   Disorders of iron metabolism**
EXCLUDES 1   *iron deficiency anemia (D50.-)*
　　　　　　 sideroblastic anemia (D64.0-D64.3)

　　　E83.10   Disorder of iron metabolism, unspecified ▽

✓6th **E83.11   Hemochromatosis**
EXCLUDES 1   ▶*GALD (P78.84)*
　　　　　　 gestational alloimmune liver disease (P78.84)
　　　　　　 neonatal hemochromatosis (P78.84)◀

　　　E83.110   Hereditary hemochromatosis   HCC
　　　　　　　　Bronzed diabetes
　　　　　　　　Pigmentary cirrhosis (of liver)
　　　　　　　　Primary (hereditary) hemochromatosis

　　　E83.111   Hemochromatosis due to repeated red
　　　　　　　　blood cell transfusions
　　　　　　　　Iron overload due to repeated red blood
　　　　　　　　　　cell transfusions
　　　　　　　　Transfusion (red blood cell) associated
　　　　　　　　　　hemochromatosis

　　　E83.118   Other hemochromatosis

　　　E83.119   Hemochromatosis, unspecified ▽

　　　E83.19   Other disorders of iron metabolism
　　　　　　　Use additional code, if applicable, for idiopathic
　　　　　　　　pulmonary hemosiderosis (J84.03)

E83.2   Disorders of zinc metabolism
Acrodermatitis enteropathica

✓5th **E83.3   Disorders of phosphorus metabolism and phosphatases**
EXCLUDES 1   *adult osteomalacia (M83.-)*
　　　　　　 osteoporosis (M80.-)

　　　E83.30   Disorder of phosphorus metabolism, unspecified ▽

　　　E83.31   Familial hypophosphatemia
　　　　　　　Vitamin D-resistant osteomalacia
　　　　　　　Vitamin D-resistant rickets
　　　　　　　EXCLUDES 1   *vitamin D-deficiency rickets (E55.0)*

　　　E83.32   Hereditary vitamin D-dependent rickets (type 1)
　　　　　　　(type 2)
　　　　　　　25-hydroxyvitamin D 1-alpha-hydroxylase deficiency
　　　　　　　Pseudovitamin D deficiency
　　　　　　　Vitamin D receptor defect

　　　E83.39   Other disorders of phosphorus metabolism
　　　　　　　Acid phosphatase deficiency
　　　　　　　Hypophosphatasia

✓5th **E83.4   Disorders of magnesium metabolism**
　　　E83.40   Disorders of magnesium metabolism, unspecified ▽
　　　E83.41   Hypermagnesemia
　　　E83.42   Hypomagnesemia
　　　E83.49   Other disorders of magnesium metabolism

✓5th **E83.5   Disorders of calcium metabolism**
EXCLUDES 1   *chondrocalcinosis (M11.1-M11.2)*
　　　　　　 hungry bone syndrome (E83.81)
　　　　　　 hyperparathyroidism (E21.0-E21.3)

　　　E83.50   Unspecified disorder of calcium metabolism ▽
　　　E83.51   Hypocalcemia
　　　E83.52   Hypercalcemia
　　　　　　　Familial hypocalciuric hypercalcemia
　　　E83.59   Other disorders of calcium metabolism
　　　　　　　Idiopathic hypercalciuria

✓5th **E83.8   Other disorders of mineral metabolism**
　　　E83.81   Hungry bone syndrome
　　　E83.89   Other disorders of mineral metabolism

E83.9   Disorder of mineral metabolism, unspecified ▽

EXCLUDES 1 Not coded here   EXCLUDES 2 Not included here   N Newborn Age: 0   P Pediatric Age: 0-17   M Maternity Age: 12-55   A Adult Age: 15-124

☑4ᵗʰ **E84   Cystic fibrosis**
   INCLUDES   mucoviscidosis
   Code also exocrine pancreatic insufficiency (K86.81)

   E84.0   Cystic fibrosis with pulmonary manifestations   HCC
     Use additional code to identify any infectious organism present, such as:
     Pseudomonas (B96.5)

   ☑5ᵗʰ **E84.1   Cystic fibrosis with intestinal manifestations**

     E84.11   Meconium ileus in cystic fibrosis   HCC N
       EXCLUDES 1   *meconium ileus not due to cystic fibrosis (P76.0)*

     E84.19   Cystic fibrosis with other intestinal manifestations   HCC
       Distal intestinal obstruction syndrome

   E84.8   Cystic fibrosis with other manifestations   HCC

   E84.9   Cystic fibrosis, unspecified   HCC ▽

☑4ᵗʰ **E85   Amyloidosis**
   EXCLUDES 1   Alzheimer's disease (G30.0-)
   EXCLUDES 2   ▶Alzheimer's disease (G30.0-)◀
   DEF: Conditions of diverse etiologies characterized by the accumulation of insoluble fibrillar proteins (amyloid) in various organs and tissues of the body, compromising vital functions.

   E85.0   Non-neuropathic heredofamilial amyloidosis   HCC
     Hereditary amyloid nephropathy
     ▶Code also associated disorders, such as:
       autoinflammatory syndromes (M04.-)◀
       EXCLUDES 2   ▶transthyretin-related (ATTR) familial amyloid cardiomyopathy (E85.4)◀

   E85.1   Neuropathic heredofamilial amyloidosis   HCC
     Amyloid polyneuropathy (Portuguese)
     ▶Transthyretin-related (ATTR) familial amyloid polyneuropathy◀
     AHA: 2012, 4Q, 99

   E85.2   Heredofamilial amyloidosis, unspecified   HCC ▽

   E85.3   Secondary systemic amyloidosis   HCC
     Hemodialysis-associated amyloidosis

   E85.4   Organ-limited amyloidosis   HCC
     Localized amyloidosis
     ▶Transthyretin-related (ATTR) familial amyloid cardiomyopathy◀

   ☑5ᵗʰ **E85.8   Other amyloidosis**

   ●   **E85.81   Light chain (AL) amyloidosis**

   ●   **E85.82   Wild-type transthyretin-related (ATTR) amyloidosis**
       Senile systemic amyloidosis (SSA)

   ●   **E85.89   Other amyloidosis**

   E85.9   Amyloidosis, unspecified   HCC

☑4ᵗʰ **E86   Volume depletion**
   Use additional code(s) for any associated disorders of electrolyte and acid-base balance (E87.-)
   EXCLUDES 1   *dehydration of newborn (P74.1)*
       hypovolemic shock NOS (R57.1)
       postprocedural hypovolemic shock (T81.19)
       traumatic hypovolemic shock (T79.4)

   E86.0   Dehydration
     AHA: 2014, 1Q, 7

   E86.1   Hypovolemia
     Depletion of volume of plasma

   E86.9   Volume depletion, unspecified   ▽
     DEF: Depletion of total body water (dehydration) and/or contraction of total intravascular plasma (hypovolemia).

☑4ᵗʰ **E87   Other disorders of fluid, electrolyte and acid-base balance**
   EXCLUDES 1   *diabetes insipidus (E23.2)*
       electrolyte imbalance associated with hyperemesis gravidarum (O21.1)
       electrolyte imbalance following ectopic or molar pregnancy (O08.5)
       familial periodic paralysis (G72.3)

   E87.0   Hyperosmolality and hypernatremia
     Sodium [Na] excess
     Sodium [Na] overload
     AHA: 2014, 1Q, 7

   E87.1   Hypo-osmolality and hyponatremia
     Sodium [Na] deficiency
     EXCLUDES 1   *syndrome of inappropriate secretion of antidiuretic hormone (E22.2)*
     AHA: 2014, 1Q, 7

   E87.2   Acidosis
     Acidosis NOS   Metabolic acidosis
     Lactic acidosis   Respiratory acidosis
     EXCLUDES 1   *diabetic acidosis—see categories E08-E10, E13 with ketoacidosis*

   E87.3   Alkalosis
     Alkalosis NOS   Respiratory alkalosis
     Metabolic alkalosis

   E87.4   Mixed disorder of acid-base balance

   E87.5   Hyperkalemia
     Potassium [K] excess   Potassium [K] overload

   E87.6   Hypokalemia
     Potassium [K] deficiency

   ☑5ᵗʰ **E87.7   Fluid overload**
     EXCLUDES 1   *edema NOS (R60.9)*
       fluid retention (R60.9)

     E87.70   Fluid overload, unspecified   ▽

     E87.71   Transfusion associated circulatory overload
       Fluid overload due to transfusion (blood) (blood components)
       TACO

     E87.79   Other fluid overload

   E87.8   Other disorders of electrolyte and fluid balance, not elsewhere classified
     Electrolyte imbalance NOS
     Hyperchloremia
     Hypochloremia

☑4ᵗʰ **E88   Other and unspecified metabolic disorders**
   Use additional codes for associated conditions
   EXCLUDES 1   *histiocytosis X (chronic) (C96.6)*

   ☑5ᵗʰ **E88.0   Disorders of plasma-protein metabolism, not elsewhere classified**
     EXCLUDES 1   *disorder of lipoprotein metabolism (E78.-)*
       monoclonal gammopathy (of undetermined significance) (D47.2)
       polyclonal hypergammaglobulinemia (D89.0)
       Waldenström's macroglobulinemia (C88.0)

     E88.01   Alpha-1-antitrypsin deficiency   HCC
       AAT deficiency

     E88.09   Other disorders of plasma-protein metabolism, not elsewhere classified
       Bisalbuminemia

   E88.1   Lipodystrophy, not elsewhere classified
     Lipodystrophy NOS
     EXCLUDES 1   *Whipple's disease (K90.81)*

   E88.2   Lipomatosis, not elsewhere classified
     Lipomatosis NOS
     Lipomatosis (Check) dolorosa [Dercum]

   E88.3   Tumor lysis syndrome
     Tumor lysis syndrome (spontaneous)
     Tumor lysis syndrome following antineoplastic drug chemotherapy
     Use additional code for adverse effect, if applicable, to identify drug (T45.1X5)
     DEF: A potentially fatal metabolic complication of tumor necrosis caused by either spontaneous or treatment-related accumulation of byproducts from dying cancer cells; symptoms include hyperkalemia, hyperphosphatemia, hypocalcemia, hyperuricemia, and hyperuricosuria.

   ☑5ᵗʰ **E88.4   Mitochondrial metabolism disorders**
     EXCLUDES 1   *disorders of pyruvate metabolism (E74.4)*
       Kearns-Sayre syndrome (H49.81)
       Leber's disease (H47.22)
       Leigh's encephalopathy (G31.82)
       Mitochondrial myopathy, NEC (G71.3)
       Reye's syndrome (G93.7)

     E88.40   Mitochondrial metabolism disorder, unspecified   HCC ▽

     E88.41   MELAS syndrome   HCC
       Mitochondrial myopathy, encephalopathy, lactic acidosis and stroke-like episodes

     E88.42   MERRF syndrome   HCC
       Myoclonic epilepsy associated with ragged-red fibers
       Code also progressive myoclonic epilepsy (G40.3-)

     E88.49   Other mitochondrial metabolism disorders   HCC

☑ Additional Character Req   ☑ⅹ7ᵗʰ Placeholder Alert   Manifestation   HCC CMS-HCC Condition   ▽ Unspecified Code   ▶◀ Revised Text   ● New Code   ▲ Revised Code Title

Chapter 4. Endocrine, Nutritional, and Metabolic Diseases *(side margin)*

√5ᵗʰ **E88.8 Other specified metabolic disorders**

    E88.81 Metabolic syndrome
        Dysmetabolic syndrome X
        Use additional codes for associated manifestations,
            such as:
        obesity (E66.-)

    E88.89 Other specified metabolic disorders `HCC`
        Launois-Bensaude adenolipomatosis
        EXCLUDES 1   *adult pulmonary Langerhans cell*
                histiocytosis (J84.82)

  E88.9 Metabolic disorder, unspecified ▽

Postprocedural endocrine and metabolic complications and disorders, not elsewhere classified (E89)

√4ᵗʰ **E89 Postprocedural endocrine and metabolic complications and disorders, not elsewhere classified**

    EXCLUDES 2   *intraoperative complications of endocrine system organ or*
           structure (E36.0-, E36.1-, E36.8)

  E89.0 Postprocedural hypothyroidism
    Postirradiation hypothyroidism
    Postsurgical hypothyroidism

  E89.1 Postprocedural hypoinsulinemia
    Postpancreatectomy hyperglycemia
    Postsurgical hypoinsulinemia

    Use additional code, if applicable, to identify:
        acquired absence of pancreas (Z90.41-)
        diabetes mellitus (postpancreatectomy) (postprocedural)
            (E13.-)
        insulin use (Z79.4)
        EXCLUDES 1   *transient postprocedural hyperglycemia (R73.9)*
                transient postprocedural hypoglycemia (E16.2)

  E89.2 Postprocedural hypoparathyroidism `HCC`
    Parathyroprival tetany

  E89.3 Postprocedural hypopituitarism `HCC`
    Postirradiation hypopituitarism

√5ᵗʰ **E89.4 Postprocedural ovarian failure**

    E89.40 Asymptomatic postprocedural ovarian failure ♀
        Postprocedural ovarian failure NOS

    E89.41 Symptomatic postprocedural ovarian failure ♀
        Symptoms such as flushing, sleeplessness, headache,
           lack of concentration, associated with
           postprocedural menopause

  E89.5 Postprocedural testicular hypofunction ♂

  E89.6 Postprocedural adrenocortical (-medullary) hypofunction `HCC`

√5ᵗʰ **E89.8 Other postprocedural endocrine and metabolic complications and disorders**

  √6ᵗʰ **E89.81 Postprocedural hemorrhage of an endocrine system organ or structure following a procedure**

    E89.810 Postprocedural hemorrhage of an endocrine system organ or structure following an endocrine system procedure

    E89.811 Postprocedural hemorrhage of an endocrine system organ or structure following other procedure

  √6ᵗʰ **E89.82 Postprocedural hematoma and seroma of an endocrine system organ or structure following a procedure**

    E89.820 Postprocedural hematoma of an endocrine system organ or structure following an endocrine system procedure

    E89.821 Postprocedural hematoma of an endocrine system organ or structure following other procedure

    E89.822 Postprocedural seroma of an endocrine system organ or structure following an endocrine system procedure

    E89.823 Postprocedural seroma of an endocrine system organ or structure following other procedure

  E89.89 Other postprocedural endocrine and metabolic complications and disorders
    Use additional code, if applicable, to further specify
        disorder

EXCLUDES 1 Not coded here   *EXCLUDES 2* Not included here   **N** Newborn Age: 0   **P** Pediatric Age: 0-17   **M** Maternity Age: 12-55   **A** Adult Age: 15-124

524   ICD-10-CM 2018

Chapter 5. Mental, Behavioral and Neurodevelopmental Disorders (F01–F99)

Chapter Specific Guidelines with Coding Examples

The chapter specific guidelines from the ICD-10-CM Official Guidelines for Coding and Reporting have been provided below. Along with these guidelines are coding examples, contained in the shaded boxes, that have been developed to help illustrate the coding and/or sequencing guidance found in these guidelines.

a. Pain disorders related to psychological factors

Assign code F45.41, for pain that is exclusively related to psychological disorders. As indicated by the Excludes 1 note under category G89, a code from category G89 should not be assigned with code F45.41.

> Chest pain determined to be persistent somatoform pain disorder
>
> **F45.41   Pain disorder exclusively related to psychological factors**
>
> *Explanation*: This pain was diagnosed as being exclusively psychological; therefore, no code from category G89 is added.

Code F45.42, Pain disorders with related psychological factors, should be used with a code from category G89, Pain, not elsewhere classified, if there is documentation of a psychological component for a patient with acute or chronic pain.

See Section I.C.6. Pain

b. Mental and behavioral disorders due to psychoactive substance use

1) In remission

Selection of codes for "in remission" for categories F10-F19, Mental and behavioral disorders due to psychoactive substance use (categories F10-F19 with -.21) requires the provider's clinical judgment. The appropriate codes for "in remission" are assigned only on the basis of provider documentation (as defined in the Official Guidelines for Coding and Reporting).

> Medical history: Alcohol dependence in remission
>
> **F10.21   Alcohol dependence, in remission**
>
> *Explanation*: The "in remission" codes are assigned when the provider documents the remission.

2) Psychoactive substance use, abuse and dependence

When the provider documentation refers to use, abuse and dependence of the same substance (e.g. alcohol, opioid, cannabis, etc.), only one code should be assigned to identify the pattern of use based on the following hierarchy:

- If both use and abuse are documented, assign only the code for abuse
  If both abuse and dependence are documented, assign only the code for dependence
- If use, abuse and dependence are all documented, assign only the code for dependence
- If both use and dependence are documented, assign only the code for dependence.

> History and physical notes cannabis dependence and ongoing cannabis abuse
>
> **F12.20   Cannabis dependence, uncomplicated**
>
> *Explanation*: In the hierarchy, the dependence code is used if both abuse and dependence are documented.

> Current problem list indicates daily opioid use with opioid abuse.
>
> **F11.10   Opioid abuse, uncomplicated**
>
> *Explanation*: In the hierarchy, the abuse code is used if both abuse and use are documented.

3) Psychoactive substance use

As with all other diagnoses, the codes for psychoactive substance use (F10.9-, F11.9-, F12.9-, F13.9-, F14.9-, F15.9-, F16.9-) should only be assigned based on provider documentation and when they meet the definition of a reportable diagnosis (see Section III, Reporting Additional Diagnoses). The codes are to be used only when the psychoactive substance use is associated with a mental or behavioral disorder, and such a relationship is documented by the provider.

> ED reports that a 27-year-old female tripped and twisted and broke her right ankle. Her friends reported that they were drinking and dancing at a nightclub.
>
> **S82.891A   Other fracture of right lower leg, initial encounter for closed fracture**
>
> **W18.40XA   Slipping, tripping and stumbling without falling, unspecified, initial encounter**
>
> **Y92.252   Music hall as the place of occurrence of the external cause**
>
> **Y93.41   Activity, dancing**
>
> *Explanation*: Note that no code was added for alcohol use or abuse. Unless it is specifically associated with a diagnosis by provider documentation and meets the definition of a reportable diagnosis, it is not assigned. However, if the documentation from the provider stated: "The patient tripped, and twisted and fractured her right ankle while dancing due to her elevated blood alcohol, consistent with her ongoing alcohol abuse," the following code would be added:
>
> **F10.10   Alcohol abuse, uncomplicated**

Chapter 5. Mental, Behavioral, and Neurodevelopmental Disorders (F01-F99)

INCLUDES disorders of psychological development
EXCLUDES 2 *symptoms, signs and abnormal clinical laboratory findings, not elsewhere classified (R00-R99)*

This chapter contains the following blocks:

F01-F09   Mental disorders due to known physiological conditions
F10-F19   Mental and behavioral disorders due to psychoactive substance use
F20-F29   Schizophrenia, schizotypal, delusional, and other non-mood psychotic disorders
F30-F39   Mood [affective] disorders
F40-F48   Anxiety, dissociative, stress-related, somatoform and other nonpsychotic mental disorders
F50-F59   Behavioral syndromes associated with physiological disturbances and physical factors
F60-F69   Disorders of adult personality and behavior
F70-F79   Intellectual disabilities
F80-F89   Pervasive and specific developmental disorders
F90-F98   Behavioral and emotional disorders with onset usually occurring in childhood and adolescence
F99   Unspecified mental disorder

Mental disorders due to known physiological conditions (F01-F09)

NOTE   This block comprises a range of mental disorders grouped together on the basis of their having in common a demonstrable etiology in cerebral disease, brain injury, or other insult leading to cerebral dysfunction. The dysfunction may be primary, as in diseases, injuries, and insults that affect the brain directly and selectively; or secondary, as in systemic diseases and disorders that attack the brain only as one of the multiple organs or systems of the body that are involved.

✓4th F01   Vascular dementia

Vascular dementia as a result of infarction of the brain due to vascular disease, including hypertensive cerebrovascular disease.
INCLUDES arteriosclerotic dementia
Code first the underlying physiological condition or sequelae of cerebrovascular disease.

✓5th F01.5   Vascular dementia

F01.50   Vascular dementia without behavioral disturbance   A
     Major neurocognitive disorder without behavioral disturbance

F01.51   Vascular dementia with behavioral disturbance   A
     Major neurocognitive disorder due to vascular disease, with behavioral disturbance
     Major neurocognitive disorder with aggressive behavior
     Major neurocognitive disorder with combative behavior
     Major neurocognitive disorder with violent behavior
     Vascular dementia with aggressive behavior
     Vascular dementia with combative behavior
     Vascular dementia with violent behavior
     Use additional code, if applicable, to identify wandering in vascular dementia (Z91.83)

✓4th F02   Dementia in other diseases classified elsewhere

INCLUDES major neurocognitive disorder in other diseases classified elsewhere
Code first the underlying physiological condition, such as:
     Alzheimer's (G30.-)
     cerebral lipidosis (E75.4)
     Creutzfeldt-Jakob disease (A81.0-)
     dementia with Lewy bodies (G31.83)
     dementia with Parkinsonism (G31.83)
     epilepsy and recurrent seizures (G40.-)
     frontotemporal dementia (G31.09)
     hepatolenticular degeneration (E83.0)
     human immunodeficiency virus [HIV] disease (B20)
     Huntington's disease (G10)
     hypercalcemia (E83.52)
     hypothyroidism, acquired (E00-E03.-)
     intoxications (T36-T65)
     Jakob-Creutzfeldt disease (A81.0-)
     multiple sclerosis (G35)
     neurosyphilis (A52.17)
     niacin deficiency [pellagra] (E52)
     Parkinson's disease (G20)
     Pick's disease (G31.01)
     polyarteritis nodosa (M30.0)
     prion disease (A81.9)
     systemic lupus erythematosus (M32.-)
     traumatic brain injury (S06.-)
     trypanosomiasis (B56.-, B57.-)
     vitamin B deficiency (E53.8)
EXCLUDES 2 *dementia in alcohol and psychoactive substance disorders (F10-F19, with .17, .27, .97)*
     vascular dementia (F01.5-)

✓5th F02.8   Dementia in other diseases classified elsewhere

AHA: 2017, 2Q, 7; 2016, 4Q, 141; 2016, 2Q, 6

F02.80   *Dementia in other diseases classified elsewhere without behavioral disturbance*
     Dementia in other diseases classified elsewhere NOS
     Major neurocognitive disorder in other diseases classified elsewhere

F02.81   *Dementia in other diseases classified elsewhere with behavioral disturbance*
     Dementia in other diseases classified elsewhere with aggressive behavior
     Dementia in other diseases classified elsewhere with combative behavior
     Dementia in other diseases classified elsewhere with violent behavior
     Major neurocognitive disorder in other diseases classified elsewhere with aggressive behavior
     Major neurocognitive disorder in other diseases classified elsewhere with combative behavior
     Major neurocognitive disorder in other diseases classified elsewhere with violent behavior
     Use additional code, if applicable, to identify wandering in dementia in conditions classified elsewhere (Z91.83)

✓4th F03   Unspecified dementia

Presenile dementia NOS
Presenile psychosis NOS
Primary degenerative dementia NOS
Senile dementia NOS
Senile dementia depressed or paranoid type
Senile psychosis NOS
EXCLUDES 1 *senility NOS (R41.81)*
EXCLUDES 2 *mild memory disturbance due to known physiological condition (F06.8)*
     senile dementia with delirium or acute confusional state (F05)

✓5th F03.9   Unspecified dementia

F03.90   Unspecified dementia without behavioral disturbance   A ▽
     Dementia NOS
     AHA: 2012, 4Q, 92

F03.91   Unspecified dementia with behavioral disturbance   A ▽
     Unspecified dementia with aggressive behavior
     Unspecified dementia with combative behavior
     Unspecified dementia with violent behavior
     Use additional code, if applicable, to identify wandering in unspecified dementia (Z91.83)

EXCLUDES 1 Not coded here   **EXCLUDES 2** Not included here   N Newborn Age: 0   P Pediatric Age: 0-17   M Maternity Age: 12-55   A Adult Age: 15-124

526   ICD-10-CM 2018

F04   Amnestic disorder due to known physiological condition
Korsakov's psychosis or syndrome, nonalcoholic
Code first the underlying physiological condition
> *EXCLUDES 1*   *amnesia NOS (R41.3)*
> *anterograde amnesia (R41.1)*
> *dissociative amnesia (F44.0)*
> *retrograde amnesia (R41.2)*
> *EXCLUDES 2*   *alcohol-induced or unspecified Korsakov's syndrome (F10.26, F10.96)*
> *Korsakov's syndrome induced by other psychoactive substances (F13.26, F13.96, F19.16, F19.26, F19.96)*

F05   Delirium due to known physiological condition
Acute or subacute brain syndrome
Acute or subacute confusional state (nonalcoholic)
Acute or subacute infective psychosis
Acute or subacute organic reaction
Acute or subacute psycho-organic syndrome
Delirium of mixed etiology
Delirium superimposed on dementia
Sundowning
Code first the underlying physiological condition
> *EXCLUDES 1*   *delirium NOS (R41.0)*
> *EXCLUDES 2*   *delirium tremens alcohol-induced or unspecified (F10.231, F10.921)*

☑4ᵗʰ **F06   Other mental disorders due to known physiological condition**
> INCLUDES   mental disorders due to endocrine disorder
> mental disorders due to exogenous hormone
> mental disorders due to exogenous toxic substance
> mental disorders due to primary cerebral disease
> mental disorders due to somatic illness
> mental disorders due to systemic disease affecting the brain

Code first the underlying physiological condition
> *EXCLUDES 1*   *unspecified dementia (F03)*
> *EXCLUDES 2*   *delirium due to known physiological condition (F05)*
> *dementia as classified in F01-F02*
> *other mental disorders associated with alcohol and other psychoactive substances (F10-F19)*

F06.0   Psychotic disorder with hallucinations due to known physiological condition
Organic hallucinatory state (nonalcoholic)
> *EXCLUDES 2*   *hallucinations and perceptual disturbance induced by alcohol and other psychoactive substances (F10-F19 with .151, .251, .951)*
> *schizophrenia (F20.-)*

F06.1   Catatonic disorder due to known physiological condition
Catatonia associated with another mental disorder
Catatonia NOS
> *EXCLUDES 1*   *catatonic stupor (R40.1)*
> *stupor NOS (R40.1)*
> *EXCLUDES 2*   *catatonic schizophrenia (F20.2)*
> *dissociative stupor (F44.2)*

F06.2   Psychotic disorder with delusions due to known physiological condition
Paranoid and paranoid-hallucinatory organic states
Schizophrenia-like psychosis in epilepsy
> *EXCLUDES 2*   *alcohol and drug-induced psychotic disorder (F10-F19 with .150, .250, .950)*
> *brief psychotic disorder (F23)*
> *delusional disorder (F22)*
> *schizophrenia (F20.-)*

☑5ᵗʰ **F06.3   Mood disorder due to known physiological condition**
> *EXCLUDES 2*   *mood disorders due to alcohol and other psychoactive substances (F10-F19 with .14, .24, .94)*
> *mood disorders, not due to known physiological condition or unspecified (F30-F39)*

F06.30   Mood disorder due to known physiological condition, unspecified ▽

F06.31   Mood disorder due to known physiological condition with depressive features
> ►Depressive disorder due to known physiological condition, with depressive features◄

F06.32   Mood disorder due to known physiological condition with major depressive-like episode
> ►Depressive disorder due to known physiological condition, with major depressive–like episode◄

F06.33   Mood disorder due to known physiological condition with manic features
> ►Bipolar and related disorder due to a known physiological condition, with manic features
> Bipolar and related disorder due to known physiological condition, with manic- or hypomanic-like episodes◄

F06.34   Mood disorder due to known physiological condition with mixed features
> ►Bipolar and related disorder due to known physiological condition, with mixed features
> Depressive disorder due to known physiological condition, with mixed features◄

F06.4   Anxiety disorder due to known physiological condition
> *EXCLUDES 2*   *anxiety disorders due to alcohol and other psychoactive substances (F10-F19 with .180, .280, .980)*
> *anxiety disorders, not due to known physiological condition or unspecified (F40.-, F41.-)*

F06.8   Other specified mental disorders due to known physiological condition
Epileptic psychosis NOS
> ►Obsessive-compulsive and related disorder due to a known physiological condition◄
Organic dissociative disorder
Organic emotionally labile [asthenic] disorder

☑4ᵗʰ **F07   Personality and behavioral disorders due to known physiological condition**
Code first the underlying physiological condition

F07.0   Personality change due to known physiological condition
Frontal lobe syndrome
Limbic epilepsy personality syndrome
Lobotomy syndrome
Organic personality disorder
Organic pseudopsychopathic personality
Organic pseudoretarded personality
Postleucotomy syndrome
Code first underlying physiological condition
> *EXCLUDES 1*   *mild cognitive impairment (G31.84)*
> *postconcussional syndrome (F07.81)*
> *postencephalitic syndrome (F07.89)*
> *signs and symptoms involving emotional state (R45.-)*
> *EXCLUDES 2*   *specific personality disorder (F60.-)*

☑5ᵗʰ **F07.8   Other personality and behavioral disorders due to known physiological condition**

F07.81   Postconcussional syndrome
Postcontusional syndrome (encephalopathy)
Post-traumatic brain syndrome, nonpsychotic
Use additional code to identify associated post-traumatic headache, if applicable (G44.3-)
> *EXCLUDES 1*   *current concussion (brain) (S06.0-)*
> *postencephalitic syndrome (F07.89)*

F07.89   Other personality and behavioral disorders due to known physiological condition
Postencephalitic syndrome
Right hemispheric organic affective disorder

F07.9   Unspecified personality and behavioral disorder due to known physiological condition ▽
Organic psychosyndrome

F09   Unspecified mental disorder due to known physiological condition ▽
Mental disorder NOS due to known physiological condition
Organic brain syndrome NOS
Organic mental disorder NOS
Organic psychosis NOS
Symptomatic psychosis NOS
Code first the underlying physiological condition
> *EXCLUDES 1*   *psychosis NOS (F29)*

Mental and behavioral disorders due to psychoactive substance use (F10-F19)

AHA: 2017, 2Q, 27

☑4ᵗʰ **F10   Alcohol related disorders**
Use additional code for blood alcohol level, if applicable (Y90.-)

☑5ᵗʰ **F10.1   Alcohol abuse**
> *EXCLUDES 1*   *alcohol dependence (F10.2-)*
> *alcohol use, unspecified (F10.9-)*
AHA: 2015, 2Q, 15

F10.10   Alcohol abuse, uncomplicated
Alcohol use disorder, mild

☑ Additional Character Req   x7ᵗʰ Placeholder Alert   Manifestation   HCC CMS-HCC Condition   ▽Unspecified Code   ►◄ Revised Text   ● New Code   ▲ Revised Code Title

●   **F10.11**   **Alcohol abuse, in remission**
Alcohol use disorder, mild, in early remission
Alcohol use disorder, mild, in sustained remission

✓6th   **F10.12**   **Alcohol abuse with intoxication**

F10.120   **Alcohol abuse with intoxication, uncomplicated**   HCC

F10.121   **Alcohol abuse with intoxication delirium**   HCC

F10.129   **Alcohol abuse with intoxication, unspecified**   HCC ▽

F10.14   **Alcohol abuse with alcohol-induced mood disorder**   HCC
Alcohol use disorder, mild, with alcohol-induced bipolar or related disorder
Alcohol use disorder, mild, with alcohol-induced depressive disorder

✓6th   **F10.15**   **Alcohol abuse with alcohol-induced psychotic disorder**

F10.150   **Alcohol abuse with alcohol-induced psychotic disorder with delusions**   HCC

F10.151   **Alcohol abuse with alcohol-induced psychotic disorder with hallucinations**   HCC
DEF: Psychosis lasting less than six months with slight or no clouding of consciousness in which auditory hallucinations predominate.

F10.159   **Alcohol abuse with alcohol-induced psychotic disorder, unspecified**   HCC ▽

✓6th   **F10.18**   **Alcohol abuse with other alcohol-induced disorders**

F10.180   **Alcohol abuse with alcohol-induced anxiety disorder**   HCC

F10.181   **Alcohol abuse with alcohol-induced sexual dysfunction**   HCC

F10.182   **Alcohol abuse with alcohol-induced sleep disorder**   HCC

F10.188   **Alcohol abuse with other alcohol-induced disorder**   HCC

F10.19   **Alcohol abuse with unspecified alcohol-induced disorder**   HCC ▽

✓5th   **F10.2**   **Alcohol dependence**
EXCLUDES 1   *alcohol abuse (F10.1-)*
alcohol use, unspecified (F10.9-)
EXCLUDES 2   *toxic effect of alcohol (T51.0-)*

F10.20   **Alcohol dependence, uncomplicated**   HCC
Alcohol use disorder, moderate
Alcohol use disorder, severe

F10.21   **Alcohol dependence, in remission**   HCC
►Alcohol use disorder, moderate, in early remission
Alcohol use disorder, moderate, in sustained remission
Alcohol use disorder, severe, in early remission
Alcohol use disorder, severe, in sustained remission◄

✓6th   **F10.22**   **Alcohol dependence with intoxication**
Acute drunkenness (in alcoholism)
EXCLUDES 2   *alcohol dependence with withdrawal (F10.23-)*

F10.220   **Alcohol dependence with intoxication, uncomplicated**   HCC

F10.221   **Alcohol dependence with intoxication delirium**   HCC

F10.229   **Alcohol dependence with intoxication, unspecified**   HCC ▽

✓6th   **F10.23**   **Alcohol dependence with withdrawal**
EXCLUDES 2   *alcohol dependence with withdrawal (F10.22-)*
AHA: 2015, 2Q, 15

F10.230   **Alcohol dependence with withdrawal, uncomplicated**   HCC

F10.231   **Alcohol dependence with withdrawal delirium**   HCC

F10.232   **Alcohol dependence with withdrawal with perceptual disturbance**   HCC

F10.239   **Alcohol dependence with withdrawal, unspecified**   HCC ▽

F10.24   **Alcohol dependence with alcohol-induced mood disorder**   HCC
Alcohol use disorder, moderate, with alcohol-induced bipolar or related disorder
Alcohol use disorder, moderate, with alcohol-induced depressive disorder
Alcohol use disorder, severe, with alcohol-induced bipolar or related disorder
Alcohol use disorder, severe, with alcohol-induced depressive disorder

✓6th   **F10.25**   **Alcohol dependence with alcohol-induced psychotic disorder**

F10.250   **Alcohol dependence with alcohol-induced psychotic disorder with delusions**   HCC

F10.251   **Alcohol dependence with alcohol-induced psychotic disorder with hallucinations**   HCC

F10.259   **Alcohol dependence with alcohol-induced psychotic disorder, unspecified**   HCC ▽

F10.26   **Alcohol dependence with alcohol-induced persisting amnestic disorder**   HCC
Alcohol use disorder, moderate, with alcohol-induced major neurocognitive disorder, amnestic-confabulatory type
Alcohol use disorder, severe, with alcohol-induced major neurocognitive disorder, amnestic-confabulatory type
DEF: Prominent and lasting reduced memory span, disordered time appreciation and confabulation, occurs in alcoholics as sequel to acute alcoholic psychosis.

F10.27   **Alcohol dependence with alcohol-induced persisting dementia**   HCC
Alcohol use disorder, moderate, with alcohol-induced major neurocognitive disorder, nonamnestic-confabulatory type
Alcohol use disorder, severe, with alcohol-induced major neurocognitive disorder, nonamnestic-confabulatory type

✓6th   **F10.28**   **Alcohol dependence with other alcohol-induced disorders**

F10.280   **Alcohol dependence with alcohol-induced anxiety disorder**   HCC

F10.281   **Alcohol dependence with alcohol-induced sexual dysfunction**   HCC

F10.282   **Alcohol dependence with alcohol-induced sleep disorder**   HCC

F10.288   **Alcohol dependence with other alcohol-induced disorder**   HCC
Alcohol use disorder, moderate, with alcohol-induced mild neurocognitive disorder
Alcohol use disorder, severe, with alcohol-induced mild neurocognitive disorder

F10.29   **Alcohol dependence with unspecified alcohol-induced disorder**   HCC ▽

✓5th   **F10.9**   **Alcohol use, unspecified**
EXCLUDES 1   *alcohol abuse (F10.1-)*
alcohol dependence (F10.2-)

✓6th   **F10.92**   **Alcohol use, unspecified with intoxication**

F10.920   **Alcohol use, unspecified with intoxication, uncomplicated**   HCC

F10.921   **Alcohol use, unspecified with intoxication delirium**   HCC

F10.929   **Alcohol use, unspecified with intoxication, unspecified**   HCC ▽

F10.94   **Alcohol use, unspecified with alcohol-induced mood disorder**   HCC
Alcohol induced bipolar or related disorder, without use disorder
Alcohol induced depressive disorder, without use disorder

✓6th   **F10.95**   **Alcohol use, unspecified with alcohol-induced psychotic disorder**

F10.950   **Alcohol use, unspecified with alcohol-induced psychotic disorder with delusions**   HCC

F10.951   **Alcohol use, unspecified with alcohol-induced psychotic disorder with hallucinations**   HCC

EXCLUDES 1 Not coded here   EXCLUDES 2 Not included here   **N** Newborn Age: 0   **P** Pediatric Age: 0-17   **M** Maternity Age: 12-55   **A** Adult Age: 15-124

F10.959   **Alcohol use, unspecified with**   HCC ▽
alcohol-induced psychotic disorder,
unspecified
Alcohol-induced psychotic disorder
without use disorder

F10.96   **Alcohol use, unspecified with alcohol-induced**   HCC
persisting amnestic disorder
Alcohol-induced major neurocognitive disorder,
amnestic-confabulatory type, without use
disorder

F10.97   **Alcohol use, unspecified with alcohol-induced**   HCC
persisting dementia
Alcohol-induced major neurocognitive disorder,
amnestic-confabulatory type, without use
disorder

√6ᵗʰ   F10.98   **Alcohol use, unspecified with other alcohol-induced**
disorders

F10.980   **Alcohol use, unspecified with**   HCC
alcohol-induced anxiety disorder
Alcohol induced anxiety disorder, without
use disorder

F10.981   **Alcohol use, unspecified with**   HCC
alcohol-induced sexual dysfunction
Alcohol induced sexual dysfunction,
without use disorder

F10.982   **Alcohol use, unspecified with**   HCC
alcohol-induced sleep disorder
Alcohol induced sleep disorder, without
use disorder

F10.988   **Alcohol use, unspecified with other**   HCC
alcohol-induced disorder
Alcohol induced mild neurocognitive
disorder, without use disorder

F10.99   **Alcohol use, unspecified with unspecified**   HCC ▽
alcohol-induced disorder

√4ᵗʰ   **F11   Opioid related disorders**

√5ᵗʰ   **F11.1   Opioid abuse**
EXCLUDES 1   *opioid dependence (F11.2-)*
opioid use, unspecified (F11.9-)

F11.10   **Opioid abuse, uncomplicated**
Opioid use disorder, mild

●   F11.11   **Opioid abuse, in remission**
Opioid use disorder, mild, in early remission
Opioid use disorder, mild, in sustained remission

√6ᵗʰ   F11.12   **Opioid abuse with intoxication**

F11.120   **Opioid abuse with intoxication,**   HCC
uncomplicated

F11.121   **Opioid abuse with intoxication**   HCC
delirium

F11.122   **Opioid abuse with intoxication**   HCC
with perceptual disturbance

F11.129   **Opioid abuse with intoxication,**   HCC ▽
unspecified

F11.14   **Opioid abuse with opioid-induced mood**   HCC
disorder
Opioid use disorder, mild, with opioid-induced
depressive disorder

√6ᵗʰ   F11.15   **Opioid abuse with opioid-induced psychotic**
disorder

F11.150   **Opioid abuse with opioid-induced**   HCC
psychotic disorder with delusions

F11.151   **Opioid abuse with opioid-induced**   HCC
psychotic disorder with hallucinations

F11.159   **Opioid abuse with opioid-induced**   HCC ▽
psychotic disorder, unspecified

√6ᵗʰ   F11.18   **Opioid abuse with other opioid-induced disorder**

F11.181   **Opioid abuse with opioid-induced**   HCC
sexual dysfunction

F11.182   **Opioid abuse with opioid-induced**   HCC
sleep disorder

F11.188   **Opioid abuse with other**   HCC
opioid-induced disorder

F11.19   **Opioid abuse with unspecified**   HCC ▽
opioid-induced disorder

√5ᵗʰ   **F11.2   Opioid dependence**
EXCLUDES 1   *opioid abuse (F11.1-)*
opioid use, unspecified (F11.9-)
EXCLUDES 2   *opioid poisoning (T40.0-T40.2-)*

F11.20   **Opioid dependence, uncomplicated**   HCC
Opioid use disorder, moderate
Opioid use disorder, severe

F11.21   **Opioid dependence, in remission**   HCC
▶Opioid use disorder, moderate, in early remission
Opioid use disorder, moderate, in sustained remission
Opioid use disorder, severe, in early remission
Opioid use disorder, severe, in sustained remission◀

√6ᵗʰ   F11.22   **Opioid dependence with intoxication**
EXCLUDES 1   *opioid dependence with withdrawal (F11.23)*

F11.220   **Opioid dependence with intoxication,**   HCC
uncomplicated

F11.221   **Opioid dependence with intoxication**   HCC
delirium

F11.222   **Opioid dependence with intoxication**   HCC
with perceptual disturbance

F11.229   **Opioid dependence with**   HCC ▽
intoxication, unspecified

F11.23   **Opioid dependence with withdrawal**   HCC
EXCLUDES 1   *opioid dependence with intoxication*
(F11.22-)

F11.24   **Opioid dependence with opioid-induced mood**   HCC
disorder
Opioid use disorder, moderate, with opioid induced
depressive disorder

√6ᵗʰ   F11.25   **Opioid dependence with opioid-induced psychotic**
disorder

F11.250   **Opioid dependence with opioid-**   HCC
induced psychotic disorder with delusions

F11.251   **Opioid dependence with**
opioid-induced psychotic disorder   HCC
with hallucinations

F11.259   **Opioid dependence with opioid-**   HCC ▽
induced psychotic disorder, unspecified

√6ᵗʰ   F11.28   **Opioid dependence with other opioid-induced**
disorder

F11.281   **Opioid dependence with opioid-**   HCC
induced sexual dysfunction

F11.282   **Opioid dependence with opioid-**   HCC
induced sleep disorder

F11.288   **Opioid dependence with other**   HCC
opioid-induced disorder

F11.29   **Opioid dependence with unspecified opioid-**   HCC ▽
induced disorder

√5ᵗʰ   **F11.9   Opioid use, unspecified**
EXCLUDES 1   *opioid abuse (F11.1-)*
opioid dependence (F11.2-)

F11.90   **Opioid use, unspecified, uncomplicated**

√6ᵗʰ   F11.92   **Opioid use, unspecified with intoxication**
EXCLUDES 1   *opioid use, unspecified with withdrawal*
(F11.93)

F11.920   **Opioid use, unspecified with**   HCC
intoxication, uncomplicated

F11.921   **Opioid use, unspecified with**   HCC
intoxication delirium
Opioid-induced delirium

F11.922   **Opioid use, unspecified with**   HCC
intoxication with perceptual disturbance

F11.929   **Opioid use, unspecified with**   HCC ▽
intoxication, unspecified

F11.93   **Opioid use, unspecified with withdrawal**   HCC
EXCLUDES 1   *opioid use, unspecified with intoxication*
(F11.92-)

F11.94   **Opioid use, unspecified with opioid-induced**   HCC
mood disorder
Opioid induced depressive disorder, without use
disorder

√6ᵗʰ   F11.95   **Opioid use, unspecified with opioid-induced**
psychotic disorder

F11.950   **Opioid use, unspecified with**   HCC
opioid-induced psychotic disorder with
delusions

☑ Additional Character Req   ✔x7ᵗʰ Placeholder Alert   Manifestation   HCC CMS-HCC Condition   ▽ Unspecified Code   ▶◀ Revised Text   ● New Code   ▲ Revised Code Title

ICD-10-CM 2018   529

Chapter 5. Mental, Behavioral and Neurodevelopmental Disorders

F11.951–F13.129

     F11.951   **Opioid use, unspecified with**   HCC
              opioid-induced psychotic disorder with
              hallucinations

     F11.959   **Opioid use, unspecified with**   HCC ▽
              opioid-induced psychotic disorder,
              unspecified

✓6th **F11.98**   **Opioid use, unspecified with other specified**
          opioid-induced disorder

     F11.981   **Opioid use, unspecified with**   HCC
              opioid-induced sexual dysfunction
                  Opioid induced sexual dysfunction, without
                     use disorder

     F11.982   **Opioid use, unspecified with**   HCC
              opioid-induced sleep disorder
                  Opioid induced sleep disorder, without use
                     disorder

     F11.988   **Opioid use, unspecified with other**   HCC
              opioid-induced disorder
                  Opioid induced anxiety disorder, without
                     use disorder

    F11.99   **Opioid use, unspecified with unspecified**   HCC ▽
          opioid-induced disorder

✓4th **F12**   **Cannabis related disorders**
      INCLUDES   marijuana

✓5th **F12.1**   **Cannabis abuse**
      EXCLUDES 1   cannabis dependence (F12.2-)
                  cannabis use, unspecified (F12.9-)

    F12.10   **Cannabis abuse, uncomplicated**
          Cannabis use disorder, mild

●   **F12.11**   **Cannabis abuse, in remission**
          Cannabis use disorder, mild, in early remission
          Cannabis use disorder, mild, in sustained remission

✓6th **F12.12**   **Cannabis abuse with intoxication**

     F12.120   **Cannabis abuse with intoxication,**   HCC
              uncomplicated

     F12.121   **Cannabis abuse with intoxication**   HCC
              delirium

     F12.122   **Cannabis abuse with intoxication**   HCC
              with perceptual disturbance

     F12.129   **Cannabis abuse with intoxication,**   HCC ▽
              unspecified

✓6th **F12.15**   **Cannabis abuse with psychotic disorder**

     F12.150   **Cannabis abuse with psychotic**   HCC
              disorder with delusions

     F12.151   **Cannabis abuse with psychotic**   HCC
              disorder with hallucinations

     F12.159   **Cannabis abuse with psychotic**   HCC ▽
              disorder, unspecified

✓6th **F12.18**   **Cannabis abuse with other cannabis-induced**
          disorder

     F12.180   **Cannabis abuse with cannabis-**   HCC
              induced anxiety disorder

     F12.188   **Cannabis abuse with other**   HCC
              cannabis-induced disorder
                Cannabis use disorder, mild, with
                  cannabis-induced sleep disorder

    F12.19   **Cannabis abuse with unspecified cannabis-**   HCC ▽
          induced disorder

✓5th **F12.2**   **Cannabis dependence**
      EXCLUDES 1   cannabis abuse (F12.1-)
                  cannabis use, unspecified (F12.9-)
      EXCLUDES 2   cannabis poisoning (T40.7-)

    F12.20   **Cannabis dependence, uncomplicated**   HCC
          Cannabis use disorder, moderate
          Cannabis use disorder, severe

    F12.21   **Cannabis dependence, in remission**   HCC
          ▶Cannabis use disorder, moderate, in early remission
          Cannabis use disorder, moderate, in sustained
            remission
          Cannabis use disorder, severe, in early remission
          Cannabis use disorder, severe, in sustained remission◀

✓6th **F12.22**   **Cannabis dependence with intoxication**

     F12.220   **Cannabis dependence with**   HCC
              intoxication, uncomplicated

     F12.221   **Cannabis dependence with**   HCC
              intoxication delirium

     F12.222   **Cannabis dependence with**   HCC
              intoxication with perceptual disturbance

     F12.229   **Cannabis dependence with**   HCC ▽
              intoxication, unspecified

✓6th **F12.25**   **Cannabis dependence with psychotic disorder**

     F12.250   **Cannabis dependence with psychotic**   HCC
              disorder with delusions

     F12.251   **Cannabis dependence with psychotic**   HCC
              disorder with hallucinations

     F12.259   **Cannabis dependence with**   HCC ▽
              psychotic disorder, unspecified

✓6th **F12.28**   **Cannabis dependence with other cannabis-induced**
          disorder

     F12.280   **Cannabis dependence with**   HCC
              cannabis-induced anxiety disorder

     F12.288   **Cannabis dependence with other**   HCC
              cannabis-induced disorder
                Cannabis use disorder, moderate, with
                  cannabis-induced sleep disorder
                Cannabis use disorder, severe, with
                  cannabis-induced sleep disorder
                Cannabis withdrawal

    F12.29   **Cannabis dependence with unspecified**   HCC ▽
          cannabis-induced disorder

✓5th **F12.9**   **Cannabis use, unspecified**
      EXCLUDES 1   cannabis abuse (F12.1-)
                  cannabis dependence (F12.2-)

    F12.90   **Cannabis use, unspecified, uncomplicated**

✓6th **F12.92**   **Cannabis use, unspecified with intoxication**

     F12.920   **Cannabis use, unspecified with**   HCC
              intoxication, uncomplicated

     F12.921   **Cannabis use, unspecified with**   HCC
              intoxication delirium

     F12.922   **Cannabis use, unspecified with**   HCC
              intoxication with perceptual disturbance

     F12.929   **Cannabis use, unspecified with**   HCC ▽
              intoxication, unspecified

✓6th **F12.95**   **Cannabis use, unspecified with psychotic disorder**

     F12.950   **Cannabis use, unspecified with**   HCC
              psychotic disorder with delusions

     F12.951   **Cannabis use, unspecified with**   HCC
              psychotic disorder with hallucinations

     F12.959   **Cannabis use, unspecified with**   HCC ▽
              psychotic disorder, unspecified
                Cannabis induced psychotic disorder,
                  without use disorder

✓6th **F12.98**   **Cannabis use, unspecified with other**
          cannabis-induced disorder

     F12.980   **Cannabis use, unspecified with**   HCC
              anxiety disorder
                Cannabis induced anxiety disorder, without
                  use disorder

     F12.988   **Cannabis use, unspecified with**   HCC
              other cannabis-induced disorder
                Cannabis induced sleep disorder, without
                  use disorder

    F12.99   **Cannabis use, unspecified with unspecified**   HCC ▽
          cannabis-induced disorder

✓4th **F13**   **Sedative, hypnotic, or anxiolytic related disorders**

✓5th **F13.1**   **Sedative, hypnotic or anxiolytic-related abuse**
      EXCLUDES 1   sedative, hypnotic or anxiolytic-related dependence
                     (F13.2-)
                  sedative, hypnotic, or anxiolytic use, unspecified
                     (F13.9-)

    F13.10   **Sedative, hypnotic or anxiolytic abuse,**
          uncomplicated
          Sedative, hypnotic, or anxiolytic use disorder, mild

●   **F13.11**   **Sedative, hypnotic or anxiolytic abuse, in remission**
          Sedative, hypnotic, or anxiolytic use disorder, mild, in
            early remission
          Sedative, hypnotic, or anxiolytic use disorder, mild, in
            sustained remission

✓6th **F13.12**   **Sedative, hypnotic or anxiolytic abuse with**
          intoxication

     F13.120   **Sedative, hypnotic or anxiolytic**   HCC
              abuse with intoxication, uncomplicated

     F13.121   **Sedative, hypnotic or anxiolytic**   HCC
              abuse with intoxication delirium

     F13.129   **Sedative, hypnotic or anxiolytic**   HCC ▽
              abuse with intoxication, unspecified

EXCLUDES 1 Not coded here   EXCLUDES 2 Not included here   **N** Newborn Age: 0   **P** Pediatric Age: 0-17   **M** Maternity Age: 12-55   **A** Adult Age: 15-124

530   ICD-10-CM 2018

F13.14   **Sedative, hypnotic or anxiolytic abuse with sedative, hypnotic or anxiolytic-induced mood disorder**   HCC
▶Sedative, hypnotic, or anxiolytic use disorder, mild, with sedative, hypnotic, or anxiolytic-induced bipolar or related disorder
Sedative, hypnotic, or anxiolytic use disorder, mild, with sedative, hypnotic, or anxiolytic-induced depressive disorder◀

✓6ᵗʰ **F13.15**   **Sedative, hypnotic or anxiolytic abuse with sedative, hypnotic or anxiolytic-induced psychotic disorder**

     F13.150   **Sedative, hypnotic or anxiolytic abuse with sedative, hypnotic or anxiolytic-induced psychotic disorder with delusions**   HCC

     F13.151   **Sedative, hypnotic or anxiolytic abuse with sedative, hypnotic or anxiolytic-induced psychotic disorder with hallucinations**   HCC

     F13.159   **Sedative, hypnotic or anxiolytic abuse with sedative, hypnotic or anxiolytic-induced psychotic disorder, unspecified**   HCC ▽

✓6ᵗʰ **F13.18**   **Sedative, hypnotic or anxiolytic abuse with other sedative, hypnotic or anxiolytic-induced disorders**

     F13.180   **Sedative, hypnotic or anxiolytic abuse with sedative, hypnotic or anxiolytic-induced anxiety disorder**   HCC

     F13.181   **Sedative, hypnotic or anxiolytic abuse with sedative, hypnotic or anxiolytic-induced sexual dysfunction**   HCC

     F13.182   **Sedative, hypnotic or anxiolytic abuse with sedative, hypnotic or anxiolytic-induced sleep disorder**   HCC

     F13.188   **Sedative, hypnotic or anxiolytic abuse with other sedative, hypnotic or anxiolytic-induced disorder**   HCC

F13.19   **Sedative, hypnotic or anxiolytic abuse with unspecified sedative, hypnotic or anxiolytic-induced disorder**   HCC ▽

✓5ᵗʰ **F13.2**   **Sedative, hypnotic or anxiolytic-related dependence**
EXCLUDES 1   *sedative, hypnotic or anxiolytic-related abuse (F13.1-)*
     sedative, hypnotic, or anxiolytic use, unspecified (F13.9-)
EXCLUDES 2   *sedative, hypnotic, or anxiolytic poisoning (T42.-)*

     F13.20   **Sedative, hypnotic or anxiolytic dependence, uncomplicated**   HCC

     F13.21   **Sedative, hypnotic or anxiolytic dependence, in remission**   HCC
▶Sedative, hypnotic or anxiolytic use disorder, moderate, in early remission
Sedative, hypnotic or anxiolytic use disorder, moderate, in sustained remission
Sedative, hypnotic or anxiolytic use disorder, severe, in early remission
Sedative, hypnotic or anxiolytic use disorder, severe, in sustained remission◀

✓6ᵗʰ **F13.22**   **Sedative, hypnotic or anxiolytic dependence with intoxication**
     EXCLUDES 1   *sedative, hypnotic or anxiolytic dependence with withdrawal (F13.23-)*

     F13.220   **Sedative, hypnotic or anxiolytic dependence with intoxication, uncomplicated**   HCC

     F13.221   **Sedative, hypnotic or anxiolytic dependence with intoxication delirium**   HCC

     F13.229   **Sedative, hypnotic or anxiolytic dependence with intoxication, unspecified**   HCC ▽

✓6ᵗʰ **F13.23**   **Sedative, hypnotic or anxiolytic dependence with withdrawal**
Sedative, hypnotic, or anxiolytic use disorder, moderate
Sedative, hypnotic, or anxiolytic use disorder, severe
     EXCLUDES 1   *sedative, hypnotic or anxiolytic dependence with intoxication (F13.22-)*

     F13.230   **Sedative, hypnotic or anxiolytic dependence with withdrawal, uncomplicated**   HCC

     F13.231   **Sedative, hypnotic or anxiolytic dependence with withdrawal delirium**   HCC

     F13.232   **Sedative, hypnotic or anxiolytic dependence with withdrawal with perceptual disturbance**   HCC
Sedative, hypnotic, or anxiolytic withdrawal with perceptual disturbances

     F13.239   **Sedative, hypnotic or anxiolytic dependence with withdrawal, unspecified**   HCC ▽
Sedative, hypnotic, or anxiolytic withdrawal without perceptual disturbances

F13.24   **Sedative, hypnotic or anxiolytic dependence with sedative, hypnotic or anxiolytic-induced mood disorder**   HCC
▶Sedative, hypnotic, or anxiolytic use disorder, moderate, with sedative, hypnotic, or anxiolytic-induced bipolar or related disorder
Sedative, hypnotic, or anxiolytic use disorder, moderate, with sedative, hypnotic, or anxiolytic-induced depressive disorder◀
Sedative, hypnotic, or anxiolytic use disorder, severe, with sedative, hypnotic, or anxiolytic-induced bipolar or related disorder
▶Sedative, hypnotic, or anxiolytic use disorder, severe, with sedative, hypnotic, or anxiolytic-induced depressive disorder◀

✓6ᵗʰ **F13.25**   **Sedative, hypnotic or anxiolytic dependence with sedative, hypnotic or anxiolytic-induced psychotic disorder**

     F13.250   **Sedative, hypnotic or anxiolytic dependence with sedative, hypnotic or anxiolytic-induced psychotic disorder with delusions**   HCC

     F13.251   **Sedative, hypnotic or anxiolytic dependence with sedative, hypnotic or anxiolytic-induced psychotic disorder with hallucinations**   HCC

     F13.259   **Sedative, hypnotic or anxiolytic dependence with sedative, hypnotic or anxiolytic-induced psychotic disorder, unspecified**   HCC ▽

F13.26   **Sedative, hypnotic or anxiolytic dependence with sedative, hypnotic or anxiolytic-induced persisting amnestic disorder**   HCC

F13.27   **Sedative, hypnotic or anxiolytic dependence with sedative, hypnotic or anxiolytic-induced persisting dementia**   HCC
▶Sedative, hypnotic, or anxiolytic use disorder, moderate, with sedative, hypnotic, or anxiolytic-induced major neurocognitive disorder◀
Sedative, hypnotic, or anxiolytic use disorder, severe, with sedative, hypnotic, or anxiolytic-induced major neurocognitive disorder

✓6ᵗʰ **F13.28**   **Sedative, hypnotic or anxiolytic dependence with other sedative, hypnotic or anxiolytic-induced disorders**

     F13.280   **Sedative, hypnotic or anxiolytic dependence with sedative, hypnotic or anxiolytic-induced anxiety disorder**   HCC

     F13.281   **Sedative, hypnotic or anxiolytic dependence with sedative, hypnotic or anxiolytic-induced sexual dysfunction**   HCC

     F13.282   **Sedative, hypnotic or anxiolytic dependence with sedative, hypnotic or anxiolytic-induced sleep disorder**   HCC

     F13.288   **Sedative, hypnotic or anxiolytic dependence with other sedative, hypnotic or anxiolytic-induced disorder**   HCC
▶Sedative, hypnotic, or anxiolytic use disorder, moderate, with sedative, hypnotic, or anxiolytic-induced mild neurocognitive disorder
Sedative, hypnotic, or anxiolytic use disorder, severe, with sedative, hypnotic, or anxiolytic-induced mild neurocognitive disorder◀

F13.29   **Sedative, hypnotic or anxiolytic dependence with unspecified sedative, hypnotic or anxiolytic-induced disorder**   HCC ▽

✓ Additional Character Req   ✓x7ᵗʰ Placeholder Alert   Manifestation   HCC CMS-HCC Condition   ▽ Unspecified Code   ▶◀ Revised Text   ● New Code   ▲ Revised Code Title

ICD-10-CM 2018   531

Chapter 5. Mental, Behavioral and Neurodevelopmental Disorders

F13.9–F14.220

√5ᵗʰ **F13.9 Sedative, hypnotic or anxiolytic-related use, unspecified**
  EXCLUDES 1 *sedative, hypnotic or anxiolytic-related abuse (F13.1-)*
    sedative, hypnotic or anxiolytic-related dependence (F13.2-)

  F13.90 Sedative, hypnotic, or anxiolytic use, unspecified, uncomplicated

√6ᵗʰ **F13.92 Sedative, hypnotic or anxiolytic use, unspecified with intoxication**
    EXCLUDES 1 *sedative, hypnotic or anxiolytic use, unspecified with withdrawal (F13.93-)*

    F13.920 Sedative, hypnotic or anxiolytic use, HCC unspecified with intoxication, uncomplicated

    F13.921 Sedative, hypnotic or anxiolytic use, HCC unspecified with intoxication delirium
      Sedative, hypnotic, or anxiolytic-induced delirium

    F13.929 Sedative, hypnotic or anxiolytic use, HCC ▽ unspecified with intoxication, unspecified

√6ᵗʰ **F13.93 Sedative, hypnotic or anxiolytic use, unspecified with withdrawal**
    EXCLUDES 1 *sedative, hypnotic or anxiolytic use, unspecified with intoxication (F13.92-)*

    F13.930 Sedative, hypnotic or anxiolytic use, HCC unspecified with withdrawal, uncomplicated

    F13.931 Sedative, hypnotic or anxiolytic use, HCC unspecified with withdrawal delirium

    F13.932 Sedative, hypnotic or anxiolytic use, HCC unspecified with withdrawal with perceptual disturbances

    F13.939 Sedative, hypnotic or anxiolytic use, HCC ▽ unspecified with withdrawal, unspecified

  F13.94 Sedative, hypnotic or anxiolytic use, HCC ▽ unspecified with sedative, hypnotic or anxiolytic-induced mood disorder
    Sedative, hypnotic, or anxiolytic-induced bipolar or related disorder, without use disorder
    Sedative, hypnotic, or anxiolytic-induced depressive disorder, without use disorder

√6ᵗʰ **F13.95 Sedative, hypnotic or anxiolytic use, unspecified with sedative, hypnotic or anxiolytic-induced psychotic disorder**
    F13.950 Sedative, hypnotic or anxiolytic use, HCC unspecified with sedative, hypnotic or anxiolytic-induced psychotic disorder with delusions

    F13.951 Sedative, hypnotic or anxiolytic use, HCC unspecified with sedative, hypnotic or anxiolytic-induced psychotic disorder with hallucinations

    F13.959 Sedative, hypnotic or anxiolytic use, HCC ▽ unspecified with sedative, hypnotic or anxiolytic-induced psychotic disorder, unspecified
      ▶Sedative, hypnotic, or anxiolytic-induced psychotic disorder, without use disorder◀

  F13.96 Sedative, hypnotic or anxiolytic use, unspecified HCC with sedative, hypnotic or anxiolytic-induced persisting amnestic disorder

  F13.97 Sedative, hypnotic or anxiolytic use, unspecified HCC with sedative, hypnotic or anxiolytic-induced persisting dementia
    ▶Sedative, hypnotic, or anxiolytic-induced major neurocognitive disorder, without use disorder◀

√6ᵗʰ **F13.98 Sedative, hypnotic or anxiolytic use, unspecified with other sedative, hypnotic or anxiolytic-induced disorders**
    F13.980 Sedative, hypnotic or anxiolytic use, HCC unspecified with sedative, hypnotic or anxiolytic-induced anxiety disorder
      ▶Sedative, hypnotic, or anxiolytic-induced anxiety disorder, without use disorder◀

    F13.981 Sedative, hypnotic or anxiolytic use, HCC unspecified with sedative, hypnotic or anxiolytic-induced sexual dysfunction
      ▶Sedative, hypnotic, or anxiolytic-induced sexual dysfunction disorder, without use disorder◀

    F13.982 Sedative, hypnotic or anxiolytic use, HCC unspecified with sedative, hypnotic or anxiolytic-induced sleep disorder
      ▶Sedative, hypnotic, or anxiolytic-induced sleep disorder, without use disorder◀

    F13.988 Sedative, hypnotic or anxiolytic use, HCC unspecified with other sedative, hypnotic or anxiolytic-induced disorder
      ▶Sedative, hypnotic, or anxiolytic-induced mild neurocognitive disorder◀

  F13.99 Sedative, hypnotic or anxiolytic use, HCC ▽ unspecified with unspecified sedative, hypnotic or anxiolytic-induced disorder

√4ᵗʰ **F14 Cocaine related disorders**
  EXCLUDES 2 *other stimulant-related disorders (F15.-)*

  √5ᵗʰ **F14.1 Cocaine abuse**
      EXCLUDES 1 *cocaine dependence (F14.2-)*
        cocaine use, unspecified (F14.9-)

    F14.10 Cocaine abuse, uncomplicated
      Cocaine use disorder, mild

    F14.11 Cocaine abuse, in remission
      Cocaine use disorder, mild, in early remission
      Cocaine use disorder, mild, in sustained remission

    √6ᵗʰ **F14.12 Cocaine abuse with intoxication**
      F14.120 Cocaine abuse with intoxication, HCC uncomplicated

      F14.121 Cocaine abuse with intoxication with HCC delirium

      F14.122 Cocaine abuse with intoxication with HCC perceptual disturbance

      F14.129 Cocaine abuse with intoxication, HCC ▽ unspecified

    F14.14 Cocaine abuse with cocaine-induced HCC mood disorder
      Cocaine use disorder, mild, with cocaine-induced bipolar or related disorder
      Cocaine use disorder, mild, with cocaine-induced depressive disorder

    √6ᵗʰ **F14.15 Cocaine abuse with cocaine-induced psychotic disorder**
      F14.150 Cocaine abuse with cocaine-induced HCC psychotic disorder with delusions

      F14.151 Cocaine abuse with cocaine-induced HCC psychotic disorder with hallucinations

      F14.159 Cocaine abuse with cocaine- HCC ▽ induced psychotic disorder, unspecified

    √6ᵗʰ **F14.18 Cocaine abuse with other cocaine-induced disorder**
      F14.180 Cocaine abuse with cocaine-induced HCC anxiety disorder

      F14.181 Cocaine abuse with cocaine-induced HCC sexual dysfunction

      F14.182 Cocaine abuse with cocaine-induced HCC sleep disorder

      F14.188 Cocaine abuse with other cocaine- HCC induced disorder
        Cocaine use disorder, mild, with cocaine-induced obsessive compulsive or related disorder

    F14.19 Cocaine abuse with unspecified cocaine- HCC ▽ induced disorder

  √5ᵗʰ **F14.2 Cocaine dependence**
      EXCLUDES 1 *cocaine abuse (F14.1-)*
        cocaine use, unspecified (F14.9-)
      EXCLUDES 2 *cocaine poisoning (T40.5-)*

    F14.20 Cocaine dependence, uncomplicated HCC
      Cocaine use disorder, moderate
      Cocaine use disorder, severe

    F14.21 Cocaine dependence, in remission HCC
      ▶Cocaine use disorder, moderate, in early remission
      Cocaine use disorder, moderate, in sustained remission
      Cocaine use disorder, severe, in early remission
      Cocaine use disorder, severe, in sustained remission◀

    √6ᵗʰ **F14.22 Cocaine dependence with intoxication**
        EXCLUDES 1 *cocaine dependence with withdrawal (F14.23)*

      F14.220 Cocaine dependence with HCC intoxication, uncomplicated

F14.221   **Cocaine dependence with intoxication delirium**   HCC

F14.222   **Cocaine dependence with intoxication with perceptual disturbance**   HCC

F14.229   **Cocaine dependence with intoxication, unspecified**   HCC ▽

F14.23   **Cocaine dependence with withdrawal**   HCC
> EXCLUDES 1   *cocaine dependence with intoxication (F14.22-)*

F14.24   **Cocaine dependence with cocaine-induced mood disorder**   HCC
> Cocaine use disorder, moderate, with cocaine-induced bipolar or related disorder
> Cocaine use disorder, moderate, with cocaine-induced depressive disorder
> Cocaine use disorder, severe, with cocaine-induced bipolar or related disorder
> Cocaine use disorder, severe, with cocaine-induced depressive disorder

✓6ᵗʰ F14.25   **Cocaine dependence with cocaine-induced psychotic disorder**

    F14.250   **Cocaine dependence with cocaine-induced psychotic disorder with delusions**   HCC

    F14.251   **Cocaine dependence with cocaine-induced psychotic disorder with hallucinations**   HCC

    F14.259   **Cocaine dependence with cocaine-induced psychotic disorder, unspecified**   HCC ▽

✓6ᵗʰ F14.28   **Cocaine dependence with other cocaine-induced disorder**

    F14.280   **Cocaine dependence with cocaine-induced anxiety disorder**   HCC

    F14.281   **Cocaine dependence with cocaine-induced sexual dysfunction**   HCC

    F14.282   **Cocaine dependence with cocaine-induced sleep disorder**   HCC

    F14.288   **Cocaine dependence with other cocaine-induced disorder**   HCC
> Cocaine use disorder, moderate, with cocaine-induced obsessive compulsive or related disorder
> Cocaine use disorder, severe, with cocaine-induced obsessive compulsive or related disorder

F14.29   **Cocaine dependence with unspecified cocaine-induced disorder**   HCC ▽

✓5ᵗʰ F14.9   **Cocaine use, unspecified**
> EXCLUDES 1   *cocaine abuse (F14.1-)*
> *cocaine dependence (F14.2-)*

F14.90   **Cocaine use, unspecified, uncomplicated**

✓6ᵗʰ F14.92   **Cocaine use, unspecified with intoxication**

    F14.920   **Cocaine use, unspecified with intoxication, uncomplicated**   HCC

    F14.921   **Cocaine use, unspecified with intoxication delirium**   HCC

    F14.922   **Cocaine use, unspecified with intoxication with perceptual disturbance**   HCC

    F14.929   **Cocaine use, unspecified with intoxication, unspecified**   HCC ▽

F14.94   **Cocaine use, unspecified with cocaine-induced mood disorder**   HCC
> Cocaine induced bipolar or related disorder, without use disorder
> Cocaine induced depressive disorder, without use disorder

✓6ᵗʰ F14.95   **Cocaine use, unspecified with cocaine-induced psychotic disorder**

    F14.950   **Cocaine use, unspecified with cocaine-induced psychotic disorder with delusions**   HCC

    F14.951   **Cocaine use, unspecified with cocaine-induced psychotic disorder with hallucinations**   HCC

    F14.959   **Cocaine use, unspecified with cocaine-induced psychotic disorder, unspecified**   HCC ▽
> Cocaine induced psychotic disorder, without use disorder

✓6ᵗʰ F14.98   **Cocaine use, unspecified with other specified cocaine-induced disorder**

    F14.980   **Cocaine use, unspecified with cocaine-induced anxiety disorder**   HCC
> Cocaine induced anxiety disorder, without use disorder

    F14.981   **Cocaine use, unspecified with cocaine-induced sexual dysfunction**   HCC
> Cocaine induced sexual dysfunction, without use disorder

    F14.982   **Cocaine use, unspecified with cocaine-induced sleep disorder**   HCC
> Cocaine induced sleep disorder, without use disorder

    F14.988   **Cocaine use, unspecified with other cocaine-induced disorder**   HCC
> Cocaine induced obsessive compulsive or related disorder

F14.99   **Cocaine use, unspecified with unspecified cocaine-induced disorder**   HCC ▽

✓4ᵗʰ **F15   Other stimulant related disorders**
> INCLUDES   amphetamine-related disorders
> caffeine
> EXCLUDES 2   *cocaine-related disorders (F14.-)*

✓5ᵗʰ F15.1   **Other stimulant abuse**
> EXCLUDES 1   *other stimulant dependence (F15.2-)*
> *other stimulant use, unspecified (F15.9-)*

F15.10   **Other stimulant abuse, uncomplicated**
> Amphetamine type substance use disorder, mild
> Other or unspecified stimulant use disorder, mild

● F15.11   **Other stimulant abuse, in remission**
> Amphetamine type substance use disorder, mild, in early remission
> Amphetamine type substance use disorder, mild, in sustained remission
> Other or unspecified stimulant use disorder, mild, in early remission
> Other or unspecified stimulant use disorder, mild, in sustained remission

✓6ᵗʰ F15.12   **Other stimulant abuse with intoxication**

    F15.120   **Other stimulant abuse with intoxication, uncomplicated**   HCC

    F15.121   **Other stimulant abuse with intoxication delirium**   HCC

    F15.122   **Other stimulant abuse with intoxication with perceptual disturbance**   HCC
> Amphetamine or other stimulant use disorder, mild, with amphetamine or other stimulant intoxication, with perceptual disturbances

    F15.129   **Other stimulant abuse with intoxication, unspecified**   HCC ▽
> Amphetamine or other stimulant use disorder, mild, with amphetamine or other stimulant intoxication, without perceptual disturbances

F15.14   **Other stimulant abuse with stimulant-induced mood disorder**   HCC
> Amphetamine or other stimulant use disorder, mild, with amphetamine or other stimulant induced bipolar or related disorder
> Amphetamine or other stimulant use disorder, mild, with amphetamine or other stimulant induced depressive disorder

✓6ᵗʰ F15.15   **Other stimulant abuse with stimulant-induced psychotic disorder**

    F15.150   **Other stimulant abuse with stimulant-induced psychotic disorder with delusions**   HCC

    F15.151   **Other stimulant abuse with stimulant-induced psychotic disorder with hallucinations**   HCC

    F15.159   **Other stimulant abuse with stimulant-induced psychotic disorder, unspecified**   HCC ▽

✓6ᵗʰ F15.18   **Other stimulant abuse with other stimulant-induced disorder**

    F15.180   **Other stimulant abuse with stimulant-induced anxiety disorder**   HCC

    F15.181   **Other stimulant abuse with stimulant-induced sexual dysfunction**   HCC

☑ Additional Character Req   ☑7ᵗʰ Placeholder Alert   Manifestation   HCC CMS-HCC Condition   ▽ Unspecified Code   ►◄ Revised Text   ● New Code   ▲ Revised Code Title

ICD-10-CM 2018   533

Chapter 5. Mental, Behavioral and Neurodevelopmental Disorders

    F15.182   **Other stimulant abuse with** HCC
         stimulant-induced sleep disorder

    F15.188   **Other stimulant abuse with other** HCC
         stimulant-induced disorder
         Amphetamine or other stimulant use
         disorder, mild, with amphetamine or
         other stimulant induced
         obsessive-compulsive or related
         disorder

F15.19   **Other stimulant abuse with unspecified** HCC ▽
     stimulant-induced disorder

✓5th **F15.2**   **Other stimulant dependence**
     EXCLUDES 1   other stimulant abuse (F15.1-)
               other stimulant use, unspecified (F15.9-)

    F15.20   **Other stimulant dependence, uncomplicated** HCC
         Amphetamine type substance use disorder, moderate
         Amphetamine type substance use disorder, severe
         Other or unspecified stimulant use disorder, moderate
         Other or unspecified stimulant use disorder, severe

    F15.21   **Other stimulant dependence, in remission** HCC
         ▶Amphetamine type substance use disorder, moderate,
         in early remission
         Amphetamine type substance use disorder, moderate,
         in sustained remission
         Amphetamine type substance use disorder, severe, in
         early remission
         Amphetamine type substance use disorder, severe, in
         sustained remission
         Other or unspecified stimulant use disorder,
         moderate, in early remission
         Other or unspecified stimulant use disorder,
         moderate, in sustained remission
         Other or unspecified stimulant use disorder, severe, in
         early remission
         Other or unspecified stimulant use disorder, severe, in
         sustained remission◀

✓6th **F15.22**   **Other stimulant dependence with intoxication**
         EXCLUDES 1   other stimulant dependence with withdrawal
                 (F15.23)

    F15.220   **Other stimulant dependence with** HCC
         intoxication, uncomplicated

    F15.221   **Other stimulant dependence with** HCC
         intoxication delirium

    F15.222   **Other stimulant dependence with** HCC
         intoxication with perceptual disturbance
         Amphetamine or other stimulant use
         disorder, moderate, with
         amphetamine or other stimulant
         intoxication, with perceptual
         disturbances
         Amphetamine or other stimulant use
         disorder, severe, with amphetamine or
         other stimulant intoxication, with
         perceptual disturbances

    F15.229   **Other stimulant dependence with** HCC ▽
         intoxication, unspecified
         Amphetamine or other stimulant use
         disorder, moderate, with
         amphetamine or other stimulant
         intoxication, without perceptual
         disturbances
         Amphetamine or other stimulant use
         disorder, severe, with amphetamine or
         other stimulant intoxication, without
         perceptual disturbances

F15.23   **Other stimulant dependence with withdrawal** HCC
     Amphetamine or other stimulant withdrawal
     EXCLUDES 1   other stimulant dependence with
                 intoxication (F15.22-)

F15.24   **Other stimulant dependence with** HCC
     stimulant-induced mood disorder
     Amphetamine or other stimulant use disorder,
     moderate, with amphetamine or other
     stimulant-induced bipolar or related disorder
     Amphetamine or other stimulant use disorder,
     moderate, with amphetamine or other stimulant
     induced depressive disorder
     Amphetamine or other stimulant use disorder, severe,
     with amphetamine or other stimulant-induced
     bipolar or related disorder
     Amphetamine or other stimulant use disorder, severe,
     with amphetamine or other stimulant-induced
     depressive disorder

✓6th **F15.25**   **Other stimulant dependence with**
     stimulant-induced psychotic disorder

    F15.250   **Other stimulant dependence with** HCC
         stimulant-induced psychotic disorder with
         delusions

    F15.251   **Other stimulant dependence with** HCC
         stimulant-induced psychotic disorder with
         hallucinations

    F15.259   **Other stimulant dependence with** HCC ▽
         stimulant-induced psychotic disorder,
         unspecified

✓6th **F15.28**   **Other stimulant dependence with other**
     stimulant-induced disorder

    F15.280   **Other stimulant dependence with** HCC
         stimulant-induced anxiety disorder

    F15.281   **Other stimulant dependence with** HCC
         stimulant-induced sexual dysfunction

    F15.282   **Other stimulant dependence with** HCC
         stimulant-induced sleep disorder

    F15.288   **Other stimulant dependence with** HCC
         other stimulant-induced disorder
         ▶Amphetamine or other stimulant use
         disorder, moderate, with
         amphetamine or other stimulant
         induced obsessive compulsive or
         related disorder
         Amphetamine or other stimulant use
         disorder, severe, with amphetamine or
         other stimulant induced obsessive
         compulsive or related disorder◀

F15.29   **Other stimulant dependence with unspecified** HCC ▽
     stimulant-induced disorder

✓5th **F15.9**   **Other stimulant use, unspecified**
     EXCLUDES 1   other stimulant abuse (F15.1-)
               other stimulant dependence (F15.2-)

    F15.90   **Other stimulant use, unspecified, uncomplicated**

✓6th **F15.92**   **Other stimulant use, unspecified with intoxication**
         EXCLUDES 1   other stimulant use, unspecified with
                 withdrawal (F15.93)

    F15.920   **Other stimulant use, unspecified with** HCC
         intoxication, uncomplicated

    F15.921   **Other stimulant use, unspecified with** HCC
         intoxication delirium
         Amphetamine or other stimulant-induced
         delirium

    F15.922   **Other stimulant use, unspecified with** HCC
         intoxication with perceptual disturbance

    F15.929   **Other stimulant use, unspecified** HCC ▽
         with intoxication, unspecified
         Caffeine intoxication

    F15.93   **Other stimulant use, unspecified with** HCC
     withdrawal
     Caffeine withdrawal
     EXCLUDES 1   other stimulant use, unspecified with
                 intoxication (F15.92-)

    F15.94   **Other stimulant use, unspecified with** HCC
     stimulant-induced mood disorder
     Amphetamine or other stimulant-induced bipolar or
     related disorder, without use disorder
     Amphetamine or other stimulant-induced depressive
     disorder, without use disorder

✓6th **F15.95**   **Other stimulant use, unspecified with**
     stimulant-induced psychotic disorder

    F15.950   **Other stimulant use, unspecified with** HCC
         stimulant-induced psychotic disorder
         with delusions

    F15.951   **Other stimulant use, unspecified with** HCC
         stimulant-induced psychotic disorder
         with hallucinations

    F15.959   **Other stimulant use, unspecified** HCC ▽
         with stimulant-induced psychotic
         disorder, unspecified
         ▶Amphetamine or other stimulant-induced
         psychotic disorder, without use
         disorder◀

EXCLUDES 1 Not coded here   EXCLUDES 2 Not included here   N Newborn Age: 0   P Pediatric Age: 0-17   M Maternity Age: 12-55   A Adult Age: 15-124

534   ICD-10-CM 2018

✓6th **F15.98** **Other stimulant use, unspecified with other stimulant-induced disorder**

     F15.980 **Other stimulant use, unspecified with** HCC **stimulant-induced anxiety disorder**
         Amphetamine or other stimulant-induced anxiety disorder, without use disorder
         Caffeine induced anxiety disorder, without use disorder

     F15.981 **Other stimulant use, unspecified with** HCC **stimulant-induced sexual dysfunction**
         Amphetamine or other stimulant-induced sexual dysfunction, without use disorder

     F15.982 **Other stimulant use, unspecified with** HCC **stimulant-induced sleep disorder**
         Amphetamine or other stimulant-induced sleep disorder, without use disorder
         Caffeine induced sleep disorder, without use disorder

     F15.988 **Other stimulant use, unspecified with** HCC **other stimulant-induced disorder**
         Amphetamine or other stimulant-induced obsessive compulsive or related disorder, without use disorder

F15.99 **Other stimulant use, unspecified with** HCC ▽ **unspecified stimulant-induced disorder**

✓4th **F16** **Hallucinogen related disorders**
     INCLUDES   ecstasy
         PCP
         phencyclidine

✓5th **F16.1** **Hallucinogen abuse**
     EXCLUDES 1   *hallucinogen dependence (F16.2-)*
         hallucinogen use, unspecified (F16.9-)

     F16.10 **Hallucinogen abuse, uncomplicated**
         Other hallucinogen use disorder, mild
         Phencyclidine use disorder, mild

●   **F16.11** **Hallucinogen abuse, in remission**
         Other hallucinogen use disorder, mild, in early remission
         Other hallucinogen use disorder, mild, in sustained remission
         Phencyclidine use disorder, mild, in early remission
         Phencyclidine use disorder, mild, in sustained remission

✓6th **F16.12** **Hallucinogen abuse with intoxication**

     F16.120 **Hallucinogen abuse with intoxication,** HCC **uncomplicated**

     F16.121 **Hallucinogen abuse with intoxication** HCC **with delirium**

     F16.122 **Hallucinogen abuse with intoxication** HCC **with perceptual disturbance**

     F16.129 **Hallucinogen abuse with** HCC ▽ **intoxication, unspecified**

F16.14 **Hallucinogen abuse with hallucinogen-induced mood disorder**
     Other hallucinogen use disorder, mild, with other hallucinogen induced bipolar or related disorder
     Other hallucinogen use disorder, mild, with other hallucinogen induced depressive disorder
     Phencyclidine use disorder, mild, with phencyclidine induced bipolar or related disorder
     Phencyclidine use disorder, mild, with phencyclidine induced depressive disorder

✓6th **F16.15** **Hallucinogen abuse with hallucinogen-induced psychotic disorder**

     F16.150 **Hallucinogen abuse with** HCC **hallucinogen-induced psychotic disorder with delusions**

     F16.151 **Hallucinogen abuse with** HCC **hallucinogen-induced psychotic disorder with hallucinations**

     F16.159 **Hallucinogen abuse with** HCC ▽ **hallucinogen-induced psychotic disorder, unspecified**

✓6th **F16.18** **Hallucinogen abuse with other hallucinogen-induced disorder**

     F16.180 **Hallucinogen abuse with** HCC **hallucinogen-induced anxiety disorder**

     F16.183 **Hallucinogen abuse with** HCC **hallucinogen persisting perception disorder (flashbacks)**

     F16.188 **Hallucinogen abuse with other** HCC **hallucinogen-induced disorder**

     F16.19 **Hallucinogen abuse with unspecified** HCC ▽ **hallucinogen-induced disorder**

✓5th **F16.2** **Hallucinogen dependence**
     EXCLUDES 1   *hallucinogen abuse (F16.1-)*
         hallucinogen use, unspecified (F16.9-)

     F16.20 **Hallucinogen dependence, uncomplicated** HCC
         Other hallucinogen use disorder, moderate
         Other hallucinogen use disorder, severe
         Phencyclidine use disorder, moderate
         Phencyclidine use disorder, severe

     F16.21 **Hallucinogen dependence, in remission** HCC
         ▶Other hallucinogen use disorder, moderate, in early remission
         Other hallucinogen use disorder, moderate, in sustained remission
         Other hallucinogen use disorder, severe, in early remission
         Other hallucinogen use disorder, severe, in sustained remission
         Phencyclidine use disorder, moderate, in early remission
         Phencyclidine use disorder, moderate, in sustained remission
         Phencyclidine use disorder, severe, in early remission
         Phencyclidine use disorder, severe, in sustained remission◀

✓6th **F16.22** **Hallucinogen dependence with intoxication**

     F16.220 **Hallucinogen dependence with** HCC **intoxication, uncomplicated**

     F16.221 **Hallucinogen dependence with** HCC **intoxication with delirium**

     F16.229 **Hallucinogen dependence with** HCC ▽ **intoxication, unspecified**

F16.24 **Hallucinogen dependence with** HCC **hallucinogen-induced mood disorder**
     Other hallucinogen use disorder, moderate, with other hallucinogen induced bipolar or related disorder
     Other hallucinogen use disorder, moderate, with other hallucinogen induced depressive disorder
     Other hallucinogen use disorder, severe, with other hallucinogen-induced bipolar or related disorder
     Other hallucinogen use disorder, severe, with other hallucinogen-induced depressive disorder
     Phencyclidine use disorder, moderate, with phencyclidine induced bipolar or related disorder
     Phencyclidine use disorder, moderate, with phencyclidine induced depressive disorder
     Phencyclidine use disorder, severe, with phencyclidine induced bipolar or related disorder
     Phencyclidine use disorder, severe, with phencyclidine-induced depressive disorder

✓6th **F16.25** **Hallucinogen dependence with hallucinogen-induced psychotic disorder**

     F16.250 **Hallucinogen dependence with** HCC **hallucinogen-induced psychotic disorder with delusions**

     F16.251 **Hallucinogen dependence with** HCC **hallucinogen-induced psychotic disorder with hallucinations**

     F16.259 **Hallucinogen dependence with** HCC ▽ **hallucinogen-induced psychotic disorder, unspecified**

✓6th **F16.28** **Hallucinogen dependence with other hallucinogen-induced disorder**

     F16.280 **Hallucinogen dependence with** HCC **hallucinogen-induced anxiety disorder**

     F16.283 **Hallucinogen dependence with** HCC **hallucinogen persisting perception disorder (flashbacks)**

     F16.288 **Hallucinogen dependence with other** HCC **hallucinogen-induced disorder**

     F16.29 **Hallucinogen dependence with unspecified** HCC ▽ **hallucinogen-induced disorder**

✓5th **F16.9** **Hallucinogen use, unspecified**
     EXCLUDES 1   *hallucinogen abuse (F16.1-)*
         hallucinogen dependence (F16.2-)

     F16.90 **Hallucinogen use, unspecified, uncomplicated**

✓ Additional Character Req   ✓x7th Placeholder Alert   Manifestation   HCC CMS-HCC Condition   ▽ Unspecified Code   ▶◀ Revised Text   ● New Code   ▲ Revised Code Title

Chapter 5. Mental, Behavioral and Neurodevelopmental Disorders

F16.92–F17.299

✓6th **F16.92 Hallucinogen use, unspecified with intoxication**

  F16.920 Hallucinogen use, unspecified with HCC
    intoxication, uncomplicated

  F16.921 Hallucinogen use, unspecified with HCC
    intoxication with delirium
      Other hallucinogen intoxication delirium

  F16.929 Hallucinogen use, unspecified with HCC ▽
    intoxication, unspecified

F16.94 Hallucinogen use, unspecified with HCC
  hallucinogen-induced mood disorder
    Other hallucinogen induced bipolar or related
      disorder, without use disorder
    Other hallucinogen induced depressive disorder,
      without use disorder
    Phencyclidine induced bipolar or related disorder,
      without use disorder
    Phencyclidine induced depressive disorder, without
      use disorder

✓6th **F16.95 Hallucinogen use, unspecified with**
  hallucinogen-induced psychotic disorder

  F16.950 Hallucinogen use, unspecified with HCC
    hallucinogen-induced psychotic disorder
    with delusions

  F16.951 Hallucinogen use, unspecified with HCC
    hallucinogen-induced psychotic disorder
    with hallucinations

  F16.959 Hallucinogen use, unspecified with HCC ▽
    hallucinogen-induced psychotic disorder,
    unspecified
      Other hallucinogen induced psychotic
        disorder, without use disorder
      Phencyclidine induced psychotic disorder,
        without use disorder

✓6th **F16.98 Hallucinogen use, unspecified with other specified**
  hallucinogen-induced disorder

  F16.980 Hallucinogen use, unspecified with HCC
    hallucinogen-induced anxiety disorder
      Other hallucinogen-induced anxiety
        disorder, without use disorder
      Phencyclidine induced anxiety disorder,
        without use disorder

  F16.983 Hallucinogen use, unspecified with HCC
    hallucinogen persisting perception
    disorder (flashbacks)

  F16.988 Hallucinogen use, unspecified with HCC
    other hallucinogen-induced disorder

F16.99 Hallucinogen use, unspecified with HCC ▽
  unspecified hallucinogen-induced disorder

✓4th **F17 Nicotine dependence**

  EXCLUDES 1   *history of tobacco dependence (Z87.891)*
      tobacco use NOS (Z72.0)

  EXCLUDES 2   *tobacco use (smoking) during pregnancy, childbirth and the*
      puerperium (O99.33-)
      toxic effect of nicotine (T65.2-)

  AHA: 2013, 4Q, 108-109

✓5th **F17.2 Nicotine dependence**

  ✓6th **F17.20 Nicotine dependence, unspecified**

    F17.200 Nicotine dependence, unspecified, ▽
      uncomplicated
        Tobacco use disorder, mild
        Tobacco use disorder, moderate
        Tobacco use disorder, severe
        AHA: 2016, 1Q, 36

    F17.201 Nicotine dependence, unspecified, in ▽
      remission
        ►Tobacco use disorder, mild, in early
          remission
        Tobacco use disorder, mild, in sustained
          remission
        Tobacco use disorder, moderate, in early
          remission
        Tobacco use disorder, moderate, in
          sustained remission
        Tobacco use disorder, severe, in early
          remission
        Tobacco use disorder, severe, in sustained
          remission◄

    F17.203 Nicotine dependence unspecified, ▽
      with withdrawal
        Tobacco withdrawal

  F17.208 Nicotine dependence, unspecified, ▽
    with other nicotine-induced disorders

  F17.209 Nicotine dependence, unspecified, ▽
    with unspecified nicotine-induced
    disorders

✓6th **F17.21 Nicotine dependence, cigarettes**

  F17.210 Nicotine dependence, cigarettes,
    uncomplicated
      AHA: 2017, 2Q, 28-29

  F17.211 Nicotine dependence, cigarettes, in
    remission
      ►Tobacco use disorder, cigarettes, mild, in
        early remission
      Tobacco use disorder, cigarettes, mild, in
        sustained remission
      Tobacco use disorder, cigarettes, moderate,
        in early remission
      Tobacco use disorder, cigarettes, moderate,
        in sustained remission
      Tobacco use disorder, cigarettes, severe, in
        early remission
      Tobacco use disorder, cigarettes, severe, in
        sustained remission◄

  F17.213 Nicotine dependence, cigarettes, with
    withdrawal

  F17.218 Nicotine dependence, cigarettes, with
    other nicotine-induced disorders

  F17.219 Nicotine dependence, cigarettes, with ▽
    unspecified nicotine-induced disorders

✓6th **F17.22 Nicotine dependence, chewing tobacco**

  F17.220 Nicotine dependence, chewing tobacco,
    uncomplicated

  F17.221 Nicotine dependence, chewing tobacco, in
    remission
      ►Tobacco use disorder, chewing tobacco,
        mild, in early remission
      Tobacco use disorder, chewing tobacco,
        mild, in sustained remission
      Tobacco use disorder, chewing tobacco,
        moderate, in early remission
      Tobacco use disorder, chewing tobacco,
        moderate, in sustained remission
      Tobacco use disorder, chewing tobacco,
        severe, in early remission
      Tobacco use disorder, chewing tobacco,
        severe, in sustained remission◄

  F17.223 Nicotine dependence, chewing tobacco,
    with withdrawal

  F17.228 Nicotine dependence, chewing tobacco,
    with other nicotine-induced disorders

  F17.229 Nicotine dependence, chewing ▽
    tobacco, with unspecified
    nicotine-induced disorders

✓6th **F17.29 Nicotine dependence, other tobacco product**

  F17.290 Nicotine dependence, other tobacco
    product, uncomplicated
      AHA: 2017, 2Q, 28-29

  F17.291 Nicotine dependence, other tobacco
    product, in remission
      ►Tobacco use disorder, other tobacco
        product, mild, in early remission
      Tobacco use disorder, other tobacco
        product, mild, in sustained remission
      Tobacco use disorder, other tobacco
        product, moderate, in early remission
      Tobacco use disorder, other tobacco
        product, moderate, in sustained
        remission
      Tobacco use disorder, other tobacco
        product, severe, in early remission
      Tobacco use disorder, other tobacco
        product, severe, in sustained
        remission◄

  F17.293 Nicotine dependence, other tobacco
    product, with withdrawal

  F17.298 Nicotine dependence, other tobacco
    product, with other nicotine-induced
    disorders

  F17.299 Nicotine dependence, other tobacco ▽
    product, with unspecified
    nicotine-induced disorders

EXCLUDES 1 Not coded here   EXCLUDES 2 Not included here   N Newborn Age: 0   P Pediatric Age: 0-17   M Maternity Age: 12-55   A Adult Age: 15-124

536   ICD-10-CM 2018

✓4ᵗʰ **F18 Inhalant related disorders**
    INCLUDES volatile solvents

✓5ᵗʰ **F18.1 Inhalant abuse**
    EXCLUDES 1 *inhalant dependence (F18.2-)*
                    inhalant use, unspecified (F18.9-)

      F18.10 Inhalant abuse, uncomplicated
          Inhalant use disorder, mild

●   **F18.11 Inhalant abuse, in remission**
          Inhalant use disorder, mild, in early remission
          Inhalant use disorder, mild, in sustained remission

✓6ᵗʰ **F18.12 Inhalant abuse with intoxication**
        F18.120 Inhalant abuse with intoxication, HCC
               uncomplicated
        F18.121 Inhalant abuse with intoxication HCC
               delirium
        F18.129 Inhalant abuse with intoxication, HCC ▽
               unspecified

      F18.14 Inhalant abuse with inhalant-induced mood HCC
          disorder
          Inhalant use disorder, mild, with inhalant induced
            depressive disorder

✓6ᵗʰ **F18.15 Inhalant abuse with inhalant-induced psychotic**
          disorder
        F18.150 Inhalant abuse with inhalant-induced HCC
               psychotic disorder with delusions
        F18.151 Inhalant abuse with inhalant-induced HCC
               psychotic disorder with hallucinations
        F18.159 Inhalant abuse with inhalant- HCC ▽
               induced psychotic disorder, unspecified

      F18.17 Inhalant abuse with inhalant-induced dementia HCC
          Inhalant use disorder, mild, with inhalant induced
            major neurocognitive disorder

✓6ᵗʰ **F18.18 Inhalant abuse with other inhalant-induced**
          disorders
        F18.180 Inhalant abuse with inhalant-induced HCC
               anxiety disorder
        F18.188 Inhalant abuse with other HCC
               inhalant-induced disorder
            Inhalant use disorder, mild, with inhalant
               induced mild neurocognitive disorder

      F18.19 Inhalant abuse with unspecified inhalant- HCC ▽
          induced disorder

✓5ᵗʰ **F18.2 Inhalant dependence**
    EXCLUDES 1 *inhalant abuse (F18.1-)*
                      inhalant use, unspecified (F18.9-)

      F18.20 Inhalant dependence, uncomplicated HCC
          Inhalant use disorder, moderate
          Inhalant use disorder, severe

      F18.21 Inhalant dependence, in remission HCC
          ▶Inhalant use disorder, moderate, in early remission
          Inhalant use disorder, moderate, in sustained
            remission
          Inhalant use disorder, severe, in early remission
          Inhalant use disorder, severe, in sustained remission◀

✓6ᵗʰ **F18.22 Inhalant dependence with intoxication**
        F18.220 Inhalant dependence with in HCC
               toxication, uncomplicated
        F18.221 Inhalant dependence with HCC
               intoxication delirium
        F18.229 Inhalant dependence with HCC ▽
               intoxication, unspecified

      F18.24 Inhalant dependence with inhalant-induced HCC
          mood disorder
          Inhalant use disorder, moderate, with inhalant
            induced depressive disorder
          Inhalant use disorder, severe, with inhalant induced
            depressive disorder

✓6ᵗʰ **F18.25 Inhalant dependence with inhalant-induced**
          psychotic disorder
        F18.250 Inhalant dependence with HCC
               inhalant-induced psychotic disorder
               with delusions
        F18.251 Inhalant dependence with HCC
               inhalant-induced psychotic disorder
               with hallucinations
        F18.259 Inhalant dependence with HCC ▽
               inhalant-induced psychotic disorder,
               unspecified

      F18.27 Inhalant dependence with inhalant-induced HCC
          dementia
          Inhalant use disorder, moderate, with inhalant
            induced major neurocognitive disorder
          Inhalant use disorder, severe, with inhalant induced
            major neurocognitive disorder

✓6ᵗʰ **F18.28 Inhalant dependence with other inhalant-induced**
          disorders
        F18.280 Inhalant dependence with HCC
               inhalant-induced anxiety disorder
        F18.288 Inhalant dependence with other HCC
               inhalant-induced disorder
            Inhalant use disorder, moderate, with
               inhalant-induced mild neurocognitive
               disorder
            Inhalant use disorder, severe, with
               inhalant-induced mild neurocognitive
               disorder

      F18.29 Inhalant dependence with unspecified HCC ▽
          inhalant-induced disorder

✓5ᵗʰ **F18.9 Inhalant use, unspecified**
    EXCLUDES 1 *inhalant abuse (F18.1-)*
                      inhalant dependence (F18.2-)

      F18.90 Inhalant use, unspecified, uncomplicated

✓6ᵗʰ **F18.92 Inhalant use, unspecified with intoxication**
        F18.920 Inhalant use, unspecified with HCC
               intoxication, uncomplicated
        F18.921 Inhalant use, unspecified with HCC
               intoxication with delirium
        F18.929 Inhalant use, unspecified with HCC ▽
               intoxication, unspecified

      F18.94 Inhalant use, unspecified with inhalant-induced HCC
          mood disorder
          Inhalant induced depressive disorder

✓6ᵗʰ **F18.95 Inhalant use, unspecified with inhalant-induced**
          psychotic disorder
        F18.950 Inhalant use, unspecified with HCC
               inhalant-induced psychotic disorder
               with delusions
        F18.951 Inhalant use, unspecified with HCC
               inhalant-induced psychotic disorder
               with hallucinations
        F18.959 Inhalant use, unspecified with HCC ▽
               inhalant-induced psychotic disorder,
               unspecified

      F18.97 Inhalant use, unspecified with inhalant- HCC
          induced persisting dementia
          Inhalant-induced major neurocognitive disorder

✓6ᵗʰ **F18.98 Inhalant use, unspecified with other**
          inhalant-induced disorders
        F18.980 Inhalant use, unspecified with HCC
               inhalant-induced anxiety disorder
        F18.988 Inhalant use, unspecified with other HCC
               inhalant-induced disorder
            Inhalant-induced mild neurocognitive
               disorder

      F18.99 Inhalant use, unspecified with unspecified HCC ▽
          inhalant-induced disorder

✓4ᵗʰ **F19 Other psychoactive substance related disorders**
    INCLUDES polysubstance drug use (indiscriminate drug use)

✓5ᵗʰ **F19.1 Other psychoactive substance abuse**
    EXCLUDES 1 *other psychoactive substance dependence (F19.2-)*
                      other psychoactive substance use, unspecified (F19.9-)

      F19.10 Other psychoactive substance abuse, uncomplicated
          Other (or unknown) substance use disorder, mild

●   **F19.11 Other psychoactive substance abuse, in remission**
          Other (or unknown) substance use disorder, mild, in
            early remission
          Other (or unknown) substance use disorder, mild, in
            sustained remission

✓6ᵗʰ **F19.12 Other psychoactive substance abuse with**
          intoxication
        F19.120 Other psychoactive substance abuse
               with intoxication, uncomplicated
        F19.121 Other psychoactive substance abuse HCC
               with intoxication delirium

✓ Additional Character Req   ✓x7ᵗʰ Placeholder Alert   Manifestation   HCC CMS-HCC Condition   ▽ Unspecified Code   ▶◀ Revised Text   ● New Code   ▲ Revised Code Title

ICD-10-CM 2018   537

F19.122   **Other psychoactive substance abuse** HCC **with intoxication with perceptual disturbances**

F19.129   **Other psychoactive substance** HCC ▽ **abuse with intoxication, unspecified**

F19.14   **Other psychoactive substance abuse with** HCC **psychoactive substance-induced mood disorder**
Other (or unknown) substance use disorder, mild, with other (or unknown) substance-induced bipolar or related disorder
Other (or unknown) substance use disorder, mild, with other (or unknown) substance-induced depressive disorder

✓6ᵗʰ **F19.15**   **Other psychoactive substance abuse with psychoactive substance-induced psychotic disorder**

    F19.150   **Other psychoactive substance abuse** HCC **with psychoactive substance-induced psychotic disorder with delusions**

    F19.151   **Other psychoactive substance abuse** HCC **with psychoactive substance-induced psychotic disorder with hallucinations**

    F19.159   **Other psychoactive substance** HCC ▽ **abuse with psychoactive substance-induced psychotic disorder, unspecified**

F19.16   **Other psychoactive substance abuse with** HCC **psychoactive substance-induced persisting amnestic disorder**

F19.17   **Other psychoactive substance abuse with** HCC **psychoactive substance-induced persisting dementia**
Other (or unknown) substance use disorder, mild, with other (or unknown) substance-induced major neurocognitive disorder

✓6ᵗʰ **F19.18**   **Other psychoactive substance abuse with other psychoactive substance-induced disorders**

    F19.180   **Other psychoactive substance abuse** HCC **with psychoactive substance-induced anxiety disorder**

    F19.181   **Other psychoactive substance abuse** HCC **with psychoactive substance-induced sexual dysfunction**

    F19.182   **Other psychoactive substance abuse** HCC **with psychoactive substance-induced sleep disorder**

    F19.188   **Other psychoactive substance abuse** HCC **with other psychoactive substance-induced disorder**
Other (or unknown) substance use disorder, mild, with other (or unknown) substance induced mild neurocognitive disorder
Other (or unknown) substance use disorder, mild, with other (or unknown) substance induced obsessive-compulsive or related disorder

F19.19   **Other psychoactive substance abuse with** HCC ▽ **unspecified psychoactive substance-induced disorder**

✓5ᵗʰ **F19.2**   **Other psychoactive substance dependence**
EXCLUDES 1   *other psychoactive substance abuse (F19.1-)*
other psychoactive substance use, unspecified (F19.9-)

F19.20   **Other psychoactive substance dependence,** HCC **uncomplicated**
Other (or unknown) substance use disorder, moderate
Other (or unknown) substance use disorder, severe

F19.21   **Other psychoactive substance dependence,** HCC **in remission**
▶Other (or unknown) substance use disorder, moderate, in early remission
Other (or unknown) substance use disorder, moderate, in sustained remission
Other (or unknown) substance use disorder, severe, in early remission
Other (or unknown) substance use, severe, in sustained remission◀

✓6ᵗʰ **F19.22**   **Other psychoactive substance dependence with intoxication**
EXCLUDES 1   *other psychoactive substance dependence with withdrawal (F19.23-)*

    F19.220   **Other psychoactive substance** HCC **dependence with intoxication, uncomplicated**

    F19.221   **Other psychoactive substance** HCC **dependence with intoxication delirium**

    F19.222   **Other psychoactive substance** HCC **dependence with intoxication with perceptual disturbance**

    F19.229   **Other psychoactive substance** HCC ▽ **dependence with intoxication, unspecified**

✓6ᵗʰ **F19.23**   **Other psychoactive substance dependence with withdrawal**
EXCLUDES 1   *other psychoactive substance dependence with intoxication (F19.22-)*

    F19.230   **Other psychoactive substance** HCC **dependence with withdrawal, uncomplicated**

    F19.231   **Other psychoactive substance** HCC **dependence with withdrawal delirium**

    F19.232   **Other psychoactive substance** HCC **dependence with withdrawal with perceptual disturbance**

    F19.239   **Other psychoactive substance** HCC ▽ **dependence with withdrawal, unspecified**

F19.24   **Other psychoactive substance dependence with** HCC **psychoactive substance-induced mood disorder**
Other (or unknown) substance use disorder, moderate, with other (or unknown) substance induced bipolar or related disorder
Other (or unknown) substance use disorder, moderate, with other (or unknown) substance induced depressive disorder
Other (or unknown) use disorder, severe, with other (or unknown) substance induced bipolar or related disorder
Other (or unknown) substance use disorder, severe, with other (or unknown) substance induced depressive disorder

✓6ᵗʰ **F19.25**   **Other psychoactive substance dependence with psychoactive substance-induced psychotic disorder**

    F19.250   **Other psychoactive substance** HCC **dependence with psychoactive substance-induced psychotic disorder with delusions**

    F19.251   **Other psychoactive substance** HCC **dependence with psychoactive substance-induced psychotic disorder with hallucinations**

    F19.259   **Other psychoactive substance** HCC ▽ **dependence with psychoactive substance-induce d psychotic disorder, unspecified**

F19.26   **Other psychoactive substance dependence** HCC **with psychoactive substance-induced persisting amnestic disorder**

F19.27   **Other psychoactive substance dependence with** HCC **psychoactive substance-induced persisting dementia**
Other (or unknown) substance use disorder, moderate, with other (or unknown) substance induced major neurocognitive disorder
Other (or unknown) substance use disorder, severe, with other (or unknown) substance induced major neurocognitive disorder

✓6ᵗʰ **F19.28**   **Other psychoactive substance dependence with other psychoactive substance-induced disorders**

    F19.280   **Other psychoactive substance** HCC **dependence with psychoactive substance-induced anxiety disorder**

    F19.281   **Other psychoactive substance** HCC **dependence with psychoactive substance-induced sexual dysfunction**

    F19.282   **Other psychoactive substance** HCC **dependence with psychoactive substance-induced sleep disorder**

EXCLUDES 1 Not coded here   EXCLUDES 2 Not included here   N Newborn Age: 0   P Pediatric Age: 0-17   M Maternity Age: 12-55   A Adult Age: 15-124

538   ICD-10-CM 2018

F19.288 Other psychoactive substance dependence with other psychoactive substance-induced disorder `HCC`
Other (or unknown) substance use disorder, moderate, with other (or unknown) substance induced mild neurocognitive disorder
Other (or unknown) substance use disorder, severe, with other (or unknown) substance induced mild neurocognitive disorder
Other (or unknown) substance use disorder, moderate, with other (or unknown) substance induced obsessive compulsive or related disorder
Other (or unknown) substance use disorder, severe, with other (or unknown) substance induced obsessive-compulsive or related disorder

F19.29 Other psychoactive substance dependence with unspecified psychoactive substance-induced disorder `HCC` ▽

`√5th` **F19.9 Other psychoactive substance use, unspecified**
`EXCLUDES 1`   other psychoactive substance abuse (F19.1-)
    other psychoactive substance dependence (F19.2-)

F19.90 Other psychoactive substance use, unspecified, uncomplicated

`√6th` **F19.92 Other psychoactive substance use, unspecified with intoxication**
`EXCLUDES 1`   other psychoactive substance use, unspecified with withdrawal (F19.93)

F19.920 Other psychoactive substance use, unspecified with intoxication, uncomplicated `HCC`

F19.921 Other psychoactive substance use, unspecified with intoxication with delirium `HCC`
Other (or unknown) substance-induced delirium

F19.922 Other psychoactive substance use, unspecified with intoxication with perceptual disturbance `HCC`

F19.929 Other psychoactive substance use, unspecified with intoxication, unspecified `HCC` ▽

`√6th` **F19.93 Other psychoactive substance use, unspecified with withdrawal**
`EXCLUDES 1`   other psychoactive substance use, unspecified with intoxication (F19.92-)

F19.930 Other psychoactive substance use, unspecified with withdrawal, uncomplicated `HCC`

F19.931 Other psychoactive substance use, unspecified with withdrawal delirium `HCC`

F19.932 Other psychoactive substance use, unspecified with withdrawal with perceptual disturbance `HCC`

F19.939 Other psychoactive substance use, unspecified with withdrawal, unspecified `HCC` ▽

F19.94 Other psychoactive substance use, unspecified with psychoactive substance-induced mood disorder `HCC`
Other (or unknown) substance-induced bipolar or related disorder, without use disorder
Other (or unknown) substance-induced depressive disorder, without use disorder

`√6th` **F19.95 Other psychoactive substance use, unspecified with psychoactive substance-induced psychotic disorder**

F19.950 Other psychoactive substance use, unspecified with psychoactive substance-induced psychotic disorder with delusions `HCC`

F19.951 Other psychoactive substance use, unspecified with psychoactive substance-induced psychotic disorder with hallucinations `HCC`

F19.959 Other psychoactive substance use, unspecified with psychoactive substance-induced psychotic disorder, unspecified `HCC` ▽
Other or unknown substance-induced psychotic disorder, without use disorder

F19.96 Other psychoactive substance use, unspecified with psychoactive substance-induced persisting amnestic disorder `HCC`

F19.97 Other psychoactive substance use, unspecified with psychoactive substance-induced persisting dementia `HCC`
Other (or unknown) substance-induced major neurocognitive disorder, without use disorder

`√6th` **F19.98 Other psychoactive substance use, unspecified with other psychoactive substance-induced disorders**

F19.980 Other psychoactive substance use, unspecified with psychoactive substance-induced anxiety disorder `HCC`
Other (or unknown) substance-induced anxiety disorder, without use disorder

F19.981 Other psychoactive substance use, unspecified with psychoactive substance-induced sexual dysfunction `HCC`
Other (or unknown) substance-induced sexual dysfunction, without use disorder

F19.982 Other psychoactive substance use, unspecified with psychoactive substance-induced sleep disorder `HCC`
Other (or unknown) substance-induced sleep disorder, without use disorder

F19.988 Other psychoactive substance use, unspecified with other psychoactive substance-induced disorder `HCC`
Other (or unknown) substance-induced mild neurocognitive disorder, without use disorder
Other (or unknown) substance-induced obsessive-compulsive or related disorder, without use disorder

F19.99 Other psychoactive substance use, unspecified with unspecified psychoactive substance-induced disorder `HCC` ▽

Schizophrenia, schizotypal, delusional, and other non-mood psychotic disorders (F20-F29)

`√4th` **F20 Schizophrenia**
`EXCLUDES 1`   brief psychotic disorder (F23)
    cyclic schizophrenia (F25.0)
    mood [affective] disorders with psychotic symptoms (F30.2, F31.2, F31.5, F31.64, F32.3, F33.3)
    schizoaffective disorder (F25.-)
    schizophrenic reaction NOS (F23)
`EXCLUDES 2`   schizophrenic reaction in:
    alcoholism (F10.15-, F10.25-, F10.95-)
    brain disease (F06.2)
    epilepsy (F06.2)
    psychoactive drug use (F11-F19 with .15, .25, .95)
    schizotypal disorder (F21)
DEF: Group of disorders with disturbances in thought (delusions, hallucinations), mood (blunted, flattened, inappropriate affect), sense of self; also bizarre, purposeless behavior, repetitious activity, or inactivity.

F20.0 Paranoid schizophrenia `HCC`
Paraphrenic schizophrenia
`EXCLUDES 1`   involutional paranoid state (F22)
    paranoia (F22)
DEF: Preoccupied with delusional suspicions and auditory hallucinations related to single theme; usually hostile, grandiose, threatening, persecutory, occasionally hypochondriacal.

F20.1 Disorganized schizophrenia `HCC`
Hebephrenic schizophrenia
Hebephrenia

F20.2 Catatonic schizophrenia `HCC`
Schizophrenic catalepsy
Schizophrenic catatonia
Schizophrenic flexibilitas cerea
`EXCLUDES 1`   catatonic stupor (R40.1)
DEF: Extreme changes in motor activity; one extreme is decreased response or reaction to the environment and the other is spontaneous activity.

☑ Additional Character Req   `√x7th` Placeholder Alert   Manifestation   `HCC` CMS-HCC Condition   ▽ Unspecified Code   ►◄ Revised Text   ● New Code   ▲ Revised Code Title

ICD-10-CM 2018   539

F20.3 Undifferentiated schizophrenia   `HCC`
Atypical schizophrenia
EXCLUDES 1   *acute schizophrenia-like psychotic disorder (F23)*
EXCLUDES 2   *post-schizophrenic depression (F32.89)*

F20.5 Residual schizophrenia   `HCC`
Restzustand (schizophrenic)
Schizophrenic residual state

✓5ᵗʰ **F20.8 Other schizophrenia**

    F20.81 Schizophreniform disorder   `HCC`
        Schizophreniform psychosis NOS

    F20.89 Other schizophrenia
        Cenesthopathic schizophrenia
        Simple schizophrenia

F20.9 Schizophrenia, unspecified   `HCC` ▽

F21 Schizotypal disorder
Borderline schizophrenia   Prodromal schizophrenia
Latent schizophrenia   Pseudoneurotic schizophrenia
Latent schizophrenic reaction   Pseudopsychopathic schizophrenia
Prepsychotic schizophrenia   Schizotypal personality disorder
EXCLUDES 2   *Asperger's syndrome (F84.5)*
            schizoid personality disorder (F60.1)

F22 Delusional disorders   `HCC`
Delusional dysmorphophobia   Paranoid psychosis
Involutional paranoid state   Paranoid state
Paranoia   Paraphrenia (late)
Paranoia querulans   Sensitiver Beziehungswahn
EXCLUDES 1   *mood [affective] disorders with psychotic symptoms (F30.2,*
            F31.2, F31.5, F31.64, F32.3, F33.3)
            paranoid schizophrenia (F20.0)
EXCLUDES 2   *paranoid personality disorder (F60.0)*
            paranoid psychosis, psychogenic (F23)
            paranoid reaction (F23)

F23 Brief psychotic disorder
Paranoid reaction
Psychogenic paranoid psychosis
EXCLUDES 2   *mood [affective] disorders with psychotic symptoms (F30.2,*
            F31.2, F31.5, F31.64, F32.3, F33.3)

F24 Shared psychotic disorder   `HCC`
Folie à deux
Induced paranoid disorder
Induced psychotic disorder

✓4ᵗʰ **F25 Schizoaffective disorders**
EXCLUDES 1   *mood [affective] disorders with psychotic symptoms (F30.2,*
            F31.2, F31.5, F31.64, F32.3, F33.3)
            schizophrenia (F20.-)

    F25.0 Schizoaffective disorder, bipolar type   `HCC`
        Cyclic schizophrenia
        Schizoaffective disorder, manic type
        Schizoaffective disorder, mixed type
        Schizoaffective psychosis, bipolar type
        ~~Schizophreniform psychosis, manic type~~

    F25.1 Schizoaffective disorder, depressive type   `HCC`
        Schizoaffective psychosis, depressive type
        ~~Schizophreniform psychosis, depressive type~~

    F25.8 Other schizoaffective disorders   `HCC`

    F25.9 Schizoaffective disorder, unspecified   `HCC` ▽
        Schizoaffective psychosis NOS

F28 Other psychotic disorder not due to a substance or known physiological condition
Chronic hallucinatory psychosis
▶Other specified schizophrenia spectrum and other psychotic disorder◀

F29 Unspecified psychosis not due to a substance or known physiological condition   ▽
Psychosis NOS
▶Unspecified schizophrenia spectrum and other psychotic disorder◀
EXCLUDES 1   *mental disorder NOS (F99)*
            unspecified mental disorder due to known physiological
            condition (F09)

Mood [affective] disorders (F30-F39)

✓4ᵗʰ **F30 Manic episode**
INCLUDES   bipolar disorder, single manic episode
           mixed affective episode
EXCLUDES 1   *bipolar disorder (F31.-)*
            major depressive disorder, recurrent (F33.-)
            major depressive disorder, single episode (F32.-)

✓5ᵗʰ **F30.1 Manic episode without psychotic symptoms**

    F30.10 Manic episode without psychotic symptoms, unspecified   `HCC` ▽

    F30.11 Manic episode without psychotic symptoms, mild   `HCC`

    F30.12 Manic episode without psychotic symptoms, moderate   `HCC`

    F30.13 Manic episode, severe, without psychotic symptoms   `HCC`

    F30.2 Manic episode, severe with psychotic symptoms   `HCC`
        Manic stupor
        Mania with mood-congruent psychotic symptoms
        Mania with mood-incongruent psychotic symptoms

    F30.3 Manic episode in partial remission   `HCC`

    F30.4 Manic episode in full remission   `HCC`

    F30.8 Other manic episodes   `HCC`
        Hypomania

    F30.9 Manic episode, unspecified   `HCC` ▽
        Mania NOS

✓4ᵗʰ **F31 Bipolar disorder**
INCLUDES   ▶bipolar I disorder
           bipolar type I disorder◀
           manic-depressive illness
           manic-depressive psychosis
           manic-depressive reaction
EXCLUDES 1   *bipolar disorder, single manic episode (F30.-)*
            major depressive disorder, single episode (F32.-)
            major depressive disorder, recurrent (F33.-)
EXCLUDES 2   *cyclothymia (F34.0)*

    F31.0 Bipolar disorder, current episode hypomanic   `HCC`

✓5ᵗʰ **F31.1 Bipolar disorder, current episode manic without psychotic features**

    F31.10 Bipolar disorder, current episode manic without psychotic features, unspecified   `HCC` ▽

    F31.11 Bipolar disorder, current episode manic without psychotic features, mild   `HCC`

    F31.12 Bipolar disorder, current episode manic without psychotic features, moderate   `HCC`

    F31.13 Bipolar disorder, current episode manic without psychotic features, severe   `HCC`

    F31.2 Bipolar disorder, current episode manic severe with psychotic features   `HCC`
        Bipolar disorder, current episode manic with mood-congruent psychotic symptoms
        Bipolar disorder, current episode manic with mood-incongruent psychotic symptoms
        ▶Bipolar I disorder, current or most recent episode manic with psychotic features◀

✓5ᵗʰ **F31.3 Bipolar disorder, current episode depressed, mild or moderate severity**

    F31.30 Bipolar disorder, current episode depressed, mild or moderate severity, unspecified   `HCC` ▽

    F31.31 Bipolar disorder, current episode depressed, mild   `HCC`

    F31.32 Bipolar disorder, current episode depressed, moderate   `HCC`

    F31.4 Bipolar disorder, current episode depressed, severe, without psychotic features   `HCC`

    F31.5 Bipolar disorder, current episode depressed, severe, with psychotic features   `HCC`
        Bipolar disorder, current episode depressed with mood-incongruent psychotic symptoms
        Bipolar disorder, current episode depressed with mood-congruent psychotic symptoms
        ▶Bipolar I disorder, current or most recent episode depressed, with psychotic features◀

✓5ᵗʰ **F31.6 Bipolar disorder, current episode mixed**

    F31.60 Bipolar disorder, current episode mixed, unspecified   `HCC` ▽

    F31.61 Bipolar disorder, current episode mixed, mild   `HCC`

EXCLUDES 1 Not coded here   *EXCLUDES 2* Not included here   N Newborn Age: 0   P Pediatric Age: 0-17   M Maternity Age: 12-55   A Adult Age: 15-124

540   ICD-10-CM 2018

F31.62 Bipolar disorder, current episode mixed, **moderate**   `HCC`

F31.63 Bipolar disorder, current episode mixed, **severe, without psychotic features**   `HCC`

F31.64 Bipolar disorder, current episode mixed, **severe, with psychotic features**   `HCC`
Bipolar disorder, current episode mixed with mood-congruent psychotic symptoms
Bipolar disorder, current episode mixed with mood-incongruent psychotic symptoms

√5ᵗʰ **F31.7** Bipolar disorder, **currently in remission**

F31.70 Bipolar disorder, **currently in remission**, most recent episode unspecified   `HCC` ▽

F31.71 Bipolar disorder, **in partial remission**, most recent episode **hypomanic**   `HCC`

F31.72 Bipolar disorder, **in full remission**, most recent episode **hypomanic**   `HCC`

F31.73 Bipolar disorder, **in partial remission**, most recent episode **manic**   `HCC`

F31.74 Bipolar disorder, **in full remission**, most recent episode **manic**   `HCC`

F31.75 Bipolar disorder, **in partial remission**, most recent episode **depressed**   `HCC`

F31.76 Bipolar disorder, **in full remission**, most recent episode **depressed**   `HCC`

F31.77 Bipolar disorder, **in partial remission**, most recent episode **mixed**   `HCC`

F31.78 Bipolar disorder, **in full remission**, most recent episode **mixed**   `HCC`

√5ᵗʰ **F31.8** Other bipolar disorders

F31.81 **Bipolar II disorder**   `HCC`
▶Bipolar disorder, type 2◀

F31.89 **Other bipolar disorder**   `HCC`
Recurrent manic episodes NOS

F31.9 Bipolar disorder, **unspecified**   `HCC` ▽
▶Manic depression◀

√4ᵗʰ **F32** Major depressive disorder, single episode

[INCLUDES] single episode of agitated depression
single episode of depressive reaction
single episode of major depression
single episode of psychogenic depression
single episode of reactive depression
single episode of vital depression

[EXCLUDES 1] bipolar disorder (F31.-)
manic episode (F30.-)
recurrent depressive disorder (F33.-)

[EXCLUDES 2] adjustment disorder (F43.2)

DEF: Mood disorder that produces depression; may exhibit as sadness, low self-esteem, or guilt feelings; other manifestations may be withdrawal from friends and family and interrupted sleep.

F32.0 Major depressive disorder, single episode, **mild**   `HCC`

F32.1 Major depressive disorder, single episode, **moderate**   `HCC`

F32.2 Major depressive disorder, single episode, **severe without psychotic features**   `HCC`

F32.3 Major depressive disorder, single episode, **severe with psychotic features**   `HCC`
Single episode of major depression with mood-congruent psychotic symptoms
Single episode of major depression with mood-incongruent psychotic symptoms
Single episode of major depression with psychotic symptoms
Single episode of psychogenic depressive psychosis
Single episode of psychotic depression
Single episode of reactive depressive psychosis

F32.4 Major depressive disorder, single episode, **in partial remission**   `HCC`

F32.5 Major depressive disorder, single episode, **in full remission**   `HCC`

√5ᵗʰ **F32.8** Other depressive episodes

F32.81 **Premenstrual dysphoric disorder**   ♀
[EXCLUDES 1] premenstrual tension syndrome (N94.3)

F32.89 **Other specified depressive episodes**
Atypical depression
Post-schizophrenic depression
Single episode of 'masked' depression NOS

F32.9 Major depressive disorder, single episode, **unspecified**   ▽
Depression NOS
Depressive disorder NOS
Major depression NOS
AHA: 2013, 4Q, 107

√4ᵗʰ **F33** Major depressive disorder, **recurrent**
Recurrent episodes of depressive reaction
Recurrent episodes of endogenous depression
Recurrent episodes of major depression
Recurrent episodes of psychogenic depression
Recurrent episodes of reactive depression
Recurrent episodes of seasonal depressive disorder
Recurrent episodes of vital depression

[EXCLUDES 1] bipolar disorder (F31.-)
manic episode (F30.-)

F33.0 Major depressive disorder, recurrent, **mild**   `HCC`

F33.1 Major depressive disorder, recurrent, **moderate**   `HCC`

F33.2 Major depressive disorder, recurrent, **severe without psychotic features**   `HCC`

F33.3 Major depressive disorder, recurrent, **severe with psychotic symptoms**   `HCC`
Endogenous depression with psychotic symptoms
▶Major depressive disorder, recurrent, with psychotic features◀
Recurrent severe episodes of major depression with mood-congruent psychotic symptoms
Recurrent severe episodes of major depression with mood-incongruent psychotic symptoms
Recurrent severe episodes of major depression with psychotic symptoms
Recurrent severe episodes of psychogenic depressive psychosis
Recurrent severe episodes of psychotic depression
Recurrent severe episodes of reactive depressive psychosis

√5ᵗʰ **F33.4** Major depressive disorder, recurrent, **in remission**

F33.40 Major depressive disorder, recurrent, in **remission, unspecified**   `HCC` ▽

F33.41 Major depressive disorder, recurrent, in **partial remission**   `HCC`

F33.42 Major depressive disorder, recurrent, in **full remission**   `HCC`

F33.8 Other recurrent depressive disorders   `HCC`
Recurrent brief depressive episodes

F33.9 Major depressive disorder, recurrent, **unspecified**   `HCC` ▽
Monopolar depression NOS

√4ᵗʰ **F34** Persistent mood [affective] disorders

F34.0 **Cyclothymic** disorder
Affective personality disorder
Cycloid personality
Cyclothymia
Cyclothymic personality

F34.1 **Dysthymic** disorder
Depressive neurosis
Depressive personality disorder
Dysthymia
Neurotic depression
Persistent anxiety depression
Persistent depressive disorder
[EXCLUDES 2] anxiety depression (mild or not persistent) (F41.8)
DEF: Depression without psychosis; less severe but persistent depression; is considered a mild to moderate chronic form of depression.

√5ᵗʰ **F34.8** Other persistent mood [affective] disorders

F34.81 **Disruptive mood dysregulation disorder**   `HCC`

F34.89 **Other specified persistent mood disorders**   `HCC`

F34.9 Persistent mood [affective] disorder, **unspecified**   `HCC` ▽

F39 Unspecified mood [affective] disorder   `HCC` ▽
Affective psychosis NOS

Anxiety, dissociative, stress-related, somatoform and other nonpsychotic mental disorders (F40-F48)

√4ᵗʰ **F40** Phobic anxiety disorders

√5ᵗʰ **F40.0** Agoraphobia
DEF: Profound anxiety or fear of leaving familiar settings like home, or being in unfamiliar locations or with strangers or crowds; may or may not be preceded by recurrent panic attacks.

F40.00 Agoraphobia, unspecified   ▽

F40.01 Agoraphobia **with panic disorder**
Panic disorder with agoraphobia
[EXCLUDES 1] panic disorder without agoraphobia (F41.0)

☑ Additional Character Req   √x7ᵗʰ Placeholder Alert   Manifestation   `HCC`CMS-HCC Condition   ▽ Unspecified Code   ▶◀ Revised Text   ● New Code   ▲ Revised Code Title

F40.02   **Agoraphobia without panic disorder**

✓5ᵗʰ **F40.1   Social phobias**
Anthropophobia
▶Social anxiety disorder◀
Social anxiety disorder of childhood
Social neurosis

F40.10   **Social phobia, unspecified** ▽

F40.11   **Social phobia, generalized**

✓5ᵗʰ **F40.2   Specific (isolated) phobias**
EXCLUDES 2   *dysmorphophobia (nondelusional) (F45.22)*
nosophobia (F45.22)

✓6ᵗʰ **F40.21   Animal type phobia**

F40.210   **Arachnophobia**
Fear of spiders

F40.218   **Other animal type phobia**

✓6ᵗʰ **F40.22   Natural environment type phobia**

F40.220   **Fear of thunderstorms**

F40.228   **Other natural environment type phobia**

✓6ᵗʰ **F40.23   Blood, injection, injury type phobia**

F40.230   **Fear of blood**

F40.231   **Fear of injections and transfusions**

F40.232   **Fear of other medical care**

F40.233   **Fear of injury**

✓6ᵗʰ **F40.24   Situational type phobia**

F40.240   **Claustrophobia**

F40.241   **Acrophobia**

F40.242   **Fear of bridges**

F40.243   **Fear of flying**

F40.248   **Other situational type phobia**

✓6ᵗʰ **F40.29   Other specified phobia**

F40.290   **Androphobia**
Fear of men

F40.291   **Gynephobia**
Fear of women

F40.298   **Other specified phobia**

F40.8   **Other phobic anxiety disorders**
Phobic anxiety disorder of childhood

F40.9   **Phobic anxiety disorder, unspecified** ▽
Phobia NOS
Phobic state NOS

✓4ᵗʰ **F41   Other anxiety disorders**
EXCLUDES 2   *anxiety in:*
acute stress reaction (F43.0)
transient adjustment reaction (F43.2)
neurasthenia (F48.8)
psychophysiologic disorders (F45.-)
separation anxiety (F93.0)

▲ **F41.0   Panic disorder [episodic paroxysmal anxiety]**
Panic attack
Panic state
EXCLUDES 1   *panic disorder with agoraphobia (F40.01)*
DEF: Neurotic disorder characterized by recurrent panic or anxiety, apprehension, fear, or terror; symptoms include shortness of breath, palpitations, dizziness, shakiness; fear of dying may persist.

F41.1   Generalized anxiety disorder
Anxiety neurosis   Anxiety state
Anxiety reaction   Overanxious disorder
EXCLUDES 2   *neurasthenia (F48.8)*

F41.3   Other mixed anxiety disorders

F41.8   Other specified anxiety disorders
Anxiety depression (mild or not persistent)
Anxiety hysteria
Mixed anxiety and depressive disorder

F41.9   Anxiety disorder, unspecified ▽
Anxiety NOS

✓4ᵗʰ **F42   Obsessive-compulsive disorder**
EXCLUDES 2   *obsessive-compulsive personality (disorder) (F60.5)*
obsessive-compulsive symptoms occurring in depression (F32-F33)
obsessive-compulsive symptoms occurring in schizophrenia (F20.-)

F42.2   Mixed obsessional thoughts and acts

F42.3   Hoarding disorder

F42.4   **Excoriation (skin-picking) disorder**
EXCLUDES 1   *factitial dermatitis (L98.1)*
other specified behavioral and emotional disorders with onset usually occurring in early childhood and adolescence (F98.8)

F42.8   **Other obsessive-compulsive disorder**
Anancastic neurosis
Obsessive-compulsive neurosis

F42.9   **Obsessive-compulsive disorder, unspecified** ▽

✓4ᵗʰ **F43   Reaction to severe stress, and adjustment disorders**

F43.0   **Acute stress reaction**
Acute crisis reaction
Acute reaction to stress
Combat and operational stress reaction
Combat fatigue
Crisis state
Psychic shock

✓5ᵗʰ **F43.1   Post-traumatic stress disorder (PTSD)**
Traumatic neurosis
DEF: Preoccupation with traumatic events beyond normal experience; i.e., rape, personal assault, etc.; also recurring flashbacks of trauma; symptoms include difficulty remembering, sleeping, or concentrating, and guilt feelings for surviving.

F43.10   **Post-traumatic stress disorder, unspecified** ▽

F43.11   **Post-traumatic stress disorder, acute**

F43.12   **Post-traumatic stress disorder, chronic**

✓5ᵗʰ **F43.2   Adjustment disorders**
Culture shock
Grief reaction
Hospitalism in children
EXCLUDES 2   *separation anxiety disorder of childhood (F93.0)*

F43.20   **Adjustment disorder, unspecified** ▽

F43.21   **Adjustment disorder with depressed mood**
AHA: 2014, 1Q, 25

F43.22   **Adjustment disorder with anxiety**

F43.23   **Adjustment disorder with mixed anxiety and depressed mood**

F43.24   **Adjustment disorder with disturbance of conduct**

F43.25   **Adjustment disorder with mixed disturbance of emotions and conduct**

F43.29   **Adjustment disorder with other symptoms**

F43.8   **Other reactions to severe stress**
Other specified trauma and stressor-related disorder

F43.9   **Reaction to severe stress, unspecified** ▽
Trauma and stressor-related disorder, NOS

✓4ᵗʰ **F44   Dissociative and conversion disorders**
INCLUDES   conversion hysteria
conversion reaction
hysteria
hysterical psychosis
EXCLUDES 2   *malingering [conscious simulation] (Z76.5)*

F44.0   **Dissociative amnesia**
EXCLUDES 1   *amnesia NOS (R41.3)*
anterograde amnesia (R41.1)
dissociative amnesia with dissociative fugue (F44.1)
retrograde amnesia (R41.2)
EXCLUDES 2   *alcohol-or other psychoactive substance-induced amnestic disorder (F10, F13, F19 with .26, .96)*
amnestic disorder due to known physiological condition (F04)
postictal amnesia in epilepsy (G40.-)

F44.1   **Dissociative fugue**
Dissociative amnesia with dissociative fugue
EXCLUDES 2   *postictal fugue in epilepsy (G40.-)*
DEF: Dissociative hysteria; identified by loss of memory, flight from familiar surroundings to a completely separate environment, episodes may last hours or days; conscious activity is not associated with perception of surroundings and there is no later memory of episode.

F44.2   **Dissociative stupor**
EXCLUDES 1   *catatonic stupor (R40.1)*
stupor NOS (R40.1)
EXCLUDES 2   *catatonic disorder due to known physiological condition (F06.1)*
depressive stupor (F32, F33)
manic stupor (F30, F31)

F44.4 Conversion disorder with motor symptom or deficit
▶Conversion disorder with abnormal movement
Conversion disorder with speech symptoms
Conversion disorder with swallowing symptoms
Conversion disorder with weakness/paralysis◄
Dissociative motor disorders
Psychogenic aphonia
Psychogenic dysphonia

F44.5 Conversion disorder with seizures or convulsions
▶Conversion disorder with attacks or seizures◄
Dissociative convulsions

F44.6 Conversion disorder with sensory symptom or deficit
▶Conversion disorder with anesthesia or sensory loss
Conversion disorder with special sensory symptoms◄
Dissociative anesthesia and sensory loss
Psychogenic deafness

F44.7 Conversion disorder with mixed symptom presentation

✓5ᵗʰ **F44.8 Other dissociative and conversion disorders**

F44.81 Dissociative identity disorder
Multiple personality disorder

F44.89 Other dissociative and conversion disorders
Ganser's syndrome
Psychogenic confusion
Psychogenic twilight state
Trance and possession disorders

F44.9 Dissociative and conversion disorder, unspecified ▽
Dissociative disorder NOS

✓4ᵗʰ **F45 Somatoform disorders**
EXCLUDES 2   *dissociative and conversion disorders (F44.-)*
factitious disorders (F68.1-)
hair-plucking (F63.3)
lalling (F80.0)
lisping (F80.0)
malingering [conscious simulation] (Z76.5)
nail-biting (F98.8)
psychological or behavioral factors associated with disorders or
diseases classified elsewhere (F54)
sexual dysfunction, not due to a substance or known
physiological condition (F52.-)
thumb-sucking (F98.8)
tic disorders (in childhood and adolescence) (F95.-)
Tourette's syndrome (F95.2)
trichotillomania (F63.3)

F45.0 Somatization disorder
Briquet's disorder
Multiple psychosomatic disorder

F45.1 Undifferentiated somatoform disorder
Somatic symptom disorder
Undifferentiated psychosomatic disorder

✓5ᵗʰ **F45.2 Hypochondriacal disorders**
EXCLUDES 2   *delusional dysmorphophobia (F22)*
fixed delusions about bodily functions or shape (F22)

F45.20 Hypochondriacal disorder, unspecified ▽

F45.21 Hypochondriasis
Hypochondriacal neurosis
Illness anxiety disorder

F45.22 Body dysmorphic disorder
Dysmorphophobia (nondelusional)
Nosophobia

F45.29 Other hypochondriacal disorders

✓5ᵗʰ **F45.4 Pain disorders related to psychological factors**
EXCLUDES 1   *pain NOS (R52)*

F45.41 Pain disorder exclusively related to psychological factors
Somatoform pain disorder (persistent)

F45.42 Pain disorder with related psychological factors
Code also associated acute or chronic pain (G89.-)

F45.8 Other somatoform disorders
Psychogenic dysmenorrhea
Psychogenic dysphagia, including "globus hystericus"
Psychogenic pruritus
Psychogenic torticollis
Somatoform autonomic dysfunction
Teeth grinding
EXCLUDES 1   *sleep related teeth grinding (G47.63)*

F45.9 Somatoform disorder, unspecified ▽
Psychosomatic disorder NOS

✓4ᵗʰ **F48 Other nonpsychotic mental disorders**

F48.1 Depersonalization-derealization syndrome

F48.2 Pseudobulbar affect
Involuntary emotional expression disorder
Code first underlying cause, if known, such as:
amyotrophic lateral sclerosis (G12.21)
multiple sclerosis (G35)
sequelae of cerebrovascular disease (I69.-)
sequelae of traumatic intracranial injury (S06.-)

F48.8 Other specified nonpsychotic mental disorders
Dhat syndrome
Neurasthenia
Occupational neurosis, including writer's cramp
Psychasthenia
Psychasthenic neurosis
Psychogenic syncope

F48.9 Nonpsychotic mental disorder, unspecified ▽
Neurosis NOS

Behavioral syndromes associated with physiological disturbances and physical factors (F50-F59)

✓4ᵗʰ **F50 Eating disorders**
EXCLUDES 1   *anorexia NOS (R63.0)*
feeding difficulties (R63.3)
▶*feeding problems of newborn (P92.-)*◄
polyphagia (R63.2)
EXCLUDES 2   *feeding disorder in infancy or childhood (F98.2-)*

✓5ᵗʰ **F50.0 Anorexia nervosa**
EXCLUDES 1   *loss of appetite (R63.0)*
psychogenic loss of appetite (F50.89)

F50.00 Anorexia nervosa, unspecified ▽

F50.01 Anorexia nervosa, restricting type

F50.02 Anorexia nervosa, binge eating/purging type
EXCLUDES 1   *bulimia nervosa (F50.2)*

F50.2 Bulimia nervosa
Bulimia NOS
Hyperorexia nervosa
EXCLUDES 1   *anorexia nervosa, binge eating/purging type (F50.02)*

✓5ᵗʰ **F50.8 Other eating disorders**
EXCLUDES 2   *pica of infancy and childhood (F98.3)*

F50.81 Binge eating disorder

● **F50.82 Avoidant/restrictive food intake disorder**

F50.89 Other specified eating disorder
Pica in adults
Psychogenic loss of appetite

F50.9 Eating disorder, unspecified ▽
Atypical anorexia nervosa
Atypical bulimia nervosa
▶Feeding or eating disorder, unspecified
Other specified feeding disorder ◄

✓4ᵗʰ **F51 Sleep disorders not due to a substance or known physiological condition**
EXCLUDES 2   *organic sleep disorders (G47.-)*

✓5ᵗʰ **F51.0 Insomnia not due to a substance or known physiological condition**
EXCLUDES 2   *alcohol related insomnia (F10.182, F10.282, F10.982)*
drug-related insomnia (F11.182, F11.282, F11.982,
F13.182, F13.282, F13.982, F14.182, F14.282,
F14.982, F15.182, F15.282, F15.982, F19.182,
F19.282, F19.982)
insomnia NOS (G47.0-)
insomnia due to known physiological condition
(G47.0-)
organic insomnia (G47.0-)
sleep deprivation (Z72.820)

F51.01 Primary insomnia
Idiopathic insomnia

F51.02 Adjustment insomnia

F51.03 Paradoxical insomnia

F51.04 Psychophysiologic insomnia

F51.05 Insomnia due to other mental disorder
Code also associated mental disorder

F51.09 Other insomnia not due to a substance or known physiological condition

✓ Additional Character Req   ✓x7ᵗʰ Placeholder Alert   Manifestation   ᴴᶜᶜ CMS-HCC Condition   ▽ Unspecified Code   ▶◄ Revised Text   ● New Code   ▲ Revised Code Title

ICD-10-CM 2018   543

Chapter 5. Mental, Behavioral and Neurodevelopmental Disorders

√5ᵗʰ **F51.1** **Hypersomnia not due to a substance or known physiological condition**

> EXCLUDES 2   *alcohol related hypersomnia (F10.182, F10.282, F10.982)*
> *drug-related hypersomnia (F11.182, F11.282, F11.982, F13.182, F13.282, F13.982, F14.182, F14.282, F14.982, F15.182, F15.282, F15.982, F19.182, F19.282, F19.982)*
> *hypersomnia NOS (G47.10)*
> *hypersomnia due to known physiological condition (G47.10)*
> *idiopathic hypersomnia (G47.11, G47.12)*
> *narcolepsy (G47.4-)*

     F51.11 **Primary hypersomnia**

     F51.12 **Insufficient sleep syndrome**
> EXCLUDES 1   *sleep deprivation (Z72.820)*

     F51.13 **Hypersomnia due to other mental disorder**
Code also associated mental disorder

     F51.19 **Other hypersomnia not due to a substance or known physiological condition**

F51.3 **Sleepwalking [somnambulism]**
▶Non–rapid eye movement sleep arousal disorders, sleepwalking type◀

F51.4 **Sleep terrors [night terrors]**
▶Non–rapid eye movement sleep arousal disorders, sleep terror type◀

F51.5 **Nightmare disorder**
Dream anxiety disorder

F51.8 **Other sleep disorders not due to a substance or known physiological condition**

F51.9 **Sleep disorder not due to a substance or known physiological condition, unspecified**   ▽
Emotional sleep disorder NOS

√4ᵗʰ **F52** **Sexual dysfunction not due to a substance or known physiological condition**
> EXCLUDES 2   *Dhat syndrome (F48.8)*

F52.0 **Hypoactive sexual desire disorder**
Lack or loss of sexual desire
▶Male hypoactive sexual desire disorder◀
Sexual anhedonia
> EXCLUDES 1   *decreased libido (R68.82)*

F52.1 **Sexual aversion disorder**
Sexual aversion and lack of sexual enjoyment

√5ᵗʰ **F52.2** **Sexual arousal disorders**
Failure of genital response

     F52.21 **Male erectile disorder**   ♂
▶Erectile disorder◀
Psychogenic impotence
> EXCLUDES 1   *impotence of organic origin (N52.-)*
> *impotence NOS (N52.-)*

     F52.22 **Female sexual arousal disorder**   ♀
▶Female sexual interest/arousal disorder◀

√5ᵗʰ **F52.3** **Orgasmic disorder**
Inhibited orgasm
Psychogenic anorgasmy

     F52.31 **Female orgasmic disorder**   ♀

     F52.32 **Male orgasmic disorder**   ♂
Delayed ejaculation

F52.4 **Premature ejaculation**   ♂

F52.5 **Vaginismus not due to a substance or known physiological condition**   ♀
Psychogenic vaginismus
> EXCLUDES 2   *vaginismus (due to a known physiological condition) (N94.2)*

DEF: Psychogenic response resulting in painful contractions of vaginal canal muscles; can be severe enough to prevent sexual intercourse.

F52.6 **Dyspareunia not due to a substance or known physiological condition**   ♀
Genito-pelvic pain or penetration disorder
Psychogenic dyspareunia
> EXCLUDES 2   *dyspareunia (due to a known physiological condition) (N94.1-)*

F52.8 **Other sexual dysfunction not due to a substance or known physiological condition**
Excessive sexual drive
Nymphomania
Satyriasis

F52.9 **Unspecified sexual dysfunction not due to a substance or known physiological condition**   ▽
Sexual dysfunction NOS

F53 **Puerperal psychosis**   M♀
Postpartum depression
> EXCLUDES 1   *mood disorders with psychotic features (F30.2, F31.2, F31.5, F31.64, F32.3, F33.3)*
> *postpartum dysphoria (O90.6)*
> *psychosis in schizophrenia, schizotypal, delusional, and other psychotic disorders (F20-F29)*

F54 **Psychological and behavioral factors associated with disorders or diseases classified elsewhere**
Psychological factors affecting physical conditions
Code first the associated physical disorder, such as:
     asthma (J45.-)
     dermatitis (L23-L25)
     gastric ulcer (K25.-)
     mucous colitis (K58.-)
     ulcerative colitis (K51.-)
     urticaria (L50.-)
> EXCLUDES 2   *tension-type headache (G44.2)*

√4ᵗʰ **F55** **Abuse of non-psychoactive substances**
> EXCLUDES 2   *abuse of psychoactive substances (F10-F19)*

F55.0 **Abuse of antacids**

F55.1 **Abuse of herbal or folk remedies**

F55.2 **Abuse of laxatives**

F55.3 **Abuse of steroids or hormones**

F55.4 **Abuse of vitamins**

F55.8 **Abuse of other non-psychoactive substances**

F59 **Unspecified behavioral syndromes associated with physiological disturbances and physical factors**   ▽
Psychogenic physiological dysfunction NOS

Disorders of adult personality and behavior (F60-F69)

√4ᵗʰ **F60** **Specific personality disorders**

F60.0 **Paranoid personality disorder**
Expansive paranoid personality (disorder)
Fanatic personality (disorder)
Paranoid personality (disorder)
Querulant personality (disorder)
Sensitive paranoid personality (disorder)
> EXCLUDES 2   *paranoia (F22)*
> *paranoia querulans (F22)*
> *paranoid psychosis (F22)*
> *paranoid schizophrenia (F20.0)*
> *paranoid state (F22)*

F60.1 **Schizoid personality disorder**
> EXCLUDES 2   *Asperger's syndrome (F84.5)*
> *delusional disorder (F22)*
> *schizoid disorder of childhood (F84.5)*
> *schizophrenia (F20.-)*
> *schizotypal disorder (F21)*

F60.2 **Antisocial personality disorder**
Amoral personality (disorder)
Asocial personality (disorder)
Dissocial personality disorder
Psychopathic personality (disorder)
Sociopathic personality (disorder)
> EXCLUDES 1   *conduct disorders (F91.-)*
> EXCLUDES 2   *borderline personality disorder (F60.3)*

F60.3 **Borderline personality disorder**
Aggressive personality (disorder)
Emotionally unstable personality disorder
Explosive personality (disorder)
> EXCLUDES 2   *antisocial personality disorder (F60.2)*

F60.4 **Histrionic personality disorder**
Hysterical personality (disorder)
Psychoinfantile personality (disorder)

F60.5 **Obsessive-compulsive personality disorder**
Anankastic personality (disorder)
Compulsive personality (disorder)
Obsessional personality (disorder)
> EXCLUDES 2   *obsessive-compulsive disorder (F42-)*

F60.6 **Avoidant personality disorder**
Anxious personality disorder

F60.7 **Dependent personality disorder**
Asthenic personality (disorder)
Inadequate personality (disorder)
Passive personality (disorder)

EXCLUDES 1 Not coded here   EXCLUDES 2 Not included here   N Newborn Age: 0   P Pediatric Age: 0-17   M Maternity Age: 12-55   A Adult Age: 15-124

544   ICD-10-CM 2018

✓5ᵗʰ **F60.8**   **Other specific personality disorders**

     F60.81   **Narcissistic personality disorder**

     F60.89   **Other specific personality disorders**
         Eccentric personality disorder
         "Haltlose" type personality disorder
         Immature personality disorder
         Passive-aggressive personality disorder
         Psychoneurotic personality disorder
         Self-defeating personality disorder

   F60.9   **Personality disorder, unspecified**   ▽
       Character disorder NOS
       Character neurosis NOS
       Pathological personality NOS

✓4ᵗʰ **F63**   **Impulse disorders**
     EXCLUDES 2   *habitual excessive use of alcohol or psychoactive substances (F10-F19)*
            impulse disorders involving sexual behavior (F65.-)

   F63.0   **Pathological gambling**
       Compulsive gambling
       ►Gambling disorder◄
       EXCLUDES 1   *gambling and betting NOS (Z72.6)*
       EXCLUDES 2   *excessive gambling by manic patients (F30, F31)*
              gambling in antisocial personality disorder (F60.2)

   F63.1   **Pyromania**
       Pathological fire-setting
       EXCLUDES 2   *fire-setting (by) (in):*
              adult with antisocial personality disorder (F60.2)
              alcohol or psychoactive substance intoxication (F10-F19)
              conduct disorders (F91.-)
              mental disorders due to known physiological condition (F01-F09)
              schizophrenia (F20.-)

   F63.2   **Kleptomania**
       Pathological stealing
       EXCLUDES 1   *shoplifting as the reason for observation for suspected mental disorder (Z03.8)*
       EXCLUDES 2   *depressive disorder with stealing (F31-F33)*
              stealing due to underlying mental condition—code to mental condition
              stealing in mental disorders due to known physiological condition (F01-F09)

   F63.3   **Trichotillomania**
       Hair plucking
       EXCLUDES 2   *other stereotyped movement disorder (F98.4)*

✓5ᵗʰ **F63.8**   **Other impulse disorders**

     F63.81   **Intermittent explosive disorder**

     F63.89   **Other impulse disorders**

   F63.9   **Impulse disorder, unspecified**   ▽
       Impulse control disorder NOS

✓4ᵗʰ **F64**   **Gender identity disorders**

   F64.0   **Transsexualism**
       Gender identity disorder in adolescence and adulthood
       Gender dysphoria in adolescents and adults

   F64.1   **Dual role transvestism**
       Use additional code to identify sex reassignment status (Z87.890)
       EXCLUDES 1   *gender identity disorder in childhood (F64.2)*
       EXCLUDES 2   *fetishistic transvestism (F65.1)*

   F64.2   **Gender identity disorder of childhood**   P
       Gender dysphoria in children
       EXCLUDES 1   *gender identity disorder in adolescence and adulthood (F64.0)*
       EXCLUDES 2   *sexual maturation disorder (F66)*

   F64.8   **Other gender identity disorders**
       ►Other specified gender dysphoria◄

   F64.9   **Gender identity disorder, unspecified**   ▽
       ►Gender dysphoria, unspecified◄
       Gender-role disorder NOS

✓4ᵗʰ **F65**   **Paraphilias**

   F65.0   **Fetishism**
       ►Fetishistic disorder◄

   F65.1   **Transvestic fetishism**
       Fetishistic transvestism
       ►Transvestic disorder◄

   F65.2   **Exhibitionism**
       ►Exhibitionistic disorder◄

   F65.3   **Voyeurism**
       ►Voyeuristic disorder◄

   F65.4   **Pedophilia**
       ►Pedophilic disorder◄

✓5ᵗʰ **F65.5**   **Sadomasochism**   ▽

     F65.50   **Sadomasochism, unspecified**

     F65.51   **Sexual masochism**
         ►Sexual masochism disorder◄

     F65.52   **Sexual sadism**
         ►Sexual sadism disorder◄

✓5ᵗʰ **F65.8**   **Other paraphilias**

     F65.81   **Frotteurism**
         ►Frotteuristic disorder◄

     F65.89   **Other paraphilias**
         Necrophilia
         ►Other specified paraphilic disorder◄

   F65.9   **Paraphilia, unspecified**   ▽
       ►Paraphilic disorder, unspecified◄
       Sexual deviation NOS

F66   **Other sexual disorders**
       Sexual maturation disorder
       Sexual relationship disorder

✓4ᵗʰ **F68**   **Other disorders of adult personality and behavior**

✓5ᵗʰ **F68.1**   **Factitious disorder**
       Compensation neurosis
       Elaboration of physical symptoms for psychological reasons
       Hospital hopper syndrome
       Münchhausen's syndrome
       Peregrinating patient
       EXCLUDES 2   *factitial dermatitis (L98.1)*
              person feigning illness (with obvious motivation) (Z76.5)

     F68.10   **Factitious disorder, unspecified**   ▽

     F68.11   **Factitious disorder with predominantly psychological signs and symptoms**

     F68.12   **Factitious disorder with predominantly physical signs and symptoms**

     F68.13   **Factitious disorder with combined psychological and physical signs and symptoms**

   F68.8   **Other specified disorders of adult personality and behavior**

F69   **Unspecified disorder of adult personality and behavior**   Ⓐ ▽

Intellectual Disabilities (F70-F79)

Code first any associated physical or developmental disorders
EXCLUDES 1   *borderline intellectual functioning, IQ above 70 to 84 (R41.83)*

F70   **Mild intellectual disabilities**
       IQ level 50-55 to approximately 70
       Mild mental subnormality

F71   **Moderate intellectual disabilities**
       IQ level 35-40 to 50-55
       Moderate mental subnormality

F72   **Severe intellectual disabilities**
       IQ 20-25 to 35-40
       Severe mental subnormality

F73   **Profound intellectual disabilities**
       IQ level below 20-25
       Profound mental subnormality

F78   **Other intellectual disabilities**

F79   **Unspecified intellectual disabilities**   ▽
       Mental deficiency NOS
       Mental subnormality NOS

✓ Additional Character Req   ✓ˣ7ᵗʰ Placeholder Alert   Manifestation   HCC CMS-HCC Condition   ▽ Unspecified Code   ►◄ Revised Text   ● New Code   ▲ Revised Code Title

ICD-10-CM 2018   545

Chapter 5. Mental, Behavioral and Neurodevelopmental Disorders

Pervasive and specific developmental disorders (F80-F89)

☑4ᵗʰ **F80   Specific developmental disorders of speech and language**

F80.0   Phonological disorder
Dyslalia
Functional speech articulation disorder
Lalling
Lisping
Phonological developmental disorder
Speech articulation developmental disorder
Speech-sound disorder

EXCLUDES 1   speech articulation impairment due to aphasia NOS (R47.01)
speech articulation impairment due to apraxia (R48.2)

EXCLUDES 2   speech articulation impairment due to hearing loss (F80.4)
speech articulation impairment due to intellectual disabilities (F70-F79)
speech articulation impairment with expressive language developmental disorder (F80.1)
speech articulation impairment with mixed receptive expressive language developmental disorder (F80.2)

F80.1   Expressive language disorder
Developmental dysphasia or aphasia, expressive type

EXCLUDES 1   dysphasia and aphasia NOS (R47.-)
mixed receptive-expressive language disorder (F80.2)

EXCLUDES 2   acquired aphasia with epilepsy [Landau-Kleffner] (G40.80-)
intellectual disabilities (F70-F79)
pervasive developmental disorders (F84.-)
selective mutism (F94.0)

F80.2   Mixed receptive-expressive language disorder
Developmental dysphasia or aphasia, receptive type
Developmental Wernicke's aphasia

EXCLUDES 1   central auditory processing disorder (H93.25)
dysphasia or aphasia NOS (R47.-)
expressive language disorder (F80.1)
expressive type dysphasia or aphasia (F80.1)
word deafness (H93.25)

EXCLUDES 2   acquired aphasia with epilepsy [Landau-Kleffner] (G40.80-)
intellectual disabilities (F70-F79)
pervasive developmental disorders (F84.-)
selective mutism (F94.0)

F80.4   Speech and language development delay due to hearing loss
Code also type of hearing loss (H90.-, H91.-)

☑5ᵗʰ **F80.8   Other developmental disorders of speech and language**
AHA: 2017, 1Q, 27

F80.81   Childhood onset fluency disorder
Cluttering NOS
Stuttering NOS

EXCLUDES 1   adult onset fluency disorder (F98.5)
fluency disorder in conditions classified elsewhere (R47.82)
fluency disorder (stuttering) following cerebrovascular disease (I69. with final characters-23)

F80.82   Social pragmatic communication disorder

EXCLUDES 1   Asperger's syndrome (F84.5)
autistic disorder (F84.0)

F80.89   Other developmental disorders of speech and language

F80.9   Developmental disorder of speech and language, unspecified   ▽
Communication disorder NOS
Language disorder NOS

☑4ᵗʰ **F81   Specific developmental disorders of scholastic skills**

F81.0   Specific reading disorder
"Backward reading"
Developmental dyslexia
▶Specific learning disorder, with impairment in reading◀
Specific reading retardation

EXCLUDES 1   alexia NOS (R48.0)
dyslexia NOS (R48.0)

DEF: Serious impairment of reading skills unexplained in relation to general intelligence and teaching processes.

F81.2   Mathematics disorder
Developmental acalculia
Developmental arithmetical disorder
Developmental Gerstmann's syndrome
▶Specific learning disorder, with impairment in mathmatics◀

EXCLUDES 1   acalculia NOS (R48.8)

EXCLUDES 2   arithmetical difficulties associated with a reading disorder (F81.0)
arithmetical difficulties associated with a spelling disorder (F81.81)
arithmetical difficulties due to inadequate teaching (Z55.8)

☑5ᵗʰ **F81.8   Other developmental disorders of scholastic skills**

F81.81   Disorder of written expression
▶Specific learning disorder, with impairment in written expression◀
Specific spelling disorder

F81.89   Other developmental disorders of scholastic skills

F81.9   Developmental disorder of scholastic skills, unspecified   ▽
Knowledge acquisition disability NOS
Learning disability NOS
Learning disorder NOS

F82   Specific developmental disorder of motor function
Clumsy child syndrome
Developmental coordination disorder
Developmental dyspraxia

EXCLUDES 1   abnormalities of gait and mobility (R26.-)
lack of coordination (R27.-)

EXCLUDES 2   lack of coordination secondary to intellectual disabilities (F70-F79)

☑4ᵗʰ **F84   Pervasive developmental disorders**
Use additional code to identify any associated medical condition and intellectual disabilities

F84.0   Autistic disorder
Autism spectrum disorder
Infantile autism
Infantile psychosis
Kanner's syndrome

EXCLUDES 1   Asperger's syndrome (F84.5)

AHA: 2017, 1Q, 27

F84.2   Rett's syndrome

EXCLUDES 1   Asperger's syndrome (F84.5)
Autistic disorder (F84.0)
Other childhood disintegrative disorder (F84.3)

F84.3   Other childhood disintegrative disorder   P
Dementia infantilis
Disintegrative psychosis
Heller's syndrome
Symbiotic psychosis
Use additional code to identify any associated neurological condition

EXCLUDES 1   Asperger's syndrome (F84.5)
Autistic disorder (F84.0)
Rett's syndrome (F84.2)

F84.5   Asperger's syndrome
Asperger's disorder
Autistic psychopathy
Schizoid disorder of childhood

F84.8   Other pervasive developmental disorders
Overactive disorder associated with intellectual disabilities and stereotyped movements

F84.9   Pervasive developmental disorder, unspecified   ▽
Atypical autism

F88   Other disorders of psychological development
Developmental agnosia
Global development delay
Other specified neurodevelopmental disorder

F89   Unspecified disorder of psychological development   ▽
Developmental disorder NOS
Neurodevelopmental disorder NOS

EXCLUDES 1 Not coded here   EXCLUDES 2 Not included here   N Newborn Age: 0   P Pediatric Age: 0-17   M Maternity Age: 12-55   A Adult Age: 15-124

Behavioral and emotional disorders with onset usually occurring in childhood and adolescence (F90-F98)

> **NOTE**   Codes within categories F90-F98 may be used regardless of the age of a patient. These disorders generally have onset within the childhood or adolescent years, but may continue throughout life or not be diagnosed until adulthood.

✓4th **F90** **Attention-deficit hyperactivity disorders**

> **INCLUDES**   attention deficit disorder with hyperactivity
> attention deficit syndrome with hyperactivity
>
> **EXCLUDES 2**   anxiety disorders (F40.-, F41.-)
> mood [affective] disorders (F30-F39)
> pervasive developmental disorders (F84.-)
> schizophrenia (F20.-)

   F90.0 **Attention-deficit hyperactivity disorder, predominantly inattentive type**
> ▶Attention-deficit/hyperactivity disorder, predominantly inattentive presentation◀

   F90.1 **Attention-deficit hyperactivity disorder, predominantly hyperactive type**
> ▶Attention-deficit/hyperactivity disorder, predominantly hyperactive impulsive presentation◀

   F90.2 **Attention-deficit hyperactivity disorder, combined type**
> ▶Attention-deficit/hyperactivity disorder, combined presentation◀

   F90.8 **Attention-deficit hyperactivity disorder, other type**

   F90.9 **Attention-deficit hyperactivity disorder, unspecified type** ▽
> Attention-deficit hyperactivity disorder of childhood or adolescence NOS
> Attention-deficit hyperactivity disorder NOS

✓4th **F91** **Conduct disorders**

> **EXCLUDES 1**   antisocial behavior (Z72.81-)
> antisocial personality disorder (F60.2)
>
> **EXCLUDES 2**   conduct problems associated with attention-deficit hyperactivity disorder (F90.-)
> mood [affective] disorders (F30-F39)
> pervasive developmental disorders (F84.-)
> schizophrenia (F20.-)

   F91.0 **Conduct disorder confined to family context**

   F91.1 **Conduct disorder, childhood-onset type**
> Unsocialized conduct disorder
> Conduct disorder, solitary aggressive type
> Unsocialized aggressive disorder

   F91.2 **Conduct disorder, adolescent-onset type**
> Socialized conduct disorder
> Conduct disorder, group type

   F91.3 **Oppositional defiant disorder**

   F91.8 **Other conduct disorders**
> Other specified conduct disorder
> Other specified disruptive disorder

   F91.9 **Conduct disorder, unspecified** ▽
> Behavioral disorder NOS
> Conduct disorder NOS
> Disruptive behavior disorder NOS
> Disruptive disorder NOS

✓4th **F93** **Emotional disorders with onset specific to childhood**

   F93.0 **Separation anxiety disorder of childhood**
> **EXCLUDES 2**   mood [affective] disorders (F30-F39)
> nonpsychotic mental disorders (F40-F48)
> phobic anxiety disorder of childhood (F40.8)
> social phobia (F40.1)

   F93.8 **Other childhood emotional disorders**
> Identity disorder
> **EXCLUDES 2**   gender identity disorder of childhood (F64.2)

   F93.9 **Childhood emotional disorder, unspecified** ▽

✓4th **F94** **Disorders of social functioning with onset specific to childhood and adolescence**

   F94.0 **Selective mutism**
> Elective mutism
> **EXCLUDES 2**   pervasive developmental disorders (F84.-)
> schizophrenia (F20.-)
> specific developmental disorders of speech and language (F80.-)
> transient mutism as part of separation anxiety in young children (F93.0)

   F94.1 **Reactive attachment disorder of childhood**
> Use additional code to identify any associated failure to thrive or growth retardation
>
> **EXCLUDES 1**   disinhibited attachment disorder of childhood (F94.1)
> normal variation in pattern of selective attachment
>
> **EXCLUDES 2**   Asperger's syndrome (F84.5)
> maltreatment syndromes (T74.-)
> sexual or physical abuse in childhood, resulting in psychosocial problems (Z62.81-)

   F94.2 **Disinhibited attachment disorder of childhood**
> Affectionless psychopathy
> Institutional syndrome
>
> **EXCLUDES 1**   reactive attachment disorder of childhood (F94.1)
>
> **EXCLUDES 2**   Asperger's syndrome (F84.5)
> attention-deficit hyperactivity disorders (F90.-)
> hospitalism in children (F43.2-)

   F94.8 **Other childhood disorders of social functioning**

   F94.9 **Childhood disorder of social functioning, unspecified** ▽

✓4th **F95** **Tic disorder**

   F95.0 **Transient tic disorder**
> Provisional tic disorder

   F95.1 **Chronic motor or vocal tic disorder**

   F95.2 **Tourette's disorder**
> Combined vocal and multiple motor tic disorder [de la Tourette]
> Tourette's syndrome

   F95.8 **Other tic disorders**

   F95.9 **Tic disorder, unspecified** ▽
> Tic NOS

✓4th **F98** **Other behavioral and emotional disorders with onset usually occurring in childhood and adolescence**

> **EXCLUDES 2**   breath-holding spells (R06.89)
> gender identity disorder of childhood (F64.2)
> Kleine-Levin syndrome (G47.13)
> obsessive-compulsive disorder (F42-)
> sleep disorders not due to a substance or known physiological condition (F51.-)

   F98.0 **Enuresis not due to a substance or known physiological condition**
> Enuresis (primary) (secondary) of nonorganic origin
> Functional enuresis
> Psychogenic enuresis
> Urinary incontinence of nonorganic origin
> **EXCLUDES 1**   enuresis NOS (R32)

   F98.1 **Encopresis not due to a substance or known physiological condition**
> Functional encopresis
> Incontinence of feces of nonorganic origin
> Psychogenic encopresis
> Use additional code to identify the cause of any coexisting constipation
> **EXCLUDES 1**   encopresis NOS (R15.-)

✓5th **F98.2** **Other feeding disorders of infancy and childhood**
> **EXCLUDES 1**   feeding difficulties (R63.3)
> **EXCLUDES 2**   anorexia nervosa and other eating disorders (F50.-)
> feeding problems of newborn (P92.-)
> pica of infancy or childhood (F98.3)

   F98.21 **Rumination disorder of infancy**

   F98.29 **Other feeding disorders of infancy and early childhood**

   F98.3 **Pica of infancy and childhood**

   F98.4 **Stereotyped movement disorders**
> Stereotype/habit disorder
> **EXCLUDES 1**   abnormal involuntary movements (R25.-)
> **EXCLUDES 2**   compulsions in obsessive-compulsive disorder (F42-)
> hair plucking (F63.3)
> movement disorders of organic origin (G20-G25)
> nail-biting (F98.8)
> nose-picking (F98.8)
> stereotypies that are part of a broader psychiatric condition (F01-F95)
> thumb-sucking (F98.8)
> tic disorders (F95.-)
> trichotillomania (F63.3)

✓ Additional Character Req   ✓x7th Placeholder Alert   Manifestation   HCC CMS-HCC Condition   ▽ Unspecified Code   ▶◀ Revised Text   ● New Code   ▲ Revised Code Title

ICD-10-CM 2018   **F90–F98.4**   **547**

F98.5   **Adult onset fluency disorder**

> *EXCLUDES 1*   *childhood onset fluency disorder (F80.81)*
> *dysphasia (R47.02)*
> *fluency disorder in conditions classified elsewhere*
>   *(R47.82)*
> *fluency disorder (stuttering) following cerebrovascular*
>   *disease (I69. with final characters -23)*
> *tic disorders (F95.-)*

F98.8   **Other specified behavioral and emotional disorders with onset usually occurring in childhood and adolescence**

    Excessive masturbation
    Nail-biting
    Nose-picking
    Thumb-sucking

F98.9   **Unspecified behavioral and emotional disorders with onset usually occurring in childhood and adolescence**   ▽

Unspecified mental disorder (F99)

F99   **Mental disorder, not otherwise specified**

    Mental illness NOS

> *EXCLUDES 1*   *unspecified mental disorder due to known physiological*
>   *condition (F09)*

EXCLUDES 1 Not coded here   *EXCLUDES 2* Not included here   **N** Newborn Age: 0   **P** Pediatric Age: 0-17   **M** Maternity Age: 12-55   **A** Adult Age: 15-124

548   ICD-10-CM 2018

Chapter 6. Diseases of the Nervous System (G00-G99)

Chapter Specific Guidelines with Coding Examples

The chapter specific guidelines from the ICD-10-CM Official Guidelines for Coding and Reporting have been provided below. Along with these guidelines are coding examples, contained in the shaded boxes, that have been developed to help illustrate the coding and/or sequencing guidance found in these guidelines.

a. Dominant/nondominant side

Codes from category G81, Hemiplegia and hemiparesis, and subcategories G83.1, Monoplegia of lower limb, G83.2, Monoplegia of upper limb, and G83.3, Monoplegia, unspecified, identify whether the dominant or nondominant side is affected. Should the affected side be documented, but not specified as dominant or nondominant, and the classification system does not indicate a default, code selection is as follows:

- For ambidextrous patients, the default should be dominant.
- If the left side is affected, the default is non-dominant.
- If the right side is affected, the default is dominant.

> Hemiplegia affecting left side of ambidextrous patient
>
> **G81.92   Hemiplegia, unspecified affecting left dominant side**
>
> *Explanation*: Documentation states that the left side is affected and dominant is used for ambidextrous persons.

> Right spastic hemiplegia, unknown whether patient is right- or left-handed
>
> **G81.11   Spastic hemiplegia affecting right dominant side**
>
> *Explanation*: Since it is unknown whether the patient is right- or left-handed, if the right side is affected, the default is dominant.

b. Pain—Category G89

1) General coding information

Codes in category G89, Pain, not elsewhere classified, may be used in conjunction with codes from other categories and chapters to provide more detail about acute or chronic pain and neoplasm-related pain, unless otherwise indicated below.

If the pain is not specified as acute or chronic, post-thoracotomy, postprocedural, or neoplasm-related, do not assign codes from category G89.

A code from category G89 should not be assigned if the underlying (definitive) diagnosis is known, unless the reason for the encounter is pain control/ management and not management of the underlying condition.

When an admission or encounter is for a procedure aimed at treating the underlying condition (e.g., spinal fusion, kyphoplasty), a code for the underlying condition (e.g., vertebral fracture, spinal stenosis) should be assigned as the principal diagnosis. No code from category G89 should be assigned.

> Elderly patient with back pain is admitted for outpatient kyphoplasty for age-related osteopathic compression fracture at vertebra T3
>
> **M80.08XA   Age-related osteoporosis with current pathological fracture, vertebra(e), initial encounter for fracture**
>
> *Explanation*: No code is assigned for the pain as it is inherent in the underlying condition being treated.

(a) Category G89 codes as principal or first-listed diagnosis

Category G89 codes are acceptable as principal diagnosis or the first-listed code:

- When pain control or pain management is the reason for the admission/encounter (e.g., a patient with displaced intervertebral disc, nerve impingement and severe back pain presents for injection of steroid into the spinal canal). The underlying cause of the pain should be reported as an additional diagnosis, if known.

> Patient presents for steroid injection in the right elbow due to chronic pain associated with primary degenerative joint disease.
>
> **G89.29   Other chronic pain**
>
> **M19.021   Primary osteoarthritis, right elbow**
>
> *Explanation*: Since the encounter is for control of pain, not treating the underlying condition, the pain code is sequenced first followed by the underlying condition. The M25 pain code is not necessary as the underlying condition code represents the specific site.

- When a patient is admitted for the insertion of a neurostimulator for pain control, assign the appropriate pain code as the principal or first-listed diagnosis. When an admission or encounter is for a procedure aimed at treating the underlying condition and a neurostimulator is inserted for pain control during the same admission/encounter, a code for the underlying condition should be assigned as the principal diagnosis and the appropriate pain code should be assigned as a secondary diagnosis.

(b) Use of category G89 codes in conjunction with site specific pain codes

(i) Assigning category G89 and site-specific pain codes

Codes from category G89 may be used in conjunction with codes that identify the site of pain (including codes from chapter 18) if the category G89 code provides additional information. For example, if the code describes the site of the pain, but does not fully describe whether the pain is acute or chronic, then both codes should be assigned.

> Patient is seen to evaluate chronic right knee pain
>
> **M25.561   Pain in right knee**
>
> **G89.29   Other chronic pain**
>
> *Explanation*: No underlying condition has been determined yet so the pain would be the reason for the visit. The M25 pain code in this instance does not fully describe the condition as it does not represent that the pain is chronic. The G89 chronic pain code is assigned to provide specificity.

(ii) Sequencing of category G89 codes with site-specific pain codes

The sequencing of category G89 codes with site-specific pain codes (including chapter 18 codes), is dependent on the circumstances of the encounter/admission as follows:

- If the encounter is for pain control or pain management, assign the code from category G89 followed by the code identifying the specific site of pain (e.g., encounter for pain management for acute neck pain from trauma is assigned code G89.11, Acute pain due to trauma, followed by code M54.2, Cervicalgia, to identify the site of pain).

> Management of acute, traumatic left shoulder pain
>
> **G89.11   Acute pain due to trauma**
>
> **M25.512   Pain in left shoulder**
>
> *Explanation*: The reason for the encounter is to manage or control the pain, not to treat or evaluate an underlying condition. The G89 pain code is assigned as the first-listed diagnosis but in this instance does not fully describe the condition as it does not include the site and laterality. The M25 pain code is added to provide this information.

- If the encounter is for any other reason except pain control or pain management, and a related definitive diagnosis has not been established (confirmed) by the provider, assign the code for the specific site of pain first, followed by the appropriate code from category G89.

Tests are performed to investigate the source of the patient's chronic epigastric abdominal pain

R10.13	Epigastric pain
G89.29	Other chronic pain

Explanation: In this instance the patient's epigastric pain is not being treated; rather the source of the pain is being investigated. A code from chapter 18 for epigastric pain is sequenced before the additional specificity of the G89 code for the chronic pain.

2) Pain due to devices, implants and grafts

See Section I.C.19. Pain due to medical devices

3) Postoperative Pain

The provider's documentation should be used to guide the coding of postoperative pain, as well as *Section III. Reporting Additional Diagnoses* and *Section IV. Diagnostic Coding and Reporting in the Outpatient Setting.*

The default for post-thoracotomy and other postoperative pain not specified as acute or chronic is the code for the acute form.

Routine or expected postoperative pain immediately after surgery should not be coded.

Pain pump dose is increased for the patient's unexpected, extreme pain post-thoracotomy

G89.12	Acute post-thoracotomy pain

Explanation: When acute or chronic is not documented, default to acute. The use of "unexpected, extreme" and the increase of medication dosage indicate that the pain was more than routine or expected.

(a) Postoperative pain not associated with specific postoperative complication

Postoperative pain not associated with a specific postoperative complication is assigned to the appropriate postoperative pain code in category G89.

(b) Postoperative pain associated with specific postoperative complication

Postoperative pain associated with a specific postoperative complication (such as painful wire sutures) is assigned to the appropriate code(s) found in Chapter 19, Injury, poisoning, and certain other consequences of external causes. If appropriate, use additional code(s) from category G89 to identify acute or chronic pain (G89.18 or G89.28).

4) Chronic pain

Chronic pain is classified to subcategory G89.2. There is no time frame defining when pain becomes chronic pain. The provider's documentation should be used to guide use of these codes.

5) Neoplasm related pain

Code G89.3 is assigned to pain documented as being related, associated or due to cancer, primary or secondary malignancy, or tumor. This code is assigned regardless of whether the pain is acute or chronic.

This code may be assigned as the principal or first-listed code when the stated reason for the admission/encounter is documented as pain control/pain management. The underlying neoplasm should be reported as an additional diagnosis.

Patient referred today for pain management due to acute pain related to malignancy of the right breast

G89.3	Neoplasm related pain (acute)(chronic)
C50.911	Malignant neoplasm of unspecified site of right female breast

Explanation: Since the encounter was for pain medication management, the pain, rather than the neoplasm, was the reason for the encounter and is sequenced first. This "neoplasm-related pain" code includes both acute and chronic pain.

When the reason for the admission/encounter is management of the neoplasm and the pain associated with the neoplasm is also documented, code G89.3 may be assigned as an additional diagnosis. It is not necessary to assign an additional code for the site of the pain.

See Section I.C.2 for instructions on the sequencing of neoplasms for all other stated reasons for the admission/encounter (except for pain control/pain management).

Patient with lung cancer presents with acute hip pain and is evaluated and found to have iliac bone metastasis

C79.51	Secondary malignant neoplasm of bone
C34.90	Malignant neoplasm of unspecified part of unspecified bronchus or lung
G89.3	Neoplasm related pain (acute)(chronic)

Explanation: The reason for the encounter was the evaluation and diagnosis of the bone metastasis, whose code would be assigned as first-listed, followed by codes for the primary neoplasm and the pain due to the iliac bone metastasis.

6) Chronic pain syndrome

Central pain syndrome (G89.0) and chronic pain syndrome (G89.4) are different than the term "chronic pain," and therefore codes should only be used when the provider has specifically documented this condition.

See Section I.C.5. Pain disorders related to psychological factors

Chapter 6. Diseases of the Nervous System (G00-G99)

EXCLUDES 2   certain conditions originating in the perinatal period (P04-P96)
certain infectious and parasitic diseases (A00-B99)
complications of pregnancy, childbirth and the puerperium (O00-O9A)
congenital malformations, deformations, and chromosomal abnormalities (Q00-Q99)
endocrine, nutritional and metabolic diseases (E00-E88)
injury, poisoning and certain other consequences of external causes (S00-T88)
neoplasms (C00-D49)
symptoms, signs and abnormal clinical and laboratory findings, not elsewhere classified (R00-R94)

This chapter contains the following blocks:

G00-G09   Inflammatory diseases of the central nervous system
G10-G14   Systemic atrophies primarily affecting the central nervous system
G20-G26   Extrapyramidal and movement disorders
G30-G32   Other degenerative diseases of the nervous system
G35-G37   Demyelinating diseases of the central nervous system
G40-G47   Episodic and paroxysmal disorders
G50-G59   Nerve, nerve root and plexus disorders
G60-G65   Polyneuropathies and other disorders of the peripheral nervous system
G70-G73   Diseases of myoneural junction and muscle
G80-G83   Cerebral palsy and other paralytic syndromes
G89-G99   Other disorders of the nervous system

Inflammatory diseases of the central nervous system (G00-G09)

✓4ᵗʰ **G00   Bacterial meningitis, not elsewhere classified**
INCLUDES   bacterial arachnoiditis
bacterial leptomeningitis
bacterial meningitis
bacterial pachymeningitis
EXCLUDES 1   ►bacterial meningoencephalitis◄ (G04.2)
►bacterial meningomyelitis◄ (G04.2)

G00.0   Hemophilus meningitis
Meningitis due to Hemophilus influenzae

G00.1   Pneumococcal meningitis
Meningtitis due to Streptococcal pneumoniae

G00.2   Streptococcal meningitis
Use additional code to further identify organism (B95.0-B95.5)

G00.3   Staphylococcal meningitis
Use additional code to further identify organism (B95.61-B95.8)

G00.8   Other bacterial meningitis
Meningitis due to Escherichia coli
Meningitis due to Friedländer's bacillus
Meningitis due to Klebsiella
Use additional code to further identify organism (B96.-)

G00.9   Bacterial meningitis, unspecified   ▽
Meningitis due to gram-negative bacteria, unspecified
Purulent meningitis NOS
Pyogenic meningitis NOS
Suppurative meningitis NOS

G01   *Meningitis in bacterial diseases classified elsewhere*
Code first underlying disease
EXCLUDES 1   meningitis (in):
gonococcal (A54.81)
leptospirosis (A27.81)
listeriosis (A32.11)
Lyme disease (A69.21)
meningococcal (A39.0)
neurosyphilis (A52.13)
tuberculosis (A17.0)
meningoencephalitis and meningomyelitis in bacterial diseases classified elsewhere (G05)

G02   *Meningitis in other infectious and parasitic diseases classified elsewhere*
Code first underlying disease, such as:
African trypanosomiasis (B56.-)
poliovirus infection (A80.-)
EXCLUDES 1   candidal meningitis (B37.5)
coccidioidomycosis meningitis (B38.4)
cryptococcal meningitis (B45.1)
herpesviral [herpes simplex] meningitis (B00.3)
infectious mononucleosis complicated by meningitis (B27.- with fourth character 2)
measles complicated by meningitis (B05.1)
meningoencephalitis and meningomyelitis in other infectious and parasitic diseases classified elsewhere (G05)
mumps meningitis (B26.1)
rubella meningitis (B06.02)
varicella [chickenpox] meningitis (B01.0)
zoster meningitis (B02.1)

✓4ᵗʰ **G03   Meningitis due to other and unspecified causes**
INCLUDES   arachnoiditis NOS
leptomeningitis NOS
meningitis NOS
pachymeningitis NOS
EXCLUDES 1   meningoencephalitis (G04.-)
meningomyelitis (G04.-)

G03.0   Nonpyogenic meningitis
Aseptic meningitis
Nonbacterial meningitis

G03.1   Chronic meningitis

G03.2   Benign recurrent meningitis [Mollaret]

G03.8   Meningitis due to other specified causes

G03.9   Meningitis, unspecified   ▽
Arachnoiditis (spinal) NOS

✓4ᵗʰ **G04   Encephalitis, myelitis and encephalomyelitis**
INCLUDES   acute ascending myelitis
meningoencephalitis
meningomyelitis
EXCLUDES 1   encephalopathy NOS (G93.40)
EXCLUDES 2   acute transverse myelitis (G37.3-)
alcoholic encephalopathy (G31.2)
benign myalgic encephalomyelitis (G93.3)
multiple sclerosis (G35)
subacute necrotizing myelitis (G37.4)
toxic encephalitis (G92)
toxic encephalopathy (G92)

✓5ᵗʰ **G04.0   Acute disseminated encephalitis and encephalomyelitis (ADEM)**
EXCLUDES 1   acute necrotizing hemorrhagic encephalopathy (G04.3-)
other noninfectious acute disseminated encephalomyelitis (noninfectious ADEM) (G04.81)

G04.00   Acute disseminated encephalitis and encephalomyelitis, unspecified   ▽

G04.01   Postinfectious acute disseminated encephalitis and encephalomyelitis (postinfectious ADEM)
EXCLUDES 1   post chickenpox encephalitis (B01.1)
post measles encephalitis (B05.0)
post measles myelitis (B05.1)

G04.02   Postimmunization acute disseminated encephalitis, myelitis and encephalomyelitis
Encephalitis, postimmunization
Encephalomyelitis, postimmunization
Use additional code to identify the vaccine (T50.A-, T50.B-, T50.Z-)

G04.1   Tropical spastic paraplegia   HCC

G04.2   Bacterial meningoencephalitis and meningomyelitis, not elsewhere classified

✓5ᵗʰ **G04.3   Acute necrotizing hemorrhagic encephalopathy**
EXCLUDES 1   acute disseminated encephalitis and encephalomyelitis (G04.0-)

G04.30   Acute necrotizing hemorrhagic encephalopathy, unspecified   ▽

G04.31   Postinfectious acute necrotizing hemorrhagic encephalopathy

G04.32   Postimmunization acute necrotizing hemorrhagic encephalopathy
Use additional code to identify the vaccine (T50.A-, T50.B-, T50.Z-)

✔ Additional Character Req   √xTᵗʰ Placeholder Alert   Manifestation   HCC CMS-HCC Condition   ▽ Unspecified Code   ►◄ Revised Text   ● New Code   ▲ Revised Code Title

ICD-10-CM 2018   551

G04.39   Other acute necrotizing hemorrhagic encephalopathy
Code also underlying etiology, if applicable

☑5ᵗʰ **G04.8   Other encephalitis, myelitis and encephalomyelitis**
Code also any associated seizure (G40.-, R56.9)

G04.81   Other encephalitis and encephalomyelitis
Noninfectious acute disseminated encephalomyelitis (noninfectious ADEM)

G04.89   Other myelitis   HCC

☑5ᵗʰ **G04.9   Encephalitis, myelitis and encephalomyelitis, unspecified**

G04.90   Encephalitis and encephalomyelitis, unspecified   ▽
Ventriculitis (cerebral) NOS

G04.91   Myelitis, unspecified   HCC ▽

☑4ᵗʰ **G05   Encephalitis, myelitis and encephalomyelitis in diseases classified elsewhere**
Code first underlying disease, such as:
human immunodeficiency virus [HIV] disease (B20)
poliovirus (A80.-)
suppurative otitis media (H66.01-H66.4)
trichinellosis (B75)

EXCLUDES 1   adenoviral encephalitis, myelitis and encephalomyelitis (A85.1)
congenital toxoplasmosis encephalitis, myelitis and encephalomyelitis (P37.1)
cytomegaloviral encephalitis, myelitis and encephalomyelitis (B25.8)
encephalitis, myelitis and encephalomyelitis (in) measles (B05.0)
encephalitis, myelitis and encephalomyelitis (in) systemic lupus erythematosus (M32.19)
enteroviral encephalitis, myelitis and encephalomyelitis (A85.0)
eosinophilic meningoencephalitis (B83.2)
herpesviral [herpes simplex] encephalitis, myelitis and encephalomyelitis (B00.4)
listerial encephalitis, myelitis and encephalomyelitis (A32.12)
meningococcal encephalitis, myelitis and encephalomyelitis (A39.81)
mumps encephalitis, myelitis and encephalomyelitis (B26.2)
postchickenpox encephalitis, myelitis and encephalomyelitis (B01.1-)
rubella encephalitis, myelitis and encephalomyelitis (B06.01)
toxoplasmosis encephalitis, myelitis and encephalomyelitis (B58.2)
zoster encephalitis, myelitis and encephalomyelitis (B02.0)

G05.3   Encephalitis and encephalomyelitis in diseases classified elsewhere
Meningoencephalitis in diseases classified elsewhere

G05.4   Myelitis in diseases classified elsewhere   HCC
Meningomyelitis in diseases classified elsewhere

☑4ᵗʰ **G06   Intracranial and intraspinal abscess and granuloma**
Use additional code (B95-B97) to identify infectious agent

G06.0   Intracranial abscess and granuloma
Brain [any part] abscess (embolic)
Cerebellar abscess (embolic)
Cerebral abscess (embolic)
Intracranial epidural abscess or granuloma
Intracranial extradural abscess or granuloma
Intracranial subdural abscess or granuloma
Otogenic abscess (embolic)

EXCLUDES 1   tuberculous intracranial abscess and granuloma (A17.81)

G06.1   Intraspinal abscess and granuloma
Abscess (embolic) of spinal cord [any part]
Intraspinal epidural abscess or granuloma
Intraspinal extradural abscess or granuloma
Intraspinal subdural abscess or granuloma

EXCLUDES 1   tuberculous intraspinal abscess and granuloma (A17.81)

G06.2   Extradural and subdural abscess, unspecified   ▽

G07   Intracranial and intraspinal abscess and granuloma in diseases classified elsewhere
Code first underlying disease, such as:
schistosomiasis granuloma of brain (B65.-)

EXCLUDES 1   abscess of brain:
amebic (A06.6)
chromomycotic (B43.1)
gonococcal (A54.82)
tuberculous (A17.81)
tuberculoma of meninges (A17.1)

G08   Intracranial and intraspinal phlebitis and thrombophlebitis
Septic embolism of intracranial or intraspinal venous sinuses and veins
Septic endophlebitis of intracranial or intraspinal venous sinuses and veins
Septic phlebitis of intracranial or intraspinal venous sinuses and veins
Septic thrombophlebitis of intracranial or intraspinal venous sinuses and veins
Septic thrombosis of intracranial or intraspinal venous sinuses and veins

EXCLUDES 1   intracranial phlebitis and thrombophlebitis complicating:
abortion, ectopic or molar pregnancy (O00-O07, O08.7)
pregnancy, childbirth and the puerperium (O22.5, O87.3)
nonpyogenic intracranial phlebitis and thrombophlebitis (I67.6)

EXCLUDES 2   intracranial phlebitis and thrombophlebitis complicating nonpyogenic intraspinal phlebitis and thrombophlebitis (G95.1)

DEF: Inflammation and formation of blood clot in a vein within the brain or spine, or their linings.

G09   Sequelae of inflammatory diseases of central nervous system
NOTE   Category G09 is to be used to indicate conditions whose primary classification is to G00-G08 as the cause of sequelae, themselves classifiable elsewhere. The "sequelae" include conditions specified as residuals.
Code first condition resulting from (sequela) of inflammatory diseases of central nervous system

Systemic atrophies primarily affecting the central nervous system (G10-G14)

G10   Huntington's disease   HCC
Huntington's chorea
Huntington's dementia
▶Code also dementia in other diseases classified elsewhere without behavioral disturbance (F02.80)◀
DEF: Genetic disease caused by degeneration of nerve cells in the brain, characterized by chronic progressive mental deterioration; dementia and death within 15 to 20 years of onset.

☑4ᵗʰ **G11   Hereditary ataxia**
EXCLUDES 2   cerebral palsy (G80.-)
hereditary and idiopathic neuropathy (G60.-)
metabolic disorders (E70-E88)

G11.0   Congenital nonprogressive ataxia   HCC

G11.1   Early-onset cerebellar ataxia   HCC
Early-onset cerebellar ataxia with essential tremor
Early-onset cerebellar ataxia with myoclonus [Hunt's ataxia]
Early-onset cerebellar ataxia with retained tendon reflexes
Friedreich's ataxia (autosomal recessive)
X-linked recessive spinocerebellar ataxia

G11.2   Late-onset cerebellar ataxia   HCC A

G11.3   Cerebellar ataxia with defective DNA repair   HCC
Ataxia telangiectasia [Louis-Bar]
EXCLUDES 2   Cockayne's syndrome (Q87.1)
other disorders of purine and pyrimidine metabolism (E79.-)
xeroderma pigmentosum (Q82.1)

G11.4   Hereditary spastic paraplegia   HCC

G11.8   Other hereditary ataxias   HCC

G11.9   Hereditary ataxia, unspecified   HCC ▽
Hereditary cerebellar ataxia NOS
Hereditary cerebellar degeneration
Hereditary cerebellar disease
Hereditary cerebellar syndrome

☑4ᵗʰ **G12   Spinal muscular atrophy and related syndromes**

G12.0   Infantile spinal muscular atrophy, type I [Werdnig-Hoffman]   HCC

G12.1   Other inherited spinal muscular atrophy   HCC
Adult form spinal muscular atrophy
Childhood form, type II spinal muscular atrophy
Distal spinal muscular atrophy
Juvenile form, type III spinal muscular atrophy [Kugelberg-Welander]
Progressive bulbar palsy of childhood [Fazio-Londe]
Scapuloperoneal form spinal muscular atrophy

☑5ᵗʰ **G12.2   Motor neuron disease**

G12.20   Motor neuron disease, unspecified   HCC ▽

G12.21   Amyotrophic lateral sclerosis   HCC A
~~Progressive spinal muscle atrophy~~

G12.22   Progressive bulbar palsy   HCC

●   **G12.23   Primary lateral sclerosis**

●   **G12.24   Familial motor neuron disease**

●   **G12.25   Progressive spinal muscle atrophy**

G12.29   **Other motor neuron disease**   `HCC`
     ~~Familial motor neuron disease~~
     ~~Primary lateral sclerosis~~

G12.8   **Other spinal muscular atrophies and related syndromes**   `HCC`

G12.9   **Spinal muscular atrophy, unspecified**   `HCC` ▽

✓4ᵗʰ **G13   Systemic atrophies primarily affecting central nervous system in diseases classified elsewhere**

   G13.0   Paraneoplastic neuromyopathy and neuropathy   `HCC`
     Carcinomatous neuromyopathy
     Sensorial paraneoplastic neuropathy [Denny Brown]
     Code first underlying neoplasm (C00-D49)

   G13.1   Other systemic atrophy primarily affecting central nervous system in neoplastic disease   `HCC`
     Paraneoplastic limbic encephalopathy
     Code first underlying neoplasm (C00-D49)

   G13.2   Systemic atrophy primarily affecting the central nervous system in myxedema
     Code first underlying disease, such as:
       hypothyroidism (E03.-)
       myxedematous congenital iodine deficiency (E00.1)

   G13.8   Systemic atrophy primarily affecting central nervous system in other diseases classified elsewhere
     Code first underlying disease

G14   Postpolio syndrome
     Postpolio myelitic syndrome
     `EXCLUDES 1`   *sequelae of poliomyelitis (B91)*

Extrapyramidal and movement disorders (G20-G26)

G20   Parkinson's disease   `HCC`
     Hemiparkinsonism
     Idiopathic Parkinsonism or Parkinson's disease
     Paralysis agitans
     Parkinsonism or Parkinson's disease NOS
     Primary Parkinsonism or Parkinson's disease
     `EXCLUDES 1`   *dementia with Parkinsonism (G31.83)*
     AHA: 2017, 2Q, 7; 2016, 2Q, 6

✓4ᵗʰ **G21   Secondary parkinsonism**
     `EXCLUDES 1`   *dementia with Parkinsonism (G31.83)*
       Huntington's disease (G10)
       Shy-Drager syndrome (G90.3)
       syphilitic Parkinsonism (A52.19)

   G21.0   **Malignant neuroleptic syndrome**
     Use additional code for adverse effect, if applicable, to identify drug (T43.3X5, T43.4X5, T43.505, T43.595)
     `EXCLUDES 1`   *neuroleptic induced parkinsonism (G21.11)*

   ✓5ᵗʰ G21.1   **Other drug-induced secondary parkinsonism**

     G21.11   **Neuroleptic induced parkinsonism**   `HCC`
       Use additional code for adverse effect, if applicable, to identify drug (T43.3X5, T43.4X5, T43.505, T43.595)
       `EXCLUDES 1`   *malignant neuroleptic syndrome (G21.0)*

     G21.19   **Other drug induced secondary parkinsonism**   `HCC`
       ▶Other medication-induced parkinsonism◀
       Use additional code for adverse effect, if applicable, to identify drug (T36-T50 with fifth or sixth character 5)

   G21.2   **Secondary parkinsonism due to other external agents**   `HCC`
     Code first (T51-T65) to identify external agent

   G21.3   **Postencephalitic parkinsonism**   `HCC`

   G21.4   **Vascular parkinsonism**   `HCC`

   G21.8   **Other secondary parkinsonism**   `HCC`

   G21.9   **Secondary parkinsonism, unspecified**   `HCC` ▽

✓4ᵗʰ **G23   Other degenerative diseases of basal ganglia**
     `EXCLUDES 2`   *multi-system degeneration of the autonomic nervous system (G90.3)*

   G23.0   **Hallervorden-Spatz disease**   `HCC`
     Pigmentary pallidal degeneration

   G23.1   **Progressive supranuclear ophthalmoplegia [Steele-Richardson-Olszewski]**   `HCC`
     Progressive supranuclear palsy

   G23.2   **Striatonigral degeneration**   `HCC`

   G23.8   **Other specified degenerative diseases of basal ganglia**   `HCC`
     Calcification of basal ganglia

   G23.9   **Degenerative disease of basal ganglia, unspecified**   `HCC` ▽

✓4ᵗʰ **G24   Dystonia**
     `INCLUDES`   dyskinesia
     `EXCLUDES 2`   *athetoid cerebral palsy (G80.3)*

   ✓5ᵗʰ G24.0   **Drug induced dystonia**
     Use additional code for adverse effect, if applicable, to identify drug (T36-T50 with fifth or sixth character5)

     G24.01   **Drug induced subacute dyskinesia**
       Drug induced blepharospasm
       Drug induced orofacial dyskinesia
       Neuroleptic induced tardive dyskinesia
       Tardive dyskinesia

     G24.02   **Drug induced acute dystonia**
       Acute dystonic reaction to drugs
       Neuroleptic induced acute dystonia

     G24.09   **Other drug induced dystonia**

   G24.1   **Genetic torsion dystonia**
     Dystonia deformans progressiva
     Dystonia musculorum deformans
     Familial torsion dystonia
     Idiopathic familial dystonia
     Idiopathic (torsion) dystonia NOS
     (Schwalbe-) Ziehen-Oppenheim disease

   G24.2   **Idiopathic nonfamilial dystonia**

   G24.3   **Spasmodic torticollis**
     `EXCLUDES 1`   *congenital torticollis (Q68.0)*
       hysterical torticollis (F44.4)
       ocular torticollis (R29.891)
       psychogenic torticollis (F45.8)
       torticollis NOS (M43.6)
       traumatic recurrent torticollis (S13.4)

   G24.4   **Idiopathic orofacial dystonia**
     Orofacial dyskinesia
     `EXCLUDES 1`   *drug induced orofacial dyskinesia (G24.01)*

   G24.5   **Blepharospasm**
     `EXCLUDES 1`   *drug induced blepharospasm (G24.01)*

   G24.8   **Other dystonia**
     Acquired torsion dystonia NOS

   G24.9   **Dystonia, unspecified**   ▽
     Dyskinesia NOS

✓4ᵗʰ **G25   Other extrapyramidal and movement disorders**
     `EXCLUDES 2`   *sleep related movement disorders (G47.6-)*

   G25.0   **Essential tremor**
     Familial tremor
     `EXCLUDES 1`   *tremor NOS (R25.1)*

   G25.1   **Drug-induced tremor**
     Use additional code for adverse effect, if applicable, to identify drug (T36-T50 with fifth or sixth character 5)

   G25.2   **Other specified forms of tremor**
     Intention tremor

   G25.3   **Myoclonus**
     Drug-induced myoclonus
     Palatal myoclonus
     Use additional code for adverse effect, if applicable, to identify drug (T36-T50 with fifth or sixth character 5)
     `EXCLUDES 1`   *facial myokymia (G51.4)*
       myoclonic epilepsy (G40.-)

   G25.4   **Drug-induced chorea**
     Use additional code for adverse effect, if applicable, to identify drug (T36-T50 with fifth or sixth character 5)

   G25.5   **Other chorea**
     Chorea NOS
     `EXCLUDES 1`   *chorea NOS with heart involvement (I02.0)*
       Huntington's chorea (G10)
       rheumatic chorea (I02.-)
       Sydenham's chorea (I02.-)

   ✓5ᵗʰ G25.6   **Drug induced tics and other tics of organic origin**

     G25.61   **Drug induced tics**
       Use additional code for adverse effect, if applicable, to identify drug (T36-T50 with fifth or sixth character 5)

     G25.69   **Other tics of organic origin**
       `EXCLUDES 1`   *habit spasm (F95.9)*
       tic NOS (F95.9)
       Tourette's syndrome (F95.2)

   ✓5ᵗʰ G25.7   **Other and unspecified drug induced movement disorders**
     Use additional code for adverse effect, if applicable, to identify drug (T36-T50 with fifth or sixth character 5)

     G25.70   **Drug induced movement disorder, unspecified**   ▽

☑ Additional Character Req   `√x7ᵗʰ` Placeholder Alert   Manifestation   `HCC` CMS-HCC Condition   ▽ Unspecified Code   ▶◀ Revised Text   ● New Code   ▲ Revised Code Title

G25.71 **Drug induced akathisia**
Drug induced acathisia
Neuroleptic induced acute akathisia
▶Tardive akathisia◀

G25.79 **Other drug induced movement disorders**

✓5th **G25.8** **Other specified extrapyramidal and movement disorders**

G25.81 **Restless legs syndrome**
DEF: Neurological disorder of unknown etiology creating an irresistible urge to move the legs, which may temporarily relieve the symptoms; is accompanied by motor restlessness and sensations of pain, burning, prickling, or tingling.

G25.82 **Stiff-man syndrome**

G25.83 **Benign shuddering attacks**

G25.89 **Other specified extrapyramidal and movement disorders**

G25.9 **Extrapyramidal and movement disorder, unspecified** ▽

G26 *Extrapyramidal and movement disorders in diseases classified elsewhere*
Code first underlying disease

Other degenerative diseases of the nervous system (G30-G32)

✓4th **G30** **Alzheimer's disease**
INCLUDES Alzheimer's dementia senile and presenile forms
Use additional code to identify:
delirium, if applicable (F05)
dementia with behavioral disturbance (F02.81)
dementia without behavioral disturbance (F02.80)
EXCLUDES 1 *senile degeneration of brain NEC (G31.1)*
senile dementia NOS (F03)
senility NOS (R41.81)
AHA: 2017, 1Q, 43

G30.0 **Alzheimer's disease with early onset**

G30.1 **Alzheimer's disease with late onset** A

G30.8 **Other Alzheimer's disease**

G30.9 **Alzheimer's disease, unspecified** ▽
AHA: 2016, 2Q, 6; 2012, 4Q, 95

✓4th **G31** **Other degenerative diseases of nervous system, not elsewhere classified**
Use additional code to identify:
dementia with behavioral disturbance (F02.81)
dementia without behavioral disturbance (F02.80)
EXCLUDES 2 *Reye's syndrome (G93.7)*

✓5th **G31.0** **Frontotemporal dementia**

G31.01 **Pick's disease**
Primary progressive aphasia
Progressive isolated aphasia
DEF: A progressive frontotemporal dementia with asymmetrical atrophy of the frontal and temporal regions of the cerebral cortex, abnormal rounded brain cells called Pick cells with the presence of abnormal staining of protein (called tau); symptoms include prominent apathy, behavioral changes such as disinhibition and restlessness, echolalia, impairment of language, memory, and intellect, increased carelessness, poor personal hygiene, and decreased attention span.

G31.09 **Other frontotemporal dementia**
Frontal dementia

G31.1 **Senile degeneration of brain, not elsewhere classified**
EXCLUDES 1 *Alzheimer's disease (G30.-)*
senility NOS (R41.81)

G31.2 **Degeneration of nervous system due to alcohol**
Alcoholic cerebellar ataxia
Alcoholic cerebellar degeneration
Alcoholic cerebral degeneration
Alcoholic encephalopathy
Dysfunction of the autonomic nervous system due to alcohol
Code also associated alcoholism (F10.-)

✓5th **G31.8** **Other specified degenerative diseases of nervous system**

G31.81 **Alpers disease**
Grey-matter degeneration

G31.82 **Leigh's disease**
Subacute necrotizing encephalopathy

G31.83 **Dementia with Lewy bodies**
Dementia with Parkinsonism
Lewy body dementia
Lewy body disease
AHA: 2017, 2Q, 7; 2016, 4Q, 141
DEF: A cerebral dementia with neurophysiologic changes, increased hippocampal volume, hypoperfusion in the occipital lobes, beta amyloid deposits with neurofibrillary tangles, and atrophy of cortex and brainstem. Hallmark neuropsychological characteristics include fluctuating cognition with pronounced variation in attention and alertness; recurrent hallucinations; and Parkinsonism.

G31.84 **Mild cognitive impairment, so stated**
▶Mild neurocognitive disorder◀
EXCLUDES 1 *age related cognitive decline (R41.81)*
altered mental status (R41.82)
cerebral degeneration (G31.9)
change in mental status (R41.82)
cognitive deficits following (sequelae of) cerebral hemorrhage or infarction (I69.01-, I69.11-, I69.21-, I69.31-, I69.81-, I69.91-)
cognitive impairment due to intracranial or head injury (S06.-)
dementia (F01.-, F02.-, F03)
mild memory disturbance (F06.8)
neurologic neglect syndrome (R41.4)
personality change, nonpsychotic (F68.8)

G31.85 **Corticobasal degeneration**

G31.89 **Other specified degenerative diseases of nervous system**

G31.9 **Degenerative disease of nervous system, unspecified** ▽

✓4th **G32** **Other degenerative disorders of nervous system in diseases classified elsewhere**

G32.0 *Subacute combined degeneration of spinal cord in diseases classified elsewhere* HCC
Dana-Putnam syndrome
Sclerosis of spinal cord (combined) (dorsolateral) (posterolateral)
Code first underlying disease, such as:
vitamin B12 deficiency (E53.8)
vitamin B12 deficiency:
anemia (D51.9)
dietary (D51.3)
pernicious (D51.0)
EXCLUDES 1 *syphilitic combined degeneration of spinal cord (A52.11)*

✓5th **G32.8** **Other specified degenerative disorders of nervous system in diseases classified elsewhere**
Code first underlying disease, such as:
amyloidosis cerebral degeneration (E85.-)
cerebral degeneration (due to) hypothyroidism (E00.0-E03.9)
cerebral degeneration (due to) neoplasm (C00-D49)
cerebral degeneration (due to) vitamin B deficiency, except thiamine (E52-E53.-)
EXCLUDES 1 *superior hemorrhagic polioencephalitis [Wernicke's encephalopathy] (E51.2)*

G32.81 *Cerebellar ataxia in diseases classified elsewhere* HCC
Code first underlying disease, such as:
celiac disease (with gluten ataxia) (K90.0)
cerebellar ataxia (in) neoplastic disease (paraneoplastic cerebellar degeneration) (C00-D49)
non-celiac gluten ataxia (M35.9)
EXCLUDES 1 *systemic atrophy primarily affecting the central nervous system in alcoholic cerebellar ataxia (G31.2)*
systemic atrophy primarily affecting the central nervous system in myxedema (G13.2)

G32.89 *Other specified degenerative disorders of nervous system in diseases classified elsewhere*
Degenerative encephalopathy in diseases classified elsewhere

Demyelinating diseases of the central nervous system (G35-G37)

G35 **Multiple sclerosis** HCC
Disseminated multiple sclerosis
Generalized multiple sclerosis
Multiple sclerosis NOS
Multiple sclerosis of brain stem
Multiple sclerosis of cord

EXCLUDES 1 Not coded here   **EXCLUDES 2** Not included here   N Newborn Age: 0   P Pediatric Age: 0-17   M Maternity Age: 12-55   A Adult Age: 15-124

554   ICD-10-CM 2018

☑4ᵗʰ **G36** **Other acute disseminated demyelination**
> EXCLUDES 1   *postinfectious encephalitis and encephalomyelitis NOS (G04.01)*

G36.0 **Neuromyelitis optica [Devic]**   HCC
> Demyelination in optic neuritis
> EXCLUDES 1   *optic neuritis NOS (H46)*

G36.1 **Acute and subacute hemorrhagic leukoencephalitis [Hurst]**   HCC

G36.8 **Other specified acute disseminated demyelination**   HCC

G36.9 **Acute disseminated demyelination, unspecified**   HCC ▽

☑4ᵗʰ **G37** **Other demyelinating diseases of central nervous system**

G37.0 **Diffuse sclerosis of central nervous system**   HCC
> Periaxial encephalitis
> Schilder's disease
> EXCLUDES 1   *X linked adrenoleukodystrophy (E71.52-)*

G37.1 **Central demyelination of corpus callosum**   HCC

G37.2 **Central pontine myelinolysis**   HCC

G37.3 **Acute transverse myelitis in demyelinating disease of central nervous system**   HCC
> Acute transverse myelitis NOS
> Acute transverse myelopathy
> EXCLUDES 1   *multiple sclerosis (G35)*
>   *neuromyelitis optica [Devic] (G36.0)*

G37.4 **Subacute necrotizing myelitis of central nervous system**   HCC

G37.5 **Concentric sclerosis [Balo] of central nervous system**   HCC

G37.8 **Other specified demyelinating diseases of central nervous system**   HCC

G37.9 **Demyelinating disease of central nervous system, unspecified**   HCC ▽

Episodic and paroxysmal disorders (G40-G47)

☑4ᵗʰ **G40** **Epilepsy and recurrent seizures**
> NOTE   The following terms are to be considered equivalent to intractable: pharmacoresistant (pharmacologically resistant), treatment resistant, refractory (medically) and poorly controlled
> EXCLUDES 1   *conversion disorder with seizures (F44.5)*
>   *convulsions NOS (R56.9)*
>   *post traumatic seizures (R56.1)*
>   *seizure (convulsive) NOS (R56.9)*
>   *seizure of newborn (P90)*
> EXCLUDES 2   *hippocampal sclerosis (G93.81)*
>   *mesial temporal sclerosis (G93.81)*
>   *temporal sclerosis (G93.81)*
>   *Todd's paralysis (G83.84)*

☑5ᵗʰ **G40.0** **Localization-related (focal) (partial) idiopathic epilepsy and epileptic syndromes with seizures of localized onset**
> Benign childhood epilepsy with centrotemporal EEG spikes
> Childhood epilepsy with occipital EEG paroxysms
> EXCLUDES 1   *adult onset localization-related epilepsy (G40.1-, G40.2-)*

☑6ᵗʰ **G40.00** **Localization-related (focal) (partial) idiopathic epilepsy and epileptic syndromes with seizures of localized onset, not intractable**
> Localization-related (focal) (partial) idiopathic epilepsy and epileptic syndromes with seizures of localized onset without intractability

G40.001 **Localization-related (focal) (partial) idiopathic epilepsy and epileptic syndromes with seizures of localized onset, not intractable, with status epilepticus**   HCC

G40.009 **Localization-related (focal) (partial) idiopathic epilepsy and epileptic syndromes with seizures of localized onset, not intractable, without status epilepticus**   HCC
> Localization-related (focal) (partial) idiopathic epilepsy and epileptic syndromes with seizures of localized onset NOS

☑6ᵗʰ **G40.01** **Localization-related (focal) (partial) idiopathic epilepsy and epileptic syndromes with seizures of localized onset, intractable**

G40.011 **Localization-related (focal) (partial) idiopathic epilepsy and epileptic syndromes with seizures of localized onset, intractable, with status epilepticus**   HCC

G40.019 **Localization-related (focal) (partial) idiopathic epilepsy and epileptic syndromes with seizures of localized onset, intractable, without status epilepticus**   HCC

☑5ᵗʰ **G40.1** **Localization-related (focal) (partial) symptomatic epilepsy and epileptic syndromes with simple partial seizures**
> Attacks without alteration of consciousness
> Epilepsia partialis continua [Kozhevnikof]
> Simple partial seizures developing into secondarily generalized seizures

☑6ᵗʰ **G40.10** **Localization-related (focal) (partial) symptomatic epilepsy and epileptic syndromes with simple partial seizures, not intractable**
> Localization-related (focal) (partial) symptomatic epilepsy and epileptic syndromes with simple partial seizures without intractability

G40.101 **Localization-related (focal) (partial) symptomatic epilepsy and epileptic syndromes with simple partial seizures, not intractable, with status epilepticus**   HCC

G40.109 **Localization-related (focal) (partial) symptomatic epilepsy and epileptic syndromes with simple partial seizures, not intractable, without status epilepticus**   HCC
> Localization-related (focal) (partial) symptomatic epilepsy and epileptic syndromes with simple partial seizures NOS

☑6ᵗʰ **G40.11** **Localization-related (focal) (partial) symptomatic epilepsy and epileptic syndromes with simple partial seizures, intractable**

G40.111 **Localization-related (focal) (partial) symptomatic epilepsy and epileptic syndromes with simple partial seizures, intractable, with status epilepticus**   HCC

G40.119 **Localization-related (focal) (partial) symptomatic epilepsy and epileptic syndromes with simple partial seizures, intractable, without status epilepticus**   HCC

☑5ᵗʰ **G40.2** **Localization-related (focal) (partial) symptomatic epilepsy and epileptic syndromes with complex partial seizures**
> Attacks with alteration of consciousness, often with automatisms
> Complex partial seizures developing into secondarily generalized seizures

☑6ᵗʰ **G40.20** **Localization-related (focal) (partial) symptomatic epilepsy and epileptic syndromes with complex partial seizures, not intractable**
> Localization-related (focal) (partial) symptomatic epilepsy and epileptic syndromes with complex partial seizures without intractability

G40.201 **Localization-related (focal) (partial) symptomatic epilepsy and epileptic syndromes with complex partial seizures, not intractable, with status epilepticus**   HCC

G40.209 **Localization-related (focal) (partial) symptomatic epilepsy and epileptic syndromes with complex partial seizures, not intractable, without status epilepticus**   HCC
> Localization-related (focal) (partial) symptomatic epilepsy and epileptic syndromes with complex partial seizures NOS

☑6ᵗʰ **G40.21** **Localization-related (focal) (partial) symptomatic epilepsy and epileptic syndromes with complex partial seizures, intractable**

G40.211 **Localization-related (focal) (partial) symptomatic epilepsy and epileptic syndromes with complex partial seizures, intractable, with status epilepticus**   HCC

G40.219 **Localization-related (focal) (partial) symptomatic epilepsy and epileptic syndromes with complex partial seizures, intractable, without status epilepticus**   HCC

☑5ᵗʰ **G40.3** **Generalized idiopathic epilepsy and epileptic syndromes**
> Code also MERRF syndrome, if applicable (E88.42)

☑6ᵗʰ **G40.30** **Generalized idiopathic epilepsy and epileptic syndromes, not intractable**
> Generalized idiopathic epilepsy and epileptic syndromes without intractability

---

G40.301   Generalized idiopathic epilepsy and epileptic syndromes, not intractable, with status epilepticus   **HCC**

G40.309   Generalized idiopathic epilepsy and epileptic syndromes, not intractable, without status epilepticus   **HCC**
     Generalized idiopathic epilepsy and epileptic syndromes NOS

✓6th **G40.31**   Generalized idiopathic epilepsy and epileptic syndromes, intractable

G40.311   Generalized idiopathic epilepsy and epileptic syndromes, intractable, with status epilepticus   **HCC**

G40.319   Generalized idiopathic epilepsy and epileptic syndromes, intractable, without status epilepticus   **HCC**

✓5th **G40.A**   Absence epileptic syndrome
     Childhood absence epilepsy [pyknolepsy]
     Juvenile absence epilepsy
     Absence epileptic syndrome, NOS

✓6th **G40.A0**   Absence epileptic syndrome, not intractable

G40.A01   Absence epileptic syndrome, not intractable, with status epilepticus   **HCC**

G40.A09   Absence epileptic syndrome, not intractable, without status epilepticus   **HCC**

✓6th **G40.A1**   Absence epileptic syndrome, intractable

G40.A11   Absence epileptic syndrome, intractable, with status epilepticus   **HCC**

G40.A19   Absence epileptic syndrome, intractable, without status epilepticus   **HCC**

✓5th **G40.B**   Juvenile myoclonic epilepsy [impulsive petit mal]

✓6th **G40.B0**   Juvenile myoclonic epilepsy, not intractable

G40.B01   Juvenile myoclonic epilepsy, not intractable, with status epilepticus   **HCC**

G40.B09   Juvenile myoclonic epilepsy, not intractable, without status epilepticus   **HCC**

✓6th **G40.B1**   Juvenile myoclonic epilepsy, intractable

G40.B11   Juvenile myoclonic epilepsy, intractable, with status epilepticus   **HCC**

G40.B19   Juvenile myoclonic epilepsy, intractable, without status epilepticus   **HCC**

✓5th **G40.4**   Other generalized epilepsy and epileptic syndromes
     Epilepsy with grand mal seizures on awakening
     Epilepsy with myoclonic absences
     Epilepsy with myoclonic-astatic seizures
     Grand mal seizure NOS
     Nonspecific atonic epileptic seizures
     Nonspecific clonic epileptic seizures
     Nonspecific myoclonic epileptic seizures
     Nonspecific tonic epileptic seizures
     Nonspecific tonic-clonic epileptic seizures
     Symptomatic early myoclonic encephalopathy

✓6th **G40.40**   Other generalized epilepsy and epileptic syndromes, not intractable
     Other generalized epilepsy and epileptic syndromes without intractability
     Other generalized epilepsy and epileptic syndromes NOS

G40.401   Other generalized epilepsy and epileptic syndromes, not intractable, with status epilepticus   **HCC**

G40.409   Other generalized epilepsy and epileptic syndromes, not intractable, without status epilepticus   **HCC**

✓6th **G40.41**   Other generalized epilepsy and epileptic syndromes, intractable

G40.411   Other generalized epilepsy and epileptic syndromes, intractable, with status epilepticus   **HCC**

G40.419   Other generalized epilepsy and epileptic syndromes, intractable, without status epilepticus   **HCC**

✓5th **G40.5**   Epileptic seizures related to external causes
     Epileptic seizures related to alcohol
     Epileptic seizures related to drugs
     Epileptic seizures related to hormonal changes
     Epileptic seizures related to sleep deprivation
     Epileptic seizures related to stress
     Code also, if applicable, associated epilepsy and recurrent seizures (G40.-)
     Use additional code for adverse effect, if applicable, to identify drug (T36-T50 with fifth or sixth character 5)

✓6th **G40.50**   Epileptic seizures related to external causes, not intractable

G40.501   Epileptic seizures related to external causes, not intractable, with status epilepticus   **HCC**

G40.509   Epileptic seizures related to external causes, not intractable, without status epilepticus   **HCC**
     Epileptic seizures related to external causes, NOS

✓5th **G40.8**   Other epilepsy and recurrent seizures
     Epilepsies and epileptic syndromes undetermined as to whether they are focal or generalized
     Landau-Kleffner syndrome

✓6th **G40.80**   Other epilepsy

G40.801   Other epilepsy, not intractable, with status epilepticus   **HCC**
     Other epilepsy without intractability with status epilepticus

G40.802   Other epilepsy, not intractable, without status epilepticus   **HCC**
     Other epilepsy NOS
     Other epilepsy without intractability without status epilepticus

G40.803   Other epilepsy, intractable, with status epilepticus   **HCC**

G40.804   Other epilepsy, intractable, without status epilepticus   **HCC**

✓6th **G40.81**   Lennox-Gastaut syndrome

G40.811   Lennox-Gastaut syndrome, not intractable, with status epilepticus   **HCC**

G40.812   Lennox-Gastaut syndrome, not intractable, without status epilepticus   **HCC**

G40.813   Lennox-Gastaut syndrome, intractable, with status epilepticus   **HCC**

G40.814   Lennox-Gastaut syndrome, intractable, without status epilepticus   **HCC**

✓6th **G40.82**   Epileptic spasms
     Infantile spasms
     Salaam attacks
     West's syndrome

G40.821   Epileptic spasms, not intractable, with status epilepticus   **HCC**

G40.822   Epileptic spasms, not intractable, without status epilepticus   **HCC**

G40.823   Epileptic spasms, intractable, with status epilepticus   **HCC**

G40.824   Epileptic spasms, intractable, without status epilepticus   **HCC**

G40.89   Other seizures   **HCC**
     EXCLUDES 1   *post traumatic seizures (R56.1)*
         recurrent seizures NOS (G40.909)
         seizure NOS (R56.9)

✓5th **G40.9**   Epilepsy, unspecified

✓6th **G40.90**   Epilepsy, unspecified, not intractable
     Epilepsy, unspecified, without intractability

G40.901   Epilepsy, unspecified, not intractable, with status epilepticus   **HCC** ▽

G40.909   Epilepsy, unspecified, not intractable, without status epilepticus   **HCC** ▽
     Epilepsy NOS
     Epileptic convulsions NOS
     Epileptic fits NOS
     Epileptic seizures NOS
     Recurrent seizures NOS
     Seizure disorder NOS

EXCLUDES 1 Not coded here   **EXCLUDES 2** Not included here   **N** Newborn Age: 0   **P** Pediatric Age: 0-17   **M** Maternity Age: 12-55   **A** Adult Age: 15-124

556   ICD-10-CM 2018

✓6ᵗʰ **G40.91** **Epilepsy, unspecified, intractable**
Intractable seizure disorder NOS

G40.911 **Epilepsy, unspecified, intractable,** ᴴᶜᶜ ▽
with status epilepticus

G40.919 **Epilepsy, unspecified, intractable,** ᴴᶜᶜ ▽
without status epilepticus

✓4ᵗʰ **G43** **Migraine**
NOTE The following terms are to be considered equivalent to
intractable: pharmacoresistant (pharmacologically resistant),
treatment resistant, refractory (medically) and poorly
controlled.
Use additional code for adverse effect, if applicable, to identify drug
(T36-T50 with fifth or sixth character 5)
EXCLUDES 1 *headache NOS (R51)*
lower half migraine (G44.00)
EXCLUDES 2 *headache syndromes (G44.-)*

✓5ᵗʰ **G43.0** **Migraine without aura**
Common migraine
EXCLUDES 1 *chronic migraine without aura (G43.7-)*

✓6ᵗʰ **G43.00** **Migraine without aura, not intractable**
Migraine without aura without mention of refractory
migraine

G43.001 **Migraine without aura, not intractable,**
with status migrainosus

G43.009 **Migraine without aura, not intractable,**
without status migrainosus
Migraine without aura NOS

✓6ᵗʰ **G43.01** **Migraine without aura, intractable**
Migraine without aura with refractory migraine

G43.011 **Migraine without aura, intractable, with**
status migrainosus

G43.019 **Migraine without aura, intractable,**
without status migrainosus

✓5ᵗʰ **G43.1** **Migraine with aura**
Basilar migraine
Classical migraine
Migraine equivalents
Migraine preceded or accompanied by transient focal
neurological phenomena
Migraine triggered seizures
Migraine with acute-onset aura
Migraine with aura without headache (migraine equivalents)
Migraine with prolonged aura
Migraine with typical aura
Retinal migraine
Code also any associated seizure (G40.-, R56.9)
EXCLUDES 1 *persistent migraine aura (G43.5-, G43.6-)*

✓6ᵗʰ **G43.10** **Migraine with aura, not intractable**
Migraine with aura without mention of refractory
migraine

G43.101 **Migraine with aura, not intractable, with**
status migrainosus

G43.109 **Migraine with aura, not intractable,**
without status migrainosus
Migraine with aura NOS

✓6ᵗʰ **G43.11** **Migraine with aura, intractable**
Migraine with aura with refractory migraine

G43.111 **Migraine with aura, intractable, with**
status migrainosus

G43.119 **Migraine with aura, intractable, without**
status migrainosus

✓5ᵗʰ **G43.4** **Hemiplegic migraine**
Familial migraine
Sporadic migraine

✓6ᵗʰ **G43.40** **Hemiplegic migraine, not intractable**
Hemiplegic migraine without refractory migraine

G43.401 **Hemiplegic migraine, not intractable, with**
status migrainosus

G43.409 **Hemiplegic migraine, not intractable,**
without status migrainosus
Hemiplegic migraine NOS

✓6ᵗʰ **G43.41** **Hemiplegic migraine, intractable**
Hemiplegic migraine with refractory migraine

G43.411 **Hemiplegic migraine, intractable, with**
status migrainosus

G43.419 **Hemiplegic migraine, intractable, without**
status migrainosus

✓5ᵗʰ **G43.5** **Persistent migraine aura without cerebral infarction**

✓6ᵗʰ **G43.50** **Persistent migraine aura without cerebral infarction,**
not intractable
Persistent migraine aura without cerebral infarction,
without refractory migraine

G43.501 **Persistent migraine aura without cerebral**
infarction, not intractable, with status
migrainosus

G43.509 **Persistent migraine aura without cerebral**
infarction, not intractable, without status
migrainosus
Persistent migraine aura NOS

✓6ᵗʰ **G43.51** **Persistent migraine aura without cerebral infarction,**
intractable
Persistent migraine aura without cerebral infarction,
with refractory migraine

G43.511 **Persistent migraine aura without cerebral**
infarction, intractable, with status
migrainosus

G43.519 **Persistent migraine aura without cerebral**
infarction, intractable, without status
migrainosus

✓5ᵗʰ **G43.6** **Persistent migraine aura with cerebral infarction**
Code also the type of cerebral infarction (I63.-)

✓6ᵗʰ **G43.60** **Persistent migraine aura with cerebral infarction,**
not intractable
Persistent migraine aura with cerebral infarction,
without refractory migraine

G43.601 **Persistent migraine aura with cerebral**
infarction, not intractable, with status
migrainosus

G43.609 **Persistent migraine aura with cerebral**
infarction, not intractable, without status
migrainosus

✓6ᵗʰ **G43.61** **Persistent migraine aura with cerebral infarction,**
intractable
Persistent migraine aura with cerebral infarction, with
refractory migraine

G43.611 **Persistent migraine aura with cerebral**
infarction, intractable, with status
migrainosus

G43.619 **Persistent migraine aura with cerebral**
infarction, intractable, without status
migrainosus

✓5ᵗʰ **G43.7** **Chronic migraine without aura**
Transformed migraine
EXCLUDES 1 *migraine without aura (G43.0-)*

✓6ᵗʰ **G43.70** **Chronic migraine without aura, not intractable**
Chronic migraine without aura, without refractory
migraine

G43.701 **Chronic migraine without aura, not**
intractable, with status migrainosus

G43.709 **Chronic migraine without aura, not**
intractable, without status migrainosus
Chronic migraine without aura NOS

✓6ᵗʰ **G43.71** **Chronic migraine without aura, intractable**
Chronic migraine without aura, with refractory
migraine

G43.711 **Chronic migraine without aura,**
intractable, with status migrainosus

G43.719 **Chronic migraine without aura,**
intractable, without status migrainosus

✓5ᵗʰ **G43.A** **Cyclical vomiting**

G43.A0 **Cyclical vomiting, not intractable**
Cyclical vomiting, without refractory migraine

G43.A1 **Cyclical vomiting, intractable**
Cyclical vomiting, with refractory migraine

✓5ᵗʰ **G43.B** **Ophthalmoplegic migraine**

G43.B0 **Ophthalmoplegic migraine, not intractable**
Ophthalmoplegic migraine, without refractory
migraine

G43.B1 **Ophthalmoplegic migraine, intractable**
Ophthalmoplegic migraine, with refractory migraine

✓5ᵗʰ **G43.C** **Periodic headache syndromes in child or adult**

G43.C0 **Periodic headache syndromes in child or adult, not**
intractable
Periodic headache syndromes in child or adult,
without refractory migraine

☑ Additional Character Req   ✓7ᵗʰ Placeholder Alert   Manifestation   ᴴᶜᶜ CMS-HCC Condition   ▽ Unspecified Code   ▶◀ Revised Text   ● New Code   ▲ Revised Code Title

G43.C1 **Periodic headache syndromes in child or adult, intractable**
Periodic headache syndromes in child or adult, with refractory migraine

✓5ᵗʰ **G43.D** **Abdominal migraine**

G43.D0 **Abdominal migraine, not intractable**
Abdominal migraine, without refractory migraine

G43.D1 **Abdominal migraine, intractable**
Abdominal migraine, with refractory migraine

✓5ᵗʰ **G43.8** **Other migraine**

✓6ᵗʰ **G43.80** **Other migraine, not intractable**
Other migraine, without refractory migraine

G43.801 **Other migraine, not intractable, with status migrainosus**

G43.809 **Other migraine, not intractable, without status migrainosus**

✓6ᵗʰ **G43.81** **Other migraine, intractable**
Other migraine, with refractory migraine

G43.811 **Other migraine, intractable, with status migrainosus**

G43.819 **Other migraine, intractable, without status migrainosus**

✓6ᵗʰ **G43.82** **Menstrual migraine, not intractable**
Menstrual headache, not intractable
Menstrual migraine, without refractory migraine
Menstrually related migraine, not intractable
Pre-menstrual headache, not intractable
Pre-menstrual migraine, not intractable
Pure menstrual migraine, not intractable
Code also associated premenstrual tension syndrome (N94.3)

G43.821 **Menstrual migraine, not intractable, with status migrainosus** ♀

G43.829 **Menstrual migraine, not intractable, without status migrainosus** ♀
Menstrual migraine NOS

✓6ᵗʰ **G43.83** **Menstrual migraine, intractable**
Menstrual headache, intractable
Menstrual migraine, with refractory migraine
Menstrually related migraine, intractable
Pre-menstrual headache, intractable
Pre-menstrual migraine, intractable
Pure menstrual migraine, intractable
Code also associated premenstrual tension syndrome (N94.3)

G43.831 **Menstrual migraine, intractable, with status migrainosus** ♀

G43.839 **Menstrual migraine, intractable, without status migrainosus** ♀

✓5ᵗʰ **G43.9** **Migraine, unspecified**

✓6ᵗʰ **G43.90** **Migraine, unspecified, not intractable**
Migraine, unspecified, without refractory migraine

G43.901 **Migraine, unspecified, not intractable, with status migrainosus** ▽
Status migrainosus NOS

G43.909 **Migraine, unspecified, not intractable, without status migrainosus** ▽
Migraine NOS

✓6ᵗʰ **G43.91** **Migraine, unspecified, intractable**
Migraine, unspecified, with refractory migraine

G43.911 **Migraine, unspecified, intractable, with status migrainosus** ▽

G43.919 **Migraine, unspecified, intractable, without status migrainosus** ▽

✓4ᵗʰ **G44** **Other headache syndromes**
EXCLUDES 1   headache NOS (R51)
EXCLUDES 2   atypical facial pain (G50.1)
headache due to lumbar puncture (G97.1)
migraines (G43.-)
trigeminal neuralgia (G50.0)

✓5ᵗʰ **G44.0** **Cluster headaches and other trigeminal autonomic cephalgias (TAC)**

✓6ᵗʰ **G44.00** **Cluster headache syndrome, unspecified**
Ciliary neuralgia
Cluster headache NOS
Histamine cephalgia
Lower half migraine
Migrainous neuralgia

G44.001 **Cluster headache syndrome, unspecified, intractable** ▽

G44.009 **Cluster headache syndrome, unspecified, not intractable** ▽
Cluster headache syndrome NOS

✓6ᵗʰ **G44.01** **Episodic cluster headache**

G44.011 **Episodic cluster headache, intractable**

G44.019 **Episodic cluster headache, not intractable**
Episodic cluster headache NOS

✓6ᵗʰ **G44.02** **Chronic cluster headache**

G44.021 **Chronic cluster headache, intractable**

G44.029 **Chronic cluster headache, not intractable**
Chronic cluster headache NOS

✓6ᵗʰ **G44.03** **Episodic paroxysmal hemicrania**
Paroxysmal hemicrania NOS

G44.031 **Episodic paroxysmal hemicrania, intractable**

G44.039 **Episodic paroxysmal hemicrania, not intractable**
Episodic paroxysmal hemicrania NOS

✓6ᵗʰ **G44.04** **Chronic paroxysmal hemicrania**

G44.041 **Chronic paroxysmal hemicrania, intractable**

G44.049 **Chronic paroxysmal hemicrania, not intractable**
Chronic paroxysmal hemicrania NOS

✓6ᵗʰ **G44.05** **Short lasting unilateral neuralgiform headache with conjunctival injection and tearing (SUNCT)**

G44.051 **Short lasting unilateral neuralgiform headache with conjunctival injection and tearing (SUNCT), intractable**

G44.059 **Short lasting unilateral neuralgiform headache with conjunctival injection and tearing (SUNCT), not intractable**
Short lasting unilateral neuralgiform headache with conjunctival injection and tearing (SUNCT) NOS

✓6ᵗʰ **G44.09** **Other trigeminal autonomic cephalgias (TAC)**

G44.091 **Other trigeminal autonomic cephalgias (TAC), intractable**

G44.099 **Other trigeminal autonomic cephalgias syndrome (TAC), not intractable**

G44.1 **Vascular headache, not elsewhere classified**
EXCLUDES 2   cluster headache (G44.0)
complicated headache syndromes (G44.5-)
drug-induced headache (G44.4-)
migraine (G43.-)
other specified headache syndromes (G44.8-)
post-traumatic headache (G44.3-)
tension-type headache (G44.2-)

✓5ᵗʰ **G44.2** **Tension-type headache**

✓6ᵗʰ **G44.20** **Tension-type headache, unspecified**

G44.201 **Tension-type headache, unspecified, intractable** ▽

G44.209 **Tension-type headache, unspecified, not intractable** ▽
Tension headache NOS

✓6ᵗʰ **G44.21** **Episodic tension-type headache**

G44.211 **Episodic tension-type headache, intractable**

G44.219 **Episodic tension-type headache, not intractable**
Episodic tension-type headache NOS

EXCLUDES 1 Not coded here   EXCLUDES 2 Not included here   N Newborn Age: 0   P Pediatric Age: 0-17   M Maternity Age: 12-55   A Adult Age: 15-124

558   ICD-10-CM 2018

☑6ᵗʰ **G44.22**   **Chronic tension-type headache**
     G44.221   **Chronic tension-type headache, intractable**
     G44.229   **Chronic tension-type headache, not intractable**
          Chronic tension-type headache NOS

☑5ᵗʰ **G44.3**   **Post-traumatic headache**
   ☑6ᵗʰ **G44.30**   **Post-traumatic headache, unspecified**
       G44.301   **Post-traumatic headache, unspecified, intractable** ▽
       G44.309   **Post-traumatic headache, unspecified, not intractable** ▽
          Post-traumatic headache NOS

   ☑6ᵗʰ **G44.31**   **Acute post-traumatic headache**
       G44.311   **Acute post-traumatic headache, intractable**
       G44.319   **Acute post-traumatic headache, not intractable**
          Acute post-traumatic headache NOS

   ☑6ᵗʰ **G44.32**   **Chronic post-traumatic headache**
       G44.321   **Chronic post-traumatic headache, intractable**
       G44.329   **Chronic post-traumatic headache, not intractable**
          Chronic post-traumatic headache NOS

☑5ᵗʰ **G44.4**   **Drug-induced headache, not elsewhere classified**
     Medication overuse headache
     Use additional code for adverse effect, if applicable, to identify drug (T36-T50 with fifth or sixth character 5)
     G44.40   **Drug-induced headache, not elsewhere classified, not intractable**
     G44.41   **Drug-induced headache, not elsewhere classified, intractable**

☑5ᵗʰ **G44.5**   **Complicated headache syndromes**
     G44.51   **Hemicrania continua**
     G44.52   **New daily persistent headache (NDPH)**
     G44.53   **Primary thunderclap headache**
     G44.59   **Other complicated headache syndrome**

☑5ᵗʰ **G44.8**   **Other specified headache syndromes**
     G44.81   **Hypnic headache**
     G44.82   **Headache associated with sexual activity**
          Orgasmic headache
          Preorgasmic headache
     G44.83   **Primary cough headache**
     G44.84   **Primary exertional headache**
     G44.85   **Primary stabbing headache**
     G44.89   **Other headache syndrome**

☑4ᵗʰ **G45**   **Transient cerebral ischemic attacks and related syndromes**
     EXCLUDES 1   neonatal cerebral ischemia (P91.0)
          transient retinal artery occlusion (H34.0-)
     G45.0   **Vertebro-basilar artery syndrome**
     G45.1   **Carotid artery syndrome (hemispheric)**
     G45.2   **Multiple and bilateral precerebral artery syndromes**
     G45.3   **Amaurosis fugax**
     G45.4   **Transient global amnesia**
         EXCLUDES 1   amnesia NOS (R41.3)
     G45.8   **Other transient cerebral ischemic attacks and related syndromes**
     G45.9   **Transient cerebral ischemic attack, unspecified** ▽
          Spasm of cerebral artery
          TIA
          Transient cerebral ischemia NOS

☑4ᵗʰ **G46**   **Vascular syndromes of brain in cerebrovascular diseases**
     Code first underlying cerebrovascular disease (I60-I69)
     G46.0   **Middle cerebral artery syndrome**
     G46.1   **Anterior cerebral artery syndrome**
     G46.2   **Posterior cerebral artery syndrome**
     G46.3   **Brain stem stroke syndrome**
          Benedikt syndrome
          Claude syndrome
          Foville syndrome
          Millard-Gubler syndrome
          Wallenberg syndrome
          Weber syndrome
     G46.4   **Cerebellar stroke syndrome**

     G46.5   **Pure motor lacunar syndrome**
     G46.6   **Pure sensory lacunar syndrome**
     G46.7   **Other lacunar syndromes**
     G46.8   **Other vascular syndromes of brain in cerebrovascular diseases**

☑4ᵗʰ **G47**   **Sleep disorders**
     EXCLUDES 2   nightmares (F51.5)
          nonorganic sleep disorders (F51.-)
          sleep terrors (F51.4)
          sleepwalking (F51.3)

   ☑5ᵗʰ **G47.0**   **Insomnia**
       EXCLUDES 2   alcohol related insomnia (F10.182, F10.282, F10.982)
          drug-related insomnia (F11.182, F11.282, F11.982, F13.182, F13.282, F13.982, F14.182, F14.282, F14.982, F15.182, F15.282, F15.982, F19.182, F19.282, F19.982)
          idiopathic insomnia (F51.01)
          insomnia due to a mental disorder (F51.05)
          insomnia not due to a substance or known physiological condition (F51.0-)
          nonorganic insomnia (F51.0-)
          primary insomnia (F51.01)
          sleep apnea (G47.3-)
       G47.00   **Insomnia, unspecified** ▽
          Insomnia NOS
       G47.01   **Insomnia due to medical condition**
          Code also associated medical condition
       G47.09   **Other insomnia**

   ☑5ᵗʰ **G47.1**   **Hypersomnia**
       EXCLUDES 2   alcohol-related hypersomnia (F10.182, F10.282, F10.982)
          drug-related hypersomnia (F11.182, F11.282, F11.982, F13.182, F13.282, F13.982, F14.182, F14.282, F14.982, F15.182, F15.282, F15.982, F19.182, F19.282, F19.982)
          hypersomnia due to a mental disorder (F51.13)
          hypersomnia not due to a substance or known physiological condition (F51.1-)
          primary hypersomnia (F51.11)
          sleep apnea (G47.3-)
       G47.10   **Hypersomnia, unspecified** ▽
          Hypersomnia NOS
       G47.11   **Idiopathic hypersomnia with long sleep time**
          Idiopathic hypersomnia NOS
       G47.12   **Idiopathic hypersomnia without long sleep time**
       G47.13   **Recurrent hypersomnia**
          Kleine-Levin syndrome
          Menstrual related hypersomnia
       G47.14   **Hypersomnia due to medical condition**
          Code also associated medical condition
       G47.19   **Other hypersomnia**

   ☑5ᵗʰ **G47.2**   **Circadian rhythm sleep disorders**
       Disorders of the sleep wake schedule
       Inversion of nyctohemeral rhythm
       Inversion of sleep rhythm
       G47.20   **Circadian rhythm sleep disorder, unspecified type** ▽
          Sleep wake schedule disorder NOS
       G47.21   **Circadian rhythm sleep disorder, delayed sleep phase type**
          Delayed sleep phase syndrome
       G47.22   **Circadian rhythm sleep disorder, advanced sleep phase type**
       G47.23   **Circadian rhythm sleep disorder, irregular sleep wake type**
          Irregular sleep-wake pattern
       G47.24   **Circadian rhythm sleep disorder, free running type**
          ▶Circadian rhythm sleep disorder, non-24-hour sleep-wake type◀
       G47.25   **Circadian rhythm sleep disorder, jet lag type**
       G47.26   **Circadian rhythm sleep disorder, shift work type**
       G47.27   *Circadian rhythm sleep disorder in conditions classified elsewhere*
          Code first underlying condition
       G47.29   **Other circadian rhythm sleep disorder**

☑ Additional Character Req   ✓ᵡ7ᵗʰ Placeholder Alert   Manifestation   HCC CMS-HCC Condition   ▽ Unspecified Code   ▶◀ Revised Text   ● New Code   ▲ Revised Code Title

ICD-10-CM 2018   **559**

☑5th **G47.3　Sleep apnea**
　　　Code also any associated underlying condition
　　　EXCLUDES 1　apnea NOS (R06.81)
　　　　　　　Cheyne-Stokes breathing (R06.3)
　　　　　　　pickwickian syndrome (E66.2)
　　　　　　　sleep apnea of newborn (P28.3)

　　G47.30　Sleep apnea, unspecified　　　▽
　　　　　Sleep apnea NOS

　　G47.31　Primary central sleep apnea
　　　　　►Idiopathic central sleep apnea◄

　　G47.32　High altitude periodic breathing

　　G47.33　Obstructive sleep apnea (adult) (pediatric)
　　　　　►Obstructive sleep apnea hypopnea◄
　　　　　EXCLUDES 1　obstructive sleep apnea of newborn (P28.3)

　　G47.34　Idiopathic sleep related nonobstructive alveolar hypoventilation
　　　　　Sleep related hypoxia

　　G47.35　Congenital central alveolar hypoventilation syndrome

　　G47.36　Sleep related hypoventilation in conditions classified elsewhere
　　　　　Sleep related hypoxemia in conditions classified elsewhere
　　　　　Code first underlying condition

　　G47.37　Central sleep apnea in conditions classified elsewhere
　　　　　Code first underlying condition

　　G47.39　Other sleep apnea

☑5th **G47.4　Narcolepsy and cataplexy**

　☑6th **G47.41　Narcolepsy**
　　　　G47.411　Narcolepsy with cataplexy
　　　　G47.419　Narcolepsy without cataplexy
　　　　　　Narcolepsy NOS

　☑6th **G47.42　Narcolepsy in conditions classified elsewhere**
　　　　Code first underlying condition
　　　　G47.421　Narcolepsy in conditions classified elsewhere with cataplexy
　　　　G47.429　Narcolepsy in conditions classified elsewhere without cataplexy

☑5th **G47.5　Parasomnia**
　　　EXCLUDES 1　alcohol induced parasomnia (F10.182, F10.282, F10.982)
　　　　　　　drug induced parasomnia (F11.182, F11.282, F11.982, F13.182, F13.282, F13.982, F14.182, F14.282, F14.982, F15.182, F15.282, F15.982, F19.182, F19.282, F19.982)
　　　　　　　parasomnia not due to a substance or known physiological condition (F51.8)

　　G47.50　Parasomnia, unspecified　　　▽
　　　　　Parasomnia NOS

　　G47.51　Confusional arousals

　　G47.52　REM sleep behavior disorder

　　G47.53　Recurrent isolated sleep paralysis

　　G47.54　Parasomnia in conditions classified elsewhere
　　　　　Code first underlying condition

　　G47.59　Other parasomnia

☑5th **G47.6　Sleep related movement disorders**
　　　EXCLUDES 2　restless legs syndrome (G25.81)

　　G47.61　Periodic limb movement disorder
　　　　　Periodic limb movement disorder

　　G47.62　Sleep related leg cramps

　　G47.63　Sleep related bruxism
　　　　　EXCLUDES 1　psychogenic bruxism (F45.8)

　　G47.69　Other sleep related movement disorders

G47.8　Other sleep disorders
　　►Other specified sleep-wake disorder◄

G47.9　Sleep disorder, unspecified　　　▽
　　Sleep disorder NOS
　　►Unspecified sleep-wake disorder◄

Trigeminal and Facial Nerve Branches

Supratrochlear nerve
Supraorbital nerve
V2 branch
Infraorbital nerve
Mental nerve
Mental foramen
V1 branch
Trigeminal nerve (CN V) branches in infratemporal fossa
V3 branch

Nerve, nerve root and plexus disorders (G50-G59)

　EXCLUDES 1　current traumatic nerve, nerve root and plexus disorders—see Injury, nerve by body region
　　　　　neuralgia NOS (M79.2)
　　　　　neuritis NOS (M79.2)
　　　　　peripheral neuritis in pregnancy (O26.82-)
　　　　　radiculitis NOS (M54.1-)

☑4th **G50　Disorders of trigeminal nerve**
　　INCLUDES　disorders of 5th cranial nerve

　　G50.0　Trigeminal neuralgia
　　　　　Syndrome of paroxysmal facial pain
　　　　　Tic douloureux

　　G50.1　Atypical facial pain

　　G50.8　Other disorders of trigeminal nerve

　　G50.9　Disorder of trigeminal nerve, unspecified　　　▽

☑4th **G51　Facial nerve disorders**
　　INCLUDES　disorders of 7th cranial nerve

　　G51.0　Bell's palsy
　　　　　Facial palsy

　　G51.1　Geniculate ganglionitis
　　　　　EXCLUDES 1　postherpetic geniculate ganglionitis (B02.21)

　　G51.2　Melkersson's syndrome
　　　　　Melkersson-Rosenthal syndrome

　　G51.3　Clonic hemifacial spasm

　　G51.4　Facial myokymia

　　G51.8　Other disorders of facial nerve

　　G51.9　Disorder of facial nerve, unspecified　　　▽

☑4th **G52　Disorders of other cranial nerves**
　　EXCLUDES 2　disorders of acoustic [8th] nerve (H93.3)
　　　　　disorders of optic [2nd] nerve (H46, H47.0)
　　　　　paralytic strabismus due to nerve palsy (H49.0-H49.2)

　　G52.0　Disorders of olfactory nerve
　　　　　Disorders of 1st cranial nerve

　　G52.1　Disorders of glossopharyngeal nerve
　　　　　Disorder of 9th cranial nerve
　　　　　Glossopharyngeal neuralgia

　　G52.2　Disorders of vagus nerve
　　　　　Disorders of pneumogastric [10th] nerve

　　G52.3　Disorders of hypoglossal nerve
　　　　　Disorders of 12th cranial nerve

　　G52.7　Disorders of multiple cranial nerves
　　　　　Polyneuritis cranialis

　　G52.8　Disorders of other specified cranial nerves

　　G52.9　Cranial nerve disorder, unspecified　　　▽

G53　*Cranial nerve disorders in diseases classified elsewhere*
　　Code first underlying disease, such as:
　　　neoplasm (C00-D49)
　　　EXCLUDES 1　multiple cranial nerve palsy in sarcoidosis (D86.82)
　　　　　　multiple cranial nerve palsy in syphilis (A52.15)
　　　　　　postherpetic geniculate ganglionitis (B02.21)
　　　　　　postherpetic trigeminal neuralgia (B02.22)

EXCLUDES 1 Not coded here　　EXCLUDES 2 Not included here　　N Newborn Age: 0　　P Pediatric Age: 0-17　　M Maternity Age: 12-55　　A Adult Age: 15-124

560　　　　　ICD-10-CM 2018

☑ 4ᵗʰ **G54** **Nerve root and plexus disorders**

    EXCLUDES 1 current traumatic nerve root and plexus disorders—see nerve injury by body region
                intervertebral disc disorders (M50-M51)
                neuralgia or neuritis NOS (M79.2)
                neuritis or radiculitis brachial NOS (M54.13)
                neuritis or radiculitis lumbar NOS (M54.16)
                neuritis or radiculitis lumbosacral NOS (M54.17)
                neuritis or radiculitis thoracic NOS (M54.14)
                radiculitis NOS (M54.10)
                radiculopathy NOS (M54.10)
                spondylosis (M47.-)

G54.0 **Brachial plexus disorders**
    Thoracic outlet syndrome
    DEF: Acquired disorder affecting the spinal nerves that send signals to the shoulder, arm, and hand; causes corresponding motor and sensory dysfunction; characterized by regional paresthesia, pain, and muscle weakness, and in severe cases paralysis.

G54.1 **Lumbosacral plexus disorders**

G54.2 **Cervical root disorders, not elsewhere classified**

G54.3 **Thoracic root disorders, not elsewhere classified**

G54.4 **Lumbosacral root disorders, not elsewhere classified**

G54.5 **Neuralgic amyotrophy**
    Parsonage-Aldren-Turner syndrome
    Shoulder-girdle neuritis
    EXCLUDES 1 neuralgic amyotrophy in diabetes mellitus (E08-E13 with .44)

G54.6 **Phantom limb syndrome with pain**   HCC

G54.7 **Phantom limb syndrome without pain**   HCC
    Phantom limb syndrome NOS

G54.8 **Other nerve root and plexus disorders**

G54.9 **Nerve root and plexus disorder, unspecified** ▽

G55 *Nerve root and plexus compressions in diseases classified elsewhere*

    Code first underlying disease, such as:
        neoplasm (C00-D49)
    EXCLUDES 1 nerve root compression (due to) (in) ankylosing spondylitis (M45.-)
                nerve root compression (due to) (in) dorsopathies (M53.-, M54.-)
                nerve root compression (due to) (in) intervertebral disc disorders (M50.1-, M51.1-)
                nerve root compression (due to) (in) spondylopathies (M46.-, M48.-)

☑ 4ᵗʰ **G56** **Mononeuropathies of upper limb**

    EXCLUDES 1 current traumatic nerve disorder—see nerve injury by body region

✓ 5ᵗʰ **G56.0** **Carpal tunnel syndrome**
    G56.00 **Carpal tunnel syndrome, unspecified upper limb** ▽
    G56.01 **Carpal tunnel syndrome, right upper limb**
    G56.02 **Carpal tunnel syndrome, left upper limb**
    G56.03 **Carpal tunnel syndrome, bilateral upper limbs**

✓ 5ᵗʰ **G56.1** **Other lesions of median nerve**
    G56.10 **Other lesions of median nerve, unspecified upper limb** ▽
    G56.11 **Other lesions of median nerve, right upper limb**
    G56.12 **Other lesions of median nerve, left upper limb**
    G56.13 **Other lesions of median nerve, bilateral upper limbs**

✓ 5ᵗʰ **G56.2** **Lesion of ulnar nerve**
    Tardy ulnar nerve palsy
    G56.20 **Lesion of ulnar nerve, unspecified upper limb** ▽
    G56.21 **Lesion of ulnar nerve, right upper limb**
    G56.22 **Lesion of ulnar nerve, left upper limb**
    G56.23 **Lesion of ulnar nerve, bilateral upper limbs**

✓ 5ᵗʰ **G56.3** **Lesion of radial nerve**
    G56.30 **Lesion of radial nerve, unspecified upper limb** ▽
    G56.31 **Lesion of radial nerve, right upper limb**
    G56.32 **Lesion of radial nerve, left upper limb**
    G56.33 **Lesion of radial nerve, bilateral upper limbs**

Nerves of Upper Limb

    Radial
    Deep branch of radial
    Ulnar
    Superficial branch of radial
    Median

✓ 5ᵗʰ **G56.4** **Causalgia of upper limb**
    Complex regional pain syndrome II of upper limb
    EXCLUDES 1 complex regional pain syndrome I of lower limb (G90.52-)
                complex regional pain syndrome I of upper limb (G90.51-)
                complex regional pain syndrome II of lower limb (G57.7-)
                reflex sympathetic dystrophy of lower limb (G90.52-)
                reflex sympathetic dystrophy of upper limb (G90.51-)
    G56.40 **Causalgia of unspecified upper limb** ▽
    G56.41 **Causalgia of right upper limb**
    G56.42 **Causalgia of left upper limb**
    G56.43 **Causalgia of bilateral upper limbs**

✓ 5ᵗʰ **G56.8** **Other specified mononeuropathies of upper limb**
    Interdigital neuroma of upper limb
    G56.80 **Other specified mononeuropathies of unspecified upper limb** ▽
    G56.81 **Other specified mononeuropathies of right upper limb**
    G56.82 **Other specified mononeuropathies of left upper limb**
    G56.83 **Other specified mononeuropathies of bilateral upper limbs**

✓ 5ᵗʰ **G56.9** **Unspecified mononeuropathy of upper limb**
    G56.90 **Unspecified mononeuropathy of unspecified upper limb** ▽
    G56.91 **Unspecified mononeuropathy of right upper limb** ▽
    G56.92 **Unspecified mononeuropathy of left upper limb** ▽
    G56.93 **Unspecified mononeuropathy of bilateral upper limbs** ▽

☑ 4ᵗʰ **G57** **Mononeuropathies of lower limb**

    EXCLUDES 1 current traumatic nerve disorder—see nerve injury by body region

✓ 5ᵗʰ **G57.0** **Lesion of sciatic nerve**
    EXCLUDES 1 sciatica NOS (M54.3-)
    EXCLUDES 2 sciatica attributed to intervertebral disc disorder (M51.1-)
    G57.00 **Lesion of sciatic nerve, unspecified lower limb** ▽
    G57.01 **Lesion of sciatic nerve, right lower limb**
    G57.02 **Lesion of sciatic nerve, left lower limb**
    G57.03 **Lesion of sciatic nerve, bilateral lower limbs**

✓ 5ᵗʰ **G57.1** **Meralgia paresthetica**
    Lateral cutaneous nerve of thigh syndrome
    G57.10 **Meralgia paresthetica, unspecified lower limb** ▽
    G57.11 **Meralgia paresthetica, right lower limb**
    G57.12 **Meralgia paresthetica, left lower limb**
    G57.13 **Meralgia paresthetica, bilateral lower limbs**

☑ Additional Character Req   ✓ x7ᵗʰ Placeholder Alert   Manifestation   HCC CMS-HCC Condition   ▽ Unspecified Code   ▶◀ Revised Text   ● New Code   ▲ Revised Code Title

Nerves of Lower Limb

Obturator nerve
Sciatic nerve
Femoral nerve
Saphenous nerve
Common fibular (peroneal) nerve
Deep fibular (peroneal) nerve
Tibial nerve
Superficial fibular (peroneal) nerve

✓5ᵗʰ G57.2 Lesion of femoral nerve
- G57.20 Lesion of femoral nerve, unspecified lower limb ▽
- G57.21 Lesion of femoral nerve, right lower limb
- G57.22 Lesion of femoral nerve, left lower limb
- G57.23 Lesion of femoral nerve, bilateral lower limbs

✓5ᵗʰ G57.3 Lesion of lateral popliteal nerve
Peroneal nerve palsy
- G57.30 Lesion of lateral popliteal nerve, unspecified lower limb ▽
- G57.31 Lesion of lateral popliteal nerve, right lower limb
- G57.32 Lesion of lateral popliteal nerve, left lower limb
- G57.33 Lesion of lateral popliteal nerve, bilateral lower limbs

✓5ᵗʰ G57.4 Lesion of medial popliteal nerve
- G57.40 Lesion of medial popliteal nerve, unspecified lower limb ▽
- G57.41 Lesion of medial popliteal nerve, right lower limb
- G57.42 Lesion of medial popliteal nerve, left lower limb
- G57.43 Lesion of medial popliteal nerve, bilateral lower limbs

✓5ᵗʰ G57.5 Tarsal tunnel syndrome
- G57.50 Tarsal tunnel syndrome, unspecified lower limb ▽
- G57.51 Tarsal tunnel syndrome, right lower limb
- G57.52 Tarsal tunnel syndrome, left lower limb
- G57.53 Tarsal tunnel syndrome, bilateral lower limbs

✓5ᵗʰ G57.6 Lesion of plantar nerve
Morton's metatarsalgia
- G57.60 Lesion of plantar nerve, unspecified lower limb ▽
- G57.61 Lesion of plantar nerve, right lower limb
- G57.62 Lesion of plantar nerve, left lower limb
- G57.63 Lesion of plantar nerve, bilateral lower limbs

✓5ᵗʰ G57.7 Causalgia of lower limb
Complex regional pain syndrome II of lower limb
> EXCLUDES 1   complex regional pain syndrome I of lower limb (G90.52-)
> complex regional pain syndrome I of upper limb (G90.51-)
> complex regional pain syndrome II of upper limb (G56.4-)
> reflex sympathetic dystrophy of lower limb (G90.52-)
> reflex sympathetic dystrophy of upper limb (G90.51-)
- G57.70 Causalgia of unspecified lower limb ▽
- G57.71 Causalgia of right lower limb
- G57.72 Causalgia of left lower limb
- G57.73 Causalgia of bilateral lower limbs

✓5ᵗʰ G57.8 Other specified mononeuropathies of lower limb
Interdigital neuroma of lower limb
- G57.80 Other specified mononeuropathies of unspecified lower limb ▽
- G57.81 Other specified mononeuropathies of right lower limb
- G57.82 Other specified mononeuropathies of left lower limb
- G57.83 Other specified mononeuropathies of bilateral lower limbs

✓5ᵗʰ G57.9 Unspecified mononeuropathy of lower limb
- G57.90 Unspecified mononeuropathy of unspecified lower limb ▽
- G57.91 Unspecified mononeuropathy of right lower limb ▽
- G57.92 Unspecified mononeuropathy of left lower limb ▽
- G57.93 Unspecified mononeuropathy of bilateral lower limbs ▽

✓4ᵗʰ G58 Other mononeuropathies
- G58.0 Intercostal neuropathy
- G58.7 Mononeuritis multiplex
- G58.8 Other specified mononeuropathies
- G58.9 Mononeuropathy, unspecified ▽

G59 *Mononeuropathy in diseases classified elsewhere*
Code first underlying disease
> EXCLUDES 1   diabetic mononeuropathy (E08-E13 with .41)
> syphilitic nerve paralysis (A52.19)
> syphilitic neuritis (A52.15)
> tuberculous mononeuropathy (A17.83)

Polyneuropathies and other disorders of the peripheral nervous system (G60-G65)

> EXCLUDES 1   neuralgia NOS (M79.2)
> neuritis NOS (M79.2)
> peripheral neuritis in pregnancy (O26.82-)
> radiculitis NOS (M54.10)

✓4ᵗʰ G60 Hereditary and idiopathic neuropathy
- **G60.0 Hereditary motor and sensory neuropathy**
  Charcôt-Marie-Tooth disease
  Déjérine-Sottas disease
  Hereditary motor and sensory neuropathy, types I-IV
  Hypertrophic neuropathy of infancy
  Peroneal muscular atrophy (axonal type) (hypertrophic type)
  Roussy-Levy syndrome
- **G60.1 Refsum's disease**
  Infantile Refsum disease
  DEF: Genetic disorder of lipid metabolism; characterized by retinitis pigmentosa, degenerative nerve disease, ataxia, and dry, rough, scaly skin.
- **G60.2 Neuropathy in association with hereditary ataxia**
- **G60.3 Idiopathic progressive neuropathy**
- **G60.8 Other hereditary and idiopathic neuropathies**
  Dominantly inherited sensory neuropathy
  Morvan's disease
  Nelaton's syndrome
  Recessively inherited sensory neuropathy
- **G60.9 Hereditary and idiopathic neuropathy, unspecified** ▽

✓4ᵗʰ G61 Inflammatory polyneuropathy
- **G61.0 Guillain-Barre syndrome**   HCC
  Acute (post-)infective polyneuritis
  Miller Fisher syndrome
  AHA: 2014, 2Q, 4
- **G61.1 Serum neuropathy**   HCC
  Use additional code for adverse effect, if applicable, to identify serum (T50.-)
- **✓5ᵗʰ G61.8 Other inflammatory polyneuropathies**
  - G61.81 Chronic inflammatory demyelinating polyneuritis   HCC
  - G61.82 Multifocal motor neuropathy   HCC
    MMN
  - G61.89 Other inflammatory polyneuropathies   HCC
- **G61.9 Inflammatory polyneuropathy, unspecified**   HCC ▽

EXCLUDES 1 Not coded here   EXCLUDES 2 Not included here   N Newborn Age: 0   P Pediatric Age: 0-17   M Maternity Age: 12-55   A Adult Age: 15-124

✓4ᵗʰ **G62 Other and unspecified polyneuropathies**

G62.0 Drug-induced polyneuropathy HCC
Use additional code for adverse effect, if applicable, to identify drug (T36-T50 with fifth or sixth character 5)

G62.1 Alcoholic polyneuropathy HCC

G62.2 Polyneuropathy due to other toxic agents HCC
Code first (T51-T65) to identify toxic agent

✓5ᵗʰ **G62.8 Other specified polyneuropathies**

G62.81 Critical illness polyneuropathy HCC
Acute motor neuropathy

G62.82 Radiation-induced polyneuropathy HCC
Use additional external cause code (W88-W90, X39.0-) to identify cause

G62.89 Other specified polyneuropathies
AHA: 2016, 2Q, 11

G62.9 Polyneuropathy, unspecified ▽
Neuropathy NOS

G63 Polyneuropathy in diseases classified elsewhere HCC
Code first underlying disease, such as:
amyloidosis (E85.-)
endocrine disease, except diabetes (E00-E07, E15-E16, E20-E34)
metabolic diseases (E70-E88)
neoplasm (C00-D49)
nutritional deficiency (E40-E64)
EXCLUDES 1   *polyneuropathy (in):*
diabetes mellitus (E08-E13 with .42)
diphtheria (A36.83)
infectious mononucleosis (B27.0-B27.9 with 1)
Lyme disease (A69.22)
mumps (B26.84)
postherpetic (B02.23)
rheumatoid arthritis (M05.33)
scleroderma (M34.83)
systemic lupus erythematosus (M32.19)
AHA: 2012, 4Q, 99

G64 Other disorders of peripheral nervous system
Disorder of peripheral nervous system NOS

✓4ᵗʰ **G65 Sequelae of inflammatory and toxic polyneuropathies**
Code first condition resulting from (sequela) of inflammatory and toxic polyneuropathies

G65.0 Sequelae of Guillain-Barré syndrome HCC

G65.1 Sequelae of other inflammatory polyneuropathy HCC

G65.2 Sequelae of toxic polyneuropathy HCC

Diseases of myoneural junction and muscle (G70-G73)

✓4ᵗʰ **G70 Myasthenia gravis and other myoneural disorders**
EXCLUDES 1   *botulism (A05.1, A48.51-A48.52)*
transient neonatal myasthenia gravis (P94.0)

✓5ᵗʰ **G70.0 Myasthenia gravis**

G70.00 Myasthenia gravis without (acute) exacerbation HCC
Myasthenia gravis NOS

G70.01 Myasthenia gravis with (acute) exacerbation HCC
Myasthenia gravis in crisis

G70.1 Toxic myoneural disorders HCC
Code first (T51-T65) to identify toxic agent

G70.2 Congenital and developmental myasthenia HCC

✓5ᵗʰ **G70.8 Other specified myoneural disorders**

G70.80 Lambert-Eaton syndrome, unspecified HCC ▽
Lambert-Eaton syndrome NOS

G70.81 Lambert-Eaton syndrome in disease classified elsewhere HCC
Code first underlying disease
EXCLUDES 1   *Lambert-Eaton syndrome in neoplastic disease (G73.1)*

G70.89 Other specified myoneural disorders HCC

G70.9 Myoneural disorder, unspecified HCC ▽

✓4ᵗʰ **G71 Primary disorders of muscles**
EXCLUDES 2   *arthrogryposis multiplex congenita (Q74.3)*
metabolic disorders (E70-E88)
myositis (M60.-)

G71.0 Muscular dystrophy HCC
Autosomal recessive, childhood type, muscular dystrophy resembling Duchenne or Becker muscular dystrophy
Benign [Becker] muscular dystrophy
Benign scapuloperoneal muscular dystrophy with early contractures [Emery-Dreifuss]
Congenital muscular dystrophy NOS
Congenital muscular dystrophy with specific morphological abnormalities of the muscle fiber
Distal muscular dystrophy
Facioscapulohumeral muscular dystrophy
Limb-girdle muscular dystrophy
Ocular muscular dystrophy
Oculopharyngeal muscular dystrophy
Scapuloperoneal muscular dystrophy
Severe [Duchenne] muscular dystrophy

✓5ᵗʰ **G71.1 Myotonic disorders**

G71.11 Myotonic muscular dystrophy HCC
Dystrophia myotonica [Steinert]
Myotonia atrophica
Myotonic dystrophy
Proximal myotonic myopathy (PROMM)
Steinert disease

G71.12 Myotonia congenita
Acetazolamide responsive myotonia congenita
Dominant myotonia congenita [Thomsen disease]
Myotonia levior
Recessive myotonia congenita [Becker disease]

G71.13 Myotonic chondrodystrophy
Chondrodystrophic myotonia
Congenital myotonic chondrodystrophy
Schwartz-Jampel disease

G71.14 Drug induced myotonia
Use additional code for adverse effect, if applicable, to identify drug (T36-T50 with fifth or sixth character 5)

G71.19 Other specified myotonic disorders
Myotonia fluctuans
Myotonia permanens
Neuromyotonia [Isaacs]
Paramyotonia congenita (of von Eulenburg)
Pseudomyotonia
Symptomatic myotonia

G71.2 Congenital myopathies HCC
Central core disease
Fiber-type disproportion
Minicore disease
Multicore disease
Myotubular (centronuclear) myopathy
Nemaline myopathy
EXCLUDES 1   *arthrogryposis multiplex congenita (Q74.3)*

G71.3 Mitochondrial myopathy, not elsewhere classified
EXCLUDES 1   *Kearns-Sayre syndrome (H49.81)*
Leber's disease (H47.21)
Leigh's encephalopathy (G31.82)
mitochondrial metabolism disorders (E88.4-)
Reye's syndrome (G93.7)

G71.8 Other primary disorders of muscles

G71.9 Primary disorder of muscle, unspecified ▽
Hereditary myopathy NOS

✓4ᵗʰ **G72 Other and unspecified myopathies**
EXCLUDES 1   *arthrogryposis multiplex congenita (Q74.3)*
dermatopolymyositis (M33.-)
ischemic infarction of muscle (M62.2-)
myositis (M60.-)
polymyositis (M33.2-)

G72.0 Drug-induced myopathy
Use additional code for adverse effect, if applicable, to identify drug (T36-T50 with fifth or sixth character 5)

G72.1 Alcoholic myopathy
Use additional code to identify alcoholism (F10.-)

G72.2 Myopathy due to other toxic agents
Code first (T51-T65) to identify toxic agent

✓ Additional Character Req   ✓7ᵗʰ Placeholder Alert   Manifestation   HCC CMS-HCC Condition   ▽ Unspecified Code   ▶◀ Revised Text   ● New Code   ▲ Revised Code Title

ICD-10-CM 2018   563

G72.3 Periodic paralysis
Familial periodic paralysis
Hyperkalemic periodic paralysis (familial)
Hypokalemic periodic paralysis (familial)
Myotonic periodic paralysis (familial)
Normokalemic paralysis (familial)
Potassium sensitive periodic paralysis
EXCLUDES 1 *paramyotonia congenita (of von Eulenburg) (G71.19)*

✓5ᵗʰ **G72.4 Inflammatory and immune myopathies, not elsewhere classified**
G72.41 Inclusion body myositis [IBM]
G72.49 Other inflammatory and immune myopathies, not elsewhere classified
Inflammatory myopathy NOS

✓5ᵗʰ **G72.8 Other specified myopathies**
G72.81 Critical illness myopathy
Acute necrotizing myopathy
Acute quadriplegic myopathy
Intensive care (ICU) myopathy
Myopathy of critical illness
G72.89 Other specified myopathies

G72.9 Myopathy, unspecified ▽

✓4ᵗʰ **G73 Disorders of myoneural junction and muscle in diseases classified elsewhere**
G73.1 Lambert-Eaton syndrome in neoplastic disease HCC
Code first underlying neoplasm (C00-D49)
EXCLUDES 1 *Lambert-Eaton syndrome not associated with neoplasm (G70.80-G70.81)*

G73.3 Myasthenic syndromes in other diseases classified elsewhere HCC
Code first underlying disease, such as:
neoplasm (C00-D49)
thyrotoxicosis (E05.-)

G73.7 Myopathy in diseases classified elsewhere
Code first underlying disease, such as:
hyperparathyroidism (E21.0, E21.3)
hypoparathyroidism (E20.-)
glycogen storage disease (E74.0)
lipid storage disorders (E75.-)
EXCLUDES 1 *myopathy in:*
rheumatoid arthritis (M05.4-)
sarcoidosis (D86.87)
scleroderma (M34.82)
sicca syndrome [Sjögren] (M35.03)
systemic lupus erythematosus (M32.19)

Cerebral palsy and other paralytic syndromes (G80-G83)

✓4ᵗʰ **G80 Cerebral palsy**
EXCLUDES 1 *hereditary spastic paraplegia (G11.4)*
G80.0 Spastic quadriplegic cerebral palsy HCC
Congenital spastic paralysis (cerebral)
G80.1 Spastic diplegic cerebral palsy HCC
Spastic cerebral palsy NOS
G80.2 Spastic hemiplegic cerebral palsy HCC
G80.3 Athetoid cerebral palsy HCC
Double athetosis (syndrome)
Dyskinetic cerebral palsy
Dystonic cerebral palsy
Vogt disease
G80.4 Ataxic cerebral palsy HCC
G80.8 Other cerebral palsy HCC
Mixed cerebral palsy syndromes
G80.9 Cerebral palsy, unspecified HCC ▽
Cerebral palsy NOS

✓4ᵗʰ **G81 Hemiplegia and hemiparesis**
NOTE This category is to be used only when hemiplegia (complete)(incomplete) is reported without further specification, or is stated to be old or longstanding but of unspecified cause. The category is also for use in multiple coding to identify these types of hemiplegia resulting from any cause.
EXCLUDES 1 *congenital cerebral palsy (G80.-)*
hemiplegia and hemiparesis due to sequela of cerebrovascular disease (I69.05-, I69.15-, I69.25-, I69.35-, I69.85-, I69.95-)
AHA: 2015, 1Q, 25

✓5ᵗʰ **G81.0 Flaccid hemiplegia**
G81.00 Flaccid hemiplegia affecting unspecified side HCC ▽
G81.01 Flaccid hemiplegia affecting right dominant side HCC
G81.02 Flaccid hemiplegia affecting left dominant side HCC
G81.03 Flaccid hemiplegia affecting right nondominant side HCC
G81.04 Flaccid hemiplegia affecting left nondominant side HCC

✓5ᵗʰ **G81.1 Spastic hemiplegia**
G81.10 Spastic hemiplegia affecting unspecified side HCC ▽
G81.11 Spastic hemiplegia affecting right dominant side HCC
G81.12 Spastic hemiplegia affecting left dominant side HCC
G81.13 Spastic hemiplegia affecting right nondominant side HCC
G81.14 Spastic hemiplegia affecting left nondominant side HCC

✓5ᵗʰ **G81.9 Hemiplegia, unspecified**
AHA: 2014, 1Q, 23
G81.90 Hemiplegia, unspecified affecting unspecified side HCC ▽
G81.91 Hemiplegia, unspecified affecting right dominant side HCC ▽
G81.92 Hemiplegia, unspecified affecting left dominant side HCC ▽
G81.93 Hemiplegia, unspecified affecting right nondominant side HCC ▽
G81.94 Hemiplegia, unspecified affecting left nondominant side HCC ▽

✓4ᵗʰ **G82 Paraplegia (paraparesis) and quadriplegia (quadriparesis)**
NOTE This category is to be used only when the listed conditions are reported without further specification, or are stated to be old or longstanding but of unspecified cause. The category is also for use in multiple coding to identify these conditions resulting from any cause.
EXCLUDES 1 *congenital cerebral palsy (G80.-)*
functional quadriplegia (R53.2)
hysterical paralysis (F44.4)

✓5ᵗʰ **G82.2 Paraplegia**
Paralysis of both lower limbs NOS
Paraparesis (lower) NOS
Paraplegia (lower) NOS
G82.20 Paraplegia, unspecified HCC ▽
G82.21 Paraplegia, complete HCC
G82.22 Paraplegia, incomplete HCC

✓5ᵗʰ **G82.5 Quadriplegia**
G82.50 Quadriplegia, unspecified HCC ▽
G82.51 Quadriplegia, C1-C4 complete HCC
G82.52 Quadriplegia, C1-C4 incomplete HCC
G82.53 Quadriplegia, C5-C7 complete HCC
G82.54 Quadriplegia, C5-C7 incomplete HCC

✓4ᵗʰ **G83 Other paralytic syndromes**
NOTE This category is to be used only when the listed conditions are reported without further specification, or are stated to be old or longstanding but of unspecified cause. The category is also for use in multiple coding to identify these conditions resulting from any cause.
INCLUDES paralysis (complete) (incomplete), except as in G80-G82
G83.0 Diplegia of upper limbs HCC
Diplegia (upper)
Paralysis of both upper limbs

✓5ᵗʰ **G83.1 Monoplegia of lower limb**
Paralysis of lower limb
EXCLUDES 1 *monoplegia of lower limbs due to sequela of cerebrovascular disease (I69.04-, I69.14-, I69.24-, I69.34-, I69.84-, I69.94-)*
G83.10 Monoplegia of lower limb affecting unspecified side HCC ▽
G83.11 Monoplegia of lower limb affecting right dominant side HCC
G83.12 Monoplegia of lower limb affecting left dominant side HCC
G83.13 Monoplegia of lower limb affecting right nondominant side HCC
G83.14 Monoplegia of lower limb affecting left nondominant side HCC

✓5ᵗʰ **G83.2 Monoplegia of upper limb**
Paralysis of upper limb
> *EXCLUDES 1*   *monoplegia of upper limbs due to sequela of cerebrovascular disease (I69.03-, I69.13-, I69.23-, I69.33-, I69.83-, I69.93-)*

     G83.20 Monoplegia of upper limb affecting unspecified side   HCC ▽

     G83.21 Monoplegia of upper limb affecting right dominant side   HCC

     G83.22 Monoplegia of upper limb affecting left dominant side   HCC

     G83.23 Monoplegia of upper limb affecting right nondominant side   HCC

     G83.24 Monoplegia of upper limb affecting left nondominant side   HCC

✓5ᵗʰ **G83.3 Monoplegia, unspecified**

     G83.30 Monoplegia, unspecified affecting unspecified side   HCC ▽

     G83.31 Monoplegia, unspecified affecting right dominant side   HCC ▽

     G83.32 Monoplegia, unspecified affecting left dominant side   HCC ▽

     G83.33 Monoplegia, unspecified affecting right nondominant side   HCC ▽

     G83.34 Monoplegia, unspecified affecting left nondominant side   HCC ▽

G83.4 Cauda equina syndrome   HCC
Neurogenic bladder due to cauda equina syndrome
> *EXCLUDES 1*   *cord bladder NOS (G95.89)*
> *neurogenic bladder NOS (N31.9)*

G83.5 Locked-in state   HCC

✓5ᵗʰ **G83.8 Other specified paralytic syndromes**
> *EXCLUDES 1*   *paralytic syndromes due to current spinal cord injury—code to spinal cord injury (S14, S24, S34)*

     G83.81 Brown-Séquard syndrome   HCC

     G83.82 Anterior cord syndrome   HCC

     G83.83 Posterior cord syndrome   HCC

     G83.84 Todd's paralysis (postepileptic)   HCC

     G83.89 Other specified paralytic syndromes   HCC

G83.9 Paralytic syndrome, unspecified   HCC ▽

Other disorders of the nervous system (G89-G99)

✓4ᵗʰ **G89 Pain, not elsewhere classified**
Code also related psychological factors associated with pain (F45.42)
> *EXCLUDES 1*   *generalized pain NOS (R52)*
> *pain disorders exclusively related to psychological factors (F45.41)*
> *pain NOS (R52)*
> *EXCLUDES 2*   *atypical face pain (G50.1)*
> *headache syndromes (G44.-)*
> *localized pain, unspecified type—code to pain by site, such as:*
>   *abdomen pain (R10.-)*
>   *back pain (M54.9)*
>   *breast pain (N64.4)*
>   *chest pain (R07.1-R07.9)*
>   *ear pain (H92.0-)*
>   *eye pain (H57.1)*
>   *headache (R51)*
>   *joint pain (M25.5-)*
>   *limb pain (M79.6-)*
>   *lumbar region pain (M54.5)*
>   *painful urination (R30.9)*
>   *pelvic and perineal pain (R10.2)*
>   *renal colic (N23)*
>   *shoulder pain (M25.51-)*
>   *spine pain (M54.-)*
>   *throat pain (R07.0)*
>   *tongue pain (K14.6)*
>   *tooth pain (K08.8)*
> *migraines (G43.-)*
> *myalgia (M79.1)*
> *pain from prosthetic devices, implants, and grafts (T82.84, T83.84, T84.84, T85.84-)*
> *phantom limb syndrome with pain (G54.6)*
> *vulvar vestibulitis (N94.810)*
> *vulvodynia (N94.81-)*

G89.0 Central pain syndrome
Déjérine-Roussy syndrome
Myelopathic pain syndrome
Thalamic pain syndrome (hyperesthetic)

✓5ᵗʰ **G89.1 Acute pain, not elsewhere classified**

     G89.11 Acute pain due to trauma

     G89.12 Acute post-thoracotomy pain
Post-thoracotomy pain NOS

     G89.18 Other acute postprocedural pain
Postoperative pain NOS
Postprocedural pain NOS

✓5ᵗʰ **G89.2 Chronic pain, not elsewhere classified**
> *EXCLUDES 1*   *causalgia, lower limb (G57.7-)*
> *causalgia, upper limb (G56.4-)*
> *central pain syndrome (G89.0)*
> *chronic pain syndrome (G89.4)*
> *complex regional pain syndrome II, lower limb (G57.7-)*
> *complex regional pain syndrome II, upper limb (G56.4-)*
> *neoplasm related chronic pain (G89.3)*
> *reflex sympathetic dystrophy (G90.5-)*

     G89.21 Chronic pain due to trauma

     G89.22 Chronic post-thoracotomy pain

     G89.28 Other chronic postprocedural pain
Other chronic postoperative pain

     G89.29 Other chronic pain

G89.3 Neoplasm related pain (acute) (chronic)
Cancer associated pain
Pain due to malignancy (primary) (secondary)
Tumor associated pain

G89.4 Chronic pain syndrome
Chronic pain associated with significant psychosocial dysfunction

✓4ᵗʰ **G90 Disorders of autonomic nervous system**
> *EXCLUDES 1*   *dysfunction of the autonomic nervous system due to alcohol (G31.2)*

✓5ᵗʰ **G90.0 Idiopathic peripheral autonomic neuropathy**

     G90.01 Carotid sinus syncope
Carotid sinus syndrome
DEF: Vagal activation caused by pressure on the carotid sinus baroreceptors; sympathetic nerve impulses may cause sinus arrest or AV block.

     G90.09 Other idiopathic peripheral autonomic neuropathy
Idiopathic peripheral autonomic neuropathy NOS

G90.1 Familial dysautonomia [Riley-Day]   HCC

G90.2 Horner's syndrome
Bernard(-Horner) syndrome
Cervical sympathetic dystrophy or paralysis

G90.3 Multi-system degeneration of the autonomic nervous system   HCC
Neurogenic orthostatic hypotension [Shy-Drager]
> *EXCLUDES 1*   *orthostatic hypotension NOS (I95.1)*

G90.4 Autonomic dysreflexia
Use additional code to identify the cause, such as:
    fecal impaction (K56.41)
    pressure ulcer (pressure area) (L89.-)
    urinary tract infection (N39.0)

✓5ᵗʰ **G90.5 Complex regional pain syndrome I (CRPS I)**
Reflex sympathetic dystrophy
> *EXCLUDES 1*   *causalgia of lower limb (G57.7-)*
> *causalgia of upper limb (G56.4-)*
> *complex regional pain syndrome II of lower limb (G57.7-)*
> *complex regional pain syndrome II of upper limb (G56.4-)*

     G90.50 Complex regional pain syndrome I, unspecified   ▽

✓6ᵗʰ   **G90.51 Complex regional pain syndrome I of upper limb**

        G90.511 Complex regional pain syndrome I of right upper limb

        G90.512 Complex regional pain syndrome I of left upper limb

        G90.513 Complex regional pain syndrome I of upper limb, bilateral

        G90.519 Complex regional pain syndrome I of unspecified upper limb   ▽

✓6ᵗʰ   **G90.52 Complex regional pain syndrome I of lower limb**

        G90.521 Complex regional pain syndrome I of right lower limb

Chapter 6. Diseases of the Nervous System

G90.522–G95.81

Hydrocephalus (Acquired)

Normal ventricles   Hydrocephalic ventricles

G90.522   **Complex regional pain syndrome I of left lower limb**

G90.523   **Complex regional pain syndrome I of lower limb, bilateral**

G90.529   **Complex regional pain syndrome I of unspecified lower limb**   ▽

G90.59   **Complex regional pain syndrome I of other specified site**

G90.8   **Other disorders of autonomic nervous system**

G90.9   **Disorder of the autonomic nervous system, unspecified**   ▽

✓4ᵗʰ **G91   Hydrocephalus**
INCLUDES   acquired hydrocephalus
EXCLUDES 1   *Arnold-Chiari syndrome with hydrocephalus (Q07.-)*
congenital hydrocephalus (Q03.-)
spina bifida with hydrocephalus (Q05.-)

G91.0   **Communicating hydrocephalus**
Secondary normal pressure hydrocephalus

G91.1   **Obstructive hydrocephalus**
DEF: Obstruction of cerebrospinal fluid passage from brain into spinal canal; characterized by headaches, drowsiness, poor coordination, urinary incontinence, nausea, vomiting, and papilledema.

G91.2   **(Idiopathic) normal pressure hydrocephalus**
Normal pressure hydrocephalus NOS

G91.3   **Post-traumatic hydrocephalus, unspecified**

G91.4   *Hydrocephalus in diseases classified elsewhere*
Code first underlying condition, such as:
congenital syphilis (A50.4-)
neoplasm (C00-D49)
EXCLUDES 1   *hydrocephalus due to congenital toxoplasmosis (P37.1)*
AHA: 2014, 3Q, 3

G91.8   **Other hydrocephalus**

G91.9   **Hydrocephalus, unspecified**   ▽

G92   Toxic encephalopathy
Toxic encephalitis
Toxic metabolic encephalopathy
▶Code first, if applicable, drug induced (T36-T50)◀
Code first (T51-T65) to identify toxic agent
AHA: 2017, 1Q, 39-40
DEF: Brain tissue degeneration due to toxic substance.

✓4ᵗʰ **G93   Other disorders of brain**
G93.0   **Cerebral cysts**
Arachnoid cyst
Porencephalic cyst, acquired
EXCLUDES 1   *acquired periventricular cysts of newborn (P91.1)*
congenital cerebral cysts (Q04.6)

G93.1   **Anoxic brain damage, not elsewhere classified**   HCC
EXCLUDES 1   *cerebral anoxia due to anesthesia during labor and delivery (O74.3)*
cerebral anoxia due to anesthesia during the puerperium (O89.2)
neonatal anoxia (P84)
DEF: Brain injury not resulting from birth trauma that is due to lack of oxygen. Brain cells, when deprived of oxygen, begin to expire after 4 minutes.

G93.2   **Benign intracranial hypertension**
EXCLUDES 1   *hypertensive encephalopathy (I67.4)*

G93.3   **Postviral fatigue syndrome**
Benign myalgic encephalomyelitis
EXCLUDES 1   *chronic fatigue syndrome NOS (R53.82)*

✓5ᵗʰ G93.4   **Other and unspecified encephalopathy**
EXCLUDES 1   *alcoholic encephalopathy (G31.2)*
encephalopathy in diseases classified elsewhere (G94)
hypertensive encephalopathy (I67.4)
toxic (metabolic) encephalopathy (G92)

G93.40   **Encephalopathy, unspecified**   ▽
AHA: 2017, 2Q, 8

G93.41   **Metabolic encephalopathy**
Septic encephalopathy
AHA: 2017, 2Q, 8; 2016, 3Q, 42; 2015, 3Q, 21

G93.49   **Other encephalopathy**
Encephalopathy NEC
AHA: 2017, 2Q, 9

G93.5   **Compression of brain**   HCC
Arnold-Chiari type 1 compression of brain
Compression of brain (stem)
Herniation of brain (stem)
EXCLUDES 1   *diffuse traumatic compression of brain (S06.2-)*
focal traumatic compression of brain (S06.3-)

G93.6   **Cerebral edema**   HCC
EXCLUDES 1   *cerebral edema due to birth injury (P11.0)*
traumatic cerebral edema (S06.1-)

G93.7   **Reye's syndrome**   P
~~Code first (T39.0-), if salicylates-induced~~
▶Code first poisoning due to salicylates, if applicable (T39.0-, with sixth character 1-4)◀
▶Use additional code for adverse effect due to salicylates, if applicable (T39.0-, with sixth character 5)◀
DEF: Rare childhood illness often developed after a viral upper respiratory infection; characterized by vomiting, elevated serum transaminase, brain swelling, disturbances of consciousness, seizures, and changes in liver and other viscera; can be fatal.

✓5ᵗʰ G93.8   **Other specified disorders of brain**
G93.81   **Temporal sclerosis**
Hippocampal sclerosis
Mesial temporal sclerosis

G93.82   **Brain death**

G93.89   **Other specified disorders of brain**
Postradiation encephalopathy

G93.9   **Disorder of brain, unspecified**   ▽

G94   Other disorders of brain in diseases classified elsewhere
Code first underlying disease
EXCLUDES 1   *encephalopathy in congenital syphilis (A50.49)*
encephalopathy in influenza (J09.X9, J10.81, J11.81)
encephalopathy in syphilis (A52.19)
hydrocephalus in diseases classified elsewhere (G91.4)

✓4ᵗʰ **G95   Other and unspecified diseases of spinal cord**
EXCLUDES 2   *myelitis (G04.-)*

G95.0   **Syringomyelia and syringobulbia**   HCC

✓5ᵗʰ G95.1   **Vascular myelopathies**
EXCLUDES 2   *intraspinal phlebitis and thrombophlebitis, except non-pyogenic (G08)*

G95.11   **Acute infarction of spinal cord (embolic) (nonembolic)**   HCC
Anoxia of spinal cord
Arterial thrombosis of spinal cord

G95.19   **Other vascular myelopathies**   HCC
Edema of spinal cord
Hematomyelia
Nonpyogenic intraspinal phlebitis and thrombophlebitis
Subacute necrotic myelopathy

✓5ᵗʰ G95.2   **Other and unspecified cord compression**
G95.20   **Unspecified cord compression**   HCC ▽

G95.29   **Other cord compression**   HCC

✓5ᵗʰ G95.8   **Other specified diseases of spinal cord**
EXCLUDES 1   *neurogenic bladder NOS (N31.9)*
neurogenic bladder due to cauda equina syndrome (G83.4)
neuromuscular dysfunction of bladder without spinal cord lesion (N31.-)

G95.81   **Conus medullaris syndrome**   HCC

    G95.89   **Other specified diseases of spinal cord**   HCC
         Cord bladder NOS
         Drug-induced myelopathy
         Radiation-induced myelopathy
         EXCLUDES 1   myelopathy NOS (G95.9)

   G95.9 **Disease of spinal cord, unspecified**   HCC ▽
         Myelopathy NOS

✓4th **G96**   **Other disorders of central nervous system**
   G96.0 **Cerebrospinal fluid leak**
         EXCLUDES 1   cerebrospinal fluid leak from spinal puncture (G97.0)
         DEF: Cerebrospinal fluid discharging from the nose or the ear; caused by fracture of frontal bone with tearing of dura mater and arachnoid; characterized by watery drainage usually from only one side of the nose or one ear, headache, vision changes, and hearing loss.

  ✓5th G96.1 **Disorders of meninges, not elsewhere classified**
       G96.11 **Dural tear**
            EXCLUDES 1   accidental puncture or laceration of dura during a procedure (G97.41)
            AHA: 2014, 4Q, 24
       G96.12 **Meningeal adhesions (cerebral) (spinal)**
       G96.19 **Other disorders of meninges, not elsewhere classified**

   G96.8 **Other specified disorders of central nervous system**
   G96.9 **Disorder of central nervous system, unspecified**   ▽

✓4th **G97**   **Intraoperative and postprocedural complications and disorders of nervous system, not elsewhere classified**
         EXCLUDES 2   intraoperative and postprocedural cerebrovascular infarction (I97.81-, I97.82-)

   G97.0 **Cerebrospinal fluid leak from spinal puncture**
   G97.1 **Other reaction to spinal and lumbar puncture**
         Headache due to lumbar puncture
   G97.2 **Intracranial hypotension following ventricular shunting**

  ✓5th G97.3 **Intraoperative hemorrhage and hematoma of a nervous system organ or structure complicating a procedure**
         EXCLUDES 1   intraoperative hemorrhage and hematoma of a nervous system organ or structure due to accidental puncture and laceration during a procedure (G97.4-)
       G97.31 **Intraoperative hemorrhage and hematoma of a nervous system organ or structure complicating a nervous system procedure**
       G97.32 **Intraoperative hemorrhage and hematoma of a nervous system organ or structure complicating other procedure**

  ✓5th G97.4 **Accidental puncture and laceration of a nervous system organ or structure during a procedure**
       G97.41 **Accidental puncture or laceration of dura during a procedure**
            Incidental (inadvertent) durotomy
            AHA: 2014, 4Q, 24
       G97.48 **Accidental puncture and laceration of other nervous system organ or structure during a nervous system procedure**
       G97.49 **Accidental puncture and laceration of other nervous system organ or structure during other procedure**

Spinal Puncture

Spinal cord
Epidural space
Subarachnoid space
Vertebra
Spinal needle

Lumbar area

  ✓5th G97.5 **Postprocedural hemorrhage of a nervous system organ or structure following a procedure**
       G97.51 **Postprocedural hemorrhage of a nervous system organ or structure following a nervous system procedure**
       G97.52 **Postprocedural hemorrhage of a nervous system organ or structure following other procedure**

  ✓5th G97.6 **Postprocedural hematoma and seroma of a nervous system organ or structure following a procedure**
       G97.61 **Postprocedural hematoma of a nervous system organ or structure following a nervous system procedure**
       G97.62 **Postprocedural hematoma of a nervous system organ or structure following other procedure**
       G97.63 **Postprocedural seroma of a nervous system organ or structure following a nervous system procedure**
       G97.64 **Postprocedural seroma of a nervous system organ or structure following other procedure**

  ✓5th G97.8 **Other intraoperative and postprocedural complications and disorders of nervous system**
         Use additional code to further specify disorder
       G97.81 **Other intraoperative complications of nervous system**
       G97.82 **Other postprocedural complications and disorders of nervous system**

✓4th **G98**   **Other disorders of nervous system not elsewhere classified**
         INCLUDES   nervous system disorder NOS
   G98.0 **Neurogenic arthritis, not elsewhere classified**
         Nonsyphilitic neurogenic arthropathy NEC
         Nonsyphilitic neurogenic spondylopathy NEC
         EXCLUDES 1   spondylopathy (in):
              syringomyelia and syringobulbia (G95.0)
              tabes dorsalis (A52.11)

   G98.8 **Other disorders of nervous system**
         Nervous system disorder NOS

✓4th **G99**   **Other disorders of nervous system in diseases classified elsewhere**
   G99.0 *Autonomic neuropathy in diseases classified elsewhere*
         Code first underlying disease, such as:
            amyloidosis (E85.-)
            gout (M1A.-, M10.-)
            hyperthyroidism (E05.-)
         EXCLUDES 1   diabetic autonomic neuropathy (E08-E13 with .43)

   G99.2 *Myelopathy in diseases classified elsewhere*   HCC
         Code first underlying disease, such as:
            neoplasm (C00-D49)
         EXCLUDES 1   myelopathy in:
              intervertebral disease (M50.0-, M51.0-)
              spondylosis (M47.0-, M47.1-)

   G99.8 *Other specified disorders of nervous system in diseases classified elsewhere*
         Code first underlying disorder, such as:
            amyloidosis (E85.-)
            avitaminosis (E56.9)
         EXCLUDES 1   nervous system involvement in:
              cysticercosis (B69.0)
              rubella (B06.0-)
              syphilis (A52.1-)

✓ Additional Character Req   ✓x7th Placeholder Alert   Manifestation   HCC CMS-HCC Condition   ▽ Unspecified Code   ▶◀ Revised Text   ● New Code   ▲ Revised Code Title
ICD-10-CM 2018   567

G95.89–G99.8

Chapter 7. Diseases of the Eye and Adnexa (H00–H59)

Chapter Specific Guidelines with Coding Examples

The chapter specific guidelines from the ICD-10-CM Official Guidelines for Coding and Reporting have been provided below. Along with these guidelines are coding examples, contained in the shaded boxes, that have been developed to help illustrate the coding and/or sequencing guidance found in these guidelines.

a. Glaucoma

1) Assigning glaucoma codes

Assign as many codes from category H40, Glaucoma, as needed to identify the type of glaucoma, the affected eye, and the glaucoma stage.

2) Bilateral glaucoma with same type and stage

When a patient has bilateral glaucoma and both eyes are documented as being the same type and stage, and there is a code for bilateral glaucoma, report only the code for the type of glaucoma, bilateral, with the seventh character for the stage.

> Bilateral mild stage primary open-angle glaucoma
>
> **H40.1131   Primary open-angle glaucoma, bilateral, mild stage**
>
> *Explanation*: In this scenario, the patient has the same type and stage of glaucoma in both eyes. As this type of glaucoma has a code for bilateral, assign only the code for the bilateral glaucoma with the seventh character for the stage.

When a patient has bilateral glaucoma and both eyes are documented as being the same type and stage, and the classification does not provide a code for bilateral glaucoma (i.e. subcategories H40.10, H40.11 and H40.20) report only one code for the type of glaucoma with the appropriate seventh character for the stage.

> Bilateral open-angle glaucoma, severe stage; not specified as to type
>
> **H40.10X3   Unspecified open-angle glaucoma, severe stage**
>
> *Explanation*: In this scenario, the patient has glaucoma of the same type and stage of both eyes, but there is no code specifically for bilateral glaucoma. Only one code is assigned with the appropriate seventh character for the stage.

3) Bilateral glaucoma stage with different types or stages

When a patient has bilateral glaucoma and each eye is documented as having a different type or stage, and the classification distinguishes laterality, assign the appropriate code for each eye rather than the code for bilateral glaucoma.

> Bilateral chronic angle-closure glaucoma; right eye Is documented as mild stage and left eye as moderate stage
>
> **H40.2211   Chronic angle-closure glaucoma, right eye, mild stage**
>
> **H40.2222   Chronic angle-closure glaucoma, left eye, moderate stage**
>
> *Explanation*: In this scenario the patient has the same type of glaucoma in both eyes, but each eye is at a different stage. Because the subcategory for this condition identifies laterality, one code is assigned for the right eye and one code is assigned for the left eye, each with the appropriate seventh character for the stage appended.

When a patient has bilateral glaucoma and each eye is documented as having a different type, and the classification does not distinguish laterality (i.e. subcategories H40.10, H40.11 and H40.20), assign one code for each type of glaucoma with the appropriate seventh character for the stage.

> Documentation relates mild, unspecified primary angle-closure glaucoma of the left eye with mild unspecified open-angle glaucoma of the right eye
>
> **H40.20X1   Unspecified primary angle-closure glaucoma, mild stage**
>
> **H40.10X1   Unspecified open-angle glaucoma, mild stage**
>
> *Explanation*: In this scenario the patient has a different type of glaucoma in each eye and the classification does not distinguish laterality. A code for each type of glaucoma is assigned, each with the appropriate seventh character for the stage.

When a patient has bilateral glaucoma and each eye is documented as having the same type, but different stage, and the classification does not distinguish laterality (i.e. subcategories H40.10, H40.11 and H40.20), assign a code for the type of glaucoma for each eye with the seventh character for the specific glaucoma stage documented for each eye.

> Bilateral open-angle glaucoma, not specified as to type; the right eye is documented to be in mild stage and the left eye as being in moderate stage
>
> **H40.10X1   Unspecified open-angle glaucoma, mild stage**
>
> **H40.10X2   Unspecified open-angle glaucoma, moderate stage**
>
> *Explanation*: In this scenario the patient has the same type of glaucoma in each eye but each eye is at a different stage, and the classification does not distinguish laterality at this subcategory level. Two codes are assigned; both codes represent the same type of glaucoma but each has a different seventh character identifying the appropriate stage for each eye.

4) Patient admitted with glaucoma and stage evolves during the admission

If a patient is admitted with glaucoma and the stage progresses during the admission, assign the code for highest stage documented.

5) Indeterminate stage glaucoma

Assignment of the seventh character "4" for "indeterminate stage" should be based on the clinical documentation. The seventh character "4" is used for glaucomas whose stage cannot be clinically determined. This seventh character should not be confused with the seventh character "0", unspecified, which should be assigned when there is no documentation regarding the stage of the glaucoma.

Chapter 7. Diseases of the Eye and Adnexa (H00–H59)

NOTE   Use an external cause code following the code for the eye condition, if applicable, to identify the cause of the eye condition.

EXCLUDES 2   certain conditions originating in the perinatal period (P04-P96)
certain infectious and parasitic diseases (A00-B99)
complications of pregnancy, childbirth and the puerperium (O00-O9A)
congenital malformations, deformations, and chromosomal abnormalities (Q00-Q99)
diabetes mellitus related eye conditions (E09.3-, E10.3-, E11.3-, E13.3-)
endocrine, nutritional and metabolic diseases (E00-E88)
injury (trauma) of eye and orbit (S05.-)
injury, poisoning and certain other consequences of external causes (S00-T88)
neoplasms (C00-D49)
symptoms, signs and abnormal clinical and laboratory findings, not elsewhere classified (R00-R94)
syphilis related eye disorders (A50.01, A50.3-, A51.43, A52.71)

This chapter contains the following blocks:

H00-H05	Disorders of eyelid, lacrimal system and orbit
H10-H11	Disorders of conjunctiva
H15-H22	Disorders of sclera, cornea, iris and ciliary body
H25-H28	Disorders of lens
H30-H36	Disorders of choroid and retina
H40-H42	Glaucoma
H43-H44	Disorders of vitreous body and globe
H46-H47	Disorders of optic nerve and visual pathways
H49-H52	Disorders of ocular muscles, binocular movement, accommodation and refraction
H53-H54	Visual disturbances and blindness
H55-H57	Other disorders of eye and adnexa
H59	Intraoperative and postprocedural complications and disorders of eye and adnexa, not elsewhere classified

Disorders of eyelid, lacrimal system and orbit (H00–H05)

EXCLUDES 2   open wound of eyelid (S01.1-)
superficial injury of eyelid (S00.1-, S00.2-)

✓4th **H00**   **Hordeolum and chalazion**

   ✓5th **H00.0**   Hordeolum (externum) (internum) of eyelid

     ✓6th **H00.01**   **Hordeolum externum**
       Hordeolum NOS
       Stye

       H00.011   **Hordeolum externum right upper eyelid**
       H00.012   **Hordeolum externum right lower eyelid**
       H00.013   **Hordeolum externum right eye, unspecified eyelid**   ▽
       H00.014   **Hordeolum externum left upper eyelid**
       H00.015   **Hordeolum externum left lower eyelid**
       H00.016   **Hordeolum externum left eye, unspecified eyelid**   ▽
       H00.019   **Hordeolum externum unspecified eye, unspecified eyelid**   ▽

     ✓6th **H00.02**   **Hordeolum internum**
       Infection of meibomian gland

       H00.021   **Hordeolum internum right upper eyelid**
       H00.022   **Hordeolum internum right lower eyelid**
       H00.023   **Hordeolum internum right eye, unspecified eyelid**   ▽
       H00.024   **Hordeolum internum left upper eyelid**
       H00.025   **Hordeolum internum left lower eyelid**
       H00.026   **Hordeolum internum left eye, unspecified eyelid**   ▽
       H00.029   **Hordeolum internum unspecified eye, unspecified eyelid**   ▽

     ✓6th **H00.03**   **Abscess of eyelid**
       Furuncle of eyelid

       H00.031   **Abscess of right upper eyelid**
       H00.032   **Abscess of right lower eyelid**
       H00.033   **Abscess of eyelid right eye, unspecified eyelid**   ▽
       H00.034   **Abscess of left upper eyelid**
       H00.035   **Abscess of left lower eyelid**
       H00.036   **Abscess of eyelid left eye, unspecified eyelid**   ▽
       H00.039   **Abscess of eyelid unspecified eye, unspecified eyelid**   ▽

   ✓5th **H00.1**   **Chalazion**
     Meibomian (gland) cyst
     EXCLUDES 2   infected meibomian gland (H00.02-)

     H00.11   **Chalazion right upper eyelid**
     H00.12   **Chalazion right lower eyelid**
     H00.13   **Chalazion right eye, unspecified eyelid**   ▽
     H00.14   **Chalazion left upper eyelid**
     H00.15   **Chalazion left lower eyelid**
     H00.16   **Chalazion left eye, unspecified eyelid**   ▽
     H00.19   **Chalazion unspecified eye, unspecified eyelid**   ▽

✓4th **H01**   **Other inflammation of eyelid**

   ✓5th **H01.0**   **Blepharitis**
     EXCLUDES 1   blepharoconjunctivitis (H10.5-)

     ✓6th **H01.00**   **Unspecified blepharitis**
       H01.001   **Unspecified blepharitis right upper eyelid**   ▽
       H01.002   **Unspecified blepharitis right lower eyelid**   ▽
       H01.003   **Unspecified blepharitis right eye, unspecified eyelid**   ▽
       H01.004   **Unspecified blepharitis left upper eyelid**   ▽
       H01.005   **Unspecified blepharitis left lower eyelid**   ▽
       H01.006   **Unspecified blepharitis left eye, unspecified eyelid**   ▽
       H01.009   **Unspecified blepharitis unspecified eye, unspecified eyelid**   ▽

     ✓6th **H01.01**   **Ulcerative blepharitis**
       H01.011   **Ulcerative blepharitis right upper eyelid**
       H01.012   **Ulcerative blepharitis right lower eyelid**
       H01.013   **Ulcerative blepharitis right eye, unspecified eyelid**   ▽
       H01.014   **Ulcerative blepharitis left upper eyelid**
       H01.015   **Ulcerative blepharitis left lower eyelid**
       H01.016   **Ulcerative blepharitis left eye, unspecified eyelid**   ▽
       H01.019   **Ulcerative blepharitis unspecified eye, unspecified eyelid**   ▽

     ✓6th **H01.02**   **Squamous blepharitis**
       H01.021   **Squamous blepharitis right upper eyelid**
       H01.022   **Squamous blepharitis right lower eyelid**
       H01.023   **Squamous blepharitis right eye, unspecified eyelid**   ▽
       H01.024   **Squamous blepharitis left upper eyelid**
       H01.025   **Squamous blepharitis left lower eyelid**
       H01.026   **Squamous blepharitis left eye, unspecified eyelid**   ▽
       H01.029   **Squamous blepharitis unspecified eye, unspecified eyelid**   ▽

   ✓5th **H01.1**   **Noninfectious dermatoses of eyelid**

     ✓6th **H01.11**   **Allergic dermatitis of eyelid**
       Contact dermatitis of eyelid
       H01.111   **Allergic dermatitis of right upper eyelid**
       H01.112   **Allergic dermatitis of right lower eyelid**
       H01.113   **Allergic dermatitis of right eye, unspecified eyelid**   ▽
       H01.114   **Allergic dermatitis of left upper eyelid**
       H01.115   **Allergic dermatitis of left lower eyelid**
       H01.116   **Allergic dermatitis of left eye, unspecified eyelid**   ▽
       H01.119   **Allergic dermatitis of unspecified eye, unspecified eyelid**   ▽

     ✓6th **H01.12**   **Discoid lupus erythematosus of eyelid**
       H01.121   **Discoid lupus erythematosus of right upper eyelid**
       H01.122   **Discoid lupus erythematosus of right lower eyelid**
       H01.123   **Discoid lupus erythematosus of right eye, unspecified eyelid**   ▽
       H01.124   **Discoid lupus erythematosus of left upper eyelid**
       H01.125   **Discoid lupus erythematosus of left lower eyelid**

EXCLUDES 1 Not coded here   **EXCLUDES 2** Not included here   **N** Newborn Age: 0   **P** Pediatric Age: 0-17   **M** Maternity Age: 12-55   **A** Adult Age: 15-124

570   ICD-10-CM 2018

H01.126 Discoid lupus erythematosus of left eye, unspecified eyelid ▽

H01.129 Discoid lupus erythematosus of unspecified eye, unspecified eyelid ▽

✓6ᵗʰ **H01.13** Eczematous dermatitis of eyelid

    H01.131 Eczematous dermatitis of right upper eyelid

    H01.132 Eczematous dermatitis of right lower eyelid

    H01.133 Eczematous dermatitis of right eye, unspecified eyelid ▽

    H01.134 Eczematous dermatitis of left upper eyelid

    H01.135 Eczematous dermatitis of left lower eyelid

    H01.136 Eczematous dermatitis of left eye, unspecified eyelid ▽

    H01.139 Eczematous dermatitis of unspecified eye, unspecified eyelid ▽

✓6ᵗʰ **H01.14** Xeroderma of eyelid

    H01.141 Xeroderma of right upper eyelid

    H01.142 Xeroderma of right lower eyelid

    H01.143 Xeroderma of right eye, unspecified eyelid ▽

    H01.144 Xeroderma of left upper eyelid

    H01.145 Xeroderma of left lower eyelid

    H01.146 Xeroderma of left eye, unspecified eyelid ▽

    H01.149 Xeroderma of unspecified eye, unspecified eyelid ▽

H01.8 Other specified inflammations of eyelid

H01.9 Unspecified inflammation of eyelid ▽
    Inflammation of eyelid NOS

✓4ᵗʰ **H02** Other disorders of eyelid

    EXCLUDES 1 congenital malformations of eyelid (Q10.0-Q10.3)

✓5ᵗʰ **H02.0** Entropion and trichiasis of eyelid

  ✓6ᵗʰ **H02.00** Unspecified entropion of eyelid

    H02.001 Unspecified entropion of right upper eyelid ▽

    H02.002 Unspecified entropion of right lower eyelid ▽

    H02.003 Unspecified entropion of right eye, unspecified eyelid ▽

    H02.004 Unspecified entropion of left upper eyelid ▽

    H02.005 Unspecified entropion of left lower eyelid ▽

    H02.006 Unspecified entropion of left eye, unspecified eyelid ▽

    H02.009 Unspecified entropion of unspecified eye, unspecified eyelid ▽

  ✓6ᵗʰ **H02.01** Cicatricial entropion of eyelid

    H02.011 Cicatricial entropion of right upper eyelid

    H02.012 Cicatricial entropion of right lower eyelid

    H02.013 Cicatricial entropion of right eye, unspecified eyelid ▽

    H02.014 Cicatricial entropion of left upper eyelid

    H02.015 Cicatricial entropion of left lower eyelid

    H02.016 Cicatricial entropion of left eye, unspecified eyelid ▽

    H02.019 Cicatricial entropion of unspecified eye, unspecified eyelid ▽

  ✓6ᵗʰ **H02.02** Mechanical entropion of eyelid

    H02.021 Mechanical entropion of right upper eyelid

    H02.022 Mechanical entropion of right lower eyelid

    H02.023 Mechanical entropion of right eye, unspecified eyelid ▽

    H02.024 Mechanical entropion of left upper eyelid

    H02.025 Mechanical entropion of left lower eyelid

    H02.026 Mechanical entropion of left eye, unspecified eyelid ▽

    H02.029 Mechanical entropion of unspecified eye, unspecified eyelid ▽

  ✓6ᵗʰ **H02.03** Senile entropion of eyelid

    H02.031 Senile entropion of right upper eyelid Ⓐ

    H02.032 Senile entropion of right lower eyelid Ⓐ

H02.033 Senile entropion of right eye, unspecified eyelid Ⓐ▽

H02.034 Senile entropion of left upper eyelid Ⓐ

H02.035 Senile entropion of left lower eyelid Ⓐ

H02.036 Senile entropion of left eye, unspecified eyelid Ⓐ▽

H02.039 Senile entropion of unspecified eye, unspecified eyelid Ⓐ▽

✓6ᵗʰ **H02.04** Spastic entropion of eyelid

    H02.041 Spastic entropion of right upper eyelid

    H02.042 Spastic entropion of right lower eyelid

    H02.043 Spastic entropion of right eye, unspecified eyelid ▽

    H02.044 Spastic entropion of left upper eyelid

    H02.045 Spastic entropion of left lower eyelid

    H02.046 Spastic entropion of left eye, unspecified eyelid ▽

    H02.049 Spastic entropion of unspecified eye, unspecified eyelid ▽

▲ ✓6ᵗʰ **H02.05** Trichiasis without entropion

▲   **H02.051** Trichiasis without entropion right upper eyelid

    H02.052 Trichiasis without entropion right lower eyelid

▲   **H02.053** Trichiasis without entropion right eye, unspecified eyelid ▽

    H02.054 Trichiasis without entropion left upper eyelid

▲   **H02.055** Trichiasis without entropion left lower eyelid

▲   **H02.056** Trichiasis without entropion left eye, unspecified eyelid ▽

▲   **H02.059** Trichiasis without entropion unspecified eye, unspecified eyelid ▽

✓5ᵗʰ **H02.1** Ectropion of eyelid

  ✓6ᵗʰ **H02.10** Unspecified ectropion of eyelid

    H02.101 Unspecified ectropion of right upper eyelid ▽

    H02.102 Unspecified ectropion of right lower eyelid ▽

    H02.103 Unspecified ectropion of right eye, unspecified eyelid ▽

    H02.104 Unspecified ectropion of left upper eyelid ▽

    H02.105 Unspecified ectropion of left lower eyelid ▽

    H02.106 Unspecified ectropion of left eye, unspecified eyelid ▽

    H02.109 Unspecified ectropion of unspecified eye, unspecified eyelid ▽

  ✓6ᵗʰ **H02.11** Cicatricial ectropion of eyelid

    H02.111 Cicatricial ectropion of right upper eyelid

    H02.112 Cicatricial ectropion of right lower eyelid

    H02.113 Cicatricial ectropion of right eye, unspecified eyelid ▽

    H02.114 Cicatricial ectropion of left upper eyelid

    H02.115 Cicatricial ectropion of left lower eyelid

    H02.116 Cicatricial ectropion of left eye, unspecified eyelid ▽

    H02.119 Cicatricial ectropion of unspecified eye, unspecified eyelid ▽

Entropion and Ectropion

Normal eyelid   Entropion   Ectropion

✓ Additional Character Req   ✓x7ᵗʰ Placeholder Alert   Manifestation   ᴴᶜᶜ CMS-HCC Condition   ▽ Unspecified Code   ►◄ Revised Text   ● New Code   ▲ Revised Code Title

ICD-10-CM 2018   571

H01.126-H02.119

Chapter 7. Diseases of the Eye and Adnexa *(left margin)*

✓6ᵗʰ **H02.12 Mechanical ectropion of eyelid**
- H02.121 Mechanical ectropion of right upper eyelid
- H02.122 Mechanical ectropion of right lower eyelid
- H02.123 Mechanical ectropion of right eye, unspecified eyelid ▽
- H02.124 Mechanical ectropion of left upper eyelid
- H02.125 Mechanical ectropion of left lower eyelid
- H02.126 Mechanical ectropion of left eye, unspecified eyelid ▽
- H02.129 Mechanical ectropion of unspecified eye, unspecified eyelid ▽

✓6ᵗʰ **H02.13 Senile ectropion of eyelid**
- H02.131 Senile ectropion of right upper eyelid [A]
- H02.132 Senile ectropion of right lower eyelid [A]
- H02.133 Senile ectropion of right eye, unspecified eyelid [A]▽
- H02.134 Senile ectropion of left upper eyelid [A]
- H02.135 Senile ectropion of left lower eyelid [A]
- H02.136 Senile ectropion of left eye, unspecified eyelid [A]▽
- H02.139 Senile ectropion of unspecified eye, unspecified eyelid [A]▽

✓6ᵗʰ **H02.14 Spastic ectropion of eyelid**
- H02.141 Spastic ectropion of right upper eyelid
- H02.142 Spastic ectropion of right lower eyelid
- H02.143 Spastic ectropion of right eye, unspecified eyelid ▽
- H02.144 Spastic ectropion of left upper eyelid
- H02.145 Spastic ectropion of left lower eyelid
- H02.146 Spastic ectropion of left eye, unspecified eyelid ▽
- H02.149 Spastic ectropion of unspecified eye, unspecified eyelid ▽

✓5ᵗʰ **H02.2 Lagophthalmos**

✓6ᵗʰ **H02.20 Unspecified lagophthalmos**
- H02.201 Unspecified lagophthalmos right upper eyelid ▽
- H02.202 Unspecified lagophthalmos right lower eyelid ▽
- H02.203 Unspecified lagophthalmos right eye, unspecified eyelid ▽
- H02.204 Unspecified lagophthalmos left upper eyelid ▽
- H02.205 Unspecified lagophthalmos left lower eyelid ▽
- H02.206 Unspecified lagophthalmos left eye, unspecified eyelid ▽
- H02.209 Unspecified lagophthalmos unspecified eye, unspecified eyelid ▽

✓6ᵗʰ **H02.21 Cicatricial lagophthalmos**
- H02.211 Cicatricial lagophthalmos right upper eyelid
- H02.212 Cicatricial lagophthalmos right lower eyelid
- H02.213 Cicatricial lagophthalmos right eye, unspecified eyelid ▽
- H02.214 Cicatricial lagophthalmos left upper eyelid
- H02.215 Cicatricial lagophthalmos left lower eyelid
- H02.216 Cicatricial lagophthalmos left eye, unspecified eyelid ▽
- H02.219 Cicatricial lagophthalmos unspecified eye, unspecified eyelid ▽

✓6ᵗʰ **H02.22 Mechanical lagophthalmos**
- H02.221 Mechanical lagophthalmos right upper eyelid
- H02.222 Mechanical lagophthalmos right lower eyelid
- H02.223 Mechanical lagophthalmos right eye, unspecified eyelid ▽
- H02.224 Mechanical lagophthalmos left upper eyelid
- H02.225 Mechanical lagophthalmos left lower eyelid
- H02.226 Mechanical lagophthalmos left eye, unspecified eyelid ▽
- H02.229 Mechanical lagophthalmos unspecified eye, unspecified eyelid ▽

✓6ᵗʰ **H02.23 Paralytic lagophthalmos**
- H02.231 Paralytic lagophthalmos right upper eyelid
- H02.232 Paralytic lagophthalmos right lower eyelid
- H02.233 Paralytic lagophthalmos right eye, unspecified eyelid ▽
- H02.234 Paralytic lagophthalmos left upper eyelid
- H02.235 Paralytic lagophthalmos left lower eyelid
- H02.236 Paralytic lagophthalmos left eye, unspecified eyelid ▽
- H02.239 Paralytic lagophthalmos unspecified eye, unspecified eyelid ▽

✓5ᵗʰ **H02.3 Blepharochalasis**
    Pseudoptosis
- H02.30 Blepharochalasis unspecified eye, unspecified eyelid ▽
- H02.31 Blepharochalasis right upper eyelid
- H02.32 Blepharochalasis right lower eyelid
- H02.33 Blepharochalasis right eye, unspecified eyelid ▽
- H02.34 Blepharochalasis left upper eyelid
- H02.35 Blepharochalasis left lower eyelid
- H02.36 Blepharochalasis left eye, unspecified eyelid ▽

✓5ᵗʰ **H02.4 Ptosis of eyelid**

✓6ᵗʰ **H02.40 Unspecified ptosis of eyelid**
- H02.401 Unspecified ptosis of right eyelid ▽
- H02.402 Unspecified ptosis of left eyelid ▽
- H02.403 Unspecified ptosis of bilateral eyelids ▽
- H02.409 Unspecified ptosis of unspecified eyelid ▽

✓6ᵗʰ **H02.41 Mechanical ptosis of eyelid**
- H02.411 Mechanical ptosis of right eyelid
- H02.412 Mechanical ptosis of left eyelid
- H02.413 Mechanical ptosis of bilateral eyelids
- H02.419 Mechanical ptosis of unspecified eyelid ▽

✓6ᵗʰ **H02.42 Myogenic ptosis of eyelid**
- H02.421 Myogenic ptosis of right eyelid
- H02.422 Myogenic ptosis of left eyelid
- H02.423 Myogenic ptosis of bilateral eyelids
- H02.429 Myogenic ptosis of unspecified eyelid ▽

✓6ᵗʰ **H02.43 Paralytic ptosis of eyelid**
    Neurogenic ptosis of eyelid
- H02.431 Paralytic ptosis of right eyelid
- H02.432 Paralytic ptosis of left eyelid
- H02.433 Paralytic ptosis of bilateral eyelids
- H02.439 Paralytic ptosis unspecified eyelid ▽

✓5ᵗʰ **H02.5 Other disorders affecting eyelid function**
    EXCLUDES 2 blepharospasm (G24.5)
            organic tic (G25.69)
            psychogenic tic (F95.-)

✓6ᵗʰ **H02.51 Abnormal innervation syndrome**
- H02.511 Abnormal innervation syndrome right upper eyelid
- H02.512 Abnormal innervation syndrome right lower eyelid
- H02.513 Abnormal innervation syndrome right eye, unspecified eyelid ▽
- H02.514 Abnormal innervation syndrome left upper eyelid
- H02.515 Abnormal innervation syndrome left lower eyelid
- H02.516 Abnormal innervation syndrome left eye, unspecified eyelid ▽
- H02.519 Abnormal innervation syndrome unspecified eye, unspecified eyelid ▽

✓6ᵗʰ **H02.52 Blepharophimosis**
    Ankyloblepharon
- H02.521 Blepharophimosis right upper eyelid
- H02.522 Blepharophimosis right lower eyelid
- H02.523 Blepharophimosis right eye, unspecified eyelid ▽
- H02.524 Blepharophimosis left upper eyelid
- H02.525 Blepharophimosis left lower eyelid
- H02.526 Blepharophimosis left eye, unspecified eyelid ▽

EXCLUDES 1 Not coded here   EXCLUDES 2 Not included here   [N] Newborn Age: 0   [P] Pediatric Age: 0-17   [M] Maternity Age: 12-55   [A] Adult Age: 15-124

572   ICD-10-CM 2018

H02.529   **Blepharophimosis unspecified eye, unspecified lid** ▽

✓6th H02.53   **Eyelid retraction**
Eyelid lag

H02.531   **Eyelid retraction right upper eyelid**

H02.532   **Eyelid retraction right lower eyelid**

H02.533   **Eyelid retraction right eye, unspecified eyelid** ▽

H02.534   **Eyelid retraction left upper eyelid**

H02.535   **Eyelid retraction left lower eyelid**

H02.536   **Eyelid retraction left eye, unspecified eyelid** ▽

H02.539   **Eyelid retraction unspecified eye, unspecified lid** ▽

H02.59   **Other disorders affecting eyelid function**
Deficient blink reflex
Sensory disorders

✓5th H02.6   **Xanthelasma of eyelid**

H02.60   **Xanthelasma of unspecified eye, unspecified eyelid** ▽

H02.61   **Xanthelasma of right upper eyelid**

H02.62   **Xanthelasma of right lower eyelid**

H02.63   **Xanthelasma of right eye, unspecified eyelid** ▽

H02.64   **Xanthelasma of left upper eyelid**

H02.65   **Xanthelasma of left lower eyelid**

H02.66   **Xanthelasma of left eye, unspecified eyelid** ▽

✓5th H02.7   **Other and unspecified degenerative disorders of eyelid and periocular area**

H02.70   **Unspecified degenerative disorders of eyelid and periocular area** ▽

✓6th H02.71   **Chloasma of eyelid and periocular area**
Dyspigmentation of eyelid
Hyperpigmentation of eyelid

H02.711   **Chloasma of right upper eyelid and periocular area**

H02.712   **Chloasma of right lower eyelid and periocular area**

H02.713   **Chloasma of right eye, unspecified eyelid and periocular area** ▽

H02.714   **Chloasma of left upper eyelid and periocular area**

H02.715   **Chloasma of left lower eyelid and periocular area**

H02.716   **Chloasma of left eye, unspecified eyelid and periocular area** ▽

H02.719   **Chloasma of unspecified eye, unspecified eyelid and periocular area** ▽

✓6th H02.72   **Madarosis of eyelid and periocular area**
Hypotrichosis of eyelid

H02.721   **Madarosis of right upper eyelid and periocular area**

H02.722   **Madarosis of right lower eyelid and periocular area**

H02.723   **Madarosis of right eye, unspecified eyelid and periocular area** ▽

H02.724   **Madarosis of left upper eyelid and periocular area**

H02.725   **Madarosis of left lower eyelid and periocular area**

H02.726   **Madarosis of left eye, unspecified eyelid and periocular area** ▽

H02.729   **Madarosis of unspecified eye, unspecified eyelid and periocular area** ▽

✓6th H02.73   **Vitiligo of eyelid and periocular area**
Hypopigmentation of eyelid

H02.731   **Vitiligo of right upper eyelid and periocular area**

H02.732   **Vitiligo of right lower eyelid and periocular area**

H02.733   **Vitiligo of right eye, unspecified eyelid and periocular area** ▽

H02.734   **Vitiligo of left upper eyelid and periocular area**

H02.735   **Vitiligo of left lower eyelid and periocular area**

H02.736   **Vitiligo of left eye, unspecified eyelid and periocular area** ▽

H02.739   **Vitiligo of unspecified eye, unspecified eyelid and periocular area**

H02.79   **Other degenerative disorders of eyelid and periocular area**

✓5th H02.8   **Other specified disorders of eyelid**

✓6th H02.81   **Retained foreign body in eyelid**
Use additional code to identify the type of retained foreign body (Z18.-)
EXCLUDES 1 *laceration of eyelid with foreign body (S01.12-)*
retained intraocular foreign body (H44.6-, H44.7-)
superficial foreign body of eyelid and periocular area (S00.25-)

H02.811   **Retained foreign body in right upper eyelid**

H02.812   **Retained foreign body in right lower eyelid**

H02.813   **Retained foreign body in right eye, unspecified eyelid** ▽

H02.814   **Retained foreign body in left upper eyelid**

H02.815   **Retained foreign body in left lower eyelid**

H02.816   **Retained foreign body in left eye, unspecified eyelid** ▽

H02.819   **Retained foreign body in unspecified eye, unspecified eyelid** ▽

✓6th H02.82   **Cysts of eyelid**
Sebaceous cyst of eyelid

H02.821   **Cysts of right upper eyelid**

H02.822   **Cysts of right lower eyelid**

H02.823   **Cysts of right eye, unspecified eyelid** ▽

H02.824   **Cysts of left upper eyelid**

H02.825   **Cysts of left lower eyelid**

H02.826   **Cysts of left eye, unspecified eyelid** ▽

H02.829   **Cysts of unspecified eye, unspecified eyelid** ▽

✓6th H02.83   **Dermatochalasis of eyelid**
DEF: Acquired form of connective tissue disorder associated with decreased elastic tissue and abnormal elastin formation, resulting in loss of elasticity of the skin of the eyelid; generally associated with aging.

H02.831   **Dermatochalasis of right upper eyelid**

H02.832   **Dermatochalasis of right lower eyelid**

H02.833   **Dermatochalasis of right eye, unspecified eyelid** ▽

H02.834   **Dermatochalasis of left upper eyelid**

H02.835   **Dermatochalasis of left lower eyelid**

H02.836   **Dermatochalasis of left eye, unspecified eyelid** ▽

H02.839   **Dermatochalasis of unspecified eye, unspecified eyelid** ▽

✓6th H02.84   **Edema of eyelid**
Hyperemia of eyelid

H02.841   **Edema of right upper eyelid**

H02.842   **Edema of right lower eyelid**

H02.843   **Edema of right eye, unspecified eyelid** ▽

H02.844   **Edema of left upper eyelid**

H02.845   **Edema of left lower eyelid**

H02.846   **Edema of left eye, unspecified eyelid** ▽

H02.849   **Edema of unspecified eye, unspecified eyelid** ▽

✓6th H02.85   **Elephantiasis of eyelid**

H02.851   **Elephantiasis of right upper eyelid**

H02.852   **Elephantiasis of right lower eyelid**

H02.853   **Elephantiasis of right eye, unspecified eyelid** ▽

H02.854   **Elephantiasis of left upper eyelid**

H02.855   **Elephantiasis of left lower eyelid**

H02.856   **Elephantiasis of left eye, unspecified eyelid** ▽

H02.859   **Elephantiasis of unspecified eye, unspecified eyelid** ▽

✓6th H02.86   **Hypertrichosis of eyelid**

H02.861   **Hypertrichosis of right upper eyelid**

H02.862   **Hypertrichosis of right lower eyelid**

H02.863   **Hypertrichosis of right eye, unspecified eyelid** ▽

✓ Additional Character Req   ✓7th Placeholder Alert   Manifestation   HCC CMS-HCC Condition   ▽ Unspecified Code   ▶◀ Revised Text   ● New Code   ▲ Revised Code Title

ICD-10-CM 2018   573

H02.864 Hypertrichosis of **left upper** eyelid
H02.865 Hypertrichosis of **left lower** eyelid
H02.866 Hypertrichosis of **left eye,** unspecified eyelid ▽
H02.869 Hypertrichosis of **unspecified eye,** unspecified eyelid ▽

✓6ᵗʰ **H02.87 Vascular anomalies of eyelid**
H02.871 Vascular anomalies of **right upper** eyelid
H02.872 Vascular anomalies of **right lower** eyelid
H02.873 Vascular anomalies of **right eye,** unspecified eyelid
H02.874 Vascular anomalies of **left upper** eyelid
H02.875 Vascular anomalies of **left lower** eyelid
H02.876 Vascular anomalies of **left eye,** unspecified eyelid ▽
H02.879 Vascular anomalies of **unspecified** eye, unspecified eyelid ▽

H02.89 Other specified disorders of eyelid
Hemorrhage of eyelid

H02.9 Unspecified disorder of eyelid ▽
Disorder of eyelid NOS

✓4ᵗʰ **H04 Disorders of lacrimal system**
EXCLUDES 1 congenital malformations of lacrimal system (Q10.4-Q10.6)

✓5ᵗʰ **H04.0 Dacryoadenitis**
✓6ᵗʰ **H04.00 Unspecified dacryoadenitis**
H04.001 Unspecified dacryoadenitis, **right** lacrimal gland ▽
H04.002 Unspecified dacryoadenitis, **left** lacrimal gland ▽
H04.003 Unspecified dacryoadenitis, **bilateral** lacrimal glands ▽
H04.009 Unspecified dacryoadenitis, **unspecified** lacrimal gland ▽

✓6ᵗʰ **H04.01 Acute dacryoadenitis**
H04.011 Acute dacryoadenitis, **right** lacrimal gland
H04.012 Acute dacryoadenitis, **left** lacrimal gland
H04.013 Acute dacryoadenitis, **bilateral** lacrimal glands
H04.019 Acute dacryoadenitis, **unspecified** lacrimal gland ▽

✓6ᵗʰ **H04.02 Chronic dacryoadenitis**
H04.021 Chronic dacryoadenitis, **right** lacrimal gland
H04.022 Chronic dacryoadenitis, **left** lacrimal gland
H04.023 Chronic dacryoadenitis, **bilateral** lacrimal glands
H04.029 Chronic dacryoadenitis, **unspecified** lacrimal gland ▽

✓6ᵗʰ **H04.03 Chronic enlargement of lacrimal gland**
H04.031 Chronic enlargement of **right** lacrimal gland
H04.032 Chronic enlargement of **left** lacrimal gland
H04.033 Chronic enlargement of **bilateral** lacrimal glands
H04.039 Chronic enlargement of **unspecified** lacrimal gland ▽

✓5ᵗʰ **H04.1 Other disorders of lacrimal gland**
✓6ᵗʰ **H04.11 Dacryops**
H04.111 Dacryops of **right** lacrimal gland
H04.112 Dacryops of **left** lacrimal gland
H04.113 Dacryops of **bilateral** lacrimal glands
H04.119 Dacryops of **unspecified** lacrimal gland ▽

✓6ᵗʰ **H04.12 Dry eye syndrome**
Tear film insufficiency, NOS
H04.121 Dry eye syndrome of **right** lacrimal gland
H04.122 Dry eye syndrome of **left** lacrimal gland
H04.123 Dry eye syndrome of **bilateral** lacrimal glands
H04.129 Dry eye syndrome of **unspecified** lacrimal gland ▽

✓6ᵗʰ **H04.13 Lacrimal cyst**
Lacrimal cystic degeneration
H04.131 Lacrimal cyst, **right** lacrimal gland
H04.132 Lacrimal cyst, **left** lacrimal gland
H04.133 Lacrimal cyst, **bilateral** lacrimal glands

H04.139 Lacrimal cyst, unspecified lacrimal gland ▽

✓6ᵗʰ **H04.14 Primary lacrimal gland atrophy**
H04.141 Primary lacrimal gland atrophy, **right** lacrimal gland
H04.142 Primary lacrimal gland atrophy, **left** lacrimal gland
H04.143 Primary lacrimal gland atrophy, **bilateral** lacrimal glands
H04.149 Primary lacrimal gland atrophy, **unspecified** lacrimal gland ▽

✓6ᵗʰ **H04.15 Secondary lacrimal gland atrophy**
H04.151 Secondary lacrimal gland atrophy, **right** lacrimal gland
H04.152 Secondary lacrimal gland atrophy, **left** lacrimal gland
H04.153 Secondary lacrimal gland atrophy, **bilateral** lacrimal glands
H04.159 Secondary lacrimal gland atrophy, **unspecified** lacrimal gland ▽

✓6ᵗʰ **H04.16 Lacrimal gland dislocation**
H04.161 Lacrimal gland dislocation, **right** lacrimal gland
H04.162 Lacrimal gland dislocation, **left** lacrimal gland
H04.163 Lacrimal gland dislocation, **bilateral** lacrimal glands
H04.169 Lacrimal gland dislocation, **unspecified** lacrimal gland ▽

H04.19 Other specified disorders of lacrimal gland

✓5ᵗʰ **H04.2 Epiphora**
✓6ᵗʰ **H04.20 Unspecified epiphora**
H04.201 Unspecified epiphora, **right** lacrimal gland ▽
H04.202 Unspecified epiphora, **left** lacrimal gland ▽
H04.203 Unspecified epiphora, **bilateral** lacrimal glands ▽
H04.209 Unspecified epiphora, **unspecified** lacrimal gland ▽

✓6ᵗʰ **H04.21 Epiphora due to excess lacrimation**
H04.211 Epiphora due to excess lacrimation, **right** lacrimal gland
H04.212 Epiphora due to excess lacrimation, **left** lacrimal gland
H04.213 Epiphora due to excess lacrimation, **bilateral** lacrimal glands
H04.219 Epiphora due to excess lacrimation, **unspecified** lacrimal gland ▽

✓6ᵗʰ **H04.22 Epiphora due to insufficient drainage**
H04.221 Epiphora due to insufficient drainage, **right** lacrimal gland
H04.222 Epiphora due to insufficient drainage, **left** lacrimal gland
H04.223 Epiphora due to insufficient drainage, **bilateral** lacrimal glands
H04.229 Epiphora due to insufficient drainage, **unspecified** lacrimal gland ▽

✓5ᵗʰ **H04.3 Acute and unspecified inflammation of lacrimal passages**
EXCLUDES 1 neonatal dacryocystitis (P39.1)
✓6ᵗʰ **H04.30 Unspecified dacryocystitis**
H04.301 Unspecified dacryocystitis of **right** lacrimal passage ▽
H04.302 Unspecified dacryocystitis of **left** lacrimal passage ▽
H04.303 Unspecified dacryocystitis of **bilateral** lacrimal passages ▽
H04.309 Unspecified dacryocystitis of **unspecified** lacrimal passage ▽

✓6ᵗʰ **H04.31 Phlegmonous dacryocystitis**
H04.311 Phlegmonous dacryocystitis of **right** lacrimal passage
H04.312 Phlegmonous dacryocystitis of **left** lacrimal passage
H04.313 Phlegmonous dacryocystitis of **bilateral** lacrimal passages

H04.319   **Phlegmonous dacryocystitis of unspecified lacrimal passage** ▽

✓6th **H04.32**   **Acute dacryocystitis**
     Acute dacryopericystitis

H04.321   **Acute dacryocystitis of right lacrimal passage**

H04.322   **Acute dacryocystitis of left lacrimal passage**

H04.323   **Acute dacryocystitis of bilateral lacrimal passages**

H04.329   **Acute dacryocystitis of unspecified lacrimal passage** ▽

✓6th **H04.33**   **Acute lacrimal canaliculitis**

H04.331   **Acute lacrimal canaliculitis of right lacrimal passage**

H04.332   **Acute lacrimal canaliculitis of left lacrimal passage**

H04.333   **Acute lacrimal canaliculitis of bilateral lacrimal passages**

H04.339   **Acute lacrimal canaliculitis of unspecified lacrimal passage** ▽

✓5th **H04.4**   **Chronic inflammation of lacrimal passages**

✓6th **H04.41**   **Chronic dacryocystitis**

H04.411   **Chronic dacryocystitis of right lacrimal passage**

H04.412   **Chronic dacryocystitis of left lacrimal passage**

H04.413   **Chronic dacryocystitis of bilateral lacrimal passages**

H04.419   **Chronic dacryocystitis of unspecified lacrimal passage** ▽

✓6th **H04.42**   **Chronic lacrimal canaliculitis**

H04.421   **Chronic lacrimal canaliculitis of right lacrimal passage**

H04.422   **Chronic lacrimal canaliculitis of left lacrimal passage**

H04.423   **Chronic lacrimal canaliculitis of bilateral lacrimal passages**

H04.429   **Chronic lacrimal canaliculitis of unspecified lacrimal passage** ▽

✓6th **H04.43**   **Chronic lacrimal mucocele**

H04.431   **Chronic lacrimal mucocele of right lacrimal passage**

H04.432   **Chronic lacrimal mucocele of left lacrimal passage**

H04.433   **Chronic lacrimal mucocele of bilateral lacrimal passages**

H04.439   **Chronic lacrimal mucocele of unspecified lacrimal passage** ▽

✓5th **H04.5**   **Stenosis and insufficiency of lacrimal passages**

✓6th **H04.51**   **Dacryolith**

H04.511   **Dacryolith of right lacrimal passage**

H04.512   **Dacryolith of left lacrimal passage**

H04.513   **Dacryolith of bilateral lacrimal passages**

H04.519   **Dacryolith of unspecified lacrimal passage** ▽

✓6th **H04.52**   **Eversion of lacrimal punctum**

H04.521   **Eversion of right lacrimal punctum**

H04.522   **Eversion of left lacrimal punctum**

H04.523   **Eversion of bilateral lacrimal punctum**

H04.529   **Eversion of unspecified lacrimal punctum** ▽

✓6th **H04.53**   **Neonatal obstruction of nasolacrimal duct**
     EXCLUDES 1   *congenital stenosis and stricture of lacrimal duct (Q10.5)*

H04.531   **Neonatal obstruction of right nasolacrimal duct** Ⓝ

H04.532   **Neonatal obstruction of left nasolacrimal duct** Ⓝ

H04.533   **Neonatal obstruction of bilateral nasolacrimal duct** Ⓝ

H04.539   **Neonatal obstruction of unspecified nasolacrimal duct** Ⓝ ▽

✓6th **H04.54**   **Stenosis of lacrimal canaliculi**

H04.541   **Stenosis of right lacrimal canaliculi**

H04.542   **Stenosis of left lacrimal canaliculi**

H04.543   **Stenosis of bilateral lacrimal canaliculi**

H04.549   **Stenosis of unspecified lacrimal canaliculi** ▽

✓6th **H04.55**   **Acquired stenosis of nasolacrimal duct**

H04.551   **Acquired stenosis of right nasolacrimal duct**

H04.552   **Acquired stenosis of left nasolacrimal duct**

H04.553   **Acquired stenosis of bilateral nasolacrimal duct**

H04.559   **Acquired stenosis of unspecified nasolacrimal duct** ▽

✓6th **H04.56**   **Stenosis of lacrimal punctum**

H04.561   **Stenosis of right lacrimal punctum**

H04.562   **Stenosis of left lacrimal punctum**

H04.563   **Stenosis of bilateral lacrimal punctum**

H04.569   **Stenosis of unspecified lacrimal punctum** ▽

✓6th **H04.57**   **Stenosis of lacrimal sac**

H04.571   **Stenosis of right lacrimal sac**

H04.572   **Stenosis of left lacrimal sac**

H04.573   **Stenosis of bilateral lacrimal sac**

H04.579   **Stenosis of unspecified lacrimal sac** ▽

✓5th **H04.6**   **Other changes of lacrimal passages**

✓6th **H04.61**   **Lacrimal fistula**

H04.611   **Lacrimal fistula right lacrimal passage**

H04.612   **Lacrimal fistula left lacrimal passage**

H04.613   **Lacrimal fistula bilateral lacrimal passages**

H04.619   **Lacrimal fistula unspecified lacrimal passage** ▽

H04.69   **Other changes of lacrimal passages**

✓5th **H04.8**   **Other disorders of lacrimal system**

✓6th **H04.81**   **Granuloma of lacrimal passages**

H04.811   **Granuloma of right lacrimal passage**

H04.812   **Granuloma of left lacrimal passage**

H04.813   **Granuloma of bilateral lacrimal passages**

H04.819   **Granuloma of unspecified lacrimal passage** ▽

H04.89   **Other disorders of lacrimal system**

H04.9   **Disorder of lacrimal system, unspecified** ▽

✓4th **H05**   **Disorders of orbit**
     EXCLUDES 1   *congenital malformation of orbit (Q10.7)*

✓5th **H05.0**   **Acute inflammation of orbit**

H05.00   **Unspecified acute inflammation of orbit** ▽

✓6th **H05.01**   **Cellulitis of orbit**
     Abscess of orbit

H05.011   **Cellulitis of right orbit**

H05.012   **Cellulitis of left orbit**

H05.013   **Cellulitis of bilateral orbits**

H05.019   **Cellulitis of unspecified orbit** ▽

✓6th **H05.02**   **Osteomyelitis of orbit**

H05.021   **Osteomyelitis of right orbit**

H05.022   **Osteomyelitis of left orbit**

H05.023   **Osteomyelitis of bilateral orbits**

H05.029   **Osteomyelitis of unspecified orbit** ▽

✓6th **H05.03**   **Periostitis of orbit**

H05.031   **Periostitis of right orbit**

H05.032   **Periostitis of left orbit**

H05.033   **Periostitis of bilateral orbits**

H05.039   **Periostitis of unspecified orbit** ▽

✓6th **H05.04**   **Tenonitis of orbit**

H05.041   **Tenonitis of right orbit**

H05.042   **Tenonitis of left orbit**

H05.043   **Tenonitis of bilateral orbits**

H05.049   **Tenonitis of unspecified orbit** ▽

✓5th **H05.1**   **Chronic inflammatory disorders of orbit**

H05.10   **Unspecified chronic inflammatory disorders of orbit** ▽

✓6th **H05.11**   **Granuloma of orbit**
     Pseudotumor (inflammatory) of orbit

H05.111   **Granuloma of right orbit**

H05.112   **Granuloma of left orbit**

H05.113   **Granuloma of bilateral orbits**

☑ Additional Character Req   ✓x7th Placeholder Alert   Manifestation   ℍℂℂ CMS-HCC Condition   ▽ Unspecified Code   ►◄ Revised Text   ● New Code   ▲ Revised Code Title

ICD-10-CM 2018   575

H05.119   Granuloma of unspecified orbit ▽

✓6th H05.12 Orbital myositis
    H05.121   Orbital myositis, right orbit
    H05.122   Orbital myositis, left orbit
    H05.123   Orbital myositis, bilateral
    H05.129   Orbital myositis, unspecified orbit ▽

✓5th H05.2 Exophthalmic conditions
    H05.20 Unspecified exophthalmos ▽
  ✓6th H05.21 Displacement (lateral) of globe
    H05.211   Displacement (lateral) of globe, right eye
    H05.212   Displacement (lateral) of globe, left eye
    H05.213   Displacement (lateral) of globe, bilateral
    H05.219   Displacement (lateral) of globe, unspecified eye ▽
  ✓6th H05.22 Edema of orbit
      Orbital congestion
    H05.221   Edema of right orbit
    H05.222   Edema of left orbit
    H05.223   Edema of bilateral orbit
    H05.229   Edema of unspecified orbit ▽
  ✓6th H05.23 Hemorrhage of orbit
    H05.231   Hemorrhage of right orbit
    H05.232   Hemorrhage of left orbit
    H05.233   Hemorrhage of bilateral orbit
    H05.239   Hemorrhage of unspecified orbit ▽
  ✓6th H05.24 Constant exophthalmos
    H05.241   Constant exophthalmos, right eye
    H05.242   Constant exophthalmos, left eye
    H05.243   Constant exophthalmos, bilateral
    H05.249   Constant exophthalmos, unspecified eye ▽
  ✓6th H05.25 Intermittent exophthalmos
    H05.251   Intermittent exophthalmos, right eye
    H05.252   Intermittent exophthalmos, left eye
    H05.253   Intermittent exophthalmos, bilateral
    H05.259   Intermittent exophthalmos, unspecified eye ▽
  ✓6th H05.26 Pulsating exophthalmos
    H05.261   Pulsating exophthalmos, right eye
    H05.262   Pulsating exophthalmos, left eye
    H05.263   Pulsating exophthalmos, bilateral
    H05.269   Pulsating exophthalmos, unspecified eye ▽

✓5th H05.3 Deformity of orbit
    EXCLUDES 1   congenital deformity of orbit (Q10.7)
                  hypertelorism (Q75.2)
    H05.30 Unspecified deformity of orbit ▽
  ✓6th H05.31 Atrophy of orbit
    H05.311   Atrophy of right orbit
    H05.312   Atrophy of left orbit
    H05.313   Atrophy of bilateral orbit
    H05.319   Atrophy of unspecified orbit ▽
  ✓6th H05.32 Deformity of orbit due to bone disease
      Code also associated bone disease
    H05.321   Deformity of right orbit due to bone disease
    H05.322   Deformity of left orbit due to bone disease
    H05.323   Deformity of bilateral orbits due to bone disease
    H05.329   Deformity of unspecified orbit due to bone disease ▽
  ✓6th H05.33 Deformity of orbit due to trauma or surgery
    H05.331   Deformity of right orbit due to trauma or surgery
    H05.332   Deformity of left orbit due to trauma or surgery
    H05.333   Deformity of bilateral orbits due to trauma or surgery
    H05.339   Deformity of unspecified orbit due to trauma or surgery ▽
  ✓6th H05.34 Enlargement of orbit
    H05.341   Enlargement of right orbit
    H05.342   Enlargement of left orbit
    H05.343   Enlargement of bilateral orbits

    H05.349   Enlargement of unspecified orbit ▽
  ✓6th H05.35 Exostosis of orbit
    H05.351   Exostosis of right orbit
    H05.352   Exostosis of left orbit
    H05.353   Exostosis of bilateral orbits
    H05.359   Exostosis of unspecified orbit ▽

✓5th H05.4 Enophthalmos
  ✓6th H05.40 Unspecified enophthalmos
    H05.401   Unspecified enophthalmos, right eye ▽
    H05.402   Unspecified enophthalmos, left eye ▽
    H05.403   Unspecified enophthalmos, bilateral ▽
    H05.409   Unspecified enophthalmos, unspecified eye ▽
  ✓6th H05.41 Enophthalmos due to atrophy of orbital tissue
    H05.411   Enophthalmos due to atrophy of orbital tissue, right eye
    H05.412   Enophthalmos due to atrophy of orbital tissue, left eye
    H05.413   Enophthalmos due to atrophy of orbital tissue, bilateral
    H05.419   Enophthalmos due to atrophy of orbital tissue, unspecified eye ▽
  ✓6th H05.42 Enophthalmos due to trauma or surgery
    H05.421   Enophthalmos due to trauma or surgery, right eye
    H05.422   Enophthalmos due to trauma or surgery, left eye
    H05.423   Enophthalmos due to trauma or surgery, bilateral
    H05.429   Enophthalmos due to trauma or surgery, unspecified eye ▽

✓5th H05.5 Retained (old) foreign body following penetrating wound of orbit
    Retrobulbar foreign body
    Use additional code to identify the type of retained foreign body (Z18.-)
    EXCLUDES 1   current penetrating wound of orbit (S05.4-)
    EXCLUDES 2   retained foreign body of eyelid (H02.81-)
                   retained intraocular foreign body (H44.6-, H44.7-)
    H05.50 Retained (old) foreign body following penetrating wound of unspecified orbit ▽
    H05.51 Retained (old) foreign body following penetrating wound of right orbit
    H05.52 Retained (old) foreign body following penetrating wound of left orbit
    H05.53 Retained (old) foreign body following penetrating wound of bilateral orbits

✓5th H05.8 Other disorders of orbit
  ✓6th H05.81 Cyst of orbit
      Encephalocele of orbit
    H05.811   Cyst of right orbit
    H05.812   Cyst of left orbit
    H05.813   Cyst of bilateral orbits
    H05.819   Cyst of unspecified orbit ▽
  ✓6th H05.82 Myopathy of extraocular muscles
    H05.821   Myopathy of extraocular muscles, right orbit
    H05.822   Myopathy of extraocular muscles, left orbit
    H05.823   Myopathy of extraocular muscles, bilateral
    H05.829   Myopathy of extraocular muscles, unspecified orbit ▽
    H05.89 Other disorders of orbit
    H05.9 Unspecified disorder of orbit ▽

Disorders of conjunctiva (H10-H11)

✓4th H10 Conjunctivitis
    EXCLUDES 1   keratoconjunctivitis (H16.2-)
  ✓5th H10.0 Mucopurulent conjunctivitis
    ✓6th H10.01 Acute follicular conjunctivitis
        H10.011   Acute follicular conjunctivitis, right eye
        H10.012   Acute follicular conjunctivitis, left eye
        H10.013   Acute follicular conjunctivitis, bilateral

EXCLUDES 1 Not coded here   EXCLUDES 2 Not included here   N Newborn Age: 0   P Pediatric Age: 0-17   M Maternity Age: 12-55   A Adult Age: 15-124

576   ICD-10-CM 2018

         H10.019   **Acute follicular conjunctivitis, unspecified eye** ▽

   ✓6ᵗʰ   H10.02   **Other mucopurulent conjunctivitis**

         H10.021   **Other mucopurulent conjunctivitis, right eye**

         H10.022   **Other mucopurulent conjunctivitis, left eye**

         H10.023   **Other mucopurulent conjunctivitis, bilateral**

         H10.029   **Other mucopurulent conjunctivitis, unspecified eye** ▽

✓5ᵗʰ   **H10.1**   **Acute atopic conjunctivitis**
      Acute papillary conjunctivitis

         H10.10   **Acute atopic conjunctivitis, unspecified eye** ▽

         H10.11   **Acute atopic conjunctivitis, right eye**

         H10.12   **Acute atopic conjunctivitis, left eye**

         H10.13   **Acute atopic conjunctivitis, bilateral**

✓5ᵗʰ   **H10.2**   **Other acute conjunctivitis**

   ✓6ᵗʰ   H10.21   **Acute toxic conjunctivitis**
        Acute chemical conjunctivitis
        Code first (T51-T65) to identify chemical and intent
        EXCLUDES 1   *burn and corrosion of eye and adnexa (T26.-)*

         H10.211   **Acute toxic conjunctivitis, right eye**

         H10.212   **Acute toxic conjunctivitis, left eye**

         H10.213   **Acute toxic conjunctivitis, bilateral**

         H10.219   **Acute toxic conjunctivitis, unspecified eye** ▽

   ✓6ᵗʰ   H10.22   **Pseudomembranous conjunctivitis**

         H10.221   **Pseudomembranous conjunctivitis, right eye**

         H10.222   **Pseudomembranous conjunctivitis, left eye**

         H10.223   **Pseudomembranous conjunctivitis, bilateral**

         H10.229   **Pseudomembranous conjunctivitis, unspecified eye** ▽

   ✓6ᵗʰ   H10.23   **Serous conjunctivitis, except viral**
        EXCLUDES 1   *viral conjunctivitis (B30.-)*

         H10.231   **Serous conjunctivitis, except viral, right eye**

         H10.232   **Serous conjunctivitis, except viral, left eye**

         H10.233   **Serous conjunctivitis, except viral, bilateral**

         H10.239   **Serous conjunctivitis, except viral, unspecified eye** ▽

✓5ᵗʰ   **H10.3**   **Unspecified acute conjunctivitis**
      EXCLUDES 1   *ophthalmia neonatorum NOS (P39.1)*

         H10.30   **Unspecified acute conjunctivitis, unspecified eye** ▽

         H10.31   **Unspecified acute conjunctivitis, right eye** ▽

         H10.32   **Unspecified acute conjunctivitis, left eye** ▽

         H10.33   **Unspecified acute conjunctivitis, bilateral** ▽

✓5ᵗʰ   **H10.4**   **Chronic conjunctivitis**

   ✓6ᵗʰ   H10.40   **Unspecified chronic conjunctivitis**

         H10.401   **Unspecified chronic conjunctivitis, right eye** ▽

         H10.402   **Unspecified chronic conjunctivitis, left eye** ▽

         H10.403   **Unspecified chronic conjunctivitis, bilateral** ▽

         H10.409   **Unspecified chronic conjunctivitis, unspecified eye** ▽

   ✓6ᵗʰ   H10.41   **Chronic giant papillary conjunctivitis**

         H10.411   **Chronic giant papillary conjunctivitis, right eye**

         H10.412   **Chronic giant papillary conjunctivitis, left eye**

         H10.413   **Chronic giant papillary conjunctivitis, bilateral**

         H10.419   **Chronic giant papillary conjunctivitis, unspecified eye** ▽

   ✓6ᵗʰ   H10.42   **Simple chronic conjunctivitis**

         H10.421   **Simple chronic conjunctivitis, right eye**

         H10.422   **Simple chronic conjunctivitis, left eye**

         H10.423   **Simple chronic conjunctivitis, bilateral**

         H10.429   **Simple chronic conjunctivitis, unspecified eye** ▽

   ✓6ᵗʰ   H10.43   **Chronic follicular conjunctivitis**

         H10.431   **Chronic follicular conjunctivitis, right eye**

         H10.432   **Chronic follicular conjunctivitis, left eye**

         H10.433   **Chronic follicular conjunctivitis, bilateral**

         H10.439   **Chronic follicular conjunctivitis, unspecified eye** ▽

     H10.44   **Vernal conjunctivitis**
        EXCLUDES 1   *vernal keratoconjunctivitis with limbar and corneal involvement (H16.26-)*

     H10.45   **Other chronic allergic conjunctivitis**

✓5ᵗʰ   **H10.5**   **Blepharoconjunctivitis**

   ✓6ᵗʰ   H10.50   **Unspecified blepharoconjunctivitis**

         H10.501   **Unspecified blepharoconjunctivitis, right eye** ▽

         H10.502   **Unspecified blepharoconjunctivitis, left eye** ▽

         H10.503   **Unspecified blepharoconjunctivitis, bilateral** ▽

         H10.509   **Unspecified blepharoconjunctivitis, unspecified eye** ▽

   ✓6ᵗʰ   H10.51   **Ligneous conjunctivitis**

         H10.511   **Ligneous conjunctivitis, right eye**

         H10.512   **Ligneous conjunctivitis, left eye**

         H10.513   **Ligneous conjunctivitis, bilateral**

         H10.519   **Ligneous conjunctivitis, unspecified eye** ▽

   ✓6ᵗʰ   H10.52   **Angular blepharoconjunctivitis**

         H10.521   **Angular blepharoconjunctivitis, right eye**

         H10.522   **Angular blepharoconjunctivitis, left eye**

         H10.523   **Angular blepharoconjunctivitis, bilateral**

         H10.529   **Angular blepharoconjunctivitis, unspecified eye** ▽

   ✓6ᵗʰ   H10.53   **Contact blepharoconjunctivitis**

         H10.531   **Contact blepharoconjunctivitis, right eye**

         H10.532   **Contact blepharoconjunctivitis, left eye**

         H10.533   **Contact blepharoconjunctivitis, bilateral**

         H10.539   **Contact blepharoconjunctivitis, unspecified eye** ▽

✓5ᵗʰ   **H10.8**   **Other conjunctivitis**

   ✓6ᵗʰ   H10.81   **Pingueculitis**
        EXCLUDES 1   *pinguecula (H11.15-)*

         H10.811   **Pingueculitis, right eye**

         H10.812   **Pingueculitis, left eye**

         H10.813   **Pingueculitis, bilateral**

         H10.819   **Pingueculitis, unspecified eye** ▽

     H10.89   **Other conjunctivitis**

   H10.9   **Unspecified conjunctivitis** ▽

✓4ᵗʰ   **H11**   **Other disorders of conjunctiva**
      EXCLUDES 1   *keratoconjunctivitis (H16.2-)*

✓5ᵗʰ   **H11.0**   **Pterygium of eye**
      EXCLUDES 1   *pseudopterygium (H11.81-)*

   ✓6ᵗʰ   H11.00   **Unspecified pterygium of eye**

         H11.001   **Unspecified pterygium of right eye** ▽

         H11.002   **Unspecified pterygium of left eye** ▽

         H11.003   **Unspecified pterygium of eye, bilateral** ▽

         H11.009   **Unspecified pterygium of unspecified eye** ▽

Pterygium

Pterygium

✓ Additional Character Req   ✓x7ᵗʰ Placeholder Alert   Manifestation   **HCC** CMS-HCC Condition   ▽ Unspecified Code   ►◄ Revised Text   ● New Code   ▲ Revised Code Title

ICD-10-CM 2018   577

✓6ᵗʰ **H11.Ø1 Amyloid pterygium**
  H11.Ø11 Amyloid pterygium of right eye
  H11.Ø12 Amyloid pterygium of left eye
  H11.Ø13 Amyloid pterygium of eye, bilateral
  H11.Ø19 Amyloid pterygium of unspecified eye ▽
✓6ᵗʰ **H11.Ø2 Central pterygium of eye**
  H11.Ø21 Central pterygium of right eye
  H11.Ø22 Central pterygium of left eye
  H11.Ø23 Central pterygium of eye, bilateral
  H11.Ø29 Central pterygium of unspecified eye ▽
✓6ᵗʰ **H11.Ø3 Double pterygium of eye**
  H11.Ø31 Double pterygium of right eye
  H11.Ø32 Double pterygium of left eye
  H11.Ø33 Double pterygium of eye, bilateral
  H11.Ø39 Double pterygium of unspecified eye ▽
✓6ᵗʰ **H11.Ø4 Peripheral pterygium of eye, stationary**
  H11.Ø41 Peripheral pterygium, stationary, right eye
  H11.Ø42 Peripheral pterygium, stationary, left eye
  H11.Ø43 Peripheral pterygium, stationary, bilateral
  H11.Ø49 Peripheral pterygium, stationary, unspecified eye ▽
✓6ᵗʰ **H11.Ø5 Peripheral pterygium of eye, progressive**
  H11.Ø51 Peripheral pterygium, progressive, right eye
  H11.Ø52 Peripheral pterygium, progressive, left eye
  H11.Ø53 Peripheral pterygium, progressive, bilateral
  H11.Ø59 Peripheral pterygium, progressive, unspecified eye ▽
✓6ᵗʰ **H11.Ø6 Recurrent pterygium of eye**
  H11.Ø61 Recurrent pterygium of right eye
  H11.Ø62 Recurrent pterygium of left eye
  H11.Ø63 Recurrent pterygium of eye, bilateral
  H11.Ø69 Recurrent pterygium of unspecified eye ▽
✓5ᵗʰ **H11.1 Conjunctival degenerations and deposits**
  EXCLUDES 2 pseudopterygium (H11.81)
  H11.1Ø Unspecified conjunctival degenerations ▽
✓6ᵗʰ **H11.11 Conjunctival deposits**
  H11.111 Conjunctival deposits, right eye
  H11.112 Conjunctival deposits, left eye
  H11.113 Conjunctival deposits, bilateral
  H11.119 Conjunctival deposits, unspecified eye ▽
✓6ᵗʰ **H11.12 Conjunctival concretions**
  H11.121 Conjunctival concretions, right eye
  H11.122 Conjunctival concretions, left eye
  H11.123 Conjunctival concretions, bilateral
  H11.129 Conjunctival concretions, unspecified eye ▽
✓6ᵗʰ **H11.13 Conjunctival pigmentations**
  Conjunctival argyrosis [argyria]
  H11.131 Conjunctival pigmentations, right eye
  H11.132 Conjunctival pigmentations, left eye
  H11.133 Conjunctival pigmentations, bilateral
  H11.139 Conjunctival pigmentations, unspecified eye ▽
✓6ᵗʰ **H11.14 Conjunctival xerosis, unspecified**
  EXCLUDES 1 xerosis of conjunctiva due to vitamin A deficiency (E5Ø.Ø, E5Ø.1)
  DEF: Abnormal dryness of conjunctiva due to lack of insufficient tears or conjunctival secretions.
  H11.141 Conjunctival xerosis, unspecified, right eye ▽
  H11.142 Conjunctival xerosis , unspecified, left eye ▽
  H11.143 Conjunctival xerosis, unspecified, bilateral ▽
  H11.149 Conjunctival xerosis, unspecified, unspecified eye ▽
✓6ᵗʰ **H11.15 Pinguecula**
  EXCLUDES 1 pingueculitis (H1Ø.81-)
  H11.151 Pinguecula, right eye

Pinguecula

Pinguecula

  H11.152 Pinguecula, left eye
  H11.153 Pinguecula, bilateral
  H11.159 Pinguecula, unspecified eye ▽
✓5ᵗʰ **H11.2 Conjunctival scars**
  ✓6ᵗʰ **H11.21 Conjunctival adhesions and strands (localized)**
    H11.211 Conjunctival adhesions and strands (localized), right eye
    H11.212 Conjunctival adhesions and strands (localized), left eye
    H11.213 Conjunctival adhesions and strands (localized), bilateral
    H11.219 Conjunctival adhesions and strands (localized), unspecified eye ▽
  ✓6ᵗʰ **H11.22 Conjunctival granuloma**
    H11.221 Conjunctival granuloma, right eye
    H11.222 Conjunctival granuloma, left eye
    H11.223 Conjunctival granuloma, bilateral
    H11.229 Conjunctival granuloma, unspecified ▽
  ✓6ᵗʰ **H11.23 Symblepharon**
    H11.231 Symblepharon, right eye
    H11.232 Symblepharon, left eye
    H11.233 Symblepharon, bilateral
    H11.239 Symblepharon, unspecified eye ▽
  ✓6ᵗʰ **H11.24 Scarring of conjunctiva**
    H11.241 Scarring of conjunctiva, right eye
    H11.242 Scarring of conjunctiva, left eye
    H11.243 Scarring of conjunctiva, bilateral
    H11.249 Scarring of conjunctiva, unspecified eye ▽
✓5ᵗʰ **H11.3 Conjunctival hemorrhage**
  Subconjunctival hemorrhage
  H11.3Ø Conjunctival hemorrhage, unspecified eye ▽
  H11.31 Conjunctival hemorrhage, right eye
  H11.32 Conjunctival hemorrhage, left eye
  H11.33 Conjunctival hemorrhage, bilateral
✓5ᵗʰ **H11.4 Other conjunctival vascular disorders and cysts**
  ✓6ᵗʰ **H11.41 Vascular abnormalities of conjunctiva**
    Conjunctival aneurysm
    H11.411 Vascular abnormalities of conjunctiva, right eye
    H11.412 Vascular abnormalities of conjunctiva, left eye
    H11.413 Vascular abnormalities of conjunctiva, bilateral
    H11.419 Vascular abnormalities of conjunctiva, unspecified eye ▽
  ✓6ᵗʰ **H11.42 Conjunctival edema**
    H11.421 Conjunctival edema, right eye
    H11.422 Conjunctival edema, left eye
    H11.423 Conjunctival edema, bilateral
    H11.429 Conjunctival edema, unspecified eye ▽
  ✓6ᵗʰ **H11.43 Conjunctival hyperemia**
    H11.431 Conjunctival hyperemia, right eye
    H11.432 Conjunctival hyperemia, left eye
    H11.433 Conjunctival hyperemia, bilateral
    H11.439 Conjunctival hyperemia, unspecified eye ▽

✓6ᵗʰ **H11.44 Conjunctival cysts**
    H11.441 Conjunctival cysts, right eye
    H11.442 Conjunctival cysts, left eye
    H11.443 Conjunctival cysts, bilateral
    H11.449 Conjunctival cysts, unspecified eye ▽
✓5ᵗʰ **H11.8 Other specified disorders of conjunctiva**
   ✓6ᵗʰ **H11.81 Pseudopterygium of conjunctiva**
    H11.811 Pseudopterygium of conjunctiva, right eye
    H11.812 Pseudopterygium of conjunctiva, left eye
    H11.813 Pseudopterygium of conjunctiva, bilateral
    H11.819 Pseudopterygium of conjunctiva, unspecified eye ▽
   ✓6ᵗʰ **H11.82 Conjunctivochalasis**
    H11.821 Conjunctivochalasis, right eye
    H11.822 Conjunctivochalasis, left eye
    H11.823 Conjunctivochalasis, bilateral
    H11.829 Conjunctivochalasis, unspecified eye ▽
   H11.89 Other specified disorders of conjunctiva
  H11.9 Unspecified disorder of conjunctiva ▽

Disorders of sclera, cornea, iris and ciliary body (H15-H22)

✓4ᵗʰ **H15 Disorders of sclera**
  ✓5ᵗʰ **H15.0 Scleritis**
   ✓6ᵗʰ **H15.00 Unspecified scleritis**
    H15.001 Unspecified scleritis, right eye ▽
    H15.002 Unspecified scleritis, left eye ▽
    H15.003 Unspecified scleritis, bilateral ▽
    H15.009 Unspecified scleritis, unspecified eye ▽
   ✓6ᵗʰ **H15.01 Anterior scleritis**
    H15.011 Anterior scleritis, right eye
    H15.012 Anterior scleritis, left eye
    H15.013 Anterior scleritis, bilateral
    H15.019 Anterior scleritis, unspecified eye ▽
   ✓6ᵗʰ **H15.02 Brawny scleritis**
    H15.021 Brawny scleritis, right eye
    H15.022 Brawny scleritis, left eye
    H15.023 Brawny scleritis, bilateral
    H15.029 Brawny scleritis, unspecified eye ▽
   ✓6ᵗʰ **H15.03 Posterior scleritis**
    Sclerotenonitis
    H15.031 Posterior scleritis, right eye
    H15.032 Posterior scleritis, left eye
    H15.033 Posterior scleritis, bilateral
    H15.039 Posterior scleritis, unspecified eye ▽
   ✓6ᵗʰ **H15.04 Scleritis with corneal involvement**
    H15.041 Scleritis with corneal involvement, right eye
    H15.042 Scleritis with corneal involvement, left eye
    H15.043 Scleritis with corneal involvement, bilateral
    H15.049 Scleritis with corneal involvement, unspecified eye ▽
   ✓6ᵗʰ **H15.05 Scleromalacia perforans**
    H15.051 Scleromalacia perforans, right eye
    H15.052 Scleromalacia perforans, left eye
    H15.053 Scleromalacia perforans, bilateral
    H15.059 Scleromalacia perforans, unspecified eye ▽
   ✓6ᵗʰ **H15.09 Other scleritis**
    Scleral abscess
    H15.091 Other scleritis, right eye
    H15.092 Other scleritis, left eye
    H15.093 Other scleritis, bilateral
    H15.099 Other scleritis, unspecified eye ▽
  ✓5ᵗʰ **H15.1 Episcleritis**
   ✓6ᵗʰ **H15.10 Unspecified episcleritis**
    H15.101 Unspecified episcleritis, right eye ▽
    H15.102 Unspecified episcleritis, left eye ▽
    H15.103 Unspecified episcleritis, bilateral ▽
    H15.109 Unspecified episcleritis, unspecified eye ▽

   ✓6ᵗʰ **H15.11 Episcleritis periodica fugax**
    H15.111 Episcleritis periodica fugax, right eye
    H15.112 Episcleritis periodica fugax, left eye
    H15.113 Episcleritis periodica fugax, bilateral
    H15.119 Episcleritis periodica fugax, unspecified eye ▽
   ✓6ᵗʰ **H15.12 Nodular episcleritis**
    H15.121 Nodular episcleritis, right eye
    H15.122 Nodular episcleritis, left eye
    H15.123 Nodular episcleritis, bilateral
    H15.129 Nodular episcleritis, unspecified eye ▽
  ✓5ᵗʰ **H15.8 Other disorders of sclera**
   EXCLUDES 2 blue sclera (Q13.5)
     degenerative myopia (H44.2-)
   ✓6ᵗʰ **H15.81 Equatorial staphyloma**
    H15.811 Equatorial staphyloma, right eye
    H15.812 Equatorial staphyloma, left eye
    H15.813 Equatorial staphyloma, bilateral
    H15.819 Equatorial staphyloma, unspecified eye ▽
   ✓6ᵗʰ **H15.82 Localized anterior staphyloma**
    H15.821 Localized anterior staphyloma, right eye
    H15.822 Localized anterior staphyloma, left eye
    H15.823 Localized anterior staphyloma, bilateral
    H15.829 Localized anterior staphyloma, unspecified eye ▽
   ✓6ᵗʰ **H15.83 Staphyloma posticum**
    H15.831 Staphyloma posticum, right eye
    H15.832 Staphyloma posticum, left eye
    H15.833 Staphyloma posticum, bilateral
    H15.839 Staphyloma posticum, unspecified eye ▽
   ✓6ᵗʰ **H15.84 Scleral ectasia**
    H15.841 Scleral ectasia, right eye
    H15.842 Scleral ectasia, left eye
    H15.843 Scleral ectasia, bilateral
    H15.849 Scleral ectasia, unspecified eye ▽
   ✓6ᵗʰ **H15.85 Ring staphyloma**
    H15.851 Ring staphyloma, right eye
    H15.852 Ring staphyloma, left eye
    H15.853 Ring staphyloma, bilateral
    H15.859 Ring staphyloma, unspecified eye ▽
   H15.89 Other disorders of sclera
  H15.9 Unspecified disorder of sclera ▽
✓4ᵗʰ **H16 Keratitis**
  ✓5ᵗʰ **H16.0 Corneal ulcer**
   ✓6ᵗʰ **H16.00 Unspecified corneal ulcer**
    H16.001 Unspecified corneal ulcer, right eye ▽
    H16.002 Unspecified corneal ulcer, left eye ▽
    H16.003 Unspecified corneal ulcer, bilateral ▽
    H16.009 Unspecified corneal ulcer, unspecified eye ▽
   ✓6ᵗʰ **H16.01 Central corneal ulcer**
    H16.011 Central corneal ulcer, right eye
    H16.012 Central corneal ulcer, left eye
    H16.013 Central corneal ulcer, bilateral
    H16.019 Central corneal ulcer, unspecified eye ▽
   ✓6ᵗʰ **H16.02 Ring corneal ulcer**
    H16.021 Ring corneal ulcer, right eye
    H16.022 Ring corneal ulcer, left eye
    H16.023 Ring corneal ulcer, bilateral
    H16.029 Ring corneal ulcer, unspecified eye ▽
   ✓6ᵗʰ **H16.03 Corneal ulcer with hypopyon**
    H16.031 Corneal ulcer with hypopyon, right eye
    H16.032 Corneal ulcer with hypopyon, left eye
    H16.033 Corneal ulcer with hypopyon, bilateral
    H16.039 Corneal ulcer with hypopyon, unspecified eye ▽
   ✓6ᵗʰ **H16.04 Marginal corneal ulcer**
    H16.041 Marginal corneal ulcer, right eye
    H16.042 Marginal corneal ulcer, left eye
    H16.043 Marginal corneal ulcer, bilateral
    H16.049 Marginal corneal ulcer, unspecified eye ▽

✓6th **H16.05 Mooren's corneal ulcer**
- H16.051 Mooren's corneal ulcer, right eye
- H16.052 Mooren's corneal ulcer, left eye
- H16.053 Mooren's corneal ulcer, bilateral
- H16.059 Mooren's corneal ulcer, unspecified eye ▽

✓6th **H16.06 Mycotic corneal ulcer**
- H16.061 Mycotic corneal ulcer, right eye
- H16.062 Mycotic corneal ulcer, left eye
- H16.063 Mycotic corneal ulcer, bilateral
- H16.069 Mycotic corneal ulcer, unspecified eye ▽

✓6th **H16.07 Perforated corneal ulcer**
- H16.071 Perforated corneal ulcer, right eye
- H16.072 Perforated corneal ulcer, left eye
- H16.073 Perforated corneal ulcer, bilateral
- H16.079 Perforated corneal ulcer, unspecified eye ▽

✓5th **H16.1 Other and unspecified superficial keratitis without conjunctivitis**

✓6th **H16.10 Unspecified superficial keratitis**
- H16.101 Unspecified superficial keratitis, right eye ▽
- H16.102 Unspecified superficial keratitis, left eye ▽
- H16.103 Unspecified superficial keratitis, bilateral ▽
- H16.109 Unspecified superficial keratitis, unspecified eye ▽

✓6th **H16.11 Macular keratitis**
Areolar keratitis
Nummular keratitis
Stellate keratitis
Striate keratitis
- H16.111 Macular keratitis, right eye
- H16.112 Macular keratitis, left eye
- H16.113 Macular keratitis, bilateral
- H16.119 Macular keratitis, unspecified eye ▽

✓6th **H16.12 Filamentary keratitis**
- H16.121 Filamentary keratitis, right eye
- H16.122 Filamentary keratitis, left eye
- H16.123 Filamentary keratitis, bilateral
- H16.129 Filamentary keratitis, unspecified eye ▽

✓6th **H16.13 Photokeratitis**
Snow blindness
Welders keratitis
- H16.131 Photokeratitis, right eye
- H16.132 Photokeratitis, left eye
- H16.133 Photokeratitis, bilateral
- H16.139 Photokeratitis, unspecified eye ▽

✓6th **H16.14 Punctate keratitis**
- H16.141 Punctate keratitis, right eye
- H16.142 Punctate keratitis, left eye
- H16.143 Punctate keratitis, bilateral
- H16.149 Punctate keratitis, unspecified eye ▽

✓5th **H16.2 Keratoconjunctivitis**

✓6th **H16.20 Unspecified keratoconjunctivitis**
Superficial keratitis with conjunctivitis NOS
- H16.201 Unspecified keratoconjunctivitis, right eye ▽
- H16.202 Unspecified keratoconjunctivitis, left eye ▽
- H16.203 Unspecified keratoconjunctivitis, bilateral ▽
- H16.209 Unspecified keratoconjunctivitis, unspecified eye ▽

✓6th **H16.21 Exposure keratoconjunctivitis**
- H16.211 Exposure keratoconjunctivitis, right eye
- H16.212 Exposure keratoconjunctivitis, left eye
- H16.213 Exposure keratoconjunctivitis, bilateral
- H16.219 Exposure keratoconjunctivitis, unspecified eye ▽

✓6th **H16.22 Keratoconjunctivitis sicca, not specified as Sjögren's**
EXCLUDES 1 Sjögren's syndrome (M35.01)
- H16.221 Keratoconjunctivitis sicca, not specified as Sjögren's, right eye

- H16.222 Keratoconjunctivitis sicca, not specified as Sjögren's, left eye
- H16.223 Keratoconjunctivitis sicca, not specified as Sjögren's, bilateral
- H16.229 Keratoconjunctivitis sicca, not specified as Sjögren's, unspecified eye ▽

✓6th **H16.23 Neurotrophic keratoconjunctivitis**
- H16.231 Neurotrophic keratoconjunctivitis, right eye
- H16.232 Neurotrophic keratoconjunctivitis, left eye
- H16.233 Neurotrophic keratoconjunctivitis, bilateral
- H16.239 Neurotrophic keratoconjunctivitis, unspecified eye ▽

✓6th **H16.24 Ophthalmia nodosa**
- H16.241 Ophthalmia nodosa, right eye
- H16.242 Ophthalmia nodosa, left eye
- H16.243 Ophthalmia nodosa, bilateral
- H16.249 Ophthalmia nodosa, unspecified eye ▽

✓6th **H16.25 Phlyctenular keratoconjunctivitis**
- H16.251 Phlyctenular keratoconjunctivitis, right eye
- H16.252 Phlyctenular keratoconjunctivitis, left eye
- H16.253 Phlyctenular keratoconjunctivitis, bilateral
- H16.259 Phlyctenular keratoconjunctivitis, unspecified eye ▽

✓6th **H16.26 Vernal keratoconjunctivitis, with limbar and corneal involvement**
EXCLUDES 1 vernal conjunctivitis without limbar and corneal involvement (H10.44)
- H16.261 Vernal keratoconjunctivitis, with limbar and corneal involvement, right eye
- H16.262 Vernal keratoconjunctivitis, with limbar and corneal involvement, left eye
- H16.263 Vernal keratoconjunctivitis, with limbar and corneal involvement, bilateral
- H16.269 Vernal keratoconjunctivitis, with limbar and corneal involvement, unspecified eye ▽

✓6th **H16.29 Other keratoconjunctivitis**
- H16.291 Other keratoconjunctivitis, right eye
- H16.292 Other keratoconjunctivitis, left eye
- H16.293 Other keratoconjunctivitis, bilateral
- H16.299 Other keratoconjunctivitis, unspecified eye ▽

✓5th **H16.3 Interstitial and deep keratitis**

✓6th **H16.30 Unspecified interstitial keratitis**
- H16.301 Unspecified interstitial keratitis, right eye ▽
- H16.302 Unspecified interstitial keratitis, left eye ▽
- H16.303 Unspecified interstitial keratitis, bilateral ▽
- H16.309 Unspecified interstitial keratitis, unspecified eye ▽

✓6th **H16.31 Corneal abscess**
- H16.311 Corneal abscess, right eye
- H16.312 Corneal abscess, left eye
- H16.313 Corneal abscess, bilateral
- H16.319 Corneal abscess, unspecified eye ▽

✓6th **H16.32 Diffuse interstitial keratitis**
Cogan's syndrome
- H16.321 Diffuse interstitial keratitis, right eye
- H16.322 Diffuse interstitial keratitis, left eye
- H16.323 Diffuse interstitial keratitis, bilateral
- H16.329 Diffuse interstitial keratitis, unspecified eye ▽

✓6th **H16.33 Sclerosing keratitis**
- H16.331 Sclerosing keratitis, right eye
- H16.332 Sclerosing keratitis, left eye
- H16.333 Sclerosing keratitis, bilateral
- H16.339 Sclerosing keratitis, unspecified eye ▽

EXCLUDES 1 Not coded here   EXCLUDES 2 Not included here   N Newborn Age: 0   P Pediatric Age: 0-17   M Maternity Age: 12-55   A Adult Age: 15-124

580   ICD-10-CM 2018

✓6ᵗʰ **H16.39** Other interstitial and deep keratitis
  H16.391 Other interstitial and deep keratitis, right eye
  H16.392 Other interstitial and deep keratitis, left eye
  H16.393 Other interstitial and deep keratitis, bilateral
  H16.399 Other interstitial and deep keratitis, unspecified eye ▽

✓5ᵗʰ **H16.4** Corneal neovascularization
  ✓6ᵗʰ **H16.40** Unspecified corneal neovascularization
    H16.401 Unspecified corneal neovascularization, right eye ▽
    H16.402 Unspecified corneal neovascularization, left eye ▽
    H16.403 Unspecified corneal neovascularization, bilateral ▽
    H16.409 Unspecified corneal neovascularization, unspecified eye ▽
  ✓6ᵗʰ **H16.41** Ghost vessels (corneal)
    H16.411 Ghost vessels (corneal), right eye
    H16.412 Ghost vessels (corneal), left eye
    H16.413 Ghost vessels (corneal), bilateral
    H16.419 Ghost vessels (corneal), unspecified eye ▽
  ✓6ᵗʰ **H16.42** Pannus (corneal)
    H16.421 Pannus (corneal), right eye
    H16.422 Pannus (corneal), left eye
    H16.423 Pannus (corneal), bilateral
    H16.429 Pannus (corneal), unspecified eye ▽
  ✓6ᵗʰ **H16.43** Localized vascularization of cornea
    H16.431 Localized vascularization of cornea, right eye
    H16.432 Localized vascularization of cornea, left eye
    H16.433 Localized vascularization of cornea, bilateral
    H16.439 Localized vascularization of cornea, unspecified eye ▽
  ✓6ᵗʰ **H16.44** Deep vascularization of cornea
    H16.441 Deep vascularization of cornea, right eye
    H16.442 Deep vascularization of cornea, left eye
    H16.443 Deep vascularization of cornea, bilateral
    H16.449 Deep vascularization of cornea, unspecified eye ▽

  H16.8 Other keratitis
  H16.9 Unspecified keratitis ▽

✓4ᵗʰ **H17** Corneal scars and opacities
  ✓5ᵗʰ **H17.0** Adherent leukoma
    H17.00 Adherent leukoma, unspecified eye ▽
    H17.01 Adherent leukoma, right eye
    H17.02 Adherent leukoma, left eye
    H17.03 Adherent leukoma, bilateral
  ✓5ᵗʰ **H17.1** Central corneal opacity
    H17.10 Central corneal opacity, unspecified eye ▽
    H17.11 Central corneal opacity, right eye
    H17.12 Central corneal opacity, left eye
    H17.13 Central corneal opacity, bilateral
  ✓5ᵗʰ **H17.8** Other corneal scars and opacities
    ✓6ᵗʰ **H17.81** Minor opacity of cornea
      Corneal nebula
      H17.811 Minor opacity of cornea, right eye
      H17.812 Minor opacity of cornea, left eye
      H17.813 Minor opacity of cornea, bilateral
      H17.819 Minor opacity of cornea, unspecified eye ▽
    ✓6ᵗʰ **H17.82** Peripheral opacity of cornea
      H17.821 Peripheral opacity of cornea, right eye
      H17.822 Peripheral opacity of cornea, left eye
      H17.823 Peripheral opacity of cornea, bilateral
      H17.829 Peripheral opacity of cornea, unspecified eye ▽
    H17.89 Other corneal scars and opacities

  H17.9 Unspecified corneal scar and opacity ▽

✓4ᵗʰ **H18** Other disorders of cornea
  ✓5ᵗʰ **H18.0** Corneal pigmentations and deposits
    ✓6ᵗʰ **H18.00** Unspecified corneal deposit
      H18.001 Unspecified corneal deposit, right eye ▽
      H18.002 Unspecified corneal deposit, left eye ▽
      H18.003 Unspecified corneal deposit, bilateral ▽
      H18.009 Unspecified corneal deposit, unspecified eye ▽
    ✓6ᵗʰ **H18.01** Anterior corneal pigmentations
      Staehli's line
      H18.011 Anterior corneal pigmentations, right eye
      H18.012 Anterior corneal pigmentations, left eye
      H18.013 Anterior corneal pigmentations, bilateral
      H18.019 Anterior corneal pigmentations, unspecified eye ▽
    ✓6ᵗʰ **H18.02** Argentous corneal deposits
      H18.021 Argentous corneal deposits, right eye
      H18.022 Argentous corneal deposits, left eye
      H18.023 Argentous corneal deposits, bilateral
      H18.029 Argentous corneal deposits, unspecified eye ▽
    ✓6ᵗʰ **H18.03** Corneal deposits in metabolic disorders
      Code also associated metabolic disorder
      H18.031 Corneal deposits in metabolic disorders, right eye
      H18.032 Corneal deposits in metabolic disorders, left eye
      H18.033 Corneal deposits in metabolic disorders, bilateral
      H18.039 Corneal deposits in metabolic disorders, unspecified eye ▽
    ✓6ᵗʰ **H18.04** Kayser-Fleischer ring
      Code also associated Wilson's disease (E83.01)
      H18.041 Kayser-Fleischer ring, right eye
      H18.042 Kayser-Fleischer ring, left eye
      H18.043 Kayser-Fleischer ring, bilateral
      H18.049 Kayser-Fleischer ring, unspecified eye ▽
    ✓6ᵗʰ **H18.05** Posterior corneal pigmentations
      Krukenberg's spindle
      H18.051 Posterior corneal pigmentations, right eye
      H18.052 Posterior corneal pigmentations, left eye
      H18.053 Posterior corneal pigmentations, bilateral
      H18.059 Posterior corneal pigmentations, unspecified eye ▽
    ✓6ᵗʰ **H18.06** Stromal corneal pigmentations
      Hematocornea
      H18.061 Stromal corneal pigmentations, right eye
      H18.062 Stromal corneal pigmentations, left eye
      H18.063 Stromal corneal pigmentations, bilateral
      H18.069 Stromal corneal pigmentations, unspecified eye ▽
  ✓5ᵗʰ **H18.1** Bullous keratopathy
    DEF: Corneal swelling due to damaged corneal endothelium; characterized by recurring, rupturing epithelial "blisters"; occurs in glaucoma, iridocyclitis and Fuchs dystrophy.
    H18.10 Bullous keratopathy, unspecified eye ▽
    H18.11 Bullous keratopathy, right eye
    H18.12 Bullous keratopathy, left eye
    H18.13 Bullous keratopathy, bilateral
  ✓5ᵗʰ **H18.2** Other and unspecified corneal edema
    H18.20 Unspecified corneal edema ▽
    ✓6ᵗʰ **H18.21** Corneal edema secondary to contact lens
      EXCLUDES 2 other corneal disorders due to contact lens (H18.82-)
      H18.211 Corneal edema secondary to contact lens, right eye
      H18.212 Corneal edema secondary to contact lens, left eye
      H18.213 Corneal edema secondary to contact lens, bilateral
      H18.219 Corneal edema secondary to contact lens, unspecified eye ▽

Chapter 7. Diseases of the Eye and Adnexa

H18.22–H18.829

✓6ᵗʰ **H18.22 Idiopathic corneal edema**
     H18.221 Idiopathic corneal edema, **right** eye
     H18.222 Idiopathic corneal edema, **left** eye
     H18.223 Idiopathic corneal edema, **bilateral**
     H18.229 Idiopathic corneal edema, **unspecified** eye ▽

✓6ᵗʰ **H18.23 Secondary corneal edema**
     H18.231 Secondary corneal edema, **right** eye
     H18.232 Secondary corneal edema, **left** eye
     H18.233 Secondary corneal edema, **bilateral**
     H18.239 Secondary corneal edema, **unspecified** eye ▽

✓5ᵗʰ **H18.3 Changes of corneal membranes**
     H18.30 Unspecified corneal membrane change ▽

✓6ᵗʰ **H18.31 Folds and rupture in Bowman's membrane**
     H18.311 Folds and rupture in Bowman's membrane, **right** eye
     H18.312 Folds and rupture in Bowman's membrane, **left** eye
     H18.313 Folds and rupture in Bowman's membrane, **bilateral**
     H18.319 Folds and rupture in Bowman's membrane, **unspecified** eye ▽

✓6ᵗʰ **H18.32 Folds in Descemet's membrane**
     H18.321 Folds in Descemet's membrane, **right** eye
     H18.322 Folds in Descemet's membrane, **left** eye
     H18.323 Folds in Descemet's membrane, **bilateral**
     H18.329 Folds in Descemet's membrane, **unspecified** eye ▽

✓6ᵗʰ **H18.33 Rupture in Descemet's membrane**
     H18.331 Rupture in Descemet's membrane, **right** eye
     H18.332 Rupture in Descemet's membrane, **left** eye
     H18.333 Rupture in Descemet's membrane, **bilateral**
     H18.339 Rupture in Descemet's membrane, **unspecified** eye ▽

✓5ᵗʰ **H18.4 Corneal degeneration**
   EXCLUDES 1   Mooren's ulcer (H16.Ø-)
               recurrent erosion of cornea (H18.83-)
     H18.40 Unspecified corneal degeneration ▽

✓6ᵗʰ **H18.41 Arcus senilis**
     Senile corneal changes
     H18.411 Arcus senilis, **right** eye
     H18.412 Arcus senilis, **left** eye
     H18.413 Arcus senilis, **bilateral**
     H18.419 Arcus senilis, **unspecified** eye ▽

✓6ᵗʰ **H18.42 Band keratopathy**
     H18.421 Band keratopathy, **right** eye
     H18.422 Band keratopathy, **left** eye
     H18.423 Band keratopathy, **bilateral**
     H18.429 Band keratopathy, **unspecified** eye ▽

     H18.43 Other calcerous corneal degeneration

✓6ᵗʰ **H18.44 Keratomalacia**
   EXCLUDES 1   keratomalacia due to vitamin A deficiency (E5Ø.4)
     H18.441 Keratomalacia, **right** eye
     H18.442 Keratomalacia, **left** eye
     H18.443 Keratomalacia, **bilateral**
     H18.449 Keratomalacia, **unspecified** eye ▽

✓6ᵗʰ **H18.45 Nodular corneal degeneration**
     H18.451 Nodular corneal degeneration, **right** eye
     H18.452 Nodular corneal degeneration, **left** eye
     H18.453 Nodular corneal degeneration, **bilateral**
     H18.459 Nodular corneal degeneration, **unspecified** eye ▽

✓6ᵗʰ **H18.46 Peripheral corneal degeneration**
     H18.461 Peripheral corneal degeneration, **right** eye
     H18.462 Peripheral corneal degeneration, **left** eye
     H18.463 Peripheral corneal degeneration, **bilateral**
     H18.469 Peripheral corneal degeneration, **unspecified** eye ▽

     H18.49 Other corneal degeneration

✓5ᵗʰ **H18.5 Hereditary corneal dystrophies**
     H18.50 Unspecified hereditary corneal dystrophies ▽
     H18.51 Endothelial corneal dystrophy
       Fuchs' dystrophy
     H18.52 Epithelial (juvenile) corneal dystrophy
     H18.53 Granular corneal dystrophy
     H18.54 Lattice corneal dystrophy
     H18.55 Macular corneal dystrophy
     H18.59 Other hereditary corneal dystrophies

✓5ᵗʰ **H18.6 Keratoconus**
✓6ᵗʰ **H18.60 Keratoconus, unspecified**
     H18.6Ø1 Keratoconus, unspecified, **right** eye ▽
     H18.6Ø2 Keratoconus, unspecified, **left** eye ▽
     H18.6Ø3 Keratoconus, unspecified, **bilateral** ▽
     H18.6Ø9 Keratoconus, unspecified, **unspecified** eye ▽

✓6ᵗʰ **H18.61 Keratoconus, stable**
     H18.611 Keratoconus, stable, **right** eye
     H18.612 Keratoconus, stable, **left** eye
     H18.613 Keratoconus, stable, **bilateral**
     H18.619 Keratoconus, stable, **unspecified** eye ▽

✓6ᵗʰ **H18.62 Keratoconus, unstable**
     Acute hydrops
     H18.621 Keratoconus, unstable, **right** eye
     H18.622 Keratoconus, unstable, **left** eye
     H18.623 Keratoconus, unstable, **bilateral**
     H18.629 Keratoconus, unstable, **unspecified** eye ▽

✓5ᵗʰ **H18.7 Other and unspecified corneal deformities**
   EXCLUDES 1   congenital malformations of cornea (Q13.3-Q13.4)
     H18.7Ø Unspecified corneal deformity ▽

✓6ᵗʰ **H18.71 Corneal ectasia**
     H18.711 Corneal ectasia, **right** eye
     H18.712 Corneal ectasia, **left** eye
     H18.713 Corneal ectasia, **bilateral**
     H18.719 Corneal ectasia, **unspecified** eye ▽

✓6ᵗʰ **H18.72 Corneal staphyloma**
     H18.721 Corneal staphyloma, **right** eye
     H18.722 Corneal staphyloma, **left** eye
     H18.723 Corneal staphyloma, **bilateral**
     H18.729 Corneal staphyloma, **unspecified** eye ▽

✓6ᵗʰ **H18.73 Descemetocele**
     H18.731 Descemetocele, **right** eye
     H18.732 Descemetocele, **left** eye
     H18.733 Descemetocele, **bilateral**
     H18.739 Descemetocele, **unspecified** eye ▽

✓6ᵗʰ **H18.79 Other corneal deformities**
     H18.791 Other corneal deformities, **right** eye
     H18.792 Other corneal deformities, **left** eye
     H18.793 Other corneal deformities, **bilateral**
     H18.799 Other corneal deformities, **unspecified** eye ▽

✓5ᵗʰ **H18.8 Other specified disorders of cornea**
✓6ᵗʰ **H18.81 Anesthesia and hypoesthesia of cornea**
     H18.811 Anesthesia and hypoesthesia of cornea, **right** eye
     H18.812 Anesthesia and hypoesthesia of cornea, **left** eye
     H18.813 Anesthesia and hypoesthesia of cornea, **bilateral**
     H18.819 Anesthesia and hypoesthesia of cornea, **unspecified** eye ▽

✓6ᵗʰ **H18.82 Corneal disorder due to contact lens**
   EXCLUDES 2   corneal edema due to contact lens (H18.21-)
     H18.821 Corneal disorder due to contact lens, **right** eye
     H18.822 Corneal disorder due to contact lens, **left** eye
     H18.823 Corneal disorder due to contact lens, **bilateral**
     H18.829 Corneal disorder due to contact lens, **unspecified** eye ▽

EXCLUDES 1 Not coded here   *EXCLUDES 2* Not included here   **N** Newborn Age: 0   **P** Pediatric Age: 0-17   **M** Maternity Age: 12-55   **A** Adult Age: 15-124

√6th **H18.83 Recurrent erosion of cornea**
- H18.831 Recurrent erosion of cornea, right eye
- H18.832 Recurrent erosion of cornea, left eye
- H18.833 Recurrent erosion of cornea, bilateral
- H18.839 Recurrent erosion of cornea, unspecified eye ▽

√6th **H18.89 Other specified disorders of cornea**
- H18.891 Other specified disorders of cornea, right eye
- H18.892 Other specified disorders of cornea, left eye
- H18.893 Other specified disorders of cornea, bilateral
- H18.899 Other specified disorders of cornea, unspecified eye ▽

H18.9 Unspecified disorder of cornea ▽

√4th **H20 Iridocyclitis**

√5th **H20.0 Acute and subacute iridocyclitis**
Acute anterior uveitis
Acute cyclitis
Acute iritis
Subacute anterior uveitis
Subacute cyclitis
Subacute iritis

EXCLUDES 1 iridocyclitis, iritis, uveitis (due to) (in) diabetes mellitus (E08-E13 with .39)
iridocyclitis, iritis, uveitis (due to) (in) diphtheria (A36.89)
iridocyclitis, iritis, uveitis (due to) (in) gonococcal (A54.32)
iridocyclitis, iritis, uveitis (due to) (in) herpes (simplex) (B00.51)
iridocyclitis, iritis, uveitis (due to) (in) herpes zoster (B02.32)
iridocyclitis, iritis, uveitis (due to) (in) late congenital syphilis (A50.39)
iridocyclitis, iritis, uveitis (due to) (in) late syphilis (A52.71)
iridocyclitis, iritis, uveitis (due to) (in) sarcoidosis (D86.83)
iridocyclitis, iritis, uveitis (due to) (in) syphilis (A51.43)
iridocyclitis, iritis, uveitis (due to) (in) toxoplasmosis (B58.09)
iridocyclitis, iritis, uveitis (due to) (in) tuberculosis (A18.54)

- H20.00 Unspecified acute and subacute iridocyclitis ▽

√6th **H20.01 Primary iridocyclitis**
- H20.011 Primary iridocyclitis, right eye
- H20.012 Primary iridocyclitis, left eye
- H20.013 Primary iridocyclitis, bilateral
- H20.019 Primary iridocyclitis, unspecified eye ▽

√6th **H20.02 Recurrent acute iridocyclitis**
- H20.021 Recurrent acute iridocyclitis, right eye
- H20.022 Recurrent acute iridocyclitis, left eye
- H20.023 Recurrent acute iridocyclitis, bilateral
- H20.029 Recurrent acute iridocyclitis, unspecified eye ▽

√6th **H20.03 Secondary infectious iridocyclitis**
- H20.031 Secondary infectious iridocyclitis, right eye
- H20.032 Secondary infectious iridocyclitis, left eye
- H20.033 Secondary infectious iridocyclitis, bilateral
- H20.039 Secondary infectious iridocyclitis, unspecified eye ▽

√6th **H20.04 Secondary noninfectious iridocyclitis**
- H20.041 Secondary noninfectious iridocyclitis, right eye
- H20.042 Secondary noninfectious iridocyclitis, left eye
- H20.043 Secondary noninfectious iridocyclitis, bilateral
- H20.049 Secondary noninfectious iridocyclitis, unspecified eye ▽

√6th **H20.05 Hypopyon**
- H20.051 Hypopyon, right eye
- H20.052 Hypopyon, left eye
- H20.053 Hypopyon, bilateral
- H20.059 Hypopyon, unspecified eye

√5th **H20.1 Chronic iridocyclitis**
Use additional code for any associated cataract (H26.21-)
EXCLUDES 2 posterior cyclitis (H30.2-)
- H20.10 Chronic iridocyclitis, unspecified eye ▽
- H20.11 Chronic iridocyclitis, right eye
- H20.12 Chronic iridocyclitis, left eye
- H20.13 Chronic iridocyclitis, bilateral

√5th **H20.2 Lens-induced iridocyclitis**
- H20.20 Lens-induced iridocyclitis, unspecified eye ▽
- H20.21 Lens-induced iridocyclitis, right eye
- H20.22 Lens-induced iridocyclitis, left eye
- H20.23 Lens-induced iridocyclitis, bilateral

√5th **H20.8 Other iridocyclitis**
EXCLUDES 2 glaucomatocyclitis crises (H40.4-)
posterior cyclitis (H30.2-)
sympathetic uveitis (H44.13-)

√6th **H20.81 Fuchs' heterochromic cyclitis**
- H20.811 Fuchs' heterochromic cyclitis, right eye
- H20.812 Fuchs' heterochromic cyclitis, left eye
- H20.813 Fuchs' heterochromic cyclitis, bilateral
- H20.819 Fuchs' heterochromic cyclitis, unspecified eye ▽

√6th **H20.82 Vogt-Koyanagi syndrome**
- H20.821 Vogt-Koyanagi syndrome, right eye
- H20.822 Vogt-Koyanagi syndrome, left eye
- H20.823 Vogt-Koyanagi syndrome, bilateral
- H20.829 Vogt-Koyanagi syndrome, unspecified eye ▽

H20.9 Unspecified iridocyclitis ▽
Uveitis NOS

√4th **H21 Other disorders of iris and ciliary body**
EXCLUDES 2 sympathetic uveitis (H44.1-)

√5th **H21.0 Hyphema**
EXCLUDES 1 traumatic hyphema (S05.1-)
- H21.00 Hyphema, unspecified eye ▽
- H21.01 Hyphema, right eye
- H21.02 Hyphema, left eye
- H21.03 Hyphema, bilateral

√5th **H21.1 Other vascular disorders of iris and ciliary body**
Neovascularization of iris or ciliary body
Rubeosis iridis
Rubeosis of iris

√6th **H21.1X Other vascular disorders of iris and ciliary body**
- H21.1X1 Other vascular disorders of iris and ciliary body, right eye
- H21.1X2 Other vascular disorders of iris and ciliary body, left eye
- H21.1X3 Other vascular disorders of iris and ciliary body, bilateral
- H21.1X9 Other vascular disorders of iris and ciliary body, unspecified eye ▽

√5th **H21.2 Degeneration of iris and ciliary body**

√6th **H21.21 Degeneration of chamber angle**
- H21.211 Degeneration of chamber angle, right eye
- H21.212 Degeneration of chamber angle, left eye
- H21.213 Degeneration of chamber angle, bilateral
- H21.219 Degeneration of chamber angle, unspecified eye ▽

Hyphema

Iris — Cornea — Hyphema

Chapter 7. Diseases of the Eye and Adnexa

√6th H21.22 Degeneration of ciliary body
- H21.221 Degeneration of ciliary body, right eye
- H21.222 Degeneration of ciliary body, left eye
- H21.223 Degeneration of ciliary body, bilateral
- H21.229 Degeneration of ciliary body, unspecified eye ▽

√6th H21.23 Degeneration of iris (pigmentary)
  Translucency of iris
- H21.231 Degeneration of iris (pigmentary), right eye
- H21.232 Degeneration of iris (pigmentary), left eye
- H21.233 Degeneration of iris (pigmentary), bilateral
- H21.239 Degeneration of iris (pigmentary), unspecified eye ▽

√6th H21.24 Degeneration of pupillary margin
- H21.241 Degeneration of pupillary margin, right eye
- H21.242 Degeneration of pupillary margin, left eye
- H21.243 Degeneration of pupillary margin, bilateral
- H21.249 Degeneration of pupillary margin, unspecified eye ▽

√6th H21.25 Iridoschisis
- H21.251 Iridoschisis, right eye
- H21.252 Iridoschisis, left eye
- H21.253 Iridoschisis, bilateral
- H21.259 Iridoschisis, unspecified eye ▽

√6th H21.26 Iris atrophy (essential) (progressive)
- H21.261 Iris atrophy (essential) (progressive), right eye
- H21.262 Iris atrophy (essential) (progressive), left eye
- H21.263 Iris atrophy (essential) (progressive), bilateral
- H21.269 Iris atrophy (essential) (progressive), unspecified eye ▽

√6th H21.27 Miotic pupillary cyst
- H21.271 Miotic pupillary cyst, right eye
- H21.272 Miotic pupillary cyst, left eye
- H21.273 Miotic pupillary cyst, bilateral
- H21.279 Miotic pupillary cyst, unspecified eye ▽
- H21.29 Other iris atrophy

√5th H21.3 Cyst of iris, ciliary body and anterior chamber
  EXCLUDES 2 miotic pupillary cyst (H21.27-)

√6th H21.30 Idiopathic cysts of iris, ciliary body or anterior chamber
  Cyst of iris, ciliary body or anterior chamber NOS
- H21.301 Idiopathic cysts of iris, ciliary body or anterior chamber, right eye
- H21.302 Idiopathic cysts of iris, ciliary body or anterior chamber, left eye
- H21.303 Idiopathic cysts of iris, ciliary body or anterior chamber, bilateral
- H21.309 Idiopathic cysts of iris, ciliary body or anterior chamber, unspecified eye ▽

√6th H21.31 Exudative cysts of iris or anterior chamber
- H21.311 Exudative cysts of iris or anterior chamber, right eye
- H21.312 Exudative cysts of iris or anterior chamber, left eye
- H21.313 Exudative cysts of iris or anterior chamber, bilateral
- H21.319 Exudative cysts of iris or anterior chamber, unspecified eye ▽

√6th H21.32 Implantation cysts of iris, ciliary body or anterior chamber
- H21.321 Implantation cysts of iris, ciliary body or anterior chamber, right eye
- H21.322 Implantation cysts of iris, ciliary body or anterior chamber, left eye
- H21.323 Implantation cysts of iris, ciliary body or anterior chamber, bilateral
- H21.329 Implantation cysts of iris, ciliary body or anterior chamber, unspecified eye ▽

√6th H21.33 Parasitic cyst of iris, ciliary body or anterior chamber
- H21.331 Parasitic cyst of iris, ciliary body or anterior chamber, right eye
- H21.332 Parasitic cyst of iris, ciliary body or anterior chamber, left eye
- H21.333 Parasitic cyst of iris, ciliary body or anterior chamber, bilateral
- H21.339 Parasitic cyst of iris, ciliary body or anterior chamber, unspecified eye ▽

√6th H21.34 Primary cyst of pars plana
- H21.341 Primary cyst of pars plana, right eye
- H21.342 Primary cyst of pars plana, left eye
- H21.343 Primary cyst of pars plana, bilateral
- H21.349 Primary cyst of pars plana, unspecified eye ▽

√6th H21.35 Exudative cyst of pars plana
  DEF: Protein, fatty-filled bullous elevation of nonpigmented outermost ciliary epithelium of pars plana; due to fluid leak from blood vessels.
- H21.351 Exudative cyst of pars plana, right eye
- H21.352 Exudative cyst of pars plana, left eye
- H21.353 Exudative cyst of pars plana, bilateral
- H21.359 Exudative cyst of pars plana, unspecified eye ▽

√5th H21.4 Pupillary membranes
  Iris bombé
  Pupillary occlusion
  Pupillary seclusion
  EXCLUDES 1 congenital pupillary membranes (Q13.8)
- H21.40 Pupillary membranes, unspecified eye ▽
- H21.41 Pupillary membranes, right eye
- H21.42 Pupillary membranes, left eye
- H21.43 Pupillary membranes, bilateral

√5th H21.5 Other and unspecified adhesions and disruptions of iris and ciliary body
  EXCLUDES 1 corectopia (Q13.2)

√6th H21.50 Unspecified adhesions of iris
  Synechia (iris) NOS
- H21.501 Unspecified adhesions of iris, right eye ▽
- H21.502 Unspecified adhesions of iris, left eye ▽
- H21.503 Unspecified adhesions of iris, bilateral ▽
- H21.509 Unspecified adhesions of iris and ciliary body, unspecified eye

√6th H21.51 Anterior synechiae (iris)
- H21.511 Anterior synechiae (iris), right eye
- H21.512 Anterior synechiae (iris), left eye
- H21.513 Anterior synechiae (iris), bilateral
- H21.519 Anterior synechiae (iris), unspecified eye ▽

√6th H21.52 Goniosynechiae
- H21.521 Goniosynechiae, right eye
- H21.522 Goniosynechiae, left eye
- H21.523 Goniosynechiae, bilateral
- H21.529 Goniosynechiae, unspecified eye ▽

√6th H21.53 Iridodialysis
- H21.531 Iridodialysis, right eye
- H21.532 Iridodialysis, left eye
- H21.533 Iridodialysis, bilateral
- H21.539 Iridodialysis, unspecified eye ▽

√6th H21.54 Posterior synechiae (iris)
- H21.541 Posterior synechiae (iris), right eye
- H21.542 Posterior synechiae (iris), left eye
- H21.543 Posterior synechiae (iris), bilateral
- H21.549 Posterior synechiae (iris), unspecified eye ▽

√6th H21.55 Recession of chamber angle
- H21.551 Recession of chamber angle, right eye
- H21.552 Recession of chamber angle, left eye
- H21.553 Recession of chamber angle, bilateral
- H21.559 Recession of chamber angle, unspecified eye ▽

EXCLUDES 1 Not coded here   EXCLUDES 2 Not included here   N Newborn Age: 0   P Pediatric Age: 0-17   M Maternity Age: 12-55   A Adult Age: 15-124

584

ICD-10-CM 2018

✓6ᵗʰ **H21.56 Pupillary abnormalities**
Deformed pupil
Ectopic pupil
Rupture of sphincter, pupil
EXCLUDES 1 *congenital deformity of pupil (Q13.2-)*
H21.561 Pupillary abnormality, right eye
H21.562 Pupillary abnormality, left eye
H21.563 Pupillary abnormality, bilateral
H21.569 Pupillary abnormality, unspecified eye ▽

✓5ᵗʰ **H21.8 Other specified disorders of iris and ciliary body**
H21.81 Floppy iris syndrome
Intraoperative floppy iris syndrome (IFIS)
Use additional code for adverse effect, if applicable, to identify drug (T36-T50 with fifth or sixth character 5)
H21.82 Plateau iris syndrome (post-iridectomy) (postprocedural)
H21.89 Other specified disorders of iris and ciliary body
H21.9 Unspecified disorder of iris and ciliary body ▽

H22 Disorders of iris and ciliary body in diseases classified elsewhere
Code first underlying disease, such as:
gout (M1A.-, M10.-)
leprosy (A30.-)
parasitic disease (B89)

Disorders of lens (H25–H28)

✓4ᵗʰ **H25 Age-related cataract**
Senile cataract
EXCLUDES 2 *capsular glaucoma with pseudoexfoliation of lens (H40.1-)*

✓5ᵗʰ **H25.0 Age-related incipient cataract**
✓6ᵗʰ **H25.01 Cortical age-related cataract**
H25.011 Cortical age-related cataract, right eye A
H25.012 Cortical age-related cataract, left eye A
H25.013 Cortical age-related cataract, bilateral A
H25.019 Cortical age-related cataract, unspecified eye A▽
✓6ᵗʰ **H25.03 Anterior subcapsular polar age-related cataract**
H25.031 Anterior subcapsular polar age-related cataract, right eye A
H25.032 Anterior subcapsular polar age-related cataract, left eye A
H25.033 Anterior subcapsular polar age-related cataract, bilateral A
H25.039 Anterior subcapsular polar age-related cataract, unspecified eye A▽
✓6ᵗʰ **H25.04 Posterior subcapsular polar age-related cataract**
H25.041 Posterior subcapsular polar age-related cataract, right eye A
H25.042 Posterior subcapsular polar age-related cataract, left eye A
H25.043 Posterior subcapsular polar age-related cataract, bilateral A
H25.049 Posterior subcapsular polar age-related cataract, unspecified eye A▽
✓6ᵗʰ **H25.09 Other age-related incipient cataract**
Coronary age-related cataract
Punctate age-related cataract
Water clefts
H25.091 Other age-related incipient cataract, right eye A
H25.092 Other age-related incipient cataract, left eye A
H25.093 Other age-related incipient cataract, bilateral A
H25.099 Other age-related incipient cataract, unspecified eye A▽
✓5ᵗʰ **H25.1 Age-related nuclear cataract**
Cataracta brunescens
Nuclear sclerosis cataract
AHA: 2016, 1Q, 36
H25.10 Age-related nuclear cataract, unspecified eye A▽
H25.11 Age-related nuclear cataract, right eye A
H25.12 Age-related nuclear cataract, left eye A
H25.13 Age-related nuclear cataract, bilateral A

Cataracts
Vitreous / Iris / Cornea / Retina / Pupil / Lens / Normal lens / Clouded lens / Lens affected by cataracts

✓5ᵗʰ **H25.2 Age-related cataract, morgagnian type**
Age-related hypermature cataract
H25.20 Age-related cataract, morgagnian type, unspecified eye A▽
H25.21 Age-related cataract, morgagnian type, right eye A
H25.22 Age-related cataract, morgagnian type, left eye A
H25.23 Age-related cataract, morgagnian type, bilateral A
✓5ᵗʰ **H25.8 Other age-related cataract**
✓6ᵗʰ **H25.81 Combined forms of age-related cataract**
H25.811 Combined forms of age-related cataract, right eye A
H25.812 Combined forms of age-related cataract, left eye A
H25.813 Combined forms of age-related cataract, bilateral A
H25.819 Combined forms of age-related cataract, unspecified eye A▽
H25.89 Other age-related cataract A
H25.9 Unspecified age-related cataract A▽
✓4ᵗʰ **H26 Other cataract**
EXCLUDES 1 *congenital cataract (Q12.0)*
✓5ᵗʰ **H26.0 Infantile and juvenile cataract**
✓6ᵗʰ **H26.00 Unspecified infantile and juvenile cataract**
H26.001 Unspecified infantile and juvenile cataract, right eye P▽
H26.002 Unspecified infantile and juvenile cataract, left eye P▽
H26.003 Unspecified infantile and juvenile cataract, bilateral P▽
H26.009 Unspecified infantile and juvenile cataract, unspecified eye P▽
✓6ᵗʰ **H26.01 Infantile and juvenile cortical, lamellar, or zonular cataract**
H26.011 Infantile and juvenile cortical, lamellar, or zonular cataract, right eye P
H26.012 Infantile and juvenile cortical, lamellar, or zonular cataract, left eye P
H26.013 Infantile and juvenile cortical, lamellar, or zonular cataract, bilateral P
H26.019 Infantile and juvenile cortical, lamellar, or zonular cataract, unspecified eye P▽
✓6ᵗʰ **H26.03 Infantile and juvenile nuclear cataract**
H26.031 Infantile and juvenile nuclear cataract, right eye P
H26.032 Infantile and juvenile nuclear cataract, left eye P
H26.033 Infantile and juvenile nuclear cataract, bilateral P
H26.039 Infantile and juvenile nuclear cataract, unspecified eye P▽

☑ Additional Character Req   ✓ₓ7ᵗʰ Placeholder Alert   Manifestation   HCC CMS-HCC Condition   ▽ Unspecified Code   ▶◀ Revised Text   ● New Code   ▲ Revised Code Title

Chapter 7. Diseases of the Eye and Adnexa (side margin)

H26.04–H27.129 (side margin)

√6th **H26.04 Anterior subcapsular polar infantile and juvenile cataract**

    H26.041 Anterior subcapsular polar infantile and juvenile cataract, right eye 🅿

    H26.042 Anterior subcapsular polar infantile and juvenile cataract, left eye 🅿

    H26.043 Anterior subcapsular polar infantile and juvenile cataract, bilateral 🅿

    H26.049 Anterior subcapsular polar infantile and juvenile cataract, unspecified eye 🅿▽

√6th **H26.05 Posterior subcapsular polar infantile and juvenile cataract**

    H26.051 Posterior subcapsular polar infantile and juvenile cataract, right eye 🅿

    H26.052 Posterior subcapsular polar infantile and juvenile cataract, left eye 🅿

    H26.053 Posterior subcapsular polar infantile and juvenile cataract, bilateral 🅿

    H26.059 Posterior subcapsular polar infantile and juvenile cataract, unspecified eye 🅿▽

√6th **H26.06 Combined forms of infantile and juvenile cataract**

    H26.061 Combined forms of infantile and juvenile cataract, right eye 🅿

    H26.062 Combined forms of infantile and juvenile cataract, left eye 🅿

    H26.063 Combined forms of infantile and juvenile cataract, bilateral 🅿

    H26.069 Combined forms of infantile and juvenile cataract, unspecified eye 🅿▽

    H26.09 Other infantile and juvenile cataract 🅿

√5th **H26.1 Traumatic cataract**

Use additional code (Chapter 20) to identify external cause

√6th **H26.10 Unspecified traumatic cataract**

    H26.101 Unspecified traumatic cataract, right eye ▽

    H26.102 Unspecified traumatic cataract, left eye ▽

    H26.103 Unspecified traumatic cataract, bilateral ▽

    H26.109 Unspecified traumatic cataract, unspecified eye ▽

√6th **H26.11 Localized traumatic opacities**

    H26.111 Localized traumatic opacities, right eye

    H26.112 Localized traumatic opacities, left eye

    H26.113 Localized traumatic opacities, bilateral

    H26.119 Localized traumatic opacities, unspecified eye ▽

√6th **H26.12 Partially resolved traumatic cataract**

    H26.121 Partially resolved traumatic cataract, right eye

    H26.122 Partially resolved traumatic cataract, left eye

    H26.123 Partially resolved traumatic cataract, bilateral

    H26.129 Partially resolved traumatic cataract, unspecified eye ▽

√6th **H26.13 Total traumatic cataract**

    H26.131 Total traumatic cataract, right eye

    H26.132 Total traumatic cataract, left eye

    H26.133 Total traumatic cataract, bilateral

    H26.139 Total traumatic cataract, unspecified eye ▽

√5th **H26.2 Complicated cataract**

    H26.20 Unspecified complicated cataract ▽

Cataracta complicata NOS

√6th **H26.21 Cataract with neovascularization**

Code also associated condition, such as:
chronic iridocyclitis (H20.1-)

    H26.211 Cataract with neovascularization, right eye

    H26.212 Cataract with neovascularization, left eye

    H26.213 Cataract with neovascularization, bilateral

    H26.219 Cataract with neovascularization, unspecified eye ▽

√6th **H26.22 Cataract secondary to ocular disorders (degenerative) (inflammatory)**

Code also associated ocular disorder

    H26.221 Cataract secondary to ocular disorders (degenerative) (inflammatory), right eye

    H26.222 Cataract secondary to ocular disorders (degenerative) (inflammatory), left eye

    H26.223 Cataract secondary to ocular disorders (degenerative) (inflammatory), bilateral

    H26.229 Cataract secondary to ocular disorders (degenerative) (inflammatory), unspecified eye ▽

√6th **H26.23 Glaucomatous flecks (subcapsular)**

Code first underlying glaucoma (H40-H42)

    H26.231 Glaucomatous flecks (subcapsular), right eye

    H26.232 Glaucomatous flecks (subcapsular), left eye

    H26.233 Glaucomatous flecks (subcapsular), bilateral

    H26.239 Glaucomatous flecks (subcapsular), unspecified eye ▽

√5th **H26.3 Drug-induced cataract**

Toxic cataract

Use additional code for adverse effect, if applicable, to identify drug (T36-T50 with fifth or sixth character 5)

    H26.30 Drug-induced cataract, unspecified eye ▽

    H26.31 Drug-induced cataract, right eye

    H26.32 Drug-induced cataract, left eye

    H26.33 Drug-induced cataract, bilateral

√5th **H26.4 Secondary cataract**

    H26.40 Unspecified secondary cataract ▽

√6th **H26.41 Soemmering's ring**

    H26.411 Soemmering's ring, right eye

    H26.412 Soemmering's ring, left eye

    H26.413 Soemmering's ring, bilateral

    H26.419 Soemmering's ring, unspecified eye ▽

√6th **H26.49 Other secondary cataract**

    H26.491 Other secondary cataract, right eye

    H26.492 Other secondary cataract, left eye

    H26.493 Other secondary cataract, bilateral

    H26.499 Other secondary cataract, unspecified eye ▽

    H26.8 Other specified cataract

    H26.9 Unspecified cataract ▽

√4th **H27 Other disorders of lens**

EXCLUDES 1 *congenital lens malformations (Q12.-)*
mechanical complications of intraocular lens implant (T85.2)
pseudophakia (Z96.1)

√5th **H27.0 Aphakia**

Acquired absence of lens
Acquired aphakia
Aphakia due to trauma

EXCLUDES 1 *cataract extraction status (Z98.4-)*
congenital absence of lens (Q12.3)
congenital aphakia (Q12.3)

    H27.00 Aphakia, unspecified eye ▽

    H27.01 Aphakia, right eye

    H27.02 Aphakia, left eye

    H27.03 Aphakia, bilateral

√5th **H27.1 Dislocation of lens**

    H27.10 Unspecified dislocation of lens ▽

√6th **H27.11 Subluxation of lens**

    H27.111 Subluxation of lens, right eye

    H27.112 Subluxation of lens, left eye

    H27.113 Subluxation of lens, bilateral

    H27.119 Subluxation of lens, unspecified eye ▽

√6th **H27.12 Anterior dislocation of lens**

    H27.121 Anterior dislocation of lens, right eye

    H27.122 Anterior dislocation of lens, left eye

    H27.123 Anterior dislocation of lens, bilateral

    H27.129 Anterior dislocation of lens, unspecified eye ▽

EXCLUDES 1 Not coded here   EXCLUDES 2 Not included here   🅝 Newborn Age: 0   🅿 Pediatric Age: 0-17   🅜 Maternity Age: 12-55   🅐 Adult Age: 15-124

586

ICD-10-CM 2018

✓6ᵗʰ **H27.13** **Posterior dislocation of lens**
    H27.131 **Posterior dislocation of lens, right eye**
    H27.132 **Posterior dislocation of lens, left eye**
    H27.133 **Posterior dislocation of lens, bilateral**
    H27.139 **Posterior dislocation of lens, unspecified eye** ▽

H27.8 **Other specified disorders of lens**
H27.9 **Unspecified disorder of lens** ▽

H28 *Cataract in diseases classified elsewhere*
  Code first underlying disease, such as:
    hypoparathyroidism (E20.-)
    myotonia (G71.1-)
    myxedema (E03.-)
    protein-calorie malnutrition (E40-E46)
    EXCLUDES 1   cataract in diabetes mellitus (E08.36, E09.36, E10.36, E11.36, E13.36)

Disorders of choroid and retina (H30-H36)

✓4ᵗʰ **H30** **Chorioretinal inflammation**
  ✓5ᵗʰ **H30.0** **Focal chorioretinal inflammation**
    Focal chorioretinitis
    Focal choroiditis
    Focal retinitis
    Focal retinochoroiditis
    ✓6ᵗʰ **H30.00** **Unspecified focal chorioretinal inflammation**
      Focal chorioretinitis NOS
      Focal choroiditis NOS
      Focal retinitis NOS
      Focal retinochoroiditis NOS
      H30.001 **Unspecified focal chorioretinal inflammation, right eye** ▽
      H30.002 **Unspecified focal chorioretinal inflammation, left eye** ▽
      H30.003 **Unspecified focal chorioretinal inflammation, bilateral** ▽
      H30.009 **Unspecified focal chorioretinal inflammation, unspecified eye** ▽
    ✓6ᵗʰ **H30.01** **Focal chorioretinal inflammation, juxtapapillary**
      H30.011 **Focal chorioretinal inflammation, juxtapapillary, right eye**
      H30.012 **Focal chorioretinal inflammation, juxtapapillary, left eye**
      H30.013 **Focal chorioretinal inflammation, juxtapapillary, bilateral**
      H30.019 **Focal chorioretinal inflammation, juxtapapillary, unspecified eye** ▽
    ✓6ᵗʰ **H30.02** **Focal chorioretinal inflammation of posterior pole**
      H30.021 **Focal chorioretinal inflammation of posterior pole, right eye**
      H30.022 **Focal chorioretinal inflammation of posterior pole, left eye**
      H30.023 **Focal chorioretinal inflammation of posterior pole, bilateral**
      H30.029 **Focal chorioretinal inflammation of posterior pole, unspecified eye** ▽
    ✓6ᵗʰ **H30.03** **Focal chorioretinal inflammation, peripheral**
      H30.031 **Focal chorioretinal inflammation, peripheral, right eye**
      H30.032 **Focal chorioretinal inflammation, peripheral, left eye**
      H30.033 **Focal chorioretinal inflammation, peripheral, bilateral**
      H30.039 **Focal chorioretinal inflammation, peripheral, unspecified eye** ▽
    ✓6ᵗʰ **H30.04** **Focal chorioretinal inflammation, macular or paramacular**
      H30.041 **Focal chorioretinal inflammation, macular or paramacular, right eye**
      H30.042 **Focal chorioretinal inflammation, macular or paramacular, left eye**
      H30.043 **Focal chorioretinal inflammation, macular or paramacular, bilateral**
      H30.049 **Focal chorioretinal inflammation, macular or paramacular, unspecified eye** ▽

  ✓5ᵗʰ **H30.1** **Disseminated chorioretinal inflammation**
    Disseminated chorioretinitis
    Disseminated choroiditis
    Disseminated retinitis
    Disseminated retinochoroiditis
    EXCLUDES 2   exudative retinopathy (H35.02-)
    ✓6ᵗʰ **H30.10** **Unspecified disseminated chorioretinal inflammation**
      Disseminated chorioretinitis NOS
      Disseminated choroiditis NOS
      Disseminated retinitis NOS
      Disseminated retinochoroiditis NOS
      H30.101 **Unspecified disseminated chorioretinal inflammation, right eye** ▽
      H30.102 **Unspecified disseminated chorioretinal inflammation, left eye** ▽
      H30.103 **Unspecified disseminated chorioretinal inflammation, bilateral** ▽
      H30.109 **Unspecified disseminated chorioretinal inflammation, unspecified eye** ▽
    ✓6ᵗʰ **H30.11** **Disseminated chorioretinal inflammation of posterior pole**
      H30.111 **Disseminated chorioretinal inflammation of posterior pole, right eye**
      H30.112 **Disseminated chorioretinal inflammation of posterior pole, left eye**
      H30.113 **Disseminated chorioretinal inflammation of posterior pole, bilateral**
      H30.119 **Disseminated chorioretinal inflammation of posterior pole, unspecified eye** ▽
    ✓6ᵗʰ **H30.12** **Disseminated chorioretinal inflammation, peripheral**
      H30.121 **Disseminated chorioretinal inflammation, peripheral right eye**
      H30.122 **Disseminated chorioretinal inflammation, peripheral, left eye**
      H30.123 **Disseminated chorioretinal inflammation, peripheral, bilateral**
      H30.129 **Disseminated chorioretinal inflammation, peripheral, unspecified eye** ▽
    ✓6ᵗʰ **H30.13** **Disseminated chorioretinal inflammation, generalized**
      H30.131 **Disseminated chorioretinal inflammation, generalized, right eye**
      H30.132 **Disseminated chorioretinal inflammation, generalized, left eye**
      H30.133 **Disseminated chorioretinal inflammation, generalized, bilateral**
      H30.139 **Disseminated chorioretinal inflammation, generalized, unspecified eye** ▽
    ✓6ᵗʰ **H30.14** **Acute posterior multifocal placoid pigment epitheliopathy**
      H30.141 **Acute posterior multifocal placoid pigment epitheliopathy, right eye**
      H30.142 **Acute posterior multifocal placoid pigment epitheliopathy, left eye**
      H30.143 **Acute posterior multifocal placoid pigment epitheliopathy, bilateral**
      H30.149 **Acute posterior multifocal placoid pigment epitheliopathy, unspecified eye** ▽

  ✓5ᵗʰ **H30.2** **Posterior cyclitis**
    Pars planitis
    H30.20 **Posterior cyclitis, unspecified eye** ▽
    H30.21 **Posterior cyclitis, right eye**
    H30.22 **Posterior cyclitis, left eye**
    H30.23 **Posterior cyclitis, bilateral**
  ✓5ᵗʰ **H30.8** **Other chorioretinal inflammations**
    ✓6ᵗʰ **H30.81** **Harada's disease**
      H30.811 **Harada's disease, right eye**
      H30.812 **Harada's disease, left eye**
      H30.813 **Harada's disease, bilateral**
      H30.819 **Harada's disease, unspecified eye** ▽

☑ Additional Character Req   ✓x7ᵗʰ Placeholder Alert   Manifestation   HCC CMS-HCC Condition   ▽ Unspecified Code   ►◄ Revised Text   ● New Code   ▲ Revised Code Title

ICD-10-CM 2018   587

Chapter 7. Diseases of the Eye and Adnexa

H27.13–H30.819

✓6th H30.89 Other chorioretinal inflammations
       H30.891   Other chorioretinal inflammations, right eye
       H30.892   Other chorioretinal inflammations, left eye
       H30.893   Other chorioretinal inflammations, bilateral
       H30.899   Other chorioretinal inflammations, unspecified eye   ▽

✓5th H30.9 Unspecified chorioretinal inflammation
     Chorioretinitis NOS   Retinitis NOS
     Choroiditis NOS   Retinochoroiditis NOS
     Neuroretinitis NOS
       H30.90   Unspecified chorioretinal inflammation, unspecified eye   ▽
       H30.91   Unspecified chorioretinal inflammation, right eye   ▽
       H30.92   Unspecified chorioretinal inflammation, left eye   ▽
       H30.93   Unspecified chorioretinal inflammation, bilateral   ▽

✓4th H31 Other disorders of choroid

✓5th H31.0 Chorioretinal scars
     EXCLUDES 2   *postsurgical chorioretinal scars (H59.81-)*
     ✓6th H31.00 Unspecified chorioretinal scars
       H31.001   Unspecified chorioretinal scars, right eye   ▽
       H31.002   Unspecified chorioretinal scars, left eye   ▽
       H31.003   Unspecified chorioretinal scars, bilateral   ▽
       H31.009   Unspecified chorioretinal scars, unspecified eye   ▽

     ✓6th H31.01 Macula scars of posterior pole (postinflammatory) (post-traumatic)
     EXCLUDES 1   *postprocedural chorioretinal scar (H59.81-)*
       H31.011   Macula scars of posterior pole (postinflammatory) (post-traumatic), right eye
       H31.012   Macula scars of posterior pole (postinflammatory) (post-traumatic), left eye
       H31.013   Macula scars of posterior pole (postinflammatory) (post-traumatic), bilateral
       H31.019   Macula scars of posterior pole (postinflammatory) (post-traumatic), unspecified eye   ▽

     ✓6th H31.02 Solar retinopathy
       H31.021   Solar retinopathy, right eye
       H31.022   Solar retinopathy, left eye
       H31.023   Solar retinopathy, bilateral
       H31.029   Solar retinopathy, unspecified eye   ▽

     ✓6th H31.09 Other chorioretinal scars
       H31.091   Other chorioretinal scars, right eye
       H31.092   Other chorioretinal scars, left eye
       H31.093   Other chorioretinal scars, bilateral
       H31.099   Other chorioretinal scars, unspecified eye   ▽

✓5th H31.1 Choroidal degeneration
     EXCLUDES 2   *angioid streaks of macula (H35.33)*
     ✓6th H31.10 Unspecified choroidal degeneration
     Choroidal sclerosis NOS
       H31.101   Choroidal degeneration, unspecified, right eye   ▽
       H31.102   Choroidal degeneration, unspecified, left eye   ▽
       H31.103   Choroidal degeneration, unspecified, bilateral   ▽
       H31.109   Choroidal degeneration, unspecified, unspecified eye   ▽

     ✓6th H31.11 Age-related choroidal atrophy
       H31.111   Age-related choroidal atrophy, right eye   Ⓐ
       H31.112   Age-related choroidal atrophy, left eye   Ⓐ
       H31.113   Age-related choroidal atrophy, bilateral   Ⓐ
       H31.119   Age-related choroidal atrophy, unspecified eye   Ⓐ ▽

✓6th H31.12 Diffuse secondary atrophy of choroid
       H31.121   Diffuse secondary atrophy of choroid, right eye
       H31.122   Diffuse secondary atrophy of choroid, left eye
       H31.123   Diffuse secondary atrophy of choroid, bilateral
       H31.129   Diffuse secondary atrophy of choroid, unspecified eye   ▽

✓5th H31.2 Hereditary choroidal dystrophy
     EXCLUDES 2   *hyperornithinemia (E72.4)*
                ornithinemia (E72.4)
       H31.20   Hereditary choroidal dystrophy, unspecified   ▽
       H31.21   Choroideremia
       H31.22   Choroidal dystrophy (central areolar) (generalized) (peripapillary)
       H31.23   Gyrate atrophy, choroid
       H31.29   Other hereditary choroidal dystrophy

✓5th H31.3 Choroidal hemorrhage and rupture
     ✓6th H31.30 Unspecified choroidal hemorrhage
       H31.301   Unspecified choroidal hemorrhage, right eye   ▽
       H31.302   Unspecified choroidal hemorrhage, left eye   ▽
       H31.303   Unspecified choroidal hemorrhage, bilateral   ▽
       H31.309   Unspecified choroidal hemorrhage, unspecified eye   ▽

     ✓6th H31.31 Expulsive choroidal hemorrhage
       H31.311   Expulsive choroidal hemorrhage, right eye
       H31.312   Expulsive choroidal hemorrhage, left eye
       H31.313   Expulsive choroidal hemorrhage, bilateral
       H31.319   Expulsive choroidal hemorrhage, unspecified eye   ▽

     ✓6th H31.32 Choroidal rupture
       H31.321   Choroidal rupture, right eye
       H31.322   Choroidal rupture, left eye
       H31.323   Choroidal rupture, bilateral
       H31.329   Choroidal rupture, unspecified eye   ▽

✓5th H31.4 Choroidal detachment
     ✓6th H31.40 Unspecified choroidal detachment
       H31.401   Unspecified choroidal detachment, right eye   ▽
       H31.402   Unspecified choroidal detachment, left eye   ▽
       H31.403   Unspecified choroidal detachment, bilateral   ▽
       H31.409   Unspecified choroidal detachment, unspecified eye   ▽

     ✓6th H31.41 Hemorrhagic choroidal detachment
       H31.411   Hemorrhagic choroidal detachment, right eye
       H31.412   Hemorrhagic choroidal detachment, left eye
       H31.413   Hemorrhagic choroidal detachment, bilateral
       H31.419   Hemorrhagic choroidal detachment, unspecified eye   ▽

     ✓6th H31.42 Serous choroidal detachment
       H31.421   Serous choroidal detachment, right eye
       H31.422   Serous choroidal detachment, left eye
       H31.423   Serous choroidal detachment, bilateral
       H31.429   Serous choroidal detachment, unspecified eye   ▽

     H31.8   Other specified disorders of choroid
     H31.9   Unspecified disorder of choroid   ▽

H32 *Chorioretinal disorders in diseases classified elsewhere*
     Code first underlying disease, such as:
       congenital toxoplasmosis (P37.1)
       histoplasmosis (B39.-)
       leprosy (A30.-)
     EXCLUDES 1   *chorioretinitis (in):*
       toxoplasmosis (acquired) (B58.01)
       tuberculosis (A18.53)

EXCLUDES 1 Not coded here   EXCLUDES 2 Not included here   Ⓝ Newborn Age: 0   Ⓟ Pediatric Age: 0-17   Ⓜ Maternity Age: 12-55   Ⓐ Adult Age: 15-124

588   ICD-10-CM 2018

Retinal Detachment

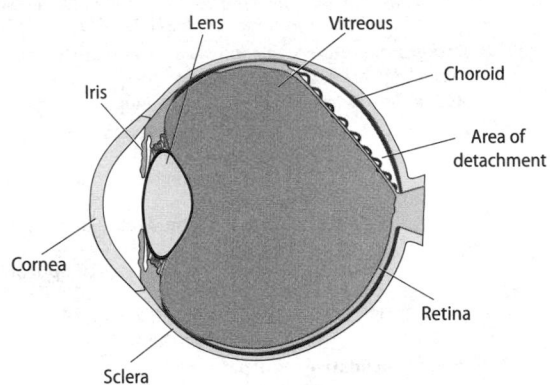

Lens Vitreous Iris Choroid Area of detachment Cornea Retina Sclera

✓4ᵗʰ **H33 Retinal detachments and breaks**
    EXCLUDES 1 *detachment of retinal pigment epithelium (H35.72-, H35.73-)*

✓5ᵗʰ **H33.0 Retinal detachment with retinal break**
    Rhegmatogenous retinal detachment
    EXCLUDES 1 *serous retinal detachment (without retinal break) (H33.2-)*

  ✓6ᵗʰ **H33.00 Unspecified retinal detachment with retinal break**
    H33.001 Unspecified retinal detachment with retinal break, right eye ▽
    H33.002 Unspecified retinal detachment with retinal break, left eye ▽
    H33.003 Unspecified retinal detachment with retinal break, bilateral ▽
    H33.009 Unspecified retinal detachment with retinal break, unspecified eye ▽

  ✓6ᵗʰ **H33.01 Retinal detachment with single break**
    H33.011 Retinal detachment with single break, right eye
    H33.012 Retinal detachment with single break, left eye
    H33.013 Retinal detachment with single break, bilateral
    H33.019 Retinal detachment with single break, unspecified eye ▽

  ✓6ᵗʰ **H33.02 Retinal detachment with multiple breaks**
    H33.021 Retinal detachment with multiple breaks, right eye
    H33.022 Retinal detachment with multiple breaks, left eye
    H33.023 Retinal detachment with multiple breaks, bilateral
    H33.029 Retinal detachment with multiple breaks, unspecified eye ▽

  ✓6ᵗʰ **H33.03 Retinal detachment with giant retinal tear**
    H33.031 Retinal detachment with giant retinal tear, right eye
    H33.032 Retinal detachment with giant retinal tear, left eye
    H33.033 Retinal detachment with giant retinal tear, bilateral
    H33.039 Retinal detachment with giant retinal tear, unspecified eye ▽

  ✓6ᵗʰ **H33.04 Retinal detachment with retinal dialysis**
    H33.041 Retinal detachment with retinal dialysis, right eye
    H33.042 Retinal detachment with retinal dialysis, left eye
    H33.043 Retinal detachment with retinal dialysis, bilateral
    H33.049 Retinal detachment with retinal dialysis, unspecified eye ▽

  ✓6ᵗʰ **H33.05 Total retinal detachment**
    H33.051 Total retinal detachment, right eye
    H33.052 Total retinal detachment, left eye
    H33.053 Total retinal detachment, bilateral
    H33.059 Total retinal detachment, unspecified eye ▽

✓5ᵗʰ **H33.1 Retinoschisis and retinal cysts**
    EXCLUDES 1 *congenital retinoschisis (Q14.1)*
      microcystoid degeneration of retina (H35.42-)

  ✓6ᵗʰ **H33.10 Unspecified retinoschisis**
    H33.101 Unspecified retinoschisis, right eye ▽
    H33.102 Unspecified retinoschisis, left eye ▽
    H33.103 Unspecified retinoschisis, bilateral ▽
    H33.109 Unspecified retinoschisis, unspecified eye ▽

  ✓6ᵗʰ **H33.11 Cyst of ora serrata**
    H33.111 Cyst of ora serrata, right eye
    H33.112 Cyst of ora serrata, left eye
    H33.113 Cyst of ora serrata, bilateral
    H33.119 Cyst of ora serrata, unspecified eye ▽

  ✓6ᵗʰ **H33.12 Parasitic cyst of retina**
    H33.121 Parasitic cyst of retina, right eye
    H33.122 Parasitic cyst of retina, left eye
    H33.123 Parasitic cyst of retina, bilateral
    H33.129 Parasitic cyst of retina, unspecified eye ▽

  ✓6ᵗʰ **H33.19 Other retinoschisis and retinal cysts**
    Pseudocyst of retina
    H33.191 Other retinoschisis and retinal cysts, right eye
    H33.192 Other retinoschisis and retinal cysts, left eye
    H33.193 Other retinoschisis and retinal cysts, bilateral
    H33.199 Other retinoschisis and retinal cysts, unspecified eye ▽

✓5ᵗʰ **H33.2 Serous retinal detachment**
    Retinal detachment NOS
    Retinal detachment without retinal break
    EXCLUDES 1 *central serous chorioretinopathy (H35.71-)*
    H33.20 Serous retinal detachment, unspecified eye ▽
    H33.21 Serous retinal detachment, right eye
    H33.22 Serous retinal detachment, left eye
    H33.23 Serous retinal detachment, bilateral

✓5ᵗʰ **H33.3 Retinal breaks without detachment**
    EXCLUDES 1 *chorioretinal scars after surgery for detachment (H59.81-)*
      peripheral retinal degeneration without break (H35.4-)

  ✓6ᵗʰ **H33.30 Unspecified retinal break**
    H33.301 Unspecified retinal break, right eye ▽
    H33.302 Unspecified retinal break, left eye ▽
    H33.303 Unspecified retinal break, bilateral ▽
    H33.309 Unspecified retinal break, unspecified eye ▽

  ✓6ᵗʰ **H33.31 Horseshoe tear of retina without detachment**
    Operculum of retina without detachment
    H33.311 Horseshoe tear of retina without detachment, right eye
    H33.312 Horseshoe tear of retina without detachment, left eye
    H33.313 Horseshoe tear of retina without detachment, bilateral
    H33.319 Horseshoe tear of retina without detachment, unspecified eye ▽

  ✓6ᵗʰ **H33.32 Round hole of retina without detachment**
    H33.321 Round hole, right eye
    H33.322 Round hole, left eye
    H33.323 Round hole, bilateral
    H33.329 Round hole, unspecified eye ▽

  ✓6ᵗʰ **H33.33 Multiple defects of retina without detachment**
    H33.331 Multiple defects of retina without detachment, right eye
    H33.332 Multiple defects of retina without detachment, left eye
    H33.333 Multiple defects of retina without detachment, bilateral
    H33.339 Multiple defects of retina without detachment, unspecified eye ▽

✓ Additional Character Req   ✓x7ᵗʰ Placeholder Alert   Manifestation   HCC CMS-HCC Condition   ▽ Unspecified Code   ►◄ Revised Text   ● New Code   ▲ Revised Code Title

ICD-10-CM 2018   589

Chapter 7. Diseases of the Eye and Adnexa

H33.4–H35.109

✓5ᵗʰ **H33.4 Traction detachment of retina**
Proliferative vitreo-retinopathy with retinal detachment

H33.40 Traction detachment of retina, unspecified eye ▽
H33.41 Traction detachment of retina, right eye
H33.42 Traction detachment of retina, left eye
H33.43 Traction detachment of retina, bilateral
H33.8 Other retinal detachments

✓4ᵗʰ **H34 Retinal vascular occlusions**
EXCLUDES 1   amaurosis fugax (G45.3)

✓5ᵗʰ **H34.0 Transient retinal artery occlusion**

H34.00 Transient retinal artery occlusion, unspecified eye ▽
H34.01 Transient retinal artery occlusion, right eye
H34.02 Transient retinal artery occlusion, left eye
H34.03 Transient retinal artery occlusion, bilateral

✓5ᵗʰ **H34.1 Central retinal artery occlusion**

H34.10 Central retinal artery occlusion, unspecified eye ▽
H34.11 Central retinal artery occlusion, right eye
H34.12 Central retinal artery occlusion, left eye
H34.13 Central retinal artery occlusion, bilateral

✓5ᵗʰ **H34.2 Other retinal artery occlusions**

✓6ᵗʰ **H34.21 Partial retinal artery occlusion**
Hollenhorst's plaque
Retinal microembolism

H34.211 Partial retinal artery occlusion, right eye
H34.212 Partial retinal artery occlusion, left eye
H34.213 Partial retinal artery occlusion, bilateral
H34.219 Partial retinal artery occlusion, unspecified eye ▽

✓6ᵗʰ **H34.23 Retinal artery branch occlusion**

H34.231 Retinal artery branch occlusion, right eye
H34.232 Retinal artery branch occlusion, left eye
H34.233 Retinal artery branch occlusion, bilateral
H34.239 Retinal artery branch occlusion, unspecified eye ▽

✓5ᵗʰ **H34.8 Other retinal vascular occlusions**

✓6ᵗʰ **H34.81 Central retinal vein occlusion**

> One of the following 7th characters is to be assigned to codes in subcategory H34.81 to designate the severity of the occlusion:
> 0   with macular edema
> 1   with retinal neovascularization
> 2   stable
>   old central retinal vein occlusion

✓7ᵗʰ **H34.811 Central retinal vein occlusion, right eye**
✓7ᵗʰ **H34.812 Central retinal vein occlusion, left eye**
✓7ᵗʰ **H34.813 Central retinal vein occlusion, bilateral**
✓7ᵗʰ **H34.819 Central retinal vein occlusion, unspecified eye** ▽

✓6ᵗʰ **H34.82 Venous engorgement**
Incipient retinal vein occlusion
Partial retinal vein occlusion

H34.821 Venous engorgement, right eye
H34.822 Venous engorgement, left eye
H34.823 Venous engorgement, bilateral
H34.829 Venous engorgement, unspecified eye ▽

✓6ᵗʰ **H34.83 Tributary (branch) retinal vein occlusion**

> One of the following 7th characters is to be assigned to codes in subcategory H34.83 to designate the severity of the occlusion:
> 0   with macular edema
> 1   with retinal neovascularization
> 2   stable
>   old tributary (branch) retinal vein occlusion

✓7ᵗʰ **H34.831 Tributary (branch) retinal vein occlusion, right eye**
✓7ᵗʰ **H34.832 Tributary (branch) retinal vein occlusion, left eye**
✓7ᵗʰ **H34.833 Tributary (branch) retinal vein occlusion, bilateral**
✓7ᵗʰ **H34.839 Tributary (branch) retinal vein occlusion, unspecified eye** ▽

H34.9 Unspecified retinal vascular occlusion ▽

✓4ᵗʰ **H35 Other retinal disorders**
EXCLUDES 2   diabetic retinal disorders (E08.311- E08.359, E09.311- E09.359, E10.311- E10.359, E11.311- E11.359, E13.311- E13.359)

✓5ᵗʰ **H35.0 Background retinopathy and retinal vascular changes**
Code also any associated hypertension (I10.-)

H35.00 Unspecified background retinopathy ▽

✓6ᵗʰ **H35.01 Changes in retinal vascular appearance**
Retinal vascular sheathing

H35.011 Changes in retinal vascular appearance, right eye
H35.012 Changes in retinal vascular appearance, left eye
H35.013 Changes in retinal vascular appearance, bilateral
H35.019 Changes in retinal vascular appearance, unspecified eye ▽

✓6ᵗʰ **H35.02 Exudative retinopathy**
Coats retinopathy

H35.021 Exudative retinopathy, right eye
H35.022 Exudative retinopathy, left eye
H35.023 Exudative retinopathy, bilateral
H35.029 Exudative retinopathy, unspecified eye ▽

✓6ᵗʰ **H35.03 Hypertensive retinopathy**

H35.031 Hypertensive retinopathy, right eye
H35.032 Hypertensive retinopathy, left eye
H35.033 Hypertensive retinopathy, bilateral
H35.039 Hypertensive retinopathy, unspecified eye ▽

✓6ᵗʰ **H35.04 Retinal micro-aneurysms, unspecified**

H35.041 Retinal micro-aneurysms, unspecified, right eye ▽
H35.042 Retinal micro-aneurysms, unspecified, left eye ▽
H35.043 Retinal micro-aneurysms, unspecified, bilateral ▽
H35.049 Retinal micro-aneurysms, unspecified, unspecified eye ▽

✓6ᵗʰ **H35.05 Retinal neovascularization, unspecified**

H35.051 Retinal neovascularization, unspecified, right eye ▽
H35.052 Retinal neovascularization, unspecified, left eye ▽
H35.053 Retinal neovascularization, unspecified, bilateral ▽
H35.059 Retinal neovascularization, unspecified, unspecified eye ▽

✓6ᵗʰ **H35.06 Retinal vasculitis**
Eales disease
Retinal perivasculitis
DEF: Sight-threatening intraocular inflammation of the retinal blood vessels; causes minimal, partial, or even complete blindness.

H35.061 Retinal vasculitis, right eye
H35.062 Retinal vasculitis, left eye
H35.063 Retinal vasculitis, bilateral
H35.069 Retinal vasculitis, unspecified eye ▽

✓6ᵗʰ **H35.07 Retinal telangiectasis**

H35.071 Retinal telangiectasis, right eye
H35.072 Retinal telangiectasis, left eye
H35.073 Retinal telangiectasis, bilateral
H35.079 Retinal telangiectasis, unspecified eye ▽

H35.09 Other intraretinal microvascular abnormalities
Retinal varices

✓5ᵗʰ **H35.1 Retinopathy of prematurity**

✓6ᵗʰ **H35.10 Retinopathy of prematurity, unspecified**
Retinopathy of prematurity NOS

H35.101 Retinopathy of prematurity, unspecified, right eye ▽
H35.102 Retinopathy of prematurity, unspecified, left eye ▽
H35.103 Retinopathy of prematurity, unspecified, bilateral ▽
H35.109 Retinopathy of prematurity, unspecified, unspecified eye ▽

EXCLUDES 1 Not coded here   *EXCLUDES 2* Not included here   **N** Newborn Age: 0   **P** Pediatric Age: 0-17   **M** Maternity Age: 12-55   **A** Adult Age: 15-124

590   ICD-10-CM 2018

✓6ᵗʰ **H35.11 Retinopathy of prematurity, stage 0**
    H35.111 Retinopathy of prematurity, stage 0, right eye
    H35.112 Retinopathy of prematurity, stage 0, left eye
    H35.113 Retinopathy of prematurity, stage 0, bilateral
    H35.119 Retinopathy of prematurity, stage 0, unspecified eye ▽

✓6ᵗʰ **H35.12 Retinopathy of prematurity, stage 1**
    H35.121 Retinopathy of prematurity, stage 1, right eye
    H35.122 Retinopathy of prematurity, stage 1, left eye
    H35.123 Retinopathy of prematurity, stage 1, bilateral
    H35.129 Retinopathy of prematurity, stage 1, unspecified eye ▽

✓6ᵗʰ **H35.13 Retinopathy of prematurity, stage 2**
    H35.131 Retinopathy of prematurity, stage 2, right eye
    H35.132 Retinopathy of prematurity, stage 2, left eye
    H35.133 Retinopathy of prematurity, stage 2, bilateral
    H35.139 Retinopathy of prematurity, stage 2, unspecified eye ▽

✓6ᵗʰ **H35.14 Retinopathy of prematurity, stage 3**
    H35.141 Retinopathy of prematurity, stage 3, right eye
    H35.142 Retinopathy of prematurity, stage 3, left eye
    H35.143 Retinopathy of prematurity, stage 3, bilateral
    H35.149 Retinopathy of prematurity, stage 3, unspecified eye ▽

✓6ᵗʰ **H35.15 Retinopathy of prematurity, stage 4**
    H35.151 Retinopathy of prematurity, stage 4, right eye
    H35.152 Retinopathy of prematurity, stage 4, left eye
    H35.153 Retinopathy of prematurity, stage 4, bilateral
    H35.159 Retinopathy of prematurity, stage 4, unspecified eye ▽

✓6ᵗʰ **H35.16 Retinopathy of prematurity, stage 5**
    H35.161 Retinopathy of prematurity, stage 5, right eye
    H35.162 Retinopathy of prematurity, stage 5, left eye
    H35.163 Retinopathy of prematurity, stage 5, bilateral
    H35.169 Retinopathy of prematurity, stage 5, unspecified eye ▽

✓6ᵗʰ **H35.17 Retrolental fibroplasia**
    H35.171 Retrolental fibroplasia, right eye
    H35.172 Retrolental fibroplasia, left eye
    H35.173 Retrolental fibroplasia, bilateral
    H35.179 Retrolental fibroplasia, unspecified eye ▽

✓5ᵗʰ **H35.2 Other non-diabetic proliferative retinopathy**
    Proliferative vitreo-retinopathy
    EXCLUDES 1   *proliferative vitreo-retinopathy with retinal detachment (H33.4-)*
    H35.20 Other non-diabetic proliferative retinopathy, unspecified eye ▽
    H35.21 Other non-diabetic proliferative retinopathy, right eye
    H35.22 Other non-diabetic proliferative retinopathy, left eye
    H35.23 Other non-diabetic proliferative retinopathy, bilateral

✓5ᵗʰ **H35.3 Degeneration of macula and posterior pole**
    H35.30 Unspecified macular degeneration 🅰▽
    Age-related macular degeneration

✓6ᵗʰ **H35.31 Nonexudative age-related macular degeneration**
    Atrophic age-related macular degeneration
    Dry age-related macular degeneration
    AHA: 2016, 4Q, 21

> One of the following 7th characters is to be assigned to codes in subcategory H35.31 to designate the stage of the disease:
> 0   stage unspecified
> 1   early dry stage
> 2   intermediate dry stage
> 3   advanced atrophic without subfoveal involvement
>   advanced dry stage
> 4   advanced atrophic with subfoveal involvement

    ✓7ᵗʰ **H35.311 Nonexudative age-related macular degeneration, right eye** 🅰
    ✓7ᵗʰ **H35.312 Nonexudative age-related macular degeneration, left eye** 🅰
    ✓7ᵗʰ **H35.313 Nonexudative age-related macular degeneration, bilateral** 🅰
    ✓7ᵗʰ **H35.319 Nonexudative age-related macular degeneration, unspecified eye** 🅰▽

✓6ᵗʰ **H35.32 Exudative age-related macular degeneration**
    Wet age-related macular degeneration

> One of the following 7th characters is to be assigned to codes in subcategory H35.32 to designate the stage of the disease:
> 0   stage unspecified
> 1   with active choroidal neovascularization
> 2   with inactive choroidal neovascularization
>   with involuted or regressed neovascularization
> 3   with inactive scar

    ✓7ᵗʰ **H35.321 Exudative age-related macular degeneration, right eye** HCC 🅰
    ✓7ᵗʰ **H35.322 Exudative age-related macular degeneration, left eye** HCC 🅰
    ✓7ᵗʰ **H35.323 Exudative age-related macular degeneration, bilateral** HCC 🅰
    ✓7ᵗʰ **H35.329 Exudative age-related macular degeneration, unspecified eye** HCC 🅰▽

    H35.33 Angioid streaks of macula
    DEF: Degeneration of choroid; characterized by broad, irregular, dark brown streaks radiating from optic disc; occurs with pseudoxanthoma elasticum or Paget's disease.

✓6ᵗʰ **H35.34 Macular cyst, hole, or pseudohole**
    H35.341 Macular cyst, hole, or pseudohole, right eye
    H35.342 Macular cyst, hole, or pseudohole, left eye
    H35.343 Macular cyst, hole, or pseudohole, bilateral
    H35.349 Macular cyst, hole, or pseudohole, unspecified eye ▽

✓6ᵗʰ **H35.35 Cystoid macular degeneration**
    EXCLUDES 1   *cystoid macular edema following cataract surgery (H59.03-)*
    H35.351 Cystoid macular degeneration, right eye
    H35.352 Cystoid macular degeneration, left eye
    H35.353 Cystoid macular degeneration, bilateral
    H35.359 Cystoid macular degeneration, unspecified eye ▽

✓6ᵗʰ **H35.36 Drusen (degenerative) of macula**
    AHA: 2017, 1Q, 51; 2016, 4Q, 21
    H35.361 Drusen (degenerative) of macula, right eye
    H35.362 Drusen (degenerative) of macula, left eye
    H35.363 Drusen (degenerative) of macula, bilateral
    H35.369 Drusen (degenerative) of macula, unspecified eye ▽

✓6ᵗʰ **H35.37 Puckering of macula**
    H35.371 Puckering of macula, right eye
    H35.372 Puckering of macula, left eye
    H35.373 Puckering of macula, bilateral
    H35.379 Puckering of macula, unspecified eye ▽

☑ Additional Character Req   ✓7ᵗʰ Placeholder Alert   Manifestation   HCC CMS-HCC Condition   ▽ Unspecified Code   ▶◀ Revised Text   ● New Code   ▲ Revised Code Title

Chapter 7. Diseases of the Eye and Adnexa

H35.38–H40.009

√6ᵗʰ **H35.38 Toxic maculopathy**
Code first poisoning due to drug or toxin, if applicable (T36-T65 with fifth or sixth character 1-4 or 6)
Use additional code for adverse effect, if applicable, to identify drug (T36-T50 with fifth or sixth character 5)

    H35.381   **Toxic maculopathy, right eye**
    H35.382   **Toxic maculopathy, left eye**
    H35.383   **Toxic maculopathy, bilateral**
    H35.389   **Toxic maculopathy, unspecified eye** ▽

√5ᵗʰ **H35.4 Peripheral retinal degeneration**
   EXCLUDES 1   hereditary retinal degeneration (dystrophy) (H35.5-)
          peripheral retinal degeneration with retinal break (H33.3-)

    H35.40   Unspecified peripheral retinal degeneration ▽

√6ᵗʰ **H35.41 Lattice degeneration of retina**
Palisade degeneration of retina
DEF: Degeneration of retina; often bilateral, usually benign; characterized by lines intersecting at irregular intervals in peripheral retina; retinal thinning and retinal holes may occur.

    H35.411   **Lattice degeneration of retina, right eye**
    H35.412   **Lattice degeneration of retina, left eye**
    H35.413   **Lattice degeneration of retina, bilateral**
    H35.419   **Lattice degeneration of retina, unspecified eye** ▽

√6ᵗʰ **H35.42 Microcystoid degeneration of retina**
    H35.421   **Microcystoid degeneration of retina, right eye**
    H35.422   **Microcystoid degeneration of retina, left eye**
    H35.423   **Microcystoid degeneration of retina, bilateral**
    H35.429   **Microcystoid degeneration of retina, unspecified eye** ▽

√6ᵗʰ **H35.43 Paving stone degeneration of retina**
    H35.431   **Paving stone degeneration of retina, right eye**
    H35.432   **Paving stone degeneration of retina, left eye**
    H35.433   **Paving stone degeneration of retina, bilateral**
    H35.439   **Paving stone degeneration of retina, unspecified eye** ▽

√6ᵗʰ **H35.44 Age-related reticular degeneration of retina**
    H35.441   **Age-related reticular degeneration of retina, right eye** 🅐
    H35.442   **Age-related reticular degeneration of retina, left eye** 🅐
    H35.443   **Age-related reticular degeneration of retina, bilateral** 🅐
    H35.449   **Age-related reticular degeneration of retina, unspecified eye** 🅐▽

√6ᵗʰ **H35.45 Secondary pigmentary degeneration**
    H35.451   **Secondary pigmentary degeneration, right eye**
    H35.452   **Secondary pigmentary degeneration, left eye**
    H35.453   **Secondary pigmentary degeneration, bilateral**
    H35.459   **Secondary pigmentary degeneration, unspecified eye** ▽

√6ᵗʰ **H35.46 Secondary vitreoretinal degeneration**
    H35.461   **Secondary vitreoretinal degeneration, right eye**
    H35.462   **Secondary vitreoretinal degeneration, left eye**
    H35.463   **Secondary vitreoretinal degeneration, bilateral**
    H35.469   **Secondary vitreoretinal degeneration, unspecified eye** ▽

√5ᵗʰ **H35.5 Hereditary retinal dystrophy**
   EXCLUDES 1   dystrophies primarily involving Bruch's membrane (H31.1-)

    H35.50   Unspecified hereditary retinal dystrophy ▽
    H35.51   Vitreoretinal dystrophy

H35.52 Pigmentary retinal dystrophy
Albipunctate retinal dystrophy
Retinitis pigmentosa
Tapetoretinal dystrophy

H35.53 Other dystrophies primarily involving the sensory retina
Stargardt's disease

H35.54 Dystrophies primarily involving the retinal pigment epithelium
Vitelliform retinal dystrophy

√5ᵗʰ **H35.6 Retinal hemorrhage**
    H35.60   Retinal hemorrhage, unspecified eye ▽
    H35.61   Retinal hemorrhage, right eye
    H35.62   Retinal hemorrhage, left eye
    H35.63   Retinal hemorrhage, bilateral

√5ᵗʰ **H35.7 Separation of retinal layers**
   EXCLUDES 1   retinal detachment (serous) (H33.2-)
          rhegmatogenous retinal detachment (H33.0-)

    H35.70   Unspecified separation of retinal layers ▽

√6ᵗʰ **H35.71 Central serous chorioretinopathy**
    H35.711   **Central serous chorioretinopathy, right eye**
    H35.712   **Central serous chorioretinopathy, left eye**
    H35.713   **Central serous chorioretinopathy, bilateral**
    H35.719   **Central serous chorioretinopathy, unspecified eye** ▽

√6ᵗʰ **H35.72 Serous detachment of retinal pigment epithelium**
    H35.721   **Serous detachment of retinal pigment epithelium, right eye**
    H35.722   **Serous detachment of retinal pigment epithelium, left eye**
    H35.723   **Serous detachment of retinal pigment epithelium, bilateral**
    H35.729   **Serous detachment of retinal pigment epithelium, unspecified eye** ▽

√6ᵗʰ **H35.73 Hemorrhagic detachment of retinal pigment epithelium**
    H35.731   **Hemorrhagic detachment of retinal pigment epithelium, right eye**
    H35.732   **Hemorrhagic detachment of retinal pigment epithelium, left eye**
    H35.733   **Hemorrhagic detachment of retinal pigment epithelium, bilateral**
    H35.739   **Hemorrhagic detachment of retinal pigment epithelium, unspecified eye** ▽

√5ᵗʰ **H35.8 Other specified retinal disorders**
   EXCLUDES 2   retinal hemorrhage (H35.6-)

    H35.81   Retinal edema
          Retinal cotton wool spots
    H35.82   Retinal ischemia
    H35.89   Other specified retinal disorders

H35.9 Unspecified retinal disorder ▽

H36 *Retinal disorders in diseases classified elsewhere*
Code first underlying disease, such as:
   lipid storage disorders (E75.-)
   sickle-cell disorders (D57.-)
   EXCLUDES 1   arteriosclerotic retinopathy (H35.0-)
          diabetic retinopathy (E08.3-, E09.3-, E10.3-, E11.3-, E13.3-)

Glaucoma (H40-H42)

√4ᵗʰ **H40 Glaucoma**
   EXCLUDES 1   absolute glaucoma (H44.51-)
          congenital glaucoma (Q15.0)
          traumatic glaucoma due to birth injury (P15.3)

√5ᵗʰ **H40.0 Glaucoma suspect**
  √6ᵗʰ **H40.00   Preglaucoma, unspecified**
      H40.001   **Preglaucoma, unspecified, right eye** ▽
      H40.002   **Preglaucoma, unspecified, left eye** ▽
      H40.003   **Preglaucoma, unspecified, bilateral** ▽
      H40.009   **Preglaucoma, unspecified, unspecified eye** ▽

EXCLUDES 1 Not coded here   *EXCLUDES 2* Not included here   🅝 Newborn Age: 0   🅟 Pediatric Age: 0-17   🅜 Maternity Age: 12-55   🅐 Adult Age: 15-124

592   ICD-10-CM 2018

✓6ᵗʰ **H40.01** **Open angle with borderline findings, low risk**
Open angle, low risk

    H40.011 Open angle with borderline findings, low risk, right eye

    H40.012 Open angle with borderline findings, low risk, left eye

    H40.013 Open angle with borderline findings, low risk, bilateral

    H40.019 Open angle with borderline findings, low risk, unspecified eye ▽

✓6ᵗʰ **H40.02** **Open angle with borderline findings, high risk**
Open angle, high risk

    H40.021 Open angle with borderline findings, high risk, right eye

    H40.022 Open angle with borderline findings, high risk, left eye

    H40.023 Open angle with borderline findings, high risk, bilateral

    H40.029 Open angle with borderline findings, high risk, unspecified eye ▽

✓6ᵗʰ **H40.03** **Anatomical narrow angle**
Primary angle closure suspect

    H40.031 Anatomical narrow angle, right eye

    H40.032 Anatomical narrow angle, left eye

    H40.033 Anatomical narrow angle, bilateral

    H40.039 Anatomical narrow angle, unspecified eye ▽

✓6ᵗʰ **H40.04** **Steroid responder**

    H40.041 Steroid responder, right eye

    H40.042 Steroid responder, left eye

    H40.043 Steroid responder, bilateral

    H40.049 Steroid responder, unspecified eye ▽

✓6ᵗʰ **H40.05** **Ocular hypertension**

    H40.051 Ocular hypertension, right eye

    H40.052 Ocular hypertension, left eye

    H40.053 Ocular hypertension, bilateral

    H40.059 Ocular hypertension, unspecified eye ▽

✓6ᵗʰ **H40.06** **Primary angle closure without glaucoma damage**

    H40.061 Primary angle closure without glaucoma damage, right eye

    H40.062 Primary angle closure without glaucoma damage, left eye

    H40.063 Primary angle closure without glaucoma damage, bilateral

    H40.069 Primary angle closure without glaucoma damage, unspecified eye ▽

✓5ᵗʰ **H40.1** **Open-angle glaucoma**

> One of the following 7th characters is to be assigned to each code in subcategories H40.10, H40.11-, H40.12-, H40.13-, and H40.14- to designate the stage of glaucoma.
> Ø   stage unspecified
> 1   mild stage
> 2   moderate stage
> 3   severe stage
> 4   indeterminate stage

✓ₓ7ᵗʰ **H40.10** Unspecified open-angle glaucoma ▽

✓6ᵗʰ **H40.11** **Primary open-angle glaucoma**
Chronic simple glaucoma

    ✓7ᵗʰ **H40.111** Primary open-angle glaucoma, right eye

    ✓7ᵗʰ **H40.112** Primary open-angle glaucoma, left eye

    ✓7ᵗʰ **H40.113** Primary open-angle glaucoma, bilateral

    ✓7ᵗʰ **H40.119** Primary open-angle glaucoma, unspecified eye ▽

✓6ᵗʰ **H40.12** **Low-tension glaucoma**

    ✓7ᵗʰ **H40.121** Low-tension glaucoma, right eye

    ✓7ᵗʰ **H40.122** Low-tension glaucoma, left eye

    ✓7ᵗʰ **H40.123** Low-tension glaucoma, bilateral

    ✓7ᵗʰ **H40.129** Low-tension glaucoma, unspecified eye ▽

✓6ᵗʰ **H40.13** **Pigmentary glaucoma**

    ✓7ᵗʰ **H40.131** Pigmentary glaucoma, right eye

    ✓7ᵗʰ **H40.132** Pigmentary glaucoma, left eye

    ✓7ᵗʰ **H40.133** Pigmentary glaucoma, bilateral

    ✓7ᵗʰ **H40.139** Pigmentary glaucoma, unspecified eye ▽

Open Angle/Angle Closure Glaucoma

✓6ᵗʰ **H40.14** **Capsular glaucoma with pseudoexfoliation of lens**

    ✓7ᵗʰ **H40.141** Capsular glaucoma with pseudoexfoliation of lens, right eye

    ✓7ᵗʰ **H40.142** Capsular glaucoma with pseudoexfoliation of lens, left eye

    ✓7ᵗʰ **H40.143** Capsular glaucoma with pseudoexfoliation of lens, bilateral

    ✓7ᵗʰ **H40.149** Capsular glaucoma with pseudoexfoliation of lens, unspecified eye ▽

✓6ᵗʰ **H40.15** **Residual stage of open-angle glaucoma**

    H40.151 Residual stage of open-angle glaucoma, right eye

    H40.152 Residual stage of open-angle glaucoma, left eye

    H40.153 Residual stage of open-angle glaucoma, bilateral

    H40.159 Residual stage of open-angle glaucoma, unspecified eye ▽

✓5ᵗʰ **H40.2** **Primary angle-closure glaucoma**

> **EXCLUDES 1**   *aqueous misdirection (H40.83-)*
> *malignant glaucoma (H40.83-)*

> One of the following 7th characters is to be assigned to each code in subcategories H40.20 and H40.22- to designate the stage of glaucoma.
> Ø   stage unspecified
> 1   mild stage
> 2   moderate stage
> 3   severe stage
> 4   indeterminate stage

✓ₓ7ᵗʰ **H40.20** Unspecified primary angle-closure glaucoma ▽

✓6ᵗʰ **H40.21** **Acute angle-closure glaucoma**
Acute angle-closure glaucoma attack
Acute angle-closure glaucoma crisis

    H40.211 Acute angle-closure glaucoma, right eye

    H40.212 Acute angle-closure glaucoma, left eye

    H40.213 Acute angle-closure glaucoma, bilateral

    H40.219 Acute angle-closure glaucoma, unspecified eye ▽

✓6ᵗʰ **H40.22** **Chronic angle-closure glaucoma**
Chronic primary angle-closure glaucoma

    ✓7ᵗʰ **H40.221** Chronic angle-closure glaucoma, right eye

    ✓7ᵗʰ **H40.222** Chronic angle-closure glaucoma, left eye

    ✓7ᵗʰ **H40.223** Chronic angle-closure glaucoma, bilateral

    ✓7ᵗʰ **H40.229** Chronic angle-closure glaucoma, unspecified eye ▽

✓6ᵗʰ **H40.23** **Intermittent angle-closure glaucoma**

    H40.231 Intermittent angle-closure glaucoma, right eye

    H40.232 Intermittent angle-closure glaucoma, left eye

    H40.233 Intermittent angle-closure glaucoma, bilateral

    H40.239 Intermittent angle-closure glaucoma, unspecified eye ▽

✓6ᵗʰ **H40.24** **Residual stage of angle-closure glaucoma**

    H40.241 Residual stage of angle-closure glaucoma, right eye

    H40.242 Residual stage of angle-closure glaucoma, left eye

✓ Additional Character Req   ✓ₓ7ᵗʰ Placeholder Alert   Manifestation   HCC CMS-HCC Condition   ▽ Unspecified Code   ►◄ Revised Text   ● New Code   ▲ Revised Code Title

ICD-10-CM 2018   593

H40.243   **Residual stage of angle-closure glaucoma, bilateral**

H40.249   **Residual stage of angle-closure glaucoma, unspecified eye** ▽

√5ᵗʰ **H40.3**   **Glaucoma secondary to eye trauma**
Code also underlying condition

> One of the following 7th characters is to be assigned to each code in subcategory H40.3- to designate the stage of glaucoma.
> Ø   stage unspecified
> 1   mild stage
> 2   moderate stage
> 3   severe stage
> 4   indeterminate stage

√x7ᵗʰ **H40.30**   **Glaucoma secondary to eye trauma, unspecified eye** ▽

√x7ᵗʰ **H40.31**   **Glaucoma secondary to eye trauma, right eye**

√x7ᵗʰ **H40.32**   **Glaucoma secondary to eye trauma, left eye**

√x7ᵗʰ **H40.33**   **Glaucoma secondary to eye trauma, bilateral**

√5ᵗʰ **H40.4**   **Glaucoma secondary to eye inflammation**
Code also underlying condition

> One of the following 7th characters is to be assigned to each code in subcategory H40.4- to designate the stage of glaucoma.
> Ø   stage unspecified
> 1   mild stage
> 2   moderate stage
> 3   severe stage
> 4   indeterminate stage

√x7ᵗʰ **H40.40**   **Glaucoma secondary to eye inflammation, unspecified eye** ▽

√x7ᵗʰ **H40.41**   **Glaucoma secondary to eye inflammation, right eye**

√x7ᵗʰ **H40.42**   **Glaucoma secondary to eye inflammation, left eye**

√x7ᵗʰ **H40.43**   **Glaucoma secondary to eye inflammation, bilateral**

√5ᵗʰ **H40.5**   **Glaucoma secondary to other eye disorders**
Code also underlying eye disorder

> One of the following 7th characters is to be assigned to each code in subcategory H40.5- to designate the stage of glaucoma.
> Ø   stage unspecified
> 1   mild stage
> 2   moderate stage
> 3   severe stage
> 4   indeterminate stage

√x7ᵗʰ **H40.50**   **Glaucoma secondary to other eye disorders, unspecified eye** ▽

√x7ᵗʰ **H40.51**   **Glaucoma secondary to other eye disorders, right eye**

√x7ᵗʰ **H40.52**   **Glaucoma secondary to other eye disorders, left eye**

√x7ᵗʰ **H40.53**   **Glaucoma secondary to other eye disorders, bilateral**

√5ᵗʰ **H40.6**   **Glaucoma secondary to drugs**
Use additional code for adverse effect, if applicable, to identify drug (T36-T50 with fifth or sixth character 5)

> One of the following 7th characters is to be assigned to each code in subcategory H40.6- to designate the stage of glaucoma.
> Ø   stage unspecified
> 1   mild stage
> 2   moderate stage
> 3   severe stage
> 4   indeterminate stage

√x7ᵗʰ **H40.60**   **Glaucoma secondary to drugs, unspecified eye** ▽

√x7ᵗʰ **H40.61**   **Glaucoma secondary to drugs, right eye**

√x7ᵗʰ **H40.62**   **Glaucoma secondary to drugs, left eye**

√x7ᵗʰ **H40.63**   **Glaucoma secondary to drugs, bilateral**

√5ᵗʰ **H40.8**   **Other glaucoma**

√6ᵗʰ **H40.81**   **Glaucoma with increased episcleral venous pressure**

H40.811   **Glaucoma with increased episcleral venous pressure, right eye**

H40.812   **Glaucoma with increased episcleral venous pressure, left eye**

H40.813   **Glaucoma with increased episcleral venous pressure, bilateral**

H40.819   **Glaucoma with increased episcleral venous pressure, unspecified eye** ▽

√6ᵗʰ **H40.82**   **Hypersecretion glaucoma**

H40.821   **Hypersecretion glaucoma, right eye**

H40.822   **Hypersecretion glaucoma, left eye**

H40.823   **Hypersecretion glaucoma, bilateral**

H40.829   **Hypersecretion glaucoma, unspecified eye** ▽

√6ᵗʰ **H40.83**   **Aqueous misdirection**
Malignant glaucoma

H40.831   **Aqueous misdirection, right eye**

H40.832   **Aqueous misdirection, left eye**

H40.833   **Aqueous misdirection, bilateral**

H40.839   **Aqueous misdirection, unspecified eye** ▽

H40.89   **Other specified glaucoma**

H40.9   **Unspecified glaucoma** ▽

H42   *Glaucoma in diseases classified elsewhere*
Code first underlying condition, such as:
    amyloidosis (E85.-)
    aniridia (Q13.1)
    ▶glaucoma (in) diabetes mellitus (E08.39, E09.39, E10.39, E11.39, E13.39)◀
    Lowe's syndrome (E72.03)
    Reiger's anomaly (Q13.81)
    specified metabolic disorder (E70-E88)

> EXCLUDES 1   *glaucoma (in) onchocerciasis (B73.02)*
>   *glaucoma (in) syphilis (A52.71)*
>   *glaucoma (in) tuberculous (A18.59)*
> EXCLUDES 2   *glaucoma (in) diabetes mellitus (E08.39, E09.39, E10.39, E11.39, E13.39)*

Disorders of vitreous body and globe (H43-H44)

√4ᵗʰ **H43**   **Disorders of vitreous body**

√5ᵗʰ **H43.0**   **Vitreous prolapse**

> EXCLUDES 1   *traumatic vitreous prolapse (S05.2-)*
>   *vitreous syndrome following cataract surgery (H59.0-)*

H43.00   **Vitreous prolapse, unspecified eye** ▽

H43.01   **Vitreous prolapse, right eye**

H43.02   **Vitreous prolapse, left eye**

H43.03   **Vitreous prolapse, bilateral**

√5ᵗʰ **H43.1**   **Vitreous hemorrhage**

H43.10   **Vitreous hemorrhage, unspecified eye**   HCC ▽

H43.11   **Vitreous hemorrhage, right eye**   HCC

H43.12   **Vitreous hemorrhage, left eye**   HCC

H43.13   **Vitreous hemorrhage, bilateral**   HCC

√5ᵗʰ **H43.2**   **Crystalline deposits in vitreous body**

H43.20   **Crystalline deposits in vitreous body, unspecified eye** ▽

H43.21   **Crystalline deposits in vitreous body, right eye**

H43.22   **Crystalline deposits in vitreous body, left eye**

H43.23   **Crystalline deposits in vitreous body, bilateral**

√5ᵗʰ **H43.3**   **Other vitreous opacities**

√6ᵗʰ **H43.31**   **Vitreous membranes and strands**

H43.311   **Vitreous membranes and strands, right eye**

H43.312   **Vitreous membranes and strands, left eye**

H43.313   **Vitreous membranes and strands, bilateral**

H43.319   **Vitreous membranes and strands, unspecified eye** ▽

√6ᵗʰ **H43.39**   **Other vitreous opacities**
Vitreous floaters

H43.391   **Other vitreous opacities, right eye**

H43.392   **Other vitreous opacities, left eye**

H43.393   **Other vitreous opacities, bilateral**

H43.399   **Other vitreous opacities, unspecified eye** ▽

√5ᵗʰ **H43.8**   **Other disorders of vitreous body**

> EXCLUDES 1   *proliferative vitreo-retinopathy with retinal detachment (H33.4-)*
> EXCLUDES 2   *vitreous abscess (H44.02-)*

√6ᵗʰ **H43.81**   **Vitreous degeneration**
Vitreous detachment

H43.811   **Vitreous degeneration, right eye**

EXCLUDES 1 Not coded here   EXCLUDES 2 Not included here   **N** Newborn Age: 0   **P** Pediatric Age: 0-17   **M** Maternity Age: 12-55   **A** Adult Age: 15-124

594   ICD-10-CM 2018

H43.812 **Vitreous degeneration, left eye**
H43.813 **Vitreous degeneration, bilateral**
H43.819 **Vitreous degeneration, unspecified eye** ▽

✓6ᵗʰ H43.82 **Vitreomacular adhesion**
Vitreomacular traction
H43.821 **Vitreomacular adhesion, right eye** Ⓐ
H43.822 **Vitreomacular adhesion, left eye** Ⓐ
H43.823 **Vitreomacular adhesion, bilateral** Ⓐ
H43.829 **Vitreomacular adhesion, unspecified** Ⓐ▽
eye

H43.89 **Other disorders of vitreous body**
H43.9 **Unspecified disorder of vitreous body** ▽

✓4ᵗʰ **H44 Disorders of globe**
INCLUDES disorders affecting multiple structures of eye

✓5ᵗʰ **H44.0 Purulent endophthalmitis**
Use additional code to identify organism
EXCLUDES 1 *bleb associated endophthalmitis (H59.4-)*

✓6ᵗʰ H44.00 **Unspecified purulent endophthalmitis**
H44.001 **Unspecified purulent endophthalmitis,** ▽
right eye
H44.002 **Unspecified purulent endophthalmitis,** ▽
left eye
H44.003 **Unspecified purulent endophthalmitis,** ▽
bilateral
H44.009 **Unspecified purulent endophthalmitis,** ▽
unspecified eye

✓6ᵗʰ H44.01 **Panophthalmitis (acute)**
H44.011 **Panophthalmitis (acute), right eye**
H44.012 **Panophthalmitis (acute), left eye**
H44.013 **Panophthalmitis (acute), bilateral**
H44.019 **Panophthalmitis (acute), unspecified** ▽
eye

✓6ᵗʰ H44.02 **Vitreous abscess (chronic)**
H44.021 **Vitreous abscess (chronic), right eye**
H44.022 **Vitreous abscess (chronic), left eye**
H44.023 **Vitreous abscess (chronic), bilateral**
H44.029 **Vitreous abscess (chronic), unspecified** ▽
eye

✓5ᵗʰ **H44.1 Other endophthalmitis**
EXCLUDES 1 *bleb associated endophthalmitis (H59.4-)*
EXCLUDES 2 *ophthalmia nodosa (H16.2-)*

✓6ᵗʰ H44.11 **Panuveitis**
DEF: Inflammation of all layers of uvea of eye, including
choroid, iris, and ciliary body; also typically involves lens,
retina, optic nerve, and vitreous; causes reduced vision
or blindness.
H44.111 **Panuveitis, right eye**
H44.112 **Panuveitis, left eye**
H44.113 **Panuveitis, bilateral**
H44.119 **Panuveitis, unspecified eye** ▽

✓6ᵗʰ H44.12 **Parasitic endophthalmitis, unspecified**
H44.121 **Parasitic endophthalmitis, unspecified,** ▽
right eye
H44.122 **Parasitic endophthalmitis, unspecified,** ▽
left eye
H44.123 **Parasitic endophthalmitis, unspecified,** ▽
bilateral
H44.129 **Parasitic endophthalmitis, unspecified,** ▽
unspecified eye

✓6ᵗʰ H44.13 **Sympathetic uveitis**
H44.131 **Sympathetic uveitis, right eye**
H44.132 **Sympathetic uveitis, left eye**
H44.133 **Sympathetic uveitis, bilateral**
H44.139 **Sympathetic uveitis, unspecified eye** ▽

H44.19 **Other endophthalmitis**

✓5ᵗʰ **H44.2 Degenerative myopia**
Malignant myopia
H44.20 **Degenerative myopia, unspecified eye** ▽
H44.21 **Degenerative myopia, right eye**
H44.22 **Degenerative myopia, left eye**
H44.23 **Degenerative myopia, bilateral**

● ✓6ᵗʰ H44.2A **Degenerative myopia with choroidal**
neovascularization
Use additional code for any associated choroid
disorders (H31.-)
● H44.2A1 **Degenerative myopia with choroidal**
neovascularization, right eye
● H44.2A2 **Degenerative myopia with choroidal**
neovascularization, left eye
● H44.2A3 **Degenerative myopia with choroidal**
neovascularization, bilateral eye
● H44.2A9 **Degenerative myopia with choroidal** ▽
neovascularization, unspecified eye

● ✓6ᵗʰ H44.2B **Degenerative myopia with macular hole**
● H44.2B1 **Degenerative myopia with macular hole,**
right eye
● H44.2B2 **Degenerative myopia with macular hole,**
left eye
● H44.2B3 **Degenerative myopia with macular hole,**
bilateral eye
● H44.2B9 **Degenerative myopia with macular** ▽
hole, unspecified eye

● ✓6ᵗʰ H44.2C **Degenerative myopia with retinal detachment**
Use additional code to identify the retinal detachment
(H33.-)
● H44.2C1 **Degenerative myopia with retinal**
detachment, right eye
● H44.2C2 **Degenerative myopia with retinal**
detachment, left eye
● H44.2C3 **Degenerative myopia with retinal**
detachment, bilateral eye
● H44.2C9 **Degenerative myopia with retinal** ▽
detachment, unspecified eye

● ✓6ᵗʰ H44.2D **Degenerative myopia with foveoschisis**
● H44.2D1 **Degenerative myopia with foveoschisis,**
right eye
● H44.2D2 **Degenerative myopia with foveoschisis,**
left eye
● H44.2D3 **Degenerative myopia with foveoschisis,**
bilateral eye
● H44.2D9 **Degenerative myopia with** ▽
foveoschisis, unspecified eye

● ✓6ᵗʰ H44.2E **Degenerative myopia with other maculopathy**
● H44.2E1 **Degenerative myopia with other**
maculopathy, right eye
● H44.2E2 **Degenerative myopia with other**
maculopathy, left eye
● H44.2E3 **Degenerative myopia with other**
maculopathy, bilateral eye
● H44.2E9 **Degenerative myopia with other** ▽
maculopathy, unspecified eye

✓5ᵗʰ **H44.3 Other and unspecified degenerative disorders of globe** ▽
H44.30 **Unspecified degenerative disorder of globe** ▽

✓6ᵗʰ H44.31 **Chalcosis**
H44.311 **Chalcosis, right eye**
H44.312 **Chalcosis, left eye**
H44.313 **Chalcosis, bilateral**
H44.319 **Chalcosis, unspecified eye** ▽

✓6ᵗʰ H44.32 **Siderosis of eye**
DEF: Iron pigment deposits within tissue of eyeball;
caused by high iron content of blood; characterized by
cataract, rust-colored anterior subcapsular deposits, iris
heterochromia, pupillary mydriasis, and depressed
electroretinogram amplitudes.
H44.321 **Siderosis of eye, right eye**
H44.322 **Siderosis of eye, left eye**
H44.323 **Siderosis of eye, bilateral**
H44.329 **Siderosis of eye, unspecified eye** ▽

✓6ᵗʰ H44.39 **Other degenerative disorders of globe**
H44.391 **Other degenerative disorders of globe,**
right eye
H44.392 **Other degenerative disorders of globe,**
left eye
H44.393 **Other degenerative disorders of globe,**
bilateral
H44.399 **Other degenerative disorders of globe,** ▽
unspecified eye

✓ Additional Character Req   ✓x7ᵗʰ Placeholder Alert   Manifestation   HCC CMS-HCC Condition   ▽ Unspecified Code   ►◄ Revised Text   ● New Code   ▲ Revised Code Title

ICD-10-CM 2018   595

Chapter 7. Diseases of the Eye and Adnexa

H44.4–H44.709

√5th **H44.4** **Hypotony of eye**

    H44.40 Unspecified hypotony of eye ▽

√6th **H44.41** Flat anterior chamber hypotony of eye

        H44.411 Flat anterior chamber hypotony of right eye

        H44.412 Flat anterior chamber hypotony of left eye

        H44.413 Flat anterior chamber hypotony of eye, bilateral

        H44.419 Flat anterior chamber hypotony of unspecified eye ▽

√6th **H44.42** Hypotony of eye due to ocular fistula

        H44.421 Hypotony of right eye due to ocular fistula

        H44.422 Hypotony of left eye due to ocular fistula

        H44.423 Hypotony of eye due to ocular fistula, bilateral

        H44.429 Hypotony of unspecified eye due to ocular fistula ▽

√6th **H44.43** Hypotony of eye due to other ocular disorders

        H44.431 Hypotony of eye due to other ocular disorders, right eye

        H44.432 Hypotony of eye due to other ocular disorders, left eye

        H44.433 Hypotony of eye due to other ocular disorders, bilateral

        H44.439 Hypotony of eye due to other ocular disorders, unspecified eye ▽

√6th **H44.44** Primary hypotony of eye

        H44.441 Primary hypotony of right eye

        H44.442 Primary hypotony of left eye

        H44.443 Primary hypotony of eye, bilateral

        H44.449 Primary hypotony of unspecified eye ▽

√5th **H44.5** **Degenerated conditions of globe**

    H44.50 Unspecified degenerated conditions of globe ▽

√6th **H44.51** Absolute glaucoma

        H44.511 Absolute glaucoma, right eye

        H44.512 Absolute glaucoma, left eye

        H44.513 Absolute glaucoma, bilateral

        H44.519 Absolute glaucoma, unspecified eye ▽

√6th **H44.52** Atrophy of globe

        Phthisis bulbi

        H44.521 Atrophy of globe, right eye

        H44.522 Atrophy of globe, left eye

        H44.523 Atrophy of globe, bilateral

        H44.529 Atrophy of globe, unspecified eye ▽

√6th **H44.53** Leucocoria

        H44.531 Leucocoria, right eye

        H44.532 Leucocoria, left eye

        H44.533 Leucocoria, bilateral

        H44.539 Leucocoria, unspecified eye ▽

√5th **H44.6** **Retained (old) intraocular foreign body, magnetic**

    Use additional code to identify magnetic foreign body (Z18.11)

    EXCLUDES 1   current intraocular foreign body (S05.-)

    EXCLUDES 2   retained foreign body in eyelid (H02.81-)

              retained (old) foreign body following penetrating wound of orbit (H05.5-)

              retained (old) intraocular foreign body, nonmagnetic (H44.7-)

√6th **H44.60** Unspecified retained (old) intraocular foreign body, magnetic

        H44.601 Unspecified retained (old) intraocular foreign body, magnetic, right eye ▽

        H44.602 Unspecified retained (old) intraocular foreign body, magnetic, left eye ▽

        H44.603 Unspecified retained (old) intraocular foreign body, magnetic, bilateral ▽

        H44.609 Unspecified retained (old) intraocular foreign body, magnetic, unspecified eye ▽

√6th **H44.61** Retained (old) magnetic foreign body in anterior chamber

        H44.611 Retained (old) magnetic foreign body in anterior chamber, right eye

        H44.612 Retained (old) magnetic foreign body in anterior chamber, left eye

        H44.613 Retained (old) magnetic foreign body in anterior chamber, bilateral

        H44.619 Retained (old) magnetic foreign body in anterior chamber, unspecified eye ▽

√6th **H44.62** Retained (old) magnetic foreign body in iris or ciliary body

        H44.621 Retained (old) magnetic foreign body in iris or ciliary body, right eye

        H44.622 Retained (old) magnetic foreign body in iris or ciliary body, left eye

        H44.623 Retained (old) magnetic foreign body in iris or ciliary body, bilateral

        H44.629 Retained (old) magnetic foreign body in iris or ciliary body, unspecified eye ▽

√6th **H44.63** Retained (old) magnetic foreign body in lens

        H44.631 Retained (old) magnetic foreign body in lens, right eye

        H44.632 Retained (old) magnetic foreign body in lens, left eye

        H44.633 Retained (old) magnetic foreign body in lens, bilateral

        H44.639 Retained (old) magnetic foreign body in lens, unspecified eye ▽

√6th **H44.64** Retained (old) magnetic foreign body in posterior wall of globe

        H44.641 Retained (old) magnetic foreign body in posterior wall of globe, right eye

        H44.642 Retained (old) magnetic foreign body in posterior wall of globe, left eye

        H44.643 Retained (old) magnetic foreign body in posterior wall of globe, bilateral

        H44.649 Retained (old) magnetic foreign body in posterior wall of globe, unspecified eye ▽

√6th **H44.65** Retained (old) magnetic foreign body in vitreous body

        H44.651 Retained (old) magnetic foreign body in vitreous body, right eye

        H44.652 Retained (old) magnetic foreign body in vitreous body, left eye

        H44.653 Retained (old) magnetic foreign body in vitreous body, bilateral

        H44.659 Retained (old) magnetic foreign body in vitreous body, unspecified eye ▽

√6th **H44.69** Retained (old) intraocular foreign body, magnetic, in other or multiple sites

        H44.691 Retained (old) intraocular foreign body, magnetic, in other or multiple sites, right eye

        H44.692 Retained (old) intraocular foreign body, magnetic, in other or multiple sites, left eye

        H44.693 Retained (old) intraocular foreign body, magnetic, in other or multiple sites, bilateral

        H44.699 Retained (old) intraocular foreign body, magnetic, in other or multiple sites, unspecified eye ▽

√5th **H44.7** **Retained (old) intraocular foreign body, nonmagnetic**

    Use additional code to identify nonmagnetic foreign body (Z18.01-Z18.10, Z18.12, Z18.2-Z18.9)

    EXCLUDES 1   current intraocular foreign body (S05.-)

    EXCLUDES 2   retained foreign body in eyelid (H02.81-)

              retained (old) foreign body following penetrating wound of orbit (H05.5-)

              retained (old) intraocular foreign body, magnetic (H44.6-)

√6th **H44.70** Unspecified retained (old) intraocular foreign body, nonmagnetic

        H44.701 Unspecified retained (old) intraocular foreign body, nonmagnetic, right eye ▽

        H44.702 Unspecified retained (old) intraocular foreign body, nonmagnetic, left eye ▽

        H44.703 Unspecified retained (old) intraocular foreign body, nonmagnetic, bilateral ▽

        H44.709 Unspecified retained (old) intraocular foreign body, nonmagnetic, unspecified eye ▽

              Retained (old) intraocular foreign body NOS

EXCLUDES 1 Not coded here   EXCLUDES 2 Not included here   N Newborn Age: 0   P Pediatric Age: 0-17   M Maternity Age: 12-55   A Adult Age: 15-124

596   ICD-10-CM 2018

✓6ᵗʰ **H44.71** Retained (nonmagnetic) (old) foreign body in anterior chamber
     H44.711 Retained (nonmagnetic) (old) foreign body in anterior chamber, right eye
     H44.712 Retained (nonmagnetic) (old) foreign body in anterior chamber, left eye
     H44.713 Retained (nonmagnetic) (old) foreign body in anterior chamber, bilateral
     H44.719 Retained (nonmagnetic) (old) foreign body in anterior chamber, unspecified eye ▽

✓6ᵗʰ **H44.72** Retained (nonmagnetic) (old) foreign body in iris or ciliary body
     H44.721 Retained (nonmagnetic) (old) foreign body in iris or ciliary body, right eye
     H44.722 Retained (nonmagnetic) (old) foreign body in iris or ciliary body, left eye
     H44.723 Retained (nonmagnetic) (old) foreign body in iris or ciliary body, bilateral
     H44.729 Retained (nonmagnetic) (old) foreign body in iris or ciliary body, unspecified eye ▽

✓6ᵗʰ **H44.73** Retained (nonmagnetic) (old) foreign body in lens
     H44.731 Retained (nonmagnetic) (old) foreign body in lens, right eye
     H44.732 Retained (nonmagnetic) (old) foreign body in lens, left eye
     H44.733 Retained (nonmagnetic) (old) foreign body in lens, bilateral
     H44.739 Retained (nonmagnetic) (old) foreign body in lens, unspecified eye ▽

✓6ᵗʰ **H44.74** Retained (nonmagnetic) (old) foreign body in posterior wall of globe
     H44.741 Retained (nonmagnetic) (old) foreign body in posterior wall of globe, right eye
     H44.742 Retained (nonmagnetic) (old) foreign body in posterior wall of globe, left eye
     H44.743 Retained (nonmagnetic) (old) foreign body in posterior wall of globe, bilateral
     H44.749 Retained (nonmagnetic) (old) foreign body in posterior wall of globe, unspecified eye ▽

✓6ᵗʰ **H44.75** Retained (nonmagnetic) (old) foreign body in vitreous body
     H44.751 Retained (nonmagnetic) (old) foreign body in vitreous body, right eye
     H44.752 Retained (nonmagnetic) (old) foreign body in vitreous body, left eye
     H44.753 Retained (nonmagnetic) (old) foreign body in vitreous body, bilateral
     H44.759 Retained (nonmagnetic) (old) foreign body in vitreous body, unspecified eye ▽

✓6ᵗʰ **H44.79** Retained (old) intraocular foreign body, nonmagnetic, in other or multiple sites
     H44.791 Retained (old) intraocular foreign body, nonmagnetic, in other or multiple sites, right eye
     H44.792 Retained (old) intraocular foreign body, nonmagnetic, in other or multiple sites, left eye
     H44.793 Retained (old) intraocular foreign body, nonmagnetic, in other or multiple sites, bilateral
     H44.799 Retained (old) intraocular foreign body, nonmagnetic, in other or multiple sites, unspecified eye ▽

✓5ᵗʰ **H44.8** Other disorders of globe
  ✓6ᵗʰ **H44.81** Hemophthalmos
     DEF: Pool of blood within eyeball, not from current injury.
     H44.811 Hemophthalmos, right eye
     H44.812 Hemophthalmos, left eye
     H44.813 Hemophthalmos, bilateral
     H44.819 Hemophthalmos, unspecified eye ▽
  ✓6ᵗʰ **H44.82** Luxation of globe
     H44.821 Luxation of globe, right eye
     H44.822 Luxation of globe, left eye
     H44.823 Luxation of globe, bilateral
     H44.829 Luxation of globe, unspecified eye ▽

H44.89 Other disorders of globe
H44.9 Unspecified disorder of globe ▽

Disorders of optic nerve and visual pathways (H46-H47)

✓4ᵗʰ **H46 Optic neuritis**
     EXCLUDES 2   ischemic optic neuropathy (H47.01-)
               neuromyelitis optica [Devic] (G36.0)

  ✓5ᵗʰ **H46.0** Optic papillitis
     H46.00 Optic papillitis, unspecified eye ▽
     H46.01 Optic papillitis, right eye
     H46.02 Optic papillitis, left eye
     H46.03 Optic papillitis, bilateral

  ✓5ᵗʰ **H46.1** Retrobulbar neuritis
     Retrobulbar neuritis NOS
     EXCLUDES 1   syphilitic retrobulbar neuritis (A52.15)
     H46.10 Retrobulbar neuritis, unspecified eye ▽
     H46.11 Retrobulbar neuritis, right eye
     H46.12 Retrobulbar neuritis, left eye
     H46.13 Retrobulbar neuritis, bilateral

  H46.2 Nutritional optic neuropathy
  H46.3 Toxic optic neuropathy
     Code first (T51-T65) to identify cause
  H46.8 Other optic neuritis
  H46.9 Unspecified optic neuritis ▽

✓4ᵗʰ **H47 Other disorders of optic [2nd] nerve and visual pathways**
  ✓5ᵗʰ **H47.0** Disorders of optic nerve, not elsewhere classified
    ✓6ᵗʰ **H47.01** Ischemic optic neuropathy
       H47.011 Ischemic optic neuropathy, right eye
       H47.012 Ischemic optic neuropathy, left eye
       H47.013 Ischemic optic neuropathy, bilateral
       H47.019 Ischemic optic neuropathy, unspecified eye ▽
    ✓6ᵗʰ **H47.02** Hemorrhage in optic nerve sheath
       H47.021 Hemorrhage in optic nerve sheath, right eye
       H47.022 Hemorrhage in optic nerve sheath, left eye
       H47.023 Hemorrhage in optic nerve sheath, bilateral
       H47.029 Hemorrhage in optic nerve sheath, unspecified eye ▽
    ✓6ᵗʰ **H47.03** Optic nerve hypoplasia
       H47.031 Optic nerve hypoplasia, right eye
       H47.032 Optic nerve hypoplasia, left eye
       H47.033 Optic nerve hypoplasia, bilateral
       H47.039 Optic nerve hypoplasia, unspecified eye ▽
    ✓6ᵗʰ **H47.09** Other disorders of optic nerve, not elsewhere classified
       Compression of optic nerve
       H47.091 Other disorders of optic nerve, not elsewhere classified, right eye
       H47.092 Other disorders of optic nerve, not elsewhere classified, left eye
       H47.093 Other disorders of optic nerve, not elsewhere classified, bilateral
       H47.099 Other disorders of optic nerve, not elsewhere classified, unspecified eye ▽

  ✓5ᵗʰ **H47.1** Papilledema
     H47.10 Unspecified papilledema ▽
     H47.11 Papilledema associated with increased intracranial pressure
     H47.12 Papilledema associated with decreased ocular pressure
     H47.13 Papilledema associated with retinal disorder
    ✓6ᵗʰ **H47.14** Foster-Kennedy syndrome
       H47.141 Foster-Kennedy syndrome, right eye
       H47.142 Foster-Kennedy syndrome, left eye
       H47.143 Foster-Kennedy syndrome, bilateral
       H47.149 Foster-Kennedy syndrome, unspecified eye ▽

  ✓5ᵗʰ **H47.2** Optic atrophy
     H47.20 Unspecified optic atrophy ▽

✓ Additional Character Req   ✓x7ᵗʰ Placeholder Alert   Manifestation   HCC CMS-HCC Condition   ▽ Unspecified Code   ►◄ Revised Text   ● New Code   ▲ Revised Code Title

ICD-10-CM 2018   597

✓6ᵗʰ H47.21 Primary optic atrophy
- H47.211 Primary optic atrophy, right eye
- H47.212 Primary optic atrophy, left eye
- H47.213 Primary optic atrophy, bilateral
- H47.219 Primary optic atrophy, unspecified eye ▽

H47.22 Hereditary optic atrophy
    Leber's optic atrophy

✓6ᵗʰ H47.23 Glaucomatous optic atrophy
- H47.231 Glaucomatous optic atrophy, right eye
- H47.232 Glaucomatous optic atrophy, left eye
- H47.233 Glaucomatous optic atrophy, bilateral
- H47.239 Glaucomatous optic atrophy, unspecified eye ▽

✓6ᵗʰ H47.29 Other optic atrophy
    Temporal pallor of optic disc
- H47.291 Other optic atrophy, right eye
- H47.292 Other optic atrophy, left eye
- H47.293 Other optic atrophy, bilateral
- H47.299 Other optic atrophy, unspecified eye ▽

✓5ᵗʰ H47.3 Other disorders of optic disc

✓6ᵗʰ H47.31 Coloboma of optic disc
- H47.311 Coloboma of optic disc, right eye
- H47.312 Coloboma of optic disc, left eye
- H47.313 Coloboma of optic disc, bilateral
- H47.319 Coloboma of optic disc, unspecified eye ▽

✓6ᵗʰ H47.32 Drusen of optic disc
- H47.321 Drusen of optic disc, right eye
- H47.322 Drusen of optic disc, left eye
- H47.323 Drusen of optic disc, bilateral
- H47.329 Drusen of optic disc, unspecified eye ▽

✓6ᵗʰ H47.33 Pseudopapilledema of optic disc
- H47.331 Pseudopapilledema of optic disc, right eye
- H47.332 Pseudopapilledema of optic disc, left eye
- H47.333 Pseudopapilledema of optic disc, bilateral
- H47.339 Pseudopapilledema of optic disc, unspecified eye ▽

✓6ᵗʰ H47.39 Other disorders of optic disc
- H47.391 Other disorders of optic disc, right eye
- H47.392 Other disorders of optic disc, left eye
- H47.393 Other disorders of optic disc, bilateral
- H47.399 Other disorders of optic disc, unspecified eye ▽

✓5ᵗʰ H47.4 Disorders of optic chiasm
    Code also underlying condition
- H47.41 Disorders of optic chiasm in (due to) inflammatory disorders
- H47.42 Disorders of optic chiasm in (due to) neoplasm
- H47.43 Disorders of optic chiasm in (due to) vascular disorders
- H47.49 Disorders of optic chiasm in (due to) other disorders

✓5ᵗʰ H47.5 Disorders of other visual pathways
    Disorders of optic tracts, geniculate nuclei and optic radiations
    Code also underlying condition

✓6ᵗʰ H47.51 Disorders of visual pathways in (due to) inflammatory disorders
- H47.511 Disorders of visual pathways in (due to) inflammatory disorders, right side
- H47.512 Disorders of visual pathways in (due to) inflammatory disorders, left side
- H47.519 Disorders of visual pathways in (due to) ▽ inflammatory disorders, unspecified side

✓6ᵗʰ H47.52 Disorders of visual pathways in (due to) neoplasm
- H47.521 Disorders of visual pathways in (due to) neoplasm, right side
- H47.522 Disorders of visual pathways in (due to) neoplasm, left side
- H47.529 Disorders of visual pathways in (due to) ▽ neoplasm, unspecified side

✓6ᵗʰ H47.53 Disorders of visual pathways in (due to) vascular disorders
- H47.531 Disorders of visual pathways in (due to) vascular disorders, right side
- H47.532 Disorders of visual pathways in (due to) vascular disorders, left side

- H47.539 Disorders of visual pathways in (due to) ▽ vascular disorders, unspecified side

✓5ᵗʰ H47.6 Disorders of visual cortex
    Code also underlying condition
    EXCLUDES 1   injury to visual cortex S04.04

✓6ᵗʰ H47.61 Cortical blindness
- H47.611 Cortical blindness, right side of brain
- H47.612 Cortical blindness, left side of brain
- H47.619 Cortical blindness, unspecified side of ▽ brain

✓6ᵗʰ H47.62 Disorders of visual cortex in (due to) inflammatory disorders
- H47.621 Disorders of visual cortex in (due to) inflammatory disorders, right side of brain
- H47.622 Disorders of visual cortex in (due to) inflammatory disorders, left side of brain
- H47.629 Disorders of visual cortex in (due to) ▽ inflammatory disorders, unspecified side of brain

✓6ᵗʰ H47.63 Disorders of visual cortex in (due to) neoplasm
- H47.631 Disorders of visual cortex in (due to) neoplasm, right side of brain
- H47.632 Disorders of visual cortex in (due to) neoplasm, left side of brain
- H47.639 Disorders of visual cortex in (due to) ▽ neoplasm, unspecified side of brain

✓6ᵗʰ H47.64 Disorders of visual cortex in (due to) vascular disorders
- H47.641 Disorders of visual cortex in (due to) vascular disorders, right side of brain
- H47.642 Disorders of visual cortex in (due to) vascular disorders, left side of brain
- H47.649 Disorders of visual cortex in (due to) ▽ vascular disorders, unspecified side of brain

H47.9 Unspecified disorder of visual pathways ▽

Disorders of ocular muscles, binocular movement, accommodation and refraction (H49-H52)

EXCLUDES 2   nystagmus and other irregular eye movements (H55)

✓4ᵗʰ H49 Paralytic strabismus
    EXCLUDES 2   internal ophthalmoplegia (H52.51-)
                  internuclear ophthalmoplegia (H51.2-)
                  progressive supranuclear ophthalmoplegia (G23.1)

✓5ᵗʰ H49.0 Third [oculomotor] nerve palsy
- H49.00 Third [oculomotor] nerve palsy, unspecified eye ▽
- H49.01 Third [oculomotor] nerve palsy, right eye
- H49.02 Third [oculomotor] nerve palsy, left eye
- H49.03 Third [oculomotor] nerve palsy, bilateral

✓5ᵗʰ H49.1 Fourth [trochlear] nerve palsy
- H49.10 Fourth [trochlear] nerve palsy, unspecified eye ▽
- H49.11 Fourth [trochlear] nerve palsy, right eye
- H49.12 Fourth [trochlear] nerve palsy, left eye
- H49.13 Fourth [trochlear] nerve palsy, bilateral

✓5ᵗʰ H49.2 Sixth [abducent] nerve palsy
- H49.20 Sixth [abducent] nerve palsy, unspecified eye ▽
- H49.21 Sixth [abducent] nerve palsy, right eye
- H49.22 Sixth [abducent] nerve palsy, left eye
- H49.23 Sixth [abducent] nerve palsy, bilateral

✓5ᵗʰ H49.3 Total (external) ophthalmoplegia
- H49.30 Total (external) ophthalmoplegia, unspecified eye ▽
- H49.31 Total (external) ophthalmoplegia, right eye
- H49.32 Total (external) ophthalmoplegia, left eye
- H49.33 Total (external) ophthalmoplegia, bilateral

✓5ᵗʰ H49.4 Progressive external ophthalmoplegia
    EXCLUDES 1   Kearns-Sayre syndrome (H49.81-)
- H49.40 Progressive external ophthalmoplegia, ▽ unspecified eye
- H49.41 Progressive external ophthalmoplegia, right eye
- H49.42 Progressive external ophthalmoplegia, left eye
- H49.43 Progressive external ophthalmoplegia, bilateral

EXCLUDES 1 Not coded here   EXCLUDES 2 Not included here   N Newborn Age: 0   P Pediatric Age: 0-17   M Maternity Age: 12-55   A Adult Age: 15-124

598   ICD-10-CM 2018

✓5th **H49.8 Other paralytic strabismus**

  ✓6th **H49.81 Kearns-Sayre syndrome**
Progressive external ophthalmoplegia with pigmentary retinopathy
Use additional code for other manifestation, such as:
heart block (I45.9)

    H49.811 **Kearns-Sayre syndrome, right eye** `HCC`
    H49.812 **Kearns-Sayre syndrome, left eye** `HCC`
    H49.813 **Kearns-Sayre syndrome, bilateral** `HCC`
    H49.819 **Kearns-Sayre syndrome, unspecified eye** `HCC` ▽

  ✓6th **H49.88 Other paralytic strabismus**
External ophthalmoplegia NOS

    H49.881 **Other paralytic strabismus, right eye**
    H49.882 **Other paralytic strabismus, left eye**
    H49.883 **Other paralytic strabismus, bilateral**
    H49.889 **Other paralytic strabismus, unspecified eye** ▽

  H49.9 Unspecified paralytic strabismus ▽

✓4th **H50 Other strabismus**

  ✓5th **H50.0 Esotropia**
Convergent concomitant strabismus
EXCLUDES 1   intermittent esotropia (H50.31-, H50.32)

    H50.00 Unspecified esotropia ▽

  ✓6th **H50.01 Monocular esotropia**
    H50.011 **Monocular esotropia, right eye**
    H50.012 **Monocular esotropia, left eye**

  ✓6th **H50.02 Monocular esotropia with A pattern**
    H50.021 **Monocular esotropia with A pattern, right eye**
    H50.022 **Monocular esotropia with A pattern, left eye**

  ✓6th **H50.03 Monocular esotropia with V pattern**
    H50.031 **Monocular esotropia with V pattern, right eye**
    H50.032 **Monocular esotropia with V pattern, left eye**

  ✓6th **H50.04 Monocular esotropia with other noncomitancies**
    H50.041 **Monocular esotropia with other noncomitancies, right eye**
    H50.042 **Monocular esotropia with other noncomitancies, left eye**

    H50.05 Alternating esotropia
    H50.06 Alternating esotropia with A pattern
    H50.07 Alternating esotropia with V pattern
    H50.08 Alternating esotropia with other noncomitancies

  ✓5th **H50.1 Exotropia**
Divergent concomitant strabismus
EXCLUDES 1   intermittent exotropia (H50.33-, H50.34)

    H50.10 Unspecified exotropia ▽

Eye Muscle Diseases

R.   L.
Monocular (one eye only) esotropia (inward)

Monocular exotropia (outward)

Monocular hypertropia (upward)

✓6th **H50.11 Monocular exotropia**
    H50.111 **Monocular exotropia, right eye**
    H50.112 **Monocular exotropia, left eye**

✓6th **H50.12 Monocular exotropia with A pattern**
    H50.121 **Monocular exotropia with A pattern, right eye**
    H50.122 **Monocular exotropia with A pattern, left eye**

✓6th **H50.13 Monocular exotropia with V pattern**
    H50.131 **Monocular exotropia with V pattern, right eye**
    H50.132 **Monocular exotropia with V pattern, left eye**

✓6th **H50.14 Monocular exotropia with other noncomitancies**
    H50.141 **Monocular exotropia with other noncomitancies, right eye**
    H50.142 **Monocular exotropia with other noncomitancies, left eye**

    H50.15 Alternating exotropia
    H50.16 Alternating exotropia with A pattern
    H50.17 Alternating exotropia with V pattern
    H50.18 Alternating exotropia with other noncomitancies

✓5th **H50.2 Vertical strabismus**
Hypertropia
    H50.21 Vertical strabismus, right eye
    H50.22 Vertical strabismus, left eye

✓5th **H50.3 Intermittent heterotropia**
    H50.30 Unspecified intermittent heterotropia ▽

  ✓6th **H50.31 Intermittent monocular esotropia**
    H50.311 **Intermittent monocular esotropia, right eye**
    H50.312 **Intermittent monocular esotropia, left eye**
    H50.32 Intermittent alternating esotropia

  ✓6th **H50.33 Intermittent monocular exotropia**
    H50.331 **Intermittent monocular exotropia, right eye**
    H50.332 **Intermittent monocular exotropia, left eye**
    H50.34 Intermittent alternating exotropia

✓5th **H50.4 Other and unspecified heterotropia**
    H50.40 Unspecified heterotropia ▽

  ✓6th **H50.41 Cyclotropia**
    H50.411 **Cyclotropia, right eye**
    H50.412 **Cyclotropia, left eye**
    H50.42 Monofixation syndrome
    H50.43 Accommodative component in esotropia

✓5th **H50.5 Heterophoria**
    H50.50 Unspecified heterophoria ▽
    H50.51 Esophoria
    H50.52 Exophoria
    H50.53 Vertical heterophoria
    H50.54 Cyclophoria
    H50.55 Alternating heterophoria

✓5th **H50.6 Mechanical strabismus**
    H50.60 Mechanical strabismus, unspecified ▽

  ✓6th **H50.61 Brown's sheath syndrome**
    H50.611 **Brown's sheath syndrome, right eye**
    H50.612 **Brown's sheath syndrome, left eye**
    H50.69 Other mechanical strabismus
Strabismus due to adhesions
Traumatic limitation of duction of eye muscle

✓5th **H50.8 Other specified strabismus**

  ✓6th **H50.81 Duane's syndrome**
    H50.811 **Duane's syndrome, right eye**
    H50.812 **Duane's syndrome, left eye**
    H50.89 Other specified strabismus

  H50.9 Unspecified strabismus ▽

✓4th **H51 Other disorders of binocular movement**
    H51.0 Palsy (spasm) of conjugate gaze

  ✓5th **H51.1 Convergence insufficiency and excess**
    H51.11 Convergence insufficiency
    H51.12 Convergence excess

✓ Additional Character Req   ✓x7th Placeholder Alert   Manifestation   `HCC` CMS-HCC Condition   ▽ Unspecified Code   ▶◀ Revised Text   ● New Code   ▲ Revised Code Title

✓5th **H51.2　Internuclear ophthalmoplegia**
　　H51.20　Internuclear ophthalmoplegia, unspecified eye　▽
　　H51.21　Internuclear ophthalmoplegia, right eye
　　H51.22　Internuclear ophthalmoplegia, left eye
　　H51.23　Internuclear ophthalmoplegia, bilateral
　H51.8　Other specified disorders of binocular movement
　H51.9　Unspecified disorder of binocular movement　▽

✓4th **H52　Disorders of refraction and accommodation**
　✓5th **H52.0　Hypermetropia**
　　　H52.00　Hypermetropia, unspecified eye　▽
　　　H52.01　Hypermetropia, right eye
　　　H52.02　Hypermetropia, left eye
　　　H52.03　Hypermetropia, bilateral
　✓5th **H52.1　Myopia**
　　　EXCLUDES 1　*degenerative myopia (H44.2-)*
　　　H52.10　Myopia, unspecified eye　▽
　　　H52.11　Myopia, right eye
　　　H52.12　Myopia, left eye
　　　H52.13　Myopia, bilateral
　✓5th **H52.2　Astigmatism**
　　✓6th **H52.20　Unspecified astigmatism**
　　　　H52.201　Unspecified astigmatism, right eye　▽
　　　　H52.202　Unspecified astigmatism, left eye　▽
　　　　H52.203　Unspecified astigmatism, bilateral　▽
　　　　H52.209　Unspecified astigmatism, unspecified eye　▽
　　✓6th **H52.21　Irregular astigmatism**
　　　　H52.211　Irregular astigmatism, right eye
　　　　H52.212　Irregular astigmatism, left eye
　　　　H52.213　Irregular astigmatism, bilateral
　　　　H52.219　Irregular astigmatism, unspecified eye　▽
　　✓6th **H52.22　Regular astigmatism**
　　　　H52.221　Regular astigmatism, right eye
　　　　H52.222　Regular astigmatism, left eye
　　　　H52.223　Regular astigmatism, bilateral
　　　　H52.229　Regular astigmatism, unspecified eye　▽
　✓5th **H52.3　Anisometropia and aniseikonia**
　　　H52.31　Anisometropia
　　　H52.32　Aniseikonia
　　H52.4　Presbyopia
　✓5th **H52.5　Disorders of accommodation**
　　✓6th **H52.51　Internal ophthalmoplegia (complete) (total)**
　　　　H52.511　Internal ophthalmoplegia (complete) (total), right eye
　　　　H52.512　Internal ophthalmoplegia (complete) (total), left eye
　　　　H52.513　Internal ophthalmoplegia (complete) (total), bilateral
　　　　H52.519　Internal ophthalmoplegia (complete) (total), unspecified eye　▽
　　✓6th **H52.52　Paresis of accommodation**
　　　　H52.521　Paresis of accommodation, right eye
　　　　H52.522　Paresis of accommodation, left eye
　　　　H52.523　Paresis of accommodation, bilateral
　　　　H52.529　Paresis of accommodation, unspecified eye　▽
　　✓6th **H52.53　Spasm of accommodation**
　　　　H52.531　Spasm of accommodation, right eye
　　　　H52.532　Spasm of accommodation, left eye
　　　　H52.533　Spasm of accommodation, bilateral
　　　　H52.539　Spasm of accommodation, unspecified eye　▽
　　H52.6　Other disorders of refraction
　　H52.7　Unspecified disorder of refraction　▽

Visual disturbances and blindness (H53-H54)

✓4th **H53　Visual disturbances**
　✓5th **H53.0　Amblyopia ex anopsia**
　　　EXCLUDES 1　*amblyopia due to vitamin A deficiency (E50.5)*
　　✓6th **H53.00　Unspecified amblyopia**
　　　　H53.001　Unspecified amblyopia, right eye　▽

　　　　H53.002　Unspecified amblyopia, left eye　▽
　　　　H53.003　Unspecified amblyopia, bilateral　▽
　　　　H53.009　Unspecified amblyopia, unspecified eye　▽
　　✓6th **H53.01　Deprivation amblyopia**
　　　　H53.011　Deprivation amblyopia, right eye
　　　　H53.012　Deprivation amblyopia, left eye
　　　　H53.013　Deprivation amblyopia, bilateral
　　　　H53.019　Deprivation amblyopia, unspecified eye　▽
　　✓6th **H53.02　Refractive amblyopia**
　　　　H53.021　Refractive amblyopia, right eye
　　　　H53.022　Refractive amblyopia, left eye
　　　　H53.023　Refractive amblyopia, bilateral
　　　　H53.029　Refractive amblyopia, unspecified eye　▽
　　✓6th **H53.03　Strabismic amblyopia**
　　　　EXCLUDES 1　*strabismus (H50.-)*
　　　　H53.031　Strabismic amblyopia, right eye
　　　　H53.032　Strabismic amblyopia, left eye
　　　　H53.033　Strabismic amblyopia, bilateral
　　　　H53.039　Strabismic amblyopia, unspecified eye　▽
　　✓6th **H53.04　Amblyopia suspect**
　　　　H53.041　Amblyopia suspect, right eye
　　　　H53.042　Amblyopia suspect, left eye
　　　　H53.043　Amblyopia suspect, bilateral
　　　　H53.049　Amblyopia suspect, unspecified eye　▽
　✓5th **H53.1　Subjective visual disturbances**
　　　EXCLUDES 1　*subjective visual disturbances due to vitamin A deficiency (E50.5)*
　　　　　　　　visual hallucinations (R44.1)
　　　H53.10　Unspecified subjective visual disturbances　▽
　　　H53.11　Day blindness
　　　　　　Hemeralopia
　　✓6th **H53.12　Transient visual loss**
　　　　Scintillating scotoma
　　　　EXCLUDES 1　*amaurosis fugax (G45.3-)*
　　　　　　　　transient retinal artery occlusion (H34.0-)
　　　　H53.121　Transient visual loss, right eye
　　　　H53.122　Transient visual loss, left eye
　　　　H53.123　Transient visual loss, bilateral
　　　　H53.129　Transient visual loss, unspecified eye　▽
　　✓6th **H53.13　Sudden visual loss**
　　　　H53.131　Sudden visual loss, right eye
　　　　H53.132　Sudden visual loss, left eye
　　　　H53.133　Sudden visual loss, bilateral
　　　　H53.139　Sudden visual loss, unspecified eye　▽
　　✓6th **H53.14　Visual discomfort**
　　　　Asthenopia　　　　Photophobia
　　　　H53.141　Visual discomfort, right eye
　　　　H53.142　Visual discomfort, left eye
　　　　H53.143　Visual discomfort, bilateral
　　　　H53.149　Visual discomfort, unspecified　▽
　　　H53.15　Visual distortions of shape and size
　　　　　　Metamorphopsia
　　　H53.16　Psychophysical visual disturbances
　　　H53.19　Other subjective visual disturbances
　　　　　　Visual halos
　　H53.2　Diplopia
　　　　Double vision
　✓5th **H53.3　Other and unspecified disorders of binocular vision**
　　　H53.30　Unspecified disorder of binocular vision　▽
　　　H53.31　Abnormal retinal correspondence
　　　H53.32　Fusion with defective stereopsis
　　　H53.33　Simultaneous visual perception without fusion
　　　H53.34　Suppression of binocular vision
　✓5th **H53.4　Visual field defects**
　　　H53.40　Unspecified visual field defects　▽
　　✓6th **H53.41　Scotoma involving central area**
　　　　Central scotoma
　　　　H53.411　Scotoma involving central area, right eye
　　　　H53.412　Scotoma involving central area, left eye
　　　　H53.413　Scotoma involving central area, bilateral

EXCLUDES 1 Not coded here　　　EXCLUDES 2 Not included here　　　N Newborn Age: 0　　　P Pediatric Age: 0-17　　　M Maternity Age: 12-55　　　A Adult Age: 15-124

600　　　　　　　　　　　　　　　　　　　　　　　　　　　　　　　　　　　ICD-10-CM 2018

H53.419   **Scotoma involving central area, unspecified eye** ▽

✓6ᵗʰ H53.42   **Scotoma of blind spot area**
     Enlarged blind spot
     H53.421   **Scotoma of blind spot area, right eye**
     H53.422   **Scotoma of blind spot area, left eye**
     H53.423   **Scotoma of blind spot area, bilateral**
     H53.429   **Scotoma of blind spot area, unspecified eye** ▽

✓6ᵗʰ H53.43   **Sector or arcuate defects**
     Arcuate scotoma
     Bjerrum scotoma
     H53.431   **Sector or arcuate defects, right eye**
     H53.432   **Sector or arcuate defects, left eye**
     H53.433   **Sector or arcuate defects, bilateral**
     H53.439   **Sector or arcuate defects, unspecified eye** ▽

✓6ᵗʰ H53.45   **Other localized visual field defect**
     Peripheral visual field defect
     Ring scotoma NOS
     Scotoma NOS
     H53.451   **Other localized visual field defect, right eye**
     H53.452   **Other localized visual field defect, left eye**
     H53.453   **Other localized visual field defect, bilateral**
     H53.459   **Other localized visual field defect, unspecified eye** ▽

✓6ᵗʰ H53.46   **Homonymous bilateral field defects**
     Homonymous hemianopia
     Homonymous hemianopsia
     Quadrant anopia
     Quadrant anopsia
     H53.461   **Homonymous bilateral field defects, right side**
     H53.462   **Homonymous bilateral field defects, left side**
     H53.469   **Homonymous bilateral field defects, unspecified side** ▽
         Homonymous bilateral field defects NOS

H53.47   **Heteronymous bilateral field defects**
     Heteronymous hemianop(s)ia

✓6ᵗʰ H53.48   **Generalized contraction of visual field**
     H53.481   **Generalized contraction of visual field, right eye**
     H53.482   **Generalized contraction of visual field, left eye**
     H53.483   **Generalized contraction of visual field, bilateral**
     H53.489   **Generalized contraction of visual field, unspecified eye** ▽

✓5ᵗʰ H53.5   **Color vision deficiencies**
     Color blindness
     EXCLUDES 2   day blindness (H53.11)
     H53.50   **Unspecified color vision deficiencies** ▽
         Color blindness NOS
     H53.51   **Achromatopsia**
         DEF: Nonprogressive genetic visual disorder; characterized by complete color blindness, decreased vision, and light sensitivity.
     H53.52   **Acquired color vision deficiency**
     H53.53   **Deuteranomaly**
         Deuteranopia
         DEF: Male-only genetic disorder; difficulty in distinguishing green and red, no shortened spectrum.
     H53.54   **Protanomaly**
         Protanopia
     H53.55   **Tritanomaly**
         Tritanopia
     H53.59   **Other color vision deficiencies**

✓5ᵗʰ H53.6   **Night blindness**
     EXCLUDES 1   night blindness due to vitamin A deficiency (E50.5)
     H53.60   **Unspecified night blindness** ▽
     H53.61   **Abnormal dark adaptation curve**
     H53.62   **Acquired night blindness**
     H53.63   **Congenital night blindness**
     H53.69   **Other night blindness**

✓5ᵗʰ H53.7   **Vision sensitivity deficiencies**
     H53.71   **Glare sensitivity**
     H53.72   **Impaired contrast sensitivity**

H53.8   **Other visual disturbances**

H53.9   **Unspecified visual disturbance** ▽

✓4ᵗʰ H54   **Blindness and low vision**
     NOTE   For definition of visual impairment categories see table below
     Code first any associated underlying cause of the blindness
     EXCLUDES 1   amaurosis fugax (G45.3)

✓5ᵗʰ H54.0   **Blindness, both eyes**
     Visual impairment categories 3, 4, 5 in both eyes
     ● **✓6ᵗʰ H54.0X**   **Blindness, both eyes, different category levels**
     ●   **✓7ᵗʰ H54.0X3**   **Blindness right eye, category 3**
     ●   H54.0X33   **Blindness right eye category 3, blindness left eye category 3**
     ●   H54.0X34   **Blindness right eye category 3, blindness left eye category 4**
     ●   H54.0X35   **Blindness right eye category 3, blindness left eye category 5**
     ●   **✓7ᵗʰ H54.0X4**   **Blindness right eye, category 4**
     ●   H54.0X43   **Blindness right eye category 4, blindness left eye category 3**
     ●   H54.0X44   **Blindness right eye category 4, blindness left eye category 4**
     ●   H54.0X45   **Blindness right eye category 4, blindness left eye category 5**
     ●   **✓7ᵗʰ H54.0X5**   **Blindness right eye, category 5**
     ●   H54.0X53   **Blindness right eye category 5, blindness left eye category 3**
     ●   H54.0X54   **Blindness right eye category 5, blindness left eye category 4**
     ●   H54.0X55   **Blindness right eye category 5, blindness left eye category 5**

✓5ᵗʰ H54.1   **Blindness, one eye, low vision other eye**
     Visual impairment categories 3, 4, 5 in one eye, with categories 1 or 2 in the other eye.
     H54.10   **Blindness, one eye, low vision other eye, unspecified eyes** ▽
     ● **✓6ᵗʰ H54.11**   **Blindness, right eye, low vision left eye**
     ●   **✓7ᵗʰ H54.113**   **Blindness right eye category 3, low vision left eye**
     ●   H54.1131   **Blindness right eye category 3, low vision left eye category 1**
     ●   H54.1132   **Blindness right eye category 3, low vision left eye category 2**
     ●   **✓7ᵗʰ H54.114**   **Blindness right eye category 4, low vision left eye**
     ●   H54.1141   **Blindness right eye category 4, low vision left eye category 1**
     ●   H54.1142   **Blindness right eye category 4, low vision left eye category 2**
     ●   **✓7ᵗʰ H54.115**   **Blindness right eye category 5, low vision left eye**
     ●   H54.1151   **Blindness right eye category 5, low vision left eye category 1**
     ●   H54.1152   **Blindness right eye category 5, low vision left eye category 2**
     ● **✓6ᵗʰ H54.12**   **Blindness, left eye, low vision right eye**
     ●   **✓7ᵗʰ H54.121**   **Low vision right eye category 1, blindness left eye**
          H54.1213   **Low vision right eye category 1, blindness left eye category 3**
     ●   H54.1214   **Low vision right eye category 1, blindness left eye category 4**
     ●   H54.1215   **Low vision right eye category 1, blindness left eye category 5**

✓ Additional Character Req   ✓x7ᵗʰ Placeholder Alert   Manifestation   HCC CMS-HCC Condition   ▽ Unspecified Code   ►◄ Revised Text   ● New Code   ▲ Revised Code Title

ICD-10-CM 2018   601

Chapter 7. Diseases of the Eye and Adnexa

- ☑7ᵗʰ **H54.122** Low vision right eye category 2, blindness left eye
  - **H54.1223** Low vision right eye category 2, blindness left eye category 3
  - **H54.1224** Low vision right eye category 2, blindness left eye category 4
  - **H54.1225** Low vision right eye category 2, blindness left eye category 5
- ☑5ᵗʰ **H54.2 Low vision, both eyes**
  Visual impairment categories 1 or 2 in both eyes
  - ☑6ᵗʰ **H54.2X Low vision, both eyes, different category levels**
    - ☑7ᵗʰ **H54.2X1 Low vision, right eye, category 1**
      - **H54.2X11** Low vision right eye category 1, low vision left eye category 1
      - **H54.2X12** Low vision right eye category 1, low vision left eye category 2
    - ☑7ᵗʰ **H54.2X2 Low vision, right eye, category 2**
      - **H54.2X21** Low vision right eye category 2, low vision left eye category 1
      - **H54.2X22** Low vision right eye category 2, low vision left eye category 2
- **H54.3 Unqualified visual loss, both eyes**
  Visual impairment category 9 in both eyes.
- ☑5ᵗʰ **H54.4 Blindness, one eye**
  Visual impairment categories 3, 4, 5 in one eye [normal vision in other eye]
  - **H54.40 Blindness, one eye, unspecified eye** ▽
  - ☑6ᵗʰ **H54.41 Blindness, right eye, normal vision left eye**
    - ☑7ᵗʰ **H54.413 Blindness, right eye, category 3**
      - **H54.413A** Blindness right eye category 3, normal vision left eye
    - ☑7ᵗʰ **H54.414 Blindness, right eye, category 4**
      - **H54.414A** Blindness right eye category 4, normal vision left eye
    - ☑7ᵗʰ **H54.415 Blindness, right eye, category 5**
      - **H54.415A** Blindness right eye category 5, normal vision left eye
  - ☑6ᵗʰ **H54.42 Blindness, left eye, normal vision right eye**
    - ☑7ᵗʰ **H54.42A Blindness, left eye, category 3-5**
      - **H54.42A3** Blindness left eye category 3, normal vision right eye
      - **H54.42A4** Blindness left eye category 4, normal vision right eye
      - **H54.42A5** Blindness left eye category 5, normal vision right eye
- ☑5ᵗʰ **H54.5 Low vision, one eye**
  Visual impairment categories 1 or 2 in one eye [normal vision in other eye]
  - **H54.50 Low vision, one eye, unspecified eye** ▽
  - ☑6ᵗʰ **H54.51 Low vision, right eye, normal vision left eye**
    - ☑7ᵗʰ **H54.511 Low vision, right eye, category 1-2**
      - **H54.511A** Low vision right eye category 1, normal vision left eye
      - **H54.512A** Low vision right eye category 2, normal vision left eye
  - ☑6ᵗʰ **H54.52 Low vision, left eye, normal vision right eye**
    - ☑7ᵗʰ **H54.52A Low vision, left eye, category 1-2**
      - **H54.52A1** Low vision left eye category 1, normal vision right eye
      - **H54.52A2** Low vision left eye category 2, normal vision right eye
- ☑5ᵗʰ **H54.6 Unqualified visual loss, one eye**
  Visual impairment category 9 in one eye [normal vision in other eye].
  - **H54.60 Unqualified visual loss, one eye, unspecified** ▽
  - **H54.61 Unqualified visual loss, right eye, normal vision left eye**

H54.62 Unqualified visual loss, left eye, normal vision right eye

H54.7 Unspecified visual loss ▽
Visual impairment category 9 NOS

H54.8 Legal blindness, as defined in USA
Blindness NOS according to USA definition
> *EXCLUDES 1* legal blindness with specification of impairment level (H54.0-H54.7)

NOTE The table below gives a classification of severity of visual impairment recommended by a WHO Study Group on the Prevention of Blindness, Geneva, 6-10 November 1972.

The term "low vision" in category H54 comprises categories 1 and 2 of the table, the term "blindness" categories 3, 4 and 5, and the term "unqualified visual loss" category 9.

If the extent of the visual field is taken into account, patients with a field no greater than 10 but greater than 5 around central fixation should be placed in category 3 and patients with a field greater than 5 around central fixation should be placed in category 4, even if the central acuity is not impaired.

Category of visual impairment	Visual acuity with best possible correction	
	Maximum less than:	Minimum equal to or better than:
1	6/18 3/10 (0.3) 20/70	6/60 1/10 (0.1) 20/200
2	6/60 1/10 (0.1) 20/200	3/60 1/20 (0.05) 20/400
3	3/60 1/200 (0.05) 20/400	1/60 (finger counting at one meter) 1/50 (0.02) 5/300 (20/1200)
4	1/60 (finger counting at one meter) 1/50 (0.02) 5/300	Light perception
5	No light perception	
9	Undetermined or unspecified	

Other disorders of eye and adnexa (H55-H57)

☑4ᵗʰ **H55 Nystagmus and other irregular eye movements**
- ☑5ᵗʰ **H55.0 Nystagmus**
  - **H55.00 Unspecified nystagmus** ▽
  - **H55.01 Congenital nystagmus**
  - **H55.02 Latent nystagmus**
  - **H55.03 Visual deprivation nystagmus**
  - **H55.04 Dissociated nystagmus**
  - **H55.09 Other forms of nystagmus**
- ☑5ᵗʰ **H55.8 Other irregular eye movements**
  - **H55.81 Saccadic eye movements**
  - **H55.89 Other irregular eye movements**

☑4ᵗʰ **H57 Other disorders of eye and adnexa**
- ☑5ᵗʰ **H57.0 Anomalies of pupillary function**
  - **H57.00 Unspecified anomaly of pupillary function** ▽
  - **H57.01 Argyll Robertson pupil, atypical**
    > *EXCLUDES 1* syphilitic Argyll Robertson pupil (A52.19)
  - **H57.02 Anisocoria**
  - **H57.03 Miosis**
  - **H57.04 Mydriasis**
  - ☑6ᵗʰ **H57.05 Tonic pupil**
    - **H57.051 Tonic pupil, right eye**
    - **H57.052 Tonic pupil, left eye**
    - **H57.053 Tonic pupil, bilateral**
    - **H57.059 Tonic pupil, unspecified eye** ▽
  - **H57.09 Other anomalies of pupillary function**
- ☑5ᵗʰ **H57.1 Ocular pain**
  - **H57.10 Ocular pain, unspecified eye** ▽
  - **H57.11 Ocular pain, right eye**
  - **H57.12 Ocular pain, left eye**
  - **H57.13 Ocular pain, bilateral**

EXCLUDES 1 Not coded here   *EXCLUDES 2* Not included here   **N** Newborn Age: 0   **P** Pediatric Age: 0-17   **M** Maternity Age: 12-55   **A** Adult Age: 15-124

602   ICD-10-CM 2018

H57.8   Other specified disorders of eye and adnexa

H57.9   Unspecified disorder of eye and adnexa   ▽

Intraoperative and postprocedural complications and disorders of eye and adnexa, not elsewhere classified (H59)

✓4ᵗʰ **H59**   **Intraoperative and postprocedural complications and disorders of eye and adnexa, not elsewhere classified**

> EXCLUDES 1   *mechanical complication of intraocular lens (T85.2)*
> *mechanical complication of other ocular prosthetic devices, implants and grafts (T85.3)*
> *pseudophakia (Z96.1)*
> *secondary cataracts (H26.4-)*

✓5ᵗʰ **H59.0**   **Disorders of the eye following cataract surgery**

   ✓6ᵗʰ **H59.01**   **Keratopathy (bullous aphakic) following cataract surgery**
     Vitreal corneal syndrome
     Vitreous (touch) syndrome

     H59.011   Keratopathy (bullous aphakic) following cataract surgery, right eye

     H59.012   Keratopathy (bullous aphakic) following cataract surgery, left eye

     H59.013   Keratopathy (bullous aphakic) following cataract surgery, bilateral

     H59.019   Keratopathy (bullous aphakic) following cataract surgery, unspecified eye   ▽

   ✓6ᵗʰ **H59.02**   **Cataract (lens) fragments in eye following cataract surgery**

     H59.021   Cataract (lens) fragments in eye following cataract surgery, right eye

     H59.022   Cataract (lens) fragments in eye following cataract surgery, left eye

     H59.023   Cataract (lens) fragments in eye following cataract surgery, bilateral

     H59.029   Cataract (lens) fragments in eye following cataract surgery, unspecified eye   ▽

   ✓6ᵗʰ **H59.03**   **Cystoid macular edema following cataract surgery**

     H59.031   Cystoid macular edema following cataract surgery, right eye

     H59.032   Cystoid macular edema following cataract surgery, left eye

     H59.033   Cystoid macular edema following cataract surgery, bilateral

     H59.039   Cystoid macular edema following cataract surgery, unspecified eye   ▽

   ✓6ᵗʰ **H59.09**   **Other disorders of the eye following cataract surgery**

     H59.091   Other disorders of the right eye following cataract surgery

     H59.092   Other disorders of the left eye following cataract surgery

     H59.093   Other disorders of the eye following cataract surgery, bilateral

     H59.099   Other disorders of unspecified eye following cataract surgery   ▽

✓5ᵗʰ **H59.1**   **Intraoperative hemorrhage and hematoma of eye and adnexa complicating a procedure**

> EXCLUDES 1   *intraoperative hemorrhage and hematoma of eye and adnexa due to accidental puncture or laceration during a procedure (H59.2-)*

   ✓6ᵗʰ **H59.11**   **Intraoperative hemorrhage and hematoma of eye and adnexa complicating an ophthalmic procedure**

     H59.111   Intraoperative hemorrhage and hematoma of right eye and adnexa complicating an ophthalmic procedure

     H59.112   Intraoperative hemorrhage and hematoma of left eye and adnexa complicating an ophthalmic procedure

     H59.113   Intraoperative hemorrhage and hematoma of eye and adnexa complicating an ophthalmic procedure, bilateral

     H59.119   Intraoperative hemorrhage and hematoma of unspecified eye and adnexa complicating an ophthalmic procedure   ▽

   ✓6ᵗʰ **H59.12**   **Intraoperative hemorrhage and hematoma of eye and adnexa complicating other procedure**

     H59.121   Intraoperative hemorrhage and hematoma of right eye and adnexa complicating other procedure

     H59.122   Intraoperative hemorrhage and hematoma of left eye and adnexa complicating other procedure

     H59.123   Intraoperative hemorrhage and hematoma of eye and adnexa complicating other procedure, bilateral

     H59.129   Intraoperative hemorrhage and hematoma of unspecified eye and adnexa complicating other procedure   ▽

✓5ᵗʰ **H59.2**   **Accidental puncture and laceration of eye and adnexa during a procedure**

   ✓6ᵗʰ **H59.21**   **Accidental puncture and laceration of eye and adnexa during an ophthalmic procedure**

     H59.211   Accidental puncture and laceration of right eye and adnexa during an ophthalmic procedure

     H59.212   Accidental puncture and laceration of left eye and adnexa during an ophthalmic procedure

     H59.213   Accidental puncture and laceration of eye and adnexa during an ophthalmic procedure, bilateral

     H59.219   Accidental puncture and laceration of unspecified eye and adnexa during an ophthalmic procedure   ▽

   ✓6ᵗʰ **H59.22**   **Accidental puncture and laceration of eye and adnexa during other procedure**

     H59.221   Accidental puncture and laceration of right eye and adnexa during other procedure

     H59.222   Accidental puncture and laceration of left eye and adnexa during other procedure

     H59.223   Accidental puncture and laceration of eye and adnexa during other procedure, bilateral

     H59.229   Accidental puncture and laceration of unspecified eye and adnexa during other procedure   ▽

✓5ᵗʰ **H59.3**   **Postprocedural hemorrhage, hematoma, and seroma of eye and adnexa following a procedure**

   ✓6ᵗʰ **H59.31**   **Postprocedural hemorrhage of eye and adnexa following an ophthalmic procedure**

     H59.311   Postprocedural hemorrhage of right eye and adnexa following an ophthalmic procedure

     H59.312   Postprocedural hemorrhage of left eye and adnexa following an ophthalmic procedure

     H59.313   Postprocedural hemorrhage of eye and adnexa following an ophthalmic procedure, bilateral

     H59.319   Postprocedural hemorrhage of unspecified eye and adnexa following an ophthalmic procedure   ▽

   ✓6ᵗʰ **H59.32**   **Postprocedural hemorrhage of eye and adnexa following other procedure**

     H59.321   Postprocedural hemorrhage of right eye and adnexa following other procedure

     H59.322   Postprocedural hemorrhage of left eye and adnexa following other procedure

     H59.323   Postprocedural hemorrhage of eye and adnexa following other procedure, bilateral

     H59.329   Postprocedural hemorrhage of unspecified eye and adnexa following other procedure   ▽

   ✓6ᵗʰ **H59.33**   **Postprocedural hematoma of eye and adnexa following an ophthalmic procedure**

     H59.331   Postprocedural hematoma of right eye and adnexa following an ophthalmic procedure

     H59.332   Postprocedural hematoma of left eye and adnexa following an ophthalmic procedure

✓ Additional Character Req   ✓ˣ7ᵗʰ Placeholder Alert   Manifestation   HCC CMS-HCC Condition   ▽ Unspecified Code   ▶◀ Revised Text   ● New Code   ▲ Revised Code Title

ICD-10-CM 2018   603

Chapter 7. Diseases of the Eye and Adnexa

       H59.333   **Postprocedural hematoma of eye and adnexa following an ophthalmic procedure, bilateral**

       H59.339   **Postprocedural hematoma of unspecified eye and adnexa following an ophthalmic procedure** ▽

✓6ᵗʰ   **H59.34**   **Postprocedural hematoma of eye and adnexa following other procedure**

       H59.341   **Postprocedural hematoma of right eye and adnexa following other procedure**

       H59.342   **Postprocedural hematoma of left eye and adnexa following other procedure**

       H59.343   **Postprocedural hematoma of eye and adnexa following other procedure, bilateral**

       H59.349   **Postprocedural hematoma of unspecified eye and adnexa following other procedure** ▽

✓6ᵗʰ   **H59.35**   **Postprocedural seroma of eye and adnexa following an ophthalmic procedure**

       H59.351   **Postprocedural seroma of right eye and adnexa following an ophthalmic procedure**

       H59.352   **Postprocedural seroma of left eye and adnexa following an ophthalmic procedure**

       H59.353   **Postprocedural seroma of eye and adnexa following an ophthalmic procedure, bilateral**

       H59.359   **Postprocedural seroma of unspecified eye and adnexa following an ophthalmic procedure** ▽

✓6ᵗʰ   **H59.36**   **Postprocedural seroma of eye and adnexa following other procedure**

       H59.361   **Postprocedural seroma of right eye and adnexa following other procedure**

       H59.362   **Postprocedural seroma of left eye and adnexa following other procedure**

       H59.363   **Postprocedural seroma of eye and adnexa following other procedure, bilateral**

       H59.369   **Postprocedural seroma of unspecified eye and adnexa following other procedure** ▽

✓5ᵗʰ   **H59.4**   **Inflammation (infection) of postprocedural bleb**

Postprocedural blebitis

EXCLUDES 1   *filtering (vitreous) bleb after glaucoma surgery status (Z98.83)*

       H59.40   **Inflammation (infection) of postprocedural bleb, unspecified** ▽

       H59.41   **Inflammation (infection) of postprocedural bleb, stage 1**

       H59.42   **Inflammation (infection) of postprocedural bleb, stage 2**

       H59.43   **Inflammation (infection) of postprocedural bleb, stage 3**

Bleb endophthalmitis

✓5ᵗʰ   **H59.8**   **Other intraoperative and postprocedural complications and disorders of eye and adnexa, not elsewhere classified**

      ✓6ᵗʰ   **H59.81**   **Chorioretinal scars after surgery for detachment**

       H59.811   **Chorioretinal scars after surgery for detachment, right eye**

       H59.812   **Chorioretinal scars after surgery for detachment, left eye**

       H59.813   **Chorioretinal scars after surgery for detachment, bilateral**

       H59.819   **Chorioretinal scars after surgery for detachment, unspecified eye** ▽

       H59.88   **Other intraoperative complications of eye and adnexa, not elsewhere classified**

       H59.89   **Other postprocedural complications and disorders of eye and adnexa, not elsewhere classified**

EXCLUDES 1 Not coded here   EXCLUDES 2 Not included here   N Newborn Age: 0   P Pediatric Age: 0-17   M Maternity Age: 12-55   A Adult Age: 15-124

Chapter 8. Diseases of the Ear and Mastoid Process (H60–H95)

Chapter Specific Coding Guidelines and Examples
Reserved for future guideline expansion.

Chapter 8. Diseases of the Ear and Mastoid Process (H60–H95)

NOTE Use an external cause code following the code for the ear condition, if applicable, to identify the cause of the ear condition.

EXCLUDES 2 certain conditions originating in the perinatal period (P04-P96)
certain infectious and parasitic diseases (A00-B99)
complications of pregnancy, childbirth and the puerperium (O00-O9A)
congenital malformations, deformations and chromosomal abnormalities (Q00-Q99)
endocrine, nutritional and metabolic diseases (E00-E88)
injury, poisoning and certain other consequences of external causes (S00-T88)
neoplasms (C00-D49)
symptoms, signs and abnormal clinical and laboratory findings, not elsewhere classified (R00-R94)

This chapter contains the following blocks:

H60-H62	Diseases of external ear
H65-H75	Diseases of middle ear and mastoid
H80-H83	Diseases of inner ear
H90-H94	Other disorders of ear
H95	Intraoperative and postprocedural complications and disorders of ear and mastoid process, not elsewhere classified

Diseases of external ear (H60–H62)

√4ᵗʰ H60 Otitis externa

√5ᵗʰ H60.0 Abscess of external ear
Boil of external ear
Carbuncle of auricle or external auditory canal
Furuncle of external ear

     H60.00   Abscess of external ear, unspecified ear ▽
     H60.01   Abscess of right external ear
     H60.02   Abscess of left external ear
     H60.03   Abscess of external ear, bilateral

√5ᵗʰ H60.1 Cellulitis of external ear
Cellulitis of auricle
Cellulitis of external auditory canal

     H60.10   Cellulitis of external ear, unspecified ear ▽
     H60.11   Cellulitis of right external ear
     H60.12   Cellulitis of left external ear
     H60.13   Cellulitis of external ear, bilateral

√5ᵗʰ H60.2 Malignant otitis externa
     H60.20   Malignant otitis externa, unspecified ear ▽
     H60.21   Malignant otitis externa, right ear
     H60.22   Malignant otitis externa, left ear
     H60.23   Malignant otitis externa, bilateral

√5ᵗʰ H60.3 Other infective otitis externa

   √6ᵗʰ H60.31 Diffuse otitis externa
     H60.311   Diffuse otitis externa, right ear
     H60.312   Diffuse otitis externa, left ear
     H60.313   Diffuse otitis externa, bilateral
     H60.319   Diffuse otitis externa, unspecified ear ▽

   √6ᵗʰ H60.32 Hemorrhagic otitis externa
     H60.321   Hemorrhagic otitis externa, right ear
     H60.322   Hemorrhagic otitis externa, left ear
     H60.323   Hemorrhagic otitis externa, bilateral
     H60.329   Hemorrhagic otitis externa, unspecified ear ▽

   √6ᵗʰ H60.33 Swimmer's ear
     DEF: Otitis externa; commonly occurs when water gets trapped in the ear after swimming.
     H60.331   Swimmer's ear, right ear
     H60.332   Swimmer's ear, left ear
     H60.333   Swimmer's ear, bilateral
     H60.339   Swimmer's ear, unspecified ear ▽

   √6ᵗʰ H60.39 Other infective otitis externa
     H60.391   Other infective otitis externa, right ear
     H60.392   Other infective otitis externa, left ear
     H60.393   Other infective otitis externa, bilateral
     H60.399   Other infective otitis externa, unspecified ear ▽

√5ᵗʰ H60.4 Cholesteatoma of external ear
Keratosis obturans of external ear (canal)

     EXCLUDES 2   cholesteatoma of middle ear (H71.-)
                   recurrent cholesteatoma of postmastoidectomy cavity (H95.0-)

     H60.40   Cholesteatoma of external ear, unspecified ear ▽
     H60.41   Cholesteatoma of right external ear
     H60.42   Cholesteatoma of left external ear
     H60.43   Cholesteatoma of external ear, bilateral

√5ᵗʰ H60.5 Acute noninfective otitis externa

   √6ᵗʰ H60.50 Unspecified acute noninfective otitis externa
     Acute otitis externa NOS
     H60.501   Unspecified acute noninfective otitis externa, right ear ▽
     H60.502   Unspecified acute noninfective otitis externa, left ear ▽
     H60.503   Unspecified acute noninfective otitis externa, bilateral ▽
     H60.509   Unspecified acute noninfective otitis externa, unspecified ear ▽

   √6ᵗʰ H60.51 Acute actinic otitis externa
     H60.511   Acute actinic otitis externa, right ear
     H60.512   Acute actinic otitis externa, left ear
     H60.513   Acute actinic otitis externa, bilateral
     H60.519   Acute actinic otitis externa, unspecified ear ▽

   √6ᵗʰ H60.52 Acute chemical otitis externa
     H60.521   Acute chemical otitis externa, right ear
     H60.522   Acute chemical otitis externa, left ear
     H60.523   Acute chemical otitis externa, bilateral
     H60.529   Acute chemical otitis externa, unspecified ear ▽

   √6ᵗʰ H60.53 Acute contact otitis externa
     H60.531   Acute contact otitis externa, right ear
     H60.532   Acute contact otitis externa, left ear
     H60.533   Acute contact otitis externa, bilateral
     H60.539   Acute contact otitis externa, unspecified ear ▽

   √6ᵗʰ H60.54 Acute eczematoid otitis externa
     H60.541   Acute eczematoid otitis externa, right ear
     H60.542   Acute eczematoid otitis externa, left ear
     H60.543   Acute eczematoid otitis externa, bilateral
     H60.549   Acute eczematoid otitis externa, unspecified ear ▽

   √6ᵗʰ H60.55 Acute reactive otitis externa
     H60.551   Acute reactive otitis externa, right ear
     H60.552   Acute reactive otitis externa, left ear
     H60.553   Acute reactive otitis externa, bilateral
     H60.559   Acute reactive otitis externa, unspecified ear ▽

   √6ᵗʰ H60.59 Other noninfective acute otitis externa
     H60.591   Other noninfective acute otitis externa, right ear
     H60.592   Other noninfective acute otitis externa, left ear
     H60.593   Other noninfective acute otitis externa, bilateral
     H60.599   Other noninfective acute otitis externa, unspecified ear ▽

√5ᵗʰ H60.6 Unspecified chronic otitis externa
     H60.60   Unspecified chronic otitis externa, unspecified ear ▽
     H60.61   Unspecified chronic otitis externa, right ear ▽
     H60.62   Unspecified chronic otitis externa, left ear ▽
     H60.63   Unspecified chronic otitis externa, bilateral ▽

√5ᵗʰ H60.8 Other otitis externa
   √6ᵗʰ H60.8X Other otitis externa
     H60.8X1   Other otitis externa, right ear
     H60.8X2   Other otitis externa, left ear
     H60.8X3   Other otitis externa, bilateral
     H60.8X9   Other otitis externa, unspecified ear ▽

√5ᵗʰ H60.9 Unspecified otitis externa
     H60.90   Unspecified otitis externa, unspecified ear ▽
     H60.91   Unspecified otitis externa, right ear ▽

EXCLUDES 1 Not coded here   *EXCLUDES 2* Not included here   **N** Newborn Age: 0   **P** Pediatric Age: 0-17   **M** Maternity Age: 12-55   **A** Adult Age: 15-124

606   ICD-10-CM 2018

H60.92   **Unspecified otitis externa, left ear**   ▽

H60.93   **Unspecified otitis externa, bilateral**   ▽

✓4ᵗʰ **H61**   **Other disorders of external ear**

   ✓5ᵗʰ **H61.0**   **Chondritis and perichondritis of external ear**
Chondrodermatitis nodularis chronica helicis
Perichondritis of auricle
Perichondritis of pinna

    ✓6ᵗʰ **H61.00**   **Unspecified perichondritis of external ear**

     H61.001   **Unspecified perichondritis of right external ear**   ▽

     H61.002   **Unspecified perichondritis of left external ear**   ▽

     H61.003   **Unspecified perichondritis of external ear, bilateral**   ▽

     H61.009   **Unspecified perichondritis of external ear, unspecified ear**   ▽

    ✓6ᵗʰ **H61.01**   **Acute perichondritis of external ear**

     H61.011   **Acute perichondritis of right external ear**

     H61.012   **Acute perichondritis of left external ear**

     H61.013   **Acute perichondritis of external ear, bilateral**

     H61.019   **Acute perichondritis of external ear, unspecified ear**   ▽

    ✓6ᵗʰ **H61.02**   **Chronic perichondritis of external ear**

     H61.021   **Chronic perichondritis of right external ear**

     H61.022   **Chronic perichondritis of left external ear**

     H61.023   **Chronic perichondritis of external ear, bilateral**

     H61.029   **Chronic perichondritis of external ear, unspecified ear**   ▽

    ✓6ᵗʰ **H61.03**   **Chondritis of external ear**
Chondritis of auricle
Chondritis of pinna
AHA: 2015, 1Q, 18
DEF: Infection that has progressed into the cartilage; presents as indurated and edematous skin over the pinna; vascular compromise occurs with tissue necrosis and deformity.

     H61.031   **Chondritis of right external ear**

     H61.032   **Chondritis of left external ear**

     H61.033   **Chondritis of external ear, bilateral**

     H61.039   **Chondritis of external ear, unspecified ear**   ▽

   ✓5ᵗʰ **H61.1**   **Noninfective disorders of pinna**
EXCLUDES 2   *cauliflower ear (M95.1-)*
              gouty tophi of ear (M1A.-)

    ✓6ᵗʰ **H61.10**   **Unspecified noninfective disorders of pinna**
Disorder of pinna NOS

     H61.101   **Unspecified noninfective disorders of pinna, right ear**   ▽

     H61.102   **Unspecified noninfective disorders of pinna, left ear**   ▽

     H61.103   **Unspecified noninfective disorders of pinna, bilateral**   ▽

     H61.109   **Unspecified noninfective disorders of pinna, unspecified ear**   ▽

    ✓6ᵗʰ **H61.11**   **Acquired deformity of pinna**
Acquired deformity of auricle
EXCLUDES 2   *cauliflower ear (M95.1-)*

     H61.111   **Acquired deformity of pinna, right ear**

     H61.112   **Acquired deformity of pinna, left ear**

     H61.113   **Acquired deformity of pinna, bilateral**

     H61.119   **Acquired deformity of pinna, unspecified ear**   ▽

    ✓6ᵗʰ **H61.12**   **Hematoma of pinna**
Hematoma of auricle

     H61.121   **Hematoma of pinna, right ear**

     H61.122   **Hematoma of pinna, left ear**

     H61.123   **Hematoma of pinna, bilateral**

     H61.129   **Hematoma of pinna, unspecified ear**   ▽

    ✓6ᵗʰ **H61.19**   **Other noninfective disorders of pinna**

     H61.191   **Noninfective disorders of pinna, right ear**

     H61.192   **Noninfective disorders of pinna, left ear**

     H61.193   **Noninfective disorders of pinna, bilateral**

     H61.199   **Noninfective disorders of pinna, unspecified ear**   ▽

   ✓5ᵗʰ **H61.2**   **Impacted cerumen**
Wax in ear

     H61.20   **Impacted cerumen, unspecified ear**   ▽

     H61.21   **Impacted cerumen, right ear**

     H61.22   **Impacted cerumen, left ear**

     H61.23   **Impacted cerumen, bilateral**

   ✓5ᵗʰ **H61.3**   **Acquired stenosis of external ear canal**
Collapse of external ear canal
EXCLUDES 1   *postprocedural stenosis of external ear canal (H95.81-)*

    ✓6ᵗʰ **H61.30**   **Acquired stenosis of external ear canal, unspecified**

     H61.301   **Acquired stenosis of right external ear canal, unspecified**   ▽

     H61.302   **Acquired stenosis of left external ear canal, unspecified**   ▽

     H61.303   **Acquired stenosis of external ear canal, unspecified, bilateral**   ▽

     H61.309   **Acquired stenosis of external ear canal, unspecified, unspecified ear**   ▽

    ✓6ᵗʰ **H61.31**   **Acquired stenosis of external ear canal secondary to trauma**

     H61.311   **Acquired stenosis of right external ear canal secondary to trauma**

     H61.312   **Acquired stenosis of left external ear canal secondary to trauma**

     H61.313   **Acquired stenosis of external ear canal secondary to trauma, bilateral**

     H61.319   **Acquired stenosis of external ear canal secondary to trauma, unspecified ear**   ▽

    ✓6ᵗʰ **H61.32**   **Acquired stenosis of external ear canal secondary to inflammation and infection**
DEF: Narrowing of the external ear canal; due to chronic inflammation or infection.

     H61.321   **Acquired stenosis of right external ear canal secondary to inflammation and infection**

     H61.322   **Acquired stenosis of left external ear canal secondary to inflammation and infection**

     H61.323   **Acquired stenosis of external ear canal secondary to inflammation and infection, bilateral**

     H61.329   **Acquired stenosis of external ear canal secondary to inflammation and infection, unspecified ear**   ▽

    ✓6ᵗʰ **H61.39**   **Other acquired stenosis of external ear canal**

     H61.391   **Other acquired stenosis of right external ear canal**

     H61.392   **Other acquired stenosis of left external ear canal**

     H61.393   **Other acquired stenosis of external ear canal, bilateral**

     H61.399   **Other acquired stenosis of external ear canal, unspecified ear**   ▽

   ✓5ᵗʰ **H61.8**   **Other specified disorders of external ear**

    ✓6ᵗʰ **H61.81**   **Exostosis of external canal**

     H61.811   **Exostosis of right external canal**

     H61.812   **Exostosis of left external canal**

     H61.813   **Exostosis of external canal, bilateral**

     H61.819   **Exostosis of external canal, unspecified ear**   ▽

    ✓6ᵗʰ **H61.89**   **Other specified disorders of external ear**

     H61.891   **Other specified disorders of right external ear**

     H61.892   **Other specified disorders of left external ear**

     H61.893   **Other specified disorders of external ear, bilateral**

     H61.899   **Other specified disorders of external ear, unspecified ear**   ▽

   ✓5ᵗʰ **H61.9**   **Disorder of external ear, unspecified**

     H61.90   **Disorder of external ear, unspecified, unspecified ear**   ▽

     H61.91   **Disorder of right external ear, unspecified**   ▽

     H61.92   **Disorder of left external ear, unspecified**   ▽

     H61.93   **Disorder of external ear, unspecified, bilateral**   ▽

✓ Additional Character Req   ✓x7ᵗʰ Placeholder Alert   Manifestation   HCC CMS-HCC Condition   ▽ Unspecified Code   ►◄ Revised Text   ● New Code   ▲ Revised Code Title

ICD-10-CM 2018   607

Chapter 8. Diseases of the Ear and Mastoid Process

✓4th **H62** **Disorders of external ear in diseases classified elsewhere**

  ✓5th **H62.4** **Otitis externa in other diseases classified elsewhere**

    Code first underlying disease, such as:
      erysipelas (A46)
      impetigo (L01.0)

      EXCLUDES 1 otitis externa (in):
          candidiasis (B37.84)
          herpes viral [herpes simplex] (B00.1)
          herpes zoster (B02.8)

    H62.40 *Otitis externa in other diseases classified elsewhere, unspecified ear* ▽

    H62.41 *Otitis externa in other diseases classified elsewhere, right ear*

    H62.42 *Otitis externa in other diseases classified elsewhere, left ear*

    H62.43 *Otitis externa in other diseases classified elsewhere, bilateral*

  ✓5th **H62.8** **Other disorders of external ear in diseases classified elsewhere**

    Code first underlying disease, such as:
      gout (M1A.-, M10.-)

    ✓6th **H62.8X** **Other disorders of external ear in diseases classified elsewhere**

      H62.8X1 *Other disorders of right external ear in diseases classified elsewhere*

      H62.8X2 *Other disorders of left external ear in diseases classified elsewhere*

      H62.8X3 *Other disorders of external ear in diseases classified elsewhere, bilateral*

      H62.8X9 *Other disorders of external ear in diseases classified elsewhere, unspecified ear* ▽

Diseases of middle ear and mastoid (H65-H75)

✓4th **H65** **Nonsuppurative otitis media**

  INCLUDES nonsuppurative otitis media with myringitis

  Use additional code for any associated perforated tympanic membrane (H72.-)

  Use additional code to identify:
    exposure to environmental tobacco smoke (Z77.22)
    exposure to tobacco smoke in the perinatal period (P96.81)
    history of tobacco dependence (Z87.891)
    occupational exposure to environmental tobacco smoke (Z57.31)
    tobacco dependence (F17.-)
    tobacco use (Z72.0)

  ✓5th **H65.0** **Acute serous otitis media**

    Acute and subacute secretory otitis

    H65.00 **Acute serous otitis media, unspecified ear** ▽

    H65.01 **Acute serous otitis media, right ear**

    H65.02 **Acute serous otitis media, left ear**

    H65.03 **Acute serous otitis media, bilateral**

    H65.04 **Acute serous otitis media, recurrent, right ear**

    H65.05 **Acute serous otitis media, recurrent, left ear**

    H65.06 **Acute serous otitis media, recurrent, bilateral**

    H65.07 **Acute serous otitis media, recurrent, unspecified ear** ▽

  ✓5th **H65.1** **Other acute nonsuppurative otitis media**

    EXCLUDES 1 otitic barotrauma (T70.0)
          otitis media (acute) NOS (H66.9)

    ✓6th **H65.11** **Acute and subacute allergic otitis media (mucoid) (sanguinous) (serous)**

      H65.111 **Acute and subacute allergic otitis media (mucoid) (sanguinous) (serous), right ear**

      H65.112 **Acute and subacute allergic otitis media (mucoid) (sanguinous) (serous), left ear**

      H65.113 **Acute and subacute allergic otitis media (mucoid) (sanguinous) (serous), bilateral**

      H65.114 **Acute and subacute allergic otitis media (mucoid) (sanguinous) (serous), recurrent, right ear**

      H65.115 **Acute and subacute allergic otitis media (mucoid) (sanguinous) (serous), recurrent, left ear**

      H65.116 **Acute and subacute allergic otitis media (mucoid) (sanguinous) (serous), recurrent, bilateral**

      H65.117 **Acute and subacute allergic otitis media (mucoid) (sanguinous) (serous), recurrent, unspecified ear** ▽

      H65.119 **Acute and subacute allergic otitis media (mucoid) (sanguinous) (serous), unspecified ear** ▽

    ✓6th **H65.19** **Other acute nonsuppurative otitis media**

      Acute and subacute mucoid otitis media
      Acute and subacute nonsuppurative otitis media NOS
      Acute and subacute sanguinous otitis media
      Acute and subacute seromucinous otitis media

      H65.191 **Other acute nonsuppurative otitis media, right ear**

      H65.192 **Other acute nonsuppurative otitis media, left ear**

      H65.193 **Other acute nonsuppurative otitis media, bilateral**

      H65.194 **Other acute nonsuppurative otitis media, recurrent, right ear**

      H65.195 **Other acute nonsuppurative otitis media, recurrent, left ear**

      H65.196 **Other acute nonsuppurative otitis media, recurrent, bilateral**

      H65.197 **Other acute nonsuppurative otitis media recurrent, unspecified ear** ▽

      H65.199 **Other acute nonsuppurative otitis media, unspecified ear** ▽

  ✓5th **H65.2** **Chronic serous otitis media**

    Chronic tubotympanal catarrh

    H65.20 **Chronic serous otitis media, unspecified ear** ▽

    H65.21 **Chronic serous otitis media, right ear**

    H65.22 **Chronic serous otitis media, left ear**

    H65.23 **Chronic serous otitis media, bilateral**

  ✓5th **H65.3** **Chronic mucoid otitis media**

    Chronic mucinous otitis media
    Chronic secretory otitis media
    Chronic transudative otitis media
    Glue ear

      EXCLUDES 1 adhesive middle ear disease (H74.1)

    H65.30 **Chronic mucoid otitis media, unspecified ear** ▽

    H65.31 **Chronic mucoid otitis media, right ear**

    H65.32 **Chronic mucoid otitis media, left ear**

    H65.33 **Chronic mucoid otitis media, bilateral**

  ✓5th **H65.4** **Other chronic nonsuppurative otitis media**

    ✓6th **H65.41** **Chronic allergic otitis media**

      H65.411 **Chronic allergic otitis media, right ear**

      H65.412 **Chronic allergic otitis media, left ear**

      H65.413 **Chronic allergic otitis media, bilateral**

      H65.419 **Chronic allergic otitis media, unspecified ear** ▽

    ✓6th **H65.49** **Other chronic nonsuppurative otitis media**

      Chronic exudative otitis media
      Chronic nonsuppurative otitis media NOS
      Chronic otitis media with effusion (nonpurulent)
      Chronic seromucinous otitis media

      H65.491 **Other chronic nonsuppurative otitis media, right ear**

      H65.492 **Other chronic nonsuppurative otitis media, left ear**

      H65.493 **Other chronic nonsuppurative otitis media, bilateral**

      H65.499 **Other chronic nonsuppurative otitis media, unspecified ear** ▽

  ✓5th **H65.9** **Unspecified nonsuppurative otitis media**

    Allergic otitis media NOS   Secretory otitis media NOS
    Catarrhal otitis media NOS   Seromucinous otitis media NOS
    Exudative otitis media NOS   Serous otitis media NOS
    Mucoid otitis media NOS   Transudative otitis media NOS
    Otitis media with effusion
      (nonpurulent) NOS

    H65.90 **Unspecified nonsuppurative otitis media, unspecified ear** ▽

    H65.91 **Unspecified nonsuppurative otitis media, right ear** ▽

    H65.92 **Unspecified nonsuppurative otitis media, left ear** ▽

    H65.93 **Unspecified nonsuppurative otitis media, bilateral** ▽

EXCLUDES 1 Not coded here   *EXCLUDES 2* Not included here   **N** Newborn Age: 0   **P** Pediatric Age: 0-17   **M** Maternity Age: 12-55   **A** Adult Age: 15-124

608   ICD-10-CM 2018

☑4ᵗʰ H66 Suppurative and unspecified otitis media

INCLUDES suppurative and unspecified otitis media with myringitis
Use additional code to identify:
exposure to environmental tobacco smoke (Z77.22)
exposure to tobacco smoke in the perinatal period (P96.81)
history of tobacco dependence (Z87.891)
occupational exposure to environmental tobacco smoke (Z57.31)
tobacco dependence (F17.-)
tobacco use (Z72.0)
AHA: 2016, 1Q, 34

☑5ᵗʰ H66.0 Acute suppurative otitis media

☑6ᵗʰ H66.00 Acute suppurative otitis media without spontaneous rupture of ear drum

- **H66.001** Acute suppurative otitis media without spontaneous rupture of ear drum, right ear
- **H66.002** Acute suppurative otitis media without spontaneous rupture of ear drum, left ear
- **H66.003** Acute suppurative otitis media without spontaneous rupture of ear drum, bilateral
- **H66.004** Acute suppurative otitis media without spontaneous rupture of ear drum, recurrent, right ear
- **H66.005** Acute suppurative otitis media without spontaneous rupture of ear drum, recurrent, left ear
- **H66.006** Acute suppurative otitis media without spontaneous rupture of ear drum, recurrent, bilateral
- **H66.007** Acute suppurative otitis media without spontaneous rupture of ear drum, recurrent, unspecified ear ▽
- **H66.009** Acute suppurative otitis media without spontaneous rupture of ear drum, unspecified ear ▽

☑6ᵗʰ H66.01 Acute suppurative otitis media with spontaneous rupture of ear drum
DEF: Sudden, severe inflammation of middle ear, with pressure causing the perforation of ear drum tissue.
- **H66.011** Acute suppurative otitis media with spontaneous rupture of ear drum, right ear
- **H66.012** Acute suppurative otitis media with spontaneous rupture of ear drum, left ear
- **H66.013** Acute suppurative otitis media with spontaneous rupture of ear drum, bilateral
- **H66.014** Acute suppurative otitis media with spontaneous rupture of ear drum, recurrent, right ear
- **H66.015** Acute suppurative otitis media with spontaneous rupture of ear drum, recurrent, left ear
- **H66.016** Acute suppurative otitis media with spontaneous rupture of ear drum, recurrent, bilateral
- **H66.017** Acute suppurative otitis media with spontaneous rupture of ear drum, recurrent, unspecified ear ▽
- **H66.019** Acute suppurative otitis media with spontaneous rupture of ear drum, unspecified ear ▽

☑5ᵗʰ H66.1 Chronic tubotympanic suppurative otitis media
Benign chronic suppurative otitis media
Chronic tubotympanic disease
Use additional code for any associated perforated tympanic membrane (H72.-)
- **H66.10** Chronic tubotympanic suppurative otitis media, unspecified ▽
- **H66.11** Chronic tubotympanic suppurative otitis media, right ear
- **H66.12** Chronic tubotympanic suppurative otitis media, left ear
- **H66.13** Chronic tubotympanic suppurative otitis media, bilateral

☑5ᵗʰ H66.2 Chronic atticoantral suppurative otitis media
Chronic atticoantral disease
Use additional code for any associated perforated tympanic membrane (H72.-)
- **H66.20** Chronic atticoantral suppurative otitis media, unspecified ear ▽
- **H66.21** Chronic atticoantral suppurative otitis media, right ear
- **H66.22** Chronic atticoantral suppurative otitis media, left ear
- **H66.23** Chronic atticoantral suppurative otitis media, bilateral

☑5ᵗʰ H66.3 Other chronic suppurative otitis media
Chronic suppurative otitis media NOS
Use additional code for any associated perforated tympanic membrane (H72.-)
EXCLUDES 1 tuberculous otitis media (A18.6)

☑6ᵗʰ H66.3X Other chronic suppurative otitis media
- **H66.3X1** Other chronic suppurative otitis media, right ear
- **H66.3X2** Other chronic suppurative otitis media, left ear
- **H66.3X3** Other chronic suppurative otitis media, bilateral
- **H66.3X9** Other chronic suppurative otitis media, unspecified ear ▽

☑5ᵗʰ H66.4 Suppurative otitis media, unspecified
Purulent otitis media NOS
Use additional code for any associated perforated tympanic membrane (H72.-)
- **H66.40** Suppurative otitis media, unspecified, unspecified ear ▽
- **H66.41** Suppurative otitis media, unspecified, right ear
- **H66.42** Suppurative otitis media, unspecified, left ear
- **H66.43** Suppurative otitis media, unspecified, bilateral

☑5ᵗʰ H66.9 Otitis media, unspecified
Otitis media NOS
Acute otitis media NOS
Chronic otitis media NOS
Use additional code for any associated perforated tympanic membrane (H72.-)
- **H66.90** Otitis media, unspecified, unspecified ear ▽
- **H66.91** Otitis media, unspecified, right ear ▽
- **H66.92** Otitis media, unspecified, left ear ▽
- **H66.93** Otitis media, unspecified, bilateral ▽

☑4ᵗʰ H67 Otitis media in diseases classified elsewhere
Code first underlying disease, such as:
viral disease NEC (B00-B34)
Use additional code for any associated perforated tympanic membrane (H72.-)
EXCLUDES 1 otitis media in:
influenza (J09.X9, J10.83, J11.83)
measles (B05.3)
scarlet fever (A38.0)
tuberculosis (A18.6)

- **H67.1** *Otitis media in diseases classified elsewhere, right ear*
- **H67.2** *Otitis media in diseases classified elsewhere, left ear*
- **H67.3** *Otitis media in diseases classified elsewhere, bilateral*
- **H67.9** *Otitis media in diseases classified elsewhere, unspecified ear* ▽

☑4ᵗʰ H68 Eustachian salpingitis and obstruction

☑5ᵗʰ H68.0 Eustachian salpingitis

☑6ᵗʰ H68.00 Unspecified Eustachian salpingitis
- **H68.001** Unspecified Eustachian salpingitis, right ear ▽
- **H68.002** Unspecified Eustachian salpingitis, left ear ▽
- **H68.003** Unspecified Eustachian salpingitis, bilateral ▽
- **H68.009** Unspecified Eustachian salpingitis, unspecified ear ▽

☑6ᵗʰ H68.01 Acute Eustachian salpingitis
- **H68.011** Acute Eustachian salpingitis, right ear
- **H68.012** Acute Eustachian salpingitis, left ear
- **H68.013** Acute Eustachian salpingitis, bilateral

H68.019 Acute Eustachian salpingitis, unspecified ear ▽

✓6ᵗʰ H68.02 Chronic Eustachian salpingitis
- **H68.021 Chronic Eustachian salpingitis, right ear**
- **H68.022 Chronic Eustachian salpingitis, left ear**
- **H68.023 Chronic Eustachian salpingitis, bilateral**
- **H68.029 Chronic Eustachian salpingitis, unspecified ear** ▽

✓5ᵗʰ H68.1 Obstruction of Eustachian tube
Stenosis of Eustachian tube   Stricture of Eustachian tube

✓6ᵗʰ H68.10 Unspecified obstruction of Eustachian tube
- **H68.101 Unspecified obstruction of Eustachian tube, right ear** ▽
- **H68.102 Unspecified obstruction of Eustachian tube, left ear** ▽
- **H68.103 Unspecified obstruction of Eustachian tube, bilateral** ▽
- **H68.109 Unspecified obstruction of Eustachian tube, unspecified ear** ▽

✓6ᵗʰ H68.11 Osseous obstruction of Eustachian tube
- **H68.111 Osseous obstruction of Eustachian tube, right ear**
- **H68.112 Osseous obstruction of Eustachian tube, left ear**
- **H68.113 Osseous obstruction of Eustachian tube, bilateral**
- **H68.119 Osseous obstruction of Eustachian tube, unspecified ear** ▽

✓6ᵗʰ H68.12 Intrinsic cartilagenous obstruction of Eustachian tube
- **H68.121 Intrinsic cartilagenous obstruction of Eustachian tube, right ear**
- **H68.122 Intrinsic cartilagenous obstruction of Eustachian tube, left ear**
- **H68.123 Intrinsic cartilagenous obstruction of Eustachian tube, bilateral**
- **H68.129 Intrinsic cartilagenous obstruction of Eustachian tube, unspecified ear** ▽

✓6ᵗʰ H68.13 Extrinsic cartilagenous obstruction of Eustachian tube
Compression of Eustachian tube
- **H68.131 Extrinsic cartilagenous obstruction of Eustachian tube, right ear**
- **H68.132 Extrinsic cartilagenous obstruction of Eustachian tube, left ear**
- **H68.133 Extrinsic cartilagenous obstruction of Eustachian tube, bilateral**
- **H68.139 Extrinsic cartilagenous obstruction of Eustachian tube, unspecified ear** ▽

✓4ᵗʰ H69 Other and unspecified disorders of Eustachian tube

✓5ᵗʰ H69.0 Patulous Eustachian tube
- **H69.00 Patulous Eustachian tube, unspecified ear** ▽
- **H69.01 Patulous Eustachian tube, right ear**
- **H69.02 Patulous Eustachian tube, left ear**
- **H69.03 Patulous Eustachian tube, bilateral**

✓5ᵗʰ H69.8 Other specified disorders of Eustachian tube
- **H69.80 Other specified disorders of Eustachian tube, unspecified ear** ▽
- **H69.81 Other specified disorders of Eustachian tube, right ear**
- **H69.82 Other specified disorders of Eustachian tube, left ear**
- **H69.83 Other specified disorders of Eustachian tube, bilateral**

✓5ᵗʰ H69.9 Unspecified Eustachian tube disorder
- **H69.90 Unspecified Eustachian tube disorder, unspecified ear** ▽
- **H69.91 Unspecified Eustachian tube disorder, right ear** ▽
- **H69.92 Unspecified Eustachian tube disorder, left ear** ▽
- **H69.93 Unspecified Eustachian tube disorder, bilateral** ▽

✓4ᵗʰ H70 Mastoiditis and related conditions

✓5ᵗʰ H70.0 Acute mastoiditis
Abscess of mastoid
Empyema of mastoid

✓6ᵗʰ H70.00 Acute mastoiditis without complications
- **H70.001 Acute mastoiditis without complications, right ear**
- **H70.002 Acute mastoiditis without complications, left ear**
- **H70.003 Acute mastoiditis without complications, bilateral**
- **H70.009 Acute mastoiditis without complications, unspecified ear** ▽

✓6ᵗʰ H70.01 Subperiosteal abscess of mastoid
- **H70.011 Subperiosteal abscess of mastoid, right ear**
- **H70.012 Subperiosteal abscess of mastoid, left ear**
- **H70.013 Subperiosteal abscess of mastoid, bilateral**
- **H70.019 Subperiosteal abscess of mastoid, unspecified ear** ▽

✓6ᵗʰ H70.09 Acute mastoiditis with other complications
- **H70.091 Acute mastoiditis with other complications, right ear**
- **H70.092 Acute mastoiditis with other complications, left ear**
- **H70.093 Acute mastoiditis with other complications, bilateral**
- **H70.099 Acute mastoiditis with other complications, unspecified ear** ▽

✓5ᵗʰ H70.1 Chronic mastoiditis
Caries of mastoid
Fistula of mastoid
EXCLUDES 1 *tuberculous mastoiditis (A18.03)*
- **H70.10 Chronic mastoiditis, unspecified ear** ▽
- **H70.11 Chronic mastoiditis, right ear**
- **H70.12 Chronic mastoiditis, left ear**
- **H70.13 Chronic mastoiditis, bilateral**

✓5ᵗʰ H70.2 Petrositis
Inflammation of petrous bone

✓6ᵗʰ H70.20 Unspecified petrositis
- **H70.201 Unspecified petrositis, right ear** ▽
- **H70.202 Unspecified petrositis, left ear** ▽
- **H70.203 Unspecified petrositis, bilateral** ▽
- **H70.209 Unspecified petrositis, unspecified ear** ▽

✓6ᵗʰ H70.21 Acute petrositis
DEF: Sudden, severe inflammation of petrous temporal bone behind the ear; associated with middle ear infection.
- **H70.211 Acute petrositis, right ear**
- **H70.212 Acute petrositis, left ear**
- **H70.213 Acute petrositis, bilateral**
- **H70.219 Acute petrositis, unspecified ear** ▽

✓6ᵗʰ H70.22 Chronic petrositis
- **H70.221 Chronic petrositis, right ear**
- **H70.222 Chronic petrositis, left ear**
- **H70.223 Chronic petrositis, bilateral**
- **H70.229 Chronic petrositis, unspecified ear** ▽

✓5ᵗʰ H70.8 Other mastoiditis and related conditions
EXCLUDES 1 *preauricular sinus and cyst (Q18.1)*
sinus, fistula, and cyst of branchial cleft (Q18.0)

✓6ᵗʰ H70.81 Postauricular fistula
- **H70.811 Postauricular fistula, right ear**
- **H70.812 Postauricular fistula, left ear**
- **H70.813 Postauricular fistula, bilateral**
- **H70.819 Postauricular fistula, unspecified ear** ▽

✓6ᵗʰ H70.89 Other mastoiditis and related conditions
- **H70.891 Other mastoiditis and related conditions, right ear**
- **H70.892 Other mastoiditis and related conditions, left ear**
- **H70.893 Other mastoiditis and related conditions, bilateral**
- **H70.899 Other mastoiditis and related conditions, unspecified ear** ▽

EXCLUDES 1 Not coded here   **EXCLUDES 2** Not included here   **N** Newborn Age: 0   **P** Pediatric Age: 0-17   **M** Maternity Age: 12-55   **A** Adult Age: 15-124

610

ICD-10-CM 2018

Chapter 8. Diseases of the Ear and Mastoid Process

Cholesteatoma of Middle Ear

Middle ear chamber

Ear drum

Cholesteatoma sac

✓5th **H70.9 Unspecified mastoiditis**
- H70.90 Unspecified mastoiditis, unspecified ear ▽
- H70.91 Unspecified mastoiditis, right ear ▽
- H70.92 Unspecified mastoiditis, left ear ▽
- H70.93 Unspecified mastoiditis, bilateral ▽

✓4th **H71 Cholesteatoma of middle ear**
> EXCLUDES 2   cholesteatoma of external ear (H60.4-)
> recurrent cholesteatoma of postmastoidectomy cavity (H95.0-)

✓5th **H71.0 Cholesteatoma of attic**
- H71.00 Cholesteatoma of attic, unspecified ear ▽
- H71.01 Cholesteatoma of attic, right ear
- H71.02 Cholesteatoma of attic, left ear
- H71.03 Cholesteatoma of attic, bilateral

✓5th **H71.1 Cholesteatoma of tympanum**
- H71.10 Cholesteatoma of tympanum, unspecified ear ▽
- H71.11 Cholesteatoma of tympanum, right ear
- H71.12 Cholesteatoma of tympanum, left ear
- H71.13 Cholesteatoma of tympanum, bilateral

✓5th **H71.2 Cholesteatoma of mastoid**
- H71.20 Cholesteatoma of mastoid, unspecified ear ▽
- H71.21 Cholesteatoma of mastoid, right ear
- H71.22 Cholesteatoma of mastoid, left ear
- H71.23 Cholesteatoma of mastoid, bilateral

✓5th **H71.3 Diffuse cholesteatosis**
- H71.30 Diffuse cholesteatosis, unspecified ear ▽
- H71.31 Diffuse cholesteatosis, right ear
- H71.32 Diffuse cholesteatosis, left ear
- H71.33 Diffuse cholesteatosis, bilateral

✓5th **H71.9 Unspecified cholesteatoma**
- H71.90 Unspecified cholesteatoma, unspecified ear ▽
- H71.91 Unspecified cholesteatoma, right ear ▽
- H71.92 Unspecified cholesteatoma, left ear ▽
- H71.93 Unspecified cholesteatoma, bilateral ▽

✓4th **H72 Perforation of tympanic membrane**
> INCLUDES   persistent post-traumatic perforation of ear drum
> postinflammatory perforation of ear drum

Code first any associated otitis media (H65.-, H66.1-, H66.2-, H66.3-, H66.4-, H66.9-, H67.-)

> EXCLUDES 1   acute suppurative otitis media with rupture of the tympanic
> membrane (H66.01-)
> traumatic rupture of ear drum (S09.2-)

✓5th **H72.0 Central perforation of tympanic membrane**
- H72.00 Central perforation of tympanic membrane, unspecified ear ▽
- H72.01 Central perforation of tympanic membrane, right ear
- H72.02 Central perforation of tympanic membrane, left ear
- H72.03 Central perforation of tympanic membrane, bilateral

✓5th **H72.1 Attic perforation of tympanic membrane**
Perforation of pars flaccida
- H72.10 Attic perforation of tympanic membrane, unspecified ear ▽

- H72.11 Attic perforation of tympanic membrane, right ear
- H72.12 Attic perforation of tympanic membrane, left ear
- H72.13 Attic perforation of tympanic membrane, bilateral

✓5th **H72.2 Other marginal perforations of tympanic membrane**
- ✓6th **H72.2X Other marginal perforations of tympanic membrane**
  - H72.2X1 Other marginal perforations of tympanic membrane, right ear
  - H72.2X2 Other marginal perforations of tympanic membrane, left ear
  - H72.2X3 Other marginal perforations of tympanic membrane, bilateral
  - H72.2X9 Other marginal perforations of tympanic membrane, unspecified ear ▽

✓5th **H72.8 Other perforations of tympanic membrane**
- ✓6th **H72.81 Multiple perforations of tympanic membrane**
  - H72.811 Multiple perforations of tympanic membrane, right ear
  - H72.812 Multiple perforations of tympanic membrane, left ear
  - H72.813 Multiple perforations of tympanic membrane, bilateral
  - H72.819 Multiple perforations of tympanic membrane, unspecified ear ▽
- ✓6th **H72.82 Total perforations of tympanic membrane**
  - H72.821 Total perforations of tympanic membrane, right ear
  - H72.822 Total perforations of tympanic membrane, left ear
  - H72.823 Total perforations of tympanic membrane, bilateral
  - H72.829 Total perforations of tympanic membrane, unspecified ear ▽

✓5th **H72.9 Unspecified perforation of tympanic membrane**
- H72.90 Unspecified perforation of tympanic membrane, unspecified ear ▽
- H72.91 Unspecified perforation of tympanic membrane, right ear ▽
- H72.92 Unspecified perforation of tympanic membrane, left ear ▽
- H72.93 Unspecified perforation of tympanic membrane, bilateral ▽

✓4th **H73 Other disorders of tympanic membrane**
✓5th **H73.0 Acute myringitis**
> EXCLUDES 1   acute myringitis with otitis media (H65, H66)

- ✓6th **H73.00 Unspecified acute myringitis**
  Acute tympanitis NOS
  - H73.001 Acute myringitis, right ear
  - H73.002 Acute myringitis, left ear
  - H73.003 Acute myringitis, bilateral
  - H73.009 Acute myringitis, unspecified ear ▽
- ✓6th **H73.01 Bullous myringitis**
  DEF: Bacterial or viral otitis media; characterized by the appearance of serous or hemorrhagic blebs on the ear drum and sudden onset of severe pain in ear.
  - H73.011 Bullous myringitis, right ear
  - H73.012 Bullous myringitis, left ear
  - H73.013 Bullous myringitis, bilateral
  - H73.019 Bullous myringitis, unspecified ear ▽
- ✓6th **H73.09 Other acute myringitis**
  - H73.091 Other acute myringitis, right ear
  - H73.092 Other acute myringitis, left ear
  - H73.093 Other acute myringitis, bilateral
  - H73.099 Other acute myringitis, unspecified ear ▽

✓5th **H73.1 Chronic myringitis**
Chronic tympanitis
> EXCLUDES 1   chronic myringitis with otitis media (H65, H66)
- H73.10 Chronic myringitis, unspecified ear ▽
- H73.11 Chronic myringitis, right ear
- H73.12 Chronic myringitis, left ear
- H73.13 Chronic myringitis, bilateral

✓5th **H73.2 Unspecified myringitis**
- H73.20 Unspecified myringitis, unspecified ear ▽
- H73.21 Unspecified myringitis, right ear ▽
- H73.22 Unspecified myringitis, left ear ▽

✓ Additional Character Req   ✓7th Placeholder Alert   Manifestation   HCC CMS-HCC Condition   ▽ Unspecified Code   ►◄ Revised Text   ● New Code   ▲ Revised Code Title

ICD-10-CM 2018   611

H70.9–H73.22

     H73.23   Unspecified myringitis, bilateral ▽

✓5ᵗʰ **H73.8**   **Other specified disorders of tympanic membrane**

   ✓6ᵗʰ **H73.81**   **Atrophic flaccid tympanic membrane**

     H73.811   Atrophic flaccid tympanic membrane, **right ear**

     H73.812   Atrophic flaccid tympanic membrane, **left ear**

     H73.813   Atrophic flaccid tympanic membrane, **bilateral**

     H73.819   Atrophic flaccid tympanic membrane, **unspecified ear** ▽

   ✓6ᵗʰ **H73.82**   **Atrophic nonflaccid tympanic membrane**

     H73.821   Atrophic nonflaccid tympanic membrane, **right ear**

     H73.822   Atrophic nonflaccid tympanic membrane, **left ear**

     H73.823   Atrophic nonflaccid tympanic membrane, **bilateral**

     H73.829   Atrophic nonflaccid tympanic membrane, **unspecified ear** ▽

   ✓6ᵗʰ **H73.89**   **Other specified disorders of tympanic membrane**

     H73.891   Other specified disorders of tympanic membrane, **right ear**

     H73.892   Other specified disorders of tympanic membrane, **left ear**

     H73.893   Other specified disorders of tympanic membrane, **bilateral**

     H73.899   Other specified disorders of tympanic membrane, **unspecified ear** ▽

✓5ᵗʰ **H73.9**   **Unspecified disorder of tympanic membrane**

   H73.90   Unspecified disorder of tympanic membrane, **unspecified ear** ▽

   H73.91   Unspecified disorder of tympanic membrane, **right ear** ▽

   H73.92   Unspecified disorder of tympanic membrane, **left ear** ▽

   H73.93   Unspecified disorder of tympanic membrane, **bilateral** ▽

✓4ᵗʰ **H74**   **Other disorders of middle ear mastoid**

     EXCLUDES 2   *mastoiditis (H70.-)*

✓5ᵗʰ **H74.0**   **Tympanosclerosis**

     DEF: Calcification of tissue in the ear drum, middle ear bones, and middle ear canal.

   H74.01   Tympanosclerosis, **right ear**

   H74.02   Tympanosclerosis, **left ear**

   H74.03   Tympanosclerosis, **bilateral**

   H74.09   Tympanosclerosis, unspecified ear ▽

✓5ᵗʰ **H74.1**   **Adhesive middle ear disease**

     Adhesive otitis

     EXCLUDES 1   *glue ear (H65.3-)*

   H74.11   Adhesive **right** middle ear disease

   H74.12   Adhesive **left** middle ear disease

   H74.13   Adhesive middle ear disease, **bilateral**

   H74.19   Adhesive middle ear disease, unspecified ear ▽

✓5ᵗʰ **H74.2**   **Discontinuity and dislocation of ear ossicles**

   H74.20   Discontinuity and dislocation of ear ossicles, unspecified ear ▽

   H74.21   Discontinuity and dislocation of **right** ear ossicles

   H74.22   Discontinuity and dislocation of **left** ear ossicles

   H74.23   Discontinuity and dislocation of ear ossicles, **bilateral**

✓5ᵗʰ **H74.3**   **Other acquired abnormalities of ear ossicles**

   ✓6ᵗʰ **H74.31**   **Ankylosis** of ear ossicles

     H74.311   Ankylosis of ear ossicles, **right ear**

     H74.312   Ankylosis of ear ossicles, **left ear**

     H74.313   Ankylosis of ear ossicles, **bilateral**

     H74.319   Ankylosis of ear ossicles, unspecified ear ▽

   ✓6ᵗʰ **H74.32**   **Partial loss** of ear ossicles

     H74.321   Partial loss of ear ossicles, **right ear**

     H74.322   Partial loss of ear ossicles, **left ear**

     H74.323   Partial loss of ear ossicles, **bilateral**

     H74.329   Partial loss of ear ossicles, unspecified ear ▽

   ✓6ᵗʰ **H74.39**   **Other acquired abnormalities of ear ossicles**

     H74.391   Other acquired abnormalities of **right** ear ossicles

     H74.392   Other acquired abnormalities of **left** ear ossicles

     H74.393   Other acquired abnormalities of ear ossicles, **bilateral**

     H74.399   Other acquired abnormalities of ear ossicles, unspecified ear ▽

✓5ᵗʰ **H74.4**   **Polyp of middle ear**

   H74.40   Polyp of middle ear, unspecified ear ▽

   H74.41   Polyp of **right** middle ear

   H74.42   Polyp of **left** middle ear

   H74.43   Polyp of middle ear, **bilateral**

✓5ᵗʰ **H74.8**   **Other specified disorders of middle ear and mastoid**

   ✓6ᵗʰ **H74.8X**   **Other specified disorders of middle ear and mastoid**

     H74.8X1   Other specified disorders of **right** middle ear and mastoid

     H74.8X2   Other specified disorders of **left** middle ear and mastoid

     H74.8X3   Other specified disorders of middle ear and mastoid, **bilateral**

     H74.8X9   Other specified disorders of middle ear and mastoid, unspecified ear ▽

✓5ᵗʰ **H74.9**   **Unspecified disorder of middle ear and mastoid**

   H74.90   Unspecified disorder of middle ear and mastoid, unspecified ear ▽

   H74.91   Unspecified disorder of **right** middle ear and mastoid ▽

   H74.92   Unspecified disorder of **left** middle ear and mastoid ▽

   H74.93   Unspecified disorder of middle ear and mastoid, **bilateral** ▽

✓4ᵗʰ **H75**   **Other disorders of middle ear and mastoid in diseases classified elsewhere**

     Code first underlying disease

✓5ᵗʰ **H75.0**   **Mastoiditis in infectious and parasitic diseases classified elsewhere**

     EXCLUDES 1   *mastoiditis (in):*
             syphilis (A52.77)
             tuberculosis (A18.03)

   H75.00   *Mastoiditis in infectious and parasitic diseases classified elsewhere, unspecified ear* ▽

   H75.01   *Mastoiditis in infectious and parasitic diseases classified elsewhere, right ear*

   H75.02   *Mastoiditis in infectious and parasitic diseases classified elsewhere, left ear*

   H75.03   *Mastoiditis in infectious and parasitic diseases classified elsewhere, bilateral*

✓5ᵗʰ **H75.8**   **Other specified disorders of middle ear and mastoid in diseases classified elsewhere**

   H75.80   *Other specified disorders of middle ear and mastoid in diseases classified elsewhere, unspecified ear* ▽

   H75.81   *Other specified disorders of right middle ear and mastoid in diseases classified elsewhere*

   H75.82   *Other specified disorders of left middle ear and mastoid in diseases classified elsewhere*

   H75.83   *Other specified disorders of middle ear and mastoid in diseases classified elsewhere, bilateral*

Diseases of inner ear (H80-H83)

✓4ᵗʰ **H80**   **Otosclerosis**

     INCLUDES   otospongiosis

✓5ᵗʰ **H80.0**   **Otosclerosis involving oval window, nonobliterative**

   H80.00   Otosclerosis involving oval window, nonobliterative, unspecified ear ▽

   H80.01   Otosclerosis involving oval window, nonobliterative, **right ear**

   H80.02   Otosclerosis involving oval window, nonobliterative, **left ear**

   H80.03   Otosclerosis involving oval window, nonobliterative, **bilateral**

EXCLUDES 1   Not coded here   EXCLUDES 2   Not included here   **N** Newborn Age: 0   **P** Pediatric Age: 0-17   **M** Maternity Age: 12-55   **A** Adult Age: 15-124

612   ICD-10-CM 2018

✓5ᵗʰ **H80.1 Otosclerosis involving oval window, obliterative**

     H80.10 Otosclerosis involving oval window, obliterative, unspecified ear ▽

     H80.11 Otosclerosis involving oval window, obliterative, right ear

     H80.12 Otosclerosis involving oval window, obliterative, left ear

     H80.13 Otosclerosis involving oval window, obliterative, bilateral

✓5ᵗʰ **H80.2 Cochlear otosclerosis**
     Otosclerosis involving otic capsule
     Otosclerosis involving round window

     H80.20 Cochlear otosclerosis, unspecified ear ▽

     H80.21 Cochlear otosclerosis, right ear

     H80.22 Cochlear otosclerosis, left ear

     H80.23 Cochlear otosclerosis, bilateral

✓5ᵗʰ **H80.8 Other otosclerosis**

     H80.80 Other otosclerosis, unspecified ear ▽

     H80.81 Other otosclerosis, right ear

     H80.82 Other otosclerosis, left ear

     H80.83 Other otosclerosis, bilateral

✓5ᵗʰ **H80.9 Unspecified otosclerosis**

     H80.90 Unspecified otosclerosis, unspecified ear ▽

     H80.91 Unspecified otosclerosis, right ear ▽

     H80.92 Unspecified otosclerosis, left ear ▽

     H80.93 Unspecified otosclerosis, bilateral ▽

✓4ᵗʰ **H81 Disorders of vestibular function**
     EXCLUDES 1 epidemic vertigo (A88.1)
              vertigo NOS (R42)

✓5ᵗʰ **H81.0 Ménière's disease**
     Labyrinthine hydrops
     Ménière's syndrome or vertigo

     H81.01 Ménière's disease, right ear

     H81.02 Ménière's disease, left ear

     H81.03 Ménière's disease, bilateral

     H81.09 Ménière's disease, unspecified ear ▽

✓5ᵗʰ **H81.1 Benign paroxysmal vertigo**

     H81.10 Benign paroxysmal vertigo, unspecified ear ▽

     H81.11 Benign paroxysmal vertigo, right ear

     H81.12 Benign paroxysmal vertigo, left ear

     H81.13 Benign paroxysmal vertigo, bilateral

✓5ᵗʰ **H81.2 Vestibular neuronitis**
     DEF: Transient benign vertigo, caused by inflammation of the vestibular nerve; characterized by response to caloric stimulation on one side, nystagmus with rhythmic movement of eyes; normal auditory function present.

     H81.20 Vestibular neuronitis, unspecified ear ▽

     H81.21 Vestibular neuronitis, right ear

     H81.22 Vestibular neuronitis, left ear

     H81.23 Vestibular neuronitis, bilateral

✓5ᵗʰ **H81.3 Other peripheral vertigo**

     ✓6ᵗʰ **H81.31 Aural vertigo**

         H81.311 Aural vertigo, right ear

         H81.312 Aural vertigo, left ear

         H81.313 Aural vertigo, bilateral

         H81.319 Aural vertigo, unspecified ear ▽

     ✓6ᵗʰ **H81.39 Other peripheral vertigo**
         Lermoyez' syndrome
         Otogenic vertigo
         Peripheral vertigo NOS

         H81.391 Other peripheral vertigo, right ear

         H81.392 Other peripheral vertigo, left ear

         H81.393 Other peripheral vertigo, bilateral

         H81.399 Other peripheral vertigo, unspecified ear ▽

✓5ᵗʰ **H81.4 Vertigo of central origin**
     Central positional nystagmus

     H81.41 Vertigo of central origin, right ear

     H81.42 Vertigo of central origin, left ear

     H81.43 Vertigo of central origin, bilateral

     H81.49 Vertigo of central origin, unspecified ear ▽

✓5ᵗʰ **H81.8 Other disorders of vestibular function**

     ✓6ᵗʰ **H81.8X Other disorders of vestibular function**

         H81.8X1 Other disorders of vestibular function, right ear

         H81.8X2 Other disorders of vestibular function, left ear

         H81.8X3 Other disorders of vestibular function, bilateral

         H81.8X9 Other disorders of vestibular function, unspecified ear ▽

✓5ᵗʰ **H81.9 Unspecified disorder of vestibular function**
     Vertiginous syndrome NOS

     H81.90 Unspecified disorder of vestibular function, unspecified ear ▽

     H81.91 Unspecified disorder of vestibular function, right ear ▽

     H81.92 Unspecified disorder of vestibular function, left ear ▽

     H81.93 Unspecified disorder of vestibular function, bilateral ▽

✓4ᵗʰ **H82 Vertiginous syndromes in diseases classified elsewhere**
     Code first underlying disease
     EXCLUDES 1 epidemic vertigo (A88.1)

     H82.1 *Vertiginous syndromes in diseases classified elsewhere, right ear*

     H82.2 *Vertiginous syndromes in diseases classified elsewhere, left ear*

     H82.3 *Vertiginous syndromes in diseases classified elsewhere, bilateral*

     H82.9 *Vertiginous syndromes in diseases classified elsewhere, unspecified ear* ▽

✓4ᵗʰ **H83 Other diseases of inner ear**

✓5ᵗʰ **H83.0 Labyrinthitis**
     DEF: Inflammation of the inner ear, or labyrinth; characterized by pus, vertigo, dizziness, nausea, and hearing loss.

     H83.01 Labyrinthitis, right ear

     H83.02 Labyrinthitis, left ear

     H83.03 Labyrinthitis, bilateral

     H83.09 Labyrinthitis, unspecified ear ▽

✓5ᵗʰ **H83.1 Labyrinthine fistula**

     H83.11 Labyrinthine fistula, right ear

     H83.12 Labyrinthine fistula, left ear

     H83.13 Labyrinthine fistula, bilateral

     H83.19 Labyrinthine fistula, unspecified ear ▽

✓5ᵗʰ **H83.2 Labyrinthine dysfunction**
     Labyrinthine hypersensitivity
     Labyrinthine hypofunction
     Labyrinthine loss of function
     DEF: Decreased function of the labyrinth sensors.

     ✓6ᵗʰ **H83.2X Labyrinthine dysfunction**

         H83.2X1 Labyrinthine dysfunction, right ear

         H83.2X2 Labyrinthine dysfunction, left ear

         H83.2X3 Labyrinthine dysfunction, bilateral

         H83.2X9 Labyrinthine dysfunction, unspecified ear ▽

✓5ᵗʰ **H83.3 Noise effects on inner ear**
     Acoustic trauma of inner ear
     Noise-induced hearing loss of inner ear

     ✓6ᵗʰ **H83.3X Noise effects on inner ear**

         H83.3X1 Noise effects on right inner ear

         H83.3X2 Noise effects on left inner ear

         H83.3X3 Noise effects on inner ear, bilateral

         H83.3X9 Noise effects on inner ear, unspecified ear ▽

✓5ᵗʰ **H83.8 Other specified diseases of inner ear**

     ✓6ᵗʰ **H83.8X Other specified diseases of inner ear**

         H83.8X1 Other specified diseases of right inner ear

         H83.8X2 Other specified diseases of left inner ear

         H83.8X3 Other specified diseases of inner ear, bilateral

         H83.8X9 Other specified diseases of inner ear, unspecified ear ▽

☑ Additional Character Req   ✓x7ᵗʰ Placeholder Alert   Manifestation   HCC CMS-HCC Condition   ▽ Unspecified Code   ▶◀ Revised Text   ● New Code   ▲ Revised Code Title

H83.9 ✓5ᵗʰ Unspecified disease of inner ear
     H83.90 Unspecified disease of inner ear, unspecified ear ▽
     H83.91 Unspecified disease of right inner ear ▽
     H83.92 Unspecified disease of left inner ear ▽
     H83.93 Unspecified disease of inner ear, bilateral ▽

Other disorders of ear (H90–H94)

✓4ᵗʰ **H90** Conductive and sensorineural hearing loss
     EXCLUDES 1   *deaf nonspeaking NEC (H91.3)*
           deafness NOS (H91.9-)
           hearing loss NOS (H91.9-)
           noise-induced hearing loss (H83.3-)
           ototoxic hearing loss (H91.0-)
           sudden (idiopathic) hearing loss (H91.2-)
     AHA: 2015, 2Q, 7
   H90.0 Conductive hearing loss, bilateral
   ✓5ᵗʰ **H90.1** Conductive hearing loss, unilateral with unrestricted hearing on the contralateral side
     H90.11 Conductive hearing loss, unilateral, right ear, with unrestricted hearing on the contralateral side
     H90.12 Conductive hearing loss, unilateral, left ear, with unrestricted hearing on the contralateral side
   H90.2 Conductive hearing loss, unspecified ▽
     Conductive deafness NOS
   H90.3 Sensorineural hearing loss, bilateral
   ✓5ᵗʰ **H90.4** Sensorineural hearing loss, unilateral with unrestricted hearing on the contralateral side
     H90.41 Sensorineural hearing loss, unilateral, right ear, with unrestricted hearing on the contralateral side
     H90.42 Sensorineural hearing loss, unilateral, left ear, with unrestricted hearing on the contralateral side
   H90.5 Unspecified sensorineural hearing loss ▽
     Central hearing loss NOS
     Congenital deafness NOS
     Neural hearing loss NOS
     Perceptive hearing loss NOS
     Sensorineural deafness NOS
     Sensory hearing loss NOS
     EXCLUDES 1   *abnormal auditory perception (H93.2-)*
           psychogenic deafness (F44.6)
   H90.6 Mixed conductive and sensorineural hearing loss, bilateral
     AHA: 2015, 2Q, 7
   ✓5ᵗʰ **H90.7** Mixed conductive and sensorineural hearing loss, unilateral with unrestricted hearing on the contralateral side
     H90.71 Mixed conductive and sensorineural hearing loss, unilateral, right ear, with unrestricted hearing on the contralateral side
     H90.72 Mixed conductive and sensorineural hearing loss, unilateral, left ear, with unrestricted hearing on the contralateral side
   H90.8 Mixed conductive and sensorineural hearing loss, unspecified ▽
   ✓5ᵗʰ **H90.A** Conductive and sensorineural hearing loss with restricted hearing on the contralateral side
     ✓6ᵗʰ **H90.A1** Conductive hearing loss, unilateral, with restricted hearing on the contralateral side
         H90.A11 Conductive hearing loss, unilateral, right ear with restricted hearing on the contralateral side
         H90.A12 Conductive hearing loss, unilateral, left ear with restricted hearing on the contralateral side
     ✓6ᵗʰ **H90.A2** Sensorineural hearing loss, unilateral, with restricted hearing on the contralateral side
         H90.A21 Sensorineural hearing loss, unilateral, right ear, with restricted hearing on the contralateral side
         H90.A22 Sensorineural hearing loss, unilateral, left ear, with restricted hearing on the contralateral side
     ✓6ᵗʰ **H90.A3** Mixed conductive and sensorineural hearing loss, unilateral with restricted hearing on the contralateral side
         H90.A31 Mixed conductive and sensorineural hearing loss, unilateral, right ear with restricted hearing on the contralateral side

         H90.A32 Mixed conductive and sensorineural hearing loss, unilateral, left ear with restricted hearing on the contralateral side

✓4ᵗʰ **H91** Other and unspecified hearing loss
     EXCLUDES 1   *abnormal auditory perception (H93.2-)*
           hearing loss as classified in H90-
           impacted cerumen (H61.2-)
           noise-induced hearing loss (H83.3-)
           psychogenic deafness (F44.6)
           transient ischemic deafness (H93.01-)
   ✓5ᵗʰ **H91.0** Ototoxic hearing loss
     Code first poisoning due to drug or toxin, if applicable (T36-T65 with fifth or sixth character 1-4 or 6)
     Use additional code for adverse effect, if applicable, to identify drug (T36-T50 with fifth or sixth character 5)
     H91.01 Ototoxic hearing loss, right ear
     H91.02 Ototoxic hearing loss, left ear
     H91.03 Ototoxic hearing loss, bilateral
     H91.09 Ototoxic hearing loss, unspecified ear ▽
   ✓5ᵗʰ **H91.1** Presbycusis
     Presbyacusia
     H91.10 Presbycusis, unspecified ear ▽
     H91.11 Presbycusis, right ear
     H91.12 Presbycusis, left ear
     H91.13 Presbycusis, bilateral
   ✓5ᵗʰ **H91.2** Sudden idiopathic hearing loss
     Sudden hearing loss NOS
     H91.20 Sudden idiopathic hearing loss, unspecified ear ▽
     H91.21 Sudden idiopathic hearing loss, right ear
     H91.22 Sudden idiopathic hearing loss, left ear
     H91.23 Sudden idiopathic hearing loss, bilateral
   H91.3 Deaf nonspeaking, not elsewhere classified
   ✓5ᵗʰ **H91.8** Other specified hearing loss
     ✓6ᵗʰ **H91.8X** Other specified hearing loss
         H91.8X1 Other specified hearing loss, right ear
         H91.8X2 Other specified hearing loss, left ear
         H91.8X3 Other specified hearing loss, bilateral
         H91.8X9 Other specified hearing loss, unspecified ear ▽
   ✓5ᵗʰ **H91.9** Unspecified hearing loss
     Deafness NOS
     High frequency deafness
     Low frequency deafness
     H91.90 Unspecified hearing loss, unspecified ear ▽
     H91.91 Unspecified hearing loss, right ear ▽
     H91.92 Unspecified hearing loss, left ear ▽
     H91.93 Unspecified hearing loss, bilateral ▽
✓4ᵗʰ **H92** Otalgia and effusion of ear
   ✓5ᵗʰ **H92.0** Otalgia
     H92.01 Otalgia, right ear
     H92.02 Otalgia, left ear
     H92.03 Otalgia, bilateral
     H92.09 Otalgia, unspecified ear ▽
   ✓5ᵗʰ **H92.1** Otorrhea
     EXCLUDES 1   *leakage of cerebrospinal fluid through ear (G96.0)*
     H92.10 Otorrhea, unspecified ear ▽
     H92.11 Otorrhea, right ear
     H92.12 Otorrhea, left ear
     H92.13 Otorrhea, bilateral
   ✓5ᵗʰ **H92.2** Otorrhagia
     EXCLUDES 1   *traumatic otorrhagia—code to injury*
     H92.20 Otorrhagia, unspecified ear ▽
     H92.21 Otorrhagia, right ear
     H92.22 Otorrhagia, left ear
     H92.23 Otorrhagia, bilateral
✓4ᵗʰ **H93** Other disorders of ear, not elsewhere classified
   ✓5ᵗʰ **H93.0** Degenerative and vascular disorders of ear
     EXCLUDES 1   *presbycusis (H91.1)*
     ✓6ᵗʰ **H93.01** Transient ischemic deafness
         H93.011 Transient ischemic deafness, right ear
         H93.012 Transient ischemic deafness, left ear

EXCLUDES 1 Not coded here   EXCLUDES 2 Not included here   **N** Newborn Age: 0   **P** Pediatric Age: 0-17   **M** Maternity Age: 12-55   **A** Adult Age: 15-124

614   ICD-10-CM 2018

      H93.013   **Transient ischemic deafness, bilateral**
      H93.019   **Transient ischemic deafness, unspecified ear** ▽

  ✓6th **H93.09**   **Unspecified degenerative and vascular disorders of ear**
      H93.091   **Unspecified degenerative and vascular disorders of right ear** ▽
      H93.092   **Unspecified degenerative and vascular disorders of left ear** ▽
      H93.093   **Unspecified degenerative and vascular disorders of ear, bilateral** ▽
      H93.099   **Unspecified degenerative and vascular disorders of unspecified ear** ▽

✓5th **H93.1**   **Tinnitus**
      H93.11   **Tinnitus, right ear**
      H93.12   **Tinnitus, left ear**
      H93.13   **Tinnitus, bilateral**
      H93.19   **Tinnitus, unspecified ear** ▽

✓5th **H93.A**   **Pulsatile Tinnitus**
      H93.A1   **Pulsatile tinnitus, right ear**
      H93.A2   **Pulsatile tinnitus, left ear**
      H93.A3   **Pulsatile tinnitus, bilateral**
      H93.A9   **Pulsatile tinnitus, unspecified ear** ▽

✓5th **H93.2**   **Other abnormal auditory perceptions**
      EXCLUDES 2   *auditory hallucinations (R44.0)*

  ✓6th **H93.21**   **Auditory recruitment**
      H93.211   **Auditory recruitment, right ear**
      H93.212   **Auditory recruitment, left ear**
      H93.213   **Auditory recruitment, bilateral**
      H93.219   **Auditory recruitment, unspecified ear** ▽

  ✓6th **H93.22**   **Diplacusis**
      H93.221   **Diplacusis, right ear**
      H93.222   **Diplacusis, left ear**
      H93.223   **Diplacusis, bilateral**
      H93.229   **Diplacusis, unspecified ear** ▽

  ✓6th **H93.23**   **Hyperacusis**
      DEF: Exceptionally acute sense of hearing caused by such conditions as Bell's palsy; this term may also refer to painful sensitivity to sounds.
      H93.231   **Hyperacusis, right ear**
      H93.232   **Hyperacusis, left ear**
      H93.233   **Hyperacusis, bilateral**
      H93.239   **Hyperacusis, unspecified ear** ▽

  ✓6th **H93.24**   **Temporary auditory threshold shift**
      H93.241   **Temporary auditory threshold shift, right ear**
      H93.242   **Temporary auditory threshold shift, left ear**
      H93.243   **Temporary auditory threshold shift, bilateral**
      H93.249   **Temporary auditory threshold shift, unspecified ear** ▽

      H93.25   **Central auditory processing disorder**
      Congenital auditory imperception
      Word deafness
      EXCLUDES 1   *mixed receptive-expressive language disorder (F80.2)*

  ✓6th **H93.29**   **Other abnormal auditory perceptions**
      H93.291   **Other abnormal auditory perceptions, right ear**
      H93.292   **Other abnormal auditory perceptions, left ear**
      H93.293   **Other abnormal auditory perceptions, bilateral**
      H93.299   **Other abnormal auditory perceptions, unspecified ear** ▽

✓5th **H93.3**   **Disorders of acoustic nerve**
      Disorder of 8th cranial nerve
      EXCLUDES 1   *acoustic neuroma (D33.3)*
             syphilitic acoustic neuritis (A52.15)

  ✓6th **H93.3X**   **Disorders of acoustic nerve**
      H93.3X1   **Disorders of right acoustic nerve**
      H93.3X2   **Disorders of left acoustic nerve**
      H93.3X3   **Disorders of bilateral acoustic nerves**
      H93.3X9   **Disorders of unspecified acoustic nerve** ▽

✓5th **H93.8**   **Other specified disorders of ear**
  ✓6th **H93.8X**   **Other specified disorders of ear**
      H93.8X1   **Other specified disorders of right ear**
      H93.8X2   **Other specified disorders of left ear**
      H93.8X3   **Other specified disorders of ear, bilateral**
      H93.8X9   **Other specified disorders of ear, unspecified ear** ▽

✓5th **H93.9**   **Unspecified disorder of ear**
      H93.90   **Unspecified disorder of ear, unspecified ear** ▽
      H93.91   **Unspecified disorder of right ear** ▽
      H93.92   **Unspecified disorder of left ear** ▽
      H93.93   **Unspecified disorder of ear, bilateral** ▽

✓4th **H94**   **Other disorders of ear in diseases classified elsewhere**
  ✓5th **H94.0**   **Acoustic neuritis in infectious and parasitic diseases classified elsewhere**
      Code first underlying disease, such as:
          parasitic disease (B65-B89)
      EXCLUDES 1   *acoustic neuritis (in):*
          herpes zoster (B02.29)
          syphilis (A52.15)

      H94.00   *Acoustic neuritis in infectious and parasitic diseases classified elsewhere, unspecified ear* ▽
      H94.01   *Acoustic neuritis in infectious and parasitic diseases classified elsewhere, right ear*
      H94.02   *Acoustic neuritis in infectious and parasitic diseases classified elsewhere, left ear*
      H94.03   *Acoustic neuritis in infectious and parasitic diseases classified elsewhere, bilateral*

  ✓5th **H94.8**   **Other specified disorders of ear in diseases classified elsewhere**
      Code first underlying disease, such as:
          congenital syphilis (A50.0)
      EXCLUDES 1   *aural myiasis (B87.4)*
          syphilitic labyrinthitis (A52.79)

      H94.80   *Other specified disorders of ear in diseases classified elsewhere, unspecified ear* ▽
      H94.81   *Other specified disorders of right ear in diseases classified elsewhere*
      H94.82   *Other specified disorders of left ear in diseases classified elsewhere*
      H94.83   *Other specified disorders of ear in diseases classified elsewhere, bilateral*

Intraoperative and postprocedural complications and disorders of ear and mastoid process, not elsewhere classified (H95)

✓4th **H95**   **Intraoperative and postprocedural complications and disorders of ear and mastoid process, not elsewhere classified**
  ✓5th **H95.0**   **Recurrent cholesteatoma of postmastoidectomy cavity**
      H95.00   **Recurrent cholesteatoma of postmastoidectomy cavity, unspecified ear** ▽
      H95.01   **Recurrent cholesteatoma of postmastoidectomy cavity, right ear**
      H95.02   **Recurrent cholesteatoma of postmastoidectomy cavity, left ear**
      H95.03   **Recurrent cholesteatoma of postmastoidectomy cavity, bilateral ears**

  ✓5th **H95.1**   **Other disorders of ear and mastoid process following mastoidectomy**
  ✓6th **H95.11**   **Chronic inflammation of postmastoidectomy cavity**
      H95.111   **Chronic inflammation of postmastoidectomy cavity, right ear**
      H95.112   **Chronic inflammation of postmastoidectomy cavity, left ear**
      H95.113   **Chronic inflammation of postmastoidectomy cavity, bilateral ears**
      H95.119   **Chronic inflammation of postmastoidectomy cavity, unspecified ear** ▽

  ✓6th **H95.12**   **Granulation of postmastoidectomy cavity**
      H95.121   **Granulation of postmastoidectomy cavity, right ear**
      H95.122   **Granulation of postmastoidectomy cavity, left ear**
      H95.123   **Granulation of postmastoidectomy cavity, bilateral ears**

✓ Additional Character Req   ✓x7th Placeholder Alert   Manifestation   HCC CMS-HCC Condition   ▽ Unspecified Code   ►◄ Revised Text   ● New Code   ▲ Revised Code Title

ICD-10-CM 2018   615

H95.129   **Granulation of postmastoidectomy** ▽
          cavity, unspecified ear

✓6ᵗʰ H95.13 **Mucosal cyst of postmastoidectomy cavity**

H95.131   **Mucosal cyst of postmastoidectomy**
          cavity, right ear

H95.132   **Mucosal cyst of postmastoidectomy**
          cavity, left ear

H95.133   **Mucosal cyst of postmastoidectomy**
          cavity, bilateral ears

H95.139   **Mucosal cyst of postmastoidectomy** ▽
          cavity, unspecified ear

✓6ᵗʰ H95.19 **Other disorders following mastoidectomy**

H95.191   **Other disorders following mastoidectomy,**
          right ear

H95.192   **Other disorders following mastoidectomy,**
          left ear

H95.193   **Other disorders following mastoidectomy,**
          bilateral ears

H95.199   **Other disorders following** ▽
          mastoidectomy, unspecified ear

✓5ᵗʰ **H95.2** **Intraoperative hemorrhage and hematoma of ear and**
       mastoid process complicating a procedure

> EXCLUDES 1   *intraoperative hemorrhage and hematoma of ear and*
>   *mastoid process due to accidental puncture or*
>   *laceration during a procedure (H95.3-)*

H95.21   **Intraoperative hemorrhage and hematoma of ear**
         and mastoid process complicating a procedure on
         the ear and mastoid process

H95.22   **Intraoperative hemorrhage and hematoma of ear**
         and mastoid process complicating other procedure

✓5ᵗʰ **H95.3** **Accidental puncture and laceration of ear and mastoid**
       process during a procedure

H95.31   **Accidental puncture and laceration of the ear and**
         mastoid process during a procedure on the ear and
         mastoid process

H95.32   **Accidental puncture and laceration of the ear and**
         mastoid process during other procedure

✓5ᵗʰ **H95.4** **Postprocedural hemorrhage of ear and mastoid process**
       following a procedure

H95.41   **Postprocedural hemorrhage of ear and mastoid**
         process following a procedure on
         the ear and mastoid process

H95.42   **Postprocedural hemorrhage of ear and mastoid**
         process following other procedure

✓5ᵗʰ **H95.5** **Postprocedural hematoma and seroma of ear and mastoid**
       process following a procedure

H95.51   **Postprocedural hematoma of ear and mastoid**
         process following a procedure on the ear and
         mastoid process

H95.52   **Postprocedural hematoma of ear and mastoid**
         process following other procedure

H95.53   **Postprocedural seroma of ear and mastoid process**
         following a procedure on the ear and mastoid
         process

H95.54   **Postprocedural seroma of ear and mastoid process**
         following other procedure

✓5ᵗʰ **H95.8** **Other intraoperative and postprocedural complications and**
       disorders of the ear and mastoid process, not elsewhere
       classified

> EXCLUDES 2   *postprocedural complications and disorders following*
>   *mastoidectomy (H95.0-, H95.1-)*

✓6ᵗʰ **H95.81** **Postprocedural stenosis of external ear canal**

H95.811   **Postprocedural stenosis of right external**
          ear canal

H95.812   **Postprocedural stenosis of left external**
          ear canal

H95.813   **Postprocedural stenosis of external ear**
          canal, bilateral

H95.819   **Postprocedural stenosis of unspecified** ▽
          external ear canal

H95.88   **Other intraoperative complications and disorders of**
         the ear and mastoid process, not elsewhere
         classified
         Use additional code, if applicable, to further specify
         disorder

H95.89   **Other postprocedural complications and disorders**
         of the ear and mastoid process, not elsewhere
         classified
         Use additional code, if applicable, to further specify
         disorder

EXCLUDES 1 Not coded here   EXCLUDES 2 Not included here   N Newborn Age: 0   P Pediatric Age: 0-17   M Maternity Age: 12-55   A Adult Age: 15-124

616   ICD-10-CM 2018

Chapter 9. Diseases of the Circulatory System (I00–I99)

Chapter Specific Guidelines with Coding Examples

The chapter specific guidelines from the ICD-10-CM Official Guidelines for Coding and Reporting have been provided below. Along with these guidelines are coding examples, contained in the shaded boxes, that have been developed to help illustrate the coding and/or sequencing guidance found in these guidelines.

a. Hypertension

The classification presumes a causal relationship between hypertension and heart involvement and between hypertension and kidney involvement, as the two conditions are linked by the term "with" in the Alphabetic Index. These conditions should be coded as related even in the absence of provider documentation explicitly linking them, unless the documentation clearly states the conditions are unrelated.

For hypertension and conditions not specifically linked by relational terms such as "with," "associated with" or "due to" in the classification, provider documentation must link the conditions in order to code them as related.

1) Hypertension with heart disease

Hypertension with heart conditions classified to I50.- or I51.4-I51.9, are assigned to a code from category I11, Hypertensive heart disease. Use an additional code from category I50, Heart failure, to identify the type of heart failure in those patients with heart failure.

The same heart conditions (I50.-, I51.4-I51.9) with hypertension are coded separately if the provider has specifically documented a different cause. Sequence according to the circumstances of the admission/encounter.

> Patient is treated for left heart failure. Patient also has a history of hypertension managed by medication.
>
> **I11.0**   **Hypertensive heart disease with heart failure**
>
> **I50.1**   **Left ventricular failure, unspecified**
>
> *Explanation*: Without a diagnostic statement to the contrary, hypertension and heart failure have an assumed causal relationship, and a combination code should be used. An additional code to identify the type of heart failure (I50.-) should also be provided.

2) Hypertensive chronic kidney disease

Assign codes from category I12, Hypertensive chronic kidney disease, when both hypertension and a condition classifiable to category N18, Chronic kidney disease (CKD), are present. CKD should not be coded as hypertensive if the physician has specifically documented a different cause.

The appropriate code from category N18 should be used as a secondary code with a code from category I12 to identify the stage of chronic kidney disease.

See Section I.C.14. Chronic kidney disease.

If a patient has hypertensive chronic kidney disease and acute renal failure, an additional code for the acute renal failure is required.

> Patient presents with stage IV chronic kidney disease (CKD). The patient also has documented hypertension secondary to primary hyperparathyroidism.
>
> **N18.4**   **Chronic kidney disease, stage 4 (severe)**
>
> **I10**   **Essential (primary) hypertension**
>
> **E21.0**   **Primary hyperparathyroidism**
>
> *Explanation*: A combination code describing a relationship between hypertension and CKD is not used due to the physician documentation identifying the primary hyperparathyroidism as the cause for the hypertension.

3) Hypertensive heart and chronic kidney disease

Assign codes from combination category I13, Hypertensive heart and chronic kidney disease, when there is hypertension with both heart and kidney involvement. If heart failure is present, assign an additional code from category I50 to identify the type of heart failure.

The appropriate code from category N18, Chronic kidney disease, should be used as a secondary code with a code from category I13 to identify the stage of chronic kidney disease.

See Section I.C.14. Chronic kidney disease.

The codes in category I13, Hypertensive heart and chronic kidney disease, are combination codes that include hypertension, heart disease and chronic kidney disease. The Includes note at I13 specifies that the

conditions included at I11 and I12 are included together in I13. If a patient has hypertension, heart disease and chronic kidney disease, then a code from I13 should be used, not individual codes for hypertension, heart disease and chronic kidney disease, or codes from I11 or I12.

For patients with both acute renal failure and chronic kidney disease, an additional code for acute renal failure is required.

> Hypertensive heart and kidney disease with congestive heart failure and stage 2 chronic kidney disease
>
> **I13.0**   **Hypertensive heart and chronic kidney disease with heart failure and stage 1 through stage 4 chronic kidney disease, or unspecified chronic kidney disease**
>
> **I50.9**   **Heart failure, unspecified**
>
> **N18.2**   **Chronic kidney disease, stage 2 (mild)**
>
> *Explanation*: Combination codes in category I13 are used to report conditions classifiable to *both* categories I11 and I12. Do not report conditions classifiable to I11 and I12 separately. Use additional codes to report type of heart failure and stage of CKD.

4) Hypertensive cerebrovascular disease

For hypertensive cerebrovascular disease, first assign the appropriate code from categories I60-I69, followed by the appropriate hypertension code.

> Rupture of cerebral aneurysm caused by malignant hypertension
>
> **I60.7**   **Nontraumatic subarachnoid hemorrhage from unspecified introcranial artery**
>
> **I10**   **Essential (primary) hypertension**
>
> *Explanation*: Hypertensive cerebrovascular disease requires two codes: the appropriate I60–I69 code followed by the appropriate hypertension code.

5) Hypertensive retinopathy

Subcategory H35.0, Background retinopathy and retinal vascular changes, should be used with a code from category I10 – I15, Hypertensive disease to include the systemic hypertension. The sequencing is based on the reason for the encounter.

> Hypertensive retinopathy of the right eye
>
> **H35.031**   **Hypertensive retinopathy, right eye**
>
> **I10**   **Essential (primary) hypertension**
>
> *Explanation*: Hypertensive retinopathy requires two codes: the appropriate subcategory H35.0 code and a code for the hypertension.

6) Hypertension, secondary

Secondary hypertension is due to an underlying condition. Two codes are required: one to identify the underlying etiology and one from category I15 to identify the hypertension. Sequencing of codes is determined by the reason for admission/encounter.

> Renovascular hypertension due to renal artery atherosclerosis
>
> **I15.0**   **Renovascular hypertension**
>
> **I70.1**   **Atherosclerosis of renal artery**
>
> *Explanation*: Secondary hypertension requires two codes: a code to identify the etiology and the appropriate I15 code.

7) Hypertension, transient

Assign code R03.0, Elevated blood pressure reading without diagnosis of hypertension, unless patient has an established diagnosis of hypertension. Assign code O13.-, Gestational [pregnancy-induced] hypertension without significant proteinuria, or O14.-, Pre-eclampsia, for transient hypertension of pregnancy.

8) Hypertension, controlled

This diagnostic statement usually refers to an existing state of hypertension under control by therapy. Assign the appropriate code from categories I10-I15, Hypertensive diseases.

9) Hypertension, uncontrolled

Uncontrolled hypertension may refer to untreated hypertension or hypertension not responding to current therapeutic regimen. In either

Chapter 9. Diseases of the Circulatory System

case, assign the appropriate code from categories I10-I15, Hypertensive diseases.

10) Hypertensive Crisis

Assign a code from category I16, Hypertensive crisis, for documented hypertensive urgency, hypertensive emergency or unspecified hypertensive crisis. Code also any identified hypertensive disease (I10-I15). The sequencing is based on the reason for the encounter.

b. Atherosclerotic coronary artery disease and angina

ICD-10-CM has combination codes for atherosclerotic heart disease with angina pectoris. The subcategories for these codes are I25.11, Atherosclerotic heart disease of native coronary artery with angina pectoris, and I25.7, Atherosclerosis of coronary artery bypass graft(s) and coronary artery of transplanted heart with angina pectoris.

When using one of these combination codes it is not necessary to use an additional code for angina pectoris. A causal relationship can be assumed in a patient with both atherosclerosis and angina pectoris, unless the documentation indicates the angina is due to something other than the atherosclerosis.

If a patient with coronary artery disease is admitted due to an acute myocardial infarction (AMI), the AMI should be sequenced before the coronary artery disease.

See Section I.C.9. Acute myocardial infarction (AMI)

> Patient is being seen for spastic angina pectoris. She also has a documented history of progressive coronary artery disease of the native vessels.
>
> **I25.111**   **Atherosclerotic heart disease of native coronary artery with angina pectoris with documented spasm**
>
> *Explanation*: Report the combination code for atherosclerotic heart disease (coronary artery disease) with angina pectoris. A causal relationship is assumed in a patient with both atherosclerosis and angina pectoris, unless the documentation indicates the angina is due to something other than the atherosclerosis. When using one of these combination codes, it is not necessary to use an additional code for angina pectoris.

c. Intraoperative and postprocedural cerebrovascular accident

Medical record documentation should clearly specify the cause- and- effect relationship between the medical intervention and the cerebrovascular accident in order to assign a code for intraoperative or postprocedural cerebrovascular accident.

Proper code assignment depends on whether it was an infarction or hemorrhage and whether it occurred intraoperatively or postoperatively. If it was a cerebral hemorrhage, code assignment depends on the type of procedure performed.

> Embolic cerebral infarction of the right middle cerebral artery that occurred during hip replacement surgery. The surgeon documented as due to the surgery.
>
> **I97.811**   **Intraoperative cerebrovascular infarction during other surgery**
>
> **I63.411**   **Cerebral infarction due to embolism of right middle cerebral artery**
>
> *Explanation*: Code assignment for intraoperative or postprocedural cerebrovascular accident is based on the provider's documentation of a cause-and-effect relationship between the condition and the procedure. Proper code assignment also depends on whether the cerebrovascular accident was an infarction or hemorrhage, occurred intraoperatively or postoperatively, and the type of procedure performed.

d. Sequelae of cerebrovascular disease

1) Category I69, Sequelae of cerebrovascular disease

Category I69 is used to indicate conditions classifiable to categories I60-I67 as the causes of sequela (neurologic deficits), themselves classified elsewhere. These "late effects" include neurologic deficits that persist after initial onset of conditions classifiable to categories I60-I67. The neurologic deficits caused by cerebrovascular disease may be present from the onset or may arise at any time after the onset of the condition classifiable to categories I60-I67.

Codes from category I69, Sequelae of cerebrovascular disease, that specify hemiplegia, hemiparesis and monoplegia identify whether the dominant or nondominant side is affected. Should the affected side be documented, but not specified as dominant or nondominant, and the classification system does not indicate a default, code selection is as follows:

- For ambidextrous patients, the default should be dominant.

- If the left side is affected, the default is non-dominant.
- If the right side is affected, the default is dominant.

2) Codes from category I69 with codes from I60-I67

Codes from category I69 may be assigned on a health care record with codes from I60-I67, if the patient has a current cerebrovascular disease and deficits from an old cerebrovascular disease.

3) Codes from category I69 and personal history of transient ischemic attack (TIA) and cerebral infarction (Z86.73)

Codes from category I69 should not be assigned if the patient does not have neurologic deficits.

See Section I.C.21. 4. History (of) for use of personal history codes

e. Acute myocardial infarction (AMI)

1) ST elevation myocardial infarction (STEMI) and non ST elevation myocardial infarction (NSTEMI)

The ICD-10-CM codes for acute myocardial infarction (AMI) identify the site, such as anterolateral wall or true posterior wall. Subcategories I21.0-I21.2 and code I21.3 are used for ST elevation myocardial infarction (STEMI). Code I21.4, Non-ST elevation (NSTEMI) myocardial infarction, is used for non ST elevation myocardial infarction (NSTEMI) and nontransmural MIs.

If NSTEMI evolves to STEMI, assign the STEMI code. If STEMI converts to NSTEMI due to thrombolytic therapy, it is still coded as STEMI.

> Acute Inferior NSTEMI evolved into STEMI
>
> **I21.19**   **ST elevation (STEMI) myocardial infarction involving other coronary artery of inferior wall**
>
> *Explanation*: If an NSTEMI converts to a STEMI, report only the STEMI code.

For encounters occurring while the myocardial infarction is equal to, or less than, four weeks old, including transfers to another acute setting or a postacute setting, and the myocardial infarction meets the definition for "other diagnoses" (see Section III, Reporting Additional Diagnoses), codes from category I21 may continue to be reported. For encounters after the 4 week time frame and the patient is still receiving care related to the myocardial infarction, the appropriate aftercare code should be assigned, rather than a code from category I21. For old or healed myocardial infarctions not requiring further care, code I25.2, Old myocardial infarction, may be assigned.

2) Acute myocardial infarction, unspecified

Code I21.3, ST elevation (STEMI) myocardial infarction of unspecified site, is the default for unspecified acute myocardial infarction. If only STEMI or transmural MI without the site is documented, assign code I21.3.

3) AMI documented as nontransmural or subendocardial but site provided

If an AMI is documented as nontransmural or subendocardial, but the site is provided, it is still coded as a subendocardial AMI.

See Section I.C.21.3 for information on coding status post administration of tPA in a different facility within the last 24 hours.

> Acute inferior subendocardial myocardial infarction (NSTEMI)
>
> **I21.4**   **Non-ST elevation (NSTEMI) myocardial infarction**
>
> *Explanation*: An AMI documented as subendocardial or nontransmural is coded as such (I21.4, I22.2), even if the site of infarction is specified.

4) Subsequent acute myocardial infarction

A code from category I22, Subsequent ST elevation (STEMI) and non ST elevation (NSTEMI) myocardial infarction, is to be used when a patient who has suffered an AMI has a new AMI within the 4 week time frame of the initial AMI. A code from category I22 must be used in conjunction with a code from category I21. The sequencing of the I22 and I21 codes depends on the circumstances of the encounter.

> Acute inferior STEMI status post acute NSTEMI two weeks ago.
>
> **I22.1**   **Subsequent ST elevation (STEMI) myocardial infarction of inferior wall**
>
> **I21.4**   **Non-ST elevation (NSTEMI) myocardial infarction**
>
> *Explanation*: A code from I22 must be used in conjunction with a code from I21 when a patient who has suffered an AMI has a new AMI within four weeks of the initial one. Category I22 is never reported alone. The guidelines for assigning the correct I22 code are the same as those for reporting the initial MI (I21). Sequencing is determined by the circumstances of the encounter.

Chapter 9. Diseases of the Circulatory System (I00-I99)

EXCLUDES 2 *certain conditions originating in the perinatal period (P04-P96)*
certain infectious and parasitic diseases (A00-B99)
complications of pregnancy, childbirth and the puerperium (O00-O9A)
congenital malformations, deformations, and chromosomal abnormalities (Q00-Q99)
endocrine, nutritional and metabolic diseases (E00-E88)
injury, poisoning and certain other consequences of external causes (S00-T88)
neoplasms (C00-D49)
symptoms, signs and abnormal clinical and laboratory findings, not elsewhere classified (R00-R94)
systemic connective tissue disorders (M30-M36)
transient cerebral ischemic attacks and related syndromes (G45.-)

This chapter contains the following blocks:

I00-I02	Acute rheumatic fever
I05-I09	Chronic rheumatic heart diseases
I10-I16	Hypertensive diseases
I20-I25	Ischemic heart diseases
I26-I28	Pulmonary heart disease and diseases of pulmonary circulation
I30-I52	Other forms of heart disease
I60-I69	Cerebrovascular diseases
I70-I79	Diseases of arteries, arterioles and capillaries
I80-I89	Diseases of veins, lymphatic vessels and lymph nodes, not elsewhere classified
I95-I99	Other and unspecified disorders of the circulatory system

Acute rheumatic fever (I00-I02)

I00   **Rheumatic fever without heart involvement**
     INCLUDES   arthritis, rheumatic, acute or subacute
     EXCLUDES 1   *rheumatic fever with heart involvement (I01.0-I01.9)*

✓4ᵗʰ **I01**   **Rheumatic fever with heart involvement**
     EXCLUDES 1   *chronic diseases of rheumatic origin (I05-I09) unless rheumatic fever is also present or there is evidence of reactivation or activity of the rheumatic process.*

     I01.0   **Acute rheumatic pericarditis**
         Any condition in I00 with pericarditis
         Rheumatic pericarditis (acute)
         EXCLUDES 1   *acute pericarditis not specified as rheumatic (I30.-)*

     I01.1   **Acute rheumatic endocarditis**
         Any condition in I00 with endocarditis or valvulitis
         Acute rheumatic valvulitis

     I01.2   **Acute rheumatic myocarditis**
         Any condition in I00 with myocarditis

     I01.8   **Other acute rheumatic heart disease**
         Any condition in I00 with other or multiple types of heart involvement
         Acute rheumatic pancarditis

     I01.9   **Acute rheumatic heart disease, unspecified**   ▽
         Any condition in I00 with unspecified type of heart involvement
         Rheumatic carditis, acute
         Rheumatic heart disease, active or acute

✓4ᵗʰ **I02**   **Rheumatic chorea**
     INCLUDES   Sydenham's chorea
     EXCLUDES 1   *chorea NOS (G25.5)*
                   Huntington's chorea (G10)

     I02.0   **Rheumatic chorea with heart involvement**
         Chorea NOS with heart involvement
         Rheumatic chorea with heart involvement of any type classifiable under I01-

     I02.9   **Rheumatic chorea without heart involvement**
         Rheumatic chorea NOS

Chronic rheumatic heart diseases (I05-I09)

✓4ᵗʰ **I05**   **Rheumatic mitral valve diseases**
     INCLUDES   conditions classifiable to both I05.0 and I05.2-I05.9, whether specified as rheumatic or not
     EXCLUDES 1   *mitral valve disease specified as nonrheumatic (I34.-)*
                   mitral valve disease with aortic and/or tricuspid valve involvement (I08.-)

     I05.0   **Rheumatic mitral stenosis**
         Mitral (valve) obstruction (rheumatic)
         DEF: Narrowing of mitral valve between left atrium and left ventricle; due to rheumatic fever; characterized by shortness of breath during or after exercise, fatigue, palpitations, chest discomfort, and swelling of feet or legs.

     I05.1   **Rheumatic mitral insufficiency**
         Rheumatic mitral incompetence
         Rheumatic mitral regurgitation
         EXCLUDES 1   *mitral insufficiency not specified as rheumatic (I34.0)*

     I05.2   **Rheumatic mitral stenosis with insufficiency**
         Rheumatic mitral stenosis with incompetence or regurgitation

     I05.8   **Other rheumatic mitral valve diseases**
         Rheumatic mitral (valve) failure

     I05.9   **Rheumatic mitral valve disease, unspecified**   ▽
         Rheumatic mitral (valve) disorder (chronic) NOS

✓4ᵗʰ **I06**   **Rheumatic aortic valve diseases**
     EXCLUDES 1   *aortic valve disease not specified as rheumatic (I35.-)*
                   aortic valve disease with mitral and/or tricuspid valve involvement (I08.-)

     I06.0   **Rheumatic aortic stenosis**
         Rheumatic aortic (valve) obstruction

     I06.1   **Rheumatic aortic insufficiency**
         Rheumatic aortic incompetence
         Rheumatic aortic regurgitation

     I06.2   **Rheumatic aortic stenosis with insufficiency**
         Rheumatic aortic stenosis with incompetence or regurgitation

     I06.8   **Other rheumatic aortic valve diseases**

     I06.9   **Rheumatic aortic valve disease, unspecified**   ▽
         Rheumatic aortic (valve) disease NOS

✓4ᵗʰ **I07**   **Rheumatic tricuspid valve diseases**
     INCLUDES   rheumatic tricuspid valve diseases specified as rheumatic or unspecified
     EXCLUDES 1   *tricuspid valve disease specified as nonrheumatic (I36.-)*
                   tricuspid valve disease with aortic and/or mitral valve involvement (I08.-)

     I07.0   **Rheumatic tricuspid stenosis**
         Tricuspid (valve) stenosis (rheumatic)

     I07.1   **Rheumatic tricuspid insufficiency**
         Tricuspid (valve) insufficiency (rheumatic)

     I07.2   **Rheumatic tricuspid stenosis and insufficiency**

     I07.8   **Other rheumatic tricuspid valve diseases**

     I07.9   **Rheumatic tricuspid valve disease, unspecified**   ▽
         Rheumatic tricuspid valve disorder NOS

✓4ᵗʰ **I08**   **Multiple valve diseases**
     INCLUDES   multiple valve diseases specified as rheumatic or unspecified
     EXCLUDES 1   *endocarditis, valve unspecified (I38)*
                   multiple valve disease specified a nonrheumatic (I34.-, I35.-, I36.-, I37.-, I38.-, Q22.-, Q23.-, Q24.8-)
                   rheumatic valve disease NOS (I09.1)

     I08.0   **Rheumatic disorders of both mitral and aortic valves**
         Involvement of both mitral and aortic valves specified as rheumatic or unspecified

     I08.1   **Rheumatic disorders of both mitral and tricuspid valves**

     I08.2   **Rheumatic disorders of both aortic and tricuspid valves**

     I08.3   **Combined rheumatic disorders of mitral, aortic and tricuspid valves**

     I08.8   **Other rheumatic multiple valve diseases**

     I08.9   **Rheumatic multiple valve disease, unspecified**   ▽

✓4ᵗʰ **I09**   **Other rheumatic heart diseases**
     I09.0   **Rheumatic myocarditis**
         EXCLUDES 1   *myocarditis not specified as rheumatic (I51.4)*

     I09.1   **Rheumatic diseases of endocardium, valve unspecified**   ▽
         Rheumatic endocarditis (chronic)
         Rheumatic valvulitis (chronic)
         EXCLUDES 1   *endocarditis, valve unspecified (I38)*

     I09.2   **Chronic rheumatic pericarditis**
         Adherent pericardium, rheumatic
         Chronic rheumatic mediastinopericarditis
         Chronic rheumatic myopericarditis
         EXCLUDES 1   *chronic pericarditis not specified as rheumatic (I31.-)*

✓5ᵗʰ   **I09.8**   **Other specified rheumatic heart diseases**
         I09.81   **Rheumatic heart failure**   HCC
              Use additional code to identify type of heart failure (I50.-)
              DEF: Decreased cardiac output, edema, and hypertension; due to rheumatic heart disease.

         I09.89   **Other specified rheumatic heart diseases**
              Rheumatic disease of pulmonary valve

     I09.9   **Rheumatic heart disease, unspecified**   ▽
         Rheumatic carditis
         EXCLUDES 1   *rheumatoid carditis (M05.31)*

☑ Additional Character Req   ✓x7ᵗʰ Placeholder Alert   Manifestation   HCC CMS-HCC Condition   ▽ Unspecified Code   ►◄ Revised Text   ● New Code   ▲ Revised Code Title

Hypertensive diseases (I1Ø-I16)

Use additional code to identify:
- exposure to environmental tobacco smoke (Z77.22)
- history of tobacco dependence (Z87.891)
- occupational exposure to environmental tobacco smoke (Z57.31)
- tobacco dependence (F17.-)
- tobacco use (Z72.Ø)

EXCLUDES 1   neonatal hypertension (P29.2)
     primary pulmonary hypertension (I27.Ø)

EXCLUDES 2   hypertensive disease complicating pregnancy, childbirth and the puerperium (O1Ø-O11, O13-O16)

I1Ø   Essential (primary) hypertension

INCLUDES   high blood pressure
     hypertension (arterial) (benign) (essential) (malignant) (primary) (systemic)

EXCLUDES 1   hypertensive disease complicating pregnancy, childbirth and the puerperium (O1Ø-O11, O13-O16)

EXCLUDES 2   essential (primary) hypertension involving vessels of brain (I6Ø-I69)
     essential (primary) hypertension involving vessels of eye (H35.Ø-)

AHA: 2016, 4Q, 27

✓4th I11   Hypertensive heart disease

INCLUDES ▶any condition in I5Ø.-, I51.4-I51.9 due to hypertension◀

I11.Ø   Hypertensive heart disease with heart failure   HCC
     Hypertensive heart failure
     Use additional code to identify type of heart failure (I5Ø.-)
     AHA: 2017, 1Q, 47

I11.9   Hypertensive heart disease without heart failure   ▽
     Hypertensive heart disease NOS

✓4th I12   Hypertensive chronic kidney disease

INCLUDES   any condition in N18- and N26- due to hypertension
     arteriosclerosis of kidney
     arteriosclerotic nephritis (chronic) (interstitial)
     hypertensive nephropathy
     nephrosclerosis

EXCLUDES 1   hypertension due to kidney disease (I15.Ø, I15.1)
     renovascular hypertension (I15.Ø)
     secondary hypertension (I15.-)

EXCLUDES 2   acute kidney failure (N17.-)

AHA: 2016, 3Q, 22

I12.Ø   Hypertensive chronic kidney disease with stage 5 chronic kidney disease or end stage renal disease   HCC
     Use additional code to identify the stage of chronic kidney disease (N18.5, N18.6)

I12.9   Hypertensive chronic kidney disease with stage 1 through stage 4 chronic kidney disease, or unspecified chronic kidney disease   ▽
     Hypertensive chronic kidney disease NOS
     Hypertensive renal disease NOS
     Use additional code to identify the stage of chronic kidney disease (N18.1-N18.4, N18.9)

✓4th I13   Hypertensive heart and chronic kidney disease

INCLUDES   any condition in I11- with any condition in I12-
     cardiorenal disease
     cardiovascular renal disease

I13.Ø   Hypertensive heart and chronic kidney disease with heart failure and stage 1 through stage 4 chronic kidney disease, or unspecified chronic kidney disease   HCC
     Use additional code to identify type of heart failure (I5Ø.-)
     Use additional code to identify stage of chronic kidney disease (N18.1-N18.4, N18.9)

✓5th I13.1   Hypertensive heart and chronic kidney disease without heart failure

     I13.1Ø   Hypertensive heart and chronic kidney disease without heart failure, with stage 1 through stage 4 chronic kidney disease, or unspecified chronic kidney disease   ▽
         Hypertensive heart disease and hypertensive chronic kidney disease NOS
         Use additional code to identify the stage of chronic kidney disease (N18.1-N18.4, N18.9)

     I13.11   Hypertensive heart and chronic kidney disease without heart failure, with stage 5 chronic kidney disease, or end stage renal disease   HCC
         Use additional code to identify the stage of chronic kidney disease (N18.5, N18.6)

I13.2   Hypertensive heart and chronic kidney disease with heart failure and with stage 5 chronic kidney disease, or end stage renal disease   HCC
     Use additional code to identify type of heart failure (I5Ø.-)
     Use additional code to identify the stage of chronic kidney disease (N18.5, N18.6)

✓4th I15   Secondary hypertension

Code also underlying condition

EXCLUDES 1   postprocedural hypertension (I97.3)

EXCLUDES 2   secondary hypertension involving vessels of brain (I6Ø-I69)
     secondary hypertension involving vessels of eye (H35.Ø-)

I15.Ø   Renovascular hypertension

I15.1   Hypertension secondary to other renal disorders
     AHA: 2016, 3Q, 22

I15.2   Hypertension secondary to endocrine disorders

I15.8   Other secondary hypertension

I15.9   Secondary hypertension, unspecified   ▽

✓4th I16   Hypertensive crisis

Code also any identified hypertensive disease (I1Ø-I15)

AHA: 2016, 4Q, 27

I16.Ø   Hypertensive urgency

I16.1   Hypertensive emergency

I16.9   Hypertensive crisis, unspecified   ▽

Ischemic heart diseases (I2Ø-I25)

Use additional code to identify presence of hypertension (I1Ø-I16)

✓4th I2Ø   Angina pectoris

Use additional code to identify:
- exposure to environmental tobacco smoke (Z77.22)
- history of tobacco dependence (Z87.891)
- occupational exposure to environmental tobacco smoke (Z57.31)
- tobacco dependence (F17.-)
- tobacco use (Z72.Ø)

EXCLUDES 1   angina pectoris with atherosclerotic heart disease of native coronary arteries (I25.1-)
     atherosclerosis of coronary artery bypass graft(s) and coronary artery of transplanted heart with angina pectoris (I25.7-)
     postinfarction angina (I23.7)

I2Ø.Ø   Unstable angina   HCC
     Accelerated angina
     Crescendo angina
     De novo effort angina
     Intermediate coronary syndrome
     Preinfarction syndrome
     Worsening effort angina
     DEF: A condition representing an intermediate stage between angina of effort and acute myocardial infarction.

I2Ø.1   Angina pectoris with documented spasm   HCC
     Angiospastic angina
     Prinzmetal angina
     Spasm-induced angina
     Variant angina

I2Ø.8   Other forms of angina pectoris   HCC
     Angina equivalent
     Angina of effort
     Coronary slow flow syndrome
     Stable angina
     Stenocardia
     Use additional code(s) for symptoms associated with angina equivalent

I2Ø.9   Angina pectoris, unspecified   HCC ▽
     Angina NOS
     Anginal syndrome
     Cardiac angina
     Ischemic chest pain

EXCLUDES 1 Not coded here   **EXCLUDES 2** Not included here   **N** Newborn Age: 0   **P** Pediatric Age: 0-17   **M** Maternity Age: 12-55   **A** Adult Age: 15-124

620   ICD-10-CM 2018

▲ ✓4ᵗʰ **I21 Acute myocardial infarction**
     INCLUDES   cardiac infarction
               coronary (artery) embolism
               coronary (artery) occlusion
               coronary (artery) rupture
               coronary (artery) thrombosis
               infarction of heart, myocardium, or ventricle
               myocardial infarction specified as acute or with a stated
                   duration of 4 weeks (28 days) or less from onset
     Use additional code, if applicable, to identify:
       exposure to environmental tobacco smoke (Z77.22)
       history of tobacco dependence (Z87.891)
       occupational exposure to environmental tobacco smoke (Z57.31)
       status post administration of tPA (rtPA) in a different facility within
           the last 24 hours prior to admission to current facility (Z92.82)
       tobacco dependence (F17.-)
       tobacco use (Z72.0)
     EXCLUDES 2   *old myocardial infarction (I25.2)*
               postmyocardial infarction syndrome (I24.1)
               ▶*subsequent type 1 myocardial infarction◀ (I22.-)*
     AHA: 2017, 1Q, 44-45; 2016, 4Q, 140; 2015, 2Q, 16; 2013, 1Q, 25; 2012, 4Q,
     96, 102-103

✓5ᵗʰ **I21.0   ST elevation (STEMI) myocardial infarction of anterior wall**
     ▶Type 1 ST elevation myocardial infarction of anterior wall◀

     I21.01   ST elevation (STEMI) myocardial infarction   HCC
             involving left main coronary artery

     I21.02   ST elevation (STEMI) myocardial infarction   HCC
             involving left anterior descending coronary artery
               ST elevation (STEMI) myocardial infarction involving
                  diagonal coronary artery
               AHA: 2013, 1Q, 25

     I21.09   ST elevation (STEMI) myocardial infarction   HCC
             involving other coronary artery of anterior wall
               Acute transmural myocardial infarction of anterior wall
               Anteroapical transmural (Q wave) infarction (acute)
               Anterolateral transmural (Q wave) infarction (acute)
               Anteroseptal transmural (Q wave) infarction (acute)
               Transmural (Q wave) infarction (acute) (of) anterior
                  (wall) NOS
               AHA: 2012, 4Q, 102-103

✓5ᵗʰ **I21.1   ST elevation (STEMI) myocardial infarction of inferior wall**
     ▶Type 1 ST elevation myocardial infarction of inferior wall◀

     I21.11   ST elevation (STEMI) myocardial infarction   HCC
             involving right coronary artery
               Inferoposterior transmural (Q wave) infarction (acute)

     I21.19   ST elevation (STEMI) myocardial infarction   HCC
             involving other coronary artery of inferior wall
               Acute transmural myocardial infarction of inferior wall
               Inferolateral transmural (Q wave) infarction (acute)
               Transmural (Q wave) infarction (acute) (of)
                  diaphragmatic wall
               Transmural (Q wave) infarction (acute) (of) inferior
                  (wall) NOS
              EXCLUDES 2   *ST elevation (STEMI) myocardial infarction*
                     involving left circumflex coronary artery
                     (I21.21)
               AHA: 2012, 4Q, 96

✓5ᵗʰ **I21.2   ST elevation (STEMI) myocardial infarction of other sites**
     ▶Type 1 ST elevation myocardial infarction of other sites◀

     I21.21   ST elevation (STEMI) myocardial infarction   HCC
             involving left circumflex coronary artery
               ST elevation (STEMI) myocardial infarction involving
                  oblique marginal coronary artery

     I21.29   ST elevation (STEMI) myocardial infarction   HCC
             involving other sites
               Acute transmural myocardial infarction of other sites
               Apical-lateral transmural (Q wave) infarction (acute)
               Basal-lateral transmural (Q wave) infarction (acute)
               High lateral transmural (Q wave) infarction (acute)
               Lateral (wall) NOS transmural (Q wave) infarction
                  (acute)
               Posterior (true) transmural (Q wave) infarction (acute)
               Posterobasal transmural (Q wave) infarction (acute)
               Posterolateral transmural (Q wave) infarction (acute)
               Posteroseptal transmural (Q wave) infarction (acute)
               Septal transmural (Q wave) infarction (acute) NOS

I21.3   ST elevation (STEMI) myocardial infarction of   HCC ▽
     unspecified site
       Acute transmural myocardial infarction of unspecified site
       ~~Myocardial infarction (acute) NOS~~
       Transmural (Q wave) myocardial infarction NOS
     ▶Type 1 ST elevation myocardial infarction of unspecified site◀

I21.4   Non-ST elevation (NSTEMI) myocardial infarction   HCC
       Acute subendocardial myocardial infarction
       Non-Q wave myocardial infarction NOS
       Nontransmural myocardial infarction NOS
     ▶Type 1 non-ST elevation myocardial infarction◀
     AHA: 2017, 1Q, 44-45

● **I21.9   Acute myocardial infarction, unspecified**   ▽
       Myocardial infarction (acute) NOS

● ✓5ᵗʰ **I21.A   Other type of myocardial infarction**

●   **I21.A1   Myocardial infarction type 2**
               Myocardial infarction due to demand ischemia
               Myocardial infarction secondary to ischemic
                  imbalance
               Code also the underlying cause, if known and
                  applicable, such as:
                  anemia (D50.0-D64.9)
                  chronic obstructive pulmonary disease (J44.-)
                  heart failure (I50.-)
                  paroxysmal tachycardia (I47.0-I47.9)
                  renal failure (N17.0-N19)
                  shock (R57.0-R57.9)

●   **I21.A9   Other myocardial infarction type**
               Myocardial infarction associated with
                  revascularization procedure
               Myocardial infarction type 3
               Myocardial infarction type 4a
               Myocardial infarction type 4b
               Myocardial infarction type 4c
               Myocardial infarction type 5
               Code first, if applicable, postprocedural myocardial
                  infarction following cardiac surgery (I97.190), or
                  postprocedural myocardial infarction during
                  cardiac surgery (I97.790)
               Code also complication, if known and applicable, such
                  as:
                  (acute) stent occlusion (T82.897-)
                  (acute) stent stenosis (T82.857-)
                  (acute) stent thrombosis (T82.867-)
                  cardiac arrest due to underlying cardiac condition
                    (I46.2)
                  complication of percutaneous coronary
                    intervention (PCI) (I97.89)
                  occlusion of coronary artery bypass graft (T82.218-)

✓4ᵗʰ **I22   Subsequent ST elevation (STEMI) and non-ST elevation (NSTEMI)**
myocardial infarction
     INCLUDES   acute myocardial infarction occurring within four weeks (28
                 days) of a previous acute myocardial infarction,
                 regardless of site
               cardiac infarction
               coronary (artery) embolism
               coronary (artery) occlusion
               coronary (artery) rupture
               coronary (artery) thrombosis
               infarction of heart, myocardium, or ventricle
               recurrent myocardial infarction
               reinfarction of myocardium
               rupture of heart, myocardium, or ventricle
               ▶subsequent type 1 myocardial infarction◀
     Use additional code, if applicable, to identify:
       exposure to environmental tobacco smoke (Z77.22)
       history of tobacco dependence (Z87.891)
       occupational exposure to environmental tobacco smoke (Z57.31)
       status post administration of tPA (rtPA) in a different facility within
          the last 24 hours prior to admission to current facility (Z92.82)
       tobacco dependence (F17.-)
       tobacco use (Z72.0)
     EXCLUDES 1   ▶*subsequent myocardial infarction, type 2 (I21.A1)*
               subsequent myocardial infarction of other type (type 3) (type 4)
                 (type 5) (I21.A9)◀
     AHA: 2017, 2Q, 11; 2013, 1Q, 25; 2012, 4Q, 97, 102-103

I22.0   Subsequent ST elevation (STEMI) myocardial infarction   HCC
     of anterior wall
       Subsequent acute transmural myocardial infarction of anterior
         wall
       Subsequent transmural (Q wave) infarction (acute)(of) anterior
         (wall) NOS
       Subsequent anteroapical transmural (Q wave) infarction (acute)
       Subsequent anterolateral transmural (Q wave) infarction (acute)
       Subsequent anteroseptal transmural (Q wave) infarction (acute)

☑ Additional Character Req   ✓x7ᵗʰ Placeholder Alert   Manifestation   HCC CMS-HCC Condition   ▽ Unspecified Code   ▶◀ Revised Text   ● New Code   ▲ Revised Code Title

ICD-10-CM 2018   621

I22.1 **Subsequent ST elevation (STEMI) myocardial infarction of inferior wall** `HCC`
Subsequent acute transmural myocardial infarction of inferior wall
Subsequent transmural (Q wave) infarction (acute)(of) diaphragmatic wall
Subsequent transmural (Q wave) infarction (acute)(of) inferior (wall) NOS
Subsequent inferolateral transmural (Q wave) infarction (acute)
Subsequent inferoposterior transmural (Q wave) infarction (acute)
AHA: 2012, 4Q, 102

I22.2 **Subsequent non-ST elevation (NSTEMI) myocardial infarction** `HCC`
Subsequent acute subendocardial myocardial infarction
Subsequent non-Q wave myocardial infarction NOS
Subsequent nontransmural myocardial infarction NOS

I22.8 **Subsequent ST elevation (STEMI) myocardial infarction of other sites** `HCC`
Subsequent acute transmural myocardial infarction of other sites
Subsequent apical-lateral transmural (Q wave) myocardial infarction (acute)
Subsequent basal-lateral transmural (Q wave) myocardial infarction (acute)
Subsequent high lateral transmural (Q wave) myocardial infarction (acute)
Subsequent transmural (Q wave) myocardial infarction (acute)(of) lateral (wall) NOS
Subsequent posterior (true)transmural (Q wave) myocardial infarction (acute)
Subsequent posterobasal transmural (Q wave) myocardial infarction (acute)
Subsequent posterolateral transmural (Q wave) myocardial infarction (acute)
Subsequent posteroseptal transmural (Q wave) myocardial infarction (acute)
Subsequent septal NOS transmural (Q wave) myocardial infarction (acute)

I22.9 **Subsequent ST elevation (STEMI) myocardial infarction of unspecified site** `HCC` ▽
Subsequent acute myocardial infarction of unspecified site
Subsequent myocardial infarction (acute) NOS

✓4th **I23** **Certain current complications following ST elevation (STEMI) and non-ST elevation (NSTEMI) myocardial infarction (within the 28 day period)**
AHA: 2017, 2Q, 11

I23.0 **Hemopericardium as current complication following acute myocardial infarction** `HCC`
EXCLUDES 1 hemopericardium not specified as current complication following acute myocardial infarction (I31.2)

I23.1 **Atrial septal defect as current complication following acute myocardial infarction** `HCC` `A`
EXCLUDES 1 acquired atrial septal defect not specified as current complication following acute myocardial infarction (I51.0)

I23.2 **Ventricular septal defect as current complication following acute myocardial infarction** `HCC` `A`
EXCLUDES 1 acquired ventricular septal defect not specified as current complication following acute myocardial infarction (I51.0)

I23.3 **Rupture of cardiac wall without hemopericardium as current complication following acute myocardial infarction** `HCC` `A`

I23.4 **Rupture of chordae tendineae as current complication following acute myocardial infarction** `HCC`
EXCLUDES 1 rupture of chordae tendineae not specified as current complication following acute myocardial infarction (I51.1)

I23.5 **Rupture of papillary muscle as current complication following acute myocardial infarction** `HCC`
EXCLUDES 1 rupture of papillary muscle not specified as current complication following acute myocardial infarction (I51.2)

I23.6 **Thrombosis of atrium, auricular appendage, and ventricle as current complications following acute myocardial infarction** `HCC` `A`
EXCLUDES 1 thrombosis of atrium, auricular appendage, and ventricle not specified as current complication following acute myocardial infarction (I51.3)

I23.7 **Postinfarction angina** `HCC` `A`
AHA: 2015, 2Q, 16

I23.8 **Other current complications following acute myocardial infarction** `HCC` `A`

✓4th **I24** **Other acute ischemic heart diseases**
EXCLUDES 1 angina pectoris (I20.-)
transient myocardial ischemia in newborn (P29.4)

I24.0 **Acute coronary thrombosis not resulting in myocardial infarction** `HCC`
Acute coronary (artery) (vein) embolism not resulting in myocardial infarction
Acute coronary (artery) (vein) occlusion not resulting in myocardial infarction
Acute coronary (artery) (vein) thromboembolism not resulting in myocardial infarction
EXCLUDES 1 atherosclerotic heart disease (I25.1-)
AHA: 2013, 1Q, 24

I24.1 **Dressler's syndrome** `HCC`
Postmyocardial infarction syndrome
EXCLUDES 1 postinfarction angina (I23.7)

I24.8 **Other forms of acute ischemic heart disease** `HCC`
EXCLUDES 1 ▶myocardial infarction due to demand ischemia (I21.A1)◀

I24.9 **Acute ischemic heart disease, unspecified** `HCC` ▽
EXCLUDES 1 ischemic heart disease (chronic) NOS (I25.9)

✓4th **I25** **Chronic ischemic heart disease**
Use additional code to identify:
chronic total occlusion of coronary artery (I25.82)
exposure to environmental tobacco smoke (Z77.22)
history of tobacco dependence (Z87.891)
occupational exposure to environmental tobacco smoke (Z57.31)
tobacco dependence (F17.-)
tobacco use (Z72.0)

✓5th **I25.1** **Atherosclerotic heart disease of native coronary artery**
Atherosclerotic cardiovascular disease
Coronary (artery) atheroma
Coronary (artery) atherosclerosis
Coronary (artery) disease
Coronary (artery) sclerosis
Use additional code, if applicable, to identify:
coronary atherosclerosis due to calcified coronary lesion (I25.84)
coronary atherosclerosis due to lipid rich plaque (I25.83)
EXCLUDES 2 atheroembolism (I75.-)
atherosclerosis of coronary artery bypass graft(s) and transplanted heart (I25.7-)

I25.10 **Atherosclerotic heart disease of native coronary artery without angina pectoris** `A`
Atherosclerotic heart disease NOS
AHA: 2015, 2Q, 16; 2012, 4Q, 92

✓6th **I25.11** **Atherosclerotic heart disease of native coronary artery with angina pectoris**

I25.110 **Atherosclerotic heart disease of native coronary artery with unstable angina pectoris** `HCC` `A`
EXCLUDES 1 unstable angina without atherosclerotic heart disease (I20.0)

I25.111 **Atherosclerotic heart disease of native coronary artery with angina pectoris with documented spasm** `HCC` `A`
EXCLUDES 1 angina pectoris with documented spasm without atherosclerotic heart disease (I20.1)

Atheromas

Atheromas (fatty tissue and/or plaque)

Lumen

I25.118   **Atherosclerotic heart disease of** `HCC` `A`
       native coronary artery with other forms of
       angina pectoris
         `EXCLUDES 1`   *other forms of angina pectoris*
            without atherosclerotic
            heart disease (I20.8)
         AHA: 2015, 2Q, 16

I25.119   **Atherosclerotic heart disease of** `HCC` `A` `▽`
       native coronary artery with unspecified
       angina pectoris
         Atherosclerotic heart disease with angina
            NOS
         Atherosclerotic heart disease with ischemic
            chest pain
         `EXCLUDES 1`   *unspecified angina pectoris*
            without atherosclerotic
            heart disease (I20.9)

I25.2   **Old myocardial infarction**
     Healed myocardial infarction
     Past myocardial infarction diagnosed by ECG or other
         investigation, but currently presenting no symptoms

I25.3   **Aneurysm of heart**
     Mural aneurysm
     Ventricular aneurysm

`✓5th` **I25.4**   **Coronary artery aneurysm and dissection**

I25.41   **Coronary artery aneurysm**
       Coronary arteriovenous fistula, acquired
       `EXCLUDES 1`   *congenital coronary (artery) aneurysm*
           (Q24.5)

I25.42   **Coronary artery dissection**
       DEF: A tear in the intimal arterial wall of a coronary
       artery resulting in the sudden intrusion of blood within
       the layers of the wall.

I25.5   **Ischemic cardiomyopathy**
       `EXCLUDES 2`   *coronary atherosclerosis (I25.1-, I25.7-)*

I25.6   **Silent myocardial ischemia**

`✓5th` **I25.7**   **Atherosclerosis of coronary artery bypass graft(s) and**
     coronary artery of transplanted heart with angina pectoris
     Use additional code, if applicable, to identify:
       coronary atherosclerosis due to calcified coronary lesion
         (I25.84)
       coronary atherosclerosis due to lipid rich plaque (I25.83)
       `EXCLUDES 1`   *atherosclerosis of bypass graft(s) of transplanted heart*
           without angina pectoris (I25.812)
         atherosclerosis of coronary artery bypass graft(s)
           without angina pectoris (I25.810)
         atherosclerosis of native coronary artery of
           transplanted heart without angina pectoris
           (I25.811)
         ~~*embolism or thrombus of coronary artery bypass*~~
           ~~*graft(s) (T82.8-)*~~

`✓6th` **I25.70**   **Atherosclerosis of coronary artery bypass graft(s),**
       unspecified, with angina pectoris

I25.700   **Atherosclerosis of coronary** `HCC` `A` `▽`
       artery bypass graft(s), unspecified, with
       unstable angina pectoris
       `EXCLUDES 1`   *unstable angina pectoris without*
           atherosclerosis of coronary
           artery bypass graft (I20.0)

I25.701   **Atherosclerosis of coronary** `HCC` `A` `▽`
       artery bypass graft(s), unspecified, with
       angina pectoris with documented spasm
       `EXCLUDES 1`   *angina pectoris with documented*
           spasm without
           atherosclerosis of coronary
           artery bypass graft (I20.1)

I25.708   **Atherosclerosis of coronary** `HCC` `A` `▽`
       artery bypass graft(s), unspecified, with
       other forms of angina pectoris
       `EXCLUDES 1`   *other forms of angina pectoris*
           without atherosclerosis of
           coronary artery bypass graft
           (I20.8)

I25.709   **Atherosclerosis of coronary** `HCC` `A` `▽`
       artery bypass graft(s), unspecified, with
       unspecified angina pectoris
       `EXCLUDES 1`   *unspecified angina pectoris*
           without atherosclerosis of
           coronary artery bypass graft
           (I20.9)

`✓6th` **I25.71**   **Atherosclerosis of autologous vein coronary artery**
       bypass graft(s) with angina pectoris

I25.710   **Atherosclerosis of autologous vein** `HCC` `A`
       coronary artery bypass graft(s) with
       unstable angina pectoris
       `EXCLUDES 1`   *unstable angina without*
           atherosclerosis of
           autologous vein coronary
           artery bypass graft(s) (I20.0)
       `EXCLUDES 2` ▶*embolism or thrombus of*
           coronary artery bypass
           graft(s) (T82.8-)◀

I25.711   **Atherosclerosis of autologous vein** `HCC` `A`
       coronary artery bypass graft(s) with
       angina pectoris with documented spasm
       `EXCLUDES 1`   *angina pectoris with documented*
           spasm without
           atherosclerosis of
           autologous vein coronary
           artery bypass graft(s) (I20.1)

I25.718   **Atherosclerosis of autologous vein** `HCC` `A`
       coronary artery bypass graft(s) with
       other forms of angina pectoris
       `EXCLUDES 1`   *other forms of angina pectoris*
           without atherosclerosis of
           autologous vein coronary
           artery bypass graft(s) (I20.8)

I25.719   **Atherosclerosis of autologous** `HCC` `A` `▽`
       vein coronary artery bypass graft(s) with
       unspecified angina pectoris
       `EXCLUDES 1`   *unspecified angina pectoris*
           without atherosclerosis of
           autologous vein coronary
           artery bypass graft(s) (I20.9)

`✓6th` **I25.72**   **Atherosclerosis of autologous artery coronary artery**
       bypass graft(s) with angina pectoris
       Atherosclerosis of internal mammary artery graft with
         angina pectoris

I25.720   **Atherosclerosis of autologous artery** `HCC` `A`
       coronary artery bypass graft(s) with
       unstable angina pectoris
       `EXCLUDES 1`   *unstable angina without*
           atherosclerosis of
           autologous artery coronary
           artery bypass graft(s) (I20.0)

I25.721   **Atherosclerosis of autologous artery** `HCC` `A`
       coronary artery bypass graft(s) with
       angina pectoris with documented spasm
       `EXCLUDES 1`   *angina pectoris with documented*
           spasm without
           atherosclerosis of
           autologous artery coronary
           artery bypass graft(s) (I20.1)

I25.728   **Atherosclerosis of autologous artery** `HCC` `A`
       coronary artery bypass graft(s) with
       other forms of angina pectoris
       `EXCLUDES 1`   *other forms of angina pectoris*
           without atherosclerosis of
           autologous artery coronary
           artery bypass graft(s) (I20.8)

I25.729   **Atherosclerosis of autologous** `HCC` `A` `▽`
       artery coronary artery bypass graft(s)
       with unspecified angina pectoris
       `EXCLUDES 1`   *unspecified angina pectoris*
           without atherosclerosis of
           autologous artery coronary
           artery bypass graft(s) (I20.9)

`✓6th` **I25.73**   **Atherosclerosis of nonautologous biological**
       coronary artery bypass graft(s) with angina pectoris

I25.730   **Atherosclerosis of nonautologous** `HCC` `A`
       biological coronary artery bypass graft(s)
       with unstable angina pectoris
       `EXCLUDES 1`   *unstable angina without*
           atherosclerosis of
           nonautologous biological
           coronary artery bypass
           graft(s) (I20.0)

✓ Additional Character Req   `✓x7th` Placeholder Alert   Manifestation   `HCC` CMS-HCC Condition   ▽ Unspecified Code   ▶◀ Revised Text   ● New Code   ▲ Revised Code Title

ICD-10-CM 2018   623

I25.731   **Atherosclerosis of nonautologous** `HCC` `A`
biological coronary artery bypass graft(s)
with angina pectoris with documented
spasm
    EXCLUDES 1   angina pectoris with documented
spasm without
atherosclerosis of
nonautologous biological
coronary artery bypass
graft(s) (I20.1)

I25.738   **Atherosclerosis of nonautologous** `HCC` `A`
biological coronary artery bypass graft(s)
with other forms of angina pectoris
    EXCLUDES 1   other forms of angina pectoris
without atherosclerosis of
nonautologous biological
coronary artery bypass
graft(s) (I20.8)

I25.739   **Atherosclerosis of nonautologous** `HCC` `A` ▽
biological coronary artery bypass graft(s)
with unspecified angina pectoris
    EXCLUDES 1   unspecified angina pectoris
without atherosclerosis of
nonautologous biological
coronary artery bypass
graft(s) (I20.9)

✓6ᵗʰ   **I25.75**   **Atherosclerosis of native coronary artery of**
transplanted heart with angina pectoris
    EXCLUDES 1   atherosclerosis of native coronary artery of
transplanted heart without angina
pectoris (I25.811)

I25.750   **Atherosclerosis of native coronary** `HCC`
artery of transplanted heart with
unstable angina

I25.751   **Atherosclerosis of native coronary** `HCC`
artery of transplanted heart with
angina pectoris with documented
spasm

I25.758   **Atherosclerosis of native coronary** `HCC`
artery of transplanted heart with
other forms of angina pectoris

I25.759   **Atherosclerosis of native coronary** `HCC` ▽
artery of transplanted heart with
unspecified angina pectoris

✓6ᵗʰ   **I25.76**   **Atherosclerosis of bypass graft of coronary artery of**
transplanted heart with angina pectoris
    EXCLUDES 1   atherosclerosis of bypass graft of coronary
artery of transplanted heart without
angina pectoris (I25.812)

I25.760   **Atherosclerosis of bypass graft of** `HCC` `A`
coronary artery of transplanted heart
with unstable angina

I25.761   **Atherosclerosis of bypass graft of** `HCC` `A`
coronary artery of transplanted heart
with angina pectoris with documented
spasm

I25.768   **Atherosclerosis of bypass graft of** `HCC` `A`
coronary artery of transplanted heart
with other forms of angina pectoris

I25.769   **Atherosclerosis of bypass graft of** `HCC` `A` ▽
coronary artery of transplanted heart
with unspecified angina pectoris

✓6ᵗʰ   **I25.79**   **Atherosclerosis of other coronary artery bypass**
graft(s) with angina pectoris

I25.790   **Atherosclerosis of other coronary** `HCC` `A`
artery bypass graft(s) with unstable
angina pectoris
    EXCLUDES 1   unstable angina without
atherosclerosis of other
coronary artery bypass
graft(s) (I20.0)

I25.791   **Atherosclerosis of other coronary** `HCC` `A`
artery bypass graft(s) with angina
pectoris with documented spasm
    EXCLUDES 1   angina pectoris with documented
spasm without
atherosclerosis of other
coronary artery bypass
graft(s) (I20.1)

I25.798   **Atherosclerosis of other coronary** `HCC` `A`
artery bypass graft(s) with other
forms of angina pectoris
    EXCLUDES 1   other forms of angina pectoris
without atherosclerosis of
other coronary artery bypass
graft(s) (I20.8)

I25.799   **Atherosclerosis of other coronary** `HCC` `A` ▽
artery bypass graft(s) with unspecified
angina pectoris
    EXCLUDES 1   unspecified angina pectoris
without atherosclerosis of
other coronary artery bypass
graft(s) (I20.9)

✓5ᵗʰ   **I25.8**   **Other forms of chronic ischemic heart disease**

✓6ᵗʰ   **I25.81**   **Atherosclerosis of other coronary vessels without**
angina pectoris
Use additional code, if applicable, to identify:
     coronary atherosclerosis due to calcified coronary
     lesion (I25.84)
     coronary atherosclerosis due to lipid rich plaque
     (I25.83)
    EXCLUDES 1   atherosclerotic heart disease of native
coronary artery without angina pectoris
(I25.10)

I25.810   **Atherosclerosis of coronary artery** `A`
bypass graft(s) without angina pectoris
Atherosclerosis of coronary artery bypass
graft NOS
    EXCLUDES 1   atherosclerosis of coronary
bypass graft(s) with angina
pectoris (I25.70--I25.73-,
I25.79-)

I25.811   **Atherosclerosis of native coronary**
artery of transplanted heart without
angina pectoris
Atherosclerosis of native coronary artery of
transplanted heart NOS
    EXCLUDES 1   atherosclerosis of native coronary
artery of transplanted heart
with angina pectoris
(I25.75-)

I25.812   **Atherosclerosis of bypass graft of** `A`
coronary artery of transplanted heart
without angina pectoris
Atherosclerosis of bypass graft of
transplanted heart NOS
    EXCLUDES 1   atherosclerosis of bypass graft of
transplanted heart with
angina pectoris (I25.76)

I25.82   **Chronic total occlusion of coronary artery**
Complete occlusion of coronary artery
Total occlusion of coronary artery
Code first coronary atherosclerosis (I25.1-, I25.7-,
I25.81-)
    EXCLUDES 1 ▶acute coronary occlusion with myocardial
infarction (I21.0-I21.9, I22.-)◀
▶acute coronary occlusion without
myocardial infarction◀ (I24.0)
    DEF: Complete blockage of coronary artery due to
plaque accumulation over an extended period of time;
results in substantial reduction of blood flow;
characterized by angina or chest pain.

I25.83   **Coronary atherosclerosis due to lipid rich plaque** `A`
Code first coronary atherosclerosis (I25.1-, I25.7-,
I25.81-)

I25.84   **Coronary atherosclerosis due to calcified coronary**
lesion
Coronary atherosclerosis due to severely calcified
coronary lesion
Code first coronary atherosclerosis (I25.1-, I25.7-,
I25.81-)

I25.89   **Other forms of chronic ischemic heart disease**

I25.9   **Chronic ischemic heart disease, unspecified** ▽
Ischemic heart disease (chronic) NOS

EXCLUDES 1 Not coded here   *EXCLUDES 2* Not included here   `N` Newborn Age: 0   `P` Pediatric Age: 0-17   `M` Maternity Age: 12-55   `A` Adult Age: 15-124

624   ICD-10-CM 2018

Pulmonary heart disease and diseases of pulmonary circulation (I26-I28)

✓4th I26   Pulmonary embolism
     INCLUDES   pulmonary (acute) (artery)(vein) infarction
                 pulmonary (acute) (artery)(vein) thromboembolism
                 pulmonary (acute) (artery)(vein) thrombosis
     EXCLUDES 2   *chronic pulmonary embolism (I27.82)*
                personal history of pulmonary embolism (Z86.711)
                pulmonary embolism complicating abortion, ectopic or molar pregnancy (O00-O07, O08.2)
                pulmonary embolism complicating pregnancy, childbirth and the puerperium (O88.-)
                pulmonary embolism due to complications of surgical and medical care (T80.0, T81.7-, T82.8-)
                pulmonary embolism due to trauma (T79.0, T79.1)
                septic (non-pulmonary) arterial embolism (I76)

     ✓5th I26.0   Pulmonary embolism with acute cor pulmonale
           I26.01   Septic pulmonary embolism with acute cor pulmonale   **HCC**
                   Code first underlying infection
           I26.02   Saddle embolus of pulmonary artery with acute cor pulmonale   **HCC**
           I26.09   Other pulmonary embolism with acute cor pulmonale   **HCC**
                   Acute cor pulmonale NOS
                   AHA: 2014, 4Q, 21

     ✓5th I26.9   Pulmonary embolism without acute cor pulmonale
           I26.90   Septic pulmonary embolism without acute cor pulmonale   **HCC**
                   Code first underlying infection
           I26.92   Saddle embolus of pulmonary artery without acute cor pulmonale   **HCC**
           I26.99   Other pulmonary embolism without acute cor pulmonale   **HCC**
                   Acute pulmonary embolism NOS
                   Pulmonary embolism NOS

✓4th I27   Other pulmonary heart diseases
     I27.0   Primary pulmonary hypertension   **HCC**
         ►Heritable pulmonary arterial hypertension
         Idiopathic pulmonary arterial hypertension
         Primary group 1 pulmonary hypertension
         Primary pulmonary arterial hypertension◄
         EXCLUDES 1   ►*persistent pulmonary hypertension of newborn (P29.30)*◄
                pulmonary hypertension NOS ►*(I27.20)*◄
                ►*secondary pulmonary arterial hypertension (I27.21)*◄
                secondary pulmonary hypertension ►*(I27.29)*◄

     I27.1   Kyphoscoliotic heart disease   **HCC**

     ✓5th I27.2   Other secondary pulmonary hypertension
         ~~Pulmonary hypertension NOS~~
         Code also associated underlying condition
         EXCLUDES 1   ►*Eisenmenger's syndrome (I27.83)*◄
         AHA: 2014, 4Q, 21
           ● **I27.20   Pulmonary hypertension, unspecified**   ▽
                   Pulmonary hypertension NOS
           ● **I27.21   Secondary pulmonary arterial hypertension**
                   (Associated) (drug-induced) (toxin-induced) pulmonary arterial hypertension NOS
                   (Associated) (drug-induced) (toxin-induced) (secondary) group 1 pulmonary hypertension
                   Code also associated conditions if applicable, or adverse effects of drugs or toxins, such as:
                     adverse effect of appetite depressants (T50.5X5)
                     congenital heart disease (Q20-Q28)
                     human immunodeficiency virus [HIV] disease (B20)
                     polymyositis (M33.2)
                     portal hypertension (K76.6)
                     rheumatoid arthritis (M05.-)
                     schistosomiasis (B65.-)
                     Sjögren syndrome (M35.0-)
                     systemic sclerosis (M34.-)
           ● **I27.22   Pulmonary hypertension due to left heart disease**
                   Group 2 pulmonary hypertension
                   Code also associated left heart disease, if known, such as:
                     multiple valve disease (I08.-)
                     rheumatic mitral valve diseases (I05.-)
                     rheumatic aortic valve diseases (I06.-)

           ● **I27.23   Pulmonary hypertension due to lung diseases and hypoxia**
                   Group 3 pulmonary hypertension
                   Code also associated lung disease, if known, such as:
                     bronchiectasis (J47.-)
                     cystic fibrosis with pulmonary manifestations (E84.0)
                     interstitial lung disease (J84.-)
                     pleural effusion (J90)
                     sleep apnea (G47.3-)
           ● **I27.24   Chronic thromboembolic pulmonary hypertension**
                   Group 4 pulmonary hypertension
                   Code also associated pulmonary embolism, if applicable (I26.-, I27.82)
           ● **I27.29   Other secondary pulmonary hypertension**
                   Group 5 pulmonary hypertension
                   Pulmonary hypertension with unclear multifactorial mechanisms
                   Pulmonary hypertension due to hematologic disorders
                   Pulmonary hypertension due to metabolic disorders
                   Pulmonary hypertension due to other systemic disorders
                   Code also other associated disorders, if known, such as:
                     chronic myeloid leukemia (C92.10- C92.22)
                     essential thrombocythemia (D47.3)
                     Gaucher disease (E75.22)
                     hypertensive chronic kidney disease with end stage renal disease (I12.0, I12.11, I13.2)
                     hyperthyroidism (E05.-)
                     hypothyroidism (E00-E03)
                     polycythemia vera (D45)
                     sarcoidosis (D86.-)
                   AHA: 2016, 2Q, 8

     ✓5th I27.8   Other specified pulmonary heart diseases
           I27.81   Cor pulmonale (chronic)   **HCC**
                   Cor pulmonale NOS
                   EXCLUDES 1   *acute cor pulmonale (I26.0-)*
                   AHA: 2014, 4Q, 21
           I27.82   Chronic pulmonary embolism   **HCC**
                   Use additional code, if applicable, for associated long-term (current) use of anticoagulants (Z79.01)
                   EXCLUDES 1   *personal history of pulmonary embolism (Z86.711)*
                   DEF: A long-standing condition commonly associated with pulmonary hypertension in which small blood clots travel to the lungs repeatedly over many weeks, months, or years, requiring continuation of established anticoagulant or thrombolytic therapy.
           I27.83   Eisenmenger's syndrome
                   Eisenmenger's complex
                   (Irreversible) Eisenmenger's disease
                   Pulmonary hypertension with right to left shunt related to congenital heart disease
                   Code also underlying heart defect, if known, such as:
                     atrial septal defect (Q21.1)
                     Eisenmenger's defect (Q21.8)
                     patent ductus arteriosus (Q25.0)
                     ventricular septal defect (Q21.0)
           I27.89   Other specified pulmonary heart diseases   **HCC**
                   ~~Eisenmenger's complex~~
                   ~~Eisenmenger's syndrome~~
                   EXCLUDES 1   ~~*Eisenmenger's defect (Q21.8)*~~

     I27.9   Pulmonary heart disease, unspecified   **HCC** ▽
         Chronic cardiopulmonary disease

✓4th I28   Other diseases of pulmonary vessels
     I28.0   Arteriovenous fistula of pulmonary vessels   **HCC**
         EXCLUDES 1   *congenital arteriovenous fistula (Q25.72)*
     I28.1   Aneurysm of pulmonary artery   **HCC**
         EXCLUDES 1   *congenital aneurysm (Q25.79)*
                     congenital arteriovenous aneurysm (Q25.72)
     I28.8   Other diseases of pulmonary vessels   **HCC**
         Pulmonary arteritis
         Pulmonary endarteritis
         Rupture of pulmonary vessels
         Stenosis of pulmonary vessels
         Stricture of pulmonary vessels
     I28.9   Disease of pulmonary vessels, unspecified   **HCC** ▽

✓ Additional Character Req   ✓x7th Placeholder Alert   Manifestation   **HCC** CMS-HCC Condition   ▽ Unspecified Code   ►◄ Revised Text   ● New Code   ▲ Revised Code Title

ICD-10-CM 2018   **625**

Chapter 9. Diseases of the Circulatory System

Other forms of heart disease (I30-I52)

✓4th I30 Acute pericarditis

INCLUDES   acute mediastinopericarditis
     acute myopericarditis
     acute pericardial effusion
     acute pleuropericarditis
     acute pneumopericarditis

EXCLUDES 1   *Dressler's syndrome (I24.1)*
     rheumatic pericarditis (acute) (I01.0)
     ▶*viral pericarditis due to Coxsakie virus (B33.23)*◀

I30.0 Acute nonspecific idiopathic pericarditis

I30.1 Infective pericarditis
     Pneumococcal pericarditis
     Pneumopyopericardium
     Purulent pericarditis
     Pyopericarditis
     Pyopericardium
     Pyopneumopericardium
     Staphylococcal pericarditis
     Streptococcal pericarditis
     Suppurative pericarditis
     Viral pericarditis
     Use additional code (B95-B97) to identify infectious agent

I30.8 Other forms of acute pericarditis

I30.9 Acute pericarditis, unspecified ▽

✓4th I31 Other diseases of pericardium

EXCLUDES 1   *diseases of pericardium specified as rheumatic (I09.2)*
     postcardiotomy syndrome (I97.0)
     traumatic injury to pericardium (S26.-)

I31.0 Chronic adhesive pericarditis
     Accretio cordis
     Adherent pericardium
     Adhesive mediastinopericarditis

I31.1 Chronic constrictive pericarditis
     Concretio cordis
     Pericardial calcification

I31.2 Hemopericardium, not elsewhere classified
EXCLUDES 1   *hemopericardium as current complication following acute myocardial infarction (I23.0)*
DEF: Presence of blood in the pericardial sac (pericardium). It can lead to potentially fatal cardiac tamponade if enough blood enters the pericardial cavity.

I31.3 Pericardial effusion (noninflammatory)
     Chylopericardium
EXCLUDES 1   *acute pericardial effusion (I30.9)*

I31.4 Cardiac tamponade
     Code first underlying cause

I31.8 Other specified diseases of pericardium
     Epicardial plaques
     Focal pericardial adhesions

I31.9 Disease of pericardium, unspecified ▽
     Pericarditis (chronic) NOS

Cardiac Tamponade

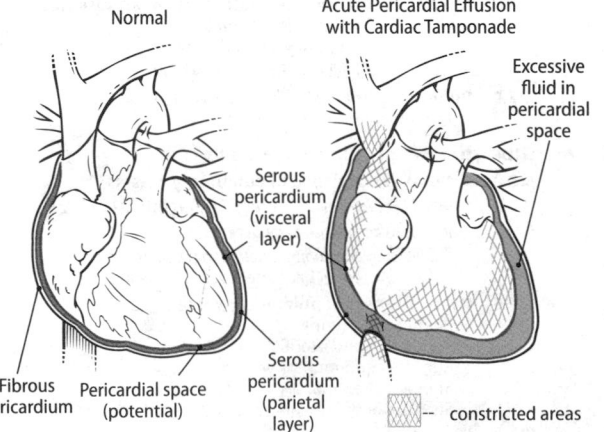

Normal

Acute Pericardial Effusion with Cardiac Tamponade

Excessive fluid in pericardial space

Serous pericardium (visceral layer)

Serous pericardium (parietal layer)

Fibrous pericardium

Pericardial space (potential)

constricted areas

I32 *Pericarditis in diseases classified elsewhere*
     Code first underlying disease
EXCLUDES 1   *pericarditis (in):*
     coxsackie (virus) (B33.23)
     gonococcal (A54.83)
     meningococcal (A39.53)
     rheumatoid (arthritis) (M05.31)
     syphilitic (A52.06)
     systemic lupus erythematosus (M32.12)
     tuberculosis (A18.84)

✓4th I33 Acute and subacute endocarditis
EXCLUDES 1   *acute rheumatic endocarditis (I01.1)*
     endocarditis NOS (I38)

I33.0 Acute and subacute infective endocarditis
     Bacterial endocarditis (acute) (subacute)
     Infective endocarditis (acute) (subacute) NOS
     Endocarditis lenta (acute) (subacute)
     Malignant endocarditis (acute) (subacute)
     Purulent endocarditis (acute) (subacute)
     Septic endocarditis (acute) (subacute)
     Ulcerative endocarditis (acute) (subacute)
     Vegetative endocarditis (acute) (subacute)
     Use additional code (B95-B97) to identify infectious agent

I33.9 Acute and subacute endocarditis, unspecified ▽
     Acute endocarditis NOS
     Acute myoendocarditis NOS
     Acute periendocarditis NOS
     Subacute endocarditis NOS
     Subacute myoendocarditis NOS
     Subacute periendocarditis NOS

✓4th I34 Nonrheumatic mitral valve disorders
EXCLUDES 1   *mitral valve disease (I05.9)*
     mitral valve failure (I05.8)
     mitral valve stenosis (I05.0)
     mitral valve disorder of unspecified cause with diseases of aortic and/or tricuspid valve(s) (I08.-)
     mitral valve disorder of unspecified cause with mitral stenosis or obstruction (I05.0)
     mitral valve disorder specified as congenital ▶(Q23.2, Q23.9)◀
     mitral valve disorder specified as rheumatic (I05.-)

I34.0 Nonrheumatic mitral (valve) insufficiency
     Nonrheumatic mitral (valve) incompetence NOS
     Nonrheumatic mitral (valve) regurgitation NOS

I34.1 Nonrheumatic mitral (valve) prolapse
     Floppy nonrheumatic mitral valve syndrome
EXCLUDES 1   *Marfan's syndrome (Q87.4-)*

I34.2 Nonrheumatic mitral (valve) stenosis

I34.8 Other nonrheumatic mitral valve disorders

I34.9 Nonrheumatic mitral valve disorder, unspecified ▽

✓4th I35 Nonrheumatic aortic valve disorders
EXCLUDES 1   *aortic valve disorder of unspecified cause but with diseases of mitral and/or tricuspid valve(s) (I08.-)*
     aortic valve disorder specified as congenital (Q23.0, Q23.1)
     aortic valve disorder specified as rheumatic (I06.-)
     hypertrophic subaortic stenosis (I42.1)

I35.0 Nonrheumatic aortic (valve) stenosis

I35.1 Nonrheumatic aortic (valve) insufficiency
     Nonrheumatic aortic (valve) incompetence NOS
     Nonrheumatic aortic (valve) regurgitation NOS

I35.2 Nonrheumatic aortic (valve) stenosis with insufficiency

I35.8 Other nonrheumatic aortic valve disorders

I35.9 Nonrheumatic aortic valve disorder, unspecified ▽

✓4th I36 Nonrheumatic tricuspid valve disorders
EXCLUDES 1   *tricuspid valve disorders of unspecified cause (I07.-)*
     tricuspid valve disorders specified as congenital (Q22.4, Q22.8, Q22.9)
     tricuspid valve disorders specified as rheumatic (I07.-)
     tricuspid valve disorders with aortic and/or mitral valve involvement (I08.-)

I36.0 Nonrheumatic tricuspid (valve) stenosis

I36.1 Nonrheumatic tricuspid (valve) insufficiency
     Nonrheumatic tricuspid (valve) incompetence
     Nonrheumatic tricuspid (valve) regurgitation

I36.2 Nonrheumatic tricuspid (valve) stenosis with insufficiency

I36.8 Other nonrheumatic tricuspid valve disorders

I36.9 Nonrheumatic tricuspid valve disorder, unspecified ▽

EXCLUDES 1 Not coded here   EXCLUDES 2 Not included here   N Newborn Age: 0   P Pediatric Age: 0-17   M Maternity Age: 12-55   A Adult Age: 15-124

626   ICD-10-CM 2018

I30–I36.9

✓4ᵗʰ **I37**   **Nonrheumatic pulmonary valve disorders**
> **EXCLUDES 1**   *pulmonary valve disorder specified as congenital (Q22.1, Q22.2, Q22.3)*
> *pulmonary valve disorder specified as rheumatic (I09.89)*

     I37.0   **Nonrheumatic pulmonary valve stenosis**

     I37.1   **Nonrheumatic pulmonary valve insufficiency**
         Nonrheumatic pulmonary valve incompetence
         Nonrheumatic pulmonary valve regurgitation

     I37.2   **Nonrheumatic pulmonary valve stenosis with insufficiency**

     I37.8   **Other nonrheumatic pulmonary valve disorders**

     I37.9   **Nonrheumatic pulmonary valve disorder, unspecified**   ▽

I38   **Endocarditis, valve unspecified**   ▽
> **INCLUDES**   endocarditis (chronic) NOS
> valvular incompetence NOS
> valvular insufficiency NOS
> valvular regurgitation NOS
> valvular stenosis NOS
> valvulitis (chronic) NOS
>
> **EXCLUDES 1**   *congenital insufficiency of cardiac valve NOS (Q24.8)*
> *congenital stenosis of cardiac valve NOS (Q24.8)*
> *endocardial fibroelastosis (I42.4)*
> *endocarditis specified as rheumatic (I09.1)*

I39   *Endocarditis and heart valve disorders in diseases classified elsewhere*
> Code first underlying disease, such as:
> Q fever (A78)
>
> **EXCLUDES 1**   *endocardial involvement in:*
> *candidiasis (B37.6)*
> *gonococcal infection (A54.83)*
> *Libman-Sacks disease (M32.11)*
> *listerosis (A32.82)*
> *meningococcal infection (A39.51)*
> *rheumatoid arthritis (M05.31)*
> *syphilis (A52.03)*
> *tuberculosis (A18.84)*
> *typhoid fever (A01.02)*

✓4ᵗʰ **I40**   **Acute myocarditis**
> **INCLUDES**   subacute myocarditis
> **EXCLUDES 1**   *acute rheumatic myocarditis (I01.2)*

     I40.0   **Infective myocarditis**
         Septic myocarditis
         Use additional code (B95-B97) to identify infectious agent

     I40.1   **Isolated myocarditis**
         Fiedler's myocarditis
         Giant cell myocarditis
         Idiopathic myocarditis

     I40.8   **Other acute myocarditis**

     I40.9   **Acute myocarditis, unspecified**   ▽

I41   *Myocarditis in diseases classified elsewhere*
> Code first underlying disease, such as:
> typhus (A75.0-A75.9)
>
> **EXCLUDES 1**   *myocarditis (in):*
> *Chagas' disease (chronic) (B57.2)*
> *acute (B57.0)*
> *coxsackie (virus) infection (B33.22)*
> *diphtheritic (A36.81)*
> *gonococcal (A54.83)*
> *influenzal (J09.X9, J10.82, J11.82)*
> *meningococcal (A39.52)*
> *mumps (B26.82)*
> *rheumatoid arthritis (M05.31)*
> *sarcoid (D86.85)*
> *syphilis (A52.06)*
> *toxoplasmosis (B58.81)*
> *tuberculous (A18.84)*

✓4ᵗʰ **I42**   **Cardiomyopathy**
> **INCLUDES**   myocardiopathy
> Code first pre-existing cardiomyopathy complicating pregnancy and puerperium (O99.4)
>
> **EXCLUDES 2**   *ischemic cardiomyopathy (I25.5)*
> *peripartum cardiomyopathy (O90.3)*
> *ventricular hypertrophy (I51.7)*

     I42.0   **Dilated cardiomyopathy**   HCC
         Congestive cardiomyopathy

     I42.1   **Obstructive hypertrophic cardiomyopathy**   HCC
         Hypertrophic subaortic stenosis (idiopathic)
         DEF: Cardiomyopathy marked by left ventricle hypertrophy, enlarged septum; results in obstructed blood flow, arrhythmias, mitral regurgitation, and sudden cardiac death.

     I42.2   **Other hypertrophic cardiomyopathy**   HCC
         Nonobstructive hypertrophic cardiomyopathy

     I42.3   **Endomyocardial (eosinophilic) disease**   HCC
         Endomyocardial (tropical) fibrosis
         Löffler's endocarditis

     I42.4   **Endocardial fibroelastosis**   HCC
         Congenital cardiomyopathy
         Elastomyofibrosis

     I42.5   **Other restrictive cardiomyopathy**   HCC
         Constrictive cardiomyopathy NOS

     I42.6   **Alcoholic cardiomyopathy**   HCC
         Code also presence of alcoholism (F10.-)

     I42.7   **Cardiomyopathy due to drug and external agent**   HCC
         Code first poisoning due to drug or toxin, if applicable (T36-T65 with fifth or sixth character 1-4 or 6)
         Use additional code for adverse effect, if applicable, to identify drug (T36-T50 with fifth or sixth character 5)

     I42.8   **Other cardiomyopathies**   HCC

     I42.9   **Cardiomyopathy, unspecified**   HCC ▽
         Cardiomyopathy (primary) (secondary) NOS

I43   *Cardiomyopathy in diseases classified elsewhere*   HCC
> Code first underlying disease, such as:
> amyloidosis (E85.-)
> glycogen storage disease (E74.0)
> gout (M10.0-)
> thyrotoxicosis (E05.0-E05.9-)
>
> **EXCLUDES 1**   *cardiomyopathy (in):*
> *coxsackie (virus) (B33.24)*
> *diphtheria (A36.81)*
> *sarcoidosis (D86.85)*
> *tuberculosis (A18.84)*

✓4ᵗʰ **I44**   **Atrioventricular and left bundle-branch block**
     I44.0   **Atrioventricular block, first degree**

     I44.1   **Atrioventricular block, second degree**
         Atrioventricular block, type I and II
         Möbitz block, type I and II
         Second degree block, type I and II
         Wenckebach's block

     I44.2   **Atrioventricular block, complete**   HCC
         Complete heart block NOS
         Third degree block

✓5ᵗʰ **I44.3**   **Other and unspecified atrioventricular block**
         Atrioventricular block NOS

         I44.30   **Unspecified atrioventricular block**   ▽

         I44.39   **Other atrioventricular block**

     I44.4   **Left anterior fascicular block**

     I44.5   **Left posterior fascicular block**

✓5ᵗʰ **I44.6**   **Other and unspecified fascicular block**

         I44.60   **Unspecified fascicular block**   ▽
            Left bundle-branch hemiblock NOS

         I44.69   **Other fascicular block**

     I44.7   **Left bundle-branch block, unspecified**   ▽

✓4ᵗʰ **I45**   **Other conduction disorders**
     I45.0   **Right fascicular block**

✓5ᵗʰ **I45.1**   **Other and unspecified right bundle-branch block**

         I45.10   **Unspecified right bundle-branch block**   ▽
            Right bundle-branch block NOS

         I45.19   **Other right bundle-branch block**

     I45.2   **Bifascicular block**

     I45.3   **Trifascicular block**

     I45.4   **Nonspecific intraventricular block**
         Bundle-branch block NOS

     I45.5   **Other specified heart block**
         Sinoatrial block
         Sinoauricular block
         EXCLUDES 1   *heart block NOS (I45.9)*

     I45.6   **Pre-excitation syndrome**
         Accelerated atrioventricular conduction
         Accessory atrioventricular conduction
         Anomalous atrioventricular excitation
         Lown-Ganong-Levine syndrome
         Pre-excitation atrioventricular conduction
         Wolff-Parkinson-White syndrome

✓ Additional Character Req   ✓x7ᵗʰ Placeholder Alert   Manifestation   HCC CMS-HCC Condition   ▽ Unspecified Code   ►◄ Revised Text   ● New Code   ▲ Revised Code Title

Conduction Disorders

Sinoatrial node (pacemaker)
Internodal tracts:
　Anterior
　Middle
　Posterior
Atrioventricular node
Atrioventricular bundle (of His)
Atrioventricular block
Accessory bundle (of Kent)
Right bundle branch
Right bundle branch block
Moderator band
Purkinje fibers

Bachmann's bundle
Left bundle branch block
Left bundle branch:
　Anterior fascicle
　Posterior fascicle
Left bundle branch hemiblock

✓5ᵗʰ I45.8　Other specified conduction disorders

　I45.81　Long QT syndrome
　　DEF: Condition characterized by recurrent syncope, malignant arrhythmias, and sudden death; characteristic prolonged Q-T interval on electrocardiogram.

　I45.89　Other specified conduction disorders
　　Atrioventricular [AV] dissociation
　　Interference dissociation
　　Isorhythmic dissociation
　　Nonparoxysmal AV nodal tachycardia
　　AHA: 2013, 2Q, 31

I45.9　Conduction disorder, unspecified ▽
　Heart block NOS
　Stokes-Adams syndrome

✓4ᵗʰ I46　Cardiac arrest
　EXCLUDES 1　*cardiogenic shock (R57.0)*

　I46.2　Cardiac arrest due to underlying cardiac condition HCC
　　Code first underlying cardiac condition

　I46.8　Cardiac arrest due to other underlying condition HCC
　　Code first underlying condition

　I46.9　Cardiac arrest, cause unspecified HCC ▽

✓4ᵗʰ I47　Paroxysmal tachycardia
　Code first tachycardia complicating:
　　abortion or ectopic or molar pregnancy (O00-O07, O08.8)
　　obstetric surgery and procedures (O75.4)
　EXCLUDES 1　*tachycardia NOS (R00.0)*
　　　sinoauricular tachycardia NOS (R00.0)
　　　sinus [sinusal] tachycardia NOS (R00.0)

　I47.0　Re-entry ventricular arrhythmia HCC

　I47.1　Supraventricular tachycardia HCC
　　Atrial (paroxysmal) tachycardia
　　Atrioventricular [AV] (paroxysmal) tachycardia
　　Atrioventricular re-entrant (nodal) tachycardia [AVNRT] [AVRT]
　　Junctional (paroxysmal) tachycardia
　　Nodal (paroxysmal) tachycardia

　I47.2　Ventricular tachycardia HCC
　　AHA: 2013, 3Q, 23

　I47.9　Paroxysmal tachycardia, unspecified HCC ▽
　　Bouveret (-Hoffman) syndrome

✓4ᵗʰ I48　Atrial fibrillation and flutter

　I48.0　Paroxysmal atrial fibrillation HCC
　I48.1　Persistent atrial fibrillation HCC
　I48.2　Chronic atrial fibrillation HCC
　　Permanent atrial fibrillation
　I48.3　Typical atrial flutter HCC
　　Type I atrial flutter
　I48.4　Atypical atrial flutter HCC
　　Type II atrial flutter

✓5ᵗʰ I48.9　Unspecified atrial fibrillation and atrial flutter
　I48.91　Unspecified atrial fibrillation HCC ▽
　I48.92　Unspecified atrial flutter HCC ▽

✓4ᵗʰ I49　Other cardiac arrhythmias
　Code first cardiac arrhythmia complicating:
　　abortion or ectopic or molar pregnancy (O00-O07, O08.8)
　　obstetric surgery and procedures (O75.4)
　EXCLUDES 1　*bradycardia NOS (R00.1)*
　　　neonatal dysrhythmia (P29.1-)
　　　sinoatrial bradycardia (R00.1)
　　　sinus bradycardia (R00.1)
　　　vagal bradycardia (R00.1)
　EXCLUDES 2　▶*bradycardia NOS (R00.1)*◀

✓5ᵗʰ I49.0　Ventricular fibrillation and flutter
　I49.01　Ventricular fibrillation HCC
　I49.02　Ventricular flutter HCC

I49.1　Atrial premature depolarization
　Atrial premature beats

I49.2　Junctional premature depolarization HCC

I49.3　Ventricular premature depolarization

✓5ᵗʰ I49.4　Other and unspecified premature depolarization
　I49.40　Unspecified premature depolarization ▽
　　Premature beats NOS
　I49.49　Other premature depolarization
　　Ectopic beats
　　Extrasystoles
　　Extrasystolic arrhythmias
　　Premature contractions

I49.5　Sick sinus syndrome HCC
　Tachycardia-bradycardia syndrome

I49.8　Other specified cardiac arrhythmias
　▶Brugada syndrome◀
　Coronary sinus rhythm disorder
　Ectopic rhythm disorder
　Nodal rhythm disorder

I49.9　Cardiac arrhythmia, unspecified ▽
　Arrhythmia (cardiac) NOS

✓4ᵗʰ I50　Heart failure
　Code first:
　　heart failure complicating abortion or ectopic or molar pregnancy (O00-O07, O08.8)
　　heart failure due to hypertension (I11.0)
　　heart failure due to hypertension with chronic kidney disease (I13.-)
　　heart failure following surgery (I97.13-)
　　obstetric surgery and procedures (O75.4)
　　rheumatic heart failure (I09.81)
　EXCLUDES 1　*neonatal cardiac failure (P29.0)*
　EXCLUDES 2　*cardiac arrest (I46.-)*
　AHA: 2017, 1Q, 47; 2014, 1Q, 25; 2013, 2Q, 33

▲ **I50.1　Left ventricular failure, unspecified** HCC ▽
　Cardiac asthma
　Edema of lung with heart disease NOS
　Edema of lung with heart failure
　Left heart failure
　Pulmonary edema with heart disease NOS
　Pulmonary edema with heart failure
　EXCLUDES 1　*edema of lung without heart disease or heart failure (J81.-)*
　　　pulmonary edema without heart disease or failure (J81.-)

✓5ᵗʰ I50.2　Systolic (congestive) heart failure
　▶Heart failure with reduced ejection fraction [HFrEF]
　Systolic left ventricular heart failure◀
　▶Code also end stage heart failure, if applicable (I50.84)◀
　AHA: 2017, 1Q, 46; 2016, 1Q, 10
　I50.20　Unspecified systolic (congestive) heart failure HCC ▽
　I50.21　Acute systolic (congestive) heart failure HCC
　I50.22　Chronic systolic (congestive) heart failure HCC
　I50.23　Acute on chronic systolic (congestive) heart failure HCC

✓5ᵗʰ I50.3　Diastolic (congestive) heart failure
　▶Diastolic left ventricular heart failure
　Heart failure with normal ejection fraction
　Heart failure with preserved ejection fraction [HFpEF]◀
　▶Code also end stage heart failure, if applicable (I50.84)◀
　EXCLUDES 1　*combined systolic (congestive) and diastolic (congestive) heart failure (I50.4-)*
　AHA: 2017, 1Q, 46; 2016, 1Q, 10

EXCLUDES 1 Not coded here　　EXCLUDES 2 Not included here　　N Newborn Age: 0　　P Pediatric Age: 0-17　　M Maternity Age: 12-55　　A Adult Age: 15-124

I50.30	**Unspecified diastolic (congestive) heart failure**	HCC ▽	
I50.31	**Acute diastolic (congestive) heart failure**	HCC	
I50.32	**Chronic diastolic (congestive) heart failure**	HCC	
I50.33	**Acute on chronic diastolic (congestive) heart failure**	HCC	

✓5ᵗʰ **I50.4** **Combined systolic (congestive) and diastolic (congestive) heart failure**
▶Combined systolic and diastolic left ventricular heart failure
Heart failure with reduced ejection fraction and diastolic dysfunction◀
▶Code also end stage heart failure, if applicable (I50.84)◀
AHA: 2017, 1Q, 46; 2016, 1Q, 10

I50.40	**Unspecified combined systolic (congestive) and diastolic (congestive) heart failure**	HCC ▽
I50.41	**Acute combined systolic (congestive) and diastolic (congestive) heart failure**	HCC
I50.42	**Chronic combined systolic (congestive) and diastolic (congestive) heart failure**	HCC
I50.43	**Acute on chronic combined systolic (congestive) and diastolic (congestive) heart failure**	HCC

● ✓5ᵗʰ **I50.8** **Other heart failure**
● ✓6ᵗʰ **I50.81** **Right heart failure**
    Right ventricular failure

●   **I50.810** **Right heart failure, unspecified** ▽
        Right heart failure without mention of left heart failure
        Right ventricular failure NOS

●   **I50.811** **Acute right heart failure**
        Acute isolated right heart failure
        Acute (isolated) right ventricular failure

●   **I50.812** **Chronic right heart failure**
        Chronic isolated right heart failure
        Chronic (isolated) right ventricular failure

●   **I50.813** **Acute on chronic right heart failure**
        Acute on chronic isolated right heart failure
        Acute on chronic (isolated) right ventricular failure
        Acute decompensation of chronic (isolated) right ventricular failure
        Acute exacerbation of chronic (isolated) right ventricular failure

●   **I50.814** **Right heart failure due to left heart failure**
        Right ventricular failure secondary to left ventricular failure
        Code also the type of left ventricular failure, if known (I50.2-I50.43)
        EXCLUDES 1   *right heart failure with but not due to left heart failure (I50.82)*

●   **I50.82** **Biventricular heart failure**
        Code also the type of left ventricular failure as systolic, diastolic, or combined, if known (I50.2-I50.43)

●   **I50.83** **High output heart failure**

●   **I50.84** **End stage heart failure**
        Stage D heart failure
        Code also the type of heart failure as systolic, diastolic, or combined, if known (I50.2-I50.43)

●   **I50.89** **Other heart failure**

I50.9 **Heart failure, unspecified**   HCC ▽
    ~~Biventricular (heart) failure NOS~~
    Cardiac, heart or myocardial failure NOS
    Congestive heart disease
    Congestive heart failure NOS
    ~~Right ventricular failure (secondary to left heart failure)~~
    EXCLUDES 2   *fluid overload (E87.70)*
    AHA: 2017, 1Q, 45-46; 2014, 4Q, 21; 2012, 4Q, 92

✓4ᵗʰ **I51** **Complications and ill-defined descriptions of heart disease**
    EXCLUDES 1   *any condition in I51.4-I51.9 due to hypertension (I11.-)*
           any condition in I51.4-I51.9 due to hypertension and chronic kidney disease (I13.-)
           heart disease specified as rheumatic (I00-I09)

I51.0 **Cardiac septal defect, acquired**   A
    Acquired septal atrial defect (old)
    Acquired septal auricular defect (old)
    Acquired septal ventricular defect (old)
    EXCLUDES 1   *cardiac septal defect as current complication following acute myocardial infarction (I23.1, I23.2)*
    DEF: Abnormal communication between opposite heart chambers due to defect of septum; not present at birth.

I51.1 **Rupture of chordae tendineae, not elsewhere classified**   HCC
    EXCLUDES 1   *rupture of chordae tendineae as current complication following acute myocardial infarction (I23.4)*

I51.2 **Rupture of papillary muscle, not elsewhere classified**   HCC
    EXCLUDES 1   *rupture of papillary muscle as current complication following acute myocardial infarction (I23.5)*

I51.3 **Intracardiac thrombosis, not elsewhere classified**
    Apical thrombosis (old)   Mural thrombosis (old)
    Atrial thrombosis (old)   Ventricular thrombosis (old)
    Auricular thrombosis (old)
    EXCLUDES 1   *intracardiac thrombosis as current complication following acute myocardial infarction (I23.6)*
    AHA: 2013, 1Q, 24

I51.4 **Myocarditis, unspecified**   HCC ▽
    Chronic (interstitial) myocarditis
    Myocardial fibrosis
    Myocarditis NOS
    EXCLUDES 1   *acute or subacute myocarditis (I40.-)*

I51.5 **Myocardial degeneration**   HCC
    Fatty degeneration of heart or myocardium
    Myocardial disease
    Senile degeneration of heart or myocardium

I51.7 **Cardiomegaly**
    Cardiac dilatation
    Cardiac hypertrophy
    Ventricular dilatation

✓5ᵗʰ **I51.8** **Other ill-defined heart diseases**
   I51.81 **Takotsubo syndrome**
        Reversible left ventricular dysfunction following sudden emotional stress
        Stress induced cardiomyopathy
        Takotsubo cardiomyopathy
        Transient left ventricular apical ballooning syndrome

   I51.89 **Other ill-defined heart diseases**
        Carditis (acute)(chronic)
        Pancarditis (acute)(chronic)

I51.9 **Heart disease, unspecified**   ▽

I52 ***Other heart disorders in diseases classified elsewhere***
    Code first underlying disease, such as:
      congenital syphilis (A50.5)
      mucopolysaccharidosis (E76.3)
      schistosomiasis (B65.0-B65.9)
    EXCLUDES 1   *heart disease (in):*
         gonococcal infection (A54.83)
         meningococcal infection (A39.50)
         rheumatoid arthritis (M05.31)
         syphilis (A52.06)

Cerebrovascular diseases (I60-I69)

Use additional code to identify presence of:
  alcohol abuse and dependence (F10.-)
  exposure to environmental tobacco smoke (Z77.22)
  history of tobacco dependence (Z87.891)
  hypertension (I10-I15)
  occupational exposure to environmental tobacco smoke (Z57.31)
  tobacco dependence (F17.-)
  tobacco use (Z72.0)
EXCLUDES 1   ~~*transient cerebral ischemic attacks and related syndromes (G45.-)*~~
        traumatic intracranial hemorrhage (S06.-)
AHA: 2014, 3Q, 5; 2012, 4Q, 91-92

✓4ᵗʰ **I60** **Nontraumatic subarachnoid hemorrhage**
    INCLUDES   ruptured cerebral aneurysm
    EXCLUDES 1   *syphilitic ruptured cerebral aneurysm (A52.05)*
    EXCLUDES 2   *sequelae of subarachnoid hemorrhage (I69.0-)*

✓5ᵗʰ **I60.0** **Nontraumatic subarachnoid hemorrhage from carotid siphon and bifurcation**
   I60.00 **Nontraumatic subarachnoid hemorrhage from unspecified carotid siphon and bifurcation**   HCC ▽
   I60.01 **Nontraumatic subarachnoid hemorrhage from right carotid siphon and bifurcation**   HCC
   I60.02 **Nontraumatic subarachnoid hemorrhage from left carotid siphon and bifurcation**   HCC

✓ Additional Character Req   ✓x7ᵗʰ Placeholder Alert   Manifestation   HCC CMS-HCC Condition   ▽ Unspecified Code   ▶◀ Revised Text   ● New Code   ▲ Revised Code Title

ICD-10-CM 2018   **629**

Chapter 9. Diseases of the Circulatory System *(left margin vertical)*

I60.1–I63.212 *(left margin vertical, bottom)*

✓5ᵗʰ **I60.1 Nontraumatic subarachnoid hemorrhage from middle cerebral artery**

     I60.10 Nontraumatic subarachnoid hemorrhage from unspecified middle cerebral artery   HCC ▽

     I60.11 Nontraumatic subarachnoid hemorrhage from right middle cerebral artery   HCC

     I60.12 Nontraumatic subarachnoid hemorrhage from left middle cerebral artery   HCC

I60.2 Nontraumatic subarachnoid hemorrhage from anterior communicating artery   HCC

✓5ᵗʰ **I60.3 Nontraumatic subarachnoid hemorrhage from posterior communicating artery**

     I60.30 Nontraumatic subarachnoid hemorrhage from unspecified posterior communicating artery   HCC ▽

     I60.31 Nontraumatic subarachnoid hemorrhage from right posterior communicating artery   HCC

     I60.32 Nontraumatic subarachnoid hemorrhage from left posterior communicating artery   HCC

I60.4 Nontraumatic subarachnoid hemorrhage from basilar artery   HCC

✓5ᵗʰ **I60.5 Nontraumatic subarachnoid hemorrhage from vertebral artery**

     I60.50 Nontraumatic subarachnoid hemorrhage from unspecified vertebral artery   HCC ▽

     I60.51 Nontraumatic subarachnoid hemorrhage from right vertebral artery   HCC

     I60.52 Nontraumatic subarachnoid hemorrhage from left vertebral artery   HCC

I60.6 Nontraumatic subarachnoid hemorrhage from other intracranial arteries   HCC

I60.7 Nontraumatic subarachnoid hemorrhage from unspecified intracranial artery   HCC ▽
Ruptured (congenital) berry aneurysm
Ruptured (congenital) cerebral aneurysm
Subarachnoid hemorrhage (nontraumatic) from cerebral artery NOS
Subarachnoid hemorrhage (nontraumatic) from communicating artery NOS
     EXCLUDES 1   berry aneurysm, nonruptured (I67.1)

I60.8 Other nontraumatic subarachnoid hemorrhage   HCC
Meningeal hemorrhage
Rupture of cerebral arteriovenous malformation

I60.9 Nontraumatic subarachnoid hemorrhage, unspecified   HCC ▽

✓4ᵗʰ **I61 Nontraumatic intracerebral hemorrhage**
     EXCLUDES 2   sequelae of intracerebral hemorrhage (I69.1-)
     AHA: 2017, 2Q, 9-10

I61.0 Nontraumatic intracerebral hemorrhage in hemisphere, subcortical   HCC
Deep intracerebral hemorrhage (nontraumatic)

I61.1 Nontraumatic intracerebral hemorrhage in hemisphere, cortical   HCC
Cerebral lobe hemorrhage (nontraumatic)
Superficial intracerebral hemorrhage (nontraumatic)

I61.2 Nontraumatic intracerebral hemorrhage in hemisphere, unspecified   HCC ▽

I61.3 Nontraumatic intracerebral hemorrhage in brain stem   HCC

I61.4 Nontraumatic intracerebral hemorrhage in cerebellum   HCC

I61.5 Nontraumatic intracerebral hemorrhage, intraventricular   HCC

I61.6 Nontraumatic intracerebral hemorrhage, multiple localized   HCC

I61.8 Other nontraumatic intracerebral hemorrhage   HCC

I61.9 Nontraumatic intracerebral hemorrhage, unspecified   HCC ▽

✓4ᵗʰ **I62 Other and unspecified nontraumatic intracranial hemorrhage**
     EXCLUDES 2   sequelae of intracranial hemorrhage (I69.2)

✓5ᵗʰ **I62.0 Nontraumatic subdural hemorrhage**

     I62.00 Nontraumatic subdural hemorrhage, unspecified   HCC ▽

     I62.01 Nontraumatic acute subdural hemorrhage   HCC

     I62.02 Nontraumatic subacute subdural hemorrhage   HCC

     I62.03 Nontraumatic chronic subdural hemorrhage   HCC

I62.1 Nontraumatic extradural hemorrhage   HCC
Nontraumatic epidural hemorrhage

I62.9 Nontraumatic intracranial hemorrhage, unspecified   HCC ▽

✓4ᵗʰ **I63 Cerebral infarction**
     INCLUDES   occlusion and stenosis of cerebral and precerebral arteries, resulting in cerebral infarction
     Use additional code, if applicable, to identify status post administration of tPA (rtPA) in a different facility within the last 24 hours prior to admission to current facility (Z92.82)
     Use additional code, if known, to indicate National Institutes of Health Stroke Scale (NIHSS) score (R29.7-)
     EXCLUDES 2   sequelae of cerebral infarction (I69.3-)
     AHA: 2017, 2Q, 9-10; 2014, 1Q, 23

✓5ᵗʰ **I63.0 Cerebral infarction due to thrombosis of precerebral arteries**

     I63.00 Cerebral infarction due to thrombosis of unspecified precerebral artery   HCC ▽

     ✓6ᵗʰ **I63.01** Cerebral infarction due to thrombosis of vertebral artery

         I63.011 Cerebral infarction due to thrombosis of right vertebral artery   HCC

         I63.012 Cerebral infarction due to thrombosis of left vertebral artery   HCC

         I63.013 Cerebral infarction due to thrombosis of bilateral vertebral arteries   HCC

         I63.019 Cerebral infarction due to thrombosis of unspecified vertebral artery   HCC ▽

     I63.02 Cerebral infarction due to thrombosis of basilar artery   HCC

     ✓6ᵗʰ **I63.03** Cerebral infarction due to thrombosis of carotid artery

         I63.031 Cerebral infarction due to thrombosis of right carotid artery   HCC

         I63.032 Cerebral infarction due to thrombosis of left carotid artery   HCC

         I63.033 Cerebral infarction due to thrombosis of bilateral carotid arteries   HCC

         I63.039 Cerebral infarction due to thrombosis of unspecified carotid artery   HCC ▽

     I63.09 Cerebral infarction due to thrombosis of other precerebral artery   HCC

✓5ᵗʰ **I63.1 Cerebral infarction due to embolism of precerebral arteries**

     I63.10 Cerebral infarction due to embolism of unspecified precerebral artery   HCC ▽

     ✓6ᵗʰ **I63.11** Cerebral infarction due to embolism of vertebral artery

         I63.111 Cerebral infarction due to embolism of right vertebral artery   HCC

         I63.112 Cerebral infarction due to embolism of left vertebral artery   HCC

         I63.113 Cerebral infarction due to embolism of bilateral vertebral arteries   HCC

         I63.119 Cerebral infarction due to embolism of unspecified vertebral artery   HCC ▽

     I63.12 Cerebral infarction due to embolism of basilar artery   HCC

     ✓6ᵗʰ **I63.13** Cerebral infarction due to embolism of carotid artery

         I63.131 Cerebral infarction due to embolism of right carotid artery   HCC

         I63.132 Cerebral infarction due to embolism of left carotid artery   HCC

         I63.133 Cerebral infarction due to embolism of bilateral carotid arteries   HCC

         I63.139 Cerebral infarction due to embolism of unspecified carotid artery   HCC ▽

     I63.19 Cerebral infarction due to embolism of other precerebral artery   HCC

✓5ᵗʰ **I63.2 Cerebral infarction due to unspecified occlusion or stenosis of precerebral arteries**

     I63.20 Cerebral infarction due to unspecified occlusion or stenosis of unspecified precerebral arteries   HCC ▽

     ✓6ᵗʰ **I63.21** Cerebral infarction due to unspecified occlusion or stenosis of vertebral arteries

▲   **I63.211** Cerebral infarction due to unspecified occlusion or stenosis of right vertebral artery   HCC

▲   **I63.212** Cerebral infarction due to unspecified occlusion or stenosis of left vertebral artery   HCC

EXCLUDES 1 Not coded here   *EXCLUDES 2* Not included here   **N** Newborn Age: 0   **P** Pediatric Age: 0-17   **M** Maternity Age: 12-55   **A** Adult Age: 15-124

630   ICD-10-CM 2018

I63.213   Cerebral infarction due to unspecified HCC occlusion or stenosis of **bilateral** vertebral arteries

I63.219   Cerebral infarction due to HCC ▽ unspecified occlusion or stenosis of unspecified vertebral arteries

▲   I63.22   **Cerebral infarction due to unspecified occlusion or stenosis of basilar artery** HCC

✓6th   I63.23   **Cerebral infarction due to unspecified occlusion or stenosis of carotid arteries**

I63.231   Cerebral infarction due to unspecified HCC occlusion or stenosis of **right** carotid arteries

I63.232   Cerebral infarction due to unspecified HCC occlusion or stenosis of **left** carotid arteries

I63.233   Cerebral infarction due to unspecified HCC occlusion or stenosis of **bilateral** carotid arteries

I63.239   Cerebral infarction due to HCC ▽ unspecified occlusion or stenosis of unspecified carotid arteries

I63.29   **Cerebral infarction due to unspecified** HCC ▽ **occlusion or stenosis of other precerebral arteries**

✓5th   I63.3   **Cerebral infarction due to thrombosis of cerebral arteries**

I63.30   **Cerebral infarction due to thrombosis of** HCC ▽ **unspecified cerebral artery**

✓6th   I63.31   **Cerebral infarction due to thrombosis of middle cerebral artery**

I63.311   Cerebral infarction due to thrombosis HCC of **right** middle cerebral artery

I63.312   Cerebral infarction due to thrombosis HCC of **left** middle cerebral artery

I63.313   Cerebral infarction due to thrombosis HCC of **bilateral** middle cerebral arteries

I63.319   Cerebral infarction due to HCC ▽ thrombosis of unspecified middle cerebral artery

✓6th   I63.32   **Cerebral infarction due to thrombosis of anterior cerebral artery**

I63.321   Cerebral infarction due to thrombosis HCC of **right** anterior cerebral artery

I63.322   Cerebral infarction due to thrombosis HCC of **left** anterior cerebral artery

▲   I63.323   Cerebral infarction due to thrombosis HCC of **bilateral** anterior cerebral arteries

I63.329   Cerebral infarction due to HCC ▽ thrombosis of unspecified anterior cerebral artery

✓6th   I63.33   **Cerebral infarction due to thrombosis of posterior cerebral artery**

I63.331   Cerebral infarction due to thrombosis HCC of **right** posterior cerebral artery

I63.332   Cerebral infarction due to thrombosis HCC of **left** posterior cerebral artery

▲   I63.333   Cerebral infarction to thrombosis of HCC **bilateral** posterior cerebral arteries

I63.339   Cerebral infarction due to HCC ▽ thrombosis of unspecified posterior cerebral artery

✓6th   I63.34   **Cerebral infarction due to thrombosis of cerebellar artery**

I63.341   Cerebral infarction due to thrombosis HCC of **right** cerebellar artery

I63.342   Cerebral infarction due to thrombosis HCC of **left** cerebellar artery

I63.343   Cerebral infarction to thrombosis of HCC **bilateral** cerebellar arteries

I63.349   Cerebral infarction due to HCC ▽ thrombosis of unspecified cerebellar artery

I63.39   **Cerebral infarction due to thrombosis of other** HCC **cerebral artery**

✓5th   I63.4   **Cerebral infarction due to embolism of cerebral arteries**

I63.40   **Cerebral infarction due to embolism of** HCC ▽ **unspecified cerebral artery**

✓6th   I63.41   **Cerebral infarction due to embolism of middle cerebral artery**

I63.411   Cerebral infarction due to embolism HCC of **right** middle cerebral artery

I63.412   Cerebral infarction due to embolism HCC of **left** middle cerebral artery

I63.413   Cerebral infarction due to embolism HCC of **bilateral** middle cerebral arteries

I63.419   Cerebral infarction due to embolism HCC ▽ of unspecified middle cerebral artery

✓6th   I63.42   **Cerebral infarction due to embolism of anterior cerebral artery**

I63.421   Cerebral infarction due to embolism HCC of **right** anterior cerebral artery

I63.422   Cerebral infarction due to embolism HCC of **left** anterior cerebral artery

I63.423   Cerebral infarction due to embolism HCC of **bilateral** anterior cerebral arteries

I63.429   Cerebral infarction due to HCC ▽ embolismof unspecified anterior cerebral artery

✓6th   I63.43   **Cerebral infarction due to embolism of posterior cerebral artery**

I63.431   Cerebral infarction due to embolism HCC of **right** posterior cerebral artery

I63.432   Cerebral infarction due to embolism HCC of **left** posterior cerebral artery

I63.433   Cerebral infarction due to embolism HCC of **bilateral** posterior cerebral arteries

I63.439   Cerebral infarction due to HCC ▽ embolism of unspecified posterior cerebral artery

✓6th   I63.44   **Cerebral infarction due to embolism of cerebellar artery**

I63.441   Cerebral infarction due to embolism HCC of **right** cerebellar artery

I63.442   Cerebral infarction due to embolism HCC of **left** cerebellar artery

I63.443   Cerebral infarction due to embolism HCC of **bilateral** cerebellar arteries

I63.449   Cerebral infarction due to HCC ▽ embolism of unspecified cerebellar artery

I63.49   **Cerebral infarction due to embolism of other** HCC **cerebral artery**

✓5th   I63.5   **Cerebral infarction due to unspecified occlusion or stenosis of cerebral arteries**

I63.50   **Cerebral infarction due to unspecified** HCC ▽ **occlusion or stenosis of unspecified cerebral artery**

✓6th   I63.51   **Cerebral infarction due to unspecified occlusion or stenosis of middle cerebral artery**

I63.511   Cerebral infarction due to unspecified HCC occlusion or stenosis of **right** middle cerebral artery

I63.512   Cerebral infarction due to unspecified HCC occlusion or stenosis of **left** middle cerebral artery

▲   I63.513   Cerebral infarction due to unspecified HCC occlusion or stenosis of **bilateral** middle cerebral arteries

I63.519   Cerebral infarction due to HCC ▽ unspecified occlusion or stenosis of unspecified middle cerebral artery

✓6th   I63.52   **Cerebral infarction due to unspecified occlusion or stenosis of anterior cerebral artery**

I63.521   Cerebral infarction due to unspecified HCC occlusion or stenosis of **right** anterior cerebral artery

I63.522   Cerebral infarction due to unspecified HCC occlusion or stenosis of **left** anterior cerebral artery

▲   I63.523   Cerebral infarction due to unspecified HCC occlusion or stenosis of **bilateral** anterior cerebral arteries

I63.529   Cerebral infarction due to HCC ▽ unspecified occlusion or stenosis of unspecified anterior cerebral artery

---

✓ Additional Character Req   ✓x7th Placeholder Alert   Manifestation   HCC CMS-HCC Condition   ▽ Unspecified Code   ►◄ Revised Text   ● New Code   ▲ Revised Code Title

ICD-10-CM 2018   631

√6ᵗʰ **I63.53 Cerebral infarction due to unspecified occlusion or stenosis of posterior cerebral artery**

    I63.531 Cerebral infarction due to unspecified HCC **occlusion or stenosis of right posterior cerebral artery**

    I63.532 Cerebral infarction due to unspecified HCC **occlusion or stenosis of left posterior cerebral artery**

    I63.533 Cerebral infarction due to unspecified HCC **occlusion or stenosis of bilateral posterior cerebral arteries**

    I63.539 Cerebral infarction due to HCC ▽ **unspecified occlusion or stenosis of unspecified posterior cerebral artery**

√6ᵗʰ **I63.54 Cerebral infarction due to unspecified occlusion or stenosis of cerebellar artery**

    I63.541 Cerebral infarction due to unspecified HCC **occlusion or stenosis of right cerebellar artery**

    I63.542 Cerebral infarction due to unspecified HCC **occlusion or stenosis of left cerebellar artery**

    I63.543 Cerebral infarction due to unspecified HCC **occlusion or stenosis of bilateral cerebellar arteries**

    I63.549 Cerebral infarction due to HCC ▽ **unspecified occlusion or stenosis of unspecified cerebellar artery**

I63.59 Cerebral infarction due to unspecified HCC ▽ **occlusion or stenosis of other cerebral artery**

I63.6 Cerebral infarction due to cerebral venous thrombosis, HCC **nonpyogenic**

I63.8 Other cerebral infarction HCC

I63.9 Cerebral infarction, unspecified HCC ▽
    Stroke NOS
    EXCLUDES 2 ▶transient cerebral ischemic attacks and related syndromes (G45.-)◀
    AHA: 2015, 1Q, 25

√4ᵗʰ **I65 Occlusion and stenosis of precerebral arteries, not resulting in cerebral infarction**
    INCLUDES   embolism of precerebral artery
       narrowing of precerebral artery
       obstruction (complete) (partial) of precerebral artery
       thrombosis of precerebral artery
    EXCLUDES 1   insufficiency, NOS, of precerebral artery (G45.-)
       insufficiency of precerebral arteries causing cerebral infarction (I63.0-I63.2)

√5ᵗʰ **I65.0 Occlusion and stenosis of vertebral artery**

    I65.01 Occlusion and stenosis of right vertebral artery

    I65.02 Occlusion and stenosis of left vertebral artery

    I65.03 Occlusion and stenosis of bilateral vertebral arteries

    I65.09 Occlusion and stenosis of unspecified ▽ **vertebral artery**

I65.1 Occlusion and stenosis of basilar artery

√5ᵗʰ **I65.2 Occlusion and stenosis of carotid artery**

    I65.21 Occlusion and stenosis of right carotid artery

    I65.22 Occlusion and stenosis of left carotid artery

    I65.23 Occlusion and stenosis of bilateral carotid arteries

    I65.29 Occlusion and stenosis of unspecified carotid ▽ **artery**

I65.8 Occlusion and stenosis of other precerebral arteries

I65.9 Occlusion and stenosis of unspecified precerebral ▽ **artery**
    Occlusion and stenosis of precerebral artery NOS

√4ᵗʰ **I66 Occlusion and stenosis of cerebral arteries, not resulting in cerebral infarction**
    INCLUDES   embolism of cerebral artery
       narrowing of cerebral artery
       obstruction (complete) (partial) of cerebral artery
       thrombosis of cerebral artery
    EXCLUDES 1   occlusion and stenosis of cerebral artery causing cerebral infarction (I63.3-I63.5)

√5ᵗʰ **I66.0 Occlusion and stenosis of middle cerebral artery**

    I66.01 Occlusion and stenosis of right middle cerebral artery

    I66.02 Occlusion and stenosis of left middle cerebral artery

    I66.03 Occlusion and stenosis of bilateral middle cerebral arteries

    I66.09 Occlusion and stenosis of unspecified middle ▽ **cerebral artery**

√5ᵗʰ **I66.1 Occlusion and stenosis of anterior cerebral artery**

    I66.11 Occlusion and stenosis of right anterior cerebral artery

    I66.12 Occlusion and stenosis of left anterior cerebral artery

    I66.13 Occlusion and stenosis of bilateral anterior cerebral arteries

    I66.19 Occlusion and stenosis of unspecified anterior ▽ **cerebral artery**

√5ᵗʰ **I66.2 Occlusion and stenosis of posterior cerebral artery**

    I66.21 Occlusion and stenosis of right posterior cerebral artery

    I66.22 Occlusion and stenosis of left posterior cerebral artery

    I66.23 Occlusion and stenosis of bilateral posterior cerebral arteries

    I66.29 Occlusion and stenosis of unspecified ▽ **posterior cerebral artery**

I66.3 Occlusion and stenosis of cerebellar arteries

I66.8 Occlusion and stenosis of other cerebral arteries
    Occlusion and stenosis of perforating arteries

I66.9 Occlusion and stenosis of unspecified cerebral artery ▽

√4ᵗʰ **I67 Other cerebrovascular diseases**
    EXCLUDES 2   sequelae of the listed conditions (I69.8)

I67.0 Dissection of cerebral arteries, nonruptured HCC
    EXCLUDES 1   ruptured cerebral artieries (I60.7)

I67.1 Cerebral aneurysm, nonruptured
    Cerebral aneurysm NOS
    Cerebral arteriovenous fistula, acquired
    Internal carotid artery aneurysm, intracranial portion
    Internal carotid artery aneurysm, NOS
    EXCLUDES 1   congenital cerebral aneurysm, nonruptured (Q28.-)
       ruptured cerebral aneurysm (I60.7)

I67.2 Cerebral atherosclerosis A
    Atheroma of cerebral and precerebral arteries

I67.3 Progressive vascular leukoencephalopathy
    Binswanger's disease

I67.4 Hypertensive encephalopathy
    EXCLUDES 2 ▶insufficiency, NOS, of precerebral arteries (G45.2)◀

Berry Aneurysm

Berry aneurysms form at the site of a weakness in an arterial wall, often at a junction

Berry aneurysm

Anterior communicating artery
Anterior cerebral artery
40%
34%
Internal carotid
Middle cerebral artery
20%
4%
Posterior cerebral artery
Posterior communicating artery
Basilar artery

Common sites of berry aneurysms in the circle of Willis arteries

EXCLUDES 1 Not coded here   EXCLUDES 2 Not included here   N Newborn Age: 0   P Pediatric Age: 0-17   M Maternity Age: 12-55   A Adult Age: 15-124

632   ICD-10-CM 2018

I67.5 Moyamoya disease
DEF: Cerebrovascular ischemia; vessels occlude and rupture, causing tiny hemorrhages at base of brain; affects predominantly Japanese people.

I67.6 Nonpyogenic thrombosis of intracranial venous system
Nonpyogenic thrombosis of cerebral vein
Nonpyogenic thrombosis of intracranial venous sinus
EXCLUDES 1   *nonpyogenic thrombosis of intracranial venous system causing infarction (I63.6)*

I67.7 Cerebral arteritis, not elsewhere classified
Granulomatous angiitis of the nervous system
EXCLUDES 1   *allergic granulomatous angiitis (M30.1)*

✓5th **I67.8 Other specified cerebrovascular diseases**
    I67.81 Acute cerebrovascular insufficiency
        Acute cerebrovascular insufficiency unspecified as to location or reversibility
    I67.82 Cerebral ischemia
        Chronic cerebral ischemia
    I67.83 Posterior reversible encephalopathy syndrome
        PRES
    ✓6th **I67.84 Cerebral vasospasm and vasoconstriction**
        I67.841 Reversible cerebrovascular vasoconstriction syndrome
            Call-Fleming syndrome
            Code first underlying condition, if applicable, such as eclampsia (O15.00-O15.9)
        I67.848 Other cerebrovascular vasospasm and vasoconstriction
    I67.89 Other cerebrovascular disease
I67.9 Cerebrovascular disease, unspecified   ▽

✓4th **I68 Cerebrovascular disorders in diseases classified elsewhere**
I68.0 Cerebral amyloid angiopathy
Code first underlying amyloidosis (E85.-)

I68.2 Cerebral arteritis in other diseases classified elsewhere
Code first underlying disease
EXCLUDES 1   *cerebral arteritis (in):*
    listerosis (A32.89)
    systemic lupus erythematosus (M32.19)
    syphilis (A52.04)
    tuberculosis (A18.89)

I68.8 Other cerebrovascular disorders in diseases classified elsewhere
Code first underlying disease
EXCLUDES 1   *syphilitic cerebral aneurysm (A52.05)*

✓4th **I69 Sequelae of cerebrovascular disease**
NOTE   Category I69 is to be used to indicate conditions in I60-I67 as the cause of sequelae. The "sequelae" include conditions specified as such or as residuals which may occur at any time after the onset of the causal condition
EXCLUDES 1   *personal history of cerebral infarction without residual deficit (Z86.73)*
    personal history of prolonged reversible ischemic neurologic deficit (PRIND) (Z86.73)
    personal history of reversible ischemic neurologcial deficit (RIND) (Z86.73)
    sequelae of traumatic intracranial injury (S06.-)
    ~~transient ischemic attack (TIA) (G45.9)~~
AHA: 2017, 1Q, 47; 2015, 1Q, 25; 2012, 4Q, 106

✓5th **I69.0 Sequelae of nontraumatic subarachnoid hemorrhage**
    I69.00 Unspecified sequelae of nontraumatic subarachnoid hemorrhage   ▽
    ✓6th **I69.01 Cognitive deficits following nontraumatic subarachnoid hemorrhage**
        I69.010 Attention and concentration deficit following nontraumatic subarachnoid hemorrhage
        I69.011 Memory deficit following nontraumatic subarachnoid hemorrhage
        I69.012 Visuospatial deficit and spatial neglect following nontraumatic subarachnoid hemorrhage
        I69.013 Psychomotor deficit following nontraumatic subarachnoid hemorrhage
        I69.014 Frontal lobe and executive function deficit following nontraumatic subarachnoid hemorrhage
        I69.015 Cognitive social or emotional deficit following nontraumatic subarachnoid hemorrhage

        I69.018 Other symptoms and signs involving cognitive functions following nontraumatic subarachnoid hemorrhage
        I69.019 Unspecified symptoms and signs   ▽ **involving cognitive functions following nontraumatic subarachnoid hemorrhage**
    ✓6th **I69.02 Speech and language deficits following nontraumatic subarachnoid hemorrhage**
        I69.020 Aphasia following nontraumatic subarachnoid hemorrhage
        I69.021 Dysphasia following nontraumatic subarachnoid hemorrhage
        I69.022 Dysarthria following nontraumatic subarachnoid hemorrhage
        I69.023 Fluency disorder following nontraumatic subarachnoid hemorrhage
            Stuttering following nontraumatic subarachnoid hemorrhage
        I69.028 Other speech and language deficits following nontraumatic subarachnoid hemorrhage
    ✓6th **I69.03 Monoplegia of upper limb following nontraumatic subarachnoid hemorrhage**
        AHA: 2017, 1Q, 47
        I69.031 Monoplegia of upper limb following HCC **nontraumatic subarachnoid hemorrhage affecting right dominant side**
        I69.032 Monoplegia of upper limb following HCC **nontraumatic subarachnoid hemorrhage affecting left dominant side**
        I69.033 Monoplegia of upper limb following HCC **nontraumatic subarachnoid hemorrhage affecting right non-dominant side**
        I69.034 Monoplegia of upper limb following HCC **nontraumatic subarachnoid hemorrhage affecting left non-dominant side**
        I69.039 Monoplegia of upper limb HCC ▽ **following nontraumatic subarachnoid hemorrhage affecting unspecified side**
    ✓6th **I69.04 Monoplegia of lower limb following nontraumatic subarachnoid hemorrhage**
        AHA: 2017, 1Q, 47
        I69.041 Monoplegia of lower limb following HCC **nontraumatic subarachnoid hemorrhage affecting right dominant side**
        I69.042 Monoplegia of lower limb following HCC **nontraumatic subarachnoid hemorrhage affecting left dominant side**
        I69.043 Monoplegia of lower limb following HCC **nontraumatic subarachnoid hemorrhage affecting right non-dominant side**
        I69.044 Monoplegia of lower limb following HCC **nontraumatic subarachnoid hemorrhage affecting left non-dominant side**
        I69.049 Monoplegia of lower limb following HCC ▽ **nontraumatic subarachnoid hemorrhage affecting unspecified side**
    ✓6th **I69.05 Hemiplegia and hemiparesis following nontraumatic subarachnoid hemorrhage**
        AHA: 2015, 1Q, 25
        I69.051 Hemiplegia and hemiparesis following HCC **nontraumatic subarachnoid hemorrhage affecting right dominant side**
        I69.052 Hemiplegia and hemiparesis following HCC **nontraumatic subarachnoid hemorrhage affecting left dominant side**
        I69.053 Hemiplegia and hemiparesis following HCC **nontraumatic subarachnoid hemorrhage affecting right non-dominant side**
        I69.054 Hemiplegia and hemiparesis following HCC **nontraumatic subarachnoid hemorrhage affecting left non-dominant side**
        I69.059 Hemiplegia and hemiparesis HCC ▽ **following nontraumatic subarachnoid hemorrhage affecting unspecified side**

✓ Additional Character Req   ✓x7th Placeholder Alert   Manifestation   HCC CMS-HCC Condition   ▽ Unspecified Code   ►◄ Revised Text   ● New Code   ▲ Revised Code Title

ICD-10-CM 2018   633

✓6th I69.06   Other paralytic syndrome following nontraumatic subarachnoid hemorrhage
Use additional code to identify type of paralytic syndrome, such as:
locked-in state (G83.5)
quadriplegia (G82.5-)

EXCLUDES 1 hemiplegia/hemiparesis following nontraumatic subarachnoid hemorrhage (I69.05-)
monoplegia of lower limb following nontraumatic subarachnoid hemorrhage (I69.04-)
monoplegia of upper limb following nontraumatic subarachnoid hemorrhage (I69.03-)

I69.061   Other paralytic syndrome following HCC
nontraumatic subarachnoid hemorrhage affecting right dominant side

I69.062   Other paralytic syndrome following HCC
nontraumatic subarachnoid hemorrhage affecting left dominant side

I69.063   Other paralytic syndrome following HCC
nontraumatic subarachnoid hemorrhage affecting right non-dominant side

I69.064   Other paralytic syndrome following HCC
nontraumatic subarachnoid hemorrhage affecting left non-dominant side

I69.065   Other paralytic syndrome following HCC
nontraumatic subarachnoid hemorrhage, bilateral

I69.069   Other paralytic syndrome following HCC ▽
nontraumatic subara chnoid hemorrhage affecting unspecified side

✓6th I69.09   Other sequelae of nontraumatic subarachnoid hemorrhage

I69.090   Apraxia following nontraumatic subarachnoid hemorrhage

I69.091   Dysphagia following nontraumatic subarachnoid hemorrhage
Use additional code to identify the type of dysphagia, if known (R13.1-)

I69.092   Facial weakness following nontraumatic subarachnoid hemorrhage
Facial droop following nontraumatic subarachnoid hemorrhage

I69.093   Ataxia following nontraumatic subarachnoid hemorrhage

I69.098   Other sequelae following nontraumatic subarachnoid hemorrhage
Alterations of sensation following nontraumatic subarachnoid hemorrhage
Disturbance of vision following nontraumatic subarachnoid hemorrhage
Use additional code to identify the sequelae

✓5th I69.1   Sequelae of nontraumatic intracerebral hemorrhage

I69.10   Unspecified sequelae of nontraumatic ▽
intracerebral hemorrhage

✓6th I69.11   Cognitive deficits following nontraumatic intracerebral hemorrhage

I69.110   Attention and concentration deficit following nontraumatic intracerebral hemorrhage

I69.111   Memory deficit following nontraumatic intracerebral hemorrhage

I69.112   Visuospatial deficit and spatial neglect following nontraumatic intracerebral hemorrhage

I69.113   Psychomotor deficit following nontraumatic intracerebral hemorrhage

I69.114   Frontal lobe and executive function deficit following nontraumatic intracerebral hemorrhage

I69.115   Cognitive social or emotional deficit following nontraumatic intracerebral hemorrhage

I69.118   Other symptoms and signs involving cognitive functions following nontraumatic intracerebral hemorrhage

I69.119   Unspecified symptoms and signs ▽
involving cognitive functions following nontraumatic intracerebral hemorrhage

✓6th I69.12   Speech and language deficits following nontraumatic intracerebral hemorrhage

I69.120   Aphasia following nontraumatic intracerebral hemorrhage

I69.121   Dysphasia following nontraumatic intracerebral hemorrhage

I69.122   Dysarthria following nontraumatic intracerebral hemorrhage

I69.123   Fluency disorder following nontraumatic intracerebral hemorrhage
Stuttering following nontraumatic intracerebral hemorrhage

I69.128   Other speech and language deficits following nontraumatic intracerebral hemorrhage

✓6th I69.13   Monoplegia of upper limb following nontraumatic intracerebral hemorrhage
AHA: 2017, 1Q, 47

I69.131   Monoplegia of upper limb following HCC
nontraumatic intracerebral hemorrhage affecting right dominant side

I69.132   Monoplegia of upper limb following HCC
nontraumatic intracerebral hemorrhage affecting left dominant side

I69.133   Monoplegia of upper limb following HCC
nontraumatic intracerebral hemorrhage affecting right non-dominant side

I69.134   Monoplegia of upper limb following HCC
nontraumatic intracerebral hemorrhage affecting left non-dominant side

I69.139   Monoplegia of upper limb HCC ▽
following nontraumatic intracerebral hemorrhage affecting unspecified side

✓6th I69.14   Monoplegia of lower limb following nontraumatic intracerebral hemorrhage
AHA: 2017, 1Q, 47

I69.141   Monoplegia of lower limb following HCC
nontraumatic intracerebral hemorrhage affecting right dominant side

I69.142   Monoplegia of lower limb following HCC
nontraumatic intracerebral hemorrhage affecting left dominant side

I69.143   Monoplegia of lower limb following HCC
nontraumatic intracerebral hemorrhage affecting right non-dominant side

I69.144   Monoplegia of lower limb following HCC
nontraumatic intracerebral hemorrhage affecting left non-dominant side

I69.149   Monoplegia of lower limb following HCC ▽
nontraumatic intracerebral hemorrhage affecting unspecified side

✓6th I69.15   Hemiplegia and hemiparesis following nontraumatic intracerebral hemorrhage
AHA: 2015, 1Q, 25

I69.151   Hemiplegia and hemiparesis following HCC
nontraumatic intracerebral hemorrhage affecting right dominant side

I69.152   Hemiplegia and hemiparesis following HCC
nontraumatic intracerebral hemorrhage affecting left dominant side

I69.153   Hemiplegia and hemiparesis following HCC
nontraumatic intracerebral hemorrhage affecting right non-dominant side

I69.154   Hemiplegia and hemiparesis following HCC
nontraumatic intracerebral hemorrhage affecting left non-dominant side

I69.159   Hemiplegia and hemiparesis HCC ▽
following nontraumatic intracerebral hemorrhage affecting unspecified side

EXCLUDES 1 Not coded here   *EXCLUDES 2* Not included here   N Newborn Age: 0   P Pediatric Age: 0-17   M Maternity Age: 12-55   A Adult Age: 15-124

634   ICD-10-CM 2018

✓6ᵗʰ **I69.16** **Other paralytic syndrome following nontraumatic intracerebral hemorrhage**
Use additional code to identify type of paralytic syndrome, such as:
    locked-in state (G83.5)
    quadriplegia (G82.5-)
    EXCLUDES 1 *hemiplegia/hemiparesis following nontraumatic intracerebral hemorrhage (I69.15-)*
          monoplegia of lower limb following nontraumatic intracerebral hemorrhage (I69.14-)
          monoplegia of upper limb following nontraumatic intracerebral hemorrhage (I69.13-)

    I69.161 **Other paralytic syndrome following** HCC **nontraumatic intracerebral hemorrhage affecting right dominant side**

    I69.162 **Other paralytic syndrome following** HCC **nontraumatic intracerebral hemorrhage affecting left dominant side**

    I69.163 **Other paralytic syndrome following** HCC **nontraumatic intracerebral hemorrhage affecting right non-dominant side**

    I69.164 **Other paralytic syndrome following** HCC **nontraumatic intracerebral hemorrhage affecting left non-dominant side**

    I69.165 **Other paralytic syndrome following** HCC **nontraumatic intracerebral hemorrhage, bilateral**

    I69.169 **Other paralytic syndrome** HCC ▽ **following nontraumatic intracerebral hemorrhage affecting unspecified side**

✓6ᵗʰ **I69.19** **Other sequelae of nontraumatic intracerebral hemorrhage**

    I69.190 **Apraxia following nontraumatic intracerebral hemorrhage**

    I69.191 **Dysphagia following nontraumatic intracerebral hemorrhage**
        Use additional code to identify the type of dysphagia, if known (R13.1-)

    I69.192 **Facial weakness following nontraumatic intracerebral hemorrhage**
        Facial droop following nontraumatic intracerebral hemorrhage

    I69.193 **Ataxia following nontraumatic intracerebral hemorrhage**

    I69.198 **Other sequelae of nontraumatic intracerebral hemorrhage**
        Alteration of sensations following nontraumatic intracerebral hemorrhage
        Disturbance of vision following nontraumatic intracerebral hemorrhage
        Use additional code to identify the sequelae

✓5ᵗʰ **I69.2** **Sequelae of other nontraumatic intracranial hemorrhage**

    I69.20 **Unspecified sequelae of other nontraumatic** ▽ **intracranial hemorrhage**

✓6ᵗʰ **I69.21** **Cognitive deficits following other nontraumatic intracranial hemorrhage**

    I69.210 **Attention and concentration deficit following other nontraumatic intracranial hemorrhage**

    I69.211 **Memory deficit following other nontraumatic intracranial hemorrhage**

    I69.212 **Visuospatial deficit and spatial neglect following other nontraumatic intracranial hemorrhage**

    I69.213 **Psychomotor deficit following other nontraumatic intracranial hemorrhage**

    I69.214 **Frontal lobe and executive function deficit following other nontraumatic intracranial hemorrhage**

    I69.215 **Cognitive social or emotional deficit following other nontraumatic intracranial hemorrhage**

    I69.218 **Other symptoms and signs involving cognitive functions following other nontraumatic intracranial hemorrhage**

    I69.219 **Unspecified symptoms and signs** ▽ **involving cognitive functions following other nontraumatic intracranial hemorrhage**

✓6ᵗʰ **I69.22** **Speech and language deficits following other nontraumatic intracranial hemorrhage**

    I69.220 **Aphasia following other nontraumatic intracranial hemorrhage**

    I69.221 **Dysphasia following other nontraumatic intracranial hemorrhage**

    I69.222 **Dysarthria following other nontraumatic intracranial hemorrhage**

    I69.223 **Fluency disorder following other nontraumatic intracranial hemorrhage**
        Stuttering following nontraumatic intracerebral hemorrhage

    I69.228 **Other speech and language deficits following other nontraumatic intracranial hemorrhage**

✓6ᵗʰ **I69.23** **Monoplegia of upper limb following other nontraumatic intracranial hemorrhage**
    AHA: 2017, 1Q, 47

    I69.231 **Monoplegia of upper limb following** HCC **other nontraumatic intracranial hemorrhage affecting right dominant side**

    I69.232 **Monoplegia of upper limb following** HCC **other nontraumatic intracranial hemorrhage affecting left dominant side**

    I69.233 **Monoplegia of upper limb following** HCC **other nontraumatic intracranial hemorrhage affecting right non-dominant side**

    I69.234 **Monoplegia of upper limb following** HCC **other nontraumatic intracranial hemorrhage affecting left non-dominant side**

    I69.239 **Monoplegia of upper limb** HCC ▽ **following other nontraumatic intracranial hemorrhage affecting unspecified side**

✓6ᵗʰ **I69.24** **Monoplegia of lower limb following other nontraumatic intracranial hemorrhage**
    AHA: 2017, 1Q, 47

    I69.241 **Monoplegia of lower limb following** HCC **other nontraumatic intracranial hemorrhage affecting right dominant side**

    I69.242 **Monoplegia of lower limb following** HCC **other nontraumatic intracranial hemorrhage affecting left dominant side**

    I69.243 **Monoplegia of lower limb following** HCC **other nontraumatic intracranial hemorrhage affecting right non-dominant side**

    I69.244 **Monoplegia of lower limb following** HCC **other nontraumatic intracranial hemorrhage affecting left non-dominant side**

    I69.249 **Monoplegia of lower limb following** HCC ▽ **other nontraumatic intracranial hemorrhage affecting unspecified side**

✓6ᵗʰ **I69.25** **Hemiplegia and hemiparesis following other nontraumatic intracranial hemorrhage**
    AHA: 2015, 1Q, 25

    I69.251 **Hemiplegia and hemiparesis following** HCC **other nontraumatic intracranial hemorrhage affecting right dominant side**

    I69.252 **Hemiplegia and hemiparesis following** HCC **other nontraumatic intracranial hemorrhage affecting left dominant side**

    I69.253 **Hemiplegia and hemiparesis following** HCC **other nontraumatic intracranial hemorrhage affecting right non-dominant side**

    I69.254 **Hemiplegia and hemiparesis following** HCC **other nontraumatic intracranial hemorrhage affecting left non-dominant side**

    I69.259 **Hemiplegia and hemiparesis** HCC ▽ **following other nontraumatic intracranial hemorrhage affecting unspecified side**

✓ Additional Character Req   ✓x7ᵗʰ Placeholder Alert   Manifestation   HCC CMS-HCC Condition   ▽ Unspecified Code   ►◄ Revised Text   ● New Code   ▲ Revised Code Title

ICD-10-CM 2018   635

☑6ᵗʰ I69.26 Other paralytic syndrome following other nontraumatic intracranial hemorrhage
Use additional code to identify type of paralytic syndrome, such as:
locked-in state (G83.5)
quadriplegia (G82.5-)
EXCLUDES 1 *hemiplegia/hemiparesis following other nontraumatic intracranial hemorrhage (I69.25-)*
monoplegia of lower limb following other nontraumatic intracranial hemorrhage (I69.24-)
monoplegia of upper limb following other nontraumatic intracranial hemorrhage (I69.23-)

I69.261 Other paralytic syndrome following HCC
other nontraumatic intracranial hemorrhage affecting right dominant side

I69.262 Other paralytic syndrome following HCC
other nontraumatic intracranial hemorrhage affecting left dominant side

I69.263 Other paralytic syndrome following HCC
other nontraumatic intracranial hemorrhage affecting right non-dominant side

I69.264 Other paralytic syndrome following HCC
other nontraumatic intracranial hemorrhage affecting left non-dominant side

I69.265 Other paralytic syndrome following HCC
other nontraumatic intracranial hemorrhage, bilateral

I69.269 Other paralytic syndrome following HCC ▽
other nontraumatic intracranial hemorrhage affecting unspecified side

☑6ᵗʰ I69.29 Other sequelae of other nontraumatic intracranial hemorrhage

I69.290 Apraxia following other nontraumatic intracranial hemorrhage

I69.291 Dysphagia following other nontraumatic intracranial hemorrhage
Use additional code to identify the type of dysphagia, if known (R13.1-)

I69.292 Facial weakness following other nontraumatic intracranial hemorrhage
Facial droop following other nontraumatic intracranial hemorrhage

I69.293 Ataxia following other nontraumatic intracranial hemorrhage

I69.298 Other sequelae of other nontraumatic intracranial hemorrhage
Alteration of sensation following other nontraumatic intracranial hemorrhage
Disturbance of vision following other nontraumatic intracranial hemorrhage
Use additional code to identify the sequelae

☑5ᵗʰ I69.3 Sequelae of cerebral infarction
Sequelae of stroke NOS
AHA: 2013, 4Q, 127-128; 2012, 4Q, 92, 94

I69.30 Unspecified sequelae of cerebral infarction   ▽

☑6ᵗʰ I69.31 Cognitive deficits following cerebral infarction

I69.310 Attention and concentration deficit following cerebral infarction

I69.311 Memory deficit following cerebral infarction

I69.312 Visuospatial deficit and spatial neglect following cerebral infarction

I69.313 Psychomotor deficit following cerebral infarction

I69.314 Frontal lobe and executive function deficit following cerebral infarction

I69.315 Cognitive social or emotional deficit following cerebral infarction

I69.318 Other symptoms and signs involving cognitive functions following cerebral infarction

I69.319 Unspecified symptoms and signs ▽
involving cognitive functions following cerebral infarction

☑6ᵗʰ I69.32 Speech and language deficits following cerebral infarction

I69.320 Aphasia following cerebral infarction

I69.321 Dysphasia following cerebral infarction
AHA: 2012, 4Q, 91

I69.322 Dysarthria following cerebral infarction
EXCLUDES 2 ▶*transient ischemic attack (TIA) (G45.9)*◀

I69.323 Fluency disorder following cerebral infarction
Stuttering following cerebral infarction

I69.328 Other speech and language deficits following cerebral infarction

☑6ᵗʰ I69.33 Monoplegia of upper limb following cerebral infarction
AHA: 2017, 1Q, 47

I69.331 Monoplegia of upper limb following HCC
cerebral infarction affecting right dominant side

I69.332 Monoplegia of upper limb following HCC
cerebral infarction affecting left dominant side

I69.333 Monoplegia of upper limb following HCC
cerebral infarction affecting right non-dominant side

I69.334 Monoplegia of upper limb following HCC
cerebral infarction affecting left non-dominant side

I69.339 Monoplegia of upper limb HCC ▽
following cerebral infarction affecting unspecified side

☑6ᵗʰ I69.34 Monoplegia of lower limb following cerebral infarction
AHA: 2017, 1Q, 47

I69.341 Monoplegia of lower limb following HCC
cerebral infarction affecting right dominant side

I69.342 Monoplegia of lower limb following HCC
cerebral infarction affecting left dominant side

I69.343 Monoplegia of lower limb following HCC
cerebral infarction affecting right non-dominant side

I69.344 Monoplegia of lower limb following HCC
cerebral infarction affecting left non-dominant side

I69.349 Monoplegia of lower limb HCC ▽
following cerebral infarction affecting unspecified side

☑6ᵗʰ I69.35 Hemiplegia and hemiparesis following cerebral infarction
AHA: 2015, 1Q, 25

I69.351 Hemiplegia and hemiparesis HCC
following cerebral infarction affecting right dominant side
EXCLUDES 2 ▶*transient ischemic attack (TIA) (G45.9)*◀

I69.352 Hemiplegia and hemiparesis HCC
following cerebral infarction affecting left dominant side

I69.353 Hemiplegia and hemiparesis HCC
following cerebral infarction affecting right non-dominant side

I69.354 Hemiplegia and hemiparesis HCC
following cerebral infarction affecting left non-dominant side
AHA: 2012, 4Q, 91

I69.359 Hemiplegia and hemiparesis HCC ▽
following cerebral infarction affecting unspecified side

☑6ᵗʰ I69.36 Other paralytic syndrome following cerebral infarction
Use additional code to identify type of paralytic syndrome, such as:
locked-in state (G83.5)
quadriplegia (G82.5-)
EXCLUDES 1 *hemiplegia/hemiparesis following cerebral infarction (I69.35-)*
monoplegia of lower limb following cerebral infarction (I69.34-)
monoplegia of upper limb following cerebral infarction (I69.33-)

EXCLUDES 1 Not coded here   *EXCLUDES 2* Not included here   **N** Newborn Age: 0   **P** Pediatric Age: 0-17   **M** Maternity Age: 12-55   **A** Adult Age: 15-124

636   ICD-10-CM 2018

I69.361 Other paralytic syndrome following cerebral infarction affecting **right dominant** side `HCC`

I69.362 Other paralytic syndrome following cerebral infarction affecting **left dominant** side `HCC`

I69.363 Other paralytic syndrome following cerebral infarction affecting **right non-dominant** side `HCC`

I69.364 Other paralytic syndrome following cerebral infarction affecting **left non-dominant** side `HCC`

I69.365 Other paralytic syndrome following cerebral infarction, **bilateral** `HCC`

I69.369 Other paralytic syndrome following cerebral infarction affecting unspecified side `HCC` ▽

✓6th **I69.39** Other sequelae of cerebral infarction

     I69.390 **Apraxia** following cerebral infarction

     I69.391 **Dysphagia** following cerebral infarction
         Use additional code to identify the type of dysphagia, if known (R13.1-)

     I69.392 **Facial weakness** following cerebral infarction
         Facial droop following cerebral infarction

     I69.393 **Ataxia** following cerebral infarction

     I69.398 **Other sequelae** of cerebral infarction
         Alteration of sensation following cerebral infarction
         Disturbance of vision following cerebral infarction
         Use additional code to identify the sequelae

✓5th **I69.8** Sequelae of other **cerebrovascular diseases**
     EXCLUDES 1   sequelae of traumatic intracranial injury (S06.-)

     I69.80 Unspecified sequelae of other cerebrovascular disease ▽

✓6th **I69.81** **Cognitive deficits** following other cerebrovascular disease

     I69.810 **Attention and concentration deficit** following other cerebrovascular disease

     I69.811 **Memory deficit** following other cerebrovascular disease

     I69.812 **Visuospatial deficit and spatial neglect** following other cerebrovascular disease

     I69.813 **Psychomotor deficit** following other cerebrovascular disease

     I69.814 **Frontal lobe and executive function deficit** following other cerebrovascular disease

     I69.815 **Cognitive social or emotional deficit** following other cerebrovascular disease

     I69.818 **Other symptoms and signs involving cognitive functions** following other cerebrovascular disease

     I69.819 **Unspecified symptoms and signs involving cognitive functions** following other cerebrovascular disease ▽

✓6th **I69.82** **Speech and language deficits** following other cerebrovascular disease

     I69.820 **Aphasia** following other cerebrovascular disease

     I69.821 **Dysphasia** following other cerebrovascular disease

     I69.822 **Dysarthria** following other cerebrovascular disease

     I69.823 **Fluency disorder** following other cerebrovascular disease
         Stuttering following other cerebrovascular disease

     I69.828 **Other speech and language deficits** following other cerebrovascular disease

✓6th **I69.83** **Monoplegia of upper limb** following other cerebrovascular disease
     AHA: 2017, 1Q, 47

     I69.831 Monoplegia of upper limb following other cerebrovascular disease affecting **right dominant** side `HCC`

     I69.832 Monoplegia of upper limb following other cerebrovascular disease affecting **left dominant** side `HCC`

I69.833 Monoplegia of upper limb following other cerebrovascular disease affecting **right non-dominant** side `HCC`

I69.834 Monoplegia of upper limb following other cerebrovascular disease affecting **left non-dominant** side `HCC`

I69.839 Monoplegia of upper limb following other cerebrovascular disease affecting unspecified side `HCC` ▽

✓6th **I69.84** **Monoplegia of lower limb** following other cerebrovascular disease
     AHA: 2017, 1Q, 47

     I69.841 Monoplegia of lower limb following other cerebrovascular disease affecting **right dominant** side `HCC`

     I69.842 Monoplegia of lower limb following other cerebrovascular disease affecting **left dominant** side `HCC`

     I69.843 Monoplegia of lower limb following other cerebrovascular disease affecting **right non-dominant** side `HCC`

     I69.844 Monoplegia of lower limb following other cerebrovascular disease affecting **left non-dominant** side `HCC`

     I69.849 Monoplegia of lower limb following other cerebrovascular disease affecting unspecified side `HCC` ▽

✓6th **I69.85** **Hemiplegia** and **hemiparesis** following other cerebrovascular disease
     AHA: 2015, 1Q, 25

     I69.851 Hemiplegia and hemiparesis following other cerebrovascular disease affecting **right dominant** side `HCC`

     I69.852 Hemiplegia and hemiparesis following other cerebrovascular disease affecting **left dominant** side `HCC`

     I69.853 Hemiplegia and hemiparesis following other cerebrovascular disease affecting **right non-dominant** side `HCC`

     I69.854 Hemiplegia and hemiparesis following other cerebrovascular disease affecting **left non-dominant** side `HCC`

     I69.859 Hemiplegia and hemiparesis following other cerebrovascular disease affecting unspecified side `HCC` ▽

✓6th **I69.86** **Other paralytic syndrome** following other cerebrovascular disease
     Use additional code to identify type of paralytic syndrome, such as:
         locked-in state (G83.5)
         quadriplegia (G82.5-)
     EXCLUDES 1   hemiplegia/hemiparesis following other cerebrovascular disease (I69.85-)
         monoplegia of lower limb following other cerebrovascular disease (I69.84-)
         monoplegia of upper limb following other cerebrovascular disease (I69.83-)

     I69.861 Other paralytic syndrome following other cerebrovascular disease affecting **right dominant** side `HCC`

     I69.862 Other paralytic syndrome following other cerebrovascular disease affecting **left dominant** side `HCC`

     I69.863 Other paralytic syndrome following other cerebrovascular disease affecting **right non-dominant** side `HCC`

     I69.864 Other paralytic syndrome following other cerebrovascular disease affecting **left non-dominant** side `HCC`

     I69.865 Other paralytic syndrome following other cerebrovascular disease, **bilateral** `HCC`

     I69.869 Other paralytic syndrome following other cerebrovascular disease affecting unspecified side `HCC` ▽

✓6th **I69.89** Other sequelae of other cerebrovascular disease

     I69.890 **Apraxia** following other cerebrovascular disease

     I69.891 **Dysphagia** following other cerebrovascular disease
         Use additional code to identify the type of dysphagia, if known (R13.1-)

✓ Additional Character Req   ✓x7th Placeholder Alert   Manifestation   `HCC` CMS-HCC Condition   ▽ Unspecified Code   ▶◀ Revised Text   ● New Code   ▲ Revised Code Title

Chapter 9. Diseases of the Circulatory System

I69.892   **Facial weakness following other cerebrovascular disease**
> Facial droop following other cerebrovascular disease

I69.893   **Ataxia following other cerebrovascular disease**

I69.898   **Other sequelae of other cerebrovascular disease**
> Alteration of sensation following other cerebrovascular disease
> Disturbance of vision following other cerebrovascular disease
> Use additional code to identify the sequelae

✓5ᵗʰ   **I69.9   Sequelae of unspecified cerebrovascular diseases**
> EXCLUDES 1   *sequelae of stroke (I69.3)*
> *sequelae of traumatic intracranial injury (S06.-)*

I69.90   **Unspecified sequelae of unspecified cerebrovascular disease** ▽

✓6ᵗʰ   I69.91   **Cognitive deficits following unspecified cerebrovascular disease**

I69.910   **Attention and concentration deficit following unspecified cerebrovascular disease** ▽

I69.911   **Memory deficit following unspecified cerebrovascular disease** ▽

I69.912   **Visuospatial deficit and spatial neglect following unspecified cerebrovascular disease** ▽

I69.913   **Psychomotor deficit following unspecified cerebrovascular disease** ▽

I69.914   **Frontal lobe and executive function deficit following unspecified cerebrovascular disease** ▽

I69.915   **Cognitive social or emotional deficit following unspecified cerebrovascular disease** ▽

I69.918   **Other symptoms and signs involving cognitive functions following unspecified cerebrovascular disease** ▽

I69.919   **Unspecified symptoms and signs involving cognitive functions following unspecified cerebrovascular disease** ▽

✓6ᵗʰ   I69.92   **Speech and language deficits following unspecified cerebrovascular disease**

I69.920   **Aphasia following unspecified cerebrovascular disease** ▽

I69.921   **Dysphasia following unspecified cerebrovascular disease** ▽

I69.922   **Dysarthria following unspecified cerebrovascular disease** ▽

I69.923   **Fluency disorder following unspecified cerebrovascular disease** ▽
> Stuttering following unspecified cerebrovascular disease

I69.928   **Other speech and language deficits following unspecified cerebrovascular disease** ▽

✓6ᵗʰ   I69.93   **Monoplegia of upper limb following unspecified cerebrovascular disease**
> AHA: 2017, 1Q, 47

I69.931   **Monoplegia of upper limb following** HCC ▽ **unspecified cerebrovascular disease affecting right dominant side**

I69.932   **Monoplegia of upper limb following** HCC ▽ **unspecified cerebrovascular disease affecting left dominant side**

I69.933   **Monoplegia of upper limb following** HCC ▽ **unspecified cerebrovascular disease affecting right non-dominant side**

I69.934   **Monoplegia of upper limb following** HCC ▽ **unspecified cerebrovascular disease affecting left non-dominant side**

I69.939   **Monoplegia of upper limb following** HCC ▽ **unspecified cerebrovascular disease affecting unspecified side**

✓6ᵗʰ   I69.94   **Monoplegia of lower limb following unspecified cerebrovascular disease**
> AHA: 2017, 1Q, 47

I69.941   **Monoplegia of lower limb following** HCC ▽ **unspecified cerebrovascular disease affecting right dominant side**

I69.942   **Monoplegia of lower limb following** HCC ▽ **unspecified cerebrovascular disease affecting left dominant side**

I69.943   **Monoplegia of lower limb following** HCC ▽ **unspecified cerebrovascular disease affecting right non-dominant side**

I69.944   **Monoplegia of lower limb following** HCC ▽ **unspecified cerebrovascular disease affecting left non-dominant side**

I69.949   **Monoplegia of lower limb following** HCC ▽ **unspecified cerebrovascular disease affecting unspecified side**

✓6ᵗʰ   I69.95   **Hemiplegia and hemiparesis following unspecified cerebrovascular disease**
> AHA: 2015, 1Q, 25

I69.951   **Hemiplegia and hemiparesis** HCC ▽ **following unspecified cerebrovascular disease affecting right dominant side**

I69.952   **Hemiplegia and hemiparesis** HCC ▽ **following unspecified cerebrovascular disease affecting left dominant side**

I69.953   **Hemiplegia and hemiparesis** HCC ▽ **following unspecified cerebrovascular disease affecting right non-dominant side**

I69.954   **Hemiplegia and hemiparesis** HCC ▽ **following unspecified cerebrovascular disease affecting left non-dominant side**

I69.959   **Hemiplegia and hemiparesis** HCC ▽ **following unspecified cerebrovascular disease affecting unspecified side**

✓6ᵗʰ   I69.96   **Other paralytic syndrome following unspecified cerebrovascular disease**
> Use additional code to identify type of paralytic syndrome, such as:
> locked-in state (G83.5)
> quadriplegia (G82.5-)
> EXCLUDES 1   *hemiplegia/hemiparesis following unspecified cerebrovascular disease (I69.95-)*
> *monoplegia of lower limb following unspecified cerebrovascular disease (I69.94-)*
> *monoplegia of upper limb following unspecified cerebrovascular disease (I69.93-)*

I69.961   **Other paralytic syndrome following** HCC ▽ **unspecified cerebrovascular disease affecting right dominant side**

I69.962   **Other paralytic syndrome following** HCC ▽ **unspecified cerebrovascular disease affecting left dominant side**

I69.963   **Other paralytic syndrome following** HCC ▽ **unspecified cerebrovascular disease affecting right non-dominant side**

I69.964   **Other paralytic syndrome following** HCC ▽ **unspecified cerebrovascular disease affecting left non-dominant side**

I69.965   **Other paralytic syndrome following** HCC ▽ **unspecified cerebrovascular disease, bilateral**

I69.969   **Other paralytic syndrome following** HCC ▽ **unspecified cerebrovascular disease affecting unspecified side**

✓6ᵗʰ   I69.99   **Other sequelae of unspecified cerebrovascular disease**

I69.990   **Apraxia following unspecified cerebrovascular disease** ▽

I69.991   **Dysphagia following unspecified cerebrovascular disease** ▽
> Use additional code to identify the type of dysphagia, if known (R13.1-)

I69.992   **Facial weakness following unspecified cerebrovascular disease** ▽
> Facial droop following unspecified cerebrovascular disease

EXCLUDES 1   Not coded here   EXCLUDES 2   Not included here   **N** Newborn Age: 0   **P** Pediatric Age: 0-17   **M** Maternity Age: 12-55   **A** Adult Age: 15-124

I69.993 **Ataxia following unspecified cerebrovascular disease** ▽

I69.998 **Other sequelae following unspecified cerebrovascular disease** ▽
Alteration in sensation following unspecified cerebrovascular disease
Disturbance of vision following unspecified cerebrovascular disease
Use additional code to identify the sequelae

Diseases of arteries, arterioles and capillaries (I70-I79)

✓4ᵗʰ **I70 Atherosclerosis**
INCLUDES   arteriolosclerosis
arterial degeneration
arteriosclerosis
arteriosclerotic vascular disease
arteriovascular degeneration
atheroma
endarteritis deformans or obliterans
senile arteritis
senile endarteritis
vascular degeneration
Use additional code to identify:
exposure to environmental tobacco smoke (Z77.22)
history of tobacco dependence (Z87.891)
occupational exposure to environmental tobacco smoke (Z57.31)
tobacco dependence (F17.-)
tobacco use (Z72.0)
EXCLUDES 2   *arteriosclerotic cardiovascular disease (I25.1-)*
arteriosclerotic heart disease (I25.1-)
atheroembolism (I75.-)
cerebral atherosclerosis (I67.2)
coronary atherosclerosis (I25.1-)
mesenteric atherosclerosis (K55.1)
precerebral atherosclerosis (I67.2)
primary pulmonary atherosclerosis (I27.0)

I70.0 **Atherosclerosis of aorta**   HCC A

I70.1 **Atherosclerosis of renal artery**   HCC A
Goldblatt's kidney
EXCLUDES 2   *atherosclerosis of renal arterioles (I12.-)*

✓5ᵗʰ **I70.2** **Atherosclerosis of native arteries of the extremities**
Mönckeberg's (medial) sclerosis
Use additional code, if applicable, to identify chronic total occlusion of artery of extremity (I70.92)
EXCLUDES 2   *atherosclerosis of bypass graft of extremities (I70.30-I70.79)*

✓6ᵗʰ **I70.20** **Unspecified atherosclerosis of native arteries of extremities**

I70.201 **Unspecified atherosclerosis of native arteries of extremities, right leg** HCC A ▽

I70.202 **Unspecified atherosclerosis of native arteries of extremities, left leg** HCC A ▽

I70.203 **Unspecified atherosclerosis of native arteries of extremities, bilateral legs** HCC A ▽

I70.208 **Unspecified atherosclerosis of native arteries of extremities, other extremity** HCC A ▽

I70.209 **Unspecified atherosclerosis of nativearteries of extremities, unspecified extremity** HCC A ▽

✓6ᵗʰ **I70.21** **Atherosclerosis of native arteries of extremities with intermittent claudication**

I70.211 **Atherosclerosis of native arteries of extremities with intermittent claudication, right leg** HCC A

I70.212 **Atherosclerosis of native arteries of extremities with intermittent claudication, left leg** HCC A

I70.213 **Atherosclerosis of native arteries of extremities with intermittent claudication, bilateral legs** HCC A

I70.218 **Atherosclerosis of native arteries of extremities with intermittent claudication, other extremity** HCC A

I70.219 **Atherosclerosis of native arteries of extremities with intermittent claudication, unspecified extremity** HCC A ▽

✓6ᵗʰ **I70.22** **Atherosclerosis of native arteries of extremities with rest pain**
INCLUDES   any condition classifiable to I70.21-

I70.221 **Atherosclerosis of native arteries of extremities with rest pain, right leg** HCC A

I70.222 **Atherosclerosis of native arteries of extremities with rest pain, left leg** HCC A

I70.223 **Atherosclerosis of native arteries of extremities with rest pain, bilateral legs** HCC A

I70.228 **Atherosclerosis of native arteries of extremities with rest pain, other extremity** HCC A

I70.229 **Atherosclerosis of native arteries of extremities with rest pain, unspecified extremity** HCC A ▽

✓6ᵗʰ **I70.23** **Atherosclerosis of native arteries of right leg with ulceration**
INCLUDES   any condition classifiable to I70.211 and I70.221
Use additional code to identify severity of ulcer (L97.-)

I70.231 **Atherosclerosis of native arteries of right leg with ulceration of thigh** HCC A

I70.232 **Atherosclerosis of native arteries of right leg with ulceration of calf** HCC A

I70.233 **Atherosclerosis of native arteries of right leg with ulceration of ankle** HCC A

I70.234 **Atherosclerosis of native arteries of right leg with ulceration of heel and midfoot** HCC A
Atherosclerosis of native arteries of right leg with ulceration of plantar surface of midfoot

I70.235 **Atherosclerosis of native arteries of right leg with ulceration of other part of foot** HCC A
Atherosclerosis of native arteries of right leg extremities with ulceration of toe

I70.238 **Atherosclerosis of native arteries of right leg with ulceration of other part of lower right leg** HCC A

I70.239 **Atherosclerosis of native arteries of right leg with ulceration of unspecified site** HCC A ▽

✓6ᵗʰ **I70.24** **Atherosclerosis of native arteries of left leg with ulceration**
INCLUDES   any condition classifiable to I70.212 and I70.222
Use additional code to identify severity of ulcer (L97.-)

I70.241 **Atherosclerosis of native arteries of left leg with ulceration of thigh** HCC A

I70.242 **Atherosclerosis of native arteries of left leg with ulceration of calf** HCC A

I70.243 **Atherosclerosis of native arteries of left leg with ulceration of ankle** HCC A

I70.244 **Atherosclerosis of native arteries of left leg with ulceration of heel and midfoot** HCC A
Atherosclerosis of native arteries of left leg with ulceration of plantar surface of midfoot

I70.245 **Atherosclerosis of native arteries of left leg with ulceration of other part of foot** HCC A
Atherosclerosis of native arteries of left leg extremities with ulceration of toe

I70.248 **Atherosclerosis of native arteries of left leg with ulceration of other part of lower left leg** HCC A

I70.249 **Atherosclerosis of native arteries of left leg with ulceration of unspecified site** HCC A ▽

I70.25 **Atherosclerosis of native arteries of other extremities with ulceration** HCC A
INCLUDES   an y condition classifiable to I70.218 and I70.228
Use additional code to identify the severity of the ulcer (L98.49-)

✓ Additional Character Req   ✓x7ᵗʰ Placeholder Alert   Manifestation   HCC CMS-HCC Condition   ▽ Unspecified Code   ▶◀ Revised Text   ● New Code   ▲ Revised Code Title

ICD-10-CM 2018   639

✓6th **I70.26** **Atherosclerosis of native arteries of extremities with gangrene**
> INCLUDES   any condition classifiable to I70.21-, I70.22-, I70.23-, I70.24-, and I70.25-
> Use additional code to identify the severity of any ulcer (L97.-, L98.49-), if applicable

I70.261 Atherosclerosis of native arteries of HCC A extremities with gangrene, right leg

I70.262 Atherosclerosis of native arteries of HCC A extremities with gangrene, left leg

I70.263 Atherosclerosis of native arteries of HCC A extremities with gangrene, bilateral legs

I70.268 Atherosclerosis of native arteries of HCC A extremities with gangrene, other extremity

I70.269 Atherosclerosis of native arteries HCC A ▽ of extremities with gangrene, unspecified extremity

✓6th **I70.29** **Other atherosclerosis of native arteries of extremities**

I70.291 Other atherosclerosis of native HCC A arteries of extremities, right leg

I70.292 Other atherosclerosis of native HCC A arteries of extremities, left leg

I70.293 Other atherosclerosis of native HCC A arteries of extremities, bilateral legs

I70.298 Other atherosclerosis of native HCC A arteries of extremities, other extremity

I70.299 Other atherosclerosis of native HCC A ▽ arteries of extremities, unspecified extremity

✓5th **I70.3** **Atherosclerosis of unspecified type of bypass graft(s) of the extremities**
> Use additional code, if applicable, to identify chronic total occlusion of artery of extremity (I70.92)
> EXCLUDES 1   embolism or thrombus of bypass graft(s) of extremities (T82.8-)

✓6th **I70.30** **Unspecified atherosclerosis of unspecified type of bypass graft(s) of the extremities**

I70.301 Unspecified atherosclerosis of HCC A ▽ unspecified type of bypass graft(s) of the extremities, right leg

I70.302 Unspecified atherosclerosis of HCC A ▽ unspecified type of bypass graft(s) of the extremities, left leg

I70.303 Unspecified atherosclerosis of HCC A ▽ unspecified type of bypass graft(s) of the extremities, bilateral legs

I70.308 Unspecified atherosclerosis of HCC A ▽ unspecified type of bypass graft(s) of the extremities, other extremity

I70.309 Unspecified atherosclerosis of HCC A ▽ unspecified type of bypass graft(s) of the extremities, unspecified extremity

✓6th **I70.31** **Atherosclerosis of unspecified type of bypass graft(s) of the extremities with intermittent claudication**

I70.311 Atherosclerosis of unspecified type HCC A of bypass graft(s) of the extremities with intermittent claudication, right leg

I70.312 Atherosclerosis of unspecified type HCC A of bypass graft(s) of the extremities with intermittent claudication, left leg

I70.313 Atherosclerosis of unspecified type HCC A of bypass graft(s) of the extremities with intermittent claudication, bilateral legs

I70.318 Atherosclerosis of unspecified type HCC A of bypass graft(s) of the extremities with intermittent claudication, other extremity

I70.319 Atherosclerosis of unspecified HCC A ▽ type of bypass graft(s) of the extremities with intermittent claudication, unspecified extremity

✓6th **I70.32** **Atherosclerosis of unspecified type of bypass graft(s) of the extremities with rest pain**
> INCLUDES   any condition classifiable to I70.31-

I70.321 Atherosclerosis of unspecified type HCC A of bypass graft(s) of the extremities with rest pain, right leg

I70.322 Atherosclerosis of unspecified type HCC A of bypass graft(s) of the extremities with rest pain, left leg

I70.323 Atherosclerosis of unspecified type HCC A of bypass graft(s) of the extremities with rest pain, bilateral legs

I70.328 Atherosclerosis of unspecified type HCC A of bypass graft(s) of the extremities with rest pain, other extremity

I70.329 Atherosclerosis of unspecified HCC A ▽ type of bypass graft(s) of the extremities with rest pain, unspecified extremity

✓6th **I70.33** **Atherosclerosis of unspecified type of bypass graft(s) of the right leg with ulceration**
> INCLUDES   any condition classifiable to I70.311 and I70.321
> Use additional code to identify severity of ulcer (L97.-)

I70.331 Atherosclerosis of unspecified type HCC A of bypass graft(s) of the right leg with ulceration of thigh

I70.332 Atherosclerosis of unspecified type HCC A of bypass graft(s) of the right leg with ulceration of calf

I70.333 Atherosclerosis of unspecified type HCC A of bypass graft(s) of the right leg with ulceration of ankle

I70.334 Atherosclerosis of unspecified type HCC A of bypass graft(s) of the right leg with ulceration of heel and midfoot
> Atherosclerosis of unspecified type of bypass graft(s) of right leg with ulceration of plantar surface of midfoot

I70.335 Atherosclerosis of unspecified type HCC A of bypass graft(s) of the right leg with ulceration of other part of foot
> Atherosclerosis of unspecified type of bypass graft(s) of the right leg with ulceration of toe

I70.338 Atherosclerosis of unspecified type HCC A of bypass graft(s) of the right leg with ulceration of other part of lower leg

I70.339 Atherosclerosis of unspecified HCC A ▽ type of bypass graft(s) of the right leg with ulceration of unspecified site

✓6th **I70.34** **Atherosclerosis of unspecified type of bypass graft(s) of the left leg with ulceration**
> INCLUDES   any condition classifiable to I70.312 and I70.322
> Use additional code to identify severity of ulcer (L97.-)

I70.341 Atherosclerosis of unspecified type HCC A of bypass graft(s) of the left leg with ulceration of thigh

I70.342 Atherosclerosis of unspecified type HCC A of bypass graft(s) of the left leg with ulceration of calf

I70.343 Atherosclerosis of unspecified type HCC A of bypass graft(s) of the left leg with ulceration of ankle

I70.344 Atherosclerosis of unspecified type HCC A of bypass graft(s) of the left leg with ulceration of heel and midfoot
> Atherosclerosis of unspecified type of bypass graft(s) of left leg with ulceration of plantar surface of midfoot

I70.345 Atherosclerosis of unspecified type HCC A of bypass graft(s) of the left leg with ulceration of other part of foot
> Atherosclerosis of unspecified type of bypass graft(s) of the left leg with ulceration of toe

I70.348 Atherosclerosis of unspecified type HCC A of bypass graft(s) of the left leg with ulceration of other part of lower leg

I70.349 Atherosclerosis of unspecified HCC A ▽ type of bypass graft(s) of the left leg with ulceration of unspecified site

I70.35   **Atherosclerosis of unspecified type of bypass** ꜱꜱ꜀ ▲
      graft(s) of other extremity with ulceration
      INCLUDES   any condition classifiable to I70.318 and
          I70.328
      Use additional code to identify severity of ulcer
      (L98.49-)

✓6ᵗʰ **I70.36**   **Atherosclerosis of unspecified type of bypass**
      graft(s) of the extremities with gangrene
      INCLUDES   any condition classifiable to I70.31-, I70.32-,
          I70.33-, I70.34-, I70.35
      Use additional code to identify the severity of any
      ulcer (L97.-, L98.49-), if applicable

     I70.361   **Atherosclerosis of unspecified type** ꜱꜱ꜀ ▲
         of bypass graft(s) of the extremities with
         gangrene, right leg

     I70.362   **Atherosclerosis of unspecified type** ꜱꜱ꜀ ▲
         of bypass graft(s) of the extremities with
         gangrene, left leg

     I70.363   **Atherosclerosis of unspecified type** ꜱꜱ꜀ ▲
         of bypass graft(s) of the extremities with
         gangrene, bilateral legs

     I70.368   **Atherosclerosis of unspecified type** ꜱꜱ꜀ ▲
         of bypass graft(s) of the extremities with
         gangrene, other extremity

     I70.369   **Atherosclerosis of unspecified** ꜱꜱ꜀ ▲ ▽
         type of bypass graft(s) of the extremities
         with gangrene, unspecified extremity

✓6ᵗʰ **I70.39**   **Other atherosclerosis of unspecified type of bypass**
      graft(s) of the extremities

     I70.391   **Other atherosclerosis of** ꜱꜱ꜀ ▲
         unspecified type of bypass graft(s)
         of the extremities, right leg

     I70.392   **Other atherosclerosis of** ꜱꜱ꜀ ▲
         unspecified type of bypass graft(s)
         of the extremities, left leg

     I70.393   **Other atherosclerosis of** ꜱꜱ꜀ ▲
         unspecified type of bypass graft(s)
         of the extremities, bilateral legs

     I70.398   **Other atherosclerosis of** ꜱꜱ꜀ ▲
         unspecified type of bypass graft(s)
         of the extremities, other extremity

     I70.399   **Other atherosclerosis of** ꜱꜱ꜀ ▲ ▽
         unspecified type of bypass graft(s)
         of the extremities, unspecified extremity

✓5ᵗʰ **I70.4**   **Atherosclerosis of autologous vein bypass graft(s) of the**
     extremities
      Use additional code, if applicable, to identify chronic total
      occlusion of artery of extremity (I70.92)

✓6ᵗʰ **I70.40**   **Unspecified atherosclerosis of autologous vein**
      bypass graft(s) of the extremities

     I70.401   **Unspecified atherosclerosis of** ꜱꜱ꜀ ▲ ▽
         autologous vein bypass graft(s) of the
         extremities, right leg

     I70.402   **Unspecified atherosclerosis of** ꜱꜱ꜀ ▲ ▽
         autologous vein bypass graft(s) of the
         extremities, left leg

     I70.403   **Unspecified atherosclerosis of** ꜱꜱ꜀ ▲ ▽
         autologous vein bypass graft(s) of the
         extremities, bilateral legs

     I70.408   **Unspecified atherosclerosis of** ꜱꜱ꜀ ▲ ▽
         autologous vein bypass graft(s) of the
         extremities, other extremity

     I70.409   **Unspecified atherosclerosis of** ꜱꜱ꜀ ▲ ▽
         autologous vein bypass graft(s) of the
         extremities, unspecified extremity

✓6ᵗʰ **I70.41**   **Atherosclerosis of autologous vein bypass graft(s) of**
      the extremities with intermittent claudication

     I70.411   **Atherosclerosis of autologous vein** ꜱꜱ꜀ ▲
         bypass graft(s) of the extremities with
         intermittent claudication, right leg

     I70.412   **Atherosclerosis of autologous vein** ꜱꜱ꜀ ▲
         bypass graft(s) of the extremities with
         intermittent claudication, left leg

     I70.413   **Atherosclerosis of autologous vein** ꜱꜱ꜀ ▲
         bypass graft(s) of the extremities with
         intermittent claudication, bilateral legs

     I70.418   **Atherosclerosis of autologous vein** ꜱꜱ꜀ ▲
         bypass graft(s) of the extremities with
         intermittent claudication, other extremity

     I70.419   **Atherosclerosis of autologous** ꜱꜱ꜀ ▲ ▽
         vein bypass graft(s) of the extremities
         with intermittent claudication,
         unspecified extremity

✓6ᵗʰ **I70.42**   **Atherosclerosis of autologous vein bypass graft(s) of**
      the extremities with rest pain
      INCLUDES   any condition classifiable to I70.41-

     I70.421   **Atherosclerosis of autologous vein** ꜱꜱ꜀ ▲
         bypass graft(s) of the extremities with
         rest pain, right leg

     I70.422   **Atherosclerosis of autologous vein** ꜱꜱ꜀ ▲
         bypass graft(s) of the extremities with
         rest pain, left leg

     I70.423   **Atherosclerosis of autologous vein** ꜱꜱ꜀ ▲
         bypass graft(s) of the extremities with
         rest pain, bilateral legs

     I70.428   **Atherosclerosis of autologous vein** ꜱꜱ꜀ ▲
         bypass graft(s) of the extremities with
         rest pain, other extremity

     I70.429   **Atherosclerosis of autologous** ꜱꜱ꜀ ▲ ▽
         vein bypass graft(s) of the extremities
         with rest pain, unspecified extremity

✓6ᵗʰ **I70.43**   **Atherosclerosis of autologous vein bypass graft(s) of**
      the right leg with ulceration
      INCLUDES   any condition classifiable to I70.411 and
          I70.421
      Use additional code to identify severity of ulcer (L97.-)

     I70.431   **Atherosclerosis of autologous vein** ꜱꜱ꜀ ▲
         bypass graft(s) of the right leg with
         ulceration of thigh

     I70.432   **Atherosclerosis of autologous vein** ꜱꜱ꜀ ▲
         bypass graft(s) of the right leg with
         ulceration of calf

     I70.433   **Atherosclerosis of autologous vein** ꜱꜱ꜀ ▲
         bypass graft(s) of the right leg with
         ulceration of ankle

     I70.434   **Atherosclerosis of autologous vein** ꜱꜱ꜀ ▲
         bypass graft(s) of the right leg with
         ulceration of heel and midfoot
          Atherosclerosis of autologous vein bypass
           graft(s) of right leg with ulceration of
           plantar surface of midfoot

     I70.435   **Atherosclerosis of autologous vein** ꜱꜱ꜀ ▲
         bypass graft(s) of the right leg with
         ulceration of other part of foot
          Atherosclerosis of autologous vein bypass
           graft(s) of right leg with ulceration of
           toe

     I70.438   **Atherosclerosis of autologous vein** ꜱꜱ꜀ ▲
         bypass graft(s) of the right leg with
         ulceration of other part of lower leg

     I70.439   **Atherosclerosis of autologous** ꜱꜱ꜀ ▲ ▽
         vein bypass graft(s) of the right leg
         with ulceration of unspecified site

✓6ᵗʰ **I70.44**   **Atherosclerosis of autologous vein bypass graft(s) of**
      the left leg with ulceration
      INCLUDES   any condition classifiable to I70.412 and
          I70.422
      Use additional code to identify severity of ulcer (L97.-)

     I70.441   **Atherosclerosis of autologous vein** ꜱꜱ꜀ ▲
         bypass graft(s) of the left leg with
         ulceration of thigh

     I70.442   **Atherosclerosis of autologous vein** ꜱꜱ꜀ ▲
         bypass graft(s) of the left leg with
         ulceration of calf

     I70.443   **Atherosclerosis of autologous vein** ꜱꜱ꜀ ▲
         bypass graft(s) of the left leg with
         ulceration of ankle

     I70.444   **Atherosclerosis of autologous vein** ꜱꜱ꜀ ▲
         bypass graft(s) of the left leg with
         ulceration of heel and midfoot
          Atherosclerosis of autologous vein bypass
           graft(s) of left leg with ulceration of
           plantar surface of midfoot

     I70.445   **Atherosclerosis of autologous vein** ꜱꜱ꜀ ▲
         bypass graft(s) of the left leg with
         ulceration of other part of foot
          Atherosclerosis of autologous vein bypass
           graft(s) of left leg with ulceration of
           toe

☑ Additional Character Req   ᵛˣ⁷ᵗʰ Placeholder Alert   Manifestation   ꜱꜱ꜀ CMS-HCC Condition   ▽ Unspecified Code   ►◄ Revised Text   ● New Code   ▲ Revised Code Title

Chapter 9. Diseases of the Circulatory System

I70.448–I70.543

I70.448 Atherosclerosis of autologous vein **HCC** **A**
bypass graft(s) of the left leg with
ulceration of other **part of lower leg**

I70.449 Atherosclerosis of autologous **HCC** **A** ▽
vein bypass graft(s) of the left leg with
ulceration of unspecified site

I70.45 Atherosclerosis of autologous vein bypass **HCC** **A**
graft(s) of other extremity with **ulceration**
[INCLUDES] any condition classifiable to I70.418,
I70.428, and I70.438
Use additional code to identify severity of ulcer
(L98.49)

✓6th **I70.46** Atherosclerosis of autologous vein bypass graft(s) of
the extremities with **gangrene**
[INCLUDES] any condition classifiable to I70.41-, I70.42-,
and I70.43-, I70.44-, I70.45
Use additional code to identify the severity of any
ulcer (L97.-, L98.49-), if applicable

I70.461 Atherosclerosis of autologous vein **HCC** **A**
bypass graft(s) of the extremities with
gangrene, **right leg**

I70.462 Atherosclerosis of autologous vein **HCC** **A**
bypass graft(s) of the extremities with
gangrene, **left leg**

I70.463 Atherosclerosis of autologous vein **HCC** **A**
bypass graft(s) of the extremities with
gangrene, **bilateral legs**

I70.468 Atherosclerosis of autologous vein **HCC** **A**
bypass graft(s) of the extremities with
gangrene, other extremity

I70.469 Atherosclerosis of autologous **HCC** **A** ▽
vein bypass graft(s) of the extremities
with gangrene, unspecified extremity

✓6th **I70.49** Other atherosclerosis of autologous vein bypass
graft(s) of the extremities

I70.491 Other atherosclerosis of autologous **HCC** **A**
vein bypass graft(s) of the extremities,
right leg

I70.492 Other atherosclerosis of autologous **HCC** **A**
vein bypass graft(s) of the extremities,
left leg

I70.493 Other atherosclerosis of autologous **HCC** **A**
vein bypass graft(s) of the extremities,
bilateral legs

I70.498 Other atherosclerosis of autologous **HCC** **A**
vein bypass graft(s) of the extremities,
other extremity

I70.499 Other atherosclerosis of **HCC** **A** ▽
autologous vein bypass graft(s) of the
extremities, unspecified extremity

✓5th **I70.5** Atherosclerosis of **nonautologous biological bypass graft(s)**
of the **extremities**
Use additional code, if applicable, to identify chronic total
occlusion of artery of extremity (I70.92)

✓6th **I70.50** Unspecified atherosclerosis of nonautologous
biological bypass graft(s) of the extremities

I70.501 Unspecified atherosclerosis of **HCC** **A** ▽
nonautologous biological bypass
graft(s) of the extremities, **right leg**

I70.502 Unspecified atherosclerosis of **HCC** **A** ▽
nonautologous biological bypass
graft(s) of the extremities, **left leg**

I70.503 Unspecified atherosclerosis of **HCC** **A** ▽
nonautologous biological bypass graft(s)
of the extremities, **bilateral legs**

I70.508 Unspecified atherosclerosis of **HCC** **A** ▽
nonautologous biological bypass graft(s)
of the extremities, other extremity

I70.509 Unspecified atherosclerosis of **HCC** **A** ▽
nonautologous biological bypass graft(s)
of the extremities, unspecified extremity

✓6th **I70.51** Atherosclerosis of nonautologous biological bypass
graft(s) of the extremities with **intermittent
claudication**

I70.511 Atherosclerosis of nonautologous **HCC** **A**
biological bypass graft(s) of the
extremities with intermittent
claudication, **right leg**

I70.512 Atherosclerosis of nonautologous **HCC** **A**
biological bypass graft(s) of the
extremities with intermittent
claudication, **left leg**

I70.513 Atherosclerosis of nonautologous **HCC** **A**
biological bypass graft(s) of the
extremities with intermittent
claudication, **bilateral legs**

I70.518 Atherosclerosis of nonautologous **HCC** **A**
biological bypass graft(s) of the
extremities with intermittent
claudication, other extremity

I70.519 Atherosclerosis of nonautologous **HCC** **A** ▽
biological bypass graft(s) of the
extremities with intermittent
claudication, unspecified extremity

✓6th **I70.52** Atherosclerosis of nonautologous biological bypass
graft(s) of the extremities with **rest pain**
[INCLUDES] any condition classifiable to I70.51-

I70.521 Atherosclerosis of nonautologous **HCC** **A**
biological bypass graft(s) of the
extremities with rest pain, **right leg**

I70.522 Atherosclerosis of nonautologous **HCC** **A**
biological bypass graft(s) of the
extremities with rest pain, **left leg**

I70.523 Atherosclerosis of nonautologous **HCC** **A**
biological bypass graft(s) of the
extremities with rest pain, **bilateral legs**

I70.528 Atherosclerosis of nonautologous **HCC** **A**
biological bypass graft(s) of the
extremities with rest pain, other extremity

I70.529 Atherosclerosis of nonautologous **HCC** **A** ▽
biological bypass graft(s) of the
extremities with rest pain, unspecified
extremity

✓6th **I70.53** Atherosclerosis of nonautologous biological bypass
graft(s) of the **right leg** with **ulceration**
[INCLUDES] any condition classifiable to I70.511 and
I70.521
Use additional code to identify severity of ulcer (L97.-)

I70.531 Atherosclerosis of nonautologous **HCC** **A**
biological bypass graft(s) of the right leg
with ulceration of **thigh**

I70.532 Atherosclerosis of nonautologous **HCC** **A**
biological bypass graft(s) of the right leg
with ulceration of **calf**

I70.533 Atherosclerosis of nonautologous **HCC** **A**
biological bypass graft(s) of the right leg
with ulceration of **ankle**

I70.534 Atherosclerosis of nonautologous **HCC** **A**
biological bypass graft(s) of the right leg
with ulceration of **heel and midfoot**
Atherosclerosis of nonautologous
biological bypass graft(s) of right leg
with ulceration of plantar surface of
midfoot

I70.535 Atherosclerosis of nonautologous **HCC** **A**
biological bypass graft(s) of the right leg
with ulceration of other **part of foot**
Atherosclerosis of nonautologous
biological bypass graft(s) of the right
leg with ulceration of toe

I70.538 Atherosclerosis of nonautologous **HCC** **A**
biological bypass graft(s) of the right leg
with ulceration of other **part of lower leg**

I70.539 Atherosclerosis of nonautologous **HCC** **A** ▽
biological bypass graft(s) of the right leg
with ulceration of unspecified site

✓6th **I70.54** Atherosclerosis of nonautologous biological bypass
graft(s) of the **left leg** with **ulceration**
[INCLUDES] any condition classifiable to I70.512 and
I70.522
Use additional code to identify severity of ulcer (L97.-)

I70.541 Atherosclerosis of nonautologous **HCC** **A**
biological bypass graft(s) of the left leg
with ulceration of **thigh**

I70.542 Atherosclerosis of nonautologous **HCC** **A**
biological bypass graft(s) of the left leg
with ulceration of **calf**

I70.543 Atherosclerosis of nonautologous **HCC** **A**
biological bypass graft(s) of the left leg
with ulceration of **ankle**

[EXCLUDES 1] Not coded here   [EXCLUDES 2] Not included here   **N** Newborn Age: 0   **P** Pediatric Age: 0-17   **M** Maternity Age: 12-55   **A** Adult Age: 15-124

642

ICD-10-CM 2018

I70.544 **Atherosclerosis of nonautologous** `HCC` `A` **biological bypass graft(s) of the left leg with ulceration of heel and midfoot**
Atherosclerosis of nonautologous biological bypass graft(s) of left leg with ulceration of plantar surface of midfoot

I70.545 **Atherosclerosis of nonautologous** `HCC` `A` **biological bypass graft(s) of the left leg with ulceration of other part of foot**
Atherosclerosis of nonautologous biological bypass graft(s) of the left leg with ulceration of toe

I70.548 **Atherosclerosis of nonautologous** `HCC` `A` **biological bypass graft(s) of the left leg with ulceration of other part of lower leg**

I70.549 **Atherosclerosis of nonautologous** `HCC` `A` `▽` **biological bypass graft(s) of the left leg with ulceration of unspecified site**

I70.55 **Atherosclerosis of nonautologous biological** `HCC` `A` **bypass graft(s) of other extremity with ulceration**
`INCLUDES` any condition classifiable to I70.518, I70.528, and I70.538
Use additional code to identify severity of ulcer (L98.49)

✓6th I70.56 **Atherosclerosis of nonautologous biological bypass graft(s) of the extremities with gangrene**
`INCLUDES` any condition classifiable to I70.51-, I70.52-, and I70.53-, I70.54-, I70.55
Use additional code to identify the severity of any ulcer (L97.-, L98.49-), if applicable

I70.561 **Atherosclerosis of nonautologous** `HCC` `A` **biological bypass graft(s) of the extremities with gangrene, right leg**

I70.562 **Atherosclerosis of nonautologous** `HCC` `A` **biological bypass graft(s) of the extremities with gangrene, left leg**

I70.563 **Atherosclerosis of nonautologous** `HCC` `A` **biological bypass graft(s) of the extremities with gangrene, bilateral legs**

I70.568 **Atherosclerosis of nonautologous** `HCC` `A` **biological bypass graft(s) of the extremities with gangrene, other extremity**

I70.569 **Atherosclerosis of nonautologous** `HCC` `A` `▽` **biological bypass graft(s) of the extremities with gangrene, unspecified extremity**

✓6th I70.59 **Other atherosclerosis of nonautologous biological bypass graft(s) of the extremities**

I70.591 **Other atherosclerosis of** `HCC` `A` **nonautologous biological bypass graft(s) of the extremities, right leg**

I70.592 **Other atherosclerosis of** `HCC` `A` **nonautologous biological bypass graft(s) of the extremities, left leg**

I70.593 **Other atherosclerosis of** `HCC` `A` **nonautologous biological bypass graft(s) of the extremities, bilateral legs**

I70.598 **Other atherosclerosis of** `HCC` `A` **nonautologous biological bypass graft(s) of the extremities, other extremity**

I70.599 **Other atherosclerosis of non-** `HCC` `A` `▽` **autologous biological bypass graft(s) of the extremities, unspecified extremity**

✓5th I70.6 **Atherosclerosis of nonbiological bypass graft(s) of the extremities**
Use additional code, if applicable, to identify chronic total occlusion of artery of extremity (I70.92)

✓6th I70.60 **Unspecified atherosclerosis of nonbiological bypass graft(s) of the extremities**

I70.601 **Unspecified atherosclerosis of** `HCC` `A` `▽` **nonbiological bypass graft(s) of the extremities, right leg**

I70.602 **Unspecified atherosclerosis of** `HCC` `A` `▽` **nonbiological bypass graft(s) of the extremities, left leg**

I70.603 **Unspecified atherosclerosis of** `HCC` `A` `▽` **nonbiological bypass graft(s) of the extremities, bilateral legs**

I70.608 **Unspecified atherosclerosis of** `HCC` `A` `▽` **nonbiological bypass graft(s) of the extremities, other extremity**

I70.609 **Unspecified atherosclerosis of** `HCC` `A` `▽` **nonbiological bypass graft(s) of the extremities, unspecified extremity**

✓6th I70.61 **Atherosclerosis of nonbiological bypass graft(s) of the extremities with intermittent claudication**

I70.611 **Atherosclerosis of nonbiological** `HCC` `A` **bypass graft(s) of the extremities with intermittent claudication, right leg**

I70.612 **Atherosclerosis of nonbiological** `HCC` `A` **bypass graft(s) of the extremities with intermittent claudication, left leg**

I70.613 **Atherosclerosis of nonbiological** `HCC` `A` **bypass graft(s) of the extremities with intermittent claudication, bilateral legs**

I70.618 **Atherosclerosis of nonbiological** `HCC` `A` **bypass graft(s) of the extremities with intermittent claudication, other extremity**

I70.619 **Atherosclerosis of nonbiological** `HCC` `A` `▽` **bypass graft(s) of the extremities with intermittent claudication, unspecified extremity**

✓6th I70.62 **Atherosclerosis of nonbiological bypass graft(s) of the extremities with rest pain**
`INCLUDES` any condition classifiable to I70.61-

I70.621 **Atherosclerosis of nonbiological** `HCC` `A` **bypass graft(s) of the extremities with rest pain, right leg**

I70.622 **Atherosclerosis of nonbiological** `HCC` `A` **bypass graft(s) of the extremities with rest pain, left leg**

I70.623 **Atherosclerosis of nonbiological** `HCC` `A` **bypass graft(s) of the extremities with rest pain, bilateral legs**

I70.628 **Atherosclerosis of nonbiological** `HCC` `A` **bypass graft(s) of the extremities with rest pain, other extremity**

I70.629 **Atherosclerosis of nonbiological** `HCC` `A` `▽` **bypass graft(s) of the extremities with rest pain, unspecified extremity**

✓6th I70.63 **Atherosclerosis of nonbiological bypass graft(s) of the right leg with ulceration**
`INCLUDES` any condition classifiable to I70.611 and I70.621
Use additional code to identify severity of ulcer (L97.-)

I70.631 **Atherosclerosis of nonbiological** `HCC` `A` **bypass graft(s) of the right leg with ulceration of thigh**

I70.632 **Atherosclerosis of nonbiological** `HCC` `A` **bypass graft(s) of the right leg with ulceration of calf**

I70.633 **Atherosclerosis of nonbiological** `HCC` `A` **bypass graft(s) of the right leg with ulceration of ankle**

I70.634 **Atherosclerosis of nonbiological** `HCC` `A` **bypass graft(s) of the right leg with ulceration of heel and midfoot**
Atherosclerosis of nonbiological bypass graft(s) of right leg with ulceration of plantar surface of midfoot

I70.635 **Atherosclerosis of nonbiological** `HCC` `A` **bypass graft(s) of the right leg with ulceration of other part of foot**
Atherosclerosis of nonbiological bypass graft(s) of the right leg with ulceration of toe

I70.638 **Atherosclerosis of nonbiological** `HCC` `A` **bypass graft(s) of the right leg with ulceration of other part of lower leg**

I70.639 **Atherosclerosis of nonbiological** `HCC` `A` `▽` **bypass graft(s) of the right leg with ulceration of unspecified site**

✓ Additional Character Req   ✓x7th Placeholder Alert   Manifestation   `HCC` CMS-HCC Condition   ▽ Unspecified Code   ►◄ Revised Text   ● New Code   ▲ Revised Code Title

ICD-10-CM 2018   643

✓6ᵗʰ **I70.64   Atherosclerosis of nonbiological bypass graft(s) of the left leg with ulceration**
INCLUDES   any condition classifiable to I70.612 and I70.622
Use additional code to identify severity of ulcer (L97.-)

I70.641   **Atherosclerosis of nonbiological** HCC A
bypass graft(s) of the left leg with ulceration of thigh

I70.642   **Atherosclerosis of nonbiological** HCC A
bypass graft(s) of the left leg with ulceration of calf

I70.643   **Atherosclerosis of nonbiological** HCC A
bypass graft(s) of the left leg with ulceration of ankle

I70.644   **Atherosclerosis of nonbiological** HCC A
bypass graft(s) of the left leg with ulceration of heel and midfoot
Atherosclerosis of nonbiological bypass graft(s) of left leg with ulceration of plantar surface of midfoot

I70.645   **Atherosclerosis of nonbiological** HCC A
bypassgraft(s) of the left leg with ulceration of other part of foot
Atherosclerosis of nonbiological bypass graft(s) of the left leg with ulceration of toe

I70.648   **Atherosclerosis of nonbiological** HCC A
bypass graft(s) of the left leg with ulceration of other part of lower leg

I70.649   **Atherosclerosis of nonbiological** HCC A ▽
bypass graft(s) of the left leg with ulceration of unspecified site

I70.65   **Atherosclerosis of nonbiological bypass** HCC A
graft(s) of other extremity with ulceration
INCLUDES   any condition classifiable to I70.618 and I70.628
Use additional code to identify severity of ulcer (L98.49)

✓6ᵗʰ **I70.66   Atherosclerosis of nonbiological bypass graft(s) of the extremities with gangrene**
INCLUDES   any condition classifiable to I70.61-, I70.62-, I70.63-, I70.64-, I70.65
Use additional code to identify the severity of any ulcer (L97.-, L98.49-), if applicable

I70.661   **Atherosclerosis of nonbiological** HCC A
bypass graft(s) of the extremities with gangrene, right leg

I70.662   **Atherosclerosis of nonbiological** HCC A
bypass graft(s) of the extremities with gangrene, left leg

I70.663   **Atherosclerosis of nonbiological** HCC A
bypass graft(s) of the extremities with gangrene, bilateral legs

I70.668   **Atherosclerosis of nonbiological** HCC A
bypass graft(s) of the extremities with gangrene, other extremity

I70.669   **Atherosclerosis of nonbiological** HCC A ▽
bypass graft(s) of the extremities with gangrene, unspecified extremity

✓6ᵗʰ **I70.69   Other atherosclerosis of nonbiological bypass graft(s) of the extremities**

I70.691   **Other atherosclerosis of** HCC A
nonbiological bypass graft(s) of the extremities, right leg

I70.692   **Other atherosclerosis of** HCC A
nonbiological bypass graft(s) of the extremities, left leg

I70.693   **Other atherosclerosis of** HCC A
nonbiological bypass graft(s) of the extremities, bilateral legs

I70.698   **Other atherosclerosis of** HCC A
nonbiological bypass graft(s) of the extremities, other extremity

I70.699   **Other atherosclerosis of non-** HCC A ▽
biological bypass graft(s) of the extremities, unspecified extremity

✓5ᵗʰ **I70.7   Atherosclerosis of other type of bypass graft(s) of the extremities**
Use additional code, if applicable, to identify chronic total occlusion of artery of extremity (I70.92)

✓6ᵗʰ **I70.70   Unspecified atherosclerosis of other type of bypass graft(s) of the extremities**

I70.701   **Unspecified atherosclerosis of** HCC A ▽
other type of bypass graft(s) of the extremities, right leg

I70.702   **Unspecified atherosclerosis of** HCC A ▽
other type of bypass graft(s) of the extremities, left leg

I70.703   **Unspecified atherosclerosis of** HCC A ▽
other type of bypass graft(s) of the extremities, bilateral legs

I70.708   **Unspecified atherosclerosis of** HCC A ▽
other type of bypass graft(s) of the extremities, other extremity

I70.709   **Unspecified atherosclerosis of** HCC A ▽
other type of bypass graft(s) of the extremities, unspecified extremity

✓6ᵗʰ **I70.71   Atherosclerosis of other type of bypass graft(s) of the extremities with intermittent claudication**

I70.711   **Atherosclerosis of other type of** HCC A
bypass graft(s) of the extremities with intermittent claudication, right leg

I70.712   **Atherosclerosis of other type of** HCC A
bypass graft(s) of the extremities with intermittent claudication, left leg

I70.713   **Atherosclerosis of other type of** HCC A
bypass graft(s) of the extremities with intermittent claudication, bilateral legs

I70.718   **Atherosclerosis of other type of** HCC A
bypass graft(s) of the extremities with intermittent claudication, other extremity

I70.719   **Atherosclerosis of other type of** HCC A ▽
bypass graft(s) of the extremities withintermittent claudication, unspecified extremity

✓6ᵗʰ **I70.72   Atherosclerosis of other type of bypass graft(s) of the extremities with rest pain**
INCLUDES   any condition classifiable to I70.71-

I70.721   **Atherosclerosis of other type of** HCC A
bypass graft(s) of the extremities with rest pain, right leg

I70.722   **Atherosclerosis of other type of** HCC A
bypass graft(s) of the extremities with rest pain, left leg

I70.723   **Atherosclerosis of other type of** HCC A
bypass graft(s) of the extremities with rest pain, bilateral legs

I70.728   **Atherosclerosis of other type of** HCC A
bypass graft(s) of the extremities with rest pain, other extremity

I70.729   **Atherosclerosis of other type of** HCC A ▽
bypass graft(s) of the extremities with rest pain, unspecified extremity

✓6ᵗʰ **I70.73   Atherosclerosis of other type of bypass graft(s) of the right leg with ulceration**
INCLUDES   any condition classifiable to I70.711 and I70.721
Use additional code to identify severity of ulcer (L97.-)

I70.731   **Atherosclerosis of other type of** HCC A
bypass graft(s) of the right leg with ulceration of thigh

I70.732   **Atherosclerosis of other type of** HCC A
bypass graft(s) of the right leg with ulceration of calf

I70.733   **Atherosclerosis of other type of** HCC A
bypass graft(s) of the right leg with ulceration of ankle

I70.734   **Atherosclerosis of other type of** HCC A
bypass graft(s) of the right leg with ulceration of heel and midfoot
Atherosclerosis of other type of bypass graft(s) of right leg with ulceration of plantar surface of midfoot

I70.735   **Atherosclerosis of other type of** `HCC` `A`
bypass graft(s) of the right leg with
ulceration of other part of foot
> Atherosclerosis of other type of bypass
> graft(s) of right leg with ulceration of
> toe

I70.738   **Atherosclerosis of other type of** `HCC` `A`
bypass graft(s) of the right leg with
ulceration of other part of lower leg

I70.739   **Atherosclerosis of other type of** `HCC` `A` ▽
bypass graft(s) of the right leg with
ulceration of unspecified site

✓6ᵗʰ **I70.74**   **Atherosclerosis of other type of bypass graft(s) of**
the left leg with ulceration
> INCLUDES   any condition classifiable to I70.712 and
> I70.722
> Use additional code to identify severity of ulcer (L97.-)

I70.741   **Atherosclerosis of other type of** `HCC` `A`
bypass graft(s) of the left leg with
ulceration of thigh

I70.742   **Atherosclerosis of other type of** `HCC` `A`
bypass graft(s) of the left leg with
ulceration of calf

I70.743   **Atherosclerosis of other type of** `HCC` `A`
bypass raft(s) of the left leg with
ulceration of ankle

I70.744   **Atherosclerosis of other type of** `HCC` `A`
bypass graft(s) of the left leg with
ulceration of heel and midfoot
> Atherosclerosis of other type of bypass
> graft(s) of left leg with ulceration of
> plantar surface of midfoot

I70.745   **Atherosclerosis of other type of** `HCC` `A`
bypass graft(s) of the left leg with
ulceration of other part of foot
> Atherosclerosis of other type of bypass
> graft(s) of left leg with ulceration of
> toe

I70.748   **Atherosclerosis of other type of** `HCC` `A`
bypass graft(s) of the left leg with
ulceration of other part of lower leg

I70.749   **Atherosclerosis of other type of** `HCC` `A` ▽
bypass graft(s) of the left leg with
ulceration of unspecified site

I70.75   **Atherosclerosis of other type of bypass** `HCC` `A`
graft(s) of other extremity with ulceration
> INCLUDES   any condition classifiable to I70.718 and
> I70.728
> Use additional code to identify severity of ulcer
> (L98.49)

✓6ᵗʰ **I70.76**   **Atherosclerosis of other type of bypass graft(s) of**
the extremities with gangrene
> INCLUDES   any condition classifiable to I70.71-, I70.72-,
> I70.73-, I70.74-, I70.75
> Use additional code to identify the severity of any
> ulcer (L97.-, L98.49-), if applicable

I70.761   **Atherosclerosis of other type of** `HCC` `A`
bypass graft(s) of the extremities
with gangrene, right leg

I70.762   **Atherosclerosis of other type of** `HCC` `A`
bypass graft(s) of the extremities
with gangrene, left leg

I70.763   **Atherosclerosis of other type of** `HCC` `A`
bypass graft(s) of the extremities
with gangrene, bilateral legs

I70.768   **Atherosclerosis of other type of** `HCC` `A`
bypass graft(s) of the extremities
with gangrene, other extremity

I70.769   **Atherosclerosis of other type of** `HCC` `A` ▽
bypass graft(s) of the extremities
with gangrene, unspecified extremity

✓6ᵗʰ **I70.79**   **Other atherosclerosis of other type of bypass graft(s)**
of the extremities

I70.791   **Other atherosclerosis of other type** `HCC` `A`
of bypass graft(s) of the extremities,
right leg

I70.792   **Other atherosclerosis of other type** `HCC` `A`
of bypass graft(s) of the extremities, left
leg

I70.793   **Other atherosclerosis of other type** `HCC` `A`
of bypass graft(s) of the extremities,
bilateral legs

I70.798   **Other atherosclerosis of other type** `HCC` `A`
of bypass graft(s) of the extremities,
other extremity

I70.799   **Other atherosclerosis of other** `HCC` `A` ▽
type of bypass graft(s) of the extremities,
unspecified extremity

I70.8   **Atherosclerosis of other arteries** `A`
> TIP: Arteriosclerosis of the iliac arteries is coded here.

✓5ᵗʰ **I70.9**   **Other and unspecified atherosclerosis**

I70.90   **Unspecified atherosclerosis** `A` ▽

I70.91   **Generalized atherosclerosis** `A`

I70.92   **Chronic total occlusion of artery of the** `HCC` `A`
extremities
> Complete occlusion of artery of the extremities
> Total occlusion of artery of the extremities
> Code first atherosclerosis of arteries of the extremities
> (I70.2-, I70.3-, I70.4-, I70.5-, I70.6-, I70.7-)

✓4ᵗʰ **I71**   **Aortic aneurysm and dissection**
> EXCLUDES 1   aortic ectasia (I77.81-)
> syphilitic aortic aneurysm (A52.01)
> traumatic aortic aneurysm (S25.09, S35.09)

✓5ᵗʰ **I71.0**   **Dissection of aorta**

I71.00   **Dissection of unspecified site of aorta** `HCC` ▽

I71.01   **Dissection of thoracic aorta** `HCC`

I71.02   **Dissection of abdominal aorta** `HCC`

I71.03   **Dissection of thoracoabdominal aorta** `HCC`

I71.1   **Thoracic aortic aneurysm, ruptured** `HCC`

I71.2   **Thoracic aortic aneurysm, without rupture** `HCC`

I71.3   **Abdominal aortic aneurysm, ruptured** `HCC`

I71.4   **Abdominal aortic aneurysm, without rupture** `HCC`

I71.5   **Thoracoabdominal aortic aneurysm, ruptured** `HCC`

I71.6   **Thoracoabdominal aortic aneurysm, without rupture** `HCC`

I71.8   **Aortic aneurysm of unspecified site, ruptured** `HCC` ▽
> Rupture of aorta NOS

I71.9   **Aortic aneurysm of unspecified site, without rupture** `HCC` ▽
> Aneurysm of aorta
> Dilatation of aorta
> Hyaline necrosis of aorta

✓4ᵗʰ **I72**   **Other aneurysm**
> INCLUDES   aneurysm (cirsoid) (false) (ruptured)
> EXCLUDES 2   acquired aneurysm (I77.0)
> aneurysm (of) aorta (I71.-)
> aneurysm (of) arteriovenous NOS (Q27.3-)
> carotid artery dissection (I77.71)
> cerebral (nonruptured) aneurysm (I67.1)
> coronary aneurysm (I25.4)
> coronary artery dissection (I25.42)
> dissection of artery NEC (I77.79)
> dissection of precerebral artery, congenital (nonruptured)
> (Q28.1)
> heart aneurysm (I25.3)
> iliac artery dissection (I77.72)
> ▶precerebral artery, congenital (nonruptured) (Q28.1)◀
> pulmonary artery aneurysm (I28.1)
> renal artery dissection (I77.73)
> retinal aneurysm (H35.0)
> ruptured cerebral aneurysm (I60.7)
> varicose aneurysm (I77.0)
> vertebral artery dissection (I77.74)

I72.0   **Aneurysm of carotid artery** `HCC`
> Aneurysm of common carotid artery
> Aneurysm of external carotid artery
> Aneurysm of internal carotid artery, extracranial portion
> EXCLUDES 1   aneurysm of internal carotid artery, intracranial
> portion (I67.1)
> aneurysm of internal carotid artery NOS (I67.1)

I72.1   **Aneurysm of artery of upper extremity** `HCC`

I72.2   **Aneurysm of renal artery** `HCC`

I72.3   **Aneurysm of iliac artery** `HCC`

I72.4   **Aneurysm of artery of lower extremity** `HCC`

I72.5   **Aneurysm of other precerebral arteries** `HCC`
> Aneurysm of basilar artery (trunk)
> EXCLUDES 2   aneurysm of carotid artery (I72.0)
> aneurysm of vertebral artery (I72.6)
> dissection of carotid artery (I77.71)
> dissection of other precerebral arteries (I77.75)
> dissection of vertebral artery (I77.74)

✓ Additional Character Req   ✓x7ᵗʰ Placeholder Alert   Manifestation   `HCC` CMS-HCC Condition   ▽ Unspecified Code   ▶◀ Revised Text   ● New Code   ▲ Revised Code Title

Aneurysm

I72.6   **Aneurysm of vertebral artery**   `HCC`
> *EXCLUDES 2*   *dissection of vertebral artery (I77.74)*

I72.8   **Aneurysm of other specified arteries**   `HCC`

I72.9   **Aneurysm of unspecified site**   `HCC` ▽

✓4th **I73**   **Other peripheral vascular diseases**
> *EXCLUDES 2*   *chilblains (T69.1)*
> *frostbite (T33- T34)*
> *immersion hand or foot (T69.0-)*
> *spasm of cerebral artery (G45.9)*

✓5th   I73.0   **Raynaud's syndrome**
> Raynaud's disease
> Raynaud's phenomenon (secondary)

     I73.00   **Raynaud's syndrome without gangrene**

     I73.01   **Raynaud's syndrome with gangrene**   `HCC`

  I73.1   **Thromboangiitis obliterans [Buerger's disease]**   `HCC`
> **DEF:** Inflammatory disease of extremity blood vessels, mainly the lower; associated with heavy tobacco use; arteries are more affected than veins; occurs primarily in young men and leads to tissue ischemia and gangrene.

✓5th   I73.8   **Other specified peripheral vascular diseases**
> *EXCLUDES 1*   *diabetic (peripheral) angiopathy (E08-E13 with .51-.52)*

     I73.81   **Erythromelalgia**   `HCC`

     I73.89   **Other specified peripheral vascular diseases**   `HCC`
> Acrocyanosis
> Erythrocyanosis
> Simple acroparesthesia [Schultze's type]
> Vasomotor acroparesthesia [Nothnagel's type]

  I73.9   **Peripheral vascular disease, unspecified**   `HCC` ▽
> Intermittent claudication
> Peripheral angiopathy NOS
> Spasm of artery
> *EXCLUDES 1*   *atherosclerosis of the extremities (I70.2--I70.7-)*

✓4th **I74**   **Arterial embolism and thrombosis**
> *INCLUDES*   embolic infarction
> embolic occlusion
> thrombotic infarction
> thrombotic occlusion
>
> Code first:
> embolism and thrombosis complicating abortion or ectopic or molar pregnancy (O00-O07, O08.2)
> embolism and thrombosis complicating pregnancy, childbirth and the puerperium (O88.-)
> *EXCLUDES 2*   *atheroembolism (I75.-)*
> *basilar embolism and thrombosis (I63.0-I63.2, I65.1)*
> *carotid embolism and thrombosis (I63.0-I63.2, I65.2)*
> *cerebral embolism and thrombosis (I63.3-I63.5, I66-)*
> *coronary embolism and thrombosis (I21-I25)*
> *mesenteric embolism and thrombosis (K55.0-)*
> *ophthalmic embolism and thrombosis (H34.-)*
> *precerebral embolism and thrombosis NOS (I63.0-I63.2, I65.9)*
> *pulmonary embolism and thrombosis (I26.-)*
> *renal embolism and thrombosis (N28.0)*
> *retinal embolism and thrombosis (H34.-)*
> *septic embolism and thrombosis (I76)*
> *vertebral embolism and thrombosis (I63.0-I63.2, I65.0)*

✓5th   I74.0   **Embolism and thrombosis of abdominal aorta**

     I74.01   **Saddle embolus of abdominal aorta**   `HCC`

     I74.09   **Other arterial embolism and thrombosis of abdominal aorta**   `HCC`
> Aortic bifurcation syndrome
> Aortoiliac obstruction
> Leriche's syndrome

✓5th   I74.1   **Embolism and thrombosis of other and unspecified parts of aorta**

     I74.10   **Embolism and thrombosis of unspecified parts of aorta**   `HCC` ▽

     I74.11   **Embolism and thrombosis of thoracic aorta**   `HCC`

     I74.19   **Embolism and thrombosis of other parts of aorta**   `HCC`

  I74.2   **Embolism and thrombosis of arteries of the upper extremities**   `HCC`

  I74.3   **Embolism and thrombosis of arteries of the lower extremities**   `HCC`

  I74.4   **Embolism and thrombosis of arteries of extremities, unspecified**   `HCC` ▽
> Peripheral arterial embolism NOS

  I74.5   **Embolism and thrombosis of iliac artery**   `HCC`

  I74.8   **Embolism and thrombosis of other arteries**   `HCC`

  I74.9   **Embolism and thrombosis of unspecified artery**   `HCC` ▽

✓4th **I75**   **Atheroembolism**
> *INCLUDES*   atherothrombotic microembolism
> cholesterol embolism

✓5th   I75.0   **Atheroembolism of extremities**

✓6th   I75.01   **Atheroembolism of upper extremity**

     I75.011   **Atheroembolism of right upper extremity**   `HCC`

     I75.012   **Atheroembolism of left upper extremity**   `HCC`

     I75.013   **Atheroembolism of bilateral upper extremities**   `HCC`

     I75.019   **Atheroembolism of unspecified upper extremity**   `HCC` ▽

✓6th   I75.02   **Atheroembolism of lower extremity**

     I75.021   **Atheroembolism of right lower extremity**   `HCC`

     I75.022   **Atheroembolism of left lower extremity**   `HCC`

     I75.023   **Atheroembolism of bilateral lower extremities**   `HCC`

     I75.029   **Atheroembolism of unspecified lower extremity**   `HCC` ▽

✓5th   I75.8   **Atheroembolism of other sites**

     I75.81   **Atheroembolism of kidney**   `HCC`
> Use additional code for any associated acute kidney failure and chronic kidney disease (N17.-, N18.-)

     I75.89   **Atheroembolism of other site**   `HCC`

I76   **Septic arterial embolism**   `HCC`
> Code first underlying infection, such as:
> infective endocarditis (I33.0)
> lung abscess (J85.-)
> Use additional code to identify the site of the embolism (I74.-)
> *EXCLUDES 2*   *septic pulmonary embolism (I26.01, I26.90)*

✓4th **I77**   **Other disorders of arteries and arterioles**
> *EXCLUDES 2*   *collagen (vascular) diseases (M30-M36)*
> *hypersensitivity angiitis (M31.0)*
> *pulmonary artery (I28.-)*

  I77.0   **Arteriovenous fistula, acquired**   `HCC`
> Aneurysmal varix
> Arteriovenous aneurysm, acquired
> *EXCLUDES 1*   *arteriovenous aneurysm NOS (Q27.3-)*
> *presence of arteriovenous shunt (fistula) for dialysis (Z99.2)*
> *traumatic—see injury of blood vessel by body region*
> *EXCLUDES 2*   *cerebral (I67.1)*
> *coronary (I25.4)*
> **DEF:** Communication between an artery and vein; caused by trauma or invasive procedures.

  I77.1   **Stricture of artery**   `HCC`
> Narrowing of artery

  I77.2   **Rupture of artery**   `HCC`
> Erosion of artery
> Fistula of artery
> Ulcer of artery
> *EXCLUDES 1*   *traumatic rupture of artery—see injury of blood vessel by body region*

  I77.3   **Arterial fibromuscular dysplasia**   `HCC`
> Fibromuscular hyperplasia (of) carotid artery
> Fibromuscular hyperplasia (of) renal artery

  I77.4   **Celiac artery compression syndrome**   `HCC`

EXCLUDES 1 Not coded here   *EXCLUDES 2* Not included here   N Newborn Age: 0   P Pediatric Age: 0-17   M Maternity Age: 12-55   A Adult Age: 15-124

646   ICD-10-CM 2018

I77.5 **Necrosis of artery** `HCC`

I77.6 **Arteritis, unspecified** `HCC` ▽
Aortitis NOS
Endarteritis NOS
EXCLUDES 1 arteritis or endarteritis:
aortic arch (M31.4)
cerebral NEC (I67.7)
coronary (I25.89)
deformans (I70.-)
giant cell (M31.5., M31.6)
obliterans (I70.-)
senile (I70.-)

✓5ᵗʰ **I77.7** **Other arterial dissection**
EXCLUDES 2 dissection of aorta (I71.0-)
dissection of coronary artery (I25.42)

  I77.70 **Dissection of unspecified artery** `HCC` ▽
  I77.71 **Dissection of carotid artery** `HCC`
  I77.72 **Dissection of iliac artery** `HCC`
  I77.73 **Dissection of renal artery** `HCC`
  I77.74 **Dissection of vertebral artery** `HCC`
  EXCLUDES 2 aneurysm of vertebral artery (I72.6)
  I77.75 **Dissection of other precerebral arteries** `HCC`
  Dissection of basilar artery (trunk)
  EXCLUDES 2 aneurysm of carotid artery (I72.0)
  aneurysm of other precerebral arteries (I72.5)
  aneurysm of vertebral artery (I72.6)
  dissection of carotid artery (I77.71)
  dissection of vertebral artery (I77.74)
  I77.76 **Dissection of artery of upper extremity** `HCC`
  I77.77 **Dissection of artery of lower extremity** `HCC`
  I77.79 **Dissection of other specified artery** `HCC`

✓5ᵗʰ **I77.8** **Other specified disorders of arteries and arterioles**
  ✓6ᵗʰ **I77.81** **Aortic ectasia**
  Ectasis aorta
  EXCLUDES 1 aortic aneurysm and dissection (I71.0-)
    I77.810 **Thoracic aortic ectasia** `HCC`
    I77.811 **Abdominal aortic ectasia** `HCC`
    I77.812 **Thoracoabdominal aortic ectasia** `HCC`
    I77.819 **Aortic ectasia, unspecified site** `HCC` ▽
  I77.89 **Other specified disorders of arteries and arterioles** `HCC`

I77.9 **Disorder of arteries and arterioles, unspecified** `HCC` ▽

✓4ᵗʰ **I78** **Diseases of capillaries**
  I78.0 **Hereditary hemorrhagic telangiectasia** `HCC`
  Rendu-Osler-Weber disease
  I78.1 **Nevus, non-neoplastic**
  Araneus nevus
  Senile nevus
  Spider nevus
  Stellar nevus
  EXCLUDES 1 nevus NOS (D22.-)
  vascular NOS (Q82.5)
  EXCLUDES 2 blue nevus (D22.-)
  flammeus nevus (Q82.5)
  hairy nevus (D22.-)
  melanocytic nevus (D22.-)
  pigmented nevus (D22.-)
  portwine nevus (Q82.5)
  sanguineous nevus (Q82.5)
  strawberry nevus (Q82.5)
  verrucous nevus (Q82.5)
  I78.8 **Other diseases of capillaries**
  I78.9 **Disease of capillaries, unspecified** ▽

✓4ᵗʰ **I79** **Disorders of arteries, arterioles and capillaries in diseases classified elsewhere**
  I79.0 **Aneurysm of aorta in diseases classified elsewhere** `HCC`
  Code first underlying disease
  EXCLUDES 1 syphilitic aneurysm (A52.01)
  I79.1 **Aortitis in diseases classified elsewhere** `HCC`
  Code first underlying disease
  EXCLUDES 1 syphilitic aortitis (A52.02)

I79.8 **Other disorders of arteries, arterioles and capillaries in diseases classified elsewhere** `HCC`
Code first underlying disease, such as:
amyloidosis (E85.-)
EXCLUDES 1 diabetic (peripheral) angiopathy (E08-E13 with .51-.52)
syphilitic endarteritis (A52.09)
tuberculous endarteritis (A18.89)

Diseases of veins, lymphatic vessels and lymph nodes, not elsewhere classified (I80-I89)

✓4ᵗʰ **I80** **Phlebitis and thrombophlebitis**
INCLUDES endophlebitis
inflammation, vein
periphlebitis
suppurative phlebitis
Code first:
phlebitis and thrombophlebitis complicating abortion, ectopic or molar pregnancy (O00-O07, O08.7)
phlebitis and thrombophlebitis complicating pregnancy, childbirth and the puerperium (O22.-, O87.-)
EXCLUDES 1 venous embolism and thrombosis of lower extremities ((I82.4-, I82.5-, I82.81-)

✓5ᵗʰ **I80.0** **Phlebitis and thrombophlebitis of superficial vessels of lower extremities**
Phlebitis and thrombophlebitis of femoropopliteal vein
  I80.00 **Phlebitis and thrombophlebitis of superficial vessels of unspecified lower extremity** ▽
  I80.01 **Phlebitis and thrombophlebitis of superficial vessels of right lower extremity**
  I80.02 **Phlebitis and thrombophlebitis of superficial vessels of left lower extremity**
  I80.03 **Phlebitis and thrombophlebitis of superficial vessels of lower extremities, bilateral**

✓5ᵗʰ **I80.1** **Phlebitis and thrombophlebitis of femoral vein**
  I80.10 **Phlebitis and thrombophlebitis of unspecified femoral vein** `HCC` ▽
  I80.11 **Phlebitis and thrombophlebitis of right femoral vein** `HCC`
  I80.12 **Phlebitis and thrombophlebitis of left femoral vein** `HCC`
  I80.13 **Phlebitis and thrombophlebitis of femoral vein, bilateral** `HCC`

✓5ᵗʰ **I80.2** **Phlebitis and thrombophlebitis of other and unspecified deep vessels of lower extremities**
  ✓6ᵗʰ **I80.20** **Phlebitis and thrombophlebitis of unspecified deep vessels of lower extremities**
    I80.201 **Phlebitis and thrombophlebitis of unspecified deep vessels of right lower extremity** `HCC`
    I80.202 **Phlebitis and thrombophlebitis of unspecified deep vessels of left lower extremity** `HCC`
    I80.203 **Phlebitis and thrombophlebitis of unspecified deep vessels of lower extremities, bilateral** `HCC`
    I80.209 **Phlebitis and thrombophlebitis of unspecified deep vessels of unspecified lower extremity** `HCC` ▽
  ✓6ᵗʰ **I80.21** **Phlebitis and thrombophlebitis of iliac vein**
    I80.211 **Phlebitis and thrombophlebitis of right iliac vein** `HCC`
    I80.212 **Phlebitis and thrombophlebitis of left iliac vein** `HCC`
    I80.213 **Phlebitis and thrombophlebitis of iliac vein, bilateral** `HCC`
    I80.219 **Phlebitis and thrombophlebitis of unspecified iliac vein** `HCC` ▽
  ✓6ᵗʰ **I80.22** **Phlebitis and thrombophlebitis of popliteal vein**
    I80.221 **Phlebitis and thrombophlebitis of right popliteal vein** `HCC`
    I80.222 **Phlebitis and thrombophlebitis of left popliteal vein** `HCC`
    I80.223 **Phlebitis and thrombophlebitis of popliteal vein, bilateral** `HCC`
    I80.229 **Phlebitis and thrombophlebitis of unspecified popliteal vein** `HCC` ▽

Chapter 9. Diseases of the Circulatory System

✓6ᵗʰ **I80.23 Phlebitis and thrombophlebitis of tibial vein**

- **I80.231** Phlebitis and thrombophlebitis of **right tibial vein** HCC
- **I80.232** Phlebitis and thrombophlebitis of **left tibial vein** HCC
- **I80.233** Phlebitis and thrombophlebitis of **tibial vein, bilateral** HCC
- **I80.239** Phlebitis and thrombophlebitis of **unspecified tibial vein** HCC ▽

✓6ᵗʰ **I80.29 Phlebitis and thrombophlebitis of other deep vessels of lower extremities**

- **I80.291** Phlebitis and thrombophlebitis of **other deep vessels of right lower extremity** HCC
- **I80.292** Phlebitis and thrombophlebitis of **other deep vessels of left lower extremity** HCC
- **I80.293** Phlebitis and thrombophlebitis of **other deep vessels of lower extremity, bilateral** HCC
- **I80.299** Phlebitis and thrombophlebitis of **other deep vessels of unspecified lower extremity** HCC ▽

I80.3 Phlebitis and thrombophlebitis of lower extremities, unspecified ▽

I80.8 Phlebitis and thrombophlebitis of other sites

I80.9 Phlebitis and thrombophlebitis of unspecified site ▽

I81 Portal vein thrombosis
Portal (vein) obstruction
EXCLUDES 2   hepatic vein thrombosis (I82.0)
phlebitis of portal vein (K75.1)

✓4ᵗʰ **I82 Other venous embolism and thrombosis**
Code first venous embolism and thrombosis complicating:
abortion, ectopic or molar pregnancy (O00-O07, O08.7)
pregnancy, childbirth and the puerperium (O22.-, O87.-)
EXCLUDES 2   venous embolism and thrombosis (of):
cerebral (I63.6, I67.6)
coronary (I21-I25)
intracranial and intraspinal, septic or NOS (G08)
intracranial, nonpyogenic (I67.6)
intraspinal, nonpyogenic (G95.1)
mesenteric (K55.0-)
portal (I81)
pulmonary (I26.-)

I82.0 Budd-Chiari syndrome HCC
Hepatic vein thrombosis
DEF: Thrombosis or other obstruction of hepatic veins; symptoms include enlarged liver, extensive collateral vessels, intractable ascites, and severe portal hypertension.

I82.1 Thrombophlebitis migrans

✓5ᵗʰ **I82.2 Embolism and thrombosis of vena cava and other thoracic veins**

✓6ᵗʰ **I82.21 Embolism and thrombosis of superior vena cava**

- **I82.210** Acute embolism and thrombosis of **superior vena cava** HCC
  Embolism and thrombosis of superior vena cava NOS
- **I82.211** Chronic embolism and thrombosis of **superior vena cava** HCC

✓6ᵗʰ **I82.22 Embolism and thrombosis of inferior vena cava**

- **I82.220** Acute embolism and thrombosis of **inferior vena cava** HCC
  Embolism and thrombosis of inferior vena cava NOS
- **I82.221** Chronic embolism and thrombosis of **inferior vena cava** HCC

✓6ᵗʰ **I82.29 Embolism and thrombosis of other thoracic veins**
Embolism and thrombosis of brachiocephalic (innominate) vein

- **I82.290** Acute embolism and thrombosis of **other thoracic veins** HCC
- **I82.291** Chronic embolism and thrombosis of **other thoracic veins** HCC

I82.3 Embolism and thrombosis of renal vein HCC

✓5ᵗʰ **I82.4 Acute embolism and thrombosis of deep veins of lower extremity**

✓6ᵗʰ **I82.40 Acute embolism and thrombosis of unspecified deep veins of lower extremity**
Deep vein thrombosis NOS
DVT NOS
EXCLUDES 1   acute embolism and thrombosis of unspecified deep veins of distal lower extremity (I82.4Z-)
acute embolism and thrombosis of unspecified deep veins of proximal lower extremity (I82.4Y-)

- **I82.401** Acute embolism and thrombosis of **unspecified deep veins of right lower extremity** HCC ▽
- **I82.402** Acute embolism and thrombosis of **unspecified deep veins of left lower extremity** HCC ▽
- **I82.403** Acute embolism and thrombosis of **unspecified deep veins of lower extremity, bilateral** HCC ▽
- **I82.409** Acute embolism and thrombosis of **unspecified deep veins of unspecified lower extremity** HCC ▽

✓6ᵗʰ **I82.41 Acute embolism and thrombosis of femoral vein**

- **I82.411** Acute embolism and thrombosis of **right femoral vein** HCC
- **I82.412** Acute embolism and thrombosis of **left femoral vein** HCC
- **I82.413** Acute embolism and thrombosis of **femoral vein, bilateral** HCC
- **I82.419** Acute embolism and thrombosis of **unspecified femoral vein** HCC ▽

✓6ᵗʰ **I82.42 Acute embolism and thrombosis of iliac vein**

- **I82.421** Acute embolism and thrombosis of **right iliac vein** HCC
- **I82.422** Acute embolism and thrombosis of **left iliac vein** HCC
- **I82.423** Acute embolism and thrombosis of **iliac vein, bilateral** HCC
- **I82.429** Acute embolism and thrombosis of **unspecified iliac vein** HCC ▽

✓6ᵗʰ **I82.43 Acute embolism and thrombosis of popliteal vein**

- **I82.431** Acute embolism and thrombosis of **right popliteal vein** HCC
- **I82.432** Acute embolism and thrombosis of **left popliteal vein** HCC
- **I82.433** Acute embolism and thrombosis of **popliteal vein, bilateral** HCC
- **I82.439** Acute embolism and thrombosis of **unspecified popliteal vein** HCC ▽

✓6ᵗʰ **I82.44 Acute embolism and thrombosis of tibial vein**

- **I82.441** Acute embolism and thrombosis of **right tibial vein** HCC
- **I82.442** Acute embolism and thrombosis of **left tibial vein** HCC
- **I82.443** Acute embolism and thrombosis of **tibial vein, bilateral** HCC
- **I82.449** Acute embolism and thrombosis of **unspecified tibial vein** HCC ▽

✓6ᵗʰ **I82.49 Acute embolism and thrombosis of other specified deep vein of lower extremity**

- **I82.491** Acute embolism and thrombosis of **other specified deep vein of right lower extremity** HCC
- **I82.492** Acute embolism and thrombosis of **other specified deep vein of left lower extremity** HCC
- **I82.493** Acute embolism and thrombosis of **other specified deep vein of lower extremity, bilateral** HCC
- **I82.499** Acute embolism and thrombosis of **other specified deep vein of unspecified lower extremity** HCC ▽

EXCLUDES 1 Not coded here   EXCLUDES 2 Not included here   N Newborn Age: 0   P Pediatric Age: 0-17   M Maternity Age: 12-55   A Adult Age: 15-124

648   ICD-10-CM 2018

✓6ᵗʰ **I82.4Y** **Acute embolism and thrombosis of unspecified deep veins of proximal lower extremity**
Acute embolism and thrombosis of deep vein of thigh NOS
Acute embolism and thrombosis of deep vein of upper leg NOS

     I82.4Y1 **Acute embolism and thrombosis of** HCC ▽ **unspecified deep veins of right proximal lower extremity**

     I82.4Y2 **Acute embolism and thrombosis of** HCC ▽ **unspecified deep veins of left proximal lower extremity**

     I82.4Y3 **Acute embolism and thrombosis of** HCC ▽ **unspecified deep veins of proximal lower extremity, bilateral**

     I82.4Y9 **Acute embolism and thrombosis of** HCC ▽ **unspecified deep veins of unspecified proximal lower extremity**

✓6ᵗʰ **I82.4Z** **Acute embolism and thrombosis of unspecified deep veins of distal lower extremity**
Acute embolism and thrombosis of deep vein of calf NOS
Acute embolism and thrombosis of deep vein of lower leg NOS

     I82.4Z1 **Acute embolism and thrombosis of** HCC ▽ **unspecified deep veins of right distal lower extremity**

     I82.4Z2 **Acute embolism and thrombosis of** HCC ▽ **unspecified deep veins of left distal lower extremity**

     I82.4Z3 **Acute embolism and thrombosis of** HCC ▽ **unspecified deep veins of distal lower extremity, bilateral**

     I82.4Z9 **Acute embolism and thrombosis of** HCC ▽ **unspecified deep veins of unspecified distal lower extremity**

✓5ᵗʰ **I82.5** **Chronic embolism and thrombosis of deep veins of lower extremity**
Use additional code, if applicable, for associated long-term (current) use of anticoagulants (Z79.01)
EXCLUDES 1   *personal history of venous embolism and thrombosis (Z86.718)*

✓6ᵗʰ **I82.50** **Chronic embolism and thrombosis of unspecified deep veins of lower extremity**
EXCLUDES 1   *chronic embolism and thrombosis of unspecified deep veins of distal lower extremity (I82.5Z-)*
chronic embolism and thrombosis of unspecified deep veins of proximal lower extremity (I82.5Y-)

     I82.501 **Chronic embolism and thrombosis** HCC ▽ **of unspecified deep veins of right lower extremity**

     I82.502 **Chronic embolism and thrombosis** HCC ▽ **of unspecified deep veins of left lower extremity**

     I82.503 **Chronic embolism and thrombosis** HCC ▽ **of unspecified deep veins of lower extremity, bilateral**

     I82.509 **Chronic embolism and thrombosis** HCC ▽ **of unspecified deep veins of unspecified lower extremity**

✓6ᵗʰ **I82.51** **Chronic embolism and thrombosis of femoral vein**

     I82.511 **Chronic embolism and thrombosis of** HCC **right femoral vein**

     I82.512 **Chronic embolism and thrombosis of** HCC **left femoral vein**

     I82.513 **Chronic embolism and thrombosis of** HCC **femoral vein, bilateral**

     I82.519 **Chronic embolism and thrombosis** HCC ▽ **of unspecified femoral vein**

✓6ᵗʰ **I82.52** **Chronic embolism and thrombosis of iliac vein**

     I82.521 **Chronic embolism and thrombosis of** HCC **right iliac vein**

     I82.522 **Chronic embolism and thrombosis of** HCC **left iliac vein**

     I82.523 **Chronic embolism and thrombosis of** HCC **iliac vein, bilateral**

     I82.529 **Chronic embolism and thrombosis** HCC ▽ **of unspecified iliac vein**

✓6ᵗʰ **I82.53** **Chronic embolism and thrombosis of popliteal vein**

     I82.531 **Chronic embolism and thrombosis of** HCC **right popliteal vein**

     I82.532 **Chronic embolism and thrombosis of** HCC **left popliteal vein**

     I82.533 **Chronic embolism and thrombosis of** HCC **popliteal vein, bilateral**

     I82.539 **Chronic embolism and thrombosis** HCC ▽ **of unspecified popliteal vein**

✓6ᵗʰ **I82.54** **Chronic embolism and thrombosis of tibial vein**

     I82.541 **Chronic embolism and thrombosis of** HCC **right tibial vein**

     I82.542 **Chronic embolism and thrombosis of** HCC **left tibial vein**

     I82.543 **Chronic embolism and thrombosis of** HCC **tibial vein, bilateral**

     I82.549 **Chronic embolism and thrombosis** HCC ▽ **of unspecified tibial vein**

✓6ᵗʰ **I82.59** **Chronic embolism and thrombosis of other specified deep vein of lower extremity**

     I82.591 **Chronic embolism and thrombosis of** HCC **other specified deep vein of right lower extremity**

     I82.592 **Chronic embolism and thrombosis of** HCC **other specified deep vein of left lower extremity**

     I82.593 **Chronic embolism and thrombosis of** HCC **other specified deep vein of lower extremity, bilateral**

     I82.599 **Chronic embolism and thrombosis** HCC ▽ **of other specified deep vein of unspecified lower extremity**

✓6ᵗʰ **I82.5Y** **Chronic embolism and thrombosis of unspecified deep veins of proximal lower extremity**
Chronic embolism and thrombosis of deep veins of thigh NOS
Chronic embolism and thrombosis of deep veins of upper leg NOS

     I82.5Y1 **Chronic embolism and thrombosis** HCC ▽ **of unspecified deep veins of right proximal lower extremity**

     I82.5Y2 **Chronic embolism and thrombosis** HCC ▽ **of unspecified deep veins of left proximal lower extremity**

     I82.5Y3 **Chronic embolism and thrombosis** HCC ▽ **of unspecified deep veins of proximal lower extremity, bilateral**

     I82.5Y9 **Chronic embolism and thrombosis** HCC ▽ **of unspecified deep veins of unspecified proximal lower extremity**

✓6ᵗʰ **I82.5Z** **Chronic embolism and thrombosis of unspecified deep veins of distal lower extremity**
Chronic embolism and thrombosis of deep veins of calf NOS
Chronic embolism and thrombosis of deep veins of lower leg NOS

     I82.5Z1 **Chronic embolism and thrombosis** HCC ▽ **of unspecified deep veins of right distal lower extremity**

     I82.5Z2 **Chronic embolism and thrombosis** HCC ▽ **of unspecified deep veins of left distal lower extremity**

     I82.5Z3 **Chronic embolism and thrombosis** HCC ▽ **of unspecified deep veins of distal lower extremity, bilateral**

     I82.5Z9 **Chronic embolism and thrombosis** HCC ▽ **of unspecified deep veins of unspecified distal lower extremity**

✓5ᵗʰ **I82.6** **Acute embolism and thrombosis of veins of upper extremity**

✓6ᵗʰ **I82.60** **Acute embolism and thrombosis of unspecified veins of upper extremity**

     I82.601 **Acute embolism and thrombosis of** ▽ **unspecified veins of right upper extremity**

     I82.602 **Acute embolism and thrombosis of** ▽ **unspecified veins of left upper extremity**

     I82.603 **Acute embolism and thrombosis of** ▽ **unspecified veins of upper extremity, bilateral**

✓ Additional Character Req   ✓ₓ7ᵗʰ Placeholder Alert   Manifestation   HCC CMS-HCC Condition   ▽ Unspecified Code   ►◄ Revised Text   ● New Code   ▲ Revised Code Title

ICD-10-CM 2018   **649**

Chapter 9. Diseases of the Circulatory System

I82.609   Acute embolism and thrombosis of unspecified veins of unspecified upper extremity   ▽

✓6ᵗʰ I82.61   Acute embolism and thrombosis of superficial veins of upper extremity
Acute embolism and thrombosis of antecubital vein
Acute embolism and thrombosis of basilic vein
Acute embolism and thrombosis of cephalic vein

I82.611   Acute embolism and thrombosis of superficial veins of right upper extremity

I82.612   Acute embolism and thrombosis of superficial veins of left upper extremity

I82.613   Acute embolism and thrombosis of superficial veins of upper extremity, bilateral

I82.619   Acute embolism and thrombosis of superficial veins of unspecified upper extremity   ▽

✓6ᵗʰ I82.62   Acute embolism and thrombosis of deep veins of upper extremity
Acute embolism and thrombosis of brachial vein
Acute embolism and thrombosis of radial vein
Acute embolism and thrombosis of ulnar vein

I82.621   Acute embolism and thrombosis of deep veins of right upper extremity   HCC

I82.622   Acute embolism and thrombosis of deep veins of left upper extremity   HCC

I82.623   Acute embolism and thrombosis of deep veins of upper extremity, bilateral   HCC

I82.629   Acute embolism and thrombosis of deep veins of unspecified upper extremity   HCC ▽

✓5ᵗʰ I82.7   Chronic embolism and thrombosis of veins of upper extremity
Use additional code, if applicable, for associated long-term (current) use of anticoagulants (Z79.01)
> EXCLUDES 1   personal history of venous embolism and thrombosis (Z86.718)

✓6ᵗʰ I82.70   Chronic embolism and thrombosis of unspecified veins of upper extremity

I82.701   Chronic embolism and thrombosis of unspecified veins of right upper extremity   ▽

I82.702   Chronic embolism and thrombosis of unspecified veins of left upper extremity   ▽

I82.703   Chronic embolism and thrombosis of unspecified veins of upper extremity, bilateral   ▽

I82.709   Chronic embolism and thrombosis of unspecified veins of unspecified upper extremity   ▽

✓6ᵗʰ I82.71   Chronic embolism and thrombosis of superficial veins of upper extremity
Chronic embolism and thrombosis of antecubital vein
Chronic embolism and thrombosis of basilic vein
Chronic embolism and thrombosis of cephalic vein

I82.711   Chronic embolism and thrombosis of superficial veins of right upper extremity

I82.712   Chronic embolism and thrombosis of superficial veins of left upper extremity

I82.713   Chronic embolism and thrombosis of superficial veins of upper extremity, bilateral

I82.719   Chronic embolism and thrombosis of superficial veins of unspecified upper extremity   ▽

✓6ᵗʰ I82.72   Chronic embolism and thrombosis of deep veins of upper extremity
Chronic embolism and thrombosis of brachial vein
Chronic embolism and thrombosis of radial vein
Chronic embolism and thrombosis of ulnar vein

I82.721   Chronic embolism and thrombosis of deep veins of right upper extremity   HCC

I82.722   Chronic embolism and thrombosis of deep veins of left upper extremity   HCC

I82.723   Chronic embolism and thrombosis of deep veins of upper extremity, bilateral   HCC

I82.729   Chronic embolism and thrombosis of deep veins of unspecified upper extremity   HCC ▽

✓5ᵗʰ I82.A   Embolism and thrombosis of axillary vein

✓6ᵗʰ I82.A1   Acute embolism and thrombosis of axillary vein

I82.A11   Acute embolism and thrombosis of right axillary vein   HCC

I82.A12   Acute embolism and thrombosis of left axillary vein   HCC

I82.A13   Acute embolism and thrombosis of axillary vein, bilateral   HCC

I82.A19   Acute embolism and thrombosis of unspecified axillary vein   HCC ▽

✓6ᵗʰ I82.A2   Chronic embolism and thrombosis of axillary vein

I82.A21   Chronic embolism and thrombosis of right axillary vein   HCC

I82.A22   Chronic embolism and thrombosis of left axillary vein   HCC

I82.A23   Chronic embolism and thrombosis of axillary vein, bilateral   HCC

I82.A29   Chronic embolism and thrombosis of unspecified axillary vein   HCC ▽

✓5ᵗʰ I82.B   Embolism and thrombosis of subclavian vein

✓6ᵗʰ I82.B1   Acute embolism and thrombosis of subclavian vein

I82.B11   Acute embolism and thrombosis of right subclavian vein   HCC

I82.B12   Acute embolism and thrombosis of left subclavian vein   HCC

I82.B13   Acute embolism and thrombosis of subclavian vein, bilateral   HCC

I82.B19   Acute embolism and thrombosis of unspecified subclavian vein   HCC ▽

✓6ᵗʰ I82.B2   Chronic embolism and thrombosis of subclavian vein

I82.B21   Chronic embolism and thrombosis of right subclavian vein   HCC

I82.B22   Chronic embolism and thrombosis of left subclavian vein   HCC

I82.B23   Chronic embolism and thrombosis of subclavian vein, bilateral   HCC

I82.B29   Chronic embolism and thrombosis of unspecified subclavian vein   HCC ▽

✓5ᵗʰ I82.C   Embolism and thrombosis of internal jugular vein

✓6ᵗʰ I82.C1   Acute embolism and thrombosis of internal jugular vein

I82.C11   Acute embolism and thrombosis of right internal jugular vein   HCC

I82.C12   Acute embolism and thrombosis of left internal jugular vein   HCC

I82.C13   Acute embolism and thrombosis of internal jugular vein, bilateral   HCC

I82.C19   Acute embolism and thrombosis of unspecified internal jugular vein   HCC ▽

✓6ᵗʰ I82.C2   Chronic embolism and thrombosis of internal jugular vein

I82.C21   Chronic embolism and thrombosis of right internal jugular vein   HCC

I82.C22   Chronic embolism and thrombosis of left internal jugular vein   HCC

I82.C23   Chronic embolism and thrombosis of internal jugular vein, bilateral   HCC

I82.C29   Chronic embolism and thrombosis of unspecified internal jugular vein   HCC ▽

✓5ᵗʰ I82.8   Embolism and thrombosis of other specified veins
Use additional code, if applicable, for associated long-term (current) use of anticoagulants (Z79.01)

✓6ᵗʰ I82.81   Embolism and thrombosis of superficial veins of lower extremities
Embolism and thrombosis of saphenous vein (greater) (lesser)

▲   **I82.811**   Embolism and thrombosis of superficial veins of right lower extremity

▲   **I82.812**   Embolism and thrombosis of superficial veins of left lower extremity

I82.813   Embolism and thrombosis of superficial veins of lower extremities, bilateral

▲   **I82.819**   Embolism and thrombosis of superficial veins of unspecified lower extremity   ▽

EXCLUDES 1   Not coded here   EXCLUDES 2   Not included here   N Newborn Age: 0   P Pediatric Age: 0-17   M Maternity Age: 12-55   A Adult Age: 15-124

650   ICD-10-CM 2018

☑6ᵗʰ I82.89 Embolism and thrombosis of other specified veins

    I82.890 Acute embolism and thrombosis of other specified veins

    I82.891 Chronic embolism and thrombosis of other specified veins

☑5ᵗʰ I82.9 Embolism and thrombosis of unspecified vein

    I82.90 Acute embolism and thrombosis of unspecified vein ▽

      Embolism of vein NOS
      Thrombosis (vein) NOS

    I82.91 Chronic embolism and thrombosis of unspecified vein ▽

☑4ᵗʰ I83 Varicose veins of lower extremities

    EXCLUDES 1   *varicose veins complicating pregnancy (O22.0-)*
             varicose veins complicating the puerperium (O87.4)

☑5ᵗʰ I83.0 Varicose veins of lower extremities with ulcer

    Use additional code to identify severity of ulcer (L97.-)

    ☑6ᵗʰ I83.00 Varicose veins of unspecified lower extremity with ulcer

      I83.001 Varicose veins of unspecified lower extremity with ulcer of thigh HCC A ▽

      I83.002 Varicose veins of unspecified lower extremity with ulcer of calf HCC A ▽

      I83.003 Varicose veins of unspecified lower extremity with ulcer of ankle HCC A ▽

      I83.004 Varicose veins of unspecified lower extremity with ulcer of heel and midfoot HCC A ▽

        Varicose veins of unspecified lower extremity with ulcer of plantar surface of midfoot

      I83.005 Varicose veins of unspecified lower extremity with ulcer other part of foot HCC A ▽

        Varicose veins of unspecified lower extremity with ulcer of toe

      I83.008 Varicose veins of unspecified lower extremity with ulcer other part of lower leg HCC A ▽

      I83.009 Varicose veins of unspecified lower extremity with ulcer of unspecified site HCC A ▽

    ☑6ᵗʰ I83.01 Varicose veins of right lower extremity with ulcer

      I83.011 Varicose veins of right lower extremity with ulcer of thigh HCC A

      I83.012 Varicose veins of right lower extremity with ulcer of calf HCC A

      I83.013 Varicose veins of right lower extremity with ulcer of ankle HCC A

      I83.014 Varicose veins of right lower extremity with ulcer of heel and midfoot HCC A

        Varicose veins of right lower extremity with ulcer of plantar surface of midfoot

      I83.015 Varicose veins of right lower extremity with ulcer other part of foot HCC A

        Varicose veins of right lower extremity with ulcer of toe

      I83.018 Varicose veins of right lower extremity with ulcer other part of lower leg HCC A

      I83.019 Varicose veins of right lower extremity with ulcer of unspecified site HCC A ▽

    ☑6ᵗʰ I83.02 Varicose veins of left lower extremity with ulcer

      I83.021 Varicose veins of left lower extremity with ulcer of thigh HCC A

      I83.022 Varicose veins of left lower extremity with ulcer of calf HCC A

      I83.023 Varicose veins of left lower extremity with ulcer of ankle HCC A

      I83.024 Varicose veins of left lower extremity with ulcer of heel and midfoot HCC A

        Varicose veins of left lower extremity with ulcer of plantar surface of midfoot

      I83.025 Varicose veins of left lower extremity with ulcer other part of foot HCC A

        Varicose veins of left lower extremity with ulcer of toe

    I83.028 Varicose veins of left lower extremity with ulcer other part of lower leg HCC A

    I83.029 Varicose veins of left lower extremity with ulcer of unspecified site HCC A ▽

☑5ᵗʰ I83.1 Varicose veins of lower extremities with inflammation

    I83.10 Varicose veins of unspecified lower extremity with inflammation A ▽

    I83.11 Varicose veins of right lower extremity with inflammation A

    I83.12 Varicose veins of left lower extremity with inflammation A

☑5ᵗʰ I83.2 Varicose veins of lower extremities with both ulcer and inflammation

    Use additional code to identify severity of ulcer (L97.-)

    ☑6ᵗʰ I83.20 Varicose veins of unspecified lower extremity with both ulcer and inflammation

      I83.201 Varicose veins of unspecified lower extremity with both ulcer of thigh and inflammation HCC A ▽

      I83.202 Varicose veins of unspecified lower extremity with both ulcer of calf and inflammation HCC A ▽

      I83.203 Varicose veins of unspecified lower extremity with both ulcer of ankle and inflammation HCC A ▽

      I83.204 Varicose veins of unspecified lower extremity with both ulcer of heel and midfoot and inflammation HCC A ▽

        Varicose veins of unspecified lower extremity with both ulcer of plantar surface of midfoot and inflammation

      I83.205 Varicose veins of unspecified lower extremity with both ulcer of other part of foot and inflammation HCC A ▽

        Varicose veins of unspecified lower extremity with both ulcer of toe and inflammation

      I83.208 Varicose veins of unspecified lower extremity with both ulcer of other part of lower extremity and inflammation HCC A ▽

      I83.209 Varicose veins of unspecified lower extremity with both ulcer of unspecified site and inflammation HCC A ▽

    ☑6ᵗʰ I83.21 Varicose veins of right lower extremity with both ulcer and inflammation

      I83.211 Varicose veins of right lower extremity with both ulcer of thigh and inflammation HCC A

      I83.212 Varicose veins of right lower extremity with both ulcer of calf and inflammation HCC A

      I83.213 Varicose veins of right lower extremity with both ulcer of ankle and inflammation HCC A

      I83.214 Varicose veins of right lower extremity with both ulcer of heel and midfoot and inflammation HCC A

        Varicose veins of right lower extremity with both ulcer of plantar surface of midfoot and inflammation

      I83.215 Varicose veins of right lower extremity with both ulcer other part of foot and inflammation HCC A

        Varicose veins of right lower extremity with both ulcer of toe and inflammation

      I83.218 Varicose veins of right lower extremity with both ulcer of other part of lower extremity and inflammation HCC A

      I83.219 Varicose veins of right lower extremity with both ulcer of unspecified site and inflammation HCC A ▽

    ☑6ᵗʰ I83.22 Varicose veins of left lower extremity with both ulcer and inflammation

      I83.221 Varicose veins of left lower extremity with both ulcer of thigh and inflammation HCC A

      I83.222 Varicose veins of left lower extremity with both ulcer of calf and inflammation HCC A

I83.223   **Varicose veins of left lower**   HCC A
       extremity with both ulcer of ankle and
       inflammation

I83.224   **Varicose veins of left lower**   HCC A
       extremity with both ulcer of heel and
       midfoot and inflammation
         Varicose veins of left lower extremity with
           both ulcer of plantar surface of
           midfoot and inflammation

I83.225   **Varicose veins of left lower**   HCC A
       extremity with both ulcer other part of
       foot and inflammation
         Varicose veins of left lower extremity with
           both ulcer of toe and inflammation

I83.228   **Varicose veins of left lower**   HCC A
       extremity with both ulcer of other part of
       lower extremity and inflammation

I83.229   **Varicose veins of left lower**   HCC A ▽
       extremity with both ulcer of unspecified
       site and inflammation

✓5ᵗʰ **I83.8   Varicose veins of lower extremities with other complications**

   ✓6ᵗʰ **I83.81   Varicose veins of lower extremities with pain**

▲   I83.811   **Varicose veins of right lower**   A
              extremity with pain

▲   I83.812   **Varicose veins of left lower extremity**   A
              with pain

     I83.813   **Varicose veins of bilateral lower**   A
              extremities with pain

▲   I83.819   **Varicose veins of unspecified lower**   A ▽
              extremity with pain

   ✓6ᵗʰ **I83.89   Varicose veins of lower extremities with other**
         complications
         Varicose veins of lower extremities with edema
         Varicose veins of lower extremities with swelling

▲   I83.891   **Varicose veins of right lower**   A
              extremity with other complications

▲   I83.892   **Varicose veins of left lower extremity**   A
              with other complications

     I83.893   **Varicose veins of bilateral lower**   A
              extremities with other complications

▲   I83.899   **Varicose veins of unspecified lower**   A ▽
              extremity with other complications

✓5ᵗʰ **I83.9   Asymptomatic varicose veins of lower extremities**
       Phlebectasia of lower extremities
       Varicose veins of lower extremities
       Varix of lower extremities

   I83.90   **Asymptomatic varicose veins of unspecified**   A ▽
         lower extremity
         Varicose veins NOS

   I83.91   **Asymptomatic varicose veins of right lower**   A
         extremity

   I83.92   **Asymptomatic varicose veins of left lower**   A
         extremity

   I83.93   **Asymptomatic varicose veins of bilateral lower**   A
         extremities

✓4ᵗʰ **I85   Esophageal varices**
       Use additional code to identify:
         alcohol abuse and dependence (F10.-)

   ✓5ᵗʰ **I85.0   Esophageal varices**
       Idiopathic esophageal varices
       Primary esophageal varices

     I85.00   **Esophageal varices without bleeding**   HCC
         Esophageal varices NOS

     I85.01   **Esophageal varices with bleeding**   HCC

   ✓5ᵗʰ **I85.1   Secondary esophageal varices**
       Esophageal varices secondary to alcoholic liver disease
       Esophageal varices secondary to cirrhosis of liver
       Esophageal varices secondary to schistosomiasis
       Esophageal varices secondary to toxic liver disease
       Code first underlying disease

     I85.10   **Secondary esophageal varices without bleeding**   HCC

     I85.11   **Secondary esophageal varices with bleeding**   HCC

✓4ᵗʰ **I86   Varicose veins of other sites**
       EXCLUDES 1   varicose veins of unspecified site (I83.9-)
       EXCLUDES 2   retinal varices (H35.0-)

   I86.0   Sublingual varices
       DEF: Distended, tortuous veins beneath tongue.

I86.1   **Scrotal varices**   ♂
       Varicocele

I86.2   **Pelvic varices**

I86.3   **Vulval varices**   ♀
       EXCLUDES 1   vulval varices complicating childbirth and the
                 puerperium (O87.8)
                 vulval varices complicating pregnancy (O22.1-)

I86.4   **Gastric varices**

I86.8   **Varicose veins of other specified sites**   A
       Varicose ulcer of nasal septum

✓4ᵗʰ **I87   Other disorders of veins**

   ✓5ᵗʰ **I87.0   Postthrombotic syndrome**
       Chronic venous hypertension due to deep vein thrombosis
       Postphlebitic syndrome
       EXCLUDES 1   chronic venous hypertension without deep vein
                 thrombosis (I87.3-)

     ✓6ᵗʰ **I87.00   Postthrombotic syndrome without complications**
         Asymptomatic postthrombotic syndrome

       I87.001   **Postthrombotic syndrome without**
               complications of right lower extremity

       I87.002   **Postthrombotic syndrome without**
               complications of left lower extremity

       I87.003   **Postthrombotic syndrome without**
               complications of bilateral lower extremity

       I87.009   **Postthrombotic syndrome without**   ▽
               complications of unspecified extremity
               Postthrombotic syndrome NOS

     ✓6ᵗʰ **I87.01   Postthrombotic syndrome with ulcer**
         Use additional code to specify site and severity of ulcer
           (L97.-)

       I87.011   **Postthrombotic syndrome with ulcer**   HCC
               of right lower extremity

       I87.012   **Postthrombotic syndrome with ulcer**   HCC
               of left lower extremity

       I87.013   **Postthrombotic syndrome with ulcer**   HCC
               of bilateral lower extremity

       I87.019   **Postthrombotic syndrome with**   HCC ▽
               ulcer of unspecified lower extremity

     ✓6ᵗʰ **I87.02   Postthrombotic syndrome with inflammation**

       I87.021   **Postthrombotic syndrome with**
               inflammation of right lower extremity

       I87.022   **Postthrombotic syndrome with**
               inflammation of left lower extremity

       I87.023   **Postthrombotic syndrome with**
               inflammation of bilateral lower extremity

       I87.029   **Postthrombotic syndrome with**   ▽
               inflammation of unspecified lower
               extremity

     ✓6ᵗʰ **I87.03   Postthrombotic syndrome with ulcer and**
         inflammation
         Use additional code to specify site and severity of ulcer
           (L97.-)

       I87.031   **Postthrombotic syndrome with ulcer**   HCC
               and inflammation of right lower extremity

       I87.032   **Postthrombotic syndrome with ulcer**   HCC
               and inflammation of left lower extremity

       I87.033   **Postthrombotic syndrome with ulcer**   HCC
               and inflammation of bilateral lower
               extremity

       I87.039   **Postthrombotic syndrome with**   HCC ▽
               ulcer and inflammation of unspecified
               lower extremity

     ✓6ᵗʰ **I87.09   Postthrombotic syndrome with other complications**

       I87.091   **Postthrombotic syndrome with other**
               complications of right lower extremity

       I87.092   **Postthrombotic syndrome with other**
               complications of left lower extremity

       I87.093   **Postthrombotic syndrome with other**
               complications of bilateral lower extremity

       I87.099   **Postthrombotic syndrome with other**   ▽
               complications of unspecified lower
               extremity

   I87.1   Compression of vein
       Stricture of vein
       Vena cava syndrome (inferior) (superior)
       EXCLUDES 2   compression of pulmonary vein (I28.8)

EXCLUDES 1 Not coded here   *EXCLUDES 2* Not included here   N Newborn Age: 0   P Pediatric Age: 0-17   M Maternity Age: 12-55   A Adult Age: 15-124

652   ICD-10-CM 2018

I87.2   **Venous insufficiency (chronic) (peripheral)**
Stasis dermatitis
EXCLUDES 1   *stasis dermatitis with varicose veins of lower extremities (I83.1-, I83.2-)*
DEF: Insufficient drainage of venous blood in any part of body; results in edema or dermatosis.

✓5ᵗʰ **I87.3**   **Chronic venous hypertension (idiopathic)**
Stasis edema
EXCLUDES 1   *chronic venous hypertension due to deep vein thrombosis (I87.0-)*
varicose veins of lower extremities (I83.-)

✓6ᵗʰ **I87.30**   **Chronic venous hypertension (idiopathic) without complications**
Asymptomatic chronic venous hypertension (idiopathic)

I87.301   **Chronic venous hypertension (idiopathic) without complications of right lower extremity**

I87.302   **Chronic venous hypertension (idiopathic) without complications of left lower extremity**

I87.303   **Chronic venous hypertension (idiopathic) without complications of bilateral lower extremity**

I87.309   **Chronic venous hypertension (idiopathic) without complications of unspecified lower extremity** ▽
Chronic venous hypertension NOS

✓6ᵗʰ **I87.31**   **Chronic venous hypertension (idiopathic) with ulcer**
Use additional code to specify site and severity of ulcer (L97.-)

I87.311   **Chronic venous hypertension (idiopathic) with ulcer of right lower extremity**   HCC

I87.312   **Chronic venous hypertension (idiopathic) with ulcer of left lower extremity**   HCC

I87.313   **Chronic venous hypertension (idiopathic) with ulcer of bilateral lower extremity**   HCC

I87.319   **Chronic venous hypertension (idiopathic) with ulcer of unspecified lower extremity**   HCC ▽

✓6ᵗʰ **I87.32**   **Chronic venous hypertension (idiopathic) with inflammation**

I87.321   **Chronic venous hypertension (idiopathic) with inflammation of right lower extremity**

I87.322   **Chronic venous hypertension (idiopathic) with inflammation of left lower extremity**

I87.323   **Chronic venous hypertension (idiopathic) with inflammation of bilateral lower extremity**

I87.329   **Chronic venous hypertension (idiopathic) with inflammation of unspecified lower extremity** ▽

✓6ᵗʰ **I87.33**   **Chronic venous hypertension (idiopathic) with ulcer and inflammation**
Use additional code to specify site and severity of ulcer (L97.-)

I87.331   **Chronic venous hypertension (idiopathic) with ulcer and inflammation of right lower extremity**   HCC

I87.332   **Chronic venous hypertension (idiopathic) with ulcer and inflammation of left lower extremity**   HCC

I87.333   **Chronic venous hypertension (idiopathic) with ulcer and inflammation of bilateral lower extremity**   HCC

I87.339   **Chronic venous hypertension (idiopathic) with ulcer and inflammation of unspecified lower extremity**   HCC ▽

✓6ᵗʰ **I87.39**   **Chronic venous hypertension (idiopathic) with other complications**

I87.391   **Chronic venous hypertension (idiopathic) with other complications of right lower extremity**

I87.392   **Chronic venous hypertension (idiopathic) with other complications of left lower extremity**

I87.393   **Chronic venous hypertension (idiopathic) with other complications of bilateral lower extremity**

I87.399   **Chronic venous hypertension (idiopathic) with other complications of unspecified lower extremity** ▽

I87.8   **Other specified disorders of veins**
Phlebosclerosis
Venofibrosis

I87.9   **Disorder of vein, unspecified** ▽

✓4ᵗʰ **I88**   **Nonspecific lymphadenitis**
EXCLUDES 1   *acute lymphadenitis, except mesenteric (L04.-)*
enlarged lymph nodes NOS (R59.-)
human immunodeficiency virus [HIV] disease resulting in generalized lymphadenopathy (B20)

I88.0   **Nonspecific mesenteric lymphadenitis**
Mesenteric lymphadenitis (acute)(chronic)

I88.1   **Chronic lymphadenitis, except mesenteric**
Adenitis
Lymphadenitis

I88.8   **Other nonspecific lymphadenitis**

I88.9   **Nonspecific lymphadenitis, unspecified** ▽
Lymphadenitis NOS

✓4ᵗʰ **I89**   **Other noninfective disorders of lymphatic vessels and lymph nodes**
EXCLUDES 1   *chylocele, tunica vaginalis (nonfilarial) NOS (N50.89)*
enlarged lymph nodes NOS (R59.-)
filarial chylocele (B74.-)
hereditary lymphedema (Q82.0)

I89.0   **Lymphedema, not elsewhere classified**
Elephantiasis (nonfilarial) NOS
Lymphangiectasis
Obliteration, lymphatic vessel
Praecox lymphedema
Secondary lymphedema
EXCLUDES 1   *postmastectomy lymphedema (I97.2)*

I89.1   **Lymphangitis**
Chronic lymphangitis
Lymphangitis NOS
Subacute lymphangitis
EXCLUDES 1   *acute lymphangitis (L03.-)*

I89.8   **Other specified noninfective disorders of lymphatic vessels and lymph nodes**
Chylocele (nonfilarial)
Chylous ascites
Chylous cyst
Lipomelanotic reticulosis
Lymph node or vessel fistula
Lymph node or vessel infarction
Lymph node or vessel rupture

I89.9   **Noninfective disorder of lymphatic vessels and lymph nodes, unspecified** ▽
Disease of lymphatic vessels NOS

Other and unspecified disorders of the circulatory system (I95-I99)

✓4ᵗʰ **I95**   **Hypotension**
EXCLUDES 1   *cardiovascular collapse (R57.9)*
maternal hypotension syndrome (O26.5-)
nonspecific low blood pressure reading NOS (R03.1)

I95.0   **Idiopathic hypotension**

I95.1   **Orthostatic hypotension**
Hypotension, postural
EXCLUDES 1   *neurogenic orthostatic hypotension [Shy-Drager] (G90.3)*
orthostatic hypotension due to drugs (I95.2)

I95.2   **Hypotension due to drugs**
Orthostatic hypotension due to drugs
Use additional code for adverse effect, if applicable, to identify drug (T36-T50 with fifth or sixth character 5)

I95.3   **Hypotension of hemodialysis**
Intra-dialytic hypotension

✓5ᵗʰ **I95.8**   **Other hypotension**

I95.81   **Postprocedural hypotension**

I95.89   **Other hypotension**
Chronic hypotension

I95.9   **Hypotension, unspecified** ▽

☑ Additional Character Req   ☑7ᵗʰ Placeholder Alert   Manifestation   HCC CMS-HCC Condition   ▽ Unspecified Code   ►◄ Revised Text   ● New Code   ▲ Revised Code Title

ICD-10-CM 2018   **653**

I96   Gangrene, not elsewhere classified   `HCC`
Gangrenous cellulitis

> `EXCLUDES 1`   gangrene in atherosclerosis of native arteries of the extremities (I70.26)
> ~~gangrene in diabetes mellitus (E08-E13 with .52)~~
> gangrene in hernia (K40.1, K40.4, K41.1, K41.4, K42.1, K43.1-, K44.1, K45.1, K46.1)
> gangrene in other peripheral vascular diseases (I73.-)
> gangrene of certain specified sites—see Alphabetical Index
> gas gangrene (A48.0)
> pyoderma gangrenosum (L88)

> `EXCLUDES 2` ▶gangrene in diabetes mellitus (E08-E13 with .52)◄

AHA: 2013, 2Q, 34

`√4th` **I97   Intraoperative and postprocedural complications and disorders of circulatory system, not elsewhere classified**

> `EXCLUDES 2`   postprocedural shock (T81.1-)

I97.0   Postcardiotomy syndrome

`√5th` **I97.1   Other postprocedural cardiac functional disturbances**

> `EXCLUDES 2`   acute pulmonary insufficiency following thoracic surgery (J95.1)
> intraoperative cardiac functional disturbances (I97.7-)

`√6th` **I97.11   Postprocedural cardiac insufficiency**

I97.110   Postprocedural cardiac insufficiency following cardiac surgery

I97.111   Postprocedural cardiac insufficiency following other surgery

`√6th` **I97.12   Postprocedural cardiac arrest**

I97.120   Postprocedural cardiac arrest following cardiac surgery

I97.121   Postprocedural cardiac arrest following other surgery

`√6th` **I97.13   Postprocedural heart failure**
Use additional code to identify the heart failure (I50.-)

I97.130   Postprocedural heart failure following cardiac surgery

I97.131   Postprocedural heart failure following other surgery

`√6th` **I97.19   Other postprocedural cardiac functional disturbances**
Use additional code, if applicable, to further specify disorder

I97.190   Other postprocedural cardiac functional disturbances following cardiac surgery
▶Use additional code, if applicable, for type 4 or type 5 myocardial infarction, to further specify disorder◄

I97.191   Other postprocedural cardiac functional disturbances following other surgery

I97.2   Postmastectomy lymphedema syndrome   `A`
Elephantiasis due to mastectomy
Obliteration of lymphatic vessels

I97.3   Postprocedural hypertension

`√5th` **I97.4   Intraoperative hemorrhage and hematoma of a circulatory system organ or structure complicating a procedure**

> `EXCLUDES 1`   intraoperative hemorrhage and hematoma of a circulatory system organ or structure due to accidental puncture and laceration during a procedure (I97.5-)

> `EXCLUDES 2`   intraoperative cerebrovascular hemorrhage complicating a procedure (G97.3-)

`√6th` **I97.41   Intraoperative hemorrhage and hematoma of a circulatory system organ or structure complicating a circulatory system procedure**

I97.410   Intraoperative hemorrhage and hematoma of a circulatory system organ or structure complicating a cardiac catheterization

I97.411   Intraoperative hemorrhage and hematoma of a circulatory system organ or structure complicating a cardiac bypass

I97.418   Intraoperative hemorrhage and hematoma of a circulatory system organ or structure complicating other circulatory system procedure

I97.42   Intraoperative hemorrhage and hematoma of a circulatory system organ or structure complicating other procedure

`√5th` **I97.5   Accidental puncture and laceration of a circulatory system organ or structure during a procedure**

> `EXCLUDES 2`   accidental puncture and laceration of brain during a procedure (G97.4-)

I97.51   Accidental puncture and laceration of a circulatory system organ or structure during a circulatory system procedure

I97.52   Accidental puncture and laceration of a circulatory system organ or structure during other procedure

`√5th` **I97.6   Postprocedural hemorrhage, hematoma and seroma of a circulatory system organ or structure following a procedure**

> `EXCLUDES 2`   postprocedural cerebrovascular hemorrhage complicating a procedure (G97.5-)

`√6th` **I97.61   Postprocedural hemorrhage of a circulatory system organ or structure following a circulatory system procedure**

I97.610   Postprocedural hemorrhage of a circulatory system organ or structure following a cardiac catheterization

I97.611   Postprocedural hemorrhage of a circulatory system organ or structure following cardiac bypass

I97.618   Postprocedural hemorrhage of a circulatory system organ or structure following other circulatory system procedure

`√6th` **I97.62   Postprocedural hemorrhage, hematoma and seroma of a circulatory system organ or structure following other procedure**

I97.620   Postprocedural hemorrhage of a circulatory system organ or structure following other procedure

I97.621   Postprocedural hematoma of a circulatory system organ or structure following other procedure

I97.622   Postprocedural seroma of a circulatory system organ or structure following procedure

`√6th` **I97.63   Postprocedural hematoma of a circulatory system organ or structure following a circulatory system procedure**

I97.630   Postprocedural hematoma of a circulatory system organ or structure following a cardiac catheterization

I97.631   Postprocedural hematoma of a circulatory system organ or structure following cardiac bypass

I97.638   Postprocedural hematoma of a circulatory system organ or structure following other circulatory system procedure

`√6th` **I97.64   Postprocedural seroma of a circulatory system organ or structure following a circulatory system procedure**

I97.640   Postprocedural seroma of a circulatory system organ or structure following a cardiac catheterization

I97.641   Postprocedural seroma of a circulatory system organ or structure following cardiac bypass

I97.648   Postprocedural seroma of a circulatory system organ or structure following other circulatory system procedure

`√5th` **I97.7   Intraoperative cardiac functional disturbances**

> `EXCLUDES 2`   acute pulmonary insufficiency following thoracic surgery (J95.1)
> postprocedural cardiac functional disturbances (I97.1-)

`√6th` **I97.71   Intraoperative cardiac arrest**

I97.710   Intraoperative cardiac arrest during cardiac surgery

I97.711   Intraoperative cardiac arrest during other surgery

`√6th` **I97.79   Other intraoperative cardiac functional disturbances**
Use additional code, if applicable, to further specify disorder

I97.790   Other intraoperative cardiac functional disturbances during cardiac surgery

I97.791   Other intraoperative cardiac functional disturbances during other surgery

`EXCLUDES 1` Not coded here   `EXCLUDES 2` Not included here   `N` Newborn Age: 0   `P` Pediatric Age: 0-17   `M` Maternity Age: 12-55   `A` Adult Age: 15-124

✓5ᵗʰ **I97.8** **Other intraoperative and postprocedural complications and disorders of the circulatory system, not elsewhere classified**
Use additional code, if applicable, to further specify disorder

     ✓6ᵗʰ **I97.81** **Intraoperative cerebrovascular infarction**

         I97.810 Intraoperative cerebrovascular infarction during **cardiac surgery**   `HCC`

         I97.811 Intraoperative cerebrovascular infarction during **other surgery**   `HCC`

     ✓6ᵗʰ **I97.82** **Postprocedural cerebrovascular infarction**

         I97.820 Postprocedural cerebrovascular infarction following **cardiac surgery**   `HCC`

         I97.821 Postprocedural cerebrovascular infarction following **other surgery**   `HCC`

     I97.88 **Other intraoperative complications of the circulatory system, not elsewhere classified**

     I97.89 **Other postprocedural complications and disorders of the circulatory system, not elsewhere classified**

✓4ᵗʰ **I99** **Other and unspecified disorders of circulatory system**

     I99.8 **Other disorder of circulatory system**

     I99.9 **Unspecified disorder of circulatory system**   ▽

☑ Additional Character Req   ✓ₓ7ᵗʰ Placeholder Alert   Manifestation   `HCC` CMS-HCC Condition   ▽ Unspecified Code   ▶◀ Revised Text   ● New Code   ▲ Revised Code Title

Chapter 10. Diseases of the Respiratory System (J00–J99)

Chapter Specific Guidelines with Coding Examples

The chapter specific guidelines from the ICD-10-CM Official Guidelines for Coding and Reporting have been provided below. Along with these guidelines are coding examples, contained in the shaded boxes, that have been developed to help illustrate the coding and/or sequencing guidance found in these guidelines.

a. Chronic obstructive pulmonary disease [COPD] and asthma

1) Acute exacerbation of chronic obstructive bronchitis and asthma

The codes in categories J44 and J45 distinguish between uncomplicated cases and those in acute exacerbation. An acute exacerbation is a worsening or a decompensation of a chronic condition. An acute exacerbation is not equivalent to an infection superimposed on a chronic condition, though an exacerbation may be triggered by an infection.

Acute streptococcal bronchitis with acute exacerbation of COPD

J20.2	**Acute bronchitis due to streptococcus**
J44.0	**Chronic obstructive pulmonary disease with acute lower respiratory infection**
J44.1	**Chronic obstructive pulmonary disease with (acute) exacerbation**

Explanation: ICD-10-CM uses combination codes to create organism-specific classifications for acute bronchitis. Category J44 codes include combination codes with severity components, which differentiate between COPD with acute lower respiratory infection (acute bronchitis), COPD with acute exacerbation, and COPD without mention of a complication (unspecified).

An acute exacerbation is a worsening or a decompensation of a chronic condition. An acute exacerbation is not equivalent to an infection superimposed on a chronic condition, though an exacerbation may be triggered by an infection, as in this example.

Exacerbation of moderate persistent asthma with status asthmaticus

J45.42	**Moderate persistent asthma with status asthmaticus**

Explanation: Category J45 Asthma includes severity-specific subcategories and fifth-character codes to distinguish between uncomplicated cases, those in acute exacerbation, and those with status asthmaticus.

b. Acute respiratory failure

1) Acute respiratory failure as principal diagnosis

A code from subcategory J96.0, Acute respiratory failure, or subcategory J96.2, Acute and chronic respiratory failure, may be assigned as a principal diagnosis when it is the condition established after study to be chiefly responsible for occasioning the admission to the hospital, and the selection is supported by the Alphabetic Index and Tabular List. However, chapter-specific coding guidelines (such as obstetrics, poisoning, HIV, newborn) that provide sequencing direction take precedence.

Acute hypoxic respiratory failure due to exacerbation of chronic obstructive bronchitis

J96.01	**Acute respiratory failure with hypoxia**
J44.1	**Chronic obstructive pulmonary disease with (acute) exacerbation**

Explanation: Category J96 classifies respiratory failure with combination codes that designate the severity and the presence of hypoxia and hypercapnia. Code J96.01 is sequenced as the first-listed diagnosis, as the reason for the encounter. Respiratory failure may be assigned as a principal diagnosis when it is the condition established after study to be chiefly responsible for occasioning the encounter and the selection is supported by the Alphabetic Index and Tabular List.

2) Acute respiratory failure as secondary diagnosis

Respiratory failure may be listed as a secondary diagnosis if it occurs after admission, or if it is present on admission, but does not meet the definition of principal diagnosis.

Acute respiratory failure due to accidental oxycodone overdose

T40.2X1A	**Poisoning by other opioids, accidental (unintentional), initial encounter**
J96.00	**Acute respiratory failure, unspecified whether with hypoxia or hypercapnia**

Explanation: Respiratory failure may be assigned as a principal diagnosis when it is the condition established after study to be chiefly responsible for occasioning the encounter, and the selection is supported by the Alphabetic Index and Tabular List. However, chapter-specific coding guidelines, such as poisoning, that provide sequencing direction take precedence. When coding a poisoning or reaction to the improper use of a medication (e.g. overdose, wrong substance given or taken in error, wrong route of administration), first assign the appropriate code from categories T36–T50. Use additional code(s) for all manifestations of the poisoning. In this instance, the respiratory failure is a manifestation of the poisoning and is sequenced as a secondary diagnosis.

3) Sequencing of acute respiratory failure and another acute condition

When a patient is admitted with respiratory failure and another acute condition, (e.g., myocardial infarction, cerebrovascular accident, aspiration pneumonia), the principal diagnosis will not be the same in every situation. This applies whether the other acute condition is a respiratory or nonrespiratory condition. Selection of the principal diagnosis will be dependent on the circumstances of admission. If both the respiratory failure and the other acute condition are equally responsible for occasioning the admission to the hospital, and there are no chapter-specific sequencing rules, the guideline regarding two or more diagnoses that equally meet the definition for principal diagnosis (*Section II, C.*) may be applied in these situations.

If the documentation is not clear as to whether acute respiratory failure and another condition are equally responsible for occasioning the admission, query the provider for clarification.

Patient presents with acute pneumococcal pneumonia and acute respiratory failure

J96.00	**Acute respiratory failure, unspecified whether with hypoxia or hypercapnia**
J13	**Pneumonia due to Streptococcus pneumoniae**

Explanation: When a patient is seen for respiratory failure and another acute condition, such as a bacterial pneumonia, the principal or first-listed diagnosis is not the same in every situation. This applies whether the other acute condition is a respiratory or nonrespiratory condition. The principal diagnosis depends on the problem chiefly responsible for the encounter.

c. Influenza due to certain identified influenza viruses

Code only confirmed cases of influenza due to certain identified influenza viruses (category J09), and due to other identified influenza virus (category J10). This is an exception to the hospital inpatient guideline Section II, H. (Uncertain Diagnosis).

In this context, "confirmation" does not require documentation of positive laboratory testing specific for avian or other novel influenza A or other identified influenza virus. However, coding should be based on the provider's diagnostic statement that the patient has avian influenza, or other novel influenza A, for category J09, or has another particular identified strain of influenza, such as H1N1 or H3N2, but not identified as novel or variant, for category J10.

If the provider records "suspected" or "possible" or "probable" avian influenza, or novel influenza, or other identified influenza, then the appropriate influenza code from category J11, Influenza due to unidentified influenza virus, should be assigned. A code from category J09, Influenza due to certain identified influenza viruses, should not be assigned nor should a code from category J10, Influenza due to other identified influenza virus.

Influenza due to avian influenza virus with pneumonia

J09.X1   Influenza due to identified novel influenza A virus with pneumonia

Explanation: Codes in category J09 Influenza due to certain identified influenza viruses should be assigned only for confirmed cases. "Confirmation" does not require positive laboratory testing of a specific influenza virus but does need to be based on the provider's diagnostic statement, which should not include terms such as "possible," "probable," or "suspected."

d. Ventilator associated pneumonia

1) Documentation of ventilator associated pneumonia

As with all procedural or postprocedural complications, code assignment is based on the provider's documentation of the relationship between the condition and the procedure.

Code J95.851, Ventilator associated pneumonia, should be assigned only when the provider has documented ventilator associated pneumonia (VAP). An additional code to identify the organism (e.g., Pseudomonas aeruginosa, code B96.5) should also be assigned. Do not assign an additional code from categories J12-J18 to identify the type of pneumonia.

Code J95.851 should not be assigned for cases where the patient has pneumonia and is on a mechanical ventilator and the provider has not specifically stated that the pneumonia is ventilator-associated pneumonia. If the documentation is unclear as to whether the patient has a pneumonia that is a complication attributable to the mechanical ventilator, query the provider.

2) Ventilator associated pneumonia develops after admission

A patient may be admitted with one type of pneumonia (e.g., code J13, Pneumonia due to Streptococcus pneumonia) and subsequently develop VAP. In this instance, the principal diagnosis would be the appropriate code from categories J12-J18 for the pneumonia diagnosed at the time of admission. Code J95.851, Ventilator associated pneumonia, would be assigned as an additional diagnosis when the provider has also documented the presence of ventilator associated pneumonia.

Chapter 10. Diseases of the Respiratory System (J00-J99)

NOTE   When a respiratory condition is described as occurring in more than one site and is not specifically indexed, it should be classified to the lower anatomic site (e.g. tracheobronchitis to bronchitis in J40).

Use additional code, where applicable, to identify:
- exposure to environmental tobacco smoke (Z77.22)
- exposure to tobacco smoke in the perinatal period (P96.81)
- history of tobacco dependence (Z87.891)
- occupational exposure to environmental tobacco smoke (Z57.31)
- tobacco dependence (F17.-)
- tobacco use (Z72.0)

EXCLUDES 2 *certain conditions originating in the perinatal period (P04-P96)*
certain infectious and parasitic diseases (A00-B99)
complications of pregnancy, childbirth and the puerperium (O00-O9A)
congenital malformations, deformations and chromosomal abnormalities (Q00-Q99)
endocrine, nutritional and metabolic diseases (E00-E88)
injury, poisoning and certain other consequences of external causes (S00-T88)
neoplasms (C00-D49)
smoke inhalation (T59.81-)
symptoms, signs and abnormal clinical and laboratory findings, not elsewhere classified (R00-R94)

This chapter contains the following blocks:

J00-J06	Acute upper respiratory infections
J09-J18	Influenza and pneumonia
J20-J22	Other acute lower respiratory infections
J30-J39	Other diseases of upper respiratory tract
J40-J47	Chronic lower respiratory diseases
J60-J70	Lung diseases due to external agents
J80-J84	Other respiratory diseases principally affecting the interstitium
J85-J86	Suppurative and necrotic conditions of the lower respiratory tract
J90-J94	Other diseases of the pleura
J95	Intraoperative and postprocedural complications and disorders of respiratory system, not elsewhere classified
J96-J99	Other diseases of the respiratory system

Acute upper respiratory infections (J00-J06)

EXCLUDES 1 *chronic obstructive pulmonary disease with acute lower respiratory infection (J44.0)*
influenza virus with other respiratory manifestations (J09.X2, J10.1, J11.1)

J00   **Acute nasopharyngitis (common cold)**
- Acute rhinitis
- Coryza (acute)
- Infective nasopharyngitis NOS
- Infective rhinitis
- Nasal catarrh, acute
- Nasopharyngitis NOS

EXCLUDES 1 *acute pharyngitis (J02.-)*
acute sore throat NOS (J02.9)
pharyngitis NOS (J02.9)
rhinitis NOS (J31.0)
sore throat NOS (J02.9)

EXCLUDES 2 *allergic rhinitis (J30.1-J30.9)*
chronic pharyngitis (J31.2)
chronic rhinitis (J31.0)
chronic sore throat (J31.2)
nasopharyngitis, chronic (J31.1)
vasomotor rhinitis (J30.0)

DEF: Acute inflammation of mucous membranes; extends from nares to pharynx; characterized by nasal obstruction, sneezing, runny nose, and sore throat.

✓4ᵗʰ J01   **Acute sinusitis**
INCLUDES   acute abscess of sinus
acute empyema of sinus
acute infection of sinus
acute inflammation of sinus
acute suppuration of sinus

Use additional code (B95-B97) to identify infectious agent
EXCLUDES 1 *sinusitis NOS (J32.9)*
EXCLUDES 2 *chronic sinusitis (J32.0-J32.8)*

✓5ᵗʰ J01.0   **Acute maxillary sinusitis**
Acute antritis
- **J01.00**   Acute maxillary sinusitis, unspecified ▽
- **J01.01**   Acute recurrent maxillary sinusitis

✓5ᵗʰ J01.1   **Acute frontal sinusitis**
- **J01.10**   Acute frontal sinusitis, unspecified ▽
- **J01.11**   Acute recurrent frontal sinusitis

✓5ᵗʰ J01.2   **Acute ethmoidal sinusitis**
- **J01.20**   Acute ethmoidal sinusitis, unspecified ▽
- **J01.21**   Acute recurrent ethmoidal sinusitis

✓5ᵗʰ J01.3   **Acute sphenoidal sinusitis**
- **J01.30**   Acute sphenoidal sinusitis, unspecified ▽
- **J01.31**   Acute recurrent sphenoidal sinusitis

✓5ᵗʰ J01.4   **Acute pansinusitis**
- **J01.40**   Acute pansinusitis, unspecified ▽
- **J01.41**   Acute recurrent pansinusitis

✓5ᵗʰ J01.8   **Other acute sinusitis**
- **J01.80**   **Other acute sinusitis**
  Acute sinusitis involving more than one sinus but not pansinusitis
- **J01.81**   **Other acute recurrent sinusitis**
  Acute recurrent sinusitis involving more than one sinus but not pansinusitis

✓5ᵗʰ J01.9   **Acute sinusitis, unspecified**
- **J01.90**   Acute sinusitis, unspecified ▽
- **J01.91**   Acute recurrent sinusitis, unspecified ▽

✓4ᵗʰ J02   **Acute pharyngitis**
INCLUDES   acute sore throat
EXCLUDES 1 *acute laryngopharyngitis (J06.0)*
peritonsillar abscess (J36)
pharyngeal abscess (J39.1)
retropharyngeal abscess (J39.0)
EXCLUDES 2 *chronic pharyngitis (J31.2)*

J02.0   **Streptococcal pharyngitis**
Septic pharyngitis
Streptococcal sore throat
EXCLUDES 2 *scarlet fever (A38.-)*

J02.8   **Acute pharyngitis due to other specified organisms**
Use additional code (B95-B97) to identify infectious agent
EXCLUDES 1 *acute pharyngitis due to coxsackie virus (B08.5)*
acute pharyngitis due to gonococcus (A54.5)
acute pharyngitis due to herpes [simplex] virus (B00.2)
acute pharyngitis due to infectious mononucleosis (B27.-)
enteroviral vesicular pharyngitis (B08.5)

J02.9   **Acute pharyngitis, unspecified** ▽
- Gangrenous pharyngitis (acute)
- Infective pharyngitis (acute) NOS
- Pharyngitis (acute) NOS
- Sore throat (acute) NOS
- Suppurative pharyngitis (acute)
- Ulcerative pharyngitis (acute)

✓4ᵗʰ J03   **Acute tonsillitis**
EXCLUDES 1 *acute sore throat (J02.-)*
hypertrophy of tonsils (J35.1)
peritonsillar abscess (J36)
sore throat NOS (J02.9)
streptococcal sore throat (J02.0)
EXCLUDES 2 *chronic tonsillitis (J35.0)*

✓5ᵗʰ J03.0   **Streptococcal tonsillitis**
- **J03.00**   Acute streptococcal tonsillitis, unspecified ▽
- **J03.01**   Acute recurrent streptococcal tonsillitis

✓5ᵗʰ J03.8   **Acute tonsillitis due to other specified organisms**
Use additional code (B95-B97) to identify infectious agent
EXCLUDES 1 *diphtheritic tonsillitis (A36.0)*
herpesviral pharyngotonsillitis (B00.2)
streptococcal tonsillitis (J03.0)
tuberculous tonsillitis (A15.8)
Vincent's tonsillitis (A69.1)
- **J03.80**   Acute tonsillitis due to other specified organisms
- **J03.81**   Acute recurrent tonsillitis due to other specified organisms

✓5ᵗʰ J03.9   **Acute tonsillitis, unspecified**
- Follicular tonsillitis (acute)
- Gangrenous tonsillitis (acute)
- Infective tonsillitis (acute)
- Tonsillitis (acute) NOS
- Ulcerative tonsillitis (acute)
- **J03.90**   Acute tonsillitis, unspecified ▽
- **J03.91**   Acute recurrent tonsillitis, unspecified ▽

✓ Additional Character Req   **✓x7ᵗʰ** Placeholder Alert   Manifestation   **HCC** CMS-HCC Condition   ▽ Unspecified Code   ►◄ Revised Text   ● New Code   ▲ Revised Code Title

ICD-10-CM 2018   **659**

Chapter 10. Diseases of the Respiratory System

✓4th **J04   Acute laryngitis and tracheitis**
> Use additional code (B95-B97) to identify infectious agent
> *EXCLUDES 1*   *acute obstructive laryngitis [croup] and epiglottitis (J05.-)*
> *EXCLUDES 2*   *laryngismus (stridulus) (J38.5)*

> **J04.0   Acute laryngitis**
> > Edematous laryngitis (acute)
> > Laryngitis (acute) NOS
> > Subglottic laryngitis (acute)
> > Suppurative laryngitis (acute)
> > Ulcerative laryngitis (acute)
> > *EXCLUDES 1*   *acute obstructive laryngitis (J05.0)*
> > *EXCLUDES 2*   *chronic laryngitis (J37.0)*

> ✓5th **J04.1   Acute tracheitis**
> > Acute viral tracheitis
> > Catarrhal tracheitis (acute)
> > Tracheitis (acute) NOS
> > *EXCLUDES 2*   *chronic tracheitis (J42)*
> > > **J04.10   Acute tracheitis without obstruction**
> > > **J04.11   Acute tracheitis with obstruction**

> **J04.2   Acute laryngotracheitis**
> > Laryngotracheitis NOS
> > Tracheitis (acute) with laryngitis (acute)
> > *EXCLUDES 1*   *acute obstructive laryngotracheitis (J05.0)*
> > *EXCLUDES 2*   *chronic laryngotracheitis (J37.1)*

> ✓5th **J04.3   Supraglottitis, unspecified**
> > **J04.30   Supraglottitis, unspecified, without obstruction** ▽
> > **J04.31   Supraglottitis, unspecified, with obstruction** ▽

✓4th **J05   Acute obstructive laryngitis [croup] and epiglottitis**
> Use additional code (B95-B97) to identify infectious agent

> **J05.0   Acute obstructive laryngitis [croup]**
> > Obstructive laryngitis (acute) NOS
> > Obstructive laryngotracheitis NOS
> > **DEF:** Acute laryngeal obstruction due to allergy, foreign body, or in the majority of cases a viral infection; symptoms include harsh, barking cough, hoarseness, and persistent high-pitched respiratory sound (stridor).

> ✓5th **J05.1   Acute epiglottitis**
> > *EXCLUDES 2*   *epiglottitis, chronic (J37.0)*
> > > **J05.10   Acute epiglottitis without obstruction**
> > > > Epiglottitis NOS
> > > **J05.11   Acute epiglottitis with obstruction**

✓4th **J06   Acute upper respiratory infections of multiple and unspecified sites**
> *EXCLUDES 1*   *acute respiratory infection NOS (J22)*
> > *streptococcal pharyngitis (J02.0)3*

> **J06.0   Acute laryngopharyngitis**

> **J06.9   Acute upper respiratory infection, unspecified** ▽
> > Upper respiratory disease, acute
> > Upper respiratory infection NOS

Influenza and pneumonia (J09-J18)

> *EXCLUDES 2*   *allergic or eosinophilic pneumonia (J82)*
> > *aspiration pneumonia NOS (J69.0)*
> > *congenital pneumonia (P23.9)*
> > *lipid pneumonia (J69.1)*
> > *meconium pneumonia (P24.01)*
> > *neonatal aspiration pneumonia (P24.-)*
> > *pneumonia due to solids and liquids (J69.-)*
> > *rheumatic pneumonia (I00)*
> > *ventilator associated pneumonia (J95.851)*

✓4th **J09   Influenza due to certain identified influenza viruses**
> *EXCLUDES 1*   ▶*influenza A/H1N1 (J10.-)*◀
> > *influenza due to other identified influenza virus (J10.-)*
> > *influenza due to unidentified influenza virus (J11.-)*
> > *seasonal influenza due to other identified influenza virus (J10.-)*
> > *seasonal influenza due to unidentified influenza virus (J11.-)*

> ✓5th **J09.X   Influenza due to identified novel influenza A virus**
> > Avian influenza
> > Bird influenza
> > Influenza A/H5N1
> > Influenza of other animal origin, not bird or swine
> > Swine influenza virus (viruses that normally cause infections in pigs)
> > **AHA:** 2016, 3Q, 10

> > **J09.X1   Influenza due to identified novel influenza A virus with pneumonia**
> > > Code also, if applicable, associated:
> > > lung abscess (J85.1)
> > > other specified type of pneumonia

> > **J09.X2   Influenza due to identified novel influenza A virus with other respiratory manifestations**
> > > Influenza due to identified novel influenza A virus NOS
> > > Influenza due to identified novel influenza A virus with laryngitis
> > > Influenza due to identified novel influenza A virus with pharyngitis
> > > Influenza due to identified novel influenza A virus with upper respiratory symptoms
> > > Use additional code, if applicable, for associated:
> > > pleural effusion (J91.8)
> > > sinusitis (J01.-)

> > **J09.X3   Influenza due to identified novel influenza A virus with gastrointestinal manifestations**
> > > Influenza due to identified novel influenza A virus gastroenteritis
> > > *EXCLUDES 1*   *'intestinal flu' [viral gastroenteritis] (A08.-)*

> > **J09.X9   Influenza due to identified novel influenza A virus with other manifestations**
> > > Influenza due to identified novel influenza A virus with encephalopathy
> > > Influenza due to identified novel influenza A virus with myocarditis
> > > Influenza due to identified novel influenza A virus with otitis media
> > > Use additional code to identify manifestation

✓4th **J10   Influenza due to other identified influenza virus**
> *EXCLUDES 1*   *influenza due to avian influenza virus (J09.X-)*
> > *influenza due to swine flu (J09.X-)*
> > *influenza due to unidentifed influenza virus (J11.-)*

> ✓5th **J10.0   Influenza due to other identified influenza virus with pneumonia**
> > Code also associated lung abscess, if applicable (J85.1)

> > **J10.00   Influenza due to other identified influenza virus with unspecified type of pneumonia** ▽

> > **J10.01   Influenza due to other identified influenza virus with the same other identified influenza virus pneumonia**

> > **J10.08   Influenza due to other identified influenza virus with other specified pneumonia**
> > > Code also other specified type of pneumonia

> **J10.1   Influenza due to other identified influenza virus with other respiratory manifestations**
> > Influenza due to other identified influenza virus NOS
> > Influenza due to other identified influenza virus with laryngitis
> > Influenza due to other identified influenza virus with pharyngitis
> > Influenza due to other identified influenza virus with upper respiratory symptoms
> > Use additional code for associated pleural effusion, if applicable (J91.8)
> > Use additional code for associated sinusitis, if applicable (J01.-)
> > **AHA:** 2016, 3Q, 10-11

> **J10.2   Influenza due to other identified influenza virus with gastrointestinal manifestations**
> > Influenza due to other identified influenza virus gastroenteritis
> > *EXCLUDES 1*   *'intestinal flu' [viral gastroenteritis] (A08.-)*

> ✓5th **J10.8   Influenza due to other identified influenza virus with other manifestations**

> > **J10.81   Influenza due to other identified influenza virus with encephalopathy**

> > **J10.82   Influenza due to other identified influenza virus with myocarditis**

> > **J10.83   Influenza due to other identified influenza virus with otitis media**
> > > Use additional code for any associated perforated tympanic membrane (H72.-)

> > **J10.89   Influenza due to other identified influenza virus with other manifestations**
> > > Use additional codes to identify the manifestations

✓4th **J11   Influenza due to unidentified influenza virus**

> ✓5th **J11.0   Influenza due to unidentified influenza virus with pneumonia**
> > Code also associated lung abscess, if applicable (J85.1)
> > **AHA:** 2016, 3Q, 11

> > **J11.00   Influenza due to unidentified influenza virus with unspecified type of pneumonia** ▽
> > > Influenza with pneumonia NOS

EXCLUDES 1 Not coded here   *EXCLUDES 2* Not included here   **N** Newborn Age: 0   **P** Pediatric Age: 0-17   **M** Maternity Age: 12-55   **A** Adult Age: 15-124

660   ICD-10-CM 2018

J11.08   **Influenza due to unidentified influenza virus with specified pneumonia**
Code also other specified type of pneumonia

J11.1   **Influenza due to unidentified influenza virus with other respiratory manifestations**
Influenza NOS
Influenzal laryngitis NOS
Influenzal pharyngitis NOS
Influenza with upper respiratory symptoms NOS
Use additional code for associated pleural effusion, if applicable (J91.8)
Use additional code for associated sinusitis, if applicable (J01.-)

J11.2   **Influenza due to unidentified influenza virus with gastrointestinal manifestations**
Influenza gastroenteritis NOS
EXCLUDES 1   *'intestinal flu' [viral gastroenteritis] (A08.-)*

✓5ᵗʰ **J11.8**   **Influenza due to unidentified influenza virus with other manifestations**

    J11.81   **Influenza due to unidentified influenza virus with encephalopathy**
Influenzal encephalopathy NOS

    J11.82   **Influenza due to unidentified influenza virus with myocarditis**
Influenzal myocarditis NOS

    J11.83   **Influenza due to unidentified influenza virus with otitis media**
Influenzal otitis media NOS
Use additional code for any associated perforated tympanic membrane (H72.-)

    J11.89   **Influenza due to unidentified influenza virus with other manifestations**
Use additional codes to identify the manifestations

✓4ᵗʰ **J12**   **Viral pneumonia, not elsewhere classified**
INCLUDES   bronchopneumonia due to viruses other than influenza viruses
Code first associated influenza, if applicable (J09.X1, J10.0-, J11.0-)
Code also associated abscess, if applicable (J85.1)
EXCLUDES 1   *aspiration pneumonia due to anesthesia during labor and delivery (O74.0)*
aspiration pneumonia due to anesthesia during pregnancy (O29)
aspiration pneumonia due to anesthesia during puerperium (O89.0)
aspiration pneumonia due to solids and liquids (J69.-)
aspiration pneumonia NOS (J69.0)
congenital pneumonia (P23.0)
congenital rubella pneumonitis (P35.0)
interstitial pneumonia NOS (J84.9)
lipid pneumonia (J69.1)
neonatal aspiration pneumonia (P24.-)
AHA: 2016, 3Q, 15; 2013, 4Q, 118

J12.0   **Adenoviral pneumonia**

J12.1   **Respiratory syncytial virus pneumonia**

J12.2   **Parainfluenza virus pneumonia**

J12.3   **Human metapneumovirus pneumonia**

✓5ᵗʰ **J12.8**   **Other viral pneumonia**

    J12.81   **Pneumonia due to SARS-associated coronavirus**
Severe acute respiratory syndrome NOS
DEF: A severe adult respiratory syndrome caused by the coronavirus, specified as inflammation of the lungs with consolidation.

    J12.89   **Other viral pneumonia**

J12.9   **Viral pneumonia, unspecified**   ▽

J13   **Pneumonia due to Streptococcus pneumoniae**   HCC
Bronchopneumonia due to S. pneumoniae
Code first associated influenza, if applicable (J09.X1, J10.0-, J11.0-)
Code also associated lung abscess, if applicable (J85.1)
EXCLUDES 1   *congenital pneumonia due to S. pneumoniae (P23.6)*
lobar pneumonia, unspecified organism (J18.1)
pneumonia due to other streptococci (J15.3-J15.4)
AHA: 2016, 3Q, 15; 2013, 4Q, 118

J14   **Pneumonia due to Hemophilus influenzae**   HCC
Bronchopneumonia due to H. influenzae
Code first associated influenza, if applicable (J09.X1, J10.0-, J11.0-)
Code also associated lung abscess, if applicable (J85.1)
EXCLUDES 1   *congenital pneumonia due to H. influenzae (P23.6)*
AHA: 2016, 3Q, 15; 2013, 4Q, 118

✓4ᵗʰ **J15**   **Bacterial pneumonia, not elsewhere classified**
INCLUDES   bronchopneumonia due to bacteria other than S. pneumoniae and H. influenzae
Code first associated influenza, if applicable (J09.X1, J10.0-, J11.0-)
Code also associated lung abscess, if applicable (J85.1)
EXCLUDES 1   *chlamydial pneumonia (J16.0)*
congenital pneumonia (P23.-)
Legionnaires' disease (A48.1)
spirochetal pneumonia (A69.8)
AHA: 2016, 3Q, 15; 2013, 4Q, 118

J15.0   **Pneumonia due to Klebsiella pneumoniae**   HCC

J15.1   **Pneumonia due to Pseudomonas**   HCC

✓5ᵗʰ **J15.2**   **Pneumonia due to staphylococcus**

    J15.20   **Pneumonia due to staphylococcus, unspecified**   HCC ▽

   ✓6ᵗʰ **J15.21**   **Pneumonia due to Staphylococcus aureus**

      J15.211   **Pneumonia due to Methicillin susceptible Staphylococcus aureus**   HCC
MSSA pneumonia
Pneumonia due to Staphylococcus aureus NOS

      J15.212   **Pneumonia due to Methicillin resistant Staphylococcus aureus**   HCC

    J15.29   **Pneumonia due to other staphylococcus**   HCC

J15.3   **Pneumonia due to streptococcus, group B**   HCC

J15.4   **Pneumonia due to other streptococci**   HCC
EXCLUDES 1   *pneumonia due to streptococcus, group B (J15.3)*
pneumonia due to Streptococcus pneumoniae (J13)

J15.5   **Pneumonia due to Escherichia coli**   HCC

▲ **J15.6**   **Pneumonia due to other Gram-negative bacteria**   HCC
▶Pneumonia due to other aerobic Gram-negative bacteria◀
Pneumonia due to Serratia marcescens

J15.7   **Pneumonia due to Mycoplasma pneumoniae**

J15.8   **Pneumonia due to other specified bacteria**   HCC

J15.9   **Unspecified bacterial pneumonia**   ▽
Pneumonia due to gram-positive bacteria

✓4ᵗʰ **J16**   **Pneumonia due to other infectious organisms, not elsewhere classified**
Code first associated influenza, if applicable (J09.X1, J10.0-, J11.0-)
Code also associated lung abscess, if applicable (J85.1)
EXCLUDES 1   *congenital pneumonia (P23.-)*
ornithosis (A70)
pneumocystosis (B59)
pneumonia NOS (J18.9)
AHA: 2016, 3Q, 15; 2013, 4Q, 118

J16.0   **Chlamydial pneumonia**

J16.8   **Pneumonia due to other specified infectious organisms**

J17   *Pneumonia in diseases classified elsewhere*
Code first underlying disease, such as:
Q fever (A78)
rheumatic fever (I00)
schistosomiasis (B65.0-B65.9)
EXCLUDES 1   *candidial pneumonia (B37.1)*
chlamydial pneumonia (J16.0)
gonorrheal pneumonia (A54.84)
histoplasmosis pneumonia (B39.0-B39.2)
measles pneumonia (B05.2)
nocardiosis pneumonia (A43.0)
pneumocystosis (B59)
pneumonia due to Pneumocystis carinii (B59)
pneumonia due to Pneumocystis jiroveci (B59)
pneumonia in actinomycosis (A42.0)
pneumonia in anthrax (A22.1)
pneumonia in ascariasis (B77.81)
pneumonia in aspergillosis (B44.0-B44.1)
pneumonia in coccidioidomycosis (B38.0-B38.2)
pneumonia in cytomegalovirus disease (B25.0)
pneumonia in toxoplasmosis (B58.3)
rubella pneumonia (B06.81)
salmonella pneumonia (A02.22)
spirochetal infection NEC with pneumonia (A69.8)
tularemia pneumonia (A21.2)
typhoid fever with pneumonia (A01.03)
varicella pneumonia (B01.2)
whooping cough with pneumonia (A37 with fifth-character 1)
AHA: 2016, 3Q, 15; 2013, 4Q, 118

☑ Additional Character Req   ✓ₓ7ᵗʰ Placeholder Alert   Manifestation   HCC CMS-HCC Condition   ▽ Unspecified Code   ▶◀ Revised Text   ● New Code   ▲ Revised Code Title

✓4ᵗʰ J18   Pneumonia, unspecified organism

Code first associated influenza, if applicable (J09.X1, J10.0-, J11.0-)

EXCLUDES 1   abscess of lung with pneumonia (J85.1)
aspiration pneumonia due to anesthesia during labor and delivery (O74.0)
aspiration pneumonia due to anesthesia during pregnancy (O29)
aspiration pneumonia due to anesthesia during puerperium (O89.0)
aspiration pneumonia due to solids and liquids (J69.-)
aspiration pneumonia NOS (J69.0)
congenital pneumonia (P23.0)
drug-induced interstitial lung disorder (J70.2-J70.4)
interstitial pneumonia NOS (J84.9)
lipid pneumonia (J69.1)
neonatal aspiration pneumonia (P24.-)
pneumonitis due to external agents (J67-J70)
pneumonitis due to fumes and vapors (J68.0)
usual interstitial pneumonia (J84.17)

AHA: 2016, 3Q, 15; 2013, 4Q, 15

J18.0   **Bronchopneumonia, unspecified organism**   ▽

    EXCLUDES 1   hypostatic bronchopneumonia (J18.2)
                lipid pneumonia (J69.1)
    EXCLUDES 2   acute bronchiolitis (J21.-)
                chronic bronchiolitis (J44.9)

J18.1   **Lobar pneumonia, unspecified organism**   HCC ▽

J18.2   **Hypostatic pneumonia, unspecified organism**   ▽

Hypostatic bronchopneumonia
Passive pneumonia

J18.8   **Other pneumonia, unspecified organism**   ▽

J18.9   **Pneumonia, unspecified organism**   ▽

    AHA: 2014, 3Q, 4; 2013, 4Q, 119; 2012, 4Q, 94

Other acute lower respiratory infections (J20-J22)

EXCLUDES 2   chronic obstructive pulmonary disease with acute lower respiratory infection (J44.0)

✓4ᵗʰ J20   Acute bronchitis

INCLUDES   acute and subacute bronchitis (with) bronchospasm
acute and subacute bronchitis (with) tracheitis
acute and subacute bronchitis (with) tracheobronchitis, acute
acute and subacute fibrinous bronchitis
acute and subacute membranous bronchitis
acute and subacute purulent bronchitis
acute and subacute septic bronchitis

    EXCLUDES 1   bronchitis NOS (J40)
                tracheobronchitis NOS (J40)
    EXCLUDES 2   acute bronchitis with bronchiectasis (J47.0)
                acute bronchitis with chronic obstructive asthma (J44.0)
                acute bronchitis with chronic obstructive pulmonary disease (J44.0)
                allergic bronchitis NOS (J45.909)
                bronchitis due to chemicals, fumes and vapors (J68.0)
                chronic bronchitis NOS (J42)
                chronic mucopurulent bronchitis (J41.1)
                chronic obstructive bronchitis (J44.-)
                chronic obstructive tracheobronchitis (J44.-)
                chronic simple bronchitis (J41.0)
                chronic tracheobronchitis (J42)

AHA: 2016, 3Q, 10, 16

DEF: Acute inflammation of main branches of bronchial tree due to infectious or irritant agents; symptoms include cough with a varied production of sputum, fever, substernal soreness, and lung rales; usually last for three to 10 days.

J20.0   **Acute bronchitis due to Mycoplasma pneumoniae**

J20.1   **Acute bronchitis due to Hemophilus influenzae**

J20.2   **Acute bronchitis due to streptococcus**

J20.3   **Acute bronchitis due to coxsackievirus**

J20.4   **Acute bronchitis due to parainfluenza virus**

J20.5   **Acute bronchitis due to respiratory syncytial virus**

J20.6   **Acute bronchitis due to rhinovirus**

J20.7   **Acute bronchitis due to echovirus**

J20.8   **Acute bronchitis due to other specified organisms**

J20.9   **Acute bronchitis, unspecified**   ▽

✓4ᵗʰ J21   Acute bronchiolitis

Acute bronchiolitis with bronchospasm

    EXCLUDES 2   respiratory bronchiolitis interstitial lung disease (J84.115)

J21.0   **Acute bronchiolitis due to respiratory syncytial virus**

J21.1   **Acute bronchiolitis due to human metapneumovirus**

J21.8   **Acute bronchiolitis due to other specified organisms**

J21.9   **Acute bronchiolitis, unspecified**   ▽

Bronchiolitis (acute)

    EXCLUDES 1   chronic bronchiolitis (J44.-)

J22   Unspecified acute lower respiratory infection   ▽

Acute (lower) respiratory (tract) infection NOS

    EXCLUDES 1   upper respiratory infection (acute) (J06.9)

Other diseases of upper respiratory tract (J30-J39)

✓4ᵗʰ J30   Vasomotor and allergic rhinitis

INCLUDES   spasmodic rhinorrhea

    EXCLUDES 1   allergic rhinitis with asthma (bronchial) (J45.909)
                rhinitis NOS (J31.0)

J30.0   **Vasomotor rhinitis**

J30.1   **Allergic rhinitis due to pollen**

Allergy NOS due to pollen
Hay fever
Pollinosis

J30.2   **Other seasonal allergic rhinitis**

J30.5   **Allergic rhinitis due to food**

✓5ᵗʰ **J30.8**   **Other allergic rhinitis**

    J30.81   **Allergic rhinitis due to animal (cat) (dog) hair and dander**

    J30.89   **Other allergic rhinitis**

          Perennial allergic rhinitis

J30.9   **Allergic rhinitis, unspecified**   ▽

✓4ᵗʰ J31   Chronic rhinitis, nasopharyngitis and pharyngitis

Use additional code to identify:
exposure to environmental tobacco smoke (Z77.22)
exposure to tobacco smoke in the perinatal period (P96.81)
history of tobacco dependence (Z87.891)
occupational exposure to environmental tobacco smoke (Z57.31)
tobacco dependence (F17.-)
tobacco use (Z72.0)

J31.0   **Chronic rhinitis**

Atrophic rhinitis (chronic)
Granulomatous rhinitis (chronic)
Hypertrophic rhinitis (chronic)
Obstructive rhinitis (chronic)
Ozena
Purulent rhinitis (chronic)
Rhinitis (chronic) NOS
Ulcerative rhinitis (chronic)

    EXCLUDES 1   allergic rhinitis (J30.1-J30.9)
                vasomotor rhinitis (J30.0)

DEF: Persistent inflammation of mucous membranes of nose; characterized by postnasal drip.

J31.1   **Chronic nasopharyngitis**

    EXCLUDES 2   acute nasopharyngitis (J00)

DEF: Persistent inflammation of mucous membranes extending from nares to pharynx; characterized by constant irritation in nasopharynx and postnasal drip.

J31.2   **Chronic pharyngitis**

Atrophic pharyngitis (chronic)
Chronic sore throat
Granular pharyngitis (chronic)
Hypertrophic pharyngitis (chronic)

    EXCLUDES 2   acute pharyngitis (J02.9)

✓4ᵗʰ J32   Chronic sinusitis

INCLUDES   sinus abscess
sinus empyema
sinus infection
sinus suppuration

Use additional code to identify:
exposure to environmental tobacco smoke (Z77.22)
exposure to tobacco smoke in the perinatal period (P96.81)
history of tobacco dependence (Z87.891)
infectious agent (B95-B97)
occupational exposure to environmental tobacco smoke (Z57.31)
tobacco dependence (F17.-)
tobacco use (Z72.0)

    EXCLUDES 2   acute sinusitis (J01.-)

J32.0   **Chronic maxillary sinusitis**

Antritis (chronic)
Maxillary sinusitis NOS

J32.1   **Chronic frontal sinusitis**

Frontal sinusitis NOS

J32.2   **Chronic ethmoidal sinusitis**

Ethmoidal sinusitis NOS

    EXCLUDES 1   Woakes' ethmoiditis (J33.1)

EXCLUDES 1 Not coded here   **EXCLUDES 2** Not included here   N Newborn Age: 0   P Pediatric Age: 0-17   M Maternity Age: 12-55   A Adult Age: 15-124

662   ICD-10-CM 2018

J32.3   **Chronic sphenoidal sinusitis**
Sphenoidal sinusitis NOS

J32.4   **Chronic pansinusitis**
Pansinusitis NOS

J32.8   **Other chronic sinusitis**
Sinusitis (chronic) involving more than one sinus but not pansinusitis

J32.9   **Chronic sinusitis, unspecified**   ▽
Sinusitis (chronic) NOS

✓4ᵗʰ **J33**   **Nasal polyp**
Use additional code to identify:
exposure to environmental tobacco smoke (Z77.22)
exposure to tobacco smoke in the perinatal period (P96.81)
history of tobacco dependence (Z87.891)
occupational exposure to environmental tobacco smoke (Z57.31)
tobacco dependence (F17.-)
tobacco use (Z72.0)
EXCLUDES 1   *adenomatous polyps (D14.0)*

J33.0   **Polyp of nasal cavity**
Choanal polyp
Nasopharyngeal polyp

J33.1   **Polypoid sinus degeneration**
Woakes' syndrome or ethmoiditis

J33.8   **Other polyp of sinus**
Accessory polyp of sinus
Ethmoidal polyp of sinus
Maxillary polyp of sinus
Sphenoidal polyp of sinus

J33.9   **Nasal polyp, unspecified**   ▽

✓4ᵗʰ **J34**   **Other and unspecified disorders of nose and nasal sinuses**
EXCLUDES 2   *varicose ulcer of nasal septum (I86.8)*

J34.0   **Abscess, furuncle and carbuncle of nose**
Cellulitis of nose
Necrosis of nose
Ulceration of nose

J34.1   **Cyst and mucocele of nose and nasal sinus**

J34.2   **Deviated nasal septum**
Deflection or deviation of septum (nasal) (acquired)
EXCLUDES 1   *congenital deviated nasal septum (Q67.4)*

J34.3   **Hypertrophy of nasal turbinates**

✓5ᵗʰ **J34.8**   **Other specified disorders of nose and nasal sinuses**

J34.81   **Nasal mucositis (ulcerative)**
Code also type of associated therapy, such as:
antineoplastic and immunosuppressive drugs (T45.1X-)
radiological procedure and radiotherapy (Y84.2)
EXCLUDES 2   *gastrointestinal mucositis (ulcerative) (K92.81)*
mucositis (ulcerative) of vagina and vulva (N76.81)
oral mucositis (ulcerative) (K12.3-)

J34.89   **Other specified disorders of nose and nasal sinuses**
Perforation of nasal septum NOS
Rhinolith

J34.9   **Unspecified disorder of nose and nasal sinuses**   ▽

✓4ᵗʰ **J35**   **Chronic diseases of tonsils and adenoids**
Use additional code to identify:
exposure to environmental tobacco smoke (Z77.22)
exposure to tobacco smoke in the perinatal period (P96.81)
history of tobacco dependence (Z87.891)
occupational exposure to environmental tobacco smoke (Z57.31)
tobacco dependence (F17.-)
tobacco use (Z72.0)

✓5ᵗʰ **J35.0**   **Chronic tonsillitis and adenoiditis**
EXCLUDES 2   *acute tonsillitis (J03.-)*

J35.01   **Chronic tonsillitis**

J35.02   **Chronic adenoiditis**

J35.03   **Chronic tonsillitis and adenoiditis**

J35.1   **Hypertrophy of tonsils**
Enlargement of tonsils
EXCLUDES 1   *hypertrophy of tonsils with tonsillitis (J35.0-)*

J35.2   **Hypertrophy of adenoids**
Enlargement of adenoids
EXCLUDES 1   *hypertrophy of adenoids with adenoiditis (J35.0-)*

J35.3   **Hypertrophy of tonsils with hypertrophy of adenoids**
EXCLUDES 1   *hypertrophy of tonsils and adenoids with tonsillitis and adenoiditis (J35.03)*

J35.8   **Other chronic diseases of tonsils and adenoids**
Adenoid vegetations
Amygdalolith
Calculus, tonsil
Cicatrix of tonsil (and adenoid)
Tonsillar tag
Ulcer of tonsil

J35.9   **Chronic disease of tonsils and adenoids, unspecified**   ▽
Disease (chronic) of tonsils and adenoids NOS

J36   **Peritonsillar abscess**
INCLUDES   abscess of tonsil
peritonsillar cellulitis
quinsy
Use additional code (B95-B97) to identify infectious agent
EXCLUDES 1   *acute tonsillitis (J03.-)*
chronic tonsillitis (J35.0)
retropharyngeal abscess (J39.0)
tonsillitis NOS (J03.9-)

✓4ᵗʰ **J37**   **Chronic laryngitis and laryngotracheitis**
Use additional code to identify:
exposure to environmental tobacco smoke (Z77.22)
exposure to tobacco smoke in the perinatal period (P96.81)
history of tobacco dependence (Z87.891)
infectious agent (B95-B97)
occupational exposure to environmental tobacco smoke (Z57.31)
tobacco dependence (F17.-)
tobacco use (Z72.0)

J37.0   **Chronic laryngitis**
Catarrhal laryngitis
Hypertrophic laryngitis
Sicca laryngitis
EXCLUDES 2   *acute laryngitis (J04.0)*
obstructive (acute) laryngitis (J05.0)

J37.1   **Chronic laryngotracheitis**
Laryngitis, chronic, with tracheitis (chronic)
Tracheitis, chronic, with laryngitis
EXCLUDES 1   *chronic tracheitis (J42)*
EXCLUDES 2   *acute laryngotracheitis (J04.2)*
acute tracheitis (J04.1)

✓4ᵗʰ **J38**   **Diseases of vocal cords and larynx, not elsewhere classified**
Use additional code to identify:
exposure to environmental tobacco smoke (Z77.22)
exposure to tobacco smoke in the perinatal period (P96.81)
history of tobacco dependence (Z87.891)
occupational exposure to environmental tobacco smoke (Z57.31)
tobacco dependence (F17.-)
tobacco use (Z72.0)
EXCLUDES 1   *congenital laryngeal stridor (P28.89)*
obstructive laryngitis (acute) (J05.0)
postprocedural subglottic stenosis (J95.5)
stridor (R06.1)
ulcerative laryngitis (J04.0)

✓5ᵗʰ **J38.0**   **Paralysis of vocal cords and larynx**
Laryngoplegia
Paralysis of glottis

J38.00   **Paralysis of vocal cords and larynx, unspecified**   ▽

J38.01   **Paralysis of vocal cords and larynx, unilateral**

J38.02   **Paralysis of vocal cords and larynx, bilateral**

J38.1   **Polyp of vocal cord and larynx**
EXCLUDES 1   *adenomatous polyps (D14.1)*

J38.2   **Nodules of vocal cords**
Chorditis (fibrinous)(nodosa)(tuberosa)
Singer's nodes
Teacher's nodes

J38.3   **Other diseases of vocal cords**
Abscess of vocal cords
Cellulitis of vocal cords
Granuloma of vocal cords
Leukokeratosis of vocal cords
Leukoplakia of vocal cords

J38.4   **Edema of larynx**
Edema (of) glottis
Subglottic edema
Supraglottic edema
EXCLUDES 1   *acute obstructive laryngitis [croup] (J05.0)*
edematous laryngitis (J04.0)

J38.5   **Laryngeal spasm**
Laryngismus (stridulus)

J38.6   **Stenosis of larynx**

✓ Additional Character Req   ✓×7ᵗʰ Placeholder Alert   Manifestation   HCC CMS-HCC Condition   ▽ Unspecified Code   ►◄ Revised Text   ● New Code   ▲ Revised Code Title

J38.7   **Other diseases of larynx**
   Abscess of larynx   Pachyderma of larynx
   Cellulitis of larynx   Perichondritis of larynx
   Disease of larynx NOS   Ulcer of larynx
   Necrosis of larynx

✓4ᵗʰ **J39**   **Other diseases of upper respiratory tract**
   EXCLUDES 1   *acute respiratory infection NOS (J22)*
               acute upper respiratory infection (J06.9)
               upper respiratory inflammation due to chemicals, gases, fumes
                  or vapors (J68.2)

J39.0   **Retropharyngeal and parapharyngeal abscess**
   Peripharyngeal abscess
   EXCLUDES 1   *peritonsillar abscess (J36)*
   DEF: Purulent infection behind pharynx and front of precerebral
   fascia; characterized by neck stiffness, cervical lymphadenopathy,
   sore throat, fever, and stridor.

J39.1   **Other abscess of pharynx**
   Cellulitis of pharynx
   Nasopharyngeal abscess

J39.2   **Other diseases of pharynx**
   Cyst of pharynx
   Edema of pharynx
   EXCLUDES 2   *chronic pharyngitis (J31.2)*
               ulcerative pharyngitis (J02.9)

J39.3   **Upper respiratory tract hypersensitivity reaction, site**   ▽
           unspecified
   EXCLUDES 1   *hypersensitivity reaction of upper respiratory tract,*
                  such as:
                     extrinsic allergic alveolitis (J67.9)
                     pneumoconiosis (J60-J67.9)

J39.8   **Other specified diseases of upper respiratory tract**

J39.9   **Disease of upper respiratory tract, unspecified**   ▽

Chronic lower respiratory diseases (J40-J47)

EXCLUDES 1   *bronchitis due to chemicals, gases, fumes and vapors (J68.0)*
EXCLUDES 2   *cystic fibrosis (E84.-)*

J40   **Bronchitis, not specified as acute or chronic**   ▽
   Bronchitis NOS
   Bronchitis with tracheitis NOS
   Catarrhal bronchitis
   Tracheobronchitis NOS
   Use additional code to identify:
      exposure to environmental tobacco smoke (Z77.22)
      exposure to tobacco smoke in the perinatal period (P96.81)
      history of tobacco dependence (Z87.891)
      occupational exposure to environmental tobacco smoke (Z57.31)
      tobacco dependence (F17.-)
      tobacco use (Z72.0)
   EXCLUDES 1   *acute bronchitis (J20.-)*
               allergic bronchitis NOS (J45.909)
               asthmatic bronchitis NOS (J45.9-)
               bronchitis due to chemicals, gases, fumes and vapors (J68.0)

✓4ᵗʰ **J41**   **Simple and mucopurulent chronic bronchitis**
   Use additional code to identify:
      exposure to environmental tobacco smoke (Z77.22)
      exposure to tobacco smoke in the perinatal period (P96.81)
      history of tobacco dependence (Z87.891)
      occupational exposure to environmental tobacco smoke (Z57.31)
      tobacco dependence (F17.-)
      tobacco use (Z72.0)
   EXCLUDES 1   *chronic bronchitis NOS (J42)*
               chronic obstructive bronchitis (J44.-)

J41.0   **Simple chronic bronchitis**   HCC
J41.1   **Mucopurulent chronic bronchitis**   HCC
J41.8   **Mixed simple and mucopurulent chronic bronchitis**   HCC

Emphysema

Healthy alveoli   Alveoli w/ Emphysema

Patent bronchiole   Collapsed bronchiole

Well-vascularized   Enlarged alveoli   Broken/fewer capillaries

Dilated alveoli   Alveolar membranes break down

Excess mucus

J42   **Unspecified chronic bronchitis**   HCC ▽
   Chronic bronchitis NOS
   Chronic tracheitis
   Chronic tracheobronchitis
   Use additional code to identify:
      exposure to environmental tobacco smoke (Z77.22)
      exposure to tobacco smoke in the perinatal period (P96.81)
      history of tobacco dependence (Z87.891)
      occupational exposure to environmental tobacco smoke (Z57.31)
      tobacco dependence (F17.-)
      tobacco use (Z72.0)
   EXCLUDES 1   *chronic asthmatic bronchitis (J44.-)*
               chronic bronchitis with airways obstruction (J44.-)
               chronic emphysematous bronchitis (J44.-)
               chronic obstructive pulmonary disease NOS (J44.9)
               simple and mucopurulent chronic bronchitis (J41.-)

✓4ᵗʰ **J43**   **Emphysema**
   Use additional code to identify:
      exposure to environmental tobacco smoke (Z77.22)
      history of tobacco dependence (Z87.891)
      occupational exposure to environmental tobacco smoke (Z57.31)
      tobacco dependence (F17.-)
      tobacco use (Z72.0)
   EXCLUDES 1   *compensatory emphysema (J98.3)*
               emphysema due to inhalation of chemicals, gases, fumes or
                  vapors (J68.4)
               emphysema with chronic (obstructive) bronchitis (J44.-)
               emphysematous (obstructive) bronchitis (J44.-)
               interstitial emphysema (J98.2)
               mediastinal emphysema (J98.2)
               neonatal interstitial emphysema (P25.0)
               surgical (subcutaneous) emphysema (T81.82)
               traumatic subcutaneous emphysema (T79.7)

J43.0   **Unilateral pulmonary emphysema [MacLeod's syndrome]**   HCC
   Swyer-James syndrome
   Unilateral emphysema
   Unilateral hyperlucent lung
   Unilateral pulmonary artery functional hypoplasia
   Unilateral transparency of lung

J43.1   **Panlobular emphysema**   HCC
   Panacinar emphysema

J43.2   **Centrilobular emphysema**   HCC
J43.8   **Other emphysema**   HCC
J43.9   **Emphysema, unspecified**   HCC ▽
   Bullous emphysema (lung)(pulmonary)
   Emphysema (lung)(pulmonary) NOS
   Emphysematous bleb
   Vesicular emphysema (lung)(pulmonary)

EXCLUDES 1 Not coded here   *EXCLUDES 2* Not included here   Ⓝ Newborn Age: 0   Ⓟ Pediatric Age: 0-17   Ⓜ Maternity Age: 12-55   Ⓐ Adult Age: 15-124

664   ICD-10-CM 2018

✓4th **J44** **Other chronic obstructive pulmonary disease**

     INCLUDES   asthma with chronic obstructive pulmonary disease
                chronic asthmatic (obstructive) bronchitis
                chronic bronchitis with airways obstruction
                chronic bronchitis with emphysema
                chronic emphysematous bronchitis
                chronic obstructive asthma
                chronic obstructive bronchitis
                chronic obstructive tracheobronchitis

     Code also type of asthma, if applicable (J45.-)
     Use additional code to identify:
       exposure to environmental tobacco smoke (Z77.22)
       history of tobacco dependence (Z87.891)
       occupational exposure to environmental tobacco smoke (Z57.31)
       tobacco dependence (F17.-)
       tobacco use (Z72.0)

     EXCLUDES 1   *bronchiectasis (J47.-)*
                chronic bronchitis NOS (J42)
                chronic simple and mucopurulent bronchitis (J41.-)
                chronic tracheitis (J42)
                chronic tracheobronchitis (J42)
                emphysema without chronic bronchitis (J43.-)

     EXCLUDES 2   ~~*lung diseases due to external agents (J60-J70)*~~
     AHA: 2017, 1Q, 25-26; 2016, 3Q, 15-16; 2013, 4Q, 109

     J44.0   **Chronic obstructive pulmonary disease with acute lower**   HCC
           respiratory infection
           ▶Code also to identify the infection◀
           ~~Use additional code to identify the infection~~
           AHA: 2017, 1Q, 24-25

     J44.1   **Chronic obstructive pulmonary disease with (acute)**   HCC
           exacerbation
           Decompensated COPD
           Decompensated COPD with (acute) exacerbation
           EXCLUDES 2   *chronic obstructive pulmonary disease [COPD] with*
                        acute bronchitis (J44.0)
                        ▶*lung diseases due to external agents (J60-J70)*◀
           AHA: 2017, 1Q, 26; 2016, 1Q, 35

     J44.9   **Chronic obstructive pulmonary disease, unspecified**   HCC ▽
           Chronic obstructive airway disease NOS
           Chronic obstructive lung disease NOS
           EXCLUDES 2 ▶*lung diseases due to external agents (J60-J70)*◀
           AHA: 2016, 1Q, 36; 2014, 4Q, 21; 2013, 4Q, 129

✓4th **J45** **Asthma**

     INCLUDES   allergic (predominantly) asthma
                allergic bronchitis nos
                allergic rhinitis with asthma
                atopic asthma
                extrinsic allergic asthma
                hay fever with asthma
                idiosyncratic asthma
                intrinsic nonallergic asthma
                nonallergic asthma

     Use additional code to identify:
       exposure to environmental tobacco smoke (Z77.22)
       exposure to tobacco smoke in the perinatal period (P96.81)
       history of tobacco dependence (Z87.891)
       occupational exposure to environmental tobacco smoke (Z57.31)
       tobacco dependence (F17.-)
       tobacco use (Z72.0)

     EXCLUDES 1   *detergent asthma (J69.8)*
                eosinophilic asthma (J82)
                ~~*lung diseases due to external agents (J60-J70)*~~
                miner's asthma (J60)
                wheezing NOS (R06.2)
                wood asthma (J67.8)

     EXCLUDES 2   *asthma with chronic obstructive pulmonary disease (J44.9)*
                chronic asthmatic (obstructive) bronchitis (J44.9)
                chronic obstructive asthma (J44.9)
     AHA: 2017, 1Q, 25-26; 2012, 4Q, 99
     DEF: Status asthmaticus: Severe, intractable episode of asthma that is
     unresponsive to normal therapeutic measures.

     ✓5th **J45.2**   **Mild intermittent asthma**
           J45.20   **Mild intermittent asthma, uncomplicated**
                 Mild intermittent asthma NOS
           J45.21   **Mild intermittent asthma with (acute) exacerbation**
           J45.22   **Mild intermittent asthma with status asthmaticus**

Asthma

Respiratory bronchiole — Smooth muscle fibres — Contraction of smooth muscle fibres

Mucus lining bronchial tubes — Extra mucus secretion in inflamed bronchial tubes — Air trapped within alveoli

Alveoli

     Normal alveoli   **Asthmatic alveoli**

     ✓5th **J45.3**   **Mild persistent asthma**
           J45.30   **Mild persistent asthma, uncomplicated**
                 Mild persistent asthma NOS
           J45.31   **Mild persistent asthma with (acute) exacerbation**
                 AHA: 2016, 1Q, 35
           J45.32   **Mild persistent asthma with status asthmaticus**

     ✓5th **J45.4**   **Moderate persistent asthma**
           J45.40   **Moderate persistent asthma, uncomplicated**
                 Moderate persistent asthma NOS
           J45.41   **Moderate persistent asthma with (acute)**
                 exacerbation
                 AHA: 2017, 1Q, 26
           J45.42   **Moderate persistent asthma with status asthmaticus**

     ✓5th **J45.5**   **Severe persistent asthma**
           J45.50   **Severe persistent asthma, uncomplicated**
                 Severe persistent asthma NOS
           J45.51   **Severe persistent asthma with (acute) exacerbation**
           J45.52   **Severe persistent asthma with status asthmaticus**

     ✓5th **J45.9**   **Other and unspecified asthma**
           ✓6th **J45.90**   **Unspecified asthma**
                 Asthmatic bronchitis NOS
                 Childhood asthma NOS
                 Late onset asthma
                 J45.901   **Unspecified asthma with (acute)**   ▽
                        exacerbation
                 J45.902   **Unspecified asthma with status**   ▽
                        asthmaticus
                 J45.909   **Unspecified asthma, uncomplicated**   ▽
                        Asthma NOS
                        EXCLUDES 2 ▶*lung diseases due to external*
                                  agents (J60-J70)◀
                        AHA: 2017, 1Q, 25

           ✓6th **J45.99**   **Other asthma**
                 J45.990   **Exercise induced bronchospasm**
                 J45.991   **Cough variant asthma**
                 J45.998   **Other asthma**

✓4th **J47** **Bronchiectasis**

     INCLUDES   bronchiolectasis
     Use additional code to identify:
       exposure to environmental tobacco smoke (Z77.22)
       exposure to tobacco smoke in the perinatal period (P96.81)
       history of tobacco dependence (Z87.891)
       occupational exposure to environmental tobacco smoke (Z57.31)
       tobacco dependence (F17.-)
       tobacco use (Z72.0)

     EXCLUDES 1   *congenital bronchiectasis (Q33.4)*
                tuberculous bronchiectasis (current disease) (A15.0)

     J47.0   **Bronchiectasis with acute lower respiratory infection**   HCC
           Bronchiectasis with acute bronchitis
           Use additional code to identify the infection

     J47.1   **Bronchiectasis with (acute) exacerbation**   HCC

     J47.9   **Bronchiectasis, uncomplicated**   HCC ▽
           Bronchiectasis NOS

✓ Additional Character Req   ✓x7th Placeholder Alert   Manifestation   HCC CMS-HCC Condition   ▽ Unspecified Code   ▶◀ Revised Text   ● New Code   ▲ Revised Code Title

ICD-10-CM 2018   **665**

Lung diseases due to external agents (J60-J70)

EXCLUDES 2   *asthma (J45.-)*
malignant neoplasm of bronchus and lung (C34.-)

J60   Coalworker's pneumoconiosis   HCC A
Anthracosilicosis
Anthracosis
Black lung disease
Coalworker's lung
EXCLUDES 1   *coalworker pneumoconiosis with tuberculosis, any type in A15 (J65)*

J61   Pneumoconiosis due to asbestos and other mineral fibers   HCC A
Asbestosis
EXCLUDES 1   *pleural plaque with asbestosis (J92.0)*
pneumoconiosis with tuberculosis, any type in A15 (J65)

✓4th **J62   Pneumoconiosis due to dust containing silica**
INCLUDES   *silicotic fibrosis (massive) of lung*
EXCLUDES 1   *pneumoconiosis with tuberculosis, any type in A15 (J65)*

   J62.0   Pneumoconiosis due to talc dust   HCC

   J62.8   Pneumoconiosis due to other dust containing silica   HCC
Silicosis NOS

✓4th **J63   Pneumoconiosis due to other inorganic dusts**
EXCLUDES 1   *pneumoconiosis with tuberculosis, any type in A15 (J65)*

   J63.0   Aluminosis (of lung)   HCC

   J63.1   Bauxite fibrosis (of lung)   HCC

   J63.2   Berylliosis   HCC

   J63.3   Graphite fibrosis (of lung)   HCC

   J63.4   Siderosis   HCC

   J63.5   Stannosis   HCC

   J63.6   Pneumoconiosis due to other specified inorganic dusts   HCC

J64   Unspecified pneumoconiosis   HCC ▽
EXCLUDES 1   *pneumonoconiosis with tuberculosis, any type in A15 (J65)*

J65   Pneumoconiosis associated with tuberculosis   HCC
Any condition in J60-J64 with tuberculosis, any type in A15
Silicotuberculosis

✓4th **J66   Airway disease due to specific organic dust**
EXCLUDES 2   *allergic alveolitis (J67.-)*
asbestosis (J61)
bagassosis (J67.1)
farmer's lung (J67.0)
hypersensitivity pneumonitis due to organic dust (J67.-)
reactive airways dysfunction syndrome (J68.3)

   J66.0   Byssinosis   HCC
Airway disease due to cotton dust

   J66.1   Flax-dressers' disease   HCC

   J66.2   Cannabinosis   HCC

   J66.8   Airway disease due to other specific organic dusts   HCC

✓4th **J67   Hypersensitivity pneumonitis due to organic dust**
INCLUDES   allergic alveolitis and pneumonitis due to inhaled organic dust and particles of fungal, actinomycetic or other origin
EXCLUDES 1   *pneumonitis due to inhalation of chemicals, gases, fumes or vapors (J68.0)*

   J67.0   Farmer's lung   HCC
Harvester's lung   Moldy hay disease
Haymaker's lung

   J67.1   Bagassosis   HCC
Bagasse disease   Bagasse pneumonitis

   J67.2   Bird fancier's lung   HCC
Budgerigar fancier's disease or lung
Pigeon fancier's disease or lung

   J67.3   Suberosis   HCC
Corkhandler's disease or lung
Corkworker's disease or lung

   J67.4   Maltworker's lung   HCC
Alveolitis due to Aspergillus clavatus

   J67.5   Mushroom-worker's lung   HCC

   J67.6   Maple-bark-stripper's lung   HCC
Alveolitis due to Cryptostroma corticale
Cryptostromosis

   J67.7   Air conditioner and humidifier lung   HCC
Allergic alveolitis due to fungal, thermophilic actinomycetes and other organisms growing in ventilation [air conditioning] systems

   J67.8   Hypersensitivity pneumonitis due to other organic dusts   HCC
Cheese-washer's lung   Furrier's lung
Coffee-worker's lung   Sequoiosis
Fish-meal worker's lung

   J67.9   Hypersensitivity pneumonitis due to unspecified organic dust   HCC ▽
Allergic alveolitis (extrinsic) NOS
Hypersensitivity pneumonitis NOS

✓4th **J68   Respiratory conditions due to inhalation of chemicals, gases, fumes and vapors**
Code first (T51-T65) to identify cause
Use additional code to identify associated respiratory conditions, such as:
acute respiratory failure (J96.0-)

   J68.0   Bronchitis and pneumonitis due to chemicals, gases, fumes and vapors   HCC
Chemical bronchitis (acute)

   J68.1   Pulmonary edema due to chemicals, gases, fumes and vapors   HCC
Chemical pulmonary edema (acute) (chronic)
EXCLUDES 1   *pulmonary edema (acute) (chronic) NOS (J81.-)*

   J68.2   Upper respiratory inflammation due to chemicals, gases, fumes and vapors, not elsewhere classified   HCC

   J68.3   Other acute and subacute respiratory conditions due to chemicals, gases, fumes and vapors   HCC
Reactive airways dysfunction syndrome

   J68.4   Chronic respiratory conditions due to chemicals, gases, fumes and vapors   HCC
Emphysema (diffuse) (chronic) due to inhalation of chemicals, gases, fumes and vapors
Obliterative bronchiolitis (chronic) (subacute) due to inhalation of chemicals, gases, fumes and vapors
Pulmonary fibrosis (chronic) due to inhalation of chemicals, gases, fumes and vapors
EXCLUDES 1   *chronic pulmonary edema due to chemicals, gases, fumes and vapors (J68.1)*

   J68.8   Other respiratory conditions due to chemicals, gases, fumes and vapors   HCC

   J68.9   Unspecified respiratory condition due to chemicals, gases, fumes and vapors   HCC ▽

✓4th **J69   Pneumonitis due to solids and liquids**
EXCLUDES 1   *neonatal aspiration syndromes (P24.-)*
postprocedural pneumonitis (J95.4)
AHA: 2017, 1Q, 24

   J69.0   Pneumonitis due to inhalation of food and vomit   HCC
Aspiration pneumonia NOS
Aspiration pneumonia (due to) food (regurgitated)
Aspiration pneumonia (due to) gastric secretions
Aspiration pneumonia (due to) milk
Aspiration pneumonia (due to) vomit
Code also any associated foreign body in respiratory tract (T17.-)
EXCLUDES 1   *chemical pneumonitis due to anesthesia (J95.4)*
obstetric aspiration pneumonia (O74.0)

   J69.1   Pneumonitis due to inhalation of oils and essences   HCC
Exogenous lipoid pneumonia
Lipid pneumonia NOS
Code first (T51-T65) to identify substance
EXCLUDES 1   *endogenous lipoid pneumonia (J84.89)*

   J69.8   Pneumonitis due to inhalation of other solids and liquids   HCC
Pneumonitis due to aspiration of blood
Pneumonitis due to aspiration of detergent
Code first (T51-T65) to identify substance

✓4th **J70   Respiratory conditions due to other external agents**

   J70.0   Acute pulmonary manifestations due to radiation   HCC
Radiation pneumonitis
Use additional code (W88-W90, X39.0-) to identify the external cause

   J70.1   Chronic and other pulmonary manifestations due to radiation   HCC
Fibrosis of lung following radiation
Use additional code (W88-W90, X39.0-) to identify the external cause

   J70.2   Acute drug-induced interstitial lung disorders   HCC
Use additional code for adverse effect, if applicable, to identify drug (T36-T50 with fifth or sixth character 5)
EXCLUDES 1   *interstitial pneumonia NOS (J84.9)*
lymphoid interstitial pneumonia (J84.2)

EXCLUDES 1 Not coded here   EXCLUDES 2 Not included here   N Newborn Age: 0   P Pediatric Age: 0-17   M Maternity Age: 12-55   A Adult Age: 15-124

666   ICD-10-CM 2018

J70.3 **Chronic drug-induced interstitial lung disorders** HCC
Use additional code for adverse effect, if applicable, to identify drug (T36-T50 with fifth or sixth character 5)
EXCLUDES 1 interstitial pneumonia NOS (J84.9)
lymphoid interstitial pneumonia (J84.2)

J70.4 **Drug-induced interstitial lung disorders, unspecified** HCC ▽
Use additional code for adverse effect, if applicable, to identify drug (T36-T50 with fifth or sixth character 5)
EXCLUDES 1 interstitial pneumonia NOS (J84.9)
lymphoid interstitial pneumonia (J84.2)

J70.5 **Respiratory conditions due to smoke inhalation** HCC
Smoke inhalation NOS
EXCLUDES 1 smoke inhalation due to chemicals, gases, fumes and vapors (J68.9)
AHA: 2013, 4Q, 121

J70.8 **Respiratory conditions due to other specified external agents** HCC
Code first (T51-T65) to identify the external agent

J70.9 **Respiratory conditions due to unspecified external agent** HCC ▽
Code first (T51-T65) to identify the external agent

Other respiratory diseases principally affecting the interstitium (J80-J84)

J80 **Acute respiratory distress syndrome** HCC
Acute respiratory distress syndrome in adult or child
Adult hyaline membrane disease
EXCLUDES 1 respiratory distress syndrome in newborn (perinatal) (P22.0)
AHA: 2017, 1Q, 26

✓4ᵗʰ **J81** **Pulmonary edema**
Use additional code to identify:
exposure to environmental tobacco smoke (Z77.22)
history of tobacco dependence (Z87.891)
occupational exposure to environmental tobacco smoke (Z57.31)
tobacco dependence (F17.-)
tobacco use (Z72.0)
EXCLUDES 1 chemical (acute) pulmonary edema (J68.1)
hypostatic pneumonia (J18.2)
passive pneumonia (J18.2)
pulmonary edema due to external agents (J60-J70)
pulmonary edema with heart disease NOS (I50.1)
pulmonary edema with heart failure (I50.1)

J81.0 **Acute pulmonary edema** HCC
Acute edema of lung

J81.1 **Chronic pulmonary edema**
Pulmonary congestion (chronic) (passive)
Pulmonary edema NOS

J82 **Pulmonary eosinophilia, not elsewhere classified** HCC
Allergic pneumonia
Eosinophilic asthma
Eosinophilic pneumonia
Löffler's pneumonia
Tropical (pulmonary) eosinophilia NOS
EXCLUDES 1 pulmonary eosinophilia due to aspergillosis (B44.-)
pulmonary eosinophilia due to drugs (J70.2-J70.4)
pulmonary eosinophilia due to specified parasitic infection (B50-B83)
pulmonary eosinophilia due to systemic connective tissue disorders (M30-M36)
pulmonary infiltrate NOS (R91.8)

✓4ᵗʰ **J84** **Other interstitial pulmonary diseases**
EXCLUDES 1 drug-induced interstitial lung disorders (J70.2-J70.4)
interstitial emphysema (J98.2)
~~lung diseases due to external agents (J60-J70)~~
EXCLUDES 2 ►lung diseases due to external agents (J60-J70)◄

✓5ᵗʰ **J84.0** **Alveolar and parieto-alveolar conditions**

J84.01 **Alveolar proteinosis** HCC
DEF: Reduced ventilation due to proteinaceous deposits on alveoli; symptoms include dyspnea, cough, chest pain, weakness, weight loss, and hemoptysis.

J84.02 **Pulmonary alveolar microlithiasis** HCC

J84.03 *Idiopathic pulmonary hemosiderosis* HCC
Essential brown induration of lung
Code first underlying disease, such as:
disorders of iron metabolism (E83.1-)
EXCLUDES 1 acute idiopathic pulmonary hemorrhage in infants [AIPHI] (R04.81)
DEF: Fibrosis of alveolar walls; marked by abnormal accumulation of iron as hemosiderin in lungs; primarily affects children; symptoms include anemia, fluid in lungs, and blood in sputum; etiology unknown.

J84.09 **Other alveolar and parieto-alveolar conditions** HCC

J84.1 **Other interstitial pulmonary diseases with fibrosis**
EXCLUDES 1 pulmonary fibrosis (chronic) due to inhalation of chemicals, gases, fumes or vapors (J68.4)
pulmonary fibrosis (chronic) following radiation (J70.1)

J84.10 **Pulmonary fibrosis, unspecified** HCC ▽
Capillary fibrosis of lung
Cirrhosis of lung (chronic) NOS
Fibrosis of lung (atrophic) (chronic) (confluent) (massive) (perialveolar) (peribronchial) NOS
Induration of lung (chronic) NOS
Postinflammatory pulmonary fibrosis

✓6ᵗʰ **J84.11** **Idiopathic interstitial pneumonia**
EXCLUDES 1 lymphoid interstitial pneumonia (J84.2)
pneumocystis pneumonia (B59)

J84.111 **Idiopathic interstitial pneumonia, not otherwise specified** HCC ▽

J84.112 **Idiopathic pulmonary fibrosis** HCC
Cryptogenic fibrosing alveolitis
Idiopathic fibrosing alveolitis

J84.113 **Idiopathic non-specific interstitial pneumonitis** HCC
EXCLUDES 1 non-specific interstitial pneumonia NOS, or due to known underlying cause (J84.89)

J84.114 **Acute interstitial pneumonitis** HCC
Hamman-Rich syndrome
EXCLUDES 1 pneumocystis pneumonia (B59)

J84.115 **Respiratory bronchiolitis interstitial lung disease** HCC

J84.116 **Cryptogenic organizing pneumonia** HCC
EXCLUDES 1 organizing pneumonia NOS, or due to known underlying cause (J84.89)

J84.117 **Desquamative interstitial pneumonia** HCC

J84.17 *Other interstitial pulmonary diseases with fibrosis* HCC *in diseases classified elsewhere*
Interstitial pneumonia (nonspecific) (usual) due to collagen vascular disease
Interstitial pneumonia (nonspecific) (usual) in diseases classified elsewhere
Organizing pneumonia due to collagen vascular disease
Organizing pneumonia in diseases classified elsewhere
Code first underlying disease, such as:
progressive systemic sclerosis (M34.0)
rheumatoid arthritis (M05.00-M06.9)
systemic lupus erythematosis (M32.0-M32.9)

J84.2 **Lymphoid interstitial pneumonia** HCC
Lymphoid interstitial pneumonitis

✓5ᵗʰ **J84.8** **Other specified interstitial pulmonary diseases**
EXCLUDES 1 exogenous lipoid pneumonia (J69.1)
unspecified lipoid pneumonia (J69.1)

J84.81 **Lymphangioleiomyomatosis** HCC ♀
Lymphangiomyomatosis

J84.82 **Adult pulmonary Langerhans cell histiocytosis** HCC ▲
Adult PLCH

J84.83 **Surfactant mutations of the lung** HCC
DEF: Genetic disorder resulting in insufficient secretion of a complex mixture of phospholipids and proteins that reduce surface tension in the alveoli following the onset of breathing to facilitate lung expansion in the newborn; leading indication for pediatric lung transplantation.

✓6ᵗʰ **J84.84** **Other interstitial lung diseases of childhood**

J84.841 **Neuroendocrine cell hyperplasia of infancy** HCC

J84.842 **Pulmonary interstitial glycogenosis** HCC

J84.843 **Alveolar capillary dysplasia with vein misalignment** HCC

J84.848 **Other interstitial lung diseases of childhood** HCC

✅ Additional Character Req   ✓x7ᵗʰ Placeholder Alert   Manifestation   HCC CMS-HCC Condition   ▽ Unspecified Code   ►◄ Revised Text   ● New Code   ▲ Revised Code Title

J84.89   **Other specified interstitial pulmonary diseases** `HCC`
    Endogenous lipoid pneumonia
    Interstitial pneumonitis
    Non-specific interstitial pneumonitis NOS
    Organizing pneumonia NOS
    Code first, if applicable:
        poisoning due to drug or toxin (T51-T65 with fifth or
            sixth character to indicate intent), for toxic
            pneumonopathy
        underlying cause of pneumonopathy, if known
    Use additional code, for adverse effect, to identify
        drug (T36-T50 with fifth or sixth character 5), if
        drug-induced
        `EXCLUDES 1`   *cryptogenic organizing pneumonia (J84.116)*
                idiopathic non-specific interstitial
                    pneumonitis (J84.113)
                lipoid pneumonia, exogenous or unspecified
                    (J69.1)
                lymphoid interstitial pneumonia (J84.2)

J84.9   **Interstitial pulmonary disease, unspecified** `HCC` ▽
    Interstitial pneumonia NOS

Suppurative and necrotic conditions of the lower respiratory tract (J85-J86)

✓4ᵗʰ **J85**   **Abscess of lung and mediastinum**
    Use additional code (B95-B97) to identify infectious agent.

J85.0   **Gangrene and necrosis of lung** `HCC`

J85.1   **Abscess of lung with pneumonia** `HCC`
    Code also the type of pneumonia

J85.2   **Abscess of lung without pneumonia** `HCC`
    Abscess of lung NOS

J85.3   **Abscess of mediastinum** `HCC`

✓4ᵗʰ **J86**   **Pyothorax**
    Use additional code (B95-B97) to identify infectious agent
    `EXCLUDES 1`   *abscess of lung (J85.-)*
               pyothorax due to tuberculosis (A15.6)

J86.0   **Pyothorax with fistula** `HCC`
    Bronchocutaneous fistula
    Bronchopleural fistula
    Hepatopleural fistula
    Mediastinal fistula
    Pleural fistula
    Thoracic fistula
    Any condition classifiable to J86.9 with fistula
    DEF: Purulent infection of respiratory cavity, with communication from cavity to another structure.

J86.9   **Pyothorax without fistula** `HCC`
    Abscess of pleura   Pyopneumothorax
    Abscess of thorax   Septic pleurisy
    Empyema (chest) (lung) (pleura)   Seropurulent pleurisy
    Fibrinopurulent pleurisy   Suppurative pleurisy
    Purulent pleurisy

Other diseases of the pleura (J90-J94)

J90   **Pleural effusion, not elsewhere classified**
    Encysted pleurisy
    Pleural effusion NOS
    Pleurisy with effusion (exudative) (serous)
    `EXCLUDES 1`   *chylous (pleural) effusion (J94.0)*
               malignant pleural effusion (J91.0))
               pleurisy NOS (R09.1)
               tuberculous pleural effusion (A15.6)

✓4ᵗʰ **J91**   **Pleural effusion in conditions classified elsewhere**
    `EXCLUDES 2`   *pleural effusion in heart failure (I50.-)*
               pleural effusion in systemic lupus erythematosus (M32.13)

J91.0   *Malignant pleural effusion*
    Code first underlying neoplasm

J91.8   *Pleural effusion in other conditions classified elsewhere*
    Code first underlying disease, such as:
        filariasis (B74.0-B74.9)
        influenza (J09.X2, J10.1, J11.1)
    AHA: 2015, 2Q, 15

Pleural Effusion

Figure labels: Right lung, Left lung, Pleura, Pleural space, Pleural effusion

---

✓4ᵗʰ **J92**   **Pleural plaque**
    `INCLUDES`   pleural thickening

J92.0   **Pleural plaque with presence of asbestos**

J92.9   **Pleural plaque without asbestos**
    Pleural plaque NOS

✓4ᵗʰ **J93**   **Pneumothorax and air leak**
    `EXCLUDES 1`   *congenital or perinatal pneumothorax (P25.1)*
               postprocedural air leak (J95.812)
               postprocedural pneumothorax (J95.811)
               traumatic pneumothorax (S27.0)
               tuberculous (current disease) pneumothorax (A15.-)
               pyopneumothorax (J86.-)

J93.0   **Spontaneous tension pneumothorax**
    DEF: Leaking air from lung into lining, causing collapse.

✓5ᵗʰ **J93.1**   **Other spontaneous pneumothorax**

    J93.11   **Primary spontaneous pneumothorax**

    J93.12   **Secondary spontaneous pneumothorax**
        Code first underlying condition, such as:
            catamenial pneumothorax due to endometriosis
                (N80.8)
            cystic fibrosis (E84.-)
            eosinophilic pneumonia (J82)
            lymphangioleiomyomatosis (J84.81)
            malignant neoplasm of bronchus and lung (C34.-)
            Marfan's syndrome (Q87.4)
            pneumonia due to Pneumocystis carinii (B59)
            secondary malignant neoplasm of lung (C78.0-)
            spontaneous rupture of the esophagus (K22.3)

✓5ᵗʰ **J93.8**   **Other pneumothorax and air leak**

    J93.81   **Chronic pneumothorax**

    J93.82   **Other air leak**
        Persistent air leak

    J93.83   **Other pneumothorax**
        Acute pneumothorax
        Spontaneous pneumothorax NOS

J93.9   **Pneumothorax, unspecified** ▽
    Pneumothorax NOS

✓4ᵗʰ **J94**   **Other pleural conditions**
    `EXCLUDES 1`   *pleurisy NOS (R09.1)*
               traumatic hemopneumothorax (S27.2)
               traumatic hemothorax (S27.1)
               tuberculous pleural conditions (current disease) (A15.-)

J94.0   **Chylous effusion**
    Chyliform effusion

J94.1   **Fibrothorax**

J94.2   **Hemothorax**
    Hemopneumothorax

J94.8   **Other specified pleural conditions**
    Hydropneumothorax
    Hydrothorax

J94.9   **Pleural condition, unspecified** ▽

`EXCLUDES 1` Not coded here   `EXCLUDES 2` Not included here   **N** Newborn Age: 0   **P** Pediatric Age: 0-17   **M** Maternity Age: 12-55   **A** Adult Age: 15-124

668   ICD-10-CM 2018

Tracheostomy

Tracheostomy
in place

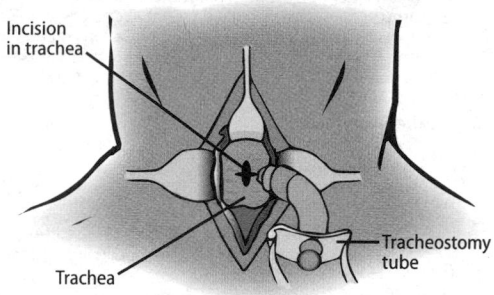

Incision
in trachea

Tracheostomy
tube

Trachea

Intraoperative and postprocedural complications and disorders of respiratory system, not elsewhere classified (J95)

✓4ᵗʰ **J95 Intraoperative and postprocedural complications and disorders of respiratory system, not elsewhere classified**

    EXCLUDES 2   *aspiration pneumonia (J69.-)*
                  emphysema (subcutaneous) resulting from a procedure (T81.82)
                  hypostatic pneumonia (J18.2)
                  pulmonary manifestations due to radiation (J70.0- J70.1)

✓5ᵗʰ **J95.0 Tracheostomy complications**

  J95.00 Unspecified tracheostomy complication HCC ▽

  J95.01 Hemorrhage from tracheostomy stoma HCC

  J95.02 Infection of tracheostomy stoma HCC
        Use additional code to identify type of infection, such as:
           cellulitis of neck ▶(L03.221)◀
           sepsis (A40, A41-)

  J95.03 Malfunction of tracheostomy stoma HCC
        Mechanical complication of tracheostomy stoma
        Obstruction of tracheostomy airway
        Tracheal stenosis due to tracheostomy

  J95.04 Tracheo-esophageal fistula following tracheostomy HCC

  J95.09 Other tracheostomy complication HCC

J95.1 Acute pulmonary insufficiency following thoracic surgery HCC
    EXCLUDES 2 *functional disturbances following cardiac surgery (I97.0, I97.1-)*

J95.2 Acute pulmonary insufficiency following nonthoracic surgery HCC
    EXCLUDES 2 *functional disturbances following cardiac surgery (I97.0, I97.1-)*

J95.3 Chronic pulmonary insufficiency following surgery HCC
    EXCLUDES 2 *functional disturbances following cardiac surgery (I97.0, I97.1-)*

J95.4 Chemical pneumonitis due to anesthesia
    Mendelson's syndrome
    Postprocedural aspiration pneumonia
    Use additional code for adverse effect, if applicable, to identify drug (T41.- with fifth or sixth character 5)
    EXCLUDES 1 *aspiration pneumonitis due to anesthesia complicating labor and delivery (O74.0)*
              aspiration pneumonitis due to anesthesia complicating pregnancy (O29)
              aspiration pneumonitis due to anesthesia complicating the puerperium (O89.01)

J95.5 Postprocedural subglottic stenosis

✓5ᵗʰ **J95.6 Intraoperative hemorrhage and hematoma of a respiratory system organ or structure complicating a procedure**
    EXCLUDES 1 *intraoperative hemorrhage and hematoma of a respiratory system organ or structure due to accidental puncture and laceration during procedure (J95.7-)*

  J95.61 Intraoperative hemorrhage and hematoma of a respiratory system organ or structure complicating a respiratory system procedure

  J95.62 Intraoperative hemorrhage and hematoma of a respiratory system organ or structure complicating other procedure

✓5ᵗʰ **J95.7 Accidental puncture and laceration of a respiratory system organ or structure during a procedure**
    EXCLUDES 2 *postprocedural pneumothorax (J95.811)*

  J95.71 Accidental puncture and laceration of a respiratory system organ or structure during a respiratory system procedure

  J95.72 Accidental puncture and laceration of a respiratory system organ or structure during other procedure

✓5ᵗʰ **J95.8 Other intraoperative and postprocedural complications and disorders of respiratory system, not elsewhere classified**

  ✓6ᵗʰ **J95.81 Postprocedural pneumothorax and air leak**
    J95.811 Postprocedural pneumothorax
    J95.812 Postprocedural air leak

  ✓6ᵗʰ **J95.82 Postprocedural respiratory failure**
    EXCLUDES 1 *respiratory failure in other conditions (J96.-)*
    J95.821 Acute postprocedural respiratory failure HCC
        Postprocedural respiratory failure NOS
    J95.822 Acute and chronic postprocedural respiratory failure HCC

  ✓6ᵗʰ **J95.83 Postprocedural hemorrhage of a respiratory system organ or structure following a procedure**
    J95.830 Postprocedural hemorrhage of a respiratory system organ or structure following a respiratory system procedure
    J95.831 Postprocedural hemorrhage of a respiratory system organ or structure following other procedure

  J95.84 Transfusion-related acute lung injury (TRALI)
    DEF: A relatively rare, but serious, pulmonary complication of blood transfusion, with acute respiratory distress, noncardiogenic pulmonary edema, cyanosis, hypoxemia, hypotension, fever, and chills.

  ✓6ᵗʰ **J95.85 Complication of respirator [ventilator]**
    J95.850 Mechanical complication of respirator HCC
        EXCLUDES 1 *encounter for respirator [ventilator] dependence during power failure (Z99.12)*
    J95.851 Ventilator associated pneumonia HCC
        Ventilator associated pneumonitis
        Use additional code to identify the organism, if known (B95.-, B96.-, B97.-)
        EXCLUDES 1 *ventilator lung in newborn (P27.8)*
        AHA: 2017, 1Q, 25
    J95.859 Other complication of respirator [ventilator] HCC

  ✓6ᵗʰ **J95.86 Postprocedural hematoma and seroma of a respiratory system organ or structure following a procedure**
    J95.860 Postprocedural hematoma of a respiratory system organ or structure following a respiratory system procedure
    J95.861 Postprocedural hematoma of a respiratory system organ or structure following other procedure
    J95.862 Postprocedural seroma of a respiratory system organ or structure following a respiratory system procedure
    J95.863 Postprocedural seroma of a respiratory system organ or structure following other procedure

  J95.88 Other intraoperative complications of respiratory system, not elsewhere classified

---

☑ Additional Character Req   ✓x7ᵗʰ Placeholder Alert   Manifestation   HCC CMS-HCC Condition   ▽ Unspecified Code   ▶◀ Revised Text   ● New Code   ▲ Revised Code Title

J95.89 **Other postprocedural complications and disorders of respiratory system, not elsewhere classified**
Use additional code to identify disorder, such as:
aspiration pneumonia (J69.-)
bacterial or viral pneumonia (J12-J18)
EXCLUDES 2 *acute pulmonary insufficiency following thoracic surgery (J95.1)*
postprocedural subglottic stenosis (J95.5)

Other diseases of the respiratory system (J96-J99)

✓4ᵗʰ J96 Respiratory failure, not elsewhere classified
EXCLUDES 1 *acute respiratory distress syndrome (J80)*
cardiorespiratory failure (R09.2)
newborn respiratory distress syndrome (P22.0)
postprocedural respiratory failure (J95.82-)
respiratory arrest (R09.2)
respiratory arrest of newborn (P28.81)
respiratory failure of newborn (P28.5)

✓5ᵗʰ J96.0 Acute respiratory failure

J96.00 **Acute respiratory failure, unspecified whether with hypoxia or hypercapnia** HCC ▽
AHA: 2016, 3Q, 14; 2013, 4Q, 121

J96.01 **Acute respiratory failure with hypoxia** HCC

J96.02 **Acute respiratory failure with hypercapnia** HCC

✓5ᵗʰ J96.1 Chronic respiratory failure

J96.10 **Chronic respiratory failure, unspecified whether with hypoxia or hypercapnia** HCC ▽
AHA: 2016, 1Q, 38; 2015, 1Q, 21

J96.11 **Chronic respiratory failure with hypoxia** HCC
AHA: 2013, 4Q, 129

J96.12 **Chronic respiratory failure with hypercapnia** HCC

✓5ᵗʰ J96.2 Acute and chronic respiratory failure
Acute on chronic respiratory failure

J96.20 **Acute and chronic respiratory failure, unspecified whether with hypoxia or hypercapnia** HCC ▽

J96.21 **Acute and chronic respiratory failure with hypoxia** HCC

J96.22 **Acute and chronic respiratory failure with hypercapnia** HCC

✓5ᵗʰ J96.9 Respiratory failure, unspecified

J96.90 **Respiratory failure, unspecified, unspecified whether with hypoxia or hypercapnia** HCC ▽

J96.91 **Respiratory failure, unspecified with hypoxia** HCC ▽

J96.92 **Respiratory failure, unspecified with hypercapnia** HCC ▽

✓4ᵗʰ J98 Other respiratory disorders
Use additional code to identify:
exposure to environmental tobacco smoke (Z77.22)
exposure to tobacco smoke in the perinatal period (P96.81)
history of tobacco dependence (Z87.891)
occupational exposure to environmental tobacco smoke (Z57.31)
tobacco dependence (F17.-)
tobacco use (Z72.0)
EXCLUDES 1 *newborn apnea (P28.4)*
newborn sleep apnea (P28.3)
EXCLUDES 2 *apnea NOS (R06.81)*
sleep apnea (G47.3-)

✓5ᵗʰ J98.0 Diseases of bronchus, not elsewhere classified

J98.01 **Acute bronchospasm**
EXCLUDES 1 *acute bronchiolitis with bronchospasm (J21.-)*
acute bronchitis with bronchospasm (J20.-)
asthma (J45.-)
exercise induced bronchospasm (J45.990)

J98.09 **Other diseases of bronchus, not elsewhere classified**
Broncholithiasis
Calcification of bronchus
Stenosis of bronchus
Tracheobronchial collapse
Tracheobronchial dyskinesia
Ulcer of bronchus

✓5ᵗʰ J98.1 Pulmonary collapse
EXCLUDES 1 *therapeutic collapse of lung status (Z98.3)*

J98.11 **Atelectasis**
EXCLUDES 1 *newborn atelectasis*
tuberculous atelectasis (current disease) (A15)

J98.19 **Other pulmonary collapse**

J98.2 Interstitial emphysema HCC
Mediastinal emphysema
EXCLUDES 1 *emphysema NOS (J43.9)*
emphysema in newborn (P25.0)
surgical emphysema (subcutaneous) (T81.82)
traumatic subcutaneous emphysema (T79.7)

J98.3 Compensatory emphysema HCC
DEF: Distention of all or part of the lung caused by disease processes or surgical intervention that decreased volume in another part of the lung; overcompensation reaction to the loss of capacity in another part of the lung; occurs in association with pneumonias, pleural effusions, atelectasis, empyema, and pneumothorax.

J98.4 Other disorders of lung
Calcification of lung
Cystic lung disease (acquired)
Lung disease NOS
Pulmolithiasis
EXCLUDES 1 *acute interstitial pneumonitis (J84.114)*
pulmonary insufficiency following surgery (J95.1-J95.2)

✓5ᵗʰ J98.5 Diseases of mediastinum, not elsewhere classified
EXCLUDES 2 *abscess of mediastinum (J85.3)*

J98.51 **Mediastinitis**
Code first:
underlying condition, if applicable, such as postoperative mediastinitis (T81.-)

J98.59 **Other diseases of mediastinum, not elsewhere classified**
Fibrosis of mediastinum
Hernia of mediastinum
Retraction of mediastinum

J98.6 Disorders of diaphragm
Diaphragmatitis
Paralysis of diaphragm
Relaxation of diaphragm
EXCLUDES 1 *congenital malformation of diaphragm NEC (Q79.1)*
congenital diaphragmatic hernia (Q79.0)
EXCLUDES 2 *diaphragmatic hernia (K44.-)*

J98.8 Other specified respiratory disorders

J98.9 Respiratory disorder, unspecified ▽
Respiratory disease (chronic) NOS

J99 *Respiratory disorders in diseases classified elsewhere* HCC
Code first underlying disease, such as:
amyloidosis (E85.-)
ankylosing spondylitis (M45)
congenital syphilis (A50.5)
cryoglobulinemia (D89.1)
early congenital syphilis (A50.0)
schistosomiasis (B65.0-B65.9)
EXCLUDES 1 *respiratory disorders in:*
amebiasis (A06.5)
blastomycosis (B40.0-B40.2)
candidiasis (B37.1)
coccidioidomycosis (B38.0-B38.2)
cystic fibrosis with pulmonary manifestations (E84.0)
dermatomyositis (M33.01, M33.11)
histoplasmosis (B39.0-B39.2)
late syphilis (A52.72, A52.73)
polymyositis (M33.21)
sicca syndrome (M35.02)
systemic lupus erythematosus (M32.13)
systemic sclerosis (M34.81)
Wegener's granulomatosis (M31.30-M31.31)

EXCLUDES 1 Not coded here   *EXCLUDES 2* Not included here   **N** Newborn Age: 0   **P** Pediatric Age: 0-17   **M** Maternity Age: 12-55   **A** Adult Age: 15-124

670   ICD-10-CM 2018

Chapter 11. Diseases of the Digestive System (K00–K95)

Chapter Specific Coding Guidelines and Examples
Reserved for future guideline expansion.

Chapter 11. Diseases of the Digestive System (K00-K95)

> EXCLUDES 2   certain conditions originating in the perinatal period (P04-P96)
> certain infectious and parasitic diseases (A00-B99)
> complications of pregnancy, childbirth and the puerperium (O00-O9A)
> congenital malformations, deformations and chromosomal abnormalities (Q00-Q99)
> endocrine, nutritional and metabolic diseases (E00-E88)
> injury, poisoning and certain other consequences of external causes (S00-T88)
> neoplasms (C00-D49)
> symptoms, signs and abnormal clinical and laboratory findings, not elsewhere classified (R00-R94)

This chapter contains the following blocks:

K00-K14	Diseases of oral cavity and salivary glands
K20-K31	Diseases of esophagus, stomach and duodenum
K35-K38	Diseases of appendix
K40-K46	Hernia
K50-K52	Noninfective enteritis and colitis
K55-K64	Other diseases of intestines
K65-K68	Diseases of peritoneum and retroperitoneum
K70-K77	Diseases of liver
K80-K87	Disorders of gallbladder, biliary tract and pancreas
K90-K95	Other diseases of the digestive system

Diseases of oral cavity and salivary glands (K00-K14)

✓4ᵗʰ K00 Disorders of tooth development and eruption
> EXCLUDES 2   embedded and impacted teeth (K01.-)

K00.0 Anodontia
Hypodontia
Oligodontia
> EXCLUDES 1   acquired absence of teeth (K08.1-)

K00.1 Supernumerary teeth
Distomolar
Fourth molar
Mesiodens
Paramolar
Supplementary teeth
> EXCLUDES 2   supernumerary roots (K00.2)

K00.2 Abnormalities of size and form of teeth
Concrescence of teeth
Dens evaginatus
Dens in dente
Dens invaginatus
Enamel pearls
Fusion of teeth
Gemination of teeth
Macrodontia
Microdontia
Peg-shaped [conical] teeth
Supernumerary roots
Taurodontism
Tuberculum paramolare
> EXCLUDES 1   abnormalities of teeth due to congenital syphilis (A50.5)
> tuberculum Carabelli, which is regarded as a normal variation and should not be coded

K00.3 Mottled teeth
Dental fluorosis
Mottling of enamel
Nonfluoride enamel opacities
> EXCLUDES 2   deposits [accretions] on teeth (K03.6)

K00.4 Disturbances in tooth formation
Aplasia and hypoplasia of cementum
Dilaceration of tooth
Enamel hypoplasia (neonatal) (postnatal) (prenatal)
Regional odontodysplasia
Turner's tooth
> EXCLUDES 1   Hutchinson's teeth and mulberry molars in congenital syphilis (A50.5)
> EXCLUDES 2   mottled teeth (K00.3)

K00.5 Hereditary disturbances in tooth structure, not elsewhere classified
Amelogenesis imperfecta
Dentinogenesis imperfecta
Odontogenesis imperfecta
Dentinal dysplasia
Shell teeth

Tooth Anatomy

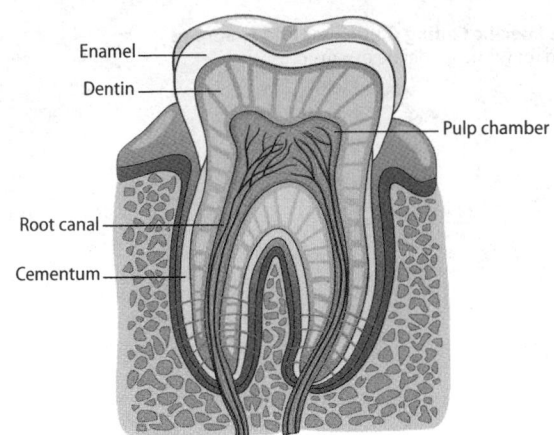

K00.6 Disturbances in tooth eruption
Dentia praecox
Natal tooth
Neonatal tooth
Premature eruption of tooth
Premature shedding of primary [deciduous] tooth
Prenatal teeth
Retained [persistent] primary tooth
> EXCLUDES 2   embedded and impacted teeth (K01.-)

K00.7 Teething syndrome

K00.8 Other disorders of tooth development
Color changes during tooth formation
Intrinsic staining of teeth NOS
> EXCLUDES 2   posteruptive color changes (K03.7)

K00.9 Disorder of tooth development, unspecified   ▽
Disorder of odontogenesis NOS

✓4ᵗʰ K01 Embedded and impacted teeth
> EXCLUDES 1   abnormal position of fully erupted teeth (M26.3-)

K01.0 Embedded teeth

K01.1 Impacted teeth

✓4ᵗʰ K02 Dental caries
> INCLUDES   caries of dentine
> dental cavities
> early childhood caries
> pre-eruptive caries
> recurrent caries (dentino enamel junction) (enamel) (to the pulp)
> tooth decay

K02.3 Arrested dental caries
Arrested coronal and root caries

✓5ᵗʰ K02.5 Dental caries on pit and fissure surface
Dental caries on chewing surface of tooth

     K02.51 Dental caries on pit and fissure surface limited to enamel
White spot lesions [initial caries] on pit and fissure surface of tooth

     K02.52 Dental caries on pit and fissure surface penetrating into dentin
Primary dental caries, cervical origin)

     K02.53 Dental caries on pit and fissure surface penetrating into pulp

✓5ᵗʰ K02.6 Dental caries on smooth surface

     K02.61 Dental caries on smooth surface limited to enamel
White spot lesions [initial caries] on smooth surface of tooth

     K02.62 Dental caries on smooth surface penetrating into dentin

     K02.63 Dental caries on smooth surface penetrating into pulp

K02.7 Dental root caries

K02.9 Dental caries, unspecified   ▽

EXCLUDES 1 Not coded here   EXCLUDES 2 Not included here   N Newborn Age: 0   P Pediatric Age: 0-17   M Maternity Age: 12-55   A Adult Age: 15-124

672   ICD-10-CM 2018

☑4ᵗʰ K03 Other diseases of hard tissues of teeth

EXCLUDES 2   bruxism (F45.8)
     dental caries (K02.-)
     teeth-grinding NOS (F45.8)

K03.0 Excessive attrition of teeth
   Approximal wear of teeth
   Occlusal wear of teeth

K03.1 Abrasion of teeth
   Dentifrice abrasion of teeth
   Habitual abrasion of teeth
   Occupational abrasion of teeth
   Ritual abrasion of teeth
   Traditional abrasion of teeth
   Wedge defect NOS

K03.2 Erosion of teeth
   Erosion of teeth due to diet
   Erosion of teeth due to drugs and medicaments
   Erosion of teeth due to persistent vomiting
   Erosion of teeth NOS
   Idiopathic erosion of teeth
   Occupational erosion of teeth

K03.3 Pathological resorption of teeth
   Internal granuloma of pulp
   Resorption of teeth (external)

K03.4 Hypercementosis
   Cementation hyperplasia

K03.5 Ankylosis of teeth

K03.6 Deposits [accretions] on teeth
   Betel deposits [accretions] on teeth
   Black deposits [accretions] on teeth
   Extrinsic staining of teeth NOS
   Green deposits [accretions] on teeth
   Materia alba deposits [accretions] on teeth
   Orange deposits [accretions] on teeth
   Staining of teeth NOS
   Subgingival dental calculus
   Supragingival dental calculus
   Tobacco deposits [accretions] on teeth

K03.7 Posteruptive color changes of dental hard tissues
   EXCLUDES 2   deposits [accretions] on teeth (K03.6)

☑5ᵗʰ K03.8 Other specified diseases of hard tissues of teeth

K03.81 Cracked tooth
   EXCLUDES 1   asymptomatic craze lines in enamel—omit code
     broken or fractured tooth due to trauma (S02.5)

K03.89 Other specified diseases of hard tissues of teeth

K03.9 Disease of hard tissues of teeth, unspecified ▽

☑4ᵗʰ K04 Diseases of pulp and periapical tissues

☑5ᵗʰ K04.0 Pulpitis
   Acute pulpitis
   Chronic (hyperplastic) (ulcerative) pulpitis

K04.01 Reversible pulpitis

K04.02 Irreversible pulpitis

K04.1 Necrosis of pulp
   Pulpal gangrene

K04.2 Pulp degeneration
   Denticles
   Pulpal calcifications
   Pulpal stones

K04.3 Abnormal hard tissue formation in pulp
   Secondary or irregular dentine

K04.4 Acute apical periodontitis of pulpal origin
   Acute apical periodontitis NOS
   EXCLUDES 1   acute periodontitis (K05.2-)
   DEF: Severe inflammation of the area surrounding the tip of a tooth's root; often secondary to infection or trauma.

K04.5 Chronic apical periodontitis
   Apical or periapical granuloma
   Apical periodontitis NOS
   EXCLUDES 1   chronic periodontitis (K05.3-)

K04.6 Periapical abscess with sinus
   Dental abscess with sinus
   Dentoalveolar abscess with sinus

K04.7 Periapical abscess without sinus
   Dental abscess without sinus
   Dentoalveolar abscess without sinus
   ~~Periapical abscess without sinus~~

K04.8 Radicular cyst
   Apical (periodontal) cyst
   Periapical cyst
   Residual radicular cyst
   EXCLUDES 2   lateral periodontal cyst (K09.0)
   DEF: Most common odontogenic cyst in tissue around tooth apex due to chronic inflammation of dental pulp.

☑5ᵗʰ K04.9 Other and unspecified diseases of pulp and periapical tissues

K04.90 Unspecified diseases of pulp and periapical tissues ▽

K04.99 Other diseases of pulp and periapical tissues

☑4ᵗʰ K05 Gingivitis and periodontal diseases

Use additional code to identify:
   alcohol abuse and dependence (F10.-)
   exposure to environmental tobacco smoke (Z77.22)
   exposure to tobacco smoke in the perinatal period (P96.81)
   history of tobacco dependence (Z87.891)
   occupational exposure to environmental tobacco smoke (Z57.31)
   tobacco dependence (F17.-)
   tobacco use (Z72.0)

☑5ᵗʰ K05.0 Acute gingivitis
   EXCLUDES 1   acute necrotizing ulcerative gingivitis (A69.1)
     herpesviral [herpes simplex] gingivostomatitis (B00.2)

K05.00 Acute gingivitis, plaque induced
   Acute gingivitis NOS
   Plaque induced gingival disease

K05.01 Acute gingivitis, non-plaque induced

☑5ᵗʰ K05.1 Chronic gingivitis
   Desquamative gingivitis (chronic)
   Gingivitis (chronic) NOS
   Hyperplastic gingivitis (chronic)
   Pregnancy associated gingivitis
   Simple marginal gingivitis (chronic)
   Ulcerative gingivitis (chronic)
   Code first, if applicable, diseases of the digestive system complicating pregnancy (O99.61-)

K05.10 Chronic gingivitis, plaque induced
   Chronic gingivitis NOS
   Gingivitis NOS

K05.11 Chronic gingivitis, non-plaque induced

☑5ᵗʰ K05.2 Aggressive periodontitis
   Acute pericoronitis
   EXCLUDES 1   acute apical periodontitis (K04.4)
     periapical abscess (K04.7)
     periapical abscess with sinus (K04.6)

K05.20 Aggressive periodontitis, unspecified ▽

☑6ᵗʰ K05.21 Aggressive periodontitis, localized
   Periodontal abscess

K05.211 Aggressive periodontitis, localized, slight

K05.212 Aggressive periodontitis, localized, moderate

K05.213 Aggressive periodontitis, localized, severe

K05.219 Aggressive periodontitis, localized, unspecified severity ▽

☑6ᵗʰ K05.22 Aggressive periodontitis, generalized

K05.221 Aggressive periodontitis, generalized, slight

K05.222 Aggressive periodontitis, generalized, moderate

K05.223 Aggressive periodontitis, generalized, severe

K05.229 Aggressive periodontitis, generalized, unspecified severity ▽

☑5ᵗʰ K05.3 Chronic periodontitis
   Chronic pericoronitis
   Complex periodontitis
   Periodontitis NOS
   Simplex periodontitis
   EXCLUDES 1   chronic apical periodontitis (K04.5)

K05.30 Chronic periodontitis, unspecified ▽

☑6ᵗʰ K05.31 Chronic periodontitis, localized

K05.311 Chronic periodontitis, localized, slight

K05.312 Chronic periodontitis, localized, moderate

☑ Additional Character Req   ☑x7ᵗʰ Placeholder Alert   Manifestation   HCC CMS-HCC Condition   ▽ Unspecified Code   ▶◀ Revised Text   ● New Code   ▲ Revised Code Title

ICD-10-CM 2018   673

Chapter 11. Diseases of the Digestive System

K05.313 – K08.403

K05.313   **Chronic periodontitis, localized, severe**

K05.319   **Chronic periodontitis, localized, unspecified severity** ▽

✓6ᵗʰ **K05.32**   **Chronic periodontitis, generalized**

K05.321   **Chronic periodontitis, generalized, slight**

K05.322   **Chronic periodontitis, generalized, moderate**

K05.323   **Chronic periodontitis, generalized, severe**

K05.329   **Chronic periodontitis, generalized, unspecified severity** ▽

K05.4   **Periodontosis**
Juvenile periodontosis

K05.5   **Other periodontal diseases**
Combined periodontic-endodontic lesion
Narrow gingival width (of periodontal soft tissue)
    EXCLUDES 2   *leukoplakia of gingiva (K13.21)*

K05.6   **Periodontal disease, unspecified** ▽

✓4ᵗʰ **K06**   **Other disorders of gingiva and edentulous alveolar ridge**
    EXCLUDES 2   *acute gingivitis (K05.0)*
               atrophy of edentulous alveolar ridge (K08.2)
               chronic gingivitis (K05.1)
               gingivitis NOS (K05.1)

✓5ᵗʰ **K06.0**   **Gingival recession**
▶Gingival recession (postinfective) (postprocedural)◀

- ✓6ᵗʰ **K06.01**   **Gingival recession, localized**

- K06.010   **Localized gingival recession, unspecified** ▽
       Localized gingival recession, NOS

- K06.011   **Localized gingival recession, minimal**

- K06.012   **Localized gingival recession, moderate**

- K06.013   **Localized gingival recession, severe**

- ✓6ᵗʰ **K06.02**   **Gingival recession, generalized**

- K06.020   **Generalized gingival recession, unspecified** ▽
       Generalized gingival recession, NOS

- K06.021   **Generalized gingival recession, minimal**

- K06.022   **Generalized gingival recession, moderate**

- K06.023   **Generalized gingival recession, severe**

K06.1   **Gingival enlargement**
Gingival fibromatosis

K06.2   **Gingival and edentulous alveolar ridge lesions associated with trauma**
Irritative hyperplasia of edentulous ridge [denture hyperplasia]
Use additional code (Chapter 20) to identify external cause or denture status (Z97.2)

K06.3   **Horizontal alveolar bone loss**

K06.8   **Other specified disorders of gingiva and edentulous alveolar ridge**
Fibrous epulis
Flabby alveolar ridge
Giant cell epulis
Peripheral giant cell granuloma of gingiva
Pyogenic granuloma of gingiva
Vertical ridge deficiency
    EXCLUDES 2   *gingival cyst (K09.0)*

K06.9   **Disorder of gingiva and edentulous alveolar ridge, unspecified** ▽

✓4ᵗʰ **K08**   **Other disorders of teeth and supporting structures**
    EXCLUDES 2   *dentofacial anomalies [including malocclusion] (M26.-)*
               disorders of jaw (M27.-)

K08.0   **Exfoliation of teeth due to systemic causes**
Code also underlying systemic condition

✓5ᵗʰ **K08.1**   **Complete loss of teeth**
Acquired loss of teeth, complete
    EXCLUDES 1   *congenital absence of teeth (K00.0)*
               exfoliation of teeth due to systemic causes (K08.0)
               partial loss of teeth (K08.4-)

✓6ᵗʰ **K08.10**   **Complete loss of teeth, unspecified cause**

K08.101   **Complete loss of teeth, unspecified cause, class I** ▽

K08.102   **Complete loss of teeth, unspecified cause, class II** ▽

K08.103   **Complete loss of teeth, unspecified cause, class III** ▽

K08.104   **Complete loss of teeth, unspecified cause, class IV** ▽

K08.109   **Complete loss of teeth, unspecified cause, unspecified class** ▽
       Edentulism NOS

✓6ᵗʰ **K08.11**   **Complete loss of teeth due to trauma**

K08.111   **Complete loss of teeth due to trauma, class I**

K08.112   **Complete loss of teeth due to trauma, class II**

K08.113   **Complete loss of teeth due to trauma, class III**

K08.114   **Complete loss of teeth due to trauma, class IV**

K08.119   **Complete loss of teeth due to trauma, unspecified class** ▽

✓6ᵗʰ **K08.12**   **Complete loss of teeth due to periodontal diseases**

K08.121   **Complete loss of teeth due to periodontal diseases, class I**

K08.122   **Complete loss of teeth due to periodontal diseases, class II**

K08.123   **Complete loss of teeth due to periodontal diseases, class III**

K08.124   **Complete loss of teeth due to periodontal diseases, class IV**

K08.129   **Complete loss of teeth due to periodontal diseases, unspecified class** ▽

✓6ᵗʰ **K08.13**   **Complete loss of teeth due to caries**

K08.131   **Complete loss of teeth due to caries, class I**

K08.132   **Complete loss of teeth due to caries, class II**

K08.133   **Complete loss of teeth due to caries, class III**

K08.134   **Complete loss of teeth due to caries, class IV**

K08.139   **Complete loss of teeth due to caries, unspecified class** ▽

✓6ᵗʰ **K08.19**   **Complete loss of teeth due to other specified cause**

K08.191   **Complete loss of teeth due to other specified cause, class I**

K08.192   **Complete loss of teeth due to other specified cause, class II**

K08.193   **Complete loss of teeth due to other specified cause, class III**

K08.194   **Complete loss of teeth due to other specified cause, class IV**

K08.199   **Complete loss of teeth due to other specified cause, unspecified class** ▽

✓5ᵗʰ **K08.2**   **Atrophy of edentulous alveolar ridge**

K08.20   **Unspecified atrophy of edentulous alveolar ridge** ▽
       Atrophy of the mandible NOS
       Atrophy of the maxilla NOS

K08.21   **Minimal atrophy of the mandible**
       Minimal atrophy of the edentulous mandible

K08.22   **Moderate atrophy of the mandible**
       Moderate atrophy of the edentulous mandible

K08.23   **Severe atrophy of the mandible**
       Severe atrophy of the edentulous mandible

K08.24   **Minimal atrophy of maxilla**
       Minimal atrophy of the edentulous maxilla

K08.25   **Moderate atrophy of the maxilla**
       Moderate atrophy of the edentulous maxilla

K08.26   **Severe atrophy of the maxilla**
       Severe atrophy of the edentulous maxilla

K08.3   **Retained dental root**

✓5ᵗʰ **K08.4**   **Partial loss of teeth**
Acquired loss of teeth, partial
    EXCLUDES 1   *complete loss of teeth (K08.1-)*
               congenital absence of teeth (K00.0)
    EXCLUDES 2   *exfoliation of teeth due to systemic causes (K08.0)*

✓6ᵗʰ **K08.40**   **Partial loss of teeth, unspecified cause**

K08.401   **Partial loss of teeth, unspecified cause, class I** ▽

K08.402   **Partial loss of teeth, unspecified cause, class II** ▽

K08.403   **Partial loss of teeth, unspecified cause, class III** ▽

EXCLUDES 1 Not coded here   EXCLUDES 2 Not included here   N Newborn Age: 0   P Pediatric Age: 0-17   M Maternity Age: 12-55   A Adult Age: 15-124

674   ICD-10-CM 2018

K08.404   Partial loss of teeth, unspecified cause, ▽
class IV

K08.409   Partial loss of teeth, unspecified ▽
cause, unspecified class
Tooth extraction status NOS

√6ᵗʰ **K08.41   Partial loss of teeth due to trauma**
K08.411   Partial loss of teeth due to trauma, class I
K08.412   Partial loss of teeth due to trauma, class II
K08.413   Partial loss of teeth due to trauma, class III
K08.414   Partial loss of teeth due to trauma, class IV
K08.419   Partial loss of teeth due to trauma, ▽
unspecified class

√6ᵗʰ **K08.42   Partial loss of teeth due to periodontal diseases**
K08.421   Partial loss of teeth due to periodontal diseases, class I
K08.422   Partial loss of teeth due to periodontal diseases, class II
K08.423   Partial loss of teeth due to periodontal diseases, class III
K08.424   Partial loss of teeth due to periodontal diseases, class IV
K08.429   Partial loss of teeth due to periodontal ▽ diseases, unspecified class

√6ᵗʰ **K08.43   Partial loss of teeth due to caries**
K08.431   Partial loss of teeth due to caries, class I
K08.432   Partial loss of teeth due to caries, class II
K08.433   Partial loss of teeth due to caries, class III
K08.434   Partial loss of teeth due to caries, class IV
K08.439   Partial loss of teeth due to caries, ▽
unspecified class

√6ᵗʰ **K08.49   Partial loss of teeth due to other specified cause**
K08.491   Partial loss of teeth due to other specified cause, class I
K08.492   Partial loss of teeth due to other specified cause, class II
K08.493   Partial loss of teeth due to other specified cause, class III
K08.494   Partial loss of teeth due to other specified cause, class IV
K08.499   Partial loss of teeth due to other ▽
specified cause, unspecified class

√5ᵗʰ **K08.5   Unsatisfactory restoration of tooth**
Defective bridge, crown, filling
Defective dental restoration
EXCLUDES 1   dental restoration status (Z98.811)
EXCLUDES 2   endosseous dental implant failure (M27.6-)
       unsatisfactory endodontic treatment (M27.5-)

K08.50   Unsatisfactory restoration of tooth, unspecified ▽
Defective dental restoration NOS

K08.51   **Open restoration margins of tooth**
Dental restoration failure of marginal integrity
Open margin on tooth restoration
Poor gingival margin to tooth restoration

K08.52   **Unrepairable overhanging of dental restorative materials**
Overhanging of tooth restoration

√6ᵗʰ **K08.53   Fractured dental restorative material**
EXCLUDES 1   cracked tooth (K03.81)
       traumatic fracture of tooth (S02.5)
K08.530   Fractured dental restorative material without loss of material
K08.531   Fractured dental restorative material with loss of material
K08.539   Fractured dental restorative material, ▽
unspecified

K08.54   **Contour of existing restoration of tooth biologically incompatible with oral health**
Dental restoration failure of periodontal anatomical integrity
Unacceptable contours of existing restoration of tooth
Unacceptable morphology of existing restoration of tooth

K08.55   **Allergy to existing dental restorative material**
Use additional code to identify the specific type of allergy

K08.56   **Poor aesthetic of existing restoration of tooth**
Dental restoration aesthetically inadequate or displeasing

K08.59   **Other unsatisfactory restoration of tooth**
Other defective dental restoration

√5ᵗʰ **K08.8   Other specified disorders of teeth and supporting structures**
K08.81   Primary occlusal trauma
K08.82   Secondary occlusal trauma
K08.89   Other specified disorders of teeth and supporting structures
Enlargement of alveolar ridge NOS
Insufficient anatomic crown height
Insufficient clinical crown length
Irregular alveolar process
Toothache NOS

K08.9   **Disorder of teeth and supporting structures, unspecified**   ▽

√4ᵗʰ **K09   Cysts of oral region, not elsewhere classified**
INCLUDES   lesions showing histological features both of aneurysmal cyst and of another fibro-osseous lesion
EXCLUDES 2   cysts of jaw (M27.0-, M27.4-)
       radicular cyst (K04.8)

K09.0   **Developmental odontogenic cysts**
Dentigerous cyst
Eruption cyst
Follicular cyst
Gingival cyst
Lateral periodontal cyst
Primordial cyst
EXCLUDES 2   keratocysts (D16.4, D16.5)
       odontogenic keratocystic tumors (D16.4, D16.5)

K09.1   **Developmental (nonodontogenic) cysts of oral region**
Cyst (of) incisive canal
Cyst (of) palatine of papilla
Globulomaxillary cyst
Median palatal cyst
Nasoalveolar cyst
Nasolabial cyst
Nasopalatine duct cyst

K09.8   **Other cysts of oral region, not elsewhere classified**
Dermoid cyst
Epidermoid cyst
Lymphoepithelial cyst
Epstein's pearl

K09.9   **Cyst of oral region, unspecified**   ▽

√4ᵗʰ **K11   Diseases of salivary glands**
Use additional code to identify:
alcohol abuse and dependence (F10.-)
exposure to environmental tobacco smoke (Z77.22)
exposure to tobacco smoke in the perinatal period (P96.81)
history of tobacco dependence (Z87.891)
occupational exposure to environmental tobacco smoke (Z57.31)
tobacco dependence (F17.-)
tobacco use (Z72.0)

K11.0   **Atrophy of salivary gland**

K11.1   **Hypertrophy of salivary gland**
DEF: Overgrowth of or enlarged salivary gland tissue; caused by infection, salivary duct blockage, autoimmune diseases, and benign and malignant tumors.

√5ᵗʰ **K11.2   Sialoadenitis**
Parotitis
EXCLUDES 1   epidemic parotitis (B26.-)
       mumps (B26.-)
       uveoparotid fever [Heerfordt] (D86.89)
K11.20   Sialoadenitis, unspecified   ▽
K11.21   Acute sialoadenitis
EXCLUDES 1   acute recurrent sialoadenitis (K11.22)
K11.22   Acute recurrent sialoadenitis
K11.23   Chronic sialoadenitis

K11.3   **Abscess of salivary gland**

K11.4   **Fistula of salivary gland**
EXCLUDES 1   congenital fistula of salivary gland (Q38.4)

K11.5   **Sialolithiasis**
Calculus of salivary gland or duct
Stone of salivary gland or duct

K11.6   **Mucocele of salivary gland**
Mucous extravasation cyst of salivary gland
Mucous retention cyst of salivary gland
Ranula

✔ Additional Character Req   ✔ˣ⁷ᵗʰ Placeholder Alert   Manifestation   HCC CMS-HCC Condition   ▽ Unspecified Code   ▶◀ Revised Text   ● New Code   ▲ Revised Code Title

K11.7   Disturbances of salivary secretion
Hypoptyalism
Ptyalism
Xerostomia
EXCLUDES 2   dry mouth NOS (R68.2)

K11.8   Other diseases of salivary glands
Benign lymphoepithelial lesion of salivary gland
Mikulicz' disease
Necrotizing sialometaplasia
Sialectasia
Stenosis of salivary duct
Stricture of salivary duct
EXCLUDES 1   sicca syndrome [Sjögren] (M35.0-)

K11.9   Disease of salivary gland, unspecified   ▽
Sialoadenopathy NOS

✓4ᵗʰ K12   Stomatitis and related lesions
Use additional code to identify:
alcohol abuse and dependence (F10.-)
exposure to environmental tobacco smoke (Z77.22)
exposure to tobacco smoke in the perinatal period (P96.81)
history of tobacco dependence (Z87.891)
occupational exposure to environmental tobacco smoke (Z57.31)
tobacco dependence (F17.-)
tobacco use (Z72.0)
EXCLUDES 1   cancrum oris (A69.0)
       cheilitis (K13.0)
       gangrenous stomatitis (A69.0)
       herpesviral [herpes simplex] gingivostomatitis (B00.2)
       noma (A69.0)

K12.0   Recurrent oral aphthae
Aphthous stomatitis (major) (minor)
Bednar's aphthae
Periadenitis mucosa necrotica recurrens
Recurrent aphthous ulcer
Stomatitis herpetiformis
DEF: Disorder of unknown etiology with small oval or round painful ulcers of the mouth marked by a grayish exudate and a red halo effect.

K12.1   Other forms of stomatitis
Stomatitis NOS   Ulcerative stomatitis
Denture stomatitis   Vesicular stomatitis
EXCLUDES 1   acute necrotizing ulcerative stomatitis (A69.1)
       Vincent's stomatitis (A69.1)

K12.2   Cellulitis and abscess of mouth
Cellulitis of mouth (floor)
Submandibular abscess
EXCLUDES 2   abscess of salivary gland (K11.3)
       abscess of tongue (K14.0)
       periapical abscess (K04.6-K04.7)
       periodontal abscess (K05.21)
       peritonsillar abscess (J36)

✓5ᵗʰ K12.3   Oral mucositis (ulcerative)
Mucositis (oral) (oropharyneal)
EXCLUDES 2   gastrointestinal mucositis (ulcerative) (K92.81)
       mucositis (ulcerative) of vagina and vulva (N76.81)
       nasal mucositis (ulcerative) (J34.81)

   K12.30   Oral mucositis (ulcerative), unspecified   ▽

   K12.31   Oral mucositis (ulcerative) due to antineoplastic therapy
Use additional code for adverse effect, if applicable, to identify antineoplastic and immunosuppressive drugs (T45.1X5)
Use additional code for other antineoplastic therapy, such as:
radiological procedure and radiotherapy (Y84.2)

   K12.32   Oral mucositis (ulcerative) due to other drugs
Use additional code for adverse effect, if applicable, to identify drug (T36-T50 with fifth or sixth character 5)

   K12.33   Oral mucositis (ulcerative) due to radiation
Use additional external cause code (W88-W90, X39.0-) to identify cause

   K12.39   Other oral mucositis (ulcerative)
Viral oral mucositis (ulcerative)

✓4ᵗʰ K13   Other diseases of lip and oral mucosa
INCLUDES   epithelial disturbances of tongue
Use additional code to identify:
alcohol abuse and dependence (F10.-)
exposure to environmental tobacco smoke (Z77.22)
exposure to tobacco smoke in the perinatal period (P96.81)
history of tobacco dependence (Z87.891)
occupational exposure to environmental tobacco smoke (Z57.31)
tobacco dependence (F17.-)
tobacco use (Z72.0)
EXCLUDES 2   certain disorders of gingiva and edentulous alveolar ridge (K05-K06)
       cysts of oral region (K09.-)
       diseases of tongue (K14.-)
       stomatitis and related lesions (K12.-)

K13.0   Diseases of lips
Abscess of lips   Exfoliative cheilitis
Angular cheilitis   Fistula of lips
Cellulitis of lips   Glandular cheilitis
Cheilitis NOS   Hypertrophy of lips
Cheilodynia   Perlèche NEC
Cheilosis
EXCLUDES 1   ariboflavinosis (E53.0)
       cheilitis due to radiation-related disorders (L55-L59)
       congenital fistula of lips (Q38.0)
       congenital hypertrophy of lips (Q18.6)
       Perlèche due to candidiasis (B37.83)
       Perlèche due to riboflavin deficiency (E53.0)

K13.1   Cheek and lip biting

✓5ᵗʰ K13.2   Leukoplakia and other disturbances of oral epithelium, including tongue
EXCLUDES 1   carcinoma in situ of oral epithelium (D00.0-)
       hairy leukoplakia (K13.3)

   K13.21   Leukoplakia of oral mucosa, including tongue
Leukokeratosis of oral mucosa
Leukoplakia of gingiva, lips, tongue
EXCLUDES 1   hairy leukoplakia (K13.3)
       leukokeratosis nicotina palati (K13.24)

   K13.22   Minimal keratinized residual ridge mucosa
Minimal keratinization of alveolar ridge mucosa

   K13.23   Excessive keratinized residual ridge mucosa
Excessive keratinization of alveolar ridge mucosa

   K13.24   Leukokeratosis nicotina palati
Smoker's palate

   K13.29   Other disturbances of oral epithelium, including tongue
Erythroplakia of mouth or tongue
Focal epithelial hyperplasia of mouth or tongue
Leukoedema of mouth or tongue
Other oral epithelium disturbances

K13.3   Hairy leukoplakia

K13.4   Granuloma and granuloma-like lesions of oral mucosa
Eosinophilic granuloma
Granuloma pyogenicum
Verrucous xanthoma

K13.5   Oral submucous fibrosis
Submucous fibrosis of tongue

K13.6   Irritative hyperplasia of oral mucosa
EXCLUDES 2   irritative hyperplasia of edentulous ridge [denture hyperplasia] (K06.2)

✓5ᵗʰ K13.7   Other and unspecified lesions of oral mucosa

   K13.70   Unspecified lesions of oral mucosa   ▽

   K13.79   Other lesions of oral mucosa
Focal oral mucinosis

EXCLUDES 1 Not coded here   *EXCLUDES 2* Not included here   **N** Newborn Age: 0   **P** Pediatric Age: 0-17   **M** Maternity Age: 12-55   **A** Adult Age: 15-124

✓4ᵗʰ K14 Diseases of tongue

Use additional code to identify:
- alcohol abuse and dependence (F10.-)
- exposure to environmental tobacco smoke (Z77.22)
- history of tobacco dependence (Z87.891)
- occupational exposure to environmental tobacco smoke (Z57.31)
- tobacco dependence (F17.-)
- tobacco use (Z72.0)

EXCLUDES 2   erythroplakia (K13.29)
     focal epithelial hyperplasia (K13.29)
     leukedema of tongue (K13.29)
     leukoplakia of tongue (K13.21)
     hairy leukoplakia (K13.3)
     macroglossia (congenital) (Q38.2)
     submucous fibrosis of tongue (K13.5)

K14.0 Glossitis
Abscess of tongue
Ulceration (traumatic) of tongue
EXCLUDES 1   atrophic glossitis (K14.4)

K14.1 Geographic tongue
Benign migratory glossitis
Glossitis areata exfoliativa

K14.2 Median rhomboid glossitis

K14.3 Hypertrophy of tongue papillae
Black hairy tongue
Coated tongue
Hypertrophy of foliate papillae
Lingua villosa nigra

K14.4 Atrophy of tongue papillae
Atrophic glossitis

K14.5 Plicated tongue
Fissured tongue
Furrowed tongue
Scrotal tongue
EXCLUDES 1   fissured tongue, congenital (Q38.3)

K14.6 Glossodynia
Glossopyrosis
Painful tongue

K14.8 Other diseases of tongue
Atrophy of tongue   Glossocele
Crenated tongue   Glossoptosis
Enlargement of tongue   Hypertrophy of tongue

K14.9 Disease of tongue, unspecified ▽
Glossopathy NOS

Diseases of esophagus, stomach and duodenum (K20-K31)

EXCLUDES 2   hiatus hernia (K44.-)

✓4ᵗʰ K20 Esophagitis

Use additional code to identify:
- alcohol abuse and dependence (F10.-)

EXCLUDES 1   erosion of esophagus (K22.1-)
     esophagitis with gastro-esophageal reflux disease (K21.0)
     reflux esophagitis (K21.0)
     ulcerative esophagitis (K22.1-)
EXCLUDES 2   eosinophilic gastritis or gastroenteritis (K52.81)

K20.0 Eosinophilic esophagitis

K20.8 Other esophagitis
Abscess of esophagus

K20.9 Esophagitis, unspecified ▽
Esophagitis NOS

✓4ᵗʰ K21 Gastro-esophageal reflux disease

EXCLUDES 1   newborn esophageal reflux (P78.83)

K21.0 Gastro-esophageal reflux disease with esophagitis
Reflux esophagitis

K21.9 Gastro-esophageal reflux disease without esophagitis
Esophageal reflux NOS
AHA: 2016, 1Q, 18

✓4ᵗʰ K22 Other diseases of esophagus

EXCLUDES 2   esophageal varices (I85.-)

K22.0 Achalasia of cardia
Achalasia NOS
Cardiospasm
EXCLUDES 1   congenital cardiospasm (Q39.5)
DEF: Esophageal motility disorder; caused by absence of esophageal peristalsis and impaired relaxation of lower esophageal sphincter; characterized by dysphagia, regurgitation, and heartburn.

✓5ᵗʰ K22.1 Ulcer of esophagus
Barrett's ulcer
Erosion of esophagus
Fungal ulcer of esophagus
Peptic ulcer of esophagus
Ulcer of esophagus due to ingestion of chemicals
Ulcer of esophagus due to ingestion of drugs and medicaments
Ulcerative esophagitis
Code first poisoning due to drug or toxin, if applicable (T36-T65 with fifth or sixth character 1-4 or 6)
Use additional code for adverse effect, if applicable, to identify drug (T36-T50 with fifth or sixth character 5)
EXCLUDES 1   Barrett's esophagus (K22.7-)

K22.10 Ulcer of esophagus without bleeding
Ulcer of esophagus NOS

K22.11 Ulcer of esophagus with bleeding
EXCLUDES 2   bleeding esophageal varices (I85.01, I85.11)

K22.2 Esophageal obstruction
Compression of esophagus
Constriction of esophagus
Stenosis of esophagus
Stricture of esophagus
EXCLUDES 1   congenital stenosis or stricture of esophagus (Q39.3)

K22.3 Perforation of esophagus
Rupture of esophagus
EXCLUDES 1   traumatic perforation of (thoracic) esophagus (S27.8-)

K22.4 Dyskinesia of esophagus
Corkscrew esophagus
Diffuse esophageal spasm
Spasm of esophagus
EXCLUDES 1   cardiospasm (K22.0)

K22.5 Diverticulum of esophagus, acquired
Esophageal pouch, acquired
EXCLUDES 1   diverticulum of esophagus (congenital) (Q39.6)

K22.6 Gastro-esophageal laceration-hemorrhage syndrome
Mallory-Weiss syndrome

✓5ᵗʰ K22.7 Barrett's esophagus
Barrett's disease
Barrett's syndrome
EXCLUDES 1   Barrett's ulcer (K22.1)
     malignant neoplasm of esophagus (C15.-)
DEF: A metaplastic disorder in which specialized columnar epithelial cells replace the normal squamous epithelial cells; secondary to chronic gastroesophageal reflux damage to the mucosa; increases risk of developing adenocarcinoma.

K22.70 Barrett's esophagus without dysplasia
Barrett's esophagus NOS

✓6ᵗʰ K22.71 Barrett's esophagus with dysplasia

K22.710 Barrett's esophagus with low grade dysplasia

K22.711 Barrett's esophagus with high grade dysplasia

K22.719 Barrett's esophagus with dysplasia, unspecified ▽

K22.8 Other specified diseases of esophagus
Hemorrhage of esophagus NOS
EXCLUDES 2   esophageal varices (I85.-)
     Paterson-Kelly syndrome (D50.1)

K22.9 Disease of esophagus, unspecified ▽

K23 Disorders of esophagus in diseases classified elsewhere

Code first underlying disease, such as:
- congenital syphilis (A50.5)

EXCLUDES 1   late syphilis (A52.79)
     megaesophagus due to Chagas' disease (B57.31)
     tuberculosis (A18.83)

✓4ᵗʰ K25 Gastric ulcer

INCLUDES   erosion (acute) of stomach
     pylorus ulcer (peptic)
     stomach ulcer (peptic)
Use additional code to identify:
- alcohol abuse and dependence (F10.-)

EXCLUDES 1   acute gastritis (K29.0-)
     peptic ulcer NOS (K27.-)

K25.0 Acute gastric ulcer with hemorrhage

K25.1 Acute gastric ulcer with perforation   HCC

K25.2 Acute gastric ulcer with both hemorrhage and perforation   HCC

K25.3 Acute gastric ulcer without hemorrhage or perforation

✓ Additional Character Req   ✓ₓ7ᵗʰ Placeholder Alert   Manifestation   HCC CMS-HCC Condition   ▽ Unspecified Code   ►◄ Revised Text   ● New Code   ▲ Revised Code Title

Gastrointestinal Ulcers

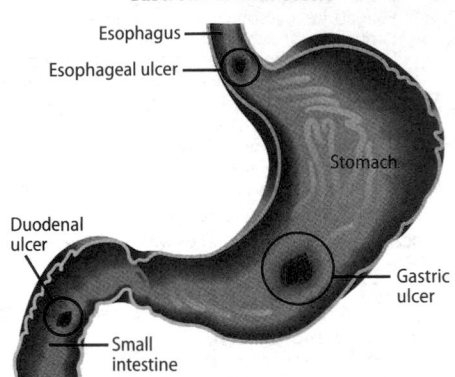

Esophagus

Esophageal ulcer

Stomach

Duodenal ulcer

Gastric ulcer

Small intestine

K25.4 Chronic or unspecified gastric ulcer with hemorrhage

K25.5 Chronic or unspecified gastric ulcer with perforation — HCC

K25.6 Chronic or unspecified gastric ulcer with both hemorrhage and perforation — HCC

K25.7 Chronic gastric ulcer without hemorrhage or perforation

K25.9 Gastric ulcer, unspecified as acute or chronic, without hemorrhage or perforation ▽

✓4ᵗʰ K26 Duodenal ulcer
> INCLUDES   erosion (acute) of duodenum
> duodenum ulcer (peptic)
> postpyloric ulcer (peptic)
> Use additional code to identify:
> alcohol abuse and dependence (F10.-)
> EXCLUDES 1 peptic ulcer NOS (K27.-)

K26.0 Acute duodenal ulcer with hemorrhage

K26.1 Acute duodenal ulcer with perforation — HCC

K26.2 Acute duodenal ulcer with both hemorrhage and perforation — HCC

K26.3 Acute duodenal ulcer without hemorrhage or perforation

K26.4 Chronic or unspecified duodenal ulcer with hemorrhage
> AHA: 2016, 1Q, 14

K26.5 Chronic or unspecified duodenal ulcer with perforation — HCC

K26.6 Chronic or unspecified duodenal ulcer with both hemorrhage and perforation — HCC

K26.7 Chronic duodenal ulcer without hemorrhage or perforation

K26.9 Duodenal ulcer, unspecified as acute or chronic, without hemorrhage or perforation ▽

✓4ᵗʰ K27 Peptic ulcer, site unspecified
> INCLUDES   gastroduodenal ulcer NOS
> peptic ulcer NOS
> Use additional code to identify:
> alcohol abuse and dependence (F10.-)
> EXCLUDES 1 peptic ulcer of newborn (P78.82)

K27.0 Acute peptic ulcer, site unspecified, with hemorrhage

K27.1 Acute peptic ulcer, site unspecified, with perforation — HCC

K27.2 Acute peptic ulcer, site unspecified, with both hemorrhage and perforation — HCC

K27.3 Acute peptic ulcer, site unspecified, without hemorrhage or perforation

K27.4 Chronic or unspecified peptic ulcer, site unspecified, with hemorrhage

K27.5 Chronic or unspecified peptic ulcer, site unspecified, with perforation — HCC

K27.6 Chronic or unspecified peptic ulcer, site unspecified, with both hemorrhage and perforation — HCC

K27.7 Chronic peptic ulcer, site unspecified, without hemorrhage or perforation

K27.9 Peptic ulcer, site unspecified, unspecified as acute or chronic, without hemorrhage or perforation ▽

✓4ᵗʰ K28 Gastrojejunal ulcer
> INCLUDES   anastomotic ulcer (peptic) or erosion
> gastrocolic ulcer (peptic) or erosion
> gastrointestinal ulcer (peptic) or erosion
> gastrojejunal ulcer (peptic) or erosion
> jejunal ulcer (peptic) or erosion
> marginal ulcer (peptic) or erosion
> stomal ulcer (peptic) or erosion
> Use additional code to identify:
> alcohol abuse and dependence (F10.-)
> EXCLUDES 1 primary ulcer of small intestine (K63.3)

K28.0 Acute gastrojejunal ulcer with hemorrhage

K28.1 Acute gastrojejunal ulcer with perforation — HCC

K28.2 Acute gastrojejunal ulcer with both hemorrhage and perforation — HCC

K28.3 Acute gastrojejunal ulcer without hemorrhage or perforation

K28.4 Chronic or unspecified gastrojejunal ulcer with hemorrhage

K28.5 Chronic or unspecified gastrojejunal ulcer with perforation — HCC

K28.6 Chronic or unspecified gastrojejunal ulcer with both hemorrhage and perforation — HCC

K28.7 Chronic gastrojejunal ulcer without hemorrhage or perforation

K28.9 Gastrojejunal ulcer, unspecified as acute or chronic, without hemorrhage or perforation ▽

✓4ᵗʰ K29 Gastritis and duodenitis
> EXCLUDES 1 eosinophilic gastritis or gastroenteritis (K52.81)
> Zollinger-Ellison syndrome (E16.4)

✓5ᵗʰ K29.0 Acute gastritis
> Use additional code to identify:
> alcohol abuse and dependence (F10.-)
> EXCLUDES 1 erosion (acute) of stomach (K25.-)

K29.00 Acute gastritis without bleeding

K29.01 Acute gastritis with bleeding

✓5ᵗʰ K29.2 Alcoholic gastritis
> Use additional code to identify:
> alcohol abuse and dependence (F10.-)

K29.20 Alcoholic gastritis without bleeding

K29.21 Alcoholic gastritis with bleeding

✓5ᵗʰ K29.3 Chronic superficial gastritis

K29.30 Chronic superficial gastritis without bleeding

K29.31 Chronic superficial gastritis with bleeding

✓5ᵗʰ K29.4 Chronic atrophic gastritis
> Gastric atrophy

K29.40 Chronic atrophic gastritis without bleeding

K29.41 Chronic atrophic gastritis with bleeding

✓5ᵗʰ K29.5 Unspecified chronic gastritis
> Chronic antral gastritis
> Chronic fundal gastritis

K29.50 Unspecified chronic gastritis without bleeding ▽

K29.51 Unspecified chronic gastritis with bleeding ▽

✓5ᵗʰ K29.6 Other gastritis
> Giant hypertrophic gastritis
> Granulomatous gastritis
> Ménétrier's disease

K29.60 Other gastritis without bleeding

K29.61 Other gastritis with bleeding

✓5ᵗʰ K29.7 Gastritis, unspecified

K29.70 Gastritis, unspecified, without bleeding ▽

K29.71 Gastritis, unspecified, with bleeding ▽

✓5ᵗʰ K29.8 Duodenitis

K29.80 Duodenitis without bleeding

K29.81 Duodenitis with bleeding

✓5ᵗʰ K29.9 Gastroduodenitis, unspecified

K29.90 Gastroduodenitis, unspecified, without bleeding ▽

K29.91 Gastroduodenitis, unspecified, with bleeding ▽

K30 Functional dyspepsia
> Indigestion
> EXCLUDES 1 dyspepsia NOS (R10.13)
> heartburn (R12)
> nervous dyspepsia (F45.8)
> neurotic dyspepsia (F45.8)
> psychogenic dyspepsia (F45.8)

EXCLUDES 1 Not coded here | EXCLUDES 2 Not included here | N Newborn Age: 0 | P Pediatric Age: 0-17 | M Maternity Age: 12-55 | A Adult Age: 15-124

678 | ICD-10-CM 2018

✓4ᵗʰ K31 Other diseases of stomach and duodenum
> INCLUDES functional disorders of stomach
> EXCLUDES 2 *diabetic gastroparesis (E08.43, E09.43, E10.43, E11.43, E13.43)*
> *diverticulum of duodenum (K57.00-K57.13)*

K31.0 Acute dilatation of stomach
Acute distention of stomach

K31.1 Adult hypertrophic pyloric stenosis   **A**
Pyloric stenosis NOS
> EXCLUDES 1 *congenital or infantile pyloric stenosis (Q40.0)*

K31.2 Hourglass stricture and stenosis of stomach
> EXCLUDES 1 *congenital hourglass stomach (Q40.2)*
> *hourglass contraction of stomach (K31.89)*

K31.3 Pylorospasm, not elsewhere classified
> EXCLUDES 1 *congenital or infantile pylorospasm (Q40.0)*
> *neurotic pylorospasm (F45.8)*
> *psychogenic pylorospasm (F45.8)*

K31.4 Gastric diverticulum
> EXCLUDES 1 *congenital diverticulum of stomach (Q40.2)*

K31.5 Obstruction of duodenum
Constriction of duodenum
Duodenal ileus (chronic)
Stenosis of duodenum
Stricture of duodenum
Volvulus of duodenum
> EXCLUDES 1 *congenital stenosis of duodenum (Q41.0)*

K31.6 Fistula of stomach and duodenum
Gastrocolic fistula
Gastrojejunocolic fistula

K31.7 Polyp of stomach and duodenum
> EXCLUDES 1 *adenomatous polyp of stomach (D13.1)*

✓5ᵗʰ K31.8 Other specified diseases of stomach and duodenum

   ✓6ᵗʰ K31.81 Angiodysplasia of stomach and duodenum

     K31.811 Angiodysplasia of stomach and duodenum with bleeding

     K31.819 Angiodysplasia of stomach and duodenum without bleeding
Angiodysplasia of stomach and duodenum NOS

   K31.82 Dieulafoy lesion (hemorrhagic) of stomach and duodenum
> EXCLUDES 2 *Dieulafoy lesion of intestine (K63.81)*

   K31.83 Achlorhydria
DEF: Absence of hydrochloric acid in gastric secretions due to gastric mucosa atrophy; unresponsive to histamines; also known as gastric anacidity.

   K31.84 Gastroparesis
Gastroparalysis
Code first underlying disease, if known, such as:
   anorexia nervosa (F50.0-)
   diabetes mellitus (E08.43, E09.43, E10.43, E11.43, E13.43)
   scleroderma (M34.-)
AHA: 2013, 4Q, 114

   K31.89 Other diseases of stomach and duodenum
AHA: 2017, 1Q, 28

K31.9 Disease of stomach and duodenum, unspecified   ▽

Diseases of appendix (K35-K38)

✓4ᵗʰ K35 Acute appendicitis

K35.2 Acute appendicitis with generalized peritonitis
Appendicitis (acute) with generalized (diffuse) peritonitis following rupture or perforation of appendix
Perforated appendix NOS
Ruptured appendix NOS

K35.3 Acute appendicitis with localized peritonitis
Acute appendicitis with or without perforation or rupture with peritonitis NOS
Acute appendicitis with or without perforation or rupture with localized peritonitis
Acute appendicitis with peritoneal abscess

✓5ᵗʰ K35.8 Other and unspecified acute appendicitis

   K35.80 Unspecified acute appendicitis   ▽
Acute appendicitis NOS
Acute appendicitis without (localized) (generalized) peritonitis

   K35.89 Other acute appendicitis

K36 Other appendicitis
Chronic appendicitis
Recurrent appendicitis

K37 Unspecified appendicitis   ▽
> EXCLUDES 1 *unspecified appendicitis with peritonitis (K35.2-K35.3)*

✓4ᵗʰ K38 Other diseases of appendix

K38.0 Hyperplasia of appendix

K38.1 Appendicular concretions
Fecalith of appendix
Stercolith of appendix

K38.2 Diverticulum of appendix

K38.3 Fistula of appendix

K38.8 Other specified diseases of appendix
Intussusception of appendix

K38.9 Disease of appendix, unspecified   ▽

Hernia (K40-K46)

> NOTE Hernia with both gangrene and obstruction is classified to hernia with gangrene.
> INCLUDES acquired hernia
> congenital [except diaphragmatic or hiatus] hernia
> recurrent hernia

✓4ᵗʰ K40 Inguinal hernia
> INCLUDES bubonocele
> direct inguinal hernia
> double inguinal hernia
> indirect inguinal hernia
> inguinal hernia NOS
> oblique inguinal hernia
> scrotal hernia

✓5ᵗʰ K40.0 Bilateral inguinal hernia, with obstruction, without gangrene
Inguinal hernia (bilateral) causing obstruction without gangrene
Incarcerated inguinal hernia (bilateral) without gangrene
Irreducible inguinal hernia (bilateral) without gangrene
Strangulated inguinal hernia (bilateral) without gangrene

   K40.00 Bilateral inguinal hernia, with obstruction, without gangrene, not specified as recurrent
Bilateral inguinal hernia, with obstruction, without gangrene NOS

   K40.01 Bilateral inguinal hernia, with obstruction, without gangrene, recurrent

✓5ᵗʰ K40.1 Bilateral inguinal hernia, with gangrene

   K40.10 Bilateral inguinal hernia, with gangrene, not specified as recurrent
Bilateral inguinal hernia, with gangrene NOS

   K40.11 Bilateral inguinal hernia, with gangrene, recurrent

✓5ᵗʰ K40.2 Bilateral inguinal hernia, without obstruction or gangrene

   K40.20 Bilateral inguinal hernia, without obstruction or gangrene, not specified as recurrent
Bilateral inguinal hernia NOS

   K40.21 Bilateral inguinal hernia, without obstruction or gangrene, recurrent

✓5ᵗʰ K40.3 Unilateral inguinal hernia, with obstruction, without gangrene
Inguinal hernia (unilateral) causing obstruction without gangrene
Incarcerated inguinal hernia (unilateral) without gangrene
Irreducible inguinal hernia (unilateral) without gangrene
Strangulated inguinal hernia (unilateral) without gangrene

   K40.30 Unilateral inguinal hernia, with obstruction, without gangrene, not specified as recurrent
Inguinal hernia, with obstruction NOS
Unilateral inguinal hernia, with obstruction, without gangrene NOS

   K40.31 Unilateral inguinal hernia, with obstruction, without gangrene, recurrent

✓5ᵗʰ K40.4 Unilateral inguinal hernia, with gangrene

   K40.40 Unilateral inguinal hernia, with gangrene, not specified as recurrent
Inguinal hernia with gangrene NOS
Unilateral inguinal hernia with gangrene NOS

   K40.41 Unilateral inguinal hernia, with gangrene, recurrent

✓5ᵗʰ K40.9 Unilateral inguinal hernia, without obstruction or gangrene

   K40.90 Unilateral inguinal hernia, without obstruction or gangrene, not specified as recurrent
Inguinal hernia NOS
Unilateral inguinal hernia NOS

   K40.91 Unilateral inguinal hernia, without obstruction or gangrene, recurrent

✓ Additional Character Req   ✓x7ᵗʰ Placeholder Alert   Manifestation   HCC CMS-HCC Condition   ▽ Unspecified Code   ►◄ Revised Text   ● New Code   ▲ Revised Code Title

ICD-10-CM 2018   **679**

Chapter 11. Diseases of the Digestive System

K41–K44.1

Hernia Sites

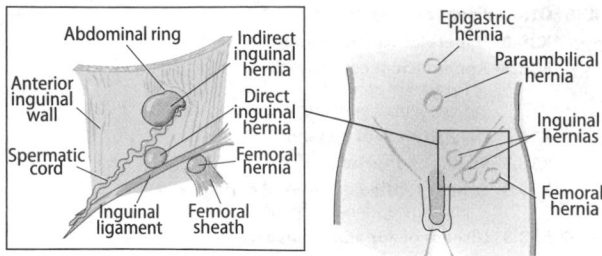

✓4ᵗʰ **K41   Femoral hernia**

✓5ᵗʰ **K41.0   Bilateral femoral hernia, with obstruction, without gangrene**
Femoral hernia (bilateral) causing obstruction, without gangrene
Incarcerated femoral hernia (bilateral), without gangrene
Irreducible femoral hernia (bilateral), without gangrene
Strangulated femoral hernia (bilateral), without gangrene

    K41.00   Bilateral femoral hernia, with obstruction, without gangrene, not specified as recurrent
Bilateral femoral hernia, with obstruction, without gangrene NOS

    K41.01   Bilateral femoral hernia, with obstruction, without gangrene, recurrent

✓5ᵗʰ **K41.1   Bilateral femoral hernia, with gangrene**

    K41.10   Bilateral femoral hernia, with gangrene, not specified as recurrent
Bilateral femoral hernia, with gangrene NOS

    K41.11   Bilateral femoral hernia, with gangrene, recurrent

✓5ᵗʰ **K41.2   Bilateral femoral hernia, without obstruction or gangrene**

    K41.20   Bilateral femoral hernia, without obstruction or gangrene, not specified as recurrent
Bilateral femoral hernia NOS

    K41.21   Bilateral femoral hernia, without obstruction or gangrene, recurrent

✓5ᵗʰ **K41.3   Unilateral femoral hernia, with obstruction, without gangrene**
Femoral hernia (unilateral) causing obstruction, without gangrene
Incarcerated femoral hernia (unilateral), without gangrene
Irreducible femoral hernia (unilateral), without gangrene
Strangulated femoral hernia (unilateral), without gangrene

    K41.30   Unilateral femoral hernia, with obstruction, without gangrene, not specified as recurrent
Femoral hernia, with obstruction NOS
Unilateral femoral hernia, with obstruction NOS

    K41.31   Unilateral femoral hernia, with obstruction, without gangrene, recurrent

✓5ᵗʰ **K41.4   Unilateral femoral hernia, with gangrene**

    K41.40   Unilateral femoral hernia, with gangrene, not specified as recurrent
Femoral hernia, with gangrene NOS
Unilateral femoral hernia, with gangrene NOS

    K41.41   Unilateral femoral hernia, with gangrene, recurrent

✓5ᵗʰ **K41.9   Unilateral femoral hernia, without obstruction or gangrene**

    K41.90   Unilateral femoral hernia, without obstruction or gangrene, not specified as recurrent
Femoral hernia NOS
Unilateral femoral hernia NOS

    K41.91   Unilateral femoral hernia, without obstruction or gangrene, recurrent

✓4ᵗʰ **K42   Umbilical hernia**
INCLUDES   paraumbilical hernia
EXCLUDES 1   *omphalocele (Q79.2)*

K42.0   Umbilical hernia with obstruction, without gangrene
Umbilical hernia causing obstruction, without gangrene
Incarcerated umbilical hernia, without gangrene
Irreducible umbilical hernia, without gangrene
Strangulated umbilical hernia, without gangrene

K42.1   Umbilical hernia with gangrene
Gangrenous umbilical hernia

K42.9   Umbilical hernia without obstruction or gangrene
Umbilical hernia NOS

✓4ᵗʰ **K43   Ventral hernia**

K43.0   Incisional hernia with obstruction, without gangrene
Incisional hernia causing obstruction, without gangrene
Incarcerated incisional hernia, without gangrene
Irreducible incisional hernia, without gangrene
Strangulated incisional hernia, without gangrene

K43.1   Incisional hernia with gangrene
Gangrenous incisional hernia

K43.2   Incisional hernia without obstruction or gangrene
Incisional hernia NOS

K43.3   Parastomal hernia with obstruction, without gangrene
Incarcerated parastomal hernia, without gangrene
Irreducible parastomal hernia, without gangrene
Parastomal hernia causing obstruction, without gangrene
Strangulated parastomal hernia, without gangrene

K43.4   Parastomal hernia with gangrene
Gangrenous parastomal hernia

K43.5   Parastomal hernia without obstruction or gangrene
Parastomal hernia NOS

K43.6   Other and unspecified ventral hernia with obstruction, without gangrene   ▽
Epigastric hernia causing obstruction, without gangrene
Hypogastric hernia causing obstruction, without gangrene
Incarcerated epigastric hernia without gangrene
Incarcerated hypogastric hernia without gangrene
Incarcerated midline hernia without gangrene
Incarcerated spigelian hernia without gangrene
Incarcerated subxiphoid hernia without gangrene
Irreducible epigastric hernia without gangrene
Irreducible hypogastric hernia without gangrene
Irreducible midline hernia without gangrene
Irreducible spigelian hernia without gangrene
Irreducible subxiphoid hernia without gangrene
Midline hernia causing obstruction, without gangrene
Spigelian hernia causing obstruction, without gangrene
Strangulated epigastric hernia without gangrene
Strangulated hypogastric hernia without gangrene
Strangulated midline hernia without gangrene
Strangulated spigelian hernia without gangrene
Strangulated subxiphoid hernia without gangrene
Subxiphoid hernia causing obstruction, without gangrene

K43.7   Other and unspecified ventral hernia with gangrene   ▽
Any condition listed under K43.6 specified as gangrenous

K43.9   Ventral hernia without obstruction or gangrene   ▽
Epigastric hernia
Ventral hernia NOS

✓4ᵗʰ **K44   Diaphragmatic hernia**
INCLUDES   hiatus hernia (esophageal) (sliding)
paraesophageal hernia
EXCLUDES 1   *congenital diaphragmatic hernia (Q79.0)*
congenital hiatus hernia (Q40.1)

K44.0   Diaphragmatic hernia with obstruction, without gangrene
Diaphragmatic hernia causing obstruction
Incarcerated diaphragmatic hernia
Irreducible diaphragmatic hernia
Strangulated diaphragmatic hernia

K44.1   Diaphragmatic hernia with gangrene
Gangrenous diaphragmatic hernia

Hiatal Hernia

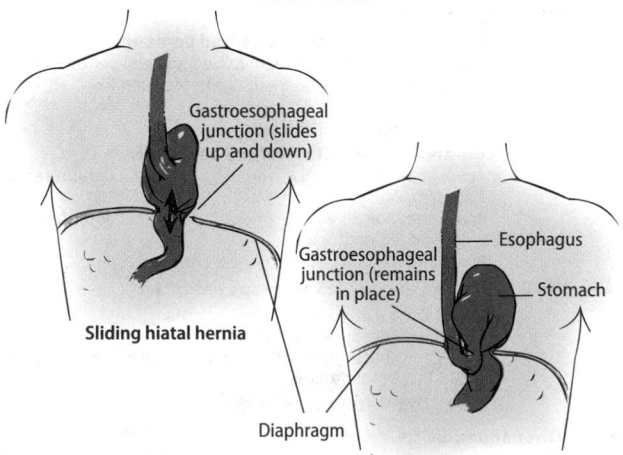

Sliding hiatal hernia

Paraesophageal hiatal hernia

EXCLUDES 1 Not coded here   EXCLUDES 2 Not included here   N Newborn Age: 0   P Pediatric Age: 0-17   M Maternity Age: 12-55   A Adult Age: 15-124

680   ICD-10-CM 2018

K44.9 **Diaphragmatic hernia without obstruction or gangrene**
Diaphragmatic hernia NOS

✓4ᵗʰ **K45** **Other abdominal hernia**
    INCLUDES   abdominal hernia, specified site NEC
             lumbar hernia
             obturator hernia
             pudendal hernia
             retroperitoneal hernia
             sciatic hernia

K45.0 **Other specified abdominal hernia with obstruction, without gangrene**
Other specified abdominal hernia causing obstruction
Other specified incarcerated abdominal hernia
Other specified irreducible abdominal hernia
Other specified strangulated abdominal hernia

K45.1 **Other specified abdominal hernia with gangrene**
Any condition listed under K45 specified as gangrenous

K45.8 **Other specified abdominal hernia without obstruction or gangrene**

✓4ᵗʰ **K46** **Unspecified abdominal hernia**
    INCLUDES   enterocele
             epiplocele
             hernia NOS
             interstitial hernia
             intestinal hernia
             intra-abdominal hernia
    EXCLUDES 1   *vaginal enterocele (N81.5)*

K46.0 **Unspecified abdominal hernia with obstruction, without gangrene** ▽
Unspecified abdominal hernia causing obstruction
Unspecified incarcerated abdominal hernia
Unspecified irreducible abdominal hernia
Unspecified strangulated abdominal hernia

K46.1 **Unspecified abdominal hernia with gangrene** ▽
Any condition listed under K46 specified as gangrenous

K46.9 **Unspecified abdominal hernia without obstruction or gangrene** ▽
Abdominal hernia NOS

Noninfective enteritis and colitis (K50-K52)

    INCLUDES   noninfective inflammatory bowel disease
    EXCLUDES 1   *irritable bowel syndrome (K58.-)*
                  megacolon (K59.3-)

✓4ᵗʰ **K50** **Crohn's disease [regional enteritis]**
    INCLUDES   granulomatous enteritis
Use additional code to identify manifestations, such as:
    pyoderma gangrenosum (L88)
    EXCLUDES 1   *ulcerative colitis (K51.-)*
    AHA: 2012, 4Q, 104

✓5ᵗʰ **K50.0** **Crohn's disease of small intestine**
Crohn's disease [regional enteritis] of duodenum
Crohn's disease [regional enteritis] of ileum
Crohn's disease [regional enteritis] of jejunum
Regional ileitis
Terminal ileitis
    EXCLUDES 1   *Crohn's disease of both small and large intestine (K50.8-)*

K50.00 **Crohn's disease of small intestine without complications** HCC

✓6ᵗʰ **K50.01** **Crohn's disease of small intestine with complications**

    K50.011 **Crohn's disease of small intestine with rectal bleeding** HCC

    K50.012 **Crohn's disease of small intestine with intestinal obstruction** HCC

    K50.013 **Crohn's disease of small intestine with fistula** HCC

    K50.014 **Crohn's disease of small intestine with abscess** HCC
             AHA: 2012, 4Q, 104

    K50.018 **Crohn's disease of small intestine with other complication** HCC

    K50.019 **Crohn's disease of small intestine with unspecified complications** HCC ▽

✓5ᵗʰ **K50.1** **Crohn's disease of large intestine**
Crohn's disease [regional enteritis] of colon
Crohn's disease [regional enteritis] of large bowel
Crohn's disease [regional enteritis] of rectum
Granulomatous colitis
Regional colitis
    EXCLUDES 1   *Crohn's disease of both small and large intestine (K50.8)*

K50.10 **Crohn's disease of large intestine without complications** HCC

✓6ᵗʰ **K50.11** **Crohn's disease of large intestine with complications**

    K50.111 **Crohn's disease of large intestine with rectal bleeding** HCC

    K50.112 **Crohn's disease of large intestine with intestinal obstruction** HCC

    K50.113 **Crohn's disease of large intestine with fistula** HCC

    K50.114 **Crohn's disease of large intestine with abscess** HCC

    K50.118 **Crohn's disease of large intestine with other complication** HCC

    K50.119 **Crohn's disease of large intestine with unspecified complications** HCC ▽

✓5ᵗʰ **K50.8** **Crohn's disease of both small and large intestine**

K50.80 **Crohn's disease of both small and large intestine without complications** HCC

✓6ᵗʰ **K50.81** **Crohn's disease of both small and large intestine with complications**

    K50.811 **Crohn's disease of both small and large intestine with rectal bleeding** HCC

    K50.812 **Crohn's disease of both small and large intestine with intestinal obstruction** HCC

    K50.813 **Crohn's disease of both small and large intestine with fistula** HCC

    K50.814 **Crohn's disease of both small and large intestine with abscess** HCC

    K50.818 **Crohn's disease of both small and large intestine with other complication** HCC

    K50.819 **Crohn's disease of both small and large intestine with unspecified complications** HCC ▽

✓5ᵗʰ **K50.9** **Crohn's disease, unspecified**

K50.90 **Crohn's disease, unspecified, without complications** HCC ▽
Crohn's disease NOS
Regional enteritis NOS

✓6ᵗʰ **K50.91** **Crohn's disease, unspecified, with complications**

    K50.911 **Crohn's disease, unspecified, with rectal bleeding** HCC ▽

    K50.912 **Crohn's disease, unspecified, with intestinal obstruction** HCC ▽

    K50.913 **Crohn's disease, unspecified, with fistula** HCC ▽

    K50.914 **Crohn's disease, unspecified, with abscess** HCC ▽

    K50.918 **Crohn's disease, unspecified, with other complication** HCC ▽

    K50.919 **Crohn's disease, unspecified, with unspecified complications** HCC ▽

✓4ᵗʰ **K51** **Ulcerative colitis**
Use additional code to identify manifestations, such as:
    pyoderma gangrenosum (L88)
    EXCLUDES 1   *Crohn's disease [regional enteritis] (K50.-)*

✓5ᵗʰ **K51.0** **Ulcerative (chronic) pancolitis**
Backwash ileitis

K51.00 **Ulcerative (chronic) pancolitis without complications** HCC
Ulcerative (chronic) pancolitis NOS

✓6ᵗʰ **K51.01** **Ulcerative (chronic) pancolitis with complications**

    K51.011 **Ulcerative (chronic) pancolitis with rectal bleeding** HCC

    K51.012 **Ulcerative (chronic) pancolitis with intestinal obstruction** HCC

    K51.013 **Ulcerative (chronic) pancolitis with fistula** HCC

    K51.014 **Ulcerative (chronic) pancolitis with abscess** HCC

Chapter 11. Diseases of the Digestive System

K51.Ø18   Ulcerative (chronic) pancolitis with other complication   HCC

K51.Ø19   Ulcerative (chronic) pancolitis with unspecified complications   HCC ▽

✓5ᵗʰ **K51.2   Ulcerative (chronic) proctitis**

     K51.2Ø   **Ulcerative (chronic) proctitis without complications**   HCC
           Ulcerative (chronic) proctitis NOS

     ✓6ᵗʰ K51.21   **Ulcerative (chronic) proctitis with complications**

         K51.211   **Ulcerative (chronic) proctitis with rectal bleeding**   HCC

         K51.212   **Ulcerative (chronic) proctitis with intestinal obstruction**   HCC

         K51.213   **Ulcerative (chronic) proctitis with fistula**   HCC

         K51.214   **Ulcerative (chronic) proctitis with abscess**   HCC

         K51.218   **Ulcerative (chronic) proctitis with other complication**   HCC

         K51.219   **Ulcerative (chronic) proctitis with unspecified complications**   HCC ▽

✓5ᵗʰ **K51.3   Ulcerative (chronic) rectosigmoiditis**

     K51.3Ø   **Ulcerative (chronic) rectosigmoiditis without complications**   HCC
           Ulcerative (chronic) rectosigmoiditis NOS

     ✓6ᵗʰ K51.31   **Ulcerative (chronic) rectosigmoiditis with complications**

         K51.311   **Ulcerative (chronic) rectosigmoiditis with rectal bleeding**   HCC

         K51.312   **Ulcerative (chronic) rectosigmoiditis with intestinal obstruction**   HCC

         K51.313   **Ulcerative (chronic) rectosigmoiditis with fistula**   HCC

         K51.314   **Ulcerative (chronic) rectosigmoiditis with abscess**   HCC

         K51.318   **Ulcerative (chronic) rectosigmoiditis with other complication**   HCC

         K51.319   **Ulcerative (chronic) rectosigmoiditis with unspecified complications**   HCC ▽

✓5ᵗʰ **K51.4   Inflammatory polyps of colon**

     EXCLUDES 1   *adenomatous polyp of colon (D12.6)*
                   polyposis of colon (D12.6)
                   polyps of colon NOS (K63.5)

     K51.4Ø   **Inflammatory polyps of colon without complications**   HCC
           Inflammatory polyps of colon NOS

     ✓6ᵗʰ K51.41   **Inflammatory polyps of colon with complications**

         K51.411   **Inflammatory polyps of colon with rectal bleeding**   HCC

         K51.412   **Inflammatory polyps of colon with intestinal obstruction**   HCC

         K51.413   **Inflammatory polyps of colon with fistula**   HCC

         K51.414   **Inflammatory polyps of colon with abscess**   HCC

         K51.418   **Inflammatory polyps of colon with other complication**   HCC

         K51.419   **Inflammatory polyps of colon with unspecified complications**   HCC ▽

✓5ᵗʰ **K51.5   Left sided colitis**
         Left hemicolitis

     K51.5Ø   **Left sided colitis without complications**   HCC
           Left sided colitis NOS

     ✓6ᵗʰ K51.51   **Left sided colitis with complications**

         K51.511   **Left sided colitis with rectal bleeding**   HCC

         K51.512   **Left sided colitis with intestinal obstruction**   HCC

         K51.513   **Left sided colitis with fistula**   HCC

         K51.514   **Left sided colitis with abscess**   HCC

         K51.518   **Left sided colitis with other complication**   HCC

         K51.519   **Left sided colitis with unspecified complications**   HCC ▽

✓5ᵗʰ **K51.8   Other ulcerative colitis**

     K51.8Ø   **Other ulcerative colitis without complications**   HCC

     ✓6ᵗʰ K51.81   **Other ulcerative colitis with complications**

         K51.811   **Other ulcerative colitis with rectal bleeding**   HCC

         K51.812   **Other ulcerative colitis with intestinal obstruction**   HCC

         K51.813   **Other ulcerative colitis with fistula**   HCC

         K51.814   **Other ulcerative colitis with abscess**   HCC

         K51.818   **Other ulcerative colitis with other complication**   HCC

         K51.819   **Other ulcerative colitis with unspecified complications**   HCC ▽

✓5ᵗʰ **K51.9   Ulcerative colitis, unspecified**

     K51.9Ø   **Ulcerative colitis, unspecified, without complications**   HCC ▽

     ✓6ᵗʰ K51.91   **Ulcerative colitis, unspecified, with complications**

         K51.911   **Ulcerative colitis, unspecified with rectal bleeding**   HCC ▽

         K51.912   **Ulcerative colitis, unspecified with intestinal obstruction**   HCC ▽

         K51.913   **Ulcerative colitis, unspecified with fistula**   HCC ▽

         K51.914   **Ulcerative colitis, unspecified with abscess**   HCC ▽

         K51.918   **Ulcerative colitis, unspecified with other complication**   HCC ▽

         K51.919   **Ulcerative colitis, unspecified with unspecified complications**   HCC ▽

✓4ᵗʰ **K52   Other and unspecified noninfective gastroenteritis and colitis**

     K52.Ø   Gastroenteritis and colitis due to radiation

     K52.1   Toxic gastroenteritis and colitis
         Drug-induced gastroenteritis and colitis
         Code first (T51-T65) to identify toxic agent
         Use additional code for adverse effect, if applicable, to identify drug (T36-T5Ø with fifth or sixth character 5)

     ✓5ᵗʰ **K52.2   Allergic and dietetic gastroenteritis and colitis**
         Food hypersensitivity gastroenteritis or colitis
         Use additional code to identify type of food allergy (Z91.Ø1-, Z91.Ø2-)

         EXCLUDES 2   *allergic eosinophilic colitis (K52.82)*
                   allergic eosinophilic esophagitis (K20.Ø)
                   allergic eosinophilic gastritis (K52.81)
                   allergic eosinophilic gastroenteritis (K52.81)
                   food protein-induced proctocolitis (K52.82)

         DEF: True immunoglobulin E (IgE)-mediated allergic reaction of the lining of the stomach, intestines, or colon to food proteins; causes nausea, vomiting, diarrhea, and abdominal cramping.

         K52.21   Food protein-induced enterocolitis syndrome
             Use additional code for hypovolemic shock, if present (R57.1)

         K52.22   Food protein-induced enteropathy

         K52.29   Other allergic and dietetic gastroenteritis and colitis
             Food hypersensitivity gastroenteritis or colitis
             Immediate gastrointestinal hypersensitivity

     K52.3   Indeterminate colitis
         Colonic inflammatory bowel disease unclassified (IBDU)
         EXCLUDES 1   *unspecified colitis (K52.9)*

     ✓5ᵗʰ **K52.8   Other specified noninfective gastroenteritis and colitis**

         K52.81   Eosinophilic gastritis or gastroenteritis
             Eosinophilic enteritis
             EXCLUDES 2   *eosinophilic esophagitis (K20.Ø)*

         K52.82   Eosinophilic colitis
             Allergic proctocolitis
             Food-induced eosinophilic proctocolitis
             Food protein-induced proctocolitis
             Milk protein-induced proctocolitis

     ✓6ᵗʰ   **K52.83   Microscopic colitis**

         K52.831   Collagenous colitis

         K52.832   Lymphocytic colitis

         K52.838   Other microscopic colitis

         K52.839   Microscopic colitis, unspecified   ▽

         K52.89   Other specified noninfective gastroenteritis and colitis

EXCLUDES 1 Not coded here   EXCLUDES 2 Not included here   N Newborn Age: 0   P Pediatric Age: 0-17   M Maternity Age: 12-55   A Adult Age: 15-124

682   ICD-10-CM 2018

K52.9 Noninfective gastroenteritis and colitis, unspecified ▽

Colitis NOS
Enteritis NOS
Gastroenteritis NOS
Ileitis NOS
Jejunitis NOS
Sigmoiditis NOS

EXCLUDES 1   diarrhea NOS (R19.7)
functional diarrhea (K59.1)
infectious gastroenteritis and colitis NOS (A09)
neonatal diarrhea (noninfective) (P78.3)
psychogenic diarrhea (F45.8)

Other diseases of intestines (K55-K64)

✓4ᵗʰ **K55 Vascular disorders of intestine**

EXCLUDES 1   necrotizing enterocolitis of newborn (P77.-)

✓5ᵗʰ **K55.0 Acute vascular disorders of intestine**   HCC

Infarction of appendices epiploicae
Mesenteric (artery) (vein) embolism
Mesenteric (artery) (vein) infarction
Mesenteric (artery) (vein) thrombosis

✓6ᵗʰ **K55.01 Acute (reversible) ischemia of small intestine**

K55.011 Focal (segmental) acute (reversible)   HCC
ischemia of small intestine

K55.012 Diffuse acute (reversible) ischemia of   HCC
small intestine

K55.019 Acute (reversible) ischemia of small   HCC ▽
intestine, extent unspecified

✓6ᵗʰ **K55.02 Acute infarction of small intestine**

Gangrene of small intestine
Necrosis of small intestine

K55.021 Focal (segmental) acute infarction of   HCC
small intestine

K55.022 Diffuse acute infarction of small   HCC
intestine

K55.029 Acute infarction of small intestine,   HCC ▽
extent unspecified

✓6ᵗʰ **K55.03 Acute (reversible) ischemia of large intestine**

Acute fulminant ischemic colitis
Subacute ischemic colitis

K55.031 Focal (segmental) acute (reversible)   HCC
ischemia of large intestine

K55.032 Diffuse acute (reversible) ischemia of   HCC
large intestine

K55.039 Acute (reversible) ischemia of large   HCC ▽
intestine, extent unspecified

✓6ᵗʰ **K55.04 Acute infarction of large intestine**

Gangrene of small intestine
Necrosis of small intestine

K55.041 Focal (segmental) acute infarction of   HCC
large intestine

K55.042 Diffuse acute infarction of large   HCC
intestine

K55.049 Acute infarction of large intestine,   HCC ▽
extent unspecified

✓6ᵗʰ **K55.05 Acute (reversible) ischemia of intestine, part**
unspecified

K55.051 Focal (segmental) acute (reversible)   HCC ▽
ischemia of intestine, part unspecified

K55.052 Diffuse acute (reversible) ischemia   HCC ▽
of intestine, part unspecified

K55.059 Acute (reversible) ischemia of   HCC ▽
intestine, part and extent unspecified

✓6ᵗʰ **K55.06 Acute infarction of intestine, part unspecified**

Acute intestinal infarction
Gangrene of intestine
Necrosis of intestine

K55.061 Focal (segmental) acute infarction   HCC ▽
of intestine, part unspecified

K55.062 Diffuse acute infarction of   HCC ▽
intestine, part unspecified

K55.069 Acute infarction of intestine, part   HCC ▽
and extent unspecified

K55.1 Chronic vascular disorders of intestine   HCC

Chronic ischemic colitis
Chronic ischemic enteritis
Chronic ischemic enterocolitis
Ischemic stricture of intestine
Mesenteric atherosclerosis
Mesenteric vascular
  insufficiency

✓5ᵗʰ **K55.2 Angiodysplasia of colon**

K55.20 Angiodysplasia of colon without hemorrhage

K55.21 Angiodysplasia of colon with hemorrhage

DEF: Small vascular abnormalities due to fragile blood
vessels in the colon; results in blood loss from the
gastrointestinal (GI) tract.

✓5ᵗʰ **K55.3 Necrotizing enterocolitis**

EXCLUDES 1   necrotizing enterocolitis of newborn (P77.-)

EXCLUDES 2   necrotizing enterocolitis due to Clostridium difficile
▶(A04.7-)◀

K55.30 Necrotizing enterocolitis, unspecified   HCC ▽

Necrotizing enterocolitis, NOS

K55.31 Stage 1 necrotizing enterocolitis   HCC

Necrotizing enterocolitis without pneumatosis,
without perforation

K55.32 Stage 2 necrotizing enterocolitis   HCC

Necrotizing enterocolitis with pneumatosis, without
perforation

K55.33 Stage 3 necrotizing enterocolitis   HCC

Necrotizing enterocolitis with perforation
Necrotizing enterocolitis with pneumatosis and
perforation

K55.8 Other vascular disorders of intestine   HCC

K55.9 Vascular disorder of intestine, unspecified   HCC ▽

Ischemic colitis
Ischemic enteritis
Ischemic enterocolitis

✓4ᵗʰ **K56 Paralytic ileus and intestinal obstruction without hernia**

EXCLUDES 1   congenital stricture or stenosis of intestine (Q41-Q42)
cystic fibrosis with meconium ileus (E84.11)
~~intestinal obstruction with hernia (K40-K46)~~
ischemic stricture of intestine (K55.1)
meconium ileus NOS (P76.0)
neonatal intestinal obstructions classifiable to P76-
obstruction of duodenum (K31.5)
postprocedural intestinal obstruction ▶(K91.3-)◀
stenosis of anus or rectum (K62.4)

K56.0 Paralytic ileus   HCC

Paralysis of bowel   Paralysis of intestine
Paralysis of colon

EXCLUDES 1   gallstone ileus (K56.3)
ileus NOS (K56.7)
obstructive ileus NOS ▶(K56.69-)◀

K56.1 Intussusception   HCC

Intussusception or invagination of bowel
Intussusception or invagination of colon
Intussusception or invagination of intestine
Intussusception or invagination of rectum

EXCLUDES 2   Intussusception of appendix (K38.8)

DEF: Intestinal obstruction due to prolapse of a bowel section into
adjacent section; occurs primarily in children; symptoms include
acute abdominal pain, vomiting, and passage of blood and mucus
from rectum.

K56.2 Volvulus   HCC

Strangulation of colon or intestine
Torsion of colon or intestine
Twist of colon or intestine

EXCLUDES 2   volvulus of duodenum (K31.5)

Volvulus

Knotted
intestine
(volvulus)

☑ Additional Character Req   ✓x7ᵗʰ Placeholder Alert   Manifestation   HCC CMS-HCC Condition   ▽ Unspecified Code   ▶◀ Revised Text   ● New Code   ▲ Revised Code Title

ICD-10-CM 2018   683

K56.3 Gallstone ileus `HCC`
     Obstruction of intestine by gallstone

✓5th **K56.4 Other impaction of intestine**

     K56.41 Fecal impaction `HCC`
        EXCLUDES 1   *constipation (K59.0-)*
                 incomplete defecation (R15.0)

     K56.49 Other impaction of intestine `HCC`

▲ ✓5th **K56.5 Intestinal adhesions [bands] with obstruction (postinfection)**
     Abdominal hernia due to adhesions with obstruction
     ▶Peritoneal adhesions [bands] with intestinal obstruction (postinfection)◀

●   **K56.50 Intestinal adhesions [bands], unspecified as to partial versus complete obstruction** ▽
        Intestinal adhesions with obstruction NOS

●   **K56.51 Intestinal adhesions [bands], with partial obstruction**
        Intestinal adhesions with incomplete obstruction

●   **K56.52 Intestinal adhesions [bands] with complete obstruction**

✓5th **K56.6 Other and unspecified intestinal obstruction**
     AHA: 2017, 2Q, 12

     ✓6th **K56.60 Unspecified intestinal obstruction**
        ~~Intestinal obstruction NOS~~
        EXCLUDES 1   *intestinal obstruction due to specified condition—code to condition*

●   **K56.600 Partial intestinal obstruction, unspecified as to cause** ▽
           Incomplete intestinal obstruction, NOS

●   **K56.601 Complete intestinal obstruction, unspecified as to cause** ▽

●   **K56.609 Unspecified intestinal obstruction, unspecified as to partial versus complete obstruction** ▽
           Intestinal obstruction NOS

     ✓6th **K56.69 Other intestinal obstruction**
        Enterostenosis NOS
        Obstructive ileus NOS
        Occlusion of colon or intestine NOS
        Stenosis of colon or intestine NOS
        Stricture of colon or intestine NOS
        EXCLUDES 1   *intestinal obstruction due to specified condition—code to condition*

●   **K56.690 Other partial intestinal obstruction**
           Other incomplete intestinal obstruction

●   **K56.691 Other complete intestinal obstruction**

●   **K56.699 Other intestinal obstruction unspecified as to partial versus complete obstruction** ▽
           Other intestinal obstruction, NEC

K56.7 Ileus, unspecified `HCC` ▽
     EXCLUDES 1   *obstructive ileus ▶(K56.69-)◀*
     EXCLUDES 2   *▶intestinal obstruction with hernia (K40-K46)◀*
     AHA: 2017, 1Q, 40

✓4th **K57 Diverticular disease of intestine**
     EXCLUDES 1   *congenital diverticulum of intestine (Q43.8)*
                  Meckel's diverticulum (Q43.0)
     EXCLUDES 2   *diverticulum of appendix (K38.2)*

✓5th **K57.0 Diverticulitis of small intestine with perforation and abscess**
     Diverticulitis of small intestine with peritonitis
     EXCLUDES 1   *diverticulitis of both small and large intestine with perforation and abscess (K57.4-)*

     K57.00 Diverticulitis of small intestine with perforation and abscess without bleeding

     K57.01 Diverticulitis of small intestine with perforation and abscess with bleeding

✓5th **K57.1 Diverticular disease of small intestine without perforation or abscess**
     EXCLUDES 1   *diverticular disease of both small and large intestine without perforation or abscess (K57.5-)*

     K57.10 Diverticulosis of small intestine without perforation or abscess without bleeding
        Diverticular disease of small intestine NOS

     K57.11 Diverticulosis of small intestine without perforation or abscess with bleeding

     K57.12 Diverticulitis of small intestine without perforation or abscess without bleeding

     K57.13 Diverticulitis of small intestine without perforation or abscess with bleeding

✓5th **K57.2 Diverticulitis of large intestine with perforation and abscess**
     Diverticulitis of colon with peritonitis
     EXCLUDES 1   *diverticulitis of both small and large intestine with perforation and abscess (K57.4-)*

     K57.20 Diverticulitis of large intestine with perforation and abscess without bleeding

     K57.21 Diverticulitis of large intestine with perforation and abscess with bleeding

✓5th **K57.3 Diverticular disease of large intestine without perforation or abscess**
     EXCLUDES 1   *diverticular disease of both small and large intestine without perforation or abscess (K57.5-)*

     K57.30 Diverticulosis of large intestine without perforation or abscess without bleeding
        Diverticular disease of colon NOS

     K57.31 Diverticulosis of large intestine without perforation or abscess with bleeding

     K57.32 Diverticulitis of large intestine without perforation or abscess without bleeding

     K57.33 Diverticulitis of large intestine without perforation or abscess with bleeding

✓5th **K57.4 Diverticulitis of both small and large intestine with perforation and abscess**
     Diverticulitis of both small and large intestine with peritonitis

     K57.40 Diverticulitis of both small and large intestine with perforation and abscess without bleeding

     K57.41 Diverticulitis of both small and large intestine with perforation and abscess with bleeding

✓5th **K57.5 Diverticular disease of both small and large intestine without perforation or abscess**

     K57.50 Diverticulosis of both small and large intestine without perforation or abscess without bleeding
        Diverticular disease of both small and large intestine NOS

     K57.51 Diverticulosis of both small and large intestine without perforation or abscess with bleeding

     K57.52 Diverticulitis of both small and large intestine without perforation or abscess without bleeding

     K57.53 Diverticulitis of both small and large intestine without perforation or abscess with bleeding

✓5th **K57.8 Diverticulitis of intestine, part unspecified, with perforation and abscess**
     Diverticulitis of intestine NOS with peritonitis

     K57.80 Diverticulitis of intestine, part unspecified, with perforation and abscess without bleeding ▽

     K57.81 Diverticulitis of intestine, part unspecified, with perforation and abscess with bleeding ▽

✓5th **K57.9 Diverticular disease of intestine, part unspecified, without perforation or abscess**

     K57.90 Diverticulosis of intestine, part unspecified, without perforation or abscess without bleeding ▽
        Diverticular disease of intestine NOS

     K57.91 Diverticulosis of intestine, part unspecified, without perforation or abscess with bleeding ▽

     K57.92 Diverticulitis of intestine, part unspecified, without perforation or abscess without bleeding ▽

     K57.93 Diverticulitis of intestine, part unspecified, without perforation or abscess with bleeding ▽

✓4th **K58 Irritable bowel syndrome**
     INCLUDES   irritable colon
                 spastic colon

     K58.0 Irritable bowel syndrome with diarrhea

     K58.1 Irritable bowel syndrome with constipation

     K58.2 Mixed irritable bowel syndrome

     K58.8 Other irritable bowel syndrome

     K58.9 Irritable bowel syndrome without diarrhea
        Irritable bowel syndrome NOS

EXCLUDES 1 Not coded here   EXCLUDES 2 Not included here   N Newborn Age: 0   P Pediatric Age: 0-17   M Maternity Age: 12-55   A Adult Age: 15-124

684   ICD-10-CM 2018

☑4ᵗʰ **K59 Other functional intestinal disorders**
> *EXCLUDES 1* change in bowel habit NOS (R19.4)
> intestinal malabsorption (K90.-)
> psychogenic intestinal disorders (F45.8)
> *EXCLUDES 2* functional disorders of stomach (K31.-)

☑5ᵗʰ **K59.0 Constipation**
> Use additional code for adverse effect, if applicable, to identify drug (T36-T50 with fifth or sixth character 5)
> *EXCLUDES 1* fecal impaction (K56.41)
> incomplete defecation (R15.0)

K59.00 Constipation, unspecified ▽

K59.01 Slow transit constipation
> **DEF:** Delay in the transit of fecal material through the colon secondary to smooth muscle dysfunction or decreased peristaltic contractions along the colon: also called colonic inertia or delayed transit.

K59.02 Outlet dysfunction constipation

K59.03 Drug induced constipation
> Use additional code for adverse effect, if applicable, to identify drug (T36-T50 with fifth or sixth character 5)

K59.04 Chronic idiopathic constipation
> Functional constipation

K59.09 Other constipation
> Chronic constipation

K59.1 Functional diarrhea
> *EXCLUDES 1* diarrhea NOS (R19.7)
> irritable bowel syndrome with diarrhea (K58.0)

K59.2 Neurogenic bowel, not elsewhere classified
> **DEF:** Disorder of bowel due to spinal cord lesion due to injury or as a complication of conditions such as multiple sclerosis (MS) or spina bifida; loss of bowel control is the primary symptom, manifested as constipation or bowel incontinence.

☑5ᵗʰ **K59.3 Megacolon, not elsewhere classified**
> Dilatation of colon
> Code first, if applicable (T51-T65) to identify toxic agent
> *EXCLUDES 1* congenital megacolon (aganglionic) (Q43.1)
> megacolon (due to) (in) Chagas' disease (B57.32)
> megacolon (due to) (in) Clostridium difficile ▶(A04.7-)◀
> megacolon (due to) (in) Hirschsprung's disease (Q43.1)

K59.31 Toxic megacolon ᴴᶜᶜ

K59.39 Other megacolon
> Megacolon NOS

K59.4 Anal spasm
> Proctalgia fugax

K59.8 Other specified functional intestinal disorders
> Atony of colon
> Pseudo-obstruction (acute) (chronic) of intestine

K59.9 Functional intestinal disorder, unspecified ▽

☑4ᵗʰ **K60 Fissure and fistula of anal and rectal regions**
> *EXCLUDES 1* fissure and fistula of anal and rectal regions with abscess or cellulitis (K61.-)
> *EXCLUDES 2* anal sphincter tear (healed) (nontraumatic) (old) (K62.81)

K60.0 Acute anal fissure

K60.1 Chronic anal fissure

K60.2 Anal fissure, unspecified ▽

K60.3 Anal fistula

K60.4 Rectal fistula
> Fistula of rectum to skin
> *EXCLUDES 1* rectovaginal fistula (N82.3)
> vesicorectal fistual (N32.1)

K60.5 Anorectal fistula

☑4ᵗʰ **K61 Abscess of anal and rectal regions**
> *INCLUDES* abscess of anal and rectal regions
> cellulitis of anal and rectal regions

K61.0 Anal abscess
> Perianal abscess
> *EXCLUDES 1* intrasphincteric abscess (K61.4)

K61.1 Rectal abscess
> Perirectal abscess
> *EXCLUDES 1* ischiorectal abscess (K61.3)
> **AHA:** 2012, 4Q, 104

K61.2 Anorectal abscess

K61.3 Ischiorectal abscess
> Abscess of ischiorectal fossa

K61.4 Intrasphincteric abscess

☑4ᵗʰ **K62 Other diseases of anus and rectum**
> *INCLUDES* anal canal
> *EXCLUDES 2* colostomy and enterostomy malfunction (K94.0-, K94.1-)
> fecal incontinence (R15.-)
> hemorrhoids (K64.-)

K62.0 Anal polyp

K62.1 Rectal polyp
> *EXCLUDES 1* adenomatous polyp (D12.8)

K62.2 Anal prolapse
> Prolapse of anal canal

K62.3 Rectal prolapse
> Prolapse of rectal mucosa

K62.4 Stenosis of anus and rectum
> Stricture of anus (sphincter)

K62.5 Hemorrhage of anus and rectum
> *EXCLUDES 1* gastrointestinal bleeding NOS (K92.2)
> melena (K92.1)
> neonatal rectal hemorrhage (P54.2)

K62.6 Ulcer of anus and rectum
> Solitary ulcer of anus and rectum
> Stercoral ulcer of anus and rectum
> *EXCLUDES 1* fissure and fistula of anus and rectum (K60.-)
> ulcerative colitis (K51.-)

K62.7 Radiation proctitis
> Use additional code to identify the type of radiation (W90.-)

☑5ᵗʰ **K62.8 Other specified diseases of anus and rectum**
> *EXCLUDES 2* ulcerative proctitis (K51.2)

K62.81 Anal sphincter tear (healed) (nontraumatic) (old)
> Tear of anus, nontraumatic
> Use additional code for any associated fecal incontinence (R15.-)
> *EXCLUDES 2* anal fissure (K60.-)
> anal sphincter tear (healed) (old) complicating delivery (O34.7-)
> traumatic tear of anal sphincter (S31.831)

K62.82 Dysplasia of anus
> Anal intraepithelial neoplasia I and II (AIN I and II) (histologically confirmed)
> Dysplasia of anus NOS
> Mild and moderate dysplasia of anus (histologically confirmed)
> *EXCLUDES 1* abnormal results from anal cytologic examination without histologic confirmation (R85.61-)
> anal intraepithelial neoplasia III (D01.3)
> carcinoma in situ of anus (D01.3)
> HGSIL of anus (R85.613)
> severe dysplasia of anus (D01.3)

K62.89 Other specified diseases of anus and rectum
> Proctitis NOS
> Use additional code for any associated fecal incontinence (R15.-)

K62.9 Disease of anus and rectum, unspecified ▽

☑4ᵗʰ **K63 Other diseases of intestine**

K63.0 Abscess of intestine
> *EXCLUDES 1* abscess of intestine with Crohn's disease (K50.014, K50.114, K50.814, K50.914)
> abscess of intestine with diverticular disease (K57.0, K57.2, K57.4, K57.8)
> abscess of intestine with ulcerative colitis (K51.014, K51.214, K51.314, K51.414, K51.514, K51.814, K51.914)
> *EXCLUDES 2* abscess of anal and rectal regions (K61.-)
> abscess of appendix (K35.3)

K63.1 Perforation of intestine (nontraumatic) ᴴᶜᶜ
> Perforation (nontraumatic) of rectum
> *EXCLUDES 1* perforation (nontraumatic) of duodenum (K26.-)
> perforation (nontraumatic) of intestine with diverticular disease (K57.0, K57.2, K57.4, K57.8)
> *EXCLUDES 2* perforation (nontraumatic) of appendix (K35.2, K35.3)

☑ Additional Character Req   ☑x7ᵗʰ Placeholder Alert   ▮Manifestation▮   ᴴᶜᶜ CMS-HCC Condition   ▽ Unspecified Code   ▶◀ Revised Text   ● New Code   ▲ Revised Code Title

K63.2 Fistula of intestine
> EXCLUDES 1   fistula of duodenum (K31.6)
>> fistula of intestine with Crohn's disease (K50.013,
>> K50.113, K50.813, K50.913)
>> fistula of intestine with ulcerative colitis (K51.013,
>> K51.213, K51.313, K51.413, K51.513, K51.813,
>> K51.913)
> EXCLUDES 2   fistula of anal and rectal regions (K60.-)
>> fistula of appendix (K38.3)
>> intestinal-genital fistula, female (N82.2-N82.4)
>> vesicointestinal fistula (N32.1)

K63.3 Ulcer of intestine
Primary ulcer of small intestine
> EXCLUDES 1   duodenal ulcer (K26.-)
>> gastrointestinal ulcer (K28.-)
>> gastrojejunal ulcer (K28.-)
>> jejunal ulcer (K28.-)
>> peptic ulcer, site unspecified (K27.-)
>> ulcer of intestine with perforation (K63.1)
>> ulcer of anus or rectum (K62.6)
>> ulcerative colitis (K51.-)

K63.4 Enteroptosis

K63.5 Polyp of colon
> EXCLUDES 1   adenomatous polyp of colon (D12.6)
>> inflammatory polyp of colon (K51.4-)
>> polyposis of colon (D12.6)
> **AHA:** 2017, 1Q, 15; 2015, 2Q, 14

✓5ᵗʰ **K63.8 Other specified diseases of intestine**
> **K63.81 Dieulafoy lesion of intestine**
>> EXCLUDES 2   Dieulafoy lesion of stomach and duodenum
>> (K31.82)

> **K63.89 Other specified diseases of intestine**
>> **AHA:** 2013, 2Q, 31

K63.9 Disease of intestine, unspecified   ▽

✓4ᵗʰ **K64 Hemorrhoids and perianal venous thrombosis**
> INCLUDES   piles
> EXCLUDES 1   hemorrhoids complicating childbirth and the puerperium
>> (O87.2)
>> hemorrhoids complicating pregnancy (O22.4)

K64.0 First degree hemorrhoids
Grade/stage I hemorrhoids
Hemorrhoids (bleeding) without prolapse outside of anal canal

K64.1 Second degree hemorrhoids
Grade/stage II hemorrhoids
Hemorrhoids (bleeding) that prolapse with straining, but retract
spontaneously

K64.2 Third degree hemorrhoids
Grade/stage III hemorrhoids
Hemorrhoids (bleeding) that prolapse with straining and require
manual replacement back inside anal cana

K64.3 Fourth degree hemorrhoids
Grade/stage IV hemorrhoids
Hemorrhoids (bleeding) with prolapsed tissue that cannot be
manually replaced

K64.4 Residual hemorrhoidal skin tags
External hemorrhoids, NOS
Skin tags of anus

Hemorrhoids

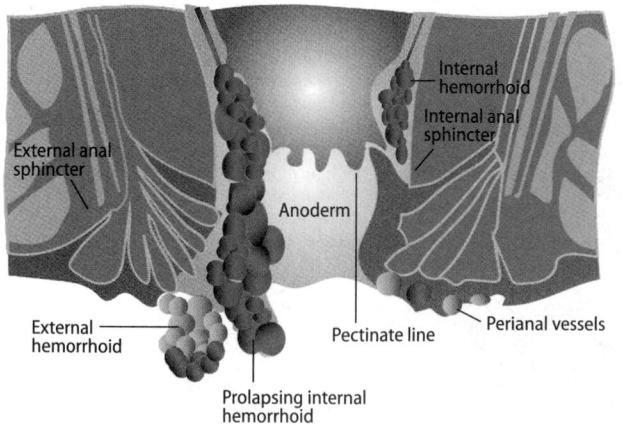

External anal sphincter
Internal hemorrhoid
Internal anal sphincter
Anoderm
Pectinate line
Perianal vessels
External hemorrhoid
Prolapsing internal hemorrhoid

K64.5 Perianal venous thrombosis
External hemorrhoids with thrombosis
Perianal hematoma
Thrombosed hemorrhoids NOS

K64.8 Other hemorrhoids
Internal hemorrhoids, without mention of degree
Prolapsed hemorrhoids, degree not specified

K64.9 Unspecified hemorrhoids   ▽
Hemorrhoids (bleeding) NOS
Hemorrhoids (bleeding) without mention of degree

Diseases of peritoneum and retroperitoneum (K65-K68)

✓4ᵗʰ **K65 Peritonitis**
Use additional code (B95-B97), to identify infectious agent
> EXCLUDES 1   acute appendicitis with generalized peritonitis (K35.2)
>> aseptic peritonitis (T81.6)
>> benign paroxysmal peritonitis (E85.0)
>> chemical peritonitis (T81.6)
>> diverticulitis of both small and large intestine with peritonitis
>> (K57.4-)
>> diverticulitis of colon with peritonitis (K57.2-)
>> diverticulitis of intestine, NOS, with peritonitis (K57.8-)
>> diverticulitis of small intestine with peritonitis (K57.0-)
>> gonococcal peritonitis (A54.85)
>> neonatal peritonitis (P78.0-P78.1)
>> pelvic peritonitis, female (N73.3-N73.5)
>> periodic familial peritonitis (E85.0)
>> peritonitis due to talc or other foreign substance (T81.6)
>> peritonitis in chlamydia (A74.81)
>> peritonitis in diphtheria (A36.89)
>> peritonitis in syphilis (late) (A52.74)
>> peritonitis in tuberculosis (A18.31)
>> peritonitis with or following abortion or ectopic or molar
>> pregnancy (O00-O07, O08.0)
>> peritonitis with or following appendicitis (K35.-)
>> peritonitis with or following diverticular disease of intestine
>> (K57.-)
>> puerperal peritonitis (O85)
>> retroperitoneal infections (K68.-)

K65.0 Generalized (acute) peritonitis   HCC
Pelvic peritonitis (acute), male
Subphrenic peritonitis (acute)
Suppurative peritonitis (acute)

K65.1 Peritoneal abscess   HCC
Abdominopelvic abscess	Subdiaphragmatic abscess
Abscess (of) omentum	Subhepatic abscess
Abscess (of) peritoneum	Subphrenic abscess
Mesenteric abscess	
Retrocecal abscess	

K65.2 Spontaneous bacterial peritonitis   HCC
> EXCLUDES 1   bacterial peritonitis NOS (K65.9)

K65.3 Choleperitonitis   HCC
Peritonitis due to bile
DEF: Inflammation of the peritoneum due to leakage of bile into
the peritoneal cavity resulting from rupture of the bile passages or
gallbladder.

K65.4 Sclerosing mesenteritis   HCC
Fat necrosis of peritoneum
(Idiopathic) sclerosing mesenteric fibrosis
Mesenteric lipodystrophy
Mesenteric panniculitis
Retractile mesenteritis

K65.8 Other peritonitis   HCC
Chronic proliferative peritonitis
Peritonitis due to urine

K65.9 Peritonitis, unspecified   HCC ▽
Bacterial peritonitis NOS
AHA: 2013, 2Q, 31

✓4ᵗʰ **K66 Other disorders of peritoneum**
> EXCLUDES 2   ascites (R18.-)
>> peritoneal effusion (chronic) (R18.8)

K66.0 Peritoneal adhesions (postprocedural) (postinfection)
Adhesions (of) abdominal (wall)	Adhesions (of) omentum
Adhesions (of) diaphragm	Adhesions (of) stomach
Adhesions (of) intestine	Adhesive bands
Adhesions (of) male pelvis	Mesenteric adhesions
> EXCLUDES 1   female pelvic adhesions [bands] (N73.6)
>> peritoneal adhesions with intestinal obstruction
>> ►(K56.5-)◄

K66.1   **Hemoperitoneum**
> **EXCLUDES 1**   *traumatic hemoperitoneum (S36.8-)*

K66.8   **Other specified disorders of peritoneum**

K66.9   **Disorder of peritoneum, unspecified**   ▽

K67   *Disorders of peritoneum in infectious diseases classified elsewhere*   HCC
> Code first underlying disease, such as:
>   congenital syphilis (A50.0)
>   helminthiasis (B65.0-B83.9)
> **EXCLUDES 1**   *peritonitis in chlamydia (A74.81)*
>   *peritonitis in diphtheria (A36.89)*
>   *peritonitis in gonococcal (A54.85)*
>   *peritonitis in syphilis (late) (A52.74)*
>   *peritonitis in tuberculosis (A18.31)*

✓4ᵗʰ **K68**   **Disorders of retroperitoneum**

   ✓5ᵗʰ **K68.1**   **Retroperitoneal abscess**

      K68.11   **Postprocedural retroperitoneal abscess**

      K68.12   **Psoas muscle abscess**   HCC

      K68.19   **Other retroperitoneal abscess**   HCC

   K68.9   **Other disorders of retroperitoneum**

Diseases of liver (K70-K77)

> **EXCLUDES 1**   *jaundice NOS (R17)*
> **EXCLUDES 2**   *hemochromatosis (E83.11-)*
>   *Reye's syndrome (G93.7)*
>   *viral hepatitis (B15-B19)*
>   *Wilson's disease (E83.0)*

✓4ᵗʰ **K70**   **Alcoholic liver disease**
> Use additional code to identify:
>   alcohol abuse and dependence (F10.-)

   K70.0   **Alcoholic fatty liver**   A

   ✓5ᵗʰ **K70.1**   **Alcoholic hepatitis**

      K70.10   **Alcoholic hepatitis without ascites**   A

      K70.11   **Alcoholic hepatitis with ascites**   A

   K70.2   **Alcoholic fibrosis and sclerosis of liver**   A

   ✓5ᵗʰ **K70.3**   **Alcoholic cirrhosis of liver**
>   Alcoholic cirrhosis NOS

      K70.30   **Alcoholic cirrhosis of liver without ascites**   HCC A

      K70.31   **Alcoholic cirrhosis of liver with ascites**   HCC A

   ✓5ᵗʰ **K70.4**   **Alcoholic hepatic failure**
>   Acute alcoholic hepatic failure
>   Alcoholic hepatic failure NOS
>   Chronic alcoholic hepatic failure
>   Subacute alcoholic hepatic failure

      K70.40   **Alcoholic hepatic failure without coma**   HCC A

      K70.41   **Alcoholic hepatic failure with coma**   HCC A

   K70.9   **Alcoholic liver disease, unspecified**   HCC A ▽

✓4ᵗʰ **K71**   **Toxic liver disease**
> **INCLUDES**   drug-induced idiosyncratic (unpredictable) liver disease
>   drug-induced toxic (predictable) liver disease
>
> Code first poisoning due to drug or toxin, if applicable (T36-T65 with fifth or sixth character 1-4 or 6)
>
> Use additional code for adverse effect, if applicable, to identify drug (T36-T50 with fifth or sixth character 5)
> **EXCLUDES 2**   *alcoholic liver disease (K70.-)*
>   *Budd-Chiari syndrome (I82.0)*

   K71.0   **Toxic liver disease with cholestasis**
>   Cholestasis with hepatocyte injury
>   "Pure" cholestasis

   ✓5ᵗʰ **K71.1**   **Toxic liver disease with hepatic necrosis**
>   Hepatic failure (acute) (chronic) due to drugs

      K71.10   **Toxic liver disease with hepatic necrosis, without coma**

      K71.11   **Toxic liver disease with hepatic necrosis, with coma**   HCC

   K71.2   **Toxic liver disease with acute hepatitis**

   K71.3   **Toxic liver disease with chronic persistent hepatitis**

   K71.4   **Toxic liver disease with chronic lobular hepatitis**

   ✓5ᵗʰ **K71.5**   **Toxic liver disease with chronic active hepatitis**
>   Toxic liver disease with lupoid hepatitis

      K71.50   **Toxic liver disease with chronic active hepatitis without ascites**

      K71.51   **Toxic liver disease with chronic active hepatitis with ascites**

   K71.6   **Toxic liver disease with hepatitis, not elsewhere classified**

   K71.7   **Toxic liver disease with fibrosis and cirrhosis of liver**

   K71.8   **Toxic liver disease with other disorders of liver**
>   Toxic liver disease with focal nodular hyperplasia
>   Toxic liver disease with hepatic granulomas
>   Toxic liver disease with peliosis hepatis
>   Toxic liver disease with veno-occlusive disease of liver

   K71.9   **Toxic liver disease, unspecified**   ▽

✓4ᵗʰ **K72**   **Hepatic failure, not elsewhere classified**
> **INCLUDES**   fulminant hepatitis NEC, with hepatic failure
>   hepatic encephalopathy NOS
>   liver (cell) necrosis with hepatic failure
>   malignant hepatitis NEC, with hepatic failure
>   yellow liver atrophy or dystrophy
> **EXCLUDES 1**   *alcoholic hepatic failure (K70.4)*
>   *hepatic failure with toxic liver disease (K71.1-)*
>   *icterus of newborn (P55-P59)*
>   *postprocedural hepatic failure (K91.82)*
> **EXCLUDES 2**   *hepatic failure complicating abortion or ectopic or molar*
>   *pregnancy (O00-O07, O08.8)*
>   *hepatic failure complicating pregnancy, childbirth and the*
>   *puerperium (O26.6-)*
>   *viral hepatitis with hepatic coma (B15-B19)*
> **AHA:** 2017, 1Q, 41

   ✓5ᵗʰ **K72.0**   **Acute and subacute hepatic failure**
>   Acute non-viral hepatitis NOS
>   **AHA:** 2015, 2Q, 17; 2014, 2Q, 13

      K72.00   **Acute and subacute hepatic failure without coma**

      K72.01   **Acute and subacute hepatic failure with coma**   HCC

   ✓5ᵗʰ **K72.1**   **Chronic hepatic failure**

      K72.10   **Chronic hepatic failure without coma**   HCC

      K72.11   **Chronic hepatic failure with coma**   HCC

   ✓5ᵗʰ **K72.9**   **Hepatic failure, unspecified**

      K72.90   **Hepatic failure, unspecified without coma**   HCC ▽
>   **AHA:** 2016, 2Q, 35

      K72.91   **Hepatic failure, unspecified with coma**   HCC ▽
>   Hepatic coma NOS

✓4ᵗʰ **K73**   **Chronic hepatitis, not elsewhere classified**
> **EXCLUDES 1**   *alcoholic hepatitis (chronic) (K70.1-)*
>   *drug-induced hepatitis (chronic) (K71.-)*
>   *granulomatous hepatitis (chronic) NEC (K75.3)*
>   *reactive, nonspecific hepatitis (chronic) (K75.2)*
>   *viral hepatitis (chronic) (B15-B19)*

   K73.0   **Chronic persistent hepatitis, not elsewhere classified**   HCC

   K73.1   **Chronic lobular hepatitis, not elsewhere classified**   HCC

   K73.2   **Chronic active hepatitis, not elsewhere classified**   HCC

   K73.8   **Other chronic hepatitis, not elsewhere classified**   HCC

   K73.9   **Chronic hepatitis, unspecified**   HCC ▽

✓4ᵗʰ **K74**   **Fibrosis and cirrhosis of liver**
> Code also, if applicable, viral hepatitis (acute) (chronic) (B15-B19)
> **EXCLUDES 1**   *alcoholic cirrhosis (of liver) (K70.3)*
>   *alcoholic fibrosis of liver (K70.2)*
>   *cardiac sclerosis of liver (K76.1)*
>   *cirrhosis (of liver) with toxic liver disease (K71.7)*
>   *congenital cirrhosis (of liver) (P78.81)*
>   *pigmentary cirrhosis (of liver) (E83.110)*

   K74.0   **Hepatic fibrosis**

   K74.1   **Hepatic sclerosis**

   K74.2   **Hepatic fibrosis with hepatic sclerosis**

   K74.3   **Primary biliary cirrhosis**   HCC
>   Chronic nonsuppurative destructive cholangitis

   K74.4   **Secondary biliary cirrhosis**   HCC

   K74.5   **Biliary cirrhosis, unspecified**   HCC ▽

   ✓5ᵗʰ **K74.6**   **Other and unspecified cirrhosis of liver**

      K74.60   **Unspecified cirrhosis of liver**   HCC ▽
>   Cirrhosis (of liver) NOS

      K74.69   **Other cirrhosis of liver**   HCC
>   Cryptogenic cirrhosis (of liver)
>   Macronodular cirrhosis (of liver)
>   Micronodular cirrhosis (of liver)
>   Mixed type cirrhosis (of liver)
>   Portal cirrhosis (of liver)
>   Postnecrotic cirrhosis (of liver)

✓ Additional Character Req   ✓ˣ⁷ᵗʰ Placeholder Alert   Manifestation   HCC CMS-HCC Condition   ▽ Unspecified Code   ►◄ Revised Text   ● New Code   ▲ Revised Code Title

☑4th **K75 Other inflammatory liver diseases**
> EXCLUDES 2 *toxic liver disease (K71.-)*

K75.0 Abscess of liver
> Cholangitic hepatic abscess
> Hematogenic hepatic abscess
> Hepatic abscess NOS
> Lymphogenic hepatic abscess
> Pylephlebitic hepatic abscess
> > EXCLUDES 1 *amebic liver abscess (A06.4)*
> > *cholangitis without liver abscess (K83.0)*
> > *pylephlebitis without liver abscess (K75.1)*
> > EXCLUDES 2 *acute or subacute hepatitis NOS (B17.9)*
> > *acute or subacute non-viral hepatitis (K72.0)*
> > *chronic hepatitis NEC (K73.8)*

K75.1 Phlebitis of portal vein
> Pylephlebitis
> > EXCLUDES 1 *pylephlebitic liver abscess (K75.0)*
> **DEF:** Inflammation of portal vein or branches; may be due to diverticulitis, perforated appendicitis, or peritonitis; symptoms include fever, chills, jaundice, sweating, and abscess in various body parts.

K75.2 Nonspecific reactive hepatitis
> > EXCLUDES 1 *acute or subacute hepatitis (K72.0-)*
> > *chronic hepatitis NEC (K73.-)*
> > *viral hepatitis (B15-B19)*

K75.3 Granulomatous hepatitis, not elsewhere classified
> > EXCLUDES 1 *acute or subacute hepatitis (K72.0-)*
> > *chronic hepatitis NEC (K73.-)*
> > *viral hepatitis (B15-B19)*

K75.4 Autoimmune hepatitis   HCC
> Lupoid hepatitis NEC

☑5th **K75.8 Other specified inflammatory liver diseases**
> **K75.81 Nonalcoholic steatohepatitis (NASH)**
> **K75.89 Other specified inflammatory liver diseases**

K75.9 Inflammatory liver disease, unspecified   ▽
> Hepatitis NOS
> > EXCLUDES 1 *acute or subacute hepatitis (K72.0-)*
> > *chronic hepatitis NEC (K73.-)*
> > *viral hepatitis (B15-B19)*
> **AHA:** 2015, 2Q, 17

☑4th **K76 Other diseases of liver**
> EXCLUDES 2 *alcoholic liver disease (K70.-)*
> *amyloid degeneration of liver (E85.-)*
> *cystic disease of liver (congenital) (Q44.6)*
> *hepatic vein thrombosis (I82.0)*
> *hepatomegaly NOS (R16.0)*
> *pigmentary cirrhosis (of liver) (E83.110)*
> *portal vein thrombosis (I81)*
> *toxic liver disease (K71.-)*

K76.0 Fatty (change of) liver, not elsewhere classified
> Nonalcoholic fatty liver disease (NAFLD)
> > EXCLUDES 1 *nonalcoholic steatohepatitis (NASH) (K75.81)*

K76.1 Chronic passive congestion of liver
> Cardiac cirrhosis
> Cardiac sclerosis

K76.2 Central hemorrhagic necrosis of liver
> > EXCLUDES 1 *liver necrosis with hepatic failure (K72.-)*

K76.3 Infarction of liver

K76.4 Peliosis hepatis
> Hepatic angiomatosis

K76.5 Hepatic veno-occlusive disease
> > EXCLUDES 1 *Budd-Chiari syndrome (I82.0)*

K76.6 Portal hypertension   HCC
> Use additional code for any associated complications, such as:
> portal hypertensive gastropathy (K31.89)

K76.7 Hepatorenal syndrome   HCC
> > EXCLUDES 1 *hepatorenal syndrome following labor and delivery (O90.4)*
> > *postprocedural hepatorenal syndrome (K91.83)*

☑5th **K76.8 Other specified diseases of liver**
> **K76.81 Hepatopulmonary syndrome**   HCC
> > Code first underlying liver disease, such as:
> > alcoholic cirrhosis of liver (K70.3-)
> > cirrhosis of liver without mention of alcohol (K74.6-)
> **K76.89 Other specified diseases of liver**
> > Cyst (simple) of liver
> > Focal nodular hyperplasia of liver
> > Hepatoptosis

K76.9 Liver disease, unspecified   ▽

K77 Liver disorders in diseases classified elsewhere
> Code first underlying disease, such as:
> amyloidosis (E85.-)
> congenital syphilis (A50.0, A50.5)
> congenital toxoplasmosis (P37.1)
> schistosomiasis (B65.0-B65.9)
> > EXCLUDES 1 *alcoholic hepatitis (K70.1-)*
> > *alcoholic liver disease (K70-.)*
> > *cytomegaloviral hepatitis (B25.1)*
> > *herpesviral [herpes simplex] hepatitis (B00.81)*
> > *infectious mononucleosis with liver disease (B27.0-B27.9 with .9)*
> > *mumps hepatitis (B26.81)*
> > *sarcoidosis with liver disease (D86.89)*
> > *secondary syphilis with liver disease (A51.45)*
> > *syphilis (late) with liver disease (A52.74)*
> > *toxoplasmosis (acquired) hepatitis (B58.1)*
> > *tuberculosis with liver disease (A18.83)*

Disorders of gallbladder, biliary tract and pancreas (K80-K87)

☑4th **K80 Cholelithiasis**
> EXCLUDES 1 *retained cholelithiasis following cholecystectomy (K91.86)*

☑5th **K80.0 Calculus of gallbladder with acute cholecystitis**
> Any condition listed in K80.2 with acute cholecystitis
> **K80.00 Calculus of gallbladder with acute cholecystitis without obstruction**
> **K80.01 Calculus of gallbladder with acute cholecystitis with obstruction**

☑5th **K80.1 Calculus of gallbladder with other cholecystitis**
> **K80.10 Calculus of gallbladder with chronic cholecystitis without obstruction**
> > Cholelithiasis with cholecystitis NOS
> **K80.11 Calculus of gallbladder with chronic cholecystitis with obstruction**
> **K80.12 Calculus of gallbladder with acute and chronic cholecystitis without obstruction**
> **K80.13 Calculus of gallbladder with acute and chronic cholecystitis with obstruction**
> **K80.18 Calculus of gallbladder with other cholecystitis without obstruction**
> **K80.19 Calculus of gallbladder with other cholecystitis with obstruction**

☑5th **K80.2 Calculus of gallbladder without cholecystitis**
> Cholecystolithiasis without cholecystitis
> Cholelithiasis (without cholecystitis)
> Colic (recurrent) of gallbladder (without cholecystitis)
> Gallstone (impacted) of cystic duct (without cholecystitis)
> Gallstone (impacted) of gallbladder (without cholecystitis)
> **K80.20 Calculus of gallbladder without cholecystitis without obstruction**
> **K80.21 Calculus of gallbladder without cholecystitis with obstruction**

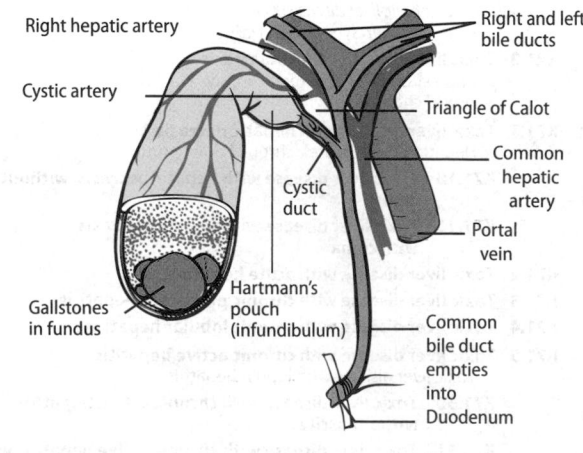

Cholelithiasis

Right hepatic artery
Cystic artery
Gallstones in fundus
Cystic duct
Hartmann's pouch (infundibulum)
Right and left bile ducts
Triangle of Calot
Common hepatic artery
Portal vein
Common bile duct empties into Duodenum

EXCLUDES 1 Not coded here   EXCLUDES 2 Not included here   N Newborn Age: 0   P Pediatric Age: 0-17   M Maternity Age: 12-55   A Adult Age: 15-124

688   ICD-10-CM 2018

☑5ᵗʰ **K80.3 Calculus of bile duct with cholangitis**
Any condition listed in K80.5 with cholangitis

    K80.30 Calculus of bile duct with cholangitis, unspecified, without obstruction ▽

    K80.31 Calculus of bile duct with cholangitis, unspecified, with obstruction ▽

    K80.32 Calculus of bile duct with acute cholangitis without obstruction

    K80.33 Calculus of bile duct with acute cholangitis with obstruction

    K80.34 Calculus of bile duct with chronic cholangitis without obstruction

    K80.35 Calculus of bile duct with chronic cholangitis with obstruction

    K80.36 Calculus of bile duct with acute and chronic cholangitis without obstruction

    K80.37 Calculus of bile duct with acute and chronic cholangitis with obstruction

☑5ᵗʰ **K80.4 Calculus of bile duct with cholecystitis**
Any condition listed in K80.5 with cholecystitis (with cholangitis)

    K80.40 Calculus of bile duct with cholecystitis, unspecified, without obstruction ▽

    K80.41 Calculus of bile duct with cholecystitis, unspecified, with obstruction ▽

    K80.42 Calculus of bile duct with acute cholecystitis without obstruction

    K80.43 Calculus of bile duct with acute cholecystitis with obstruction

    K80.44 Calculus of bile duct with chronic cholecystitis without obstruction

    K80.45 Calculus of bile duct with chronic cholecystitis with obstruction

    K80.46 Calculus of bile duct with acute and chronic cholecystitis without obstruction

    K80.47 Calculus of bile duct with acute and chronic cholecystitis with obstruction

☑5ᵗʰ **K80.5 Calculus of bile duct without cholangitis or cholecystitis**
Choledocholithiasis (without cholangitis or cholecystitis)
Gallstone (impacted) of bile duct NOS (without cholangitis or cholecystitis)
Gallstone (impacted) of common duct (without cholangitis or cholecystitis)
Gallstone (impacted) of hepatic duct (without cholangitis or cholecystitis)
Hepatic cholelithiasis (without cholangitis or cholecystitis)
Hepatic colic (recurrent) (without cholangitis or cholecystitis)

    K80.50 Calculus of bile duct without cholangitis or cholecystitis without obstruction

    K80.51 Calculus of bile duct without cholangitis or cholecystitis with obstruction

☑5ᵗʰ **K80.6 Calculus of gallbladder and bile duct with cholecystitis**

    K80.60 Calculus of gallbladder and bile duct with cholecystitis, unspecified, without obstruction ▽

    K80.61 Calculus of gallbladder and bile duct with cholecystitis, unspecified, with obstruction ▽

    K80.62 Calculus of gallbladder and bile duct with acute cholecystitis without obstruction

    K80.63 Calculus of gallbladder and bile duct with acute cholecystitis with obstruction

    K80.64 Calculus of gallbladder and bile duct with chronic cholecystitis without obstruction

    K80.65 Calculus of gallbladder and bile duct with chronic cholecystitis with obstruction

    K80.66 Calculus of gallbladder and bile duct with acute and chronic cholecystitis without obstruction

    K80.67 Calculus of gallbladder and bile duct with acute and chronic cholecystitis with obstruction

☑5ᵗʰ **K80.7 Calculus of gallbladder and bile duct without cholecystitis**

    K80.70 Calculus of gallbladder and bile duct without cholecystitis without obstruction

    K80.71 Calculus of gallbladder and bile duct without cholecystitis with obstruction

☑5ᵗʰ **K80.8 Other cholelithiasis**

    K80.80 Other cholelithiasis without obstruction

    K80.81 Other cholelithiasis with obstruction

☑4ᵗʰ **K81 Cholecystitis**
  EXCLUDES 1 cholecystitis with cholelithiasis (K80.-)

  K81.0 Acute cholecystitis
Abscess of gallbladder
Angiocholecystitis
Emphysematous (acute) cholecystitis
Empyema of gallbladder
Gangrene of gallbladder
Gangrenous cholecystitis
Suppurative cholecystitis

  K81.1 Chronic cholecystitis

  K81.2 Acute cholecystitis with chronic cholecystitis

  K81.9 Cholecystitis, unspecified ▽

☑4ᵗʰ **K82 Other diseases of gallbladder**
  EXCLUDES 1 nonvisualization of gallbladder (R93.2)
          postcholecystectomy syndrome (K91.5)

  K82.0 Obstruction of gallbladder
Occlusion of cystic duct or gallbladder without cholelithiasis
Stenosis of cystic duct or gallbladder without cholelithiasis
Stricture of cystic duct or gallbladder without cholelithiasis
  EXCLUDES 1 obstruction of gallbladder with cholelithiasis (K80.-)

  K82.1 Hydrops of gallbladder
Mucocele of gallbladder

  K82.2 Perforation of gallbladder
Rupture of cystic duct or gallbladder

  K82.3 Fistula of gallbladder
Cholecystocolic fistula
Cholecystoduodenal fistula

  K82.4 Cholesterolosis of gallbladder
Strawberry gallbladder
  EXCLUDES 1 cholesterolosis of gallbladder with cholecystitis (K81.-)
          cholesterolosis of gallbladder with cholelithiasis (K80.-)

  K82.8 Other specified diseases of gallbladder
Adhesions of cystic duct or gallbladder
Atrophy of cystic duct or gallbladder
Cyst of cystic duct or gallbladder
Dyskinesia of cystic duct or gallbladder
Hypertrophy of cystic duct or gallbladder
Nonfunctioning of cystic duct or gallbladder
Ulcer of cystic duct or gallbladder

  K82.9 Disease of gallbladder, unspecified ▽

☑4ᵗʰ **K83 Other diseases of biliary tract**
  EXCLUDES 1 postcholecystectomy syndrome (K91.5)
  EXCLUDES 2 conditions involving the gallbladder (K81-K82)
          conditions involving the cystic duct (K81-K82)

  K83.0 Cholangitis
Ascending cholangitis
Cholangitis NOS
Primary cholangitis
Recurrent cholangitis
Sclerosing cholangitis
Secondary cholangitis
Stenosing cholangitis
Suppurative cholangitis
  EXCLUDES 1 cholangitic liver abscess (K75.0)
          cholangitis with choledocholithiasis (K80.3-, K80.4-)
          chronic nonsuppurative destructive cholangitis (K74.3)

  K83.1 Obstruction of bile duct
Occlusion of bile duct without cholelithiasis
Stenosis of bile duct without cholelithiasis
Stricture of bile duct without cholelithiasis
  EXCLUDES 1 congenital obstruction of bile duct (Q44.3)
          obstruction of bile duct with cholelithiasis (K80.-)
  AHA: 2016, 1Q, 18

  K83.2 Perforation of bile duct
Rupture of bile duct

  K83.3 Fistula of bile duct
Choledochoduodenal fistula

  K83.4 Spasm of sphincter of Oddi

  K83.5 Biliary cyst

  K83.8 Other specified diseases of biliary tract
Adhesions of biliary tract
Atrophy of biliary tract
Hypertrophy of biliary tract
Ulcer of biliary tract

  K83.9 Disease of biliary tract, unspecified ▽

☑ Additional Character Req Vx7ᵗʰ Placeholder Alert Manifestation HCC CMS-HCC Condition ▽ Unspecified Code ▶◀ Revised Text ● New Code ▲ Revised Code Title

ICD-10-CM 2018 **689**

✔4ᵗʰ **K85　Acute pancreatitis**
　INCLUDES　acute (recurrent) pancreatitis
　　　　　　subacute pancreatitis

✔5ᵗʰ **K85.0　Idiopathic acute pancreatitis**
　K85.00　Idiopathic acute pancreatitis without necrosis or infection
　K85.01　Idiopathic acute pancreatitis with uninfected necrosis
　K85.02　Idiopathic acute pancreatitis with infected necrosis

✔5ᵗʰ **K85.1　Biliary acute pancreatitis**
　Gallstone pancreatitis
　K85.10　Biliary acute pancreatitis without necrosis or infection
　K85.11　Biliary acute pancreatitis with uninfected necrosis
　K85.12　Biliary acute pancreatitis with infected necrosis

✔5ᵗʰ **K85.2　Alcohol induced acute pancreatitis**
　EXCLUDES 2　alcohol induced chronic pancreatitis (K86.0)
　K85.20　Alcohol induced acute pancreatitis without necrosis or infection
　K85.21　Alcohol induced acute pancreatitis with uninfected necrosis
　K85.22　Alcohol induced acute pancreatitis with infected necrosis

✔5ᵗʰ **K85.3　Drug induced acute pancreatitis**
　Use additional code for adverse effect, if applicable, to identify drug (T36-T50 with fifth or sixth character 5)
　Use additional code to identify drug abuse and dependence (F11. – F17.-)
　K85.30　Drug induced acute pancreatitis without necrosis or infection
　K85.31　Drug induced acute pancreatitis with uninfected necrosis
　K85.32　Drug induced acute pancreatitis with infected necrosis

✔5ᵗʰ **K85.8　Other acute pancreatitis**
　K85.80　Other acute pancreatitis without necrosis or infection
　K85.81　Other acute pancreatitis with uninfected necrosis
　K85.82　Other acute pancreatitis with infected necrosis

✔5ᵗʰ **K85.9　Acute pancreatitis, unspecified**
　Pancreatitis NOS
　K85.90　Acute pancreatitis without necrosis or infection, unspecified　▽
　K85.91　Acute pancreatitis with uninfected necrosis, unspecified　▽
　K85.92　Acute pancreatitis with infected necrosis, unspecified　▽

✔4ᵗʰ **K86　Other diseases of pancreas**
　EXCLUDES 2　fibrocystic disease of pancreas (E84.-)
　　　　　　islet cell tumor (of pancreas) (D13.7)
　　　　　　pancreatic steatorrhea (K90.3)

　K86.0　Alcohol-induced chronic pancreatitis　HCC
　Use additional code to identify:
　　alcohol abuse and dependence (F10.-)
　Code also exocrine pancreatic insufficiency (K86.81)
　EXCLUDES 2　alcohol induced acute pancreatitis (K85.2-)

　K86.1　Other chronic pancreatitis　HCC
　Chronic pancreatitis NOS
　Infectious chronic pancreatitis
　Recurrent chronic pancreatitis
　Relapsing chronic pancreatitis
　Code also exocrine pancreatic insufficiency (K86.81)

　K86.2　Cyst of pancreas
　K86.3　Pseudocyst of pancreas

✔5ᵗʰ **K86.8　Other specified diseases of pancreas**
　K86.81　Exocrine pancreatic insufficiency
　K86.89　Other specified diseases of pancreas
　　Aseptic pancreatic necrosis, unrelated to acute pancreatitis
　　Atrophy of pancreas
　　Calculus of pancreas
　　Cirrhosis of pancreas
　　Fibrosis of pancreas
　　Pancreatic fat necrosis, unrelated to acute pancreatitis
　　Pancreatic infantilism
　　Pancreatic necrosis NOS, unrelated to acute pancreatitis

K86.9　Disease of pancreas, unspecified　▽

K87　Disorders of gallbladder, biliary tract and pancreas in diseases classified elsewhere
　Code first underlying disease
　EXCLUDES 1　cytomegaloviral pancreatitis (B25.2)
　　　　　　mumps pancreatitis (B26.3)
　　　　　　syphilitic gallbladder (A52.74)
　　　　　　syphilitic pancreas (A52.74)
　　　　　　tuberculosis of gallbladder (A18.83)
　　　　　　tuberculosis of pancreas (A18.83)

Other diseases of the digestive system (K90-K95)

✔4ᵗʰ **K90　Intestinal malabsorption**
　EXCLUDES 1　intestinal malabsorption following gastrointestinal surgery (K91.2)

　K90.0　Celiac disease
　Celiac disease with steatorrhea
　►Celiac gluten-sensitive enteropathy◄
　Nontropical sprue
　Use additional code for associated disorders including:
　　dermatitis herpetiformis (L13.0)
　　gluten ataxia (G32.81)
　Code also exocrine pancreatic insufficiency (K86.81)
　DEF: Malabsorption syndrome due to gluten consumption; symptoms include fetid, bulky, frothy, oily stools, distended abdomen, gas, asthenia, electrolyte depletion, and vitamin B, D, and K deficiency.

　K90.1　Tropical sprue
　Sprue NOS
　Tropical steatorrhea

　K90.2　Blind loop syndrome, not elsewhere classified
　Blind loop syndrome NOS
　EXCLUDES 1　congenital blind loop syndrome (Q43.8)
　　　　　　postsurgical blind loop syndrome (K91.2)

　K90.3　Pancreatic steatorrhea

✔5ᵗʰ **K90.4　Other malabsorption due to intolerance**
　EXCLUDES 2　►celiac gluten-sensitive enteropathy◄ (K90.0)
　　　　　　lactose intolerance (E73.-)
　K90.41　Non-celiac gluten sensitivity
　　Gluten sensitivity NOS
　　Non-celiac gluten sensitive enteropathy
　K90.49　Malabsorption due to intolerance, not elsewhere classified
　　Malabsorption due to intolerance to carbohydrate
　　Malabsorption due to intolerance to fat
　　Malabsorption due to intolerance to protein
　　Malabsorption due to intolerance to starch

✔5ᵗʰ **K90.8　Other intestinal malabsorption**
　K90.81　Whipple's disease
　K90.89　Other intestinal malabsorption
　K90.9　Intestinal malabsorption, unspecified　▽

✔4ᵗʰ **K91　Intraoperative and postprocedural complications and disorders of digestive system, not elsewhere classified**
　EXCLUDES 2　complications of artificial opening of digestive system (K94.-)
　　　　　　complications of bariatric procedures (K95.-)
　　　　　　gastrojejunal ulcer (K28.-)
　　　　　　postprocedural (radiation) retroperitoneal abscess (K68.11)
　　　　　　radiation colitis (K52.0)
　　　　　　radiation gastroenteritis (K52.0)
　　　　　　radiation proctitis (K62.7)

　K91.0　Vomiting following gastrointestinal surgery
　K91.1　Postgastric surgery syndromes
　Dumping syndrome
　Postgastrectomy syndrome
　Postvagotomy syndrome

　K91.2　Postsurgical malabsorption, not elsewhere classified
　Postsurgical blind loop syndrome
　EXCLUDES 1　malabsorption osteomalacia in adults (M83.2)
　　　　　　malabsorption osteoporosis, postsurgical (M80.8-, M81.8)

✔5ᵗʰ **K91.3　Postprocedural intestinal obstruction**
　AHA: 2017, 1Q, 40
　K91.30　Postprocedural intestinal obstruction, unspecified as to partial versus complete　▽
　　Postprocedural intestinal obstruction NOS
　K91.31　Postprocedural partial intestinal obstruction
　　Postprocedural incomplete intestinal obstruction
　K91.32　Postprocedural complete intestinal obstruction

K91.5   **Postcholecystectomy syndrome**

✓5ᵗʰ **K91.6**   **Intraoperative hemorrhage and hematoma of a digestive system organ or structure complicating a procedure**
> EXCLUDES 1   *intraoperative hemorrhage and hematoma of a digestive system organ or structure due to accidental puncture and laceration during a procedure (K91.7-)*

     K91.61   **Intraoperative hemorrhage and hematoma of a digestive system organ or structure complicating a digestive system procedure**

     K91.62   **Intraoperative hemorrhage and hematoma of a digestive system organ or structure complicating other procedure**

✓5ᵗʰ **K91.7**   **Accidental puncture and laceration of a digestive system organ or structure during a procedure**

     K91.71   **Accidental puncture and laceration of a digestive system organ or structure during a digestive system procedure**

     K91.72   **Accidental puncture and laceration of a digestive system organ or structure during other procedure**

✓5ᵗʰ **K91.8**   **Other intraoperative and postprocedural complications and disorders of digestive system**

     K91.81   **Other intraoperative complications of digestive system**

     K91.82   **Postprocedural hepatic failure**

     K91.83   **Postprocedural hepatorenal syndrome**

     ✓6ᵗʰ **K91.84**   **Postprocedural hemorrhage of a digestive system organ or structure following a procedure**

         K91.840   **Postprocedural hemorrhage of a digestive system organ or structure following a digestive system procedure**
             AHA: 2016, 1Q, 15

         K91.841   **Postprocedural hemorrhage of a digestive system organ or structure following other procedure**

     ✓6ᵗʰ **K91.85**   **Complications of intestinal pouch**

         K91.850   **Pouchitis**   HCC
             Inflammation of internal ileoanal pouch
             DEF: Inflammatory complication of an existing surgically created ileoanal pouch, resulting in multiple GI complaints, including diarrhea, abdominal pain, rectal bleeding, fecal urgency, or incontinence.

         K91.858   **Other complications of intestinal pouch**   HCC

     K91.86   **Retained cholelithiasis following cholecystectomy**

     ✓6ᵗʰ **K91.87**   **Postprocedural hematoma and seroma of a digestive system organ or structure following a procedure**

         K91.870   **Postprocedural hematoma of a digestive system organ or structure following a digestive system procedure**

         K91.871   **Postprocedural hematoma of a digestive system organ or structure following other procedure**

         K91.872   **Postprocedural seroma of a digestive system organ or structure following a digestive system procedure**

         K91.873   **Postprocedural seroma of a digestive system organ or structure following other procedure**

     K91.89   **Other postprocedural complications and disorders of digestive system**
         Use additional code, if applicable, to further specify disorder
> EXCLUDES 2   *postprocedural retroperitoneal abscess (K68.11)*

         AHA: 2017, 1Q, 40

✓4ᵗʰ **K92**   **Other diseases of digestive system**
> EXCLUDES 1   *neonatal gastrointestinal hemorrhage (P54.0-P54.3)*

K92.0   **Hematemesis**

K92.1   **Melena**
> EXCLUDES 1   *occult blood in feces (R19.5)*

K92.2   **Gastrointestinal hemorrhage, unspecified**   ▽
Gastric hemorrhage NOS
Intestinal hemorrhage NOS
> EXCLUDES 1   *acute hemorrhagic gastritis (K29.01)*
> *hemorrhage of anus and rectum (K62.5)*
> *angiodysplasia of stomach with hemorrhage (K31.811)*
> *diverticular disease with hemorrhage (K57.-)*
> *gastritis and duodenitis with hemorrhage (K29.-)*
> *peptic ulcer with hemorrhage (K25-K28)*

✓5ᵗʰ **K92.8**   **Other specified diseases of the digestive system**

     K92.81   **Gastrointestinal mucositis (ulcerative)**
         Code also type of associated therapy, such as:
         antineoplastic and immunosuppressive drugs (T45.1X-)
         radiological procedure and radiotherapy (Y84.2)
> EXCLUDES 2   *mucositis (ulcerative) of vagina and vulva (N76.81)*
> *nasal mucositis (ulcerative) (J34.81)*
> *oral mucositis (ulcerative) (K12.3-)*

     K92.89   **Other specified diseases of the digestive system**

K92.9   **Disease of digestive system, unspecified**   ▽

✓4ᵗʰ **K94**   **Complications of artificial openings of the digestive system**

✓5ᵗʰ **K94.0**   **Colostomy complications**

     K94.00   **Colostomy complication, unspecified**   HCC ▽

     K94.01   **Colostomy hemorrhage**   HCC

     K94.02   **Colostomy infection**   HCC
         Use additional code to specify type of infection, such as:
         cellulitis of abdominal wall (L03.311)
         sepsis (A40-, A41-)

     K94.03   **Colostomy malfunction**   HCC
         Mechanical complication of colostomy

     K94.09   **Other complications of colostomy**   HCC

✓5ᵗʰ **K94.1**   **Enterostomy complications**

     K94.10   **Enterostomy complication, unspecified**   HCC ▽

     K94.11   **Enterostomy hemorrhage**   HCC

     K94.12   **Enterostomy infection**   HCC
         Use additional code to specify type of infection, such as:
         cellulitis of abdominal wall (L03.311)
         sepsis (A40-, A41-)

     K94.13   **Enterostomy malfunction**   HCC
         Mechanical complication of enterostomy

     K94.19   **Other complications of enterostomy**   HCC

✓5ᵗʰ **K94.2**   **Gastrostomy complications**

     K94.20   **Gastrostomy complication, unspecified**   HCC ▽

     K94.21   **Gastrostomy hemorrhage**   HCC

     K94.22   **Gastrostomy infection**   HCC
         Use additional code to specify type of infection, such as:
         cellulitis of abdominal wall (L03.311)
         sepsis (A40-, A41-)

     K94.23   **Gastrostomy malfunction**   HCC
         Mechanical complication of gastrostomy

     K94.29   **Other complications of gastrostomy**   HCC

✓5ᵗʰ **K94.3**   **Esophagostomy complications**

     K94.30   **Esophagostomy complications, unspecified**   HCC ▽

     K94.31   **Esophagostomy hemorrhage**   HCC

     K94.32   **Esophagostomy infection**   HCC
         Use additional code to identify the infection

     K94.33   **Esophagostomy malfunction**   HCC
         Mechanical complication of esophagostomy

     K94.39   **Other complications of esophagostomy**   HCC

✓4ᵗʰ **K95**   **Complications of bariatric procedures**

✓5ᵗʰ **K95.0**   **Complications of gastric band procedure**

     K95.01   **Infection due to gastric band procedure**
         Use additional code to specify type of infection or organism, such as:
         bacterial and viral infectious agents (B95.-, B96.-)
         cellulitis of abdominal wall (L03.311)
         sepsis (A40.-, A41.-)

     K95.09   **Other complications of gastric band procedure**
         Use additional code, if applicable, to further specify complication

---

☑ Additional Character Req   ✓7ᵗʰ Placeholder Alert   Manifestation   HCC CMS-HCC Condition   ▽ Unspecified Code   ►◄ Revised Text   ● New Code   ▲ Revised Code Title

ICD-10-CM 2018   691

√5ᵗʰ **K95.8** **Complications of other bariatric procedure**

> EXCLUDES 1   *complications of gastric band surgery (K95.0-)*

K95.81 **Infection due to other bariatric procedure**
> Use additional code to specify type of infection or organism, such as:
> bacterial and viral infectious agents (B95.-, B96.-)
> cellulitis of abdominal wall (L03.311)
> sepsis (A40.-, A41.-)

K95.89 **Other complications of other bariatric procedure**
> Use additional code, if applicable, to further specify complication

EXCLUDES 1 Not coded here   EXCLUDES 2 Not included here   N Newborn Age: 0   P Pediatric Age: 0-17   M Maternity Age: 12-55   A Adult Age: 15-124

692   ICD-10-CM 2018

Chapter 12. Diseases of the Skin and Subcutaneous Tissue (L00–L99)

Chapter Specific Guidelines with Coding Examples

The chapter specific guidelines from the ICD-10-CM Official Guidelines for Coding and Reporting have been provided below. Along with these guidelines are coding examples, contained in the shaded boxes, that have been developed to help illustrate the coding and/or sequencing guidance found in these guidelines.

a. Pressure ulcer stage codes

1) Pressure ulcer stages

Codes from category L89, Pressure ulcer, identify the site of the pressure ulcer as well as the stage of the ulcer.

The ICD-10-CM classifies pressure ulcer stages based on severity, which is designated by stages 1-4, unspecified stage and unstageable.

Assign as many codes from category L89 as needed to identify all the pressure ulcers the patient has, if applicable.

> Stage 3 pressure ulcer left ankle, 6 x 7 cm that invades the fascia; stage 2 pressure ulcer of left hip
>
> **L89.523**   **Pressure ulcer of left ankle, stage 3**
>
> **L89.222**   **Pressure ulcer of left hip, stage 2**
>
> *Explanation:* Patient has a left ankle pressure ulcer documented as stage 3 and a left hip pressure ulcer documented as stage 2. Combination codes from category L89 Pressure ulcer, identify the site of the pressure ulcer as well as the stage. Assign as many codes from category L89 as needed to identify all the pressure ulcers the patient has.

2) Unstageable pressure ulcers

Assignment of the code for unstageable pressure ulcer (L89.--0) should be based on the clinical documentation. These codes are used for pressure ulcers whose stage cannot be clinically determined (e.g., the ulcer is covered by eschar or has been treated with a skin or muscle graft) and pressure ulcers that are documented as deep tissue injury but not documented as due to trauma. This code should not be confused with the codes for unspecified stage (L89.--9). When there is no documentation regarding the stage of the pressure ulcer, assign the appropriate code for unspecified stage (L89.--9).

> Pressure ulcer of the right lower back documented as unstageable due to the presence of thick eschar covering the ulcer
>
> **L89.130**   **Pressure ulcer of right lower back, unstageable**
>
> *Explanation:* Codes for unstageable pressure ulcers are assigned when the stage cannot be clinically determined (e.g., the ulcer is covered by eschar or has been treated with a skin or muscle graft).

3) Documented pressure ulcer stage

Assignment of the pressure ulcer stage code should be guided by clinical documentation of the stage or documentation of the terms found in the Alphabetic Index. For clinical terms describing the stage that are not found in the Alphabetic Index, and there is no documentation of the stage, the provider should be queried.

> Left heel pressure ulcer with partial thickness skin loss involving the dermis
>
> **L89.622**   **Pressure ulcer of left heel, stage 2**
>
> *Explanation:* Code assignment for the pressure ulcer stage should be guided by either the clinical documentation of the stage or the documentation of terms found in the Alphabetic Index. The clinical documentation describing the left heel pressure ulcer "partial thickness skin loss involving the dermis" matches the ICD-10-CM index parenthetical description for stage 2 "(abrasion, blister, partial thickness skin loss involving epidermis and/or dermis)."

4) Patients admitted with pressure ulcers documented as healed

No code is assigned if the documentation states that the pressure ulcer is completely healed.

> Patient receiving follow-up examination of a completely healed pressure ulcer of the foot
>
> **Z09**   **Encounter for follow-up examination after completed treatment for conditions other than malignant neoplasm**
>
> **Z87.2**   **Personal history of diseases of the skin and subcutaneous tissue**
>
> *Explanation:* Assign only codes for the reason for the encounter and the personal history of the pressure ulcer. Personal history code Z87.2 includes conditions classifiable to L00–L99 such as pressure ulcer. No code is assigned for a pressure ulcer documented as completely healed.

5) Patients admitted with pressure ulcers documented as healing

Pressure ulcers described as healing should be assigned the appropriate pressure ulcer stage code based on the documentation in the medical record. If the documentation does not provide information about the stage of the healing pressure ulcer, assign the appropriate code for unspecified stage.

If the documentation is unclear as to whether the patient has a current (new) pressure ulcer or if the patient is being treated for a healing pressure ulcer, query the provider.

For ulcers that were present on admission but healed at the time of discharge, assign the code for the site and stage of the pressure ulcer at the time of admission.

6) Patient admitted with pressure ulcer evolving into another stage during the admission

If a patient is admitted with a pressure ulcer at one stage and it progresses to a higher stage, two separate codes should be assigned: one code for the site and stage of the ulcer on admission and a second code for the same ulcer site and the highest stage reported during the stay.

Chapter 12. Diseases of the Skin and Subcutaneous Tissue (L00-L99)

EXCLUDES 2   certain conditions originating in the perinatal period (P04-P96)
certain infectious and parasitic diseases (A00-B99)
complications of pregnancy, childbirth and the puerperium (O00-O9A)
congenital malformations, deformations, and chromosomal abnormalities (Q00-Q99)
endocrine, nutritional and metabolic diseases (E00-E88)
lipomelanotic reticulosis (I89.8)
neoplasms (C00-D49)
symptoms, signs and abnormal clinical and laboratory findings, not elsewhere classified (R00-R94)
systemic connective tissue disorders (M30-M36)
viral warts (B07.-)

This chapter contains the following blocks:

L00-L08   Infections of the skin and subcutaneous tissue
L10-L14   Bullous disorders
L20-L30   Dermatitis and eczema
L40-L45   Papulosquamous disorders
L49-L54   Urticaria and erythema
L55-L59   Radiation-related disorders of the skin and subcutaneous tissue
L60-L75   Disorders of skin appendages
L76   Intraoperative and postprocedural complications of skin and subcutaneous tissue
L80-L99   Other disorders of the skin and subcutaneous tissue

Infections of the skin and subcutaneous tissue (L00-L08)

Use additional code (B95-B97) to identify infectious agent

EXCLUDES 2   hordeolum (H00.0)
infective dermatitis (L30.3)
local infections of skin classified in Chapter 1
lupus panniculitis (L93.2)
panniculitis NOS (M79.3)
panniculitis of neck and back (M54.0-)
perlèche NOS (K13.0)
perlèche due to candidiasis (B37.0)
perlèche due to riboflavin deficiency (E53.0)
pyogenic granuloma (L98.0)
relapsing panniculitis [Weber-Christian] (M35.6)
viral warts (B07.-)
zoster (B02.-)

L00   Staphylococcal scalded skin syndrome

Ritter's disease
Use additional code to identify percentage of skin exfoliation (L49.-)

EXCLUDES 1   bullous impetigo (L01.03)
pemphigus neonatorum (L01.03)
toxic epidermal necrolysis [Lyell] (L51.2)

DEF: Infectious skin disease of children younger than 5 years marked by eruptions ranging from a few localized blisters to widespread, easily ruptured, fine vesicles and bullae affecting almost the entire body; results in exfoliation of large planes of skin and leaves raw areas.

✓4ᵗʰ L01   Impetigo

EXCLUDES 1   impetigo herpetiformis (L40.1)

✓5ᵗʰ L01.0   Impetigo

Impetigo contagiosa
Impetigo vulgaris

     L01.00   **Impetigo, unspecified**   ▽
         Impetigo NOS

     L01.01   **Non-bullous impetigo**

     L01.02   **Bockhart's impetigo**
         Impetigo follicularis
         Perifolliculitis NOS
         Superficial pustular perifolliculitis

     L01.03   **Bullous impetigo**
         Impetigo neonatorum
         Pemphigus neonatorum

     L01.09   **Other impetigo**
         Ulcerative impetigo

    L01.1   **Impetiginization of other dermatoses**

✓4ᵗʰ L02   Cutaneous abscess, furuncle and carbuncle

Use additional code to identify organism (B95-B96)

EXCLUDES 2   abscess of anus and rectal regions (K61.-)
abscess of female genital organs (external) (N76.4)
abscess of male genital organs (external) (N48.2, N49-)

✓5ᵗʰ L02.0   Cutaneous abscess, furuncle and carbuncle of face

EXCLUDES 2   abscess of ear, external (H60.0)
abscess of eyelid (H00.0)
abscess of head [any part, except face] (L02.8)
abscess of lacrimal gland (H04.0)
abscess of lacrimal passages (H04.3)
abscess of mouth (K12.2)
abscess of nose (J34.0)
abscess of orbit (H05.0)
submandibular abscess (K12.2)

    L02.01   **Cutaneous abscess of face**

    L02.02   **Furuncle of face**
        Boil of face
        Folliculitis of face

    L02.03   **Carbuncle of face**

✓5ᵗʰ L02.1   Cutaneous abscess, furuncle and carbuncle of neck

    L02.11   **Cutaneous abscess of neck**

    L02.12   **Furuncle of neck**
        Boil of neck
        Folliculitis of neck

    L02.13   **Carbuncle of neck**

✓5ᵗʰ L02.2   Cutaneous abscess, furuncle and carbuncle of trunk

EXCLUDES 1   non-newborn omphalitis (L08.82)
omphalitis of newborn (P38.-)

EXCLUDES 2   abscess of breast (N61.1)
abscess of buttocks (L02.3)
abscess of female external genital organs (N76.4)
abscess of hip (L02.4)
abscess of male external genital organs (N48.2, N49-)

   ✓6ᵗʰ **L02.21**   **Cutaneous abscess of trunk**

     L02.211   **Cutaneous abscess of abdominal wall**

     L02.212   **Cutaneous abscess of back [any part, except buttock]**

     L02.213   **Cutaneous abscess of chest wall**

     L02.214   **Cutaneous abscess of groin**

     L02.215   **Cutaneous abscess of perineum**

     L02.216   **Cutaneous abscess of umbilicus**

     L02.219   **Cutaneous abscess of trunk, unspecified**   ▽

   ✓6ᵗʰ **L02.22**   **Furuncle of trunk**
        Boil of trunk
        Folliculitis of trunk

     L02.221   **Furuncle of abdominal wall**

     L02.222   **Furuncle of back [any part, except buttock]**

     L02.223   **Furuncle of chest wall**

     L02.224   **Furuncle of groin**

     L02.225   **Furuncle of perineum**

     L02.226   **Furuncle of umbilicus**

     L02.229   **Furuncle of trunk, unspecified**   ▽

   ✓6ᵗʰ **L02.23**   **Carbuncle of trunk**

     L02.231   **Carbuncle of abdominal wall**

     L02.232   **Carbuncle of back [any part, except buttock]**

     L02.233   **Carbuncle of chest wall**

     L02.234   **Carbuncle of groin**

     L02.235   **Carbuncle of perineum**

     L02.236   **Carbuncle of umbilicus**

     L02.239   **Carbuncle of trunk, unspecified**   ▽

✓5ᵗʰ L02.3   Cutaneous abscess, furuncle and carbuncle of buttock

EXCLUDES 1   pilonidal cyst with abscess (L05.01)

    L02.31   **Cutaneous abscess of buttock**
        Cutaneous abscess of gluteal region

    L02.32   **Furuncle of buttock**
        Boil of buttock
        Folliculitis of buttock
        Furuncle of gluteal region

    L02.33   **Carbuncle of buttock**
        Carbuncle of gluteal region

EXCLUDES 1   Not coded here   EXCLUDES 2   Not included here   N Newborn Age: 0   P Pediatric Age: 0-17   M Maternity Age: 12-55   A Adult Age: 15-124

694   ICD-10-CM 2018

√5th **L02.4 Cutaneous abscess, furuncle and carbuncle of limb**
EXCLUDES 2 *cutaneous abscess, furuncle and carbuncle of groin (L02.214, L02.224, L02.234)*
cutaneous abscess, furuncle and carbuncle of hand (L02.5-)
cutaneous abscess, furuncle and carbuncle of foot (L02.6-)

√6th **L02.41 Cutaneous abscess of limb**
L02.411 Cutaneous abscess of right axilla
L02.412 Cutaneous abscess of left axilla
L02.413 Cutaneous abscess of right upper limb
L02.414 Cutaneous abscess of left upper limb
L02.415 Cutaneous abscess of right lower limb
L02.416 Cutaneous abscess of left lower limb
L02.419 Cutaneous abscess of limb, unspecified ▽

√6th **L02.42 Furuncle of limb**
Boil of limb
Folliculitis of limb
L02.421 Furuncle of right axilla
L02.422 Furuncle of left axilla
L02.423 Furuncle of right upper limb
L02.424 Furuncle of left upper limb
L02.425 Furuncle of right lower limb
L02. Furuncle of left lower limb
L02.429 Furuncle of limb, unspecified ▽

√6th **L02.43 Carbuncle of limb**
L02.431 Carbuncle of right axilla
L02.432 Carbuncle of left axilla
L02.433 Carbuncle of right upper limb
L02.434 Carbuncle of left upper limb
L02.435 Carbuncle of right lower limb
L02.436 Carbuncle of left lower limb
L02.439 Carbuncle of limb, unspecified ▽

√5th **L02.5 Cutaneous abscess, furuncle and carbuncle of hand**
√6th **L02.51 Cutaneous abscess of hand**
L02.511 Cutaneous abscess of right hand
L02.512 Cutaneous abscess of left hand
L02.519 Cutaneous abscess of unspecified hand ▽

√6th **L02.52 Furuncle hand**
Boil of hand
Folliculitis of hand
L02.521 Furuncle right hand
L02.522 Furuncle left hand
L02.529 Furuncle unspecified hand ▽

√6th **L02.53 Carbuncle of hand**
L02.531 Carbuncle of right hand
L02.532 Carbuncle of left hand
L02.539 Carbuncle of unspecified hand ▽

√5th **L02.6 Cutaneous abscess, furuncle and carbuncle of foot**
√6th **L02.61 Cutaneous abscess of foot**
L02.611 Cutaneous abscess of right foot
L02.612 Cutaneous abscess of left foot
L02.619 Cutaneous abscess of unspecified foot ▽

√6th **L02.62 Furuncle of foot**
Boil of foot
Folliculitis of foot
L02.621 Furuncle of right foot
L02.622 Furuncle of left foot
L02.629 Furuncle of unspecified foot ▽

√6th **L02.63 Carbuncle of foot**
L02.631 Carbuncle of right foot
L02.632 Carbuncle of left foot
L02.639 Carbuncle of unspecified foot ▽

√5th **L02.8 Cutaneous abscess, furuncle and carbuncle of other sites**
√6th **L02.81 Cutaneous abscess of other sites**
L02.811 Cutaneous abscess of head [any part, except face]
L02.818 Cutaneous abscess of other sites

√6th **L02.82 Furuncle of other sites**
Boil of other sites
Folliculitis of other sites
L02.821 Furuncle of head [any part, except face]
L02.828 Furuncle of other sites

√6th **L02.83 Carbuncle of other sites**
L02.831 Carbuncle of head [any part, except face]
L02.838 Carbuncle of other sites

√5th **L02.9 Cutaneous abscess, furuncle and carbuncle, unspecified**
L02.91 Cutaneous abscess, unspecified ▽
L02.92 Furuncle, unspecified ▽
Boil NOS
Furunculosis NOS
L02.93 Carbuncle, unspecified ▽

√4th **L03 Cellulitis and acute lymphangitis**
EXCLUDES 2 *cellulitis of anal and rectal region (K61.-)*
cellulitis of external auditory canal (H60.1)
cellulitis of eyelid (H00.03-)
cellulitis of female external genital organs (N76.4)
cellulitis of lacrimal apparatus (H04.3)
cellulitis of male external genital organs (N48.2, N49-)
cellulitis of mouth (K12.2)
cellulitis of nose (J34.0)
eosinophilic cellulitis [Wells] (L98.3)
febrile neutrophilic dermatosis [Sweet] (L98.2)
lymphangitis (chronic) (subacute) (I89.1)

√5th **L03.0 Cellulitis and acute lymphangitis of finger and toe**
Infection of nail
Onychia
Paronychia
Perionychia

√6th **L03.01 Cellulitis of finger**
Felon
Whitlow
EXCLUDES 1 *herpetic whitlow (B00.89)*
DEF: Felon: Superficial bacterial skin infection at the tip of the finger.
L03.011 Cellulitis of right finger
L03.012 Cellulitis of left finger
L03.019 Cellulitis of unspecified finger ▽

√6th **L03.02 Acute lymphangitis of finger**
Hangnail with lymphangitis of finger
L03.021 Acute lymphangitis of right finger
L03.022 Acute lymphangitis of left finger
L03.029 Acute lymphangitis of unspecified finger ▽

√6th **L03.03 Cellulitis of toe**
L03.031 Cellulitis of right toe
L03.032 Cellulitis of left toe
L03.039 Cellulitis of unspecified toe ▽

√6th **L03.04 Acute lymphangitis of toe**
Hangnail with lymphangitis of toe
L03.041 Acute lymphangitis of right toe
L03.042 Acute lymphangitis of left toe
L03.049 Acute lymphangitis of unspecified toe ▽

√5th **L03.1 Cellulitis and acute lymphangitis of other parts of limb**
√6th **L03.11 Cellulitis of other parts of limb**
EXCLUDES 2 *cellulitis of fingers (L03.01-)*
cellulitis of toes (L03.03-)
groin (L03.314)
L03.111 Cellulitis of right axilla
L03.112 Cellulitis of left axilla
L03.113 Cellulitis of right upper limb
L03.114 Cellulitis of left upper limb
L03.115 Cellulitis of right lower limb
L03.116 Cellulitis of left lower limb
L03.119 Cellulitis of unspecified part of limb ▽

√6th **L03.12 Acute lymphangitis of other parts of limb**
EXCLUDES 2 *acute lymphangitis of fingers (L03.02-)*
acute lymphangitis of groin (L03.324)
acute lymphangitis of toes (L03.04-)
L03.121 Acute lymphangitis of right axilla
L03.122 Acute lymphangitis of left axilla
L03.123 Acute lymphangitis of right upper limb
L03.124 Acute lymphangitis of left upper limb
L03.125 Acute lymphangitis of right lower limb
L03.126 Acute lymphangitis of left lower limb
L03.129 Acute lymphangitis of unspecified part of limb ▽

Chapter 12. Diseases of the Skin and Subcutaneous Tissue

✓5ᵗʰ L03.2   **Cellulitis and acute lymphangitis of face and neck**

     ✓6ᵗʰ L03.21   **Cellulitis and acute lymphangitis of face**

         L03.211   **Cellulitis of face**
            EXCLUDES 2   *abscess of orbit (H05.01-)*
                cellulitis of ear (H60.1-)
                cellulitis of eyelid (H00.03-)
                cellulitis of head (L03.811)
                cellulitis of lacrimal apparatus
                   (H04.3)
                cellulitis of lip (K13.0)
                cellulitis of mouth (K12.2)
                cellulitis of nose (internal) (J34.0)
                cellulitis of orbit (H05.01-)
                cellulitis of scalp (L03.811)
            AHA: 2013, 4Q, 123

         L03.212   **Acute lymphangitis of face**

         L03.213   **Periorbital cellulitis**
            Preseptal cellulitis

     ✓6ᵗʰ L03.22   **Cellulitis and acute lymphangitis of neck**

         L03.221   **Cellulitis of neck**

         L03.222   **Acute lymphangitis of neck**

✓5ᵗʰ L03.3   **Cellulitis and acute lymphangitis of trunk**

     ✓6ᵗʰ L03.31   **Cellulitis of trunk**
           EXCLUDES 2   *cellulitis of anal and rectal regions (K61.-)*
               cellulitis of breast NOS (N61.0)
               cellulitis of female external genital organs
                  (N76.4)
               cellulitis of male external genital organs
                  (N48.2, N49-)
               omphalitis of newborn (P38.-)
               puerperal cellulitis of breast (O91.2)

         L03.311   **Cellulitis of abdominal wall**
            EXCLUDES 2   *cellulitis of umbilicus (L03.316)*
                 cellulitis of groin (L03.314)

         L03.312   **Cellulitis of back [any part except buttock]**

         L03.313   **Cellulitis of chest wall**

         L03.314   **Cellulitis of groin**

         L03.315   **Cellulitis of perineum**

         L03.316   **Cellulitis of umbilicus**

         L03.317   **Cellulitis of buttock**

         L03.319   **Cellulitis of trunk, unspecified**   ▽

     ✓6ᵗʰ L03.32   **Acute lymphangitis of trunk**

         L03.321   **Acute lymphangitis of abdominal wall**

         L03.322   **Acute lymphangitis of back [any part except buttock]**

         L03.323   **Acute lymphangitis of chest wall**

         L03.324   **Acute lymphangitis of groin**

         L03.325   **Acute lymphangitis of perineum**

         L03.326   **Acute lymphangitis of umbilicus**

         L03.327   **Acute lymphangitis of buttock**

         L03.329   **Acute lymphangitis of trunk, unspecified**   ▽

✓5ᵗʰ L03.8   **Cellulitis and acute lymphangitis of other sites**

     ✓6ᵗʰ L03.81   **Cellulitis of other sites**

         L03.811   **Cellulitis of head [any part, except face]**
            Cellulitis of scalp
            EXCLUDES 2   *cellulitis of face (L03.211)*

         L03.818   **Cellulitis of other sites**

     ✓6ᵗʰ L03.89   **Acute lymphangitis of other sites**

         L03.891   **Acute lymphangitis of head [any part, except face]**

         L03.898   **Acute lymphangitis of other sites**

✓5ᵗʰ L03.9   **Cellulitis and acute lymphangitis, unspecified**

     L03.90   **Cellulitis, unspecified**   ▽

     L03.91   **Acute lymphangitis, unspecified**   ▽
         EXCLUDES 1   *lymphangitis NOS (I89.1)*

✓4ᵗʰ L04   **Acute lymphadenitis**
     INCLUDES   abscess (acute) of lymph nodes, except mesenteric
            acute lymphadenitis, except mesenteric
     EXCLUDES 1   *chronic or subacute lymphadenitis, except mesenteric (I88.1)*
            enlarged lymph nodes (R59.-)
            human immunodeficiency virus [HIV] disease resulting in
               generalized lymphadenopathy (B20)
            lymphadenitis NOS (I88.9)
            nonspecific mesenteric lymphadenitis (I88.0)

     L04.0   **Acute lymphadenitis of face, head and neck**

Pilonidal Cyst

     Skin

     Fistula

     Pilonidal cyst

     Fat

     Bone

     L04.1   **Acute lymphadenitis of trunk**

     L04.2   **Acute lymphadenitis of upper limb**
         Acute lymphadenitis of axilla
         Acute lymphadenitis of shoulder

     L04.3   **Acute lymphadenitis of lower limb**
         Acute lymphadenitis of hip
         EXCLUDES 2   *acute lymphadenitis of groin (L04.1)*

     L04.8   **Acute lymphadenitis of other sites**

     L04.9   **Acute lymphadenitis, unspecified**   ▽

✓4ᵗʰ L05   **Pilonidal cyst and sinus**

     ✓5ᵗʰ L05.0   **Pilonidal cyst and sinus with abscess**

         L05.01   **Pilonidal cyst with abscess**
            Pilonidal abscess
            Pilonidal dimple with abscess
            Postanal dimple with abscess
            EXCLUDES 2   *congenital sacral dimple (Q82.6)*
                 parasacral dimple (Q82.6)

         L05.02   **Pilonidal sinus with abscess**
            Coccygeal fistula with abscess
            Coccygeal sinus with abscess
            Pilonidal fistula with abscess

     ✓5ᵗʰ L05.9   **Pilonidal cyst and sinus without abscess**

         L05.91   **Pilonidal cyst without abscess**
            Pilonidal dimple
            Postanal dimple
            Pilonidal cyst NOS
            EXCLUDES 2   *congenital sacral dimple (Q82.6)*
                 parasacral dimple (Q82.6)

         L05.92   **Pilonidal sinus without abscess**
            Coccygeal fistula
            Coccygeal sinus without abscess
            Pilonidal fistula

✓4ᵗʰ L08   **Other local infections of skin and subcutaneous tissue**

     L08.0   **Pyoderma**
         Dermatitis gangrenosa
         Purulent dermatitis
         Septic dermatitis
         Suppurative dermatitis
         EXCLUDES 1   *pyoderma gangrenosum (L88)*
                 pyoderma vegetans (L08.81)

     L08.1   **Erythrasma**

     ✓5ᵗʰ L08.8   **Other specified local infections of the skin and subcutaneous tissue**

         L08.81   **Pyoderma vegetans**
            EXCLUDES 1   *pyoderma gangrenosum (L88)*
                 pyoderma NOS (L08.0)

         L08.82   **Omphalitis not of newborn**
            EXCLUDES 1   *omphalitis of newborn (P38.-)*

         L08.89   **Other specified local infections of the skin and subcutaneous tissue**

     L08.9   **Local infection of the skin and subcutaneous tissue, unspecified**   ▽

EXCLUDES 1 Not coded here   EXCLUDES 2 Not included here   N Newborn Age: 0   P Pediatric Age: 0-17   M Maternity Age: 12-55   A Adult Age: 15-124

L03.2–L08.9

696   ICD-10-CM 2018

Bullous disorders (L10-L14)

EXCLUDES 1   *benign familial pemphigus [Hailey-Hailey] (Q82.8)*
staphylococcal scalded skin syndrome (L00)
toxic epidermal necrolysis [Lyell] (L51.2)

✓4ᵗʰ L10   Pemphigus
EXCLUDES 1   *pemphigus neonatorum (L01.03)*

L10.0   **Pemphigus vulgaris**

L10.1   **Pemphigus vegetans**

L10.2   **Pemphigus foliaceous**

L10.3   **Brazilian pemphigus [fogo selvagem]**

L10.4   **Pemphigus erythematosus**
Senear-Usher syndrome

L10.5   **Drug-induced pemphigus**
Use additional code for adverse effect, if applicable, to identify drug (T36-T50 with fifth or sixth character 5)

✓5ᵗʰ **L10.8**   **Other pemphigus**

     L10.81   **Paraneoplastic pemphigus**

     L10.89   **Other pemphigus**

L10.9   **Pemphigus, unspecified** ▽

✓4ᵗʰ L11   Other acantholytic disorders

L11.0   **Acquired keratosis follicularis**
EXCLUDES 1   *keratosis follicularis (congenital) [Darier-White] (Q82.8)*

L11.1   **Transient acantholytic dermatosis [Grover]**

L11.8   **Other specified acantholytic disorders**

L11.9   **Acantholytic disorder, unspecified** ▽

✓4ᵗʰ L12   Pemphigoid
EXCLUDES 1   *herpes gestationis (O26.4-)*
impetigo herpetiformis (L40.1)

L12.0   **Bullous pemphigoid**

L12.1   **Cicatricial pemphigoid**
Benign mucous membrane pemphigoid
DEF: Chronic autoimmune disease characterized by subepidermal blistering lesions of mucosa, including the conjunctiva; seen predominantly in the elderly; produces adhesions and scarring.

L12.2   **Chronic bullous disease of childhood** P
Juvenile dermatitis herpetiformis

✓5ᵗʰ **L12.3**   **Acquired epidermolysis bullosa**
EXCLUDES 1   *epidermolysis bullosa (congenital) (Q81.-)*

     L12.30   **Acquired epidermolysis bullosa, unspecified** HCC ▽

     L12.31   **Epidermolysis bullosa due to drug** HCC
Use additional code for adverse effect, if applicable, to identify drug (T36-T50 with fifth or sixth character 5)

     L12.35   **Other acquired epidermolysis bullosa** HCC

L12.8   **Other pemphigoid**

L12.9   **Pemphigoid, unspecified** ▽

✓4ᵗʰ L13   Other bullous disorders

L13.0   **Dermatitis herpetiformis**
Duhring's disease
Hydroa herpetiformis
EXCLUDES 1   *juvenile dermatitis herpetiformis (L12.2)*
senile dermatitis herpetiformis (L12.0)
DEF: Skin disease to which people are genetically predisposed resulting from an immunological response to gluten; seen as an extremely pruritic eruption of various lesions that frequently heal, leaving hyperpigmentation or hypopigmentation and occasionally scarring; usually associated with an asymptomatic gluten-sensitive enteropathy.

L13.1   **Subcorneal pustular dermatitis**
Sneddon-Wilkinson disease

L13.8   **Other specified bullous disorders**

L13.9   **Bullous disorder, unspecified** ▽

L14   *Bullous disorders in diseases classified elsewhere*
Code first underlying disease

Dermatitis and eczema (L20-L30)

NOTE   In this block the terms dermatitis and eczema are used synonymously and interchangeably.

EXCLUDES 2   *chronic (childhood) granulomatous disease (D71)*
dermatitis gangrenosa (L08.0)
dermatitis herpetiformis (L13.0)
dry skin dermatitis (L85.3)
factitial dermatitis (L98.1)
perioral dermatitis (L71.0)
radiation-related disorders of the skin and subcutaneous tissue (L55-L59)
stasis dermatitis (I87.2)

✓4ᵗʰ L20   Atopic dermatitis

L20.0   **Besnier's prurigo**

✓5ᵗʰ **L20.8**   **Other atopic dermatitis**
EXCLUDES 2   *circumscribed neurodermatitis (L28.0)*

     L20.81   **Atopic neurodermatitis**
Diffuse neurodermatitis

     L20.82   **Flexural eczema**

     L20.83   **Infantile (acute) (chronic) eczema** P

     L20.84   **Intrinsic (allergic) eczema**

     L20.89   **Other atopic dermatitis**

L20.9   **Atopic dermatitis, unspecified** ▽

✓4ᵗʰ L21   Seborrheic dermatitis
EXCLUDES 2   *infective dermatitis (L30.3)*
seborrheic keratosis (L82.-)

L21.0   **Seborrhea capitis** P
Cradle cap

L21.1   **Seborrheic infantile dermatitis** P

L21.8   **Other seborrheic dermatitis**

L21.9   **Seborrheic dermatitis, unspecified** ▽
Seborrhea NOS

L22   Diaper dermatitis
Diaper erythema
Diaper rash
Psoriasiform diaper rash

✓4ᵗʰ L23   Allergic contact dermatitis
EXCLUDES 1   *allergy NOS (T78.40)*
contact dermatitis NOS (L25.9)
dermatitis NOS (L30.9)
EXCLUDES 2   *dermatitis due to substances taken internally (L27.-)*
dermatitis of eyelid (H01.1-)
diaper dermatitis (L22)
eczema of external ear (H60.5-)
irritant contact dermatitis (L24.-)
perioral dermatitis (L71.0)
radiation-related disorders of the skin and subcutaneous tissue (L55-L59)

L23.0   **Allergic contact dermatitis due to metals**
Allergic contact dermatitis due to chromium
Allergic contact dermatitis due to nickel

L23.1   **Allergic contact dermatitis due to adhesives**

L23.2   **Allergic contact dermatitis due to cosmetics**

L23.3   **Allergic contact dermatitis due to drugs in contact with skin**
Use additional code for adverse effect, if applicable, to identify drug (T36-T50 with fifth or sixth character 5)
EXCLUDES 2   *dermatitis due to ingested drugs and medicaments (L27.0-L27.1)*

L23.4   **Allergic contact dermatitis due to dyes**

L23.5   **Allergic contact dermatitis due to other chemical products**
Allergic contact dermatitis due to cement
Allergic contact dermatitis due to insecticide
Allergic contact dermatitis due to plastic
Allergic contact dermatitis due to rubber

L23.6   **Allergic contact dermatitis due to food in contact with the skin**
EXCLUDES 2   *dermatitis due to ingested food (L27.2)*

L23.7   **Allergic contact dermatitis due to plants, except food**
EXCLUDES 2   *allergy NOS due to pollen (J30.1)*

✓5ᵗʰ **L23.8**   **Allergic contact dermatitis due to other agents**

     L23.81   **Allergic contact dermatitis due to animal (cat) (dog) dander**
Allergic contact dermatitis due to animal (cat) (dog) hair

     L23.89   **Allergic contact dermatitis due to other agents**

✓ Additional Character Req   ✓x7ᵗʰ Placeholder Alert   Manifestation   HCC CMS-HCC Condition   ▽ Unspecified Code   ▶◀ Revised Text   ● New Code   ▲ Revised Code Title

L23.9   Allergic contact dermatitis, unspecified cause ▽
Allergic contact eczema NOS

✓4ᵗʰ **L24   Irritant contact dermatitis**
EXCLUDES 1   *allergy NOS (T78.40)*
contact dermatitis NOS (L25.9)
dermatitis NOS (L30.9)
EXCLUDES 2   *allergic contact dermatitis (L23.-)*
dermatitis due to substances taken internally (L27.-)
dermatitis of eyelid (H01.1-)
diaper dermatitis (L22)
eczema of external ear (H60.5-)
perioral dermatitis (L71.0)
radiation-related disorders of the skin and subcutaneous tissue (L55-L59)

L24.0   Irritant contact dermatitis due to detergents
L24.1   Irritant contact dermatitis due to oils and greases
L24.2   Irritant contact dermatitis due to solvents
Irritant contact dermatitis due to chlorocompound
Irritant contact dermatitis due to cyclohexane
Irritant contact dermatitis due to ester
Irritant contact dermatitis due to glycol
Irritant contact dermatitis due to hydrocarbon
Irritant contact dermatitis due to ketone
L24.3   Irritant contact dermatitis due to cosmetics
L24.4   Irritant contact dermatitis due to drugs in contact with skin
Use additional code for adverse effect, if applicable, to identify drug (T36-T50 with fifth or sixth character 5)
L24.5   Irritant contact dermatitis due to other chemical products
Irritant contact dermatitis due to cement
Irritant contact dermatitis due to insecticide
Irritant contact dermatitis due to plastic
Irritant contact dermatitis due to rubber
L24.6   Irritant contact dermatitis due to food in contact with skin
EXCLUDES 2   *dermatitis due to ingested food (L27.2)*
L24.7   Irritant contact dermatitis due to plants, except food
EXCLUDES 2   *allergy NOS to pollen (J30.1)*
✓5ᵗʰ **L24.8   Irritant contact dermatitis due to other agents**
L24.81   Irritant contact dermatitis due to metals
Irritant contact dermatitis due to chromium
Irritant contact dermatitis due to nickel
L24.89   Irritant contact dermatitis due to other agents
Irritant contact dermatitis due to dyes
L24.9   Irritant contact dermatitis, unspecified cause ▽
Irritant contact eczema NOS

✓4ᵗʰ **L25   Unspecified contact dermatitis**
EXCLUDES 1   *allergic contact dermatitis (L23.-)*
allergy NOS (T78.40)
dermatitis NOS (L30.9)
irritant contact dermatitis (L24.-)
EXCLUDES 2   *dermatitis due to ingested substances (L27.-)*
dermatitis of eyelid (H01.1-)
eczema of external ear (H60.5-)
perioral dermatitis (L71.0)
radiation-related disorders of the skin and subcutaneous tissue (L55-L59)

L25.0   Unspecified contact dermatitis due to cosmetics ▽
L25.1   Unspecified contact dermatitis due to drugs in contact with skin ▽
Use additional code for adverse effect, if applicable, to identify drug (T36-T50 with fifth or sixth character 5)
EXCLUDES 2   *dermatitis due to ingested drugs and medicaments (L27.0-L27.1)*
L25.2   Unspecified contact dermatitis due to dyes ▽
L25.3   Unspecified contact dermatitis due to other chemical products ▽
Unspecified contact dermatitis due to cement
Unspecified contact dermatitis due to insecticide
L25.4   Unspecified contact dermatitis due to food in contact with skin ▽
EXCLUDES 2   *dermatitis due to ingested food (L27.2)*
L25.5   Unspecified contact dermatitis due to plants, except food ▽
EXCLUDES 1   *nettle rash (L50.9)*
EXCLUDES 2   *allergy NOS due to pollen (J30.1)*
L25.8   Unspecified contact dermatitis due to other agents ▽
L25.9   Unspecified contact dermatitis, unspecified cause ▽
Contact dermatitis (occupational) NOS
Contact eczema (occupational) NOS

L26   Exfoliative dermatitis
Hebra's pityriasis
EXCLUDES 1   *Ritter's disease (L00)*

✓4ᵗʰ **L27   Dermatitis due to substances taken internally**
EXCLUDES 1   *allergy NOS (T78.40)*
EXCLUDES 2   *adverse food reaction, except dermatitis (T78.0-T78.1)*
contact dermatitis (L23-L25)
drug photoallergic response (L56.1)
drug phototoxic response (L56.0)
urticaria (L50.-)
L27.0   Generalized skin eruption due to drugs and medicaments taken internally
Use additional code for adverse effect, if applicable, to identify drug (T36-T50 with fifth or sixth character 5)
L27.1   Localized skin eruption due to drugs and medicaments taken internally
Use additional code for adverse effect, if applicable, to identify drug (T36-T50 with fifth or sixth character 5)
L27.2   Dermatitis due to ingested food
EXCLUDES 2   *dermatitis due to food in contact with skin (L23.6, L24.6, L25.4)*
L27.8   Dermatitis due to other substances taken internally
L27.9   Dermatitis due to unspecified substance taken internally ▽

✓4ᵗʰ **L28   Lichen simplex chronicus and prurigo**
L28.0   Lichen simplex chronicus
Circumscribed neurodermatitis
Lichen NOS
L28.1   Prurigo nodularis
L28.2   Other prurigo
Prurigo NOS
Prurigo Hebra
Prurigo mitis
Urticaria papulosa

✓4ᵗʰ **L29   Pruritus**
EXCLUDES 1   *neurotic excoriation (L98.1)*
psychogenic pruritus (F45.8)
L29.0   Pruritus ani
L29.1   Pruritus scroti ♂
L29.2   Pruritus vulvae ♀
L29.3   Anogenital pruritus, unspecified ▽
L29.8   Other pruritus
L29.9   Pruritus, unspecified ▽
Itch NOS

✓4ᵗʰ **L30   Other and unspecified dermatitis**
EXCLUDES 2   *contact dermatitis (L23-L25)*
dry skin dermatitis (L85.3)
small plaque parapsoriasis (L41.3)
stasis dermatitis (I87.2)
L30.0   Nummular dermatitis
L30.1   Dyshidrosis [pompholyx]
L30.2   Cutaneous autosensitization
Candidid [levurid]
Dermatophytid
Eczematid
L30.3   Infective dermatitis
Infectious eczematoid dermatitis
L30.4   Erythema intertrigo
L30.5   Pityriasis alba
L30.8   Other specified dermatitis
L30.9   Dermatitis, unspecified ▽
Eczema NOS

Papulosquamous disorders (L40-L45)

✓4ᵗʰ **L40   Psoriasis**
L40.0   Psoriasis vulgaris
Nummular psoriasis
Plaque psoriasis
L40.1   Generalized pustular psoriasis
Impetigo herpetiformis
Von Zumbusch's disease
L40.2   Acrodermatitis continua
L40.3   Pustulosis palmaris et plantaris
L40.4   Guttate psoriasis

✓5th **L40.5 Arthropathic psoriasis**
    L40.50 Arthropathic psoriasis, unspecified HCC ▽
    L40.51 Distal interphalangeal psoriatic arthropathy HCC
    L40.52 Psoriatic arthritis mutilans HCC
    L40.53 Psoriatic spondylitis HCC
    L40.54 Psoriatic juvenile arthropathy HCC
    L40.59 Other psoriatic arthropathy HCC
  L40.8 Other psoriasis
    Flexural psoriasis
  L40.9 Psoriasis, unspecified ▽

✓4th **L41 Parapsoriasis**
  EXCLUDES 1   *poikiloderma vasculare atrophicans (L94.5)*
  L41.0 Pityriasis lichenoides et varioliformis acuta
    Mucha-Habermann disease
  L41.1 Pityriasis lichenoides chronica
  L41.3 Small plaque parapsoriasis
  L41.4 Large plaque parapsoriasis
  L41.5 Retiform parapsoriasis
  L41.8 Other parapsoriasis
  L41.9 Parapsoriasis, unspecified ▽

L42 Pityriasis rosea

✓4th **L43 Lichen planus**
  EXCLUDES 1   *lichen planopilaris (L66.1)*
  L43.0 Hypertrophic lichen planus
  L43.1 Bullous lichen planus
  L43.2 Lichenoid drug reaction
    Use additional code for adverse effect, if applicable, to identify drug (T36-T50 with fifth or sixth character 5)
  L43.3 Subacute (active) lichen planus
    Lichen planus tropicus
  L43.8 Other lichen planus
  L43.9 Lichen planus, unspecified ▽

✓4th **L44 Other papulosquamous disorders**
  L44.0 Pityriasis rubra pilaris
  L44.1 Lichen nitidus
    DEF: Chronic, inflammatory, asymptomatic skin disorder, characterized by numerous glistening, flat-topped, discrete, skin-colored micropapules, most often on the penis, lower abdomen, inner thighs, wrists, forearms, breasts and buttocks.
  L44.2 Lichen striatus
  L44.3 Lichen ruber moniliformis
  L44.4 Infantile papular acrodermatitis [Gianotti-Crosti] P
  L44.8 Other specified papulosquamous disorders
  L44.9 Papulosquamous disorder, unspecified ▽

L45 *Papulosquamous disorders in diseases classified elsewhere*
  Code first underlying disease

Urticaria and erythema (L49-L54)
EXCLUDES 1   *Lyme disease (A69.2-)*
    rosacea (L71.-)

✓4th **L49 Exfoliation due to erythematous conditions according to extent of body surface involved**
  Code first erythematous condition causing exfoliation, such as:
    Ritter's disease (L00)
    (Staphylococcal) scalded skin syndrom (L00)
    Stevens-Johnson syndrome (L51.1)
    Stevens-Johnson syndrome-toxic epidermal necrolysis overlap syndrome (L51.3)
    toxic epidermal necrolysis (L51.2)
  L49.0 Exfoliation due to erythematous condition involving less than 10 percent of body surface
    Exfoliation due to erythematous condition NOS
  L49.1 Exfoliation due to erythematous condition involving 10-19 percent of body surface
  L49.2 Exfoliation due to erythematous condition involving 20-29 percent of body surface
  L49.3 Exfoliation due to erythematous condition involving 30-39 percent of body surface
  L49.4 Exfoliation due to erythematous condition involving 40-49 percent of body surface
  L49.5 Exfoliation due to erythematous condition involving 50-59 percent of body surface

  L49.6 Exfoliation due to erythematous condition involving 60-69 percent of body surface
  L49.7 Exfoliation due to erythematous condition involving 70-79 percent of body surface
  L49.8 Exfoliation due to erythematous condition involving 80-89 percent of body surface
  L49.9 Exfoliation due to erythematous condition involving 90 or more percent of body surface

✓4th **L50 Urticaria**
  EXCLUDES 1   *allergic contact dermatitis (L23.-)*
    angioneurotic edema (T78.3)
    giant urticaria (T78.3)
    hereditary angio-edema (D84.1)
    Quincke's edema (T78.3)
    serum urticaria (T80.6-)
    solar urticaria (L56.3)
    urticaria neonatorum (P83.8)
    urticaria papulosa (L28.2)
    urticaria pigmentosa (Q82.2)
  L50.0 Allergic urticaria
  L50.1 Idiopathic urticaria
  L50.2 Urticaria due to cold and heat
    EXCLUDES 2   *familial cold urticaria (M04.2)*
  L50.3 Dermatographic urticaria
  L50.4 Vibratory urticaria
  L50.5 Cholinergic urticaria
  L50.6 Contact urticaria
  L50.8 Other urticaria
    Chronic urticaria
    Recurrent periodic urticaria
  L50.9 Urticaria, unspecified ▽

✓4th **L51 Erythema multiforme**
  Use additional code for adverse effect, if applicable, to identify drug (T36-T50 with fifth or sixth character 5)
  Use additional code to identify associated manifestations, such as:
    arthropathy associated with dermatological disorders (M14.8-)
    conjunctival edema (H11.42)
    conjunctivitis (H10.22-)
    corneal scars and opacities (H17.-)
    corneal ulcer (H16.0-)
    edema of eyelid (H02.84)
    inflammation of eyelid (H01.8)
    keratoconjunctivitis sicca (H16.22-)
    mechanical lagophthalmos (H02.22-)
    stomatitis (K12.-)
    symblepharon (H11.23-)
  Use additional code to identify percentage of skin exfoliation (L49.-)
  EXCLUDES 1   *staphylococcal scalded skin syndrome (L00)*
    Ritter's disease (L00)
  L51.0 Nonbullous erythema multiforme
  L51.1 Stevens-Johnson syndrome HCC
  L51.2 Toxic epidermal necrolysis [Lyell] HCC
  L51.3 Stevens-Johnson syndrome-toxic epidermal necrolysis overlap syndrome HCC
    SJS-TEN overlap syndrome
  L51.8 Other erythema multiforme
  L51.9 Erythema multiforme, unspecified ▽
    Erythema iris
    Erythema multiforme major NOS
    Erythema multiforme minor NOS
    Herpes iris

L52 Erythema nodosum
  EXCLUDES 1   *tuberculous erythema nodosum (A18.4)*
  DEF: A form of panniculitis (inflammation of the fat layer beneath the skin) of particularly women, usually seen as a hypersensitivity reaction to infections, drugs, sarcoidosis, and specific enteropathies; the acute stage is associated with fever, malaise, and arthralgia; the lesions are pink to blue in color as tender nodules and are found on the front of the legs below the knees.

✓4th **L53 Other erythematous conditions**
  EXCLUDES 1   *erythema ab igne (L59.0)*
    erythema due to external agents in contact with skin (L23-L25)
    erythema intertrigo (L30.4)
  L53.0 Toxic erythema
    Code first poisoning due to drug or toxin, if applicable (T36-T65 with fifth or sixth character 1-4 or 6)
    Use additional code for adverse effect, if applicable, to identify drug (T36-T50 with fifth or sixth character 5)
    EXCLUDES 1   *neonatal erythema toxicum (P83.1)*

✓ Additional Character Req   ✓x7th Placeholder Alert   Manifestation   HCC CMS-HCC Condition   ▽ Unspecified Code   ►◄ Revised Text   ● New Code   ▲ Revised Code Title

ICD-10-CM 2018   699

Chapter 12. Diseases of the Skin and Subcutaneous Tissue

   L53.1   **Erythema annulare centrifugum**

   L53.2   **Erythema marginatum**

   L53.3   **Other chronic figurate erythema**

   L53.8   **Other specified erythematous conditions**

   L53.9   **Erythematous condition, unspecified** ▽
            Erythema NOS
            Erythroderma NOS

  L54   *Erythema in diseases classified elsewhere*
        Code first underlying disease

Radiation-related disorders of the skin and subcutaneous tissue (L55-L59)

✓4ᵗʰ **L55** **Sunburn**

   L55.0   **Sunburn of first degree**

   L55.1   **Sunburn of second degree**

   L55.2   **Sunburn of third degree**

   L55.9   **Sunburn, unspecified** ▽

✓4ᵗʰ **L56** **Other acute skin changes due to ultraviolet radiation**
     Use additional code to identify the source of the ultraviolet radiation (W89, X32)

   L56.0   **Drug phototoxic response**
        Use additional code for adverse effect, if applicable, to identify drug (T36-T50 with fifth or sixth character 5)

   L56.1   **Drug photoallergic response**
        Use additional code for adverse effect, if applicable, to identify drug (T36-T50 with fifth or sixth character 5)

   L56.2   **Photocontact dermatitis [berloque dermatitis]**

   L56.3   **Solar urticaria**

   L56.4   **Polymorphous light eruption**

   L56.5   **Disseminated superficial actinic porokeratosis (DSAP)**
        DEF: Autosomal dominant skin condition occurring in sun-exposed areas of the skin (particularly the arms and legs); characterized by superficial annular, keratotic, brownish-red spots or thickenings with depressed centers and sharp, ridged borders; may evolve into squamous cell carcinoma.

   L56.8   **Other specified acute skin changes due to ultraviolet radiation**

   L56.9   **Acute skin change due to ultraviolet radiation, unspecified** ▽

✓4ᵗʰ **L57** **Skin changes due to chronic exposure to nonionizing radiation**
     Use additional code to identify the source of the ultraviolet radiation ▶(W89)◀

   L57.0   **Actinic keratosis**
        Keratosis NOS
        Senile keratosis
        Solar keratosis

   L57.1   **Actinic reticuloid**

   L57.2   **Cutis rhomboidalis nuchae**

   L57.3   **Poikiloderma of Civatte**

   L57.4   **Cutis laxa senilis**
        Elastosis senilis

   L57.5   **Actinic granuloma**

   L57.8   **Other skin changes due to chronic exposure to nonionizing radiation**
        Farmer's skin
        Sailor's skin
        Solar dermatitis

   L57.9   **Skin changes due to chronic exposure to nonionizing radiation, unspecified** ▽

✓4ᵗʰ **L58** **Radiodermatitis**
     Use additional code to identify the source of the radiation (W88, W90)

   L58.0   **Acute radiodermatitis**

   L58.1   **Chronic radiodermatitis**

   L58.9   **Radiodermatitis, unspecified** ▽

✓4ᵗʰ **L59** **Other disorders of skin and subcutaneous tissue related to radiation**

   L59.0   **Erythema ab igne [dermatitis ab igne]**

   L59.8   **Other specified disorders of the skin and subcutaneous tissue related to radiation**
        AHA: 2017, 1Q, 33

   L59.9   **Disorder of the skin and subcutaneous tissue related to radiation, unspecified** ▽

Nail Disorders

Normal

Koilonychia

Beau's Lines

Disorders of skin appendages (L60-L75)

  EXCLUDES 1   *congenital malformations of integument (Q84.-)*

✓4ᵗʰ **L60** **Nail disorders**
     EXCLUDES 2   *clubbing of nails (R68.3)*
                   onychia and paronychia (L03.0-)

   L60.0   **Ingrowing nail**

   L60.1   **Onycholysis**

   L60.2   **Onychogryphosis**

   L60.3   **Nail dystrophy**

   L60.4   **Beau's lines**

   L60.5   **Yellow nail syndrome**

   L60.8   **Other nail disorders**

   L60.9   **Nail disorder, unspecified** ▽

  L62   *Nail disorders in diseases classified elsewhere*
        Code first underlying disease, such as:
        pachydermoperiostosis (M89.4-)

✓4ᵗʰ **L63** **Alopecia areata**

   L63.0   **Alopecia (capitis) totalis**

   L63.1   **Alopecia universalis**

   L63.2   **Ophiasis**

   L63.8   **Other alopecia areata**

   L63.9   **Alopecia areata, unspecified** ▽

✓4ᵗʰ **L64** **Androgenic alopecia**
     INCLUDES   male-pattern baldness

   L64.0   **Drug-induced androgenic alopecia**
        Use additional code for adverse effect, if applicable, to identify drug (T36-T50 with fifth or sixth character 5)

   L64.8   **Other androgenic alopecia**

   L64.9   **Androgenic alopecia, unspecified** ▽

✓4ᵗʰ **L65** **Other nonscarring hair loss**
     Use additional code for adverse effect, if applicable, to identify drug (T36-T50 with fifth or sixth character 5)
     EXCLUDES 1   *trichotillomania (F63.3)*

   L65.0   **Telogen effluvium**
        DEF: A form of nonscarring alopecia characterized by shedding of hair from premature telogen development in follicles due to stress, including shock, childbirth, surgery, drugs, or weight loss.

   L65.1   **Anagen effluvium**

   L65.2   **Alopecia mucinosa**

   L65.8   **Other specified nonscarring hair loss**

   L65.9   **Nonscarring hair loss, unspecified** ▽
        Alopecia NOS

✓4ᵗʰ **L66** **Cicatricial alopecia [scarring hair loss]**

   L66.0   **Pseudopelade**

   L66.1   **Lichen planopilaris**
        Follicular lichen planus

   L66.2   **Folliculitis decalvans**

   L66.3   **Perifolliculitis capitis abscedens**

   L66.4   **Folliculitis ulerythematosa reticulata**

   L66.8   **Other cicatricial alopecia**
        AHA: 2015, 1Q, 19

   L66.9   **Cicatricial alopecia, unspecified** ▽

EXCLUDES 1 Not coded here   EXCLUDES 2 Not included here   N Newborn Age: 0   P Pediatric Age: 0-17   M Maternity Age: 12-55   A Adult Age: 15-124

700   ICD-10-CM 2018

☑4ᵗʰ **L67 Hair color and hair shaft abnormalities**
> EXCLUDES 1   monilethrix (Q84.1)
> pili annulati (Q84.1)
> telogen effluvium (L65.0)

L67.0 Trichorrhexis nodosa

L67.1 Variations in hair color
> Canities
> Greyness, hair (premature)
> Heterochromia of hair
> Poliosis circumscripta, acquired
> Poliosis NOS

L67.8 Other hair color and hair shaft abnormalities
> Fragilitas crinium

L67.9 Hair color and hair shaft abnormality, unspecified ▽

☑4ᵗʰ **L68 Hypertrichosis**
> INCLUDES   excess hair
> EXCLUDES 1   congenital hypertrichosis (Q84.2)
> persistent lanugo (Q84.2)

L68.0 Hirsutism

L68.1 Acquired hypertrichosis lanuginosa

L68.2 Localized hypertrichosis

L68.3 Polytrichia

L68.8 Other hypertrichosis

L68.9 Hypertrichosis, unspecified ▽

☑4ᵗʰ **L70 Acne**
> EXCLUDES 2   acne keloid (L73.0)

L70.0 Acne vulgaris

L70.1 Acne conglobata

L70.2 Acne varioliformis
> Acne necrotica miliaris
> **DEF:** Rare form of acne characterized by development of persistent brown papulo-pustules followed by scar formation; usually on the brow and temporoparietal part of the scalp.

L70.3 Acne tropica

L70.4 Infantile acne P

L70.5 Acné excoriée
> Acné excoriée des jeunes filles
> Picker's acne

L70.8 Other acne

L70.9 Acne, unspecified ▽

☑4ᵗʰ **L71 Rosacea**
> Use additional code for adverse effect, if applicable, to identify drug (T36-T50 with fifth or sixth character 5)

L71.0 Perioral dermatitis

L71.1 Rhinophyma

L71.8 Other rosacea

L71.9 Rosacea, unspecified ▽

☑4ᵗʰ **L72 Follicular cysts of skin and subcutaneous tissue**

L72.0 Epidermal cyst

✓5ᵗʰ **L72.1 Pilar and trichodermal cyst**

     L72.11 Pilar cyst

     L72.12 Trichodermal cyst
> Trichilemmal (proliferating) cyst

L72.2 Steatocystoma multiplex

L72.3 Sebaceous cyst
> EXCLUDES 2   pilar cyst (L72.11)
> trichilemmal (proliferating) cyst (L72.12)

L72.8 Other follicular cysts of the skin and subcutaneous tissue

L72.9 Follicular cyst of the skin and subcutaneous tissue, unspecified ▽

☑4ᵗʰ **L73 Other follicular disorders**

L73.0 Acne keloid

L73.1 Pseudofolliculitis barbae

L73.2 Hidradenitis suppurativa

L73.8 Other specified follicular disorders
> Sycosis barbae

L73.9 Follicular disorder, unspecified ▽

☑4ᵗʰ **L74 Eccrine sweat disorders**
> EXCLUDES 2   generalized hyperhidrosis (R61)

L74.0 Miliaria rubra

L74.1 Miliaria crystallina

L74.2 Miliaria profunda
> Miliaria tropicalis

L74.3 Miliaria, unspecified ▽

L74.4 Anhidrosis
> Hypohidrosis

✓5ᵗʰ **L74.5 Focal hyperhidrosis**

   ✓6ᵗʰ **L74.51 Primary focal hyperhidrosis**

     L74.510 Primary focal hyperhidrosis, axilla

     L74.511 Primary focal hyperhidrosis, face

     L74.512 Primary focal hyperhidrosis, palms

     L74.513 Primary focal hyperhidrosis, soles

     L74.519 Primary focal hyperhidrosis, unspecified ▽

     L74.52 Secondary focal hyperhidrosis
> Frey's syndrome

L74.8 Other eccrine sweat disorders

L74.9 Eccrine sweat disorder, unspecified ▽
> Sweat gland disorder NOS

☑4ᵗʰ **L75 Apocrine sweat disorders**
> EXCLUDES 1   dyshidrosis (L30.1)
> hidradenitis suppurativa (L73.2)

L75.0 Bromhidrosis

L75.1 Chromhidrosis

L75.2 Apocrine miliaria
> Fox-Fordyce disease
> **DEF:** Chronic, usually pruritic disease evidenced by small follicular papular eruptions, especially in the axillary and pubic areas; develops from the closure and rupture of the affected apocrine glands' intraepidermal portion of the ducts.

L75.8 Other apocrine sweat disorders

L75.9 Apocrine sweat disorder, unspecified ▽

Intraoperative and postprocedural complications of skin and subcutaneous tissue (L76)

☑4ᵗʰ **L76 Intraoperative and postprocedural complications of skin and subcutaneous tissue**

✓5ᵗʰ **L76.0 Intraoperative hemorrhage and hematoma of skin and subcutaneous tissue complicating a procedure**
> EXCLUDES 1   intraoperative hemorrhage and hematoma of skin and subcutaneous tissue due to accidental puncture and laceration during a procedure (L76.1-)

     L76.01 Intraoperative hemorrhage and hematoma of skin and subcutaneous tissue complicating a dermatologic procedure

     L76.02 Intraoperative hemorrhage and hematoma of skin and subcutaneous tissue complicating other procedure

✓5ᵗʰ **L76.1 Accidental puncture and laceration of skin and subcutaneous tissue during a procedure**

     L76.11 Accidental puncture and laceration of skin and subcutaneous tissue during a dermatologic procedure

     L76.12 Accidental puncture and laceration of skin and subcutaneous tissue during other procedure

✓5ᵗʰ **L76.2 Postprocedural hemorrhage of skin and subcutaneous tissue following a procedure**

     L76.21 Postprocedural hemorrhage of skin and subcutaneous tissue following a dermatologic procedure

     L76.22 Postprocedural hemorrhage of skin and subcutaneous tissue following other procedure

✓5ᵗʰ **L76.3 Postprocedural hematoma and seroma of skin and subcutaneous tissue following a procedure**

     L76.31 Postprocedural hematoma of skin and subcutaneous tissue following a dermatologic procedure

     L76.32 Postprocedural hematoma of skin and subcutaneous tissue following other procedure

     L76.33 Postprocedural seroma of skin and subcutaneous tissue following a dermatologic procedure

     L76.34 Postprocedural seroma of skin and subcutaneous tissue following other procedure

✓5ᵗʰ **L76.8 Other intraoperative and postprocedural complications of skin and subcutaneous tissue**
> Use additional code, if applicable, to further specify disorder

     L76.81 Other intraoperative complications of skin and subcutaneous tissue

     L76.82 Other postprocedural complications of skin and subcutaneous tissue

Other disorders of the skin and subcutaneous tissue (L80-L99)

L80 Vitiligo
- **EXCLUDES 2** vitiligo of eyelids (H02.73-)
- vitiligo of vulva (N90.89)
- **DEF:** Persistent, progressive development of nonpigmented white patches on otherwise normal skin.

✓4ᵗʰ L81 Other disorders of pigmentation
- **EXCLUDES 1** birthmark NOS (Q82.5)
- Peutz-Jeghers syndrome (Q85.8)
- **EXCLUDES 2** nevus—see Alphabetical Index

L81.0 Postinflammatory hyperpigmentation

L81.1 Chloasma

L81.2 Freckles

L81.3 Café au lait spots

L81.4 Other melanin hyperpigmentation
- Lentigo

L81.5 Leukoderma, not elsewhere classified

L81.6 Other disorders of diminished melanin formation

L81.7 Pigmented purpuric dermatosis
- Angioma serpiginosum

L81.8 Other specified disorders of pigmentation
- Iron pigmentation
- Tattoo pigmentation

L81.9 Disorder of pigmentation, unspecified ▽

✓4ᵗʰ L82 Seborrheic keratosis
- **INCLUDES** basal cell papilloma
- dermatosis papulosa nigra
- Leser-Trélat disease
- **EXCLUDES 2** seborrheic dermatitis (L21.-)

L82.0 Inflamed seborrheic keratosis

L82.1 Other seborrheic keratosis
- Seborrheic keratosis NOS

L83 Acanthosis nigricans
- Confluent and reticulated papillomatosis
- **DEF:** Diffuse, velvety hyperplasia of the spinous skin layer of the axilla and other body folds marked by gray, brown, or black pigmentation; in adult form often associated with malignant acanthosis nigricans in a benign, nevoid form relatively generalized.

L84 Corns and callosities
- Callus
- Clavus

✓4ᵗʰ L85 Other epidermal thickening
- **EXCLUDES 2** hypertrophic disorders of the skin (L91.-)

L85.0 Acquired ichthyosis
- **EXCLUDES 1** congenital ichthyosis (Q80.-)

L85.1 Acquired keratosis [keratoderma] palmaris et plantaris
- **EXCLUDES 1** inherited keratosis palmaris et plantaris (Q82.8)

L85.2 Keratosis punctata (palmaris et plantaris)

L85.3 Xerosis cutis
- Dry skin dermatitis

L85.8 Other specified epidermal thickening
- Cutaneous horn

L85.9 Epidermal thickening, unspecified ▽

L86 Keratoderma in diseases classified elsewhere
- Code first underlying disease, such as:
- Reiter's disease (M02.3-)
- **EXCLUDES 1** gonococcal keratoderma (A54.89)
- gonococcal keratosis (A54.89)
- keratoderma due to vitamin A deficiency (E50.8)
- keratosis due to vitamin A deficiency (E50.8)
- xeroderma due to vitamin A deficiency (E50.8)

✓4ᵗʰ L87 Transepidermal elimination disorders
- **EXCLUDES 1** granuloma annulare (perforating) (L92.0)

L87.0 Keratosis follicularis et parafollicularis in cutem penetrans
- Hyperkeratosis follicularis penetrans
- Kyrle disease

L87.1 Reactive perforating collagenosis

L87.2 Elastosis perforans serpiginosa

L87.8 Other transepidermal elimination disorders

L87.9 Transepidermal elimination disorder, unspecified ▽

L88 Pyoderma gangrenosum
- Phagedenic pyoderma
- **EXCLUDES 1** dermatitis gangrenosa (L08.0)
- **DEF:** Persistent debilitating skin disease characterized by irregular, boggy, blue-red ulcerations, with central healing and undermined edges.

Four Stages of Pressure Ulcer

Epidermis
Dermis
Subcutaneous tissue

Stage 1
Persistent focal erythema

Stage 2
Abrasion, blister, partial thickness skin loss involving epidermis and/or dermis

Superficial fascia
Muscle
Deep fascia
Bone

Stage 3
Full thickness skin loss involving damage or necrosis of subcutaneous tissue

Stage 4
Necrosis of soft tissues through to underlying muscle, tendon, or bone

✓4ᵗʰ L89 Pressure ulcer
- **INCLUDES** bed sore
- decubitus ulcer
- plaster ulcer
- pressure area
- pressure sore
- Code first any associated gangrene (I96)
- **EXCLUDES 2** decubitus (trophic) ulcer of cervix (uteri) (N86)
- diabetic ulcers (E08.621, E08.622, E09.621, E09.622, E10.621, E10.622, E11.621, E11.622, E13.621, E13.622)
- non-pressure chronic ulcer of skin (L97.-)
- skin infections (L00-L08)
- varicose ulcer (I83.0, I83.2)
- **AHA:** 2017, 1Q, 49; 2016, 4Q, 143

✓5ᵗʰ L89.0 Pressure ulcer of elbow

✓6ᵗʰ L89.00 Pressure ulcer of unspecified elbow

L89.000 Pressure ulcer of unspecified elbow, HCC ▽ unstageable

L89.001 Pressure ulcer of unspecified elbow, ▽ stage 1
- Healing pressure ulcer of unspecified elbow, stage 1
- Pressure pre-ulcer skin changes limited to persistent focal edema, unspecified elbow

L89.002 Pressure ulcer of unspecified elbow, ▽ stage 2
- Healing pressure ulcer of unspecified elbow, stage 2
- Pressure ulcer with abrasion, blister, partial thickness skin loss involving epidermis and/or dermis, unspecified elbow

L89.003 Pressure ulcer of unspecified HCC ▽ elbow, stage 3
- Healing pressure ulcer of unspecified elbow, stage 3
- Pressure ulcer with full thickness skin loss involving damage or necrosis of subcutaneous tissue, unspecified elbow

L89.004 Pressure ulcer of unspecified HCC ▽ elbow, stage 4
- Healing pressure ulcer of unspecified elbow, stage 4
- Pressure ulcer with necrosis of soft tissues through to underlying muscle, tendon, or bone, unspecified elbow

L89.009 Pressure ulcer of unspecified elbow, ▽ unspecified stage
- Healing pressure ulcer of elbow NOS
- Healing pressure ulcer of unspecified elbow, unspecified stage

✓6ᵗʰ L89.01 Pressure ulcer of right elbow

L89.010 Pressure ulcer of right elbow, HCC unstageable

EXCLUDES 1 Not coded here   EXCLUDES 2 Not included here   N Newborn Age: 0   P Pediatric Age: 0-17   M Maternity Age: 12-55   A Adult Age: 15-124

702   ICD-10-CM 2018

L89.011   **Pressure ulcer of right elbow, stage 1**
Healing pressure ulcer of right elbow, stage 1
Pressure pre-ulcer skin changes limited to persistent focal edema, right elbow

L89.012   **Pressure ulcer of right elbow, stage 2**
Healing pressure ulcer of right elbow, stage 2
Pressure ulcer with abrasion, blister, partial thickness skin loss involving epidermis and/or dermis, right elbow

L89.013   **Pressure ulcer of right elbow, stage 3**   HCC
Healing pressure ulcer of right elbow, stage 3
Pressure ulcer with full thickness skin loss involving damage or necrosis of subcutaneous tissue, right elbow

L89.014   **Pressure ulcer of right elbow, stage 4**   HCC
Healing pressure ulcer of right elbow, stage 4
Pressure ulcer with necrosis of soft tissues through to underlying muscle, tendon, or bone, right elbow

L89.019   **Pressure ulcer of right elbow, unspecified stage**   ▽
Healing pressure right of elbow NOS
▶Healing pressure ulcer of right elbow, unspecified stage◀

✓6ᵗʰ   L89.02   **Pressure ulcer of left elbow**

L89.020   **Pressure ulcer of left elbow, unstageable**   HCC

L89.021   **Pressure ulcer of left elbow, stage 1**
Healing pressure ulcer of left elbow, stage 1
Pressure pre-ulcer skin changes limited to persistent focal edema, left elbow

L89.022   **Pressure ulcer of left elbow, stage 2**
Healing pressure ulcer of left elbow, stage 2
Pressure ulcer with abrasion, blister, partial thickness skin loss involving epidermis and/or dermis, left elbow

L89.023   **Pressure ulcer of left elbow, stage 3**   HCC
Healing pressure ulcer of left elbow, stage 3
Pressure ulcer with full thickness skin loss involving damage or necrosis of subcutaneous tissue, left elbow

L89.024   **Pressure ulcer of left elbow, stage 4**   HCC
Healing pressure ulcer of left elbow, stage 4
Pressure ulcer with necrosis of soft tissues through to underlying muscle, tendon, or bone, left elbow

L89.029   **Pressure ulcer of left elbow, unspecified stage**   ▽
Healing pressure ulcer of left of elbow NOS
▶Healing pressure ulcer of left elbow, unspecified stage◀

✓5ᵗʰ   L89.1   **Pressure ulcer of back**

✓6ᵗʰ   L89.10   **Pressure ulcer of unspecified part of back**

L89.100   **Pressure ulcer of unspecified part of back, unstageable**   HCC ▽

L89.101   **Pressure ulcer of unspecified part of back, stage 1**   ▽
Healing pressure ulcer of unspecified part of back, stage 1
Pressure pre-ulcer skin changes limited to persistent focal edema, unspecified part of back

L89.102   **Pressure ulcer of unspecified part of back, stage 2**   ▽
Healing pressure ulcer of unspecified part of back, stage 2
Pressure ulcer with abrasion, blister, partial thickness skin loss involving epidermis and/or dermis, unspecified part of back

L89.103   **Pressure ulcer of unspecified part of back, stage 3**   HCC ▽
Healing pressure ulcer of unspecified part of back, stage 3
Pressure ulcer with full thickness skin loss involving damage or necrosis of subcutaneous tissue, unspecified part of back

L89.104   **Pressure ulcer of unspecified part of back, stage 4**   HCC ▽
Healing pressure ulcer of unspecified part of back, stage 4
Pressure ulcer with necrosis of soft tissues through to underlying muscle, tendon, or bone, unspecified part of back

L89.109   **Pressure ulcer of unspecified part of back, unspecified stage**   ▽
Healing pressure ulcer of unspecified part of back NOS
Healing pressure ulcer of unspecified part of back, unspecified stage

✓6ᵗʰ   L89.11   **Pressure ulcer of right upper back**
Pressure ulcer of right shoulder blade

L89.110   **Pressure ulcer of right upper back, unstageable**   HCC

L89.111   **Pressure ulcer of right upper back, stage 1**
Healing pressure ulcer of right upper back, stage 1
Pressure pre-ulcer skin changes limited to persistent focal edema, right upper back

L89.112   **Pressure ulcer of right upper back, stage 2**
Healing pressure ulcer of right upper back, stage 2
Pressure ulcer with abrasion, blister, partial thickness skin loss involving epidermis and/or dermis, right upper back

L89.113   **Pressure ulcer of right upper back, stage 3**   HCC
Healing pressure ulcer of right upper back, stage 3
Pressure ulcer with full thickness skin loss involving damage or necrosis of subcutaneous tissue, right upper back

L89.114   **Pressure ulcer of right upper back, stage 4**   HCC
Healing pressure ulcer of right upper back, stage 4
Pressure ulcer with necrosis of soft tissues through to underlying muscle, tendon, or bone, right upper back

L89.119   **Pressure ulcer of right upper back, unspecified stage**   ▽
Healing pressure ulcer of right upper back NOS
Healing pressure ulcer of right upper back, unspecified stage

✓6ᵗʰ   L89.12   **Pressure ulcer of left upper back**
Pressure ulcer of left shoulder blade

L89.120   **Pressure ulcer of left upper back, unstageable**   HCC

L89.121   **Pressure ulcer of left upper back, stage 1**
Healing pressure ulcer of left upper back, stage 1
Pressure pre-ulcer skin changes limited to persistent focal edema, left upper back

L89.122   **Pressure ulcer of left upper back, stage 2**
Healing pressure ulcer of left upper back, stage 2
Pressure ulcer with abrasion, blister, partial thickness skin loss involving epidermis and/or dermis, left upper back

L89.123   **Pressure ulcer of left upper back, stage 3**   HCC
Healing pressure ulcer of left upper back, stage 3
Pressure ulcer with full thickness skin loss involving damage or necrosis of subcutaneous tissue, left upper back

L89.124   **Pressure ulcer of left upper back, stage 4**   HCC
Healing pressure ulcer of left upper back, stage 4
Pressure ulcer with necrosis of soft tissues through to underlying muscle, tendon, or bone, left upper back

---

☑ Additional Character Req   ✓x7ᵗʰ Placeholder Alert   Manifestation   HCC CMS-HCC Condition   ▽ Unspecified Code   ▶◀ Revised Text   ● New Code   ▲ Revised Code Title

L89.129 **Pressure ulcer of left upper back, unspecified stage** ▽
  Healing pressure ulcer of left upper back NOS
  Healing pressure ulcer of left upper back, unspecified stage

✓6ᵗʰ **L89.13** **Pressure ulcer of right lower back**

L89.130 **Pressure ulcer of right lower back, unstageable** HCC

L89.131 **Pressure ulcer of right lower back, stage 1**
  Healing pressure ulcer of right lower back, stage 1
  Pressure pre-ulcer skin changes limited to persistent focal edema, right lower back

L89.132 **Pressure ulcer of right lower back, stage 2**
  Healing pressure ulcer of right lower back, stage 2
  Pressure ulcer with abrasion, blister, partial thickness skin loss involving epidermis and/or dermis, right lower back

L89.133 **Pressure ulcer of right lower back, stage 3** HCC
  Healing pressure ulcer of right lower back, stage 3
  Pressure ulcer with full thickness skin loss involving damage or necrosis of subcutaneous tissue, right lower back

L89.134 **Pressure ulcer of right lower back, stage 4** HCC
  Healing pressure ulcer of right lower back, stage 4
  Pressure ulcer with necrosis of soft tissues through to underlying muscle, tendon, or bone, right lower back

L89.139 **Pressure ulcer of right lower back, unspecified stage** ▽
  Healing pressure ulcer of right lower back NOS
  Healing pressure ulcer of right lower back, unspecified stage

✓6ᵗʰ **L89.14** **Pressure ulcer of left lower back**

L89.140 **Pressure ulcer of left lower back, unstageable** HCC

L89.141 **Pressure ulcer of left lower back, stage 1**
  Healing pressure ulcer of left lower back, stage 1
  Pressure pre-ulcer skin changes limited to persistent focal edema, left lower back

L89.142 **Pressure ulcer of left lower back, stage 2**
  Healing pressure ulcer of left lower back, stage 2
  Pressure ulcer with abrasion, blister, partial thickness skin loss involving epidermis and/or dermis, left lower back

L89.143 **Pressure ulcer of left lower back, stage 3** HCC
  Healing pressure ulcer of left lower back, stage 3
  Pressure ulcer with full thickness skin loss involving damage or necrosis of subcutaneous tissue, left lower back

L89.144 **Pressure ulcer of left lower back, stage 4** HCC
  Healing pressure ulcer of left lower back, stage 4
  Pressure ulcer with necrosis of soft tissues through to underlying muscle, tendon, or bone, left lower back

L89.149 **Pressure ulcer of left lower back, unspecified stage** ▽
  Healing pressure ulcer of left lower back NOS
  Healing pressure ulcer of left lower back, unspecified stage

✓6ᵗʰ **L89.15** **Pressure ulcer of sacral region**
  Pressure ulcer of coccyx
  Pressure ulcer of tailbone

L89.150 **Pressure ulcer of sacral region, unstageable** HCC

L89.151 **Pressure ulcer of sacral region, stage 1**
  Healing pressure ulcer of sacral region, stage 1
  Pressure pre-ulcer skin changes limited to persistent focal edema, sacral region

L89.152 **Pressure ulcer of sacral region, stage 2**
  Healing pressure ulcer of sacral region, stage 2
  Pressure ulcer with abrasion, blister, partial thickness skin loss involving epidermis and/or dermis, sacral region

L89.153 **Pressure ulcer of sacral region, stage 3** HCC
  Healing pressure ulcer of sacral region, stage 3
  Pressure ulcer with full thickness skin loss involving damage or necrosis of subcutaneous tissue, sacral region

L89.154 **Pressure ulcer of sacral region, stage 4** HCC
  Healing pressure ulcer of sacral region, stage 4
  Pressure ulcer with necrosis of soft tissues through to underlying muscle, tendon, or bone, sacral region

L89.159 **Pressure ulcer of sacral region, unspecified stage** ▽
  Healing pressure ulcer of sacral region NOS
  Healing pressure ulcer of sacral region, unspecified stage

✓5ᵗʰ **L89.2** **Pressure ulcer of hip**

✓6ᵗʰ **L89.20** **Pressure ulcer of unspecified hip**

L89.200 **Pressure ulcer of unspecified hip, unstageable** HCC ▽

L89.201 **Pressure ulcer of unspecified hip, stage 1** ▽
  Healing pressure ulcer of unspecified hip, stage 1
  Pressure pre-ulcer skin changes limited to persistent focal edema, unspecified hip

L89.202 **Pressure ulcer of unspecified hip, stage 2** ▽
  Healing pressure ulcer of unspecified hip, stage 2
  Pressure ulcer with abrasion, blister, partial thickness skin loss involving epidermis and/or dermis, unspecified hip

L89.203 **Pressure ulcer of unspecified hip, stage 3** HCC ▽
  Healing pressure ulcer of unspecified hip, stage 3
  Pressure ulcer with full thickness skin loss involving damage or necrosis of subcutaneous tissue, unspecified hip

L89.204 **Pressure ulcer of unspecified hip, stage 4** HCC ▽
  Healing pressure ulcer of unspecified hip, stage 4
  Pressure ulcer with necrosis of soft tissues through to underlying muscle, tendon, or bone, unspecified hip

L89.209 **Pressure ulcer of unspecified hip, unspecified stage** ▽
  Healing pressure ulcer of unspecified hip NOS
  Healing pressure ulcer of unspecified hip, unspecified stage

✓6ᵗʰ **L89.21** **Pressure ulcer of right hip**

L89.210 **Pressure ulcer of right hip, unstageable** HCC

L89.211 **Pressure ulcer of right hip, stage 1**
  Healing pressure ulcer of right hip, stage 1
  Pressure pre-ulcer skin changes limited to persistent focal edema, right hip

L89.212 **Pressure ulcer of right hip, stage 2**
  Healing pressure ulcer of right hip, stage 2
  Pressure ulcer with abrasion, blister, partial thickness skin loss involving epidermis and/or dermis, right hip

L89.213 **Pressure ulcer of right hip, stage 3** HCC
  Healing pressure ulcer of right hip, stage 3
  Pressure ulcer with full thickness skin loss involving damage or necrosis of subcutaneous tissue, right hip

EXCLUDES 1 Not coded here　　　**EXCLUDES 2** Not included here　　　**N** Newborn Age: 0　　　**P** Pediatric Age: 0-17　　　**M** Maternity Age: 12-55　　　**A** Adult Age: 15-124

704　　　　ICD-10-CM 2018

L89.214 **Pressure ulcer of right hip, stage 4** `HCC`
    Healing pressure ulcer of right hip, stage 4
    Pressure ulcer with necrosis of soft tissues through to underlying muscle, tendon, or bone, right hip

L89.219 **Pressure ulcer of right hip, unspecified stage** ▽
    Healing pressure ulcer of right hip NOS
    Healing pressure ulcer of right hip, unspecified stage

✓6th **L89.22** **Pressure ulcer of left hip**

L89.220 **Pressure ulcer of left hip, unstageable** `HCC`

L89.221 **Pressure ulcer of left hip, stage 1**
    Healing pressure ulcer of left hip, stage 1
    Pressure pre-ulcer skin changes limited to persistent focal edema, left hip

L89.222 **Pressure ulcer of left hip, stage 2**
    Healing pressure ulcer of left hip, stage 2
    Pressure ulcer with abrasion, blister, partial thickness skin loss involving epidermis and/or dermis, left hip

L89.223 **Pressure ulcer of left hip, stage 3** `HCC`
    Healing pressure ulcer of left hip, stage 3
    Pressure ulcer with full thickness skin loss involving damage or necrosis of subcutaneous tissue, left hip

L89.224 **Pressure ulcer of left hip, stage 4** `HCC`
    Healing pressure ulcer of left hip, stage 4
    Pressure ulcer with necrosis of soft tissues through to underlying muscle, tendon, or bone, left hip

L89.229 **Pressure ulcer of left hip, unspecified stage** ▽
    Healing pressure ulcer of left hip NOS
    Healing pressure ulcer of left hip, unspecified stage

✓5th **L89.3** **Pressure ulcer of buttock**

✓6th **L89.30** **Pressure ulcer of unspecified buttock**

L89.300 **Pressure ulcer of unspecified buttock, unstageable** `HCC` ▽

L89.301 **Pressure ulcer of unspecified buttock, stage 1** ▽
    Healing pressure ulcer of unspecified buttock, stage 1
    Pressure pre-ulcer skin changes limited to persistent focal edema, unspecified buttock

L89.302 **Pressure ulcer of unspecified buttock, stage 2** ▽
    Healing pressure ulcer of unspecified buttock, stage 2
    Pressure ulcer with abrasion, blister, partial thickness skin loss involving epidermis and/or dermis, unspecified buttock

L89.303 **Pressure ulcer of unspecified buttock, stage 3** `HCC` ▽
    Healing pressure ulcer of unspecified buttock, stage 3
    Pressure ulcer with full thickness skin loss involving damage or necrosis of subcutaneous tissue, unspecified buttock

L89.304 **Pressure ulcer of unspecified buttock, stage 4** `HCC` ▽
    Healing pressure ulcer of unspecified buttock, stage 4
    Pressure ulcer with necrosis of soft tissues through to underlying muscle, tendon, or bone, unspecified buttock

L89.309 **Pressure ulcer of unspecified buttock, unspecified stage** ▽
    Healing pressure ulcer of unspecified buttock NOS
    Healing pressure ulcer of unspecified buttock, unspecified stage

✓6th **L89.31** **Pressure ulcer of right buttock**

L89.310 **Pressure ulcer of right buttock, unstageable** `HCC`

L89.311 **Pressure ulcer of right buttock, stage 1**
    Healing pressure ulcer of right buttock, stage 1
    Pressure pre-ulcer skin changes limited to persistent focal edema, right buttock

L89.312 **Pressure ulcer of right buttock, stage 2**
    Healing pressure ulcer of right buttock, stage 2
    Pressure ulcer with abrasion, blister, partial thickness skin loss involving epidermis and/or dermis, right buttock

L89.313 **Pressure ulcer of right buttock, stage 3** `HCC`
    Healing pressure ulcer of right buttock, stage 3
    Pressure ulcer with full thickness skin loss involving damage or necrosis of subcutaneous tissue, right buttock

L89.314 **Pressure ulcer of right buttock, stage 4** `HCC`
    Healing pressure ulcer of right buttock, stage 4
    Pressure ulcer with necrosis of soft tissues through to underlying muscle, tendon, or bone, right buttock

L89.319 **Pressure ulcer of right buttock, unspecified stage** ▽
    Healing pressure ulcer of right buttock NOS
    Healing pressure ulcer of right buttock, unspecified stage

✓6th **L89.32** **Pressure ulcer of left buttock**

L89.320 **Pressure ulcer of left buttock, unstageable** `HCC`

L89.321 **Pressure ulcer of left buttock, stage 1**
    Healing pressure ulcer of left buttock, stage 1
    Pressure pre-ulcer skin changes limited to persistent focal edema, left buttock

L89.322 **Pressure ulcer of left buttock, stage 2**
    Healing pressure ulcer of left buttock, stage 2
    Pressure ulcer with abrasion, blister, partial thickness skin loss involving epidermis and/or dermis, left buttock

L89.323 **Pressure ulcer of left buttock, stage 3** `HCC`
    Healing pressure ulcer of left buttock, stage 3
    Pressure ulcer with full thickness skin loss involving damage or necrosis of subcutaneous tissue, left buttock

L89.324 **Pressure ulcer of left buttock, stage 4** `HCC`
    Healing pressure ulcer of left buttock, stage 4
    Pressure ulcer with necrosis of soft tissues through to underlying muscle, tendon, or bone, left buttock

L89.329 **Pressure ulcer of left buttock, unspecified stage** ▽
    Healing pressure ulcer of left buttock NOS
    Healing pressure ulcer of left buttock, unspecified stage

✓5th **L89.4** **Pressure ulcer of contiguous site of back, buttock and hip**

L89.40 **Pressure ulcer of contiguous site of back, buttock and hip, unspecified stage** ▽
    Healing pressure ulcer of contiguous site of back, buttock and hip NOS
    Healing pressure ulcer of contiguous site of back, buttock and hip, unspecified stage

L89.41 **Pressure ulcer of contiguous site of back, buttock and hip, stage 1**
    Healing pressure ulcer of contiguous site of back, buttock and hip, stage 1
    Pressure pre-ulcer skin changes limited to persistent focal edema, contiguous site of back, buttock and hip

L89.42 **Pressure ulcer of contiguous site of back, buttock and hip, stage 2**
    Healing pressure ulcer of contiguous site of back, buttock and hip, stage 2
    Pressure ulcer with abrasion, blister, partial thickness skin loss involving epidermis and/or dermis, contiguous site of back, buttock and hip

---

☑ Additional Character Req   ✓x7th Placeholder Alert   Manifestation   `HCC` CMS-HCC Condition   ▽ Unspecified Code   ►◄ Revised Text   ● New Code   ▲ Revised Code Title

ICD-10-CM 2018   **705**

L89.43 **Pressure ulcer of contiguous site of back, buttock and hip, stage 3** `HCC`
Healing pressure ulcer of contiguous site of back, buttock and hip, stage 3
Pressure ulcer with full thickness skin loss involving damage or necrosis of subcutaneous tissue, contiguous site of back, buttock and hip

L89.44 **Pressure ulcer of contiguous site of back, buttock and hip, stage 4** `HCC`
Healing pressure ulcer of contiguous site of back, buttock and hip, stage 4
Pressure ulcer with necrosis of soft tissues through to underlying muscle, tendon, or bone, contiguous site of back, buttock and hip

L89.45 **Pressure ulcer of contiguous site of back, buttock and hip, unstageable** `HCC`

☑5ᵗʰ **L89.5** **Pressure ulcer of ankle**

☑6ᵗʰ **L89.50** **Pressure ulcer of unspecified ankle**

L89.500 **Pressure ulcer of unspecified ankle, unstageable** `HCC` ▽

L89.501 **Pressure ulcer of unspecified ankle, stage 1** ▽
Healing pressure ulcer of unspecified ankle, stage 1
Pressure pre-ulcer skin changes limited to persistent focal edema, unspecified ankle

L89.502 **Pressure ulcer of unspecified ankle, stage 2** ▽
Healing pressure ulcer of unspecified ankle, stage 2
Pressure ulcer with abrasion, blister, partial thickness skin loss involving epidermis and/or dermis, unspecified ankle

L89.503 **Pressure ulcer of unspecified ankle, stage 3** `HCC` ▽
Healing pressure ulcer of unspecified ankle, stage 3
Pressure ulcer with full thickness skin loss involving damage or necrosis of subcutaneous tissue, unspecified ankle

L89.504 **Pressure ulcer of unspecified ankle, stage 4** `HCC` ▽
Healing pressure ulcer of unspecified ankle, stage 4
Pressure ulcer with necrosis of soft tissues through to underlying muscle, tendon, or bone, unspecified ankle

L89.509 **Pressure ulcer of unspecified ankle, unspecified stage** ▽
Healing pressure ulcer of unspecified ankle NOS
Healing pressure ulcer of unspecified ankle, unspecified stage

☑6ᵗʰ **L89.51** **Pressure ulcer of right ankle**

L89.510 **Pressure ulcer of right ankle, unstageable** `HCC`

L89.511 **Pressure ulcer of right ankle, stage 1**
Healing pressure ulcer of right ankle, stage 1
Pressure pre-ulcer skin changes limited to persistent focal edema, right ankle

L89.512 **Pressure ulcer of right ankle, stage 2**
Healing pressure ulcer of right ankle, stage 2
Pressure ulcer with abrasion, blister, partial thickness skin loss involving epidermis and/or dermis, right ankle

L89.513 **Pressure ulcer of right ankle, stage 3** `HCC`
Healing pressure ulcer of right ankle, stage 3
Pressure ulcer with full thickness skin loss involving damage or necrosis of subcutaneous tissue, right ankle

L89.514 **Pressure ulcer of right ankle, stage 4** `HCC`
Healing pressure ulcer of right ankle, stage 4
Pressure ulcer with necrosis of soft tissues through to underlying muscle, tendon, or bone, right ankle

L89.519 **Pressure ulcer of right ankle, unspecified stage** ▽
Healing pressure ulcer of right ankle NOS
Healing pressure ulcer of right ankle, unspecified stage

☑6ᵗʰ **L89.52** **Pressure ulcer of left ankle**

L89.520 **Pressure ulcer of left ankle, unstageable** `HCC`

L89.521 **Pressure ulcer of left ankle, stage 1**
Healing pressure ulcer of left ankle, stage 1
Pressure pre-ulcer skin changes limited to persistent focal edema, left ankle

L89.522 **Pressure ulcer of left ankle, stage 2**
Healing pressure ulcer of left ankle, stage 2
Pressure ulcer with abrasion, blister, partial thickness skin loss involving epidermis and/or dermis, left ankle

L89.523 **Pressure ulcer of left ankle, stage 3** `HCC`
Healing pressure ulcer of left ankle, stage 3
Pressure ulcer with full thickness skin loss involving damage or necrosis of subcutaneous tissue, left ankle

L89.524 **Pressure ulcer of left ankle, stage 4** `HCC`
Healing pressure ulcer of left ankle, stage 4
Pressure ulcer with necrosis of soft tissues through to underlying muscle, tendon, or bone, left ankle

L89.529 **Pressure ulcer of left ankle, unspecified stage** ▽
Healing pressure ulcer of left ankle NOS
Healing pressure ulcer of left ankle, unspecified stage

☑5ᵗʰ **L89.6** **Pressure ulcer of heel**

☑6ᵗʰ **L89.60** **Pressure ulcer of unspecified heel**

L89.600 **Pressure ulcer of unspecified heel, unstageable** `HCC` ▽

L89.601 **Pressure ulcer of unspecified heel, stage 1** ▽
Healing pressure ulcer of unspecified heel, stage 1
Pressure pre-ulcer skin changes limited to persistent focal edema, unspecified heel

L89.602 **Pressure ulcer of unspecified heel, stage 2** ▽
Healing pressure ulcer of unspecified heel, stage 2
Pressure ulcer with abrasion, blister, partial thickness skin loss involving epidermis and/or dermis, unspecified heel

L89.603 **Pressure ulcer of unspecified heel, stage 3** `HCC` ▽
Healing pressure ulcer of unspecified heel, stage 3
Pressure ulcer with full thickness skin loss involving damage or necrosis of subcutaneous tissue, unspecified heel

L89.604 **Pressure ulcer of unspecified heel, stage 4** `HCC` ▽
Healing pressure ulcer of unspecified heel, stage 4
Pressure ulcer with necrosis of soft tissues through to underlying muscle, tendon, or bone, unspecified heel

L89.609 **Pressure ulcer of unspecified heel, unspecified stage** ▽
Healing pressure ulcer of unspecified heel NOS
Healing pressure ulcer of unspecified heel, unspecified stage

☑6ᵗʰ **L89.61** **Pressure ulcer of right heel**

L89.610 **Pressure ulcer of right heel, unstageable** `HCC`

L89.611 **Pressure ulcer of right heel, stage 1**
Healing pressure ulcer of right heel, stage 1
Pressure pre-ulcer skin changes limited to persistent focal edema, right heel

EXCLUDES 1 Not coded here | **EXCLUDES 2** Not included here | **N** Newborn Age: 0 | **P** Pediatric Age: 0-17 | **M** Maternity Age: 12-55 | **A** Adult Age: 15-124

706
ICD-10-CM 2018

L89.612 Pressure ulcer of right heel, stage 2
Healing pressure ulcer of right heel, stage 2
Pressure ulcer with abrasion, blister, partial thickness skin loss involving epidermis and/or dermis, right heel

L89.613 Pressure ulcer of right heel, stage 3 `HCC`
Healing pressure ulcer of right heel, stage 3
Pressure ulcer with full thickness skin loss involving damage or necrosis of subcutaneous tissue, right heel

L89.614 Pressure ulcer of right heel, stage 4 `HCC`
Healing pressure ulcer of right heel, stage 4
Pressure ulcer with necrosis of soft tissues through to underlying muscle, tendon, or bone, right heel

L89.619 Pressure ulcer of right heel, unspecified stage ▽
Healing pressure ulcer of right heel NOS
▶Healing pressure ulcer of right heel, unspecified stage◀

✓6ᵗʰ **L89.62 Pressure ulcer of left heel**

L89.620 Pressure ulcer of left heel, unstageable `HCC`

L89.621 Pressure ulcer of left heel, stage 1
Healing pressure ulcer of left heel, stage 1
Pressure pre-ulcer skin changes limited to persistent focal edema, left heel

L89.622 Pressure ulcer of left heel, stage 2
Healing pressure ulcer of left heel, stage 2
Pressure ulcer with abrasion, blister, partial thickness skin loss involving epidermis and/or dermis, left heel

L89.623 Pressure ulcer of left heel, stage 3 `HCC`
Healing pressure ulcer of left heel, stage 3
Pressure ulcer with full thickness skin loss involving damage or necrosis of subcutaneous tissue, left heel

L89.624 Pressure ulcer of left heel, stage 4 `HCC`
Healing pressure ulcer of left heel, stage 4
Pressure ulcer with necrosis of soft tissues through to underlying muscle, tendon, or bone, left heel

L89.629 Pressure ulcer of left heel, unspecified stage ▽
Healing pressure ulcer of left heel NOS
Healing pressure ulcer of left heel, unspecified stage

✓5ᵗʰ **L89.8 Pressure ulcer of other site**

✓6ᵗʰ **L89.81 Pressure ulcer of head**
Pressure ulcer of face

L89.810 Pressure ulcer of head, unstageable `HCC`

L89.811 Pressure ulcer of head, stage 1
Healing pressure ulcer of head, stage 1
Pressure pre-ulcer skin changes limited to persistent focal edema, head

L89.812 Pressure ulcer of head, stage 2
Healing pressure ulcer of head, stage 2
Pressure ulcer with abrasion, blister, partial thickness skin loss involving epidermis and/or dermis, head

L89.813 Pressure ulcer of head, stage 3 `HCC`
Healing pressure ulcer of head, stage 3
Pressure ulcer with full thickness skin loss involving damage or necrosis of subcutaneous tissue, head

L89.814 Pressure ulcer of head, stage 4 `HCC`
Healing pressure ulcer of head, stage 4
Pressure ulcer with necrosis of soft tissues through to underlying muscle, tendon, or bone, head

L89.819 Pressure ulcer of head, unspecified stage ▽
Healing pressure ulcer of head NOS
Healing pressure ulcer of head, unspecified stage

✓6ᵗʰ **L89.89 Pressure ulcer of other site**

L89.890 Pressure ulcer of other site, unstageable `HCC`

L89.891 Pressure ulcer of other site, stage 1
Healing pressure ulcer of other site, stage 1
Pressure pre-ulcer skin changes limited to persistent focal edema, other site

L89.892 Pressure ulcer of other site, stage 2
Healing pressure ulcer of other site, stage 2
Pressure ulcer with abrasion, blister, partial thickness skin loss involving epidermis and/or dermis, other site

L89.893 Pressure ulcer of other site, stage 3 `HCC`
Healing pressure ulcer of other site, stage 3
Pressure ulcer with full thickness skin loss involving damage or necrosis of subcutaneous tissue, other site

L89.894 Pressure ulcer of other site, stage 4 `HCC`
Healing pressure ulcer of other site, stage 4
Pressure ulcer with necrosis of soft tissues through to underlying muscle, tendon, or bone, other site

L89.899 Pressure ulcer of other site, unspecified stage ▽
Healing pressure ulcer of other site NOS
Healing pressure ulcer of other site, unspecified stage

✓5ᵗʰ **L89.9 Pressure ulcer of unspecified site**

L89.90 Pressure ulcer of unspecified site, unspecified stage ▽
Healing pressure ulcer of unspecified site NOS
Healing pressure ulcer of unspecified site, unspecified stage

L89.91 Pressure ulcer of unspecified site, stage 1 ▽
Healing pressure ulcer of unspecified site, stage 1
Pressure pre-ulcer skin changes limited to persistent focal edema, unspecified site

L89.92 Pressure ulcer of unspecified site, stage 2 ▽
Healing pressure ulcer of unspecified site, stage 2
Pressure ulcer with abrasion, blister, partial thickness skin loss involving epidermis and/or dermis, unspecified site

L89.93 Pressure ulcer of unspecified site, stage 3 `HCC` ▽
Healing pressure ulcer of unspecified site, stage 3
Pressure ulcer with full thickness skin loss involving damage or necrosis of subcutaneous tissue, unspecified site

L89.94 Pressure ulcer of unspecified site, stage 4 `HCC` ▽
Healing pressure ulcer of unspecified site, stage 4
Pressure ulcer with necrosis of soft tissues through to underlying muscle, tendon, or bone, unspecified site

L89.95 Pressure ulcer of unspecified site, unstageable `HCC` ▽

✓4ᵗʰ **L90 Atrophic disorders of skin**

L90.0 Lichen sclerosus et atrophicus
EXCLUDES 2 *lichen sclerosus of external female genital organs (N90.4)*
lichen sclerosus of external male genital organs (N48.0)

L90.1 Anetoderma of Schweninger-Buzzi

L90.2 Anetoderma of Jadassohn-Pellizzari

L90.3 Atrophoderma of Pasini and Pierini

L90.4 Acrodermatitis chronica atrophicans

L90.5 Scar conditions and fibrosis of skin
Adherent scar (skin)
Cicatrix
Disfigurement of skin due to scar
Fibrosis of skin NOS
Scar NOS
EXCLUDES 2 *hypertrophic scar (L91.0)*
keloid scar (L91.0)
AHA: 2016, 2Q, 5; 2015, 1Q, 19

L90.6 Striae atrophicae

L90.8 Other atrophic disorders of skin

L90.9 Atrophic disorder of skin, unspecified ▽

Chapter 12. Diseases of the Skin and Subcutaneous Tissue   L91–L97.125

L91 Hypertrophic disorders of skin

L91.0 Hypertrophic scar
Keloid
Keloid scar
EXCLUDES 2   acne keloid (L73.0)
scar NOS (L90.5)
DEF: Overgrowth of scar tissue due to excess amounts of collagen during connective tissue repair; occurs mainly on upper trunk, face.

L91.8 Other hypertrophic disorders of the skin

L91.9 Hypertrophic disorder of the skin, unspecified ▽

L92 Granulomatous disorders of skin and subcutaneous tissue
EXCLUDES 2   actinic granuloma (L57.5)

L92.0 Granuloma annulare
Perforating granuloma annulare

L92.1 Necrobiosis lipoidica, not elsewhere classified
EXCLUDES 1   necrobiosis lipoidica associated with diabetes mellitus (E08-E13 with .620)

L92.2 Granuloma faciale [eosinophilic granuloma of skin]

L92.3 Foreign body granuloma of the skin and subcutaneous tissue
Use additional code to identify the type of retained foreign body (Z18.-)

L92.8 Other granulomatous disorders of the skin and subcutaneous tissue

L92.9 Granulomatous disorder of the skin and subcutaneous tissue, unspecified ▽
EXCLUDES 2 ▶umbilical granuloma (P83.81)◀

L93 Lupus erythematosus
Use additional code for adverse effect, if applicable, to identify drug (T36-T50 with fifth or sixth character 5)
EXCLUDES 1   lupus exedens (A18.4)
lupus vulgaris (A18.4)
scleroderma (M34.-)
systemic lupus erythematosus (M32.-)

L93.0 Discoid lupus erythematosus
Lupus erythematosus NOS

L93.1 Subacute cutaneous lupus erythematosus

L93.2 Other local lupus erythematosus
Lupus erythematosus profundus
Lupus panniculitis

L94 Other localized connective tissue disorders
EXCLUDES 1   systemic connective tissue disorders (M30-M36)

L94.0 Localized scleroderma [morphea]
Circumscribed scleroderma

L94.1 Linear scleroderma
En coup de sabre lesion

L94.2 Calcinosis cutis

L94.3 Sclerodactyly

L94.4 Gottron's papules

L94.5 Poikiloderma vasculare atrophicans

L94.6 Ainhum

L94.8 Other specified localized connective tissue disorders

L94.9 Localized connective tissue disorder, unspecified ▽

L95 Vasculitis limited to skin, not elsewhere classified
EXCLUDES 1   angioma serpiginosum (L81.7)
Henoch(-Schönlein) purpura (D69.0)
hypersensitivity angiitis (M31.0)
lupus panniculitis (L93.2)
panniculitis NOS (M79.3)
panniculitis of neck and back (M54.0-)
polyarteritis nodosa (M30.0)
relapsing panniculitis (M35.6)
rheumatoid vasculitis (M05.2)
serum sickness (T80.6-)
urticaria (L50.-)
Wegener's granulomatosis (M31.3-)

L95.0 Livedoid vasculitis
Atrophie blanche (en plaque)

L95.1 Erythema elevatum diutinum

L95.8 Other vasculitis limited to the skin

L95.9 Vasculitis limited to the skin, unspecified ▽

L97 Non-pressure chronic ulcer of lower limb, not elsewhere classified
INCLUDES   chronic ulcer of skin of lower limb NOS
non-healing ulcer of skin
non-infected sinus of skin
trophic ulcer NOS
tropical ulcer NOS
ulcer of skin of lower limb NOS
Code first any associated underlying condition, such as:
any associated gangrene (I96)
atherosclerosis of the lower extremities (I70.23-, I70.24-, I70.33-, I70.34-, I70.43-, I70.44-, I70.53-, I70.54-, I70.63-, I70.64-, I70.73-, I70.74-)
chronic venous hypertension (I87.31-, I87.33-)
diabetic ulcers (E08.621, E08.622, E09.621, E09.622, E10.621, E10.622, E11.621, E11.622, E13.621, E13.622)
postphlebitic syndrome (I87.01-, I87.03-)
postthrombotic syndrome (I87.01-, I87.03-)
varicose ulcer (I83.0-, I83.2-)
EXCLUDES 2   pressure ulcer (pressure area) (L89.-)
skin infections (L00-L08)
specific infections classified to A00-B99

L97.1 Non-pressure chronic ulcer of thigh

L97.10 Non-pressure chronic ulcer of unspecified thigh

L97.101 Non-pressure chronic ulcer of unspecified thigh limited to breakdown of skin   HCC ▽

L97.102 Non-pressure chronic ulcer of unspecified thigh with fat layer exposed   HCC ▽

L97.103 Non-pressure chronic ulcer of unspecified thigh with necrosis of muscle   HCC ▽

L97.104 Non-pressure chronic ulcer of unspecified thigh with necrosis of bone   HCC ▽

L97.105 Non-pressure chronic ulcer of unspecified thigh with muscle involvement without evidence of necrosis ▽

L97.106 Non-pressure chronic ulcer of unspecified thigh with bone involvement without evidence of necrosis ▽

L97.108 Non-pressure chronic ulcer of unspecified thigh with other specified severity ▽

L97.109 Non-pressure chronic ulcer of unspecified thigh with unspecified severity   HCC ▽

L97.11 Non-pressure chronic ulcer of right thigh

L97.111 Non-pressure chronic ulcer of right thigh limited to breakdown of skin   HCC

L97.112 Non-pressure chronic ulcer of right thigh with fat layer exposed   HCC

L97.113 Non-pressure chronic ulcer of right high with necrosis of muscle   HCC

L97.114 Non-pressure chronic ulcer of right thigh with necrosis of bone   HCC

L97.115 Non-pressure chronic ulcer of right thigh with muscle involvement without evidence of necrosis

L97.116 Non-pressure chronic ulcer of right thigh with bone involvement without evidence of necrosis

L97.118 Non-pressure chronic ulcer of right thigh with other specified severity

L97.119 Non-pressure chronic ulcer of right thigh with unspecified severity   HCC ▽

L97.12 Non-pressure chronic ulcer of left thigh

L97.121 Non-pressure chronic ulcer of left thigh limited to breakdown of skin   HCC

L97.122 Non-pressure chronic ulcer of left thigh with fat layer exposed   HCC

L97.123 Non-pressure chronic ulcer of left thigh with necrosis of muscle   HCC

L97.124 Non-pressure chronic ulcer of left thigh with necrosis of bone   HCC

L97.125 Non-pressure chronic ulcer of left thigh with muscle involvement without evidence of necrosis

EXCLUDES 1 Not coded here   EXCLUDES 2 Not included here   N Newborn Age: 0   P Pediatric Age: 0-17   M Maternity Age: 12-55   A Adult Age: 15-124

708   ICD-10-CM 2018

- **L97.126** Non-pressure chronic ulcer of left thigh with bone involvement without evidence of necrosis
- **L97.128** Non-pressure chronic ulcer of left thigh with other specified severity
- **L97.129** Non-pressure chronic ulcer of left thigh with unspecified severity HCC ▽

✓5th **L97.2** Non-pressure chronic ulcer of calf
  ✓6th **L97.20** Non-pressure chronic ulcer of unspecified calf
  - **L97.201** Non-pressure chronic ulcer of unspecified calf limited to breakdown of skin HCC ▽
  - **L97.202** Non-pressure chronic ulcer of unspecified calf with fat layer exposed HCC ▽
  - **L97.203** Non-pressure chronic ulcer of unspecified calf with necrosis of muscle HCC ▽
  - **L97.204** Non-pressure chronic ulcer of unspecified calf with necrosis of bone HCC ▽
  - **L97.205** Non-pressure chronic ulcer of unspecified calf with muscle involvement without evidence of necrosis ▽
  - **L97.206** Non-pressure chronic ulcer of unspecified calf with bone involvement without evidence of necrosis ▽
  - **L97.208** Non-pressure chronic ulcer of unspecified calf with other specified severity ▽
  - **L97.209** Non-pressure chronic ulcer of unspecified calf with unspecified severity HCC ▽
  ✓6th **L97.21** Non-pressure chronic ulcer of right calf
  - **L97.211** Non-pressure chronic ulcer of right calf limited to breakdown of skin HCC
  - **L97.212** Non-pressure chronic ulcer of right calf with fat layer exposed HCC
  - **L97.213** Non-pressure chronic ulcer of right calf with necrosis of muscle HCC
  - **L97.214** Non-pressure chronic ulcer of right calf with necrosis of bone HCC
  - **L97.215** Non-pressure chronic ulcer of right calf with muscle involvement without evidence of necrosis
  - **L97.216** Non-pressure chronic ulcer of right calf with bone involvement without evidence of necrosis
  - **L97.218** Non-pressure chronic ulcer of right calf with other specified severity
  - **L97.219** Non-pressure chronic ulcer of right calf with unspecified severity HCC ▽
  ✓6th **L97.22** Non-pressure chronic ulcer of left calf
  - **L97.221** Non-pressure chronic ulcer of left calf limited to breakdown of skin HCC
  - **L97.222** Non-pressure chronic ulcer of left calf with fat layer exposed HCC
  - **L97.223** Non-pressure chronic ulcer of left calf with necrosis of muscle HCC
  - **L97.224** Non-pressure chronic ulcer of left calf with necrosis of bone HCC
  - **L97.225** Non-pressure chronic ulcer of left calf with muscle involvement without evidence of necrosis
  - **L97.226** Non-pressure chronic ulcer of left calf with bone involvement without evidence of necrosis
  - **L97.228** Non-pressure chronic ulcer of left calf with other specified severity
  - **L97.229** Non-pressure chronic ulcer of left calf with unspecified severity HCC ▽

✓5th **L97.3** Non-pressure chronic ulcer of ankle
  ✓6th **L97.30** Non-pressure chronic ulcer of unspecified ankle
  - **L97.301** Non-pressure chronic ulcer of unspecified ankle limited to breakdown of skin HCC ▽
  - **L97.302** Non-pressure chronic ulcer of unspecified ankle with fat layer exposed HCC ▽
  - **L97.303** Non-pressure chronic ulcer of unspecified ankle with necrosis of muscle HCC ▽
  - **L97.304** Non-pressure chronic ulcer of unspecified ankle with necrosis of bone HCC ▽
  - **L97.305** Non-pressure chronic ulcer of unspecified ankle with muscle involvement without evidence of necrosis ▽
  - **L97.306** Non-pressure chronic ulcer of unspecified ankle with bone involvement without evidence of necrosis ▽
  - **L97.308** Non-pressure chronic ulcer of unspecified ankle with other specified severity ▽
  - **L97.309** Non-pressure chronic ulcer of unspecified ankle with unspecified severity HCC ▽
  ✓6th **L97.31** Non-pressure chronic ulcer of right ankle
  - **L97.311** Non-pressure chronic ulcer of right ankle limited to breakdown of skin HCC
  - **L97.312** Non-pressure chronic ulcer of right ankle with fat layer exposed HCC
  - **L97.313** Non-pressure chronic ulcer of right ankle with necrosis of muscle HCC
  - **L97.314** Non-pressure chronic ulcer of right ankle with necrosis of bone HCC
  - **L97.315** Non-pressure chronic ulcer of right ankle with muscle involvement without evidence of necrosis
  - **L97.316** Non-pressure chronic ulcer of right ankle with bone involvement without evidence of necrosis
  - **L97.318** Non-pressure chronic ulcer of right ankle with other specified severity
  - **L97.319** Non-pressure chronic ulcer of right ankle with unspecified severity HCC ▽
  ✓6th **L97.32** Non-pressure chronic ulcer of left ankle
  - **L97.321** Non-pressure chronic ulcer of left ankle limited to breakdown of skin HCC
  - **L97.322** Non-pressure chronic ulcer of left ankle with fat layer exposed HCC
  - **L97.323** Non-pressure chronic ulcer of left ankle with necrosis of muscle HCC
  - **L97.324** Non-pressure chronic ulcer of left ankle with necrosis of bone HCC
  - **L97.325** Non-pressure chronic ulcer of left ankle with muscle involvement without evidence of necrosis
  - **L97.326** Non-pressure chronic ulcer of left ankle with bone involvement without evidence of necrosis
  - **L97.328** Non-pressure chronic ulcer of left ankle with other specified severity
  - **L97.329** Non-pressure chronic ulcer of left ankle with unspecified severity HCC ▽

✓5th **L97.4** Non-pressure chronic ulcer of heel and midfoot
  Non-pressure chronic ulcer of plantar surface of midfoot
  ✓6th **L97.40** Non-pressure chronic ulcer of unspecified heel and midfoot
  - **L97.401** Non-pressure chronic ulcer of unspecified heel and midfoot limited to breakdown of skin HCC ▽
  - **L97.402** Non-pressure chronic ulcer of unspecified heel and midfoot with fat layer exposed HCC ▽
  - **L97.403** Non-pressure chronic ulcer of unspecified heel and midfoot with necrosis of muscle HCC ▽
  - **L97.404** Non-pressure chronic ulcer of unspecified heel and midfoot with necrosis of bone HCC ▽
  - **L97.405** Non-pressure chronic ulcer of unspecified heel and midfoot with muscle involvement without evidence of necrosis ▽
  - **L97.406** Non-pressure chronic ulcer of unspecified heel and midfoot with bone involvement without evidence of necrosis ▽

✓ Additional Character Req   ✗7th Placeholder Alert   Manifestation   HCC CMS-HCC Condition   ▽ Unspecified Code   ▶◀ Revised Text   ● New Code   ▲ Revised Code Title

ICD-10-CM 2018   709

L97.408 Non-pressure chronic ulcer of unspecified heel and midfoot with other specified severity ▽

L97.409 Non-pressure chronic ulcer of unspecified heel and midfoot with unspecified severity   HCC ▽

✓6th **L97.41** Non-pressure chronic ulcer of right heel and midfoot

L97.411 Non-pressure chronic ulcer of right heel and midfoot limited to breakdown of skin   HCC

L97.412 Non-pressure chronic ulcer of right heel and midfoot with fat layer exposed   HCC

L97.413 Non-pressure chronic ulcer of right heel and midfoot with necrosis of muscle   HCC

L97.414 Non-pressure chronic ulcer of right heel and midfoot with necrosis of bone   HCC

L97.415 Non-pressure chronic ulcer of right heel and midfoot with muscle involvement without evidence of necrosis

L97.416 Non-pressure chronic ulcer of right heel and midfoot with bone involvement without evidence of necrosis

L97.418 Non-pressure chronic ulcer of right heel and midfoot with other specified severity

L97.419 Non-pressure chronic ulcer of right heel and midfoot with unspecified severity   HCC ▽

✓6th **L97.42** Non-pressure chronic ulcer of left heel and midfoot

L97.421 Non-pressure chronic ulcer of left heel and midfoot limited to breakdown of skin   HCC
     AHA: 2016, 1Q, 12

L97.422 Non-pressure chronic ulcer of left heel and midfoot with fat layer exposed   HCC

L97.423 Non-pressure chronic ulcer of left heel and midfoot with necrosis of muscle   HCC

L97.424 Non-pressure chronic ulcer of left heel and midfoot with necrosis of bone   HCC

L97.425 Non-pressure chronic ulcer of left heel and midfoot with muscle involvement without evidence of necrosis

L97.426 Non-pressure chronic ulcer of left heel and midfoot with bone involvement without evidence of necrosis

L97.428 Non-pressure chronic ulcer of left heel and midfoot with other specified severity

L97.429 Non-pressure chronic ulcer of left heel and midfoot with unspecified severity   HCC ▽

✓5th **L97.5** Non-pressure chronic ulcer of other part of foot
Non-pressure chronic ulcer of toe

✓6th **L97.50** Non-pressure chronic ulcer of other part of unspecified foot

L97.501 Non-pressure chronic ulcer of other part of unspecified foot limited to breakdown of skin   HCC ▽

L97.502 Non-pressure chronic ulcer of other part of unspecified foot with fat layer exposed   HCC ▽

L97.503 Non-pressure chronic ulcer of other part of unspecified foot with necrosis of muscle   HCC ▽

L97.504 Non-pressure chronic ulcer of other part of unspecified foot with necrosis of bone   HCC ▽

L97.505 Non-pressure chronic ulcer of other part of unspecified foot with muscle involvement without evidence of necrosis ▽

L97.506 Non-pressure chronic ulcer of other part of unspecified foot with bone involvement without evidence of necrosis ▽

L97.508 Non-pressure chronic ulcer of other part of unspecified foot with other specified severity ▽

L97.509 Non-pressure chronic ulcer of other part of unspecified foot with unspecified severity   HCC ▽

✓6th **L97.51** Non-pressure chronic ulcer of other part of right foot

L97.511 Non-pressure chronic ulcer of other part of right foot limited to breakdown of skin   HCC

L97.512 Non-pressure chronic ulcer of other part of right foot with fat layer exposed   HCC

L97.513 Non-pressure chronic ulcer of other part of right foot with necrosis of muscle   HCC

L97.514 Non-pressure chronic ulcer of other part of right foot with necrosis of bone   HCC

L97.515 Non-pressure chronic ulcer of other part of right foot with muscle involvement without evidence of necrosis

L97.516 Non-pressure chronic ulcer of other part of right foot with bone involvement without evidence of necrosis

L97.518 Non-pressure chronic ulcer of other part of right foot with other specified severity

L97.519 Non-pressure chronic ulcer of other part of right foot with unspecified severity   HCC ▽

✓6th **L97.52** Non-pressure chronic ulcer of other part of left foot

L97.521 Non-pressure chronic ulcer of other part of left foot limited to breakdown of skin   HCC

L97.522 Non-pressure chronic ulcer of other part of left foot with fat layer exposed   HCC

L97.523 Non-pressure chronic ulcer of other part of left foot with necrosis of muscle   HCC

L97.524 Non-pressure chronic ulcer of other part of left foot with necrosis of bone   HCC

L97.525 Non-pressure chronic ulcer of other part of left foot with muscle involvement without evidence of necrosis

L97.526 Non-pressure chronic ulcer of other part of left foot with bone involvement without evidence of necrosis

L97.528 Non-pressure chronic ulcer of other part of left foot with other specified severity

L97.529 Non-pressure chronic ulcer of other part of left foot with unspecified severity   HCC ▽

✓5th **L97.8** Non-pressure chronic ulcer of other part of lower leg

✓6th **L97.80** Non-pressure chronic ulcer of other part of unspecified lower leg

L97.801 Non-pressure chronic ulcer of other part of unspecified lower leg limited to breakdown of skin   HCC ▽

L97.802 Non-pressure chronic ulcer of other part of unspecified lower leg with fat layer exposed   HCC ▽

L97.803 Non-pressure chronic ulcer of other part of unspecified lower leg with necrosis of muscle   HCC ▽

L97.804 Non-pressure chronic ulcer of other part of unspecified lower leg with necrosis of bone   HCC ▽

L97.805 Non-pressure chronic ulcer of other part of unspecified lower leg with muscle involvement without evidence of necrosis ▽

L97.806 Non-pressure chronic ulcer of other part of unspecified lower leg with bone involvement without evidence of necrosis ▽

L97.808 Non-pressure chronic ulcer of other part of unspecified lower leg with other specified severity ▽

L97.809 Non-pressure chronic ulcer of other part of unspecified lower leg with unspecified severity   HCC ▽

✓6th **L97.81** Non-pressure chronic ulcer of other part of right lower leg

L97.811 Non-pressure chronic ulcer of other part of right lower leg limited to breakdown of skin   HCC

L97.812 Non-pressure chronic ulcer of other part of right lower leg with fat layer exposed   HCC

EXCLUDES 1 Not coded here   **EXCLUDES 2** Not included here   **N** Newborn Age: 0   **P** Pediatric Age: 0-17   **M** Maternity Age: 12-55   **A** Adult Age: 15-124

710   ICD-10-CM 2018

L97.813   Non-pressure chronic ulcer of other **HCC** part of right lower leg with necrosis of muscle

L97.814   Non-pressure chronic ulcer of other **HCC** part of right lower leg with necrosis of bone

●   L97.815   Non-pressure chronic ulcer of other part of right lower leg with muscle involvement without evidence of necrosis

●   L97.816   Non-pressure chronic ulcer of other part of right lower leg with bone involvement without evidence of necrosis

●   L97.818   Non-pressure chronic ulcer of other part of right lower leg with other specified severity

L97.819   Non-pressure chronic ulcer of other **HCC** ▽ part of right lower leg with unspecified severity

√6ᵗʰ L97.82   **Non-pressure chronic ulcer of other part of left lower leg**

L97.821   Non-pressure chronic ulcer of other **HCC** part of left lower leg limited to breakdown of skin

L97.822   Non-pressure chronic ulcer of other **HCC** part of left lower leg with fat layer exposed

L97.823   Non-pressure chronic ulcer of other **HCC** part of left lower leg with necrosis of muscle

L97.824   Non-pressure chronic ulcer of other **HCC** part of left lower leg with necrosis of bone

●   L97.825   Non-pressure chronic ulcer of other part of left lower leg with muscle involvement without evidence of necrosis

●   L97.826   Non-pressure chronic ulcer of other part of left lower leg with bone involvement without evidence of necrosis

●   L97.828   Non-pressure chronic ulcer of other part of left lower leg with other specified severity

L97.829   Non-pressure chronic ulcer of **HCC** ▽ other part of left lower leg with unspecified severity

√5ᵗʰ L97.9   **Non-pressure chronic ulcer of unspecified part of lower leg**

√6ᵗʰ L97.90   **Non-pressure chronic ulcer of unspecified part of unspecified lower leg**

L97.901   Non-pressure chronic ulcer of **HCC** ▽ unspecified part of unspecified lower leg limited to breakdown of skin

L97.902   Non-pressure chronic ulcer of **HCC** ▽ unspecified part of unspecified lower leg with fat layer exposed

L97.903   Non-pressure chronic ulcer of **HCC** ▽ unspecified part of unspecified lower leg with necrosis of muscle

L97.904   Non-pressure chronic ulcer of **HCC** ▽ unspecified part of unspecified lower leg with necrosis of bone

●   L97.905   Non-pressure chronic ulcer of ▽ unspecified part of unspecified lower leg with muscle involvement without evidence of necrosis

●   L97.906   Non-pressure chronic ulcer of ▽ unspecified part of unspecified lower leg with bone involvement without evidence of necrosis

●   L97.908   Non-pressure chronic ulcer of ▽ unspecified part of unspecified lower leg with other specified severity

L97.909   Non-pressure chronic ulcer of **HCC** ▽ unspecified part of unspecified lower leg with unspecified severity

√6ᵗʰ L97.91   **Non-pressure chronic ulcer of unspecified part of right lower leg**

L97.911   Non-pressure chronic ulcer of **HCC** ▽ unspecified part of right lower leg limited to breakdown of skin

L97.912   Non-pressure chronic ulcer of **HCC** ▽ unspecified part of right lower leg with fat layer exposed

L97.913   Non-pressure chronic ulcer of **HCC** ▽ unspecified part of right lower leg with necrosis of muscle

L97.914   Non-pressure chronic ulcer of **HCC** ▽ unspecified part of right lower leg with necrosis of bone

●   L97.915   Non-pressure chronic ulcer of ▽ unspecified part of right lower leg with muscle involvement without evidence of necrosis

●   L97.916   Non-pressure chronic ulcer of ▽ unspecified part of right lower leg with bone involvement without evidence of necrosis

●   L97.918   Non-pressure chronic ulcer of ▽ unspecified part of right lower leg with other specified severity

L97.919   Non-pressure chronic ulcer of **HCC** ▽ unspecified part of right lower leg with unspecified severity

√6ᵗʰ L97.92   **Non-pressure chronic ulcer of unspecified part of left lower leg**

L97.921   Non-pressure chronic ulcer of **HCC** ▽ unspecified part of left lower leg limited to breakdown of skin

L97.922   Non-pressure chronic ulcer of **HCC** ▽ unspecified part of left lower leg with fat layer exposed

L97.923   Non-pressure chronic ulcer of **HCC** ▽ unspecified part of left lower leg with necrosis of muscle

L97.924   Non-pressure chronic ulcer of **HCC** ▽ unspecified part of left lower leg with necrosis of bone

●   L97.925   Non-pressure chronic ulcer of ▽ unspecified part of left lower leg with muscle involvement without evidence of necrosis

●   L97.926   Non-pressure chronic ulcer of ▽ unspecified part of left lower leg with bone involvement without evidence of necrosis

●   L97.928   Non-pressure chronic ulcer of ▽ unspecified part of left lower leg with other specified severity

L97.929   Non-pressure chronic ulcer of **HCC** ▽ unspecified part of left lower leg with unspecified severity

√4ᵗʰ L98   **Other disorders of skin and subcutaneous tissue, not elsewhere classified**

L98.0   **Pyogenic granuloma**

     EXCLUDES 2   pyogenic granuloma of gingiva (K06.8)
         pyogenic granuloma of maxillary alveolar ridge (K04.5)
         pyogenic granuloma of oral mucosa (K13.4)

     DEF: Solitary polypoid capillary hemangioma often associated with local irritation, trauma, and superimposed inflammation; located on the skin and gingival or oral mucosa; they bleed easily and may ulcerate and form crusted sores.

L98.1   **Factitial dermatitis**

     Neurotic excoriation

     EXCLUDES 1   excoriation (skin-picking) disorder (F42.4)

     DEF: Self-inflicted skin lesions to satisfy an unconscious psychological or emotional need; methods used to injure the skin include deep excoriations with a sharp instrument, scarification with a knife, or the application of caustic chemicals and burning, sometimes with a cigarette.

L98.2   **Febrile neutrophilic dermatosis [Sweet]**

L98.3   **Eosinophilic cellulitis [Wells]**

√5ᵗʰ L98.4   **Non-pressure chronic ulcer of skin, not elsewhere classified**

     Chronic ulcer of skin NOS
     Tropical ulcer NOS
     Ulcer of skin NOS

     EXCLUDES 2   pressure ulcer (pressure area) (L89.-)
         gangrene (I96)
         skin infections (L00-L08)
         specific infections classified to A00-B99
         ulcer of lower limb NEC (L97.-)
         varicose ulcer (I83.0-I82.2)

√6ᵗʰ L98.41   **Non-pressure chronic ulcer of buttock**

L98.411   Non-pressure chronic ulcer of buttock **HCC** limited to breakdown of skin

---

☑ Additional Character Req   √x7ᵗʰ Placeholder Alert   Manifestation   **HCC** CMS-HCC Condition   ▽ Unspecified Code   ►◄ Revised Text   ● New Code   ▲ Revised Code Title

ICD-10-CM 2018   **711**

L98.412 Non-pressure chronic ulcer of buttock `HCC` with fat layer exposed

L98.413 Non-pressure chronic ulcer of buttock `HCC` with necrosis of muscle

L98.414 Non-pressure chronic ulcer of buttock `HCC` with necrosis of bone

● **L98.415** Non-pressure chronic ulcer of buttock with muscle involvement without evidence of necrosis

● **L98.416** Non-pressure chronic ulcer of buttock with bone involvement without evidence of necrosis

● **L98.418** Non-pressure chronic ulcer of buttock with other specified severity

L98.419 Non-pressure chronic ulcer of buttock with unspecified severity `HCC` ▽

✓6ᵗʰ **L98.42** Non-pressure chronic ulcer of back

L98.421 Non-pressure chronic ulcer of back `HCC` limited to breakdown of skin

L98.422 Non-pressure chronic ulcer of back `HCC` with fat layer exposed

L98.423 Non-pressure chronic ulcer of back `HCC` with necrosis of muscle

L98.424 Non-pressure chronic ulcer of back `HCC` with necrosis of bone

● **L98.425** Non-pressure chronic ulcer of back with muscle involvement without evidence of necrosis

● **L98.426** Non-pressure chronic ulcer of back with bone involvement without evidence of necrosis

● **L98.428** Non-pressure chronic ulcer of back with other specified severity

L98.429 Non-pressure chronic ulcer of back `HCC` ▽ with unspecified severity

✓6ᵗʰ **L98.49** Non-pressure chronic ulcer of skin of other sites
Non-pressure chronic ulcer of skin NOS

L98.491 Non-pressure chronic ulcer of skin of `HCC` other sites limited to breakdown of skin

L98.492 Non-pressure chronic ulcer of skin of `HCC` other sites with fat layer exposed

L98.493 Non-pressure chronic ulcer of skin of `HCC` other sites with necrosis of muscle

L98.494 Non-pressure chronic ulcer of skin of `HCC` other sites with necrosis of bone

● **L98.495** Non-pressure chronic ulcer of other sites with muscle involvement without evidence of necrosis

● **L98.496** Non-pressure chronic ulcer of other sites with bone involvement without evidence of necrosis

● **L98.498** Non-pressure chronic ulcer of other sites with other specified severity

L98.499 Non-pressure chronic ulcer of skin `HCC` ▽ of other sites with unspecified severity

L98.5 Mucinosis of the skin
Focal mucinosis
Lichen myxedematosus
Reticular erythematous mucinosis
EXCLUDES 1   focal oral mucinosis (K13.79)
       myxedema (E03.9)

L98.6 Other infiltrative disorders of the skin and subcutaneous tissue
EXCLUDES 1   hyalinosis cutis et mucosae (E78.89)

L98.7 Excessive and redundant skin and subcutaneous tissue
Loose or sagging skin following bariatric surgery weight loss
Loose or sagging skin following dietary weight loss
Loose or sagging skin, NOS
EXCLUDES 2   acquired excess or redundant skin of eyelid (H02.3-)
       congenital excess or redundant skin of eyelid (Q10.3)
       skin changes due to chronic exposure to nonionizing
       radiation (L57.-)

L98.8 Other specified disorders of the skin and subcutaneous tissue
AHA: 2013, 2Q, 32

L98.9 Disorder of the skin and subcutaneous tissue, unspecified ▽

L99 *Other disorders of skin and subcutaneous tissue in diseases classified elsewhere*
Code first underlying disease, such as:
amyloidosis (E85.-)
EXCLUDES 1   skin disorders in diabetes (E08-E13 with .62)
       skin disorders in gonorrhea (A54.89)
       skin disorders in syphilis (A51.31, A52.79)

EXCLUDES 1 Not coded here   *EXCLUDES 2* Not included here   N Newborn Age: 0   P Pediatric Age: 0-17   M Maternity Age: 12-55   A Adult Age: 15-124

712   ICD-10-CM 2018

Chapter 13. Diseases of the Musculoskeletal System and Connective Tissue (M00–M99)

Chapter Specific Guidelines with Coding Examples

The chapter specific guidelines from the ICD-10-CM Official Guidelines for Coding and Reporting have been provided below. Along with these guidelines are coding examples, contained in the shaded boxes, that have been developed to help illustrate the coding and/or sequencing guidance found in these guidelines.

a. Site and laterality

Most of the codes within Chapter 13 have site and laterality designations. The site represents the bone, joint or the muscle involved. For some conditions where more than one bone, joint or muscle is usually involved, such as osteoarthritis, there is a "multiple sites" code available. For categories where no multiple site code is provided and more than one bone, joint or muscle is involved, multiple codes should be used to indicate the different sites involved.

> Olecranon bursitis of the left elbow
>
> **M70.22**   **Olecranon bursitis, left elbow**
>
> *Explanation:* Most of the codes within chapter 13 have site and laterality designations. The site represents the bone, joint, or the muscle involved.

> Rheumatoid arthritis of multiple sites without rheumatoid factor
>
> **M06.09**   **Rheumatoid arthritis without rheumatoid factor, multiple sites**
>
> *Explanation:* For some conditions where more than one bone, joint or muscle is usually involved, such as osteoarthritis, there is a "multiple sites" code available.

> Adolescent scoliosis in the upper thoracic region and the lumbar vertebrae
>
> **M41.124**   **Adolescent idiopathic scoliosis, thoracic region**
>
> **M41.126**   **Adolescent idiopathic scoliosis, lumbar region**
>
> *Explanation:* For categories without a multiple site code and more than one bone, joint, or muscle is involved, multiple codes should be used to indicate the different sites involved.

1) Bone versus joint

For certain conditions, the bone may be affected at the upper or lower end, (e.g., avascular necrosis of bone, M87, Osteoporosis, M80, M81). Though the portion of the bone affected may be at the joint, the site designation will be the bone, not the joint.

> Idiopathic avascular necrosis of the femoral head of the left hip joint
>
> **M87.052**   **Idiopathic aseptic necrosis of left femur**
>
> *Explanation:* For certain conditions such as avascular necrosis, the bone may be affected at the joint, but the site designation is the bone, not the joint.

b. Acute traumatic versus chronic or recurrent musculoskeletal conditions

Many musculoskeletal conditions are a result of previous injury or trauma to a site, or are recurrent conditions. Bone, joint or muscle conditions that are the result of a healed injury are usually found in chapter 13. Recurrent bone, joint or muscle conditions are also usually found in chapter 13. Any current, acute injury should be coded to the appropriate injury code from chapter 19. Chronic or recurrent conditions should generally be coded with a code from chapter 13. If it is difficult to determine from the documentation in the record which code is best to describe a condition, query the provider.

> Acute traumatic bucket handle tear of right medial meniscus
>
> **S83.211A**   **Bucket-handle tear of medial meniscus, current injury, right knee, initial encounter**
>
> *Explanation:* Any current, acute injury is not coded in chapter 13. It should instead be coded to the appropriate injury code from chapter 19.

> Old bucket handle tear of right medial meniscus
>
> **M23.203**   **Derangement of unspecified medial meniscus due to old tear or injury, right knee**
>
> *Explanation:* Chronic or recurrent conditions should generally be coded with a code from chapter 13.

c. Coding of Pathologic Fractures

7th character A is for use as long as the patient is receiving active treatment for the fracture. Examples of active treatment are: surgical treatment, emergency department encounter, evaluation and continuing treatment by the same or a different physician. While the patient may be seen by a new or different provider over the course of treatment for a pathological fracture, assignment of the 7th character is based on whether the patient is undergoing active treatment and not whether the provider is seeing the patient for the first time.

> Pathologic fracture of left foot, unknown cause, currently under active treatment by a follow-up provider
>
> **M84.475A**   **Pathological fracture, left foot, initial encounter for fracture**
>
> *Explanation:* Seventh character A is for use as long as the patient is receiving active treatment for a pathologic fracture. Examples of active treatment are surgical treatment, emergency department encounter, evaluation, and continuing treatment by the same or a different physician.
>
> The seventh character is based on whether the patient is undergoing active treatment and not whether the provider is seeing the patient for the first time.

7th character D is to be used for encounters after the patient has completed active treatment. The other 7th characters, listed under each subcategory in the Tabular List, are to be used for subsequent encounters for routine care of fractures during the healing and recovery phase as well as treatment of problems associated with the healing, such as malunions, nonunions, and sequelae.

Care for complications of surgical treatment for fracture repairs during the healing or recovery phase should be coded with the appropriate complication codes.

See Section I.C.19. Coding of traumatic fractures.

d. Osteoporosis

Osteoporosis is a systemic condition, meaning that all bones of the musculoskeletal system are affected. Therefore, site is not a component of the codes under category M81, Osteoporosis without current pathological fracture. The site codes under category M80, Osteoporosis with current pathological fracture, identify the site of the fracture, not the osteoporosis.

1) Osteoporosis without pathological fracture

Category M81, Osteoporosis without current pathological fracture, is for use for patients with osteoporosis who do not currently have a pathologic fracture due to the osteoporosis, even if they have had a fracture in the past. For patients with a history of osteoporosis fractures, status code Z87.310, Personal history of (healed) osteoporosis fracture, should follow the code from M81.

> Age-related osteoporosis with healed osteoporotic fracture of the lumbar vertebra
>
> **M81.0**   **Age-related osteoporosis without current pathological fracture**
>
> **Z87.310**   **Personal history of (healed) osteoporosis fracture**
>
> *Explanation:* Category M81 is used for patients with osteoporosis who do not currently have a pathologic fracture due to the osteoporosis. To report a previous (healed) fracture, status code Z87.310 Personal history of (healed) osteoporosis fracture, should follow the code from M81.

2) Osteoporosis with current pathological fracture

Category M80, Osteoporosis with current pathological fracture, is for patients who have a current pathologic fracture at the time of an encounter. The codes under M80 identify the site of the fracture. A code from category M80, not a traumatic fracture code, should be used for any patient with known osteoporosis who suffers a fracture, even if the patient had a minor fall or trauma, if that fall or trauma would not usually break a normal, healthy bone.

> Disuse osteoporosis with current fracture of right shoulder sustained lifting a grocery bag, initial encounter
>
> **M80.811A**   **Other osteoporosis with current pathological fracture, right shoulder, initial encounter for fracture**
>
> *Explanation:* A code from category M80, not a traumatic fracture code, should be used for any patient with known osteoporosis who suffers a fracture, even if the patient had a minor fall or trauma, if that fall or trauma would not usually break a normal, healthy bone.

Muscle/Tendon Table

ICD-10-CM categorizes certain muscles and tendons in the upper and lower extremities by their action (e.g., extension, flexion), their anatomical location (e.g., posterior, anterior), and/or whether they are intrinsic or extrinsic to a certain anatomical area. The Muscle/Tendon Table is provided at the beginning of chapters 13 and 19 as a resource to help users when code selection depends on one or more of these characteristics. A **TIP** has been placed at those categories and/or subcategories that relate to this table. Please note that this table is not all-inclusive, and proper code assignment should be based on the provider's documentation.

Body Region	Muscle	Extensor Tendon	Flexor Tendon	Other Tendon
Shoulder				
	Deltoid	Posterior deltoid	Anterior deltoid	
	Rotator cuff			
	Infraspinatus			Infraspinatus
	Subscapularis			Subscapularis
	Supraspinatus			Supraspinatus
	Teres minor			Teres minor
	Teres major	Teres major		
Upper arm				
	Anterior muscles			
	Biceps brachii — long head		Biceps brachii — long head	
	Biceps brachii — short head		Biceps brachii — short head	
	Brachialis		Brachialis	
	Coracobrachialis		Coracobrachialis	
	Posterior muscles			
	Triceps brachii	Triceps brachii		
Forearm				
	Anterior muscles			
	Flexors			
	Deep			
	Flexor digitorum profundus		Flexor digitorum profundus	
	Flexor pollicis longus		Flexor pollicis longus	
	Intermediate			
	Flexor digitorum superficialis		Flexor digitorum superficialis	
	Superficial			
	Flexor carpi radialis		Flexor carpi radialis	
	Flexor carpi ulnaris		Flexor carpi ulnaris	
	Palmaris longus		Palmaris longus	
	Pronators			
	Pronator quadratus			Pronator quadratus
	Pronator teres			Pronator teres
	Posterior muscles			
	Extensors			
	Deep			
	Abductor pollicis longus			Abductor pollicis longus
	Extensor indicis	Extensor indicis		
	Extensor pollicis brevis	Extensor pollicis brevis		
	Extensor pollicis longus	Extensor pollicis longus		
	Superficial			
	Brachioradialis			Brachioradialis
	Extensor carpi radialis brevis	Extensor carpi radialis brevis		
	Extensor carpi radialis longus	Extensor carpi radialis longus		
	Extensor carpi ulnaris	Extensor carpi ulnaris		
	Extensor digiti minimi	Extensor digiti minimi		
	Extensor digitorum	Extensor digitorum		
	Anconeus	Anconeus		
	Supinator			Supinator

Body Region	Muscle	Extensor Tendon	Flexor Tendon	Other Tendon
Hand				
Extrinsic — attach to a site in the forearm as well as a site in the hand with action related to hand movement at the wrist				
	Extensor carpi radialis brevis	Extensor carpi radialis brevis		
	Extensor carpi radialis longus	Extensor carpie radialis longus		
	Extensor carpi ulnaris	Extensor carpi ulnaris		
	Flexor carpi radialis		Flexor carpi radialis	
	Flexor carpi ulnaris		Flexor carpi ulnaris	
	Flexor digitorum superficialis		Flexor digitorum superficialis	
	Palmaris longus		Palmaris longus	
Extrinsic — attach to a site in the forearm as well as a site in the hand with action in the hand related to finger movement				
	Adductor pollicis longus			Adductor pollicis longus
	Extensor digiti minimi	Extensor digiti minimi		
	Extensor digitorum	Extensor digitorum		
	Extensor indicis	Extensor indicis		
	Flexor digitorum profundus		Flexor digitorum profundus	
	Flexor digitorum superficialis		Flexor digitorum superficialis	
Extrinsic — attach to a site in the forearm as well as a site in the hand with action in the hand related to thumb movement				
	Extensor pollicis brevis	Extensor pollicis brevis		
	Extensor pollicis longus	Extensor pollicis longus		
	Flexor pollicis longus		Flexor pollicis longus	
Intrinsic — found within the hand only				
	Adductor pollicis			Adductor pollicis
	Dorsal interossei	Dorsal interossei	Dorsal interossei	
	Lumbricals	Lumbricals	Lumbricals	
	Palmaris brevis			Palmaris brevis
	Palmar interossei	Palmar interossei	Palmar interossei	
	Hypothenar muscles			
	Abductor digiti minimi			Abductor digiti minimi
	Flexor digiti minimi brevis		Flexor digiti minimi brevis	
	Oppenens digiti minimi		Oppenens digiti minimi	
	Thenar muscles			
	Abductor pollicis brevis			Abductor pollicis brevis
	Flexor pollicis brevis		Flexor pollicis brevis	
	Oppenens pollicis		Oppenens pollicis	
Thigh				
	Anterior muscles			
	Iliopsoas		Iliopsoas	
	Pectineus		Pectineus	
	Quadriceps	Quadriceps		
	Rectus femoris	Rectus femoris — Extends knee	Rectus femoris — Flexes hip	
	Vastus intermedius	Vastus intermedius		
	Vastus lateralis	Vastus lateralis		
	Vastus medialis	Vastus medialis		
	Sartorius		Sartorius	
	Medial muscles			
	Adductor brevis			Adductor brevis
	Adductor longus			Adductor longus
	Adductor magnus			Adductor magnus
	Gracilis			Gracilis
	Obturator externus			Obturator externus
	Posterior muscles			
	Hamstring	Hamstring — Extends hip	Hamstring — Flexes knee	
	Biceps femoris	Biceps femoris	Biceps femoris	
	Semimembranosus	Semimembranosus	Semimembranosus	
	Semitendinosus	Semitendinosus	Semitendinosus	

Chapter 13. Diseases of the Musculoskeletal System and Connective Tissue

Body Region	Muscle	Extensor Tendon	Flexor Tendon	Other Tendon
Lower leg				
	Anterior muscles			
	Extensor digitorum longus	Extensor digitorum longus		
	Extensor hallucis longus	Extensor hallucis longus		
	Fibularis (peroneus) tertius	Fibularis (peroneus) tertius		
	Tibialis anterior	Tibialis anterior		Tibialis anterior
	Lateral muscles			
	Fibularis (peroneus) brevis		Fibularis (peroneus) brevis	
	Fibularis (peroneus) longus		Fibularis (peroneus) longus	
	Posterior muscles			
	Deep			
	Flexor digitorum longus		Flexor digitorum longus	
	Flexor hallucis longus		Flexor hallucis longus	
	Popliteus		Popliteus	
	Tibialis posterior		Tibialis posterior	
	Superficial			
	Gastrocnemius		Gastrocnemius	
	Plantaris		Plantaris	
	Soleus		Soleus	
				Calcaneal (Achilles)
Ankle/Foot				
Extrinsic — attach to a site in the lower leg as well as a site in the foot with action related to foot movement at the ankle				
	Plantaris		Plantaris	
	Soleus		Soleus	
	Tibialis anterior	Tibialis anterior		
	Tibialis posterior		Tibialis posterior	
Extrinsic — attach to a site in the lower leg as well as a site in the foot with action in the foot related to toe movement				
	Extensor digitorum longus	Extensor digitorum longus		
	Extensor hallicus longus	Extensor hallucis longus		
	Flexor digitorum longus		Flexor digitorum longus	
	Flexor hallucis longus		Flexor hallucis longus	
Intrinsic — found within the ankle/foot only				
	Dorsal muscles			
	Extensor digitorum brevis	Extensor digitorum brevis		
	Extensor hallucis brevis	Extensor hallucis brevis		
	Plantar muscles			
	Abductor digiti minimi		Abductor digiti minimi	
	Abductor hallucis		Abductor hallucis	
	Dorsal interossei	Dorsal interossei	Dorsal interossei	
	Flexor digiti minimi brevis		Flexor digiti minimi brevis	
	Flexor digitorum brevis		Flexor digitorum brevis	
	Flexor hallucis brevis		Flexor hallucis brevis	
	Lumbricals	Lumbricals	Lumbricals	
	Quadratus plantae		Quadratus plantae	
	Plantar interossei	Plantar interossei	Plantar interossei	

Chapter 13. Diseases of the Musculoskeletal System and Connective Tissue (M00-M99)

NOTE   Use an external cause code following the code for the musculoskeletal condition, if applicable, to identify the cause of the musculoskeletal condition.

EXCLUDES 2   *arthropathic psoriasis (L40.5-)*
certain conditions originating in the perinatal period (P04-P96)
certain infectious and parasitic diseases (A00-B99)
compartment syndrome (traumatic) (T79.A-)
complications of pregnancy, childbirth and the puerperium (O00-O9A)
congenital malformations, deformations, and chromosomal abnormalities (Q00-Q99)
endocrine, nutritional and metabolic diseases (E00-E88)
injury, poisoning and certain other consequences of external causes (S00-T88)
neoplasms (C00-D49)
symptoms, signs and abnormal clinical and laboratory findings, not elsewhere classified (R00-R94)

This chapter contains the following blocks:
M00-M02   Infectious arthropathies
~~M04~~   ~~Autoinflammatory syndromes~~
M05-M14   Inflammatory polyarthropathies
M15-M19   Osteoarthritis
M20-M25   Other joint disorders
M26-M27   Dentofacial anomalies [including malocclusion] and other disorders of jaw
M30-M36   Systemic connective tissue disorders
M40-M43   Deforming dorsopathies
M45-M49   Spondylopathies
M50-M54   Other dorsopathies
M60-M63   Disorders of muscles
M65-M67   Disorders of synovium and tendon
M70-M79   Other soft tissue disorders
M80-M85   Disorders of bone density and structure
M86-M90   Other osteopathies
M91-M94   Chondropathies
M95   Other disorders of the musculoskeletal system and connective tissue
M96   Intraoperative and postprocedural complications and disorders of musculoskeletal system, not elsewhere classified
~~M97~~   ~~Periprosthetic fracture around internal prosthetic joint~~
M99   Biomechanical lesions, not elsewhere classified

ARTHROPATHIES (M00-M25)

INCLUDES   disorders affecting predominantly peripheral (limb) joints

Infectious arthropathies (M00-M02)

NOTE   This block comprises arthropathies due to microbiological agents. Distinction is made between the following types of etiological relationship:

a) direct infection of joint, where organisms invade synovial tissue and microbial antigen is present in the joint;

b) indirect infection, which may be of two types: a reactive arthropathy, where microbial infection of the body is established but neither organisms nor antigens can be identified in the joint, and a postinfective arthropathy, where microbial antigen is present but recovery of an organism is inconstant and evidence of local multiplication is lacking.

√4ᵗʰ **M00 Pyogenic arthritis**

√5ᵗʰ   **M00.0 Staphylococcal arthritis and polyarthritis**
     Use additional code (B95.61-B95.8) to identify bacterial agent
     EXCLUDES 2   *infection and inflammatory reaction due to internal joint prosthesis (T84.5-)*

     M00.00 Staphylococcal arthritis, unspecified joint   HCC ▽

√6ᵗʰ   **M00.01 Staphylococcal arthritis, shoulder**
     M00.011 Staphylococcal arthritis, right shoulder   HCC
     M00.012 Staphylococcal arthritis, left shoulder   HCC
     M00.019 Staphylococcal arthritis, unspecified shoulder   HCC ▽

√6ᵗʰ   **M00.02 Staphylococcal arthritis, elbow**
     M00.021 Staphylococcal arthritis, right elbow   HCC
     M00.022 Staphylococcal arthritis, left elbow   HCC
     M00.029 Staphylococcal arthritis, unspecified elbow   HCC ▽

√6ᵗʰ   **M00.03 Staphylococcal arthritis, wrist**
     Staphylococcal arthritis of carpal bones
     M00.031 Staphylococcal arthritis, right wrist   HCC
     M00.032 Staphylococcal arthritis, left wrist   HCC
     M00.039 Staphylococcal arthritis, unspecified wrist   HCC ▽

√6ᵗʰ   **M00.04 Staphylococcal arthritis, hand**
     Staphylococcal arthritis of metacarpus and phalanges
     M00.041 Staphylococcal arthritis, right hand   HCC
     M00.042 Staphylococcal arthritis, left hand   HCC
     M00.049 Staphylococcal arthritis, unspecified hand   HCC ▽

√6ᵗʰ   **M00.05 Staphylococcal arthritis, hip**
     M00.051 Staphylococcal arthritis, right hip   HCC
     M00.052 Staphylococcal arthritis, left hip   HCC
     M00.059 Staphylococcal arthritis, unspecified hip   HCC ▽

√6ᵗʰ   **M00.06 Staphylococcal arthritis, knee**
     M00.061 Staphylococcal arthritis, right knee   HCC
     M00.062 Staphylococcal arthritis, left knee   HCC
     M00.069 Staphylococcal arthritis, unspecified knee   HCC ▽

√6ᵗʰ   **M00.07 Staphylococcal arthritis, ankle and foot**
     Staphylococcal arthritis, tarsus, metatarsus and phalanges
     M00.071 Staphylococcal arthritis, right ankle and foot   HCC
     M00.072 Staphylococcal arthritis, left ankle and foot   HCC
     M00.079 Staphylococcal arthritis, unspecified ankle and foot   HCC ▽

     M00.08 Staphylococcal arthritis, vertebrae   HCC
     M00.09 Staphylococcal polyarthritis   HCC

√5ᵗʰ   **M00.1 Pneumococcal arthritis and polyarthritis**
     M00.10 Pneumococcal arthritis, unspecified joint   HCC ▽

√6ᵗʰ   **M00.11 Pneumococcal arthritis, shoulder**
     M00.111 Pneumococcal arthritis, right shoulder HCC
     M00.112 Pneumococcal arthritis, left shoulder   HCC
     M00.119 Pneumococcal arthritis, unspecified shoulder   HCC ▽

√6ᵗʰ   **M00.12 Pneumococcal arthritis, elbow**
     M00.121 Pneumococcal arthritis, right elbow   HCC
     M00.122 Pneumococcal arthritis, left elbow   HCC
     M00.129 Pneumococcal arthritis, unspecified elbow   HCC ▽

√6ᵗʰ   **M00.13 Pneumococcal arthritis, wrist**
     Pneumococcal arthritis of carpal bones
     M00.131 Pneumococcal arthritis, right wrist   HCC
     M00.132 Pneumococcal arthritis, left wrist   HCC
     M00.139 Pneumococcal arthritis, unspecified wrist   HCC ▽

√6ᵗʰ   **M00.14 Pneumococcal arthritis, hand**
     Pneumococcal arthritis of metacarpus and phalanges
     M00.141 Pneumococcal arthritis, right hand   HCC
     M00.142 Pneumococcal arthritis, left hand   HCC
     M00.149 Pneumococcal arthritis, unspecified hand   HCC ▽

√6ᵗʰ   **M00.15 Pneumococcal arthritis, hip**
     M00.151 Pneumococcal arthritis, right hip   HCC
     M00.152 Pneumococcal arthritis, left hip   HCC
     M00.159 Pneumococcal arthritis, unspecified hip   HCC ▽

√6ᵗʰ   **M00.16 Pneumococcal arthritis, knee**
     M00.161 Pneumococcal arthritis, right knee   HCC
     M00.162 Pneumococcal arthritis, left knee   HCC
     M00.169 Pneumococcal arthritis, unspecified knee   HCC ▽

√6ᵗʰ   **M00.17 Pneumococcal arthritis, ankle and foot**
     Pneumococcal arthritis, tarsus, metatarsus and phalanges
     M00.171 Pneumococcal arthritis, right ankle and foot   HCC
     M00.172 Pneumococcal arthritis, left ankle and foot   HCC

☑ Additional Character Req   √x7ᵗʰ Placeholder Alert   Manifestation   HCC CMS-HCC Condition   ▽ Unspecified Code   ►◄ Revised Text   ● New Code   ▲ Revised Code Title

M00.179 **Pneumococcal arthritis, unspecified ankle and foot** HCC ▽

M00.18 **Pneumococcal arthritis, vertebrae** HCC

M00.19 **Pneumococcal polyarthritis** HCC

✓5ᵗʰ M00.2 **Other streptococcal arthritis and polyarthritis**
Use additional code (B95.0-B95.2, B95.4-B95.5) to identify bacterial agent

M00.20 **Other streptococcal arthritis, unspecified joint** HCC ▽

✓6ᵗʰ M00.21 **Other streptococcal arthritis, shoulder**
M00.211 **Other streptococcal arthritis, right shoulder** HCC
M00.212 **Other streptococcal arthritis, left shoulder** HCC
M00.219 **Other streptococcal arthritis, unspecified shoulder** HCC ▽

✓6ᵗʰ M00.22 **Other streptococcal arthritis, elbow**
M00.221 **Other streptococcal arthritis, right elbow** HCC
M00.222 **Other streptococcal arthritis, left elbow** HCC
M00.229 **Other streptococcal arthritis, unspecified elbow** HCC ▽

✓6ᵗʰ M00.23 **Other streptococcal arthritis, wrist**
Other streptococcal arthritis of carpal bones
M00.231 **Other streptococcal arthritis, right wrist** HCC
M00.232 **Other streptococcal arthritis, left wrist** HCC
M00.239 **Other streptococcal arthritis, unspecified wrist** HCC ▽

✓6ᵗʰ M00.24 **Other streptococcal arthritis, hand**
Other streptococcal arthritis metacarpus and phalanges
M00.241 **Other streptococcal arthritis, right hand** HCC
M00.242 **Other streptococcal arthritis, left hand** HCC
M00.249 **Other streptococcal arthritis, unspecified hand** HCC ▽

✓6ᵗʰ M00.25 **Other streptococcal arthritis, hip**
M00.251 **Other streptococcal arthritis, right hip** HCC
M00.252 **Other streptococcal arthritis, left hip** HCC
M00.259 **Other streptococcal arthritis, unspecified hip** HCC ▽

✓6ᵗʰ M00.26 **Other streptococcal arthritis, knee**
M00.261 **Other streptococcal arthritis, right knee** HCC
M00.262 **Other streptococcal arthritis, left knee** HCC
M00.269 **Other streptococcal arthritis, unspecified knee** HCC ▽

✓6ᵗʰ M00.27 **Other streptococcal arthritis, ankle and foot**
Other streptococcal arthritis, tarsus, metatarsus and phalanges
M00.271 **Other streptococcal arthritis, right ankle and foot** HCC
M00.272 **Other streptococcal arthritis, left ankle and foot** HCC
M00.279 **Other streptococcal arthritis, unspecified ankle and foot** HCC ▽

M00.28 **Other streptococcal arthritis, vertebrae** HCC

M00.29 **Other streptococcal polyarthritis** HCC

✓5ᵗʰ M00.8 **Arthritis and polyarthritis due to other bacteria**
Use additional code (B96) to identify bacteria

M00.80 **Arthritis due to other bacteria, unspecified joint** HCC ▽

✓6ᵗʰ M00.81 **Arthritis due to other bacteria, shoulder**
M00.811 **Arthritis due to other bacteria, right shoulder** HCC
M00.812 **Arthritis due to other bacteria, left shoulder** HCC
M00.819 **Arthritis due to other bacteria, unspecified shoulder** HCC ▽

✓6ᵗʰ M00.82 **Arthritis due to other bacteria, elbow**
M00.821 **Arthritis due to other bacteria, right elbow** HCC
M00.822 **Arthritis due to other bacteria, left elbow** HCC
M00.829 **Arthritis due to other bacteria, unspecified elbow** HCC ▽

✓6ᵗʰ M00.83 **Arthritis due to other bacteria, wrist**
Arthritis due to other bacteria, carpal bones
M00.831 **Arthritis due to other bacteria, right wrist** HCC
M00.832 **Arthritis due to other bacteria, left wrist** HCC
M00.839 **Arthritis due to other bacteria, unspecified wrist** HCC ▽

✓6ᵗʰ M00.84 **Arthritis due to other bacteria, hand**
Arthritis due to other bacteria, metacarpus and phalanges
M00.841 **Arthritis due to other bacteria, right hand** HCC
M00.842 **Arthritis due to other bacteria, left hand** HCC
M00.849 **Arthritis due to other bacteria, unspecified hand** HCC ▽

✓6ᵗʰ M00.85 **Arthritis due to other bacteria, hip**
M00.851 **Arthritis due to other bacteria, right hip** HCC
M00.852 **Arthritis due to other bacteria, left hip** HCC
M00.859 **Arthritis due to other bacteria, unspecified hip** HCC ▽

✓6ᵗʰ M00.86 **Arthritis due to other bacteria, knee**
M00.861 **Arthritis due to other bacteria, right knee** HCC
M00.862 **Arthritis due to other bacteria, left knee** HCC
M00.869 **Arthritis due to other bacteria, unspecified knee** HCC ▽

✓6ᵗʰ M00.87 **Arthritis due to other bacteria, ankle and foot**
Arthritis due to other bacteria, tarsus, metatarsus, and phalanges
M00.871 **Arthritis due to other bacteria, right ankle and foot** HCC
M00.872 **Arthritis due to other bacteria, left ankle and foot** HCC
M00.879 **Arthritis due to other bacteria, unspecified ankle and foot** HCC ▽

M00.88 **Arthritis due to other bacteria, vertebrae** HCC

M00.89 **Polyarthritis due to other bacteria** HCC

M00.9 **Pyogenic arthritis, unspecified** HCC ▽
Infective arthritis NOS

✓4ᵗʰ M01 **Direct infections of joint in infectious and parasitic diseases classified elsewhere**
Code first underlying disease, such as:
leprosy [Hansen's disease] (A30.-)
mycoses (B35-B49)
O'nyong-nyong fever (A92.1)
paratyphoid fever (A01.1-A01.4)

EXCLUDES 1   *arthropathy in Lyme disease (A69.23)*
gonococcal arthritis (A54.42)
meningococcal arthritis (A39.83)
mumps arthritis (B26.85)
postinfective arthropathy (M02.-)
postmeningococcal arthritis (A39.84)
reactive arthritis (M02.3)
rubella arthritis (B06.82)
sarcoidosis arthritis (D86.86)
typhoid fever arthritis (A01.04)
tuberculosis arthritis (A18.01-A18.02)

✓5ᵗʰ M01.X **Direct infection of joint in infectious and parasitic diseases classified elsewhere**

M01.X0 *Direct infection of unspecified joint in infectious and parasitic diseases classified elsewhere* HCC ▽

✓6ᵗʰ M01.X1 **Direct infection of shoulder joint in infectious and parasitic diseases classified elsewhere**

M01.X11 *Direct infection of right shoulder in infectious and parasitic diseases classified elsewhere* HCC

EXCLUDES 1 Not coded here   EXCLUDES 2 Not included here   N Newborn Age: 0   P Pediatric Age: 0-17   M Maternity Age: 12-55   A Adult Age: 15-124

M01.X12 *Direct infection of left shoulder in infectious and parasitic diseases classified elsewhere* `HCC`

M01.X19 *Direct infection of unspecified shoulder in infectious and parasitic diseases classified elsewhere* `HCC` ▽

✓6ᵗʰ M01.X2 **Direct infection of elbow in infectious and parasitic diseases classified elsewhere**

M01.X21 *Direct infection of right elbow in infectious and parasitic diseases classified elsewhere* `HCC`

M01.X22 *Direct infection of left elbow in infectious and parasitic diseases classified elsewhere* `HCC`

M01.X29 *Direct infection of unspecified elbow in infectious and parasitic diseases classified elsewhere* `HCC` ▽

✓6ᵗʰ M01.X3 **Direct infection of wrist in infectious and parasitic diseases classified elsewhere**
Direct infection of carpal bones in infectious and parasitic diseases classified elsewhere

M01.X31 *Direct infection of right wrist in infectious and parasitic diseases classified elsewhere* `HCC`

M01.X32 *Direct infection of left wrist in infectious and parasitic diseases classified elsewhere* `HCC`

M01.X39 *Direct infection of unspecified wrist in infectious and parasitic diseases classified elsewhere* `HCC` ▽

✓6ᵗʰ M01.X4 **Direct infection of hand in infectious and parasitic diseases classified elsewhere**
Direct infection of metacarpus and phalanges in infectious and parasitic diseases classified elsewhere

M01.X41 *Direct infection of right hand in infectious and parasitic diseases classified elsewhere* `HCC`

M01.X42 *Direct infection of left hand in infectious and parasitic diseases classified elsewhere* `HCC`

M01.X49 *Direct infection of unspecified hand in infectious and parasitic diseases classified elsewhere* `HCC` ▽

✓6ᵗʰ M01.X5 **Direct infection of hip in infectious and parasitic diseases classified elsewhere**

M01.X51 *Direct infection of right hip in infectious and parasitic diseases classified elsewhere* `HCC`

M01.X52 *Direct infection of left hip in infectious and parasitic diseases classified elsewhere* `HCC`

M01.X59 *Direct infection of unspecified hip in infectious and parasitic diseases classified elsewhere* `HCC` ▽

✓6ᵗʰ M01.X6 **Direct infection of knee in infectious and parasitic diseases classified elsewhere**

M01.X61 *Direct infection of right knee in infectious and parasitic diseases classified elsewhere* `HCC`

M01.X62 *Direct infection of left knee in infectious and parasitic diseases classified elsewhere* `HCC`

M01.X69 *Direct infection of unspecified knee in infectious and parasitic diseases classified elsewhere* `HCC` ▽

✓6ᵗʰ M01.X7 **Direct infection of ankle and foot in infectious and parasitic diseases classified elsewhere**
Direct infection of tarsus, metatarsus and phalanges in infectious and parasitic diseases classified elsewhere

M01.X71 *Direct infection of right ankle and foot in infectious and parasitic diseases classified elsewhere* `HCC`

M01.X72 *Direct infection of left ankle and foot in infectious and parasitic diseases classified elsewhere* `HCC`

M01.X79 *Direct infection of unspecified ankle and foot in infectious and parasitic diseases classified elsewhere* `HCC` ▽

M01.X8 *Direct infection of vertebrae in infectious and parasitic diseases classified elsewhere* `HCC`

M01.X9 *Direct infection of multiple joints in infectious and parasitic diseases classified elsewhere* `HCC`

✓4ᵗʰ **M02 Postinfective and reactive arthropathies**
Code first underlying disease, such as:
congenital syphilis [Clutton's joints] (A50.5)
enteritis due to Yersinia enterocolitica (A04.6)
infective endocarditis (I33.0)
viral hepatitis (B15-B19)

EXCLUDES 1 *Behçet's disease (M35.2)*
direct infections of joint in infectious and parasitic diseases classified elsewhere (M01.-)
postmeningococcal arthritis (A39.84)
mumps arthritis (B26.85)
rheumatic fever (I00)
rubella arthritis (B06.82)
syphilis arthritis (late) (A52.77)
tabetic arthropathy [Charcôt's] (A52.16)

✓5ᵗʰ **M02.0 Arthropathy following intestinal bypass**

M02.00 **Arthropathy following intestinal bypass, unspecified site** ▽

✓6ᵗʰ M02.01 **Arthropathy following intestinal bypass, shoulder**

M02.011 **Arthropathy following intestinal bypass, right shoulder**

M02.012 **Arthropathy following intestinal bypass, left shoulder**

M02.019 **Arthropathy following intestinal bypass, unspecified shoulder** ▽

✓6ᵗʰ M02.02 **Arthropathy following intestinal bypass, elbow**

M02.021 **Arthropathy following intestinal bypass, right elbow**

M02.022 **Arthropathy following intestinal bypass, left elbow**

M02.029 **Arthropathy following intestinal bypass, unspecified elbow** ▽

✓6ᵗʰ M02.03 **Arthropathy following intestinal bypass, wrist**
Arthropathy following intestinal bypass, carpal bones

M02.031 **Arthropathy following intestinal bypass, right wrist**

M02.032 **Arthropathy following intestinal bypass, left wrist**

M02.039 **Arthropathy following intestinal bypass, unspecified wrist** ▽

✓6ᵗʰ M02.04 **Arthropathy following intestinal bypass, hand**
Arthropathy following intestinal bypass, metacarpals and phalanges

M02.041 **Arthropathy following intestinal bypass, right hand**

M02.042 **Arthropathy following intestinal bypass, left hand**

M02.049 **Arthropathy following intestinal bypass, unspecified hand** ▽

✓6ᵗʰ M02.05 **Arthropathy following intestinal bypass, hip**

M02.051 **Arthropathy following intestinal bypass, right hip**

M02.052 **Arthropathy following intestinal bypass, left hip**

M02.059 **Arthropathy following intestinal bypass, unspecified hip** ▽

✓6ᵗʰ M02.06 **Arthropathy following intestinal bypass, knee**

M02.061 **Arthropathy following intestinal bypass, right knee**

M02.062 **Arthropathy following intestinal bypass, left knee**

M02.069 **Arthropathy following intestinal bypass, unspecified knee** ▽

✓6ᵗʰ M02.07 **Arthropathy following intestinal bypass, ankle and foot**
Arthropathy following intestinal bypass, tarsus, metatarsus and phalanges

M02.071 **Arthropathy following intestinal bypass, right ankle and foot**

M02.072 **Arthropathy following intestinal bypass, left ankle and foot**

M02.079 **Arthropathy following intestinal bypass, unspecified ankle and foot** ▽

M02.08 **Arthropathy following intestinal bypass, vertebrae**

☑ Additional Character Req   ✓x7ᵗʰ Placeholder Alert   Manifestation   `HCC` CMS-HCC Condition   ▽ Unspecified Code   ►◄ Revised Text   ● New Code   ▲ Revised Code Title

M02.09 Arthropathy following intestinal bypass, multiple sites

✓5th **M02.1** Postdysenteric arthropathy

  M02.10 Postdysenteric arthropathy, unspecified site **HCC** ▽

  ✓6th **M02.11** Postdysenteric arthropathy, shoulder

    M02.111 Postdysenteric arthropathy, right shoulder **HCC**

    M02.112 Postdysenteric arthropathy, left shoulder **HCC**

    M02.119 Postdysenteric arthropathy, unspecified shoulder **HCC** ▽

  ✓6th **M02.12** Postdysenteric arthropathy, elbow

    M02.121 Postdysenteric arthropathy, right elbow **HCC**

    M02.122 Postdysenteric arthropathy, left elbow **HCC**

    M02.129 Postdysenteric arthropathy, unspecified elbow **HCC** ▽

  ✓6th **M02.13** Postdysenteric arthropathy, wrist
    Postdysenteric arthropathy, carpal bones

    M02.131 Postdysenteric arthropathy, right wrist **HCC**

    M02.132 Postdysenteric arthropathy, left wrist **HCC**

    M02.139 Postdysenteric arthropathy, unspecified wrist **HCC** ▽

  ✓6th **M02.14** Postdysenteric arthropathy, hand
    Postdysenteric arthropathy, metacarpus and phalanges

    M02.141 Postdysenteric arthropathy, right hand **HCC**

    M02.142 Postdysenteric arthropathy, left hand **HCC**

    M02.149 Postdysenteric arthropathy, unspecified hand **HCC** ▽

  ✓6th **M02.15** Postdysenteric arthropathy, hip

    M02.151 Postdysenteric arthropathy, right hip **HCC**

    M02.152 Postdysenteric arthropathy, left hip **HCC**

    M02.159 Postdysenteric arthropathy, unspecified hip **HCC** ▽

  ✓6th **M02.16** Postdysenteric arthropathy, knee

    M02.161 Postdysenteric arthropathy, right knee **HCC**

    M02.162 Postdysenteric arthropathy, left knee **HCC**

    M02.169 Postdysenteric arthropathy, unspecified knee **HCC** ▽

  ✓6th **M02.17** Postdysenteric arthropathy, ankle and foot
    Postdysenteric arthropathy, tarsus, metatarsus and phalanges

    M02.171 Postdysenteric arthropathy, right ankle and foot **HCC**

    M02.172 Postdysenteric arthropathy, left ankle and foot **HCC**

    M02.179 Postdysenteric arthropathy, unspecified ankle and foot **HCC** ▽

  M02.18 Postdysenteric arthropathy, vertebrae **HCC**

  M02.19 Postdysenteric arthropathy, multiple sites **HCC**

✓5th **M02.2** Postimmunization arthropathy

  M02.20 Postimmunization arthropathy, unspecified site ▽

  ✓6th **M02.21** Postimmunization arthropathy, shoulder

    M02.211 Postimmunization arthropathy, right shoulder

    M02.212 Postimmunization arthropathy, left shoulder

    M02.219 Postimmunization arthropathy, unspecified shoulder ▽

  ✓6th **M02.22** Postimmunization arthropathy, elbow

    M02.221 Postimmunization arthropathy, right elbow

    M02.222 Postimmunization arthropathy, left elbow

    M02.229 Postimmunization arthropathy, unspecified elbow ▽

  ✓6th **M02.23** Postimmunization arthropathy, wrist
    Postimmunization arthropathy, carpal bones

    M02.231 Postimmunization arthropathy, right wrist

    M02.232 Postimmunization arthropathy, left wrist

    M02.239 Postimmunization arthropathy, unspecified wrist ▽

  ✓6th **M02.24** Postimmunization arthropathy, hand
    Postimmunization arthropathy, metacarpus and phalanges

    M02.241 Postimmunization arthropathy, right hand

    M02.242 Postimmunization arthropathy, left hand

    M02.249 Postimmunization arthropathy, unspecified hand ▽

  ✓6th **M02.25** Postimmunization arthropathy, hip

    M02.251 Postimmunization arthropathy, right hip

    M02.252 Postimmunization arthropathy, left hip

    M02.259 Postimmunization arthropathy, unspecified hip ▽

  ✓6th **M02.26** Postimmunization arthropathy, knee

    M02.261 Postimmunization arthropathy, right knee

    M02.262 Postimmunization arthropathy, left knee

    M02.269 Postimmunization arthropathy, unspecified knee ▽

  ✓6th **M02.27** Postimmunization arthropathy, ankle and foot
    Postimmunization arthropathy, tarsus, metatarsus and phalanges

    M02.271 Postimmunization arthropathy, right ankle and foot

    M02.272 Postimmunization arthropathy, left ankle and foot

    M02.279 Postimmunization arthropathy, unspecified ankle and foot ▽

  M02.28 Postimmunization arthropathy, vertebrae

  M02.29 Postimmunization arthropathy, multiple sites

✓5th **M02.3** Reiter's disease
  Reactive arthritis

  M02.30 Reiter's disease, unspecified site **HCC** ▽

  ✓6th **M02.31** Reiter's disease, shoulder

    M02.311 Reiter's disease, right shoulder **HCC**

    M02.312 Reiter's disease, left shoulder **HCC**

    M02.319 Reiter's disease, unspecified shoulder **HCC** ▽

  ✓6th **M02.32** Reiter's disease, elbow

    M02.321 Reiter's disease, right elbow **HCC**

    M02.322 Reiter's disease, left elbow **HCC**

    M02.329 Reiter's disease, unspecified elbow **HCC** ▽

  ✓6th **M02.33** Reiter's disease, wrist
    Reiter's disease, carpal bones

    M02.331 Reiter's disease, right wrist **HCC**

    M02.332 Reiter's disease, left wrist **HCC**

    M02.339 Reiter's disease, unspecified wrist **HCC** ▽

  ✓6th **M02.34** Reiter's disease, hand
    Reiter's disease, metacarpus and phalanges

    M02.341 Reiter's disease, right hand **HCC**

    M02.342 Reiter's disease, left hand **HCC**

    M02.349 Reiter's disease, unspecified hand **HCC** ▽

  ✓6th **M02.35** Reiter's disease, hip

    M02.351 Reiter's disease, right hip **HCC**

    M02.352 Reiter's disease, left hip **HCC**

    M02.359 Reiter's disease, unspecified hip **HCC** ▽

  ✓6th **M02.36** Reiter's disease, knee

    M02.361 Reiter's disease, right knee **HCC**

    M02.362 Reiter's disease, left knee **HCC**

    M02.369 Reiter's disease, unspecified knee **HCC** ▽

  ✓6th **M02.37** Reiter's disease, ankle and foot
    Reiter's disease, tarsus, metatarsus and phalanges

    M02.371 Reiter's disease, right ankle and foot **HCC**

    M02.372 Reiter's disease, left ankle and foot **HCC**

    M02.379 Reiter's disease, unspecified ankle and foot **HCC** ▽

  M02.38 Reiter's disease, vertebrae **HCC**

EXCLUDES 1 Not coded here   **EXCLUDES 2** Not included here   **N** Newborn Age: 0   **P** Pediatric Age: 0-17   **M** Maternity Age: 12-55   **A** Adult Age: 15-124

720　　　ICD-10-CM 2018

      M02.39   Reiter's disease, **multiple sites**   HCC

✓5th   **M02.8**   Other **reactive** arthropathies

      M02.80   *Other reactive arthropathies, unspecified site*   HCC ▽

✓6th   **M02.81**   Other reactive arthropathies, **shoulder**

      M02.811   *Other reactive arthropathies, right shoulder*   HCC

      M02.812   *Other reactive arthropathies, left shoulder*   HCC

      M02.819   *Other reactive arthropathies, unspecified shoulder*   HCC ▽

✓6th   **M02.82**   Other reactive arthropathies, **elbow**

      M02.821   *Other reactive arthropathies, right elbow*   HCC

      M02.822   *Other reactive arthropathies, left elbow*   HCC

      M02.829   *Other reactive arthropathies, unspecified elbow*   HCC ▽

✓6th   **M02.83**   Other reactive arthropathies, **wrist**

      Other reactive arthropathies, carpal bones

      M02.831   *Other reactive arthropathies, right wrist*   HCC

      M02.832   *Other reactive arthropathies, left wrist*   HCC

      M02.839   *Other reactive arthropathies, unspecified wrist*   HCC ▽

✓6th   **M02.84**   Other reactive arthropathies, **hand**

      Other reactive arthropathies, metacarpus and phalanges

      M02.841   *Other reactive arthropathies, right hand*   HCC

      M02.842   *Other reactive arthropathies, left hand*   HCC

      M02.849   *Other reactive arthropathies, unspecified hand*   HCC ▽

✓6th   **M02.85**   Other reactive arthropathies, **hip**

      M02.851   *Other reactive arthropathies, right hip*   HCC

      M02.852   *Other reactive arthropathies, left hip*   HCC

      M02.859   *Other reactive arthropathies, unspecified hip*   HCC ▽

✓6th   **M02.86**   Other reactive arthropathies, **knee**

      M02.861   *Other reactive arthropathies, right knee*   HCC

      M02.862   *Other reactive arthropathies, left knee*   HCC

      M02.869   *Other reactive arthropathies, unspecified knee*   HCC ▽

✓6th   **M02.87**   Other reactive arthropathies, **ankle and foot**

      Other reactive arthropathies, tarsus, metatarsus and phalanges

      M02.871   *Other reactive arthropathies, right ankle and foot*   HCC

      M02.872   *Other reactive arthropathies, left ankle and foot*   HCC

      M02.879   *Other reactive arthropathies, unspecified ankle and foot*   HCC ▽

      M02.88   *Other reactive arthropathies, vertebrae*   HCC

      M02.89   *Other reactive arthropathies, multiple sites*   HCC

    M02.9   *Reactive arthropathy, unspecified*   HCC ▽

Autoinflammatory syndromes (M04)

✓4th   **M04**   **Autoinflammatory syndromes**

      EXCLUDES 2   *Crohn's disease (K50.-)*

    M04.1   **Periodic fever syndromes**   HCC

      Familial Mediterranean fever

      Hyperimmunoglobin D syndrome

      Mevalonate kinase deficiency

      Tumor necrosis factor receptor associated periodic syndrome [TRAPS]

    M04.2   **Cryopyrin-associated periodic syndromes**   HCC

      Chronic infantile neurological, cutaneous and articular syndrome [CINCA]

      Familial cold autoinflammatory syndrome

      Familial cold urticaria

      Muckle-Wells syndrome

      Neonatal onset multisystemic inflammatory disorder [NOMID]

    M04.8   **Other autoinflammatory syndromes**   HCC

      Blau syndrome

      Deficiency of interleukin 1 receptor antagonist [DIRA]

      Majeed syndrome

      Periodic fever, aphthous stomatitis, pharyngitis, and adenopathy syndrome [PFAPA]

      Pyogenic arthritis, pyoderma gangrenosum, and acne syndrome [PAPA]

    M04.9   **Autoinflammatory syndrome, unspecified**   HCC ▽

Inflammatory polyarthropathies (M05-M14)

✓4th   **M05**   **Rheumatoid arthritis with rheumatoid factor**

      EXCLUDES 1   *rheumatic fever (I00)*

          juvenile rheumatoid arthritis (M08.-)

          rheumatoid arthritis of spine (M45.-)

      DEF: Autoimmune systemic disease that causes chronic inflammation of joints and other areas of the body, manifested by inflammatory changes in articular structures and synovial membranes, atrophy, and loss in bone density.

✓5th   **M05.0**   **Felty's syndrome**

      Rheumatoid arthritis with splenoadenomegaly and leukopenia

      M05.00   Felty's syndrome, unspecified site   HCC ▽

✓6th   **M05.01**   Felty's syndrome, **shoulder**

      M05.011   Felty's syndrome, **right shoulder**   HCC

      M05.012   Felty's syndrome, **left shoulder**   HCC

      M05.019   Felty's syndrome, **unspecified shoulder**   HCC ▽

✓6th   **M05.02**   Felty's syndrome, **elbow**

      M05.021   Felty's syndrome, **right elbow**   HCC

      M05.022   Felty's syndrome, **left elbow**   HCC

      M05.029   Felty's syndrome, **unspecified elbow**   HCC ▽

✓6th   **M05.03**   Felty's syndrome, **wrist**

      Felty's syndrome, carpal bones

      M05.031   Felty's syndrome, **right wrist**   HCC

      M05.032   Felty's syndrome, **left wrist**   HCC

      M05.039   Felty's syndrome, **unspecified wrist**   HCC ▽

✓6th   **M05.04**   Felty's syndrome, **hand**

      Felty's syndrome, metacarpus and phalanges

      M05.041   Felty's syndrome, **right hand**   HCC

      M05.042   Felty's syndrome, **left hand**   HCC

      M05.049   Felty's syndrome, **unspecified hand**   HCC ▽

✓6th   **M05.05**   Felty's syndrome, **hip**

      M05.051   Felty's syndrome, **right hip**   HCC

      M05.052   Felty's syndrome, **left hip**   HCC

      M05.059   Felty's syndrome, **unspecified hip**   HCC ▽

✓6th   **M05.06**   Felty's syndrome, **knee**

      M05.061   Felty's syndrome, **right knee**   HCC

      M05.062   Felty's syndrome, **left knee**   HCC

      M05.069   Felty's syndrome, **unspecified knee**   HCC ▽

✓6th   **M05.07**   Felty's syndrome, **ankle and foot**

      Felty's syndrome, tarsus, metatarsus and phalanges

      M05.071   Felty's syndrome, **right ankle and foot**   HCC

      M05.072   Felty's syndrome, **left ankle and foot**   HCC

      M05.079   Felty's syndrome, **unspecified ankle and foot**   HCC ▽

      M05.09   Felty's syndrome, **multiple sites**   HCC

✓5th   **M05.1**   **Rheumatoid lung disease with rheumatoid arthritis**

      DEF: Lung disorders associated with rheumatoid arthritis.

      M05.10   Rheumatoid lung disease with rheumatoid arthritis of unspecified site   HCC ▽

✓6th   **M05.11**   Rheumatoid lung disease with rheumatoid arthritis of **shoulder**

      M05.111   Rheumatoid lung disease with rheumatoid arthritis of **right shoulder**   HCC

      M05.112   Rheumatoid lung disease with rheumatoid arthritis of **left shoulder**   HCC

      M05.119   Rheumatoid lung disease with rheumatoid arthritis of unspecified **shoulder**   HCC ▽

✓ Additional Character Req   ✓x7th Placeholder Alert   Manifestation   HCC CMS-HCC Condition   ▽ Unspecified Code   ►◄ Revised Text   ● New Code   ▲ Revised Code Title

√6ᵗʰ **M05.12 Rheumatoid lung disease with rheumatoid arthritis of elbow**

    M05.121 Rheumatoid lung disease with rheumatoid arthritis of right elbow HCC

    M05.122 Rheumatoid lung disease with rheumatoid arthritis of left elbow HCC

    M05.129 Rheumatoid lung disease with rheumatoid arthritis of unspecified elbow HCC ▽

√6ᵗʰ **M05.13 Rheumatoid lung disease with rheumatoid arthritis of wrist**
    Rheumatoid lung disease with rheumatoid arthritis, carpal bones

    M05.131 Rheumatoid lung disease with rheumatoid arthritis of right wrist HCC

    M05.132 Rheumatoid lung disease with rheumatoid arthritis of left wrist HCC

    M05.139 Rheumatoid lung disease with rheumatoid arthritis of unspecified wrist HCC ▽

√6ᵗʰ **M05.14 Rheumatoid lung disease with rheumatoid arthritis of hand**
    Rheumatoid lung disease with rheumatoid arthritis, metacarpus and phalanges

    M05.141 Rheumatoid lung disease with rheumatoid arthritis of right hand HCC

    M05.142 Rheumatoid lung disease with rheumatoid arthritis of left hand HCC

    M05.149 Rheumatoid lung disease with rheumatoid arthritis of unspecified hand HCC ▽

√6ᵗʰ **M05.15 Rheumatoid lung disease with rheumatoid arthritis of hip**

    M05.151 Rheumatoid lung disease with rheumatoid arthritis of right hip HCC

    M05.152 Rheumatoid lung disease with rheumatoid arthritis of left hip HCC

    M05.159 Rheumatoid lung disease with rheumatoid arthritis of unspecified hip HCC ▽

√6ᵗʰ **M05.16 Rheumatoid lung disease with rheumatoid arthritis of knee**

    M05.161 Rheumatoid lung disease with rheumatoid arthritis of right knee HCC

    M05.162 Rheumatoid lung disease with rheumatoid arthritis of left knee HCC

    M05.169 Rheumatoid lung disease with rheumatoid arthritis of unspecified knee HCC ▽

√6ᵗʰ **M05.17 Rheumatoid lung disease with rheumatoid arthritis of ankle and foot**
    Rheumatoid lung disease with rheumatoid arthritis, tarsus, metatarsus and phalanges

    M05.171 Rheumatoid lung disease with rheumatoid arthritis of right ankle and foot HCC

    M05.172 Rheumatoid lung disease with rheumatoid arthritis of left ankle and foot HCC

    M05.179 Rheumatoid lung disease with rheumatoid arthritis of unspecified ankle and foot HCC ▽

    M05.19 Rheumatoid lung disease with rheumatoid arthritis of multiple sites HCC

√5ᵗʰ **M05.2 Rheumatoid vasculitis with rheumatoid arthritis**

    M05.20 Rheumatoid vasculitis with rheumatoid arthritis of unspecified site HCC ▽

√6ᵗʰ **M05.21 Rheumatoid vasculitis with rheumatoid arthritis of shoulder**

    M05.211 Rheumatoid vasculitis with rheumatoid arthritis of right shoulder HCC

    M05.212 Rheumatoid vasculitis with rheumatoid arthritis of left shoulder HCC

    M05.219 Rheumatoid vasculitis with rheumatoid arthritis of unspecified shoulder HCC ▽

√6ᵗʰ **M05.22 Rheumatoid vasculitis with rheumatoid arthritis of elbow**

    M05.221 Rheumatoid vasculitis with rheumatoid arthritis of right elbow HCC

    M05.222 Rheumatoid vasculitis with rheumatoid arthritis of left elbow HCC

    M05.229 Rheumatoid vasculitis with rheumatoid arthritis of unspecified elbow HCC ▽

√6ᵗʰ **M05.23 Rheumatoid vasculitis with rheumatoid arthritis of wrist**
    Rheumatoid vasculitis with rheumatoid arthritis, carpal bones

    M05.231 Rheumatoid vasculitis with rheumatoid arthritis of right wrist HCC

    M05.232 Rheumatoid vasculitis with rheumatoid arthritis of left wrist HCC

    M05.239 Rheumatoid vasculitis with rheumatoid arthritis of unspecified wrist HCC ▽

√6ᵗʰ **M05.24 Rheumatoid vasculitis with rheumatoid arthritis of hand**
    Rheumatoid vasculitis with rheumatoid arthritis, metacarpus and phalanges

    M05.241 Rheumatoid vasculitis with rheumatoid arthritis of right hand HCC

    M05.242 Rheumatoid vasculitis with rheumatoid arthritis of left hand HCC

    M05.249 Rheumatoid vasculitis with rheumatoid arthritis of unspecified hand HCC ▽

√6ᵗʰ **M05.25 Rheumatoid vasculitis with rheumatoid arthritis of hip**

    M05.251 Rheumatoid vasculitis with rheumatoid arthritis of right hip HCC

    M05.252 Rheumatoid vasculitis with rheumatoid arthritis of left hip HCC

    M05.259 Rheumatoid vasculitis with rheumatoid arthritis of unspecified hip HCC ▽

√6ᵗʰ **M05.26 Rheumatoid vasculitis with rheumatoid arthritis of knee**

    M05.261 Rheumatoid vasculitis with rheumatoid arthritis of right knee HCC

    M05.262 Rheumatoid vasculitis with rheumatoid arthritis of left knee HCC

    M05.269 Rheumatoid vasculitis with rheumatoid arthritis of unspecified knee HCC ▽

√6ᵗʰ **M05.27 Rheumatoid vasculitis with rheumatoid arthritis of ankle and foot**
    Rheumatoid vasculitis with rheumatoid arthritis, tarsus, metatarsus and phalanges

    M05.271 Rheumatoid vasculitis with rheumatoid arthritis of right ankle and foot HCC

    M05.272 Rheumatoid vasculitis with rheumatoid arthritis of left ankle and foot HCC

    M05.279 Rheumatoid vasculitis with rheumatoid arthritis of unspecified ankle and foot HCC ▽

    M05.29 Rheumatoid vasculitis with rheumatoid arthritis of multiple sites HCC

√5ᵗʰ **M05.3 Rheumatoid heart disease with rheumatoid arthritis**
    Rheumatoid carditis
    Rheumatoid endocarditis
    Rheumatoid myocarditis
    Rheumatoid pericarditis

    M05.30 Rheumatoid heart disease with rheumatoid arthritis of unspecified site HCC ▽

√6ᵗʰ **M05.31 Rheumatoid heart disease with rheumatoid arthritis of shoulder**

    M05.311 Rheumatoid heart disease with rheumatoid arthritis of right shoulder HCC

    M05.312 Rheumatoid heart disease with rheumatoid arthritis of left shoulder HCC

    M05.319 Rheumatoid heart disease with rheumatoid arthritis of unspecified shoulder HCC ▽

EXCLUDES 1 Not coded here   *EXCLUDES 2* Not included here   N Newborn Age: 0   P Pediatric Age: 0-17   M Maternity Age: 12-55   A Adult Age: 15-124

722   ICD-10-CM 2018

M05.12–M05.319

Chapter 13. Diseases of the Musculoskeletal System and Connective Tissue

√6ᵗʰ **M05.32 Rheumatoid heart disease with rheumatoid arthritis of elbow**
- M05.321 Rheumatoid heart disease with rheumatoid arthritis of right elbow HCC
- M05.322 Rheumatoid heart disease with rheumatoid arthritis of left elbow HCC
- M05.329 Rheumatoid heart disease with rheumatoid arthritis of unspecified elbow HCC ▽

√6ᵗʰ **M05.33 Rheumatoid heart disease with rheumatoid arthritis of wrist**
  Rheumatoid heart disease with rheumatoid arthritis, carpal bones
- M05.331 Rheumatoid heart disease with rheumatoid arthritis of right wrist HCC
- M05.332 Rheumatoid heart disease with rheumatoid arthritis of left wrist HCC
- M05.339 Rheumatoid heart disease with rheumatoid arthritis of unspecified wrist HCC ▽

√6ᵗʰ **M05.34 Rheumatoid heart disease with rheumatoid arthritis of hand**
  Rheumatoid heart disease with rheumatoid arthritis, metacarpus and phalanges
- M05.341 Rheumatoid heart disease with rheumatoid arthritis of right hand HCC
- M05.342 Rheumatoid heart disease with rheumatoid arthritis of left hand HCC
- M05.349 Rheumatoid heart disease with rheumatoid arthritis of unspecified hand HCC ▽

√6ᵗʰ **M05.35 Rheumatoid heart disease with rheumatoid arthritis of hip**
- M05.351 Rheumatoid heart disease with rheumatoid arthritis of right hip HCC
- M05.352 Rheumatoid heart disease with rheumatoid arthritis of left hip HCC
- M05.359 Rheumatoid heart disease with rheumatoid arthritis of unspecified hip HCC ▽

√6ᵗʰ **M05.36 Rheumatoid heart disease with rheumatoid arthritis of knee**
- M05.361 Rheumatoid heart disease with rheumatoid arthritis of right knee HCC
- M05.362 Rheumatoid heart disease with rheumatoid arthritis of left knee HCC
- M05.369 Rheumatoid heart disease with rheumatoid arthritis of unspecified knee HCC ▽

√6ᵗʰ **M05.37 Rheumatoid heart disease with rheumatoid arthritis of ankle and foot**
  Rheumatoid heart disease with rheumatoid arthritis, tarsus, metatarsus and phalanges
- M05.371 Rheumatoid heart disease with rheumatoid arthritis of right ankle and foot HCC
- M05.372 Rheumatoid heart disease with rheumatoid arthritis of left ankle and foot HCC
- M05.379 Rheumatoid heart disease with rheumatoid arthritis of unspecified ankle and foot HCC ▽

M05.39 Rheumatoid heart disease with rheumatoid arthritis of multiple sites HCC

√5ᵗʰ **M05.4 Rheumatoid myopathy with rheumatoid arthritis**
M05.40 Rheumatoid myopathy with rheumatoid arthritis of unspecified site HCC ▽

√6ᵗʰ **M05.41 Rheumatoid myopathy with rheumatoid arthritis of shoulder**
- M05.411 Rheumatoid myopathy with rheumatoid arthritis of right shoulder HCC
- M05.412 Rheumatoid myopathy with rheumatoid arthritis of left shoulder HCC
- M05.419 Rheumatoid myopathy with rheumatoid arthritis of unspecified shoulder HCC ▽

√6ᵗʰ **M05.42 Rheumatoid myopathy with rheumatoid arthritis of elbow**
- M05.421 Rheumatoid myopathy with rheumatoid arthritis of right elbow HCC
- M05.422 Rheumatoid myopathy with rheumatoid arthritis of left elbow HCC
- M05.429 Rheumatoid myopathy with rheumatoid arthritis of unspecified elbow HCC ▽

√6ᵗʰ **M05.43 Rheumatoid myopathy with rheumatoid arthritis of wrist**
  Rheumatoid myopathy with rheumatoid arthritis, carpal bones
- M05.431 Rheumatoid myopathy with rheumatoid arthritis of right wrist HCC
- M05.432 Rheumatoid myopathy with rheumatoid arthritis of left wrist HCC
- M05.439 Rheumatoid myopathy with rheumatoid arthritis of unspecified wrist HCC ▽

√6ᵗʰ **M05.44 Rheumatoid myopathy with rheumatoid arthritis of hand**
  Rheumatoid myopathy with rheumatoid arthritis, metacarpus and phalanges
- M05.441 Rheumatoid myopathy with rheumatoid arthritis of right hand HCC
- M05.442 Rheumatoid myopathy with rheumatoid arthritis of left hand HCC
- M05.449 Rheumatoid myopathy with rheumatoid arthritis of unspecified hand HCC ▽

√6ᵗʰ **M05.45 Rheumatoid myopathy with rheumatoid arthritis of hip**
- M05.451 Rheumatoid myopathy with rheumatoid arthritis of right hip HCC
- M05.452 Rheumatoid myopathy with rheumatoid arthritis of left hip HCC
- M05.459 Rheumatoid myopathy with rheumatoid arthritis of unspecified hip HCC ▽

√6ᵗʰ **M05.46 Rheumatoid myopathy with rheumatoid arthritis of knee**
- M05.461 Rheumatoid myopathy with rheumatoid arthritis of right knee HCC
- M05.462 Rheumatoid myopathy with rheumatoid arthritis of left knee HCC
- M05.469 Rheumatoid myopathy with rheumatoid arthritis of unspecified knee HCC ▽

√6ᵗʰ **M05.47 Rheumatoid myopathy with rheumatoid arthritis of ankle and foot**
  Rheumatoid myopathy with rheumatoid arthritis, tarsus, metatarsus and phalanges
- M05.471 Rheumatoid myopathy with rheumatoid arthritis of right ankle and foot HCC
- M05.472 Rheumatoid myopathy with rheumatoid arthritis of left ankle and foot HCC
- M05.479 Rheumatoid myopathy with rheumatoid arthritis of unspecified ankle and foot HCC ▽

M05.49 Rheumatoid myopathy with rheumatoid arthritis of multiple sites HCC

√5ᵗʰ **M05.5 Rheumatoid polyneuropathy with rheumatoid arthritis**
M05.50 Rheumatoid polyneuropathy with rheumatoid arthritis of unspecified site HCC ▽

√6ᵗʰ **M05.51 Rheumatoid polyneuropathy with rheumatoid arthritis of shoulder**
- M05.511 Rheumatoid polyneuropathy with rheumatoid arthritis of right shoulder HCC
- M05.512 Rheumatoid polyneuropathy with rheumatoid arthritis of left shoulder HCC
- M05.519 Rheumatoid polyneuropathy with rheumatoid arthritis of unspecified shoulder HCC ▽

Chapter 13. Diseases of the Musculoskeletal System and Connective Tissue

√6th **M05.52 Rheumatoid polyneuropathy with rheumatoid arthritis of elbow**
- **M05.521** Rheumatoid polyneuropathy with rheumatoid arthritis of **right** elbow   HCC
- **M05.522** Rheumatoid polyneuropathy with rheumatoid arthritis of **left** elbow   HCC
- **M05.529** Rheumatoid polyneuropathy with rheumatoid arthritis of unspecified elbow   HCC ▽

√6th **M05.53 Rheumatoid polyneuropathy with rheumatoid arthritis of wrist**
Rheumatoid polyneuropathy with rheumatoid arthritis, carpal bones
- **M05.531** Rheumatoid polyneuropathy with rheumatoid arthritis of **right** wrist   HCC
- **M05.532** Rheumatoid polyneuropathy with rheumatoid arthritis of **left** wrist   HCC
- **M05.539** Rheumatoid polyneuropathy with rheumatoid arthritis of unspecified wrist   HCC ▽

√6th **M05.54 Rheumatoid polyneuropathy with rheumatoid arthritis of hand**
Rheumatoid polyneuropathy with rheumatoid arthritis, metacarpus and phalanges
- **M05.541** Rheumatoid polyneuropathy with rheumatoid arthritis of **right** hand   HCC
- **M05.542** Rheumatoid polyneuropathy with rheumatoid arthritis of **left** hand   HCC
- **M05.549** Rheumatoid polyneuropathy with rheumatoid arthritis of unspecified hand   HCC ▽

√6th **M05.55 Rheumatoid polyneuropathy with rheumatoid arthritis of hip**
- **M05.551** Rheumatoid polyneuropathy with rheumatoid arthritis of **right** hip   HCC
- **M05.552** Rheumatoid polyneuropathy with rheumatoid arthritis of **left** hip   HCC
- **M05.559** Rheumatoid polyneuropathy with rheumatoid arthritls of unspecified hip   HCC ▽

√6th **M05.56 Rheumatoid polyneuropathy with rheumatoid arthritis of knee**
- **M05.561** Rheumatoid polyneuropathy with rheumatoid arthritis of **right** knee   HCC
- **M05.562** Rheumatoid polyneuropathy with rheumatoid arthritis of **left** knee   HCC
- **M05.569** Rheumatoid polyneuropathy with rheumatoid arthritis of unspecified knee   HCC ▽

√6th **M05.57 Rheumatoid polyneuropathy with rheumatoid arthritis of ankle and foot**
Rheumatoid polyneuropathy with rheumatoid arthritis, tarsus, metatarsus and phalanges
- **M05.571** Rheumatoid polyneuropathy with rheumatoid arthritis of **right** ankle and foot   HCC
- **M05.572** Rheumatoid polyneuropathy with rheumatoid arthritis of **left** ankle and foot   HCC
- **M05.579** Rheumatoid polyneuropathy with rheumatoid arthritis of unspecified ankle and foot   HCC ▽

M05.59 Rheumatoid polyneuropathy with rheumatoid arthritis of multiple sites   HCC

√6th **M05.6 Rheumatoid arthritis with involvement of other organs and systems**
- **M05.60 Rheumatoid arthritis of unspecified site with involvement of other organs and systems**   HCC ▽
- √6th **M05.61 Rheumatoid arthritis of shoulder with involvement of other organs and systems**
  - **M05.611** Rheumatoid arthritis of **right** shoulder with involvement of other organs and systems   HCC
  - **M05.612** Rheumatoid arthritis of **left** shoulder with involvement of other organs and systems   HCC
  - **M05.619** Rheumatoid arthritis of unspecified shoulder with involvement of other organs and systems   HCC ▽

√6th **M05.62 Rheumatoid arthritis of elbow with involvement of other organs and systems**
- **M05.621** Rheumatoid arthritis of **right** elbow with involvement of other organs and systems   HCC
- **M05.622** Rheumatoid arthritis of **left** elbow with involvement of other organs and systems   HCC
- **M05.629** Rheumatoid arthritis of unspecified elbow with involvement of other organs and systems   HCC ▽

√6th **M05.63 Rheumatoid arthritis of wrist with involvement of other organs and systems**
Rheumatoid arthritis of carpal bones with involvement of other organs and systems
- **M05.631** Rheumatoid arthritis of **right** wrist with involvement of other organs and systems   HCC
- **M05.632** Rheumatoid arthritis of **left** wrist with involvement of other organs and systems   HCC
- **M05.639** Rheumatoid arthritis of unspecified wrist with involvement of other organs and systems   HCC ▽

√6th **M05.64 Rheumatoid arthritis of hand with involvement of other organs and systems**
Rheumatoid arthritis of metacarpus and phalanges with involvement of other organs and systems
- **M05.641** Rheumatoid arthritis of **right** hand with involvement of other organs and systems   HCC
- **M05.642** Rheumatoid arthritis of **left** hand with involvement of other organs and systems   HCC
- **M05.649** Rheumatoid arthritis of unspecified hand with involvement of other organs and systems   HCC ▽

√6th **M05.65 Rheumatoid arthritis of hip with involvement of other organs and systems**
- **M05.651** Rheumatoid arthritis of **right** hip with involvement of other organs and systems   HCC
- **M05.652** Rheumatoid arthritis of **left** hip with involvement of other organs and systems   HCC
- **M05.659** Rheumatoid arthritis of unspecified hip with involvement of other organs and systems   HCC ▽

√6th **M05.66 Rheumatoid arthritis of knee with involvement of other organs and systems**
- **M05.661** Rheumatoid arthritis of **right** knee with involvement of other organs and systems   HCC
- **M05.662** Rheumatoid arthritis of **left** knee with involvement of other organs and systems   HCC
- **M05.669** Rheumatoid arthritis of unspecified knee with involvement of other organs and systems   HCC ▽

√6th **M05.67 Rheumatoid arthritis of ankle and foot with involvement of other organs and systems**
Rheumatoid arthritis of tarsus, metatarsus and phalanges with involvement of other organs and systems
- **M05.671** Rheumatoid arthritis of **right** ankle and foot with involvement of other organs and systems   HCC
- **M05.672** Rheumatoid arthritis of **left** ankle and foot with involvement of other organs and systems   HCC
- **M05.679** Rheumatoid arthritis of unspecified ankle and foot with involvement of other organs and systems   HCC ▽

M05.69 Rheumatoid arthritis of multiple sites with involvement of other organs and systems   HCC

√5th **M05.7 Rheumatoid arthritis with rheumatoid factor without organ or systems involvement**
- **M05.70 Rheumatoid arthritis with rheumatoid factor of unspecified site without organ or systems involvement**   HCC ▽

EXCLUDES 1 Not coded here   EXCLUDES 2 Not included here   N Newborn Age: 0   P Pediatric Age: 0-17   M Maternity Age: 12-55   A Adult Age: 15-124

724   ICD-10-CM 2018

M05.52–M05.70   Chapter 13. Diseases of the Musculoskeletal System and Connective Tissue

✓6ᵗʰ **M05.71** Rheumatoid arthritis with rheumatoid factor of **shoulder** without organ or systems involvement

     M05.711 Rheumatoid arthritis with rheumatoid factor of **right** shoulder without organ or systems involvement   `HCC`

     M05.712 Rheumatoid arthritis with rheumatoid factor of **left** shoulder without organ or systems involvement   `HCC`

     M05.719 Rheumatoid arthritis with rheumatoid factor of unspecified shoulder without organ or systems involvement   `HCC` ▽

✓6ᵗʰ **M05.72** Rheumatoid arthritis with rheumatoid factor of **elbow** without organ or systems involvement

     M05.721 Rheumatoid arthritis with rheumatoid factor of **right** elbow without organ or systems involvement   `HCC`

     M05.722 Rheumatoid arthritis with rheumatoid factor of **left** elbow without organ or systems involvement   `HCC`

     M05.729 Rheumatoid arthritis with rheumatoid factor of unspecified elbow without organ or systems involvement   `HCC` ▽

✓6ᵗʰ **M05.73** Rheumatoid arthritis with rheumatoid factor of **wrist** without organ or systems involvement

     M05.731 Rheumatoid arthritis with rheumatoid factor of **right** wrist without organ or systems involvement   `HCC`

     M05.732 Rheumatoid arthritis with rheumatoid factor of **left** wrist without organ or systems involvement   `HCC`

     M05.739 Rheumatoid arthritis with rheumatoid factor of unspecified wrist without organ or systems involvement   `HCC` ▽

✓6ᵗʰ **M05.74** Rheumatoid arthritis with rheumatoid factor of **hand** without organ or systems involvement

     M05.741 Rheumatoid arthritis with rheumatoid factor of **right** hand without organ or systems involvement   `HCC`

     M05.742 Rheumatoid arthritis with rheumatoid factor of **left** hand without organ or systems involvement   `HCC`

     M05.749 Rheumatoid arthritis with factor of rheumatoid unspecified hand without organ or systems involvement   `HCC` ▽

✓6ᵗʰ **M05.75** Rheumatoid arthritis with rheumatoid factor of **hip** without organ or systems involvement

     M05.751 Rheumatoid arthritis with rheumatoid factor of **right** hip without organ or systems involvement   `HCC`

     M05.752 Rheumatoid arthritis with rheumatoid factor of **left** hip without organ or systems involvement   `HCC`

     M05.759 Rheumatoid arthritis with rheumatoid factor of unspecified hip without organ or systems involvement   `HCC` ▽

✓6ᵗʰ **M05.76** Rheumatoid arthritis with rheumatoid factor of **knee** without organ or systems involvement

     M05.761 Rheumatoid arthritis with rheumatoid factor of **right** knee without organ or systems involvement   `HCC`

     M05.762 Rheumatoid arthritis with rheumatoid factor of **left** knee without organ or systems involvement   `HCC`

     M05.769 Rheumatoid arthritis with rheumatoidfactor of unspecified knee without organ or systems involvement   `HCC` ▽

✓6ᵗʰ **M05.77** Rheumatoid arthritis with rheumatoid factor of **ankle and foot** without organ or systems involvement

     M05.771 Rheumatoid arthritis with rheumatoid factor of **right** ankle and foot without organ or systems involvement   `HCC`

     M05.772 Rheumatoid arthritis with rheumatoid factor of **left** ankle and foot without organ or systems involvement   `HCC`

     M05.779 Rheumatoid arthritis with rheumatoid factor of unspecified ankle and foot without organ or systems involvement   `HCC` ▽

M05.79 Rheumatoid arthritis with rheumatoid factor of **multiple sites** without organ or systems involvement   `HCC`

✓5ᵗʰ **M05.8** Other rheumatoid arthritis **with rheumatoid factor**

     M05.80 Other rheumatoid arthritis with rheumatoid factor of unspecified site   `HCC` ▽

✓6ᵗʰ **M05.81** Other rheumatoid arthritis with rheumatoid factor of **shoulder**

     M05.811 Other rheumatoid arthritis with rheumatoid factor of **right** shoulder   `HCC`

     M05.812 Other rheumatoid arthritis with rheumatoid factor of **left** shoulder   `HCC`

     M05.819 Other rheumatoid arthritis with rheumatoid factor of unspecified shoulder   `HCC` ▽

✓6ᵗʰ **M05.82** Other rheumatoid arthritis with rheumatoid factor of **elbow**

     M05.821 Other rheumatoid arthritis with rheumatoid factor of **right** elbow   `HCC`

     M05.822 Other rheumatoid arthritis with rheumatoid factor of **left** elbow   `HCC`

     M05.829 Other rheumatoid arthritis with rheumatoid factor of unspecified elbow   `HCC` ▽

✓6ᵗʰ **M05.83** Other rheumatoid arthritis with rheumatoid factor of **wrist**

     M05.831 Other rheumatoid arthritis with rheumatoid factor of **right** wrist   `HCC`

     M05.832 Other rheumatoid arthritis with rheumatoid factor of **left** wrist   `HCC`

     M05.839 Other rheumatoid arthritis with rheumatoid factor of unspecified wrist   `HCC` ▽

✓6ᵗʰ **M05.84** Other rheumatoid arthritis with rheumatoid factor of **hand**

     M05.841 Other rheumatoid arthritis with rheumatoid factor of **right** hand   `HCC`

     M05.842 Other rheumatoid arthritis with rheumatoid factor of **left** hand   `HCC`

     M05.849 Other rheumatoid arthritis with rheumatoid factor of unspecified hand   `HCC` ▽

✓6ᵗʰ **M05.85** Other rheumatoid arthritis with rheumatoid factor of **hip**

     M05.851 Other rheumatoid arthritis with rheumatoid factor of **right** hip   `HCC`

     M05.852 Other rheumatoid arthritis with rheumatoid factor of **left** hip   `HCC`

     M05.859 Other rheumatoid arthritis with rheumatoid factor of unspecified hip   `HCC` ▽

✓6ᵗʰ **M05.86** Other rheumatoid arthritis with rheumatoid factor of **knee**

     M05.861 Other rheumatoid arthritis with rheumatoid factor of **right** knee   `HCC`

     M05.862 Other rheumatoid arthritis with rheumatoid factor of **left** knee   `HCC`

     M05.869 Other rheumatoid arthritis with rheumatoid factor of unspecified knee   `HCC` ▽

✓6ᵗʰ **M05.87** Other rheumatoid arthritis with rheumatoid factor of **ankle and foot**

     M05.871 Other rheumatoid arthritis with rheumatoid factor of **right** ankle and foot   `HCC`

     M05.872 Other rheumatoid arthritis with rheumatoid factor of **left** ankle and foot   `HCC`

     M05.879 Other rheumatoid arthritis with rheumatoid factor of unspecified ankle and foot   `HCC` ▽

     M05.89 Other rheumatoid arthritis with rheumatoid factor of **multiple sites**   `HCC`

M05.9 Rheumatoid arthritis with rheumatoid factor, unspecified   `HCC` ▽

✓4ᵗʰ **M06 Other rheumatoid arthritis**

     DEF: Autoimmune systemic disease that causes chronic inflammation of joints and other areas of the body, manifested by inflammatory changes in articular structures and synovial membranes, atrophy, and loss in bone density.

✓5ᵗʰ **M06.0** Rheumatoid arthritis **without rheumatoid factor**

     M06.00 Rheumatoid arthritis without rheumatoid factor, unspecified site   `HCC` ▽

☑ Additional Character Req   ✓ₓ7ᵗʰ Placeholder Alert   Manifestation   `HCC` CMS-HCC Condition   ▽ Unspecified Code   ▶◀ Revised Text   ● New Code   ▲ Revised Code Title

ICD-10-CM 2018   725

√6ᵗʰ **M06.01** Rheumatoid arthritis without rheumatoid factor, **shoulder**

     M06.011 Rheumatoid arthritis without rheumatoid factor, **right** shoulder `HCC`

     M06.012 Rheumatoid arthritis without rheumatoid factor, **left** shoulder `HCC`

     M06.019 Rheumatoid arthritis without rheumatoid factor, unspecified shoulder `HCC` ▽

√6ᵗʰ **M06.02** Rheumatoid arthritis without rheumatoid factor, **elbow**

     M06.021 Rheumatoid arthritis without rheumatoid factor, **right** elbow `HCC`

     M06.022 Rheumatoid arthritis without rheumatoid factor, **left** elbow `HCC`

     M06.029 Rheumatoid arthritis without rheumatoid factor, unspecified elbow `HCC` ▽

√6ᵗʰ **M06.03** Rheumatoid arthritis without rheumatoid factor, **wrist**

     M06.031 Rheumatoid arthritis without rheumatoid factor, **right** wrist `HCC`

     M06.032 Rheumatoid arthritis without rheumatoid factor, **left** wrist `HCC`

     M06.039 Rheumatoid arthritis without rheumatoid factor, unspecified wrist `HCC` ▽

√6ᵗʰ **M06.04** Rheumatoid arthritis without rheumatoid factor, **hand**

     M06.041 Rheumatoid arthritis without rheumatoid factor, **right** hand `HCC`

     M06.042 Rheumatoid arthritis without rheumatoid factor, **left** hand `HCC`

     M06.049 Rheumatoid arthritis without rheumatoid factor, unspecified hand `HCC` ▽

√6ᵗʰ **M06.05** Rheumatoid arthritis without rheumatoid factor, **hip**

     M06.051 Rheumatoid arthritis without rheumatoid factor, **right** hip `HCC`

     M06.052 Rheumatoid arthritis without rheumatoid factor, **left** hip `HCC`

     M06.059 Rheumatoid arthritis without rheumatoid factor, unspecified hip `HCC` ▽

√6ᵗʰ **M06.06** Rheumatoid arthritis without rheumatoid factor, **knee**

     M06.061 Rheumatoid arthritis without rheumatoid factor, **right** knee `HCC`

     M06.062 Rheumatoid arthritis without rheumatoid factor, **left** knee `HCC`

     M06.069 Rheumatoid arthritis without rheumatoid factor, unspecified knee `HCC` ▽

√6ᵗʰ **M06.07** Rheumatoid arthritis without rheumatoid factor, **ankle and foot**

     M06.071 Rheumatoid arthritis without rheumatoid factor, **right** ankle and foot `HCC`

     M06.072 Rheumatoid arthritis without rheumatoid factor, **left** ankle and foot `HCC`

     M06.079 Rheumatoid arthritis without rheumatoid factor, unspecified ankle and foot `HCC` ▽

     M06.08 Rheumatoid arthritis without rheumatoid factor, **vertebrae** `HCC`

     M06.09 Rheumatoid arthritis without rheumatoid factor, **multiple sites** `HCC`

M06.1 **Adult-onset Still's** disease `HCC` `A`

     EXCLUDES 1   Still's disease NOS (M08.2-)

√5ᵗʰ **M06.2** **Rheumatoid bursitis**

     M06.20 Rheumatoid bursitis, unspecified site `HCC` ▽

√6ᵗʰ **M06.21** Rheumatoid bursitis, **shoulder**

     M06.211 Rheumatoid bursitis, **right** shoulder `HCC`

     M06.212 Rheumatoid bursitis, **left** shoulder `HCC`

     M06.219 Rheumatoid bursitis, unspecified shoulder `HCC` ▽

√6ᵗʰ **M06.22** Rheumatoid bursitis, **elbow**

     M06.221 Rheumatoid bursitis, **right** elbow `HCC`

     M06.222 Rheumatoid bursitis, **left** elbow `HCC`

     M06.229 Rheumatoid bursitis, unspecified elbow `HCC` ▽

√6ᵗʰ **M06.23** Rheumatoid bursitis, **wrist**

     M06.231 Rheumatoid bursitis, **right** wrist `HCC`

     M06.232 Rheumatoid bursitis, **left** wrist `HCC`

     M06.239 Rheumatoid bursitis, unspecified wrist `HCC` ▽

√6ᵗʰ **M06.24** Rheumatoid bursitis, **hand**

     M06.241 Rheumatoid bursitis, **right** hand `HCC`

     M06.242 Rheumatoid bursitis, **left** hand `HCC`

     M06.249 Rheumatoid bursitis, unspecified hand `HCC` ▽

√6ᵗʰ **M06.25** Rheumatoid bursitis, **hip**

     M06.251 Rheumatoid bursitis, **right** hip `HCC`

     M06.252 Rheumatoid bursitis, **left** hip `HCC`

     M06.259 Rheumatoid bursitis, unspecified hip `HCC` ▽

√6ᵗʰ **M06.26** Rheumatoid bursitis, **knee**

     M06.261 Rheumatoid bursitis, **right** knee `HCC`

     M06.262 Rheumatoid bursitis, **left** knee `HCC`

     M06.269 Rheumatoid bursitis, unspecified knee `HCC` ▽

√6ᵗʰ **M06.27** Rheumatoid bursitis, **ankle and foot**

     M06.271 Rheumatoid bursitis, **right** ankle and foot `HCC`

     M06.272 Rheumatoid bursitis, **left** ankle and foot `HCC`

     M06.279 Rheumatoid bursitis, unspecified ankle and foot `HCC` ▽

     M06.28 Rheumatoid bursitis, **vertebrae** `HCC`

     M06.29 Rheumatoid bursitis, **multiple sites** `HCC`

√5ᵗʰ **M06.3** **Rheumatoid nodule**

     M06.30 Rheumatoid nodule, unspecified site `HCC` ▽

√6ᵗʰ **M06.31** Rheumatoid nodule, **shoulder**

     M06.311 Rheumatoid nodule, **right** shoulder `HCC`

     M06.312 Rheumatoid nodule, **left** shoulder `HCC`

     M06.319 Rheumatoid nodule, unspecified shoulder `HCC` ▽

√6ᵗʰ **M06.32** Rheumatoid nodule, **elbow**

     M06.321 Rheumatoid nodule, **right** elbow `HCC`

     M06.322 Rheumatoid nodule, **left** elbow `HCC`

     M06.329 Rheumatoid nodule, unspecified elbow `HCC` ▽

√6ᵗʰ **M06.33** Rheumatoid nodule, **wrist**

     M06.331 Rheumatoid nodule, **right** wrist `HCC`

     M06.332 Rheumatoid nodule, **left** wrist `HCC`

     M06.339 Rheumatoid nodule, unspecified wrist `HCC` ▽

√6ᵗʰ **M06.34** Rheumatoid nodule, **hand**

     M06.341 Rheumatoid nodule, **right** hand `HCC`

     M06.342 Rheumatoid nodule, **left** hand `HCC`

     M06.349 Rheumatoid nodule, unspecified hand `HCC` ▽

√6ᵗʰ **M06.35** Rheumatoid nodule, **hip**

     M06.351 Rheumatoid nodule, **right** hip `HCC`

     M06.352 Rheumatoid nodule, **left** hip `HCC`

     M06.359 Rheumatoid nodule, unspecified hip `HCC` ▽

√6ᵗʰ **M06.36** Rheumatoid nodule, **knee**

     M06.361 Rheumatoid nodule, **right** knee `HCC`

     M06.362 Rheumatoid nodule, **left** knee `HCC`

     M06.369 Rheumatoid nodule, unspecified knee `HCC` ▽

√6ᵗʰ **M06.37** Rheumatoid nodule, **ankle and foot**

     M06.371 Rheumatoid nodule, **right** ankle and foot `HCC`

     M06.372 Rheumatoid nodule, **left** ankle and foot `HCC`

     M06.379 Rheumatoid nodule, unspecified and ankle foot `HCC` ▽

     M06.38 Rheumatoid nodule, **vertebrae** `HCC`

     M06.39 Rheumatoid nodule, **multiple sites** `HCC`

M06.4 Inflammatory polyarthropathy `HCC`

     EXCLUDES 1   polyarthritis NOS (M13.0)

EXCLUDES 1 Not coded here   *EXCLUDES 2* Not included here   **N** Newborn Age: 0   **P** Pediatric Age: 0-17   **M** Maternity Age: 12-55   **A** Adult Age: 15-124

✓5ᵗʰ **M06.8 Other specified rheumatoid arthritis**

M06.80 Other specified rheumatoid arthritis, unspecified site   HCC ▽

✓6ᵗʰ **M06.81** Other specified rheumatoid arthritis, **shoulder**

M06.811 Other specified rheumatoid arthritis, **right** shoulder   HCC

M06.812 Other specified rheumatoid arthritis, **left** shoulder   HCC

M06.819 Other specified rheumatoid arthritis, unspecified shoulder   HCC ▽

✓6ᵗʰ **M06.82** Other specified rheumatoid arthritis, **elbow**

M06.821 Other specified rheumatoid arthritis, **right** elbow   HCC

M06.822 Other specified rheumatoid arthritis, **left** elbow   HCC

M06.829 Other specified rheumatoid arthritis, unspecified elbow   HCC ▽

✓6ᵗʰ **M06.83** Other specified rheumatoid arthritis, **wrist**

M06.831 Other specified rheumatoid arthritis, **right** wrist   HCC

M06.832 Other specified rheumatoid arthritis, **left** wrist   HCC

M06.839 Other specified rheumatoid arthritis, unspecified wrist   HCC ▽

✓6ᵗʰ **M06.84** Other specified rheumatoid arthritis, **hand**

M06.841 Other specified rheumatoid arthritis, **right** hand   HCC

M06.842 Other specified rheumatoid arthritis, **left** hand   HCC

M06.849 Other specified rheumatoid arthritis, unspecified hand   HCC ▽

✓6ᵗʰ **M06.85** Other specified rheumatoid arthritis, **hip**

M06.851 Other specified rheumatoid arthritis, **right** hip   HCC

M06.852 Other specified rheumatoid arthritis, **left** hip   HCC

M06.859 Other specified rheumatoid arthritis, unspecified hip   HCC ▽

✓6ᵗʰ **M06.86** Other specified rheumatoid arthritis, **knee**

M06.861 Other specified rheumatoid arthritis, **right** knee   HCC

M06.862 Other specified rheumatoid arthritis, **left** knee   HCC

M06.869 Other specified rheumatoid arthritis, unspecified knee   HCC ▽

✓6ᵗʰ **M06.87** Other specified rheumatoid arthritis, **ankle and foot**

M06.871 Other specified rheumatoid arthritis, **right** ankle and foot   HCC

M06.872 Other specified rheumatoid arthritis, **left** ankle and foot   HCC

M06.879 Other specified rheumatoid arthritis, unspecified ankle and foot   HCC ▽

M06.88 Other specified rheumatoid arthritis, **vertebrae**   HCC

M06.89 Other specified rheumatoid arthritis, **multiple sites**   HCC

M06.9 Rheumatoid arthritis, unspecified   HCC ▽
DEF: Autoimmune systemic disease that causes chronic inflammation of joints and other areas of the body, manifested by inflammatory changes in articular structures and synovial membranes, atrophy, and loss in bone density.

✓4ᵗʰ **M07 Enteropathic arthropathies**
Code also associated enteropathy, such as:
     regional enteritis [Crohn's disease] (K50.-)
     ulcerative colitis (K51.-)
     EXCLUDES 1   *psoriatic arthropathies (L40.5-)*

✓5ᵗʰ **M07.6 Enteropathic arthropathies**

M07.60 Enteropathic arthropathies, unspecified site   ▽

✓6ᵗʰ **M07.61** Enteropathic arthropathies, **shoulder**

M07.611 Enteropathic arthropathies, **right** shoulder

M07.612 Enteropathic arthropathies, **left** shoulder

M07.619 Enteropathic arthropathies, unspecified shoulder   ▽

✓6ᵗʰ **M07.62** Enteropathic arthropathies, **elbow**

M07.621 Enteropathic arthropathies, **right** elbow

M07.622 Enteropathic arthropathies, **left** elbow

M07.629 Enteropathic arthropathies, unspecified elbow   ▽

✓6ᵗʰ **M07.63** Enteropathic arthropathies, **wrist**

M07.631 Enteropathic arthropathies, **right** wrist

M07.632 Enteropathic arthropathies, **left** wrist

M07.639 Enteropathic arthropathies, unspecified wrist   ▽

✓6ᵗʰ **M07.64** Enteropathic arthropathies, **hand**

M07.641 Enteropathic arthropathies, **right** hand

M07.642 Enteropathic arthropathies, **left** hand

M07.649 Enteropathic arthropathies, unspecified hand   ▽

✓6ᵗʰ **M07.65** Enteropathic arthropathies, **hip**

M07.651 Enteropathic arthropathies, **right** hip

M07.652 Enteropathic arthropathies, **left** hip

M07.659 Enteropathic arthropathies, unspecified hip   ▽

✓6ᵗʰ **M07.66** Enteropathic arthropathies, **knee**

M07.661 Enteropathic arthropathies, **right** knee

M07.662 Enteropathic arthropathies, **left** knee

M07.669 Enteropathic arthropathies, unspecified knee   ▽

✓6ᵗʰ **M07.67** Enteropathic arthropathies, **ankle and foot**

M07.671 Enteropathic arthropathies, **right** ankle and foot

M07.672 Enteropathic arthropathies, **left** ankle and foot

M07.679 Enteropathic arthropathies, unspecified ankle and foot   ▽

M07.68 Enteropathic arthropathies, **vertebrae**

M07.69 Enteropathic arthropathies, **multiple sites**

✓4ᵗʰ **M08 Juvenile arthritis**
Code also any associated underlying condition, such as:
     regional enteritis [Crohn's disease] (K50.-)
     ulcerative colitis (K51.-)
     EXCLUDES 1   *arthropathy in Whipple's disease (M14.8)*
                 Felty's syndrome (M05.0)
                 juvenile dermatomyositis (M33.0-)
                 psoriatic juvenile arthropathy (L40.54)

✓5ᵗʰ **M08.0 Unspecified juvenile rheumatoid arthritis**
Juvenile rheumatoid arthritis with or without rheumatoid factor

M08.00 Unspecified juvenile rheumatoid arthritis of unspecified site   HCC ▽

✓6ᵗʰ **M08.01** Unspecified juvenile rheumatoid arthritis, **shoulder**

M08.011 Unspecified juvenile rheumatoid arthritis, **right** shoulder   HCC ▽

M08.012 Unspecified juvenile rheumatoid arthritis, **left** shoulder   HCC ▽

M08.019 Unspecified juvenile rheumatoid arthritis, unspecified shoulder   HCC ▽

✓6ᵗʰ **M08.02** Unspecified juvenile rheumatoid arthritis of elbow

M08.021 Unspecified juvenile rheumatoid arthritis, **right** elbow   HCC ▽

M08.022 Unspecified juvenile rheumatoid arthritis, **left** elbow   HCC ▽

M08.029 Unspecified juvenile rheumatoid arthritis, unspecified elbow   HCC ▽

✓6ᵗʰ **M08.03** Unspecified juvenile rheumatoid arthritis, **wrist**

M08.031 Unspecified juvenile rheumatoid arthritis, **right** wrist   HCC ▽

M08.032 Unspecified juvenile rheumatoid arthritis, **left** wrist   HCC ▽

M08.039 Unspecified juvenile rheumatoid arthritis, unspecified wrist   HCC ▽

✓6ᵗʰ **M08.04** Unspecified juvenile rheumatoid arthritis, **hand**

M08.041 Unspecified juvenile rheumatoid arthritis, **right** hand   HCC ▽

M08.042 Unspecified juvenile rheumatoid arthritis, **left** hand   HCC ▽

M08.049 Unspecified juvenile rheumatoid arthritis, unspecified hand   HCC ▽

✓6ᵗʰ **M08.05** Unspecified juvenile rheumatoid arthritis, **hip**

M08.051 Unspecified juvenile rheumatoid arthritis, **right** hip   HCC ▽

M08.052 Unspecified juvenile rheumatoid arthritis, **left hip** `HCC` ▽

M08.059 Unspecified juvenile rheumatoid arthritis, **unspecified hip** `HCC` ▽

✓6ᵗʰ **M08.06** Unspecified juvenile rheumatoid arthritis, **knee** ▽

    M08.061 Unspecified juvenile rheumatoid arthritis, **right knee** `HCC` ▽

    M08.062 Unspecified juvenile rheumatoid arthritis, **left knee** `HCC` ▽

    M08.069 Unspecified juvenile rheumatoid arthritis, **unspecified knee** `HCC` ▽

✓6ᵗʰ **M08.07** Unspecified juvenile rheumatoid arthritis, **ankle and foot** ▽

    M08.071 Unspecified juvenile rheumatoid arthritis, **right ankle and foot** `HCC` ▽

    M08.072 Unspecified juvenile rheumatoid arthritis, **left ankle and foot** `HCC` ▽

    M08.079 Unspecified juvenile rheumatoid arthritis, **unspecified ankle and foot** `HCC` ▽

M08.08 Unspecified juvenile rheumatoid arthritis, **vertebrae** `HCC` ▽

M08.09 Unspecified juvenile rheumatoid arthritis, **multiple sites** `HCC` ▽

M08.1 Juvenile **ankylosing spondylitis** `HCC`

    EXCLUDES 1   ankylosing spondylitis in adults (M45.0-)

✓5ᵗʰ **M08.2** Juvenile **rheumatoid arthritis with systemic onset**

    Still's disease NOS

    EXCLUDES 1   adult-onset Still's disease (M06.1-)

    M08.20 Juvenile rheumatoid arthritis with systemic onset, **unspecified site** `HCC` ▽

    ✓6ᵗʰ **M08.21** Juvenile rheumatoid arthritis with systemic onset, **shoulder**

        M08.211 Juvenile rheumatoid arthritis with systemic onset, **right shoulder** `HCC`

        M08.212 Juvenile rheumatoid arthritis with systemic onset, **left shoulder** `HCC`

        M08.219 Juvenile rheumatoid arthritis with systemic onset, **unspecified shoulder** `HCC` ▽

    ✓6ᵗʰ **M08.22** Juvenile rheumatoid arthritis with systemic onset, **elbow**

        M08.221 Juvenile rheumatoid arthritis with systemic onset, **right elbow** `HCC`

        M08.222 Juvenile rheumatoid arthritis with systemic onset, **left elbow** `HCC`

        M08.229 Juvenile rheumatoid arthritis with systemic onset, **unspecified elbow** `HCC` ▽

    ✓6ᵗʰ **M08.23** Juvenile rheumatoid arthritis with systemic onset, **wrist**

        M08.231 Juvenile rheumatoid arthritis with systemic onset, **right wrist** `HCC`

        M08.232 Juvenile rheumatoid arthritis with systemic onset, **left wrist** `HCC`

        M08.239 Juvenile rheumatoid arthritis with systemic onset, **unspecified wrist** `HCC` ▽

    ✓6ᵗʰ **M08.24** Juvenile rheumatoid arthritis with systemic onset, **hand**

        M08.241 Juvenile rheumatoid arthritis with systemic onset, **right hand** `HCC`

        M08.242 Juvenile rheumatoid arthritis with systemic onset, **left hand** `HCC`

        M08.249 Juvenile rheumatoid arthritis with systemic onset, **unspecified hand** `HCC` ▽

    ✓6ᵗʰ **M08.25** Juvenile rheumatoid arthritis with systemic onset, **hip**

        M08.251 Juvenile rheumatoid arthritis with systemic onset, **right hip** `HCC`

        M08.252 Juvenile rheumatoid arthritis with systemic onset, **left hip** `HCC`

        M08.259 Juvenile rheumatoid arthritis with systemic onset, **unspecified hip** `HCC` ▽

    ✓6ᵗʰ **M08.26** Juvenile rheumatoid arthritis with systemic onset, **knee**

        M08.261 Juvenile rheumatoid arthritis with systemic onset, **right knee** `HCC`

        M08.262 Juvenile rheumatoid arthritis with systemic onset, **left knee** `HCC`

        M08.269 Juvenile rheumatoid arthritis with systemic onset, **unspecified knee** `HCC` ▽

    ✓6ᵗʰ **M08.27** Juvenile rheumatoid arthritis with systemic onset, **ankle and foot**

        M08.271 Juvenile rheumatoid arthritis with systemic onset, **right ankle and foot** `HCC`

        M08.272 Juvenile rheumatoid arthritis with systemic onset, **left ankle and foot** `HCC`

        M08.279 Juvenile rheumatoid arthritis with systemic onset, **unspecified ankle and foot** `HCC` ▽

    M08.28 Juvenile rheumatoid arthritis with systemic onset, **vertebrae** `HCC`

    M08.29 Juvenile rheumatoid arthritis with systemic onset, **multiple sites** `HCC`

M08.3 Juvenile rheumatoid polyarthritis (seronegative) `HCC`

✓5ᵗʰ **M08.4** Pauciarticular juvenile rheumatoid arthritis

    M08.40 Pauciarticular juvenile rheumatoid arthritis, **unspecified site** `HCC` ▽

    ✓6ᵗʰ **M08.41** Pauciarticular juvenile rheumatoid arthritis, **shoulder**

        M08.411 Pauciarticular juvenile rheumatoid arthritis, **right shoulder** `HCC`

        M08.412 Pauciarticular juvenile rheumatoid arthritis, **left shoulder** `HCC`

        M08.419 Pauciarticular juvenile rheumatoid arthritis, **unspecified shoulder** `HCC` ▽

    ✓6ᵗʰ **M08.42** Pauciarticular juvenile rheumatoid arthritis, **elbow**

        M08.421 Pauciarticular juvenile rheumatoid arthritis, **right elbow** `HCC`

        M08.422 Pauciarticular juvenile rheumatoid arthritis, **left elbow** `HCC`

        M08.429 Pauciarticular juvenile rheumatoid arthritis, **unspecified elbow** `HCC` ▽

    ✓6ᵗʰ **M08.43** Pauciarticular juvenile rheumatoid arthritis, **wrist**

        M08.431 Pauciarticular juvenile rheumatoid arthritis, **right wrist** `HCC`

        M08.432 Pauciarticular juvenile rheumatoid arthritis, **left wrist** `HCC`

        M08.439 Pauciarticular juvenile rheumatoid arthritis, **unspecified wrist** `HCC` ▽

    ✓6ᵗʰ **M08.44** Pauciarticular juvenile rheumatoid arthritis, **hand**

        M08.441 Pauciarticular juvenile rheumatoid arthritis, **right hand** `HCC`

        M08.442 Pauciarticular juvenile rheumatoid arthritis, **left hand** `HCC`

        M08.449 Pauciarticular juvenile rheumatoid arthritis, **unspecified hand** `HCC` ▽

    ✓6ᵗʰ **M08.45** Pauciarticular juvenile rheumatoid arthritis, **hip**

        M08.451 Pauciarticular juvenile rheumatoid arthritis, **right hip** `HCC`

        M08.452 Pauciarticular juvenile rheumatoid arthritis, **left hip** `HCC`

        M08.459 Pauciarticular juvenile rheumatoid arthritis, **unspecified hip** `HCC` ▽

    ✓6ᵗʰ **M08.46** Pauciarticular juvenile rheumatoid arthritis, **knee**

        M08.461 Pauciarticular juvenile rheumatoid arthritis, **right knee** `HCC`

        M08.462 Pauciarticular juvenile rheumatoid arthritis, **left knee** `HCC`

        M08.469 Pauciarticular juvenile rheumatoid arthritis, **unspecified knee** `HCC` ▽

    ✓6ᵗʰ **M08.47** Pauciarticular juvenile rheumatoid arthritis, **ankle and foot**

        M08.471 Pauciarticular juvenile rheumatoid arthritis, **right ankle and foot** `HCC`

        M08.472 Pauciarticular juvenile rheumatoid arthritis, **left ankle and foot** `HCC`

        M08.479 Pauciarticular juvenile rheumatoid arthritis, **unspecified ankle and foot** `HCC` ▽

    M08.48 Pauciarticular juvenile rheumatoid arthritis, **vertebrae** `HCC`

✓5ᵗʰ **M08.8** Other juvenile arthritis

    M08.80 Other juvenile arthritis, **unspecified site** `HCC` ▽

    ✓6ᵗʰ **M08.81** Other juvenile arthritis, **shoulder**

        M08.811 Other juvenile arthritis, **right shoulder** `HCC`

        M08.812 Other juvenile arthritis, **left shoulder** `HCC`

        M08.819 Other juvenile arthritis, **unspecified shoulder** `HCC` ▽

EXCLUDES 1 Not coded here   *EXCLUDES 2* Not included here   N Newborn Age: 0   P Pediatric Age: 0-17   M Maternity Age: 12-55   A Adult Age: 15-124

✓6ᵗʰ **M08.82** Other juvenile arthritis, **elbow**

     M08.821 Other juvenile arthritis, **right** elbow   HCC

     M08.822 Other juvenile arthritis, **left** elbow   HCC

     M08.829 Other juvenile arthritis, unspecified HCC ▽
          elbow

✓6ᵗʰ **M08.83** Other juvenile arthritis, **wrist**

     M08.831 Other juvenile arthritis, **right** wrist   HCC

     M08.832 Other juvenile arthritis, **left** wrist   HCC

     M08.839 Other juvenile arthritis, unspecified HCC ▽
          wrist

✓6ᵗʰ **M08.84** Other juvenile arthritis, **hand**

     M08.841 Other juvenile arthritis, **right** hand   HCC

     M08.842 Other juvenile arthritis, **left** hand   HCC

     M08.849 Other juvenile arthritis, unspecified HCC ▽
          hand

✓6ᵗʰ **M08.85** Other juvenile arthritis, **hip**

     M08.851 Other juvenile arthritis, **right** hip   HCC

     M08.852 Other juvenile arthritis, **left** hip   HCC

     M08.859 Other juvenile arthritis,   HCC ▽
          unspecified hip

✓6ᵗʰ **M08.86** Other juvenile arthritis, **knee**

     M08.861 Other juvenile arthritis, **right** knee   HCC

     M08.862 Other juvenile arthritis, **left** knee   HCC

     M08.869 Other juvenile arthritis,   HCC ▽
          unspecified knee

✓6ᵗʰ **M08.87** Other juvenile arthritis, **ankle and foot**

     M08.871 Other juvenile arthritis, **right** ankle   HCC
          and foot

     M08.872 Other juvenile arthritis, **left** ankle   HCC
          and foot

     M08.879 Other juvenile arthritis,   HCC ▽
          unspecified ankle and foot

     M08.88 Other juvenile arthritis, other specified site   HCC
          Other juvenile arthritis, vertebrae

     M08.89 Other juvenile arthritis, **multiple sites**   HCC

✓5ᵗʰ **M08.9** Juvenile arthritis, **unspecified**

     EXCLUDES 1   *juvenile rheumatoid arthritis, unspecified (M08.0-)*

     M08.90 Juvenile arthritis, unspecified,   HCC ▽
          unspecified site

✓6ᵗʰ **M08.91** Juvenile arthritis, unspecified, **shoulder**

     M08.911 Juvenile arthritis, unspecified, **right** HCC ▽
          shoulder

     M08.912 Juvenile arthritis, unspecified, **left** HCC ▽
          shoulder

     M08.919 Juvenile arthritis, unspecified,   HCC ▽
          unspecified shoulder

✓6ᵗʰ **M08.92** Juvenile arthritis, unspecified, **elbow**

     M08.921 Juvenile arthritis, unspecified,   HCC ▽
          right elbow

     M08.922 Juvenile arthritis, unspecified,   HCC ▽
          left elbow

     M08.929 Juvenile arthritis, unspecified,   HCC ▽
          unspecified elbow

✓6ᵗʰ **M08.93** Juvenile arthritis, unspecified, **wrist**

     M08.931 Juvenile arthritis, unspecified,   HCC ▽
          right wrist

     M08.932 Juvenile arthritis, unspecified,   HCC ▽
          left wrist

     M08.939 Juvenile arthritis, unspecified,   HCC ▽
          unspecified wrist

✓6ᵗʰ **M08.94** Juvenile arthritis, unspecified, **hand**

     M08.941 Juvenile arthritis, unspecified,   HCC ▽
          right hand

     M08.942 Juvenile arthritis, unspecified,   HCC ▽
          left hand

     M08.949 Juvenile arthritis, unspecified,   HCC ▽
          unspecified hand

✓6ᵗʰ **M08.95** Juvenile arthritis, unspecified, **hip**

     M08.951 Juvenile arthritis, unspecified,   HCC ▽
          right hip

     M08.952 Juvenile arthritis, unspecified,   HCC ▽
          left hip

     M08.959 Juvenile arthritis, unspecified,   HCC ▽
          unspecified hip

✓6ᵗʰ **M08.96** Juvenile arthritis, unspecified, **knee**

     M08.961 Juvenile arthritis, unspecified,   HCC ▽
          right knee

     M08.962 Juvenile arthritis, unspecified,   HCC ▽
          left knee

     M08.969 Juvenile arthritis, unspecified,   HCC ▽
          unspecified knee

✓6ᵗʰ **M08.97** Juvenile arthritis, unspecified, **ankle and foot**

     M08.971 Juvenile arthritis, unspecified,   HCC ▽
          right ankle and foot

     M08.972 Juvenile arthritis, unspecified,   HCC ▽
          left ankle and foot

     M08.979 Juvenile arthritis, unspecified,   HCC ▽
          unspecified ankle and foot

     M08.98 Juvenile arthritis, unspecified, **vertebrae**   HCC ▽

     M08.99 Juvenile arthritis, unspecified, **multiple sites**   HCC ▽

✓4ᵗʰ **M1A Chronic gout**

     Use additional code to identify:
         autonomic neuropathy in diseases classified elsewhere (G99.0)
         calculus of urinary tract in diseases classified elsewhere (N22)
         cardiomyopathy in diseases classified elsewhere (I43)
         disorders of external ear in diseases classified elsewhere (H61.1-,
           H62.8-)
         disorders of iris and ciliary body in diseases classified elsewhere (H22)
         glomerular disorders in diseases classified elsewhere (N08)

     EXCLUDES 1   *gout NOS (M10.-)*
     EXCLUDES 2   *acute gout (M10.-)*

     The appropriate 7th character is to be added to each code
     from category M1A.
     0   without tophus (tophi)
     1   with tophus (tophi)

✓5ᵗʰ **M1A.0** **Idiopathic** chronic gout
     Chronic gouty bursitis   Primary chronic gout

   ✓x7ᵗʰ **M1A.00** Idiopathic chronic gout, unspecified site   ▽

   ✓6ᵗʰ **M1A.01** Idiopathic chronic gout, **shoulder**

     ✓7ᵗʰ M1A.011 Idiopathic chronic gout, **right** shoulder

     ✓7ᵗʰ M1A.012 Idiopathic chronic gout, **left** shoulder

     ✓7ᵗʰ M1A.019 Idiopathic chronic gout, unspecified   ▽
          shoulder

   ✓6ᵗʰ **M1A.02** Idiopathic chronic gout, **elbow**

     ✓7ᵗʰ M1A.021 Idiopathic chronic gout, **right** elbow

     ✓7ᵗʰ M1A.022 Idiopathic chronic gout, **left** elbow

     ✓7ᵗʰ M1A.029 Idiopathic chronic gout, unspecified   ▽
          elbow

   ✓6ᵗʰ **M1A.03** Idiopathic chronic gout, **wrist**

     ✓7ᵗʰ M1A.031 Idiopathic chronic gout, **right** wrist

     ✓7ᵗʰ M1A.032 Idiopathic chronic gout, **left** wrist

     ✓7ᵗʰ M1A.039 Idiopathic chronic gout, unspecified   ▽
          wrist

   ✓6ᵗʰ **M1A.04** Idiopathic chronic gout, **hand**

     ✓7ᵗʰ M1A.041 Idiopathic chronic gout, **right** hand

     ✓7ᵗʰ M1A.042 Idiopathic chronic gout, **left** hand

     ✓7ᵗʰ M1A.049 Idiopathic chronic gout, unspecified   ▽
          hand

   ✓6ᵗʰ **M1A.05** Idiopathic chronic gout, **hip**

     ✓7ᵗʰ M1A.051 Idiopathic chronic gout, **right** hip

     ✓7ᵗʰ M1A.052 Idiopathic chronic gout, **left** hip

     ✓7ᵗʰ M1A.059 Idiopathic chronic gout, unspecified hip ▽

   ✓6ᵗʰ **M1A.06** Idiopathic chronic gout, **knee**

     ✓7ᵗʰ M1A.061 Idiopathic chronic gout, **right** knee

     ✓7ᵗʰ M1A.062 Idiopathic chronic gout, **left** knee

     ✓7ᵗʰ M1A.069 Idiopathic chronic gout, unspecified   ▽
          knee

   ✓6ᵗʰ **M1A.07** Idiopathic chronic gout, **ankle and foot**

     ✓7ᵗʰ M1A.071 Idiopathic chronic gout, **right** ankle and
          foot

     ✓7ᵗʰ M1A.072 Idiopathic chronic gout, **left** ankle and
          foot

     ✓7ᵗʰ M1A.079 Idiopathic chronic gout, unspecified   ▽
          ankle and foot

   ✓x7ᵗʰ **M1A.08** Idiopathic chronic gout, **vertebrae**

   ✓x7ᵗʰ **M1A.09** Idiopathic chronic gout, **multiple sites**

✔ Additional Character Req   ✓x7ᵗʰ Placeholder Alert   Manifestation   HCC CMS-HCC Condition   ▽ Unspecified Code   ▶◀ Revised Text   ● New Code   ▲ Revised Code Title

ICD-10-CM 2018   729

√5ᵗʰ **M1A.1** **Lead-induced** chronic gout
Code first toxic effects of lead and its compounds (T56.Ø-)

√7ᵗʰ **M1A.1Ø** Lead-induced chronic gout, unspecified site ▽

√6ᵗʰ **M1A.11** Lead-induced chronic gout, **shoulder**

√7ᵗʰ **M1A.111** Lead-induced chronic gout, **right** shoulder

√7ᵗʰ **M1A.112** Lead-induced chronic gout, **left** shoulder

√7ᵗʰ **M1A.119** Lead-induced chronic gout, ▽
unspecified shoulder

√6ᵗʰ **M1A.12** Lead-induced chronic gout, **elbow**

√7ᵗʰ **M1A.121** Lead-induced chronic gout, **right** elbow

√7ᵗʰ **M1A.122** Lead-induced chronic gout, **left** elbow

√7ᵗʰ **M1A.129** Lead-induced chronic gout, ▽
unspecified elbow

√6ᵗʰ **M1A.13** Lead-induced chronic gout, **wrist**

√7ᵗʰ **M1A.131** Lead-induced chronic gout, **right** wrist

√7ᵗʰ **M1A.132** Lead-induced chronic gout, **left** wrist

√7ᵗʰ **M1A.139** Lead-induced chronic gout, ▽
unspecified wrist

√6ᵗʰ **M1A.14** Lead-induced chronic gout, **hand**

√7ᵗʰ **M1A.141** Lead-induced chronic gout, **right** hand

√7ᵗʰ **M1A.142** Lead-induced chronic gout, **left** hand

√7ᵗʰ **M1A.149** Lead-induced chronic gout, ▽
unspecified hand

√6ᵗʰ **M1A.15** Lead-induced chronic gout, **hip**

√7ᵗʰ **M1A.151** Lead-induced chronic gout, **right** hip

√7ᵗʰ **M1A.152** Lead-induced chronic gout, **left** hip

√7ᵗʰ **M1A.159** Lead-induced chronic gout, ▽
unspecified hip

√6ᵗʰ **M1A.16** Lead-induced chronic gout, **knee**

√7ᵗʰ **M1A.161** Lead-induced chronic gout, **right** knee

√7ᵗʰ **M1A.162** Lead-induced chronic gout, **left** knee

√7ᵗʰ **M1A.169** Lead-induced chronic gout, ▽
unspecified knee

√6ᵗʰ **M1A.17** Lead-induced chronic gout, **ankle and foot**

√7ᵗʰ **M1A.171** Lead-induced chronic gout, **right** ankle
and foot

√7ᵗʰ **M1A.172** Lead-induced chronic gout, **left** ankle and
foot

√7ᵗʰ **M1A.179** Lead-induced chronic gout, ▽
unspecified ankle and foot

√x7ᵗʰ **M1A.18** Lead-induced chronic gout, **vertebrae**

√x7ᵗʰ **M1A.19** Lead-induced chronic gout, **multiple sites**

√5ᵗʰ **M1A.2** **Drug-induced** chronic gout
Use additional code for adverse effect, if applicable, to identify
drug (T36-T5Ø with fifth or sixth character 5)

√x7ᵗʰ **M1A.2Ø** Drug-induced chronic gout, unspecified site ▽

√6ᵗʰ **M1A.21** Drug-induced chronic gout, **shoulder**

√7ᵗʰ **M1A.211** Drug-induced chronic gout, **right** shoulder

√7ᵗʰ **M1A.212** Drug-induced chronic gout, **left** shoulder

√7ᵗʰ **M1A.219** Drug-induced chronic gout, ▽
unspecified shoulder

√6ᵗʰ **M1A.22** Drug-induced chronic gout, **elbow**

√7ᵗʰ **M1A.221** Drug-induced chronic gout, **right** elbow

√7ᵗʰ **M1A.222** Drug-induced chronic gout, **left** elbow

√7ᵗʰ **M1A.229** Drug-induced chronic gout, ▽
unspecified elbow

√6ᵗʰ **M1A.23** Drug-induced chronic gout, **wrist**

√7ᵗʰ **M1A.231** Drug-induced chronic gout, **right** wrist

√7ᵗʰ **M1A.232** Drug-induced chronic gout, **left** wrist

√7ᵗʰ **M1A.239** Drug-induced chronic gout, ▽
unspecified wrist

√6ᵗʰ **M1A.24** Drug-induced chronic gout, **hand**

√7ᵗʰ **M1A.241** Drug-induced chronic gout, **right** hand

√7ᵗʰ **M1A.242** Drug-induced chronic gout, **left** hand

√7ᵗʰ **M1A.249** Drug-induced chronic gout, ▽
unspecified hand

√6ᵗʰ **M1A.25** Drug-induced chronic gout, **hip**

√7ᵗʰ **M1A.251** Drug-induced chronic gout, **right** hip

√7ᵗʰ **M1A.252** Drug-induced chronic gout, **left** hip

√7ᵗʰ **M1A.259** Drug-induced chronic gout, ▽
unspecified hip

√6ᵗʰ **M1A.26** Drug-induced chronic gout, **knee**

√7ᵗʰ **M1A.261** Drug-induced chronic gout, **right** knee

√7ᵗʰ **M1A.262** Drug-induced chronic gout, **left** knee

√7ᵗʰ **M1A.269** Drug-induced chronic gout, ▽
unspecified knee

√6ᵗʰ **M1A.27** Drug-induced chronic gout, **ankle and foot**

√7ᵗʰ **M1A.271** Drug-induced chronic gout, **right** ankle
and foot

√7ᵗʰ **M1A.272** Drug-induced chronic gout, **left** ankle and
foot

√7ᵗʰ **M1A.279** Drug-induced chronic gout, ▽
unspecified ankle and foot

√x7ᵗʰ **M1A.28** Drug-induced chronic gout, **vertebrae**

√x7ᵗʰ **M1A.29** Drug-induced chronic gout, **multiple sites**

√5ᵗʰ **M1A.3** Chronic gout **due to renal impairment**
Code first associated renal disease

√x7ᵗʰ **M1A.3Ø** Chronic gout due to renal impairment, ▽
unspecified site

√6ᵗʰ **M1A.31** Chronic gout due to renal impairment, **shoulder**

√7ᵗʰ **M1A.311** Chronic gout due to renal impairment,
right shoulder

√7ᵗʰ **M1A.312** Chronic gout due to renal impairment, **left**
shoulder

√7ᵗʰ **M1A.319** Chronic gout due to renal impairment, ▽
unspecified shoulder

√6ᵗʰ **M1A.32** Chronic gout due to renal impairment, **elbow**

√7ᵗʰ **M1A.321** Chronic gout due to renal impairment,
right elbow

√7ᵗʰ **M1A.322** Chronic gout due to renal impairment, **left**
elbow

√7ᵗʰ **M1A.329** Chronic gout due to renal impairment, ▽
unspecified elbow

√6ᵗʰ **M1A.33** Chronic gout due to renal impairment, **wrist**

√7ᵗʰ **M1A.331** Chronic gout due to renal impairment,
right wrist

√7ᵗʰ **M1A.332** Chronic gout due to renal impairment,
left wrist

√7ᵗʰ **M1A.339** Chronic gout due to renal impairment, ▽
unspecified wrist

√6ᵗʰ **M1A.34** Chronic gout due to renal impairment, **hand**

√7ᵗʰ **M1A.341** Chronic gout due to renal impairment,
right hand

√7ᵗʰ **M1A.342** Chronic gout due to renal impairment,
left hand

√7ᵗʰ **M1A.349** Chronic gout due to renal impairment, ▽
unspecified hand

√6ᵗʰ **M1A.35** Chronic gout due to renal impairment, **hip**

√7ᵗʰ **M1A.351** Chronic gout due to renal impairment,
right hip

√7ᵗʰ **M1A.352** Chronic gout due to renal impairment,
left hip

√7ᵗʰ **M1A.359** Chronic gout due to renal impairment, ▽
unspecified hip

√6ᵗʰ **M1A.36** Chronic gout due to renal impairment, **knee**

√7ᵗʰ **M1A.361** Chronic gout due to renal impairment,
right knee

√7ᵗʰ **M1A.362** Chronic gout due to renal impairment,
left knee

√7ᵗʰ **M1A.369** Chronic gout due to renal impairment, ▽
unspecified knee

√6ᵗʰ **M1A.37** Chronic gout due to renal impairment, **ankle and
foot**

√7ᵗʰ **M1A.371** Chronic gout due to renal impairment,
right ankle and foot

√7ᵗʰ **M1A.372** Chronic gout due to renal impairment,
left ankle and foot

√7ᵗʰ **M1A.379** Chronic gout due to renal impairment, ▽
unspecified ankle and foot

√x7ᵗʰ **M1A.38** Chronic gout due to renal impairment, **vertebrae**

√x7ᵗʰ **M1A.39** Chronic gout due to renal impairment, **multiple sites**

EXCLUDES 1 Not coded here   **EXCLUDES 2** Not included here   **N** Newborn Age: 0   **P** Pediatric Age: 0-17   **M** Maternity Age: 12-55   **A** Adult Age: 15-124

730   ICD-10-CM 2018

✓5ᵗʰ **M1A.4** **Other secondary chronic gout**
      Code first associated condition

  ✓×7ᵗʰ **M1A.40** Other secondary chronic gout, unspecified site ▽

  ✓6ᵗʰ **M1A.41** Other secondary chronic gout, **shoulder**
    ✓7ᵗʰ **M1A.411** Other secondary chronic gout, **right shoulder**
    ✓7ᵗʰ **M1A.412** Other secondary chronic gout, **left shoulder**
    ✓7ᵗʰ **M1A.419** Other secondary chronic gout, unspecified shoulder ▽

  ✓6ᵗʰ **M1A.42** Other secondary chronic gout, **elbow**
    ✓7ᵗʰ **M1A.421** Other secondary chronic gout, **right** elbow
    ✓7ᵗʰ **M1A.422** Other secondary chronic gout, **left** elbow
    ✓7ᵗʰ **M1A.429** Other secondary chronic gout, unspecified elbow ▽

  ✓6ᵗʰ **M1A.43** Other secondary chronic gout, **wrist**
    ✓7ᵗʰ **M1A.431** Other secondary chronic gout, **right** wrist
    ✓7ᵗʰ **M1A.432** Other secondary chronic gout, **left** wrist
    ✓7ᵗʰ **M1A.439** Other secondary chronic gout, unspecified wrist ▽

  ✓6ᵗʰ **M1A.44** Other secondary chronic gout, **hand**
    ✓7ᵗʰ **M1A.441** Other secondary chronic gout, **right** hand
    ✓7ᵗʰ **M1A.442** Other secondary chronic gout, **left** hand
    ✓7ᵗʰ **M1A.449** Other secondary chronic gout, unspecified hand ▽

  ✓6ᵗʰ **M1A.45** Other secondary chronic gout, **hip**
    ✓7ᵗʰ **M1A.451** Other secondary chronic gout, **right** hip
    ✓7ᵗʰ **M1A.452** Other secondary chronic gout, **left** hip
    ✓7ᵗʰ **M1A.459** Other secondary chronic gout, unspecified hip ▽

  ✓6ᵗʰ **M1A.46** Other secondary chronic gout, **knee**
    ✓7ᵗʰ **M1A.461** Other secondary chronic gout, **right** knee
    ✓7ᵗʰ **M1A.462** Other secondary chronic gout, **left** knee
    ✓7ᵗʰ **M1A.469** Other secondary chronic gout, unspecified knee ▽

  ✓6ᵗʰ **M1A.47** Other secondary chronic gout, **ankle and foot**
    ✓7ᵗʰ **M1A.471** Other secondary chronic gout, **right** ankle and foot
    ✓7ᵗʰ **M1A.472** Other secondary chronic gout, **left** ankle and foot
    ✓7ᵗʰ **M1A.479** Other secondary chronic gout, unspecified ankle and foot ▽

  ✓×7ᵗʰ **M1A.48** Other secondary chronic gout, **vertebrae**
  ✓×7ᵗʰ **M1A.49** Other secondary chronic gout, **multiple sites**

✓×7ᵗʰ **M1A.9** **Chronic gout, unspecified** ▽

✓4ᵗʰ **M10** **Gout**
    Acute gout   Gout flare
    Gout attack   Podagra
    Use additional code to identify:
      autonomic neuropathy in diseases classified elsewhere (G99.0)
      calculus of urinary tract in diseases classified elsewhere (N22)
      cardiomyopathy in diseases classified elsewhere (I43)
      disorders of external ear in diseases classified elsewhere (H61.1-, H62.8-)
      disorders of iris and ciliary body in diseases classified elsewhere (H22)
      glomerular disorders in diseases classified elsewhere (N08)
    EXCLUDES 2 chronic gout (M1A.-)
    DEF: Purine and pyrimidine metabolic disorders; manifested by hyperuricemia and recurrent acute inflammatory arthritis; monosodium urate or monohydrate crystals may be deposited in and around the joints, leading to joint destruction and severe crippling.

  ✓5ᵗʰ **M10.0** **Idiopathic gout**
    Gouty bursitis
    Primary gout

    M10.00 Idiopathic gout, unspecified site ▽

  ✓6ᵗʰ **M10.01** Idiopathic gout, **shoulder**
    M10.011 Idiopathic gout, **right** shoulder
    M10.012 Idiopathic gout, **left** shoulder
    M10.019 Idiopathic gout, unspecified shoulder ▽

  ✓6ᵗʰ **M10.02** Idiopathic gout, **elbow**
    M10.021 Idiopathic gout, **right** elbow
    M10.022 Idiopathic gout, **left** elbow
    M10.029 Idiopathic gout, unspecified elbow ▽

  ✓6ᵗʰ **M10.03** Idiopathic gout, **wrist**
    M10.031 Idiopathic gout, **right wrist**
    M10.032 Idiopathic gout, **left wrist**
    M10.039 Idiopathic gout, **unspecified wrist** ▽

  ✓6ᵗʰ **M10.04** Idiopathic gout, **hand**
    M10.041 Idiopathic gout, **right hand**
    M10.042 Idiopathic gout, **left hand**
    M10.049 Idiopathic gout, **unspecified hand** ▽

  ✓6ᵗʰ **M10.05** Idiopathic gout, **hip**
    M10.051 Idiopathic gout, **right hip**
    M10.052 Idiopathic gout, **left hip**
    M10.059 Idiopathic gout, **unspecified hip** ▽

  ✓6ᵗʰ **M10.06** Idiopathic gout, **knee**
    M10.061 Idiopathic gout, **right knee**
    M10.062 Idiopathic gout, **left knee**
    M10.069 Idiopathic gout, **unspecified knee** ▽

  ✓6ᵗʰ **M10.07** Idiopathic gout, **ankle and foot**
    M10.071 Idiopathic gout, **right ankle and foot**
    M10.072 Idiopathic gout, **left ankle and foot**
    M10.079 Idiopathic gout, **unspecified ankle and foot** ▽

    M10.08 Idiopathic gout, **vertebrae**
    M10.09 Idiopathic gout, **multiple sites**

  ✓5ᵗʰ **M10.1** **Lead-induced gout**
    Code first toxic effects of lead and its compounds (T56.0-)

    M10.10 Lead-induced gout, unspecified site ▽

  ✓6ᵗʰ **M10.11** Lead-induced gout, **shoulder**
    M10.111 Lead-induced gout, **right shoulder**
    M10.112 Lead-induced gout, **left shoulder**
    M10.119 Lead-induced gout, unspecified shoulder ▽

  ✓6ᵗʰ **M10.12** Lead-induced gout, **elbow**
    M10.121 Lead-induced gout, **right elbow**
    M10.122 Lead-induced gout, **left elbow**
    M10.129 Lead-induced gout, **unspecified elbow** ▽

  ✓6ᵗʰ **M10.13** Lead-induced gout, **wrist**
    M10.131 Lead-induced gout, **right wrist**
    M10.132 Lead-induced gout, **left wrist**
    M10.139 Lead-induced gout, **unspecified wrist** ▽

  ✓6ᵗʰ **M10.14** Lead-induced gout, **hand**
    M10.141 Lead-induced gout, **right hand**
    M10.142 Lead-induced gout, **left hand**
    M10.149 Lead-induced gout, **unspecified hand** ▽

  ✓6ᵗʰ **M10.15** Lead-induced gout, **hip**
    M10.151 Lead-induced gout, **right hip**
    M10.152 Lead-induced gout, **left hip**
    M10.159 Lead-induced gout, **unspecified hip** ▽

  ✓6ᵗʰ **M10.16** Lead-induced gout, **knee**
    M10.161 Lead-induced gout, **right knee**
    M10.162 Lead-induced gout, **left knee**
    M10.169 Lead-induced gout, **unspecified knee** ▽

  ✓6ᵗʰ **M10.17** Lead-induced gout, **ankle and foot**
    M10.171 Lead-induced gout, **right ankle and foot**
    M10.172 Lead-induced gout, **left ankle and foot**
    M10.179 Lead-induced gout, **unspecified ankle and foot** ▽

    M10.18 Lead-induced gout, **vertebrae**
    M10.19 Lead-induced gout, **multiple sites**

  ✓5ᵗʰ **M10.2** **Drug-induced gout**
    Use additional code for adverse effect, if applicable, to identify drug (T36-T50 with fifth or sixth character 5)

    M10.20 Drug-induced gout, unspecified site ▽

  ✓6ᵗʰ **M10.21** Drug-induced gout, **shoulder**
    M10.211 Drug-induced gout, **right shoulder**
    M10.212 Drug-induced gout, **left shoulder**
    M10.219 Drug-induced gout, unspecified shoulder ▽

  ✓6ᵗʰ **M10.22** Drug-induced gout, **elbow**
    M10.221 Drug-induced gout, **right elbow**
    M10.222 Drug-induced gout, **left elbow**
    M10.229 Drug-induced gout, unspecified elbow ▽

✓ Additional Character Req   ✓×7ᵗʰ Placeholder Alert   Manifestation   HCC CMS-HCC Condition   ▽ Unspecified Code   ►◄ Revised Text   ● New Code   ▲ Revised Code Title

✓6ᵗʰ **M10.23 Drug-induced gout, wrist**
- M10.231 Drug-induced gout, **right** wrist
- M10.232 Drug-induced gout, **left** wrist
- M10.239 Drug-induced gout, unspecified wrist ▽

✓6ᵗʰ **M10.24 Drug-induced gout, hand**
- M10.241 Drug-induced gout, **right** hand
- M10.242 Drug-induced gout, **left** hand
- M10.249 Drug-induced gout, unspecified hand ▽

✓6ᵗʰ **M10.25 Drug-induced gout, hip**
- M10.251 Drug-induced gout, **right** hip
- M10.252 Drug-induced gout, **left** hip
- M10.259 Drug-induced gout, unspecified hip ▽

✓6ᵗʰ **M10.26 Drug-induced gout, knee**
- M10.261 Drug-induced gout, **right** knee
- M10.262 Drug-induced gout, **left** knee
- M10.269 Drug-induced gout, unspecified knee ▽

✓6ᵗʰ **M10.27 Drug-induced gout, ankle and foot**
- M10.271 Drug-induced gout, **right** ankle and foot
- M10.272 Drug-induced gout, **left** ankle and foot
- M10.279 Drug-induced gout, unspecified ankle and foot ▽

M10.28 Drug-induced gout, vertebrae

M10.29 Drug-induced gout, multiple sites

✓5ᵗʰ **M10.3 Gout due to renal impairment**
Code first associated renal disease
- **M10.30 Gout due to renal impairment, unspecified site** ▽

✓6ᵗʰ **M10.31 Gout due to renal impairment, shoulder**
- M10.311 Gout due to renal impairment, **right** shoulder
- M10.312 Gout due to renal impairment, **left** shoulder
- M10.319 Gout due to renal impairment, unspecified shoulder ▽

✓6ᵗʰ **M10.32 Gout due to renal impairment, elbow**
- M10.321 Gout due to renal impairment, **right** elbow
- M10.322 Gout due to renal impairment, **left** elbow
- M10.329 Gout due to renal impairment, unspecified elbow ▽

✓6ᵗʰ **M10.33 Gout due to renal impairment, wrist**
- M10.331 Gout due to renal impairment, **right** wrist
- M10.332 Gout due to renal impairment, **left** wrist
- M10.339 Gout due to renal impairment, unspecified wrist ▽

✓6ᵗʰ **M10.34 Gout due to renal impairment, hand**
- M10.341 Gout due to renal impairment, **right** hand
- M10.342 Gout due to renal impairment, **left** hand
- M10.349 Gout due to renal impairment, unspecified hand ▽

✓6ᵗʰ **M10.35 Gout due to renal impairment, hip**
- M10.351 Gout due to renal impairment, **right** hip
- M10.352 Gout due to renal impairment, **left** hip
- M10.359 Gout due to renal impairment, unspecified hip ▽

✓6ᵗʰ **M10.36 Gout due to renal impairment, knee**
- M10.361 Gout due to renal impairment, **right** knee
- M10.362 Gout due to renal impairment, **left** knee
- M10.369 Gout due to renal impairment, unspecified knee ▽

✓6ᵗʰ **M10.37 Gout due to renal impairment, ankle and foot**
- M10.371 Gout due to renal impairment, **right** ankle and foot
- M10.372 Gout due to renal impairment, **left** ankle and foot
- M10.379 Gout due to renal impairment, unspecified ankle and foot ▽

M10.38 Gout due to renal impairment, vertebrae

M10.39 Gout due to renal impairment, multiple sites

✓5ᵗʰ **M10.4 Other secondary gout**
Code first associated condition
- **M10.40 Other secondary gout, unspecified site** ▽

✓6ᵗʰ **M10.41 Other secondary gout, shoulder**
- M10.411 Other secondary gout, **right** shoulder
- M10.412 Other secondary gout, **left** shoulder
- M10.419 Other secondary gout, unspecified shoulder ▽

✓6ᵗʰ **M10.42 Other secondary gout, elbow**
- M10.421 Other secondary gout, **right** elbow
- M10.422 Other secondary gout, **left** elbow
- M10.429 Other secondary gout, unspecified elbow ▽

✓6ᵗʰ **M10.43 Other secondary gout, wrist**
- M10.431 Other secondary gout, **right** wrist
- M10.432 Other secondary gout, **left** wrist
- M10.439 Other secondary gout, unspecified wrist ▽

✓6ᵗʰ **M10.44 Other secondary gout, hand**
- M10.441 Other secondary gout, **right** hand
- M10.442 Other secondary gout, **left** hand
- M10.449 Other secondary gout, unspecified hand ▽

✓6ᵗʰ **M10.45 Other secondary gout, hip**
- M10.451 Other secondary gout, **right** hip
- M10.452 Other secondary gout, **left** hip
- M10.459 Other secondary gout, unspecified hip ▽

✓6ᵗʰ **M10.46 Other secondary gout, knee**
- M10.461 Other secondary gout, **right** knee
- M10.462 Other secondary gout, **left** knee
- M10.469 Other secondary gout, unspecified knee ▽

✓6ᵗʰ **M10.47 Other secondary gout, ankle and foot**
- M10.471 Other secondary gout, **right** ankle and foot
- M10.472 Other secondary gout, **left** ankle and foot
- M10.479 Other secondary gout, unspecified ankle and foot ▽

M10.48 Other secondary gout, vertebrae

M10.49 Other secondary gout, multiple sites

M10.9 Gout, unspecified ▽
Gout NOS

✓4ᵗʰ **M11 Other crystal arthropathies**

✓5ᵗʰ **M11.0 Hydroxyapatite deposition disease**
- **M11.00 Hydroxyapatite deposition disease, unspecified site** ▽

✓6ᵗʰ **M11.01 Hydroxyapatite deposition disease, shoulder**
- M11.011 Hydroxyapatite deposition disease, **right** shoulder
- M11.012 Hydroxyapatite deposition disease, **left** shoulder
- M11.019 Hydroxyapatite deposition disease, unspecified shoulder ▽

✓6ᵗʰ **M11.02 Hydroxyapatite deposition disease, elbow**
- M11.021 Hydroxyapatite deposition disease, **right** elbow
- M11.022 Hydroxyapatite deposition disease, **left** elbow
- M11.029 Hydroxyapatite deposition disease, unspecified elbow ▽

✓6ᵗʰ **M11.03 Hydroxyapatite deposition disease, wrist**
- M11.031 Hydroxyapatite deposition disease, **right** wrist
- M11.032 Hydroxyapatite deposition disease, **left** wrist
- M11.039 Hydroxyapatite deposition disease, unspecified wrist ▽

✓6ᵗʰ **M11.04 Hydroxyapatite deposition disease, hand**
- M11.041 Hydroxyapatite deposition disease, **right** hand
- M11.042 Hydroxyapatite deposition disease, **left** hand
- M11.049 Hydroxyapatite deposition disease, unspecified hand ▽

✓6ᵗʰ **M11.05 Hydroxyapatite deposition disease, hip**
- M11.051 Hydroxyapatite deposition disease, **right** hip
- M11.052 Hydroxyapatite deposition disease, **left** hip
- M11.059 Hydroxyapatite deposition disease, unspecified hip ▽

EXCLUDES 1 Not coded here   **EXCLUDES 2** Not included here   **N** Newborn Age: 0   **P** Pediatric Age: 0-17   **M** Maternity Age: 12-55   **A** Adult Age: 15-124

732   ICD-10-CM 2018

√6ᵗʰ **M11.06 Hydroxyapatite deposition disease, knee**
    M11.061 Hydroxyapatite deposition disease, **right knee**
    M11.062 Hydroxyapatite deposition disease, **left knee**
    M11.069 Hydroxyapatite deposition disease, unspecified knee ▽

√6ᵗʰ **M11.07 Hydroxyapatite deposition disease, ankle and foot**
    M11.071 Hydroxyapatite deposition disease, **right ankle and foot**
    M11.072 Hydroxyapatite deposition disease, **left ankle and foot**
    M11.079 Hydroxyapatite deposition disease, unspecified ankle and foot ▽

    M11.08 Hydroxyapatite deposition disease, **vertebrae**
    M11.09 Hydroxyapatite deposition disease, **multiple sites**

√5ᵗʰ **M11.1 Familial chondrocalcinosis**
    M11.10 Familial chondrocalcinosis, unspecified site ▽

√6ᵗʰ **M11.11 Familial chondrocalcinosis, shoulder**
    M11.111 Familial chondrocalcinosis, **right shoulder**
    M11.112 Familial chondrocalcinosis, **left shoulder**
    M11.119 Familial chondrocalcinosis, unspecified shoulder ▽

√6ᵗʰ **M11.12 Familial chondrocalcinosis, elbow**
    M11.121 Familial chondrocalcinosis, **right elbow**
    M11.122 Familial chondrocalcinosis, **left elbow**
    M11.129 Familial chondrocalcinosis, unspecified elbow ▽

√6ᵗʰ **M11.13 Familial chondrocalcinosis, wrist**
    M11.131 Familial chondrocalcinosis, **right wrist**
    M11.132 Familial chondrocalcinosis, **left wrist**
    M11.139 Familial chondrocalcinosis, unspecified wrist ▽

√6ᵗʰ **M11.14 Familial chondrocalcinosis, hand**
    M11.141 Familial chondrocalcinosis, **right hand**
    M11.142 Familial chondrocalcinosis, **left hand**
    M11.149 Familial chondrocalcinosis, unspecified hand ▽

√6ᵗʰ **M11.15 Familial chondrocalcinosis, hip**
    M11.151 Familial chondrocalcinosis, **right hip**
    M11.152 Familial chondrocalcinosis, **left hip**
    M11.159 Familial chondrocalcinosis, unspecified hip ▽

√6ᵗʰ **M11.16 Familial chondrocalcinosis, knee**
    M11.161 Familial chondrocalcinosis, **right knee**
    M11.162 Familial chondrocalcinosis, **left knee**
    M11.169 Familial chondrocalcinosis, unspecified knee ▽

√6ᵗʰ **M11.17 Familial chondrocalcinosis, ankle and foot**
    M11.171 Familial chondrocalcinosis, **right ankle and foot**
    M11.172 Familial chondrocalcinosis, **left ankle and foot**
    M11.179 Familial chondrocalcinosis, unspecified ankle and foot ▽

    M11.18 Familial chondrocalcinosis, **vertebrae**
    M11.19 Familial chondrocalcinosis, **multiple sites**

√5ᵗʰ **M11.2 Other chondrocalcinosis**
    Chondrocalcinosis NOS
    M11.20 Other chondrocalcinosis, unspecified site ▽

√6ᵗʰ **M11.21 Other chondrocalcinosis, shoulder**
    M11.211 Other chondrocalcinosis, **right shoulder**
    M11.212 Other chondrocalcinosis, **left shoulder**
    M11.219 Other chondrocalcinosis, unspecified shoulder ▽

√6ᵗʰ **M11.22 Other chondrocalcinosis, elbow**
    M11.221 Other chondrocalcinosis, **right elbow**
    M11.222 Other chondrocalcinosis, **left elbow**
    M11.229 Other chondrocalcinosis, unspecified elbow ▽

√6ᵗʰ **M11.23 Other chondrocalcinosis, wrist**
    M11.231 Other chondrocalcinosis, **right wrist**
    M11.232 Other chondrocalcinosis, **left wrist**

    M11.239 Other chondrocalcinosis, unspecified wrist ▽

√6ᵗʰ **M11.24 Other chondrocalcinosis, hand**
    M11.241 Other chondrocalcinosis, **right hand**
    M11.242 Other chondrocalcinosis, **left hand**
    M11.249 Other chondrocalcinosis, unspecified hand ▽

√6ᵗʰ **M11.25 Other chondrocalcinosis, hip**
    M11.251 Other chondrocalcinosis, **right hip**
    M11.252 Other chondrocalcinosis, **left hip**
    M11.259 Other chondrocalcinosis, unspecified hip ▽

√6ᵗʰ **M11.26 Other chondrocalcinosis, knee**
    M11.261 Other chondrocalcinosis, **right knee**
    M11.262 Other chondrocalcinosis, **left knee**
    M11.269 Other chondrocalcinosis, unspecified knee ▽

√6ᵗʰ **M11.27 Other chondrocalcinosis, ankle and foot**
    M11.271 Other chondrocalcinosis, **right ankle and foot**
    M11.272 Other chondrocalcinosis, **left ankle and foot**
    M11.279 Other chondrocalcinosis, unspecified ankle and foot ▽

    M11.28 Other chondrocalcinosis, **vertebrae**
    M11.29 Other chondrocalcinosis, **multiple sites**

√5ᵗʰ **M11.8 Other specified crystal arthropathies**
    M11.80 Other specified crystal arthropathies, unspecified site ▽

√6ᵗʰ **M11.81 Other specified crystal arthropathies, shoulder**
    M11.811 Other specified crystal arthropathies, **right shoulder**
    M11.812 Other specified crystal arthropathies, left shoulder
    M11.819 Other specified crystal arthropathies, unspecified shoulder ▽

√6ᵗʰ **M11.82 Other specified crystal arthropathies, elbow**
    M11.821 Other specified crystal arthropathies, **right elbow**
    M11.822 Other specified crystal arthropathies, **left elbow**
    M11.829 Other specified crystal arthropathies, unspecified elbow ▽

√6ᵗʰ **M11.83 Other specified crystal arthropathies, wrist**
    M11.831 Other specified crystal arthropathies, **right wrist**
    M11.832 Other specified crystal arthropathies, **left wrist**
    M11.839 Other specified crystal arthropathies, unspecified wrist ▽

√6ᵗʰ **M11.84 Other specified crystal arthropathies, hand**
    M11.841 Other specified crystal arthropathies, **right hand**
    M11.842 Other specified crystal arthropathies, **left hand**
    M11.849 Other specified crystal arthropathies, unspecified hand ▽

√6ᵗʰ **M11.85 Other specified crystal arthropathies, hip**
    M11.851 Other specified crystal arthropathies, **right hip**
    M11.852 Other specified crystal arthropathies, **left hip**
    M11.859 Other specified crystal arthropathies, unspecified hip ▽

√6ᵗʰ **M11.86 Other specified crystal arthropathies, knee**
    M11.861 Other specified crystal arthropathies, **right knee**
    M11.862 Other specified crystal arthropathies, **left knee**
    M11.869 Other specified crystal arthropathies, unspecified knee ▽

√6ᵗʰ **M11.87 Other specified crystal arthropathies, ankle and foot**
    M11.871 Other specified crystal arthropathies, **right ankle and foot**
    M11.872 Other specified crystal arthropathies, left ankle and foot

---

☑ Additional Character Req   ✓X7ᵗʰ Placeholder Alert   Manifestation   HCC CMS-HCC Condition   ▽ Unspecified Code   ▶◀ Revised Text   ● New Code   ▲ Revised Code Title

      M11.879 Other specified crystal arthropathies, unspecified ankle and foot ▽

    M11.88 Other specified crystal arthropathies, vertebrae

    M11.89 Other specified crystal arthropathies, multiple sites

  M11.9 Crystal arthropathy, unspecified ▽

✓4ᵗʰ **M12** **Other and unspecified arthropathy**

    EXCLUDES 1   arthrosis (M15-M19)
                  cricoarytenoid arthropathy (J38.7)

  ✓5ᵗʰ **M12.0** Chronic postrheumatic arthropathy [Jaccoud]

      M12.00 Chronic postrheumatic arthropathy [Jaccoud], HCC ▽ unspecified site

    ✓6ᵗʰ **M12.01** Chronic postrheumatic arthropathy [Jaccoud], shoulder

        M12.011 Chronic postrheumatic arthropathy [Jaccoud], **right shoulder** HCC

        M12.012 Chronic postrheumatic arthropathy [Jaccoud], **left shoulder** HCC

        M12.019 Chronic postrheumatic arthropathy HCC ▽ [Jaccoud], unspecified shoulder

    ✓6ᵗʰ **M12.02** Chronic postrheumatic arthropathy [Jaccoud], elbow

        M12.021 Chronic postrheumatic arthropathy [Jaccoud], **right elbow** HCC

        M12.022 Chronic postrheumatic arthropathy [Jaccoud], **left elbow** HCC

        M12.029 Chronic postrheumatic arthropathy HCC ▽ [Jaccoud], unspecified elbow

    ✓6ᵗʰ **M12.03** Chronic postrheumatic arthropathy [Jaccoud], wrist

        M12.031 Chronic postrheumatic arthropathy [Jaccoud], **right wrist** HCC

        M12.032 Chronic postrheumatic arthropathy [Jaccoud], **left wrist** HCC

        M12.039 Chronic postrheumatic arthropathy HCC ▽ [Jaccoud], unspecified wrist

    ✓6ᵗʰ **M12.04** Chronic postrheumatic arthropathy [Jaccoud], hand

        M12.041 Chronic postrheumatic arthropathy [Jaccoud], **right hand** HCC

        M12.042 Chronic postrheumatic arthropathy [Jaccoud], **left hand** HCC

        M12.049 Chronic postrheumatic arthropathy HCC ▽ [Jaccoud], unspecified hand

    ✓6ᵗʰ **M12.05** Chronic postrheumatic arthropathy [Jaccoud], hip

        M12.051 Chronic postrheumatic arthropathy [Jaccoud], **right hip** HCC

        M12.052 Chronic postrheumatic arthropathy [Jaccoud], **left hip** HCC

        M12.059 Chronic postrheumatic arthropathy HCC ▽ [Jaccoud], unspecified hip

    ✓6ᵗʰ **M12.06** Chronic postrheumatic arthropathy [Jaccoud], knee

        M12.061 Chronic postrheumatic arthropathy [Jaccoud], **right knee** HCC

        M12.062 Chronic postrheumatic arthropathy [Jaccoud], **left knee** HCC

        M12.069 Chronic postrheumatic arthropathy HCC ▽ [Jaccoud], unspecified knee

    ✓6ᵗʰ **M12.07** Chronic postrheumatic arthropathy [Jaccoud], ankle and foot

        M12.071 Chronic postrheumatic arthropathy [Jaccoud], **right ankle and foot** HCC

        M12.072 Chronic postrheumatic arthropathy [Jaccoud], **left ankle and foot** HCC

        M12.079 Chronic postrheumatic arthropathy HCC ▽ [Jaccoud], unspecified ankle and foot

      M12.08 Chronic postrheumatic arthropathy [Jaccoud], HCC other specified site

        Chronic postrheumatic arthropathy [Jaccoud], vertebrae

      M12.09 Chronic postrheumatic arthropathy [Jaccoud], HCC multiple sites

  ✓5ᵗʰ **M12.1** Kaschin-Beck disease

      Osteochondroarthrosis deformans endemica

    M12.10 Kaschin-Beck disease, unspecified site ▽

    ✓6ᵗʰ **M12.11** Kaschin-Beck disease, shoulder

        M12.111 Kaschin-Beck disease, **right shoulder**

        M12.112 Kaschin-Beck disease, **left shoulder**

        M12.119 Kaschin-Beck disease, unspecified ▽ shoulder

    ✓6ᵗʰ **M12.12** Kaschin-Beck disease, elbow

        M12.121 Kaschin-Beck disease, **right elbow**

        M12.122 Kaschin-Beck disease, **left elbow**

        M12.129 Kaschin-Beck disease, unspecified ▽ elbow

    ✓6ᵗʰ **M12.13** Kaschin-Beck disease, wrist

        M12.131 Kaschin-Beck disease, **right wrist**

        M12.132 Kaschin-Beck disease, **left wrist**

        M12.139 Kaschin-Beck disease, unspecified wrist ▽

    ✓6ᵗʰ **M12.14** Kaschin-Beck disease, hand

        M12.141 Kaschin-Beck disease, **right hand**

        M12.142 Kaschin-Beck disease, **left hand**

        M12.149 Kaschin-Beck disease, unspecified hand ▽

    ✓6ᵗʰ **M12.15** Kaschin-Beck disease, hip

        M12.151 Kaschin-Beck disease, **right hip**

        M12.152 Kaschin-Beck disease, **left hip**

        M12.159 Kaschin-Beck disease, unspecified hip ▽

    ✓6ᵗʰ **M12.16** Kaschin-Beck disease, knee

        M12.161 Kaschin-Beck disease, **right knee**

        M12.162 Kaschin-Beck disease, **left knee**

        M12.169 Kaschin-Beck disease, unspecified ▽ knee

    ✓6ᵗʰ **M12.17** Kaschin-Beck disease, ankle and foot

        M12.171 Kaschin-Beck disease, **right ankle and foot**

        M12.172 Kaschin-Beck disease, **left ankle and foot**

        M12.179 Kaschin-Beck disease, unspecified a ▽ nkle and foot

    M12.18 Kaschin-Beck disease, vertebrae

    M12.19 Kaschin-Beck disease, multiple sites

  ✓5ᵗʰ **M12.2** Villonodular synovitis (pigmented)

    M12.20 Villonodular synovitis (pigmented), unspecified ▽ site

    ✓6ᵗʰ **M12.21** Villonodular synovitis (pigmented), shoulder

        M12.211 Villonodular synovitis (pigmented), right shoulder

        M12.212 Villonodular synovitis (pigmented), left shoulder

        M12.219 Villonodular synovitis (pigmented), ▽ unspecified shoulder

    ✓6ᵗʰ **M12.22** Villonodular synovitis (pigmented), elbow

        M12.221 Villonodular synovitis (pigmented), right elbow

        M12.222 Villonodular synovitis (pigmented), left elbow

        M12.229 Villonodular synovitis (pigmented), ▽ unspecified elbow

    ✓6ᵗʰ **M12.23** Villonodular synovitis (pigmented), wrist

        M12.231 Villonodular synovitis (pigmented), right wrist

        M12.232 Villonodular synovitis (pigmented), left wrist

        M12.239 Villonodular synovitis (pigmented), ▽ unspecified wrist

    ✓6ᵗʰ **M12.24** Villonodular synovitis (pigmented), hand

        M12.241 Villonodular synovitis (pigmented), right hand

        M12.242 Villonodular synovitis (pigmented), left hand

        M12.249 Villonodular synovitis (pigmented), ▽ unspecified hand

    ✓6ᵗʰ **M12.25** Villonodular synovitis (pigmented), hip

        M12.251 Villonodular synovitis (pigmented), right hip

        M12.252 Villonodular synovitis (pigmented), left hip

        M12.259 Villonodular synovitis (pigmented), ▽ unspecified hip

    ✓6ᵗʰ **M12.26** Villonodular synovitis (pigmented), knee

        M12.261 Villonodular synovitis (pigmented), right knee

        M12.262 Villonodular synovitis (pigmented), left knee

        M12.269 Villonodular synovitis (pigmented), ▽ unspecified knee

---

EXCLUDES 1 Not coded here   EXCLUDES 2 Not included here   N Newborn Age: 0   P Pediatric Age: 0-17   M Maternity Age: 12-55   A Adult Age: 15-124

✓6ᵗʰ **M12.27 Villonodular synovitis (pigmented), ankle and foot**

 M12.271 Villonodular synovitis (pigmented), **right ankle and foot**

 M12.272 Villonodular synovitis (pigmented), **left ankle and foot**

 M12.279 Villonodular synovitis (pigmented), unspecified ankle and foot ▽

M12.28 Villonodular synovitis (pigmented), other specified site
 Villonodular synovitis (pigmented), vertebrae

M12.29 Villonodular synovitis (pigmented), multiple sites

✓5ᵗʰ **M12.3 Palindromic rheumatism**

M12.30 Palindromic rheumatism, unspecified site ▽

✓6ᵗʰ **M12.31 Palindromic rheumatism, shoulder**

 M12.311 Palindromic rheumatism, **right shoulder**

 M12.312 Palindromic rheumatism, **left shoulder**

 M12.319 Palindromic rheumatism, unspecified shoulder ▽

✓6ᵗʰ **M12.32 Palindromic rheumatism, elbow**

 M12.321 Palindromic rheumatism, **right elbow**

 M12.322 Palindromic rheumatism, **left elbow**

 M12.329 Palindromic rheumatism, unspecified elbow ▽

✓6ᵗʰ **M12.33 Palindromic rheumatism, wrist**

 M12.331 Palindromic rheumatism, **right wrist**

 M12.332 Palindromic rheumatism, **left wrist**

 M12.339 Palindromic rheumatism, unspecified wrist ▽

✓6ᵗʰ **M12.34 Palindromic rheumatism, hand**

 M12.341 Palindromic rheumatism, **right hand**

 M12.342 Palindromic rheumatism, **left hand**

 M12.349 Palindromic rheumatism, unspecified hand ▽

✓6ᵗʰ **M12.35 Palindromic rheumatism, hip**

 M12.351 Palindromic rheumatism, **right hip**

 M12.352 Palindromic rheumatism, **left hip**

 M12.359 Palindromic rheumatism, unspecified hip ▽

✓6ᵗʰ **M12.36 Palindromic rheumatism, knee**

 M12.361 Palindromic rheumatism, **right knee**

 M12.362 Palindromic rheumatism, **left knee**

 M12.369 Palindromic rheumatism, unspecified knee ▽

✓6ᵗʰ **M12.37 Palindromic rheumatism, ankle and foot**

 M12.371 Palindromic rheumatism, **right ankle and foot**

 M12.372 Palindromic rheumatism, **left ankle and foot**

 M12.379 Palindromic rheumatism, unspecified ankle and foot ▽

M12.38 Palindromic rheumatism, other specified site
 Palindromic rheumatism, vertebrae

M12.39 Palindromic rheumatism, multiple sites

✓5ᵗʰ **M12.4 Intermittent hydrarthrosis**

M12.40 Intermittent hydrarthrosis, unspecified site ▽

✓6ᵗʰ **M12.41 Intermittent hydrarthrosis, shoulder**

 M12.411 Intermittent hydrarthrosis, **right shoulder**

 M12.412 Intermittent hydrarthrosis, **left shoulder**

 M12.419 Intermittent hydrarthrosis, unspecified shoulder ▽

✓6ᵗʰ **M12.42 Intermittent hydrarthrosis, elbow**

 M12.421 Intermittent hydrarthrosis, **right elbow**

 M12.422 Intermittent hydrarthrosis, **left elbow**

 M12.429 Intermittent hydrarthrosis, unspecified elbow ▽

✓6ᵗʰ **M12.43 Intermittent hydrarthrosis, wrist**

 M12.431 Intermittent hydrarthrosis, **right wrist**

 M12.432 Intermittent hydrarthrosis, **left wrist**

 M12.439 Intermittent hydrarthrosis, unspecified wrist ▽

✓6ᵗʰ **M12.44 Intermittent hydrarthrosis, hand**

 M12.441 Intermittent hydrarthrosis, **right hand**

 M12.442 Intermittent hydrarthrosis, **left hand**

 M12.449 Intermittent hydrarthrosis, unspecified hand ▽

✓6ᵗʰ **M12.45 Intermittent hydrarthrosis, hip**

 M12.451 Intermittent hydrarthrosis, **right hip**

 M12.452 Intermittent hydrarthrosis, **left hip**

 M12.459 Intermittent hydrarthrosis, unspecified hip ▽

✓6ᵗʰ **M12.46 Intermittent hydrarthrosis, knee**

 M12.461 Intermittent hydrarthrosis, **right knee**

 M12.462 Intermittent hydrarthrosis, **left knee**

 M12.469 Intermittent hydrarthrosis, unspecified knee ▽

✓6ᵗʰ **M12.47 Intermittent hydrarthrosis, ankle and foot**

 M12.471 Intermittent hydrarthrosis, **right ankle and foot**

 M12.472 Intermittent hydrarthrosis, **left ankle and foot**

 M12.479 Intermittent hydrarthrosis, unspecified ankle and foot ▽

M12.48 Intermittent hydrarthrosis, other site

M12.49 Intermittent hydrarthrosis, multiple sites

✓5ᵗʰ **M12.5 Traumatic arthropathy**

 EXCLUDES 1 *current injury-see Alphabetic Index*
  post-traumatic osteoarthritis NOS (M19.1-)
  post-traumatic osteoarthritis of first carpometacarpal joint (M18.2-M18.3)
  post-traumatic osteoarthritis of hip (M16.4-M16.5)
  post-traumatic osteoarthritis of knee (M17.2-M17.3)
  post-traumatic osteoarthritis of other single joints (M19.1-)

 AHA: 2015, 1Q, 17

M12.50 Traumatic arthropathy, unspecified site ▽

✓6ᵗʰ **M12.51 Traumatic arthropathy, shoulder**

 M12.511 Traumatic arthropathy, **right shoulder**

 M12.512 Traumatic arthropathy, **left shoulder**

 M12.519 Traumatic arthropathy, unspecified shoulder ▽

✓6ᵗʰ **M12.52 Traumatic arthropathy, elbow**

 M12.521 Traumatic arthropathy, **right elbow**

 M12.522 Traumatic arthropathy, **left elbow**

 M12.529 Traumatic arthropathy, unspecified elbow ▽

✓6ᵗʰ **M12.53 Traumatic arthropathy, wrist**

 M12.531 Traumatic arthropathy, **right wrist**

 M12.532 Traumatic arthropathy, **left wrist**

 M12.539 Traumatic arthropathy, unspecified wrist ▽

✓6ᵗʰ **M12.54 Traumatic arthropathy, hand**

 M12.541 Traumatic arthropathy, **right hand**

 M12.542 Traumatic arthropathy, **left hand**

 M12.549 Traumatic arthropathy, unspecified hand ▽

✓6ᵗʰ **M12.55 Traumatic arthropathy, hip**

 M12.551 Traumatic arthropathy, **right hip**

 M12.552 Traumatic arthropathy, **left hip**

 M12.559 Traumatic arthropathy, unspecified hip ▽

✓6ᵗʰ **M12.56 Traumatic arthropathy, knee**

 M12.561 Traumatic arthropathy, **right knee**

 M12.562 Traumatic arthropathy, **left knee**

 M12.569 Traumatic arthropathy, unspecified knee ▽

✓6ᵗʰ **M12.57 Traumatic arthropathy, ankle and foot**

 M12.571 Traumatic arthropathy, **right ankle and foot**

 M12.572 Traumatic arthropathy, **left ankle and foot**

 M12.579 Traumatic arthropathy, unspecified ankle and foot ▽

M12.58 Traumatic arthropathy, other specified site
 Traumatic arthropathy, vertebrae

M12.59 Traumatic arthropathy, multiple sites

✓5ᵗʰ **M12.8 Other specific arthropathies, not elsewhere classified**
 Transient arthropathy

M12.80 Other specific arthropathies, not elsewhere classified, unspecified site ▽

☑ Additional Character Req   ✓x7ᵗʰ Placeholder Alert   Manifestation   ʜᴄᴄ CMS-HCC Condition   ▽ Unspecified Code   ►◄ Revised Text   ● New Code   ▲ Revised Code Title

ICD-10-CM 2018   735

M12.81 Other specific arthropathies, not elsewhere classified, **shoulder**
M12.811 Other specific arthropathies, not elsewhere classified, **right**shoulder
M12.812 Other specific arthropathies, not elsewhere classified, **left**shoulder
M12.819 Other specific arthropathies, not elsewhere classified, unspecified shoulder ▽

M12.82 Other specific arthropathies, not elsewhere classified, **elbow**
M12.821 Other specific arthropathies, not elsewhere classified, **right**elbow
M12.822 Other specific arthropathies, not elsewhere classified, **left**elbow
M12.829 Other specific arthropathies, not elsewhere classified, unspecified elbow ▽

M12.83 Other specific arthropathies, not elsewhere classified, **wrist**
M12.831 Other specific arthropathies, not elsewhere classified, **right**wrist
M12.832 Other specific arthropathies, not elsewhere classified, **left**wrist
M12.839 Other specific arthropathies, not elsewhere classified, unspecified wrist ▽

M12.84 Other specific arthropathies, not elsewhere classified, **hand**
M12.841 Other specific arthropathies, not elsewhere classified, **right**hand
M12.842 Other specific arthropathies, not elsewhere classified, **left**hand
M12.849 Other specific arthropathies, not elsewhere classified, unspecified hand ▽

M12.85 Other specific arthropathies, not elsewhere classified, **hip**
M12.851 Other specific arthropathies, not elsewhere classified, **right**hip
M12.852 Other specific arthropathies, not elsewhere classified, **left**hip
M12.859 Other specific arthropathies, not elsewhere classified, unspecified hip ▽

M12.86 Other specific arthropathies, not elsewhere classified, **knee**
M12.861 Other specific arthropathies, not elsewhere classified, **right**knee
M12.862 Other specific arthropathies, not elsewhere classified, **left**knee
M12.869 Other specific arthropathies, not elsewhere classified, unspecified knee ▽

M12.87 Other specific arthropathies, not elsewhere classified, **ankle and foot**
M12.871 Other specific arthropathies, not elsewhere classified, **right**ankle and foot
M12.872 Other specific arthropathies, not elsewhere classified, **left**ankle and foot
M12.879 Other specific arthropathies, not elsewhere classified, unspecified ankle and foot ▽

M12.88 Other specific arthropathies, not elsewhere classified, other specified site
Other specific arthropathies, not elsewhere classified, vertebrae

M12.89 Other specific arthropathies, not elsewhere classified, **multiple sites**

M12.9 Arthropathy, unspecified ▽

M13 Other arthritis
EXCLUDES 1 arthrosis (M15-M19)
osteoarthritis (M15-M19)

M13.0 Polyarthritis, unspecified ▽

M13.1 Monoarthritis, not elsewhere classified
M13.10 Monoarthritis, not elsewhere classified, unspecified site ▽
M13.11 Monoarthritis, not elsewhere classified, **shoulder**
M13.111 Monoarthritis, not elsewhere classified, **right**shoulder
M13.112 Monoarthritis, not elsewhere classified, **left**shoulder

M13.119 Monoarthritis, not elsewhere classified, unspecified shoulder ▽
M13.12 Monoarthritis, not elsewhere classified, **elbow**
M13.121 Monoarthritis, not elsewhere classified, **right**elbow
M13.122 Monoarthritis, not elsewhere classified, **left**elbow
M13.129 Monoarthritis, not elsewhere classified, unspecified elbow ▽
M13.13 Monoarthritis, not elsewhere classified, **wrist**
M13.131 Monoarthritis, not elsewhere classified, **right**wrist
M13.132 Monoarthritis, not elsewhere classified, **left**wrist
M13.139 Monoarthritis, not elsewhere classified, unspecified wrist ▽
M13.14 Monoarthritis, not elsewhere classified, **hand**
M13.141 Monoarthritis, not elsewhere classified, **right**hand
M13.142 Monoarthritis, not elsewhere classified, **left**hand
M13.149 Monoarthritis, not elsewhere classified, unspecified hand ▽
M13.15 Monoarthritis, not elsewhere classified, **hip**
M13.151 Monoarthritis, not elsewhere classified, **right**hip
M13.152 Monoarthritis, not elsewhere classified, **left**hip
M13.159 Monoarthritis, not elsewhere classified, unspecified hip ▽
M13.16 Monoarthritis, not elsewhere classified, **knee**
M13.161 Monoarthritis, not elsewhere classified, **right**knee
M13.162 Monoarthritis, not elsewhere classified, **left**knee
M13.169 Monoarthritis, not elsewhere classified, unspecified knee ▽
M13.17 Monoarthritis, not elsewhere classified, **ankle and foot**
M13.171 Monoarthritis, not elsewhere classified, **right**ankle and foot
M13.172 Monoarthritis, not elsewhere classified, **left**ankle and foot
M13.179 Monoarthritis, not elsewhere classified, unspecified ankle and foot ▽

M13.8 Other specified arthritis
Allergic arthritis
EXCLUDES 1 osteoarthritis (M15-M19)
M13.80 Other specified arthritis, unspecified site ▽
M13.81 Other specified arthritis, **shoulder**
M13.811 Other specified arthritis, **right**shoulder
M13.812 Other specified arthritis, **left**shoulder
M13.819 Other specified arthritis, unspecified shoulder ▽
M13.82 Other specified arthritis, **elbow**
M13.821 Other specified arthritis, **right**elbow
M13.822 Other specified arthritis, **left**elbow
M13.829 Other specified arthritis, unspecified elbow ▽
M13.83 Other specified arthritis, **wrist**
M13.831 Other specified arthritis, **right**wrist
M13.832 Other specified arthritis, **left**wrist
M13.839 Other specified arthritis, unspecified wrist ▽
M13.84 Other specified arthritis, **hand**
M13.841 Other specified arthritis, **right**hand
M13.842 Other specified arthritis, **left**hand
M13.849 Other specified arthritis, unspecified hand ▽
M13.85 Other specified arthritis, **hip**
M13.851 Other specified arthritis, **right**hip
M13.852 Other specified arthritis, **left**hip
M13.859 Other specified arthritis, unspecified hip ▽

✓6ᵗʰ **M13.86 Other specified arthritis, knee**
    M13.861 Other specified arthritis, right knee
    M13.862 Other specified arthritis, left knee
    M13.869 Other specified arthritis, unspecified ▽
        knee

✓6ᵗʰ **M13.87 Other specified arthritis, ankle and foot**
    M13.871 Other specified arthritis, right ankle and
        foot
    M13.872 Other specified arthritis, left ankle and
        foot
    M13.879 Other specified arthritis, unspecified ▽
        ankle and foot

   M13.88 Other specified arthritis, other site

   M13.89 Other specified arthritis, multiple sites

✓4ᵗʰ **M14 Arthropathies in other diseases classified elsewhere**
   EXCLUDES 1 arthropathy in:
      diabetes mellitus (E08-E13 with .61-)
      hematological disorders (M36.2-M36.3)
      hypersensitivity reactions (M36.4)
      neoplastic disease (M36.1)
      neurosyphillis (A52.16)
      sarcoidosis (D86.86)
     enteropathic arthropathies (M07.-)
     juvenile psoriatic arthropathy (L40.54)
     lipoid dermatoarthritis (E78.81)

✓5ᵗʰ **M14.6 Charcôt's joint**
   Neuropathic arthropathy
   EXCLUDES 1 Charcôt's joint in diabetes mellitus (E08-E13 with .610)
          Charcôt's joint in tabes dorsalis (A52.16)

   M14.60 Charcôt's joint, unspecified site ▽

✓6ᵗʰ **M14.61 Charcôt's joint, shoulder**
    M14.611 Charcôt's joint, right shoulder
    M14.612 Charcôt's joint, left shoulder
    M14.619 Charcôt's joint, unspecified shoulder ▽

✓6ᵗʰ **M14.62 Charcôt's joint, elbow**
    M14.621 Charcôt's joint, right elbow
    M14.622 Charcôt's joint, left elbow
    M14.629 Charcôt's joint, unspecified elbow ▽

✓6ᵗʰ **M14.63 Charcôt's joint, wrist**
    M14.631 Charcôt's joint, right wrist
    M14.632 Charcôt's joint, left wrist
    M14.639 Charcôt's joint, unspecified wrist ▽

✓6ᵗʰ **M14.64 Charcôt's joint, hand**
    M14.641 Charcôt's joint, right hand
    M14.642 Charcôt's joint, left hand
    M14.649 Charcôt's joint, unspecified hand ▽

✓6ᵗʰ **M14.65 Charcôt's joint, hip**
    M14.651 Charcôt's joint, right hip
    M14.652 Charcôt's joint, left hip
    M14.659 Charcôt's joint, unspecified hip ▽

✓6ᵗʰ **M14.66 Charcôt's joint, knee**
    M14.661 Charcôt's joint, right knee
    M14.662 Charcôt's joint, left knee
    M14.669 Charcôt's joint, unspecified knee ▽

✓6ᵗʰ **M14.67 Charcôt's joint, ankle and foot**
    M14.671 Charcôt's joint, right ankle and foot
    M14.672 Charcôt's joint, left ankle and foot
    M14.679 Charcôt's joint, unspecified ankle ▽
        and foot

   M14.68 Charcôt's joint, vertebrae

   M14.69 Charcôt's joint, multiple sites

✓5ᵗʰ **M14.8 Arthropathies in other specified diseases classified elsewhere**
   Code first underlying disease, such as:
     amyloidosis (E85.-)
     erythema multiforme (L51.-)
     erythema nodosum (L52)
     hemochromatosis (E83.11-)
     hyperparathyroidism (E21.-)
     hypothyroidism (E00-E03)
     sickle-cell disorders (D57.-)
     thyrotoxicosis [hyperthyroidism] (E05.-)
     Whipple's disease (K90.81)

   M14.80 Arthropathies in other specified diseases ▽
        classified elsewhere, unspecified site

✓6ᵗʰ **M14.81 Arthropathies in other specified diseases classified elsewhere, shoulder**
    M14.811 Arthropathies in other specified diseases
        classified elsewhere, right shoulder
    M14.812 Arthropathies in other specified diseases
        classified elsewhere, left shoulder
    M14.819 Arthropathies in other specified diseases ▽
        classified elsewhere, unspecified shoulder

✓6ᵗʰ **M14.82 Arthropathies in other specified diseases classified elsewhere, elbow**
    M14.821 Arthropathies in other specified diseases
        classified elsewhere, right elbow
    M14.822 Arthropathies in other specified diseases
        classified elsewhere, left elbow
    M14.829 Arthropathies in other specified diseases ▽
        classified elsewhere, unspecified elbow

✓6ᵗʰ **M14.83 Arthropathies in other specified diseases classified elsewhere, wrist**
    M14.831 Arthropathies in other specified diseases
        classified elsewhere, right wrist
    M14.832 Arthropathies in other specified diseases
        classified elsewhere, left wrist
    M14.839 Arthropathies in other specified diseases ▽
        classified elsewhere, unspecified wrist

✓6ᵗʰ **M14.84 Arthropathies in other specified diseases classified elsewhere, hand**
    M14.841 Arthropathies in other specified diseases
        classified elsewhere, right hand
    M14.842 Arthropathies in other specified diseases
        classified elsewhere, left hand
    M14.849 Arthropathies in other specified diseases ▽
        classified elsewhere, unspecified hand

✓6ᵗʰ **M14.85 Arthropathies in other specified diseases classified elsewhere, hip**
    M14.851 Arthropathies in other specified diseases
        classified elsewhere, right hip
    M14.852 Arthropathies in other specified diseases
        classified elsewhere, left hip
    M14.859 Arthropathies in other specified diseases ▽
        classified elsewhere, unspecified hip

✓6ᵗʰ **M14.86 Arthropathies in other specified diseases classified elsewhere, knee**
    M14.861 Arthropathies in other specified diseases
        classified elsewhere, right knee
    M14.862 Arthropathies in other specified diseases
        classified elsewhere, left knee
    M14.869 Arthropathies in other specified diseases ▽
        classified elsewhere, unspecified knee

✓6ᵗʰ **M14.87 Arthropathies in other specified diseases classified elsewhere, ankle and foot**
    M14.871 Arthropathies in other specified diseases
        classified elsewhere, right ankle and foot
    M14.872 Arthropathies in other specified diseases
        classified elsewhere, left ankle and foot
    M14.879 Arthropathies in other specified diseases ▽
        classified elsewhere, unspecified ankle
        and foot

   M14.88 Arthropathies in other specified diseases classified elsewhere, vertebrae

   M14.89 Arthropathies in other specified diseases classified elsewhere, multiple sites

Osteoarthritis (M15-M19)
   EXCLUDES 2 osteoarthritis of spine (M47.-)

✓4ᵗʰ **M15 Polyosteoarthritis**
   INCLUDES arthritis of multiple sites
   EXCLUDES 1 bilateral involvement of single joint (M16-M19)

   M15.0 Primary generalized (osteo)arthritis

   M15.1 Heberden's nodes (with arthropathy)
     Interphalangeal distal osteoarthritis

   M15.2 Bouchard's nodes (with arthropathy)
     Juxtaphalangeal distal osteoarthritis

   M15.3 Secondary multiple arthritis
     Post-traumatic polyosteoarthritis

   M15.4 Erosive (osteo)arthritis

   M15.8 Other polyosteoarthritis

☑ Additional Character Req   ✓7ᵗʰ Placeholder Alert   Manifestation   HCC CMS-HCC Condition   ▽ Unspecified Code   ►◄ Revised Text   ● New Code   ▲ Revised Code Title

M15.9 Polyosteoarthritis, unspecified ▽
  Generalized osteoarthritis NOS

✓4ᵗʰ M16 Osteoarthritis of hip
  AHA: 2016, 4Q, 146
  M16.0 Bilateral primary osteoarthritis of hip
  ✓5ᵗʰ M16.1 Unilateral primary osteoarthritis of hip
    Primary osteoarthritis of hip NOS
    M16.10 Unilateral primary osteoarthritis, unspecified hip ▽
    M16.11 Unilateral primary osteoarthritis, right hip
    M16.12 Unilateral primary osteoarthritis, left hip
  M16.2 Bilateral osteoarthritis resulting from hip dysplasia
  ✓5ᵗʰ M16.3 Unilateral osteoarthritis resulting from hip dysplasia
    Dysplastic osteoarthritis of hip NOS
    M16.30 Unilateral osteoarthritis resulting from hip dysplasia, unspecified hip ▽
    M16.31 Unilateral osteoarthritis resulting from hip dysplasia, right hip
    M16.32 Unilateral osteoarthritis resulting from hip dysplasia, left hip
  M16.4 Bilateral post-traumatic osteoarthritis of hip
  ✓5ᵗʰ M16.5 Unilateral post-traumatic osteoarthritis of hip
    Post-traumatic osteoarthritis of hip NOS
    M16.50 Unilateral post-traumatic osteoarthritis, unspecified hip ▽
    M16.51 Unilateral post-traumatic osteoarthritis, right hip
    M16.52 Unilateral post-traumatic osteoarthritis, left hip
  M16.6 Other bilateral secondary osteoarthritis of hip
  M16.7 Other unilateral secondary osteoarthritis of hip
    Secondary osteoarthritis of hip NOS
  M16.9 Osteoarthritis of hip, unspecified ▽

✓4ᵗʰ M17 Osteoarthritis of knee
  AHA: 2016, 4Q, 146-147
  M17.0 Bilateral primary osteoarthritis of knee
  ✓5ᵗʰ M17.1 Unilateral primary osteoarthritis of knee
    Primary osteoarthritis of knee NOS
    M17.10 Unilateral primary osteoarthritis, unspecified knee ▽
    M17.11 Unilateral primary osteoarthritis, right knee
    M17.12 Unilateral primary osteoarthritis, left knee
  M17.2 Bilateral post-traumatic osteoarthritis of knee
  ✓5ᵗʰ M17.3 Unilateral post-traumatic osteoarthritis of knee
    Post-traumatic osteoarthritis of knee NOS
    M17.30 Unilateral post-traumatic osteoarthritis, unspecified knee ▽
    M17.31 Unilateral post-traumatic osteoarthritis, right knee
    M17.32 Unilateral post-traumatic osteoarthritis, left knee
  M17.4 Other bilateral secondary osteoarthritis of knee
  M17.5 Other unilateral secondary osteoarthritis of knee
    Secondary osteoarthritis of knee NOS
  M17.9 Osteoarthritis of knee, unspecified ▽

✓4ᵗʰ M18 Osteoarthritis of first carpometacarpal joint
  M18.0 Bilateral primary osteoarthritis of first carpometacarpal joints
  ✓5ᵗʰ M18.1 Unilateral primary osteoarthritis of first carpometacarpal joint
    Primary osteoarthritis of first carpometacarpal joint NOS
    M18.10 Unilateral primary osteoarthritis of first carpometacarpal joint, unspecified hand ▽
    M18.11 Unilateral primary osteoarthritis of first carpometacarpal joint, right hand
    M18.12 Unilateral primary osteoarthritis of first carpometacarpal joint, left hand
  M18.2 Bilateral post-traumatic osteoarthritis of first carpometacarpal joints
  ✓5ᵗʰ M18.3 Unilateral post-traumatic osteoarthritis of first carpometacarpal joint
    Post-traumatic osteoarthritis of first carpometacarpal joint NOS
    M18.30 Unilateral post-traumatic osteoarthritis of first carpometacarpal joint, unspecified hand ▽
    M18.31 Unilateral post-traumatic osteoarthritis of first carpometacarpal joint, right hand
    M18.32 Unilateral post-traumatic osteoarthritis of first carpometacarpal joint, left hand

M18.4 Other bilateral secondary osteoarthritis of first carpometacarpal joints
✓5ᵗʰ M18.5 Other unilateral secondary osteoarthritis of first carpometacarpal joint
  Secondary osteoarthritis of first carpometacarpal joint NOS
  M18.50 Other unilateral secondary osteoarthritis of first carpometacarpal joint, unspecified hand ▽
  M18.51 Other unilateral secondary osteoarthritis of first carpometacarpal joint, right hand
  M18.52 Other unilateral secondary osteoarthritis of first carpometacarpal joint, left hand
M18.9 Osteoarthritis of first carpometacarpal joint, unspecified ▽

✓4ᵗʰ M19 Other and unspecified osteoarthritis
  EXCLUDES 1 polyarthritis (M15.-)
  EXCLUDES 2 arthrosis of spine (M47.-)
    hallux rigidus (M20.2)
    osteoarthritis of spine (M47.-)
  ✓5ᵗʰ M19.0 Primary osteoarthritis of other joints
    AHA: 2016, 4Q, 145
    ✓6ᵗʰ M19.01 Primary osteoarthritis, shoulder
      M19.011 Primary osteoarthritis, right shoulder
      M19.012 Primary osteoarthritis, left shoulder
      M19.019 Primary osteoarthritis, unspecified shoulder ▽
    ✓6ᵗʰ M19.02 Primary osteoarthritis, elbow
      M19.021 Primary osteoarthritis, right elbow
      M19.022 Primary osteoarthritis, left elbow
      M19.029 Primary osteoarthritis, unspecified elbow ▽
    ✓6ᵗʰ M19.03 Primary osteoarthritis, wrist
      M19.031 Primary osteoarthritis, right wrist
      M19.032 Primary osteoarthritis, left wrist
      M19.039 Primary osteoarthritis, unspecified wrist ▽
    ✓6ᵗʰ M19.04 Primary osteoarthritis, hand
      EXCLUDES 2 primary osteoarthritis of first carpometacarpal joint (M18.0-, M18.1-)
      M19.041 Primary osteoarthritis, right hand
      M19.042 Primary osteoarthritis, left hand
      M19.049 Primary osteoarthritis, unspecified hand ▽
    ✓6ᵗʰ M19.07 Primary osteoarthritis ankle and foot
      M19.071 Primary osteoarthritis, right ankle and foot
      M19.072 Primary osteoarthritis, left ankle and foot
      M19.079 Primary osteoarthritis, unspecified ankle and foot ▽
  ✓5ᵗʰ M19.1 Post-traumatic osteoarthritis of other joints
    ✓6ᵗʰ M19.11 Post-traumatic osteoarthritis, shoulder
      M19.111 Post-traumatic osteoarthritis, right shoulder
      M19.112 Post-traumatic osteoarthritis, left shoulder
      M19.119 Post-traumatic osteoarthritis, unspecified shoulder ▽
    ✓6ᵗʰ M19.12 Post-traumatic osteoarthritis, elbow
      M19.121 Post-traumatic osteoarthritis, right elbow
      M19.122 Post-traumatic osteoarthritis, left elbow
      M19.129 Post-traumatic osteoarthritis, unspecified elbow ▽
    ✓6ᵗʰ M19.13 Post-traumatic osteoarthritis, wrist
      M19.131 Post-traumatic osteoarthritis, right wrist
      M19.132 Post-traumatic osteoarthritis, left wrist
      M19.139 Post-traumatic osteoarthritis, unspecified wrist ▽
    ✓6ᵗʰ M19.14 Post-traumatic osteoarthritis, hand
      EXCLUDES 2 post-traumatic osteoarthritis of first carpometacarpal joint (M18.2-, M18.3-)
      M19.141 Post-traumatic osteoarthritis, right hand
      M19.142 Post-traumatic osteoarthritis, left hand
      M19.149 Post-traumatic osteoarthritis, unspecified hand ▽

✓6ᵗʰ **M19.17 Post-traumatic osteoarthritis, ankle and foot**
    M19.171   Post-traumatic osteoarthritis, **right** ankle and foot
    M19.172   Post-traumatic osteoarthritis, **left** ankle and foot
    M19.179   Post-traumatic osteoarthritis, unspecified ankle and foot ▽

✓5ᵗʰ **M19.2 Secondary osteoarthritis of other joints**
   ✓6ᵗʰ **M19.21 Secondary osteoarthritis, shoulder**
     M19.211   Secondary osteoarthritis, **right** shoulder
     M19.212   Secondary osteoarthritis, **left** shoulder
     M19.219   Secondary osteoarthritis, unspecified shoulder ▽

   ✓6ᵗʰ **M19.22 Secondary osteoarthritis, elbow**
     M19.221   Secondary osteoarthritis, **right** elbow
     M19.222   Secondary osteoarthritis, **left** elbow
     M19.229   Secondary osteoarthritis, unspecified elbow ▽

   ✓6ᵗʰ **M19.23 Secondary osteoarthritis, wrist**
     M19.231   Secondary osteoarthritis, **right** wrist
     M19.232   Secondary osteoarthritis, **left** wrist
     M19.239   Secondary osteoarthritis, unspecified wrist ▽

   ✓6ᵗʰ **M19.24 Secondary osteoarthritis, hand**
     M19.241   Secondary osteoarthritis, **right** hand
     M19.242   Secondary osteoarthritis, **left** hand
     M19.249   Secondary osteoarthritis, unspecified hand ▽

   ✓6ᵗʰ **M19.27 Secondary osteoarthritis, ankle and foot**
     M19.271   Secondary osteoarthritis, **right** ankle and foot
     M19.272   Secondary osteoarthritis, **left** ankle and foot
     M19.279   Secondary osteoarthritis, unspecified ankle and foot ▽

✓5ᵗʰ **M19.9 Osteoarthritis, unspecified site**
    M19.90   **Unspecified osteoarthritis, unspecified site** ▽
      Arthrosis NOSOsteoarthritis NOS
      Arthritis NOS
      AHA: 2016, 4Q, 147
    M19.91   **Primary osteoarthritis, unspecified site** ▽
      Primary osteoarthritis NOS
    M19.92   **Post-traumatic osteoarthritis, unspecified site** ▽
      Post-traumatic osteoarthritis NOS
    M19.93   **Secondary osteoarthritis, unspecified site** ▽
      Secondary osteoarthritis NOS

Other joint disorders (M20–M25)

EXCLUDES 2   *joints of the spine (M40-M54)*

✓4ᵗʰ **M20 Acquired deformities of fingers and toes**
   EXCLUDES 1   *acquired absence of fingers and toes (Z89.-)*
          congenital absence of fingers and toes (Q71.3-, Q72.3-)
          congenital deformities and malformations of fingers and toes (Q66-, Q68-Q70, Q74-)

✓5ᵗʰ **M20.0 Deformity of finger(s)**
   EXCLUDES 1   *clubbing of fingers (R68.3)*
          palmar fascial fibromatosis [Dupuytren] (M72.0)
          trigger finger (M65.3)

   ✓6ᵗʰ **M20.00 Unspecified deformity of finger(s)**
     M20.001   Unspecified deformity of **right** finger(s) ▽
     M20.002   Unspecified deformity of **left** finger(s) ▽
     M20.009   Unspecified deformity of unspecified finger(s) ▽

   ✓6ᵗʰ **M20.01 Mallet finger**
     M20.011   Mallet finger of **right** finger(s)
     M20.012   Mallet finger of **left** finger(s)
     M20.019   Mallet finger of unspecified finger(s) ▽

   ✓6ᵗʰ **M20.02 Boutonnière deformity**
      DEF: A deformity of the finger caused by flexion of the proximal interphalangeal joint and hyperextension of the distal joint; results from rheumatoid arthritis, osteoarthritis, or injury; also called buttonhole deformity.
     M20.021   Boutonnière deformity of **right** finger(s)
     M20.022   Boutonnière deformity of **left** finger(s)

     M20.029   Boutonnière deformity of unspecified finger(s) ▽

   ✓6ᵗʰ **M20.03 Swan-neck deformity**
      DEF: Flexed distal and hyperextended proximal interphalangeal joint; most commonly caused by rheumatoid arthritis.
     M20.031   Swan-neck deformity of **right** finger(s)
     M20.032   Swan-neck deformity of **left** finger(s)
     M20.039   Swan-neck deformity of unspecified finger(s) ▽

   ✓6ᵗʰ **M20.09 Other deformity of finger(s)**
     M20.091   Other deformity of **right** finger(s)
     M20.092   Other deformity of **left** finger(s)
     M20.099   Other deformity of finger(s), unspecified finger(s) ▽

✓5ᵗʰ **M20.1 Hallux valgus (acquired)**
   EXCLUDES 2   *bunion (M21.6-)*
    M20.10   Hallux valgus (acquired), unspecified foot ▽
    M20.11   Hallux valgus (acquired), **right** foot
    M20.12   Hallux valgus (acquired), **left** foot

✓5ᵗʰ **M20.2 Hallux rigidus**
    M20.20   Hallux rigidus, unspecified foot ▽
    M20.21   Hallux rigidus, **right** foot
    M20.22   Hallux rigidus, **left** foot

✓5ᵗʰ **M20.3 Hallux varus (acquired)**
    M20.30   Hallux varus (acquired), unspecified foot ▽
    M20.31   Hallux varus (acquired), **right** foot
    M20.32   Hallux varus (acquired), **left** foot

✓5ᵗʰ **M20.4 Other hammer toe(s) (acquired)**
    M20.40   Other hammer toe(s) (acquired), unspecified foot ▽
    M20.41   Other hammer toe(s) (acquired), **right** foot
    M20.42   Other hammer toe(s) (acquired), **left** foot

✓5ᵗʰ **M20.5 Other deformities of toe(s) (acquired)**
   ✓6ᵗʰ **M20.5X Other deformities of toe(s) (acquired)**
     M20.5X1   Other deformities of toe(s) (acquired), **right** foot
     M20.5X2   Other deformities of toe(s) (acquired), **left** foot
     M20.5X9   Other deformities of toe(s) (acquired), unspecified foot ▽

✓5ᵗʰ **M20.6 Acquired deformities of toe(s), unspecified**
    M20.60   Acquired deformities of toe(s), unspecified, unspecified foot ▽
    M20.61   Acquired deformities of toe(s), unspecified, **right** foot ▽
    M20.62   Acquired deformities of toe(s), unspecified, **left** foot ▽

Hallux Valgus

Hallux valgus
Medial eminence of metatarsal bone
Right foot

✓ Additional Character Req   ✓x7ᵗʰ Placeholder Alert   Manifestation   HCC CMS-HCC Condition   ▽ Unspecified Code   ▶◀ Revised Text   ● New Code   ▲ Revised Code Title

ICD-10-CM 2018   739

Genu Valga (knock-knee)

Genu Varus (bowleg)

✓4ᵗʰ **M21 Other acquired deformities of limbs**

     EXCLUDES 1   *acquired absence of limb (Z89.-)*
                congenital absence of limbs (Q71-Q73)
                congenital deformities and malformations of limbs (Q65-Q66,
                Q68-Q74)

     EXCLUDES 2   *acquired deformities of fingers or toes (M20.-)*
                coxa plana (M91.2)

✓5ᵗʰ **M21.0 Valgus deformity, not elsewhere classified**

     EXCLUDES 1   *metatarsus valgus (Q66.6)*
                talipes calcaneovalgus (Q66.4)

     M21.00 Valgus deformity, not elsewhere classified, ▽
          unspecified site

     ✓6ᵗʰ **M21.02 Valgus deformity, not elsewhere classified, elbow**
          Cubitus valgus

          M21.021 Valgus deformity, not elsewhere
              classified, right elbow

          M21.022 Valgus deformity, not elsewhere
              classified, left elbow

          M21.029 Valgus deformity, not elsewhere ▽
              classified, unspecified elbow

     ✓6ᵗʰ **M21.05 Valgus deformity, not elsewhere classified, hip**

          M21.051 Valgus deformity, not elsewhere
              classified, right hip

          M21.052 Valgus deformity, not elsewhere
              classified, left hip

          M21.059 Valgus deformity, not elsewhere ▽
              classified, unspecified hip

     ✓6ᵗʰ **M21.06 Valgus deformity, not elsewhere classified, knee**
          Genu valgum
          Knock knee

          M21.061 Valgus deformity, not elsewhere
              classified, right knee

          M21.062 Valgus deformity, not elsewhere
              classified, left knee

          M21.069 Valgus deformity, not elsewhere ▽
              classified, unspecified knee

     ✓6ᵗʰ **M21.07 Valgus deformity, not elsewhere classified, ankle**

          M21.071 Valgus deformity, not elsewhere
              classified, right ankle

          M21.072 Valgus deformity, not elsewhere
              classified, left ankle

          M21.079 Valgus deformity, not elsewhere ▽
              classified, unspecified ankle

✓5ᵗʰ **M21.1 Varus deformity, not elsewhere classified**

     EXCLUDES 1   *metatarsus varus (Q66.22)*
                tibia vara (M92.5)

     M21.10 Varus deformity, not elsewhere classified, ▽
          unspecified site

     ✓6ᵗʰ **M21.12 Varus deformity, not elsewhere classified, elbow**
          Cubitus varus, elbow

          M21.121 Varus deformity, not elsewhere classified,
              right elbow

          M21.122 Varus deformity, not elsewhere classified,
              left elbow

          M21.129 Varus deformity, not elsewhere ▽
              classified, unspecified elbow

     ✓6ᵗʰ **M21.15 Varus deformity, not elsewhere classified, hip**

          M21.151 Varus deformity, not elsewhere classified,
              right hip

          M21.152 Varus deformity, not elsewhere classified,
              left hip

          M21.159 Varus deformity, not elsewhere ▽
              classified, unspecified

     ✓6ᵗʰ **M21.16 Varus deformity, not elsewhere classified, knee**
          Bow leg
          Genu varum

          M21.161 Varus deformity, not elsewhere classified,
              right knee

          M21.162 Varus deformity, not elsewhere classified,
              left knee

          M21.169 Varus deformity, not elsewhere ▽
              classified, unspecified knee

     ✓6ᵗʰ **M21.17 Varus deformity, not elsewhere classified, ankle**

          M21.171 Varus deformity, not elsewhere classified,
              right ankle

          M21.172 Varus deformity, not elsewhere classified,
              left ankle

          M21.179 Varus deformity, not elsewhere ▽
              classified, unspecified ankle

✓5ᵗʰ **M21.2 Flexion deformity**

     M21.20 Flexion deformity, unspecified site ▽

     ✓6ᵗʰ **M21.21 Flexion deformity, shoulder**

          M21.211 Flexion deformity, right shoulder
          M21.212 Flexion deformity, left shoulder
          M21.219 Flexion deformity, unspecified ▽
              shoulder

     ✓6ᵗʰ **M21.22 Flexion deformity, elbow**

          M21.221 Flexion deformity, right elbow
          M21.222 Flexion deformity, left elbow
          M21.229 Flexion deformity, unspecified elbow ▽

     ✓6ᵗʰ **M21.23 Flexion deformity, wrist**

          M21.231 Flexion deformity, right wrist
          M21.232 Flexion deformity, left wrist
          M21.239 Flexion deformity, unspecified wrist ▽

     ✓6ᵗʰ **M21.24 Flexion deformity, finger joints**

          M21.241 Flexion deformity, right finger joints
          M21.242 Flexion deformity, left finger joints
          M21.249 Flexion deformity, unspecified finger ▽
              joints

     ✓6ᵗʰ **M21.25 Flexion deformity, hip**

          M21.251 Flexion deformity, right hip
          M21.252 Flexion deformity, left hip
          M21.259 Flexion deformity, unspecified hip ▽

EXCLUDES 1 Not coded here   EXCLUDES 2 Not included here   N Newborn Age: 0   P Pediatric Age: 0-17   M Maternity Age: 12-55   A Adult Age: 15-124

740   ICD-10-CM 2018

✓6ᵗʰ **M21.26** Flexion deformity, **knee**
     M21.261 Flexion deformity, **right** knee
     M21.262 Flexion deformity, **left** knee
     M21.269 Flexion deformity, unspecified knee ▽

✓6ᵗʰ **M21.27** Flexion deformity, **ankle and toes**
     M21.271 Flexion deformity, **right** ankle and toes
     M21.272 Flexion deformity, **left** ankle and toes
     M21.279 Flexion deformity, unspecified ankle ▽ and toes

✓5ᵗʰ **M21.3 Wrist or foot drop** (acquired)

✓6ᵗʰ **M21.33 Wrist drop** (acquired)
     M21.331 Wrist drop, **right** wrist
     M21.332 Wrist drop, **left** wrist
     M21.339 Wrist drop, unspecified wrist ▽

✓6ᵗʰ **M21.37 Foot drop** (acquired)
     M21.371 Foot drop, **right** foot
     M21.372 Foot drop, **left** foot
     M21.379 Foot drop, unspecified foot ▽

✓5ᵗʰ **M21.4 Flat foot** [pes planus] (acquired)
     EXCLUDES 1   congenital pes planus (Q66.5-)
     M21.40 Flat foot [pes planus] (acquired), unspecified foot ▽
     M21.41 Flat foot [pes planus] (acquired), **right** foot
     M21.42 Flat foot [pes planus] (acquired), **left** foot

✓5ᵗʰ **M21.5 Acquired clawhand, clubhand, clawfoot and clubfoot**
     EXCLUDES 1   clubfoot, not specified as acquired (Q66.89)

✓6ᵗʰ **M21.51 Acquired clawhand**
     M21.511 Acquired clawhand, **right** hand
     M21.512 Acquired clawhand, **left** hand
     M21.519 Acquired clawhand, unspecified hand ▽

✓6ᵗʰ **M21.52 Acquired clubhand**
     M21.521 Acquired clubhand, **right** hand
     M21.522 Acquired clubhand, **left** hand
     M21.529 Acquired clubhand, unspecified hand ▽

✓6ᵗʰ **M21.53 Acquired clawfoot**
     DEF: High foot arch with hyperextended toes at metatarsophalangeal joint and flexed toes at distal joints.
     M21.531 Acquired clawfoot, **right** foot
     M21.532 Acquired clawfoot, **left** foot
     M21.539 Acquired clawfoot, unspecified foot ▽

✓6ᵗʰ **M21.54 Acquired clubfoot**
     M21.541 Acquired clubfoot, **right** foot
     M21.542 Acquired clubfoot, **left** foot
     M21.549 Acquired clubfoot, unspecified foot ▽

✓5ᵗʰ **M21.6 Other acquired deformities of foot**
     EXCLUDES 2   deformities of toe (acquired) (M20.1-M20.6-)

✓6ᵗʰ **M21.61 Bunion**
     M21.611 Bunion of **right** foot
     M21.612 Bunion of **left** foot
     M21.619 Bunion of unspecified foot ▽

✓6ᵗʰ **M21.62 Bunionette**
     M21.621 Bunionette of **right** foot
     M21.622 Bunionette of **left** foot
     M21.629 Bunionette of unspecified foot ▽

✓6ᵗʰ **M21.6X Other acquired deformities of foot**
     M21.6X1 Other acquired deformities of **right** foot
     M21.6X2 Other acquired deformities of **left** foot
     M21.6X9 Other acquired deformities of unspecified foot ▽

✓5ᵗʰ **M21.7 Unequal limb length** (acquired)
     NOTE   The site used should correspond to the shorter limb.
     M21.70 Unequal limb length (acquired), unspecified site ▽

✓6ᵗʰ **M21.72 Unequal limb length** (acquired), **humerus**
     M21.721 Unequal limb length (acquired), **right** humerus
     M21.722 Unequal limb length (acquired), **left** humerus
     M21.729 Unequal limb length (acquired), unspecified humerus ▽

✓6ᵗʰ **M21.73 Unequal limb length** (acquired), **ulna and radius**
     M21.731 Unequal limb length (acquired), **right** ulna
     M21.732 Unequal limb length (acquired), **left** ulna

     M21.733 Unequal limb length (acquired), **right radius**
     M21.734 Unequal limb length (acquired), **left radius**
     M21.739 Unequal limb length (acquired), unspecified ulna and radius ▽

✓6ᵗʰ **M21.75 Unequal limb length** (acquired), **femur**
     M21.751 Unequal limb length (acquired), **right** femur
     M21.752 Unequal limb length (acquired), **left** femur
     M21.759 Unequal limb length (acquired), unspecified femur ▽

✓6ᵗʰ **M21.76 Unequal limb length** (acquired), **tibia and fibula**
     M21.761 Unequal limb length (acquired), **right tibia**
     M21.762 Unequal limb length (acquired), **left tibia**
     M21.763 Unequal limb length (acquired), **right fibula**
     M21.764 Unequal limb length (acquired), **left fibula**
     M21.769 Unequal limb length (acquired), unspecified tibia and fibula ▽

✓5ᵗʰ **M21.8 Other specified acquired deformities of limbs**
     EXCLUDES 2   coxa plana (M91.2)
     M21.80 Other specified acquired deformities of unspecified limb ▽

✓6ᵗʰ **M21.82 Other specified acquired deformities of upper arm**
     M21.821 Other specified acquired deformities of **right** upper arm
     M21.822 Other specified acquired deformities of **left** upper arm
     M21.829 Other specified acquired deformities of unspecified upper arm ▽

✓6ᵗʰ **M21.83 Other specified acquired deformities of forearm**
     M21.831 Other specified acquired deformities of **right** forearm
     M21.832 Other specified acquired deformities of **left** forearm
     M21.839 Other specified acquired deformities of unspecified forearm ▽

✓6ᵗʰ **M21.85 Other specified acquired deformities of thigh**
     M21.851 Other specified acquired deformities of **right** thigh
     M21.852 Other specified acquired deformities of **left** thigh
     M21.859 Other specified acquired deformities of unspecified thigh ▽

✓6ᵗʰ **M21.86 Other specified acquired deformities of lower leg**
     M21.861 Other specified acquired deformities of **right** lower leg
     M21.862 Other specified acquired deformities of **left** lower leg
     M21.869 Other specified acquired deformities of unspecified lower leg ▽

✓5ᵗʰ **M21.9 Unspecified acquired deformity of limb and hand**
     M21.90 Unspecified acquired deformity of unspecified limb ▽

✓6ᵗʰ **M21.92 Unspecified acquired deformity of upper arm**
     M21.921 Unspecified acquired deformity of **right** upper arm ▽
     M21.922 Unspecified acquired deformity of **left** upper arm ▽
     M21.929 Unspecified acquired deformity of unspecified upper arm ▽

✓6ᵗʰ **M21.93 Unspecified acquired deformity of forearm**
     M21.931 Unspecified acquired deformity of **right** forearm ▽
     M21.932 Unspecified acquired deformity of **left** forearm ▽
     M21.939 Unspecified acquired deformity of unspecified forearm ▽

✓6ᵗʰ **M21.94 Unspecified acquired deformity of hand**
     M21.941 Unspecified acquired deformity of hand, **right** hand ▽
     M21.942 Unspecified acquired deformity of hand, **left** hand ▽
     M21.949 Unspecified acquired deformity of hand, unspecified hand ▽

☑ Additional Character Req   ✓x7ᵗʰ Placeholder Alert   Manifestation   HCC CMS-HCC Condition   ▽ Unspecified Code   ▶◀ Revised Text   ● New Code   ▲ Revised Code Title

ICD-10-CM 2018   741

√6ᵗʰ **M21.95** Unspecified acquired deformity of **thigh**

M21.951 Unspecified acquired deformity of **right** thigh ▽

M21.952 Unspecified acquired deformity of **left** thigh ▽

M21.959 Unspecified acquired deformity of unspecified thigh ▽

√6ᵗʰ **M21.96** Unspecified acquired deformity of **lower leg**

M21.961 Unspecified acquired deformity of **right** lower leg ▽

M21.962 Unspecified acquired deformity of **left** lower leg ▽

M21.969 Unspecified acquired deformity of unspecified lower leg ▽

√4ᵗʰ **M22 Disorder of patella**

EXCLUDES1   traumatic dislocation of patella (S83.0-)

√5ᵗʰ **M22.0** **Recurrent dislocation** of patella

M22.00 Recurrent dislocation of patella, unspecified knee ▽

M22.01 Recurrent dislocation of patella, **right** knee

M22.02 Recurrent dislocation of patella, **left** knee

√5ᵗʰ **M22.1** **Recurrent subluxation** of patella
Incomplete dislocation of patella

M22.10 Recurrent subluxation of patella, unspecified knee ▽

M22.11 Recurrent subluxation of patella, **right** knee

M22.12 Recurrent subluxation of patella, **left** knee

√5ᵗʰ **M22.2** **Patellofemoral** disorders

√6ᵗʰ **M22.2X** Patellofemoral disorders

M22.2X1 Patellofemoral disorders, **right** knee

M22.2X2 Patellofemoral disorders, **left** knee

M22.2X9 Patellofemoral disorders, unspecified knee ▽

√5ᵗʰ **M22.3** Other derangements of patella

√6ᵗʰ **M22.3X** Other derangements of patella

M22.3X1 Other derangements of patella, **right** knee

M22.3X2 Other derangements of patella, **left** knee

M22.3X9 Other derangements of patella, unspecified knee ▽

√5ᵗʰ **M22.4** **Chondromalacia** patellae

M22.40 Chondromalacia patellae, unspecified knee ▽

M22.41 Chondromalacia patellae, **right** knee

M22.42 Chondromalacia patellae, **left** knee

√5ᵗʰ **M22.8** Other disorders of patella

√6ᵗʰ **M22.8X** Other disorders of patella

M22.8X1 Other disorders of patella, **right** knee

M22.8X2 Other disorders of patella, **left** knee

M22.8X9 Other disorders of patella, unspecified knee ▽

√5ᵗʰ **M22.9** Unspecified disorder of patella

M22.90 Unspecified disorder of patella, unspecified knee ▽

M22.91 Unspecified disorder of patella, **right** knee ▽

M22.92 Unspecified disorder of patella, **left** knee ▽

√4ᵗʰ **M23 Internal derangement of knee**

EXCLUDES1   ankylosis (M24.66)
current injury—see injury of knee and lower leg (S80-S89)
deformity of knee (M21.-)
osteochondritis dissecans (M93.2)
recurrent dislocation or subluxation of joints (M24.4)
recurrent dislocation or subluxation of patella (M22.0-M22.1)

√5ᵗʰ **M23.0** Cystic meniscus

√6ᵗʰ **M23.00** Cystic meniscus, unspecified meniscus
Cystic meniscus, unspecified lateral meniscus
Cystic meniscus, unspecified medial meniscus

M23.000 Cystic meniscus, unspecified **lateral** meniscus, **right** knee

M23.001 Cystic meniscus, unspecified **lateral** meniscus, **left** knee

M23.002 Cystic meniscus, unspecified **lateral** meniscus, unspecified knee ▽

M23.003 Cystic meniscus, unspecified **medial** meniscus, **right** knee

M23.004 Cystic meniscus, unspecified **medial** meniscus, **left** knee

M23.005 Cystic meniscus, unspecified **medial** meniscus, unspecified knee ▽

M23.006 Cystic meniscus, unspecified meniscus, **right** knee

M23.007 Cystic meniscus, unspecified meniscus, **left** knee

M23.009 Cystic meniscus, unspecified meniscus, unspecified knee ▽

√6ᵗʰ **M23.01** Cystic meniscus, **anterior horn of medial** meniscus

M23.011 Cystic meniscus, anterior horn of medial meniscus, **right** knee

M23.012 Cystic meniscus, anterior horn of medial meniscus, **left** knee

M23.019 Cystic meniscus, anterior horn of medial meniscus, unspecified knee ▽

√6ᵗʰ **M23.02** Cystic meniscus, **posterior horn of medial** meniscus

M23.021 Cystic meniscus, posterior horn of medial meniscus, **right** knee

M23.022 Cystic meniscus, posterior horn of medial meniscus, **left** knee

M23.029 Cystic meniscus, posterior horn of medial meniscus, unspecified knee ▽

√6ᵗʰ **M23.03** Cystic meniscus, **other medial** meniscus

M23.031 Cystic meniscus, other medial meniscus, **right** knee

M23.032 Cystic meniscus, other medial meniscus, **left** knee

M23.039 Cystic meniscus, other medial meniscus, unspecified knee ▽

√6ᵗʰ **M23.04** Cystic meniscus, **anterior horn of lateral** meniscus

M23.041 Cystic meniscus, anterior horn of lateral meniscus, **right** knee

M23.042 Cystic meniscus, anterior horn of lateral meniscus, **left** knee

M23.049 Cystic meniscus, anterior horn of lateral meniscus, unspecified knee ▽

√6ᵗʰ **M23.05** Cystic meniscus, **posterior horn of lateral** meniscus

M23.051 Cystic meniscus, posterior horn of lateral meniscus, **right** knee

M23.052 Cystic meniscus, posterior horn of lateral meniscus, **left** knee

M23.059 Cystic meniscus, posterior horn of lateral meniscus, unspecified knee ▽

√6ᵗʰ **M23.06** Cystic meniscus, **other lateral** meniscus

M23.061 Cystic meniscus, other lateral meniscus, **right** knee

M23.062 Cystic meniscus, other lateral meniscus, **left** knee

M23.069 Cystic meniscus, other lateral meniscus, unspecified knee ▽

√5ᵗʰ **M23.2** Derangement of meniscus due to old tear or injury
Old bucket-handle tear

√6ᵗʰ **M23.20** Derangement of unspecified meniscus due to old tear or injury
Derangement of unspecified lateral meniscus due to old tear or injury
Derangement of unspecified medial meniscus due to old tear or injury

M23.200 Derangement of unspecified **lateral** meniscus due to old tear or injury, **right** knee ▽

M23.201 Derangement of unspecified **lateral** meniscus due to old tear or injury, **left** knee ▽

M23.202 Derangement of unspecified **lateral** meniscus due to old tear or injury, unspecified knee ▽

M23.203 Derangement of unspecified **medial** meniscus due to old tear or injury, **right** knee ▽

M23.204 Derangement of unspecified **medial** meniscus due to old tear or injury, **left** knee ▽

EXCLUDES1 Not coded here   EXCLUDES2 Not included here   N Newborn Age: 0   P Pediatric Age: 0-17   M Maternity Age: 12-55   A Adult Age: 15-124

742   ICD-10-CM 2018

M21.95–M23.204

Derangement of Meniscus

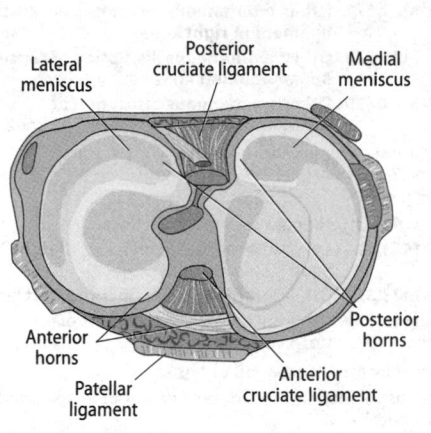

Lateral meniscus
Posterior cruciate ligament
Medial meniscus
Anterior horns
Posterior horns
Patellar ligament
Anterior cruciate ligament

Overhead view of right knee

Bucket handle tear

Radial tear

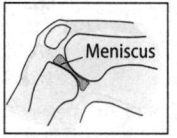

Meniscus

M23.205   Derangement of unspecified **medial** meniscus due to old tear or injury, unspecified knee ▽

M23.206   Derangement of unspecified meniscus due to old tear or injury, **right** knee ▽

M23.207   Derangement of unspecified meniscus due to old tear or injury, **left** knee ▽

M23.209   Derangement of unspecified meniscus due to old tear or injury, unspecified knee ▽

√6ᵗʰ **M23.21** Derangement of **anterior horn of medial** meniscus due to old tear or injury

   M23.211   Derangement of anterior horn of medial meniscus due to old tear or injury, **right** knee

   M23.212   Derangement of anterior horn of medial meniscus due to old tear or injury, **left** knee

   M23.219   Derangement of anterior horn of medial meniscus due to old tear or injury, unspecified knee ▽

√6ᵗʰ **M23.22** Derangement of **posterior horn of medial** meniscus due to old tear or injury

   M23.221   Derangement of posterior horn of medial meniscus due to old tear or injury, **right** knee

   M23.222   Derangement of posterior horn of medial meniscus due to old tear or injury, **left** knee

   M23.229   Derangement of posterior horn of medial meniscus due to old tear or injury, unspecified knee ▽

√6ᵗʰ **M23.23** Derangement of **other medial** meniscus due to old tear or injury

   M23.231   Derangement of other medial meniscus due to old tear or injury, **right** knee

   M23.232   Derangement of other medial meniscus due to old tear or injury, **left** knee

   M23.239   Derangement of other medial meniscus due to old tear or injury, unspecified knee ▽

√6ᵗʰ **M23.24** Derangement of **anterior horn of lateral** meniscus due to old tear or injury

   M23.241   Derangement of anterior horn of lateral meniscus due to old tear or injury, **right** knee

   M23.242   Derangement of anterior horn of lateral meniscus due to old tear or injury, **left** knee

   M23.249   Derangement of anterior horn of lateral meniscus due to old tear or injury, unspecified knee ▽

√6ᵗʰ **M23.25** Derangement of **posterior horn of lateral** meniscus due to old tear or injury

   M23.251   Derangement of posterior horn of lateral meniscus due to old tear or injury, **right** knee

   M23.252   Derangement of posterior horn of lateral meniscus due to old tear or injury, **left** knee

   M23.259   Derangement of posterior horn of lateral meniscus due to old tear or injury, unspecified knee ▽

√6ᵗʰ **M23.26** Derangement of **other lateral** meniscus due to old tear or injury

   M23.261   Derangement of other lateral meniscus due to old tear or injury, **right** knee

   M23.262   Derangement of other lateral meniscus due to old tear or injury, **left** knee

   M23.269   Derangement of other lateral meniscus ▽ due to old tear or injury, unspecified knee

√5ᵗʰ **M23.3** Other meniscus derangements

   Degenerate meniscus
   Detached meniscus
   Retained meniscus

√6ᵗʰ **M23.30** Other meniscus derangements, unspecified meniscus

   Other meniscus derangements, unspecified lateral meniscus
   Other meniscus derangements, unspecified medial meniscus

   M23.300   Other meniscus derangements, unspecified **lateral** meniscus, right knee ▽

   M23.301   Other meniscus derangements, unspecified **lateral** meniscus, **left** knee ▽

   M23.302   Other meniscus derangements, unspecified **lateral** meniscus, unspecified knee ▽

   M23.303   Other meniscus derangements, unspecified **medial** meniscus, right knee ▽

   M23.304   Other meniscus derangements, unspecified **medial** meniscus, **left** knee ▽

   M23.305   Other meniscus derangements, unspecified **medial** meniscus, unspecified knee ▽

   M23.306   Other meniscus derangements, unspecified meniscus, **right** knee ▽

   M23.307   Other meniscus derangements, unspecified meniscus, **left** knee ▽

   M23.309   Other meniscus derangements, unspecified meniscus, unspecified knee ▽

√6ᵗʰ **M23.31** Other meniscus derangements, **anterior horn of medial** meniscus

   M23.311   Other meniscus derangements, anterior horn of medial meniscus, **right** knee

   M23.312   Other meniscus derangements, anterior horn of medial meniscus, **left** knee

   M23.319   Other meniscus derangements, anterior horn of medial meniscus, unspecified knee ▽

√6ᵗʰ **M23.32** Other meniscus derangements, **posterior horn of medial** meniscus

   M23.321   Other meniscus derangements, posterior horn of medial meniscus, **right** knee

   M23.322   Other meniscus derangements, posterior horn of medial meniscus, **left** knee

   M23.329   Other meniscus derangements, posterior horn of medial meniscus, unspecified knee ▽

√6ᵗʰ **M23.33** Other meniscus derangements, **other medial** meniscus

   M23.331   Other meniscus derangements, other medial meniscus, **right** knee

   M23.332   Other meniscus derangements, other medial meniscus, **left** knee

   M23.339   Other meniscus derangements, other medial meniscus, unspecified knee ▽

√6ᵗʰ **M23.34** Other meniscus derangements, **anterior horn of lateral** meniscus

   M23.341   Other meniscus derangements, anterior horn of lateral meniscus, **right** knee

---

✔ Additional Character Req   √7ᵗʰ Placeholder Alert   Manifestation   HCC CMS-HCC Condition   ▽ Unspecified Code   ►◄ Revised Text   ● New Code   ▲ Revised Code Title

ICD-10-CM 2018   743

Chapter 13. Diseases of the Musculoskeletal System and Connective Tissue

M23.342–M24.119

M23.342   Other meniscus derangements, anterior horn of lateral meniscus, **left** knee

M23.349   Other meniscus derangements, anterior horn of lateral meniscus, unspecified knee ▽

✓6th **M23.35**   Other meniscus derangements, **posterior horn of lateral** meniscus

    M23.351   Other meniscus derangements, posterior horn of lateral meniscus, **right** knee

    M23.352   Other meniscus derangements, posterior horn of lateral meniscus, **left** knee

    M23.359   Other meniscus derangements, posterior horn of lateral meniscus, unspecified knee ▽

✓6th **M23.36**   Other meniscus derangements, **other lateral** meniscus

    M23.361   Other meniscus derangements, other lateral meniscus, **right** knee

    M23.362   Other meniscus derangements, other lateral meniscus, **left** knee

    M23.369   Other meniscus derangements, other lateral meniscus, unspecified knee ▽

✓5th **M23.4**   Loose body in knee

    M23.40   Loose body in knee, unspecified knee ▽

    M23.41   Loose body in knee, **right** knee

    M23.42   Loose body in knee, **left** knee

✓5th **M23.5**   Chronic instability of knee

    M23.50   Chronic instability of knee, unspecified knee ▽

    M23.51   Chronic instability of knee, **right** knee

    M23.52   Chronic instability of knee, **left** knee

✓5th **M23.6**   Other spontaneous disruption of ligament(s) of knee

   ✓6th **M23.60**   Other spontaneous disruption of unspecified ligament of knee

     M23.601   Other spontaneous disruption of unspecified ligament of **right** knee ▽

     M23.602   Other spontaneous disruption of unspecified ligament of **left** knee ▽

     M23.609   Other spontaneous disruption of unspecified ligament of unspecified knee ▽

   ✓6th **M23.61**   Other spontaneous disruption of **anterior cruciate** ligament of knee

     M23.611   Other spontaneous disruption of anterior cruciate ligament of **right** knee

     M23.612   Other spontaneous disruption of anterior cruciate ligament of **left** knee

     M23.619   Other spontaneous disruption of anterior cruciate ligament of unspecified knee ▽

   ✓6th **M23.62**   Other spontaneous disruption of **posterior cruciate** ligament of knee

     M23.621   Other spontaneous disruption of posterior cruciate ligament of **right** knee

     M23.622   Other spontaneous disruption of posterior cruciate ligament of **left** knee

     M23.629   Other spontaneous disruption of posterior cruciate ligament of unspecified knee ▽

   ✓6th **M23.63**   Other spontaneous disruption of **medial collateral** ligament of knee

     M23.631   Other spontaneous disruption of medial collateral ligament of **right** knee

     M23.632   Other spontaneous disruption of medial collateral ligament of **left** knee

     M23.639   Other spontaneous disruption of medial collateral ligament of unspecified knee ▽

   ✓6th **M23.64**   Other spontaneous disruption of **lateral collateral** ligament of knee

     M23.641   Other spontaneous disruption of lateral collateral ligament of **right** knee

     M23.642   Other spontaneous disruption of lateral collateral ligament of **left** knee

     M23.649   Other spontaneous disruption of lateral collateral ligament of unspecified knee ▽

   ✓6th **M23.67**   Other spontaneous disruption of **capsular** ligament of knee

     M23.671   Other spontaneous disruption of capsular ligament of **right** knee

     M23.672   Other spontaneous disruption of capsular ligament of **left** knee

     M23.679   Other spontaneous disruption of capsular ligament of unspecified knee ▽

✓5th **M23.8**   Other internal derangements of knee
    Laxity of ligament of knee
    Snapping knee

   ✓6th **M23.8X**   Other internal derangements of knee

     M23.8X1   Other internal derangements of **right** knee

     M23.8X2   Other internal derangements of **left** knee

     M23.8X9   Other internal derangements of unspecified knee ▽

✓5th **M23.9**   Unspecified internal derangement of knee

    M23.90   Unspecified internal derangement of unspecified knee ▽

    M23.91   Unspecified internal derangement of **right** knee ▽

    M23.92   Unspecified internal derangement of **left** knee ▽

✓4th **M24**   **Other specific joint derangements**

   EXCLUDES 1   *current injury—see injury of joint by body region*

   EXCLUDES 2   *ganglion (M67.4)*
      snapping knee (M23.8-)
      temporomandibular joint disorders (M26.6-)

✓5th **M24.0**   Loose body in joint

   EXCLUDES 2   *loose body in knee (M23.4)*

    M24.00   Loose body in unspecified joint ▽

   ✓6th **M24.01**   Loose body in **shoulder**

     M24.011   Loose body in **right** shoulder

     M24.012   Loose body in **left** shoulder

     M24.019   Loose body in unspecified shoulder ▽

   ✓6th **M24.02**   Loose body in **elbow**

     M24.021   Loose body in **right** elbow

     M24.022   Loose body in **left** elbow

     M24.029   Loose body in unspecified elbow ▽

   ✓6th **M24.03**   Loose body in **wrist**

     M24.031   Loose body in **right** wrist

     M24.032   Loose body in **left** wrist

     M24.039   Loose body in unspecified wrist ▽

   ✓6th **M24.04**   Loose body in **finger joints**

     M24.041   Loose body in **right** finger joint(s)

     M24.042   Loose body in **left** finger joint(s)

     M24.049   Loose body in unspecified finger joint(s) ▽

   ✓6th **M24.05**   Loose body in **hip**

     M24.051   Loose body in **right** hip

     M24.052   Loose body in **left** hip

     M24.059   Loose body in unspecified hip ▽

   ✓6th **M24.07**   Loose body in **ankle and toe joints**

     M24.071   Loose body in **right** ankle

     M24.072   Loose body in **left** ankle

     M24.073   Loose body in unspecified ankle ▽

     M24.074   Loose body in **right toe joint(s)**

     M24.075   Loose body in **left toe joint(s)**

     M24.076   Loose body in unspecified toe joints ▽

    M24.08   Loose body, other site

✓5th **M24.1**   Other articular cartilage disorders

   EXCLUDES 2   *chondrocalcinosis (M11.1, M11.2-)*
      internal derangement of knee (M23.-)
      metastatic calcification (E83.5)
      ochronosis (E70.2)

    M24.10   Other articular cartilage disorders, unspecified site ▽

   ✓6th **M24.11**   Other articular cartilage disorders, **shoulder**

     M24.111   Other articular cartilage disorders, **right** shoulder

     M24.112   Other articular cartilage disorders, **left** shoulder

     M24.119   Other articular cartilage disorders, unspecified shoulder ▽

EXCLUDES 1 Not coded here   EXCLUDES 2 Not included here   N Newborn Age: 0   P Pediatric Age: 0-17   M Maternity Age: 12-55   A Adult Age: 15-124

744

ICD-10-CM 2018

✓6th **M24.12** **Other articular cartilage disorders, elbow**

    M24.121 Other articular cartilage disorders, **right** elbow

    M24.122 Other articular cartilage disorders, **left** elbow

    M24.129 Other articular cartilage disorders, unspecified elbow ▽

✓6th **M24.13** **Other articular cartilage disorders, wrist**

    M24.131 Other articular cartilage disorders, **right** wrist

    M24.132 Other articular cartilage disorders, **left** wrist

    M24.139 Other articular cartilage disorders, unspecified wrist ▽

✓6th **M24.14** **Other articular cartilage disorders, hand**

    M24.141 Other articular cartilage disorders, **right** hand

    M24.142 Other articular cartilage disorders, **left** hand

    M24.149 Other articular cartilage disorders, unspecified hand ▽

✓6th **M24.15** **Other articular cartilage disorders, hip**

    M24.151 Other articular cartilage disorders, **right** hip

    M24.152 Other articular cartilage disorders, **left** hip

    M24.159 Other articular cartilage disorders, unspecified hip ▽

✓6th **M24.17** **Other articular cartilage disorders, ankle and foot**

    M24.171 Other articular cartilage disorders, **right** ankle

    M24.172 Other articular cartilage disorders, **left** ankle

    M24.173 Other articular cartilage disorders, unspecified ankle ▽

    M24.174 Other articular cartilage disorders, **right** foot

    M24.175 Other articular cartilage disorders, **left** foot

    M24.176 Other articular cartilage disorders, unspecified foot ▽

✓5th **M24.2** **Disorder of ligament**

    Instability secondary to old ligament injury

    Ligamentous laxity NOS

    EXCLUDES 1   *familial ligamentous laxity (M35.7)*

    EXCLUDES 2   *internal derangement of knee (M23.5-M23.89)*

    M24.20 Disorder of ligament, unspecified site ▽

✓6th **M24.21** **Disorder of ligament, shoulder**

    M24.211 Disorder of ligament, **right** shoulder

    M24.212 Disorder of ligament, **left** shoulder

    M24.219 Disorder of ligament, unspecified shoulder ▽

✓6th **M24.22** **Disorder of ligament, elbow**

    M24.221 Disorder of ligament, **right** elbow

    M24.222 Disorder of ligament, **left** elbow

    M24.229 Disorder of ligament, unspecified elbow ▽

✓6th **M24.23** **Disorder of ligament, wrist**

    M24.231 Disorder of ligament, **right** wrist

    M24.232 Disorder of ligament, **left** wrist

    M24.239 Disorder of ligament, unspecified wrist ▽

✓6th **M24.24** **Disorder of ligament, hand**

    M24.241 Disorder of ligament, **right** hand

    M24.242 Disorder of ligament, **left** hand

    M24.249 Disorder of ligament, unspecified hand ▽

✓6th **M24.25** **Disorder of ligament, hip**

    M24.251 Disorder of ligament, **right** hip

    M24.252 Disorder of ligament, **left** hip

    M24.259 Disorder of ligament, unspecified hip ▽

✓6th **M24.27** **Disorder of ligament, ankle and foot**

    M24.271 Disorder of ligament, **right ankle**

    M24.272 Disorder of ligament, **left ankle**

    M24.273 Disorder of ligament, **unspecified ankle** ▽

    M24.274 Disorder of ligament, **right foot**

    M24.275 Disorder of ligament, **left foot**

    M24.276 Disorder of ligament, **unspecified foot** ▽

    M24.28 Disorder of ligament, **vertebrae**

✓5th **M24.3** **Pathological dislocation of joint, not elsewhere classified**

    EXCLUDES 1   *congenital dislocation or displacement of joint—see congenital malformations and deformations of the musculoskeletal system (Q65-Q79)*

    current injury—see injury of joints and ligaments by body region

    recurrent dislocation of joint (M24.4-)

    M24.30 Pathological dislocation of unspecified joint, not elsewhere classified ▽

✓6th **M24.31** **Pathological dislocation of shoulder, not elsewhere classified**

    M24.311 Pathological dislocation of **right** shoulder, not elsewhere classified

    M24.312 Pathological dislocation of **left** shoulder, not elsewhere classified

    M24.319 Pathological dislocation of unspecified shoulder, not elsewhere classified ▽

✓6th **M24.32** **Pathological dislocation of elbow, not elsewhere classified**

    M24.321 Pathological dislocation of **right** elbow, not elsewhere classified

    M24.322 Pathological dislocation of **left** elbow, not elsewhere classified

    M24.329 Pathological dislocation of unspecified elbow, not elsewhere classified ▽

✓6th **M24.33** **Pathological dislocation of wrist, not elsewhere classified**

    M24.331 Pathological dislocation of **right** wrist, not elsewhere classified

    M24.332 Pathological dislocation of **left** wrist, not elsewhere classified

    M24.339 Pathological dislocation of unspecified wrist, not elsewhere classified ▽

✓6th **M24.34** **Pathological dislocation of hand, not elsewhere classified**

    M24.341 Pathological dislocation of **right** hand, not elsewhere classified

    M24.342 Pathological dislocation of **left** hand, not elsewhere classified

    M24.349 Pathological dislocation of unspecified hand, not elsewhere classified ▽

✓6th **M24.35** **Pathological dislocation of hip, not elsewhere classified**

    M24.351 Pathological dislocation of **right** hip, not elsewhere classified

    M24.352 Pathological dislocation of **left** hip, not elsewhere classified

    M24.359 Pathological dislocation of unspecified hip, not elsewhere classified ▽

✓6th **M24.36** **Pathological dislocation of knee, not elsewhere classified**

    M24.361 Pathological dislocation of **right** knee, not elsewhere classified

    M24.362 Pathological dislocation of **left** knee, not elsewhere classified

    M24.369 Pathological dislocation of unspecified knee, not elsewhere classified ▽

✓6th **M24.37** **Pathological dislocation of ankle and foot, not elsewhere classified**

    M24.371 Pathological dislocation of **right ankle**, not elsewhere classified

    M24.372 Pathological dislocation of **left ankle**, not elsewhere classified

    M24.373 Pathological dislocation of unspecified ankle, not elsewhere classified ▽

    M24.374 Pathological dislocation of **right foot**, not elsewhere classified

    M24.375 Pathological dislocation of **left foot**, not elsewhere classified

    M24.376 Pathological dislocation of unspecified foot, not elsewhere classified ▽

✓5ᵗʰ **M24.4 Recurrent dislocation of joint**
　　　　Recurrent subluxation of joint
　　　　EXCLUDES 2　　*recurrent dislocation of patella (M22.0-M22.1)*
　　　　　　　　　　recurrent vertebral dislocation (M43.3-, M43.4, M43.5-)
　　　　M24.40 Recurrent dislocation, unspecified joint ▽
　✓6ᵗʰ **M24.41 Recurrent dislocation, shoulder**
　　　　　　M24.411 Recurrent dislocation, right shoulder
　　　　　　M24.412 Recurrent dislocation, left shoulder
　　　　　　M24.419 Recurrent dislocation, unspecified ▽
　　　　　　　　　　shoulder
　✓6ᵗʰ **M24.42 Recurrent dislocation, elbow**
　　　　　　M24.421 Recurrent dislocation, right elbow
　　　　　　M24.422 Recurrent dislocation, left elbow
　　　　　　M24.429 Recurrent dislocation, unspecified ▽
　　　　　　　　　　elbow
　✓6ᵗʰ **M24.43 Recurrent dislocation, wrist**
　　　　　　M24.431 Recurrent dislocation, right wrist
　　　　　　M24.432 Recurrent dislocation, left wrist
　　　　　　M24.439 Recurrent dislocation, unspecified wrist ▽
　✓6ᵗʰ **M24.44 Recurrent dislocation, hand and finger(s)**
　　　　　　M24.441 Recurrent dislocation, right hand
　　　　　　M24.442 Recurrent dislocation, left hand
　　　　　　M24.443 Recurrent dislocation, unspecified hand ▽
　　　　　　M24.444 Recurrent dislocation, right finger
　　　　　　M24.445 Recurrent dislocation, left finger
　　　　　　M24.446 Recurrent dislocation, unspecified ▽
　　　　　　　　　　finger
　✓6ᵗʰ **M24.45 Recurrent dislocation, hip**
　　　　　　M24.451 Recurrent dislocation, right hip
　　　　　　M24.452 Recurrent dislocation, left hip
　　　　　　M24.459 Recurrent dislocation, unspecified hip ▽
　✓6ᵗʰ **M24.46 Recurrent dislocation, knee**
　　　　　　M24.461 Recurrent dislocation, right knee
　　　　　　M24.462 Recurrent dislocation, left knee
　　　　　　M24.469 Recurrent dislocation, unspecified knee ▽
　✓6ᵗʰ **M24.47 Recurrent dislocation, ankle, foot and toes**
　　　　　　M24.471 Recurrent dislocation, right ankle
　　　　　　M24.472 Recurrent dislocation, left ankle
　　　　　　M24.473 Recurrent dislocation, unspecified ▽
　　　　　　　　　　ankle
　　　　　　M24.474 Recurrent dislocation, right foot
　　　　　　M24.475 Recurrent dislocation, left foot
　　　　　　M24.476 Recurrent dislocation, unspecified foot ▽
　　　　　　M24.477 Recurrent dislocation, right toe(s)
　　　　　　M24.478 Recurrent dislocation, left toe(s)
　　　　　　M24.479 Recurrent dislocation, unspecified ▽
　　　　　　　　　　toe(s)
✓5ᵗʰ **M24.5 Contracture of joint**
　　　　EXCLUDES 1　　*contracture of muscle without contracture of joint*
　　　　　　　　　　　(M62.4-)
　　　　　　　　　contracture of tendon (sheath) without contracture of
　　　　　　　　　　joint (M62.4-)
　　　　　　　　　Dupuytren's contracture (M72.0)
　　　　EXCLUDES 2　　*acquired deformities of limbs (M20-M21)*
　　　　AHA: 2016, 2Q, 6
　　　　M24.50 Contracture, unspecified joint ▽
　✓6ᵗʰ **M24.51 Contracture, shoulder**
　　　　　　M24.511 Contracture, right shoulder
　　　　　　M24.512 Contracture, left shoulder
　　　　　　M24.519 Contracture, unspecified shoulder ▽
　✓6ᵗʰ **M24.52 Contracture, elbow**
　　　　　　M24.521 Contracture, right elbow
　　　　　　M24.522 Contracture, left elbow
　　　　　　M24.529 Contracture, unspecified elbow ▽
　✓6ᵗʰ **M24.53 Contracture, wrist**
　　　　　　M24.531 Contracture, right wrist
　　　　　　M24.532 Contracture, left wrist
　　　　　　M24.539 Contracture, unspecified wrist ▽
　✓6ᵗʰ **M24.54 Contracture, hand**
　　　　　　M24.541 Contracture, right hand
　　　　　　M24.542 Contracture, left hand
　　　　　　M24.549 Contracture, unspecified hand ▽

✓6ᵗʰ **M24.55 Contracture, hip**
　　　　M24.551 Contracture, right hip
　　　　M24.552 Contracture, left hip
　　　　M24.559 Contracture, unspecified hip ▽
✓6ᵗʰ **M24.56 Contracture, knee**
　　　　M24.561 Contracture, right knee
　　　　M24.562 Contracture, left knee
　　　　M24.569 Contracture, unspecified knee ▽
✓6ᵗʰ **M24.57 Contracture, ankle and foot**
　　　　M24.571 Contracture, right ankle
　　　　M24.572 Contracture, left ankle
　　　　M24.573 Contracture, unspecified ankle ▽
　　　　M24.574 Contracture, right foot
　　　　M24.575 Contracture, left foot
　　　　M24.576 Contracture, unspecified foot ▽
✓5ᵗʰ **M24.6 Ankylosis of joint**
　　　　EXCLUDES 1　　*stiffness of joint without ankylosis (M25.6-)*
　　　　EXCLUDES 2　　*spine (M43.2-)*
　　　　M24.60 Ankylosis, unspecified joint ▽
✓6ᵗʰ **M24.61 Ankylosis, shoulder**
　　　　M24.611 Ankylosis, right shoulder
　　　　M24.612 Ankylosis, left shoulder
　　　　M24.619 Ankylosis, unspecified shoulder ▽
✓6ᵗʰ **M24.62 Ankylosis, elbow**
　　　　M24.621 Ankylosis, right elbow
　　　　M24.622 Ankylosis, left elbow
　　　　M24.629 Ankylosis, unspecified elbow ▽
✓6ᵗʰ **M24.63 Ankylosis, wrist**
　　　　M24.631 Ankylosis, right wrist
　　　　M24.632 Ankylosis, left wrist
　　　　M24.639 Ankylosis, unspecified wrist ▽
✓6ᵗʰ **M24.64 Ankylosis, hand**
　　　　M24.641 Ankylosis, right hand
　　　　M24.642 Ankylosis, left hand
　　　　M24.649 Ankylosis, unspecified hand ▽
✓6ᵗʰ **M24.65 Ankylosis, hip**
　　　　M24.651 Ankylosis, right hip
　　　　M24.652 Ankylosis, left hip
　　　　M24.659 Ankylosis, unspecified hip ▽
✓6ᵗʰ **M24.66 Ankylosis, knee**
　　　　M24.661 Ankylosis, right knee
　　　　M24.662 Ankylosis, left knee
　　　　M24.669 Ankylosis, unspecified knee ▽
✓6ᵗʰ **M24.67 Ankylosis, ankle and foot**
　　　　M24.671 Ankylosis, right ankle
　　　　M24.672 Ankylosis, left ankle
　　　　M24.673 Ankylosis, unspecified ankle ▽
　　　　M24.674 Ankylosis, right foot
　　　　M24.675 Ankylosis, left foot
　　　　M24.676 Ankylosis, unspecified foot ▽
M24.7 Protrusio acetabuli
✓5ᵗʰ **M24.8 Other specific joint derangements, not elsewhere classified**
　　　　EXCLUDES 2　　*iliotibial band syndrome (M76.3)*
　　　　M24.80 Other specific joint derangements of unspecified ▽
　　　　　　　　joint, not elsewhere classified
✓6ᵗʰ **M24.81 Other specific joint derangements of shoulder, not**
　　　　　　elsewhere classified
　　　　M24.811 Other specific joint derangements of right
　　　　　　　　shoulder, not elsewhere classified
　　　　M24.812 Other specific joint derangements of left
　　　　　　　　shoulder, not elsewhere classified
　　　　M24.819 Other specific joint derangements of ▽
　　　　　　　　unspecified shoulder, not elsewhere
　　　　　　　　classified
✓6ᵗʰ **M24.82 Other specific joint derangements of elbow, not**
　　　　　　elsewhere classified
　　　　M24.821 Other specific joint derangements of
　　　　　　　　right elbow, not elsewhere classified
　　　　M24.822 Other specific joint derangements of
　　　　　　　　left elbow, not elsewhere classified
　　　　M24.829 Other specific joint derangements of ▽
　　　　　　　　unspecified elbow, not elsewhere
　　　　　　　　classified

✓6ᵗʰ **M24.83** Other specific joint derangements of **wrist,** not elsewhere classified
    M24.831 Other specific joint derangements of **right** wrist, not elsewhere classified
    M24.832 Other specific joint derangements of **left** wrist, not elsewhere classified
    M24.839 Other specific joint derangements of unspecified wrist, not elsewhere classified ▽

✓6ᵗʰ **M24.84** Other specific joint derangements of **hand,** not elsewhere classified
    M24.841 Other specific joint derangements of **right** hand, not elsewhere classified
    M24.842 Other specific joint derangements of **left** hand, not elsewhere classified
    M24.849 Other specific joint derangements of unspecified hand, not elsewhere classified ▽

✓6ᵗʰ **M24.85** Other specific joint derangements of **hip,** not elsewhere classified
    Irritable hip
    M24.851 Other specific joint derangements of **right** hip, not elsewhere classified
    M24.852 Other specific joint derangements of **left** hip, not elsewhere classified
    M24.859 Other specific joint derangements of unspecified hip, not elsewhere classified ▽

✓6ᵗʰ **M24.87** Other specific joint derangements of **ankle and foot,** not elsewhere classified
    M24.871 Other specific joint derangements of **right ankle,** not elsewhere classified
    M24.872 Other specific joint derangements of **left ankle,** not elsewhere classified
    M24.873 Other specific joint derangements of unspecified ankle, not elsewhere classified ▽
    M24.874 Other specific joint derangements of **right foot,** not elsewhere classified
    M24.875 Other specific joint derangements **left foot,** not elsewhere classified
    M24.876 Other specific joint derangements of unspecified foot, not elsewhere classified ▽

M24.9 Joint derangement, unspecified ▽

✓4ᵗʰ **M25** Other joint disorder, not elsewhere classified
    EXCLUDES 2   *abnormality of gait and mobility (R26.-)*
            acquired deformities of limb (M20-M21)
            calcification of bursa (M71.4-)
            calcification of shoulder (joint) (M75.3)
            calcification of tendon (M65.2-)
            difficulty in walking (R26.2)
            temporomandibular joint disorder (M26.6-)

✓5ᵗʰ **M25.0** Hemarthrosis
    EXCLUDES 1   *current injury—see injury of joint by body region*
            hemophilic arthropathy (M36.2)
    M25.00 Hemarthrosis, unspecified joint ▽

✓6ᵗʰ **M25.01** Hemarthrosis, **shoulder**
    M25.011 Hemarthrosis, **right** shoulder
    M25.012 Hemarthrosis, **left** shoulder
    M25.019 Hemarthrosis, unspecified shoulder ▽

✓6ᵗʰ **M25.02** Hemarthrosis, **elbow**
    M25.021 Hemarthrosis, **right** elbow
    M25.022 Hemarthrosis, **left** elbow
    M25.029 Hemarthrosis, unspecified elbow ▽

✓6ᵗʰ **M25.03** Hemarthrosis, **wrist**
    M25.031 Hemarthrosis, **right** wrist
    M25.032 Hemarthrosis, **left** wrist
    M25.039 Hemarthrosis, unspecified wrist ▽

✓6ᵗʰ **M25.04** Hemarthrosis, **hand**
    M25.041 Hemarthrosis, **right** hand
    M25.042 Hemarthrosis, **left** hand
    M25.049 Hemarthrosis, unspecified hand ▽

✓6ᵗʰ **M25.05** Hemarthrosis, **hip**
    M25.051 Hemarthrosis, **right** hip
    M25.052 Hemarthrosis, **left** hip
    M25.059 Hemarthrosis, unspecified hip ▽

✓6ᵗʰ **M25.06** Hemarthrosis, **knee**
    M25.061 Hemarthrosis, **right** knee
    M25.062 Hemarthrosis, **left** knee

M25.069 Hemarthrosis, unspecified knee ▽

✓6ᵗʰ **M25.07** Hemarthrosis, **ankle and foot**
    M25.071 Hemarthrosis, **right ankle**
    M25.072 Hemarthrosis, **left ankle**
    M25.073 Hemarthrosis, unspecified ankle ▽
    M25.074 Hemarthrosis, **right foot**
    M25.075 Hemarthrosis, **left foot**
    M25.076 Hemarthrosis, unspecified foot ▽

M25.08 Hemarthrosis, other specified site
    Hemarthrosis, vertebrae

✓5ᵗʰ **M25.1** Fistula of joint
    M25.10 Fistula, unspecified joint ▽

✓6ᵗʰ **M25.11** Fistula, **shoulder**
    M25.111 Fistula, **right shoulder**
    M25.112 Fistula, **left shoulder**
    M25.119 Fistula, unspecified shoulder ▽

✓6ᵗʰ **M25.12** Fistula, **elbow**
    M25.121 Fistula, **right elbow**
    M25.122 Fistula, **left elbow**
    M25.129 Fistula, unspecified elbow ▽

✓6ᵗʰ **M25.13** Fistula, **wrist**
    M25.131 Fistula, **right wrist**
    M25.132 Fistula, **left wrist**
    M25.139 Fistula, unspecified wrist ▽

✓6ᵗʰ **M25.14** Fistula, **hand**
    M25.141 Fistula, **right hand**
    M25.142 Fistula, **left hand**
    M25.149 Fistula, unspecified hand ▽

✓6ᵗʰ **M25.15** Fistula, **hip**
    M25.151 Fistula, **right hip**
    M25.152 Fistula, **left hip**
    M25.159 Fistula, unspecified hip ▽

✓6ᵗʰ **M25.16** Fistula, **knee**
    M25.161 Fistula, **right knee**
    M25.162 Fistula, **left knee**
    M25.169 Fistula, unspecified knee ▽

✓6ᵗʰ **M25.17** Fistula, **ankle and foot**
    M25.171 Fistula, **right ankle**
    M25.172 Fistula, **left ankle**
    M25.173 Fistula, unspecified ankle ▽
    M25.174 Fistula, **right foot**
    M25.175 Fistula, **left foot**
    M25.176 Fistula, unspecified foot ▽

M25.18 Fistula, other specified site
    Fistula, vertebrae

✓5ᵗʰ **M25.2** Flail joint
    M25.20 Flail joint, unspecified joint ▽

✓6ᵗʰ **M25.21** Flail joint, **shoulder**
    M25.211 Flail joint, **right shoulder**
    M25.212 Flail joint, **left shoulder**
    M25.219 Flail joint, unspecified shoulder ▽

✓6ᵗʰ **M25.22** Flail joint, **elbow**
    M25.221 Flail joint, **right elbow**
    M25.222 Flail joint, **left elbow**
    M25.229 Flail joint, unspecified elbow ▽

✓6ᵗʰ **M25.23** Flail joint, **wrist**
    M25.231 Flail joint, **right wrist**
    M25.232 Flail joint, **left wrist**
    M25.239 Flail joint, unspecified wrist ▽

✓6ᵗʰ **M25.24** Flail joint, **hand**
    M25.241 Flail joint, **right hand**
    M25.242 Flail joint, **left hand**
    M25.249 Flail joint, unspecified hand ▽

✓6ᵗʰ **M25.25** Flail joint, **hip**
    M25.251 Flail joint, **right hip**
    M25.252 Flail joint, **left hip**
    M25.259 Flail joint, unspecified hip ▽

✓6ᵗʰ **M25.26** Flail joint, **knee**
    M25.261 Flail joint, **right knee**
    M25.262 Flail joint, **left knee**
    M25.269 Flail joint, unspecified knee ▽

☑ Additional Character Req   ✓x7ᵗʰ Placeholder Alert   Manifestation   HCC CMS-HCC Condition   ▽ Unspecified Code   ▶◀ Revised Text   ● New Code   ▲ Revised Code Title

√6ᵗʰ **M25.27** **Flail joint, ankle and foot**
     M25.271 Flail joint, **right** ankle and foot
     M25.272 Flail joint, **left** ankle and foot
     M25.279 Flail joint, unspecified ankle and foot ▽
M25.28 **Flail joint, other site**

√5ᵗʰ **M25.3** **Other instability of joint**
     EXCLUDES 1   *instability of joint secondary to old ligament injury*
          (M24.2-)
          instability of joint secondary to removal of joint
          prosthesis (M96.8-)
     EXCLUDES 2   *spinal instabilities (M53.2-)*
M25.30 **Other instability, unspecified joint** ▽
√6ᵗʰ **M25.31** **Other instability, shoulder**
     M25.311 Other instability, **right** shoulder
     M25.312 Other instability, **left** shoulder
     M25.319 Other instability, unspecified shoulder ▽
√6ᵗʰ **M25.32** **Other instability, elbow**
     M25.321 Other instability, **right** elbow
     M25.322 Other instability, **left** elbow
     M25.329 Other instability, unspecified elbow ▽
√6ᵗʰ **M25.33** **Other instability, wrist**
     M25.331 Other instability, **right** wrist
     M25.332 Other instability, **left** wrist
     M25.339 Other instability, unspecified wrist ▽
√6ᵗʰ **M25.34** **Other instability, hand**
     M25.341 Other instability, **right** hand
     M25.342 Other instability, **left** hand
     M25.349 Other instability, unspecified hand ▽
√6ᵗʰ **M25.35** **Other instability, hip**
     M25.351 Other instability, **right** hip
     M25.352 Other instability, **left** hip
     M25.359 Other instability, unspecified hip ▽
√6ᵗʰ **M25.36** **Other instability, knee**
     M25.361 Other instability, **right** knee
     M25.362 Other instability, **left** knee
     M25.369 Other instability, unspecified knee ▽
√6ᵗʰ **M25.37** **Other instability, ankle and foot**
     M25.371 Other instability, **right** ankle
     M25.372 Other instability, **left** ankle
     M25.373 Other instability, unspecified ankle ▽
     M25.374 Other instability, **right** foot
     M25.375 Other instability, **left** foot
     M25.376 Other instability, unspecified foot ▽

√5ᵗʰ **M25.4** **Effusion of joint**
     EXCLUDES 1   *hydrarthrosis in yaws (A66.6)*
          intermittent hydrarthrosis (M12.4-)
          other infective (teno)synovitis (M65.1-)
M25.40 **Effusion, unspecified joint** ▽
√6ᵗʰ **M25.41** **Effusion, shoulder**
     M25.411 Effusion, **right** shoulder
     M25.412 Effusion, **left** shoulder
     M25.419 Effusion, unspecified shoulder ▽
√6ᵗʰ **M25.42** **Effusion, elbow**
     M25.421 Effusion, **right** elbow
     M25.422 Effusion, **left** elbow
     M25.429 Effusion, unspecified elbow ▽
√6ᵗʰ **M25.43** **Effusion, wrist**
     M25.431 Effusion, **right** wrist
     M25.432 Effusion, **left** wrist
     M25.439 Effusion, unspecified wrist ▽
√6ᵗʰ **M25.44** **Effusion, hand**
     M25.441 Effusion, **right** hand
     M25.442 Effusion, **left** hand
     M25.449 Effusion, unspecified hand ▽
√6ᵗʰ **M25.45** **Effusion, hip**
     M25.451 Effusion, **right** hip
     M25.452 Effusion, **left** hip
     M25.459 Effusion, unspecified hip ▽
√6ᵗʰ **M25.46** **Effusion, knee**
     M25.461 Effusion, **right** knee
     M25.462 Effusion, **left** knee
     M25.469 Effusion, unspecified knee ▽

√6ᵗʰ **M25.47** **Effusion, ankle and foot**
     M25.471 Effusion, **right** ankle
     M25.472 Effusion, **left** ankle
     M25.473 Effusion, unspecified ankle ▽
     M25.474 Effusion, **right** foot
     M25.475 Effusion, **left** foot
     M25.476 Effusion, unspecified foot ▽
M25.48 **Effusion, other site**

√5ᵗʰ **M25.5** **Pain in joint**
     EXCLUDES 2   *pain in hand (M79.64-)*
          pain in fingers (M79.64-)
          pain in foot (M79.67-)
          pain in limb (M79.6-)
          pain in toes (M79.67-)
M25.50 **Pain in unspecified joint** ▽
√6ᵗʰ **M25.51** **Pain in shoulder**
     M25.511 Pain in **right** shoulder
     M25.512 Pain in **left** shoulder
     M25.519 Pain in unspecified shoulder ▽
√6ᵗʰ **M25.52** **Pain in elbow**
     M25.521 Pain in **right** elbow
     M25.522 Pain in **left** elbow
     M25.529 Pain in unspecified elbow ▽
√6ᵗʰ **M25.53** **Pain in wrist**
     M25.531 Pain in **right** wrist
     M25.532 Pain in **left** wrist
     M25.539 Pain in unspecified wrist ▽
√6ᵗʰ **M25.54** **Pain in joints of hand**
     M25.541 Pain in joints of **right** hand
     M25.542 Pain in joints of **left** hand
     M25.549 Pain in joints of unspecified hand ▽
          Pain in joints of hand NOS
√6ᵗʰ **M25.55** **Pain in hip**
     M25.551 Pain in **right** hip
     M25.552 Pain in **left** hip
     M25.559 Pain in unspecified hip ▽
√6ᵗʰ **M25.56** **Pain in knee**
     M25.561 Pain in **right** knee
     M25.562 Pain in **left** knee
     M25.569 Pain in unspecified knee ▽
√6ᵗʰ **M25.57** **Pain in ankle and joints of foot**
     M25.571 Pain in **right** ankle and joints of right foot
     M25.572 Pain in **left** ankle and joints of left foot
     M25.579 Pain in unspecified ankle and joints of ▽
          unspecified foot

√5ᵗʰ **M25.6** **Stiffness of joint, not elsewhere classified**
     EXCLUDES 1   *ankylosis of joint (M24.6-)*
          contracture of joint (M24.5-)
M25.60 **Stiffness of unspecified joint, not elsewhere** ▽
     classified
√6ᵗʰ **M25.61** **Stiffness of shoulder, not elsewhere classified**
     M25.611 Stiffness of **right** shoulder, not elsewhere
          classified
     M25.612 Stiffness of **left** shoulder, not elsewhere
          classified
     M25.619 Stiffness of unspecified shoulder, not ▽
          elsewhere classified
√6ᵗʰ **M25.62** **Stiffness of elbow, not elsewhere classified**
     M25.621 Stiffness of **right** elbow, not elsewhere
          classified
     M25.622 Stiffness of **left** elbow, not elsewhere
          classified
     M25.629 Stiffness of unspecified elbow, not ▽
          elsewhere classified
√6ᵗʰ **M25.63** **Stiffness of wrist, not elsewhere classified**
     M25.631 Stiffness of **right** wrist, not elsewhere
          classified
     M25.632 Stiffness of **left** wrist, not elsewhere
          classified
     M25.639 Stiffness of unspecified wrist, not ▽
          elsewhere classified

EXCLUDES 1 Not coded here   *EXCLUDES 2* Not included here   N Newborn Age: 0   P Pediatric Age: 0-17   M Maternity Age: 12-55   A Adult Age: 15-124

748   ICD-10-CM 2018

✓6ᵗʰ **M25.64 Stiffness of hand, not elsewhere classified**
     M25.641 Stiffness of right hand, not elsewhere classified
     M25.642 Stiffness of left hand, not elsewhere classified
     M25.649 Stiffness of unspecified hand, not elsewhere classified ▽

✓6ᵗʰ **M25.65 Stiffness of hip, not elsewhere classified**
     M25.651 Stiffness of right hip, not elsewhere classified
     M25.652 Stiffness of left hip, not elsewhere classified
     M25.659 Stiffness of unspecified hip, not elsewhere classified ▽

✓6ᵗʰ **M25.66 Stiffness of knee, not elsewhere classified**
     M25.661 Stiffness of right knee, not elsewhere classified
     M25.662 Stiffness of left knee, not elsewhere classified
     M25.669 Stiffness of unspecified knee, not elsewhere classified ▽

✓6ᵗʰ **M25.67 Stiffness of ankle and foot, not elsewhere classified**
     M25.671 Stiffness of right ankle, not elsewhere classified
     M25.672 Stiffness of left ankle, not elsewhere classified
     M25.673 Stiffness of unspecified ankle, not elsewhere classified ▽
     M25.674 Stiffness of right foot, not elsewhere classified
     M25.675 Stiffness of left foot, not elsewhere classified
     M25.676 Stiffness of unspecified foot, not elsewhere classified ▽

✓5ᵗʰ **M25.7 Osteophyte**
     M25.70 Osteophyte, unspecified joint ▽

✓6ᵗʰ **M25.71 Osteophyte, shoulder**
     M25.711 Osteophyte, right shoulder
     M25.712 Osteophyte, left shoulder
     M25.719 Osteophyte, unspecified shoulder ▽

✓6ᵗʰ **M25.72 Osteophyte, elbow**
     M25.721 Osteophyte, right elbow
     M25.722 Osteophyte, left elbow
     M25.729 Osteophyte, unspecified elbow ▽

✓6ᵗʰ **M25.73 Osteophyte, wrist**
     M25.731 Osteophyte, right wrist
     M25.732 Osteophyte, left wrist
     M25.739 Osteophyte, unspecified wrist ▽

✓6ᵗʰ **M25.74 Osteophyte, hand**
     M25.741 Osteophyte, right hand
     M25.742 Osteophyte, left hand
     M25.749 Osteophyte, unspecified hand ▽

✓6ᵗʰ **M25.75 Osteophyte, hip**
     M25.751 Osteophyte, right hip
     M25.752 Osteophyte, left hip
     M25.759 Osteophyte, unspecified hip ▽

✓6ᵗʰ **M25.76 Osteophyte, knee**
     M25.761 Osteophyte, right knee
     M25.762 Osteophyte, left knee
     M25.769 Osteophyte, unspecified knee ▽

✓6ᵗʰ **M25.77 Osteophyte, ankle and foot**
     M25.771 Osteophyte, right ankle
     M25.772 Osteophyte, left ankle
     M25.773 Osteophyte, unspecified ankle ▽
     M25.774 Osteophyte, right foot
     M25.775 Osteophyte, left foot
     M25.776 Osteophyte, unspecified foot ▽
     M25.78 Osteophyte, vertebrae

✓5ᵗʰ **M25.8 Other specified joint disorders**
     M25.80 Other specified joint disorders, unspecified joint ▽

✓6ᵗʰ **M25.81 Other specified joint disorders, shoulder**
     M25.811 Other specified joint disorders, right shoulder

M25.812 Other specified joint disorders, left shoulder
M25.819 Other specified joint disorders, unspecified shoulder ▽

✓6ᵗʰ **M25.82 Other specified joint disorders, elbow**
     M25.821 Other specified joint disorders, right elbow
     M25.822 Other specified joint disorders, left elbow
     M25.829 Other specified joint disorders, unspecified elbow ▽

✓6ᵗʰ **M25.83 Other specified joint disorders, wrist**
     M25.831 Other specified joint disorders, right wrist
     M25.832 Other specified joint disorders, left wrist
     M25.839 Other specified joint disorders, unspecifiedwrist ▽

✓6ᵗʰ **M25.84 Other specified joint disorders, hand**
     M25.841 Other specified joint disorders, right hand
     M25.842 Other specified joint disorders, left hand
     M25.849 Other specified joint disorders, unspecified hand ▽

✓6ᵗʰ **M25.85 Other specified joint disorders, hip**
     AHA: 2014, 4Q, 25
     M25.851 Other specified joint disorders, right hip
     M25.852 Other specified joint disorders, left hip
     M25.859 Other specified joint disorders, unspecified hip ▽

✓6ᵗʰ **M25.86 Other specified joint disorders, knee**
     M25.861 Other specified joint disorders, right knee
     M25.862 Other specified joint disorders, left knee
     M25.869 Other specified joint disorders, unspecified knee ▽

✓6ᵗʰ **M25.87 Other specified joint disorders, ankle and foot**
     M25.871 Other specified joint disorders, right ankle and foot
     M25.872 Other specified joint disorders, left ankle and foot
     M25.879 Other specified joint disorders, unspecified ankle and foot ▽

M25.9 Joint disorder, unspecified ▽

Dentofacial anomalies [including malocclusion] and other disorders of jaw (M26-M27)

EXCLUDES 1 hemifacial atrophy or hypertrophy (Q67.4)
unilateral condylar hyperplasia or hypoplasia (M27.8)

✓4ᵗʰ **M26 Dentofacial anomalies [including malocclusion]**

✓5ᵗʰ **M26.0 Major anomalies of jaw size**
     EXCLUDES 1 acromegaly (E22.0)
         Robin's syndrome (Q87.0)
     M26.00 Unspecified anomaly of jaw size ▽
     M26.01 Maxillary hyperplasia
     M26.02 Maxillary hypoplasia
         AHA: 2014, 3Q, 23
     M26.03 Mandibular hyperplasia
     M26.04 Mandibular hypoplasia
     M26.05 Macrogenia
     M26.06 Microgenia
     M26.07 Excessive tuberosity of jaw
         Entire maxillary tuberosity
     M26.09 Other specified anomalies of jaw size

✓5ᵗʰ **M26.1 Anomalies of jaw-cranial base relationship**
     M26.10 Unspecified anomaly of jaw-cranial base relationship ▽
     M26.11 Maxillary asymmetry
     M26.12 Other jaw asymmetry
     M26.19 Other specified anomalies of jaw-cranial base relationship

✓5ᵗʰ **M26.2 Anomalies of dental arch relationship**
     M26.20 Unspecified anomaly of dental arch relationship ▽

✓6ᵗʰ **M26.21 Malocclusion, Angle's class**
     M26.211 Malocclusion, Angle's class I
         Neutro-occlusion
     M26.212 Malocclusion, Angle's class II
         Disto-occlusion Division I
         Disto-occlusion Division II

☑ Additional Character Req   ✓x7ᵗʰ Placeholder Alert   Manifestation   **HCC** CMS-HCC Condition   ▽ Unspecified Code   ▶◀ Revised Text   ● New Code   ▲ Revised Code Title

ICD-10-CM 2018   749

M26.213 Malocclusion, Angle's class III
Mesio-occlusion

M26.219 Malocclusion, Angle's class, unspecified ▽

✓6ᵗʰ **M26.22 Open occlusal relationship**

M26.220 Open anterior occlusal relationship
Anterior openbite

M26.221 Open posterior occlusal relationship
Posterior openbite

M26.23 Excessive horizontal overlap
Excessive horizontal overjet

M26.24 Reverse articulation
Crossbite (anterior) (posterior)

M26.25 Anomalies of interarch distance

M26.29 Other anomalies of dental arch relationship
Midline deviation of dental arch
Overbite (excessive) deep
Overbite (excessive) horizontal
Overbite (excessive) vertical
Posterior lingual occlusion of mandibular teeth

✓5ᵗʰ **M26.3 Anomalies of tooth position of fully erupted tooth or teeth**
EXCLUDES 2 embedded and impacted teeth (K01.-)

M26.30 Unspecified anomaly of tooth position of fully ▽
erupted tooth or teeth
Abnormal spacing of fully erupted tooth or teeth NOS
Displacement of fully erupted tooth or teeth NOS
Transposition of fully erupted tooth or teeth NOS

M26.31 Crowding of fully erupted teeth

M26.32 Excessive spacing of fully erupted teeth
Diastema of fully erupted tooth or teeth NOS

M26.33 Horizontal displacement of fully erupted tooth or
teeth
Tipped tooth or teeth
Tipping of fully erupted tooth

M26.34 Vertical displacement of fully erupted tooth or teeth
Extruded tooth
Infraeruption of tooth or teeth
Supraeruption of tooth or teeth

M26.35 Rotation of fully erupted tooth or teeth

M26.36 Insufficient interocclusal distance of fully erupted
teeth (ridge)
Lack of adequate intermaxillary vertical dimension of
fully erupted teeth

M26.37 Excessive interocclusal distance of fully erupted
teeth
Excessive intermaxillary vertical dimension of fully
erupted teeth
Loss of occlusal vertical dimension of fully erupted
teeth

M26.39 Other anomalies of tooth position of fully erupted
tooth or teeth

M26.4 Malocclusion, unspecified ▽

✓5ᵗʰ **M26.5 Dentofacial functional abnormalities**
EXCLUDES 1 bruxism (F45.8)
teeth-grinding NOS (F45.8)

M26.50 Dentofacial functional abnormalities, unspecified ▽

M26.51 Abnormal jaw closure

M26.52 Limited mandibular range of motion

M26.53 Deviation in opening and closing of the mandible

M26.54 Insufficient anterior guidance
Insufficient anterior occlusal guidance

M26.55 Centric occlusion maximum intercuspation
discrepancy
EXCLUDES 1 centric occlusion NOS (M26.59)

M26.56 Non-working side interference
Balancing side interference

M26.57 Lack of posterior occlusal support

M26.59 Other dentofacial functional abnormalities
Centric occlusion (of teeth) NOS
Malocclusion due to abnormal swallowing
Malocclusion due to mouth breathing
Malocclusion due to tongue, lip or finger habits

Temporomandibular Joint

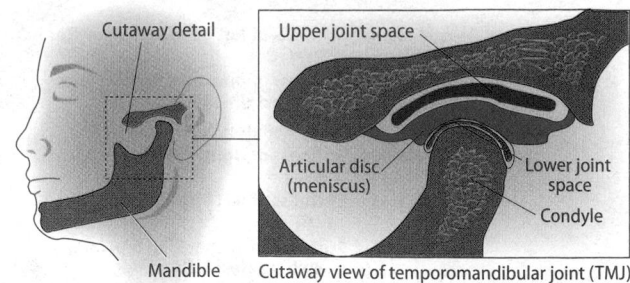

Cutaway detail · Upper joint space · Articular disc (meniscus) · Lower joint space · Condyle · Mandible
Cutaway view of temporomandibular joint (TMJ)

✓5ᵗʰ **M26.6 Temporomandibular joint disorders**
EXCLUDES 2 current temporomandibular joint dislocation (S03.0)
current temporomandibular joint sprain (S03.4)

✓6ᵗʰ **M26.60 Temporomandibular joint disorder, unspecified**

M26.601 Right temporomandibular joint ▽
disorder, unspecified

M26.602 Left temporomandibular joint ▽
disorder, unspecified

M26.603 Bilateral temporomandibular joint ▽
disorder, unspecified

M26.609 Unspecified temporomandibular joint ▽
disorder, unspecified side
Temporomandibular joint disorder NOS

✓6ᵗʰ **M26.61 Adhesions and ankylosis of temporomandibular**
joint

M26.611 Adhesions and ankylosis of right
temporomandibular joint

M26.612 Adhesions and ankylosis of left
temporomandibular joint

M26.613 Adhesions and ankylosis of bilateral
temporomandibular joint

M26.619 Adhesions and ankylosis of ▽
temporomandibular joint,
unspecified side

✓6ᵗʰ **M26.62 Arthralgia of temporomandibular joint**

M26.621 Arthralgia of right temporomandibular
joint

M26.622 Arthralgia of left temporomandibular
joint

M26.623 Arthralgia of bilateral
temporomandibular joint

M26.629 Arthralgia of temporomandibular ▽
joint, unspecified side

✓6ᵗʰ **M26.63 Articular disc disorder of temporomandibular joint**

M26.631 Articular disc disorder of right
temporomandibular joint

M26.632 Articular disc disorder of left
temporomandibular joint

M26.633 Articular disc disorder of bilateral
temporomandibular joint

M26.639 Articular disc disorder of ▽
temporomandibular joint,
unspecified side

M26.69 Other specified disorders of temporomandibular
joint

✓5ᵗʰ **M26.7 Dental alveolar anomalies**

M26.70 Unspecified alveolar anomaly ▽

M26.71 Alveolar maxillary hyperplasia

M26.72 Alveolar mandibular hyperplasia

M26.73 Alveolar maxillary hypoplasia

M26.74 Alveolar mandibular hypoplasia

M26.79 Other specified alveolar anomalies

✓5ᵗʰ **M26.8 Other dentofacial anomalies**

M26.81 Anterior soft tissue impingement
Anterior soft tissue impingement on teeth

M26.82 Posterior soft tissue impingement
Posterior soft tissue impingement on teeth

M26.89 Other dentofacial anomalies

M26.9 Dentofacial anomaly, unspecified ▽

EXCLUDES 1 Not coded here   EXCLUDES 2 Not included here   N Newborn Age: 0   P Pediatric Age: 0-17   M Maternity Age: 12-55   A Adult Age: 15-124

☑️4ᵗʰ M27 Other diseases of jaws

M27.0 Developmental disorders of jaws
Latent bone cyst of jaw   Torus mandibularis
Stafne's cyst   Torus palatinus

M27.1 Giant cell granuloma, central
Giant cell granuloma NOS
EXCLUDES 1   peripheral giant cell granuloma (K06.8)

M27.2 Inflammatory conditions of jaws
Osteitis of jaw(s)   Periostitis jaw(s)
Osteomyelitis (neonatal) jaw(s)   Sequestrum of jaw bone
Osteoradionecrosis jaw(s)
Use additional code (W88-W90, X39.0) to identify radiation, if radiation-induced
EXCLUDES 2   osteonecrosis of jaw due to drug (M87.180)

M27.3 Alveolitis of jaws
Alveolar osteitis   Dry socket

☑️5ᵗʰ M27.4 Other and unspecified cysts of jaw
EXCLUDES 1   cysts of oral region (K09.-)
     latent bone cyst of jaw (M27.0)
     Stafne's cyst (M27.0)

     M27.40 Unspecified cyst of jaw ▽
         Cyst of jaw NOS

     M27.49 Other cysts of jaw
         Aneurysmal cyst of jaw
         Hemorrhagic cyst of jaw
         Traumatic cyst of jaw

☑️5ᵗʰ M27.5 Periradicular pathology associated with previous endodontic treatment

     M27.51 Perforation of root canal space due to endodontic treatment

     M27.52 Endodontic overfill

     M27.53 Endodontic underfill

     M27.59 Other periradicular pathology associated with previous endodontic treatment

☑️5ᵗʰ M27.6 Endosseous dental implant failure

     M27.61 Osseointegration failure of dental implant
         Hemorrhagic complications of dental implant placement
         Iatrogenic osseointegration failure of dental implant
         Osseointegration failure of dental implant due to complications of systemic disease
         Osseointegration failure of dental implant due to poor bone quality
         Pre-integration failure of dental implant NOS
         Pre-osseointegration failure of dental implant

     M27.62 Post-osseointegration biological failure of dental implant
         Failure of dental implant due to lack of attached gingiva
         Failure of dental implant due to occlusal trauma (caused by poor prosthetic design)
         Failure of dental implant due to parafunctional habits
         Failure of dental implant due to periodontal infection (peri-implantitis)
         Failure of dental implant due to poor oral hygiene
         Iatrogenic post-osseointegration failure of dental implant
         Post-osseointegration failure of dental implant due to complications of systemic disease

     M27.63 Post-osseointegration mechanical failure of dental implant
         Failure of dental prosthesis causing loss of dental implant
         Fracture of dental implant
         EXCLUDES 2   cracked tooth (K03.81)
             fractured dental restorative material with loss of material (K08.531)
             fractured dental restorative material without loss of material (K08.530)
             fractured tooth (S02.5)

     M27.69 Other endosseous dental implant failure
         Dental implant failure NOS

M27.8 Other specified diseases of jaws
Cherubism   Unilateral condylar hyperplasia
Exostosis   Unilateral condylar hypoplasia
Fibrous dysplasia
EXCLUDES 1   jaw pain (R68.84)

M27.9 Disease of jaws, unspecified ▽

Systemic connective tissue disorders (M30-M36)

INCLUDES   autoimmune disease NOS
     collagen (vascular) disease NOS
     systemic autoimmune disease
     systemic collagen (vascular) disease
EXCLUDES 1   autoimmune disease, single organ or single cell-type—code to relevant condition category

☑️4ᵗʰ M30 Polyarteritis nodosa and related conditions
EXCLUDES 1   microscopic polyarteritis (M31.7)

     M30.0 Polyarteritis nodosa `HCC`

     M30.1 Polyarteritis with lung involvement [Churg-Strauss] `HCC`
         Allergic granulomatosis angiitis

     M30.2 Juvenile polyarteritis `HCC`

     M30.3 Mucocutaneous lymph node syndrome [Kawasaki] `HCC`

     M30.8 Other conditions related to polyarteritis nodosa `HCC`
         Polyangiitis overlap syndrome

☑️4ᵗʰ M31 Other necrotizing vasculopathies

     M31.0 Hypersensitivity angiitis `HCC`
         Goodpasture's syndrome

     M31.1 Thrombotic microangiopathy `HCC`
         Thrombotic thrombocytopenic purpura

     M31.2 Lethal midline granuloma `HCC`

     ☑️5ᵗʰ M31.3 Wegener's granulomatosis
         Necrotizing respiratory granulomatosis

         M31.30 Wegener's granulomatosis without renal involvement `HCC`
             Wegener's granulomatosis NOS

         M31.31 Wegener's granulomatosis with renal involvement `HCC`

     M31.4 Aortic arch syndrome [Takayasu] `HCC`

     M31.5 Giant cell arteritis with polymyalgia rheumatica `HCC`

     M31.6 Other giant cell arteritis `HCC`

     M31.7 Microscopic polyangiitis `HCC`
         Microscopic polyarteritis
         EXCLUDES 1   polyarteritis nodosa (M30.0)

     M31.8 Other specified necrotizing vasculopathies `HCC`
         Hypocomplementemic vasculitis
         Septic vasculitis

     M31.9 Necrotizing vasculopathy, unspecified `HCC` ▽

☑️4ᵗʰ M32 Systemic lupus erythematosus (SLE)
EXCLUDES 1   lupus erythematosus (discoid) (NOS) (L93.0)

     M32.0 Drug-induced systemic lupus erythematosus `HCC`
         Use additional code for adverse effect, if applicable, to identify drug (T36-T50 with fifth or sixth character 5)

     ☑️5ᵗʰ M32.1 Systemic lupus erythematosus with organ or system involvement

         M32.10 Systemic lupus erythematosus, organ or system involvement unspecified `HCC` ▽

         M32.11 Endocarditis in systemic lupus erythematosus `HCC`
             Libman-Sacks disease

         M32.12 Pericarditis in systemic lupus erythematosus `HCC`
             Lupus pericarditis

         M32.13 Lung involvement in systemic lupus erythematosus `HCC`
             Pleural effusion due to systemic lupus erythematosus

         M32.14 Glomerular disease in systemic lupus erythematosus `HCC`
             Lupus renal disease NOS
             AHA: 2013, 4Q, 125

         M32.15 Tubulo-interstitial nephropathy in systemic lupus erythematosus `HCC`

         M32.19 Other organ or system involvement in systemic lupus erythematosus `HCC`

     M32.8 Other forms of systemic lupus erythematosus `HCC`

     M32.9 Systemic lupus erythematosus, unspecified `HCC` ▽
         SLE NOS
         Systemic lupus erythematosus NOS
         Systemic lupus erythematosus without organ involvement

☑️4ᵗʰ M33 Dermatopolymyositis

▲   **☑️5ᵗʰ M33.0 Juvenile dermatomyositis**

▲   **M33.00 Juvenile dermatomyositis, organ involvement unspecified** `HCC` ▽

▲   **M33.01 Juvenile dermatomyositis with respiratory involvement** `HCC`

▲   **M33.02 Juvenile dermatomyositis with myopathy** `HCC`

☑️ Additional Character Req   ☑️x7ᵗʰ Placeholder Alert   Manifestation   `HCC` CMS-HCC Condition   ▽ Unspecified Code   ►◄ Revised Text   ● New Code   ▲ Revised Code Title

●   **M33.03**   **Juvenile dermatomyositis without myopathy**

▲   **M33.09**   **Juvenile dermatomyositis with other organ involvement**   `HCC`

▲   ✓5ᵗʰ   **M33.1**   **Other dermatomyositis**
      ▶Adult dermatomyositis◀

▲   **M33.10**   **Other dermatomyositis, organ involvement unspecified**   `HCC` ▽

▲   **M33.11**   **Other dermatomyositis with respiratory involvement**   `HCC`

▲   **M33.12**   **Other dermatomyositis with myopathy**   `HCC`

●   **M33.13**   **Other dermatomyositis without myopathy**
        Dermatomyositis NOS

▲   **M33.19**   **Other dermatomyositis with other organ involvement**   `HCC`

✓5ᵗʰ   **M33.2**   **Polymyositis**

      M33.20   **Polymyositis, organ involvement unspecified**   `HCC` ▽

      M33.21   **Polymyositis with respiratory involvement**   `HCC`

      M33.22   **Polymyositis with myopathy**   `HCC`

      M33.29   **Polymyositis with other organ involvement**   `HCC`

✓5ᵗʰ   **M33.9**   **Dermatopolymyositis, unspecified**

      M33.90   **Dermatopolymyositis, unspecified, organ involvement unspecified**   `HCC` ▽

      M33.91   **Dermatopolymyositis, unspecified with respiratory involvement**   `HCC` ▽

      M33.92   **Dermatopolymyositis, unspecified with myopathy**   `HCC` ▽

●   **M33.93**   **Dermatopolymyositis, unspecified without myopathy**   ▽

      M33.99   **Dermatopolymyositis, unspecified with other organ involvement**   `HCC` ▽

✓4ᵗʰ   **M34**   **Systemic sclerosis [scleroderma]**
      EXCLUDES 1   circumscribed scleroderma (L94.0)
              neonatal scleroderma (P83.8)

      M34.0   **Progressive systemic sclerosis**   `HCC`

      M34.1   **CR(E)ST syndrome**   `HCC`
        Combination of calcinosis, Raynaud's phenomenon, esophageal dysfunction, sclerodactyly, telangiectasia

      M34.2   **Systemic sclerosis induced by drug and chemical**   `HCC`
        Code first poisoning due to drug or toxin, if applicable (T36-T65 with fifth or sixth character 1-4 or 6)
        Use additional code for adverse effect, if applicable, to identify drug (T36-T50 with fifth or sixth character 5)

✓5ᵗʰ   **M34.8**   **Other forms of systemic sclerosis**

      M34.81   **Systemic sclerosis with lung involvement**   `HCC`

      M34.82   **Systemic sclerosis with myopathy**   `HCC`

      M34.83   **Systemic sclerosis with polyneuropathy**   `HCC`

      M34.89   **Other systemic sclerosis**   `HCC`

      M34.9   **Systemic sclerosis, unspecified**   `HCC` ▽

✓4ᵗʰ   **M35**   **Other systemic involvement of connective tissue**
      EXCLUDES 1   reactive perforating collagenosis (L87.1)

✓5ᵗʰ   **M35.0**   **Sicca syndrome [Sjögren]**
      DEF: Autoimmune disease; associated with keratoconjunctivitis, laryngopharyngitis, rhinitis, dry mouth, enlarged parotid gland, and chronic polyarthritis.

      M35.00   **Sicca syndrome, unspecified**   `HCC` ▽

      M35.01   **Sicca syndrome with keratoconjunctivitis**   `HCC`

      M35.02   **Sicca syndrome with lung involvement**   `HCC`

      M35.03   **Sicca syndrome with myopathy**   `HCC`

      M35.04   **Sicca syndrome with tubulo-interstitial nephropathy**   `HCC`
        Renal tubular acidosis in sicca syndrome

      M35.09   **Sicca syndrome with other organ involvement**   `HCC`

      M35.1   **Other overlap syndromes**   `HCC`
        Mixed connective tissue disease
        EXCLUDES 1   polyangiitis overlap syndrome (M30.8)

      M35.2   **Behçet's disease**   `HCC`

      M35.3   **Polymyalgia rheumatica**   `HCC`
        EXCLUDES 1   polymyalgia rheumatica with giant cell arteritis (M31.5)

      M35.4   **Diffuse (eosinophilic) fasciitis**

      M35.5   **Multifocal fibrosclerosis**   `HCC`

      M35.6   **Relapsing panniculitis [Weber-Christian]**
        EXCLUDES 1   lupus panniculitis (L93.2)
              panniculitis NOS (M79.3-)

      M35.7   **Hypermobility syndrome**
        Familial ligamentous laxity
        EXCLUDES 1   Ehlers-Danlos syndrome (Q79.6)
              ligamentous laxity, NOS (M24.2-)

      M35.8   **Other specified systemic involvement of connective tissue**   `HCC`

      M35.9   **Systemic involvement of connective tissue, unspecified**   `HCC` ▽
        Autoimmune disease (systemic) NOS
        Collagen (vascular) disease NOS

✓4ᵗʰ   **M36**   **Systemic disorders of connective tissue in diseases classified elsewhere**
      EXCLUDES 2   arthropathies in diseases classified elsewhere (M14.-)

      M36.0   *Dermato(poly)myositis in neoplastic disease*   `HCC`
        Code first underlying neoplasm (C00-D49)

      M36.1   *Arthropathy in neoplastic disease*
        Code first underlying neoplasm, such as:
          leukemia (C91-C95)
          malignant histiocytosis (C96.A)
          multiple myeloma (C90.0)

      M36.2   *Hemophilic arthropathy*
        Hemarthrosis in hemophilic arthropathy
        Code first underlying disease, such as:
          factor VIII deficiency (D66)
            with vascular defect (D68.0)
          factor IX deficiency (D67)
          hemophilia (classical) (D66)
          hemophilia B (D67)
          hemophilia C (D68.1)

      M36.3   *Arthropathy in other blood disorders*

      M36.4   *Arthropathy in hypersensitivity reactions classified elsewhere*
        Code first underlying disease, such as:
          Henoch (-Schönlein) purpura (D69.0)
          serum sickness (T80.6-)

      M36.8   *Systemic disorders of connective tissue in other diseases classified elsewhere*   `HCC`
        Code first underlying disease, such as:
          alkaptonuria (E70.2)
          hypogammaglobulinemia (D80.-)
          ochronosis (E70.2)

Dorsopathies (M40-M54)

Deforming dorsopathies (M40-M43)

✓4ᵗʰ   **M40**   **Kyphosis and lordosis**
      EXCLUDES 1   congenital kyphosis and lordosis (Q76.4)
              kyphoscoliosis (M41.-)
              postprocedural kyphosis and lordosis (M96.-)

✓5ᵗʰ   **M40.0**   **Postural kyphosis**
      EXCLUDES 1   osteochondrosis of spine (M42.-)

      M40.00   **Postural kyphosis, site unspecified**   ▽

      M40.03   **Postural kyphosis, cervicothoracic region**

      M40.04   **Postural kyphosis, thoracic region**

      M40.05   **Postural kyphosis, thoracolumbar region**

✓5ᵗʰ   **M40.1**   **Other secondary kyphosis**

      M40.10   **Other secondary kyphosis, site unspecified**   ▽

      M40.12   **Other secondary kyphosis, cervical region**

      M40.13   **Other secondary kyphosis, cervicothoracic region**

      M40.14   **Other secondary kyphosis, thoracic region**

      M40.15   **Other secondary kyphosis, thoracolumbar region**

✓5ᵗʰ   **M40.2**   **Other and unspecified kyphosis**

   ✓6ᵗʰ   **M40.20**   **Unspecified kyphosis**

        M40.202   **Unspecified kyphosis, cervical region**   ▽

        M40.203   **Unspecified kyphosis, cervicothoracic region**   ▽

        M40.204   **Unspecified kyphosis, thoracic region**   ▽

        M40.205   **Unspecified kyphosis, thoracolumbar region**   ▽

        M40.209   **Unspecified kyphosis, site unspecified**   ▽

   ✓6ᵗʰ   **M40.29**   **Other kyphosis**

        M40.292   **Other kyphosis, cervical region**

        M40.293   **Other kyphosis, cervicothoracic region**

        M40.294   **Other kyphosis, thoracic region**

        M40.295   **Other kyphosis, thoracolumbar region**

        M40.299   **Other kyphosis, site unspecified**   ▽

EXCLUDES 1 Not coded here   *EXCLUDES 2* Not included here   **N** Newborn Age: 0   **P** Pediatric Age: 0-17   **M** Maternity Age: 12-55   **A** Adult Age: 15-124

752   ICD-10-CM 2018

Kyphosis and Lordosis

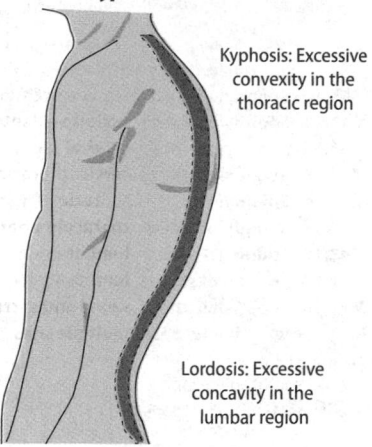

Kyphosis: Excessive
convexity in the
thoracic region

Lordosis: Excessive
concavity in the
lumbar region

✓5ᵗʰ **M40.3 Flatback syndrome**
  M40.30 Flatback syndrome, site unspecified ▽
  M40.35 Flatback syndrome, **thoracolumbar** region
  M40.36 Flatback syndrome, **lumbar** region
  M40.37 Flatback syndrome, **lumbosacral** region
✓5ᵗʰ **M40.4 Postural lordosis**
    Acquired lordosis
  M40.40 Postural lordosis, site unspecified ▽
  M40.45 Postural lordosis, **thoracolumbar** region
  M40.46 Postural lordosis, **lumbar** region
  M40.47 Postural lordosis, **lumbosacral** region
✓5ᵗʰ **M40.5 Lordosis, unspecified**
  M40.50 Lordosis, unspecified, site unspecified ▽
  M40.55 Lordosis, unspecified, **thoracolumbar** region
  M40.56 Lordosis, unspecified, **lumbar** region
  M40.57 Lordosis, unspecified, **lumbosacral** region

✓4ᵗʰ **M41 Scoliosis**
    INCLUDES kyphoscoliosis
    EXCLUDES 1 *congenital scoliosis due to bony malformation (Q76.3)*
          congenital scoliosis NOS (Q67.5)
          kyphoscoliotic heart disease (I27.1)
          postprocedural scoliosis (M96.-)
          postural congenital scoliosis (Q67.5)
✓5ᵗʰ **M41.0 Infantile idiopathic scoliosis**
    AHA: 2014, 4Q, 26
  M41.00 Infantile idiopathic scoliosis, site unspecified ▽
  M41.02 Infantile idiopathic scoliosis, **cervical** region
  M41.03 Infantile idiopathic scoliosis, **cervicothoracic** region
  M41.04 Infantile idiopathic scoliosis, **thoracic** region
  M41.05 Infantile idiopathic scoliosis, **thoracolumbar** region
  M41.06 Infantile idiopathic scoliosis, **lumbar** region
  M41.07 Infantile idiopathic scoliosis, **lumbosacral** region
  M41.08 Infantile idiopathic scoliosis, **sacral and sacrococcygeal** region
✓5ᵗʰ **M41.1 Juvenile and adolescent idiopathic scoliosis**
  ✓6ᵗʰ **M41.11** **Juvenile idiopathic scoliosis**
      AHA: 2014, 4Q, 28
    M41.112 Juvenile idiopathic scoliosis, **cervical** region
    M41.113 Juvenile idiopathic scoliosis, **cervicothoracic** region
    M41.114 Juvenile idiopathic scoliosis, **thoracic** region
    M41.115 Juvenile idiopathic scoliosis, **thoracolumbar** region
    M41.116 Juvenile idiopathic scoliosis, **lumbar** region
    M41.117 Juvenile idiopathic scoliosis, **lumbosacral** region
    M41.119 Juvenile idiopathic scoliosis, site unspecified ▽

Scoliosis

Lateral curvature of spine

  ✓6ᵗʰ **M41.12** **Adolescent scoliosis**
    M41.122 Adolescent idiopathic scoliosis, **cervical** region
    M41.123 Adolescent idiopathic scoliosis, **cervicothoracic** region
    M41.124 Adolescent idiopathic scoliosis, **thoracic** region
    M41.125 Adolescent idiopathic scoliosis, **thoracolumbar** region
    M41.126 Adolescent idiopathic scoliosis, **lumbar** region
    M41.127 Adolescent idiopathic scoliosis, **lumbosacral** region
    M41.129 Adolescent idiopathic scoliosis, site unspecified ▽
✓5ᵗʰ **M41.2 Other idiopathic scoliosis**
  M41.20 Other idiopathic scoliosis, site unspecified ▽
  M41.22 Other idiopathic scoliosis, **cervical** region
  M41.23 Other idiopathic scoliosis, **cervicothoracic** region
  M41.24 Other idiopathic scoliosis, **thoracic** region
  M41.25 Other idiopathic scoliosis, **thoracolumbar** region
  M41.26 Other idiopathic scoliosis, **lumbar** region
  M41.27 Other idiopathic scoliosis, **lumbosacral** region
✓5ᵗʰ **M41.3 Thoracogenic scoliosis**
  M41.30 Thoracogenic scoliosis, site unspecified ▽
  M41.34 Thoracogenic scoliosis, **thoracic** region
  M41.35 Thoracogenic scoliosis, **thoracolumbar** region
✓5ᵗʰ **M41.4 Neuromuscular scoliosis**
    Scoliosis secondary to cerebral palsy, Friedreich's ataxia,
      poliomyelitis and other neuromuscular disorders
    Code also underlying condition
    AHA: 2014, 4Q, 27
  M41.40 Neuromuscular scoliosis, site unspecified ▽
  M41.41 Neuromuscular scoliosis, **occipito-atlanto-axial** region
  M41.42 Neuromuscular scoliosis, **cervical** region
  M41.43 Neuromuscular scoliosis, **cervicothoracic** region
  M41.44 Neuromuscular scoliosis, **thoracic** region
  M41.45 Neuromuscular scoliosis, **thoracolumbar** region
  M41.46 Neuromuscular scoliosis, **lumbar** region
  M41.47 Neuromuscular scoliosis, **lumbosacral** region
✓5ᵗʰ **M41.5 Other secondary scoliosis**
  M41.50 Other secondary scoliosis, site unspecified ▽
  M41.52 Other secondary scoliosis, **cervical** region
  M41.53 Other secondary scoliosis, **cervicothoracic** region
  M41.54 Other secondary scoliosis, **thoracic** region
  M41.55 Other secondary scoliosis, **thoracolumbar** region
  M41.56 Other secondary scoliosis, **lumbar** region
  M41.57 Other secondary scoliosis, **lumbosacral** region

Chapter 13. Diseases of the Musculoskeletal System and Connective Tissue

M40.3-M41.57

✓5ᵗʰ M41.8 Other forms of scoliosis
- M41.80 Other forms of scoliosis, site unspecified ▽
- M41.82 Other forms of scoliosis, **cervical region**
- M41.83 Other forms of scoliosis, **cervicothoracic region**
- M41.84 Other forms of scoliosis, **thoracic region**
- M41.85 Other forms of scoliosis, **thoracolumbar region**
- M41.86 Other forms of scoliosis, **lumbar region**
- M41.87 Other forms of scoliosis, **lumbosacral region**

M41.9 Scoliosis, unspecified ▽

✓4ᵗʰ M42 Spinal osteochondrosis

✓5ᵗʰ M42.0 Juvenile osteochondrosis of spine
Calvé's disease
Scheuermann's disease
EXCLUDES 1   postural kyphosis (M40.0)
- M42.00 Juvenile osteochondrosis of spine, site unspecified ▽
- M42.01 Juvenile osteochondrosis of spine, **occipito-atlanto-axial region**
- M42.02 Juvenile osteochondrosis of spine, **cervical region**
- M42.03 Juvenile osteochondrosis of spine, **cervicothoracic region**
- M42.04 Juvenile osteochondrosis of spine, **thoracic region**
- M42.05 Juvenile osteochondrosis of spine, **thoracolumbar region**
- M42.06 Juvenile osteochondrosis of spine, **lumbar region**
- M42.07 Juvenile osteochondrosis of spine, **lumbosacral region**
- M42.08 Juvenile osteochondrosis of spine, **sacral and sacrococcygeal region**
- M42.09 Juvenile osteochondrosis of spine, **multiple sites in spine**

✓5ᵗʰ M42.1 Adult osteochondrosis of spine
- M42.10 Adult osteochondrosis of spine, site unspecified Ⓐ▽
- M42.11 Adult osteochondrosis of spine, **occipito-atlanto-axial region** Ⓐ
- M42.12 Adult osteochondrosis of spine, **cervical region** Ⓐ
- M42.13 Adult osteochondrosis of spine, **cervicothoracic region** Ⓐ
- M42.14 Adult osteochondrosis of spine, **thoracic region** Ⓐ
- M42.15 Adult osteochondrosis of spine, **thoracolumbar region** Ⓐ
- M42.16 Adult osteochondrosis of spine, **lumbar region** Ⓐ
- M42.17 Adult osteochondrosis of spine, **lumbosacral region** Ⓐ
- M42.18 Adult osteochondrosis of spine, **sacral and sacrococcygeal region** Ⓐ
- M42.19 Adult osteochondrosis of spine, **multiple sites in spine** Ⓐ

M42.9 Spinal osteochondrosis, unspecified ▽

✓4ᵗʰ M43 Other deforming dorsopathies
EXCLUDES 1   congenital spondylolysis and spondylolisthesis (Q76.2)
hemivertebra (Q76.3-Q76.4)
Klippel-Feil syndrome (Q76.1)
lumbarization and sacralization (Q76.4)
platyspondylisis (Q76.4)
spina bifida occulta (Q76.0)
spinal curvature in osteoporosis (M80.-)
spinal curvature in Paget's disease of bone [osteitis deformans] (M88.-)

✓5ᵗʰ M43.0 Spondylolysis
EXCLUDES 1   congenital spondylolysis (Q76.2)
spondylolisthesis (M43.1)
- M43.00 Spondylolysis, site unspecified ▽
- M43.01 Spondylolysis, **occipito-atlanto-axial region**
- M43.02 Spondylolysis, **cervical region**
- M43.03 Spondylolysis, **cervicothoracic region**
- M43.04 Spondylolysis, **thoracic region**
- M43.05 Spondylolysis, **thoracolumbar region**
- M43.06 Spondylolysis, **lumbar region**
- M43.07 Spondylolysis, **lumbosacral region**
- M43.08 Spondylolysis, **sacral and sacrococcygeal region**
- M43.09 Spondylolysis, **multiple sites in spine**

✓5ᵗʰ M43.1 Spondylolisthesis
EXCLUDES 1   acute traumatic of lumbosacral region (S33.1)
acute traumatic of sites other than lumbosacral— code to Fracture, vertebra, by region
congenital spondylolisthesis (Q76.2)
- M43.10 Spondylolisthesis, site unspecified ▽
- M43.11 Spondylolisthesis, **occipito-atlanto-axial region**
- M43.12 Spondylolisthesis, **cervical region**
- M43.13 Spondylolisthesis, **cervicothoracic region**
- M43.14 Spondylolisthesis, **thoracic region**
- M43.15 Spondylolisthesis, **thoracolumbar region**
- M43.16 Spondylolisthesis, **lumbar region**
- M43.17 Spondylolisthesis, **lumbosacral region**
- M43.18 Spondylolisthesis, **sacral and sacrococcygeal region**
- M43.19 Spondylolisthesis, **multiple sites in spine**

✓5ᵗʰ M43.2 Fusion of spine
Ankylosis of spinal joint
EXCLUDES 1   ankylosing spondylitis (M45.0-)
congenital fusion of spine (Q76.4)
EXCLUDES 2   arthrodesis status (Z98.1)
pseudoarthrosis after fusion or arthrodesis (M96.0)
- M43.20 Fusion of spine, site unspecified ▽
- M43.21 Fusion of spine, **occipito-atlanto-axial region**
- M43.22 Fusion of spine, **cervical region**
- M43.23 Fusion of spine, **cervicothoracic region**
- M43.24 Fusion of spine, **thoracic region**
- M43.25 Fusion of spine, **thoracolumbar region**
- M43.26 Fusion of spine, **lumbar region**
- M43.27 Fusion of spine, **lumbosacral region**
- M43.28 Fusion of spine, **sacral and sacrococcygeal region**

M43.3 Recurrent atlantoaxial dislocation with myelopathy

M43.4 Other recurrent atlantoaxial dislocation

✓5ᵗʰ M43.5 Other recurrent vertebral dislocation
EXCLUDES 1   biomechanical lesions NEC (M99.-)
- **✓6ᵗʰ M43.5X Other recurrent vertebral dislocation**
  - M43.5X2 Other recurrent vertebral dislocation, **cervical region**
  - M43.5X3 Other recurrent vertebral dislocation, **cervicothoracic region**
  - M43.5X4 Other recurrent vertebral dislocation, **thoracic region**
  - M43.5X5 Other recurrent vertebral dislocation, **thoracolumbar region**
  - M43.5X6 Other recurrent vertebral dislocation, **lumbar region**
  - M43.5X7 Other recurrent vertebral dislocation, **lumbosacral region**
  - M43.5X8 Other recurrent vertebral dislocation, **sacral and sacrococcygeal region**
  - M43.5X9 Other recurrent vertebral dislocation, site unspecified ▽

M43.6 Torticollis
EXCLUDES 1   congenital (sternomastoid) torticollis (Q68.0)
current injury—see Injury, of spine, by body region
ocular torticollis (R29.891)
psychogenic torticollis (F45.8)
spasmodic torticollis (G24.3)
torticollis due to birth injury (P15.2)

✓5ᵗʰ M43.8 Other specified deforming dorsopathies
EXCLUDES 2   kyphosis and lordosis (M40.-)
scoliosis (M41.-)
- **✓6ᵗʰ M43.8X Other specified deforming dorsopathies**
  - M43.8X1 Other specified deforming dorsopathies, **occipito-atlanto-axial region**
  - M43.8X2 Other specified deforming dorsopathies, **cervical region**
  - M43.8X3 Other specified deforming dorsopathies, **cervicothoracic region**
  - M43.8X4 Other specified deforming dorsopathies, **thoracic region**
  - M43.8X5 Other specified deforming dorsopathies, **thoracolumbar region**
  - M43.8X6 Other specified deforming dorsopathies, **lumbar region**
  - M43.8X7 Other specified deforming dorsopathies, **lumbosacral region**

M43.8X8 Other specified deforming dorsopathies, sacral and sacrococcygeal region

M43.8X9 Other specified deforming dorsopathies, site unspecified ▽

M43.9 Deforming dorsopathy, unspecified ▽
Curvature of spine NOS

Spondylopathies (M45-M49)

✓4ᵗʰ **M45 Ankylosing spondylitis**
Rheumatoid arthritis of spine
EXCLUDES 1 arthropathy in Reiter's disease (M02.3-)
juvenile (ankylosing) spondylitis (M08.1)
EXCLUDES 2 Behçet's disease (M35.2)

M45.0 Ankylosing spondylitis of multiple sites in spine HCC

M45.1 Ankylosing spondylitis of occipito-atlanto-axial region HCC

M45.2 Ankylosing spondylitis of cervical region HCC

M45.3 Ankylosing spondylitis of cervicothoracic region HCC

M45.4 Ankylosing spondylitis of thoracic region HCC

M45.5 Ankylosing spondylitis of thoracolumbar region HCC

M45.6 Ankylosing spondylitis lumbar region HCC

M45.7 Ankylosing spondylitis of lumbosacral region HCC

M45.8 Ankylosing spondylitis sacral and sacrococcygeal region HCC

M45.9 Ankylosing spondylitis of unspecified sites in spine HCC ▽

✓4ᵗʰ **M46 Other inflammatory spondylopathies**

✓5ᵗʰ **M46.0 Spinal enthesopathy**
Disorder of ligamentous or muscular attachments of spine

M46.00 Spinal enthesopathy, site unspecified HCC ▽

M46.01 Spinal enthesopathy, occipito-atlanto-axial region HCC

M46.02 Spinal enthesopathy, cervical region HCC

M46.03 Spinal enthesopathy, cervicothoracic region HCC

M46.04 Spinal enthesopathy, thoracic region HCC

M46.05 Spinal enthesopathy, thoracolumbar region HCC

M46.06 Spinal enthesopathy, lumbar region HCC

M46.07 Spinal enthesopathy, lumbosacral region HCC

M46.08 Spinal enthesopathy, sacral and sacrococcygeal region HCC

M46.09 Spinal enthesopathy, multiple sites in spine HCC

M46.1 Sacroiliitis, not elsewhere classified HCC
DEF: Inflammation of sacroiliac joint (situated at juncture of sacrum and hip); characterized by pain in buttocks or lower back that can extend down one or both legs.

✓5ᵗʰ **M46.2 Osteomyelitis of vertebra**

M46.20 Osteomyelitis of vertebra, site unspecified HCC ▽

M46.21 Osteomyelitis of vertebra, occipito-atlanto-axial region HCC

M46.22 Osteomyelitis of vertebra, cervical region HCC

M46.23 Osteomyelitis of vertebra, cervicothoracic region HCC

M46.24 Osteomyelitis of vertebra, thoracic region HCC

M46.25 Osteomyelitis of vertebra, thoracolumbar region HCC

M46.26 Osteomyelitis of vertebra, lumbar region HCC

M46.27 Osteomyelitis of vertebra, lumbosacral region HCC

M46.28 Osteomyelitis of vertebra, sacral and sacrococcygeal region HCC

✓5ᵗʰ **M46.3 Infection of intervertebral disc (pyogenic)**
Use additional code (B95-B97) to identify infectious agent

M46.30 Infection of intervertebral disc (pyogenic), site unspecified HCC ▽

M46.31 Infection of intervertebral disc (pyogenic), occipito-atlanto-axial region HCC

M46.32 Infection of intervertebral disc (pyogenic), cervical region HCC

M46.33 Infection of intervertebral disc (pyogenic), cervicothoracic region HCC

M46.34 Infection of intervertebral disc (pyogenic), thoracic region HCC

M46.35 Infection of intervertebral disc (pyogenic), thoracolumbar region HCC

M46.36 Infection of intervertebral disc (pyogenic), lumbar region HCC

M46.37 Infection of intervertebral disc (pyogenic), lumbosacral region HCC

M46.38 Infection of intervertebral disc (pyogenic), sacral and sacrococcygeal region HCC

M46.39 Infection of intervertebral disc (pyogenic), multiple sites in spine HCC

✓5ᵗʰ **M46.4 Discitis, unspecified**

M46.40 Discitis, unspecified, site unspecified ▽

M46.41 Discitis, unspecified, occipito-atlanto-axial region ▽

M46.42 Discitis, unspecified, cervical region ▽

M46.43 Discitis, unspecified, cervicothoracic region ▽

M46.44 Discitis, unspecified, thoracic region ▽

M46.45 Discitis, unspecified, thoracolumbar region ▽

M46.46 Discitis, unspecified, lumbar region ▽

M46.47 Discitis, unspecified, lumbosacral region ▽

M46.48 Discitis, unspecified, sacral and sacrococcygeal region ▽

M46.49 Discitis, unspecified, multiple sites in spine ▽

✓5ᵗʰ **M46.5 Other infective spondylopathies**

M46.50 Other infective spondylopathies, site unspecified HCC ▽

M46.51 Other infective spondylopathies, occipito-atlanto-axial region HCC

M46.52 Other infective spondylopathies, cervical region HCC

M46.53 Other infective spondylopathies, cervicothoracic region HCC

M46.54 Other infective spondylopathies, thoracic region HCC

M46.55 Other infective spondylopathies, thoracolumbar region HCC

M46.56 Other infective spondylopathies, lumbar region HCC

M46.57 Other infective spondylopathies, lumbosacral region HCC

M46.58 Other infective spondylopathies, sacral and sacrococcygeal region HCC

M46.59 Other infective spondylopathies, multiple sites in spine HCC

✓5ᵗʰ **M46.8 Other specified inflammatory spondylopathies**

M46.80 Other specified inflammatory spondylopathies, site unspecified HCC ▽

M46.81 Other specified inflammatory spondylopathies, occipito-atlanto-axial region HCC

M46.82 Other specified inflammatory spondylopathies, cervical region HCC

M46.83 Other specified inflammatory spondylopathies, cervicothoracic region HCC

M46.84 Other specified inflammatory spondylopathies, thoracic region HCC

M46.85 Other specified inflammatory spondylopathies, thoracolumbar region HCC

M46.86 Other specified inflammatory spondylopathies, lumbar region HCC

M46.87 Other specified inflammatory spondylopathies, lumbosacral region HCC

M46.88 Other specified inflammatory spondylopathies, sacral and sacrococcygeal region HCC

M46.89 Other specified inflammatory spondylopathies, multiple sites in spine HCC

✓5ᵗʰ **M46.9 Unspecified inflammatory spondylopathy**

M46.90 Unspecified inflammatory spondylopathy, site unspecified HCC ▽

M46.91 Unspecified inflammatory spondylopathy, occipito-atlanto-axial region HCC ▽

M46.92 Unspecified inflammatory spondylopathy, cervical region HCC ▽

M46.93 Unspecified inflammatory spondylopathy, cervicothoracic region HCC ▽

M46.94 Unspecified inflammatory spondylopathy, thoracic region HCC ▽

M46.95 Unspecified inflammatory spondylopathy, thoracolumbar region HCC ▽

M46.96 Unspecified inflammatory spondylopathy, lumbar region HCC ▽

M46.97 Unspecified inflammatory spondylopathy, lumbosacral region HCC ▽

M46.98   Unspecified inflammatory spondylopathy, **sacral and sacrococcygeal** region   `HCC` ▽

M46.99   Unspecified inflammatory spondylopathy, **multiple sites in spine**   `HCC` ▽

✓4ᵗʰ **M47 Spondylosis**

INCLUDES   arthrosis or osteoarthritis of spine
degeneration of facet joints

✓5ᵗʰ **M47.0 Anterior spinal and vertebral artery compression syndromes**

   ✓6ᵗʰ **M47.01**   **Anterior spinal artery** compression syndromes

     M47.011   Anterior spinal artery compression syndromes, **occipito-atlanto-axial** region

     M47.012   Anterior spinal artery compression syndromes, **cervical** region

     M47.013   Anterior spinal artery compression syndromes, **cervicothoracic** region

     M47.014   Anterior spinal artery compression syndromes, **thoracic** region

     M47.015   Anterior spinal artery compression syndromes, **thoracolumbar** region

     M47.016   Anterior spinal artery compression syndromes, **lumbar** region

     M47.019   Anterior spinal artery compression syndromes, **site unspecified** ▽

   ✓6ᵗʰ **M47.02**   **Vertebral artery** compression syndromes

     M47.021   Vertebral artery compression syndromes, **occipito-atlanto-axial** region

     M47.022   Vertebral artery compression syndromes, **cervical** region

     M47.029   Vertebral artery compression syndromes, **site unspecified** ▽

✓5ᵗʰ **M47.1 Other spondylosis with myelopathy**

Spondylogenic compression of spinal cord

EXCLUDES 1   vertebral subluxation (M43.3-M43.5X9)

   M47.10   Other spondylosis with myelopathy, **site unspecified** ▽

   M47.11   Other spondylosis with myelopathy, **occipito-atlanto-axial** region

   M47.12   Other spondylosis with myelopathy, **cervical** region

   M47.13   Other spondylosis with myelopathy, **cervicothoracic** region

   M47.14   Other spondylosis with myelopathy, **thoracic** region

   M47.15   Other spondylosis with myelopathy, **thoracolumbar** region

   M47.16   Other spondylosis with myelopathy, **lumbar** region

✓5ᵗʰ **M47.2 Other spondylosis with radiculopathy**

   M47.20   Other spondylosis with radiculopathy, **site unspecified** ▽

   M47.21   Other spondylosis with radiculopathy, **occipito-atlanto-axial** region

   M47.22   Other spondylosis with radiculopathy, **cervical** region

   M47.23   Other spondylosis with radiculopathy, **cervicothoracic** region

   M47.24   Other spondylosis with radiculopathy, **thoracic** region

   M47.25   Other spondylosis with radiculopathy, **thoracolumbar** region

   M47.26   Other spondylosis with radiculopathy, **lumbar** region

   M47.27   Other spondylosis with radiculopathy, **lumbosacral** region

   M47.28   Other spondylosis with radiculopathy, **sacral and sacrococcygeal** region

✓5ᵗʰ **M47.8 Other spondylosis**

   ✓6ᵗʰ **M47.81**   Spondylosis **without myelopathy or radiculopathy**

     M47.811   Spondylosis without myelopathy or radiculopathy, **occipito-atlanto-axial** region

     M47.812   Spondylosis without myelopathy or radiculopathy, **cervical** region

     M47.813   Spondylosis without myelopathy or radiculopathy, **cervicothoracic** region

     M47.814   Spondylosis without myelopathy or radiculopathy, **thoracic** region

     M47.815   Spondylosis without myelopathy or radiculopathy, **thoracolumbar** region

     M47.816   Spondylosis without myelopathy or radiculopathy, **lumbar** region

     M47.817   Spondylosis without myelopathy or radiculopathy, **lumbosacral** region

     M47.818   Spondylosis without myelopathy or radiculopathy, **sacral and sacrococcygeal** region

     M47.819   Spondylosis without myelopathy or radiculopathy, **site unspecified** ▽

   ✓6ᵗʰ **M47.89**   **Other spondylosis**

     M47.891   Other spondylosis, **occipito-atlanto-axial** region

     M47.892   Other spondylosis, **cervical** region

     M47.893   Other spondylosis, **cervicothoracic** region

     M47.894   Other spondylosis, **thoracic** region

     M47.895   Other spondylosis, **thoracolumbar** region

     M47.896   Other spondylosis, **lumbar** region

     M47.897   Other spondylosis, **lumbosacral** region

     M47.898   Other spondylosis, **sacral and sacrococcygeal** region

     M47.899   Other spondylosis, site unspecified ▽

   M47.9 Spondylosis, unspecified ▽

✓4ᵗʰ **M48 Other spondylopathies**

✓5ᵗʰ **M48.0 Spinal stenosis**

Caudal stenosis

   M48.00   Spinal stenosis, **site unspecified** ▽

   M48.01   Spinal stenosis, **occipito-atlanto-axial** region

   M48.02   Spinal stenosis, **cervical** region

   M48.03   Spinal stenosis, **cervicothoracic** region

   M48.04   Spinal stenosis, **thoracic** region

   M48.05   Spinal stenosis, **thoracolumbar** region

   ✓6ᵗʰ **M48.06**   Spinal stenosis, **lumbar** region

     DEF: Spinal canal narrowing in the lumbar area with nerve root compression, causing muscle pain, fatigue, and weakness during extension of the lumbar spine; pain is relieved by sitting or bending.

     ●   **M48.061**   Spinal stenosis, lumbar region **without neurogenic claudication**

       Spinal stenosis, lumbar region NOS

     ●   **M48.062**   Spinal stenosis, lumbar region **with neurogenic claudication**

   M48.07   Spinal stenosis, **lumbosacral** region

   M48.08   Spinal stenosis, **sacral and sacrococcygeal** region

✓5ᵗʰ **M48.1 Ankylosing hyperostosis [Forestier]**

Diffuse idiopathic skeletal hyperostosis [DISH]

   M48.10   Ankylosing hyperostosis [Forestier], **site unspecified** ▽

   M48.11   Ankylosing hyperostosis [Forestier], **occipito-atlanto-axial** region

   M48.12   Ankylosing hyperostosis [Forestier], **cervical** region

   M48.13   Ankylosing hyperostosis [Forestier], **cervicothoracic** region

   M48.14   Ankylosing hyperostosis [Forestier], **thoracic** region

   M48.15   Ankylosing hyperostosis [Forestier], **thoracolumbar** region

   M48.16   Ankylosing hyperostosis [Forestier], **lumbar** region

   M48.17   Ankylosing hyperostosis [Forestier], **lumbosacral** region

   M48.18   Ankylosing hyperostosis [Forestier], **sacral and sacrococcygeal** region

   M48.19   Ankylosing hyperostosis [Forestier], **multiple sites in spine**

✓5ᵗʰ **M48.2 Kissing spine**

   M48.20   Kissing spine, site unspecified ▽

   M48.21   Kissing spine, **occipito-atlanto-axial** region

   M48.22   Kissing spine, **cervical** region

   M48.23   Kissing spine, **cervicothoracic** region

   M48.24   Kissing spine, **thoracic** region

   M48.25   Kissing spine, **thoracolumbar** region

   M48.26   Kissing spine, **lumbar** region

   M48.27   Kissing spine, **lumbosacral** region

EXCLUDES 1 Not coded here   EXCLUDES 2 Not included here   N Newborn Age: 0   P Pediatric Age: 0-17   M Maternity Age: 12-55   A Adult Age: 15-124

756   ICD-10-CM 2018

✓5ᵗʰ **M48.3 Traumatic spondylopathy**

    M48.30 Traumatic spondylopathy, site unspecified ▽

    M48.31 Traumatic spondylopathy, occipito-atlanto-axial region

    M48.32 Traumatic spondylopathy, cervical region

    M48.33 Traumatic spondylopathy, cervicothoracic region

    M48.34 Traumatic spondylopathy, thoracic region

    M48.35 Traumatic spondylopathy, thoracolumbar region

    M48.36 Traumatic spondylopathy, lumbar region

    M48.37 Traumatic spondylopathy, lumbosacral region

    M48.38 Traumatic spondylopathy, sacral and sacrococcygeal region

✓5ᵗʰ **M48.4 Fatigue fracture of vertebra**

    Stress fracture of vertebra

    EXCLUDES 1   *pathological fracture NOS (M84.4-)*

        pathological fracture of vertebra due to neoplasm (M84.58)

        pathological fracture of vertebra due to other diagnosis (M84.68)

        pathological fracture of vertebra due to osteoporosis (M80.-)

        traumatic fracture of vertebrae (S12.0-S12.3-, S22.0-, S32.0-)

> The appropriate 7th character is to be added to each code from subcategory M48.4.
> A   initial encounter for fracture
> D   subsequent encounter for fracture with routine healing
> G   subsequent encounter for fracture with delayed healing
> S   sequela of fracture

  ✓x7ᵗʰ **M48.40 Fatigue fracture of vertebra, site unspecified** ▽

  ✓x7ᵗʰ **M48.41 Fatigue fracture of vertebra, occipito-atlanto-axial region**

  ✓x7ᵗʰ **M48.42 Fatigue fracture of vertebra, cervical region**

  ✓x7ᵗʰ **M48.43 Fatigue fracture of vertebra, cervicothoracic region**

  ✓x7ᵗʰ **M48.44 Fatigue fracture of vertebra, thoracic region**

  ✓x7ᵗʰ **M48.45 Fatigue fracture of vertebra, thoracolumbar region**

  ✓x7ᵗʰ **M48.46 Fatigue fracture of vertebra, lumbar region**

  ✓x7ᵗʰ **M48.47 Fatigue fracture of vertebra, lumbosacral region**

  ✓x7ᵗʰ **M48.48 Fatigue fracture of vertebra, sacral and sacrococcygeal region**

✓5ᵗʰ **M48.5 Collapsed vertebra, not elsewhere classified**

    Collapsed vertebra NOS

    Compression fracture of vertebra NOS

    Wedging of vertebra NOS

    EXCLUDES 1   *current injury—see Injury of spine, by body region*

        fatigue fracture of vertebra (M48.4)

        pathological fracture of vertebra due to neoplasm (M84.58)

        pathological fracture of vertebra due to other diagnosis (M84.68)

        pathological fracture of vertebra due to osteoporosis (M80.-)

        pathological fracture NOS (M84.4-)

        stress fracture of vertebra (M48.4-)

        traumatic fracture of vertebra (S12-, S22-, S32-)

> The appropriate 7th character is to be added to each code from subcategory M48.5.
> A   initial encounter for fracture
> D   subsequent encounter for fracture with routine healing
> G   subsequent encounter for fracture with delayed healing
> S   sequela of fracture

¹ ✓x7ᵗʰ **M48.50 Collapsed vertebra, not elsewhere classified, site unspecified** `HCC` ▽

¹ ✓x7ᵗʰ **M48.51 Collapsed vertebra, not elsewhere classified, occipito-atlanto-axial region** `HCC`

¹ ✓x7ᵗʰ **M48.52 Collapsed vertebra, not elsewhere classified, cervical region** `HCC`

¹ ✓x7ᵗʰ **M48.53 Collapsed vertebra, not elsewhere classified, cervicothoracic region** `HCC`

¹ ✓x7ᵗʰ **M48.54 Collapsed vertebra, not elsewhere classified, thoracic region** `HCC`

¹ ✓x7ᵗʰ **M48.55 Collapsed vertebra, not elsewhere classified, thoracolumbar region** `HCC`

¹ ✓x7ᵗʰ **M48.56 Collapsed vertebra, not elsewhere classified, lumbar region** `HCC`

¹ ✓x7ᵗʰ **M48.57 Collapsed vertebra, not elsewhere classified, lumbosacral region** `HCC`

¹ ✓x7ᵗʰ **M48.58 Collapsed vertebra, not elsewhere classified, sacral and sacrococcygeal region** `HCC`

✓5ᵗʰ **M48.8 Other specified spondylopathies**

    Ossification of posterior longitudinal ligament

  ✓6ᵗʰ **M48.8X Other specified spondylopathies**

    M48.8X1 Other specified spondylopathies, occipito-atlanto-axial region `HCC`

    M48.8X2 Other specified spondylopathies, cervical region `HCC`

    M48.8X3 Other specified spondylopathies, cervicothoracic region `HCC`

    M48.8X4 Other specified spondylopathies, thoracic region `HCC`

    M48.8X5 Other specified spondylopathies, thoracolumbar region `HCC`

    M48.8X6 Other specified spondylopathies, lumbar region `HCC`

    M48.8X7 Other specified spondylopathies, lumbosacral region `HCC`

    M48.8X8 Other specified spondylopathies, sacral and sacrococcygeal region `HCC`

    M48.8X9 Other specified spondylopathies, site unspecified `HCC` ▽

  M48.9 Spondylopathy, unspecified ▽

✓4ᵗʰ **M49 Spondylopathies in diseases classified elsewhere**

    INCLUDES   curvature of spine in diseases classified elsewhere

        deformity of spine in diseases classified elsewhere

        kyphosis in diseases classified elsewhere

        scoliosis in diseases classified elsewhere

        spondylopathy in diseases classified elsewhere

    Code first underlying disease, such as:

      brucellosis (A23.-)

      Charcôt-Marie-Tooth disease (G60.0)

      enterobacterial infections (A01-A04)

      osteitis fibrosa cystica (E21.0)

    EXCLUDES 1   *curvature of spine in tuberculosis [Pott's] (A18.01)*

        enteropathic arthropathies (M07.-)

        gonococcal spondylitis (A54.41)

        neuropathic [tabes dorsalis] spondylitis (A52.11)

        neuropathic spondylopathy in syringomyelia (G95.0)

        neuropathic spondylopathy in tabes dorsalis (A52.11)

        nonsyphilitic neuropathic spondylopathy NEC (G98.0)

        spondylitis in syphilis (acquired) (A52.77)

        tuberculous spondylitis (A18.01)

        typhoid fever spondylitis (A01.05)

✓5ᵗʰ **M49.8 Spondylopathy in diseases classified elsewhere**

    M49.80 Spondylopathy in diseases classified elsewhere, site unspecified `HCC` ▽

    M49.81 Spondylopathy in diseases classified elsewhere, occipito-atlanto-axial region `HCC`

    M49.82 Spondylopathy in diseases classified elsewhere, cervical region `HCC`

    M49.83 Spondylopathy in diseases classified elsewhere, cervicothoracic region `HCC`

    M49.84 Spondylopathy in diseases classified elsewhere, thoracic region `HCC`

    M49.85 Spondylopathy in diseases classified elsewhere, thoracolumbar region `HCC`

    M49.86 Spondylopathy in diseases classified elsewhere, lumbar region `HCC`

    M49.87 Spondylopathy in diseases classified elsewhere, lumbosacral region `HCC`

    M49.88 Spondylopathy in diseases classified elsewhere, sacral and sacrococcygeal region `HCC`

    M49.89 Spondylopathy in diseases classified elsewhere, multiple sites in spine `HCC`

---

¹ HCC with 7th character indicating initial encounter (A, B or C - specific to category).

✓ Additional Character Req   ✓x7ᵗʰ Placeholder Alert   Manifestation   `HCC` CMS-HCC Condition   ▽ Unspecified Code   ▶◀ Revised Text   ● New Code   ▲ Revised Code Title

ICD-10-CM 2018   757

Other dorsopathies (M50-M54)

EXCLUDES 1   current injury—see injury of spine by body region
discitis NOS (M46.4-)

✓4th **M50 Cervical disc disorders**

NOTE   Code to the most superior level of disorder.

INCLUDES   cervicothoracic disc disorders with cervicalgia
cervicothoracic disc disorders

AHA: 2016, 1Q, 17

✓5th **M50.0 Cervical disc disorder with myelopathy**

M50.00 Cervical disc disorder with myelopathy, unspecified cervical region ▽

M50.01 Cervical disc disorder with myelopathy, high cervical region
C2-C3 disc disorder with myelopathy
C3-C4 disc disorder with myelopathy

✓6th **M50.02 Cervical disc disorder with myelopathy, mid-cervical region**

M50.020 Cervical disc disorder with myelopathy, mid-cervical region, unspecified level ▽

M50.021 Cervical disc disorder at C4-C5 level with myelopathy
C4-C5 disc disorder with myelopathy

M50.022 Cervical disc disorder at C5-C6 level with myelopathy
C5-C6 disc disorder with myelopathy

M50.023 Cervical disc disorder at C6-C7 level with myelopathy
C6-C7 disc disorder with myelopathy

M50.03 Cervical disc disorder with myelopathy, cervicothoracic region
C7-T1 disc disorder with myelopathy

✓5th **M50.1 Cervical disc disorder with radiculopathy**

EXCLUDES 2   brachial radiculitis NOS (M54.13)

M50.10 Cervical disc disorder with radiculopathy, unspecified cervical region ▽

M50.11 Cervical disc disorder with radiculopathy, high cervical region
C2-C3 disc disorder with radiculopathy
C3 radiculopathy due to disc disorder
C3-C4 disc disorder with radiculopathy
C4 radiculopathy due to disc disorder

✓6th **M50.12 Cervical disc disorder with radiculopathy, mid-cervical region**

M50.120 Mid-cervical disc disorder, unspecified ▽

M50.121 Cervical disc disorder at C4-C5 level with radiculopathy
C4-C5 disc disorder with radiculopathy
C5 radiculopathy due to disc disorder

M50.122 Cervical disc disorder at C5-C6 level with radiculopathy
C5-C6 disc disorder with radiculopathy
C6 radiculopathy due to disc disorder

M50.123 Cervical disc disorder at C6-C7 level with radiculopathy
C6-C7 disc disorder with radiculopathy
C7 radiculopathy due to disc disorder

M50.13 Cervical disc disorder with radiculopathy, cervicothoracic region
C7-T1 disc disorder with radiculopathy
C8 radiculopathy due to disc disorder

✓5th **M50.2 Other cervical disc displacement**

M50.20 Other cervical disc displacement, unspecified cervical region ▽

M50.21 Other cervical disc displacement, high cervical region
Other C2-C3 cervical disc displacement
Other C3-C4 cervical disc displacement

✓6th **M50.22 Other cervical disc displacement, mid-cervical region**

M50.220 Other cervical disc displacement, mid-cervical region, unspecified level ▽

M50.221 Other cervical disc displacement at C4-C5 level
Other C4-C5 cervical disc displacement

M50.222 Other cervical disc displacement at C5-C6 level
Other C5-C6 cervical disc displacement

M50.223 Other cervical disc displacement at C6-C7 level
Other C6-C7 cervical disc displacement

M50.23 Other cervical disc displacement, cervicothoracic region
Other C7-T1 cervical disc displacement

✓5th **M50.3 Other cervical disc degeneration**

M50.30 Other cervical disc degeneration, unspecified cervical region ▽

M50.31 Other cervical disc degeneration, high cervical region
Other C2-C3 cervical disc degeneration
Other C3-C4 cervical disc degeneration

✓6th **M50.32 Other cervical disc degeneration, mid-cervical region**

M50.320 Other cervical disc degeneration, mid-cervical region, unspecified level ▽

M50.321 Other cervical disc degeneration at C4-C5 level
Other C4-C5 cervical disc degeneration

M50.322 Other cervical disc degeneration at C5-C6 level
Other C5-C6 cervical disc degeneration

M50.323 Other cervical disc degeneration at C6-C7 level
Other C6-C7 cervical disc degeneration

M50.33 Other cervical disc degeneration, cervicothoracic region
Other C7-T1 cervical disc degeneration

✓5th **M50.8 Other cervical disc disorders**

M50.80 Other cervical disc disorders, unspecified cervical region ▽

M50.81 Other cervical disc disorders, high cervical region
Other C2-C3 cervical disc disorders
Other C3-C4 cervical disc disorders

✓6th **M50.82 Other cervical disc disorders, mid-cervical region**

M50.820 Other cervical disc disorders, mid-cervical region, unspecified level ▽

M50.821 Other cervical disc disorders at C4-C5 level
Other C4-C5 cervical disc disorders

M50.822 Other cervical disc disorders at C5-C6 level
Other C5-C6 cervical disc disorders

M50.823 Other cervical disc disorders at C6-C7 level
Other C6-C7 cervical disc disorders

M50.83 Other cervical disc disorders, cervicothoracic region
Other C7-T1 cervical disc disorders

✓5th **M50.9 Cervical disc disorder, unspecified**

M50.90 Cervical disc disorder, unspecified, unspecified cervical region ▽

M50.91 Cervical disc disorder, unspecified, high cervical region ▽
C2-C3 cervical disc disorder, unspecified
C3-C4 cervical disc disorder, unspecified

✓6th **M50.92 Cervical disc disorder, unspecified, mid-cervical region**

M50.920 Unspecified cervical disc disorder, mid-cervical region, unspecified level ▽

M50.921 Unspecified cervical disc disorder at C4-C5 level ▽
Unspecified C4-C5 cervical disc disorder

M50.922 Unspecified cervical disc disorder at C5-C6 level ▽
Unspecified C5-C6 cervical disc disorder

M50.923 Unspecified cervical disc disorder at C6-C7 level ▽
Unspecified C6-C7 cervical disc disorder

M50.93 Cervical disc disorder, unspecified, cervicothoracic region ▽
C7-T1 cervical disc disorder, unspecified

✓4th **M51 Thoracic, thoracolumbar, and lumbosacral intervertebral disc disorders**

EXCLUDES 2   cervical and cervicothoracic disc disorders (M50.-)
sacral and sacrococcygeal disorders (M53.3)

✓5th **M51.0 Thoracic, thoracolumbar and lumbosacral intervertebral disc disorders with myelopathy**

M51.04 Intervertebral disc disorders with myelopathy, thoracic region

EXCLUDES 1 Not coded here   EXCLUDES 2 Not included here   N Newborn Age: 0   P Pediatric Age: 0-17   M Maternity Age: 12-55   A Adult Age: 15-124

758   ICD-10-CM 2018

M51.05   Intervertebral disc disorders with myelopathy, **thoracolumbar** region

M51.06   Intervertebral disc disorders with myelopathy, **lumbar** region

✓5ᵗʰ **M51.1**   **Thoracic, thoracolumbar and lumbosacral intervertebral disc disorders with radiculopathy**
Sciatica due to intervertebral disc disorder
> EXCLUDES 1   *lumbar radiculitis NOS (M54.16)*
> *sciatica NOS (M54.3)*

M51.14   Intervertebral disc disorders with radiculopathy, **thoracic** region

M51.15   Intervertebral disc disorders with radiculopathy, **thoracolumbar** region

M51.16   Intervertebral disc disorders with radiculopathy, **lumbar** region

M51.17   Intervertebral disc disorders with radiculopathy, **lumbosacral** region

✓5ᵗʰ **M51.2**   **Other thoracic, thoracolumbar and lumbosacral intervertebral disc displacement**
Lumbago due to displacement of intervertebral disc

M51.24   Other intervertebral disc displacement, **thoracic** region

M51.25   Other intervertebral disc displacement, **thoracolumbar** region

M51.26   Other intervertebral disc displacement, **lumbar** region

M51.27   Other intervertebral disc displacement, **lumbosacral** region

✓5ᵗʰ **M51.3**   **Other thoracic, thoracolumbar and lumbosacral intervertebral disc degeneration**
AHA: 2013, 3Q, 22

M51.34   Other intervertebral disc degeneration, **thoracic** region

M51.35   Other intervertebral disc degeneration, **thoracolumbar** region

M51.36   Other intervertebral disc degeneration, **lumbar** region

M51.37   Other intervertebral disc degeneration, **lumbosacral** region

✓5ᵗʰ **M51.4**   **Schmorl's nodes**
DEF: Irregular bone defect in the margin of the vertebral body; causes herniation into end plate of vertebral body.

M51.44   Schmorl's nodes, **thoracic** region

M51.45   Schmorl's nodes, **thoracolumbar** region

M51.46   Schmorl's nodes, **lumbar** region

M51.47   Schmorl's nodes, **lumbosacral** region

✓5ᵗʰ **M51.8**   **Other thoracic, thoracolumbar and lumbosacral intervertebral disc disorders**

M51.84   Other intervertebral disc disorders, **thoracic** region

M51.85   Other intervertebral disc disorders, **thoracolumbar** region

M51.86   Other intervertebral disc disorders, **lumbar** region

M51.87   Other intervertebral disc disorders, **lumbosacral** region

M51.9   Unspecified thoracic, thoracolumbar and lumbosacral intervertebral disc disorder   ▽

✓4ᵗʰ **M53**   **Other and unspecified dorsopathies, not elsewhere classified**

M53.0   **Cervicocranial syndrome**
Posterior cervical sympathetic syndrome

M53.1   **Cervicobrachial syndrome**
> EXCLUDES 2   *cervical disc disorder (M50.-)*
> *thoracic outlet syndrome (G54.0)*

✓5ᵗʰ **M53.2**   **Spinal instabilities**

✓6ᵗʰ **M53.2X**   **Spinal instabilities**

M53.2X1   Spinal instabilities, **occipito-atlanto-axial** region

M53.2X2   Spinal instabilities, **cervical** region

M53.2X3   Spinal instabilities, **cervicothoracic** region

M53.2X4   Spinal instabilities, **thoracic** region

M53.2X5   Spinal instabilities, **thoracolumbar** region

M53.2X6   Spinal instabilities, **lumbar** region

M53.2X7   Spinal instabilities, **lumbosacral** region

M53.2X8   Spinal instabilities, **sacral and sacrococcygeal** region

---

Displacement Intervertebral Disc

Normal Top View   Herniated Top View

Labels: Lamina, Ligamentum flavum, Disc annulus, Nucleus pulposus, Nucleus pulposus, Herniates through annulus, Spinal cord, Spinal nerve

---

M53.2X9   Spinal instabilities, site unspecified   ▽

M53.3   **Sacrococcygeal disorders, not elsewhere classified**
Coccygodynia

✓5ᵗʰ **M53.8**   **Other specified dorsopathies**

M53.80   Other specified dorsopathies, site unspecified   ▽

M53.81   Other specified dorsopathies, occipito-atlanto-axial region

M53.82   Other specified dorsopathies, cervical region

M53.83   Other specified dorsopathies, cervicothoracic region

M53.84   Other specified dorsopathies, thoracic region

M53.85   Other specified dorsopathies, thoracolumbar region

M53.86   Other specified dorsopathies, lumbar region

M53.87   Other specified dorsopathies, lumbosacral region

M53.88   Other specified dorsopathies, sacral and sacrococcygeal region

M53.9   **Dorsopathy, unspecified**   ▽

✓4ᵗʰ **M54**   **Dorsalgia**
> EXCLUDES 1   *psychogenic dorsalgia (F45.41)*

✓5ᵗʰ **M54.0**   **Panniculitis affecting regions of neck and back**
> EXCLUDES 1   *lupus panniculitis (L93.2)*
> *panniculitis NOS (M79.3)*
> *relapsing [Weber-Christian] panniculitis (M35.6)*

M54.00   Panniculitis affecting regions of neck and back, site unspecified   ▽

M54.01   Panniculitis affecting regions of neck and back, occipito-atlanto-axial region

M54.02   Panniculitis affecting regions of neck and back, cervical region

M54.03   Panniculitis affecting regions of neck and back, cervicothoracic region

M54.04   Panniculitis affecting regions of neck and back, thoracic region

M54.05   Panniculitis affecting regions of neck and back, thoracolumbar region

M54.06   Panniculitis affecting regions of neck and back, lumbar region

M54.07   Panniculitis affecting regions of neck and back, lumbosacral region

M54.08   Panniculitis affecting regions of neck and back, sacral and sacrococcygeal region

M54.09   Panniculitis affecting regions, neck and back, multiple sites in spine

✓5ᵗʰ **M54.1**   **Radiculopathy**
Brachial neuritis or radiculitis NOS
Lumbar neuritis or radiculitis NOS
Lumbosacral neuritis or radiculitis NOS
Thoracic neuritis or radiculitis NOS
Radiculitis NOS
> EXCLUDES 1   *neuralgia and neuritis NOS (M79.2)*
> *radiculopathy with cervical disc disorder (M50.1)*
> *radiculopathy with lumbar and other intervertebral disc disorder (M51.1-)*
> *radiculopathy with spondylosis (M47.2-)*

M54.10   Radiculopathy, site unspecified   ▽

M54.11   Radiculopathy, occipito-atlanto-axial region

M54.12   Radiculopathy, cervical region

M54.13   Radiculopathy, cervicothoracic region

M54.14   Radiculopathy, thoracic region

☑ Additional Character Req   ✓7ᵗʰ Placeholder Alert   Manifestation   HCC CMS-HCC Condition   ▽ Unspecified Code   ►◄ Revised Text   ● New Code   ▲ Revised Code Title

ICD-10-CM 2018   759

M54.15　Radiculopathy, thoracolumbar region
M54.16　Radiculopathy, lumbar region
M54.17　Radiculopathy, lumbosacral region
M54.18　Radiculopathy, sacral and sacrococcygeal region

M54.2　**Cervicalgia**
　　EXCLUDES 1　cervicalgia due to intervertebral cervical disc disorder (M50.-)

✓5th M54.3　**Sciatica**
　　EXCLUDES 1　lesion of sciatic nerve (G57.0)
　　　　sciatica due to intervertebral disc disorder (M51.1-)
　　　　sciatica with lumbago (M54.4-)
　　M54.30　Sciatica, unspecified side　▽
　　M54.31　Sciatica, right side
　　M54.32　Sciatica, left side

✓5th M54.4　**Lumbago with sciatica**
　　EXCLUDES 1　lumbago with sciatica due to intervertebral disc disorder (M51.1-)
　　AHA: 2016, 2Q, 7
　　M54.40　Lumbago with sciatica, unspecified side　▽
　　M54.41　Lumbago with sciatica, right side
　　M54.42　Lumbago with sciatica, left side

M54.5　**Low back pain**
　　Loin pain
　　Lumbago NOS
　　EXCLUDES 1　low back strain (S39.012)
　　　　lumbago due to intervertebral disc displacement (M51.2-)
　　　　lumbago with sciatica (M54.4-)

M54.6　**Pain in thoracic spine**
　　EXCLUDES 1　pain in thoracic spine due to intervertebral disc disorder (M51.-)

✓5th M54.8　**Other dorsalgia**
　　EXCLUDES 1　dorsalgia in thoracic region (M54.6)
　　　　low back pain (M54.5)
　　M54.81　Occipital neuralgia
　　M54.89　Other dorsalgia

M54.9　**Dorsalgia, unspecified**　▽
　　Backache NOS　　　Back pain NOS

SOFT TISSUE DISORDERS (M60-M79)

Disorders of muscles (M60-M63)

EXCLUDES 1　dermatopolymyositis (M33.-)
　　muscular dystrophies and myopathies (G71-G72)
　　myopathy in amyloidosis (E85.-)
　　myopathy in polyarteritis nodosa (M30.0)
　　myopathy in rheumatoid arthritis (M05.32)
　　myopathy in scleroderma (M34.-)
　　myopathy in Sjögren's syndrome (M35.03)
　　myopathy in systemic lupus erythematosus (M32.-)

✓4th **M60　Myositis**
　　EXCLUDES 2　inclusion body myositis [IBM] (G72.41)

✓5th M60.0　**Infective myositis**
　　Tropical pyomyositis
　　Use additional code (B95-B97) to identify infectious agent

　✓6th M60.00　**Infective myositis, unspecified site**
　　　M60.000　Infective myositis, unspecified right arm
　　　　Infective myositis, right upper limb NOS
　　　M60.001　Infective myositis, unspecified left arm
　　　　Infective myositis, left upper limb NOS
　　　M60.002　Infective myositis, unspecified arm　▽
　　　　Infective myositis, upper limb NOS
　　　M60.003　Infective myositis, unspecified right leg
　　　　Infective myositis, right lower limb NOS
　　　M60.004　Infective myositis, unspecified left leg
　　　　Infective myositis, left lower limb NOS
　　　M60.005　Infective myositis, unspecified leg　▽
　　　　Infective myositis, lower limb NOS
　　　M60.009　Infective myositis, unspecified site　▽

　✓6th M60.01　**Infective myositis, shoulder**
　　　M60.011　Infective myositis, right shoulder
　　　M60.012　Infective myositis, left shoulder
　　　M60.019　Infective myositis, unspecified shoulder▽

　✓6th M60.02　**Infective myositis, upper arm**
　　　M60.021　Infective myositis, right upper arm

M60.022　Infective myositis, left upper arm
M60.029　Infective myositis, unspecified upper arm　▽

✓6th M60.03　**Infective myositis, forearm**
　M60.031　Infective myositis, right forearm
　M60.032　Infective myositis, left forearm
　M60.039　Infective myositis, unspecified forearm　▽

✓6th M60.04　**Infective myositis, hand and fingers**
　M60.041　Infective myositis, right hand
　M60.042　Infective myositis, left hand
　M60.043　Infective myositis, unspecified hand　▽
　M60.044　Infective myositis, right finger(s)
　M60.045　Infective myositis, left finger(s)
　M60.046　Infective myositis, unspecified finger(s)▽

✓6th M60.05　**Infective myositis, thigh**
　M60.051　Infective myositis, right thigh
　M60.052　Infective myositis, left thigh
　M60.059　Infective myositis, unspecified thigh　▽

✓6th M60.06　**Infective myositis, lower leg**
　M60.061　Infective myositis, right lower leg
　M60.062　Infective myositis, left lower leg
　M60.069　Infective myositis, unspecified lower leg　▽

✓6th M60.07　**Infective myositis, ankle, foot and toes**
　M60.070　Infective myositis, right ankle
　M60.071　Infective myositis, left ankle
　M60.072　Infective myositis, unspecified ankle　▽
　M60.073　Infective myositis, right foot
　M60.074　Infective myositis, left foot
　M60.075　Infective myositis, unspecified foot　▽
　M60.076　Infective myositis, right toe(s)
　M60.077　Infective myositis, left toe(s)
　M60.078　Infective myositis, unspecified toe(s)　▽

M60.08　Infective myositis, other site
M60.09　Infective myositis, multiple sites

✓5th M60.1　**Interstitial myositis**
　M60.10　Interstitial myositis of unspecified site　▽

　✓6th M60.11　**Interstitial myositis, shoulder**
　　M60.111　Interstitial myositis, right shoulder
　　M60.112　Interstitial myositis, left shoulder
　　M60.119　Interstitial myositis, unspecified shoulder　▽

　✓6th M60.12　**Interstitial myositis, upper arm**
　　M60.121　Interstitial myositis, right upper arm
　　M60.122　Interstitial myositis, left upper arm
　　M60.129　Interstitial myositis, unspecified upper arm　▽

　✓6th M60.13　**Interstitial myositis, forearm**
　　M60.131　Interstitial myositis, right forearm
　　M60.132　Interstitial myositis, left forearm
　　M60.139　Interstitial myositis, unspecified forearm　▽

　✓6th M60.14　**Interstitial myositis, hand**
　　M60.141　Interstitial myositis, right hand
　　M60.142　Interstitial myositis, left hand
　　M60.149　Interstitial myositis, unspecified hand　▽

　✓6th M60.15　**Interstitial myositis, thigh**
　　M60.151　Interstitial myositis, right thigh
　　M60.152　Interstitial myositis, left thigh
　　M60.159　Interstitial myositis, unspecified thigh　▽

　✓6th M60.16　**Interstitial myositis, lower leg**
　　M60.161　Interstitial myositis, right lower leg
　　M60.162　Interstitial myositis, left lower leg
　　M60.169　Interstitial myositis, unspecified lower leg　▽

　✓6th M60.17　**Interstitial myositis, ankle and foot**
　　M60.171　Interstitial myositis, right ankle and foot
　　M60.172　Interstitial myositis, left ankle and foot
　　M60.179　Interstitial myositis, unspecified ankle and foot　▽

M60.18　Interstitial myositis, other site
M60.19　Interstitial myositis, multiple sites

EXCLUDES 1 Not coded here　　*EXCLUDES 2* Not included here　　N Newborn Age: 0　　P Pediatric Age: 0-17　　M Maternity Age: 12-55　　A Adult Age: 15-124

760　　　　ICD-10-CM 2018

✓5ᵗʰ **M60.2 Foreign body granuloma of soft tissue, not elsewhere classified**

> Use additional code to identify the type of retained foreign body (Z18.-)
>
> EXCLUDES 1   *foreign body granuloma of skin and subcutaneous tissue (L92.3)*

     M60.20   Foreign body granuloma of soft tissue, not elsewhere classified, unspecified site ▽

✓6ᵗʰ   M60.21   Foreign body granuloma of soft tissue, not elsewhere classified, **shoulder**

     M60.211   Foreign body granuloma of soft tissue, not elsewhere classified, **right shoulder**

     M60.212   Foreign body granuloma of soft tissue, not elsewhere classified, **left shoulder**

     M60.219   Foreign body granuloma of soft tissue, not elsewhere classified, unspecified shoulder ▽

✓6ᵗʰ   M60.22   Foreign body granuloma of soft tissue, not elsewhere classified, **upper arm**

     M60.221   Foreign body granuloma of soft tissue, not elsewhere classified, **right upper arm**

     M60.222   Foreign body granuloma of soft tissue, not elsewhere classified, **left upper arm**

     M60.229   Foreign body granuloma of soft tissue, not elsewhere classified, unspecified upper arm ▽

✓6ᵗʰ   M60.23   Foreign body granuloma of soft tissue, not elsewhere classified, **forearm**

     M60.231   Foreign body granuloma of soft tissue, not elsewhere classified, **right forearm**

     M60.232   Foreign body granuloma of soft tissue, not elsewhere classified, **left forearm**

     M60.239   Foreign body granuloma of soft tissue, not elsewhere classified, unspecified forearm ▽

✓6ᵗʰ   M60.24   Foreign body granuloma of soft tissue, not elsewhere classified, **hand**

     M60.241   Foreign body granuloma of soft tissue, not elsewhere classified, **right hand**

     M60.242   Foreign body granuloma of soft tissue, not elsewhere classified, **left hand**

     M60.249   Foreign body granuloma of soft tissue, not elsewhere classified, unspecified hand ▽

✓6ᵗʰ   M60.25   Foreign body granuloma of soft tissue, not elsewhere classified, **thigh**

     M60.251   Foreign body granuloma of soft tissue, not elsewhere classified, **right thigh**

     M60.252   Foreign body granuloma of soft tissue, not elsewhere classified, **left thigh**

     M60.259   Foreign body granuloma of soft tissue, not elsewhere classified, unspecified thigh ▽

✓6ᵗʰ   M60.26   Foreign body granuloma of soft tissue, not elsewhere classified, **lower leg**

     M60.261   Foreign body granuloma of soft tissue, not elsewhere classified, **right lower leg**

     M60.262   Foreign body granuloma of soft tissue, not elsewhere classified, **left lower leg**

     M60.269   Foreign body granuloma of soft tissue, not elsewhere classified, unspecified lower leg ▽

✓6ᵗʰ   M60.27   Foreign body granuloma of soft tissue, not elsewhere classified, **ankle and foot**

     M60.271   Foreign body granuloma of soft tissue, not elsewhere classified, **right ankle and foot**

     M60.272   Foreign body granuloma of soft tissue, not elsewhere classified, **left ankle and foot**

     M60.279   Foreign body granuloma of soft tissue, not elsewhere classified, unspecified ankle and foot ▽

     M60.28   Foreign body granuloma of soft tissue, not elsewhere classified, other site

✓5ᵗʰ **M60.8 Other myositis**

     M60.80   Other myositis, unspecified site ▽

✓6ᵗʰ   M60.81   Other myositis **shoulder**

     M60.811   Other myositis, **right shoulder**

     M60.812   Other myositis, **left shoulder**

     M60.819   Other myositis, unspecified shoulder ▽

✓6ᵗʰ   M60.82   Other myositis, **upper arm**

     M60.821   Other myositis, **right upper arm**

     M60.822   Other myositis, **left upper arm**

     M60.829   Other myositis, unspecified upper arm ▽

✓6ᵗʰ   M60.83   Other myositis, **forearm**

     M60.831   Other myositis, **right forearm**

     M60.832   Other myositis, **left forearm**

     M60.839   Other myositis, unspecified forearm ▽

✓6ᵗʰ   M60.84   Other myositis, **hand**

     M60.841   Other myositis, **right hand**

     M60.842   Other myositis, **left hand**

     M60.849   Other myositis, unspecified hand ▽

✓6ᵗʰ   M60.85   Other myositis, **thigh**

     M60.851   Other myositis, **right thigh**

     M60.852   Other myositis, **left thigh**

     M60.859   Other myositis, unspecified thigh ▽

✓6ᵗʰ   M60.86   Other myositis, **lower leg**

     M60.861   Other myositis, **right lower leg**

     M60.862   Other myositis, **left lower leg**

     M60.869   Other myositis, unspecified lower leg ▽

✓6ᵗʰ   M60.87   Other myositis, **ankle and foot**

     M60.871   Other myositis, **right ankle and foot**

     M60.872   Other myositis, **left ankle and foot**

     M60.879   Other myositis, unspecified ankle and foot ▽

     M60.88   Other myositis, other site

     M60.89   Other myositis, multiple sites

     M60.9 Myositis, unspecified ▽

✓4ᵗʰ **M61 Calcification and ossification of muscle**

✓5ᵗʰ **M61.0 Myositis ossificans traumatica**

     M61.00   Myositis ossificans traumatica, unspecified site ▽

✓6ᵗʰ   M61.01   Myositis ossificans traumatica, **shoulder**

     M61.011   Myositis ossificans traumatica, **right shoulder**

     M61.012   Myositis ossificans traumatica, **left shoulder**

     M61.019   Myositis ossificans traumatica, unspecified shoulder ▽

✓6ᵗʰ   M61.02   Myositis ossificans traumatica, **upper arm**

     M61.021   Myositis ossificans traumatica, **right upper arm**

     M61.022   Myositis ossificans traumatica, **left upper arm**

     M61.029   Myositis ossificans traumatica, unspecified upper arm ▽

✓6ᵗʰ   M61.03   Myositis ossificans traumatica, **forearm**

     M61.031   Myositis ossificans traumatica, **right forearm**

     M61.032   Myositis ossificans traumatica, **left forearm**

     M61.039   Myositis ossificans traumatica, unspecified forearm ▽

✓6ᵗʰ   M61.04   Myositis ossificans traumatica, **hand**

     M61.041   Myositis ossificans traumatica, **right hand**

     M61.042   Myositis ossificans traumatica, **left hand**

     M61.049   Myositis ossificans traumatica, unspecified hand ▽

✓6ᵗʰ   M61.05   Myositis ossificans traumatica, **thigh**

     M61.051   Myositis ossificans traumatica, **right thigh**

     M61.052   Myositis ossificans traumatica, **left thigh**

     M61.059   Myositis ossificans traumatica, unspecified thigh ▽

✓6ᵗʰ   M61.06   Myositis ossificans traumatica, **lower leg**

     M61.061   Myositis ossificans traumatica, **right lower leg**

     M61.062   Myositis ossificans traumatica, **left lower leg**

     M61.069   Myositis ossificans traumatica, unspecified lower leg ▽

✓6ᵗʰ   M61.07   Myositis ossificans traumatica, **ankle and foot**

     M61.071   Myositis ossificans traumatica, **right ankle and foot**

☑ Additional Character Req   ✓x7ᵗʰ Placeholder Alert   Manifestation   HCC CMS-HCC Condition   ▽ Unspecified Code   ▶◀ Revised Text   ● New Code   ▲ Revised Code Title

M61.072   Myositis ossificans traumatica, **left** ankle and foot
M61.079   Myositis ossificans traumatica, unspecified ankle and foot ▽

M61.08   Myositis ossificans traumatica, **other site**
M61.09   Myositis ossificans traumatica, **multiple sites**

√5ᵗʰ M61.1   Myositis ossificans **progressiva**
            Fibrodysplasia ossificans progressiva

M61.10   Myositis ossificans progressiva, unspecified site ▽

√6ᵗʰ M61.11   Myositis ossificans progressiva, **shoulder**
M61.111   Myositis ossificans progressiva, **right** shoulder
M61.112   Myositis ossificans progressiva, **left** shoulder
M61.119   Myositis ossificans progressiva, unspecified shoulder ▽

√6ᵗʰ M61.12   Myositis ossificans progressiva, **upper arm**
M61.121   Myositis ossificans progressiva, **right** upper arm
M61.122   Myositis ossificans progressiva, **left** upper arm
M61.129   Myositis ossificans progressiva, unspecified arm ▽

√6ᵗʰ M61.13   Myositis ossificans progressiva, **forearm**
M61.131   Myositis ossificans progressiva, **right** forearm
M61.132   Myositis ossificans progressiva, **left** forearm
M61.139   Myositis ossificans progressiva, unspecified forearm ▽

√6ᵗʰ M61.14   Myositis ossificans progressiva, **hand and finger(s)**
M61.141   Myositis ossificans progressiva, **right hand**
M61.142   Myositis ossificans progressiva, **left hand**
M61.143   Myositis ossificans progressiva, unspecified hand ▽
M61.144   Myositis ossificans progressiva, **right finger(s)**
M61.145   Myositis ossificans progressiva, **left finger(s)**
M61.146   Myositis ossificans progressiva, unspecified finger(s) ▽

√6ᵗʰ M61.15   Myositis ossificans progressiva, **thigh**
M61.151   Myositis ossificans progressiva, **right** thigh
M61.152   Myositis ossificans progressiva, **left** thigh
M61.159   Myositis ossificans progressiva, unspecified thigh ▽

√6ᵗʰ M61.16   Myositis ossificans progressiva, **lower leg**
M61.161   Myositis ossificans progressiva, **right** lower leg
M61.162   Myositis ossificans progressiva, **left** lower leg
M61.169   Myositis ossificans progressiva, unspecified lower leg ▽

√6ᵗʰ M61.17   Myositis ossificans progressiva, **ankle, foot and toe(s)**
M61.171   Myositis ossificans progressiva, **right** ankle
M61.172   Myositis ossificans progressiva, **left** ankle
M61.173   Myositis ossificans progressiva, unspecified ankle ▽
M61.174   Myositis ossificans progressiva, **right foot**
M61.175   Myositis ossificans progressiva, **left foot**
M61.176   Myositis ossificans progressiva, unspecified foot ▽
M61.177   Myositis ossificans progressiva, **right toe(s)**
M61.178   Myositis ossificans progressiva, **left toe(s)**
M61.179   Myositis ossificans progressiva, unspecified toe(s) ▽

M61.18   Myositis ossificans progressiva, **other site**
M61.19   Myositis ossificans progressiva, **multiple sites**

√5ᵗʰ M61.2   Paralytic calcification and ossification of muscle
            Myositis ossificans associated with quadriplegia or paraplegia

M61.20   Paralytic calcification and ossification of muscle, unspecified site ▽

√6ᵗʰ M61.21   Paralytic calcification and ossification of muscle, **shoulder**
M61.211   Paralytic calcification and ossification of muscle, **right shoulder**
M61.212   Paralytic calcification and ossification of muscle, **left shoulder**
M61.219   Paralytic calcification and ossification of muscle, unspecified shoulder ▽

√6ᵗʰ M61.22   Paralytic calcification and ossification of muscle, **upper arm**
M61.221   Paralytic calcification and ossification of muscle, **right upper arm**
M61.222   Paralytic calcification and ossification of muscle, **left upper arm**
M61.229   Paralytic calcification and ossification of muscle, unspecified upper arm ▽

√6ᵗʰ M61.23   Paralytic calcification and ossification of muscle, **forearm**
M61.231   Paralytic calcification and ossification of muscle, **right forearm**
M61.232   Paralytic calcification and ossification of muscle, **left forearm**
M61.239   Paralytic calcification and ossification of muscle, unspecified forearm ▽

√6ᵗʰ M61.24   Paralytic calcification and ossification of muscle, **hand**
M61.241   Paralytic calcification and ossification of muscle, **right** hand
M61.242   Paralytic calcification and ossification of muscle, **left** hand
M61.249   Paralytic calcification and ossification of muscle, unspecified hand ▽

√6ᵗʰ M61.25   Paralytic calcification and ossification of muscle, **thigh**
M61.251   Paralytic calcification and ossification of muscle, **right** thigh
M61.252   Paralytic calcification and ossification of muscle, **left** thigh
M61.259   Paralytic calcification and ossification of muscle, unspecified thigh ▽

√6ᵗʰ M61.26   Paralytic calcification and ossification of muscle, **lower leg**
M61.261   Paralytic calcification and ossification of muscle, **right** lower leg
M61.262   Paralytic calcification and ossification of muscle, **left** lower leg
M61.269   Paralytic calcification and ossification of muscle, unspecified lower leg ▽

√6ᵗʰ M61.27   Paralytic calcification and ossification of muscle, **ankle and foot**
M61.271   Paralytic calcification and ossification of muscle, **right** ankle and foot
M61.272   Paralytic calcification and ossification of muscle, **left** ankle and foot
M61.279   Paralytic calcification and ossification of muscle, unspecified ankle and foot ▽

M61.28   Paralytic calcification and ossification of muscle, **other site**
M61.29   Paralytic calcification and ossification of muscle, **multiple sites**

√5ᵗʰ M61.3   Calcification and ossification of muscles **associated with burns**
            Myositis ossificans associated with burns

M61.30   Calcification and ossification of muscles associated with burns, unspecified site ▽

√6ᵗʰ M61.31   Calcification and ossification of muscles associated with burns, **shoulder**
M61.311   Calcification and ossification of muscles associated with burns, **right** shoulder
M61.312   Calcification and ossification of muscles associated with burns, **left** shoulder
M61.319   Calcification and ossification of muscles associated with burns, unspecified shoulder ▽

√6ᵗʰ M61.32   Calcification and ossification of muscles associated with burns, **upper arm**
M61.321   Calcification and ossification of muscles associated with burns, **right upper arm**

EXCLUDES 1 Not coded here   EXCLUDES 2 Not included here   N Newborn Age: 0   P Pediatric Age: 0-17   M Maternity Age: 12-55   A Adult Age: 15-124

762   ICD-10-CM 2018

M61.322   Calcification and ossification of muscles associated with burns, **left** upper arm

M61.329   Calcification and ossification of muscles associated with burns, unspecified upper arm ▽

✓6th **M61.33**   Calcification and ossification of muscles associated with burns, **forearm**

M61.331   Calcification and ossification of muscles associated with burns, **right** forearm

M61.332   Calcification and ossification of muscles associated with burns, **left** forearm

M61.339   Calcification and ossification of muscles associated with burns, unspecified forearm ▽

✓6th **M61.34**   Calcification and ossification of muscles associated with burns, **hand**

M61.341   Calcification and ossification of muscles associated with burns, **right** hand

M61.342   Calcification and ossification of muscles associated with burns, **left** hand

M61.349   Calcification and ossification of muscles associated with burns, unspecified hand ▽

✓6th **M61.35**   Calcification and ossification of muscles associated with burns, **thigh**

M61.351   Calcification and ossification of muscles associated with burns, **right** thigh

M61.352   Calcification and ossification of muscles associated with burns, **left** thigh

M61.359   Calcification and ossification of muscles associated with burns, unspecified thigh ▽

✓6th **M61.36**   Calcification and ossification of muscles associated with burns, **lower leg**

M61.361   Calcification and ossification of muscles associated with burns, **right** lower leg

M61.362   Calcification and ossification of muscles associated with burns, **left** lower leg

M61.369   Calcification and ossification of muscles associated with burns, unspecified lower leg ▽

✓6th **M61.37**   Calcification and ossification of muscles associated with burns, **ankle and foot**

M61.371   Calcification and ossification of muscles associated with burns, **right** ankle and foot

M61.372   Calcification and ossification of muscles associated with burns, **left** ankle and foot

M61.379   Calcification and ossification of muscles associated with burns, unspecified ankle and foot ▽

M61.38   Calcification and ossification of muscles associated with burns, other site

M61.39   Calcification and ossification of muscles associated with burns, **multiple sites**

✓5th **M61.4**   Other **calcification** of muscle

EXCLUDES 1   *calcific tendinitis NOS (M65.2-)*
calcific tendinitis of shoulder (M75.3)

M61.40   Other calcification of muscle, unspecified site ▽

✓6th **M61.41**   Other calcification of muscle, **shoulder**

M61.411   Other calcification of muscle, **right** shoulder

M61.412   Other calcification of muscle, **left** shoulder

M61.419   Other calcification of muscle, unspecified shoulder ▽

✓6th **M61.42**   Other calcification of muscle, **upper arm**

M61.421   Other calcification of muscle, **right** upper arm

M61.422   Other calcification of muscle, **left** upper arm

M61.429   Other calcification of muscle, unspecified upper arm ▽

✓6th **M61.43**   Other calcification of muscle, **forearm**

M61.431   Other calcification of muscle, **right** forearm

M61.432   Other calcification of muscle, **left** forearm

M61.439   Other calcification of muscle, unspecified forearm ▽

✓6th **M61.44**   Other calcification of muscle, **hand**

M61.441   Other calcification of muscle, right hand

M61.442   Other calcification of muscle, left hand

M61.449   Other calcification of muscle, unspecified hand ▽

✓6th **M61.45**   Other calcification of muscle, **thigh**

M61.451   Other calcification of muscle, right thigh

M61.452   Other calcification of muscle, left thigh

M61.459   Other calcification of muscle, unspecified thigh ▽

✓6th **M61.46**   Other calcification of muscle, **lower leg**

M61.461   Other calcification of muscle, right lower leg

M61.462   Other calcification of muscle, left lower leg

M61.469   Other calcification of muscle, unspecified lower leg ▽

✓6th **M61.47**   Other calcification of muscle, **ankle and foot**

M61.471   Other calcification of muscle, right ankle and foot

M61.472   Other calcification of muscle, left ankle and foot

M61.479   Other calcification of muscle, unspecified ankle and foot ▽

M61.48   Other calcification of muscle, other site

M61.49   Other calcification of muscle, **multiple sites**

✓5th **M61.5**   Other **ossification** of muscle

M61.50   Other ossification of muscle, unspecified site ▽

✓6th **M61.51**   Other ossification of muscle, **shoulder**

M61.511   Other ossification of muscle, right shoulder

M61.512   Other ossification of muscle, left shoulder

M61.519   Other ossification of muscle, unspecified shoulder ▽

✓6th **M61.52**   Other ossification of muscle, **upper arm**

M61.521   Other ossification of muscle, right upper arm

M61.522   Other ossification of muscle, left upper arm

M61.529   Other ossification of muscle, unspecified upper arm ▽

✓6th **M61.53**   Other ossification of muscle, **forearm**

M61.531   Other ossification of muscle, **right forearm**

M61.532   Other ossification of muscle, **left forearm**

M61.539   Other ossification of muscle, unspecified forearm ▽

✓6th **M61.54**   Other ossification of muscle, **hand**

M61.541   Other ossification of muscle, right hand

M61.542   Other ossification of muscle, left hand

M61.549   Other ossification of muscle, unspecified hand ▽

✓6th **M61.55**   Other ossification of muscle, **thigh**

M61.551   Other ossification of muscle, right thigh

M61.552   Other ossification of muscle, left thigh

M61.559   Other ossification of muscle, unspecified thigh ▽

✓6th **M61.56**   Other ossification of muscle, **lower leg**

M61.561   Other ossification of muscle, right lower leg

M61.562   Other ossification of muscle, left lower leg

M61.569   Other ossification of muscle, unspecified lower leg ▽

✓6th **M61.57**   Other ossification of muscle, **ankle and foot**

M61.571   Other ossification of muscle, right ankle and foot

M61.572   Other ossification of muscle, left ankle and foot

M61.579   Other ossification of muscle, unspecified ankle and foot ▽

M61.58   Other ossification of muscle, other site

M61.59   Other ossification of muscle, **multiple sites**

M61.9   Calcification and ossification of muscle, unspecified ▽

☑ Additional Character Req   ✓x7th Placeholder Alert   Manifestation   HCC CMS-HCC Condition   ▽ Unspecified Code   ►◄ Revised Text   ● New Code   ▲ Revised Code Title

✓4th M62 Other disorders of muscle

EXCLUDES 1   alcoholic myopathy (G72.1)
cramp and spasm (R25.2)
drug-induced myopathy (G72.0)
myalgia (M79.1)
stiff-man syndrome (G25.82)

EXCLUDES 2   nontraumatic hematoma of muscle (M79.81)

✓5th M62.0 Separation of muscle (nontraumatic)
Diastasis of muscle

EXCLUDES 1   diastasis recti complicating pregnancy, labor and delivery (O71.8)
traumatic separation of muscle—see strain of muscle by body region

M62.00   Separation of muscle (nontraumatic), unspecified site ▽

✓6th **M62.01 Separation of muscle (nontraumatic), shoulder**
- M62.011   Separation of muscle (nontraumatic), right shoulder
- M62.012   Separation of muscle (nontraumatic), left shoulder
- M62.019   Separation of muscle (nontraumatic), unspecified shoulder ▽

✓6th **M62.02 Separation of muscle (nontraumatic), upper arm**
- M62.021   Separation of muscle (nontraumatic), right upper arm
- M62.022   Separation of muscle (nontraumatic), left upper arm
- M62.029   Separation of muscle (nontraumatic), unspecified upper arm ▽

✓6th **M62.03 Separation of muscle (nontraumatic), forearm**
- M62.031   Separation of muscle (nontraumatic), right forearm
- M62.032   Separation of muscle (nontraumatic), left forearm
- M62.039   Separation of muscle (nontraumatic), unspecified forearm ▽

✓6th **M62.04 Separation of muscle (nontraumatic), hand**
- M62.041   Separation of muscle (nontraumatic), right hand
- M62.042   Separation of muscle (nontraumatic), left hand
- M62.049   Separation of muscle (nontraumatic), unspecified hand ▽

✓6th **M62.05 Separation of muscle (nontraumatic), thigh**
- M62.051   Separation of muscle (nontraumatic), right thigh
- M62.052   Separation of muscle (nontraumatic), left thigh
- M62.059   Separation of muscle (nontraumatic), unspecified thigh ▽

✓6th **M62.06 Separation of muscle (nontraumatic), lower leg**
- M62.061   Separation of muscle (nontraumatic), right lower leg
- M62.062   Separation of muscle (nontraumatic), left lower leg
- M62.069   Separation of muscle (nontraumatic), unspecified lower leg ▽

✓6th **M62.07 Separation of muscle (nontraumatic), ankle and foot**
- M62.071   Separation of muscle (nontraumatic), right ankle and foot
- M62.072   Separation of muscle (nontraumatic), left ankle and foot
- M62.079   Separation of muscle (nontraumatic), unspecified ankle and foot ▽

M62.08   Separation of muscle (nontraumatic), other site

✓5th M62.1 Other rupture of muscle (nontraumatic)

EXCLUDES 1   traumatic rupture of muscle—see strain of muscle by body region

EXCLUDES 2   rupture of tendon (M66.-)

M62.10   Other rupture of muscle (nontraumatic), unspecified site ▽

✓6th **M62.11 Other rupture of muscle (nontraumatic), shoulder**
- M62.111   Other rupture of muscle (nontraumatic), right shoulder
- M62.112   Other rupture of muscle (nontraumatic), left shoulder

- M62.119   Other rupture of muscle (nontraumatic), unspecified shoulder ▽

✓6th **M62.12 Other rupture of muscle (nontraumatic), upper arm**
- M62.121   Other rupture of muscle (nontraumatic), right upper arm
- M62.122   Other rupture of muscle (nontraumatic), left upper arm
- M62.129   Other rupture of muscle (nontraumatic), unspecified upper arm ▽

✓6th **M62.13 Other rupture of muscle (nontraumatic), forearm**
- M62.131   Other rupture of muscle (nontraumatic), right forearm
- M62.132   Other rupture of muscle (nontraumatic), left forearm
- M62.139   Other rupture of muscle (nontraumatic), unspecified forearm ▽

✓6th **M62.14 Other rupture of muscle (nontraumatic), hand**
- M62.141   Other rupture of muscle (nontraumatic), right hand
- M62.142   Other rupture of muscle (nontraumatic), left hand
- M62.149   Other rupture of muscle (nontraumatic), unspecified hand ▽

✓6th **M62.15 Other rupture of muscle (nontraumatic), thigh**
- M62.151   Other rupture of muscle (nontraumatic), right thigh
- M62.152   Other rupture of muscle (nontraumatic), left thigh
- M62.159   Other rupture of muscle (nontraumatic), unspecified thigh ▽

✓6th **M62.16 Other rupture of muscle (nontraumatic), lower leg**
- M62.161   Other rupture of muscle (nontraumatic), right lower leg
- M62.162   Other rupture of muscle (nontraumatic), left lower leg
- M62.169   Other rupture of muscle (nontraumatic), unspecified lower leg ▽

✓6th **M62.17 Other rupture of muscle (nontraumatic), ankle and foot**
- M62.171   Other rupture of muscle (nontraumatic), right ankle and foot
- M62.172   Other rupture of muscle (nontraumatic), left ankle and foot
- M62.179   Other rupture of muscle (nontraumatic), unspecified ankle and foot ▽

M62.18   Other rupture of muscle (nontraumatic), other site

✓5th M62.2 Nontraumatic ischemic infarction of muscle

EXCLUDES 1   compartment syndrome (traumatic) (T79.A-)
nontraumatic compartment syndrome (M79.A-)
rhabdomyolysis (M62.82)
traumatic ischemia of muscle (T79.6)
Volkmann's ischemic contracture (T79.6)

M62.20   Nontraumatic ischemic infarction of muscle, unspecified site ▽

✓6th **M62.21 Nontraumatic ischemic infarction of muscle, shoulder**
- M62.211   Nontraumatic ischemic infarction of muscle, right shoulder
- M62.212   Nontraumatic ischemic infarction of muscle, left shoulder
- M62.219   Nontraumatic ischemic infarction of muscle, unspecified shoulder ▽

✓6th **M62.22 Nontraumatic ischemic infarction of muscle, upper arm**
- M62.221   Nontraumatic ischemic infarction of muscle, right upper arm
- M62.222   Nontraumatic ischemic infarction of muscle, left upper arm
- M62.229   Nontraumatic ischemic infarction of muscle, unspecified upper arm ▽

✓6th **M62.23 Nontraumatic ischemic infarction of muscle, forearm**
- M62.231   Nontraumatic ischemic infarction of muscle, right forearm
- M62.232   Nontraumatic ischemic infarction of muscle, left forearm
- M62.239   Nontraumatic ischemic infarction of muscle, unspecified forearm ▽

EXCLUDES 1 Not coded here   **EXCLUDES 2** Not included here   **N** Newborn Age: 0   **P** Pediatric Age: 0-17   **M** Maternity Age: 12-55   **A** Adult Age: 15-124

764   ICD-10-CM 2018

Chapter 13. Diseases of the Musculoskeletal System and Connective Tissue

M62.24–M62.81

✓6ᵗʰ M62.24 Nontraumatic ischemic infarction of muscle, hand
- M62.241 Nontraumatic ischemic infarction of muscle, **right** hand
- M62.242 Nontraumatic ischemic infarction of muscle, **left** hand
- M62.249 Nontraumatic ischemic infarction of muscle, unspecified hand ▽

✓6ᵗʰ M62.25 Nontraumatic ischemic infarction of muscle, thigh
- M62.251 Nontraumatic ischemic infarction of muscle, **right** thigh
- M62.252 Nontraumatic ischemic infarction of muscle, **left** thigh
- M62.259 Nontraumatic ischemic infarction of muscle, unspecified thigh ▽

✓6ᵗʰ M62.26 Nontraumatic ischemic infarction of muscle, lower leg
- M62.261 Nontraumatic ischemic infarction of muscle, **right** lower leg
- M62.262 Nontraumatic ischemic infarction of muscle, **left** lower leg
- M62.269 Nontraumatic ischemic infarction of muscle, unspecified lower leg ▽

✓6ᵗʰ M62.27 Nontraumatic ischemic infarction of muscle, ankle and foot
- M62.271 Nontraumatic ischemic infarction of muscle, **right** ankle and foot
- M62.272 Nontraumatic ischemic infarction of muscle, **left** ankle and foot
- M62.279 Nontraumatic ischemic infarction of muscle, unspecified ankle and foot ▽

- M62.28 Nontraumatic ischemic infarction of muscle, other site

M62.3 Immobility syndrome (paraplegic)

✓5ᵗʰ M62.4 Contracture of muscle
Contracture of tendon (sheath)
EXCLUDES1   contracture of joint (M24.5-)
- M62.40 Contracture of muscle, unspecified site ▽
- **✓6ᵗʰ M62.41 Contracture of muscle, shoulder**
  - M62.411 Contracture of muscle, **right** shoulder
  - M62.412 Contracture of muscle, **left** shoulder
  - M62.419 Contracture of muscle, unspecified shoulder ▽
- **✓6ᵗʰ M62.42 Contracture of muscle, upper arm**
  - M62.421 Contracture of muscle, **right** upper arm
  - M62.422 Contracture of muscle, **left** upper arm
  - M62.429 Contracture of muscle, unspecified upper arm ▽
- **✓6ᵗʰ M62.43 Contracture of muscle, forearm**
  - M62.431 Contracture of muscle, **right** forearm
  - M62.432 Contracture of muscle, **left** forearm
  - M62.439 Contracture of muscle, unspecified forearm ▽
- **✓6ᵗʰ M62.44 Contracture of muscle, hand**
  - M62.441 Contracture of muscle, **right** hand
  - M62.442 Contracture of muscle, **left** hand
  - M62.449 Contracture of muscle, unspecified hand ▽
- **✓6ᵗʰ M62.45 Contracture of muscle, thigh**
  - M62.451 Contracture of muscle, **right** thigh
  - M62.452 Contracture of muscle, **left** thigh
  - M62.459 Contracture of muscle, unspecified thigh ▽
- **✓6ᵗʰ M62.46 Contracture of muscle, lower leg**
  - M62.461 Contracture of muscle, **right** lower leg
  - M62.462 Contracture of muscle, **left** lower leg
  - M62.469 Contracture of muscle, unspecified lower leg ▽
- **✓6ᵗʰ M62.47 Contracture of muscle, ankle and foot**
  - M62.471 Contracture of muscle, **right** ankle and foot
  - M62.472 Contracture of muscle, **left** ankle and foot
  - M62.479 Contracture of muscle, unspecified ankle and foot ▽
- M62.48 Contracture of muscle, other site
- M62.49 Contracture of muscle, **multiple sites**

✓5ᵗʰ M62.5 Muscle wasting and atrophy, not elsewhere classified
Disuse atrophy NEC
EXCLUDES1   neuralgic amyotrophy (G54.5)
progressive muscular atrophy ▶(G12.21)◀
sarcopenia (M62.84)
EXCLUDES2   pelvic muscle wasting (N81.84)
- M62.50 Muscle wasting and atrophy, not elsewhere classified, unspecified site ▽
- **✓6ᵗʰ M62.51 Muscle wasting and atrophy, not elsewhere classified, shoulder**
  - M62.511 Muscle wasting and atrophy, not elsewhere classified, **right** shoulder
  - M62.512 Muscle wasting and atrophy, not elsewhere classified, **left** shoulder
  - M62.519 Muscle wasting and atrophy, not elsewhere classified, unspecified shoulder ▽
- **✓6ᵗʰ M62.52 Muscle wasting and atrophy, not elsewhere classified, upper arm**
  - M62.521 Muscle wasting and atrophy, not elsewhere classified, **right** upper arm
  - M62.522 Muscle wasting and atrophy, not elsewhere classified, **left** upper arm
  - M62.529 Muscle wasting and atrophy, not elsewhere classified, unspecified upper arm ▽
- **✓6ᵗʰ M62.53 Muscle wasting and atrophy, not elsewhere classified, forearm**
  - M62.531 Muscle wasting and atrophy, not elsewhere classified, **right** forearm
  - M62.532 Muscle wasting and atrophy, not elsewhere classified, **left** forearm
  - M62.539 Muscle wasting and atrophy, not elsewhere classified, unspecified forearm ▽
- **✓6ᵗʰ M62.54 Muscle wasting and atrophy, not elsewhere classified, hand**
  - M62.541 Muscle wasting and atrophy, not elsewhere classified, **right** hand
  - M62.542 Muscle wasting and atrophy, not elsewhere classified, **left** hand
  - M62.549 Muscle wasting and atrophy, not elsewhere classified, unspecified hand ▽
- **✓6ᵗʰ M62.55 Muscle wasting and atrophy, not elsewhere classified, thigh**
  - M62.551 Muscle wasting and atrophy, not elsewhere classified, **right** thigh
  - M62.552 Muscle wasting and atrophy, not elsewhere classified, **left** thigh
  - M62.559 Muscle wasting and atrophy, not elsewhere classified, unspecified thigh ▽
- **✓6ᵗʰ M62.56 Muscle wasting and atrophy, not elsewhere classified, lower leg**
  - M62.561 Muscle wasting and atrophy, not elsewhere classified, **right** lower leg
  - M62.562 Muscle wasting and atrophy, not elsewhere classified, **left** lower leg
  - M62.569 Muscle wasting and atrophy, not elsewhere classified, unspecified lower leg ▽
- **✓6ᵗʰ M62.57 Muscle wasting and atrophy, not elsewhere classified, ankle and foot**
  - M62.571 Muscle wasting and atrophy, not elsewhere classified, **right** ankle and foot
  - M62.572 Muscle wasting and atrophy, not elsewhere classified, **left** ankle and foot
  - M62.579 Muscle wasting and atrophy, not elsewhere classified, unspecified ankle and foot ▽
- M62.58 Muscle wasting and atrophy, not elsewhere classified, other site
- M62.59 Muscle wasting and atrophy, not elsewhere classified, **multiple sites**

✓5ᵗʰ M62.8 Other specified disorders of muscle
EXCLUDES2   nontraumatic hematoma of muscle (M79.81)
- M62.81 Muscle weakness (generalized)
  EXCLUDES1   muscle weakness in sarcopenia (M62.84)

M62.82 Rhabdomyolysis
EXCLUDES 1 *traumatic rhabdomyolysis (T79.6)*
DEF: Rapid disintegration or destruction of skeletal muscle caused by direct or indirect injury; resulting in the excretion of muscle protein myoglobin into the urine.

√6th **M62.83 Muscle spasm**
M62.830 Muscle spasm of **back**
M62.831 Muscle spasm of **calf**
Charley-horse
M62.838 Other muscle spasm

M62.84 Sarcopenia
Age-related sarcopenia
Code first underlying disease, if applicable, such as:
disorders of myoneural junction and muscle disease in diseases classified elsewhere (G73.-)
other and unspecified myopathies (G72.-)
primary disorders of muscles (G71.-)

M62.89 Other specified disorders of muscle
Muscle (sheath) hernia

M62.9 Disorder of muscle, unspecified ▽

√4th **M63 Disorders of muscle in diseases classified elsewhere**
Code first underlying disease, such as:
leprosy (A30.-)
neoplasm (C49-, C79.89, D21-, D48.1)
schistosomiasis (B65.-)
trichinellosis (B75)
EXCLUDES 1 *myopathy in cysticercosis (B69.81)*
myopathy in endocrine diseases (G73.7)
myopathy in metabolic diseases (G73.7)
myopathy in sarcoidosis (D86.87)
myopathy in secondary syphilis (A51.49)
myopathy in syphilis (late) (A52.78)
myopathy in toxoplasmosis (B58.82)
myopathy in tuberculosis (A18.09)

√5th **M63.8 Disorders of muscle in diseases classified elsewhere**
M63.80 *Disorders of muscle in diseases classified elsewhere, unspecified site* ▽
√6th **M63.81 Disorders of muscle in diseases classified elsewhere, shoulder**
M63.811 *Disorders of muscle in diseases classified elsewhere, right shoulder*
M63.812 *Disorders of muscle in diseases classified elsewhere, left shoulder*
M63.819 *Disorders of muscle in diseases classified elsewhere, unspecified shoulder* ▽
√6th **M63.82 Disorders of muscle in diseases classified elsewhere, upper arm**
M63.821 *Disorders of muscle in diseases classified elsewhere, right upper arm*
M63.822 *Disorders of muscle in diseases classified elsewhere, left upper arm*
M63.829 *Disorders of muscle in diseases classified elsewhere, unspecified upper arm* ▽
√6th **M63.83 Disorders of muscle in diseases classified elsewhere, forearm**
M63.831 *Disorders of muscle in diseases classified elsewhere, right forearm*
M63.832 *Disorders of muscle in diseases classified elsewhere, left forearm*
M63.839 *Disorders of muscle in diseases classified elsewhere, unspecified forearm* ▽
√6th **M63.84 Disorders of muscle in diseases classified elsewhere, hand**
M63.841 *Disorders of muscle in diseases classified elsewhere, right hand*
M63.842 *Disorders of muscle in diseases classified elsewhere, left hand*
M63.849 *Disorders of muscle in diseases classified elsewhere, unspecified hand* ▽
√6th **M63.85 Disorders of muscle in diseases classified elsewhere, thigh**
M63.851 *Disorders of muscle in diseases classified elsewhere, right thigh*
M63.852 *Disorders of muscle in diseases classified elsewhere, left thigh*
M63.859 *Disorders of muscle in diseases classified elsewhere, unspecified thigh* ▽

√6th **M63.86 Disorders of muscle in diseases classified elsewhere, lower leg**
M63.861 *Disorders of muscle in diseases classified elsewhere, right lower leg*
M63.862 *Disorders of muscle in diseases classified elsewhere, left lower leg*
M63.869 *Disorders of muscle in diseases classified elsewhere, unspecified lower leg* ▽
√6th **M63.87 Disorders of muscle in diseases classified elsewhere, ankle and foot**
M63.871 *Disorders of muscle in diseases classified elsewhere, right ankle and foot*
M63.872 *Disorders of muscle in diseases classified elsewhere, left ankle and foot*
M63.879 *Disorders of muscle in diseases classified elsewhere, unspecified ankle and foot* ▽
M63.88 *Disorders of muscle in diseases classified elsewhere, other site*
M63.89 *Disorders of muscle in diseases classified elsewhere, multiple sites*

Disorders of synovium and tendon (M65-M67)

√4th **M65 Synovitis and tenosynovitis**
EXCLUDES 1 *chronic crepitant synovitis of hand and wrist (M70.0-)*
current injury—see injury of ligament or tendon by body region
soft tissue disorders related to use, overuse and pressure (M70.-)

√5th **M65.0 Abscess of tendon sheath**
Use additional code (B95-B96) to identify bacterial agent.
M65.00 Abscess of tendon sheath, unspecified site ▽
√6th **M65.01 Abscess of tendon sheath, shoulder**
M65.011 Abscess of tendon sheath, **right** shoulder
M65.012 Abscess of tendon sheath, **left** shoulder
M65.019 Abscess of tendon sheath, unspecified shoulder ▽
√6th **M65.02 Abscess of tendon sheath, upper arm**
M65.021 Abscess of tendon sheath, **right** upper arm
M65.022 Abscess of tendon sheath, **left** upper arm
M65.029 Abscess of tendon sheath, unspecified upper arm ▽
√6th **M65.03 Abscess of tendon sheath, forearm**
M65.031 Abscess of tendon sheath, **right** forearm
M65.032 Abscess of tendon sheath, **left** forearm
M65.039 Abscess of tendon sheath, unspecified forearm ▽
√6th **M65.04 Abscess of tendon sheath, hand**
M65.041 Abscess of tendon sheath, **right** hand
M65.042 Abscess of tendon sheath, **left** hand
M65.049 Abscess of tendon sheath, unspecified hand ▽
√6th **M65.05 Abscess of tendon sheath, thigh**
M65.051 Abscess of tendon sheath, **right** thigh
M65.052 Abscess of tendon sheath, **left** thigh
M65.059 Abscess of tendon sheath, unspecified thigh ▽
√6th **M65.06 Abscess of tendon sheath, lower leg**
M65.061 Abscess of tendon sheath, **right** lower leg
M65.062 Abscess of tendon sheath, **left** lower leg
M65.069 Abscess of tendon sheath, unspecified lower leg ▽
√6th **M65.07 Abscess of tendon sheath, ankle and foot**
M65.071 Abscess of tendon sheath, **right** ankle and foot
M65.072 Abscess of tendon sheath, **left** ankle and foot
M65.079 Abscess of tendon sheath, unspecified ankle and foot ▽
M65.08 Abscess of tendon sheath, other site

√5th **M65.1 Other infective (teno)synovitis**
M65.10 Other infective (teno)synovitis, unspecified site ▽
√6th **M65.11 Other infective (teno)synovitis, shoulder**
M65.111 Other infective (teno)synovitis, **right** shoulder
M65.112 Other infective (teno)synovitis, **left** shoulder

M65.119   Other infective (teno)synovitis, unspecified shoulder ▽

☑6ᵗʰ   **M65.12**   Other infective (teno)synovitis, **elbow**
    M65.121   Other infective (teno)synovitis, **right** elbow
    M65.122   Other infective (teno)synovitis, **left** elbow
    M65.129   Other infective (teno)synovitis, unspecified elbow ▽

☑6ᵗʰ   **M65.13**   Other infective (teno)synovitis, **wrist**
    M65.131   Other infective (teno)synovitis, **right** wrist
    M65.132   Other infective (teno)synovitis, **left** wrist
    M65.139   Other infective (teno)synovitis, unspecified wrist ▽

☑6ᵗʰ   **M65.14**   Other infective (teno)synovitis, **hand**
    M65.141   Other infective (teno)synovitis, **right** hand
    M65.142   Other infective (teno)synovitis, **left** hand
    M65.149   Other infective (teno)synovitis, unspecified hand ▽

☑6ᵗʰ   **M65.15**   Other infective (teno)synovitis, **hip**
    M65.151   Other infective (teno)synovitis, **right** hip
    M65.152   Other infective (teno)synovitis, **left** hip
    M65.159   Other infective (teno)synovitis, unspecified hip ▽

☑6ᵗʰ   **M65.16**   Other infective (teno)synovitis, **knee**
    M65.161   Other infective (teno)synovitis, **right** knee
    M65.162   Other infective (teno)synovitis, **left** knee
    M65.169   Other infective (teno)synovitis, unspecified knee ▽

☑6ᵗʰ   **M65.17**   Other infective (teno)synovitis, **ankle and foot**
    M65.171   Other infective (teno)synovitis, **right** ankle and foot
    M65.172   Other infective (teno)synovitis, **left** ankle and foot
    M65.179   Other infective (teno)synovitis, unspecified ankle and foot ▽

    M65.18   Other infective (teno)synovitis, other site
    M65.19   Other infective (teno)synovitis, **multiple sites**

☑5ᵗʰ   **M65.2**   **Calcific tendinitis**
    EXCLUDES 1   *tendinitis as classified in M75-M77*
             calcified tendinitis of shoulder (M75.3)

    M65.20   Calcific tendinitis, unspecified site ▽

☑6ᵗʰ   **M65.22**   Calcific tendinitis, **upper arm**
    M65.221   Calcific tendinitis, **right** upper arm
    M65.222   Calcific tendinitis, **left** upper arm
    M65.229   Calcific tendinitis, unspecified upper arm ▽

☑6ᵗʰ   **M65.23**   Calcific tendinitis, **forearm**
    M65.231   Calcific tendinitis, **right** forearm
    M65.232   Calcific tendinitis, **left** forearm
    M65.239   Calcific tendinitis, unspecified forearm ▽

☑6ᵗʰ   **M65.24**   Calcific tendinitis, **hand**
    M65.241   Calcific tendinitis, **right** hand
    M65.242   Calcific tendinitis, **left** hand
    M65.249   Calcific tendinitis, unspecified hand ▽

☑6ᵗʰ   **M65.25**   Calcific tendinitis, **thigh**
    M65.251   Calcific tendinitis, **right** thigh
    M65.252   Calcific tendinitis, **left** thigh
    M65.259   Calcific tendinitis, unspecified thigh ▽

☑6ᵗʰ   **M65.26**   Calcific tendinitis, **lower leg**
    M65.261   Calcific tendinitis, **right** lower leg
    M65.262   Calcific tendinitis, **left** lower leg
    M65.269   Calcific tendinitis, unspecified lower leg ▽

☑6ᵗʰ   **M65.27**   Calcific tendinitis, **ankle and foot**
    M65.271   Calcific tendinitis, **right** ankle and foot
    M65.272   Calcific tendinitis, **left** ankle and foot
    M65.279   Calcific tendinitis, unspecified ankle and foot ▽

    M65.28   Calcific tendinitis, other site
    M65.29   Calcific tendinitis, **multiple sites**

☑5ᵗʰ   **M65.3**   **Trigger finger**
    Nodular tendinous disease
    M65.30   Trigger finger, unspecified finger ▽

☑6ᵗʰ   **M65.31**   Trigger **thumb**
    M65.311   Trigger thumb, **right** thumb
    M65.312   Trigger thumb, **left** thumb
    M65.319   Trigger thumb, unspecified thumb ▽

☑6ᵗʰ   **M65.32**   Trigger finger, **index finger**
    M65.321   Trigger finger, **right** index finger
    M65.322   Trigger finger, **left** index finger
    M65.329   Trigger finger, unspecified index finger ▽

☑6ᵗʰ   **M65.33**   Trigger finger, **middle finger**
    M65.331   Trigger finger, **right** middle finger
    M65.332   Trigger finger, **left** middle finger
    M65.339   Trigger finger, unspecified middle finger ▽

☑6ᵗʰ   **M65.34**   Trigger finger, **ring finger**
    M65.341   Trigger finger, **right** ring finger
    M65.342   Trigger finger, **left** ring finger
    M65.349   Trigger finger, unspecified ring finger ▽

☑6ᵗʰ   **M65.35**   Trigger finger, **little finger**
    M65.351   Trigger finger, **right** little finger
    M65.352   Trigger finger, **left** little finger
    M65.359   Trigger finger, unspecified little finger ▽

M65.4   **Radial styloid tenosynovitis [de Quervain]**

☑5ᵗʰ   **M65.8**   **Other synovitis and tenosynovitis**
    M65.80   Other synovitis and tenosynovitis, unspecified site ▽

☑6ᵗʰ   **M65.81**   Other synovitis and tenosynovitis, **shoulder**
    M65.811   Other synovitis and tenosynovitis, **right** shoulder
    M65.812   Other synovitis and tenosynovitis, **left** shoulder
    M65.819   Other synovitis and tenosynovitis, unspecified shoulder ▽

☑6ᵗʰ   **M65.82**   Other synovitis and tenosynovitis, **upper arm**
    M65.821   Other synovitis and tenosynovitis, **right** upper arm
    M65.822   Other synovitis and tenosynovitis, **left** upper arm
    M65.829   Other synovitis and tenosynovitis, unspecified upper arm ▽

☑6ᵗʰ   **M65.83**   Other synovitis and tenosynovitis, **forearm**
    M65.831   Other synovitis and tenosynovitis, **right** forearm
    M65.832   Other synovitis and tenosynovitis, **left** forearm
    M65.839   Other synovitis and tenosynovitis, unspecified forearm ▽

☑6ᵗʰ   **M65.84**   Other synovitis and tenosynovitis, **hand**
    M65.841   Other synovitis and tenosynovitis, **right** hand
    M65.842   Other synovitis and tenosynovitis, **left** hand
    M65.849   Other synovitis and tenosynovitis, unspecified hand ▽

☑6ᵗʰ   **M65.85**   Other synovitis and tenosynovitis, **thigh**
    M65.851   Other synovitis and tenosynovitis, **right** thigh
    M65.852   Other synovitis and tenosynovitis, **left** thigh
    M65.859   Other synovitis and tenosynovitis, unspecified thigh ▽

☑6ᵗʰ   **M65.86**   Other synovitis and tenosynovitis, **lower leg**
    M65.861   Other synovitis and tenosynovitis, **right** lower leg
    M65.862   Other synovitis and tenosynovitis, **left** lower leg
    M65.869   Other synovitis and tenosynovitis, unspecified lower leg ▽

☑6ᵗʰ   **M65.87**   Other synovitis and tenosynovitis, **ankle and foot**
    M65.871   Other synovitis and tenosynovitis, **right** ankle and foot
    M65.872   Other synovitis and tenosynovitis, **left** ankle and foot
    M65.879   Other synovitis and tenosynovitis, unspecified ankle and foot ▽

☑ Additional Character Req   ☑×7ᵗʰ Placeholder Alert   Manifestation   HCC CMS-HCC Condition   ▽ Unspecified Code   ►◄ Revised Text   ● New Code   ▲ Revised Code Title

M65.88 Other synovitis and tenosynovitis, other site
M65.89 Other synovitis and tenosynovitis, **multiple sites**
M65.9 Synovitis and tenosynovitis, unspecified ▽

✓4th M66 Spontaneous rupture of synovium and tendon
  INCLUDES rupture that occurs when a normal force is applied to tissues that are inferred to have less than normal strength
  EXCLUDES 2 rotator cuff syndrome (M75.1-)
  rupture where an abnormal force is applied to normal tissue—see injury of tendon by body region

M66.0 Rupture of popliteal cyst

✓5th M66.1 Rupture of synovium
Rupture of synovial cyst
  EXCLUDES 2 rupture of popliteal cyst (M66.0)
M66.10 Rupture of synovium, unspecified joint ▽
✓6th M66.11 Rupture of synovium, shoulder
M66.111 Rupture of synovium, **right** shoulder
M66.112 Rupture of synovium, **left** shoulder
M66.119 Rupture of synovium, unspecified shoulder ▽
✓6th M66.12 Rupture of synovium, elbow
M66.121 Rupture of synovium, **right** elbow
M66.122 Rupture of synovium, **left** elbow
M66.129 Rupture of synovium, unspecified elbow ▽
✓6th M66.13 Rupture of synovium, wrist
M66.131 Rupture of synovium, **right** wrist
M66.132 Rupture of synovium, **left** wrist
M66.139 Rupture of synovium, unspecified wrist ▽
✓6th M66.14 Rupture of synovium, hand and fingers
M66.141 Rupture of synovium, **right hand**
M66.142 Rupture of synovium, **left hand**
M66.143 Rupture of synovium, unspecified hand ▽
M66.144 Rupture of synovium, **right finger(s)**
M66.145 Rupture of synovium, **left finger(s)**
M66.146 Rupture of synovium, unspecified finger(s) ▽
✓6th M66.15 Rupture of synovium, hip
M66.151 Rupture of synovium, **right** hip
M66.152 Rupture of synovium, **left** hip
M66.159 Rupture of synovium, unspecified hip ▽
✓6th M66.17 Rupture of synovium, ankle, foot and toes
M66.171 Rupture of synovium, **right** ankle
M66.172 Rupture of synovium, **left** ankle
M66.173 Rupture of synovium, unspecified ankle ▽
M66.174 Rupture of synovium, **right foot**
M66.175 Rupture of synovium, **left foot**
M66.176 Rupture of synovium, unspecified foot ▽
M66.177 Rupture of synovium, **right toe(s)**
M66.178 Rupture of synovium, **left toe(s)**
M66.179 Rupture of synovium, unspecified toe(s) ▽
M66.18 Rupture of synovium, other site

✓5th M66.2 Spontaneous rupture of extensor tendons
TIP: Refer to the Muscle/Tendon table at the beginning of this chapter.
M66.20 Spontaneous rupture of extensor tendons, unspecified site ▽
✓6th M66.21 Spontaneous rupture of extensor tendons, shoulder
M66.211 Spontaneous rupture of extensor tendons, **right** shoulder
M66.212 Spontaneous rupture of extensor tendons, **left** shoulder
M66.219 Spontaneous rupture of extensor tendons, unspecified shoulder ▽
✓6th M66.22 Spontaneous rupture of extensor tendons, upper arm
M66.221 Spontaneous rupture of extensor tendons, **right** upper arm
M66.222 Spontaneous rupture of extensor tendons, **left** upper arm
M66.229 Spontaneous rupture of extensor tendons, unspecified upper arm ▽

✓6th M66.23 Spontaneous rupture of extensor tendons, forearm
M66.231 Spontaneous rupture of extensor tendons, **right** forearm
M66.232 Spontaneous rupture of extensor tendons, **left** forearm
M66.239 Spontaneous rupture of extensor tendons, unspecified forearm ▽
✓6th M66.24 Spontaneous rupture of extensor tendons, hand
M66.241 Spontaneous rupture of extensor tendons, **right** hand
M66.242 Spontaneous rupture of extensor tendons, **left** hand
M66.249 Spontaneous rupture of extensor tendons, unspecified hand ▽
✓6th M66.25 Spontaneous rupture of extensor tendons, thigh
M66.251 Spontaneous rupture of extensor tendons, **right** thigh
M66.252 Spontaneous rupture of extensor tendons, **left** thigh
M66.259 Spontaneous rupture of extensor tendons, unspecified thigh ▽
✓6th M66.26 Spontaneous rupture of extensor tendons, lower leg
M66.261 Spontaneous rupture of extensor tendons, **right** lower leg
M66.262 Spontaneous rupture of extensor tendons, **left** lower leg
M66.269 Spontaneous rupture of extensor tendons, unspecified lower leg ▽
✓6th M66.27 Spontaneous rupture of extensor tendons, ankle and foot
M66.271 Spontaneous rupture of extensor tendons, **right** ankle and foot
M66.272 Spontaneous rupture of extensor tendons, **left** ankle and foot
M66.279 Spontaneous rupture of extensor tendons, unspecified ankle and foot ▽
M66.28 Spontaneous rupture of extensor tendons, other site
M66.29 Spontaneous rupture of extensor tendons, **multiple sites**

✓5th M66.3 Spontaneous rupture of flexor tendons
TIP: Refer to the Muscle/Tendon table at the beginning of this chapter.
M66.30 Spontaneous rupture of flexor tendons, unspecified site ▽
✓6th M66.31 Spontaneous rupture of flexor tendons, shoulder
M66.311 Spontaneous rupture of flexor tendons, **right** shoulder
M66.312 Spontaneous rupture of flexor tendons, **left** shoulder
M66.319 Spontaneous rupture of flexor tendons, unspecified shoulder ▽
✓6th M66.32 Spontaneous rupture of flexor tendons, upper arm
M66.321 Spontaneous rupture of flexor tendons, **right** upper arm
M66.322 Spontaneous rupture of flexor tendons, **left** upper arm
M66.329 Spontaneous rupture of flexor tendons, unspecified upper arm ▽
✓6th M66.33 Spontaneous rupture of flexor tendons, forearm
M66.331 Spontaneous rupture of flexor tendons, **right** forearm
M66.332 Spontaneous rupture of flexor tendons, **left** forearm
M66.339 Spontaneous rupture of flexor tendons, unspecified forearm ▽
✓6th M66.34 Spontaneous rupture of flexor tendons, hand
M66.341 Spontaneous rupture of flexor tendons, **right** hand
M66.342 Spontaneous rupture of flexor tendons, **left** hand
M66.349 Spontaneous rupture of flexor tendons, unspecified hand ▽
✓6th M66.35 Spontaneous rupture of flexor tendons, thigh
M66.351 Spontaneous rupture of flexor tendons, **right** thigh
M66.352 Spontaneous rupture of flexor tendons, **left** thigh

M66.359   Spontaneous rupture of flexor tendons, unspecified thigh ▽

✓6ᵗʰ **M66.36**   **Spontaneous rupture of flexor tendons, lower leg**

M66.361   Spontaneous rupture of flexor tendons, **right lower leg**

M66.362   Spontaneous rupture of flexor tendons, **left lower leg**

M66.369   Spontaneous rupture of flexor tendons, unspecified lower leg ▽

✓6ᵗʰ **M66.37**   **Spontaneous rupture of flexor tendons, ankle and foot**

M66.371   Spontaneous rupture of flexor tendons, **right ankle and foot**

M66.372   Spontaneous rupture of flexor tendons, **left ankle and foot**

M66.379   Spontaneous rupture of flexor tendons, unspecified ankle and foot ▽

M66.38   Spontaneous rupture of flexor tendons, other site

M66.39   Spontaneous rupture of flexor tendons, multiple sites

✓5ᵗʰ **M66.8**   **Spontaneous rupture of other tendons**

TIP: Refer to the Muscle/Tendon table at the beginning of this chapter.

M66.80   Spontaneous rupture of other tendons, unspecified site ▽

✓6ᵗʰ **M66.81**   **Spontaneous rupture of other tendons, shoulder**

M66.811   Spontaneous rupture of other tendons, **right shoulder**

M66.812   Spontaneous rupture of other tendons, **left shoulder**

M66.819   Spontaneous rupture of other tendons, unspecified shoulder ▽

✓6ᵗʰ **M66.82**   **Spontaneous rupture of other tendons, upper arm**

M66.821   Spontaneous rupture of other tendons, **right upper arm**

M66.822   Spontaneous rupture of other tendons, **left upper arm**

M66.829   Spontaneous rupture of other tendons, unspecified upper arm ▽

✓6ᵗʰ **M66.83**   **Spontaneous rupture of other tendons, forearm**

M66.831   Spontaneous rupture of other tendons, **right forearm**

M66.832   Spontaneous rupture of other tendons, **left forearm**

M66.839   Spontaneous rupture of other tendons, unspecified forearm ▽

✓6ᵗʰ **M66.84**   **Spontaneous rupture of other tendons, hand**

M66.841   Spontaneous rupture of other tendons, **right hand**

M66.842   Spontaneous rupture of other tendons, **left hand**

M66.849   Spontaneous rupture of other tendons, unspecified hand ▽

✓6ᵗʰ **M66.85**   **Spontaneous rupture of other tendons, thigh**

M66.851   Spontaneous rupture of other tendons, **right thigh**

M66.852   Spontaneous rupture of other tendons, **left thigh**

M66.859   Spontaneous rupture of other tendons, unspecified thigh ▽

✓6ᵗʰ **M66.86**   **Spontaneous rupture of other tendons, lower leg**

M66.861   Spontaneous rupture of other tendons, **right lower leg**

M66.862   Spontaneous rupture of other tendons, **left lower leg**

M66.869   Spontaneous rupture of other tendons, unspecified lower leg ▽

✓6ᵗʰ **M66.87**   **Spontaneous rupture of other tendons, ankle and foot**

M66.871   Spontaneous rupture of other tendons, **right ankle and foot**

M66.872   Spontaneous rupture of other tendons, **left ankle and foot**

M66.879   Spontaneous rupture of other tendons, unspecified ankle and foot ▽

M66.88   Spontaneous rupture of other tendons, other

M66.89   Spontaneous rupture of other tendons, multiple sites

M66.9   Spontaneous rupture of unspecified tendon ▽

Rupture at musculotendinous junction, nontraumatic

✓4ᵗʰ **M67**   **Other disorders of synovium and tendon**

EXCLUDES 1   *palmar fascial fibromatosis [Dupuytren] (M72.0)*
tendinitis NOS (M77.9-)
xanthomatosis localized to tendons (E78.2)

✓5ᵗʰ **M67.0**   **Short Achilles tendon (acquired)**

M67.00   Short Achilles tendon (acquired), unspecified ankle ▽

M67.01   Short Achilles tendon (acquired), right ankle

M67.02   Short Achilles tendon (acquired), left ankle

✓5ᵗʰ **M67.2**   **Synovial hypertrophy, not elsewhere classified**

EXCLUDES 1   *villonodular synovitis (pigmented) (M12.2-)*

M67.20   Synovial hypertrophy, not elsewhere classified, unspecified site ▽

✓6ᵗʰ **M67.21**   **Synovial hypertrophy, not elsewhere classified, shoulder**

M67.211   Synovial hypertrophy, not elsewhere classified, **right shoulder**

M67.212   Synovial hypertrophy, not elsewhere classified, **left shoulder**

M67.219   Synovial hypertrophy, not elsewhere classified, unspecified shoulder ▽

✓6ᵗʰ **M67.22**   **Synovial hypertrophy, not elsewhere classified, upper arm**

M67.221   Synovial hypertrophy, not elsewhere classified, **right upper arm**

M67.222   Synovial hypertrophy, not elsewhere classified, **left upper arm**

M67.229   Synovial hypertrophy, not elsewhere classified, unspecified upper arm ▽

✓6ᵗʰ **M67.23**   **Synovial hypertrophy, not elsewhere classified, forearm**

M67.231   Synovial hypertrophy, not elsewhere classified, **right forearm**

M67.232   Synovial hypertrophy, not elsewhere classified, **left forearm**

M67.239   Synovial hypertrophy, not elsewhere classified, unspecified forearm ▽

✓6ᵗʰ **M67.24**   **Synovial hypertrophy, not elsewhere classified, hand**

M67.241   Synovial hypertrophy, not elsewhere classified, **right hand**

M67.242   Synovial hypertrophy, not elsewhere classified, **left hand**

M67.249   Synovial hypertrophy, not elsewhere classified, unspecified hand ▽

✓6ᵗʰ **M67.25**   **Synovial hypertrophy, not elsewhere classified, thigh**

M67.251   Synovial hypertrophy, not elsewhere classified, **right thigh**

M67.252   Synovial hypertrophy, not elsewhere classified, **left thigh**

M67.259   Synovial hypertrophy, not elsewhere classified, unspecified thigh ▽

✓6ᵗʰ **M67.26**   **Synovial hypertrophy, not elsewhere classified, lower leg**

M67.261   Synovial hypertrophy, not elsewhere classified, **right lower leg**

M67.262   Synovial hypertrophy, not elsewhere classified, **left lower leg**

M67.269   Synovial hypertrophy, not elsewhere classified, unspecified lower leg ▽

✓6ᵗʰ **M67.27**   **Synovial hypertrophy, not elsewhere classified, ankle and foot**

M67.271   Synovial hypertrophy, not elsewhere classified, **right ankle and foot**

M67.272   Synovial hypertrophy, not elsewhere classified, **left ankle and foot**

M67.279   Synovial hypertrophy, not elsewhere classified, unspecified ankle and foot ▽

M67.28   Synovial hypertrophy, not elsewhere classified, other site

M67.29   Synovial hypertrophy, not elsewhere classified, multiple sites

✓ Additional Character Req   ✓⁷ᵗʰ Placeholder Alert   Manifestation   **HCC** CMS-HCC Condition   ▽ Unspecified Code   ▶◀ Revised Text   ● New Code   ▲ Revised Code Title

ICD-10-CM 2018   769

✓5ᵗʰ M67.3 Transient synovitis
　　Toxic synovitis
　　　EXCLUDES 1　palindromic rheumatism (M12.3-)
　　M67.30 Transient synovitis, unspecified site ▽
　✓6ᵗʰ M67.31 Transient synovitis, shoulder
　　　M67.311 Transient synovitis, right shoulder
　　　M67.312 Transient synovitis, left shoulder
　　　M67.319 Transient synovitis, unspecified ▽
　　　　　shoulder
　✓6ᵗʰ M67.32 Transient synovitis, elbow
　　　M67.321 Transient synovitis, right elbow
　　　M67.322 Transient synovitis, left elbow
　　　M67.329 Transient synovitis, unspecified elbow ▽
　✓6ᵗʰ M67.33 Transient synovitis, wrist
　　　M67.331 Transient synovitis, right wrist
　　　M67.332 Transient synovitis, left wrist
　　　M67.339 Transient synovitis, unspecified wrist ▽
　✓6ᵗʰ M67.34 Transient synovitis, hand
　　　M67.341 Transient synovitis, right hand
　　　M67.342 Transient synovitis, left hand
　　　M67.349 Transient synovitis, unspecified hand ▽
　✓6ᵗʰ M67.35 Transient synovitis, hip
　　　M67.351 Transient synovitis, right hip
　　　M67.352 Transient synovitis, left hip
　　　M67.359 Transient synovitis, unspecified hip ▽
　✓6ᵗʰ M67.36 Transient synovitis, knee
　　　M67.361 Transient synovitis, right knee
　　　M67.362 Transient synovitis, left knee
　　　M67.369 Transient synovitis, unspecified knee ▽
　✓6ᵗʰ M67.37 Transient synovitis, ankle and foot
　　　M67.371 Transient synovitis, right ankle and foot
　　　M67.372 Transient synovitis, left ankle and foot
　　　M67.379 Transient synovitis, unspecified ▽
　　　　　ankle and foot
　　M67.38 Transient synovitis, other site
　　M67.39 Transient synovitis, multiple sites
✓5ᵗʰ M67.4 Ganglion
　　Ganglion of joint or tendon (sheath)
　　　EXCLUDES 1　ganglion in yaws (A66.6)
　　　EXCLUDES 2　cyst of bursa (M71.2-M71.3)
　　　　　cyst of synovium (M71.2-M71.3)
　　M67.40 Ganglion, unspecified site ▽
　✓6ᵗʰ M67.41 Ganglion, shoulder
　　　M67.411 Ganglion, right shoulder
　　　M67.412 Ganglion, left shoulder
　　　M67.419 Ganglion, unspecified shoulder ▽
　✓6ᵗʰ M67.42 Ganglion, elbow
　　　M67.421 Ganglion, right elbow
　　　M67.422 Ganglion, left elbow
　　　M67.429 Ganglion, unspecified elbow ▽
　✓6ᵗʰ M67.43 Ganglion, wrist
　　　M67.431 Ganglion, right wrist
　　　M67.432 Ganglion, left wrist
　　　M67.439 Ganglion, unspecified wrist ▽
　✓6ᵗʰ M67.44 Ganglion, hand
　　　M67.441 Ganglion, right hand
　　　M67.442 Ganglion, left hand
　　　M67.449 Ganglion, unspecified hand ▽
　✓6ᵗʰ M67.45 Ganglion, hip
　　　M67.451 Ganglion, right hip
　　　M67.452 Ganglion, left hip
　　　M67.459 Ganglion, unspecified hip ▽
　✓6ᵗʰ M67.46 Ganglion, knee
　　　M67.461 Ganglion, right knee
　　　M67.462 Ganglion, left knee
　　　M67.469 Ganglion, unspecified knee ▽

Ganglion of Wrist

Extensor
tendon sheaths

Ganglion of wrist
(fluid-filled sac)

　✓6ᵗʰ M67.47 Ganglion, ankle and foot
　　　M67.471 Ganglion, right ankle and foot
　　　M67.472 Ganglion, left ankle and foot
　　　M67.479 Ganglion, unspecified ankle and foot ▽
　　M67.48 Ganglion, other site
　　M67.49 Ganglion, multiple sites
✓5ᵗʰ M67.5 Plica syndrome
　　Plica knee
　　M67.50 Plica syndrome, unspecified knee ▽
　　M67.51 Plica syndrome, right knee
　　M67.52 Plica syndrome, left knee
✓5ᵗʰ M67.8 Other specified disorders of synovium and tendon
　　M67.80 Other specified disorders of synovium and ▽
　　　　tendon, unspecified site
　✓6ᵗʰ M67.81 Other specified disorders of synovium and tendon, shoulder
　　　M67.811 Other specified disorders of synovium, right shoulder
　　　M67.812 Other specified disorders of synovium, left shoulder
　　　M67.813 Other specified disorders of tendon, right shoulder
　　　M67.814 Other specified disorders of tendon, left shoulder
　　　M67.819 Other specified disorders of synovium ▽
　　　　　and tendon, unspecified shoulder
　✓6ᵗʰ M67.82 Other specified disorders of synovium and tendon, elbow
　　　M67.821 Other specified disorders of synovium, right elbow
　　　M67.822 Other specified disorders of synovium, left elbow
　　　M67.823 Other specified disorders of tendon, right elbow
　　　M67.824 Other specified disorders of tendon, left elbow
　　　M67.829 Other specified disorders of synovium ▽
　　　　　and tendon, unspecified elbow
　✓6ᵗʰ M67.83 Other specified disorders of synovium and tendon, wrist
　　　M67.831 Other specified disorders of synovium, right wrist
　　　M67.832 Other specified disorders of synovium, left wrist
　　　M67.833 Other specified disorders of tendon, right wrist
　　　M67.834 Other specified disorders of tendon, left wrist
　　　M67.839 Other specified disorders of synovium ▽
　　　　　and tendon, unspecified forearm

✓6ᵗʰ **M67.84 Other specified disorders of synovium and tendon, hand**
    M67.841 Other specified disorders of synovium, right hand
    M67.842 Other specified disorders of synovium, left hand
    M67.843 Other specified disorders of tendon, right hand
    M67.844 Other specified disorders of tendon, left hand
    M67.849 Other specified disorders of synovium and tendon, unspecified hand ▽

✓6ᵗʰ **M67.85 Other specified disorders of synovium and tendon, hip**
    M67.851 Other specified disorders of synovium, right hip
    M67.852 Other specified disorders of synovium, left hip
    M67.853 Other specified disorders of tendon, right hip
    M67.854 Other specified disorders of tendon, left hip
    M67.859 Other specified disorders of synovium and tendon, unspecified hip ▽

✓6ᵗʰ **M67.86 Other specified disorders of synovium and tendon, knee**
    M67.861 Other specified disorders of synovium, right knee
    M67.862 Other specified disorders of synovium, left knee
    M67.863 Other specified disorders of tendon, right knee
    M67.864 Other specified disorders of tendon, left knee
    M67.869 Other specified disorders of synovium and tendon, unspecified knee ▽

✓6ᵗʰ **M67.87 Other specified disorders of synovium and tendon, ankle and foot**
    M67.871 Other specified disorders of synovium, right ankle and foot
    M67.872 Other specified disorders of synovium, left ankle and foot
    M67.873 Other specified disorders of tendon, right ankle and foot
    M67.874 Other specified disorders of tendon, left ankle and foot
    M67.879 Other specified disorders of synovium and tendon, unspecified ankle and foot ▽

M67.88 Other specified disorders of synovium and tendon, other site

M67.89 Other specified disorders of synovium and tendon, multiple sites

✓5ᵗʰ **M67.9 Unspecified disorder of synovium and tendon**
    M67.90 Unspecified disorder of synovium and tendon, unspecified site ▽

✓6ᵗʰ **M67.91 Unspecified disorder of synovium and tendon, shoulder**
    M67.911 Unspecified disorder of synovium and tendon, right shoulder ▽
    M67.912 Unspecified disorder of synovium and tendon, left shoulder ▽
    M67.919 Unspecified disorder of synovium and tendon, unspecified shoulder ▽

✓6ᵗʰ **M67.92 Unspecified disorder of synovium and tendon, upper arm**
    M67.921 Unspecified disorder of synovium and tendon, right upper arm ▽
    M67.922 Unspecified disorder of synovium and tendon, left upper arm ▽
    M67.929 Unspecified disorder of synovium and tendon, unspecified upper arm ▽

✓6ᵗʰ **M67.93 Unspecified disorder of synovium and tendon, forearm**
    M67.931 Unspecified disorder of synovium and tendon, right forearm ▽
    M67.932 Unspecified disorder of synovium and tendon, left forearm ▽

    M67.939 Unspecified disorder of synovium and tendon, unspecified forearm ▽

✓6ᵗʰ **M67.94 Unspecified disorder of synovium and tendon, hand**
    M67.941 Unspecified disorder of synovium and tendon, right hand ▽
    M67.942 Unspecified disorder of synovium and tendon, left hand ▽
    M67.949 Unspecified disorder of synovium and tendon, unspecified hand ▽

✓6ᵗʰ **M67.95 Unspecified disorder of synovium and tendon, thigh**
    M67.951 Unspecified disorder of synovium and tendon, right thigh ▽
    M67.952 Unspecified disorder of synovium and tendon, left thigh ▽
    M67.959 Unspecified disorder of synovium and tendon, unspecified thigh ▽

✓6ᵗʰ **M67.96 Unspecified disorder of synovium and tendon, lower leg**
    M67.961 Unspecified disorder of synovium and tendon, right lower leg ▽
    M67.962 Unspecified disorder of synovium and tendon, left lower leg ▽
    M67.969 Unspecified disorder of synovium and tendon, unspecified lower leg ▽

✓6ᵗʰ **M67.97 Unspecified disorder of synovium and tendon, ankle and foot**
    M67.971 Unspecified disorder of synovium and tendon, right ankle and foot ▽
    M67.972 Unspecified disorder of synovium and tendon, left ankle and foot ▽
    M67.979 Unspecified disorder of synovium and tendon, unspecified ankle and foot ▽

M67.98 Unspecified disorder of synovium and tendon, other site ▽

M67.99 Unspecified disorder of synovium and tendon, multiple sites ▽

Other soft tissue disorders (M70-M79)

✓4ᵗʰ **M70 Soft tissue disorders related to use, overuse and pressure**
    INCLUDES soft tissue disorders of occupational origin
    Use additional external cause code to identify activity causing disorder (Y93.-)
    EXCLUDES 1 bursitis NOS (M71.9-)
    EXCLUDES 2 bursitis of shoulder (M75.5)
        enthesopathies (M76-M77)
        pressure ulcer (pressure area) (L89.-)

✓5ᵗʰ **M70.0 Crepitant synovitis (acute) (chronic) of hand and wrist**
    ✓6ᵗʰ **M70.03 Crepitant synovitis (acute) (chronic), wrist**
        M70.031 Crepitant synovitis (acute) (chronic), right wrist
        M70.032 Crepitant synovitis (acute) (chronic), left wrist
        M70.039 Crepitant synovitis (acute) (chronic), unspecified wrist ▽
    ✓6ᵗʰ **M70.04 Crepitant synovitis (acute) (chronic), hand**
        M70.041 Crepitant synovitis (acute) (chronic), right hand
        M70.042 Crepitant synovitis (acute) (chronic), left hand
        M70.049 Crepitant synovitis (acute) (chronic), unspecified hand ▽

✓5ᵗʰ **M70.1 Bursitis of hand**
    M70.10 Bursitis, unspecified hand ▽
    M70.11 Bursitis, right hand
    M70.12 Bursitis, left hand

✓5ᵗʰ **M70.2 Olecranon bursitis**
    M70.20 Olecranon bursitis, unspecified elbow ▽
    M70.21 Olecranon bursitis, right elbow
    M70.22 Olecranon bursitis, left elbow

✓5ᵗʰ **M70.3 Other bursitis of elbow**
    M70.30 Other bursitis of elbow, unspecified elbow ▽
    M70.31 Other bursitis of elbow, right elbow
    M70.32 Other bursitis of elbow, left elbow

✓ Additional Character Req   ✓ˣ7ᵗʰ Placeholder Alert   Manifestation   HCC CMS-HCC Condition   ▽ Unspecified Code   ▶◀ Revised Text   ● New Code   ▲ Revised Code Title

ICD-10-CM 2018   771

✓5ᵗʰ **M70.4 Prepatellar** bursitis
     M70.40   Prepatellar bursitis, unspecified knee   ▽
     M70.41   Prepatellar bursitis, **right** knee
     M70.42   Prepatellar bursitis, **left** knee

✓5ᵗʰ **M70.5 Other bursitis of knee**
     M70.50   Other bursitis of knee, unspecified knee   ▽
     M70.51   Other bursitis of knee, **right** knee
     M70.52   Other bursitis of knee, **left** knee

✓5ᵗʰ **M70.6 Trochanteric** bursitis
     Trochanteric tendinitis
     M70.60   Trochanteric bursitis, unspecified hip   ▽
     M70.61   Trochanteric bursitis, **right** hip
     M70.62   Trochanteric bursitis, **left** hip

✓5ᵗʰ **M70.7 Other bursitis of hip**
     Ischial bursitis
     M70.70   Other bursitis of hip, unspecified hip   ▽
     M70.71   Other bursitis of hip, **right** hip
     M70.72   Other bursitis of hip, **left** hip

✓5ᵗʰ **M70.8 Other soft tissue disorders related to use, overuse and pressure**
     M70.80   Other soft tissue disorders related to use,   ▽
         overuse and pressure of unspecified site

    ✓6ᵗʰ M70.81   Other soft tissue disorders related to use, overuse and pressure of **shoulder**
         M70.811   Other soft tissue disorders related to use, overuse and pressure, **right** shoulder
         M70.812   Other soft tissue disorders related to use, overuse and pressure, **left** shoulder
         M70.819   Other soft tissue disorders related to   ▽ use, overuse and pressure, unspecified shoulder

    ✓6ᵗʰ M70.82   Other soft tissue disorders related to use, overuse and pressure of **upper arm**
         M70.821   Other soft tissue disorders related to use, overuse and pressure, **right** upper arm
         M70.822   Other soft tissue disorders related to use, overuse and pressure, **left** upper arm
         M70.829   Other soft tissue disorders related to   ▽ use, overuse and pressure, unspecified upper arms

    ✓6ᵗʰ M70.83   Other soft tissue disorders related to use, overuse and pressure of **forearm**
         M70.831   Other soft tissue disorders related to use, overuse and pressure, **right** forearm
         M70.832   Other soft tissue disorders related to use, overuse and pressure, **left** forearm
         M70.839   Other soft tissue disorders related to   ▽ use, overuse and pressure, unspecified forearm

    ✓6ᵗʰ M70.84   Other soft tissue disorders related to use, overuse and pressure of **hand**
         M70.841   Other soft tissue disorders related to use, overuse and pressure, **right** hand
         M70.842   Other soft tissue disorders related to use, overuse and pressure, **left** hand
         M70.849   Other soft tissue disorders related to   ▽ use, overuse and pressure, unspecified hand

    ✓6ᵗʰ M70.85   Other soft tissue disorders related to use, overuse and pressure of **thigh**
         M70.851   Other soft tissue disorders related to use, overuse and pressure, **right** thigh
         M70.852   Other soft tissue disorders related to use, overuse and pressure, **left** thigh
         M70.859   Other soft tissue disorders related to   ▽ use, overuse and pressure, unspecified thigh

    ✓6ᵗʰ M70.86   Other soft tissue disorders related to use, overuse and pressure **lower leg**
         M70.861   Other soft tissue disorders related to use, overuse and pressure, **right** lower leg
         M70.862   Other soft tissue disorders related to use, overuse and pressure, **left** lower leg
         M70.869   Other soft tissue disorders related to   ▽ use, overuse and pressure, unspecified leg

    ✓6ᵗʰ M70.87   Other soft tissue disorders related to use, overuse and pressure of **ankle and foot**
         M70.871   Other soft tissue disorders related to use, overuse and pressure, **right** ankle and foot
         M70.872   Other soft tissue disorders related to use, overuse and pressure, **left** ankle and foot
         M70.879   Other soft tissue disorders related to   ▽ use, overuse and pressure, unspecified ankle and foot

     M70.88   Other soft tissue disorders related to use, overuse and pressure other site

     M70.89   Other soft tissue disorders related to use, overuse and pressure **multiple sites**

✓5ᵗʰ **M70.9 Unspecified soft tissue disorder related to use, overuse and pressure**
     M70.90   Unspecified soft tissue disorder related to use,   ▽ overuse and pressure of unspecified site

    ✓6ᵗʰ M70.91   Unspecified soft tissue disorder related to use, overuse and pressure of **shoulder**
         M70.911   Unspecified soft tissue disorder related ▽ to use, overuse and pressure, **right** shoulder
         M70.912   Unspecified soft tissue disorder related ▽ to use, overuse and pressure, **left** shoulder
         M70.919   Unspecified soft tissue disorder related ▽ to use, overuse and pressure, unspecified shoulder

    ✓6ᵗʰ M70.92   Unspecified soft tissue disorder related to use, overuse and pressure of **upper arm**
         M70.921   Unspecified soft tissue disorder related ▽ to use, overuse and pressure, **right** upper arm
         M70.922   Unspecified soft tissue disorder related ▽ to use, overuse and pressure, **left** upper arm
         M70.929   Unspecified soft tissue disorder related ▽ to use, overuse and pressure, unspecified upper arm

    ✓6ᵗʰ M70.93   Unspecified soft tissue disorder related to use, overuse and pressure of **forearm**
         M70.931   Unspecified soft tissue disorder related ▽ to use, overuse and pressure, **right** forearm
         M70.932   Unspecified soft tissue disorder related ▽ to use, overuse and pressure, **left** forearm
         M70.939   Unspecified soft tissue disorder related ▽ to use, overuse and pressure, unspecified forearm

    ✓6ᵗʰ M70.94   Unspecified soft tissue disorder related to use, overuse and pressure of **hand**
         M70.941   Unspecified soft tissue disorder related ▽ to use, overuse and pressure, **right** hand
         M70.942   Unspecified soft tissue disorder related ▽ to use, overuse and pressure, **left** hand
         M70.949   Unspecified soft tissue disorder related ▽ to use, overuse and pressure, unspecified hand

    ✓6ᵗʰ M70.95   Unspecified soft tissue disorder related to use, overuse and pressure of **thigh**
         M70.951   Unspecified soft tissue disorder related ▽ to use, overuse and pressure, **right** thigh
         M70.952   Unspecified soft tissue disorder related ▽ to use, overuse and pressure, **left** thigh
         M70.959   Unspecified soft tissue disorder related ▽ to use, overuse and pressure, unspecified thigh

    ✓6ᵗʰ M70.96   Unspecified soft tissue disorder related to use, overuse and pressure **lower leg**
         M70.961   Unspecified soft tissue disorder related ▽ to use, overuse and pressure, **right** lower leg
         M70.962   Unspecified soft tissue disorder related ▽ to use, overuse and pressure, **left** lower leg
         M70.969   Unspecified soft tissue disorder related ▽ to use, overuse and pressure, unspecified lower leg

EXCLUDES 1 Not coded here   **EXCLUDES 2** Not included here   **N** Newborn Age: 0   **P** Pediatric Age: 0-17   **M** Maternity Age: 12-55   **A** Adult Age: 15-124

772   ICD-10-CM 2018

☑6ᵗʰ **M70.97 Unspecified soft tissue disorder related to use, overuse and pressure of ankle and foot**
     M70.971 Unspecified soft tissue disorder related ▽ to use, overuse and pressure, right ankle and foot
     M70.972 Unspecified soft tissue disorder related ▽ to use, overuse and pressure, left ankle and foot
     M70.979 Unspecified soft tissue disorder related ▽ to use, overuse and pressure, unspecified ankle and foot
     M70.98 Unspecified soft tissue disorder related to use, ▽ **overuse and pressure other**
     M70.99 Unspecified soft tissue disorder related to use, ▽ **overuse and pressure multiple sites**

☑4ᵗʰ **M71 Other bursopathies**
     EXCLUDES 1   *bunion (M20.1)*
                 bursitis related to use, overuse or pressure (M70.-)
                 enthesopathies (M76-M77)

☑5ᵗʰ **M71.0 Abscess of bursa**
     Use additional code (B95.-, B96.-) to identify causative organism
     M71.00 Abscess of bursa, unspecified site ▽
     ☑6ᵗʰ **M71.01 Abscess of bursa, shoulder**
         M71.011 Abscess of bursa, right shoulder
         M71.012 Abscess of bursa, left shoulder
         M71.019 Abscess of bursa, unspecified shoulder ▽
     ☑6ᵗʰ **M71.02 Abscess of bursa, elbow**
         M71.021 Abscess of bursa, right elbow
         M71.022 Abscess of bursa, left elbow
         M71.029 Abscess of bursa, unspecified elbow ▽
     ☑6ᵗʰ **M71.03 Abscess of bursa, wrist**
         M71.031 Abscess of bursa, right wrist
         M71.032 Abscess of bursa, left wrist
         M71.039 Abscess of bursa, unspecified wrist ▽
     ☑6ᵗʰ **M71.04 Abscess of bursa, hand**
         M71.041 Abscess of bursa, right hand
         M71.042 Abscess of bursa, left hand
         M71.049 Abscess of bursa, unspecified hand ▽
     ☑6ᵗʰ **M71.05 Abscess of bursa, hip**
         M71.051 Abscess of bursa, right hip
         M71.052 Abscess of bursa, left hip
         M71.059 Abscess of bursa, unspecified hip ▽
     ☑6ᵗʰ **M71.06 Abscess of bursa, knee**
         M71.061 Abscess of bursa, right knee
         M71.062 Abscess of bursa, left knee
         M71.069 Abscess of bursa, unspecified knee ▽
     ☑6ᵗʰ **M71.07 Abscess of bursa, ankle and foot**
         M71.071 Abscess of bursa, right ankle and foot
         M71.072 Abscess of bursa, left ankle and foot
         M71.079 Abscess of bursa, unspecified ankle ▽ and foot
     M71.08 Abscess of bursa, other site
     M71.09 Abscess of bursa, multiple sites

☑5ᵗʰ **M71.1 Other infective bursitis**
     Use additional code (B95.-, B96.-) to identify causative organism
     M71.10 Other infective bursitis, unspecified site ▽
     ☑6ᵗʰ **M71.11 Other infective bursitis, shoulder**
         M71.111 Other infective bursitis, right shoulder
         M71.112 Other infective bursitis, left shoulder
         M71.119 Other infective bursitis, unspecified ▽ shoulder
     ☑6ᵗʰ **M71.12 Other infective bursitis, elbow**
         M71.121 Other infective bursitis, right elbow
         M71.122 Other infective bursitis, left elbow
         M71.129 Other infective bursitis, unspecified ▽ elbow
     ☑6ᵗʰ **M71.13 Other infective bursitis, wrist**
         M71.131 Other infective bursitis, right wrist
         M71.132 Other infective bursitis, left wrist
         M71.139 Other infective bursitis, unspecified ▽ wrist

☑6ᵗʰ **M71.14 Other infective bursitis, hand**
     M71.141 Other infective bursitis, right hand
     M71.142 Other infective bursitis, left hand
     M71.149 Other infective bursitis, unspecified ▽ hand
☑6ᵗʰ **M71.15 Other infective bursitis, hip**
     M71.151 Other infective bursitis, right hip
     M71.152 Other infective bursitis, left hip
     M71.159 Other infective bursitis, unspecified hip ▽
☑6ᵗʰ **M71.16 Other infective bursitis, knee**
     M71.161 Other infective bursitis, right knee
     M71.162 Other infective bursitis, left knee
     M71.169 Other infective bursitis, unspecified ▽ knee
☑6ᵗʰ **M71.17 Other infective bursitis, ankle and foot**
     M71.171 Other infective bursitis, right ankle and foot
     M71.172 Other infective bursitis, left ankle and foot
     M71.179 Other infective bursitis, unspecified ▽ ankle and foot
     M71.18 Other infective bursitis, other site
     M71.19 Other infective bursitis, multiple sites

☑5ᵗʰ **M71.2 Synovial cyst of popliteal space [Baker]**
     EXCLUDES 1   *synovial cyst of popliteal space with rupture (M66.0)*
     M71.20 Synovial cyst of popliteal space [Baker], ▽ **unspecified knee**
     M71.21 Synovial cyst of popliteal space [Baker], right knee
     M71.22 Synovial cyst of popliteal space [Baker], left knee

☑5ᵗʰ **M71.3 Other bursal cyst**
     Synovial cyst NOS
     EXCLUDES 1   *synovial cyst with rupture (M66.1-)*
     M71.30 Other bursal cyst, unspecified site ▽
     ☑6ᵗʰ **M71.31 Other bursal cyst, shoulder**
         M71.311 Other bursal cyst, right shoulder
         M71.312 Other bursal cyst, left shoulder
         M71.319 Other bursal cyst, unspecified shoulder ▽
     ☑6ᵗʰ **M71.32 Other bursal cyst, elbow**
         M71.321 Other bursal cyst, right elbow
         M71.322 Other bursal cyst, left elbow
         M71.329 Other bursal cyst, unspecified elbow ▽
     ☑6ᵗʰ **M71.33 Other bursal cyst, wrist**
         M71.331 Other bursal cyst, right wrist
         M71.332 Other bursal cyst, left wrist
         M71.339 Other bursal cyst, unspecified wrist ▽
     ☑6ᵗʰ **M71.34 Other bursal cyst, hand**
         M71.341 Other bursal cyst, right hand
         M71.342 Other bursal cyst, left hand
         M71.349 Other bursal cyst, unspecified hand ▽

Baker's Cyst

Baker's cyst connected to knee joint synovial cavity

☑ Additional Character Req   ☑7ᵗʰ Placeholder Alert   Manifestation   HCC CMS-HCC Condition   ▽ Unspecified Code   ▶◀ Revised Text   ● New Code   ▲ Revised Code Title

ICD-10-CM 2018   773

√6ᵗʰ **M71.35 Other bursal cyst, hip**
    M71.351 Other bursal cyst, **right** hip
    M71.352 Other bursal cyst, **left** hip
    M71.359 Other bursal cyst, **unspecified** hip ▽

√6ᵗʰ **M71.37 Other bursal cyst, ankle and foot**
    M71.371 Other bursal cyst, **right** ankle and foot
    M71.372 Other bursal cyst, **left** ankle and foot
    M71.379 Other bursal cyst, **unspecified** ankle and foot ▽

    M71.38 Other bursal cyst, other site
    M71.39 Other bursal cyst, multiple sites

√5ᵗʰ **M71.4 Calcium deposit in bursa**
    EXCLUDES 2   *calcium deposit in bursa of shoulder (M75.3)*
    M71.40 Calcium deposit in bursa, unspecified site ▽

√6ᵗʰ **M71.42 Calcium deposit in bursa, elbow**
    M71.421 Calcium deposit in bursa, **right** elbow
    M71.422 Calcium deposit in bursa, **left** elbow
    M71.429 Calcium deposit in bursa, **unspecified** elbow ▽

√6ᵗʰ **M71.43 Calcium deposit in bursa, wrist**
    M71.431 Calcium deposit in bursa, **right** wrist
    M71.432 Calcium deposit in bursa, **left** wrist
    M71.439 Calcium deposit in bursa, **unspecified** wrist ▽

√6ᵗʰ **M71.44 Calcium deposit in bursa, hand**
    M71.441 Calcium deposit in bursa, **right** hand
    M71.442 Calcium deposit in bursa, **left** hand
    M71.449 Calcium deposit in bursa, **unspecified** hand ▽

√6ᵗʰ **M71.45 Calcium deposit in bursa, hip**
    M71.451 Calcium deposit in bursa, **right** hip
    M71.452 Calcium deposit in bursa, **left** hip
    M71.459 Calcium deposit in bursa, **unspecified** hip ▽

√6ᵗʰ **M71.46 Calcium deposit in bursa, knee**
    M71.461 Calcium deposit in bursa, **right** knee
    M71.462 Calcium deposit in bursa, **left** knee
    M71.469 Calcium deposit in bursa, **unspecified** knee ▽

√6ᵗʰ **M71.47 Calcium deposit in bursa, ankle and foot**
    M71.471 Calcium deposit in bursa, **right** ankle and foot
    M71.472 Calcium deposit in bursa, **left** ankle and foot
    M71.479 Calcium deposit in bursa, **unspecified** ankle and foot ▽

    M71.48 Calcium deposit in bursa, other site
    M71.49 Calcium deposit in bursa, multiple sites

√5ᵗʰ **M71.5 Other bursitis, not elsewhere classified**
    EXCLUDES 1   *bursitis NOS (M71.9-)*
    EXCLUDES 2   *bursitis of shoulder (M75.5)*
               bursitis of tibial collateral [Pellegrini-Stieda] (M76.4-)

    M71.50 Other bursitis, not elsewhere classified, unspecified site ▽

√6ᵗʰ **M71.52 Other bursitis, not elsewhere classified, elbow**
    M71.521 Other bursitis, not elsewhere classified, **right** elbow
    M71.522 Other bursitis, not elsewhere classified, **left** elbow
    M71.529 Other bursitis, not elsewhere classified, **unspecified** elbow ▽

√6ᵗʰ **M71.53 Other bursitis, not elsewhere classified, wrist**
    M71.531 Other bursitis, not elsewhere classified, **right** wrist
    M71.532 Other bursitis, not elsewhere classified, **left** wrist
    M71.539 Other bursitis, not elsewhere classified, **unspecified** wrist ▽

√6ᵗʰ **M71.54 Other bursitis, not elsewhere classified, hand**
    M71.541 Other bursitis, not elsewhere classified, **right** hand
    M71.542 Other bursitis, not elsewhere classified, **left** hand

    M71.549 Other bursitis, not elsewhere classified, **unspecified** hand ▽

√6ᵗʰ **M71.55 Other bursitis, not elsewhere classified, hip**
    M71.551 Other bursitis, not elsewhere classified, **right** hip
    M71.552 Other bursitis, not elsewhere classified, **left** hip
    M71.559 Other bursitis, not elsewhere classified, **unspecified** hip ▽

√6ᵗʰ **M71.56 Other bursitis, not elsewhere classified, knee**
    M71.561 Other bursitis, not elsewhere classified, **right** knee
    M71.562 Other bursitis, not elsewhere classified, **left** knee
    M71.569 Other bursitis, not elsewhere classified, **unspecified** knee ▽

√6ᵗʰ **M71.57 Other bursitis, not elsewhere classified, ankle and foot**
    M71.571 Other bursitis, not elsewhere classified, **right** ankle and foot
    M71.572 Other bursitis, not elsewhere classified, **left** ankle and foot
    M71.579 Other bursitis, not elsewhere classified, **unspecified** ankle and foot ▽

    M71.58 Other bursitis, not elsewhere classified, other site

√5ᵗʰ **M71.8 Other specified bursopathies**
    M71.80 Other specified bursopathies, unspecified site ▽

√6ᵗʰ **M71.81 Other specified bursopathies, shoulder**
    M71.811 Other specified bursopathies, **right** shoulder
    M71.812 Other specified bursopathies, **left** shoulder
    M71.819 Other specified bursopathies, **unspecified** shoulder ▽

√6ᵗʰ **M71.82 Other specified bursopathies, elbow**
    M71.821 Other specified bursopathies, **right** elbow
    M71.822 Other specified bursopathies, **left** elbow
    M71.829 Other specified bursopathies, **unspecified** elbow ▽

√6ᵗʰ **M71.83 Other specified bursopathies, wrist**
    M71.831 Other specified bursopathies, **right** wrist
    M71.832 Other specified bursopathies, **left** wrist
    M71.839 Other specified bursopathies, **unspecified** wrist ▽

√6ᵗʰ **M71.84 Other specified bursopathies, hand**
    M71.841 Other specified bursopathies, **right** hand
    M71.842 Other specified bursopathies, **left** hand
    M71.849 Other specified bursopathies, **unspecified** hand ▽

√6ᵗʰ **M71.85 Other specified bursopathies, hip**
    M71.851 Other specified bursopathies, **right** hip
    M71.852 Other specified bursopathies, **left** hip
    M71.859 Other specified bursopathies, **unspecified** hip ▽

√6ᵗʰ **M71.86 Other specified bursopathies, knee**
    M71.861 Other specified bursopathies, **right** knee
    M71.862 Other specified bursopathies, **left** knee
    M71.869 Other specified bursopathies, **unspecified** knee ▽

√6ᵗʰ **M71.87 Other specified bursopathies, ankle and foot**
    M71.871 Other specified bursopathies, **right** ankle and foot
    M71.872 Other specified bursopathies, **left** ankle and foot
    M71.879 Other specified bursopathies, **unspecified** ankle and foot ▽

    M71.88 Other specified bursopathies, other site
    M71.89 Other specified bursopathies, multiple sites

    M71.9 Bursopathy, unspecified ▽
    Bursitis NOS

EXCLUDES 1 Not coded here   EXCLUDES 2 Not included here   N Newborn Age: 0   P Pediatric Age: 0-17   M Maternity Age: 12-55   A Adult Age: 15-124

774   ICD-10-CM 2018

✓4ᵗʰ M72 Fibroblastic disorders
     EXCLUDES 2   *retroperitoneal fibromatosis (D48.3)*

     M72.0 Palmar fascial fibromatosis [Dupuytren]   A
         DEF: Dupuytren's contracture: Flexion deformity of finger, due to shortened, thickened fibrosing of palmar fascia; cause unknown; associated with long-standing epilepsy.

     M72.1 Knuckle pads

     M72.2 Plantar fascial fibromatosis
         Plantar fasciitis
         DEF: Rapid-growing and multiplanar nodular swellings and pain in the foot; not associated with contractures.

     M72.4 Pseudosarcomatous fibromatosis
         Nodular fasciitis

     M72.6 Necrotizing fasciitis   HCC
         Use additional code (B95.-, B96.-) to identify causative organism

     M72.8 Other fibroblastic disorders
         Abscess of fascia
         Fasciitis NEC
         Other infective fasciitis
         Use additional code to (B95.-, B96.-) identify causative organism
         EXCLUDES 1   *diffuse (eosinophilic) fasciitis (M35.4)*
                    necrotizing fasciitis (M72.6)
                    nodular fasciitis (M72.4)
                    perirenal fasciitis NOS (N13.5)
                    perirenal fasciitis with infection (N13.6)
                    plantar fasciitis (M72.2)

     M72.9 Fibroblastic disorder, unspecified   ▽
         Fasciitis NOS
         Fibromatosis NOS

✓4ᵗʰ M75 Shoulder lesions
     EXCLUDES 2   *shoulder-hand syndrome (M89.0-)*

     ✓5ᵗʰ M75.0 Adhesive capsulitis of shoulder
         Frozen shoulder
         Periarthritis of shoulder
         AHA: 2015, 2Q, 23

         M75.00 Adhesive capsulitis of unspecified shoulder   ▽
         M75.01 Adhesive capsulitis of right shoulder
         M75.02 Adhesive capsulitis of left shoulder

     ✓5ᵗʰ M75.1 Rotator cuff tear or rupture, not specified as traumatic
         Rotator cuff syndrome
         Supraspinatus syndrome
         Supraspinatus tear or rupture, not specified as traumatic
         EXCLUDES 1   *tear of rotator cuff, traumatic (S46.01-)*

         ✓6ᵗʰ M75.10 Unspecified rotator cuff tear or rupture, not specified as traumatic
             M75.100 Unspecified rotator cuff tear or rupture ▽ **of unspecified shoulder, not specified as traumatic**
             M75.101 Unspecified rotator cuff tear or rupture ▽ **of right shoulder, not specified as traumatic**
             M75.102 Unspecified rotator cuff tear or rupture ▽ **of left shoulder, not specified as traumatic**

         ✓6ᵗʰ M75.11 Incomplete rotator cuff tear or rupture not specified as traumatic
             M75.110 Incomplete rotator cuff tear or rupture ▽ **of unspecified shoulder, not specified as traumatic**
             M75.111 Incomplete rotator cuff tear or rupture of right shoulder, not specified as traumatic
             M75.112 Incomplete rotator cuff tear or rupture of left shoulder, not specified as traumatic

         ✓6ᵗʰ M75.12 Complete rotator cuff tear or rupture not specified as traumatic
             M75.120 Complete rotator cuff tear or rupture ▽ **of unspecified shoulder, not specified as traumatic**
             M75.121 Complete rotator cuff tear or rupture of right shoulder, not specified as traumatic
             M75.122 Complete rotator cuff tear or rupture of left shoulder, not specified as traumatic

     ✓5ᵗʰ M75.2 Bicipital tendinitis
         M75.20 Bicipital tendinitis, unspecified shoulder   ▽
         M75.21 Bicipital tendinitis, right shoulder
         M75.22 Bicipital tendinitis, left shoulder

     ✓5ᵗʰ M75.3 Calcific tendinitis of shoulder
         Calcified bursa of shoulder
         M75.30 Calcific tendinitis of unspecified shoulder   ▽
         M75.31 Calcific tendinitis of right shoulder
         M75.32 Calcific tendinitis of left shoulder

     ✓5ᵗʰ M75.4 Impingement syndrome of shoulder
         M75.40 Impingement syndrome of unspecified shoulder   ▽
         M75.41 Impingement syndrome of right shoulder
         M75.42 Impingement syndrome of left shoulder

     ✓5ᵗʰ M75.5 Bursitis of shoulder
         M75.50 Bursitis of unspecified shoulder   ▽
         M75.51 Bursitis of right shoulder
         M75.52 Bursitis of left shoulder

     ✓5ᵗʰ M75.8 Other shoulder lesions
         M75.80 Other shoulder lesions, unspecified shoulder   ▽
         M75.81 Other shoulder lesions, right shoulder
         M75.82 Other shoulder lesions, left shoulder

     ✓5ᵗʰ M75.9 Shoulder lesion, unspecified
         M75.90 Shoulder lesion, unspecified, unspecified   ▽ **shoulder**
         M75.91 Shoulder lesion, unspecified, right shoulder   ▽
         M75.92 Shoulder lesion, unspecified, left shoulder   ▽

✓4ᵗʰ M76 Enthesopathies, lower limb, excluding foot
     EXCLUDES 2   *bursitis due to use, overuse and pressure (M70.-)*
                    enthesopathies of ankle and foot (M77.5-)

     ✓5ᵗʰ M76.0 Gluteal tendinitis
         M76.00 Gluteal tendinitis, unspecified hip   ▽
         M76.01 Gluteal tendinitis, right hip
         M76.02 Gluteal tendinitis, left hip

     ✓5ᵗʰ M76.1 Psoas tendinitis
         M76.10 Psoas tendinitis, unspecified hip   ▽
         M76.11 Psoas tendinitis, right hip
         M76.12 Psoas tendinitis, left hip

     ✓5ᵗʰ M76.2 Iliac crest spur
         M76.20 Iliac crest spur, unspecified hip   ▽
         M76.21 Iliac crest spur, right hip
         M76.22 Iliac crest spur, left hip

     ✓5ᵗʰ M76.3 Iliotibial band syndrome
         M76.30 Iliotibial band syndrome, unspecified leg   ▽
         M76.31 Iliotibial band syndrome, right leg
         M76.32 Iliotibial band syndrome, left leg

     ✓5ᵗʰ M76.4 Tibial collateral bursitis [Pellegrini-Stieda]
         M76.40 Tibial collateral bursitis [Pellegrini-Stieda],   ▽ **unspecified leg**
         M76.41 Tibial collateral bursitis [Pellegrini-Stieda], right leg
         M76.42 Tibial collateral bursitis [Pellegrini-Stieda], left leg

     ✓5ᵗʰ M76.5 Patellar tendinitis
         M76.50 Patellar tendinitis, unspecified knee   ▽
         M76.51 Patellar tendinitis, right knee
         M76.52 Patellar tendinitis, left knee

     ✓5ᵗʰ M76.6 Achilles tendinitis
         Achilles bursitis
         M76.60 Achilles tendinitis, unspecified leg   ▽
         M76.61 Achilles tendinitis, right leg
         M76.62 Achilles tendinitis, left leg

     ✓5ᵗʰ M76.7 Peroneal tendinitis
         M76.70 Peroneal tendinitis, unspecified leg   ▽
         M76.71 Peroneal tendinitis, right leg
         M76.72 Peroneal tendinitis, left leg

     ✓5ᵗʰ M76.8 Other specified enthesopathies of lower limb, excluding foot
         ✓6ᵗʰ M76.81 Anterior tibial syndrome
             M76.811 Anterior tibial syndrome, right leg
             M76.812 Anterior tibial syndrome, left leg
             M76.819 Anterior tibial syndrome, unspecified   ▽ **leg**

         ✓6ᵗʰ M76.82 Posterior tibial tendinitis
             M76.821 Posterior tibial tendinitis, right leg
             M76.822 Posterior tibial tendinitis, left leg
             M76.829 Posterior tibial tendinitis, unspecified   ▽ **leg**

✔ Additional Character Req   ✓x7ᵗʰ Placeholder Alert   Manifestation   HCC CMS-HCC Condition   ▽ Unspecified Code   ►◄ Revised Text   ● New Code   ▲ Revised Code Title

√6th M76.89 Other specified enthesopathies of lower limb, excluding foot

     M76.891 Other specified enthesopathies of right lower limb, excluding foot

     M76.892 Other specified enthesopathies of left lower limb, excluding foot

     M76.899 Other specified enthesopathies of unspecified lower limb, excluding foot ▽

M76.9 Unspecified enthesopathy, lower limb, excluding foot ▽

√4th M77 Other enthesopathies

EXCLUDES 1   *bursitis NOS (M71.9-)*

EXCLUDES 2   *bursitis due to use, overuse and pressure (M70.-)*
     osteophyte (M25.7)
     spinal enthesopathy (M46.0-)

√5th M77.0 Medial epicondylitis

     M77.00 Medial epicondylitis, unspecified elbow ▽

     M77.01 Medial epicondylitis, right elbow

     M77.02 Medial epicondylitis, left elbow

√5th M77.1 Lateral epicondylitis

     Tennis elbow

     M77.10 Lateral epicondylitis, unspecified elbow ▽

     M77.11 Lateral epicondylitis, right elbow

     M77.12 Lateral epicondylitis, left elbow

√5th M77.2 Periarthritis of wrist

     M77.20 Periarthritis, unspecified wrist ▽

     M77.21 Periarthritis, right wrist

     M77.22 Periarthritis, left wrist

√5th M77.3 Calcaneal spur

     DEF: Overgrowth of calcaneus bone on underside of the heel; causes pain on walking; due to chronic avulsion injury of plantar fascia from calcaneus.

     M77.30 Calcaneal spur, unspecified foot ▽

     M77.31 Calcaneal spur, right foot

     M77.32 Calcaneal spur, left foot

√5th M77.4 Metatarsalgia

EXCLUDES 1   *Morton's metatarsalgia (G57.6)*

     M77.40 Metatarsalgia, unspecified foot ▽

     M77.41 Metatarsalgia, right foot

     M77.42 Metatarsalgia, left foot

√5th M77.5 Other enthesopathy of foot

     M77.50 Other enthesopathy of unspecified foot ▽

     M77.51 Other enthesopathy of right foot

     M77.52 Other enthesopathy of left foot

M77.8 Other enthesopathies, not elsewhere classified

M77.9 Enthesopathy, unspecified ▽

     Bone spur NOS   Periarthritis NOS
     Capsulitis NOS   Tendinitis NOS

√4th M79 Other and unspecified soft tissue disorders, not elsewhere classified

EXCLUDES 1   *psychogenic rheumatism (F45.8)*
     soft tissue pain, psychogenic (F45.41)

M79.0 Rheumatism, unspecified ▽

EXCLUDES 1   *fibromyalgia (M79.7)*
     palindromic rheumatism (M12.3-)

M79.1 Myalgia

     Myofascial pain syndrome

EXCLUDES 1   *fibromyalgia (M79.7)*
     myositis (M60.-)

M79.2 Neuralgia and neuritis, unspecified ▽

EXCLUDES 1   *brachial radiculitis NOS (M54.1)*
     lumbosacral radiculitis NOS (M54.1)
     mononeuropathies (G56-G58)
     radiculitis NOS (M54.1)
     sciatica (M54.3-M54.4)

M79.3 Panniculitis, unspecified ▽

EXCLUDES 1   *lupus panniculitis (L93.2)*
     neck and back panniculitis (M54.0-)
     relapsing [Weber-Christian] panniculitis (M35.6)

M79.4 Hypertrophy of (infrapatellar) fat pad

M79.5 Residual foreign body in soft tissue

EXCLUDES 1   *foreign body granuloma of skin and subcutaneous tissue (L92.3)*
     foreign body granuloma of soft tissue (M60.2-)

√6th M79.6 Pain in limb, hand, foot, fingers and toes

EXCLUDES 2   *pain in joint (M25.5-)*

√6th M79.60 Pain in limb, unspecified

     M79.601 Pain in right arm
         Pain in right upper limb NOS

     M79.602 Pain in left arm
         Pain in left upper limb NOS

     M79.603 Pain in arm, unspecified ▽
         Pain in upper limb NOS

     M79.604 Pain in right leg
         Pain in right lower limb NOS

     M79.605 Pain in left leg
         Pain in left lower limb NOS

     M79.606 Pain in leg, unspecified ▽
         Pain in lower limb NOS

     M79.609 Pain in unspecified limb ▽
         Pain in limb NOS

√6th M79.62 Pain in upper arm

     Pain in axillary region

     M79.621 Pain in right upper arm

     M79.622 Pain in left upper arm

     M79.629 Pain in unspecified upper arm ▽

√6th M79.63 Pain in forearm

     M79.631 Pain in right forearm

     M79.632 Pain in left forearm

     M79.639 Pain in unspecified forearm ▽

√6th M79.64 Pain in hand and fingers

     M79.641 Pain in right hand

     M79.642 Pain in left hand

     M79.643 Pain in unspecified hand ▽

     M79.644 Pain in right finger(s)

     M79.645 Pain in left finger(s)

     M79.646 Pain in unspecified finger(s) ▽

√6th M79.65 Pain in thigh

     M79.651 Pain in right thigh

     M79.652 Pain in left thigh

     M79.659 Pain in unspecified thigh ▽

√6th M79.66 Pain in lower leg

     M79.661 Pain in right lower leg

     M79.662 Pain in left lower leg

     M79.669 Pain in unspecified lower leg ▽

√6th M79.67 Pain in foot and toes

     M79.671 Pain in right foot

     M79.672 Pain in left foot

     M79.673 Pain in unspecified foot ▽

     M79.674 Pain in right toe(s)

     M79.675 Pain in left toe(s)

     M79.676 Pain in unspecified toe(s) ▽

M79.7 Fibromyalgia

     Fibromyositis   Myofibrositis
     Fibrositis

√5th M79.A Nontraumatic compartment syndrome

     Code first, if applicable, associated postprocedural complication

EXCLUDES 1   *compartment syndrome NOS (T79.A-)*
     fibromyalgia (M79.7)
     nontraumatic ischemic infarction of muscle (M62.2-)
     traumatic compartment syndrome (T79.A-)

√6th M79.A1 Nontraumatic compartment syndrome of upper extremity

     Nontraumatic compartment syndrome of shoulder, arm, forearm, wrist, hand, and fingers

     M79.A11 Nontraumatic compartment syndrome of right upper extremity

     M79.A12 Nontraumatic compartment syndrome of left upper extremity

     M79.A19 Nontraumatic compartment syndrome ▽ of unspecified upper extremity

√6th M79.A2 Nontraumatic compartment syndrome of lower extremity

     Nontraumatic compartment syndrome of hip, buttock, thigh, leg, foot, and toes

     M79.A21 Nontraumatic compartment syndrome of right lower extremity

     M79.A22 Nontraumatic compartment syndrome of left lower extremity

EXCLUDES 1 Not coded here   EXCLUDES 2 Not included here   N Newborn Age: 0   P Pediatric Age: 0-17   M Maternity Age: 12-55   A Adult Age: 15-124

776   ICD-10-CM 2018

      M79.A29   **Nontraumatic compartment syndrome** ▽
              of unspecified lower extremity

    M79.A3   **Nontraumatic compartment syndrome of abdomen**

    M79.A9   **Nontraumatic compartment syndrome of other sites**

✓5ᵗʰ **M79.8**   **Other specified soft tissue disorders**

    M79.81   **Nontraumatic hematoma of soft tissue**
        Nontraumatic hematoma of muscle
        Nontraumatic seroma of muscle and soft tissue

    M79.89   **Other specified soft tissue disorders**
        Polyalgia

  M79.9   **Soft tissue disorder, unspecified**   ▽

OSTEOPATHIES AND CHONDROPATHIES (M80-M94)

Disorders of bone density and structure (M80-M85)

✓4ᵗʰ **M80**   **Osteoporosis with current pathological fracture**
    INCLUDES   osteoporosis with current fragility fracture
    Use additional code to identify major osseous defect, if applicable
    (M89.7-)
      EXCLUDES 1   *collapsed vertebra NOS (M48.5)*
              pathological fracture NOS (M84.4)
              wedging of vertebra NOS (M48.5)
      EXCLUDES 2   *personal history of (healed) osteoporosis fracture (Z87.310)*

    The appropriate 7th character is to be added to each code from
    category M80.
    A   initial encounter for fracture
    D   subsequent encounter for fracture with routine healing
    G   subsequent encounter for fracture with delayed healing
    K   subsequent encounter for fracture with nonunion
    P   subsequent encounter for fracture with malunion
    S   sequela

✓5ᵗʰ **M80.0**   **Age-related osteoporosis with current pathological fracture**
      Involutional osteoporosis with current pathological fracture
      Osteoporosis NOS with current pathological fracture
      Postmenopausal osteoporosis with current pathological fracture
      Senile osteoporosis with current pathological fracture

    ✓x7ᵗʰ **M80.00**   **Age-related osteoporosis with current**   A ▽
           pathological fracture, unspecified site

    ✓6ᵗʰ **M80.01**   **Age-related osteoporosis with current pathological**
           fracture, shoulder

      ✓7ᵗʰ **M80.011**   **Age-related osteoporosis with current**   A
             pathological fracture, right shoulder

      ✓7ᵗʰ **M80.012**   **Age-related osteoporosis with current**   A
             pathological fracture, left shoulder

      ✓7ᵗʰ **M80.019**   **Age-related osteoporosis with**   A ▽
             current pathological fracture,
             unspecified shoulder

    ✓6ᵗʰ **M80.02**   **Age-related osteoporosis with current pathological**
           fracture, humerus

      ✓7ᵗʰ **M80.021**   **Age-related osteoporosis with current**   A
             pathological fracture, right humerus

      ✓7ᵗʰ **M80.022**   **Age-related osteoporosis with current**   A
             pathological fracture, left humerus

      ✓7ᵗʰ **M80.029**   **Age-related osteoporosis with**   A ▽
             current pathological fracture,
             unspecified humerus

    ✓6ᵗʰ **M80.03**   **Age-related osteoporosis with current pathological**
           fracture, forearm
        Age-related osteoporosis with current pathological
          fracture of wrist

      ✓7ᵗʰ **M80.031**   **Age-related osteoporosis with current**   A
             pathological fracture, right forearm

      ✓7ᵗʰ **M80.032**   **Age-related osteoporosis with current**   A
             pathological fracture, left forearm

      ✓7ᵗʰ **M80.039**   **Age-related osteoporosis with**   A ▽
             current pathological fracture,
             unspecified forearm

    ✓6ᵗʰ **M80.04**   **Age-related osteoporosis with current pathological**
           fracture, hand

      ✓7ᵗʰ **M80.041**   **Age-related osteoporosis with current**   A
             pathological fracture, right hand

      ✓7ᵗʰ **M80.042**   **Age-related osteoporosis with current**   A
             pathological fracture, left hand

      ✓7ᵗʰ **M80.049**   **Age-related osteoporosis with**   A ▽
             current pathological fracture,
             unspecified hand

    ✓6ᵗʰ **M80.05**   **Age-related osteoporosis with current pathological**
           fracture, femur
        Age-related osteoporosis with current pathological
          fracture of hip

    ¹ ✓7ᵗʰ **M80.051**   **Age-related osteoporosis with**   HCC A
             current pathological fracture,
             right femur

    ¹ ✓7ᵗʰ **M80.052**   **Age-related osteoporosis with**   HCC A
             current pathological fracture,
             left femur

    ¹ ✓7ᵗʰ **M80.059**   **Age-related osteoporosis with**   HCC A ▽
             current pathological fracture,
             unspecified femur

    ✓6ᵗʰ **M80.06**   **Age-related osteoporosis with current pathological**
           fracture, lower leg

      ✓7ᵗʰ **M80.061**   **Age-related osteoporosis with current**   A
             pathological fracture, right lower leg

      ✓7ᵗʰ **M80.062**   **Age-related osteoporosis with current**   A
             pathological fracture, left lower leg

      ✓7ᵗʰ **M80.069**   **Age-related osteoporosis with**   A ▽
             current pathological fracture,
             unspecified lower leg

    ✓6ᵗʰ **M80.07**   **Age-related osteoporosis with current pathological**
           fracture, ankle and foot

      ✓7ᵗʰ **M80.071**   **Age-related osteoporosis with current**   A
             pathological fracture, right ankle and foot

      ✓7ᵗʰ **M80.072**   **Age-related osteoporosis with current**   A
             pathological fracture, left ankle and foot

      ✓7ᵗʰ **M80.079**   **Age-related osteoporosis with**   A ▽
             current pathological fracture,
             unspecified ankle and foot

  ¹ ✓x7ᵗʰ **M80.08**   **Age-related osteoporosis with current**   HCC A
        pathological fracture, vertebra(e)

✓6ᵗʰ **M80.8**   **Other osteoporosis with current pathological fracture**
      Drug-induced osteoporosis with current pathological fracture
      Idiopathic osteoporosis with current pathological fracture
      Osteoporosis of disuse with current pathological fracture
      Postoophorectomy osteoporosis with current pathological
        fracture
      Postsurgical malabsorption osteoporosis with current
        pathological fracture
      Post-traumatic osteoporosis with current pathological fracture
      Use additional code for adverse effect, if applicable, to identify
        drug (T36-T50 with fifth or sixth character 5)

    ✓x7ᵗʰ **M80.80**   **Other osteoporosis with current pathological**   ▽
           fracture, unspecified site

    ✓6ᵗʰ **M80.81**   **Other osteoporosis with pathological fracture,**
           shoulder

      ✓7ᵗʰ **M80.811**   **Other osteoporosis with current**
             pathological fracture, right shoulder

      ✓7ᵗʰ **M80.812**   **Other osteoporosis with current**
             pathological fracture, left shoulder

      ✓7ᵗʰ **M80.819**   **Other osteoporosis with current**   ▽
             pathological fracture, unspecified
             shoulder

    ✓6ᵗʰ **M80.82**   **Other osteoporosis with current pathological**
           fracture, humerus

      ✓7ᵗʰ **M80.821**   **Other osteoporosis with current**
             pathological fracture, right humerus

      ✓7ᵗʰ **M80.822**   **Other osteoporosis with current**
             pathological fracture, left humerus

      ✓7ᵗʰ **M80.829**   **Other osteoporosis with current**   ▽
             pathological fracture, unspecified
             humerus

    ✓6ᵗʰ **M80.83**   **Other osteoporosis with current pathological**
           fracture, forearm
        Other osteoporosis with current pathological fracture
          of wrist

      ✓7ᵗʰ **M80.831**   **Other osteoporosis with current**
             pathological fracture, right forearm

      ✓7ᵗʰ **M80.832**   **Other osteoporosis with current**
             pathological fracture, left forearm

      ✓7ᵗʰ **M80.839**   **Other osteoporosis with current**   ▽
             pathological fracture, unspecified forearm

---

¹   HCC with 7th character indicating initial encounter (A, B or C - specific to category).

☑ Additional Character Req   ✓x7ᵗʰ Placeholder Alert   Manifestation   HCC CMS-HCC Condition   ▽ Unspecified Code   ▶◀ Revised Text   ● New Code   ▲ Revised Code Title

ICD-10-CM 2018   777

√6ᵗʰ M80.84 Other osteoporosis with current pathological fracture, hand

√7ᵗʰ M80.841 Other osteoporosis with current pathological fracture, **right** hand

√7ᵗʰ M80.842 Other osteoporosis with current pathological fracture, **left** hand

√7ᵗʰ M80.849 Other osteoporosis with current pathological fracture, unspecified hand ▽

√6ᵗʰ M80.85 Other osteoporosis with current pathological fracture, femur
Other osteoporosis with current pathological fracture of hip

1 √7ᵗʰ M80.851 Other osteoporosis with current pathological fracture, **right** femur HCC

1 √7ᵗʰ M80.852 Other osteoporosis with current pathological fracture, **left** femur HCC

1 √7ᵗʰ M80.859 Other osteoporosis with current pathological fracture, unspecified femur HCC ▽

√6ᵗʰ M80.86 Other osteoporosis with current pathological fracture, lower leg

√7ᵗʰ M80.861 Other osteoporosis with current pathological fracture, **right** lower leg

√7ᵗʰ M80.862 Other osteoporosis with current pathological fracture, **left** lower leg

√7ᵗʰ M80.869 Other osteoporosis with current pathological fracture, unspecified lower leg ▽

√6ᵗʰ M80.87 Other osteoporosis with current pathological fracture, ankle and foot

√7ᵗʰ M80.871 Other osteoporosis with current pathological fracture, **right** ankle and foot

√7ᵗʰ M80.872 Other osteoporosis with current pathological fracture, **left** ankle and foot

√7ᵗʰ M80.879 Other osteoporosis with current pathological fracture, unspecified ankle and foot ▽

1 √x7ᵗʰ M80.88 Other osteoporosis with current pathological fracture, **vertebra(e)** HCC

√4ᵗʰ M81 Osteoporosis without current pathological fracture
Use additional code to identify:
major osseous defect, if applicable (M89.7-)
personal history of (healed) osteoporosis fracture, if applicable (Z87.310)
EXCLUDES 1 *osteoporosis with current pathological fracture (M80.-)*
Sudeck's atrophy (M89.0)

M81.0 Age-related osteoporosis without current pathological fracture A
Involutional osteoporosis without current pathological fracture
Osteoporosis NOS
Postmenopausal osteoporosis without current pathological fracture
Senile osteoporosis without current pathological fracture

M81.6 Localized osteoporosis [Lequesne]
EXCLUDES 1 *Sudeck's atrophy (M89.0)*

M81.8 Other osteoporosis without current pathological fracture
Drug-induced osteoporosis without current pathological fracture
Idiopathic osteoporosis without current pathological fracture
Osteoporosis of disuse without current pathological fracture
Postoophorectomy osteoporosis without current pathological fracture
Postsurgical malabsorption osteoporosis without current pathological fracture
Post-traumatic osteoporosis without current pathological fracture
Use additional code for adverse effect, if applicable, to identify drug (T36-T50 with fifth or sixth character 5)

√4ᵗʰ M83 Adult osteomalacia
EXCLUDES 1 *infantile and juvenile osteomalacia (E55.0)*
renal osteodystrophy (N25.0)
rickets (active) (E55.0)
rickets (active) sequelae (E64.3)
vitamin D-resistant osteomalacia (E83.3)
vitamin D-resistant rickets (active) (E83.3)

M83.0 Puerperal osteomalacia M♀

M83.1 Senile osteomalacia A

M83.2 Adult osteomalacia due to malabsorption A
Postsurgical malabsorption osteomalacia in adults

M83.3 Adult osteomalacia due to malnutrition A

M83.4 Aluminum bone disease

M83.5 Other drug-induced osteomalacia in adults A
Use additional code for adverse effect, if applicable, to identify drug (T36-T50 with fifth or sixth character 5)

M83.8 Other adult osteomalacia A

M83.9 Adult osteomalacia, unspecified A ▽

√4ᵗʰ M84 Disorder of continuity of bone
EXCLUDES 2 *traumatic fracture of bone-see fracture, by site*

√5ᵗʰ M84.3 Stress fracture
Fatigue fracture   Stress fracture NOS
March fracture   Stress reaction
Use additional external cause code(s) to identify the cause of the stress fracture
EXCLUDES 1 *pathological fracture NOS (M84.4-)*
pathological fracture due to osteoporosis (M80.-)
traumatic fracture (S12-, S22-, S32-, S42-, S52-, S62-, S72-, S82-, S92-)
EXCLUDES 2 *personal history of (healed) stress (fatigue) fracture (Z87.312)*
stress fracture of vertebra (M48.4-)

The appropriate 7th character is to be added to each code from subcategory M84.3.
A   initial encounter for fracture
D   subsequent encounter for fracture with routine healing
G   subsequent encounter for fracture with delayed healing
K   subsequent encounter for fracture with nonunion
P   subsequent encounter for fracture with malunion
S   sequela

√x7ᵗʰ M84.30 Stress fracture, unspecified site ▽

√6ᵗʰ M84.31 Stress fracture, shoulder
√7ᵗʰ M84.311 Stress fracture, **right** shoulder
√7ᵗʰ M84.312 Stress fracture, **left** shoulder
√7ᵗʰ M84.319 Stress fracture, unspecified shoulder ▽

√6ᵗʰ M84.32 Stress fracture, humerus
√7ᵗʰ M84.321 Stress fracture, **right** humerus
√7ᵗʰ M84.322 Stress fracture, **left** humerus
√7ᵗʰ M84.329 Stress fracture, unspecified humerus ▽

√6ᵗʰ M84.33 Stress fracture, ulna and radius
√7ᵗʰ M84.331 Stress fracture, **right** ulna
√7ᵗʰ M84.332 Stress fracture, **left** ulna
√7ᵗʰ M84.333 Stress fracture, **right** radius
√7ᵗʰ M84.334 Stress fracture, **left** radius
√7ᵗʰ M84.339 Stress fracture, unspecified ulna and radius ▽

√6ᵗʰ M84.34 Stress fracture, hand and fingers
√7ᵗʰ M84.341 Stress fracture, **right** hand
√7ᵗʰ M84.342 Stress fracture, **left** hand
√7ᵗʰ M84.343 Stress fracture, unspecified hand ▽
√7ᵗʰ M84.344 Stress fracture, **right** finger(s)
√7ᵗʰ M84.345 Stress fracture, **left** finger(s)
√7ᵗʰ M84.346 Stress fracture, unspecified finger(s) ▽

√6ᵗʰ M84.35 Stress fracture, pelvis and femur
Stress fracture, hip
√7ᵗʰ M84.350 Stress fracture, **pelvis**
√7ᵗʰ M84.351 Stress fracture, **right** femur
√7ᵗʰ M84.352 Stress fracture, **left** femur
√7ᵗʰ M84.353 Stress fracture, unspecified femur ▽
√7ᵗʰ M84.359 Stress fracture, hip, unspecified ▽

√6ᵗʰ M84.36 Stress fracture, tibia and fibula
√7ᵗʰ M84.361 Stress fracture, **right** tibia
√7ᵗʰ M84.362 Stress fracture, **left** tibia
√7ᵗʰ M84.363 Stress fracture, **right** fibula
√7ᵗʰ M84.364 Stress fracture, **left** fibula
√7ᵗʰ M84.369 Stress fracture, unspecified tibia and fibula ▽

---

1 HCC with 7th character indicating initial encounter (A, B or C - specific to category).

EXCLUDES 1 Not coded here   *EXCLUDES 2* Not included here   N Newborn Age: 0   P Pediatric Age: 0-17   M Maternity Age: 12-55   A Adult Age: 15-124

778   ICD-10-CM 2018

Chapter 13. Diseases of the Musculoskeletal System and Connective Tissue

☑6ᵗʰ **M84.37 Stress fracture, ankle, foot and toes**
     ✓7ᵗʰ **M84.371 Stress fracture, right ankle**
     ✓7ᵗʰ **M84.372 Stress fracture, left ankle**
     ✓7ᵗʰ **M84.373 Stress fracture, unspecified ankle** ▽
     ✓7ᵗʰ **M84.374 Stress fracture, right foot**
     ✓7ᵗʰ **M84.375 Stress fracture, left foot**
     ✓7ᵗʰ **M84.376 Stress fracture, unspecified foot** ▽
     ✓7ᵗʰ **M84.377 Stress fracture, right toe(s)**
     ✓7ᵗʰ **M84.378 Stress fracture, left toe(s)**
     ✓7ᵗʰ **M84.379 Stress fracture, unspecified toe(s)** ▽

✓x7ᵗʰ **M84.38 Stress fracture, other site**
     EXCLUDES 2   stress fracture of vertebra (M48.4-)

✓5ᵗʰ **M84.4 Pathological fracture, not elsewhere classified**
     Chronic fracture
     Pathological fracture NOS
     EXCLUDES 1   collapsed vertebra NEC (M48.5)
         pathological fracture in neoplastic disease (M84.5-)
         pathological fracture in osteoporosis (M80.-)
         pathological fracture from other disease (M84.6-)
         stress fracture (M84.3-)
         traumatic fracture (S12.-, S22.-, S32.-, S42.-, S52.-,
         S62.-, S72.-, S82.-, S92.-)
     EXCLUDES 2   personal history of (healed) pathological fracture
         (Z87.311)

> The appropriate 7th character is to be added to each code
> from subcategory M84.4.
> A   initial encounter for fracture
> D   subsequent encounter for fracture with routine healing
> G   subsequent encounter for fracture with delayed healing
> K   subsequent encounter for fracture with nonunion
> P   subsequent encounter for fracture with malunion
> S   sequela

✓x7ᵗʰ **M84.40 Pathological fracture, unspecified site** ▽
✓6ᵗʰ **M84.41 Pathological fracture, shoulder**
     ✓7ᵗʰ **M84.411 Pathological fracture, right shoulder**
     ✓7ᵗʰ **M84.412 Pathological fracture, left shoulder**
     ✓7ᵗʰ **M84.419 Pathological fracture, unspecified** ▽
         shoulder
✓6ᵗʰ **M84.42 Pathological fracture, humerus**
     ✓7ᵗʰ **M84.421 Pathological fracture, right humerus**
     ✓7ᵗʰ **M84.422 Pathological fracture, left humerus**
     ✓7ᵗʰ **M84.429 Pathological fracture, unspecified** ▽
         humerus
✓6ᵗʰ **M84.43 Pathological fracture, ulna and radius**
     ✓7ᵗʰ **M84.431 Pathological fracture, right ulna**
     ✓7ᵗʰ **M84.432 Pathological fracture, left ulna**
     ✓7ᵗʰ **M84.433 Pathological fracture, right radius**
     ✓7ᵗʰ **M84.434 Pathological fracture, left radius**
     ✓7ᵗʰ **M84.439 Pathological fracture, unspecified ulna** ▽
         and radius
✓6ᵗʰ **M84.44 Pathological fracture, hand and fingers**
     ✓7ᵗʰ **M84.441 Pathological fracture, right hand**
     ✓7ᵗʰ **M84.442 Pathological fracture, left hand**
     ✓7ᵗʰ **M84.443 Pathological fracture, unspecified hand** ▽
     ✓7ᵗʰ **M84.444 Pathological fracture, right finger(s)**
     ✓7ᵗʰ **M84.445 Pathological fracture, left finger(s)**
     ✓7ᵗʰ **M84.446 Pathological fracture, unspecified** ▽
         finger(s)
✓6ᵗʰ **M84.45 Pathological fracture, femur and pelvis**
     1 ✓7ᵗʰ **M84.451 Pathological fracture, right femur** HCC
     1 ✓7ᵗʰ **M84.452 Pathological fracture, left femur** HCC
     1 ✓7ᵗʰ **M84.453 Pathological fracture, unspecified** HCC ▽
         femur
     ✓7ᵗʰ **M84.454 Pathological fracture, pelvis**
     1 ✓7ᵗʰ **M84.459 Pathological fracture, hip,** HCC ▽
         unspecified
✓6ᵗʰ **M84.46 Pathological fracture, tibia and fibula**
     ✓7ᵗʰ **M84.461 Pathological fracture, right tibia**
     ✓7ᵗʰ **M84.462 Pathological fracture, left tibia**
     ✓7ᵗʰ **M84.463 Pathological fracture, right fibula**
     ✓7ᵗʰ **M84.464 Pathological fracture, left fibula**

     ✓7ᵗʰ **M84.469 Pathological fracture, unspecified** ▽
         tibia and fibula
✓6ᵗʰ **M84.47 Pathological fracture, ankle, foot and toes**
     ✓7ᵗʰ **M84.471 Pathological fracture, right ankle**
     ✓7ᵗʰ **M84.472 Pathological fracture, left ankle**
     ✓7ᵗʰ **M84.473 Pathological fracture, unspecified ankle** ▽
     ✓7ᵗʰ **M84.474 Pathological fracture, right foot**
     ✓7ᵗʰ **M84.475 Pathological fracture, left foot**
     ✓7ᵗʰ **M84.476 Pathological fracture, unspecified foot** ▽
     ✓7ᵗʰ **M84.477 Pathological fracture, right toe(s)**
     ✓7ᵗʰ **M84.478 Pathological fracture, left toe(s)**
     ✓7ᵗʰ **M84.479 Pathological fracture, unspecified** ▽
         toe(s)

✓x7ᵗʰ **M84.48 Pathological fracture, other site**
✓5ᵗʰ **M84.5 Pathological fracture in neoplastic disease**
     Code also underlying neoplasm

> The appropriate 7th character is to be added to each code
> from subcategory M84.5.
> A   initial encounter for fracture
> D   subsequent encounter for fracture with routine healing
> G   subsequent encounter for fracture with delayed healing
> K   subsequent encounter for fracture with nonunion
> P   subsequent encounter for fracture with malunion
> S   sequela

✓x7ᵗʰ **M84.50 Pathological fracture in neoplastic disease,** ▽
     unspecified site
✓6ᵗʰ **M84.51 Pathological fracture in neoplastic disease, shoulder**
     ✓7ᵗʰ **M84.511 Pathological fracture in neoplastic**
         disease, right shoulder
     ✓7ᵗʰ **M84.512 Pathological fracture in neoplastic**
         disease, left shoulder
     ✓7ᵗʰ **M84.519 Pathological fracture in neoplastic** ▽
         disease, unspecified shoulder
✓6ᵗʰ **M84.52 Pathological fracture in neoplastic disease, humerus**
     ✓7ᵗʰ **M84.521 Pathological fracture in neoplastic**
         disease, right humerus
     ✓7ᵗʰ **M84.522 Pathological fracture in neoplastic**
         disease, left humerus
     ✓7ᵗʰ **M84.529 Pathological fracture in neoplastic** ▽
         disease, unspecified humerus
✓6ᵗʰ **M84.53 Pathological fracture in neoplastic disease,**
     ulna and radius
     ✓7ᵗʰ **M84.531 Pathological fracture in neoplastic**
         disease, right ulna
     ✓7ᵗʰ **M84.532 Pathological fracture in neoplastic**
         disease, left ulna
     ✓7ᵗʰ **M84.533 Pathological fracture in neoplastic**
         disease, right radius
     ✓7ᵗʰ **M84.534 Pathological fracture in neoplastic**
         disease, left radius
     ✓7ᵗʰ **M84.539 Pathological fracture in neoplastic** ▽
         disease, unspecified ulna and radius
✓6ᵗʰ **M84.54 Pathological fracture in neoplastic disease, hand**
     ✓7ᵗʰ **M84.541 Pathological fracture in neoplastic**
         disease, right hand
     ✓7ᵗʰ **M84.542 Pathological fracture in neoplastic**
         disease, left hand
     ✓7ᵗʰ **M84.549 Pathological fracture in neoplastic** ▽
         disease, unspecified hand
✓6ᵗʰ **M84.55 Pathological fracture in neoplastic disease,**
     pelvis and femur
     ✓7ᵗʰ **M84.550 Pathological fracture in neoplastic**
         disease, pelvis
     1 ✓7ᵗʰ **M84.551 Pathological fracture in neoplastic** HCC
         disease, right femur
     1 ✓7ᵗʰ **M84.552 Pathological fracture in neoplastic** HCC
         disease, left femur
     1 ✓7ᵗʰ **M84.553 Pathological fracture in neoplastic** HCC ▽
         disease, unspecified femur
     1 ✓7ᵗʰ **M84.559 Pathological fracture in neoplastic** HCC ▽
         disease, hip, unspecified

---

1   HCC with 7th character indicating initial encounter (A, B or C - specific to category).

☑ Additional Character Req   ✓x7ᵗʰ Placeholder Alert   Manifestation   HCC CMS-HCC Condition   ▽Unspecified Code   ►◄ Revised Text   ● New Code   ▲ Revised Code Title

ICD-10-CM 2018   779

Chapter 13. Diseases of the Musculoskeletal System and Connective Tissue *(side margin)*

M84.56–M84.759 *(side margin)*

✓6ᵗʰ **M84.56 Pathological fracture in neoplastic disease, tibia and fibula**

  ✓7ᵗʰ **M84.561** Pathological fracture in neoplastic disease, **right tibia**

  ✓7ᵗʰ **M84.562** Pathological fracture in neoplastic disease, **left tibia**

  ✓7ᵗʰ **M84.563** Pathological fracture in neoplastic disease, **right fibula**

  ✓7ᵗʰ **M84.564** Pathological fracture in neoplastic disease, **left fibula**

  ✓7ᵗʰ **M84.569** Pathological fracture in neoplastic disease, unspecified tibia and fibula ▽

✓6ᵗʰ **M84.57 Pathological fracture in neoplastic disease, ankle and foot**

  ✓7ᵗʰ **M84.571** Pathological fracture in neoplastic disease, **right ankle**

  ✓7ᵗʰ **M84.572** Pathological fracture in neoplastic disease, **left ankle**

  ✓7ᵗʰ **M84.573** Pathological fracture in neoplastic disease, unspecified ankle ▽

  ✓7ᵗʰ **M84.574** Pathological fracture in neoplastic disease, **right foot**

  ✓7ᵗʰ **M84.575** Pathological fracture in neoplastic disease, **left foot**

  ✓7ᵗʰ **M84.576** Pathological fracture in neoplastic disease, unspecified foot ▽

✓x7ᵗʰ **M84.58 Pathological fracture in neoplastic disease, other specified site**

    Pathological fracture in neoplastic disease, vertebrae

✓5ᵗʰ **M84.6 Pathological fracture in other disease**

  Code also underlying condition

  EXCLUDES 1   pathological fracture in osteoporosis (M80.-)

> The appropriate 7th character is to be added to each code from subcategory M84.6.
> A   initial encounter for fracture
> D   subsequent encounter for fracture with routine healing
> G   subsequent encounter for fracture with delayed healing
> K   subsequent encounter for fracture with nonunion
> P   subsequent encounter for fracture with malunion
> S   sequela

✓x7ᵗʰ **M84.60 Pathological fracture in other disease, unspecified site** ▽

✓6ᵗʰ **M84.61 Pathological fracture in other disease, shoulder**

  ✓7ᵗʰ **M84.611** Pathological fracture in other disease, **right shoulder**

  ✓7ᵗʰ **M84.612** Pathological fracture in other disease, **left shoulder**

  ✓7ᵗʰ **M84.619** Pathological fracture in other disease, unspecified shoulder ▽

✓6ᵗʰ **M84.62 Pathological fracture in other disease, humerus**

  ✓7ᵗʰ **M84.621** Pathological fracture in other disease, **right humerus**

  ✓7ᵗʰ **M84.622** Pathological fracture in other disease, **left humerus**

  ✓7ᵗʰ **M84.629** Pathological fracture in other disease, unspecified humerus ▽

✓6ᵗʰ **M84.63 Pathological fracture in other disease, ulna and radius**

  ✓7ᵗʰ **M84.631** Pathological fracture in other disease, **right ulna**

  ✓7ᵗʰ **M84.632** Pathological fracture in other disease, **left ulna**

  ✓7ᵗʰ **M84.633** Pathological fracture in other disease, **right radius**

  ✓7ᵗʰ **M84.634** Pathological fracture in other disease, **left radius**

  ✓7ᵗʰ **M84.639** Pathological fracture in other disease, unspecified ulna and radius ▽

✓6ᵗʰ **M84.64 Pathological fracture in other disease, hand**

  ✓7ᵗʰ **M84.641** Pathological fracture in other disease, **right hand**

  ✓7ᵗʰ **M84.642** Pathological fracture in other disease, **left hand**

  ✓7ᵗʰ **M84.649** Pathological fracture in other disease, unspecified hand ▽

✓6ᵗʰ **M84.65 Pathological fracture in other disease, pelvis and femur**

  ✓7ᵗʰ **M84.650** Pathological fracture in other disease, pelvis

  [1] ✓7ᵗʰ **M84.651** Pathological fracture in other disease, **right femur** HCC

  [1] ✓7ᵗʰ **M84.652** Pathological fracture in other disease, **left femur** HCC

  [1] ✓7ᵗʰ **M84.653** Pathological fracture in other disease, unspecified femur HCC ▽

  [1] ✓7ᵗʰ **M84.659** Pathological fracture in other disease, hip, unspecified HCC ▽

✓6ᵗʰ **M84.66 Pathological fracture in other disease, tibia and fibula**

  ✓7ᵗʰ **M84.661** Pathological fracture in other disease, **right tibia**

  ✓7ᵗʰ **M84.662** Pathological fracture in other disease, **left tibia**

  ✓7ᵗʰ **M84.663** Pathological fracture in other disease, **right fibula**

  ✓7ᵗʰ **M84.664** Pathological fracture in other disease, **left fibula**

  ✓7ᵗʰ **M84.669** Pathological fracture in other disease, unspecified tibia and fibula ▽

✓6ᵗʰ **M84.67 Pathological fracture in other disease, ankle and foot**

  ✓7ᵗʰ **M84.671** Pathological fracture in other disease, **right ankle**

  ✓7ᵗʰ **M84.672** Pathological fracture in other disease, **left ankle**

  ✓7ᵗʰ **M84.673** Pathological fracture in other disease, unspecified ankle ▽

  ✓7ᵗʰ **M84.674** Pathological fracture in other disease, **right foot**

  ✓7ᵗʰ **M84.675** Pathological fracture in other disease, **left foot**

  ✓7ᵗʰ **M84.676** Pathological fracture in other disease, unspecified foot ▽

✓x7ᵗʰ **M84.68 Pathological fracture in other disease, other site**

✓5ᵗʰ **M84.7 Nontraumatic fracture, not elsewhere classified**

✓6ᵗʰ **M84.75 Atypical femoral fracture**

> The appropriate 7th character is to be added to each code from subcategory M84.75.
> A   initial encounter for fracture
> D   subsequent encounter for fracture with routine healing
> G   subsequent encounter for fracture with delayed healing
> K   subsequent encounter for fracture with nonunion
> P   subsequent encounter for fracture with malunion
> S   sequela

  ✓7ᵗʰ **M84.750** Atypical femoral fracture, unspecified ▽

  ✓7ᵗʰ **M84.751** Incomplete atypical femoral fracture, right leg

  ✓7ᵗʰ **M84.752** Incomplete atypical femoral fracture, left leg

  ✓7ᵗʰ **M84.753** Incomplete atypical femoral fracture, unspecified leg ▽

  [1] ✓7ᵗʰ **M84.754** Complete transverse atypical femoral fracture, right leg HCC

  [1] ✓7ᵗʰ **M84.755** Complete transverse atypical femoral fracture, left leg HCC

  [1] ✓7ᵗʰ **M84.756** Complete transverse atypical femoral fracture, unspecified leg HCC ▽

  [1] ✓7ᵗʰ **M84.757** Complete oblique atypical femoral fracture, right leg HCC

  [1] ✓7ᵗʰ **M84.758** Complete oblique atypical femoral fracture, left leg HCC

  [1] ✓7ᵗʰ **M84.759** Complete oblique atypical femoral fracture, unspecified leg HCC ▽

---

[1] HCC with 7th character indicating initial encounter (A, B or C - specific to category).

EXCLUDES 1 Not coded here   *EXCLUDES 2* Not included here   **N** Newborn Age: 0   **P** Pediatric Age: 0-17   **M** Maternity Age: 12-55   **A** Adult Age: 15-124

☑5ᵗʰ **M84.8** Other disorders of continuity of bone

     M84.80 Other disorders of continuity of bone, unspecified site ▽

     ☑6ᵗʰ **M84.81** Other disorders of continuity of bone, **shoulder**

         M84.811 Other disorders of continuity of bone, **right shoulder**

         M84.812 Other disorders of continuity of bone, **left shoulder**

         M84.819 Other disorders of continuity of bone, unspecified shoulder ▽

     ☑6ᵗʰ **M84.82** Other disorders of continuity of bone, **humerus**

         M84.821 Other disorders of continuity of bone, **right humerus**

         M84.822 Other disorders of continuity of bone, **left humerus**

         M84.829 Other disorders of continuity of bone, unspecified humerus ▽

     ☑6ᵗʰ **M84.83** Other disorders of continuity of bone, **ulna and radius**

         M84.831 Other disorders of continuity of bone, **right ulna**

         M84.832 Other disorders of continuity of bone, **left ulna**

         M84.833 Other disorders of continuity of bone, **right radius**

         M84.834 Other disorders of continuity of bone, **left radius**

         M84.839 Other disorders of continuity of bone, unspecified ulna and radius ▽

     ☑6ᵗʰ **M84.84** Other disorders of continuity of bone, **hand**

         M84.841 Other disorders of continuity of bone, **right hand**

         M84.842 Other disorders of continuity of bone, **left hand**

         M84.849 Other disorders of continuity of bone, unspecified hand ▽

     ☑6ᵗʰ **M84.85** Other disorders of continuity of bone, **pelvic region and thigh**

         M84.851 Other disorders of continuity of bone, **right pelvic region and thigh**

         M84.852 Other disorders of continuity of bone, **left pelvic region and thigh**

         M84.859 Other disorders of continuity of bone, unspecified pelvic region and thigh ▽

     ☑6ᵗʰ **M84.86** Other disorders of continuity of bone, **tibia and fibula**

         M84.861 Other disorders of continuity of bone, **right tibia**

         M84.862 Other disorders of continuity of bone, **left tibia**

         M84.863 Other disorders of continuity of bone, **right fibula**

         M84.864 Other disorders of continuity of bone, **left fibula**

         M84.869 Other disorders of continuity of bone, unspecified tibia and fibula ▽

     ☑6ᵗʰ **M84.87** Other disorders of continuity of bone, **ankle and foot**

         M84.871 Other disorders of continuity of bone, **right ankle and foot**

         M84.872 Other disorders of continuity of bone, **left ankle and foot**

         M84.879 Other disorders of continuity of bone, unspecified ankle and foot ▽

     M84.88 Other disorders of continuity of bone, other site

     M84.9 Disorder of continuity of bone, unspecified ▽

☑4ᵗʰ **M85** **Other disorders of bone density and structure**

     EXCLUDES 1   osteogenesis imperfecta (Q78.0)

                osteopetrosis (Q78.2)

                osteopoikilosis (Q78.8)

                polyostotic fibrous dysplasia (Q78.1)

     ☑5ᵗʰ **M85.0** Fibrous dysplasia (monostotic)

         EXCLUDES 2   fibrous dysplasia of jaw (M27.8)

         M85.00 Fibrous dysplasia (monostotic), unspecified site ▽

         ☑6ᵗʰ **M85.01** Fibrous dysplasia (monostotic), **shoulder**

             M85.011 Fibrous dysplasia (monostotic), **right shoulder**

             M85.012 Fibrous dysplasia (monostotic), **left shoulder**

             M85.019 Fibrous dysplasia (monostotic), unspecified shoulder ▽

         ☑6ᵗʰ **M85.02** Fibrous dysplasia (monostotic), **upper arm**

             M85.021 Fibrous dysplasia (monostotic), **right upper arm**

             M85.022 Fibrous dysplasia (monostotic), **left upper arm**

             M85.029 Fibrous dysplasia (monostotic), unspecified upper arm ▽

         ☑6ᵗʰ **M85.03** Fibrous dysplasia (monostotic), **forearm**

             M85.031 Fibrous dysplasia (monostotic), **right forearm**

             M85.032 Fibrous dysplasia (monostotic), **left forearm**

             M85.039 Fibrous dysplasia (monostotic), unspecified forearm ▽

         ☑6ᵗʰ **M85.04** Fibrous dysplasia (monostotic), **hand**

             M85.041 Fibrous dysplasia (monostotic), **right hand**

             M85.042 Fibrous dysplasia (monostotic), **left hand**

             M85.049 Fibrous dysplasia (monostotic), unspecified hand ▽

         ☑6ᵗʰ **M85.05** Fibrous dysplasia (monostotic), **thigh**

             M85.051 Fibrous dysplasia (monostotic), **right thigh**

             M85.052 Fibrous dysplasia (monostotic), **left thigh**

             M85.059 Fibrous dysplasia (monostotic), unspecified thigh ▽

         ☑6ᵗʰ **M85.06** Fibrous dysplasia (monostotic), **lower leg**

             M85.061 Fibrous dysplasia (monostotic), **right lower leg**

             M85.062 Fibrous dysplasia (monostotic), **left lower leg**

             M85.069 Fibrous dysplasia (monostotic), unspecified lower leg ▽

         ☑6ᵗʰ **M85.07** Fibrous dysplasia (monostotic), **ankle and foot**

             M85.071 Fibrous dysplasia (monostotic), **right ankle and foot**

             M85.072 Fibrous dysplasia (monostotic), **left ankle and foot**

             M85.079 Fibrous dysplasia (monostotic), unspecified ankle and foot ▽

         M85.08 Fibrous dysplasia (monostotic), other site

         M85.09 Fibrous dysplasia (monostotic), **multiple sites**

     ☑5ᵗʰ **M85.1** Skeletal fluorosis

         M85.10 Skeletal fluorosis, unspecified site ▽

         ☑6ᵗʰ **M85.11** Skeletal fluorosis, **shoulder**

             M85.111 Skeletal fluorosis, **right** shoulder

             M85.112 Skeletal fluorosis, **left** shoulder

             M85.119 Skeletal fluorosis, unspecified shoulder ▽

         ☑6ᵗʰ **M85.12** Skeletal fluorosis, **upper arm**

             M85.121 Skeletal fluorosis, **right** upper arm

             M85.122 Skeletal fluorosis, **left** upper arm

             M85.129 Skeletal fluorosis, unspecified upper arm ▽

         ☑6ᵗʰ **M85.13** Skeletal fluorosis, **forearm**

             M85.131 Skeletal fluorosis, **right** forearm

             M85.132 Skeletal fluorosis, **left** forearm

             M85.139 Skeletal fluorosis, unspecified forearm ▽

         ☑6ᵗʰ **M85.14** Skeletal fluorosis, **hand**

             M85.141 Skeletal fluorosis, **right** hand

             M85.142 Skeletal fluorosis, **left** hand

             M85.149 Skeletal fluorosis, unspecified hand ▽

         ☑6ᵗʰ **M85.15** Skeletal fluorosis, **thigh**

             M85.151 Skeletal fluorosis, **right** thigh

             M85.152 Skeletal fluorosis, **left** thigh

             M85.159 Skeletal fluorosis, unspecified thigh ▽

         ☑6ᵗʰ **M85.16** Skeletal fluorosis, **lower leg**

             M85.161 Skeletal fluorosis, **right** lower leg

             M85.162 Skeletal fluorosis, **left** lower leg

             M85.169 Skeletal fluorosis, unspecified lower leg ▽

☑ Additional Character Req   ✓x7ᵗʰ Placeholder Alert   Manifestation   HCC CMS-HCC Condition   ▽ Unspecified Code   ▶◀ Revised Text   ● New Code   ▲ Revised Code Title

✓6ᵗʰ **M85.17 Skeletal fluorosis, ankle and foot**
    M85.171 Skeletal fluorosis, right ankle and foot
    M85.172 Skeletal fluorosis, left ankle and foot
    M85.179 Skeletal fluorosis, unspecified ankle and foot ▽
  M85.18 Skeletal fluorosis, other site
  M85.19 Skeletal fluorosis, multiple sites
M85.2 Hyperostosis of skull
    DEF: Abnormal bone growth on inner aspect of cranial bones.
✓5ᵗʰ **M85.3 Osteitis condensans**
  M85.30 Osteitis condensans, unspecified site ▽
  ✓6ᵗʰ **M85.31 Osteitis condensans, shoulder**
    M85.311 Osteitis condensans, right shoulder
    M85.312 Osteitis condensans, left shoulder
    M85.319 Osteitis condensans, unspecified shoulder ▽
  ✓6ᵗʰ **M85.32 Osteitis condensans, upper arm**
    M85.321 Osteitis condensans, right upper arm
    M85.322 Osteitis condensans, left upper arm
    M85.329 Osteitis condensans, unspecified upper arm ▽
  ✓6ᵗʰ **M85.33 Osteitis condensans, forearm**
    M85.331 Osteitis condensans, right forearm
    M85.332 Osteitis condensans, left forearm
    M85.339 Osteitis condensans, unspecified forearm ▽
  ✓6ᵗʰ **M85.34 Osteitis condensans, hand**
    M85.341 Osteitis condensans, right hand
    M85.342 Osteitis condensans, left hand
    M85.349 Osteitis condensans, unspecified hand ▽
  ✓6ᵗʰ **M85.35 Osteitis condensans, thigh**
    M85.351 Osteitis condensans, right thigh
    M85.352 Osteitis condensans, left thigh
    M85.359 Osteitis condensans, unspecified thigh ▽
  ✓6ᵗʰ **M85.36 Osteitis condensans, lower leg**
    M85.361 Osteitis condensans, right lower leg
    M85.362 Osteitis condensans, left lower leg
    M85.369 Osteitis condensans, unspecified lower leg ▽
  ✓6ᵗʰ **M85.37 Osteitis condensans, ankle and foot**
    M85.371 Osteitis condensans, right ankle and foot
    M85.372 Osteitis condensans, left ankle and foot
    M85.379 Osteitis condensans, unspecified ankle and foot ▽
  M85.38 Osteitis condensans, other site
  M85.39 Osteitis condensans, multiple sites
✓5ᵗʰ **M85.4 Solitary bone cyst**
    EXCLUDES 2   *solitary cyst of jaw (M27.4)*
  M85.40 Solitary bone cyst, unspecified site ▽
  ✓6ᵗʰ **M85.41 Solitary bone cyst, shoulder**
    M85.411 Solitary bone cyst, right shoulder
    M85.412 Solitary bone cyst, left shoulder
    M85.419 Solitary bone cyst, unspecified shoulder ▽
  ✓6ᵗʰ **M85.42 Solitary bone cyst, humerus**
    M85.421 Solitary bone cyst, right humerus
    M85.422 Solitary bone cyst, left humerus
    M85.429 Solitary bone cyst, unspecified humerus ▽
  ✓6ᵗʰ **M85.43 Solitary bone cyst, ulna and radius**
    M85.431 Solitary bone cyst, right ulna and radius
    M85.432 Solitary bone cyst, left ulna and radius
    M85.439 Solitary bone cyst, unspecified ulna and radius ▽
  ✓6ᵗʰ **M85.44 Solitary bone cyst, hand**
    M85.441 Solitary bone cyst, right hand
    M85.442 Solitary bone cyst, left hand
    M85.449 Solitary bone cyst, unspecified hand ▽
  ✓6ᵗʰ **M85.45 Solitary bone cyst, pelvis**
    M85.451 Solitary bone cyst, right pelvis
    M85.452 Solitary bone cyst, left pelvis
    M85.459 Solitary bone cyst, unspecified pelvis ▽

✓6ᵗʰ **M85.46 Solitary bone cyst, tibia and fibula**
    M85.461 Solitary bone cyst, right tibia and fibula
    M85.462 Solitary bone cyst, left tibia and fibula
    M85.469 Solitary bone cyst, unspecified tibia and fibula ▽
  ✓6ᵗʰ **M85.47 Solitary bone cyst, ankle and foot**
    M85.471 Solitary bone cyst, right ankle and foot
    M85.472 Solitary bone cyst, left ankle and foot
    M85.479 Solitary bone cyst, unspecified ankle and foot ▽
  M85.48 Solitary bone cyst, other site
✓5ᵗʰ **M85.5 Aneurysmal bone cyst**
    EXCLUDES 2   *aneurysmal cyst of jaw (M27.4)*
    DEF: Solitary bone lesion, bulges into periosteum; marked by calcified rim.
  M85.50 Aneurysmal bone cyst, unspecified site ▽
  ✓6ᵗʰ **M85.51 Aneurysmal bone cyst, shoulder**
    M85.511 Aneurysmal bone cyst, right shoulder
    M85.512 Aneurysmal bone cyst, left shoulder
    M85.519 Aneurysmal bone cyst, unspecified shoulder ▽
  ✓6ᵗʰ **M85.52 Aneurysmal bone cyst, upper arm**
    M85.521 Aneurysmal bone cyst, right upper arm
    M85.522 Aneurysmal bone cyst, left upper arm
    M85.529 Aneurysmal bone cyst, unspecified upper arm ▽
  ✓6ᵗʰ **M85.53 Aneurysmal bone cyst, forearm**
    M85.531 Aneurysmal bone cyst, right forearm
    M85.532 Aneurysmal bone cyst, left forearm
    M85.539 Aneurysmal bone cyst, unspecified forearm ▽
  ✓6ᵗʰ **M85.54 Aneurysmal bone cyst, hand**
    M85.541 Aneurysmal bone cyst, right hand
    M85.542 Aneurysmal bone cyst, left hand
    M85.549 Aneurysmal bone cyst, unspecified hand ▽
  ✓6ᵗʰ **M85.55 Aneurysmal bone cyst, thigh**
    M85.551 Aneurysmal bone cyst, right thigh
    M85.552 Aneurysmal bone cyst, left thigh
    M85.559 Aneurysmal bone cyst, unspecified thigh ▽
  ✓6ᵗʰ **M85.56 Aneurysmal bone cyst, lower leg**
    M85.561 Aneurysmal bone cyst, right lower leg
    M85.562 Aneurysmal bone cyst, left lower leg
    M85.569 Aneurysmal bone cyst, unspecified lower leg ▽
  ✓6ᵗʰ **M85.57 Aneurysmal bone cyst, ankle and foot**
    M85.571 Aneurysmal bone cyst, right ankle and foot
    M85.572 Aneurysmal bone cyst, left ankle and foot
    M85.579 Aneurysmal bone cyst, unspecified ankle and foot ▽
  M85.58 Aneurysmal bone cyst, other site
  M85.59 Aneurysmal bone cyst, multiple sites
✓5ᵗʰ **M85.6 Other cyst of bone**
    EXCLUDES 1   *cyst of jaw NEC (M27.4)*
      osteitis fibrosa cystica generalisata [von Recklinghausen's disease of bone] (E21.0)
  M85.60 Other cyst of bone, unspecified site ▽
  ✓6ᵗʰ **M85.61 Other cyst of bone, shoulder**
    M85.611 Other cyst of bone, right shoulder
    M85.612 Other cyst of bone, left shoulder
    M85.619 Other cyst of bone, unspecified shoulder ▽
  ✓6ᵗʰ **M85.62 Other cyst of bone, upper arm**
    M85.621 Other cyst of bone, right upper arm
    M85.622 Other cyst of bone, left upper arm
    M85.629 Other cyst of bone, unspecified upper arm ▽
  ✓6ᵗʰ **M85.63 Other cyst of bone, forearm**
    M85.631 Other cyst of bone, right forearm
    M85.632 Other cyst of bone, left forearm
    M85.639 Other cyst of bone, unspecified forearm ▽

EXCLUDES 1 Not coded here   EXCLUDES 2 Not included here   N Newborn Age: 0   P Pediatric Age: 0-17   M Maternity Age: 12-55   A Adult Age: 15-124

782   ICD-10-CM 2018

√6ᵗʰ **M85.64** Other cyst of bone, **hand**
    M85.641 Other cyst of bone, **right** hand
    M85.642 Other cyst of bone, **left** hand
    M85.649 Other cyst of bone, unspecified hand ▽

√6ᵗʰ **M85.65** Other cyst of bone, **thigh**
    M85.651 Other cyst of bone, **right** thigh
    M85.652 Other cyst of bone, **left** thigh
    M85.659 Other cyst of bone, unspecified thigh ▽

√6ᵗʰ **M85.66** Other cyst of bone, **lower leg**
    M85.661 Other cyst of bone, **right** lower leg
    M85.662 Other cyst of bone, **left** lower leg
    M85.669 Other cyst of bone, unspecified lower leg ▽

√6ᵗʰ **M85.67** Other cyst of bone, **ankle and foot**
    M85.671 Other cyst of bone, **right** ankle and foot
    M85.672 Other cyst of bone, **left** ankle and foot
    M85.679 Other cyst of bone, unspecified ankle and foot ▽

  M85.68 Other cyst of bone, other site
  M85.69 Other cyst of bone, **multiple sites**

√5ᵗʰ **M85.8** Other specified disorders of bone density and structure
  Hyperostosis of bones, except skull
  Osteosclerosis, acquired
    EXCLUDES 1 diffuse idiopathic skeletal hyperostosis [DISH] (M48.1)
      osteosclerosis congenita (Q77.4)
      osteosclerosis fragilitas (generalista) (Q78.2)
      osteosclerosis myelofibrosis (D75.81)

  M85.80 Other specified disorders of bone density and structure, unspecified site ▽

√6ᵗʰ **M85.81** Other specified disorders of bone density and structure, **shoulder**
    M85.811 Other specified disorders of bone density and structure, **right** shoulder
    M85.812 Other specified disorders of bone density and structure, **left** shoulder
    M85.819 Other specified disorders of bone density and structure, unspecified shoulder ▽

√6ᵗʰ **M85.82** Other specified disorders of bone density and structure, **upper arm**
    M85.821 Other specified disorders of bone density and structure, **right** upper arm
    M85.822 Other specified disorders of bone density and structure, **left** upper arm
    M85.829 Other specified disorders of bone density and structure, unspecified upper arm ▽

√6ᵗʰ **M85.83** Other specified disorders of bone density and structure, **forearm**
    M85.831 Other specified disorders of bone density and structure, **right** forearm
    M85.832 Other specified disorders of bone density and structure, **left** forearm
    M85.839 Other specified disorders of bone density and structure, unspecified forearm ▽

√6ᵗʰ **M85.84** Other specified disorders of bone density and structure, **hand**
    M85.841 Other specified disorders of bone density and structure, **right** hand
    M85.842 Other specified disorders of bone density and structure, **left** hand
    M85.849 Other specified disorders of bone density and structure, unspecified hand ▽

√6ᵗʰ **M85.85** Other specified disorders of bone density and structure, **thigh**
    M85.851 Other specified disorders of bone density and structure, **right** thigh
    M85.852 Other specified disorders of bone density and structure, **left** thigh
    M85.859 Other specified disorders of bone density and structure, unspecified thigh ▽

√6ᵗʰ **M85.86** Other specified disorders of bone density and structure, **lower leg**
    M85.861 Other specified disorders of bone density and structure, **right** lower leg

    M85.862 Other specified disorders of bone density and structure, **left** lower leg
    M85.869 Other specified disorders of bone density and structure, unspecified lower leg ▽

√6ᵗʰ **M85.87** Other specified disorders of bone density and structure, **ankle and foot**
    M85.871 Other specified disorders of bone density and structure, **right** ankle and foot
    M85.872 Other specified disorders of bone density and structure, **left** ankle and foot
    M85.879 Other specified disorders of bone density and structure, unspecified ankle and foot ▽

  M85.88 Other specified disorders of bone density and structure, other site
  M85.89 Other specified disorders of bone density and structure, **multiple sites**

  M85.9 Disorder of bone density and structure, unspecified ▽

Other osteopathies (M86-M9Ø)
EXCLUDES 1 postprocedural osteopathies (M96.-)

√4ᵗʰ **M86 Osteomyelitis**
  Use additional code (B95-B97) to identify infectious agent
  Use additional code to identify major osseous defect, if applicable (M89.7-)
    EXCLUDES 1 osteomyelitis due to:
      echinococcus (B67.2)
      gonococcus (A54.43)
      salmonella (AØ2.24)
    EXCLUDES 2 ostemyelitis of:
      orbit (HØ5.Ø-)
      petrous bone (H7Ø.2-)
      vertebra (M46.2-)

√5ᵗʰ **M86.Ø Acute hematogenous osteomyelitis**
  M86.ØØ Acute hematogenous osteomyelitis, unspecified site HCC ▽

√6ᵗʰ **M86.Ø1** Acute hematogenous osteomyelitis, **shoulder**
    M86.Ø11 Acute hematogenous osteomyelitis, **right** shoulder HCC
    M86.Ø12 Acute hematogenous osteomyelitis, **left** shoulder HCC
    M86.Ø19 Acute hematogenous osteomyelitis, unspecified shoulder HCC ▽

√6ᵗʰ **M86.Ø2** Acute hematogenous osteomyelitis, **humerus**
    M86.Ø21 Acute hematogenous osteomyelitis, **right** humerus HCC
    M86.Ø22 Acute hematogenous osteomyelitis, **left** humerus HCC
    M86.Ø29 Acute hematogenous osteomyelitis, unspecified humerus HCC ▽

√6ᵗʰ **M86.Ø3** Acute hematogenous osteomyelitis, **radius and ulna**
    M86.Ø31 Acute hematogenous osteomyelitis, **right** radius and ulna HCC
    M86.Ø32 Acute hematogenous osteomyelitis, **left** radius and ulna HCC
    M86.Ø39 Acute hematogenous osteomyelitis, unspecified radius and ulna HCC ▽

√6ᵗʰ **M86.Ø4** Acute hematogenous osteomyelitis, **hand**
    M86.Ø41 Acute hematogenous osteomyelitis, **right** hand HCC
    M86.Ø42 Acute hematogenous osteomyelitis, **left** hand HCC
    M86.Ø49 Acute hematogenous osteomyelitis, unspecified hand HCC ▽

√6ᵗʰ **M86.Ø5** Acute hematogenous osteomyelitis, **femur**
    M86.Ø51 Acute hematogenous osteomyelitis, **right** femur HCC
    M86.Ø52 Acute hematogenous osteomyelitis, **left** femur HCC
    M86.Ø59 Acute hematogenous osteomyelitis, unspecified femur HCC ▽

✓ Additional Character Req   ✓x7ᵗʰ Placeholder Alert   Manifestation   HCC CMS-HCC Condition   ▽ Unspecified Code   ▶◀ Revised Text   ● New Code   ▲ Revised Code Title

ICD-10-CM 2018   783

M85.64-M86.Ø59

✓6ᵗʰ **M86.06 Acute hematogenous osteomyelitis, tibia and fibula**
- **M86.061 Acute hematogenous osteomyelitis, right tibia and fibula** HCC
- **M86.062 Acute hematogenous osteomyelitis, left tibia and fibula** HCC
- **M86.069 Acute hematogenous osteomyelitis, unspecified tibia and fibula** HCC ▽

✓6ᵗʰ **M86.07 Acute hematogenous osteomyelitis, ankle and foot**
- **M86.071 Acute hematogenous osteomyelitis, right ankle and foot** HCC
- **M86.072 Acute hematogenous osteomyelitis, left ankle and foot** HCC
- **M86.079 Acute hematogenous osteomyelitis, unspecified ankle and foot** HCC ▽

M86.08 Acute hematogenous osteomyelitis, other sites HCC

M86.09 Acute hematogenous osteomyelitis, multiple sites HCC

✓5ᵗʰ **M86.1 Other acute osteomyelitis**
- **M86.10 Other acute osteomyelitis, unspecified site** HCC ▽

✓6ᵗʰ **M86.11 Other acute osteomyelitis, shoulder**
- **M86.111 Other acute osteomyelitis, right shoulder** HCC
- **M86.112 Other acute osteomyelitis, left shoulder** HCC
- **M86.119 Other acute osteomyelitis, unspecified shoulder** HCC ▽

✓6ᵗʰ **M86.12 Other acute osteomyelitis, humerus**
- **M86.121 Other acute osteomyelitis, right humerus** HCC
- **M86.122 Other acute osteomyelitis, left humerus** HCC
- **M86.129 Other acute osteomyelitis, unspecified humerus** HCC ▽

✓6ᵗʰ **M86.13 Other acute osteomyelitis, radius and ulna**
- **M86.131 Other acute osteomyelitis, right radius and ulna** HCC
- **M86.132 Other acute osteomyelitis, left radius and ulna** HCC
- **M86.139 Other acute osteomyelitis, unspecified radius and ulna** HCC ▽

✓6ᵗʰ **M86.14 Other acute osteomyelitis, hand**
- **M86.141 Other acute osteomyelitis, right hand** HCC
- **M86.142 Other acute osteomyelitis, left hand** HCC
- **M86.149 Other acute osteomyelitis, unspecified hand** HCC ▽

✓6ᵗʰ **M86.15 Other acute osteomyelitis, femur**
- **M86.151 Other acute osteomyelitis, right femur** HCC
- **M86.152 Other acute osteomyelitis, left femur** HCC
- **M86.159 Other acute osteomyelitis, unspecified femur** HCC ▽

✓6ᵗʰ **M86.16 Other acute osteomyelitis, tibia and fibula**
- **M86.161 Other acute osteomyelitis, right tibia and fibula** HCC
- **M86.162 Other acute osteomyelitis, left tibia and fibula** HCC
- **M86.169 Other acute osteomyelitis, unspecified tibia and fibula** HCC ▽

✓6ᵗʰ **M86.17 Other acute osteomyelitis, ankle and foot**
- **M86.171 Other acute osteomyelitis, right ankle and foot** HCC
- **M86.172 Other acute osteomyelitis, left ankle and foot** HCC
- **M86.179 Other acute osteomyelitis, unspecified ankle and foot** HCC ▽

M86.18 Other acute osteomyelitis, other site HCC

M86.19 Other acute osteomyelitis, multiple sites HCC

✓5ᵗʰ **M86.2 Subacute osteomyelitis**
- **M86.20 Subacute osteomyelitis, unspecified site** HCC ▽

✓5ᵗʰ **M86.21 Subacute osteomyelitis, shoulder**
- **M86.211 Subacute osteomyelitis, right shoulder** HCC
- **M86.212 Subacute osteomyelitis, left shoulder** HCC
- **M86.219 Subacute osteomyelitis, unspecified shoulder** HCC ▽

✓6ᵗʰ **M86.22 Subacute osteomyelitis, humerus**
- **M86.221 Subacute osteomyelitis, right humerus** HCC
- **M86.222 Subacute osteomyelitis, left humerus** HCC
- **M86.229 Subacute osteomyelitis, unspecified humerus** HCC ▽

✓6ᵗʰ **M86.23 Subacute osteomyelitis, radius and ulna**
- **M86.231 Subacute osteomyelitis, right radius and ulna** HCC
- **M86.232 Subacute osteomyelitis, left radius and ulna** HCC
- **M86.239 Subacute osteomyelitis, unspecified radius and ulna** HCC ▽

✓6ᵗʰ **M86.24 Subacute osteomyelitis, hand**
- **M86.241 Subacute osteomyelitis, right hand** HCC
- **M86.242 Subacute osteomyelitis, left hand** HCC
- **M86.249 Subacute osteomyelitis, unspecified hand** HCC ▽

✓6ᵗʰ **M86.25 Subacute osteomyelitis, femur**
- **M86.251 Subacute osteomyelitis, right femur** HCC
- **M86.252 Subacute osteomyelitis, left femur** HCC
- **M86.259 Subacute osteomyelitis, unspecified femur** HCC ▽

✓6ᵗʰ **M86.26 Subacute osteomyelitis, tibia and fibula**
- **M86.261 Subacute osteomyelitis, right tibia and fibula** HCC
- **M86.262 Subacute osteomyelitis, left tibia and fibula** HCC
- **M86.269 Subacute osteomyelitis, unspecified tibia and fibula** HCC ▽

✓6ᵗʰ **M86.27 Subacute osteomyelitis, ankle and foot**
- **M86.271 Subacute osteomyelitis, right ankle and foot** HCC
- **M86.272 Subacute osteomyelitis, left ankle and foot** HCC
- **M86.279 Subacute osteomyelitis, unspecified ankle and foot** HCC ▽

M86.28 Subacute osteomyelitis, other site HCC

M86.29 Subacute osteomyelitis, multiple sites HCC

✓5ᵗʰ **M86.3 Chronic multifocal osteomyelitis**
- **M86.30 Chronic multifocal osteomyelitis, unspecified site** HCC ▽

✓6ᵗʰ **M86.31 Chronic multifocal osteomyelitis, shoulder**
- **M86.311 Chronic multifocal osteomyelitis, right shoulder** HCC
- **M86.312 Chronic multifocal osteomyelitis, left shoulder** HCC
- **M86.319 Chronic multifocal osteomyelitis, unspecified shoulder** HCC ▽

✓6ᵗʰ **M86.32 Chronic multifocal osteomyelitis, humerus**
- **M86.321 Chronic multifocal osteomyelitis, right humerus** HCC
- **M86.322 Chronic multifocal osteomyelitis, left humerus** HCC
- **M86.329 Chronic multifocal osteomyelitis, unspecified humerus** HCC ▽

✓6ᵗʰ **M86.33 Chronic multifocal osteomyelitis, radius and ulna**
- **M86.331 Chronic multifocal osteomyelitis, right radius and ulna** HCC
- **M86.332 Chronic multifocal osteomyelitis, left radius and ulna** HCC
- **M86.339 Chronic multifocal osteomyelitis, unspecified radius and ulna** HCC ▽

✓6ᵗʰ **M86.34 Chronic multifocal osteomyelitis, hand**
- **M86.341 Chronic multifocal osteomyelitis, right hand** HCC
- **M86.342 Chronic multifocal osteomyelitis, left hand** HCC
- **M86.349 Chronic multifocal osteomyelitis, unspecified hand** HCC ▽

EXCLUDES 1 Not coded here   EXCLUDES 2 Not included here   N Newborn Age: 0   P Pediatric Age: 0-17   M Maternity Age: 12-55   A Adult Age: 15-124

784   ICD-10-CM 2018

✓6ᵗʰ **M86.35** Chronic multifocal osteomyelitis, femur

     M86.351 Chronic multifocal osteomyelitis, right femur   HCC

     M86.352 Chronic multifocal osteomyelitis, left femur   HCC

     M86.359 Chronic multifocal osteomyelitis, unspecified femur   HCC ▽

✓6ᵗʰ **M86.36** Chronic multifocal osteomyelitis, tibia and fibula

     M86.361 Chronic multifocal osteomyelitis, right tibia and fibula   HCC

     M86.362 Chronic multifocal osteomyelitis, left tibia and fibula   HCC

     M86.369 Chronic multifocal osteomyelitis, unspecified tibia and fibula   HCC ▽

✓6ᵗʰ **M86.37** Chronic multifocal osteomyelitis, ankle and foot

     M86.371 Chronic multifocal osteomyelitis, right ankle and foot   HCC

     M86.372 Chronic multifocal osteomyelitis, left ankle and foot   HCC

     M86.379 Chronic multifocal osteomyelitis, unspecified ankle and foot   HCC ▽

M86.38 Chronic multifocal osteomyelitis, other site   HCC

M86.39 Chronic multifocal osteomyelitis, multiple sites   HCC

✓5ᵗʰ **M86.4** Chronic osteomyelitis with draining sinus

     M86.40 Chronic osteomyelitis with draining sinus, unspecified site   HCC ▽

✓6ᵗʰ **M86.41** Chronic osteomyelitis with draining sinus, shoulder

     M86.411 Chronic osteomyelitis with draining sinus, right shoulder   HCC

     M86.412 Chronic osteomyelitis with draining sinus, left shoulder   HCC

     M86.419 Chronic osteomyelitis with draining sinus, unspecified shoulder   HCC ▽

✓6ᵗʰ **M86.42** Chronic osteomyelitis with draining sinus, humerus

     M86.421 Chronic osteomyelitis with draining sinus, right humerus   HCC

     M86.422 Chronic osteomyelitis with draining sinus, left humerus   HCC

     M86.429 Chronic osteomyelitis with draining sinus, unspecified humerus   HCC ▽

✓6ᵗʰ **M86.43** Chronic osteomyelitis with draining sinus, radius and ulna

     M86.431 Chronic osteomyelitis with draining sinus, right radius and ulna   HCC

     M86.432 Chronic osteomyelitis with draining sinus, left radius and ulna   HCC

     M86.439 Chronic osteomyelitis with draining sinus, unspecified radius and ulna   HCC ▽

✓6ᵗʰ **M86.44** Chronic osteomyelitis with draining sinus, hand

     M86.441 Chronic osteomyelitis with draining sinus, right hand   HCC

     M86.442 Chronic osteomyelitis with draining sinus, left hand   HCC

     M86.449 Chronic osteomyelitis with draining sinus, unspecified hand   HCC ▽

✓6ᵗʰ **M86.45** Chronic osteomyelitis with draining sinus, femur

     M86.451 Chronic osteomyelitis with draining sinus, right femur   HCC

     M86.452 Chronic osteomyelitis with draining sinus, left femur   HCC

     M86.459 Chronic osteomyelitis with draining sinus, unspecified femur   HCC ▽

✓6ᵗʰ **M86.46** Chronic osteomyelitis with draining sinus, tibia and fibula

     M86.461 Chronic osteomyelitis with draining sinus, right tibia and fibula   HCC

     M86.462 Chronic osteomyelitis with draining sinus, left tibia and fibula   HCC

     M86.469 Chronic osteomyelitis with draining sinus, unspecified tibia and fibula   HCC ▽

✓6ᵗʰ **M86.47** Chronic osteomyelitis with draining sinus, ankle and foot

     M86.471 Chronic osteomyelitis with draining sinus, right ankle and foot   HCC

     M86.472 Chronic osteomyelitis with draining sinus, left ankle and foot   HCC

     M86.479 Chronic osteomyelitis with draining sinus, unspecified ankle and foot   HCC ▽

M86.48 Chronic osteomyelitis with draining sinus, other site   HCC

M86.49 Chronic osteomyelitis with draining sinus, multiple sites   HCC

✓5ᵗʰ **M86.5** Other chronic hematogenous osteomyelitis

     M86.50 Other chronic hematogenous osteomyelitis, unspecified site   HCC ▽

✓6ᵗʰ **M86.51** Other chronic hematogenous osteomyelitis, shoulder

     M86.511 Other chronic hematogenous osteomyelitis, right shoulder   HCC

     M86.512 Other chronic hematogenous osteomyelitis, left shoulder   HCC

     M86.519 Other chronic hematogenous osteomyelitis, unspecified shoulder   HCC ▽

✓6ᵗʰ **M86.52** Other chronic hematogenous osteomyelitis, humerus

     M86.521 Other chronic hematogenous osteomyelitis, right humerus   HCC

     M86.522 Other chronic hematogenous osteomyelitis, left humerus   HCC

     M86.529 Other chronic hematogenous osteomyelitis, unspecified humerus   HCC ▽

✓6ᵗʰ **M86.53** Other chronic hematogenous osteomyelitis, radius and ulna

     M86.531 Other chronic hematogenous osteomyelitis, right radius and ulna   HCC

     M86.532 Other chronic hematogenous osteomyelitis, left radius and ulna   HCC

     M86.539 Other chronic hematogenous osteomyelitis, unspecified radius and ulna   HCC ▽

✓6ᵗʰ **M86.54** Other chronic hematogenous osteomyelitis, hand

     M86.541 Other chronic hematogenous osteomyelitis, right hand   HCC

     M86.542 Other chronic hematogenous osteomyelitis, left hand   HCC

     M86.549 Other chronic hematogenous osteomyelitis, unspecified hand   HCC ▽

✓6ᵗʰ **M86.55** Other chronic hematogenous osteomyelitis, femur

     M86.551 Other chronic hematogenous osteomyelitis, right femur   HCC

     M86.552 Other chronic hematogenous osteomyelitis, left femur   HCC

     M86.559 Other chronic hematogenous osteomyelitis, unspecified femur   HCC ▽

✓6ᵗʰ **M86.56** Other chronic hematogenous osteomyelitis, tibia and fibula

     M86.561 Other chronic hematogenous osteomyelitis, right tibia and fibula   HCC

     M86.562 Other chronic hematogenous osteomyelitis, left tibia and fibula   HCC

     M86.569 Other chronic hematogenous osteomyelitis, unspecified tibia and fibula   HCC ▽

✓6ᵗʰ **M86.57** Other chronic hematogenous osteomyelitis, ankle and foot

     M86.571 Other chronic hematogenous osteomyelitis, right ankle and foot   HCC

     M86.572 Other chronic hematogenous osteomyelitis, left ankle and foot   HCC

     M86.579 Other chronic hematogenous osteomyelitis, unspecified ankle and foot   HCC ▽

M86.58 Other chronic hematogenous osteomyelitis, other site   HCC

M86.59 Other chronic hematogenous osteomyelitis, multiple sites   HCC

✓5ᵗʰ **M86.6** Other chronic osteomyelitis

     M86.60 Other chronic osteomyelitis, unspecified site   HCC ▽

✓5ᵗʰ **M86.61** Other chronic osteomyelitis, shoulder

     M86.611 Other chronic osteomyelitis, right shoulder   HCC

     M86.612 Other chronic osteomyelitis, left shoulder   HCC

     M86.619 Other chronic osteomyelitis, unspecified shoulder   HCC ▽

✓ Additional Character Req   ✓x7ᵗʰ Placeholder Alert   Manifestation   HCC CMS-HCC Condition   ▽ Unspecified Code   ►◄ Revised Text   ● New Code   ▲ Revised Code Title

ICD-10-CM 2018   785

✓6ᵗʰ **M86.62 Other chronic osteomyelitis, humerus**
    M86.621 Other chronic osteomyelitis, right `HCC`
         humerus
    M86.622 Other chronic osteomyelitis, left `HCC`
         humerus
    M86.629 Other chronic osteomyelitis, `HCC` ▽
         unspecified humerus

✓6ᵗʰ **M86.63 Other chronic osteomyelitis, radius and ulna**
    M86.631 Other chronic osteomyelitis, right `HCC`
         radius and ulna
    M86.632 Other chronic osteomyelitis, left `HCC`
         radius and ulna
    M86.639 Other chronic osteomyelitis, `HCC` ▽
         unspecified radius and ulna

✓6ᵗʰ **M86.64 Other chronic osteomyelitis, hand**
    M86.641 Other chronic osteomyelitis, right `HCC`
         hand
    M86.642 Other chronic osteomyelitis, left `HCC`
         hand
    M86.649 Other chronic osteomyelitis, `HCC` ▽
         unspecified hand

✓6ᵗʰ **M86.65 Other chronic osteomyelitis, thigh**
    M86.651 Other chronic osteomyelitis, `HCC`
         right thigh
    M86.652 Other chronic osteomyelitis, `HCC`
         left thigh
    M86.659 Other chronic osteomyelitis, `HCC` ▽
         unspecified thigh

✓6ᵗʰ **M86.66 Other chronic osteomyelitis, tibia and fibula**
    M86.661 Other chronic osteomyelitis, `HCC`
         right tibia and fibula
    M86.662 Other chronic osteomyelitis, left `HCC`
         tibia and fibula
    M86.669 Other chronic osteomyelitis, `HCC` ▽
         unspecified tibia and fibula

✓6ᵗʰ **M86.67 Other chronic osteomyelitis, ankle and foot**
    M86.671 Other chronic osteomyelitis, right `HCC`
         ankle and foot
         AHA: 2016, 1Q, 13
    M86.672 Other chronic osteomyelitis, left `HCC`
         ankle and foot
    M86.679 Other chronic osteomyelitis, `HCC` ▽
         unspecified ankle and foot

  M86.68 Other chronic osteomyelitis, other site `HCC`
  M86.69 Other chronic osteomyelitis, multiple sites `HCC`

✓5ᵗʰ **M86.8 Other osteomyelitis**
    Brodie's abscess

✓6ᵗʰ **M86.8X Other osteomyelitis**
    M86.8X0 Other osteomyelitis, multiple sites `HCC`
    M86.8X1 Other osteomyelitis, shoulder `HCC`
    M86.8X2 Other osteomyelitis, upper arm `HCC`
    M86.8X3 Other osteomyelitis, forearm `HCC`
    M86.8X4 Other osteomyelitis, hand `HCC`
    M86.8X5 Other osteomyelitis, thigh `HCC`
    M86.8X6 Other osteomyelitis, lower leg `HCC`
    M86.8X7 Other osteomyelitis, ankle and foot `HCC`
    M86.8X8 Other osteomyelitis, other site `HCC`
    M86.8X9 Other osteomyelitis, unspecified `HCC` ▽
         sites

M86.9 Osteomyelitis, unspecified `HCC` ▽
    Infection of bone NOS
    Periostitis without osteomyelitis

✓4ᵗʰ **M87 Osteonecrosis**
  `INCLUDES` avascular necrosis of bone
  Use additional code to identify major osseous defect, if applicable
  (M89.7-)
  `EXCLUDES 1` juvenile osteonecrosis (M91-M92)
         osteochondropathies (M90-M93)

✓5ᵗʰ **M87.0 Idiopathic aseptic necrosis of bone**
  M87.00 Idiopathic aseptic necrosis of unspecified `HCC` ▽
         bone

✓6ᵗʰ **M87.01 Idiopathic aseptic necrosis of shoulder**
    Idiopathic aseptic necrosis of clavicle and scapula
    M87.011 Idiopathic aseptic necrosis of right `HCC`
         shoulder

    M87.012 Idiopathic aseptic necrosis of left `HCC`
         shoulder
    M87.019 Idiopathic aseptic necrosis of `HCC` ▽
         unspecified shoulder

✓6ᵗʰ **M87.02 Idiopathic aseptic necrosis of humerus**
    M87.021 Idiopathic aseptic necrosis of right `HCC`
         humerus
    M87.022 Idiopathic aseptic necrosis of left `HCC`
         humerus
    M87.029 Idiopathic aseptic necrosis of `HCC` ▽
         unspecified humerus

✓6ᵗʰ **M87.03 Idiopathic aseptic necrosis of radius, ulna and carpus**
    M87.031 Idiopathic aseptic necrosis of `HCC`
         right radius
    M87.032 Idiopathic aseptic necrosis of `HCC`
         left radius
    M87.033 Idiopathic aseptic necrosis of `HCC` ▽
         unspecified radius
    M87.034 Idiopathic aseptic necrosis of `HCC`
         right ulna
    M87.035 Idiopathic aseptic necrosis of `HCC`
         left ulna
    M87.036 Idiopathic aseptic necrosis of `HCC` ▽
         unspecified ulna
    M87.037 Idiopathic aseptic necrosis of `HCC`
         right carpus
    M87.038 Idiopathic aseptic necrosis of `HCC`
         left carpus
    M87.039 Idiopathic aseptic necrosis of `HCC` ▽
         unspecified carpus

✓6ᵗʰ **M87.04 Idiopathic aseptic necrosis of hand and fingers**
    Idiopathic aseptic necrosis of metacarpals and
    phalanges of hands
    M87.041 Idiopathic aseptic necrosis of `HCC`
         right hand
    M87.042 Idiopathic aseptic necrosis of `HCC`
         left hand
    M87.043 Idiopathic aseptic necrosis of `HCC` ▽
         unspecified hand
    M87.044 Idiopathic aseptic necrosis of right `HCC`
         finger(s)
    M87.045 Idiopathic aseptic necrosis of `HCC`
         left finger(s)
    M87.046 Idiopathic aseptic necrosis of `HCC` ▽
         unspecified finger(s)

✓6ᵗʰ **M87.05 Idiopathic aseptic necrosis of pelvis and femur**
    M87.050 Idiopathic aseptic necrosis of pelvis `HCC`
    M87.051 Idiopathic aseptic necrosis of `HCC`
         right femur
    M87.052 Idiopathic aseptic necrosis of `HCC`
         left femur
    M87.059 Idiopathic aseptic necrosis of `HCC` ▽
         unspecified femur
         Idiopathic aseptic necrosis of hip NOS

✓6ᵗʰ **M87.06 Idiopathic aseptic necrosis of tibia and fibula**
    M87.061 Idiopathic aseptic necrosis of `HCC`
         right tibia
    M87.062 Idiopathic aseptic necrosis of `HCC`
         left tibia
    M87.063 Idiopathic aseptic necrosis of `HCC` ▽
         unspecified tibia
    M87.064 Idiopathic aseptic necrosis of `HCC`
         right fibula
    M87.065 Idiopathic aseptic necrosis of `HCC`
         left fibula
    M87.066 Idiopathic aseptic necrosis of `HCC` ▽
         unspecified fibula

✓6ᵗʰ **M87.07 Idiopathic aseptic necrosis of ankle, foot and toes**
    Idiopathic aseptic necrosis of metatarsus, tarsus, and
    phalanges of toes
    M87.071 Idiopathic aseptic necrosis of `HCC`
         right ankle
    M87.072 Idiopathic aseptic necrosis of `HCC`
         left ankle
    M87.073 Idiopathic aseptic necrosis of `HCC` ▽
         unspecified ankle
    M87.074 Idiopathic aseptic necrosis of `HCC`
         right foot

M87.075 Idiopathic aseptic necrosis of **left foot** `HCC`

M87.076 Idiopathic aseptic necrosis of **unspecified foot** `HCC` ▽

M87.077 Idiopathic aseptic necrosis of **right toe(s)** `HCC`

M87.078 Idiopathic aseptic necrosis of **left toe(s)** `HCC`

M87.079 Idiopathic aseptic necrosis of **unspecified toe(s)** `HCC` ▽

M87.08 Idiopathic aseptic necrosis of bone, other site' `HCC`

M87.09 Idiopathic aseptic necrosis of bone, **multiple sites** `HCC`

✓5th **M87.1 Osteonecrosis due to drugs**

Use additional code for adverse effect, if applicable, to identify drug (T36-T50 with fifth or sixth character 5)

M87.10 Osteonecrosis due to drugs, unspecified bone `HCC` ▽

✓6th **M87.11 Osteonecrosis due to drugs, shoulder**

M87.111 Osteonecrosis due to drugs, **right shoulder** `HCC`

M87.112 Osteonecrosis due to drugs, **left shoulder** `HCC`

M87.119 Osteonecrosis due to drugs, **unspecified shoulder** `HCC` ▽

✓6th **M87.12 Osteonecrosis due to drugs, humerus**

M87.121 Osteonecrosis due to drugs, **right humerus** `HCC`

M87.122 Osteonecrosis due to drugs, **left humerus** `HCC`

M87.129 Osteonecrosis due to drugs, **unspecified humerus** `HCC` ▽

✓6th **M87.13 Osteonecrosis due to drugs of radius, ulna and carpus**

M87.131 Osteonecrosis due to drugs of **right radius** `HCC`

M87.132 Osteonecrosis due to drugs of **left radius** `HCC`

M87.133 Osteonecrosis due to drugs of **unspecified radius** `HCC` ▽

M87.134 Osteonecrosis due to drugs of **right ulna** `HCC`

M87.135 Osteonecrosis due to drugs of **left ulna** `HCC`

M87.136 Osteonecrosis due to drugs of **unspecified ulna** `HCC` ▽

M87.137 Osteonecrosis due to drugs of **right carpus** `HCC`

M87.138 Osteonecrosis due to drugs of **left carpus** `HCC`

M87.139 Osteonecrosis due to drugs of **unspecified carpus** `HCC` ▽

✓6th **M87.14 Osteonecrosis due to drugs, hand and fingers**

M87.141 Osteonecrosis due to drugs, **right hand** `HCC`

M87.142 Osteonecrosis due to drugs, **left hand** `HCC`

M87.143 Osteonecrosis due to drugs, **unspecified hand** `HCC` ▽

M87.144 Osteonecrosis due to drugs, **right finger(s)** `HCC`

M87.145 Osteonecrosis due to drugs, **left finger(s)** `HCC`

M87.146 Osteonecrosis due to drugs, **unspecified finger(s)** `HCC` ▽

✓6th **M87.15 Osteonecrosis due to drugs, pelvis and femur**

M87.150 Osteonecrosis due to drugs, **pelvis** `HCC`

M87.151 Osteonecrosis due to drugs, **right femur** `HCC`

M87.152 Osteonecrosis due to drugs, **left femur** `HCC`

M87.159 Osteonecrosis due to drugs, **unspecified femur** `HCC` ▽

✓6th **M87.16 Osteonecrosis due to drugs, tibia and fibula**

M87.161 Osteonecrosis due to drugs, **right tibia** `HCC`

M87.162 Osteonecrosis due to drugs, **left tibia** `HCC`

M87.163 Osteonecrosis due to drugs, **unspecified tibia** `HCC` ▽

M87.164 Osteonecrosis due to drugs, **right fibula** `HCC`

M87.165 Osteonecrosis due to drugs, **left fibula** `HCC`

M87.166 Osteonecrosis due to drugs, **unspecified fibula** `HCC` ▽

✓6th **M87.17 Osteonecrosis due to drugs, ankle, foot and toes**

M87.171 Osteonecrosis due to drugs, **right ankle** `HCC`

M87.172 Osteonecrosis due to drugs, **left ankle** `HCC`

M87.173 Osteonecrosis due to drugs, **unspecified ankle** `HCC` ▽

M87.174 Osteonecrosis due to drugs, **right foot** `HCC`

M87.175 Osteonecrosis due to drugs, **left foot** `HCC`

M87.176 Osteonecrosis due to drugs, **unspecified foot** `HCC` ▽

M87.177 Osteonecrosis due to drugs, **right toe(s)** `HCC`

M87.178 Osteonecrosis due to drugs, **left toe(s)** `HCC`

M87.179 Osteonecrosis due to drugs, **unspecified toe(s)** `HCC` ▽

✓6th **M87.18 Osteonecrosis due to drugs, other site**

M87.180 Osteonecrosis due to drugs, jaw `HCC`

M87.188 Osteonecrosis due to drugs, other site `HCC`

M87.19 Osteonecrosis due to drugs, **multiple sites** `HCC`

✓5th **M87.2 Osteonecrosis due to previous trauma**

M87.20 Osteonecrosis due to previous trauma, unspecified bone `HCC` ▽

✓6th **M87.21 Osteonecrosis due to previous trauma, shoulder**

M87.211 Osteonecrosis due to previous trauma, **right** shoulder `HCC`

M87.212 Osteonecrosis due to previous trauma, **left shoulder** `HCC`

M87.219 Osteonecrosis due to previous trauma, unspecified shoulder `HCC` ▽

✓6th **M87.22 Osteonecrosis due to previous trauma, humerus**

M87.221 Osteonecrosis due to previous trauma, **right humerus** `HCC`

M87.222 Osteonecrosis due to previous trauma, **left humerus** `HCC`

M87.229 Osteonecrosis due to previous trauma, unspecified humerus `HCC` ▽

✓6th **M87.23 Osteonecrosis due to previous trauma of radius, ulna and carpus**

M87.231 Osteonecrosis due to previous trauma of **right radius** `HCC`

M87.232 Osteonecrosis due to previous trauma of **left radius** `HCC`

M87.233 Osteonecrosis due to previous trauma of unspecified radius `HCC` ▽

M87.234 Osteonecrosis due to previous trauma of **right ulna** `HCC`

M87.235 Osteonecrosis due to previous trauma of **left ulna** `HCC`

M87.236 Osteonecrosis due to previous trauma of unspecified ulna `HCC` ▽

M87.237 Osteonecrosis due to previous trauma of **right carpus** `HCC`

M87.238 Osteonecrosis due to previous trauma of **left carpus** `HCC`

M87.239 Osteonecrosis due to previous trauma of unspecified carpus `HCC` ▽

✓6th **M87.24 Osteonecrosis due to previous trauma, hand and fingers**

M87.241 Osteonecrosis due to previous trauma, **right hand** `HCC`

M87.242 Osteonecrosis due to previous trauma, **left hand** `HCC`

M87.243 Osteonecrosis due to previous trauma, unspecified hand `HCC` ▽

✔ Additional Character Req   ✓x7th Placeholder Alert   Manifestation   `HCC` CMS-HCC Condition   ▽ Unspecified Code   ▶◀ Revised Text   ● New Code   ▲ Revised Code Title

M87.244 Osteonecrosis due to previous trauma, right finger(s) `HCC`

M87.245 Osteonecrosis due to previous trauma, left finger(s) `HCC`

M87.246 Osteonecrosis due to previous trauma, unspecified finger(s) `HCC` ▽

☑6ᵗʰ M87.25 Osteonecrosis due to previous trauma, pelvis and femur

    M87.250 Osteonecrosis due to previous trauma, pelvis `HCC`

    M87.251 Osteonecrosis due to previous trauma, right femur `HCC`

    M87.252 Osteonecrosis due to previous trauma, left femur `HCC`

    M87.256 Osteonecrosis due to previous trauma, unspecified femur `HCC` ▽

☑6ᵗʰ M87.26 Osteonecrosis due to previous trauma, tibia and fibula

    M87.261 Osteonecrosis due to previous trauma, right tibia `HCC`

    M87.262 Osteonecrosis due to previous trauma, left tibia `HCC`

    M87.263 Osteonecrosis due to previous trauma, unspecified tibia `HCC` ▽

    M87.264 Osteonecrosis due to previous trauma, right fibula `HCC`

    M87.265 Osteonecrosis due to previous trauma, left fibula `HCC`

    M87.266 Osteonecrosis due to previous trauma, unspecified fibula `HCC` ▽

☑6ᵗʰ M87.27 Osteonecrosis due to previous trauma, ankle, foot and toes

    M87.271 Osteonecrosis due to previous trauma, right ankle `HCC`

    M87.272 Osteonecrosis due to previous trauma, left ankle `HCC`

    M87.273 Osteonecrosis due to previous trauma, unspecified ankle `HCC` ▽

    M87.274 Osteonecrosis due to previous trauma, right foot `HCC`

    M87.275 Osteonecrosis due to previous trauma, left foot `HCC`

    M87.276 Osteonecrosis due to previous trauma, unspecified foot `HCC` ▽

    M87.277 Osteonecrosis due to previous trauma, right toe(s) `HCC`

    M87.278 Osteonecrosis due to previous trauma, left toe(s) `HCC`

    M87.279 Osteonecrosis due to previous trauma, unspecified toe(s) `HCC` ▽

M87.28 Osteonecrosis due to previous trauma, other site `HCC`

M87.29 Osteonecrosis due to previous trauma, multiple sites `HCC`

☑5ᵗʰ M87.3 Other secondary osteonecrosis

    M87.30 Other secondary osteonecrosis, unspecified bone `HCC` ▽

☑6ᵗʰ M87.31 Other secondary osteonecrosis, shoulder

    M87.311 Other secondary osteonecrosis, right shoulder `HCC`

    M87.312 Other secondary osteonecrosis, left shoulder `HCC`

    M87.319 Other secondary osteonecrosis, unspecified shoulder `HCC` ▽

☑6ᵗʰ M87.32 Other secondary osteonecrosis, humerus

    M87.321 Other secondary osteonecrosis, right humerus `HCC`

    M87.322 Other secondary osteonecrosis, left humerus `HCC`

    M87.329 Other secondary osteonecrosis, unspecified humerus `HCC` ▽

☑6ᵗʰ M87.33 Other secondary osteonecrosis of radius, ulna and carpus

    M87.331 Other secondary osteonecrosis of right radius `HCC`

    M87.332 Other secondary osteonecrosis of left radius `HCC`

    M87.333 Other secondary osteonecrosis of unspecified radius `HCC` ▽

    M87.334 Other secondary osteonecrosis of right ulna `HCC`

    M87.335 Other secondary osteonecrosis of left ulna `HCC`

    M87.336 Other secondary osteonecrosis of unspecified ulna `HCC` ▽

    M87.337 Other secondary osteonecrosis of right carpus `HCC`

    M87.338 Other secondary osteonecrosis of left carpus `HCC`

    M87.339 Other secondary osteonecrosis of unspecified carpus `HCC` ▽

☑6ᵗʰ M87.34 Other secondary osteonecrosis, hand and fingers

    M87.341 Other secondary osteonecrosis, right hand `HCC`

    M87.342 Other secondary osteonecrosis, left hand `HCC`

    M87.343 Other secondary osteonecrosis, unspecified hand `HCC` ▽

    M87.344 Other secondary osteonecrosis, right finger(s) `HCC`

    M87.345 Other secondary osteonecrosis, left finger(s) `HCC`

    M87.346 Other secondary osteonecrosis, unspecified finger(s) `HCC` ▽

☑6ᵗʰ M87.35 Other secondary osteonecrosis, pelvis and femur

    M87.350 Other secondary osteonecrosis, pelvis `HCC`

    M87.351 Other secondary osteonecrosis, right femur `HCC`

    M87.352 Other secondary osteonecrosis, left femur `HCC`

    M87.353 Other secondary osteonecrosis, unspecified femur `HCC` ▽

☑6ᵗʰ M87.36 Other secondary osteonecrosis, tibia and fibula

    M87.361 Other secondary osteonecrosis, right tibia `HCC`

    M87.362 Other secondary osteonecrosis, left tibia `HCC`

    M87.363 Other secondary osteonecrosis, unspecified tibia `HCC` ▽

    M87.364 Other secondary osteonecrosis, right fibula `HCC`

    M87.365 Other secondary osteonecrosis, left fibula `HCC`

    M87.366 Other secondary osteonecrosis, unspecified fibula `HCC` ▽

☑6ᵗʰ M87.37 Other secondary osteonecrosis, ankle and foot

    M87.371 Other secondary osteonecrosis, right ankle `HCC`

    M87.372 Other secondary osteonecrosis, left ankle `HCC`

    M87.373 Other secondary osteonecrosis, unspecified ankle `HCC` ▽

    M87.374 Other secondary osteonecrosis, right foot `HCC`

    M87.375 Other secondary osteonecrosis, left foot `HCC`

    M87.376 Other secondary osteonecrosis, unspecified foot `HCC` ▽

    M87.377 Other secondary osteonecrosis, right toe(s) `HCC`

    M87.378 Other secondary osteonecrosis, left toe(s) `HCC`

    M87.379 Other secondary osteonecrosis, unspecified toe(s) `HCC` ▽

M87.38 Other secondary osteonecrosis, other site `HCC`

M87.39 Other secondary osteonecrosis, multiple sites `HCC`

☑5ᵗʰ M87.8 Other osteonecrosis

    M87.80 Other osteonecrosis, unspecified bone `HCC` ▽

☑6ᵗʰ M87.81 Other osteonecrosis, shoulder

    M87.811 Other osteonecrosis, right shoulder `HCC`

    M87.812 Other osteonecrosis, left shoulder `HCC`

    M87.819 Other osteonecrosis, unspecified shoulder `HCC` ▽

✓6ᵗʰ **M87.82 Other osteonecrosis, humerus**
     M87.821 Other osteonecrosis, **right** humerus   `HCC`
     M87.822 Other osteonecrosis, **left** humerus   `HCC`
     M87.829 Other osteonecrosis, **unspecified** humerus   `HCC` ▽

✓6ᵗʰ **M87.83 Other osteonecrosis of radius, ulna and carpus**
     M87.831 Other osteonecrosis of **right** radius   `HCC`
     M87.832 Other osteonecrosis of **left** radius   `HCC`
     M87.833 Other osteonecrosis of **unspecified** radius   `HCC` ▽
     M87.834 Other osteonecrosis of **right** ulna   `HCC`
     M87.835 Other osteonecrosis of **left** ulna   `HCC`
     M87.836 Other osteonecrosis of **unspecified** ulna   `HCC` ▽
     M87.837 Other osteonecrosis of **right** carpus   `HCC`
     M87.838 Other osteonecrosis of **left** carpus   `HCC`
     M87.839 Other osteonecrosis of **unspecified** carpus   `HCC` ▽

✓6ᵗʰ **M87.84 Other osteonecrosis, hand and fingers**
     M87.841 Other osteonecrosis, **right** hand   `HCC`
     M87.842 Other osteonecrosis, **left** hand   `HCC`
     M87.843 Other osteonecrosis, **unspecified** hand   `HCC` ▽
     M87.844 Other osteonecrosis, **right** finger(s)   `HCC`
     M87.845 Other osteonecrosis, **left** finger(s)   `HCC`
     M87.849 Other osteonecrosis, **unspecified** finger(s)   `HCC` ▽

✓6ᵗʰ **M87.85 Other osteonecrosis, pelvis and femur**
     M87.850 Other osteonecrosis, **pelvis**   `HCC`
     M87.851 Other osteonecrosis, **right** femur   `HCC`
     M87.852 Other osteonecrosis, **left** femur   `HCC`
     M87.859 Other osteonecrosis, **unspecified** femur   `HCC` ▽

✓6ᵗʰ **M87.86 Other osteonecrosis, tibia and fibula**
     M87.861 Other osteonecrosis, **right** tibia   `HCC`
     M87.862 Other osteonecrosis, **left** tibia   `HCC`
     M87.863 Other osteonecrosis, **unspecified** tibia   `HCC` ▽
     M87.864 Other osteonecrosis, **right** fibula   `HCC`
     M87.865 Other osteonecrosis, **left** fibula   `HCC`
     M87.869 Other osteonecrosis, **unspecified** fibula   `HCC` ▽

✓6ᵗʰ **M87.87 Other osteonecrosis, ankle, foot and toes**
     M87.871 Other osteonecrosis, **right** ankle   `HCC`
     M87.872 Other osteonecrosis, **left** ankle   `HCC`
     M87.873 Other osteonecrosis, **unspecified** ankle   `HCC` ▽
     M87.874 Other osteonecrosis, **right** foot   `HCC`
     M87.875 Other osteonecrosis, **left** foot   `HCC`
     M87.876 Other osteonecrosis, **unspecified** foot   `HCC` ▽
     M87.877 Other osteonecrosis, **right** toe(s)   `HCC`
     M87.878 Other osteonecrosis, **left** toe(s)   `HCC`
     M87.879 Other osteonecrosis, **unspecified** toe(s)   `HCC` ▽

     M87.88 Other osteonecrosis, other site   `HCC`
     M87.89 Other osteonecrosis, **multiple sites**   `HCC`

M87.9 Osteonecrosis, unspecified   `HCC` ▽
     Necrosis of bone NOS

✓4ᵗʰ **M88 Osteitis deformans [Paget's disease of bone]**
     EXCLUDES 1   osteitis deformans in neoplastic disease (M90.6)

M88.0 Osteitis deformans of skull

M88.1 Osteitis deformans of vertebrae

✓5ᵗʰ **M88.8 Osteitis deformans of other bones**

✓6ᵗʰ **M88.81 Osteitis deformans of shoulder**
     M88.811 Osteitis deformans of **right** shoulder
     M88.812 Osteitis deformans of **left** shoulder
     M88.819 Osteitis deformans of unspecified shoulder ▽

✓6ᵗʰ **M88.82 Osteitis deformans of upper arm**
     M88.821 Osteitis deformans of **right** upper arm
     M88.822 Osteitis deformans of **left** upper arm
     M88.829 Osteitis deformans of unspecified upper arm ▽

✓6ᵗʰ **M88.83 Osteitis deformans of forearm**
     M88.831 Osteitis deformans of **right** forearm
     M88.832 Osteitis deformans of **left** forearm
     M88.839 Osteitis deformans of unspecified forearm ▽

✓6ᵗʰ **M88.84 Osteitis deformans of hand**
     M88.841 Osteitis deformans of **right** hand
     M88.842 Osteitis deformans of **left** hand
     M88.849 Osteitis deformans of unspecified hand ▽

✓6ᵗʰ **M88.85 Osteitis deformans of thigh**
     M88.851 Osteitis deformans of **right** thigh
     M88.852 Osteitis deformans of **left** thigh
     M88.859 Osteitis deformans of unspecified thigh ▽

✓6ᵗʰ **M88.86 Osteitis deformans of lower leg**
     M88.861 Osteitis deformans of **right** lower leg
     M88.862 Osteitis deformans of **left** lower leg
     M88.869 Osteitis deformans of unspecified lower leg ▽

✓6ᵗʰ **M88.87 Osteitis deformans of ankle and foot**
     M88.871 Osteitis deformans of **right** ankle and foot
     M88.872 Osteitis deformans of **left** ankle and foot
     M88.879 Osteitis deformans of unspecified ankle and foot ▽

     M88.88 Osteitis deformans of other bones
         EXCLUDES 2   osteitis deformans of skull (M88.0)
                 osteitis deformans of vertebrae (M88.1)

     M88.89 Osteitis deformans of **multiple sites**

M88.9 Osteitis deformans of unspecified bone ▽

✓4ᵗʰ **M89 Other disorders of bone**

✓5ᵗʰ **M89.0 Algoneurodystrophy**
     Shoulder-hand syndrome
     Sudeck's atrophy
     EXCLUDES 1   causalgia, lower limb (G57.7-)
                 causalgia, upper limb (G56.4-)
                 complex regional pain syndrome II, lower limb (G57.7-)
                 complex regional pain syndrome II, upper limb (G56.4-)
                 reflex sympathetic dystrophy (G90.5-)

     M89.00 Algoneurodystrophy, unspecified site ▽

✓6ᵗʰ **M89.01 Algoneurodystrophy, shoulder**
     M89.011 Algoneurodystrophy, **right** shoulder
     M89.012 Algoneurodystrophy, **left** shoulder
     M89.019 Algoneurodystrophy, **unspecified** shoulder ▽

✓6ᵗʰ **M89.02 Algoneurodystrophy, upper arm**
     M89.021 Algoneurodystrophy, **right** upper arm
     M89.022 Algoneurodystrophy, **left** upper arm
     M89.029 Algoneurodystrophy, **unspecified** upper arm ▽

✓6ᵗʰ **M89.03 Algoneurodystrophy, forearm**
     M89.031 Algoneurodystrophy, **right** forearm
     M89.032 Algoneurodystrophy, **left** forearm
     M89.039 Algoneurodystrophy, **unspecified** forearm ▽

✓6ᵗʰ **M89.04 Algoneurodystrophy, hand**
     M89.041 Algoneurodystrophy, **right** hand
     M89.042 Algoneurodystrophy, **left** hand
     M89.049 Algoneurodystrophy, **unspecified** hand ▽

✓6ᵗʰ **M89.05 Algoneurodystrophy, thigh**
     M89.051 Algoneurodystrophy, **right** thigh
     M89.052 Algoneurodystrophy, **left** thigh
     M89.059 Algoneurodystrophy, **unspecified** thigh ▽

✓6ᵗʰ **M89.06 Algoneurodystrophy, lower leg**
     M89.061 Algoneurodystrophy, **right** lower leg
     M89.062 Algoneurodystrophy, **left** lower leg
     M89.069 Algoneurodystrophy, **unspecified** lower leg ▽

✓6ᵗʰ **M89.07 Algoneurodystrophy, ankle and foot**
     M89.071 Algoneurodystrophy, **right** ankle and foot
     M89.072 Algoneurodystrophy, **left** ankle and foot
     M89.079 Algoneurodystrophy, **unspecified** ankle and foot ▽

     M89.08 Algoneurodystrophy, other site
     M89.09 Algoneurodystrophy, **multiple sites**

✓ Additional Character Req   ✓x7ᵗʰ Placeholder Alert   Manifestation   `HCC` CMS-HCC Condition   ▽ Unspecified Code   ▶◀ Revised Text   ● New Code   ▲ Revised Code Title

✓5ᵗʰ **M89.1 Physeal arrest**
    Arrest of growth plate   Growth plate arrest
    Epiphyseal arrest

  ✓6ᵗʰ **M89.12 Physeal arrest, humerus**
    M89.121 Complete physeal arrest, right proximal humerus
    M89.122 Complete physeal arrest, left proximal humerus
    M89.123 Partial physeal arrest, right proximal humerus
    M89.124 Partial physeal arrest, left proximal humerus
    M89.125 Complete physeal arrest, right distal humerus
    M89.126 Complete physeal arrest, left distal humerus
    M89.127 Partial physeal arrest, right distal humerus
    M89.128 Partial physeal arrest, left distal humerus
    M89.129 Physeal arrest, humerus, unspecified ▽

  ✓6ᵗʰ **M89.13 Physeal arrest, forearm**
    M89.131 Complete physeal arrest, right distal radius
    M89.132 Complete physeal arrest, left distal radius
    M89.133 Partial physeal arrest, right distal radius
    M89.134 Partial physeal arrest, left distal radius
    M89.138 Other physeal arrest of forearm
    M89.139 Physeal arrest, forearm, unspecified ▽

  ✓6ᵗʰ **M89.15 Physeal arrest, femur**
    M89.151 Complete physeal arrest, right proximal femur
    M89.152 Complete physeal arrest, left proximal femur
    M89.153 Partial physeal arrest, right proximal femur
    M89.154 Partial physeal arrest, left proximal femur
    M89.155 Complete physeal arrest, right distal femur
    M89.156 Complete physeal arrest, left distal femur
    M89.157 Partial physeal arrest, right distal femur
    M89.158 Partial physeal arrest, left distal femur
    M89.159 Physeal arrest, femur, unspecified ▽

  ✓6ᵗʰ **M89.16 Physeal arrest, lower leg**
    M89.160 Complete physeal arrest, right proximal tibia
    M89.161 Complete physeal arrest, left proximal tibia
    M89.162 Partial physeal arrest, right proximal tibia
    M89.163 Partial physeal arrest, left proximal tibia
    M89.164 Complete physeal arrest, right distal tibia
    M89.165 Complete physeal arrest, left distal tibia
    M89.166 Partial physeal arrest, right distal tibia
    M89.167 Partial physeal arrest, left distal tibia
    M89.168 Other physeal arrest of lower leg
    M89.169 Physeal arrest, lower leg, unspecified ▽

    M89.18 Physeal arrest, other site

✓5ᵗʰ **M89.2 Other disorders of bone development and growth**
    M89.20 Other disorders of bone development and growth, unspecified site ▽

  ✓6ᵗʰ **M89.21 Other disorders of bone development and growth, shoulder**
    M89.211 Other disorders of bone development and growth, right shoulder
    M89.212 Other disorders of bone development and growth, left shoulder
    M89.219 Other disorders of bone development and growth, unspecified shoulder ▽

  ✓6ᵗʰ **M89.22 Other disorders of bone development and growth, humerus**
    M89.221 Other disorders of bone development and growth, right humerus
    M89.222 Other disorders of bone development and growth, left humerus
    M89.229 Other disorders of bone development and growth, unspecified humerus ▽

✓6ᵗʰ **M89.23 Other disorders of bone development and growth, ulna and radius**
    M89.231 Other disorders of bone development and growth, right ulna
    M89.232 Other disorders of bone development and growth, left ulna
    M89.233 Other disorders of bone development and growth, right radius
    M89.234 Other disorders of bone development and growth, left radius
    M89.239 Other disorders of bone development and growth, unspecified ulna and radius ▽

✓6ᵗʰ **M89.24 Other disorders of bone development and growth, hand**
    M89.241 Other disorders of bone development and growth, right hand
    M89.242 Other disorders of bone development and growth, left hand
    M89.249 Other disorders of bone development and growth, unspecified hand ▽

✓6ᵗʰ **M89.25 Other disorders of bone development and growth, femur**
    M89.251 Other disorders of bone development and growth, right femur
    M89.252 Other disorders of bone development and growth, left femur
    M89.259 Other disorders of bone development and growth, unspecified femur ▽

✓6ᵗʰ **M89.26 Other disorders of bone development and growth, tibia and fibula**
    M89.261 Other disorders of bone development and growth, right tibia
    M89.262 Other disorders of bone development and growth, left tibia
    M89.263 Other disorders of bone development and growth, right fibula
    M89.264 Other disorders of bone development and growth, left fibula
    M89.269 Other disorders of bone development and growth, unspecified lower leg ▽

✓6ᵗʰ **M89.27 Other disorders of bone development and growth, ankle and foot**
    M89.271 Other disorders of bone development and growth, right ankle and foot
    M89.272 Other disorders of bone development and growth, left ankle and foot
    M89.279 Other disorders of bone development and growth, unspecified ankle and foot ▽

    M89.28 Other disorders of bone development and growth, other site

    M89.29 Other disorders of bone development and growth, multiple sites

✓5ᵗʰ **M89.3 Hypertrophy of bone**
    M89.30 Hypertrophy of bone, unspecified site ▽

  ✓6ᵗʰ **M89.31 Hypertrophy of bone, shoulder**
    M89.311 Hypertrophy of bone, right shoulder
    M89.312 Hypertrophy of bone, left shoulder
    M89.319 Hypertrophy of bone, unspecified shoulder ▽

  ✓6ᵗʰ **M89.32 Hypertrophy of bone, humerus**
    M89.321 Hypertrophy of bone, right humerus
    M89.322 Hypertrophy of bone, left humerus
    M89.329 Hypertrophy of bone, unspecified humerus ▽

  ✓6ᵗʰ **M89.33 Hypertrophy of bone, ulna and radius**
    M89.331 Hypertrophy of bone, right ulna
    M89.332 Hypertrophy of bone, left ulna
    M89.333 Hypertrophy of bone, right radius
    M89.334 Hypertrophy of bone, left radius
    M89.339 Hypertrophy of bone, unspecified ulna and radius ▽

  ✓6ᵗʰ **M89.34 Hypertrophy of bone, hand**
    M89.341 Hypertrophy of bone, right hand
    M89.342 Hypertrophy of bone, left hand
    M89.349 Hypertrophy of bone, unspecified hand ▽

EXCLUDES 1 Not coded here   **EXCLUDES 2** Not included here   **N** Newborn Age: 0   **P** Pediatric Age: 0-17   **M** Maternity Age: 12-55   **A** Adult Age: 15-124

790   ICD-10-CM 2018

✓6ᵗʰ **M89.35 Hypertrophy of bone, femur**
     M89.351 Hypertrophy of bone, right femur
     M89.352 Hypertrophy of bone, left femur
     M89.359 Hypertrophy of bone, unspecified femur ▽

✓6ᵗʰ **M89.36 Hypertrophy of bone, tibia and fibula**
     M89.361 Hypertrophy of bone, right tibia
     M89.362 Hypertrophy of bone, left tibia
     M89.363 Hypertrophy of bone, right fibula
     M89.364 Hypertrophy of bone, left fibula
     M89.369 Hypertrophy of bone, unspecified tibia and fibula ▽

✓6ᵗʰ **M89.37 Hypertrophy of bone, ankle and foot**
     M89.371 Hypertrophy of bone, right ankle and foot
     M89.372 Hypertrophy of bone, left ankle and foot
     M89.379 Hypertrophy of bone, unspecified ankle and foot ▽

     M89.38 Hypertrophy of bone, other site
     M89.39 Hypertrophy of bone, multiple sites

✓5ᵗʰ **M89.4 Other hypertrophic osteoarthropathy**
     Marie-Bamberger disease   Pachydermoperiostosis
     M89.40 Other hypertrophic osteoarthropathy, unspecified site ▽

✓6ᵗʰ **M89.41 Other hypertrophic osteoarthropathy, shoulder**
     M89.411 Other hypertrophic osteoarthropathy, right shoulder
     M89.412 Other hypertrophic osteoarthropathy, left shoulder
     M89.419 Other hypertrophic osteoarthropathy, unspecified shoulder ▽

✓6ᵗʰ **M89.42 Other hypertrophic osteoarthropathy, upper arm**
     M89.421 Other hypertrophic osteoarthropathy, right upper arm
     M89.422 Other hypertrophic osteoarthropathy, left upper arm
     M89.429 Other hypertrophic osteoarthropathy, unspecified upper arm ▽

✓6ᵗʰ **M89.43 Other hypertrophic osteoarthropathy, forearm**
     M89.431 Other hypertrophic osteoarthropathy, right forearm
     M89.432 Other hypertrophic osteoarthropathy, left forearm
     M89.439 Other hypertrophic osteoarthropathy, unspecified forearm ▽

✓6ᵗʰ **M89.44 Other hypertrophic osteoarthropathy, hand**
     M89.441 Other hypertrophic osteoarthropathy, right hand
     M89.442 Other hypertrophic osteoarthropathy, left hand
     M89.449 Other hypertrophic osteoarthropathy, unspecified hand ▽

✓6ᵗʰ **M89.45 Other hypertrophic osteoarthropathy, thigh**
     M89.451 Other hypertrophic osteoarthropathy, right thigh
     M89.452 Other hypertrophic osteoarthropathy, left thigh
     M89.459 Other hypertrophic osteoarthropathy, unspecified thigh ▽

✓6ᵗʰ **M89.46 Other hypertrophic osteoarthropathy, lower leg**
     M89.461 Other hypertrophic osteoarthropathy, right lower leg
     M89.462 Other hypertrophic osteoarthropathy, left lower leg
     M89.469 Other hypertrophic osteoarthropathy, unspecified lower leg ▽

✓6ᵗʰ **M89.47 Other hypertrophic osteoarthropathy, ankle and foot**
     M89.471 Other hypertrophic osteoarthropathy, right ankle and foot
     M89.472 Other hypertrophic osteoarthropathy, left ankle and foot
     M89.479 Other hypertrophic osteoarthropathy, unspecified ankle and foot ▽

     M89.48 Other hypertrophic osteoarthropathy, other site
     M89.49 Other hypertrophic osteoarthropathy, multiple sites

✓5ᵗʰ **M89.5 Osteolysis**
     Use additional code to identify major osseous defect, if applicable (M89.7-)
     EXCLUDES 2   periprosthetic osteolysis of internal prosthetic joint (T84.Ø5-)
     M89.5Ø Osteolysis, unspecified site ▽

✓6ᵗʰ **M89.51 Osteolysis, shoulder**
     M89.511 Osteolysis, right shoulder
     M89.512 Osteolysis, left shoulder
     M89.519 Osteolysis, unspecified shoulder ▽

✓6ᵗʰ **M89.52 Osteolysis, upper arm**
     M89.521 Osteolysis, right upper arm
     M89.522 Osteolysis, left upper arm
     M89.529 Osteolysis, unspecified upper arm ▽

✓6ᵗʰ **M89.53 Osteolysis, forearm**
     M89.531 Osteolysis, right forearm
     M89.532 Osteolysis, left forearm
     M89.539 Osteolysis, unspecified forearm ▽

✓6ᵗʰ **M89.54 Osteolysis, hand**
     M89.541 Osteolysis, right hand
     M89.542 Osteolysis, left hand
     M89.549 Osteolysis, unspecified hand

✓6ᵗʰ **M89.55 Osteolysis, thigh**
     M89.551 Osteolysis, right thigh
     M89.552 Osteolysis, left thigh
     M89.559 Osteolysis, unspecified thigh ▽

✓6ᵗʰ **M89.56 Osteolysis, lower leg**
     M89.561 Osteolysis, right lower leg
     M89.562 Osteolysis, left lower leg
     M89.569 Osteolysis, unspecified lower leg ▽

✓6ᵗʰ **M89.57 Osteolysis, ankle and foot**
     M89.571 Osteolysis, right ankle and foot
     M89.572 Osteolysis, left ankle and foot
     M89.579 Osteolysis, unspecified ankle and foot ▽

     M89.58 Osteolysis, other site
     M89.59 Osteolysis, multiple sites

✓5ᵗʰ **M89.6 Osteopathy after poliomyelitis**
     Use additional code (B91) to identify previous poliomyelitis
     EXCLUDES 1   postpolio syndrome (G14)
     M89.6Ø Osteopathy after poliomyelitis, unspecified site   HCC ▽

✓6ᵗʰ **M89.61 Osteopathy after poliomyelitis, shoulder**
     M89.611 Osteopathy after poliomyelitis, right shoulder   HCC
     M89.612 Osteopathy after poliomyelitis, left shoulder   HCC
     M89.619 Osteopathy after poliomyelitis, unspecified shoulder   HCC ▽

✓6ᵗʰ **M89.62 Osteopathy after poliomyelitis, upper arm**
     M89.621 Osteopathy after poliomyelitis, right upper arm   HCC
     M89.622 Osteopathy after poliomyelitis, left upper arm   HCC
     M89.629 Osteopathy after poliomyelitis, unspecified upper arm   HCC ▽

✓6ᵗʰ **M89.63 Osteopathy after poliomyelitis, forearm**
     M89.631 Osteopathy after poliomyelitis, right forearm   HCC
     M89.632 Osteopathy after poliomyelitis, left forearm   HCC
     M89.639 Osteopathy after poliomyelitis, unspecified forearm   HCC ▽

✓6ᵗʰ **M89.64 Osteopathy after poliomyelitis, hand**
     M89.641 Osteopathy after poliomyelitis, right hand   HCC
     M89.642 Osteopathy after poliomyelitis, left hand   HCC
     M89.649 Osteopathy after poliomyelitis, unspecified hand   HCC ▽

✓6ᵗʰ **M89.65 Osteopathy after poliomyelitis, thigh**
     M89.651 Osteopathy after poliomyelitis, right thigh   HCC
     M89.652 Osteopathy after poliomyelitis, left thigh   HCC

✓ Additional Character Req   ✓×7ᵗʰ Placeholder Alert   Manifestation   HCC CMS-HCC Condition   ▽ Unspecified Code   ►◄ Revised Text   ● New Code   ▲ Revised Code Title

ICD-10-CM 2018   **791**

M89.659   Osteopathy after poliomyelitis, unspecified thigh   `HCC` ▽

✓6ᵗʰ M89.66   **Osteopathy after poliomyelitis, lower leg**

    M89.661   Osteopathy after poliomyelitis, right lower leg   `HCC`

    M89.662   Osteopathy after poliomyelitis, left lower leg   `HCC`

    M89.669   Osteopathy after poliomyelitis, unspecified lower leg   `HCC` ▽

✓6ᵗʰ M89.67   **Osteopathy after poliomyelitis, ankle and foot**

    M89.671   Osteopathy after poliomyelitis, right ankle and foot   `HCC`

    M89.672   Osteopathy after poliomyelitis, left ankle and foot   `HCC`

    M89.679   Osteopathy after poliomyelitis, unspecified ankle and foot   `HCC` ▽

   M89.68   Osteopathy after poliomyelitis, other site   `HCC`

   M89.69   Osteopathy after poliomyelitis, multiple sites   `HCC`

✓5ᵗʰ M89.7   **Major osseous defect**

    Code first underlying disease, if known, such as:
     aseptic necrosis of bone (M87.-)
     malignant neoplasm of bone (C40.-)
     osteolysis (M89.5)
     osteomyelitis (M86.-)
     osteonecrosis (M87.-)
     osteoporosis (M80.-, M81.-)
     periprosthetic osteolysis (T84.05-)

   M89.70   **Major osseous defect, unspecified site** ▽

✓6ᵗʰ M89.71   **Major osseous defect, shoulder region**
     Major osseous defect clavicle or scapula

    M89.711   Major osseous defect, right shoulder region

    M89.712   Major osseous defect, left shoulder region

    M89.719   Major osseous defect, unspecified shoulder region ▽

✓6ᵗʰ M89.72   **Major osseous defect, humerus**

    M89.721   Major osseous defect, right humerus

    M89.722   Major osseous defect, left humerus

    M89.729   Major osseous defect, unspecified humerus ▽

✓6ᵗʰ M89.73   **Major osseous defect, forearm**
     Major osseous defect of radius and ulna

    M89.731   Major osseous defect, right forearm

    M89.732   Major osseous defect, left forearm

    M89.739   Major osseous defect, unspecified forearm ▽

✓6ᵗʰ M89.74   **Major osseous defect, hand**
     Major osseous defect of carpus, fingers, metacarpus

    M89.741   Major osseous defect, right hand

    M89.742   Major osseous defect, left hand

    M89.749   Major osseous defect, unspecified hand ▽

✓6ᵗʰ M89.75   **Major osseous defect, pelvic region and thigh**
     Major osseous defect of femur and pelvis

    M89.751   Major osseous defect, right pelvic region and thigh

    M89.752   Major osseous defect, left pelvic region and thigh

    M89.759   Major osseous defect, unspecified pelvic region and thigh ▽

✓6ᵗʰ M89.76   **Major osseous defect, lower leg**
     Major osseous defect of fibula and tibia

    M89.761   Major osseous defect, right lower leg

    M89.762   Major osseous defect, left lower leg

    M89.769   Major osseous defect, unspecified lower leg ▽

✓6ᵗʰ M89.77   **Major osseous defect, ankle and foot**
     Major osseous defect of metatarsus, tarsus, toes

    M89.771   Major osseous defect, right ankle and foot

    M89.772   Major osseous defect, left ankle and foot

    M89.779   Major osseous defect, unspecified ankle and foot ▽

   M89.78   Major osseous defect, other site

   M89.79   Major osseous defect, multiple sites

✓5ᵗʰ M89.8   **Other specified disorders of bone**
     Infantile cortical hyperostoses
     Post-traumatic subperiosteal ossification

✓6ᵗʰ M89.8X   **Other specified disorders of bone**

    M89.8X0   Other specified disorders of bone, multiple sites

    M89.8X1   Other specified disorders of bone, shoulder

    M89.8X2   Other specified disorders of bone, upper arm

    M89.8X3   Other specified disorders of bone, forearm

    M89.8X4   Other specified disorders of bone, hand

    M89.8X5   Other specified disorders of bone, thigh

    M89.8X6   Other specified disorders of bone, lower leg

    M89.8X7   Other specified disorders of bone, ankle and foot

    M89.8X8   Other specified disorders of bone, other site

    M89.8X9   Other specified disorders of bone, unspecified site ▽

   M89.9   Disorder of bone, unspecified ▽

✓4ᵗʰ **M90 Osteopathies in diseases classified elsewhere**

   `EXCLUDES 1`   *osteochondritis, osteomyelitis, and osteopathy (in):*
     cryptococcosis (B45.3)
     diabetes mellitus (E08-E13 with .69-)
     gonococcal (A54.43)
     neurogenic syphilis (A52.11)
     renal osteodystrophy (N25.0)
     salmonellosis (A02.24)
     secondary syphilis (A51.46)
     syphilis (late) (A52.77)

✓5ᵗʰ M90.5   **Osteonecrosis in diseases classified elsewhere**
     Code first underlying disease, such as:
     caisson disease (T70.3)
     hemoglobinopathy (D50-D64)

   M90.50   *Osteonecrosis in diseases classified elsewhere, unspecified site*   `HCC` ▽

✓6ᵗʰ M90.51   **Osteonecrosis in diseases classified elsewhere, shoulder**

    M90.511   *Osteonecrosis in diseases classified elsewhere, right shoulder*   `HCC`

    M90.512   *Osteonecrosis in diseases classified elsewhere, left shoulder*   `HCC`

    M90.519   *Osteonecrosis in diseases classified elsewhere, unspecified shoulder*   `HCC` ▽

✓6ᵗʰ M90.52   **Osteonecrosis in diseases classified elsewhere, upper arm**

    M90.521   *Osteonecrosis in diseases classified elsewhere, right upper arm*   `HCC`

    M90.522   *Osteonecrosis in diseases classified elsewhere, left upper arm*   `HCC`

    M90.529   *Osteonecrosis in diseases classified elsewhere, unspecified upper arm*   `HCC` ▽

✓6ᵗʰ M90.53   **Osteonecrosis in diseases classified elsewhere, forearm**

    M90.531   *Osteonecrosis in diseases classified elsewhere, right forearm*   `HCC`

    M90.532   *Osteonecrosis in diseases classified elsewhere, left forearm*   `HCC`

    M90.539   *Osteonecrosis in diseases classified elsewhere, unspecified forearm*   `HCC` ▽

✓6ᵗʰ M90.54   **Osteonecrosis in diseases classified elsewhere, hand**

    M90.541   *Osteonecrosis in diseases classified elsewhere, right hand*   `HCC`

    M90.542   *Osteonecrosis in diseases classified elsewhere, left hand*   `HCC`

    M90.549   *Osteonecrosis in diseases classified elsewhere, unspecified hand*   `HCC` ▽

✓6ᵗʰ M90.55   **Osteonecrosis in diseases classified elsewhere, thigh**

    M90.551   *Osteonecrosis in diseases classified elsewhere, right thigh*   `HCC`

    M90.552   *Osteonecrosis in diseases classified elsewhere, left thigh*   `HCC`

    M90.559   *Osteonecrosis in diseases classified elsewhere, unspecified thigh*   `HCC` ▽

`EXCLUDES 1` Not coded here   `EXCLUDES 2` Not included here   **N** Newborn Age: 0   **P** Pediatric Age: 0-17   **M** Maternity Age: 12-55   **A** Adult Age: 15-124

792
ICD-10-CM 2018

✓6ᵗʰ **M90.56 Osteonecrosis in diseases classified elsewhere, lower leg**
   M90.561 Osteonecrosis in diseases classified elsewhere, right lower leg HCC
   M90.562 Osteonecrosis in diseases classified elsewhere, left lower leg HCC
   M90.569 Osteonecrosis in diseases classified elsewhere, unspecified lower leg HCC ▽

✓6ᵗʰ **M90.57 Osteonecrosis in diseases classified elsewhere, ankle and foot**
   M90.571 Osteonecrosis in diseases classified elsewhere, right ankle and foot HCC
   M90.572 Osteonecrosis in diseases classified elsewhere, left ankle and foot HCC
   M90.579 Osteonecrosis in diseases classified elsewhere, unspecified ankle and foot HCC ▽

M90.58 Osteonecrosis in diseases classified elsewhere, other site HCC

M90.59 Osteonecrosis in diseases classified elsewhere, multiple sites HCC

✓5ᵗʰ **M90.6 Osteitis deformans in neoplastic diseases**
  Osteitis deformans in malignant neoplasm of bone
  Code first the neoplasm (C40-, C41-)
  EXCLUDES 1   *osteitis deformans [Paget's disease of bone] (M88.-)*

M90.60 Osteitis deformans in neoplastic diseases, unspecified site ▽

✓6ᵗʰ **M90.61 Osteitis deformans in neoplastic diseases, shoulder**
  M90.611 Osteitis deformans in neoplastic diseases, right shoulder
  M90.612 Osteitis deformans in neoplastic diseases, left shoulder
  M90.619 Osteitis deformans in neoplastic diseases, unspecified shoulder ▽

✓6ᵗʰ **M90.62 Osteitis deformans in neoplastic diseases, upper arm**
  M90.621 Osteitis deformans in neoplastic diseases, right upper arm
  M90.622 Osteitis deformans in neoplastic diseases, left upper arm
  M90.629 Osteitis deformans in neoplastic diseases, unspecified upper arm ▽

✓6ᵗʰ **M90.63 Osteitis deformans in neoplastic diseases, forearm**
  M90.631 Osteitis deformans in neoplastic diseases, right forearm
  M90.632 Osteitis deformans in neoplastic diseases, left forearm
  M90.639 Osteitis deformans in neoplastic diseases, unspecified forearm ▽

✓6ᵗʰ **M90.64 Osteitis deformans in neoplastic diseases, hand**
  M90.641 Osteitis deformans in neoplastic diseases, right hand
  M90.642 Osteitis deformans in neoplastic diseases, left hand
  M90.649 Osteitis deformans in neoplastic diseases, unspecified hand ▽

✓6ᵗʰ **M90.65 Osteitis deformans in neoplastic diseases, thigh**
  M90.651 Osteitis deformans in neoplastic diseases, right thigh
  M90.652 Osteitis deformans in neoplastic diseases, left thigh
  M90.659 Osteitis deformans in neoplastic diseases, unspecified thigh ▽

✓6ᵗʰ **M90.66 Osteitis deformans in neoplastic diseases, lower leg**
  M90.661 Osteitis deformans in neoplastic diseases, right lower leg
  M90.662 Osteitis deformans in neoplastic diseases, left lower leg
  M90.669 Osteitis deformans in neoplastic diseases, unspecified lower leg ▽

✓6ᵗʰ **M90.67 Osteitis deformans in neoplastic diseases, ankle and foot**
  M90.671 Osteitis deformans in neoplastic diseases, right ankle and foot
  M90.672 Osteitis deformans in neoplastic diseases, left ankle and foot
  M90.679 Osteitis deformans in neoplastic diseases, unspecified ankle and foot ▽

M90.68 Osteitis deformans in neoplastic diseases, other site

M90.69 Osteitis deformans in neoplastic diseases, multiple sites

✓5ᵗʰ **M90.8 Osteopathy in diseases classified elsewhere**
  Code first underlying disease, such as:
  rickets (E55.0)
  vitamin-D-resistant rickets (E83.3)

M90.80 Osteopathy in diseases classified elsewhere, unspecified site ▽

✓6ᵗʰ **M90.81 Osteopathy in diseases classified elsewhere, shoulder**
  M90.811 Osteopathy in diseases classified elsewhere, right shoulder
  M90.812 Osteopathy in diseases classified elsewhere, left shoulder
  M90.819 Osteopathy in diseases classified elsewhere, unspecified shoulder ▽

✓6ᵗʰ **M90.82 Osteopathy in diseases classified elsewhere, upper arm**
  M90.821 Osteopathy in diseases classified elsewhere, right upper arm
  M90.822 Osteopathy in diseases classified elsewhere, left upper arm
  M90.829 Osteopathy in diseases classified elsewhere, unspecified upper arm ▽

✓6ᵗʰ **M90.83 Osteopathy in diseases classified elsewhere, forearm**
  M90.831 Osteopathy in diseases classified elsewhere, right forearm
  M90.832 Osteopathy in diseases classified elsewhere, left forearm
  M90.839 Osteopathy in diseases classified elsewhere, unspecified forearm ▽

✓6ᵗʰ **M90.84 Osteopathy in diseases classified elsewhere, hand**
  M90.841 Osteopathy in diseases classified elsewhere, right hand
  M90.842 Osteopathy in diseases classified elsewhere, left hand
  M90.849 Osteopathy in diseases classified elsewhere, unspecified hand ▽

✓6ᵗʰ **M90.85 Osteopathy in diseases classified elsewhere, thigh**
  M90.851 Osteopathy in diseases classified elsewhere, right thigh
  M90.852 Osteopathy in diseases classified elsewhere, left thigh
  M90.859 Osteopathy in diseases classified elsewhere, unspecified thigh ▽

✓6ᵗʰ **M90.86 Osteopathy in diseases classified elsewhere, lower leg**
  M90.861 Osteopathy in diseases classified elsewhere, right lower leg
  M90.862 Osteopathy in diseases classified elsewhere, left lower leg
  M90.869 Osteopathy in diseases classified elsewhere, unspecified lower leg ▽

✓6ᵗʰ **M90.87 Osteopathy in diseases classified elsewhere, ankle and foot**
  M90.871 Osteopathy in diseases classified elsewhere, right ankle and foot
  M90.872 Osteopathy in diseases classified elsewhere, left ankle and foot
  M90.879 Osteopathy in diseases classified elsewhere, unspecified ankle and foot ▽

M90.88 Osteopathy in diseases classified elsewhere, other site

M90.89 Osteopathy in diseases classified elsewhere, multiple sites

Chondropathies (M91-M94)

EXCLUDES 1   *postprocedural chondropathies (M96.-)*

✓4ᵗʰ **M91 Juvenile osteochondrosis of hip and pelvis**
  EXCLUDES 1   *slipped upper femoral epiphysis (nontraumatic) (M93.0)*

M91.0 Juvenile osteochondrosis of pelvis
  Osteochondrosis (juvenile) of acetabulum
  Osteochondrosis (juvenile) of iliac crest [Buchanan]
  Osteochondrosis (juvenile) of ischiopubic synchondrosis [van Neck]
  Osteochondrosis (juvenile) of symphysis pubis [Pierson]

✔ Additional Character Req   ✓x7ᵗʰ Placeholder Alert   Manifestation   HCC CMS-HCC Condition   ▽ Unspecified Code   ►◄ Revised Text   ● New Code   ▲ Revised Code Title

ICD-10-CM 2018   793

✓5ᵗʰ **M91.1 Juvenile osteochondrosis of head of femur [Legg-Calvé-Perthes]**

     M91.10 Juvenile osteochondrosis of head of femur [Legg-Calvé-Perthes], unspecified leg ▽

     M91.11 Juvenile osteochondrosis of head of femur [Legg-Calvé-Perthes], right leg

     M91.12 Juvenile osteochondrosis of head of femur [Legg-Calvé-Perthes], left leg

✓5ᵗʰ **M91.2 Coxa plana**

     Hip deformity due to previous juvenile osteochondrosis

     M91.20 Coxa plana, unspecified hip ▽

     M91.21 Coxa plana, right hip

     M91.22 Coxa plana, left hip

✓5ᵗʰ **M91.3 Pseudocoxalgia**

     M91.30 Pseudocoxalgia, unspecified hip ▽

     M91.31 Pseudocoxalgia, right hip

     M91.32 Pseudocoxalgia, left hip

✓5ᵗʰ **M91.4 Coxa magna**

     M91.40 Coxa magna, unspecified hip ▽

     M91.41 Coxa magna, right hip

     M91.42 Coxa magna, left hip

✓5ᵗʰ **M91.8 Other juvenile osteochondrosis of hip and pelvis**

     Juvenile osteochondrosis after reduction of congenital dislocation of hip

     M91.80 Other juvenile osteochondrosis of hip and pelvis, unspecified leg ▽

     M91.81 Other juvenile osteochondrosis of hip and pelvis, right leg

     M91.82 Other juvenile osteochondrosis of hip and pelvis, left leg

✓5ᵗʰ **M91.9 Juvenile osteochondrosis of hip and pelvis, unspecified**

     M91.90 Juvenile osteochondrosis of hip and pelvis, unspecified, unspecified leg ▽

     M91.91 Juvenile osteochondrosis of hip and pelvis, unspecified, right leg ▽

     M91.92 Juvenile osteochondrosis of hip and pelvis, unspecified, left leg ▽

✓4ᵗʰ **M92 Other juvenile osteochondrosis**

✓5ᵗʰ **M92.0 Juvenile osteochondrosis of humerus**

     Osteochondrosis (juvenile) of capitulum of humerus [Panner]
     Osteochondrosis (juvenile) of head of humerus [Haas]

     M92.00 Juvenile osteochondrosis of humerus, unspecified arm ▽

     M92.01 Juvenile osteochondrosis of humerus, right arm

     M92.02 Juvenile osteochondrosis of humerus, left arm

✓5ᵗʰ **M92.1 Juvenile osteochondrosis of radius and ulna**

     Osteochondrosis (juvenile) of lower ulna [Burns]
     Osteochondrosis (juvenile) of radial head [Brailsford]

     M92.10 Juvenile osteochondrosis of radius and ulna, unspecified arm ▽

     M92.11 Juvenile osteochondrosis of radius and ulna, right arm

     M92.12 Juvenile osteochondrosis of radius and ulna, left arm

✓5ᵗʰ **M92.2 Juvenile osteochondrosis, hand**

     ✓6ᵗʰ **M92.20** Unspecified juvenile osteochondrosis, hand

         M92.201 Unspecified juvenile osteochondrosis, right hand ▽

         M92.202 Unspecified juvenile osteochondrosis, left hand ▽

         M92.209 Unspecified juvenile osteochondrosis, unspecified hand ▽

     ✓6ᵗʰ **M92.21** Osteochondrosis (juvenile) of carpal lunate [Kienböck]

         M92.211 Osteochondrosis (juvenile) of carpal lunate [Kienböck], right hand

         M92.212 Osteochondrosis (juvenile) of carpal lunate [Kienböck], left hand

         M92.219 Osteochondrosis (juvenile) of carpal lunate [Kienböck], unspecified hand ▽

     ✓6ᵗʰ **M92.22** Osteochondrosis (juvenile) of metacarpal heads [Mauclaire]

         M92.221 Osteochondrosis (juvenile) of metacarpal heads [Mauclaire], right hand

         M92.222 Osteochondrosis (juvenile) of metacarpal heads [Mauclaire], left hand

         M92.229 Osteochondrosis (juvenile) of metacarpal heads [Mauclaire], unspecified hand ▽

     ✓6ᵗʰ **M92.29** Other juvenile osteochondrosis, hand

         M92.291 Other juvenile osteochondrosis, right hand

         M92.292 Other juvenile osteochondrosis, left hand

         M92.299 Other juvenile osteochondrosis, unspecified hand ▽

✓5ᵗʰ **M92.3 Other juvenile osteochondrosis, upper limb**

     M92.30 Other juvenile osteochondrosis, unspecified upper limb ▽

     M92.31 Other juvenile osteochondrosis, right upper limb

     M92.32 Other juvenile osteochondrosis, left upper limb

✓5ᵗʰ **M92.4 Juvenile osteochondrosis of patella**

     Osteochondrosis (juvenile) of primary patellar center [Köhler]
     Osteochondrosis (juvenile) of secondary patellar centre [Sinding Larsen]

     M92.40 Juvenile osteochondrosis of patella, unspecified knee ▽

     M92.41 Juvenile osteochondrosis of patella, right knee

     M92.42 Juvenile osteochondrosis of patella, left knee

✓5ᵗʰ **M92.5 Juvenile osteochondrosis of tibia and fibula**

     Osteochondrosis (juvenile) of proximal tibia [Blount]
     Osteochondrosis (juvenile) of tibial tubercle [Osgood-Schlatter]
     Tibia vara

     M92.50 Juvenile osteochondrosis of tibia and fibula, unspecified leg ▽

     M92.51 Juvenile osteochondrosis of tibia and fibula, right leg

     M92.52 Juvenile osteochondrosis of tibia and fibula, left leg

✓5ᵗʰ **M92.6 Juvenile osteochondrosis of tarsus**

     Osteochondrosis (juvenile) of calcaneum [Sever]
     Osteochondrosis (juvenile) of os tibiale externum [Haglund]
     Osteochondrosis (juvenile) of talus [Diaz]
     Osteochondrosis (juvenile) of tarsal navicular [Köhler]

     M92.60 Juvenile osteochondrosis of tarsus, unspecified ankle ▽

     M92.61 Juvenile osteochondrosis of tarsus, right ankle

     M92.62 Juvenile osteochondrosis of tarsus, left ankle

✓5ᵗʰ **M92.7 Juvenile osteochondrosis of metatarsus**

     Osteochondrosis (juvenile) of fifth metatarsus [Iselin]
     Osteochondrosis (juvenile) of second metatarsus [Freiberg]

     M92.70 Juvenile osteochondrosis of metatarsus, unspecified foot ▽

     M92.71 Juvenile osteochondrosis of metatarsus, right foot

     M92.72 Juvenile osteochondrosis of metatarsus, left foot

     M92.8 Other specified juvenile osteochondrosis

     Calcaneal apophysitis

     M92.9 Juvenile osteochondrosis, unspecified ▽

     Juvenile apophysitis NOS
     Juvenile epiphysitis NOS
     Juvenile osteochondritis NOS
     Juvenile osteochondrosis NOS

✓4ᵗʰ **M93 Other osteochondropathies**

     EXCLUDES 2   osteochondrosis of spine (M42.-)

✓5ᵗʰ **M93.0 Slipped upper femoral epiphysis (nontraumatic)**

     Use additional code for associated chondrolysis (M94.3)

     ✓6ᵗʰ **M93.00** Unspecified slipped upper femoral epiphysis (nontraumatic)

         M93.001 Unspecified slipped upper femoral epiphysis (nontraumatic), right hip ▽

         M93.002 Unspecified slipped upper femoral epiphysis (nontraumatic), left hip ▽

         M93.003 Unspecified slipped upper femoral epiphysis (nontraumatic), unspecified hip ▽

     ✓6ᵗʰ **M93.01** Acute slipped upper femoral epiphysis (nontraumatic)

         M93.011 Acute slipped upper femoral epiphysis (nontraumatic), right hip

         M93.012 Acute slipped upper femoral epiphysis (nontraumatic), left hip

         M93.013 Acute slipped upper femoral epiphysis (nontraumatic), unspecified hip ▽

EXCLUDES 1 Not coded here   **EXCLUDES 2** Not included here   **N** Newborn Age: 0   **P** Pediatric Age: 0-17   **M** Maternity Age: 12-55   **A** Adult Age: 15-124

794   ICD-10-CM 2018

☑6ᵗʰ **M93.02** **Chronic slipped upper femoral epiphysis (nontraumatic)**
     M93.021 **Chronic slipped upper femoral epiphysis (nontraumatic), right hip**
     M93.022 **Chronic slipped upper femoral epiphysis (nontraumatic), left hip**
     M93.023 **Chronic slipped upper femoral epiphysis (nontraumatic), unspecified hip** ▽

☑6ᵗʰ **M93.03** **Acute on chronic slipped upper femoral epiphysis (nontraumatic)**
     M93.031 **Acute on chronic slipped upper femoral epiphysis (nontraumatic), right hip**
     M93.032 **Acute on chronic slipped upper femoral epiphysis (nontraumatic), left hip**
     M93.033 **Acute on chronic slipped upper femoral epiphysis (nontraumatic), unspecified hip** ▽

M93.1 **Kienböck's disease of adults** 🄰
     Adult osteochondrosis of carpal lunates

☑5ᵗʰ **M93.2** **Osteochondritis dissecans**
     M93.20 **Osteochondritis dissecans of unspecified site** ▽

☑6ᵗʰ **M93.21** **Osteochondritis dissecans of shoulder**
     M93.211 **Osteochondritis dissecans, right shoulder**
     M93.212 **Osteochondritis dissecans, left shoulder**
     M93.219 **Osteochondritis dissecans, unspecified shoulder** ▽

☑6ᵗʰ **M93.22** **Osteochondritis dissecans of elbow**
     M93.221 **Osteochondritis dissecans, right elbow**
     M93.222 **Osteochondritis dissecans, left elbow**
     M93.229 **Osteochondritis dissecans, unspecified elbow** ▽

☑6ᵗʰ **M93.23** **Osteochondritis dissecans of wrist**
     M93.231 **Osteochondritis dissecans, right wrist**
     M93.232 **Osteochondritis dissecans, left wrist**
     M93.239 **Osteochondritis dissecans, unspecified wrist** ▽

☑6ᵗʰ **M93.24** **Osteochondritis dissecans of joints of hand**
     M93.241 **Osteochondritis dissecans, joints of right hand**
     M93.242 **Osteochondritis dissecans, joints of left hand**
     M93.249 **Osteochondritis dissecans, joints of unspecified hand** ▽

☑6ᵗʰ **M93.25** **Osteochondritis dissecans of hip**
     M93.251 **Osteochondritis dissecans, right hip**
     M93.252 **Osteochondritis dissecans, left hip**
     M93.259 **Osteochondritis dissecans, unspecified hip** ▽

☑6ᵗʰ **M93.26** **Osteochondritis dissecans knee**
     M93.261 **Osteochondritis dissecans, right knee**
     M93.262 **Osteochondritis dissecans, left knee**
     M93.269 **Osteochondritis dissecans, unspecified knee** ▽

☑6ᵗʰ **M93.27** **Osteochondritis dissecans of ankle and joints of foot**
     M93.271 **Osteochondritis dissecans, right ankle and joints of right foot**
     M93.272 **Osteochondritis dissecans, left ankle and joints of left foot**
     M93.279 **Osteochondritis dissecans, unspecified ankle and joints of foot** ▽

     M93.28 **Osteochondritis dissecans other site**
     M93.29 **Osteochondritis dissecans multiple sites**

☑5ᵗʰ **M93.8** **Other specified osteochondropathies**
     M93.80 **Other specified osteochondropathies of unspecified site** ▽

☑6ᵗʰ **M93.81** **Other specified osteochondropathies of shoulder**
     M93.811 **Other specified osteochondropathies, right shoulder**
     M93.812 **Other specified osteochondropathies, left shoulder**
     M93.819 **Other specified osteochondropathies, unspecified shoulder** ▽

☑6ᵗʰ **M93.82** **Other specified osteochondropathies of upper arm**
     M93.821 **Other specified osteochondropathies, right upper arm**
     M93.822 **Other specified osteochondropathies, left upper arm**
     M93.829 **Other specified osteochondropathies, unspecified upper arm** ▽

☑6ᵗʰ **M93.83** **Other specified osteochondropathies of forearm**
     M93.831 **Other specified osteochondropathies, right forearm**
     M93.832 **Other specified osteochondropathies, left forearm**
     M93.839 **Other specified osteochondropathies, unspecified forearm** ▽

☑6ᵗʰ **M93.84** **Other specified osteochondropathies of hand**
     M93.841 **Other specified osteochondropathies, right hand**
     M93.842 **Other specified osteochondropathies, left hand**
     M93.849 **Other specified osteochondropathies, unspecified hand** ▽

☑6ᵗʰ **M93.85** **Other specified osteochondropathies of thigh**
     M93.851 **Other specified osteochondropathies, right thigh**
     M93.852 **Other specified osteochondropathies, left thigh**
     M93.859 **Other specified osteochondropathies, unspecified thigh** ▽

☑6ᵗʰ **M93.86** **Other specified osteochondropathies lower leg**
     M93.861 **Other specified osteochondropathies, right lower leg**
     M93.862 **Other specified osteochondropathies, left lower leg**
     M93.869 **Other specified osteochondropathies, unspecified lower leg** ▽

☑6ᵗʰ **M93.87** **Other specified osteochondropathies of ankle and foot**
     M93.871 **Other specified osteochondropathies, right ankle and foot**
     M93.872 **Other specified osteochondropathies, left ankle and foot**
     M93.879 **Other specified osteochondropathies, unspecified ankle and foot** ▽

     M93.88 **Other specified osteochondropathies other site**
     M93.89 **Other specified osteochondropathies multiple sites**

☑5ᵗʰ **M93.9** **Osteochondropathy, unspecified**
     Apophysitis NOS   Osteochondritis NOS
     Epiphysitis NOS   Osteochondrosis NOS

     M93.90 **Osteochondropathy, unspecified of unspecified site** ▽

☑6ᵗʰ **M93.91** **Osteochondropathy, unspecified of shoulder**
     M93.911 **Osteochondropathy, unspecified, right shoulder** ▽
     M93.912 **Osteochondropathy, unspecified, left shoulder** ▽
     M93.919 **Osteochondropathy, unspecified, unspecified shoulder** ▽

☑6ᵗʰ **M93.92** **Osteochondropathy, unspecified of upper arm**
     M93.921 **Osteochondropathy, unspecified, right upper arm** ▽
     M93.922 **Osteochondropathy, unspecified, left upper arm** ▽
     M93.929 **Osteochondropathy, unspecified, unspecified upper arm** ▽

☑6ᵗʰ **M93.93** **Osteochondropathy, unspecified of forearm**
     M93.931 **Osteochondropathy, unspecified, right forearm** ▽
     M93.932 **Osteochondropathy, unspecified, left forearm** ▽
     M93.939 **Osteochondropathy, unspecified, unspecified forearm** ▽

☑6ᵗʰ **M93.94** **Osteochondropathy, unspecified of hand**
     M93.941 **Osteochondropathy, unspecified, right hand** ▽
     M93.942 **Osteochondropathy, unspecified, left hand** ▽
     M93.949 **Osteochondropathy, unspecified, unspecified hand** ▽

☑ Additional Character Req   ☑ˣ⁷ᵗʰ Placeholder Alert   Manifestation   HCC CMS-HCC Condition   ▽ Unspecified Code   ►◄ Revised Text   ● New Code   ▲ Revised Code Title

√6ᵗʰ M93.95 Osteochondropathy, unspecified of thigh
- M93.951 Osteochondropathy, unspecified, **right thigh** ▽
- M93.952 Osteochondropathy, unspecified, **left thigh** ▽
- M93.959 Osteochondropathy, unspecified, unspecified thigh ▽

√6ᵗʰ M93.96 Osteochondropathy, unspecified lower leg
- M93.961 Osteochondropathy, unspecified, **right lower leg** ▽
- M93.962 Osteochondropathy, unspecified, **left lower leg** ▽
- M93.969 Osteochondropathy, unspecified, unspecified lower leg ▽

√6ᵗʰ M93.97 Osteochondropathy, unspecified of ankle and foot
- M93.971 Osteochondropathy, unspecified, **right ankle and foot** ▽
- M93.972 Osteochondropathy, unspecified, **left ankle and foot** ▽
- M93.979 Osteochondropathy, unspecified, unspecified ankle and foot ▽

M93.98 Osteochondropathy, unspecified other site ▽
M93.99 Osteochondropathy, unspecified **multiple sites** ▽

√4ᵗʰ M94 Other disorders of cartilage
M94.0 Chondrocostal junction syndrome [Tietze]
    Costochondritis
M94.1 Relapsing polychondritis

√5ᵗʰ M94.2 Chondromalacia
    EXCLUDES 1   chondromalacia patellae (M22.4)
- M94.20 Chondromalacia, unspecified site ▽
- **√6ᵗʰ M94.21 Chondromalacia, shoulder**
  - M94.211 Chondromalacia, **right** shoulder
  - M94.212 Chondromalacia, **left** shoulder
  - M94.219 Chondromalacia, unspecified shoulder ▽
- **√6ᵗʰ M94.22 Chondromalacia, elbow**
  - M94.221 Chondromalacia, **right** elbow
  - M94.222 Chondromalacia, **left** elbow
  - M94.229 Chondromalacia, unspecified elbow ▽
- **√6ᵗʰ M94.23 Chondromalacia, wrist**
  - M94.231 Chondromalacia, **right** wrist
  - M94.232 Chondromalacia, **left** wrist
  - M94.239 Chondromalacia, unspecified wrist ▽
- **√6ᵗʰ M94.24 Chondromalacia, joints of hand**
  - M94.241 Chondromalacia, joints of **right** hand
  - M94.242 Chondromalacia, joints of **left** hand
  - M94.249 Chondromalacia, joints of unspecified hand ▽
- **√6ᵗʰ M94.25 Chondromalacia, hip**
  - M94.251 Chondromalacia, **right** hip
  - M94.252 Chondromalacia, **left** hip
  - M94.259 Chondromalacia, unspecified hip ▽
- **√6ᵗʰ M94.26 Chondromalacia, knee**
  - M94.261 Chondromalacia, **right** knee
  - M94.262 Chondromalacia, **left** knee
  - M94.269 Chondromalacia, unspecified knee ▽
- **√6ᵗʰ M94.27 Chondromalacia, ankle and joints of foot**
  - M94.271 Chondromalacia, **right** ankle and joints of right foot
  - M94.272 Chondromalacia, **left** ankle and joints of left foot
  - M94.279 Chondromalacia, unspecified ankle and joints of foot ▽
- M94.28 Chondromalacia, other site
- M94.29 Chondromalacia, **multiple sites**

√5ᵗʰ M94.3 Chondrolysis
    Code first any associated slipped upper femoral epiphysis (nontraumatic) (M93.0-)
- **√6ᵗʰ M94.35 Chondrolysis, hip**
  - M94.351 Chondrolysis, **right hip**
  - M94.352 Chondrolysis, **left hip**
  - M94.359 Chondrolysis, unspecified hip ▽

√5ᵗʰ M94.8 Other specified disorders of cartilage
- **√6ᵗʰ M94.8X Other specified disorders of cartilage**
  - M94.8X0 Other specified disorders of cartilage, **multiple sites**
  - M94.8X1 Other specified disorders of cartilage, **shoulder**
  - M94.8X2 Other specified disorders of cartilage, **upper arm**
  - M94.8X3 Other specified disorders of cartilage, **forearm**
  - M94.8X4 Other specified disorders of cartilage, **hand**
  - M94.8X5 Other specified disorders of cartilage, **thigh**
  - M94.8X6 Other specified disorders of cartilage, **lower leg**
  - M94.8X7 Other specified disorders of cartilage, **ankle and foot**
  - M94.8X8 Other specified disorders of cartilage, **other site**
  - M94.8X9 Other specified disorders of cartilage, **unspecified sites** ▽

M94.9 Disorder of cartilage, unspecified ▽

Other disorders of the musculoskeletal system and connective tissue (M95)

√4ᵗʰ M95 Other acquired deformities of musculoskeletal system and connective tissue
    EXCLUDES 2   acquired absence of limbs and organs (Z89-Z90)
         acquired deformities of limbs (M20-M21)
         congenital malformations and deformations of the musculoskeletal system (Q65-Q79)
         deforming dorsopathies (M40-M43)
         dentofacial anomalies [including malocclusion] (M26.-)
         postprocedural musculoskeletal disorders (M96.-)

M95.0 Acquired deformity of nose
    EXCLUDES 2   deviated nasal septum (J34.2)

√5ᵗʰ M95.1 Cauliflower ear
    EXCLUDES 2   other acquired deformities of ear (H61.1)
    DEF: Acquired deformity of the external ear; due to injury, subsequent perichondritis.
- M95.10 Cauliflower ear, unspecified ear ▽
- M95.11 Cauliflower ear, **right** ear
- M95.12 Cauliflower ear, **left** ear

M95.2 Other acquired **deformity of head**
M95.3 Acquired **deformity of neck**
M95.4 Acquired **deformity of chest and rib**
    AHA: 2014, 4Q, 26-27
M95.5 Acquired **deformity of pelvis**
    EXCLUDES 1   maternal care for known or suspected disproportion (O33.-)
M95.8 Other specified acquired deformities of musculoskeletal system
M95.9 Acquired deformity of musculoskeletal system, unspecified ▽

Intraoperative and postprocedural complications and disorders of musculoskeletal system, not elsewhere classified (M96)

√4ᵗʰ M96 Intraoperative and postprocedural complications and disorders of musculoskeletal system, not elsewhere classified
    EXCLUDES 2   arthropathy following intestinal bypass (M02.0-)
         complications of internal orthopedic prosthetic devices, implants and grafts (T84.-)
         disorders associated with osteoporosis (M80)
         periprosthetic fracture around internal prosthetic joint (M97.-)
         presence of functional implants and other devices (Z96-Z97)

M96.0 **Pseudarthrosis after fusion or arthrodesis**
M96.1 **Postlaminectomy syndrome, not elsewhere classified**
M96.2 **Postradiation kyphosis**
M96.3 **Postlaminectomy kyphosis**
M96.4 **Postsurgical lordosis**
M96.5 **Postradiation scoliosis**

EXCLUDES 1 Not coded here   EXCLUDES 2 Not included here   N Newborn Age: 0   P Pediatric Age: 0-17   M Maternity Age: 12-55   A Adult Age: 15-124

√5ᵗʰ **M96.6 Fracture of bone following insertion of orthopedic implant, joint prosthesis, or bone plate**
Intraoperative fracture of bone during insertion of orthopedic implant, joint prosthesis, or bone plate
EXCLUDES 2   *complication of internal orthopedic devices, implants or grafts (T84.-)*

   √6ᵗʰ **M96.62 Fracture of humerus following insertion of orthopedic implant, joint prosthesis, or bone plate**
     M96.621 Fracture of humerus following insertion of orthopedic implant, joint prosthesis, or bone plate, right arm   HCC
     M96.622 Fracture of humerus following insertion of orthopedic implant, joint prosthesis, or bone plate, left arm   HCC
     M96.629 Fracture of humerus following insertion of orthopedic implant, joint prosthesis, or bone plate, unspecified arm   HCC ▽

   √6ᵗʰ **M96.63 Fracture of radius or ulna following insertion of orthopedic implant, joint prosthesis, or bone plate**
     M96.631 Fracture of radius or ulna following insertion of orthopedic implant, joint prosthesis, or bone plate, right arm   HCC
     M96.632 Fracture of radius or ulna following insertion of orthopedic implant, joint prosthesis, or bone plate, left arm   HCC
     M96.639 Fracture of radius or ulna following insertion of orthopedic implant, joint prosthesis, or bone plate, unspecified arm   HCC ▽

   M96.65 Fracture of pelvis following insertion of orthopedic implant, joint prosthesis, or bone plate   HCC

   √6ᵗʰ **M96.66 Fracture of femur following insertion of orthopedic implant, joint prosthesis, or bone plate**
     M96.661 Fracture of femur following insertion of orthopedic implant, joint prosthesis, or bone plate, right leg   HCC
     M96.662 Fracture of femur following insertion of orthopedic implant, joint prosthesis, or bone plate, left leg   HCC
     M96.669 Fracture of femur following insertion of orthopedic implant, joint prosthesis, or bone plate, unspecified leg   HCC ▽

   √6ᵗʰ **M96.67 Fracture of tibia or fibula following insertion of orthopedic implant, joint prosthesis, or bone plate**
     M96.671 Fracture of tibia or fibula following insertion of orthopedic implant, joint prosthesis, or bone plate, right leg   HCC
     M96.672 Fracture of tibia or fibula following insertion of orthopedic implant, joint prosthesis, or bone plate, left leg   HCC
     M96.679 Fracture of tibia or fibula following insertion of orthopedic implant, joint prosthesis, or bone plate, unspecified leg   HCC ▽

   M96.69 Fracture of other bone following insertion of orthopedic implant, joint prosthesis, or bone plate   HCC

√5ᵗʰ **M96.8 Other intraoperative and postprocedural complications and disorders of musculoskeletal system, not elsewhere classified**

   √6ᵗʰ **M96.81 Intraoperative hemorrhage and hematoma of a musculoskeletal structure complicating a procedure**
     EXCLUDES 1   *intraoperative hemorrhage and hematoma of a musculoskeletal structure due to accidental puncture and laceration during a procedure (M96.82-)*
     M96.810 Intraoperative hemorrhage and hematoma of a musculoskeletal structure complicating a musculoskeletal system procedure
     M96.811 Intraoperative hemorrhage and hematoma of a musculoskeletal structure complicating other procedure

   √6ᵗʰ **M96.82 Accidental puncture and laceration of a musculoskeletal structure during a procedure**
     M96.820 Accidental puncture and laceration of a musculoskeletal structure during a musculoskeletal system procedure
     M96.821 Accidental puncture and laceration of a musculoskeletal structure during other procedure

   √6ᵗʰ **M96.83 Postprocedural hemorrhage of a musculoskeletal structure following a procedure**
     M96.830 Postprocedural hemorrhage of a musculoskeletal structure following a musculoskeletal system procedure
     M96.831 Postprocedural hemorrhage of a musculoskeletal structure following other procedure

   √6ᵗʰ **M96.84 Postprocedural hematoma and seroma of a musculoskeletal structure following a procedure**
     M96.840 Postprocedural hematoma of a musculoskeletal structure following a musculoskeletal system procedure
     M96.841 Postprocedural hematoma of a musculoskeletal structure following other procedure
     M96.842 Postprocedural seroma of a musculoskeletal structure following a musculoskeletal system procedure
     M96.843 Postprocedural seroma of a musculoskeletal structure following other procedure

   M96.89 Other intraoperative and postprocedural complications and disorders of the musculoskeletal system
     Instability of joint secondary to removal of joint prosthesis
     Use additional code, if applicable, to further specify disorder

Periprosthetic fracture around internal prosthetic joint (M97)

√4ᵗʰ **M97 Periprosthetic fracture around internal prosthetic joint**
     EXCLUDES 2   *breakage (fracture) of prosthetic joint (T84.01-)*
               fracture of bone following insertion of orthopedic implant, joint prosthesis or bone plate (M96.6-)

> The appropriate 7th character is to be added to each code from category M97.
> A   initial encounter
> D   subsequent encounter
> S   sequela

√5ᵗʰ **M97.0 Periprosthetic fracture around internal prosthetic hip joint**
   [1] √x7ᵗʰ **M97.01 Periprosthetic fracture around internal prosthetic right hip joint**   HCC
   [1] √x7ᵗʰ **M97.02 Periprosthetic fracture around internal prosthetic left hip joint**   HCC

√5ᵗʰ **M97.1 Periprosthetic fracture around internal prosthetic knee joint**
   √x7ᵗʰ **M97.11 Periprosthetic fracture around internal prosthetic right knee joint**
   √x7ᵗʰ **M97.12 Periprosthetic fracture around internal prosthetic left knee joint**

√5ᵗʰ **M97.2 Periprosthetic fracture around internal prosthetic ankle joint**
   √x7ᵗʰ **M97.21 Periprosthetic fracture around internal prosthetic right ankle joint**
   √x7ᵗʰ **M97.22 Periprosthetic fracture around internal prosthetic left ankle joint**

√5ᵗʰ **M97.3 Periprosthetic fracture around internal prosthetic shoulder joint**
   √x7ᵗʰ **M97.31 Periprosthetic fracture around internal prosthetic right shoulder joint**
   √x7ᵗʰ **M97.32 Periprosthetic fracture around internal prosthetic left shoulder joint**

√5ᵗʰ **M97.4 Periprosthetic fracture around internal prosthetic elbow joint**
   √x7ᵗʰ **M97.41 Periprosthetic fracture around internal prosthetic right elbow joint**
   √x7ᵗʰ **M97.42 Periprosthetic fracture around internal prosthetic left elbow joint**

√x7ᵗʰ **M97.8 Periprosthetic fracture around other internal prosthetic joint**
   Periprosthetic fracture around internal prosthetic finger joint
   Periprosthetic fracture around internal prosthetic spinal joint
   Periprosthetic fracture around internal prosthetic toe joint
   Periprosthetic fracture around internal prosthetic wrist joint
   Use additional code to identify the joint (Z96.6-)

√x7ᵗʰ **M97.9 Periprosthetic fracture around unspecified internal prosthetic joint**   ▽

---

[1] HCC with 7th character indicating initial encounter (A, B or C - specific to category).

✔ Additional Character Req   √x7ᵗʰ Placeholder Alert   Manifestation   HCC CMS-HCC Condition   ▽ Unspecified Code   ►◄ Revised Text   ● New Code   ▲ Revised Code Title

Biomechanical lesions, not elsewhere classified (M99)

✓4ᵗʰ M99 Biomechanical lesions, not elsewhere classified

> **NOTE** This category should not be used if the condition can be classified elsewhere.

✓5ᵗʰ M99.0 Segmental and somatic dysfunction

- M99.00 Segmental and somatic dysfunction of **head region**
- M99.01 Segmental and somatic dysfunction of **cervical region**
- M99.02 Segmental and somatic dysfunction of **thoracic region**
- M99.03 Segmental and somatic dysfunction of **lumbar region**
- M99.04 Segmental and somatic dysfunction of **sacral region**
- M99.05 Segmental and somatic dysfunction of **pelvic region**
- M99.06 Segmental and somatic dysfunction of **lower extremity**
- M99.07 Segmental and somatic dysfunction of **upper extremity**
- M99.08 Segmental and somatic dysfunction of **rib cage**
- M99.09 Segmental and somatic dysfunction of **abdomen and other regions**

✓5ᵗʰ M99.1 Subluxation complex (vertebral)

- M99.10 Subluxation complex (vertebral) of **head region**
- M99.11 Subluxation complex (vertebral) of **cervical** region
- M99.12 Subluxation complex (vertebral) of **thoracic** region
- M99.13 Subluxation complex (vertebral) of **lumbar** region
- M99.14 Subluxation complex (vertebral) of **sacral** region
- M99.15 Subluxation complex (vertebral) of **pelvic** region
- M99.16 Subluxation complex (vertebral) of **lower extremity**
- M99.17 Subluxation complex (vertebral) of **upper extremity**
- M99.18 Subluxation complex (vertebral) of **rib cage**
- M99.19 Subluxation complex (vertebral) of **abdomen and other regions**

✓5ᵗʰ M99.2 Subluxation stenosis of neural canal

- M99.20 Subluxation stenosis of neural canal of **head region**
- M99.21 Subluxation stenosis of neural canal of **cervical region**
- M99.22 Subluxation stenosis of neural canal of **thoracic region**
- M99.23 Subluxation stenosis of neural canal of **lumbar region**
- M99.24 Subluxation stenosis of neural canal of **sacral region**
- M99.25 Subluxation stenosis of neural canal of **pelvic region**
- M99.26 Subluxation stenosis of neural canal of **lower extremity**
- M99.27 Subluxation stenosis of neural canal of **upper extremity**
- M99.28 Subluxation stenosis of neural canal of **rib cage**
- M99.29 Subluxation stenosis of neural canal of **abdomen and other regions**

✓5ᵗʰ M99.3 Osseous stenosis of neural canal

- M99.30 Osseous stenosis of neural canal of **head region**
- M99.31 Osseous stenosis of neural canal of **cervical region**
- M99.32 Osseous stenosis of neural canal of **thoracic region**
- M99.33 Osseous stenosis of neural canal of **lumbar region**
- M99.34 Osseous stenosis of neural canal of **sacral region**
- M99.35 Osseous stenosis of neural canal of **pelvic region**
- M99.36 Osseous stenosis of neural canal of **lower extremity**
- M99.37 Osseous stenosis of neural canal of **upper extremity**
- M99.38 Osseous stenosis of neural canal of **rib cage**
- M99.39 Osseous stenosis of neural canal of **abdomen and other regions**

✓5ᵗʰ M99.4 Connective tissue stenosis of neural canal

- M99.40 Connective tissue stenosis of neural canal of **head region**
- M99.41 Connective tissue stenosis of neural canal of **cervical region**
- M99.42 Connective tissue stenosis of neural canal of **thoracic region**
- M99.43 Connective tissue stenosis of neural canal of **lumbar region**
- M99.44 Connective tissue stenosis of neural canal of **sacral region**
- M99.45 Connective tissue stenosis of neural canal of **pelvic region**
- M99.46 Connective tissue stenosis of neural canal of **lower extremity**
- M99.47 Connective tissue stenosis of neural canal of **upper extremity**
- M99.48 Connective tissue stenosis of neural canal of **rib cage**
- M99.49 Connective tissue stenosis of neural canal of **abdomen and other** regions

✓5ᵗʰ M99.5 Intervertebral disc stenosis of neural canal

- M99.50 Intervertebral disc stenosis of neural canal of **head region**
- M99.51 Intervertebral disc stenosis of neural canal of **cervical region**
- M99.52 Intervertebral disc stenosis of neural canal of **thoracic region**
- M99.53 Intervertebral disc stenosis of neural canal of **lumbar region**
- M99.54 Intervertebral disc stenosis of neural canal of **sacral region**
- M99.55 Intervertebral disc stenosis of neural canal of **pelvic region**
- M99.56 Intervertebral disc stenosis of neural canal of **lower extremity**
- M99.57 Intervertebral disc stenosis of neural canal of **upper extremity**
- M99.58 Intervertebral disc stenosis of neural canal of **rib cage**
- M99.59 Intervertebral disc stenosis of neural canal of **abdomen and other** regions

✓5ᵗʰ M99.6 Osseous and subluxation stenosis of intervertebral foramina

- M99.60 Osseous and subluxation stenosis of intervertebral foramina of **head region**
- M99.61 Osseous and subluxation stenosis of intervertebral foramina of **cervical region**
- M99.62 Osseous and subluxation stenosis of intervertebral foramina of **thoracic region**
- M99.63 Osseous and subluxation stenosis of intervertebral foramina of **lumbar region**
- M99.64 Osseous and subluxation stenosis of intervertebral foramina of **sacral region**
- M99.65 Osseous and subluxation stenosis of intervertebral foramina of **pelvic region**
- M99.66 Osseous and subluxation stenosis of intervertebral foramina of **lower extremity**
- M99.67 Osseous and subluxation stenosis of intervertebral foramina of **upper extremity**
- M99.68 Osseous and subluxation stenosis of intervertebral foramina of **rib cage**
- M99.69 Osseous and subluxation stenosis of intervertebral foramina of **abdomen and other** regions

✓5ᵗʰ M99.7 Connective tissue and disc stenosis of intervertebral foramina

- M99.70 Connective tissue and disc stenosis of intervertebral foramina of **head region**
- M99.71 Connective tissue and disc stenosis of intervertebral foramina of **cervical region**
- M99.72 Connective tissue and disc stenosis of intervertebral foramina of **thoracic region**
- M99.73 Connective tissue and disc stenosis of intervertebral foramina of **lumbar region**
- M99.74 Connective tissue and disc stenosis of intervertebral foramina of **sacral region**
- M99.75 Connective tissue and disc stenosis of intervertebral foramina of **pelvic region**

EXCLUDES 1 Not coded here   **EXCLUDES 2** Not included here   **N** Newborn Age: 0   **P** Pediatric Age: 0-17   **M** Maternity Age: 12-55   **A** Adult Age: 15-124

798   ICD-10-CM 2018

M99.76 Connective tissue and disc stenosis of intervertebral foramina of **lower extremity**

M99.77 Connective tissue and disc stenosis of intervertebral foramina of **upper extremity**

M99.78 Connective tissue and disc stenosis of intervertebral foramina of **rib cage**

M99.79 Connective tissue and disc stenosis of intervertebral foramina of **abdomen and other regions**

 M99.8 Other biomechanical lesions

M99.80 Other biomechanical lesions of **head region**

M99.81 Other biomechanical lesions of **cervical region**

M99.82 Other biomechanical lesions of **thoracic region**

M99.83 Other biomechanical lesions of **lumbar region**

M99.84 Other biomechanical lesions of **sacral region**

M99.85 Other biomechanical lesions of **pelvic region**

M99.86 Other biomechanical lesions of **lower extremity**

M99.87 Other biomechanical lesions of **upper extremity**

M99.88 Other biomechanical lesions of **rib cage**

M99.89 Other biomechanical lesions of **abdomen and other regions**

M99.9 Biomechanical lesion, unspecified   ▽

☑ Additional Character Req   ✓x7ʰ Placeholder Alert   Manifestation   HCC CMS-HCC Condition   ▽ Unspecified Code   ▶◀ Revised Text   ● New Code   ▲ Revised Code Title

Chapter 14. Diseases of Genitourinary System (NØØ–N99)

Chapter Specific Guidelines with Coding Examples

The chapter specific guidelines from the ICD-10-CM Official Guidelines for Coding and Reporting have been provided below. Along with these guidelines are coding examples, contained in the shaded boxes, that have been developed to help illustrate the coding and/or sequencing guidance found in these guidelines.

a. Chronic kidney disease

1) Stages of chronic kidney disease (CKD)

The ICD-10-CM classifies CKD based on severity. The severity of CKD is designated by stages 1-5. Stage 2, code N18.2, equates to mild CKD; stage 3, code N18.3, equates to moderate CKD; and stage 4, code N18.4, equates to severe CKD. Code N18.6, End stage renal disease (ESRD), is assigned when the provider has documented end-stage-renal disease (ESRD).

If both a stage of CKD and ESRD are documented, assign code N18.6 only.

> Stage 5 chronic kidney disease with ESRD requiring chronic dialysis
>
> **N18.6   End stage renal disease**
>
> **Z99.2   Dependence on renal dialysis**
>
> *Explanation:* The diagnostic statement indicates the patient has chronic kidney disease, documented both as stage 5 and as ESRD requiring chronic dialysis. Code N18.6 End stage renal disease (ESRD), is assigned when the provider has documented end-stage-renal disease (ESRD). If both a stage of CKD and ESRD are documented, assign code N18.6 only.

2) Chronic kidney disease and kidney transplant status

Patients who have undergone kidney transplant may still have some form of chronic kidney disease (CKD) because the kidney transplant may not fully restore kidney function. Therefore, the presence of CKD alone does not constitute a transplant complication. Assign the appropriate N18 code for the patient's stage of CKD and code Z94.Ø, Kidney transplant status. If a transplant complication such as failure or rejection or other transplant complication is documented, see section I.C.19.g for information on coding complications of a kidney transplant. If the documentation is unclear as to whether the patient has a complication of the transplant, query the provider.

> Patient with residual chronic kidney disease stage 1 after kidney transplant
>
> **N18.1   Chronic kidney disease, stage 1**
>
> **Z94.Ø   Kidney transplant status**
>
> *Explanation:* Patients who have undergone kidney transplant may still have some form of chronic kidney disease (CKD) because the kidney transplant may not fully restore kidney function. The presence of CKD alone does not constitute a transplant complication. Assign the appropriate N18 code for the patient's stage of CKD and code Z94.Ø Kidney transplant status.

3) Chronic kidney disease with other conditions

Patients with CKD may also suffer from other serious conditions, most commonly diabetes mellitus and hypertension. The sequencing of the CKD code in relationship to codes for other contributing conditions is based on the conventions in the Tabular List.

See I.C.9. Hypertensive chronic kidney disease.

See I.C.19. Chronic kidney disease and kidney transplant complications.

> Type 1 diabetic chronic kidney disease, stage 2
>
> **E1Ø.22   Type 1 diabetes mellitus with diabetic chronic kidney disease**
>
> **N18.2   Chronic kidney disease, stage 2 (mild)**
>
> *Explanation:* Patients with CKD may also suffer from other serious conditions such as diabetes mellitus. The sequencing of the CKD code in relationship to codes for other contributing conditions is based on the conventions in the Tabular List. Diabetic CKD code E1Ø.22 includes an instructional note to "Use additional code to identify stage of chronic kidney disease (N18.1–N18.6)," thus providing sequencing direction.

Chapter 14. Diseases of the Genitourinary System (N00-N99)

EXCLUDES 2	certain conditions originating in the perinatal period (P04-P96)

certain conditions originating in the perinatal period (P04-P96)
certain infectious and parasitic diseases (A00-B99)
complications of pregnancy, childbirth and the puerperium (O00-O9A)
congenital malformations, deformations and chromosomal abnormalities (Q00-Q99)
endocrine, nutritional and metabolic diseases (E00-E88)
injury, poisoning and certain other consequences of external causes (S00-T88)
neoplasms (C00-D49)
symptoms, signs and abnormal clinical and laboratory findings, not elsewhere classified (R00-R94)

This chapter contains the following blocks:

N00-N08   Glomerular diseases
N10-N16   Renal tubulo-interstitial diseases
N17-N19   Acute kidney failure and chronic kidney disease
N20-N23   Urolithiasis
N25-N29   Other disorders of kidney and ureter
N30-N39   Other diseases of the urinary system
N40-N53   Diseases of male genital organs
N60-N65   Disorders of breast
N70-N77   Inflammatory diseases of female pelvic organs
N80-N98   Noninflammatory disorders of female genital tract
N99   Intraoperative and postprocedural complications and disorders of genitourinary system, not elsewhere classified

Glomerular diseases (N00-N08)

Code also any associated kidney failure (N17-N19)

EXCLUDES 1   hypertensive chronic kidney disease (I12.-)

✓4th N00 Acute nephritic syndrome
INCLUDES   acute glomerular disease
acute glomerulonephritis
acute nephritis

EXCLUDES 1   acute tubulo-interstitial nephritis (N10)
nephritic syndrome NOS (N05.-)

N00.0 Acute nephritic syndrome with minor glomerular abnormality
Acute nephritic syndrome with minimal change lesion

N00.1 Acute nephritic syndrome with focal and segmental glomerular lesions
Acute nephritic syndrome with focal and segmental hyalinosis
Acute nephritic syndrome with focal and segmental sclerosis
Acute nephritic syndrome with focal glomerulonephritis

N00.2 Acute nephritic syndrome with diffuse membranous glomerulonephritis

N00.3 Acute nephritic syndrome with diffuse mesangial proliferative glomerulonephritis

N00.4 Acute nephritic syndrome with diffuse endocapillary proliferative glomerulonephritis

N00.5 Acute nephritic syndrome with diffuse mesangiocapillary glomerulonephritis
Acute nephritic syndrome with membranoproliferative glomerulonephritis, types 1 and 3, or NOS

N00.6 Acute nephritic syndrome with dense deposit disease
Acute nephritic syndrome with membranoproliferative glomerulonephritis, type 2

N00.7 Acute nephritic syndrome with diffuse crescentic glomerulonephritis
Acute nephritic syndrome with extracapillary glomerulonephritis

N00.8 Acute nephritic syndrome with other morphologic changes
Acute nephritic syndrome with proliferative glomerulonephritis NOS

N00.9 Acute nephritic syndrome with unspecified morphologic ▽ changes

✓4th N01 Rapidly progressive nephritic syndrome
INCLUDES   rapidly progressive glomerular disease
rapidly progressive glomerulonephritis
rapidly progressive nephritis

EXCLUDES 1   nephritic syndrome NOS (N05.-)

N01.0 Rapidly progressive nephritic syndrome with minor glomerular abnormality
Rapidly progressive nephritic syndrome with minimal change lesion

N01.1 Rapidly progressive nephritic syndrome with focal and segmental glomerular lesions
Rapidly progressive nephritic syndrome with focal and segmental hyalinosis
Rapidly progressive nephritic syndrome with focal and segmental sclerosis
Rapidly progressive nephritic syndrome with focal glomerulonephritis

N01.2 Rapidly progressive nephritic syndrome with diffuse membranous glomerulonephritis

N01.3 Rapidly progressive nephritic syndrome with diffuse mesangial proliferative glomerulonephritis

N01.4 Rapidly progressive nephritic syndrome with diffuse endocapillary proliferative glomerulonephritis

N01.5 Rapidly progressive nephritic syndrome with diffuse mesangiocapillary glomerulonephritis
Rapidly progressive nephritic syndrome with membranoproliferative glomerulonephritis, types 1 and 3, or NOS

N01.6 Rapidly progressive nephritic syndrome with dense deposit disease
Rapidly progressive nephritic syndrome with membranoproliferative glomerulonephritis, type 2

N01.7 Rapidly progressive nephritic syndrome with diffuse crescentic glomerulonephritis
Rapidly progressive nephritic syndrome with extracapillary glomerulonephritis

N01.8 Rapidly progressive nephritic syndrome with other morphologic changes
Rapidly progressive nephritic syndrome with proliferative glomerulonephritis NOS

N01.9 Rapidly progressive nephritic syndrome with unspecified ▽ morphologic changes

✓4th N02 Recurrent and persistent hematuria
EXCLUDES 1   acute cystitis with hematuria (N30.01)
hematuria NOS (R31.9)
hematuria not associated with specified morphologic lesions (R31.-)

N02.0 Recurrent and persistent hematuria with minor glomerular abnormality
Recurrent and persistent hematuria with minimal change lesion

N02.1 Recurrent and persistent hematuria with focal and segmental glomerular lesions
Recurrent and persistent hematuria with focal and segmental hyalinosis
Recurrent and persistent hematuria with focal and segmental sclerosis
Recurrent and persistent hematuria with focal glomerulonephritis

N02.2 Recurrent and persistent hematuria with diffuse membranous glomerulonephritis

N02.3 Recurrent and persistent hematuria with diffuse mesangial proliferative glomerulonephritis

N02.4 Recurrent and persistent hematuria with diffuse endocapillary proliferative glomerulonephritis

N02.5 Recurrent and persistent hematuria with diffuse mesangiocapillary glomerulonephritis
Recurrent and persistent hematuria with membranoproliferative glomerulonephritis, types 1 and 3, or NOS

N02.6 Recurrent and persistent hematuria with dense deposit disease
Recurrent and persistent hematuria with membranoproliferative glomerulonephritis, type 2

N02.7 Recurrent and persistent hematuria with diffuse crescentic glomerulonephritis
Recurrent and persistent hematuria with extracapillary glomerulonephritis

N02.8 Recurrent and persistent hematuria with other morphologic changes
Recurrent and persistent hematuria with proliferative glomerulonephritis NOS

N02.9 Recurrent and persistent hematuria with unspecified ▽ morphologic changes
AHA: 2017, 2Q, 5

| EXCLUDES 1 Not coded here | EXCLUDES 2 Not included here | N Newborn Age: 0 | P Pediatric Age: 0-17 | M Maternity Age: 12-55 | A Adult Age: 15-124 |

802   ICD-10-CM 2018

☑4ᵗʰ **N03 Chronic nephritic syndrome**
     INCLUDES   chronic glomerular disease
                  chronic glomerulonephritis
                  chronic nephritis
     EXCLUDES 1   *chronic tubulo-interstitial nephritis (N11.-)*
                  diffuse sclerosing glomerulonephritis (N05.8-)
                  nephritic syndrome NOS (N05.-)
     DEF: Slow, progressive type of nephritis characterized by inflammation of the capillary loops in the glomeruli of the kidney, which leads to renal failure.

     N03.0 Chronic nephritic syndrome with minor glomerular abnormality
           Chronic nephritic syndrome with minimal change lesion

     N03.1 Chronic nephritic syndrome with focal and segmental glomerular lesions
           Chronic nephritic syndrome with focal and segmental hyalinosis
           Chronic nephritic syndrome with focal and segmental sclerosis
           Chronic nephritic syndrome with focal glomerulonephritis

     N03.2 Chronic nephritic syndrome with diffuse membranous glomerulonephritis

     N03.3 Chronic nephritic syndrome with diffuse mesangial proliferative glomerulonephritis

     N03.4 Chronic nephritic syndrome with diffuse endocapillary proliferative glomerulonephritis

     N03.5 Chronic nephritic syndrome with diffuse mesangiocapillary glomerulonephritis
           Chronic nephritic syndrome with membranoproliferative glomerulonephritis, types 1 and 3, or NOS

     N03.6 Chronic nephritic syndrome with dense deposit disease
           Chronic nephritic syndrome with membranoproliferative glomerulonephritis, type 2

     N03.7 Chronic nephritic syndrome with diffuse crescentic glomerulonephritis
           Chronic nephritic syndrome with extracapillary glomerulonephritis

     N03.8 Chronic nephritic syndrome with other morphologic changes
           Chronic nephritic syndrome with proliferative glomerulonephritis NOS

     N03.9 Chronic nephritic syndrome with unspecified morphologic changes ▽

☑4ᵗʰ **N04 Nephrotic syndrome**
     INCLUDES   congenital nephrotic syndrome
                  lipoid nephrosis

     N04.0 Nephrotic syndrome with minor glomerular abnormality
           Nephrotic syndrome with minimal change lesion

     N04.1 Nephrotic syndrome with focal and segmental glomerular lesions
           Nephrotic syndrome with focal and segmental hyalinosis
           Nephrotic syndrome with focal and segmental sclerosis
           Nephrotic syndrome with focal glomerulonephritis

     N04.2 Nephrotic syndrome with diffuse membranous glomerulonephritis

     N04.3 Nephrotic syndrome with diffuse mesangial proliferative glomerulonephritis

     N04.4 Nephrotic syndrome with diffuse endocapillary proliferative glomerulonephritis

     N04.5 Nephrotic syndrome with diffuse mesangiocapillary glomerulonephritis
           Nephrotic syndrome with membranoproliferative glomerulonephritis, types 1 and 3, or NOS

     N04.6 Nephrotic syndrome with dense deposit disease
           Nephrotic syndrome with membranoproliferative glomerulonephritis, type 2

     N04.7 Nephrotic syndrome with diffuse crescentic glomerulonephritis
           Nephrotic syndrome with extracapillary glomerulonephritis

     N04.8 Nephrotic syndrome with other morphologic changes
           Nephrotic syndrome with proliferative glomerulonephritis NOS

     N04.9 Nephrotic syndrome with unspecified morphologic changes ▽

☑4ᵗʰ **N05 Unspecified nephritic syndrome**
     INCLUDES   glomerular disease NOS
                  glomerulonephritis NOS
                  nephritis NOS
                  nephropathy NOS and renal disease NOS with morphological lesion specified in .0-.8
     EXCLUDES 1   *nephropathy NOS with no stated morphological lesion (N28.9)*
                  renal disease NOS with no stated morphological lesion (N28.9)
                  tubulo-interstitial nephritis NOS (N12)

     N05.0 Unspecified nephritic syndrome with minor glomerular abnormality ▽
           Unspecified nephritic syndrome with minimal change lesion

     N05.1 Unspecified nephritic syndrome with focal and segmental glomerular lesions ▽
           Unspecified nephritic syndrome with focal and segmental hyalinosis
           Unspecified nephritic syndrome with focal and segmental sclerosis
           Unspecified nephritic syndrome with focal glomerulonephritis

     N05.2 Unspecified nephritic syndrome with diffuse membranous glomerulonephritis ▽

     N05.3 Unspecified nephritic syndrome with diffuse mesangial proliferative glomerulonephritis ▽

     N05.4 Unspecified nephritic syndrome with diffuse endocapillary proliferative glomerulonephritis ▽

     N05.5 Unspecified nephritic syndrome with diffuse mesangiocapillary glomerulonephritis ▽
           Unspecified nephritic syndrome with membranoproliferative glomerulonephritis, types 1 and 3, or NOS

     N05.6 Unspecified nephritic syndrome with dense deposit disease ▽
           Unspecified nephritic syndrome with membranoproliferative glomerulonephritis, type 2

     N05.7 Unspecified nephritic syndrome with diffuse crescentic glomerulonephritis ▽
           Unspecified nephritic syndrome with extracapillary glomerulonephritis

     N05.8 Unspecified nephritic syndrome with other morphologic changes ▽
           Unspecified nephritic syndrome with proliferative glomerulonephritis NOS

     N05.9 Unspecified nephritic syndrome with unspecified morphologic changes ▽

☑4ᵗʰ **N06 Isolated proteinuria with specified morphological lesion**
     EXCLUDES 1   *proteinuria not associated with specific morphologic lesions (R80.0)*

     N06.0 Isolated proteinuria with minor glomerular abnormality
           Isolated proteinuria with minimal change lesion

     N06.1 Isolated proteinuria with focal and segmental glomerular lesions
           Isolated proteinuria with focal and segmental hyalinosis
           Isolated proteinuria with focal and segmental sclerosis
           Isolated proteinuria with focal glomerulonephritis

     N06.2 Isolated proteinuria with diffuse membranous glomerulonephritis

     N06.3 Isolated proteinuria with diffuse mesangial proliferative glomerulonephritis

     N06.4 Isolated proteinuria with diffuse endocapillary proliferative glomerulonephritis

     N06.5 Isolated proteinuria with diffuse mesangiocapillary glomerulonephritis
           Isolated proteinuria with membranoproliferative glomerulonephritis, types 1 and 3, or NOS

     N06.6 Isolated proteinuria with dense deposit disease
           Isolated proteinuria with membranoproliferative glomerulonephritis, type 2

     N06.7 Isolated proteinuria with diffuse crescentic glomerulonephritis
           Isolated proteinuria with extracapillary glomerulonephritis

     N06.8 Isolated proteinuria with other morphologic lesion
           Isolated proteinuria with proliferative glomerulonephritis NOS

     N06.9 Isolated proteinuria with unspecified morphologic lesion ▽

☑ Additional Character Req   ✔x7ᵗʰ Placeholder Alert   Manifestation   HCC CMS-HCC Condition   ▽ Unspecified Code   ►◄ Revised Text   ● New Code   ▲ Revised Code Title

ICD-10-CM 2018   803

☑4ᵗʰ N07 Hereditary nephropathy, not elsewhere classified

EXCLUDES 2   Alport's syndrome (Q87.81-)
              hereditary amyloid nephropathy (E85.-)
              nail patella syndrome (Q87.2)
              non-neuropathic heredofamilial amyloidosis (E85.-)

N07.0 Hereditary nephropathy, not elsewhere classified with minor glomerular abnormality
Hereditary nephropathy, not elsewhere classified with minimal change lesion

N07.1 Hereditary nephropathy, not elsewhere classified with focal and segmental glomerular lesions
Hereditary nephropathy, not elsewhere classified with focal and segmental hyalinosis
Hereditary nephropathy, not elsewhere classified with focal and segmental sclerosis
Hereditary nephropathy, not elsewhere classified with focal glomerulonephritis

N07.2 Hereditary nephropathy, not elsewhere classified with diffuse membranous glomerulonephritis

N07.3 Hereditary nephropathy, not elsewhere classified with diffuse mesangial proliferative glomerulonephritis

N07.4 Hereditary nephropathy, not elsewhere classified with diffuse endocapillary proliferative glomerulonephritis

N07.5 Hereditary nephropathy, not elsewhere classified with diffuse mesangiocapillary glomerulonephritis
Hereditary nephropathy, not elsewhere classified with membranoproliferative glomerulonephritis, types 1 and 3, or NOS

N07.6 Hereditary nephropathy, not elsewhere classified with dense deposit disease
Hereditary nephropathy, not elsewhere classified with membranoproliferative glomerulonephritis, type 2

N07.7 Hereditary nephropathy, not elsewhere classified with diffuse crescentic glomerulonephritis
Hereditary nephropathy, not elsewhere classified with extracapillary glomerulonephritis

N07.8 Hereditary nephropathy, not elsewhere classified with other morphologic lesions
Hereditary nephropathy, not elsewhere classified with proliferative glomerulonephritis NOS

N07.9 Hereditary nephropathy, not elsewhere classified with unspecified morphologic lesions   ▽

N08 *Glomerular disorders in diseases classified elsewhere*
Glomerulonephritis
Nephritis
Nephropathy
Code first underlying disease, such as:
amyloidosis (E85.-)
congenital syphilis (A50.5)
cryoglobulinemia (D89.1)
disseminated intravascular coagulation (D65)
gout (M1A.-, M10.-)
microscopic polyangiitis (M31.7)
multiple myeloma (C90.0-)
sepsis (A40.0-A41.9)
sickle-cell disease (D57.0-D57.8)

EXCLUDES 1   glomerulonephritis, nephritis and nephropathy (in):
              antiglomerular basement membrane disease (M31.0)
              diabetes (E08-E13 with .21)
              gonococcal (A54.21)
              Goodpasture's syndrome (M31.0)
              hemolytic-uremic syndrome (D59.3)
              lupus (M32.14)
              mumps (B26.83)
              syphilis (A52.75)
              systemic lupus erythematosus (M32.14)
              Wegener's granulomatosis (M31.31)
              pyelonephritis in diseases classified elsewhere (N16)
              renal tubulo-interstitial disorders classified elsewhere (N16)

Renal tubulo-interstitial diseases (N10-N16)

INCLUDES   pyelonephritis
EXCLUDES 1 pyeloureteritis cystica (N28.85)

N10 Acute pyelonephritis
Acute infectious interstitial nephritis
Acute pyelitis
Acute tubulo-interstitial nephritis
Hemoglobin nephrosis
Myoglobin nephrosis
Use additional code (B95-B97), to identify infectious agent

☑4ᵗʰ N11 Chronic tubulo-interstitial nephritis

INCLUDES   chronic infectious interstitial nephritis
            chronic pyelitis
            chronic pyelonephritis
Use additional code (B95-B97), to identify infectious agent

N11.0 Nonobstructive reflux-associated chronic pyelonephritis
Pyelonephritis (chronic) associated with (vesicoureteral) reflux
EXCLUDES 1   vesicoureteral reflux NOS (N13.70)

N11.1 Chronic obstructive pyelonephritis
Pyelonephritis (chronic) associated with anomaly of pelviureteric junction
Pyelonephritis (chronic) associated with anomaly of pyeloureteric junction
Pyelonephritis (chronic) associated with crossing of vessel
Pyelonephritis (chronic) associated with kinking of ureter
Pyelonephritis (chronic) associated with obstruction of ureter
Pyelonephritis (chronic) associated with stricture of pelviureteric junction
Pyelonephritis (chronic) associated with stricture of ureter
EXCLUDES 1   calculous pyelonephritis (N20.9)
              obstructive uropathy (N13.-)

N11.8 Other chronic tubulo-interstitial nephritis
Nonobstructive chronic pyelonephritis NOS

N11.9 Chronic tubulo-interstitial nephritis, unspecified   ▽
Chronic interstitial nephritis NOS
Chronic pyelitis NOS
Chronic pyelonephritis NOS

N12 Tubulo-interstitial nephritis, not specified as acute or chronic
Interstitial nephritis NOS
Pyelitis NOS
Pyelonephritis NOS
EXCLUDES 1   calculous pyelonephritis (N20.9)

☑4ᵗʰ N13 Obstructive and reflux uropathy
EXCLUDES 2   calculus of kidney and ureter without hydronephrosis (N20.-)
              congenital obstructive defects of renal pelvis and ureter (Q62.0-Q62.3)
              hydronephrosis with ureteropelvic junction obstruction ▶(Q62.11)◀
              obstructive pyelonephritis (N11.1)

N13.0 Hydronephrosis with ureteropelvic junction obstruction
Hydronephrosis due to acquired occlusion of ureteropelvic junction
EXCLUDES 2   hydronephrosis with ureteropelvic junction obstruction due to calculus (N13.2)

N13.1 Hydronephrosis with ureteral stricture, not elsewhere classified
EXCLUDES 1   hydronephrosis with ureteral stricture with infection (N13.6)

N13.2 Hydronephrosis with renal and ureteral calculous obstruction
EXCLUDES 1   hydronephrosis with renal and ureteral calculous obstruction with infection (N13.6)

Hydronephrosis/UPJ Obstruction

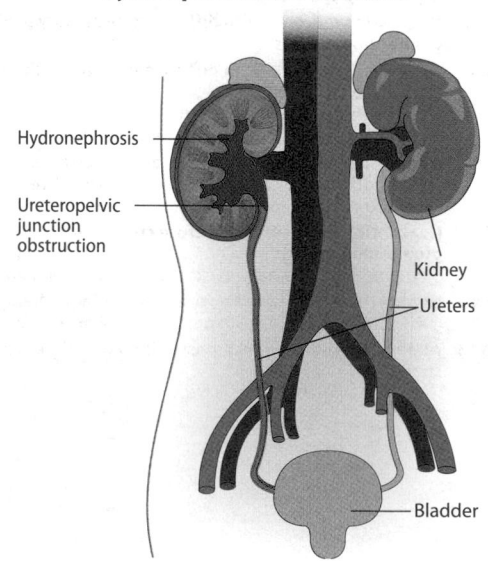

Hydronephrosis

Ureteropelvic junction obstruction

Kidney

Ureters

Bladder

EXCLUDES 1 Not coded here   EXCLUDES 2 Not included here   Ⓝ Newborn Age: 0   Ⓟ Pediatric Age: 0-17   Ⓜ Maternity Age: 12-55   Ⓐ Adult Age: 15-124

804   ICD-10-CM 2018

Vesicoureteral Reflux

Kidneys

Ureters

Bladder

Normal flow of urine   Urine flowing the wrong way (VUR)

✓5ᵗʰ **N13.3 Other and unspecified hydronephrosis**
     EXCLUDES 1   *hydronephrosis with infection (N13.6)*
     N13.30 Unspecified hydronephrosis ▽
     N13.39 Other hydronephrosis

N13.4 Hydroureter
     EXCLUDES 1   *congenital hydroureter (Q62.3-)*
              hydroureter with infection (N13.6)
              vesicoureteral-reflux with hydroureter (N13.73-)

N13.5 Crossing vessel and stricture of ureter without hydronephrosis
     Kinking and stricture of ureter without hydronephrosis
     EXCLUDES 1   *crossing vessel and stricture of ureter without hydronephrosis with infection (N13.6)*

N13.6 Pyonephrosis
     Conditions in N13.0-N13.5 with infection
     Obstructive uropathy with infection
     Use additional code (B95-B97), to identify infectious agent

✓5ᵗʰ **N13.7 Vesicoureteral-reflux**
     EXCLUDES 1   *reflux-associated pyelonephritis (N11.0)*
     N13.70 Vesicoureteral-reflux, unspecified ▽
          Vesicoureteral-reflux NOS
     N13.71 Vesicoureteral-reflux without reflux nephropathy
     ✓6ᵗʰ **N13.72 Vesicoureteral-reflux with reflux nephropathy without hydroureter**
          N13.721 Vesicoureteral-reflux with reflux nephropathy without hydroureter, unilateral
          N13.722 Vesicoureteral-reflux with reflux nephropathy without hydroureter, bilateral
          N13.729 Vesicoureteral-reflux with reflux nephropathy without hydroureter, unspecified ▽
     ✓6ᵗʰ **N13.73 Vesicoureteral-reflux with reflux nephropathy with hydroureter**
          N13.731 Vesicoureteral-reflux with reflux nephropathy with hydroureter, unilateral
          N13.732 Vesicoureteral-reflux with reflux nephropathy with hydroureter, bilateral
          N13.739 Vesicoureteral-reflux with reflux nephropathy with hydroureter, unspecified ▽

N13.8 Other obstructive and reflux uropathy
     Urinary tract obstruction due to specified cause
     Code first, if applicable, any causal condition, such as: enlarged prostate (N40.1)

N13.9 Obstructive and reflux uropathy, unspecified ▽
     Urinary tract obstruction NOS

✓4ᵗʰ **N14 Drug- and heavy-metal-induced tubulo-interstitial and tubular conditions**
     Code first poisoning due to drug or toxin, if applicable (T36-T65 with fifth or sixth character 1-4 or 6)
     Use additional code for adverse effect, if applicable, to identify drug (T36-T50 with fifth or sixth character 5)
     N14.0 Analgesic nephropathy
     N14.1 Nephropathy induced by other drugs, medicaments and biological substances

     N14.2 Nephropathy induced by unspecified drug, medicament or biological substance ▽
     N14.3 Nephropathy induced by heavy metals
     N14.4 Toxic nephropathy, not elsewhere classified

✓4ᵗʰ **N15 Other renal tubulo-interstitial diseases**
     N15.0 Balkan nephropathy
          Balkan endemic nephropathy
     N15.1 Renal and perinephric abscess
     N15.8 Other specified renal tubulo-interstitial diseases
     N15.9 Renal tubulo-interstitial disease, unspecified ▽
          Infection of kidney NOS
          EXCLUDES 1   *urinary tract infection NOS (N39.0)*

N16   **Renal tubulo-interstitial disorders in diseases classified elsewhere**
     Pyelonephritis
     Tubulo-interstitial nephritis
     Code first underlying disease, such as:
         brucellosis (A23.0-A23.9)
         cryoglobulinemia (D89.1)
         glycogen storage disease (E74.0)
         leukemia (C91-C95)
         lymphoma (C81.0-C85.9, C96.0-C96.9)
         multiple myeloma (C90.0-)
         sepsis (A40.0-A41.9)
         Wilson's disease (E83.0)
     EXCLUDES 1   *diphtheritic pyelonephritis and tubulo-interstitial nephritis (A36.84)*
          pyelonephritis and tubulo-interstitial nephritis in candidiasis (B37.49)
          pyelonephritis and tubulo-interstitial nephritis in cystinosis (E72.04)
          pyelonephritis and tubulo-interstitial nephritis in salmonella infection (A02.25)
          pyelonephritis and tubulo-interstitial nephritis in sarcoidosis (D86.84)
          pyelonephritis and tubulo-interstitial nephritis in sicca syndrome [Sjogren's] (M35.04)
          pyelonephritis and tubulo-interstitial nephritis in systemic lupus erythematosus (M32.15)
          pyelonephritis and tubulo-interstitial nephritis in toxoplasmosis (B58.83)
          renal tubular degeneration in diabetes (E08-E13 with .29)
          syphilitic pyelonephritis and tubulo-interstitial nephritis (A52.75)

Acute kidney failure and chronic kidney disease (N17-N19)

     EXCLUDES 2   *congenital renal failure (P96.0)*
          drug- and heavy-metal-induced tubulo-interstitial and tubular conditions (N14.-)
          extrarenal uremia (R39.2)
          hemolytic-uremic syndrome (D59.3)
          hepatorenal syndrome (K76.7)
          postpartum hepatorenal syndrome (O90.4)
          posttraumatic renal failure (T79.5)
          prerenal uremia (R39.2)
          renal failure complicating abortion or ectopic or molar pregnancy (O00-O07, O08.4)
          renal failure following labor and delivery (O90.4)
          renal failure postprocedural (N99.0)

✓4ᵗʰ **N17 Acute kidney failure**
     Code also associated underlying condition
     EXCLUDES 1   *posttraumatic renal failure (T79.5)*
     AHA: 2013, 4Q, 124
     N17.0 Acute kidney failure with tubular necrosis   **HCC**
          Acute tubular necrosis
          Renal tubular necrosis
          Tubular necrosis NOS
     N17.1 Acute kidney failure with acute cortical necrosis   **HCC**
          Acute cortical necrosis
          Cortical necrosis NOS
          Renal cortical necrosis
     N17.2 Acute kidney failure with medullary necrosis   **HCC**
          Medullary [papillary] necrosis NOS
          Acute medullary [papillary] necrosis
          Renal medullary [papillary] necrosis
     N17.8 Other acute kidney failure   **HCC**
     N17.9 Acute kidney failure, unspecified   **HCC** ▽
          Acute kidney injury (nontraumatic)
          EXCLUDES 2   *traumatic kidney injury (S37.0-)*

☑ Additional Character Req   √x7ᵗʰ Placeholder Alert   Manifestation   **HCC** CMS-HCC Condition   ▽ Unspecified Code   ►◄ Revised Text   ● New Code   ▲ Revised Code Title

ICD-10-CM 2018   805

Chapter 14. Diseases of Genitourinary System

N18–N28.89

✓4ᵗʰ **N18 Chronic kidney disease (CKD)**
Code first any associated:
diabetic chronic kidney disease (E08.22, E09.22, E10.22, E11.22, E13.22)
hypertensive chronic kidney disease (I12.-, I13-)
Use additional code to identify kidney transplant status, if applicable, (Z94.0)
AHA: 2013, 1Q, 24

N18.1 Chronic kidney disease, stage 1

N18.2 Chronic kidney disease, stage 2 (mild)

N18.3 Chronic kidney disease, stage 3 (moderate)

N18.4 Chronic kidney disease, stage 4 (severe)   HCC

N18.5 Chronic kidney disease, stage 5   HCC
EXCLUDES 1   chronic kidney disease, stage 5 requiring chronic dialysis (N18.6)
DEF: End-stage renal disease (ESRD) with GFR value of 15 ml/min or less not yet requiring chronic dialysis.

N18.6 End stage renal disease   HCC
Chronic kidney disease requiring chronic dialysis
Use additional code to identify dialysis status (Z99.2)
AHA: 2016, 3Q, 22; 2016, 1Q, 12; 2013, 4Q, 124-125

N18.9 Chronic kidney disease, unspecified   ▽
Chronic renal disease
Chronic renal failure NOS
Chronic renal insufficiency
▶Chronic uremia NOS
Diffuse sclerosing glomerulonephritis NOS◀

N19 Unspecified kidney failure   ▽
Uremia NOS
EXCLUDES 1   acute kidney failure (N17.-)
chronic kidney disease (N18.-)
chronic uremia (N18.9)
extrarenal uremia (R39.2)
prerenal uremia (R39.2)
renal insufficiency (acute) (N28.9)
uremia of newborn (P96.0)

Urolithiasis (N20-N23)

AHA: 2017, 1Q, 5; 2015, 2Q, 8

✓4ᵗʰ **N20 Calculus of kidney and ureter**
Calculous pyelonephritis
EXCLUDES 1   nephrocalcinosis (E83.5)
that with hydronephrosis (N13.2)

N20.0 Calculus of kidney
Nephrolithiasis NOS
Renal calculus
Renal stone
Staghorn calculus
Stone in kidney

N20.1 Calculus of ureter
Ureteric stone
AHA: 2016, 3Q, 22

N20.2 Calculus of kidney with calculus of ureter

N20.9 Urinary calculus, unspecified   ▽

✓4ᵗʰ **N21 Calculus of lower urinary tract**
Calculus of lower urinary tract with cystitis and urethritis

N21.0 Calculus in bladder
Calculus in diverticulum of bladder
Urinary bladder stone
EXCLUDES 2   staghorn calculus (N20.0)

N21.1 Calculus in urethra
EXCLUDES 2   calculus of prostate (N42.0)

N21.8 Other lower urinary tract calculus

N21.9 Calculus of lower urinary tract, unspecified   ▽
EXCLUDES 1   calculus of urinary tract NOS (N20.9)

N22 Calculus of urinary tract in diseases classified elsewhere
Code first underlying disease, such as:
gout (M1A.-, M10.-)
schistosomiasis (B65.0-B65.9)

N23 Unspecified renal colic   ▽

Other disorders of kidney and ureter (N25-N29)

EXCLUDES 2   disorders of kidney and ureter with urolithiasis (N20-N23)

✓4ᵗʰ **N25 Disorders resulting from impaired renal tubular function**
EXCLUDES 1   metabolic disorders classifiable to E70-E88

N25.0 Renal osteodystrophy
Azotemic osteodystrophy
Phosphate-losing tubular disorders
Renal rickets
Renal short stature
EXCLUDES 2 ▶metabolic disorders classifiable to E70-E88◀

N25.1 Nephrogenic diabetes insipidus   HCC
EXCLUDES 1   diabetes insipidus NOS (E23.2)
DEF: Type of diabetes due to inability of renal tubules to reabsorb water back into the body; not responsive to vasopressin (antidiuretic hormone); characterized by excessive thirst and excessive urine production; may develop into chronic renal insufficiency.

✓5ᵗʰ **N25.8 Other disorders resulting from impaired renal tubular function**

N25.81 Secondary hyperparathyroidism of renal origin   HCC
EXCLUDES 1   secondary hyperparathyroidism, non-renal (E21.1)
EXCLUDES 2 ▶metabolic disorders classifiable to E70-E88◀
DEF: Parathyroid dysfunction caused by chronic renal failure; phosphate clearance is impaired, phosphate is released from bone, vitamin D is not produced, intestinal calcium absorption is low, and blood levels of calcium are lowered, causing excessive production of parathyroid hormone.

N25.89 Other disorders resulting from impaired renal tubular function
Hypokalemic nephropathy
Lightwood-Albright syndrome
Renal tubular acidosis NOS

N25.9 Disorder resulting from impaired renal tubular function, unspecified   ▽

✓4ᵗʰ **N26 Unspecified contracted kidney**
EXCLUDES 1   contracted kidney due to hypertension (I12.-)
diffuse sclerosing glomerulonephritis (N05.8-)
hypertensive nephrosclerosis (arteriolar) (arteriosclerotic) (I12.-)
small kidney of unknown cause (N27.-)

N26.1 Atrophy of kidney (terminal)

N26.2 Page kidney

N26.9 Renal sclerosis, unspecified   ▽

✓4ᵗʰ **N27 Small kidney of unknown cause**
INCLUDES   oligonephronia

N27.0 Small kidney, unilateral

N27.1 Small kidney, bilateral

N27.9 Small kidney, unspecified   ▽

✓4ᵗʰ **N28 Other disorders of kidney and ureter, not elsewhere classified**

N28.0 Ischemia and infarction of kidney   HCC
Renal artery embolism   Renal artery thrombosis
Renal artery obstruction   Renal infarct
Renal artery occlusion
EXCLUDES 1   atherosclerosis of renal artery (extrarenal part) (I70.1)
congenital stenosis of renal artery (Q27.1)
Goldblatt's kidney (I70.1)

N28.1 Cyst of kidney, acquired
▶Cyst (multiple) (solitary) of kidney (acquired)◀
EXCLUDES 1   cystic kidney disease (congenital) (Q61.-)

✓5ᵗʰ **N28.8 Other specified disorders of kidney and ureter**
EXCLUDES 1   hydroureter (N13.4)
ureteric stricture with hydronephrosis (N13.1)
ureteric stricture without hydronephrosis (N13.5)

N28.81 Hypertrophy of kidney

N28.82 Megaloureter

N28.83 Nephroptosis

N28.84 Pyelitis cystica

N28.85 Pyeloureteritis cystica

N28.86 Ureteritis cystica

N28.89 Other specified disorders of kidney and ureter

EXCLUDES 1 Not coded here   *EXCLUDES 2* Not included here   N Newborn Age: 0   P Pediatric Age: 0-17   M Maternity Age: 12-55   A Adult Age: 15-124

806   ICD-10-CM 2018

N28.9 **Disorder of kidney and ureter, unspecified** ▽
Nephropathy NOS
Renal disease (acute) NOS
Renal insufficiency (acute)
> *EXCLUDES 1* *chronic renal insufficiency (N18.9)*
> *unspecified nephritic syndrome (N05.-)*
AHA: 2016, 1Q, 13

N29 *Other disorders of kidney and ureter in diseases classified elsewhere*
Code first underlying disease, such as:
amyloidosis (E85.-)
nephrocalcinosis (E83.5)
schistosomiasis (B65.0-B65.9)
> *EXCLUDES 1* *disorders of kidney and ureter in:*
> *cystinosis (E72.0)*
> *gonorrhea (A54.21)*
> *syphilis (A52.75)*
> *tuberculosis (A18.11)*

Other diseases of the urinary system (N30-N39)

> *EXCLUDES 1* *urinary infection (complicating):*
> *abortion or ectopic or molar pregnancy (-O07, O08.8)*
> *pregnancy, childbirth and the puerperium (O23-, O75.3, O86.2-)*

✓4th **N30** **Cystitis**
Use additional code to identify infectious agent (B95-B97)
> *EXCLUDES 1* *prostatocystitis (N41.3)*
AHA: 2017, 1Q, 6

✓5th **N30.0** **Acute cystitis**
> *EXCLUDES 1* *irradiation cystitis (N30.4-)*
> *trigonitis (N30.3-)*

N30.00 **Acute cystitis without hematuria**
N30.01 **Acute cystitis with hematuria**

✓5th **N30.1** **Interstitial cystitis (chronic)**
N30.10 **Interstitial cystitis (chronic) without hematuria**
N30.11 **Interstitial cystitis (chronic) with hematuria**

✓5th **N30.2** **Other chronic cystitis**
N30.20 **Other chronic cystitis without hematuria**
N30.21 **Other chronic cystitis with hematuria**

✓5th **N30.3** **Trigonitis**
Urethrotrigonitis
N30.30 **Trigonitis without hematuria**
N30.31 **Trigonitis with hematuria**

✓5th **N30.4** **Irradiation cystitis**
N30.40 **Irradiation cystitis without hematuria**
N30.41 **Irradiation cystitis with hematuria**

✓5th **N30.8** **Other cystitis**
Abscess of bladder
N30.80 **Other cystitis without hematuria**
N30.81 **Other cystitis with hematuria**

✓5th **N30.9** **Cystitis, unspecified**
N30.90 **Cystitis, unspecified without hematuria** ▽
N30.91 **Cystitis, unspecified with hematuria** ▽

✓4th **N31** **Neuromuscular dysfunction of bladder, not elsewhere classified**
Use additional code to identify any associated urinary incontinence (N39.3-N39.4-)
> *EXCLUDES 1* *cord bladder NOS (G95.89)*
> *neurogenic bladder due to cauda equina syndrome (G83.4)*
> *neuromuscular dysfunction due to spinal cord lesion (G95.89)*

N31.0 **Uninhibited neuropathic bladder, not elsewhere classified**
N31.1 **Reflex neuropathic bladder, not elsewhere classified**
N31.2 **Flaccid neuropathic bladder, not elsewhere classified**
Atonic (motor) (sensory) neuropathic bladder
Autonomous neuropathic bladder
Nonreflex neuropathic bladder
N31.8 **Other neuromuscular dysfunction of bladder**
N31.9 **Neuromuscular dysfunction of bladder, unspecified** ▽
Neurogenic bladder dysfunction NOS

✓4th **N32** **Other disorders of bladder**
> *EXCLUDES 2* *calculus of bladder (N21.0)*
> *cystocele (N81.1-)*
> *hernia or prolapse of bladder, female (N81.1-)*

N32.0 **Bladder-neck obstruction**
Bladder-neck stenosis (acquired)
> *EXCLUDES 1* *congenital bladder-neck obstruction (Q64.3-)*
DEF: Bladder outlet and vesicourethral obstruction; occurs as a consequence of benign prostatic hypertrophy or prostatic cancer; may also occur in either sex due to strictures, radiation, cystoscopy, catheterization, injury, infection, blood clots, bladder cancer, impaction, or other disease that compresses the bladder neck.

N32.1 **Vesicointestinal fistula**
Vesicorectal fistula

N32.2 **Vesical fistula, not elsewhere classified**
> *EXCLUDES 1* *fistula between bladder and female genital tract (N82.0-N82.1)*

N32.3 **Diverticulum of bladder**
> *EXCLUDES 1* *congenital diverticulum of bladder (Q64.6)*
> *diverticulitis of bladder (N30.8-)*

✓5th **N32.8** **Other specified disorders of bladder**
N32.81 **Overactive bladder**
Detrusor muscle hyperactivity
> *EXCLUDES 1* *frequent urination due to specified bladder condition—code to condition*
DEF: Sudden involuntary contractions of the muscular wall of bladder; results in sudden, strong urge to urinate.

N32.89 **Other specified disorders of bladder**
Bladder hemorrhage
Bladder hypertrophy
Calcified bladder
Contracted bladder

N32.9 **Bladder disorder, unspecified** ▽

N33 *Bladder disorders in diseases classified elsewhere*
Code first underlying disease, such as:
schistosomiasis (B65.0-B65.9)
> *EXCLUDES 1* *bladder disorder in syphilis (A52.76)*
> *bladder disorder in tuberculosis (A18.12)*
> *candidal cystitis (B37.41)*
> *chlamydial cystitis (A56.01)*
> *cystitis in gonorrhea (A54.01)*
> *cystitis in neurogenic bladder (N31.-)*
> *diphtheritic cystitis (A36.85)*
> *neurogenic bladder (N31.-)*
> *syphilitic cystitis (A52.76)*
> *trichomonal cystitis (A59.03)*

✓4th **N34** **Urethritis and urethral syndrome**
Use additional code (B95-B97), to identify infectious agent
> *EXCLUDES 2* *Reiter's disease (M02.3-)*
> *urethritis in diseases with a predominantly sexual mode of transmission (A50-A64)*
> *urethrotrigonitis (N30.3-)*
AHA: 2017, 1Q, 6

N34.0 **Urethral abscess**
Abscess (of) Cowper's gland
Abscess (of) Littrés gland
Abscess (of) urethral (gland)
Periurethral abscess
> *EXCLUDES 1* *urethral caruncle (N36.2)*

N34.1 **Nonspecific urethritis**
Nongonococcal urethritis
Nonvenereal urethritis

N34.2 **Other urethritis**
Meatitis, urethral
Postmenopausal urethritis
Ulcer of urethra (meatus)
Urethritis NOS

N34.3 **Urethral syndrome, unspecified** ▽

✓4th **N35** **Urethral stricture**
> *EXCLUDES 1* *congenital urethral stricture (Q64.3-)*
> *postprocedural urethral stricture (N99.1-)*

✓5th **N35.0** **Post-traumatic urethral stricture**
Urethral stricture due to injury
> *EXCLUDES 1* *postprocedural urethral stricture (N99.1-)*

✓6th **N35.01** **Post-traumatic urethral stricture, male**
N35.010 **Post-traumatic urethral stricture, male, meatal** ♂
N35.011 **Post-traumatic bulbous urethral stricture**
N35.012 **Post-traumatic membranous urethral stricture**
N35.013 **Post-traumatic anterior urethral stricture**

N35.014 Post-traumatic urethral stricture, male, unspecified ♂▽

✓6ᵗʰ **N35.02 Post-traumatic urethral stricture, female**

N35.021 Urethral stricture due to childbirth ♀

N35.028 Other post-traumatic urethral stricture, female ♀

✓5ᵗʰ **N35.1 Postinfective urethral stricture, not elsewhere classified**
　EXCLUDES 1　urethral stricture associated with schistosomiasis (B65-, N29)
　　gonococcal urethral stricture (A54.01)
　　syphilitic urethral stricture (A52.76)

✓6ᵗʰ **N35.11 Postinfective urethral stricture, not elsewhere classified, male**

N35.111 Postinfective urethral stricture, not elsewhere classified, male, meatal ♂

▲ **N35.112 Postinfective bulbous urethral stricture, not elsewhere classified, male**

▲ **N35.113 Postinfective membranous urethral stricture, not elsewhere classified, male**

▲ **N35.114 Postinfective anterior urethral stricture, not elsewhere classified, male**

N35.119 Postinfective urethral stricture, not elsewhere classified, male, unspecified ♂▽

N35.12 Postinfective urethral stricture, not elsewhere classified, female ♀

N35.8 Other urethral stricture
　EXCLUDES 1　postprocedural urethral stricture (N99.1-)

N35.9 Urethral stricture, unspecified ▽

✓4ᵗʰ **N36 Other disorders of urethra**

N36.0 Urethral fistula
　Urethroperineal fistula
　Urethrorectal fistula
　Urinary fistula NOS
　EXCLUDES 1　urethroscrotal fistula (N50.89)
　　urethrovaginal fistula (N82.1)
　　urethrovesicovaginal fistula (N82.1)

N36.1 Urethral diverticulum

N36.2 Urethral caruncle

✓5ᵗʰ **N36.4 Urethral functional and muscular disorders**
　Use additional code to identify associated urinary stress incontinence (N39.3)

N36.41 Hypermobility of urethra
N36.42 Intrinsic sphincter deficiency (ISD)
N36.43 Combined hypermobility of urethra and intrinsic sphincter deficiency
N36.44 Muscular disorders of urethra
　Bladder sphincter dyssynergy

N36.5 Urethral false passage

N36.8 Other specified disorders of urethra
　EXCLUDES 1　congenital urethrocele (Q64.7)
　　female urethrocele (N81.0)

N36.9 Urethral disorder, unspecified ▽

N37 Urethral disorders in diseases classified elsewhere
　Code first underlying disease
　EXCLUDES 1　urethritis (in):
　　candidal infection (B37.41)
　　chlamydial (A56.01)
　　gonorrhea (A54.01)
　　syphilis (A52.76)
　　trichomonal infection (A59.03)
　　tuberculosis (A18.13)

✓4ᵗʰ **N39 Other disorders of urinary system**
　EXCLUDES 2　hematuria NOS (R31.-)
　　recurrent or persistent hematuria (N02.-)
　　recurrent or persistent hematuria with specified morphological lesion (N02.-)
　　proteinuria NOS (R80.-)

N39.0 Urinary tract infection, site not specified ▽
　Use additional code (B95-B97), to identify infectious agent
　EXCLUDES 1　candidiasis of urinary tract (B37.4-)
　　neonatal urinary tract infection (P39.3)
　　urinary tract infection of specified site, such as:
　　　cystitis (N30.-)
　　　urethritis (N34.-)
　AHA: 2017, 1Q, 6; 2012, 4Q, 94

N39.3 Stress incontinence (female) (male)
　Code also any associated overactive bladder (N32.81)
　EXCLUDES 1　mixed incontinence (N39.46)

✓5ᵗʰ **N39.4 Other specified urinary incontinence**
　Code also any associated overactive bladder (N32.81)
　EXCLUDES 1　enuresis NOS (R32)
　　functional urinary incontinence (R39.81)
　　urinary incontinence associated with cognitive impairment (R39.81)
　　urinary incontinence NOS (R32)
　　urinary incontinence of nonorganic origin (F98.0)

N39.41 Urge incontinence
　EXCLUDES 1　mixed incontinence (N39.46)

N39.42 Incontinence without sensory awareness
　Insensible (urinary) incontinence

N39.43 Post-void dribbling
N39.44 Nocturnal enuresis
N39.45 Continuous leakage
N39.46 Mixed incontinence
　Urge and stress incontinence

✓6ᵗʰ **N39.49 Other specified urinary incontinence**
N39.490 Overflow incontinence
N39.491 Coital incontinence
N39.492 Postural (urinary) incontinence
N39.498 Other specified urinary incontinence
　Reflex incontinence
　Total incontinence

N39.8 Other specified disorders of urinary system
N39.9 Disorder of urinary system, unspecified ▽

Diseases of male genital organs (N40-N53)

✓4ᵗʰ **N40 Benign prostatic hyperplasia**
　INCLUDES　adenofibromatous hypertrophy of prostate
　　benign hypertrophy of the prostate
　　benign prostatic hypertrophy
　　BPH
　　enlarged prostate
　　nodular prostate
　　polyp of prostate
　EXCLUDES 1　benign neoplasms of prostate (adenoma, benign) (fibroadenoma) (fibroma) (myoma) (D29.1)
　EXCLUDES 2　malignant neoplasm of prostate (C61)

N40.0 Benign prostatic hyperplasia without lower urinary tract symptoms 🅰♂
　Enlarged prostate NOS
　Enlarged prostate without LUTS

N40.1 Benign prostatic hyperplasia with lower urinary tract symptoms 🅰♂
　Enlarged prostate with LUTS
　Use additional code for associated symptoms, when specified:
　　incomplete bladder emptying (R39.14)
　　nocturia (R35.1)
　　straining on urination (R39.16)
　　urinary frequency (R35.0)
　　urinary hesitancy (R39.11)
　　urinary incontinence (N39.4-)
　　urinary obstruction (N13.8)
　　urinary retention (R33.8)
　　urinary urgency (R39.15)
　　weak urinary stream (R39.12)

N40.2 Nodular prostate without lower urinary tract symptoms 🅰♂
　Nodular prostate without LUTS

N40.3 Nodular prostate with lower urinary tract symptoms 🅰♂
　Use additional code for associated symptoms, when specified:
　　incomplete bladder emptying (R39.14)
　　nocturia (R35.1)
　　straining on urination (R39.16)
　　urinary frequency (R35.0)
　　urinary hesitancy (R39.11)
　　urinary incontinence (N39.4-)
　　urinary obstruction (N13.8)
　　urinary retention (R33.8)
　　urinary urgency (R39.15)
　　weak urinary stream (R39.12)

✓4ᵗʰ **N41 Inflammatory diseases of prostate**
　Use additional code (B95-B97), to identify infectious agent

N41.0 Acute prostatitis 🅰♂
N41.1 Chronic prostatitis 🅰♂

N41.2   **Abscess of prostate**   A♂

N41.3   **Prostatocystitis**   A♂

N41.4   **Granulomatous prostatitis**   A♂

N41.8   **Other inflammatory diseases of prostate**   A♂

N41.9   **Inflammatory disease of prostate, unspecified**   A♂▽
     Prostatitis NOS

✓4ᵗʰ **N42**   **Other and unspecified disorders of prostate**

N42.0   **Calculus of prostate**   A♂
     Prostatic stone
     DEF: Formation of small, solid stone often composed of calcium carbonate or calcium phosphate in the prostate gland.

N42.1   **Congestion and hemorrhage of prostate**   A♂
     EXCLUDES 1   enlarged prostate (N40.-)
                 hematuria (R31.-)
                 hyperplasia of prostate (N40.-)
                 inflammatory diseases of prostate (N41.-)

✓5ᵗʰ **N42.3**   **Dysplasia of prostate**

     N42.30   **Unspecified dysplasia of prostate**   ♂▽

     N42.31   **Prostatic intraepithelial neoplasia**   ♂
             PIN
             Prostatic intraepithelial neoplasia I (PIN I)
             Prostatic intraepithelial neoplasia II (PIN II)
             EXCLUDES 1   prostatic intraepithelial neoplasia III (PIN III) (D07.5)
             DEF: Abnormality of shape and size of the intraepithelial tissues of the prostate; premalignant condition characterized by stalks and absence of a basilar cell layer; synonyms are intraductal dysplasia, large acinar atypical hyperplasia, atypical primary hyperplasia, hyperplasia with malignant changes, marked atypia, or duct-acinar dysplasia.

     N42.32   **Atypical small acinar proliferation of prostate**   ♂

     N42.39   **Other dysplasia of prostate**   ♂

✓5ᵗʰ **N42.8**   **Other specified disorders of prostate**

     N42.81   **Prostatodynia syndrome**   A♂
             Painful prostate syndrome

     N42.82   **Prostatosis syndrome**   A♂

     N42.83   **Cyst of prostate**   A♂

     N42.89   **Other specified disorders of prostate**   A♂

N42.9   **Disorder of prostate, unspecified**   A♂▽

✓4ᵗʰ **N43**   **Hydrocele and spermatocele**
     INCLUDES   hydrocele of spermatic cord, testis or tunica vaginalis
     EXCLUDES 1   congenital hydrocele (P83.5)

N43.0   **Encysted hydrocele**   ♂

N43.1   **Infected hydrocele**   ♂
     Use additional code (B95-B97), to identify infectious agent

N43.2   **Other hydrocele**   ♂

N43.3   **Hydrocele, unspecified**   ♂▽

✓5ᵗʰ **N43.4**   **Spermatocele of epididymis**
     Spermatic cyst

     N43.40   **Spermatocele of epididymis, unspecified**   ♂▽

     N43.41   **Spermatocele of epididymis, single**   ♂

     N43.42   **Spermatocele of epididymis, multiple**   ♂

Hydrocele

Normal   Noncommunicating hydrocele   Communicating hydrocele   Hydrocele of the cord

---

✓4ᵗʰ **N44**   **Noninflammatory disorders of testis**

✓5ᵗʰ **N44.0**   **Torsion of testis**

     N44.00   **Torsion of testis, unspecified**   ♂▽

     N44.01   **Extravaginal torsion of spermatic cord**   ♂
             DEF: Torsion of the spermatic cord just below the tunica vaginalis attachments.

     N44.02   **Intravaginal torsion of spermatic cord**   ♂
             Torsion of spermatic cord NOS

     N44.03   **Torsion of appendix testis**   ♂

     N44.04   **Torsion of appendix epididymis**   ♂

N44.1   **Cyst of tunica albuginea testis**   ♂

N44.2   **Benign cyst of testis**   ♂

N44.8   **Other noninflammatory disorders of the testis**   ♂

✓4ᵗʰ **N45**   **Orchitis and epididymitis**
     Use additional code (B95-B97), to identify infectious agent

N45.1   **Epididymitis**   ♂

N45.2   **Orchitis**   ♂

N45.3   **Epididymo-orchitis**   ♂

N45.4   **Abscess of epididymis or testis**   ♂

✓4ᵗʰ **N46**   **Male infertility**
     EXCLUDES 1   vasectomy status (Z98.52)

✓5ᵗʰ **N46.0**   **Azoospermia**
     Absolute male infertility
     Male infertility due to germinal (cell) aplasia
     Male infertility due to spermatogenic arrest (complete)

     N46.01   **Organic azoospermia**   A♂
             Azoospermia NOS

     ✓6ᵗʰ **N46.02**   **Azoospermia due to extratesticular causes**
             Code also associated cause

         N46.021   **Azoospermia due to drug therapy**   A♂

         N46.022   **Azoospermia due to infection**   A♂

         N46.023   **Azoospermia due to obstruction of efferent ducts**   A♂

         N46.024   **Azoospermia due to radiation**   A♂

         N46.025   **Azoospermia due to systemic disease**   A♂

         N46.029   **Azoospermia due to other extratesticular causes**   A♂

✓5ᵗʰ **N46.1**   **Oligospermia**
     Male infertility due to germinal cell desquamation
     Male infertility due to hypospermatogenesis
     Male infertility due to incomplete spermatogenic arrest

     N46.11   **Organic oligospermia**   A♂
             Oligospermia NOS

     ✓6ᵗʰ **N46.12**   **Oligospermia due to extratesticular causes**
             Code also associated cause

         N46.121   **Oligospermia due to drug therapy**   A♂

         N46.122   **Oligospermia due to infection**   A♂

         N46.123   **Oligospermia due to obstruction of efferent ducts**   A♂

         N46.124   **Oligospermia due to radiation**   A♂

         N46.125   **Oligospermia due to systemic disease**   A♂

         N46.129   **Oligospermia due to other extratesticular causes**   A♂

N46.8   **Other male infertility**   A♂

N46.9   **Male infertility, unspecified**   A♂▽

✓4ᵗʰ **N47**   **Disorders of prepuce**

N47.0   **Adherent prepuce, newborn**   N♂

N47.1   **Phimosis**   ♂

N47.2   **Paraphimosis**   ♂

N47.3   **Deficient foreskin**   ♂

N47.4   **Benign cyst of prepuce**   ♂

N47.5   **Adhesions of prepuce and glans penis**   ♂

N47.6   **Balanoposthitis**   ♂
     Use additional code (B95-B97), to identify infectious agent
     EXCLUDES 1   balanitis (N48.1)

N47.7   **Other inflammatory diseases of prepuce**   ♂
     Use additional code (B95-B97), to identify infectious agent

N47.8   **Other disorders of prepuce**   ♂

✓ Additional Character Req   ✓7ᵗʰ Placeholder Alert   Manifestation   HCC CMS-HCC Condition   ▽ Unspecified Code   ►◄ Revised Text   ● New Code   ▲ Revised Code Title

ICD-10-CM 2018   809

✓4th **N48 Other disorders of penis**

N48.0 Leukoplakia of penis ♂
Balanitis xerotica obliterans
Kraurosis of penis
Lichen sclerosus of external male genital organs
EXCLUDES 1   *carcinoma in situ of penis (D07.4)*

N48.1 Balanitis ♂
Use additional code (B95-B97), to identify infectious agent
EXCLUDES 1   *amebic balanitis (A06.8)*
balanitis xerotica obliterans (N48.0)
candidal balanitis (B37.42)
gonococcal balanitis (A54.23)
herpesviral [herpes simplex] balanitis (A60.01)

✓5th **N48.2 Other inflammatory disorders of penis**
Use additional code (B95-B97), to identify infectious agent
EXCLUDES 1   *balanitis (N48.1)*
balanitis xerotica obliterans (N48.0)
balanoposthitis (N47.6)

     N48.21 Abscess of corpus cavernosum and penis ♂
     N48.22 Cellulitis of corpus cavernosum and penis ♂
     N48.29 Other inflammatory disorders of penis ♂

✓5th **N48.3 Priapism**
Painful erection
Code first underlying cause

     N48.30 Priapism, unspecified ♂▽
     N48.31 Priapism due to trauma ♂
     N48.32 Priapism due to disease classified elsewhere ♂
     N48.33 Priapism, drug-induced ♂
     N48.39 Other priapism ♂

N48.5 Ulcer of penis ♂

N48.6 Induration penis plastica ♂
Peyronie's disease
Plastic induration of penis

✓5th **N48.8 Other specified disorders of penis**
     N48.81 Thrombosis of superficial vein of penis ♂
     N48.82 Acquired torsion of penis ♂
         Acquired torsion of penis NOS
         EXCLUDES 1   *congenital torsion of penis (Q55.63)*
     N48.83 Acquired buried penis ♂
         EXCLUDES 1   *congenital hidden penis (Q55.64)*
     N48.89 Other specified disorders of penis ♂

N48.9 Disorder of penis, unspecified ♂▽

✓4th **N49 Inflammatory disorders of male genital organs, not elsewhere classified**
Use additional code (B95-B97), to identify infectious agent
EXCLUDES 1   *inflammation of penis (N48.1, N48.2-)*
orchitis and epididymitis (N45.-)

N49.0 Inflammatory disorders of seminal vesicle ♂
Vesiculitis NOS

N49.1 Inflammatory disorders of spermatic cord, tunica vaginalis and vas deferens ♂
Vasitis

N49.2 Inflammatory disorders of scrotum ♂

N49.3 Fournier gangrene ♂

N49.8 Inflammatory disorders of other specified male genital organs ♂
Inflammation of multiple sites in male genital organs

N49.9 Inflammatory disorder of unspecified male genital organ ♂▽
Abscess of unspecified male genital organ
Boil of unspecified male genital organ
Carbuncle of unspecified male genital organ
Cellulitis of unspecified male genital organ

✓4th **N50 Other and unspecified disorders of male genital organs**
EXCLUDES 2   *torsion of testis (N44.0-)*

N50.0 Atrophy of testis ♂

N50.1 Vascular disorders of male genital organs ♂
Hematocele, NOS, of male genital organs
Hemorrhage of male genital organs
Thrombosis of male genital organs

N50.3 Cyst of epididymis ♂

✓5th **N50.8 Other specified disorders of male genital organs**
     ✓6th **N50.81 Testicular pain**
         N50.811 Right testicular pain ♂
         N50.812 Left testicular pain ♂

         N50.819 Testicular pain, unspecified ♂▽
     N50.82 Scrotal pain ♂
     N50.89 Other specified disorders of the male genital organs ♂
         Atrophy of scrotum, seminal vesicle, spermatic cord, tunica vaginalis and vas deferens
         Chylocele, tunica vaginalis (nonfilarial) NOS
         Edema of scrotum, seminal vesicle, spermatic cord, testis, tunica vaginalis and vas deferens
         Hypertrophy of scrotum, seminal vesicle, spermatic cord, testis, tunica vaginalis and vas deferens
         Stricture of spermatic cord, tunica vaginalis, and vas deferens
         Ulcer of scrotum, seminal vesicle, spermatic cord, testis, tunica vaginalis and vas deferens
         Urethroscrotal fistula

N50.9 Disorder of male genital organs, unspecified ♂▽

N51 Disorders of male genital organs in diseases classified elsewhere ♂
Code first underlying disease, such as:
filariasis (B74.0-B74.9)
EXCLUDES 1   *amebic balanitis (A06.8)*
candidal balanitis (B37.42)
gonococcal balanitis (A54.23)
gonococcal prostatitis (A54.22)
herpesviral [herpes simplex] balanitis (A60.01)
trichomonal prostatitis (A59.02)
tuberculous prostatitis (A18.14)

✓4th **N52 Male erectile dysfunction**
EXCLUDES 1   *psychogenic impotence (F52.21)*

✓5th **N52.0 Vasculogenic erectile dysfunction**
     N52.01 Erectile dysfunction due to arterial insufficiency Ⓐ♂
     N52.02 Corporo-venous occlusive erectile dysfunction Ⓐ♂
     N52.03 Combined arterial insufficiency and corporo-venous occlusive erectile dysfunction Ⓐ♂

N52.1 Erectile dysfunction due to diseases classified elsewhere Ⓐ♂
Code first underlying disease

N52.2 Drug-induced erectile dysfunction Ⓐ♂

✓5th **N52.3 Postprocedural erectile dysfunction**
     N52.31 Erectile dysfunction following radical prostatectomy Ⓐ♂
     N52.32 Erectile dysfunction following radical cystectomy Ⓐ♂
     N52.33 Erectile dysfunction following urethral surgery Ⓐ♂
     N52.34 Erectile dysfunction following simple prostatectomy Ⓐ♂
     N52.35 Erectile dysfunction following radiation therapy Ⓐ♂
     N52.36 Erectile dysfunction following interstitial seed therapy Ⓐ♂
     N52.37 Erectile dysfunction following prostate ablative therapy Ⓐ♂
         Erectile dysfunction following cryotherapy
         Erectile dysfunction following other prostate ablative therapies
         Erectile dysfunction following ultrasound ablative therapies
     N52.39 Other and unspecified postprocedural erectile dysfunction Ⓐ♂▽

N52.8 Other male erectile dysfunction Ⓐ♂

N52.9 Male erectile dysfunction, unspecified Ⓐ♂▽
Impotence NOS

✓4th **N53 Other male sexual dysfunction**
EXCLUDES 1   *psychogenic sexual dysfunction (F52.-)*

✓5th **N53.1 Ejaculatory dysfunction**
EXCLUDES 1   *premature ejaculation (F52.4)*
     N53.11 Retarded ejaculation ♂
     N53.12 Painful ejaculation ♂
     N53.13 Anejaculatory orgasm ♂
     N53.14 Retrograde ejaculation ♂
         DEF: A form of male sexual dysfunction in which the semen enters the bladder instead of going out through the urethra during ejaculation.
     N53.19 Other ejaculatory dysfunction ♂
         Ejaculatory dysfunction NOS

N53.8 Other male sexual dysfunction ♂

N53.9 Unspecified male sexual dysfunction ♂▽

EXCLUDES 1 Not coded here   *EXCLUDES 2* Not included here   Ⓝ Newborn Age: 0   Ⓟ Pediatric Age: 0-17   Ⓜ Maternity Age: 12-55   Ⓐ Adult Age: 15-124

810   ICD-10-CM 2018

Disorders of breast (N60-N65)

EXCLUDES 1   disorders of breast associated with childbirth (O91-O92)

✓4ᵗʰ **N60 Benign mammary dysplasia**
     INCLUDES   fibrocystic mastopathy

   ✓5ᵗʰ **N60.0 Solitary cyst of breast**
       Cyst of breast

     N60.01 Solitary cyst of right breast

     N60.02 Solitary cyst of left breast

     N60.09 Solitary cyst of unspecified breast ▽

   ✓5ᵗʰ **N60.1 Diffuse cystic mastopathy**
       Cystic breast
       Fibrocystic disease of breast
       EXCLUDES 1   diffuse cystic mastopathy with epithelial proliferation (N60.3-)

     N60.11 Diffuse cystic mastopathy of right breast A

     N60.12 Diffuse cystic mastopathy of left breast A

     N60.19 Diffuse cystic mastopathy of unspecified breast A▽

   ✓5ᵗʰ **N60.2 Fibroadenosis of breast**
       Adenofibrosis of breast
       EXCLUDES 2   fibroadenoma of breast (D24.-)

     N60.21 Fibroadenosis of right breast

     N60.22 Fibroadenosis of left breast

     N60.29 Fibroadenosis of unspecified breast ▽

   ✓5ᵗʰ **N60.3 Fibrosclerosis of breast**
       Cystic mastopathy with epithelial proliferation

     N60.31 Fibrosclerosis of right breast

     N60.32 Fibrosclerosis of left breast

     N60.39 Fibrosclerosis of unspecified breast ▽

   ✓5ᵗʰ **N60.4 Mammary duct ectasia**

     N60.41 Mammary duct ectasia of right breast

     N60.42 Mammary duct ectasia of left breast

     N60.49 Mammary duct ectasia of unspecified breast ▽

   ✓5ᵗʰ **N60.8 Other benign mammary dysplasias**

     N60.81 Other benign mammary dysplasias of right breast

     N60.82 Other benign mammary dysplasias of left breast

     N60.89 Other benign mammary dysplasias of unspecified breast ▽

   ✓5ᵗʰ **N60.9 Unspecified benign mammary dysplasia**

     N60.91 Unspecified benign mammary dysplasia of right breast ▽

     N60.92 Unspecified benign mammary dysplasia of left breast ▽

     N60.99 Unspecified benign mammary dysplasia of unspecified breast ▽

✓4ᵗʰ **N61 Inflammatory disorders of breast**
     EXCLUDES 1   inflammatory carcinoma of breast (C50.9)
         inflammatory disorder of breast associated with childbirth (O91.-)
         neonatal infective mastitis (P39.0)
         thrombophlebitis of breast [Mondor's disease] (I80.8)

   N61.0 Mastitis without abscess
       Infective mastitis (acute) (nonpuerperal) (subacute)
       Mastitis (acute) (nonpuerperal) (subacute) NOS
       Cellulitis (acute) (nonpuerperal) (subacute) of breast NOS
       Cellulitis (acute) (nonpuerperal) (subacute) of nipple NOS

   N61.1 Abscess of the breast and nipple
       Abscess (acute) (chronic) (nonpuerperal) of areola
       Abscess (acute) (chronic) (nonpuerperal) of breast
       Carbuncle of breast
       Mastitis with abscess

N62 Hypertrophy of breast
     Gynecomastia
     Hypertrophy of breast NOS
     Massive pubertal hypertrophy of breast
     EXCLUDES 1   breast engorgement of newborn (P83.4)
         disproportion of reconstructed breast (N65.1)

✓4ᵗʰ **N63 Unspecified lump in breast**
     Nodule(s) NOS in breast

●   **N63.0 Unspecified lump in unspecified breast** ▽

●   ✓5ᵗʰ **N63.1 Unspecified lump in the right breast**

●   **N63.10 Unspecified lump in the right breast, unspecified quadrant** ▽

●   **N63.11 Unspecified lump in the right breast, upper outer quadrant** ▽

●   **N63.12 Unspecified lump in the right breast, upper inner quadrant** ▽

●   **N63.13 Unspecified lump in the right breast, lower outer quadrant** ▽

●   **N63.14 Unspecified lump in the right breast, lower inner quadrant** ▽

●   ✓5ᵗʰ **N63.2 Unspecified lump in the left breast**

●   **N63.20 Unspecified lump in the left breast, unspecified quadrant** ▽

●   **N63.21 Unspecified lump in the left breast, upper outer quadrant** ▽

●   **N63.22 Unspecified lump in the left breast, upper inner quadrant** ▽

●   **N63.23 Unspecified lump in the left breast, lower outer quadrant** ▽

●   **N63.24 Unspecified lump in the left breast, lower inner quadrant** ▽

●   ✓5ᵗʰ **N63.3 Unspecified lump in axillary tail**

     N63.31 Unspecified lump in axillary tail of the right breast ▽

     N63.32 Unspecified lump in axillary tail of the left breast ▽

●   ✓5ᵗʰ **N63.4 Unspecified lump in breast, subareolar**

●   **N63.41 Unspecified lump in right breast, subareolar** ▽

●   **N63.42 Unspecified lump in left breast, subareolar** ▽

✓4ᵗʰ **N64 Other disorders of breast**
     EXCLUDES 2   mechanical complication of breast prosthesis and implant (T85.4-)

   N64.0 Fissure and fistula of nipple

   N64.1 Fat necrosis of breast
       Fat necrosis (segmental) of breast
       Code first breast necrosis due to breast graft (T85.898)

   N64.2 Atrophy of breast

   N64.3 Galactorrhea not associated with childbirth

   N64.4 Mastodynia

   ✓5ᵗʰ **N64.5 Other signs and symptoms in breast**
       EXCLUDES 2   abnormal findings on diagnostic imaging of breast (R92.-)

     N64.51 Induration of breast

     N64.52 Nipple discharge
         EXCLUDES 1   abnormal findings in nipple discharge (R89.-)

     N64.53 Retraction of nipple

     N64.59 Other signs and symptoms in breast

   ✓5ᵗʰ **N64.8 Other specified disorders of breast**

     N64.81 Ptosis of breast A
         EXCLUDES 1   ptosis of native breast in relation to reconstructed breast (N65.1)

     N64.82 Hypoplasia of breast A
       Micromastia
         EXCLUDES 1   congenital absence of breast (Q83.0)
           hypoplasia of native breast in relation to reconstructed breast (N65.1)

     N64.89 Other specified disorders of breast
       Galactocele
       Subinvolution of breast (postlactational)

   N64.9 Disorder of breast, unspecified ▽

✓4ᵗʰ **N65 Deformity and disproportion of reconstructed breast**

   N65.0 Deformity of reconstructed breast A
       Contour irregularity in reconstructed breast
       Excess tissue in reconstructed breast
       Misshapen reconstructed breast

   N65.1 Disproportion of reconstructed breast A
       Breast asymmetry between native breast and reconstructed breast
       Disproportion between native breast and reconstructed breast

---

☑ Additional Character Req   ✓x7ᵗʰ Placeholder Alert   Manifestation   HCC CMS-HCC Condition   ▽ Unspecified Code   ►◄ Revised Text   ● New Code   ▲ Revised Code Title

ICD-10-CM 2018   811

Chapter 14. Diseases of Genitourinary System

Inflammatory diseases of female pelvic organs (N70-N77)

> EXCLUDES 1   inflammatory diseases of female pelvic organs complicating:
> abortion or ectopic or molar pregnancy (O00-O07, O08.0)
> pregnancy, childbirth and the puerperium (O23-, O75.3, O85, O86-)

✓4th **N70 Salpingitis and oophoritis**

   INCLUDES   abscess (of) fallopian tube
            abscess (of) ovary
            pyosalpinx
            salpingo-oophoritis
            tubo-ovarian abscess
            tubo-ovarian inflammatory disease

   Use additional code (B95-B97), to identify infectious agent

> EXCLUDES 1   gonococcal infection (A54.24)
> tuberculous infection (A18.17)

✓5th **N70.0 Acute salpingitis and oophoritis**

     N70.01   **Acute salpingitis** ♀
     N70.02   **Acute oophoritis** ♀
     N70.03   **Acute salpingitis and oophoritis** ♀

✓5th **N70.1 Chronic salpingitis and oophoritis**

     Hydrosalpinx

     N70.11   **Chronic salpingitis** ♀
     N70.12   **Chronic oophoritis** ♀
     N70.13   **Chronic salpingitis and oophoritis** ♀

✓5th **N70.9 Salpingitis and oophoritis, unspecified**

     N70.91   **Salpingitis, unspecified** ♀ ▽
     N70.92   **Oophoritis, unspecified** ♀▽
     N70.93   **Salpingitis and oophoritis, unspecified** ♀ ▽

✓4th **N71 Inflammatory disease of uterus, except cervix**

   INCLUDES   endo (myo) metritis   pyometra
            metritis   uterine abscess
            myometritis

   Use additional code (B95-B97), to identify infectious agent

> EXCLUDES 1   hyperplastic endometritis (N85.0-)
> infection of uterus following delivery (O85, O86.-)

     N71.0   **Acute inflammatory disease of uterus** ♀
     N71.1   **Chronic inflammatory disease of uterus** ♀
     N71.9   **Inflammatory disease of uterus, unspecified** ♀ ▽

N72 Inflammatory disease of cervix uteri ♀

   INCLUDES   cervicitis (with or without erosion or ectropion)
            endocervicitis (with or without erosion or ectropion)
            exocervicitis (with or without erosion or ectropion)

   Use additional code (B95-B97), to identify infectious agent

> EXCLUDES 1   erosion and ectropion of cervix without cervicitis (N86)

✓4th **N73 Other female pelvic inflammatory diseases**

   Use additional code (B95-B97), to identify infectious agent

     N73.0   **Acute parametritis and pelvic cellulitis** ♀

       Abscess of broad ligament
       Abscess of parametrium
       Pelvic cellulitis, female
       DEF: Parametritis: Inflammation of the parametrium; pelvic cellulitis is a synonym for parametritis.

     N73.1   **Chronic parametritis and pelvic cellulitis** ♀

       Any condition in N73.0 specified as chronic

> EXCLUDES 1   tuberculous parametritis and pelvic cellulitis (A18.17)

     N73.2   **Unspecified parametritis and pelvic cellulitis** ♀ ▽

       Any condition in N73.0 unspecified whether acute or chronic

     N73.3   **Female acute pelvic peritonitis** ♀
     N73.4   **Female chronic pelvic peritonitis** ♀

> EXCLUDES 1   tuberculous pelvic (female) peritonitis (A18.17)

     N73.5   **Female pelvic peritonitis, unspecified** ♀▽
     N73.6   **Female pelvic peritoneal adhesions (postinfective)** ♀

> EXCLUDES 2   postprocedural pelvic peritoneal adhesions (N99.4)

       AHA: 2014, 1Q, 6

     N73.8   **Other specified female pelvic inflammatory diseases** ♀
     N73.9   **Female pelvic inflammatory disease, unspecified** ♀ ▽

       Female pelvic infection or inflammation NOS

N74 Female pelvic inflammatory disorders in diseases classified elsewhere ♀

   Code first underlying disease

> EXCLUDES 1   chlamydial cervicitis (A56.02)
> chlamydial pelvic inflammatory disease (A56.11)
> gonococcal cervicitis (A54.03)
> gonococcal pelvic inflammatory disease (A54.24)
> herpesviral [herpes simplex] cervicitis (A60.03)
> herpesviral [herpes simplex] pelvic inflammatory disease (A60.09)
> syphilitic cervicitis (A52.76)
> syphilitic pelvic inflammatory disease (A52.76)
> trichomonal cervicitis (A59.09)
> tuberculous cervicitis (A18.16)
> tuberculous pelvic inflammatory disease (A18.17)

✓4th **N75 Diseases of Bartholin's gland**

     N75.0   **Cyst of Bartholin's gland** ♀
     N75.1   **Abscess of Bartholin's gland** ♀
     N75.8   **Other diseases of Bartholin's gland** ♀

       Bartholinitis

     N75.9   **Disease of Bartholin's gland, unspecified** ♀ ▽

✓4th **N76 Other inflammation of vagina and vulva**

   Use additional code (B95-B97), to identify infectious agent

> EXCLUDES 2   senile (atrophic) vaginitis (N95.2)
> vulvar vestibulitis (N94.810)

     N76.0   **Acute vaginitis** ♀

       Acute vulvovaginitis
       Vaginitis NOS
       Vulvovaginitis NOS

     N76.1   **Subacute and chronic vaginitis** ♀

       Chronic vulvovaginitis
       Subacute vulvovaginitis

     N76.2   **Acute vulvitis** ♀

       Vulvitis NOS

     N76.3   **Subacute and chronic vulvitis** ♀
     N76.4   **Abscess of vulva** ♀

       Furuncle of vulva

     N76.5   **Ulceration of vagina** ♀
     N76.6   **Ulceration of vulva** ♀

✓5th **N76.8 Other specified inflammation of vagina and vulva**

     N76.81   **Mucositis (ulcerative) of vagina and vulva** ♀

       Code also type of associated therapy, such as:
         antineoplastic and immunosuppressive drugs (T45.1X-)
         radiological procedure and radiotherapy (Y84.2)

> EXCLUDES 2   gastrointestinal mucositis (ulcerative) (K92.81)
> nasal mucositis (ulcerative) (J34.81)
> oral mucositis (ulcerative) (K12.3-)

     N76.89   **Other specified inflammation of vagina and vulva** ♀

✓4th **N77 Vulvovaginal ulceration and inflammation in diseases classified elsewhere**

     N77.0   **Ulceration of vulva in diseases classified elsewhere** ♀

       Code first underlying disease, such as:
       Behçet's disease (M35.2)

> EXCLUDES 1   ulceration of vulva in gonococcal infection (A54.02)
> ulceration of vulva in herpesviral [herpes simplex] infection (A60.04)
> ulceration of vulva in syphilis (A51.0)
> ulceration of vulva in tuberculosis (A18.18)

     N77.1   **Vaginitis, vulvitis and vulvovaginitis in diseases classified elsewhere** ♀

       Code first underlying disease, such as:
       pinworm (B80)

> EXCLUDES 1   candidal vulvovaginitis (B37.3)
> chlamydial vulvovaginitis (A56.02)
> gonococcal vulvovaginitis (A54.02)
> herpesviral [herpes simplex] vulvovaginitis (A60.04)
> trichomonal vulvovaginitis (A59.01)
> tuberculous vulvovaginitis (A18.18)
> vulvovaginitis in early syphilis (A51.0)
> vulvovaginitis in late syphilis (A52.76)

EXCLUDES 1 Not coded here   EXCLUDES 2 Not included here   N Newborn Age: 0   P Pediatric Age: 0-17   M Maternity Age: 12-55   A Adult Age: 15-124

812   ICD-10-CM 2018

N70–N77.1

Types of Pelvic Organ Prolapse

Urethrocele   Cystocele

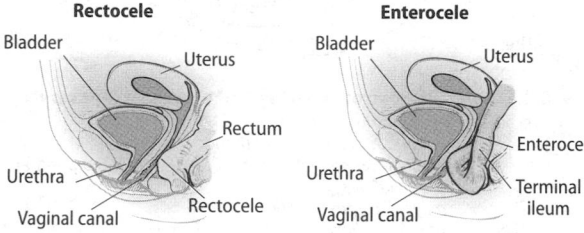

Rectocele   Enterocele

Noninflammatory disorders of female genital tract (N80-N98)

✓4ᵗʰ N80 Endometriosis

N80.0 Endometriosis of uterus ♀
Adenomyosis
EXCLUDES 1   stromal endometriosis (D39.0)

N80.1 Endometriosis of ovary ♀

N80.2 Endometriosis of fallopian tube ♀

N80.3 Endometriosis of pelvic peritoneum ♀

N80.4 Endometriosis of rectovaginal septum and vagina ♀

N80.5 Endometriosis of intestine ♀

N80.6 Endometriosis in cutaneous scar ♀

N80.8 Other endometriosis ♀
►Endometriosis of thorax◄

N80.9 Endometriosis, unspecified ♀ ▽

✓4ᵗʰ N81 Female genital prolapse

EXCLUDES 1   genital prolapse complicating pregnancy, labor or delivery (O34.5-)
prolapse and hernia of ovary and fallopian tube (N83.4-)
prolapse of vaginal vault after hysterectomy (N99.3)

N81.0 Urethrocele ♀
EXCLUDES 1   urethrocele with cystocele (N81.1-)
urethrocele with prolapse of uterus (N81.2-N81.4)

✓5ᵗʰ N81.1 Cystocele
Cystocele with urethrocele
Cystourethrocele
EXCLUDES 1   cystocele with prolapse of uterus (N81.2-N81.4)

N81.10 Cystocele, unspecified ♀ ▽
Prolapse of (anterior) vaginal wall NOS

N81.11 Cystocele, midline ♀

N81.12 Cystocele, lateral ♀
Paravaginal cystocele
DEF: Detachment of the lateral support connections of the vagina at the arcus tendineus fasciae pelvis (ATFP) results in bladder drop; bladder herniates into the vagina laterally.

N81.2 Incomplete uterovaginal prolapse ♀
First degree uterine prolapse
Prolapse of cervix NOS
Second degree uterine prolapse
EXCLUDES 1 ►cervical stump prolapse◄ (N81.85)

N81.3 Complete uterovaginal prolapse ♀
Procidentia (uteri) NOS
Third degree uterine prolapse

N81.4 Uterovaginal prolapse, unspecified ♀ ▽
Prolapse of uterus NOS

N81.5 Vaginal enterocele ♀
EXCLUDES 1   enterocele with prolapse of uterus (N81.2-N81.4)

N81.6 Rectocele ♀
Prolapse of posterior vaginal wall
Use additional code for any associated fecal incontinence, if applicable (R15.-)
EXCLUDES 2   perineocele (N81.81)
rectal prolapse (K62.3)
rectocele with prolapse of uterus (N81.2-N81.4)

✓5ᵗʰ N81.8 Other female genital prolapse

N81.81 Perineocele ♀

N81.82 Incompetence or weakening of pubocervical tissue ♀

N81.83 Incompetence or weakening of rectovaginal tissue ♀

N81.84 Pelvic muscle wasting ♀
Disuse atrophy of pelvic muscles and anal sphincter

N81.85 Cervical stump prolapse ♀

N81.89 Other female genital prolapse ♀
Deficient perineum
Old laceration of muscles of pelvic floor

N81.9 Female genital prolapse, unspecified ♀ ▽

✓4ᵗʰ N82 Fistulae involving female genital tract
EXCLUDES 1   vesicointestinal fistulae (N32.1)

N82.0 Vesicovaginal fistula ♀

N82.1 Other female urinary-genital tract fistulae ♀
Cervicovesical fistula
Ureterovaginal fistula
Urethrovaginal fistula
Uteroureteric fistula
Uterovesical fistula

N82.2 Fistula of vagina to small intestine ♀

N82.3 Fistula of vagina to large intestine ♀
Rectovaginal fistula

N82.4 Other female intestinal-genital tract fistulae ♀
Intestinouterine fistula

N82.5 Female genital tract-skin fistulae ♀
Uterus to abdominal wall fistula
Vaginoperineal fistula

N82.8 Other female genital tract fistulae ♀

N82.9 Female genital tract fistula, unspecified ♀ ▽

✓4ᵗʰ N83 Noninflammatory disorders of ovary, fallopian tube and broad ligament
EXCLUDES 2   hydrosalpinx (N70.1-)

✓5ᵗʰ N83.0 Follicular cyst of ovary
Cyst of graafian follicle
Hemorrhagic follicular cyst (of ovary)

N83.00 Follicular cyst of ovary, unspecified side ♀ ▽

N83.01 Follicular cyst of right ovary ♀

N83.02 Follicular cyst of left ovary ♀

✓5ᵗʰ N83.1 Corpus luteum cyst
Hemorrhagic corpus luteum cyst

N83.10 Corpus luteum cyst of ovary, unspecified side ♀ ▽

N83.11 Corpus luteum cyst of right ovary ♀

N83.12 Corpus luteum cyst of left ovary ♀

✓5ᵗʰ N83.2 Other and unspecified ovarian cysts
EXCLUDES 1   developmental ovarian cyst (Q50.1)
neoplastic ovarian cyst (D27.-)
polycystic ovarian syndrome (E28.2)
Stein-Leventhal syndrome (E28.2)

✓6ᵗʰ N83.20 Unspecified ovarian cysts

N83.201 Unspecified ovarian cyst, right side ♀ ▽

N83.202 Unspecified ovarian cyst, left side ♀ ▽

N83.209 Unspecified ovarian cyst, unspecified side ♀ ▽
Ovarian cyst, NOS

✓6ᵗʰ N83.29 Other ovarian cysts
Retention cyst of ovary
Simple cyst of ovary

N83.291 Other ovarian cyst, right side ♀

N83.292 Other ovarian cyst, left side ♀

N83.299 Other ovarian cyst, unspecified side ♀ ▽

✓5ᵗʰ N83.3 Acquired atrophy of ovary and fallopian tube

✓6ᵗʰ N83.31 Acquired atrophy of ovary

N83.311 Acquired atrophy of right ovary ♀

N83.312 Acquired atrophy of left ovary ♀

Chapter 14. Diseases of Genitourinary System

         N83.319   **Acquired atrophy of ovary, unspecified side** ♀▽
            Acquired atrophy of ovary, NOS

   ✓6ᵗʰ **N83.32**   **Acquired atrophy of fallopian tube**
         N83.321   **Acquired atrophy of right fallopian tube** ♀
         N83.322   **Acquired atrophy of left fallopian tube** ♀
         N83.329   **Acquired atrophy of fallopian tube, unspecified side** ♀▽
            Acquired atrophy of fallopian tube, NOS

   ✓6ᵗʰ **N83.33**   **Acquired atrophy of ovary and fallopian tube**
         N83.331   **Acquired atrophy of right ovary and fallopian tube** ♀
         N83.332   **Acquired atrophy of left ovary and fallopian tube** ♀
         N83.339   **Acquired atrophy of ovary and fallopian tube, unspecified side** ♀▽
            Acquired atrophy of ovary and fallopian tube, NOS

✓5ᵗʰ **N83.4**   **Prolapse and hernia of ovary and fallopian tube**
         N83.40   **Prolapse and hernia of ovary and fallopian tube, unspecified side** ♀▽
            Prolapse and hernia of ovary and fallopian tube, NOS
         N83.41   **Prolapse and hernia of right ovary and fallopian tube** ♀
         N83.42   **Prolapse and hernia of left ovary and fallopian tube** ♀

✓5ᵗʰ **N83.5**   **Torsion of ovary, ovarian pedicle and fallopian tube**
         Torsion of accessory tube
   ✓6ᵗʰ **N83.51**   **Torsion of ovary and ovarian pedicle**
         N83.511   **Torsion of right ovary and ovarian pedicle** ♀
         N83.512   **Torsion of left ovary and ovarian pedicle** ♀
         N83.519   **Torsion of ovary and ovarian pedicle, unspecified side** ♀▽
            Torsion of ovary and ovarian pedicle, NOS
   ✓6ᵗʰ **N83.52**   **Torsion of fallopian tube**
         Torsion of hydatid of Morgagni
         N83.521   **Torsion of right fallopian tube** ♀
         N83.522   **Torsion of left fallopian tube** ♀
         N83.529   **Torsion of fallopian tube, unspecified side** ♀▽
            Torsion of fallopian tube, NOS
         N83.53   **Torsion of ovary, ovarian pedicle and fallopian tube** ♀

N83.6   **Hematosalpinx** ♀
     EXCLUDES 1   *hematosalpinx (with) (in):*
         hematocolpos (N89.7)
         hematometra (N85.7)
         tubal pregnancy (O00.1-)

N83.7   **Hematoma of broad ligament** ♀

N83.8   **Other noninflammatory disorders of ovary, fallopian tube and broad ligament** ♀
     Broad ligament laceration syndrome [Allen-Masters]

N83.9   **Noninflammatory disorder of ovary, fallopian tube and broad ligament, unspecified** ♀▽

✓4ᵗʰ **N84**   **Polyp of female genital tract**
     EXCLUDES 1   *adenomatous polyp (D28.-)*
         placental polyp (O90.89)

N84.0   **Polyp of corpus uteri** ♀
     Polyp of endometrium
     Polyp of uterus NOS
     EXCLUDES 1   *polypoid endometrial hyperplasia (N85.0-)*

N84.1   **Polyp of cervix uteri** ♀
     Mucous polyp of cervix

N84.2   **Polyp of vagina** ♀

N84.3   **Polyp of vulva** ♀
     Polyp of labia

N84.8   **Polyp of other parts of female genital tract** ♀

N84.9   **Polyp of female genital tract, unspecified** ♀▽

Inversion of Uterus

Uterus

✓4ᵗʰ **N85**   **Other noninflammatory disorders of uterus, except cervix**
     EXCLUDES 1   *endometriosis (N80.-)*
         inflammatory diseases of uterus (N71.-)
         noninflammatory disorders of cervix, except malposition (N86-N88)
         polyp of corpus uteri (N84.0)
         uterine prolapse (N81.-)

   ✓5ᵗʰ **N85.0**   **Endometrial hyperplasia**
         N85.00   **Endometrial hyperplasia, unspecified** ♀▽
            Hyperplasia (adenomatous) (cystic) (glandular) of endometrium
            Hyperplastic endometritis
         N85.01   **Benign endometrial hyperplasia** ♀
            Endometrial hyperplasia (complex) (simple) without atypia
         N85.02   **Endometrial intraepithelial neoplasia [EIN]** ♀
            Endometrial hyperplasia with atypia
            EXCLUDES 1   *malignant neoplasm of endometrium (with endometrial intraepithelial neoplasia [EIN]) (C54.1)*

N85.2   **Hypertrophy of uterus** ♀
     Bulky or enlarged uterus
     EXCLUDES 1   *puerperal hypertrophy of uterus (O90.89)*

N85.3   **Subinvolution of uterus** ♀
     EXCLUDES 1   *puerperal subinvolution of uterus (O90.89)*

N85.4   **Malposition of uterus** ♀
     Anteversion of uterus   Retroversion of uterus
     Retroflexion of uterus
     EXCLUDES 1   *malposition of uterus complicating pregnancy, labor or delivery (O34.5-, O65.5)*

N85.5   **Inversion of uterus** ♀
     EXCLUDES 1   *current obstetric trauma (O71.2)*
         postpartum inversion of uterus (O71.2)

N85.6   **Intrauterine synechiae** ♀

N85.7   **Hematometra** ♀
     Hematosalpinx with hematometra
     EXCLUDES 1   *hematometra with hematocolpos (N89.7)*
     DEF: Accumulation of blood within the uterus.

N85.8   **Other specified noninflammatory disorders of uterus** ♀
     Atrophy of uterus, acquired
     Fibrosis of uterus NOS

N85.9   **Noninflammatory disorder of uterus, unspecified** ♀▽
     Disorder of uterus NOS

N86   **Erosion and ectropion of cervix uteri** ♀
     Decubitus (trophic) ulcer of cervix
     Eversion of cervix
     EXCLUDES 1   *erosion and ectropion of cervix with cervicitis (N72)*

✓4ᵗʰ **N87**   **Dysplasia of cervix uteri**
     EXCLUDES 1   *abnormal results from cervical cytologic examination without histologic confirmation (R87.61-)*
         carcinoma in situ of cervix uteri (D06.-)
         cervical intraepithelial neoplasia III [CIN III] (D06.-)
         HGSIL of cervix (R87.613)
         severe dysplasia of cervix uteri (D06.-)

N87.0   **Mild cervical dysplasia** ♀
     Cervical intraepithelial neoplasia I [CIN I]

N87.1   **Moderate cervical dysplasia** ♀
     Cervical intraepithelial neoplasia II [CIN II]

N87.9   **Dysplasia of cervix uteri, unspecified** ♀▽
     Anaplasia of cervix   Cervical dysplasia NOS
     Cervical atypism

EXCLUDES 1 Not coded here   **EXCLUDES 2** Not included here   **N** Newborn Age: 0   **P** Pediatric Age: 0-17   **M** Maternity Age: 12-55   **A** Adult Age: 15-124

814   ICD-10-CM 2018

N83.319–N87.9

☑4ᵗʰ **N88** **Other noninflammatory disorders of cervix uteri**
    EXCLUDES 2   *inflammatory disease of cervix (N72)*
             polyp of cervix (N84.1)

N88.0   **Leukoplakia of cervix uteri** ♀

N88.1   **Old laceration of cervix uteri** ♀
    Adhesions of cervix
    EXCLUDES 1   *current obstetric trauma (O71.3)*

N88.2   **Stricture and stenosis of cervix uteri** ♀
    EXCLUDES 1   *stricture and stenosis of cervix uteri complicating labor*
                 (O65.5)

N88.3   **Incompetence of cervix uteri** ♀
    Investigation and management of (suspected) cervical
    incompetence in a nonpregnant woman
    EXCLUDES 1   *cervical incompetence complicating pregnancy*
                 (O34.3-)

N88.4   **Hypertrophic elongation of cervix uteri** ♀

N88.8   **Other specified noninflammatory disorders of cervix uteri** ♀
    EXCLUDES 1   *current obstetric trauma (O71.3)*

N88.9   **Noninflammatory disorder of cervix uteri, unspecified** ♀ ▽

☑4ᵗʰ **N89** **Other noninflammatory disorders of vagina**
    EXCLUDES 1   *abnormal results from vaginal cytologic examination without*
                 histologic confirmation (R87.62-)
             carcinoma in situ of vagina (D07.2)
             HGSIL of vagina (R87.623)
             inflammation of vagina (N76.-)
             senile (atrophic) vaginitis (N95.2)
             severe dysplasia of vagina (D07.2)
             trichomonal leukorrhea (A59.00)
             vaginal intraepithelial neoplasia [VAIN], grade III (D07.2)

N89.0   **Mild vaginal dysplasia** ♀
    Vaginal intraepithelial neoplasia [VAIN], grade I

N89.1   **Moderate vaginal dysplasia** ♀
    Vaginal intraepithelial neoplasia [VAIN], grade II

N89.3   **Dysplasia of vagina, unspecified** ♀ ▽

N89.4   **Leukoplakia of vagina** ♀

N89.5   **Stricture and atresia of vagina** ♀
    Vaginal adhesions
    Vaginal stenosis
    EXCLUDES 1   *congenital atresia or stricture (Q52.4)*
                 postprocedural adhesions of vagina (N99.2)

N89.6   **Tight hymenal ring** ♀
    Rigid hymen
    Tight introitus
    EXCLUDES 1   *imperforate hymen (Q52.3)*

N89.7   **Hematocolpos** ♀
    Hematocolpos with hematometra or hematosalpinx

N89.8   **Other specified noninflammatory disorders of vagina** ♀
    Leukorrhea NOS
    Old vaginal laceration
    Pessary ulcer of vagina
    EXCLUDES 1   *current obstetric trauma (O70-, O71.4, O71.7-O71.8)*
                 old laceration involving muscles of pelvic floor (N81.8)

N89.9   **Noninflammatory disorder of vagina, unspecified** ♀ ▽

☑4ᵗʰ **N90** **Other noninflammatory disorders of vulva and perineum**
    EXCLUDES 1   *anogenital (venereal) warts (A63.0)*
             carcinoma in situ of vulva (D07.1)
             condyloma acuminatum (A63.0)
             current obstetric trauma (O70-, O71.7-O71.8)
             inflammation of vulva (N76.-)
             severe dysplasia of vulva (D07.1)
             vulvar intraepithelial neoplasm III [VIN III] (D07.1)

N90.0   **Mild vulvar dysplasia** ♀
    Vulvar intraepithelial neoplasia [VIN], grade I

N90.1   **Moderate vulvar dysplasia** ♀
    Vulvar intraepithelial neoplasia [VIN], grade II

N90.3   **Dysplasia of vulva, unspecified** ♀ ▽

N90.4   **Leukoplakia of vulva** ♀
    Dystrophy of vulva
    Kraurosis of vulva
    Lichen sclerosus of external female genital organs

N90.5   **Atrophy of vulva** ♀
    Stenosis of vulva

☑5ᵗʰ **N90.6**   **Hypertrophy of vulva** ♀

    N90.60   **Unspecified hypertrophy of vulva** ♀ ▽
            Unspecified hypertrophy of labia

    N90.61   **Childhood asymmetric labium majus** ♀
            enlargement
            CALME

    N90.69   **Other specified hypertrophy of vulva** ♀
            Other specified hypertrophy of labia

N90.7   **Vulvar cyst** ♀

☑5ᵗʰ **N90.8**   **Other specified noninflammatory disorders of vulva and perineum**

    ☑6ᵗʰ **N90.81**   **Female genital mutilation status**
            Female genital cutting status

         N90.810   **Female genital mutilation status,** ♀ ▽
               unspecified
               Female genital cutting status, unspecified
               Female genital mutilation status NOS

         N90.811   **Female genital mutilation Type I status** ♀
               Clitorectomy status
               Female genital cutting Type I status

         N90.812   **Female genital mutilation Type II status** ♀
               Clitorectomy with excision of labia minora
               status
               Female genital cutting Type II status

         N90.813   **Female genital mutilation Type III status** ♀
               Female genital cutting Type III status
               Infibulation status

         N90.818   **Other female genital mutilation status** ♀
               Female genital cutting Type IV status
               Female genital mutilation Type IV status
               Other female genital cutting status

    N90.89   **Other specified noninflammatory disorders of**
            vulva and perineum
            Adhesions of vulva   Hypertrophy of clitoris

N90.9   **Noninflammatory disorder of vulva and perineum,** ♀ ▽
    unspecified

☑4ᵗʰ **N91** **Absent, scanty and rare menstruation**
    EXCLUDES 1   *ovarian dysfunction (E28.-)*

N91.0   **Primary amenorrhea** ♀

N91.1   **Secondary amenorrhea** ♀

N91.2   **Amenorrhea, unspecified** ♀ ▽

N91.3   **Primary oligomenorrhea** ♀

N91.4   **Secondary oligomenorrhea** ♀

N91.5   **Oligomenorrhea, unspecified** ♀ ▽
    Hypomenorrhea NOS

☑4ᵗʰ **N92** **Excessive, frequent and irregular menstruation**
    EXCLUDES 1   *postmenopausal bleeding (N95.0)*
             precocious puberty (menstruation) (E30.1)

N92.0   **Excessive and frequent menstruation with regular cycle** ♀
    Heavy periods NOS
    Menorrhagia NOS
    Polymenorrhea

N92.1   **Excessive and frequent menstruation with irregular cycle** ♀
    Irregular intermenstrual bleeding
    Irregular, shortened intervals between menstrual bleeding
    Menometrorrhagia
    Metrorrhagia

N92.2   **Excessive menstruation at puberty** P♀
    Excessive bleeding associated with onset of menstrual periods
    Pubertal menorrhagia
    Puberty bleeding

N92.3   **Ovulation bleeding** ♀
    Regular intermenstrual bleeding

N92.4   **Excessive bleeding in the premenopausal period** ♀
    Climacteric menorrhagia or metrorrhagia
    Menopausal menorrhagia or metrorrhagia
    Preclimacteric menorrhagia or metrorrhagia
    Premenopausal menorrhagia or metrorrhagia

N92.5   **Other specified irregular menstruation** ♀

N92.6   **Irregular menstruation, unspecified** ♀ ▽
    Irregular bleeding NOS
    Irregular periods NOS
    EXCLUDES 1   *irregular menstruation with:*
             lengthened intervals or scanty bleeding
               (N91.3-N91.5)
             shortened intervals or excessive bleeding (N92.1)

☑ Additional Character Req   ✔x7ᵗʰ Placeholder Alert   Manifestation   HCC CMS-HCC Condition   ▽ Unspecified Code   ►◄ Revised Text   ● New Code   ▲ Revised Code Title

ICD-10-CM 2018   815

☑4th **N93 Other abnormal uterine and vaginal bleeding**
> EXCLUDES 1   *neonatal vaginal hemorrhage (P54.6)*
> *precocious puberty (menstruation) (E30.1)*
> *pseudomenses (P54.6)*

    N93.0 Postcoital and contact bleeding ♀

    N93.1 Pre-pubertal vaginal bleeding ♀

    N93.8 Other specified abnormal uterine and vaginal bleeding ♀
> Dysfunctional or functional uterine or vaginal bleeding NOS

    N93.9 Abnormal uterine and vaginal bleeding, unspecified ♀▽

☑4th **N94 Pain and other conditions associated with female genital organs and menstrual cycle**

    N94.0 Mittelschmerz ♀
> **DEF:** One-sided, lower abdominal pain occurring between menstrual periods; associated with ovulation.

    ☑5th **N94.1 Dyspareunia**
> EXCLUDES 1   *psychogenic dyspareunia (F52.6)*

        N94.10 Unspecified dyspareunia ♀▽

        N94.11 Superficial (introital) dyspareunia ♀

        N94.12 Deep dyspareunia ♀

        N94.19 Other specified dyspareunia ♀

    N94.2 Vaginismus ♀
> EXCLUDES 1   *psychogenic vaginismus (F52.5)*

    N94.3 Premenstrual tension syndrome ♀
> ~~Premenstrual dysphoric disorder~~
> Code also associated menstrual migraine (G43.82-, G43.83-)
> EXCLUDES 1   *premenstrual dysphoric disorder (F32.81)*

    N94.4 Primary dysmenorrhea ♀

    N94.5 Secondary dysmenorrhea ♀

    N94.6 Dysmenorrhea, unspecified ♀▽
> EXCLUDES 1   *psychogenic dysmenorrhea (F45.8)*

    ☑5th **N94.8 Other specified conditions associated with female genital organs and menstrual cycle**

        ☑6th **N94.81 Vulvodynia**

            N94.810 Vulvar vestibulitis ♀

            N94.818 Other vulvodynia ♀

            N94.819 Vulvodynia, unspecified ♀▽
> Vulvodynia NOS

        N94.89 Other specified conditions associated with female genital organs and menstrual cycle ♀

    N94.9 Unspecified condition associated with female genital organs and menstrual cycle ♀▽

☑4th **N95 Menopausal and other perimenopausal disorders**
> Menopausal and other perimenopausal disorders due to naturally occurring (age-related) menopause and perimenopause
> EXCLUDES 1   *excessive bleeding in the premenopausal period (N92.4)*
> *menopausal and perimenopausal disorders due to artificial or premature menopause (E89.4-, E28.31-)*
> *premature menopause (E28.31-)*
> EXCLUDES 2   *postmenopausal osteoporosis (M81.0-)*
> *postmenopausal osteoporosis with current pathological fracture (M80.0-)*
> *postmenopausal urethritis (N34.2)*

    N95.0 Postmenopausal bleeding ♀

    N95.1 Menopausal and female climacteric states ♀
> Symptoms such as flushing, sleeplessness, headache, lack of concentration, associated with natural (age-related) menopause
> Use additional code for associated symptoms
> EXCLUDES 1   *asymptomatic menopausal state (Z78.0)*
> *symptoms associated with artificial menopause (E89.41)*
> *symptoms associated with premature menopause (E28.310)*

    N95.2 Postmenopausal atrophic vaginitis ♀
> Senile (atrophic) vaginitis

    N95.8 Other specified menopausal and perimenopausal disorders ♀

    N95.9 Unspecified menopausal and perimenopausal disorder ♀▽

N96 Recurrent pregnancy loss ♀
> Investigation or care in a nonpregnant woman with history of recurrent pregnancy loss
> EXCLUDES 1   *recurrent pregnancy loss with current pregnancy (O26.2-)*

☑4th **N97 Female infertility**
> INCLUDES   inability to achieve a pregnancy
> sterility, female NOS
> EXCLUDES 1   *female infertility associated with:*
> *hypopituitarism (E23.0)*
> *Stein-Leventhal syndrome (E28.2)*
> EXCLUDES 2   *incompetence of cervix uteri (N88.3)*
> **DEF:** Infertility: Inability to conceive for at least one year with regular intercourse.
> **DEF:** Primary infertility: Infertility occurring in patients who have never conceived.
> **DEF:** Secondary infertility: Infertility occurring in patients who have previously conceived.

    N97.0 Female infertility associated with anovulation ♀

    N97.1 Female infertility of tubal origin ♀
> Female infertility associated with congenital anomaly of tube
> Female infertility due to tubal block
> Female infertility due to tubal occlusion
> Female infertility due to tubal stenosis

    N97.2 Female infertility of uterine origin ♀
> Female infertility associated with congenital anomaly of uterus
> Female infertility due to nonimplantation of ovum

    N97.8 Female infertility of other origin ♀

    N97.9 Female infertility, unspecified ♀▽

☑4th **N98 Complications associated with artificial fertilization**

    N98.0 Infection associated with artificial insemination ♀

    N98.1 Hyperstimulation of ovaries ♀
> Hyperstimulation of ovaries NOS
> Hyperstimulation of ovaries associated with induced ovulation

    N98.2 Complications of attempted introduction of fertilized ovum following in vitro fertilization ♀

    N98.3 Complications of attempted introduction of embryo in embryo transfer ♀

    N98.8 Other complications associated with artificial fertilization ♀

    N98.9 Complication associated with artificial fertilization, unspecified ♀▽

Intraoperative and postprocedural complications and disorders of genitourinary system, not elsewhere classified (N99)

☑4th **N99 Intraoperative and postprocedural complications and disorders of genitourinary system, not elsewhere classified**
> EXCLUDES 2   *irradiation cystitis (N30.4-)*
> *postoophorectomy osteoporosis with current pathological fracture (M80.8-)*
> *postoophorectomy osteoporosis without current pathological fracture (M81.8)*

    N99.0 Postprocedural (acute) (chronic) kidney failure
> Use additional code to type of kidney disease

    ☑5th **N99.1 Postprocedural urethral stricture**
> Postcatheterization urethral stricture

        ☑6th **N99.11 Postprocedural urethral stricture, male**

            N99.110 Postprocedural urethral stricture, male, meatal ♂

    ▲   **N99.111 Postprocedural bulbous urethral stricture, male** ♂

    ▲   **N99.112 Postprocedural membranous urethral stricture, male** ♂

    ▲   **N99.113 Postprocedural anterior bulbous urethral stricture, male** ♂

            N99.114 Postprocedural urethral stricture, male, unspecified ♂▽

            N99.115 Postprocedural fossa navicularis urethral stricture ♂

        N99.12 Postprocedural urethral stricture, female ♀

    N99.2 Postprocedural adhesions of vagina ♀

    N99.3 Prolapse of vaginal vault after hysterectomy ♀

    N99.4 Postprocedural pelvic peritoneal adhesions
> EXCLUDES 2   *pelvic peritoneal adhesions NOS (N73.6)*
> *postinfective pelvic peritoneal adhesions (N73.6)*

EXCLUDES 1 Not coded here   EXCLUDES 2 Not included here   N Newborn Age: 0   P Pediatric Age: 0-17   M Maternity Age: 12-55   A Adult Age: 15-124

816   ICD-10-CM 2018

✓5ᵗʰ **N99.5 Complications of stoma of urinary tract**
     EXCLUDES 2   *mechanical complication of urinary catheter (T83.0-)*

    ✓6ᵗʰ **N99.51 Complication of cystostomy**
         N99.510 **Cystostomy hemorrhage**   HCC
         N99.511 **Cystostomy infection**   HCC
         N99.512 **Cystostomy malfunction**   HCC
         N99.518 **Other cystostomy complication**   HCC

    ✓6ᵗʰ **N99.52 Complication of incontinent external stoma of urinary tract**
         N99.520 **Hemorrhage of incontinent external stoma of urinary tract**   HCC
         N99.521 **Infection of incontinent external stoma of urinary tract**   HCC
         N99.522 **Malfunction of incontinent external stoma of urinary tract**   HCC
         N99.523 **Herniation of incontinent stoma of urinary tract**   HCC
         N99.524 **Stenosis of incontinent stoma of urinary tract**   HCC
         N99.528 **Other complication of incontinent external stoma of urinary tract**   HCC

    ✓6ᵗʰ **N99.53 Complication of continent stoma of urinary tract**
         N99.530 **Hemorrhage of continent stoma of urinary tract**   HCC
         N99.531 **Infection of continent stoma of urinary tract**   HCC
         N99.532 **Malfunction of continent stoma of urinary tract**   HCC
         N99.533 **Herniation of continent stoma of urinary tract**   HCC
         N99.534 **Stenosis of continent stoma of urinary tract**   HCC
         N99.538 **Other complication of continent stoma of urinary tract**   HCC

✓5ᵗʰ **N99.6 Intraoperative hemorrhage and hematoma of a genitourinary system organ or structure complicating a procedure**
     EXCLUDES 1   *intraoperative hemorrhage and hematoma of a genitourinary system organ or structure due to accidental puncture or laceration during a procedure (N99.7-)*

     N99.61 **Intraoperative hemorrhage and hematoma of a genitourinary system organ or structure complicating a genitourinary system procedure**

     N99.62 **Intraoperative hemorrhage and hematoma of a genitourinary system organ or structure complicating other procedure**

✓5ᵗʰ **N99.7 Accidental puncture and laceration of a genitourinary system organ or structure during a procedure**

     N99.71 **Accidental puncture and laceration of a genitourinary system organ or structure during a genitourinary system procedure**

     N99.72 **Accidental puncture and laceration of a genitourinary system organ or structure during other procedure**

✓5ᵗʰ **N99.8 Other intraoperative and postprocedural complications and disorders of genitourinary system**

     N99.81 **Other intraoperative complications of genitourinary system**

    ✓6ᵗʰ **N99.82 Postprocedural hemorrhage of a genitourinary system organ or structure following a procedure**
         N99.820 **Postprocedural hemorrhage of a genitourinary system organ or structure following a genitourinary system procedure**
         N99.821 **Postprocedural hemorrhage of a genitourinary system organ or structure following other procedure**

     N99.83 **Residual ovary syndrome**   ♀

    ✓6ᵗʰ **N99.84 Postprocedural hematoma and seroma of a genitourinary system organ or structure following a procedure**
         N99.840 **Postprocedural hematoma of a genitourinary system organ or structure following a genitourinary system procedure**
         N99.841 **Postprocedural hematoma of a genitourinary system organ or structure following other procedure**
         N99.842 **Postprocedural seroma of a genitourinary system organ or structure following a genitourinary system procedure**
         N99.843 **Postprocedural seroma of a genitourinary system organ or structure following other procedure**

     N99.89 **Other postprocedural complications and disorders of genitourinary system**

☑ Additional Character Req   ✓x7ᵗʰ Placeholder Alert   Manifestation   HCC CMS-HCC Condition   ▽ Unspecified Code   ►◄ Revised Text   ● New Code   ▲ Revised Code Title

Chapter 15. Pregnancy, Childbirth, and the Puerperium (O00–O9A)

Chapter Specific Guidelines with Coding Examples

The chapter specific guidelines from the ICD-10-CM Official Guidelines for Coding and Reporting have been provided below. Along with these guidelines are coding examples, contained in the shaded boxes, that have been developed to help illustrate the coding and/or sequencing guidance found in these guidelines.

a. General rules for obstetric cases

1) Codes from Chapter 15 and sequencing priority

Obstetric cases require codes from chapter 15, codes in the range O00-O9A, Pregnancy, Childbirth, and the Puerperium. Chapter 15 codes have sequencing priority over codes from other chapters. Additional codes from other chapters may be used in conjunction with chapter 15 codes to further specify conditions. Should the provider document that the pregnancy is incidental to the encounter, then code Z33.1, Pregnant state, incidental, should be used in place of any chapter 15 codes. It is the provider's responsibility to state that the condition being treated is not affecting the pregnancy.

> Bladder abscess in pregnant patient at 25 weeks' gestation
>
> **O23.12**   **Infections of bladder in pregnancy, second trimester**
>
> **N30.80**   **Other cystitis without hematuria**
>
> **Z3A.25**   **25 weeks gestation of pregnancy**
>
> *Explanation:* The documentation does not indicate that the pregnancy is incidental or in any way unaffected by the bladder abscess; therefore, an obstetrics code should be sequenced first. An additional code was provided to identify the specific bladder condition as this information is not called out specifically in the obstetrics code.

2) Chapter 15 codes used only on the maternal record

Chapter 15 codes are to be used only on the maternal record, never on the record of the newborn.

3) Final character for trimester

The majority of codes in Chapter 15 have a final character indicating the trimester of pregnancy. The timeframes for the trimesters are indicated at the beginning of the chapter. If trimester is not a component of a code, it is because the condition always occurs in a specific trimester, or the concept of trimester of pregnancy is not applicable. Certain codes have characters for only certain trimesters because the condition does not occur in all trimesters, but it may occur in more than just one. Assignment of the final character for trimester should be based on the provider's documentation of the trimester (or number of weeks) for the current admission/encounter. This applies to the assignment of trimester for pre-existing conditions as well as those that develop during or are due to the pregnancy. The provider's documentation of the number of weeks may be used to assign the appropriate code identifying the trimester.

Whenever delivery occurs during the current admission, and there is an "in childbirth" option for the obstetric complication being coded, the "in childbirth" code should be assigned.

> Pregnant patient at 21 weeks' gestation admitted with excessive vomiting
>
> **O21.2**   **Late vomiting of pregnancy**
>
> **Z3A.21**   **21 weeks gestation of pregnancy**
>
> *Explanation:* Category O21 classifies vomiting in pregnancy. Although code selection is based on whether the vomiting is before or after 20 completed weeks, these codes are not further classified by trimester. If vomiting only in the second trimester was documented, the provider should be queried for the specific week of gestation, as this will affect code selection.

4) Selection of trimester for inpatient admissions that encompass more than one trimester

In instances when a patient is admitted to a hospital for complications of pregnancy during one trimester and remains in the hospital into a subsequent trimester, the trimester character for the antepartum complication code should be assigned on the basis of the trimester when the complication developed, not the trimester of the discharge. If the condition developed prior to the current admission/encounter or represents a pre-existing condition, the trimester character for the trimester at the time of the admission/encounter should be assigned.

5) Unspecified trimester

Each category that includes codes for trimester has a code for "unspecified trimester." The "unspecified trimester" code should rarely be used, such as when the documentation in the record is insufficient to determine the trimester and it is not possible to obtain clarification.

6) 7th character for fetus identification

Where applicable, a 7th character is to be assigned for certain categories (O31, O32, O33.3 - O33.6, O35, O36, O40, O41, O60.1, O60.2, O64, and O69) to identify the fetus for which the complication code applies.

Assign 7th character "0":

- For single gestations
- When the documentation in the record is insufficient to determine the fetus affected and it is not possible to obtain clarification.
- When it is not possible to clinically determine which fetus is affected.

> Maternal patient with twin gestations is seen after ultrasound identifies fetus B to be in breech presentation
>
> **O32.1XX2**   **Maternal care for breech presentation, fetus 2**
>
> *Explanation:* The documentation indicates that although there are two fetuses, only one fetus is determined to be in breech presentation. Whether fetus 2 or fetus B is used, the coder can assign the seventh character of 2 to identify the second fetus as the one in breech.

b. Selection of OB principal or first-listed diagnosis

1) Routine outpatient prenatal visits

For routine outpatient prenatal visits when no complications are present, a code from category Z34, Encounter for supervision of normal pregnancy, should be used as the first-listed diagnosis. These codes should not be used in conjunction with chapter 15 codes.

2) *Supervision of high-risk pregnancy*

Codes from category O09, Supervision of high-risk pregnancy, are intended for use only during the prenatal period. For complications during the labor or delivery episode as a result of a high-risk pregnancy, assign the applicable complication codes from Chapter 15. If there are no complications during the labor or delivery episode, assign code O80, Encounter for full-term uncomplicated delivery.

For routine prenatal outpatient visits for patients with high-risk pregnancies, a code from category O09, Supervision of high-risk pregnancy, should be used as the first-listed diagnosis. Secondary chapter 15 codes may be used in conjunction with these codes if appropriate.

> 36-year-old seen in labor with second child at 39 weeks' gestation, delivered a healthy baby, delivery complicated by tear of fourchette that was repaired
>
> **O70.0**   **First degree perineal laceration during delivery**
>
> **Z3A.39**   **39 weeks gestation of pregnancy**
>
> **Z37.0**   **Single live birth**
>
> Explanation: Although this patient is over 35 and having her second child (elderly multigravida), do not append a code from subcategory O09.52-. A code describing the tear of the fourchette, which complicated the delivery, should be used in addition to the applicable Z codes.

3) Episodes when no delivery occurs

In episodes when no delivery occurs, the principal diagnosis should correspond to the principal complication of the pregnancy which necessitated the encounter. Should more than one complication exist, all of which are treated or monitored, any of the complications codes may be sequenced first.

4) When a delivery occurs

When an obstetric patient is admitted and delivers during that admission, the condition that prompted the admission should be sequenced as the principal diagnosis. If multiple conditions prompted the admission, sequence the one most related to the delivery as the principal diagnosis. A code for any complication of the delivery should be assigned as an additional diagnosis. In cases of cesarean delivery, if the patient was admitted with a condition that resulted in the performance of a cesarean procedure, that condition should be selected as the principal diagnosis. If the reason for the admission was unrelated to the condition resulting in the cesarean delivery, the condition related to the reason for the admission should be selected as the principal diagnosis.

> Maternal patient with diet-controlled gestational diabetes was seen at 38 weeks' gestation in obstructed labor due to footling presentation; cesarean performed for the malpresentation
>
> | O64.8XX0 | Obstructed labor due to other malposition and malpresentation, not applicable or unspecified |
> |---|---|
> | O24.420 | Gestational diabetes mellitus in childbirth, diet controlled |
> | Z3A.38 | 38 weeks gestation of pregnancy |
> | Z37.0 | Single live birth |
>
> *Explanation:* The obstructed labor necessitated the cesarean procedure.

5) Outcome of delivery

A code from category Z37, Outcome of delivery, should be included on every maternal record when a delivery has occurred. These codes are not to be used on subsequent records or on the newborn record.

c. Pre-existing conditions versus conditions due to the pregnancy

Certain categories in Chapter 15 distinguish between conditions of the mother that existed prior to pregnancy (pre-existing) and those that are a direct result of pregnancy. When assigning codes from Chapter 15, it is important to assess if a condition was pre-existing prior to pregnancy or developed during or due to the pregnancy in order to assign the correct code.

Categories that do not distinguish between pre-existing and pregnancy-related conditions may be used for either. It is acceptable to use codes specifically for the puerperium with codes complicating pregnancy and childbirth if a condition arises postpartum during the delivery encounter.

d. Pre-existing hypertension in pregnancy

Category O10, Pre-existing hypertension complicating pregnancy, childbirth and the puerperium, includes codes for hypertensive heart and hypertensive chronic kidney disease. When assigning one of the O10 codes that includes hypertensive heart disease or hypertensive chronic kidney disease, it is necessary to add a secondary code from the appropriate hypertension category to specify the type of heart failure or chronic kidney disease.

See Section I.C.9. Hypertension.

e. Fetal conditions affecting the management of the mother

1) Codes from categories O35 and O36

Codes from categories O35, Maternal care for known or suspected fetal abnormality and damage, and O36, Maternal care for other fetal problems, are assigned only when the fetal condition is actually responsible for modifying the management of the mother, i.e., by requiring diagnostic studies, additional observation, special care, or termination of pregnancy. The fact that the fetal condition exists does not justify assigning a code from this series to the mother's record.

> A patient with twin gestation is seen for spotting 15 weeks into her pregnancy; the doctors also suspect fetal hydrocephalus. Patient is instructed to return in one week for additional diagnostic testing, sooner if the problem worsens.
>
> | O35.0XX0 | Maternal care for (suspected) central nervous system malformation in fetus, not applicable or unspecified |
> |---|---|
> | O26.852 | Spotting complicating pregnancy, second trimester |
> | Z3A.15 | 15 weeks gestation of pregnancy |
>
> *Explanation:* Whether the fetal hydrocephalus was suspected or confirmed, an additional code is warranted for this condition since documentation indicates the patient is to return sooner than her routine visit for further testing.

2) In utero surgery

In cases when surgery is performed on the fetus, a diagnosis code from category O35, Maternal care for known or suspected fetal abnormality and damage, should be assigned identifying the fetal condition. Assign the appropriate procedure code for the procedure performed.

No code from Chapter 16, the perinatal codes, should be used on the mother's record to identify fetal conditions. Surgery performed in utero on a fetus is still to be coded as an obstetric encounter.

f. HIV infection in pregnancy, childbirth and the puerperium

During pregnancy, childbirth or the puerperium, a patient admitted because of an HIV-related illness should receive a principal diagnosis from subcategory O98.7-, Human immunodeficiency [HIV] disease complicating pregnancy, childbirth and the puerperium, followed by the code(s) for the HIV-related illness(es).

Patients with asymptomatic HIV infection status admitted during pregnancy, childbirth, or the puerperium should receive codes of O98.7- and Z21, Asymptomatic human immunodeficiency virus [HIV] infection status.

> A previously asymptomatic HIV patient who is 13 weeks pregnant is evaluated for HIV-related candidal bronchitis
>
> | O98.711 | Human immunodeficiency virus [HIV] disease complicating pregnancy, first trimester |
> |---|---|
> | B20 | Human immunodeficiency virus [HIV] disease |
> | B37.1 | Candidal bronchitis |
> | Z3A.13 | 13 weeks gestation of pregnancy |
>
> *Explanation:* Because candidal bronchitis is an AIDS-related condition, this patient is now considered to have HIV disease. An obstetrics code indicating that HIV is complicating the pregnancy is coded first, followed by B20 for HIV disease as well as a code for the candidal bronchitis.

g. Diabetes mellitus in pregnancy

Diabetes mellitus is a significant complicating factor in pregnancy. Pregnant women who are diabetic should be assigned a code from category O24, Diabetes mellitus in pregnancy, childbirth, and the puerperium, first, followed by the appropriate diabetes code(s) (E08-E13) from Chapter 4.

h. Long term use of insulin and oral hypoglycemics

Code Z79.4, Long-term (current) use of insulin, or code Z79.84, Long-term (current) use of oral hypoglycemic drugs, should also be assigned if the diabetes mellitus is being treated with insulin or oral medications. If the patient is treated with both oral medications and insulin, only the code for insulin-controlled should be assigned.

i. Gestational (pregnancy induced) diabetes

Gestational (pregnancy induced) diabetes can occur during the second and third trimester of pregnancy in women who were not diabetic prior to pregnancy. Gestational diabetes can cause complications in the pregnancy similar to those of pre-existing diabetes mellitus. It also puts the woman at greater risk of developing diabetes after the pregnancy. Codes for gestational diabetes are in subcategory O24.4, Gestational diabetes mellitus. No other code from category O24, Diabetes mellitus in pregnancy, childbirth, and the puerperium, should be used with a code from O24.4.

The codes under subcategory O24.4 include diet controlled, insulin controlled, and controlled by oral hypoglycemic drugs. If a patient with gestational diabetes is treated with both diet and insulin, only the code for insulin-controlled is required. If a patient with gestational diabetes is treated with both diet and oral hypoglycemic medications, only the code for "controlled by oral hypoglycemic drugs" is required. Code Z79.4, Long-term (current) use of insulin or code Z79.84, Long-term (current) use of oral hypoglycemic drugs, should not be assigned with codes from subcategory O24.4.

An abnormal glucose tolerance in pregnancy is assigned a code from subcategory O99.81, Abnormal glucose complicating pregnancy, childbirth, and the puerperium.

j. Sepsis and septic shock complicating abortion, pregnancy, childbirth and the puerperium

When assigning a chapter 15 code for sepsis complicating abortion, pregnancy, childbirth, and the puerperium, a code for the specific type of infection should be assigned as an additional diagnosis. If severe sepsis is present, a code from subcategory R65.2, Severe sepsis, and code(s) for associated organ dysfunction(s) should also be assigned as additional diagnoses.

Patient is seen several days after a miscarriage with sepsis; cultures return MSSA

O03.87	Sepsis following complete or unspecified spontaneous abortion
B95.61	Methicillin susceptible Staphylococcus aureus infection as the cause of diseases classified elsewhere

Explanation: The type of infection that caused this patient to become septic was methicillin susceptible *Staphylococcus aureus* (MSSA), which as a secondary code helps capture all aspects related to this patient's septic condition.

k. Puerperal sepsis

Code O85, Puerperal sepsis, should be assigned with a secondary code to identify the causal organism (e.g., for a bacterial infection, assign a code from category B95-B96, Bacterial infections in conditions classified elsewhere). A code from category A40, Streptococcal sepsis, or A41, Other sepsis, should not be used for puerperal sepsis. If applicable, use additional codes to identify severe sepsis (R65.2-) and any associated acute organ dysfunction.

l. Alcohol and tobacco use during pregnancy, childbirth and the puerperium

1) Alcohol use during pregnancy, childbirth and the puerperium

Codes under subcategory O99.31, Alcohol use complicating pregnancy, childbirth, and the puerperium, should be assigned for any pregnancy case when a mother uses alcohol during the pregnancy or postpartum. A secondary code from category F10, Alcohol related disorders, should also be assigned to identify manifestations of the alcohol use.

2) Tobacco use during pregnancy, childbirth and the puerperium

Codes under subcategory O99.33, Smoking (tobacco) complicating pregnancy, childbirth, and the puerperium, should be assigned for any pregnancy case when a mother uses any type of tobacco product during the pregnancy or postpartum. A secondary code from category F17, Nicotine dependence, should also be assigned to identify the type of nicotine dependence.

m. Poisoning, toxic effects, adverse effects and underdosing in a pregnant patient

A code from subcategory O9A.2, Injury, poisoning and certain other consequences of external causes complicating pregnancy, childbirth, and the puerperium, should be sequenced first, followed by the appropriate injury, poisoning, toxic effect, adverse effect or underdosing code, and then the additional code(s) that specifies the condition caused by the poisoning, toxic effect, adverse effect or underdosing.

See Section I.C.19. Adverse effects, poisoning, underdosing and toxic effects.

Patient treated for accidental carbon monoxide poisoning from a gas heating implement; the patient is 18 weeks' pregnant

O9A.212	Injury, poisoning and certain other consequences of external causes complicating pregnancy, second trimester
T58.11XA	Toxic effect of carbon monoxide from utility gas, accidental (unintentional), initial encounter
Z3A.18	18 weeks gestation of pregnancy

Explanation: Although the carbon monoxide poisoning is the reason for the encounter, a code from the obstetrics chapter must be sequenced first. Chapter 15 codes have sequencing priority over codes from other chapters.

n. Normal delivery, code O80

1) Encounter for full term uncomplicated delivery

Code O80 should be assigned when a woman is admitted for a full-term normal delivery and delivers a single, healthy infant without any complications antepartum, during the delivery, or postpartum during the delivery episode. Code O80 is always a principal diagnosis. It is not to be used if any other code from chapter 15 is needed to describe a current complication of the antenatal, delivery, or perinatal period. Additional codes from other chapters may be used with code O80 if they are not related to or are in any way complicating the pregnancy.

2) Uncomplicated delivery with resolved antepartum complication

Code O80 may be used if the patient had a complication at some point during the pregnancy, but the complication is not present at the time of the admission for delivery.

Patient presents in labor at 39 weeks' gestation and delivers a healthy newborn; patient had abnormal glucose levels in her first trimester, which have since resolved

O80	Encounter for full-term uncomplicated delivery
Z37.0	Single live birth

Explanation: The abnormal glucose levels during the first trimester cannot be coded if they are not affecting the patient's current trimester. Without additional complications associated with the pregnancy, fetus, or mother, code O80 is appropriate.

3) Outcome of delivery for O80

Z37.0, Single live birth, is the only outcome of delivery code appropriate for use with O80.

o. The peripartum and postpartum periods

1) Peripartum and postpartum periods

The postpartum period begins immediately after delivery and continues for six weeks following delivery. The peripartum period is defined as the last month of pregnancy to five months postpartum.

2) Peripartum and postpartum complication

A postpartum complication is any complication occurring within the six-week period.

3) Pregnancy-related complications after 6 week period

Chapter 15 codes may also be used to describe pregnancy-related complications after the peripartum or postpartum period if the provider documents that a condition is pregnancy related.

Patient referred for varicose veins. She had a baby boy three months ago; the varicose veins started to appear one month ago. The doctor attributes the patient's pregnancy as the cause of the varicose veins, which continue to be painful and bother the patient. She is seeking surgical relief.

O87.4	Varicose veins of the lower extremity in the puerperium

Explanation: Although the varicose veins occurred several months after the delivery of the newborn, the doctor attributed the varicose veins to pregnancy and therefore a code from chapter 15 is appropriate.

4) Admission for routine postpartum care following delivery outside hospital

When the mother delivers outside the hospital prior to admission and is admitted for routine postpartum care and no complications are noted, code Z39.0, Encounter for care and examination of mother immediately after delivery, should be assigned as the principal diagnosis.

5) Pregnancy associated cardiomyopathy

Pregnancy associated cardiomyopathy, code O90.3, is unique in that it may be diagnosed in the third trimester of pregnancy but may continue to progress months after delivery. For this reason, it is referred to as peripartum cardiomyopathy. Code O90.3 is only for use when the cardiomyopathy develops as a result of pregnancy in a woman who did not have pre-existing heart disease.

p. Code O94, Sequelae of complication of pregnancy, childbirth, and the puerperium

1) Code O94

Code O94, Sequelae of complication of pregnancy, childbirth, and the puerperium, is for use in those cases when an initial complication of a pregnancy develops a sequelae requiring care or treatment at a future date.

2) After the initial postpartum period

This code may be used at any time after the initial postpartum period.

3) Sequencing of code O94

This code, like all sequela codes, is to be sequenced following the code describing the sequelae of the complication.

q. Termination of pregnancy and spontaneous abortions

1) Abortion with liveborn fetus

When an attempted termination of pregnancy results in a liveborn fetus, assign code Z33.2, Encounter for elective termination of pregnancy and a code from category Z37, Outcome of Delivery.

2) Retained products of conception following an abortion

Subsequent encounters for retained products of conception following a spontaneous abortion or elective termination of pregnancy are assigned the appropriate code from category O03, Spontaneous abortion, or codes O07.4, Failed attempted termination of pregnancy without complication and Z33.2, Encounter for elective termination of pregnancy. This advice is appropriate even when the patient was discharged previously with a discharge diagnosis of complete abortion.

> Patient was seen two days ago for complete spontaneous abortion but returns today for urinary tract infection (UTI) with ultrasound showing retained products of conception
>
> **O03.38   Urinary tract infection following incomplete spontaneous abortion**
>
> *Explanation:* Although the diagnosis from the patient's previous stay indicated that the patient had a complete abortion, it is now determined that there were actually retained products of conception (POC). An abortion with retained POC is considered incomplete and in this case resulted in the patient developing a UTI.

3) Complications leading to abortion

Codes from Chapter 15 may be used as additional codes to identify any documented complications of the pregnancy in conjunction with codes in categories in O07 and O08.

r. Abuse in a pregnant patient

For suspected or confirmed cases of abuse of a pregnant patient, a code(s) from subcategories O9A.3, Physical abuse complicating pregnancy, childbirth, and the puerperium, O9A.4, Sexual abuse complicating pregnancy, childbirth, and the puerperium, and O9A.5, Psychological abuse complicating pregnancy, childbirth, and the puerperium, should be sequenced first, followed by the appropriate codes (if applicable) to identify any associated current injury due to physical abuse, sexual abuse, and the perpetrator of abuse.

See Section I.C.19. Adult and child abuse, neglect and other maltreatment.

Chapter 15. Pregnancy, Childbirth and the Puerperium (O00-O9A)

NOTE CODES FROM THIS CHAPTER ARE FOR USE ONLY ON MATERNAL RECORDS, NEVER ON NEWBORN RECORDS.

Codes from this chapter are for use for conditions related to or aggravated by the pregnancy, childbirth, or by the puerperium (maternal causes or obstetric causes).

NOTE Trimesters are counted from the first day of the last menstrual period. They are defined as follows:

1st trimester- less than 14 weeks 0 days
2nd trimester- 14 weeks 0 days to less than 28 weeks 0 days
3rd trimester- 28 weeks 0 days until delivery.

Use additional code from category Z3A, Weeks of gestation, to identify the specific week of the pregnancy, if known

EXCLUDES 1 *supervision of normal pregnancy (Z34.-)*
EXCLUDES 2 *mental and behavioral disorders associated with the puerperium (F53)*
obstetrical tetanus (A34)
postpartum necrosis of pituitary gland (E23.0)
puerperal osteomalacia (M83.0)

AHA: 2016, 1Q, 3-5; 2014, 3Q, 17

This chapter contains the following blocks:

O00-O08   Pregnancy with abortive outcome
O09   Supervision of high risk pregnancy
O10-O16   Edema, proteinuria and hypertensive disorders in pregnancy, childbirth and the puerperium
O20-O29   Other maternal disorders predominantly related to pregnancy
O30-O48   Maternal care related to the fetus and amniotic cavity and possible delivery problems
O60-O77   Complications of labor and delivery
O80, O82 Encounter for delivery
O85-O92   Complications predominantly related to the puerperium
O94-O9A   Other obstetric conditions, not elsewhere classified

Pregnancy with abortive outcome (O00-O08)

EXCLUDES 1 *continuing pregnancy in multiple gestation after abortion of one fetus or more (O31.1-, O31.3-)*

✓4th O00 Ectopic pregnancy
INCLUDES ruptured ectopic pregnancy
Use additional code from category O08 to identify any associated complication
AHA: 2014, 3Q, 17
DEF: Implantation of fertilized egg outside the uterus, usually in fallopian tube or abdomen; requires emergency treatment.

✓5th O00.0 Abdominal pregnancy
  EXCLUDES 1 *maternal care for viable fetus in abdominal pregnancy (O36.7-)*

  O00.00 Abdominal pregnancy without intrauterine pregnancy Ⓜ♀
    Abdominal pregnancy NOS

  O00.01 Abdominal pregnancy with intrauterine pregnancy Ⓜ♀

✓5th O00.1 Tubal pregnancy
  Fallopian pregnancy
  Rupture of (fallopian) tube due to pregnancy
  Tubal abortion

  ✓6th O00.10 Tubal pregnancy without intrauterine pregnancy
    Tubal pregnancy NOS

●   **O00.101 Right tubal pregnancy without intrauterine pregnancy**

●   **O00.102 Left tubal pregnancy without intrauterine pregnancy**

●   **O00.109 Unspecified tubal pregnancy without intrauterine pregnancy** ▽

  ✓6th O00.11 Tubal pregnancy with intrauterine pregnancy

●   **O00.111 Right tubal pregnancy with intrauterine pregnancy**

●   **O00.112 Left tubal pregnancy with intrauterine pregnancy**

●   **O00.119 Unspecified tubal pregnancy with intrauterine pregnancy** ▽

  ✓5th O00.2 Ovarian pregnancy

  ✓6th O00.20 Ovarian pregnancy without intrauterine pregnancy
    Ovarian pregnancy NOS

●   **O00.201 Right ovarian pregnancy without intrauterine pregnancy**

●   **O00.202 Left ovarian pregnancy without intrauterine pregnancy**

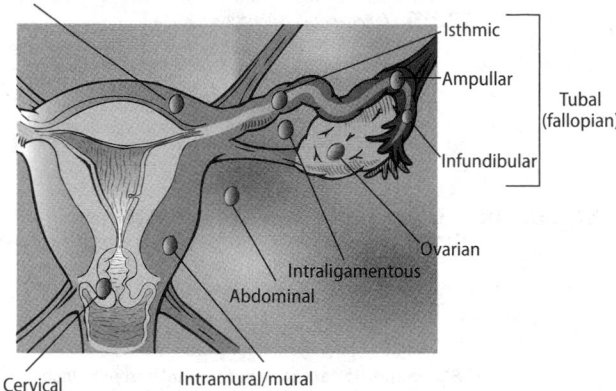

Ectopic Pregnancy

Cornual/interstitial — Isthmic — Ampullar — Tubal (fallopian) — Infundibular — Ovarian — Intraligamentous — Abdominal — Cervical — Intramural/mural

●   **O00.209 Unspecified ovarian pregnancy without intrauterine pregnancy** ▽

  ✓6th O00.21 Ovarian pregnancy with intrauterine pregnancy

●   **O00.211 Right ovarian pregnancy with intrauterine pregnancy**

●   **O00.212 Left ovarian pregnancy with intrauterine pregnancy**

●   **O00.219 Unspecified ovarian pregnancy with intrauterine pregnancy** ▽

✓5th O00.8 Other ectopic pregnancy
  Cervical pregnancy
  Cornual pregnancy
  Intraligamentous pregnancy
  Mural pregnancy

  O00.80 Other ectopic pregnancy without intrauterine pregnancy Ⓜ♀
    Other ectopic pregnancy NOS

  O00.81 Other ectopic pregnancy with intrauterine pregnancy Ⓜ♀

✓5th O00.9 Ectopic pregnancy, unspecified

  O00.90 Unspecified ectopic pregnancy without intrauterine pregnancy Ⓜ♀▽
    Ectopic pregnancy NOS

  O00.91 Unspecified ectopic pregnancy with intrauterine pregnancy Ⓜ♀▽

✓4th O01 Hydatidiform mole
Use additional code from category O08 to identify any associated complication
EXCLUDES 1 *chorioadenoma (destruens) (D39.2)*
malignant hydatidiform mole (D39.2)
AHA: 2014, 3Q, 17
DEF: Abnormal product of pregnancy; marked by mass of cysts resembling bunch of grapes due to chorionic villi proliferation and dissolution; must be surgically removed.

O01.0 Classical hydatidiform mole Ⓜ♀
  Complete hydatidiform mole

O01.1 Incomplete and partial hydatidiform mole Ⓜ♀

O01.9 Hydatidiform mole, unspecified Ⓜ♀▽
  Trophoblastic disease NOS
  Vesicular mole NOS

✓4th O02 Other abnormal products of conception
Use additional code from category O08 to identify any associated complication
EXCLUDES 1 *papyraceous fetus (O31.0-)*
AHA: 2014, 3Q, 17

O02.0 Blighted ovum and nonhydatidiform mole Ⓜ♀
  Carneous mole
  Fleshy mole
  Intrauterine mole NOS
  Molar pregnancy NEC
  Pathological ovum

✔ Additional Character Req   ✔7th Placeholder Alert   Manifestation   **HCC** CMS-HCC Condition   ▽Unspecified Code   ►◄ Revised Text   ● New Code   ▲ Revised Code Title

O02.1 Missed abortion   M♀
Early fetal death, before completion of 20 weeks of gestation, with retention of dead fetus
> EXCLUDES 1   *failed induced abortion (O07.-)*
> *fetal death (intrauterine) (late) (O36.4)*
> *missed abortion with blighted ovum (O02.0)*
> *missed abortion with hydatidiform mole (O01.-)*
> *missed abortion with nonhydatidiform (O02.0)*
> *missed abortion with other abnormal products of conception (O02.8-)*
> *missed delivery (O36.4)*
> *stillbirth (P95)*

✓5th **O02.8 Other specified abnormal products of conception**
> EXCLUDES 1   *abnormal products of conception with blighted ovum (O02.0)*
> *abnormal products of conception with hydatidiform mole (O01.-)*
> *abnormal products of conception with nonhydatidiform mole (O02.0)*

O02.81 Inappropriate change in quantitative human chorionic gonadotropin (hCG) in early pregnancy   M♀
Biochemical pregnancy
Chemical pregnancy
Inappropriate level of quantitative human chorionic gonadotropin (hCG) for gestational age in early pregnancy

O02.89 Other abnormal products of conception   M♀
O02.9 Abnormal product of conception, unspecified   M♀▽

✓4th **O03 Spontaneous abortion**
> NOTE   Incomplete abortion includes retained products of conception following spontaneous abortion
> INCLUDES   miscarriage

O03.0 Genital tract and pelvic infection following incomplete spontaneous abortion   M♀
Endometritis following incomplete spontaneous abortion
Oophoritis following incomplete spontaneous abortion
Parametritis following incomplete spontaneous abortion
Pelvic peritonitis following incomplete spontaneous abortion
Salpingitis following incomplete spontaneous abortion
Salpingo-oophoritis following incomplete spontaneous abortion
> EXCLUDES 1   *sepsis following incomplete spontaneous abortion (O03.37)*
> *urinary tract infection following incomplete spontaneous abortion (O03.38)*

O03.1 Delayed or excessive hemorrhage following incomplete spontaneous abortion   M♀
Afibrinogenemia following incomplete spontaneous abortion
Defibrination syndrome following incomplete spontaneous abortion
Hemolysis following incomplete spontaneous abortion
Intravascular coagulation following incomplete spontaneous abortion

O03.2 Embolism following incomplete spontaneous abortion   M♀
Air embolism following incomplete spontaneous abortion
Amniotic fluid embolism following incomplete spontaneous abortion
Blood-clot embolism following incomplete spontaneous abortion
Embolism NOS following incomplete spontaneous abortion
Fat embolism following incomplete spontaneous abortion
Pulmonary embolism following incomplete spontaneous abortion
Pyemic embolism following incomplete spontaneous abortion
Septic or septicopyemic embolism following incomplete spontaneous abortion
Soap embolism following incomplete spontaneous abortion

✓5th **O03.3 Other and unspecified complications following incomplete spontaneous abortion**

O03.30 Unspecified complication following incomplete spontaneous abortion   M♀▽

O03.31 Shock following incomplete spontaneous abortion   M♀
Circulatory collapse following incomplete spontaneous abortion
Shock (postprocedural) following incomplete spontaneous abortion
> EXCLUDES 1   *shock due to infection following incomplete spontaneous abortion (O03.37)*

O03.32 Renal failure following incomplete spontaneous abortion   M♀
Kidney failure (acute) following incomplete spontaneous abortion
Oliguria following incomplete spontaneous abortion
Renal shutdown following incomplete spontaneous abortion
Renal tubular necrosis following incomplete spontaneous abortion
Uremia following incomplete spontaneous abortion

O03.33 Metabolic disorder following incomplete spontaneous abortion   M♀

O03.34 Damage to pelvic organs following incomplete spontaneous abortion   M♀
Laceration, perforation, tear or chemical damage of bladder following incomplete spontaneous abortion
Laceration, perforation, tear or chemical damage of bowel following incomplete spontaneous abortion
Laceration, perforation, tear or chemical damage of broad ligament following incomplete spontaneous abortion
Laceration, perforation, tear or chemical damage of cervix following incomplete spontaneous abortion
Laceration, perforation, tear or chemical damage of periurethral tissue following incomplete spontaneous abortion
Laceration, perforation, tear or chemical damage of uterus following incomplete spontaneous abortion
Laceration, perforation, tear or chemical damage of vagina following incomplete spontaneous abortion

O03.35 Other venous complications following incomplete spontaneous abortion   M♀
O03.36 Cardiac arrest following incomplete spontaneousabortion   M♀
O03.37 Sepsis following incomplete spontaneous abortion   M♀
Use additional code to identify infectious agent (B95-B97)
Use additional code to identify severe sepsis, if applicable (R65.2-)
> EXCLUDES 1   *septic or septicopyemic embolism following incomplete spontaneous abortion (O03.2)*

O03.38 Urinary tract infection following incomplete spontaneous abortion   M♀
Cystitis following incomplete spontaneous abortion
O03.39 Incomplete spontaneous abortion with other complications   M♀
O03.4 Incomplete spontaneous abortion without complication   M♀
O03.5 Genital tract and pelvic infection following complete or unspecified spontaneous abortion   M♀
Endometritis following complete or unspecified spontaneous abortion
Oophoritis following complete or unspecified spontaneous abortion
Parametritis following complete or unspecified spontaneous abortion
Pelvic peritonitis following complete or unspecified spontaneous abortion
Salpingitis following complete or unspecified spontaneous abortion
Salpingo-oophoritis following complete or unspecified spontaneous abortion
> EXCLUDES 1   *sepsis following complete or unspecified spontaneous abortion (O03.87)*
> *urinary tract infection following complete or unspecified spontaneous abortion (O03.88)*

O03.6 Delayed or excessive hemorrhage following complete or unspecified spontaneous abortion   M♀
Afibrinogenemia following complete or unspecified spontaneous abortion
Defibrination syndrome following complete or unspecified spontaneous abortion
Hemolysis following complete or unspecified spontaneous abortion
Intravascular coagulation following complete or unspecified spontaneous abortion

O03.7 Embolism following complete or unspecified Ⓜ♀
spontaneous abortion
Air embolism following complete or unspecified spontaneous abortion
Amniotic fluid embolism following complete or unspecified spontaneous abortion
Blood-clot embolism following complete or unspecified spontaneous abortion
Embolism NOS following complete or unspecified spontaneous abortion
Fat embolism following complete or unspecified spontaneous abortion
Pulmonary embolism following complete or unspecified spontaneous abortion
Pyemic embolism following complete or unspecified spontaneous abortion
Septic or septicopyemic embolism following complete or unspecified spontaneous abortion
Soap embolism following complete or unspecified spontaneous abortion

✓5ᵗʰ O03.8 Other and unspecified complications following complete or unspecified spontaneous abortion

O03.80 Unspecified complication following Ⓜ♀▽
complete or unspecified spontaneous abortion

O03.81 Shock following complete or unspecified Ⓜ♀
spontaneous abortion
Circulatory collapse following complete or unspecified spontaneous abortion
Shock (postprocedural) following complete or unspecified spontaneous abortion
EXCLUDES 1 *shock due to infection following complete or unspecified spontaneous abortion (O03.87)*

O03.82 Renal failure following complete or unspecified Ⓜ♀
spontaneous abortion
Kidney failure (acute) following complete or unspecified spontaneous abortion
Oliguria following complete or unspecified spontaneous abortion
Renal shutdown following complete or unspecified spontaneous abortion
Renal tubular necrosis following complete or unspecified spontaneous abortion
Uremia following complete or unspecified spontaneous abortion

O03.83 Metabolic disorder following complete or Ⓜ♀
unspecified spontaneous abortion

O03.84 Damage to pelvic organs following complete or Ⓜ♀
unspecified spontaneous abortion
Laceration, perforation, tear or chemical damage of bladder following complete or unspecified spontaneous abortion
Laceration, perforation, tear or chemical damage of bowel following complete or unspecified spontaneous abortion
Laceration, perforation, tear or chemical damage of broad ligament following complete or unspecified spontaneous abortion
Laceration, perforation, tear or chemical damage of cervix following complete or unspecified spontaneous abortion
Laceration, perforation, tear or chemical damage of periurethral tissue following complete or unspecified spontaneous abortion
Laceration, perforation, tear or chemical damage of uterus following complete or unspecified spontaneous abortion
Laceration, perforation, tear or chemical damage of vagina following complete or unspecified spontaneous abortion

O03.85 Other venous complications following complete Ⓜ♀
or unspecified spontaneous abortion

O03.86 Cardiac arrest following complete or unspecified Ⓜ♀
spontaneous abortion

O03.87 Sepsis following complete or unspecified Ⓜ♀
spontaneous abortion
Use additional code to identify infectious agent (B95-B97)
Use additional code to identify severe sepsis, if applicable (R65.2-)
EXCLUDES 1 *septic or septicopyemic embolism following complete or unspecified spontaneous abortion (O03.7)*

O03.88 Urinary tract infection following complete or Ⓜ♀
unspecified spontaneous abortion
Cystitis following complete or unspecified spontaneous abortion

O03.89 Complete or unspecified spontaneous abortion Ⓜ♀
with other complications

O03.9 Complete or unspecified spontaneous abortion Ⓜ♀▽
without complication
Miscarriage NOS
Spontaneous abortion NOS

✓4ᵗʰ O04 Complications following (induced) termination of pregnancy
INCLUDES complications following (induced) termination of pregnancy
EXCLUDES 1 *encounter for elective termination of pregnancy, uncomplicated (Z33.2)*
failed attempted termination of pregnancy (O07.-)

O04.5 Genital tract and pelvic infection following (induced) Ⓜ♀
termination of pregnancy
Endometritis following (induced) termination of pregnancy
Oophoritis following (induced) termination of pregnancy
Parametritis following (induced) termination of pregnancy
Pelvic peritonitis following (induced) termination of pregnancy
Salpingitis following (induced) termination of pregnancy
Salpingo-oophoritis following (induced) termination of pregnancy
EXCLUDES 1 *sepsis following (induced) termination of pregnancy (O04.87)*
urinary tract infection following (induced) termination of pregnancy (O04.88)

O04.6 Delayed or excessive hemorrhage following (induced) Ⓜ♀
termination of pregnancy
Afibrinogenemia following (induced) termination of pregnancy
Defibrination syndrome following (induced) termination of pregnancy
Hemolysis following (induced) termination of pregnancy
Intravascular coagulation following (induced) termination of pregnancy

O04.7 Embolism following (induced) termination of pregnancy Ⓜ♀
Air embolism following (induced) termination of pregnancy
Amniotic fluid embolism following (induced) termination of pregnancy
Blood-clot embolism following (induced) termination of pregnancy
Embolism NOS following (induced) termination of pregnancy
Fat embolism following (induced) termination of pregnancy
Pulmonary embolism following (induced) termination of pregnancy
Pyemic embolism following (induced) termination of pregnancy
Septic or septicopyemic embolism following (induced) termination of pregnancy
Soap embolism following (induced) termination of pregnancy

✓5ᵗʰ O04.8 (Induced) termination of pregnancy with other and unspecified complications

O04.80 (Induced) termination of pregnancy with Ⓜ♀▽
unspecified complications

O04.81 Shock following (induced) termination of Ⓜ♀
pregnancy
Circulatory collapse following (induced) termination of pregnancy
Shock (postprocedural) following (induced) termination of pregnancy
EXCLUDES 1 *shock due to infection following (induced) termination of pregnancy (O04.87)*

O04.82 Renal failure following (induced) termination Ⓜ♀
of pregnancy
Kidney failure (acute) following (induced) termination of pregnancy
Oliguria following (induced) termination of pregnancy
Renal shutdown following (induced) termination of pregnancy
Renal tubular necrosis following (induced) termination of pregnancy
Uremia following (induced) termination of pregnancy

O04.83 Metabolic disorder following (induced) Ⓜ♀
termination of pregnancy

☑ Additional Character Req   ✓x7ᵗʰ Placeholder Alert   Manifestation   ᴴᶜᶜ CMS-HCC Condition   ▽ Unspecified Code   ►◄ Revised Text   ● New Code   ▲ Revised Code Title

O04.84   **Damage to pelvic organs following (induced) termination of pregnancy**   Ⓜ♀

Laceration, perforation, tear or chemical damage of bladder following (induced) termination of pregnancy

Laceration, perforation, tear or chemical damage of bowel following (induced) termination of pregnancy

Laceration, perforation, tear or chemical damage of broad ligament following (induced) termination of pregnancy

Laceration, perforation, tear or chemical damage of cervix following (induced) termination of pregnancy

Laceration, perforation, tear or chemical damage of periurethral tissue following (induced) termination of pregnancy

Laceration, perforation, tear or chemical damage of uterus following (induced) termination of pregnancy

Laceration, perforation, tear or chemical damage of vagina following (induced) termination of pregnancy

O04.85   **Other venous complications following (induced) termination of pregnancy**   Ⓜ♀

O04.86   **Cardiac arrest following (induced) termination of pregnancy**   Ⓜ♀

O04.87   **Sepsis following (induced) termination of pregnancy**   Ⓜ♀

Use additional code to identify infectious agent (B95-B97)

Use additional code to identify severe sepsis, if applicable (R65.2-)

> **EXCLUDES 1**   *septic or septicopyemic embolism following (induced) termination of pregnancy (O04.7)*

O04.88   **Urinary tract infection following (induced) termination of pregnancy**   Ⓜ♀

Cystitis following (induced) termination of pregnancy

O04.89   **(Induced) termination of pregnancy with other complications**   Ⓜ♀

☑4ᵗʰ O07   Failed attempted termination of pregnancy

> **INCLUDES**   failure of attempted induction of termination of pregnancy
> incomplete elective abortion

> **EXCLUDES 1**   *incomplete spontaneous abortion (O03.0-)*

O07.0   **Genital tract and pelvic infection following failed attempted termination of pregnancy**   Ⓜ♀

Endometritis following failed attempted termination of pregnancy

Oophoritis following failed attempted termination of pregnancy

Parametritis following failed attempted termination of pregnancy

Pelvic peritonitis following failed attempted termination of pregnancy

Salpingitis following failed attempted termination of pregnancy

Salpingo-oophoritis following failed attempted termination of pregnancy

> **EXCLUDES 1**   *sepsis following failed attempted termination of pregnancy (O07.37)*
> *urinary tract infection following failed attempted termination of pregnancy (O07.38)*

O07.1   **Delayed or excessive hemorrhage following failed attempted termination of pregnancy**   Ⓜ♀

Afibrinogenemia following failed attempted termination of pregnancy

Defibrination syndrome following failed attempted termination of pregnancy

Hemolysis following failed attempted termination of pregnancy

Intravascular coagulation following failed attempted termination of pregnancy

O07.2   **Embolism following failed attempted termination of pregnancy**   Ⓜ♀

Air embolism following failed attempted termination of pregnancy

Amniotic fluid embolism following failed attempted termination of pregnancy

Blood-clot embolism following failed attempted termination of pregnancy

Embolism NOS following failed attempted termination of pregnancy

Fat embolism following failed attempted termination of pregnancy

Pulmonary embolism following failed attempted termination of pregnancy

Pyemic embolism following failed attempted termination of pregnancy

Septic or septicopyemic embolism following failed attempted termination of pregnancy

Soap embolism following failed attempted termination of pregnancy

☑5ᵗʰ O07.3   Failed attempted termination of pregnancy with other and unspecified complications

O07.30   **Failed attempted termination of pregnancy with unspecified complications**   Ⓜ♀ ▽

O07.31   **Shock following failed attempted termination of pregnancy**   Ⓜ♀

Circulatory collapse following failed attempted termination of pregnancy

Shock (postprocedural) following failed attempted termination of pregnancy

> **EXCLUDES 1**   *shock due to infection following failed attempted termination of pregnancy (O07.37)*

O07.32   **Renal failure following failed attempted termination of pregnancy**   Ⓜ♀

Kidney failure (acute) following failed attempted termination of pregnancy

Oliguria following failed attempted termination of pregnancy

Renal shutdown following failed attempted termination of pregnancy

Renal tubular necrosis following failed attempted termination of pregnancy

Uremia following failed attempted termination of pregnancy

O07.33   **Metabolic disorder following failed attempted termination of pregnancy**   Ⓜ♀

O07.34   **Damage to pelvic organs following failed attempted termination of pregnancy**   Ⓜ♀

Laceration, perforation, tear or chemical damage of bladder following failed attempted termination of pregnancy

Laceration, perforation, tear or chemical damage of bowel following failed attempted termination of pregnancy

Laceration, perforation, tear or chemical damage of broad ligament following failed attempted termination of pregnancy

Laceration, perforation, tear or chemical damage of cervix following failed attempted termination of pregnancy

Laceration, perforation, tear or chemical damage of periurethral tissue following failed attempted termination of pregnancy

Laceration, perforation, tear or chemical damage of uterus following failed attempted termination of pregnancy

Laceration, perforation, tear or chemical damage of vagina following failed attempted termination of pregnancy

O07.35   **Other venous complications following failed attempted termination of pregnancy**   Ⓜ♀

O07.36   **Cardiac arrest following failed attempted termination of pregnancy**   Ⓜ♀

O07.37   **Sepsis following failed attempted termination of pregnancy**   Ⓜ♀

Use additional code to identify infectious agent (B95-B97)

Use additional code to identify severe sepsis, if applicable (R65.2-)

> **EXCLUDES 1**   *septic or septicopyemic embolism following failed attempted termination of pregnancy (O07.2)*

EXCLUDES 1 Not coded here   **EXCLUDES 2** Not included here   Ⓝ Newborn Age: 0   Ⓟ Pediatric Age: 0-17   Ⓜ Maternity Age: 12-55   Ⓐ Adult Age: 15-124

826   ICD-10-CM 2018

O07.38 **Urinary tract infection following failed attempted termination of pregnancy** Ⓜ♀
Cystitis following failed attempted termination of pregnancy

O07.39 **Failed attempted termination of pregnancy with other complications** Ⓜ♀

O07.4 **Failed attempted termination of pregnancy without complication** Ⓜ♀

✓4ᵗʰ **O08 Complications following ectopic and molar pregnancy**
This category is for use with categories O00-O02 to identify any associated complications

O08.0 **Genital tract and pelvic infection following ectopic and molar pregnancy** Ⓜ♀
Endometritis following ectopic and molar pregnancy
Oophoritis following ectopic and molar pregnancy
Parametritis following ectopic and molar pregnancy
Pelvic peritonitis following ectopic and molar pregnancy
Salpingitis following ectopic and molar pregnancy
Salpingo-oophoritis following ectopic and molar pregnancy
EXCLUDES 1 *sepsis following ectopic and molar pregnancy (O08.82)*
urinary tract infection (O08.83)

O08.1 **Delayed or excessive hemorrhage following ectopic and molar pregnancy** Ⓜ♀
Afibrinogenemia following ectopic and molar pregnancy
Defibrination syndrome following ectopic and molar pregnancy
Hemolysis following ectopic and molar pregnancy
Intravascular coagulation following ectopic and molar pregnancy
EXCLUDES 1 *delayed or excessive hemorrhage due to incomplete abortion (O03.1)*

O08.2 **Embolism following ectopic and molar pregnancy** Ⓜ♀
Air embolism following ectopic and molar pregnancy
Amniotic fluid embolism following ectopic and molar pregnancy
Blood-clot embolism following ectopic and molar pregnancy
Embolism NOS following ectopic and molar pregnancy
Fat embolism following ectopic and molar pregnancy
Pulmonary embolism following ectopic and molar pregnancy
Pyemic embolism following ectopic and molar pregnancy
Septic or septicopyemic embolism following ectopic and molar pregnancy
Soap embolism following ectopic and molar pregnancy

O08.3 **Shock following ectopic and molar pregnancy** Ⓜ♀
Circulatory collapse following ectopic and molar pregnancy
Shock (postprocedural) following ectopic and molar pregnancy
EXCLUDES 1 *shock due to infection following ectopic and molar pregnancy (O08.82)*

O08.4 **Renal failure following ectopic and molar pregnancy** Ⓜ♀
Kidney failure (acute) following ectopic and molar pregnancy
Oliguria following ectopic and molar pregnancy
Renal shutdown following ectopic and molar pregnancy
Renal tubular necrosis following ectopic and molar pregnancy
Uremia following ectopic and molar pregnancy

O08.5 **Metabolic disorders following an ectopic and molar pregnancy** Ⓜ♀

O08.6 **Damage to pelvic organs and tissues following an ectopic and molar pregnancy** Ⓜ♀
Laceration, perforation, tear or chemical damage of bladder following an ectopic and molar pregnancy
Laceration, perforation, tear or chemical damage of bowel following an ectopic and molar pregnancy
Laceration, perforation, tear or chemical damage of broad ligament following an ectopic and molar pregnancy
Laceration, perforation, tear or chemical damage of cervix following an ectopic and molar pregnancy
Laceration, perforation, tear or chemical damage of periurethral tissue following an ectopic and molar pregnancy
Laceration, perforation, tear or chemical damage of uterus following an ectopic and molar pregnancy
Laceration, perforation, tear or chemical damage of vagina following an ectopic and molar pregnancy

O08.7 **Other venous complications following an ectopic and molar pregnancy** Ⓜ♀

✓5ᵗʰ O08.8 **Other complications following an ectopic and molar pregnancy**
O08.81 **Cardiac arrest following an ectopic and molar pregnancy** Ⓜ♀
O08.82 **Sepsis following ectopic and molar pregnancy** Ⓜ♀
Use additional code to identify infectious agent (B95-B97)
Use additional code to identify severe sepsis, if applicable (R65.2-)
EXCLUDES 1 *septic or septicopyemic embolism following ectopic and molar pregnancy (O08.2)*

O08.83 **Urinary tract infection following an ectopic and molar pregnancy** Ⓜ♀
Cystitis following an ectopic and molar pregnancy

O08.89 **Other complications following an ectopic and molar pregnancy** Ⓜ♀

O08.9 **Unspecified complication following an ectopic and molar pregnancy** Ⓜ♀▽

Supervision of high risk pregnancy (O09)

✓4ᵗʰ **O09 Supervision of high risk pregnancy**
AHA: 2016, 4Q, 150

✓5ᵗʰ O09.0 **Supervision of pregnancy with history of infertility**
O09.00 **Supervision of pregnancy with history of infertility, unspecified trimester** Ⓜ♀▽
O09.01 **Supervision of pregnancy with history of infertility, first trimester** Ⓜ♀
O09.02 **Supervision of pregnancy with history of infertility, second trimester** Ⓜ♀
O09.03 **Supervision of pregnancy with history of infertility, third trimester** Ⓜ♀

✓5ᵗʰ O09.1 **Supervision of pregnancy with history of ectopic pregnancy**
O09.10 **Supervision of pregnancy with history of ectopic pregnancy, unspecified trimester** Ⓜ♀▽
O09.11 **Supervision of pregnancy with history of ectopic pregnancy, first trimester** Ⓜ♀
O09.12 **Supervision of pregnancy with history of ectopic pregnancy, second trimester** Ⓜ♀
O09.13 **Supervision of pregnancy with history of ectopic pregnancy, third trimester** Ⓜ♀

✓5ᵗʰ O09.A **Supervision of pregnancy with history of molar pregnancy**
O09.A0 **Supervision of pregnancy with history of molar pregnancy, unspecified trimester** Ⓜ♀▽
O09.A1 **Supervision of pregnancy with history of molar pregnancy, first trimester** Ⓜ♀
O09.A2 **Supervision of pregnancy with history of molar pregnancy, second trimester** Ⓜ♀
O09.A3 **Supervision of pregnancy with history of molar pregnancy, third trimester** Ⓜ♀

✓5ᵗʰ O09.2 **Supervision of pregnancy with other poor reproductive or obstetric history**
EXCLUDES 2 *pregnancy care for patient with history of recurrent pregnancy loss (O26.2-)*
✓6ᵗʰ O09.21 **Supervision of pregnancy with history of pre-term labor**
O09.211 **Supervision of pregnancy with history of pre-term labor, first trimester** Ⓜ♀
O09.212 **Supervision of pregnancy with history of pre-term labor, second trimester** Ⓜ♀
O09.213 **Supervision of pregnancy with history of pre-term labor, third trimester** Ⓜ♀
O09.219 **Supervision of pregnancy with history of pre-term labor, unspecified trimester** Ⓜ♀▽
✓6ᵗʰ O09.29 **Supervision of pregnancy with other poor reproductive or obstetric history**
Supervision of pregnancy with history of neonatal death
Supervision of pregnancy with history of stillbirth
O09.291 **Supervision of pregnancy with other poor reproductive or obstetric history, first trimester** Ⓜ♀
O09.292 **Supervision of pregnancy with other poor reproductive or obstetric history, second trimester** Ⓜ♀
O09.293 **Supervision of pregnancy with other poor reproductive or obstetric history, third trimester** Ⓜ♀
O09.299 **Supervision of pregnancy with other poor reproductive or obstetric history, unspecified trimester** Ⓜ♀▽

✓5ᵗʰ O09.3 **Supervision of pregnancy with insufficient antenatal care**
Supervision of concealed pregnancy
Supervision of hidden pregnancy
O09.30 **Supervision of pregnancy with insufficient antenatal care, unspecified trimester** Ⓜ♀▽
O09.31 **Supervision of pregnancy with insufficient antenatal care, first trimester** Ⓜ♀

O09.32 **Supervision of pregnancy with insufficient antenatal care, second trimester** ⬜♀

O09.33 **Supervision of pregnancy with insufficient antenatal care, third trimester** ⬜♀

✓5ᵗʰ O09.4 **Supervision of pregnancy with grand multiparity**

O09.40 **Supervision of pregnancy with grand multiparity, unspecified trimester** ⬜♀▽

O09.41 **Supervision of pregnancy with grand multiparity, first trimester** ⬜♀

O09.42 **Supervision of pregnancy with grand multiparity, second trimester** ⬜♀

O09.43 **Supervision of pregnancy with grand multiparity, third trimester** ⬜♀

✓5ᵗʰ O09.5 **Supervision of elderly primigravida and multigravida**
Pregnancy for a female 35 years and older at expected date of delivery

   ✓6ᵗʰ O09.51 **Supervision of elderly primigravida**

O09.511 **Supervision of elderly primigravida, first trimester** ⬜♀

O09.512 **Supervision of elderly primigravida, second trimester** ⬜♀

O09.513 **Supervision of elderly primigravida, third trimester** ⬜♀

O09.519 **Supervision of elderly primigravida, unspecified trimester** ⬜♀▽

   ✓6ᵗʰ O09.52 **Supervision of elderly multigravida**

O09.521 **Supervision of elderly multigravida, first trimester** ⬜♀

O09.522 **Supervision of elderly multigravida, second trimester** ⬜♀

O09.523 **Supervision of elderly multigravida, third trimester** ⬜♀

O09.529 **Supervision of elderly multigravida, unspecified trimester** ⬜♀▽

✓5ᵗʰ O09.6 **Supervision of young primigravida and multigravida**
Supervision of pregnancy for a female less than 16 years old at expected date of delivery

   ✓6ᵗʰ O09.61 **Supervision of young primigravida**

O09.611 **Supervision of young primigravida, first trimester** ⬜♀

O09.612 **Supervision of young primigravida, second trimester** ⬜♀

O09.613 **Supervision of young primigravida, third trimester** ⬜♀

O09.619 **Supervision of young primigravida, unspecified trimester** ⬜♀▽

   ✓6ᵗʰ O09.62 **Supervision of young multigravida**

O09.621 **Supervision of young multigravida, first trimester** ⬜♀

O09.622 **Supervision of young multigravida, second trimester** ⬜♀

O09.623 **Supervision of young multigravida, third trimester** ⬜♀

O09.629 **Supervision of young multigravida, unspecified trimester** ⬜♀▽

✓5ᵗʰ O09.7 **Supervision of high risk pregnancy due to social problems**

O09.70 **Supervision of high risk pregnancy due to social problems, unspecified trimester** ⬜♀▽

O09.71 **Supervision of high risk pregnancy due to social problems, first trimester** ⬜♀

O09.72 **Supervision of high risk pregnancy due to social problems, second trimester** ⬜♀

O09.73 **Supervision of high risk pregnancy due to social problems, third trimester** ⬜♀

✓5ᵗʰ O09.8 **Supervision of other high risk pregnancies**

   ✓6ᵗʰ O09.81 **Supervision of pregnancy resulting from assisted reproductive technology**
Supervision of pregnancy resulting from in-vitro fertilization
EXCLUDES 2 *gestational carrier status (Z33.3)*

O09.811 **Supervision of pregnancy resulting from assisted reproductive technology, first trimester** ⬜♀

O09.812 **Supervision of pregnancy resulting from assisted reproductive technology, second trimester** ⬜♀

O09.813 **Supervision of pregnancy resulting from assisted reproductive technology, third trimester** ⬜♀

O09.819 **Supervision of pregnancy resulting from assisted reproductive technology, unspecified trimester** ⬜♀▽

   ✓6ᵗʰ O09.82 **Supervision of pregnancy with history of in utero procedure during previous pregnancy**

O09.821 **Supervision of pregnancy with history of in utero procedure during previous pregnancy, first trimester** ⬜♀

O09.822 **Supervision of pregnancy with history of in utero procedure during previous pregnancy, second trimester** ⬜♀

O09.823 **Supervision of pregnancy with history of in utero procedure during previous pregnancy, third trimester** ⬜♀

O09.829 **Supervision of pregnancy with history of in utero procedure during previous pregnancy, unspecified trimester** ⬜♀▽
EXCLUDES 1 *supervision of pregnancy affected by in utero procedure during current pregnancy (O35.7)*

   ✓6ᵗʰ O09.89 **Supervision of other high risk pregnancies**

O09.891 **Supervision of other high risk pregnancies, first trimester** ⬜♀

O09.892 **Supervision of other high risk pregnancies, second trimester** ⬜♀

O09.893 **Supervision of other high risk pregnancies, third trimester** ⬜♀

O09.899 **Supervision of other high risk pregnancies, unspecified trimester** ♀

✓5ᵗʰ O09.9 **Supervision of high risk pregnancy, unspecified**

O09.90 **Supervision of high risk pregnancy, unspecified, unspecified trimester** ⬜♀▽

O09.91 **Supervision of high risk pregnancy, unspecified, first trimester** ⬜♀▽

O09.92 **Supervision of high risk pregnancy, unspecified, second trimester** ⬜♀▽

O09.93 **Supervision of high risk pregnancy, unspecified, third trimester** ⬜♀▽

Edema, proteinuria and hypertensive disorders in pregnancy, childbirth and the puerperium (O10-O16)

✓4ᵗʰ O10 **Pre-existing hypertension complicating pregnancy, childbirth and the puerperium**
Pre-existing hypertension with pre-existing proteinuria complicating pregnancy, childbirth and the puerperium
EXCLUDES 2 *pre-existing hypertension with superimposed pre-eclampsia complicating pregnancy, childbirth and the puerperium (O11.-)*

✓5ᵗʰ O10.0 **Pre-existing essential hypertension complicating pregnancy, childbirth and the puerperium**
Any condition in I10 specified as a reason for obstetric care during pregnancy, childbirth or the puerperium

   ✓6ᵗʰ O10.01 **Pre-existing essential hypertension complicating pregnancy**

O10.011 **Pre-existing essential hypertension complicating pregnancy, first trimester** ⬜♀

O10.012 **Pre-existing essential hypertension complicating pregnancy, second trimester** ⬜♀

O10.013 **Pre-existing essential hypertension complicating pregnancy, third trimester** ⬜♀

O10.019 **Pre-existing essential hypertension complicating pregnancy, unspecified trimester** ⬜♀▽

O10.02 **Pre-existing essential hypertension complicating childbirth** ⬜♀

O10.03 **Pre-existing essential hypertension complicating the puerperium** ⬜♀

EXCLUDES 1 Not coded here   EXCLUDES 2 Not included here   N Newborn Age: 0   P Pediatric Age: 0-17   M Maternity Age: 12-55   A Adult Age: 15-124

828

ICD-10-CM 2018

✓5ᵗʰ **O10.1** **Pre-existing hypertensive heart disease complicating pregnancy, childbirth and the puerperium**
Any condition in I11 specified as a reason for obstetric care during pregnancy, childbirth or the puerperium
Use additional code from I11 to identify the type of hypertensive heart disease

   ✓6ᵗʰ **O10.11** **Pre-existing hypertensive heart disease complicating pregnancy**

      O10.111 Pre-existing hypertensive heart disease complicating pregnancy, first trimester   Ⓜ♀

      O10.112 Pre-existing hypertensive heart disease complicating pregnancy, second trimester   Ⓜ♀

      O10.113 Pre-existing hypertensive heart disease complicating pregnancy, third trimester   Ⓜ♀

      O10.119 Pre-existing hypertensive heart disease complicating pregnancy, unspecified trimester   Ⓜ♀▽

   O10.12 Pre-existing hypertensive heart disease complicating childbirth   Ⓜ♀

   O10.13 Pre-existing hypertensive heart disease complicating the puerperium   Ⓜ♀

✓5ᵗʰ **O10.2** **Pre-existing hypertensive chronic kidney disease complicating pregnancy, childbirth and the puerperium**
Any condition in I12 specified as a reason for obstetric care during pregnancy, childbirth or the puerperium
Use additional code from I12 to identify the type of hypertensive chronic kidney disease

   ✓6ᵗʰ **O10.21** **Pre-existing hypertensive chronic kidney disease complicating pregnancy**

      O10.211 Pre-existing hypertensive chronic kidney disease complicating pregnancy, first trimester   Ⓜ♀

      O10.212 Pre-existing hypertensive chronic kidney disease complicating pregnancy, second trimester   Ⓜ♀

      O10.213 Pre-existing hypertensive chronic kidney disease complicating pregnancy, third trimester   Ⓜ♀

      O10.219 Pre-existing hypertensive chronic kidney disease complicating pregnancy, unspecified trimester   Ⓜ♀▽

   O10.22 Pre-existing hypertensive chronic kidney disease complicating childbirth   Ⓜ♀

   O10.23 Pre-existing hypertensive chronic kidney disease complicating the puerperium   Ⓜ♀

✓5ᵗʰ **O10.3** **Pre-existing hypertensive heart and chronic kidney disease complicating pregnancy, childbirth and the puerperium**
Any condition in I13 specified as a reason for obstetric care during pregnancy, childbirth or the puerperium
Use additional code from I13 to identify the type of hypertensive heart and chronic kidney disease

   ✓6ᵗʰ **O10.31** **Pre-existing hypertensive heart and chronic kidney disease complicating pregnancy**

      O10.311 Pre-existing hypertensive heart and chronic kidney disease complicating pregnancy, first trimester   Ⓜ♀

      O10.312 Pre-existing hypertensive heart and chronic kidney disease complicating pregnancy, second trimester   Ⓜ♀

      O10.313 Pre-existing hypertensive heart and chronic kidney disease complicating pregnancy, third trimester   Ⓜ♀

      O10.319 Pre-existing hypertensive heart and chronic kidney disease complicating pregnancy, unspecified trimester   Ⓜ♀▽

   O10.32 Pre-existing hypertensive heart and chronic kidney disease complicating childbirth   Ⓜ♀

   O10.33 Pre-existing hypertensive heart and chronic kidney disease complicating the puerperium   Ⓜ♀

✓5ᵗʰ **O10.4** **Pre-existing secondary hypertension complicating pregnancy, childbirth and the puerperium**
Any condition in I15 specified as a reason for obstetric care during pregnancy, childbirth or the puerperium
Use additional code from I15 to identify the type of secondary hypertension

   ✓6ᵗʰ **O10.41** **Pre-existing secondary hypertension complicating pregnancy**

      O10.411 Pre-existing secondary hypertension complicating pregnancy, first trimester   Ⓜ♀

      O10.412 Pre-existing secondary hypertension complicating pregnancy, second trimester   Ⓜ♀

      O10.413 Pre-existing secondary hypertension complicating pregnancy, third trimester   Ⓜ♀

      O10.419 Pre-existing secondary hypertension complicating pregnancy, unspecified trimester   Ⓜ♀▽

   O10.42 Pre-existing secondary hypertension complicating childbirth   Ⓜ♀

   O10.43 Pre-existing secondary hypertension complicating the puerperium   Ⓜ♀

✓5ᵗʰ **O10.9** **Unspecified pre-existing hypertension complicating pregnancy, childbirth and the puerperium**

   ✓6ᵗʰ **O10.91** **Unspecified pre-existing hypertension complicating pregnancy**

      O10.911 Unspecified pre-existing hypertension complicating pregnancy, first trimester   Ⓜ♀▽

      O10.912 Unspecified pre-existing hypertension complicating pregnancy, second trimester   Ⓜ♀▽

      O10.913 Unspecified pre-existing hypertension complicating pregnancy, third trimester   Ⓜ♀▽

      O10.919 Unspecified pre-existing hypertension complicating pregnancy, unspecified trimester   Ⓜ♀▽

   O10.92 Unspecified pre-existing hypertension complicating childbirth   Ⓜ♀▽

   O10.93 Unspecified pre-existing hypertension complicating the puerperium   Ⓜ♀▽

✓4ᵗʰ **O11** **Pre-existing hypertension with pre-eclampsia**
   INCLUDES   conditions in O10 complicated by pre-eclampsia
               pre-eclampsia superimposed pre-existing hypertension
Use additional code from O10 to identify the type of hypertension

   O11.1 Pre-existing hypertension with pre-eclampsia, first trimester   Ⓜ♀

   O11.2 Pre-existing hypertension with pre-eclampsia, second trimester   Ⓜ♀

   O11.3 Pre-existing hypertension with pre-eclampsia, third trimester   Ⓜ♀

   O11.4 Pre-existing hypertension with pre-eclampsia, complicating childbirth   Ⓜ♀

   O11.5 Pre-existing hypertension with pre-eclampsia, complicating the puerperium   Ⓜ♀

   O11.9 Pre-existing hypertension with pre-eclampsia, unspecified trimester   Ⓜ♀▽

✓4ᵗʰ **O12** **Gestational [pregnancy-induced] edema and proteinuria without hypertension**

   ✓5ᵗʰ **O12.0** **Gestational edema**

      O12.00 Gestational edema, unspecified trimester   Ⓜ♀▽

      O12.01 Gestational edema, first trimester   Ⓜ♀

      O12.02 Gestational edema, second trimester   Ⓜ♀

      O12.03 Gestational edema, third trimester   Ⓜ♀

      O12.04 Gestational edema, complicating childbirth   Ⓜ♀

      O12.05 Gestational edema, complicating the puerperium   Ⓜ♀

   ✓5ᵗʰ **O12.1** **Gestational proteinuria**

      O12.10 Gestational proteinuria, unspecified trimester   Ⓜ♀▽

      O12.11 Gestational proteinuria, first trimester   Ⓜ♀

      O12.12 Gestational proteinuria, second trimester   Ⓜ♀

      O12.13 Gestational proteinuria, third trimester   Ⓜ♀

      O12.14 Gestational proteinuria, complicating childbirth   Ⓜ♀

✓ Additional Character Req   ✓x7ᵗʰ Placeholder Alert   Manifestation   HCC CMS-HCC Condition   ▽ Unspecified Code   ▶◀ Revised Text   ● New Code   ▲ Revised Code Title

O12.15　Gestational proteinuria, complicating the puerperium ＭＱ

✓5th O12.2　Gestational edema with proteinuria

O12.20　Gestational edema with proteinuria, unspecified trimester ＭＱ▽

O12.21　Gestational edema with proteinuria, first trimester ＭＱ

O12.22　Gestational edema with proteinuria, second trimester ＭＱ

O12.23　Gestational edema with proteinuria, third trimester ＭＱ

O12.24　Gestational edema with proteinuria, complicating childbirth ＭＱ

O12.25　Gestational edema with proteinuria, complicating the puerperium ＭＱ

✓4th O13　Gestational [pregnancy-induced] hypertension without significant proteinuria

INCLUDES　gestational hypertension NOS
transient hypertension of pregnancy

AHA: 2016, 1Q, 5

O13.1　Gestational [pregnancy-induced] hypertension without significant proteinuria, first trimester ＭＱ

O13.2　Gestational [pregnancy-induced] hypertension without significant proteinuria, second trimester ＭＱ

O13.3　Gestational [pregnancy-induced] hypertension without significant proteinuria, third trimester ＭＱ

O13.4　Gestational [pregnancy-induced] hypertension without significant proteinuria, complicating childbirth ＭＱ

O13.5　Gestational [pregnancy-induced] hypertension without significant proteinuria, complicating the puerperium ＭＱ

O13.9　Gestational [pregnancy-induced] hypertension without significant proteinuria, unspecified trimester ＭＱ▽

✓4th O14　Pre-eclampsia

EXCLUDES 1　pre-existing hypertension with pre-eclampsia (O11)

✓5th O14.0　Mild to moderate pre-eclampsia

O14.00　Mild to moderate pre-eclampsia, unspecified trimester ＭＱ▽

O14.02　Mild to moderate pre-eclampsia, second trimester ＭＱ

O14.03　Mild to moderate pre-eclampsia, third trimester ＭＱ

O14.04　Mild to moderate pre-eclampsia, complicating childbirth ＭＱ

O14.05　Mild to moderate pre-eclampsia, complicating the puerperium ＭＱ

✓5th O14.1　Severe pre-eclampsia

EXCLUDES 1　HELLP syndrome (O14.2-)

O14.10　Severe pre-eclampsia, unspecified trimester ＭＱ▽

O14.12　Severe pre-eclampsia, second trimester ＭＱ

O14.13　Severe pre-eclampsia, third trimester ＭＱ

O14.14　Severe pre-eclampsia complicating childbirth ＭＱ

O14.15　Severe pre-eclampsia, complicating the puerperium ＭＱ

✓5th O14.2　HELLP syndrome

Severe pre-eclampsia with hemolysis, elevated liver enzymes and low platelet count (HELLP)

O14.20　HELLP syndrome (HELLP), unspecified trimester ＭＱ▽

O14.22　HELLP syndrome (HELLP), second trimester ＭＱ

O14.23　HELLP syndrome (HELLP), third trimester ＭＱ

O14.24　HELLP syndrome, complicating childbirth ＭＱ

O14.25　HELLP syndrome, complicating the puerperium ＭＱ

✓5th O14.9　Unspecified pre-eclampsia

O14.90　Unspecified pre-eclampsia, unspecified trimester ＭＱ▽

O14.92　Unspecified pre-eclampsia, second trimester ＭＱ▽

O14.93　Unspecified pre-eclampsia, third trimester ＭＱ▽

O14.94　Unspecified pre-eclampsia, complicating childbirth ＭＱ▽

O14.95　Unspecified pre-eclampsia, complicating the puerperium ＭＱ▽

✓4th O15　Eclampsia

INCLUDES　convulsions following conditions in O10-O14 and O16

✓5th O15.0　Eclampsia complicating pregnancy

O15.00　Eclampsia complicating pregnancy, unspecified trimester ＭＱ▽

O15.02　Eclampsia complicating pregnancy, second trimester ＭＱ

O15.03　Eclampsia complicating pregnancy, third trimester ＭＱ

O15.1　Eclampsia complicating labor ＭＱ

O15.2　Eclampsia complicating the puerperium ＭＱ

O15.9　Eclampsia, unspecified as to time period ＭＱ▽
Eclampsia NOS

✓4th O16　Unspecified maternal hypertension

O16.1　Unspecified maternal hypertension, first trimester ＭＱ▽

O16.2　Unspecified maternal hypertension, second trimester ＭＱ▽

O16.3　Unspecified maternal hypertension, third trimester ＭＱ▽

O16.4　Unspecified maternal hypertension, complicating childbirth ＭＱ▽

O16.5　Unspecified maternal hypertension, complicating the puerperium ＭＱ▽

O16.9　Unspecified maternal hypertension, unspecified trimester ＭＱ▽

Other maternal disorders predominantly related to pregnancy (O20-O29)

EXCLUDES 2　maternal care related to the fetus and amniotic cavity and possible delivery problems (O30-O48)
maternal diseases classifiable elsewhere but complicating pregnancy, labor and delivery, and the puerperium (O98-O99)

✓4th O20　Hemorrhage in early pregnancy

INCLUDES　hemorrhage before completion of 20 weeks gestation

EXCLUDES 1　pregnancy with abortive outcome (O00-O08)

O20.0　Threatened abortion ＭＱ
Hemorrhage specified as due to threatened abortion
DEF: Bloody discharge during pregnancy; cervix may be dilated and pregnancy threatened, but the pregnancy is not terminated.

O20.8　Other hemorrhage in early pregnancy ＭＱ

O20.9　Hemorrhage in early pregnancy, unspecified ＭＱ▽

✓4th O21　Excessive vomiting in pregnancy

O21.0　Mild hyperemesis gravidarum ＭＱ
Hyperemesis gravidarum, mild or unspecified, starting before the end of the 20th week of gestation

O21.1　Hyperemesis gravidarum with metabolic disturbance ＭＱ
Hyperemesis gravidarum, starting before the end of the 20th week of gestation, with metabolic disturbance such as carbohydrate depletion
Hyperemesis gravidarum, starting before the end of the 20th week of gestation, with metabolic disturbance such as dehydration
Hyperemesis gravidarum, starting before the end of the 20th week of gestation, with metabolic disturbance such as electrolyte imbalance

O21.2　Late vomiting of pregnancy ＭＱ
Excessive vomiting starting after 20 completed weeks of gestation

O21.8　Other vomiting complicating pregnancy ＭＱ
Vomiting due to diseases classified elsewhere, complicating pregnancy
Use additional code, to identify cause

O21.9　Vomiting of pregnancy, unspecified ＭＱ▽

✓4th O22　Venous complications and hemorrhoids in pregnancy

EXCLUDES 1　venous complications of:
abortion NOS (O03.9)
ectopic or molar pregnancy (O08.7)
failed attempted abortion (O07.35)
induced abortion (O04.85)
spontaneous abortion (O03.89)

EXCLUDES 2　obstetric pulmonary embolism (O88.-)
venous complications and hemorrhoids of childbirth and the puerperium (O87.-)

✓5th O22.0　Varicose veins of lower extremity in pregnancy
Varicose veins NOS in pregnancy
DEF: Distended, tortuous veins of lower extremities associated with pregnancy.

O22.00　Varicose veins of lower extremity in pregnancy, unspecified trimester ＭＱ▽

EXCLUDES 1　Not coded here　　EXCLUDES 2　Not included here　　Ｎ Newborn Age: 0　　Ｐ Pediatric Age: 0-17　　Ｍ Maternity Age: 12-55　　Ａ Adult Age: 15-124

830

ICD-10-CM 2018

O22.01 Varicose veins of lower extremity in pregnancy, Ⓜ♀
first trimester

O22.02 Varicose veins of lower extremity in pregnancy, Ⓜ♀
second trimester

O22.03 Varicose veins of lower extremity in pregnancy, Ⓜ♀
third trimester

√5ᵗʰ **O22.1 Genital varices in pregnancy**
Perineal varices in pregnancy
Vaginal varices in pregnancy
Vulval varices in pregnancy

O22.10 Genital varices in pregnancy, unspecified Ⓜ♀▽
trimester

O22.11 Genital varices in pregnancy, first trimester Ⓜ♀

O22.12 Genital varices in pregnancy, second trimester Ⓜ♀

O22.13 Genital varices in pregnancy, third trimester Ⓜ♀

√5ᵗʰ **O22.2 Superficial thrombophlebitis in pregnancy**
Phlebitis in pregnancy NOS
Thrombophlebitis of legs in pregnancy
Thrombosis in pregnancy NOS
Use additional code to identify the superficial thrombophlebitis
(I80.0-)

O22.20 Superficial thrombophlebitis in pregnancy, Ⓜ♀▽
unspecified trimester

O22.21 Superficial thrombophlebitis in pregnancy, Ⓜ♀
first trimester

O22.22 Superficial thrombophlebitis in pregnancy, Ⓜ♀
second trimester

O22.23 Superficial thrombophlebitis in pregnancy, Ⓜ♀
third trimester

√5ᵗʰ **O22.3 Deep phlebothrombosis in pregnancy**
Deep vein thrombosis, antepartum
Use additional code to identify the deep vein thrombosis (I82.4-,
I82.5-, I82.62-, I82.72-)
Use additional code, if applicable, for associated long-term
(current) use of anticoagulants (Z79.01)

O22.30 Deep phlebothrombosis in pregnancy, Ⓜ♀▽
unspecified trimester

O22.31 Deep phlebothrombosis in pregnancy, Ⓜ♀
first trimester

O22.32 Deep phlebothrombosis in pregnancy, Ⓜ♀
second trimester

O22.33 Deep phlebothrombosis in pregnancy, Ⓜ♀
third trimester

√5ᵗʰ **O22.4 Hemorrhoids in pregnancy**

O22.40 Hemorrhoids in pregnancy, unspecified Ⓜ♀▽
trimester

O22.41 Hemorrhoids in pregnancy, first trimester Ⓜ♀

O22.42 Hemorrhoids in pregnancy, second trimester Ⓜ♀

O22.43 Hemorrhoids in pregnancy, third trimester Ⓜ♀

√5ᵗʰ **O22.5 Cerebral venous thrombosis in pregnancy**
Cerebrovenous sinus thrombosis in pregnancy

O22.50 Cerebral venous thrombosis in pregnancy, Ⓜ♀▽
unspecified trimester

O22.51 Cerebral venous thrombosis in pregnancy, Ⓜ♀
first trimester

O22.52 Cerebral venous thrombosis in pregnancy, Ⓜ♀
second trimester

O22.53 Cerebral venous thrombosis in pregnancy, Ⓜ♀
third trimester

√5ᵗʰ **O22.8 Other venous complications in pregnancy**

√6ᵗʰ **O22.8X Other venous complications in pregnancy**

O22.8X1 Other venous complications in Ⓜ♀
pregnancy, first trimester

O22.8X2 Other venous complications in Ⓜ♀
pregnancy, second trimester

O22.8X3 Other venous complications in Ⓜ♀
pregnancy, third trimester

O22.8X9 Other venous complications in Ⓜ♀▽
pregnancy, unspecified trimester

√5ᵗʰ **O22.9 Venous complication in pregnancy, unspecified**
Gestational phlebitis NOS
Gestational phlebopathy NOS
Gestational thrombosis NOS

O22.90 Venous complication in pregnancy, Ⓜ♀▽
unspecified, unspecified trimester

O22.91 Venous complication in pregnancy, Ⓜ♀▽
unspecified, first trimester

O22.92 Venous complication in pregnancy, Ⓜ♀▽
unspecified, second trimester

O22.93 Venous complication in pregnancy, Ⓜ♀▽
unspecified, third trimester

√4ᵗʰ **O23 Infections of genitourinary tract in pregnancy**
Use additional code to identify organism (B95.-, B96.-)
EXCLUDES 2   gonococcal infections complicating pregnancy, childbirth and
the puerperium (O98.2)
infections with a predominantly sexual mode of transmission
NOS complicating pregnancy, childbirth and the
puerperium (O98.3)
syphilis complicating pregnancy, childbirth and the puerperium
(O98.1)
tuberculosis of genitourinary system complicating pregnancy,
childbirth and the puerperium (O98.0)
venereal disease NOS complicating pregnancy, childbirth and
the puerperium (O98.3)

√5ᵗʰ **O23.0 Infections of kidney in pregnancy**
Pyelonephritis in pregnancy

O23.00 Infections of kidney in pregnancy, unspecified Ⓜ♀▽
trimester

O23.01 Infections of kidney in pregnancy, first trimester Ⓜ♀

O23.02 Infections of kidney in pregnancy, second Ⓜ♀
trimester

O23.03 Infections of kidney in pregnancy, third Ⓜ♀
trimester

√5ᵗʰ **O23.1 Infections of bladder in pregnancy**

O23.10 Infections of bladder in pregnancy, Ⓜ♀▽
unspecified trimester

O23.11 Infections of bladder in pregnancy, Ⓜ♀
first trimester

O23.12 Infections of bladder in pregnancy, Ⓜ♀
second trimester

O23.13 Infections of bladder in pregnancy, Ⓜ♀
third trimester

√5ᵗʰ **O23.2 Infections of urethra in pregnancy**

O23.20 Infections of urethra in pregnancy, Ⓜ♀▽
unspecified trimester

O23.21 Infections of urethra in pregnancy, Ⓜ♀
first trimester

O23.22 Infections of urethra in pregnancy, Ⓜ♀
second trimester

O23.23 Infections of urethra in pregnancy, Ⓜ♀
third trimester

√5ᵗʰ **O23.3 Infections of other parts of urinary tract in pregnancy**

O23.30 Infections of other parts of urinary tract in Ⓜ♀▽
pregnancy, unspecified trimester

O23.31 Infections of other parts of urinary tract in Ⓜ♀
pregnancy, first trimester

O23.32 Infections of other parts of urinary tract in Ⓜ♀
pregnancy, second trimester

O23.33 Infections of other parts of urinary tract in ♀
pregnancy, third trimester

√5ᵗʰ **O23.4 Unspecified infection of urinary tract in pregnancy**

O23.40 Unspecified infection of urinary tract in Ⓜ♀▽
pregnancy, unspecified trimester

O23.41 Unspecified infection of urinary tract in Ⓜ♀▽
pregnancy, first trimester

O23.42 Unspecified infection of urinary tract in Ⓜ♀▽
pregnancy, second trimester

O23.43 Unspecified infection of urinary tract in Ⓜ♀▽
pregnancy, third trimester

√5ᵗʰ **O23.5 Infections of the genital tract in pregnancy**

√6ᵗʰ **O23.51 Infection of cervix in pregnancy**

O23.511 Infections of cervix in pregnancy, Ⓜ♀
first trimester

O23.512 Infections of cervix in pregnancy, Ⓜ♀
second trimester

O23.513 Infections of cervix in pregnancy, Ⓜ♀
third trimester

O23.519 Infections of cervix in pregnancy, Ⓜ♀▽
unspecified trimester

O23.52 Salpingo-oophoritis in pregnancy
Oophoritis in pregnancy
Salpingitis in pregnancy

O23.521 **Salpingo-oophoritis in pregnancy, first trimester** Ⓜ♀

O23.522 **Salpingo-oophoritis in pregnancy, second trimester** Ⓜ♀

O23.523 **Salpingo-oophoritis in pregnancy, third trimester** Ⓜ♀

O23.529 **Salpingo-oophoritis in pregnancy, unspecified trimester** Ⓜ♀▽

O23.59 Infection of other part of genital tract in pregnancy

O23.591 **Infection of other part of genital tract in pregnancy, first trimester** Ⓜ♀

O23.592 **Infection of other part of genital tract in pregnancy, second trimester** Ⓜ♀

O23.593 **Infection of other part of genital tract in pregnancy, third trimester** Ⓜ♀

O23.599 **Infection of other part of genital tract in pregnancy, unspecified trimester** Ⓜ♀▽

O23.9 Unspecified genitourinary tract infection in pregnancy
Genitourinary tract infection in pregnancy NOS

O23.90 **Unspecified genitourinary tract infection in pregnancy, unspecified trimester** Ⓜ♀▽

O23.91 **Unspecified genitourinary tract infection in pregnancy, first trimester** Ⓜ♀▽

O23.92 **Unspecified genitourinary tract infection in pregnancy, second trimester** Ⓜ♀▽

O23.93 **Unspecified genitourinary tract infection in pregnancy, third trimester** Ⓜ♀▽

O24 Diabetes mellitus in pregnancy, childbirth and the puerperium

O24.0 Pre-existing type 1 diabetes mellitus, in pregnancy, childbirth and the puerperium
Juvenile onset diabetes mellitus, in pregnancy, childbirth and the puerperium
Ketosis-prone diabetes mellitus in pregnancy, childbirth and the puerperium
Use additional code from category E10 to further identify any manifestations

O24.01 Pre-existing type 1 diabetes mellitus, in pregnancy

O24.011 **Pre-existing type 1 diabetes mellitus, in pregnancy, first trimester** Ⓜ♀

O24.012 **Pre-existing type 1 diabetes mellitus, in pregnancy, second trimester** Ⓜ♀

O24.013 **Pre-existing type 1 diabetes mellitus, in pregnancy, third trimester** Ⓜ♀

O24.019 **Pre-existing type 1 diabetes mellitus, in pregnancy, unspecified trimester** Ⓜ♀▽

O24.02 **Pre-existing type 1 diabetes mellitus, in childbirth** Ⓜ♀

O24.03 **Pre-existing type 1 diabetes mellitus, in the puerperium** Ⓜ♀

O24.1 Pre-existing type 2 diabetes mellitus, in pregnancy, childbirth and the puerperium
Insulin-resistant diabetes mellitus in pregnancy, childbirth and the puerperium
Use additional code (for):
from category E11 to further identify any manifestations
long-term (current) use of insulin (Z79.4)

O24.11 Pre-existing type 2 diabetes mellitus, in pregnancy

O24.111 **Pre-existing type 2 diabetes mellitus, in pregnancy, first trimester** Ⓜ♀

O24.112 **Pre-existing type 2 diabetes mellitus, in pregnancy, second trimester** Ⓜ♀

O24.113 **Pre-existing type 2 diabetes mellitus, in pregnancy, third trimester** Ⓜ♀

O24.119 **Pre-existing type 2 diabetes mellitus, in pregnancy, unspecified trimester** Ⓜ♀▽

O24.12 **Pre-existing type 2 diabetes mellitus, in childbirth** Ⓜ♀

O24.13 **Pre-existing type 2 diabetes mellitus, in the puerperium** Ⓜ♀

O24.3 Unspecified pre-existing diabetes mellitus in pregnancy, childbirth and the puerperium
Use additional code (for):
from category E11 to further identify any manifestation
long-term (current) use of insulin (Z79.4)

O24.31 Unspecified pre-existing diabetes mellitus in pregnancy

O24.311 **Unspecified pre-existing diabetes mellitus in pregnancy, first trimester** Ⓜ♀▽

O24.312 **Unspecified pre-existing diabetes mellitus in pregnancy, second trimester** Ⓜ♀▽

O24.313 **Unspecified pre-existing diabetes mellitus in pregnancy, third trimester** Ⓜ♀▽

O24.319 **Unspecified pre-existing diabetes mellitus in pregnancy, unspecified trimester** Ⓜ♀▽

O24.32 **Unspecified pre-existing diabetes mellitus in childbirth** Ⓜ♀▽

O24.33 **Unspecified pre-existing diabetes mellitus in the puerperium** Ⓜ♀▽

O24.4 Gestational diabetes mellitus
Diabetes mellitus arising in pregnancy
Gestational diabetes mellitus NOS

O24.41 Gestational diabetes mellitus in pregnancy

O24.410 **Gestational diabetes mellitus in pregnancy, diet controlled** Ⓜ♀

O24.414 **Gestational diabetes mellitus in pregnancy, insulin controlled** Ⓜ♀

O24.415 **Gestational diabetes mellitus in pregnancy, controlled by oral hypoglycemic drugs**
Gestational diabetes mellitus in pregnancy, controlled by oral antidiabetic drugs

O24.419 **Gestational diabetes mellitus in pregnancy, unspecified control** Ⓜ♀▽
AHA: 2015, 4Q, 34

O24.42 Gestational diabetes mellitus in childbirth
AHA: 2016, 1Q, 5

O24.420 **Gestational diabetes mellitus in childbirth, diet controlled** Ⓜ♀

O24.424 **Gestational diabetes mellitus in childbirth, insulin controlled** Ⓜ♀

O24.425 **Gestational diabetes mellitus in childbirth, controlled by oral hypoglycemic drugs** Ⓜ♀
Gestational diabetes mellitus in childbirth, controlled by oral antidiabetic drugs

O24.429 **Gestational diabetes mellitus in childbirth, unspecified control** Ⓜ♀▽
AHA: 2015, 4Q, 34

O24.43 Gestational diabetes mellitus in the puerperium

O24.430 **Gestational diabetes mellitus in the puerperium, diet controlled** Ⓜ♀

O24.434 **Gestational diabetes mellitus in the puerperium, insulin controlled** Ⓜ♀

O24.435 **Gestational diabetes mellitus in puerperium, controlled by oral hypoglycemic drugs** Ⓜ♀
Gestational diabetes mellitus in puerperium, controlled by oral antidiabetic drugs

O24.439 **Gestational diabetes mellitus in the puerperium, unspecified control** Ⓜ♀▽
AHA: 2015, 4Q, 34

O24.8 Other pre-existing diabetes mellitus in pregnancy, childbirth, and the puerperium
Use additional code (for):
from categories E08, E09 and E13 to further identify any manifestation
long-term (current) use of insulin (Z79.4)

O24.81 Other pre-existing diabetes mellitus in pregnancy

O24.811 **Other pre-existing diabetes mellitus in pregnancy, first trimester** Ⓜ♀

O24.812 **Other pre-existing diabetes mellitus in pregnancy, second trimester** Ⓜ♀

O24.813 **Other pre-existing diabetes mellitus in pregnancy, third trimester** Ⓜ♀

O24.819 **Other pre-existing diabetes mellitus in pregnancy, unspecified trimester** Ⓜ♀▽

EXCLUDES 1 Not coded here   **EXCLUDES 2** Not included here   Ⓝ Newborn Age: 0   Ⓟ Pediatric Age: 0-17   Ⓜ Maternity Age: 12-55   Ⓐ Adult Age: 15-124

832   ICD-10-CM 2018

O24.82 **Other pre-existing diabetes mellitus in childbirth** Ⓜ♀

O24.83 **Other pre-existing diabetes mellitus in the puerperium** Ⓜ♀

√5ᵗʰ O24.9 **Unspecified diabetes mellitus in pregnancy, childbirth and the puerperium**
     Use additional code for long-term (current) use of insulin (Z79.4)

     √6ᵗʰ O24.91 **Unspecified diabetes mellitus in pregnancy**

         O24.911 **Unspecified diabetes mellitus in pregnancy, first trimester** Ⓜ♀▽

         O24.912 **Unspecified diabetes mellitus in pregnancy, second trimester** Ⓜ♀▽

         O24.913 **Unspecified diabetes mellitus in pregnancy, third trimester** Ⓜ♀▽

         O24.919 **Unspecified diabetes mellitus in pregnancy, unspecified trimester** Ⓜ♀▽

     O24.92 **Unspecified diabetes mellitus in childbirth** Ⓜ♀▽

     O24.93 **Unspecified diabetes mellitus in the puerperium** Ⓜ♀▽

√4ᵗʰ O25 **Malnutrition in pregnancy, childbirth and the puerperium**

     √5ᵗʰ O25.1 **Malnutrition in pregnancy**

         O25.10 **Malnutrition in pregnancy, unspecified trimester** Ⓜ♀▽

         O25.11 **Malnutrition in pregnancy, first trimester** Ⓜ♀

         O25.12 **Malnutrition in pregnancy, second trimester** Ⓜ♀

         O25.13 **Malnutrition in pregnancy, third trimester** Ⓜ♀

     O25.2 **Malnutrition in childbirth** Ⓜ♀

     O25.3 **Malnutrition in the puerperium** Ⓜ♀

√4ᵗʰ O26 **Maternal care for other conditions predominantly related to pregnancy**

     √5ᵗʰ O26.0 **Excessive weight gain in pregnancy**
         EXCLUDES 2   gestational edema (O12.0, O12.2)

         O26.00 **Excessive weight gain in pregnancy, unspecified trimester** Ⓜ♀▽

         O26.01 **Excessive weight gain in pregnancy, first trimester** Ⓜ♀

         O26.02 **Excessive weight gain in pregnancy, second trimester** Ⓜ♀

         O26.03 **Excessive weight gain in pregnancy, third trimester** Ⓜ♀

     √5ᵗʰ O26.1 **Low weight gain in pregnancy**

         O26.10 **Low weight gain in pregnancy, unspecified trimester** Ⓜ♀▽

         O26.11 **Low weight gain in pregnancy, first trimester** Ⓜ♀

         O26.12 **Low weight gain in pregnancy, second trimester** Ⓜ♀

         O26.13 **Low weight gain in pregnancy, third trimester** Ⓜ♀

     √5ᵗʰ O26.2 **Pregnancy care for patient with recurrent pregnancy loss**

         O26.20 **Pregnancy care for patient with recurrent pregnancy loss, unspecified trimester** Ⓜ♀▽

         O26.21 **Pregnancy care for patient with recurrent pregnancy loss, first trimester** Ⓜ♀

         O26.22 **Pregnancy care for patient with recurrent pregnancy loss, second trimester** Ⓜ♀

         O26.23 **Pregnancy care for patient with recurrent pregnancy loss, third trimester** Ⓜ♀

     √5ᵗʰ O26.3 **Retained intrauterine contraceptive device in pregnancy**

         O26.30 **Retained intrauterine contraceptive device in pregnancy, unspecified trimester** Ⓜ♀▽

         O26.31 **Retained intrauterine contraceptive device in pregnancy, first trimester** Ⓜ♀

         O26.32 **Retained intrauterine contraceptive device in pregnancy, second trimester** Ⓜ♀

         O26.33 **Retained intrauterine contraceptive device in pregnancy, third trimester** Ⓜ♀

     √5ᵗʰ O26.4 **Herpes gestationis**

         O26.40 **Herpes gestationis, unspecified trimester** Ⓜ♀▽

         O26.41 **Herpes gestationis, first trimester** Ⓜ♀

         O26.42 **Herpes gestationis, second trimester** Ⓜ♀

         O26.43 **Herpes gestationis, third trimester** Ⓜ♀

√5ᵗʰ O26.5 **Maternal hypotension syndrome**
     Supine hypotensive syndrome

     O26.50 **Maternal hypotension syndrome, unspecified trimester** Ⓜ♀▽

     O26.51 **Maternal hypotension syndrome, first trimester** Ⓜ♀

     O26.52 **Maternal hypotension syndrome, second trimester** Ⓜ♀

     O26.53 **Maternal hypotension syndrome, third trimester** Ⓜ♀

√5ᵗʰ O26.6 **Liver and biliary tract disorders in pregnancy, childbirth and the puerperium**
     Use additional code to identify the specific disorder
     EXCLUDES 2   hepatorenal syndrome following labor and delivery (O90.4)

     √6ᵗʰ O26.61 **Liver and biliary tract disorders in pregnancy**

         O26.611 **Liver and biliary tract disorders in pregnancy, first trimester** Ⓜ♀

         O26.612 **Liver and biliary tract disorders in pregnancy, second trimester** Ⓜ♀

         O26.613 **Liver and biliary tract disorders in pregnancy, third trimester** Ⓜ♀

         O26.619 **Liver and biliary tract disorders in pregnancy, unspecified trimester** Ⓜ♀▽

     O26.62 **Liver and biliary tract disorders in childbirth** Ⓜ♀

     O26.63 **Liver and biliary tract disorders in the puerperium** Ⓜ♀

√5ᵗʰ O26.7 **Subluxation of symphysis (pubis) in pregnancy, childbirth and the puerperium**
     EXCLUDES 1   traumatic separation of symphysis (pubis) during childbirth (O71.6)

     √6ᵗʰ O26.71 **Subluxation of symphysis (pubis) in pregnancy**

         O26.711 **Subluxation of symphysis (pubis) in pregnancy, first trimester** Ⓜ♀

         O26.712 **Subluxation of symphysis (pubis) in pregnancy, second trimester** Ⓜ♀

         O26.713 **Subluxation of symphysis (pubis) in pregnancy, third trimester** Ⓜ♀

         O26.719 **Subluxation of symphysis (pubis) in pregnancy, unspecified trimester** Ⓜ♀▽

     O26.72 **Subluxation of symphysis (pubis) in childbirth** Ⓜ♀

     O26.73 **Subluxation of symphysis (pubis) in the puerperium** Ⓜ♀

√5ᵗʰ O26.8 **Other specified pregnancy related conditions**

     √6ᵗʰ O26.81 **Pregnancy related exhaustion and fatigue**

         O26.811 **Pregnancy related exhaustion and fatigue, first trimester** Ⓜ♀

         O26.812 **Pregnancy related exhaustion and fatigue, second trimester** Ⓜ♀

         O26.813 **Pregnancy related exhaustion and fatigue, third trimester** Ⓜ♀

         O26.819 **Pregnancy related exhaustion and fatigue, unspecified trimester** Ⓜ♀▽

     √6ᵗʰ O26.82 **Pregnancy related peripheral neuritis**

         O26.821 **Pregnancy related peripheral neuritis, first trimester** Ⓜ♀

         O26.822 **Pregnancy related peripheral neuritis, second trimester** Ⓜ♀

         O26.823 **Pregnancy related peripheral neuritis, third trimester** Ⓜ♀

         O26.829 **Pregnancy related peripheral neuritis, unspecified trimester** Ⓜ♀▽

     √6ᵗʰ O26.83 **Pregnancy related renal disease**
         Use additional code to identify the specific disorder

         O26.831 **Pregnancy related renal disease, first trimester** Ⓜ♀

         O26.832 **Pregnancy related renal disease, second trimester** Ⓜ♀

         O26.833 **Pregnancy related renal disease, third trimester** Ⓜ♀

         O26.839 **Pregnancy related renal disease, unspecified trimester** Ⓜ♀▽

☑ Additional Character Req   √x7ᵗʰ Placeholder Alert   Manifestation   ℍℂℂ CMS-HCC Condition   ▽ Unspecified Code   ►◄ Revised Text   ● New Code   ▲ Revised Code Title

ICD-10-CM 2018   833

O24.82–O26.839

✓6th **O26.84** **Uterine size-date discrepancy complicating pregnancy**
> EXCLUDES 1 *encounter for suspected problem with fetal growth ruled out (Z03.74)*

O26.841 Uterine size-date discrepancy, first trimester ♏♀

O26.842 Uterine size-date discrepancy, second trimester ♏♀

O26.843 Uterine size-date discrepancy, third trimester ♏♀

O26.849 Uterine size-date discrepancy, unspecified trimester ♏♀▽

✓6th **O26.85** **Spotting complicating pregnancy**

O26.851 Spotting complicating pregnancy, first trimester ♏♀

O26.852 Spotting complicating pregnancy, second trimester ♏♀

O26.853 Spotting complicating pregnancy, third trimester ♏♀

O26.859 Spotting complicating pregnancy, unspecified trimester ♏♀▽

O26.86 **Pruritic urticarial papules and plaques of pregnancy (PUPPP)** ♏♀
Polymorphic eruption of pregnancy

✓6th **O26.87** **Cervical shortening**
> EXCLUDES 1 *encounter for suspected cervical shortening ruled out (Z03.75)*

> **DEF:** A cervix that has shortened to < 25 mm before the 24th week of pregnancy; warning sign for impending premature delivery; treated by cervical cerclage placement or progesterone.

O26.872 Cervical shortening, second trimester ♏♀

O26.873 Cervical shortening, third trimester ♏♀

O26.879 Cervical shortening, unspecified trimester ♏♀▽

✓6th **O26.89** **Other specified pregnancy related conditions**
> AHA: 2015, 3Q, 40

O26.891 Other specified pregnancy related conditions, first trimester ♏♀

O26.892 Other specified pregnancy related conditions, second trimester ♏♀

O26.893 Other specified pregnancy related conditions, third trimester ♏♀

O26.899 Other specified pregnancy related conditions, unspecified trimester ♏♀▽

✓5th **O26.9** **Pregnancy related conditions, unspecified**

O26.90 Pregnancy related conditions, unspecified, unspecified trimester ♏♀▽

O26.91 Pregnancy related conditions, unspecified, first trimester ♏♀▽

O26.92 Pregnancy related conditions, unspecified, second trimester ♏♀▽

O26.93 Pregnancy related conditions, unspecified, third trimester ♏♀▽

✓4th **O28** **Abnormal findings on antenatal screening of mother**
> EXCLUDES 1 *diagnostic findings classified elsewhere—see Alphabetical Index*

O28.0 **Abnormal hematological finding on antenatal screening of mother** ♏♀

O28.1 **Abnormal biochemical finding on antenatal screening of mother** ♏♀

O28.2 **Abnormal cytological finding on antenatal screening of mother** ♏♀

O28.3 **Abnormal ultrasonic finding on antenatal screening of mother** ♏♀

O28.4 **Abnormal radiological finding on antenatal screening of mother** ♏♀

O28.5 **Abnormal chromosomal and genetic finding on antenatal screening of mother** ♏♀

O28.8 **Other abnormal findings on antenatal screening of mother** ♏♀

O28.9 **Unspecified abnormal findings on antenatal screening of mother** ♏♀▽

✓4th **O29** **Complications of anesthesia during pregnancy**
> INCLUDES maternal complications arising from the administration of a general, regional or local anesthetic, analgesic or other sedation during pregnancy

> Use additional code, if necessary, to identify the complication

> EXCLUDES 2 *complications of anesthesia during labor and delivery (O74.-)*
> *complications of anesthesia during the puerperium (O89.-)*

✓5th **O29.0** **Pulmonary complications of anesthesia during pregnancy**

✓6th **O29.01** **Aspiration pneumonitis due to anesthesia during pregnancy**
Inhalation of stomach contents or secretions NOS due to anesthesia during pregnancy
Mendelson's syndrome due to anesthesia during pregnancy

O29.011 Aspiration pneumonitis due to anesthesia during pregnancy, first trimester ♏♀

O29.012 Aspiration pneumonitis due to anesthesia during pregnancy, second trimester ♏♀

O29.013 Aspiration pneumonitis due to anesthesia during pregnancy, third trimester ♏♀

O29.019 Aspiration pneumonitis due to anesthesia during pregnancy, unspecified trimester ♏♀▽

✓6th **O29.02** **Pressure collapse of lung due to anesthesia during pregnancy**

O29.021 Pressure collapse of lung due to anesthesia during pregnancy, first trimester ♏♀

O29.022 Pressure collapse of lung due to anesthesia during pregnancy, second trimester ♏♀

O29.023 Pressure collapse of lung due to anesthesia during pregnancy, third trimester ♏♀

O29.029 Pressure collapse of lung due to anesthesia during pregnancy, unspecified trimester ♏♀▽

✓6th **O29.09** **Other pulmonary complications of anesthesia during pregnancy**

O29.091 Other pulmonary complications of anesthesia during pregnancy, first trimester ♏♀

O29.092 Other pulmonary complications of anesthesia during pregnancy, second trimester ♏♀

O29.093 Other pulmonary complications of anesthesia during pregnancy, third trimester ♏♀

O29.099 Other pulmonary complications of anesthesia during pregnancy, unspecified trimester ♏♀▽

✓5th **O29.1** **Cardiac complications of anesthesia during pregnancy**

✓6th **O29.11** **Cardiac arrest due to anesthesia during pregnancy**

O29.111 Cardiac arrest due to anesthesia during pregnancy, first trimester ♏♀

O29.112 Cardiac arrest due to anesthesia during pregnancy, second trimester ♏♀

O29.113 Cardiac arrest due to anesthesia during pregnancy, third trimester ♏♀

O29.119 Cardiac arrest due to anesthesia during pregnancy, unspecified trimester ♏♀▽

✓6th **O29.12** **Cardiac failure due to anesthesia during pregnancy**

O29.121 Cardiac failure due to anesthesia during pregnancy, first trimester ♏♀

O29.122 Cardiac failure due to anesthesia during pregnancy, second trimester ♏♀

O29.123 Cardiac failure due to anesthesia during pregnancy, third trimester ♏♀

O29.129 Cardiac failure due to anesthesia during pregnancy, unspecified trimester ♏♀▽

✓6th **O29.19** Other cardiac complications of anesthesia during pregnancy

  O29.191 Other cardiac complications of anesthesia during pregnancy, first trimester M♀

  O29.192 Other cardiac complications of anesthesia during pregnancy, second trimester M♀

  O29.193 Other cardiac complications of anesthesia during pregnancy, third trimester M♀

  O29.199 Other cardiac complications of anesthesia during pregnancy, unspecified trimester M♀▽

✓5th **O29.2** Central nervous system complications of anesthesia during pregnancy

  ✓6th **O29.21** Cerebral anoxia due to anesthesia during pregnancy

    O29.211 Cerebral anoxia due to anesthesia during pregnancy, first trimester M♀

    O29.212 Cerebral anoxia due to anesthesia during pregnancy, second trimester M♀

    O29.213 Cerebral anoxia due to anesthesia during pregnancy, third trimester M♀

    O29.219 Cerebral anoxia due to anesthesia during pregnancy, unspecified trimester M♀▽

  ✓6th **O29.29** Other central nervous system complications of anesthesia during pregnancy

    O29.291 Other central nervous system complications of anesthesia during pregnancy, first trimester M♀

    O29.292 Other central nervous system complications of anesthesia during pregnancy, second trimester M♀

    O29.293 Other central nervous system complications of anesthesia during pregnancy, third trimester M♀

    O29.299 Other central nervous system complications of anesthesia during pregnancy, unspecified trimester M♀▽

✓5th **O29.3** Toxic reaction to local anesthesia during pregnancy

  ✓6th **O29.3X** Toxic reaction to local anesthesia during pregnancy

    O29.3X1 Toxic reaction to local anesthesia during pregnancy, first trimester M♀

    O29.3X2 Toxic reaction to local anesthesia during pregnancy, second trimester M♀

    O29.3X3 Toxic reaction to local anesthesia during pregnancy, third trimester M♀

    O29.3X9 Toxic reaction to local anesthesia during pregnancy, unspecified trimester M♀▽

✓5th **O29.4** Spinal and epidural anesthesia induced headache during pregnancy

  O29.40 Spinal and epidural anesthesia induced headache during pregnancy, unspecified trimester M♀▽

  O29.41 Spinal and epidural anesthesia induced headache during pregnancy, first trimester M♀

  O29.42 Spinal and epidural anesthesia induced headache during pregnancy, second trimester M♀

  O29.43 Spinal and epidural anesthesia induced headache during pregnancy, third trimester M♀

✓5th **O29.5** Other complications of spinal and epidural anesthesia during pregnancy

  ✓6th **O29.5X** Other complications of spinal and epidural anesthesia during pregnancy

    O29.5X1 Other complications of spinal and epidural anesthesia during pregnancy, first trimester M♀

    O29.5X2 Other complications of spinal and epidural anesthesia during pregnancy, second trimester M♀

    O29.5X3 Other complications of spinal and epidural anesthesia during pregnancy, third trimester M♀

    O29.5X9 Other complications of spinal and epidural anesthesia during pregnancy, unspecified trimester M♀▽

✓5th **O29.6** Failed or difficult intubation for anesthesia during pregnancy

  O29.60 Failed or difficult intubation for anesthesia during pregnancy, unspecified trimester M♀▽

  O29.61 Failed or difficult intubation for anesthesia during pregnancy, first trimester M♀

  O29.62 Failed or difficult intubation for anesthesia during pregnancy, second trimester M♀

  O29.63 Failed or difficult intubation for anesthesia during pregnancy, third trimester M♀

✓5th **O29.8** Other complications of anesthesia during pregnancy

  ✓6th **O29.8X** Other complications of anesthesia during pregnancy

    O29.8X1 Other complications of anesthesia during pregnancy, first trimester M♀

    O29.8X2 Other complications of anesthesia during pregnancy, second trimester M♀

    O29.8X3 Other complications of anesthesia during pregnancy, third trimester M♀

    O29.8X9 Other complications of anesthesia during pregnancy, unspecified trimester M♀▽

✓5th **O29.9** Unspecified complication of anesthesia during pregnancy

  O29.90 Unspecified complication of anesthesia during pregnancy, unspecified trimester M♀▽

  O29.91 Unspecified complication of anesthesia during pregnancy, first trimester M♀▽

  O29.92 Unspecified complication of anesthesia during pregnancy, second trimester M♀▽

  O29.93 Unspecified complication of anesthesia during pregnancy, third trimester M♀▽

Maternal care related to the fetus and amniotic cavity and possible delivery problems (O30-O48)

✓4th **O30 Multiple gestation**

Code also any complications specific to multiple gestation

✓5th **O30.0** Twin pregnancy

  ✓6th **O30.00** Twin pregnancy, unspecified number of placenta and unspecified number of amniotic sacs

    O30.001 Twin pregnancy, unspecified number of placenta and unspecified number of amniotic sacs, first trimester M♀▽

    O30.002 Twin pregnancy, unspecified number of placenta and unspecified number of amniotic sacs, second trimester M♀▽

    O30.003 Twin pregnancy, unspecified number of placenta and unspecified number of amniotic sacs, third trimester M♀▽

    O30.009 Twin pregnancy, unspecified number of placenta and unspecified number of amniotic sacs, unspecified trimester M♀▽

  ✓6th **O30.01** Twin pregnancy, monochorionic/monoamniotic

Twin pregnancy, one placenta, one amniotic sac

EXCLUDES 1   conjoined twins (O30.02-)

    O30.011 Twin pregnancy, monochorionic/monoamniotic, first trimester M♀

    O30.012 Twin pregnancy, monochorionic/monoamniotic, second trimester M♀

    O30.013 Twin pregnancy, monochorionic/monoamniotic, third trimester M♀

    O30.019 Twin pregnancy, monochorionic/monoamniotic, unspecified trimester M♀▽

Twin Gestation – Monochorionic/Monoamniotic

- 1 Chorionic sac
- 1 Amniotic sac
- 2 Fetuses
- 2 Umbilical cords
- 1 Placenta

✓ Additional Character Req   ✓x7th Placeholder Alert   Manifestation   HCC CMS-HCC Condition   ▽ Unspecified Code   ►◄ Revised Text   ● New Code   ▲ Revised Code Title

ICD-10-CM 2018   835

Chapter 15. Pregnancy, Childbirth, and the Puerperium

Twin Gestation – Monochorionic/Diamniotic

1 Chorionic sac
2 Amniotic sacs
2 Fetuses
2 Umbilical cords
1 Placenta

Twin Gestation – Dichorionic/Diamniotic

2 Chorionic sacs
2 Amniotic sacs
2 Fetuses
2 Umbilical cords
2 Placentas

✓6ᵗʰ **O30.02** **Conjoined twin pregnancy**
     O30.021   Conjoined twin pregnancy, first trimester   Ⓜ♀
     O30.022   Conjoined twin pregnancy, second trimester   Ⓜ♀
     O30.023   Conjoined twin pregnancy, third trimester   Ⓜ♀
     O30.029   Conjoined twin pregnancy, unspecified trimester   Ⓜ♀▽

✓6ᵗʰ **O30.03** **Twin pregnancy, monochorionic/diamniotic**
     Twin pregnancy, one placenta, two amniotic sacs
     O30.031   Twin pregnancy, monochorionic/diamniotic, first trimester   Ⓜ♀
     O30.032   Twin pregnancy, monochorionic/diamniotic, second trimester   Ⓜ♀
     O30.033   Twin pregnancy, monochorionic/diamniotic, third trimester   Ⓜ♀
     O30.039   Twin pregnancy, monochorionic/diamniotic, unspecified trimester   Ⓜ♀▽

✓6ᵗʰ **O30.04** **Twin pregnancy, dichorionic/diamniotic**
     Twin pregnancy, two placentae, two amniotic sacs
     O30.041   Twin pregnancy, dichorionic/diamniotic, first trimester   Ⓜ♀
     O30.042   Twin pregnancy, dichorionic/diamniotic, second trimester   Ⓜ♀
     O30.043   Twin pregnancy, dichorionic/diamniotic, third trimester   Ⓜ♀
     O30.049   Twin pregnancy, dichorionic/diamniotic, unspecified trimester   Ⓜ♀▽

✓6ᵗʰ **O30.09** **Twin pregnancy, unable to determine number of placenta and number of amniotic sacs**
     O30.091   Twin pregnancy, unable to determine number of placenta and number of amniotic sacs, first trimester   Ⓜ♀
     O30.092   Twin pregnancy, unable to determine number of placenta and number of amniotic sacs, second trimester   Ⓜ♀
     O30.093   Twin pregnancy, unable to determine number of placenta and number of amniotic sacs, third trimester   Ⓜ♀

     O30.099   Twin pregnancy, unable to determine number of placenta and number of amniotic sacs, unspecified trimester   Ⓜ♀▽

✓5ᵗʰ **O30.1** **Triplet pregnancy**
   ✓6ᵗʰ **O30.10** **Triplet pregnancy, unspecified number of placenta and unspecified number of amniotic sacs**
     AHA: 2016, 2Q, 8
     O30.101   Triplet pregnancy, unspecified number of placenta and unspecified number of amniotic sacs, first trimester   Ⓜ♀▽
     O30.102   Triplet pregnancy, unspecified number of placenta and unspecified number of amniotic sacs, second trimester   Ⓜ♀▽
     O30.103   Triplet pregnancy, unspecified number of placenta and unspecified number of amniotic sacs, third trimester   Ⓜ♀▽
     O30.109   Triplet pregnancy, unspecified number of placenta and unspecified number of amniotic sacs, unspecified trimester   Ⓜ♀▽

   ✓6ᵗʰ **O30.11** **Triplet pregnancy with two or more monochorionic fetuses**
     O30.111   Triplet pregnancy with two or more monochorionic fetuses, first trimester   Ⓜ♀
     O30.112   Triplet pregnancy with two or more monochorionic fetuses, second trimester   Ⓜ♀
     O30.113   Triplet pregnancy with two or more monochorionic fetuses, third trimester   Ⓜ♀
     O30.119   Triplet pregnancy with two or more monochorionic fetuses, unspecified trimester   Ⓜ♀▽

   ✓6ᵗʰ **O30.12** **Triplet pregnancy with two or more monoamniotic fetuses**
     O30.121   Triplet pregnancy with two or more monoamniotic fetuses, first trimester   Ⓜ♀
     O30.122   Triplet pregnancy with two or more monoamniotic fetuses, second trimester   Ⓜ♀
     O30.123   Triplet pregnancy with two or more monoamniotic fetuses, third trimester   Ⓜ♀
     O30.129   Triplet pregnancy with two or more monoamniotic fetuses, unspecified trimester   Ⓜ♀▽

   ✓6ᵗʰ **O30.19** **Triplet pregnancy, unable to determine number of placenta and number of amniotic sacs**
     O30.191   Triplet pregnancy, unable to determine number of placenta and number of amniotic sacs, first trimester   Ⓜ♀
     O30.192   Triplet pregnancy, unable to determine number of placenta and number of amniotic sacs, second trimester   Ⓜ♀
     O30.193   Triplet pregnancy, unable to determine number of placenta and number of amniotic sacs, third trimester   Ⓜ♀
     O30.199   Triplet pregnancy, unable to determine number of placenta and number of amniotic sacs, unspecified trimester   Ⓜ♀▽

✓5ᵗʰ **O30.2** **Quadruplet pregnancy**
   ✓6ᵗʰ **O30.20** **Quadruplet pregnancy, unspecified number of placenta and unspecified number of amniotic sacs**
     O30.201   Quadruplet pregnancy, unspecified number of placenta and unspecified number of amniotic sacs, first trimester   Ⓜ♀▽
     O30.202   Quadruplet pregnancy, unspecified number of placenta and unspecified number of amniotic sacs, second trimester   Ⓜ♀▽

O30.203 Quadruplet pregnancy, unspecified Ⓜ♀▽
number of placenta and unspecified
number of amniotic sacs, third trimester

O30.209 Quadruplet pregnancy, unspecified Ⓜ♀▽
number of placenta and unspecified
number of amniotic sacs, unspecified
trimester

✓6ᵗʰ **O30.21** **Quadruplet pregnancy with two or more**
monochorionic fetuses

O30.211 Quadruplet pregnancy with two or Ⓜ♀
more monochorionic fetuses, first
trimester

O30.212 Quadruplet pregnancy with two or Ⓜ♀
more monochorionic fetuses, second
trimester

O30.213 Quadruplet pregnancy with two or Ⓜ♀
more monochorionic fetuses, third
trimester

O30.219 Quadruplet pregnancy with two or Ⓜ♀▽
more monochorionic fetuses,
unspecified trimester

✓6ᵗʰ **O30.22** **Quadruplet pregnancy with two or more**
monoamniotic fetuses

O30.221 Quadruplet pregnancy with two or Ⓜ♀
more monoamniotic fetuses, first
trimester

O30.222 Quadruplet pregnancy with two or Ⓜ♀
more monoamniotic fetuses, second
trimester

O30.223 Quadruplet pregnancy with two or Ⓜ♀
more monoamniotic fetuses, third
trimester

O30.229 Quadruplet pregnancy with two or Ⓜ♀▽
more monoamniotic fetuses,
unspecified trimester

✓6ᵗʰ **O30.29** **Quadruplet pregnancy, unable to determine number**
of placenta and number of amniotic sacs

O30.291 Quadruplet pregnancy, unable to Ⓜ♀
determine number of placenta and
number of amniotic sacs, first
trimester

O30.292 Quadruplet pregnancy, unable to Ⓜ♀
determine number of placenta and
number of amniotic sacs, second
trimester

O30.293 Quadruplet pregnancy, unable to Ⓜ♀
determine number of placenta and
number of amniotic sacs, third
trimester

O30.299 Quadruplet pregnancy, unable to Ⓜ♀▽
determine number of placenta and
number of amniotic sacs, unspecified

✓5ᵗʰ **O30.8** **Other specified multiple gestation**
Multiple gestation pregnancy greater than quadruplets

✓6ᵗʰ **O30.80** **Other specified multiple gestation, unspecified**
number of placenta and unspecified number of
amniotic sacs

O30.801 Other specified multiple gestation, Ⓜ♀▽
unspecified number of placenta and
unspecified number of amniotic sacs,
first trimester

O30.802 Other specified multiple gestation, Ⓜ♀▽
unspecified number of placenta and
unspecified number of amniotic sacs,
second trimester

O30.803 Other specified multiple gestation, Ⓜ♀▽
unspecified number of placenta and
unspecified number of amniotic sacs,
third trimester

O30.809 Other specified multiple Ⓜ♀▽
gestation, unspecified number of placenta
and unspecified number of amniotic sacs,
unspecified trimester

✓6ᵗʰ **O30.81** **Other specified multiple gestation with two or more**
monochorionic fetuses

O30.811 Other specified multiple gestation Ⓜ♀
with two or more monochorionic
fetuses, first trimester

O30.812 Other specified multiple gestation Ⓜ♀
with two or more monochorionic
fetuses, second trimester

O30.813 Other specified multiple gestation Ⓜ♀
with two or more monochorionic
fetuses, third trimester

O30.819 Other specified multiple gestation Ⓜ♀▽
with two or more monochorionic
fetuses, unspecified trimester

✓6ᵗʰ **O30.82** **Other specified multiple gestation with two or more**
monoamniotic fetuses

O30.821 Other specified multiple gestation Ⓜ♀
with two or more monoamniotic
fetuses, first trimester

O30.822 Other specified multiple gestation Ⓜ♀
with two or more monoamniotic
fetuses, second trimester

O30.823 Other specified multiple gestation Ⓜ♀
with two or more monoamniotic
fetuses, third trimester

O30.829 Other specified multiple gestation Ⓜ♀▽
with two or more monoamniotic
fetuses, unspecified trimester

✓6ᵗʰ **O30.89** **Other specified multiple gestation, unable to**
determine number of placenta and number of
amniotic sacs

O30.891 Other specified multiple gestation, Ⓜ♀
unable to determine number of
placenta and number of amniotic sacs,
first trimester

O30.892 Other specified multiple gestation, Ⓜ♀
unable to determine number of placenta
and number of amniotic sacs, second
trimester

O30.893 Other specified multiple gestation, Ⓜ♀
unable to determine number of placenta
and number of amniotic sacs, third
trimester

O30.899 Other specified multiple gestation, Ⓜ♀▽
unable to determine number of
placenta and number of amniotic
sacs, unspecified trimester

✓5ᵗʰ **O30.9** **Multiple gestation, unspecified**
Multiple pregnancy NOS

O30.90 Multiple gestation, unspecified, unspecified Ⓜ♀▽
trimester

O30.91 Multiple gestation, unspecified, first trimester Ⓜ♀▽

O30.92 Multiple gestation, unspecified, second Ⓜ♀▽
trimester

O30.93 Multiple gestation, unspecified, third Ⓜ♀▽
trimester

✓4ᵗʰ **O31** **Complications specific to multiple gestation**

EXCLUDES 2 *delayed delivery of second twin, triplet, etc. (O63.2)*
malpresentation of one fetus or more (O32.9)
placental transfusion syndromes (O43.0-)

AHA: 2012, 4Q, 107

One of the following 7th characters is to be assigned to each code
under category O31. 7th character Ø is for single gestations and
multiple gestations where the fetus is unspecified. 7th characters 1
through 9 are for cases of multiple gestations to identify the fetus for
which the code applies. The appropriate code from category O30,
Multiple gestation, must also be assigned when assigning a code
from category O31 that has a 7th character of 1 through 9.

Ø	not applicable or unspecified	4	fetus 4
1	fetus 1	5	fetus 5
2	fetus 2	9	other fetus
3	fetus 3		

✓5ᵗʰ **O31.0** **Papyraceous fetus**
Fetus compressus

✓x7ᵗʰ O31.00 Papyraceous fetus, unspecified trimester Ⓜ♀▽

✓x7ᵗʰ O31.01 Papyraceous fetus, first trimester Ⓜ♀

✓x7ᵗʰ O31.02 Papyraceous fetus, second trimester Ⓜ♀

✓x7ᵗʰ O31.03 Papyraceous fetus, third trimester Ⓜ♀

✓5ᵗʰ **O31.1** **Continuing pregnancy after spontaneous abortion of one**
fetus or more

✓x7ᵗʰ O31.10 Continuing pregnancy after spontaneous Ⓜ♀▽
abortion of one fetus or more, unspecified
trimester

✓x7ᵗʰ O31.11 Continuing pregnancy after spontaneous Ⓜ♀
abortion of one fetus or more, first trimester

✓ Additional Character Req   ✓x7ᵗʰ Placeholder Alert   Manifestation   ᴴᶜᶜ CMS-HCC Condition   ▽ Unspecified Code   ►◄ Revised Text   ● New Code   ▲ Revised Code Title

ICD-10-CM 2018   837

√x7th O31.12 Continuing pregnancy after spontaneous abortion of one fetus or more, second trimester   M♀

√x7th O31.13 Continuing pregnancy after spontaneous abortion of one fetus or more, third trimester   M♀

√5th O31.2 Continuing pregnancy after intrauterine death of one fetus or more

√x7th O31.20 Continuing pregnancy after intrauterine death of one fetus or more, unspecified trimester   M♀▽

√x7th O31.21 Continuing pregnancy after intrauterine death of one fetus or more, first trimester   M♀

√x7th O31.22 Continuing pregnancy after intrauterine death of one fetus or more, second trimester   M♀

√x7th O31.23 Continuing pregnancy after intrauterine death of one fetus or more, third trimester   M♀

√5th O31.3 Continuing pregnancy after elective fetal reduction of one fetus or more

Continuing pregnancy after selective termination of one fetus or more

√x7th O31.30 Continuing pregnancy after elective fetal reduction of one fetus or more, unspecified trimester   M♀▽

√x7th O31.31 Continuing pregnancy after elective fetal reduction of one fetus or more, first trimester   M♀

√x7th O31.32 Continuing pregnancy after elective fetal reduction of one fetus or more, second trimester   M♀

√x7th O31.33 Continuing pregnancy after elective fetal reduction of one fetus or more, third trimester   M♀

√5th O31.8 Other complications specific to multiple gestation

√6th O31.8X Other complications specific to multiple gestation

√7th O31.8X1 Other complications specific to multiple gestation, first trimester   M♀

√7th O31.8X2 Other complications specific to multiple gestation, second trimester   M♀

√7th O31.8X3 Other complications specific to multiple gestation, third trimester   M♀

√7th O31.8X9 Other complications specific to multiple gestation, unspecified trimester   M♀▽

√4th O32 Maternal care for malpresentation of fetus

INCLUDES the listed conditions as a reason for observation, hospitalization or other obstetric care of the mother, or for cesarean delivery before onset of labor

EXCLUDES 1 *malpresentation of fetus with obstructed labor (O64.-)*

AHA: 2012, 4Q, 107

> One of the following 7th characters is to be assigned to each code under category O32. 7th character 0 is for single gestations and multiple gestations where the fetus is unspecified. 7th characters 1 through 9 are for cases of multiple gestations to identify the fetus for which the code applies. The appropriate code from category O30, Multiple gestation, must also be assigned when assigning a code from category O32 that has a 7th character of 1 through 9.
> | 0 | not applicable or unspecified | 4 | fetus 4 |
> | 1 | fetus 1 | 5 | fetus 5 |
> | 2 | fetus 2 | 9 | other fetus |
> | 3 | fetus 3 | | |

Fetal Malpresentation

Breech

Shoulder (arm prolapse)

Mother's pelvis

Face (mentum)

Compound (extremity together with head)

Oblique

√x7th O32.0 Maternal care for unstable lie   M♀

√x7th O32.1 Maternal care for breech presentation   M♀
Maternal care for buttocks presentation
Maternal care for complete breech
Maternal care for frank breech
EXCLUDES 1 *footling presentation (O32.8)*
incomplete breech (O32.8)
DEF: Fetus presentation in a longitudinal lie with the buttocks or feet closest to birth canal; may require external cephalic version or cesarean delivery.

√x7th O32.2 Maternal care for transverse and oblique lie   M♀
Maternal care for oblique presentation
Maternal care for transverse presentation

√x7th O32.3 Maternal care for face, brow and chin presentation   M♀

√x7th O32.4 Maternal care for high head at term   M♀
Maternal care for failure of head to enter pelvic brim

√x7th O32.6 Maternal care for compound presentation   M♀

√x7th O32.8 Maternal care for other malpresentation of fetus   M♀
Maternal care for footling presentation
Maternal care for incomplete breech

√x7th O32.9 Maternal care for malpresentation of fetus, unspecified   M♀▽

√4th O33 Maternal care for disproportion

INCLUDES the listed conditions as a reason for observation, hospitalization or other obstetric care of the mother, or for cesarean delivery before onset of labor

EXCLUDES 1 *disproportion with obstructed labor (O65-O66)*

O33.0 Maternal care for disproportion due to deformity of maternal pelvic bones   M♀
Maternal care for disproportion due to pelvic deformity causing disproportion NOS

O33.1 Maternal care for disproportion due to generally contracted pelvis   M♀
Maternal care for disproportion due to contracted pelvis NOS causing disproportion

O33.2 Maternal care for disproportion due to inlet contraction of pelvis   M♀
Maternal care for disproportion due to inlet contraction (pelvis) causing disproportion

√x7th O33.3 Maternal care for disproportion due to outlet contraction of pelvis   M♀
Maternal care for disproportion due to mid-cavity contraction (pelvis)
Maternal care for disproportion due to outlet contraction (pelvis)

> One of the following 7th characters is to be assigned to code O33.3. 7th character 0 is for single gestations and multiple gestations where the fetus is unspecified. 7th characters 1 through 9 are for cases of multiple gestations to identify the fetus for which the code applies. The appropriate code from category O30, Multiple gestation, must also be assigned when assigning code O33.3 with a 7th character of 1 through 9.
> | 0 | not applicable or unspecified | 4 | fetus 4 |
> | 1 | fetus 1 | 5 | fetus 5 |
> | 2 | fetus 2 | 9 | other fetus |
> | 3 | fetus 3 | | |

√x7th O33.4 Maternal care for disproportion of mixed maternal and fetal origin   M♀

> One of the following 7th characters is to be assigned to code O33.4. 7th character 0 is for single gestations and multiple gestations where the fetus is unspecified. 7th characters 1 through 9 are for cases of multiple gestations to identify the fetus for which the code applies. The appropriate code from category O30, Multiple gestation, must also be assigned when assigning code O33.4 with a 7th character of 1 through 9.
> | 0 | not applicable or unspecified | 4 | fetus 4 |
> | 1 | fetus 1 | 5 | fetus 5 |
> | 2 | fetus 2 | 9 | other fetus |
> | 3 | fetus 3 | | |

EXCLUDES 1 Not coded here   EXCLUDES 2 Not included here   N Newborn Age: 0   P Pediatric Age: 0-17   M Maternity Age: 12-55   A Adult Age: 15-124

838   ICD-10-CM 2018

✓x7ᵗʰ **O33.5 Maternal care for disproportion due to unusually large** Ⓜ♀
fetus
Maternal care for disproportion due to disproportion of fetal
origin with normally formed fetus
Maternal care for disproportion due to fetal disproportion NOS

> One of the following 7th characters is to be assigned to code
> O33.5. 7th character Ø is for single gestations and multiple
> gestations where the fetus is unspecified. 7th characters 1
> through 9 are for cases of multiple gestations to identify the
> fetus for which the code applies. The appropriate code from
> category O30, Multiple gestation, must also be assigned when
> assigning code O33.5 with a 7th character of 1 through 9.
> | | | | |
> |---|---|---|---|
> | Ø | not applicable or unspecified | 4 | fetus 4 |
> | 1 | fetus 1 | 5 | fetus 5 |
> | 2 | fetus 2 | 9 | other fetus |
> | 3 | fetus 3 | | |

✓x7ᵗʰ **O33.6 Maternal care for disproportion due to hydrocephalic** Ⓜ♀
fetus

> One of the following 7th characters is to be assigned to code
> O33.6. 7th character Ø is for single gestations and multiple
> gestations where the fetus is unspecified. 7th characters 1
> through 9 are for cases of multiple gestations to identify the
> fetus for which the code applies. The appropriate code from
> category O30, Multiple gestation, must also be assigned when
> assigning code O33.6 with a 7th character of 1 through 9.
> | | | | |
> |---|---|---|---|
> | Ø | not applicable or unspecified | 4 | fetus 4 |
> | 1 | fetus 1 | 5 | fetus 5 |
> | 2 | fetus 2 | 9 | other fetus |
> | 3 | fetus 3 | | |

✓x7ᵗʰ **O33.7 Maternal care for disproportion due to other fetal** Ⓜ♀
deformities
Maternal care for disproportion due to fetal ascites
Maternal care for disproportion due to fetal hydrops
Maternal care for disproportion due to fetal meningomyelocele
Maternal care for disproportion due to fetal sacral teratoma
Maternal care for disproportion due to fetal tumor
EXCLUDES 1   *obstructed labor due to other fetal deformities (O66.3)*

> One of the following 7th characters is to be assigned to code
> O33.7. 7th character Ø is for single gestations and multiple
> gestations where the fetus is unspecified. 7th characters 1
> through 9 are for cases of multiple gestations to identify the
> fetus for which the code applies. The appropriate code from
> category O30, Multiple gestation, must also be assigned when
> assigning code O33.7 with a 7th character of 1 through 9.
> | | | | |
> |---|---|---|---|
> | Ø | not applicable or unspecified | 4 | fetus 4 |
> | 1 | fetus 1 | 5 | fetus 5 |
> | 2 | fetus 2 | 9 | other fetus |
> | 3 | fetus 3 | | |

O33.8 Maternal care for disproportion of other origin Ⓜ♀

O33.9 Maternal care for disproportion, unspecified Ⓜ♀▽
Maternal care for disproportion due to cephalopelvic
disproportion NOS
Maternal care for disproportion due to fetopelvic disproportion
NOS

✓4ᵗʰ **O34 Maternal care for abnormality of pelvic organs**
INCLUDES   the listed conditions as a reason for hospitalization or other
obstetric care of the mother, or for cesarean delivery
before onset of labor
Code first any associated obstructed labor (O65.5)
Use additional code for specific condition

✓5ᵗʰ **O34.0 Maternal care for congenital malformation of uterus**
Maternal care for double uterus
Maternal care for uterus bicornis

O34.00 Maternal care for unspecified congenital Ⓜ♀▽
malformation of uterus, unspecified trimester

O34.01 Maternal care for unspecified congenital Ⓜ♀▽
malformation of uterus, first trimester

O34.02 Maternal care for unspecified congenital Ⓜ♀▽
malformation of uterus, second trimester

O34.03 Maternal care for unspecified congenital Ⓜ♀▽
malformation of uterus, third trimester

✓5ᵗʰ **O34.1 Maternal care for benign tumor of corpus uteri**
EXCLUDES 2   *maternal care for benign tumor of cervix (O34.4-)*
maternal care for malignant neoplasm of uterus
(O9A.1-)

O34.10 Maternal care for benign tumor of corpus Ⓜ♀▽
uteri, unspecified trimester

O34.11 Maternal care for benign tumor of corpus uteri, Ⓜ♀
first trimester

O34.12 Maternal care for benign tumor of corpus uteri, Ⓜ♀
second trimester

O34.13 Maternal care for benign tumor of corpus uteri, Ⓜ♀
third trimester

✓5ᵗʰ **O34.2 Maternal care due to uterine scar from previous surgery**

✓6ᵗʰ **O34.21 Maternal care for scar from previous cesarean**
delivery

O34.211 Maternal care for low transverse scar Ⓜ♀
from previous cesarean delivery

O34.212 Maternal care for vertical scar from Ⓜ♀
previous cesarean delivery
Maternal care for classical scar from
previous cesarean delivery

O34.219 Maternal care for unspecified type Ⓜ♀▽
scar from previous cesarean delivery
Maternal care due to uterine scar from
other transmural uterine incision

O34.29 Maternal care due to uterine scar from other Ⓜ♀
previous surgery
Maternal care due to uterine scar from other
transmural uterine incision

✓5ᵗʰ **O34.3 Maternal care for cervical incompetence**
Maternal care for cerclage with or without cervical
incompetence
Maternal care for Shirodkar suture with or without cervical
incompetence
DEF: Inadequate functioning of cervix marked by abnormal
widening during pregnancy and causing premature birth or
miscarriage.

O34.30 Maternal care for cervical incompetence, Ⓜ♀▽
unspecified trimester

O34.31 Maternal care for cervical incompetence, first Ⓜ♀
trimester

O34.32 Maternal care for cervical incompetence, second Ⓜ♀
trimester

O34.33 Maternal care for cervical incompetence, third Ⓜ♀
trimester

✓5ᵗʰ **O34.4 Maternal care for other abnormalities of cervix**

O34.40 Maternal care for other abnormalities of Ⓜ♀▽
cervix, unspecified trimester

O34.41 Maternal care for other abnormalities of cervix, Ⓜ♀
first trimester

O34.42 Maternal care for other abnormalities of cervix, Ⓜ♀
second trimester

O34.43 Maternal care for other abnormalities of cervix, Ⓜ♀
third trimester

✓5ᵗʰ **O34.5 Maternal care for other abnormalities of gravid uterus**

✓6ᵗʰ **O34.51 Maternal care for incarceration of gravid uterus**

O34.511 Maternal care for incarceration of Ⓜ♀
gravid uterus, first trimester

O34.512 Maternal care for incarceration of Ⓜ♀
gravid uterus, second trimester

O34.513 Maternal care for incarceration of Ⓜ♀
gravid uterus, third trimester

O34.519 Maternal care for incarceration of Ⓜ♀▽
gravid uterus, unspecified trimester

✓6ᵗʰ **O34.52 Maternal care for prolapse of gravid uterus**

O34.521 Maternal care for prolapse of gravid Ⓜ♀
uterus, first trimester

O34.522 Maternal care for prolapse of gravid Ⓜ♀
uterus, second trimester

O34.523 Maternal care for prolapse of gravid Ⓜ♀
uterus, third trimester

O34.529 Maternal care for prolapse of gravid Ⓜ♀▽
uterus, unspecified trimester

✓6ᵗʰ **O34.53 Maternal care for retroversion of gravid uterus**

O34.531 Maternal care for retroversion of Ⓜ♀
gravid uterus, first trimester

O34.532 Maternal care for retroversion of Ⓜ♀
gravid uterus, second trimester

O34.533 Maternal care for retroversion of Ⓜ♀
gravid uterus, third trimester

O34.539 Maternal care for retroversion of Ⓜ♀▽
gravid uterus, unspecified trimester

✓6ᵗʰ **O34.59 Maternal care for other abnormalities of gravid**
uterus

O34.591 Maternal care for other abnormalities Ⓜ♀
of gravid uterus, first trimester

☑ Additional Character Req   ✓x7ᵗʰ Placeholder Alert   Manifestation   HCC CMS-HCC Condition   ▽ Unspecified Code   ►◄ Revised Text   ● New Code   ▲ Revised Code Title

ICD-10-CM 2018   839

Chapter 15. Pregnancy, Childbirth, and the Puerperium

O34.592–O36.113

O34.592   **Maternal care for other abnormalities** Ⓜ♀
     of gravid uterus, second trimester

O34.593   **Maternal care for other abnormalities** Ⓜ♀
     of gravid uterus, third trimester

O34.599   **Maternal care for other** Ⓜ♀▽
     abnormalities of gravid uterus,
     unspecified trimester

✓5th **O34.6   Maternal care for abnormality of vagina**

     EXCLUDES 2   *maternal care for vaginal varices in pregnancy (O22.1-)*

O34.60   **Maternal care for abnormality of vagina,** Ⓜ♀▽
     unspecified trimester

O34.61   **Maternal care for abnormality of vagina, first** Ⓜ♀
     trimester

O34.62   **Maternal care for abnormality of vagina, second** Ⓜ♀
     trimester

O34.63   **Maternal care for abnormality of vagina, third** Ⓜ♀
     trimester

✓5th **O34.7   Maternal care for abnormality of vulva and perineum**

     EXCLUDES 2   *maternal care for perineal and vulval varices in pregnancy (O22.1-)*

O34.70   **Maternal care for abnormality of vulva and** Ⓜ♀▽
     perineum, unspecified trimester

O34.71   **Maternal care for abnormality of vulva and** Ⓜ♀
     perineum, first trimester

O34.72   **Maternal care for abnormality of vulva and** Ⓜ♀
     perineum, second trimester

O34.73   **Maternal care for abnormality of vulva and** Ⓜ♀
     perineum, third trimester

✓5th **O34.8   Maternal care for other abnormalities of pelvic organs**

O34.80   **Maternal care for other abnormalities of** Ⓜ♀▽
     pelvic organs, unspecified trimester

O34.81   **Maternal care for other abnormalities of pelvic** Ⓜ♀
     organs, first trimester

O34.82   **Maternal care for other abnormalities of pelvic** Ⓜ♀
     organs, second trimester

O34.83   **Maternal care for other abnormalities of pelvic** Ⓜ♀
     organs, third trimester

✓5th **O34.9   Maternal care for abnormality of pelvic organ, unspecified**

O34.90   **Maternal care for abnormality of pelvic** Ⓜ♀▽
     organ,unspecified, unspecified trimester

O34.91   **Maternal care for abnormality of pelvic** Ⓜ♀▽
     organ, unspecified, first trimester

O34.92   **Maternal care for abnormality of pelvic** Ⓜ♀▽
     organ, unspecified, second trimester

O34.93   **Maternal care for abnormality of pelvic** Ⓜ♀▽
     organ, unspecified, third trimester

✓4th **O35   Maternal care for known or suspected fetal abnormality and damage**

     INCLUDES   the listed conditions in the fetus as a reason for hospitalization or other obstetric care to the mother, or for termination of pregnancy

     Code also any associated maternal condition

     EXCLUDES 1   *encounter for suspected maternal and fetal conditions ruled out (Z03.7-)*

One of the following 7th characters is to be assigned to each code under category O35. 7th character Ø is for single gestations and multiple gestations where the fetus is unspecified. 7th characters 1 through 9 are for cases of multiple gestations to identify the fetus for which the code applies. The appropriate code from category O30, Multiple gestation, must also be assigned when assigning a code from category O35 that has a 7th character of 1 through 9.

Ø	not applicable or unspecified	4	fetus 4
1	fetus 1	5	fetus 5
2	fetus 2	9	other fetus
3	fetus 3		

✓x7th **O35.0   Maternal care for (suspected) central nervous system** Ⓜ♀
     malformation in fetus

     Maternal care for fetal anencephaly
     Maternal care for fetal hydrocephalus
     Maternal care for fetal spina bifida

     EXCLUDES 2   *chromosomal abnormality in fetus (O35.1)*

✓x7th **O35.1   Maternal care for (suspected) chromosomal abnormality** Ⓜ♀
     in fetus

✓x7th **O35.2   Maternal care for (suspected) hereditary disease in fetus** Ⓜ♀

     EXCLUDES 2   *chromosomal abnormality in fetus (O35.1)*

✓x7th **O35.3   Maternal care for (suspected) damage to fetus from viral** Ⓜ♀
     disease in mother

     Maternal care for damage to fetus from maternal cytomegalovirus infection
     Maternal care for damage to fetus from maternal rubella

✓x7th **O35.4   Maternal care for (suspected) damage to fetus from** Ⓜ♀
     alcohol

✓x7th **O35.5   Maternal care for (suspected) damage to fetus by drugs** Ⓜ♀

     Maternal care for damage to fetus from drug addiction

✓x7th **O35.6   Maternal care for (suspected) damage to fetus by** Ⓜ♀
     radiation

✓x7th **O35.7   Maternal care for (suspected) damage to fetus by other** Ⓜ♀
     medical procedures

     Maternal care for damage to fetus by amniocentesis
     Maternal care for damage to fetus by biopsy procedures
     Maternal care for damage to fetus by hematological investigation
     Maternal care for damage to fetus by intrauterine contraceptive device
     Maternal care for damage to fetus by intrauterine surgery

✓x7th **O35.8   Maternal care for other (suspected) fetal abnormality** Ⓜ♀
     and damage

     Maternal care for damage to fetus from maternal listeriosis
     Maternal care for damage to fetus from maternal toxoplasmosis

✓x7th **O35.9   Maternal care for (suspected) fetal abnormality and** Ⓜ♀▽
     damage, unspecified

✓4th **O36   Maternal care for other fetal problems**

     INCLUDES   the listed conditions in the fetus as a reason for hospitalization or other obstetric care of the mother, or for termination of pregnancy

     EXCLUDES 1   *encounter for suspected maternal and fetal conditions ruled out (Z03.7-)*
                  placental transfusion syndromes (O43.0-)

     EXCLUDES 2   *labor and delivery complicated by fetal stress (O77.-)*

     AHA: 2015, 3Q, 40

One of the following 7th characters is to be assigned to each code under category O36. 7th character Ø is for single gestations and multiple gestations where the fetus is unspecified. 7th characters 1 through 9 are for cases of multiple gestations to identify the fetus for which the code applies. The appropriate code from category O30, Multiple gestation, must also be assigned when assigning a code from category O36 that has a 7th character of 1 through 9.

Ø	not applicable or unspecified	4	fetus 4
1	fetus 1	5	fetus 5
2	fetus 2	9	other fetus
3	fetus 3		

✓5th **O36.0   Maternal care for rhesus isoimmunization**

     Maternal care for Rh incompatibility (with hydrops fetalis)

✓6th **O36.01   Maternal care for anti-D [Rh] antibodies**

     AHA: 2014, 4Q, 17

     ✓7th **O36.011   Maternal care for anti-D [Rh]** Ⓜ♀
            antibodies, first trimester

     ✓7th **O36.012   Maternal care for anti-D [Rh]** Ⓜ♀
            antibodies, second trimester

     ✓7th **O36.013   Maternal care for anti-D [Rh]** Ⓜ♀
            antibodies, third trimester

     ✓7th **O36.019   Maternal care for anti-D [Rh]** Ⓜ♀▽
            antibodies, unspecified trimester

✓6th **O36.09   Maternal care for other rhesus isoimmunization**

     ✓7th **O36.091   Maternal care for other rhesus** Ⓜ♀
            isoimmunization, first trimester

     ✓7th **O36.092   Maternal care for other rhesus** Ⓜ♀
            isoimmunization, second trimester

     ✓7th **O36.093   Maternal care for other rhesus** Ⓜ♀
            isoimmunization, third trimester

     ✓7th **O36.099   Maternal care for other rhesus** Ⓜ♀▽
            isoimmunization, unspecified trimester

✓5th **O36.1   Maternal care for other isoimmunization**

     Maternal care for ABO isoimmunization

✓6th **O36.11   Maternal care for Anti-A sensitization**

     Maternal care for isoimmunization NOS (with hydrops fetalis)

     ✓7th **O36.111   Maternal care for Anti-A sensitization,** Ⓜ♀
            first trimester

     ✓7th **O36.112   Maternal care for Anti-A sensitization,** Ⓜ♀
            second trimester

     ✓7th **O36.113   Maternal care for Anti-A sensitization,** Ⓜ♀
            third trimester

| EXCLUDES 1 Not coded here | EXCLUDES 2 Not included here | Ⓝ Newborn Age: 0 | Ⓟ Pediatric Age: 0-17 | Ⓜ Maternity Age: 12-55 | Ⓐ Adult Age: 15-124 |

840   ICD-10-CM 2018

√7ᵗʰ **O36.119 Maternal care for Anti-A** Ⓜ♀▽
         sensitization, unspecified trimester

√6ᵗʰ **O36.19 Maternal care for other isoimmunization**
         Maternal care for Anti-B sensitization

     √7ᵗʰ **O36.191 Maternal care for other** Ⓜ♀
            isoimmunization, first trimester

     √7ᵗʰ **O36.192 Maternal care for other** Ⓜ♀
            isoimmunization, second trimester

     √7ᵗʰ **O36.193 Maternal care for other** Ⓜ♀
            isoimmunization, third trimester

     √7ᵗʰ **O36.199 Maternal care for other** Ⓜ♀▽
            isoimmunization, unspecified trimester

√5ᵗʰ **O36.2 Maternal care for hydrops fetalis**
     Maternal care for hydrops fetalis NOS
     Maternal care for hydrops fetalis not associated with
       isoimmunization
     EXCLUDES 1   hydrops fetalis associated with ABO isoimmunization
            (O36.1-)
            hydrops fetalis associated with rhesus
               isoimmunization (O36.0-)

     √x7ᵗʰ **O36.20 Maternal care for hydrops fetalis, unspecified** Ⓜ♀▽
            trimester

     √x7ᵗʰ **O36.21 Maternal care for hydrops fetalis, first** Ⓜ♀
            trimester

     √x7ᵗʰ **O36.22 Maternal care for hydrops fetalis, second** Ⓜ♀
            trimester

     √x7ᵗʰ **O36.23 Maternal care for hydrops fetalis, third** Ⓜ♀
            trimester

√x7ᵗʰ **O36.4 Maternal care for intrauterine death** Ⓜ♀
     Maternal care for intrauterine fetal death NOS
     Maternal care for intrauterine fetal death after completion of 20
       weeks of gestation
     Maternal care for late fetal death
     Maternal care for missed delivery
     EXCLUDES 1   missed abortion (O02.1)
            stillbirth (P95)

√5ᵗʰ **O36.5 Maternal care for known or suspected poor fetal growth**

     √6ᵗʰ **O36.51 Maternal care for known or suspected placental**
            insufficiency

         √7ᵗʰ **O36.511 Maternal care for known or suspected** Ⓜ♀
                placental insufficiency, first trimester

         √7ᵗʰ **O36.512 Maternal care for known or suspected** Ⓜ♀
                placental insufficiency, second trimester

         √7ᵗʰ **O36.513 Maternal care for known or suspected** Ⓜ♀
                placental insufficiency, third trimester

         √7ᵗʰ **O36.519 Maternal care for known or** Ⓜ♀▽
                suspected placental insufficiency,
                unspecified trimester

     √6ᵗʰ **O36.59 Maternal care for other known or suspected poor**
            fetal growth
         Maternal care for known or suspected light-for-dates
            NOS
         Maternal care for known or suspected small-for-dates
            NOS

         √7ᵗʰ **O36.591 Maternal care for other known or** Ⓜ♀
                suspected poor fetal growth, first
                trimester

         √7ᵗʰ **O36.592 Maternal care for other known or** Ⓜ♀
                suspected poor fetal growth, second
                trimester

         √7ᵗʰ **O36.593 Maternal care for other known or** Ⓜ♀
                suspected poor fetal growth, third
                trimester

         √7ᵗʰ **O36.599 Maternal care for other known or** Ⓜ♀▽
                suspected poor fetal growth,
                unspecified trimester

√5ᵗʰ **O36.6 Maternal care for excessive fetal growth**
     Maternal care for known or suspected large-for-dates

     √x7ᵗʰ **O36.60 Maternal care for excessive fetal growth,** Ⓜ♀▽
            unspecified trimester

     √x7ᵗʰ **O36.61 Maternal care for excessive fetal growth,** Ⓜ♀
            first trimester

     √x7ᵗʰ **O36.62 Maternal care for excessive fetal growth,** Ⓜ♀
            second trimester

     √x7ᵗʰ **O36.63 Maternal care for excessive fetal growth,** Ⓜ♀
            third trimester

√5ᵗʰ **O36.7 Maternal care for viable fetus in abdominal pregnancy**

     √x7ᵗʰ **O36.70 Maternal care for viable fetus in abdominal** Ⓜ♀▽
            pregnancy, unspecified trimester

     √x7ᵗʰ **O36.71 Maternal care for viable fetus in abdominal** Ⓜ♀
            pregnancy, first trimester

     √x7ᵗʰ **O36.72 Maternal care for viable fetus in abdominal** Ⓜ♀
            pregnancy, second trimester

     √x7ᵗʰ **O36.73 Maternal care for viable fetus in abdominal** Ⓜ♀
            pregnancy, third trimester

√5ᵗʰ **O36.8 Maternal care for other specified fetal problems**

     √x7ᵗʰ **O36.80 Pregnancy with inconclusive fetal viability** Ⓜ♀
         Encounter to determine fetal viability of pregnancy

     √6ᵗʰ **O36.81 Decreased fetal movements**

         √7ᵗʰ **O36.812 Decreased fetal movements, second** Ⓜ♀
                trimester

         √7ᵗʰ **O36.813 Decreased fetal movements, third** Ⓜ♀
                trimester

         √7ᵗʰ **O36.819 Decreased fetal movements,** Ⓜ♀
                unspecified trimester

     √6ᵗʰ **O36.82 Fetal anemia and thrombocytopenia**

         √7ᵗʰ **O36.821 Fetal anemia and thrombocytopenia,** Ⓜ♀
                first trimester

         √7ᵗʰ **O36.822 Fetal anemia and thrombocytopenia,** Ⓜ♀
                second trimester

         √7ᵗʰ **O36.823 Fetal anemia and thrombocytopenia,** Ⓜ♀
                third trimester

         √7ᵗʰ **O36.829 Fetal anemia and** Ⓜ♀
                thrombocytopenia, unspecified trimester

●   √6ᵗʰ **O36.83 Maternal care for abnormalities of the fetal heart**
            rate or rhythm

●   √7ᵗʰ **O36.831 Maternal care for abnormalities of the**
                fetal heart rate or rhythm, first trimester

●   √7ᵗʰ **O36.832 Maternal care for abnormalities of the**
                fetal heart rate or rhythm, second
                trimester

●   √7ᵗʰ **O36.833 Maternal care for abnormalities of the**
                fetal heart rate or rhythm, third trimester

●   √7ᵗʰ **O36.839 Maternal care for abnormalities of the** ▽
                fetal heart rate or rhythm, unspecified
                trimester

     √6ᵗʰ **O36.89 Maternal care for other specified fetal problems**

         √7ᵗʰ **O36.891 Maternal care for other specified fetal** Ⓜ♀
                problems, first trimester

         √7ᵗʰ **O36.892 Maternal care for other specified fetal** Ⓜ♀
                problems, second trimester

         √7ᵗʰ **O36.893 Maternal care for other specified fetal** Ⓜ♀
                problems, third trimester

         √7ᵗʰ **O36.899 Maternal care for other specified** Ⓜ♀▽
                fetal problems, unspecified trimester

√5ᵗʰ **O36.9 Maternal care for fetal problem, unspecified**

     √x7ᵗʰ **O36.90 Maternal care for fetal problem, unspecified,** Ⓜ♀▽
            unspecified trimester

     √x7ᵗʰ **O36.91 Maternal care for fetal problem, unspecified,** Ⓜ♀▽
            first trimester

     √x7ᵗʰ **O36.92 Maternal care for fetal problem, unspecified,** Ⓜ♀▽
            second trimester

     √x7ᵗʰ **O36.93 Maternal care for fetal problem, unspecified,** Ⓜ♀▽
            third trimester

√4ᵗʰ **O40 Polyhydramnios**
     Hydramnios
     EXCLUDES 1   encounter for suspected maternal and fetal conditions ruled out
            (Z03.7-)
     AHA: 2016, 1Q, 4

> One of the following 7th characters is to be assigned to each code
> under category O40. 7th character 0 is for single gestations and
> multiple gestations where the fetus is unspecified. 7th characters 1
> through 9 are for cases of multiple gestations to identify the fetus
> for which the code applies. The appropriate code from category
> O30, Multiple gestation, must also be assigned when assigning a
> code from category O40 that has a 7th character of 1 through 9.
> 0   not applicable or unspecified   4   fetus 4
> 1   fetus 1   5   fetus 5
> 2   fetus 2   9   other fetus
> 3   fetus 3

√x7ᵗʰ **O40.1 Polyhydramnios, first trimester** Ⓜ♀

☑ Additional Character Req   √x7ᵗʰ Placeholder Alert   Manifestation   ᴴᶜᶜ CMS-HCC Condition   ▽ Unspecified Code   ▶◀ Revised Text   ● New Code   ▲ Revised Code Title

ICD-10-CM 2018   841

√x7ᵗʰ **O40.2** **Polyhydramnios, second trimester** Ⓜ♀

√x7ᵗʰ **O40.3** **Polyhydramnios, third trimester** Ⓜ♀

√x7ᵗʰ **O40.9** **Polyhydramnios, unspecified trimester** Ⓜ♀▽

√4ᵗʰ **O41** **Other disorders of amniotic fluid and membranes**

    EXCLUDES 1   encounter for suspected maternal and fetal conditions ruled out (Z03.7-)

One of the following 7th characters is to be assigned to each code under category O41. 7th character Ø is for single gestations and multiple gestations where the fetus is unspecified. 7th characters 1 through 9 are for cases of multiple gestations to identify the fetus for which the code applies. The appropriate code from category O30, Multiple gestation, must also be assigned when assigning a code from category O41 that has a 7th character of 1 through 9.

Ø	not applicable or unspecified	4	fetus 4
1	fetus 1	5	fetus 5
2	fetus 2	9	other fetus
3	fetus 3		

√5ᵗʰ **O41.0** **Oligohydramnios**

    Oligohydramnios without rupture of membranes

√x7ᵗʰ **O41.00** **Oligohydramnios, unspecified trimester** Ⓜ♀▽

√x7ᵗʰ **O41.01** **Oligohydramnios, first trimester** Ⓜ♀

√x7ᵗʰ **O41.02** **Oligohydramnios, second trimester** Ⓜ♀

√x7ᵗʰ **O41.03** **Oligohydramnios, third trimester** Ⓜ♀

√5ᵗʰ **O41.1** **Infection of amniotic sac and membranes**

√6ᵗʰ **O41.10** **Infection of amniotic sac and membranes, unspecified**

√7ᵗʰ **O41.101** **Infection of amniotic sac and membranes, unspecified, first trimester** Ⓜ♀▽

√7ᵗʰ **O41.102** **Infection of amniotic sac and membranes, unspecified, second trimester** Ⓜ♀▽

√7ᵗʰ **O41.103** **Infection of amniotic sac and membranes, unspecified, third trimester** Ⓜ♀▽

√7ᵗʰ **O41.109** **Infection of amniotic sac and membranes, unspecified, unspecified trimester** Ⓜ♀▽

√6ᵗʰ **O41.12** **Chorioamnionitis**

√7ᵗʰ **O41.121** **Chorioamnionitis, first trimester** Ⓜ♀

√7ᵗʰ **O41.122** **Chorioamnionitis, second trimester** Ⓜ♀

√7ᵗʰ **O41.123** **Chorioamnionitis, third trimester** Ⓜ♀

√7ᵗʰ **O41.129** **Chorioamnionitis, unspecified trimester** Ⓜ♀▽

√6ᵗʰ **O41.14** **Placentitis**

√7ᵗʰ **O41.141** **Placentitis, first trimester** Ⓜ♀

√7ᵗʰ **O41.142** **Placentitis, second trimester** Ⓜ♀

√7ᵗʰ **O41.143** **Placentitis, third trimester** Ⓜ♀

√7ᵗʰ **O41.149** **Placentitis, unspecified trimester** Ⓜ♀▽

√5ᵗʰ **O41.8** **Other specified disorders of amniotic fluid and membranes**

√6ᵗʰ **O41.8X** **Other specified disorders of amniotic fluid and membranes**

√7ᵗʰ **O41.8X1** **Other specified disorders of amniotic fluid and membranes, first trimester** Ⓜ♀

√7ᵗʰ **O41.8X2** **Other specified disorders of amniotic fluid and membranes, second trimester** Ⓜ♀

√7ᵗʰ **O41.8X3** **Other specified disorders of amniotic fluid and membranes, third trimester** Ⓜ♀

√7ᵗʰ **O41.8X9** **Other specified disorders of amniotic fluid and membranes, unspecified trimester** Ⓜ♀▽

√5ᵗʰ **O41.9** **Disorder of amniotic fluid and membranes, unspecified**

√x7ᵗʰ **O41.90** **Disorder of amniotic fluid and membranes, unspecified, unspecified trimester** Ⓜ♀▽

√x7ᵗʰ **O41.91** **Disorder of amniotic fluid and membranes, unspecified, first trimester** Ⓜ♀▽

√x7ᵗʰ **O41.92** **Disorder of amniotic fluid and membranes, unspecified, second trimester** Ⓜ♀▽

√x7ᵗʰ **O41.93** **Disorder of amniotic fluid and membranes, unspecified, third trimester** Ⓜ♀▽

√4ᵗʰ **O42** **Premature rupture of membranes**

    AHA: 2016, 1Q, 3

√5ᵗʰ **O42.0** **Premature rupture of membranes, onset of labor within 24 hours of rupture**

O42.00 **Premature rupture of membranes, onset of labor within 24 hours of rupture, unspecified weeks of gestation** Ⓜ♀▽

√6ᵗʰ **O42.01** **Preterm premature rupture of membranes, onset of labor within 24 hours of rupture**

    Premature rupture of membranes before 37 completed weeks of gestation

O42.011 **Preterm premature rupture of membranes, onset of labor within 24 hours of rupture, first trimester** Ⓜ♀

O42.012 **Preterm premature rupture of membranes, onset of labor within 24 hours of rupture, second trimester** Ⓜ♀

O42.013 **Preterm premature rupture of membranes, onset of labor within 24 hours of rupture, third trimester** Ⓜ♀

O42.019 **Preterm premature rupture of membranes, onset of labor within 24 hours of rupture, unspecified trimester** Ⓜ♀▽

O42.02 **Full-term premature rupture of membranes, onset of labor within 24 hours of rupture** Ⓜ♀

    Premature rupture of membranes at or after 37 completed weeks of gestation, onset of labor within 24 hours of rupture

√5ᵗʰ **O42.1** **Premature rupture of membranes, onset of labor more than 24 hours following rupture**

    AHA: 2016, 1Q, 5

O42.10 **Premature rupture of membranes, onset of labor more than 24 hours following rupture, unspecified weeks of gestation** Ⓜ♀▽

√6ᵗʰ **O42.11** **Preterm premature rupture of membranes, onset of labor more than 24 hours following rupture**

    Premature rupture of membranes before 37 completed weeks of gestation

O42.111 **Preterm premature rupture of membranes, onset of labor more than 24 hours following rupture, first trimester** Ⓜ♀

O42.112 **Preterm premature rupture of membranes, onset of labor more than 24 hours following rupture, second trimester** Ⓜ♀

O42.113 **Preterm premature rupture of membranes, onset of labor more than 24 hours following rupture, third trimester** Ⓜ♀

O42.119 **Preterm premature rupture of membranes, onset of labor more than 24 hours following rupture, unspecified trimester** Ⓜ♀▽

O42.12 **Full-term premature rupture of membranes, onset of labor more than 24 hours following rupture** Ⓜ♀

    Premature rupture of membranes at or after 37 completed weeks of gestation, onset of labor within 24 hours of rupture

√5ᵗʰ **O42.9** **Premature rupture of membranes, unspecified as to length of time between rupture and onset of labor**

O42.90 **Premature rupture of membranes, unspecified as to length of time between rupture and onset of labor, unspecified weeks of gestation** Ⓜ♀▽

√6ᵗʰ **O42.91** **Preterm premature rupture of membranes, unspecified as to length of time between rupture and onset of labor**

    Premature rupture of membranes before 37 completed weeks of gestation

O42.911 **Preterm premature rupture of membranes, unspecified as to length of time between rupture and onset of labor, first trimester** Ⓜ♀▽

O42.912 **Preterm premature rupture of membranes, unspecified as to length of time between rupture and onset of labor, second trimester** Ⓜ♀

O42.913 **Preterm premature rupture of membranes, unspecified as to length of time between rupture and onset of labor, third trimester** Ⓜ♀▽

| EXCLUDES 1 Not coded here | EXCLUDES 2 Not included here | N Newborn Age: 0 | P Pediatric Age: 0-17 | M Maternity Age: 12-55 | A Adult Age: 15-124 |

842   ICD-10-CM 2018

Twin to Twin Transfusion Syndrome (TTTS)

Healthy twins   Twins with TTTS

O42.919 Preterm premature rupture of membranes, unspecified as to length of time between rupture and onset of labor, unspecified trimester M♀▽

O42.92 Full-term premature rupture of membranes, unspecified as to length of time between rupture and onset of labor M♀▽
Premature rupture of membranes at or after 37 completed weeks of gestation, unspecified as to length of time between rupture and onset of labor

O43 Placental disorders ✓4th
EXCLUDES 2   maternal care for poor fetal growth due to placental insufficiency (O36.5-)
placenta previa (O44.-)
placental polyp (O90.89)
placentitis (O41.14-)
premature separation of placenta [abruptio placentae] (O45.-)

✓5th **O43.0 Placental transfusion syndromes**

✓6th **O43.01 Fetomaternal placental transfusion syndrome**
Maternofetal placental transfusion syndrome

O43.011 Fetomaternal placental transfusion syndrome, first trimester M♀

O43.012 Fetomaternal placental transfusion syndrome, second trimester M♀

O43.013 Fetomaternal placental transfusion syndrome, third trimester M♀

O43.019 Fetomaternal placental transfusion syndrome, unspecified trimester M♀▽

✓6th **O43.02 Fetus-to-fetus placental transfusion syndrome**

O43.021 Fetus-to-fetus placental transfusion syndrome, first trimester M♀

O43.022 Fetus-to-fetus placental transfusion syndrome, second trimester M♀

O43.023 Fetus-to-fetus placental transfusion syndrome, third trimester M♀

O43.029 Fetus-to-fetus placental transfusion syndrome, unspecified trimester M♀▽

✓5th **O43.1 Malformation of placenta**

✓6th **O43.10 Malformation of placenta, unspecified**
Abnormal placenta NOS

O43.101 Malformation of placenta, unspecified, first trimester M♀▽

O43.102 Malformation of placenta, unspecified, second trimester M♀ ▽

O43.103 Malformation of placenta, unspecified, third trimester M♀▽

O43.109 Malformation of placenta, unspecified, unspecified trimester M♀▽

✓6th **O43.11 Circumvallate placenta**

O43.111 Circumvallate placenta, first trimester M♀

O43.112 Circumvallate placenta, second trimester M♀

O43.113 Circumvallate placenta, third trimester M♀

O43.119 Circumvallate placenta, unspecified trimester M♀▽

✓6th **O43.12 Velamentous insertion of umbilical cord** M♀

O43.121 Velamentous insertion of umbilical cord, first trimester M♀

O43.122 Velamentous insertion of umbilical cord, second trimester M♀

O43.123 Velamentous insertion of umbilical cord, third trimester M♀

O43.129 Velamentous insertion of umbilical cord, unspecified trimester M♀▽

✓6th **O43.19 Other malformation of placenta**

O43.191 Other malformation of placenta, first trimester M♀

O43.192 Other malformation of placenta, second trimester M♀

O43.193 Other malformation of placenta, third trimester M♀

O43.199 Other malformation of placenta, unspecified trimester M♀▽

✓5th **O43.2 Morbidly adherent placenta**
Code also associated third stage postpartum hemorrhage, if applicable (O72.0)
EXCLUDES 1   retained placenta (O73.-)

✓6th **O43.21 Placenta accreta**

O43.211 Placenta accreta, first trimester M♀

O43.212 Placenta accreta, second trimester M♀

O43.213 Placenta accreta, third trimester M♀

O43.219 Placenta accreta, unspecified trimester M♀▽

✓6th **O43.22 Placenta increta**

O43.221 Placenta increta, first trimester M♀

O43.222 Placenta increta, second trimester M♀

O43.223 Placenta increta, third trimester M♀

O43.229 Placenta increta, unspecified trimester M♀▽

✓6th **O43.23 Placenta percreta**

O43.231 Placenta percreta, first trimester M♀

O43.232 Placenta percreta, second trimester M♀

O43.233 Placenta percreta, third trimester M♀

O43.239 Placenta percreta, unspecified trimester M♀▽

✓5th **O43.8 Other placental disorders**

✓6th **O43.81 Placental infarction**

O43.811 Placental infarction, first trimester M♀

O43.812 Placental infarction, second trimester M♀

O43.813 Placental infarction, third trimester M♀

O43.819 Placental infarction, unspecified trimester M♀▽

✓6th **O43.89 Other placental disorders**
Placental dysfunction

O43.891 Other placental disorders, first trimester M♀

O43.892 Other placental disorders, second trimester M♀

O43.893 Other placental disorders, third trimester M♀

O43.899 Other placental disorders, unspecified trimester M♀▽

✓5th **O43.9 Unspecified placental disorder**

O43.90 Unspecified placental disorder, unspecified trimester M♀▽

O43.91 Unspecified placental disorder, first trimester M♀▽

O43.92 Unspecified placental disorder, second trimester M♀▽

O43.93 Unspecified placental disorder, third trimester M♀▽

✓4th **O44 Placenta previa**
DEF: Placenta implanted in lower segment of uterus; commonly causes hemorrhage in the last trimester of pregnancy.

✓5th **O44.0 Complete placenta previa NOS or without hemorrhage**
Placenta previa NOS

O44.00 Complete placenta previa NOS or without hemorrhage, unspecified trimester M♀▽

O44.01 Complete placenta previa NOS or without hemorrhage, first trimester M♀

     O44.02   Complete placenta previa NOS or without hemorrhage, second trimester   Ⓜ♀

     O44.03   Complete placenta previa NOS or without hemorrhage, third trimester   Ⓜ♀

✓5ᵗʰ **O44.1**   Complete placenta previa with hemorrhage

     EXCLUDES 1   labor and delivery complicated by hemorrhage from vasa previa (O69.4)

     O44.10   Complete placenta previa with hemorrhage, unspecified trimester   Ⓜ♀▽

     O44.11   Complete placenta previa with hemorrhage, first trimester   Ⓜ♀

     O44.12   Complete placenta previa with hemorrhage, second trimester   Ⓜ♀

     O44.13   Complete placenta previa with hemorrhage, third trimester   Ⓜ♀

✓5ᵗʰ **O44.2**   Partial placenta previa without hemorrhage
     Marginal placenta previa, NOS or without hemorrhage

     O44.20   Partial placenta previa NOS or without hemorrhage, unspecified trimester   Ⓜ♀▽

     O44.21   Partial placenta previa NOS or without hemorrhage, first trimester   Ⓜ♀

     O44.22   Partial placenta previa NOS or without hemorrhage, second trimester   Ⓜ♀

     O44.23   Partial placenta previa NOS or without hemorrhage, third trimester   Ⓜ♀

✓5ᵗʰ **O44.3**   Partial placenta previa with hemorrhage
     Marginal placenta previa with hemorrhage

     O44.30   Partial placenta previa with hemorrhage, unspecified trimester   Ⓜ♀▽

     O44.31   Partial placenta previa with hemorrhage, first trimester   Ⓜ♀

     O44.32   Partial placenta previa with hemorrhage, second trimester   Ⓜ♀

     O44.33   Partial placenta previa with hemorrhage, third trimester   Ⓜ♀

✓5ᵗʰ **O44.4**   Low lying placenta NOS or without hemorrhage
     Low implantation of placenta NOS or without hemorrhage

     O44.40   Low lying placenta NOS or without hemorrhage, unspecified trimester   Ⓜ♀▽

     O44.41   Low lying placenta NOS or without hemorrhage, first trimester   Ⓜ♀

     O44.42   Low lying placenta NOS or without hemorrhage, second trimester   Ⓜ♀

     O44.43   Low lying placenta NOS or without hemorrhage, third trimester   Ⓜ♀

✓5ᵗʰ **O44.5**   Low lying placenta with hemorrhage
     Low implantation of placenta with hemorrhage

     O44.50   Low lying placenta with hemorrhage, unspecified trimester   Ⓜ♀▽

     O44.51   Low lying placenta with hemorrhage, first trimester   Ⓜ♀

     O44.52   Low lying placenta with hemorrhage, second trimester   Ⓜ♀

     O44.53   Low lying placenta with hemorrhage, third trimester   Ⓜ♀

✓4ᵗʰ **O45**   **Premature separation of placenta [abruptio placentae]**

✓5ᵗʰ **O45.0**   Premature separation of placenta with coagulation defect

     ✓6ᵗʰ **O45.00**   Premature separation of placenta with coagulation defect, unspecified

         O45.001   Premature separation of placenta with coagulation defect, unspecified, first trimester   Ⓜ♀▽

         O45.002   Premature separation of placenta with coagulation defect, unspecified, second trimester   Ⓜ♀▽

         O45.003   Premature separation of placenta with coagulation defect, unspecified, third trimester   Ⓜ♀▽

         O45.009   Premature separation of placenta with coagulation defect, unspecified, unspecified trimester   Ⓜ♀▽

     ✓6ᵗʰ **O45.01**   Premature separation of placenta with afibrinogenemia
         Premature separation of placenta with hypofibrinogenemia

         O45.011   Premature separation of placenta with afibrinogenemia, first trimester   Ⓜ♀

         O45.012   Premature separation of placenta with afibrinogenemia, second trimester   Ⓜ♀

         O45.013   Premature separation of placenta with afibrinogenemia, third trimester   Ⓜ♀

         O45.019   Premature separation of placenta with afibrinogenemia, unspecified trimester   Ⓜ♀▽

     ✓6ᵗʰ **O45.02**   Premature separation of placenta with disseminated intravascular coagulation

         O45.021   Premature separation of placenta with disseminated intravascular coagulation, first trimester   Ⓜ♀

         O45.022   Premature separation of placenta with disseminated intravascular coagulation, second trimester   Ⓜ♀

         O45.023   Premature separation of placenta with disseminated intravascular coagulation, third trimester   Ⓜ♀

         O45.029   Premature separation of placenta with disseminated intravascular coagulation, unspecified trimester   Ⓜ♀▽

     ✓6ᵗʰ **O45.09**   Premature separation of placenta with other coagulation defect

         O45.091   Premature separation of placenta with other coagulation defect, first trimester   Ⓜ♀

         O45.092   Premature separation of placenta with other coagulation defect, second trimester   Ⓜ♀

         O45.093   Premature separation of placenta with other coagulation defect, third trimester   Ⓜ♀

         O45.099   Premature separation of placenta with other coagulation defect, unspecified trimester   Ⓜ♀▽

✓5ᵗʰ **O45.8**   Other premature separation of placenta

     ✓6ᵗʰ **O45.8X**   Other premature separation of placenta

         O45.8X1   Other premature separation of placenta, first trimester   Ⓜ♀

         O45.8X2   Other premature separation of placenta, second trimester   Ⓜ♀

         O45.8X3   Other premature separation of placenta, third trimester   Ⓜ♀

         O45.8X9   Other premature separation of placenta, unspecified trimester   Ⓜ♀▽

✓5ᵗʰ **O45.9**   Premature separation of placenta, unspecified
     Abruptio placentae NOS

     O45.90   Premature separation of placenta, unspecified, unspecified trimester   Ⓜ♀▽

     O45.91   Premature separation of placenta, unspecified, first trimester   Ⓜ♀▽

     O45.92   Premature separation of placenta, unspecified, second trimester   Ⓜ♀▽

     O45.93   Premature separation of placenta, unspecified, third trimester   Ⓜ♀▽

✓4ᵗʰ **O46**   **Antepartum hemorrhage, not elsewhere classified**

     EXCLUDES 1   hemorrhage in early pregnancy (O20.-)
         intrapartum hemorrhage NEC (O67.-)
         placenta previa (O44.-)
         premature separation of placenta [abruptio placentae] (O45.-)

     DEF: Uterine hemorrhage prior to delivery; not related to placenta previa or abruptio placentae.

✓5ᵗʰ **O46.0**   Antepartum hemorrhage with coagulation defect

     ✓6ᵗʰ **O46.00**   Antepartum hemorrhage with coagulation defect, unspecified

         O46.001   Antepartum hemorrhage with coagulation defect, unspecified, first trimester   Ⓜ♀▽

         O46.002   Antepartum hemorrhage with coagulation defect, unspecified, second trimester   Ⓜ♀▽

         O46.003   Antepartum hemorrhage with coagulation defect, unspecified, third trimester   Ⓜ♀▽

         O46.009   Antepartum hemorrhage with coagulation defect, unspecified, unspecified trimester   Ⓜ♀▽

EXCLUDES 1 Not coded here   *EXCLUDES 2* Not included here   Ⓝ Newborn Age: 0   Ⓟ Pediatric Age: 0-17   Ⓜ Maternity Age: 12-55   Ⓐ Adult Age: 15-124

844   ICD-10-CM 2018

✓6ᵗʰ **O46.01 Antepartum hemorrhage with afibrinogenemia**
Antepartum hemorrhage with hypofibrinogenemia

     O46.011 Antepartum hemorrhage with afibrinogenemia, first trimester Ⓜ♀

     O46.012 Antepartum hemorrhage with afibrinogenemia, second trimester Ⓜ♀

     O46.013 Antepartum hemorrhage with afibrinogenemia, third trimester Ⓜ♀

     O46.019 Antepartum hemorrhage with afibrinogenemia, unspecified trimester Ⓜ♀▽

✓6ᵗʰ **O46.02 Antepartum hemorrhage with disseminated intravascular coagulation**

     O46.021 Antepartum hemorrhage with disseminated intravascular coagulation, first trimester Ⓜ♀

     O46.022 Antepartum hemorrhage with disseminated intravascular coagulation, second trimester Ⓜ♀

     O46.023 Antepartum hemorrhage with disseminated intravascular coagulation, third trimester Ⓜ♀

     O46.029 Antepartum hemorrhage with disseminated intravascular coagulation, unspecified trimester Ⓜ♀▽

✓6ᵗʰ **O46.09 Antepartum hemorrhage with other coagulation defect**

     O46.091 Antepartum hemorrhage with other coagulation defect, first trimester Ⓜ♀

     O46.092 Antepartum hemorrhage with other coagulation defect, second trimester Ⓜ♀

     O46.093 Antepartum hemorrhage with other coagulation defect, third trimester Ⓜ♀

     O46.099 Antepartum hemorrhage with other coagulation defect, unspecified trimester Ⓜ♀▽

✓5ᵗʰ **O46.8 Other antepartum hemorrhage**

     ✓6ᵗʰ **O46.8X Other antepartum hemorrhage**

       O46.8X1 Other antepartum hemorrhage, first trimester Ⓜ♀

       O46.8X2 Other antepartum hemorrhage, second trimester Ⓜ♀

       O46.8X3 Other antepartum hemorrhage, third trimester Ⓜ♀

       O46.8X9 Other antepartum hemorrhage, unspecified trimester Ⓜ♀▽

✓5ᵗʰ **O46.9 Antepartum hemorrhage, unspecified**

     O46.90 Antepartum hemorrhage, unspecified, unspecified trimester Ⓜ♀▽

     O46.91 Antepartum hemorrhage, unspecified, first trimester Ⓜ♀▽

     O46.92 Antepartum hemorrhage, unspecified, second trimester Ⓜ♀▽

     O46.93 Antepartum hemorrhage, unspecified, third trimester Ⓜ♀▽

✓4ᵗʰ **O47 False labor**
     INCLUDES Braxton Hicks contractions
            threatened labor
     EXCLUDES 1 *preterm labor (O60.-)*

✓5ᵗʰ **O47.0 False labor before 37 completed weeks of gestation**

     O47.00 False labor before 37 completed weeks of gestation, unspecified trimester Ⓜ♀▽

     O47.02 False labor before 37 completed weeks of gestation, second trimester Ⓜ♀

     O47.03 False labor before 37 completed weeks of gestation, third trimester Ⓜ♀

     O47.1 False labor at or after 37 completed weeks of gestation Ⓜ♀

     O47.9 False labor, unspecified Ⓜ♀▽

✓4ᵗʰ **O48 Late pregnancy**

     O48.0 Post-term pregnancy Ⓜ♀
       Pregnancy over 40 completed weeks to 42 completed weeks gestation

     O48.1 Prolonged pregnancy Ⓜ♀
       Pregnancy which has advanced beyond 42 completed weeks gestation
       AHA: 2016, 1Q, 5

Complications of labor and delivery (O60-O77)

✓4ᵗʰ **O60 Preterm labor**
     INCLUDES onset (spontaneous) of labor before 37 completed weeks of gestation
     EXCLUDES 1 *false labor (O47.0-)*
            threatened labor NOS (O47.0-)

✓5ᵗʰ **O60.0 Preterm labor without delivery**

     O60.00 Preterm labor without delivery, unspecified trimester Ⓜ♀▽

     O60.02 Preterm labor without delivery, second trimester Ⓜ♀

     O60.03 Preterm labor without delivery, third trimester Ⓜ♀

✓5ᵗʰ **O60.1 Preterm labor with preterm delivery**
     AHA: 2016, 2Q, 10

> One of the following 7th characters is to be assigned to each code under subcategory O60.1. 7th character Ø is for single gestations and multiple gestations where the fetus is unspecified. 7th characters 1 through 9 are for cases of multiple gestations to identify the fetus for which the code applies. The appropriate code from category O30, Multiple gestation, must also be assigned when assigning a code from subcategory O60.1 that has a 7th character of 1 through 9.
> Ø   not applicable or unspecified   4   fetus 4
> 1   fetus 1   5   fetus 5
> 2   fetus 2   9   other fetus
> 3   fetus 3

     ✓x7ᵗʰ **O60.10 Preterm labor with preterm delivery, unspecified trimester** Ⓜ♀▽
       Preterm labor with delivery NOS

     ✓x7ᵗʰ **O60.12 Preterm labor second trimester with preterm delivery second trimester** Ⓜ♀

     ✓x7ᵗʰ **O60.13 Preterm labor second trimester with preterm delivery third trimester** Ⓜ♀

     ✓x7ᵗʰ **O60.14 Preterm labor third trimester with preterm delivery third trimester** Ⓜ♀

✓5ᵗʰ **O60.2 Term delivery with preterm labor**

> One of the following 7th characters is to be assigned to each code under subcategory O60.2. 7th character Ø is for single gestations and multiple gestations where the fetus is unspecified. 7th characters 1 through 9 are for cases of multiple gestations to identify the fetus for which the code applies. The appropriate code from category O30, Multiple gestation, must also be assigned when assigning a code from subcategory O60.2 that has a 7th character of 1 through 9.
> Ø   not applicable or unspecified   4   fetus 4
> 1   fetus 1   5   fetus 5
> 2   fetus 2   9   other fetus
> 3   fetus 3

     ✓x7ᵗʰ **O60.20 Term delivery with preterm labor, unspecified trimester** Ⓜ♀▽

     ✓x7ᵗʰ **O60.22 Term delivery with preterm labor, second trimester** Ⓜ♀

     ✓x7ᵗʰ **O60.23 Term delivery with preterm labor, third trimester** Ⓜ♀

✓4ᵗʰ **O61 Failed induction of labor**

     O61.0 Failed medical induction of labor Ⓜ♀
       Failed induction (of labor) by oxytocin
       Failed induction (of labor) by prostaglandins

     O61.1 Failed instrumental induction of labor Ⓜ♀
       Failed mechanical induction (of labor)
       Failed surgical induction (of labor)

     O61.8 Other failed induction of labor Ⓜ♀

     O61.9 Failed induction of labor, unspecified Ⓜ♀▽

✓4ᵗʰ **O62 Abnormalities of forces of labor**

     O62.0 Primary inadequate contractions Ⓜ♀
       Failure of cervical dilatation
       Primary hypotonic uterine dysfunction
       Uterine inertia during latent phase of labor

     O62.1 Secondary uterine inertia Ⓜ♀
       Arrested active phase of labor
       Secondary hypotonic uterine dysfunction

✓ Additional Character Req   ✓x7ᵗʰ Placeholder Alert   Manifestation   HCC CMS-HCC Condition   ▽ Unspecified Code   ►◄ Revised Text   ● New Code   ▲ Revised Code Title

ICD-10-CM 2018   845

Chapter 15. Pregnancy, Childbirth, and the Puerperium

O62.2–O66.9

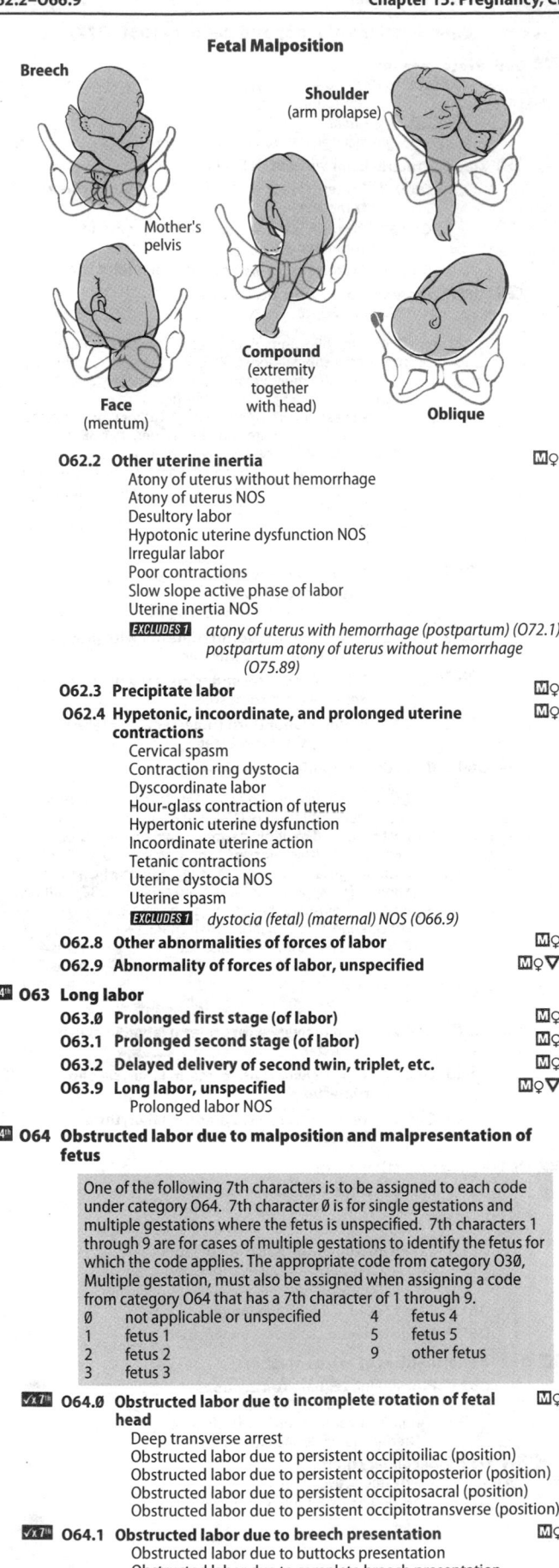

Fetal Malposition

Breech

Mother's pelvis

Shoulder (arm prolapse)

Face (mentum)

Compound (extremity together with head)

Oblique

O62.2 Other uterine inertia   Ⓜ♀
- Atony of uterus without hemorrhage
- Atony of uterus NOS
- Desultory labor
- Hypotonic uterine dysfunction NOS
- Irregular labor
- Poor contractions
- Slow slope active phase of labor
- Uterine inertia NOS
  > EXCLUDES 1   *atony of uterus with hemorrhage (postpartum) (O72.1)*
  > *postpartum atony of uterus without hemorrhage (O75.89)*

O62.3 Precipitate labor   Ⓜ♀

O62.4 Hypetonic, incoordinate, and prolonged uterine contractions   Ⓜ♀
- Cervical spasm
- Contraction ring dystocia
- Dyscoordinate labor
- Hour-glass contraction of uterus
- Hypertonic uterine dysfunction
- Incoordinate uterine action
- Tetanic contractions
- Uterine dystocia NOS
- Uterine spasm
  > EXCLUDES 1   *dystocia (fetal) (maternal) NOS (O66.9)*

O62.8 Other abnormalities of forces of labor   Ⓜ♀

O62.9 Abnormality of forces of labor, unspecified   Ⓜ♀▽

✓4ᵗʰ **O63 Long labor**

O63.0 Prolonged first stage (of labor)   Ⓜ♀

O63.1 Prolonged second stage (of labor)   Ⓜ♀

O63.2 Delayed delivery of second twin, triplet, etc.   Ⓜ♀

O63.9 Long labor, unspecified   Ⓜ♀▽
- Prolonged labor NOS

✓4ᵗʰ **O64 Obstructed labor due to malposition and malpresentation of fetus**

> One of the following 7th characters is to be assigned to each code under category O64. 7th character 0 is for single gestations and multiple gestations where the fetus is unspecified. 7th characters 1 through 9 are for cases of multiple gestations to identify the fetus for which the code applies. The appropriate code from category O30, Multiple gestation, must also be assigned when assigning a code from category O64 that has a 7th character of 1 through 9.
>
> | 0 | not applicable or unspecified | 4 | fetus 4 |
> |---|---|---|---|
> | 1 | fetus 1 | 5 | fetus 5 |
> | 2 | fetus 2 | 9 | other fetus |
> | 3 | fetus 3 | | |

✓x7ᵗʰ **O64.0 Obstructed labor due to incomplete rotation of fetal head**   Ⓜ♀
- Deep transverse arrest
- Obstructed labor due to persistent occipitoiliac (position)
- Obstructed labor due to persistent occipitoposterior (position)
- Obstructed labor due to persistent occipitosacral (position)
- Obstructed labor due to persistent occipitotransverse (position)

✓x7ᵗʰ **O64.1 Obstructed labor due to breech presentation**   Ⓜ♀
- Obstructed labor due to buttocks presentation
- Obstructed labor due to complete breech presentation
- Obstructed labor due to frank breech presentation

✓x7ᵗʰ **O64.2 Obstructed labor due to face presentation**   Ⓜ♀
- Obstructed labor due to chin presentation

✓x7ᵗʰ **O64.3 Obstructed labor due to brow presentation**   Ⓜ♀

✓x7ᵗʰ **O64.4 Obstructed labor due to shoulder presentation**   Ⓜ♀
- Prolapsed arm
  > EXCLUDES 1   *impacted shoulders (O66.0)*
  > *shoulder dystocia (O66.0)*

✓x7ᵗʰ **O64.5 Obstructed labor due to compound presentation**   Ⓜ♀

✓x7ᵗʰ **O64.8 Obstructed labor due to other malposition and malpresentation**   Ⓜ♀
- Obstructed labor due to footling presentation
- Obstructed labor due to incomplete breech presentation

✓x7ᵗʰ **O64.9 Obstructed labor due to malposition and malpresentation, unspecified**   Ⓜ♀▽

✓4ᵗʰ **O65 Obstructed labor due to maternal pelvic abnormality**

O65.0 Obstructed labor due to deformed pelvis   Ⓜ♀

O65.1 Obstructed labor due to generally contracted pelvis   Ⓜ♀

O65.2 Obstructed labor due to pelvic inlet contraction   Ⓜ♀

O65.3 Obstructed labor due to pelvic outlet and mid-cavity contraction   Ⓜ♀

O65.4 Obstructed labor due to fetopelvic disproportion, unspecified   Ⓜ♀▽
  > EXCLUDES 1   *dystocia due to abnormality of fetus (O66.2-O66.3)*

O65.5 Obstructed labor due to abnormality of maternal pelvic organs   Ⓜ♀
- Obstructed labor due to conditions listed In O34-
- Use additional code to identify abnormality of pelvic organs (O34.-)

O65.8 Obstructed labor due to other maternal pelvic abnormalities   Ⓜ♀

O65.9 Obstructed labor due to maternal pelvic abnormality, unspecified   Ⓜ♀▽

✓4ᵗʰ **O66 Other obstructed labor**

O66.0 Obstructed labor due to shoulder dystocia   Ⓜ♀
- Impacted shoulders
- **DEF:** Obstructed labor due to impacted fetal shoulders; emergency condition that may require cesarean section, forceps delivery, vacuum extraction, or simphysiotomy.

O66.1 Obstructed labor due to locked twins   Ⓜ♀

O66.2 Obstructed labor due to unusually large fetus   Ⓜ♀

O66.3 Obstructed labor due to other abnormalities of fetus   Ⓜ♀
- Dystocia due to fetal ascites
- Dystocia due to fetal hydrops
- Dystocia due to fetal meningomyelocele
- Dystocia due to fetal sacral teratoma
- Dystocia due to fetal tumor
- Dystocia due to hydrocephalic fetus
- Use additional code to identify cause of obstruction

✓5ᵗʰ **O66.4 Failed trial of labor**

O66.40 Failed trial of labor, unspecified   Ⓜ♀▽

O66.41 Failed attempted vaginal birth after previous cesarean delivery   Ⓜ♀
- Code first rupture of uterus, if applicable (O71.0-, O71.1)

O66.5 Attempted application of vacuum extractor and forceps   Ⓜ♀
- Attempted application of vacuum or forceps, with subsequent delivery by forceps or cesarean delivery

O66.6 Obstructed labor due to other multiple fetuses   Ⓜ♀

O66.8 Other specified obstructed labor   Ⓜ♀
- Use additional code to identify cause of obstruction

O66.9 Obstructed labor, unspecified   Ⓜ♀▽
- Dystocia NOS
- Fetal dystocia NOS
- Maternal dystocia NOS

EXCLUDES 1 Not coded here   EXCLUDES 2 Not included here   Ⓝ Newborn Age: 0   Ⓟ Pediatric Age: 0-17   Ⓜ Maternity Age: 12-55   Ⓐ Adult Age: 15-124

846   ICD-10-CM 2018

✅4ᵗʰ **O67 Labor and delivery complicated by intrapartum hemorrhage, not elsewhere classified**

>EXCLUDES1 *antepartum hemorrhage NEC (O46.-)*
>*placenta previa (O44.-)*
>*premature separation of placenta [abruptio placentae] (O45.-)*
>
>EXCLUDES2 *postpartum hemorrhage (O72.-)*

O67.0 Intrapartum hemorrhage with coagulation defect M♀

Intrapartum hemorrhage (excessive) associated with afibrinogenemia

Intrapartum hemorrhage (excessive) associated with disseminated intravascular coagulation

Intrapartum hemorrhage (excessive) associated with hyperfibrinolysis

Intrapartum hemorrhage (excessive) associated with hypofibrinogenemia

O67.8 Other intrapartum hemorrhage M♀

Excessive intrapartum hemorrhage

O67.9 Intrapartum hemorrhage, unspecified M♀▽

O68 Labor and delivery complicated by abnormality of fetal acid-base balance M♀

Fetal acidemia complicating labor and delivery

Fetal acidosis complicating labor and delivery

Fetal alkalosis complicating labor and delivery

Fetal metabolic acidemia complicating labor and delivery

>EXCLUDES1 *fetal stress NOS (O77.9)*
>*labor and delivery complicated by electrocardiographic evidence of fetal stress (O77.8)*
>*labor and delivery complicated by ultrasonic evidence of fetal stress (O77.8)*
>
>EXCLUDES2 *abnormality in fetal heart rate or rhythm (O76)*
>*labor and delivery complicated by meconium in amniotic fluid (O77.0)*

✅4ᵗʰ **O69 Labor and delivery complicated by umbilical cord complications**

AHA: 2016, 1Q, 5

> One of the following 7th characters is to be assigned to each code under category O69. 7th character 0 is for single gestations and multiple gestations where the fetus is unspecified. 7th characters 1 through 9 are for cases of multiple gestations to identify the fetus for which the code applies. The appropriate code from category O30, Multiple gestation, must also be assigned when assigning a code from category O69 that has a 7th character of 1 through 9.
>
> 0 not applicable or unspecified   4 fetus 4
> 1 fetus 1   5 fetus 5
> 2 fetus 2   9 other fetus
> 3 fetus 3

✅x7ᵗʰ **O69.0 Labor and delivery complicated by prolapse of cord** M♀

DEF: Abnormal presentation of fetus; marked by protruding umbilical cord during labor; can cause fetal death.

✅x7ᵗʰ **O69.1 Labor and delivery complicated by cord around neck, with compression** M♀

>EXCLUDES1 *labor and delivery complicated by cord around neck, without compression (O69.81)*

✅x7ᵗʰ **O69.2 Labor and delivery complicated by other cord entanglement, with compression** M♀

Labor and delivery complicated by compression of cord NOS

Labor and delivery complicated by entanglement of cords of twins in monoamniotic sac

Labor and delivery complicated by knot in cord

>EXCLUDES1 *labor and delivery complicated by other cord entanglement, without compression (O69.82)*

✅x7ᵗʰ **O69.3 Labor and delivery complicated by short cord** M♀

✅x7ᵗʰ **O69.4 Labor and delivery complicated by vasa previa** M♀

Labor and delivery complicated by hemorrhage from vasa previa

✅x7ᵗʰ **O69.5 Labor and delivery complicated by vascular lesion of cord** M♀

Labor and delivery complicated by cord bruising

Labor and delivery complicated by cord hematoma

Labor and delivery complicated by thrombosis of umbilical vessels

✅5ᵗʰ **O69.8 Labor and delivery complicated by other cord complications**

✅x7ᵗʰ **O69.81 Labor and delivery complicated by cord around neck, without compression** M♀

AHA: 2016, 1Q, 5

✅x7ᵗʰ **O69.82 Labor and delivery complicated by other cord entanglement, without compression** M♀

✅x7ᵗʰ **O69.89 Labor and delivery complicated by other cord complications** M♀

✅x7ᵗʰ **O69.9 Labor and delivery complicated by cord complication, unspecified** M♀▽

✅4ᵗʰ **O70 Perineal laceration during delivery**

Episiotomy extended by laceration

>EXCLUDES1 *obstetric high vaginal laceration alone (O71.4)*

AHA: 2016, 2Q, 34; 2016, 1Q, 3-4, 5

O70.0 First degree perineal laceration during delivery M♀

Perineal laceration, rupture or tear involving fourchette during delivery

Perineal laceration, rupture or tear involving labia during delivery

Perineal laceration, rupture or tear involving skin during delivery

Perineal laceration, rupture or tear involving vagina during delivery

Perineal laceration, rupture or tear involving vulva during delivery

Slight perineal laceration, rupture or tear during delivery

O70.1 Second degree perineal laceration during delivery M♀

Perineal laceration, rupture or tear during delivery as in O70.0, also involving pelvic floor

Perineal laceration, rupture or tear during delivery as in O70.0, also involving perineal muscles

Perineal laceration, rupture or tear during delivery as in O70.0, also involving vaginal muscles

>EXCLUDES1 *perineal laceration involving anal sphincter (O70.2)*

✅5ᵗʰ **O70.2 Third degree perineal laceration during delivery**

Perineal laceration, rupture or tear during delivery as in O70.1, also involving anal sphincter

Perineal laceration, rupture or tear during delivery as in O70.1, also involving rectovaginal septum

Perineal laceration, rupture or tear during delivery as in O70.1, also involving sphincter NOS

>EXCLUDES1 *anal sphincter tear during delivery without third degree perineal laceration (O70.4)*
>*perineal laceration involving anal or rectal mucosa (O70.3)*

O70.20 Third degree perineal laceration during delivery, unspecified M♀▽

O70.21 Third degree perineal laceration during delivery, IIIa M♀

Third degree perineal laceration during delivery with less than 50% of external anal sphincter (EAS) thickness torn

O70.22 Third degree perineal laceration during delivery, IIIb M♀

Third degree perineal laceration during delivery with more than 50% external anal sphincter (EAS) thickness torn

O70.23 Third degree perineal laceration during delivery, IIIc M♀

Third degree perineal laceration during delivery with both external anal sphincter (EAS) and internal anal sphincter (IAS) torn

O70.3 Fourth degree perineal laceration during delivery M♀

Perineal laceration, rupture or tear during delivery as in O70.2, also involving anal mucosa

Perineal laceration, rupture or tear during delivery as in O70.2, also involving rectal mucosa

O70.4 Anal sphincter tear complicating delivery, not associated with third degree laceration M♀

>EXCLUDES1 *anal sphincter tear with third degree perineal laceration (O70.2)*

O70.9 Perineal laceration during delivery, unspecified M♀▽

✅4ᵗʰ **O71 Other obstetric trauma**

INCLUDES obstetric damage from instruments

✅5ᵗʰ **O71.0 Rupture of uterus (spontaneous) before onset of labor**

>EXCLUDES1 *disruption of (current) cesarean delivery wound (O90.0)*
>*laceration of uterus, NEC (O71.81)*

O71.00 Rupture of uterus before onset of labor, unspecified trimester M♀▽

O71.02 Rupture of uterus before onset of labor, second trimester M♀

O71.03 Rupture of uterus before onset of labor, third trimester M♀

O71.1 Rupture of uterus during labor M♀

Rupture of uterus not stated as occurring before onset of labor

>EXCLUDES1 *disruption of cesarean delivery wound (O90.0)*
>*laceration of uterus, NEC (O71.81)*

O71.2 Postpartum inversion of uterus M♀

O71.3 Obstetric laceration of cervix M♀

Annular detachment of cervix

✅ Additional Character Req   ✅x7ᵗʰ Placeholder Alert   Manifestation   HCC CMS-HCC Condition   ▽ Unspecified Code   ►◄ Revised Text   ● New Code   ▲ Revised Code Title

ICD-10-CM 2018   847

Chapter 15. Pregnancy, Childbirth, and the Puerperium

O71.4 Obstetric high vaginal laceration alone Ⓜ♀
Laceration of vaginal wall without perineal laceration
EXCLUDES 1 obstetric high vaginal laceration with perineal laceration (O70.-)
AHA: 2016, 1Q, 5

O71.5 Other obstetric injury to pelvic organs Ⓜ♀
Obstetric injury to bladder
Obstetric injury to urethra
EXCLUDES 2 obstetric periurethral trauma (O71.82)
AHA: 2014, 4Q, 18

O71.6 Obstetric damage to pelvic joints and ligaments Ⓜ♀
Obstetric avulsion of inner symphyseal cartilage
Obstetric damage to coccyx
Obstetric traumatic separation of symphysis (pubis)

O71.7 Obstetric hematoma of pelvis Ⓜ♀
Obstetric hematoma of perineum
Obstetric hematoma of vagina
Obstetric hematoma of vulva

O71.8 Other specified obstetric trauma
O71.81 Laceration of uterus, not elsewhere classified Ⓜ♀
O71.82 Other specified trauma to perineum and vulva Ⓜ♀
Obstetric periurethral trauma
AHA: 2016, 1Q, 4; 2014, 4Q, 18
O71.89 Other specified obstetric trauma Ⓜ♀

O71.9 Obstetric trauma, unspecified Ⓜ♀▽

O72 Postpartum hemorrhage
INCLUDES hemorrhage after delivery of fetus or infant
O72.0 Third-stage hemorrhage Ⓜ♀
Hemorrhage associated with retained, trapped or adherent placenta
Retained placenta NOS
Code also type of adherent placenta (O43.2-)

O72.1 Other immediate postpartum hemorrhage Ⓜ♀
Hemorrhage following delivery of placenta
Postpartum hemorrhage (atonic) NOS
Uterine atony with hemorrhage
EXCLUDES 1 uterine atony NOS (O62.2)
uterine atony without hemorrhage (O62.2)
postpartum atony of uterus without hemorrhage (O75.89)
AHA: 2016, 1Q, 4

O72.2 Delayed and secondary postpartum hemorrhage Ⓜ♀
Hemorrhage associated with retained portions of placenta or membranes after the first 24 hours following delivery of placenta
Retained products of conception NOS, following delivery

O72.3 Postpartum coagulation defects Ⓜ♀
Postpartum afibrinogenemia
Postpartum fibrinolysis

O73 Retained placenta and membranes, without hemorrhage
EXCLUDES 1 placenta accreta (O43.21-)
placenta increta (O43.22-)
placenta percreta (O43.23-)
DEF: Postpartum condition resulting from failure to expel placental membrane tissues due to failed contractions of uterine wall.

O73.0 Retained placenta without hemorrhage Ⓜ♀
Adherent placenta, without hemorrhage
Trapped placenta without hemorrhage

O73.1 Retained portions of placenta and membranes, without hemorrhage Ⓜ♀
Retained products of conception following delivery, without hemorrhage

O74 Complications of anesthesia during labor and delivery
INCLUDES maternal complications arising from the administration of a general, regional or local anesthetic, analgesic or other sedation during labor and delivery
Use additional code, if applicable, to identify specific complication

O74.0 Aspiration pneumonitis due to anesthesia during labor and delivery Ⓜ♀
Inhalation of stomach contents or secretions NOS due to anesthesia during labor and delivery
Mendelson's syndrome due to anesthesia during labor and delivery

O74.1 Other pulmonary complications of anesthesia during labor and delivery Ⓜ♀

O74.2 Cardiac complications of anesthesia during labor and delivery Ⓜ♀

O74.3 Central nervous system complications of anesthesia during labor and delivery Ⓜ♀

O74.4 Toxic reaction to local anesthesia during labor and delivery Ⓜ♀

O74.5 Spinal and epidural anesthesia-induced headache during labor and delivery Ⓜ♀

O74.6 Other complications of spinal and epidural anesthesia during labor and delivery Ⓜ♀

O74.7 Failed or difficult intubation for anesthesia during labor and delivery Ⓜ♀

O74.8 Other complications of anesthesia during labor and delivery Ⓜ♀

O74.9 Complication of anesthesia during labor and delivery, unspecified Ⓜ♀▽

O75 Other complications of labor and delivery, not elsewhere classified
EXCLUDES 2 puerperal (postpartum) infection (O86.-)
puerperal (postpartum) sepsis (O85)

O75.0 Maternal distress during labor and delivery Ⓜ♀

O75.1 Shock during or following labor and delivery Ⓜ♀
Obstetric shock following labor and delivery

O75.2 Pyrexia during labor, not elsewhere classified Ⓜ♀

O75.3 Other infection during labor Ⓜ♀
Sepsis during labor
Use additional code (B95-B97), to identify infectious agent

O75.4 Other complications of obstetric surgery and procedures Ⓜ♀
Cardiac arrest following obstetric surgery or procedures
Cardiac failure following obstetric surgery or procedures
Cerebral anoxia following obstetric surgery or procedures
Pulmonary edema following obstetric surgery or procedures
Use additional code to identify specific complication
EXCLUDES 2 complications of anesthesia during labor and delivery (O74.-)
disruption of obstetrical (surgical) wound (O90.0-O90.1)
hematoma of obstetrical (surgical) wound (O90.2)
infection of obstetrical (surgical) wound (O86.0)

O75.5 Delayed delivery after artificial rupture of membranes Ⓜ♀

O75.8 Other specified complications of labor and delivery
O75.81 Maternal exhaustion complicating labor and delivery Ⓜ♀
O75.82 Onset (spontaneous) of labor after 37 completed weeks of gestation but before 39 completed weeks gestation, with delivery by (planned) cesarean section Ⓜ♀
Delivery by (planned) cesarean section occurring after 37 completed weeks of gestation but before 39 completed weeks gestation due to (spontaneous) onset of labor
Code first to specify reason for planned cesarean section such as:
cephalopelvic disproportion (normally formed fetus) (O33.9)
previous cesarean delivery (O34.21)
O75.89 Other specified complications of labor and delivery Ⓜ♀

O75.9 Complication of labor and delivery, unspecified Ⓜ♀▽

O76 Abnormality in fetal heart rate and rhythm complicating labor and delivery Ⓜ♀
Depressed fetal heart rate tones complicating labor and delivery
Fetal bradycardia complicating labor and delivery
Fetal heart rate abnormal variability complicating labor and delivery
Fetal heart rate decelerations complicating labor and delivery
Fetal heart rate irregularity complicating labor and delivery
Fetal tachycardia complicating labor and delivery
Non-reassuring fetal heart rate or rhythm complicating labor and delivery
EXCLUDES 1 fetal stress NOS (O77.9)
labor and delivery complicated by electrocardiographic evidence of fetal stress (O77.8)
labor and delivery complicated by ultrasonic evidence of fetal stress (O77.8)
EXCLUDES 2 fetal metabolic acidemia (O68)
other fetal stress (O77.0-O77.1)
AHA: 2013, 4Q, 118

O77 Other fetal stress complicating labor and delivery
O77.0 Labor and delivery complicated by meconium in amniotic fluid Ⓜ♀
AHA: 2013, 4Q, 117-118
O77.1 Fetal stress in labor or delivery due to drug administration Ⓜ♀

EXCLUDES 1 Not coded here   *EXCLUDES 2* Not included here   Ⓝ Newborn Age: 0   Ⓟ Pediatric Age: 0-17   Ⓜ Maternity Age: 12-55   Ⓐ Adult Age: 15-124

O77.8 Labor and delivery complicated by other evidence of fetal stress   Ⓜ♀
Labor and delivery complicated by electrocardiographic evidence of fetal stress
Labor and delivery complicated by ultrasonic evidence of fetal stress
> EXCLUDES 1   *abnormality in fetal heart rate or rhythm (O76)*
> *abnormality of fetal acid-base balance (O68)*
> *fetal metabolic acidemia (O68)*

O77.9 Labor and delivery complicated by fetal stress, unspecified   Ⓜ♀▽
> EXCLUDES 1   *abnormality in fetal heart rate or rhythm (O76)*
> *abnormality of fetal acid-base balance (O68)*
> *fetal metabolic acidemia (O68)*

Encounter for delivery (O80, O82)

O80 Encounter for full-term uncomplicated delivery   Ⓜ♀
> NOTE   Delivery requiring minimal or no assistance, with or without episiotomy, without fetal manipulation [e.g., rotation version] or instrumentation [forceps] of a spontaneous, cephalic, vaginal, full-term, single, live-born infant. This code is for use as a single diagnosis code and is not to be used with any other code from chapter 15.

Use additional code to indicate outcome of delivery (Z37.0)
AHA: 2016, 4Q, 150; 2014, 2Q, 9

O82 Encounter for cesarean delivery without indication   Ⓜ♀
Use additional code to indicate outcome of delivery (Z37.0)

Complications predominantly related to the puerperium (O85-O92)

> EXCLUDES 2   *mental and behavioral disorders associated with the puerperium (F53)*
> *obstetrical tetanus (A34)*
> *puerperal osteomalacia (M83.0)*

O85 Puerperal sepsis   Ⓜ♀
Postpartum sepsis
Puerperal peritonitis
Puerperal pyemia
Use additional code (B95-B97), to identify infectious agent
Use additional code (R65.2-) to identify severe sepsis, if applicable
> EXCLUDES 1   *fever of unknown origin following delivery (O86.4)*
> *genital tract infection following delivery (O86.1-)*
> *obstetric pyemic and septic embolism (O88.3-)*
> *puerperal septic thrombophlebitis (O86.81)*
> *urinary tract infection following delivery (O86.2-)*
> EXCLUDES 2   *sepsis during labor (O75.3)*

✓4ᵗʰ O86 Other puerperal infections
Use additional code (B95-B97), to identify infectious agent
> EXCLUDES 2   *infection during labor (O75.3)*
> *obstetrical tetanus (A34)*

O86.0 Infection of obstetric surgical wound   Ⓜ♀
Infected cesarean delivery wound following delivery
Infected perineal repair following delivery

✓5ᵗʰ O86.1 Other infection of genital tract following delivery
   O86.11 Cervicitis following delivery   Ⓜ♀
   O86.12 Endometritis following delivery   Ⓜ♀
   O86.13 Vaginitis following delivery   Ⓜ♀
   O86.19 Other infection of genital tract following delivery   Ⓜ♀

✓5ᵗʰ O86.2 Urinary tract infection following delivery
   O86.20 Urinary tract infection following delivery, unspecified   Ⓜ♀▽
     Puerperal urinary tract infection NOS
   O86.21 Infection of kidney following delivery   Ⓜ♀
   O86.22 Infection of bladder following delivery   Ⓜ♀
     Infection of urethra following delivery
   O86.29 Other urinary tract infection following delivery   Ⓜ♀

O86.4 Pyrexia of unknown origin following delivery   Ⓜ♀
Puerperal infection NOS following delivery
Puerperal pyrexia NOS following delivery
> EXCLUDES 2   *pyrexia during labor (O75.2)*
DEF: Fever of unknown origin experienced by the mother after childbirth.

✓5ᵗʰ O86.8 Other specified puerperal infections
   O86.81 Puerperal septic thrombophlebitis   Ⓜ♀
   O86.89 Other specified puerperal infections   Ⓜ♀

✓4ᵗʰ O87 Venous complications and hemorrhoids in the puerperium
> INCLUDES   venous complications in labor, delivery and the puerperium
> EXCLUDES 2   *obstetric embolism (O88.-)*
> *puerperal septic thrombophlebitis (O86.81)*
> *venous complications in pregnancy (O22.-)*

O87.0 Superficial thrombophlebitis in the puerperium   Ⓜ♀
Puerperal phlebitis NOS
Puerperal thrombosis NOS

O87.1 Deep phlebothrombosis in the puerperium   Ⓜ♀
Deep vein thrombosis, postpartum
Pelvic thrombophlebitis, postpartum
Use additional code to identify the deep vein thrombosis (I82.4-, I82.5-, I82.62-, I82.72-)
Use additional code, if applicable, for associated long-term (current) use of anticoagulants (Z79.01)

O87.2 Hemorrhoids in the puerperium   Ⓜ♀

O87.3 Cerebral venous thrombosis in the puerperium   Ⓜ♀
Cerebrovenous sinus thrombosis in the puerperium

O87.4 Varicose veins of lower extremity in the puerperium   Ⓜ♀

O87.8 Other venous complications in the puerperium   Ⓜ♀
Genital varices in the puerperium

O87.9 Venous complication in the puerperium, unspecified   Ⓜ♀▽
Puerperal phlebopathy NOS

✓4ᵗʰ O88 Obstetric embolism
> EXCLUDES 1   *embolism complicating abortion NOS (O03.2)*
> *embolism complicating ectopic or molar pregnancy (O08.2)*
> *embolism complicating failed attempted abortion (O07.2)*
> *embolism complicating induced abortion (O04.7)*
> *embolism complicating spontaneous abortion (O03.2, O03.7)*

✓5ᵗʰ O88.0 Obstetric air embolism
DEF: Sudden blocking of pulmonary artery or right ventricle with air or nitrogen bubbles.
   ✓6ᵗʰ O88.01 Obstetric air embolism in pregnancy
     O88.011 Air embolism in pregnancy, first trimester   Ⓜ♀
     O88.012 Air embolism in pregnancy, second trimester   Ⓜ♀
     O88.013 Air embolism in pregnancy, third trimester   Ⓜ♀
     O88.019 Air embolism in pregnancy, unspecified trimester   Ⓜ♀▽
   O88.02 Air embolism in childbirth   Ⓜ♀
   O88.03 Air embolism in the puerperium   Ⓜ♀

✓5ᵗʰ O88.1 Amniotic fluid embolism
Anaphylactoid syndrome in pregnancy
   ✓6ᵗʰ O88.11 Amniotic fluid embolism in pregnancy
     O88.111 Amniotic fluid embolism in pregnancy, first trimester   Ⓜ♀
     O88.112 Amniotic fluid embolism in pregnancy, second trimester   Ⓜ♀
     O88.113 Amniotic fluid embolism in pregnancy, third trimester   Ⓜ♀
     O88.119 Amniotic fluid embolism in pregnancy, unspecified trimester   Ⓜ♀▽
   O88.12 Amniotic fluid embolism in childbirth   Ⓜ♀
   O88.13 Amniotic fluid embolism in the puerperium   Ⓜ♀

✓5ᵗʰ O88.2 Obstetric thromboembolism
   ✓6ᵗʰ O88.21 Thromboembolism in pregnancy
     Obstetric (pulmonary) embolism NOS
     O88.211 Thromboembolism in pregnancy, first trimester   Ⓜ♀
     O88.212 Thromboembolism in pregnancy, second trimester   Ⓜ♀
     O88.213 Thromboembolism in pregnancy, third trimester   Ⓜ♀
     O88.219 Thromboembolism in pregnancy, unspecified trimester   Ⓜ♀▽
   O88.22 Thromboembolism in childbirth   Ⓜ♀
   O88.23 Thromboembolism in the puerperium   Ⓜ♀
     Puerperal (pulmonary) embolism NOS

✓5ᵗʰ O88.3 Obstetric pyemic and septic embolism
   ✓6ᵗʰ O88.31 Pyemic and septic embolism in pregnancy
     O88.311 Pyemic and septic embolism in pregnancy, first trimester   Ⓜ♀
     O88.312 Pyemic and septic embolism in pregnancy, second trimester   Ⓜ♀

☑ Additional Character Req   ☑7ᵗʰ Placeholder Alert   Manifestation   HCC CMS-HCC Condition   ▽ Unspecified Code   ►◄ Revised Text   ● New Code   ▲ Revised Code Title

O88.313 Pyemic and septic embolism in pregnancy, third trimester Ⓜ♀

O88.319 Pyemic and septic embolism in pregnancy, unspecified trimester Ⓜ♀▽

O88.32 Pyemic and septic embolism in childbirth Ⓜ♀

O88.33 Pyemic and septic embolism in the puerperium Ⓜ♀

✓5ᵗʰ **O88.8** Other obstetric embolism
Obstetric fat embolism

✓6ᵗʰ **O88.81** Other embolism in pregnancy

O88.811 Other embolism in pregnancy, first trimester Ⓜ♀

O88.812 Other embolism in pregnancy, second trimester Ⓜ♀

O88.813 Other embolism in pregnancy, third trimester Ⓜ♀

O88.819 Other embolism in pregnancy, unspecified trimester Ⓜ♀▽

O88.82 Other embolism in childbirth Ⓜ♀

O88.83 Other embolism in the puerperium Ⓜ♀

✓4ᵗʰ **O89** Complications of anesthesia during the puerperium
INCLUDES maternal complications arising from the administration of a general, regional or local anesthetic, analgesic or other sedation during the puerperium
Use additional code, if applicable, to identify specific complication

✓5ᵗʰ **O89.0** Pulmonary complications of anesthesia during the puerperium

O89.01 Aspiration pneumonitis due to anesthesia during the puerperium Ⓜ♀
Inhalation of stomach contents or secretions NOS due to anesthesia during the puerperium
Mendelson's syndrome due to anesthesia during the puerperium

O89.09 Other pulmonary complications of anesthesia during the puerperium Ⓜ♀

O89.1 Cardiac complications of anesthesia during the puerperium Ⓜ♀

O89.2 Central nervous system complications of anesthesia during the puerperium Ⓜ♀

O89.3 Toxic reaction to local anesthesia during the puerperium Ⓜ♀

O89.4 Spinal and epidural anesthesia-induced headache during the puerperium Ⓜ♀

O89.5 Other complications of spinal and epidural anesthesia during the puerperium Ⓜ♀

O89.6 Failed or difficult intubation for anesthesia during the puerperium Ⓜ♀

O89.8 Other complications of anesthesia during the puerperium Ⓜ♀

O89.9 Complication of anesthesia during the puerperium, unspecified Ⓜ♀▽

✓4ᵗʰ **O90** Complications of the puerperium, not elsewhere classified

O90.0 Disruption of cesarean delivery wound Ⓜ♀
Dehiscence of cesarean delivery wound
EXCLUDES 1 rupture of uterus (spontaneous) before onset of labor (O71.0-)
rupture of uterus during labor (O71.1)

O90.1 Disruption of perineal obstetric wound Ⓜ♀
Disruption of wound of episiotomy
Disruption of wound of perineal laceration
Secondary perineal tear

O90.2 Hematoma of obstetric wound Ⓜ♀

O90.3 Peripartum cardiomyopathy Ⓜ♀
Conditions in I42- arising during pregnancy and the puerperium
EXCLUDES 1 pre-existing heart disease complicating pregnancy and the puerperium (O99.4-)
DEF: Any structural or functional abnormality of the ventricular myocardium, noninflammatory disease of obscure or unknown etiology with onset during the postpartum period.

O90.4 Postpartum acute kidney failure Ⓜ♀
Hepatorenal syndrome following labor and delivery

O90.5 Postpartum thyroiditis Ⓜ♀

O90.6 Postpartum mood disturbance Ⓜ♀
Postpartum blues
Postpartum dysphoria
Postpartum sadness
EXCLUDES 1 postpartum depression (F53)
puerperal psychosis (F53)

✓5ᵗʰ **O90.8** Other complications of the puerperium, not elsewhere classified

O90.81 Anemia of the puerperium Ⓜ♀
Postpartum anemia NOS
EXCLUDES 1 pre-existing anemia complicating the puerperium (O99.03)

O90.89 Other complications of the puerperium, not elsewhere classified Ⓜ♀
Placental polyp

O90.9 Complication of the puerperium, unspecified Ⓜ♀▽

✓4ᵗʰ **O91** Infections of breast associated with pregnancy, the puerperium and lactation
Use additional code to identify infection

✓5ᵗʰ **O91.0** Infection of nipple associated with pregnancy, the puerperium and lactation

✓6ᵗʰ **O91.01** Infection of nipple associated with pregnancy
Gestational abscess of nipple

O91.011 Infection of nipple associated with pregnancy, first trimester Ⓜ♀

O91.012 Infection of nipple associated with pregnancy, second trimester Ⓜ♀

O91.013 Infection of nipple associated with pregnancy, third trimester Ⓜ♀

O91.019 Infection of nipple associated with pregnancy, unspecified trimester Ⓜ♀▽

O91.02 Infection of nipple associated with the puerperium Ⓜ♀
Puerperal abscess of nipple

O91.03 Infection of nipple associated with lactation Ⓜ♀
Abscess of nipple associated with lactation

✓5ᵗʰ **O91.1** Abscess of breast associated with pregnancy, the puerperium and lactation

✓6ᵗʰ **O91.11** Abscess of breast associated with pregnancy
Gestational mammary abscess
Gestational purulent mastitis
Gestational subareolar abscess

O91.111 Abscess of breast associated with pregnancy, first trimester Ⓜ♀

O91.112 Abscess of breast associated with pregnancy, second trimester Ⓜ♀

O91.113 Abscess of breast associated with pregnancy, third trimester Ⓜ♀

O91.119 Abscess of breast associated with pregnancy, unspecified trimester Ⓜ♀▽

O91.12 Abscess of breast associated with the puerperium Ⓜ♀
Puerperal mammary abscess
Puerperal purulent mastitis
Puerperal subareolar abscess

O91.13 Abscess of breast associated with lactation Ⓜ♀
Mammary abscess associated with lactation
Purulent mastitis associated with lactation
Subareolar abscess associated with lactation

✓5ᵗʰ **O91.2** Nonpurulent mastitis associated with pregnancy, the puerperium and lactation

✓6ᵗʰ **O91.21** Nonpurulent mastitis associated with pregnancy
Gestational interstitial mastitis
Gestational lymphangitis of breast
Gestational mastitis NOS
Gestational parenchymatous mastitis

O91.211 Nonpurulent mastitis associated with pregnancy, first trimester Ⓜ♀

O91.212 Nonpurulent mastitis associated with pregnancy, second trimester Ⓜ♀

O91.213 Nonpurulent mastitis associated with pregnancy, third trimester Ⓜ♀

O91.219 Nonpurulent mastitis associated with pregnancy, unspecified trimester Ⓜ♀▽

O91.22 Nonpurulent mastitis associated with the puerperium Ⓜ♀
Puerperal interstitial mastitis
Puerperal lymphangitis of breast
Puerperal mastitis NOS
Puerperal parenchymatous mastitis

O91.23 Nonpurulent mastitis associated with lactation Ⓜ♀
Interstitial mastitis associated with lactation
Lymphangitis of breast associated with lactation
Mastitis NOS associated with lactation
Parenchymatous mastitis associated with lactation

√4ᵗʰ O92 Other disorders of breast and disorders of lactation associated with pregnancy and the puerperium

√5ᵗʰ O92.0 Retracted nipple associated with pregnancy, the puerperium, and lactation

    √6ᵗʰ O92.01 Retracted nipple associated with pregnancy

        O92.011 Retracted nipple associated with pregnancy, first trimester Ⓜ♀

        O92.012 Retracted nipple associated with pregnancy, second trimester Ⓜ♀

        O92.013 Retracted nipple associated with pregnancy, third trimester Ⓜ♀

        O92.019 Retracted nipple associated with pregnancy, unspecified trimester Ⓜ♀▽

    O92.02 Retracted nipple associated with the puerperium Ⓜ♀

    O92.03 Retracted nipple associated with lactation Ⓜ♀

√5ᵗʰ O92.1 Cracked nipple associated with pregnancy, the puerperium, and lactation
    Fissure of nipple, gestational or puerperal

    √6ᵗʰ O92.11 Cracked nipple associated with pregnancy

        O92.111 Cracked nipple associated with pregnancy, first trimester Ⓜ♀

        O92.112 Cracked nipple associated with pregnancy, second trimester Ⓜ♀

        O92.113 Cracked nipple associated with pregnancy, third trimester Ⓜ♀

        O92.119 Cracked nipple associated with pregnancy, unspecified trimester Ⓜ♀▽

    O92.12 Cracked nipple associated with the puerperium Ⓜ♀

    O92.13 Cracked nipple associated with lactation Ⓜ♀

√5ᵗʰ O92.2 Other and unspecified disorders of breast associated with pregnancy and the puerperium

    O92.20 Unspecified disorder of breast associated with pregnancy and the puerperium Ⓜ♀▽

    O92.29 Other disorders of breast associated with pregnancy and the puerperium Ⓜ♀

O92.3 Agalactia Ⓜ♀
    Primary agalactia
    EXCLUDES 1 elective agalactia (O92.5)
        secondary agalactia (O92.5)
        therapeutic agalactia (O92.5)
    DEF: Absence of milk secretion in a female after delivery.

O92.4 Hypogalactia Ⓜ♀

O92.5 Suppressed lactation Ⓜ♀
    Elective agalactia
    Secondary agalactia
    Therapeutic agalactia
    EXCLUDES 1 primary agalactia (O92.3)

O92.6 Galactorrhea Ⓜ♀
    DEF: Excessive or persistent milk secretion by breast; may occur in absence of nursing.

√5ᵗʰ O92.7 Other and unspecified disorders of lactation

    O92.70 Unspecified disorders of lactation Ⓜ♀▽

    O92.79 Other disorders of lactation Ⓜ♀
        Puerperal galactocele

Other obstetric conditions, not elsewhere classified (O94-O9A)

O94 Sequelae of complication of pregnancy, childbirth, and the puerperium Ⓜ♀
    NOTE This category is to be used to indicate conditions in O00-O77.-, O85-O94 and O98-O9A.- as the cause of late effects. The sequelae include conditions specified as such, or as late effects, which may occur at any time after the puerperium.
    Code first condition resulting from (sequela) of complication of pregnancy, childbirth, and the puerperium

√4ᵗʰ O98 Maternal infectious and parasitic diseases classifiable elsewhere but complicating pregnancy, childbirth and the puerperium
    INCLUDES the listed conditions when complicating the pregnant state, when aggravated by the pregnancy, or as a reason for obstetric care
    Use additional code (Chapter 1), to identify specific infectious or parasitic disease
    EXCLUDES 2 herpes gestationis (O26.4-)
        infectious carrier state (O99.82-, O99.83-)
        obstetrical tetanus (A34)
        puerperal infection (O86.-)
        puerperal sepsis (O85)
        when the reason for maternal care is that the disease is known or suspected to have affected the fetus (O35-O36)

√5ᵗʰ O98.0 Tuberculosis complicating pregnancy, childbirth and the puerperium
    Conditions in A15-A19

    √6ᵗʰ O98.01 Tuberculosis complicating pregnancy

        O98.011 Tuberculosis complicating pregnancy, first trimester Ⓜ♀

        O98.012 Tuberculosis complicating pregnancy, second trimester Ⓜ♀

        O98.013 Tuberculosis complicating pregnancy, third trimester Ⓜ♀

        O98.019 Tuberculosis complicating pregnancy, unspecified trimester Ⓜ♀▽

    O98.02 Tuberculosis complicating childbirth Ⓜ♀

    O98.03 Tuberculosis complicating the puerperium Ⓜ♀

√5ᵗʰ O98.1 Syphilis complicating pregnancy, childbirth and the puerperium
    Conditions in A50-A53

    √6ᵗʰ O98.11 Syphilis complicating pregnancy

        O98.111 Syphilis complicating pregnancy, first trimester Ⓜ♀

        O98.112 Syphilis complicating pregnancy, second trimester Ⓜ♀

        O98.113 Syphilis complicating pregnancy, third trimester Ⓜ♀

        O98.119 Syphilis complicating pregnancy, unspecified trimester Ⓜ♀▽

    O98.12 Syphilis complicating childbirth Ⓜ♀

    O98.13 Syphilis complicating the puerperium Ⓜ♀

√5ᵗʰ O98.2 Gonorrhea complicating pregnancy, childbirth and the puerperium
    Conditions in A54-

    √6ᵗʰ O98.21 Gonorrhea complicating pregnancy

        O98.211 Gonorrhea complicating pregnancy, first trimester Ⓜ♀

        O98.212 Gonorrhea complicating pregnancy, second trimester Ⓜ♀

        O98.213 Gonorrhea complicating pregnancy, third trimester Ⓜ♀

        O98.219 Gonorrhea complicating pregnancy, ▽ unspecified trimester Ⓜ♀

    O98.22 Gonorrhea complicating childbirth Ⓜ♀

    O98.23 Gonorrhea complicating the puerperium Ⓜ♀

√5ᵗʰ O98.3 Other infections with a predominantly sexual mode of transmission complicating pregnancy, childbirth and the puerperium
    Conditions in A55-A64

    √6ᵗʰ O98.31 Other infections with a predominantly sexual mode of transmission complicating pregnancy

        O98.311 Other infections with a predominantly sexual mode of transmission complicating pregnancy, first trimester Ⓜ♀

        O98.312 Other infections with a predominantly sexual mode of transmission complicating pregnancy, second trimester Ⓜ♀

        O98.313 Other infections with a predominantly sexual mode of transmission complicating pregnancy, third trimester Ⓜ♀

        O98.319 Other infections with a predominantly sexual mode of transmission complicating pregnancy, unspecified trimester Ⓜ♀▽

☑ Additional Character Req   √×7ᵗʰ Placeholder Alert   Manifestation   HCC CMS-HCC Condition   ▽ Unspecified Code   ►◄ Revised Text   ● New Code   ▲ Revised Code Title

ICD-10-CM 2018

851

O98.32 Other infections with a predominantly sexual mode of transmission complicating childbirth   Ⓜ♀

O98.33 Other infections with a predominantly sexual mode of transmission complicating the puerperium   Ⓜ♀

✓5ᵗʰ **O98.4 Viral hepatitis complicating pregnancy, childbirth and the puerperium**
Conditions in B15-B19

✓6ᵗʰ **O98.41** Viral hepatitis complicating pregnancy

O98.411 Viral hepatitis complicating pregnancy, first trimester   Ⓜ♀

O98.412 Viral hepatitis complicating pregnancy, second trimester   Ⓜ♀

O98.413 Viral hepatitis complicating pregnancy, third trimester   Ⓜ♀

O98.419 Viral hepatitis complicating pregnancy, unspecified trimester   Ⓜ♀▽

O98.42 Viral hepatitis complicating childbirth   Ⓜ♀

O98.43 Viral hepatitis complicating the puerperium   Ⓜ♀

✓5ᵗʰ **O98.5 Other viral diseases complicating pregnancy, childbirth and the puerperium**
Conditions in A80-B09, B25-B34, R87.81-, R87.82-
EXCLUDES 1   human immunodeficiency virus [HIV] disease complicating pregnancy, childbirth and the puerperium (O98.7-)

✓6ᵗʰ **O98.51** Other viral diseases complicating pregnancy

O98.511 Other viral diseases complicating pregnancy, first trimester   Ⓜ♀

O98.512 Other viral diseases complicating pregnancy, second trimester   Ⓜ♀

O98.513 Other viral diseases complicating pregnancy, third trimester   Ⓜ♀

O98.519 Other viral diseases complicating pregnancy, unspecified trimester   Ⓜ♀▽

O98.52 Other viral diseases complicating childbirth   Ⓜ♀

O98.53 Other viral diseases complicating the puerperium   Ⓜ♀

✓5ᵗʰ **O98.6 Protozoal diseases complicating pregnancy, childbirth and the puerperium**
Conditions in B50-B64

✓6ᵗʰ **O98.61** Protozoal diseases complicating pregnancy

O98.611 Protozoal diseases complicating pregnancy, first trimester   Ⓜ♀

O98.612 Protozoal diseases complicating pregnancy, second trimester   Ⓜ♀

O98.613 Protozoal diseases complicating pregnancy, third trimester   Ⓜ♀

O98.619 Protozoal diseases complicating pregnancy, unspecified trimester   Ⓜ♀▽

O98.62 Protozoal diseases complicating childbirth   Ⓜ♀

O98.63 Protozoal diseases complicating the puerperium   Ⓜ♀

✓5ᵗʰ **O98.7 Human immunodeficiency virus [HIV] disease complicating pregnancy, childbirth and the puerperium**
Use additional code to identify the type of HIV disease:
acquired immune deficiency syndrome (AIDS) (B20)
asymptomatic HIV status (Z21)
HIV positive NOS (Z21)
symptomatic HIV disease (B20)

✓6ᵗʰ **O98.71** Human immunodeficiency virus [HIV] disease complicating pregnancy

O98.711 Human immunodeficiency virus [HIV] disease complicating pregnancy, first trimester   Ⓜ♀

O98.712 Human immunodeficiency virus [HIV] disease complicating pregnancy, second trimester   Ⓜ♀

O98.713 Human immunodeficiency virus [HIV] disease complicating pregnancy, third trimester   Ⓜ♀

O98.719 Human immunodeficiency virus [HIV] disease complicating pregnancy, unspecified trimester   Ⓜ♀▽

O98.72 Human immunodeficiency virus [HIV] disease complicating childbirth   Ⓜ♀

O98.73 Human immunodeficiency virus [HIV] disease complicating the puerperium   Ⓜ♀

✓5ᵗʰ **O98.8 Other maternal infectious and parasitic diseases complicating pregnancy, childbirth and the puerperium**

✓6ᵗʰ **O98.81** Other maternal infectious and parasitic diseases complicating pregnancy

O98.811 Other maternal infectious and parasitic diseases complicating pregnancy, first trimester   Ⓜ♀

O98.812 Other maternal infectious and parasitic diseases complicating pregnancy, second trimester   Ⓜ♀

O98.813 Other maternal infectious and parasitic diseases complicating pregnancy, third trimester   Ⓜ♀

O98.819 Other maternal infectious and parasitic diseases complicating pregnancy, unspecified trimester   Ⓜ♀▽

O98.82 Other maternal infectious and parasitic diseases complicating childbirth   Ⓜ♀

O98.83 Other maternal infectious and parasitic diseases complicating the puerperium   Ⓜ♀

✓5ᵗʰ **O98.9 Unspecified maternal infectious and parasitic disease complicating pregnancy, childbirth and the puerperium**

✓6ᵗʰ **O98.91** Unspecified maternal infectious and parasitic disease complicating pregnancy

O98.911 Unspecified maternal infectious and parasitic disease complicating pregnancy, first trimester   Ⓜ♀▽

O98.912 Unspecified maternal infectious and parasitic disease complicating pregnancy, second trimester   Ⓜ♀▽

O98.913 Unspecified maternal infectious and parasitic disease complicating pregnancy, third trimester   Ⓜ♀▽

O98.919 Unspecified maternal infectious and parasitic disease complicating pregnancy, unspecified trimester   Ⓜ♀▽

O98.92 Unspecified maternal infectious and parasitic disease complicating childbirth   Ⓜ♀▽

O98.93 Unspecified maternal infectious and parasitic disease complicating the puerperium   Ⓜ♀▽

✓4ᵗʰ **O99 Other maternal diseases classifiable elsewhere but complicating pregnancy, childbirth and the puerperium**
INCLUDES   conditions which complicate the pregnant state, are aggravated by the pregnancy or are a main reason for obstetric care
Use additional code to identify specific condition
EXCLUDES 2   when the reason for maternal care is that the condition is known or suspected to have affected the fetus (O35-O36)

✓5ᵗʰ **O99.0 Anemia complicating pregnancy, childbirth and the puerperium**
Conditions in D50-D64
EXCLUDES 1   anemia arising in the puerperium (O90.81)
postpartum anemia NOS (O90.81)

✓6ᵗʰ **O99.01** Anemia complicating pregnancy
AHA: 2016, 1Q, 4

O99.011 Anemia complicating pregnancy, first trimester   Ⓜ♀

O99.012 Anemia complicating pregnancy, second trimester   Ⓜ♀

O99.013 Anemia complicating pregnancy, third trimester   Ⓜ♀

O99.019 Anemia complicating pregnancy, unspecified trimester   Ⓜ♀▽

O99.02 Anemia complicating childbirth   Ⓜ♀

O99.03 Anemia complicating the puerperium   Ⓜ♀
EXCLUDES 1   postpartum anemia not pre-existing prior to delivery (O90.81)

✓5ᵗʰ **O99.1 Other diseases of the blood and blood-forming organs and certain disorders involving the immune mechanism complicating pregnancy, childbirth and the puerperium**
Conditions in D65-D89
EXCLUDES 1 ▶hemorrhage with coagulation defects (O45.-, O46.0-, O67.0, O72.3)◀
EXCLUDES 2   hemorrhage with coagulation defects (O45.-, O46.0-, O67.0, O72.3)

EXCLUDES 1 Not coded here   EXCLUDES 2 Not included here   Ⓝ Newborn Age: 0   Ⓟ Pediatric Age: 0-17   Ⓜ Maternity Age: 12-55   Ⓐ Adult Age: 15-124

852   ICD-10-CM 2018

√6ᵗʰ **O99.11** **Other diseases of the blood and blood-forming organs and certain disorders involving the immune mechanism complicating pregnancy**

    O99.111 **Other diseases of the blood and blood-forming organs and certain disorders involving the immune mechanism complicating pregnancy, first trimester** Ⓜ♀

    O99.112 **Other diseases of the blood and blood-forming organs and certain disorders involving the immune mechanism complicating pregnancy, second trimester** Ⓜ♀

    O99.113 **Other diseases of the blood and blood-forming organs and certain disorders involving the immune mechanism complicating pregnancy, third trimester** Ⓜ♀

    O99.119 **Other diseases of the blood and blood-forming organs and certain disorders involving the immune mechanism complicating pregnancy, unspecified trimester** Ⓜ♀▽

O99.12 **Other diseases of the blood and blood-forming organs and certain disorders involving the immune mechanism complicating childbirth** Ⓜ♀

O99.13 **Other diseases of the blood and blood-forming organs and certain disorders involving the immune mechanism complicating the puerperium** Ⓜ♀

√5ᵗʰ **O99.2** **Endocrine, nutritional and metabolic diseases complicating pregnancy, childbirth and the puerperium**
    Conditions in E00-E88
    EXCLUDES 2   *diabetes mellitus (O24.-)*
         malnutrition (O25.-)
         postpartum thyroiditis (O90.5)

√6ᵗʰ **O99.21** **Obesity complicating pregnancy, childbirth, and the puerperium**
    Use additional code to identify the type of obesity (E66.-)

    O99.210 **Obesity complicating pregnancy, unspecified trimester** Ⓜ♀▽

    O99.211 **Obesity complicating pregnancy, first trimester** Ⓜ♀

    O99.212 **Obesity complicating pregnancy, second trimester** Ⓜ♀

    O99.213 **Obesity complicating pregnancy, third trimester** Ⓜ♀

    O99.214 **Obesity complicating childbirth** Ⓜ♀

    O99.215 **Obesity complicating the puerperium** Ⓜ♀

√6ᵗʰ **O99.28** **Other endocrine, nutritional and metabolic diseases complicating pregnancy, childbirth and the puerperium**

    O99.280 **Endocrine, nutritional and metabolic diseases complicating pregnancy, unspecified trimester** Ⓜ♀▽

    O99.281 **Endocrine, nutritional and metabolic diseases complicating pregnancy, first trimester** Ⓜ♀

    O99.282 **Endocrine, nutritional and metabolic diseases complicating pregnancy, second trimester** Ⓜ♀

    O99.283 **Endocrine, nutritional and metabolic diseases complicating pregnancy, third trimester** Ⓜ♀

    O99.284 **Endocrine, nutritional and metabolic diseases complicating childbirth** Ⓜ♀

    O99.285 **Endocrine, nutritional and metabolic diseases complicating the puerperium** Ⓜ♀

√5ᵗʰ **O99.3** **Mental disorders and diseases of the nervous system complicating pregnancy, childbirth and the puerperium**

√6ᵗʰ **O99.31** **Alcohol use complicating pregnancy, childbirth, and the puerperium**
    Use additional code(s) from F10 to identify manifestations of the alcohol use

    O99.310 **Alcohol use complicating pregnancy, unspecified trimester** Ⓜ♀▽

    O99.311 **Alcohol use complicating pregnancy, first trimester** Ⓜ♀

    O99.312 **Alcohol use complicating pregnancy, second trimester** Ⓜ♀

    O99.313 **Alcohol use complicating pregnancy, third trimester** Ⓜ♀

    O99.314 **Alcohol use complicating childbirth** Ⓜ♀

    O99.315 **Alcohol use complicating the puerperium** Ⓜ♀

√6ᵗʰ **O99.32** **Drug use complicating pregnancy, childbirth, and the puerperium**
    Use additional code(s) from F11-F16 and F18-F19 to identify manifestations of the drug use

    O99.320 **Drug use complicating pregnancy, unspecified trimester** Ⓜ♀▽

    O99.321 **Drug use complicating pregnancy, first trimester** Ⓜ♀

    O99.322 **Drug use complicating pregnancy, second trimester** Ⓜ♀

    O99.323 **Drug use complicating pregnancy, third trimester** Ⓜ♀

    O99.324 **Drug use complicating childbirth** Ⓜ♀

    O99.325 **Drug use complicating the puerperium** Ⓜ♀

√6ᵗʰ **O99.33** **Tobacco use disorder complicating pregnancy, childbirth, and the puerperium**
    Smoking complicating pregnancy, childbirth, and the puerperium
    Use additional code from category F17 to identify type of tobacco nicotine dependence

    O99.330 **Smoking (tobacco) complicating pregnancy, unspecified trimester** Ⓜ♀▽

    O99.331 **Smoking (tobacco) complicating pregnancy, first trimester** Ⓜ♀

    O99.332 **Smoking (tobacco) complicating pregnancy, second trimester** Ⓜ♀

    O99.333 **Smoking (tobacco) complicating pregnancy, third trimester** Ⓜ♀

    O99.334 **Smoking (tobacco) complicating childbirth** Ⓜ♀

    O99.335 **Smoking (tobacco) complicating the puerperium** Ⓜ♀

√6ᵗʰ **O99.34** **Other mental disorders complicating pregnancy, childbirth, and the puerperium**
    Conditions in F01-F09 and F20-F99
    EXCLUDES 2   *postpartum mood disturbance (O90.6)*
         postnatal psychosis (F53)
         puerperal psychosis (F53)

    O99.340 **Other mental disorders complicating pregnancy, unspecified trimester** Ⓜ♀▽

    O99.341 **Other mental disorders complicating pregnancy, first trimester** Ⓜ♀

    O99.342 **Other mental disorders complicating pregnancy, second trimester** Ⓜ♀

    O99.343 **Other mental disorders complicating pregnancy, third trimester** Ⓜ♀

    O99.344 **Other mental disorders complicating childbirth** Ⓜ♀

    O99.345 **Other mental disorders complicating the puerperium** Ⓜ♀

√6ᵗʰ **O99.35** **Diseases of the nervous system complicating pregnancy, childbirth, and the puerperium**
    Conditions in G00-G99
    EXCLUDES 2   *pregnancy related peripheral neuritis (O26.8-)*

    O99.350 **Diseases of the nervous system complicating pregnancy, unspecified trimester** Ⓜ♀▽

    O99.351 **Diseases of the nervous system complicating pregnancy, first trimester** Ⓜ♀

    O99.352 **Diseases of the nervous system complicating pregnancy, second trimester** Ⓜ♀

    O99.353 **Diseases of the nervous system complicating pregnancy, third trimester** Ⓜ♀

    O99.354 **Diseases of the nervous system complicating childbirth** Ⓜ♀

    O99.355 **Diseases of the nervous system complicating the puerperium** Ⓜ♀

☑ Additional Character Req   √x7ᵗʰ Placeholder Alert   Manifestation   ᴴᶜᶜ CMS-HCC Condition   ▽ Unspecified Code   ►◄ Revised Text   ● New Code   ▲ Revised Code Title

Chapter 15. Pregnancy, Childbirth, and the Puerperium

☑5ᵗʰ **O99.4 Diseases of the circulatory system complicating pregnancy, childbirth and the puerperium**
Conditions in I00-I99

     EXCLUDES 1   *peripartum cardiomyopathy (O90.3)*
     EXCLUDES 2   *hypertensive disorders (O10-O16)*
              obstetric embolism (O88.-)
              venous complications and cerebrovenous sinus thrombosis in labor, childbirth and the puerperium (O87.-)
              venous complications and cerebrovenous sinus thrombosis in pregnancy (O22.-)

     AHA: 2016, 2Q, 8

   ☑6ᵗʰ **O99.41 Diseases of the circulatory system complicating pregnancy**
       O99.411 Diseases of the circulatory system complicating pregnancy, first trimester Ⓜ♀
       O99.412 Diseases of the circulatory system complicating pregnancy, second trimester Ⓜ♀
       O99.413 Diseases of the circulatory system complicating pregnancy, third trimester Ⓜ♀
       O99.419 Diseases of the circulatory system complicating pregnancy, unspecified trimester Ⓜ♀▽

     O99.42 Diseases of the circulatory system complicating childbirth Ⓜ♀

     O99.43 Diseases of the circulatory system complicating the puerperium Ⓜ♀

☑5ᵗʰ **O99.5 Diseases of the respiratory system complicating pregnancy, childbirth and the puerperium**
Conditions in J00-J99

   ☑6ᵗʰ **O99.51 Diseases of the respiratory system complicating pregnancy**
       O99.511 Diseases of the respiratory system complicating pregnancy, first trimester Ⓜ♀
       O99.512 Diseases of the respiratory system complicating pregnancy, second trimester Ⓜ♀
       O99.513 Diseases of the respiratory system complicating pregnancy, third trimester Ⓜ♀
       O99.519 Diseases of the respiratory system complicating pregnancy, unspecified trimester Ⓜ♀▽

     O99.52 Diseases of the respiratory system complicating childbirth Ⓜ♀

     O99.53 Diseases of the respiratory system complicating the puerperium Ⓜ♀

☑5ᵗʰ **O99.6 Diseases of the digestive system complicating pregnancy, childbirth and the puerperium**
Conditions in K00-K93

     EXCLUDES 2   *hemorrhoids in pregnancy (O22.4-)*
              liver and biliary tract disorders in pregnancy, childbirth and the puerperium (O26.6-)

   ☑6ᵗʰ **O99.61 Diseases of the digestive system complicating pregnancy**
       AHA: 2016, 1Q, 4
       O99.611 Diseases of the digestive system complicating pregnancy, first trimester Ⓜ♀
       O99.612 Diseases of the digestive system complicating pregnancy, second trimester Ⓜ♀
       O99.613 Diseases of the digestive system complicating pregnancy, third trimester Ⓜ♀
       O99.619 Diseases of the digestive system complicating pregnancy, unspecified trimester Ⓜ♀▽

     O99.62 Diseases of the digestive system complicating childbirth Ⓜ♀

     O99.63 Diseases of the digestive system complicating the puerperium Ⓜ♀

☑5ᵗʰ **O99.7 Diseases of the skin and subcutaneous tissue complicating pregnancy, childbirth and the puerperium**
Conditions in L00-L99

     EXCLUDES 2   *herpes gestationis (O26.4)*
              pruritic urticarial papules and plaques of pregnancy (PUPPP) (O26.86)

   ☑6ᵗʰ **O99.71 Diseases of the skin and subcutaneous tissue complicating pregnancy**
       O99.711 Diseases of the skin and subcutaneous tissue complicating pregnancy, first trimester Ⓜ♀
       O99.712 Diseases of the skin and subcutaneous tissue complicating pregnancy, second trimester Ⓜ♀
       O99.713 Diseases of the skin and subcutaneous tissue complicating pregnancy, third trimester Ⓜ♀
       O99.719 Diseases of the skin and subcutaneous tissue complicating pregnancy, unspecified trimester Ⓜ♀▽

     O99.72 Diseases of the skin and subcutaneous tissue complicating childbirth Ⓜ♀

     O99.73 Diseases of the skin and subcutaneous tissue complicating the puerperium Ⓜ♀

☑5ᵗʰ **O99.8 Other specified diseases and conditions complicating pregnancy, childbirth and the puerperium**
Conditions in D00-D48, H00-H95, M00-N99, and Q00-Q99
Use additional code to identify condition

     EXCLUDES 2   *genitourinary infections in pregnancy (O23.-)*
              infection of genitourinary tract following delivery (O86.1-O86.3)
              malignant neoplasm complicating pregnancy, childbirth and the puerperium (O9A.1-)
              maternal care for known or suspected abnormality of maternal pelvic organs (O34.-)
              postpartum acute kidney failure (O90.4)
              traumatic injuries in pregnancy (O9A.2)

   ☑6ᵗʰ **O99.81 Abnormal glucose complicating pregnancy, childbirth and the puerperium**
       EXCLUDES 1   *gestational diabetes (O24.4-)*
       O99.810 Abnormal glucose complicating pregnancy Ⓜ♀
       O99.814 Abnormal glucose complicating childbirth Ⓜ♀
       O99.815 Abnormal glucose complicating the puerperium Ⓜ♀

   ☑6ᵗʰ **O99.82 Streptococcus B carrier state complicating pregnancy, childbirth and the puerperium**
       EXCLUDES 1   *carrier of streptococcus group B (GBS) in a nonpregnant woman (Z22.330)*
       O99.820 Streptococcus B carrier state complicating pregnancy Ⓜ♀
       O99.824 Streptococcus B carrier state complicating childbirth Ⓜ♀
       O99.825 Streptococcus B carrier state complicating the puerperium Ⓜ♀

   ☑6ᵗʰ **O99.83 Other infection carrier state complicating pregnancy, childbirth and the puerperium**
       Use additional code to identify the carrier state (Z22.-)
       O99.830 Other infection carrier state complicating pregnancy Ⓜ♀
       O99.834 Other infection carrier state complicating childbirth Ⓜ♀
       O99.835 Other infection carrier state complicating the puerperium Ⓜ♀

   ☑6ᵗʰ **O99.84 Bariatric surgery status complicating pregnancy, childbirth and the puerperium**
       Gastric banding status complicating pregnancy, childbirth and the puerperium
       Gastric bypass status for obesity complicating pregnancy, childbirth and the puerperium
       Obesity surgery status complicating pregnancy, childbirth and the puerperium
       O99.840 Bariatric surgery status complicating pregnancy, unspecified trimester Ⓜ♀▽
       O99.841 Bariatric surgery status complicating pregnancy, first trimester Ⓜ♀
       O99.842 Bariatric surgery status complicating pregnancy, second trimester Ⓜ♀

EXCLUDES 1 Not coded here   EXCLUDES 2 Not included here   Ⓝ Newborn Age: 0   Ⓟ Pediatric Age: 0-17   Ⓜ Maternity Age: 12-55   Ⓐ Adult Age: 15-124

854   ICD-10-CM 2018

O99.843   **Bariatric surgery status complicating** Ⓜ♀ **pregnancy, third trimester**

O99.844   **Bariatric surgery status complicating** Ⓜ♀ **childbirth**

O99.845   **Bariatric surgery status complicating** Ⓜ♀ **the puerperium**

O99.89   **Other specified diseases and conditions** Ⓜ♀ **complicating pregnancy, childbirth and the puerperium**

√4ᵗʰ **O9A**   **Maternal malignant neoplasms, traumatic injuries and abuse classifiable elsewhere but complicating pregnancy, childbirth and the puerperium**

√5ᵗʰ **O9A.1**   **Malignant neoplasm complicating pregnancy, childbirth and the puerperium**
Conditions in C00-C96
Use additional code to identify neoplasm
EXCLUDES 2   *maternal care for benign tumor of corpus uteri (O34.1-)*
          maternal care for benign tumor of cervix (O34.4-)
AHA: 2015, 3Q, 19

√6ᵗʰ **O9A.11**   **Malignant neoplasm complicating pregnancy**

O9A.111   **Malignant neoplasm complicating** Ⓜ♀ **pregnancy, first trimester**

O9A.112   **Malignant neoplasm complicating** Ⓜ♀ **pregnancy, second trimester**

O9A.113   **Malignant neoplasm complicating** Ⓜ♀ **pregnancy, third trimester**

O9A.119   **Malignant neoplasm complicating** Ⓜ♀▽ **pregnancy, unspecified trimester**

O9A.12   **Malignant neoplasm complicating childbirth** Ⓜ♀

O9A.13   **Malignant neoplasm complicating the** Ⓜ♀ **puerperium**

√5ᵗʰ **O9A.2**   **Injury, poisoning and certain other consequences of external causes complicating pregnancy, childbirth and the puerperium**
Conditions in S00-T88, except T74 and T76
Use additional code(s) to identify the injury or poisoning
EXCLUDES 2   *physical, sexual and psychological abuse complicating pregnancy, childbirth and the puerperium (O9A.3-, O9A.4-, O9A.5-)*

√6ᵗʰ **O9A.21**   **Injury, poisoning and certain other consequences of external causes complicating pregnancy**

O9A.211   **Injury, poisoning and certain other** Ⓜ♀ **consequences of external causes complicating pregnancy, first trimester**

O9A.212   **Injury, poisoning and certain other** Ⓜ♀ **consequences of external causes complicating pregnancy, second trimester**

O9A.213   **Injury, poisoning and certain other** Ⓜ♀ **consequences of external causes complicating pregnancy, third trimester**

O9A.219   **Injury, poisoning and certain other** Ⓜ♀▽ **consequences of external causes complicating pregnancy, unspecified trimester**

O9A.22   **Injury, poisoning and certain other** Ⓜ♀ **consequences of external causes complicating childbirth**

O9A.23   **Injury, poisoning and certain other** Ⓜ♀ **consequencesof external causes complicating the puerperium**

√5ᵗʰ **O9A.3**   **Physical abuse complicating pregnancy, childbirth and the puerperium**
Conditions in T74.11 or T76.11
Use additional code (if applicable):
     to identify any associated current injury due to physical abuse
     to identify the perpetrator of abuse (Y07.-)
EXCLUDES 2   *sexual abuse complicating pregnancy, childbirth and the puerperium (O9A.4)*

√6ᵗʰ **O9A.31**   **Physical abuse complicating pregnancy**

O9A.311   **Physical abuse complicating** Ⓜ♀ **pregnancy, first trimester**

O9A.312   **Physical abuse complicating** Ⓜ♀ **pregnancy,second trimester**

O9A.313   **Physical abuse complicating** Ⓜ♀ **pregnancy, third trimester**

O9A.319   **Physical abuse complicating** Ⓜ♀▽ **pregnancy,unspecified trimester**

O9A.32   **Physical abuse complicating childbirth** Ⓜ♀

O9A.33   **Physical abuse complicating the puerperium** Ⓜ♀

√5ᵗʰ **O9A.4**   **Sexual abuse complicating pregnancy, childbirth and the puerperium**
Conditions in T74.21 or T76.21
Use additional code (if applicable):
     to identify any associated current injury due to sexual abuse
     to identify the perpetrator of abuse (Y07.-)

√6ᵗʰ **O9A.41**   **Sexual abuse complicating pregnancy**

O9A.411   **Sexual abuse complicating** Ⓜ♀ **pregnancy, first trimester**

O9A.412   **Sexual abuse complicating pregnancy,** Ⓜ♀ **second trimester**

O9A.413   **Sexual abuse complicating** Ⓜ♀ **pregnancy, third trimester**

O9A.419   **Sexual abuse complicating** Ⓜ♀▽ **pregnancy, unspecified trimester**

O9A.42   **Sexual abuse complicating childbirth** Ⓜ♀

O9A.43   **Sexual abuse complicating the puerperium** Ⓜ♀

√5ᵗʰ **O9A.5**   **Psychological abuse complicating pregnancy, childbirth and the puerperium**
Conditions in T74.31 or T76.31
Use additional code to identify the perpetrator of abuse (Y07.-)

√6ᵗʰ **O9A.51**   **Psychological abuse complicating pregnancy**

O9A.511   **Psychological abuse complicating** Ⓜ♀ **pregnancy, first trimester**

O9A.512   **Psychological abuse complicating** Ⓜ♀ **pregnancy, second trimester**

O9A.513   **Psychological abuse complicating** Ⓜ♀ **pregnancy, third trimester**

O9A.519   **Psychological abuse complicating** Ⓜ♀▽ **pregnancy, unspecified trimester**

O9A.52   **Psychological abuse complicating childbirth** Ⓜ♀

O9A.53   **Psychological abuse complicating the** Ⓜ♀ **puerperium**

Chapter 16. Certain Conditions Originating in the Perinatal Period (P00–P96)

Chapter Specific Guidelines with Coding Examples

The chapter specific guidelines from the ICD-10-CM Official Guidelines for Coding and Reporting have been provided below. Along with these guidelines are coding examples, contained in the shaded boxes, that have been developed to help illustrate the coding and/or sequencing guidance found in these guidelines.

For coding and reporting purposes the perinatal period is defined as before birth through the 28th day following birth. The following guidelines are provided for reporting purposes

a. General perinatal rules

1) Use of Chapter 16 codes

Codes in this chapter are <u>never</u> for use on the maternal record. Codes from Chapter 15, the obstetric chapter, are never permitted on the newborn record. Chapter 16 codes may be used throughout the life of the patient if the condition is still present.

2) Principal diagnosis for birth record

When coding the birth episode in a newborn record, assign a code from category Z38, Liveborn infants according to place of birth and type of delivery, as the principal diagnosis. A code from category Z38 is assigned only once, to a newborn at the time of birth. If a newborn is transferred to another institution, a code from category Z38 should not be used at the receiving hospital.

A code from category Z38 is used only on the newborn record, not on the mother's record.

3) Use of codes from other chapters with codes from Chapter 16

Codes from other chapters may be used with codes from chapter 16 if the codes from the other chapters provide more specific detail. Codes for signs and symptoms may be assigned when a definitive diagnosis has not been established. If the reason for the encounter is a perinatal condition, the code from chapter 16 should be sequenced first.

4) Use of Chapter 16 codes after the perinatal period

Should a condition originate in the perinatal period, and continue throughout the life of the patient, the perinatal code should continue to be used regardless of the patient's age.

> A 7-year-old patient with history of birth injury that resulted in Erb's palsy is seen for subscapularis release
>
> **P14.0**   **Erb's paralysis due to birth injury**
>
> *Explanation:* Although in this instance Erb's palsy is specifically related to a birth injury, it has not resolved and continues to be a health concern. A perinatal code is appropriate even though this patient is beyond the perinatal period.

5) Birth process or community acquired conditions

If a newborn has a condition that may be either due to the birth process or community acquired and the documentation does not indicate which it is, the default is due to the birth process and the code from Chapter 16 should be used. If the condition is community-acquired, a code from Chapter 16 should not be assigned.

6) Code all clinically significant conditions

All clinically significant conditions noted on routine newborn examination should be coded. A condition is clinically significant if it requires:

clinical evaluation; or

therapeutic treatment; or

diagnostic procedures; or

extended length of hospital stay; or

increased nursing care and/or monitoring; or

has implications for future health care needs

Note: The perinatal guidelines listed above are the same as the general coding guidelines for "additional diagnoses", except for the final point regarding implications for future health care needs. Codes should be assigned for conditions that have been specified by the provider as having implications for future health care needs.

b. Observation and evaluation of newborns for suspected conditions not found

1)
Assign a code from category Z05, Observation and evaluation of newborns and infants for suspected conditions ruled out, to identify those instances when a healthy newborn is evaluated for a suspected condition that is determined after study not to be present. Do not use a code from category Z05 when the patient has identified signs or symptoms of a suspected problem; in such cases code the sign or symptom.

2)
A code from category Z05 may also be assigned as a principal or first-listed code for readmissions or encounters when the code from category Z38 code no longer applies. Codes from category Z05 are for use only for healthy newborns and infants for which no condition after study is found to be present.

3) Z05 on a birth record

A code from category Z05 is to be used as a secondary code after the code from category Z38, Liveborn infants according to place of birth and type of delivery.

> Newborn delivered via vaginal delivery; previous ultrasounds showed what appeared to be an abnormality of the right kidney. Kidney function tests were performed and ultrasounds taken and any genitourinary conditions ruled out.
>
> **Z38.00**   **Single liveborn infant, delivered vaginally**
>
> **Z05.6**   **Observation and evaluation of newborn for suspected genitourinary condition ruled out**
>
> Explanation: The newborn had no signs or symptoms of kidney or other genitourinary condition but was evaluated after delivery due to the abnormal prenatal ultrasound findings. A Z code describing the type and place of birth should be coded first, followed by a Z05 category code for the work performed to rule out a suspected genitourinary condition.

c. Coding additional perinatal diagnoses

1) Assigning codes for conditions that require treatment

Assign codes for conditions that require treatment or further investigation, prolong the length of stay, or require resource utilization.

2) Codes for conditions specified as having implications for future health care needs

Assign codes for conditions that have been specified by the provider as having implications for future health care needs.

Note: This guideline should not be used for adult patients.

> An abnormal noise was heard in the left hip of a post-term newborn during a physical examination. The pediatrician would like to follow the patient after discharge as a hip click can be an early sign of hip dysplasia. The newborn was delivered via cesarean at 41 weeks.
>
> **Z38.01**   **Single liveborn infant, delivered by cesarean**
>
> **P08.21**   **Post-term newborn**
>
> **R29.4**   **Clicking hip**
>
> *Explanation:* The abnormal hip noise or click is appended as a secondary diagnosis not only because it is an abnormal finding upon examination, but also due to its potential to be part of a bigger health issue. The hip dysplasia has not yet been diagnosed and does not warrant a code at this time.

d. Prematurity and fetal growth retardation

Providers utilize different criteria in determining prematurity. A code for prematurity should not be assigned unless it is documented. Assignment of codes in categories P05, Disorders of newborn related to slow fetal growth and fetal malnutrition, and P07, Disorders of newborn related to short gestation and low birth weight, not elsewhere classified, should be based on the recorded birth weight and estimated gestational age. Codes from category P05 should not be assigned with codes from category P07.

When both birth weight and gestational age are available, two codes from category P07 should be assigned, with the code for birth weight sequenced before the code for gestational age.

e. Low birth weight and immaturity status

Codes from category P07, Disorders of newborn related to short gestation and low birth weight, not elsewhere classified, are for use for a child or adult who was premature or had a low birth weight as a newborn and this is affecting the patient's current health status.

See Section I.C.21. Factors influencing health status and contact with health services, Status.

A 35-year-old patient, who weighed 659 grams at birth, is seen for heart disease documented as being a consequence of the low birth weight

I51.9   Heart disease, unspecified

P07.02   Extremely low birth weight newborn, 500–749 grams

Explanation: A code from subcategories P07.0- and P07.1- is appropriate, regardless of the age of the patient, as long as the documentation provides a clear link between the patient's current illness and the low birth weight.

f. Bacterial sepsis of newborn

Category P36, Bacterial sepsis of newborn, includes congenital sepsis. If a perinate is documented as having sepsis without documentation of congenital or community acquired, the default is congenital and a code from category P36 should be assigned. If the P36 code includes the causal organism, an additional code from category B95, Streptococcus, Staphylococcus, and Enterococcus as the cause of diseases classified elsewhere, or B96, Other bacterial agents as the cause of diseases classified elsewhere, should not be assigned. If the P36 code does not include the causal organism, assign an additional code from category B96. If applicable, use additional codes to identify severe sepsis (R65.2-) and any associated acute organ dysfunction.

A full-term infant develops severe sepsis 24 hours after discharge from the hospital and is readmitted; cultures identified *E. coli* as the infective agent

P36.4   Sepsis of newborn due to Escherichia coli

R65.20   Severe sepsis without septic shock

Explanation: Even though this newborn was discharged and could have acquired *E. coli* from his/her external environment, due to the lack of documentation specifying specifically how this pathogen was acquired, the default is to code the *E. coli* sepsis as congenital. A code from chapter 1, "Certain Infectious and Parasitic Diseases," is not required because the perinatal sepsis code identifies both the sepsis and the bacteria causing the sepsis.

g. Stillbirth

Code P95, Stillbirth, is only for use in institutions that maintain separate records for stillbirths. No other code should be used with P95. Code P95 should not be used on the mother's record.

Chapter 16. Certain Conditions Originating in the Perinatal Period (P00-P96)

NOTE   Codes from this chapter are for use on newborn records only, never on maternal records.

INCLUDES   conditions that have their origin in the fetal or perinatal period (before birth through the first 28 days after birth) even if morbidity occurs later

EXCLUDES 2   congenital malformations, deformations and chromosomal abnormalities (Q00-Q99)
endocrine, nutritional and metabolic diseases (E00-E88)
injury, poisoning and certain other consequences of external causes (S00-T88)
neoplasms (C00-D49)
tetanus neonatorum (A33)

This chapter contains the following blocks:

P00-P04	Newborn affected by maternal factors and by complications of pregnancy, labor, and delivery
P05-P08	Disorders of newborn related to length of gestation and fetal growth
P09	Abnormal findings on neonatal screening
P10-P15	Birth trauma
P19-P29	Respiratory and cardiovascular disorders specific to the perinatal period
P35-P39	Infections specific to the perinatal period
P50-P61	Hemorrhagic and hematological disorders of newborn
P70-P74	Transitory endocrine and metabolic disorders specific to newborn
P76-P78	Digestive system disorders of newborn
P80-P83	Conditions involving the integument and temperature regulation of newborn
P84	Other problems with newborn
P90-P96	Other disorders originating in the perinatal period

Newborn affected by maternal factors and by complications of pregnancy, labor, and delivery (P00-P04)

NOTE   These codes are for use when the listed maternal conditions are specified as the cause of confirmed morbidity or potential morbidity which have their origin in the perinatal period (before birth through the first 28 days after birth).

✓4ᵗʰ P00   Newborn affected by maternal conditions that may be unrelated to present pregnancy

Code first any current condition in newborn

EXCLUDES 2   encounter for observation of newborn for suspected diseases and conditions ruled out (Z05.-)
newborn affected by maternal complications of pregnancy (P01.-)
newborn affected by maternal endocrine and metabolic disorders (P70-P74)
newborn affected by noxious substances transmitted via placenta or breast milk (P04.-)

P00.0   Newborn affected by maternal hypertensive disorders
Newborn affected by maternal conditions classifiable to O10-O11, O13-O16

P00.1   Newborn affected by maternal renal and urinary tract diseases
Newborn affected by maternal conditions classifiable to N00-N39

P00.2   Newborn affected by maternal infectious and parasitic diseases
Newborn affected by maternal infectious disease classifiable to A00-B99, J09 and J10

EXCLUDES 1   ~~infections specific to the perinatal period (P35-P39)~~
maternal genital tract or other localized infections (P00.8)

EXCLUDES 2 ▶ infections specific to the perinatal period (P35-P39)◀
AHA: 2015, 3Q, 20

P00.3   Newborn affected by other maternal circulatory and respiratory diseases
Newborn affected by maternal conditions classifiable to I00-I99, J00-J99, Q20-Q34 and not included in P00.0, P00.2

P00.4   Newborn affected by maternal nutritional disorders
Newborn affected by maternal disorders classifiable to E40-E64
Maternal malnutrition NOS

P00.5   Newborn affected by maternal injury
Newborn affected by maternal conditions classifiable to O9A.2-

P00.6   Newborn affected by surgical procedure on mother
Newborn affected by amniocentesis

EXCLUDES 1   Cesarean delivery for present delivery (P03.4)
damage to placenta from amniocentesis, Cesarean delivery or surgical induction (P02.1)
previous surgery to uterus or pelvic organs (P03.89)

EXCLUDES 2   newborn affected by complication of (fetal) intrauterine procedure (P96.5)

P00.7   Newborn affected by other medical procedures on mother, not elsewhere classified
Newborn affected by radiation to mother

EXCLUDES 1   damage to placenta from amniocentesis, cesarean delivery or surgical induction (P02.1)
newborn affected by other complications of labor and delivery (P03.-)

✓5ᵗʰ P00.8   Newborn affected by other maternal conditions

P00.81   Newborn affected by periodontal disease in mother

P00.89   Newborn affected by other maternal conditions
Newborn affected by conditions classifiable to T80-T88
Newborn affected by maternal genital tract or other localized infections
Newborn affected by maternal systemic lupus erythematosus

P00.9   Newborn affected by unspecified maternal condition ▽

✓4ᵗʰ P01   Newborn affected by maternal complications of pregnancy

Code first any current condition in newborn

EXCLUDES 2   encounter for observation of newborn for suspected diseases and conditions ruled out (Z05.-)

P01.0   Newborn affected by incompetent cervix

P01.1   Newborn affected by premature rupture of membranes

P01.2   Newborn affected by oligohydramnios
EXCLUDES 1   oligohydramnios due to premature rupture of membranes (P01.1)
DEF: Low amniotic fluid level, resulting in underdeveloped organs in the fetus.

P01.3   Newborn affected by polyhydramnios
Newborn affected by hydramnios

P01.4   Newborn affected by ectopic pregnancy
Newborn affected by abdominal pregnancy

P01.5   Newborn affected by multiple pregnancy
Newborn affected by triplet (pregnancy)
Newborn affected by twin (pregnancy)

P01.6   Newborn affected by maternal death

P01.7   Newborn affected by malpresentation before labor
Newborn affected by breech presentation before labor
Newborn affected by external version before labor
Newborn affected by face presentation before labor
Newborn affected by transverse lie before labor
Newborn affected by unstable lie before labor

P01.8   Newborn affected by other maternal complications of pregnancy

P01.9   Newborn affected by maternal complication of pregnancy, unspecified ▽

✓4ᵗʰ P02   Newborn affected by complications of placenta, cord and membranes

Code first any current condition in newborn

EXCLUDES 2   encounter for observation of newborn for suspected diseases and conditions ruled out (Z05.-)

P02.0   Newborn affected by placenta previa
DEF: Placenta developed in lower segment of uterus; can cause hemorrhaging leading to preterm delivery.

P02.1   Newborn affected by other forms of placental separation and hemorrhage
Newborn affected by abruptio placenta
Newborn affected by accidental hemorrhage
Newborn affected by antepartum hemorrhage
Newborn affected by damage to placenta from amniocentesis, cesarean delivery or surgical induction
Newborn affected by maternal blood loss
Newborn affected by premature separation of placenta

✓5ᵗʰ P02.2   Newborn affected by other and unspecified morphological and functional abnormalities of placenta

P02.20   Newborn affected by unspecified morphological ▽ **and functional abnormalities of placenta**

| ✓ Additional Character Req | ✓x7ᵗʰ Placeholder Alert | Manifestation | HCC CMS-HCC Condition | ▽ Unspecified Code | ▶◀ Revised Text | ● New Code | ▲ Revised Code Title |

ICD-10-CM 2018   859

P02.29   **Newborn affected by other morphological and functional abnormalities of placenta**
Newborn affected by placental dysfunction
Newborn affected by placental infarction
Newborn affected by placental insufficiency

P02.3   **Newborn affected by placental transfusion syndromes**
Newborn affected by placental and cord abnormalities resulting in twin-to-twin or other transplacental transfusion

P02.4   **Newborn affected by prolapsed cord**

P02.5   **Newborn affected by other compression of umbilical cord**
Newborn affected by umbilical cord (tightly) around neck
Newborn affected by entanglement of umbilical cord
Newborn affected by knot in umbilical cord

✓5ᵗʰ P02.6   **Newborn affected by other and unspecified conditions of umbilical cord**

    P02.60   **Newborn affected by unspecified conditions of umbilical cord**   ▽

    P02.69   **Newborn affected by other conditions of umbilical cord**
Newborn affected by short umbilical cord
Newborn affected by vasa previa
EXCLUDES 1   *newborn affected by single umbilical artery (Q27.0)*

P02.7   **Newborn affected by chorioamnionitis**
Newborn affected by amnionitis
Newborn affected by membranitis
Newborn affected by placentitis
DEF: Inflammation of the fetal membranes due to maternal infection; characterized by fetal tachycardia, respiratory distress, apnea, weak cries, and poor sucking.

P02.8   **Newborn affected by other abnormalities of membranes**

P02.9   **Newborn affected by abnormality of membranes, unspecified**   ▽

✓4ᵗʰ P03   **Newborn affected by other complications of labor and delivery**
Code first any current condition in newborn
EXCLUDES 2   *encounter for observation of newborn for suspected diseases and conditions ruled out (Z05.-)*

P03.0   **Newborn affected by breech delivery and extraction**

P03.1   **Newborn affected by other malpresentation, malposition and disproportion during labor and delivery**
Newborn affected by contracted pelvis
Newborn affected by conditions classifiable to O64-O66
Newborn affected by persistent occipitoposterior
Newborn affected by transverse lie

Forceps Assisted Birth

Forceps extractor

Vacuum Assisted Birth

Vacuum extractor

P03.2   **Newborn affected by forceps delivery**

P03.3   **Newborn affected by delivery by vacuum extractor [ventouse]**

P03.4   **Newborn affected by Cesarean delivery**

P03.5   **Newborn affected by precipitate delivery**
Newborn affected by rapid second stage

P03.6   **Newborn affected by abnormal uterine contractions**
Newborn affected by conditions classifiable to O62-, except O62.3
Newborn affected by hypertonic labor
Newborn affected by uterine inertia

✓5ᵗʰ P03.8   **Newborn affected by other specified complications of labor and delivery**

    ✓6ᵗʰ P03.81   **Newborn affected by abnormality in fetal (intrauterine) heart rate or rhythm**
EXCLUDES 1   *neonatal cardiac dysrhythmia (P29.1-)*

      P03.810   **Newborn affected by abnormality in fetal (intrauterine) heart rate or rhythm before the onset of labor**

      P03.811   **Newborn affected by abnormality in fetal (intrauterine) heart rate or rhythm during labor**

      P03.819   **Newborn affected by abnormality in fetal (intrauterine) heart rate or rhythm, unspecified as to time of onset**   ▽

    P03.82   **Meconium passage during delivery**
EXCLUDES 1   *meconium aspiration (P24.00, P24.01)*
meconium staining (P96.83)
DEF: Fetal intestinal activity that increases in response to a fetomaternal distressed state during delivery; the anal sphincter relaxes, and meconium is passed into the amniotic fluid.

    P03.89   **Newborn affected by other specified complications of labor and delivery**
Newborn affected by abnormality of maternal soft tissues
Newborn affected by conditions classifiable to O60-O75 and by procedures used in labor and delivery not included in P02.- and P03.0-P03.6
Newborn affected by induction of labor

P03.9   **Newborn affected by complication of labor and delivery, unspecified**   ▽

✓4ᵗʰ P04   **Newborn affected by noxious substances transmitted via placenta or breast milk**
INCLUDES   nonteratogenic effects of substances transmitted via placenta
EXCLUDES 2   *congenital malformations (Q00-Q99)*
encounter for observation of newborn for suspected diseases and conditions ruled out (Z05.-)
neonatal jaundice from excessive hemolysis due to drugs or toxins transmitted from mother (P58.4)
newborn in contact with and (suspected) exposures hazardous to health not transmitted via placenta or breast milk (Z77.-)

P04.0   **Newborn affected by maternal anesthesia and analgesia in pregnancy, labor and delivery**
Newborn affected by reactions and intoxications from maternal opiates and tranquilizers administered during labor and delivery

P04.1   **Newborn affected by other maternal medication**
Newborn affected by cancer chemotherapy
Newborn affected by cytotoxic drugs
EXCLUDES 1   *dysmorphism due to warfarin (Q86.2)*
fetal hydantoin syndrome (Q86.1)
maternal use of drugs of addiction (P04.4-)

P04.2   **Newborn affected by maternal use of tobacco**
Newborn affected by exposure in utero to tobacco smoke
EXCLUDES 2   *newborn exposure to environmental tobacco smoke (P96.81)*

P04.3   **Newborn affected by maternal use of alcohol**
EXCLUDES 1   *fetal alcohol syndrome (Q86.0)*

✓5ᵗʰ P04.4   **Newborn affected by maternal use of drugs of addiction**

    P04.41   **Newborn affected by maternal use of cocaine**
"Crack baby"

    P04.49   **Newborn affected by maternal use of other drugs of addiction**
EXCLUDES 2   *newborn affected by maternal anesthesia and analgesia (P04.0)*
withdrawal symptoms from maternal use of drugs of addiction (P96.1)

P04.5   **Newborn affected by maternal use of nutritional chemical substances**

P04.6   **Newborn affected by maternal exposure to environmental chemical substances**

P04.8   **Newborn affected by other maternal noxious substances**

P04.9   **Newborn affected by maternal noxious substance, unspecified** ▽

Disorders of newborn related to length of gestation and fetal growth (P05-P08)

✓4ᵗʰ **P05   Disorders of newborn related to slow fetal growth and fetal malnutrition**

✓5ᵗʰ   **P05.0   Newborn light for gestational age**
Newborn light-for-dates
Weight below but length above 10th percentile for gestational age

P05.00   **Newborn light for gestational age, unspecified weight** ▽

P05.01   **Newborn light for gestational age, less than 500 grams**

P05.02   **Newborn light for gestational age, 500-749 grams**

P05.03   **Newborn light for gestational age, 750-999 grams**

P05.04   **Newborn light for gestational age, 1000-1249 grams**

P05.05   **Newborn light for gestational age, 1250-1499 grams**

P05.06   **Newborn light for gestational age, 1500-1749 grams**

P05.07   **Newborn light for gestational age, 1750-1999 grams**

P05.08   **Newborn light for gestational age, 2000-2499 grams**

P05.09   **Newborn light for gestational age, 2500 grams and over**
Newborn light for gestational age, other

✓5ᵗʰ   **P05.1   Newborn small for gestational age**
Newborn small-and-light-for-dates
Newborn small-for-dates
Weight and length below 10th percentile for gestational age

P05.10   **Newborn small for gestational age, unspecified weight** ▽

P05.11   **Newborn small for gestational age, less than 500 grams**

P05.12   **Newborn small for gestational age, 500-749 grams**

P05.13   **Newborn small for gestational age, 750-999 grams**

P05.14   **Newborn small for gestational age, 1000-1249 grams**

P05.15   **Newborn small for gestational age, 1250-1499 grams**

P05.16   **Newborn small for gestational age, 1500-1749 grams**

P05.17   **Newborn small for gestational age, 1750-1999 grams**

P05.18   **Newborn small for gestational age, 2000-2499 grams**

P05.19   **Newborn small for gestational age, other**
Newborn small for gestational age, 2500 grams and over

P05.2   **Newborn affected by fetal (intrauterine) malnutrition not light or small for gestational age**
Infant, not light or small for gestational age, showing signs of fetal malnutrition, such as dry, peeling skin and loss of subcutaneous tissue
EXCLUDES 1   *newborn affected by fetal malnutrition with light for gestational age (P05.0-)*
newborn affected by fetal malnutrition with small for gestational age (P05.1-)

P05.9   **Newborn affected by slow intrauterine growth, unspecified** ▽
Newborn affected by fetal growth retardation NOS

✓4ᵗʰ **P07   Disorders of newborn related to short gestation and low birth weight, not elsewhere classified**
NOTE   When both birth weight and gestational age of the newborn are available, both should be coded with birth weight sequenced before gestational age
INCLUDES   the listed conditions, without further specification, as the cause of morbidity or additional care, in newborn

✓5ᵗʰ   **P07.0   Extremely low birth weight newborn**
Newborn birth weight 999 g. or less
EXCLUDES 1   *low birth weight due to slow fetal growth and fetal malnutrition (P05.-)*

P07.00   **Extremely low birth weight newborn, unspecified weight** ▽

P07.01   **Extremely low birth weight newborn, less than 500 grams**

P07.02   **Extremely low birth weight newborn, 500-749 grams**

P07.03   **Extremely low birth weight newborn, 750-999 grams**

✓5ᵗʰ   **P07.1   Other low birth weight newborn**
Newborn birth weight 1000-2499 g.
EXCLUDES 1   *low birth weight due to slow fetal growth and fetal malnutrition (P05.-)*

P07.10   **Other low birth weight newborn, unspecified weight** ▽

P07.14   **Other low birth weight newborn, 1000-1249 grams**

P07.15   **Other low birth weight newborn, 1250-1499 grams**

P07.16   **Other low birth weight newborn, 1500-1749 grams**

P07.17   **Other low birth weight newborn, 1750-1999 grams**

P07.18   **Other low birth weight newborn, 2000-2499 grams**

✓5ᵗʰ   **P07.2   Extreme immaturity of newborn**
Less than 28 completed weeks (less than 196 completed days) of gestation.

P07.20   **Extreme immaturity of newborn, unspecified weeks of gestation** ▽
Gestational age less than 28 completed weeks NOS

P07.21   **Extreme immaturity of newborn, gestational age less than 23 completed weeks**
Extreme immaturity of newborn, gestational age less than 23 weeks, 0 days

P07.22   **Extreme immaturity of newborn, gestational age 23 completed weeks**
Extreme immaturity of newborn, gestational age 23 weeks, 0 days through 23 weeks, 6 days

P07.23   **Extreme immaturity of newborn, gestational age 24 completed weeks**
Extreme immaturity of newborn, gestational age 24 weeks, 0 days through 24 weeks, 6 days

P07.24   **Extreme immaturity of newborn, gestational age 25 completed weeks**
Extreme immaturity of newborn, gestational age 25 weeks, 0 days through 25 weeks, 6 days

P07.25   **Extreme immaturity of newborn, gestational age 26 completed weeks**
Extreme immaturity of newborn, gestational age 26 weeks, 0 days through 26 weeks, 6 days

P07.26   **Extreme immaturity of newborn, gestational age 27 completed weeks**
Extreme immaturity of newborn, gestational age 27 weeks, 0 days through 27 weeks, 6 days

✓5ᵗʰ   **P07.3   Preterm [premature] newborn [other]**
28 completed weeks or more but less than 37 completed weeks (196 completed days but less than 259 completed days) of gestation
Prematurity NOS

P07.30   **Preterm newborn, unspecified weeks of gestation** ▽

P07.31   **Preterm newborn, gestational age 28 completed weeks**
Preterm newborn, gestational age 28 weeks, 0 days through 28 weeks, 6 days

P07.32   **Preterm newborn, gestational age 29 completed weeks**
Preterm newborn, gestational age 29 weeks, 0 days through 29 weeks, 6 days

P07.33   **Preterm newborn, gestational age 30 completed weeks**
Preterm newborn, gestational age 30 weeks, 0 days through 30 weeks, 6 days

---

☑ Additional Character Req   ☑x7ᵗʰ Placeholder Alert   Manifestation   HCC CMS-HCC Condition   ▽ Unspecified Code   ▶◀ Revised Text   ● New Code   ▲ Revised Code Title

P07.34 **Preterm newborn, gestational age 31 completed weeks**
Preterm newborn, gestational age 31 weeks, 0 days through 31 weeks, 6 days

P07.35 **Preterm newborn, gestational age 32 completed weeks**
Preterm newborn, gestational age 32 weeks, 0 days through 32 weeks, 6 days

P07.36 **Preterm newborn, gestational age 33 completed weeks**
Preterm newborn, gestational age 33 weeks, 0 days through 33 weeks, 6 days

P07.37 **Preterm newborn, gestational age 34 completed weeks**
Preterm newborn, gestational age 34 weeks, 0 days through 34 weeks, 6 days

P07.38 **Preterm newborn, gestational age 35 completed weeks**
Preterm newborn, gestational age 35 weeks, 0 days through 35 weeks, 6 days

P07.39 **Preterm newborn, gestational age 36 completed weeks**
Preterm newborn, gestational age 36 weeks, 0 days through 36 weeks, 6 days

✓4ᵗʰ **P08** **Disorders of newborn related to long gestation and high birth weight**

> **NOTE** When both birth weight and gestational age of the newborn are available, priority of assignment should be given to birth weight
>
> **INCLUDES** the listed conditions, without further specification, as causes of morbidity or additional care, in newborn

P08.0 **Exceptionally large newborn baby**
Usually implies a birth weight of 4500 g. or more
> **EXCLUDES 1** *syndrome of infant of diabetic mother (P70.1)*
> *syndrome of infant of mother with gestational diabetes (P70.0)*

P08.1 **Other heavy for gestational age newborn**
Other newborn heavy- or large-for-dates regardless of period of gestation
Usually implies a birth weight of 4000 g. to 4499 g.
> **EXCLUDES 1** *newborn with a birth weight of 4500 or more (P08.0)*
> *syndrome of infant of diabetic mother (P70.1)*
> *syndrome of infant of mother with gestational diabetes (P70.0).*

✓5ᵗʰ **P08.2** **Late newborn, not heavy for gestational age**
AHA: 2014, 1Q, 14

    P08.21 **Post-term newborn**
Newborn with gestation period over 40 completed weeks to 42 completed weeks

    P08.22 **Prolonged gestation of newborn**
Newborn with gestation period over 42 completed weeks (294 days or more), not heavy- or large-for-dates.
Postmaturity NOS

Abnormal findings on neonatal screening (P09)

P09 **Abnormal findings on neonatal screening**
Use additional code to identify signs, symptoms and conditions associated with the screening
> **EXCLUDES 2** *nonspecific serologic evidence of human immunodeficiency virus [HIV] (R75)*

Birth trauma (P10-P15)

✓4ᵗʰ **P10** **Intracranial laceration and hemorrhage due to birth injury**
> **EXCLUDES 1** *intracranial hemorrhage of newborn NOS (P52.9)*
> *intracranial hemorrhage of newborn due to anoxia or hypoxia (P52.-)*
> *nontraumatic intracranial hemorrhage of newborn (P52.-)*

P10.0 **Subdural hemorrhage due to birth injury**
Subdural hematoma (localized) due to birth injury
> **EXCLUDES 1** *subdural hemorrhage accompanying tentorial tear (P10.4)*

P10.1 **Cerebral hemorrhage due to birth injury**

P10.2 **Intraventricular hemorrhage due to birth injury**

P10.3 **Subarachnoid hemorrhage due to birth injury**

P10.4 **Tentorial tear due to birth injury**

P10.8 **Other intracranial lacerations and hemorrhages due to birth injury**

Birth Injuries to Scalp

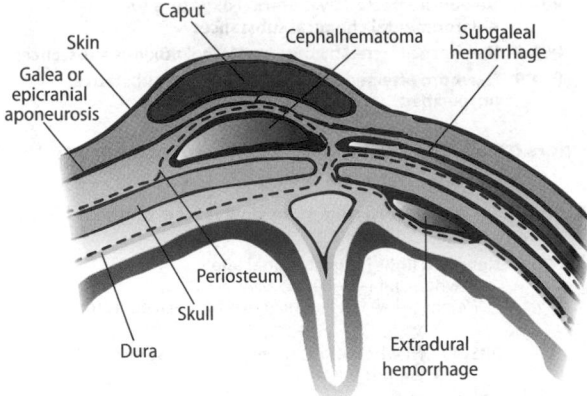

P10.9 **Unspecified intracranial laceration and hemorrhage due to birth injury** ▽

✓4ᵗʰ **P11** **Other birth injuries to central nervous system**

P11.0 **Cerebral edema due to birth injury**

P11.1 **Other specified brain damage due to birth injury**

P11.2 **Unspecified brain damage due to birth injury** ▽

P11.3 **Birth injury to facial nerve**
Facial palsy due to birth injury

P11.4 **Birth injury to other cranial nerves**

P11.5 **Birth injury to spine and spinal cord**
Fracture of spine due to birth injury

P11.9 **Birth injury to central nervous system, unspecified** ▽

✓4ᵗʰ **P12** **Birth injury to scalp**

P12.0 **Cephalhematoma due to birth injury**

P12.1 **Chignon (from vacuum extraction) due to birth injury**

P12.2 **Epicranial subaponeurotic hemorrhage due to birth injury**
Subgaleal hemorrhage

P12.3 **Bruising of scalp due to birth injury**

P12.4 **Injury of scalp of newborn due to monitoring equipment**
Sampling incision of scalp of newborn
Scalp clip (electrode) injury of newborn

✓5ᵗʰ **P12.8** **Other birth injuries to scalp**

    P12.81 **Caput succedaneum**

    P12.89 **Other birth injuries to scalp**

P12.9 **Birth injury to scalp, unspecified** ▽

✓4ᵗʰ **P13** **Birth injury to skeleton**
> **EXCLUDES 2** *birth injury to spine (P11.5)*

P13.0 **Fracture of skull due to birth injury**

P13.1 **Other birth injuries to skull**
> **EXCLUDES 1** *cephalhematoma (P12.0)*

P13.2 **Birth injury to femur**

P13.3 **Birth injury to other long bones**

P13.4 **Fracture of clavicle due to birth injury**

P13.8 **Birth injuries to other parts of skeleton**

P13.9 **Birth injury to skeleton, unspecified** ▽

✓4ᵗʰ **P14** **Birth injury to peripheral nervous system**

P14.0 **Erb's paralysis due to birth injury**

P14.1 **Klumpke's paralysis due to birth injury**

P14.2 **Phrenic nerve paralysis due to birth injury**

P14.3 **Other brachial plexus birth injuries**

P14.8 **Birth injuries to other parts of peripheral nervous system**

P14.9 **Birth injury to peripheral nervous system, unspecified** ▽

✓4ᵗʰ **P15** **Other birth injuries**

P15.0 **Birth injury to liver**
Rupture of liver due to birth injury

P15.1 **Birth injury to spleen**
Rupture of spleen due to birth injury

P15.2 **Sternomastoid injury due to birth injury**

P15.3 **Birth injury to eye**
Subconjunctival hemorrhage due to birth injury
Traumatic glaucoma due to birth injury

EXCLUDES 1 Not coded here   **EXCLUDES 2** Not included here   **N** Newborn Age: 0   **P** Pediatric Age: 0-17   **M** Maternity Age: 12-55   **A** Adult Age: 15-124

862   ICD-10-CM 2018

P15.4 Birth injury to face
Facial congestion due to birth injury

P15.5 Birth injury to external genitalia

P15.6 Subcutaneous fat necrosis due to birth injury

P15.8 Other specified birth injuries
TIP: Use for any injury of newborn from scalpel.

P15.9 Birth injury, unspecified ▽

Respiratory and cardiovascular disorders specific to the perinatal period (P19-P29)

☑4ᵗʰ **P19 Metabolic acidemia in newborn**
[INCLUDES] metabolic acidemia in newborn

P19.0 Metabolic acidemia in newborn first noted before onset of labor

P19.1 Metabolic acidemia in newborn first noted during labor

P19.2 Metabolic acidemia noted at birth

P19.9 Metabolic acidemia, unspecified ▽

☑4ᵗʰ **P22 Respiratory distress of newborn**
EXCLUDES 1   *respiratory arrest of newborn (P28.81)*
respiratory failure of newborn NOS (P28.5)

P22.0 Respiratory distress syndrome of newborn
Cardiorespiratory distress syndrome of newborn
Hyaline membrane disease
Idiopathic respiratory distress syndrome [IRDS or RDS] of newborn
Pulmonary hypoperfusion syndrome
Respiratory distress syndrome, type I
DEF: Severe chest contractions upon air intake and expiratory grunting; infant appears blue due to oxygen deficiency and has rapid respiratory rate; formerly called hyaline membrane disease.

P22.1 Transient tachypnea of newborn
Idiopathic tachypnea of newborn
Respiratory distress syndrome, type II
Wet lung syndrome
DEF: Rapid, labored breathing of newborn; short-term problem that begins after birth and lasts about three days.

P22.8 Other respiratory distress of newborn

P22.9 Respiratory distress of newborn, unspecified ▽

☑4ᵗʰ **P23 Congenital pneumonia**
[INCLUDES] infective pneumonia acquired in utero or during birth
EXCLUDES 1 *neonatal pneumonia resulting from aspiration (P24.-)*

P23.0 Congenital pneumonia due to viral agent
Use additional code (B97) to identify organism
EXCLUDES 1   *congenital rubella pneumonitis (P35.0)*

P23.1 Congenital pneumonia due to Chlamydia

P23.2 Congenital pneumonia due to staphylococcus

P23.3 Congenital pneumonia due to streptococcus, group B

P23.4 Congenital pneumonia due to Escherichia coli

P23.5 Congenital pneumonia due to Pseudomonas

P23.6 Congenital pneumonia due to other bacterial agents
Congenital pneumonia due to Hemophilus influenzae
Congenital pneumonia due to Klebsiella pneumoniae
Congenital pneumonia due to Mycoplasma
Congenital pneumonia due to Streptococcus, except group B
Use additional code (B95-B96) to identify organism

P23.8 Congenital pneumonia due to other organisms

P23.9 Congenital pneumonia, unspecified ▽

☑4ᵗʰ **P24 Neonatal aspiration**
[INCLUDES] aspiration in utero and during delivery

☑5ᵗʰ **P24.0 Meconium aspiration**
EXCLUDES 1   *meconium passage (without aspiration) during delivery (P03.82)*
meconium staining (P96.83)

P24.00 Meconium aspiration without respiratory symptoms
Meconium aspiration NOS

P24.01 Meconium aspiration with respiratory symptoms
Meconium aspiration pneumonia
Meconium aspiration pneumonitis
Meconium aspiration syndrome NOS
Use additional code to identify any secondary pulmonary hypertension, if applicable ▶(I27.2-)◀
DEF: Aspiration of fetal intestinal material during or prior to delivery; usually a complication of placental insufficiency, causing pneumonitis and bronchial obstruction (inflammatory reaction of lungs).

☑5ᵗʰ **P24.1 Neonatal aspiration of (clear) amniotic fluid and mucus**
Neonatal aspiration of liquor (amnii)

P24.10 Neonatal aspiration of (clear) amniotic fluid and mucus without respiratory symptoms
Neonatal aspiration of amniotic fluid and mucus NOS

P24.11 Neonatal aspiration of (clear) amniotic fluid and mucus with respiratory symptoms
Neonatal aspiration of amniotic fluid and mucus with pneumonia
Neonatal aspiration of amniotic fluid and mucus with pneumonitis
Use additional code to identify any secondary pulmonary hypertension, if applicable ▶(I27.2-)◀

☑5ᵗʰ **P24.2 Neonatal aspiration of blood**

P24.20 Neonatal aspiration of blood without respiratory symptoms
Neonatal aspiration of blood NOS

P24.21 Neonatal aspiration of blood with respiratory symptoms
Neonatal aspiration of blood with pneumonia
Neonatal aspiration of blood with pneumonitis
Use additional code to identify any secondary pulmonary hypertension, if applicable ▶(I27.2-)◀

☑5ᵗʰ **P24.3 Neonatal aspiration of milk and regurgitated food**
Neonatal aspiration of stomach contents

P24.30 Neonatal aspiration of milk and regurgitated food without respiratory symptoms
Neonatal aspiration of milk and regurgitated food NOS

P24.31 Neonatal aspiration of milk and regurgitated food with respiratory symptoms
Neonatal aspiration of milk and regurgitated food with pneumonia
Neonatal aspiration of milk and regurgitated food with pneumonitis
Use additional code to identify any secondary pulmonary hypertension, if applicable ▶(I27.2-)◀

☑5ᵗʰ **P24.8 Other neonatal aspiration**

P24.80 Other neonatal aspiration without respiratory symptoms
Neonatal aspiration NEC

P24.81 Other neonatal aspiration with respiratory symptoms
Neonatal aspiration pneumonia NEC
Neonatal aspiration with pneumonitis NEC
Neonatal aspiration with pneumonia NOS
Neonatal aspiration with pneumonitis NOS
Use additional code to identify any secondary pulmonary hypertension, if applicable ▶(I27.2-)◀

P24.9 Neonatal aspiration, unspecified ▽

☑4ᵗʰ **P25 Interstitial emphysema and related conditions originating in the perinatal period**

P25.0 Interstitial emphysema originating in the perinatal period

P25.1 Pneumothorax originating in the perinatal period

P25.2 Pneumomediastinum originating in the perinatal period

P25.3 Pneumopericardium originating in the perinatal period

P25.8 Other conditions related to interstitial emphysema originating in the perinatal period

☑4ᵗʰ **P26 Pulmonary hemorrhage originating in the perinatal period**
EXCLUDES 1   *acute idiopathic hemorrhage in infants over 28 days old (R04.81)*

P26.0 Tracheobronchial hemorrhage originating in the perinatal period

P26.1 Massive pulmonary hemorrhage originating in the perinatal period

P26.8 Other pulmonary hemorrhages originating in the perinatal period

P26.9 Unspecified pulmonary hemorrhage originating in the perinatal period ▽

☑4ᵗʰ **P27 Chronic respiratory disease originating in the perinatal period**
EXCLUDES 1   *respiratory distress of newborn (P22.0-P22.9)*
EXCLUDES 2 ▶*respiratory distress of newborn (P22.0-P22.9)*◀

P27.0 Wilson-Mikity syndrome
Pulmonary dysmaturity

P27.1 Bronchopulmonary dysplasia originating in the perinatal period

☑ Additional Character Req   x7ᵗʰ Placeholder Alert   Manifestation   HCC CMS-HCC Condition   ▽ Unspecified Code   ▶◀ Revised Text   ● New Code   ▲ Revised Code Title

ICD-10-CM 2018   863

P27.8 **Other chronic respiratory diseases originating in the perinatal period**
Congenital pulmonary fibrosis
Ventilator lung in newborn

P27.9 **Unspecified chronic respiratory disease originating in the perinatal period** ▽

√4ᵗʰ **P28** **Other respiratory conditions originating in the perinatal period**
EXCLUDES 1 congenital malformations of the respiratory system (Q30-Q34)

P28.0 **Primary atelectasis of newborn**
Primary failure to expand terminal respiratory units
Pulmonary hypoplasia associated with short gestation
Pulmonary immaturity NOS

√5ᵗʰ **P28.1** **Other and unspecified atelectasis of newborn**

P28.10 **Unspecified atelectasis of newborn** ▽
Atelectasis of newborn NOS

P28.11 **Resorption atelectasis without respiratory distress syndrome**
EXCLUDES 1 resorption atelectasis with respiratory distress syndrome (P22.0)

P28.19 **Other atelectasis of newborn**
Partial atelectasis of newborn
Secondary atelectasis of newborn

P28.2 **Cyanotic attacks of newborn**
EXCLUDES 1 apnea of newborn (P28.3-P28.4)

P28.3 **Primary sleep apnea of newborn**
Central sleep apnea of newborn
Obstructive sleep apnea of newborn
Sleep apnea of newborn NOS
DEF: Unexplained cessation of breathing when a neonate makes no respiratory effort for 20 seconds or longer, or when neonate's breathing cessation is accompanied by cyanosis, bradycardia, or hypotonia.

P28.4 **Other apnea of newborn**
Apnea of prematurity
Obstructive apnea of newborn
EXCLUDES 1 obstructive sleep apnea of newborn (P28.3)

P28.5 **Respiratory failure of newborn**
EXCLUDES 1 respiratory arrest of newborn (P28.81)
respiratory distress of newborn (P22.0-)

√5ᵗʰ **P28.8** **Other specified respiratory conditions of newborn**

P28.81 **Respiratory arrest of newborn**

P28.89 **Other specified respiratory conditions of newborn**
Congenital laryngeal stridor
Sniffles in newborn
Snuffles in newborn
EXCLUDES 1 early congenital syphilitic rhinitis (A50.05)

P28.9 **Respiratory condition of newborn, unspecified** ▽
Respiratory depression in newborn

√4ᵗʰ **P29** **Cardiovascular disorders originating in the perinatal period**
EXCLUDES 1 congenital malformations of the circulatory system (Q20-Q28)

P29.0 **Neonatal cardiac failure**

√5ᵗʰ **P29.1** **Neonatal cardiac dysrhythmia**

P29.11 **Neonatal tachycardia**

P29.12 **Neonatal bradycardia**

P29.2 **Neonatal hypertension**

√5ᵗʰ **P29.3** **Persistent fetal circulation**
~~Delayed closure of ductus arteriosus~~
~~(Persistent) pulmonary hypertension of newborn~~

● **P29.30** **Pulmonary hypertension of newborn**
Persistent pulmonary hypertension of newborn

● **P29.38** **Other persistent fetal circulation**
Delayed closure of ductus arteriosus

P29.4 **Transient myocardial ischemia in newborn**

√5ᵗʰ **P29.8** **Other cardiovascular disorders originating in the perinatal period**

P29.81 **Cardiac arrest of newborn**

P29.89 **Other cardiovascular disorders originating in the perinatal period**
AHA: 2014, 4Q, 23

P29.9 **Cardiovascular disorder originating in the perinatal period, unspecified** ▽

Infections specific to the perinatal period (P35-P39)

Infections acquired in utero, during birth via the umbilicus, or during the first 28 days after birth

EXCLUDES 2 asymptomatic human immunodeficiency virus [HIV] infection status (Z21)
congenital gonococcal infection (A54.-)
congenital pneumonia (P23.-)
congenital syphilis (A50.-)
human immunodeficiency virus [HIV] disease (B20)
infant botulism (A48.51)
infectious diseases not specific to the perinatal period (A00-B99, J09, J10-)
intestinal infectious disease (A00-A09)
laboratory evidence of human immunodeficiency virus [HIV] (R75)
tetanus neonatorum (A33)

√4ᵗʰ **P35** **Congenital viral diseases**
INCLUDES infections acquired in utero or during birth

P35.0 **Congenital rubella syndrome**
Congenital rubella pneumonitis

P35.1 **Congenital cytomegalovirus infection**

P35.2 **Congenital herpesviral [herpes simplex] infection**

P35.3 **Congenital viral hepatitis**

P35.8 **Other congenital viral diseases**
Congenital varicella [chickenpox]

P35.9 **Congenital viral disease, unspecified** ▽

√4ᵗʰ **P36** **Bacterial sepsis of newborn**
INCLUDES congenital sepsis
Use additional code(s), if applicable, to identify severe sepsis (R65.2-) and associated acute organ dysfunction(s)

P36.0 **Sepsis of newborn due to streptococcus, group B** HCC

√5ᵗʰ **P36.1** **Sepsis of newborn due to other and unspecified streptococci**

P36.10 **Sepsis of newborn due to unspecified streptococci** HCC ▽

P36.19 **Sepsis of newborn due to other streptococci** HCC

P36.2 **Sepsis of newborn due to Staphylococcus aureus** HCC

√5ᵗʰ **P36.3** **Sepsis of newborn due to other and unspecified staphylococci**

P36.30 **Sepsis of newborn due to unspecified staphylococci** HCC ▽

P36.39 **Sepsis of newborn due to other staphylococci** HCC

P36.4 **Sepsis of newborn due to Escherichia coli** HCC

P36.5 **Sepsis of newborn due to anaerobes** HCC

P36.8 **Other bacterial sepsis of newborn** HCC
Use additional code from category B96 to identify organism

P36.9 **Bacterial sepsis of newborn, unspecified** HCC ▽

√4ᵗʰ **P37** **Other congenital infectious and parasitic diseases**
EXCLUDES 2 congenital syphilis (A50.-)
infectious neonatal diarrhea (A00-A09)
necrotizing enterocolitis in newborn (P77.-)
noninfectious neonatal diarrhea (P78.3)
ophthalmia neonatorum due to gonococcus (A54.31)
tetanus neonatorum (A33)

P37.0 **Congenital tuberculosis**

P37.1 **Congenital toxoplasmosis**
Hydrocephalus due to congenital toxoplasmosis

P37.2 **Neonatal (disseminated) listeriosis**

P37.3 **Congenital falciparum malaria**

P37.4 **Other congenital malaria**

P37.5 **Neonatal candidiasis**

P37.8 **Other specified congenital infectious and parasitic diseases**

P37.9 **Congenital infectious or parasitic disease, unspecified** ▽

√4ᵗʰ **P38** **Omphalitis of newborn**
EXCLUDES 1 omphalitis not of newborn (L08.82)
tetanus omphalitis (A33)
umbilical hemorrhage of newborn (P51.-)

P38.1 **Omphalitis with mild hemorrhage**

P38.9 **Omphalitis without hemorrhage**
Omphalitis of newborn NOS

EXCLUDES 1 Not coded here   EXCLUDES 2 Not included here   N Newborn Age: 0   P Pediatric Age: 0-17   M Maternity Age: 12-55   A Adult Age: 15-124

864   ICD-10-CM 2018

✓4ᵗʰ **P39 Other infections specific to the perinatal period**
Use additional code to identify organism or specific infection

P39.0 Neonatal infective mastitis
EXCLUDES 1   *breast engorgement of newborn (P83.4)*
       noninfective mastitis of newborn (P83.4)

P39.1 Neonatal conjunctivitis and dacryocystitis
Neonatal chlamydial conjunctivitis
Ophthalmia neonatorum NOS
EXCLUDES 1   *gonococcal conjunctivitis (A54.31)*

P39.2 Intra-amniotic infection affecting newborn, not elsewhere classified

P39.3 Neonatal urinary tract infection

P39.4 Neonatal skin infection
Neonatal pyoderma
EXCLUDES 1   *pemphigus neonatorum (L00)*
       staphylococcal scalded skin syndrome (L00)

P39.8 Other specified infections specific to the perinatal period

P39.9 Infection specific to the perinatal period, unspecified ▽

Hemorrhagic and hematological disorders of newborn (P50-P61)

EXCLUDES 1   *congenital stenosis and stricture of bile ducts (Q44.3)*
       Crigler-Najjar syndrome (E80.5)
       Dubin-Johnson syndrome (E80.6)
       Gilbert syndrome (E80.4)
       hereditary hemolytic anemias (D55-D58)

✓4ᵗʰ **P50 Newborn affected by intrauterine (fetal) blood loss**
EXCLUDES 1   *congenital anemia from intrauterine (fetal) blood loss (P61.3)*

P50.0 Newborn affected by intrauterine (fetal) blood loss from vasa previa

P50.1 Newborn affected by intrauterine (fetal) blood loss from ruptured cord

P50.2 Newborn affected by intrauterine (fetal) blood loss from placenta

P50.3 Newborn affected by hemorrhage into co-twin

P50.4 Newborn affected by hemorrhage into maternal circulation

P50.5 Newborn affected by intrauterine (fetal) blood loss from cut end of co-twin's cord

P50.8 Newborn affected by other intrauterine (fetal) blood loss

P50.9 Newborn affected by intrauterine (fetal) blood loss, unspecified ▽
Newborn affected by fetal hemorrhage NOS

✓4ᵗʰ **P51 Umbilical hemorrhage of newborn**
EXCLUDES 1   *omphalitis with mild hemorrhage (P38.1)*
       umbilical hemorrhage from cut end of co-twins cord (P50.5)

P51.0 Massive umbilical hemorrhage of newborn

P51.8 Other umbilical hemorrhages of newborn
Slipped umbilical ligature NOS

P51.9 Umbilical hemorrhage of newborn, unspecified ▽

✓4ᵗʰ **P52 Intracranial nontraumatic hemorrhage of newborn**
INCLUDES   intracranial hemorrhage due to anoxia or hypoxia
EXCLUDES 1   *intracranial hemorrhage due to birth injury (P10.-)*
       intracranial hemorrhage due to other injury (S06.-)

P52.0 Intraventricular (nontraumatic) hemorrhage, grade 1, of newborn
Subependymal hemorrhage (without intraventricular extension)
Bleeding into germinal matrix

P52.1 Intraventricular (nontraumatic) hemorrhage, grade 2, of newborn
Subependymal hemorrhage with intraventricular extension
Bleeding into ventricle

✓5ᵗʰ **P52.2 Intraventricular (nontraumatic) hemorrhage, grade 3 and grade 4, of newborn**

     P52.21 Intraventricular (nontraumatic) hemorrhage, grade 3, of newborn
         Subependymal hemorrhage with intraventricular extension with enlargement of ventricle

     P52.22 Intraventricular (nontraumatic) hemorrhage, grade 4, of newborn
         Bleeding into cerebral cortex
         Subependymal hemorrhage with intracerebral extension

P52.3 Unspecified intraventricular (nontraumatic) hemorrhage of newborn ▽

P52.4 Intracerebral (nontraumatic) hemorrhage of newborn

P52.5 Subarachnoid (nontraumatic) hemorrhage of newborn

P52.6 Cerebellar (nontraumatic) and posterior fossa hemorrhage of newborn

P52.8 Other intracranial (nontraumatic) hemorrhages of newborn

P52.9 Intracranial (nontraumatic) hemorrhage of newborn, unspecified ▽

P53 Hemorrhagic disease of newborn
Vitamin K deficiency of newborn

✓4ᵗʰ **P54 Other neonatal hemorrhages**
EXCLUDES 1   *newborn affected by (intrauterine) blood loss (P50.-)*
       pulmonary hemorrhage originating in the perinatal period (P26.-)

P54.0 Neonatal hematemesis
EXCLUDES 1   *neonatal hematemesis due to swallowed maternal blood (P78.2)*

P54.1 Neonatal melena
EXCLUDES 1   *neonatal melena due to swallowed maternal blood (P78.2)*

P54.2 Neonatal rectal hemorrhage

P54.3 Other neonatal gastrointestinal hemorrhage

P54.4 Neonatal adrenal hemorrhage

P54.5 Neonatal cutaneous hemorrhage
Neonatal bruising
Neonatal ecchymoses
Neonatal petechiae
Neonatal superficial hematomata
EXCLUDES 2   *bruising of scalp due to birth injury (P12.3)*
       cephalhematoma due to birth injury (P12.0)

P54.6 Neonatal vaginal hemorrhage ♀
Neonatal pseudomenses

P54.8 Other specified neonatal hemorrhages

P54.9 Neonatal hemorrhage, unspecified ▽

✓4ᵗʰ **P55 Hemolytic disease of newborn**

P55.0 Rh isoimmunization of newborn
DEF: Incompatible Rh fetal-maternal blood grouping; prematurely destroys red blood cells; characterized by jaundice, asphyxia, pulmonary hypertension, edema, respiratory distress, kernicterus, and coagulopathies; detected by Coombs test.

P55.1 ABO isoimmunization of newborn
AHA: 2015, 3Q, 20

P55.8 Other hemolytic diseases of newborn

P55.9 Hemolytic disease of newborn, unspecified ▽

✓4ᵗʰ **P56 Hydrops fetalis due to hemolytic disease**
EXCLUDES 1   *hydrops fetalis NOS (P83.2)*

P56.0 Hydrops fetalis due to isoimmunization

✓5ᵗʰ **P56.9 Hydrops fetalis due to other and unspecified hemolytic disease**

     P56.90 Hydrops fetalis due to unspecified hemolytic disease ▽

     P56.99 Hydrops fetalis due to other hemolytic disease

✓4ᵗʰ **P57 Kernicterus**

P57.0 Kernicterus due to isoimmunization
DEF: Complication of erythroblastosis fetalis associated with severe neural symptoms, high blood bilirubin levels and nerve cell destruction; results in bilirubin-pigmented gray matter of central nervous system.

P57.8 Other specified kernicterus
EXCLUDES 1   *Crigler-Najjar syndrome (E80.5)*

P57.9 Kernicterus, unspecified ▽

✓4ᵗʰ **P58 Neonatal jaundice due to other excessive hemolysis**
EXCLUDES 1   *jaundice due to isoimmunization (P55-P57)*

P58.0 Neonatal jaundice due to bruising

P58.1 Neonatal jaundice due to bleeding

P58.2 Neonatal jaundice due to infection

P58.3 Neonatal jaundice due to polycythemia

✓5ᵗʰ **P58.4 Neonatal jaundice due to drugs or toxins transmitted from mother or given to newborn**
Code first poisoning due to drug or toxin, if applicable (T36-T65 with fifth or sixth character 1-4 or 6)
Use additional code for adverse effect, if applicable, to identify drug (T36-T50 with fifth or sixth character 5)

     P58.41 Neonatal jaundice due to drugs or toxins transmitted from mother

     P58.42 Neonatal jaundice due to drugs or toxins given to newborn

✔ Additional Character Req   ✓7ᵗʰ Placeholder Alert   Manifestation   HCC CMS-HCC Condition   ▽ Unspecified Code   ►◄ Revised Text   ● New Code   ▲ Revised Code Title

ICD-10-CM 2018   **865**

Chapter 16. Certain Conditions Originating in the Perinatal Period

P58.5–P77.2

P58.5   **Neonatal jaundice due to swallowed maternal blood**

P58.8   **Neonatal jaundice due to other specified excessive hemolysis**

P58.9   **Neonatal jaundice due to excessive hemolysis, unspecified**   ▽

✓4ᵗʰ **P59**   **Neonatal jaundice from other and unspecified causes**
> EXCLUDES 1   *jaundice due to inborn errors of metabolism (E70-E88)*
> *kernicterus (P57.-)*

P59.0   **Neonatal jaundice associated with preterm delivery**
Hyperbilirubinemia of prematurity
Jaundice due to delayed conjugation associated with preterm delivery

P59.1   **Inspissated bile syndrome**

✓5ᵗʰ **P59.2**   **Neonatal jaundice from other and unspecified hepatocellular damage**
> EXCLUDES 1   *congenital viral hepatitis (P35.3)*

     P59.20   **Neonatal jaundice from unspecified hepatocellular damage**   ▽

     P59.29   **Neonatal jaundice from other hepatocellular damage**
         Neonatal giant cell hepatitis
         Neonatal (idiopathic) hepatitis

P59.3   **Neonatal jaundice from breast milk inhibitor**

P59.8   **Neonatal jaundice from other specified causes**

P59.9   **Neonatal jaundice, unspecified**   ▽
Neonatal physiological jaundice (intense)(prolonged) NOS
AHA: 2015, 3Q, 20

P60   **Disseminated intravascular coagulation of newborn**
Defibrination syndrome of newborn

✓4ᵗʰ **P61**   **Other perinatal hematological disorders**
> EXCLUDES 1   *transient hypogammaglobulinemia of infancy (D80.7)*

P61.0   **Transient neonatal thrombocytopenia**
Neonatal thrombocytopenia due to exchange transfusion
Neonatal thrombocytopenia due to idiopathic maternal thrombocytopenia
Neonatal thrombocytopenia due to isoimmunization
DEF: Temporary decrease in blood platelets of newborn; secondary to placental insufficiency.

P61.1   **Polycythemia neonatorum**
DEF: Abnormal increase of total red blood cells of newborn; results in hyperviscosity, which slows the flow of blood through small blood vessels.

P61.2   **Anemia of prematurity**

P61.3   **Congenital anemia from fetal blood loss**

P61.4   **Other congenital anemias, not elsewhere classified**
Congenital anemia NOS

P61.5   **Transient neonatal neutropenia**
> EXCLUDES 1   *congenital neutropenia (nontransient) (D70.0)*
DEF: Low blood neutrophil counts of newborn; occurs due to maternal hypertension, sepsis, twin-twin transfusion, alloimmunization, and hemolytic disease.

P61.6   **Other transient neonatal disorders of coagulation**

P61.8   **Other specified perinatal hematological disorders**

P61.9   **Perinatal hematological disorder, unspecified**   ▽

Transitory endocrine and metabolic disorders specific to newborn (P70-P74)

> INCLUDES   transitory endocrine and metabolic disturbances caused by the infant's response to maternal endocrine and metabolic factors, or its adjustment to extrauterine environment

✓4ᵗʰ **P70**   **Transitory disorders of carbohydrate metabolism specific to newborn**

P70.0   **Syndrome of infant of mother with gestational diabetes**
Newborn (with hypoglycemia) affected by maternal gestational diabetes
> EXCLUDES 1   *newborn (with hypoglycemia) affected by maternal (pre-existing) diabetes mellitus (P70.1)*
> *syndrome of infant of a diabetic mother (P70.1)*

P70.1   **Syndrome of infant of a diabetic mother**
Newborn (with hypoglycemia) affected by maternal (pre-existing) diabetes mellitus
> EXCLUDES 1   *newborn (with hypoglycemia) affected by maternal gestational diabetes (P70.0)*
> *syndrome of infant of mother with gestational diabetes (P70.0)*

P70.2   **Neonatal diabetes mellitus**

P70.3   **Iatrogenic neonatal hypoglycemia**

P70.4   **Other neonatal hypoglycemia**
Transitory neonatal hypoglycemia

P70.8   **Other transitory disorders of carbohydrate metabolism of newborn**

P70.9   **Transitory disorder of carbohydrate metabolism of newborn, unspecified**   ▽

✓4ᵗʰ **P71**   **Transitory neonatal disorders of calcium and magnesium metabolism**

P71.0   **Cow's milk hypocalcemia in newborn**

P71.1   **Other neonatal hypocalcemia**
> EXCLUDES 1   *neonatal hypoparathyroidism (P71.4)*

P71.2   **Neonatal hypomagnesemia**

P71.3   **Neonatal tetany without calcium or magnesium deficiency**
Neonatal tetany NOS

P71.4   **Transitory neonatal hypoparathyroidism**

P71.8   **Other transitory neonatal disorders of calcium and magnesium metabolism**

P71.9   **Transitory neonatal disorder of calcium and magnesium metabolism, unspecified**   ▽

✓4ᵗʰ **P72**   **Other transitory neonatal endocrine disorders**
> EXCLUDES 1   *congenital hypothyroidism with or without goiter (E03.0-E03.1)*
> *dyshormogenetic goiter (E07.1)*
> *Pendred's syndrome (E07.1)*

P72.0   **Neonatal goiter, not elsewhere classified**
Transitory congenital goiter with normal functioning

P72.1   **Transitory neonatal hyperthyroidism**
Neonatal thyrotoxicosis

P72.2   **Other transitory neonatal disorders of thyroid function, not elsewhere classified**
Transitory neonatal hypothyroidism

P72.8   **Other specified transitory neonatal endocrine disorders**

P72.9   **Transitory neonatal endocrine disorder, unspecified**   ▽

✓4ᵗʰ **P74**   **Other transitory neonatal electrolyte and metabolic disturbances**

P74.0   **Late metabolic acidosis of newborn**
> EXCLUDES 1   *(fetal) metabolic acidosis of newborn (P19)*

P74.1   **Dehydration of newborn**

P74.2   **Disturbances of sodium balance of newborn**

P74.3   **Disturbances of potassium balance of newborn**

P74.4   **Other transitory electrolyte disturbances of newborn**

P74.5   **Transitory tyrosinemia of newborn**

P74.6   **Transitory hyperammonemia of newborn**

P74.8   **Other transitory metabolic disturbances of newborn**
Amino-acid metabolic disorders described as transitory

P74.9   **Transitory metabolic disturbance of newborn, unspecified**   ▽

Digestive system disorders of newborn (P76-P78)

✓4ᵗʰ **P76**   **Other intestinal obstruction of newborn**

P76.0   **Meconium plug syndrome**
Meconium ileus NOS
> EXCLUDES 1   *meconium ileus in cystic fibrosis (E84.11)*

P76.1   **Transitory ileus of newborn**
> EXCLUDES 1   *Hirschsprung's disease (Q43.1)*

P76.2   **Intestinal obstruction due to inspissated milk**

P76.8   **Other specified intestinal obstruction of newborn**
> EXCLUDES 1   *intestinal obstruction classifiable to K56-*

P76.9   **Intestinal obstruction of newborn, unspecified**   ▽

✓4ᵗʰ **P77**   **Necrotizing enterocolitis of newborn**
DEF: Serious intestinal infection and inflammation in preterm infants; severity is measured by stages and may progress to life-threatening perforation or peritonitis; resection surgical treatment may be necessary.

P77.1   **Stage 1 necrotizing enterocolitis in newborn**
Necrotizing enterocolitis without pneumatosis, without perforation
DEF: Broad-spectrum symptoms with nonspecific signs, including feeding intolerance, abdominal distention, bradycardia, and metabolic abnormalities.

P77.2   **Stage 2 necrotizing enterocolitis in newborn**
Necrotizing enterocolitis with pneumatosis, without perforation
DEF: Radiographic confirmation of necrotizing enterocolitis showing intestinal dilatation, fixed loops of bowels, pneumatosis intestinalis, metabolic acidosis, and thrombocytopenia.

EXCLUDES 1 Not coded here   EXCLUDES 2 Not included here   N Newborn Age: 0   P Pediatric Age: 0-17   M Maternity Age: 12-55   A Adult Age: 15-124

866   ICD-10-CM 2018

P77.3 **Stage 3 necrotizing enterocolitis in newborn**
Necrotizing enterocolitis with perforation
Necrotizing enterocolitis with pneumatosis and perforation
DEF: Advanced stage in which infant demonstrates signs of bowel perforation, septic shock, metabolic acidosis, ascites, disseminated intravascular coagulopathy, neutropenia.

P77.9 **Necrotizing enterocolitis in newborn, unspecified** ▽
Necrotizing enterocolitis in newborn, NOS

✓4ᵗʰ **P78 Other perinatal digestive system disorders**
> EXCLUDES 1   cystic fibrosis (E84.0-E84.9)
>   neonatal gastrointestinal hemorrhages (P54.0-P54.3)

P78.0 **Perinatal intestinal perforation**
Meconium peritonitis

P78.1 **Other neonatal peritonitis**
Neonatal peritonitis NOS

P78.2 **Neonatal hematemesis and melena due to swallowed maternal blood**

P78.3 **Noninfective neonatal diarrhea**
Neonatal diarrhea NOS

✓5ᵗʰ P78.8 **Other specified perinatal digestive system disorders**

P78.81 **Congenital cirrhosis (of liver)**

P78.82 **Peptic ulcer of newborn**

P78.83 **Newborn esophageal reflux**
Neonatal esophageal reflux

●   P78.84 **Gestational alloimmune liver disease**
GALD
Neonatal hemochromatosis
> EXCLUDES 1   hemochromatosis (E83.11-)

P78.89 **Other specified perinatal digestive system disorders**

P78.9 **Perinatal digestive system disorder, unspecified** ▽

Conditions involving the integument and temperature regulation of newborn (P80-P83)

✓4ᵗʰ **P80 Hypothermia of newborn**

P80.0 **Cold injury syndrome**
Severe and usually chronic hypothermia associated with a pink flushed appearance, edema and neurological and biochemical abnormalities.
> EXCLUDES 1   mild hypothermia of newborn (P80.8)

P80.8 **Other hypothermia of newborn**
Mild hypothermia of newborn

P80.9 **Hypothermia of newborn, unspecified** ▽

✓4ᵗʰ **P81 Other disturbances of temperature regulation of newborn**

P81.0 **Environmental hyperthermia of newborn**

P81.8 **Other specified disturbances of temperature regulation of newborn**

P81.9 **Disturbance of temperature regulation of newborn, unspecified** ▽
Fever of newborn NOS

✓4ᵗʰ **P83 Other conditions of integument specific to newborn**
> EXCLUDES 1   congenital malformations of skin and integument (Q80-Q84)
>   hydrops fetalis due to hemolytic disease (P56.-)
>   neonatal skin infection (P39.4)
>   staphylococcal scalded skin syndrome (L00)
> EXCLUDES 2   cradle cap (L21.0)
>   diaper [napkin] dermatitis (L22)

P83.0 **Sclerema neonatorum**
DEF: Diffuse, rapidly progressing white, waxy, nonpitting hardening of tissue, usually of legs and feet that is life-threatening; found in preterm or debilitated infants; unknown etiology.

P83.1 **Neonatal erythema toxicum**

P83.2 **Hydrops fetalis not due to hemolytic disease**
Hydrops fetalis NOS
DEF: Severe, life-threatening problem of newborn characterized by severe edema of entire body; unrelated to immune response.

✓5ᵗʰ P83.3 **Other and unspecified edema specific to newborn**

P83.30 **Unspecified edema specific to newborn** ▽

P83.39 **Other edema specific to newborn**

P83.4 **Breast engorgement of newborn**
Noninfective mastitis of newborn

P83.5 **Congenital hydrocele** ♂

P83.6 **Umbilical polyp of newborn**

✓5ᵗʰ P83.8 **Other specified conditions of integument specific to newborn**
Bronze baby syndrome
Neonatal scleroderma
Urticaria neonatorum

●   P83.81 **Umbilical granuloma**
> EXCLUDES 2   granulomatous disorder of the skin and subcutaneous tissue, unspecified (L92.9)

●   P83.88 **Other specified conditions of integument specific to newborn**
Bronze baby syndrome
Neonatal scleroderma
Urticaria neonatorum

P83.9 **Condition of the integument specific to newborn, unspecified** ▽

Other problems with newborn (P84)

P84 Other problems with newborn
Acidemia of newborn
Acidosis of newborn
Anoxia of newborn NOS
Asphyxia of newborn NOS
Hypercapnia of newborn
Hypoxemia of newborn
Hypoxia of newborn NOS
Mixed metabolic and respiratory acidosis of newborn
> EXCLUDES 1   intracranial hemorrhage due to anoxia or hypoxia (P52.-)
>   hypoxic ischemic encephalopathy [HIE] (P91.6-)
>   late metabolic acidosis of newborn (P74.0)

Other disorders originating in the perinatal period (P90-P96)

P90 Convulsions of newborn
> EXCLUDES 1   benign myoclonic epilepsy in infancy (G40.3-)
>   benign neonatal convulsions (familial) (G40.3-)

✓4ᵗʰ **P91 Other disturbances of cerebral status of newborn**

P91.0 **Neonatal cerebral ischemia**

P91.1 **Acquired periventricular cysts of newborn**

P91.2 **Neonatal cerebral leukomalacia**
Periventricular leukomalacia

P91.3 **Neonatal cerebral irritability**

P91.4 **Neonatal cerebral depression**

P91.5 **Neonatal coma**

✓5ᵗʰ P91.6 **Hypoxic ischemic encephalopathy [HIE]**
> EXCLUDES 1   ►neonatal cerebral depression (P91.4)
>   neonatal cerebral irritability (P91.3)
>   neonatal coma (P91.5)◄

P91.60 **Hypoxic ischemic encephalopathy [HIE], unspecified** ▽

P91.61 **Mild hypoxic ischemic encephalopathy [HIE]**

P91.62 **Moderate hypoxic ischemic encephalopathy [HIE]**

P91.63 **Severe hypoxic ischemic encephalopathy [HIE]**

✓5ᵗʰ P91.8 **Other specified disturbances of cerebral status of newborn**

●   ✓6ᵗʰ P91.81 **Neonatal encephalopathy**

●   P91.811 **Neonatal encephalopathy in diseases classified elsewhere**
Code first underlying condition, if known, such as:
congenital cirrhosis (of liver) (P78.71)
intracranial nontraumatic hemorrhage of newborn (P52.-)
kernicterus (P57.-)

●   P91.819 **Neonatal encephalopathy, unspecified** ▽

●   P91.88 **Other specified disturbances of cerebral status of newborn**

P91.9 **Disturbance of cerebral status of newborn, unspecified** ▽

✓4ᵗʰ **P92 Feeding problems of newborn**
> EXCLUDES 1   ►eating disorders (F50.-)◄
>   feeding problems in child over 28 days old (R63.3)
AHA: 2016, 3Q, 19

✓5ᵗʰ P92.0 **Vomiting of newborn**
> EXCLUDES 1   vomiting of child over 28 days old (R11.-)

P92.01 **Bilious vomiting of newborn**
> EXCLUDES 1   bilious vomiting in child over 28 days old (R11.14)

P92.09 **Other vomiting of newborn**
> EXCLUDES 1   regurgitation of food in newborn (P92.1)

☑ Additional Character Req   ✓x7ᵗʰ Placeholder Alert   Manifestation   HCC CMS-HCC Condition   ▽ Unspecified Code   ►◄ Revised Text   ● New Code   ▲ Revised Code Title

P92.1   **Regurgitation and rumination of newborn**

P92.2   **Slow feeding of newborn**

P92.3   **Underfeeding of newborn**

P92.4   **Overfeeding of newborn**

P92.5   **Neonatal difficulty in feeding at breast**
AHA: 2017, 1Q, 28

P92.6   **Failure to thrive in newborn**
EXCLUDES 1   *failure to thrive in child over 28 days old (R62.51)*

P92.8   **Other feeding problems of newborn**

P92.9   **Feeding problem of newborn, unspecified**   ▽

✓4ᵗʰ **P93**   **Reactions and intoxications due to drugs administered to newborn**
INCLUDES   reactions and intoxications due to drugs administered to fetus affecting newborn
EXCLUDES 1   *jaundice due to drugs or toxins transmitted from mother or given to newborn (P58.4-)*
reactions and intoxications from maternal opiates, tranquilizers and other medication (P04.0-P04.1, P04.4)
withdrawal symptoms from maternal use of drugs of addiction (P96.1)
withdrawal symptoms from therapeutic use of drugs in newborn (P96.2)

P93.0   **Grey baby syndrome**
Grey syndrome from chloramphenicol administration in newborn

P93.8   **Other reactions and intoxications due to drugs administered to newborn**
Use additional code for adverse effect, if applicable, to identify drug (T36-T50 with fifth or sixth character 5)

✓4ᵗʰ **P94**   **Disorders of muscle tone of newborn**

P94.0   **Transient neonatal myasthenia gravis**
EXCLUDES 1   *myasthenia gravis (G70.0)*

P94.1   **Congenital hypertonia**

P94.2   **Congenital hypotonia**
Floppy baby syndrome, unspecified

P94.8   **Other disorders of muscle tone of newborn**

P94.9   **Disorder of muscle tone of newborn, unspecified**   ▽

P95   **Stillbirth**
Deadborn fetus NOS
Fetal death of unspecified cause
Stillbirth NOS
EXCLUDES 1   *maternal care for intrauterine death (O36.4)*
missed abortion (O02.1)
outcome of delivery, stillbirth (Z37.1, Z37.3, Z37.4, Z37.7)

✓4ᵗʰ **P96**   **Other conditions originating in the perinatal period**

P96.0   **Congenital renal failure**
Uremia of newborn

P96.1   **Neonatal withdrawal symptoms from maternal use of drugs of addiction**
Drug withdrawal syndrome in infant of dependent mother
Neonatal abstinence syndrome
EXCLUDES 1   *reactions and intoxications from maternal opiates and tranquilizers administered during labor and delivery (P04.0)*

P96.2   **Withdrawal symptoms from therapeutic use of drugs in newborn**

P96.3   **Wide cranial sutures of newborn**
Neonatal craniotabes

P96.5   **Complication to newborn due to (fetal) intrauterine procedure**
EXCLUDES 2   *newborn affected by amniocentesis (P00.6)*

✓5ᵗʰ **P96.8**   **Other specified conditions originating in the perinatal period**

P96.81   **Exposure to (parental) (environmental) tobacco smoke in the perinatal period**
EXCLUDES 2   *newborn affected by in utero exposure to tobacco (P04.2)*
exposure to environmental tobacco smoke after the perinatal period (Z77.22)

P96.82   **Delayed separation of umbilical cord**

P96.83   **Meconium staining**
EXCLUDES 1   *meconium aspiration (P24.00, P24.01)*
meconium passage during delivery (P03.82)

P96.89   **Other specified conditions originating in the perinatal period**
Use additional code to specify condition

P96.9   **Condition originating in the perinatal period, unspecified**   ▽
Congenital debility NOS

EXCLUDES 1 Not coded here   EXCLUDES 2 Not included here   N Newborn Age: 0   P Pediatric Age: 0-17   M Maternity Age: 12-55   A Adult Age: 15-124

868   ICD-10-CM 2018

Chapter 17. Congenital Malformations, Deformations, and Chromosomal Abnormalities (Q00–Q99)

Chapter Specific Guidelines with Coding Examples

The chapter specific guidelines from the ICD-10-CM Official Guidelines for Coding and Reporting have been provided below. Along with these guidelines are coding examples, contained in the shaded boxes, that have been developed to help illustrate the coding and/or sequencing guidance found in these guidelines.

Assign an appropriate code(s) from categories Q00-Q99, Congenital malformations, deformations, and chromosomal abnormalities when a malformation/deformation or chromosomal abnormality is documented. A malformation/deformation/or chromosomal abnormality may be the principal/first-listed diagnosis on a record or a secondary diagnosis.

When a malformation/deformation/or chromosomal abnormality does not have a unique code assignment, assign additional code(s) for any manifestations that may be present.

When the code assignment specifically identifies the malformation/deformation/or chromosomal abnormality, manifestations that are an inherent component of the anomaly should not be coded separately. Additional codes should be assigned for manifestations that are not an inherent component.

8-day-old infant with tetralogy of Fallot and pulmonary stenosis

Q21.3   Tetralogy of Fallot

Explanation: Pulmonary stenosis is inherent in the disease process of tetralogy of Fallot. When the code assignment specifically identifies the malformation/deformation/or chromosomal abnormality, manifestations that are inherent components of the anomaly should not be coded separately.

7-month-old infant with Down syndrome and common atrioventricular canal

Q90.9   Down syndrome, unspecified

Q21.2   Atrioventricular septal defect

Explanation: While a common atrioventricular canal is often associated with patients with Down syndrome, this manifestation is not an inherent component and may be reported separately. When the code assignment specifically identifies the anomaly, manifestations that are inherent components of the condition should not be coded separately. Additional codes should be assigned for manifestations that are not inherent components.

Codes from Chapter 17 may be used throughout the life of the patient. If a congenital malformation or deformity has been corrected, a personal history code should be used to identify the history of the malformation or deformity. Although present at birth, malformation/deformation/or chromosomal abnormality may not be identified until later in life. Whenever the condition is diagnosed by the physician, it is appropriate to assign a code from codes Q00-Q99. For the birth admission, the appropriate code from category Z38, Liveborn infants, according to place of birth and type of delivery, should be sequenced as the principal diagnosis, followed by any congenital anomaly codes, Q00- Q99.

Three-year-old with history of corrected ventricular septal defect

Z87.74   Personal history of (corrected) congenital malformations of heart and circulatory system

Explanation: If a congenital malformation or deformity has been corrected, a personal history code should be used to identify the history of the malformation or deformity.

Forty-year-old man with headaches diagnosed with congenital arteriovenous malformation by brain scan

Q28.2   Arteriovenous malformation of cerebral vessels

Explanation: Although present at birth, malformations may not be identified until later in life. Whenever the condition is diagnosed by the physician, it is appropriate to assign a code from the range Q00–Q99.

Newborn with anencephaly delivered vaginally in hospital

Z38.00   Single liveborn infant, delivered vaginally

Q00.0   Anencephaly

Explanation: For the birth admission, the appropriate code from category Z38 Liveborn infants, according to place of birth and type of delivery, should be sequenced as the principal diagnosis, followed by any congenital anomaly codes, Q00–Q99.

Chapter 17. Congenital Malformations, Deformations and Chromosomal Abnormalities(Q00-Q99)

NOTE   Codes from this chapter are not for use on maternal or fetal records.

EXCLUDES 2 *inborn errors of metabolism (E70-E88)*

This chapter contains the following blocks:

Q00-Q07   Congenital malformations of the nervous system
Q10-Q18   Congenital malformations of eye, ear, face and neck
Q20-Q28   Congenital malformations of the circulatory system
Q30-Q34   Congenital malformations of the respiratory system
Q35-Q37   Cleft lip and cleft palate
Q38-Q45   Other congenital malformations of the digestive system
Q50-Q56   Congenital malformations of genital organs
Q60-Q64   Congenital malformations of the urinary system
Q65-Q79   Congenital malformations and deformations of the musculoskeletal system
Q80-Q89   Other congenital malformations
Q90-Q99   Chromosomal abnormalities, not elsewhere classified

Congenital malformations of the nervous system (Q00-Q07)

√4th **Q00   Anencephaly and similar malformations**

Q00.0   Anencephaly   HCC
   Acephaly
   Acrania
   Amyelencephaly
   Hemianencephaly
   Hemicephaly

Q00.1   Craniorachischisis   HCC

Q00.2   Iniencephaly   HCC

√4th **Q01   Encephalocele**
   INCLUDES   Arnold-Chiari syndrome, type III
               encephalocystocele
               encephalomyelocele
               hydroencephalocele
               hydromeningocele, cranial
               meningocele, cerebral
               meningoencephalocele
   EXCLUDES 1 *Meckel-Gruber syndrome (Q61.9)*

Q01.0   Frontal encephalocele   HCC

Q01.1   Nasofrontal encephalocele   HCC

Q01.2   Occipital encephalocele   HCC

Q01.8   Encephalocele of other sites   HCC

Q01.9   Encephalocele, unspecified   HCC ▽

Q02   Microcephaly   HCC
   INCLUDES   hydromicrocephaly
               micrencephalon
   EXCLUDES 1 *Meckel-Gruber syndrome (Q61.9)*

√4th **Q03   Congenital hydrocephalus**
   INCLUDES   hydrocephalus in newborn
   EXCLUDES 1 *Arnold-Chiari syndrome, type II (Q07.0-)*
               acquired hydrocephalus (G91.-)
               hydrocephalus due to congenital toxoplasmosis (P37.1)
               hydrocephalus with spina bifida (Q05.0-Q05.4)

Q03.0   Malformations of aqueduct of Sylvius   HCC
   Anomaly of aqueduct of Sylvius
   Obstruction of aqueduct of Sylvius, congenital
   Stenosis of aqueduct of Sylvius

Q03.1   Atresia of foramina of Magendie and Luschkaq HCC
   Dandy-Walker syndrome

Congenital Hydrocephalus

Normal ventricles   Hydrocephalic ventricles

Q03.8   Other congenital hydrocephalus   HCC

Q03.9   Congenital hydrocephalus, unspecified   HCC ▽

√4th **Q04   Other congenital malformations of brain**
   EXCLUDES 1 *cyclopia (Q87.0)*
               macrocephaly (Q75.3)

Q04.0   Congenital malformations of corpus callosum   HCC
   Agenesis of corpus callosum

Q04.1   Arhinencephaly   HCC

Q04.2   Holoprosencephaly   HCC

Q04.3   Other reduction deformities of brain   HCC
   Absence of part of brain
   Agenesis of part of brain
   Agyria
   Aplasia of part of brain
   Hydranencephaly
   Hypoplasia of part of brain
   Lissencephaly
   Microgyria
   Pachygyria
   EXCLUDES 1 *congenital malformations of corpus callosum (Q04.0)*

Q04.4   Septo-optic dysplasia of brain   HCC

Q04.5   Megalencephaly   HCC

Q04.6   Congenital cerebral cysts   HCC
   Porencephaly
   Schizencephaly
   EXCLUDES 1 *acquired porencephalic cyst (G93.0)*

Q04.8   Other specified congenital malformations of brain HCC
   Arnold-Chiari syndrome, type IV
   Macrogyria

Q04.9   Congenital malformation of brain, unspecified HCC ▽
   Congenital anomaly NOS of brain
   Congenital deformity NOS of brain
   Congenital disease or lesion NOS of brain
   Multiple anomalies NOS of brain, congenital

√4th **Q05   Spina bifida**
   INCLUDES   hydromeningocele (spinal)
               meningocele (spinal)
               meningomyelocele
               myelocele
               myelomeningocele
               rachischisis
               spina bifida (aperta)(cystica)
               syringomyelocele

   Use additional code for any associated paraplegia (paraparesis) (G82.2-)
   EXCLUDES 1 *Arnold-Chiari syndrome, type II (Q07.0-)*
               spina bifida occulta (Q76.0)

Q05.0   Cervical spina bifida with hydrocephalus   HCC

Q05.1   Thoracic spina bifida with hydrocephalus   HCC
   Dorsal spina bifida with hydrocephalus
   Thoracolumbar spina bifida with hydrocephalus

Q05.2   Lumbar spina bifida with hydrocephalus   HCC
   Lumbosacral spina bifida with hydrocephalus

Q05.3   Sacral spina bifida with hydrocephalus   HCC

Q05.4   Unspecified spina bifida with hydrocephalus   HCC ▽

Q05.5   Cervical spina bifida without hydrocephalus   HCC

Q05.6   Thoracic spina bifida without hydrocephalus   HCC
   Dorsal spina bifida NOS
   Thoracolumbar spina bifida NOS

Q05.7   Lumbar spina bifida without hydrocephalus   HCC
   Lumbosacral spina bifida NOS

Q05.8   Sacral spina bifida without hydrocephalus   HCC

Q05.9   Spina bifida, unspecified   HCC ▽

Spina Bifida

Spina bifida occulta   Meningocele   Myelomeningocele

EXCLUDES 1 Not coded here   *EXCLUDES 2* Not included here   N Newborn Age: 0   P Pediatric Age: 0-17   M Maternity Age: 12-55   A Adult Age: 15-124

870   ICD-10-CM 2018

✓4ᵗʰ **Q06 Other congenital malformations of spinal cord**

Q06.0 Amyelia   HCC

Q06.1 Hypoplasia and dysplasia of spinal cord   HCC
Atelomyelia
Myelatelia
Myelodysplasia of spinal cord

Q06.2 Diastematomyelia   HCC
DEF: Rare congenital anomaly often associated with spina bifida; the spinal cord is separated into longitudinal halves by a bony, cartilaginous or fibrous septum, each half surrounded by a dural sac.

Q06.3 Other congenital cauda equina malformations   HCC

Q06.4 Hydromyelia   HCC
Hydrorachis

Q06.8 Other specified congenital malformations of spinal cord   HCC

Q06.9 Congenital malformation of spinal cord, unspecified   HCC ▽
Congenital anomaly NOS of spinal cord
Congenital deformity NOS of spinal cord
Congenital disease or lesion NOS of spinal cord

✓4ᵗʰ **Q07 Other congenital malformations of nervous system**
EXCLUDES 2   congenital central alveolar hypoventilation syndrome (G47.35)
familial dysautonomia [Riley-Day] (G90.1)
neurofibromatosis (nonmalignant) (Q85.0-)

✓5ᵗʰ **Q07.0 Arnold-Chiari syndrome**
Arnold-Chiari syndrome, type II
EXCLUDES 1   Arnold-Chiari syndrome, type III (Q01.-)
Arnold-Chiari syndrome, type IV (Q04.8)

Q07.00 Arnold-Chiari syndrome without spina bifida or hydrocephalus   HCC

Q07.01 Arnold-Chiari syndrome with spina bifida   HCC

Q07.02 Arnold-Chiari syndrome with hydrocephalus   HCC

Q07.03 Arnold-Chiari syndrome with spina bifida and hydrocephalus   HCC

Q07.8 Other specified congenital malformations of nervous system   HCC
Agenesis of nerve
Displacement of brachial plexus
Jaw-winking syndrome
Marcus Gunn's syndrome

Q07.9 Congenital malformation of nervous system, unspecified   HCC ▽
Congenital anomaly NOS of nervous system
Congenital deformity NOS of nervous system
Congenital disease or lesion NOS of nervous system

Congenital malformations of eye, ear, face and neck (Q10-Q18)
EXCLUDES 2   cleft lip and cleft palate (Q35-Q37)
congenital malformation of cervical spine (Q05.0, Q05.5, Q67.5, Q76.0-Q76.4)
congenital malformation of larynx (Q31.-)
congenital malformation of lip NEC (Q38.0)
congenital malformation of nose (Q30.-)
congenital malformation of parathyroid gland (Q89.2)
congenital malformation of thyroid gland (Q89.2)

✓4ᵗʰ **Q10 Congenital malformations of eyelid, lacrimal apparatus and orbit**
EXCLUDES 1   cryptophthalmos NOS (Q11.2)
cryptophthalmos syndrome (Q87.0)

Q10.0 Congenital ptosis
DEF: Congenital drooping of eyelid; mostly idiopathic, but may occur genetically.

Q10.1 Congenital ectropion

Q10.2 Congenital entropion

Q10.3 Other congenital malformations of eyelid
Ablepharon
Blepharophimosis, congenital
Coloboma of eyelid
Congenital absence or agenesis of cilia
Congenital absence or agenesis of eyelid
Congenital accessory eyelid
Congenital accessory eye muscle
Congenital malformation of eyelid NOS

Q10.4 Absence and agenesis of lacrimal apparatus
Congenital absence of punctum lacrimale

Q10.5 Congenital stenosis and stricture of lacrimal duct

Q10.6 Other congenital malformations of lacrimal apparatus
Congenital malformation of lacrimal apparatus NOS

Q10.7 Congenital malformation of orbit

Coloboma of Lens

Coloboma

✓4ᵗʰ **Q11 Anophthalmos, microphthalmos and macrophthalmos**

Q11.0 Cystic eyeball

Q11.1 Other anophthalmos
Anophthalmos NOS
Agenesis of eye
Aplasia of eye

Q11.2 Microphthalmos
Cryptophthalmos NOS
Dysplasia of eye
Hypoplasia of eye
Rudimentary eye
EXCLUDES 1   cryptophthalmos syndrome (Q87.0)

Q11.3 Macrophthalmos
EXCLUDES 1   macrophthalmos in congenital glaucoma (Q15.0)

✓4ᵗʰ **Q12 Congenital lens malformations**

Q12.0 Congenital cataract

Q12.1 Congenital displaced lens

Q12.2 Coloboma of lens

Q12.3 Congenital aphakia

Q12.4 Spherophakia

Q12.8 Other congenital lens malformations
Microphakia

Q12.9 Congenital lens malformation, unspecified   ▽

✓4ᵗʰ **Q13 Congenital malformations of anterior segment of eye**

Q13.0 Coloboma of iris
Coloboma NOS

Q13.1 Absence of iris
Aniridia
Use additional code for associated glaucoma (H42)
DEF: Incompletely formed or absent iris; affects both eyes; dominant trait.

Q13.2 Other congenital malformations of iris
Anisocoria, congenital
Atresia of pupil
Congenital malformation of iris NOS
Corectopia

Q13.3 Congenital corneal opacity

Q13.4 Other congenital corneal malformations
Congenital malformation of cornea NOS
Microcornea
Peter's anomaly

Q13.5 Blue sclera

✓5ᵗʰ **Q13.8 Other congenital malformations of anterior segment of eye**

Q13.81 Rieger's anomaly
Use additional code for associated glaucoma (H42)

Q13.89 Other congenital malformations of anterior segment of eye

Q13.9 Congenital malformation of anterior segment of eye, unspecified   ▽

✓4ᵗʰ **Q14 Congenital malformations of posterior segment of eye**
EXCLUDES 2   optic nerve hypoplasia (H47.03-)

Q14.0 Congenital malformation of vitreous humor
Congenital vitreous opacity

Q14.1 Congenital malformation of retina
Congenital retinal aneurysm

Q14.2 Congenital malformation of optic disc
Coloboma of optic disc

Q14.3 Congenital malformation of choroid

Q14.8 Other congenital malformations of posterior segment of eye
Coloboma of the fundus

✓ Additional Character Req   ✓x7ᵗʰ Placeholder Alert   Manifestation   HCC CMS-HCC Condition   ▽ Unspecified Code   ►◄ Revised Text   ● New Code   ▲ Revised Code Title

Q14.9   **Congenital malformation of posterior segment of eye, unspecified** ▽

✓4th **Q15**   **Other congenital malformations of eye**
> EXCLUDES 1   *congenital nystagmus (H55.01)*
> *ocular albinism (E70.31-)*
> *optic nerve hypoplasia (H47.03-)*
> *retinitis pigmentosa (H35.52)*

Q15.0   **Congenital glaucoma**
Axenfeld's anomaly
Buphthalmos
Glaucoma of childhood
Glaucoma of newborn
Hydrophthalmos
Keratoglobus, congenital, with glaucoma
Macrocornea with glaucoma
Macrophthalmos in congenital glaucoma
Megalocornea with glaucoma

Q15.8   **Other specified congenital malformations of eye**

Q15.9   **Congenital malformation of eye, unspecified** ▽
Congenital anomaly of eye
Congenital deformity of eye

✓4th **Q16**   **Congenital malformations of ear causing impairment of hearing**
> EXCLUDES 1   *congenital deafness (H90.-)*

Q16.0   **Congenital absence of (ear) auricle**

Q16.1   **Congenital absence, atresia and stricture of auditory canal (external)**
Congenital atresia or stricture of osseous meatus

Q16.2   **Absence of eustachian tube**

Q16.3   **Congenital malformation of ear ossicles**
Congenital fusion of ear ossicles

Q16.4   **Other congenital malformations of middle ear**
Congenital malformation of middle ear NOS

Q16.5   **Congenital malformation of inner ear**
Congenital anomaly of membranous labyrinth
Congenital anomaly of organ of Corti

Q16.9   **Congenital malformation of ear causing impairment of hearing, unspecified** ▽
Congenital absence of ear NOS

✓4th **Q17**   **Other congenital malformations of ear**
> EXCLUDES 1   *congenital malformations of ear with impairment of hearing (Q16.0- Q16.9)*
> *preauricular sinus (Q18.1)*

Q17.0   **Accessory auricle**
Accessory tragus
Polyotia
Preauricular appendage or tag
Supernumerary ear
Supernumerary lobule

Q17.1   **Macrotia**
DEF: Birth defect characterized by abnormal enlargement of the pinna of the ear.

Q17.2   **Microtia**

Q17.3   **Other misshapen ear**
Pointed ear

Q17.4   **Misplaced ear**
Low-set ears
> EXCLUDES 1   *cervical auricle (Q18.2)*

Q17.5   **Prominent ear**
Bat ear

Q17.8   **Other specified congenital malformations of ear**
Congenital absence of lobe of ear

Q17.9   **Congenital malformation of ear, unspecified** ▽
Congenital anomaly of ear NOS

✓4th **Q18**   **Other congenital malformations of face and neck**
> EXCLUDES 1   *cleft lip and cleft palate (Q35-Q37)*
> *conditions classified to Q67.0-Q67.4*
> *congenital malformations of skull and face bones (Q75.-)*
> *cyclopia (Q87.0)*
> *dentofacial anomalies [including malocclusion] (M26.-)*
> *malformation syndromes affecting facial appearance (Q87.0)*
> *persistent thyroglossal duct (Q89.2)*

Q18.0   **Sinus, fistula and cyst of branchial cleft**
Branchial vestige

Q18.1   **Preauricular sinus and cyst**
Fistula of auricle, congenital
Cervicoaural fistula

Q18.2   **Other branchial cleft malformations**
Branchial cleft malformation NOS
Cervical auricle
Otocephaly

Q18.3   **Webbing of neck**
Pterygium colli
DEF: Congenital malformation characterized by thick, triangular skinfold that stretches from the lateral side of the neck across the shoulder; associated with genetic conditions Turner's and Noonan's syndromes.

Q18.4   **Macrostomia**
DEF: Rare congenital craniofacial bilateral or unilateral anomaly of mouth due to malformed maxillary and mandibular processes; results in abnormally large mouth extending towards ear.

Q18.5   **Microstomia**

Q18.6   **Macrocheilia**
Hypertrophy of lip, congenital

Q18.7   **Microcheilia**

Q18.8   **Other specified congenital malformations of face and neck**
Medial cyst of face and neck
Medial fistula of face and neck
Medial sinus of face and neck

Q18.9   **Congenital malformation of face and neck, unspecified** ▽
Congenital anomaly NOS of face and neck

Congenital malformations of the circulatory system (Q20-Q28)

✓4th **Q20**   **Congenital malformations of cardiac chambers and connections**
> EXCLUDES 1   *dextrocardia with situs inversus (Q89.3)*
> *mirror-image atrial arrangement with situs inversus (Q89.3)*

Q20.0   **Common arterial trunk**
Persistent truncus arteriosus
> EXCLUDES 1   *aortic septal defect (Q21.4)*

Q20.1   **Double outlet right ventricle**
Taussig-Bing syndrome

Q20.2   **Double outlet left ventricle**

Q20.3   **Discordant ventriculoarterial connection**
Dextrotransposition of aorta
Transposition of great vessels (complete)

Q20.4   **Double inlet ventricle**
Common ventricle
Cor triloculare biatriatum
Single ventricle

Q20.5   **Discordant atrioventricular connection**
Corrected transposition
Levotransposition
Ventricular inversion

Q20.6   **Isomerism of atrial appendages**
Isomerism of atrial appendages with asplenia or polysplenia

Q20.8   **Other congenital malformations of cardiac chambers and connections**
Cor binoculare

Q20.9   **Congenital malformation of cardiac chambers and connections, unspecified** ▽

✓4th **Q21**   **Congenital malformations of cardiac septa**
> EXCLUDES 1   *acquired cardiac septal defect (I51.0)*

Q21.0   **Ventricular septal defect**
Roger's disease

Ventricular Septal Defect

EXCLUDES 1 Not coded here   EXCLUDES 2 Not included here   **N** Newborn Age: 0   **P** Pediatric Age: 0-17   **M** Maternity Age: 12-55   **A** Adult Age: 15-124

872   ICD-10-CM 2018

Atrial Septal Defect

Atrioventricular Septal Defect

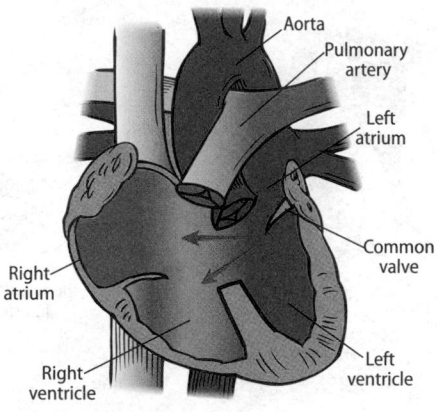

Q21.1 Atrial septal defect
Coronary sinus defect
Patent or persistent foramen ovale
Patent or persistent ostium secundum defect (type II)
Patent or persistent sinus venosus defect

Q21.2 Atrioventricular septal defect
Common atrioventricular canal
Endocardial cushion defect
Ostium primum atrial septal defect (type I)

Q21.3 Tetralogy of Fallot
Ventricular septal defect with pulmonary stenosis or atresia, dextroposition of aorta and hypertrophy of right ventricle.
AHA: 2014, 3Q, 16

Q21.4 Aortopulmonary septal defect
Aortic septal defect   Aortopulmonary window

Q21.8 Other congenital malformations of cardiac septa
Eisenmenger's defect
Pentalogy of Fallot
▶Code also if applicable:
Eisenmenger's complex (I27.83)
Eisenmenger's syndrome (I27.83)◀
EXCLUDES 1 ~~Eisenmenger's complex (I27.8)~~
~~Eisenmenger's syndrome (I27.8)~~

Q21.9 Congenital malformation of cardiac septum, unspecified ▽
Septal (heart) defect NOS

√4ᵗʰ Q22 Congenital malformations of pulmonary and tricuspid valves

Q22.0 Pulmonary valve atresia

Q22.1 Congenital pulmonary valve stenosis
DEF: Stenosis of opening between pulmonary artery and right ventricle; causes obstructed blood outflow from right ventricle.

Q22.2 Congenital pulmonary valve insufficiency
Congenital pulmonary valve regurgitation

Q22.3 Other congenital malformations of pulmonary valve
Congenital malformation of pulmonary valve NOS
Supernumerary cusps of pulmonary valve

Q22.4 Congenital tricuspid stenosis
Congenital tricuspid atresia

Q22.5 Ebstein's anomaly
DEF: Malformation of the tricuspid valve characterized by septal and posterior leaflets attaching to the wall of the right ventricle; causes the right ventricle to fuse with the atrium into a large right atrium and a small ventricle; leads to heart failure and abnormal cardiac rhythm.

Q22.6 Hypoplastic right heart syndrome

Q22.8 Other congenital malformations of tricuspid valve

Q22.9 Congenital malformation of tricuspid valve, unspecified ▽

√4ᵗʰ Q23 Congenital malformations of aortic and mitral valves

Q23.0 Congenital stenosis of aortic valve
Congenital aortic atresia
Congenital aortic stenosis NOS
EXCLUDES 1 congenital stenosis of aortic valve in hypoplastic left heart syndrome (Q23.4)
congenital subaortic stenosis (Q24.4)
supravalvular aortic stenosis (congenital) (Q25.3)

Q23.1 Congenital insufficiency of aortic valve
Bicuspid aortic valve
Congenital aortic insufficiency

Q23.2 Congenital mitral stenosis
Congenital mitral atresia
DEF: Congenital stenosis of mitral valve orifice between left atrium and ventricle; at the supravalvular, valvular, or subvalvular levels; causes obstruction to left ventricular filling.

Q23.3 Congenital mitral insufficiency

Q23.4 Hypoplastic left heart syndrome

Q23.8 Other congenital malformations of aortic and mitral valves

Q23.9 Congenital malformation of aortic and mitral valves, unspecified ▽

√4ᵗʰ Q24 Other congenital malformations of heart
EXCLUDES 1 endocardial fibroelastosis (I42.4)

Q24.0 Dextrocardia
EXCLUDES 1 dextrocardia with situs inversus (Q89.3)
isomerism of atrial appendages (with asplenia or polysplenia) (Q20.6)
mirror-image atrial arrangement with situs inversus (Q89.3)

Q24.1 Levocardia

Q24.2 Cor triatriatum

Q24.3 Pulmonary infundibular stenosis
Subvalvular pulmonic stenosis

Q24.4 Congenital subaortic stenosis
DEF: Congenital heart defect characterized by stenosis of left ventricular outflow tract due to fibrous tissue ring or septal hypertrophy below aortic valve.

Q24.5 Malformation of coronary vessels
Congenital coronary (artery) aneurysm

Q24.6 Congenital heart block

Q24.8 Other specified congenital malformations of heart
Congenital diverticulum of left ventricle
Congenital malformation of myocardium
Congenital malformation of pericardium
Malposition of heart
Uhl's disease

Q24.9 Congenital malformation of heart, unspecified ▽
Congenital anomaly of heart
Congenital disease of heart

√4ᵗʰ Q25 Congenital malformations of great arteries

Q25.0 Patent ductus arteriosus
Patent ductus Botallo   Persistent ductus arteriosus

Q25.1 Coarctation of aorta
Coarctation of aorta (preductal) (postductal)
Stenosis of Aorta

√5ᵗʰ Q25.2 Atresia of aorta

Q25.21 Interruption of Aortic Arch
Atresia of aortic arch

Q25.29 Other atresia of aorta
Atresia of aorta

Q25.3 Supravalvular aortic stenosis
EXCLUDES 1 congenital aortic stenosis NOS (Q23.0)
congenital stenosis of aortic valve (Q23.0)

Patent Ductus Arteriosus

Aortic Arch Anomalies

Double aortic arch   Right aortic arch

✓5ᵗʰ **Q25.4** **Other congenital malformations of aorta**
EXCLUDES 1 *hypoplasia of aorta in hypoplastic left heart syndrome (Q23.4)*

Q25.40 **Congenital malformation of aorta unspecified** ▽

Q25.41 **Absence and aplasia of aorta**

Q25.42 **Hypoplasia of aorta**

Q25.43 **Congenital aneurysm of aorta**
Congenital aneurysm of aortic root
Congenital aneurysm of aortic sinus

Q25.44 **Congenital dilation of aorta**

Q25.45 **Double aortic arch**
Vascular ring of aorta

Q25.46 **Tortuous aortic arch**
Persistent convolutions of aortic arch

Q25.47 **Right aortic arch**
Persistent right aortic arch

Q25.48 **Anomalous origin of subclavian artery**

Q25.49 **Other congenital malformations of aorta**
▶Aortic arch
Bovine arch◀

Q25.5 **Atresia of pulmonary artery**

Q25.6 **Stenosis of pulmonary artery**
Supravalvular pulmonary stenosis

✓5ᵗʰ **Q25.7** **Other congenital malformations of pulmonary artery**

Q25.71 **Coarctation of pulmonary artery**

Q25.72 **Congenital pulmonary arteriovenous malformation**
Congenital pulmonary arteriovenous aneurysm

Q25.79 **Other congenital malformations of pulmonary artery**
Aberrant pulmonary artery
Agenesis of pulmonary artery
Congenital aneurysm of pulmonary artery
Congenital anomaly of pulmonary artery
Hypoplasia of pulmonary artery

Q25.8 **Other congenital malformations of other great arteries**

Q25.9 **Congenital malformation of great arteries, unspecified** ▽

✓4ᵗʰ **Q26** **Congenital malformations of great veins**

Q26.0 **Congenital stenosis of vena cava**
Congenital stenosis of vena cava (inferior)(superior)

Q26.1 **Persistent left superior vena cava**

Q26.2 **Total anomalous pulmonary venous connection**
Total anomalous pulmonary venous return [TAPVR], subdiaphragmatic
Total anomalous pulmonary venous return [TAPVR], supradiaphragmatic

Q26.3 **Partial anomalous pulmonary venous connection**
Partial anomalous pulmonary venous return

Q26.4 **Anomalous pulmonary venous connection, unspecified** ▽

Q26.5 **Anomalous portal venous connection**

Q26.6 **Portal vein-hepatic artery fistula**

Q26.8 **Other congenital malformations of great veins**
Absence of vena cava (inferior) (superior)
Azygos continuation of inferior vena cava
Persistent left posterior cardinal vein
Scimitar syndrome

Q26.9 **Congenital malformation of great vein, unspecified** ▽
Congenital anomaly of vena cava (inferior) (superior) NOS

✓4ᵗʰ **Q27** **Other congenital malformations of peripheral vascular system**
EXCLUDES 2 *anomalies of cerebral and precerebral vessels (Q28.0-Q28.3)*
anomalies of coronary vessels (Q24.5)
anomalies of pulmonary artery (Q25.5-Q25.7)
congenital retinal aneurysm (Q14.1)
hemangioma and lymphangioma (D18.-)

Q27.0 **Congenital absence and hypoplasia of umbilical artery**
Single umbilical artery

Q27.1 **Congenital renal artery stenosis**

Q27.2 **Other congenital malformations of renal artery**
Congenital malformation of renal artery NOS
Multiple renal arteries

✓5ᵗʰ **Q27.3** **Arteriovenous malformation (peripheral)**
Arteriovenous aneurysm
EXCLUDES 1 *acquired arteriovenous aneurysm (I77.0)*
EXCLUDES 2 *arteriovenous malformation of cerebral vessels (Q28.2)*
arteriovenous malformation of precerebral vessels (Q28.0)

Q27.30 **Arteriovenous malformation, site unspecified** ▽

Q27.31 **Arteriovenous malformation of vessel of upper limb**

Q27.32 **Arteriovenous malformation of vessel of lower limb**

Q27.33 **Arteriovenous malformation of digestive system vessel**

Q27.34 **Arteriovenous malformation of renal vessel**

Q27.39 **Arteriovenous malformation, other site**

Q27.4 **Congenital phlebectasia**

Q27.8 **Other specified congenital malformations of peripheral vascular system**
Absence of peripheral vascular system
Atresia of peripheral vascular system
Congenital aneurysm (peripheral)
Congenital stricture, artery
Congenital varix
EXCLUDES 1 *arteriovenous malformation (Q27.3-)*

Q27.9 **Congenital malformation of peripheral vascular system, unspecified** ▽
Anomaly of artery or vein NOS

EXCLUDES 1 Not coded here   EXCLUDES 2 Not included here   N Newborn Age: 0   P Pediatric Age: 0-17   M Maternity Age: 12-55   A Adult Age: 15-124

874   ICD-10-CM 2018

☑4ᵗʰ **Q28   Other congenital malformations of circulatory system**
> EXCLUDES 1   *congenital aneurysm NOS (Q27.8)*
> *congenital coronary aneurysm (Q24.5)*
> *ruptured cerebral arteriovenous malformation (I60.8)*
> *ruptured malformation of precerebral vessels (I72.0)*
> EXCLUDES 2   *congenital peripheral aneurysm (Q27.8)*
> *congenital pulmonary aneurysm (Q25.79)*
> *congenital retinal aneurysm (Q14.1)*

Q28.0   Arteriovenous malformation of precerebral vessels
Congenital arteriovenous precerebral aneurysm (nonruptured)

Q28.1   Other malformations of precerebral vessels
Congenital malformation of precerebral vessels NOS
Congenital precerebral aneurysm (nonruptured)

Q28.2   Arteriovenous malformation of cerebral vessels
Arteriovenous malformation of brain NOS
Congenital arteriovenous cerebral aneurysm (nonruptured)

Q28.3   Other malformations of cerebral vessels
Congenital cerebral aneurysm (nonruptured)
Congenital malformation of cerebral vessels NOS
Developmental venous anomaly

Q28.8   Other specified congenital malformations of circulatory system
Congenital aneurysm, specified site NEC
Spinal vessel anomaly

Q28.9   Congenital malformation of circulatory system, unspecified ▽

Congenital malformations of the respiratory system (Q30-Q34)

☑4ᵗʰ **Q30   Congenital malformations of nose**
> EXCLUDES 1   *congenital deviation of nasal septum (Q67.4)*

Q30.0   Choanal atresia
Atresia of nares (anterior) (posterior)
Congenital stenosis of nares (anterior) (posterior)

Q30.1   Agenesis and underdevelopment of nose
Congenital absent of nose

Q30.2   Fissured, notched and cleft nose

Q30.3   Congenital perforated nasal septum

Q30.8   Other congenital malformations of nose
Accessory nose
Congenital anomaly of nasal sinus wall

Q30.9   Congenital malformation of nose, unspecified ▽

☑4ᵗʰ **Q31   Congenital malformations of larynx**
> EXCLUDES 1   *congenital laryngeal stridor NOS (P28.89)*

Q31.0   Web of larynx
Glottic web of larynx
Subglottic web of larynx
Web of larynx NOS
DEF: Congenital malformation of larynx; marked by thin, translucent, or thick, fibrotic membrane-like structure between vocal folds; characterized by shortness of breath, and stridor.

Q31.1   Congenital subglottic stenosis

Q31.2   Laryngeal hypoplasia

Q31.3   Laryngocele

Q31.5   Congenital laryngomalacia

Q31.8   Other congenital malformations of larynx
Absence of larynx
Agenesis of larynx
Atresia of larynx
Congenital cleft thyroid cartilage
Congenital fissure of epiglottis
Congenital stenosis of larynx NEC
Posterior cleft of cricoid cartilage

Q31.9   Congenital malformation of larynx, unspecified ▽

☑4ᵗʰ **Q32   Congenital malformations of trachea and bronchus**
> EXCLUDES 1   *congenital bronchiectasis (Q33.4)*

Q32.0   Congenital tracheomalacia

Q32.1   Other congenital malformations of trachea
Atresia of trachea
Congenital anomaly of tracheal cartilage
Congenital dilatation of trachea
Congenital malformation of trachea
Congenital stenosis of trachea
Congenital tracheocele

Q32.2   Congenital bronchomalacia

Q32.3   Congenital stenosis of bronchus

Q32.4   Other congenital malformations of bronchus
Absence of bronchus
Agenesis of bronchus
Atresia of bronchus
Congenital diverticulum of bronchus
Congenital malformation of bronchus NOS

☑4ᵗʰ **Q33   Congenital malformations of lung**

Q33.0   Congenital cystic lung
Congenital cystic lung disease
Congenital honeycomb lung
Congenital polycystic lung disease
> EXCLUDES 1   *cystic fibrosis (E84.0)*
> *cystic lung disease, acquired or unspecified (J98.4)*

Q33.1   Accessory lobe of lung
Azygos lobe (fissured), lung

Q33.2   Sequestration of lung

Q33.3   Agenesis of lung
Congenital absence of lung (lobe)

Q33.4   Congenital bronchiectasis

Q33.5   Ectopic tissue in lung

Q33.6   Congenital hypoplasia and dysplasia of lung
> EXCLUDES 1   *pulmonary hypoplasia associated with short gestation (P28.0)*

Q33.8   Other congenital malformations of lung

Q33.9   Congenital malformation of lung, unspecified ▽

☑4ᵗʰ **Q34   Other congenital malformations of respiratory system**
> EXCLUDES 2   *congenital central alveolar hypoventilation syndrome (G47.35)*

Q34.0   Anomaly of pleura

Q34.1   Congenital cyst of mediastinum

Q34.8   Other specified congenital malformations of respiratory system
Atresia of nasopharynx

Q34.9   Congenital malformation of respiratory system, unspecified ▽
Congenital absence of respiratory system
Congenital anomaly of respiratory system NOS

Cleft lip and cleft palate (Q35-Q37)

Use additional code to identify associated malformation of the nose (Q30.2)
> EXCLUDES 1   *Robin's syndrome (Q87.0)*

☑4ᵗʰ **Q35   Cleft palate**
> INCLUDES   fissure of palate
> palatoschisis
> EXCLUDES 1   *cleft palate with cleft lip (Q37.-)*

Q35.1   Cleft hard palate

Q35.3   Cleft soft palate

Q35.5   Cleft hard palate with cleft soft palate

Q35.7   Cleft uvula

Q35.9   Cleft palate, unspecified ▽
Cleft palate NOS

☑4ᵗʰ **Q36   Cleft lip**
> INCLUDES   cheiloschisis
> congenital fissure of lip
> harelip
> labium leporinum
> EXCLUDES 1   *cleft lip with cleft palate (Q37.-)*

Q36.0   Cleft lip, bilateral

Q36.1   Cleft lip, median

Q36.9   Cleft lip, unilateral
Cleft lip NOS

Cleft Palate

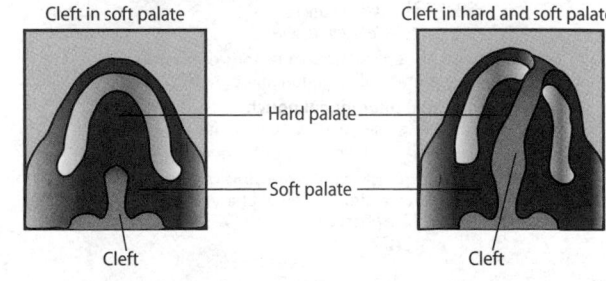
Cleft in soft palate   Cleft in hard and soft palate
Hard palate
Soft palate
Cleft   Cleft

☑ Additional Character Req   ☑x7ᵗʰ Placeholder Alert   Manifestation   HCC CMS-HCC Condition   ▽ Unspecified Code   ►◄ Revised Text   ● New Code   ▲ Revised Code Title

ICD-10-CM 2018   **875**

Cleft Lip

Unilateral incomplete   Unilateral complete   Bilateral complete

✓4th **Q37   Cleft palate with cleft lip**
   INCLUDES cheilopalatoschisis

   Q37.0   Cleft hard palate with bilateral cleft lip

   Q37.1   Cleft hard palate with unilateral cleft lip
      Cleft hard palate with cleft lip NOS

   Q37.2   Cleft soft palate with bilateral cleft lip

   Q37.3   Cleft soft palate with unilateral cleft lip
      Cleft soft palate with cleft lip NOS

   Q37.4   Cleft hard and soft palate with bilateral cleft lip

   Q37.5   Cleft hard and soft palate with unilateral cleft lip
      Cleft hard and soft palate with cleft lip NOS

   Q37.8   Unspecified cleft palate with bilateral cleft lip   ▽

   Q37.9   Unspecified cleft palate with unilateral cleft lip   ▽
      Cleft palate with cleft lip NOS

Other congenital malformations of the digestive system (Q38-Q45)

✓4th **Q38   Other congenital malformations of tongue, mouth and pharynx**
      EXCLUDES 1 dentofacial anomalies (M26.-)
         macrostomia (Q18.4)
         microstomia (Q18.5)

   Q38.0   Congenital malformations of lips, not elsewhere classified
      Congenital fistula of lip
      Congenital malformation of lip NOS
      Van der Woude's syndrome
      EXCLUDES 1 cleft lip (Q36.-)
         cleft lip with cleft palate (Q37.-)
         macrocheilia (Q18.6)
         microcheilia (Q18.7)

   Q38.1   Ankyloglossia
      Tongue tie

   Q38.2   Macroglossia
      Congenital hypertrophy of tongue

   Q38.3   Other congenital malformations of tongue
      Aglossia
      Bifid tongue
      Congenital adhesion of tongue
      Congenital fissure of tongue
      Congenital malformation of tongue NOS
      Double tongue
      Hypoglossia
      Hypoplasia of tongue
      Microglossia

   Q38.4   Congenital malformations of salivary glands and ducts
      Atresia of salivary glands and ducts
      Congenital absence of salivary glands and ducts
      Congenital accessory salivary glands and ducts
      Congenital fistula of salivary gland

   Q38.5   Congenital malformations of palate, not elsewhere classified
      Congenital absence of uvula
      Congenital malformation of palate NOS
      Congenital high arched palate
      EXCLUDES 1 cleft palate (Q35.-)
         cleft palate with cleft lip (Q37.-)

   Q38.6   Other congenital malformations of mouth
      Congenital malformation of mouth NOS

   Q38.7   Congenital pharyngeal pouch
      Congenital diverticulum of pharynx
      EXCLUDES 1 pharyngeal pouch syndrome (D82.1)

   Q38.8   Other congenital malformations of pharynx
      Congenital malformation of pharynx NOS
      Imperforate pharynx

✓4th **Q39   Congenital malformations of esophagus**

   Q39.0   Atresia of esophagus without fistula
      Atresia of esophagus NOS

   Q39.1   Atresia of esophagus with tracheo-esophageal fistula
      Atresia of esophagus with broncho-esophageal fistula

   Q39.2   Congenital tracheo-esophageal fistula without atresia
      Congenital tracheo-esophageal fistula NOS

   Q39.3   Congenital stenosis and stricture of esophagus

   Q39.4   Esophageal web

   Q39.5   Congenital dilatation of esophagus
      Congenital cardiospasm

   Q39.6   Congenital diverticulum of esophagus
      Congenital esophageal pouch

   Q39.8   Other congenital malformations of esophagus
      Congenital absence of esophagus
      Congenital displacement of esophagus
      Congenital duplication of esophagus

   Q39.9   Congenital malformation of esophagus, unspecified   ▽

✓4th **Q40   Other congenital malformations of upper alimentary tract**

   Q40.0   Congenital hypertrophic pyloric stenosis
      Congenital or infantile constriction
      Congenital or infantile hypertrophy
      Congenital or infantile spasm
      Congenital or infantile stenosis
      Congenital or infantile stricture

   Q40.1   Congenital hiatus hernia
      Congenital displacement of cardia through esophageal hiatus
      EXCLUDES 1 congenital diaphragmatic hernia (Q79.0)

   Q40.2   Other specified congenital malformations of stomach
      Congenital displacement of stomach
      Congenital diverticulum of stomach
      Congenital hourglass stomach
      Congenital duplication of stomach
      Megalogastria
      Microgastria

   Q40.3   Congenital malformation of stomach, unspecified   ▽

   Q40.8   Other specified congenital malformations of upper alimentary tract

   Q40.9   Congenital malformation of upper alimentary tract, unspecified   ▽
      Congenital anomaly of upper alimentary tract
      Congenital deformity of upper alimentary tract

✓4th **Q41   Congenital absence, atresia and stenosis of small intestine**
      INCLUDES congenital obstruction, occlusion or stricture of small intestine or intestine NOS
      EXCLUDES 1 cystic fibrosis with intestinal manifestation (E84.11)
         meconium ileus NOS (without cystic fibrosis) (P76.0)

   Q41.0   Congenital absence, atresia and stenosis of duodenum

   Q41.1   Congenital absence, atresia and stenosis of jejunum
      Apple peel syndrome
      Imperforate jejunum

   Q41.2   Congenital absence, atresia and stenosis of ileum

   Q41.8   Congenital absence, atresia and stenosis of other specified parts of small intestine

   Q41.9   Congenital absence, atresia and stenosis of small intestine, part unspecified   ▽
      Congenital absence, atresia and stenosis of intestine NOS

✓4th **Q42   Congenital absence, atresia and stenosis of large intestine**
      INCLUDES congenital obstruction, occlusion and stricture of large intestine

   Q42.0   Congenital absence, atresia and stenosis of rectum with fistula

   Q42.1   Congenital absence, atresia and stenosis of rectum without fistula
      Imperforate rectum

   Q42.2   Congenital absence, atresia and stenosis of anus with fistula

   Q42.3   Congenital absence, atresia and stenosis of anus without fistula
      Imperforate anus

   Q42.8   Congenital absence, atresia and stenosis of other parts of large intestine

   Q42.9   Congenital absence, atresia and stenosis of large intestine, part unspecified   ▽

EXCLUDES 1 Not coded here   EXCLUDES 2 Not included here   N Newborn Age: 0   P Pediatric Age: 0-17   M Maternity Age: 12-55   A Adult Age: 15-124

876   ICD-10-CM 2018

✓4ᵗʰ **Q43　Other congenital malformations of intestine**

　Q43.0　Meckel's diverticulum (displaced) (hypertrophic)
　　Persistent omphalomesenteric duct
　　Persistent vitelline duct

　Q43.1　Hirschsprung's disease
　　Aganglionosis
　　Congenital (aganglionic) megacolon

　Q43.2　Other congenital functional disorders of colon
　　Congenital dilatation of colon

　Q43.3　Congenital malformations of intestinal fixation
　　Congenital omental, anomalous adhesions [bands]
　　Congenital peritoneal adhesions [bands]
　　Incomplete rotation of cecum and colon
　　Insufficient rotation of cecum and colon
　　Jackson's membrane
　　Malrotation of colon
　　Rotation failure of cecum and colon
　　Universal mesentery

　Q43.4　Duplication of intestine

　Q43.5　Ectopic anus

　Q43.6　Congenital fistula of rectum and anus
　　EXCLUDES 1　congenital fistula of anus with absence, atresia and
　　　　　　　　stenosis (Q42.2)
　　　　　　　congenital fistula of rectum with absence, atresia and
　　　　　　　　stenosis (Q42.0)
　　　　　　　congenital rectovaginal fistula (Q52.2)
　　　　　　　congenital urethrorectal fistula (Q64.73)
　　　　　　　pilonidal fistula or sinus (L05.-)

　Q43.7　Persistent cloaca
　　Cloaca NOS

　Q43.8　Other specified congenital malformations of intestine
　　Congenital blind loop syndrome
　　Congenital diverticulitis, colon
　　Congenital diverticulum, intestine
　　Dolichocolon
　　Megaloappendix
　　Megaloduodenum
　　Microcolon
　　Transposition of appendix
　　Transposition of colon
　　Transposition of intestine
　　AHA: 2013, 2Q, 31

　Q43.9　Congenital malformation of intestine, unspecified　▽

✓4ᵗʰ **Q44　Congenital malformations of gallbladder, bile ducts and liver**

　Q44.0　Agenesis, aplasia and hypoplasia of gallbladder
　　Congenital absence of gallbladder

　Q44.1　Other congenital malformations of gallbladder
　　Congenital malformation of gallbladder NOS
　　Intrahepatic gallbladder

　Q44.2　Atresia of bile ducts

　Q44.3　Congenital stenosis and stricture of bile ducts

　Q44.4　Choledochal cyst

　Q44.5　Other congenital malformations of bile ducts
　　Accessory hepatic duct
　　Biliary duct duplication
　　Congenital malformation of bile duct NOS
　　Cystic duct duplication

　Q44.6　Cystic disease of liver
　　Fibrocystic disease of liver

　Q44.7　Other congenital malformations of liver
　　Accessory liver
　　Alagille's syndrome
　　Congenital absence of liver
　　Congenital hepatomegaly
　　Congenital malformation of liver NOS

✓4ᵗʰ **Q45　Other congenital malformations of digestive system**
　　EXCLUDES 2　congenital diaphragmatic hernia (Q79.0)
　　　　　　　congenital hiatus hernia (Q40.1)

　Q45.0　Agenesis, aplasia and hypoplasia of pancreas
　　Congenital absence of pancreas

　Q45.1　Annular pancreas

　Q45.2　Congenital pancreatic cyst

　Q45.3　Other congenital malformations of pancreas and pancreatic duct
　　Accessory pancreas
　　Congenital malformation of pancreas or pancreatic duct NOS
　　EXCLUDES 1　congenital diabetes mellitus (E10.-)
　　　　　　　cystic fibrosis (E84.0-E84.9)
　　　　　　　fibrocystic disease of pancreas (E84.-)
　　　　　　　neonatal diabetes mellitus (P70.2)

　Q45.8　Other specified congenital malformations of digestive system
　　Absence (complete) (partial) of alimentary tract NOS
　　Duplication of digestive system
　　Malposition, congenital of digestive system

　Q45.9　Congenital malformation of digestive system, unspecified　▽
　　Congenital anomaly of digestive system
　　Congenital deformity of digestive system

Congenital malformations of genital organs (Q50-Q56)

　EXCLUDES 1　androgen insensitivity syndrome (E34.5-)
　　　　　　　syndromes associated with anomalies in the number and form of
　　　　　　　chromosomes (Q90-Q99)

✓4ᵗʰ **Q50　Congenital malformations of ovaries, fallopian tubes and broad ligaments**

　✓5ᵗʰ **Q50.0　Congenital absence of ovary**
　　　EXCLUDES 1　Turner's syndrome (Q96.-)

　　Q50.01　Congenital absence of ovary, unilateral　♀
　　Q50.02　Congenital absence of ovary, bilateral　♀

　Q50.1　Developmental ovarian cyst　♀

　Q50.2　Congenital torsion of ovary　♀

　✓5ᵗʰ **Q50.3　Other congenital malformations of ovary**

　　Q50.31　Accessory ovary　♀

　　Q50.32　Ovarian streak　♀
　　　46, XX with streak gonads

　　Q50.39　Other congenital malformation of ovary　♀
　　　Congenital malformation of ovary NOS

　Q50.4　Embryonic cyst of fallopian tube　♀
　　Fimbrial cyst

　Q50.5　Embryonic cyst of broad ligament　♀
　　Epoophoron cyst
　　Parovarian cyst

　Q50.6　Other congenital malformations of fallopian tube and broad ligament　♀
　　Absence of fallopian tube and broad ligament
　　Accessory fallopian tube and broad ligament
　　Atresia of fallopian tube and broad ligament
　　Congenital malformation of fallopian tube or broad ligament NOS

✓4ᵗʰ **Q51　Congenital malformations of uterus and cervix**

　Q51.0　Agenesis and aplasia of uterus　♀
　　Congenital absence of uterus

　✓5ᵗʰ **Q51.1　Doubling of uterus with doubling of cervix and vagina**

　　Q51.10　Doubling of uterus with doubling of cervix and vagina without obstruction　♀
　　　Doubling of uterus with doubling of cervix and vagina NOS

　　Q51.11　Doubling of uterus with doubling of cervix and vagina with obstruction　♀

　Q51.2　Other doubling of uterus　♀
　　Doubling of uterus NOS
　　Septate uterus, complete or partial

　Q51.3　Bicornate uterus　♀
　　Bicornate uterus, complete or partial

　Q51.4　Unicornate uterus　♀
　　Unicornate uterus with or without a separate uterine horn
　　Uterus with only one functioning horn

　Q51.5　Agenesis and aplasia of cervix　♀
　　Congenital absence of cervix

　Q51.6　Embryonic cyst of cervix　♀

　Q51.7　Congenital fistulae between uterus and digestive and urinary tracts　♀

　✓5ᵗʰ **Q51.8　Other congenital malformations of uterus and cervix**

　　✓6ᵗʰ **Q51.81　Other congenital malformations of uterus**

　　　Q51.810　Arcuate uterus　♀
　　　　Arcuatus uterus

　　　Q51.811　Hypoplasia of uterus　♀

　　　Q51.818　Other congenital malformations of uterus　♀
　　　　Müllerian anomaly of uterus NEC

　　✓6ᵗʰ **Q51.82　Other congenital malformations of cervix**

　　　Q51.820　Cervical duplication　♀
　　　Q51.821　Hypoplasia of cervix　♀
　　　Q51.828　Other congenital malformations of cervix　♀

　Q51.9　Congenital malformation of uterus and cervix, unspecified　♀▽

✓ Additional Character Req　✓x7ᵗʰ Placeholder Alert　Manifestation　HCC CMS-HCC Condition　▽ Unspecified Code　▶◀ Revised Text　● New Code　▲ Revised Code Title

Chapter 17. Congenital Malformations, Deformations, and Chromosomal Abnormalities

Q52–Q55.9

✓4ᵗʰ **Q52 Other congenital malformations of female genitalia**

    Q52.0 Congenital absence of vagina ♀
        Vaginal agenesis, total or partial

  ✓5ᵗʰ **Q52.1 Doubling of vagina**
        EXCLUDES 1   doubling of vagina with doubling of uterus and cervix (Q51.1-)

        Q52.10 Doubling of vagina, unspecified ♀▽
            Septate vagina NOS

        Q52.11 Transverse vaginal septum ♀

    ✓6ᵗʰ **Q52.12 Longitudinal vaginal septum**
            Q52.120 Longitudinal vaginal septum, nonobstructing
            Q52.121 Longitudinal vaginal septum, obstructing, right side ♀
            Q52.122 Longitudinal vaginal septum, obstructing, left side ♀
            Q52.123 Longitudinal vaginal septum, microperforate, right side ♀
            Q52.124 Longitudinal vaginal septum, microperforate, left side ♀
            Q52.129 Other and unspecified longitudinal vaginal septum ♀▽

    Q52.2 Congenital rectovaginal fistula ♀
        EXCLUDES 1   cloaca (Q43.7)

    Q52.3 Imperforate hymen
        DEF: Obstructive anomaly of vagina, characterized by complete closure of membranous fold around external opening of vagina, obstructing the vaginal introitus.

    Q52.4 Other congenital malformations of vagina ♀
        Canal of Nuck cyst, congenital
        Congenital malformation of vagina NOS
        Embryonic vaginal cyst
        Gartner's duct cyst

    Q52.5 Fusion of labia ♀

    Q52.6 Congenital malformation of clitoris ♀

  ✓5ᵗʰ **Q52.7 Other and unspecified congenital malformations of vulva**
        Q52.70 Unspecified congenital malformations of vulva ♀▽
            Congenital malformation of vulva NOS
        Q52.71 Congenital absence of vulva ♀
        Q52.79 Other congenital malformations of vulva ♀
            Congenital cyst of vulva

    Q52.8 Other specified congenital malformations of female genitalia ♀

    Q52.9 Congenital malformation of female genitalia, unspecified ♀▽

✓4ᵗʰ **Q53 Undescended and ectopic testicle**

  ✓5ᵗʰ **Q53.0 Ectopic testis**
        Q53.00 Ectopic testis, unspecified ♂▽
        Q53.01 Ectopic testis, unilateral ♂
        Q53.02 Ectopic testes, bilateral ♂

  ✓5ᵗʰ **Q53.1 Undescended testicle, unilateral**
        Q53.10 Unspecified undescended testicle, unilateral ♂▽
    ✓6ᵗʰ **Q53.11 Abdominal testis, unilateral**
            ● **Q53.111 Unilateral intraabdominal testis**
            ● **Q53.112 Unilateral inguinal testis**
        ● **Q53.12 Ectopic perineal testis, unilateral** ♂
        ● **Q53.13 Unilateral high scrotal testis**

  ✓5ᵗʰ **Q53.2 Undescended testicle, bilateral**
        Q53.20 Undescended testicle, unspecified, bilateral ♂▽
    ✓6ᵗʰ **Q53.21 Abdominal testis, bilateral**
            ● **Q53.211 Bilateral intraabdominal testes**
            ● **Q53.212 Bilateral inguinal testes**
        ● **Q53.22 Ectopic perineal testis, bilateral** ♂
        ● **Q53.23 Bilateral high scrotal testes**

    Q53.9 Undescended testicle, unspecified ♂▽
        Cryptorchism NOS

✓4ᵗʰ **Q54 Hypospadias**
    EXCLUDES 1   epispadias (Q64.0)
    DEF: Abnormal opening of urethra on the ventral (underside) surface of the penis.

    Q54.0 Hypospadias, balanic ♂
        Hypospadias, coronal
        Hypospadias, glandular

    Q54.1 Hypospadias, penile ♂

Hypospadias and Epispadias

Hypospadias (ventral view) labels: Balanic (glanular, coronal) hypospadias; Subcoronal hypospadias; Penile hypospadias; Scrotal hypospadias; Scrotum; Penile raphe; Penoscrotal hypospadius; Scrotal raphe; Perineal hypospadias

Epispadias (dorsal view) labels: Normal external urethral orifice; Glans penis; Foreskin (retracted); Epispadias

    Q54.2 Hypospadias, penoscrotal ♂
    Q54.3 Hypospadias, perineal ♂
    Q54.4 Congenital chordee ♂
        Chordee without hypospadias
    Q54.8 Other hypospadias ♂
        Hypospadias with intersex state
    Q54.9 Hypospadias, unspecified ♂▽

✓4ᵗʰ **Q55 Other congenital malformations of male genital organs**
    EXCLUDES 1   congenital hydrocele (P83.5)
               hypospadias (Q54.-)

    Q55.0 Absence and aplasia of testis ♂
        Monorchism

    Q55.1 Hypoplasia of testis and scrotum ♂
        Fusion of testes

  ✓5ᵗʰ **Q55.2 Other and unspecified congenital malformations of testis and scrotum**
        Q55.20 Unspecified congenital malformations of testis and scrotum ♂▽
            Congenital malformation of testis or scrotum NOS
        Q55.21 Polyorchism ♂
        Q55.22 Retractile testis ♂
        Q55.23 Scrotal transposition ♂
        Q55.29 Other congenital malformations of testis and scrotum ♂

    Q55.3 Atresia of vas deferens ♂
        Code first any associated cystic fibrosis (E84.-)

    Q55.4 Other congenital malformations of vas deferens, epididymis, seminal vesicles and prostate ♂
        Absence or aplasia of prostate
        Absence or aplasia of spermatic cord
        Congenital malformation of vas deferens, epididymis, seminal vesicles or prostate NOS

    Q55.5 Congenital absence and aplasia of penis ♂

  ✓5ᵗʰ **Q55.6 Other congenital malformations of penis**
        Q55.61 Curvature of penis (lateral) ♂
        Q55.62 Hypoplasia of penis ♂
            Micropenis
        Q55.63 Congenital torsion of penis ♂
            EXCLUDES 1   acquired torsion of penis (N48.82)
        Q55.64 Hidden penis
            Buried penis
            Concealed penis
            EXCLUDES 1   acquired buried penis (N48.83)
        Q55.69 Other congenital malformation of penis ♂
            Congenital malformation of penis NOS

    Q55.7 Congenital vasocutaneous fistula ♂

    Q55.8 Other specified congenital malformations of male genital organs ♂

    Q55.9 Congenital malformation of male genital organ, unspecified ♂▽
        Congenital anomaly of male genital organ
        Congenital deformity of male genital organ

EXCLUDES 1 Not coded here   EXCLUDES 2 Not included here   N Newborn Age: 0   P Pediatric Age: 0-17   M Maternity Age: 12-55   A Adult Age: 15-124

878   ICD-10-CM 2018

✓4th **Q56 Indeterminate sex and pseudohermaphroditism**
> *EXCLUDES 1* 46, XX true hermaphrodite (Q99.1)
> androgen insensitivity syndrome (E34.5-)
> chimera 46, XX/46, XY true hermaphrodite (Q99.0)
> female pseudohermaphroditism with adrenocortical disorder
> (E25.-)
> pseudohermaphroditism with specified chromosomal anomaly
> (Q96-Q99)
> pure gonadal dysgenesis (Q99.1)

Q56.0 Hermaphroditism, not elsewhere classified
Ovotestis

Q56.1 Male pseudohermaphroditism, not elsewhere classified   ♂
46, XY with streak gonads
Male pseudohermaphroditism NOS

Q56.2 Female pseudohermaphroditism, not elsewhere classified   ♀
Female pseudohermaphroditism NOS

Q56.3 Pseudohermaphroditism, unspecified   ▽

Q56.4 Indeterminate sex, unspecified   ▽
Ambiguous genitalia

Congenital malformations of the urinary system (Q60-Q64)

✓4th **Q60 Renal agenesis and other reduction defects of kidney**
> *INCLUDES* congenital absence of kidney
> congenital atrophy of kidney
> infantile atrophy of kidney

Q60.0 Renal agenesis, unilateral

Q60.1 Renal agenesis, bilateral

Q60.2 Renal agenesis, unspecified   ▽

Q60.3 Renal hypoplasia, unilateral

Q60.4 Renal hypoplasia, bilateral

Q60.5 Renal hypoplasia, unspecified   ▽

Q60.6 Potter's syndrome

✓4th **Q61 Cystic kidney disease**
> *EXCLUDES 1* acquired cyst of kidney (N28.1)
> Potter's syndrome (Q60.6)

✓5th **Q61.0 Congenital renal cyst**

Q61.00 Congenital renal cyst, unspecified   ▽
Cyst of kidney NOS (congenital)

Q61.01 Congenital single renal cyst

Q61.02 Congenital multiple renal cysts

✓5th **Q61.1 Polycystic kidney, infantile type**
Polycystic kidney, autosomal recessive

Q61.11 Cystic dilatation of collecting ducts

Q61.19 Other polycystic kidney, infantile type

Q61.2 Polycystic kidney, adult type
Polycystic kidney, autosomal dominant

Q61.3 Polycystic kidney, unspecified   ▽
AHA: 2016, 3Q, 22

Q61.4 Renal dysplasia
Multicystic dysplastic kidney
Multicystic kidney (development)
Multicystic kidney disease
Multicystic renal dysplasia
> *EXCLUDES 1* polycystic kidney disease (Q61.11-Q61.3)

Q61.5 Medullary cystic kidney
Nephronopthisis
Sponge kidney NOS
DEF: Sponge kidney: Dilated collecting tubules; usually
asymptomatic but calcinosis in tubules may cause renal
insufficiency.

Q61.8 Other cystic kidney diseases
Fibrocystic kidney
Fibrocystic renal degeneration or disease

Q61.9 Cystic kidney disease, unspecified   ▽
Meckel-Gruber syndrome

✓4th **Q62 Congenital obstructive defects of renal pelvis and congenital malformations of ureter**

Q62.0 Congenital hydronephrosis

✓5th **Q62.1 Congenital occlusion of ureter**
Atresia and stenosis of ureter

Q62.10 Congenital occlusion of ureter, unspecified   ▽

Q62.11 Congenital occlusion of ureteropelvic junction

Q62.12 Congenital occlusion of ureterovesical orifice

Q62.2 Congenital megaureter
Congenital dilatation of ureter

✓5th **Q62.3 Other obstructive defects of renal pelvis and ureter**

Q62.31 Congenital ureterocele, orthotopic

Q62.32 Cecoureterocele
Ectopic ureterocele

Q62.39 Other obstructive defects of renal pelvis and ureter
Ureteropelvic junction obstruction NOS

Q62.4 Agenesis of ureter
Congenital absence ureter

Q62.5 Duplication of ureter
Accessory ureter
Double ureter

✓5th **Q62.6 Malposition of ureter**

Q62.60 Malposition of ureter, unspecified   ▽

Q62.61 Deviation of ureter

Q62.62 Displacement of ureter

Q62.63 Anomalous implantation of ureter
Ectopia of ureter
Ectopic ureter

Q62.69 Other malposition of ureter

Q62.7 Congenital vesico-uretero-renal reflux

Q62.8 Other congenital malformations of ureter
Anomaly of ureter NOS

✓4th **Q63 Other congenital malformations of kidney**
> *EXCLUDES 1* congenital nephrotic syndrome (N04.-)

Q63.0 Accessory kidney

Q63.1 Lobulated, fused and horseshoe kidney

Q63.2 Ectopic kidney
Congenital displaced kidney
Malrotation of kidney

Q63.3 Hyperplastic and giant kidney
Compensatory hypertrophy of kidney

Q63.8 Other specified congenital malformations of kidney
Congenital renal calculi

Q63.9 Congenital malformation of kidney, unspecified   ▽

✓4th **Q64 Other congenital malformations of urinary system**

Q64.0 Epispadias   ♂
> *EXCLUDES 1* hypospadias (Q54.-)

✓5th **Q64.1 Exstrophy of urinary bladder**

Q64.10 Exstrophy of urinary bladder, unspecified   ▽
Ectopia vesicae

▲   **Q64.11 Supravesical fissure of urinary bladder**

Q64.12 Cloacal exstrophy of urinary bladder

Q64.19 Other exstrophy of urinary bladder
Extroversion of bladder

Q64.2 Congenital posterior urethral valves

✓5th **Q64.3 Other atresia and stenosis of urethra and bladder neck**

Q64.31 Congenital bladder neck obstruction
Congenital obstruction of vesicourethral orifice

Q64.32 Congenital stricture of urethra

Q64.33 Congenital stricture of urinary meatus

Q64.39 Other atresia and stenosis of urethra and bladder neck
Atresia and stenosis of urethra and bladder neck NOS

Q64.4 Malformation of urachus
Cyst of urachus
Patent urachus
Prolapse of urachus

Q64.5 Congenital absence of bladder and urethra

Q64.6 Congenital diverticulum of bladder

✓5th **Q64.7 Other and unspecified congenital malformations of bladder and urethra**
> *EXCLUDES 1* congenital prolapse of bladder (mucosa) (Q79.4)

Q64.70 Unspecified congenital malformation of bladder and urethra   ▽
Malformation of bladder or urethra NOS

Q64.71 Congenital prolapse of urethra

Q64.72 Congenital prolapse of urinary meatus

Q64.73 Congenital urethrorectal fistula

Q64.74 Double urethra

Q64.75 Double urinary meatus

Q64.79 Other congenital malformations of bladder and urethra

Q64.8 Other specified congenital malformations of urinary system

---

✔ Additional Character Req   ✔x7th Placeholder Alert   Manifestation   HCC CMS-HCC Condition   ▽ Unspecified Code   ►◄ Revised Text   ● New Code   ▲ Revised Code Title

Q64.9 Congenital malformation of urinary system, unspecified ▽
Congenital anomaly NOS of urinary system
Congenital deformity NOS of urinary system

Congenital malformations and deformations of the musculoskeletal system (Q65-Q79)

✓4ᵗʰ **Q65 Congenital deformities of hip**
     EXCLUDES 1   clicking hip (R29.4)

✓5ᵗʰ **Q65.0 Congenital dislocation of hip, unilateral**

     Q65.00 Congenital dislocation of unspecified hip, unilateral ▽

     Q65.01 Congenital dislocation of right hip, unilateral

     Q65.02 Congenital dislocation of left hip, unilateral

Q65.1 Congenital dislocation of hip, bilateral

Q65.2 Congenital dislocation of hip, unspecified ▽

✓5ᵗʰ **Q65.3 Congenital partial dislocation of hip, unilateral**

     Q65.30 Congenital partial dislocation of unspecified hip, unilateral ▽

     Q65.31 Congenital partial dislocation of right hip, unilateral

     Q65.32 Congenital partial dislocation of left hip, unilateral

Q65.4 Congenital partial dislocation of hip, bilateral

Q65.5 Congenital partial dislocation of hip, unspecified ▽

Q65.6 Congenital unstable hip
     Congenital dislocatable hip

✓5ᵗʰ **Q65.8 Other congenital deformities of hip**

     Q65.81 Congenital coxa valga

     Q65.82 Congenital coxa vara

     Q65.89 Other specified congenital deformities of hip
         Anteversion of femoral neck
         Congenital acetabular dysplasia

Q65.9 Congenital deformity of hip, unspecified ▽

✓4ᵗʰ **Q66 Congenital deformities of feet**
     EXCLUDES 1   reduction defects of feet (Q72.-)
         valgus deformities (acquired) (M21.0-)
         varus deformities (acquired) (M21.1-)

Q66.0 Congenital talipes equinovarus

Q66.1 Congenital talipes calcaneovarus

✓5ᵗʰ **Q66.2 Congenital metatarsus (primus) varus**

     Q66.21 Congenital metatarsus primus varus

     Q66.22 Congenital metatarsus adductus
         Congenital metatarsus varus

Q66.3 Other congenital varus deformities of feet
     Hallux varus, congenital

Q66.4 Congenital talipes calcaneovalgus

✓5ᵗʰ **Q66.5 Congenital pes planus**
     Congenital flat foot
     Congenital rigid flat foot
     Congenital spastic (everted) flat foot
     EXCLUDES 1   pes planus, acquired (M21.4)

     Q66.50 Congenital pes planus, unspecified foot ▽

     Q66.51 Congenital pes planus, right foot

     Q66.52 Congenital pes planus, left foot

Q66.6 Other congenital valgus deformities of feet
     Congenital metatarsus valgus

Q66.7 Congenital pes cavus

✓5ᵗʰ **Q66.8 Other congenital deformities of feet**

     Q66.80 Congenital vertical talus deformity, unspecified foot ▽

     Q66.81 Congenital vertical talus deformity, right foot

     Q66.82 Congenital vertical talus deformity, left foot

     Q66.89 Other specified congenital deformities of feet
         Congenital asymmetric talipes
         Congenital clubfoot NOS
         Congenital talipes NOS
         Congenital tarsal coalition
         Hammer toe, congenital

Q66.9 Congenital deformity of feet, unspecified ▽

✓4ᵗʰ **Q67 Congenital musculoskeletal deformities of head, face, spine and chest**
     EXCLUDES 1   congenital malformation syndromes classified to Q87-
         Potter's syndrome (Q60.6)

Q67.0 Congenital facial asymmetry

Q67.1 Congenital compression facies

Q67.2 Dolichocephaly

Q67.3 Plagiocephaly

Q67.4 Other congenital deformities of skull, face and jaw
     Congenital depressions in skull
     Congenital hemifacial atrophy or hypertrophy
     Deviation of nasal septum, congenital
     Squashed or bent nose, congenital
     EXCLUDES 1   dentofacial anomalies [including malocclusion]
         (M26.-)
         syphilitic saddle nose (A50.5)

Q67.5 Congenital deformity of spine
     Congenital postural scoliosis
     Congenital scoliosis NOS
     EXCLUDES 1   infantile idiopathic scoliosis (M41.0)
         scoliosis due to congenital bony malformation (Q76.3
     AHA: 2014, 4Q, 26

Q67.6 Pectus excavatum
     Congenital funnel chest

Q67.7 Pectus carinatum
     Congenital pigeon chest

Q67.8 Other congenital deformities of chest
     Congenital deformity of chest wall NOS

✓4ᵗʰ **Q68 Other congenital musculoskeletal deformities**
     EXCLUDES 1   reduction defects of limb(s) (Q71-Q73)
     EXCLUDES 2   congenital myotonic chondrodystrophy (G71.13)

Q68.0 Congenital deformity of sternocleidomastoid muscle
     Congenital contracture of sternocleidomastoid (muscle)
     Congenital (sternomastoid) torticollis
     Sternomastoid tumor (congenital)

Q68.1 Congenital deformity of finger(s) and hand
     Congenital clubfinger
     Spade-like hand (congenital)

Q68.2 Congenital deformity of knee
     Congenital dislocation of knee
     Congenital genu recurvatum

Q68.3 Congenital bowing of femur
     EXCLUDES 1   anteversion of femur (neck) (Q65.89)

Q68.4 Congenital bowing of tibia and fibula

Q68.5 Congenital bowing of long bones of leg, unspecified ▽

Q68.6 Discoid meniscus

Q68.8 Other specified congenital musculoskeletal deformities
     Congenital deformity of clavicle
     Congenital deformity of elbow
     Congenital deformity of forearm
     Congenital deformity of scapula
     Congenital deformity of wrist
     Congenital dislocation of elbow
     Congenital dislocation of shoulder
     Congenital dislocation of wrist

✓4ᵗʰ **Q69 Polydactyly**

Q69.0 Accessory finger(s)

Q69.1 Accessory thumb(s)

Q69.2 Accessory toe(s)
     Accessory hallux

Q69.9 Polydactyly, unspecified ▽
     Supernumerary digit(s) NOS

✓4ᵗʰ **Q70 Syndactyly**

✓5ᵗʰ **Q70.0 Fused fingers**
     Complex syndactyly of fingers with synostosis

     Q70.00 Fused fingers, unspecified hand ▽

     Q70.01 Fused fingers, right hand

     Q70.02 Fused fingers, left hand

     Q70.03 Fused fingers, bilateral

✓5ᵗʰ **Q70.1 Webbed fingers**
     Simple syndactyly of fingers without synostosis

     Q70.10 Webbed fingers, unspecified hand ▽

     Q70.11 Webbed fingers, right hand

     Q70.12 Webbed fingers, left hand

     Q70.13 Webbed fingers, bilateral

✓5ᵗʰ **Q70.2 Fused toes**
     Complex syndactyly of toes with synostosis

     Q70.20 Fused toes, unspecified foot ▽

     Q70.21 Fused toes, right foot

     Q70.22 Fused toes, left foot

     Q70.23 Fused toes, bilateral

EXCLUDES 1 Not coded here   EXCLUDES 2 Not included here   N Newborn Age: 0   P Pediatric Age: 0-17   M Maternity Age: 12-55   A Adult Age: 15-124

880   ICD-10-CM 2018

✓5ᵗʰ **Q70.3 Webbed toes**
Simple syndactyly of toes without synostosis
    Q70.30   Webbed toes, unspecified foot   ▽
    Q70.31   Webbed toes, right foot
    Q70.32   Webbed toes, left foot
    Q70.33   Webbed toes, bilateral
   Q70.4 Polysyndactyly, unspecified   ▽
     EXCLUDES 1   specified syndactyly of hand and feet—code to specified conditions (Q70.0-Q70.3-)
   Q70.9 Syndactyly, unspecified   ▽
Symphalangy NOS

✓4ᵗʰ **Q71 Reduction defects of upper limb**

✓5ᵗʰ **Q71.0 Congenital complete absence of upper limb**
    Q71.00   Congenital complete absence of unspecified   ▽
              upper limb
    Q71.01   Congenital complete absence of right upper limb
    Q71.02   Congenital complete absence of left upper limb
    Q71.03   Congenital complete absence of upper limb, bilateral

✓5ᵗʰ **Q71.1 Congenital absence of upper arm and forearm with hand present**
    Q71.10   Congenital absence of unspecified upper arm   ▽
              and forearm with hand present
    Q71.11   Congenital absence of right upper arm and forearm with hand present
    Q71.12   Congenital absence of left upper arm and forearm with hand present
    Q71.13   Congenital absence of upper arm and forearm with hand present, bilateral

✓5ᵗʰ **Q71.2 Congenital absence of both forearm and hand**
    Q71.20   Congenital absence of both forearm and hand,   ▽
              unspecified upper limb
    Q71.21   Congenital absence of both forearm and hand, right upper limb
    Q71.22   Congenital absence of both forearm and hand, left upper limb
    Q71.23   Congenital absence of both forearm and hand, bilateral

✓5ᵗʰ **Q71.3 Congenital absence of hand and finger**
    Q71.30   Congenital absence of unspecified hand   ▽
              and finger
    Q71.31   Congenital absence of right hand and finger
    Q71.32   Congenital absence of left hand and finger
    Q71.33   Congenital absence of hand and finger, bilateral

✓5ᵗʰ **Q71.4 Longitudinal reduction defect of radius**
Clubhand (congenital)
Radial clubhand
    Q71.40   Longitudinal reduction defect of unspecified   ▽
              radius
    Q71.41   Longitudinal reduction defect of right radius
    Q71.42   Longitudinal reduction defect of left radius
    Q71.43   Longitudinal reduction defect of radius, bilateral

✓5ᵗʰ **Q71.5 Longitudinal reduction defect of ulna**
    Q71.50   Longitudinal reduction defect of unspecified ulna   ▽
    Q71.51   Longitudinal reduction defect of right ulna
    Q71.52   Longitudinal reduction defect of left ulna
    Q71.53   Longitudinal reduction defect of ulna, bilateral

✓5ᵗʰ **Q71.6 Lobster-claw hand**
    Q71.60   Lobster-claw hand, unspecified hand   ▽
    Q71.61   Lobster-claw right hand
    Q71.62   Lobster-claw left hand
    Q71.63   Lobster-claw hand, bilateral

✓5ᵗʰ **Q71.8 Other reduction defects of upper limb**
    ✓6ᵗʰ **Q71.81 Congenital shortening of upper limb**
        Q71.811   Congenital shortening of right upper limb
        Q71.812   Congenital shortening of left upper limb
        Q71.813   Congenital shortening of upper limb, bilateral
        Q71.819   Congenital shortening of unspecified   ▽
                  upper limb

    ✓6ᵗʰ **Q71.89 Other reduction defects of upper limb**
        Q71.891   Other reduction defects of right upper limb
        Q71.892   Other reduction defects of left upper limb
        Q71.893   Other reduction defects of upper limb, bilateral
        Q71.899   Other reduction defects of unspecified   ▽
                  upper limb

✓5ᵗʰ **Q71.9 Unspecified reduction defect of upper limb**
    Q71.90   Unspecified reduction defect of unspecified   ▽
              upper limb
    Q71.91   Unspecified reduction defect of right upper limb   ▽
    Q71.92   Unspecified reduction defect of left upper limb   ▽
    Q71.93   Unspecified reduction defect of upper limb,   ▽
              bilateral

✓4ᵗʰ **Q72 Reduction defects of lower limb**

✓5ᵗʰ **Q72.0 Congenital complete absence of lower limb**
    Q72.00   Congenital complete absence of unspecified   ▽
              lower limb
    Q72.01   Congenital complete absence of right lower limb
    Q72.02   Congenital complete absence of left lower limb
    Q72.03   Congenital complete absence of lower limb, bilateral

✓5ᵗʰ **Q72.1 Congenital absence of thigh and lower leg with foot present**
    Q72.10   Congenital absence of unspecified thigh and   ▽
              lower leg with foot present
    Q72.11   Congenital absence of right thigh and lower leg with foot present
    Q72.12   Congenital absence of left thigh and lower leg with foot present
    Q72.13   Congenital absence of thigh and lower leg with foot present, bilateral

✓5ᵗʰ **Q72.2 Congenital absence of both lower leg and foot**
    Q72.20   Congenital absence of both lower leg and foot,   ▽
              unspecified lower limb
    Q72.21   Congenital absence of both lower leg and foot, right lower limb
    Q72.22   Congenital absence of both lower leg and foot, left lower limb
    Q72.23   Congenital absence of both lower leg and foot, bilateral

✓5ᵗʰ **Q72.3 Congenital absence of foot and toe(s)**
    Q72.30   Congenital absence of unspecified foot and toe(s) ▽
    Q72.31   Congenital absence of right foot and toe(s)
    Q72.32   Congenital absence of left foot and toe(s)
    Q72.33   Congenital absence of foot and toe(s), bilateral

✓5ᵗʰ **Q72.4 Longitudinal reduction defect of femur**
Proximal femoral focal deficiency
    Q72.40   Longitudinal reduction defect of unspecified   ▽
              femur
    Q72.41   Longitudinal reduction defect of right femur
    Q72.42   Longitudinal reduction defect of left femur
    Q72.43   Longitudinal reduction defect of femur, bilateral

✓5ᵗʰ **Q72.5 Longitudinal reduction defect of tibia**
    Q72.50   Longitudinal reduction defect of unspecified tibia ▽
    Q72.51   Longitudinal reduction defect of right tibia
    Q72.52   Longitudinal reduction defect of left tibia
    Q72.53   Longitudinal reduction defect of tibia, bilateral

✓5ᵗʰ **Q72.6 Longitudinal reduction defect of fibula**
    Q72.60   Longitudinal reduction defect of unspecified   ▽
              fibula
    Q72.61   Longitudinal reduction defect of right fibula
    Q72.62   Longitudinal reduction defect of left fibula
    Q72.63   Longitudinal reduction defect of fibula, bilateral

✓5ᵗʰ **Q72.7 Split foot**
    Q72.70   Split foot, unspecified lower limb   ▽
    Q72.71   Split foot, right lower limb
    Q72.72   Split foot, left lower limb
    Q72.73   Split foot, bilateral

✓5ᵗʰ **Q72.8 Other reduction defects of lower limb**
    ✓6ᵗʰ **Q72.81 Congenital shortening of lower limb**
        Q72.811   Congenital shortening of right lower limb
        Q72.812   Congenital shortening of left lower limb

✔ Additional Character Req   ✔7ᵗʰ Placeholder Alert   Manifestation   HCC CMS-HCC Condition   ▽ Unspecified Code   ►◄ Revised Text   ● New Code   ▲ Revised Code Title

ICD-10-CM 2018   881

Q72.813 Congenital shortening of lower limb, bilateral

Q72.819 Congenital shortening of unspecified lower limb ▽

✓6ᵗʰ **Q72.89 Other reduction defects of lower limb**

    Q72.891 Other reduction defects of right lower limb

    Q72.892 Other reduction defects of left lower limb

    Q72.893 Other reduction defects of lower limb, bilateral

    Q72.899 Other reduction defects of unspecified lower limb ▽

✓5ᵗʰ **Q72.9 Unspecified reduction defect of lower limb**

    Q72.90 Unspecified reduction defect of unspecified lower limb ▽

    Q72.91 Unspecified reduction defect of right lower limb ▽

    Q72.92 Unspecified reduction defect of left lower limb ▽

    Q72.93 Unspecified reduction defect of lower limb, bilateral ▽

✓4ᵗʰ **Q73 Reduction defects of unspecified limb**

Q73.0 Congenital absence of unspecified limb(s) ▽
    Amelia NOS

Q73.1 Phocomelia, unspecified limb(s) ▽
    Phocomelia NOS

Q73.8 Other reduction defects of unspecified limb(s) ▽
    Longitudinal reduction deformity of unspecified limb(s)
    Ectromelia of limb NOS
    Hemimelia of limb NOS
    Reduction defect of limb NOS

✓4ᵗʰ **Q74 Other congenital malformations of limb(s)**
    EXCLUDES 1 polydactyly (Q69.-)
        reduction defect of limb (Q71-Q73)
        syndactyly (Q70.-)

Q74.0 Other congenital malformations of upper limb(s), including shoulder girdle
    Accessory carpal bones
    Cleidocranial dysostosis
    Congenital pseudarthrosis of clavicle
    Macrodactylia (fingers)
    Madelung's deformity
    Radioulnar synostosis
    Sprengel's deformity
    Triphalangeal thumb

Q74.1 Congenital malformation of knee
    Congenital absence of patella
    Congenital dislocation of patella
    Congenital genu valgum
    Congenital genu varum
    Rudimentary patella
    EXCLUDES 1 congenital dislocation of knee (Q68.2)
        congenital genu recurvatum (Q68.2)
        nail patella syndrome (Q87.2)

Q74.2 Other congenital malformations of lower limb(s), including pelvic girdle
    Congenital fusion of sacroiliac joint
    Congenital malformation of ankle joint
    Congenital malformation of sacroiliac joint
    EXCLUDES 1 anteversion of femur (neck) (Q65.89)

Q74.3 Arthrogryposis multiplex congenita

Q74.8 Other specified congenital malformations of limb(s)

Q74.9 Unspecified congenital malformation of limb(s) ▽
    Congenital anomaly of limb(s) NOS

✓4ᵗʰ **Q75 Other congenital malformations of skull and face bones**
    EXCLUDES 1 congenital malformation of face NOS (Q18.-)
        congenital malformation syndromes classified to Q87.-
        dentofacial anomalies [including malocclusion] (M26.-)
        musculoskeletal deformities of head and face (Q67.0-Q67.4)
        skull defects associated with congenital anomalies of brain such as:
        anencephaly (Q00.0)
        encephalocele (Q01.-)
        hydrocephalus (Q03.-)
        microcephaly (Q02)

Q75.0 Craniosynostosis
    Acrocephaly
    Imperfect fusion of skull
    Oxycephaly
    Trigonocephaly

Q75.1 Craniofacial dysostosis
    Crouzon's disease

Q75.2 Hypertelorism

Q75.3 Macrocephaly

Q75.4 Mandibulofacial dysostosis
    Franceschetti syndrome
    Treacher Collins syndrome

Q75.5 Oculomandibular dysostosis

Q75.8 Other specified congenital malformations of skull and face bones
    Absence of skull bone, congenital
    Congenital deformity of forehead
    Platybasia

Q75.9 Congenital malformation of skull and face bones, unspecified ▽
    Congenital anomaly of face bones NOS
    Congenital anomaly of skull NOS

✓4ᵗʰ **Q76 Congenital malformations of spine and bony thorax**
    EXCLUDES 1 congenital musculoskeletal deformities of spine and chest (Q67.5-Q67.8)

Q76.0 Spina bifida occulta
    EXCLUDES 1 meningocele (spinal) (Q05.-)
        spina bifida (aperta) (cystica) (Q05.-)

Q76.1 Klippel-Feil syndrome
    Cervical fusion syndrome

Q76.2 Congenital spondylolisthesis
    Congenital spondylolysis
    EXCLUDES 1 spondylolisthesis (acquired) (M43.1-)
        spondylolysis (acquired) (M43.0-)

Q76.3 Congenital scoliosis due to congenital bony malformation
    Hemivertebra fusion or failure of segmentation with scoliosis

✓5ᵗʰ **Q76.4 Other congenital malformations of spine, not associated with scoliosis**

✓6ᵗʰ **Q76.41 Congenital kyphosis**

    Q76.411 Congenital kyphosis, occipito-atlanto-axial region

    Q76.412 Congenital kyphosis, cervical region

    Q76.413 Congenital kyphosis, cervicothoracic region

    Q76.414 Congenital kyphosis, thoracic region

    Q76.415 Congenital kyphosis, thoracolumbar region

    Q76.419 Congenital kyphosis, unspecified region ▽

✓6ᵗʰ **Q76.42 Congenital lordosis**

    Q76.425 Congenital lordosis, thoracolumbar region

    Q76.426 Congenital lordosis, lumbar region

    Q76.427 Congenital lordosis, lumbosacral region

    Q76.428 Congenital lordosis, sacral and sacrococcygeal region

    Q76.429 Congenital lordosis, unspecified region ▽

    Q76.49 Other congenital malformations of spine, not associated with scoliosis
        Congenital absence of vertebra NOS
        Congenital fusion of spine NOS
        Congenital malformation of lumbosacral (joint) (region) NOS
        Congenital malformation of spine NOS
        Hemivertebra NOS
        Malformation of spine NOS
        Platyspondylisis NOS
        Supernumerary vertebra NOS

Q76.5 Cervical rib
    Supernumerary rib in cervical region

Q76.6 Other congenital malformations of ribs
    Accessory rib
    Congenital absence of rib
    Congenital fusion of ribs
    Congenital malformation of ribs NOS
    EXCLUDES 1 short rib syndrome (Q77.2)

Q76.7 Congenital malformation of sternum
    Congenital absence of sternum
    Sternum bifidum

Q76.8 Other congenital malformations of bony thorax

Q76.9 Congenital malformation of bony thorax, unspecified ▽

EXCLUDES 1 Not coded here   *EXCLUDES 2* Not included here   N Newborn Age: 0   P Pediatric Age: 0-17   M Maternity Age: 12-55   A Adult Age: 15-124

882   ICD-10-CM 2018

☑4ᵗʰ **Q77 Osteochondrodysplasia with defects of growth of tubular bones and spine**

    EXCLUDES 1 *mucopolysaccharidosis (E76.0-E76.3)*

    EXCLUDES 2 *congenital myotonic chondrodystrophy (G71.13)*

  Q77.0 Achondrogenesis
    Hypochondrogenesis

  Q77.1 Thanatophoric short stature

  Q77.2 Short rib syndrome
    Asphyxiating thoracic dysplasia [Jeune]

  Q77.3 Chondrodysplasia punctata
    EXCLUDES 1 *Rhizomelic chondrodysplasia punctata (E71.43)*

  Q77.4 Achondroplasia
    Hypochondroplasia
    Osteosclerosis congenita

  Q77.5 Diastrophic dysplasia

  Q77.6 Chondroectodermal dysplasia
    Ellis-van Creveld syndrome

  Q77.7 Spondyloepiphyseal dysplasia

  Q77.8 Other osteochondrodysplasia with defects of growth of tubular bones and spine

  Q77.9 Osteochondrodysplasia with defects of growth of tubular bones and spine, unspecified ▽

☑4ᵗʰ **Q78 Other osteochondrodysplasias**

    EXCLUDES 2 *congenital myotonic chondrodystrophy (G71.13)*

  Q78.0 Osteogenesis imperfecta
    Fragilitas ossium
    Osteopsathyrosis

  Q78.1 Polyostotic fibrous dysplasia
    Albright(-McCune)(-Sternberg) syndrome

  Q78.2 Osteopetrosis
    Albers-Schönberg syndrome
    Osteosclerosis NOS

  Q78.3 Progressive diaphyseal dysplasia
    Camurati-Engelmann syndrome

  Q78.4 Enchondromatosis
    Maffucci's syndrome
    Ollier's disease

  Q78.5 Metaphyseal dysplasia
    Pyle's syndrome

  Q78.6 Multiple congenital exostoses
    Diaphyseal aclasis

  Q78.8 Other specified osteochondrodysplasias
    Osteopoikilosis

  Q78.9 Osteochondrodysplasia, unspecified ▽
    Chondrodystrophy NOS
    Osteodystrophy NOS

☑4ᵗʰ **Q79 Congenital malformations of musculoskeletal system, not elsewhere classified**

    EXCLUDES 2 *congenital (sternomastoid) torticollis (Q68.0)*

  Q79.0 Congenital diaphragmatic hernia
    EXCLUDES 1 *congenital hiatus hernia (Q40.1)*

  Q79.1 Other congenital malformations of diaphragm
    Absence of diaphragm
    Congenital malformation of diaphragm NOS
    Eventration of diaphragm

  Q79.2 Exomphalos
    Omphalocele
    EXCLUDES 1 *umbilical hernia (K42.-)*

  Q79.3 Gastroschisis

  Q79.4 Prune belly syndrome
    Congenital prolapse of bladder mucosa
    Eagle-Barrett syndrome

☑5ᵗʰ   **Q79.5 Other congenital malformations of abdominal wall**
    EXCLUDES 1 *umbilical hernia (K42.-)*

    Q79.51 Congenital hernia of bladder

    Q79.59 Other congenital malformations of abdominal wall

  Q79.6 Ehlers-Danlos syndrome
    DEF: Connective tissue disorder that causes hyperextended skin and joints; results in fragile blood vessels with bleeding, poor wound healing, and subcutaneous pseudotumors.

Gastroschisis

Herniated small bowel (gastroschisis)
Rectus abdominus m.
Umbilicus
distal
proximal
skin
Defect

  Q79.8 Other congenital malformations of musculoskeletal system
    Absence of muscle
    Absence of tendon
    Accessory muscle
    Amyotrophia congenita
    Congenital constricting bands
    Congenital shortening of tendon
    Poland syndrome

  Q79.9 Congenital malformation of musculoskeletal system, unspecified ▽
    Congenital anomaly of musculoskeletal system NOS
    Congenital deformity of musculoskeletal system NOS

Other congenital malformations (Q80-Q89)

☑4ᵗʰ **Q80 Congenital ichthyosis**

    EXCLUDES 1 *Refsum's disease (G60.1)*

  Q80.0 Ichthyosis vulgaris

  Q80.1 X-linked ichthyosis

  Q80.2 Lamellar ichthyosis
    Collodion baby

  Q80.3 Congenital bullous ichthyosiform erythroderma

  Q80.4 Harlequin fetus

  Q80.8 Other congenital ichthyosis

  Q80.9 Congenital ichthyosis, unspecified ▽

☑4ᵗʰ **Q81 Epidermolysis bullosa**

  Q81.0 Epidermolysis bullosa simplex
    EXCLUDES 1 *Cockayne's syndrome (Q87.1)*

  Q81.1 Epidermolysis bullosa letalis
    Herlitz' syndrome

  Q81.2 Epidermolysis bullosa dystrophica

  Q81.8 Other epidermolysis bullosa

  Q81.9 Epidermolysis bullosa, unspecified ▽

☑4ᵗʰ **Q82 Other congenital malformations of skin**

    EXCLUDES 1 *acrodermatitis enteropathica (E83.2)*
            congenital erythropoietic porphyria (E80.0)
            pilonidal cyst or sinus (L05.-)
            Sturge-Weber (-Dimitri) syndrome (Q85.8)

  Q82.0 Hereditary lymphedema

  Q82.1 Xeroderma pigmentosum

▲   **Q82.2 Congenital cutaneous mastocytosis**
    ▶Congenital diffuse cutaneous mastocytosis
    Congenital maculopapular cutaneous mastocytosis
    Congenital urticaria pigmentosa◀
    Urticaria pigmentosa
    EXCLUDES 1 ▶*cutaneous mastocytosis NOS (D47.01)*
            diffuse cutaneous mastocytosis (with onset after newborn period) (D47.01)◀
            malignant mastocytosis ▶(C96.2-)◀
            ▶*systemic mastocytosis (D47.02)*
            urticaria pigmentosa (non-congenital) (with onset after newborn period) (D47.01)◀

  Q82.3 Incontinentia pigmenti

  Q82.4 Ectodermal dysplasia (anhidrotic)
    EXCLUDES 1 *Ellis-van Creveld syndrome (Q77.6)*

☑ Additional Character Req   ☑7ᵗʰ Placeholder Alert   Manifestation   HCC CMS-HCC Condition   ▽ Unspecified Code   ▶◀ Revised Text   ● New Code   ▲ Revised Code Title

Chapter 17. Congenital Malformations, Deformations, and Chromosomal Abnormalities

Q82.5 Congenital non-neoplastic nevus
Birthmark NOS   Strawberry Nevus
Flammeus Nevus   Vascular Nevus NOS
Portwine Nevus   Verrucous Nevus
Sanguineous Nevus

  EXCLUDES 2   *araneus nevus (I78.1)*
              café au lait spots (L81.3)
              lentigo (L81.4)
              melanocytic nevus (D22.-)
              nevus NOS (D22.-)
              pigmented nevus (D22.-)
              spider nevus (I78.1)
              stellar nevus (I78.1)

Q82.6 Congenital sacral dimple
Parasacral dimple

  EXCLUDES 2   *pilonidal cyst with abscess (L05.01)*
              pilonidal cyst without abscess (L05.91)

Q82.8 Other specified congenital malformations of skin
Abnormal palmar creases
Accessory skin tags
Benign familial pemphigus [Hailey-Hailey]
Congenital poikiloderma
Cutis laxa (hyperelastica)
Dermatoglyphic anomalies
Inherited keratosis palmaris et plantaris
Keratosis follicularis [Darier-White]

  EXCLUDES 1   *Ehlers-Danlos syndrome (Q79.6)*
AHA: 2016, 1Q, 17

Q82.9 Congenital malformation of skin, unspecified   ▽

✓4ᵗʰ **Q83 Congenital malformations of breast**

  EXCLUDES 2   *absence of pectoral muscle (Q79.8)*
              hypoplasia of breast (N64.82)
              micromastia (N64.82)

Q83.0 Congenital absence of breast with absent nipple

Q83.1 Accessory breast
Supernumerary breast

Q83.2 Absent nipple

Q83.3 Accessory nipple
Supernumerary nipple

Q83.8 Other congenital malformations of breast

Q83.9 Congenital malformation of breast, unspecified   ▽

✓4ᵗʰ **Q84 Other congenital malformations of integument**

Q84.0 Congenital alopecia
Congenital atrichosis

Q84.1 Congenital morphological disturbances of hair, not elsewhere classified
Beaded hair
Monilethrix
Pili annulati

  EXCLUDES 1   *Menkes' kinky hair syndrome (E83.0)*

Q84.2 Other congenital malformations of hair
Congenital hypertrichosis
Congenital malformation of hair NOS
Persistent lanugo

Q84.3 Anonychia

  EXCLUDES 1   *nail patella syndrome (Q87.2)*

Q84.4 Congenital leukonychia

Q84.5 Enlarged and hypertrophic nails
Congenital onychauxis
Pachyonychia

Q84.6 Other congenital malformations of nails
Congenital clubnail
Congenital koilonychia
Congenital malformation of nail NOS

Q84.8 Other specified congenital malformations of integument
Aplasia cutis congenita

Q84.9 Congenital malformation of integument, unspecified   ▽
Congenital anomaly of integument NOS
Congenital deformity of integument NOS

✓4ᵗʰ **Q85 Phakomatoses, not elsewhere classified**

  EXCLUDES 1   *ataxia telangiectasia [Louis-Bar] (G11.3)*
              familial dysautonomia [Riley-Day] (G90.1)

✓5ᵗʰ **Q85.0 Neurofibromatosis (nonmalignant)**

Q85.00 Neurofibromatosis, unspecified   HCC ▽

Q85.01 Neurofibromatosis, type 1   HCC
Von Recklinghausen disease

Q85.02 Neurofibromatosis, type 2   HCC
Acoustic neurofibromatosis
DEF: Inherited condition with cutaneous lesions, benign tumors of peripheral nerves, and bilateral 8th nerve masses.

Q85.03 Schwannomatosis   HCC
DEF: A genetic mutation (SMARCB1/INI1) causing multiple benign tumors along nerve pathways; characterized by the exception of 8th cranial nerve involvement.

Q85.09 Other neurofibromatosis   HCC

Q85.1 Tuberous sclerosis   HCC
Bourneville's disease
Epiloia

Q85.8 Other phakomatoses, not elsewhere classified   HCC
Peutz-Jeghers Syndrome
Sturge-Weber(-Dimitri) syndrome
von Hippel-Lindau syndrome

  EXCLUDES 1   *Meckel-Gruber syndrome (Q61.9)*

Q85.9 Phakomatosis, unspecified   HCC ▽
Hamartosis NOS

✓4ᵗʰ **Q86 Congenital malformation syndromes due to known exogenous causes, not elsewhere classified**

  EXCLUDES 2   *iodine-deficiency-related hypothyroidism (E00-E02)*
              nonteratogenic effects of substances transmitted via placenta or breast milk (P04.-)

Q86.0 Fetal alcohol syndrome (dysmorphic)

Q86.1 Fetal hydantoin syndrome
Meadow's syndrome

Q86.2 Dysmorphism due to warfarin

Q86.8 Other congenital malformation syndromes due to known exogenous causes

✓4ᵗʰ **Q87 Other specified congenital malformation syndromes affecting multiple systems**
Use additional code(s) to identify all associated manifestations

Q87.0 Congenital malformation syndromes predominantly affecting facial appearance
Acrocephalopolysyndactyly   Moebius syndrome
Acrocephalosyndactyly [Apert]   Oro-facial-digital
  syndrome
Cryptophthalmos syndrome   Robin syndrome
Cyclopia   Whistling face
Goldenhar syndrome

Q87.1 Congenital malformation syndromes predominantly associated with short stature
Aarskog syndrome   Robinow-Silverman-Smith
Cockayne syndrome   syndrome
De Lange syndrome   Russell-Silver syndrome
Dubowitz syndrome   Seckel syndrome
Noonan syndrome
Prader-Willi syndrome

  EXCLUDES 1   *Ellis-van Creveld syndrome (Q77.6)*
              Smith-Lemli-Opitz syndrome (E78.72)

Q87.2 Congenital malformation syndromes predominantly involving limbs
Holt-Oram syndrome
Klippel-Trenaunay-Weber syndrome
Nail patella syndrome
Rubinstein-Taybi syndrome
Sirenomelia syndrome
Thrombocytopenia with absent radius [TAR] syndrome
VATER syndrome

Q87.3 Congenital malformation syndromes involving early overgrowth
Beckwith-Wiedemann syndrome
Sotos syndrome
Weaver syndrome

✓5ᵗʰ **Q87.4 Marfan's syndrome**

Q87.40 Marfan's syndrome, unspecified   ▽

✓6ᵗʰ **Q87.41 Marfan's syndrome with cardiovascular manifestations**

Q87.410 Marfan's syndrome with aortic dilation

Q87.418 Marfan's syndrome with other cardiovascular manifestations

Q87.42 Marfan's syndrome with ocular manifestations

Q87.43 Marfan's syndrome with skeletal manifestation

Q87.5 Other congenital malformation syndromes with other skeletal changes

EXCLUDES 1 Not coded here   EXCLUDES 2 Not included here   N Newborn Age: 0   P Pediatric Age: 0-17   M Maternity Age: 12-55   A Adult Age: 15-124

884   ICD-10-CM 2018

✓5ᵗʰ **Q87.8　Other specified congenital malformation syndromes, not elsewhere classified**
　　EXCLUDES 1　*Zellweger syndrome (E71.51Ø)*

　　Q87.81　Alport syndrome
　　　　Use additional code to identify stage of chronic kidney disease (N18.1-N18.6)

　　Q87.82　Arterial tortuosity syndrome

　　Q87.89　Other specified congenital malformation syndromes, not elsewhere classified
　　　　Laurence-Moon (-Bardet)-Biedl syndrome

✓4ᵗʰ **Q89　Other congenital malformations, not elsewhere classified**

　✓5ᵗʰ **Q89.Ø　Congenital absence and malformations of spleen**
　　EXCLUDES 1　*isomerism of atrial appendages (with asplenia or polysplenia) (Q2Ø.6)*

　　Q89.Ø1　Asplenia (congenital)

　　Q89.Ø9　Congenital malformations of spleen
　　　　Congenital splenomegaly

　Q89.1　Congenital malformations of adrenal gland
　　EXCLUDES 1　*adrenogenital disorders (E25.-)*
　　　　congenital adrenal hyperplasia (E25.Ø)

　Q89.2　Congenital malformations of other endocrine glands
　　　Congenital malformation of parathyroid or thyroid gland
　　　Persistent thyroglossal duct
　　　Thyroglossal cyst
　　EXCLUDES 1　*congenital goiter (EØ3.Ø)*
　　　　congenital hypothyroidism (EØ3.1)

　Q89.3　Situs inversus
　　　Dextrocardia with situs inversus
　　　Mirror-image atrial arrangement with situs inversus
　　　Situs inversus or transversus abdominalis
　　　Situs inversus or transversus thoracis
　　　Transposition of abdominal viscera
　　　Transposition of thoracic viscera
　　EXCLUDES 1　*dextrocardia NOS (Q24.Ø)*

　Q89.4　Conjoined twins
　　　Craniopagus　　　　　Pygopagus
　　　Dicephaly　　　　　　Thoracopagus

　Q89.7　Multiple congenital malformations, not elsewhere classified
　　　Multiple congenital anomalies NOS
　　　Multiple congenital deformities NOS
　　EXCLUDES 1　*congenital malformation syndromes affecting multiple systems (Q87.-)*

　Q89.8　Other specified congenital malformations
　　　Use additional code(s) to identify all associated manifestations

　Q89.9　Congenital malformation, unspecified　　▽
　　　Congenital anomaly NOS
　　　Congenital deformity NOS

Chromosomal abnormalities, not elsewhere classified (Q9Ø-Q99)
　　EXCLUDES 2　*mitochondrial metabolic disorders (E88.4-)*

✓4ᵗʰ **Q9Ø　Down syndrome**
　　Use additional code(s) to identify any associated physical conditions and degree of intellectual disabilities (F7Ø-F79)

　Q9Ø.Ø　Trisomy 21, nonmosaicism (meiotic nondisjunction)

　Q9Ø.1　Trisomy 21, mosaicism (mitotic nondisjunction)

　Q9Ø.2　Trisomy 21, translocation

　Q9Ø.9　Down syndrome, unspecified　　▽
　　　Trisomy 21 NOS

✓4ᵗʰ **Q91　Trisomy 18 and Trisomy 13**

　Q91.Ø　Trisomy 18, nonmosaicism (meiotic nondisjunction)

　Q91.1　Trisomy 18, mosaicism (mitotic nondisjunction)

　Q91.2　Trisomy 18, translocation

　Q91.3　Trisomy 18, unspecified　　▽

　Q91.4　Trisomy 13, nonmosaicism (meiotic nondisjunction)

　Q91.5　Trisomy 13, mosaicism (mitotic nondisjunction)

　Q91.6　Trisomy 13, translocation

　Q91.7　Trisomy 13, unspecified　　▽

✓4ᵗʰ **Q92　Other trisomies and partial trisomies of the autosomes, not elsewhere classified**
　　INCLUDES　unbalanced translocations and insertions
　　EXCLUDES 1　*trisomies of chromosomes 13, 18, 21 (Q9Ø-Q91)*

　Q92.Ø　Whole chromosome trisomy, nonmosaicism (meiotic nondisjunction)

　Q92.1　Whole chromosome trisomy, mosaicism (mitotic nondisjunction)

　Q92.2　Partial trisomy
　　　Less than whole arm duplicated
　　　Whole arm or more duplicated
　　EXCLUDES 1　*partial trisomy due to unbalanced translocation (Q92.5)*

　Q92.5　Duplications with other complex rearrangements
　　　Partial trisomy due to unbalanced translocations
　　　Code also any associated deletions due to unbalanced translocations, inversions and insertions (Q93.7)

　✓5ᵗʰ **Q92.6　Marker chromosomes**
　　　Trisomies due to dicentrics
　　　Trisomies due to extra rings
　　　Trisomies due to isochromosomes
　　　Individual with marker heterochromatin

　　Q92.61　Marker chromosomes in normal individual

　　Q92.62　Marker chromosomes in abnormal individual

　Q92.7　Triploidy and polyploidy

　Q92.8　Other specified trisomies and partial trisomies of autosomes
　　　Duplications identified by fluorescence in situ hybridization (FISH)
　　　Duplications identified by in situ hybridization (ISH)
　　　Duplications seen only at prometaphase

　Q92.9　Trisomy and partial trisomy of autosomes, unspecified　　▽

✓4ᵗʰ **Q93　Monosomies and deletions from the autosomes, not elsewhere classified**

　Q93.Ø　Whole chromosome monosomy, nonmosaicism (meiotic nondisjunction)

　Q93.1　Whole chromosome monosomy, mosaicism (mitotic nondisjunction)

　Q93.2　Chromosome replaced with ring, dicentric or isochromosome

　Q93.3　Deletion of short arm of chromosome 4
　　　Wolff-Hirschorn syndrome

　Q93.4　Deletion of short arm of chromosome 5
　　　Cri-du-chat syndrome

　Q93.5　Other deletions of part of a chromosome
　　　Angelman syndrome

　Q93.7　Deletions with other complex rearrangements
　　　Deletions due to unbalanced translocations, inversions and insertions
　　　Code also any associated duplications due to unbalanced translocations, inversions and insertions (Q92.5)

　✓5ᵗʰ **Q93.8　Other deletions from the autosomes**

　　Q93.81　Velo-cardio-facial syndrome
　　　　Deletion 22q11.2
　　　　DEF: Microdeletion syndrome affecting multiple organs; characteristic cleft palate, heart defects, elongated face with almond-shaped eyes, wide nose, small ears, weak immune system, weak musculature, hypothyroidism, short stature, and scoliosis; deletion at q11.2 on the long arm of the chromosome 22.

　　Q93.88　Other microdeletions
　　　　Miller-Dieker syndrome
　　　　Smith-Magenis syndrome

　　Q93.89　Other deletions from the autosomes
　　　　Deletions identified by fluorescence in situ hybridization (FISH)
　　　　Deletions identified by in situ hybridization (ISH)
　　　　Deletions seen only at prometaphase

　Q93.9　Deletion from autosomes, unspecified　　▽

✓4ᵗʰ **Q95　Balanced rearrangements and structural markers, not elsewhere classified**
　　INCLUDES　Robertsonian and balanced reciprocal translocations and insertions

　Q95.Ø　Balanced translocation and insertion in normal individual

　Q95.1　Chromosome inversion in normal individual

　Q95.2　Balanced autosomal rearrangement in abnormal individual

　Q95.3　Balanced sex/autosomal rearrangement in abnormal individual

　Q95.5　Individual with autosomal fragile site

　Q95.8　Other balanced rearrangements and structural markers

　Q95.9　Balanced rearrangement and structural marker, unspecified　　▽

✓4ᵗʰ **Q96　Turner's syndrome**
　　EXCLUDES 1　*Noonan syndrome (Q87.1)*

　Q96.Ø　Karyotype 45, X　　♀

　Q96.1　Karyotype 46, X iso (Xq)　　♀
　　　Karyotype 46, isochromosome Xq

✓ Additional Character Req　　✓ˣ⁷ᵗʰ Placeholder Alert　　Manifestation　　**HCC** CMS-HCC Condition　　▽ Unspecified Code　　►◄ Revised Text　　● New Code　　▲ Revised Code Title

ICD-10-CM 2018　　**885**

Q96.2 Karyotype 46, X with abnormal sex chromosome, except iso (Xq) ♀
    Karyotype 46, X with abnormal sex chromosome, except isochromosome Xq

Q96.3 Mosaicism, 45, X/46, XX or XY ♀

Q96.4 Mosaicism, 45, X/other cell line(s) with abnormal sex chromosome ♀

Q96.8 Other variants of Turner's syndrome ♀

Q96.9 Turner's syndrome, unspecified ♀▽

☑4ᵗʰ **Q97** Other sex chromosome abnormalities, female phenotype, not elsewhere classified
    EXCLUDES 1   Turner's syndrome (Q96.-)

Q97.0 Karyotype 47, XXX ♀

Q97.1 Female with more than three X chromosomes ♀

Q97.2 Mosaicism, lines with various numbers of X chromosomes ♀

Q97.3 Female with 46, XY karyotype ♀

Q97.8 Other specified sex chromosome abnormalities, female phenotype ♀

Q97.9 Sex chromosome abnormality, female phenotype, unspecified ♀▽

☑4ᵗʰ **Q98** Other sex chromosome abnormalities, male phenotype, not elsewhere classified

Q98.0 Klinefelter syndrome karyotype 47, XXY ♂

Q98.1 Klinefelter syndrome, male with more than two X chromosomes ♂

Q98.3 Other male with 46, XX karyotype ♂

Q98.4 Klinefelter syndrome, unspecified ♂▽

Q98.5 Karyotype 47, XYY

Q98.6 Male with structurally abnormal sex chromosome ♂

Q98.7 Male with sex chromosome mosaicism ♂

Q98.8 Other specified sex chromosome abnormalities, male phenotype ♂

Q98.9 Sex chromosome abnormality, male phenotype, unspecified ♂▽

☑4ᵗʰ **Q99** Other chromosome abnormalities, not elsewhere classified

Q99.0 Chimera 46, XX/46, XY
    Chimera 46, XX/46, XY true hermaphrodite

Q99.1 46, XX true hermaphrodite
    46, XX with streak gonads   Pure gonadal dysgenesis
    46, XY with streak gonads

Q99.2 Fragile X chromosome
    Fragile X syndrome

Q99.8 Other specified chromosome abnormalities

Q99.9 Chromosomal abnormality, unspecified ▽

Chapter 18. Symptoms, Signs, and Abnormal Clinical and Laboratory Findings, Not Elsewhere Classified (R00–R99)

Chapter Specific Guidelines with Coding Examples

The chapter specific guidelines from the ICD-10-CM Official Guidelines for Coding and Reporting have been provided below. Along with these guidelines are coding examples, contained in the shaded boxes, that have been developed to help illustrate the coding and/or sequencing guidance found in these guidelines.

Chapter 18 includes symptoms, signs, abnormal results of clinical or other investigative procedures, and ill-defined conditions regarding which no diagnosis classifiable elsewhere is recorded. Signs and symptoms that point to a specific diagnosis have been assigned to a category in other chapters of the classification.

a. Use of symptom codes

Codes that describe symptoms and signs are acceptable for reporting purposes when a related definitive diagnosis has not been established (confirmed) by the provider.

> Tenderness and localized pain in the right upper quadrant; based on presentation, probable gallstones
>
> **R10.11   Right upper quadrant pain**
>
> **R10.811   Right upper quadrant abdominal tenderness**
>
> *Explanation:* Codes that describe symptoms such as abdominal pain are acceptable for reporting purposes when the provider has not established (confirmed) a definitive diagnosis.

b. Use of a symptom code with a definitive diagnosis code

Codes for signs and symptoms may be reported in addition to a related definitive diagnosis when the sign or symptom is not routinely associated with that diagnosis, such as the various signs and symptoms associated with complex syndromes. The definitive diagnosis code should be sequenced before the symptom code.

Signs or symptoms that are associated routinely with a disease process should not be assigned as additional codes, unless otherwise instructed by the classification.

> Pneumonia with hemoptysis
>
> **J18.9   Pneumonia, unspecified organism**
>
> **R04.2   Hemoptysis**
>
> *Explanation:* Codes for signs and symptoms may be reported in addition to a related definitive diagnosis when the sign or symptom is not routinely associated with that diagnosis.

> Abdominal pain due to acute appendicitis
>
> **K35.80   Unspecified acute appendicitis**
>
> *Explanation:* Codes for signs or symptoms routinely associated with a disease process should not be assigned unless the classification instructs otherwise.

c. Combination codes that include symptoms

ICD-10-CM contains a number of combination codes that identify both the definitive diagnosis and common symptoms of that diagnosis. When using one of these combination codes, an additional code should not be assigned for the symptom.

> IBS with diarrhea
>
> **K58.0   Irritable bowel syndrome, with diarrhea**
>
> *Explanation:* When a combination code identifies both the definitive diagnosis and the symptom, an additional code should not be assigned for the symptom.

d. Repeated falls

Code R29.6, Repeated falls, is for use for encounters when a patient has recently fallen and the reason for the fall is being investigated.

Code Z91.81, History of falling, is for use when a patient has fallen in the past and is at risk for future falls. When appropriate, both codes R29.6 and Z91.81 may be assigned together.

e. Coma scale

The coma scale codes (R40.2-) can be used in conjunction with traumatic brain injury codes, acute cerebrovascular disease or sequelae of cerebrovascular disease codes. These codes are primarily for use by trauma registries, but they may be used in any setting where this information is collected. The coma scale may also be used to assess the status of the central nervous system for other non-trauma conditions, such as monitoring patients in the intensive care unit regardless of medical condition. The coma scale codes should be sequenced after the diagnosis code(s).

These codes, one from each subcategory, are needed to complete the scale. The 7th character indicates when the scale was recorded. The 7th character should match for all three codes.

At a minimum, report the initial score documented on presentation at your facility. This may be a score from the emergency medicine technician (EMT) or in the emergency department. If desired, a facility may choose to capture multiple coma scale scores.

Assign code R40.24, Glasgow coma scale, total score, when only the total score is documented in the medical record and not the individual score(s).

> 36-year-old man found down after unknown injury with skull fracture and with concussion and loss of consciousness of unknown duration. Upon hospital admission, the patient was evaluated with the following Glasgow coma scores:
>
> Eye-opening response—3: eyes open to speech
>
> Verbal response—3: random speech with no conversational exchange
>
> Motor response—4: pulls limb away from painful stimulus
>
> **S02.0XXA   Fracture of vault of skull, initial encounter for closed fracture**
>
> **S06.0X9A   Concussion with loss of consciousness of unspecified duration, initial encounter**
>
> **R40.2133   Coma scale, eyes open, to sound, at hospital admission**
>
> **R40.2233   Coma scale, best verbal response, inappropriate words, at hospital admission**
>
> **R40.2343   Coma scale, best motor response, flexion withdrawal, at hospital admission**
>
> *Explanation:* When individual scores for the Glasgow coma scale are documented, one code from each category is needed to complete the scale. The seventh character indicates when the scale was recorded and should match for all three codes. Assign a code from subcategory R40.24-Glasgow coma scale, total score, when only the total and not the individual score(s) is documented.

f. Functional quadriplegia

Functional quadriplegia (code R53.2) is the lack of ability to use one's limbs or to ambulate due to extreme debility. It is not associated with neurologic deficit or injury, and code R53.2 should not be used for cases of neurologic quadriplegia. It should only be assigned if functional quadriplegia is specifically documented in the medical record.

g. SIRS due to non-infectious process

The systemic inflammatory response syndrome (SIRS) can develop as a result of certain non-infectious disease processes, such as trauma, malignant neoplasm, or pancreatitis. When SIRS is documented with a noninfectious condition, and no subsequent infection is documented, the code for the underlying condition, such as an injury, should be assigned, followed by code R65.10, Systemic inflammatory response syndrome (SIRS) of non-infectious origin without acute organ dysfunction, or code R65.11, Systemic inflammatory response syndrome (SIRS) of non-infectious origin with acute organ dysfunction. If an associated acute organ dysfunction is documented, the appropriate code(s) for the specific type of organ dysfunction(s) should be assigned in addition to code R65.11. If acute organ dysfunction is documented, but it cannot be determined if the acute organ dysfunction is associated with SIRS or due to another condition (e.g., directly due to the trauma), the provider should be queried.

Systemic inflammatory response syndrome (SIRS) due to acute gallstone pancreatitis

K85.1Ø **Biliary acute pancreatitis without necrosis or infection**

R65.1Ø **Systemic inflammatory response syndrome (SIRS) of noninfectious origin without acute organ dysfunction**

Explanation: When SIRS is documented with a noninfectious condition without subsequent infection documented, the code for the underlying condition such as pancreatitis should be assigned followed by the appropriate code for SIRS of noninfectious origin, either with or without associated organ dysfunction.

h. Death NOS

Code R99, Ill-defined and unknown cause of mortality, is only for use in the very limited circumstance when a patient who has already died is brought into an emergency department or other healthcare facility and is pronounced dead upon arrival. It does not represent the discharge disposition of death.

i. NIHSS stroke scale

The NIH stroke scale (NIHSS) codes (R29.7- -) can be used in conjunction with acute stroke codes (I63) to identify the patient's neurological status and the severity of the stroke. The stroke scale codes should be sequenced after the acute stroke diagnosis code(s).

At a minimum, report the initial score documented. If desired, a facility may choose to capture multiple stroke scale scores.

See Section I.B.14. for information concerning the medical record documentation that may be used for assignment of the NIHSS codes.

h. Death NOS

Chapter 18. Symptoms, Signs and Abnormal Clinical and Laboratory Findings, Not Elsewhere Classified (R00-R99)

NOTE This chapter includes symptoms, signs, abnormal results of clinical or other investigative procedures, and ill-defined conditions regarding which no diagnosis classifiable elsewhere is recorded.

Signs and symptoms that point rather definitely to a given diagnosis have been assigned to a category in other chapters of the classification. In general, categories in this chapter include the less well-defined conditions and symptoms that, without the necessary study of the case to establish a final diagnosis, point perhaps equally to two or more diseases or to two or more systems of the body. Practically all categories in the chapter could be designated "not otherwise specified", "unknown etiology" or "transient". The Alphabetical Index should be consulted to determine which symptoms and signs are to be allocated here and which to other chapters. The residual subcategories, numbered .8, are generally provided for other relevant symptoms that cannot be allocated elsewhere in the classification.

The conditions and signs or symptoms included in categories R00-R94 consist of:

(a) cases for which no more specific diagnosis can be made even after all the facts bearing on the case have been investigated;

(b) signs or symptoms existing at the time of initial encounter that proved to be transient and whose causes could not be determined;

(c) provisional diagnosis in a patient who failed to return for further investigation or care;

(d) cases referred elsewhere for investigation or treatment before the diagnosis was made;

(e) cases in which a more precise diagnosis was not available for any other reason;

(f) certain symptoms, for which supplementary information is provided, that represent important problems in medical care in their own right.

EXCLUDES 2 *abnormal findings on antenatal screening of mother (O28.-)*
certain conditions originating in the perinatal period (P04-P96)
signs and symptoms classified in the body system chapters
signs and symptoms of breast (N63, N64.5)

AHA: 2017, 1Q, 6, 7

This chapter contains the following blocks:

R00-R09	Symptoms and signs involving the circulatory and respiratory systems
R10-R19	Symptoms and signs involving the digestive system and abdomen
R20-R23	Symptoms and signs involving the skin and subcutaneous tissue
R25-R29	Symptoms and signs involving the nervous and musculoskeletal systems
R30-R39	Symptoms and signs involving the genitourinary system
R40-R46	Symptoms and signs involving cognition, perception, emotional state and behavior
R47-R49	Symptoms and signs involving speech and voice
R50-R69	General symptoms and signs
R70-R79	Abnormal findings on examination of blood, without diagnosis
R80-R82	Abnormal findings on examination of urine, without diagnosis
R83-R89	Abnormal findings on examination of other body fluids, substances and tissues, without diagnosis
R90-R94	Abnormal findings on diagnostic imaging and in function studies, without diagnosis
R97	Abnormal tumor markers
R99	Ill-defined and unknown cause of mortality

Symptoms and signs involving the circulatory and respiratory systems (R00-R09)

✓4ᵗʰ R00 Abnormalities of heart beat

EXCLUDES 1 *abnormalities originating in the perinatal period (P29.1-)*
EXCLUDES 2 *specified arrhythmias (I47-I49)*

R00.0 Tachycardia, unspecified ▽
Rapid heart beat
Sinoauricular tachycardia NOS
Sinus [sinusal] tachycardia NOS
EXCLUDES 1 *neonatal tachycardia (P29.11)*
paroxysmal tachycardia (I47.-)
DEF: Excessively rapid heart rate of more than 100 beats per minute.

R00.1 Bradycardia, unspecified ▽
Sinoatrial bradycardia
Sinus bradycardia
Slow heart beat
Vagal bradycardia
Use additional code for adverse effect, if applicable, to identify drug (T36-T50 with fifth or sixth character 5)
EXCLUDES 1 *neonatal bradycardia (P29.12)*

R00.2 Palpitations
Awareness of heart beat

R00.8 Other abnormalities of heart beat

R00.9 Unspecified abnormalities of heart beat ▽

✓4ᵗʰ R01 Cardiac murmurs and other cardiac sounds
EXCLUDES 1 *cardiac murmurs and sounds originating in the perinatal period (P29.8)*

R01.0 Benign and innocent cardiac murmurs
Functional cardiac murmur

R01.1 Cardiac murmur, unspecified ▽
Cardiac bruit NOS
Heart murmur NOS
Systolic murmur NOS

R01.2 Other cardiac sounds
Cardiac dullness, increased or decreased
Precordial friction

✓4ᵗʰ R03 Abnormal blood-pressure reading, without diagnosis

R03.0 Elevated blood-pressure reading, without diagnosis of hypertension
NOTE This category is to be used to record an episode of elevated blood pressure in a patient in whom no formal diagnosis of hypertension has been made, or as an isolated incidental finding.

R03.1 Nonspecific low blood-pressure reading
EXCLUDES 1 *hypotension (I95.-)*
maternal hypotension syndrome (O26.5-)
neurogenic orthostatic hypotension (G90.3)

✓4ᵗʰ R04 Hemorrhage from respiratory passages

R04.0 Epistaxis
Hemorrhage from nose
Nosebleed

R04.1 Hemorrhage from throat
EXCLUDES 2 *hemoptysis (R04.2)*

R04.2 Hemoptysis
Blood-stained sputum
Cough with hemorrhage
AHA: 2013, 4Q, 118

✓5ᵗʰ R04.8 Hemorrhage from other sites in respiratory passages

R04.81 Acute idiopathic pulmonary hemorrhage in infants 🅿
AIPHI
Acute idiopathic hemorrhage in infants over 28 days old
EXCLUDES 1 *perinatal pulmonary hemorrhage (P26.-)*
von Willebrand's disease (D68.0)

R04.89 Hemorrhage from other sites in respiratory passages
Pulmonary hemorrhage NOS

R04.9 Hemorrhage from respiratory passages, unspecified ▽

R05 Cough
EXCLUDES 1 *cough with hemorrhage (R04.2)*
smoker's cough (J41.0)
AHA: 2016, 2Q, 33

✓4ᵗʰ R06 Abnormalities of breathing
EXCLUDES 1 *acute respiratory distress syndrome (J80)*
respiratory arrest (R09.2)
respiratory arrest of newborn (P28.81)
respiratory distress syndrome of newborn (P22.-)
respiratory failure (J96.-)
respiratory failure of newborn (P28.5)

✓5ᵗʰ R06.0 Dyspnea
EXCLUDES 1 *tachypnea NOS (R06.82)*
transient tachypnea of newborn (P22.1)

R06.00 Dyspnea, unspecified ▽
AHA: 2017, 1Q, 26

R06.01 Orthopnea

R06.02 Shortness of breath

● **R06.03 Acute respiratory distress**

R06.09 Other forms of dyspnea

Chapter 18. Symptoms, Signs, and Abnormal Clinical and Laboratory Findings, Not Elsewhere Classified

R00–R06.09

R06.1 Stridor
> EXCLUDES 1   *congenital laryngeal stridor (P28.89)*
> *laryngismus (stridulus) (J38.5)*

R06.2 Wheezing
> EXCLUDES 1   *asthma (J45.-)*
>
> **AHA:** 2016, 2Q, 33
> **DEF:** High-pitched whistling sound during breathing due to stenosis of respiratory passageway; associated with asthma, sleep apnea, bronchiectasis, bronchiolitis, COPD, and pleural effusion.

R06.3 Periodic breathing
> Cheyne-Stokes breathing

R06.4 Hyperventilation
> EXCLUDES 1   *psychogenic hyperventilation (F45.8)*

R06.5 Mouth breathing
> EXCLUDES 2   *dry mouth NOS (R68.2)*

R06.6 Hiccough
> EXCLUDES 1   *psychogenic hiccough (F45.8)*

R06.7 Sneezing

✓5th **R06.8 Other abnormalities of breathing**

> **R06.81 Apnea, not elsewhere classified**
> Apnea NOS
> > EXCLUDES 1   *apnea (of) newborn (P28.4)*
> > *sleep apnea (G47.3-)*
> > *sleep apnea of newborn (primary) (P28.3)*
>
> **R06.82 Tachypnea, not elsewhere classified**
> Tachypnea NOS
> > EXCLUDES 1   *transitory tachypnea of newborn (P22.1)*
>
> **R06.83 Snoring**
>
> **R06.89 Other abnormalities of breathing**
> Breath-holding (spells)
> Sighing

R06.9 Unspecified abnormalities of breathing   ▽

✓4th **R07 Pain in throat and chest**
> EXCLUDES 1   *epidemic myalgia (B33.0)*
> EXCLUDES 2   *jaw pain (R68.84)*
> *pain in breast (N64.4)*

> **R07.0 Pain in throat**
> > EXCLUDES 1   *chronic sore throat (J31.2)*
> > *sore throat (acute) NOS (J02.9)*
> > EXCLUDES 2   *dysphagia (R13.1-)*
> > *pain in neck (M54.2)*
>
> **R07.1 Chest pain on breathing**
> Painful respiration
>
> **R07.2 Precordial pain**
>
> ✓5th **R07.8 Other chest pain**
> > **R07.81 Pleurodynia**
> > Pleurodynia NOS
> > > EXCLUDES 1   *epidemic pleurodynia (B33.0)*
> >
> > **R07.82 Intercostal pain**
> >
> > **R07.89 Other chest pain**
> > Anterior chest-wall pain NOS
>
> **R07.9 Chest pain, unspecified**   ▽

✓4th **R09 Other symptoms and signs involving the circulatory and respiratory system**
> EXCLUDES 1   *acute respiratory distress syndrome (J80)*
> *respiratory arrest of newborn (P28.81)*
> *respiratory distress syndrome of newborn (P22.0)*
> *respiratory failure (J96.-)*
> *respiratory failure of newborn (P28.5)*

> ✓5th **R09.0 Asphyxia and hypoxemia**
> > EXCLUDES 1   *asphyxia due to carbon monoxide (T58.-)*
> > *asphyxia due to foreign body in respiratory tract (T17.-)*
> > *birth (intrauterine) asphyxia (P84)*
> > ~~*hypercapnia (R06.4)*~~
> > *hyperventilation (R06.4)*
> > *traumatic asphyxia (T71.-)*
> > EXCLUDES 2   ▶*hypercapnia (R06.89)*◀
> >
> > **R09.01 Asphyxia**
> >
> > **R09.02 Hypoxemia**
>
> **R09.1 Pleurisy**
> > EXCLUDES 1   *pleurisy with effusion (J90)*

R09.2 Respiratory arrest   HCC
> Cardiorespiratory failure
> > EXCLUDES 1   *cardiac arrest (I46.-)*
> > *respiratory arrest of newborn (P28.81)*
> > *respiratory distress of newborn (P22.0)*
> > *respiratory failure (J96.-)*
> > *respiratory failure of newborn (P28.5)*
> > *respiratory insufficiency (R06.89)*
> > *respiratory insufficiency of newborn (P28.5)*

R09.3 Abnormal sputum
> Abnormal amount of sputum
> Abnormal color of sputum
> Abnormal odor of sputum
> Excessive sputum
> > EXCLUDES 1   *blood-stained sputum (R04.2)*

✓5th **R09.8 Other specified symptoms and signs involving the circulatory and respiratory systems**

> **R09.81 Nasal congestion**
>
> **R09.82 Postnasal drip**
>
> **R09.89 Other specified symptoms and signs involving the circulatory and respiratory systems**
> Abnormal chest percussion
> Bruit (arterial)
> Chest tympany
> Choking sensation
> Feeling of foreign body in throat
> Friction sounds in chest
> Rales
> Weak pulse
> > EXCLUDES 2   *foreign body in throat (T17.2-)*
> > *wheezing (R06.2)*

Symptoms and signs involving the digestive system and abdomen (R10-R19)

> EXCLUDES 2   *congenital or infantile pylorospasm (Q40.0)*
> *gastrointestinal hemorrhage (K92.0-K92.2)*
> *intestinal obstruction (K56.-)*
> *newborn gastrointestinal hemorrhage (P54.0-P54.3)*
> *newborn intestinal obstruction (P76.-)*
> *pylorospasm (K31.3)*
> *signs and symptoms involving the urinary system (R30-R39)*
> *symptoms referable to female genital organs (N94.-)*
> *symptoms referable to male genital organs (N48-N50)*

✓4th **R10 Abdominal and pelvic pain**
> EXCLUDES 1   *renal colic (N23)*
> EXCLUDES 2   *dorsalgia (M54.-)*
> *flatulence and related conditions (R14.-)*

> **R10.0 Acute abdomen**
> Severe abdominal pain (generalized) (with abdominal rigidity)
> > EXCLUDES 1   *abdominal rigidity NOS (R19.3)*
> > *generalized abdominal pain NOS (R10.84)*
> > *localized abdominal pain (R10.1-R10.3-)*

Abdominal Pain

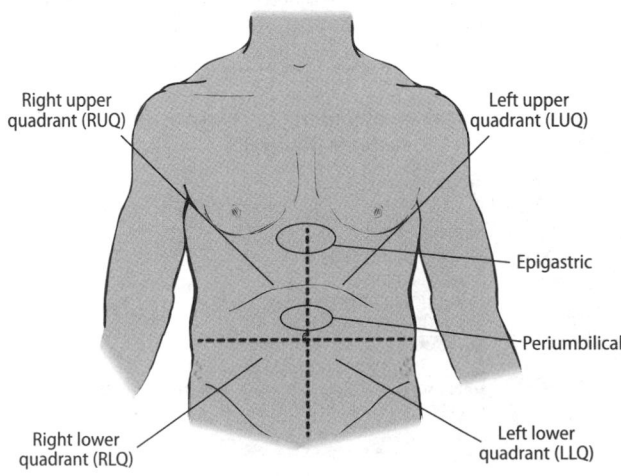

Right upper quadrant (RUQ)
Left upper quadrant (LUQ)
Epigastric
Periumbilical
Right lower quadrant (RLQ)
Left lower quadrant (LLQ)

EXCLUDES 1 Not coded here   EXCLUDES 2 Not included here   N Newborn Age: 0   P Pediatric Age: 0-17   M Maternity Age: 12-55   A Adult Age: 15-124

√5ᵗʰ **R10.1** Pain **localized to upper abdomen** ▽
     R10.10   Upper abdominal pain, unspecified
     R10.11   **Right** upper quadrant pain
     R10.12   **Left** upper quadrant pain
     R10.13   **Epigastric** pain
         Dyspepsia
         EXCLUDES 1   *functional dyspepsia (K30)*

R10.2 **Pelvic and perineal pain**
     EXCLUDES 1   *vulvodynia (N94.81)*

√5ᵗʰ **R10.3** Pain **localized to other parts of lower abdomen** ▽
     R10.30   Lower abdominal pain, unspecified
     R10.31   **Right** lower quadrant pain
     R10.32   **Left** lower quadrant pain
     R10.33   **Periumbilical** pain

√5ᵗʰ **R10.8** Other abdominal pain
     √6ᵗʰ **R10.81**   Abdominal **tenderness**
         Abdominal tenderness NOS
         R10.811   **Right upper** quadrant abdominal tenderness
         R10.812   **Left upper** quadrant abdominal tenderness
         R10.813   **Right lower** quadrant abdominal tenderness
         R10.814   **Left lower** quadrant abdominal tenderness
         R10.815   **Periumbilic** abdominal tenderness
         R10.816   **Epigastric** abdominal tenderness
         R10.817   **Generalized** abdominal tenderness
         R10.819   Abdominal tenderness, unspecified site ▽
     √6ᵗʰ **R10.82**   **Rebound** abdominal tenderness
         R10.821   **Right upper** quadrant rebound abdominal tenderness
         R10.822   **Left upper** quadrant rebound abdominal tenderness
         R10.823   **Right lower** quadrant rebound abdominal tenderness
         R10.824   **Left lower** quadrant rebound abdominal tenderness
         R10.825   **Periumbilic** rebound abdominal tenderness
         R10.826   **Epigastric** rebound abdominal tenderness
         R10.827   **Generalized** rebound abdominal tenderness
         R10.829   Rebound abdominal tenderness, unspecified site ▽
     R10.83   **Colic**   P
         Colic NOS
         Infantile colic
         EXCLUDES 1   *colic in adult and child over 12 months old (R10.84)*
         DEF: Inconsolable crying in an otherwise well-fed and healthy infant for more than three hours a day, three days a week, for more than three weeks.
     R10.84   **Generalized** abdominal pain
         EXCLUDES 1   *generalized abdominal pain associated with acute abdomen (R10.0)*

R10.9 Unspecified abdominal pain ▽

√4ᵗʰ **R11** **Nausea and vomiting**
     EXCLUDES 1   *cyclical vomiting associated with migraine (G43.A-)*
         excessive vomiting in pregnancy (O21.-)
         hematemesis (K92.0)
         neonatal hematemesis (P54.0)
         newborn vomiting (P92.0-)
         psychogenic vomiting (F50.89)
         vomiting associated with bulimia nervosa (F50.2)
         vomiting following gastrointestinal surgery (K91.0)
     AHA: 2017, 1Q, 28
     R11.0 **Nausea**
         Nausea NOS
         Nausea without vomiting
     √5ᵗʰ **R11.1** **Vomiting**
         R11.10   **Vomiting, unspecified** ▽
             Vomiting NOS
         R11.11   **Vomiting without nausea**
         R11.12   **Projectile** vomiting
         R11.13   **Vomiting of fecal matter**

Swallowing Function

Oral phase   Oropharyngeal phase

Pharyngeal phase   Pharyngoesophageal phase

         R11.14   **Bilious** vomiting
             Bilious emesis
     R11.2 **Nausea with vomiting, unspecified** ▽
         Persistent nausea with vomiting NOS

R12 **Heartburn**
     EXCLUDES 1   *dyspepsia NOS (R10.13)*
         functional dyspepsia (K30)

√4ᵗʰ **R13** **Aphagia and dysphagia**
     R13.0 **Aphagia**
         Inability to swallow
         EXCLUDES 1   *psychogenic aphagia (F50.9)*
     √5ᵗʰ **R13.1** **Dysphagia**
         Code first, if applicable, dysphagia following cerebrovascular disease (I69. with final characters -91)
         EXCLUDES 1   *psychogenic dysphagia (F45.8)*
         R13.10   **Dysphagia, unspecified** ▽
             Difficulty in swallowing NOS
         R13.11   Dysphagia, **oral phase**
         R13.12   Dysphagia, **oropharyngeal** phase
         R13.13   Dysphagia, **pharyngeal** phase
         R13.14   Dysphagia, **pharyngoesophageal** phase
         R13.19   **Other dysphagia**
             Cervical dysphagia
             Neurogenic dysphagia

√4ᵗʰ **R14** **Flatulence and related conditions**
     EXCLUDES 1   *psychogenic aerophagy (F45.8)*
     R14.0 **Abdominal distension (gaseous)**
         Bloating
         Tympanites (abdominal) (intestinal)
     R14.1 **Gas pain**
     R14.2 **Eructation**
     R14.3 **Flatulence**

√4ᵗʰ **R15** **Fecal incontinence**
     INCLUDES   encopresis NOS
     EXCLUDES 1   *fecal incontinence of nonorganic origin (F98.1)*
     R15.0 **Incomplete defecation**
         EXCLUDES 1   *constipation (K59.0-)*
         fecal impaction (K56.41)
     R15.1 **Fecal smearing**
         Fecal soiling
     R15.2 **Fecal urgency**
     R15.9 **Full incontinence of feces**
         Fecal incontinence NOS

√4ᵗʰ **R16** **Hepatomegaly and splenomegaly, not elsewhere classified**
     R16.0 **Hepatomegaly, not elsewhere classified**
         Hepatomegaly NOS
     R16.1 **Splenomegaly, not elsewhere classified**
         Splenomegaly NOS
     R16.2 **Hepatomegaly with splenomegaly, not elsewhere classified**
         Hepatosplenomegaly NOS

R17 **Unspecified jaundice** ▽
     EXCLUDES 1   *neonatal jaundice (P55, P57-P59)*

✔ Additional Character Req   √x7ᵗʰ Placeholder Alert   Manifestation   **HCC** CMS-HCC Condition   ▽ Unspecified Code   ►◄ Revised Text   ● New Code   ▲ Revised Code Title

✓4th R18 Ascites
> INCLUDES fluid in peritoneal cavity
> EXCLUDES 1 ascites in alcoholic cirrhosis (K70.31)
> ascites in alcoholic hepatitis (K70.11)
> ascites in toxic liver disease with chronic active hepatitis (K71.51)

R18.0 Malignant ascites
> Code first malignancy, such as:
> malignant neoplasm of ovary (C56.-)
> secondary malignant neoplasm of retroperitoneum and peritoneum (C78.6)

R18.8 Other ascites
> Ascites NOS
> Peritoneal effusion (chronic)

✓4th R19 Other symptoms and signs involving the digestive system and abdomen
> EXCLUDES 1 acute abdomen (R10.0)

✓5th R19.0 Intra-abdominal and pelvic swelling, mass and lump
> EXCLUDES 1 abdominal distension (gaseous) (R14.-)
> ascites (R18.-)

R19.00 Intra-abdominal and pelvic swelling, mass and lump, unspecified site ▽

R19.01 Right upper quadrant abdominal swelling, mass and lump

R19.02 Left upper quadrant abdominal swelling, mass and lump

R19.03 Right lower quadrant abdominal swelling, mass and lump

R19.04 Left lower quadrant abdominal swelling, mass and lump

R19.05 Periumbilic swelling, mass or lump
> Diffuse or generalized umbilical swelling or mass

R19.06 Epigastric swelling, mass or lump

R19.07 Generalized intra-abdominal and pelvic swelling, mass and lump
> Diffuse or generalized intra-abdominal swelling or mass NOS
> Diffuse or generalized pelvic swelling or mass NOS

R19.09 Other intra-abdominal and pelvic swelling, mass and lump

✓5th R19.1 Abnormal bowel sounds

R19.11 Absent bowel sounds

R19.12 Hyperactive bowel sounds

R19.15 Other abnormal bowel sounds
> Abnormal bowel sounds NOS

R19.2 Visible peristalsis
> Hyperperistalsis
> **DEF:** Visible movements of muscular attempts to move food through the digestive tract; due to pyloric obstruction, stomach obstruction, or intestinal obstruction.

✓5th R19.3 Abdominal rigidity
> EXCLUDES 1 abdominal rigidity with severe abdominal pain (R10.0)

R19.30 Abdominal rigidity, unspecified site ▽

R19.31 Right upper quadrant abdominal rigidity

R19.32 Left upper quadrant abdominal rigidity

R19.33 Right lower quadrant abdominal rigidity

R19.34 Left lower quadrant abdominal rigidity

R19.35 Periumbilic abdominal rigidity

R19.36 Epigastric abdominal rigidity

R19.37 Generalized abdominal rigidity

R19.4 Change in bowel habit
> EXCLUDES 1 constipation (K59.0-)
> functional diarrhea (K59.1)

R19.5 Other fecal abnormalities
> Abnormal stool color
> Bulky stools
> Mucus in stools
> Occult blood in feces
> Occult blood in stools
> EXCLUDES 1 melena (K92.1)
> neonatal melena (P54.1)

R19.6 Halitosis

R19.7 Diarrhea, unspecified ▽
> Diarrhea NOS
> EXCLUDES 1 functional diarrhea (K59.1)
> neonatal diarrhea (P78.3)
> psychogenic diarrhea (F45.8)

R19.8 Other specified symptoms and signs involving the digestive system and abdomen

Symptoms and signs involving the skin and subcutaneous tissue (R20-R23)
> EXCLUDES 2 symptoms relating to breast (N64.4-N64.5)

✓4th R20 Disturbances of skin sensation
> EXCLUDES 1 dissociative anesthesia and sensory loss (F44.6)
> psychogenic disturbances (F45.8)

R20.0 Anesthesia of skin

R20.1 Hypoesthesia of skin

R20.2 Paresthesia of skin
> Formication
> Pins and needles
> Tingling skin
> EXCLUDES 1 acroparesthesia (I73.8)

R20.3 Hyperesthesia

R20.8 Other disturbances of skin sensation

R20.9 Unspecified disturbances of skin sensation ▽

R21 Rash and other nonspecific skin eruption
> INCLUDES rash NOS
> EXCLUDES 1 specified type of rash—code to condition
> vesicular eruption (R23.8)

✓4th R22 Localized swelling, mass and lump of skin and subcutaneous tissue
> INCLUDES subcutaneous nodules (localized)(superficial)
> EXCLUDES 1 abnormal findings on diagnostic imaging (R90-R93)
> edema (R60.-)
> enlarged lymph nodes (R59.-)
> localized adiposity (E65)
> swelling of joint (M25.4-)

R22.0 Localized swelling, mass and lump, head

R22.1 Localized swelling, mass and lump, neck

R22.2 Localized swelling, mass and lump, trunk
> EXCLUDES 1 intra-abdominal or pelvic mass and lump (R19.0-)
> intra-abdominal or pelvic swelling (R19.0-)
> EXCLUDES 2 breast mass and lump (N63)

✓5th R22.3 Localized swelling, mass and lump, upper limb

R22.30 Localized swelling, mass and lump, unspecified upper limb ▽

R22.31 Localized swelling, mass and lump, right upper limb

R22.32 Localized swelling, mass and lump, left upper limb

R22.33 Localized swelling, mass and lump, upper limb, bilateral

✓5th R22.4 Localized swelling, mass and lump, lower limb

R22.40 Localized swelling, mass and lump, unspecified lower limb ▽

R22.41 Localized swelling, mass and lump, right lower limb

R22.42 Localized swelling, mass and lump, left lower limb

R22.43 Localized swelling, mass and lump, lower limb, bilateral

R22.9 Localized swelling, mass and lump, unspecified ▽

✓4th R23 Other skin changes

R23.0 Cyanosis
> EXCLUDES 1 acrocyanosis (I73.8)
> cyanotic attacks of newborn (P28.2)
> **DEF:** Bluish or purplish discoloration of the skin due to inadequate oxygen level of blood.

R23.1 Pallor
> Clammy skin

R23.2 Flushing
> Excessive blushing
> Code first, if applicable, menopausal and female climacteric states (N95.1)

R23.3 Spontaneous ecchymoses
> Petechiae
> EXCLUDES 1 ecchymoses of newborn (P54.5)
> purpura (D69.-)

R23.4 Changes in skin texture
> Desquamation of skin
> Induration of skin
> Scaling of skin
> EXCLUDES 1 epidermal thickening NOS (L85.9)

R23.8 Other skin changes

R23.9 Unspecified skin changes ▽

Symptoms and signs involving the nervous and musculoskeletal systems (R25-R29)

☑4ᵗʰ R25 Abnormal involuntary movements
> EXCLUDES 1   specific movement disorders (G20-G26)
> stereotyped movement disorders (F98.4)
> tic disorders (F95.-)

R25.0 Abnormal head movements

R25.1 Tremor, unspecified ▽
> EXCLUDES 1   chorea NOS (G25.5)
> essential tremor (G25.0)
> hysterical tremor (F44.4)
> intention tremor (G25.2)

R25.2 Cramp and spasm
> EXCLUDES 2   carpopedal spasm (R29.0)
> charley-horse (M62.831)
> infantile spasms (G40.4-)
> muscle spasm of back (M62.830)
> muscle spasm of calf (M62.831)

R25.3 Fasciculation
> Twitching NOS

R25.8 Other abnormal involuntary movements

R25.9 Unspecified abnormal involuntary movements ▽

☑4ᵗʰ R26 Abnormalities of gait and mobility
> EXCLUDES 1   ataxia NOS (R27.0)
> hereditary ataxia (G11.-)
> locomotor (syphilitic) ataxia (A52.11)
> immobility syndrome (paraplegic) (M62.3)

R26.0 Ataxic gait
> Staggering gait

R26.1 Paralytic gait
> Spastic gait

R26.2 Difficulty in walking, not elsewhere classified
> EXCLUDES 1   falling (R29.6)
> unsteadiness on feet (R26.81)
> **AHA:** 2016, 2Q, 7

☑5ᵗʰ R26.8 Other abnormalities of gait and mobility

R26.81 Unsteadiness on feet

R26.89 Other abnormalities of gait and mobility

R26.9 Unspecified abnormalities of gait and mobility ▽

☑4ᵗʰ R27 Other lack of coordination
> EXCLUDES 1   ataxic gait (R26.0)
> hereditary ataxia (G11.-)
> vertigo NOS (R42)

R27.0 Ataxia, unspecified ▽
> EXCLUDES 1   ataxia following cerebrovascular disease (I69. with final characters -93)

R27.8 Other lack of coordination

R27.9 Unspecified lack of coordination ▽

☑4ᵗʰ R29 Other symptoms and signs involving the nervous and musculoskeletal systems

R29.0 Tetany
> Carpopedal spasm
> EXCLUDES 1   hysterical tetany (F44.5)
> neonatal tetany (P71.3)
> parathyroid tetany (E20.9)
> post-thyroidectomy tetany (E89.2)

R29.1 Meningismus

R29.2 Abnormal reflex
> EXCLUDES 2   abnormal pupillary reflex (H57.0)
> hyperactive gag reflex (J39.2)
> vasovagal reaction or syncope (R55)

R29.3 Abnormal posture

R29.4 Clicking hip
> EXCLUDES 1   congenital deformities of hip (Q65.-)

R29.5 Transient paralysis
> Code first any associated spinal cord injury (S14.0, S14.1-, S24.0, S24.1-, S34.0-, S34.1-)
> EXCLUDES 1   transient ischemic attack (G45.9)

R29.6 Repeated falls
> Falling
> Tendency to fall
> EXCLUDES 2   at risk for falling (Z91.81)
> history of falling (Z91.81)
> **AHA:** 2016, 2Q, 6

☑5ᵗʰ R29.7 National Institutes of Health Stroke Scale (NIHSS) Score
> Code first the type of cerebral infarction (I63.-)

☑6ᵗʰ R29.70 NIHSS score 0-9

R29.700	NIHSS score 0
R29.701	NIHSS score 1
R29.702	NIHSS score 2
R29.703	NIHSS score 3
R29.704	NIHSS score 4
R29.705	NIHSS score 5
R29.706	NIHSS score 6
R29.707	NIHSS score 7
R29.708	NIHSS score 8
R29.709	NIHSS score 9

☑6ᵗʰ R29.71 NIHSS score 10-19

R29.710	NIHSS score 10
R29.711	NIHSS score 11
R29.712	NIHSS score 12
R29.713	NIHSS score 13
R29.714	NIHSS score 14
R29.715	NIHSS score 15
R29.716	NIHSS score 16
R29.717	NIHSS score 17
R29.718	NIHSS score 18
R29.719	NIHSS score 19

☑6ᵗʰ R29.72 NIHSS score 20-29

R29.720	NIHSS score 20
R29.721	NIHSS score 21
R29.722	NIHSS score 22
R29.723	NIHSS score 23
R29.724	NIHSS score 24
R29.725	NIHSS score 25
R29.726	NIHSS score 26
R29.727	NIHSS score 27
R29.728	NIHSS score 28
R29.729	NIHSS score 29

☑6ᵗʰ R29.73 NIHSS score 30-39

R29.730	NIHSS score 30
R29.731	NIHSS score 31
R29.732	NIHSS score 32
R29.733	NIHSS score 33
R29.734	NIHSS score 34
R29.735	NIHSS score 35
R29.736	NIHSS score 36
R29.737	NIHSS score 37
R29.738	NIHSS score 38
R29.739	NIHSS score 39

☑6ᵗʰ R29.74 NIHSS score 40-42

R29.740	NIHSS score 40
R29.741	NIHSS score 41
R29.742	NIHSS score 42

☑5ᵗʰ R29.8 Other symptoms and signs involving the nervous and musculoskeletal systems

☑6ᵗʰ R29.81 Other symptoms and signs involving the nervous system

R29.810 Facial weakness
> Facial droop
> EXCLUDES 1   Bell's palsy (G51.0)
> facial weakness following cerebrovascular disease (I69. with final characters -92)

R29.818 Other symptoms and signs involving the nervous system

☑6ᵗʰ R29.89 Other symptoms and signs involving the musculoskeletal system
> EXCLUDES 2   pain in limb (M79.6-)

R29.890 Loss of height
> EXCLUDES 1   osteoporosis (M80-M81)

☑ Additional Character Req   ✔x7ᵗʰ Placeholder Alert   Manifestation   HCC CMS-HCC Condition   ▽ Unspecified Code   ►◄ Revised Text   ● New Code   ▲ Revised Code Title

ICD-10-CM 2018   893

R29.891   **Ocular torticollis**
    EXCLUDES 1   congenital (sternomastoid)
        torticollis Q68.0
        psychogenic torticollis (F45.8)
        spasmodic torticollis (G24.3)
        torticollis due to birth injury
        (P15.8)
        torticollis NOS M43.6
    DEF: Abnormal head posture as a result of a
    contracted state of cervical muscles to
    correct a visual disturbance, either double
    vision or a visual field defect.

R29.898   **Other symptoms and signs involving the
musculoskeletal system**

**R29.9   Unspecified symptoms and signs involving the nervous and
musculoskeletal systems**

R29.90   **Unspecified symptoms and signs involving the
nervous system**　▽

R29.91   **Unspecified symptoms and signs involving the
musculoskeletal system**　▽

Symptoms and signs involving
the genitourinary system (R30-R39)

R30   Pain associated with micturition
    EXCLUDES 1   psychogenic pain associated with micturition (F45.8)

R30.0   **Dysuria**
    Strangury

R30.1   **Vesical tenesmus**

R30.9   **Painful micturition, unspecified**　▽
    Painful urination NOS

R31   Hematuria
    EXCLUDES 1   hematuria included with underlying conditions, such as:
        acute cystitis with hematuria (N30.01)
        recurrent and persistent hematuria in glomerular diseases
        (N02.-)
    AHA: 2017, 1Q, 17

R31.0   **Gross hematuria**

R31.1   **Benign essential microscopic hematuria**

R31.2   **Other microscopic hematuria**

R31.21   **Asymptomatic microscopic hematuria**
    AMH

R31.29   **Other microscopic hematuria**

R31.9   **Hematuria, unspecified**　▽

R32   Unspecified urinary incontinence　▽
    Enuresis NOS
    EXCLUDES 1   functional urinary incontinence (R39.81)
        nonorganic enuresis (F98.0)
        stress incontinence and other specified urinary incontinence
        (N39.3-N39.4-)
        urinary incontinence associated with cognitive impairment
        (R39.81)

R33   Retention of urine
    EXCLUDES 1   psychogenic retention of urine (F45.8)

R33.0   **Drug induced retention of urine**
    Use additional code for adverse effect, if applicable, to identify
    drug (T36-T50 with fifth or sixth character 5)

R33.8   **Other retention of urine**
    Code first, if applicable, any causal condition, such as:
    enlarged prostate (N40.1)

R33.9   **Retention of urine, unspecified**　▽

R34   Anuria and oliguria
    EXCLUDES 1   anuria and oliguria complicating abortion or ectopic or molar
        pregnancy (O00-O07, O08.4)
        anuria and oliguria complicating pregnancy (O26.83-)
        anuria and oliguria complicating the puerperium (O90.4)

R35   Polyuria
    Code first, if applicable, any causal condition, such as:
    enlarged prostate (N40.1)
    EXCLUDES 1   psychogenic polyuria (F45.8)

R35.0   **Frequency of micturition**

R35.1   **Nocturia**

R35.8   **Other polyuria**
    Polyuria NOS

R36   Urethral discharge

R36.0   **Urethral discharge without blood**

R36.1   **Hematospermia**　♂

R36.9   **Urethral discharge, unspecified**　▽
    Penile discharge NOS
    Urethrorrhea

R37   **Sexual dysfunction, unspecified**　▽

**R39   Other and unspecified symptoms and signs involving the
genitourinary system**

R39.0   **Extravasation of urine**

R39.1   **Other difficulties with micturition**
    Code first, if applicable, any causal condition, such as:
    enlarged prostate (N40.1)

R39.11   **Hesitancy of micturition**

R39.12   **Poor urinary stream**
    Weak urinary steam

R39.13   **Splitting of urinary stream**

R39.14   **Feeling of incomplete bladder emptying**

R39.15   **Urgency of urination**
    EXCLUDES 1   urge incontinence (N39.41, N39.46)

R39.16   **Straining to void**

R39.19   **Other difficulties with micturition**

R39.191   **Need to immediately re-void**

R39.192   **Position dependent micturition**

R39.198   **Other difficulties with micturition**

R39.2   **Extrarenal uremia**
    Prerenal uremia
    EXCLUDES 1   uremia NOS (N19)

R39.8   **Other symptoms and signs involving the genitourinary
system**

R39.81   **Functional urinary incontinence**
    Urinary incontinence due to cognitive impairment, or
    severe physical disability or immobility
    EXCLUDES 1   stress incontinence and other specified
        urinary incontinence (N39.3-N39.4-)
        urinary incontinence NOS (R32)

R39.82   **Chronic bladder pain**

•　R39.83   **Unilateral non-palpable testicle**

•　R39.84   **Bilateral non-palpable testicles**

R39.89   **Other symptoms and signs involving the
genitourinary system**

R39.9   **Unspecified symptoms and signs involving the
genitourinary system**　▽

Symptoms and signs involving cognition, perception,
emotional state and behavior (R40-R46)

    EXCLUDES 2   symptoms and signs constituting part of a pattern of mental disorder
    (F01-F99)

R40   Somnolence, stupor and coma
    EXCLUDES 1   neonatal coma (P91.5)
        somnolence, stupor and coma in diabetes (E08-E13)
        somnolence, stupor and coma in hepatic failure (K72.-)
        somnolence, stupor and coma in hypoglycemia (nondiabetic)
        (E15)

R40.0   **Somnolence**
    Drowsiness
    EXCLUDES 1   coma (R40.2-)

R40.1   **Stupor**
    Catatonic stupor
    Semicoma
    EXCLUDES 1   catatonic schizophrenia (F20.2)
        coma (R40.2-)
        depressive stupor (F31-F33)
        dissociative stupor (F44.2)
        manic stupor (F30.2)

R40.2   **Coma**
    Code first any associated:
    fracture of skull (S02.-)
    intracranial injury (S06.-)
    NOTE　One code from each subcategory, R40.21-R40.23, is
    required to complete the coma scale
    AHA: 2015, 2Q, 17; 2014, 1Q, 19

R40.20   **Unspecified coma**　HCG ▽
    Coma NOS
    Unconsciousness NOS

✓⁶ᵗʰ R40.21 Coma scale, eyes open

> The following appropriate 7th character is to be added to subcategories R40.21-, R40.22-, R40.23-, and R40.24-.
> Ø   unspecified time
> 1   in the field [EMT or ambulance]
> 2   at arrival to emergency department
> 3   at hospital admission
> 4   24 hours or more after hospital admission

    ✓⁷ᵗʰ R40.211 Coma scale, eyes open, **never**   HCC
    ✓⁷ᵗʰ R40.212 Coma scale, eyes open, **to pain**   HCC
    ✓⁷ᵗʰ R40.213 Coma scale, eyes open, **to sound**
    ✓⁷ᵗʰ R40.214 Coma scale, eyes open, **spontaneous**

✓⁶ᵗʰ R40.22 Coma scale, best verbal response

    ✓⁷ᵗʰ R40.221 Coma scale, best verbal response, **none**   HCC
    ✓⁷ᵗʰ R40.222 Coma scale, best verbal response, **incomprehensible words**   HCC
          ▶Incomprehensible sounds (2-5 years of age)
          Moans/grunts to pain; restless (< 2 years old)◀
    ✓⁷ᵗʰ R40.223 Coma scale, best verbal response, **inappropriate words**
          ▶Inappropriate crying or screaming (< 2 years of age)
          Screaming (2-5 years of age)
    ✓⁷ᵗʰ R40.224 Coma scale, best verbal response, **confused conversation**
          ▶Inappropriate words (2-5 years of age)
          Irritable cries (< 2 years of age)◀
    ✓⁷ᵗʰ R40.225 Coma scale, best verbal response, **oriented**
          ▶Cooing or babbling or crying appropriately (< 2 years of age)
          Uses appropriate words (2- 5 years of age)◀

✓⁶ᵗʰ R40.23 Coma scale, best motor response

    ✓⁷ᵗʰ R40.231 Coma scale, best motor response, **none**   HCC
    ✓⁷ᵗʰ R40.232 Coma scale, best motor response, **extension**   HCC
          ▶Abnormal extensor posturing to pain or noxious stimuli (< 2 years of age)
          Extensor posturing to pain or noxious stimuli (2-5 years of age)◀
    ✓⁷ᵗʰ R40.233 Coma scale, best motor response, **abnormal**
          ▶Abnormal flexure posturing to pain or noxious stimuli (Ø-5 years of age)
          Flexion/decorticate posturing (< 2 years of age)◀
    ✓⁷ᵗʰ R40.234 Coma scale, best motor response, **flexion withdrawal**   HCC
          ▶Withdraws from pain or noxious stimuli (Ø-5 years of age)◀
    ✓⁷ᵗʰ R40.235 Coma scale, best motor response, **localizes pain**
          ▶Localizes pain (2-5 years of age)
          Withdraws to touch (< 2 years of age)◀
    ✓⁷ᵗʰ R40.236 Coma scale, best motor response, **obeys commands**
          ▶Normal or spontaneous movement (< 2 years of age)
          Obeys commands (2-5 years of age)◀

✓⁶ᵗʰ R40.24 Glasgow coma scale, total score
          NOTE   Assign a code from subcategory R40.24, when only the total coma score is documented

    ✓⁷ᵗʰ R40.241 Glasgow coma scale **score 13-15**
    ✓⁷ᵗʰ R40.242 Glasgow coma scale **score 9-12**
    ✓⁷ᵗʰ R40.243 Glasgow coma scale **score 3-8**   HCC
    ✓⁷ᵗʰ R40.244 **Other coma, without documented Glasgow coma scale score, or with partial score reported**   HCC

R40.3 Persistent vegetative state   HCC
          DEF: Persistent wakefulness without consciousness due to nonfunctioning cerebral cortex.

R40.4 Transient alteration of awareness

✓⁴ᵗʰ R41 Other symptoms and signs involving cognitive functions and awareness
          EXCLUDES 1   dissociative [conversion] disorders (F44.-)
                        mild cognitive impairment, so stated (G31.84)

    R41.0 Disorientation, unspecified   ▽
          Confusion NOS
          Delirium NOS
    R41.1 Anterograde amnesia
    R41.2 Retrograde amnesia
    R41.3 Other amnesia
          Amnesia NOS
          Memory loss NOS
          EXCLUDES 1   amnestic disorder due to known physiologic condition (F04)
                        amnestic syndrome due to psychoactive substance use (F10-F19 with 5th character .6)
                        mild memory disturbance due to known physiological condition (F06.8)
                        transient global amnesia (G45.4)
    R41.4 Neurologic neglect syndrome
          Asomatognosia
          Hemi-akinesia
          Hemi-inattention
          Hemispatial neglect
          Left-sided neglect
          Sensory neglect
          Visuospatial neglect
          EXCLUDES 1   visuospatial deficit (R41.842)

✓⁵ᵗʰ R41.8 Other symptoms and signs involving cognitive functions and awareness

    R41.81 Age-related cognitive decline   A
          Senility NOS
    R41.82 Altered mental status, unspecified   ▽
          Change in mental status NOS
          EXCLUDES 1   altered level of consciousness (R40.-)
                        altered mental status due to known condition—code to condition
                        delirium NOS (R41.Ø)
          AHA: 2012, 4Q, 97
    R41.83 Borderline intellectual functioning
          IQ level 71 to 84
          EXCLUDES 1   intellectual disabilities (F70-F79)
    ✓⁶ᵗʰ R41.84 Other specified cognitive deficit
          EXCLUDES 1   cognitive deficits as sequelae of cerebrovascular disease (I69.01-, I69.11-, I69.21-, I69.31-, I69.81-, I69.91-)
          R41.840 Attention and concentration deficit
                EXCLUDES 1   attention-deficit hyperactivity disorders (F90.-)
          R41.841 Cognitive communication deficit
          R41.842 Visuospatial deficit
          R41.843 Psychomotor deficit
          R41.844 Frontal lobe and executive function deficit
    R41.89 Other symptoms and signs involving cognitive functions and awareness
          Anosognosia

    R41.9 Unspecified symptoms and signs involving cognitive functions and awareness   ▽
          ▶Unspecified neurocognitive disorder◀

R42 Dizziness and giddiness
          Light-headedness
          Vertigo NOS
          EXCLUDES 1   vertiginous syndromes (H81.-)
                        vertigo from infrasound (T75.23)

✓⁴ᵗʰ R43 Disturbances of smell and taste

    R43.0 Anosmia
    R43.1 Parosmia
    R43.2 Parageusia
    R43.8 Other disturbances of smell and taste
          Mixed disturbance of smell and taste
    R43.9 Unspecified disturbances of smell and taste   ▽

✓ Additional Character Req   ✓x⁷ᵗʰ Placeholder Alert   Manifestation   HCC CMS-HCC Condition   ▽ Unspecified Code   ▶◀ Revised Text   ● New Code   ▲ Revised Code Title

☑ 4ᵗʰ R44 Other symptoms and signs involving general sensations and perceptions

EXCLUDES 1 alcoholic hallucinations (F1.5)
hallucinations in drug psychosis (F11-F19 with .5)
hallucinations in mood disorders with psychotic symptoms (F30.2, F31.5, F32.3, F33.3)
hallucinations in schizophrenia, schizotypal and delusional disorders (F20-F29)

EXCLUDES 2 disturbances of skin sensation (R20.-)

R44.0 **Auditory** hallucinations

R44.1 **Visual** hallucinations

R44.2 **Other hallucinations**

R44.3 **Hallucinations, unspecified**   ▽

R44.8 **Other symptoms and signs involving general sensations and perceptions**

R44.9 **Unspecified symptoms and signs involving general sensations and perceptions**   ▽

☑ 4ᵗʰ R45 Symptoms and signs involving emotional state

R45.0 **Nervousness**
Nervous tension

R45.1 **Restlessness and agitation**

R45.2 **Unhappiness**

R45.3 **Demoralization and apathy**
EXCLUDES 1 anhedonia (R45.84)

R45.4 **Irritability and anger**

R45.5 **Hostility**

R45.6 **Violent behavior**

R45.7 **State of emotional shock and stress, unspecified**   ▽

☑ 5ᵗʰ R45.8 Other symptoms and signs involving emotional state

R45.81 **Low self-esteem**

R45.82 **Worries**

R45.83 **Excessive crying of child, adolescent or adult**
EXCLUDES 1 excessive crying of infant (baby) R68.11

R45.84 **Anhedonia**

☑ 6ᵗʰ R45.85 Homicidal and suicidal ideations
EXCLUDES 1 suicide attempt (T14.91)

R45.850 **Homicidal ideations**

R45.851 **Suicidal ideations**
DEF: Thoughts of committing suicide; no actual attempt of suicide has been made.

R45.86 **Emotional lability**

R45.87 **Impulsiveness**

R45.89 **Other symptoms and signs involving emotional state**

☑ 4ᵗʰ R46 Symptoms and signs involving appearance and behavior

EXCLUDES 1 appearance and behavior in schizophrenia, schizotypal and delusional disorders (F20-F29)
mental and behavioral disorders (F01-F99)

R46.0 **Very low level of personal hygiene**

R46.1 **Bizarre personal appearance**

R46.2 **Strange and inexplicable behavior**

R46.3 **Overactivity**

R46.4 **Slowness and poor responsiveness**
EXCLUDES 1 stupor (R40.1)

R46.5 **Suspiciousness and marked evasiveness**

R46.6 **Undue concern and preoccupation with stressful events**

R46.7 **Verbosity and circumstantial detail obscuring reason for contact**

☑ 5ᵗʰ R46.8 Other symptoms and signs involving appearance and behavior

R46.81 **Obsessive-compulsive behavior**
EXCLUDES 1 obsessive-compulsive disorder (F42-)

R46.89 **Other symptoms and signs involving appearance and behavior**

Symptoms and signs involving speech and voice (R47-R49)

☑ 4ᵗʰ R47 Speech disturbances, not elsewhere classified

EXCLUDES 1 autism (F84.0)
cluttering (F80.81)
specific developmental disorders of speech and language (F80.-)
stuttering (F80.81)

☑ 5ᵗʰ R47.0 Dysphasia and aphasia

R47.01 **Aphasia**
EXCLUDES 1 aphasia following cerebrovascular disease (I69. with final characters -20)
progressive isolated aphasia (G31.01)

R47.02 **Dysphasia**
EXCLUDES 1 dysphasia following cerebrovascular disease (I69. with final characters -21)

R47.1 **Dysarthria and anarthria**
EXCLUDES 1 dysarthria following cerebrovascular disease (I69. with final characters -22)

☑ 5ᵗʰ R47.8 Other speech disturbances
EXCLUDES 1 dysarthria following cerebrovascular disease (I69. with final characters -28)

R47.81 **Slurred speech**

R47.82 *Fluency disorder in conditions classified elsewhere*
Stuttering in conditions classified elsewhere
Code first underlying disease or condition, such as:
Parkinson's disease (G20)
EXCLUDES 1 adult onset fluency disorder (F98.5)
childhood onset fluency disorder (F80.81)
fluency disorder (stuttering) following cerebrovascular disease (I69. with final characters-23)

R47.89 **Other speech disturbances**

R47.9 **Unspecified speech disturbances**   ▽

☑ 4ᵗʰ R48 Dyslexia and other symbolic dysfunctions, not elsewhere classified

EXCLUDES 1 specific developmental disorders of scholastic skills (F81.-)

R48.0 **Dyslexia and alexia**

R48.1 **Agnosia**
Astereognosia (astereognosis)
Autotopagnosia
EXCLUDES 1 visual object agnosia (R48.3)

R48.2 **Apraxia**
EXCLUDES 1 apraxia following cerebrovascular disease (I69. with final characters -90)

R48.3 **Visual agnosia**
Prosopagnosia
Simultanagnosia (asimultagnosia)

R48.8 **Other symbolic dysfunctions**
Acalculia
Agraphia
AHA: 2017, 1Q, 27

R48.9 **Unspecified symbolic dysfunctions**   ▽

☑ 4ᵗʰ R49 Voice and resonance disorders

EXCLUDES 1 psychogenic voice and resonance disorders (F44.4)

R49.0 **Dysphonia**
Hoarseness

R49.1 **Aphonia**
Loss of voice

☑ 5ᵗʰ R49.2 Hypernasality and hyponasality

R49.21 **Hypernasality**

R49.22 **Hyponasality**

R49.8 **Other voice and resonance disorders**

R49.9 **Unspecified voice and resonance disorder**   ▽
Change in voice NOS
Resonance disorder NOS

EXCLUDES 1 Not coded here   EXCLUDES 2 Not included here   N Newborn Age: 0   P Pediatric Age: 0-17   M Maternity Age: 12-55   A Adult Age: 15-124

896   ICD-10-CM 2018

General symptoms and signs (R50-R69)

✓4ᵗʰ R50 Fever of other and unknown origin
> EXCLUDES 1 chills without fever (R68.83)
> febrile convulsions (R56.0-)
> fever of unknown origin during labor (O75.2)
> fever of unknown origin in newborn (P81.9)
> hypothermia due to illness (R68.0)
> malignant hyperthermia due to anesthesia (T88.3)
> puerperal pyrexia NOS (O86.4)

R50.2 Drug induced fever
Use additional code for adverse effect, if applicable, to identify drug (T36-T50 with fifth or sixth character 5)
> EXCLUDES 1 postvaccination (postimmunization) fever (R50.83)

✓5ᵗʰ R50.8 Other specified fever

R50.81 Fever presenting with conditions classified elsewhere
Code first underlying condition when associated fever is present, such as with:
leukemia (C91-C95)
neutropenia (D70.-)
sickle-cell disease (D57.-)
AHA: 2014, 4Q, 22

R50.82 Postprocedural fever
> EXCLUDES 1 postprocedural infection (T81.4-)
> posttransfusion fever (R50.84)
> postvaccination (postimmunization) fever (R50.83)

R50.83 Postvaccination fever
Postimmunization fever

R50.84 Febrile nonhemolytic transfusion reaction
FNHTR
Posttransfusion fever

R50.9 Fever, unspecified ▽
Fever NOS
Fever of unknown origin [FUO]
Fever with chills
Fever with rigors
Hyperpyrexia NOS
Persistent fever
Pyrexia NOS

R51 Headache
Facial pain NOS
> EXCLUDES 1 atypical face pain (G50.1)
> migraine and other headache syndromes (G43-G44)
> trigeminal neuralgia (G50.0)

R52 Pain, unspecified ▽
Acute pain NOS
Generalized pain NOS
Pain NOS
> EXCLUDES 1 acute and chronic pain, not elsewhere classified (G89.-)
> localized pain, unspecified type—code to pain by site, such as:
> abdomen pain (R10.-)
> back pain (M54.9)
> breast pain (N64.4)
> chest pain (R07.1-R07.9)
> ear pain (H92.0-)
> eye pain (H57.1)
> headache (R51)
> joint pain (M25.5-)
> limb pain (M79.6-)
> lumbar region pain (M54.5)
> pelvic and perineal pain (R10.2)
> renal colic (N23)
> shoulder pain (M25.51-)
> spine pain (M54.-)
> throat pain (R07.0)
> tongue pain (K14.6)
> tooth pain (K08.8)
> pain disorders exclusively related to psychological factors (F45.41)

✓4ᵗʰ R53 Malaise and fatigue

R53.0 Neoplastic (malignant) related fatigue
Code first associated neoplasm

R53.1 Weakness
Asthenia NOS
> EXCLUDES 1 age-related weakness (R54)
> muscle weakness (M62.8-)
> sarcopenia (M62.84)
> senile asthenia (R54)
AHA: 2017, 1Q, 7; 2015, 1Q, 25

R53.2 Functional quadriplegia HCC
Complete immobility due to severe physical disability or frailty
> EXCLUDES 1 frailty NOS (R54)
> hysterical paralysis (F44.4)
> immobility syndrome (M62.3)
> neurologic quadriplegia (G82.5-)
> quadriplegia (G82.50)
AHA: 2016, 2Q, 6
DEF: Inability to move due to a nonphysiological condition, such as dementia; no mental ability to move independently; typically found in severely demented patients.

✓5ᵗʰ R53.8 Other malaise and fatigue
> EXCLUDES 1 combat exhaustion and fatigue (F43.0)
> congenital debility (P96.9)
> ~~exhaustion and fatigue due to depressive episode (F32.-)~~
> exhaustion and fatigue due to excessive exertion (T73.3)
> exhaustion and fatigue due to exposure (T73.2)
> exhaustion and fatigue due to heat (T67.-)
> exhaustion and fatigue due to pregnancy (O26.8-)
> exhaustion and fatigue due to recurrent depressive episode (F33)
> exhaustion and fatigue due to senile debility (R54)

R53.81 Other malaise
Chronic debility
Debility NOS
General physical deterioration
Malaise NOS
Nervous debility
> EXCLUDES 1 age-related physical debility (R54)

R53.82 Chronic fatigue, unspecified ▽
Chronic fatigue syndrome NOS
> EXCLUDES 1 postviral fatigue syndrome (G93.3)

R53.83 Other fatigue
Fatigue NOS
Lack of energy
Lethargy
Tiredness
> EXCLUDES 2 ►exhaustion and fatigue due to depressive episode (F32.-)◄

R54 Age-related physical debility 🅰
Frailty
Old age
Senescence
Senile asthenia
Senile debility
> EXCLUDES 1 age-related cognitive decline (R41.81)
> sarcopenia (M62.84)
> senile psychosis (F03)
> senility NOS (R41.81)

R55 Syncope and collapse
Blackout
Fainting
Vasovagal attack
> EXCLUDES 1 cardiogenic shock (R57.0)
> carotid sinus syncope (G90.01)
> heat syncope (T67.1)
> neurocirculatory asthenia (F45.8)
> neurogenic orthostatic hypotension (G90.3)
> orthostatic hypotension (I95.1)
> postprocedural shock (T81.1-)
> psychogenic syncope (F48.8)
> shock NOS (R57.9)
> shock complicating or following abortion or ectopic or molar pregnancy (O00-O07, O08.3)
> shock complicating or following labor and delivery (O75.1)
> Stokes-Adams attack (I45.9)
> unconsciousness NOS (R40.2-)

✓4ᵗʰ R56 Convulsions, not elsewhere classified
> EXCLUDES 1 dissociative convulsions and seizures (F44.5)
> epileptic convulsions and seizures (G40.-)
> newborn convulsions and seizures (P90)

✓5ᵗʰ R56.0 Febrile convulsions

R56.00 Simple febrile convulsions HCC
Febrile convulsion NOS
Febrile seizure NOS

R56.01 Complex febrile convulsions HCC
Atypical febrile seizure
Complex febrile seizure
Complicated febrile seizure
> EXCLUDES 1 status epilepticus (G40.901)

R56.1 Post traumatic seizures   HCC
> EXCLUDES 1   *post traumatic epilepsy (G40.-)*

R56.9 Unspecified convulsions   HCC ▽
Convulsion disorder
Fit NOS
Recurrent convulsions
Seizure(s) (convulsive) NOS

✓4ᵗʰ **R57 Shock, not elsewhere classified**
> EXCLUDES 1   *anaphylactic shock NOS (T78.2)*
> *anaphylactic reaction or shock due to adverse food reaction (T78.0-)*
> *anaphylactic shock due to adverse effect of correct drug or medicament properly administered (T88.6)*
> *anaphylactic shock due to serum (T80.5-)*
> *anesthetic shock (T88.3)*
> *electric shock (T75.4)*
> *obstetric shock (O75.1)*
> *postprocedural shock (T81.1-)*
> *psychic shock (F43.0)*
> ~~*septic shock (R65.21)*~~
> *shock complicating or following ectopic or molar pregnancy (O00-O07, O08.3)*
> *shock due to lightning (T75.01)*
> *traumatic shock (T79.4)*
> *toxic shock syndrome (A48.3)*

R57.0 Cardiogenic shock   HCC
> EXCLUDES 2   ▶*septic shock (R65.21)*◀
> **DEF:** Associated with myocardial infarction, cardiac tamponade, and massive pulmonary embolism; symptoms include mental confusion, reduced blood pressure, tachycardia, pallor, and cold, clammy skin.

R57.1 Hypovolemic shock   HCC

R57.8 Other shock   HCC

R57.9 Shock, unspecified   HCC ▽
Failure of peripheral circulation NOS

R58 Hemorrhage, not elsewhere classified
Hemorrhage NOS
> EXCLUDES 1   *hemorrhage included with underlying conditions, such as:*
> *acute duodenal ulcer with hemorrhage (K26.0)*
> *acute gastritis with bleeding (K29.01)*
> *ulcerative enterocolitis with rectal bleeding (K51.01)*

✓4ᵗʰ **R59 Enlarged lymph nodes**
> INCLUDES   swollen glands
> EXCLUDES 1   *acute lymphadenitis (L04.-)*
> *chronic lymphadenitis (I88.1)*
> *lymphadenitis NOS (I88.9)*
> *mesenteric (acute) (chronic) lymphadenitis (I88.0)*

R59.0 Localized enlarged lymph nodes

R59.1 Generalized enlarged lymph nodes
Lymphadenopathy NOS

R59.9 Enlarged lymph nodes, unspecified   ▽

✓4ᵗʰ **R60 Edema, not elsewhere classified**
> EXCLUDES 1   *angioneurotic edema (T78.3)*
> *ascites (R18.-)*
> *cerebral edema (G93.6)*
> *cerebral edema due to birth injury (P11.0)*
> *edema of larynx (J38.4)*
> *edema of nasopharynx (J39.2)*
> *edema of pharynx (J39.2)*
> *gestational edema (O12.0-)*
> *hereditary edema (Q82.0)*
> *hydrops fetalis NOS (P83.2)*
> *hydrothorax (J94.8)*
> ~~*nutritional edema (E40-E46)*~~
> *hydrops fetalis NOS (P83.2)*
> *newborn edema (P83.3)*
> *pulmonary edema (J81.-)*

R60.0 Localized edema

R60.1 Generalized edema
> EXCLUDES 2   ▶*nutritional edema (E40-E46)*◀

R60.9 Edema, unspecified   ▽
Fluid retention NOS

R61 Generalized hyperhidrosis
Excessive sweating
Night sweats
Secondary hyperhidrosis
Code first, if applicable, menopausal and female climacteric states (N95.1)
> EXCLUDES 1   *focal (primary) (secondary) hyperhidrosis (L74.5-)*
> *Frey's syndrome (L74.52)*
> *localized (primary) (secondary) hyperhidrosis (L74.5-)*

✓4ᵗʰ **R62 Lack of expected normal physiological development in childhood and adults**
> EXCLUDES 1   *delayed puberty (E30.0)*
> *gonadal dysgenesis (Q99.1)*
> *hypopituitarism (E23.0)*

R62.0 Delayed milestone in childhood   P
Delayed attainment of expected physiological developmental stage
Late talker
Late walker

✓5ᵗʰ **R62.5 Other and unspecified lack of expected normal physiological development in childhood**
> EXCLUDES 1   *HIV disease resulting in failure to thrive (B20)*
> *physical retardation due to malnutrition (E45)*

R62.50 Unspecified lack of expected normal   ▽
physiological development in childhood
Infantilism NOS

R62.51 Failure to thrive (child)   P
Failure to gain weight
> EXCLUDES 1   *failure to thrive in child under 28 days old (P92.6)*
> **DEF:** Organic failure to thrive (FTT): Acute or chronic illness that interferes with nutritional intake, absorption, metabolism excretion, and energy requirements; nonorganic FTT is a symptom of neglect or abuse.

R62.52 Short stature (child)
Lack of growth
Physical retardation
Short stature NOS
> EXCLUDES 1   *short stature due to endocrine disorder (E34.3)*

R62.59 Other lack of expected normal physiological development in childhood

R62.7 Adult failure to thrive   A

✓4ᵗʰ **R63 Symptoms and signs concerning food and fluid intake**
> EXCLUDES 1   *bulimia NOS (F50.2)*
> *eating disorders of nonorganic origin (F50.-)*
> *malnutrition (E40-E46)*

R63.0 Anorexia
Loss of appetite
> EXCLUDES 1   *anorexia nervosa (F50.0-)*
> *loss of appetite of nonorganic origin (F50.89)*

R63.1 Polydipsia
Excessive thirst

R63.2 Polyphagia
Excessive eating
Hyperalimentation NOS

R63.3 Feeding difficulties
Feeding problem (elderly) (infant) NOS
▶Picky eater◀
> EXCLUDES 1   ▶*eating disorders (F50.-)*◀
> *feeding problems of newborn (P92.-)*
> *infant feeding disorder of nonorganic origin (F98.2-)*
> **AHA:** 2017, 1Q, 28; 2016, 3Q, 19

R63.4 Abnormal weight loss

R63.5 Abnormal weight gain
> EXCLUDES 1   *excessive weight gain in pregnancy (O26.0-)*
> *obesity (E66.-)*

R63.6 Underweight
Use additional code to identify body mass index (BMI), if known (Z68.-)
> EXCLUDES 1   *abnormal weight loss (R63.4)*
> *anorexia nervosa (F50.0-)*
> *malnutrition (E40-E46)*

R63.8 Other symptoms and signs concerning food and fluid intake

R64 Cachexia   HCC
Wasting syndrome
Code first underlying condition, if known
> EXCLUDES 1   *abnormal weight loss (R63.4)*
> *nutritional marasmus (E41)*

EXCLUDES 1 Not coded here   EXCLUDES 2 Not included here   N Newborn Age: 0   P Pediatric Age: 0-17   M Maternity Age: 12-55   A Adult Age: 15-124

898   ICD-10-CM 2018

☑4ᵗʰ **R65** **Symptoms and signs specifically associated with systemic inflammation and infection**

☑5ᵗʰ **R65.1** **Systemic inflammatory response syndrome [SIRS] of non-infectious origin**

Code first underlying condition, such as:
heatstroke (T67.0)
injury and trauma (S00-T88)
EXCLUDES 1   sepsis—code to infection
           severe sepsis (R65.2)

R65.10 **Systemic inflammatory response syndrome [SIRS] of non-infectious origin without acute organ dysfunction**   HCC
Systemic inflammatory response syndrome (SIRS) NOS

R65.11 **Systemic inflammatory response syndrome [SIRS] of non-infectious origin with acute organ dysfunction**   HCC
Use additional code to identify specific acute organ dysfunction, such as:
acute kidney failure (N17.-)
acute respiratory failure (J96.0-)
critical illness myopathy (G72.81)
critical illness polyneuropathy (G62.81)
disseminated intravascular coagulopathy [DIC] (D65)
encephalopathy (metabolic) (septic) (G93.41)
hepatic failure (K72.0-)

☑5ᵗʰ **R65.2** **Severe sepsis**
Infection with associated acute organ dysfunction
Sepsis with acute organ dysfunction
Sepsis with multiple organ dysfunction
Systemic inflammatory response syndrome due to infectious process with acute organ dysfunction
Code first underlying infection, such as:
infection following a procedure (T81.4-)
infections following infusion, transfusion and therapeutic injection (T80.2-)
puerperal sepsis (O85)
sepsis following complete or unspecified spontaneous abortion (O03.87)
sepsis following ectopic and molar pregnancy (O08.82)
sepsis following incomplete spontaneous abortion (O03.37)
sepsis following (induced) termination of pregnancy (O04.87)
sepsis NOS (A41.9)
Use additional code to identify specific acute organ dysfunction, such as:
acute kidney failure (N17.-)
acute respiratory failure (J96.0-)
critical illness myopathy (G72.81)
critical illness polyneuropathy (G62.81)
disseminated intravascular coagulopathy [DIC] (D65)
encephalopathy (metabolic) (septic) (G93.41)
hepatic failure (K72.0-)
AHA: 2016, 3Q, 8

R65.20 **Severe sepsis without septic shock**   HCC
Severe sepsis NOS
AHA: 2016, 3Q, 14; 2013, 4Q, 119

R65.21 **Severe sepsis with septic shock**   HCC

☑4ᵗʰ **R68** **Other general symptoms and signs**

R68.0 **Hypothermia, not associated with low environmental temperature**
EXCLUDES 1   hypothermia NOS (accidental) (T68)
           hypothermia due to anesthesia (T88.51)
           hypothermia due to low environmental temperature (T68)
           newborn hypothermia (P80.-)

☑5ᵗʰ **R68.1** **Nonspecific symptoms peculiar to infancy**
EXCLUDES 1   colic, infantile (R10.83)
           neonatal cerebral irritability (P91.3)
           teething syndrome (K00.7)

R68.11 **Excessive crying of infant (baby)**   P
EXCLUDES 1   excessive crying of child, adolescent, or adult (R45.83)

R68.12 **Fussy infant (baby)**   P
Irritable infant

R68.13 **Apparent life threatening event in infant (ALTE)**   P
Apparent life threatening event in newborn
▶Brief resolved unexplained event (BRUE)◀
Code first confirmed diagnosis, if known
Use additional code(s) for associated signs and symptoms if no confirmed diagnosis established, or if signs and symptoms are not associated routinely with confirmed diagnosis, or provide additional information for cause of ALTE

R68.19 **Other nonspecific symptoms peculiar to infancy**   P

R68.2 **Dry mouth, unspecified**   ▽
EXCLUDES 1   dry mouth due to dehydration (E86.0)
           dry mouth due to sicca syndrome [Sjögren] (M35.0-)
           salivary gland hyposecretion (K11.7)

R68.3 **Clubbing of fingers**
Clubbing of nails
DEF: Enlarged soft tissue of distal fingers; usually occurs in heart and lung diseases.
EXCLUDES 1   congenital clubfinger (Q68.1)

☑5ᵗʰ **R68.8** **Other general symptoms and signs**

R68.81 **Early satiety**
DEF: The premature feeling of being full after eating only a small amount of food; mechanism of satiety is multifactorial.

R68.82 **Decreased libido**   A
Decreased sexual desire

R68.83 **Chills (without fever)**
Chills NOS
EXCLUDES 1   chills with fever (R50.9)

R68.84 **Jaw pain**
Mandibular pain
Maxilla pain
EXCLUDES 1   temporomandibular joint arthralgia (M26.62-)

R68.89 **Other general symptoms and signs**

R69 **Illness, unspecified**   ▽
Unknown and unspecified cases of morbidity

Abnormal findings on examination of blood, without diagnosis (R70-R79)

EXCLUDES 2   abnormal findings on antenatal screening of mother (O28.-)
           abnormalities of lipids (E78.-)
           abnormalities of platelets and thrombocytes (D69.-)
           abnormalities of white blood cells classified elsewhere (D70-D72)
           coagulation hemorrhagic disorders (D65-D68)
           diagnostic abnormal findings classified elsewhere—see Alphabetical Index
           hemorrhagic and hematological disorders of newborn (P50-P61)

☑4ᵗʰ **R70** **Elevated erythrocyte sedimentation rate and abnormality of plasma viscosity**

R70.0 **Elevated erythrocyte sedimentation rate**

R70.1 **Abnormal plasma viscosity**

☑4ᵗʰ **R71** **Abnormality of red blood cells**
EXCLUDES 1   anemias (D50-D64)
           anemia of premature infant (P61.2)
           benign (familial) polycythemia (D75.0)
           congenital anemias (P61.2-P61.4)
           newborn anemia due to isoimmunization (P55.-)
           polycythemia neonatorum (P61.1)
           polycythemia NOS (D75.1)
           polycythemia vera (D45)
           secondary polycythemia (D75.1)

R71.0 **Precipitous drop in hematocrit**
Drop (precipitous) in hemoglobin
Drop in hematocrit

R71.8 **Other abnormality of red blood cells**
Abnormal red-cell morphology NOS
Abnormal red-cell volume NOS
Anisocytosis
Poikilocytosis

☑ Additional Character Req   ☑x7ᵗʰ Placeholder Alert   Manifestation   HCC CMS-HCC Condition   ▽ Unspecified Code   ▶◀ Revised Text   ● New Code   ▲ Revised Code Title

ICD-10-CM 2018   **899**

☑4ᵗʰ **R73** **Elevated blood glucose level**
     EXCLUDES 1   diabetes mellitus (E08-E13)
         diabetes mellitus in pregnancy, childbirth and the puerperium
           (O24.-)
         neonatal disorders (P70.0-P70.2)
         postsurgical hypoinsulinemia (E89.1)

     ☑5ᵗʰ **R73.0** **Abnormal glucose**
         EXCLUDES 1   abnormal glucose in pregnancy (O99.81-)
            diabetes mellitus (E08-E13)
            dysmetabolic syndrome X (E88.81)
            gestational diabetes (O24.4-)
            glycosuria (R81)
            hypoglycemia (E16.2)

         R73.01 **Impaired fasting glucose**
            Elevated fasting glucose

         R73.02 **Impaired glucose tolerance (oral)**
            Elevated glucose tolerance

         R73.03 **Prediabetes**
            Latent diabetes

         R73.09 **Other abnormal glucose**
            Abnormal glucose NOS
            Abnormal non-fasting glucose tolerance

     R73.9 **Hyperglycemia, unspecified** ▽

☑4ᵗʰ **R74** **Abnormal serum enzyme levels**
     R74.0 **Nonspecific elevation of levels of transaminase and lactic acid dehydrogenase [LDH]**

     R74.8 **Abnormal levels of other serum enzymes**
         Abnormal level of acid phosphatase
         Abnormal level of alkaline phosphatase
         Abnormal level of amylase
         Abnormal level of lipase [triacylglycerol lipase]

     R74.9 **Abnormal serum enzyme level, unspecified** ▽

R75 **Inconclusive laboratory evidence of human immunodeficiency virus [HIV]**
     Nonconclusive HIV-test finding in infants
     EXCLUDES 1   asymptomatic human immunodeficiency virus [HIV] infection
           status (Z21)
         human immunodeficiency virus [HIV] disease (B20)

☑4ᵗʰ **R76** **Other abnormal immunological findings in serum**
     R76.0 **Raised antibody titer**
         EXCLUDES 1   isoimmunization in pregnancy (O36.0-O36.1)
            isoimmunization affecting newborn (P55.-)

     ☑5ᵗʰ **R76.1** **Nonspecific reaction to test for tuberculosis**
         R76.11 **Nonspecific reaction to tuberculin skin test without active tuberculosis**
            Abnormal result of Mantoux test
            PPD positive
            Tuberculin (skin test) positive
            Tuberculin (skin test) reactor
            EXCLUDES 1   nonspecific reaction to cell mediated
               immunity measurement of gamma
               interferon antigen response without
               active tuberculosis (R76.12)

         R76.12 **Nonspecific reaction to cell mediated immunity measurement of gamma interferon antigen response without active tuberculosis**
            Nonspecific reaction to QuantiFERON-TB test (QFT) without active tuberculosis
            EXCLUDES 1   nonspecific reaction to tuberculin skin test
               without active tuberculosis (R76.11)
               positive tuberculin skin test (R76.11)

     R76.8 **Other specified abnormal immunological findings in serum**
         Raised level of immunoglobulins NOS

     R76.9 **Abnormal immunological finding in serum, unspecified** ▽

☑4ᵗʰ **R77** **Other abnormalities of plasma proteins**
     EXCLUDES 1   disorders of plasma-protein metabolism (E88.0)

     R77.0 **Abnormality of albumin**
     R77.1 **Abnormality of globulin**
         Hyperglobulinemia NOS
     R77.2 **Abnormality of alphafetoprotein**
     R77.8 **Other specified abnormalities of plasma proteins**
     R77.9 **Abnormality of plasma protein, unspecified** ▽

☑4ᵗʰ **R78** **Findings of drugs and other substances, not normally found in blood**
     Use additional code to identify any retained foreign body, if applicable (Z18.-)
     EXCLUDES 1   mental or behavioral disorders due to psychoactive substance
           use (F10-F19)

     R78.0 **Finding of alcohol in blood**
         Use additional external cause code (Y90.-), for detail regarding alcohol level

     R78.1 **Finding of opiate drug in blood**
     R78.2 **Finding of cocaine in blood**
     R78.3 **Finding of hallucinogen in blood**
     R78.4 **Finding of other drugs of addictive potential in blood**
     R78.5 **Finding of other psychotropic drug in blood**
     R78.6 **Finding of steroid agent in blood**

     ☑5ᵗʰ **R78.7** **Finding of abnormal level of heavy metals in blood**
         R78.71 **Abnormal lead level in blood**
            EXCLUDES 1   lead poisoning (T56.0-)

         R78.79 **Finding of abnormal level of heavy metals in blood**

     ☑5ᵗʰ **R78.8** **Finding of other specified substances, not normally found in blood**
         R78.81 **Bacteremia**
            EXCLUDES 1   sepsis—code to specified infection
            DEF: Laboratory finding of bacteria in the blood in the absence of two or more signs of sepsis; transient in nature, it progresses to septicemia with severe infectious process.

         R78.89 **Finding of other specified substances, not normally found in blood**
            Finding of abnormal level of lithium in blood

     R78.9 **Finding of unspecified substance, not normally found in blood** ▽

☑4ᵗʰ **R79** **Other abnormal findings of blood chemistry**
     Use additional code to identify any retained foreign body, if applicable (Z18.-)
     EXCLUDES 1   ~~abnormality of fluid, electrolyte or acid-base balance (E86-E87)~~
         asymptomatic hyperuricemia (E79.0)
         hyperglycemia NOS (R73.9)
         hypoglycemia NOS (E16.2)
         neonatal hypoglycemia (P70.3-P70.4)
         specific findings indicating disorder of amino-acid metabolism
           (E70-E72)
         specific findings indicating disorder of carbohydrate
           metabolism (E73-E74)
         specific findings indicating disorder of lipid metabolism (E75.-)

     R79.0 **Abnormal level of blood mineral**
         Abnormal blood level of cobalt
         Abnormal blood level of copper
         Abnormal blood level of iron
         Abnormal blood level of magnesium
         Abnormal blood level of mineral NEC
         Abnormal blood level of zinc
         EXCLUDES 1   abnormal level of lithium (R78.89)
            disorders of mineral metabolism (E83.-)
            neonatal hypomagnesemia (P71.2)
            nutritional mineral deficiency (E58-E61)

     R79.1 **Abnormal coagulation profile**
         Abnormal or prolonged bleeding time
         Abnormal or prolonged coagulation time
         Abnormal or prolonged partial thromboplastin time [PTT]
         Abnormal or prolonged prothrombin time [PT]
         EXCLUDES 1   coagulation defects (D68.-)
         EXCLUDES 2 ▶abnormality of fluid, electrolyte or acid-base balance
           (E86-E87)◀

     ☑5ᵗʰ **R79.8** **Other specified abnormal findings of blood chemistry**
         R79.81 **Abnormal blood-gas level**
         R79.82 **Elevated C-reactive protein [CRP]**
         R79.89 **Other specified abnormal findings of blood chemistry**

     R79.9 **Abnormal finding of blood chemistry, unspecified** ▽

EXCLUDES 1 Not coded here   *EXCLUDES 2* Not included here   **N** Newborn Age: 0   **P** Pediatric Age: 0-17   **M** Maternity Age: 12-55   **A** Adult Age: 15-124

900   ICD-10-CM 2018

Abnormal findings on examination of urine, without diagnosis (R80-R82)

EXCLUDES 1   abnormal findings on antenatal screening of mother (O28.-)
diagnostic abnormal findings classified elsewhere—see Alphabetical Index
specific findings indicating disorder of amino-acid metabolism (E70-E72)
specific findings indicating disorder of carbohydrate metabolism (E73-E74)

✓4th **R80 Proteinuria**
    EXCLUDES 1   gestational proteinuria (O12.1-)

R80.0 Isolated proteinuria
    Idiopathic proteinuria
    EXCLUDES 1   isolated proteinuria with specific morphological lesion (N06.-)

R80.1 Persistent proteinuria, unspecified ▽

R80.2 Orthostatic proteinuria, unspecified ▽
    Postural proteinuria

R80.3 Bence Jones proteinuria

R80.8 Other proteinuria

R80.9 Proteinuria, unspecified ▽
    Albuminuria NOS

R81 Glycosuria
    EXCLUDES 1   renal glycosuria (E74.8)

✓4th **R82 Other and unspecified abnormal findings in urine**
    INCLUDES   chromoabnormalities in urine
    Use additional code to identify any retained foreign body, if applicable (Z18.-)
    EXCLUDES 2   hematuria (R31.-)

R82.0 Chyluria
    EXCLUDES 1   filarial chyluria (B74.-)

R82.1 Myoglobinuria

R82.2 Biliuria

R82.3 Hemoglobinuria
    EXCLUDES 1   hemoglobinuria due to hemolysis from external causes NEC (D59.6)
           hemoglobinuria due to paroxysmal nocturnal [Marchiafava-Micheli] (D59.5)
    DEF: Free hemoglobin in blood due to rapid hemolysis of red blood cells; causes include burns, crushed injury, sickle cell anemia, thalassemia, parasitic infections, or kidney infections.

R82.4 Acetonuria
    Ketonuria
    DEF: Excessive excretion of acetone in urine; commonly occurs in diabetic acidosis.

R82.5 Elevated urine levels of drugs, medicaments and biological substances
    Elevated urine levels of catecholamines
    Elevated urine levels of indoleacetic acid
    Elevated urine levels of 17-ketosteroids
    Elevated urine levels of steroids

R82.6 Abnormal urine levels of substances chiefly nonmedicinal as to source
    Abnormal urine level of heavy metals

✓5th **R82.7 Abnormal findings on microbiological examination of urine**
    EXCLUDES 1   colonization status (Z22.-)

R82.71 Bacteriuria

R82.79 Other abnormal findings on microbiological examination of urine
    Positive culture findings of urine

R82.8 Abnormal findings on cytological and histological examination of urine

✓5th **R82.9 Other and unspecified abnormal findings in urine**

R82.90 Unspecified abnormal findings in urine ▽

R82.91 Other chromoabnormalities of urine
    Chromoconversion (dipstick)
    Idiopathic dipstick converts positive for blood with no cellular forms in sediment
    EXCLUDES 1   hemoglobinuria (R82.3)
           myoglobinuria (R82.1)

R82.99 Other abnormal findings in urine
    Cells and casts in urine
    Crystalluria
    Melanuria

Cerebrospinal Fluid

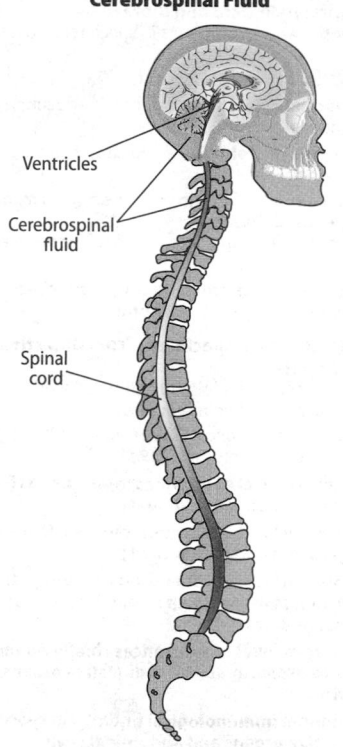

Ventricles

Cerebrospinal fluid

Spinal cord

Abnormal findings on examination of other body fluids, substances and tissues, without diagnosis (R83-R89)

EXCLUDES 1   abnormal findings on antenatal screening of mother (O28.-)
diagnostic abnormal findings classified elsewhere—see Alphabetical Index

EXCLUDES 2   abnormal findings on examination of blood, without diagnosis (R70-R79)
abnormal findings on examination of urine, without diagnosis (R80-R82)
abnormal tumor markers (R97.-)

R83.3 Abnormal level of substances chiefly nonmedicinal as to source in cerebrospinal fluid

✓4th **R83 Abnormal findings in cerebrospinal fluid**

R83.0 Abnormal level of enzymes in cerebrospinal fluid

R83.1 Abnormal level of hormones in cerebrospinal fluid

R83.2 Abnormal level of other drugs, medicaments and biological substances in cerebrospinal fluid

R83.4 Abnormal immunological findings in cerebrospinal fluid

R83.5 Abnormal microbiological findings in cerebrospinal fluid
    Positive culture findings in cerebrospinal fluid
    EXCLUDES 1   colonization status (Z22.-)

R83.6 Abnormal cytological findings in cerebrospinal fluid

R83.8 Other abnormal findings in cerebrospinal fluid
    Abnormal chromosomal findings in cerebrospinal fluid

R83.9 Unspecified abnormal finding in cerebrospinal fluid ▽

✓4th **R84 Abnormal findings in specimens from respiratory organs and thorax**
    INCLUDES   abnormal findings in bronchial washings
    abnormal findings in nasal secretions
    abnormal findings in pleural fluid
    abnormal findings in sputum
    abnormal findings in throat scrapings
    EXCLUDES 1   blood-stained sputum (R04.2)

R84.0 Abnormal level of enzymes in specimens from respiratory organs and thorax

R84.1 Abnormal level of hormones in specimens from respiratory organs and thorax

R84.2 Abnormal level of other drugs, medicaments and biological substances in specimens from respiratory organs and thorax

R84.3 Abnormal level of substances chiefly nonmedicinal as to source in specimens from respiratory organs and thorax

R84.4 Abnormal immunological findings in specimens from respiratory organs and thorax

R84.5   **Abnormal microbiological findings in specimens from respiratory organs and thorax**
Positive culture findings in specimens from respiratory organs and thorax
EXCLUDES 1   *colonization status (Z22.-)*

R84.6   **Abnormal cytological findings in specimens from respiratory organs and thorax**

R84.7   **Abnormal histological findings in specimens from respiratory organs and thorax**

R84.8   **Other abnormal findings in specimens from respiratory organs and thorax**
Abnormal chromosomal findings in specimens from respiratory organs and thorax

R84.9   **Unspecified abnormal finding in specimens from respiratory organs and thorax**   ▽

✓4ᵗʰ **R85**   **Abnormal findings in specimens from digestive organs and abdominal cavity**
INCLUDES   abnormal findings in peritoneal fluid
abnormal findings in saliva
EXCLUDES 1   *cloudy peritoneal dialysis effluent (R88.0)*
fecal abnormalities (R19.5)

R85.0   **Abnormal level of enzymes in specimens from digestive organs and abdominal cavity**

R85.1   **Abnormal level of hormones in specimens from digestive organs and abdominal cavity**

R85.2   **Abnormal level of other drugs, medicaments and biological substances in specimens from digestive organs and abdominal cavity**

R85.3   **Abnormal level of substances chiefly nonmedicinal as to source in specimens from digestive organs and abdominal cavity**

R85.4   **Abnormal immunological findings in specimens from digestive organs and abdominal cavity**

R85.5   **Abnormal microbiological findings in specimens from digestive organs and abdominal cavity**
Positive culture findings in specimens from digestive organs and abdominal cavity
EXCLUDES 1   *colonization status (Z22.-)*

✓5ᵗʰ R85.6   **Abnormal cytological findings in specimens from digestive organs and abdominal cavity**

✓6ᵗʰ   R85.61   **Abnormal cytologic smear of anus**
EXCLUDES 1   *abnormal cytological findings in specimens from other digestive organs and abdominal cavity (R85.69)*
anal intraepithelial neoplasia I [AIN I] (K62.82)
anal intraepithelial neoplasia II [AIN II] (K62.82)
anal intraepithelial neoplasia III [AIN III] (D01.3)
carcinoma in situ of anus (histologically confirmed) (D01.3)
dysplasia (mild) (moderate) of anus (histologically confirmed) (K62.82)
severe dysplasia of anus (histologically confirmed) (D01.3)
EXCLUDES 2   *anal high risk human papillomavirus (HPV) DNA test positive (R85.81)*
anal low risk human papillomavirus (HPV) DNA test positive (R85.82)

R85.610   **Atypical squamous cells of undetermined significance on cytologic smear of anus [ASC-US]**

R85.611   **Atypical squamous cells cannot exclude high grade squamous intraepithelial lesion on cytologic smear of anus [ASC-H]**

R85.612   **Low grade squamous intraepithelial lesion on cytologic smear of anus [LGSIL]**

R85.613   **High grade squamous intraepithelial lesion on cytologic smear of anus [HGSIL]**

R85.614   **Cytologic evidence of malignancy on smear of anus**

R85.615   **Unsatisfactory cytologic smear of anus**
Inadequate sample of cytologic smear of anus

R85.616   **Satisfactory anal smear but lacking transformation zone**

R85.618   **Other abnormal cytological findings on specimens from anus**

R85.619   **Unspecified abnormal cytological findings in specimens from anus**   ▽
Abnormal anal cytology NOS
Atypical glandular cells of anus NOS

R85.69   **Abnormal cytological findings in specimens from other digestive organs and abdominal cavity**

R85.7   **Abnormal histological findings in specimens from digestive organs and abdominal cavity**

✓5ᵗʰ R85.8   **Other abnormal findings in specimens from digestive organs and abdominal cavity**

R85.81   **Anal high risk human papillomavirus [HPV] DNA test positive**
EXCLUDES 1   *anogenital warts due to human papillomavirus (HPV) (A63.0)*
condyloma acuminatum (A63.0)

R85.82   **Anal low risk human papillomavirus [HPV] DNA test positive**
Use additional code for associated human papillomavirus (B97.7)

R85.89   **Other abnormal findings in specimens from digestive organs and abdominal cavity**
Abnormal chromosomal findings in specimens from digestive organs and abdominal cavity

R85.9   **Unspecified abnormal finding in specimens from digestive organs and abdominal cavity**   ▽

✓4ᵗʰ **R86**   **Abnormal findings in specimens from male genital organs**
INCLUDES   abnormal findings in prostatic secretions
abnormal findings in semen, seminal fluid
abnormal spermatozoa
EXCLUDES 1   *azoospermia (N46.0-)*
oligospermia (N46.1-)

R86.0   **Abnormal level of enzymes in specimens from male genital organs**   ♂

R86.1   **Abnormal level of hormones in specimens from male genital organs**   ♂

R86.2   **Abnormal level of other drugs, medicaments and biological ♂ substances in specimens from male genital organs**

R86.3   **Abnormal level of substances chiefly nonmedicinal as to source in specimens from male genital organs**   ♂

R86.4   **Abnormal immunological findings in specimens from male ♂ genital organs**

R86.5   **Abnormal microbiological findings in specimens from male ♂ genital organs**
Positive culture findings in specimens from male genital organs
EXCLUDES 1   *colonization status (Z22.-)*

R86.6   **Abnormal cytological findings in specimens from male genital organs**   ♂

R86.7   **Abnormal histological findings in specimens from male genital organs**   ♂

R86.8   **Other abnormal findings in specimens from male genital organs**   ♂
Abnormal chromosomal findings in specimens from male genital organs

R86.9   **Unspecified abnormal finding in specimens from male genital organs**   ♂▽

✓4ᵗʰ **R87**   **Abnormal findings in specimens from female genital organs**
INCLUDES   abnormal findings in secretion and smears from cervix uteri
abnormal findings in secretion and smears from vagina
abnormal findings in secretion and smears from vulva

R87.0   **Abnormal level of enzymes in specimens from female genital organs**   ♀

R87.1   **Abnormal level of hormones in specimens from female genital organs**   ♀

R87.2   **Abnormal level of other drugs, medicaments and biological substances in specimens from female genital organs**   ♀

R87.3   **Abnormal level of substances chiefly nonmedicinal as to source in specimens from female genital organs**   ♀

R87.4   **Abnormal immunological findings in specimens from female genital organs**   ♀

R87.5   **Abnormal microbiological findings in specimens from female genital organs**   ♀
Positive culture findings in specimens from female genital organs
EXCLUDES 1   *colonization status (Z22.-)*

✓5th **R87.6** **Abnormal cytological findings in specimens from female genital organs**

    ✓6th **R87.61** **Abnormal cytological findings in specimens from cervix uteri**

      EXCLUDES 1   *abnormal cytological findings in specimens from other female genital organs (R87.69)*

          abnormal cytological findings in specimens from vagina (R87.62-)

          carcinoma in situ of cervix uteri (histologically confirmed) (D06.-)

          cervical intraepithelial neoplasia I [CIN I] (N87.0)

          cervical intraepithelial neoplasia II [CIN II] (N87.1)

          cervical intraepithelial neoplasia III [CIN III] (D06.-)

          dysplasia (mild) (moderate) of cervix uteri (histologically confirmed) (N87.-)

          severe dysplasia of cervix uteri (histologically confirmed) (D06.-)

      EXCLUDES 2   *cervical high risk human papillomavirus (HPV) DNA test positive (R87.810)*

          cervical low risk human papillomavirus (HPV) DNA test positive (R87.820)

    R87.610 **Atypical squamous cells of undetermined significance on cytologic smear of cervix [ASC-US]** ♀

    R87.611 **Atypical squamous cells cannot exclude high grade squamous intraepithelial lesion on cytologic smear of cervix [ASC-H]** ♀

    R87.612 **Low grade squamous intraepithelial lesion on cytologic smear of cervix [LGSIL]** ♀

    R87.613 **High grade squamous intraepithelial lesion on cytologic smear of cervix [HGSIL]** ♀

    R87.614 **Cytologic evidence of malignancy on smear of cervix** ♀

    R87.615 **Unsatisfactory cytologic smear of cervix** ♀
        Inadequate sample of cytologic smear of cervix

    R87.616 **Satisfactory cervical smear but lacking transformation zone** ♀

    R87.618 **Other abnormal cytological findings on specimens from cervix uteri** ♀

    R87.619 **Unspecified abnormal cytological findings in specimens from cervix uteri** ♀ ▽
        Abnormal cervical cytology NOS
        Abnormal Papanicolaou smear of cervix NOS
        Abnormal thin preparation smear of cervix NOS
        Atypical endocervial cells of cervix NOS
        Atypical endometrial cells of cervix NOS
        Atypical glandular cells of cervix NOS

    ✓6th **R87.62** **Abnormal cytological findings in specimens from vagina**
      Use additional code to identify acquired absence of uterus and cervix, if applicable (Z90.71-)

      EXCLUDES 1   *abnormal cytological findings in specimens from cervix uteri (R87.61-)*

          abnormal cytological findings in specimens from other female genital organs (R87.69)

          carcinoma in situ of vagina (histologically confirmed) (D07.2)

          dysplasia (mild) (moderate) of vagina (histologically confirmed) (N89.-)

          severe dysplasia of vagina (histologically confirmed) (D07.2)

          vaginal intraepithelial neoplasia I [VAIN I] (N89.0)

          vaginal intraepithelial neoplasia II [VAIN II] (N89.1)

          vaginal intraepithelial neoplasia III [VAIN III] (D07.2)

      EXCLUDES 2   *vaginal high risk human papillomavirus (HPV) DNA test positive (R87.811)*

          vaginal low risk human papillomavirus (HPV) DNA test positive (R87.821)

    R87.620 **Atypical squamous cells of undetermined significance on cytologic smear of vagina [ASC-US]** ♀

    R87.621 **Atypical squamous cells cannot exclude high grade squamous intraepithelial lesion on cytologic smear of vagina [ASC-H]** ♀

    R87.622 **Low grade squamous intraepithelial lesion on cytologic smear of vagina [LGSIL]** ♀

    R87.623 **High grade squamous intraepithelial lesion on cytologic smear of vagina [HGSIL]** ♀

    R87.624 **Cytologic evidence of malignancy on smear of vagina** ♀

    R87.625 **Unsatisfactory cytologic smear of vagina** ♀
        Inadequate sample of cytologic smear of vagina

    R87.628 **Other abnormal cytological findings on specimens from vagina** ♀

    R87.629 **Unspecified abnormal cytological findings in specimens from vagina** ♀ ▽
        Abnormal Papanicolaou smear of vagina NOS
        Abnormal thin preparation smear of vagina NOS
        Abnormal vaginal cytology NOS
        Atypical endocervical cells of vagina NOS
        Atypical endometrial cells of vagina NOS
        Atypical glandular cells of vagina NOS

    R87.69 **Abnormal cytological findings in specimens from other female genital organs** ♀
      Abnormal cytological findings in specimens from female genital organs NOS

      EXCLUDES 1   *dysplasia of vulva (histologically confirmed) (N90.0-N90.3)*

R87.7 **Abnormal histological findings in specimens from female genital organs** ♀

      EXCLUDES 1   *carcinoma in situ (histologically confirmed) of female genital organs (D06-D07.3)*

          cervical intraepithelial neoplasia I [CIN I] (N87.0)

          cervical intraepithelial neoplasia II [CIN II] (N87.1)

          cervical intraepithelial neoplasia III [CIN III] (D06.-)

          dysplasia (mild) (moderate) of cervix uteri (histologically confirmed) (N87.-)

          dysplasia (mild) (moderate) of vagina (histologically confirmed) (N89.-)

          severe dysplasia of cervix uteri (histologically confirmed) (D06.-)

          severe dysplasia of vagina (histologically confirmed) (D07.2)

          vaginal intraepithelial neoplasia I [VAIN I] (N89.0)

          vaginal intraepithelial neoplasia II [VAIN II] (N89.1)

          vaginal intraepithelial neoplasia III [VAIN III] (D07.2)

✓5th **R87.8** **Other abnormal findings in specimens from female genital organs**

    ✓6th **R87.81** **High risk human papillomavirus [HPV] DNA test positive from female genital organs**

      EXCLUDES 1   *anogenital warts due to human papillomavirus (HPV) (A63.0)*

          condyloma acuminatum (A63.0)

    R87.810 **Cervical high risk human papillomavirus [HPV] DNA test positive** ♀

    R87.811 **Vaginal high risk human papillomavirus [HPV] DNA test positive** ♀

    ✓6th **R87.82** **Low risk human papillomavirus [HPV] DNA test positive from female genital organs**
      Use additional code for associated human papillomavirus (B97.7)

    R87.820 **Cervical low risk human papillomavirus [HPV] DNA test positive** ♀

    R87.821 **Vaginal low risk human papillomavirus [HPV] DNA test positive** ♀

    R87.89 **Other abnormal findings in specimens from female genital organs** ♀
      Abnormal chromosomal findings in specimens from female genital organs

R87.9 **Unspecified abnormal finding in specimens from female genital organs** ♀ ▽

☑ Additional Character Req   ✓x7th Placeholder Alert   Manifestation   HCC CMS-HCC Condition   ▽ Unspecified Code   ►◄ Revised Text   ● New Code   ▲ Revised Code Title

ICD-10-CM 2018   903

✓4ᵗʰ **R88** **Abnormal findings in other body fluids and substances**
     R88.0 Cloudy (hemodialysis) (peritoneal) dialysis effluent
     R88.8 Abnormal findings in other body fluids and substances

✓4ᵗʰ **R89** **Abnormal findings in specimens from other organs, systems and tissues**
     INCLUDES   abnormal findings in nipple discharge
              abnormal findings in synovial fluid
              abnormal findings in wound secretions

     R89.0 Abnormal level of **enzymes** in specimens from other organs, systems and tissues

     R89.1 Abnormal level of **hormones** in specimens from other organs, systems and tissues

     R89.2 Abnormal level of other drugs, medicaments and biological substances in specimens from other organs, systems and tissues

     R89.3 Abnormal level of **substances chiefly nonmedicinal** as to source in specimens from other organs, systems and tissues

     R89.4 Abnormal **immunological** findings in specimens from other organs, systems and tissues

     R89.5 Abnormal **microbiological** findings in specimens from other organs, systems and tissues
         Positive culture findings in specimens from other organs, systems and tissues
         EXCLUDES 1   *colonization status (Z22.-)*

     R89.6 Abnormal **cytological** findings in specimens from other organs, systems and tissues

     R89.7 Abnormal **histological** findings in specimens from other organs, systems and tissues

     R89.8 Other abnormal findings in specimens from other organs, systems and tissues
         Abnormal chromosomal findings in specimens from other organs, systems and tissues

     R89.9 Unspecified abnormal finding in specimens from other organs, systems and tissues   ▽

Abnormal findings on diagnostic imaging and in function studies, without diagnosis (R90-R94)

     INCLUDES   nonspecific abnormal findings on diagnostic imaging by computerized axial tomography [CAT scan]
              nonspecific abnormal findings on diagnostic imaging by magnetic resonance imaging [MRI][NMR]
              nonspecific abnormal findings on diagnostic imaging by positron emission tomography [PET scan]
              nonspecific abnormal findings on diagnostic imaging by thermography
              nonspecific abnormal findings on diagnostic imaging by ultrasound [echogram]
              nonspecific abnormal findings on diagnostic imaging by X-ray examination
     EXCLUDES 1   *abnormal findings on antenatal screening of mother (O28.-)*
              diagnostic abnormal findings classified elsewhere—see Alphabetical Index

✓4ᵗʰ **R90** **Abnormal findings on diagnostic imaging of central nervous system**
     R90.0 **Intracranial** space-occupying lesion found on diagnostic imaging of central nervous system

     ✓5ᵗʰ **R90.8** Other abnormal findings on diagnostic imaging of central nervous system
         R90.81 **Abnormal echoencephalogram**
         R90.82 White matter disease, unspecified   ▽
         R90.89 Other abnormal findings on diagnostic imaging of central nervous system
              Other cerebrovascular abnormality found on diagnostic imaging of central nervous system

✓4ᵗʰ **R91** **Abnormal findings on diagnostic imaging of lung**
     R91.1 Solitary pulmonary nodule
         Coin lesion lung
         Solitary pulmonary nodule, subsegmental branch of the bronchial tree

     R91.8 Other nonspecific abnormal finding of lung field
         Lung mass NOS found on diagnostic imaging of lung
         Pulmonary infiltrate NOS
         Shadow, lung

✓4ᵗʰ **R92** **Abnormal and inconclusive findings on diagnostic imaging of breast**
     R92.0 Mammographic **microcalcification** found on diagnostic imaging of breast
         EXCLUDES 2   *mammographic calcification (calculus) found on diagnostic imaging of breast (R92.1)*
         DEF: Calcium and cellular debris deposits in the breast that cannot be felt but can be detected on a mammogram; can be a sign of cancer, benign conditions, or changes in the breast tissue as a result of inflammation, injury, or obstructed duct.

     R92.1 Mammographic **calcification** found on diagnostic imaging of breast
         Mammographic calculus found on diagnostic imaging of breast

     R92.2 **Inconclusive** mammogram
         Dense breasts NOS
         Inconclusive mammogram NEC
         Inconclusive mammography due to dense breasts
         Inconclusive mammography NEC
         AHA: 2015, 1Q, 24

     R92.8 Other abnormal and inconclusive findings on diagnostic imaging of breast

✓4ᵗʰ **R93** **Abnormal findings on diagnostic imaging of other body structures**
     R93.0 Abnormal findings on diagnostic imaging of **skull and head**, not elsewhere classified
         EXCLUDES 1   *intracranial space-occupying lesion found on diagnostic imaging (R90.0)*

     R93.1 Abnormal findings on diagnostic imaging of **heart and coronary** circulation
         Abnormal echocardiogram NOS
         Abnormal heart shadow

     R93.2 Abnormal findings on diagnostic imaging of **liver and biliary tract**
         Nonvisualization of gallbladder

     R93.3 Abnormal findings on diagnostic imaging of other parts of digestive tract

     ✓5ᵗʰ **R93.4** Abnormal findings on diagnostic imaging of **urinary organs**
         EXCLUDES 2   *hypertrophy of kidney (N28.81)*
         R93.41 Abnormal radiologic findings on diagnostic imaging of **renal pelvis, ureter, or bladder**
              Filling defect of bladder found on diagnostic imaging
              Filling defect of renal pelvis found on diagnostic imaging
              Filling defect of ureter found on diagnostic imaging

         ✓6ᵗʰ **R93.42** Abnormal radiologic findings on diagnositic imaging of **kidney**
              R93.421 Abnormal radiologic findings on diagnositic imaging of **right** kidney
              R93.422 Abnormal radiologic findings on diagnositic imaging of **left** kidney
              R93.429 Abnormal radiologic findings on   ▽ diagnositic imaging of unspecified kidney

         R93.49 Abnormal radiologic findings on diagnositic imaging of other urinary organs

     R93.5 Abnormal findings on diagnostic imaging of other abdominal regions, including retroperitoneum

     R93.6 Abnormal findings on diagnostic imaging of **limbs**
         EXCLUDES 2   *abnormal finding in skin and subcutaneous tissue (R93.8)*

     R93.7 Abnormal findings on diagnostic imaging of other parts of musculoskeletal system
         EXCLUDES 2   *abnormal findings on diagnostic imaging of skull (R93.0)*

     R93.8 Abnormal findings on diagnostic imaging of other specified body structures
         Abnormal finding by radioisotope localization of placenta
         Abnormal radiological finding in skin and subcutaneous tissue
         Mediastinal shift

     R93.9 Diagnostic imaging inconclusive due to **excess body fat of patient**

✓4ᵗʰ **R94** **Abnormal results of function studies**
     INCLUDES   abnormal results of radionuclide [radioisotope] uptake studies
              abnormal results of scintigraphy

     ✓5ᵗʰ **R94.0** Abnormal results of function studies of **central nervous system**
         R94.01 Abnormal **electroencephalogram** [EEG]
         R94.02 Abnormal **brain scan**

EXCLUDES 1 Not coded here   EXCLUDES 2 Not included here   N Newborn Age: 0   P Pediatric Age: 0-17   M Maternity Age: 12-55   A Adult Age: 15-124

904   ICD-10-CM 2018

R94.09   **Abnormal results of other function studies of central nervous system**

☑5ᵗʰ   **R94.1**   **Abnormal results of function studies of peripheral nervous system and special senses**

     ☑6ᵗʰ   **R94.11**   **Abnormal results of function studies of eye**

         R94.110   **Abnormal electro-oculogram [EOG]**

         R94.111   **Abnormal electroretinogram [ERG]**
             Abnormal retinal function study

         R94.112   **Abnormal visually evoked potential [VEP]**

         R94.113   **Abnormal oculomotor study**

         R94.118   **Abnormal results of other function studies of eye**

     ☑6ᵗʰ   **R94.12**   **Abnormal results of function studies of ear and other special senses**
         AHA: 2016, 3Q, 17

         R94.120   **Abnormal auditory function study**

         R94.121   **Abnormal vestibular function study**

         R94.128   **Abnormal results of other function studies of ear and other special senses**

     ☑6ᵗʰ   **R94.13**   **Abnormal results of function studies of peripheral nervous system**

         R94.130   **Abnormal response to nerve stimulation, unspecified**   ▽

         R94.131   **Abnormal electromyogram [EMG]**
             EXCLUDES 1   *electromyogram of eye (R94.113)*

         R94.138   **Abnormal results of other function studies of peripheral nervous system**

  R94.2   **Abnormal results of pulmonary function studies**
     Reduced ventilatory capacity
     Reduced vital capacity

☑5ᵗʰ   **R94.3**   **Abnormal results of cardiovascular function studies**

     R94.30   **Abnormal result of cardiovascular function study, unspecified**   ▽

     R94.31   **Abnormal electrocardiogram [ECG] [EKG]**
         EXCLUDES 1   *long QT syndrome (I45.81)*

     R94.39   **Abnormal result of other cardiovascular function study**
         Abnormal electrophysiological intracardiac studies
         Abnormal phonocardiogram
         Abnormal vectorcardiogram

  R94.4   **Abnormal results of kidney function studies**
     Abnormal renal function test

  R94.5   **Abnormal results of liver function studies**

  R94.6   **Abnormal results of thyroid function studies**

  R94.7   **Abnormal results of other endocrine function studies**
     EXCLUDES 2   *abnormal glucose (R73.0-)*

  R94.8   **Abnormal results of function studies of other organs and systems**
     Abnormal basal metabolic rate [BMR]
     Abnormal bladder function test
     Abnormal splenic function test

Abnormal tumor markers (R97)

☑4ᵗʰ   **R97**   **Abnormal tumor markers**
     Elevated tumor associated antigens [TAA]
     Elevated tumor specific antigens [TSA]

  R97.0   **Elevated carcinoembryonic antigen [CEA]**

  R97.1   **Elevated cancer antigen 125 [CA 125]**   ♀

☑5ᵗʰ   **R97.2**   **Elevated prostate specific antigen [PSA]**

     R97.20   **Elevated prostate specific antigen [PSA]**   Ⓐ♂

     R97.21   **Rising PSA following treatment for malignant neoplasm of prostate**   Ⓐ♂

  R97.8   **Other abnormal tumor markers**

Ill-defined and unknown cause of mortality (R99)

  R99   **Ill-defined and unknown cause of mortality**   ▽
     Death (unexplained) NOS
     Unspecified cause of mortality

☑ Additional Character Req   ✓×7ᵗʰ Placeholder Alert   Manifestation   HCC CMS-HCC Condition   ▽ Unspecified Code   ►◄ Revised Text   ● New Code   ▲ Revised Code Title

Chapter 19. Injury, Poisoning, and Certain Other Consequences of External Causes (SØØ–T88)

Chapter Specific Guidelines with Coding Examples

The chapter specific guidelines from the ICD-10-CM Official Guidelines for Coding and Reporting have been provided below. Along with these guidelines are coding examples, contained in the shaded boxes, that have been developed to help illustrate the coding and/or sequencing guidance found in these guidelines.

a. Application of 7th characters in Chapter 19

Most categories in chapter 19 have a 7th character requirement for each applicable code. Most categories in this chapter have three 7th character values (with the exception of fractures): A, initial encounter, D, subsequent encounter and S, sequela. Categories for traumatic fractures have additional 7th character values. While the patient may be seen by a new or different provider over the course of treatment for an injury, assignment of the 7th character is based on whether the patient is undergoing active treatment and not whether the provider is seeing the patient for the first time.

For complication codes, active treatment refers to treatment for the condition described by the code, even though it may be related to an earlier precipitating problem. For example, code T84.50XA, Infection and inflammatory reaction due to unspecified internal joint prosthesis, initial encounter, is used when active treatment is provided for the infection, even though the condition relates to the prosthetic device, implant or graft that was placed at a previous encounter.

7th character "A", initial encounter is used for each encounter where the patient is receiving active treatment for the condition.

> Patient evaluated after fall from a skateboard onto the sidewalk, x-rays identify a nondisplaced fracture to the distal pole of the right scaphoid bone. The patient is placed in a cast.
>
> | S62.Ø14A | Nondisplaced fracture of distal pole of navicular [scaphoid] bone of right wrist, initial encounter for closed fracture |
> |---|---|
> | VØØ.131A | Fall from skateboard, initial encounter |
> | Y93.51 | Activity, roller skating (inline) and skateboarding |
> | Y92.48Ø | Sidewalk as the place of occurrence of the external cause |
> | Y99.8 | Other external cause status |
>
> *Explanation:* This fracture would be coded with a seventh character A for initial encounter because the patient received x-rays to identify the site of the fracture and treatment was rendered; this would be considered active treatment.

7th character "D" subsequent encounter is used for encounters after the patient has completed active treatment of the condition and is receiving routine care for the condition during the healing or recovery phase.

> Patient seen in follow-up after fall from a skateboard onto the sidewalk resulted in casting of the right arm. X-rays are taken to evaluate how well the nondisplaced fracture to the distal pole of the right scaphoid bone is healing. The physician feels the fracture is healing appropriately; no adjustments to the cast are made.
>
> | S62.Ø14D | Nondisplaced fracture of distal pole of navicular [scaphoid] bone of right wrist, subsequent encounter for fracture with routine healing |
> |---|---|
> | VØØ.131D | Fall from skateboard, subsequent encounter |
>
> *Explanation:* This fracture would be coded with a seventh character D for subsequent encounter, whether the same physician who provided the initial cast application or a different physician is now seeing the patient. Although the patient received x-rays, the intent of the x-rays was to assess how the fracture was healing. There was no active treatment rendered and the visit is therefore considered a subsequent encounter.

The aftercare Z codes should not be used for aftercare for conditions such as injuries or poisonings, where 7th characters are provided to identify subsequent care. For example, for aftercare of an injury, assign the acute injury code with the 7th character "D" (subsequent encounter).

7th character "S", sequela, is for use for complications or conditions that arise as a direct result of a condition, such as scar formation after a burn.

The scars are sequelae of the burn. When using 7th character "S", it is necessary to use both the injury code that precipitated the sequela and the code for the sequela itself. The "S" is added only to the injury code, not the sequela code. The 7th character "S" identifies the injury responsible for the sequela. The specific type of sequela (e.g. scar) is sequenced first, followed by the injury code.

See Section I.B.1Ø Sequelae, (Late Effects)

> Patient with a history of a nondisplaced fracture to the distal pole of the right scaphoid bone due to a fall from a skateboard is seen for evaluation of arthritis to the right wrist that has developed as a consequence of the traumatic fracture.
>
> | M12.531 | Traumatic arthropathy, right wrist |
> |---|---|
> | S62.Ø14S | Nondisplaced fracture of distal pole of navicular [scaphoid] bone of right wrist, sequela |
> | VØØ.131S | Fall from skateboard, sequela |
>
> *Explanation:* The code identifying the specific sequela condition (traumatic arthritis) should be coded first followed by the injury that instigated the development of the sequela (fracture). The scaphoid fracture injury code is given a 7th character S for sequela to represent its role as the inciting injury. The fracture has healed and is not being managed or treated on this admit and therefore is not applicable as a first listed or principal diagnosis. However, it is directly related to the development of the arthritis and should be appended as a secondary code to signify this cause and effect relationship.

b. Coding of injuries

When coding injuries, assign separate codes for each injury unless a combination code is provided, in which case the combination code is assigned. Code TØ7, Unspecified multiple injuries should not be assigned in the inpatient setting unless information for a more specific code is not available. Traumatic injury codes (SØØ–T14.9) are not to be used for normal, healing surgical wounds or to identify complications of surgical wounds.

> 11-year-old girl fell from her horse, resulting in a laceration to her right forearm with several large pieces of wooden fragments embedded in the wound as well as abrasions to her right ear; in addition, her right shoulder was dislocated
>
> | S43.ØØ4A | Unspecified dislocation of right shoulder joint, initial encounter |
> |---|---|
> | S51.821A | Laceration with foreign body of right forearm, initial encounter |
> | SØØ.411A | Abrasion of right ear, initial encounter |
> | V8Ø.Ø1ØA | Animal-rider injured by fall from or being thrown from horse in noncollision accident, initial encounter |
> | Y93.52 | Activity, horseback riding |
>
> *Explanation:* Each separate injury should be reported. The patient's injury to the forearm is reported with one combination code that captures both the laceration and the foreign body.

The code for the most serious injury, as determined by the provider and the focus of treatment, is sequenced first.

1) Superficial injuries

Superficial injuries such as abrasions or contusions are not coded when associated with more severe injuries of the same site.

2) Primary injury with damage to nerves/blood vessels

When a primary injury results in minor damage to peripheral nerves or blood vessels, the primary injury is sequenced first with additional code(s) for injuries to nerves and spinal cord (such as category SØ4), and/or injury to blood vessels (such as category S15). When the primary injury is to the blood vessels or nerves, that injury should be sequenced first.

c. Coding of traumatic fractures

The principles of multiple coding of injuries should be followed in coding fractures. Fractures of specified sites are coded individually by site in accordance with both the provisions within categories SØ2, S12, S22, S32, S42, S49, S52, S59, S62, S72, S79, S82, S89, S92 and the level of detail furnished by medical record content.

A fracture not indicated as open or closed should be coded to closed. A fracture not indicated whether displaced or not displaced should be coded to displaced.

More specific guidelines are as follows:

1) Initial vs. subsequent encounter for fractures

Traumatic fractures are coded using the appropriate 7th character for initial encounter (A, B, C) for each encounter where the patient is receiving active treatment for the fracture. The appropriate 7th character for initial encounter should also be assigned for a patient who delayed seeking treatment for the fracture or nonunion.

Fractures are coded using the appropriate 7th character for subsequent care for encounters after the patient has completed active treatment of the fracture and is receiving routine care for the fracture during the healing or recovery phase.

Care for complications of surgical treatment for fracture repairs during the healing or recovery phase should be coded with the appropriate complication codes.

Care of complications of fractures, such as malunion and nonunion, should be reported with the appropriate 7th character for subsequent care with nonunion (K, M, N,) or subsequent care with malunion (P, Q, R).

Malunion/nonunion: The appropriate 7th character for initial encounter should also be assigned for a patient who delayed seeking treatment for the fracture or nonunion.

Female patient fell during a forest hiking excursion almost six months ago and until recently did not feel she needed to seek medical attention for her left ankle pain; x-rays show nonunion of lateral malleolus and surgery has been scheduled

S82.62XA	Displaced fracture of lateral malleolus of left fibula, initial encounter for closed fracture
W01.0XXA	Fall on same level from slipping, tripping and stumbling without subsequent striking against object, initial encounter
Y92.821	Forest as place of occurrence of the external cause
Y93.01	Activity, walking, marching and hiking
Y99.8	Other external cause status

Explanation: A seventh character of A is used for the lateral malleolus nonunion fracture to signify that the fracture is receiving active treatment. The delayed care for the fracture has resulted in a nonunion, but capturing the nonunion in the seventh character is trumped by the provision of active care.

The open fracture designations in the assignment of the 7th character for fractures of the forearm, femur and lower leg, including ankle are based on the Gustilo open fracture classification. When the Gustilo classification type is not specified for an open fracture, the 7th character for open fracture type I or II should be assigned (B, E, H, M, Q).

A code from category M80, not a traumatic fracture code, should be used for any patient with known osteoporosis who suffers a fracture, even if the patient had a minor fall or trauma, if that fall or trauma would not usually break a normal, healthy bone.

See Section I.C.13. Osteoporosis.

The aftercare Z codes should not be used for aftercare for traumatic fractures. For aftercare of a traumatic fracture, assign the acute fracture code with the appropriate 7th character.

2) Multiple fractures sequencing

Multiple fractures are sequenced in accordance with the severity of the fracture.

d. Coding of burns and corrosions

The ICD-10-CM makes a distinction between burns and corrosions. The burn codes are for thermal burns, except sunburns, that come from a heat source, such as a fire or hot appliance. The burn codes are also for burns resulting from electricity and radiation. Corrosions are burns due to chemicals. The guidelines are the same for burns and corrosions.

Current burns (T20-T25) are classified by depth, extent and by agent (X code). Burns are classified by depth as first degree (erythema), second degree (blistering), and third degree (full-thickness involvement). Burns of the eye and internal organs (T26-T28) are classified by site, but not by degree.

1) Sequencing of burn and related condition codes

Sequence first the code that reflects the highest degree of burn when more than one burn is present.

---

a. When the reason for the admission or encounter is for treatment of external multiple burns, sequence first the code that reflects the burn of the highest degree.

b. When a patient has both internal and external burns, the circumstances of admission govern the selection of the principal diagnosis or first-listed diagnosis.

c. When a patient is admitted for burn injuries and other related conditions such as smoke inhalation and/or respiratory failure, the circumstances of admission govern the selection of the principal or first-listed diagnosis.

Patient referred for minor first-degree burns to multiple sites of her right and left hands as well as severe smoke inhalation. While she was sleeping at home, a candle on her dresser lit the bedroom curtains on fire.

T59.811A	Toxic effect of smoke, accidental (unintentional), initial encounter
J70.5	Respiratory conditions due to smoke inhalation
T23.191A	Burn of first degree of multiple sites of right wrist and hand, initial encounter
T23.192A	Burn of first degree of multiple sites of left wrist and hand, initial encounter
X08.8XXA	Exposure to other specified smoke, fire and flames, initial encounter
Y99.8	Other exteranl cause status
Y92.003	Bedroom of unspecified non-institutional (private) residence as the place of occurrence of the external cause
Y93.84	Activity, sleeping

Explanation: Based on the documentation, the inhalation injury is more severe than the first-degree burns and is sequenced first. The burns to the hands are appended as secondary diagnoses.

2) Burns of the same local site

Classify burns of the same local site (three-character category level, T20-T28) but of different degrees to the subcategory identifying the highest degree recorded in the diagnosis.

10-year-old male patient is treated for third-degree burns of his right palm and second-degree burns of multiple right fingers; right thumb not affected

T23.351A	Burn of third degree of right palm, initial encounter

Explanation: Although there is a code for second-degree burns of multiple fingers, not including the thumb (T23.131-), this code falls in the same three-digit category that the third-degree burn of the right palm falls under, category T23. Only the subcategory identifying the highest degree is captured when different burn degrees are classified to a single category.

Patient is treated for third-degree burns of the scalp as well as second-degree burns to the back of the right hand

T20.35XA	Burn of third degree of scalp [any part], initial encounter
T23.261A	Burn of second degree of back of right hand, initial encounter

Explanation: Since burns to the hand and scalp are classified to two different three-digit categories, both burns may be reported as they represent distinct sites.

3) Non-healing burns

Non-healing burns are coded as acute burns.

Necrosis of burned skin should be coded as a non-healed burn.

4) Infected burn

For any documented infected burn site, use an additional code for the infection.

5) Assign separate codes for each burn site

When coding burns, assign separate codes for each burn site. Category T30, Burn and corrosion, body region unspecified is extremely vague and should rarely be used.

6) Burns and corrosions classified according to extent of body surface involved

Assign codes from category T31, Burns classified according to extent of body surface involved, or T32, Corrosions classified according to extent of body surface involved, when the site of the burn is not specified or when there is a need for additional data. It is advisable to use category T31 as additional coding when needed to provide data for evaluating burn mortality, such as that needed by burn units. It is also advisable to use category T31 as an additional code for reporting purposes when there is mention of a third-degree burn involving 20 percent or more of the body surface.

Categories T31 and T32 are based on the classic "rule of nines" in estimating body surface involved: head and neck are assigned nine percent, each arm nine percent, each leg 18 percent, the anterior trunk 18 percent, posterior trunk 18 percent, and genitalia one percent. Providers may change these percentage assignments where necessary to accommodate infants and children who have proportionately larger heads than adults, and patients who have large buttocks, thighs, or abdomen that involve burns.

> Patient seen for dressing change after he accidentally spilled acetic acid on himself two days ago. The second-degree burns to his right thigh, covering about 3 percent of his body surface, are healing appropriately.
>
> **T54.2X1D**   **Toxic effect of corrosive acids and acid-like substances, accidental (unintentional), subsequent encounter**
>
> **T24.611D**   **Corrosion of second degree of right thigh, subsequent encounter**
>
> **T32.0**   **Corrosions involving less than 10% of body surface**
>
> *Explanation:* Code T32.0 provides additional information as to how much of the patient's body was affected by the corrosive substance.

7) Encounters for treatment of sequela of burns

Encounters for the treatment of the late effects of burns or corrosions (i.e., scars or joint contractures) should be coded with a burn or corrosion code with the 7th character "S" for sequela.

8) Sequelae with a late effect code and current burn

When appropriate, both a code for a current burn or corrosion with 7th character "A" or "D" and a burn or corrosion code with 7th character "S" may be assigned on the same record (when both a current burn and sequelae of an old burn exist). Burns and corrosions do not heal at the same rate and a current healing wound may still exist with sequela of a healed burn or corrosion.

See Section I.B.10 Sequela (Late Effects)

> Female patient seen for second-degree burn to the left ear; she also has significant scarring on her left elbow from a third-degree burn from childhood
>
> **T20.212A**   **Burn of second degree of left ear [any part, except ear drum], initial encounter**
>
> **L90.5**   **Scar conditions and fibrosis of skin**
>
> **T22.322S**   **Burn of third degree of left elbow, sequela**
>
> *Explanation:* The patient is being seen for management of a current second-degree burn, which is reflected in the code by appending the seventh character of A, indicating active treatment or management of this burn. The elbow scarring is a sequela of a previous third-degree burn. The sequela condition precedes the original burn injury, which is appended with a seventh character of S.

9) Use of an external cause code with burns and corrosions

An external cause code should be used with burns and corrosions to identify the source and intent of the burn, as well as the place where it occurred.

e. Adverse effects, poisoning, underdosing and toxic effects

Codes in categories T36-T65 are combination codes that include the substance that was taken as well as the intent. No additional external cause code is required for poisonings, toxic effects, adverse effects and underdosing codes.

1) Do not code directly from the Table of Drugs

Do not code directly from the Table of Drugs and Chemicals. Always refer back to the Tabular List.

2) Use as many codes as necessary to describe

Use as many codes as necessary to describe completely all drugs, medicinal or biological substances.

3) If the same code would describe the causative agent

If the same code would describe the causative agent for more than one adverse reaction, poisoning, toxic effect or underdosing, assign the code only once.

4) If two or more drugs, medicinal or biological substances

If two or more drugs, medicinal or biological substances are reported, code each individually unless a combination code is listed in the Table of Drugs and Chemicals.

5) The occurrence of drug toxicity is classified in ICD-10-CM as follows:

(a) Adverse effect

When coding an adverse effect of a drug that has been correctly prescribed and properly administered, assign the appropriate code for the nature of the adverse effect followed by the appropriate code for the adverse effect of the drug (T36-T50). The code for the drug should have a 5th or 6th character "5" (for example T36.0X5-) Examples of the nature of an adverse effect are tachycardia, delirium, gastrointestinal hemorrhaging, vomiting, hypokalemia, hepatitis, renal failure, or respiratory failure.

> Patient seen for stomach pain and jaundice, indicated by physician as possible side-effects of Inderal, recently started for hypertension. Inderal was discontinued and the patient switched to Atenolol instead.
>
> **R10.9**   **Unspecified abdominal pain**
>
> **R17**   **Unspecified jaundice**
>
> **T44.7X5A**   **Adverse effect of beta-adrenoreceptor antagonists, initial encounter**
>
> **I10**   **Essential (primary) hypertension**
>
> *Explanation:* The side-effects caused by the drug are listed first, followed by the code for the adverse effect of the drug to capture the specific drug that was used.

(b) Poisoning

When coding a poisoning or reaction to the improper use of a medication (e.g., overdose, wrong substance given or taken in error, wrong route of administration), first assign the appropriate code from categories T36-T50. The poisoning codes have an associated intent as their 5th or 6th character (accidental, intentional self-harm, assault and undetermined. If the intent of the poisoning is unknown or unspecified, code the intent as accidental intent. The undetermined intent is only for use if the documentation in the record specifies that the intent cannot be determined. Use additional code(s) for all manifestations of poisonings.

If there is also a diagnosis of abuse or dependence of the substance, the abuse or dependence is assigned as an additional code.

Examples of poisoning include:

(i) Error was made in drug prescription

Errors made in drug prescription or in the administration of the drug by provider, nurse, patient, or other person.

(ii) Overdose of a drug intentionally taken

If an overdose of a drug was intentionally taken or administered and resulted in drug toxicity, it would be coded as a poisoning.

(iii) Nonprescribed drug taken with correctly prescribed and properly administered drug

If a nonprescribed drug or medicinal agent was taken in combination with a correctly prescribed and properly administered drug, any drug toxicity or other reaction resulting from the interaction of the two drugs would be classified as a poisoning.

(iv) Interaction of drug(s) and alcohol

When a reaction results from the interaction of a drug(s) and alcohol, this would be classified as poisoning.

See Section I.C.4. if poisoning is the result of insulin pump malfunctions.

(c) Underdosing

Underdosing refers to taking less of a medication than is prescribed by a provider or a manufacturer's instruction. For underdosing, assign the code from categories T36-T50 (fifth or sixth character "6").

Codes for underdosing should never be assigned as principal or first-listed codes. If a patient has a relapse or exacerbation of the medical

Chapter 19. Injury, Poisoning, and Certain Other Consequences of External Causes

condition for which the drug is prescribed because of the reduction in dose, then the medical condition itself should be coded.

Noncompliance (Z91.12-, Z91.13-) or complication of care (Y63.6-Y63.9) codes are to be used with an underdosing code to indicate intent, if known.

> Patient referred for atrial fibrillation with history of chronic atrial fibrillation for which she is prescribed amiodarone. Financial concerns have left the patient unable to pay for her prescriptions and she has been skipping her amiodarone dose every other day to offset the cost.
>
> | I48.2 | Chronic atrial fibrillation |
> |---|---|
> | T46.2X6A | Underdosing of other antidysrhythmic drugs, initial encounter |
> | Z91.12Ø | Patient's intentional underdosing of medication regimen due to financial hardship |
>
> *Explanation:* By skipping her amiodarone pill every other day, the patient's atrial fibrillation returned. The condition for which the drug was being taken is reported first, followed by an underdosing code to show that the patient was not adhering to her prescription regiment. The Z code helps elaborate on the patient's social and/or economic circumstances that led to the patient taking less then what she was prescribed.

(d) Toxic effects

When a harmful substance is ingested or comes in contact with a person, this is classified as a toxic effect. The toxic effect codes are in categories T51-T65.

Toxic effect codes have an associated intent: accidental, intentional self-harm, assault and undetermined.

f. Adult and child abuse, neglect and other maltreatment

Sequence first the appropriate code from categories T74.- (Adult and child abuse, neglect and other maltreatment, confirmed) or T76.- (Adult and child abuse, neglect and other maltreatment, suspected) for abuse, neglect and other maltreatment, followed by any accompanying mental health or injury code(s).

If the documentation in the medical record states abuse or neglect it is coded as confirmed (T74.-). It is coded as suspected if it is documented as suspected (T76.-).

For cases of confirmed abuse or neglect an external cause code from the assault section (X92-Y09) should be added to identify the cause of any physical injuries. A perpetrator code (Y07) should be added when the perpetrator of the abuse is known. For suspected cases of abuse or neglect, do not report external cause or perpetrator code.

If a suspected case of abuse, neglect or mistreatment is ruled out during an encounter code Z04.71, Encounter for examination and observation following alleged physical adult abuse, ruled out, or code Z04.72, Encounter for examination and observation following alleged child physical abuse, ruled out, should be used, not a code from T76.

If a suspected case of alleged rape or sexual abuse is ruled out during an encounter code Z04.41, Encounter for examination and observation following alleged adult rape or code Z04.42, Encounter for examination and observation following alleged child rape, should be used, not a code from T76.

See Section I.C.15. Abuse in a pregnant patient.

g. Complications of care

1) General guidelines for complications of care

(a) Documentation of complications of care

See Section I.B.16. for information on documentation of complications of care.

2) Pain due to medical devices

Pain associated with devices, implants or grafts left in a surgical site (for example painful hip prosthesis) is assigned to the appropriate code(s) found in Chapter 19, Injury, poisoning, and certain other consequences of external causes. Specific codes for pain due to medical devices are found in the T code section of the ICD-10-CM. Use additional code(s) from category G89 to identify acute or chronic pain due to presence of the device, implant or graft (G89.18 or G89.28).

> Chronic left breast pain secondary to breast implant
>
> | T85.848A | Pain due to other internal prosthetic devices, implants and grafts, initial encounter |
> |---|---|
> | N64.4 | Mastodynia |
> | G89.28 | Other chronic postprocedural pain |
>
> *Explanation:* As the pain is a complication related to the breast implant, the complication code is sequenced first. The T code does not describe the site or type of pain, so additional codes may be appended to indicate that the patient is experiencing chronic pain in the breast.

3) Transplant complications

(a) Transplant complications other than kidney

Codes under category T86, Complications of transplanted organs and tissues, are for use for both complications and rejection of transplanted organs. A transplant complication code is only assigned if the complication affects the function of the transplanted organ. Two codes are required to fully describe a transplant complication: the appropriate code from category T86 and a secondary code that identifies the complication.

Pre-existing conditions or conditions that develop after the transplant are not coded as complications unless they affect the function of the transplanted organs.

See I.C.21. for transplant organ removal status

See I.C.2. for malignant neoplasm associated with transplanted organ.

(b) Kidney transplant complications

Patients who have undergone kidney transplant may still have some form of chronic kidney disease (CKD) because the kidney transplant may not fully restore kidney function. Code T86.1- should be assigned for documented complications of a kidney transplant, such as transplant failure or rejection or other transplant complication. Code T86.1- should not be assigned for post kidney transplant patients who have chronic kidney (CKD) unless a transplant complication such as transplant failure or rejection is documented. If the documentation is unclear as to whether the patient has a complication of the transplant, query the provider.

Conditions that affect the function of the transplanted kidney, other than CKD, should be assigned a code from subcategory T86.1, Complications of transplanted organ, Kidney, and a secondary code that identifies the complication.

For patients with CKD following a kidney transplant, but who do not have a complication such as failure or rejection, *see section I.C.14. Chronic kidney disease and kidney transplant status.*

> Patient seen for chronic kidney disease stage 2; history of successful kidney transplant with no complications identified
>
> | N18.2 | Chronic kidney disease, stage 2 (mild) |
> |---|---|
> | Z94.Ø | Kidney transplant status |
>
> *Explanation:* This patient's stage 2 CKD is not indicated as being due to the transplanted kidney but instead is just the residual disease the patient had prior to the transplant.

4) Complication codes that include the external cause

As with certain other T codes, some of the complications of care codes have the external cause included in the code. The code includes the nature of the complication as well as the type of procedure that caused the complication. No external cause code indicating the type of procedure is necessary for these codes.

5) Complications of care codes within the body system chapters

Intraoperative and postprocedural complication codes are found within the body system chapters with codes specific to the organs and structures of that body system. These codes should be sequenced first, followed by a code(s) for the specific complication, if applicable.

> During a spinal fusion procedure, the surgeon inadvertently punctured the dura. The midline durotomy was repaired, and the fusion procedure was completed.
>
> | G97.41 | Accidental puncture or laceration of dura during a procedure |
> |---|---|
>
> *Explanation:* The accidental durotomy is not coded to an injury code in chapter 19 but instead is categorized to the nervous system chapter.

Muscle/Tendon Table

ICD-10-CM categorizes certain muscles and tendons in the upper and lower extremities by their action (e.g., extension, flexion), their anatomical location (e.g., posterior, anterior), and/or whether they are intrinsic or extrinsic to a certain anatomical area. The Muscle/Tendon Table is provided at the beginning of chapters 13 and 19 as a resource to help users when code selection depends on one or more of these characteristics. A **TIP** has been placed at those categories and/or subcategories that relate to this table. Please note that this table is not all-inclusive, and proper code assignment should be based on the provider's documentation.

Body Region	Muscle	Extensor Tendon	Flexor Tendon	Other Tendon
Shoulder				
	Deltoid	Posterior deltoid	Anterior deltoid	
	Rotator cuff			
	Infraspinatus			Infraspinatus
	Subscapularis			Subscapularis
	Supraspinatus			Supraspinatus
	Teres minor			Teres minor
	Teres major	Teres major		
Upper arm				
	Anterior muscles			
	Biceps brachii — long head		Biceps brachii — long head	
	Biceps brachii — short head		Biceps brachii — short head	
	Brachialis		Brachialis	
	Coracobrachialis		Coracobrachialis	
	Posterior muscles			
	Triceps brachii	Triceps brachii		
Forearm				
	Anterior muscles			
	Flexors			
	Deep			
	Flexor digitorum profundus		Flexor digitorum profundus	
	Flexor pollicis longus		Flexor pollicis longus	
	Intermediate			
	Flexor digitorum superficialis		Flexor digitorum superficialis	
	Superficial			
	Flexor carpi radialis		Flexor carpi radialis	
	Flexor carpi ulnaris		Flexor carpi ulnaris	
	Palmaris longus		Palmaris longus	
	Pronators			
	Pronator quadratus			Pronator quadratus
	Pronator teres			Pronator teres
	Posterior muscles			
	Extensors			
	Deep			
	Abductor pollicis longus			Abductor pollicis longus
	Extensor indicis	Extensor indicis		
	Extensor pollicis brevis	Extensor pollicis brevis		
	Extensor pollicis longus	Extensor pollicis longus		
	Superficial			
	Brachioradialis			Brachioradialis
	Extensor carpi radialis brevis	Extensor carpi radialis brevis		
	Extensor carpi radialis longus	Extensor carpi radialis longus		
	Extensor carpi ulnaris	Extensor carpi ulnaris		
	Extensor digiti minimi	Extensor digiti minimi		
	Extensor digitorum	Extensor digitorum		
	Anconeus	Anconeus		
	Supinator			Supinator

Chapter 19. Injury, Poisoning, and Certain Other Consequences of External Causes

Body Region	Muscle	Extensor Tendon	Flexor Tendon	Other Tendon
Hand				
Extrinsic — attach to a site in the forearm as well as a site in the hand with action related to hand movement at the wrist				
	Extensor carpi radialis brevis	Extensor carpi radialis brevis		
	Extensor carpi radialis longus	Extensor carpie radialis longus		
	Extensor carpi ulnaris	Extensor carpi ulnaris		
	Flexor carpi radialis		Flexor carpi radialis	
	Flexor carpi ulnaris		Flexor carpi ulnaris	
	Flexor digitorum superficialis		Flexor digitorum superficialis	
	Palmaris longus		Palmaris longus	
Extrinsic — attach to a site in the forearm as well as a site in the hand with action in the hand related to finger movement				
	Adductor pollicis longus			Adductor pollicis longus
	Extensor digiti minimi	Extensor digiti minimi		
	Extensor digitorum	Extensor digitorum		
	Extensor indicis	Extensor indicis		
	Flexor digitorum profundus		Flexor digitorum profundus	
	Flexor digitorum superficialis		Flexor digitorum superficialis	
Extrinsic — attach to a site in the forearm as well as a site in the hand with action in the hand related to thumb movement				
	Extensor pollicis brevis	Extensor pollicis brevis		
	Extensor pollicis longus	Extensor pollicis longus		
	Flexor pollicis longus		Flexor pollicis longus	
Intrinsic — found within the hand only				
	Adductor pollicis			Adductor pollicis
	Dorsal interossei	Dorsal interossei	Dorsal interossei	
	Lumbricals	Lumbricals	Lumbricals	
	Palmaris brevis			Palmaris brevis
	Palmar interossei	Palmar interossei	Palmar interossei	
	Hypothenar muscles			
	Abductor digiti minimi			Abductor digiti minimi
	Flexor digiti minimi brevis		Flexor digiti minimi brevis	
	Oppenens digiti minimi		Oppenens digiti minimi	
	Thenar muscles			
	Abductor pollicis brevis			Abductor pollicis brevis
	Flexor pollicis brevis		Flexor pollicis brevis	
	Oppenens pollicis		Oppenens pollicis	
Thigh				
	Anterior muscles			
	Iliopsoas		Iliopsoas	
	Pectineus		Pectineus	
	Quadriceps	Quadriceps		
	Rectus femoris	Rectus femoris — Extends knee	Rectus femoris — Flexes hip	
	Vastus intermedius	Vastus intermedius		
	Vastus lateralis	Vastus lateralis		
	Vastus medialis	Vastus medialis		
	Sartorius		Sartorius	
	Medial muscles			
	Adductor brevis			Adductor brevis
	Adductor longus			Adductor longus
	Adductor magnus			Adductor magnus
	Gracilis			Gracilis
	Obturator externus			Obturator externus
	Posterior muscles			
	Hamstring	Hamstring — Extends hip	Hamstring — Flexes knee	
	Biceps femoris	Biceps femoris	Biceps femoris	
	Semimembranosus	Semimembranosus	Semimembranosus	
	Semitendinosus	Semitendinosus	Semitendinosus	

Body Region	Muscle	Extensor Tendon	Flexor Tendon	Other Tendon
Lower leg				
	Anterior muscles			
	Extensor digitorum longus	Extensor digitorum longus		
	Extensor hallucis longus	Extensor hallucis longus		
	Fibularis (peroneus) tertius	Fibularis (peroneus) tertius		
	Tibialis anterior	Tibialis anterior		Tibialis anterior
	Lateral muscles			
	Fibularis (peroneus) brevis		Fibularis (peroneus) brevis	
	Fibularis (peroneus) longus		Fibularis (peroneus) longus	
	Posterior muscles			
	Deep			
	Flexor digitorum longus		Flexor digitorum longus	
	Flexor hallucis longus		Flexor hallucis longus	
	Popliteus		Popliteus	
	Tibialis posterior		Tibialis posterior	
	Superficial			
	Gastrocnemius		Gastrocnemius	
	Plantaris		Plantaris	
	Soleus		Soleus	
				Calcaneal (Achilles)
Ankle/Foot				
Extrinsic — attach to a site in the lower leg as well as a site in the foot with action related to foot movement at the ankle				
	Plantaris		Plantaris	
	Soleus		Soleus	
	Tibialis anterior	Tibialis anterior		
	Tibialis posterior		Tibialis posterior	
Extrinsic — attach to a site in the lower leg as well as a site in the foot with action in the foot related to toe movement				
	Extensor digitorum longus	Extensor digitorum longus		
	Extensor hallicus longus	Extensor hallicus longus		
	Flexor digitorum longus		Flexor digitorum longus	
	Flexor hallucis longus		Flexor hallucis longus	
Intrinsic — found within the ankle/foot only				
	Dorsal muscles			
	Extensor digitorum brevis	Extensor digitorum brevis		
	Extensor hallucis brevis	Extensor hallucis brevis		
	Plantar muscles			
	Abductor digiti minimi		Abductor digiti minimi	
	Abductor hallucis		Abductor hallucis	
	Dorsal interossei	Dorsal interossei	Dorsal interossei	
	Flexor digiti minimi brevis		Flexor digiti minimi brevis	
	Flexor digitorum brevis		Flexor digitorum brevis	
	Flexor hallucis brevis		Flexor hallucis brevis	
	Lumbricals	Lumbricals	Lumbricals	
	Quadratus plantae		Quadratus plantae	
	Plantar interossei	Plantar interossei	Plantar interossei	

Chapter 19. Injury, Poisoning and Certain Other Consequences of External Causes (S00-T88)

NOTE   Use secondary code(s) from Chapter 20, External causes of morbidity, to indicate cause of injury. Codes within the T section that include the external cause do not require an additional external cause code.

Use additional code to identify any retained foreign body, if applicable (Z18.-)

EXCLUDES 1   birth trauma (P10-P15)
        obstetric trauma (O70-O71)

NOTE   The chapter uses the S-section for coding different types of injuries related to single body regions and the T-section to cover injuries to unspecified body regions as well as poisoning and certain other consequences of external causes.

AHA: 2016, 2Q, 3-7; 2015, 4Q, 35-38; 2015, 3Q, 37-39, 40; 2015, 2Q, 6; 2015, 1Q, 3-21

This chapter contains the following blocks:

S00-S09	Injuries to the head
S10-S19	Injuries to the neck
S20-S29	Injuries to the thorax
S30-S39	Injuries to the abdomen, lower back, lumbar spine, pelvis and external genitals
S40-S49	Injuries to the shoulder and upper arm
S50-S59	Injuries to the elbow and forearm
S60-S69	Injuries to the wrist, hand and fingers
S70-S79	Injuries to the hip and thigh
S80-S89	Injuries to the knee and lower leg
S90-S99	Injuries to the ankle and foot
T07	Injuries involving multiple body regions
T14	Injury of unspecified body region
T15-T19	Effects of foreign body entering through natural orifice
T20-T25	Burns and corrosions of external body surface, specified by site
T26-T28	Burns and corrosions confined to eye and internal organs
T30-T32	Burns and corrosions of multiple and unspecified body regions
T33-T34	Frostbite
T36-T50	Poisoning by, adverse effect of and underdosing of drugs, medicaments and biological substances
T51-T65	Toxic effects of substances chiefly nonmedicinal as to source
T66-T78	Other and unspecified effects of external causes
T79	Certain early complications of trauma
T80-T88	Complications of surgical and medical care, not elsewhere classified

Injuries to the head (S00-S09)

INCLUDES   injuries of ear
        injuries of eye
        injuries of face [any part]
        injuries of gum
        injuries of jaw
        injuries of oral cavity
        injuries of palate
        injuries of periocular area
        injuries of scalp
        injuries of temporomandibular joint area
        injuries of tongue
        injuries of tooth

Code also for any associated infection

EXCLUDES 2   burns and corrosions (T20-T32)
        effects of foreign body in ear (T16)
        effects of foreign body in larynx (T17.3)
        effects of foreign body in mouth NOS (T18.0)
        effects of foreign body in nose (T17.0-T17.1)
        effects of foreign body in pharynx (T17.2)
        effects of foreign body on external eye (T15.-)
        frostbite (T33-T34)
        insect bite or sting, venomous (T63.4)

√4th S00 Superficial injury of head

EXCLUDES 1   diffuse cerebral contusion (S06.2-)
        focal cerebral contusion (S06.3-)
        injury of eye and orbit (S05.-)
        open wound of head (S01.-)

> The appropriate 7th character is to be added to each code from category S00.
> A   initial encounter
> D   subsequent encounter
> S   sequela

√5th S00.0 Superficial injury of scalp

√x7th S00.00 Unspecified superficial injury of scalp   ▽

√x7th S00.01 Abrasion of scalp

√x7th S00.02 Blister (nonthermal) of scalp

√x7th S00.03 Contusion of scalp
       Bruise of scalp
       Hematoma of scalp

√x7th S00.04 External constriction of part of scalp

√x7th S00.05 Superficial foreign body of scalp
       Splinter in the scalp

√x7th S00.06 Insect bite (nonvenomous) of scalp

√x7th S00.07 Other superficial bite of scalp
     EXCLUDES 1   open bite of scalp (S01.05)

√5th S00.1 Contusion of eyelid and periocular area
       Black eye
     EXCLUDES 2   contusion of eyeball and orbital tissues (S05.1)

√x7th S00.10 Contusion of unspecified eyelid and periocular area   ▽

√x7th S00.11 Contusion of right eyelid and periocular area

√x7th S00.12 Contusion of left eyelid and periocular area

√5th S00.2 Other and unspecified superficial injuries of eyelid and periocular area
     EXCLUDES 2   superficial injury of conjunctiva and cornea (S05.0-)

√6th S00.20 Unspecified superficial injury of eyelid and periocular area

     √7th S00.201 Unspecified superficial injury of right eyelid and periocular area   ▽

     √7th S00.202 Unspecified superficial injury of left eyelid and periocular area   ▽

     √7th S00.209 Unspecified superficial injury of unspecified eyelid and periocular area   ▽

√6th S00.21 Abrasion of eyelid and periocular area

     √7th S00.211 Abrasion of right eyelid and periocular area

     √7th S00.212 Abrasion of left eyelid and periocular area

     √7th S00.219 Abrasion of unspecified eyelid and periocular area   ▽

√6th S00.22 Blister (nonthermal) of eyelid and periocular area

     √7th S00.221 Blister (nonthermal) of right eyelid and periocular area

     √7th S00.222 Blister (nonthermal) of left eyelid and periocular area

     √7th S00.229 Blister (nonthermal) of unspecified eyelid and periocular area   ▽

√6th S00.24 External constriction of eyelid and periocular area

     √7th S00.241 External constriction of right eyelid and periocular area

     √7th S00.242 External constriction of left eyelid and periocular area

     √7th S00.249 External constriction of unspecified eyelid and periocular area   ▽

√6th S00.25 Superficial foreign body of eyelid and periocular area
       Splinter of eyelid and periocular area
     EXCLUDES 2   retained foreign body in eyelid (H02.81-)

     √7th S00.251 Superficial foreign body of right eyelid and periocular area

     √7th S00.252 Superficial foreign body of left eyelid and periocular area

     √7th S00.259 Superficial foreign body of unspecified eyelid and periocular area   ▽

√6th S00.26 Insect bite (nonvenomous) of eyelid and periocular area

     √7th S00.261 Insect bite (nonvenomous) of right eyelid and periocular area

     √7th S00.262 Insect bite (nonvenomous) of left eyelid and periocular area

     √7th S00.269 Insect bite (nonvenomous) of unspecified eyelid and periocular area   ▽

√6th S00.27 Other superficial bite of eyelid and periocular area
     EXCLUDES 1   open bite of eyelid and periocular area (S01.15)

     √7th S00.271 Other superficial bite of right eyelid and periocular area

     √7th S00.272 Other superficial bite of left eyelid and periocular area

     √7th S00.279 Other superficial bite of unspecified eyelid and periocular area   ▽

EXCLUDES 1 Not coded here   **EXCLUDES 2** Not included here   **N** Newborn Age: 0   **P** Pediatric Age: 0-17   **M** Maternity Age: 12-55   **A** Adult Age: 15-124

914   ICD-10-CM 2018

✓5ᵗʰ **S00.3 Superficial injury of nose**

  ✓x7ᵗʰ **S00.30 Unspecified superficial injury of nose** ▽

  ✓x7ᵗʰ **S00.31 Abrasion of nose**

  ✓x7ᵗʰ **S00.32 Blister (nonthermal) of nose**

  ✓x7ᵗʰ **S00.33 Contusion of nose**
    Bruise of nose
    Hematoma of nose

  ✓x7ᵗʰ **S00.34 External constriction of nose**

  ✓x7ᵗʰ **S00.35 Superficial foreign body of nose**
    Splinter in the nose

  ✓x7ᵗʰ **S00.36 Insect bite (nonvenomous) of nose**

  ✓x7ᵗʰ **S00.37 Other superficial bite of nose**
    EXCLUDES 1 open bite of nose (S01.25)

✓5ᵗʰ **S00.4 Superficial injury of ear**

  ✓6ᵗʰ **S00.40 Unspecified superficial injury of ear**

    ✓7ᵗʰ **S00.401 Unspecified superficial injury of right ear** ▽

    ✓7ᵗʰ **S00.402 Unspecified superficial injury of left ear** ▽

    ✓7ᵗʰ **S00.409 Unspecified superficial injury of unspecified ear** ▽

  ✓6ᵗʰ **S00.41 Abrasion of ear**

    ✓7ᵗʰ **S00.411 Abrasion of right ear**

    ✓7ᵗʰ **S00.412 Abrasion of left ear**

    ✓7ᵗʰ **S00.419 Abrasion of unspecified ear** ▽

  ✓6ᵗʰ **S00.42 Blister (nonthermal) of ear**

    ✓7ᵗʰ **S00.421 Blister (nonthermal) of right ear**

    ✓7ᵗʰ **S00.422 Blister (nonthermal) of left ear**

    ✓7ᵗʰ **S00.429 Blister (nonthermal) of unspecified ear** ▽

  ✓6ᵗʰ **S00.43 Contusion of ear**
    Bruise of ear
    Hematoma of ear

    ✓7ᵗʰ **S00.431 Contusion of right ear**

    ✓7ᵗʰ **S00.432 Contusion of left ear**

    ✓7ᵗʰ **S00.439 Contusion of unspecified ear** ▽

  ✓6ᵗʰ **S00.44 External constriction of ear**

    ✓7ᵗʰ **S00.441 External constriction of right ear**

    ✓7ᵗʰ **S00.442 External constriction of left ear**

    ✓7ᵗʰ **S00.449 External constriction of unspecified ear** ▽

  ✓6ᵗʰ **S00.45 Superficial foreign body of ear**
    Splinter in the ear

    ✓7ᵗʰ **S00.451 Superficial foreign body of right ear**

    ✓7ᵗʰ **S00.452 Superficial foreign body of left ear**

    ✓7ᵗʰ **S00.459 Superficial foreign body of unspecified ear** ▽

  ✓6ᵗʰ **S00.46 Insect bite (nonvenomous) of ear**

    ✓7ᵗʰ **S00.461 Insect bite (nonvenomous) of right ear**

    ✓7ᵗʰ **S00.462 Insect bite (nonvenomous) of left ear**

    ✓7ᵗʰ **S00.469 Insect bite (nonvenomous) of unspecified ear** ▽

  ✓6ᵗʰ **S00.47 Other superficial bite of ear**
    EXCLUDES 1 open bite of ear (S01.35)

    ✓7ᵗʰ **S00.471 Other superficial bite of right ear**

    ✓7ᵗʰ **S00.472 Other superficial bite of left ear**

    ✓7ᵗʰ **S00.479 Other superficial bite of unspecified ear** ▽

✓5ᵗʰ **S00.5 Superficial injury of lip and oral cavity**

  ✓6ᵗʰ **S00.50 Unspecified superficial injury of lip and oral cavity**

    ✓7ᵗʰ **S00.501 Unspecified superficial injury of lip** ▽

    ✓7ᵗʰ **S00.502 Unspecified superficial injury of oral cavity** ▽

  ✓6ᵗʰ **S00.51 Abrasion of lip and oral cavity**

    ✓7ᵗʰ **S00.511 Abrasion of lip**

    ✓7ᵗʰ **S00.512 Abrasion of oral cavity**

  ✓6ᵗʰ **S00.52 Blister (nonthermal) of lip and oral cavity**

    ✓7ᵗʰ **S00.521 Blister (nonthermal) of lip**

    ✓7ᵗʰ **S00.522 Blister (nonthermal) of oral cavity**

  ✓6ᵗʰ **S00.53 Contusion of lip and oral cavity**

    ✓7ᵗʰ **S00.531 Contusion of lip**
      Bruise of lip
      ▶Hematoma of lip◀

    ✓7ᵗʰ **S00.532 Contusion of oral cavity**
      ▶Bruise of oral cavity◀
      Hematoma of oral cavity

  ✓6ᵗʰ **S00.54 External constriction of lip and oral cavity**

    ✓7ᵗʰ **S00.541 External constriction of lip**

    ✓7ᵗʰ **S00.542 External constriction of oral cavity**

  ✓6ᵗʰ **S00.55 Superficial foreign body of lip and oral cavity**

    ✓7ᵗʰ **S00.551 Superficial foreign body of lip**
      Splinter of lip and oral cavity

    ✓7ᵗʰ **S00.552 Superficial foreign body of oral cavity**
      Splinter of lip and oral cavity

  ✓6ᵗʰ **S00.56 Insect bite (nonvenomous) of lip and oral cavity**

    ✓7ᵗʰ **S00.561 Insect bite (nonvenomous) of lip**

    ✓7ᵗʰ **S00.562 Insect bite (nonvenomous) of oral cavity**

  ✓6ᵗʰ **S00.57 Other superficial bite of lip and oral cavity**

    ✓7ᵗʰ **S00.571 Other superficial bite of lip**
      EXCLUDES 1 open bite of lip (S01.551)

    ✓7ᵗʰ **S00.572 Other superficial bite of oral cavity**
      EXCLUDES 1 open bite of oral cavity (S01.552)

✓5ᵗʰ **S00.8 Superficial injury of other parts of head**
  Superfical injuries of face [any part]

  ✓x7ᵗʰ **S00.80 Unspecified superficial injury of other part of head** ▽

  ✓x7ᵗʰ **S00.81 Abrasion of other part of head**

  ✓x7ᵗʰ **S00.82 Blister (nonthermal) of other part of head**

  ✓x7ᵗʰ **S00.83 Contusion of other part of head**
    Bruise of other part of head
    Hematoma of other part of head

  ✓x7ᵗʰ **S00.84 External constriction of other part of head**

  ✓x7ᵗʰ **S00.85 Superficial foreign body of other part of head**
    Splinter in other part of head

  ✓x7ᵗʰ **S00.86 Insect bite (nonvenomous) of other part of head**

  ✓x7ᵗʰ **S00.87 Other superficial bite of other part of head**
    EXCLUDES 1 open bite of other part of head (S01.85)

✓5ᵗʰ **S00.9 Superficial injury of unspecified part of head**

  ✓x7ᵗʰ **S00.90 Unspecified superficial injury of unspecified part of head** ▽

  ✓x7ᵗʰ **S00.91 Abrasion of unspecified part of head** ▽

  ✓x7ᵗʰ **S00.92 Blister (nonthermal) of unspecified part of head** ▽

  ✓x7ᵗʰ **S00.93 Contusion of unspecified part of head** ▽
    Bruise of head
    Hematoma of head

  ✓x7ᵗʰ **S00.94 External constriction of unspecified part of head** ▽

  ✓x7ᵗʰ **S00.95 Superficial foreign body of unspecified part of head** ▽
    Splinter of head

  ✓x7ᵗʰ **S00.96 Insect bite (nonvenomous) of unspecified part of head** ▽

  ✓x7ᵗʰ **S00.97 Other superficial bite of unspecified part of head** ▽
    EXCLUDES 1 open bite of head (S01.95)

✓4ᵗʰ **S01 Open wound of head**
  Code also any associated:
    injury of cranial nerve (S04.-)
    injury of muscle and tendon of head (S09.1-)
    intracranial injury (S06.-)
    wound infection
  EXCLUDES 1 open skull fracture (S02- with 7th character B)
  EXCLUDES 2 injury of eye and orbit (S05.-)
          traumatic amputation of part of head (S08.-)

> The appropriate 7th character is to be added to each code from category S01.
> A   initial encounter
> D   subsequent encounter
> S   sequela

✓5ᵗʰ **S01.0 Open wound of scalp**
  EXCLUDES 1 avulsion of scalp (S08.0)

  ✓x7ᵗʰ **S01.00 Unspecified open wound of scalp** ▽

  ✓x7ᵗʰ **S01.01 Laceration without foreign body of scalp**

✓ Additional Character Req   ✓x7ᵗʰ Placeholder Alert   Manifestation   HCC CMS-HCC Condition   ▽ Unspecified Code   ▶◀ Revised Text   ● New Code   ▲ Revised Code Title

ICD-10-CM 2018   915

√x7ᵗʰ   **S01.02**   **Laceration with foreign body of scalp**

√x7ᵗʰ   **S01.03**   **Puncture wound without foreign body of scalp**

√x7ᵗʰ   **S01.04**   **Puncture wound with foreign body of scalp**

√x7ᵗʰ   **S01.05**   **Open bite of scalp**
Bite of scalp NOS
EXCLUDES 1   superficial bite of scalp (S00.06, S00.07-)

√5ᵗʰ   **S01.1**   **Open wound of eyelid and periocular area**
Open wound of eyelid and periocular area with or without involvement of lacrimal passages

    √6ᵗʰ   **S01.10**   **Unspecified open wound of eyelid and periocular area**

       √7ᵗʰ   **S01.101**   Unspecified open wound of right eyelid and periocular area   ▽

       √7ᵗʰ   **S01.102**   Unspecified open wound of left eyelid and periocular area   ▽

       √7ᵗʰ   **S01.109**   Unspecified open wound of unspecified eyelid and periocular area   ▽

    √6ᵗʰ   **S01.11**   **Laceration without foreign body of eyelid and periocular area**

       √7ᵗʰ   **S01.111**   Laceration without foreign body of right eyelid and periocular area

       √7ᵗʰ   **S01.112**   Laceration without foreign body of left eyelid and periocular area

       √7ᵗʰ   **S01.119**   Laceration without foreign body of unspecified eyelid and periocular area   ▽

    √6ᵗʰ   **S01.12**   **Laceration with foreign body of eyelid and periocular area**

       √7ᵗʰ   **S01.121**   Laceration with foreign body of right eyelid and periocular area

       √7ᵗʰ   **S01.122**   Laceration with foreign body of left eyelid and periocular area

       √7ᵗʰ   **S01.129**   Laceration with foreign body of unspecified eyelid and periocular area   ▽

    √6ᵗʰ   **S01.13**   **Puncture wound without foreign body of eyelid and periocular area**

       √7ᵗʰ   **S01.131**   Puncture wound without foreign body of right eyelid and periocular area

       √7ᵗʰ   **S01.132**   Puncture wound without foreign body of left eyelid and periocular area

       √7ᵗʰ   **S01.139**   Puncture wound without foreign body of unspecified eyelid and periocular area   ▽

    √6ᵗʰ   **S01.14**   **Puncture wound with foreign body of eyelid and periocular area**

       √7ᵗʰ   **S01.141**   Puncture wound with foreign body of right eyelid and periocular area

       √7ᵗʰ   **S01.142**   Puncture wound with foreign body of left eyelid and periocular area

       √7ᵗʰ   **S01.149**   Puncture wound with foreign body of unspecified eyelid and periocular area   ▽

    √6ᵗʰ   **S01.15**   **Open bite of eyelid and periocular area**
Bite of eyelid and periocular area NOS
EXCLUDES 1   superficial bite of eyelid and periocular area (S00.26, S00.27)

       √7ᵗʰ   **S01.151**   Open bite of right eyelid and periocular area

       √7ᵗʰ   **S01.152**   Open bite of left eyelid and periocular area

       √7ᵗʰ   **S01.159**   Open bite of unspecified eyelid and periocular area   ▽

√5ᵗʰ   **S01.2**   **Open wound of nose**

    √x7ᵗʰ   **S01.20**   **Unspecified open wound of nose**   ▽

    √x7ᵗʰ   **S01.21**   **Laceration without foreign body of nose**

    √x7ᵗʰ   **S01.22**   **Laceration with foreign body of nose**

    √x7ᵗʰ   **S01.23**   **Puncture wound without foreign body of nose**

    √x7ᵗʰ   **S01.24**   **Puncture wound with foreign body of nose**

    √x7ᵗʰ   **S01.25**   **Open bite of nose**
Bite of nose NOS
EXCLUDES 1   superficial bite of nose (S00.36, S00.37)

√5ᵗʰ   **S01.3**   **Open wound of ear**

    √6ᵗʰ   **S01.30**   **Unspecified open wound of ear**

       √7ᵗʰ   **S01.301**   Unspecified open wound of right ear   ▽

       √7ᵗʰ   **S01.302**   Unspecified open wound of left ear   ▽

       √7ᵗʰ   **S01.309**   Unspecified open wound of unspecified ear   ▽

    √6ᵗʰ   **S01.31**   **Laceration without foreign body of ear**

       √7ᵗʰ   **S01.311**   Laceration without foreign body of right ear

       √7ᵗʰ   **S01.312**   Laceration without foreign body of left ear

       √7ᵗʰ   **S01.319**   Laceration without foreign body of unspecified ear   ▽

    √6ᵗʰ   **S01.32**   **Laceration with foreign body of ear**

       √7ᵗʰ   **S01.321**   Laceration with foreign body of right ear

       √7ᵗʰ   **S01.322**   Laceration with foreign body of left ear

       √7ᵗʰ   **S01.329**   Laceration with foreign body of unspecified ear   ▽

    √6ᵗʰ   **S01.33**   **Puncture wound without foreign body of ear**

       √7ᵗʰ   **S01.331**   Puncture wound without foreign body of right ear

       √7ᵗʰ   **S01.332**   Puncture wound without foreign body of left ear

       √7ᵗʰ   **S01.339**   Puncture wound without foreign body of unspecified ear   ▽

    √6ᵗʰ   **S01.34**   **Puncture wound with foreign body of ear**

       √7ᵗʰ   **S01.341**   Puncture wound with foreign body of right ear

       √7ᵗʰ   **S01.342**   Puncture wound with foreign body of left ear

       √7ᵗʰ   **S01.349**   Puncture wound with foreign body of unspecified ear   ▽

    √6ᵗʰ   **S01.35**   **Open bite of ear**
Bite of ear NOS
EXCLUDES 1   superficial bite of ear (S00.46, S00.47)

       √7ᵗʰ   **S01.351**   Open bite of right ear

       √7ᵗʰ   **S01.352**   Open bite of left ear

       √7ᵗʰ   **S01.359**   Open bite of unspecified ear   ▽

√5ᵗʰ   **S01.4**   **Open wound of cheek and temporomandibular area**

    √6ᵗʰ   **S01.40**   **Unspecified open wound of cheek and temporomandibular area**

       √7ᵗʰ   **S01.401**   Unspecified open wound of right cheek and temporomandibular area   ▽

       √7ᵗʰ   **S01.402**   Unspecified open wound of left cheek and temporomandibular area   ▽

       √7ᵗʰ   **S01.409**   Unspecified open wound of unspecified cheek and temporomandibular area   ▽

    √6ᵗʰ   **S01.41**   **Laceration without foreign body of cheek and temporomandibular area**

       √7ᵗʰ   **S01.411**   Laceration without foreign body of right cheek and temporomandibular area

       √7ᵗʰ   **S01.412**   Laceration without foreign body of left cheek and temporomandibular area

       √7ᵗʰ   **S01.419**   Laceration without foreign body of unspecified cheek and temporomandibular area   ▽

    √6ᵗʰ   **S01.42**   **Laceration with foreign body of cheek and temporomandibular area**

       √7ᵗʰ   **S01.421**   Laceration with foreign body of right cheek and temporomandibular area

       √7ᵗʰ   **S01.422**   Laceration with foreign body of left cheek and temporomandibular area

       √7ᵗʰ   **S01.429**   Laceration with foreign body of unspecified cheek and temporomandibular area   ▽

    √6ᵗʰ   **S01.43**   **Puncture wound without foreign body of cheek and temporomandibular area**

       √7ᵗʰ   **S01.431**   Puncture wound without foreign body of right cheek and temporomandibular area

       √7ᵗʰ   **S01.432**   Puncture wound without foreign body of left cheek and temporomandibular area

       √7ᵗʰ   **S01.439**   Puncture wound without foreign body of unspecified cheek and temporomandibular area   ▽

    √6ᵗʰ   **S01.44**   **Puncture wound with foreign body of cheek and temporomandibular area**

       √7ᵗʰ   **S01.441**   Puncture wound with foreign body of right cheek and temporomandibular area

EXCLUDES 1 Not coded here   *EXCLUDES 2* Not included here   **N** Newborn Age: 0   **P** Pediatric Age: 0-17   **M** Maternity Age: 12-55   **A** Adult Age: 15-124

916   ICD-10-CM 2018

☑7ᵗʰ **S01.442 Puncture wound with foreign body of left cheek and temporomandibular area**

☑7ᵗʰ **S01.449 Puncture wound with foreign body of unspecified cheek and temporomandibular area** ▽

☑6ᵗʰ **S01.45 Open bite of cheek and temporomandibular area**
Bite of cheek and temporomandibular area NOS
EXCLUDES 2   superficial bite of cheek and temporomandibular area (S00.86, S00.87)

☑7ᵗʰ **S01.451 Open bite of right cheek and temporomandibular area**

☑7ᵗʰ **S01.452 Open bite of left cheek and temporomandibular area**

☑7ᵗʰ **S01.459 Open bite of unspecified cheek and temporomandibular area** ▽

☑5ᵗʰ **S01.5 Open wound of lip and oral cavity**
EXCLUDES 2   tooth dislocation (S03.2)
         tooth fracture (S02.5)

☑6ᵗʰ **S01.50 Unspecified open wound of lip and oral cavity**

☑7ᵗʰ **S01.501 Unspecified open wound of lip** ▽

☑7ᵗʰ **S01.502 Unspecified open wound of oral cavity** ▽

☑6ᵗʰ **S01.51 Laceration of lip and oral cavity without foreign body**

☑7ᵗʰ **S01.511 Laceration without foreign body of lip**

☑7ᵗʰ **S01.512 Laceration without foreign body of oral cavity**

☑6ᵗʰ **S01.52 Laceration of lip and oral cavity with foreign body**

☑7ᵗʰ **S01.521 Laceration with foreign body of lip**

☑7ᵗʰ **S01.522 Laceration with foreign body of oral cavity**

☑6ᵗʰ **S01.53 Puncture wound of lip and oral cavity without foreign body**

☑7ᵗʰ **S01.531 Puncture wound without foreign body of lip**

☑7ᵗʰ **S01.532 Puncture wound without foreign body of oral cavity**

☑6ᵗʰ **S01.54 Puncture wound of lip and oral cavity with foreign body**

☑7ᵗʰ **S01.541 Puncture wound with foreign body of lip**

☑7ᵗʰ **S01.542 Puncture wound with foreign body of oral cavity**

☑6ᵗʰ **S01.55 Open bite of lip and oral cavity**

☑7ᵗʰ **S01.551 Open bite of lip**
Bite of lip NOS
EXCLUDES 1   superficial bite of lip (S00.571)

☑7ᵗʰ **S01.552 Open bite of oral cavity**
Bite of oral cavity NOS
EXCLUDES 1   superficial bite of oral cavity (S00.572)

☑5ᵗʰ **S01.8 Open wound of other parts of head**

☑x7ᵗʰ **S01.80 Unspecified open wound of other part of head** ▽

☑x7ᵗʰ **S01.81 Laceration without foreign body of other part of head**

☑x7ᵗʰ **S01.82 Laceration with foreign body of other part of head**

☑x7ᵗʰ **S01.83 Puncture wound without foreign body of other part of head**

☑x7ᵗʰ **S01.84 Puncture wound with foreign body of other part of head**

☑x7ᵗʰ **S01.85 Open bite of other part of head**
Bite of other part of head NOS
EXCLUDES 1   superficial bite of other part of head ▶(S00.87)◀

☑5ᵗʰ **S01.9 Open wound of unspecified part of head**

☑x7ᵗʰ **S01.90 Unspecified open wound of unspecified part of head** ▽

☑x7ᵗʰ **S01.91 Laceration without foreign body of unspecified part of head** ▽

☑x7ᵗʰ **S01.92 Laceration with foreign body of unspecified part of head** ▽

☑x7ᵗʰ **S01.93 Puncture wound without foreign body of unspecified part of head** ▽

☑x7ᵗʰ **S01.94 Puncture wound with foreign body of unspecified part of head** ▽

☑x7ᵗʰ **S01.95 Open bite of unspecified part of head** ▽
Bite of head NOS
EXCLUDES 1   superficial bite of head NOS (S00.97)

☑4ᵗʰ **S02 Fracture of skull and facial bones**
NOTE   A fracture not indicated as open or closed should be coded to closed.
Code also any associated intracranial injury (S06.-).
AHA: 2017, 1Q, 42

> The appropriate 7th character is to be added to each code from category S02.
> A   initial encounter for closed fracture
> B   initial encounter for open fracture
> D   subsequent encounter for fracture with routine healing
> G   subsequent encounter for fracture with delayed healing
> K   subsequent encounter for fracture with nonunion
> S   sequela

² ☑x7ᵗʰ **S02.0 Fracture of vault of skull** HCC
Fracture of frontal bone
Fracture of parietal bone

☑5ᵗʰ **S02.1 Fracture of base of skull**
EXCLUDES 1   orbit NOS (S02.8)
EXCLUDES 2   orbital floor (S02.3-)

☑6ᵗʰ **S02.10 Unspecified fracture of base of skull**

² ☑7ᵗʰ **S02.101 Fracture of base of skull, right side** HCC

² ☑7ᵗʰ **S02.102 Fracture of base of skull, left side** HCC

² ☑7ᵗʰ **S02.109 Fracture of base of skull, unspecified side** HCC ▽

☑6ᵗʰ **S02.11 Fracture of occiput**

² ☑7ᵗʰ **S02.110 Type I occipital condyle fracture, unspecified side** HCC ▽

² ☑7ᵗʰ **S02.111 Type II occipital condyle fracture, unspecified side** HCC ▽

² ☑7ᵗʰ **S02.112 Type III occipital condyle fracture, unspecified side** HCC ▽

² ☑7ᵗʰ **S02.113 Unspecified occipital condyle fracture** HCC ▽

² ☑7ᵗʰ **S02.118 Other fracture of occiput, unspecified side** HCC ▽

² ☑7ᵗʰ **S02.119 Unspecified fracture of occiput** HCC ▽

² ☑7ᵗʰ **S02.11A Type I occipital condyle fracture, right side** HCC

² ☑7ᵗʰ **S02.11B Type I occipital condyle fracture, left side** HCC

² ☑7ᵗʰ **S02.11C Type II occipital condyle fracture, right side** HCC

² ☑7ᵗʰ **S02.11D Type II occipital condyle fracture, left side** HCC

² ☑7ᵗʰ **S02.11E Type III occipital condyle fracture, right side** HCC

² ☑7ᵗʰ **S02.11F Type III occipital condyle fracture, left side** HCC

² ☑7ᵗʰ **S02.11G Other fracture of occiput, right side** HCC

² ☑7ᵗʰ **S02.11H Other fracture of occiput, left side** HCC

² ☑x7ᵗʰ **S02.19 Other fracture of base of skull** HCC
Fracture of anterior fossa of base of skull
Fracture of ethmoid sinus
Fracture of frontal sinus
Fracture of middle fossa of base of skull
Fracture of orbital roof
Fracture of posterior fossa of base of skull
Fracture of sphenoid
Fracture of temporal bone

☑x7ᵗʰ **S02.2 Fracture of nasal bones**

☑5ᵗʰ **S02.3 Fracture of orbital floor**
EXCLUDES 1   orbit NOS (S02.8)
EXCLUDES 2   orbital roof (S02.1-)

² ☑x7ᵗʰ **S02.30 Fracture of orbital floor, unspecified side** HCC ▽

² ☑x7ᵗʰ **S02.31 Fracture of orbital floor, right side** HCC

² ☑x7ᵗʰ **S02.32 Fracture of orbital floor, left side** HCC

---

²   HCC with 7th character indicating initial encounter (A or B - specific to category) OR sequela.

| ☑ Additional Character Req | ☑x7ᵗʰ Placeholder Alert | Manifestation | HCC CMS-HCC Condition | ▽ Unspecified Code | ▶◀ Revised Text | ● New Code | ▲ Revised Code Title |

LeFort Fracture Types

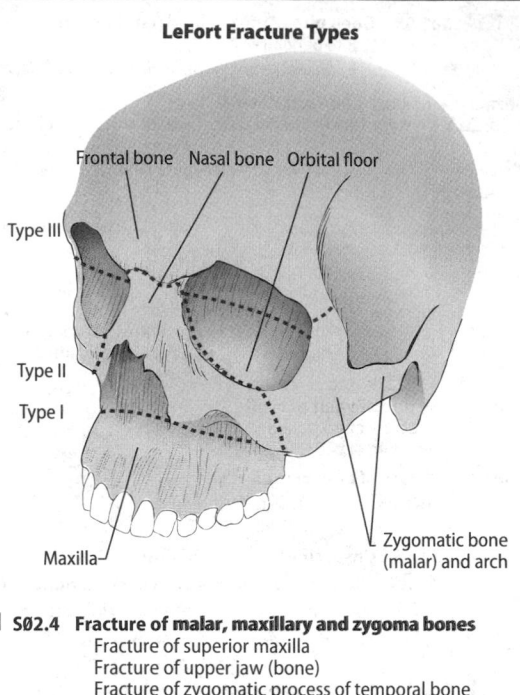

Frontal bone   Nasal bone   Orbital floor

Type III

Type II

Type I

Maxilla

Zygomatic bone (malar) and arch

√5ᵗʰ **S02.4   Fracture of malar, maxillary and zygoma bones**
  Fracture of superior maxilla
  Fracture of upper jaw (bone)
  Fracture of zygomatic process of temporal bone

  √6ᵗʰ **S02.40   Fracture of malar, maxillary and zygoma bones, unspecified**
    2 √7ᵗʰ **S02.400   Malar fracture, unspecified side** HCC ▽
    2 √7ᵗʰ **S02.401   Maxillary fracture, unspecified side** HCC ▽
    2 √7ᵗʰ **S02.402   Zygomatic fracture, unspecified side** HCC ▽
    2 √7ᵗʰ **S02.40A   Malar fracture, right side** HCC
    2 √7ᵗʰ **S02.40B   Malar fracture, left side** HCC
    2 √7ᵗʰ **S02.40C   Maxillary fracture, right side** HCC
    2 √7ᵗʰ **S02.40D   Maxillary fracture, left side** HCC
    2 √7ᵗʰ **S02.40E   Zygomatic fracture, right side** HCC
    2 √7ᵗʰ **S02.40F   Zygomatic fracture, left side** HCC

  √6ᵗʰ **S02.41   LeFort fracture**
    2 √7ᵗʰ **S02.411   LeFort I fracture** HCC
    2 √7ᵗʰ **S02.412   LeFort II fracture** HCC
    2 √7ᵗʰ **S02.413   LeFort III fracture** HCC
  2 √x7ᵗʰ **S02.42   Fracture of alveolus of maxilla** HCC

√x7ᵗʰ **S02.5   Fracture of tooth (traumatic)**
  Broken tooth
  EXCLUDES 1 cracked tooth (nontraumatic) (K03.81)

√5ᵗʰ **S02.6   Fracture of mandible**
  Fracture of lower jaw (bone)

  √6ᵗʰ **S02.60   Fracture of mandible, unspecified**
    2 √7ᵗʰ **S02.600   Fracture of unspecified part of body of mandible, unspecified side** HCC ▽
    2 √7ᵗʰ **S02.601   Fracture of unspecified part of body of right mandible** HCC ▽
    2 √7ᵗʰ **S02.602   Fracture of unspecified part of body of left mandible** HCC ▽
    2 √7ᵗʰ **S02.609   Fracture of mandible, unspecified** HCC ▽

  √6ᵗʰ **S02.61   Fracture of condylar process of mandible**
    2 √7ᵗʰ **S02.610   Fracture of condylar process of mandible, unspecified side** HCC ▽
    2 √7ᵗʰ **S02.611   Fracture of condylar process of right mandible** HCC
    2 √7ᵗʰ **S02.612   Fracture of condylar process of left mandible** HCC

  √6ᵗʰ **S02.62   Fracture of subcondylar process of mandible**
    2 √7ᵗʰ **S02.620   Fracture of subcondylar process of mandible, unspecified side** HCC ▽
    2 √7ᵗʰ **S02.621   Fracture of subcondylar process of right mandible** HCC
    2 √7ᵗʰ **S02.622   Fracture of subcondylar process of left mandible** HCC

  √6ᵗʰ **S02.63   Fracture of coronoid process of mandible**
    2 √7ᵗʰ **S02.630   Fracture of coronoid process of mandible, unspecified side** HCC ▽
    2 √7ᵗʰ **S02.631   Fracture of coronoid process of right mandible** HCC
    2 √7ᵗʰ **S02.632   Fracture of coronoid process of left mandible** HCC

  √6ᵗʰ **S02.64   Fracture of ramus of mandible**
    2 √7ᵗʰ **S02.640   Fracture of ramus of mandible, unspecified side** HCC ▽
    2 √7ᵗʰ **S02.641   Fracture of ramus of right mandible** HCC
    2 √7ᵗʰ **S02.642   Fracture of ramus of left mandible** HCC

  √6ᵗʰ **S02.65   Fracture of angle of mandible**
    2 √7ᵗʰ **S02.650   Fracture of angle of mandible, unspecified side** HCC ▽
    2 √7ᵗʰ **S02.651   Fracture of angle of right mandible** HCC
    2 √7ᵗʰ **S02.652   Fracture of angle of left mandible** HCC
  2 √x7ᵗʰ **S02.66   Fracture of symphysis of mandible** HCC

  √6ᵗʰ **S02.67   Fracture of alveolus of mandible**
    2 √7ᵗʰ **S02.670   Fracture of alveolus of mandible, unspecified side** HCC ▽
    2 √7ᵗʰ **S02.671   Fracture of alveolus of right mandible** HCC
    2 √7ᵗʰ **S02.672   Fracture of alveolus of left mandible** HCC
  2 √x7ᵗʰ **S02.69   Fracture of mandible of other specified site** HCC

√5ᵗʰ **S02.8   Fractures of other specified skull and facial bones**
  Fracture of orbit NOS
  Fracture of palate
  EXCLUDES 1 fracture of orbital floor (S02.3-)
           fracture of orbital roof (S02.1-)
  2 √x7ᵗʰ **S02.80   Fracture of other specified skull and facial bones, unspecified side** HCC ▽
  2 √x7ᵗʰ **S02.81   Fracture of other specified skull and facial bones, right side** HCC
  2 √x7ᵗʰ **S02.82   Fracture of other specified skull and facial bones, left side** HCC

√5ᵗʰ **S02.9   Fracture of unspecified skull and facial bones**
  2 √x7ᵗʰ **S02.91   Unspecified fracture of skull** HCC ▽
  2 √x7ᵗʰ **S02.92   Unspecified fracture of facial bones** HCC ▽

√4ᵗʰ **S03   Dislocation and sprain of joints and ligaments of head**
  INCLUDES avulsion of joint (capsule) or ligament of head
           laceration of cartilage, joint (capsule) or ligament of head
           sprain of cartilage, joint (capsule) or ligament of head
           traumatic hemarthrosis of joint or ligament of head
           traumatic rupture of joint or ligament of head
           traumatic subluxation of joint or ligament of head
           traumatic tear of joint or ligament of head
  Code also any associated open wound
  EXCLUDES 2 strain of muscle or tendon of head (S09.1)

  The appropriate 7th character is to be added to each code from category S03.
  A   initial encounter
  D   subsequent encounter
  S   sequela

  √5ᵗʰ **S03.0   Dislocation of jaw**
    Dislocation of jaw (cartilage) (meniscus)
    Dislocation of mandible
    Dislocation of temporomandibular (joint)
    √7ᵗʰ **S03.00   Dislocation of jaw, unspecified side** ▽
    √7ᵗʰ **S03.01   Dislocation of jaw, right side**
    √7ᵗʰ **S03.02   Dislocation of jaw, left side**
    √7ᵗʰ **S03.03   Dislocation of jaw, bilateral**
  √x7ᵗʰ **S03.1   Dislocation of septal cartilage of nose**
  √x7ᵗʰ **S03.2   Dislocation of tooth**
  √5ᵗʰ **S03.4   Sprain of jaw**
    Sprain of temporomandibular (joint) (ligament)
    √7ᵗʰ **S03.40   Sprain of jaw, unspecified side** ▽
    √7ᵗʰ **S03.41   Sprain of jaw, right side**
    √7ᵗʰ **S03.42   Sprain of jaw, left side**
    √7ᵗʰ **S03.43   Sprain of jaw, bilateral**
  √x7ᵗʰ **S03.8   Sprain of joints and ligaments of other parts of head**
  √x7ᵗʰ **S03.9   Sprain of joints and ligaments of unspecified parts of head** ▽

---

2   HCC with 7th character indicating initial encounter (A or B - specific to category) OR sequela.

☑4ᵗʰ **S04 Injury of cranial nerve**

The selection of side should be based on the side of the body being affected

Codes first any associated intracranial injury (S06.-)

Code also any associated:
    open wound of head (S01.-)
    skull fracture (S02.-)

> The appropriate 7th character is to be added to each code from category S04.
> A   initial encounter
> D   subsequent encounter
> S   sequela

☑5ᵗʰ **S04.0 Injury of optic nerve and pathways**

Use additional code to identify any visual field defect or blindness ▶(H53.4-, H54.-)◀

  ☑6ᵗʰ **S04.01 Injury of optic nerve**
    Injury of 2nd cranial nerve

    ☑7ᵗʰ **S04.011 Injury of optic nerve, right eye**

    ☑7ᵗʰ **S04.012 Injury of optic nerve, left eye**

    ☑7ᵗʰ **S04.019 Injury of optic nerve, unspecified eye** ▽
        Injury of optic nerve NOS

  ☑x7ᵗʰ **S04.02 Injury of optic chiasm**

  ☑6ᵗʰ **S04.03 Injury of optic tract and pathways**
    Injury of optic radiation

▲   ☑7ᵗʰ **S04.031 Injury of optic tract and pathways, right side**

▲   ☑7ᵗʰ **S04.032 Injury of optic tract and pathways, left side**

▲   ☑7ᵗʰ **S04.039 Injury of optic tract and pathways, unspecified side** ▽
        Injury of optic tract and pathways NOS

  ☑6ᵗʰ **S04.04 Injury of visual cortex**

▲   ☑7ᵗʰ **S04.041 Injury of visual cortex, right side**

▲   ☑7ᵗʰ **S04.042 Injury of visual cortex, left side**

▲   ☑7ᵗʰ **S04.049 Injury of visual cortex, unspecified side** ▽
        Injury of visual cortex NOS

☑5ᵗʰ **S04.1 Injury of oculomotor nerve**
  Injury of 3rd cranial nerve

  ☑x7ᵗʰ **S04.10 Injury of oculomotor nerve, unspecified side** ▽

  ☑x7ᵗʰ **S04.11 Injury of oculomotor nerve, right side**

  ☑x7ᵗʰ **S04.12 Injury of oculomotor nerve, left side**

☑5ᵗʰ **S04.2 Injury of trochlear nerve**
  Injury of 4th cranial nerve

  ☑x7ᵗʰ **S04.20 Injury of trochlear nerve, unspecified side** ▽

  ☑x7ᵗʰ **S04.21 Injury of trochlear nerve, right side**

  ☑x7ᵗʰ **S04.22 Injury of trochlear nerve, left side**

☑5ᵗʰ **S04.3 Injury of trigeminal nerve**
  Injury of 5th cranial nerve

  ☑x7ᵗʰ **S04.30 Injury of trigeminal nerve, unspecified side** ▽

  ☑x7ᵗʰ **S04.31 Injury of trigeminal nerve, right side**

  ☑x7ᵗʰ **S04.32 Injury of trigeminal nerve, left side**

☑5ᵗʰ **S04.4 Injury of abducent nerve**
  Injury of 6th cranial nerve

  ☑x7ᵗʰ **S04.40 Injury of abducent nerve, unspecified side** ▽

  ☑x7ᵗʰ **S04.41 Injury of abducent nerve, right side**

  ☑x7ᵗʰ **S04.42 Injury of abducent nerve, left side**

☑5ᵗʰ **S04.5 Injury of facial nerve**
  Injury of 7th cranial nerve

  ☑x7ᵗʰ **S04.50 Injury of facial nerve, unspecified side** ▽

  ☑x7ᵗʰ **S04.51 Injury of facial nerve, right side**

  ☑x7ᵗʰ **S04.52 Injury of facial nerve, left side**

☑5ᵗʰ **S04.6 Injury of acoustic nerve**
  Injury of auditory nerve
  Injury of 8th cranial nerve

  ☑x7ᵗʰ **S04.60 Injury of acoustic nerve, unspecified side** ▽

  ☑x7ᵗʰ **S04.61 Injury of acoustic nerve, right side**

  ☑x7ᵗʰ **S04.62 Injury of acoustic nerve, left side**

☑5ᵗʰ **S04.7 Injury of accessory nerve**
  Injury of 11th cranial nerve

  ☑x7ᵗʰ **S04.70 Injury of accessory nerve, unspecified side** ▽

  ☑x7ᵗʰ **S04.71 Injury of accessory nerve, right side**

  ☑x7ᵗʰ **S04.72 Injury of accessory nerve, left side**

☑5ᵗʰ **S04.8 Injury of other cranial nerves**

  ☑6ᵗʰ **S04.81 Injury of olfactory [1st] nerve**

    ☑7ᵗʰ **S04.811 Injury of olfactory [1st] nerve, right side**

    ☑7ᵗʰ **S04.812 Injury of olfactory [1st] nerve, left side**

    ☑7ᵗʰ **S04.819 Injury of olfactory [1st] nerve, unspecified side** ▽

  ☑6ᵗʰ **S04.89 Injury of other cranial nerves**
    Injury of vagus [10th] nerve

    ☑7ᵗʰ **S04.891 Injury of other cranial nerves, right side**

    ☑7ᵗʰ **S04.892 Injury of other cranial nerves, left side**

    ☑7ᵗʰ **S04.899 Injury of other cranial nerves, unspecified side** ▽

☑x7ᵗʰ **S04.9 Injury of unspecified cranial nerve** ▽

☑4ᵗʰ **S05 Injury of eye and orbit**

  INCLUDES   open wound of eye and orbit

  EXCLUDES 2   2nd cranial [optic] nerve injury (S04.0-)
    3rd cranial [oculomotor] nerve injury (S04.1-)
    open wound of eyelid and periocular area (S01.1-)
    orbital bone fracture (S02.1-, S02.3-, S02.8-)
    superficial injury of eyelid (S00.1-S00.2)

> The appropriate 7th character is to be added to each code from category S05.
> A   initial encounter
> D   subsequent encounter
> S   sequela

☑5ᵗʰ **S05.0 Injury of conjunctiva and corneal abrasion without foreign body**

  EXCLUDES 1   foreign body in conjunctival sac (T15.1)
    foreign body in cornea (T15.0)

  ☑x7ᵗʰ **S05.00 Injury of conjunctiva and corneal abrasion without foreign body, unspecified eye** ▽

  ☑x7ᵗʰ **S05.01 Injury of conjunctiva and corneal abrasion without foreign body, right eye**

  ☑x7ᵗʰ **S05.02 Injury of conjunctiva and corneal abrasion without foreign body, left eye**

☑5ᵗʰ **S05.1 Contusion of eyeball and orbital tissues**
  Traumatic hyphema

  EXCLUDES 2   black eye NOS (S00.1)
    contusion of eyelid and periocular area (S00.1)

  ☑x7ᵗʰ **S05.10 Contusion of eyeball and orbital tissues, unspecified eye** ▽

  ☑x7ᵗʰ **S05.11 Contusion of eyeball and orbital tissues, right eye**

  ☑x7ᵗʰ **S05.12 Contusion of eyeball and orbital tissues, left eye**

☑5ᵗʰ **S05.2 Ocular laceration and rupture with prolapse or loss of intraocular tissue**

  ☑x7ᵗʰ **S05.20 Ocular laceration and rupture with prolapse or loss of intraocular tissue, unspecified eye** ▽

  ☑x7ᵗʰ **S05.21 Ocular laceration and rupture with prolapse or loss of intraocular tissue, right eye**

  ☑x7ᵗʰ **S05.22 Ocular laceration and rupture with prolapse or loss of intraocular tissue, left eye**

☑5ᵗʰ **S05.3 Ocular laceration without prolapse or loss of intraocular tissue**
  Laceration of eye NOS
  DEF: Tear in ocular tissue without displacing structures; due to blunt trauma; characterized by pain, redness, and decreased vision.

  ☑x7ᵗʰ **S05.30 Ocular laceration without prolapse or loss of intraocular tissue, unspecified eye** ▽

  ☑x7ᵗʰ **S05.31 Ocular laceration without prolapse or loss of intraocular tissue, right eye**

  ☑x7ᵗʰ **S05.32 Ocular laceration without prolapse or loss of intraocular tissue, left eye**

☑5ᵗʰ **S05.4 Penetrating wound of orbit with or without foreign body**

  EXCLUDES 2   retained (old) foreign body following penetrating wound in orbit (H05.5-)

  ☑x7ᵗʰ **S05.40 Penetrating wound of orbit with or without foreign body, unspecified eye** ▽

  ☑x7ᵗʰ **S05.41 Penetrating wound of orbit with or without foreign body, right eye**

  ☑x7ᵗʰ **S05.42 Penetrating wound of orbit with or without foreign body, left eye**

☑ Additional Character Req   ☑x7ᵗʰ Placeholder Alert   Manifestation   HCC CMS-HCC Condition   ▽ Unspecified Code   ▶◀ Revised Text   ● New Code   ▲ Revised Code Title

✓5th S05.5 Penetrating wound with foreign body of eyeball
EXCLUDES 2   retained (old) intraocular foreign body (H44.6-, H44.7)

✓x7th **S05.50 Penetrating wound with foreign body of unspecified eyeball** ▽

✓x7th **S05.51 Penetrating wound with foreign body of right eyeball**

✓x7th **S05.52 Penetrating wound with foreign body of left eyeball**

✓5th S05.6 Penetrating wound without foreign body of eyeball
Ocular penetration NOS

✓x7th **S05.60 Penetrating wound without foreign body of unspecified eyeball** ▽

✓x7th **S05.61 Penetrating wound without foreign body of right eyeball**

✓x7th **S05.62 Penetrating wound without foreign body of left eyeball**

✓5th S05.7 Avulsion of eye
Traumatic enucleation

✓x7th **S05.70 Avulsion of unspecified eye** ▽

✓x7th **S05.71 Avulsion of right eye**

✓x7th **S05.72 Avulsion of left eye**

✓5th S05.8 Other injuries of eye and orbit
Lacrimal duct injury

✓6th **S05.8X Other injuries of eye and orbit**

✓7th **S05.8X1 Other injuries of right eye and orbit**

✓7th **S05.8X2 Other injuries of left eye and orbit**

✓7th **S05.8X9 Other injuries of unspecified eye and orbit** ▽

✓5th S05.9 Unspecified injury of eye and orbit
Injury of eye NOS

✓x7th **S05.90 Unspecified injury of unspecified eye and orbit** ▽

✓x7th **S05.91 Unspecified injury of right eye and orbit** ▽

✓x7th **S05.92 Unspecified injury of left eye and orbit** ▽

✓4th S06 Intracranial injury
NOTE   ▶7th characters D and S do not apply to codes in category S06 with 6th character 7 – death due to brain injury prior to regaining consciousness, or 8 – death due to other cause prior to regaining consciousness◀
INCLUDES   traumatic brain injury
Code also any associated:
    open wound of head (S01.-)
    skull fracture (S02.-)
EXCLUDES 1   head injury NOS (S09.90)
AHA: 2017, 1Q, 42; 2015, 3Q, 37

> The appropriate 7th character is to be added to each code from category S06.
> A   initial encounter
> D   subsequent encounter
> S   sequela

✓5th S06.0 Concussion
Commotio cerebri
EXCLUDES 1   concussion with intracranial injuries classified in subcategories S06.1- to S06.6-, S06.81-, S06.82- code to specified intracranial injury

✓6th **S06.0X Concussion**

3 ✓7th **S06.0X0 Concussion without loss of consciousness** HCC

3 ✓7th **S06.0X1 Concussion with loss of consciousness of 30 minutes or less** HCC

3 ✓7th **S06.0X9 Concussion with loss of consciousness of unspecified duration** HCC ▽
Concussion NOS

✓5th S06.1 Traumatic cerebral edema
Diffuse traumatic cerebral edema
Focal traumatic cerebral edema

✓6th **S06.1X Traumatic cerebral edema**

2 ✓7th **S06.1X0 Traumatic cerebral edema without loss of consciousness** HCC

2 ✓7th **S06.1X1 Traumatic cerebral edema with loss of consciousness of 30 minutes or less** HCC

2 ✓7th **S06.1X2 Traumatic cerebral edema with loss of consciousness of 31 minutes to 59 minutes** HCC

2 ✓7th **S06.1X3 Traumatic cerebral edema with loss of consciousness of 1 hour to 5 hours 59 minutes** HCC

2 ✓7th **S06.1X4 Traumatic cerebral edema with loss of consciousness of 6 hours to 24 hours** HCC

2 ✓7th **S06.1X5 Traumatic cerebral edema with loss of consciousness greater than 24 hours with return to pre-existing conscious level** HCC

2 ✓7th **S06.1X6 Traumatic cerebral edema with loss of consciousness greater than 24 hours without return to pre-existing conscious level with patient surviving** HCC

✓7th **S06.1X7 Traumatic cerebral edema with loss of consciousness of any duration with death due to brain injury prior to regaining consciousness**

✓7th **S06.1X8 Traumatic cerebral edema with loss of consciousness of any duration with death due to other cause prior to regaining consciousness**

2 ✓7th **S06.1X9 Traumatic cerebral edema with loss of consciousness of unspecified duration** HCC ▽
Traumatic cerebral edema NOS

✓5th S06.2 Diffuse traumatic brain injury
Diffuse axonal brain injury
EXCLUDES 1   traumatic diffuse cerebral edema (S06.1X-)

✓6th **S06.2X Diffuse traumatic brain injury**

2 ✓7th **S06.2X0 Diffuse traumatic brain injury without loss of consciousness** HCC

2 ✓7th **S06.2X1 Diffuse traumatic brain injury with loss of consciousness of 30 minutes or less** HCC

2 ✓7th **S06.2X2 Diffuse traumatic brain injury with loss of consciousness of 31 minutes to 59 minutes** HCC

2 ✓7th **S06.2X3 Diffuse traumatic brain injury with loss of consciousness of 1 hour to 5 hours 59 minutes** HCC

2 ✓7th **S06.2X4 Diffuse traumatic brain injury with loss of consciousness of 6 hours to 24 hours** HCC

2 ✓7th **S06.2X5 Diffuse traumatic brain injury with loss of consciousness greater than 24 hours with return to pre-existing conscious levels** HCC

2 ✓7th **S06.2X6 Diffuse traumatic brain injury with loss of consciousness greater than 24 hours without return to pre-existing conscious level with patient surviving** HCC

✓7th **S06.2X7 Diffuse traumatic brain injury with loss of consciousness of any duration with death due to brain injury prior to regaining consciousness**

✓7th **S06.2X8 Diffuse traumatic brain injury with loss of consciousness of any duration with death due to other cause prior to regaining consciousness**

2 ✓7th **S06.2X9 Diffuse traumatic brain injury with loss of consciousness of unspecified duration** HCC ▽
Diffuse traumatic brain injury NOS

✓5th S06.3 Focal traumatic brain injury
EXCLUDES 1   any condition classifiable to S06.4-S06.6
    focal cerebral edema (S06.1)

✓6th **S06.30 Unspecified focal traumatic brain injury**

2 ✓7th **S06.300 Unspecified focal traumatic brain injury without loss of consciousness** HCC ▽

2 ✓7th **S06.301 Unspecified focal traumatic brain injury with loss of consciousness of 30 minutes or less** HCC ▽

2 ✓7th **S06.302 Unspecified focal traumatic brain injury with loss of consciousness of 31 minutes to 59 minutes** HCC ▽

2 ✓7th **S06.303 Unspecified focal traumatic brain injury with loss of consciousness of 1 hour to 5 hours 59 minutes** HCC ▽

---

2   HCC with 7th character indicating initial encounter (A or B - specific to category) OR sequela.
3   HCC with 7th character indicating sequela.

2 ✓7ᵗʰ **S06.304** **Unspecified focal traumatic brain injury with loss of consciousness of 6 hours to 24 hours** HCC ▽

2 ✓7ᵗʰ **S06.305** **Unspecified focal traumatic brain injury with loss of consciousness greater than 24 hours with return to pre-existing conscious level** HCC ▽

2 ✓7ᵗʰ **S06.306** **Unspecified focal traumatic brain injury with loss of consciousness greater than 24 hours without return to pre-existing conscious level with patient surviving** HCC ▽

✓7ᵗʰ **S06.307** **Unspecified focal traumatic brain injury with loss of consciousness of any duration with death due to brain injury prior to regaining consciousness** ▽

✓7ᵗʰ **S06.308** **Unspecified focal traumatic brain injury with loss of consciousness of any duration with death due to other cause prior to regaining consciousness** ▽

2 ✓7ᵗʰ **S06.309** **Unspecified focal traumatic brain injury with loss of consciousness of unspecified duration** HCC ▽
     Unspecified focal traumatic brain injury NOS

✓6ᵗʰ **S06.31** **Contusion and laceration of right cerebrum**

2 ✓7ᵗʰ **S06.310** **Contusion and laceration of right cerebrum without loss of consciousness** HCC

2 ✓7ᵗʰ **S06.311** **Contusion and laceration of right cerebrum with loss of consciousness of 30 minutes or less** HCC

2 ✓7ᵗʰ **S06.312** **Contusion and laceration of right cerebrum with loss of consciousness of 31 minutes to 59 minutes** HCC

2 ✓7ᵗʰ **S06.313** **Contusion and laceration of right cerebrum with loss of consciousness of 1 hour to 5 hours 59 minutes** HCC

2 ✓7ᵗʰ **S06.314** **Contusion and laceration of right cerebrum with loss of consciousness of 6 hours to 24 hours** HCC

2 ✓7ᵗʰ **S06.315** **Contusion and laceration of right cerebrum with loss of consciousness greater than 24 hours with return to pre-existing conscious level** HCC

2 ✓7ᵗʰ **S06.316** **Contusion and laceration of right cerebrum with loss of consciousness greater than 24 hours without return to pre-existing conscious level with patient surviving** HCC

✓7ᵗʰ **S06.317** **Contusion and laceration of right cerebrum with loss of consciousness of any duration with death due to brain injury prior to regaining consciousness**

✓7ᵗʰ **S06.318** **Contusion and laceration of right cerebrum with loss of consciousness of any duration with death due to other cause prior to regaining consciousness**

2 ✓7ᵗʰ **S06.319** **Contusion and laceration of right cerebrum with loss of consciousness of unspecified duration** HCC ▽
     Contusion and laceration of right cerebrum NOS

✓6ᵗʰ **S06.32** **Contusion and laceration of left cerebrum**

2 ✓7ᵗʰ **S06.320** **Contusion and laceration of left cerebrum without loss of consciousness** HCC

2 ✓7ᵗʰ **S06.321** **Contusion and laceration of left cerebrum with loss of consciousness of 30 minutes or less** HCC

2 ✓7ᵗʰ **S06.322** **Contusion and laceration of left cerebrum with loss of consciousness of 31 minutes to 59 minutes** HCC

2 ✓7ᵗʰ **S06.323** **Contusion and laceration of left cerebrum with loss of consciousness of 1 hour to 5 hours 59 minutes** HCC

2 ✓7ᵗʰ **S06.324** **Contusion and laceration of left cerebrum with loss of consciousness of 6 hours to 24 hours** HCC

2 ✓7ᵗʰ **S06.325** **Contusion and laceration of left cerebrum with loss of consciousness greater than 24 hours with return to pre-existing conscious level** HCC

2 ✓7ᵗʰ **S06.326** **Contusion and laceration of left cerebrum with loss of consciousness greater than 24 hours without return to pre-existing conscious level with patient surviving** HCC

✓7ᵗʰ **S06.327** **Contusion and laceration of left cerebrum with loss of consciousness of any duration with death due to brain injury prior to regaining consciousness**

✓7ᵗʰ **S06.328** **Contusion and laceration of left cerebrum with loss of consciousness of any duration with death due to other cause prior to regaining consciousness**

2 ✓7ᵗʰ **S06.329** **Contusion and laceration of left cerebrum with loss of consciousness of unspecified duration** HCC ▽
     Contusion and laceration of left cerebrum NOS

✓6ᵗʰ **S06.33** **Contusion and laceration of cerebrum, unspecified**

2 ✓7ᵗʰ **S06.330** **Contusion and laceration of cerebrum, unspecified, without loss of consciousness** HCC ▽

2 ✓7ᵗʰ **S06.331** **Contusion and laceration of cerebrum, unspecified, with loss of consciousness of 30 minutes or less** HCC ▽

2 ✓7ᵗʰ **S06.332** **Contusion and laceration of cerebrum, unspecified, with loss of consciousness of 31 minutes to 59 minutes** HCC ▽

2 ✓7ᵗʰ **S06.333** **Contusion and laceration of cerebrum, unspecified, with loss of consciousness of 1 hour to 5 hours 59 minutes** HCC ▽

2 ✓7ᵗʰ **S06.334** **Contusion and laceration of cerebrum, unspecified, with loss of consciousness of 6 hours to 24 hours** HCC ▽

2 ✓7ᵗʰ **S06.335** **Contusion and laceration of cerebrum, unspecified, with loss of consciousness greater than 24 hours with return to pre-existing conscious level** HCC ▽

2 ✓7ᵗʰ **S06.336** **Contusion and laceration of cerebrum, unspecified, with loss of consciousness greater than 24 hours without return to pre-existing conscious level with patient surviving** HCC ▽

✓7ᵗʰ **S06.337** **Contusion and laceration of cerebrum, unspecified, with loss of consciousness of any duration with death due to brain injury prior to regaining consciousness** ▽

✓7ᵗʰ **S06.338** **Contusion and laceration of cerebrum, unspecified, with loss of consciousness of any duration with death due to other cause prior to regaining consciousness** ▽

2 ✓7ᵗʰ **S06.339** **Contusion and laceration of cerebrum, unspecified, with loss of consciousness of unspecified duration** HCC ▽
     Contusion and laceration of cerebrum NOS

✓6ᵗʰ **S06.34** **Traumatic hemorrhage of right cerebrum**
     Traumatic intracerebral hemorrhage and hematoma of right cerebrum

2 ✓7ᵗʰ **S06.340** **Traumatic hemorrhage of right cerebrum without loss of consciousness** HCC

2 ✓7ᵗʰ **S06.341** **Traumatic hemorrhage of right cerebrum with loss of consciousness of 30 minutes or less** HCC

2 ✓7ᵗʰ **S06.342** **Traumatic hemorrhage of right cerebrum with loss of consciousness of 31 minutes to 59 minutes** HCC

2 ✓7ᵗʰ **S06.343** **Traumatic hemorrhage of right cerebrum with loss of consciousness of 1 hours to 5 hours 59 minutes** HCC

2 ✓7ᵗʰ **S06.344** **Traumatic hemorrhage of right cerebrum with loss of consciousness of 6 hours to 24 hours** HCC

---

2   HCC with 7th character indicating initial encounter (A or B - specific to category) OR sequela.

☑ Additional Character Req   ✓ₓ7ᵗʰ Placeholder Alert   Manifestation   HCC CMS-HCC Condition   ▽ Unspecified Code   ▶◀ Revised Text   ● New Code   ▲ Revised Code Title

2 ✓7ᵗʰ **S06.345** Traumatic hemorrhage of right [HCC]
cerebrum with loss of consciousness
**greater than 24 hours with return to
pre-existing conscious level**

2 ✓7ᵗʰ **S06.346** Traumatic hemorrhage of right [HCC]
cerebrum with loss of consciousness
**greater than 24 hours without return to
pre-existing conscious level with patient
surviving**

✓7ᵗʰ **S06.347** Traumatic hemorrhage of right cerebrum
with loss of consciousness of **any duration
with death due to brain injury prior to
regaining consciousness**

✓7ᵗʰ **S06.348** Traumatic hemorrhage of right cerebrum
with loss of consciousness of **any duration
with death due to other cause prior to
regaining consciousness**

2 ✓7ᵗʰ **S06.349** Traumatic hemorrhage of right [HCC] ▽
cerebrum with loss of consciousness of
unspecified duration
Traumatic hemorrhage of right cerebrum
NOS

✓6ᵗʰ **S06.35** Traumatic hemorrhage of **left cerebrum**
Traumatic intracerebral hemorrhage and hematoma
of left cerebrum

2 ✓7ᵗʰ **S06.350** Traumatic hemorrhage of left [HCC]
cerebrum **without loss of consciousness**

2 ✓7ᵗʰ **S06.351** Traumatic hemorrhage of left [HCC]
cerebrum with loss of consciousness
of 30 minutes or less

2 ✓7ᵗʰ **S06.352** Traumatic hemorrhage of left [HCC]
cerebrum with loss of consciousness
of 31 minutes to 59 minutes

2 ✓7ᵗʰ **S06.353** Traumatic hemorrhage of left [HCC]
cerebrum with loss of consciousness
of 1 hours to 5 hours 59 minutes

2 ✓7ᵗʰ **S06.354** Traumatic hemorrhage of left [HCC]
cerebrum with loss of consciousness
of 6 hours to 24 hours

2 ✓7ᵗʰ **S06.355** Traumatic hemorrhage of left [HCC]
cerebrum with loss of consciousness
**greater than 24 hours with return to
pre-existing conscious level**

2 ✓7ᵗʰ **S06.356** Traumatic hemorrhage of left [HCC]
cerebrum with loss of consciousness
**greater than 24 hours without return
to pre-existing conscious level with
patient surviving**

✓7ᵗʰ **S06.357** Traumatic hemorrhage of left cerebrum
with loss of consciousness of **any duration
with death due to brain injury prior to
regaining consciousness**

✓7ᵗʰ **S06.358** Traumatic hemorrhage of left cerebrum
with loss of consciousness of **any duration
with death due to other cause prior to
regaining consciousness**

2 ✓7ᵗʰ **S06.359** Traumatic hemorrhage of left [HCC] ▽
cerebrum with loss of consciousness
of **unspecified duration**
Traumatic hemorrhage of left cerebrum
NOS

✓6ᵗʰ **S06.36** Traumatic hemorrhage of **cerebrum, unspecified**
Traumatic intracerebral hemorrhage and hematoma,
unspecified

2 ✓7ᵗʰ **S06.360** Traumatic hemorrhage of [HCC] ▽
cerebrum, unspecified, **without
loss of consciousness**

2 ✓7ᵗʰ **S06.361** Traumatic hemorrhage of [HCC] ▽
cerebrum, unspecified, with loss of
consciousness **of 30 minutes or less**

2 ✓7ᵗʰ **S06.362** Traumatic hemorrhage of [HCC] ▽
cerebrum, unspecified, with loss of
consciousness **of 31 minutes to
59 minutes**

2 ✓7ᵗʰ **S06.363** Traumatic hemorrhage of [HCC] ▽
cerebrum, unspecified, with loss of
consciousness of **1 hours to
5 hours 59 minutes**

2 ✓7ᵗʰ **S06.364** Traumatic hemorrhage of [HCC] ▽
cerebrum, unspecified, with loss of
consciousness **of 6 hours to 24 hours**

2 ✓7ᵗʰ **S06.365** Traumatic hemorrhage of [HCC] ▽
cerebrum, unspecified, with loss of
consciousness **greater than 24 hours
with return to pre-existing conscious level**

2 ✓7ᵗʰ **S06.366** Traumatic hemorrhage of [HCC] ▽
cerebrum, unspecified, with loss of
consciousness **greater than 24 hours
without return to pre-existing conscious
level with patient surviving**

✓7ᵗʰ **S06.367** Traumatic hemorrhage of ▽
cerebrum, unspecified, with loss of
consciousness of **any duration with death
due to brain injury prior to regaining
consciousness**

✓7ᵗʰ **S06.368** Traumatic hemorrhage of ▽
cerebrum, unspecified, with loss of
consciousness of **any duration with
death due to other cause prior to
regaining consciousness**

2 ✓7ᵗʰ **S06.369** Traumatic hemorrhage of [HCC] ▽
cerebrum, unspecified, with loss of
consciousness of **unspecified duration**
Traumatic hemorrhage of cerebrum NOS

✓6ᵗʰ **S06.37** Contusion, laceration, and hemorrhage of
cerebellum

2 ✓7ᵗʰ **S06.370** Contusion, laceration, and [HCC]
hemorrhage of cerebellum **without
loss of consciousness**

2 ✓7ᵗʰ **S06.371** Contusion, laceration, and [HCC]
hemorrhage of cerebellum with loss
of consciousness **of 30 minutes or less**

2 ✓7ᵗʰ **S06.372** Contusion, laceration, and [HCC]
hemorrhage of cerebellum with
loss of consciousness **of 31 minutes
to 59 minutes**

2 ✓7ᵗʰ **S06.373** Contusion, laceration, and [HCC]
hemorrhage of cerebellum with
loss of consciousness **of 1 hour to
5 hours 59 minutes**

2 ✓7ᵗʰ **S06.374** Contusion, laceration, and [HCC]
hemorrhage of cerebellum with
loss of consciousness **of 6 hours
to 24 hours**

2 ✓7ᵗʰ **S06.375** Contusion, laceration, and [HCC]
hemorrhage of cerebellum with
loss of consciousness **greater than
24 hours with return to pre-existing
conscious level**

2 ✓7ᵗʰ **S06.376** Contusion, laceration, and [HCC]
hemorrhage of cerebellum with loss
of consciousness **greater than 24 hours
without return to pre-existing conscious
level with patient surviving**

✓7ᵗʰ **S06.377** Contusion, laceration, and hemorrhage of
cerebellum with loss of consciousness of
**any duration with death due to brain
injury prior to regaining consciousness**

✓7ᵗʰ **S06.378** Contusion, laceration, and hemorrhage of
cerebellum with loss of consciousness of
**any duration with death due to other
cause prior to regaining consciousness**

2 ✓7ᵗʰ **S06.379** Contusion, laceration, and [HCC] ▽
hemorrhage of cerebellum with loss
of consciousness of **unspecified duration**
Contusion, laceration, and hemorrhage of
cerebellum NOS

✓6ᵗʰ **S06.38** Contusion, laceration, and hemorrhage of **brainstem**

2 ✓7ᵗʰ **S06.380** Contusion, laceration, and [HCC]
hemorrhage of brainstem **without
loss of consciousness**

2 ✓7ᵗʰ **S06.381** Contusion, laceration, and [HCC]
hemorrhage of brainstem with loss of
consciousness **of 30 minutes or less**

2 ✓7ᵗʰ **S06.382** Contusion, laceration, and [HCC]
hemorrhage of brainstem with loss of
consciousness **of 31 minutes to 59 minutes**

---

2 HCC with 7th character indicating initial encounter (A or B - specific to category) OR sequela.

| EXCLUDES 1 Not coded here | EXCLUDES 2 Not included here | N Newborn Age: 0 | P Pediatric Age: 0-17 | M Maternity Age: 12-55 | A Adult Age: 15-124 |

2 ✓7ᵗʰ S06.383 Contusion, laceration, and hemorrhage of brainstem with loss of consciousness of 1 hour to 5 hours 59 minutes HCC

2 ✓7ᵗʰ S06.384 Contusion, laceration, and hemorrhage of brainstem with loss of consciousness of 6 hours to 24 hours HCC

2 ✓7ᵗʰ S06.385 Contusion, laceration, and hemorrhage of brainstem with loss of consciousness greater than 24 hours with return to pre-existing conscious level HCC

2 ✓7ᵗʰ S06.386 Contusion, laceration, and hemorrhage of brainstem with loss of consciousness greater than 24 hours without return to pre-existing conscious level with patient surviving HCC

✓7ᵗʰ S06.387 Contusion, laceration, and hemorrhage of brainstem with loss of consciousness of any duration with death due to brain injury prior to regaining consciousness

✓7ᵗʰ S06.388 Contusion, laceration, and hemorrhage of brainstem with loss of consciousness of any duration with death due to other cause prior to regaining consciousness

2 ✓7ᵗʰ S06.389 Contusion, laceration, and hemorrhage of brainstem with loss of consciousness of unspecified duration HCC ▽
Contusion, laceration, and hemorrhage of brainstem NOS

✓5ᵗʰ S06.4 Epidural hemorrhage
Extradural hemorrhage NOS
Extradural hemorrhage (traumatic)

✓6ᵗʰ S06.4X Epidural hemorrhage

2 ✓7ᵗʰ S06.4X0 Epidural hemorrhage without loss of consciousness HCC

2 ✓7ᵗʰ S06.4X1 Epidural hemorrhage with loss of consciousness of 30 minutes or less HCC

2 ✓7ᵗʰ S06.4X2 Epidural hemorrhage with loss of consciousness of 31 minutes to 59 minutes HCC

2 ✓7ᵗʰ S06.4X3 Epidural hemorrhage with loss of consciousness of 1 hour to 5 hours 59 minutes HCC

2 ✓7ᵗʰ S06.4X4 Epidural hemorrhage with loss of consciousness of 6 hours to 24 hours HCC

2 ✓7ᵗʰ S06.4X5 Epidural hemorrhage with loss of consciousness greater than 24 hours with return to pre-existing conscious level HCC

2 ✓7ᵗʰ S06.4X6 Epidural hemorrhage with loss of consciousness greater than 24 hours without return to pre-existing conscious level with patient surviving HCC

✓7ᵗʰ S06.4X7 Epidural hemorrhage with loss of consciousness of any duration with death due to brain injury prior to regaining consciousness

✓7ᵗʰ S06.4X8 Epidural hemorrhage with loss of consciousness of any duration with death due to other causes prior to regaining consciousness

2 ✓7ᵗʰ S06.4X9 Epidural hemorrhage with loss of consciousness of unspecified duration HCC ▽
Epidural hemorrhage NOS

✓5ᵗʰ S06.5 Traumatic subdural hemorrhage

✓6ᵗʰ S06.5X Traumatic subdural hemorrhage

2 ✓7ᵗʰ S06.5X0 Traumatic subdural hemorrhage without loss of consciousness HCC

2 ✓7ᵗʰ S06.5X1 Traumatic subdural hemorrhage with loss of consciousness of 30 minutes or less HCC

2 ✓7ᵗʰ S06.5X2 Traumatic subdural hemorrhage with loss of consciousness of 31 minutes to 59 minutes HCC

2 ✓7ᵗʰ S06.5X3 Traumatic subdural hemorrhage with loss of consciousness of 1 hour to 5 hours 59 minutes HCC

2 ✓7ᵗʰ S06.5X4 Traumatic subdural hemorrhage with loss of consciousness of 6 hours to 24 hours HCC

2 ✓7ᵗʰ S06.5X5 Traumatic subdural hemorrhage with loss of consciousness greater than 24 hours with return to pre-existing conscious level HCC

2 ✓7ᵗʰ S06.5X6 Traumatic subdural hemorrhage with loss of consciousness greater than 24 hours without return to pre-existing conscious level with patient surviving HCC

✓7ᵗʰ S06.5X7 Traumatic subdural hemorrhage with loss of consciousness of any duration with death due to brain injury before regaining consciousness

✓7ᵗʰ S06.5X8 Traumatic subdural hemorrhage with loss of consciousness of any duration with death due to other cause before regaining consciousness

2 ✓7ᵗʰ S06.5X9 Traumatic subdural hemorrhage with loss of consciousness of unspecified duration HCC ▽
Traumatic subdural hemorrhage NOS

✓5ᵗʰ S06.6 Traumatic subarachnoid hemorrhage

✓6ᵗʰ S06.6X Traumatic subarachnoid hemorrhage

2 ✓7ᵗʰ S06.6X0 Traumatic subarachnoid hemorrhage without loss of consciousness HCC

2 ✓7ᵗʰ S06.6X1 Traumatic subarachnoid hemorrhage with loss of consciousness of 30 minutes or less HCC

2 ✓7ᵗʰ S06.6X2 Traumatic subarachnoid hemorrhage with loss of consciousness of 31 minutes to 59 minutes HCC

2 ✓7ᵗʰ S06.6X3 Traumatic subarachnoid hemorrhage with loss of consciousness of 1 hour to 5 hours 59 minutes HCC

2 ✓7ᵗʰ S06.6X4 Traumatic subarachnoid hemorrhage with loss of consciousness of 6 hours to 24 hours HCC

2 ✓7ᵗʰ S06.6X5 Traumatic subarachnoid hemorrhage with loss of consciousness greater than 24 hours with return to pre-existing conscious level HCC

2 ✓7ᵗʰ S06.6X6 Traumatic subarachnoid hemorrhage with loss of consciousness greater than 24 hours without return to pre-existing conscious level with patient surviving HCC

✓7ᵗʰ S06.6X7 Traumatic subarachnoid hemorrhage with loss of consciousness of any duration with death due to brain injury prior to regaining consciousness

✓7ᵗʰ S06.6X8 Traumatic subarachnoid hemorrhage with loss of consciousness of any duration with death due to other cause prior to regaining consciousness

2 ✓7ᵗʰ S06.6X9 Traumatic subarachnoid hemorrhage with loss of consciousness of unspecified duration HCC ▽
Traumatic subarachnoid hemorrhage NOS

✓5ᵗʰ S06.8 Other specified intracranial injuries

✓6ᵗʰ S06.81 Injury of right internal carotid artery, intracranial portion, not elsewhere classified

2 ✓7ᵗʰ S06.810 Injury of right internal carotid artery, intracranial portion, not elsewhere classified without loss of consciousness HCC

2 ✓7ᵗʰ S06.811 Injury of right internal carotid artery, intracranial portion, not elsewhere classified with loss of consciousness of 30 minutes or less HCC

2 ✓7ᵗʰ S06.812 Injury of right internal carotid artery, intracranial portion, not elsewhere classified with loss of consciousness of 31 minutes to 59 minutes HCC

2 ✓7ᵗʰ S06.813 Injury of right internal carotid artery, intracranial portion, not elsewhere classified with loss of consciousness of 1 hour to 5 hours 59 minutes HCC

---

2   HCC with 7th character indicating initial encounter (A or B - specific to category) OR sequela.

✓ Additional Character Req   ✓x7ᵗʰ Placeholder Alert   Manifestation   HCC CMS-HCC Condition   ▽ Unspecified Code   ►◄ Revised Text   ● New Code   ▲ Revised Code Title

Chapter 19. Injury, Poisoning, and Certain Other Consequences of External Causes

2 √7ᵗʰ **S06.814** **Injury of right internal carotid artery, intracranial portion, not elsewhere classified with loss of consciousness of 6 hours to 24 hours** HCC

2 √7ᵗʰ **S06.815** **Injury of right internal carotid artery, intracranial portion, not elsewhere classified with loss of consciousness greater than 24 hours with return to pre-existing conscious level** HCC

2 √7ᵗʰ **S06.816** **Injury of right internal carotid artery, intracranial portion, not elsewhere classified with loss of consciousness greater than 24 hours without return to pre-existing conscious level with patient surviving** HCC

√7ᵗʰ **S06.817** **Injury of right internal carotid artery, intracranial portion, not elsewhere classified with loss of consciousness of any duration with death due to brain injury prior to regaining consciousness**

√7ᵗʰ **S06.818** **Injury of right internal carotid artery, intracranial portion, not elsewhere classified with loss of consciousness of any duration with death due to other cause prior to regaining consciousness**

2 √7ᵗʰ **S06.819** **Injury of right internal carotid artery, intracranial portion, not elsewhere classified with loss of consciousness of unspecified duration** HCC ▽
Injury of right internal carotid artery, intracranial portion, not elsewhere classified NOS

√6ᵗʰ **S06.82** **Injury of left internal carotid artery, intracranial portion, not elsewhere classified**

2 √7ᵗʰ **S06.820** **Injury of left internal carotid artery, intracranial portion, not elsewhere classified without loss of consciousness** HCC

2 √7ᵗʰ **S06.821** **Injury of left internal carotid artery, intracranial portion, not elsewhere classified with loss of consciousness of 30 minutes or less** HCC

2 √7ᵗʰ **S06.822** **Injury of left internal carotid artery, intracranial portion, not elsewhere classified with loss of consciousness of 31 minutes to 59 minutes** HCC

2 √7ᵗʰ **S06.823** **Injury of left internal carotid artery, intracranial portion, not elsewhere classified with loss of consciousness of 1 hour to 5 hours 59 minutes** HCC

2 √7ᵗʰ **S06.824** **Injury of left internal carotid artery, intracranial portion, not elsewhere classified with loss of consciousness of 6 hours to 24 hours** HCC

2 √7ᵗʰ **S06.825** **Injury of left internal carotid artery, intracranial portion, not elsewhere classified with loss of consciousness greater than 24 hours with return to pre-existing conscious level** HCC

2 √7ᵗʰ **S06.826** **Injury of left internal carotid artery, intracranial portion, not elsewhere classified with loss of consciousness greater than 24 hours without return to pre-existing conscious level with patient surviving** HCC

√7ᵗʰ **S06.827** **Injury of left internal carotid artery, intracranial portion, not elsewhere classified with loss of consciousness of any duration with death due to brain injury prior to regaining consciousness**

√7ᵗʰ **S06.828** **Injury of left internal carotid artery, intracranial portion, not elsewhere classified with loss of consciousness of any duration with death due to other cause prior to regaining consciousness**

2 √7ᵗʰ **S06.829** **Injury of left internal carotid artery, intracranial portion, not elsewhere classified with loss of consciousness of unspecified duration** HCC ▽
Injury of left internal carotid artery, intracranial portion, not elsewhere classified NOS

√6ᵗʰ **S06.89** **Other specified intracranial injury**
EXCLUDES 1 concussion (S06.0X-)

2 √7ᵗʰ **S06.890** **Other specified intracranial injury without loss of consciousness** HCC

2 √7ᵗʰ **S06.891** **Other specified intracranial injury with loss of consciousness of 30 minutes or less** HCC

2 √7ᵗʰ **S06.892** **Other specified intracranial injury with loss of consciousness of 31 minutes to 59 minutes** HCC

2 √7ᵗʰ **S06.893** **Other specified intracranial injury with loss of consciousness of 1 hour to 5 hours 59 minutes** HCC

2 √7ᵗʰ **S06.894** **Other specified intracranial injury with loss of consciousness of 6 hours to 24 hours** HCC

2 √7ᵗʰ **S06.895** **Other specified intracranial injury with loss of consciousness greater t han 24 hours with return to pre-existing conscious level** HCC

2 √7ᵗʰ **S06.896** **Other specified intracranial injury with loss of consciousness greater than 24 hours without return to pre-existing conscious level with patient surviving** HCC

√7ᵗʰ **S06.897** **Other specified intracranial injury with loss of consciousness of any duration with death due to brain injury prior to regaining consciousness**

√7ᵗʰ **S06.898** **Other specified intracranial injury with loss of consciousness of any duration with death due to other cause prior to regaining consciousness**

2 √7ᵗʰ **S06.899** **Other specified intracranial injury with loss of consciousness of unspecified duration** HCC ▽

√5ᵗʰ **S06.9** **Unspecified intracranial injury**
Brain injury NOS
Head injury NOS with loss of consciousness
Traumatic brain injury NOS
EXCLUDES 1 conditions classifiable to S06.0- to S06.8- code to specified intracranial injury
head injury NOS (S09.90)

√6ᵗʰ **S06.9X** **Unspecified intracranial injury**

2 √7ᵗʰ **S06.9X0** **Unspecified intracranial injury without loss of consciousness** HCC ▽

2 √7ᵗʰ **S06.9X1** **Unspecified intracranial injury with loss of consciousness of 30 minutes or less** HCC ▽

2 √7ᵗʰ **S06.9X2** **Unspecified intracranial injury with loss of consciousness of 31 minutes to 59 minutes** HCC ▽

2 √7ᵗʰ **S06.9X3** **Unspecified intracranial injury with loss of consciousness of 1 hour to 5 hours 59 minutes** HCC ▽

2 √7ᵗʰ **S06.9X4** **Unspecified intracranial injury with loss of consciousness of 6 hours to 24 hours** HCC ▽

2 √7ᵗʰ **S06.9X5** **Unspecified intracranial injury with loss of consciousness greater than 24 hours with return to pre-existing conscious level** HCC ▽

2 √7ᵗʰ **S06.9X6** **Unspecified intracranial injury with loss of consciousness greater than 24 hours without return to pre-existing conscious level with patient surviving** HCC ▽

√7ᵗʰ **S06.9X7** **Unspecified intracranial injury with loss of consciousness of any duration with death due to brain injury prior to regaining consciousness** ▽

√7ᵗʰ **S06.9X8** **Unspecified intracranial injury with loss of consciousness of any duration with death due to other cause prior to regaining consciousness** ▽

2 √7ᵗʰ **S06.9X9** **Unspecified intracranial injury with loss of consciousness of unspecified duration** HCC ▽

---

2   HCC with 7th character indicating initial encounter (A or B - specific to category) OR sequela.

EXCLUDES 1 Not coded here   *EXCLUDES 2* Not included here   N Newborn Age: 0   P Pediatric Age: 0-17   M Maternity Age: 12-55   A Adult Age: 15-124

924   ICD-10-CM 2018

☑4th **S07** **Crushing injury of head**
> Use additional code for all associated injuries, such as:
> intracranial injuries (S06.-)
> skull fractures (S02.-)

> The appropriate 7th character is to be added to each code from category S07.
> A   initial encounter
> D   subsequent encounter
> S   sequela

☑x7th **S07.0** **Crushing injury of face**
☑x7th **S07.1** **Crushing injury of skull**
☑x7th **S07.8** **Crushing injury of other parts of head**
☑x7th **S07.9** **Crushing injury of head, part unspecified** ▽

☑4th **S08** **Avulsion and traumatic amputation of part of head**
> An amputation not identified as partial or complete should be coded to complete

> The appropriate 7th character is to be added to each code from category S08.
> A   initial encounter
> D   subsequent encounter
> S   sequela

☑x7th **S08.0** **Avulsion of scalp**
☑5th **S08.1** **Traumatic amputation of ear**
    ☑6th **S08.11** **Complete traumatic amputation of ear**
        ☑7th **S08.111** **Complete traumatic amputation of right ear**
        ☑7th **S08.112** **Complete traumatic amputation of left ear**
        ☑7th **S08.119** **Complete traumatic amputation of unspecified ear** ▽
    ☑6th **S08.12** **Partial traumatic amputation of ear**
        ☑7th **S08.121** **Partial traumatic amputation of right ear**
        ☑7th **S08.122** **Partial traumatic amputation of left ear**
        ☑7th **S08.129** **Partial traumatic amputation of unspecified ear** ▽
☑5th **S08.8** **Traumatic amputation of other parts of head**
    ☑6th **S08.81** **Traumatic amputation of nose**
        ☑7th **S08.811** **Complete traumatic amputation of nose**
        ☑7th **S08.812** **Partial traumatic amputation of nose**
    ☑x7th **S08.89** **Traumatic amputation of other parts of head**

☑4th **S09** **Other and unspecified injuries of head**
> The appropriate 7th character is to be added to each code from category S09.
> A   initial encounter
> D   subsequent encounter
> S   sequela

☑x7th **S09.0** **Injury of blood vessels of head, not elsewhere classified**
    EXCLUDES1 *injury of cerebral blood vessels (S06.-)*
        injury of precerebral blood vessels (S15.-)
☑5th **S09.1** **Injury of muscle and tendon of head**
    Code also any associated open wound (S01.-)
    EXCLUDES2 *sprain to joints and ligament of head (S03.9)*
    ☑x7th **S09.10** **Unspecified injury of muscle and tendon of head** ▽
        Injury of muscle and tendon of head NOS
    ☑x7th **S09.11** **Strain of muscle and tendon of head**
    ☑x7th **S09.12** **Laceration of muscle and tendon of head**
    ☑x7th **S09.19** **Other specified injury of muscle and tendon of head**
☑5th **S09.2** **Traumatic rupture of ear drum**
    EXCLUDES1 *traumatic rupture of ear drum due to blast injury (S09.31-)*
    ☑x7th **S09.20** **Traumatic rupture of unspecified ear drum** ▽
    ☑x7th **S09.21** **Traumatic rupture of right ear drum**
    ☑x7th **S09.22** **Traumatic rupture of left ear drum**
☑5th **S09.3** **Other specified and unspecified injury of middle and inner ear**
    EXCLUDES1 *injury to ear NOS (S09.91-)*
    EXCLUDES2 *injury to external ear (S00.4-, S01.3-, S08.1-)*
    ☑6th **S09.30** **Unspecified injury of middle and inner ear**
        ☑7th **S09.301** **Unspecified injury of right middle and inner ear** ▽

        ☑7th **S09.302** **Unspecified injury of left middle and inner ear** ▽
        ☑7th **S09.309** **Unspecified injury of unspecified middle and inner ear** ▽
    ☑6th **S09.31** **Primary blast injury of ear**
        Blast injury of ear NOS
        ☑7th **S09.311** **Primary blast injury of right ear**
        ☑7th **S09.312** **Primary blast injury of left ear**
        ☑7th **S09.313** **Primary blast injury of ear, bilateral**
        ☑7th **S09.319** **Primary blast injury of unspecified ear**
    ☑6th **S09.39** **Other specified injury of middle and inner ear**
        Secondary blast injury to ear
        ☑7th **S09.391** **Other specified injury of right middle and inner ear**
        ☑7th **S09.392** **Other specified injury of left middle and inner ear**
        ☑7th **S09.399** **Other specified injury of unspecified middle and inner ear** ▽
☑x7th **S09.8** **Other specified injuries of head**
☑5th **S09.9** **Unspecified injury of face and head**
    ☑x7th **S09.90** **Unspecified injury of head** ▽
        Head injury NOS
        EXCLUDES1 *brain injury NOS (S06.9-)*
            head injury NOS with loss of consciousness (S06.9-)
            intracranial injury NOS (S06.9-)
    ☑x7th **S09.91** **Unspecified injury of ear** ▽
        Injury of ear NOS
    ☑x7th **S09.92** **Unspecified injury of nose** ▽
        Injury of nose NOS
    ☑x7th **S09.93** **Unspecified injury of face** ▽
        Injury of face NOS

Injuries to the neck (S10-S19)

INCLUDES injuries of nape
    injuries of supraclavicular region
    injuries of throat
EXCLUDES2 *burns and corrosions (T20-T32)*
    effects of foreign body in esophagus (T18.1)
    effects of foreign body in larynx (T17.3)
    effects of foreign body in pharynx (T17.2)
    effects of foreign body in trachea (T17.4)
    frostbite (T33-T34)
    insect bite or sting, venomous (T63.4)

☑4th **S10** **Superficial injury of neck**
> The appropriate 7th character is to be added to each code from category S10.
> A   initial encounter
> D   subsequent encounter
> S   sequela

☑x7th **S10.0** **Contusion of throat**
    Contusion of cervical esophagus
    Contusion of larynx
    Contusion of pharynx
    Contusion of trachea
☑5th **S10.1** **Other and unspecified superficial injuries of throat**
    ☑x7th **S10.10** **Unspecified superficial injuries of throat** ▽
    ☑x7th **S10.11** **Abrasion of throat**
    ☑x7th **S10.12** **Blister (nonthermal) of throat**
    ☑x7th **S10.14** **External constriction of part of throat**
    ☑x7th **S10.15** **Superficial foreign body of throat**
        Splinter in the throat
    ☑x7th **S10.16** **Insect bite (nonvenomous) of throat**
    ☑x7th **S10.17** **Other superficial bite of throat**
        EXCLUDES1 *open bite of throat (S11.85)*
☑5th **S10.8** **Superficial injury of other specified parts of neck**
    ☑x7th **S10.80** **Unspecified superficial injury of other specified part of neck** ▽
    ☑x7th **S10.81** **Abrasion of other specified part of neck**
    ☑x7th **S10.82** **Blister (nonthermal) of other specified part of neck**
    ☑x7th **S10.83** **Contusion of other specified part of neck**
    ☑x7th **S10.84** **External constriction of other specified part of neck**

☑ Additional Character Req   ☑x7th Placeholder Alert   Manifestation   HCC CMS-HCC Condition   ▽ Unspecified Code   ►◄ Revised Text   ● New Code   ▲ Revised Code Title

ICD-10-CM 2018   925

√x7ᵗʰ **S10.85** **Superficial foreign body** of other specified part of neck
Splinter in other specified part of neck

√x7ᵗʰ **S10.86** **Insect bite** of other specified part of neck

√x7ᵗʰ **S10.87** **Other superficial bite** of other specified part of neck
EXCLUDES 1   *open bite of other specified parts of neck (S11.85)*

√5ᵗʰ **S10.9** **Superficial injury of unspecified part of neck**

√x7ᵗʰ **S10.90** **Unspecified superficial injury** of unspecified part of neck   ▽

√x7ᵗʰ **S10.91** **Abrasion** of unspecified part of neck   ▽

√x7ᵗʰ **S10.92** **Blister** (nonthermal) of unspecified part of neck   ▽

√x7ᵗʰ **S10.93** **Contusion** of unspecified part of neck   ▽

√x7ᵗʰ **S10.94** **External constriction** of unspecified part of neck   ▽

√x7ᵗʰ **S10.95** **Superficial foreign body** of unspecified part of neck   ▽

√x7ᵗʰ **S10.96** **Insect bite** of unspecified part of neck   ▽

√x7ᵗʰ **S10.97** **Other superficial bite** of unspecified part of neck   ▽

√4ᵗʰ **S11** **Open wound of neck**
Code also any associated:
spinal cord injury (S14.0, S14.1-)
wound infection
EXCLUDES 2   *open fracture of vertebra (S12- with 7th character B)*

> The appropriate 7th character is to be added to each code from category S11.
> A   initial encounter
> D   subsequent encounter
> S   sequela

√5ᵗʰ **S11.0** **Open wound of larynx and trachea**

√6ᵗʰ **S11.01** **Open wound of larynx**
EXCLUDES 2   *open wound of vocal cord (S11.03)*

√7ᵗʰ **S11.011** **Laceration without foreign body of larynx**

√7ᵗʰ **S11.012** **Laceration with foreign body of larynx**

√7ᵗʰ **S11.013** **Puncture wound without foreign body of larynx**

√7ᵗʰ **S11.014** **Puncture wound with foreign body of larynx**

√7ᵗʰ **S11.015** **Open bite of larynx**
Bite of larynx NOS

√7ᵗʰ **S11.019** **Unspecified open wound of larynx**   ▽

√6ᵗʰ **S11.02** **Open wound of trachea**
Open wound of cervical trachea
Open wound of trachea NOS
EXCLUDES 2   *open wound of thoracic trachea (S27.5-)*

√7ᵗʰ **S11.021** **Laceration without foreign body of trachea**

√7ᵗʰ **S11.022** **Laceration with foreign body of trachea**

√7ᵗʰ **S11.023** **Puncture wound without foreign body of trachea**

√7ᵗʰ **S11.024** **Puncture wound with foreign body of trachea**

√7ᵗʰ **S11.025** **Open bite of trachea**
Bite of trachea NOS

√7ᵗʰ **S11.029** **Unspecified open wound of trachea**   ▽

√6ᵗʰ **S11.03** **Open wound of vocal cord**

√7ᵗʰ **S11.031** **Laceration without foreign body of vocal cord**

√7ᵗʰ **S11.032** **Laceration with foreign body of vocal cord**

√7ᵗʰ **S11.033** **Puncture wound without foreign body of vocal cord**

√7ᵗʰ **S11.034** **Puncture wound with foreign body of vocal cord**

√7ᵗʰ **S11.035** **Open bite of vocal cord**
Bite of vocal cord NOS

√7ᵗʰ **S11.039** **Unspecified open wound of vocal cord**   ▽

√5ᵗʰ **S11.1** **Open wound of thyroid gland**

√x7ᵗʰ **S11.10** **Unspecified open wound of thyroid gland**   ▽

√x7ᵗʰ **S11.11** **Laceration without foreign body of thyroid gland**

√x7ᵗʰ **S11.12** **Laceration with foreign body of thyroid gland**

√x7ᵗʰ **S11.13** **Puncture wound without foreign body of thyroid gland**

√x7ᵗʰ **S11.14** **Puncture wound with foreign body of thyroid gland**

√x7ᵗʰ **S11.15** **Open bite of thyroid gland**
Bite of thyroid gland NOS

√5ᵗʰ **S11.2** **Open wound of pharynx and cervical esophagus**
EXCLUDES 1   *open wound of esophagus NOS (S27.8-)*

√x7ᵗʰ **S11.20** **Unspecified open wound of pharynx and cervical esophagus**   ▽

√x7ᵗʰ **S11.21** **Laceration without foreign body of pharynx and cervical esophagus**

√x7ᵗʰ **S11.22** **Laceration with foreign body of pharynx and cervical esophagus**

√x7ᵗʰ **S11.23** **Puncture wound without foreign body of pharynx and cervical esophagus**

√x7ᵗʰ **S11.24** **Puncture wound with foreign body of pharynx and cervical esophagus**

√x7ᵗʰ **S11.25** **Open bite of pharynx and cervical esophagus**
Bite of pharynx and cervical esophagus NOS

√5ᵗʰ **S11.8** **Open wound of other specified parts of neck**

√x7ᵗʰ **S11.80** **Unspecified open wound of other specified part of neck**   ▽

√x7ᵗʰ **S11.81** **Laceration without foreign body of other specified part of neck**

√x7ᵗʰ **S11.82** **Laceration with foreign body of other specified part of neck**

√x7ᵗʰ **S11.83** **Puncture wound without foreign body of other specified part of neck**

√x7ᵗʰ **S11.84** **Puncture wound with foreign body of other specified part of neck**

√x7ᵗʰ **S11.85** **Open bite of other specified part of neck**
Bite of other specified part of neck NOS
EXCLUDES 1   *superficial bite of other specified part of neck (S10.87)*

√x7ᵗʰ **S11.89** **Other open wound of other specified part of neck**

√5ᵗʰ **S11.9** **Open wound of unspecified part of neck**

√x7ᵗʰ **S11.90** **Unspecified open wound of unspecified part of neck**   ▽

√x7ᵗʰ **S11.91** **Laceration without foreign body of unspecified part of neck**   ▽

√x7ᵗʰ **S11.92** **Laceration with foreign body of unspecified part of neck**   ▽

√x7ᵗʰ **S11.93** **Puncture wound without foreign body of unspecified part of neck**   ▽

√x7ᵗʰ **S11.94** **Puncture wound with foreign body of unspecified part of neck**   ▽

√x7ᵗʰ **S11.95** **Open bite of unspecified part of neck**   ▽
Bite of neck NOS
EXCLUDES 1   *superficial bite of neck (S10.97)*

√4ᵗʰ **S12** **Fracture of cervical vertebra and other parts of neck**
NOTE   A fracture not indicated as nondisplaced or displaced should be coded to displaced.
A fracture not indicated as open or closed should be coded to closed.
INCLUDES   fracture of cervical neural arch
fracture of cervical spine
fracture of cervical spinous process
fracture of cervical transverse process
fracture of cervical vertebral arch
fracture of neck
Code first any associated cervical spinal cord injury (S14.0, S14.1-)
AHA: 2015, 3Q, 37-39

> The appropriate 7th character is to be added to all codes from subcategories S12.0-S12.6.
> A   initial encounter for closed fracture
> B   initial encounter for open fracture
> D   subsequent encounter for fracture with routine healing
> G   subsequent encounter for fracture with delayed healing
> K   subsequent encounter for fracture with nonunion
> S   sequela

√5ᵗʰ **S12.0** **Fracture of first cervical vertebra**
Atlas

√6ᵗʰ **S12.00** **Unspecified fracture of first cervical vertebra**

[1] √7ᵗʰ **S12.000** **Unspecified displaced fracture of first cervical vertebra**   HCC ▽

---

[1] HCC with 7th character indicating initial encounter (A, B or C - specific to category).

EXCLUDES 1 Not coded here   EXCLUDES 2 Not included here   N Newborn Age: 0   P Pediatric Age: 0-17   M Maternity Age: 12-55   A Adult Age: 15-124

926   ICD-10-CM 2018

1 ✓7ᵗʰ **S12.001** Unspecified **nondisplaced** fracture of first cervical vertebra `HCC` ▽

1 ✓x7ᵗʰ **S12.01** **Stable burst** fracture of first cervical vertebra `HCC`

1 ✓x7ᵗʰ **S12.02** **Unstable burst** fracture of first cervical vertebra `HCC`

✓6ᵗʰ **S12.03** **Posterior arch** fracture of first cervical vertebra

1 ✓7ᵗʰ **S12.030** **Displaced** posterior arch fracture of first cervical vertebra `HCC`

1 ✓7ᵗʰ **S12.031** **Nondisplaced** posterior arch fracture of first cervical vertebra `HCC`

✓6ᵗʰ **S12.04** **Lateral mass** fracture of first cervical vertebra

1 ✓7ᵗʰ **S12.040** **Displaced** lateral mass fracture of first cervical vertebra `HCC`

1 ✓7ᵗʰ **S12.041** **Nondisplaced** lateral mass fracture of first cervical vertebra `HCC`

✓6ᵗʰ **S12.09** Other fracture of first cervical vertebra

1 ✓7ᵗʰ **S12.090** Other **displaced** fracture of first cervical vertebra `HCC`

1 ✓7ᵗʰ **S12.091** Other **nondisplaced** fracture of first cervical vertebra `HCC`

✓5ᵗʰ **S12.1** Fracture of **second** cervical vertebra
Axis

✓6ᵗʰ **S12.10** Unspecified fracture of second cervical vertebra

1 ✓7ᵗʰ **S12.100** Unspecified **displaced** fracture of second cervical vertebra `HCC` ▽

1 ✓7ᵗʰ **S12.101** Unspecified **nondisplaced** fracture of second cervical vertebra `HCC` ▽

✓6ᵗʰ **S12.11** **Type II dens** fracture

1 ✓7ᵗʰ **S12.110** **Anterior displaced** Type II dens fracture `HCC`

1 ✓7ᵗʰ **S12.111** **Posterior displaced** Type II dens fracture `HCC`

1 ✓7ᵗʰ **S12.112** **Nondisplaced** Type II dens fracture `HCC`

✓6ᵗʰ **S12.12** Other dens fracture

1 ✓7ᵗʰ **S12.120** Other **displaced** dens fracture `HCC`

1 ✓7ᵗʰ **S12.121** Other **nondisplaced** dens fracture `HCC`

✓6ᵗʰ **S12.13** Unspecified traumatic **spondylolisthesis** of second cervical vertebra

1 ✓7ᵗʰ **S12.130** Unspecified traumatic **displaced** spondylolisthesis of second cervical vertebra `HCC` ▽

1 ✓7ᵗʰ **S12.131** Unspecified traumatic **nondisplaced** spondylolisthesis of second cervical vertebra `HCC` ▽

1 ✓x7ᵗʰ **S12.14** **Type III** traumatic **spondylolisthesis** of second cervical vertebra `HCC`

✓6ᵗʰ **S12.15** Other traumatic **spondylolisthesis** of second cervical vertebra

1 ✓7ᵗʰ **S12.150** Other traumatic **displaced** spondylolisthesis of second cervical vertebra `HCC`

1 ✓7ᵗʰ **S12.151** Other traumatic **nondisplaced** spondylolisthesis of second cervical vertebra `HCC`

✓6ᵗʰ **S12.19** Other fracture of second cervical vertebra

1 ✓7ᵗʰ **S12.190** Other **displaced** fracture of second cervical vertebra `HCC`

1 ✓7ᵗʰ **S12.191** Other **nondisplaced** fracture of second cervical vertebra `HCC`

✓5ᵗʰ **S12.2** Fracture of **third** cervical vertebra

✓6ᵗʰ **S12.20** Unspecified fracture of third cervical vertebra

1 ✓7ᵗʰ **S12.200** Unspecified **displaced** fracture of third cervical vertebra `HCC` ▽

1 ✓7ᵗʰ **S12.201** Unspecified **nondisplaced** fracture of third cervical vertebra `HCC` ▽

✓6ᵗʰ **S12.23** Unspecified traumatic **spondylolisthesis** of third cervical vertebra

1 ✓7ᵗʰ **S12.230** Unspecified traumatic **displaced** spondylolisthesis of third cervical vertebra `HCC` ▽

1 ✓7ᵗʰ **S12.231** Unspecified traumatic **nondisplaced** spondylolisthesis of third cervical vertebra `HCC` ▽

1 ✓x7ᵗʰ **S12.24** **Type III** traumatic **spondylolisthesis** of third cervical vertebra `HCC`

✓6ᵗʰ **S12.25** Other traumatic spondylolisthesis of third cervical vertebra

1 ✓7ᵗʰ **S12.250** Other traumatic **displaced** spondylolisthesis of third cervical vertebra `HCC`

1 ✓7ᵗʰ **S12.251** Other traumatic **nondisplaced** spondylolisthesis of third cervical vertebra `HCC`

✓6ᵗʰ **S12.29** Other fracture of third cervical vertebra

1 ✓7ᵗʰ **S12.290** Other **displaced** fracture of third cervical vertebra `HCC`

1 ✓7ᵗʰ **S12.291** Other **nondisplaced** fracture of third cervical vertebra `HCC`

✓5ᵗʰ **S12.3** Fracture of **fourth** cervical vertebra

✓6ᵗʰ **S12.30** Unspecified fracture of fourth cervical vertebra

1 ✓7ᵗʰ **S12.300** Unspecified **displaced** fracture of fourth cervical vertebra `HCC` ▽

1 ✓7ᵗʰ **S12.301** Unspecified **nondisplaced** fracture of fourth cervical vertebra `HCC` ▽

✓6ᵗʰ **S12.33** Unspecified traumatic **spondylolisthesis** of fourth cervical vertebra

1 ✓7ᵗʰ **S12.330** Unspecified traumatic **displaced** spondylolisthesis of fourth cervical vertebra `HCC` ▽

1 ✓7ᵗʰ **S12.331** Unspecified traumatic **nondisplaced** spondylolisthesis of fourth cervical vertebra `HCC` ▽

1 ✓x7ᵗʰ **S12.34** **Type III** traumatic **spondylolisthesis** of fourth cervical vertebra `HCC`

✓6ᵗʰ **S12.35** Other traumatic spondylolisthesis of fourth cervical vertebra

1 ✓7ᵗʰ **S12.350** Other traumatic **displaced** spondylolisthesis of fourth cervical vertebra `HCC`

1 ✓7ᵗʰ **S12.351** Other traumatic **nondisplaced** spondylolisthesis of fourth cervical vertebra `HCC`

✓6ᵗʰ **S12.39** Other fracture of fourth cervical vertebra

1 ✓7ᵗʰ **S12.390** Other **displaced** fracture of fourth cervical vertebra `HCC`

1 ✓7ᵗʰ **S12.391** Other **nondisplaced** fracture of fourth cervical vertebra `HCC`

✓5ᵗʰ **S12.4** Fracture of **fifth** cervical vertebra

✓6ᵗʰ **S12.40** Unspecified fracture of fifth cervical vertebra

1 ✓7ᵗʰ **S12.400** Unspecified **displaced** fracture of fifth cervical vertebra `HCC` ▽

1 ✓7ᵗʰ **S12.401** Unspecified **nondisplaced** fracture of fifth cervical vertebra `HCC` ▽

✓6ᵗʰ **S12.43** Unspecified traumatic **spondylolisthesis** of fifth cervical vertebra

1 ✓7ᵗʰ **S12.430** Unspecified traumatic **displaced** spondylolisthesis of fifth cervical vertebra `HCC` ▽

1 ✓7ᵗʰ **S12.431** Unspecified traumatic **nondisplaced** spondylolisthesis of fifth cervical vertebra `HCC` ▽

1 ✓x7ᵗʰ **S12.44** **Type III** traumatic **spondylolisthesis** of fifth cervical vertebra `HCC`

✓6ᵗʰ **S12.45** Other traumatic **spondylolisthesis** of fifth cervical vertebra

1 ✓7ᵗʰ **S12.450** Other traumatic **displaced** spondylolisthesis of fifth cervical vertebra `HCC`

1 ✓7ᵗʰ **S12.451** Other traumatic **nondisplaced** spondylolisthesis of fifth cervical vertebra `HCC`

✓6ᵗʰ **S12.49** Other fracture of fifth cervical vertebra

1 ✓7ᵗʰ **S12.490** Other **displaced** fracture of fifth cervical vertebra `HCC`

1 ✓7ᵗʰ **S12.491** Other **nondisplaced** fracture of fifth cervical vertebra `HCC`

---

1 HCC with 7th character indicating initial encounter (A, B or C - specific to category).

✓ Additional Character Req   ✓7ᵗʰ Placeholder Alert   Manifestation   `HCC` CMS-HCC Condition   ▽ Unspecified Code   ►◄ Revised Text   ● New Code   ▲ Revised Code Title

Chapter 19. Injury, Poisoning, and Certain Other Consequences of External Causes *(left margin)*

S12.5–S13.4 *(left margin bottom)*

✓5ᵗʰ S12.5   Fracture of sixth cervical vertebra

✓6ᵗʰ **S12.50**   Unspecified fracture of sixth cervical vertebra

1   ✓7ᵗʰ **S12.500**   Unspecified displaced fracture of sixth cervical vertebra   HCC ▽

1   ✓7ᵗʰ **S12.501**   Unspecified nondisplaced fracture of sixth cervical vertebra   HCC ▽

✓6ᵗʰ **S12.53**   Unspecified traumatic spondylolisthesis of sixth cervical vertebra

1   ✓7ᵗʰ **S12.530**   Unspecified traumatic displaced spondylolisthesis of sixth cervical vertebra   HCC ▽

1   ✓7ᵗʰ **S12.531**   Unspecified traumatic nondisplaced spondylolisthesis of sixth cervical vertebra   HCC ▽

1   ✓x7ᵗʰ **S12.54**   Type III traumatic spondylolisthesis of sixth cervical vertebra   HCC

✓6ᵗʰ **S12.55**   Other traumatic spondylolisthesis of sixth cervical vertebra

1   ✓7ᵗʰ **S12.550**   Other traumatic displaced spondylolisthesis of sixth cervical vertebra   HCC

1   ✓7ᵗʰ **S12.551**   Other traumatic nondisplaced spondylolisthesis of sixth cervical vertebra   HCC

✓6ᵗʰ **S12.59**   Other fracture of sixth cervical vertebra

1   ✓7ᵗʰ **S12.590**   Other displaced fracture of sixth cervical vertebra   HCC

1   ✓7ᵗʰ **S12.591**   Other nondisplaced fracture of sixth cervical vertebra   HCC

✓5ᵗʰ S12.6   Fracture of seventh cervical vertebra

✓6ᵗʰ **S12.60**   Unspecified fracture of seventh cervical vertebra

1   ✓7ᵗʰ **S12.600**   Unspecified displaced fracture of seventh cervical vertebra   HCC ▽

1   ✓7ᵗʰ **S12.601**   Unspecified nondisplaced fracture of seventh cervical vertebra   HCC ▽

✓6ᵗʰ **S12.63**   Unspecified traumatic spondylolisthesis of seventh cervical vertebra

1   ✓7ᵗʰ **S12.630**   Unspecified traumatic displaced spondylolisthesis of seventh cervical vertebra   HCC ▽

1   ✓7ᵗʰ **S12.631**   Unspecified traumatic nondisplaced spondylolisthesis of seventh cervical vertebra   HCC ▽

1   ✓x7ᵗʰ **S12.64**   Type III traumatic spondylolisthesis of seventh cervical vertebra   HCC

✓6ᵗʰ **S12.65**   Other traumatic spondylolisthesis of seventh cervical vertebra

1   ✓7ᵗʰ **S12.650**   Other traumatic displaced spondylolisthesis of seventh cervical vertebra   HCC

1   ✓7ᵗʰ **S12.651**   Other traumatic nondisplaced spondylolisthesis of seventh cervical vertebra   HCC

✓6ᵗʰ **S12.69**   Other fracture of seventh cervical vertebra

1   ✓7ᵗʰ **S12.690**   Other displaced fracture of seventh cervical vertebra   HCC

1   ✓7ᵗʰ **S12.691**   Other nondisplaced fracture of seventh cervical vertebra   HCC

1   ✓x7ᵗʰ S12.8   Fracture of other parts of neck   HCC

Hyoid bone   Thyroid cartilage
Larynx   Trachea

> The appropriate 7th character is to be added to code S12.8.
> A   initial encounter
> D   subsequent encounter
> S   sequela

1   ✓x7ᵗʰ S12.9   Fracture of neck, unspecified   HCC ▽

Fracture of cervical spine NOS
Fracture of cervical vertebra NOS
Fracture of neck NOS

> The appropriate 7th character is to be added to code S12.9.
> A   initial encounter
> D   subsequent encounter
> S   sequela

✓4ᵗʰ S13   Dislocation and sprain of joints and ligaments at neck level

INCLUDES   avulsion of joint or ligament at neck level
laceration of cartilage, joint or ligament at neck level
sprain of cartilage, joint or ligament at neck level
traumatic hemarthrosis of joint or ligament at neck level
traumatic rupture of joint or ligament at neck level
traumatic subluxation of joint or ligament at neck level
traumatic tear of joint or ligament at neck level

Code also any associated open wound

EXCLUDES 2   strain of muscle or tendon at neck level (S16.1)

> The appropriate 7th character is to be added to each code from category S13.
> A   initial encounter
> D   subsequent encounter
> S   sequela

✓x7ᵗʰ **S13.0**   Traumatic rupture of cervical intervertebral disc

EXCLUDES 1   rupture or displacement (nontraumatic) of cervical intervertebral disc NOS (M50.-)

✓5ᵗʰ **S13.1**   Subluxation and dislocation of cervical vertebrae

Code also any associated:
   open wound of neck (S11.-)
   spinal cord injury (S14.1-)

EXCLUDES 2   fracture of cervical vertebrae (S12.0--S12.3-)

✓6ᵗʰ **S13.10**   Subluxation and dislocation of unspecified cervical vertebrae

✓7ᵗʰ **S13.100**   Subluxation of unspecified cervical vertebrae   ▽

✓7ᵗʰ **S13.101**   Dislocation of unspecified cervical vertebrae   ▽

✓6ᵗʰ **S13.11**   Subluxation and dislocation of C0/C1 cervical vertebrae

Subluxation and dislocation of atlantooccipital joint
Subluxation and dislocation of atloidooccipital joint
Subluxation and dislocation of occipitoatloid joint

✓7ᵗʰ **S13.110**   Subluxation of C0/C1 cervical vertebrae

✓7ᵗʰ **S13.111**   Dislocation of C0/C1 cervical vertebrae

✓6ᵗʰ **S13.12**   Subluxation and dislocation of C1/C2 cervical vertebrae

Subluxation and dislocation of atlantoaxial joint

✓7ᵗʰ **S13.120**   Subluxation of C1/C2 cervical vertebrae

✓7ᵗʰ **S13.121**   Dislocation of C1/C2 cervical vertebrae

✓6ᵗʰ **S13.13**   Subluxation and dislocation of C2/C3 cervical vertebrae

✓7ᵗʰ **S13.130**   Subluxation of C2/C3 cervical vertebrae

✓7ᵗʰ **S13.131**   Dislocation of C2/C3 cervical vertebrae

✓6ᵗʰ **S13.14**   Subluxation and dislocation of C3/C4 cervical vertebrae

✓7ᵗʰ **S13.140**   Subluxation of C3/C4 cervical vertebrae

✓7ᵗʰ **S13.141**   Dislocation of C3/C4 cervical vertebrae

✓6ᵗʰ **S13.15**   Subluxation and dislocation of C4/C5 cervical vertebrae

✓7ᵗʰ **S13.150**   Subluxation of C4/C5 cervical vertebrae

✓7ᵗʰ **S13.151**   Dislocation of C4/C5 cervical vertebrae

✓6ᵗʰ **S13.16**   Subluxation and dislocation of C5/C6 cervical vertebrae

✓7ᵗʰ **S13.160**   Subluxation of C5/C6 cervical vertebrae

✓7ᵗʰ **S13.161**   Dislocation of C5/C6 cervical vertebrae

✓6ᵗʰ **S13.17**   Subluxation and dislocation of C6/C7 cervical vertebrae

✓7ᵗʰ **S13.170**   Subluxation of C6/C7 cervical vertebrae

✓7ᵗʰ **S13.171**   Dislocation of C6/C7 cervical vertebrae

✓6ᵗʰ **S13.18**   Subluxation and dislocation of C7/T1 cervical vertebrae

✓7ᵗʰ **S13.180**   Subluxation of C7/T1 cervical vertebrae

✓7ᵗʰ **S13.181**   Dislocation of C7/T1 cervical vertebrae

✓5ᵗʰ **S13.2**   Dislocation of other and unspecified parts of neck

✓x7ᵗʰ **S13.20**   Dislocation of unspecified parts of neck   ▽

✓x7ᵗʰ **S13.29**   Dislocation of other parts of neck

✓x7ᵗʰ **S13.4**   Sprain of ligaments of cervical spine

Sprain of anterior longitudinal (ligament), cervical
Sprain of atlanto-axial (joints)
Sprain of atlanto-occipital (joints)
Whiplash injury of cervical spine

---

1   HCC with 7th character indicating initial encounter (A, B or C - specific to category).

EXCLUDES 1 Not coded here   **EXCLUDES 2** Not included here   N Newborn Age: 0   P Pediatric Age: 0-17   M Maternity Age: 12-55   A Adult Age: 15-124

928   ICD-10-CM 2018

√7th **S13.5   Sprain of thyroid region**
Sprain of cricoarytenoid (joint) (ligament)
Sprain of cricothyroid (joint) (ligament)
Sprain of thyroid cartilage

√7th **S13.8   Sprain of joints and ligaments of other parts of neck**

√7th **S13.9   Sprain of joints and ligaments of unspecified parts of neck** ▽

√4th **S14   Injury of nerves and spinal cord at neck level**
> **NOTE**   Code to highest level of cervical cord injury.

Code also any associated:
   fracture of cervical vertebra (S12.0- -S12.6-)
   open wound of neck (S11.-)
   transient paralysis (R29.5)

> The appropriate 7th character is to be added to each code from category S14.
> A   initial encounter
> D   subsequent encounter
> S   sequela

√7th **S14.0   Concussion and edema of cervical spinal cord**   HCC

√5th **S14.1   Other and unspecified injuries of cervical spinal cord**

  √6th **S14.10   Unspecified injury of cervical spinal cord**

    √7th **S14.101   Unspecified injury at C1 level of cervical spinal cord**   HCC ▽

    √7th **S14.102   Unspecified injury at C2 level of cervical spinal cord**   HCC ▽

    √7th **S14.103   Unspecified injury at C3 level of cervical spinal cord**   HCC ▽

    √7th **S14.104   Unspecified injury at C4 level of cervical spinal cord**   HCC ▽

    √7th **S14.105   Unspecified injury at C5 level of cervical spinal cord**   HCC ▽

    √7th **S14.106   Unspecified injury at C6 level of cervical spinal cord**   HCC ▽

    √7th **S14.107   Unspecified injury at C7 level of cervical spinal cord**   HCC ▽

    √7th **S14.108   Unspecified injury at C8 level of cervical spinal cord**   HCC ▽

    √7th **S14.109   Unspecified injury at unspecified level of cervical spinal cord**   HCC ▽
       Injury of cervical spinal cord NOS

  √6th **S14.11   Complete lesion of cervical spinal cord**

    √7th **S14.111   Complete lesion at C1 level of cervical spinal cord**   HCC

    √7th **S14.112   Complete lesion at C2 level of cervical spinal cord**   HCC

    √7th **S14.113   Complete lesion at C3 level of cervical spinal cord**   HCC

    √7th **S14.114   Complete lesion at C4 level of cervical spinal cord**   HCC

    √7th **S14.115   Complete lesion at C5 level of cervical spinal cord**   HCC

    √7th **S14.116   Complete lesion at C6 level of cervical spinal cord**   HCC

    √7th **S14.117   Complete lesion at C7 level of cervical spinal cord**   HCC

    √7th **S14.118   Complete lesion at C8 level of cervical spinal cord**   HCC

    √7th **S14.119   Complete lesion at unspecified level of cervical spinal cord**   HCC ▽

  √6th **S14.12   Central cord syndrome of cervical spinal cord**

    √7th **S14.121   Central cord syndrome at C1 level of cervical spinal cord**   HCC

    √7th **S14.122   Central cord syndrome at C2 level of cervical spinal cord**   HCC

    √7th **S14.123   Central cord syndrome at C3 level of cervical spinal cord**   HCC

    √7th **S14.124   Central cord syndrome at C4 level of cervical spinal cord**   HCC

    √7th **S14.125   Central cord syndrome at C5 level of cervical spinal cord**   HCC

    √7th **S14.126   Central cord syndrome at C6 level of cervical spinal cord**   HCC

    √7th **S14.127   Central cord syndrome at C7 level of cervical spinal cord**   HCC

    √7th **S14.128   Central cord syndrome at C8 level of cervical spinal cord**   HCC

    √7th **S14.129   Central cord syndrome at unspecified level of cervical spinal cord**   HCC ▽

  √6th **S14.13   Anterior cord syndrome of cervical spinal cord**

    √7th **S14.131   Anterior cord syndrome at C1 level of cervical spinal cord**   HCC

    √7th **S14.132   Anterior cord syndrome at C2 level of cervical spinal cord**   HCC

    √7th **S14.133   Anterior cord syndrome at C3 level of cervical spinal cord**   HCC

    √7th **S14.134   Anterior cord syndrome at C4 level of cervical spinal cord**   HCC

    √7th **S14.135   Anterior cord syndrome at C5 level of cervical spinal cord**   HCC

    √7th **S14.136   Anterior cord syndrome at C6 level of cervical spinal cord**   HCC

    √7th **S14.137   Anterior cord syndrome at C7 level of cervical spinal cord**   HCC

    √7th **S14.138   Anterior cord syndrome at C8 level of cervical spinal cord**   HCC

    √7th **S14.139   Anterior cord syndrome at unspecified level of cervical spinal cord**   HCC ▽

  √6th **S14.14   Brown-Séquard syndrome of cervical spinal cord**

    √7th **S14.141   Brown-Séquard syndrome at C1 level of cervical spinal cord**   HCC

    √7th **S14.142   Brown-Séquard syndrome at C2 level of cervical spinal cord**   HCC

    √7th **S14.143   Brown-Séquard syndrome at C3 level of cervical spinal cord**   HCC

    √7th **S14.144   Brown-Séquard syndrome at C4 level of cervical spinal cord**   HCC

    √7th **S14.145   Brown-Séquard syndrome at C5 level of cervical spinal cord**   HCC

    √7th **S14.146   Brown-Séquard syndrome at C6 level of cervical spinal cord**   HCC

    √7th **S14.147   Brown-Séquard syndrome at C7 level of cervical spinal cord**   HCC

    √7th **S14.148   Brown-Séquard syndrome at C8 level of cervical spinal cord**   HCC

    √7th **S14.149   Brown-Séquard syndrome at unspecified level of cervical spinal cord**   HCC ▽

  √6th **S14.15   Other incomplete lesions of cervical spinal cord**
    Incomplete lesion of cervical spinal cord NOS
    Posterior cord syndrome of cervical spinal cord

    √7th **S14.151   Other incomplete lesion at C1 level of cervical spinal cord**   HCC

    √7th **S14.152   Other incomplete lesion at C2 level of cervical spinal cord**   HCC

    √7th **S14.153   Other incomplete lesion at C3 level of cervical spinal cord**   HCC

    √7th **S14.154   Other incomplete lesion at C4 level of cervical spinal cord**   HCC

    √7th **S14.155   Other incomplete lesion at C5 level of cervical spinal cord**   HCC

    √7th **S14.156   Other incomplete lesion at C6 level of cervical spinal cord**   HCC

    √7th **S14.157   Other incomplete lesion at C7 level of cervical spinal cord**   HCC

    √7th **S14.158   Other incomplete lesion at C8 level of cervical spinal cord**   HCC

    √7th **S14.159   Other incomplete lesion at unspecified level of cervical spinal cord**   HCC ▽

√7th **S14.2   Injury of nerve root of cervical spine**

√7th **S14.3   Injury of brachial plexus**

√7th **S14.4   Injury of peripheral nerves of neck**

√7th **S14.5   Injury of cervical sympathetic nerves**

√7th **S14.8   Injury of other specified nerves of neck**

√7th **S14.9   Injury of unspecified nerves of neck**   ▽

☑ Additional Character Req   √x7th Placeholder Alert   Manifestation   HCC CMS-HCC Condition   ▽ Unspecified Code   ►◄ Revised Text   ● New Code   ▲ Revised Code Title

√4th S15 Injury of blood vessels at neck level

Code also any associated open wound (S11.-)

> The appropriate 7th character is to be added to each code from category S15.
> A   initial encounter
> D   subsequent encounter
> S   sequela

√5th S15.0 Injury of carotid artery of neck

Injury of carotid artery (common) (external) (internal, extracranial portion)
Injury of carotid artery NOS

> *EXCLUDES 1*   injury of internal carotid artery, intracranial portion (S06.8)

√6th S15.00 Unspecified injury of carotid artery

- √7th **S15.001** Unspecified injury of right carotid artery ▽
- √7th **S15.002** Unspecified injury of left carotid artery ▽
- √7th **S15.009** Unspecified injury of unspecified carotid artery ▽

√6th S15.01 Minor laceration of carotid artery

Incomplete transection of carotid artery
Laceration of carotid artery NOS
Superficial laceration of carotid artery

- √7th **S15.011** Minor laceration of right carotid artery
- √7th **S15.012** Minor laceration of left carotid artery
- √7th **S15.019** Minor laceration of unspecified carotid artery ▽

√6th S15.02 Major laceration of carotid artery

Complete transection of carotid artery
Traumatic rupture of carotid artery

- √7th **S15.021** Major laceration of right carotid artery
- √7th **S15.022** Major laceration of left carotid artery
- √7th **S15.029** Major laceration of unspecified carotid artery ▽

√6th S15.09 Other specified injury of carotid artery

- √7th **S15.091** Other specified injury of right carotid artery
- √7th **S15.092** Other specified injury of left carotid artery
- √7th **S15.099** Other specified injury of unspecified carotid artery ▽

√5th S15.1 Injury of vertebral artery

√6th S15.10 Unspecified injury of vertebral artery

- √7th **S15.101** Unspecified injury of right vertebral artery ▽
- √7th **S15.102** Unspecified injury of left vertebral artery ▽
- √7th **S15.109** Unspecified injury of unspecified vertebral artery ▽

√6th S15.11 Minor laceration of vertebral artery

Incomplete transection of vertebral artery
Laceration of vertebral artery NOS
Superficial laceration of vertebral artery

- √7th **S15.111** Minor laceration of right vertebral artery
- √7th **S15.112** Minor laceration of left vertebral artery
- √7th **S15.119** Minor laceration of unspecified vertebral artery ▽

√6th S15.12 Major laceration of vertebral artery

Complete transection of vertebral artery
Traumatic rupture of vertebral artery

- √7th **S15.121** Major laceration of right vertebral artery
- √7th **S15.122** Major laceration of left vertebral artery
- √7th **S15.129** Major laceration of unspecified vertebral artery ▽

√6th S15.19 Other specified injury of vertebral artery

- √7th **S15.191** Other specified injury of right vertebral artery
- √7th **S15.192** Other specified injury of left vertebral artery
- √7th **S15.199** Other specified injury of unspecified vertebral artery ▽

√5th S15.2 Injury of external jugular vein

√6th S15.20 Unspecified injury of external jugular vein

- √7th **S15.201** Unspecified injury of right external jugular vein ▽
- √7th **S15.202** Unspecified injury of left external jugular vein ▽
- √7th **S15.209** Unspecified injury of unspecified external jugular vein ▽

√6th S15.21 Minor laceration of external jugular vein

Incomplete transection of external jugular vein
Laceration of external jugular vein NOS
Superficial laceration of external jugular vein

- √7th **S15.211** Minor laceration of right external jugular vein
- √7th **S15.212** Minor laceration of left external jugular vein
- √7th **S15.219** Minor laceration of unspecified external jugular vein ▽

√6th S15.22 Major laceration of external jugular vein

Complete transection of external jugular vein
Traumatic rupture of external jugular vein

- √7th **S15.221** Major laceration of right external jugular vein
- √7th **S15.222** Major laceration of left external jugular vein
- √7th **S15.229** Major laceration of unspecified external jugular vein ▽

√6th S15.29 Other specified injury of external jugular vein

- √7th **S15.291** Other specified injury of right external jugular vein
- √7th **S15.292** Other specified injury of left external jugular vein
- √7th **S15.299** Other specified injury of unspecified external jugular vein

√5th S15.3 Injury of internal jugular vein

√6th S15.30 Unspecified injury of internal jugular vein

- √7th **S15.301** Unspecified injury of right internal jugular vein ▽
- √7th **S15.302** Unspecified injury of left internal jugular vein ▽
- √7th **S15.309** Unspecified injury of unspecified internal jugular vein ▽

√6th S15.31 Minor laceration of internal jugular vein

Incomplete transection of internal jugular vein
Laceration of internal jugular vein NOS
Superficial laceration of internal jugular vein

- √7th **S15.311** Minor laceration of right internal jugular vein
- √7th **S15.312** Minor laceration of left internal jugular vein
- √7th **S15.319** Minor laceration of unspecified internal jugular vein ▽

√6th S15.32 Major laceration of internal jugular vein

Complete transection of internal jugular vein
Traumatic rupture of internal jugular vein

- √7th **S15.321** Major laceration of right internal jugular vein
- √7th **S15.322** Major laceration of left internal jugular vein
- √7th **S15.329** Major laceration of unspecified internal jugular vein ▽

√6th S15.39 Other specified injury of internal jugular vein

- √7th **S15.391** Other specified injury of right internal jugular vein
- √7th **S15.392** Other specified injury of left internal jugular vein
- √7th **S15.399** Other specified injury of unspecified internal jugular vein ▽

√x7th **S15.8 Injury of other specified blood vessels at neck level**

√x7th **S15.9 Injury of unspecified blood vessel at neck level** ▽

EXCLUDES 1 Not coded here   *EXCLUDES 2* Not included here   **N** Newborn Age: 0   **P** Pediatric Age: 0-17   **M** Maternity Age: 12-55   **A** Adult Age: 15-124

930   ICD-10-CM 2018

☑4ᵗʰ **S16 Injury of muscle, fascia and tendon at neck level**
Code also any associated open wound (S11.-)
EXCLUDES 2 sprain of joint or ligament at neck level (S13.9)

The appropriate 7th character is to be added to each code from category S16.
A   initial encounter
D   subsequent encounter
S   sequela

√x7ᵗʰ **S16.1 Strain of muscle, fascia and tendon at neck level**

√x7ᵗʰ **S16.2 Laceration of muscle, fascia and tendon at neck level**

√x7ᵗʰ **S16.8 Other specified injury of muscle, fascia and tendon at neck level**

√x7ᵗʰ **S16.9 Unspecified injury of muscle, fascia and tendon at neck level** ▽

☑4ᵗʰ **S17 Crushing injury of neck**
Use additional code for all associated injuries, such as:
injury of blood vessels (S15.-)
open wound of neck (S11.-)
spinal cord injury (S14.0, S14.1-)
vertebral fracture (S12.0- -S12.3-)

The appropriate 7th character is to be added to each code from category S17.
A   initial encounter
D   subsequent encounter
S   sequela

√x7ᵗʰ **S17.0 Crushing injury of larynx and trachea**

√x7ᵗʰ **S17.8 Crushing injury of other specified parts of neck**

√x7ᵗʰ **S17.9 Crushing injury of neck, part unspecified** ▽

☑4ᵗʰ **S19 Other specified and unspecified injuries of neck**

The appropriate 7th character is to be added to each code from category S19.
A   initial encounter
D   subsequent encounter
S   sequela

√5ᵗʰ **S19.8 Other specified injuries of neck**

√x7ᵗʰ **S19.80 Other specified injuries of unspecified part of neck** ▽

√x7ᵗʰ **S19.81 Other specified injuries of larynx**

√x7ᵗʰ **S19.82 Other specified injuries of cervical trachea**
EXCLUDES 2 other specified injury of thoracic trachea (S27.5-)

√x7ᵗʰ **S19.83 Other specified injuries of vocal cord**

√x7ᵗʰ **S19.84 Other specified injuries of thyroid gland**

√x7ᵗʰ **S19.85 Other specified injuries of pharynx and cervical esophagus**

√x7ᵗʰ **S19.89 Other specified injuries of other specified part of neck**

√x7ᵗʰ **S19.9 Unspecified injury of neck** ▽

Injuries to the thorax (S20-S29)

INCLUDES injuries of breast
injuries of chest (wall)
injuries of interscapular area
EXCLUDES 2 burns and corrosions (T20-T32)
effects of foreign body in bronchus (T17.5)
effects of foreign body in esophagus (T18.1)
effects of foreign body in lung (T17.8)
effects of foreign body in trachea (T17.4)
frostbite (T33-T34)
injuries of axilla
injuries of clavicle
injuries of scapular region
injuries of shoulder
insect bite or sting, venomous (T63.4)

☑4ᵗʰ **S20 Superficial injury of thorax**

The appropriate 7th character is to be added to each code from category S20.
A   initial encounter
D   subsequent encounter
S   sequela

√5ᵗʰ **S20.0 Contusion of breast**

√x7ᵗʰ **S20.00 Contusion of breast, unspecified breast** ▽

√x7ᵗʰ **S20.01 Contusion of right breast**

√x7ᵗʰ **S20.02 Contusion of left breast**

√5ᵗʰ **S20.1 Other and unspecified superficial injuries of breast**

√6ᵗʰ **S20.10 Unspecified superficial injuries of breast**

√7ᵗʰ **S20.101 Unspecified superficial injuries of breast, right breast** ▽

√7ᵗʰ **S20.102 Unspecified superficial injuries of breast, left breast** ▽

√7ᵗʰ **S20.109 Unspecified superficial injuries of breast, unspecified breast** ▽

√6ᵗʰ **S20.11 Abrasion of breast**

√7ᵗʰ **S20.111 Abrasion of breast, right breast**

√7ᵗʰ **S20.112 Abrasion of breast, left breast**

√7ᵗʰ **S20.119 Abrasion of breast, unspecified breast** ▽

√6ᵗʰ **S20.12 Blister (nonthermal) of breast**

√7ᵗʰ **S20.121 Blister (nonthermal) of breast, right breast**

√7ᵗʰ **S20.122 Blister (nonthermal) of breast, left breast**

√7ᵗʰ **S20.129 Blister (nonthermal) of breast, unspecified breast** ▽

√6ᵗʰ **S20.14 External constriction of part of breast**

√7ᵗʰ **S20.141 External constriction of part of breast, right breast**

√7ᵗʰ **S20.142 External constriction of part of breast, left breast**

√7ᵗʰ **S20.149 External constriction of part of breast, unspecified breast** ▽

√6ᵗʰ **S20.15 Superficial foreign body of breast**
Splinter in the breast

√7ᵗʰ **S20.151 Superficial foreign body of breast, right breast**

√7ᵗʰ **S20.152 Superficial foreign body of breast, left breast**

√7ᵗʰ **S20.159 Superficial foreign body of breast, unspecified breast** ▽

√6ᵗʰ **S20.16 Insect bite (nonvenomous) of breast**

√7ᵗʰ **S20.161 Insect bite (nonvenomous) of breast, right breast**

√7ᵗʰ **S20.162 Insect bite (nonvenomous) of breast, left breast**

√7ᵗʰ **S20.169 Insect bite (nonvenomous) of breast, unspecified breast** ▽

√6ᵗʰ **S20.17 Other superficial bite of breast**
EXCLUDES 1 open bite of breast (S21.05-)

√7ᵗʰ **S20.171 Other superficial bite of breast, right breast**

√7ᵗʰ **S20.172 Other superficial bite of breast, left breast**

√7ᵗʰ **S20.179 Other superficial bite of breast, unspecified breast** ▽

√5ᵗʰ **S20.2 Contusion of thorax**

√x7ᵗʰ **S20.20 Contusion of thorax, unspecified** ▽

√6ᵗʰ **S20.21 Contusion of front wall of thorax**

√7ᵗʰ **S20.211 Contusion of right front wall of thorax**

√7ᵗʰ **S20.212 Contusion of left front wall of thorax**

√7ᵗʰ **S20.219 Contusion of unspecified front wall of thorax** ▽

√6ᵗʰ **S20.22 Contusion of back wall of thorax**

√7ᵗʰ **S20.221 Contusion of right back wall of thorax**

√7ᵗʰ **S20.222 Contusion of left back wall of thorax**

√7ᵗʰ **S20.229 Contusion of unspecified back wall of thorax** ▽

√5ᵗʰ **S20.3 Other and unspecified superficial injuries of front wall of thorax**

√6ᵗʰ **S20.30 Unspecified superficial injuries of front wall of thorax**

√7ᵗʰ **S20.301 Unspecified superficial injuries of right front wall of thorax** ▽

√7ᵗʰ **S20.302 Unspecified superficial injuries of left front wall of thorax** ▽

√7ᵗʰ **S20.309 Unspecified superficial injuries of unspecified front wall of thorax** ▽

√6ᵗʰ **S20.31 Abrasion of front wall of thorax**

√7ᵗʰ **S20.311 Abrasion of right front wall of thorax**

√7ᵗʰ **S20.312 Abrasion of left front wall of thorax**

√7ᵗʰ **S20.319** Abrasion of unspecified front wall of thorax ▽

√6ᵗʰ **S20.32** Blister (nonthermal) of front wall of thorax

   √7ᵗʰ **S20.321** Blister (nonthermal) of right front wall of thorax

   √7ᵗʰ **S20.322** Blister (nonthermal) of left front wall of thorax

   √7ᵗʰ **S20.329** Blister (nonthermal) of unspecified front wall of thorax ▽

√6ᵗʰ **S20.34** External constriction of front wall of thorax

   √7ᵗʰ **S20.341** External constriction of right front wall of thorax

   √7ᵗʰ **S20.342** External constriction of left front wall of thorax

   √7ᵗʰ **S20.349** External constriction of unspecified front wall of thorax ▽

√6ᵗʰ **S20.35** Superficial foreign body of front wall of thorax
Splinter in front wall of thorax

   √7ᵗʰ **S20.351** Superficial foreign body of right front wall of thorax

   √7ᵗʰ **S20.352** Superficial foreign body of left front wall of thorax

   √7ᵗʰ **S20.359** Superficial foreign body of unspecified front wall of thorax ▽

√6ᵗʰ **S20.36** Insect bite (nonvenomous) of front wall of thorax

   √7ᵗʰ **S20.361** Insect bite (nonvenomous) of right front wall of thorax

   √7ᵗʰ **S20.362** Insect bite (nonvenomous) of left front wall of thorax

   √7ᵗʰ **S20.369** Insect bite (nonvenomous) of unspecified front wall of thorax ▽

√6ᵗʰ **S20.37** Other superficial bite of front wall of thorax
EXCLUDES 1   open bite of front wall of thorax (S21.14)

   √7ᵗʰ **S20.371** Other superficial bite of right front wall of thorax

   √7ᵗʰ **S20.372** Other superficial bite of left front wall of thorax

   √7ᵗʰ **S20.379** Other superficial bite of unspecified front wall of thorax ▽

√5ᵗʰ **S20.4** Other and unspecified superficial injuries of back wall of thorax

√6ᵗʰ **S20.40** Unspecified superficial injuries of back wall of thorax

   √7ᵗʰ **S20.401** Unspecified superficial injuries of right back wall of thorax ▽

   √7ᵗʰ **S20.402** Unspecified superficial injuries of left back wall of thorax ▽

   √7ᵗʰ **S20.409** Unspecified superficial injuries of unspecified back wall of thorax ▽

√6ᵗʰ **S20.41** Abrasion of back wall of thorax

   √7ᵗʰ **S20.411** Abrasion of right back wall of thorax

   √7ᵗʰ **S20.412** Abrasion of left back wall of thorax

   √7ᵗʰ **S20.419** Abrasion of unspecified back wall of thorax ▽

√6ᵗʰ **S20.42** Blister (nonthermal) of back wall of thorax

   √7ᵗʰ **S20.421** Blister (nonthermal) of right back wall of thorax

   √7ᵗʰ **S20.422** Blister (nonthermal) of left back wall of thorax

   √7ᵗʰ **S20.429** Blister (nonthermal) of unspecified back wall of thorax ▽

√6ᵗʰ **S20.44** External constriction of back wall of thorax

   √7ᵗʰ **S20.441** External constriction of right back wall of thorax

   √7ᵗʰ **S20.442** External constriction of left back wall of thorax

   √7ᵗʰ **S20.449** External constriction of unspecified back wall of thorax ▽

√6ᵗʰ **S20.45** Superficial foreign body of back wall of thorax
Splinter of back wall of thorax

   √7ᵗʰ **S20.451** Superficial foreign body of right back wall of thorax

√7ᵗʰ **S20.452** Superficial foreign body of left back wall of thorax

√7ᵗʰ **S20.459** Superficial foreign body of unspecified back wall of thorax ▽

√6ᵗʰ **S20.46** Insect bite (nonvenomous) of back wall of thorax

   √7ᵗʰ **S20.461** Insect bite (nonvenomous) of right back wall of thorax

   √7ᵗʰ **S20.462** Insect bite (nonvenomous) of left back wall of thorax

   √7ᵗʰ **S20.469** Insect bite (nonvenomous) of unspecified back wall of thorax ▽

√6ᵗʰ **S20.47** Other superficial bite of back wall of thorax
EXCLUDES 1   open bite of back wall of thorax (S21.24)

   √7ᵗʰ **S20.471** Other superficial bite of right back wall of thorax

   √7ᵗʰ **S20.472** Other superficial bite of left back wall of thorax

   √7ᵗʰ **S20.479** Other superficial bite of unspecified back wall of thorax ▽

√5ᵗʰ **S20.9** Superficial injury of unspecified parts of thorax
EXCLUDES 1   contusion of thorax NOS (S20.20)

√×7ᵗʰ **S20.90** Unspecified superficial injury of unspecified parts of thorax ▽
Superficial injury of thoracic wall NOS

√×7ᵗʰ **S20.91** Abrasion of unspecified parts of thorax ▽

√×7ᵗʰ **S20.92** Blister (nonthermal) of unspecified parts of thorax ▽

√×7ᵗʰ **S20.94** External constriction of unspecified parts of thorax ▽

√×7ᵗʰ **S20.95** Superficial foreign body of unspecified parts of thorax ▽
Splinter in thorax NOS

√×7ᵗʰ **S20.96** Insect bite (nonvenomous) of unspecified parts of thorax ▽

√×7ᵗʰ **S20.97** Other superficial bite of unspecified parts of thorax ▽
EXCLUDES 1   open bite of thorax NOS (S21.95)

√4ᵗʰ **S21** **Open wound of thorax**
Code also any associated injury, such as:
  injury of heart (S26.-)
  injury of intrathoracic organs (S27.-)
  rib fracture (S22.3-, S22.4-)
  spinal cord injury (S24.0-, S24.1-)
  traumatic hemopneumothorax (S27.3)
  traumatic hemothorax (S27.1)
  traumatic pneumothorax (S27.0)
  wound infection
EXCLUDES 1   traumatic amputation (partial) of thorax (S28.1)

> The appropriate 7th character is to be added to each code from category S21.
> A   initial encounter
> D   subsequent encounter
> S   sequela

√5ᵗʰ **S21.0** Open wound of breast

√6ᵗʰ **S21.00** Unspecified open wound of breast

   √7ᵗʰ **S21.001** Unspecified open wound of right breast ▽

   √7ᵗʰ **S21.002** Unspecified open wound of left breast ▽

   √7ᵗʰ **S21.009** Unspecified open wound of unspecified breast ▽

√6ᵗʰ **S21.01** Laceration without foreign body of breast

   √7ᵗʰ **S21.011** Laceration without foreign body of right breast

   √7ᵗʰ **S21.012** Laceration without foreign body of left breast

   √7ᵗʰ **S21.019** Laceration without foreign body of unspecified breast ▽

√6ᵗʰ **S21.02** Laceration with foreign body of breast

   √7ᵗʰ **S21.021** Laceration with foreign body of right breast

   √7ᵗʰ **S21.022** Laceration with foreign body of left breast

   √7ᵗʰ **S21.029** Laceration with foreign body of unspecified breast ▽

EXCLUDES 1 Not coded here   EXCLUDES 2 Not included here   N Newborn Age: 0   P Pediatric Age: 0-17   M Maternity Age: 12-55   A Adult Age: 15-124

932   ICD-10-CM 2018

√6ᵗʰ **S21.03** **Puncture wound without foreign body** of breast

    √7ᵗʰ **S21.031** **Puncture wound without foreign body** of **right** breast

    √7ᵗʰ **S21.032** **Puncture wound without foreign body** of **left** breast

    √7ᵗʰ **S21.039** **Puncture wound without foreign body of unspecified breast**   ▽

√6ᵗʰ **S21.04** **Puncture wound with foreign body** of breast

    √7ᵗʰ **S21.041** **Puncture wound with foreign body of right breast**

    √7ᵗʰ **S21.042** **Puncture wound with foreign body of left breast**

    √7ᵗʰ **S21.049** **Puncture wound with foreign body of unspecified breast**   ▽

√6ᵗʰ **S21.05** **Open bite** of breast

    Bite of breast NOS

    EXCLUDES 1   superficial bite of breast (S20.17)

    √7ᵗʰ **S21.051** **Open bite of right breast**

    √7ᵗʰ **S21.052** **Open bite of left breast**

    √7ᵗʰ **S21.059** **Open bite of unspecified breast**   ▽

√5ᵗʰ **S21.1** **Open wound of front wall of thorax without penetration** into thoracic cavity

    Open wound of chest without penetration into thoracic cavity

√6ᵗʰ **S21.10** **Unspecified open wound of front wall of thorax without penetration into thoracic cavity**

    √7ᵗʰ **S21.101** **Unspecified open wound of right front wall of thorax without penetration into thoracic cavity** ▽

    √7ᵗʰ **S21.102** **Unspecified open wound of left front wall of thorax without penetration into thoracic cavity** ▽

    √7ᵗʰ **S21.109** **Unspecified open wound of unspecified front wall of thorax without penetration into thoracic cavity** ▽

√6ᵗʰ **S21.11** **Laceration without foreign body** of front wall of thorax without penetration into thoracic cavity

    √7ᵗʰ **S21.111** **Laceration without foreign body of right front wall of thorax without penetration into thoracic cavity**

    √7ᵗʰ **S21.112** **Laceration without foreign body of left front wall of thorax without penetration into thoracic cavity**

    √7ᵗʰ **S21.119** **Laceration without foreign body of unspecified front wall of thorax without penetration into thoracic cavity** ▽

√6ᵗʰ **S21.12** **Laceration with foreign body** of front wall of thorax without penetration into thoracic cavity

    √7ᵗʰ **S21.121** **Laceration with foreign body of right front wall of thorax without penetration into thoracic cavity**

    √7ᵗʰ **S21.122** **Laceration with foreign body of left front wall of thorax without penetration into thoracic cavity**

    √7ᵗʰ **S21.129** **Laceration with foreign body of unspecified front wall of thorax without penetration into thoracic cavity** ▽

√6ᵗʰ **S21.13** **Puncture wound without foreign body** of front wall of thorax without penetration into thoracic cavity

    √7ᵗʰ **S21.131** **Puncture wound without foreign body of right front wall of thorax without penetration into thoracic cavity**

    √7ᵗʰ **S21.132** **Puncture wound without foreign body of left front wall of thorax without penetration into thoracic cavity**

    √7ᵗʰ **S21.139** **Puncture wound without foreign body of unspecified front wall of thorax without penetration into thoracic cavity** ▽

√6ᵗʰ **S21.14** **Puncture wound with foreign body** of front wall of thorax without penetration into thoracic cavity

    √7ᵗʰ **S21.141** **Puncture wound with foreign body of right front wall of thorax without penetration into thoracic cavity**

    √7ᵗʰ **S21.142** **Puncture wound with foreign body of left front wall of thorax without penetration into thoracic cavity**

√7ᵗʰ **S21.149** **Puncture wound with foreign body of unspecified front wall of thorax without penetration into thoracic cavity** ▽

√6ᵗʰ **S21.15** **Open bite** of front wall of thorax without penetration into thoracic cavity

    Bite of front wall of thorax NOS

    EXCLUDES 1   superficial bite of front wall of thorax (S20.37)

    √7ᵗʰ **S21.151** **Open bite of right front wall of thorax without penetration into thoracic cavity**

    √7ᵗʰ **S21.152** **Open bite of left front wall of thorax without penetration into thoracic cavity**

    √7ᵗʰ **S21.159** **Open bite of unspecified front wall of thorax without penetration into thoracic cavity** ▽

√5ᵗʰ **S21.2** **Open wound of back wall of thorax without penetration** into thoracic cavity

√6ᵗʰ **S21.20** **Unspecified open wound of back wall of thorax without penetration into thoracic cavity**

    √7ᵗʰ **S21.201** **Unspecified open wound of right back wall of thorax without penetration into thoracic cavity** ▽

    √7ᵗʰ **S21.202** **Unspecified open wound of left back wall of thorax without penetration into thoracic cavity** ▽

    √7ᵗʰ **S21.209** **Unspecified open wound of unspecified back wall of thorax without penetration into thoracic cavity** ▽

√6ᵗʰ **S21.21** **Laceration without foreign body** of back wall of thorax without penetration into thoracic cavity

    √7ᵗʰ **S21.211** **Laceration without foreign body of right back wall of thorax without penetration into thoracic cavity**

    √7ᵗʰ **S21.212** **Laceration without foreign body of left back wall of thorax without penetration into thoracic cavity**

    √7ᵗʰ **S21.219** **Laceration without foreign body of unspecified back wall of thorax without penetration into thoracic cavity** ▽

√6ᵗʰ **S21.22** **Laceration with foreign body** of back wall of thorax without penetration into thoracic cavity

    √7ᵗʰ **S21.221** **Laceration with foreign body of right back wall of thorax without penetration into thoracic cavity**

    √7ᵗʰ **S21.222** **Laceration with foreign body of left back wall of thorax without penetration into thoracic cavity**

    √7ᵗʰ **S21.229** **Laceration with foreign body of unspecified back wall of thorax without penetration into thoracic cavity** ▽

√5ᵗʰ **S21.23** **Puncture wound without foreign body** of back wall of thorax without penetration into thoracic cavity

    √7ᵗʰ **S21.231** **Puncture wound without foreign body of right back wall of thorax without penetration into thoracic cavity**

    √7ᵗʰ **S21.232** **Puncture wound without foreign body of left back wall of thorax without penetration into thoracic cavity**

    √7ᵗʰ **S21.239** **Puncture wound without foreign body of unspecified back wall of thorax without penetration into thoracic cavity** ▽

√6ᵗʰ **S21.24** **Puncture wound with foreign body** of back wall of thorax without penetration into thoracic cavity

    √7ᵗʰ **S21.241** **Puncture wound with foreign body of right back wall of thorax without penetration into thoracic cavity**

    √7ᵗʰ **S21.242** **Puncture wound with foreign body of left back wall of thorax without penetration into thoracic cavity**

    √7ᵗʰ **S21.249** **Puncture wound with foreign body of unspecified back wall of thorax without penetration into thoracic cavity** ▽

☑ Additional Character Req   √x7ᵗʰ Placeholder Alert   Manifestation   HCC CMS-HCC Condition   ▽ Unspecified Code   ▶◀ Revised Text   ● New Code   ▲ Revised Code Title

ICD-10-CM 2018   933

√6ᵗʰ **S21.25** **Open bite** of back wall of thorax without penetration into thoracic cavity
Bite of back wall of thorax NOS
EXCLUDES 1   *superficial bite of back wall of thorax (S20.47)*

   √7ᵗʰ **S21.251** Open bite of **right** back wall of thorax without penetration into thoracic cavity

   √7ᵗʰ **S21.252** Open bite of **left** back wall of thorax without penetration into thoracic cavity

   √7ᵗʰ **S21.259** Open bite of unspecified back wall of thorax without penetration into thoracic cavity ▽

√5ᵗʰ **S21.3** Open wound of **front wall of thorax with penetration** into thoracic cavity
Open wound of chest with penetration into thoracic cavity

  √6ᵗʰ **S21.30** Unspecified open wound of front wall of thorax with penetration into thoracic cavity

   √7ᵗʰ **S21.301** Unspecified open wound of **right** front wall of thorax with penetration into thoracic cavity ▽

   √7ᵗʰ **S21.302** Unspecified open wound of **left** front wall of thorax with penetration into thoracic cavity ▽

   √7ᵗʰ **S21.309** Unspecified open wound of unspecified front wall of thorax with penetration into thoracic cavity ▽

  √6ᵗʰ **S21.31** **Laceration without foreign body** of front wall of thorax with penetration into thoracic cavity

   √7ᵗʰ **S21.311** Laceration without foreign body of **right** front wall of thorax with penetration into thoracic cavity

   √7ᵗʰ **S21.312** Laceration without foreign body of **left** front wall of thorax with penetration into thoracic cavity

   √7ᵗʰ **S21.319** Laceration without foreign body of unspecified front wall of thorax with penetration into thoracic cavity ▽

  √6ᵗʰ **S21.32** **Laceration with foreign body** of front wall of thorax with penetration into thoracic cavity

   √7ᵗʰ **S21.321** Laceration with foreign body of **right** front wall of thorax with penetration into thoracic cavity

   √7ᵗʰ **S21.322** Laceration with foreign body of **left** front wall of thorax with penetration into thoracic cavity

   √7ᵗʰ **S21.329** Laceration with foreign body of unspecified front wall of thorax with penetration into thoracic cavity ▽

  √6ᵗʰ **S21.33** **Puncture wound without foreign body** of front wall of thorax with penetration into thoracic cavity

   √7ᵗʰ **S21.331** Puncture wound without foreign body of **right** front wall of thorax with penetration into thoracic cavity

   √7ᵗʰ **S21.332** Puncture wound without foreign body of **left** front wall of thorax with penetration into thoracic cavity

   √7ᵗʰ **S21.339** Puncture wound without foreign body of unspecified front wall of thorax with penetration into thoracic cavity ▽

  √6ᵗʰ **S21.34** **Puncture wound with foreign body** of front wall of thorax with penetration into thoracic cavity

   √7ᵗʰ **S21.341** Puncture wound with foreign body of **right** front wall of thorax with penetration into thoracic cavity

   √7ᵗʰ **S21.342** Puncture wound with foreign body of **left** front wall of thorax with penetration into thoracic cavity

   √7ᵗʰ **S21.349** Puncture wound with foreign body of unspecified front wall of thorax with penetration into thoracic cavity ▽

  √6ᵗʰ **S21.35** **Open bite** of front wall of thorax with penetration into thoracic cavity
EXCLUDES 1   *superficial bite of front wall of thorax (S20.37)*

   √7ᵗʰ **S21.351** Open bite of **right** front wall of thorax with penetration into thoracic cavity

   √7ᵗʰ **S21.352** Open bite of **left** front wall of thorax with penetration into thoracic cavity

   √7ᵗʰ **S21.359** Open bite of unspecified front wall of thorax with penetration into thoracic cavity ▽

√5ᵗʰ **S21.4** Open wound of **back wall of thorax with penetration** into thoracic cavity

  √6ᵗʰ **S21.40** Unspecified open wound of back wall of thorax with penetration into thoracic cavity

   √7ᵗʰ **S21.401** Unspecified open wound of **right** back wall of thorax with penetration into thoracic cavity ▽

   √7ᵗʰ **S21.402** Unspecified open wound of **left** back wall of thorax with penetration into thoracic cavity ▽

   √7ᵗʰ **S21.409** Unspecified open wound of unspecified back wall of thorax with penetration into thoracic cavity ▽

  √6ᵗʰ **S21.41** **Laceration without foreign body** of back wall of thorax with penetration into thoracic cavity

   √7ᵗʰ **S21.411** Laceration without foreign body of **right** back wall of thorax with penetration into thoracic cavity

   √7ᵗʰ **S21.412** Laceration without foreign body of **left** back wall of thorax with penetration into thoracic cavity

   √7ᵗʰ **S21.419** Laceration without foreign body of unspecified back wall of thorax with penetration into thoracic cavity ▽

  √6ᵗʰ **S21.42** **Laceration with foreign body** of back wall of thorax with penetration into thoracic cavity

   √7ᵗʰ **S21.421** Laceration with foreign body of **right** back wall of thorax with penetration into thoracic cavity

   √7ᵗʰ **S21.422** Laceration with foreign body of **left** back wall of thorax with penetration into thoracic cavity

   √7ᵗʰ **S21.429** Laceration with foreign body of unspecified back wall of thorax with penetration into thoracic cavity ▽

  √6ᵗʰ **S21.43** **Puncture wound without foreign body** of back wall of thorax with penetration into thoracic cavity

   √7ᵗʰ **S21.431** Puncture wound without foreign body of **right** back wall of thorax with penetration into thoracic cavity

   √7ᵗʰ **S21.432** Puncture wound without foreign body of **left** back wall of thorax with penetration into thoracic cavity

   √7ᵗʰ **S21.439** Puncture wound without foreign body of unspecified back wall of thorax with penetration into thoracic cavity ▽

  √6ᵗʰ **S21.44** **Puncture wound with foreign body** of back wall of thorax with penetration into thoracic cavity

   √7ᵗʰ **S21.441** Puncture wound with foreign body of **right** back wall of thorax with penetration into thoracic cavity

   √7ᵗʰ **S21.442** Puncture wound with foreign body of **left** back wall of thorax with penetration into thoracic cavity

   √7ᵗʰ **S21.449** Puncture wound with foreign body of unspecified back wall of thorax with penetration into thoracic cavity ▽

  √6ᵗʰ **S21.45** **Open bite** of back wall of thorax with penetration into thoracic cavity
Bite of back wall of thorax NOS
EXCLUDES 1   *superficial bite of back wall of thorax (S20.47)*

   √7ᵗʰ **S21.451** Open bite of **right** back wall of thorax with penetration into thoracic cavity

   √7ᵗʰ **S21.452** Open bite of **left** back wall of thorax with penetration into thoracic cavity

   √7ᵗʰ **S21.459** Open bite of unspecified back wall of thorax with penetration into thoracic cavity ▽

√5ᵗʰ **S21.9** Open wound of unspecified part of thorax
Open wound of thoracic wall NOS

  √×7ᵗʰ **S21.90** Unspecified open wound of unspecified part of thorax ▽

  √×7ᵗʰ **S21.91** **Laceration without foreign body** of unspecified part of thorax ▽

EXCLUDES 1 Not coded here   **EXCLUDES 2** Not included here   **N** Newborn Age: 0   **P** Pediatric Age: 0-17   **M** Maternity Age: 12-55   **A** Adult Age: 15-124

✓x7ᵗʰ **S21.92** **Laceration with foreign body of unspecified part of thorax** ▽

✓x7ᵗʰ **S21.93** **Puncture wound without foreign body of unspecified part of thorax** ▽

✓x7ᵗʰ **S21.94** **Puncture wound with foreign body of unspecified part of thorax** ▽

✓x7ᵗʰ **S21.95** **Open bite of unspecified part of thorax** ▽
       EXCLUDES 1   superficial bite of thorax (S20.97)

✓4ᵗʰ **S22** **Fracture of rib(s), sternum and thoracic spine**
     NOTE   A fracture not indicated as nondisplaced or displaced should be coded to displaced.
             A fracture not indicated as open or closed should be coded to closed.
     INCLUDES   fracture of thoracic neural arch
             fracture of thoracic spinous process
             fracture of thoracic transverse process
             fracture of thoracic vertebra
             fracture of thoracic vertebral arch
     Code first any associated:
       injury of intrathoracic organ (S27.-)
       spinal cord injury (S24.0-, S24.1-)
     EXCLUDES 1   transection of thorax (S28.1)
     EXCLUDES 2   fracture of clavicle (S42.0-)
                 fracture of scapula (S42.1-)
     AHA: 2015, 3Q, 37-39

> The appropriate 7th character is to be added to each code from category S22.
> A   initial encounter for closed fracture
> B   initial encounter for open fracture
> D   subsequent encounter for fracture with routine healing
> G   subsequent encounter for fracture with delayed healing
> K   subsequent encounter for fracture with nonunion
> S   sequela

✓5ᵗʰ **S22.0** **Fracture of thoracic vertebra**

✓6ᵗʰ **S22.00** **Fracture of unspecified thoracic vertebra**
   1 ✓7ᵗʰ **S22.000** **Wedge compression fracture of unspecified thoracic vertebra** HCC ▽
   1 ✓7ᵗʰ **S22.001** **Stable burst fracture of unspecified thoracic vertebra** HCC ▽
   1 ✓7ᵗʰ **S22.002** **Unstable burst fracture of unspecified thoracic vertebra** HCC ▽
   1 ✓7ᵗʰ **S22.008** **Other fracture of unspecified thoracic vertebra** HCC ▽
   1 ✓7ᵗʰ **S22.009** **Unspecified fracture of unspecified thoracic vertebra** HCC ▽

✓6ᵗʰ **S22.01** **Fracture of first thoracic vertebra**
   1 ✓7ᵗʰ **S22.010** **Wedge compression fracture of first thoracic vertebra** HCC
   1 ✓7ᵗʰ **S22.011** **Stable burst fracture of first thoracic vertebra** HCC
   1 ✓7ᵗʰ **S22.012** **Unstable burst fracture of first thoracic vertebra** HCC
   1 ✓7ᵗʰ **S22.018** **Other fracture of first thoracic vertebra** HCC
   1 ✓7ᵗʰ **S22.019** **Unspecified fracture of first thoracic vertebra** HCC ▽

✓6ᵗʰ **S22.02** **Fracture of second thoracic vertebra**
   1 ✓7ᵗʰ **S22.020** **Wedge compression fracture of second thoracic vertebra** HCC
   1 ✓7ᵗʰ **S22.021** **Stable burst fracture of second thoracic vertebra** HCC
   1 ✓7ᵗʰ **S22.022** **Unstable burst fracture of second thoracic vertebra** HCC
   1 ✓7ᵗʰ **S22.028** **Other fracture of second thoracic vertebra** HCC
   1 ✓7ᵗʰ **S22.029** **Unspecified fracture of second thoracic vertebra** HCC ▽

✓6ᵗʰ **S22.03** **Fracture of third thoracic vertebra**
   1 ✓7ᵗʰ **S22.030** **Wedge compression fracture of third thoracic vertebra** HCC
   1 ✓7ᵗʰ **S22.031** **Stable burst fracture of third thoracic vertebra** HCC
   1 ✓7ᵗʰ **S22.032** **Unstable burst fracture of third thoracic vertebra** HCC

1 ✓7ᵗʰ **S22.038** **Other fracture of third thoracic vertebra** HCC

1 ✓7ᵗʰ **S22.039** **Unspecified fracture of third thoracic vertebra** HCC ▽

✓6ᵗʰ **S22.04** **Fracture of fourth thoracic vertebra**
   1 ✓7ᵗʰ **S22.040** **Wedge compression fracture of fourth thoracic vertebra** HCC
   1 ✓7ᵗʰ **S22.041** **Stable burst fracture of fourth thoracic vertebra** HCC
   1 ✓7ᵗʰ **S22.042** **Unstable burst fracture of fourth thoracic vertebra** HCC
   1 ✓7ᵗʰ **S22.048** **Other fracture of fourth thoracic vertebra** HCC
   1 ✓7ᵗʰ **S22.049** **Unspecified fracture of fourth thoracic vertebra** HCC ▽

✓6ᵗʰ **S22.05** **Fracture of T5-T6 vertebra**
   1 ✓7ᵗʰ **S22.050** **Wedge compression fracture of T5-T6 vertebra** HCC
   1 ✓7ᵗʰ **S22.051** **Stable burst fracture of T5-T6 vertebra** HCC
   1 ✓7ᵗʰ **S22.052** **Unstable burst fracture of T5-T6 vertebra** HCC
   1 ✓7ᵗʰ **S22.058** **Other fracture of T5-T6 vertebra** HCC
   1 ✓7ᵗʰ **S22.059** **Unspecified fracture of T5-T6 vertebra** HCC ▽

✓6ᵗʰ **S22.06** **Fracture of T7-T8 vertebra**
   1 ✓7ᵗʰ **S22.060** **Wedge compression fracture of T7-T8 vertebra** HCC
   1 ✓7ᵗʰ **S22.061** **Stable burst fracture of T7-T8 vertebra** HCC
   1 ✓7ᵗʰ **S22.062** **Unstable burst fracture of T7-T8 vertebra** HCC
   1 ✓7ᵗʰ **S22.068** **Other fracture of T7-T8 thoracic vertebra** HCC
   1 ✓7ᵗʰ **S22.069** **Unspecified fracture of T7-T8 vertebra** HCC ▽

✓6ᵗʰ **S22.07** **Fracture of T9-T10 vertebra**
   1 ✓7ᵗʰ **S22.070** **Wedge compression fracture of T9-T10 vertebra** HCC
   1 ✓7ᵗʰ **S22.071** **Stable burst fracture of T9-T10 vertebra** HCC
   1 ✓7ᵗʰ **S22.072** **Unstable burst fracture of T9-T10 vertebra** HCC
   1 ✓7ᵗʰ **S22.078** **Other fracture of T9-T10 vertebra** HCC
   1 ✓7ᵗʰ **S22.079** **Unspecified fracture of T9-T10 vertebra** HCC ▽

✓6ᵗʰ **S22.08** **Fracture of T11-T12 vertebra**
   1 ✓7ᵗʰ **S22.080** **Wedge compression fracture of T11-T12 vertebra** HCC
   1 ✓7ᵗʰ **S22.081** **Stable burst fracture of T11-T12 vertebra** HCC
   1 ✓7ᵗʰ **S22.082** **Unstable burst fracture of T11-T12 vertebra** HCC
   1 ✓7ᵗʰ **S22.088** **Other fracture of T11-T12 vertebra** HCC
   1 ✓7ᵗʰ **S22.089** **Unspecified fracture of T11-T12 vertebra** HCC ▽

✓5ᵗʰ **S22.2** **Fracture of sternum**
     DEF: Break in flat bone (breast bone) in anterior thorax; caused by blunt trauma to anterior chest.

✓x7ᵗʰ **S22.20** **Unspecified fracture of sternum** ▽

✓x7ᵗʰ **S22.21** **Fracture of manubrium**

✓x7ᵗʰ **S22.22** **Fracture of body of sternum**

✓x7ᵗʰ **S22.23** **Sternal manubrial dissociation**

✓x7ᵗʰ **S22.24** **Fracture of xiphoid process**

✓5ᵗʰ **S22.3** **Fracture of one rib**

✓x7ᵗʰ **S22.31** **Fracture of one rib, right side**

✓x7ᵗʰ **S22.32** **Fracture of one rib, left side**

✓x7ᵗʰ **S22.39** **Fracture of one rib, unspecified side** ▽

✓5ᵗʰ **S22.4** **Multiple fractures of ribs**
     Fractures of two or more ribs
     EXCLUDES 1   flail chest (S22.5-)

✓x7ᵗʰ **S22.41** **Multiple fractures of ribs, right side**

---

1   HCC with 7th character indicating initial encounter (A, B or C - specific to category).

✓ Additional Character Req   ✓x7ᵗʰ Placeholder Alert   Manifestation   HCC CMS-HCC Condition   ▽ Unspecified Code   ►◄ Revised Text   ● New Code   ▲ Revised Code Title

√x7ᵗʰ **S22.42** **Multiple fractures of ribs, left side**

√x7ᵗʰ **S22.43** **Multiple fractures of ribs, bilateral**

√x7ᵗʰ **S22.49** **Multiple fractures of ribs, unspecified side** ▽

√x7ᵗʰ **S22.5** **Flail chest**

√x7ᵗʰ **S22.9** **Fracture of bony thorax, part unspecified** ▽

√4ᵗʰ **S23** **Dislocation and sprain of joints and ligaments of thorax**

INCLUDES   avulsion of joint or ligament of thorax
laceration of cartilage, joint or ligament of thorax
sprain of cartilage, joint or ligament of thorax
traumatic hemarthrosis of joint or ligament of thorax
traumatic rupture of joint or ligament of thorax
traumatic subluxation of joint or ligament of thorax
traumatic tear of joint or ligament of thorax

Code also any associated open wound

EXCLUDES 2   *dislocation, sprain of sternoclavicular joint (S43.2, S43.6)*
strain of muscle or tendon of thorax (S29.01-)

> The appropriate 7th character is to be added to each code from category S23.
> A   initial encounter
> D   subsequent encounter
> S   sequela

√x7ᵗʰ **S23.0** **Traumatic rupture of thoracic intervertebral disc**

EXCLUDES 1   *rupture or displacement (nontraumatic) of thoracic intervertebral disc NOS (M51- with fifth character 4)*

√5ᵗʰ **S23.1** **Subluxation and dislocation of thoracic vertebra**

Code also any associated
open wound of thorax (S21.-)
spinal cord injury (S24.0-, S24.1-)

EXCLUDES 2   *fracture of thoracic vertebrae (S22.0-)*

√6ᵗʰ **S23.10** **Subluxation and dislocation of unspecified thoracic vertebra**

√7ᵗʰ **S23.100** **Subluxation of unspecified thoracic vertebra** ▽

√7ᵗʰ **S23.101** **Dislocation of unspecified thoracic vertebra** ▽

√6ᵗʰ **S23.11** **Subluxation and dislocation of T1/T2 thoracic vertebra**

√7ᵗʰ **S23.110** **Subluxation of T1/T2 thoracic vertebra**

√7ᵗʰ **S23.111** **Dislocation of T1/T2 thoracic vertebra**

√6ᵗʰ **S23.12** **Subluxation and dislocation of T2/T3-T3/T4 thoracic vertebra**

√7ᵗʰ **S23.120** **Subluxation of T2/T3 thoracic vertebra**

√7ᵗʰ **S23.121** **Dislocation of T2/T3 thoracic vertebra**

√7ᵗʰ **S23.122** **Subluxation of T3/T4 thoracic vertebra**

√7ᵗʰ **S23.123** **Dislocation of T3/T4 thoracic vertebra**

√6ᵗʰ **S23.13** **Subluxation and dislocation of T4/T5-T5/T6 thoracic vertebra**

√7ᵗʰ **S23.130** **Subluxation of T4/T5 thoracic vertebra**

√7ᵗʰ **S23.131** **Dislocation of T4/T5 thoracic vertebra**

√7ᵗʰ **S23.132** **Subluxation of T5/T6 thoracic vertebra**

√7ᵗʰ **S23.133** **Dislocation of T5/T6 thoracic vertebra**

√6ᵗʰ **S23.14** **Subluxation and dislocation of T6/T7-T7/T8 thoracic vertebra**

√7ᵗʰ **S23.140** **Subluxation of T6/T7 thoracic vertebra**

√7ᵗʰ **S23.141** **Dislocation of T6/T7 thoracic vertebra**

√7ᵗʰ **S23.142** **Subluxation of T7/T8 thoracic vertebra**

√7ᵗʰ **S23.143** **Dislocation of T7/T8 thoracic vertebra**

√6ᵗʰ **S23.15** **Subluxation and dislocation of T8/T9-T9/T10 thoracic vertebra**

√7ᵗʰ **S23.150** **Subluxation of T8/T9 thoracic vertebra**

√7ᵗʰ **S23.151** **Dislocation of T8/T9 thoracic vertebra**

√7ᵗʰ **S23.152** **Subluxation of T9/T10 thoracic vertebra**

√7ᵗʰ **S23.153** **Dislocation of T9/T10 thoracic vertebra**

√6ᵗʰ **S23.16** **Subluxation and dislocation of T10/T11-T11/T12 thoracic vertebra**

√7ᵗʰ **S23.160** **Subluxation of T10/T11 thoracic vertebra**

√7ᵗʰ **S23.161** **Dislocation of T10/T11 thoracic vertebra**

√7ᵗʰ **S23.162** **Subluxation of T11/T12 thoracic vertebra**

√7ᵗʰ **S23.163** **Dislocation of T11/T12 thoracic vertebra**

√6ᵗʰ **S23.17** **Subluxation and dislocation of T12/L1 thoracic vertebra**

√7ᵗʰ **S23.170** **Subluxation of T12/L1 thoracic vertebra**

√7ᵗʰ **S23.171** **Dislocation of T12/L1 thoracic vertebra**

√5ᵗʰ **S23.2** **Dislocation of other and unspecified parts of thorax**

√x7ᵗʰ **S23.20** **Dislocation of unspecified part of thorax** ▽

√x7ᵗʰ **S23.29** **Dislocation of other parts of thorax**

√x7ᵗʰ **S23.3** **Sprain of ligaments of thoracic spine**

√5ᵗʰ **S23.4** **Sprain of ribs and sternum**

√x7ᵗʰ **S23.41** **Sprain of ribs**

√6ᵗʰ **S23.42** **Sprain of sternum**

√7ᵗʰ **S23.420** **Sprain of sternoclavicular (joint) (ligament)**

√7ᵗʰ **S23.421** **Sprain of chondrosternal joint**

√7ᵗʰ **S23.428** **Other sprain of sternum**

√7ᵗʰ **S23.429** **Unspecified sprain of sternum** ▽

√x7ᵗʰ **S23.8** **Sprain of other specified parts of thorax**

√x7ᵗʰ **S23.9** **Sprain of unspecified parts of thorax** ▽

√4ᵗʰ **S24** **Injury of nerves and spinal cord at thorax level**

NOTE   Code to highest level of thoracic spinal cord injury.
Injuries to the spinal cord (S24.0 and S24.1) refer to the cord level and not bone level injury, and can affect nerve roots at and below the level given.

Code also any associated:
fracture of thoracic vertebra (S22.0-)
open wound of thorax (S21.-)
transient paralysis (R29.5)

EXCLUDES 2   *injury of brachial plexus (S14.3)*

> The appropriate 7th character is to be added to each code from category S24.
> A   initial encounter
> D   subsequent encounter
> S   sequela

√x7ᵗʰ **S24.0** **Concussion and edema of thoracic spinal cord** HCC

√5ᵗʰ **S24.1** **Other and unspecified injuries of thoracic spinal cord**

√6ᵗʰ **S24.10** **Unspecified injury of thoracic spinal cord**

√7ᵗʰ **S24.101** **Unspecified injury at T1 level of thoracic spinal cord** HCC ▽

√7ᵗʰ **S24.102** **Unspecified injury at T2-T6 level of thoracic spinal cord** HCC ▽

√7ᵗʰ **S24.103** **Unspecified injury at T7-T10 level of thoracic spinal cord** HCC ▽

√7ᵗʰ **S24.104** **Unspecified injury at T11-T12 level of thoracic spinal cord** HCC ▽

√7ᵗʰ **S24.109** **Unspecified injury at unspecified level of thoracic spinal cord** HCC ▽
Injury of thoracic spinal cord NOS

√6ᵗʰ **S24.11** **Complete lesion of thoracic spinal cord**

√7ᵗʰ **S24.111** **Complete lesion at T1 level of thoracic spinal cord** HCC

√7ᵗʰ **S24.112** **Complete lesion at T2-T6 level of thoracic spinal cord** HCC

√7ᵗʰ **S24.113** **Complete lesion at T7-T10 level of thoracic spinal cord** HCC

√7ᵗʰ **S24.114** **Complete lesion at T11-T12 level of thoracic spinal cord** HCC

√7ᵗʰ **S24.119** **Complete lesion at unspecified level of thoracic spinal cord** HCC ▽

√6ᵗʰ **S24.13** **Anterior cord syndrome of thoracic spinal cord**

√7ᵗʰ **S24.131** **Anterior cord syndrome at T1 level of thoracic spinal cord** HCC

√7ᵗʰ **S24.132** **Anterior cord syndrome at T2-T6 level of thoracic spinal cord** HCC

√7ᵗʰ **S24.133** **Anterior cord syndrome at T7-T10 level of thoracic spinal cord** HCC

√7ᵗʰ **S24.134** **Anterior cord syndrome at T11-T12 level of thoracic spinal cord** HCC

√7ᵗʰ **S24.139** **Anterior cord syndrome at unspecified level of thoracic spinal cord** HCC ▽

√6ᵗʰ **S24.14** **Brown-Séquard syndrome of thoracic spinal cord**

√7ᵗʰ **S24.141** **Brown-Séquard syndrome at T1 level of thoracic spinal cord** HCC

EXCLUDES 1 Not coded here   EXCLUDES 2 Not included here   N Newborn Age: 0   P Pediatric Age: 0-17   M Maternity Age: 12-55   A Adult Age: 15-124

936   ICD-10-CM 2018

√7ᵗʰ **S24.142 Brown-Séquard syndrome at T2-T6 level of thoracic spinal cord** HCC

√7ᵗʰ **S24.143 Brown-Séquard syndrome at T7-T10 level of thoracic spinal cord** HCC

√7ᵗʰ **S24.144 Brown-Séquard syndrome at T11-T12 level of thoracic spinal cord** HCC

√7ᵗʰ **S24.149 Brown-Séquard syndrome at unspecified level of thoracic spinal cord** HCC ▽

√6ᵗʰ **S24.15 Other incomplete lesions of thoracic spinal cord**
Incomplete lesion of thoracic spinal cord NOS
Posterior cord syndrome of thoracic spinal cord

√7ᵗʰ **S24.151 Other incomplete lesion at T1 level of thoracic spinal cord** HCC

√7ᵗʰ **S24.152 Other incomplete lesion at T2-T6 level of thoracic spinal cord** HCC

√7ᵗʰ **S24.153 Other incomplete lesion at T7-T10 level of thoracic spinal cord** HCC

√7ᵗʰ **S24.154 Other incomplete lesion at T11-T12 level of thoracic spinal cord** HCC

√7ᵗʰ **S24.159 Other incomplete lesion at unspecified level of thoracic spinal cord** HCC ▽

√x7ᵗʰ **S24.2 Injury of nerve root of thoracic spine**

√x7ᵗʰ **S24.3 Injury of peripheral nerves of thorax**

√x7ᵗʰ **S24.4 Injury of thoracic sympathetic nervous system**
Injury of cardiac plexus
Injury of esophageal plexus
Injury of pulmonary plexus
Injury of stellate ganglion
Injury of thoracic sympathetic ganglion

√x7ᵗʰ **S24.8 Injury of other specified nerves of thorax**

√x7ᵗʰ **S24.9 Injury of unspecified nerve of thorax** ▽

√4ᵗʰ **S25 Injury of blood vessels of thorax**
Code also any associated open wound (S21.-)

The appropriate 7th character is to be added to each code from category S25.
A initial encounter
D subsequent encounter
S sequela

√5ᵗʰ **S25.0 Injury of thoracic aorta**
Injury of aorta NOS

√x7ᵗʰ **S25.00 Unspecified injury of thoracic aorta** ▽

√x7ᵗʰ **S25.01 Minor laceration of thoracic aorta**
Incomplete transection of thoracic aorta
Laceration of thoracic aorta NOS
Superficial laceration of thoracic aorta

√x7ᵗʰ **S25.02 Major laceration of thoracic aorta**
Complete transection of thoracic aorta
Traumatic rupture of thoracic aorta

√x7ᵗʰ **S25.09 Other specified injury of thoracic aorta**

√5ᵗʰ **S25.1 Injury of innominate or subclavian artery**

√6ᵗʰ **S25.10 Unspecified injury of innominate or subclavian artery**

√7ᵗʰ **S25.101 Unspecified injury of right innominate or subclavian artery** ▽

√7ᵗʰ **S25.102 Unspecified injury of left innominate or subclavian artery** ▽

√7ᵗʰ **S25.109 Unspecified injury of unspecified innominate or subclavian artery** ▽

√6ᵗʰ **S25.11 Minor laceration of innominate or subclavian artery**
Incomplete transection of innominate or subclavian artery
Laceration of innominate or subclavian artery NOS
Superficial laceration of innominate or subclavian artery

√7ᵗʰ **S25.111 Minor laceration of right innominate or subclavian artery**

√7ᵗʰ **S25.112 Minor laceration of left innominate or subclavian artery**

√7ᵗʰ **S25.119 Minor laceration of unspecified innominate or subclavian artery** ▽

√6ᵗʰ **S25.12 Major laceration of Innominate or subclavian artery**
Complete transection of innominate or subclavian artery
Traumatic rupture of innominate or subclavian artery

√7ᵗʰ **S25.121 Major laceration of right innominate or subclavian artery**

√7ᵗʰ **S25.122 Major laceration of left innominate or subclavian artery**

√7ᵗʰ **S25.129 Major laceration of unspecified innominate or subclavian artery** ▽

√6ᵗʰ **S25.19 Other specified injury of innominate or subclavian artery**

√7ᵗʰ **S25.191 Other specified injury of right innominate or subclavian artery**

√7ᵗʰ **S25.192 Other specified injury of left innominate or subclavian artery**

√7ᵗʰ **S25.199 Other specified injury of unspecified innominate or subclavian artery** ▽

√5ᵗʰ **S25.2 Injury of superior vena cava**
Injury of vena cava NOS

√x7ᵗʰ **S25.20 Unspecified injury of superior vena cava** ▽

√x7ᵗʰ **S25.21 Minor laceration of superior vena cava**
Incomplete transection of superior vena cava
Laceration of superior vena cava NOS
Superficial laceration of superior vena cava

√x7ᵗʰ **S25.22 Major laceration of superior vena cava**
Complete transection of superior vena cava
Traumatic rupture of superior vena cava

√x7ᵗʰ **S25.29 Other specified injury of superior vena cava**

√5ᵗʰ **S25.3 Injury of innominate or subclavian vein**

√6ᵗʰ **S25.30 Unspecified injury of innominate or subclavian vein**

√7ᵗʰ **S25.301 Unspecified injury of right innominate or subclavian vein** ▽

√7ᵗʰ **S25.302 Unspecified injury of left innominate or subclavian vein** ▽

√7ᵗʰ **S25.309 Unspecified injury of unspecified innominate or subclavian vein** ▽

√6ᵗʰ **S25.31 Minor laceration of innominate or subclavian vein**
Incomplete transection of innominate or subclavian vein
Laceration of innominate or subclavian vein NOS
Superficial laceration of innominate or subclavian vein

√7ᵗʰ **S25.311 Minor laceration of right innominate or subclavian vein**

√7ᵗʰ **S25.312 Minor laceration of left innominate or subclavian vein**

√7ᵗʰ **S25.319 Minor laceration of unspecified innominate or subclavian vein** ▽

√6ᵗʰ **S25.32 Major laceration of innominate or subclavian vein**
Complete transection of innominate or subclavian vein
Traumatic rupture of innominate or subclavian vein

√7ᵗʰ **S25.321 Major laceration of right innominate or subclavian vein**

√7ᵗʰ **S25.322 Major laceration of left innominate or subclavian vein**

√7ᵗʰ **S25.329 Major laceration of unspecified innominate or subclavian vein** ▽

√6ᵗʰ **S25.39 Other specified injury of innominate or subclavian vein**

√7ᵗʰ **S25.391 Other specified injury of right innominate or subclavian vein**

√7ᵗʰ **S25.392 Other specified injury of left innominate or subclavian vein**

√7ᵗʰ **S25.399 Other specified injury of unspecified innominate or subclavian vein** ▽

√5ᵗʰ **S25.4 Injury of pulmonary blood vessels**

√6ᵗʰ **S25.40 Unspecified injury of pulmonary blood vessels**

√7ᵗʰ **S25.401 Unspecified injury of right pulmonary blood vessels** ▽

√7ᵗʰ **S25.402 Unspecified injury of left pulmonary blood vessels** ▽

√7ᵗʰ **S25.409 Unspecified injury of unspecified pulmonary blood vessels** ▽

✓6ᵗʰ **S25.41 Minor laceration of pulmonary blood vessels**
Incomplete transection of pulmonary blood vessels
Laceration of pulmonary blood vessels NOS
Superficial laceration of pulmonary blood vessels

     ✓7ᵗʰ **S25.411 Minor laceration of right pulmonary blood vessels**

     ✓7ᵗʰ **S25.412 Minor laceration of left pulmonary blood vessels**

     ✓7ᵗʰ **S25.419 Minor laceration of unspecified pulmonary blood vessels** ▽

✓6ᵗʰ **S25.42 Major laceration of pulmonary blood vessels**
Complete transection of pulmonary blood vessels
Traumatic rupture of pulmonary blood vessels

     ✓7ᵗʰ **S25.421 Major laceration of right pulmonary blood vessels**

     ✓7ᵗʰ **S25.422 Major laceration of left pulmonary blood vessels**

     ✓7ᵗʰ **S25.429 Major laceration of unspecified pulmonary blood vessels** ▽

✓6ᵗʰ **S25.49 Other specified injury of pulmonary blood vessels**

     ✓7ᵗʰ **S25.491 Other specified injury of right pulmonary blood vessels**

     ✓7ᵗʰ **S25.492 Other specified injury of left pulmonary blood vessels**

     ✓7ᵗʰ **S25.499 Other specified injury of unspecified pulmonary blood vessels** ▽

✓5ᵗʰ **S25.5 Injury of intercostal blood vessels**

   ✓6ᵗʰ **S25.50 Unspecified injury of intercostal blood vessels**

     ✓7ᵗʰ **S25.501 Unspecified injury of intercostal blood vessels, right side** ▽

     ✓7ᵗʰ **S25.502 Unspecified injury of intercostal blood vessels, left side** ▽

     ✓7ᵗʰ **S25.509 Unspecified injury of intercostal blood vessels, unspecified side** ▽

   ✓6ᵗʰ **S25.51 Laceration of intercostal blood vessels**

     ✓7ᵗʰ **S25.511 Laceration of intercostal blood vessels, right side**

     ✓7ᵗʰ **S25.512 Laceration of intercostal blood vessels, left side**

     ✓7ᵗʰ **S25.519 Laceration of intercostal blood vessels, unspecified side** ▽

   ✓6ᵗʰ **S25.59 Other specified injury of intercostal blood vessels**

     ✓7ᵗʰ **S25.591 Other specified injury of intercostal blood vessels, right side**

     ✓7ᵗʰ **S25.592 Other specified injury of intercostal blood vessels, left side**

     ✓7ᵗʰ **S25.599 Other specified injury of intercostal blood vessels, unspecified side** ▽

✓5ᵗʰ **S25.8 Injury of other blood vessels of thorax**
Injury of azygos vein
Injury of mammary artery or vein

   ✓6ᵗʰ **S25.80 Unspecified injury of other blood vessels of thorax**

     ✓7ᵗʰ **S25.801 Unspecified injury of other blood vessels of thorax, right side** ▽

     ✓7ᵗʰ **S25.802 Unspecified injury of other blood vessels of thorax, left side** ▽

     ✓7ᵗʰ **S25.809 Unspecified injury of other blood vessels of thorax, unspecified side** ▽

   ✓6ᵗʰ **S25.81 Laceration of other blood vessels of thorax**

     ✓7ᵗʰ **S25.811 Laceration of other blood vessels of thorax, right side**

     ✓7ᵗʰ **S25.812 Laceration of other blood vessels of thorax, left side**

     ✓7ᵗʰ **S25.819 Laceration of other blood vessels of thorax, unspecified side** ▽

   ✓6ᵗʰ **S25.89 Other specified injury of other blood vessels of thorax**

     ✓7ᵗʰ **S25.891 Other specified injury of other blood vessels of thorax, right side**

     ✓7ᵗʰ **S25.892 Other specified injury of other blood vessels of thorax, left side**

     ✓7ᵗʰ **S25.899 Other specified injury of other blood vessels of thorax, unspecified side** ▽

✓5ᵗʰ **S25.9 Injury of unspecified blood vessel of thorax**

   ✓x7ᵗʰ **S25.90 Unspecified injury of unspecified blood vessel of thorax** ▽

   ✓x7ᵗʰ **S25.91 Laceration of unspecified blood vessel of thorax** ▽

   ✓x7ᵗʰ **S25.99 Other specified injury of unspecified blood vessel of thorax** ▽

✓4ᵗʰ **S26 Injury of heart**
Code also any associated:
open wound of thorax (S21.-)
traumatic hemopneumothorax (S27.2)
traumatic hemothorax (S27.1)
traumatic pneumothorax (S27.0)

> The appropriate 7th character is to be added to each code from category S26.
> A   initial encounter
> D   subsequent encounter
> S   sequela

✓5ᵗʰ **S26.0 Injury of heart with hemopericardium**

   ✓x7ᵗʰ **S26.00 Unspecified injury of heart with hemopericardium** ▽

   ✓x7ᵗʰ **S26.01 Contusion of heart with hemopericardium**

   ✓6ᵗʰ **S26.02 Laceration of heart with hemopericardium**

     ✓7ᵗʰ **S26.020 Mild laceration of heart with hemopericardium**
Laceration of heart without penetration of heart chamber

     ✓7ᵗʰ **S26.021 Moderate laceration of heart with hemopericardium**
Laceration of heart with penetration of heart chamber

     ✓7ᵗʰ **S26.022 Major laceration of heart with hemopericardium**
Laceration of heart with penetration of multiple heart chambers

   ✓x7ᵗʰ **S26.09 Other injury of heart with hemopericardium**

✓5ᵗʰ **S26.1 Injury of heart without hemopericardium**

   ✓x7ᵗʰ **S26.10 Unspecified injury of heart without hemopericardium** ▽

   ✓x7ᵗʰ **S26.11 Contusion of heart without hemopericardium**

   ✓x7ᵗʰ **S26.12 Laceration of heart without hemopericardium**

   ✓x7ᵗʰ **S26.19 Other injury of heart without hemopericardium**

✓5ᵗʰ **S26.9 Injury of heart, unspecified with or without hemopericardium**

   ✓x7ᵗʰ **S26.90 Unspecified injury of heart, unspecified with or without hemopericardium** ▽

   ✓x7ᵗʰ **S26.91 Contusion of heart, unspecified with or without hemopericardium** ▽
DEF: Bruising within the heart muscle with no mention of open wound; usually caused by blunt chest trauma in motor vehicle accidents, falling from great heights, or receiving CPR.

   ✓x7ᵗʰ **S26.92 Laceration of heart, unspecified with or without hemopericardium** ▽
Laceration of heart NOS

   ✓x7ᵗʰ **S26.99 Other injury of heart, unspecified with or without hemopericardium** ▽

✓4ᵗʰ **S27 Injury of other and unspecified intrathoracic organs**
Code also any associated open wound of thorax (S21.-)
EXCLUDES 2   injury of cervical esophagus (S10-S19)
             injury of trachea (cervical) (S10-S19)

> The appropriate 7th character is to be added to each code from category S27.
> A   initial encounter
> D   subsequent encounter
> S   sequela

✓x7ᵗʰ **S27.0 Traumatic pneumothorax**
EXCLUDES 1   spontaneous pneumothorax (J93.-)

✓x7ᵗʰ **S27.1 Traumatic hemothorax**

✓x7ᵗʰ **S27.2 Traumatic hemopneumothorax**

✓5ᵗʰ **S27.3 Other and unspecified injuries of lung**

   ✓6ᵗʰ **S27.30 Unspecified injury of lung**

     ✓7ᵗʰ **S27.301 Unspecified injury of lung, unilateral** ▽

     ✓7ᵗʰ **S27.302 Unspecified injury of lung, bilateral** ▽

     ✓7ᵗʰ **S27.309 Unspecified injury of lung, unspecified** ▽

EXCLUDES 1 Not coded here   **EXCLUDES 2** Not included here   **N** Newborn Age: 0   **P** Pediatric Age: 0-17   **M** Maternity Age: 12-55   **A** Adult Age: 15-124

938   ICD-10-CM 2018

✓6ᵗʰ **S27.31** **Primary blast injury of lung**
Blast injury of lung NOS

  ✓7ᵗʰ **S27.311** **Primary blast injury of lung, unilateral**

  ✓7ᵗʰ **S27.312** **Primary blast injury of lung, bilateral**

  ✓7ᵗʰ **S27.319** **Primary blast injury of lung, unspecified** ▽

✓6ᵗʰ **S27.32** **Contusion of lung**
DEF: Bruising of lung without mention of open wound.

  ✓7ᵗʰ **S27.321** **Contusion of lung, unilateral**

  ✓7ᵗʰ **S27.322** **Contusion of lung, bilateral**

  ✓7ᵗʰ **S27.329** **Contusion of lung, unspecified** ▽

✓6ᵗʰ **S27.33** **Laceration of lung**

  ✓7ᵗʰ **S27.331** **Laceration of lung, unilateral**

  ✓7ᵗʰ **S27.332** **Laceration of lung, bilateral**

  ✓7ᵗʰ **S27.339** **Laceration of lung, unspecified** ▽

✓6ᵗʰ **S27.39** **Other injuries of lung**
Secondary blast injury of lung

  ✓7ᵗʰ **S27.391** **Other injuries of lung, unilateral**

  ✓7ᵗʰ **S27.392** **Other injuries of lung, bilateral**

  ✓7ᵗʰ **S27.399** **Other injuries of lung, unspecified** ▽

✓5ᵗʰ **S27.4** **Injury of bronchus**

✓6ᵗʰ **S27.40** **Unspecified injury of bronchus**

  ✓7ᵗʰ **S27.401** **Unspecified injury of bronchus, unilateral** ▽

  ✓7ᵗʰ **S27.402** **Unspecified injury of bronchus, bilateral** ▽

  ✓7ᵗʰ **S27.409** **Unspecified injury of bronchus, unspecified** ▽

✓6ᵗʰ **S27.41** **Primary blast injury of bronchus**
Blast injury of bronchus NOS

  ✓7ᵗʰ **S27.411** **Primary blast injury of bronchus, unilateral**

  ✓7ᵗʰ **S27.412** **Primary blast injury of bronchus, bilateral**

  ✓7ᵗʰ **S27.419** **Primary blast injury of bronchus, unspecified** ▽

✓6ᵗʰ **S27.42** **Contusion of bronchus**

  ✓7ᵗʰ **S27.421** **Contusion of bronchus, unilateral**

  ✓7ᵗʰ **S27.422** **Contusion of bronchus, bilateral**

  ✓7ᵗʰ **S27.429** **Contusion of bronchus, unspecified** ▽

✓6ᵗʰ **S27.43** **Laceration of bronchus**

  ✓7ᵗʰ **S27.431** **Laceration of bronchus, unilateral**

  ✓7ᵗʰ **S27.432** **Laceration of bronchus, bilateral**

  ✓7ᵗʰ **S27.439** **Laceration of bronchus, unspecified** ▽

✓6ᵗʰ **S27.49** **Other injury of bronchus**
Secondary blast injury of bronchus

  ✓7ᵗʰ **S27.491** **Other injury of bronchus, unilateral**

  ✓7ᵗʰ **S27.492** **Other injury of bronchus, bilateral**

  ✓7ᵗʰ **S27.499** **Other injury of bronchus, unspecified** ▽

✓5ᵗʰ **S27.5** **Injury of thoracic trachea**

✓x7ᵗʰ **S27.50** **Unspecified injury of thoracic trachea** ▽

✓x7ᵗʰ **S27.51** **Primary blast injury of thoracic trachea**
Blast injury of thoracic trachea NOS

✓x7ᵗʰ **S27.52** **Contusion of thoracic trachea**

✓x7ᵗʰ **S27.53** **Laceration of thoracic trachea**

✓x7ᵗʰ **S27.59** **Other injury of thoracic trachea**
Secondary blast injury of thoracic trachea

✓5ᵗʰ **S27.6** **Injury of pleura**

✓x7ᵗʰ **S27.60** **Unspecified injury of pleura** ▽

✓x7ᵗʰ **S27.63** **Laceration of pleura**

✓x7ᵗʰ **S27.69** **Other injury of pleura**

✓5ᵗʰ **S27.8** **Injury of other specified intrathoracic organs**

✓6ᵗʰ **S27.80** **Injury of diaphragm**

  ✓7ᵗʰ **S27.802** **Contusion of diaphragm**

  ✓7ᵗʰ **S27.803** **Laceration of diaphragm**

  ✓7ᵗʰ **S27.808** **Other injury of diaphragm**

  ✓7ᵗʰ **S27.809** **Unspecified injury of diaphragm** ▽

✓6ᵗʰ **S27.81** **Injury of esophagus (thoracic part)**

  ✓7ᵗʰ **S27.812** **Contusion of esophagus (thoracic part)**

  ✓7ᵗʰ **S27.813** **Laceration of esophagus (thoracic part)**

  ✓7ᵗʰ **S27.818** **Other injury of esophagus (thoracic part)**

  ✓7ᵗʰ **S27.819** **Unspecified injury of esophagus (thoracic part)** ▽

✓6ᵗʰ **S27.89** **Injury of other specified intrathoracic organs**
Injury of lymphatic thoracic duct
Injury of thymus gland

  ✓7ᵗʰ **S27.892** **Contusion of other specified intrathoracic organs**

  ✓7ᵗʰ **S27.893** **Laceration of other specified intrathoracic organs**

  ✓7ᵗʰ **S27.898** **Other injury of other specified intrathoracic organs**

  ✓7ᵗʰ **S27.899** **Unspecified injury of other specified intrathoracic organs** ▽

✓x7ᵗʰ **S27.9** **Injury of unspecified intrathoracic organ** ▽

✓4ᵗʰ **S28** **Crushing injury of thorax, and traumatic amputation of part of thorax**

> The appropriate 7th character is to be added to each code from category S28.
> A   initial encounter
> D   subsequent encounter
> S   sequela

✓x7ᵗʰ **S28.0** **Crushed chest**
Use additional code for all associated injuries
EXCLUDES 1   flail chest (S22.5)

✓x7ᵗʰ **S28.1** **Traumatic amputation (partial) of part of thorax, except breast**

✓5ᵗʰ **S28.2** **Traumatic amputation of breast**

✓6ᵗʰ **S28.21** **Complete traumatic amputation of breast**
Traumatic amputation of breast NOS

  ✓7ᵗʰ **S28.211** **Complete traumatic amputation of right breast**

  ✓7ᵗʰ **S28.212** **Complete traumatic amputation of left breast**

  ✓7ᵗʰ **S28.219** **Complete traumatic amputation of unspecified breast** ▽

✓6ᵗʰ **S28.22** **Partial traumatic amputation of breast**

  ✓7ᵗʰ **S28.221** **Partial traumatic amputation of right breast**

  ✓7ᵗʰ **S28.222** **Partial traumatic amputation of left breast**

  ✓7ᵗʰ **S28.229** **Partial traumatic amputation of unspecified breast** ▽

✓4ᵗʰ **S29** **Other and unspecified injuries of thorax**
Code also any associated open wound (S21.-)

> The appropriate 7th character is to be added to each code from category S29.
> A   initial encounter
> D   subsequent encounter
> S   sequela

✓5ᵗʰ **S29.0** **Injury of muscle and tendon at thorax level**

✓6ᵗʰ **S29.00** **Unspecified injury of muscle and tendon of thorax**

  ✓7ᵗʰ **S29.001** **Unspecified injury of muscle and tendon of front wall of thorax** ▽

  ✓7ᵗʰ **S29.002** **Unspecified injury of muscle and tendon of back wall of thorax** ▽

  ✓7ᵗʰ **S29.009** **Unspecified injury of muscle and tendon of unspecified wall of thorax** ▽

✓6ᵗʰ **S29.01** **Strain of muscle and tendon of thorax**

  ✓7ᵗʰ **S29.011** **Strain of muscle and tendon of front wall of thorax**

  ✓7ᵗʰ **S29.012** **Strain of muscle and tendon of back wall of thorax**

  ✓7ᵗʰ **S29.019** **Strain of muscle and tendon of unspecified wall of thorax** ▽

✓6ᵗʰ **S29.02** **Laceration of muscle and tendon of thorax**

  ✓7ᵗʰ **S29.021** **Laceration of muscle and tendon of front wall of thorax**

  ✓7ᵗʰ **S29.022** **Laceration of muscle and tendon of back wall of thorax**

  ✓7ᵗʰ **S29.029** **Laceration of muscle and tendon of unspecified wall of thorax** ▽

✓ Additional Character Req   ✓x7ᵗʰ Placeholder Alert   Manifestation   HCC CMS-HCC Condition   ▽ Unspecified Code   ▶◀ Revised Text   ● New Code   ▲ Revised Code Title

ICD-10-CM 2018   939

√6ᵗʰ **S29.09**   **Other injury of muscle and tendon of thorax**

    √7ᵗʰ **S29.091**   **Other injury of muscle and tendon of front wall of thorax**

    √7ᵗʰ **S29.092**   **Other injury of muscle and tendon of back wall of thorax**

    √7ᵗʰ **S29.099**   **Other injury of muscle and tendon of unspecified wall of thorax** ▽

√x7ᵗʰ **S29.8**   **Other specified injuries of thorax**

√x7ᵗʰ **S29.9**   **Unspecified injury of thorax** ▽

Injuries to the abdomen, lower back, lumbar spine, pelvis and external genitals (S30-S39)

INCLUDES   injuries to the abdominal wall
injuries to the anus
injuries to the buttock
injuries to the external genitalia
injuries to the flank
injuries to the groin

EXCLUDES 2   *burns and corrosions (T20-T32)*
effects of foreign body in anus and rectum (T18.5)
effects of foreign body in genitourinary tract (T19.-)
effects of foreign body in stomach, small intestine and colon (T18.2-T18.4)
frostbite (T33-T34)
insect bite or sting, venomous (T63.4)

√4ᵗʰ **S30**   **Superficial injury of abdomen, lower back, pelvis and external genitals**

    EXCLUDES 2   *superficial injury of hip (S70.-)*

> The appropriate 7th character is to be added to each code from category S30.
> A   initial encounter
> D   subsequent encounter
> S   sequela

√x7ᵗʰ **S30.0**   **Contusion of lower back and pelvis**
    Contusion of buttock

√x7ᵗʰ **S30.1**   **Contusion of abdominal wall**
    Contusion of flank   Contusion of groin

√5ᵗʰ **S30.2**   **Contusion of external genital organs**

    √6ᵗʰ **S30.20**   **Contusion of unspecified external genital organ**

       √7ᵗʰ **S30.201**   **Contusion of unspecified external genital organ, male** ♂▽

       √7ᵗʰ **S30.202**   **Contusion of unspecified external genital organ, female** ♀▽

    √x7ᵗʰ **S30.21**   **Contusion of penis** ♂

    √x7ᵗʰ **S30.22**   **Contusion of scrotum and testes** ♂

    √x7ᵗʰ **S30.23**   **Contusion of vagina and vulva** ♀

√x7ᵗʰ **S30.3**   **Contusion of anus**

√5ᵗʰ **S30.8**   **Other superficial injuries of abdomen, lower back, pelvis and external genitals**

    √6ᵗʰ **S30.81**   **Abrasion of abdomen, lower back, pelvis and external genitals**

       √7ᵗʰ **S30.810**   **Abrasion of lower back and pelvis**

       √7ᵗʰ **S30.811**   **Abrasion of abdominal wall**

       √7ᵗʰ **S30.812**   **Abrasion of penis** ♂

       √7ᵗʰ **S30.813**   **Abrasion of scrotum and testes** ♂

       √7ᵗʰ **S30.814**   **Abrasion of vagina and vulva** ♀

       √7ᵗʰ **S30.815**   **Abrasion of unspecified external genital organs, male** ♂▽

       √7ᵗʰ **S30.816**   **Abrasion of unspecified external genital organs, female** ♀▽

       √7ᵗʰ **S30.817**   **Abrasion of anus**

    √6ᵗʰ **S30.82**   **Blister (nonthermal) of abdomen, lower back, pelvis and external genitals**

       √7ᵗʰ **S30.820**   **Blister (nonthermal) of lower back and pelvis**

       √7ᵗʰ **S30.821**   **Blister (nonthermal) of abdominal wall**

       √7ᵗʰ **S30.822**   **Blister (nonthermal) of penis** ♂

       √7ᵗʰ **S30.823**   **Blister (nonthermal) of scrotum and testes** ♂

       √7ᵗʰ **S30.824**   **Blister (nonthermal) of vagina and vulva** ♀

       √7ᵗʰ **S30.825**   **Blister (nonthermal) of unspecified external genital organs, male** ♂▽

       √7ᵗʰ **S30.826**   **Blister (nonthermal) of unspecified external genital organs, female** ♀▽

       √7ᵗʰ **S30.827**   **Blister (nonthermal) of anus**

    √6ᵗʰ **S30.84**   **External constriction of abdomen, lower back, pelvis and external genitals**

       √7ᵗʰ **S30.840**   **External constriction of lower back and pelvis**

       √7ᵗʰ **S30.841**   **External constriction of abdominal wall**

       √7ᵗʰ **S30.842**   **External constriction of penis** ♂
          Hair tourniquet syndrome of penis
          Use additional cause code to identify the constricting item (W49.0-)

       √7ᵗʰ **S30.843**   **External constriction of scrotum and testes** ♂

       √7ᵗʰ **S30.844**   **External constriction of vagina and vulva** ♀

       √7ᵗʰ **S30.845**   **External constriction of unspecified external genital organs, male** ♂▽

       √7ᵗʰ **S30.846**   **External constriction of unspecified external genital organs, female** ♀▽

    √6ᵗʰ **S30.85**   **Superficial foreign body of abdomen, lower back, pelvis and external genitals**
       Splinter in the abdomen, lower back, pelvis and external genitals

       √7ᵗʰ **S30.850**   **Superficial foreign body of lower back and pelvis**

       √7ᵗʰ **S30.851**   **Superficial foreign body of abdominal wall**

       √7ᵗʰ **S30.852**   **Superficial foreign body of penis** ♂

       √7ᵗʰ **S30.853**   **Superficial foreign body of scrotum and testes** ♂

       √7ᵗʰ **S30.854**   **Superficial foreign body of vagina and vulva** ♀

       √7ᵗʰ **S30.855**   **Superficial foreign body of unspecified external genital organs, male** ♂▽

       √7ᵗʰ **S30.856**   **Superficial foreign body of unspecified external genital organs, female** ♀▽

       √7ᵗʰ **S30.857**   **Superficial foreign body of anus**

    √6ᵗʰ **S30.86**   **Insect bite (nonvenomous) of abdomen, lower back, pelvis and external genitals**

       √7ᵗʰ **S30.860**   **Insect bite (nonvenomous) of lower back and pelvis**

       √7ᵗʰ **S30.861**   **Insect bite (nonvenomous) of abdominal wall**

       √7ᵗʰ **S30.862**   **Insect bite (nonvenomous) of penis** ♂

       √7ᵗʰ **S30.863**   **Insect bite (nonvenomous) of scrotum and testes** ♂

       √7ᵗʰ **S30.864**   **Insect bite (nonvenomous) of vagina and vulva** ♀

       √7ᵗʰ **S30.865**   **Insect bite (nonvenomous) of unspecified external genital organs, male** ♂▽

       √7ᵗʰ **S30.866**   **Insect bite (nonvenomous) of unspecified external genital organs, female** ♀▽

       √7ᵗʰ **S30.867**   **Insect bite (nonvenomous) of anus**

    √6ᵗʰ **S30.87**   **Other superficial bite of abdomen, lower back, pelvis and external genitals**
       EXCLUDES 1   *open bite of abdomen, lower back, pelvis and external genitals (S31.05, S31.15, S31.25, S31.35, S31.45, S31.55)*

       √7ᵗʰ **S30.870**   **Other superficial bite of lower back and pelvis**

       √7ᵗʰ **S30.871**   **Other superficial bite of abdominal wall**

       √7ᵗʰ **S30.872**   **Other superficial bite of penis** ♂

       √7ᵗʰ **S30.873**   **Other superficial bite of scrotum and testes** ♂

       √7ᵗʰ **S30.874**   **Other superficial bite of vagina and vulva** ♀

       √7ᵗʰ **S30.875**   **Other superficial bite of unspecified external genital organs, male** ♂▽

       √7ᵗʰ **S30.876**   **Other superficial bite of unspecified external genital organs, female** ♀▽

       √7ᵗʰ **S30.877**   **Other superficial bite of anus**

EXCLUDES 1 Not coded here   EXCLUDES 2 Not included here   N Newborn Age: 0   P Pediatric Age: 0-17   M Maternity Age: 12-55   A Adult Age: 15-124

√5ᵗʰ **S30.9** **Unspecified superficial injury of abdomen, lower back, pelvis and external genitals**

√x7ᵗʰ **S30.91** **Unspecified superficial injury of lower back and pelvis** ▽

√x7ᵗʰ **S30.92** **Unspecified superficial injury of abdominal wall** ▽

√x7ᵗʰ **S30.93** **Unspecified superficial injury of penis** ♂▽

√x7ᵗʰ **S30.94** **Unspecified superficial injury of scrotum and testes** ♂▽

√x7ᵗʰ **S30.95** **Unspecified superficial injury of vagina and vulva** ♀▽

√x7ᵗʰ **S30.96** **Unspecified superficial injury of unspecified external genital organs, male** ♂▽

√x7ᵗʰ **S30.97** **Unspecified superficial injury of unspecified external genital organs, female** ♀▽

√x7ᵗʰ **S30.98** **Unspecified superficial injury of anus** ▽

√4ᵗʰ **S31** **Open wound of abdomen, lower back, pelvis and external genitals**

Code also any associated:
spinal cord injury (S24.0, S24.1-, S34.0-, S34.1-)
wound infection

EXCLUDES 1 *traumatic amputation of part of abdomen, lower back and pelvis (S38.2-, S38.3)*

EXCLUDES 2 *open wound of hip (S71.00-S71.02)*
open fracture of pelvis (S32.1- -S32.9 with 7th character B)

> The appropriate 7th character is to be added to each code from category S31.
> A   initial encounter
> D   subsequent encounter
> S   sequela

√5ᵗʰ **S31.0** **Open wound of lower back and pelvis**

√6ᵗʰ **S31.00** **Unspecified open wound of lower back and pelvis**

√7ᵗʰ **S31.000** **Unspecified open wound of lower back and pelvis without penetration into retroperitoneum** ▽
Unspecified open wound of lower back and pelvis NOS

√7ᵗʰ **S31.001** **Unspecified open wound of lower back and pelvis with penetration into retroperitoneum** ▽

√6ᵗʰ **S31.01** **Laceration without foreign body of lower back and pelvis**

√7ᵗʰ **S31.010** **Laceration without foreign body of lower back and pelvis without penetration into retroperitoneum**
Laceration without foreign body of lower back and pelvis NOS

√7ᵗʰ **S31.011** **Laceration without foreign body of lower back and pelvis with penetration into retroperitoneum**

√6ᵗʰ **S31.02** **Laceration with foreign body of lower back and pelvis**

√7ᵗʰ **S31.020** **Laceration with foreign body of lower back and pelvis without penetration into retroperitoneum**
Laceration with foreign body of lower back and pelvis NOS

√7ᵗʰ **S31.021** **Laceration with foreign body of lower back and pelvis with penetration into retroperitoneum**

√6ᵗʰ **S31.03** **Puncture wound without foreign body of lower back and pelvis**

√7ᵗʰ **S31.030** **Puncture wound without foreign body of lower back and pelvis without penetration into retroperitoneum**
Puncture wound without foreign body of lower back and pelvis NOS

√7ᵗʰ **S31.031** **Puncture wound without foreign body of lower back and pelvis with penetration into retroperitoneum**

√6ᵗʰ **S31.04** **Puncture wound with foreign body of lower back and pelvis**

√7ᵗʰ **S31.040** **Puncture wound with foreign body of lower back and pelvis without penetration into retroperitoneum**
Puncture wound with foreign body of lower back and pelvis NOS

√7ᵗʰ **S31.041** **Puncture wound with foreign body of lower back and pelvis with penetration into retroperitoneum**

√6ᵗʰ **S31.05** **Open bite of lower back and pelvis**
Bite of lower back and pelvis NOS

EXCLUDES 1 *superficial bite of lower back and pelvis (S30.860, S30.870)*

√7ᵗʰ **S31.050** **Open bite of lower back and pelvis without penetration into retroperitoneum**
Open bite of lower back and pelvis NOS

√7ᵗʰ **S31.051** **Open bite of lower back and pelvis with penetration into retroperitoneum**

√5ᵗʰ **S31.1** **Open wound of abdominal wall without penetration into peritoneal cavity**
Open wound of abdominal wall NOS

EXCLUDES 2 *open wound of abdominal wall with penetration into peritoneal cavity (S31.6-)*

√6ᵗʰ **S31.10** **Unspecified open wound of abdominal wall without penetration into peritoneal cavity**

√7ᵗʰ **S31.100** **Unspecified open wound of abdominal wall, right upper quadrant without penetration into peritoneal cavity** ▽

√7ᵗʰ **S31.101** **Unspecified open wound of abdominal wall, left upper quadrant without penetration into peritoneal cavity** ▽

√7ᵗʰ **S31.102** **Unspecified open wound of abdominal wall, epigastric region without penetration into peritoneal cavity** ▽

√7ᵗʰ **S31.103** **Unspecified open wound of abdominal wall, right lower quadrant without penetration into peritoneal cavity** ▽

√7ᵗʰ **S31.104** **Unspecified open wound of abdominal wall, left lower quadrant without penetration into peritoneal cavity** ▽

√7ᵗʰ **S31.105** **Unspecified open wound of abdominal wall, periumbilic region without penetration into peritoneal cavity** ▽

√7ᵗʰ **S31.109** **Unspecified open wound of abdominal wall, unspecified quadrant without penetration into peritoneal cavity** ▽
Unspecified open wound of abdominal wall NOS

√6ᵗʰ **S31.11** **Laceration without foreign body of abdominal wall without penetration into peritoneal cavity**

√7ᵗʰ **S31.110** **Laceration without foreign body of abdominal wall, right upper quadrant without penetration into peritoneal cavity**

√7ᵗʰ **S31.111** **Laceration without foreign body of abdominal wall, left upper quadrant without penetration into peritoneal cavity**

√7ᵗʰ **S31.112** **Laceration without foreign body of abdominal wall, epigastric region without penetration into peritoneal cavity**

√7ᵗʰ **S31.113** **Laceration without foreign body of abdominal wall, right lower quadrant without penetration into peritoneal cavity**

√7ᵗʰ **S31.114** **Laceration without foreign body of abdominal wall, left lower quadrant without penetration into peritoneal cavity**

√7ᵗʰ **S31.115** **Laceration without foreign body of abdominal wall, periumbilic region without penetration into peritoneal cavity**

√7ᵗʰ **S31.119** **Laceration without foreign body of abdominal wall, unspecified quadrant without penetration into peritoneal cavity** ▽

√6ᵗʰ **S31.12** **Laceration with foreign body of abdominal wall without penetration into peritoneal cavity**

√7ᵗʰ **S31.120** **Laceration of abdominal wall with foreign body, right upper quadrant without penetration into peritoneal cavity**

√7ᵗʰ **S31.121** **Laceration of abdominal wall with foreign body, left upper quadrant without penetration into peritoneal cavity**

√7ᵗʰ **S31.122** **Laceration of abdominal wall with foreign body, epigastric region without penetration into peritoneal cavity**

√7ᵗʰ **S31.123** **Laceration of abdominal wall with foreign body, right lower quadrant without penetration into peritoneal cavity**

☑ Additional Character Req   √x7ᵗʰ Placeholder Alert   Manifestation   **HCC** CMS-HCC Condition   ▽ Unspecified Code   ▶◀ Revised Text   ● New Code   ▲ Revised Code Title

ICD-10-CM 2018   **941**

√7th **S31.124** Laceration of abdominal wall with foreign body, left lower quadrant without penetration into peritoneal cavity

√7th **S31.125** Laceration of abdominal wall with foreign body, periumbilic region without penetration into peritoneal cavity

√7th **S31.129** Laceration of abdominal wall with foreign body, unspecified quadrant without penetration into peritoneal cavity ▽

√6th **S31.13** Puncture wound of abdominal wall without foreign body without penetration into peritoneal cavity

√7th **S31.130** Puncture wound of abdominal wall without foreign body, right upper quadrant without penetration into peritoneal cavity

√7th **S31.131** Puncture wound of abdominal wall without foreign body, left upper quadrant without penetration into peritoneal cavity

√7th **S31.132** Puncture wound of abdominal wall without foreign body, epigastric region without penetration into peritoneal cavity

√7th **S31.133** Puncture wound of abdominal wall without foreign body, right lower quadrant without penetration into peritoneal cavity

√7th **S31.134** Puncture wound of abdominal wall without foreign body, left lower quadrant without penetration into peritoneal cavity

√7th **S31.135** Puncture wound of abdominal wall without foreign body, periumbilic region without penetration into peritoneal cavity

√7th **S31.139** Puncture wound of abdominal wall without foreign body, unspecified quadrant without penetration into peritoneal cavity ▽

√6th **S31.14** Puncture wound of abdominal wall with foreign body without penetration into peritoneal cavity

√7th **S31.140** Puncture wound of abdominal wall with foreign body, right upper quadrant without penetration into peritoneal cavity

√7th **S31.141** Puncture wound of abdominal wall with foreign body, left upper quadrant without penetration into peritoneal cavity

√7th **S31.142** Puncture wound of abdominal wall with foreign body, epigastric region without penetration into peritoneal cavity

√7th **S31.143** Puncture wound of abdominal wall with foreign body, right lower quadrant without penetration into peritoneal cavity

√7th **S31.144** Puncture wound of abdominal wall with foreign body, left lower quadrant without penetration into peritoneal cavity

√7th **S31.145** Puncture wound of abdominal wall with foreign body, periumbilic region without penetration into peritoneal cavity

√7th **S31.149** Puncture wound of abdominal wall with foreign body, unspecified quadrant without penetration into peritoneal cavity ▽

√6th **S31.15** Open bite of abdominal wall without penetration into peritoneal cavity
Bite of abdominal wall NOS
EXCLUDES 1   superficial bite of abdominal wall (S30.871)

√7th **S31.150** Open bite of abdominal wall, right upper quadrant without penetration into peritoneal cavity

√7th **S31.151** Open bite of abdominal wall, left upper quadrant without penetration into peritoneal cavity

√7th **S31.152** Open bite of abdominal wall, epigastric region without penetration into peritoneal cavity

√7th **S31.153** Open bite of abdominal wall, right lower quadrant without penetration into peritoneal cavity

√7th **S31.154** Open bite of abdominal wall, left lower quadrant without penetration into peritoneal cavity

√7th **S31.155** Open bite of abdominal wall, periumbilic region without penetration into peritoneal cavity

√7th **S31.159** Open bite of abdominal wall, unspecified quadrant without penetration into peritoneal cavity ▽

√5th **S31.2** Open wound of penis

√x7th **S31.20** Unspecified open wound of penis   ♂▽

√x7th **S31.21** Laceration without foreign body of penis   ♂

√x7th **S31.22** Laceration with foreign body of penis   ♂

√x7th **S31.23** Puncture wound without foreign body of penis   ♂

√x7th **S31.24** Puncture wound with foreign body of penis   ♂

√x7th **S31.25** Open bite of penis   ♂
Bite of penis NOS
EXCLUDES 1   superficial bite of penis (S30.862, S30.872)

√5th **S31.3** Open wound of scrotum and testes

√x7th **S31.30** Unspecified open wound of scrotum and testes   ♂▽

√x7th **S31.31** Laceration without foreign body of scrotum and testes   ♂

√x7th **S31.32** Laceration with foreign body of scrotum and testes   ♂

√x7th **S31.33** Puncture wound without foreign body of scrotum and testes   ♂

√x7th **S31.34** Puncture wound with foreign body of scrotum and testes   ♂

√x7th **S31.35** Open bite of scrotum and testes   ♂
Bite of scrotum and testes NOS
EXCLUDES 1   superficial bite of scrotum and testes (S30.863, S30.873)

√5th **S31.4** Open wound of vagina and vulva
EXCLUDES 1   injury to vagina and vulva during delivery (O70-, O71.4)

√x7th **S31.40** Unspecified open wound of vagina and vulva   ♀▽

√x7th **S31.41** Laceration without foreign body of vagina and vulva   ♀

√x7th **S31.42** Laceration with foreign body of vagina and vulva   ♀

√x7th **S31.43** Puncture wound without foreign body of vagina and vulva   ♀

√x7th **S31.44** Puncture wound with foreign body of vagina and vulva   ♀

√x7th **S31.45** Open bite of vagina and vulva   ♀
Bite of vagina and vulva NOS
EXCLUDES 1   superficial bite of vagina and vulva (S30.864, S30.874)

√6th **S31.5** Open wound of unspecified external genital organs
EXCLUDES 1   traumatic amputation of external genital organs (S38.21, S38.22)

√6th **S31.50** Unspecified open wound of unspecified external genital organs

√7th **S31.501** Unspecified open wound of unspecified external genital organs, male   ♂▽

√7th **S31.502** Unspecified open wound of unspecified external genital organs, female   ♀▽

√6th **S31.51** Laceration without foreign body of unspecified external genital organs

√7th **S31.511** Laceration without foreign body of unspecified external genital organs, male   ♂▽

√7th **S31.512** Laceration without foreign body of unspecified external genital organs, female   ♀▽

√6th **S31.52** Laceration with foreign body of unspecified external genital organs

√7th **S31.521** Laceration with foreign body of unspecified external genital organs, male   ♂▽

√7th **S31.522** Laceration with foreign body of unspecified external genital organs, female   ♀▽

√6ᵗʰ **S31.53** **Puncture wound without foreign body of unspecified external genital organs**

     √7ᵗʰ **S31.531** Puncture wound without foreign body of unspecified external genital organs, male ♂▽

     √7ᵗʰ **S31.532** Puncture wound without foreign body of unspecified external genital organs, female ♀▽

√6ᵗʰ **S31.54** **Puncture wound with foreign body of unspecified external genital organs**

     √7ᵗʰ **S31.541** Puncture wound with foreign body of unspecified external genital organs, male ♂▽

     √7ᵗʰ **S31.542** Puncture wound with foreign body of unspecified external genital organs, female ♀▽

√6ᵗʰ **S31.55** **Open bite of unspecified external genital organs**
     Bite of unspecified external genital organs NOS
     EXCLUDES 1   *superficial bite of unspecified external genital organs (S30.865, S30.866, S30.875, S30.876)*

     √7ᵗʰ **S31.551** Open bite of unspecified external genital organs, male ♂▽

     √7ᵗʰ **S31.552** Open bite of unspecified external genital organs, female ♀▽

√5ᵗʰ **S31.6** **Open wound of abdominal wall with penetration into peritoneal cavity**

     √6ᵗʰ **S31.60** **Unspecified open wound of abdominal wall with penetration into peritoneal cavity**

         √7ᵗʰ **S31.600** Unspecified open wound of abdominal wall, right upper quadrant with penetration into peritoneal cavity ▽

         √7ᵗʰ **S31.601** Unspecified open wound of abdominal wall, left upper quadrant with penetration into peritoneal cavity ▽

         √7ᵗʰ **S31.602** Unspecified open wound of abdominal wall, epigastric region with penetration into peritoneal cavity ▽

         √7ᵗʰ **S31.603** Unspecified open wound of abdominal wall, right lower quadrant with penetration into peritoneal cavity ▽

         √7ᵗʰ **S31.604** Unspecified open wound of abdominal wall, left lower quadrant with penetration into peritoneal cavity ▽

         √7ᵗʰ **S31.605** Unspecified open wound of abdominal wall, periumbilic region with penetration into peritoneal cavity ▽

         √7ᵗʰ **S31.609** Unspecified open wound of abdominal wall, unspecified quadrant with penetration into peritoneal cavity ▽

     √6ᵗʰ **S31.61** **Laceration without foreign body of abdominal wall with penetration into peritoneal cavity**

         √7ᵗʰ **S31.610** Laceration without foreign body of abdominal wall, right upper quadrant with penetration into peritoneal cavity

         √7ᵗʰ **S31.611** Laceration without foreign body of abdominal wall, left upper quadrant with penetration into peritoneal cavity

         √7ᵗʰ **S31.612** Laceration without foreign body of abdominal wall, epigastric region with penetration into peritoneal cavity

         √7ᵗʰ **S31.613** Laceration without foreign body of abdominal wall, right lower quadrant with penetration into peritoneal cavity

         √7ᵗʰ **S31.614** Laceration without foreign body of abdominal wall, left lower quadrant with penetration into peritoneal cavity

         √7ᵗʰ **S31.615** Laceration without foreign body of abdominal wall, periumbilic region with penetration into peritoneal cavity

         √7ᵗʰ **S31.619** Laceration without foreign body of abdominal wall, unspecified quadrant with penetration into peritoneal cavity ▽

     √6ᵗʰ **S31.62** **Laceration with foreign body of abdominal wall with penetration into peritoneal cavity**

         √7ᵗʰ **S31.620** Laceration with foreign body of abdominal wall, right upper quadrant with penetration into peritoneal cavity

         √7ᵗʰ **S31.621** Laceration with foreign body of abdominal wall, left upper quadrant with penetration into peritoneal cavity

         √7ᵗʰ **S31.622** Laceration with foreign body of abdominal wall, epigastric region with penetration into peritoneal cavity

         √7ᵗʰ **S31.623** Laceration with foreign body of abdominal wall, right lower quadrant with penetration into peritoneal cavity

         √7ᵗʰ **S31.624** Laceration with foreign body of abdominal wall, left lower quadrant with penetration into peritoneal cavity

         √7ᵗʰ **S31.625** Laceration with foreign body of abdominal wall, periumbilic region with penetration into peritoneal cavity

         √7ᵗʰ **S31.629** Laceration with foreign body of abdominal wall, unspecified quadrant with penetration into peritoneal cavity ▽

     √6ᵗʰ **S31.63** **Puncture wound without foreign body of abdominal wall with penetration into peritoneal cavity**

         √7ᵗʰ **S31.630** Puncture wound without foreign body of abdominal wall, right upper quadrant with penetration into peritoneal cavity

         √7ᵗʰ **S31.631** Puncture wound without foreign body of abdominal wall, left upper quadrant with penetration into peritoneal cavity

         √7ᵗʰ **S31.632** Puncture wound without foreign body of abdominal wall, epigastric region with penetration into peritoneal cavity

         √7ᵗʰ **S31.633** Puncture wound without foreign body of abdominal wall, right lower quadrant with penetration into peritoneal cavity

         √7ᵗʰ **S31.634** Puncture wound without foreign body of abdominal wall, left lower quadrant with penetration into peritoneal cavity

         √7ᵗʰ **S31.635** Puncture wound without foreign body of abdominal wall, periumbilic region with penetration into peritoneal cavity

         √7ᵗʰ **S31.639** Puncture wound without foreign body of abdominal wall, unspecified quadrant with penetration into peritoneal cavity ▽

     √6ᵗʰ **S31.64** **Puncture wound with foreign body of abdominal wall with penetration into peritoneal cavity**

         √7ᵗʰ **S31.640** Puncture wound with foreign body of abdominal wall, right upper quadrant with penetration into peritoneal cavity

         √7ᵗʰ **S31.641** Puncture wound with foreign body of abdominal wall, left upper quadrant with penetration into peritoneal cavity

         √7ᵗʰ **S31.642** Puncture wound with foreign body of abdominal wall, epigastric region with penetration Into peritoneal cavity

         √7ᵗʰ **S31.643** Puncture wound with foreign body of abdominal wall, right lower quadrant with penetration into peritoneal cavity

         √7ᵗʰ **S31.644** Puncture wound with foreign body of abdominal wall, left lower quadrant with penetration into peritoneal cavity

         √7ᵗʰ **S31.645** Puncture wound with foreign body of abdominal wall, periumbilic region with penetration into peritoneal cavity

         √7ᵗʰ **S31.649** Puncture wound with foreign body of abdominal wall, unspecified quadrant with penetration into peritoneal cavity ▽

     √6ᵗʰ **S31.65** **Open bite of abdominal wall with penetration into peritoneal cavity**
     EXCLUDES 1   *superficial bite of abdominal wall (S30.861, S30.871)*

         √7ᵗʰ **S31.650** Open bite of abdominal wall, right upper quadrant with penetration into peritoneal cavity

         √7ᵗʰ **S31.651** Open bite of abdominal wall, left upper quadrant with penetration into peritoneal cavity

         √7ᵗʰ **S31.652** Open bite of abdominal wall, epigastric region with penetration into peritoneal cavity

☑ Additional Character Req   ⱽˣ⁷ᵗʰ Placeholder Alert   Manifestation   ʜᴄᴄ CMS-HCC Condition   ▽ Unspecified Code   ▶◀ Revised Text   ● New Code   ▲ Revised Code Title

ICD-10-CM 2018   **943**

✓7ᵗʰ S31.653 Open bite of abdominal wall, **right lower quadrant** with penetration into peritoneal cavity

✓7ᵗʰ S31.654 Open bite of abdominal wall, **left lower quadrant** with penetration into peritoneal cavity

✓7ᵗʰ S31.655 Open bite of abdominal wall, **periumbilic region** with penetration into peritoneal cavity

✓7ᵗʰ S31.659 Open bite of abdominal wall, unspecified quadrant with penetration into peritoneal cavity ▽

✓5ᵗʰ S31.8 Open wound of other parts of abdomen, lower back and pelvis

  ✓6ᵗʰ S31.80 Open wound of unspecified buttock

    ✓7ᵗʰ S31.801 Laceration without foreign body of unspecified buttock ▽

    ✓7ᵗʰ S31.802 Laceration with foreign body of unspecified buttock ▽

    ✓7ᵗʰ S31.803 Puncture wound without foreign body of unspecified buttock ▽

    ✓7ᵗʰ S31.804 Puncture wound with foreign body of unspecified buttock ▽

    ✓7ᵗʰ S31.805 Open bite of unspecified buttock ▽
       Bite of buttock NOS
       EXCLUDES 1   superficial bite of buttock (S30.870)

    ✓7ᵗʰ S31.809 Unspecified open wound of unspecified buttock ▽

  ✓6ᵗʰ S31.81 Open wound of right buttock

    ✓7ᵗʰ S31.811 Laceration without foreign body of right buttock

    ✓7ᵗʰ S31.812 Laceration with foreign body of right buttock

    ✓7ᵗʰ S31.813 Puncture wound without foreign body of right buttock

    ✓7ᵗʰ S31.814 Puncture wound with foreign body of right buttock

    ✓7ᵗʰ S31.815 Open bite of right buttock
       Bite of right buttock NOS
       EXCLUDES 1   superficial bite of buttock (S30.870)

    ✓7ᵗʰ S31.819 Unspecified open wound of right buttock ▽

  ✓6ᵗʰ S31.82 Open wound of left buttock

    ✓7ᵗʰ S31.821 Laceration without foreign body of left buttock

    ✓7ᵗʰ S31.822 Laceration with foreign body of left buttock

    ✓7ᵗʰ S31.823 Puncture wound without foreign body of left buttock

    ✓7ᵗʰ S31.824 Puncture wound with foreign body of left buttock

    ✓7ᵗʰ S31.825 Open bite of left buttock
       Bite of left buttock NOS
       EXCLUDES 1   superficial bite of buttock (S30.870)

    ✓7ᵗʰ S31.829 Unspecified open wound of left buttock ▽

  ✓6ᵗʰ S31.83 Open wound of anus

    ✓7ᵗʰ S31.831 Laceration without foreign body of anus

    ✓7ᵗʰ S31.832 Laceration with foreign body of anus

    ✓7ᵗʰ S31.833 Puncture wound without foreign body of anus

    ✓7ᵗʰ S31.834 Puncture wound with foreign body of anus

    ✓7ᵗʰ S31.835 Open bite of anus
       Bite of anus NOS
       EXCLUDES 1   superficial bite of anus (S30.877)

    ✓7ᵗʰ S31.839 Unspecified open wound of anus ▽

✓4ᵗʰ S32 Fracture of lumbar spine and pelvis

NOTE   A fracture not indicated as displaced or nondisplaced should be coded to displaced.
A fracture not indicated as opened or closed should be coded to closed.

INCLUDES   fracture of lumbosacral neural arch
fracture of lumbosacral spinous process
fracture of lumbosacral transverse process
fracture of lumbosacral vertebra
fracture of lumbosacral vertebral arch

Code first any associated spinal cord and spinal nerve injury (S34.-)

EXCLUDES 1   transection of abdomen (S38.3)
EXCLUDES 2   fracture of hip NOS (S72.0-)

AHA: 2015, 3Q, 37-39; 2012, 4Q, 93

> The appropriate 7th character is to be added to each code from category S32.
> A   initial encounter for closed fracture
> B   initial encounter for open fracture
> D   subsequent encounter for fracture with routine healing
> G   subsequent encounter for fracture with delayed healing
> K   subsequent encounter for fracture with nonunion
> S   sequela

✓5ᵗʰ S32.0 Fracture of lumbar vertebra
   Fracture of lumbar spine NOS

  ✓6ᵗʰ S32.00 Fracture of unspecified lumbar vertebra

    1 **✓7ᵗʰ S32.000** Wedge compression fracture of unspecified lumbar vertebra   HCC ▽

    1 **✓7ᵗʰ S32.001** Stable burst fracture of unspecified lumbar vertebra   HCC ▽

    1 **✓7ᵗʰ S32.002** Unstable burst fracture of unspecified lumbar vertebra   HCC ▽

    1 **✓7ᵗʰ S32.008** Other fracture of unspecified lumbar vertebra   HCC ▽

    1 **✓7ᵗʰ S32.009** Unspecified fracture of unspecified lumbar vertebra   HCC ▽

  ✓6ᵗʰ S32.01 Fracture of first lumbar vertebra

    1 **✓7ᵗʰ S32.010** Wedge compression fracture of first lumbar vertebra   HCC

    1 **✓7ᵗʰ S32.011** Stable burst fracture of first lumbar vertebra   HCC

    1 **✓7ᵗʰ S32.012** Unstable burst fracture of first lumbar vertebra   HCC

    1 **✓7ᵗʰ S32.018** Other fracture of first lumbar vertebra   HCC

    1 **✓7ᵗʰ S32.019** Unspecified fracture of first lumbar vertebra   HCC ▽

  ✓6ᵗʰ S32.02 Fracture of second lumbar vertebra

    1 **✓7ᵗʰ S32.020** Wedge compression fracture of second lumbar vertebra   HCC

    1 **✓7ᵗʰ S32.021** Stable burst fracture of second lumbar vertebra   HCC

    1 **✓7ᵗʰ S32.022** Unstable burst fracture of second lumbar vertebra   HCC

    1 **✓7ᵗʰ S32.028** Other fracture of second lumbar vertebra   HCC

    1 **✓7ᵗʰ S32.029** Unspecified fracture of second lumbar vertebra   HCC ▽

  ✓6ᵗʰ S32.03 Fracture of third lumbar vertebra

    1 **✓7ᵗʰ S32.030** Wedge compression fracture of third lumbar vertebra   HCC

    1 **✓7ᵗʰ S32.031** Stable burst fracture of third lumbar vertebra   HCC

    1 **✓7ᵗʰ S32.032** Unstable burst fracture of third lumbar vertebra   HCC

    1 **✓7ᵗʰ S32.038** Other fracture of third lumbar vertebra   HCC

    1 **✓7ᵗʰ S32.039** Unspecified fracture of third lumbar vertebra   HCC ▽

  ✓6ᵗʰ S32.04 Fracture of fourth lumbar vertebra

    1 **✓7ᵗʰ S32.040** Wedge compression fracture of fourth lumbar vertebra   HCC

    1 **✓7ᵗʰ S32.041** Stable burst fracture of fourth lumbar vertebra   HCC

    1 **✓7ᵗʰ S32.042** Unstable burst fracture of fourth lumbar vertebra   HCC

---

1   HCC with 7th character indicating initial encounter (A, B or C - specific to category).

EXCLUDES 1 Not coded here   *EXCLUDES 2* Not included here   N Newborn Age: 0   P Pediatric Age: 0-17   M Maternity Age: 12-55   A Adult Age: 15-124

944   ICD-10-CM 2018

1 ✓7ᵗʰ **S32.048** Other fracture of fourth lumbar vertebra `HCC`

1 ✓7ᵗʰ **S32.049** Unspecified fracture of fourth lumbar vertebra `HCC` ▽

✓6ᵗʰ **S32.05** Fracture of fifth lumbar vertebra

1 ✓7ᵗʰ **S32.050** **Wedge compression** fracture of fifth lumbar vertebra `HCC`

1 ✓7ᵗʰ **S32.051** **Stable burst** fracture of fifth lumbar vertebra `HCC`

1 ✓7ᵗʰ **S32.052** **Unstable burst** fracture of fifth lumbar vertebra `HCC`

1 ✓7ᵗʰ **S32.058** Other fracture of fifth lumbar vertebra `HCC`

1 ✓7ᵗʰ **S32.059** **Unspecified** fracture of fifth lumbar vertebra `HCC` ▽

✓5ᵗʰ **S32.1** Fracture of sacrum

> `NOTE` For vertical fractures, code to most medial fracture extension.
> Use two codes if both a vertical and transverse fracture are present.

> Code also any associated fracture of pelvic ring (S32.8-)

1 ✓x7ᵗʰ **S32.10** Unspecified fracture of sacrum `HCC` ▽

✓6ᵗʰ **S32.11** **Zone I** fracture of sacrum
Vertical sacral ala fracture of sacrum

1 ✓7ᵗʰ **S32.110** **Nondisplaced** Zone I fracture of sacrum `HCC`

1 ✓7ᵗʰ **S32.111** **Minimally displaced** Zone I fracture of sacrum `HCC`

1 ✓7ᵗʰ **S32.112** **Severely displaced** Zone I fracture of sacrum `HCC`

1 ✓7ᵗʰ **S32.119** **Unspecified** Zone I fracture of sacrum `HCC` ▽

✓6ᵗʰ **S32.12** **Zone II** fracture of sacrum
Vertical foraminal region fracture of sacrum

1 ✓7ᵗʰ **S32.120** **Nondisplaced** Zone II fracture of sacrum `HCC`

1 ✓7ᵗʰ **S32.121** **Minimally displaced** Zone II fracture of sacrum `HCC`

1 ✓7ᵗʰ **S32.122** **Severely displaced** Zone II fracture of sacrum `HCC`

1 ✓7ᵗʰ **S32.129** **Unspecified** Zone II fracture of sacrum `HCC` ▽

Vertical Sacral Fracture Zones

Zones: 1 2 3

Transverse Sacral Fracture Types

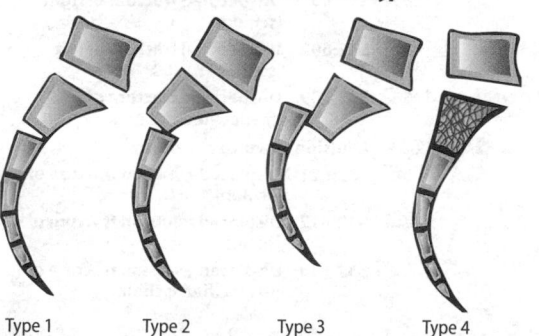

Type 1   Type 2   Type 3   Type 4

✓6ᵗʰ **S32.13** **Zone III** fracture of sacrum
Vertical fracture into spinal canal region of sacrum

1 ✓7ᵗʰ **S32.130** **Nondisplaced** Zone III fracture of sacrum `HCC`

1 ✓7ᵗʰ **S32.131** **Minimally displaced** Zone III fracture of sacrum `HCC`

1 ✓7ᵗʰ **S32.132** **Severely displaced** Zone III fracture of sacrum `HCC`

1 ✓7ᵗʰ **S32.139** **Unspecified** Zone III fracture of sacrum `HCC` ▽

1 ✓x7ᵗʰ **S32.14** **Type 1** fracture of sacrum `HCC`
Transverse flexion fracture of sacrum without displacement

1 ✓x7ᵗʰ **S32.15** **Type 2** fracture of sacrum `HCC`
Transverse flexion fracture of sacrum with posterior displacement

1 ✓x7ᵗʰ **S32.16** **Type 3** fracture of sacrum `HCC`
Transverse extension fracture of sacrum with anterior displacement

1 ✓x7ᵗʰ **S32.17** **Type 4** fracture of sacrum `HCC`
Transverse segmental comminution of upper sacrum

1 ✓x7ᵗʰ **S32.19** Other fracture of sacrum `HCC`

1 ✓x7ᵗʰ **S32.2** Fracture of coccyx `HCC`

✓5ᵗʰ **S32.3** Fracture of ilium

> `EXCLUDES 1` fracture of ilium with associated disruption of pelvic ring (S32.8-)

✓6ᵗʰ **S32.30** Unspecified fracture of ilium

1 ✓7ᵗʰ **S32.301** Unspecified fracture of **right** ilium `HCC` ▽

1 ✓7ᵗʰ **S32.302** Unspecified fracture of **left** ilium `HCC` ▽

1 ✓7ᵗʰ **S32.309** Unspecified fracture of unspecified ilium `HCC` ▽

✓6ᵗʰ **S32.31** **Avulsion** fracture of ilium

1 ✓7ᵗʰ **S32.311** **Displaced** avulsion fracture of **right** ilium `HCC`

1 ✓7ᵗʰ **S32.312** **Displaced** avulsion fracture of **left** ilium `HCC`

1 ✓7ᵗʰ **S32.313** **Displaced** avulsion fracture of unspecified ilium `HCC` ▽

1 ✓7ᵗʰ **S32.314** **Nondisplaced** avulsion fracture of **right** ilium `HCC`

1 ✓7ᵗʰ **S32.315** **Nondisplaced** avulsion fracture of **left** ilium `HCC`

1 ✓7ᵗʰ **S32.316** **Nondisplaced** avulsion fracture of unspecified ilium `HCC` ▽

✓6ᵗʰ **S32.39** Other fracture of ilium

1 ✓7ᵗʰ **S32.391** Other fracture of **right** ilium `HCC`

1 ✓7ᵗʰ **S32.392** Other fracture of **left** ilium `HCC`

1 ✓7ᵗʰ **S32.399** Other fracture of unspecified ilium `HCC` ▽

✓5ᵗʰ **S32.4** Fracture of acetabulum
Code also any associated fracture of pelvic ring (S32.8-)
AHA: 2016, 3Q, 16

✓6ᵗʰ **S32.40** Unspecified fracture of acetabulum

1 ✓7ᵗʰ **S32.401** Unspecified fracture of **right** acetabulum `HCC` ▽

1 ✓7ᵗʰ **S32.402** Unspecified fracture of **left** acetabulum `HCC` ▽

1 ✓7ᵗʰ **S32.409** Unspecified fracture of unspecified acetabulum `HCC` ▽

✓6ᵗʰ **S32.41** Fracture of **anterior wall** of acetabulum

1 ✓7ᵗʰ **S32.411** **Displaced** fracture of anterior wall of **right** acetabulum `HCC`

1 ✓7ᵗʰ **S32.412** **Displaced** fracture of anterior wall of **left** acetabulum `HCC`

1 ✓7ᵗʰ **S32.413** **Displaced** fracture of anterior wall of unspecified acetabulum `HCC` ▽

1 ✓7ᵗʰ **S32.414** **Nondisplaced** fracture of anterior wall of **right** acetabulum `HCC`

1 ✓7ᵗʰ **S32.415** **Nondisplaced** fracture of anterior wall of **left** acetabulum `HCC`

1 ✓7ᵗʰ **S32.416** **Nondisplaced** fracture of anterior wall of unspecified acetabulum `HCC` ▽

---

1 HCC with 7th character indicating initial encounter (A, B or C - specific to category).

☑ Additional Character Req   ✓x7ᵗʰ Placeholder Alert   Manifestation   `HCC` CMS-HCC Condition   ▽ Unspecified Code   ►◄ Revised Text   ● New Code   ▲ Revised Code Title

Chapter 19. Injury, Poisoning, and Certain Other Consequences of External Causes

S32.42–S32.613

✓6ᵗʰ **S32.42 Fracture of posterior wall of acetabulum**
- 1 ✓7ᵗʰ S32.421 Displaced fracture of posterior wall of right acetabulum `HCC`
- 1 ✓7ᵗʰ S32.422 Displaced fracture of posterior wall of left acetabulum `HCC`
- 1 ✓7ᵗʰ S32.423 Displaced fracture of posterior wall of unspecified acetabulum `HCC` ▽
- 1 ✓7ᵗʰ S32.424 Nondisplaced fracture of posterior wall of right acetabulum `HCC`
- 1 ✓7ᵗʰ S32.425 Nondisplaced fracture of posterior wall of left acetabulum `HCC`
- 1 ✓7ᵗʰ S32.426 Nondisplaced fracture of posterior wall of unspecified acetabulum `HCC` ▽

✓6ᵗʰ **S32.43 Fracture of anterior column [iliopubic] of acetabulum**
- 1 ✓7ᵗʰ S32.431 Displaced fracture of anterior column [iliopubic] of right acetabulum `HCC`
- 1 ✓7ᵗʰ S32.432 Displaced fracture of anterior column [iliopubic] of left acetabulum `HCC`
- 1 ✓7ᵗʰ S32.433 Displaced fracture of anterior column [iliopubic] of unspecified acetabulum `HCC` ▽
- 1 ✓7ᵗʰ S32.434 Nondisplaced fracture of anterior column [iliopubic] of right acetabulum `HCC`
- 1 ✓7ᵗʰ S32.435 Nondisplaced fracture of anterior column [iliopubic] of left acetabulum `HCC`
- 1 ✓7ᵗʰ S32.436 Nondisplaced fracture of anterior column [iliopubic] of unspecified acetabulum `HCC` ▽

✓6ᵗʰ **S32.44 Fracture of posterior column [ilioischial] of acetabulum**
- 1 ✓7ᵗʰ S32.441 Displaced fracture of posterior column [ilioischial] of right acetabulum `HCC`
- 1 ✓7ᵗʰ S32.442 Displaced fracture of posterior column [ilioischial] of left acetabulum `HCC`
- 1 ✓7ᵗʰ S32.443 Displaced fracture of posterior column [ilioischial] of unspecified acetabulum `HCC` ▽
- 1 ✓7ᵗʰ S32.444 Nondisplaced fracture of posterior column [ilioischial] of right acetabulum `HCC`
- 1 ✓7ᵗʰ S32.445 Nondisplaced fracture of posterior column [ilioischial] of left acetabulum `HCC`
- 1 ✓7ᵗʰ S32.446 Nondisplaced fracture of posterior column [ilioischial] of unspecified acetabulum `HCC` ▽

✓6ᵗʰ **S32.45 Transverse fracture of acetabulum**
- 1 ✓7ᵗʰ S32.451 Displaced transverse fracture of right acetabulum `HCC`
- 1 ✓7ᵗʰ S32.452 Displaced transverse fracture of left acetabulum `HCC`
- 1 ✓7ᵗʰ S32.453 Displaced transverse fracture of unspecified acetabulum `HCC` ▽
- 1 ✓7ᵗʰ S32.454 Nondisplaced transverse fracture of right acetabulum `HCC`
- 1 ✓7ᵗʰ S32.455 Nondisplaced transverse fracture of left acetabulum `HCC`
- 1 ✓7ᵗʰ S32.456 Nondisplaced transverse fracture of unspecified acetabulum `HCC` ▽

✓6ᵗʰ **S32.46 Associated transverse-posterior fracture of acetabulum**
- 1 ✓7ᵗʰ S32.461 Displaced associated transverse-posterior fracture of right acetabulum `HCC`
- 1 ✓7ᵗʰ S32.462 Displaced associated transverse-posterior fracture of left acetabulum `HCC`
- 1 ✓7ᵗʰ S32.463 Displaced associated transverse-posterior fracture of unspecified acetabulum `HCC` ▽
- 1 ✓7ᵗʰ S32.464 Nondisplaced associated transverse posterior fracture of right acetabulum `HCC`
- 1 ✓7ᵗʰ S32.465 Nondisplaced associated transverse-posterior fracture of left acetabulum `HCC`
- 1 ✓7ᵗʰ S32.466 Nondisplaced associated transverse-posterior fracture of unspecified acetabulum `HCC` ▽

✓6ᵗʰ **S32.47 Fracture of medial wall of acetabulum**
- 1 ✓7ᵗʰ S32.471 Displaced fracture of medial wall of right acetabulum `HCC`
- 1 ✓7ᵗʰ S32.472 Displaced fracture of medial wall of left acetabulum `HCC`
- 1 ✓7ᵗʰ S32.473 Displaced fracture of medial wall of unspecified acetabulum `HCC` ▽
- 1 ✓7ᵗʰ S32.474 Nondisplaced fracture of medial wall of right acetabulum `HCC`
- 1 ✓7ᵗʰ S32.475 Nondisplaced fracture of medial wall of left acetabulum `HCC`
- 1 ✓7ᵗʰ S32.476 Nondisplaced fracture of medial wall of unspecified acetabulum `HCC` ▽

✓6ᵗʰ **S32.48 Dome fracture of acetabulum**
- 1 ✓7ᵗʰ S32.481 Displaced dome fracture of right acetabulum `HCC`
- 1 ✓7ᵗʰ S32.482 Displaced dome fracture of left acetabulum `HCC`
- 1 ✓7ᵗʰ S32.483 Displaced dome fracture of unspecified acetabulum `HCC` ▽
- 1 ✓7ᵗʰ S32.484 Nondisplaced dome fracture of right acetabulum `HCC`
- 1 ✓7ᵗʰ S32.485 Nondisplaced dome fracture of left acetabulum `HCC`
- 1 ✓7ᵗʰ S32.486 Nondisplaced dome fracture of unspecified acetabulum `HCC` ▽

✓6ᵗʰ **S32.49 Other specified fracture of acetabulum**
- 1 ✓7ᵗʰ S32.491 Other specified fracture of right acetabulum `HCC`
- 1 ✓7ᵗʰ S32.492 Other specified fracture of left acetabulum `HCC`
- 1 ✓7ᵗʰ S32.499 Other specified fracture of unspecified acetabulum `HCC` ▽

✓5ᵗʰ **S32.5 Fracture of pubis**
> *EXCLUDES 1* *fracture of pubis with associated disruption of pelvic ring (S32.8-)*

✓6ᵗʰ **S32.50 Unspecified fracture of pubis**
- 1 ✓7ᵗʰ S32.501 Unspecified fracture of right pubis `HCC` ▽
- 1 ✓7ᵗʰ S32.502 Unspecified fracture of left pubis `HCC` ▽
- 1 ✓7ᵗʰ S32.509 Unspecified fracture of unspecified pubis `HCC` ▽

✓6ᵗʰ **S32.51 Fracture of superior rim of pubis**
- 1 ✓7ᵗʰ S32.511 Fracture of superior rim of right pubis `HCC`
- 1 ✓7ᵗʰ S32.512 Fracture of superior rim of left pubis `HCC`
- 1 ✓7ᵗʰ S32.519 Fracture of superior rim of unspecified pubis `HCC` ▽

✓6ᵗʰ **S32.59 Other specified fracture of pubis**
- 1 ✓7ᵗʰ S32.591 Other specified fracture of right pubis `HCC`
- 1 ✓7ᵗʰ S32.592 Other specified fracture of left pubis `HCC`
- 1 ✓7ᵗʰ S32.599 Other specified fracture of unspecified pubis `HCC` ▽

✓5ᵗʰ **S32.6 Fracture of ischium**
> *EXCLUDES 1* *fracture of ischium with associated disruption of pelvic ring (S32.8-)*

✓6ᵗʰ **S32.60 Unspecified fracture of ischium**
- 1 ✓7ᵗʰ S32.601 Unspecified fracture of right ischium `HCC` ▽
- 1 ✓7ᵗʰ S32.602 Unspecified fracture of left ischium `HCC` ▽
- 1 ✓7ᵗʰ S32.609 Unspecified fracture of unspecified ischium `HCC` ▽

✓6ᵗʰ **S32.61 Avulsion fracture of ischium**
- 1 ✓7ᵗʰ S32.611 Displaced avulsion fracture of right ischium `HCC`
- 1 ✓7ᵗʰ S32.612 Displaced avulsion fracture of left ischium `HCC`
- 1 ✓7ᵗʰ S32.613 Displaced avulsion fracture of unspecified ischium `HCC` ▽

---

1 HCC with 7th character indicating initial encounter (A, B or C - specific to category).

EXCLUDES 1 Not coded here *EXCLUDES 2* Not included here **N** Newborn Age: 0 **P** Pediatric Age: 0-17 **M** Maternity Age: 12-55 **A** Adult Age: 15-124

946 ICD-10-CM 2018

[1] ✓7ᵗʰ **S32.614** **Nondisplaced avulsion fracture of right ischium** HCC

[1] ✓7ᵗʰ **S32.615** **Nondisplaced avulsion fracture of left ischium** HCC

[1] ✓7ᵗʰ **S32.616** **Nondisplaced avulsion fracture of unspecified ischium** HCC ▽

✓6ᵗʰ **S32.69** **Other specified fracture of ischium**

[1] ✓7ᵗʰ **S32.691** **Other specified fracture of right ischium** HCC

[1] ✓7ᵗʰ **S32.692** **Other specified fracture of left ischium** HCC

[1] ✓7ᵗʰ **S32.699** **Other specified fracture of unspecified ischium** HCC ▽

✓5ᵗʰ **S32.8** **Fracture of other parts of pelvis**
Code also any associated:
fracture of acetabulum (S32.4-)
sacral fracture (S32.1-)

✓6ᵗʰ **S32.81** **Multiple fractures of pelvis with disruption of pelvic ring**
Multiple pelvic fractures with disruption of pelvic circle

[1] ✓7ᵗʰ **S32.810** **Multiple fractures of pelvis with stable disruption of pelvic ring** HCC

[1] ✓7ᵗʰ **S32.811** **Multiple fractures of pelvis with unstable disruption of pelvic ring** HCC

[1] ✓x7ᵗʰ **S32.82** **Multiple fractures of pelvis without disruption of pelvic ring** HCC
Multiple pelvic fractures without disruption of pelvic circle

[1] ✓x7ᵗʰ **S32.89** **Fracture of other parts of pelvis** HCC

[1] ✓x7ᵗʰ **S32.9** **Fracture of unspecified parts of lumbosacral spine and pelvis** HCC ▽
Fracture of lumbosacral spine NOS
Fracture of pelvis NOS
AHA: 2012, 4Q, 93

Fractures Disrupting Pelvic Circle

Pelvic circle

Stable

Unstable
(two-place fracture)

Iliac crest

Anterior superior iliac spine

Ischial spine

Acetabulum

Femur

Ilium

L5

Sacrum

Coccyx

Pubis

Pubic symphysis

Ischium

Pelvic Bones

✓4ᵗʰ **S33** **Dislocation and sprain of joints and ligaments of lumbar spine and pelvis**
INCLUDES avulsion of joint or ligament of lumbar spine and pelvis
laceration of cartilage, joint or ligament of lumbar spine and pelvis
sprain of cartilage, joint or ligament of lumbar spine and pelvis
traumatic hemarthrosis of joint or ligament of lumbar spine and pelvis
traumatic rupture of joint or ligament of lumbar spine and pelvis
traumatic subluxation of joint or ligament of lumbar spine and pelvis
traumatic tear of joint or ligament of lumbar spine and pelvis
Code also any associated open wound
EXCLUDES 1 nontraumatic rupture or displacement of lumbar intervertebral disc NOS (M51.-)
obstetric damage to pelvic joints and ligaments (O71.6)
EXCLUDES 2 dislocation and sprain of joints and ligaments of hip (S73.-)
strain of muscle of lower back and pelvis (S39.01-)

> The appropriate 7th character is to be added to each code from category S33.
> A   initial encounter
> D   subsequent encounter
> S   sequela

✓x7ᵗʰ **S33.0** **Traumatic rupture of lumbar intervertebral disc**
EXCLUDES 1 rupture or displacement (nontraumatic) of lumbar intervertebral disc NOS (M51- with fifth character 6)

✓5ᵗʰ **S33.1** **Subluxation and dislocation of lumbar vertebra**
Code also any associated:
open wound of abdomen, lower back and pelvis (S31)
spinal cord injury (S24.0, S24.1-, S34.0-, S34.1-)
EXCLUDES 2 fracture of lumbar vertebrae (S32.0-)

✓6ᵗʰ **S33.10** **Subluxation and dislocation of unspecified lumbar vertebra**

✓7ᵗʰ **S33.100** **Subluxation of unspecified lumbar vertebra** ▽

✓7ᵗʰ **S33.101** **Dislocation of unspecified lumbar vertebra** ▽

✓6ᵗʰ **S33.11** **Subluxation and dislocation of L1/L2 lumbar vertebra**

✓7ᵗʰ **S33.110** **Subluxation of L1/L2 lumbar vertebra**

✓7ᵗʰ **S33.111** **Dislocation of L1/L2 lumbar vertebra**

✓6ᵗʰ **S33.12** **Subluxation and dislocation of L2/L3 lumbar vertebra**

✓7ᵗʰ **S33.120** **Subluxation of L2/L3 lumbar vertebra**

✓7ᵗʰ **S33.121** **Dislocation of L2/L3 lumbar vertebra**

✓6ᵗʰ **S33.13** **Subluxation and dislocation of L3/L4 lumbar vertebra**

✓7ᵗʰ **S33.130** **Subluxation of L3/L4 lumbar vertebra**

✓7ᵗʰ **S33.131** **Dislocation of L3/L4 lumbar vertebra**

✓6ᵗʰ **S33.14** **Subluxation and dislocation of L4/L5 lumbar vertebra**

✓7ᵗʰ **S33.140** **Subluxation of L4/L5 lumbar vertebra**

✓7ᵗʰ **S33.141** **Dislocation of L4/L5 lumbar vertebra**

✓x7ᵗʰ **S33.2** **Dislocation of sacroiliac and sacrococcygeal joint**

✓5ᵗʰ **S33.3** **Dislocation of other and unspecified parts of lumbar spine and pelvis**

✓x7ᵗʰ **S33.30** **Dislocation of unspecified parts of lumbar spine and pelvis** ▽

✓x7ᵗʰ **S33.39** **Dislocation of other parts of lumbar spine and pelvis**

✓x7ᵗʰ **S33.4** **Traumatic rupture of symphysis pubis**

✓x7ᵗʰ **S33.5** **Sprain of ligaments of lumbar spine**

✓x7ᵗʰ **S33.6** **Sprain of sacroiliac joint**

✓x7ᵗʰ **S33.8** **Sprain of other parts of lumbar spine and pelvis**

✓x7ᵗʰ **S33.9** **Sprain of unspecified parts of lumbar spine and pelvis** ▽

---

[1] HCC with 7th character indicating initial encounter (A, B or C - specific to category).

✓ Additional Character Req   ✓x7ᵗʰ Placeholder Alert   Manifestation   HCC CMS-HCC Condition   ▽ Unspecified Code   ►◄ Revised Text   ● New Code   ▲ Revised Code Title

√4ᵗʰ **S34 Injury of lumbar and sacral spinal cord and nerves at abdomen, lower back and pelvis level**

> **NOTE** Code to highest level of lumbar cord injury.
> Injuries to the spinal cord (S34.0 and S34.1) refer to the cord level and not bone level injury, and can affect nerve roots at and below the level given.
>
> **Code also any associated:**
> fracture of vertebra (S22.0-, S32.0-)
> open wound of abdomen, lower back and pelvis (S31.-)
> transient paralysis (R29.5)

> The appropriate 7th character is to be added to each code from category S34.
> A   initial encounter
> D   subsequent encounter
> S   sequela

√5ᵗʰ **S34.0 Concussion and edema of lumbar and sacral spinal cord**

√x7ᵗʰ **S34.01 Concussion and edema of lumbar spinal cord** HCC

√x7ᵗʰ **S34.02 Concussion and edema of sacral spinal cord** HCC
Concussion and edema of conus medullaris

√5ᵗʰ **S34.1 Other and unspecified injury of lumbar and sacral spinal cord**

√6ᵗʰ **S34.10 Unspecified injury to lumbar spinal cord**

√7ᵗʰ **S34.101 Unspecified injury to L1 level of lumbar spinal cord** HCC ▽
Unspecified injury to lumbar spinal cord level 1

√7ᵗʰ **S34.102 Unspecified injury to L2 level of lumbar spinal cord** HCC ▽
Unspecified injury to lumbar spinal cord level 2

√7ᵗʰ **S34.103 Unspecified injury to L3 level of lumbar spinal cord** HCC ▽
Unspecified injury to lumbar spinal cord level 3

√7ᵗʰ **S34.104 Unspecified injury to L4 level of lumbar spinal cord** HCC ▽
Unspecified injury to lumbar spinal cord level 4

√7ᵗʰ **S34.105 Unspecified injury to L5 level of lumbar spinal cord** HCC ▽
Unspecified injury to lumbar spinal cord level 5

√7ᵗʰ **S34.109 Unspecified injury to unspecified level of lumbar spinal cord** HCC ▽

√6ᵗʰ **S34.11 Complete lesion of lumbar spinal cord**

√7ᵗʰ **S34.111 Complete lesion of L1 level of lumbar spinal cord** HCC
Complete lesion of lumbar spinal cord level 1

√7ᵗʰ **S34.112 Complete lesion of L2 level of lumbar spinal cord** HCC
Complete lesion of lumbar spinal cord level 2

√7ᵗʰ **S34.113 Complete lesion of L3 level of lumbar spinal cord** HCC
Complete lesion of lumbar spinal cord level 3

√7ᵗʰ **S34.114 Complete lesion of L4 level of lumbar spinal cord** HCC
Complete lesion of lumbar spinal cord level 4

√7ᵗʰ **S34.115 Complete lesion of L5 level of lumbar spinal cord** HCC
Complete lesion of lumbar spinal cord level 5

√7ᵗʰ **S34.119 Complete lesion of unspecified level of lumbar spinal cord** HCC ▽

√6ᵗʰ **S34.12 Incomplete lesion of lumbar spinal cord**

√7ᵗʰ **S34.121 Incomplete lesion of L1 level of lumbar spinal cord** HCC
Incomplete lesion of lumbar spinal cord level 1

√7ᵗʰ **S34.122 Incomplete lesion of L2 level of lumbar spinal cord** HCC
Incomplete lesion of lumbar spinal cord level 2

√7ᵗʰ **S34.123 Incomplete lesion of L3 level of lumbar spinal cord** HCC
Incomplete lesion of lumbar spinal cord level 3

√7ᵗʰ **S34.124 Incomplete lesion of L4 level of lumbar spinal cord** HCC
Incomplete lesion of lumbar spinal cord level 4

√7ᵗʰ **S34.125 Incomplete lesion of L5 level of lumbar spinal cord** HCC
Incomplete lesion of lumbar spinal cord level 5

√7ᵗʰ **S34.129 Incomplete lesion of unspecified level of lumbar spinal cord** HCC ▽

√6ᵗʰ **S34.13 Other and unspecified injury to sacral spinal cord**
Other injury to conus medullaris

√7ᵗʰ **S34.131 Complete lesion of sacral spinal cord** HCC
Complete lesion of conus medullaris

√7ᵗʰ **S34.132 Incomplete lesion of sacral spinal cord** HCC
Incomplete lesion of conus medullaris

√7ᵗʰ **S34.139 Unspecified injury to sacral spinal cord** HCC ▽
Unspecified injury of conus medullaris

√5ᵗʰ **S34.2 Injury of nerve root of lumbar and sacral spine**

√x7ᵗʰ **S34.21 Injury of nerve root of lumbar spine**

√x7ᵗʰ **S34.22 Injury of nerve root of sacral spine**

[1] √x7ᵗʰ **S34.3 Injury of cauda equina** HCC

√x7ᵗʰ **S34.4 Injury of lumbosacral plexus**

√x7ᵗʰ **S34.5 Injury of lumbar, sacral and pelvic sympathetic nerves**
Injury of celiac ganglion or plexus
Injury of hypogastric plexus
Injury of mesenteric plexus (inferior) (superior)
Injury of splanchnic nerve

√x7ᵗʰ **S34.6 Injury of peripheral nerve(s) at abdomen, lower back and pelvis level**

√x7ᵗʰ **S34.8 Injury of other nerves at abdomen, lower back and pelvis level**

√x7ᵗʰ **S34.9 Injury of unspecified nerves at abdomen, lower back and pelvis level** ▽

√4ᵗʰ **S35 Injury of blood vessels at abdomen, lower back and pelvis level**
Code also any associated open wound (S31.-)

> The appropriate 7th character is to be added to each code from category S35.
> A   initial encounter
> D   subsequent encounter
> S   sequela

√5ᵗʰ **S35.0 Injury of abdominal aorta**
> **EXCLUDES 1** injury of aorta NOS (S25.0)

√x7ᵗʰ **S35.00 Unspecified injury of abdominal aorta** ▽

√x7ᵗʰ **S35.01 Minor laceration of abdominal aorta**
Incomplete transection of abdominal aorta
Laceration of abdominal aorta NOS
Superficial laceration of abdominal aorta

√x7ᵗʰ **S35.02 Major laceration of abdominal aorta**
Complete transection of abdominal aorta
Traumatic rupture of abdominal aorta

√x7ᵗʰ **S35.09 Other injury of abdominal aorta**

√5ᵗʰ **S35.1 Injury of inferior vena cava**
Injury of hepatic vein
> **EXCLUDES 1** injury of vena cava NOS (S25.2)

√x7ᵗʰ **S35.10 Unspecified injury of inferior vena cava** ▽

√x7ᵗʰ **S35.11 Minor laceration of inferior vena cava**
Incomplete transection of inferior vena cava
Laceration of inferior vena cava NOS
Superficial laceration of inferior vena cava

√x7ᵗʰ **S35.12 Major laceration of inferior vena cava**
Complete transection of inferior vena cava
Traumatic rupture of inferior vena cava

√x7ᵗʰ **S35.19 Other injury of inferior vena cava**

---

[1] HCC with 7th character indicating initial encounter (A, B or C - specific to category).

√5ᵗʰ **S35.2** **Injury of celiac or mesenteric artery and branches**

√6ᵗʰ **S35.21** **Injury of celiac artery**

√7ᵗʰ **S35.211** **Minor laceration of celiac artery**
Incomplete transection of celiac artery
Laceration of celiac artery NOS
Superficial laceration of celiac artery

√7ᵗʰ **S35.212** **Major laceration of celiac artery**
Complete transection of celiac artery
Traumatic rupture of celiac artery

√7ᵗʰ **S35.218** **Other injury of celiac artery**

√7ᵗʰ **S35.219** **Unspecified injury of celiac artery** ▽

√6ᵗʰ **S35.22** **Injury of superior mesenteric artery**

√7ᵗʰ **S35.221** **Minor laceration of superior mesenteric artery**
Incomplete transection of superior mesenteric artery
Laceration of superior mesenteric artery NOS
Superficial laceration of superior mesenteric artery

√7ᵗʰ **S35.222** **Major laceration of superior mesenteric artery**
Complete transection of superior mesenteric artery
Traumatic rupture of superior mesenteric artery

√7ᵗʰ **S35.228** **Other injury of superior mesenteric artery**

√7ᵗʰ **S35.229** **Unspecified injury of superior mesenteric artery** ▽

√6ᵗʰ **S35.23** **Injury of inferior mesenteric artery**

√7ᵗʰ **S35.231** **Minor laceration of inferior mesenteric artery**
Incomplete transection of inferior mesenteric artery
Laceration of inferior mesenteric artery NOS
Superficial laceration of inferior mesenteric artery

√7ᵗʰ **S35.232** **Major laceration of inferior mesenteric artery**
Complete transection of inferior mesenteric artery
Traumatic rupture of inferior mesenteric artery

√7ᵗʰ **S35.238** **Other injury of inferior mesenteric artery**

√7ᵗʰ **S35.239** **Unspecified injury of inferior mesenteric artery** ▽

√6ᵗʰ **S35.29** **Injury of branches of celiac and mesenteric artery**
Injury of gastric artery
Injury of gastroduodenal artery
Injury of hepatic artery
Injury of splenic artery

√7ᵗʰ **S35.291** **Minor laceration of branches of celiac and mesenteric artery**
Incomplete transection of branches of celiac and mesenteric artery
Laceration of branches of celiac and mesenteric artery NOS
Superficial laceration of branches of celiac and mesenteric artery

√7ᵗʰ **S35.292** **Major laceration of branches of celiac and mesenteric artery**
Complete transection of branches of celiac and mesenteric artery
Traumatic rupture of branches of celiac and mesenteric artery

√7ᵗʰ **S35.298** **Other injury of branches of celiac and mesenteric artery**

√7ᵗʰ **S35.299** **Unspecified injury of branches of celiac and mesenteric artery** ▽

√5ᵗʰ **S35.3** **Injury of portal or splenic vein and branches**

√6ᵗʰ **S35.31** **Injury of portal vein**

√7ᵗʰ **S35.311** **Laceration of portal vein**

√7ᵗʰ **S35.318** **Other specified injury of portal vein**

√7ᵗʰ **S35.319** **Unspecified injury of portal vein** ▽

√6ᵗʰ **S35.32** **Injury of splenic vein**

√7ᵗʰ **S35.321** **Laceration of splenic vein**

√7ᵗʰ **S35.328** **Other specified injury of splenic vein**

√7ᵗʰ **S35.329** **Unspecified injury of splenic vein** ▽

√6ᵗʰ **S35.33** **Injury of superior mesenteric vein**

√7ᵗʰ **S35.331** **Laceration of superior mesenteric vein**

√7ᵗʰ **S35.338** **Other specified injury of superior mesenteric vein**

√7ᵗʰ **S35.339** **Unspecified injury of superior mesenteric vein** ▽

√6ᵗʰ **S35.34** **Injury of inferior mesenteric vein**

√7ᵗʰ **S35.341** **Laceration of inferior mesenteric vein**

√7ᵗʰ **S35.348** **Other specified injury of inferior mesenteric vein**

√7ᵗʰ **S35.349** **Unspecified injury of inferior mesenteric vein** ▽

√5ᵗʰ **S35.4** **Injury of renal blood vessels**

√6ᵗʰ **S35.40** **Unspecified injury of renal blood vessel**

√7ᵗʰ **S35.401** **Unspecified injury of right renal artery** ▽

√7ᵗʰ **S35.402** **Unspecified injury of left renal artery** ▽

√7ᵗʰ **S35.403** **Unspecified injury of unspecified renal artery** ▽

√7ᵗʰ **S35.404** **Unspecified injury of right renal vein** ▽

√7ᵗʰ **S35.405** **Unspecified injury of left renal vein** ▽

√7ᵗʰ **S35.406** **Unspecified injury of unspecified renal vein** ▽

√6ᵗʰ **S35.41** **Laceration of renal blood vessel**

√7ᵗʰ **S35.411** **Laceration of right renal artery**

√7ᵗʰ **S35.412** **Laceration of left renal artery**

√7ᵗʰ **S35.413** **Laceration of unspecified renal artery** ▽

√7ᵗʰ **S35.414** **Laceration of right renal vein**

√7ᵗʰ **S35.415** **Laceration of left renal vein**

√7ᵗʰ **S35.416** **Laceration of unspecified renal vein** ▽

√6ᵗʰ **S35.49** **Other specified injury of renal blood vessel**

√7ᵗʰ **S35.491** **Other specified injury of right renal artery**

√7ᵗʰ **S35.492** **Other specified injury of left renal artery**

√7ᵗʰ **S35.493** **Other specified injury of unspecified renal artery** ▽

√7ᵗʰ **S35.494** **Other specified injury of right renal vein**

√7ᵗʰ **S35.495** **Other specified injury of left renal vein**

√7ᵗʰ **S35.496** **Other specified injury of unspecified renal vein** ▽

√5ᵗʰ **S35.5** **Injury of iliac blood vessels**

√x7ᵗʰ **S35.50** **Injury of unspecified iliac blood vessel(s)** ▽

√6ᵗʰ **S35.51** **Injury of iliac artery or vein**
Injury of hypogastric artery or vein

√7ᵗʰ **S35.511** **Injury of right iliac artery**

√7ᵗʰ **S35.512** **Injury of left iliac artery**

√7ᵗʰ **S35.513** **Injury of unspecified iliac artery** ▽

√7ᵗʰ **S35.514** **Injury of right iliac vein**

√7ᵗʰ **S35.515** **Injury of left iliac vein**

√7ᵗʰ **S35.516** **Injury of unspecified iliac vein** ▽

√6ᵗʰ **S35.53** **Injury of uterine artery or vein**

√7ᵗʰ **S35.531** **Injury of right uterine artery** ♀

√7ᵗʰ **S35.532** **Injury of left uterine artery** ♀

√7ᵗʰ **S35.533** **Injury of unspecified uterine artery** ♀▽

√7ᵗʰ **S35.534** **Injury of right uterine vein** ♀

√7ᵗʰ **S35.535** **Injury of left uterine vein** ♀

√7ᵗʰ **S35.536** **Injury of unspecified uterine vein** ♀▽

√x7ᵗʰ **S35.59** **Injury of other iliac blood vessels**

√5ᵗʰ **S35.8** **Injury of other blood vessels at abdomen, lower back and pelvis level**
Injury of ovarian artery or vein

√6ᵗʰ **S35.8X** **Injury of other blood vessels at abdomen, lower back and pelvis level**

√7ᵗʰ **S35.8X1** **Laceration of other blood vessels at abdomen, lower back and pelvis level**

√7ᵗʰ **S35.8X8** **Other specified injury of other blood vessels at abdomen, lower back and pelvis level**

√7ᵗʰ **S35.8X9** **Unspecified injury of other blood vessels at abdomen, lower back and pelvis level** ▽

✔ Additional Character Req   √x7ᵗʰ Placeholder Alert   Manifestation   **HCC** CMS-HCC Condition   ▽ Unspecified Code   ►◄ Revised Text   ● New Code   ▲ Revised Code Title

ICD-10-CM 2018   949

√5ᵗʰ **S35.9 Injury of unspecified blood vessel at abdomen, lower back and pelvis level**

- √x7ᵗʰ **S35.90 Unspecified injury of unspecified blood vessel at abdomen, lower back and pelvis level** ▽
- √x7ᵗʰ **S35.91 Laceration of unspecified blood vessel at abdomen, lower back and pelvis level** ▽
- √x7ᵗʰ **S35.99 Other specified injury of unspecified blood vessel at abdomen, lower back and pelvis level** ▽

√4ᵗʰ **S36 Injury of intra-abdominal organs**

Code also any associated open wound (S31.-)

> The appropriate 7th character is to be added to each code from category S36.
> A   initial encounter
> D   subsequent encounter
> S   sequela

√5ᵗʰ **S36.0 Injury of spleen**
     AHA: 2015, 2Q, 36; 2015, 1Q, 10

- √x7ᵗʰ **S36.00 Unspecified injury of spleen** ▽
- √6ᵗʰ **S36.02 Contusion of spleen**
  - 7ᵗʰ **S36.020 Minor contusion of spleen**
    Contusion of spleen less than 2 cm
  - 7ᵗʰ **S36.021 Major contusion of spleen**
    Contusion of spleen greater than 2 cm
  - 7ᵗʰ **S36.029 Unspecified contusion of spleen** ▽
- √6ᵗʰ **S36.03 Laceration of spleen**
  - 7ᵗʰ **S36.030 Superficial (capsular) laceration of spleen**
    Laceration of spleen less than 1cm
    Minor laceration of spleen
  - 7ᵗʰ **S36.031 Moderate laceration of spleen**
    Laceration of spleen 1 to 3 cm
  - 7ᵗʰ **S36.032 Major laceration of spleen**
    Avulsion of spleen
    Laceration of spleen greater than 3 cm
    Massive laceration of spleen
    Multiple moderate lacerations of spleen
    Stellate laceration of spleen
  - 7ᵗʰ **S36.039 Unspecified laceration of spleen** ▽
- √x7ᵗʰ **S36.09 Other injury of spleen**

√5ᵗʰ **S36.1 Injury of liver and gallbladder and bile duct**

- √6ᵗʰ **S36.11 Injury of liver**
  - 7ᵗʰ **S36.112 Contusion of liver**
  - 7ᵗʰ **S36.113 Laceration of liver, unspecified degree** ▽
  - 7ᵗʰ **S36.114 Minor laceration of liver**
    Laceration involving capsule only, or, without significant involvement of hepatic parenchyma [i.e., less than 1cm deep]
  - 7ᵗʰ **S36.115 Moderate laceration of liver**
    Laceration involving parenchyma but without major disruption of parenchyma [i.e., less than 10 cm long and less than 3 cm deep]
  - 7ᵗʰ **S36.116 Major laceration of liver**
    Laceration with significant disruption of hepatic parenchyma [i.e., greater than 10 cm long and 3 cm deep]
    Multiple moderate lacerations, with or without hematoma
    Stellate laceration of liver
  - 7ᵗʰ **S36.118 Other injury of liver**
  - 7ᵗʰ **S36.119 Unspecified injury of liver** ▽
- √6ᵗʰ **S36.12 Injury of gallbladder**
  - 7ᵗʰ **S36.122 Contusion of gallbladder**
  - 7ᵗʰ **S36.123 Laceration of gallbladder**
  - 7ᵗʰ **S36.128 Other injury of gallbladder**
  - 7ᵗʰ **S36.129 Unspecified injury of gallbladder** ▽
- √x7ᵗʰ **S36.13 Injury of bile duct**

√5ᵗʰ **S36.2 Injury of pancreas**

- √6ᵗʰ **S36.20 Unspecified injury of pancreas**
  - 7ᵗʰ **S36.200 Unspecified injury of head of pancreas** ▽
  - 7ᵗʰ **S36.201 Unspecified injury of body of pancreas** ▽
  - 7ᵗʰ **S36.202 Unspecified injury of tail of pancreas** ▽
  - 7ᵗʰ **S36.209 Unspecified injury of unspecified part of pancreas** ▽

√6ᵗʰ **S36.22 Contusion of pancreas**

- 7ᵗʰ **S36.220 Contusion of head of pancreas**
- 7ᵗʰ **S36.221 Contusion of body of pancreas**
- 7ᵗʰ **S36.222 Contusion of tail of pancreas**
- 7ᵗʰ **S36.229 Contusion of unspecified part of pancreas** ▽

√6ᵗʰ **S36.23 Laceration of pancreas, unspecified degree**

- 7ᵗʰ **S36.230 Laceration of head of pancreas, unspecified degree** ▽
- 7ᵗʰ **S36.231 Laceration of body of pancreas, unspecified degree** ▽
- 7ᵗʰ **S36.232 Laceration of tail of pancreas, unspecified degree** ▽
- 7ᵗʰ **S36.239 Laceration of unspecified part of pancreas, unspecified degree** ▽

√6ᵗʰ **S36.24 Minor laceration of pancreas**

- 7ᵗʰ **S36.240 Minor laceration of head of pancreas**
- 7ᵗʰ **S36.241 Minor laceration of body of pancreas**
- 7ᵗʰ **S36.242 Minor laceration of tail of pancreas**
- 7ᵗʰ **S36.249 Minor laceration of unspecified part of pancreas** ▽

√6ᵗʰ **S36.25 Moderate laceration of pancreas**

- 7ᵗʰ **S36.250 Moderate laceration of head of pancreas**
- 7ᵗʰ **S36.251 Moderate laceration of body of pancreas**
- 7ᵗʰ **S36.252 Moderate laceration of tail of pancreas**
- 7ᵗʰ **S36.259 Moderate laceration of unspecified part of pancreas** ▽

√6ᵗʰ **S36.26 Major laceration of pancreas**

- 7ᵗʰ **S36.260 Major laceration of head of pancreas**
- 7ᵗʰ **S36.261 Major laceration of body of pancreas**
- 7ᵗʰ **S36.262 Major laceration of tail of pancreas**
- 7ᵗʰ **S36.269 Major laceration of unspecified part of pancreas** ▽

√6ᵗʰ **S36.29 Other injury of pancreas**

- 7ᵗʰ **S36.290 Other injury of head of pancreas**
- 7ᵗʰ **S36.291 Other injury of body of pancreas**
- 7ᵗʰ **S36.292 Other injury of tail of pancreas**
- 7ᵗʰ **S36.299 Other injury of unspecified part of pancreas** ▽

√5ᵗʰ **S36.3 Injury of stomach**

- √x7ᵗʰ **S36.30 Unspecified injury of stomach** ▽
- √x7ᵗʰ **S36.32 Contusion of stomach**
- √x7ᵗʰ **S36.33 Laceration of stomach**
- √x7ᵗʰ **S36.39 Other injury of stomach**

√5ᵗʰ **S36.4 Injury of small intestine**

- √6ᵗʰ **S36.40 Unspecified injury of small intestine**
  - 7ᵗʰ **S36.400 Unspecified injury of duodenum** ▽
  - 7ᵗʰ **S36.408 Unspecified injury of other part of small intestine** ▽
  - 7ᵗʰ **S36.409 Unspecified injury of unspecified part of small intestine** ▽
- √6ᵗʰ **S36.41 Primary blast injury of small intestine**
  Blast injury of small intestine NOS
  - 7ᵗʰ **S36.410 Primary blast injury of duodenum**
  - 7ᵗʰ **S36.418 Primary blast injury of other part of small intestine**
  - 7ᵗʰ **S36.419 Primary blast injury of unspecified part of small intestine** ▽
- √6ᵗʰ **S36.42 Contusion of small intestine**
  - 7ᵗʰ **S36.420 Contusion of duodenum**
  - 7ᵗʰ **S36.428 Contusion of other part of small intestine**
  - 7ᵗʰ **S36.429 Contusion of unspecified part of small intestine** ▽
- √6ᵗʰ **S36.43 Laceration of small intestine**
  - 7ᵗʰ **S36.430 Laceration of duodenum**
  - 7ᵗʰ **S36.438 Laceration of other part of small intestine**
  - 7ᵗʰ **S36.439 Laceration of unspecified part of small intestine** ▽

√6ᵗʰ **S36.49 Other injury of small intestine**
  √7ᵗʰ **S36.490 Other injury of duodenum**
  √7ᵗʰ **S36.498 Other injury of other part of small intestine**
  √7ᵗʰ **S36.499 Other injury of unspecified part of small intestine** ▽

√5ᵗʰ **S36.5 Injury of colon**
  EXCLUDES 2 *injury of rectum (S36.6-)*
  √6ᵗʰ **S36.50 Unspecified injury of colon**
    √7ᵗʰ **S36.500 Unspecified injury of ascending [right] colon**
    √7ᵗʰ **S36.501 Unspecified injury of transverse colon** ▽
    √7ᵗʰ **S36.502 Unspecified injury of descending [left] colon** ▽
    √7ᵗʰ **S36.503 Unspecified injury of sigmoid colon** ▽
    √7ᵗʰ **S36.508 Unspecified injury of other part of colon** ▽
    √7ᵗʰ **S36.509 Unspecified injury of unspecified part of colon** ▽
  √6ᵗʰ **S36.51 Primary blast injury of colon**
    Blast injury of colon NOS
    √7ᵗʰ **S36.510 Primary blast injury of ascending [right] colon**
    √7ᵗʰ **S36.511 Primary blast injury of transverse colon**
    √7ᵗʰ **S36.512 Primary blast injury of descending [left] colon**
    √7ᵗʰ **S36.513 Primary blast injury of sigmoid colon**
    √7ᵗʰ **S36.518 Primary blast injury of other part of colon**
    √7ᵗʰ **S36.519 Primary blast injury of unspecified part of colon** ▽
  √6ᵗʰ **S36.52 Contusion of colon**
    √7ᵗʰ **S36.520 Contusion of ascending [right] colon**
    √7ᵗʰ **S36.521 Contusion of transverse colon**
    √7ᵗʰ **S36.522 Contusion of descending [left] colon**
    √7ᵗʰ **S36.523 Contusion of sigmoid colon**
    √7ᵗʰ **S36.528 Contusion of other part of colon**
    √7ᵗʰ **S36.529 Contusion of unspecified part of colon** ▽
  √6ᵗʰ **S36.53 Laceration of colon**
    √7ᵗʰ **S36.530 Laceration of ascending [right] colon**
    √7ᵗʰ **S36.531 Laceration of transverse colon**
    √7ᵗʰ **S36.532 Laceration of descending [left] colon**
    √7ᵗʰ **S36.533 Laceration of sigmoid colon**
    √7ᵗʰ **S36.538 Laceration of other part of colon**
    √7ᵗʰ **S36.539 Laceration of unspecified part of colon** ▽
  √6ᵗʰ **S36.59 Other injury of colon**
    Secondary blast injury of colon
    √7ᵗʰ **S36.590 Other injury of ascending [right] colon**
    √7ᵗʰ **S36.591 Other injury of transverse colon**
    √7ᵗʰ **S36.592 Other injury of descending [left] colon**
    √7ᵗʰ **S36.593 Other injury of sigmoid colon**
    √7ᵗʰ **S36.598 Other injury of other part of colon**
    √7ᵗʰ **S36.599 Other injury of unspecified part of colon** ▽

√5ᵗʰ **S36.6 Injury of rectum**
  √x7ᵗʰ **S36.60 Unspecified injury of rectum** ▽
  √x7ᵗʰ **S36.61 Primary blast injury of rectum**
    Blast injury of rectum NOS
  √x7ᵗʰ **S36.62 Contusion of rectum**
  √x7ᵗʰ **S36.63 Laceration of rectum**
  √x7ᵗʰ **S36.69 Other injury of rectum**
    Secondary blast injury of rectum

√5ᵗʰ **S36.8 Injury of other intra-abdominal organs**
  √x7ᵗʰ **S36.81 Injury of peritoneum**
  √6ᵗʰ **S36.89 Injury of other intra-abdominal organs**
    Injury of retroperitoneum
    √7ᵗʰ **S36.892 Contusion of other intra-abdominal organs**
    √7ᵗʰ **S36.893 Laceration of other intra-abdominal organs**
    √7ᵗʰ **S36.898 Other injury of other intra-abdominal organs**

    √7ᵗʰ **S36.899 Unspecified injury of other intra-abdominal organs** ▽
√5ᵗʰ **S36.9 Injury of unspecified intra-abdominal organ**
  √x7ᵗʰ **S36.90 Unspecified injury of unspecified intra-abdominal organ** ▽
  √x7ᵗʰ **S36.92 Contusion of unspecified intra-abdominal organ** ▽
  √x7ᵗʰ **S36.93 Laceration of unspecified intra-abdominal organ** ▽
  √x7ᵗʰ **S36.99 Other injury of unspecified intra-abdominal organ** ▽

√4ᵗʰ **S37 Injury of urinary and pelvic organs**
  Code also any associated open wound (S31.-)
  EXCLUDES 1 *obstetric trauma to pelvic organs (O71.-)*
  EXCLUDES 2 *injury of peritoneum (S36.81)*
         injury of retroperitoneum (S36.89-)

  The appropriate 7th character is to be added to each code from category S37.
  A   initial encounter
  D   subsequent encounter
  S   sequela

√5ᵗʰ **S37.0 Injury of kidney**
  EXCLUDES 2 *acute kidney injury (nontraumatic) (N17.9)*
  √6ᵗʰ **S37.00 Unspecified injury of kidney**
    √7ᵗʰ **S37.001 Unspecified injury of right kidney** ▽
    √7ᵗʰ **S37.002 Unspecified injury of left kidney** ▽
    √7ᵗʰ **S37.009 Unspecified injury of unspecified kidney** ▽
  √6ᵗʰ **S37.01 Minor contusion of kidney**
    Contusion of kidney less than 2 cm
    Contusion of kidney NOS
    √7ᵗʰ **S37.011 Minor contusion of right kidney**
    √7ᵗʰ **S37.012 Minor contusion of left kidney**
    √7ᵗʰ **S37.019 Minor contusion of unspecified kidney** ▽
  √6ᵗʰ **S37.02 Major contusion of kidney**
    Contusion of kidney greater than 2 cm
    √7ᵗʰ **S37.021 Major contusion of right kidney**
    √7ᵗʰ **S37.022 Major contusion of left kidney**
    √7ᵗʰ **S37.029 Major contusion of unspecified kidney** ▽
  √6ᵗʰ **S37.03 Laceration of kidney, unspecified degree**
    √7ᵗʰ **S37.031 Laceration of right kidney, unspecified degree** ▽
    √7ᵗʰ **S37.032 Laceration of left kidney, unspecified degree** ▽
    √7ᵗʰ **S37.039 Laceration of unspecified kidney, unspecified degree** ▽
  √6ᵗʰ **S37.04 Minor laceration of kidney**
    Laceration of kidney less than 1 cm
    √7ᵗʰ **S37.041 Minor laceration of right kidney**
    √7ᵗʰ **S37.042 Minor laceration of left kidney**
    √7ᵗʰ **S37.049 Minor laceration of unspecified kidney** ▽
  √6ᵗʰ **S37.05 Moderate laceration of kidney**
    Laceration of kidney 1 to 3 cm
    √7ᵗʰ **S37.051 Moderate laceration of right kidney**
    √7ᵗʰ **S37.052 Moderate laceration of left kidney**
    √7ᵗʰ **S37.059 Moderate laceration of unspecified kidney** ▽
  √6ᵗʰ **S37.06 Major laceration of kidney**
    Avulsion of kidney
    Laceration of kidney greater than 3 cm
    Massive laceration of kidney
    Multiple moderate lacerations of kidney
    Stellate laceration of kidney
    √7ᵗʰ **S37.061 Major laceration of right kidney**
    √7ᵗʰ **S37.062 Major laceration of left kidney**
    √7ᵗʰ **S37.069 Major laceration of unspecified kidney** ▽
  √6ᵗʰ **S37.09 Other injury of kidney**
    √7ᵗʰ **S37.091 Other injury of right kidney**
    √7ᵗʰ **S37.092 Other injury of left kidney**
    √7ᵗʰ **S37.099 Other injury of unspecified kidney** ▽
√5ᵗʰ **S37.1 Injury of ureter**
  √x7ᵗʰ **S37.10 Unspecified injury of ureter** ▽
  √x7ᵗʰ **S37.12 Contusion of ureter**
  √x7ᵗʰ **S37.13 Laceration of ureter**

☑ Additional Character Req   √x7ᵗʰ Placeholder Alert   Manifestation   HCC CMS-HCC Condition   ▽ Unspecified Code   ►◄ Revised Text   ● New Code   ▲ Revised Code Title

ICD-10-CM 2018

951

Chapter 19. Injury, Poisoning, and Certain Other Consequences of External Causes   S36.49–S37.13

√x7ᵗʰ **S37.19** Other injury of ureter

√5ᵗʰ **S37.2 Injury of bladder**

    √x7ᵗʰ **S37.20** Unspecified injury of bladder ▽

    √x7ᵗʰ **S37.22** **Contusion** of bladder

    √x7ᵗʰ **S37.23** **Laceration** of bladder

    √x7ᵗʰ **S37.29** Other injury of bladder

√5ᵗʰ **S37.3 Injury of urethra**

    √x7ᵗʰ **S37.30** Unspecified injury of urethra ▽

    √x7ᵗʰ **S37.32** **Contusion** of urethra

    √x7ᵗʰ **S37.33** **Laceration** of urethra

    √x7ᵗʰ **S37.39** Other injury of urethra

√5ᵗʰ **S37.4 Injury of ovary**

    √6ᵗʰ **S37.40** Unspecified injury of ovary

       √7ᵗʰ **S37.401** Unspecified injury of ovary, **unilateral** ♀▽

       √7ᵗʰ **S37.402** Unspecified injury of ovary, **bilateral** ♀▽

       √7ᵗʰ **S37.409** Unspecified injury of ovary, unspecified ♀▽

    √6ᵗʰ **S37.42** **Contusion** of ovary

       √7ᵗʰ **S37.421** Contusion of ovary, **unilateral** ♀

       √7ᵗʰ **S37.422** Contusion of ovary, **bilateral** ♀

       √7ᵗʰ **S37.429** Contusion of ovary, unspecified ♀▽

    √6ᵗʰ **S37.43** **Laceration** of ovary

       √7ᵗʰ **S37.431** Laceration of ovary, **unilateral** ♀

       √7ᵗʰ **S37.432** Laceration of ovary, **bilateral** ♀

       √7ᵗʰ **S37.439** Laceration of ovary, unspecified ♀▽

    √6ᵗʰ **S37.49** Other injury of ovary

       √7ᵗʰ **S37.491** Other injury of ovary, **unilateral** ♀

       √7ᵗʰ **S37.492** Other injury of ovary, **bilateral** ♀

       √7ᵗʰ **S37.499** Other injury of ovary, unspecified ♀▽

√5ᵗʰ **S37.5 Injury of fallopian tube**

    √6ᵗʰ **S37.50** Unspecified injury of fallopian tube

       √7ᵗʰ **S37.501** Unspecified injury of fallopian tube, **unilateral** ♀▽

       √7ᵗʰ **S37.502** Unspecified injury of fallopian tube, **bilateral** ♀▽

       √7ᵗʰ **S37.509** Unspecified injury of fallopian tube, unspecified ♀▽

    √6ᵗʰ **S37.51** **Primary blast** injury of fallopian tube

       Blast injury of fallopian tube NOS

       √7ᵗʰ **S37.511** Primary blast injury of fallopian tube, **unilateral** ♀

       √7ᵗʰ **S37.512** Primary blast injury of fallopian tube, **bilateral** ♀

       √7ᵗʰ **S37.519** Primary blast injury of fallopian tube, unspecified ♀▽

    √6ᵗʰ **S37.52** **Contusion** of fallopian tube

       √7ᵗʰ **S37.521** Contusion of fallopian tube, **unilateral** ♀

       √7ᵗʰ **S37.522** Contusion of fallopian tube, **bilateral** ♀

       √7ᵗʰ **S37.529** Contusion of fallopian tube, unspecified ♀▽

    √6ᵗʰ **S37.53** **Laceration** of fallopian tube

       √7ᵗʰ **S37.531** Laceration of fallopian tube, **unilateral** ♀

       √7ᵗʰ **S37.532** Laceration of fallopian tube, **bilateral** ♀

       √7ᵗʰ **S37.539** Laceration of fallopian tube, unspecified ♀▽

    √6ᵗʰ **S37.59** Other injury of fallopian tube

       Secondary blast injury of fallopian tube

       √7ᵗʰ **S37.591** Other injury of fallopian tube, **unilateral** ♀

       √7ᵗʰ **S37.592** Other injury of fallopian tube, **bilateral** ♀

       √7ᵗʰ **S37.599** Other injury of fallopian tube, unspecified ♀▽

√5ᵗʰ **S37.6 Injury of uterus**

    EXCLUDES 1   injury to gravid uterus (O9A.2-)

               injury to uterus during delivery (O71.-)

    √x7ᵗʰ **S37.60** Unspecified injury of uterus ♀▽

    √x7ᵗʰ **S37.62** **Contusion** of uterus ♀

    √x7ᵗʰ **S37.63** **Laceration** of uterus ♀

    √x7ᵗʰ **S37.69** Other injury of uterus ♀

√5ᵗʰ **S37.8 Injury of other urinary and pelvic organs**

    √6ᵗʰ **S37.81** Injury of **adrenal gland**

       √7ᵗʰ **S37.812** **Contusion** of adrenal gland

       √7ᵗʰ **S37.813** **Laceration** of adrenal gland

       √7ᵗʰ **S37.818** Other injury of adrenal gland

       √7ᵗʰ **S37.819** Unspecified injury of adrenal gland ▽

    √6ᵗʰ **S37.82** Injury of **prostate**

       √7ᵗʰ **S37.822** **Contusion** of prostate ♂

       √7ᵗʰ **S37.823** **Laceration** of prostate ♂

       √7ᵗʰ **S37.828** Other injury of prostate ♂

       √7ᵗʰ **S37.829** Unspecified injury of prostate ♂▽

    √6ᵗʰ **S37.89** Injury of other urinary and pelvic organ

       √7ᵗʰ **S37.892** **Contusion** of other urinary and pelvic organ

       √7ᵗʰ **S37.893** **Laceration** of other urinary and pelvic organ

       √7ᵗʰ **S37.898** Other injury of other urinary and pelvic organ

       √7ᵗʰ **S37.899** Unspecified injury of other urinary and pelvic organ ▽

√5ᵗʰ **S37.9 Injury of unspecified urinary and pelvic organ**

    √x7ᵗʰ **S37.90** Unspecified injury of unspecified urinary and pelvic organ ▽

    √x7ᵗʰ **S37.92** **Contusion** of unspecified urinary and pelvic organ ▽

    √x7ᵗʰ **S37.93** **Laceration** of unspecified urinary and pelvic organ ▽

    √x7ᵗʰ **S37.99** Other injury of unspecified urinary and pelvic organ ▽

√4ᵗʰ **S38 Crushing injury and traumatic amputation of abdomen, lower back, pelvis and external genitals**

    An amputation not identified as partial or complete should be coded to complete.

> The appropriate 7th character is to be added to each code from category S38.
> A   Initial encounter
> D   subsequent encounter
> S   sequela

√5ᵗʰ **S38.0 Crushing injury of external genital organs**

    Use additional code for any associated injuries

    √6ᵗʰ **S38.00** Crushing injury of unspecified external genital organs

       √7ᵗʰ **S38.001** Crushing injury of unspecified external genital organs, **male** ♂▽

       √7ᵗʰ **S38.002** Crushing injury of unspecified external genital organs, **female** ♀▽

    √x7ᵗʰ **S38.01** Crushing injury of **penis** ♂

    √x7ᵗʰ **S38.02** Crushing injury of **scrotum and testis** ♂

    √x7ᵗʰ **S38.03** Crushing injury of **vulva** ♀

√x7ᵗʰ **S38.1 Crushing injury of abdomen, lower back, and pelvis**

    Use additional code for all associated injuries, such as:

       fracture of thoracic or lumbar spine and pelvis (S22.0-, S32-)

       injury to intra-abdominal organs (S36.-)

       injury to urinary and pelvic organs (S37.-)

       open wound of abdominal wall (S31.-)

       spinal cord injury (S34.0, S34.1-)

    EXCLUDES 2   crushing injury of external genital organs (S38.0-)

√5ᵗʰ **S38.2 Traumatic amputation of external genital organs**

    √6ᵗʰ **S38.21** Traumatic amputation of **female** external genital organs

       Traumatic amputation of clitoris

       Traumatic amputation of labium (majus) (minus)

       Traumatic amputation of vulva

       √7ᵗʰ **S38.211** **Complete** traumatic amputation of female external genital organs ♀

       √7ᵗʰ **S38.212** **Partial** traumatic amputation of female external genital organs ♀

    √6ᵗʰ **S38.22** Traumatic amputation of **penis**

       √7ᵗʰ **S38.221** **Complete** traumatic amputation of penis ♂

       √7ᵗʰ **S38.222** **Partial** traumatic amputation of penis ♂

EXCLUDES 1 Not coded here   *EXCLUDES 2* Not included here   N Newborn Age: 0   P Pediatric Age: 0-17   M Maternity Age: 12-55   A Adult Age: 15-124

952   ICD-10-CM 2018

✓6ᵗʰ **S38.23** Traumatic amputation of scrotum and testis

     ✓7ᵗʰ **S38.231** **Complete** traumatic amputation of   ♂
                   scrotum and testis

     ✓7ᵗʰ **S38.232** **Partial** traumatic amputation of   ♂
                   scrotum and testis

✓x7ᵗʰ **S38.3** Transection (partial) of abdomen

✓4ᵗʰ **S39** **Other and unspecified injuries of abdomen, lower back, pelvis and external genitals**

     Code also any associated open wound (S31.-)

     EXCLUDES 2   *sprain of joints and ligaments of lumbar spine and pelvis (S33.-)*

     The appropriate 7th character is to be added to each code from category S39.
     A   initial encounter
     D   subsequent encounter
     S   sequela

   ✓5ᵗʰ **S39.0** **Injury of muscle, fascia and tendon of abdomen, lower back and pelvis**

     ✓6ᵗʰ **S39.00** **Unspecified injury of muscle, fascia and tendon of abdomen, lower back and pelvis**

       ✓7ᵗʰ **S39.001** **Unspecified injury of muscle, fascia** ▽
                   and tendon of abdomen

       ✓7ᵗʰ **S39.002** **Unspecified injury of muscle, fascia** ▽
                   and tendon of lower back

       ✓7ᵗʰ **S39.003** **Unspecified injury of muscle, fascia** ▽
                   and tendon of pelvis

     ✓6ᵗʰ **S39.01** **Strain of muscle, fascia and tendon of abdomen, lower back and pelvis**

       ✓7ᵗʰ **S39.011** **Strain of muscle, fascia and tendon of abdomen**

       ✓7ᵗʰ **S39.012** **Strain of muscle, fascia and tendon of lower back**

       ✓7ᵗʰ **S39.013** **Strain of muscle, fascia and tendon of pelvis**

     ✓6ᵗʰ **S39.02** **Laceration of muscle, fascia and tendon of abdomen, lower back and pelvis**

       ✓7ᵗʰ **S39.021** **Laceration of muscle, fascia and tendon of abdomen**

       ✓7ᵗʰ **S39.022** **Laceration of muscle, fascia and tendon of lower back**

       ✓7ᵗʰ **S39.023** **Laceration of muscle, fascia and tendon of pelvis**

     ✓6ᵗʰ **S39.09** **Other injury of muscle, fascia and tendon of abdomen, lower back and pelvis**

       ✓7ᵗʰ **S39.091** **Other injury of muscle, fascia and tendon of abdomen**

       ✓7ᵗʰ **S39.092** **Other injury of muscle, fascia and tendon of lower back**

       ✓7ᵗʰ **S39.093** **Other injury of muscle, fascia and tendon of pelvis**

   ✓5ᵗʰ **S39.8** **Other specified injuries of abdomen, lower back, pelvis and external genitals**

     ✓x7ᵗʰ **S39.81** **Other specified injuries of abdomen**

     ✓x7ᵗʰ **S39.82** **Other specified injuries of lower back**

     ✓x7ᵗʰ **S39.83** **Other specified injuries of pelvis**

     ✓6ᵗʰ **S39.84** **Other specified injuries of external genitals**

       ✓7ᵗʰ **S39.840** **Fracture of corpus cavernosum penis**   ♂

       ✓7ᵗʰ **S39.848** **Other specified injuries of external genitals**

   ✓5ᵗʰ **S39.9** **Unspecified injury of abdomen, lower back, pelvis and external genitals**

     ✓x7ᵗʰ **S39.91** **Unspecified injury of abdomen**   ▽

     ✓x7ᵗʰ **S39.92** **Unspecified injury of lower back**   ▽

     ✓x7ᵗʰ **S39.93** **Unspecified injury of pelvis**   ▽

     ✓x7ᵗʰ **S39.94** **Unspecified injury of external genitals** ▽

Injuries to the shoulder and upper arm (S40-S49)

INCLUDES   injuries of axilla
            injuries of scapular region

EXCLUDES 2   *burns and corrosions (T20-T32)*
            frostbite (T33-T34)
            injuries of elbow (S50-S59)
            insect bite or sting, venomous (T63.4)

✓4ᵗʰ **S40** **Superficial injury of shoulder and upper arm**

     The appropriate 7th character is to be added to each code from category S40.
     A   initial encounter
     D   subsequent encounter
     S   sequela

   ✓5ᵗʰ **S40.0** **Contusion of shoulder and upper arm**

     ✓6ᵗʰ **S40.01** **Contusion of shoulder**

       ✓7ᵗʰ **S40.011** **Contusion of right shoulder**

       ✓7ᵗʰ **S40.012** **Contusion of left shoulder**

       ✓7ᵗʰ **S40.019** **Contusion of unspecified shoulder** ▽

     ✓6ᵗʰ **S40.02** **Contusion of upper arm**

       ✓7ᵗʰ **S40.021** **Contusion of right upper arm**

       ✓7ᵗʰ **S40.022** **Contusion of left upper arm**

       ✓7ᵗʰ **S40.029** **Contusion of unspecified upper arm** ▽

   ✓5ᵗʰ **S40.2** **Other superficial injuries of shoulder**

     ✓6ᵗʰ **S40.21** **Abrasion of shoulder**

       ✓7ᵗʰ **S40.211** **Abrasion of right shoulder**

       ✓7ᵗʰ **S40.212** **Abrasion of left shoulder**

       ✓7ᵗʰ **S40.219** **Abrasion of unspecified shoulder** ▽

     ✓6ᵗʰ **S40.22** **Blister (nonthermal) of shoulder**

       ✓7ᵗʰ **S40.221** **Blister (nonthermal) of right shoulder**

       ✓7ᵗʰ **S40.222** **Blister (nonthermal) of left shoulder**

       ✓7ᵗʰ **S40.229** **Blister (nonthermal) of unspecified** ▽
                   shoulder

     ✓6ᵗʰ **S40.24** **External constriction of shoulder**

       ✓7ᵗʰ **S40.241** **External constriction of right shoulder**

       ✓7ᵗʰ **S40.242** **External constriction of left shoulder**

       ✓7ᵗʰ **S40.249** **External constriction of unspecified** ▽
                   shoulder

     ✓6ᵗʰ **S40.25** **Superficial foreign body of shoulder**
            Splinter in the shoulder

       ✓7ᵗʰ **S40.251** **Superficial foreign body of right shoulder**

       ✓7ᵗʰ **S40.252** **Superficial foreign body of left shoulder**

       ✓7ᵗʰ **S40.259** **Superficial foreign body of** ▽
                   unspecified shoulder

     ✓6ᵗʰ **S40.26** **Insect bite (nonvenomous) of shoulder**

       ✓7ᵗʰ **S40.261** **Insect bite (nonvenomous) of right**
                   shoulder

       ✓7ᵗʰ **S40.262** **Insect bite (nonvenomous) of left shoulder**

       ✓7ᵗʰ **S40.269** **Insect bite (nonvenomous) of** ▽
                   unspecified shoulder

     ✓6ᵗʰ **S40.27** **Other superficial bite of shoulder**
          EXCLUDES 1   *open bite of shoulder (S41.05)*

       ✓7ᵗʰ **S40.271** **Other superficial bite of right shoulder**

       ✓7ᵗʰ **S40.272** **Other superficial bite of left shoulder**

       ✓7ᵗʰ **S40.279** **Other superficial bite of unspecified** ▽
                   shoulder

   ✓5ᵗʰ **S40.8** **Other superficial injuries of upper arm**

     ✓6ᵗʰ **S40.81** **Abrasion of upper arm**

       ✓7ᵗʰ **S40.811** **Abrasion of right upper arm**

       ✓7ᵗʰ **S40.812** **Abrasion of left upper arm**

       ✓7ᵗʰ **S40.819** **Abrasion of unspecified upper arm** ▽

     ✓6ᵗʰ **S40.82** **Blister (nonthermal) of upper arm**

       ✓7ᵗʰ **S40.821** **Blister (nonthermal) of right upper arm**

       ✓7ᵗʰ **S40.822** **Blister (nonthermal) of left upper arm**

       ✓7ᵗʰ **S40.829** **Blister (nonthermal) of unspecified** ▽
                   upper arm

     ✓6ᵗʰ **S40.84** **External constriction of upper arm**

       ✓7ᵗʰ **S40.841** **External constriction of right upper arm**

       ✓7ᵗʰ **S40.842** **External constriction of left upper arm**

       ✓7ᵗʰ **S40.849** **External constriction of unspecified** ▽
                   upper arm

✓6ᵗʰ **S40.85** Superficial foreign body of upper arm
Splinter in the upper arm

  ✓7ᵗʰ **S40.851** Superficial foreign body of right upper arm

  ✓7ᵗʰ **S40.852** Superficial foreign body of left upper arm

  ✓7ᵗʰ **S40.859** Superficial foreign body of unspecified ▽ upper arm

✓6ᵗʰ **S40.86** Insect bite (nonvenomous) of upper arm

  ✓7ᵗʰ **S40.861** Insect bite (nonvenomous) of right upper arm

  ✓7ᵗʰ **S40.862** Insect bite (nonvenomous) of left upper arm

  ✓7ᵗʰ **S40.869** Insect bite (nonvenomous) of ▽ unspecified upper arm

✓6ᵗʰ **S40.87** Other superficial bite of upper arm
  EXCLUDES 1 *open bite of upper arm (S41.14)*
  EXCLUDES 2 *other superficial bite of shoulder (S40.27-)*

  ✓7ᵗʰ **S40.871** Other superficial bite of right upper arm

  ✓7ᵗʰ **S40.872** Other superficial bite of left upper arm

  ✓7ᵗʰ **S40.879** Other superficial bite of unspecified ▽ upper arm

✓5ᵗʰ **S40.9** Unspecified superficial injury of shoulder and upper arm

✓6ᵗʰ **S40.91** Unspecified superficial injury of shoulder

  ✓7ᵗʰ **S40.911** Unspecified superficial injury of right ▽ shoulder

  ✓7ᵗʰ **S40.912** Unspecified superficial injury of left ▽ shoulder

  ✓7ᵗʰ **S40.919** Unspecified superficial injury of ▽ unspecified shoulder

✓6ᵗʰ **S40.92** Unspecified superficial injury of upper arm

  ✓7ᵗʰ **S40.921** Unspecified superficial injury of right ▽ upper arm

  ✓7ᵗʰ **S40.922** Unspecified superficial injury of left ▽ upper arm

  ✓7ᵗʰ **S40.929** Unspecified superficial injury of ▽ unspecified upper arm

✓4ᵗʰ **S41** Open wound of shoulder and upper arm
Code also any associated wound infection
  EXCLUDES 1 *traumatic amputation of shoulder and upper arm (S48.-)*
  EXCLUDES 2 *open fracture of shoulder and upper arm (S42.- with 7th character B or C)*

> The appropriate 7th character is to be added to each code from category S41.
> A   initial encounter
> D   subsequent encounter
> S   sequela

✓5ᵗʰ **S41.0** Open wound of shoulder

✓6ᵗʰ **S41.00** Unspecified open wound of shoulder

  ✓7ᵗʰ **S41.001** Unspecified open wound of right ▽ shoulder

  ✓7ᵗʰ **S41.002** Unspecified open wound of left ▽ shoulder

  ✓7ᵗʰ **S41.009** Unspecified open wound of ▽ unspecified shoulder

✓6ᵗʰ **S41.01** Laceration without foreign body of shoulder

  ✓7ᵗʰ **S41.011** Laceration without foreign body of right shoulder

  ✓7ᵗʰ **S41.012** Laceration without foreign body of left shoulder

  ✓7ᵗʰ **S41.019** Laceration without foreign body of ▽ unspecified shoulder

✓6ᵗʰ **S41.02** Laceration with foreign body of shoulder

  ✓7ᵗʰ **S41.021** Laceration with foreign body of right shoulder

  ✓7ᵗʰ **S41.022** Laceration with foreign body of left shoulder

  ✓7ᵗʰ **S41.029** Laceration with foreign body of ▽ unspecified shoulder

✓6ᵗʰ **S41.03** Puncture wound without foreign body of shoulder

  ✓7ᵗʰ **S41.031** Puncture wound without foreign body of right shoulder

  ✓7ᵗʰ **S41.032** Puncture wound without foreign body of left shoulder

  ✓7ᵗʰ **S41.039** Puncture wound without foreign ▽ body of unspecified shoulder

✓6ᵗʰ **S41.04** Puncture wound with foreign body of shoulder

  ✓7ᵗʰ **S41.041** Puncture wound with foreign body of right shoulder

  ✓7ᵗʰ **S41.042** Puncture wound with foreign body of left shoulder

  ✓7ᵗʰ **S41.049** Puncture wound with foreign body of ▽ unspecified shoulder

✓6ᵗʰ **S41.05** Open bite of shoulder
Bite of shoulder NOS
  EXCLUDES 1 *superficial bite of shoulder (S40.27)*

  ✓7ᵗʰ **S41.051** Open bite of right shoulder

  ✓7ᵗʰ **S41.052** Open bite of left shoulder

  ✓7ᵗʰ **S41.059** Open bite of unspecified shoulder ▽

✓5ᵗʰ **S41.1** Open wound of upper arm

✓6ᵗʰ **S41.10** Unspecified open wound of upper arm
AHA: 2016, 3Q, 24

  ✓7ᵗʰ **S41.101** Unspecified open wound of right ▽ upper arm

  ✓7ᵗʰ **S41.102** Unspecified open wound of left ▽ upper arm

  ✓7ᵗʰ **S41.109** Unspecified open wound of ▽ unspecified upper arm

✓6ᵗʰ **S41.11** Laceration without foreign body of upper arm

  ✓7ᵗʰ **S41.111** Laceration without foreign body of right upper arm

  ✓7ᵗʰ **S41.112** Laceration without foreign body of left upper arm

  ✓7ᵗʰ **S41.119** Laceration without foreign body of ▽ unspecified upper arm

✓6ᵗʰ **S41.12** Laceration with foreign body of upper arm

  ✓7ᵗʰ **S41.121** Laceration with foreign body of right upper arm

  ✓7ᵗʰ **S41.122** Laceration with foreign body of left upper arm

  ✓7ᵗʰ **S41.129** Laceration with foreign body of ▽ unspecified upper arm

✓6ᵗʰ **S41.13** Puncture wound without foreign body of upper arm
AHA: 2016, 3Q, 24

  ✓7ᵗʰ **S41.131** Puncture wound without foreign body of right upper arm

  ✓7ᵗʰ **S41.132** Puncture wound without foreign body of left upper arm

  ✓7ᵗʰ **S41.139** Puncture wound without foreign ▽ body of unspecified upper arm

✓6ᵗʰ **S41.14** Puncture wound with foreign body of upper arm
AHA: 2016, 3Q, 24

  ✓7ᵗʰ **S41.141** Puncture wound with foreign body of right upper arm

  ✓7ᵗʰ **S41.142** Puncture wound with foreign body of left upper arm

  ✓7ᵗʰ **S41.149** Puncture wound with foreign body ▽ of unspecified upper arm

✓6ᵗʰ **S41.15** Open bite of upper arm
Bite of upper arm NOS
  EXCLUDES 1 *superficial bite of upper arm (S40.87)*

  ✓7ᵗʰ **S41.151** Open bite of right upper arm

  ✓7ᵗʰ **S41.152** Open bite of left upper arm

  ✓7ᵗʰ **S41.159** Open bite of unspecified upper arm ▽

EXCLUDES 1 Not coded here   EXCLUDES 2 Not included here   N Newborn Age: 0   P Pediatric Age: 0-17   M Maternity Age: 12-55   A Adult Age: 15-124

954   ICD-10-CM 2018

✓4th **S42 Fracture of shoulder and upper arm**

NOTE A fracture not indicated as displaced or nondisplaced should be coded to displaced.
A fracture not indicated as open or closed should be coded to closed.

EXCLUDES 1 *traumatic amputation of shoulder and upper arm (S48.-)*
AHA: 2015, 3Q, 37-39

> The appropriate 7th character is to be added to all codes from category S42 [unless otherwise indicated].
> A   initial encounter for closed fracture
> B   initial encounter for open fracture
> D   subsequent encounter for fracture with routine healing
> G   subsequent encounter for fracture with delayed healing
> K   subsequent encounter for fracture with nonunion
> P   subsequent encounter for fracture with malunion
> S   sequela

✓5th **S42.0 Fracture of clavicle**

✓6th **S42.00 Fracture of unspecified part of clavicle**

✓7th **S42.001 Fracture of unspecified part of right** ▽
clavicle

✓7th **S42.002 Fracture of unspecified part of left** ▽
clavicle

✓7th **S42.009 Fracture of unspecified part of** ▽
unspecified clavicle
AHA: 2012, 4Q, 93

✓6th **S42.01 Fracture of sternal end of clavicle**

✓7th **S42.011 Anterior displaced fracture of sternal end**
of right clavicle

✓7th **S42.012 Anterior displaced fracture of sternal end**
of left clavicle

✓7th **S42.013 Anterior displaced fracture of sternal** ▽
end of unspecified clavicle
Displaced fracture of sternal end of clavicle
NOS

✓7th **S42.014 Posterior displaced fracture of sternal end**
of right clavicle

✓7th **S42.015 Posterior displaced fracture of sternal end**
of left clavicle

✓7th **S42.016 Posterior displaced fracture of sternal** ▽
end of unspecified clavicle

✓7th **S42.017 Nondisplaced fracture of sternal end of**
right clavicle

✓7th **S42.018 Nondisplaced fracture of sternal end of**
left clavicle

✓7th **S42.019 Nondisplaced fracture of sternal end of** ▽
unspecified clavicle

✓6th **S42.02 Fracture of shaft of clavicle**

✓7th **S42.021 Displaced fracture of shaft of right clavicle**

✓7th **S42.022 Displaced fracture of shaft of left clavicle**

✓7th **S42.023 Displaced fracture of shaft of** ▽
unspecified clavicle

✓7th **S42.024 Nondisplaced fracture of shaft of right**
clavicle

✓7th **S42.025 Nondisplaced fracture of shaft of left**
clavicle

✓7th **S42.026 Nondisplaced fracture of shaft of** ▽
unspecified clavicle

✓6th **S42.03 Fracture of lateral end of clavicle**
Fracture of acromial end of clavicle

✓7th **S42.031 Displaced fracture of lateral end of right**
clavicle

✓7th **S42.032 Displaced fracture of lateral end of left**
clavicle

✓7th **S42.033 Displaced fracture of lateral end of** ▽
unspecified clavicle

✓7th **S42.034 Nondisplaced fracture of lateral end of**
right clavicle

✓7th **S42.035 Nondisplaced fracture of lateral end of left**
clavicle

✓7th **S42.036 Nondisplaced fracture of lateral end of** ▽
unspecified clavicle

✓5th **S42.1 Fracture of scapula**

✓6th **S42.10 Fracture of unspecified part of scapula**

✓7th **S42.101 Fracture of unspecified part of scapula,** ▽
right shoulder

✓7th **S42.102 Fracture of unspecified part of scapula,** ▽
left shoulder

✓7th **S42.109 Fracture of unspecified part of scapula,** ▽
unspecified shoulder

✓6th **S42.11 Fracture of body of scapula**

✓7th **S42.111 Displaced fracture of body of scapula,**
right shoulder

✓7th **S42.112 Displaced fracture of body of scapula, left**
shoulder

✓7th **S42.113 Displaced fracture of body of scapula,** ▽
unspecified shoulder

✓7th **S42.114 Nondisplaced fracture of body of scapula,**
right shoulder

✓7th **S42.115 Nondisplaced fracture of body of scapula,**
left shoulder

✓7th **S42.116 Nondisplaced fracture of body of** ▽
scapula, unspecified shoulder

✓6th **S42.12 Fracture of acromial process**

✓7th **S42.121 Displaced fracture of acromial process,**
right shoulder

✓7th **S42.122 Displaced fracture of acromial process, left**
shoulder

✓7th **S42.123 Displaced fracture of acromial process,** ▽
unspecified shoulder

✓7th **S42.124 Nondisplaced fracture of acromial**
process, right shoulder

✓7th **S42.125 Nondisplaced fracture of acromial**
process, left shoulder

✓7th **S42.126 Nondisplaced fracture of acromial** ▽
process, unspecified shoulder

✓6th **S42.13 Fracture of coracoid process**

✓7th **S42.131 Displaced fracture of coracoid process,**
right shoulder

✓7th **S42.132 Displaced fracture of coracoid process,**
left shoulder

✓7th **S42.133 Displaced fracture of coracoid process,** ▽
unspecified shoulder

✓7th **S42.134 Nondisplaced fracture of coracoid process,**
right shoulder

✓7th **S42.135 Nondisplaced fracture of coracoid process,**
left shoulder

✓7th **S42.136 Nondisplaced fracture of coracoid** ▽
process, unspecified shoulder

✓6th **S42.14 Fracture of glenoid cavity of scapula**

✓7th **S42.141 Displaced fracture of glenoid cavity of**
scapula, right shoulder

✓7th **S42.142 Displaced fracture of glenoid cavity of**
scapula, left shoulder

✓7th **S42.143 Displaced fracture of glenoid cavity of** ▽
scapula, unspecified shoulder

✓7th **S42.144 Nondisplaced fracture of glenoid cavity of**
scapula, right shoulder

✓7th **S42.145 Nondisplaced fracture of glenoid cavity of**
scapula, left shoulder

✓7th **S42.146 Nondisplaced fracture of glenoid** ▽
cavity of scapula, unspecified shoulder

✓6th **S42.15 Fracture of neck of scapula**

✓7th **S42.151 Displaced fracture of neck of scapula, right**
shoulder

✓7th **S42.152 Displaced fracture of neck of scapula, left**
shoulder

✓7th **S42.153 Displaced fracture of neck of scapula,** ▽
unspecified shoulder

✓7th **S42.154 Nondisplaced fracture of neck of scapula,**
right shoulder

✓7th **S42.155 Nondisplaced fracture of neck of scapula,**
left shoulder

✓7th **S42.156 Nondisplaced fracture of neck of** ▽
scapula, unspecified shoulder

✓6th **S42.19 Fracture of other part of scapula**

✓7th **S42.191 Fracture of other part of scapula, right**
shoulder

✓7th **S42.192 Fracture of other part of scapula, left**
shoulder

☑ Additional Character Req   ☑x7th Placeholder Alert   Manifestation   HCC CMS-HCC Condition   ▽ Unspecified Code   ►◄ Revised Text   ● New Code   ▲ Revised Code Title

ICD-10-CM 2018   955

√ 6ᵗʰ **S42.199** **Fracture of other part of scapula, unspecified shoulder** ▽

√ 6ᵗʰ **S42.2** **Fracture of upper end of humerus**
Fracture of proximal end of humerus
EXCLUDES 2   *fracture of shaft of humerus (S42.3-)*
        physeal fracture of upper end of humerus (S49.0-)

√ 6ᵗʰ **S42.20** **Unspecified fracture of upper end of humerus**

√ 7ᵗʰ **S42.201** **Unspecified fracture of upper end of right humerus** ▽

√ 7ᵗʰ **S42.202** **Unspecified fracture of upper end of left humerus** ▽

√ 7ᵗʰ **S42.209** **Unspecified fracture of upper end of unspecified humerus** ▽

√ 6ᵗʰ **S42.21** **Unspecified fracture of surgical neck of humerus**
Fracture of neck of humerus NOS

√ 7ᵗʰ **S42.211** **Unspecified displaced fracture of surgical neck of right humerus** ▽

√ 7ᵗʰ **S42.212** **Unspecified displaced fracture of surgical neck of left humerus** ▽

√ 7ᵗʰ **S42.213** **Unspecified displaced fracture of surgical neck of unspecified humerus** ▽

√ 7ᵗʰ **S42.214** **Unspecified nondisplaced fracture of surgical neck of right humerus** ▽

√ 7ᵗʰ **S42.215** **Unspecified nondisplaced fracture of surgical neck of left humerus** ▽

√ 7ᵗʰ **S42.216** **Unspecified nondisplaced fracture of surgical neck of unspecified humerus** ▽

√ 6ᵗʰ **S42.22** **2-part fracture of surgical neck of humerus**

√ 7ᵗʰ **S42.221** **2-part displaced fracture of surgical neck of right humerus**

√ 7ᵗʰ **S42.222** **2-part displaced fracture of surgical neck of left humerus**

√ 7ᵗʰ **S42.223** **2-part displaced fracture of surgical neck of unspecified humerus** ▽

√ 7ᵗʰ **S42.224** **2-part nondisplaced fracture of surgical neck of right humerus**

√ 7ᵗʰ **S42.225** **2-part nondisplaced fracture of surgical neck of left humerus**

√ 7ᵗʰ **S42.226** **2-part nondisplaced fracture of surgical neck of unspecified humerus** ▽

√ 6ᵗʰ **S42.23** **3-part fracture of surgical neck of humerus**

√ 7ᵗʰ **S42.231** **3-part fracture of surgical neck of right humerus**

√ 7ᵗʰ **S42.232** **3-part fracture of surgical neck of left humerus**

√ 7ᵗʰ **S42.239** **3-part fracture of surgical neck of unspecified humerus** ▽

√ 6ᵗʰ **S42.24** **4-part fracture of surgical neck of humerus**

√ 7ᵗʰ **S42.241** **4-part fracture of surgical neck of right humerus**

√ 7ᵗʰ **S42.242** **4-part fracture of surgical neck of left humerus**

√ 7ᵗʰ **S42.249** **4-part fracture of surgical neck of unspecified humerus** ▽

√ 6ᵗʰ **S42.25** **Fracture of greater tuberosity of humerus**

√ 7ᵗʰ **S42.251** **Displaced fracture of greater tuberosity of right humerus**

√ 7ᵗʰ **S42.252** **Displaced fracture of greater tuberosity of left humerus**

√ 7ᵗʰ **S42.253** **Displaced fracture of greater tuberosity of unspecified humerus** ▽

√ 7ᵗʰ **S42.254** **Nondisplaced fracture of greater tuberosity of right humerus**

√ 7ᵗʰ **S42.255** **Nondisplaced fracture of greater tuberosity of left humerus**

√ 7ᵗʰ **S42.256** **Nondisplaced fracture of greater tuberosity of unspecified humerus** ▽

√ 6ᵗʰ **S42.26** **Fracture of lesser tuberosity of humerus**

√ 7ᵗʰ **S42.261** **Displaced fracture of lesser tuberosity of right humerus**

√ 7ᵗʰ **S42.262** **Displaced fracture of lesser tuberosity of left humerus**

√ 7ᵗʰ **S42.263** **Displaced fracture of lesser tuberosity of unspecified humerus** ▽

√ 7ᵗʰ **S42.264** **Nondisplaced fracture of lesser tuberosity of right humerus**

√ 7ᵗʰ **S42.265** **Nondisplaced fracture of lesser tuberosity of left humerus**

√ 7ᵗʰ **S42.266** **Nondisplaced fracture of lesser tuberosity of unspecified humerus** ▽

√ 6ᵗʰ **S42.27** **Torus fracture of upper end of humerus**

> The appropriate 7th character is to be added to all codes in subcategory S42.27.
> A   initial encounter for closed fracture
> D   subsequent encounter for fracture with routine healing
> G   subsequent encounter for fracture with delayed healing
> K   subsequent encounter for fracture with nonunion
> P   subsequent encounter for fracture with malunion
> S   sequela

√ 7ᵗʰ **S42.271** **Torus fracture of upper end of right humerus**

√ 7ᵗʰ **S42.272** **Torus fracture of upper end of left humerus**

√ 7ᵗʰ **S42.279** **Torus fracture of upper end of unspecified humerus** ▽

√ 6ᵗʰ **S42.29** **Other fracture of upper end of humerus**
Fracture of anatomical neck of humerus
Fracture of articular head of humerus

√ 7ᵗʰ **S42.291** **Other displaced fracture of upper end of right humerus**

√ 7ᵗʰ **S42.292** **Other displaced fracture of upper end of left humerus**

√ 7ᵗʰ **S42.293** **Other displaced fracture of upper end of unspecified humerus** ▽

√ 7ᵗʰ **S42.294** **Other nondisplaced fracture of upper end of right humerus**

√ 7ᵗʰ **S42.295** **Other nondisplaced fracture of upper end of left humerus**

√ 7ᵗʰ **S42.296** **Other nondisplaced fracture of upper end of unspecified humerus** ▽

√ 5ᵗʰ **S42.3** **Fracture of shaft of humerus**
Fracture of humerus NOS
Fracture of upper arm NOS
EXCLUDES 2   *physeal fractures of upper end of humerus (S49.0-)*
        physeal fractures of lower end of humerus (S49.1-)

√ 6ᵗʰ **S42.30** **Unspecified fracture of shaft of humerus**

√ 7ᵗʰ **S42.301** **Unspecified fracture of shaft of humerus, right arm** ▽

√ 7ᵗʰ **S42.302** **Unspecified fracture of shaft of humerus, left arm** ▽

√ 7ᵗʰ **S42.309** **Unspecified fracture of shaft of humerus, unspecified arm** ▽

√ 6ᵗʰ **S42.31** **Greenstick fracture of shaft of humerus**

> The appropriate 7th character is to be added to all codes in subcategory S42.31.
> A   initial encounter for closed fracture
> D   subsequent encounter for fracture with routine healing
> G   subsequent encounter for fracture with delayed healing
> K   subsequent encounter for fracture with nonunion
> P   subsequent encounter for fracture with malunion
> S   sequela

√ 7ᵗʰ **S42.311** **Greenstick fracture of shaft of humerus, right arm**

√ 7ᵗʰ **S42.312** **Greenstick fracture of shaft of humerus, left arm**

√ 7ᵗʰ **S42.319** **Greenstick fracture of shaft of humerus, unspecified arm** ▽

√ 6ᵗʰ **S42.32** **Transverse fracture of shaft of humerus**

√ 7ᵗʰ **S42.321** **Displaced transverse fracture of shaft of humerus, right arm**

√ 7ᵗʰ **S42.322** **Displaced transverse fracture of shaft of humerus, left arm**

√7ᵗʰ **S42.323** **Displaced** transverse fracture of shaft of humerus, unspecified arm ▽

√7ᵗʰ **S42.324** **Nondisplaced** transverse fracture of shaft of humerus, **right** arm

√7ᵗʰ **S42.325** **Nondisplaced** transverse fracture of shaft of humerus, **left** arm

√7ᵗʰ **S42.326** **Nondisplaced** transverse fracture of shaft of humerus, unspecified arm ▽

√6ᵗʰ **S42.33** **Oblique** fracture of shaft of humerus

√7ᵗʰ **S42.331** **Displaced** oblique fracture of shaft of humerus, **right** arm

√7ᵗʰ **S42.332** **Displaced** oblique fracture of shaft of humerus, **left** arm

√7ᵗʰ **S42.333** **Displaced** oblique fracture of shaft of humerus, unspecified arm ▽

√7ᵗʰ **S42.334** **Nondisplaced** oblique fracture of shaft of humerus, **right** arm

√7ᵗʰ **S42.335** **Nondisplaced** oblique fracture of shaft of humerus, **left** arm

√7ᵗʰ **S42.336** **Nondisplaced** oblique fracture of shaft of humerus, unspecified arm ▽

√6ᵗʰ **S42.34** **Spiral** fracture of shaft of humerus

√7ᵗʰ **S42.341** **Displaced** spiral fracture of shaft of humerus, **right** arm

√7ᵗʰ **S42.342** **Displaced** spiral fracture of shaft of humerus, **left** arm

√7ᵗʰ **S42.343** **Displaced** spiral fracture of shaft of humerus, unspecified arm ▽

√7ᵗʰ **S42.344** **Nondisplaced** spiral fracture of shaft of humerus, **right** arm

√7ᵗʰ **S42.345** **Nondisplaced** spiral fracture of shaft of humerus, **left** arm

√7ᵗʰ **S42.346** **Nondisplaced** spiral fracture of shaft of humerus, unspecified arm ▽

√6ᵗʰ **S42.35** **Comminuted** fracture of shaft of humerus

√7ᵗʰ **S42.351** **Displaced** comminuted fracture of shaft of humerus, **right** arm

√7ᵗʰ **S42.352** **Displaced** comminuted fracture of shaft of humerus, **left** arm

√7ᵗʰ **S42.353** **Displaced** comminuted fracture of shaft of humerus, unspecified arm ▽

√7ᵗʰ **S42.354** **Nondisplaced** comminuted fracture of shaft of humerus, **right** arm

√7ᵗʰ **S42.355** **Nondisplaced** comminuted fracture of shaft of humerus, **left** arm

√7ᵗʰ **S42.356** **Nondisplaced** comminuted fracture of shaft of humerus, unspecified arm ▽

√6ᵗʰ **S42.36** **Segmental** fracture of shaft of humerus

√7ᵗʰ **S42.361** **Displaced** segmental fracture of shaft of humerus, **right** arm

√7ᵗʰ **S42.362** **Displaced** segmental fracture of shaft of humerus, **left** arm

√7ᵗʰ **S42.363** **Displaced** segmental fracture of shaft of humerus, unspecified arm ▽

√7ᵗʰ **S42.364** **Nondisplaced** segmental fracture of shaft of humerus, **right** arm

√7ᵗʰ **S42.365** **Nondisplaced** segmental fracture of shaft of humerus, **left** arm

√7ᵗʰ **S42.366** **Nondisplaced** segmental fracture of shaft of humerus, unspecified arm ▽

√6ᵗʰ **S42.39** **Other** fracture of shaft of humerus

√7ᵗʰ **S42.391** **Other** fracture of shaft of **right** humerus

√7ᵗʰ **S42.392** **Other** fracture of shaft of **left** humerus

√7ᵗʰ **S42.399** **Other** fracture of shaft of unspecified humerus ▽

√5ᵗʰ **S42.4** **Fracture of lower end of humerus**
Fracture of distal end of humerus
EXCLUDES 2 fracture of shaft of humerus (S42.3-)
physeal fracture of lower end of humerus (S49.1-)

√6ᵗʰ **S42.40** **Unspecified fracture of lower end of humerus**
Fracture of elbow NOS

√7ᵗʰ **S42.401** **Unspecified** fracture of lower end of **right** humerus ▽

√7ᵗʰ **S42.402** **Unspecified** fracture of lower end of **left** humerus ▽

√7ᵗʰ **S42.409** **Unspecified** fracture of lower end of unspecified humerus ▽

√6ᵗʰ **S42.41** **Simple supracondylar** fracture without intercondylar fracture of humerus

√7ᵗʰ **S42.411** **Displaced** simple supracondylar fracture without intercondylar fracture of **right** humerus

√7ᵗʰ **S42.412** **Displaced** simple supracondylar fracture without intercondylar fracture of **left** humerus

√7ᵗʰ **S42.413** **Displaced** simple supracondylar fracture without intercondylar fracture of unspecified humerus ▽

√7ᵗʰ **S42.414** **Nondisplaced** simple supracondylar fracture without intercondylar fracture of **right** humerus

√7ᵗʰ **S42.415** **Nondisplaced** simple supracondylar fracture without intercondylar fracture of **left** humerus

√7ᵗʰ **S42.416** **Nondisplaced** simple supracondylar fracture without intercondylar fracture of unspecified humerus ▽

√6ᵗʰ **S42.42** **Comminuted supracondylar** fracture without intercondylar fracture of humerus

√7ᵗʰ **S42.421** **Displaced** comminuted supracondylar fracture without intercondylar fracture of **right** humerus

√7ᵗʰ **S42.422** **Displaced** comminuted supracondylar fracture without intercondylar fracture of **left** humerus

√7ᵗʰ **S42.423** **Displaced** comminuted supracondylar ▽ fracture without intercondylar fracture of unspecified humerus

√7ᵗʰ **S42.424** **Nondisplaced** comminuted supracondylar fracture without intercondylar fracture of **right** humerus

√7ᵗʰ **S42.425** **Nondisplaced** comminuted supracondylar fracture without intercondylar fracture of **left** humerus

√7ᵗʰ **S42.426** **Nondisplaced** comminuted supracondylar fracture without intercondylar fracture of unspecified humerus ▽

√6ᵗʰ **S42.43** **Fracture (avulsion) of lateral epicondyle of humerus**

√7ᵗʰ **S42.431** **Displaced** fracture (avulsion) of lateral epicondyle of **right** humerus

√7ᵗʰ **S42.432** **Displaced** fracture (avulsion) of lateral epicondyle of **left** humerus

√7ᵗʰ **S42.433** **Displaced** fracture (avulsion) of lateral ▽ epicondyle of unspecified humerus

√7ᵗʰ **S42.434** **Nondisplaced** fracture (avulsion) of lateral epicondyle of **right** humerus

√7ᵗʰ **S42.435** **Nondisplaced** fracture (avulsion) of lateral epicondyle of **left** humerus

√7ᵗʰ **S42.436** **Nondisplaced** fracture (avulsion) of ▽ lateral epicondyle of unspecified humerus

√6ᵗʰ **S42.44** **Fracture (avulsion) of medial epicondyle of humerus**

S42.441 **Displaced** fracture (avulsion) of medial epicondyle of **right** humerus

√7ᵗʰ **S42.442** **Displaced** fracture (avulsion) of medial epicondyle of **left** humerus

√7ᵗʰ **S42.443** **Displaced** fracture (avulsion) of medial ▽ epicondyle of unspecified humerus

√7ᵗʰ **S42.444** **Nondisplaced** fracture (avulsion) of medial epicondyle of **right** humerus

√7ᵗʰ **S42.445** **Nondisplaced** fracture (avulsion) of medial epicondyle of **left** humerus

√7ᵗʰ **S42.446** **Nondisplaced** fracture (avulsion) of ▽ medial epicondyle of unspecified humerus

√7ᵗʰ **S42.447** **Incarcerated** fracture (avulsion) of medial epicondyle of **right** humerus

√7ᵗʰ **S42.448** **Incarcerated** fracture (avulsion) of medial epicondyle of **left** humerus

√7ᵗʰ **S42.449** **Incarcerated** fracture (avulsion) of ▽ medial epicondyle of unspecified humerus

---

☑ Additional Character Req   √x7ᵗʰ Placeholder Alert   Manifestation   HCC CMS-HCC Condition   ▽ Unspecified Code   ►◄ Revised Text   ● New Code   ▲ Revised Code Title

Chapter 19. Injury, Poisoning, and Certain Other Consequences of External Causes

S42.45–S43.083

√6ᵗʰ **S42.45** **Fracture of lateral condyle of humerus**
Fracture of capitellum of humerus

√7ᵗʰ **S42.451** **Displaced fracture of lateral condyle of right humerus**

√7ᵗʰ **S42.452** **Displaced fracture of lateral condyle of left humerus**

√7ᵗʰ **S42.453** **Displaced fracture of lateral condyle of unspecified humerus** ▽

√7ᵗʰ **S42.454** **Nondisplaced fracture of lateral condyle of right humerus**

√7ᵗʰ **S42.455** **Nondisplaced fracture of lateral condyle of left humerus**

√7ᵗʰ **S42.456** **Nondisplaced fracture of lateral condyle of unspecified humerus** ▽

√6ᵗʰ **S42.46** **Fracture of medial condyle of humerus**
Trochlea fracture of humerus

√7ᵗʰ **S42.461** **Displaced fracture of medial condyle of right humerus**

√7ᵗʰ **S42.462** **Displaced fracture of medial condyle of left humerus**

√7ᵗʰ **S42.463** **Displaced fracture of medial condyle of unspecified humerus** ▽

√7ᵗʰ **S42.464** **Nondisplaced fracture of medial condyle of right humerus**

√7ᵗʰ **S42.465** **Nondisplaced fracture of medial condyle of left humerus**

√7ᵗʰ **S42.466** **Nondisplaced fracture of medial condyle of unspecified humerus** ▽

√6ᵗʰ **S42.47** **Transcondylar fracture of humerus**

√7ᵗʰ **S42.471** **Displaced transcondylar fracture of right humerus**

√7ᵗʰ **S42.472** **Displaced transcondylar fracture of left humerus**

√7ᵗʰ **S42.473** **Displaced transcondylar fracture of unspecified humerus** ▽

√7ᵗʰ **S42.474** **Nondisplaced transcondylar fracture of right humerus**

√7ᵗʰ **S42.475** **Nondisplaced transcondylar fracture of left humerus**

√7ᵗʰ **S42.476** **Nondisplaced transcondylar fracture of unspecified humerus** ▽

√6ᵗʰ **S42.48** **Torus fracture of lower end of humerus**

> The appropriate 7th character is to be added to all codes in subcategory S42.48.
> A   initial encounter for closed fracture
> D   subsequent encounter for fracture with routine healing
> G   subsequent encounter for fracture with delayed healing
> K   subsequent encounter for fracture with nonunion
> P   subsequent encounter for fracture with malunion
> S   sequela

√7ᵗʰ **S42.481** **Torus fracture of lower end of right humerus**

√7ᵗʰ **S42.482** **Torus fracture of lower end of left humerus**

√7ᵗʰ **S42.489** **Torus fracture of lower end of unspecified humerus** ▽

√6ᵗʰ **S42.49** **Other fracture of lower end of humerus**

√7ᵗʰ **S42.491** **Other displaced fracture of lower end of right humerus**

√7ᵗʰ **S42.492** **Other displaced fracture of lower end of left humerus**

√7ᵗʰ **S42.493** **Other displaced fracture of lower end of unspecified humerus** ▽

√7ᵗʰ **S42.494** **Other nondisplaced fracture of lower end of right humerus**

√7ᵗʰ **S42.495** **Other nondisplaced fracture of lower end of left humerus**

√7ᵗʰ **S42.496** **Other nondisplaced fracture of lower end of unspecified humerus** ▽

√5ᵗʰ **S42.9** **Fracture of shoulder girdle, part unspecified**
Fracture of shoulder NOS

√x7ᵗʰ **S42.90** **Fracture of unspecified shoulder girdle, part unspecified** ▽

√x7ᵗʰ **S42.91** **Fracture of right shoulder girdle, part unspecified** ▽

√x7ᵗʰ **S42.92** **Fracture of left shoulder girdle, part unspecified** ▽

√4ᵗʰ **S43** **Dislocation and sprain of joints and ligaments of shoulder girdle**
[INCLUDES] avulsion of joint or ligament of shoulder girdle
laceration of cartilage, joint or ligament of shoulder girdle
sprain of cartilage, joint or ligament of shoulder girdle
traumatic hemarthrosis of joint or ligament of shoulder girdle
traumatic rupture of joint or ligament of shoulder girdle
traumatic subluxation of joint or ligament of shoulder girdle
traumatic tear of joint or ligament of shoulder girdle

Code also any associated open wound

EXCLUDES 2   *strain of muscle, fascia and tendon of shoulder and upper arm (S46.-)*

> The appropriate 7th character is to be added to each code from category S43.
> A   initial encounter
> D   subsequent encounter
> S   sequela

√5ᵗʰ **S43.0** **Subluxation and dislocation of shoulder joint**
Dislocation of glenohumeral joint
Subluxation of glenohumeral joint

√6ᵗʰ **S43.00** **Unspecified subluxation and dislocation of shoulder joint**
Dislocation of humerus NOS
Subluxation of humerus NOS

√7ᵗʰ **S43.001** **Unspecified subluxation of right shoulder joint** ▽

√7ᵗʰ **S43.002** **Unspecified subluxation of left shoulder joint** ▽

√7ᵗʰ **S43.003** **Unspecified subluxation of unspecified shoulder joint** ▽

√7ᵗʰ **S43.004** **Unspecified dislocation of right shoulder joint** ▽

√7ᵗʰ **S43.005** **Unspecified dislocation of left shoulder joint** ▽

√7ᵗʰ **S43.006** **Unspecified dislocation of unspecified shoulder joint** ▽

√6ᵗʰ **S43.01** **Anterior subluxation and dislocation of humerus**

√7ᵗʰ **S43.011** **Anterior subluxation of right humerus**

√7ᵗʰ **S43.012** **Anterior subluxation of left humerus**

√7ᵗʰ **S43.013** **Anterior subluxation of unspecified humerus** ▽

√7ᵗʰ **S43.014** **Anterior dislocation of right humerus**

√7ᵗʰ **S43.015** **Anterior dislocation of left humerus**

√7ᵗʰ **S43.016** **Anterior dislocation of unspecified humerus** ▽

√6ᵗʰ **S43.02** **Posterior subluxation and dislocation of humerus**

√7ᵗʰ **S43.021** **Posterior subluxation of right humerus**

√7ᵗʰ **S43.022** **Posterior subluxation of left humerus**

√7ᵗʰ **S43.023** **Posterior subluxation of unspecified humerus** ▽

√7ᵗʰ **S43.024** **Posterior dislocation of right humerus**

√7ᵗʰ **S43.025** **Posterior dislocation of left humerus**

√7ᵗʰ **S43.026** **Posterior dislocation of unspecified humerus** ▽

√6ᵗʰ **S43.03** **Inferior subluxation and dislocation of humerus**

√7ᵗʰ **S43.031** **Inferior subluxation of right humerus**

√7ᵗʰ **S43.032** **Inferior subluxation of left humerus**

√7ᵗʰ **S43.033** **Inferior subluxation of unspecified humerus** ▽

√7ᵗʰ **S43.034** **Inferior dislocation of right humerus**

√7ᵗʰ **S43.035** **Inferior dislocation of left humerus**

√7ᵗʰ **S43.036** **Inferior dislocation of unspecified humerus** ▽

√6ᵗʰ **S43.08** **Other subluxation and dislocation of shoulder joint**

√7ᵗʰ **S43.081** **Other subluxation of right shoulder joint**

√7ᵗʰ **S43.082** **Other subluxation of left shoulder joint**

√7ᵗʰ **S43.083** **Other subluxation of unspecified shoulder joint** ▽

EXCLUDES 1 Not coded here   *EXCLUDES 2* Not included here   **N** Newborn Age: 0   **P** Pediatric Age: 0-17   **M** Maternity Age: 12-55   **A** Adult Age: 15-124

√7ᵗʰ **S43.084** Other dislocation of right shoulder joint

√7ᵗʰ **S43.085** Other dislocation of left shoulder joint

√7ᵗʰ **S43.086** Other dislocation of unspecified shoulder joint ▽

√5ᵗʰ **S43.1** Subluxation and dislocation of acromioclavicular joint

√6ᵗʰ **S43.10** Unspecified dislocation of acromioclavicular joint

√7ᵗʰ **S43.101** Unspecified dislocation of right acromioclavicular joint ▽

√7ᵗʰ **S43.102** Unspecified dislocation of left acromioclavicular joint ▽

√7ᵗʰ **S43.109** Unspecified dislocation of unspecified acromioclavicular joint ▽

√6ᵗʰ **S43.11** Subluxation of acromioclavicular joint

√7ᵗʰ **S43.111** Subluxation of right acromioclavicular joint

√7ᵗʰ **S43.112** Subluxation of left acromioclavicular joint

√7ᵗʰ **S43.119** Subluxation of unspecified acromioclavicular joint ▽

√6ᵗʰ **S43.12** Dislocation of acromioclavicular joint, 100%-200% displacement

√7ᵗʰ **S43.121** Dislocation of right acromioclavicular joint, 100%-200% displacement

√7ᵗʰ **S43.122** Dislocation of left acromioclavicular joint, 100%-200% displacement

√7ᵗʰ **S43.129** Dislocation of unspecified acromioclavicular joint, 100%-200% displacement ▽

√6ᵗʰ **S43.13** Dislocation of acromioclavicular joint, greater than 200% displacement

√7ᵗʰ **S43.131** Dislocation of right acromioclavicular joint, greater than 200% displacement

√7ᵗʰ **S43.132** Dislocation of left acromioclavicular joint, greater than 200% displacement

√7ᵗʰ **S43.139** Dislocation of unspecified acromioclavicular joint, greater than 200% displacement ▽

√6ᵗʰ **S43.14** Inferior dislocation of acromioclavicular joint

√7ᵗʰ **S43.141** Inferior dislocation of right acromioclavicular joint

√7ᵗʰ **S43.142** Inferior dislocation of left acromioclavicular joint

√7ᵗʰ **S43.149** Inferior dislocation of unspecified acromioclavicular joint ▽

√6ᵗʰ **S43.15** Posterior dislocation of acromioclavicular joint

√7ᵗʰ **S43.151** Posterior dislocation of right acromioclavicular joint

√7ᵗʰ **S43.152** Posterior dislocation of left acromioclavicular joint

√7ᵗʰ **S43.159** Posterior dislocation of unspecified acromioclavicular joint ▽

√5ᵗʰ **S43.2** Subluxation and dislocation of sternoclavicular joint

√6ᵗʰ **S43.20** Unspecified subluxation and dislocation of sternoclavicular joint

√7ᵗʰ **S43.201** Unspecified subluxation of right sternoclavicular joint ▽

√7ᵗʰ **S43.202** Unspecified subluxation of left sternoclavicular joint ▽

√7ᵗʰ **S43.203** Unspecified subluxation of unspecified sternoclavicular joint ▽

√7ᵗʰ **S43.204** Unspecified dislocation of right sternoclavicular joint ▽

√7ᵗʰ **S43.205** Unspecified dislocation of left sternoclavicular joint ▽

√7ᵗʰ **S43.206** Unspecified dislocation of unspecified sternoclavicular joint ▽

√6ᵗʰ **S43.21** Anterior subluxation and dislocation of sternoclavicular joint

√7ᵗʰ **S43.211** Anterior subluxation of right sternoclavicular joint

√7ᵗʰ **S43.212** Anterior subluxation of left sternoclavicular joint

√7ᵗʰ **S43.213** Anterior subluxation of unspecified sternoclavicular joint ▽

√7ᵗʰ **S43.214** Anterior dislocation of right sternoclavicular joint

√7ᵗʰ **S43.215** Anterior dislocation of left sternoclavicular joint

√7ᵗʰ **S43.216** Anterior dislocation of unspecified sternoclavicular joint ▽

√6ᵗʰ **S43.22** Posterior subluxation and dislocation of sternoclavicular joint

√7ᵗʰ **S43.221** Posterior subluxation of right sternoclavicular joint

√7ᵗʰ **S43.222** Posterior subluxation of left sternoclavicular joint

√7ᵗʰ **S43.223** Posterior subluxation of unspecified sternoclavicular joint ▽

√7ᵗʰ **S43.224** Posterior dislocation of right sternoclavicular joint

√7ᵗʰ **S43.225** Posterior dislocation of left sternoclavicular joint

√7ᵗʰ **S43.226** Posterior dislocation of unspecified sternoclavicular joint ▽

√5ᵗʰ **S43.3** Subluxation and dislocation of other and unspecified parts of shoulder girdle

√6ᵗʰ **S43.30** Subluxation and dislocation of unspecified parts of shoulder girdle

Dislocation of shoulder girdle NOS
Subluxation of shoulder girdle NOS

√7ᵗʰ **S43.301** Subluxation of unspecified parts of right shoulder girdle ▽

√7ᵗʰ **S43.302** Subluxation of unspecified parts of left shoulder girdle ▽

√7ᵗʰ **S43.303** Subluxation of unspecified parts of unspecified shoulder girdle ▽

√7ᵗʰ **S43.304** Dislocation of unspecified parts of right shoulder girdle ▽

√7ᵗʰ **S43.305** Dislocation of unspecified parts of left shoulder girdle ▽

√7ᵗʰ **S43.306** Dislocation of unspecified parts of unspecified shoulder girdle ▽

√6ᵗʰ **S43.31** Subluxation and dislocation of scapula

√7ᵗʰ **S43.311** Subluxation of right scapula

√7ᵗʰ **S43.312** Subluxation of left scapula

√7ᵗʰ **S43.313** Subluxation of unspecified scapula ▽

√7ᵗʰ **S43.314** Dislocation of right scapula

√7ᵗʰ **S43.315** Dislocation of left scapula

√7ᵗʰ **S43.316** Dislocation of unspecified scapula ▽

√6ᵗʰ **S43.39** Subluxation and dislocation of other parts of shoulder girdle

√7ᵗʰ **S43.391** Subluxation of other parts of right shoulder girdle

√7ᵗʰ **S43.392** Subluxation of other parts of left shoulder girdle

√7ᵗʰ **S43.393** Subluxation of other parts of unspecified shoulder girdle ▽

√7ᵗʰ **S43.394** Dislocation of other parts of right shoulder girdle

√7ᵗʰ **S43.395** Dislocation of other parts of left shoulder girdle

√7ᵗʰ **S43.396** Dislocation of other parts of unspecified shoulder girdle ▽

√5ᵗʰ **S43.4** Sprain of shoulder joint

√6ᵗʰ **S43.40** Unspecified sprain of shoulder joint

√7ᵗʰ **S43.401** Unspecified sprain of right shoulder joint ▽

√7ᵗʰ **S43.402** Unspecified sprain of left shoulder joint ▽

√7ᵗʰ **S43.409** Unspecified sprain of unspecified shoulder joint ▽

√6ᵗʰ **S43.41** Sprain of coracohumeral (ligament)

√7ᵗʰ **S43.411** Sprain of right coracohumeral (ligament)

√7ᵗʰ **S43.412** Sprain of left coracohumeral (ligament)

√7ᵗʰ **S43.419** Sprain of unspecified coracohumeral (ligament) ▽

✔ Additional Character Req   √7ᵗʰ Placeholder Alert   Manifestation   HCC CMS-HCC Condition   ▽ Unspecified Code   ►◄ Revised Text   ● New Code   ▲ Revised Code Title

ICD-10-CM 2018   959

√6ᵗʰ **S43.42   Sprain of rotator cuff capsule**
   EXCLUDES 1   rotator cuff syndrome (complete)
                (incomplete), not specified as traumatic
                (M75.1-)
   EXCLUDES 2   injury of tendon of rotator cuff (S46.0-)

√7ᵗʰ **S43.421   Sprain of right rotator cuff capsule**

√7ᵗʰ **S43.422   Sprain of left rotator cuff capsule**

√7ᵗʰ **S43.429   Sprain of unspecified rotator cuff** ▽
           capsule

√6ᵗʰ **S43.43   Superior glenoid labrum lesion**
   SLAP lesion
   DEF: Detachment injury of the superior aspect of the
   glenoid labrum, which is the ring of fibrocartilage
   attached to the rim of the glenoid cavity of the scapula.

√7ᵗʰ **S43.431   Superior glenoid labrum lesion of right**
           shoulder

√7ᵗʰ **S43.432   Superior glenoid labrum lesion of left**
           shoulder

√7ᵗʰ **S43.439   Superior glenoid labrum lesion of** ▽
           unspecified shoulder

√6ᵗʰ **S43.49   Other sprain of shoulder joint**

√7ᵗʰ **S43.491   Other sprain of right shoulder joint**

√7ᵗʰ **S43.492   Other sprain of left shoulder joint**

√7ᵗʰ **S43.499   Other sprain of unspecified shoulder** ▽
           joint

√5ᵗʰ **S43.5   Sprain of acromioclavicular joint**
   Sprain of acromioclavicular ligament

√x7ᵗʰ **S43.50   Sprain of unspecified acromioclavicular joint** ▽

√x7ᵗʰ **S43.51   Sprain of right acromioclavicular joint**

√x7ᵗʰ **S43.52   Sprain of left acromioclavicular joint**

√5ᵗʰ **S43.6   Sprain of sternoclavicular joint**

√x7ᵗʰ **S43.60   Sprain of unspecified sternoclavicular joint** ▽

√x7ᵗʰ **S43.61   Sprain of right sternoclavicular joint**

√x7ᵗʰ **S43.62   Sprain of left sternoclavicular joint**

√5ᵗʰ **S43.8   Sprain of other specified parts of shoulder girdle**

√x7ᵗʰ **S43.80   Sprain of other specified parts of unspecified** ▽
           shoulder girdle

√x7ᵗʰ **S43.81   Sprain of other specified parts of right shoulder**
           girdle

√x7ᵗʰ **S43.82   Sprain of other specified parts of left shoulder girdle**

√5ᵗʰ **S43.9   Sprain of unspecified parts of shoulder girdle**

√x7ᵗʰ **S43.90   Sprain of unspecified parts of unspecified** ▽
           shoulder girdle
           Sprain of shoulder girdle NOS

√x7ᵗʰ **S43.91   Sprain of unspecified parts of right shoulder** ▽
           girdle

√x7ᵗʰ **S43.92   Sprain of unspecified parts of left shoulder girdle** ▽

√4ᵗʰ **S44   Injury of nerves at shoulder and upper arm level**
   Code also any associated open wound (S41.-)
   EXCLUDES 2   injury of brachial plexus (S14.3-)

   The appropriate 7th character is to be added to each code from
   category S44.
   A   initial encounter
   D   subsequent encounter
   S   sequela

√5ᵗʰ **S44.0   Injury of ulnar nerve at upper arm level**
   EXCLUDES 1   ulnar nerve NOS (S54.0)

√x7ᵗʰ **S44.00   Injury of ulnar nerve at upper arm level,** ▽
           unspecified arm

√x7ᵗʰ **S44.01   Injury of ulnar nerve at upper arm level, right arm**

√x7ᵗʰ **S44.02   Injury of ulnar nerve at upper arm level, left arm**

√5ᵗʰ **S44.1   Injury of median nerve at upper arm level**
   EXCLUDES 1   median nerve NOS (S54.1)

√x7ᵗʰ **S44.10   Injury of median nerve at upper arm level,** ▽
           unspecified arm

√x7ᵗʰ **S44.11   Injury of median nerve at upper arm level, right arm**

√x7ᵗʰ **S44.12   Injury of median nerve at upper arm level, left arm**

√5ᵗʰ **S44.2   Injury of radial nerve at upper arm level**
   EXCLUDES 1   radial nerve NOS (S54.2)

√x7ᵗʰ **S44.20   Injury of radial nerve at upper arm level,** ▽
           unspecified arm

√x7ᵗʰ **S44.21   Injury of radial nerve at upper arm level, right arm**

√x7ᵗʰ **S44.22   Injury of radial nerve at upper arm level, left arm**

√5ᵗʰ **S44.3   Injury of axillary nerve**

√x7ᵗʰ **S44.30   Injury of axillary nerve, unspecified arm** ▽

√x7ᵗʰ **S44.31   Injury of axillary nerve, right arm**

√x7ᵗʰ **S44.32   Injury of axillary nerve, left arm**

√5ᵗʰ **S44.4   Injury of musculocutaneous nerve**

√x7ᵗʰ **S44.40   Injury of musculocutaneous nerve, unspecified** ▽
           arm

√x7ᵗʰ **S44.41   Injury of musculocutaneous nerve, right arm**

√x7ᵗʰ **S44.42   Injury of musculocutaneous nerve, left arm**

√5ᵗʰ **S44.5   Injury of cutaneous sensory nerve at shoulder and upper arm**
   level

√x7ᵗʰ **S44.50   Injury of cutaneous sensory nerve at shoulder** ▽
           and upper arm level, unspecified arm

√x7ᵗʰ **S44.51   Injury of cutaneous sensory nerve at shoulder and**
           upper arm level, right arm

√x7ᵗʰ **S44.52   Injury of cutaneous sensory nerve at shoulder and**
           upper arm level, left arm

√5ᵗʰ **S44.8   Injury of other nerves at shoulder and upper arm level**

√6ᵗʰ **S44.8X   Injury of other nerves at shoulder and upper arm**
           level

√7ᵗʰ **S44.8X1   Injury of other nerves at shoulder and**
            upper arm level, right arm

√7ᵗʰ **S44.8X2   Injury of other nerves at shoulder and**
            upper arm level, left arm

√7ᵗʰ **S44.8X9   Injury of other nerves at shoulder and** ▽
            upper arm level, unspecified arm

√5ᵗʰ **S44.9   Injury of unspecified nerve at shoulder and upper arm level**

√x7ᵗʰ **S44.90   Injury of unspecified nerve at shoulder and** ▽
           upper arm level, unspecified arm

√x7ᵗʰ **S44.91   Injury of unspecified nerve at shoulder and** ▽
           upper arm level, right arm

√x7ᵗʰ **S44.92   Injury of unspecified nerve at shoulder and** ▽
           upper arm level, left arm

√4ᵗʰ **S45   Injury of blood vessels at shoulder and upper arm level**
   Code also any associated open wound (S41.-)
   EXCLUDES 2   injury of subclavian artery (S25.1)
                injury of subclavian vein (S25.3)

   The appropriate 7th character is to be added to each code from
   category S45.
   A   initial encounter
   D   subsequent encounter
   S   sequela

√5ᵗʰ **S45.0   Injury of axillary artery**

√6ᵗʰ **S45.00   Unspecified injury of axillary artery**

√7ᵗʰ **S45.001   Unspecified injury of axillary artery,** ▽
            right side

√7ᵗʰ **S45.002   Unspecified injury of axillary artery,** ▽
            left side

√7ᵗʰ **S45.009   Unspecified injury of axillary artery,** ▽
            unspecified side

√6ᵗʰ **S45.01   Laceration of axillary artery**

√7ᵗʰ **S45.011   Laceration of axillary artery, right side**

√7ᵗʰ **S45.012   Laceration of axillary artery, left side**

√7ᵗʰ **S45.019   Laceration of axillary artery,** ▽
            unspecified side

√6ᵗʰ **S45.09   Other specified injury of axillary artery**

√7ᵗʰ **S45.091   Other specified injury of axillary artery,**
            right side

√7ᵗʰ **S45.092   Other specified injury of axillary artery,**
            left side

√7ᵗʰ **S45.099   Other specified injury of axillary** ▽
            artery, unspecified side

√5ᵗʰ **S45.1   Injury of brachial artery**

√6ᵗʰ **S45.10   Unspecified injury of brachial artery**

√7ᵗʰ **S45.101   Unspecified injury of brachial artery,** ▽
            right side

√7ᵗʰ **S45.102   Unspecified injury of brachial artery,** ▽
            left side

√7ᵗʰ **S45.109   Unspecified injury of brachial artery,** ▽
            unspecified side

√6ᵗʰ **S45.11** **Laceration of brachial artery**

√7ᵗʰ S45.111 Laceration of brachial artery, right side

√7ᵗʰ S45.112 Laceration of brachial artery, left side

√7ᵗʰ S45.119 Laceration of brachial artery, unspecified side ▽

√6ᵗʰ **S45.19** **Other specified injury of brachial artery**

√7ᵗʰ S45.191 Other specified injury of brachial artery, right side

√7ᵗʰ S45.192 Other specified injury of brachial artery, left side

√7ᵗʰ S45.199 Other specified injury of brachial artery, unspecified side ▽

√5ᵗʰ **S45.2** **Injury of axillary or brachial vein**

√6ᵗʰ **S45.20** **Unspecified injury of axillary or brachial vein**

√7ᵗʰ S45.201 Unspecified injury of axillary or brachial vein, right side ▽

√7ᵗʰ S45.202 Unspecified injury of axillary or brachial vein, left side ▽

√7ᵗʰ S45.209 Unspecified injury of axillary or brachial vein, unspecified side ▽

√6ᵗʰ **S45.21** **Laceration of axillary or brachial vein**

√7ᵗʰ S45.211 Laceration of axillary or brachial vein, right side

√7ᵗʰ S45.212 Laceration of axillary or brachial vein, left side

√7ᵗʰ S45.219 Laceration of axillary or brachial vein, unspecified side ▽

√6ᵗʰ **S45.29** **Other specified injury of axillary or brachial vein**

√7ᵗʰ S45.291 Other specified injury of axillary or brachial vein, right side

√7ᵗʰ S45.292 Other specified injury of axillary or brachial vein, left side

√7ᵗʰ S45.299 Other specified injury of axillary or brachial vein, unspecified side ▽

√5ᵗʰ **S45.3** **Injury of superficial vein at shoulder and upper arm level**

√6ᵗʰ **S45.30** **Unspecified injury of superficial vein at shoulder and upper arm level**

√7ᵗʰ S45.301 Unspecified injury of superficial vein at shoulder and upper arm level, right arm ▽

√7ᵗʰ S45.302 Unspecified injury of superficial vein at shoulder and upper arm level, left arm ▽

√7ᵗʰ S45.309 Unspecified injury of superficial vein at shoulder and upper arm level, unspecified arm ▽

√6ᵗʰ **S45.31** **Laceration of superficial vein at shoulder and upper arm level**

√7ᵗʰ S45.311 Laceration of superficial vein at shoulder and upper arm level, right arm

√7ᵗʰ S45.312 Laceration of superficial vein at shoulder and upper arm level, left arm

√7ᵗʰ S45.319 Laceration of superficial vein at shoulder and upper arm level, unspecified arm ▽

√6ᵗʰ **S45.39** **Other specified injury of superficial vein at shoulder and upper arm level**

√7ᵗʰ S45.391 Other specified injury of superficial vein at shoulder and upper arm level, right arm

√7ᵗʰ S45.392 Other specified injury of superficial vein at shoulder and upper arm level, left arm

√7ᵗʰ S45.399 Other specified injury of superficial vein at shoulder and upper arm level, unspecified arm ▽

√5ᵗʰ **S45.8** **Injury of other specified blood vessels at shoulder and upper arm level**

√6ᵗʰ **S45.80** **Unspecified injury of other specified blood vessels at shoulder and upper arm level**

√7ᵗʰ S45.801 Unspecified injury of other specified blood vessels at shoulder and upper arm level, right arm ▽

√7ᵗʰ S45.802 Unspecified injury of other specified blood vessels at shoulder and upper arm level, left arm ▽

√7ᵗʰ S45.809 Unspecified injury of other specified blood vessels at shoulder and upper arm level, unspecified arm ▽

√6ᵗʰ **S45.81** **Laceration of other specified blood vessels at shoulder and upper arm level**

√7ᵗʰ S45.811 Laceration of other specified blood vessels at shoulder and upper arm level, right arm

√7ᵗʰ S45.812 Laceration of other specified blood vessels at shoulder and upper arm level, left arm

√7ᵗʰ S45.819 Laceration of other specified blood vessels at shoulder and upper arm level, unspecified arm ▽

√6ᵗʰ **S45.89** **Other specified injury of other specified blood vessels at shoulder and upper arm level**

√7ᵗʰ S45.891 Other specified injury of other specified blood vessels at shoulder and upper arm level, right arm

√7ᵗʰ S45.892 Other specified injury of other specified blood vessels at shoulder and upper arm level, left arm

√7ᵗʰ S45.899 Other specified injury of other specified blood vessels at shoulder and upper arm level, unspecified arm ▽

√5ᵗʰ **S45.9** **Injury of unspecified blood vessel at shoulder and upper arm level**

√6ᵗʰ **S45.90** **Unspecified injury of unspecified blood vessel at shoulder and upper arm level**

√7ᵗʰ S45.901 Unspecified injury of unspecified blood vessel at shoulder and upper arm level, right arm ▽

√7ᵗʰ S45.902 Unspecified injury of unspecified blood vessel at shoulder and upper arm level, left arm ▽

√7ᵗʰ S45.909 Unspecified injury of unspecified blood vessel at shoulder and upper arm level, unspecified arm ▽

√6ᵗʰ **S45.91** **Laceration of unspecified blood vessel at shoulder and upper arm level**

√7ᵗʰ S45.911 Laceration of unspecified blood vessel at shoulder and upper arm level, right arm ▽

√7ᵗʰ S45.912 Laceration of unspecified blood vessel at shoulder and upper arm level, left arm ▽

√7ᵗʰ S45.919 Laceration of unspecified blood vessel at shoulder and upper arm level, unspecified arm ▽

√6ᵗʰ **S45.99** **Other specified injury of unspecified blood vessel at shoulder and upper arm level**

√7ᵗʰ S45.991 Other specified injury of unspecified blood vessel at shoulder and upper arm level, right arm ▽

√7ᵗʰ S45.992 Other specified injury of unspecified blood vessel at shoulder and upper arm level, left arm ▽

√7ᵗʰ S45.999 Other specified injury of unspecified blood vessel at shoulder and upper arm level, unspecified arm ▽

√4ᵗʰ **S46** **Injury of muscle, fascia and tendon at shoulder and upper arm level**

Code also any associated open wound (S41.-)

EXCLUDES 2   *injury of muscle, fascia and tendon at elbow (S56.-)*
sprain of joints and ligaments of shoulder girdle (S43.9)

TIP: Refer to the Muscle/Tendon table at the beginning of this chapter.

The appropriate 7th character is to be added to each code from category S46.
A   initial encounter
D   subsequent encounter
S   sequela

√5ᵗʰ **S46.0** **Injury of muscle(s) and tendon(s) of the rotator cuff of shoulder**

√6ᵗʰ **S46.00** **Unspecified injury of muscle(s) and tendon(s) of the rotator cuff of shoulder**

√7ᵗʰ S46.001 Unspecified injury of muscle(s) and tendon(s) of the rotator cuff of right shoulder ▽

√7ᵗʰ S46.002 Unspecified injury of muscle(s) and tendon(s) of the rotator cuff of left shoulder ▽

✔ Additional Character Req   ✔×7ᵗʰ Placeholder Alert   Manifestation   HCC CMS-HCC Condition   ▽ Unspecified Code   ►◄ Revised Text   ● New Code   ▲ Revised Code Title

ICD-10-CM 2018   961

√7ᵗʰ **S46.009** Unspecified injury of muscle(s) and ▽
tendon(s) of the rotator cuff of unspecified
shoulder

√6ᵗʰ **S46.01** **Strain** of muscle(s) and tendon(s) of the rotator cuff
of shoulder

√7ᵗʰ **S46.011** Strain of muscle(s) and tendon(s) of the
rotator cuff of **right** shoulder

√7ᵗʰ **S46.012** Strain of muscle(s) and tendon(s) of the
rotator cuff of **left** shoulder

√7ᵗʰ **S46.019** Strain of muscle(s) and tendon(s) of ▽
the rotator cuff of unspecified shoulder

√6ᵗʰ **S46.02** **Laceration** of muscle(s) and tendon(s) of the rotator
cuff of shoulder

√7ᵗʰ **S46.021** Laceration of muscle(s) and tendon(s) of
the rotator cuff of **right** shoulder

√7ᵗʰ **S46.022** Laceration of muscle(s) and tendon(s) of
the rotator cuff of **left** shoulder

√7ᵗʰ **S46.029** Laceration of muscle(s) and tendon(s) ▽
of the rotator cuff of unspecified shoulder

√6ᵗʰ **S46.09** **Other injury** of muscle(s) and tendon(s) of the
rotator cuff of shoulder

√7ᵗʰ **S46.091** Other injury of muscle(s) and tendon(s) of
the rotator cuff of **right** shoulder

√7ᵗʰ **S46.092** Other injury of muscle(s) and tendon(s) of
the rotator cuff of **left** shoulder

√7ᵗʰ **S46.099** Other injury of muscle(s) and tendon(s) ▽
of the rotator cuff of unspecified shoulder

√5ᵗʰ **S46.1** Injury of muscle, fascia and tendon of **long head of biceps**

√6ᵗʰ **S46.10** Unspecified injury of muscle, fascia and tendon of
long head of biceps

√7ᵗʰ **S46.101** Unspecified injury of muscle, fascia and ▽
tendon of long head of biceps, **right** arm

√7ᵗʰ **S46.102** Unspecified injury of muscle, fascia and ▽
tendon of long head of biceps, **left** arm

√7ᵗʰ **S46.109** Unspecified injury of muscle, fascia and ▽
tendon of long head of biceps, unspecified
arm

√6ᵗʰ **S46.11** **Strain** of muscle, fascia and tendon of long head of
biceps

√7ᵗʰ **S46.111** Strain of muscle, fascia and tendon of long
head of biceps, **right** arm

√7ᵗʰ **S46.112** Strain of muscle, fascia and tendon of long
head of biceps, **left** arm

√7ᵗʰ **S46.119** Strain of muscle, fascia and tendon of ▽
long head of biceps, unspecified arm

√6ᵗʰ **S46.12** **Laceration** of muscle, fascia and tendon of long head
of biceps

√7ᵗʰ **S46.121** Laceration of muscle, fascia and tendon of
long head of biceps, **right** arm

√7ᵗʰ **S46.122** Laceration of muscle, fascia and tendon of
long head of biceps, **left** arm

√7ᵗʰ **S46.129** Laceration of muscle, fascia and tendon ▽
of long head of biceps, unspecified arm

√6ᵗʰ **S46.19** **Other injury** of muscle, fascia and tendon of long
head of biceps

√7ᵗʰ **S46.191** Other injury of muscle, fascia and tendon
of long head of biceps, **right** arm

√7ᵗʰ **S46.192** Other injury of muscle, fascia and tendon
of long head of biceps, **left** arm

√7ᵗʰ **S46.199** Other injury of muscle, fascia and ▽
tendon of long head of biceps,
unspecified arm

√5ᵗʰ **S46.2** Injury of muscle, fascia and tendon of other parts of biceps

√6ᵗʰ **S46.20** Unspecified injury of muscle, fascia and tendon of
other parts of biceps

√7ᵗʰ **S46.201** Unspecified injury of muscle, fascia and ▽
tendon of other parts of biceps, **right** arm

√7ᵗʰ **S46.202** Unspecified injury of muscle, fascia and ▽
tendon of other parts of biceps, **left** arm

√7ᵗʰ **S46.209** Unspecified injury of muscle, fascia and ▽
tendon of other parts of biceps,
unspecified arm

√6ᵗʰ **S46.21** **Strain** of muscle, fascia and tendon of other parts of
biceps

√7ᵗʰ **S46.211** Strain of muscle, fascia and tendon of
other parts of biceps, **right** arm

√7ᵗʰ **S46.212** Strain of muscle, fascia and tendon of
other parts of biceps, **left** arm

√7ᵗʰ **S46.219** Strain of muscle, fascia and tendon of ▽
other parts of biceps, unspecified arm

√6ᵗʰ **S46.22** **Laceration** of muscle, fascia and tendon of other
parts of biceps

√7ᵗʰ **S46.221** Laceration of muscle, fascia and tendon of
other parts of biceps, **right** arm

√7ᵗʰ **S46.222** Laceration of muscle, fascia and tendon of
other parts of biceps, **left** arm

√7ᵗʰ **S46.229** Laceration of muscle, fascia and tendon ▽
of other parts of biceps, unspecified arm

√6ᵗʰ **S46.29** **Other injury** of muscle, fascia and tendon of other
parts of biceps

√7ᵗʰ **S46.291** Other injury of muscle, fascia and tendon
of other parts of biceps, **right** arm

√7ᵗʰ **S46.292** Other injury of muscle, fascia and tendon
of other parts of biceps, **left** arm

√7ᵗʰ **S46.299** Other injury of muscle, fascia and ▽
tendon of other parts of biceps,
unspecified arm

√5ᵗʰ **S46.3** Injury of muscle, fascia and tendon of **triceps**

√6ᵗʰ **S46.30** Unspecified injury of muscle, fascia and tendon of
triceps

√7ᵗʰ **S46.301** Unspecified injury of muscle, fascia ▽
and tendon of triceps, **right** arm

√7ᵗʰ **S46.302** Unspecified injury of muscle, fascia ▽
and tendon of triceps, **left** arm

√7ᵗʰ **S46.309** Unspecified injury of muscle, fascia ▽
and tendon of triceps, unspecified arm

√6ᵗʰ **S46.31** **Strain** of muscle, fascia and tendon of triceps

√7ᵗʰ **S46.311** Strain of muscle, fascia and tendon of
triceps, **right** arm

√7ᵗʰ **S46.312** Strain of muscle, fascia and tendon of
triceps, **left** arm

√7ᵗʰ **S46.319** Strain of muscle, fascia and tendon ▽
of triceps, unspecified arm

√6ᵗʰ **S46.32** **Laceration** of muscle, fascia and tendon of triceps

√7ᵗʰ **S46.321** Laceration of muscle, fascia and tendon
of triceps, **right** arm

√7ᵗʰ **S46.322** Laceration of muscle, fascia and tendon
of triceps, **left** arm

√7ᵗʰ **S46.329** Laceration of muscle, fascia and tendon ▽
of triceps, unspecified arm

√6ᵗʰ **S46.39** **Other injury** of muscle, fascia and tendon of triceps

√7ᵗʰ **S46.391** Other injury of muscle, fascia and tendon
of triceps, **right** arm

√7ᵗʰ **S46.392** Other injury of muscle, fascia and tendon
of triceps, **left** arm

√7ᵗʰ **S46.399** Other injury of muscle, fascia and ▽
tendon of triceps, unspecified arm

√5ᵗʰ **S46.8** Injury of other muscles, fascia and tendons at shoulder and
upper arm level

√6ᵗʰ **S46.80** Unspecified injury of other muscles, fascia and
tendons at shoulder and upper arm level

√7ᵗʰ **S46.801** Unspecified injury of other muscles, ▽
fascia and tendons at shoulder and
upper arm level, **right** arm

√7ᵗʰ **S46.802** Unspecified injury of other muscles, ▽
fascia and tendons at shoulder and
upper arm level, **left** arm

√7ᵗʰ **S46.809** Unspecified injury of other muscles, ▽
fascia and tendons at shoulder and
upper arm level, unspecified arm

√6ᵗʰ **S46.81** **Strain** of other muscles, fascia and tendons at
shoulder and upper arm level

√7ᵗʰ **S46.811** Strain of other muscles, fascia and
tendons at shoulder and upper arm
level, **right** arm

√7ᵗʰ **S46.812** Strain of other muscles, fascia and
tendons at shoulder and upper arm
level, **left** arm

EXCLUDES 1 Not coded here   EXCLUDES 2 Not included here   N Newborn Age: 0   P Pediatric Age: 0–17   M Maternity Age: 12–55   A Adult Age: 15–124

962   ICD-10-CM 2018

☑7ᵗʰ **S46.819** Strain of other muscles, fascia and tendons at shoulder and upper arm level, unspecified arm ▽

☑6ᵗʰ **S46.82** Laceration of other muscles, fascia and tendons at shoulder and upper arm level

☑7ᵗʰ **S46.821** Laceration of other muscles, fascia and tendons at shoulder and upper arm level, right arm

☑7ᵗʰ **S46.822** Laceration of other muscles, fascia and tendons at shoulder and upper arm level, left arm

☑7ᵗʰ **S46.829** Laceration of other muscles, fascia and tendons at shoulder and upper arm level, unspecified arm ▽

☑6ᵗʰ **S46.89** Other injury of other muscles, fascia and tendons at shoulder and upper arm level

☑7ᵗʰ **S46.891** Other injury of other muscles, fascia and tendons at shoulder and upper arm level, right arm

☑7ᵗʰ **S46.892** Other injury of other muscles, fascia and tendons at shoulder and upper arm level, left arm

☑7ᵗʰ **S46.899** Other injury of other muscles, fascia and tendons at shoulder and upper arm level, unspecified arm ▽

☑5ᵗʰ **S46.9** Injury of unspecified muscle, fascia and tendon at shoulder and upper arm level

☑6ᵗʰ **S46.90** Unspecified injury of unspecified muscle, fascia and tendon at shoulder and upper arm level

☑7ᵗʰ **S46.901** Unspecified injury of unspecified muscle, fascia and tendon at shoulder and upper arm level, right arm ▽

☑7ᵗʰ **S46.902** Unspecified injury of unspecified muscle, fascia and tendon at shoulder and upper arm level, left arm ▽

☑7ᵗʰ **S46.909** Unspecified injury of unspecified muscle, fascia and tendon at shoulder and upper arm level, unspecified arm ▽

☑6ᵗʰ **S46.91** Strain of unspecified muscle, fascia and tendon at shoulder and upper arm level

☑7ᵗʰ **S46.911** Strain of unspecified muscle, fascia and tendon at shoulder and upper arm level, right arm ▽

☑7ᵗʰ **S46.912** Strain of unspecified muscle, fascia and tendon at shoulder and upper arm level, left arm ▽

☑7ᵗʰ **S46.919** Strain of unspecified muscle, fascia and tendon at shoulder and upper arm level, unspecified arm ▽

☑6ᵗʰ **S46.92** Laceration of unspecified muscle, fascia and tendon at shoulder and upper arm level

☑7ᵗʰ **S46.921** Laceration of unspecified muscle, fascia and tendon at shoulder and upper arm level, right arm ▽

☑7ᵗʰ **S46.922** Laceration of unspecified muscle, fascia and tendon at shoulder and upper arm level, left arm ▽

☑7ᵗʰ **S46.929** Laceration of unspecified muscle, fascia and tendon at shoulder and upper arm level, unspecified arm ▽

☑6ᵗʰ **S46.99** Other injury of unspecified muscle, fascia and tendon at shoulder and upper arm level

☑7ᵗʰ **S46.991** Other injury of unspecified muscle, fascia and tendon at shoulder and upper arm level, right arm ▽

☑7ᵗʰ **S46.992** Other injury of unspecified muscle, fascia and tendon at shoulder and upper arm level, left arm ▽

☑7ᵗʰ **S46.999** Other injury of unspecified muscle, fascia and tendon at shoulder and upper arm level, unspecified arm ▽

☑4ᵗʰ **S47** **Crushing injury of shoulder and upper arm**
Use additional code for all associated injuries
EXCLUDES 2 *crushing injury of elbow (S57.0-)*

> The appropriate 7th character is to be added to each code from category S47.
> A   initial encounter
> D   subsequent encounter
> S   sequela

☑x7ᵗʰ **S47.1** Crushing injury of right shoulder and upper arm

☑x7ᵗʰ **S47.2** Crushing injury of left shoulder and upper arm

☑x7ᵗʰ **S47.9** Crushing injury of shoulder and upper arm, unspecified arm ▽

☑4ᵗʰ **S48** **Traumatic amputation of shoulder and upper arm**
An amputation not identified as partial or complete should be coded to complete.
EXCLUDES 1 *traumatic amputation at elbow level (S58.0)*

> The appropriate 7th character is to be added to each code from category S48.
> A   initial encounter
> D   subsequent encounter
> S   sequela

☑5ᵗʰ **S48.0** Traumatic amputation at shoulder joint

☑6ᵗʰ **S48.01** Complete traumatic amputation at shoulder joint

2 ☑7ᵗʰ **S48.011** Complete traumatic amputation at right shoulder joint   HCC

2 ☑7ᵗʰ **S48.012** Complete traumatic amputation at left shoulder joint   HCC

2 ☑7ᵗʰ **S48.019** Complete traumatic amputation at unspecified shoulder joint   HCC ▽

☑6ᵗʰ **S48.02** Partial traumatic amputation at shoulder joint

2 ☑7ᵗʰ **S48.021** Partial traumatic amputation at right shoulder joint   HCC

2 ☑7ᵗʰ **S48.022** Partial traumatic amputation at left shoulder joint   HCC

2 ☑7ᵗʰ **S48.029** Partial traumatic amputation at unspecified shoulder joint   HCC ▽

☑5ᵗʰ **S48.1** Traumatic amputation at level between shoulder and elbow

☑6ᵗʰ **S48.11** Complete traumatic amputation at level between shoulder and elbow

2 ☑7ᵗʰ **S48.111** Complete traumatic amputation at level between right shoulder and elbow   HCC

2 ☑7ᵗʰ **S48.112** Complete traumatic amputation at level between left shoulder and elbow   HCC

2 ☑7ᵗʰ **S48.119** Complete traumatic amputation at level between unspecified shoulder and elbow   HCC ▽

☑6ᵗʰ **S48.12** Partial traumatic amputation at level between shoulder and elbow

2 ☑7ᵗʰ **S48.121** Partial traumatic amputation at level between right shoulder and elbow   HCC

2 ☑7ᵗʰ **S48.122** Partial traumatic amputation at level between left shoulder and elbow   HCC

2 ☑7ᵗʰ **S48.129** Partial traumatic amputation at level between unspecified shoulder and elbow   HCC ▽

☑5ᵗʰ **S48.9** Traumatic amputation of shoulder and upper arm, level unspecified

☑6ᵗʰ **S48.91** Complete traumatic amputation of shoulder and upper arm, level unspecified

2 ☑7ᵗʰ **S48.911** Complete traumatic amputation of right shoulder and upper arm, level unspecified   HCC ▽

2 ☑7ᵗʰ **S48.912** Complete traumatic amputation of leftshoulder and upper arm, level unspecified   HCC ▽

2 ☑7ᵗʰ **S48.919** Complete traumatic amputation of unspecified shoulder and upper arm, level unspecified   HCC ▽

☑6ᵗʰ **S48.92** Partial traumatic amputation of shoulder and upper arm, level unspecified

2 ☑7ᵗʰ **S48.921** Partial traumatic amputation of right shoulder and upper arm, level unspecified   HCC ▽

---

2   HCC with 7th character indicating initial encounter (A or B - specific to category) OR sequela.

☑ Additional Character Req   ☑x7ᵗʰ Placeholder Alert   Manifestation   HCC CMS-HCC Condition   ▽ Unspecified Code   ►◄ Revised Text   ● New Code   ▲ Revised Code Title

2 ✓7th S48.922 **Partial traumatic amputation of left shoulder and upper arm, level unspecified** HCC ▽

2 ✓7th S48.929 **Partial traumatic amputation of unspecified shoulder and upper arm, level unspecified** HCC ▽

✓4th **S49 Other and unspecified injuries of shoulder and upper arm**

The appropriate 7th character is to be added to each code from subcategories S49.0 and S49.1.
A initial encounter for closed fracture
D subsequent encounter for fracture with routine healing
G subsequent encounter for fracture with delayed healing
K subsequent encounter for fracture with nonunion
P subsequent encounter for fracture with malunion
S sequela

✓5th **S49.0 Physeal fracture of upper end of humerus**

✓6th S49.00 **Unspecified physeal fracture of upper end of humerus**

✓7th S49.001 **Unspecified physeal fracture of upper end of humerus, right arm** ▽

✓7th S49.002 **Unspecified physeal fracture of upper end of humerus, left arm** ▽

✓7th S49.009 **Unspecified physeal fracture of upper end of humerus, unspecified arm** ▽

✓6th S49.01 **Salter-Harris Type I physeal fracture of upper end of humerus**

✓7th S49.011 **Salter-Harris Type I physeal fracture of upper end of humerus, right arm**

✓7th S49.012 **Salter-Harris Type I physeal fracture of upper end of humerus, left arm**

✓7th S49.019 **Salter-Harris Type I physeal fracture of upper end of humerus, unspecified arm** ▽

✓6th S49.02 **Salter-Harris Type II physeal fracture of upper end of humerus**

✓7th S49.021 **Salter-Harris Type II physeal fracture of upper end of humerus, right arm**

✓7th S49.022 **Salter-Harris Type II physeal fracture of upper end of humerus, left arm**

✓7th S49.029 **Salter-Harris Type II physeal fracture of upper end of humerus, unspecified arm** ▽

✓6th S49.03 **Salter-Harris Type III physeal fracture of upper end of humerus**

✓7th S49.031 **Salter-Harris Type III physeal fracture of upper end of humerus, right arm**

✓7th S49.032 **Salter-Harris Type III physeal fracture of upper end of humerus, left arm**

✓7th S49.039 **Salter-Harris Type III physeal fracture of upper end of humerus, unspecified arm** ▽

✓6th S49.04 **Salter-Harris Type IV physeal fracture of upper end of humerus**

✓7th S49.041 **Salter-Harris Type IV physeal fracture of upper end of humerus, right arm**

✓7th S49.042 **Salter-Harris Type IV physeal fracture of upper end of humerus, left arm**

✓7th S49.049 **Salter-Harris Type IV physeal fracture of upper end of humerus, unspecified arm** ▽

✓6th S49.09 **Other physeal fracture of upper end of humerus**

✓7th S49.091 **Other physeal fracture of upper end of humerus, right arm**

✓7th S49.092 **Other physeal fracture of upper end of humerus, left arm**

✓7th S49.099 **Other physeal fracture of upper end of humerus, unspecified arm** ▽

✓5th **S49.1 Physeal fracture of lower end of humerus**

✓6th S49.10 **Unspecified physeal fracture of lower end of humerus**

✓7th S49.101 **Unspecified physeal fracture of lower end of humerus, right arm** ▽

✓7th S49.102 **Unspecified physeal fracture of lower end of humerus, left arm** ▽

✓7th S49.109 **Unspecified physeal fracture of lower end of humerus, unspecified arm** ▽

✓6th S49.11 **Salter-Harris Type I physeal fracture of lower end of humerus**

✓7th S49.111 **Salter-Harris Type I physeal fracture of lower end of humerus, right arm**

✓7th S49.112 **Salter-Harris Type I physeal fracture of lower end of humerus, left arm**

✓7th S49.119 **Salter-Harris Type I physeal fracture of lower end of humerus, unspecified arm** ▽

✓6th S49.12 **Salter-Harris Type II physeal fracture of lower end of humerus**

✓7th S49.121 **Salter-Harris Type II physeal fracture of lower end of humerus, right arm**

✓7th S49.122 **Salter-Harris Type II physeal fracture of lower end of humerus, left arm**

✓7th S49.129 **Salter-Harris Type II physeal fracture of lower end of humerus, unspecified arm** ▽

✓6th S49.13 **Salter Harris Type III physeal fracture of lower end of humerus**

✓7th S49.131 **Salter-Harris Type III physeal fracture of lower end of humerus, right arm**

✓7th S49.132 **Salter-Harris Type III physeal fracture of lower end of humerus, left arm**

✓7th S49.139 **Salter-Harris Type III physeal fracture of lower end of humerus, unspecified arm** ▽

✓6th S49.14 **Salter-Harris Type IV physeal fracture of lower end of humerus**

✓7th S49.141 **Salter-Harris Type IV physeal fracture of lower end of humerus, right arm**

✓7th S49.142 **Salter-Harris Type IV physeal fracture of lower end of humerus, left arm**

✓7th S49.149 **Salter-Harris Type IV physeal fracture of lower end of humerus, unspecified arm** ▽

✓6th S49.19 **Other physeal fracture of lower end of humerus**

✓7th S49.191 **Other physeal fracture of lower end of humerus, right arm**

✓7th S49.192 **Other physeal fracture of lower end of humerus, left arm**

✓7th S49.199 **Other physeal fracture of lower end of humerus, unspecified arm** ▽

✓5th **S49.8 Other specified injuries of shoulder and upper arm**

The appropriate 7th character is to be added to each code in subcategory S49.8.
A initial encounter
D subsequent encounter
S sequela

✓x7th S49.80 **Other specified injuries of shoulder and upper arm, unspecified arm** ▽

✓x7th S49.81 **Other specified injuries of right shoulder and upper arm**

✓x7th S49.82 **Other specified injuries of left shoulder and upper arm**

✓5th **S49.9 Unspecified injury of shoulder and upper arm**

The appropriate 7th character is to be added to each code in subcategory S49.9.
A initial encounter
D subsequent encounter
S sequela

✓x7th S49.90 **Unspecified injury of shoulder and upper arm, unspecified arm** ▽

✓x7th S49.91 **Unspecified injury of right shoulder and upper arm** ▽

✓x7th S49.92 **Unspecified injury of left shoulder and upper arm** ▽

2 HCC with 7th character indicating initial encounter (A or B - specific to category) OR sequela.

EXCLUDES 1 Not coded here   EXCLUDES 2 Not included here   N Newborn Age: 0   P Pediatric Age: 0-17   M Maternity Age: 12-55   A Adult Age: 15-124

964   ICD-10-CM 2018

S48.922–S49.92

Injuries to the elbow and forearm (S50-S59)

EXCLUDES 2   burns and corrosions (T20-T32)
        frostbite (T33-T34)
        injuries of wrist and hand (S60-S69)
        insect bite or sting, venomous (T63.4)

√4ᵗʰ **S50   Superficial injury of elbow and forearm**

     EXCLUDES 2   superficial injury of wrist and hand (S60.-)

> The appropriate 7th character is to be added to each code from category S50.
> A   initial encounter
> D   subsequent encounter
> S   sequela

√5ᵗʰ **S50.0   Contusion of elbow**

   √x7ᵗʰ **S50.00   Contusion of unspecified elbow** ▽

   √x7ᵗʰ **S50.01   Contusion of right elbow**

   √x7ᵗʰ **S50.02   Contusion of left elbow**

√5ᵗʰ **S50.1   Contusion of forearm**

   √x7ᵗʰ **S50.10   Contusion of unspecified forearm** ▽

   √x7ᵗʰ **S50.11   Contusion of right forearm**

   √x7ᵗʰ **S50.12   Contusion of left forearm**

√5ᵗʰ **S50.3   Other superficial injuries of elbow**

   √6ᵗʰ **S50.31   Abrasion of elbow**

     √7ᵗʰ **S50.311   Abrasion of right elbow**

     √7ᵗʰ **S50.312   Abrasion of left elbow**

     √7ᵗʰ **S50.319   Abrasion of unspecified elbow** ▽

   √6ᵗʰ **S50.32   Blister (nonthermal) of elbow**

     √7ᵗʰ **S50.321   Blister (nonthermal) of right elbow**

     √7ᵗʰ **S50.322   Blister (nonthermal) of left elbow**

     √7ᵗʰ **S50.329   Blister (nonthermal) of unspecified elbow** ▽

   √6ᵗʰ **S50.34   External constriction of elbow**

     √7ᵗʰ **S50.341   External constriction of right elbow**

     √7ᵗʰ **S50.342   External constriction of left elbow**

     √7ᵗʰ **S50.349   External constriction of unspecified elbow** ▽

   √6ᵗʰ **S50.35   Superficial foreign body of elbow**
       Splinter in the elbow

     √7ᵗʰ **S50.351   Superficial foreign body of right elbow**

     √7ᵗʰ **S50.352   Superficial foreign body of left elbow**

     √7ᵗʰ **S50.359   Superficial foreign body of unspecified elbow** ▽

   √6ᵗʰ **S50.36   Insect bite (nonvenomous) of elbow**

     √7ᵗʰ **S50.361   Insect bite (nonvenomous) of right elbow**

     √7ᵗʰ **S50.362   Insect bite (nonvenomous) of left elbow**

     √7ᵗʰ **S50.369   Insect bite (nonvenomous) of unspecified elbow** ▽

   √6ᵗʰ **S50.37   Other superficial bite of elbow**
       EXCLUDES 1   open bite of elbow (S51.05)

     √7ᵗʰ **S50.371   Other superficial bite of right elbow**

     √7ᵗʰ **S50.372   Other superficial bite of left elbow**

     √7ᵗʰ **S50.379   Other superficial bite of unspecified elbow** ▽

√5ᵗʰ **S50.8   Other superficial injuries of forearm**

   √6ᵗʰ **S50.81   Abrasion of forearm**

     √7ᵗʰ **S50.811   Abrasion of right forearm**

     √7ᵗʰ **S50.812   Abrasion of left forearm**

     √7ᵗʰ **S50.819   Abrasion of unspecified forearm** ▽

   √6ᵗʰ **S50.82   Blister (nonthermal) of forearm**

     √7ᵗʰ **S50.821   Blister (nonthermal) of right forearm**

     √7ᵗʰ **S50.822   Blister (nonthermal) of left forearm**

     √7ᵗʰ **S50.829   Blister (nonthermal) of unspecified forearm** ▽

   √6ᵗʰ **S50.84   External constriction of forearm**

     √7ᵗʰ **S50.841   External constriction of right forearm**

     √7ᵗʰ **S50.842   External constriction of left forearm**

     √7ᵗʰ **S50.849   External constriction of unspecified forearm** ▽

   √6ᵗʰ **S50.85   Superficial foreign body of forearm**
       Splinter in the forearm

     √7ᵗʰ **S50.851   Superficial foreign body of right forearm**

     √7ᵗʰ **S50.852   Superficial foreign body of left forearm**

     √7ᵗʰ **S50.859   Superficial foreign body of unspecified forearm** ▽

   √6ᵗʰ **S50.86   Insect bite (nonvenomous) of forearm**

     √7ᵗʰ **S50.861   Insect bite (nonvenomous) of right forearm**

     √7ᵗʰ **S50.862   Insect bite (nonvenomous) of left forearm**

     √7ᵗʰ **S50.869   Insect bite (nonvenomous) of unspecified forearm** ▽

   √6ᵗʰ **S50.87   Other superficial bite of forearm**
       EXCLUDES 1   open bite of forearm (S51.85)

     √7ᵗʰ **S50.871   Other superficial bite of right forearm**

     √7ᵗʰ **S50.872   Other superficial bite of left forearm**

     √7ᵗʰ **S50.879   Other superficial bite of unspecified forearm** ▽

√5ᵗʰ **S50.9   Unspecified superficial injury of elbow and forearm**

   √6ᵗʰ **S50.90   Unspecified superficial injury of elbow**

     √7ᵗʰ **S50.901   Unspecified superficial injury of right elbow** ▽

     √7ᵗʰ **S50.902   Unspecified superficial injury of left elbow** ▽

     √7ᵗʰ **S50.909   Unspecified superficial injury of unspecified elbow** ▽

   √6ᵗʰ **S50.91   Unspecified superficial injury of forearm**

     √7ᵗʰ **S50.911   Unspecified superficial injury of right forearm** ▽

     √7ᵗʰ **S50.912   Unspecified superficial injury of left forearm** ▽

     √7ᵗʰ **S50.919   Unspecified superficial injury of unspecified forearm** ▽

√4ᵗʰ **S51   Open wound of elbow and forearm**
     Code also any associated wound infection
     EXCLUDES 1   open fracture of elbow and forearm (S52- with open fracture 7th character)
         traumatic amputation of elbow and forearm (S58.-)
     EXCLUDES 2   open wound of wrist and hand (S61.-)

> The appropriate 7th character is to be added to each code from category S51.
> A   initial encounter
> D   subsequent encounter
> S   sequela

√5ᵗʰ **S51.0   Open wound of elbow**

   √6ᵗʰ **S51.00   Unspecified open wound of elbow**

     √7ᵗʰ **S51.001   Unspecified open wound of right elbow** ▽
          AHA: 2012, 4Q, 108

     √7ᵗʰ **S51.002   Unspecified open wound of left elbow** ▽

     √7ᵗʰ **S51.009   Unspecified open wound of unspecified elbow** ▽
          Open wound of elbow NOS

   √6ᵗʰ **S51.01   Laceration without foreign body of elbow**

     √7ᵗʰ **S51.011   Laceration without foreign body of right elbow**

     √7ᵗʰ **S51.012   Laceration without foreign body of left elbow**

     √7ᵗʰ **S51.019   Laceration without foreign body of unspecified elbow** ▽

   √6ᵗʰ **S51.02   Laceration with foreign body of elbow**

     √7ᵗʰ **S51.021   Laceration with foreign body of right elbow**

     √7ᵗʰ **S51.022   Laceration with foreign body of left elbow**

     √7ᵗʰ **S51.029   Laceration with foreign body of unspecified elbow** ▽

   √6ᵗʰ **S51.03   Puncture wound without foreign body of elbow**

     √7ᵗʰ **S51.031   Puncture wound without foreign body of right elbow**

     √7ᵗʰ **S51.032   Puncture wound without foreign body of left elbow**

     √7ᵗʰ **S51.039   Puncture wound without foreign body of unspecified elbow** ▽

☑ Additional Character Req   √x7ᵗʰ Placeholder Alert   Manifestation   HCC CMS-HCC Condition   ▽ Unspecified Code   ▶◀ Revised Text   ● New Code   ▲ Revised Code Title

ICD-10-CM 2018   965

Chapter 19. Injury, Poisoning, and Certain Other Consequences of External Causes

✓6ᵗʰ **S51.04** **Puncture wound with foreign body** of elbow

     ✓7ᵗʰ **S51.041** **Puncture wound with foreign body of right** elbow

     ✓7ᵗʰ **S51.042** **Puncture wound with foreign body of left** elbow

     ✓7ᵗʰ **S51.049** **Puncture wound with foreign body of unspecified elbow** ▽

✓6ᵗʰ **S51.05** **Open bite** of elbow

     Bite of elbow NOS

     EXCLUDES 1   *superficial bite of elbow (S50.36, S50.37)*

     ✓7ᵗʰ **S51.051** **Open bite, right** elbow

     ✓7ᵗʰ **S51.052** **Open bite, left** elbow

     ✓7ᵗʰ **S51.059** **Open bite, unspecified elbow** ▽

✓5ᵗʰ **S51.8** **Open wound of forearm**

     EXCLUDES 2   *open wound of elbow (S51.0-)*

     ✓6ᵗʰ **S51.80** **Unspecified open wound of forearm**

       AHA: 2016, 3Q, 24

       ✓7ᵗʰ **S51.801** **Unspecified open wound of right forearm** ▽

       ✓7ᵗʰ **S51.802** **Unspecified open wound of left forearm** ▽

       ✓7ᵗʰ **S51.809** **Unspecified open wound of unspecified forearm** ▽

         Open wound of forearm NOS

     ✓6ᵗʰ **S51.81** **Laceration without foreign body** of forearm

       ✓7ᵗʰ **S51.811** **Laceration without foreign body of right forearm**

       ✓7ᵗʰ **S51.812** **Laceration without foreign body of left forearm**

       ✓7ᵗʰ **S51.819** **Laceration without foreign body of unspecified forearm** ▽

     ✓6ᵗʰ **S51.82** **Laceration with foreign body** of forearm

       ✓7ᵗʰ **S51.821** **Laceration with foreign body of right forearm**

       ✓7ᵗʰ **S51.822** **Laceration with foreign body of left forearm**

       ✓7ᵗʰ **S51.829** **Laceration with foreign body of unspecified forearm** ▽

     ✓6ᵗʰ **S51.83** **Puncture wound without foreign body** of forearm

       AHA: 2016, 3Q, 24

       ✓7ᵗʰ **S51.831** **Puncture wound without foreign body of right forearm**

       ✓7ᵗʰ **S51.832** **Puncture wound without foreign body of left forearm**

       ✓7ᵗʰ **S51.839** **Puncture wound without foreign body of unspecified forearm** ▽

     ✓6ᵗʰ **S51.84** **Puncture wound with foreign body** of forearm

       AHA: 2016, 3Q, 24

       ✓7ᵗʰ **S51.841** **Puncture wound with foreign body of right forearm**

       ✓7ᵗʰ **S51.842** **Puncture wound with foreign body of left forearm**

       ✓7ᵗʰ **S51.849** **Puncture wound with foreign body of unspecified forearm** ▽

     ✓6ᵗʰ **S51.85** **Open bite** of forearm

       Bite of forearm NOS

       EXCLUDES 1   *superficial bite of forearm (S50.86, S50.87)*

       ✓7ᵗʰ **S51.851** **Open bite of right** forearm

       ✓7ᵗʰ **S51.852** **Open bite of left** forearm

       ✓7ᵗʰ **S51.859** **Open bite of unspecified forearm** ▽

✓4ᵗʰ **S52** **Fracture of forearm**

     NOTE   A fracture not indicated as displaced or nondisplaced should be coded to displaced.

         A fracture not indicated as open or closed should be coded to closed.

         The open fracture designations are based on the Gustilo open fracture classification.

     EXCLUDES 1   *traumatic amputation of forearm (S58.-)*

     EXCLUDES 2   *fracture at wrist and hand level (S62.-)*

     AHA: 2016, 1Q, 33; 2015, 3Q, 37-39

> The appropriate 7th character is to be added to all codes from category S52 [unless otherwise indicated].
> A   initial encounter for closed fracture
> B   initial encounter for open fracture type I or II
>   initial encounter for open fracture NOS
> C   initial encounter for open fracture type IIIA, IIIB, or IIIC
> D   subsequent encounter for closed fracture with routine healing
> E   subsequent encounter for open fracture type I or II with routine healing
> F   subsequent encounter for open fracture type IIIA, IIIB, or IIIC with routine healing
> G   subsequent encounter for closed fracture with delayed healing
> H   subsequent encounter for open fracture type I or II with delayed healing
> J   subsequent encounter for open fracture type IIIA, IIIB, or IIIC with delayed healing
> K   subsequent encounter for closed fracture with nonunion
> M   subsequent encounter for open fracture type I or II with nonunion
> N   subsequent encounter for open fracture type IIIA, IIIB, or IIIC with nonunion
> P   subsequent encounter for closed fracture with malunion
> Q   subsequent encounter for open fracture type I or II with malunion
> R   subsequent encounter for open fracture type IIIA, IIIB, or IIIC with malunion
> S   sequela

✓5ᵗʰ **S52.0** **Fracture of upper end of ulna**

     Fracture of proximal end of ulna

     EXCLUDES 2   *fracture of elbow NOS (S42.40-)*

         fractures of shaft of ulna (S52.2-)

     ✓6ᵗʰ **S52.00** **Unspecified fracture of upper end of ulna**

       ✓7ᵗʰ **S52.001** **Unspecified fracture of upper end of right ulna** ▽

       ✓7ᵗʰ **S52.002** **Unspecified fracture of upper end of left ulna** ▽

       ✓7ᵗʰ **S52.009** **Unspecified fracture of upper end of unspecified ulna** ▽

     ✓6ᵗʰ **S52.01** **Torus** fracture of upper end of ulna

> The appropriate 7th character is to be added to all codes in subcategory S52.01.
> A   initial encounter for closed fracture
> D   subsequent encounter for fracture with routine healing
> G   subsequent encounter for fracture with delayed healing
> K   subsequent encounter for fracture with nonunion
> P   subsequent encounter for fracture with malunion
> S   sequela

       ✓7ᵗʰ **S52.011** **Torus fracture of upper end of right ulna**

       ✓7ᵗʰ **S52.012** **Torus fracture of upper end of left ulna**

       ✓7ᵗʰ **S52.019** **Torus fracture of upper end of unspecified ulna** ▽

     ✓6ᵗʰ **S52.02** **Fracture of olecranon process without intraarticular extension of ulna**

       ✓7ᵗʰ **S52.021** **Displaced fracture of olecranon process without intraarticular extension of right ulna**

       ✓7ᵗʰ **S52.022** **Displaced fracture of olecranon process without intraarticular extension of left ulna**

       ✓7ᵗʰ **S52.023** **Displaced fracture of olecranon process without intraarticular extension of unspecified ulna** ▽

EXCLUDES 1 Not coded here   EXCLUDES 2 Not included here   N Newborn Age: 0   P Pediatric Age: 0-17   M Maternity Age: 12-55   A Adult Age: 15-124

966   ICD-10-CM 2018

S51.04–S52.023

☑7ᵗʰ **S52.024** **Nondisplaced fracture of olecranon process without intraarticular extension of right ulna**

☑7ᵗʰ **S52.025** **Nondisplaced fracture of olecranon process without intraarticular extension of left ulna**

☑7ᵗʰ **S52.026** **Nondisplaced fracture of olecranon process without intraarticular extension of unspecified ulna** ▽

☑6ᵗʰ **S52.03** **Fracture of olecranon process with intraarticular extension of ulna**

☑7ᵗʰ **S52.031** **Displaced fracture of olecranon process with intraarticular extension of right ulna**

☑7ᵗʰ **S52.032** **Displaced fracture of olecranon process with intraarticular extension of left ulna**

☑7ᵗʰ **S52.033** **Displaced fracture of olecranon process with intraarticular extension of unspecified ulna** ▽

☑7ᵗʰ **S52.034** **Nondisplaced fracture of olecranon process with intraarticular extension of right ulna**

☑7ᵗʰ **S52.035** **Nondisplaced fracture of olecranon process with intraarticular extension of left ulna**

☑7ᵗʰ **S52.036** **Nondisplaced fracture of olecranon process with intraarticular extension of unspecified ulna** ▽

☑6ᵗʰ **S52.04** **Fracture of coronoid process of ulna**

☑7ᵗʰ **S52.041** **Displaced fracture of coronoid process of right ulna**

☑7ᵗʰ **S52.042** **Displaced fracture of coronoid process of left ulna**

☑7ᵗʰ **S52.043** **Displaced fracture of coronoid process of unspecified ulna** ▽

☑7ᵗʰ **S52.044** **Nondisplaced fracture of coronoid process of right ulna**

☑7ᵗʰ **S52.045** **Nondisplaced fracture of coronoid process of left ulna**

☑7ᵗʰ **S52.046** **Nondisplaced fracture of coronoid process of unspecified ulna** ▽

☑6ᵗʰ **S52.09** **Other fracture of upper end of ulna**

☑7ᵗʰ **S52.091** **Other fracture of upper end of right ulna**

☑7ᵗʰ **S52.092** **Other fracture of upper end of left ulna**

☑7ᵗʰ **S52.099** **Other fracture of upper end of unspecified ulna** ▽

☑5ᵗʰ **S52.1** **Fracture of upper end of radius**
Fracture of proximal end of radius

EXCLUDES 2   physeal fractures of upper end of radius (S59.2-)
fracture of shaft of radius (S52.3-)

☑6ᵗʰ **S52.10** **Unspecified fracture of upper end of radius**

☑7ᵗʰ **S52.101** **Unspecified fracture of upper end of right radius** ▽

☑7ᵗʰ **S52.102** **Unspecified fracture of upper end of left radius** ▽

☑7ᵗʰ **S52.109** **Unspecified fracture of upper end of unspecified radius** ▽

☑6ᵗʰ **S52.11** **Torus fracture of upper end of radius**

> The appropriate 7th character is to be added to all codes in subcategory S52.11.
> A   initial encounter for closed fracture
> D   subsequent encounter for fracture with routine healing
> G   subsequent encounter for fracture with delayed healing
> K   subsequent encounter for fracture with nonunion
> P   subsequent encounter for fracture with malunion
> S   sequela

☑7ᵗʰ **S52.111** **Torus fracture of upper end of right radius**

☑7ᵗʰ **S52.112** **Torus fracture of upper end of left radius**

☑7ᵗʰ **S52.119** **Torus fracture of upper end of unspecified radius** ▽

☑6ᵗʰ **S52.12** **Fracture of head of radius**

☑7ᵗʰ **S52.121** **Displaced fracture of head of right radius**

☑7ᵗʰ **S52.122** **Displaced fracture of head of left radius**

☑7ᵗʰ **S52.123** **Displaced fracture of head of unspecified radius** ▽

☑7ᵗʰ **S52.124** **Nondisplaced fracture of head of right radius**

☑7ᵗʰ **S52.125** **Nondisplaced fracture of head of left radius**

☑7ᵗʰ **S52.126** **Nondisplaced fracture of head of unspecified radius** ▽

☑6ᵗʰ **S52.13** **Fracture of neck of radius**

☑7ᵗʰ **S52.131** **Displaced fracture of neck of right radius**

☑7ᵗʰ **S52.132** **Displaced fracture of neck of left radius**

☑7ᵗʰ **S52.133** **Displaced fracture of neck of unspecified radius** ▽

☑7ᵗʰ **S52.134** **Nondisplaced fracture of neck of right radius**

☑7ᵗʰ **S52.135** **Nondisplaced fracture of neck of left radius**

☑7ᵗʰ **S52.136** **Nondisplaced fracture of neck of unspecified radius** ▽

☑6ᵗʰ **S52.18** **Other fracture of upper end of radius**

☑7ᵗʰ **S52.181** **Other fracture of upper end of right radius**

☑7ᵗʰ **S52.182** **Other fracture of upper end of left radius**

☑7ᵗʰ **S52.189** **Other fracture of upper end of unspecified radius** ▽

☑5ᵗʰ **S52.2** **Fracture of shaft of ulna**

☑6ᵗʰ **S52.20** **Unspecified fracture of shaft of ulna**
Fracture of ulna NOS

☑7ᵗʰ **S52.201** **Unspecified fracture of shaft of right ulna** ▽

☑7ᵗʰ **S52.202** **Unspecified fracture of shaft of left ulna** ▽

☑7ᵗʰ **S52.209** **Unspecified fracture of shaft of unspecified ulna** ▽

☑6ᵗʰ **S52.21** **Greenstick fracture of shaft of ulna**

> The appropriate 7th character is to be added to all codes in subcategory S52.21.
> A   initial encounter for closed fracture
> D   subsequent encounter for fracture with routine healing
> G   subsequent encounter for fracture with delayed healing
> K   subsequent encounter for fracture with nonunion
> P   subsequent encounter for fracture with malunion
> S   sequela

☑7ᵗʰ **S52.211** **Greenstick fracture of shaft of right ulna**

☑7ᵗʰ **S52.212** **Greenstick fracture of shaft of left ulna**

☑7ᵗʰ **S52.219** **Greenstick fracture of shaft of unspecified ulna** ▽

☑6ᵗʰ **S52.22** **Transverse fracture of shaft of ulna**

☑7ᵗʰ **S52.221** **Displaced transverse fracture of shaft of right ulna**

☑7ᵗʰ **S52.222** **Displaced transverse fracture of shaft of left ulna**

☑7ᵗʰ **S52.223** **Displaced transverse fracture of shaft of unspecified ulna** ▽

☑7ᵗʰ **S52.224** **Nondisplaced transverse fracture of shaft of right ulna**

☑7ᵗʰ **S52.225** **Nondisplaced transverse fracture of shaft of left ulna**

☑7ᵗʰ **S52.226** **Nondisplaced transverse fracture of shaft of unspecified ulna** ▽

☑6ᵗʰ **S52.23** **Oblique fracture of shaft of ulna**

☑7ᵗʰ **S52.231** **Displaced oblique fracture of shaft of right ulna**

☑7ᵗʰ **S52.232** **Displaced oblique fracture of shaft of left ulna**

☑7ᵗʰ **S52.233** **Displaced oblique fracture of shaft of unspecified ulna** ▽

☑ Additional Character Req   ☑7ᵗʰ Placeholder Alert   Manifestation   HCC CMS-HCC Condition   ▽ Unspecified Code   ►◄ Revised Text   ● New Code   ▲ Revised Code Title

  ✓7ᵗʰ **S52.234 Nondisplaced oblique fracture of shaft of right ulna**

  ✓7ᵗʰ **S52.235 Nondisplaced oblique fracture of shaft of left ulna**

  ✓7ᵗʰ **S52.236 Nondisplaced oblique fracture of shaft of unspecified ulna** ▽

✓6ᵗʰ **S52.24 Spiral fracture of shaft of ulna**

  ✓7ᵗʰ **S52.241 Displaced spiral fracture of shaft of ulna, right arm**

  ✓7ᵗʰ **S52.242 Displaced spiral fracture of shaft of ulna, left arm**

  ✓7ᵗʰ **S52.243 Displaced spiral fracture of shaft of ulna, unspecified arm** ▽

  ✓7ᵗʰ **S52.244 Nondisplaced spiral fracture of shaft of ulna, right arm**

  ✓7ᵗʰ **S52.245 Nondisplaced spiral fracture of shaft of ulna, left arm**

  ✓7ᵗʰ **S52.246 Nondisplaced spiral fracture of shaft of ulna, unspecified arm** ▽

✓6ᵗʰ **S52.25 Comminuted fracture of shaft of ulna**

  ✓7ᵗʰ **S52.251 Displaced comminuted fracture of shaft of ulna, right arm**

  ✓7ᵗʰ **S52.252 Displaced comminuted fracture of shaft of ulna, left arm**

  ✓7ᵗʰ **S52.253 Displaced comminuted fracture of shaft of ulna, unspecified arm** ▽

  ✓7ᵗʰ **S52.254 Nondisplaced comminuted fracture of shaft of ulna, right arm**

  ✓7ᵗʰ **S52.255 Nondisplaced comminuted fracture of shaft of ulna, left arm**

  ✓7ᵗʰ **S52.256 Nondisplaced comminuted fracture of shaft of ulna, unspecified arm** ▽

✓6ᵗʰ **S52.26 Segmental fracture of shaft of ulna**

  ✓7ᵗʰ **S52.261 Displaced segmental fracture of shaft of ulna, right arm**

  ✓7ᵗʰ **S52.262 Displaced segmental fracture of shaft of ulna, left arm**

  ✓7ᵗʰ **S52.263 Displaced segmental fracture of shaft of ulna, unspecified arm** ▽

  ✓7ᵗʰ **S52.264 Nondisplaced segmental fracture of shaft of ulna, right arm**

  ✓7ᵗʰ **S52.265 Nondisplaced segmental fracture of shaft of ulna, left arm**

  ✓7ᵗʰ **S52.266 Nondisplaced segmental fracture of shaft of ulna, unspecified arm** ▽

✓6ᵗʰ **S52.27 Monteggia's fracture of ulna**
  Fracture of upper shaft of ulna with dislocation of radial head

  ✓7ᵗʰ **S52.271 Monteggia's fracture of right ulna**

  ✓7ᵗʰ **S52.272 Monteggia's fracture of left ulna**

  ✓7ᵗʰ **S52.279 Monteggia's fracture of unspecified ulna** ▽

✓6ᵗʰ **S52.28 Bent bone of ulna**

  ✓7ᵗʰ **S52.281 Bent bone of right ulna**

  ✓7ᵗʰ **S52.282 Bent bone of left ulna**

  ✓7ᵗʰ **S52.283 Bent bone of unspecified ulna** ▽

✓6ᵗʰ **S52.29 Other fracture of shaft of ulna**

  ✓7ᵗʰ **S52.291 Other fracture of shaft of right ulna**

  ✓7ᵗʰ **S52.292 Other fracture of shaft of left ulna**

  ✓7ᵗʰ **S52.299 Other fracture of shaft of unspecified ulna** ▽

✓5ᵗʰ **S52.3 Fracture of shaft of radius**

✓6ᵗʰ **S52.30 Unspecified fracture of shaft of radius**

  ✓7ᵗʰ **S52.301 Unspecified fracture of shaft of right radius** ▽

  ✓7ᵗʰ **S52.302 Unspecified fracture of shaft of left radius** ▽

  ✓7ᵗʰ **S52.309 Unspecified fracture of shaft of unspecified radius** ▽

✓6ᵗʰ **S52.31 Greenstick fracture of shaft of radius**

> The appropriate 7th character is to be added to all codes in subcategory S52.31.
> A initial encounter for closed fracture
> D subsequent encounter for fracture with routine healing
> G subsequent encounter for fracture with delayed healing
> K subsequent encounter for fracture with nonunion
> P subsequent encounter for fracture with malunion
> S sequela

  ✓7ᵗʰ **S52.311 Greenstick fracture of shaft of radius, right arm**

  ✓7ᵗʰ **S52.312 Greenstick fracture of shaft of radius, left arm**

  ✓7ᵗʰ **S52.319 Greenstick fracture of shaft of radius, unspecified arm** ▽

✓6ᵗʰ **S52.32 Transverse fracture of shaft of radius**

  ✓7ᵗʰ **S52.321 Displaced transverse fracture of shaft of right radius**

  ✓7ᵗʰ **S52.322 Displaced transverse fracture of shaft of left radius**

  ✓7ᵗʰ **S52.323 Displaced transverse fracture of shaft of unspecified radius** ▽

  ✓7ᵗʰ **S52.324 Nondisplaced transverse fracture of shaft of right radius**

  ✓7ᵗʰ **S52.325 Nondisplaced transverse fracture of shaft of left radius**

  ✓7ᵗʰ **S52.326 Nondisplaced transverse fracture of shaft of unspecified radius** ▽

✓6ᵗʰ **S52.33 Oblique fracture of shaft of radius**

  ✓7ᵗʰ **S52.331 Displaced oblique fracture of shaft of right radius**

  ✓7ᵗʰ **S52.332 Displaced oblique fracture of shaft of left radius**

  ✓7ᵗʰ **S52.333 Displaced oblique fracture of shaft of unspecified radius** ▽

  ✓7ᵗʰ **S52.334 Nondisplaced oblique fracture of shaft of right radius**

  ✓7ᵗʰ **S52.335 Nondisplaced oblique fracture of shaft of left radius**

  ✓7ᵗʰ **S52.336 Nondisplaced oblique fracture of shaft of unspecified radius** ▽

✓6ᵗʰ **S52.34 Spiral fracture of shaft of radius**

  ✓7ᵗʰ **S52.341 Displaced spiral fracture of shaft of radius, right arm**

  ✓7ᵗʰ **S52.342 Displaced spiral fracture of shaft of radius, left arm**

  ✓7ᵗʰ **S52.343 Displaced spiral fracture of shaft of radius, unspecified arm** ▽

  ✓7ᵗʰ **S52.344 Nondisplaced spiral fracture of shaft of radius, right arm**

  ✓7ᵗʰ **S52.345 Nondisplaced spiral fracture of shaft of radius, left arm**

  ✓7ᵗʰ **S52.346 Nondisplaced spiral fracture of shaft of radius, unspecified arm** ▽

✓6ᵗʰ **S52.35 Comminuted fracture of shaft of radius**

  ✓7ᵗʰ **S52.351 Displaced comminuted fracture of shaft of radius, right arm**

  ✓7ᵗʰ **S52.352 Displaced comminuted fracture of shaft of radius, left arm**

  ✓7ᵗʰ **S52.353 Displaced comminuted fracture of shaft of radius, unspecified arm** ▽

  ✓7ᵗʰ **S52.354 Nondisplaced comminuted fracture of shaft of radius, right arm**

  ✓7ᵗʰ **S52.355 Nondisplaced comminuted fracture of shaft of radius, left arm**

  ✓7ᵗʰ **S52.356 Nondisplaced comminuted fracture of shaft of radius, unspecified arm** ▽

✓6ᵗʰ **S52.36 Segmental fracture of shaft of radius**

  ✓7ᵗʰ **S52.361 Displaced segmental fracture of shaft of radius, right arm**

EXCLUDES 1 Not coded here EXCLUDES 2 Not included here N Newborn Age: 0 P Pediatric Age: 0-17 M Maternity Age: 12-55 A Adult Age: 15-124

968 ICD-10-CM 2018

√7ᵗʰ **S52.362** Displaced segmental fracture of shaft of radius, left arm

√7ᵗʰ **S52.363** Displaced segmental fracture of shaft of radius, unspecified arm ▽

√7ᵗʰ **S52.364** Nondisplaced segmental fracture of shaft of radius, right arm

√7ᵗʰ **S52.365** Nondisplaced segmental fracture of shaft of radius, left arm

√7ᵗʰ **S52.366** Nondisplaced segmental fracture of shaft of radius, unspecified arm ▽

√6ᵗʰ **S52.37** Galeazzi's fracture
Fracture of lower shaft of radius with radioulnar joint dislocation

√7ᵗʰ **S52.371** Galeazzi's fracture of right radius

√7ᵗʰ **S52.372** Galeazzi's fracture of left radius

√7ᵗʰ **S52.379** Galeazzi's fracture of unspecified radius ▽

√6ᵗʰ **S52.38** Bent bone of radius

√7ᵗʰ **S52.381** Bent bone of right radius

√7ᵗʰ **S52.382** Bent bone of left radius

√7ᵗʰ **S52.389** Bent bone of unspecified radius ▽

√6ᵗʰ **S52.39** Other fracture of shaft of radius

√7ᵗʰ **S52.391** Other fracture of shaft of radius, right arm

√7ᵗʰ **S52.392** Other fracture of shaft of radius, left arm

√7ᵗʰ **S52.399** Other fracture of shaft of radius, unspecified arm ▽

√5ᵗʰ **S52.5** Fracture of lower end of radius
Fracture of distal end of radius
EXCLUDES 2 *physeal fractures of lower end of radius (S59.2-)*
DEF: Fracture of distal end of radius above the wrist; most commonly caused by fall onto an outstretched hand.

√6ᵗʰ **S52.50** Unspecified fracture of the lower end of radius

√7ᵗʰ **S52.501** Unspecified fracture of the lower end of right radius ▽

√7ᵗʰ **S52.502** Unspecified fracture of the lower end of left radius ▽

√7ᵗʰ **S52.509** Unspecified fracture of the lower end of unspecified radius ▽

√6ᵗʰ **S52.51** Fracture of radial styloid process

√7ᵗʰ **S52.511** Displaced fracture of right radial styloid process

√7ᵗʰ **S52.512** Displaced fracture of left radial styloid process

√7ᵗʰ **S52.513** Displaced fracture of unspecified radial styloid process ▽

√7ᵗʰ **S52.514** Nondisplaced fracture of right radial styloid process

√7ᵗʰ **S52.515** Nondisplaced fracture of left radial styloid process

√7ᵗʰ **S52.516** Nondisplaced fracture of unspecified radial styloid process ▽

√6ᵗʰ **S52.52** Torus fracture of lower end of radius

> The appropriate 7th character is to be added to all codes in subcategory S52.52.
> A   initial encounter for closed fracture
> D   subsequent encounter for fracture with routine healing
> G   subsequent encounter for fracture with delayed healing
> K   subsequent encounter for fracture with nonunion
> P   subsequent encounter for fracture with malunion
> S   sequela

√7ᵗʰ **S52.521** Torus fracture of lower end of right radius

√7ᵗʰ **S52.522** Torus fracture of lower end of left radius

√7ᵗʰ **S52.529** Torus fracture of lower end of unspecified radius ▽

√6ᵗʰ **S52.53** Colles' fracture
AHA: 2016, 2Q, 4

√7ᵗʰ **S52.531** Colles' fracture of right radius

√7ᵗʰ **S52.532** Colles' fracture of left radius

√7ᵗʰ **S52.539** Colles' fracture of unspecified radius ▽

√6ᵗʰ **S52.54** Smith's fracture

√7ᵗʰ **S52.541** Smith's fracture of right radius

√7ᵗʰ **S52.542** Smith's fracture of left radius

√7ᵗʰ **S52.549** Smith's fracture of unspecified radius ▽

√6ᵗʰ **S52.55** Other extraarticular fracture of lower end of radius

√7ᵗʰ **S52.551** Other extraarticular fracture of lower end of right radius

√7ᵗʰ **S52.552** Other extraarticular fracture of lower end of left radius

√7ᵗʰ **S52.559** Other extraarticular fracture of lower end of unspecified radius ▽

√6ᵗʰ **S52.56** Barton's fracture

√7ᵗʰ **S52.561** Barton's fracture of right radius

√7ᵗʰ **S52.562** Barton's fracture of left radius

√7ᵗʰ **S52.569** Barton's fracture of unspecified radius ▽

√6ᵗʰ **S52.57** Other intraarticular fracture of lower end of radius

√7ᵗʰ **S52.571** Other intraarticular fracture of lower end of right radius

√7ᵗʰ **S52.572** Other intraarticular fracture of lower end of left radius

√7ᵗʰ **S52.579** Other intraarticular fracture of lower end of unspecified radius ▽

√6ᵗʰ **S52.59** Other fractures of lower end of radius

√7ᵗʰ **S52.591** Other fractures of lower end of right radius

√7ᵗʰ **S52.592** Other fractures of lower end of left radius

√7ᵗʰ **S52.599** Other fractures of lower end of unspecified radius ▽

√5ᵗʰ **S52.6** Fracture of lower end of ulna

√6ᵗʰ **S52.60** Unspecified fracture of lower end of ulna

√7ᵗʰ **S52.601** Unspecified fracture of lower end of right ulna ▽

√7ᵗʰ **S52.602** Unspecified fracture of lower end of left ulna ▽

√7ᵗʰ **S52.609** Unspecified fracture of lower end of unspecified ulna ▽

√6ᵗʰ **S52.61** Fracture of ulna styloid process

√7ᵗʰ **S52.611** Displaced fracture of right ulna styloid process

√7ᵗʰ **S52.612** Displaced fracture of left ulna styloid process

√7ᵗʰ **S52.613** Displaced fracture of unspecified ulna styloid process ▽

√7ᵗʰ **S52.614** Nondisplaced fracture of right ulna styloid process

√7ᵗʰ **S52.615** Nondisplaced fracture of left ulna styloid process

√7ᵗʰ **S52.616** Nondisplaced fracture of unspecified ulna styloid process ▽

√6ᵗʰ **S52.62** Torus fracture of lower end of ulna

> The appropriate 7th character is to be added to all codes in subcategory S52.62.
> A   initial encounter for closed fracture
> D   subsequent encounter for fracture with routine healing
> G   subsequent encounter for fracture with delayed healing
> K   subsequent encounter for fracture with nonunion
> P   subsequent encounter for fracture with malunion
> S   sequela

√7ᵗʰ **S52.621** Torus fracture of lower end of right ulna

√7ᵗʰ **S52.622** Torus fracture of lower end of left ulna

√7ᵗʰ **S52.629** Torus fracture of lower end of unspecified ulna ▽

√6ᵗʰ **S52.69** Other fracture of lower end of ulna

√7ᵗʰ **S52.691** Other fracture of lower end of right ulna

√7ᵗʰ **S52.692** Other fracture of lower end of left ulna

√7ᵗʰ **S52.699** Other fracture of lower end of unspecified ulna ▽

☑ Additional Character Req   √x7ᵗʰ Placeholder Alert   Manifestation   HCC CMS-HCC Condition   ▽ Unspecified Code   ►◄ Revised Text   ● New Code   ▲ Revised Code Title

√5ᵗʰ S52.9 Unspecified fracture of forearm

     √x7ᵗʰ S52.90 Unspecified fracture of unspecified forearm ▽

     √x7ᵗʰ S52.91 Unspecified fracture of right forearm ▽

     √x7ᵗʰ S52.92 Unspecified fracture of left forearm ▽

√4ᵗʰ S53 Dislocation and sprain of joints and ligaments of elbow

     INCLUDES avulsion of joint or ligament of elbow
         laceration of cartilage, joint or ligament of elbow
         sprain of cartilage, joint or ligament of elbow
         traumatic hemarthrosis of joint or ligament of elbow
         traumatic rupture of joint or ligament of elbow
         traumatic subluxation of joint or ligament of elbow
         traumatic tear of joint or ligament of elbow

     Code also any associated open wound

     EXCLUDES 2 *strain of muscle, fascia and tendon at forearm level (S56.-)*

> The appropriate 7th character is to be added to each code from category S53.
> A   initial encounter
> D   subsequent encounter
> S   sequela

√5ᵗʰ S53.0 Subluxation and dislocation of radial head
     Dislocation of radiohumeral joint
     Subluxation of radiohumeral joint
     EXCLUDES 1 *Monteggia's fracture-dislocation (S52.27-)*

     √6ᵗʰ S53.00 Unspecified subluxation and dislocation of radial head

         √7ᵗʰ S53.001 Unspecified subluxation of right radial head ▽

         √7ᵗʰ S53.002 Unspecified subluxation of left radial head ▽

         √7ᵗʰ S53.003 Unspecified subluxation of unspecified radial head ▽

         √7ᵗʰ S53.004 Unspecified dislocation of right radial head ▽

         √7ᵗʰ S53.005 Unspecified dislocation of left radial head ▽

         √7ᵗʰ S53.006 Unspecified dislocation of unspecified radial head ▽

     √6ᵗʰ S53.01 Anterior subluxation and dislocation of radial head
         Anteriomedial subluxation and dislocation of radial head

         √7ᵗʰ S53.011 Anterior subluxation of right radial head

         √7ᵗʰ S53.012 Anterior subluxation of left radial head

         √7ᵗʰ S53.013 Anterior subluxation of unspecified radial head ▽

         √7ᵗʰ S53.014 Anterior dislocation of right radial head

         √7ᵗʰ S53.015 Anterior dislocation of left radial head

         √7ᵗʰ S53.016 Anterior dislocation of unspecified radial head ▽

     √6ᵗʰ S53.02 Posterior subluxation and dislocation of radial head
         Posteriolateral subluxation and dislocation of radial head

         √7ᵗʰ S53.021 Posterior subluxation of right radial head

         √7ᵗʰ S53.022 Posterior subluxation of left radial head

         √7ᵗʰ S53.023 Posterior subluxation of unspecified radial head ▽

         √7ᵗʰ S53.024 Posterior dislocation of right radial head

         √7ᵗʰ S53.025 Posterior dislocation of left radial head

         √7ᵗʰ S53.026 Posterior dislocation of unspecified radial head ▽

     √6ᵗʰ S53.03 Nursemaid's elbow

         √7ᵗʰ S53.031 Nursemaid's elbow, right elbow

         √7ᵗʰ S53.032 Nursemaid's elbow, left elbow

         √7ᵗʰ S53.033 Nursemaid's elbow, unspecified elbow ▽

     √6ᵗʰ S53.09 Other subluxation and dislocation of radial head

         √7ᵗʰ S53.091 Other subluxation of right radial head

         √7ᵗʰ S53.092 Other subluxation of left radial head

         √7ᵗʰ S53.093 Other subluxation of unspecified radial head ▽

         √7ᵗʰ S53.094 Other dislocation of right radial head

         √7ᵗʰ S53.095 Other dislocation of left radial head

         √7ᵗʰ S53.096 Other dislocation of unspecified radial head ▽

√5ᵗʰ S53.1 Subluxation and dislocation of ulnohumeral joint
     Subluxation and dislocation of elbow NOS
     EXCLUDES 1 *dislocation of radial head alone (S53.0-)*

     √6ᵗʰ S53.10 Unspecified subluxation and dislocation of ulnohumeral joint

         √7ᵗʰ S53.101 Unspecified subluxation of right ulnohumeral joint ▽

         √7ᵗʰ S53.102 Unspecified subluxation of left ulnohumeral joint ▽

         √7ᵗʰ S53.103 Unspecified subluxation of unspecified ulnohumeral joint ▽

         √7ᵗʰ S53.104 Unspecified dislocation of right ulnohumeral joint ▽

         √7ᵗʰ S53.105 Unspecified dislocation of left ulnohumeral joint ▽

         √7ᵗʰ S53.106 Unspecified dislocation of unspecified ulnohumeral joint ▽

     √6ᵗʰ S53.11 Anterior subluxation and dislocation of ulnohumeral joint

         √7ᵗʰ S53.111 Anterior subluxation of right ulnohumeral joint

         √7ᵗʰ S53.112 Anterior subluxation of left ulnohumeral joint

         √7ᵗʰ S53.113 Anterior subluxation of unspecified ulnohumeral joint

         √7ᵗʰ S53.114 Anterior dislocation of right ulnohumeral joint
             AHA: 2012, 4Q, 108

         √7ᵗʰ S53.115 Anterior dislocation of left ulnohumeral joint

         √7ᵗʰ S53.116 Anterior dislocation of unspecified ulnohumeral joint ▽

     √6ᵗʰ S53.12 Posterior subluxation and dislocation of ulnohumeral joint

         √7ᵗʰ S53.121 Posterior subluxation of right ulnohumeral joint

         √7ᵗʰ S53.122 Posterior subluxation of left ulnohumeral joint

         √7ᵗʰ S53.123 Posterior subluxation of unspecified ulnohumeral joint ▽

         √7ᵗʰ S53.124 Posterior dislocation of right ulnohumeral joint

         √7ᵗʰ S53.125 Posterior dislocation of left ulnohumeral joint

         √7ᵗʰ S53.126 Posterior dislocation of unspecified ulnohumeral joint ▽

     √6ᵗʰ S53.13 Medial subluxation and dislocation of ulnohumeral joint

         √7ᵗʰ S53.131 Medial subluxation of right ulnohumeral joint

         √7ᵗʰ S53.132 Medial subluxation of left ulnohumeral joint

         √7ᵗʰ S53.133 Medial subluxation of unspecified ulnohumeral joint ▽

         √7ᵗʰ S53.134 Medial dislocation of right ulnohumeral joint

         √7ᵗʰ S53.135 Medial dislocation of left ulnohumeral joint

         √7ᵗʰ S53.136 Medial dislocation of unspecified ulnohumeral joint ▽

     √6ᵗʰ S53.14 Lateral subluxation and dislocation of ulnohumeral joint

         √7ᵗʰ S53.141 Lateral subluxation of right ulnohumeral joint

         √7ᵗʰ S53.142 Lateral subluxation of left ulnohumeral joint

         √7ᵗʰ S53.143 Lateral subluxation of unspecified ulnohumeral joint ▽

         √7ᵗʰ S53.144 Lateral dislocation of right ulnohumeral joint

         √7ᵗʰ S53.145 Lateral dislocation of left ulnohumeral joint

         √7ᵗʰ S53.146 Lateral dislocation of unspecified ulnohumeral joint ▽

EXCLUDES 1 Not coded here   **EXCLUDES 2** Not included here   **N** Newborn Age: 0   **P** Pediatric Age: 0-17   **M** Maternity Age: 12-55   **A** Adult Age: 15-124

970   ICD-10-CM 2018

√6th **S53.19** **Other subluxation and dislocation of ulnohumeral joint**

     √7th **S53.191** **Other subluxation of right ulnohumeral joint**

     √7th **S53.192** **Other subluxation of left ulnohumeral joint**

     √7th **S53.193** **Other subluxation of unspecified ulnohumeral joint** ▽

     √7th **S53.194** **Other dislocation of right ulnohumeral joint**

     √7th **S53.195** **Other dislocation of left ulnohumeral joint**

     √7th **S53.196** **Other dislocation of unspecified ulnohumeral joint** ▽

√6th **S53.2** **Traumatic rupture of radial collateral ligament**

     EXCLUDES 1   *sprain of radial collateral ligament NOS (S53.43-)*

     √x7th **S53.20** **Traumatic rupture of unspecified radial collateral ligament** ▽

     √x7th **S53.21** **Traumatic rupture of right radial collateral ligament**

     √x7th **S53.22** **Traumatic rupture of left radial collateral ligament**

√5th **S53.3** **Traumatic rupture of ulnar collateral ligament**

     EXCLUDES 1   *sprain of ulnar collateral ligament (S53.44-)*

     √x7th **S53.30** **Traumatic rupture of unspecified ulnar collateral ligament** ▽

     √x7th **S53.31** **Traumatic rupture of right ulnar collateral ligament**

     √x7th **S53.32** **Traumatic rupture of left ulnar collateral ligament**

√5th **S53.4** **Sprain of elbow**

     EXCLUDES 2   *traumatic rupture of radial collateral ligament (S53.2-)*
               traumatic rupture of ulnar collateral ligament (S53.3-)

     √6th **S53.40** **Unspecified sprain of elbow**

         √7th **S53.401** **Unspecified sprain of right elbow** ▽

         √7th **S53.402** **Unspecified sprain of left elbow** ▽

         √7th **S53.409** **Unspecified sprain of unspecified elbow** ▽
               Sprain of elbow NOS

     √6th **S53.41** **Radiohumeral (joint) sprain**

         √7th **S53.411** **Radiohumeral (joint) sprain of right elbow**

         √7th **S53.412** **Radiohumeral (joint) sprain of left elbow**

         √7th **S53.419** **Radiohumeral (joint) sprain of unspecified elbow** ▽

     √6th **S53.42** **Ulnohumeral (joint) sprain**

         √7th **S53.421** **Ulnohumeral (joint) sprain of right elbow**

         √7th **S53.422** **Ulnohumeral (joint) sprain of left elbow**

         √7th **S53.429** **Ulnohumeral (joint) sprain of unspecified elbow** ▽

     √6th **S53.43** **Radial collateral ligament sprain**

         √7th **S53.431** **Radial collateral ligament sprain of right elbow**

         √7th **S53.432** **Radial collateral ligament sprain of left elbow**

         √7th **S53.439** **Radial collateral ligament sprain of unspecified elbow** ▽

     √6th **S53.44** **Ulnar collateral ligament sprain**

         √7th **S53.441** **Ulnar collateral ligament sprain of right elbow**

         √7th **S53.442** **Ulnar collateral ligament sprain of left elbow**

         √7th **S53.449** **Ulnar collateral ligament sprain of unspecified elbow** ▽

     √6th **S53.49** **Other sprain of elbow**

         √7th **S53.491** **Other sprain of right elbow**

         √7th **S53.492** **Other sprain of left elbow**

         √7th **S53.499** **Other sprain of unspecified elbow** ▽

√4th **S54** **Injury of nerves at forearm level**

     Code also any associated open wound (S51.-)

     EXCLUDES 2   *injury of nerves at wrist and hand level (S64.-)*

     The appropriate 7th character is to be added to each code from category S54.
     A   initial encounter
     D   subsequent encounter
     S   sequela

√5th **S54.0** **Injury of ulnar nerve at forearm level**
          Injury of ulnar nerve NOS

     √x7th **S54.00** **Injury of ulnar nerve at forearm level, unspecified arm** ▽

     √x7th **S54.01** **Injury of ulnar nerve at forearm level, right arm**

     √x7th **S54.02** **Injury of ulnar nerve at forearm level, left arm**

√5th **S54.1** **Injury of median nerve at forearm level**
          Injury of median nerve NOS

     √x7th **S54.10** **Injury of median nerve at forearm level, unspecified arm** ▽

     √x7th **S54.11** **Injury of median nerve at forearm level, right arm**

     √x7th **S54.12** **Injury of median nerve at forearm level, left arm**

√5th **S54.2** **Injury of radial nerve at forearm level**
          Injury of radial nerve NOS

     √x7th **S54.20** **Injury of radial nerve at forearm level, unspecified arm** ▽

     √x7th **S54.21** **Injury of radial nerve at forearm level, right arm**

     √x7th **S54.22** **Injury of radial nerve at forearm level, left arm**

√5th **S54.3** **Injury of cutaneous sensory nerve at forearm level**

     √x7th **S54.30** **Injury of cutaneous sensory nerve at forearm level, unspecified arm** ▽

     √x7th **S54.31** **Injury of cutaneous sensory nerve at forearm level, right arm**

     √x7th **S54.32** **Injury of cutaneous sensory nerve at forearm level, left arm**

√5th **S54.8** **Injury of other nerves at forearm level**

     √6th **S54.8X** **Injury of other nerves at forearm level**

         √7th **S54.8X1** **Injury of other nerves at forearm level, right arm**

         √7th **S54.8X2** **Injury of other nerves at forearm level, left arm**

         √7th **S54.8X9** **Injury of other nerves at forearm level, unspecified arm** ▽

√5th **S54.9** **Injury of unspecified nerve at forearm level**

     √x7th **S54.90** **Injury of unspecified nerve at forearm level, unspecified arm** ▽

     √x7th **S54.91** **Injury of unspecified nerve at forearm level, right arm** ▽

     √x7th **S54.92** **Injury of unspecified nerve at forearm level, left arm** ▽

√4th **S55** **Injury of blood vessels at forearm level**

     Code also any associated open wound (S51.-)

     EXCLUDES 2   *injury of blood vessels at wrist and hand level (S65.-)*
               injury of brachial vessels (S45.1-S45.2)

     The appropriate 7th character is to be added to each code from category S55.
     A   initial encounter
     D   subsequent encounter
     S   sequela

√5th **S55.0** **Injury of ulnar artery at forearm level**

     √6th **S55.00** **Unspecified injury of ulnar artery at forearm level**

         √7th **S55.001** **Unspecified injury of ulnar artery at forearm level, right arm** ▽

         √7th **S55.002** **Unspecified injury of ulnar artery at forearm level, left arm** ▽

         √7th **S55.009** **Unspecified injury of ulnar artery at forearm level, unspecified arm** ▽

     √6th **S55.01** **Laceration of ulnar artery at forearm level**

         √7th **S55.011** **Laceration of ulnar artery at forearm level, right arm**

         √7th **S55.012** **Laceration of ulnar artery at forearm level, left arm**

         √7th **S55.019** **Laceration of ulnar artery at forearm level, unspecified arm** ▽

✓ Additional Character Req   √x7th Placeholder Alert   Manifestation   HCC CMS-HCC Condition   ▽ Unspecified Code   ►◄ Revised Text   ● New Code   ▲ Revised Code Title

ICD-10-CM 2018   971

Chapter 19. Injury, Poisoning, and Certain Other Consequences of External Causes

S55.09–S56.091

✓6ᵗʰ **S55.09** Other specified injury of ulnar artery at forearm level

     ✓7ᵗʰ **S55.091** Other specified injury of ulnar artery at forearm level, right arm

     ✓7ᵗʰ **S55.092** Other specified injury of ulnar artery at forearm level, left arm

     ✓7ᵗʰ **S55.099** Other specified injury of ulnar artery at forearm level, unspecified arm ▽

✓5ᵗʰ **S55.1** Injury of radial artery at forearm level

     ✓6ᵗʰ **S55.10** Unspecified injury of radial artery at forearm level

       ✓7ᵗʰ **S55.101** Unspecified injury of radial artery at forearm level, right arm ▽

       ✓7ᵗʰ **S55.102** Unspecified injury of radial artery at forearm level, left arm ▽

       ✓7ᵗʰ **S55.109** Unspecified injury of radial artery at forearm level, unspecified arm ▽

     ✓6ᵗʰ **S55.11** Laceration of radial artery at forearm level

       ✓7ᵗʰ **S55.111** Laceration of radial artery at forearm level, right arm

       ✓7ᵗʰ **S55.112** Laceration of radial artery at forearm level, left arm

       ✓7ᵗʰ **S55.119** Laceration of radial artery at forearm level, unspecified arm ▽

     ✓6ᵗʰ **S55.19** Other specified injury of radial artery at forearm level

       ✓7ᵗʰ **S55.191** Other specified injury of radial artery at forearm level, right arm

       ✓7ᵗʰ **S55.192** Other specified injury of radial artery at forearm level, left arm

       ✓7ᵗʰ **S55.199** Other specified injury of radial artery at forearm level, unspecified arm ▽

✓5ᵗʰ **S55.2** Injury of vein at forearm level

     ✓6ᵗʰ **S55.20** Unspecified injury of vein at forearm level

       ✓7ᵗʰ **S55.201** Unspecified injury of vein at forearm level, right arm ▽

       ✓7ᵗʰ **S55.202** Unspecified injury of vein at forearm level, left arm ▽

       ✓7ᵗʰ **S55.209** Unspecified injury of vein at forearm level, unspecified arm ▽

     ✓6ᵗʰ **S55.21** Laceration of vein at forearm level

       ✓7ᵗʰ **S55.211** Laceration of vein at forearm level, right arm

       ✓7ᵗʰ **S55.212** Laceration of vein at forearm level, left arm

       ✓7ᵗʰ **S55.219** Laceration of vein at forearm level, unspecified arm ▽

     ✓6ᵗʰ **S55.29** Other specified injury of vein at forearm level

       ✓7ᵗʰ **S55.291** Other specified injury of vein at forearm level, right arm

       ✓7ᵗʰ **S55.292** Other specified injury of vein at forearm level, left arm

       ✓7ᵗʰ **S55.299** Other specified injury of vein at forearm level, unspecified arm ▽

✓5ᵗʰ **S55.8** Injury of other blood vessels at forearm level

     ✓6ᵗʰ **S55.80** Unspecified injury of other blood vessels at forearm level

       ✓7ᵗʰ **S55.801** Unspecified injury of other blood vessels at forearm level, right arm ▽

       ✓7ᵗʰ **S55.802** Unspecified injury of other blood vessels at forearm level, left arm ▽

       ✓7ᵗʰ **S55.809** Unspecified injury of other blood vessels at forearm level, unspecified arm ▽

     ✓6ᵗʰ **S55.81** Laceration of other blood vessels at forearm level

       ✓7ᵗʰ **S55.811** Laceration of other blood vessels at forearm level, right arm

       ✓7ᵗʰ **S55.812** Laceration of other blood vessels at forearm level, left arm

       ✓7ᵗʰ **S55.819** Laceration of other blood vessels at forearm level, unspecified arm ▽

     ✓6ᵗʰ **S55.89** Other specified injury of other blood vessels at forearm level

       ✓7ᵗʰ **S55.891** Other specified injury of other blood vessels at forearm level, right arm

       ✓7ᵗʰ **S55.892** Other specified injury of other blood vessels at forearm level, left arm

       ✓7ᵗʰ **S55.899** Other specified injury of other blood vessels at forearm level, unspecified arm ▽

✓5ᵗʰ **S55.9** Injury of unspecified blood vessel at forearm level

     ✓6ᵗʰ **S55.90** Unspecified injury of unspecified blood vessel at forearm level

       ✓7ᵗʰ **S55.901** Unspecified injury of unspecified blood vessel at forearm level, right arm ▽

       ✓7ᵗʰ **S55.902** Unspecified injury of unspecified blood vessel at forearm level, left arm ▽

       ✓7ᵗʰ **S55.909** Unspecified injury of unspecified blood vessel at forearm level, unspecified arm ▽

     ✓6ᵗʰ **S55.91** Laceration of unspecified blood vessel at forearm level

       ✓7ᵗʰ **S55.911** Laceration of unspecified blood vessel at forearm level, right arm ▽

       ✓7ᵗʰ **S55.912** Laceration of unspecified blood vessel at forearm level, left arm ▽

       ✓7ᵗʰ **S55.919** Laceration of unspecified blood vessel at forearm level, unspecified arm ▽

     ✓6ᵗʰ **S55.99** Other specified injury of unspecified blood vessel at forearm level

       ✓7ᵗʰ **S55.991** Other specified injury of unspecified blood vessel at forearm level, right arm ▽

       ✓7ᵗʰ **S55.992** Other specified injury of unspecified blood vessel at forearm level, left arm ▽

       ✓7ᵗʰ **S55.999** Other specified injury of unspecified blood vessel at forearm level, unspecified arm ▽

✓4ᵗʰ **S56 Injury of muscle, fascia and tendon at forearm level**

     Code also any associated open wound (S51.-)

     EXCLUDES 2   injury of muscle, fascia and tendon at or below wrist (S66.-)
              sprain of joints and ligaments of elbow (S53.4-)

     TIP: Refer to the Muscle/Tendon table at the beginning of this chapter.

     The appropriate 7th character is to be added to each code from category S56.
     A   initial encounter
     D   subsequent encounter
     S   sequela

     ✓5ᵗʰ **S56.0** Injury of flexor muscle, fascia and tendon of thumb at forearm level

       ✓6ᵗʰ **S56.00** Unspecified injury of flexor muscle, fascia and tendon of thumb at forearm level

         ✓7ᵗʰ **S56.001** Unspecified injury of flexor muscle, fascia and tendon of right thumb at forearm level ▽

         ✓7ᵗʰ **S56.002** Unspecified injury of flexor muscle, fascia and tendon of left thumb at forearm level ▽

         ✓7ᵗʰ **S56.009** Unspecified injury of flexor muscle, fascia and tendon of unspecified thumb at forearm level ▽

       ✓6ᵗʰ **S56.01** Strain of flexor muscle, fascia and tendon of thumb at forearm level

         ✓7ᵗʰ **S56.011** Strain of flexor muscle, fascia and tendon of right thumb at forearm level

         ✓7ᵗʰ **S56.012** Strain of flexor muscle, fascia and tendon of left thumb at forearm level

         ✓7ᵗʰ **S56.019** Strain of flexor muscle, fascia and tendon of unspecified thumb at forearm level ▽

       ✓6ᵗʰ **S56.02** Laceration of flexor muscle, fascia and tendon of thumb at forearm level

         ✓7ᵗʰ **S56.021** Laceration of flexor muscle, fascia and tendon of right thumb at forearm level

         ✓7ᵗʰ **S56.022** Laceration of flexor muscle, fascia and tendon of left thumb at forearm level

         ✓7ᵗʰ **S56.029** Laceration of flexor muscle, fascia and tendon of unspecified thumb at forearm level ▽

       ✓6ᵗʰ **S56.09** Other injury of flexor muscle, fascia and tendon of thumb at forearm level

         ✓7ᵗʰ **S56.091** Other injury of flexor muscle, fascia and tendon of right thumb at forearm level

EXCLUDES 1 Not coded here   *EXCLUDES 2* Not included here   **N** Newborn Age: 0   **P** Pediatric Age: 0-17   **M** Maternity Age: 12-55   **A** Adult Age: 15-124

972   ICD-10-CM 2018

☑7ᵗʰ **S56.092** Other injury of flexor muscle, fascia and tendon of left thumb at forearm level

☑7ᵗʰ **S56.099** Other injury of flexor muscle, fascia and tendon of unspecified thumb at forearm level ▽

☑5ᵗʰ **S56.1** Injury of flexor muscle, fascia and tendon of other and unspecified finger at forearm level

   ☑6ᵗʰ **S56.10** Unspecified injury of flexor muscle, fascia and tendon of other and unspecified finger at forearm level

      ☑7ᵗʰ **S56.101** Unspecified injury of flexor muscle, fascia and tendon of right index finger at forearm level ▽

      ☑7ᵗʰ **S56.102** Unspecified injury of flexor muscle, fascia and tendon of left index finger at forearm level ▽

      ☑7ᵗʰ **S56.103** Unspecified injury of flexor muscle, fascia and tendon of right middle finger at forearm level ▽

      ☑7ᵗʰ **S56.104** Unspecified injury of flexor muscle, fascia and tendon of left middle finger at forearm level ▽

      ☑7ᵗʰ **S56.105** Unspecified injury of flexor muscle, fascia and tendon of right ring finger at forearm level ▽

      ☑7ᵗʰ **S56.106** Unspecified injury of flexor muscle, fascia and tendon of left ring finger at forearm level ▽

      ☑7ᵗʰ **S56.107** Unspecified injury of flexor muscle, fascia and tendon of right little finger at forearm level ▽

      ☑7ᵗʰ **S56.108** Unspecified injury of flexor muscle, fascia and tendon of left little finger at forearm level ▽

      ☑7ᵗʰ **S56.109** Unspecified injury of flexor muscle, fascia and tendon of unspecified finger at forearm level ▽

   ☑6ᵗʰ **S56.11** Strain of flexor muscle, fascia and tendon of other and unspecified finger at forearm level

      ☑7ᵗʰ **S56.111** Strain of flexor muscle, fascia and tendon of right index finger at forearm level

      ☑7ᵗʰ **S56.112** Strain of flexor muscle, fascia and tendon of left index finger at forearm level

      ☑7ᵗʰ **S56.113** Strain of flexor muscle, fascia and tendon of right middle finger at forearm level

      ☑7ᵗʰ **S56.114** Strain of flexor muscle, fascia and tendon of left middle finger at forearm level

      ☑7ᵗʰ **S56.115** Strain of flexor muscle, fascia and tendon of right ring finger at forearm level

      ☑7ᵗʰ **S56.116** Strain of flexor muscle, fascia and tendon of left ring finger at forearm level

      ☑7ᵗʰ **S56.117** Strain of flexor muscle, fascia and tendon of right little finger at forearm level

      ☑7ᵗʰ **S56.118** Strain of flexor muscle, fascia and tendon of left little finger at forearm level

      ☑7ᵗʰ **S56.119** Strain of flexor muscle, fascia and tendon of finger of unspecified finger at forearm level ▽

   ☑6ᵗʰ **S56.12** Laceration of flexor muscle, fascia and tendon of other and unspecified finger at forearm level

      ☑7ᵗʰ **S56.121** Laceration of flexor muscle, fascia and tendon of right index finger at forearm level

      ☑7ᵗʰ **S56.122** Laceration of flexor muscle, fascia and tendon of left index finger at forearm level

      ☑7ᵗʰ **S56.123** Laceration of flexor muscle, fascia and tendon of right middle finger at forearm level

      ☑7ᵗʰ **S56.124** Laceration of flexor muscle, fascia and tendon of left middle finger at forearm level

      ☑7ᵗʰ **S56.125** Laceration of flexor muscle, fascia and tendon of right ring finger at forearm level

      ☑7ᵗʰ **S56.126** Laceration of flexor muscle, fascia and tendon of left ring finger at forearm level

☑7ᵗʰ **S56.127** Laceration of flexor muscle, fascia and tendon of right little finger at forearm level

☑7ᵗʰ **S56.128** Laceration of flexor muscle, fascia and tendon of left little finger at forearm level

☑7ᵗʰ **S56.129** Laceration of flexor muscle, fascia and tendon of unspecified finger at forearm level ▽

   ☑6ᵗʰ **S56.19** Other injury of flexor muscle, fascia and tendon of other and unspecified finger at forearm level

      ☑7ᵗʰ **S56.191** Other injury of flexor muscle, fascia and tendon of right index finger at forearm level

      ☑7ᵗʰ **S56.192** Other injury of flexor muscle, fascia and tendon of left index finger at forearm level

      ☑7ᵗʰ **S56.193** Other injury of flexor muscle, fascia and tendon of right middle finger at forearm level

      ☑7ᵗʰ **S56.194** Other injury of flexor muscle, fascia and tendon of left middle finger at forearm level

      ☑7ᵗʰ **S56.195** Other injury of flexor muscle, fascia and tendon of right ring finger at forearm level

      ☑7ᵗʰ **S56.196** Other injury of flexor muscle, fascia and tendon of left ring finger at forearm level

      ☑7ᵗʰ **S56.197** Other injury of flexor muscle, fascia and tendon of right little finger at forearm level

      ☑7ᵗʰ **S56.198** Other injury of flexor muscle, fascia and tendon of left little finger at forearm level

      ☑7ᵗʰ **S56.199** Other injury of flexor muscle, fascia and tendon of unspecified finger at forearm level ▽

☑5ᵗʰ **S56.2** Injury of other flexor muscle, fascia and tendon at forearm level

   ☑6ᵗʰ **S56.20** Unspecified injury of other flexor muscle, fascia and tendon at forearm level

      ☑7ᵗʰ **S56.201** Unspecified injury of other flexor muscle, fascia and tendon at forearm level, right arm ▽

      ☑7ᵗʰ **S56.202** Unspecified injury of other flexor muscle, fascia and tendon at forearm level, left arm ▽

      ☑7ᵗʰ **S56.209** Unspecified injury of other flexor muscle, fascia and tendon at forearm level, unspecified arm ▽

   ☑6ᵗʰ **S56.21** Strain of other flexor muscle, fascia and tendon at forearm level

      ☑7ᵗʰ **S56.211** Strain of other flexor muscle, fascia and tendon at forearm level, right arm

      ☑7ᵗʰ **S56.212** Strain of other flexor muscle, fascia and tendon at forearm level, left arm

      ☑7ᵗʰ **S56.219** Strain of other flexor muscle, fascia and tendon at forearm level, unspecified arm ▽

   ☑6ᵗʰ **S56.22** Laceration of other flexor muscle, fascia and tendon at forearm level

      ☑7ᵗʰ **S56.221** Laceration of other flexor muscle, fascia and tendon at forearm level, right arm

      ☑7ᵗʰ **S56.222** Laceration of other flexor muscle, fascia and tendon at forearm level, left arm

      ☑7ᵗʰ **S56.229** Laceration of other flexor muscle, fascia and tendon at forearm level, unspecified arm ▽

   ☑6ᵗʰ **S56.29** Other injury of other flexor muscle, fascia and tendon at forearm level

      ☑7ᵗʰ **S56.291** Other injury of other flexor muscle, fascia and tendon at forearm level, right arm

      ☑7ᵗʰ **S56.292** Other injury of other flexor muscle, fascia and tendon at forearm level, left arm

      ☑7ᵗʰ **S56.299** Other injury of other flexor muscle, fascia and tendon at forearm level, unspecified arm ▽

☑ Additional Character Req   ☑7ᵗʰ Placeholder Alert   Manifestation   HCC CMS-HCC Condition   ▽ Unspecified Code   ►◄ Revised Text   ● New Code   ▲ Revised Code Title

✓5ᵗʰ **S56.3** **Injury of extensor or abductor muscles, fascia and tendons of thumb at forearm level**

  ✓6ᵗʰ **S56.30** **Unspecified injury of extensor or abductor muscles, fascia and tendons of thumb at forearm level**

    ✓7ᵗʰ **S56.301** Unspecified injury of extensor or abductor muscles, fascia and tendons of right thumb at forearm level ▽

    ✓7ᵗʰ **S56.302** Unspecified injury of extensor or abductor muscles, fascia and tendons of left thumb at forearm level ▽

    ✓7ᵗʰ **S56.309** Unspecified injury of extensor or abductor muscles, fascia and tendons of unspecified thumb at forearm level ▽

  ✓6ᵗʰ **S56.31** **Strain of extensor or abductor muscles, fascia and tendons of thumb at forearm level**

    ✓7ᵗʰ **S56.311** Strain of extensor or abductor muscles, fascia and tendons of right thumb at forearm level

    ✓7ᵗʰ **S56.312** Strain of extensor or abductor muscles, fascia and tendons of left thumb at forearm level

    ✓7ᵗʰ **S56.319** Strain of extensor or abductor muscles, fascia and tendons of unspecified thumb at forearm level ▽

  ✓6ᵗʰ **S56.32** **Laceration of extensor or abductor muscles, fascia and tendons of thumb at forearm level**

    ✓7ᵗʰ **S56.321** Laceration of extensor or abductor muscles, fascia and tendons of right thumb at forearm level

    ✓7ᵗʰ **S56.322** Laceration of extensor or abductor muscles, fascia and tendons of left thumb at forearm level

    ✓7ᵗʰ **S56.329** Laceration of extensor or abductor muscles, fascia and tendons of unspecified thumb at forearm level ▽

  ✓6ᵗʰ **S56.39** **Other injury of extensor or abductor muscles, fascia and tendons of thumb at forearm level**

    ✓7ᵗʰ **S56.391** Other injury of extensor or abductor muscles, fascia and tendons of right thumb at forearm level

    ✓7ᵗʰ **S56.392** Other injury of extensor or abductor muscles, fascia and tendons of left thumb at forearm level

    ✓7ᵗʰ **S56.399** Other injury of extensor or abductor muscles, fascia and tendons of unspecified thumb at forearm level ▽

✓5ᵗʰ **S56.4** **Injury of extensor muscle, fascia and tendon of other and unspecified finger at forearm level**

  ✓6ᵗʰ **S56.40** **Unspecified injury of extensor muscle, fascia and tendon of other and unspecified finger at forearm level**

    ✓7ᵗʰ **S56.401** Unspecified injury of extensor muscle, fascia and tendon of right index finger at forearm level ▽

    ✓7ᵗʰ **S56.402** Unspecified injury of extensor muscle, fascia and tendon of left index finger at forearm level ▽

    ✓7ᵗʰ **S56.403** Unspecified injury of extensor muscle, fascia and tendon of right middle finger at forearm level ▽

    ✓7ᵗʰ **S56.404** Unspecified injury of extensor muscle, fascia and tendon of left middle finger at forearm level ▽

    ✓7ᵗʰ **S56.405** Unspecified injury of extensor muscle, fascia and tendon of right ring finger at forearm level ▽

    ✓7ᵗʰ **S56.406** Unspecified injury of extensor muscle, fascia and tendon of left ring finger at forearm level ▽

    ✓7ᵗʰ **S56.407** Unspecified injury of extensor muscle, fascia and tendon of right little finger at forearm level ▽

    ✓7ᵗʰ **S56.408** Unspecified injury of extensor muscle, fascia and tendon of left little finger at forearm level ▽

    ✓7ᵗʰ **S56.409** Unspecified injury of extensor muscle, fascia and tendon of unspecified finger at forearm level ▽

✓6ᵗʰ **S56.41** **Strain of extensor muscle, fascia and tendon of other and unspecified finger at forearm level**

    ✓7ᵗʰ **S56.411** Strain of extensor muscle, fascia and tendon of right index finger at forearm level

    ✓7ᵗʰ **S56.412** Strain of extensor muscle, fascia and tendon of left index finger at forearm level

    ✓7ᵗʰ **S56.413** Strain of extensor muscle, fascia and tendon of right middle finger at forearm level

    ✓7ᵗʰ **S56.414** Strain of extensor muscle, fascia and tendon of left middle finger at forearm level

    ✓7ᵗʰ **S56.415** Strain of extensor muscle, fascia and tendon of right ring finger at forearm level

    ✓7ᵗʰ **S56.416** Strain of extensor muscle, fascia and tendon of left ring finger at forearm level

    ✓7ᵗʰ **S56.417** Strain of extensor muscle, fascia and tendon of right little finger at forearm level

    ✓7ᵗʰ **S56.418** Strain of extensor muscle, fascia and tendon of left little finger at forearm level

    ✓7ᵗʰ **S56.419** Strain of extensor muscle, fascia and tendon of finger, unspecified finger at forearm level ▽

  ✓6ᵗʰ **S56.42** **Laceration of extensor muscle, fascia and tendon of other and unspecified finger at forearm level**

    ✓7ᵗʰ **S56.421** Laceration of extensor muscle, fascia and tendon of right index finger at forearm level

    ✓7ᵗʰ **S56.422** Laceration of extensor muscle, fascia and tendon of left index finger at forearm level

    ✓7ᵗʰ **S56.423** Laceration of extensor muscle, fascia and tendon of right middle finger at forearm level

    ✓7ᵗʰ **S56.424** Laceration of extensor muscle, fascia and tendon of left middle finger at forearm level

    ✓7ᵗʰ **S56.425** Laceration of extensor muscle, fascia and tendon of right ring finger at forearm level

    ✓7ᵗʰ **S56.426** Laceration of extensor muscle, fascia and tendon of left ring finger at forearm level

    ✓7ᵗʰ **S56.427** Laceration of extensor muscle, fascia and tendon of right little finger at forearm level

    ✓7ᵗʰ **S56.428** Laceration of extensor muscle, fascia and tendon of left little finger at forearm level

    ✓7ᵗʰ **S56.429** Laceration of extensor muscle, fascia and tendon of unspecified finger at forearm level ▽

  ✓6ᵗʰ **S56.49** **Other injury of extensor muscle, fascia and tendon of other and unspecified finger at forearm level**

    ✓7ᵗʰ **S56.491** Other injury of extensor muscle, fascia and tendon of right index finger at forearm level

    ✓7ᵗʰ **S56.492** Other injury of extensor muscle, fascia and tendon of left index finger at forearm level

    ✓7ᵗʰ **S56.493** Other injury of extensor muscle, fascia and tendon of right middle finger at forearm level

    ✓7ᵗʰ **S56.494** Other injury of extensor muscle, fascia and tendon of left middle finger at forearm level

    ✓7ᵗʰ **S56.495** Other injury of extensor muscle, fascia and tendon of right ring finger at forearm level

    ✓7ᵗʰ **S56.496** Other injury of extensor muscle, fascia and tendon of left ring finger at forearm level

    ✓7ᵗʰ **S56.497** Other injury of extensor muscle, fascia and tendon of right little finger at forearm level

    ✓7ᵗʰ **S56.498** Other injury of extensor muscle, fascia and tendon of left little finger at forearm level

    ✓7ᵗʰ **S56.499** Other injury of extensor muscle, fascia and tendon of unspecified finger at forearm level ▽

EXCLUDES 1 Not coded here   **EXCLUDES 2** Not included here   **N** Newborn Age: 0   **P** Pediatric Age: 0-17   **M** Maternity Age: 12-55   **A** Adult Age: 15-124

974   ICD-10-CM 2018

✓5ᵗʰ **S56.5**   **Injury of other extensor muscle, fascia and tendon at forearm level**

    ✓6ᵗʰ **S56.50**   **Unspecified injury of other extensor muscle, fascia and tendon at forearm level**

       ✓7ᵗʰ **S56.501**   **Unspecified injury of other extensor muscle, fascia and tendon at forearm level, right arm** ▽

       ✓7ᵗʰ **S56.502**   **Unspecified injury of other extensor muscle, fascia and tendon at forearm level, left arm** ▽

       ✓7ᵗʰ **S56.509**   **Unspecified injury of other extensor muscle, fascia and tendon at forearm level, unspecified arm** ▽

    ✓6ᵗʰ **S56.51**   **Strain of other extensor muscle, fascia and tendon at forearm level**

       ✓7ᵗʰ **S56.511**   **Strain of other extensor muscle, fascia and tendon at forearm level, right arm**

       ✓7ᵗʰ **S56.512**   **Strain of other extensor muscle, fascia and tendon at forearm level, left arm**

       ✓7ᵗʰ **S56.519**   **Strain of other extensor muscle, fascia and tendon at forearm level, unspecified arm** ▽

    ✓6ᵗʰ **S56.52**   **Laceration of other extensor muscle, fascia and tendon at forearm level**

       ✓7ᵗʰ **S56.521**   **Laceration of other extensor muscle, fascia and tendon at forearm level, right arm**

       ✓7ᵗʰ **S56.522**   **Laceration of other extensor muscle, fascia and tendon at forearm level, left arm**

       ✓7ᵗʰ **S56.529**   **Laceration of other extensor muscle, fascia and tendon at forearm level, unspecified arm** ▽

    ✓6ᵗʰ **S56.59**   **Other injury of other extensor muscle, fascia and tendon at forearm level**

       ✓7ᵗʰ **S56.591**   **Other injury of other extensor muscle, fascia and tendon at forearm level, right arm**

       ✓7ᵗʰ **S56.592**   **Other injury of other extensor muscle, fascia and tendon at forearm level, left arm**

       ✓7ᵗʰ **S56.599**   **Other injury of other extensor muscle, fascia and tendon at forearm level, unspecified arm** ▽

✓5ᵗʰ **S56.8**   **Injury of other muscles, fascia and tendons at forearm level**

    ✓6ᵗʰ **S56.80**   **Unspecified injury of other muscles, fascia and tendons at forearm level**

       ✓7ᵗʰ **S56.801**   **Unspecified injury of other muscles, fascia and tendons at forearm level, right arm** ▽

       ✓7ᵗʰ **S56.802**   **Unspecified injury of other muscles, fascia and tendons at forearm level, left arm** ▽

       ✓7ᵗʰ **S56.809**   **Unspecified injury of other muscles, fascia and tendons at forearm level, unspecified arm** ▽

    ✓6ᵗʰ **S56.81**   **Strain of other muscles, fascia and tendons at forearm level**

       ✓7ᵗʰ **S56.811**   **Strain of other muscles, fascia and tendons at forearm level, right arm**

       ✓7ᵗʰ **S56.812**   **Strain of other muscles, fascia and tendons at forearm level, left arm**

       ✓7ᵗʰ **S56.819**   **Strain of other muscles, fascia and tendons at forearm level, unspecified arm** ▽

    ✓6ᵗʰ **S56.82**   **Laceration of other muscles, fascia and tendons at forearm level**

       ✓7ᵗʰ **S56.821**   **Laceration of other muscles, fascia and tendons at forearm level, right arm**

       ✓7ᵗʰ **S56.822**   **Laceration of other muscles, fascia and tendons at forearm level, left arm**

       ✓7ᵗʰ **S56.829**   **Laceration of other muscles, fascia and tendons at forearm level, unspecified arm** ▽

    ✓6ᵗʰ **S56.89**   **Other injury of other muscles, fascia and tendons at forearm level**

       ✓7ᵗʰ **S56.891**   **Other injury of other muscles, fascia and tendons at forearm level, right arm**

       ✓7ᵗʰ **S56.892**   **Other injury of other muscles, fascia and tendons at forearm level, left arm**

       ✓7ᵗʰ **S56.899**   **Other injury of other muscles, fascia and tendons at forearm level, unspecified arm** ▽

✓5ᵗʰ **S56.9**   **Injury of unspecified muscles, fascia and tendons at forearm level**

    ✓6ᵗʰ **S56.90**   **Unspecified injury of unspecified muscles, fascia and tendons at forearm level**

       ✓7ᵗʰ **S56.901**   **Unspecified injury of unspecified muscles, fascia and tendons at forearm level, right arm** ▽

       ✓7ᵗʰ **S56.902**   **Unspecified injury of unspecified muscles, fascia and tendons at forearm level, left arm** ▽

       ✓7ᵗʰ **S56.909**   **Unspecified injury of unspecified muscles, fascia and tendons at forearm level, unspecified arm** ▽

    ✓6ᵗʰ **S56.91**   **Strain of unspecified muscles, fascia and tendons at forearm level**

       ✓7ᵗʰ **S56.911**   **Strain of unspecified muscles, fascia and tendons at forearm level, right arm** ▽

       ✓7ᵗʰ **S56.912**   **Strain of unspecified muscles, fascia and tendons at forearm level, left arm** ▽

       ✓7ᵗʰ **S56.919**   **Strain of unspecified muscles, fascia and tendons at forearm level, unspecified arm** ▽

    ✓6ᵗʰ **S56.92**   **Laceration of unspecified muscles, fascia and tendons at forearm level**

       ✓7ᵗʰ **S56.921**   **Laceration of unspecified muscles, fascia and tendons at forearm level, right arm** ▽

       ✓7ᵗʰ **S56.922**   **Laceration of unspecified muscles, fascia and tendons at forearm level, left arm** ▽

       ✓7ᵗʰ **S56.929**   **Laceration of unspecified muscles, fascia and tendons at forearm level, unspecified arm** ▽

    ✓6ᵗʰ **S56.99**   **Other injury of unspecified muscles, fascia and tendons at forearm level**

       ✓7ᵗʰ **S56.991**   **Other injury of unspecified muscles, fascia and tendons at forearm level, right arm** ▽

       ✓7ᵗʰ **S56.992**   **Other injury of unspecified muscles, fascia and tendons at forearm level, left arm** ▽

       ✓7ᵗʰ **S56.999**   **Other injury of unspecified muscles, fascia and tendons at forearm level, unspecified arm** ▽

✓4ᵗʰ **S57**   **Crushing injury of elbow and forearm**

    Use additional code(s) for all associated injuries

    EXCLUDES 2   *crushing injury of wrist and hand (S67.-)*

    The appropriate 7th character is to be added to each code from category S57.
    A   initial encounter
    D   subsequent encounter
    S   sequela

    ✓5ᵗʰ **S57.0**   **Crushing injury of elbow**

       ✓x7ᵗʰ **S57.00**   **Crushing injury of unspecified elbow** ▽

       ✓x7ᵗʰ **S57.01**   **Crushing injury of right elbow**

       ✓x7ᵗʰ **S57.02**   **Crushing injury of left elbow**

    ✓5ᵗʰ **S57.8**   **Crushing injury of forearm**

       ✓x7ᵗʰ **S57.80**   **Crushing injury of unspecified forearm** ▽

       ✓x7ᵗʰ **S57.81**   **Crushing injury of right forearm**

       ✓x7ᵗʰ **S57.82**   **Crushing injury of left forearm**

☑ Additional Character Req   ✓x7ᵗʰ Placeholder Alert   Manifestation   HCC CMS-HCC Condition   ▽ Unspecified Code   ►◄ Revised Text   ● New Code   ▲ Revised Code Title

ICD-10-CM 2018   975

✓4ᵗʰ S58 Traumatic amputation of elbow and forearm

An amputation not identified as partial or complete should be coded to complete.

EXCLUDES 1   *traumatic amputation of wrist and hand (S68.-)*

The appropriate 7th character is to be added to each code from category S58.
A   initial encounter
D   subsequent encounter
S   sequela

✓5ᵗʰ S58.Ø Traumatic amputation at elbow level

   ✓6ᵗʰ S58.Ø1 Complete traumatic amputation at elbow level

     2 ✓7ᵗʰ **S58.Ø11 Complete traumatic amputation at elbow level, right arm** HCC

     2 ✓7ᵗʰ **S58.Ø12 Complete traumatic amputation at elbow level, left arm** HCC

     2 ✓7ᵗʰ **S58.Ø19 Complete traumatic amputation at elbow level, unspecified arm** HCC ▽

   ✓6ᵗʰ S58.Ø2 Partial traumatic amputation at elbow level

     2 ✓7ᵗʰ **S58.Ø21 Partial traumatic amputation at elbow level, right arm** HCC

     2 ✓7ᵗʰ **S58.Ø22 Partial traumatic amputation at elbow level, left arm** HCC

     2 ✓7ᵗʰ **S58.Ø29 Partial traumatic amputation at elbow level, unspecified arm** HCC ▽

✓5ᵗʰ S58.1 Traumatic amputation at level between elbow and wrist

   ✓6ᵗʰ S58.11 Complete traumatic amputation at level between elbow and wrist

     2 ✓7ᵗʰ **S58.111 Complete traumatic amputation at level between elbow and wrist, right arm** HCC

     2 ✓7ᵗʰ **S58.112 Complete traumatic amputation at level between elbow and wrist, left arm** HCC

     2 ✓7ᵗʰ **S58.119 Complete traumatic amputation at level between elbow and wrist, unspecified arm** HCC ▽

   ✓6ᵗʰ S58.12 Partial traumatic amputation at level between elbow and wrist

     2 ✓7ᵗʰ **S58.121 Partial traumatic amputation at level between elbow and wrist, right arm** HCC

     2 ✓7ᵗʰ **S58.122 Partial traumatic amputation at level between elbow and wrist, left arm** HCC

     2 ✓7ᵗʰ **S58.129 Partial traumatic amputation at level between elbow and wrist, unspecified arm** HCC ▽

✓5ᵗʰ S58.9 Traumatic amputation of forearm, level unspecified

EXCLUDES 1   *traumatic amputation of wrist (S68.-)*

   ✓6ᵗʰ S58.91 Complete traumatic amputation of forearm, level unspecified

     2 ✓7ᵗʰ **S58.911 Complete traumatic amputation of right forearm, level unspecified** HCC ▽

     2 ✓7ᵗʰ **S58.912 Complete traumatic amputation of left forearm, level unspecified** HCC ▽

     2 ✓7ᵗʰ **S58.919 Complete traumatic amputation of unspecified forearm, level unspecified** HCC ▽

   ✓6ᵗʰ S58.92 Partial traumatic amputation of forearm, level unspecified

     2 ✓7ᵗʰ **S58.921 Partial traumatic amputation of right forearm, level unspecified** HCC ▽

     2 ✓7ᵗʰ **S58.922 Partial traumatic amputation of left forearm, level unspecified** HCC ▽

     2 ✓7ᵗʰ **S58.929 Partial traumatic amputation of unspecified forearm, level unspecified** HCC ▽

✓4ᵗʰ S59 Other and unspecified injuries of elbow and forearm

EXCLUDES 2   *other and unspecified injuries of wrist and hand (S69.-)*

AHA: 2015, 3Q, 37-39

The appropriate 7th character is to be added to each code from subcategories S59.Ø, S59.1, and S59.2.
A   initial encounter for closed fracture
D   subsequent encounter for fracture with routine healing
G   subsequent encounter for fracture with delayed healing
K   subsequent encounter for fracture with nonunion
P   subsequent encounter for fracture with malunion
S   sequela

✓5ᵗʰ S59.Ø Physeal fracture of lower end of ulna

   ✓6ᵗʰ S59.ØØ Unspecified physeal fracture of lower end of ulna

     ✓7ᵗʰ **S59.ØØ1 Unspecified physeal fracture of lower end of ulna, right arm** ▽

     ✓7ᵗʰ **S59.ØØ2 Unspecified physeal fracture of lower end of ulna, left arm** ▽

     ✓7ᵗʰ **S59.ØØ9 Unspecified physeal fracture of lower end of ulna, unspecified arm** ▽

   ✓6ᵗʰ S59.Ø1 Salter-Harris Type I physeal fracture of lower end of ulna

     ✓7ᵗʰ **S59.Ø11 Salter-Harris Type I physeal fracture of lower end of ulna, right arm**

     ✓7ᵗʰ **S59.Ø12 Salter-Harris Type I physeal fracture of lower end of ulna, left arm**

     ✓7ᵗʰ **S59.Ø19 Salter-Harris Type I physeal fracture of lower end of ulna, unspecified arm** ▽

   ✓6ᵗʰ S59.Ø2 Salter-Harris Type II physeal fracture of lower end of ulna

     ✓7ᵗʰ **S59.Ø21 Salter-Harris Type II physeal fracture of lower end of ulna, right arm**

     ✓7ᵗʰ **S59.Ø22 Salter-Harris Type II physeal fracture of lower end of ulna, left arm**

     ✓7ᵗʰ **S59.Ø29 Salter-Harris Type II physeal fracture of lower end of ulna, unspecified arm** ▽

   ✓6ᵗʰ S59.Ø3 Salter-Harris Type III physeal fracture of lower end of ulna

     ✓7ᵗʰ **S59.Ø31 Salter-Harris Type III physeal fracture of lower end of ulna, right arm**

     ✓7ᵗʰ **S59.Ø32 Salter-Harris Type III physeal fracture of lower end of ulna, left arm**

     ✓7ᵗʰ **S59.Ø39 Salter-Harris Type III physeal fracture of lower end of ulna, unspecified arm** ▽

   ✓6ᵗʰ S59.Ø4 Salter-Harris Type IV physeal fracture of lower end of ulna

     ✓7ᵗʰ **S59.Ø41 Salter-Harris Type IV physeal fracture of lower end of ulna, right arm**

     ✓7ᵗʰ **S59.Ø42 Salter-Harris Type IV physeal fracture of lower end of ulna, left arm**

     ✓7ᵗʰ **S59.Ø49 Salter-Harris Type IV physeal fracture of lower end of ulna, unspecified arm** ▽

   ✓6ᵗʰ S59.Ø9 Other physeal fracture of lower end of ulna

     ✓7ᵗʰ **S59.Ø91 Other physeal fracture of lower end of ulna, right arm**

     ✓7ᵗʰ **S59.Ø92 Other physeal fracture of lower end of ulna, left arm**

     ✓7ᵗʰ **S59.Ø99 Other physeal fracture of lower end of ulna, unspecified arm** ▽

✓5ᵗʰ S59.1 Physeal fracture of upper end of radius

   ✓6ᵗʰ S59.1Ø Unspecified physeal fracture of upper end of radius

     ✓7ᵗʰ **S59.1Ø1 Unspecified physeal fracture of upper end of radius, right arm** ▽

     ✓7ᵗʰ **S59.1Ø2 Unspecified physeal fracture of upper end of radius, left arm** ▽

     ✓7ᵗʰ **S59.1Ø9 Unspecified physeal fracture of upper end of radius, unspecified arm** ▽

   ✓6ᵗʰ S59.11 Salter-Harris Type I physeal fracture of upper end of radius

     ✓7ᵗʰ **S59.111 Salter-Harris Type I physeal fracture of upper end of radius, right arm**

     ✓7ᵗʰ **S59.112 Salter-Harris Type I physeal fracture of upper end of radius, left arm**

     ✓7ᵗʰ **S59.119 Salter-Harris Type I physeal fracture of upper end of radius, unspecified arm** ▽

---

2   HCC with 7th character indicating initial encounter (A or B - specific to category) OR sequela.

EXCLUDES 1 Not coded here   EXCLUDES 2 Not included here   N Newborn Age: 0   P Pediatric Age: 0-17   M Maternity Age: 12-55   A Adult Age: 15-124

976   ICD-10-CM 2018

√6ᵗʰ **S59.12** **Salter-Harris Type II physeal fracture of upper end of radius**

    √7ᵗʰ **S59.121** Salter-Harris Type II physeal fracture of upper end of radius, right arm

    √7ᵗʰ **S59.122** Salter-Harris Type II physeal fracture of upper end of radius, left arm

    √7ᵗʰ **S59.129** Salter-Harris Type II physeal fracture of upper end of radius, unspecified arm ▽

√6ᵗʰ **S59.13** **Salter-Harris Type III physeal fracture of upper end of radius**

    √7ᵗʰ **S59.131** Salter-Harris Type III physeal fracture of upper end of radius, right arm

    √7ᵗʰ **S59.132** Salter-Harris Type III physeal fracture of upper end of radius, left arm

    √7ᵗʰ **S59.139** Salter-Harris Type III physeal fracture of upper end of radius, unspecified arm ▽

√6ᵗʰ **S59.14** **Salter-Harris Type IV physeal fracture of upper end of radius**

    √7ᵗʰ **S59.141** Salter-Harris Type IV physeal fracture of upper end of radius, right arm

    √7ᵗʰ **S59.142** Salter-Harris Type IV physeal fracture of upper end of radius, left arm

    √7ᵗʰ **S59.149** Salter-Harris Type IV physeal fracture of upper end of radius, unspecified arm ▽

√6ᵗʰ **S59.19** **Other physeal fracture of upper end of radius**

    √7ᵗʰ **S59.191** Other physeal fracture of upper end of radius, right arm

    √7ᵗʰ **S59.192** Other physeal fracture of upper end of radius, left arm

    √7ᵗʰ **S59.199** Other physeal fracture of upper end of radius, unspecified arm ▽

√5ᵗʰ **S59.2** **Physeal fracture of lower end of radius**

√6ᵗʰ **S59.20** **Unspecified physeal fracture of lower end of radius**

    √7ᵗʰ **S59.201** Unspecified physeal fracture of lower end of radius, right arm ▽

    √7ᵗʰ **S59.202** Unspecified physeal fracture of lower end of radius, left arm ▽

    √7ᵗʰ **S59.209** Unspecified physeal fracture of lower end of radius, unspecified arm ▽

√6ᵗʰ **S59.21** **Salter-Harris Type I physeal fracture of lower end of radius**

    √7ᵗʰ **S59.211** Salter-Harris Type I physeal fracture of lower end of radius, right arm

    √7ᵗʰ **S59.212** Salter-Harris Type I physeal fracture of lower end of radius, left arm

    √7ᵗʰ **S59.219** Salter-Harris Type I physeal fracture of lower end of radius, unspecified arm ▽

√6ᵗʰ **S59.22** **Salter-Harris Type II physeal fracture of lower end of radius**

    √7ᵗʰ **S59.221** Salter-Harris Type II physeal fracture of lower end of radius, right arm

    √7ᵗʰ **S59.222** Salter-Harris Type II physeal fracture of lower end of radius, left arm

    √7ᵗʰ **S59.229** Salter-Harris Type II physeal fracture of lower end of radius, unspecified arm ▽

√6ᵗʰ **S59.23** **Salter-Harris Type III physeal fracture of lower end of radius**

    √7ᵗʰ **S59.231** Salter-Harris Type III physeal fracture of lower end of radius, right arm

    √7ᵗʰ **S59.232** Salter-Harris Type III physeal fracture of lower end of radius, left arm

    √7ᵗʰ **S59.239** Salter-Harris Type III physeal fracture of lower end of radius, unspecified arm ▽

√6ᵗʰ **S59.24** **Salter-Harris Type IV physeal fracture of lower end of radius**

    √7ᵗʰ **S59.241** Salter-Harris Type IV physeal fracture of lower end of radius, right arm

    √7ᵗʰ **S59.242** Salter-Harris Type IV physeal fracture of lower end of radius, left arm

    √7ᵗʰ **S59.249** Salter-Harris Type IV physeal fracture of lower end of radius, unspecified arm ▽

√6ᵗʰ **S59.29** **Other physeal fracture of lower end of radius**

    √7ᵗʰ **S59.291** Other physeal fracture of lower end of radius, right arm

√7ᵗʰ **S59.292** Other physeal fracture of lower end of radius, left arm

√7ᵗʰ **S59.299** Other physeal fracture of lower end of radius, unspecified arm ▽

√5ᵗʰ **S59.8** **Other specified injuries of elbow and forearm**

> The appropriate 7th character is to be added to each code in subcategory S59.8.
> A   initial encounter
> D   subsequent encounter
> S   sequela

√6ᵗʰ **S59.80** **Other specified injuries of elbow**

    √7ᵗʰ **S59.801** Other specified injuries of right elbow

    √7ᵗʰ **S59.802** Other specified injuries of left elbow

    √7ᵗʰ **S59.809** Other specified injuries of unspecified elbow ▽

√6ᵗʰ **S59.81** **Other specified injuries of forearm**

    √7ᵗʰ **S59.811** Other specified injuries right forearm

    √7ᵗʰ **S59.812** Other specified injuries left forearm

    √7ᵗʰ **S59.819** Other specified injuries unspecified forearm ▽

√5ᵗʰ **S59.9** **Unspecified injury of elbow and forearm**

> The appropriate 7th character is to be added to each code in subcategory S59.9.
> A   initial encounter
> D   subsequent encounter
> S   sequela

√6ᵗʰ **S59.90** **Unspecified injury of elbow**

    √7ᵗʰ **S59.901** Unspecified injury of right elbow ▽

    √7ᵗʰ **S59.902** Unspecified injury of left elbow ▽

    √7ᵗʰ **S59.909** Unspecified injury of unspecified elbow ▽

√6ᵗʰ **S59.91** **Unspecified injury of forearm**

    √7ᵗʰ **S59.911** Unspecified injury of right forearm ▽

    √7ᵗʰ **S59.912** Unspecified injury of left forearm ▽

    √7ᵗʰ **S59.919** Unspecified injury of unspecified forearm ▽

Injuries to the wrist, hand and fingers (S60-S69)

EXCLUDES 2   *burns and corrosions (T20-T32)*
frostbite (T33-T34)
insect bite or sting, venomous (T63.4)

√4ᵗʰ **S60** **Superficial injury of wrist, hand and fingers**

> The appropriate 7th character is to be added to each code from category S60.
> A   initial encounter
> D   subsequent encounter
> S   sequela

√5ᵗʰ **S60.0** **Contusion of finger without damage to nail**

    EXCLUDES 1 *contusion involving nail (matrix) (S60.1)*

    √x7ᵗʰ **S60.00** **Contusion of unspecified finger without damage to nail** ▽
        Contusion of finger(s) NOS

    √6ᵗʰ **S60.01** **Contusion of thumb without damage to nail**

        √7ᵗʰ **S60.011** Contusion of right thumb without damage to nail

        √7ᵗʰ **S60.012** Contusion of left thumb without damage to nail

        √7ᵗʰ **S60.019** Contusion of unspecified thumb without damage to nail ▽

    √6ᵗʰ **S60.02** **Contusion of index finger without damage to nail**

        √7ᵗʰ **S60.021** Contusion of right index finger without damage to nail

        √7ᵗʰ **S60.022** Contusion of left index finger without damage to nail

        √7ᵗʰ **S60.029** Contusion of unspecified index finger without damage to nail ▽

    √6ᵗʰ **S60.03** **Contusion of middle finger without damage to nail**

        √7ᵗʰ **S60.031** Contusion of right middle finger without damage to nail

        √7ᵗʰ **S60.032** Contusion of left middle finger without damage to nail

---

☑ Additional Character Req   √x7ᵗʰ Placeholder Alert   Manifestation   HCC CMS-HCC Condition   ▽ Unspecified Code   ▶◀ Revised Text   ● New Code   ▲ Revised Code Title

✓7th **S60.039** Contusion of unspecified middle finger without damage to nail ▽

✓6th **S60.04** Contusion of ring finger without damage to nail
    ✓7th **S60.041** Contusion of right ring finger without damage to nail
    ✓7th **S60.042** Contusion of left ring finger without damage to nail
    ✓7th **S60.049** Contusion of unspecified ring finger without damage to nail ▽

✓6th **S60.05** Contusion of little finger without damage to nail
    ✓7th **S60.051** Contusion of right little finger without damage to nail
    ✓7th **S60.052** Contusion of left little finger without damage to nail
    ✓7th **S60.059** Contusion of unspecified little finger without damage to nail ▽

✓5th **S60.1** Contusion of finger with damage to nail
    ✓x7th **S60.10** Contusion of unspecified finger with damage to nail ▽
    ✓6th **S60.11** Contusion of thumb with damage to nail
      ✓7th **S60.111** Contusion of right thumb with damage to nail
      ✓7th **S60.112** Contusion of left thumb with damage to nail
      ✓7th **S60.119** Contusion of unspecified thumb with damage to nail ▽
    ✓6th **S60.12** Contusion of index finger with damage to nail
      ✓7th **S60.121** Contusion of right index finger with damage to nail
      ✓7th **S60.122** Contusion of left index finger with damage to nail
      ✓7th **S60.129** Contusion of unspecified index finger with damage to nail ▽
    ✓6th **S60.13** Contusion of middle finger with damage to nail
      ✓7th **S60.131** Contusion of right middle finger with damage to nail
      ✓7th **S60.132** Contusion of left middle finger with damage to nail
      ✓7th **S60.139** Contusion of unspecified middle finger with damage to nail ▽
    ✓6th **S60.14** Contusion of ring finger with damage to nail
      ✓7th **S60.141** Contusion of right ring finger with damage to nail
      ✓7th **S60.142** Contusion of left ring finger with damage to nail
      ✓7th **S60.149** Contusion of unspecified ring finger with damage to nail ▽
    ✓6th **S60.15** Contusion of little finger with damage to nail
      ✓7th **S60.151** Contusion of right little finger with damage to nail
      ✓7th **S60.152** Contusion of left little finger with damage to nail
      ✓7th **S60.159** Contusion of unspecified little finger with damage to nail ▽

✓5th **S60.2** Contusion of wrist and hand
    EXCLUDES 2   contusion of fingers (S60.0-, S60.1-)
    ✓6th **S60.21** Contusion of wrist
      ✓7th **S60.211** Contusion of right wrist
      ✓7th **S60.212** Contusion of left wrist
      ✓7th **S60.219** Contusion of unspecified wrist ▽
    ✓6th **S60.22** Contusion of hand
      ✓7th **S60.221** Contusion of right hand
      ✓7th **S60.222** Contusion of left hand
      ✓7th **S60.229** Contusion of unspecified hand ▽

✓5th **S60.3** Other superficial injuries of thumb
    ✓6th **S60.31** Abrasion of thumb
      ✓7th **S60.311** Abrasion of right thumb
      ✓7th **S60.312** Abrasion of left thumb
      ✓7th **S60.319** Abrasion of unspecified thumb ▽
    ✓6th **S60.32** Blister (nonthermal) of thumb
      ✓7th **S60.321** Blister (nonthermal) of right thumb
      ✓7th **S60.322** Blister (nonthermal) of left thumb

✓7th **S60.329** Blister (nonthermal) of unspecified thumb ▽

✓6th **S60.34** External constriction of thumb
    Hair tourniquet syndrome of thumb
    Use additional cause code to identify the constricting item (W49.0-)
    ✓7th **S60.341** External constriction of right thumb
    ✓7th **S60.342** External constriction of left thumb
    ✓7th **S60.349** External constriction of unspecified thumb ▽

✓6th **S60.35** Superficial foreign body of thumb
    Splinter in the thumb
    ✓7th **S60.351** Superficial foreign body of right thumb
    ✓7th **S60.352** Superficial foreign body of left thumb
    ✓7th **S60.359** Superficial foreign body of unspecified thumb ▽

✓6th **S60.36** Insect bite (nonvenomous) of thumb
    ✓7th **S60.361** Insect bite (nonvenomous) of right thumb
    ✓7th **S60.362** Insect bite (nonvenomous) of left thumb
    ✓7th **S60.369** Insect bite (nonvenomous) of unspecified thumb ▽

✓6th **S60.37** Other superficial bite of thumb
    EXCLUDES 1   open bite of thumb (S61.05-, S61.15-)
    ✓7th **S60.371** Other superficial bite of right thumb
    ✓7th **S60.372** Other superficial bite of left thumb
    ✓7th **S60.379** Other superficial bite of unspecified thumb ▽

✓6th **S60.39** Other superficial injuries of thumb
    ✓7th **S60.391** Other superficial injuries of right thumb
    ✓7th **S60.392** Other superficial injuries of left thumb
    ✓7th **S60.399** Other superficial injuries of unspecified thumb ▽

✓5th **S60.4** Other superficial injuries of other fingers
    ✓6th **S60.41** Abrasion of fingers
      ✓7th **S60.410** Abrasion of right index finger
      ✓7th **S60.411** Abrasion of left index finger
      ✓7th **S60.412** Abrasion of right middle finger
      ✓7th **S60.413** Abrasion of left middle finger
      ✓7th **S60.414** Abrasion of right ring finger
      ✓7th **S60.415** Abrasion of left ring finger
      ✓7th **S60.416** Abrasion of right little finger
      ✓7th **S60.417** Abrasion of left little finger
      ✓7th **S60.418** Abrasion of other finger
        Abrasion of specified finger with unspecified laterality
      ✓7th **S60.419** Abrasion of unspecified finger ▽
    ✓6th **S60.42** Blister (nonthermal) of fingers
      ✓7th **S60.420** Blister (nonthermal) of right index finger
      ✓7th **S60.421** Blister (nonthermal) of left index finger
      ✓7th **S60.422** Blister (nonthermal) of right middle finger
      ✓7th **S60.423** Blister (nonthermal) of left middle finger
      ✓7th **S60.424** Blister (nonthermal) of right ring finger
      ✓7th **S60.425** Blister (nonthermal) of left ring finger
      ✓7th **S60.426** Blister (nonthermal) of right little finger
      ✓7th **S60.427** Blister (nonthermal) of left little finger
      ✓7th **S60.428** Blister (nonthermal) of other finger
        Blister (nonthermal) of specified finger with unspecified laterality
      ✓7th **S60.429** Blister (nonthermal) of unspecified finger ▽
    ✓6th **S60.44** External constriction of fingers
    Hair tourniquet syndrome of finger
    Use additional cause code to identify the constricting item (W49.0-)
      ✓7th **S60.440** External constriction of right index finger
      ✓7th **S60.441** External constriction of left index finger
      ✓7th **S60.442** External constriction of right middle finger
      ✓7th **S60.443** External constriction of left middle finger
      ✓7th **S60.444** External constriction of right ring finger
      ✓7th **S60.445** External constriction of left ring finger

EXCLUDES 1 Not coded here   EXCLUDES 2 Not included here   N Newborn Age: 0   P Pediatric Age: 0-17   M Maternity Age: 12-55   A Adult Age: 15-124

978

ICD-10-CM 2018

√7th **S60.446** **External constriction of right little finger**

√7th **S60.447** **External constriction of left little finger**

√7th **S60.448** **External constriction of other finger**
External constriction of specified finger with unspecified laterality

√7th **S60.449** **External constriction of unspecified finger** ▽

√6th **S60.45** **Superficial foreign body of fingers**
Splinter in the finger(s)

√7th **S60.450** **Superficial foreign body of right index finger**

√7th **S60.451** **Superficial foreign body of left index finger**

√7th **S60.452** **Superficial foreign body of right middle finger**

√7th **S60.453** **Superficial foreign body of left middle finger**

√7th **S60.454** **Superficial foreign body of right ring finger**

√7th **S60.455** **Superficial foreign body of left ring finger**

√7th **S60.456** **Superficial foreign body of right little finger**

√7th **S60.457** **Superficial foreign body of left little finger**

√7th **S60.458** **Superficial foreign body of other finger**
Superficial foreign body of specified finger with unspecified laterality

√7th **S60.459** **Superficial foreign body of unspecified finger** ▽

√6th **S60.46** **Insect bite (nonvenomous) of fingers**

√7th **S60.460** **Insect bite (nonvenomous) of right index finger**

√7th **S60.461** **Insect bite (nonvenomous) of left index finger**

√7th **S60.462** **Insect bite (nonvenomous) of right middle finger**

√7th **S60.463** **Insect bite (nonvenomous) of left middle finger**

√7th **S60.464** **Insect bite (nonvenomous) of right ring finger**

√7th **S60.465** **Insect bite (nonvenomous) of left ring finger**

√7th **S60.466** **Insect bite (nonvenomous) of right little finger**

√7th **S60.467** **Insect bite (nonvenomous) of left little finger**

√7th **S60.468** **Insect bite (nonvenomous) of other finger**
Insect bite (nonvenomous) of specified finger with unspecified laterality

√7th **S60.469** **Insect bite (nonvenomous) of unspecified finger** ▽

√6th **S60.47** **Other superficial bite of fingers**
EXCLUDES 1   *open bite of fingers (S61.25-, S61.35-)*

√7th **S60.470** **Other superficial bite of right index finger**

√7th **S60.471** **Other superficial bite of left index finger**

√7th **S60.472** **Other superficial bite of right middle finger**

√7th **S60.473** **Other superficial bite of left middle finger**

√7th **S60.474** **Other superficial bite of right ring finger**

√7th **S60.475** **Other superficial bite of left ring finger**

√7th **S60.476** **Other superficial bite of right little finger**

√7th **S60.477** **Other superficial bite of left little finger**

√7th **S60.478** **Other superficial bite of other finger**
Other superficial bite of specified finger with unspecified laterality

√7th **S60.479** **Other superficial bite of unspecified finger** ▽

√5th **S60.5** **Other superficial injuries of hand**
EXCLUDES 2   *superficial injuries of fingers (S60.3-, S60.4-)*

√6th **S60.51** **Abrasion of hand**

√7th **S60.511** **Abrasion of right hand**

√7th **S60.512** **Abrasion of left hand**

√7th **S60.519** **Abrasion of unspecified hand** ▽

√6th **S60.52** **Blister (nonthermal) of hand**

√7th **S60.521** **Blister (nonthermal) of right hand**

√7th **S60.522** **Blister (nonthermal) of left hand**

√7th **S60.529** **Blister (nonthermal) of unspecified hand** ▽

√6th **S60.54** **External constriction of hand**

√7th **S60.541** **External constriction of right hand**

√7th **S60.542** **External constriction of left hand**

√7th **S60.549** **External constriction of unspecified hand** ▽

√6th **S60.55** **Superficial foreign body of hand**
Splinter in the hand

√7th **S60.551** **Superficial foreign body of right hand**

√7th **S60.552** **Superficial foreign body of left hand**

√7th **S60.559** **Superficial foreign body of unspecified hand** ▽

√6th **S60.56** **Insect bite (nonvenomous) of hand**

√7th **S60.561** **Insect bite (nonvenomous) of right hand**

√7th **S60.562** **Insect bite (nonvenomous) of left hand**

√7th **S60.569** **Insect bite (nonvenomous) of unspecified hand** ▽

√6th **S60.57** **Other superficial bite of hand**
EXCLUDES 1   *open bite of hand (S61.45-)*

√7th **S60.571** **Other superficial bite of hand of right hand**

√7th **S60.572** **Other superficial bite of hand of left hand**

√7th **S60.579** **Other superficial bite of hand of unspecified hand** ▽

√5th **S60.8** **Other superficial injuries of wrist**

√6th **S60.81** **Abrasion of wrist**

√7th **S60.811** **Abrasion of right wrist**

√7th **S60.812** **Abrasion of left wrist**

√7th **S60.819** **Abrasion of unspecified wrist** ▽

√6th **S60.82** **Blister (nonthermal) of wrist**

√7th **S60.821** **Blister (nonthermal) of right wrist**

√7th **S60.822** **Blister (nonthermal) of left wrist**

√7th **S60.829** **Blister (nonthermal) of unspecified wrist** ▽

√6th **S60.84** **External constriction of wrist**

√7th **S60.841** **External constriction of right wrist**

√7th **S60.842** **External constriction of left wrist**

√7th **S60.849** **External constriction of unspecified wrist** ▽

√6th **S60.85** **Superficial foreign body of wrist**
Splinter in the wrist

√7th **S60.851** **Superficial foreign body of right wrist**

√7th **S60.852** **Superficial foreign body of left wrist**

√7th **S60.859** **Superficial foreign body of unspecified wrist** ▽

√6th **S60.86** **Insect bite (nonvenomous) of wrist**

√7th **S60.861** **Insect bite (nonvenomous) of right wrist**

√7th **S60.862** **Insect bite (nonvenomous) of left wrist**

√7th **S60.869** **Insect bite (nonvenomous) of unspecified wrist** ▽

√6th **S60.87** **Other superficial bite of wrist**
EXCLUDES 1   *open bite of wrist (S61.55)*

√7th **S60.871** **Other superficial bite of right wrist**

√7th **S60.872** **Other superficial bite of left wrist**

√7th **S60.879** **Other superficial bite of unspecified wrist** ▽

√5th **S60.9** **Unspecified superficial injury of wrist, hand and fingers**

√6th **S60.91** **Unspecified superficial injury of wrist**

√7th **S60.911** **Unspecified superficial injury of right wrist** ▽

√7th **S60.912** **Unspecified superficial injury of left wrist** ▽

√7th **S60.919** **Unspecified superficial injury of unspecified wrist** ▽

√6th **S60.92** **Unspecified superficial injury of hand**

√7th **S60.921** **Unspecified superficial injury of right hand** ▽

☑ Additional Character Req   √x7th Placeholder Alert   Manifestation   HCC CMS-HCC Condition   ▽ Unspecified Code   ►◄ Revised Text   ● New Code   ▲ Revised Code Title

√7ᵗʰ **S60.922** Unspecified superficial injury of left hand ▽

√7ᵗʰ **S60.929** Unspecified superficial injury of unspecified hand ▽

√6ᵗʰ **S60.93** **Unspecified superficial injury of thumb**

√7ᵗʰ **S60.931** Unspecified superficial injury of right thumb ▽

√7ᵗʰ **S60.932** Unspecified superficial injury of left thumb ▽

√7ᵗʰ **S60.939** Unspecified superficial injury of unspecified thumb ▽

√6ᵗʰ **S60.94** **Unspecified superficial injury of other fingers**

√7ᵗʰ **S60.940** Unspecified superficial injury of right index finger ▽

√7ᵗʰ **S60.941** Unspecified superficial injury of left index finger ▽

√7ᵗʰ **S60.942** Unspecified superficial injury of right middle finger ▽

√7ᵗʰ **S60.943** Unspecified superficial injury of left middle finger ▽

√7ᵗʰ **S60.944** Unspecified superficial injury of right ring finger ▽

√7ᵗʰ **S60.945** Unspecified superficial injury of left ring finger ▽

√7ᵗʰ **S60.946** Unspecified superficial injury of right little finger ▽

√7ᵗʰ **S60.947** Unspecified superficial injury of left little finger ▽

√7ᵗʰ **S60.948** Unspecified superficial injury of other finger ▽
Unspecified superficial injury of specified finger with unspecified laterality

√7ᵗʰ **S60.949** Unspecified superficial injury of unspecified finger ▽

√4ᵗʰ **S61** **Open wound of wrist, hand and fingers**
Code also any associated wound infection
EXCLUDES 1 open fracture of wrist, hand and finger (S62- with 7th character B)
traumatic amputation of wrist and hand (S68.-)

> The appropriate 7th character is to be added to each code from category S61.
> A   initial encounter
> D   subsequent encounter
> S   sequela

√5ᵗʰ **S61.0** **Open wound of thumb without damage to nail**
EXCLUDES 1 open wound of thumb with damage to nail (S61.1-)

√6ᵗʰ **S61.00** **Unspecified open wound of thumb without damage to nail**

√7ᵗʰ **S61.001** Unspecified open wound of right thumb without damage to nail ▽

√7ᵗʰ **S61.002** Unspecified open wound of left thumb without damage to nail ▽

√7ᵗʰ **S61.009** Unspecified open wound of unspecified thumb without damage to nail ▽

√6ᵗʰ **S61.01** **Laceration without foreign body of thumb without damage to nail**

√7ᵗʰ **S61.011** Laceration without foreign body of right thumb without damage to nail

√7ᵗʰ **S61.012** Laceration without foreign body of left thumb without damage to nail

√7ᵗʰ **S61.019** Laceration without foreign body of unspecified thumb without damage to nail ▽

√6ᵗʰ **S61.02** **Laceration with foreign body of thumb without damage to nail**

√7ᵗʰ **S61.021** Laceration with foreign body of right thumb without damage to nail

√7ᵗʰ **S61.022** Laceration with foreign body of left thumb without damage to nail

√7ᵗʰ **S61.029** Laceration with foreign body of unspecified thumb without damage to nail ▽

√6ᵗʰ **S61.03** **Puncture wound without foreign body of thumb without damage to nail**

√7ᵗʰ **S61.031** Puncture wound without foreign body of right thumb without damage to nail

√7ᵗʰ **S61.032** Puncture wound without foreign body of left thumb without damage to nail

√7ᵗʰ **S61.039** Puncture wound without foreign body of unspecified thumb without damage to nail ▽

√6ᵗʰ **S61.04** **Puncture wound with foreign body of thumb without damage to nail**

√7ᵗʰ **S61.041** Puncture wound with foreign body of right thumb without damage to nail

√7ᵗʰ **S61.042** Puncture wound with foreign body of left thumb without damage to nail

√7ᵗʰ **S61.049** Puncture wound with foreign body of unspecified thumb without damage to nail ▽

√6ᵗʰ **S61.05** **Open bite of thumb without damage to nail**
Bite of thumb NOS
EXCLUDES 1 superficial bite of thumb (S60.36-, S60.37-)

√7ᵗʰ **S61.051** Open bite of right thumb without damage to nail

√7ᵗʰ **S61.052** Open bite of left thumb without damage to nail

√7ᵗʰ **S61.059** Open bite of unspecified thumb without damage to nail ▽

√5ᵗʰ **S61.1** **Open wound of thumb with damage to nail**

√6ᵗʰ **S61.10** **Unspecified open wound of thumb with damage to nail**

√7ᵗʰ **S61.101** Unspecified open wound of right thumb with damage to nail ▽

√7ᵗʰ **S61.102** Unspecified open wound of left thumb with damage to nail ▽

√7ᵗʰ **S61.109** Unspecified open wound of unspecified thumb with damage to nail ▽

√6ᵗʰ **S61.11** **Laceration without foreign body of thumb with damage to nail**

√7ᵗʰ **S61.111** Laceration without foreign body of right thumb with damage to nail

√7ᵗʰ **S61.112** Laceration without foreign body of left thumb with damage to nail

√7ᵗʰ **S61.119** Laceration without foreign body of unspecified thumb with damage to nail ▽

√6ᵗʰ **S61.12** **Laceration with foreign body of thumb with damage to nail**

√7ᵗʰ **S61.121** Laceration with foreign body of right thumb with damage to nail

√7ᵗʰ **S61.122** Laceration with foreign body of left thumb with damage to nail

√7ᵗʰ **S61.129** Laceration with foreign body of unspecified thumb with damage to nail ▽

√6ᵗʰ **S61.13** **Puncture wound without foreign body of thumb with damage to nail**

√7ᵗʰ **S61.131** Puncture wound without foreign body of right thumb with damage to nail

√7ᵗʰ **S61.132** Puncture wound without foreign body of left thumb with damage to nail

√7ᵗʰ **S61.139** Puncture wound without foreign body of unspecified thumb with damage to nail ▽

√6ᵗʰ **S61.14** **Puncture wound with foreign body of thumb with damage to nail**

√7ᵗʰ **S61.141** Puncture wound with foreign body of right thumb with damage to nail

√7ᵗʰ **S61.142** Puncture wound with foreign body of left thumb with damage to nail

√7ᵗʰ **S61.149** Puncture wound with foreign body of unspecified thumb with damage to nail ▽

√6ᵗʰ **S61.15** **Open bite of thumb with damage to nail**
Bite of thumb with damage to nail NOS
EXCLUDES 1 superficial bite of thumb (S60.36-, S60.37-)

√7ᵗʰ **S61.151** Open bite of right thumb with damage to nail

√7ᵗʰ **S61.152** Open bite of left thumb with damage to nail

√7ᵗʰ **S61.159** **Open bite of unspecified thumb with damage to nail** ▽

√5ᵗʰ **S61.2** **Open wound of other finger without damage to nail**
> EXCLUDES 1   *open wound of finger involving nail (matrix) (S61.3-)*
> EXCLUDES 2   *open wound of thumb without damage to nail (S61.0-)*

√6ᵗʰ **S61.20** **Unspecified open wound of other finger without damage to nail**

√7ᵗʰ **S61.200** **Unspecified open wound of right index finger without damage to nail** ▽

√7ᵗʰ **S61.201** **Unspecified open wound of left index finger without damage to nail** ▽

√7ᵗʰ **S61.202** **Unspecified open wound of right middle finger without damage to nail** ▽

√7ᵗʰ **S61.203** **Unspecified open wound of left middle finger without damage to nail** ▽

√7ᵗʰ **S61.204** **Unspecified open wound of right ring finger without damage to nail** ▽

√7ᵗʰ **S61.205** **Unspecified open wound of left ring finger without damage to nail** ▽

√7ᵗʰ **S61.206** **Unspecified open wound of right little finger without damage to nail** ▽

√7ᵗʰ **S61.207** **Unspecified open wound of left little finger without damage to nail** ▽

√7ᵗʰ **S61.208** **Unspecified open wound of other finger without damage to nail** ▽
> Unspecified open wound of specified finger with unspecified laterality without damage to nail

√7ᵗʰ **S61.209** **Unspecified open wound of unspecified finger without damage to nail** ▽

√6ᵗʰ **S61.21** **Laceration without foreign body of finger without damage to nail**

√7ᵗʰ **S61.210** **Laceration without foreign body of right index finger without damage to nail**

√7ᵗʰ **S61.211** **Laceration without foreign body of left index finger without damage to nail**

√7ᵗʰ **S61.212** **Laceration without foreign body of right middle finger without damage to nail**

√7ᵗʰ **S61.213** **Laceration without foreign body of left middle finger without damage to nail**

√7ᵗʰ **S61.214** **Laceration without foreign body of right ring finger without damage to nail**

√7ᵗʰ **S61.215** **Laceration without foreign body of left ring finger without damage to nail**

√7ᵗʰ **S61.216** **Laceration without foreign body of right little finger without damage to nail**

√7ᵗʰ **S61.217** **Laceration without foreign body of left little finger without damage to nail**

√7ᵗʰ **S61.218** **Laceration without foreign body of other finger without damage to nail**
> Laceration without foreign body of specified finger with unspecified laterality without damage to nail

√7ᵗʰ **S61.219** **Laceration without foreign body of unspecified finger without damage to nail** ▽

√6ᵗʰ **S61.22** **Laceration with foreign body of finger without damage to nail**

√7ᵗʰ **S61.220** **Laceration with foreign body of right index finger without damage to nail**

√7ᵗʰ **S61.221** **Laceration with foreign body of left index finger without damage to nail**

√7ᵗʰ **S61.222** **Laceration with foreign body of right middle finger without damage to nail**

√7ᵗʰ **S61.223** **Laceration with foreign body of left middle finger without damage to nail**

√7ᵗʰ **S61.224** **Laceration with foreign body of right ring finger without damage to nail**

√7ᵗʰ **S61.225** **Laceration with foreign body of left ring finger without damage to nail**

√7ᵗʰ **S61.226** **Laceration with foreign body of right little finger without damage to nail**

√7ᵗʰ **S61.227** **Laceration with foreign body of left little finger without damage to nail**

√7ᵗʰ **S61.228** **Laceration with foreign body of other finger without damage to nail**
> Laceration with foreign body of specified finger with unspecified laterality without damage to nail

√7ᵗʰ **S61.229** **Laceration with foreign body of unspecified finger without damage to nail** ▽

√6ᵗʰ **S61.23** **Puncture wound without foreign body of finger without damage to nail**

√7ᵗʰ **S61.230** **Puncture wound without foreign body of right index finger without damage to nail**

√7ᵗʰ **S61.231** **Puncture wound without foreign body of left index finger without damage to nail**

√7ᵗʰ **S61.232** **Puncture wound without foreign body of right middle finger without damage to nail**

√7ᵗʰ **S61.233** **Puncture wound without foreign body of left middle finger without damage to nail**

√7ᵗʰ **S61.234** **Puncture wound without foreign body of right ring finger without damage to nail**

√7ᵗʰ **S61.235** **Puncture wound without foreign body of left ring finger without damage to nail**

√7ᵗʰ **S61.236** **Puncture wound without foreign body of right little finger without damage to nail**

√7ᵗʰ **S61.237** **Puncture wound without foreign body of left little finger without damage to nail**

√7ᵗʰ **S61.238** **Puncture wound without foreign body of other finger without damage to nail**
> Puncture wound without foreign body of specified finger with unspecified laterality without damage to nail

√7ᵗʰ **S61.239** **Puncture wound without foreign body of unspecified finger without damage to nail** ▽

√6ᵗʰ **S61.24** **Puncture wound with foreign body of finger without damage to nail**

√7ᵗʰ **S61.240** **Puncture wound with foreign body of right index finger without damage to nail**

√7ᵗʰ **S61.241** **Puncture wound with foreign body of left index finger without damage to nail**

√7ᵗʰ **S61.242** **Puncture wound with foreign body of right middle finger without damage to nail**

√7ᵗʰ **S61.243** **Puncture wound with foreign body of left middle finger without damage to nail**

√7ᵗʰ **S61.244** **Puncture wound with foreign body of right ring finger without damage to nail**

√7ᵗʰ **S61.245** **Puncture wound with foreign body of left ring finger without damage to nail**

√7ᵗʰ **S61.246** **Puncture wound with foreign body of right little finger without damage to nail**

√7ᵗʰ **S61.247** **Puncture wound with foreign body of left little finger without damage to nail**

√7ᵗʰ **S61.248** **Puncture wound with foreign body of other finger without damage to nail**
> Puncture wound with foreign body of specified finger with unspecified laterality without damage to nail

√7ᵗʰ **S61.249** **Puncture wound with foreign body of unspecified finger without damage to nail** ▽

√6ᵗʰ **S61.25** **Open bite of finger without damage to nail**
> Bite of finger without damage to nail NOS
> EXCLUDES 1   *superficial bite of finger (S60.46-, S60.47-)*

√7ᵗʰ **S61.250** **Open bite of right index finger without damage to nail**

√7ᵗʰ **S61.251** **Open bite of left index finger without damage to nail**

√7ᵗʰ **S61.252** **Open bite of right middle finger without damage to nail**

√7ᵗʰ **S61.253** **Open bite of left middle finger without damage to nail**

√7ᵗʰ **S61.254** **Open bite of right ring finger without damage to nail**

√7ᵗʰ **S61.255** **Open bite of left ring finger without damage to nail**

✓ Additional Character Req   √x7ᵗʰ Placeholder Alert   Manifestation   HCC CMS-HCC Condition   ▽ Unspecified Code   ▶◀ Revised Text   ● New Code   ▲ Revised Code Title

ICD-10-CM 2018   981

☑7ᵗʰ **S61.256 Open bite of right little finger without damage to nail**

☑7ᵗʰ **S61.257 Open bite of left little finger without damage to nail**

☑7ᵗʰ **S61.258 Open bite of other finger without damage to nail**
Open bite of specified finger with unspecified laterality without damage to nail

☑7ᵗʰ **S61.259 Open bite of unspecified finger without damage to nail** ▽

☑5ᵗʰ **S61.3 Open wound of other finger with damage to nail**

   ☑6ᵗʰ **S61.30 Unspecified open wound of finger with damage to nail**

      ☑7ᵗʰ **S61.300 Unspecified open wound of right index finger with damage to nail** ▽

      ☑7ᵗʰ **S61.301 Unspecified open wound of left index finger with damage to nail** ▽

      ☑7ᵗʰ **S61.302 Unspecified open wound of right middle finger with damage to nail** ▽

      ☑7ᵗʰ **S61.303 Unspecified open wound of left middle finger with damage to nail** ▽

      ☑7ᵗʰ **S61.304 Unspecified open wound of right ring finger with damage to nail** ▽

      ☑7ᵗʰ **S61.305 Unspecified open wound of left ring finger with damage to nail** ▽

      ☑7ᵗʰ **S61.306 Unspecified open wound of right little finger with damage to nail** ▽

      ☑7ᵗʰ **S61.307 Unspecified open wound of left little finger with damage to nail** ▽

      ☑7ᵗʰ **S61.308 Unspecified open wound of other finger with damage to nail** ▽
Unspecified open wound of specified finger with unspecified laterality with damage to nail

      ☑7ᵗʰ **S61.309 Unspecified open wound of unspecified finger with damage to nail** ▽

   ☑6ᵗʰ **S61.31 Laceration without foreign body of finger with damage to nail**

      ☑7ᵗʰ **S61.310 Laceration without foreign body of right index finger with damage to nail**

      ☑7ᵗʰ **S61.311 Laceration without foreign body of left index finger with damage to nail**

      ☑7ᵗʰ **S61.312 Laceration without foreign body of right middle finger with damage to nail**

      ☑7ᵗʰ **S61.313 Laceration without foreign body of left middle finger with damage to nail**

      ☑7ᵗʰ **S61.314 Laceration without foreign body of right ring finger with damage to nail**

      ☑7ᵗʰ **S61.315 Laceration without foreign body of left ring finger with damage to nail**

      ☑7ᵗʰ **S61.316 Laceration without foreign body of right little finger with damage to nail**

      ☑7ᵗʰ **S61.317 Laceration without foreign body of left little finger with damage to nail**

      ☑7ᵗʰ **S61.318 Laceration without foreign body of other finger with damage to nail**
Laceration without foreign body of specified finger with unspecified laterality with damage to nail

      ☑7ᵗʰ **S61.319 Laceration without foreign body of unspecified finger with damage to nail** ▽

   ☑6ᵗʰ **S61.32 Laceration with foreign body of finger with damage to nail**

      ☑7ᵗʰ **S61.320 Laceration with foreign body of right index finger with damage to nail**

      ☑7ᵗʰ **S61.321 Laceration with foreign body of left index finger with damage to nail**

      ☑7ᵗʰ **S61.322 Laceration with foreign body of right middle finger with damage to nail**

      ☑7ᵗʰ **S61.323 Laceration with foreign body of left middle finger with damage to nail**

      ☑7ᵗʰ **S61.324 Laceration with foreign body of right ring finger with damage to nail**

      ☑7ᵗʰ **S61.325 Laceration with foreign body of left ring finger with damage to nail**

☑7ᵗʰ **S61.326 Laceration with foreign body of right little finger with damage to nail**

☑7ᵗʰ **S61.327 Laceration with foreign body of left little finger with damage to nail**

☑7ᵗʰ **S61.328 Laceration with foreign body of other finger with damage to nail**
Laceration with foreign body of specified finger with unspecified laterality with damage to nail

☑7ᵗʰ **S61.329 Laceration with foreign body of unspecified finger with damage to nail** ▽

☑6ᵗʰ **S61.33 Puncture wound without foreign body of finger with damage to nail**

   ☑7ᵗʰ **S61.330 Puncture wound without foreign body of right index finger with damage to nail**

   ☑7ᵗʰ **S61.331 Puncture wound without foreign body of left index finger with damage to nail**

   ☑7ᵗʰ **S61.332 Puncture wound without foreign body of right middle finger with damage to nail**

   ☑7ᵗʰ **S61.333 Puncture wound without foreign body of left middle finger with damage to nail**

   ☑7ᵗʰ **S61.334 Puncture wound without foreign body of right ring finger with damage to nail**

   ☑7ᵗʰ **S61.335 Puncture wound without foreign body of left ring finger with damage to nail**

   ☑7ᵗʰ **S61.336 Puncture wound without foreign body of right little finger with damage to nail**

   ☑7ᵗʰ **S61.337 Puncture wound without foreign body of left little finger with damage to nail**

   ☑7ᵗʰ **S61.338 Puncture wound without foreign body of other finger with damage to nail**
Puncture wound without foreign body of specified finger with unspecified laterality with damage to nail

   ☑7ᵗʰ **S61.339 Puncture wound without foreign body of unspecified finger with damage to nail** ▽

☑6ᵗʰ **S61.34 Puncture wound with foreign body of finger with damage to nail**

   ☑7ᵗʰ **S61.340 Puncture wound with foreign body of right index finger with damage to nail**

   ☑7ᵗʰ **S61.341 Puncture wound with foreign body of left index finger with damage to nail**

   ☑7ᵗʰ **S61.342 Puncture wound with foreign body of right middle finger with damage to nail**

   ☑7ᵗʰ **S61.343 Puncture wound with foreign body of left middle finger with damage to nail**

   ☑7ᵗʰ **S61.344 Puncture wound with foreign body of right ring finger with damage to nail**

   ☑7ᵗʰ **S61.345 Puncture wound with foreign body of left ring finger with damage to nail**

   ☑7ᵗʰ **S61.346 Puncture wound with foreign body of right little finger with damage to nail**

   ☑7ᵗʰ **S61.347 Puncture wound with foreign body of left little finger with damage to nail**

   ☑7ᵗʰ **S61.348 Puncture wound with foreign body of other finger with damage to nail**
Puncture wound with foreign body of specified finger with unspecified laterality with damage to nail

   ☑7ᵗʰ **S61.349 Puncture wound with foreign body of unspecified finger with damage to nail** ▽

☑6ᵗʰ **S61.35 Open bite of finger with damage to nail**
Bite of finger with damage to nail NOS
EXCLUDES 1 superficial bite of finger (S60.46-, S60.47-)

   ☑7ᵗʰ **S61.350 Open bite of right index finger with damage to nail**

   ☑7ᵗʰ **S61.351 Open bite of left index finger with damage to nail**

   ☑7ᵗʰ **S61.352 Open bite of right middle finger with damage to nail**

   ☑7ᵗʰ **S61.353 Open bite of left middle finger with damage to nail**

   ☑7ᵗʰ **S61.354 Open bite of right ring finger with damage to nail**

   ☑7ᵗʰ **S61.355 Open bite of left ring finger with damage to nail**

EXCLUDES 1 Not coded here   **EXCLUDES 2** Not included here   **N** Newborn Age: 0   **P** Pediatric Age: 0-17   **M** Maternity Age: 12-55   **A** Adult Age: 15-124

982   ICD-10-CM 2018

✓7ᵗʰ   **S61.356**   **Open bite of right little finger with damage to nail**

✓7ᵗʰ   **S61.357**   **Open bite of left little finger with damage to nail**

✓7ᵗʰ   **S61.358**   **Open bite of other finger with damage to nail**
> Open bite of specified finger with unspecified laterality with damage to nail

✓7ᵗʰ   **S61.359**   **Open bite of unspecified finger with damage to nail** ▽

✓5ᵗʰ   **S61.4**   **Open wound of hand**

  ✓6ᵗʰ   **S61.40**   **Unspecified open wound of hand**

    ✓7ᵗʰ   **S61.401**   **Unspecified open wound of right hand** ▽

    ✓7ᵗʰ   **S61.402**   **Unspecified open wound of left hand** ▽

    ✓7ᵗʰ   **S61.409**   **Unspecified open wound of unspecified hand** ▽

  ✓6ᵗʰ   **S61.41**   **Laceration without foreign body of hand**

    ✓7ᵗʰ   **S61.411**   **Laceration without foreign body of right hand**

    ✓7ᵗʰ   **S61.412**   **Laceration without foreign body of left hand**

    ✓7ᵗʰ   **S61.419**   **Laceration without foreign body of unspecified hand** ▽

  ✓6ᵗʰ   **S61.42**   **Laceration with foreign body of hand**

    ✓7ᵗʰ   **S61.421**   **Laceration with foreign body of right hand**

    ✓7ᵗʰ   **S61.422**   **Laceration with foreign body of left hand**

    ✓7ᵗʰ   **S61.429**   **Laceration with foreign body of unspecified hand** ▽

  ✓6ᵗʰ   **S61.43**   **Puncture wound without foreign body of hand**

    ✓7ᵗʰ   **S61.431**   **Puncture wound without foreign body of right hand**

    ✓7ᵗʰ   **S61.432**   **Puncture wound without foreign body of left hand**

    ✓7ᵗʰ   **S61.439**   **Puncture wound without foreign body of unspecified hand** ▽

  ✓6ᵗʰ   **S61.44**   **Puncture wound with foreign body of hand**

    ✓7ᵗʰ   **S61.441**   **Puncture wound with foreign body of right hand**

    ✓7ᵗʰ   **S61.442**   **Puncture wound with foreign body of left hand**

    ✓7ᵗʰ   **S61.449**   **Puncture wound with foreign body of unspecified hand** ▽

  ✓6ᵗʰ   **S61.45**   **Open bite of hand**
> Bite of hand NOS
> **EXCLUDES 1**   *superficial bite of hand (S60.56-, S60.57-)*

    ✓7ᵗʰ   **S61.451**   **Open bite of right hand**

    ✓7ᵗʰ   **S61.452**   **Open bite of left hand**

    ✓7ᵗʰ   **S61.459**   **Open bite of unspecified hand** ▽

✓5ᵗʰ   **S61.5**   **Open wound of wrist**

  ✓6ᵗʰ   **S61.50**   **Unspecified open wound of wrist**

    ✓7ᵗʰ   **S61.501**   **Unspecified open wound of right wrist** ▽

    ✓7ᵗʰ   **S61.502**   **Unspecified open wound of left wrist** ▽

    ✓7ᵗʰ   **S61.509**   **Unspecified open wound of unspecified wrist** ▽

  ✓6ᵗʰ   **S61.51**   **Laceration without foreign body of wrist**

    ✓7ᵗʰ   **S61.511**   **Laceration without foreign body of right wrist**

    ✓7ᵗʰ   **S61.512**   **Laceration without foreign body of left wrist**

    ✓7ᵗʰ   **S61.519**   **Laceration without foreign body of unspecified wrist** ▽

  ✓6ᵗʰ   **S61.52**   **Laceration with foreign body of wrist**

    ✓7ᵗʰ   **S61.521**   **Laceration with foreign body of right wrist**

    ✓7ᵗʰ   **S61.522**   **Laceration with foreign body of left wrist**

    ✓7ᵗʰ   **S61.529**   **Laceration with foreign body of unspecified wrist** ▽

  ✓6ᵗʰ   **S61.53**   **Puncture wound without foreign body of wrist**

    ✓7ᵗʰ   **S61.531**   **Puncture wound without foreign body of right wrist**

    ✓7ᵗʰ   **S61.532**   **Puncture wound without foreign body of left wrist**

✓7ᵗʰ   **S61.539**   **Puncture wound without foreign body of unspecified wrist** ▽

✓6ᵗʰ   **S61.54**   **Puncture wound with foreign body of wrist**

  ✓7ᵗʰ   **S61.541**   **Puncture wound with foreign body of right wrist**

  ✓7ᵗʰ   **S61.542**   **Puncture wound with foreign body of left wrist**

  ✓7ᵗʰ   **S61.549**   **Puncture wound with foreign body of unspecified wrist** ▽

✓6ᵗʰ   **S61.55**   **Open bite of wrist**
> Bite of wrist NOS
> **EXCLUDES 1**   *superficial bite of wrist (S60.86-, S60.87-)*

  ✓7ᵗʰ   **S61.551**   **Open bite of right wrist**

  ✓7ᵗʰ   **S61.552**   **Open bite of left wrist**

  ✓7ᵗʰ   **S61.559**   **Open bite of unspecified wrist** ▽

✓4ᵗʰ   **S62**   **Fracture at wrist and hand level**
> **NOTE**   A fracture not indicated as displaced or nondisplaced should be coded to displaced.
> A fracture not indicated as open or closed should be coded to closed.
> **EXCLUDES 1**   *traumatic amputation of wrist and hand (S68.-)*
> **EXCLUDES 2**   *fracture of distal parts of ulna and radius (S52.-)*
> **AHA:** 2015, 3Q, 37-39

> The appropriate 7th character is to be added to each code from category S62.
> A   initial encounter for closed fracture
> B   initial encounter for open fracture
> D   subsequent encounter for fracture with routine healing
> G   subsequent encounter for fracture with delayed healing
> K   subsequent encounter for fracture with nonunion
> P   subsequent encounter for fracture with malunion
> S   sequela

✓5ᵗʰ   **S62.0**   **Fracture of navicular [scaphoid] bone of wrist**

  ✓6ᵗʰ   **S62.00**   **Unspecified fracture of navicular [scaphoid] bone of wrist**

    ✓7ᵗʰ   **S62.001**   **Unspecified fracture of navicular [scaphoid] bone of right wrist** ▽

    ✓7ᵗʰ   **S62.002**   **Unspecified fracture of navicular [scaphoid] bone of left wrist** ▽
> **AHA:** 2012, 4Q, 106

    ✓7ᵗʰ   **S62.009**   **Unspecified fracture of navicular [scaphoid] bone of unspecified wrist** ▽

  ✓6ᵗʰ   **S62.01**   **Fracture of distal pole of navicular [scaphoid] bone of wrist**
> Fracture of volar tuberosity of navicular [scaphoid] bone of wrist

    ✓7ᵗʰ   **S62.011**   **Displaced fracture of distal pole of navicular [scaphoid] bone of right wrist**

    ✓7ᵗʰ   **S62.012**   **Displaced fracture of distal pole of navicular [scaphoid] bone of left wrist**

    ✓7ᵗʰ   **S62.013**   **Displaced fracture of distal pole of navicular [scaphoid] bone of unspecified wrist** ▽

    ✓7ᵗʰ   **S62.014**   **Nondisplaced fracture of distal pole of navicular [scaphoid] bone of right wrist**

    ✓7ᵗʰ   **S62.015**   **Nondisplaced fracture of distal pole of navicular [scaphoid] bone of left wrist**

    ✓7ᵗʰ   **S62.016**   **Nondisplaced fracture of distal pole of navicular [scaphoid] bone of unspecified wrist** ▽

  ✓6ᵗʰ   **S62.02**   **Fracture of middle third of navicular [scaphoid] bone of wrist**

    ✓7ᵗʰ   **S62.021**   **Displaced fracture of middle third of navicular [scaphoid] bone of right wrist**

    ✓7ᵗʰ   **S62.022**   **Displaced fracture of middle third of navicular [scaphoid] bone of left wrist**

    ✓7ᵗʰ   **S62.023**   **Displaced fracture of middle third of navicular [scaphoid] bone of unspecified wrist** ▽

    ✓7ᵗʰ   **S62.024**   **Nondisplaced fracture of middle third of navicular [scaphoid] bone of right wrist**

    ✓7ᵗʰ   **S62.025**   **Nondisplaced fracture of middle third of navicular [scaphoid] bone of left wrist**

    ✓7ᵗʰ   **S62.026**   **Nondisplaced fracture of middle third of navicular [scaphoid] bone of unspecified wrist** ▽

☑ Additional Character Req   ✓ₓ7ᵗʰ Placeholder Alert   Manifestation   HCC CMS-HCC Condition   ▽ Unspecified Code   ►◄ Revised Text   ● New Code   ▲ Revised Code Title

ICD-10-CM 2018   983

√6ᵗʰ **S62.03**   **Fracture of proximal third of navicular [scaphoid] bone of wrist**

√7ᵗʰ **S62.031**   Displaced fracture of proximal third of navicular [scaphoid] bone of right wrist

√7ᵗʰ **S62.032**   Displaced fracture of proximal third of navicular [scaphoid] bone of left wrist

√7ᵗʰ **S62.033**   Displaced fracture of proximal third of ▽ navicular [scaphoid] bone of unspecified wrist

√7ᵗʰ **S62.034**   Nondisplaced fracture of proximal third of navicular [scaphoid] bone of right wrist

√7ᵗʰ **S62.035**   Nondisplaced fracture of proximal third of navicular [scaphoid] bone of left wrist

√7ᵗʰ **S62.036**   Nondisplaced fracture of proximal ▽ third of navicular [scaphoid] bone of unspecified wrist

√5ᵗʰ **S62.1**   **Fracture of other and unspecified carpal bone(s)**

EXCLUDES 2   *fracture of scaphoid of wrist (S62.0-)*

√6ᵗʰ **S62.10**   **Fracture of unspecified carpal bone**
Fracture of wrist NOS

√7ᵗʰ **S62.101**   Fracture of unspecified carpal bone, ▽ right wrist

√7ᵗʰ **S62.102**   Fracture of unspecified carpal bone, ▽ left wrist
AHA: 2012, 4Q, 95

√7ᵗʰ **S62.109**   Fracture of unspecified carpal bone, ▽ unspecified wrist

√6ᵗʰ **S62.11**   **Fracture of triquetrum [cuneiform] bone of wrist**

√7ᵗʰ **S62.111**   Displaced fracture of triquetrum [cuneiform] bone, right wrist

√7ᵗʰ **S62.112**   Displaced fracture of triquetrum [cuneiform] bone, left wrist

√7ᵗʰ **S62.113**   Displaced fracture of triquetrum ▽ [cuneiform] bone, unspecified wrist

√7ᵗʰ **S62.114**   Nondisplaced fracture of triquetrum [cuneiform] bone, right wrist

√7ᵗʰ **S62.115**   Nondisplaced fracture of triquetrum [cuneiform] bone, left wrist

√7ᵗʰ **S62.116**   Nondisplaced fracture of triquetrum ▽ [cuneiform] bone, unspecified wrist

√6ᵗʰ **S62.12**   **Fracture of lunate [semilunar]**

√7ᵗʰ **S62.121**   Displaced fracture of lunate [semilunar], right wrist

√7ᵗʰ **S62.122**   Displaced fracture of lunate [semilunar], left wrist

√7ᵗʰ **S62.123**   Displaced fracture of lunate ▽ [semilunar], unspecified wrist

√7ᵗʰ **S62.124**   Nondisplaced fracture of lunate [semilunar], right wrist

√7ᵗʰ **S62.125**   Nondisplaced fracture of lunate [semilunar], left wrist

√7ᵗʰ **S62.126**   Nondisplaced fracture of lunate ▽ [semilunar], unspecified wrist

√6ᵗʰ **S62.13**   **Fracture of capitate [os magnum] bone**

√7ᵗʰ **S62.131**   Displaced fracture of capitate [os magnum] bone, right wrist

√7ᵗʰ **S62.132**   Displaced fracture of capitate [os magnum] bone, left wrist

√7ᵗʰ **S62.133**   Displaced fracture of capitate [os ▽ magnum] bone, unspecified wrist

√7ᵗʰ **S62.134**   Nondisplaced fracture of capitate [os magnum] bone, right wrist

√7ᵗʰ **S62.135**   Nondisplaced fracture of capitate [os magnum] bone, left wrist

√7ᵗʰ **S62.136**   Nondisplaced fracture of capitate [os ▽ magnum] bone, unspecified wrist

√6ᵗʰ **S62.14**   **Fracture of body of hamate [unciform] bone**
Fracture of hamate [unciform] bone NOS

√7ᵗʰ **S62.141**   Displaced fracture of body of hamate [unciform] bone, right wrist

√7ᵗʰ **S62.142**   Displaced fracture of body of hamate [unciform] bone, left wrist

√7ᵗʰ **S62.143**   Displaced fracture of body of hamate ▽ [unciform] bone, unspecified wrist

√7ᵗʰ **S62.144**   Nondisplaced fracture of body of hamate [unciform] bone, right wrist

√7ᵗʰ **S62.145**   Nondisplaced fracture of body of hamate [unciform] bone, left wrist

√7ᵗʰ **S62.146**   Nondisplaced fracture of body of ▽ hamate [unciform] bone, unspecified wrist

√6ᵗʰ **S62.15**   **Fracture of hook process of hamate [unciform] bone**
Fracture of unciform process of hamate [unciform] bone

√7ᵗʰ **S62.151**   Displaced fracture of hook process of hamate [unciform] bone, right wrist

√7ᵗʰ **S62.152**   Displaced fracture of hook process of hamate [unciform] bone, left wrist

√7ᵗʰ **S62.153**   Displaced fracture of hook process of ▽ hamate [unciform] bone, unspecified wrist

√7ᵗʰ **S62.154**   Nondisplaced fracture of hook process of hamate [unciform] bone, right wrist

√7ᵗʰ **S62.155**   Nondisplaced fracture of hook process of hamate [unciform] bone, left wrist

√7ᵗʰ **S62.156**   Nondisplaced fracture of hook process ▽ of hamate [unciform] bone, unspecified wrist

√6ᵗʰ **S62.16**   **Fracture of pisiform**

√7ᵗʰ **S62.161**   Displaced fracture of pisiform, right wrist

√7ᵗʰ **S62.162**   Displaced fracture of pisiform, left wrist

√7ᵗʰ **S62.163**   Displaced fracture of pisiform, ▽ unspecified wrist

√7ᵗʰ **S62.164**   Nondisplaced fracture of pisiform, right wrist

√7ᵗʰ **S62.165**   Nondisplaced fracture of pisiform, left wrist

√7ᵗʰ **S62.166**   Nondisplaced fracture of pisiform, ▽ unspecified wrist

√6ᵗʰ **S62.17**   **Fracture of trapezium [larger multangular]**

√7ᵗʰ **S62.171**   Displaced fracture of trapezium [larger multangular], right wrist

√7ᵗʰ **S62.172**   Displaced fracture of trapezium [larger multangular], left wrist

√7ᵗʰ **S62.173**   Displaced fracture of trapezium [larger ▽ multangular], unspecified wrist

√7ᵗʰ **S62.174**   Nondisplaced fracture of trapezium [larger multangular], right wrist

√7ᵗʰ **S62.175**   Nondisplaced fracture of trapezium [larger multangular], left wrist

√7ᵗʰ **S62.176**   Nondisplaced fracture of trapezium ▽ [larger multangular], unspecified wrist

√6ᵗʰ **S62.18**   **Fracture of trapezoid [smaller multangular]**

√7ᵗʰ **S62.181**   Displaced fracture of trapezoid [smaller multangular], right wrist

√7ᵗʰ **S62.182**   Displaced fracture of trapezoid [smaller multangular], left wrist

√7ᵗʰ **S62.183**   Displaced fracture of trapezoid ▽ [smaller multangular], unspecified wrist

√7ᵗʰ **S62.184**   Nondisplaced fracture of trapezoid [smaller multangular], right wrist

√7ᵗʰ **S62.185**   Nondisplaced fracture of trapezoid [smaller multangular], left wrist

√7ᵗʰ **S62.186**   Nondisplaced fracture of trapezoid ▽ [smaller multangular], unspecified wrist

√5ᵗʰ **S62.2**   **Fracture of first metacarpal bone**

√6ᵗʰ **S62.20**   **Unspecified fracture of first metacarpal bone**

√7ᵗʰ **S62.201**   Unspecified fracture of first metacarpal ▽ bone, right hand

√7ᵗʰ **S62.202**   Unspecified fracture of first metacarpal ▽ bone, left hand

√7ᵗʰ **S62.209**   Unspecified fracture of first metacarpal ▽ bone, unspecified hand

√6ᵗʰ **S62.21**   **Bennett's fracture**

√7ᵗʰ **S62.211**   Bennett's fracture, right hand

√7ᵗʰ **S62.212**   Bennett's fracture, left hand

√7ᵗʰ **S62.213**   Bennett's fracture, unspecified hand ▽

EXCLUDES 1 Not coded here   EXCLUDES 2 Not included here   **N** Newborn Age: 0   **P** Pediatric Age: 0-17   **M** Maternity Age: 12-55   **A** Adult Age: 15-124

√6ᵗʰ **S62.22 Rolando's fracture**

√7ᵗʰ **S62.221 Displaced Rolando's fracture, right hand**

√7ᵗʰ **S62.222 Displaced Rolando's fracture, left hand**

√7ᵗʰ **S62.223 Displaced Rolando's fracture, unspecified hand** ▽

√7ᵗʰ **S62.224 Nondisplaced Rolando's fracture, right hand**

√7ᵗʰ **S62.225 Nondisplaced Rolando's fracture, left hand**

√7ᵗʰ **S62.226 Nondisplaced Rolando's fracture, unspecified hand** ▽

√6ᵗʰ **S62.23 Other fracture of base of first metacarpal bone** ▲

√7ᵗʰ **S62.231 Other displaced fracture of base of first metacarpal bone, right hand**

√7ᵗʰ **S62.232 Other displaced fracture of base of first metacarpal bone, left hand**

√7ᵗʰ **S62.233 Other displaced fracture of base of first metacarpal bone, unspecified hand** ▽

√7ᵗʰ **S62.234 Other nondisplaced fracture of base of first metacarpal bone, right hand**

√7ᵗʰ **S62.235 Other nondisplaced fracture of base of first metacarpal bone, left hand**

√7ᵗʰ **S62.236 Other nondisplaced fracture of base of first metacarpal bone, unspecified hand** ▽

√6ᵗʰ **S62.24 Fracture of shaft of first metacarpal bone** ▲

√7ᵗʰ **S62.241 Displaced fracture of shaft of first metacarpal bone, right hand**

√7ᵗʰ **S62.242 Displaced fracture of shaft of first metacarpal bone, left hand**

√7ᵗʰ **S62.243 Displaced fracture of shaft of first metacarpal bone, unspecified hand** ▽

√7ᵗʰ **S62.244 Nondisplaced fracture of shaft of first metacarpal bone, right hand**

√7ᵗʰ **S62.245 Nondisplaced fracture of shaft of first metacarpal bone, left hand**

√7ᵗʰ **S62.246 Nondisplaced fracture of shaft of first metacarpal bone, unspecified hand** ▽

√6ᵗʰ **S62.25 Fracture of neck of first metacarpal bone**

√7ᵗʰ **S62.251 Displaced fracture of neck of first metacarpal bone, right hand**

√7ᵗʰ **S62.252 Displaced fracture of neck of first metacarpal bone, left hand**

√7ᵗʰ **S62.253 Displaced fracture of neck of first metacarpal bone, unspecified hand** ▽

√7ᵗʰ **S62.254 Nondisplaced fracture of neck of first metacarpal bone, right hand**

√7ᵗʰ **S62.255 Nondisplaced fracture of neck of first metacarpal bone, left hand**

√7ᵗʰ **S62.256 Nondisplaced fracture of neck of first metacarpal bone, unspecified hand** ▽

√6ᵗʰ **S62.29 Other fracture of first metacarpal bone**

√7ᵗʰ **S62.291 Other fracture of first metacarpal bone, right hand**

√7ᵗʰ **S62.292 Other fracture of first metacarpal bone, left hand**

√7ᵗʰ **S62.299 Other fracture of first metacarpal bone, unspecified hand** ▽

√5ᵗʰ **S62.3 Fracture of other and unspecified metacarpal bone**

EXCLUDES 2 *fracture of first metacarpal bone (S62.2-)*

√6ᵗʰ **S62.30 Unspecified fracture of other metacarpal bone**

√7ᵗʰ **S62.300 Unspecified fracture of second metacarpal bone, right hand** ▽

√7ᵗʰ **S62.301 Unspecified fracture of second metacarpal bone, left hand** ▽

√7ᵗʰ **S62.302 Unspecified fracture of third metacarpal bone, right hand** ▽

√7ᵗʰ **S62.303 Unspecified fracture of third metacarpal bone, left hand** ▽

√7ᵗʰ **S62.304 Unspecified fracture of fourth metacarpal bone, right hand** ▽

√7ᵗʰ **S62.305 Unspecified fracture of fourth metacarpal bone, left hand** ▽

√7ᵗʰ **S62.306 Unspecified fracture of fifth metacarpal bone, right hand** ▽

√7ᵗʰ **S62.307 Unspecified fracture of fifth metacarpal bone, left hand** ▽

√7ᵗʰ **S62.308 Unspecified fracture of other metacarpal bone** ▽
Unspecified fracture of specified metacarpal bone with unspecified laterality

√7ᵗʰ **S62.309 Unspecified fracture of unspecified metacarpal bone** ▽

√6ᵗʰ **S62.31 Displaced fracture of base of other metacarpal bone**

√7ᵗʰ **S62.310 Displaced fracture of base of second metacarpal bone, right hand**

√7ᵗʰ **S62.311 Displaced fracture of base of second metacarpal bone, left hand**

√7ᵗʰ **S62.312 Displaced fracture of base of third metacarpal bone, right hand**

√7ᵗʰ **S62.313 Displaced fracture of base of third metacarpal bone, left hand**

√7ᵗʰ **S62.314 Displaced fracture of base of fourth metacarpal bone, right hand**

√7ᵗʰ **S62.315 Displaced fracture of base of fourth metacarpal bone, left hand**

√7ᵗʰ **S62.316 Displaced fracture of base of fifth metacarpal bone, right hand**

√7ᵗʰ **S62.317 Displaced fracture of base of fifth metacarpal bone, left hand**

√7ᵗʰ **S62.318 Displaced fracture of base of other metacarpal bone**
Displaced fracture of base of specified metacarpal bone with unspecified laterality

√7ᵗʰ **S62.319 Displaced fracture of base of unspecified metacarpal bone** ▽

√6ᵗʰ **S62.32 Displaced fracture of shaft of other metacarpal bone**

√7ᵗʰ **S62.320 Displaced fracture of shaft of second metacarpal bone, right hand**

√7ᵗʰ **S62.321 Displaced fracture of shaft of second metacarpal bone, left hand**

√7ᵗʰ **S62.322 Displaced fracture of shaft of third metacarpal bone, right hand**

√7ᵗʰ **S62.323 Displaced fracture of shaft of third metacarpal bone, left hand**

√7ᵗʰ **S62.324 Displaced fracture of shaft of fourth metacarpal bone, right hand**

√7ᵗʰ **S62.325 Displaced fracture of shaft of fourth metacarpal bone, left hand**

√7ᵗʰ **S62.326 Displaced fracture of shaft of fifth metacarpal bone, right hand**

√7ᵗʰ **S62.327 Displaced fracture of shaft of fifth metacarpal bone, left hand**

√7ᵗʰ **S62.328 Displaced fracture of shaft of other metacarpal bone**
Displaced fracture of shaft of specified metacarpal bone with unspecified laterality

√7ᵗʰ **S62.329 Displaced fracture of shaft of unspecified metacarpal bone** ▽

√6ᵗʰ **S62.33 Displaced fracture of neck of other metacarpal bone**

√7ᵗʰ **S62.330 Displaced fracture of neck of second metacarpal bone, right hand**

√7ᵗʰ **S62.331 Displaced fracture of neck of second metacarpal bone, left hand**

√7ᵗʰ **S62.332 Displaced fracture of neck of third metacarpal bone, right hand**

√7ᵗʰ **S62.333 Displaced fracture of neck of third metacarpal bone, left hand**

√7ᵗʰ **S62.334 Displaced fracture of neck of fourth metacarpal bone, right hand**

√7ᵗʰ **S62.335 Displaced fracture of neck of fourth metacarpal bone, left hand**

√7ᵗʰ **S62.336 Displaced fracture of neck of fifth metacarpal bone, right hand**

√7ᵗʰ **S62.337 Displaced fracture of neck of fifth metacarpal bone, left hand**

☑ Additional Character Req   √x7ᵗʰ Placeholder Alert   Manifestation   HCC CMS-HCC Condition   ▽ Unspecified Code   ►◄ Revised Text   ● New Code   ▲ Revised Code Title

ICD-10-CM 2018   985

√7ᵗʰ **S62.338** **Displaced fracture of neck of other metacarpal bone**
Displaced fracture of neck of specified metacarpal bone with unspecified laterality

√7ᵗʰ **S62.339** **Displaced fracture of neck of unspecified metacarpal bone** ▽

√6ᵗʰ **S62.34** **Nondisplaced fracture of base of other metacarpal bone**

√7ᵗʰ **S62.340** **Nondisplaced fracture of base of second metacarpal bone, right hand**

√7ᵗʰ **S62.341** **Nondisplaced fracture of base of second metacarpal bone, left hand**

√7ᵗʰ **S62.342** **Nondisplaced fracture of base of third metacarpal bone, right hand**

√7ᵗʰ **S62.343** **Nondisplaced fracture of base of third metacarpal bone, left hand**

√7ᵗʰ **S62.344** **Nondisplaced fracture of base of fourth metacarpal bone, right hand**

√7ᵗʰ **S62.345** **Nondisplaced fracture of base of fourth metacarpal bone, left hand**

√7ᵗʰ **S62.346** **Nondisplaced fracture of base of fifth metacarpal bone, right hand**

√7ᵗʰ **S62.347** **Nondisplaced fracture of base of fifth metacarpal bone, left hand**

√7ᵗʰ **S62.348** **Nondisplaced fracture of base of other metacarpal bone**
Nondisplaced fracture of base of specified metacarpal bone with unspecified laterality

√7ᵗʰ **S62.349** **Nondisplaced fracture of base of unspecified metacarpal bone** ▽

√6ᵗʰ **S62.35** **Nondisplaced fracture of shaft of other metacarpal bone**

√7ᵗʰ **S62.350** **Nondisplaced fracture of shaft of second metacarpal bone, right hand**

√7ᵗʰ **S62.351** **Nondisplaced fracture of shaft of second metacarpal bone, left hand**

√7ᵗʰ **S62.352** **Nondisplaced fracture of shaft of third metacarpal bone, right hand**

√7ᵗʰ **S62.353** **Nondisplaced fracture of shaft of third metacarpal bone, left hand**

√7ᵗʰ **S62.354** **Nondisplaced fracture of shaft of fourth metacarpal bone, right hand**

√7ᵗʰ **S62.355** **Nondisplaced fracture of shaft of fourth metacarpal bone, left hand**

√7ᵗʰ **S62.356** **Nondisplaced fracture of shaft of fifth metacarpal bone, right hand**

√7ᵗʰ **S62.357** **Nondisplaced fracture of shaft of fifth metacarpal bone, left hand**

√7ᵗʰ **S62.358** **Nondisplaced fracture of shaft of other metacarpal bone**
Nondisplaced fracture of shaft of specified metacarpal bone with unspecified laterality

√7ᵗʰ **S62.359** **Nondisplaced fracture of shaft of unspecified metacarpal bone** ▽

√6ᵗʰ **S62.36** **Nondisplaced fracture of neck of other metacarpal bone**

√7ᵗʰ **S62.360** **Nondisplaced fracture of neck of second metacarpal bone, right hand**

√7ᵗʰ **S62.361** **Nondisplaced fracture of neck of second metacarpal bone, left hand**

√7ᵗʰ **S62.362** **Nondisplaced fracture of neck of third metacarpal bone, right hand**

√7ᵗʰ **S62.363** **Nondisplaced fracture of neck of third metacarpal bone, left hand**

√7ᵗʰ **S62.364** **Nondisplaced fracture of neck of fourth metacarpal bone, right hand**

√7ᵗʰ **S62.365** **Nondisplaced fracture of neck of fourth metacarpal bone, left hand**

√7ᵗʰ **S62.366** **Nondisplaced fracture of neck of fifth metacarpal bone, right hand**

√7ᵗʰ **S62.367** **Nondisplaced fracture of neck of fifth metacarpal bone, left hand**

√7ᵗʰ **S62.368** **Nondisplaced fracture of neck of other metacarpal bone**
Nondisplaced fracture of neck of specified metacarpal bone with unspecified laterality

√7ᵗʰ **S62.369** **Nondisplaced fracture of neck of unspecified metacarpal bone** ▽

√6ᵗʰ **S62.39** **Other fracture of other metacarpal bone**

√7ᵗʰ **S62.390** **Other fracture of second metacarpal bone, right hand**

√7ᵗʰ **S62.391** **Other fracture of second metacarpal bone, left hand**

√7ᵗʰ **S62.392** **Other fracture of third metacarpal bone, right hand**

√7ᵗʰ **S62.393** **Other fracture of third metacarpal bone, left hand**

√7ᵗʰ **S62.394** **Other fracture of fourth metacarpal bone, right hand**

√7ᵗʰ **S62.395** **Other fracture of fourth metacarpal bone, left hand**

√7ᵗʰ **S62.396** **Other fracture of fifth metacarpal bone, right hand**

√7ᵗʰ **S62.397** **Other fracture of fifth metacarpal bone, left hand**

√7ᵗʰ **S62.398** **Other fracture of other metacarpal bone**
Other fracture of specified metacarpal bone with unspecified laterality

√7ᵗʰ **S62.399** **Other fracture of unspecified metacarpal bone** ▽

√5ᵗʰ **S62.5** **Fracture of thumb**

√6ᵗʰ **S62.50** **Fracture of unspecified phalanx of thumb**

√7ᵗʰ **S62.501** **Fracture of unspecified phalanx of right thumb** ▽

√7ᵗʰ **S62.502** **Fracture of unspecified phalanx of left thumb** ▽

√7ᵗʰ **S62.509** **Fracture of unspecified phalanx of unspecified thumb** ▽

√6ᵗʰ **S62.51** **Fracture of proximal phalanx of thumb**

√7ᵗʰ **S62.511** **Displaced fracture of proximal phalanx of right thumb**

√7ᵗʰ **S62.512** **Displaced fracture of proximal phalanx of left thumb**

√7ᵗʰ **S62.513** **Displaced fracture of proximal phalanx of unspecified thumb** ▽

√7ᵗʰ **S62.514** **Nondisplaced fracture of proximal phalanx of right thumb**

√7ᵗʰ **S62.515** **Nondisplaced fracture of proximal phalanx of left thumb**

√7ᵗʰ **S62.516** **Nondisplaced fracture of proximal phalanx of unspecified thumb** ▽

√6ᵗʰ **S62.52** **Fracture of distal phalanx of thumb**

√7ᵗʰ **S62.521** **Displaced fracture of distal phalanx of right thumb**

√7ᵗʰ **S62.522** **Displaced fracture of distal phalanx of left thumb**

√7ᵗʰ **S62.523** **Displaced fracture of distal phalanx of unspecified thumb** ▽

√7ᵗʰ **S62.524** **Nondisplaced fracture of distal phalanx of right thumb**

√7ᵗʰ **S62.525** **Nondisplaced fracture of distal phalanx of left thumb**

√7ᵗʰ **S62.526** **Nondisplaced fracture of distal phalanx of unspecified thumb** ▽

√5ᵗʰ **S62.6** **Fracture of other and unspecified finger(s)**
EXCLUDES 2   fracture of thumb (S62.5-)

√6ᵗʰ **S62.60** **Fracture of unspecified phalanx of finger**

√7ᵗʰ **S62.600** **Fracture of unspecified phalanx of right index finger** ▽

√7ᵗʰ **S62.601** **Fracture of unspecified phalanx of left index finger** ▽

√7ᵗʰ **S62.602** **Fracture of unspecified phalanx of right middle finger** ▽

√7ᵗʰ **S62.603** **Fracture of unspecified phalanx of left middle finger** ▽

EXCLUDES 1 Not coded here   EXCLUDES 2 Not included here   N Newborn Age: 0   P Pediatric Age: 0-17   M Maternity Age: 12-55   A Adult Age: 15-124

986   ICD-10-CM 2018

√7ᵗʰ **S62.604** **Fracture of unspecified phalanx of right ring finger** ▽

√7ᵗʰ **S62.605** **Fracture of unspecified phalanx of left ring finger** ▽

√7ᵗʰ **S62.606** **Fracture of unspecified phalanx of right little finger** ▽

√7ᵗʰ **S62.607** **Fracture of unspecified phalanx of left little finger** ▽

√7ᵗʰ **S62.608** **Fracture of unspecified phalanx of other finger** ▽
Fracture of unspecified phalanx of specified finger with unspecified laterality

√7ᵗʰ **S62.609** **Fracture of unspecified phalanx of unspecified finger** ▽

√6ᵗʰ **S62.61** **Displaced fracture of proximal phalanx of finger**

√7ᵗʰ **S62.610** **Displaced fracture of proximal phalanx of right index finger**

√7ᵗʰ **S62.611** **Displaced fracture of proximal phalanx of left index finger**

√7ᵗʰ **S62.612** **Displaced fracture of proximal phalanx of right middle finger**

√7ᵗʰ **S62.613** **Displaced fracture of proximal phalanx of left middle finger**

√7ᵗʰ **S62.614** **Displaced fracture of proximal phalanx of right ring finger**

√7ᵗʰ **S62.615** **Displaced fracture of proximal phalanx of left ring finger**

√7ᵗʰ **S62.616** **Displaced fracture of proximal phalanx of right little finger**

√7ᵗʰ **S62.617** **Displaced fracture of proximal phalanx of left little finger**

√7ᵗʰ **S62.618** **Displaced fracture of proximal phalanx of other finger** ▲ ▲
Displaced fracture of proximal phalanx of specified finger with unspecified laterality

√7ᵗʰ **S62.619** **Displaced fracture of proximal phalanx of unspecified finger** ▽ ▲

▲ √6ᵗʰ **S62.62** **Displaced fracture of middle phalanx of finger** ▲

▲ √7ᵗʰ **S62.620** **Displaced fracture of middle phalanx of right index finger**

▲ √7ᵗʰ **S62.621** **Displaced fracture of middle phalanx of left index finger**

▲ √7ᵗʰ **S62.622** **Displaced fracture of middle phalanx of right middle finger**

▲ √7ᵗʰ **S62.623** **Displaced fracture of middle phalanx of left middle finger**

▲ √7ᵗʰ **S62.624** **Displaced fracture of middle phalanx of right ring finger**

▲ √7ᵗʰ **S62.625** **Displaced fracture of middle phalanx of left ring finger**

√7ᵗʰ **S62.626** **Displaced fracture of medial phalanx of right little finger**

√7ᵗʰ **S62.627** **Displaced fracture of medial phalanx of left little finger**

√7ᵗʰ **S62.628** **Displaced fracture of medial phalanx of other finger**
Displaced fracture of medial phalanx of specified finger with unspecified laterality

√7ᵗʰ **S62.629** **Displaced fracture of medial phalanx of unspecified finger** ▽

√6ᵗʰ **S62.63** **Displaced fracture of distal phalanx of finger**

√7ᵗʰ **S62.630** **Displaced fracture of distal phalanx of right index finger**

√7ᵗʰ **S62.631** **Displaced fracture of distal phalanx of left index finger**

√7ᵗʰ **S62.632** **Displaced fracture of distal phalanx of right middle finger**

√7ᵗʰ **S62.633** **Displaced fracture of distal phalanx of left middle finger**

√7ᵗʰ **S62.634** **Displaced fracture of distal phalanx of right ring finger**

√7ᵗʰ **S62.635** **Displaced fracture of distal phalanx of left ring finger**

√7ᵗʰ **S62.636** **Displaced fracture of distal phalanx of right little finger**

√7ᵗʰ **S62.637** **Displaced fracture of distal phalanx of left little finger**

√7ᵗʰ **S62.638** **Displaced fracture of distal phalanx of other finger**
Displaced fracture of distal phalanx of specified finger with unspecified laterality

√7ᵗʰ **S62.639** **Displaced fracture of distal phalanx of unspecified finger** ▽

√6ᵗʰ **S62.64** **Nondisplaced fracture of proximal phalanx of finger**

√7ᵗʰ **S62.640** **Nondisplaced fracture of proximal phalanx of right index finger**

√7ᵗʰ **S62.641** **Nondisplaced fracture of proximal phalanx of left index finger**

√7ᵗʰ **S62.642** **Nondisplaced fracture of proximal phalanx of right middle finger**

√7ᵗʰ **S62.643** **Nondisplaced fracture of proximal phalanx of left middle finger**

√7ᵗʰ **S62.644** **Nondisplaced fracture of proximal phalanx of right ring finger**

√7ᵗʰ **S62.645** **Nondisplaced fracture of proximal phalanx of left ring finger**

√7ᵗʰ **S62.646** **Nondisplaced fracture of proximal phalanx of right little finger**

√7ᵗʰ **S62.647** **Nondisplaced fracture of proximal phalanx of left little finger**

√7ᵗʰ **S62.648** **Nondisplaced fracture of proximal phalanx of other finger**
Nondisplaced fracture of proximal phalanx of specified finger with unspecified laterality

√7ᵗʰ **S62.649** **Nondisplaced fracture of proximal phalanx of unspecified finger** ▽

√6ᵗʰ **S62.65** **Nondisplaced fracture of middle phalanx of finger**

√7ᵗʰ **S62.650** **Nondisplaced fracture of middle phalanx of right index finger**

√7ᵗʰ **S62.651** **Nondisplaced fracture of middle phalanx of left index finger**

√7ᵗʰ **S62.652** **Nondisplaced fracture of middle phalanx of right middle finger**

√7ᵗʰ **S62.653** **Nondisplaced fracture of middle phalanx of left middle finger**

√7ᵗʰ **S62.654** **Nondisplaced fracture of medial phalanx of right ring finger**

√7ᵗʰ **S62.655** **Nondisplaced fracture of medial phalanx of left ring finger**

√7ᵗʰ **S62.656** **Nondisplaced fracture of medial phalanx of right little finger**

√7ᵗʰ **S62.657** **Nondisplaced fracture of medial phalanx of left little finger**

√7ᵗʰ **S62.658** **Nondisplaced fracture of medial phalanx of other finger**
Nondisplaced fracture of medial phalanx of specified finger with unspecified laterality

√7ᵗʰ **S62.659** **Nondisplaced fracture of medial phalanx of unspecified finger** ▽

√6ᵗʰ **S62.66** **Nondisplaced fracture of distal phalanx of finger**

√7ᵗʰ **S62.660** **Nondisplaced fracture of distal phalanx of right index finger**

√7ᵗʰ **S62.661** **Nondisplaced fracture of distal phalanx of left index finger**

√7ᵗʰ **S62.662** **Nondisplaced fracture of distal phalanx of right middle finger**

√7ᵗʰ **S62.663** **Nondisplaced fracture of distal phalanx of left middle finger**

√7ᵗʰ **S62.664** **Nondisplaced fracture of distal phalanx of right ring finger**

√7ᵗʰ **S62.665** **Nondisplaced fracture of distal phalanx of left ring finger**

√7ᵗʰ **S62.666** **Nondisplaced fracture of distal phalanx of right little finger**

√7ᵗʰ **S62.667** **Nondisplaced fracture of distal phalanx of left little finger**

☑ Additional Character Req   √x7ᵗʰ Placeholder Alert   Manifestation   ᴴᶜᶜ CMS-HCC Condition   ▽ Unspecified Code   ▶◀ Revised Text   ● New Code   ▲ Revised Code Title

ICD-10-CM 2018   987

☑7th **S62.668** **Nondisplaced fracture of distal phalanx of other finger**
  Nondisplaced fracture of distal phalanx of specified finger with unspecified laterality

☑7th **S62.669** **Nondisplaced fracture of distal phalanx of unspecified finger** ▽

☑5th **S62.9** **Unspecified fracture of wrist and hand**

  ☑x7th **S62.90** **Unspecified fracture of unspecified wrist and hand** ▽

  ☑x7th **S62.91** **Unspecified fracture of right wrist and hand** ▽

  ☑x7th **S62.92** **Unspecified fracture of left wrist and hand** ▽

☑4th **S63** **Dislocation and sprain of joints and ligaments at wrist and hand level**

  INCLUDES avulsion of joint or ligament at wrist and hand level
  laceration of cartilage, joint or ligament at wrist and hand level
  sprain of cartilage, joint or ligament at wrist and hand level
  traumatic hemarthrosis of joint or ligament at wrist and hand level
  traumatic rupture of joint or ligament at wrist and hand level
  traumatic subluxation of joint or ligament at wrist and hand level
  traumatic tear of joint or ligament at wrist and hand level

  Code also any associated open wound

  EXCLUDES 2 strain of muscle, fascia and tendon of wrist and hand (S66.-)

  The appropriate 7th character is to be added to each code from category S63.
  A   initial encounter
  D   subsequent encounter
  S   sequela

  ☑5th **S63.0** **Subluxation and dislocation of wrist and hand joints**

    ☑6th **S63.00** **Unspecified subluxation and dislocation of wrist and hand**
      Dislocation of carpal bone NOS
      Dislocation of distal end of radius NOS
      Subluxation of carpal bone NOS
      Subluxation of distal end of radius NOS

      ☑7th **S63.001** **Unspecified subluxation of right wrist and hand** ▽

      ☑7th **S63.002** **Unspecified subluxation of left wrist and hand** ▽

      ☑7th **S63.003** **Unspecified subluxation of unspecified wrist and hand** ▽

      ☑7th **S63.004** **Unspecified dislocation of right wrist and hand** ▽

      ☑7th **S63.005** **Unspecified dislocation of left wrist and hand** ▽

      ☑7th **S63.006** **Unspecified dislocation of unspecified wrist and hand** ▽

    ☑6th **S63.01** **Subluxation and dislocation of distal radioulnar joint**

      ☑7th **S63.011** **Subluxation of distal radioulnar joint of right wrist**

      ☑7th **S63.012** **Subluxation of distal radioulnar joint of left wrist**

      ☑7th **S63.013** **Subluxation of distal radioulnar joint of unspecified wrist** ▽

      ☑7th **S63.014** **Dislocation of distal radioulnar joint of right wrist**

      ☑7th **S63.015** **Dislocation of distal radioulnar joint of left wrist**

      ☑7th **S63.016** **Dislocation of distal radioulnar joint of unspecified wrist** ▽

    ☑6th **S63.02** **Subluxation and dislocation of radiocarpal joint**

      ☑7th **S63.021** **Subluxation of radiocarpal joint of right wrist**

      ☑7th **S63.022** **Subluxation of radiocarpal joint of left wrist**

      ☑7th **S63.023** **Subluxation of radiocarpal joint of unspecified wrist** ▽

      ☑7th **S63.024** **Dislocation of radiocarpal joint of right wrist**

      ☑7th **S63.025** **Dislocation of radiocarpal joint of left wrist**

☑7th **S63.026** **Dislocation of radiocarpal joint of unspecified wrist** ▽

☑6th **S63.03** **Subluxation and dislocation of midcarpal joint**

  ☑7th **S63.031** **Subluxation of midcarpal joint of right wrist**

  ☑7th **S63.032** **Subluxation of midcarpal joint of left wrist**

  ☑7th **S63.033** **Subluxation of midcarpal joint of unspecified wrist** ▽

  ☑7th **S63.034** **Dislocation of midcarpal joint of right wrist**

  ☑7th **S63.035** **Dislocation of midcarpal joint of left wrist**

  ☑7th **S63.036** **Dislocation of midcarpal joint of unspecified wrist** ▽

☑6th **S63.04** **Subluxation and dislocation of carpometacarpal joint of thumb**

  EXCLUDES 2 interphalangeal subluxation and dislocation of thumb (S63.1-)

  ☑7th **S63.041** **Subluxation of carpometacarpal joint of right thumb**

  ☑7th **S63.042** **Subluxation of carpometacarpal joint of left thumb**

  ☑7th **S63.043** **Subluxation of carpometacarpal joint of unspecified thumb** ▽

  ☑7th **S63.044** **Dislocation of carpometacarpal joint of right thumb**

  ☑7th **S63.045** **Dislocation of carpometacarpal joint of left thumb**

  ☑7th **S63.046** **Dislocation of carpometacarpal joint of unspecified thumb** ▽

☑6th **S63.05** **Subluxation and dislocation of other carpometacarpal joint**

  EXCLUDES 2 subluxation and dislocation of carpometacarpal joint of thumb (S63.04-)

  ☑7th **S63.051** **Subluxation of other carpometacarpal joint of right hand**

  ☑7th **S63.052** **Subluxation of other carpometacarpal joint of left hand**

  ☑7th **S63.053** **Subluxation of other carpometacarpal joint of unspecified hand** ▽

  ☑7th **S63.054** **Dislocation of other carpometacarpal joint of right hand**

  ☑7th **S63.055** **Dislocation of other carpometacarpal joint of left hand**

  ☑7th **S63.056** **Dislocation of other carpometacarpal joint of unspecified hand** ▽

☑6th **S63.06** **Subluxation and dislocation of metacarpal (bone), proximal end**

  ☑7th **S63.061** **Subluxation of metacarpal (bone), proximal end of right hand**

  ☑7th **S63.062** **Subluxation of metacarpal (bone), proximal end of left hand**

  ☑7th **S63.063** **Subluxation of metacarpal (bone), proximal end of unspecified hand** ▽

  ☑7th **S63.064** **Dislocation of metacarpal (bone), proximal end of right hand**

  ☑7th **S63.065** **Dislocation of metacarpal (bone), proximal end of left hand**

  ☑7th **S63.066** **Dislocation of metacarpal (bone), proximal end of unspecified hand** ▽

☑6th **S63.07** **Subluxation and dislocation of distal end of ulna**

  ☑7th **S63.071** **Subluxation of distal end of right ulna**

  ☑7th **S63.072** **Subluxation of distal end of left ulna**

  ☑7th **S63.073** **Subluxation of distal end of unspecified ulna** ▽

  ☑7th **S63.074** **Dislocation of distal end of right ulna**

  ☑7th **S63.075** **Dislocation of distal end of left ulna**

  ☑7th **S63.076** **Dislocation of distal end of unspecified ulna** ▽

☑6th **S63.09** **Other subluxation and dislocation of wrist and hand**

  ☑7th **S63.091** **Other subluxation of right wrist and hand**

  ☑7th **S63.092** **Other subluxation of left wrist and hand**

  ☑7th **S63.093** **Other subluxation of unspecified wrist and hand** ▽

  ☑7th **S63.094** **Other dislocation of right wrist and hand**

     √7ᵗʰ   **S63.095**   Other dislocation of left wrist and hand

     √7ᵗʰ   **S63.096**   Other dislocation of unspecified wrist and hand ▽

√5ᵗʰ   **S63.1**   **Subluxation and dislocation of thumb**

   √6ᵗʰ   **S63.10**   Unspecified subluxation and dislocation of thumb

     √7ᵗʰ   **S63.101**   Unspecified subluxation of right thumb ▽

     √7ᵗʰ   **S63.102**   Unspecified subluxation of left thumb ▽

     √7ᵗʰ   **S63.103**   Unspecified subluxation of unspecified thumb ▽

     √7ᵗʰ   **S63.104**   Unspecified dislocation of right thumb ▽

     √7ᵗʰ   **S63.105**   Unspecified dislocation of left thumb ▽

     √7ᵗʰ   **S63.106**   Unspecified dislocation of unspecified thumb ▽

   √6ᵗʰ   **S63.11**   Subluxation and dislocation of metacarpophalangeal joint of thumb

     √7ᵗʰ   **S63.111**   Subluxation of metacarpophalangeal joint of right thumb

     √7ᵗʰ   **S63.112**   Subluxation of metacarpophalangeal joint of left thumb

     √7ᵗʰ   **S63.113**   Subluxation of metacarpophalangeal joint of unspecified thumb ▽

     √7ᵗʰ   **S63.114**   Dislocation of metacarpophalangeal joint of right thumb

     √7ᵗʰ   **S63.115**   Dislocation of metacarpophalangeal joint of left thumb

     √7ᵗʰ   **S63.116**   Dislocation of metacarpophalangeal joint of unspecified thumb ▽

▲   √6ᵗʰ   **S63.12**   Subluxation and dislocation of interphalangeal joint of thumb

▲   √7ᵗʰ   **S63.121**   Subluxation of interphalangeal joint of right thumb

▲   √7ᵗʰ   **S63.122**   Subluxation of interphalangeal joint of left thumb

▲   √7ᵗʰ   **S63.123**   Subluxation of interphalangeal joint of unspecified thumb ▽

▲   √7ᵗʰ   **S63.124**   Dislocation of interphalangeal joint of right thumb

▲   √7ᵗʰ   **S63.125**   Dislocation of interphalangeal joint of left thumb

▲   √7ᵗʰ   **S63.126**   Dislocation of interphalangeal joint of unspecified thumb ▽

   √6ᵗʰ   ~~**S63.13**   Subluxation and dislocation of proximal interphalangeal joint of thumb~~

     √7ᵗʰ   ~~**S63.131**   Subluxation of proximal interphalangeal joint of right thumb~~

     √7ᵗʰ   ~~**S63.132**   Subluxation of proximal interphalangeal joint of left thumb~~

     √7ᵗʰ   ~~**S63.133**   Subluxation of proximal interphalangeal joint of unspecified thumb~~

     √7ᵗʰ   ~~**S63.134**   Dislocation of proximal interphalangeal joint of right thumb~~

     √7ᵗʰ   ~~**S63.135**   Dislocation of proximal interphalangeal joint of left thumb~~

     √7ᵗʰ   ~~**S63.136**   Dislocation of proximal interphalangeal joint of unspecified thumb~~

   √6ᵗʰ   ~~**S63.14**   Subluxation and dislocation of distal interphalangeal joint of thumb~~

     √7ᵗʰ   ~~**S63.141**   Subluxation of distal interphalangeal joint of right thumb~~

     √7ᵗʰ   ~~**S63.142**   Subluxation of distal interphalangeal joint of left thumb~~

     √7ᵗʰ   ~~**S63.143**   Subluxation of distal interphalangeal joint of unspecified thumb~~

     √7ᵗʰ   ~~**S63.144**   Dislocation of distal interphalangeal joint of right thumb~~

     √7ᵗʰ   ~~**S63.145**   Dislocation of distal interphalangeal joint of left thumb~~

     √7ᵗʰ   ~~**S63.146**   Dislocation of distal interphalangeal joint of unspecified thumb~~

√5ᵗʰ   **S63.2**   **Subluxation and dislocation of other finger(s)**

    EXCLUDES 2   *subluxation and dislocation of thumb (S63.1-)*

   √6ᵗʰ   **S63.20**   Unspecified subluxation of other finger

     √7ᵗʰ   **S63.200**   Unspecified subluxation of right index finger ▽

     √7ᵗʰ   **S63.201**   Unspecified subluxation of left index finger ▽

     √7ᵗʰ   **S63.202**   Unspecified subluxation of right middle finger ▽

     √7ᵗʰ   **S63.203**   Unspecified subluxation of left middle finger ▽

     √7ᵗʰ   **S63.204**   Unspecified subluxation of right ring finger ▽

     √7ᵗʰ   **S63.205**   Unspecified subluxation of left ring finger ▽

     √7ᵗʰ   **S63.206**   Unspecified subluxation of right little finger ▽

     √7ᵗʰ   **S63.207**   Unspecified subluxation of left little finger ▽

     √7ᵗʰ   **S63.208**   Unspecified subluxation of other finger ▽
        Unspecified subluxation of specified finger with unspecified laterality

     √7ᵗʰ   **S63.209**   Unspecified subluxation of unspecified finger ▽

   √6ᵗʰ   **S63.21**   Subluxation of metacarpophalangeal joint of finger

     √7ᵗʰ   **S63.210**   Subluxation of metacarpophalangeal joint of right index finger

     √7ᵗʰ   **S63.211**   Subluxation of metacarpophalangeal joint of left index finger

     √7ᵗʰ   **S63.212**   Subluxation of metacarpophalangeal joint of right middle finger

     √7ᵗʰ   **S63.213**   Subluxation of metacarpophalangeal joint of left middle finger

     √7ᵗʰ   **S63.214**   Subluxation of metacarpophalangeal joint of right ring finger

     √7ᵗʰ   **S63.215**   Subluxation of metacarpophalangeal joint of left ring finger

     √7ᵗʰ   **S63.216**   Subluxation of metacarpophalangeal joint of right little finger

     √7ᵗʰ   **S63.217**   Subluxation of metacarpophalangeal joint of left little finger

     √7ᵗʰ   **S63.218**   Subluxation of metacarpophalangeal joint of other finger
        Subluxation of metacarpophalangeal joint of specified finger with unspecified laterality

     √7ᵗʰ   **S63.219**   Subluxation of metacarpophalangeal joint of unspecified finger ▽

   √6ᵗʰ   **S63.22**   Subluxation of unspecified interphalangeal joint of finger

     √7ᵗʰ   **S63.220**   Subluxation of unspecified interphalangeal joint of right index finger ▽

     √7ᵗʰ   **S63.221**   Subluxation of unspecified interphalangeal joint of left index finger ▽

     √7ᵗʰ   **S63.222**   Subluxation of unspecified interphalangeal joint of right middle finger ▽

     √7ᵗʰ   **S63.223**   Subluxation of unspecified interphalangeal joint of left middle finger ▽

     √7ᵗʰ   **S63.224**   Subluxation of unspecified interphalangeal joint of right ring finger ▽

     √7ᵗʰ   **S63.225**   Subluxation of unspecified interphalangeal joint of left ring finger ▽

     √7ᵗʰ   **S63.226**   Subluxation of unspecified interphalangeal joint of right little finger ▽

     √7ᵗʰ   **S63.227**   Subluxation of unspecified interphalangeal joint of left little finger ▽

     √7ᵗʰ   **S63.228**   Subluxation of unspecified interphalangeal joint of other finger ▽
        Subluxation of unspecified interphalangeal joint of specified finger with unspecified laterality

     √7ᵗʰ   **S63.229**   Subluxation of unspecified interphalangeal joint of unspecified finger ▽

☑ Additional Character Req   √x7ᵗʰ Placeholder Alert   Manifestation   HCC CMS-HCC Condition   ▽ Unspecified Code   ►◄ Revised Text   ● New Code   ▲ Revised Code Title

ICD-10-CM 2018   989

√6ᵗʰ **S63.23 Subluxation of proximal interphalangeal joint of finger**

√7ᵗʰ **S63.230 Subluxation of proximal interphalangeal joint of right index finger**

√7ᵗʰ **S63.231 Subluxation of proximal interphalangeal joint of left index finger**

√7ᵗʰ **S63.232 Subluxation of proximal interphalangeal joint of right middle finger**

√7ᵗʰ **S63.233 Subluxation of proximal interphalangeal joint of left middle finger**

√7ᵗʰ **S63.234 Subluxation of proximal interphalangeal joint of right ring finger**

√7ᵗʰ **S63.235 Subluxation of proximal interphalangeal joint of left ring finger**

√7ᵗʰ **S63.236 Subluxation of proximal interphalangeal joint of right little finger**

√7ᵗʰ **S63.237 Subluxation of proximal interphalangeal joint of left little finger**

√7ᵗʰ **S63.238 Subluxation of proximal interphalangeal joint of other finger**
Subluxation of proximal interphalangeal joint of specified finger with unspecified laterality

√7ᵗʰ **S63.239 Subluxation of proximal inter-phalangeal joint of unspecified finger** ▽

√6ᵗʰ **S63.24 Subluxation of distal interphalangeal joint of finger**

√7ᵗʰ **S63.240 Subluxation of distal interphalangeal joint of right index finger**

√7ᵗʰ **S63.241 Subluxation of distal interphalangeal joint of left index finger**

√7ᵗʰ **S63.242 Subluxation of distal interphalangeal joint of right middle finger**

√7ᵗʰ **S63.243 Subluxation of distal interphalangeal joint of left middle finger**

√7ᵗʰ **S63.244 Subluxation of distal interphalangeal joint of right ring finger**

√7ᵗʰ **S63.245 Subluxation of distal interphalangeal joint of left ring finger**

√7ᵗʰ **S63.246 Subluxation of distal interphalangeal joint of right little finger**

√7ᵗʰ **S63.247 Subluxation of distal interphalangeal joint of left little finger**

√7ᵗʰ **S63.248 Subluxation of distal interphalangeal joint of other finger**
Subluxation of distal interphalangeal joint of specified finger with unspecified laterality

√7ᵗʰ **S63.249 Subluxation of distal interphalangeal joint of unspecified finger** ▽

√6ᵗʰ **S63.25 Unspecified dislocation of other finger**

√7ᵗʰ **S63.250 Unspecified dislocation of right index finger** ▽

√7ᵗʰ **S63.251 Unspecified dislocation of left index finger** ▽

√7ᵗʰ **S63.252 Unspecified dislocation of right middle finger** ▽

√7ᵗʰ **S63.253 Unspecified dislocation of left middle finger** ▽

√7ᵗʰ **S63.254 Unspecified dislocation of right ring finger** ▽

√7ᵗʰ **S63.255 Unspecified dislocation of left ring finger** ▽

√7ᵗʰ **S63.256 Unspecified dislocation of right little finger** ▽

√7ᵗʰ **S63.257 Unspecified dislocation of left little finger** ▽

√7ᵗʰ **S63.258 Unspecified dislocation of other finger** ▽
Unspecified dislocation of specified finger with unspecified laterality

√7ᵗʰ **S63.259 Unspecified dislocation of unspecified finger** ▽
▶Unspecified dislocation of unspecified finger with unspecified laterality◀

√6ᵗʰ **S63.26 Dislocation of metacarpophalangeal joint of finger**

√7ᵗʰ **S63.260 Dislocation of metacarpophalangeal joint of right index finger**

√7ᵗʰ **S63.261 Dislocation of metacarpophalangeal joint of left index finger**

√7ᵗʰ **S63.262 Dislocation of metacarpophalangeal joint of right middle finger**

√7ᵗʰ **S63.263 Dislocation of metacarpophalangeal joint of left middle finger**

√7ᵗʰ **S63.264 Dislocation of metacarpophalangeal joint of right ring finger**

√7ᵗʰ **S63.265 Dislocation of metacarpophalangeal joint of left ring finger**

√7ᵗʰ **S63.266 Dislocation of metacarpophalangeal joint of right little finger**

√7ᵗʰ **S63.267 Dislocation of metacarpophalangeal joint of left little finger**

√7ᵗʰ **S63.268 Dislocation of metacarpophalangeal joint of other finger**
Dislocation of metacarpophalangeal joint of specified finger with unspecified laterality

√7ᵗʰ **S63.269 Dislocation of metacarpophalangeal joint of unspecified finger** ▽

√6ᵗʰ **S63.27 Dislocation of unspecified interphalangeal joint of finger**

√7ᵗʰ **S63.270 Dislocation of unspecified interphalangeal joint of right index finger** ▽

√7ᵗʰ **S63.271 Dislocation of unspecified interphalangeal joint of left index finger** ▽

√7ᵗʰ **S63.272 Dislocation of unspecified interphalangeal joint of right middle finger** ▽

√7ᵗʰ **S63.273 Dislocation of unspecified interphalangeal joint of left middle finger** ▽

√7ᵗʰ **S63.274 Dislocation of unspecified interphalangeal joint of right ring finger** ▽

√7ᵗʰ **S63.275 Dislocation of unspecified interphalangeal joint of left ring finger** ▽

√7ᵗʰ **S63.276 Dislocation of unspecified interphalangeal joint of right little finger** ▽

√7ᵗʰ **S63.277 Dislocation of unspecified interphalangeal joint of left little finger** ▽

√7ᵗʰ **S63.278 Dislocation of unspecified interphalangeal joint of other finger** ▽
Dislocation of unspecified interphalangeal joint of specified finger with unspecified laterality

√7ᵗʰ **S63.279 Dislocation of unspecified interphalangeal joint of unspecified finger** ▽
▶Dislocation of unspecified interphalangeal joint of unspecified finger without specified laterality◀

√6ᵗʰ **S63.28 Dislocation of proximal interphalangeal joint of finger**

√7ᵗʰ **S63.280 Dislocation of proximal interphalangeal joint of right index finger**

√7ᵗʰ **S63.281 Dislocation of proximal interphalangeal joint of left index finger**

√7ᵗʰ **S63.282 Dislocation of proximal interphalangeal joint of right middle finger**

√7ᵗʰ **S63.283 Dislocation of proximal interphalangeal joint of left middle finger**

√7ᵗʰ **S63.284 Dislocation of proximal interphalangeal joint of right ring finger**

√7ᵗʰ **S63.285 Dislocation of proximal interphalangeal joint of left ring finger**

√7ᵗʰ **S63.286 Dislocation of proximal interphalangeal joint of right little finger**

√7ᵗʰ **S63.287 Dislocation of proximal interphalangeal joint of left little finger**

√7ᵗʰ **S63.288 Dislocation of proximal interphalangeal joint of other finger**
Dislocation of proximal interphalangeal joint of specified finger with unspecified laterality

√7ᵗʰ **S63.289 Dislocation of proximal inter-phalangeal joint of unspecified finger** ▽

EXCLUDES 1 Not coded here   EXCLUDES 2 Not included here   N Newborn Age: 0   P Pediatric Age: 0-17   M Maternity Age: 12-55   A Adult Age: 15-124

990   ICD-10-CM 2018

✓6ᵗʰ S63.29 Dislocation of distal Interphalangeal joint of finger

> **✓7ᵗʰ S63.290 Dislocation of distal interphalangeal joint of right index finger**
>
> **✓7ᵗʰ S63.291 Dislocation of distal interphalangeal joint of left index finger**
>
> **✓7ᵗʰ S63.292 Dislocation of distal interphalangeal joint of right middle finger**
>
> **✓7ᵗʰ S63.293 Dislocation of distal interphalangeal joint of left middle finger**
>
> **✓7ᵗʰ S63.294 Dislocation of distal interphalangeal joint of right ring finger**
>
> **✓7ᵗʰ S63.295 Dislocation of distal interphalangeal joint of left ring finger**
>
> **✓7ᵗʰ S63.296 Dislocation of distal interphalangeal joint of right little finger**
>
> **✓7ᵗʰ S63.297 Dislocation of distal interphalangeal joint of left little finger**
>
> **✓7ᵗʰ S63.298 Dislocation of distal interphalangeal joint of other finger**
>> Dislocation of distal interphalangeal joint of specified finger with unspecified laterality
>
> **✓7ᵗʰ S63.299 Dislocation of distal interphalangeal joint of unspecified finger** ▽

✓5ᵗʰ S63.3 Traumatic rupture of ligament of wrist

> **✓6ᵗʰ S63.30 Traumatic rupture of unspecified ligament of wrist**
>
> > **✓7ᵗʰ S63.301 Traumatic rupture of unspecified ligament of right wrist** ▽
> >
> > **✓7ᵗʰ S63.302 Traumatic rupture of unspecified ligament of left wrist** ▽
> >
> > **✓7ᵗʰ S63.309 Traumatic rupture of unspecified ligament of unspecified wrist** ▽
>
> **✓6ᵗʰ S63.31 Traumatic rupture of collateral ligament of wrist**
>
> > **✓7ᵗʰ S63.311 Traumatic rupture of collateral ligament of right wrist**
> >
> > **✓7ᵗʰ S63.312 Traumatic rupture of collateral ligament of left wrist**
> >
> > **✓7ᵗʰ S63.319 Traumatic rupture of collateral ligament of unspecified wrist** ▽
>
> **✓6ᵗʰ S63.32 Traumatic rupture of radiocarpal ligament**
>
> > **✓7ᵗʰ S63.321 Traumatic rupture of right radiocarpal ligament**
> >
> > **✓7ᵗʰ S63.322 Traumatic rupture of left radiocarpal ligament**
> >
> > **✓7ᵗʰ S63.329 Traumatic rupture of unspecified radiocarpal ligament** ▽
>
> **✓6ᵗʰ S63.33 Traumatic rupture of ulnocarpal (palmar) ligament**
>
> > **✓7ᵗʰ S63.331 Traumatic rupture of right ulnocarpal (palmar) ligament**
> >
> > **✓7ᵗʰ S63.332 Traumatic rupture of left ulnocarpal (palmar) ligament**
> >
> > **✓7ᵗʰ S63.339 Traumatic rupture of unspecified ulnocarpal (palmar) ligament** ▽
>
> **✓6ᵗʰ S63.39 Traumatic rupture of other ligament of wrist**
>
> > **✓7ᵗʰ S63.391 Traumatic rupture of other ligament of right wrist**
> >
> > **✓7ᵗʰ S63.392 Traumatic rupture of other ligament of left wrist**
> >
> > **✓7ᵗʰ S63.399 Traumatic rupture of other ligament of unspecified wrist** ▽

✓5ᵗʰ S63.4 Traumatic rupture of ligament of finger at metacarpophalangeal and interphalangeal joint(s)

> **✓6ᵗʰ S63.40 Traumatic rupture of unspecified ligament of finger at metacarpophalangeal and interphalangeal joint**
>
> > **✓7ᵗʰ S63.400 Traumatic rupture of unspecified ligament of right index finger at metacarpo- phalangeal and interphalangeal joint** ▽
> >
> > **✓7ᵗʰ S63.401 Traumatic rupture of unspecified ligament of left index finger at metacarpophalangeal and interphalangeal joint** ▽
> >
> > **✓7ᵗʰ S63.402 Traumatic rupture of unspecified ligament of right middle finger at metacarpophalangeal and interphalangeal joint** ▽

> > **✓7ᵗʰ S63.403 Traumatic rupture of unspecified ligament of left middle finger at metacarpo- phalangeal and interphalangeal joint** ▽
> >
> > **✓7ᵗʰ S63.404 Traumatic rupture of unspecified ligament of right ring finger at metacarpophalangeal and interphalangeal joint** ▽
> >
> > **✓7ᵗʰ S63.405 Traumatic rupture of unspecified ligament of left ring finger at metacarpophalangeal and interphalangeal joint** ▽
> >
> > **✓7ᵗʰ S63.406 Traumatic rupture of unspecified ligament of right little finger at metacarpophalangeal and interphalangeal joint** ▽
> >
> > **✓7ᵗʰ S63.407 Traumatic rupture of unspecified ligament of left little finger at metacarpophalangeal and interphalangeal joint** ▽
> >
> > **✓7ᵗʰ S63.408 Traumatic rupture of unspecified ligament of other finger at metacarpophalangeal and interphalangeal joint** ▽
> >> Traumatic rupture of unspecified ligament of specified finger with unspecified laterality at metacarpophalangeal and interphalangeal joint
> >
> > **✓7ᵗʰ S63.409 Traumatic rupture of unspecified ligament of unspecified finger at metacarpophalangeal and interphalangeal joint** ▽
>
> **✓6ᵗʰ S63.41 Traumatic rupture of collateral ligament of finger at metacarpophalangeal and interphalangeal joint**
>
> > **✓7ᵗʰ S63.410 Traumatic rupture of collateral ligament of right index finger at metacarpo-phalangeal and interphalangeal joint**
> >
> > **✓7ᵗʰ S63.411 Traumatic rupture of collateral ligament of left index finger at metacarpo-phalangeal and interphalangeal joint**
> >
> > **✓7ᵗʰ S63.412 Traumatic rupture of collateral ligament of right middle finger at metacarpo-phalangeal and interphalangeal joint**
> >
> > **✓7ᵗʰ S63.413 Traumatic rupture of collateral ligament of left middle finger at metacarpo-phalangeal and interphalangeal joint**
> >
> > **✓7ᵗʰ S63.414 Traumatic rupture of collateral ligament of right ring finger at metacarpo-phalangeal and interphalangeal joint**
> >
> > **✓7ᵗʰ S63.415 Traumatic rupture of collateral ligament of left ring finger at metacarpophalangeal and interphalangeal joint**
> >
> > **✓7ᵗʰ S63.416 Traumatic rupture of collateral ligament of right little finger at metacarpo-phalangeal and interphalangeal joint**
> >
> > **✓7ᵗʰ S63.417 Traumatic rupture of collateral ligament of left little finger at metacarpo-phalangeal and interphalangeal joint**
> >
> > **✓7ᵗʰ S63.418 Traumatic rupture of collateral ligament of other finger at metacarpophalangeal and interphalangeal joint**
> >> Traumatic rupture of collateral ligament of specified finger with unspecified laterality at metacarpophalangeal and interphalangeal joint
> >
> > **✓7ᵗʰ S63.419 Traumatic rupture of collateral ligament of unspecified finger at metacarpophalangeal and interphalangeal joint** ▽
>
> **✓6ᵗʰ S63.42 Traumatic rupture of palmar ligament of finger at metacarpophalangeal and interphalangeal joint**
>
> > **✓7ᵗʰ S63.420 Traumatic rupture of palmar ligament of right index finger at metacarpo-phalangeal and interphalangeal joint**
> >
> > **✓7ᵗʰ S63.421 Traumatic rupture of palmar ligament of left index finger at metacarpophalangeal and interphalangeal joint**
> >
> > **✓7ᵗʰ S63.422 Traumatic rupture of palmar ligament of right middle finger at metacarpo-phalangeal and interphalangeal joint**

✓ Additional Character Req   ✓×7ᵗʰ Placeholder Alert   Manifestation   HCC CMS-HCC Condition   ▽ Unspecified Code   ►◄ Revised Text   ● New Code   ▲ Revised Code Title

ICD-10-CM 2018   991

√7ᵗʰ **S63.423** Traumatic rupture of palmar ligament of left middle finger at metacarpophalangeal and interphalangeal joint

√7ᵗʰ **S63.424** Traumatic rupture of palmar ligament of right ring finger at metacarpophalangeal and interphalangeal joint

√7ᵗʰ **S63.425** Traumatic rupture of palmar ligament of left ring finger at metacarpophalangeal and interphalangeal joint

√7ᵗʰ **S63.426** Traumatic rupture of palmar ligament of right little finger at metacarpophalangeal and interphalangeal joint

√7ᵗʰ **S63.427** Traumatic rupture of palmar ligament of left little finger at metacarpophalangeal and interphalangeal joint

√7ᵗʰ **S63.428** Traumatic rupture of palmar ligament of other finger at metacarpophalangeal and interphalangeal joint
Traumatic rupture of palmar ligament of specified finger with unspecified laterality at metacarpophalangeal and interphalangeal joint

√7ᵗʰ **S63.429** Traumatic rupture of palmar ligament of unspecified finger at metacarpophalangeal and interphalangeal joint ▽

√6ᵗʰ **S63.43** Traumatic rupture of volar plate of finger at metacarpophalangeal and interphalangeal joint

√7ᵗʰ **S63.430** Traumatic rupture of volar plate of right index finger at metacarpophalangeal and interphalangeal joint

√7ᵗʰ **S63.431** Traumatic rupture of volar plate of left index finger at metacarpophalangeal and interphalangeal joint

√7ᵗʰ **S63.432** Traumatic rupture of volar plate of right middle finger at metacarpophalangeal and interphalangeal joint

√7ᵗʰ **S63.433** Traumatic rupture of volar plate of left middle finger at metacarpophalangeal and interphalangeal joint

√7ᵗʰ **S63.434** Traumatic rupture of volar plate of right ring finger at metacarpophalangeal and interphalangeal joint

√7ᵗʰ **S63.435** Traumatic rupture of volar plate of left ring finger at metacarpophalangeal and interphalangeal joint

√7ᵗʰ **S63.436** Traumatic rupture of volar plate of right little finger at metacarpophalangeal and interphalangeal joint

√7ᵗʰ **S63.437** Traumatic rupture of volar plate of left little finger at metacarpophalangeal and interphalangeal joint

√7ᵗʰ **S63.438** Traumatic rupture of volar plate of other finger at metacarpophalangeal and interphalangeal joint
Traumatic rupture of volar plate of specified finger with unspecified laterality at metacarpophalangeal and interphalangeal joint

√7ᵗʰ **S63.439** Traumatic rupture of volar plate of unspecified finger at metacarpophalangeal and interphalangeal joint ▽

√6ᵗʰ **S63.49** Traumatic rupture of other ligament of finger at metacarpophalangeal and interphalangeal joint

√7ᵗʰ **S63.490** Traumatic rupture of other ligament of right index finger at metacarpophalangeal and interphalangeal joint

√7ᵗʰ **S63.491** Traumatic rupture of other ligament of left index finger at metacarpophalangeal and interphalangeal joint

√7ᵗʰ **S63.492** Traumatic rupture of other ligament of right middle finger at metacarpophalangeal and interphalangeal joint

√7ᵗʰ **S63.493** Traumatic rupture of other ligament of left middle finger at metacarpophalangeal and interphalangeal joint

√7ᵗʰ **S63.494** Traumatic rupture of other ligament of right ring finger at metacarpophalangeal and interphalangeal joint

√7ᵗʰ **S63.495** Traumatic rupture of other ligament of left ring finger at metacarpophalangeal and interphalangeal joint

√7ᵗʰ **S63.496** Traumatic rupture of other ligament of right little finger at metacarpophalangeal and interphalangeal joint

√7ᵗʰ **S63.497** Traumatic rupture of other ligament of left little finger at metacarpophalangeal and interphalangeal joint

√7ᵗʰ **S63.498** Traumatic rupture of other ligament of other finger at metacarpophalangeal and interphalangeal joint
Traumatic rupture of ligament of specified finger with unspecified laterality at metacarpophalangeal and interphalangeal joint

√7ᵗʰ **S63.499** Traumatic rupture of other ligament of unspecified finger at metacarpophalangeal and interphalangeal joint ▽

√5ᵗʰ **S63.5** Other and unspecified sprain of wrist

√6ᵗʰ **S63.50** Unspecified sprain of wrist

√7ᵗʰ **S63.501** Unspecified sprain of right wrist ▽

√7ᵗʰ **S63.502** Unspecified sprain of left wrist ▽

√7ᵗʰ **S63.509** Unspecified sprain of unspecified wrist ▽

√6ᵗʰ **S63.51** Sprain of carpal (joint)

√7ᵗʰ **S63.511** Sprain of carpal joint of right wrist

√7ᵗʰ **S63.512** Sprain of carpal joint of left wrist

√7ᵗʰ **S63.519** Sprain of carpal joint of unspecified wrist ▽

√6ᵗʰ **S63.52** Sprain of radiocarpal joint
EXCLUDES 1   traumatic rupture of radiocarpal ligament (S63.32-)

√7ᵗʰ **S63.521** Sprain of radiocarpal joint of right wrist

√7ᵗʰ **S63.522** Sprain of radiocarpal joint of left wrist

√7ᵗʰ **S63.529** Sprain of radiocarpal joint of unspecified wrist ▽

√6ᵗʰ **S63.59** Other specified sprain of wrist

√7ᵗʰ **S63.591** Other specified sprain of right wrist

√7ᵗʰ **S63.592** Other specified sprain of left wrist

√7ᵗʰ **S63.599** Other specified sprain of unspecified wrist ▽

√5ᵗʰ **S63.6** Other and unspecified sprain of finger(s)
EXCLUDES 1   traumatic rupture of ligament of finger at metacarpophalangeal and interphalangeal joint(s) (S63.4-)

√6ᵗʰ **S63.60** Unspecified sprain of thumb

√7ᵗʰ **S63.601** Unspecified sprain of right thumb ▽

√7ᵗʰ **S63.602** Unspecified sprain of left thumb ▽

√7ᵗʰ **S63.609** Unspecified sprain of unspecified thumb ▽

√6ᵗʰ **S63.61** Unspecified sprain of other and unspecified finger(s)

√7ᵗʰ **S63.610** Unspecified sprain of right index finger ▽

√7ᵗʰ **S63.611** Unspecified sprain of left index finger ▽

√7ᵗʰ **S63.612** Unspecified sprain of right middle finger ▽

√7ᵗʰ **S63.613** Unspecified sprain of left middle finger ▽

√7ᵗʰ **S63.614** Unspecified sprain of right ring finger ▽

√7ᵗʰ **S63.615** Unspecified sprain of left ring finger ▽

√7ᵗʰ **S63.616** Unspecified sprain of right little finger ▽

√7ᵗʰ **S63.617** Unspecified sprain of left little finger ▽

√7ᵗʰ **S63.618** Unspecified sprain of other finger ▽
Unspecified sprain of specified finger with unspecified laterality

√7ᵗʰ **S63.619** Unspecified sprain of unspecified finger ▽

√6ᵗʰ **S63.62** Sprain of interphalangeal joint of thumb

√7ᵗʰ **S63.621** Sprain of interphalangeal joint of right thumb

EXCLUDES 1 Not coded here   **EXCLUDES 2** Not included here   **N** Newborn Age: 0   **P** Pediatric Age: 0-17   **M** Maternity Age: 12-55   **A** Adult Age: 15-124

992   ICD-10-CM 2018

√7ᵗʰ **S63.622** Sprain of interphalangeal joint of left thumb

√7ᵗʰ **S63.629** Sprain of interphalangeal joint of unspecified thumb ▽

√6ᵗʰ **S63.63** Sprain of interphalangeal joint of other and unspecified finger(s)

√7ᵗʰ **S63.630** Sprain of interphalangeal joint of right index finger

√7ᵗʰ **S63.631** Sprain of interphalangeal joint of left index finger

√7ᵗʰ **S63.632** Sprain of interphalangeal joint of right middle finger

√7ᵗʰ **S63.633** Sprain of interphalangeal joint of left middle finger

√7ᵗʰ **S63.634** Sprain of interphalangeal joint of right ring finger

√7ᵗʰ **S63.635** Sprain of interphalangeal joint of left ring finger

√7ᵗʰ **S63.636** Sprain of interphalangeal joint of right little finger

√7ᵗʰ **S63.637** Sprain of interphalangeal joint of left little finger

√7ᵗʰ **S63.638** Sprain of interphalangeal joint of other finger

√7ᵗʰ **S63.639** Sprain of interphalangeal joint of unspecified finger ▽

√6ᵗʰ **S63.64** Sprain of metacarpophalangeal joint of thumb

√7ᵗʰ **S63.641** Sprain of metacarpophalangeal joint of right thumb

√7ᵗʰ **S63.642** Sprain of metacarpophalangeal joint of left thumb

√7ᵗʰ **S63.649** Sprain of metacarpophalangeal joint of unspecified thumb ▽

√6ᵗʰ **S63.65** Sprain of metacarpophalangeal joint of other and unspecified finger(s)

√7ᵗʰ **S63.650** Sprain of metacarpophalangeal joint of right index finger

√7ᵗʰ **S63.651** Sprain of metacarpophalangeal joint of left index finger

√7ᵗʰ **S63.652** Sprain of metacarpophalangeal joint of right middle finger

√7ᵗʰ **S63.653** Sprain of metacarpophalangeal joint of left middle finger

√7ᵗʰ **S63.654** Sprain of metacarpophalangeal joint of right ring finger

√7ᵗʰ **S63.655** Sprain of metacarpophalangeal joint of left ring finger

√7ᵗʰ **S63.656** Sprain of metacarpophalangeal joint of right little finger

√7ᵗʰ **S63.657** Sprain of metacarpophalangeal joint of left little finger

√7ᵗʰ **S63.658** Sprain of metacarpophalangeal joint of other finger
　　　Sprain of metacarpophalangeal joint of specified finger with unspecified laterality

√7ᵗʰ **S63.659** Sprain of metacarpophalangeal joint of unspecified finger ▽

√6ᵗʰ **S63.68** Other sprain of thumb

√7ᵗʰ **S63.681** Other sprain of right thumb

√7ᵗʰ **S63.682** Other sprain of left thumb

√7ᵗʰ **S63.689** Other sprain of unspecified thumb ▽

√6ᵗʰ **S63.69** Other sprain of other and unspecified finger(s)

√7ᵗʰ **S63.690** Other sprain of right index finger

√7ᵗʰ **S63.691** Other sprain of left index finger

√7ᵗʰ **S63.692** Other sprain of right middle finger

√7ᵗʰ **S63.693** Other sprain of left middle finger

√7ᵗʰ **S63.694** Other sprain of right ring finger

√7ᵗʰ **S63.695** Other sprain of left ring finger

√7ᵗʰ **S63.696** Other sprain of right little finger

√7ᵗʰ **S63.697** Other sprain of left little finger

√7ᵗʰ **S63.698** Other sprain of other finger
　　　Other sprain of specified finger with unspecified laterality

√7ᵗʰ **S63.699** Other sprain of unspecified finger ▽

√5ᵗʰ **S63.8** Sprain of other part of wrist and hand

√6ᵗʰ **S63.8X** Sprain of other part of wrist and hand

√7ᵗʰ **S63.8X1** Sprain of other part of right wrist and hand

√7ᵗʰ **S63.8X2** Sprain of other part of left wrist and hand

√7ᵗʰ **S63.8X9** Sprain of other part of unspecified wrist and hand ▽

√5ᵗʰ **S63.9** Sprain of unspecified part of wrist and hand

√x7ᵗʰ **S63.90** Sprain of unspecified part of unspecified wrist and hand ▽

√x7ᵗʰ **S63.91** Sprain of unspecified part of right wrist and hand ▽

√x7ᵗʰ **S63.92** Sprain of unspecified part of left wrist and hand ▽

√4ᵗʰ **S64** **Injury of nerves at wrist and hand level**
Code also any associated open wound (S61.-)

> The appropriate 7th character is to be added to each code from category S64.
> A　initial encounter
> D　subsequent encounter
> S　sequela

√5ᵗʰ **S64.0** Injury of ulnar nerve at wrist and hand level

√x7ᵗʰ **S64.00** Injury of ulnar nerve at wrist and hand level of unspecified arm ▽

√x7ᵗʰ **S64.01** Injury of ulnar nerve at wrist and hand level of right arm

√x7ᵗʰ **S64.02** Injury of ulnar nerve at wrist and hand level of left arm

√5ᵗʰ **S64.1** Injury of median nerve at wrist and hand level

√x7ᵗʰ **S64.10** Injury of median nerve at wrist and hand level of unspecified arm ▽

√x7ᵗʰ **S64.11** Injury of median nerve at wrist and hand level of right arm

√x7ᵗʰ **S64.12** Injury of median nerve at wrist and hand level of left arm

√5ᵗʰ **S64.2** Injury of radial nerve at wrist and hand level

√x7ᵗʰ **S64.20** Injury of radial nerve at wrist and hand level of unspecified arm ▽

√x7ᵗʰ **S64.21** Injury of radial nerve at wrist and hand level of right arm

√x7ᵗʰ **S64.22** Injury of radial nerve at wrist and hand level of left arm

√5ᵗʰ **S64.3** Injury of digital nerve of thumb

√x7ᵗʰ **S64.30** Injury of digital nerve of unspecified thumb ▽

√x7ᵗʰ **S64.31** Injury of digital nerve of right thumb

√x7ᵗʰ **S64.32** Injury of digital nerve of left thumb

√5ᵗʰ **S64.4** Injury of digital nerve of other and unspecified finger

√x7ᵗʰ **S64.40** Injury of digital nerve of unspecified finger ▽

√6ᵗʰ **S64.49** Injury of digital nerve of other finger

√7ᵗʰ **S64.490** Injury of digital nerve of right index finger

√7ᵗʰ **S64.491** Injury of digital nerve of left index finger

√7ᵗʰ **S64.492** Injury of digital nerve of right middle finger

√7ᵗʰ **S64.493** Injury of digital nerve of left middle finger

√7ᵗʰ **S64.494** Injury of digital nerve of right ring finger

√7ᵗʰ **S64.495** Injury of digital nerve of left ring finger

√7ᵗʰ **S64.496** Injury of digital nerve of right little finger

√7ᵗʰ **S64.497** Injury of digital nerve of left little finger

√7ᵗʰ **S64.498** Injury of digital nerve of other finger
　　　Injury of digital nerve of specified finger with unspecified laterality

√5ᵗʰ **S64.8** Injury of other nerves at wrist and hand level

√6ᵗʰ **S64.8X** Injury of other nerves at wrist and hand level

√7ᵗʰ **S64.8X1** Injury of other nerves at wrist and hand level of right arm

√7ᵗʰ **S64.8X2** Injury of other nerves at wrist and hand level of left arm

√7ᵗʰ **S64.8X9** Injury of other nerves at wrist and hand level of unspecified arm ▽

☑ Additional Character Req　　√x7ᵗʰ Placeholder Alert　　Manifestation　　**HCC** CMS-HCC Condition　　▽ Unspecified Code　　►◄ Revised Text　　● New Code　　▲ Revised Code Title

√5ᵗʰ **S64.9 Injury of unspecified nerve at wrist and hand level**

√x 7ᵗʰ **S64.90** Injury of unspecified nerve at wrist and hand level of unspecified arm ▽

√x 7ᵗʰ **S64.91** Injury of unspecified nerve at wrist and hand level of right arm ▽

√x 7ᵗʰ **S64.92** Injury of unspecified nerve at wrist and hand level of left arm ▽

√4ᵗʰ **S65 Injury of blood vessels at wrist and hand level**

Code also any associated open wound (S61.-)

> The appropriate 7th character is to be added to each code from category S65.
> A   initial encounter
> D   subsequent encounter
> S   sequela

√5ᵗʰ **S65.0 Injury of ulnar artery at wrist and hand level**

√6ᵗʰ **S65.00** Unspecified injury of ulnar artery at wrist and hand level

√7ᵗʰ **S65.001** Unspecified injury of ulnar artery at wrist and hand level of right arm ▽

√7ᵗʰ **S65.002** Unspecified injury of ulnar artery at wrist and hand level of left arm ▽

√7ᵗʰ **S65.009** Unspecified injury of ulnar artery at wrist and hand level of unspecified arm ▽

√6ᵗʰ **S65.01** Laceration of ulnar artery at wrist and hand level

√7ᵗʰ **S65.011** Laceration of ulnar artery at wrist and hand level of right arm

√7ᵗʰ **S65.012** Laceration of ulnar artery at wrist and hand level of left arm

√7ᵗʰ **S65.019** Laceration of ulnar artery at wrist and hand level of unspecified arm ▽

√6ᵗʰ **S65.09** Other specified injury of ulnar artery at wrist and hand level

√7ᵗʰ **S65.091** Other specified injury of ulnar artery at wrist and hand level of right arm

√7ᵗʰ **S65.092** Other specified injury of ulnar artery at wrist and hand level of left arm

√7ᵗʰ **S65.099** Other specified injury of ulnar artery at wrist and hand level of unspecified arm ▽

√5ᵗʰ **S65.1 Injury of radial artery at wrist and hand level**

√6ᵗʰ **S65.10** Unspecified injury of radial artery at wrist and hand level

√7ᵗʰ **S65.101** Unspecified injury of radial artery at wrist and hand level of right arm ▽

√7ᵗʰ **S65.102** Unspecified injury of radial artery at wrist and hand level of left arm ▽

√7ᵗʰ **S65.109** Unspecified injury of radial artery at wrist and hand level of unspecified arm ▽

√6ᵗʰ **S65.11** Laceration of radial artery at wrist and hand level

√7ᵗʰ **S65.111** Laceration of radial artery at wrist and hand level of right arm

√7ᵗʰ **S65.112** Laceration of radial artery at wrist and hand level of left arm

√7ᵗʰ **S65.119** Laceration of radial artery at wrist and hand level of unspecified arm ▽

√6ᵗʰ **S65.19** Other specified injury of radial artery at wrist and hand level

√7ᵗʰ **S65.191** Other specified injury of radial artery at wrist and hand level of right arm

√7ᵗʰ **S65.192** Other specified injury of radial artery at wrist and hand level of left arm

√7ᵗʰ **S65.199** Other specified injury of radial artery at wrist and hand level of unspecified arm ▽

√5ᵗʰ **S65.2 Injury of superficial palmar arch**

√6ᵗʰ **S65.20** Unspecified injury of superficial palmar arch

√7ᵗʰ **S65.201** Unspecified injury of superficial palmar arch of right hand ▽

√7ᵗʰ **S65.202** Unspecified injury of superficial palmar arch of left hand ▽

√7ᵗʰ **S65.209** Unspecified injury of superficial palmar arch of unspecified hand ▽

√6ᵗʰ **S65.21** Laceration of superficial palmar arch

√7ᵗʰ **S65.211** Laceration of superficial palmar arch of right hand

√7ᵗʰ **S65.212** Laceration of superficial palmar arch of left hand

√7ᵗʰ **S65.219** Laceration of superficial palmar arch of unspecified hand ▽

√6ᵗʰ **S65.29** Other specified injury of superficial palmar arch

√7ᵗʰ **S65.291** Other specified injury of superficial palmar arch of right hand

√7ᵗʰ **S65.292** Other specified injury of superficial palmar arch of left hand

√7ᵗʰ **S65.299** Other specified injury of superficial palmar arch of unspecified hand ▽

√5ᵗʰ **S65.3 Injury of deep palmar arch**

√6ᵗʰ **S65.30** Unspecified injury of deep palmar arch

√7ᵗʰ **S65.301** Unspecified injury of deep palmar arch of right hand ▽

√7ᵗʰ **S65.302** Unspecified injury of deep palmar arch of left hand ▽

√7ᵗʰ **S65.309** Unspecified injury of deep palmar arch of unspecified hand ▽

√6ᵗʰ **S65.31** Laceration of deep palmar arch

√7ᵗʰ **S65.311** Laceration of deep palmar arch of right hand

√7ᵗʰ **S65.312** Laceration of deep palmar arch of left hand

√7ᵗʰ **S65.319** Laceration of deep palmar arch of unspecified hand ▽

√6ᵗʰ **S65.39** Other specified injury of deep palmar arch

√7ᵗʰ **S65.391** Other specified injury of deep palmar arch of right hand

√7ᵗʰ **S65.392** Other specified injury of deep palmar arch of left hand

√7ᵗʰ **S65.399** Other specified injury of deep palmar arch of unspecified hand ▽

√5ᵗʰ **S65.4 Injury of blood vessel of thumb**

√6ᵗʰ **S65.40** Unspecified injury of blood vessel of thumb

√7ᵗʰ **S65.401** Unspecified injury of blood vessel of right thumb ▽

√7ᵗʰ **S65.402** Unspecified injury of blood vessel of left thumb ▽

√7ᵗʰ **S65.409** Unspecified injury of blood vessel of unspecified thumb ▽

√6ᵗʰ **S65.41** Laceration of blood vessel of thumb

√7ᵗʰ **S65.411** Laceration of blood vessel of right thumb

√7ᵗʰ **S65.412** Laceration of blood vessel of left thumb

√7ᵗʰ **S65.419** Laceration of blood vessel of unspecified thumb ▽

√6ᵗʰ **S65.49** Other specified injury of blood vessel of thumb

√7ᵗʰ **S65.491** Other specified injury of blood vessel of right thumb

√7ᵗʰ **S65.492** Other specified injury of blood vessel of left thumb

√7ᵗʰ **S65.499** Other specified injury of blood vessel of unspecified thumb ▽

√5ᵗʰ **S65.5 Injury of blood vessel of other and unspecified finger**

√6ᵗʰ **S65.50** Unspecified injury of blood vessel of other and unspecified finger

√7ᵗʰ **S65.500** Unspecified injury of blood vessel of right index finger ▽

√7ᵗʰ **S65.501** Unspecified injury of blood vessel of left index finger ▽

√7ᵗʰ **S65.502** Unspecified injury of blood vessel of right middle finger ▽

√7ᵗʰ **S65.503** Unspecified injury of blood vessel of left middle finger ▽

√7ᵗʰ **S65.504** Unspecified injury of blood vessel of right ring finger ▽

√7ᵗʰ **S65.505** Unspecified injury of blood vessel of left ring finger ▽

√7ᵗʰ **S65.506** Unspecified injury of blood vessel of right little finger ▽

√7ᵗʰ **S65.507** Unspecified injury of blood vessel of left little finger ▽

EXCLUDES 1 Not coded here   EXCLUDES 2 Not included here   N Newborn Age: 0   P Pediatric Age: 0-17   M Maternity Age: 12-55   A Adult Age: 15-124

√7ᵗʰ **S65.508 Unspecified injury of blood vessel of other finger** ▽
Unspecified injury of blood vessel of specified finger with unspecified laterality

√7ᵗʰ **S65.509 Unspecified injury of blood vessel of unspecified finger** ▽

√6ᵗʰ **S65.51 Laceration of blood vessel of other and unspecified finger**

√7ᵗʰ **S65.510 Laceration of blood vessel of right index finger**

√7ᵗʰ **S65.511 Laceration of blood vessel of left index finger**

√7ᵗʰ **S65.512 Laceration of blood vessel of right middle finger**

√7ᵗʰ **S65.513 Laceration of blood vessel of left middle finger**

√7ᵗʰ **S65.514 Laceration of blood vessel of right ring finger**

√7ᵗʰ **S65.515 Laceration of blood vessel of left ring finger**

√7ᵗʰ **S65.516 Laceration of blood vessel of right little finger**

√7ᵗʰ **S65.517 Laceration of blood vessel of left little finger**

√7ᵗʰ **S65.518 Laceration of blood vessel of other finger**
Laceration of blood vessel of specified finger with unspecified laterality

√7ᵗʰ **S65.519 Laceration of blood vessel of unspecified finger** ▽

√6ᵗʰ **S65.59 Other specified injury of blood vessel of other and unspecified finger**

√7ᵗʰ **S65.590 Other specified injury of blood vessel of right index finger**

√7ᵗʰ **S65.591 Other specified injury of blood vessel of left index finger**

√7ᵗʰ **S65.592 Other specified injury of blood vessel of right middle finger**

√7ᵗʰ **S65.593 Other specified injury of blood vessel of left middle finger**

√7ᵗʰ **S65.594 Other specified injury of blood vessel of right ring finger**

√7ᵗʰ **S65.595 Other specified injury of blood vessel of left ring finger**

√7ᵗʰ **S65.596 Other specified injury of blood vessel of right little finger**

√7ᵗʰ **S65.597 Other specified injury of blood vessel of left little finger**

√7ᵗʰ **S65.598 Other specified injury of blood vessel of other finger**
Other specified injury of blood vessel of specified finger with unspecified laterality

√7ᵗʰ **S65.599 Other specified injury of blood vessel of unspecified finger** ▽

√5ᵗʰ **S65.8 Injury of other blood vessels at wrist and hand level**

√6ᵗʰ **S65.80 Unspecified injury of other blood vessels at wrist and hand level**

√7ᵗʰ **S65.801 Unspecified injury of other blood vessels at wrist and hand level of right arm** ▽

√7ᵗʰ **S65.802 Unspecified injury of other blood vessels at wrist and hand level of left arm** ▽

√7ᵗʰ **S65.809 Unspecified injury of other blood vessels at wrist and hand level of unspecified arm** ▽

√6ᵗʰ **S65.81 Laceration of other blood vessels at wrist and hand level**

√7ᵗʰ **S65.811 Laceration of other blood vessels at wrist and hand level of right arm**

√7ᵗʰ **S65.812 Laceration of other blood vessels at wrist and hand level of left arm**

√7ᵗʰ **S65.819 Laceration of other blood vessels at wrist and hand level of unspecified arm** ▽

√6ᵗʰ **S65.89 Other specified injury of other blood vessels at wrist and hand level**

√7ᵗʰ **S65.891 Other specified injury of other blood vessels at wrist and hand level of right arm**

√7ᵗʰ **S65.892 Other specified injury of other blood vessels at wrist and hand level of left arm**

√7ᵗʰ **S65.899 Other specified injury of other blood vessels at wrist and hand level of unspecified arm** ▽

√5ᵗʰ **S65.9 Injury of unspecified blood vessel at wrist and hand level**

√6ᵗʰ **S65.90 Unspecified injury of unspecified blood vessel at wrist and hand level**

√7ᵗʰ **S65.901 Unspecified injury of unspecified blood vessel at wrist and hand level of right arm** ▽

√7ᵗʰ **S65.902 Unspecified injury of unspecified blood vessel at wrist and hand level of left arm** ▽

√7ᵗʰ **S65.909 Unspecified injury of unspecified blood vessel at wrist and hand level of unspecified arm** ▽

√6ᵗʰ **S65.91 Laceration of unspecified blood vessel at wrist and hand level**

√7ᵗʰ **S65.911 Laceration of unspecified blood vessel at wrist and hand level of right arm** ▽

√7ᵗʰ **S65.912 Laceration of unspecified blood vessel at wrist and hand level of left arm** ▽

√7ᵗʰ **S65.919 Laceration of unspecified blood vessel at wrist and hand level of unspecified arm** ▽

√6ᵗʰ **S65.99 Other specified injury of unspecified blood vessel at wrist and hand level**

√7ᵗʰ **S65.991 Other specified injury of unspecified blood vessel at wrist and hand of right arm** ▽

√7ᵗʰ **S65.992 Other specified injury of unspecified blood vessel at wrist and hand of left arm** ▽

√7ᵗʰ **S65.999 Other specified injury of unspecified blood vessel at wrist and hand of unspecified arm** ▽

√4ᵗʰ **S66 Injury of muscle, fascia and tendon at wrist and hand level**
Code also any associated open wound (S61.-)
EXCLUDES 2   sprain of joints and ligaments of wrist and hand (S63.-)
TIP: Refer to the Muscle/Tendon table at the beginning of this chapter.

> The appropriate 7th character is to be added to each code from category S66.
> A   initial encounter
> D   subsequent encounter
> S   sequela

√5ᵗʰ **S66.0 Injury of long flexor muscle, fascia and tendon of thumb at wrist and hand level**

√6ᵗʰ **S66.00 Unspecified injury of long flexor muscle, fascia and tendon of thumb at wrist and hand level**

√7ᵗʰ **S66.001 Unspecified injury of long flexor muscle, fascia and tendon of right thumb at wrist and hand level** ▽

√7ᵗʰ **S66.002 Unspecified injury of long flexor muscle, fascia and tendon of left thumb at wrist and hand level** ▽

√7ᵗʰ **S66.009 Unspecified injury of long flexor muscle, fascia and tendon of unspecified thumb at wrist and hand level** ▽

√6ᵗʰ **S66.01 Strain of long flexor muscle, fascia and tendon of thumb at wrist and hand level**

√7ᵗʰ **S66.011 Strain of long flexor muscle, fascia and tendon of right thumb at wrist and hand level**

√7ᵗʰ **S66.012 Strain of long flexor muscle, fascia and tendon of left thumb at wrist and hand level**

√7ᵗʰ **S66.019 Strain of long flexor muscle, fascia and tendon of unspecified thumb at wrist and hand level** ▽

☑ Additional Character Req   ⬛√ₓ7ᵗʰ Placeholder Alert   Manifestation   ᴴᶜᶜ CMS-HCC Condition   ▽ Unspecified Code   ▶◀ Revised Text   ● New Code   ▲ Revised Code Title

ICD-10-CM 2018   995

√6ᵗʰ **S66.02** **Laceration of long flexor muscle, fascia and tendon of thumb at wrist and hand level**

√7ᵗʰ **S66.021** **Laceration of long flexor muscle, fascia and tendon of right thumb at wrist and hand level**

√7ᵗʰ **S66.022** **Laceration of long flexor muscle, fascia and tendon of left thumb at wrist and hand level**

√7ᵗʰ **S66.029** **Laceration of long flexor muscle, fascia and tendon of unspecified thumb at wrist and hand level** ▽

√6ᵗʰ **S66.09** **Other specified injury of long flexor muscle, fascia and tendon of thumb at wrist and hand level**

√7ᵗʰ **S66.091** **Other specified injury of long flexor muscle, fascia and tendon of right thumb at wrist and hand level**

√7ᵗʰ **S66.092** **Other specified injury of long flexor muscle, fascia and tendon of left thumb at wrist and hand level**

√7ᵗʰ **S66.099** **Other specified injury of long flexor muscle, fascia and tendon of unspecified thumb at wrist and hand level** ▽

√5ᵗʰ **S66.1** **Injury of flexor muscle, fascia and tendon of other and unspecified finger at wrist and hand level**

EXCLUDES 2 *Injury of long flexor muscle, fascia and tendon of thumb at wrist and hand level (S66.0-)*

√6ᵗʰ **S66.10** **Unspecified injury of flexor muscle, fascia and tendon of other and unspecified finger at wrist and hand level**

√7ᵗʰ **S66.100** **Unspecified injury of flexor muscle, fascia and tendon of right index finger at wrist and hand level** ▽

√7ᵗʰ **S66.101** **Unspecified injury of flexor muscle, fascia and tendon of left index finger at wrist and hand level** ▽

√7ᵗʰ **S66.102** **Unspecified injury of flexor muscle, fascia and tendon of right middle finger at wrist and hand level** ▽

√7ᵗʰ **S66.103** **Unspecified injury of flexor muscle, fascia and tendon of left middle finger at wrist and hand level** ▽

√7ᵗʰ **S66.104** **Unspecified injury of flexor muscle, fascia and tendon of right ring finger at wrist and hand level** ▽

√7ᵗʰ **S66.105** **Unspecified injury of flexor muscle, fascia and tendon of left ring finger at wrist and hand level** ▽

√7ᵗʰ **S66.106** **Unspecified injury of flexor muscle, fascia and tendon of right little finger at wrist and hand level** ▽

√7ᵗʰ **S66.107** **Unspecified injury of flexor muscle, fascia and tendon of left little finger at wrist and hand level** ▽

√7ᵗʰ **S66.108** **Unspecified injury of flexor muscle, fascia and tendon of other finger at wrist and hand level** ▽

Unspecified injury of flexor muscle, fascia and tendon of specified finger with unspecified laterality at wrist and hand level

√7ᵗʰ **S66.109** **Unspecified injury of flexor muscle, ascia and tendon of unspecified finger at wrist and hand level** ▽

√6ᵗʰ **S66.11** **Strain of flexor muscle, fascia and tendon of other and unspecified finger at wrist and hand level**

√7ᵗʰ **S66.110** **Strain of flexor muscle, fascia and tendon of right index finger at wrist and hand level**

√7ᵗʰ **S66.111** **Strain of flexor muscle, fascia and tendon of left index finger at wrist and hand level**

√7ᵗʰ **S66.112** **Strain of flexor muscle, fascia and tendon of right middle finger at wrist and hand level**

√7ᵗʰ **S66.113** **Strain of flexor muscle, fascia and tendon of left middle finger at wrist and hand level**

√7ᵗʰ **S66.114** **Strain of flexor muscle, fascia and tendon of right ring finger at wrist and hand level**

√7ᵗʰ **S66.115** **Strain of flexor muscle, fascia and tendon of left ring finger at wrist and hand level**

√7ᵗʰ **S66.116** **Strain of flexor muscle, fascia and tendon of right little finger at wrist and hand level**

√7ᵗʰ **S66.117** **Strain of flexor muscle, fascia and tendon of left little finger at wrist and hand level**

√7ᵗʰ **S66.118** **Strain of flexor muscle, fascia and tendon of other finger at wrist and hand level**

Strain of flexor muscle, fascia and tendon of specified finger with unspecified laterality at wrist and hand level

√7ᵗʰ **S66.119** **Strain of flexor muscle, fascia and tendon of unspecified finger at wrist and hand level** ▽

√6ᵗʰ **S66.12** **Laceration of flexor muscle, fascia and tendon of other and unspecified finger at wrist and hand level**

√7ᵗʰ **S66.120** **Laceration of flexor muscle, fascia and tendon of right index finger at wrist and hand level**

√7ᵗʰ **S66.121** **Laceration of flexor muscle, fascia and tendon of left index finger at wrist and hand level**

√7ᵗʰ **S66.122** **Laceration of flexor muscle, fascia and tendon of right middle finger at wrist and hand level**

√7ᵗʰ **S66.123** **Laceration of flexor muscle, fascia and tendon of left middle finger at wrist and hand level**

√7ᵗʰ **S66.124** **Laceration of flexor muscle, fascia and tendon of right ring finger at wrist and hand level**

√7ᵗʰ **S66.125** **Laceration of flexor muscle, fascia and tendon of left ring finger at wrist and hand level**

√7ᵗʰ **S66.126** **Laceration of flexor muscle, fascia and tendon of right little finger at wrist and hand level**

√7ᵗʰ **S66.127** **Laceration of flexor muscle, fascia and tendon of left little finger at wrist and hand level**

√7ᵗʰ **S66.128** **Laceration of flexor muscle, fascia and tendon of other finger at wrist and hand level**

Laceration of flexor muscle, fascia and tendon of specified finger with unspecified laterality at wrist and hand level

√7ᵗʰ **S66.129** **Laceration of flexor muscle, fascia and tendon of unspecified finger at wrist and hand level** ▽

√6ᵗʰ **S66.19** **Other injury of flexor muscle, fascia and tendon of other and unspecified finger at wrist and hand level**

√7ᵗʰ **S66.190** **Other injury of flexor muscle, fascia and tendon of right index finger at wrist and hand level**

√7ᵗʰ **S66.191** **Other injury of flexor muscle, fascia and tendon of left index finger at wrist and hand level**

√7ᵗʰ **S66.192** **Other injury of flexor muscle, fascia and tendon of right middle finger at wrist and hand level**

√7ᵗʰ **S66.193** **Other injury of flexor muscle, fascia and tendon of left middle finger at wrist and hand level**

√7ᵗʰ **S66.194** **Other injury of flexor muscle, fascia and tendon of right ring finger at wrist and hand level**

√7ᵗʰ **S66.195** **Other injury of flexor muscle, fascia and tendon of left ring finger at wrist and hand level**

√7ᵗʰ **S66.196** **Other injury of flexor muscle, fascia and tendon of right little finger at wrist and hand level**

√7ᵗʰ **S66.197** **Other injury of flexor muscle, fascia and tendon of left little finger at wrist and hand level**

√7ᵗʰ **S66.198** **Other injury of flexor muscle, fascia and tendon of other finger at wrist and hand level**
Other injury of flexor muscle, fascia and tendon of specified finger with unspecified laterality at wrist and hand level

√7ᵗʰ **S66.199** **Other injury of flexor muscle, fascia and tendon of unspecified finger at wrist and hand level** ▽

√5ᵗʰ **S66.2** **Injury of extensor muscle, fascia and tendon of thumb at wrist and hand level**

√6ᵗʰ **S66.20** **Unspecified injury of extensor muscle, fascia and tendon of thumb at wrist and hand level**

√7ᵗʰ **S66.201** **Unspecified injury of extensor muscle, fascia and tendon of right thumb at wrist and hand level** ▽

√7ᵗʰ **S66.202** **Unspecified injury of extensor muscle, fascia and tendon of left thumb at wrist and hand level** ▽

√7ᵗʰ **S66.209** **Unspecified injury of extensor muscle, fascia and tendon of unspecified thumb at wrist and hand level** ▽

√6ᵗʰ **S66.21** **Strain of extensor muscle, fascia and tendon of thumb at wrist and hand level**

√7ᵗʰ **S66.211** **Strain of extensor muscle, fascia and tendon of right thumb at wrist and hand level**

√7ᵗʰ **S66.212** **Strain of extensor muscle, fascia and tendon of left thumb at wrist and hand level**

√7ᵗʰ **S66.219** **Strain of extensor muscle, fascia and tendon of unspecified thumb at wrist and hand level** ▽

√6ᵗʰ **S66.22** **Laceration of extensor muscle, fascia and tendon of thumb at wrist and hand level**

√7ᵗʰ **S66.221** **Laceration of extensor muscle, fascia and tendon of right thumb at wrist and hand level**

√7ᵗʰ **S66.222** **Laceration of extensor muscle, fascia and tendon of left thumb at wrist and hand level**

√7ᵗʰ **S66.229** **Laceration of extensor muscle, fascia and tendon of unspecified thumb at wrist and hand level** ▽

√6ᵗʰ **S66.29** **Other specified injury of extensor muscle, fascia and tendon of thumb at wrist and hand level**

√7ᵗʰ **S66.291** **Other specified injury of extensor muscle, fascia and tendon of right thumb at wrist and hand level**

√7ᵗʰ **S66.292** **Other specified injury of extensor muscle, fascia and tendon of left thumb at wrist and hand level**

√7ᵗʰ **S66.299** **Other specified injury of extensor muscle, fascia and tendon of unspecified thumb at wrist and hand level** ▽

√5ᵗʰ **S66.3** **Injury of extensor muscle, fascia and tendon of other and unspecified finger at wrist and hand level**
EXCLUDES 2 *Injury of extensor muscle, fascia and tendon of thumb at wrist and hand level (S66.2-)*

√6ᵗʰ **S66.30** **Unspecified injury of extensor muscle, fascia and tendon of other and unspecified finger at wrist and hand level**

√7ᵗʰ **S66.300** **Unspecified injury of extensor muscle, fascia and tendon of right index finger at wrist and hand level** ▽

√7ᵗʰ **S66.301** **Unspecified injury of extensor muscle, fascia and tendon of left index finger at wrist and hand level** ▽

√7ᵗʰ **S66.302** **Unspecified injury of extensor muscle, fascia and tendon of right middle finger at wrist and hand level** ▽

√7ᵗʰ **S66.303** **Unspecified injury of extensor muscle, fascia and tendon of left middle finger at wrist and hand level** ▽

√7ᵗʰ **S66.304** **Unspecified injury of extensor muscle, fascia and tendon of right ring finger at wrist and hand level** ▽

√7ᵗʰ **S66.305** **Unspecified injury of extensor muscle, fascia and tendon of left ring finger at wrist and hand level** ▽

√7ᵗʰ **S66.306** **Unspecified injury of extensor muscle, fascia and tendon of right little finger at wrist and hand level** ▽

√7ᵗʰ **S66.307** **Unspecified injury of extensor muscle, fascia and tendon of left little finger at wrist and hand level** ▽

√7ᵗʰ **S66.308** **Unspecified injury of extensor muscle, fascia and tendon of other finger at wrist and hand level** ▽
Unspecified injury of extensor muscle, fascia and tendon of specified finger with unspecified laterality at wrist and hand level

√7ᵗʰ **S66.309** **Unspecified injury of extensor muscle, fascia and tendon of unspecified finger at wrist and hand level** ▽

√6ᵗʰ **S66.31** **Strain of extensor muscle, fascia and tendon of other and unspecified finger at wrist and hand level**

√7ᵗʰ **S66.310** **Strain of extensor muscle, fascia and tendon of right index finger at wrist and hand level**

√7ᵗʰ **S66.311** **Strain of extensor muscle, fascia and tendon of left index finger at wrist and hand level**

√7ᵗʰ **S66.312** **Strain of extensor muscle, fascia and tendon of right middle finger at wrist and hand level**

√7ᵗʰ **S66.313** **Strain of extensor muscle, fascia and tendon of left middle finger at wrist and hand level**

√7ᵗʰ **S66.314** **Strain of extensor muscle, fascia and tendon of right ring finger at wrist and hand level**

√7ᵗʰ **S66.315** **Strain of extensor muscle, fascia and tendon of left ring finger at wrist and hand level**

√7ᵗʰ **S66.316** **Strain of extensor muscle, fascia and tendon of right little finger at wrist and hand level**

√7ᵗʰ **S66.317** **Strain of extensor muscle, fascia and tendon of left little finger at wrist and hand level**

√7ᵗʰ **S66.318** **Strain of extensor muscle, fascia and tendon of other finger at wrist and hand level**
Strain of extensor muscle, fascia and tendon of specified finger with unspecified laterality at wrist and hand level

√7ᵗʰ **S66.319** **Strain of extensor muscle, fascia and tendon of unspecified finger at wrist and hand level** ▽

√6ᵗʰ **S66.32** **Laceration of extensor muscle, fascia and tendon of other and unspecified finger at wrist and hand level**

√7ᵗʰ **S66.320** **Laceration of extensor muscle, fascia and tendon of right index finger at wrist and hand level**

√7ᵗʰ **S66.321** **Laceration of extensor muscle, fascia and tendon of left index finger at wrist and hand level**

√7ᵗʰ **S66.322** **Laceration of extensor muscle, fascia and tendon of right middle finger at wrist and hand level**

√7ᵗʰ **S66.323** **Laceration of extensor muscle, fascia and tendon of left middle finger at wrist and hand level**

√7ᵗʰ **S66.324** **Laceration of extensor muscle, fascia and tendon of right ring finger at wrist and hand level**

√7ᵗʰ **S66.325** **Laceration of extensor muscle, fascia and tendon of left ring finger at wrist and hand level**

√7ᵗʰ **S66.326** **Laceration of extensor muscle, fascia and tendon of right little finger at wrist and hand level**

✔ Additional Character Req   √x7ᵗʰ Placeholder Alert   Manifestation   HCC CMS-HCC Condition   ▽ Unspecified Code   ►◄ Revised Text   ● New Code   ▲ Revised Code Title

✓7th **S66.327** **Laceration of extensor muscle, fascia and tendon of left little finger at wrist and hand level**

✓7th **S66.328** **Laceration of extensor muscle, fascia and tendon of other finger at wrist and hand level**

Laceration of extensor muscle, fascia and tendon of specified finger with unspecified laterality at wrist and hand level

✓7th **S66.329** **Laceration of extensor muscle, fascia and tendon of unspecified finger at wrist and hand level** ▽

✓6th **S66.39** **Other injury of extensor muscle, fascia and tendon of other and unspecified finger at wrist and hand level**

✓7th **S66.390** **Other injury of extensor muscle, fascia and tendon of right index finger at wrist and hand level**

✓7th **S66.391** **Other injury of extensor muscle, fascia and tendon of left index finger at wrist and hand level**

✓7th **S66.392** **Other injury of extensor muscle, fascia and tendon of right middle finger at wrist and hand level**

✓7th **S66.393** **Other injury of extensor muscle, fascia and tendon of left middle finger at wrist and hand level**

✓7th **S66.394** **Other injury of extensor muscle, fascia and tendon of right ring finger at wrist and hand level**

✓7th **S66.395** **Other injury of extensor muscle, fascia and tendon of left ring finger at wrist and hand level**

✓7th **S66.396** **Other injury of extensor muscle, fascia and tendon of right little finger at wrist and hand level**

✓7th **S66.397** **Other injury of extensor muscle, fascia and tendon of left little finger at wrist and hand level**

✓7th **S66.398** **Other injury of extensor muscle, fascia and tendon of other finger at wrist and hand level**

Other injury of extensor muscle, fascia and tendon of specified finger with unspecified laterality at wrist and hand level

✓7th **S66.399** **Other injury of extensor muscle, fascia and tendon of unspecified finger at wrist and hand level** ▽

✓5th **S66.4** **Injury of intrinsic muscle, fascia and tendon of thumb at wrist and hand level**

✓6th **S66.40** **Unspecified injury of intrinsic muscle, fascia and tendon of thumb at wrist and hand level**

✓7th **S66.401** **Unspecified injury of intrinsic muscle, fascia and tendon of right thumb at wrist and hand level** ▽

✓7th **S66.402** **Unspecified injury of intrinsic muscle, fascia and tendon of left thumb at wrist and hand level** ▽

✓7th **S66.409** **Unspecified injury of intrinsic muscle, fascia and tendon of unspecified thumb at wrist and hand level** ▽

✓6th **S66.41** **Strain of intrinsic muscle, fascia and tendon of thumb at wrist and hand level**

✓7th **S66.411** **Strain of intrinsic muscle, fascia and tendon of right thumb at wrist and hand level**

✓7th **S66.412** **Strain of intrinsic muscle, fascia and tendon of left thumb at wrist and hand level**

✓7th **S66.419** **Strain of intrinsic muscle, fascia and tendon of unspecified thumb at wrist and hand level** ▽

✓6th **S66.42** **Laceration of intrinsic muscle, fascia and tendon of thumb at wrist and hand level**

✓7th **S66.421** **Laceration of intrinsic muscle, fascia and tendon of right thumb at wrist and hand level**

✓7th **S66.422** **Laceration of intrinsic muscle, fascia and tendon of left thumb at wrist and hand level**

✓7th **S66.429** **Laceration of intrinsic muscle, fascia and tendon of unspecified thumb at wrist and hand level** ▽

✓6th **S66.49** **Other specified injury of intrinsic muscle, fascia and tendon of thumb at wrist and hand level**

✓7th **S66.491** **Other specified injury of intrinsic muscle, fascia and tendon of right thumb at wrist and hand level**

✓7th **S66.492** **Other specified injury of intrinsic muscle, fascia and tendon of left thumb at wrist and hand level**

✓7th **S66.499** **Other specified injury of intrinsic muscle, fascia and tendon of unspecified thumb at wrist and hand level** ▽

✓5th **S66.5** **Injury of intrinsic muscle, fascia and tendon of other and unspecified finger at wrist and hand level**

EXCLUDES 2   injury of intrinsic muscle, fascia and tendon of thumb at wrist and hand level (S66.4-)

✓6th **S66.50** **Unspecified injury of intrinsic muscle, fascia and tendon of other and unspecified finger at wrist and hand level**

✓7th **S66.500** **Unspecified injury of intrinsic muscle, fascia and tendon of right index finger at wrist and hand level** ▽

✓7th **S66.501** **Unspecified injury of intrinsic muscle, fascia and tendon of left index finger at wrist and hand level** ▽

✓7th **S66.502** **Unspecified injury of intrinsic muscle, fascia and tendon of right middle finger at wrist and hand level** ▽

✓7th **S66.503** **Unspecified injury of intrinsic muscle, fascia and tendon of left middle finger at wrist and hand level** ▽

✓7th **S66.504** **Unspecified injury of intrinsic muscle, fascia and tendon of right ring finger at wrist and hand level** ▽

✓7th **S66.505** **Unspecified injury of intrinsic muscle, fascia and tendon of left ring finger at wrist and hand level** ▽

✓7th **S66.506** **Unspecified injury of intrinsic muscle, fascia and tendon of right little finger at wrist and hand level** ▽

✓7th **S66.507** **Unspecified injury of intrinsic muscle, fascia and tendon of left little finger at wrist and hand level** ▽

✓7th **S66.508** **Unspecified injury of intrinsic muscle, fascia and tendon of other finger at wrist and hand level** ▽

Unspecified injury of intrinsic muscle, fascia and tendon of specified finger with unspecified laterality at wrist and hand level

✓7th **S66.509** **Unspecified injury of intrinsic muscle, fascia and tendon of unspecified finger at wrist and hand level** ▽

✓6th **S66.51** **Strain of intrinsic muscle, fascia and tendon of other and unspecified finger at wrist and hand level**

✓7th **S66.510** **Strain of intrinsic muscle, fascia and tendon of right index finger at wrist and hand level**

✓7th **S66.511** **Strain of intrinsic muscle, fascia and tendon of left index finger at wrist and hand level**

✓7th **S66.512** **Strain of intrinsic muscle, fascia and tendon of right middle finger at wrist and hand level**

✓7th **S66.513** **Strain of intrinsic muscle, fascia and tendon of left middle finger at wrist and hand level**

✓7th **S66.514** **Strain of intrinsic muscle, fascia and tendon of right ring finger at wrist and hand level**

✓7th **S66.515** **Strain of intrinsic muscle, fascia and tendon of left ring finger at wrist and hand level**

EXCLUDES 1 Not coded here   EXCLUDES 2 Not included here   N Newborn Age: 0   P Pediatric Age: 0-17   M Maternity Age: 12-55   A Adult Age: 15-124

998   ICD-10-CM 2018

√7ᵗʰ **S66.516** **Strain of intrinsic muscle, fascia and tendon of right little finger at wrist and hand level**

√7ᵗʰ **S66.517** **Strain of intrinsic muscle, fascia and tendon of left little finger at wrist and hand level**

√7ᵗʰ **S66.518** **Strain of intrinsic muscle, fascia and tendon of other finger at wrist and hand level**

Strain of intrinsic muscle, fascia and tendon of specified finger with unspecified laterality at wrist and hand level

√7ᵗʰ **S66.519** **Strain of intrinsic muscle, fascia and tendon of unspecified finger at wrist and hand level** ▽

√6ᵗʰ **S66.52** **Laceration of intrinsic muscle, fascia and tendon of other and unspecified finger at wrist and hand level**

√7ᵗʰ **S66.520** **Laceration of intrinsic muscle, fascia and tendon of right index finger at wrist and hand level**

√7ᵗʰ **S66.521** **Laceration of intrinsic muscle, fascia and tendon of left index finger at wrist and hand level**

√7ᵗʰ **S66.522** **Laceration of intrinsic muscle, fascia and tendon of right middle finger at wrist and hand level**

√7ᵗʰ **S66.523** **Laceration of intrinsic muscle, fascia and tendon of left middle finger at wrist and hand level**

√7ᵗʰ **S66.524** **Laceration of intrinsic muscle, fascia and tendon of right ring finger at wrist and hand level**

√7ᵗʰ **S66.525** **Laceration of intrinsic muscle, fascia and tendon of left ring finger at wrist and hand level**

√7ᵗʰ **S66.526** **Laceration of intrinsic muscle, fascia and tendon of right little finger at wrist and hand level**

√7ᵗʰ **S66.527** **Laceration of intrinsic muscle, fascia and tendon of left little finger at wrist and hand level**

√7ᵗʰ **S66.528** **Laceration of intrinsic muscle, fascia and tendon of other finger at wrist and hand level**

Laceration of intrinsic muscle, fascia and tendon of specified finger with unspecified laterality at wrist and hand level

√7ᵗʰ **S66.529** **Laceration of intrinsic muscle, fascia and tendon of unspecified finger at wrist and hand level** ▽

√6ᵗʰ **S66.59** **Other injury of intrinsic muscle, fascia and tendon of other and unspecified finger at wrist and hand level**

√7ᵗʰ **S66.590** **Other injury of intrinsic muscle, fascia and tendon of right index finger at wrist and hand level**

√7ᵗʰ **S66.591** **Other injury of intrinsic muscle, fascia and tendon of left index finger at wrist and hand level**

√7ᵗʰ **S66.592** **Other injury of intrinsic muscle, fascia and tendon of right middle finger at wrist and hand level**

√7ᵗʰ **S66.593** **Other injury of intrinsic muscle, fascia and tendon of left middle finger at wrist and hand level**

√7ᵗʰ **S66.594** **Other injury of intrinsic muscle, fascia and tendon of right ring finger at wrist and hand level**

√7ᵗʰ **S66.595** **Other injury of intrinsic muscle, fascia and tendon of left ring finger at wrist and hand level**

√7ᵗʰ **S66.596** **Other injury of intrinsic muscle, fascia and tendon of right little finger at wrist and hand level**

√7ᵗʰ **S66.597** **Other injury of intrinsic muscle, fascia and tendon of left little finger at wrist and hand level**

√7ᵗʰ **S66.598** **Other injury of intrinsic muscle, fascia and tendon of other finger at wrist and hand level**

Other injury of intrinsic muscle, fascia and tendon of specified finger with unspecified laterality at wrist and hand level

√7ᵗʰ **S66.599** **Other injury of intrinsic muscle, fascia and tendon of unspecified finger at wrist and hand level** ▽

√5ᵗʰ **S66.8** **Injury of other specified muscles, fascia and tendons at wrist and hand level**

√6ᵗʰ **S66.80** **Unspecified injury of other specified muscles, fascia and tendons at wrist and hand level**

√7ᵗʰ **S66.801** **Unspecified injury of other specified muscles, fascia and tendons at wrist and hand level, right hand** ▽

√7ᵗʰ **S66.802** **Unspecified injury of other specified muscles, fascia and tendons at wrist and hand level, left hand** ▽

√7ᵗʰ **S66.809** **Unspecified injury of other specified muscles, fascia and tendons at wrist and hand level, unspecified hand** ▽

√6ᵗʰ **S66.81** **Strain of other specified muscles, fascia and tendons at wrist and hand level**

√7ᵗʰ **S66.811** **Strain of other specified muscles, fascia and tendons at wrist and hand level, right hand**

√7ᵗʰ **S66.812** **Strain of other specified muscles, fascia and tendons at wrist and hand level, left hand**

√7ᵗʰ **S66.819** **Strain of other specified muscles, fascia and tendons at wrist and hand level, unspecified hand** ▽

√6ᵗʰ **S66.82** **Laceration of other specified muscles, fascia and tendons at wrist and hand level**

√7ᵗʰ **S66.821** **Laceration of other specified muscles, fascia and tendons at wrist and hand level, right hand**

√7ᵗʰ **S66.822** **Laceration of other specified muscles, fascia and tendons at wrist and hand level, left hand**

√7ᵗʰ **S66.829** **Laceration of other specified muscles, fascia and tendons at wrist and hand level, unspecified hand** ▽

√6ᵗʰ **S66.89** **Other injury of other specified muscles, fascia and tendons at wrist and hand level**

√7ᵗʰ **S66.891** **Other injury of other specified muscles, fascia and tendons at wrist and hand level, right hand**

√7ᵗʰ **S66.892** **Other injury of other specified muscles, fascia and tendons at wrist and hand level, left hand**

√7ᵗʰ **S66.899** **Other injury of other specified muscles, fascia and tendons at wrist and hand level, unspecified hand** ▽

√5ᵗʰ **S66.9** **Injury of unspecified muscle, fascia and tendon at wrist and hand level**

√6ᵗʰ **S66.90** **Unspecified injury of unspecified muscle, fascia and tendon at wrist and hand level**

√7ᵗʰ **S66.901** **Unspecified injury of unspecified muscle, fascia and tendon at wrist and hand level, right hand** ▽

√7ᵗʰ **S66.902** **Unspecified injury of unspecified muscle, fascia and tendon at wrist and hand level, left hand** ▽

√7ᵗʰ **S66.909** **Unspecified injury of unspecified muscle, fascia and tendon at wrist and hand level, unspecified hand** ▽

√6ᵗʰ **S66.91** **Strain of unspecified muscle, fascia and tendon at wrist and hand level**

√7ᵗʰ **S66.911** **Strain of unspecified muscle, fascia and tendon at wrist and hand level, right hand** ▽

√7ᵗʰ **S66.912** **Strain of unspecified muscle, fascia and tendon at wrist and hand level, left hand** ▽

✔ Additional Character Req   √x7ᵗʰ Placeholder Alert   Manifestation   **HCC** CMS-HCC Condition   ▽ Unspecified Code   ►◄ Revised Text   ● New Code   ▲ Revised Code Title

√7ᵗʰ **S66.919** Strain of unspecified muscle, fascia and tendon at wrist and hand level, unspecified hand ▽

√6ᵗʰ **S66.92** Laceration of unspecified muscle, fascia and tendon at wrist and hand level

√7ᵗʰ **S66.921** Laceration of unspecified muscle, fascia and tendon at wrist and hand level, right hand ▽

√7ᵗʰ **S66.922** Laceration of unspecified muscle, fascia and tendon at wrist and hand level, left hand ▽

√7ᵗʰ **S66.929** Laceration of unspecified muscle, fascia and tendon at wrist and hand level, unspecified hand ▽

√6ᵗʰ **S66.99** Other injury of unspecified muscle, fascia and tendon at wrist and hand level

√7ᵗʰ **S66.991** Other injury of unspecified muscle, fascia and tendon at wrist and hand level, right hand ▽

√7ᵗʰ **S66.992** Other injury of unspecified muscle, fascia and tendon at wrist and hand level, left hand ▽

√7ᵗʰ **S66.999** Other injury of unspecified muscle, fascia and tendon at wrist and hand level, unspecified hand ▽

√4ᵗʰ **S67** **Crushing injury of wrist, hand and fingers**
Use additional code for all associated injuries, such as:
   fracture of wrist and hand (S62.-)
   open wound of wrist and hand (S61.-)

> The appropriate 7th character is to be added to each code from category S67.
> A   initial encounter
> D   subsequent encounter
> S   sequela

√5ᵗʰ **S67.0** Crushing injury of thumb

√x7ᵗʰ **S67.00** Crushing injury of unspecified thumb ▽

√x7ᵗʰ **S67.01** Crushing injury of right thumb

√x7ᵗʰ **S67.02** Crushing injury of left thumb

√5ᵗʰ **S67.1** Crushing injury of other and unspecified finger(s)
   EXCLUDES 2   crushing injury of thumb (S67.0-)

√x7ᵗʰ **S67.10** Crushing injury of unspecified finger(s) ▽

√6ᵗʰ **S67.19** Crushing injury of other finger(s)

√7ᵗʰ **S67.190** Crushing injury of right index finger

√7ᵗʰ **S67.191** Crushing injury of left index finger

√7ᵗʰ **S67.192** Crushing injury of right middle finger

√7ᵗʰ **S67.193** Crushing injury of left middle finger

√7ᵗʰ **S67.194** Crushing injury of right ring finger

√7ᵗʰ **S67.195** Crushing injury of left ring finger

√7ᵗʰ **S67.196** Crushing injury of right little finger

√7ᵗʰ **S67.197** Crushing injury of left little finger

√7ᵗʰ **S67.198** Crushing injury of other finger
   Crushing injury of specified finger with unspecified laterality

√5ᵗʰ **S67.2** Crushing injury of hand
   EXCLUDES 2   crushing injury of fingers (S67.1-)
            crushing injury of thumb (S67.0-)

√x7ᵗʰ **S67.20** Crushing injury of unspecified hand ▽

√x7ᵗʰ **S67.21** Crushing injury of right hand

√x7ᵗʰ **S67.22** Crushing injury of left hand

√5ᵗʰ **S67.3** Crushing injury of wrist

√x7ᵗʰ **S67.30** Crushing injury of unspecified wrist ▽

√x7ᵗʰ **S67.31** Crushing injury of right wrist

√x7ᵗʰ **S67.32** Crushing injury of left wrist

√5ᵗʰ **S67.4** Crushing injury of wrist and hand
   EXCLUDES 1   crushing injury of hand alone (S67.2-)
            crushing injury of wrist alone (S67.3-)
   EXCLUDES 2   crushing injury of fingers (S67.1-)
            crushing injury of thumb (S67.0-)

√x7ᵗʰ **S67.40** Crushing injury of unspecified wrist and hand ▽

√x7ᵗʰ **S67.41** Crushing injury of right wrist and hand

√x7ᵗʰ **S67.42** Crushing injury of left wrist and hand

√5ᵗʰ **S67.9** Crushing injury of unspecified part(s) of wrist, hand and fingers

√x7ᵗʰ **S67.90** Crushing injury of unspecified part(s) of unspecified wrist, hand and fingers ▽

√x7ᵗʰ **S67.91** Crushing injury of unspecified part(s) of right wrist, hand and fingers ▽

√x7ᵗʰ **S67.92** Crushing injury of unspecified part(s) of left wrist, hand and fingers ▽

√4ᵗʰ **S68** **Traumatic amputation of wrist, hand and fingers**
An amputation not identified as partial or complete should be coded to complete.

> The appropriate 7th character is to be added to each code from category S68.
> A   initial encounter
> D   subsequent encounter
> S   sequela

√5ᵗʰ **S68.0** Traumatic metacarpophalangeal amputation of thumb
   Traumatic amputation of thumb NOS

√6ᵗʰ **S68.01** Complete traumatic metacarpophalangeal amputation of thumb

³ √7ᵗʰ **S68.011** Complete traumatic metacarpophalangeal amputation of right thumb HCC

³ √7ᵗʰ **S68.012** Complete traumatic metacarpophalangeal amputation of left thumb HCC

³ √7ᵗʰ **S68.019** Complete traumatic metacarpophalangeal amputation of unspecified thumb HCC ▽

√6ᵗʰ **S68.02** Partial traumatic metacarpophalangeal amputation of thumb

³ √7ᵗʰ **S68.021** Partial traumatic metacarpophalangeal amputation of right thumb HCC

³ √7ᵗʰ **S68.022** Partial traumatic metacarpophalangeal amputation of left thumb HCC

³ √7ᵗʰ **S68.029** Partial traumatic metacarpophalangeal amputation of unspecified thumb HCC ▽

√5ᵗʰ **S68.1** Traumatic metacarpophalangeal amputation of other and unspecified finger
   Traumatic amputation of finger NOS
   EXCLUDES 2   traumatic metacarpophalangeal amputation of thumb (S68.0-)

√6ᵗʰ **S68.11** Complete traumatic metacarpophalangeal amputation of other and unspecified finger

³ √7ᵗʰ **S68.110** Complete traumatic metacarpophalangeal amputation of right index finger HCC

³ √7ᵗʰ **S68.111** Complete traumatic metacarpophalangeal amputation of left index finger HCC

³ √7ᵗʰ **S68.112** Complete traumatic metacarpophalangeal amputation of right middle finger HCC

³ √7ᵗʰ **S68.113** Complete traumatic metacarpophalangeal amputation of left middle finger HCC

³ √7ᵗʰ **S68.114** Complete traumatic metacarpophalangeal amputation of right ring finger HCC

³ √7ᵗʰ **S68.115** Complete traumatic metacarpophalangeal amputation of left ring finger HCC

³ √7ᵗʰ **S68.116** Complete traumatic metacarpophalangeal amputation of right little finger HCC

³ √7ᵗʰ **S68.117** Complete traumatic metacarpophalangeal amputation of left little finger HCC

³ √7ᵗʰ **S68.118** Complete traumatic metacarpophalangeal amputation of other finger
   Complete traumatic metacarpophalangeal amputation of specified finger with unspecified laterality HCC

³ √7ᵗʰ **S68.119** Complete traumatic metacarpophalangeal amputation of unspecified finger HCC ▽

---

³   HCC with 7th character indicating sequela.

EXCLUDES 1 Not coded here   EXCLUDES 2 Not included here   N Newborn Age: 0   P Pediatric Age: 0-17   M Maternity Age: 12-55   A Adult Age: 15-124

1000   ICD-10-CM 2018

☑6ᵗʰ **S68.12 Partial traumatic metacarpophalangeal amputation of other and unspecified finger**

3 ☑7ᵗʰ **S68.120 Partial traumatic metacarpophalangeal amputation of right index finger** HCC

3 ☑7ᵗʰ **S68.121 Partial traumatic metacarpophalangeal amputation of left index finger** HCC

3 ☑7ᵗʰ **S68.122 Partial traumatic metacarpophalangeal amputation of right middle finger** HCC

3 ☑7ᵗʰ **S68.123 Partial traumatic metacarpophalangeal amputation of left middle finger** HCC

3 ☑7ᵗʰ **S68.124 Partial traumatic metacarpophalangeal amputation of right ring finger** HCC

3 ☑7ᵗʰ **S68.125 Partial traumatic metacarpophalangeal amputation of left ring finger** HCC

3 ☑7ᵗʰ **S68.126 Partial traumatic metacarpophalangeal amputation of right little finger** HCC

3 ☑7ᵗʰ **S68.127 Partial traumatic metacarpophalangeal amputation of left little finger** HCC

3 ☑7ᵗʰ **S68.128 Partial traumatic metacarpophalangeal amputation of other finger** HCC
Partial traumatic metacarpophalangeal amputation of specified finger with unspecified laterality

3 ☑7ᵗʰ **S68.129 Partial traumatic metacarpophalangeal amputation of unspecified finger** HCC ▽

☑5ᵗʰ **S68.4 Traumatic amputation of hand at wrist level**
Traumatic amputation of hand NOS
Traumatic amputation of wrist

☑6ᵗʰ **S68.41 Complete traumatic amputation of hand at wrist level**

2 ☑7ᵗʰ **S68.411 Complete traumatic amputation of right hand at wrist level** HCC

2 ☑7ᵗʰ **S68.412 Complete traumatic amputation of left hand at wrist level** HCC

2 ☑7ᵗʰ **S68.419 Complete traumatic amputation of unspecified hand at wrist level** HCC ▽

☑6ᵗʰ **S68.42 Partial traumatic amputation of hand at wrist level**

2 ☑7ᵗʰ **S68.421 Partial traumatic amputation of right hand at wrist level** HCC

2 ☑7ᵗʰ **S68.422 Partial traumatic amputation of left hand at wrist level** HCC

2 ☑7ᵗʰ **S68.429 Partial traumatic amputation of unspecified hand at wrist level** HCC ▽

☑5ᵗʰ **S68.5 Traumatic transphalangeal amputation of thumb**
Traumatic interphalangeal joint amputation of thumb

☑6ᵗʰ **S68.51 Complete traumatic transphalangeal amputation of thumb**

3 ☑7ᵗʰ **S68.511 Complete traumatic transphalangeal amputation of right thumb** HCC

3 ☑7ᵗʰ **S68.512 Complete traumatic transphalangeal amputation of left thumb** HCC

3 ☑7ᵗʰ **S68.519 Complete traumatic transphalangeal amputation of unspecified thumb** HCC ▽

☑6ᵗʰ **S68.52 Partial traumatic transphalangeal amputation of thumb**

3 ☑7ᵗʰ **S68.521 Partial traumatic transphalangeal amputation of right thumb** HCC

3 ☑7ᵗʰ **S68.522 Partial traumatic transphalangeal amputation of left thumb** HCC

3 ☑7ᵗʰ **S68.529 Partial traumatic transphalangeal amputation of unspecified thumb** HCC ▽

☑5ᵗʰ **S68.6 Traumatic transphalangeal amputation of other and unspecified finger**

☑6ᵗʰ **S68.61 Complete traumatic transphalangeal amputation of other and unspecified finger(s)**

3 ☑7ᵗʰ **S68.610 Complete traumatic transphalangeal amputation of right index finger** HCC

3 ☑7ᵗʰ **S68.611 Complete traumatic transphalangeal amputation of left index finger** HCC

3 ☑7ᵗʰ **S68.612 Complete traumatic transphalangeal amputation of right middle finger** HCC

3 ☑7ᵗʰ **S68.613 Complete traumatic transphalangeal amputation of left middle finger** HCC

3 ☑7ᵗʰ **S68.614 Complete traumatic transphalangeal amputation of right ring finger** HCC

3 ☑7ᵗʰ **S68.615 Complete traumatic transphalangeal amputation of left ring finger** HCC

3 ☑7ᵗʰ **S68.616 Complete traumatic transphalangeal amputation of right little finger** HCC

3 ☑7ᵗʰ **S68.617 Complete traumatic transphalangeal amputation of left little finger** HCC

3 ☑7ᵗʰ **S68.618 Complete traumatic transphalangeal amputation of other finger** HCC
Complete traumatic transphalangeal amputation of specified finger with unspecified laterality

3 ☑7ᵗʰ **S68.619 Complete traumatic transphalangeal amputation of unspecified finger** HCC ▽

☑6ᵗʰ **S68.62 Partial traumatic transphalangeal amputation of other and unspecified finger**

3 ☑7ᵗʰ **S68.620 Partial traumatic transphalangeal amputation of right index finger** HCC

3 ☑7ᵗʰ **S68.621 Partial traumatic transphalangeal amputation of left index finger** HCC

3 ☑7ᵗʰ **S68.622 Partial traumatic transphalangeal amputation of right middle finger** HCC

3 ☑7ᵗʰ **S68.623 Partial traumatic transphalangeal amputation of left middle finger** HCC

3 ☑7ᵗʰ **S68.624 Partial traumatic transphalangeal amputation of right ring finger** HCC

3 ☑7ᵗʰ **S68.625 Partial traumatic transphalangeal amputation of left ring finger** HCC

3 ☑7ᵗʰ **S68.626 Partial traumatic transphalangeal amputation of right little finger** HCC

3 ☑7ᵗʰ **S68.627 Partial traumatic transphalangeal amputation of left little finger** HCC

3 ☑7ᵗʰ **S68.628 Partial traumatic transphalangeal amputation of other finger** HCC
Partial traumatic transphalangeal amputation of specified finger with unspecified laterality

3 ☑7ᵗʰ **S68.629 Partial traumatic transphalangeal amputation of unspecified finger** HCC ▽

☑5ᵗʰ **S68.7 Traumatic transmetacarpal amputation of hand**

☑6ᵗʰ **S68.71 Complete traumatic transmetacarpal amputation of hand**

2 ☑7ᵗʰ **S68.711 Complete traumatic transmetacarpal amputation of right hand** HCC

2 ☑7ᵗʰ **S68.712 Complete traumatic transmetacarpal amputation of left hand** HCC

2 ☑7ᵗʰ **S68.719 Complete traumatic transmetacarpal amputation of unspecified hand** HCC ▽

☑6ᵗʰ **S68.72 Partial traumatic transmetacarpal amputation of hand**

2 ☑7ᵗʰ **S68.721 Partial traumatic transmetacarpal amputation of right hand** HCC

2 ☑7ᵗʰ **S68.722 Partial traumatic transmetacarpal amputation of left hand** HCC

2 ☑7ᵗʰ **S68.729 Partial traumatic transmetacarpal amputation of unspecified hand** HCC ▽

---

2 HCC with 7th character indicating initial encounter (A or B - specific to category) OR sequela.
3 HCC with 7th character indicating sequela.

☑ Additional Character Req   ☑7ᵗʰ Placeholder Alert   Manifestation   HCC CMS-HCC Condition   ▽ Unspecified Code   ►◄ Revised Text   ● New Code   ▲ Revised Code Title

✓4th S69 Other and unspecified injuries of wrist, hand and finger(s)

> The appropriate 7th character is to be added to each code from category S69.
> A   initial encounter
> D   subsequent encounter
> S   sequela

✓5th **S69.8** Other specified injuries of wrist, hand and finger(s)

    ✓x7th **S69.80** Other specified injuries of unspecified wrist, hand and finger(s) ▽

    ✓x7th **S69.81** Other specified injuries of right wrist, hand and finger(s)

    ✓x7th **S69.82** Other specified injuries of left wrist, hand and finger(s)

✓5th **S69.9** Unspecified injury of wrist, hand and finger(s)

    ✓x7th **S69.90** Unspecified injury of unspecified wrist, hand and finger(s) ▽

    ✓x7th **S69.91** Unspecified injury of right wrist, hand and finger(s) ▽

    ✓x7th **S69.92** Unspecified injury of left wrist, hand and finger(s) ▽

Injuries to the hip and thigh (S70-S79)

EXCLUDES 2   burns and corrosions (T20-T32)
           frostbite (T33-T34)
           snake bite (T63.0-)
           venomous insect bite or sting (T63.4-)

✓4th S70 Superficial injury of hip and thigh

> The appropriate 7th character is to be added to each code from category S70.
> A   initial encounter
> D   subsequent encounter
> S   sequela

✓5th **S70.0** Contusion of hip

    ✓x7th **S70.00** Contusion of unspecified hip ▽

    ✓x7th **S70.01** Contusion of right hip

    ✓x7th **S70.02** Contusion of left hip

✓5th **S70.1** Contusion of thigh

    ✓x7th **S70.10** Contusion of unspecified thigh ▽

    ✓x7th **S70.11** Contusion of right thigh

    ✓x7th **S70.12** Contusion of left thigh

✓5th **S70.2** Other superficial injuries of hip

    ✓6th **S70.21** Abrasion of hip

       ✓7th **S70.211** Abrasion, right hip

       ✓7th **S70.212** Abrasion, left hip

       ✓7th **S70.219** Abrasion, unspecified hip ▽

    ✓6th **S70.22** Blister (nonthermal) of hip

       ✓7th **S70.221** Blister (nonthermal), right hip

       ✓7th **S70.222** Blister (nonthermal), left hip

       ✓7th **S70.229** Blister (nonthermal), unspecified hip ▽

    ✓6th **S70.24** External constriction of hip

       ✓7th **S70.241** External constriction, right hip

       ✓7th **S70.242** External constriction, left hip

       ✓7th **S70.249** External constriction, unspecified hip ▽

    ✓6th **S70.25** Superficial foreign body of hip
        Splinter in the hip

       ✓7th **S70.251** Superficial foreign body, right hip

       ✓7th **S70.252** Superficial foreign body, left hip

       ✓7th **S70.259** Superficial foreign body, unspecified hip ▽

    ✓6th **S70.26** Insect bite (nonvenomous) of hip

       ✓7th **S70.261** Insect bite (nonvenomous), right hip

       ✓7th **S70.262** Insect bite (nonvenomous), left hip

       ✓7th **S70.269** Insect bite (nonvenomous), unspecified hip ▽

    ✓6th **S70.27** Other superficial bite of hip
       EXCLUDES 1   open bite of hip (S71.05-)

       ✓7th **S70.271** Other superficial bite of hip, right hip

       ✓7th **S70.272** Other superficial bite of hip, left hip

       ✓7th **S70.279** Other superficial bite of hip, unspecified hip ▽

✓5th **S70.3** Other superficial injuries of thigh

    ✓6th **S70.31** Abrasion of thigh

       ✓7th **S70.311** Abrasion, right thigh

       ✓7th **S70.312** Abrasion, left thigh

       ✓7th **S70.319** Abrasion, unspecified thigh ▽

    ✓6th **S70.32** Blister (nonthermal) of thigh

       ✓7th **S70.321** Blister (nonthermal), right thigh

       ✓7th **S70.322** Blister (nonthermal), left thigh

       ✓7th **S70.329** Blister (nonthermal), unspecified thigh ▽

    ✓6th **S70.34** External constriction of thigh

       ✓7th **S70.341** External constriction, right thigh

       ✓7th **S70.342** External constriction, left thigh

       ✓7th **S70.349** External constriction, unspecified thigh ▽

    ✓6th **S70.35** Superficial foreign body of thigh
        Splinter in the thigh

       ✓7th **S70.351** Superficial foreign body, right thigh

       ✓7th **S70.352** Superficial foreign body, left thigh

       ✓7th **S70.359** Superficial foreign body, unspecified thigh ▽

    ✓6th **S70.36** Insect bite (nonvenomous) of thigh

       ✓7th **S70.361** Insect bite (nonvenomous), right thigh

       ✓7th **S70.362** Insect bite (nonvenomous), left thigh

       ✓7th **S70.369** Insect bite (nonvenomous), unspecified thigh ▽

    ✓6th **S70.37** Other superficial bite of thigh
       EXCLUDES 1   open bite of thigh (S71.15)

       ✓7th **S70.371** Other superficial bite of right thigh

       ✓7th **S70.372** Other superficial bite of left thigh

       ✓7th **S70.379** Other superficial bite of unspecified thigh ▽

✓5th **S70.9** Unspecified superficial injury of hip and thigh

    ✓6th **S70.91** Unspecified superficial injury of hip

       ✓7th **S70.911** Unspecified superficial injury of right hip ▽

       ✓7th **S70.912** Unspecified superficial injury of left hip ▽

       ✓7th **S70.919** Unspecified superficial injury of unspecified hip ▽

    ✓6th **S70.92** Unspecified superficial injury of thigh

       ✓7th **S70.921** Unspecified superficial injury of right thigh ▽

       ✓7th **S70.922** Unspecified superficial injury of left thigh ▽

       ✓7th **S70.929** Unspecified superficial injury of unspecified thigh ▽

✓4th S71 Open wound of hip and thigh

Code also any associated wound infection
EXCLUDES 1   open fracture of hip and thigh (S72.-)
           traumatic amputation of hip and thigh (S78.-)
EXCLUDES 2   bite of venomous animal (T63.-)
           open wound of ankle, foot and toes (S91.-)
           open wound of knee and lower leg (S81.-)

> The appropriate 7th character is to be added to each code from category S71.
> A   initial encounter
> D   subsequent encounter
> S   sequela

✓5th **S71.0** Open wound of hip

    ✓6th **S71.00** Unspecified open wound of hip

       ✓7th **S71.001** Unspecified open wound, right hip ▽

       ✓7th **S71.002** Unspecified open wound, left hip ▽

       ✓7th **S71.009** Unspecified open wound, unspecified hip ▽

    ✓6th **S71.01** Laceration without foreign body of hip

       ✓7th **S71.011** Laceration without foreign body, right hip

       ✓7th **S71.012** Laceration without foreign body, left hip

       ✓7th **S71.019** Laceration without foreign body, unspecified hip ▽

    ✓6th **S71.02** Laceration with foreign body of hip

       ✓7th **S71.021** Laceration with foreign body, right hip

       ✓7th **S71.022** Laceration with foreign body, left hip

EXCLUDES 1 Not coded here   EXCLUDES 2 Not included here   N Newborn Age: 0   P Pediatric Age: 0-17   M Maternity Age: 12-55   A Adult Age: 15-124

1002   ICD-10-CM 2018

✓7ᵗʰ **S71.029** Laceration with foreign body, unspecified hip ▽

✓6ᵗʰ **S71.03** **Puncture wound without foreign body** of hip

  ✓7ᵗʰ **S71.031** **Puncture wound without foreign body, right hip**

  ✓7ᵗʰ **S71.032** **Puncture wound without foreign body, left hip**

  ✓7ᵗʰ **S71.039** **Puncture wound without foreign body, unspecified hip** ▽

✓6ᵗʰ **S71.04** **Puncture wound with foreign body** of hip

  ✓7ᵗʰ **S71.041** **Puncture wound with foreign body, right hip**

  ✓7ᵗʰ **S71.042** **Puncture wound with foreign body, left hip**

  ✓7ᵗʰ **S71.049** **Puncture wound with foreign body, unspecified hip** ▽

✓6ᵗʰ **S71.05** **Open bite of hip**
Bite of hip NOS
   EXCLUDES 1   superficial bite of hip (S70.26, S70.27)

  ✓7ᵗʰ **S71.051** **Open bite, right hip**

  ✓7ᵗʰ **S71.052** **Open bite, left hip**

  ✓7ᵗʰ **S71.059** **Open bite, unspecified hip** ▽

✓5ᵗʰ **S71.1** **Open wound of thigh**

  ✓6ᵗʰ **S71.10** **Unspecified open wound of thigh**
AHA: 2016, 3Q, 24

   ✓7ᵗʰ **S71.101** **Unspecified open wound, right thigh** ▽

   ✓7ᵗʰ **S71.102** **Unspecified open wound, left thigh** ▽

   ✓7ᵗʰ **S71.109** **Unspecified open wound, unspecified thigh** ▽

  ✓6ᵗʰ **S71.11** **Laceration without foreign body of thigh**

   ✓7ᵗʰ **S71.111** **Laceration without foreign body, right thigh**

   ✓7ᵗʰ **S71.112** **Laceration without foreign body, left thigh**

   ✓7ᵗʰ **S71.119** **Laceration without foreign body, unspecified thigh** ▽

  ✓6ᵗʰ **S71.12** **Laceration with foreign body of thigh**

   ✓7ᵗʰ **S71.121** **Laceration with foreign body, right thigh**

   ✓7ᵗʰ **S71.122** **Laceration with foreign body, left thigh**

   ✓7ᵗʰ **S71.129** **Laceration with foreign body, unspecified thigh** ▽

  ✓6ᵗʰ **S71.13** **Puncture wound without foreign body of thigh**
AHA: 2016, 3Q, 24

   ✓7ᵗʰ **S71.131** **Puncture wound without foreign body, right thigh**

   ✓7ᵗʰ **S71.132** **Puncture wound without foreign body, left thigh**

   ✓7ᵗʰ **S71.139** **Puncture wound without foreign body, unspecified thigh** ▽

  ✓6ᵗʰ **S71.14** **Puncture wound with foreign body of thigh**
AHA: 2016, 3Q, 24

   ✓7ᵗʰ **S71.141** **Puncture wound with foreign body, right thigh**

   ✓7ᵗʰ **S71.142** **Puncture wound with foreign body, left thigh**

   ✓7ᵗʰ **S71.149** **Puncture wound with foreign body, unspecified thigh** ▽

  ✓6ᵗʰ **S71.15** **Open bite of thigh**
Bite of thigh NOS
   EXCLUDES 1   superficial bite of thigh (S70.37-)

   ✓7ᵗʰ **S71.151** **Open bite, right thigh**

   ✓7ᵗʰ **S71.152** **Open bite, left thigh**

   ✓7ᵗʰ **S71.159** **Open bite, unspecified thigh** ▽

✓4ᵗʰ **S72** **Fracture of femur**
  NOTE   A fracture not indicated as displaced or nondisplaced should be coded to displaced.
The open fracture designations are based on the Gustilo open fracture classification.
A fracture not indicated as open or closed should be coded to closed.
  EXCLUDES 1   traumatic amputation of hip and thigh (S78.-)
  EXCLUDES 2   fracture of lower leg and ankle (S82.-)
fracture of foot (S92.-)
periprosthetic fracture of prosthetic implant of hip ▶(M97.0-)◀
AHA: 2016, 1Q, 33; 2015, 3Q, 37-39; 2015, 1Q, 17; 2013, 4Q, 128

The appropriate 7th character is to be added to all codes from category S72 [unless otherwise indicated].
A   initial encounter for closed fracture
B   initial encounter for open fracture type I or II
    initial encounter for open fracture NOS
C   initial encounter for open fracture type IIIA, IIIB, or IIIC
D   subsequent encounter for closed fracture with routine healing
E   subsequent encounter for open fracture type I or II with routine healing
F   subsequent encounter for open fracture type IIIA, IIIB, or IIIC with routine healing
G   subsequent encounter for closed fracture with delayed healing
H   subsequent encounter for open fracture type I or II with delayed healing
J   subsequent encounter for open fracture type IIIA, IIIB, or IIIC with delayed healing
K   subsequent encounter for closed fracture with nonunion
M   subsequent encounter for open fracture type I or II with nonunion
N   subsequent encounter for open fracture type IIIA, IIIB, or IIIC with nonunion
P   subsequent encounter for closed fracture with malunion
Q   subsequent encounter for open fracture type I or II with malunion
R   subsequent encounter for open fracture type IIIA, IIIB, or IIIC with malunion
S   sequela

✓5ᵗʰ **S72.0** **Fracture of head and neck of femur**
  EXCLUDES 2   physeal fracture of upper end of femur (S79.0-)
AHA: 2016, 3Q, 16

  ✓6ᵗʰ **S72.00** **Fracture of unspecified part of neck of femur**
Fracture of hip NOS
Fracture of neck of femur NOS

   [1] ✓7ᵗʰ **S72.001** **Fracture of unspecified part of neck of right femur** HCC ▽

   [1] ✓7ᵗʰ **S72.002** **Fracture of unspecified part of neck of left femur** HCC ▽

   [1] ✓7ᵗʰ **S72.009** **Fracture of unspecified part of neck of unspecified femur** HCC ▽

  ✓6ᵗʰ **S72.01** **Unspecified intracapsular fracture of femur**
Subcapital fracture of femur

   [1] ✓7ᵗʰ **S72.011** **Unspecified intracapsular fracture of right femur** HCC ▽

   [1] ✓7ᵗʰ **S72.012** **Unspecified intracapsular fracture of left femur** HCC ▽

   [1] ✓7ᵗʰ **S72.019** **Unspecified intracapsular fracture of unspecified femur** HCC ▽

  ✓6ᵗʰ **S72.02** **Fracture of epiphysis (separation) (upper) of femur**
Transepiphyseal fracture of femur
   EXCLUDES 1   capital femoral epiphyseal fracture (pediatric) of femur (S79.01-)
Salter-Harris Type I physeal fracture of upper end of femur (S79.01-)

   [1] ✓7ᵗʰ **S72.021** **Displaced fracture of epiphysis (separation) (upper) of right femur** HCC

   [1] ✓7ᵗʰ **S72.022** **Displaced fracture of epiphysis (separation) (upper) of left femur** HCC

   [1] ✓7ᵗʰ **S72.023** **Displaced fracture of epiphysis (separation) (upper) of unspecified femur** HCC ▽

   [1] ✓7ᵗʰ **S72.024** **Nondisplaced fracture of epiphysis (separation) (upper) of right femur** HCC

   [1] ✓7ᵗʰ **S72.025** **Nondisplaced fracture of epiphysis (separation) (upper) of left femur** HCC

---

[1]   HCC with 7th character indicating initial encounter (A, B or C - specific to category).

✓ Additional Character Req   ✓x7ᵗʰ Placeholder Alert   Manifestation   HCC CMS-HCC Condition   ▽ Unspecified Code   ▶◀ Revised Text   ● New Code   ▲ Revised Code Title

ICD-10-CM 2018   **1003**

¹ ✓7ᵗʰ **S72.026** Nondisplaced fracture of epiphysis (separation) (upper) of unspecified femur `HCC` ▽

✓6ᵗʰ **S72.03** Midcervical fracture of femur
Transcervical fracture of femur NOS

¹ ✓7ᵗʰ **S72.031** Displaced midcervical fracture of right femur `HCC`

¹ ✓7ᵗʰ **S72.032** Displaced midcervical fracture of left femur `HCC`

¹ ✓7ᵗʰ **S72.033** Displaced midcervical fracture of unspecified femur `HCC` ▽

¹ ✓7ᵗʰ **S72.034** Nondisplaced midcervical fracture of right femur `HCC`

¹ ✓7ᵗʰ **S72.035** Nondisplaced midcervical fracture of left femur `HCC`

¹ ✓7ᵗʰ **S72.036** Nondisplaced midcervical fracture of unspecified femur `HCC` ▽

✓6ᵗʰ **S72.04** Fracture of base of neck of femur
Cervicotrochanteric fracture of femur

¹ ✓7ᵗʰ **S72.041** Displaced fracture of base of neck of right femur `HCC`

¹ ✓7ᵗʰ **S72.042** Displaced fracture of base of neck of left femur `HCC`

¹ ✓7ᵗʰ **S72.043** Displaced fracture of base of neck of unspecified femur `HCC` ▽

¹ ✓7ᵗʰ **S72.044** Nondisplaced fracture of base of neck of right femur `HCC`

¹ ✓7ᵗʰ **S72.045** Nondisplaced fracture of base of neck of left femur `HCC`

¹ ✓7ᵗʰ **S72.046** Nondisplaced fracture of base of neck of unspecified femur `HCC` ▽

✓6ᵗʰ **S72.05** Unspecified fracture of head of femur
Fracture of head of femur NOS

¹ ✓7ᵗʰ **S72.051** Unspecified fracture of head of right femur `HCC` ▽

¹ ✓7ᵗʰ **S72.052** Unspecified fracture of head of left femur `HCC` ▽

¹ ✓7ᵗʰ **S72.059** Unspecified fracture of head of unspecified femur `HCC` ▽

✓6ᵗʰ **S72.06** Articular fracture of head of femur

¹ ✓7ᵗʰ **S72.061** Displaced articular fracture of head of right femur `HCC`

¹ ✓7ᵗʰ **S72.062** Displaced articular fracture of head of left femur `HCC`

¹ ✓7ᵗʰ **S72.063** Displaced articular fracture of head of unspecified femur `HCC` ▽

¹ ✓7ᵗʰ **S72.064** Nondisplaced articular fracture of head of right femur `HCC`

¹ ✓7ᵗʰ **S72.065** Nondisplaced articular fracture of head of left femur `HCC`

¹ ✓7ᵗʰ **S72.066** Nondisplaced articular fracture of head of unspecified femur `HCC` ▽

✓6ᵗʰ **S72.09** Other fracture of head and neck of femur

¹ ✓7ᵗʰ **S72.091** Other fracture of head and neck of right femur `HCC`

¹ ✓7ᵗʰ **S72.092** Other fracture of head and neck of left femur `HCC`

¹ ✓7ᵗʰ **S72.099** Other fracture of head and neck of unspecified femur `HCC` ▽

✓5ᵗʰ **S72.1** Pertrochanteric fracture
AHA: 2016, 3Q, 16

✓6ᵗʰ **S72.10** Unspecified trochanteric fracture of femur
Fracture of trochanter NOS

¹ ✓7ᵗʰ **S72.101** Unspecified trochanteric fracture of right femur `HCC` ▽

¹ ✓7ᵗʰ **S72.102** Unspecified trochanteric fracture of left femur `HCC` ▽

¹ ✓7ᵗʰ **S72.109** Unspecified trochanteric fracture of unspecified femur `HCC` ▽

✓6ᵗʰ **S72.11** Fracture of greater trochanter of femur

¹ ✓7ᵗʰ **S72.111** Displaced fracture of greater trochanter of right femur `HCC`

¹ ✓7ᵗʰ **S72.112** Displaced fracture of greater trochanter of left femur `HCC`

¹ ✓7ᵗʰ **S72.113** Displaced fracture of greater trochanter of unspecified femur `HCC` ▽

¹ ✓7ᵗʰ **S72.114** Nondisplaced fracture of greater trochanter of right femur `HCC`

¹ ✓7ᵗʰ **S72.115** Nondisplaced fracture of greater trochanter of left femur `HCC`

¹ ✓7ᵗʰ **S72.116** Nondisplaced fracture of greater trochanter of unspecified femur `HCC` ▽

✓6ᵗʰ **S72.12** Fracture of lesser trochanter of femur

¹ ✓7ᵗʰ **S72.121** Displaced fracture of lesser trochanter of right femur `HCC`

¹ ✓7ᵗʰ **S72.122** Displaced fracture of lesser trochanter of left femur `HCC`

¹ ✓7ᵗʰ **S72.123** Displaced fracture of lesser trochanter of unspecified femur `HCC` ▽

¹ ✓7ᵗʰ **S72.124** Nondisplaced fracture of lesser trochanter of right femur `HCC`

¹ ✓7ᵗʰ **S72.125** Nondisplaced fracture of lesser trochanter of left femur `HCC`

¹ ✓7ᵗʰ **S72.126** Nondisplaced fracture of lesser trochanter of unspecified femur `HCC` ▽

✓6ᵗʰ **S72.13** Apophyseal fracture of femur
EXCLUDES 1 chronic (nontraumatic) slipped upper femoral epiphysis (M93.0-)

¹ ✓7ᵗʰ **S72.131** Displaced apophyseal fracture of right femur `HCC`

¹ ✓7ᵗʰ **S72.132** Displaced apophyseal fracture of left femur `HCC`

¹ ✓7ᵗʰ **S72.133** Displaced apophyseal fracture of unspecified femur `HCC` ▽

¹ ✓7ᵗʰ **S72.134** Nondisplaced apophyseal fracture of right femur `HCC`

¹ ✓7ᵗʰ **S72.135** Nondisplaced apophyseal fracture of left femur `HCC`

¹ ✓7ᵗʰ **S72.136** Nondisplaced apophyseal fracture of unspecified femur `HCC` ▽

✓6ᵗʰ **S72.14** Intertrochanteric fracture of femur

¹ ✓7ᵗʰ **S72.141** Displaced intertrochanteric fracture of right femur `HCC`

¹ ✓7ᵗʰ **S72.142** Displaced intertrochanteric fracture of left femur `HCC`

¹ ✓7ᵗʰ **S72.143** Displaced intertrochanteric fracture of unspecified femur `HCC` ▽

¹ ✓7ᵗʰ **S72.144** Nondisplaced intertrochanteric fracture of right femur `HCC`

¹ ✓7ᵗʰ **S72.145** Nondisplaced intertrochanteric fracture of left femur `HCC`

¹ ✓7ᵗʰ **S72.146** Nondisplaced intertrochanteric fracture of unspecified femur `HCC` ▽

✓5ᵗʰ **S72.2** Subtrochanteric fracture of femur

¹ ✓x7ᵗʰ **S72.21** Displaced subtrochanteric fracture of right femur `HCC`

¹ ✓x7ᵗʰ **S72.22** Displaced subtrochanteric fracture of left femur `HCC`

¹ ✓x7ᵗʰ **S72.23** Displaced subtrochanteric fracture of unspecified femur `HCC` ▽

¹ ✓x7ᵗʰ **S72.24** Nondisplaced subtrochanteric fracture of right femur `HCC`

¹ ✓x7ᵗʰ **S72.25** Nondisplaced subtrochanteric fracture of left femur `HCC`

¹ ✓x7ᵗʰ **S72.26** Nondisplaced subtrochanteric fracture of unspecified femur `HCC` ▽

✓5ᵗʰ **S72.3** Fracture of shaft of femur

✓6ᵗʰ **S72.30** Unspecified fracture of shaft of femur

¹ ✓7ᵗʰ **S72.301** Unspecified fracture of shaft of right femur `HCC` ▽

¹ ✓7ᵗʰ **S72.302** Unspecified fracture of shaft of left femur `HCC` ▽

¹ ✓7ᵗʰ **S72.309** Unspecified fracture of shaft of unspecified femur `HCC` ▽

✓6ᵗʰ **S72.32** Transverse fracture of shaft of femur

¹ ✓7ᵗʰ **S72.321** Displaced transverse fracture of shaft of right femur `HCC`

---

¹ HCC with 7th character indicating initial encounter (A, B or C - specific to category).

EXCLUDES 1 Not coded here   **EXCLUDES 2** Not included here   **N** Newborn Age: 0   **P** Pediatric Age: 0-17   **M** Maternity Age: 12-55   **A** Adult Age: 15-124

1004   ICD-10-CM 2018

[1] ✓7th	S72.322	Displaced transverse fracture of shaft of left femur	HCC
[1] ✓7th	S72.323	Displaced transverse fracture of shaft of unspecified femur	HCC ▽
[1] ✓7th	S72.324	Nondisplaced transverse fracture of shaft of right femur	HCC
[1] ✓7th	S72.325	Nondisplaced transverse fracture of shaft of left femur	HCC
[1] ✓7th	S72.326	Nondisplaced transverse fracture of shaft of unspecified femur	HCC ▽

✓6th   **S72.33**   Oblique fracture of shaft of femur

[1] ✓7th	S72.331	Displaced oblique fracture of shaft of right femur	HCC
[1] ✓7th	S72.332	Displaced oblique fracture of shaft of left femur	HCC
[1] ✓7th	S72.333	Displaced oblique fracture of shaft of unspecified femur	HCC ▽
[1] ✓7th	S72.334	Nondisplaced oblique fracture of shaft of right femur	HCC
[1] ✓7th	S72.335	Nondisplaced oblique fracture of shaft of left femur	HCC
[1] ✓7th	S72.336	Nondisplaced oblique fracture of shaft of unspecified femur	HCC ▽

✓6th   **S72.34**   Spiral fracture of shaft of femur

[1] ✓7th	S72.341	Displaced spiral fracture of shaft of right femur	HCC
[1] ✓7th	S72.342	Displaced spiral fracture of shaft of left femur	HCC
[1] ✓7th	S72.343	Displaced spiral fracture of shaft of unspecified femur	HCC ▽
[1] ✓7th	S72.344	Nondisplaced spiral fracture of shaft of right femur	HCC
[1] ✓7th	S72.345	Nondisplaced spiral fracture of shaft of left femur	HCC
[1] ✓7th	S72.346	Nondisplaced spiral fracture of shaft of unspecified femur	HCC ▽

✓6th   **S72.35**   Comminuted fracture of shaft of femur

[1] ✓7th	S72.351	Displaced comminuted fracture of shaft of right femur	HCC
[1] ✓7th	S72.352	Displaced comminuted fracture of shaft of left femur	HCC
[1] ✓7th	S72.353	Displaced comminuted fracture of shaft of unspecified femur	HCC ▽
[1] ✓7th	S72.354	Nondisplaced comminuted fracture of shaft of right femur	HCC
[1] ✓7th	S72.355	Nondisplaced comminuted fracture of shaft of left femur	HCC
[1] ✓7th	S72.356	Nondisplaced comminuted fracture of shaft of unspecified femur	HCC ▽

✓6th   **S72.36**   Segmental fracture of shaft of femur

[1] ✓7th	S72.361	Displaced segmental fracture of shaft of right femur	HCC
[1] ✓7th	S72.362	Displaced segmental fracture of shaft of left femur	HCC
[1] ✓7th	S72.363	Displaced segmental fracture of shaft of unspecified femur	HCC ▽
[1] ✓7th	S72.364	Nondisplaced segmental fracture of shaft of right femur	HCC
[1] ✓7th	S72.365	Nondisplaced segmental fracture of shaft of left femur	HCC
[1] ✓7th	S72.366	Nondisplaced segmental fracture of shaft of unspecified femur	HCC ▽

✓6th   **S72.39**   Other fracture of shaft of femur

[1] ✓7th	S72.391	Other fracture of shaft of right femur	HCC
[1] ✓7th	S72.392	Other fracture of shaft of left femur	HCC
[1] ✓7th	S72.399	Other fracture of shaft of unspecified femur	HCC ▽

✓5th   **S72.4**   Fracture of lower end of femur
Fracture of distal end of femur
EXCLUDES 2   fracture of shaft of femur (S72.3-)
          physeal fracture of lower end of femur (S79.1-)

✓6th   **S72.40**   Unspecified fracture of lower end of femur

[1] ✓7th	S72.401	Unspecified fracture of lower end of right femur	HCC ▽

[1] ✓7th	S72.402	Unspecified fracture of lower end of left femur	HCC ▽
[1] ✓7th	S72.409	Unspecified fracture of lower end of unspecified femur	HCC ▽

✓6th   **S72.41**   Unspecified condyle fracture of lower end of femur
Condyle fracture of femur NOS

[1] ✓7th	S72.411	Displaced unspecified condyle fracture of lower end of right femur	HCC ▽
[1] ✓7th	S72.412	Displaced unspecified condyle fracture of lower end of left femur	HCC ▽
[1] ✓7th	S72.413	Displaced unspecified condyle fracture of lower end of unspecified femur	HCC ▽
[1] ✓7th	S72.414	Nondisplaced unspecified condyle fracture of lower end of right femur	HCC ▽
[1] ✓7th	S72.415	Nondisplaced unspecified condyle fracture of lower end of left femur	HCC ▽
[1] ✓7th	S72.416	Nondisplaced unspecified condyle fracture of lower end of unspecified femur	HCC ▽

✓6th   **S72.42**   Fracture of lateral condyle of femur

[1] ✓7th	S72.421	Displaced fracture of lateral condyle of right femur	HCC
[1] ✓7th	S72.422	Displaced fracture of lateral condyle of left femur	HCC
[1] ✓7th	S72.423	Displaced fracture of lateral condyle of unspecified femur	HCC ▽
[1] ✓7th	S72.424	Nondisplaced fracture of lateral condyle of right femur	HCC
[1] ✓7th	S72.425	Nondisplaced fracture of lateral condyle of left femur	HCC
[1] ✓7th	S72.426	Nondisplaced fracture of lateral condyle of unspecified femur	HCC ▽

✓6th   **S72.43**   Fracture of medial condyle of femur

[1] ✓7th	S72.431	Displaced fracture of medial condyle of right femur	HCC
[1] ✓7th	S72.432	Displaced fracture of medial condyle of left femur	HCC
[1] ✓7th	S72.433	Displaced fracture of medial condyle of unspecified femur	HCC ▽
[1] ✓7th	S72.434	Nondisplaced fracture of medial condyle of right femur	HCC
[1] ✓7th	S72.435	Nondisplaced fracture of medial condyle of left femur	HCC
[1] ✓7th	S72.436	Nondisplaced fracture of medial condyle of unspecified femur	HCC ▽

✓6th   **S72.44**   Fracture of lower epiphysis (separation) of femur
EXCLUDES 1   *Salter-Harris Type I physeal fracture of lower end of femur (S79.11-)*

[1] ✓7th	S72.441	Displaced fracture of lower epiphysis (separation) of right femur	HCC
[1] ✓7th	S72.442	Displaced fracture of lower epiphysis (separation) of left femur	HCC
[1] ✓7th	S72.443	Displaced fracture of lower epiphysis (separation) of unspecified femur	HCC ▽
[1] ✓7th	S72.444	Nondisplaced fracture of lower epiphysis (separation) of right femur	HCC
[1] ✓7th	S72.445	Nondisplaced fracture of lower epiphysis (separation) of left femur	HCC
[1] ✓7th	S72.446	Nondisplaced fracture of lower epiphysis (separation) of unspecified femur	HCC ▽

✓6th   **S72.45**   Supracondylar fracture without intracondylar extension of lower end of femur
Supracondylar fracture of lower end of femur NOS
EXCLUDES 1   *supracondylar fracture with intracondylar extension of lower end of femur (S72.46-)*

[1] ✓7th	S72.451	Displaced supracondylar fracture without intracondylar extension of lower end of right femur	HCC
[1] ✓7th	S72.452	Displaced supracondylar fracture without intracondylar extension of lower end of left femur	HCC

---

[1]   HCC with 7th character indicating initial encounter (A, B or C - specific to category).

✓ Additional Character Req   ✓x7th Placeholder Alert   Manifestation   HCC CMS-HCC Condition   ▽ Unspecified Code   ▶◀ Revised Text   ● New Code   ▲ Revised Code Title

1 ✓7ᵗʰ **S72.453** **Displaced supracondylar fracture** HCC ▽
without intracondylar extension of
lower end of unspecified femur

1 ✓7ᵗʰ **S72.454** **Nondisplaced supracondylar fracture** HCC
without intracondylar extension of
lower end of **right** femur

1 ✓7ᵗʰ **S72.455** **Nondisplaced supracondylar fracture** HCC
without intracondylar extension of
lower end of **left** femur

1 ✓7ᵗʰ **S72.456** **Nondisplaced supracondylar** HCC ▽
fracture without intracondylar
extension of lower end of unspecified
femur

✓6ᵗʰ **S72.46** **Supracondylar fracture with intracondylar extension**
of lower end of femur

EXCLUDES 1   *supracondylar fracture without*
intracondylar extension of lower end of
femur
(S72.45-)

1 ✓7ᵗʰ **S72.461** **Displaced supracondylar fracture** HCC
with intracondylar extension of
lower end of **right** femur

1 ✓7ᵗʰ **S72.462** **Displaced supracondylar fracture** HCC
with intracondylar extension of
lower end of **left** femur

1 ✓7ᵗʰ **S72.463** **Displaced supracondylar fracture** HCC ▽
with intracondylar extension of
lower end of unspecified femur

1 ✓7ᵗʰ **S72.464** **Nondisplaced supracondylar fracture** HCC
with intracondylar extension of
lower end of **right** femur

1 ✓7ᵗʰ **S72.465** **Nondisplaced supracondylar fracture** HCC
with intracondylar extension of
lower end of **left** femur

1 ✓7ᵗʰ **S72.466** **Nondisplaced supracondylar** HCC ▽
fracture with intracondylar extension
of lower end of unspecified femur

✓6ᵗʰ **S72.47** **Torus fracture of lower end of femur**

The appropriate 7th character is to be added to all
codes in subcategory S72.47.
A   initial encounter for closed fracture
D   subsequent encounter for fracture with
routine healing
G   subsequent encounter for fracture with
delayed healing
K   subsequent encounter for fracture with
nonunion
P   subsequent encounter for fracture with
malunion
S   sequela

1 ✓7ᵗʰ **S72.471** **Torus fracture of lower end of** HCC
right femur

1 ✓7ᵗʰ **S72.472** **Torus fracture of lower end of** HCC
left femur

1 ✓7ᵗʰ **S72.479** **Torus fracture of lower end of** HCC ▽
unspecified femur

✓6ᵗʰ **S72.49** **Other fracture of lower end of femur**

1 ✓7ᵗʰ **S72.491** **Other fracture of lower end of** HCC
right femur

1 ✓7ᵗʰ **S72.492** **Other fracture of lower end of** HCC
left femur

1 ✓7ᵗʰ **S72.499** **Other fracture of lower end of** HCC ▽
unspecified femur

✓5ᵗʰ **S72.8** **Other fracture of femur**

✓6ᵗʰ **S72.8X** **Other fracture of femur**

1 ✓7ᵗʰ **S72.8X1** **Other fracture of right femur** HCC

1 ✓7ᵗʰ **S72.8X2** **Other fracture of left femur** HCC

1 ✓7ᵗʰ **S72.8X9** **Other fracture of unspecified** HCC ▽
femur

✓5ᵗʰ **S72.9** **Unspecified fracture of femur**
Fracture of thigh NOS
Fracture of upper leg NOS
EXCLUDES 1   *fracture of hip NOS (S72.00-, S72.01-)*

1 ✓x7ᵗʰ **S72.90** **Unspecified fracture of unspecified femur** HCC ▽
AHA: 2012, 4Q, 93

1 ✓x7ᵗʰ **S72.91** **Unspecified fracture of right femur** HCC ▽

1 ✓x7ᵗʰ **S72.92** **Unspecified fracture of left femur** HCC ▽

✓4ᵗʰ **S73** **Dislocation and sprain of joint and ligaments of hip**
INCLUDES   avulsion of joint or ligament of hip
laceration of cartilage, joint or ligament of hip
sprain of cartilage, joint or ligament of hip
traumatic hemarthrosis of joint or ligament of hip
traumatic rupture of joint or ligament of hip
traumatic subluxation of joint or ligament of hip
traumatic tear of joint or ligament of hip
Code also any associated open wound
EXCLUDES 2   *strain of muscle, fascia and tendon of hip and thigh (S76.-)*

The appropriate 7th character is to be added to each code from
category S73.
A   initial encounter
D   subsequent encounter
S   sequela

✓5ᵗʰ **S73.0** **Subluxation and dislocation of hip**
EXCLUDES 2   *dislocation and subluxation of hip prosthesis (T84.020,*
T84.021)

✓6ᵗʰ **S73.00** **Unspecified subluxation and dislocation of hip**
Dislocation of hip NOS
Subluxation of hip NOS

1 ✓7ᵗʰ **S73.001** **Unspecified subluxation of right hip** HCC ▽

1 ✓7ᵗʰ **S73.002** **Unspecified subluxation of left hip** HCC ▽

1 ✓7ᵗʰ **S73.003** **Unspecified subluxation of** HCC ▽
unspecified hip

1 ✓7ᵗʰ **S73.004** **Unspecified dislocation of right hip** HCC ▽

1 ✓7ᵗʰ **S73.005** **Unspecified dislocation of left hip** HCC ▽

1 ✓7ᵗʰ **S73.006** **Unspecified dislocation of** HCC ▽
unspecified hip

✓6ᵗʰ **S73.01** **Posterior subluxation and dislocation of hip**

1 ✓7ᵗʰ **S73.011** **Posterior subluxation of right hip** HCC

1 ✓7ᵗʰ **S73.012** **Posterior subluxation of left hip** HCC

1 ✓7ᵗʰ **S73.013** **Posterior subluxation of** HCC ▽
unspecified hip

1 ✓7ᵗʰ **S73.014** **Posterior dislocation of right hip** HCC

1 ✓7ᵗʰ **S73.015** **Posterior dislocation of left hip** HCC

1 ✓7ᵗʰ **S73.016** **Posterior dislocation of** HCC ▽
unspecified hip

✓6ᵗʰ **S73.02** **Obturator subluxation and dislocation of hip**

1 ✓7ᵗʰ **S73.021** **Obturator subluxation of right hip** HCC

1 ✓7ᵗʰ **S73.022** **Obturator subluxation of left hip** HCC

1 ✓7ᵗʰ **S73.023** **Obturator subluxation of** HCC ▽
unspecified hip

1 ✓7ᵗʰ **S73.024** **Obturator dislocation of right hip** HCC

1 ✓7ᵗʰ **S73.025** **Obturator dislocation of left hip** HCC

1 ✓7ᵗʰ **S73.026** **Obturator dislocation of** HCC ▽
unspecified hip

▲ ✓6ᵗʰ **S73.03** **Other anterior subluxation and dislocation of hip**

1 ✓7ᵗʰ **S73.031** **Other anterior subluxation of** HCC
right hip

1 ✓7ᵗʰ **S73.032** **Other anterior subluxation of** HCC
left hip

1 ✓7ᵗʰ **S73.033** **Other anterior subluxation of** HCC ▽
unspecified hip

1 ✓7ᵗʰ **S73.034** **Other anterior dislocation of** HCC
right hip

1 ✓7ᵗʰ **S73.035** **Other anterior dislocation of** HCC
left hip

1 ✓7ᵗʰ **S73.036** **Other anterior dislocation of** HCC ▽
unspecified hip

▲ ✓6ᵗʰ **S73.04** **Central subluxation and dislocation of hip**

1 ✓7ᵗʰ **S73.041** **Central subluxation of right hip** HCC

1 ✓7ᵗʰ **S73.042** **Central subluxation of left hip** HCC

1 ✓7ᵗʰ **S73.043** **Central subluxation of unspecified** HCC ▽
hip

---

1 HCC with 7th character indicating initial encounter (A, B or C - specific to category).

EXCLUDES 1 Not coded here   EXCLUDES 2 Not included here   N Newborn Age: 0   P Pediatric Age: 0-17   M Maternity Age: 12-55   A Adult Age: 15-124

1006   ICD-10-CM 2018

1 ✓7ᵗʰ **S73.044** **Central dislocation of right hip** HCC

1 ✓7ᵗʰ **S73.045** **Central dislocation of left hip** HCC

1 ✓7ᵗʰ **S73.046** **Central dislocation of unspecified hip** HCC ▽

✓5ᵗʰ **S73.1** **Sprain of hip**
AHA: 2014, 4Q, 25

  ✓6ᵗʰ **S73.10** **Unspecified sprain of hip**

    ✓7ᵗʰ **S73.101** **Unspecified sprain of right hip** ▽

    ✓7ᵗʰ **S73.102** **Unspecified sprain of left hip** ▽

    ✓7ᵗʰ **S73.109** **Unspecified sprain of unspecified hip** ▽

  ✓6ᵗʰ **S73.11** **Iliofemoral ligament sprain of hip**

    ✓7ᵗʰ **S73.111** **Iliofemoral ligament sprain of right hip**

    ✓7ᵗʰ **S73.112** **Iliofemoral ligament sprain of left hip**

    ✓7ᵗʰ **S73.119** **Iliofemoral ligament sprain of unspecified hip** ▽

  ✓6ᵗʰ **S73.12** **Ischiocapsular (ligament) sprain of hip**

    ✓7ᵗʰ **S73.121** **Ischiocapsular ligament sprain of right hip**

    ✓7ᵗʰ **S73.122** **Ischiocapsular ligament sprain of left hip**

    ✓7ᵗʰ **S73.129** **Ischiocapsular ligament sprain of unspecified hip** ▽

  ✓6ᵗʰ **S73.19** **Other sprain of hip**

    ✓7ᵗʰ **S73.191** **Other sprain of right hip**

    ✓7ᵗʰ **S73.192** **Other sprain of left hip**

    ✓7ᵗʰ **S73.199** **Other sprain of unspecified hip** ▽

✓4ᵗʰ **S74** **Injury of nerves at hip and thigh level**
Code also any associated open wound (S71.-)
EXCLUDES 2 *injury of nerves at ankle and foot level (S94.-)*
    injury of nerves at lower leg level (S84.-)

> The appropriate 7th character is to be added to each code from category S74.
> A initial encounter
> D subsequent encounter
> S sequela

✓5ᵗʰ **S74.0** **Injury of sciatic nerve at hip and thigh level**

  ✓×7ᵗʰ **S74.00** **Injury of sciatic nerve at hip and thigh level, unspecified leg** ▽

  ✓×7ᵗʰ **S74.01** **Injury of sciatic nerve at hip and thigh level, right leg**

  ✓×7ᵗʰ **S74.02** **Injury of sciatic nerve at hip and thigh level, left leg**

✓5ᵗʰ **S74.1** **Injury of femoral nerve at hip and thigh level**

  ✓×7ᵗʰ **S74.10** **Injury of femoral nerve at hip and thigh level, unspecified leg** ▽

  ✓×7ᵗʰ **S74.11** **Injury of femoral nerve at hip and thigh level, right leg**

  ✓×7ᵗʰ **S74.12** **Injury of femoral nerve at hip and thigh level, left leg**

✓5ᵗʰ **S74.2** **Injury of cutaneous sensory nerve at hip and thigh level**

  ✓×7ᵗʰ **S74.20** **Injury of cutaneous sensory nerve at hip and thigh level, unspecified leg** ▽

  ✓×7ᵗʰ **S74.21** **Injury of cutaneous sensory nerve at hip and high level, right leg**

  ✓×7ᵗʰ **S74.22** **Injury of cutaneous sensory nerve at hip and thigh level, left leg**

✓5ᵗʰ **S74.8** **Injury of other nerves at hip and thigh level**

  ✓6ᵗʰ **S74.8X** **Injury of other nerves at hip and thigh level**

    ✓7ᵗʰ **S74.8X1** **Injury of other nerves at hip and thigh level, right leg**

    ✓7ᵗʰ **S74.8X2** **Injury of other nerves at hip and thigh level, left leg**

    ✓7ᵗʰ **S74.8X9** **Injury of other nerves at hip and thigh level, unspecified leg** ▽

✓5ᵗʰ **S74.9** **Injury of unspecified nerve at hip and thigh level**

  ✓×7ᵗʰ **S74.90** **Injury of unspecified nerve at hip and thigh level, unspecified leg** ▽

  ✓×7ᵗʰ **S74.91** **Injury of unspecified nerve at hip and thigh level, right leg** ▽

  ✓×7ᵗʰ **S74.92** **Injury of unspecified nerve at hip and thigh level, left leg** ▽

✓4ᵗʰ **S75** **Injury of blood vessels at hip and thigh level**
Code also any associated open wound (S71.-)
EXCLUDES 2 *injury of blood vessels at lower leg level (S85.-)*
    injury of popliteal artery (S85.0)

> The appropriate 7th character is to be added to each code from category S75.
> A initial encounter
> D subsequent encounter
> S sequela

✓5ᵗʰ **S75.0** **Injury of femoral artery**

  ✓6ᵗʰ **S75.00** **Unspecified injury of femoral artery**

    ✓7ᵗʰ **S75.001** **Unspecified injury of femoral artery, right leg** ▽

    ✓7ᵗʰ **S75.002** **Unspecified injury of femoral artery, left leg** ▽

    ✓7ᵗʰ **S75.009** **Unspecified injury of femoral artery, unspecified leg** ▽

  ✓6ᵗʰ **S75.01** **Minor laceration of femoral artery**
Incomplete transection of femoral artery
Laceration of femoral artery NOS
Superficial laceration of femoral artery

    ✓7ᵗʰ **S75.011** **Minor laceration of femoral artery, right leg**

    ✓7ᵗʰ **S75.012** **Minor laceration of femoral artery, left leg**

    ✓7ᵗʰ **S75.019** **Minor laceration of femoral artery, unspecified leg** ▽

  ✓6ᵗʰ **S75.02** **Major laceration of femoral artery**
Complete transection of femoral artery
Traumatic rupture of femoral artery

    ✓7ᵗʰ **S75.021** **Major laceration of femoral artery, right leg**

    ✓7ᵗʰ **S75.022** **Major laceration of femoral artery, left leg**

    ✓7ᵗʰ **S75.029** **Major laceration of femoral artery, unspecified leg** ▽

  ✓6ᵗʰ **S75.09** **Other specified injury of femoral artery**

    ✓7ᵗʰ **S75.091** **Other specified injury of femoral artery, right leg**

    ✓7ᵗʰ **S75.092** **Other specified injury of femoral artery, left leg**

    ✓7ᵗʰ **S75.099** **Other specified injury of femoral artery, unspecified leg** ▽

✓5ᵗʰ **S75.1** **Injury of femoral vein at hip and thigh level**

  ✓6ᵗʰ **S75.10** **Unspecified injury of femoral vein at hip and thigh level**

    ✓7ᵗʰ **S75.101** **Unspecified injury of femoral vein at hip and thigh level, right leg** ▽

    ✓7ᵗʰ **S75.102** **Unspecified injury of femoral vein at hip and thigh level, left leg** ▽

    ✓7ᵗʰ **S75.109** **Unspecified injury of femoral vein at hip and thigh level, unspecified leg** ▽

  ✓6ᵗʰ **S75.11** **Minor laceration of femoral vein at hip and thigh level**
Incomplete transection of femoral vein at hip and thigh level
Laceration of femoral vein at hip and thigh level NOS
Superficial laceration of femoral vein at hip and thigh level

    ✓7ᵗʰ **S75.111** **Minor laceration of femoral vein at hip and thigh level, right leg**

    ✓7ᵗʰ **S75.112** **Minor laceration of femoral vein at hip and thigh level, left leg**

    ✓7ᵗʰ **S75.119** **Minor laceration of femoral vein at hip and thigh level, unspecified leg** ▽

  ✓6ᵗʰ **S75.12** **Major laceration of femoral vein at hip and thigh level**
Complete transection of femoral vein at hip and thigh level
Traumatic rupture of femoral vein at hip and thigh level

    ✓7ᵗʰ **S75.121** **Major laceration of femoral vein at hip and thigh level, right leg**

    ✓7ᵗʰ **S75.122** **Major laceration of femoral vein at hip and thigh level, left leg**

    ✓7ᵗʰ **S75.129** **Major laceration of femoral vein at hip and thigh level, unspecified leg** ▽

---

1 HCC with 7th character indicating initial encounter (A, B or C - specific to category).

✓ Additional Character Req   ✓×7ᵗʰ Placeholder Alert   Manifestation   HCC CMS-HCC Condition   ▽ Unspecified Code   ►◄ Revised Text   ● New Code   ▲ Revised Code Title

ICD-10-CM 2018   1007

√6ᵗʰ **S75.19 Other specified injury of femoral vein at hip and thigh level**

    √7ᵗʰ **S75.191 Other specified injury of femoral vein at hip and thigh level, right leg**

    √7ᵗʰ **S75.192 Other specified injury of femoral vein at hip and thigh level, left leg**

    √7ᵗʰ **S75.199 Other specified injury of femoral vein at hip and thigh level, unspecified leg** ▽

√5ᵗʰ **S75.2 Injury of greater saphenous vein at hip and thigh level**

    EXCLUDES 1   *greater saphenous vein NOS (S85.3)*

   √6ᵗʰ **S75.20 Unspecified injury of greater saphenous vein at hip and thigh level**

    √7ᵗʰ **S75.201 Unspecified injury of greater saphenous vein at hip and thigh level, right leg** ▽

    √7ᵗʰ **S75.202 Unspecified injury of greater saphenous vein at hip and thigh level, left leg** ▽

    √7ᵗʰ **S75.209 Unspecified injury of greater saphenous vein at hip and thigh level, unspecified leg** ▽

   √6ᵗʰ **S75.21 Minor laceration of greater saphenous vein at hip and thigh level**

    Incomplete transection of greater saphenous vein at hip and thigh level

    Laceration of greater saphenous vein at hip and thigh level NOS

    Superficial laceration of greater saphenous vein at hip and thigh level

    √7ᵗʰ **S75.211 Minor laceration of greater saphenous vein at hip and thigh level, right leg**

    √7ᵗʰ **S75.212 Minor laceration of greater saphenous vein at hip and thigh level, left leg**

    √7ᵗʰ **S75.219 Minor laceration of greater saphenous vein at hip and thigh level, unspecified leg** ▽

   √6ᵗʰ **S75.22 Major laceration of greater saphenous vein at hip and thigh level**

    Complete transection of greater saphenous vein at hip and thigh level

    Traumatic rupture of greater saphenous vein at hip and thigh level

    √7ᵗʰ **S75.221 Major laceration of greater saphenous vein at hip and thigh level, right leg**

    √7ᵗʰ **S75.222 Major laceration of greater saphenous vein at hip and thigh level, left leg**

    √7ᵗʰ **S75.229 Major laceration of greater saphenous vein at hip and thigh level, unspecified leg** ▽

   √6ᵗʰ **S75.29 Other specified injury of greater saphenous vein at hip and thigh level**

    √7ᵗʰ **S75.291 Other specified injury of greater saphenous vein at hip and thigh level, right leg**

    √7ᵗʰ **S75.292 Other specified injury of greater saphenous vein at hip and thigh level, left leg**

    √7ᵗʰ **S75.299 Other specified injury of greater saphenous vein at hip and thigh level, unspecified leg** ▽

√5ᵗʰ **S75.8 Injury of other blood vessels at hip and thigh level**

   √6ᵗʰ **S75.80 Unspecified injury of other blood vessels at hip and thigh level**

    √7ᵗʰ **S75.801 Unspecified injury of other blood vessels at hip and thigh level, right leg** ▽

    √7ᵗʰ **S75.802 Unspecified injury of other blood vessels at hip and thigh level, left leg** ▽

    √7ᵗʰ **S75.809 Unspecified injury of other blood vessels at hip and thigh level, unspecified leg** ▽

   √6ᵗʰ **S75.81 Laceration of other blood vessels at hip and thigh level**

    √7ᵗʰ **S75.811 Laceration of other blood vessels at hip and thigh level, right leg**

    √7ᵗʰ **S75.812 Laceration of other blood vessels at hip and thigh level, left leg**

    √7ᵗʰ **S75.819 Laceration of other blood vessels at hip and thigh level, unspecified leg** ▽

   √6ᵗʰ **S75.89 Other specified injury of other blood vessels at hip and thigh level**

    √7ᵗʰ **S75.891 Other specified injury of other blood vessels at hip and thigh level, right leg**

    √7ᵗʰ **S75.892 Other specified injury of other blood vessels at hip and thigh level, left leg**

    √7ᵗʰ **S75.899 Other specified injury of other blood vessels at hip and thigh level, unspecified leg** ▽

√5ᵗʰ **S75.9 Injury of unspecified blood vessel at hip and thigh level**

   √6ᵗʰ **S75.90 Unspecified injury of unspecified blood vessel at hip and thigh level**

    √7ᵗʰ **S75.901 Unspecified injury of unspecified blood vessel at hip and thigh level, right leg** ▽

    √7ᵗʰ **S75.902 Unspecified injury of unspecified blood vessel at hip and thigh level, left leg** ▽

    √7ᵗʰ **S75.909 Unspecified injury of unspecified blood vessel at hip and thigh level, unspecified leg** ▽

   √6ᵗʰ **S75.91 Laceration of unspecified blood vessel at hip and thigh level**

    √7ᵗʰ **S75.911 Laceration of unspecified blood vessel at hip and thigh level, right leg** ▽

    √7ᵗʰ **S75.912 Laceration of unspecified blood vessel at hip and thigh level, left leg** ▽

    √7ᵗʰ **S75.919 Laceration of unspecified blood vessel at hip and thigh level, unspecified leg** ▽

   √6ᵗʰ **S75.99 Other specified injury of unspecified blood vessel at hip and thigh level**

    √7ᵗʰ **S75.991 Other specified injury of unspecified blood vessel at hip and thigh level, right leg** ▽

    √7ᵗʰ **S75.992 Other specified injury of unspecified blood vessel at hip and thigh level, left leg** ▽

    √7ᵗʰ **S75.999 Other specified injury of unspecified blood vessel at hip and thigh level, unspecified leg** ▽

√4ᵗʰ **S76 Injury of muscle, fascia and tendon at hip and thigh level**

   Code also any associated open wound (S71.-)

   EXCLUDES 2   *injury of muscle, fascia and tendon at lower leg level (S86)*
          sprain of joint and ligament of hip (S73.1)

   TIP: Refer to the Muscle/Tendon table at the beginning of this chapter.

> The appropriate 7th character is to be added to each code from category S76.
> A   initial encounter
> D   subsequent encounter
> S   sequela

√5ᵗʰ **S76.0 Injury of muscle, fascia and tendon of hip**

   √6ᵗʰ **S76.00 Unspecified injury of muscle, fascia and tendon of hip**

    √7ᵗʰ **S76.001 Unspecified injury of muscle, fascia and tendon of right hip** ▽

    √7ᵗʰ **S76.002 Unspecified injury of muscle, fascia and tendon of left hip** ▽

    √7ᵗʰ **S76.009 Unspecified injury of muscle, fascia and tendon of unspecified hip** ▽

   √6ᵗʰ **S76.01 Strain of muscle, fascia and tendon of hip**

    √7ᵗʰ **S76.011 Strain of muscle, fascia and tendon of right hip**

    √7ᵗʰ **S76.012 Strain of muscle, fascia and tendon of left hip**

    √7ᵗʰ **S76.019 Strain of muscle, fascia and tendon of unspecified hip** ▽

   √6ᵗʰ **S76.02 Laceration of muscle, fascia and tendon of hip**

    √7ᵗʰ **S76.021 Laceration of muscle, fascia and tendon of right hip**

    √7ᵗʰ **S76.022 Laceration of muscle, fascia and tendon of left hip**

    √7ᵗʰ **S76.029 Laceration of muscle, fascia and tendon of unspecified hip** ▽

EXCLUDES 1 Not coded here   EXCLUDES 2 Not included here   N Newborn Age: 0   P Pediatric Age: 0-17   M Maternity Age: 12-55   A Adult Age: 15-124

1008   ICD-10-CM 2018

√6ᵗʰ **S76.09** **Other specified injury of muscle, fascia and tendon of hip**

    √7ᵗʰ **S76.091** Other specified injury of muscle, fascia and tendon of right hip

    √7ᵗʰ **S76.092** Other specified injury of muscle, fascia and tendon of left hip

    √7ᵗʰ **S76.099** Other specified injury of muscle, fascia ▽ and tendon of unspecified hip

√5ᵗʰ **S76.1** **Injury of quadriceps muscle, fascia and tendon**
Injury of patellar ligament (tendon)

    √6ᵗʰ **S76.10** **Unspecified injury of quadriceps muscle, fascia and tendon**

       √7ᵗʰ **S76.101** Unspecified injury of right quadriceps ▽ muscle, fascia and tendon

       √7ᵗʰ **S76.102** Unspecified injury of left quadriceps ▽ muscle, fascia and tendon

       √7ᵗʰ **S76.109** Unspecified injury of unspecified ▽ quadriceps muscle, fascia and tendon

    √6ᵗʰ **S76.11** **Strain of quadriceps muscle, fascia and tendon**

       √7ᵗʰ **S76.111** Strain of right quadriceps muscle, fascia and tendon

       √7ᵗʰ **S76.112** Strain of left quadriceps muscle, fascia and tendon

       √7ᵗʰ **S76.119** Strain of unspecified quadriceps ▽ muscle, fascia and tendon

    √6ᵗʰ **S76.12** **Laceration of quadriceps muscle, fascia and tendon**

       √7ᵗʰ **S76.121** Laceration of right quadriceps muscle, fascia and tendon

       √7ᵗʰ **S76.122** Laceration of left quadriceps muscle, fascia and tendon

       √7ᵗʰ **S76.129** Laceration of unspecified quadriceps ▽ muscle, fascia and tendon

    √6ᵗʰ **S76.19** **Other specified injury of quadriceps muscle, fascia and tendon**

       √7ᵗʰ **S76.191** Other specified injury of right quadriceps muscle, fascia and tendon

       √7ᵗʰ **S76.192** Other specified injury of left quadriceps muscle, fascia and tendon

       √7ᵗʰ **S76.199** Other specified injury of unspecified ▽ quadriceps muscle, fascia and tendon

√5ᵗʰ **S76.2** **Injury of adductor muscle, fascia and tendon of thigh**

    √6ᵗʰ **S76.20** **Unspecified injury of adductor muscle, fascia and tendon of thigh**

       √7ᵗʰ **S76.201** Unspecified injury of adductor muscle, ▽ fascia and tendon of right thigh

       √7ᵗʰ **S76.202** Unspecified injury of adductor muscle, ▽ fascia and tendon of left thigh

       √7ᵗʰ **S76.209** Unspecified injury of adductor muscle, ▽ fascia and tendon of unspecified thigh

    √6ᵗʰ **S76.21** **Strain of adductor muscle, fascia and tendon of thigh**

       √7ᵗʰ **S76.211** Strain of adductor muscle, fascia and tendon of right thigh

       √7ᵗʰ **S76.212** Strain of adductor muscle, fascia and tendon of left thigh

       √7ᵗʰ **S76.219** Strain of adductor muscle, fascia and ▽ tendon of unspecified thigh

    √6ᵗʰ **S76.22** **Laceration of adductor muscle, fascia and tendon of thigh**

       √7ᵗʰ **S76.221** Laceration of adductor muscle, fascia and tendon of right thigh

       √7ᵗʰ **S76.222** Laceration of adductor muscle, fascia and tendon of left thigh

       √7ᵗʰ **S76.229** Laceration of adductor muscle, fascia ▽ and tendon of unspecified thigh

    √6ᵗʰ **S76.29** **Other injury of adductor muscle, fascia and tendon of thigh**

       √7ᵗʰ **S76.291** Other injury of adductor muscle, fascia and tendon of right thigh

       √7ᵗʰ **S76.292** Other injury of adductor muscle, fascia and tendon of left thigh

       √7ᵗʰ **S76.299** Other injury of adductor muscle, fascia ▽ and tendon of unspecified thigh

√5ᵗʰ **S76.3** **Injury of muscle, fascia and tendon of the posterior muscle group at thigh level**

    √6ᵗʰ **S76.30** **Unspecified injury of muscle, fascia and tendon of the posterior muscle group at thigh level**

       √7ᵗʰ **S76.301** Unspecified injury of muscle, fascia ▽ and tendon of the posterior muscle group at thigh level, right thigh

       √7ᵗʰ **S76.302** Unspecified injury of muscle, fascia ▽ and tendon of the posterior muscle group at thigh level, left thigh

       √7ᵗʰ **S76.309** Unspecified injury of muscle, fascia ▽ and tendon of the posterior muscle group at thigh level, unspecified thigh

    √6ᵗʰ **S76.31** **Strain of muscle, fascia and tendon of the posterior muscle group at thigh level**

       √7ᵗʰ **S76.311** Strain of muscle, fascia and tendon of the posterior muscle group at thigh level, right thigh

       √7ᵗʰ **S76.312** Strain of muscle, fascia and tendon of the posterior muscle group at thigh level, left thigh

       √7ᵗʰ **S76.319** Strain of muscle, fascia and tendon of ▽ the posterior muscle group at thigh level, unspecified thigh

    √6ᵗʰ **S76.32** **Laceration of muscle, fascia and tendon of the posterior muscle group at thigh level**

       √7ᵗʰ **S76.321** Laceration of muscle, fascia and tendon of the posterior muscle group at thigh level, right thigh

       √7ᵗʰ **S76.322** Laceration of muscle, fascia and tendon of the posterior muscle group at thigh level, left thigh

       √7ᵗʰ **S76.329** Laceration of muscle, fascia and ▽ tendon of the posterior muscle group at thigh level, unspecified thigh

    √6ᵗʰ **S76.39** **Other specified injury of muscle, fascia and tendon of the posterior muscle group at thigh level**

       √7ᵗʰ **S76.391** Other specified injury of muscle, fascia and tendon of the posterior muscle group at thigh level, right thigh

       √7ᵗʰ **S76.392** Other specified injury of muscle, fascia and tendon of the posterior muscle group at thigh level, left thigh

       √7ᵗʰ **S76.399** Other specified injury of muscle, fascia ▽ and tendon of the posterior muscle group at thigh level, unspecified thigh

√5ᵗʰ **S76.8** **Injury of other specified muscles, fascia and tendons at thigh level**

    √6ᵗʰ **S76.80** **Unspecified injury of other specified muscles, fascia and tendons at thigh level**

       √7ᵗʰ **S76.801** Unspecified injury of other specified ▽ muscles, fascia and tendons at thigh level, right thigh

       √7ᵗʰ **S76.802** Unspecified injury of other specified ▽ muscles, fascia and tendons at thigh level, left thigh

       √7ᵗʰ **S76.809** Unspecified injury of other specified ▽ muscles, fascia and tendons at thigh level, unspecified thigh

    √6ᵗʰ **S76.81** **Strain of other specified muscles, fascia and tendons at thigh level**

       √7ᵗʰ **S76.811** Strain of other specified muscles, fascia and tendons at thigh level, right thigh

       √7ᵗʰ **S76.812** Strain of other specified muscles, fascia and tendons at thigh level, left thigh

       √7ᵗʰ **S76.819** Strain of other specified muscles, ▽ fascia and tendons at thigh level, unspecified thigh

    √6ᵗʰ **S76.82** **Laceration of other specified muscles, fascia and tendons at thigh level**

       √7ᵗʰ **S76.821** Laceration of other specified muscles, fascia and tendons at thigh level, right thigh

       √7ᵗʰ **S76.822** Laceration of other specified muscles, fascia and tendons at thigh level, left thigh

---

☑ Additional Character Req   ✔x7ᵗʰ Placeholder Alert   Manifestation   HCC CMS-HCC Condition   ▽ Unspecified Code   ►◄ Revised Text   ● New Code   ▲ Revised Code Title

√7ʰ S76.829 Laceration of other specified muscles, fascia and tendons at thigh level, unspecified thigh ▽

√6ʰ S76.89 Other injury of other specified muscles, fascia and tendons at thigh level

     √7ʰ S76.891 Other injury of other specified muscles, fascia and tendons at thigh level, right thigh

     √7ʰ S76.892 Other injury of other specified muscles, fascia and tendons at thigh level, left thigh

     √7ʰ S76.899 Other injury of other specified muscles, fascia and tendons at thigh level, unspecified thigh ▽

√5ʰ S76.9 Injury of unspecified muscles, fascia and tendons at thigh level

   √6ʰ S76.90 Unspecified injury of unspecified muscles, fascia and tendons at thigh level

     √7ʰ S76.901 Unspecified injury of unspecified muscles, fascia and tendons at thigh level, right thigh ▽

     √7ʰ S76.902 Unspecified injury of unspecified muscles, fascia and tendons at thigh level, left thigh ▽

     √7ʰ S76.909 Unspecified injury of unspecified muscles, fascia and tendons at thigh level, unspecified thigh ▽

   √6ʰ S76.91 Strain of unspecified muscles, fascia and tendons at thigh level

     √7ʰ S76.911 Strain of unspecified muscles, fascia and tendons at thigh level, right thigh ▽

     √7ʰ S76.912 Strain of unspecified muscles, fascia and tendons at thigh level, left thigh ▽

     √7ʰ S76.919 Strain of unspecified muscles, fascia and tendons at thigh level, unspecified thigh ▽

   √6ʰ S76.92 Laceration of unspecified muscles, fascia and tendons at thigh level

     √7ʰ S76.921 Laceration of unspecified muscles, fascia and tendons at thigh level, right thigh ▽

     √7ʰ S76.922 Laceration of unspecified muscles, fascia and tendons at thigh level, left thigh ▽

     √7ʰ S76.929 Laceration of unspecified muscles, fascia and tendons at thigh level, unspecified thigh ▽

   √6ʰ S76.99 Other specified injury of unspecified muscles, fascia and tendons at thigh level

     √7ʰ S76.991 Other specified injury of unspecified muscles, fascia and tendons at thigh level, right thigh ▽

     √7ʰ S76.992 Other specified injury of unspecified muscles, fascia and tendons at thigh level, left thigh ▽

     √7ʰ S76.999 Other specified injury of unspecified muscles, fascia and tendons at thigh level, unspecified thigh ▽

√4ʰ S77 Crushing injury of hip and thigh

Use additional code(s) for all associated injuries

EXCLUDES 2 crushing injury of ankle and foot (S97.-)
crushing injury of lower leg (S87.-)

> The appropriate 7th character is to be added to each code from category S77.
> A   initial encounter
> D   subsequent encounter
> S   sequela

√5ʰ S77.0 Crushing injury of hip

   √×7ʰ S77.00 Crushing injury of unspecified hip ▽

   √×7ʰ S77.01 Crushing injury of right hip

   √×7ʰ S77.02 Crushing injury of left hip

√5ʰ S77.1 Crushing injury of thigh

   √×7ʰ S77.10 Crushing injury of unspecified thigh ▽

   √×7ʰ S77.11 Crushing injury of right thigh

   √×7ʰ S77.12 Crushing injury of left thigh

√5ʰ S77.2 Crushing injury of hip with thigh

   √×7ʰ S77.20 Crushing injury of unspecified hip with thigh ▽

   √×7ʰ S77.21 Crushing injury of right hip with thigh

   √×7ʰ S77.22 Crushing injury of left hip with thigh

√4ʰ S78 Traumatic amputation of hip and thigh

An amputation not identified as partial or complete should be coded to complete.

EXCLUDES 1 traumatic amputation of knee (S88.0-)

> The appropriate 7th character is to be added to each code from category S78.
> A   initial encounter
> D   subsequent encounter
> S   sequela

√5ʰ S78.0 Traumatic amputation at hip joint

   √6ʰ S78.01 Complete traumatic amputation at hip joint

     √7ʰ S78.011 Complete traumatic amputation at right hip joint HCC

     √7ʰ S78.012 Complete traumatic amputation at left hip joint HCC

     √7ʰ S78.019 Complete traumatic amputation at unspecified hip joint HCC ▽

   √6ʰ S78.02 Partial traumatic amputation at hip joint

     √7ʰ S78.021 Partial traumatic amputation at right hip joint HCC

     √7ʰ S78.022 Partial traumatic amputation at left hip joint HCC

     √7ʰ S78.029 Partial traumatic amputation at unspecified hip joint HCC ▽

√5ʰ S78.1 Traumatic amputation at level between hip and knee

EXCLUDES 1 traumatic amputation of knee (S88.0-)

   √6ʰ S78.11 Complete traumatic amputation at level between hip and knee

     √7ʰ S78.111 Complete traumatic amputation at level between right hip and knee HCC

     √7ʰ S78.112 Complete traumatic amputation at level between left hip and knee HCC

     √7ʰ S78.119 Complete traumatic amputation at level between unspecified hip and knee HCC ▽

   √6ʰ S78.12 Partial traumatic amputation at level between hip and knee

     √7ʰ S78.121 Partial traumatic amputation at level between right hip and knee HCC

     √7ʰ S78.122 Partial traumatic amputation at level between left hip and knee HCC

     √7ʰ S78.129 Partial traumatic amputation at level between unspecified hip and knee HCC ▽

√5ʰ S78.9 Traumatic amputation of hip and thigh, level unspecified

   √6ʰ S78.91 Complete traumatic amputation of hip and thigh, level unspecified

     √7ʰ S78.911 Complete traumatic amputation of right hip and thigh, level unspecified HCC ▽

     √7ʰ S78.912 Complete traumatic amputation of left hip and thigh, level unspecified HCC ▽

     √7ʰ S78.919 Complete traumatic amputation of unspecified hip and thigh, level unspecified HCC ▽

   √6ʰ S78.92 Partial traumatic amputation of hip and thigh, level unspecified

     √7ʰ S78.921 Partial traumatic amputation of right hip and thigh, level unspecified HCC ▽

     √7ʰ S78.922 Partial traumatic amputation of left hip and thigh, level unspecified HCC ▽

     √7ʰ S78.929 Partial traumatic amputation of unspecified hip and thigh, level unspecified HCC ▽

EXCLUDES 1 Not coded here   *EXCLUDES 2* Not included here   N Newborn Age: 0   P Pediatric Age: 0-17   M Maternity Age: 12-55   A Adult Age: 15-124

1010   ICD-10-CM 2018

✓4th **S79 Other and unspecified injuries of hip and thigh**
> **NOTE** A fracture not indicated as open or closed should be coded to closed.
> **AHA:** 2015, 3Q, 37-39

The appropriate 7th character is to be added to each code from subcategory S79.0 and S79.1.
A   initial encounter for closed fracture
D   subsequent encounter for fracture with routine healing
G   subsequent encounter for fracture with delayed healing
K   subsequent encounter for fracture with nonunion
P   subsequent encounter for fracture with malunion
S   sequela

✓5th **S79.0 Physeal fracture of upper end of femur**
> **EXCLUDES 1** apophyseal fracture of upper end of femur (S72.13-)
> nontraumatic slipped upper femoral epiphysis (M93.0-)

✓6th **S79.00 Unspecified physeal fracture of upper end of femur**
1 ✓7th **S79.001 Unspecified physeal fracture of upper end of right femur** HCC ▽
1 ✓7th **S79.002 Unspecified physeal fracture of upper end of left femur** HCC ▽
1 ✓7th **S79.009 Unspecified physeal fracture of upper end of unspecified femur** HCC ▽

✓6th **S79.01 Salter-Harris Type I physeal fracture of upper end of femur**
> Acute on chronic slipped capital femoral epiphysis (traumatic)
> Acute slipped capital femoral epiphysis (traumatic)
> Capital femoral epiphyseal fracture
> **EXCLUDES 1** chronic slipped upper femoral epiphysis (nontraumatic) (M93.02-)

1 ✓7th **S79.011 Salter-Harris Type I physeal fracture of upper end of right femur** HCC
1 ✓7th **S79.012 Salter-Harris Type I physeal fracture of upper end of left femur** HCC
1 ✓7th **S79.019 Salter-Harris Type I physeal fracture of upper end of unspecified femur** HCC ▽

✓6th **S79.09 Other physeal fracture of upper end of femur**
1 ✓7th **S79.091 Other physeal fracture of upper end of right femur** HCC
1 ✓7th **S79.092 Other physeal fracture of upper end of left femur** HCC
1 ✓7th **S79.099 Other physeal fracture of upper end of unspecified femur** HCC ▽

✓5th **S79.1 Physeal fracture of lower end of femur**

✓6th **S79.10 Unspecified physeal fracture of lower end of femur**
1 ✓7th **S79.101 Unspecified physeal fracture of lower end of right femur** HCC ▽
1 ✓7th **S79.102 Unspecified physeal fracture of lower end of left femur** HCC ▽
1 ✓7th **S79.109 Unspecified physeal fracture of lower end of unspecified femur** HCC ▽

✓6th **S79.11 Salter-Harris Type I physeal fracture of lower end of femur**
1 ✓7th **S79.111 Salter-Harris Type I physeal fracture of lower end of right femur** HCC
1 ✓7th **S79.112 Salter-Harris Type I physeal fracture of lower end of left femur** HCC
1 ✓7th **S79.119 Salter-Harris Type I physeal fracture of lower end of unspecified femur** HCC ▽

✓6th **S79.12 Salter-Harris Type II physeal fracture of lower end of femur**
1 ✓7th **S79.121 Salter-Harris Type II physeal fracture of lower end of right femur** HCC
1 ✓7th **S79.122 Salter-Harris Type II physeal fracture of lower end of left femur** HCC
1 ✓7th **S79.129 Salter-Harris Type II physeal fracture of lower end of unspecified femur** HCC ▽

✓6th **S79.13 Salter-Harris Type III physeal fracture of lower end of femur**
1 ✓7th **S79.131 Salter-Harris Type III physeal fracture of lower end of right femur** HCC
1 ✓7th **S79.132 Salter-Harris Type III physeal fracture of lower end of left femur** HCC
1 ✓7th **S79.139 Salter-Harris Type III physeal fracture of lower end of unspecified femur** HCC ▽

✓6th **S79.14 Salter-Harris Type IV physeal fracture of lower end of femur**
1 ✓7th **S79.141 Salter-Harris Type IV physeal fracture of lower end of right femur** HCC
1 ✓7th **S79.142 Salter-Harris Type IV physeal fracture of lower end of left femur** HCC
1 ✓7th **S79.149 Salter-Harris Type IV physeal fracture of lower end of unspecified femur** HCC ▽

✓6th **S79.19 Other physeal fracture of lower end of femur**
1 ✓7th **S79.191 Other physeal fracture of lower end of right femur** HCC
1 ✓7th **S79.192 Other physeal fracture of lower end of left femur** HCC
1 ✓7th **S79.199 Other physeal fracture of lower end of unspecified femur** HCC ▽

✓5th **S79.8 Other specified injuries of hip and thigh**

The appropriate 7th character is to be added to each code in subcategory S79.8.
A   initial encounter
D   subsequent encounter
S   sequela

✓6th **S79.81 Other specified injuries of hip**
✓7th **S79.811 Other specified injuries of right hip**
✓7th **S79.812 Other specified injuries of left hip**
✓7th **S79.819 Other specified injuries of unspecified hip** ▽

✓6th **S79.82 Other specified injuries of thigh**
✓7th **S79.821 Other specified injuries of right thigh**
✓7th **S79.822 Other specified injuries of left thigh**
✓7th **S79.829 Other specified injuries of unspecified thigh** ▽

✓5th **S79.9 Unspecified injury of hip and thigh**

The appropriate 7th character is to be added to each code in subcategory S79.9.
A   initial encounter
D   subsequent encounter
S   sequela

✓6th **S79.91 Unspecified injury of hip**
✓7th **S79.911 Unspecified injury of right hip** ▽
✓7th **S79.912 Unspecified injury of left hip** ▽
✓7th **S79.919 Unspecified injury of unspecified hip** ▽

✓6th **S79.92 Unspecified injury of thigh**
✓7th **S79.921 Unspecified injury of right thigh** ▽
✓7th **S79.922 Unspecified injury of left thigh** ▽
✓7th **S79.929 Unspecified injury of unspecified thigh** ▽

---

1 HCC with 7th character indicating initial encounter (A, B or C - specific to category).

Injuries to the knee and lower leg (S80-S89)

EXCLUDES 2   burns and corrosions (T20-T32)
frostbite (T33-T34)
injuries of ankle and foot, except fracture of ankle and malleolus (S90-S99)
insect bite or sting, venomous (T63.4)

S80   Superficial injury of knee and lower leg

EXCLUDES 2   superficial injury of ankle and foot (S90.-)

> The appropriate 7th character is to be added to each code from category S80.
> A   initial encounter
> D   subsequent encounter
> S   sequela

S80.0   Contusion of knee
- S80.00   Contusion of unspecified knee   ▽
- S80.01   Contusion of right knee
- S80.02   Contusion of left knee

S80.1   Contusion of lower leg
- S80.10   Contusion of unspecified lower leg   ▽
- S80.11   Contusion of right lower leg
- S80.12   Contusion of left lower leg

S80.2   Other superficial injuries of knee
- S80.21   Abrasion of knee
  - S80.211   Abrasion, right knee
  - S80.212   Abrasion, left knee
  - S80.219   Abrasion, unspecified knee   ▽
- S80.22   Blister (nonthermal) of knee
  - S80.221   Blister (nonthermal), right knee
  - S80.222   Blister (nonthermal), left knee
  - S80.229   Blister (nonthermal), unspecified knee   ▽
- S80.24   External constriction of knee
  - S80.241   External constriction, right knee
  - S80.242   External constriction, left knee
  - S80.249   External constriction, unspecified knee   ▽
- S80.25   Superficial foreign body of knee
  Splinter in the knee
  - S80.251   Superficial foreign body, right knee
  - S80.252   Superficial foreign body, left knee
  - S80.259   Superficial foreign body, unspecified knee   ▽
- S80.26   Insect bite (nonvenomous) of knee
  - S80.261   Insect bite (nonvenomous), right knee
  - S80.262   Insect bite (nonvenomous), left knee
  - S80.269   Insect bite (nonvenomous), unspecified knee   ▽
- S80.27   Other superficial bite of knee
  EXCLUDES 1   open bite of knee (S81.05-)
  - S80.271   Other superficial bite of right knee
  - S80.272   Other superficial bite of left knee
  - S80.279   Other superficial bite of unspecified knee   ▽

S80.8   Other superficial injuries of lower leg
- S80.81   Abrasion of lower leg
  - S80.811   Abrasion, right lower leg
  - S80.812   Abrasion, left lower leg
  - S80.819   Abrasion, unspecified lower leg   ▽
- S80.82   Blister (nonthermal) of lower leg
  - S80.821   Blister (nonthermal), right lower leg
  - S80.822   Blister (nonthermal), left lower leg
  - S80.829   Blister (nonthermal), unspecified lower leg   ▽
- S80.84   External constriction of lower leg
  - S80.841   External constriction, right lower leg
  - S80.842   External constriction, left lower leg
  - S80.849   External constriction, unspecified lower leg   ▽

- S80.85   Superficial foreign body of lower leg
  Splinter in the lower leg
  - S80.851   Superficial foreign body, right lower leg
  - S80.852   Superficial foreign body, left lower leg
  - S80.859   Superficial foreign body, unspecified lower leg   ▽
- S80.86   Insect bite (nonvenomous) of lower leg
  - S80.861   Insect bite (nonvenomous), right lower leg
  - S80.862   Insect bite (nonvenomous), left lower leg
  - S80.869   Insect bite (nonvenomous), unspecified lower leg   ▽
- S80.87   Other superficial bite of lower leg
  EXCLUDES 1   open bite of lower leg (S81.85-)
  - S80.871   Other superficial bite, right lower leg
  - S80.872   Other superficial bite, left lower leg
  - S80.879   Other superficial bite, unspecified lower leg   ▽

S80.9   Unspecified superficial injury of knee and lower leg
- S80.91   Unspecified superficial injury of knee
  - S80.911   Unspecified superficial injury of right knee   ▽
  - S80.912   Unspecified superficial injury of left knee   ▽
  - S80.919   Unspecified superficial injury of unspecified knee   ▽
- S80.92   Unspecified superficial injury of lower leg
  - S80.921   Unspecified superficial injury of right lower leg   ▽
  - S80.922   Unspecified superficial injury of left lower leg   ▽
  - S80.929   Unspecified superficial injury of unspecified lower leg   ▽

S81   Open wound of knee and lower leg

Code also any associated wound infection

EXCLUDES 1   open fracture of knee and lower leg (S82.-)
traumatic amputation of lower leg (S88.-)

EXCLUDES 2   open wound of ankle and foot (S91.-)

> The appropriate 7th character is to be added to each code from category S81.
> A   initial encounter
> D   subsequent encounter
> S   sequela

S81.0   Open wound of knee
- S81.00   Unspecified open wound of knee
  - S81.001   Unspecified open wound, right knee   ▽
  - S81.002   Unspecified open wound, left knee   ▽
  - S81.009   Unspecified open wound, unspecified knee   ▽
- S81.01   Laceration without foreign body of knee
  - S81.011   Laceration without foreign body, right knee
  - S81.012   Laceration without foreign body, left knee
  - S81.019   Laceration without foreign body, unspecified knee   ▽
- S81.02   Laceration with foreign body of knee
  - S81.021   Laceration with foreign body, right knee
  - S81.022   Laceration with foreign body, left knee
  - S81.029   Laceration with foreign body, unspecified knee   ▽
- S81.03   Puncture wound without foreign body of knee
  - S81.031   Puncture wound without foreign body, right knee
  - S81.032   Puncture wound without foreign body, left knee
  - S81.039   Puncture wound without foreign body, unspecified knee   ▽

EXCLUDES 1   Not coded here   EXCLUDES 2   Not included here   N Newborn Age: 0   P Pediatric Age: 0-17   M Maternity Age: 12-55   A Adult Age: 15-124

1012   ICD-10-CM 2018

✓6ᵗʰ **S81.04 Puncture wound with foreign body of knee**

     ✓7ᵗʰ **S81.041 Puncture wound with foreign body, right knee**

     ✓7ᵗʰ **S81.042 Puncture wound with foreign body, left knee**

     ✓7ᵗʰ **S81.049 Puncture wound with foreign body, unspecified knee** ▽

✓6ᵗʰ **S81.05 Open bite of knee**
     Bite of knee NOS
     EXCLUDES 1   *superficial bite of knee (S80.27-)*

     ✓7ᵗʰ **S81.051 Open bite, right knee**

     ✓7ᵗʰ **S81.052 Open bite, left knee**

     ✓7ᵗʰ **S81.059 Open bite, unspecified knee** ▽

✓5ᵗʰ **S81.8 Open wound of lower leg**

     ✓6ᵗʰ **S81.80 Unspecified open wound of lower leg**
     AHA: 2016, 3Q, 24

         ✓7ᵗʰ **S81.801 Unspecified open wound, right lower leg** ▽

         ✓7ᵗʰ **S81.802 Unspecified open wound, left lower leg** ▽

         ✓7ᵗʰ **S81.809 Unspecified open wound, unspecified lower leg** ▽

     ✓6ᵗʰ **S81.81 Laceration without foreign body of lower leg**

         ✓7ᵗʰ **S81.811 Laceration without foreign body, right lower leg**

         ✓7ᵗʰ **S81.812 Laceration without foreign body, left lower leg**

         ✓7ᵗʰ **S81.819 Laceration without foreign body, unspecified lower leg** ▽

     ✓6ᵗʰ **S81.82 Laceration with foreign body of lower leg**

         ✓7ᵗʰ **S81.821 Laceration with foreign body, right lower leg**

         ✓7ᵗʰ **S81.822 Laceration with foreign body, left lower leg**

         ✓7ᵗʰ **S81.829 Laceration with foreign body, unspecified lower leg** ▽

     ✓6ᵗʰ **S81.83 Puncture wound without foreign body of lower leg**
     AHA: 2016, 3Q, 24

         ✓7ᵗʰ **S81.831 Puncture wound without foreign body, right lower leg**

         ✓7ᵗʰ **S81.832 Puncture wound without foreign body, left lower leg**

         ✓7ᵗʰ **S81.839 Puncture wound without foreign body, unspecified lower leg** ▽

     ✓6ᵗʰ **S81.84 Puncture wound with foreign body of lower leg**
     AHA: 2016, 3Q, 24

         ✓7ᵗʰ **S81.841 Puncture wound with foreign body, right lower leg**

         ✓7ᵗʰ **S81.842 Puncture wound with foreign body, left lower leg**

         ✓7ᵗʰ **S81.849 Puncture wound with foreign body, unspecified lower leg** ▽

     ✓6ᵗʰ **S81.85 Open bite of lower leg**
     Bite of lower leg NOS
     EXCLUDES 1   *superficial bite of lower leg (S80.86-, S80.87-)*

         ✓7ᵗʰ **S81.851 Open bite, right lower leg**

         ✓7ᵗʰ **S81.852 Open bite, left lower leg**

         ✓7ᵗʰ **S81.859 Open bite, unspecified lower leg** ▽

✓4ᵗʰ **S82 Fracture of lower leg, including ankle**

     NOTE A fracture not indicated as displaced or nondisplaced should be coded to displaced.
     A fracture not designated as open or closed should be coded to closed.
     The open fracture designations are based on the Gustilo open fracture classification.

     INCLUDES fracture of malleolus

     EXCLUDES 1 *traumatic amputation of lower leg (S88.-)*

     EXCLUDES 2 *fracture of foot, except ankle (S92.-)*
     periprosthetic fracture of prosthetic implant of knee ▶(M97.0-)◀

     AHA: 2016, 1Q, 33; 2015, 3Q, 37-39

The appropriate 7th character is to be added to all codes from category S82 [unless otherwise indicated].

A   initial encounter for closed fracture
B   initial encounter for open fracture type I or II
     initial encounter for open fracture NOS
C   initial encounter for open fracture type IIIA, IIIB, or IIIC
D   subsequent encounter for closed fracture with routine healing
E   subsequent encounter for open fracture type I or II with routine healing
F   subsequent encounter for open fracture type IIIA, IIIB, or IIIC with routine healing
G   subsequent encounter for closed fracture with delayed healing
H   subsequent encounter for open fracture type I or II with delayed healing
J   subsequent encounter for open fracture type IIIA, IIIB or IIIC with delayed healing
K   subsequent encounter for closed fracture with nonunion
M   subsequent encounter for open fracture type I or II with nonunion
N   subsequent encounter for open fracture type IIIA, IIIB or IIIC with nonunion
P   subsequent encounter for closed fracture with malunion
Q   subsequent encounter for open fracture type I or II with malunion
R   subsequent encounter for open fracture type IIIA, IIIB or IIIC with malunion
S   sequela

✓5ᵗʰ **S82.0 Fracture of patella**
     Knee cap

     ✓6ᵗʰ **S82.00 Unspecified fracture of patella**

         ✓7ᵗʰ **S82.001 Unspecified fracture of right patella** ▽

         S82.002 Unspecified fracture of left patella ▽

         ✓7ᵗʰ **S82.009 Unspecified fracture of unspecified patella** ▽

     ✓6ᵗʰ **S82.01 Osteochondral fracture of patella**

         ✓7ᵗʰ **S82.011 Displaced osteochondral fracture of right patella**

         ✓7ᵗʰ **S82.012 Displaced osteochondral fracture of left patella**

         ✓7ᵗʰ **S82.013 Displaced osteochondral fracture of unspecified patella** ▽

         ✓7ᵗʰ **S82.014 Nondisplaced osteochondral fracture of right patella**

         ✓7ᵗʰ **S82.015 Nondisplaced osteochondral fracture of left patella**

         ✓7ᵗʰ **S82.016 Nondisplaced osteochondral fracture of unspecified patella** ▽

     ✓6ᵗʰ **S82.02 Longitudinal fracture of patella**

         ✓7ᵗʰ **S82.021 Displaced longitudinal fracture of right patella**

         ✓7ᵗʰ **S82.022 Displaced longitudinal fracture of left patella**

         ✓7ᵗʰ **S82.023 Displaced longitudinal fracture of unspecified patella** ▽

         ✓7ᵗʰ **S82.024 Nondisplaced longitudinal fracture of right patella**

         ✓7ᵗʰ **S82.025 Nondisplaced longitudinal fracture of left patella**

         ✓7ᵗʰ **S82.026 Nondisplaced longitudinal fracture of unspecified patella** ▽

     ✓6ᵗʰ **S82.03 Transverse fracture of patella**

         ✓7ᵗʰ **S82.031 Displaced transverse fracture of right patella**

         ✓7ᵗʰ **S82.032 Displaced transverse fracture of left patella**

☑ Additional Character Req   ✓x7ᵗʰ Placeholder Alert   Manifestation   HCC CMS-HCC Condition   ▽ Unspecified Code   ▶◀ Revised Text   ● New Code   ▲ Revised Code Title

ICD-10-CM 2018   1013

√7ᵗʰ **S82.Ø33** **Displaced transverse fracture of** ▽
             unspecified patella

√7ᵗʰ **S82.Ø34** **Nondisplaced transverse fracture of right**
             patella

√7ᵗʰ **S82.Ø35** **Nondisplaced transverse fracture of left**
             patella

√7ᵗʰ **S82.Ø36** **Nondisplaced transverse fracture of** ▽
             unspecified patella

√6ᵗʰ **S82.Ø4** **Comminuted fracture of patella**

√7ᵗʰ **S82.Ø41** **Displaced comminuted fracture of right**
             patella

√7ᵗʰ **S82.Ø42** **Displaced comminuted fracture of left**
             patella

√7ᵗʰ **S82.Ø43** **Displaced comminuted fracture of** ▽
             unspecified patella

√7ᵗʰ **S82.Ø44** **Nondisplaced comminuted fracture of**
             right patella

√7ᵗʰ **S82.Ø45** **Nondisplaced comminuted fracture of left**
             patella

√7ᵗʰ **S82.Ø46** **Nondisplaced comminuted fracture of** ▽
             unspecified patella

√6ᵗʰ **S82.Ø9** **Other fracture of patella**

√7ᵗʰ **S82.Ø91** **Other fracture of right patella**

√7ᵗʰ **S82.Ø92** **Other fracture of left patella**

√7ᵗʰ **S82.Ø99** **Other fracture of unspecified patella** ▽

√5ᵗʰ **S82.1** **Fracture of upper end of tibia**
        Fracture of proximal end of tibia
        EXCLUDES 2   *fracture of shaft of tibia (S82.2-)*
                     physeal fracture of upper end of tibia (S89.Ø-)

√6ᵗʰ **S82.1Ø** **Unspecified fracture of upper end of tibia**

√7ᵗʰ **S82.1Ø1** **Unspecified fracture of upper end of** ▽
             right tibia

√7ᵗʰ **S82.1Ø2** **Unspecified fracture of upper end of** ▽
             left tibia

√7ᵗʰ **S82.1Ø9** **Unspecified fracture of upper end of** ▽
             unspecified tibia

√6ᵗʰ **S82.11** **Fracture of tibial spine**

√7ᵗʰ **S82.111** **Displaced fracture of right tibial spine**

√7ᵗʰ **S82.112** **Displaced fracture of left tibial spine**

√7ᵗʰ **S82.113** **Displaced fracture of unspecified tibial** ▽
             spine

√7ᵗʰ **S82.114** **Nondisplaced fracture of right tibial spine**

√7ᵗʰ **S82.115** **Nondisplaced fracture of left tibial spine**

√7ᵗʰ **S82.116** **Nondisplaced fracture of unspecified** ▽
             tibial spine

√6ᵗʰ **S82.12** **Fracture of lateral condyle of tibia**

√7ᵗʰ **S82.121** **Displaced fracture of lateral condyle of**
             right tibia

√7ᵗʰ **S82.122** **Displaced fracture of lateral condyle of left**
             tibia

√7ᵗʰ **S82.123** **Displaced fracture of lateral condyle of** ▽
             unspecified tibia

√7ᵗʰ **S82.124** **Nondisplaced fracture of lateral condyle**
             of right tibia

√7ᵗʰ **S82.125** **Nondisplaced fracture of lateral condyle**
             of left tibia

√7ᵗʰ **S82.126** **Nondisplaced fracture of lateral** ▽
             condyle of unspecified tibia

√6ᵗʰ **S82.13** **Fracture of medial condyle of tibia**

√7ᵗʰ **S82.131** **Displaced fracture of medial condyle of**
             right tibia

√7ᵗʰ **S82.132** **Displaced fracture of medial condyle of**
             left tibia

√7ᵗʰ **S82.133** **Displaced fracture of medial condyle** ▽
             of unspecified tibia

√7ᵗʰ **S82.134** **Nondisplaced fracture of medial condyle**
             of right tibia

√7ᵗʰ **S82.135** **Nondisplaced fracture of medial condyle**
             of left tibia

√7ᵗʰ **S82.136** **Nondisplaced fracture of medial** ▽
             condyle of unspecified tibia

√6ᵗʰ **S82.14** **Bicondylar fracture of tibia**
        Fracture of tibial plateau NOS

√7ᵗʰ **S82.141** **Displaced bicondylar fracture of right tibia**

√7ᵗʰ **S82.142** **Displaced bicondylar fracture of left tibia**

√7ᵗʰ **S82.143** **Displaced bicondylar fracture of** ▽
             unspecified tibia

√7ᵗʰ **S82.144** **Nondisplaced bicondylar fracture of right**
             tibia

√7ᵗʰ **S82.145** **Nondisplaced bicondylar fracture of left**
             tibia

√7ᵗʰ **S82.146** **Nondisplaced bicondylar fracture of** ▽
             unspecified tibia

√6ᵗʰ **S82.15** **Fracture of tibial tuberosity**

√7ᵗʰ **S82.151** **Displaced fracture of right tibial**
             tuberosity

√7ᵗʰ **S82.152** **Displaced fracture of left tibial tuberosity**

√7ᵗʰ **S82.153** **Displaced fracture of unspecified** ▽
             tibial tuberosity

√7ᵗʰ **S82.154** **Nondisplaced fracture of right tibial**
             tuberosity

√7ᵗʰ **S82.155** **Nondisplaced fracture of left tibial**
             tuberosity

√7ᵗʰ **S82.156** **Nondisplaced fracture of unspecified** ▽
             tibial tuberosity

√6ᵗʰ **S82.16** **Torus fracture of upper end of tibia**

> The appropriate 7th character is to be added to all
> codes in subcategory S82.16.
> A   initial encounter for closed fracture
> D   subsequent encounter for fracture with routine
>   healing
> G   subsequent encounter for fracture with delayed
>   healing
> K   subsequent encounter for fracture with
>   nonunion
> P   subsequent encounter for fracture with
>   malunion
> S   sequela

√7ᵗʰ **S82.161** **Torus fracture of upper end of right tibia**

√7ᵗʰ **S82.162** **Torus fracture of upper end of left tibia**

√7ᵗʰ **S82.169** **Torus fracture of upper end of** ▽
             unspecified tibia

√6ᵗʰ **S82.19** **Other fracture of upper end of tibia**

√7ᵗʰ **S82.191** **Other fracture of upper end of right tibia**

√7ᵗʰ **S82.192** **Other fracture of upper end of left tibia**

√7ᵗʰ **S82.199** **Other fracture of upper end of** ▽
             unspecified tibia

√5ᵗʰ **S82.2** **Fracture of shaft of tibia**

√6ᵗʰ **S82.2Ø** **Unspecified fracture of shaft of tibia**
        Fracture of tibia NOS

√7ᵗʰ **S82.2Ø1** **Unspecified fracture of shaft of right** ▽
             tibia

√7ᵗʰ **S82.2Ø2** **Unspecified fracture of shaft of left** ▽
             tibia

√7ᵗʰ **S82.2Ø9** **Unspecified fracture of shaft of** ▽
             unspecified tibia

√6ᵗʰ **S82.22** **Transverse fracture of shaft of tibia**

√7ᵗʰ **S82.221** **Displaced transverse fracture of shaft of**
             right tibia

√7ᵗʰ **S82.222** **Displaced transverse fracture of shaft of**
             left tibia

√7ᵗʰ **S82.223** **Displaced transverse fracture of shaft** ▽
             of unspecified tibia

√7ᵗʰ **S82.224** **Nondisplaced transverse fracture of shaft**
             of right tibia

√7ᵗʰ **S82.225** **Nondisplaced transverse fracture of shaft**
             of left tibia

√7ᵗʰ **S82.226** **Nondisplaced transverse fracture of** ▽
             shaft of unspecified tibia

√6ᵗʰ **S82.23** **Oblique fracture of shaft of tibia**

√7ᵗʰ **S82.231** **Displaced oblique fracture of shaft of right**
             tibia

√7ᵗʰ **S82.232** **Displaced oblique fracture of shaft of left**
             tibia

EXCLUDES 1 Not coded here   *EXCLUDES 2* Not included here   **N** Newborn Age: 0   **P** Pediatric Age: 0-17   **M** Maternity Age: 12-55   **A** Adult Age: 15-124

1014   ICD-10-CM 2018

√7ᵗʰ **S82.233** **Displaced oblique fracture of shaft of** ▽
unspecified tibia

√7ᵗʰ **S82.234** **Nondisplaced oblique fracture of shaft of**
right tibia

√7ᵗʰ **S82.235** **Nondisplaced oblique fracture of shaft of**
left tibia

√7ᵗʰ **S82.236** **Nondisplaced oblique fracture of shaft** ▽
of unspecified tibia

√6ᵗʰ **S82.24** **Spiral fracture of shaft of tibia**
Toddler fracture

√7ᵗʰ **S82.241** **Displaced spiral fracture of shaft of right**
tibia

√7ᵗʰ **S82.242** **Displaced spiral fracture of shaft of left**
tibia

√7ᵗʰ **S82.243** **Displaced spiral fracture of shaft of** ▽
unspecified tibia

√7ᵗʰ **S82.244** **Nondisplaced spiral fracture of shaft of**
right tibia

√7ᵗʰ **S82.245** **Nondisplaced spiral fracture of shaft of**
left tibia

√7ᵗʰ **S82.246** **Nondisplaced spiral fracture of shaft** ▽
of unspecified tibia

√6ᵗʰ **S82.25** **Comminuted fracture of shaft of tibia**

√7ᵗʰ **S82.251** **Displaced comminuted fracture of shaft of**
right tibia

√7ᵗʰ **S82.252** **Displaced comminuted fracture of shaft of**
left tibia

√7ᵗʰ **S82.253** **Displaced comminuted fracture of** ▽
shaft of unspecified tibia

√7ᵗʰ **S82.254** **Nondisplaced comminuted fracture of**
shaft of right tibia

√7ᵗʰ **S82.255** **Nondisplaced comminuted fracture of**
shaft of left tibia

√7ᵗʰ **S82.256** **Nondisplaced comminuted fracture of** ▽
shaft of unspecified tibia

√6ᵗʰ **S82.26** **Segmental fracture of shaft of tibia**

√7ᵗʰ **S82.261** **Displaced segmental fracture of shaft of**
right tibia

√7ᵗʰ **S82.262** **Displaced segmental fracture of shaft of**
left tibia

√7ᵗʰ **S82.263** **Displaced segmental fracture of shaft** ▽
of unspecified tibia

√7ᵗʰ **S82.264** **Nondisplaced segmental fracture of shaft**
of right tibia

√7ᵗʰ **S82.265** **Nondisplaced segmental fracture of shaft**
of left tibia

√7ᵗʰ **S82.266** **Nondisplaced segmental fracture of** ▽
shaft of unspecified tibia

√6ᵗʰ **S82.29** **Other fracture of shaft of tibia**

√7ᵗʰ **S82.291** **Other fracture of shaft of right tibia**

√7ᵗʰ **S82.292** **Other fracture of shaft of left tibia**

√7ᵗʰ **S82.299** **Other fracture of shaft of unspecified** ▽
tibia

√5ᵗʰ **S82.3** **Fracture of lower end of tibia**
EXCLUDES 1   *bimalleolar fracture of lower leg (S82.84-)*
fracture of medial malleolus alone (S82.5-)
Maisonneuve's fracture (S82.86-)
pilon fracture of distal tibia (S82.87-)
trimalleolar fractures of lower leg (S82.85-)

√6ᵗʰ **S82.30** **Unspecified fracture of lower end of tibia**

√7ᵗʰ **S82.301** **Unspecified fracture of lower end of** ▽
right tibia

√7ᵗʰ **S82.302** **Unspecified fracture of lower end of** ▽
left tibia

√7ᵗʰ **S82.309** **Unspecified fracture of lower end of** ▽
unspecified tibia

√6ᵗʰ **S82.31** **Torus fracture of lower end of tibia**

The appropriate 7th character is to be added to all
codes in subcategory S82.31.
A   initial encounter for closed fracture
D   subsequent encounter for fracture with routine
     healing
G   subsequent encounter for fracture with
     delayed healing
K   subsequent encounter for fracture with
     nonunion
P   subsequent encounter for fracture with
     malunion
S   sequela

√7ᵗʰ **S82.311** **Torus fracture of lower end of right tibia**

√7ᵗʰ **S82.312** **Torus fracture of lower end of left tibia**

√7ᵗʰ **S82.319** **Torus fracture of lower end of** ▽
unspecified tibia

√6ᵗʰ **S82.39** **Other fracture of lower end of tibia**
AHA: 2015, 1Q, 25

√7ᵗʰ **S82.391** **Other fracture of lower end of right tibia**

√7ᵗʰ **S82.392** **Other fracture of lower end of left tibia**

√7ᵗʰ **S82.399** **Other fracture of lower end of** ▽
unspecified tibia

√5ᵗʰ **S82.4** **Fracture of shaft of fibula**
EXCLUDES 2   *fracture of lateral malleolus alone (S82.6-)*

√6ᵗʰ **S82.40** **Unspecified fracture of shaft of fibula**

√7ᵗʰ **S82.401** **Unspecified fracture of shaft of right** ▽
fibula

√7ᵗʰ **S82.402** **Unspecified fracture of shaft of left** ▽
fibula

√7ᵗʰ **S82.409** **Unspecified fracture of shaft of** ▽
unspecified fibula

√6ᵗʰ **S82.42** **Transverse fracture of shaft of fibula**

√7ᵗʰ **S82.421** **Displaced transverse fracture of shaft of**
right fibula

√7ᵗʰ **S82.422** **Displaced transverse fracture of shaft of**
left fibula

√7ᵗʰ **S82.423** **Displaced transverse fracture of shaft** ▽
of unspecified fibula

√7ᵗʰ **S82.424** **Nondisplaced transverse fracture of shaft**
of right fibula

√7ᵗʰ **S82.425** **Nondisplaced transverse fracture of shaft**
of left fibula

√7ᵗʰ **S82.426** **Nondisplaced transverse fracture of** ▽
shaft of unspecified fibula

√6ᵗʰ **S82.43** **Oblique fracture of shaft of fibula**

√7ᵗʰ **S82.431** **Displaced oblique fracture of shaft of right**
fibula

√7ᵗʰ **S82.432** **Displaced oblique fracture of shaft of left**
fibula

√7ᵗʰ **S82.433** **Displaced oblique fracture of shaft of** ▽
unspecified fibula

√7ᵗʰ **S82.434** **Nondisplaced oblique fracture of shaft of**
right fibula

√7ᵗʰ **S82.435** **Nondisplaced oblique fracture of shaft of**
left fibula

√7ᵗʰ **S82.436** **Nondisplaced oblique fracture of shaft** ▽
of unspecified fibula

√6ᵗʰ **S82.44** **Spiral fracture of shaft of fibula**

√7ᵗʰ **S82.441** **Displaced spiral fracture of shaft of right**
fibula

√7ᵗʰ **S82.442** **Displaced spiral fracture of shaft of left**
fibula

√7ᵗʰ **S82.443** **Displaced spiral fracture of shaft of** ▽
unspecified fibula

√7ᵗʰ **S82.444** **Nondisplaced spiral fracture of shaft of**
right fibula

√7ᵗʰ **S82.445** **Nondisplaced spiral fracture of shaft of**
left fibula

√7ᵗʰ **S82.446** **Nondisplaced spiral fracture of shaft of** ▽
unspecified fibula

√6ᵗʰ **S82.45** **Comminuted fracture of shaft of fibula**

√7ᵗʰ **S82.451** **Displaced comminuted fracture of shaft of**
right fibula

✔ Additional Character Req   √x7ᵗʰ Placeholder Alert   Manifestation   HCC CMS-HCC Condition   ▽ Unspecified Code   ►◄ Revised Text   ● New Code   ▲ Revised Code Title

ICD-10-CM 2018   1015

✓7ᵗʰ	**S82.452**	**Displaced comminuted fracture of shaft of left fibula**
✓7ᵗʰ	**S82.453**	**Displaced comminuted fracture of shaft of unspecified fibula** ▽
✓7ᵗʰ	**S82.454**	**Nondisplaced comminuted fracture of shaft of right fibula**
✓7ᵗʰ	**S82.455**	**Nondisplaced comminuted fracture of shaft of left fibula**
✓7ᵗʰ	**S82.456**	**Nondisplaced comminuted fracture of shaft of unspecified fibula** ▽

✓6ᵗʰ **S82.46** **Segmental fracture of shaft of fibula**

✓7ᵗʰ	**S82.461**	**Displaced segmental fracture of shaft of right fibula**
✓7ᵗʰ	**S82.462**	**Displaced segmental fracture of shaft of left fibula**
✓7ᵗʰ	**S82.463**	**Displaced segmental fracture of shaft of unspecified fibula** ▽
✓7ᵗʰ	**S82.464**	**Nondisplaced segmental fracture of shaft of right fibula**
✓7ᵗʰ	**S82.465**	**Nondisplaced segmental fracture of shaft of left fibula**
✓7ᵗʰ	**S82.466**	**Nondisplaced segmental fracture of shaft of unspecified fibula** ▽

✓6ᵗʰ **S82.49** **Other fracture of shaft of fibula**

✓7ᵗʰ	**S82.491**	**Other fracture of shaft of right fibula**
✓7ᵗʰ	**S82.492**	**Other fracture of shaft of left fibula**
✓7ᵗʰ	**S82.499**	**Other fracture of shaft of unspecified fibula** ▽

✓5ᵗʰ **S82.5** **Fracture of medial malleolus**

    EXCLUDES 1   *pilon fracture of distal tibia (S82.87-)*
                 Salter-Harris type III of lower end of tibia (S89.13-)
                 Salter-Harris type IV of lower end of tibia (S89.14-)

✓x7ᵗʰ	**S82.51**	**Displaced fracture of medial malleolus of right tibia**
✓x7ᵗʰ	**S82.52**	**Displaced fracture of medial malleolus of left tibia**
✓x7ᵗʰ	**S82.53**	**Displaced fracture of medial malleolus of unspecified tibia** ▽
✓x7ᵗʰ	**S82.54**	**Nondisplaced fracture of medial malleolus of right tibia**
✓x7ᵗʰ	**S82.55**	**Nondisplaced fracture of medial malleolus of left tibia**
✓x7ᵗʰ	**S82.56**	**Nondisplaced fracture of medial malleolus of unspecified tibia** ▽

✓5ᵗʰ **S82.6** **Fracture of lateral malleolus**

    EXCLUDES 1   *pilon fracture of distal tibia (S82.87-)*

✓x7ᵗʰ	**S82.61**	**Displaced fracture of lateral malleolus of right fibula**
✓x7ᵗʰ	**S82.62**	**Displaced fracture of lateral malleolus of left fibula**
✓x7ᵗʰ	**S82.63**	**Displaced fracture of lateral malleolus of unspecified fibula** ▽
✓x7ᵗʰ	**S82.64**	**Nondisplaced fracture of lateral malleolus of right fibula**
✓x7ᵗʰ	**S82.65**	**Nondisplaced fracture of lateral malleolus of left fibula**
✓x7ᵗʰ	**S82.66**	**Nondisplaced fracture of lateral malleolus of unspecified fibula** ▽

✓5ᵗʰ **S82.8** **Other fractures of lower leg**

✓6ᵗʰ **S82.81** **Torus fracture of upper end of fibula**

> The appropriate 7th character is to be added to all codes in subcategory S82.81.
> A   initial encounter for closed fracture
> D   subsequent encounter for fracture with routine healing
> G   subsequent encounter for fracture with delayed healing
> K   subsequent encounter for fracture with nonunion
> P   subsequent encounter for fracture with malunion
> S   sequela

✓7ᵗʰ	**S82.811**	**Torus fracture of upper end of right fibula**
✓7ᵗʰ	**S82.812**	**Torus fracture of upper end of left fibula**
✓7ᵗʰ	**S82.819**	**Torus fracture of upper end of unspecified fibula** ▽

✓6ᵗʰ **S82.82** **Torus fracture of lower end of fibula**

> The appropriate 7th character is to be added to all codes in subcategory S82.82.
> A   initial encounter for closed fracture
> D   subsequent encounter for fracture with routine healing
> G   subsequent encounter for fracture with delayed healing
> K   subsequent encounter for fracture with nonunion
> P   subsequent encounter for fracture with malunion
> S   sequela

✓7ᵗʰ	**S82.821**	**Torus fracture of lower end of right fibula**
✓7ᵗʰ	**S82.822**	**Torus fracture of lower end of left fibula**
✓7ᵗʰ	**S82.829**	**Torus fracture of lower end of unspecified fibula** ▽

✓6ᵗʰ **S82.83** **Other fracture of upper and lower end of fibula**
    AHA: 2015, 1Q, 25

✓7ᵗʰ	**S82.831**	**Other fracture of upper and lower end of right fibula**
✓7ᵗʰ	**S82.832**	**Other fracture of upper and lower end of left fibula**
✓7ᵗʰ	**S82.839**	**Other fracture of upper and lower end of unspecified fibula** ▽

✓6ᵗʰ **S82.84** **Bimalleolar fracture of lower leg**

✓7ᵗʰ	**S82.841**	**Displaced bimalleolar fracture of right lower leg**
✓7ᵗʰ	**S82.842**	**Displaced bimalleolar fracture of left lower leg**
✓7ᵗʰ	**S82.843**	**Displaced bimalleolar fracture of unspecified lower leg** ▽
✓7ᵗʰ	**S82.844**	**Nondisplaced bimalleolar fracture of right lower leg**
✓7ᵗʰ	**S82.845**	**Nondisplaced bimalleolar fracture of left lower leg**
✓7ᵗʰ	**S82.846**	**Nondisplaced bimalleolar fracture of unspecified lower leg** ▽

✓6ᵗʰ **S82.85** **Trimalleolar fracture of lower leg**

✓7ᵗʰ	**S82.851**	**Displaced trimalleolar fracture of right lower leg**
✓7ᵗʰ	**S82.852**	**Displaced trimalleolar fracture of left lower leg**
✓7ᵗʰ	**S82.853**	**Displaced trimalleolar fracture of unspecified lower leg** ▽

Right Bimalleolar Fracture

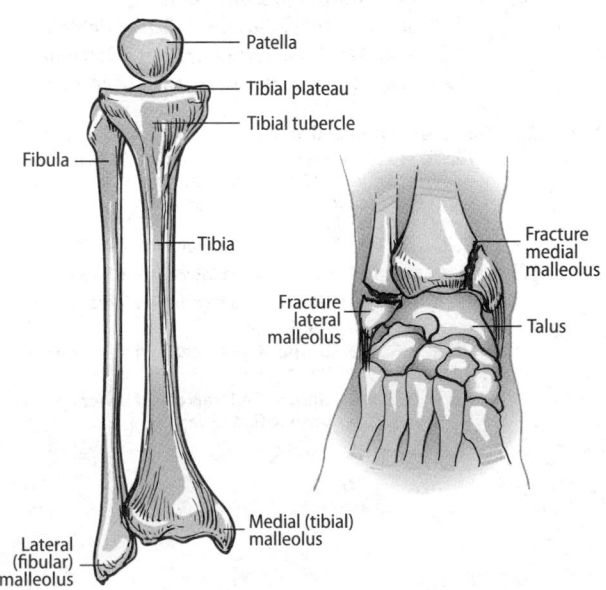

Patella
Tibial plateau
Tibial tubercle
Fibula
Tibia
Fracture medial malleolus
Fracture lateral malleolus
Talus
Medial (tibial) malleolus
Lateral (fibular) malleolus

EXCLUDES 1 Not coded here   EXCLUDES 2 Not included here   N Newborn Age: 0   P Pediatric Age: 0-17   M Maternity Age: 12-55   A Adult Age: 15-124

1016   ICD-10-CM 2018

√7ᵗʰ **S82.854** **Nondisplaced trimalleolar fracture of right lower leg**

√7ᵗʰ **S82.855** **Nondisplaced trimalleolar fracture of left lower leg**

√7ᵗʰ **S82.856** **Nondisplaced trimalleolar fracture of unspecified lower leg** ▽

√6ᵗʰ **S82.86** **Maisonneuve's fracture**

√7ᵗʰ **S82.861** **Displaced Maisonneuve's fracture of right leg**

√7ᵗʰ **S82.862** **Displaced Maisonneuve's fracture of left leg**

√7ᵗʰ **S82.863** **Displaced Maisonneuve's fracture of unspecified leg** ▽

√7ᵗʰ **S82.864** **Nondisplaced Maisonneuve's fracture of right leg**

√7ᵗʰ **S82.865** **Nondisplaced Maisonneuve's fracture of left leg**

√7ᵗʰ **S82.866** **Nondisplaced Maisonneuve's fracture of unspecified leg** ▽

√6ᵗʰ **S82.87** **Pilon fracture of tibia**

√7ᵗʰ **S82.871** **Displaced pilon fracture of right tibia**

√7ᵗʰ **S82.872** **Displaced pilon fracture of left tibia**

√7ᵗʰ **S82.873** **Displaced pilon fracture of unspecified tibia** ▽

√7ᵗʰ **S82.874** **Nondisplaced pilon fracture of right tibia**

√7ᵗʰ **S82.875** **Nondisplaced pilon fracture of left tibia**

√7ᵗʰ **S82.876** **Nondisplaced pilon fracture of unspecified tibia**

√6ᵗʰ **S82.89** **Other fractures of lower leg**
Fracture of ankle NOS

√7ᵗʰ **S82.891** **Other fracture of right lower leg**

√7ᵗʰ **S82.892** **Other fracture of left lower leg**

√7ᵗʰ **S82.899** **Other fracture of unspecified lower leg** ▽

√5ᵗʰ **S82.9** **Unspecified fracture of lower leg**

√x7ᵗʰ **S82.90** **Unspecified fracture of unspecified lower leg** ▽

√x7ᵗʰ **S82.91** **Unspecified fracture of right lower leg** ▽

√x7ᵗʰ **S82.92** **Unspecified fracture of left lower leg** ▽

√4ᵗʰ **S83** **Dislocation and sprain of joints and ligaments of knee**

INCLUDES   avulsion of joint or ligament of knee
laceration of cartilage, joint or ligament of knee
sprain of cartilage, joint or ligament of knee
traumatic hemarthrosis of joint or ligament of knee
traumatic rupture of joint or ligament of knee
traumatic subluxation of joint or ligament of knee
traumatic tear of joint or ligament of knee

Code also any associated open wound

EXCLUDES 1   *derangement of patella (M22.0-M22.3)*
injury of patellar ligament (tendon) (S76.1-)
internal derangement of knee (M23.-)
old dislocation of knee (M24.36)
pathological dislocation of knee (M24.36)
recurrent dislocation of knee (M22.0)

EXCLUDES 2   *strain of muscle, fascia and tendon of lower leg (S86.-)*

The appropriate 7th character is to be added to each code from category S83.
A   initial encounter
D   subsequent encounter
S   sequela

√5ᵗʰ **S83.0** **Subluxation and dislocation of patella**

√6ᵗʰ **S83.00** **Unspecified subluxation and dislocation of patella**

√7ᵗʰ **S83.001** **Unspecified subluxation of right patella** ▽

√7ᵗʰ **S83.002** **Unspecified subluxation of left patella** ▽

√7ᵗʰ **S83.003** **Unspecified subluxation of unspecified patella** ▽

√7ᵗʰ **S83.004** **Unspecified dislocation of right patella** ▽

√7ᵗʰ **S83.005** **Unspecified dislocation of left patella** ▽

√7ᵗʰ **S83.006** **Unspecified dislocation of unspecified patella** ▽

√6ᵗʰ **S83.01** **Lateral subluxation and dislocation of patella**

√7ᵗʰ **S83.011** **Lateral subluxation of right patella**

√7ᵗʰ **S83.012** **Lateral subluxation of left patella**

√7ᵗʰ **S83.013** **Lateral subluxation of unspecified patella** ▽

√7ᵗʰ **S83.014** **Lateral dislocation of right patella**

√7ᵗʰ **S83.015** **Lateral dislocation of left patella**

√7ᵗʰ **S83.016** **Lateral dislocation of unspecified patella** ▽

√6ᵗʰ **S83.09** **Other subluxation and dislocation of patella**

√7ᵗʰ **S83.091** **Other subluxation of right patella**

√7ᵗʰ **S83.092** **Other subluxation of left patella**

√7ᵗʰ **S83.093** **Other subluxation of unspecified patella** ▽

√7ᵗʰ **S83.094** **Other dislocation of right patella**

√7ᵗʰ **S83.095** **Other dislocation of left patella**

√7ᵗʰ **S83.096** **Other dislocation of unspecified patella** ▽

√5ᵗʰ **S83.1** **Subluxation and dislocation of knee**

EXCLUDES 2   *instability of knee prosthesis (T84.022, T84.023)*

√6ᵗʰ **S83.10** **Unspecified subluxation and dislocation of knee**

√7ᵗʰ **S83.101** **Unspecified subluxation of right knee** ▽

√7ᵗʰ **S83.102** **Unspecified subluxation of left knee** ▽

√7ᵗʰ **S83.103** **Unspecified subluxation of unspecified knee** ▽

√7ᵗʰ **S83.104** **Unspecified dislocation of right knee** ▽

√7ᵗʰ **S83.105** **Unspecified dislocation of left knee** ▽

√7ᵗʰ **S83.106** **Unspecified dislocation of unspecified knee** ▽

√6ᵗʰ **S83.11** **Anterior subluxation and dislocation of proximal end of tibia**
Posterior subluxation and dislocation of distal end of femur

√7ᵗʰ **S83.111** **Anterior subluxation of proximal end of tibia, right knee**

√7ᵗʰ **S83.112** **Anterior subluxation of proximal end of tibia, left knee**

√7ᵗʰ **S83.113** **Anterior subluxation of proximal end of tibia, unspecified knee** ▽

√7ᵗʰ **S83.114** **Anterior dislocation of proximal end of tibia, right knee**

√7ᵗʰ **S83.115** **Anterior dislocation of proximal end of tibia, left knee**

√7ᵗʰ **S83.116** **Anterior dislocation of proximal end of tibia, unspecified knee** ▽

√6ᵗʰ **S83.12** **Posterior subluxation and dislocation of proximal end of tibia**
Anterior dislocation of distal end of femur

√7ᵗʰ **S83.121** **Posterior subluxation of proximal end of tibia, right knee**

√7ᵗʰ **S83.122** **Posterior subluxation of proximal end of tibia, left knee**

√7ᵗʰ **S83.123** **Posterior subluxation of proximal end of tibia, unspecified knee** ▽

√7ᵗʰ **S83.124** **Posterior dislocation of proximal end of tibia, right knee**

√7ᵗʰ **S83.125** **Posterior dislocation of proximal end of tibia, left knee**

√7ᵗʰ **S83.126** **Posterior dislocation of proximal end of tibia, unspecified knee** ▽

√6ᵗʰ **S83.13** **Medial subluxation and dislocation of proximal end of tibia**

√7ᵗʰ **S83.131** **Medial subluxation of proximal end of tibia, right knee**

√7ᵗʰ **S83.132** **Medial subluxation of proximal end of tibia, left knee**

√7ᵗʰ **S83.133** **Medial subluxation of proximal end of tibia, unspecified knee** ▽

√7ᵗʰ **S83.134** **Medial dislocation of proximal end of tibia, right knee**

√7ᵗʰ **S83.135** **Medial dislocation of proximal end of tibia, left knee**

√7ᵗʰ **S83.136** **Medial dislocation of proximal end of tibia, unspecified knee** ▽

√ Additional Character Req   √x7ᵗʰ Placeholder Alert   Manifestation   HCC CMS-HCC Condition   ▽ Unspecified Code   ▶◀ Revised Text   ● New Code   ▲ Revised Code Title

√6ᵗʰ **S83.14** **Lateral subluxation and dislocation of proximal end of tibia**

    √7ᵗʰ **S83.141** **Lateral subluxation of proximal end of tibia, right knee**

    √7ᵗʰ **S83.142** **Lateral subluxation of proximal end of tibia, left knee**

    √7ᵗʰ **S83.143** **Lateral subluxation of proximal end of tibia, unspecified knee** ▽

    √7ᵗʰ **S83.144** **Lateral dislocation of proximal end of tibia, right knee**

    √7ᵗʰ **S83.145** **Lateral dislocation of proximal end of tibia, left knee**

    √7ᵗʰ **S83.146** **Lateral dislocation of proximal end of tibia, unspecified knee** ▽

√6ᵗʰ **S83.19** **Other subluxation and dislocation of knee**

    √7ᵗʰ **S83.191** **Other subluxation of right knee**

    √7ᵗʰ **S83.192** **Other subluxation of left knee**

    √7ᵗʰ **S83.193** **Other subluxation of unspecified knee** ▽

    √7ᵗʰ **S83.194** **Other dislocation of right knee**

    √7ᵗʰ **S83.195** **Other dislocation of left knee**

    √7ᵗʰ **S83.196** **Other dislocation of unspecified knee** ▽

√5ᵗʰ **S83.2** **Tear of meniscus, current injury**

    EXCLUDES 1   old bucket-handle tear (M23.2)

    √6ᵗʰ **S83.20** **Tear of unspecified meniscus, current injury**
      Tear of meniscus of knee NOS

      √7ᵗʰ **S83.200** **Bucket-handle tear of unspecified meniscus, current injury, right knee** ▽

      √7ᵗʰ **S83.201** **Bucket-handle tear of unspecified meniscus, current injury, left knee** ▽

      √7ᵗʰ **S83.202** **Bucket-handle tear of unspecified meniscus, current injury, unspecified knee** ▽

      √7ᵗʰ **S83.203** **Other tear of unspecified meniscus, current injury, right knee** ▽

      √7ᵗʰ **S83.204** **Other tear of unspecified meniscus, current injury, left knee** ▽

      √7ᵗʰ **S83.205** **Other tear of unspecified meniscus, current injury, unspecified knee** ▽

      √7ᵗʰ **S83.206** **Unspecified tear of unspecified meniscus, current injury, right knee** ▽

      √7ᵗʰ **S83.207** **Unspecified tear of unspecified meniscus, current injury, left knee** ▽

      √7ᵗʰ **S83.209** **Unspecified tear of unspecified meniscus, current injury, unspecified knee** ▽

    √6ᵗʰ **S83.21** **Bucket-handle tear of medial meniscus, current injury**

      √7ᵗʰ **S83.211** **Bucket-handle tear of medial meniscus, current injury, right knee**

      √7ᵗʰ **S83.212** **Bucket-handle tear of medial meniscus, current injury, left knee**

      √7ᵗʰ **S83.219** **Bucket-handle tear of medial meniscus, current injury, unspecified knee** ▽

    √6ᵗʰ **S83.22** **Peripheral tear of medial meniscus, current injury**

      √7ᵗʰ **S83.221** **Peripheral tear of medial meniscus, current injury, right knee**

      √7ᵗʰ **S83.222** **Peripheral tear of medial meniscus, current injury, left knee**

      √7ᵗʰ **S83.229** **Peripheral tear of medial meniscus, current injury, unspecified knee** ▽

    √6ᵗʰ **S83.23** **Complex tear of medial meniscus, current injury**

      √7ᵗʰ **S83.231** **Complex tear of medial meniscus, current injury, right knee**

      √7ᵗʰ **S83.232** **Complex tear of medial meniscus, current injury, left knee**

      √7ᵗʰ **S83.239** **Complex tear of medial meniscus, current injury, unspecified knee** ▽

    √6ᵗʰ **S83.24** **Other tear of medial meniscus, current injury**

      √7ᵗʰ **S83.241** **Other tear of medial meniscus, current injury, right knee**

      √7ᵗʰ **S83.242** **Other tear of medial meniscus, current injury, left knee**

      √7ᵗʰ **S83.249** **Other tear of medial meniscus, current injury, unspecified knee** ▽

    √6ᵗʰ **S83.25** **Bucket-handle tear of lateral meniscus, current injury**

      √7ᵗʰ **S83.251** **Bucket-handle tear of lateral meniscus, current injury, right knee**

      √7ᵗʰ **S83.252** **Bucket-handle tear of lateral meniscus, current injury, left knee**

      √7ᵗʰ **S83.259** **Bucket-handle tear of lateral meniscus, current injury, unspecified knee** ▽

    √6ᵗʰ **S83.26** **Peripheral tear of lateral meniscus, current injury**

      √7ᵗʰ **S83.261** **Peripheral tear of lateral meniscus, current injury, right knee**

      √7ᵗʰ **S83.262** **Peripheral tear of lateral meniscus, current injury, left knee**

      √7ᵗʰ **S83.269** **Peripheral tear of lateral meniscus, current injury, unspecified knee** ▽

    √6ᵗʰ **S83.27** **Complex tear of lateral meniscus, current injury**

      √7ᵗʰ **S83.271** **Complex tear of lateral meniscus, current injury, right knee**

      √7ᵗʰ **S83.272** **Complex tear of lateral meniscus, current injury, left knee**

      √7ᵗʰ **S83.279** **Complex tear of lateral meniscus, current injury, unspecified knee** ▽

    √6ᵗʰ **S83.28** **Other tear of lateral meniscus, current injury**

      √7ᵗʰ **S83.281** **Other tear of lateral meniscus, current injury, right knee**

      √7ᵗʰ **S83.282** **Other tear of lateral meniscus, current injury, left knee**

      √7ᵗʰ **S83.289** **Other tear of lateral meniscus, current injury, unspecified knee** ▽

√5ᵗʰ **S83.3** **Tear of articular cartilage of knee, current**

    √x7ᵗʰ **S83.30** **Tear of articular cartilage of unspecified knee, current** ▽

    √x7ᵗʰ **S83.31** **Tear of articular cartilage of right knee, current**

    √x7ᵗʰ **S83.32** **Tear of articular cartilage of left knee, current**

√5ᵗʰ **S83.4** **Sprain of collateral ligament of knee**

    √6ᵗʰ **S83.40** **Sprain of unspecified collateral ligament of knee**

      √7ᵗʰ **S83.401** **Sprain of unspecified collateral ligament of right knee** ▽

      √7ᵗʰ **S83.402** **Sprain of unspecified collateral ligament of left knee** ▽

      √7ᵗʰ **S83.409** **Sprain of unspecified collateral ligament of unspecified knee** ▽

    √6ᵗʰ **S83.41** **Sprain of medial collateral ligament of knee**
      Sprain of tibial collateral ligament

      √7ᵗʰ **S83.411** **Sprain of medial collateral ligament of right knee**

      √7ᵗʰ **S83.412** **Sprain of medial collateral ligament of left knee**

      √7ᵗʰ **S83.419** **Sprain of medial collateral ligament of unspecified knee** ▽

    √6ᵗʰ **S83.42** **Sprain of lateral collateral ligament of knee**
      Sprain of fibular collateral ligament

      √7ᵗʰ **S83.421** **Sprain of lateral collateral ligament of right knee**

      √7ᵗʰ **S83.422** **Sprain of lateral collateral ligament of left knee**

      √7ᵗʰ **S83.429** **Sprain of lateral collateral ligament of unspecified knee** ▽

√5ᵗʰ **S83.5** **Sprain of cruciate ligament of knee**
    AHA: 2016, 2Q, 3

    √6ᵗʰ **S83.50** **Sprain of unspecified cruciate ligament of knee**

      √7ᵗʰ **S83.501** **Sprain of unspecified cruciate ligament of right knee** ▽

      √7ᵗʰ **S83.502** **Sprain of unspecified cruciate ligament of left knee** ▽

      √7ᵗʰ **S83.509** **Sprain of unspecified cruciate ligament of unspecified knee** ▽

    √6ᵗʰ **S83.51** **Sprain of anterior cruciate ligament of knee**

      √7ᵗʰ **S83.511** **Sprain of anterior cruciate ligament of right knee**

      √7ᵗʰ **S83.512** **Sprain of anterior cruciate ligament of left knee**

EXCLUDES 1 Not coded here   *EXCLUDES 2* Not included here   N Newborn Age: 0   P Pediatric Age: 0-17   M Maternity Age: 12-55   A Adult Age: 15-124

1018   ICD-10-CM 2018

☑7ᵗʰ **S83.519** Sprain of anterior cruciate ligament of ▽
unspecified knee

☑6ᵗʰ **S83.52** Sprain of **posterior** cruciate ligament of knee

☑7ᵗʰ **S83.521** Sprain of posterior cruciate ligament of
right knee

☑7ᵗʰ **S83.522** Sprain of posterior cruciate ligament of
left knee

☑7ᵗʰ **S83.529** Sprain of posterior cruciate ligament of ▽
unspecified knee

☑5ᵗʰ **S83.6** Sprain of the superior tibiofibular joint and ligament

☑x7ᵗʰ **S83.60** Sprain of the superior tibiofibular joint and ▽
ligament, unspecified knee

☑x7ᵗʰ **S83.61** Sprain of the superior tibiofibular joint and
ligament, right knee

☑x7ᵗʰ **S83.62** Sprain of the superior tibiofibular joint and
ligament, left knee

☑5ᵗʰ **S83.8** Sprain of other specified parts of knee

☑6ᵗʰ **S83.8X** Sprain of other specified parts of knee

☑7ᵗʰ **S83.8X1** Sprain of other specified parts of right
knee

☑7ᵗʰ **S83.8X2** Sprain of other specified parts of left knee

☑7ᵗʰ **S83.8X9** Sprain of other specified parts of ▽
unspecified knee

☑5ᵗʰ **S83.9** Sprain of unspecified site of knee

☑x7ᵗʰ **S83.90** Sprain of unspecified site of unspecified knee ▽

☑x7ᵗʰ **S83.91** Sprain of unspecified site of right knee ▽

☑x7ᵗʰ **S83.92** Sprain of unspecified site of left knee ▽

☑4ᵗʰ **S84** **Injury of nerves at lower leg level**

Code also any associated open wound (S81.-)

EXCLUDES 2 injury of nerves at ankle and foot level (S94.-)

The appropriate 7th character is to be added to each code from
category S84.
A   initial encounter
D   subsequent encounter
S   sequela

☑5ᵗʰ **S84.0** Injury of tibial nerve at lower leg level

☑x7ᵗʰ **S84.00** Injury of tibial nerve at lower leg level, ▽
unspecified leg

☑x7ᵗʰ **S84.01** Injury of tibial nerve at lower leg level, right leg

☑x7ᵗʰ **S84.02** Injury of tibial nerve at lower leg level, left leg

☑5ᵗʰ **S84.1** Injury of peroneal nerve at lower leg level

☑x7ᵗʰ **S84.10** Injury of peroneal nerve at lower leg level, ▽
unspecified leg

☑x7ᵗʰ **S84.11** Injury of peroneal nerve at lower leg level, right leg

☑x7ᵗʰ **S84.12** Injury of peroneal nerve at lower leg level, left leg

☑5ᵗʰ **S84.2** Injury of cutaneous sensory nerve at lower leg level

☑x7ᵗʰ **S84.20** Injury of cutaneous sensory nerve at lower leg ▽
level, unspecified leg

☑x7ᵗʰ **S84.21** Injury of cutaneous sensory nerve at lower leg level,
right leg

☑x7ᵗʰ **S84.22** Injury of cutaneous sensory nerve at lower leg level,
left leg

☑5ᵗʰ **S84.8** Injury of other nerves at lower leg level

☑6ᵗʰ **S84.80** Injury of other nerves at lower leg level

☑7ᵗʰ **S84.801** Injury of other nerves at lower leg level,
right leg

☑7ᵗʰ **S84.802** Injury of other nerves at lower leg level,
left leg

☑7ᵗʰ **S84.809** Injury of other nerves at lower leg level, ▽
unspecified leg

☑5ᵗʰ **S84.9** Injury of unspecified nerve at lower leg level

☑x7ᵗʰ **S84.90** Injury of unspecified nerve at lower leg level, ▽
unspecified leg

☑x7ᵗʰ **S84.91** Injury of unspecified nerve at lower leg level, ▽
right leg

☑x7ᵗʰ **S84.92** Injury of unspecified nerve at lower leg level, ▽
left leg

☑4ᵗʰ **S85** **Injury of blood vessels at lower leg level**

Code also any associated open wound (S81.-)

EXCLUDES 2 injury of blood vessels at ankle and foot level (S95.-)

The appropriate 7th character is to be added to each code from
category S85.
A   initial encounter
D   subsequent encounter
S   sequela

☑5ᵗʰ **S85.0** Injury of popliteal artery

☑6ᵗʰ **S85.00** Unspecified injury of popliteal artery

☑7ᵗʰ **S85.001** Unspecified injury of popliteal artery, ▽
right leg

☑7ᵗʰ **S85.002** Unspecified injury of popliteal artery, ▽
left leg

☑7ᵗʰ **S85.009** Unspecified injury of popliteal artery, ▽
unspecified leg

☑6ᵗʰ **S85.01** Laceration of popliteal artery

☑7ᵗʰ **S85.011** Laceration of popliteal artery, right leg

☑7ᵗʰ **S85.012** Laceration of popliteal artery, left leg

☑7ᵗʰ **S85.019** Laceration of popliteal artery, ▽
unspecified leg

☑6ᵗʰ **S85.09** Other specified injury of popliteal artery

☑7ᵗʰ **S85.091** Other specified injury of popliteal artery,
right leg

☑7ᵗʰ **S85.092** Other specified injury of popliteal artery,
left leg

☑7ᵗʰ **S85.099** Other specified injury of popliteal ▽
artery, unspecified leg

☑5ᵗʰ **S85.1** Injury of tibial artery

☑6ᵗʰ **S85.10** Unspecified injury of unspecified tibial artery
Injury of tibial artery NOS

☑7ᵗʰ **S85.101** Unspecified injury of unspecified tibial ▽
artery, right leg

☑7ᵗʰ **S85.102** Unspecified injury of unspecified tibial ▽
artery, left leg

☑7ᵗʰ **S85.109** Unspecified injury of unspecified tibial ▽
artery, unspecified leg

☑6ᵗʰ **S85.11** Laceration of unspecified tibial artery

☑7ᵗʰ **S85.111** Laceration of unspecified tibial artery, ▽
right leg

☑7ᵗʰ **S85.112** Laceration of unspecified tibial artery, ▽
left leg

☑7ᵗʰ **S85.119** Laceration of unspecified tibial artery, ▽
unspecified leg

☑6ᵗʰ **S85.12** Other specified injury of unspecified tibial artery

☑7ᵗʰ **S85.121** Other specified injury of unspecified ▽
tibial artery, right leg

☑7ᵗʰ **S85.122** Other specified injury of unspecified ▽
tibial artery, left leg

☑7ᵗʰ **S85.129** Other specified injury of unspecified ▽
tibial artery, unspecified leg

☑6ᵗʰ **S85.13** Unspecified injury of anterior tibial artery

☑7ᵗʰ **S85.131** Unspecified injury of anterior tibial ▽
artery, right leg

☑7ᵗʰ **S85.132** Unspecified injury of anterior tibial ▽
artery, left leg

☑7ᵗʰ **S85.139** Unspecified injury of anterior tibial ▽
artery, unspecified leg

☑6ᵗʰ **S85.14** Laceration of anterior tibial artery

☑7ᵗʰ **S85.141** Laceration of anterior tibial artery, right
leg

☑7ᵗʰ **S85.142** Laceration of anterior tibial artery, left leg

☑7ᵗʰ **S85.149** Laceration of anterior tibial artery, ▽
unspecified leg

☑6ᵗʰ **S85.15** Other specified injury of anterior tibial artery

☑7ᵗʰ **S85.151** Other specified injury of anterior tibial
artery, right leg

☑7ᵗʰ **S85.152** Other specified injury of anterior tibial
artery, left leg

☑7ᵗʰ **S85.159** Other specified injury of anterior tibial ▽
artery, unspecified leg

☑ Additional Character Req   ☑x7ᵗʰ Placeholder Alert   Manifestation   HCC CMS-HCC Condition   ▽ Unspecified Code   ►◄ Revised Text   ● New Code   ▲ Revised Code Title

ICD-10-CM 2018   1019

√6ᵗʰ **S85.16** Unspecified injury of posterior tibial artery
- √7ᵗʰ **S85.161** Unspecified injury of posterior tibial artery, right leg ▽
- √7ᵗʰ **S85.162** Unspecified injury of posterior tibial artery, left leg ▽
- √7ᵗʰ **S85.169** Unspecified injury of posterior tibial artery, unspecified leg ▽

√6ᵗʰ **S85.17** Laceration of posterior tibial artery
- √7ᵗʰ **S85.171** Laceration of posterior tibial artery, right leg
- √7ᵗʰ **S85.172** Laceration of posterior tibial artery, left leg
- √7ᵗʰ **S85.179** Laceration of posterior tibial artery, unspecified leg ▽

√6ᵗʰ **S85.18** Other specified injury of posterior tibial artery
- √7ᵗʰ **S85.181** Other specified injury of posterior tibial artery, right leg
- √7ᵗʰ **S85.182** Other specified injury of posterior tibial artery, left leg
- √7ᵗʰ **S85.189** Other specified injury of posterior tibial artery, unspecified leg ▽

√5ᵗʰ **S85.2** Injury of peroneal artery
√6ᵗʰ **S85.20** Unspecified injury of peroneal artery
- √7ᵗʰ **S85.201** Unspecified injury of peroneal artery, right leg ▽
- √7ᵗʰ **S85.202** Unspecified injury of peroneal artery, left leg ▽
- √7ᵗʰ **S85.209** Unspecified injury of peroneal artery, unspecified leg ▽

√6ᵗʰ **S85.21** Laceration of peroneal artery
- √7ᵗʰ **S85.211** Laceration of peroneal artery, right leg
- √7ᵗʰ **S85.212** Laceration of peroneal artery, left leg
- √7ᵗʰ **S85.219** Laceration of peroneal artery, unspecified leg ▽

√6ᵗʰ **S85.29** Other specified injury of peroneal artery
- √7ᵗʰ **S85.291** Other specified injury of peroneal artery, right leg
- √7ᵗʰ **S85.292** Other specified injury of peroneal artery, left leg
- √7ᵗʰ **S85.299** Other specified injury of peroneal artery, unspecified leg ▽

√5ᵗʰ **S85.3** Injury of greater saphenous vein at lower leg level
Injury of greater saphenous vein NOS
Injury of saphenous vein NOS
√6ᵗʰ **S85.30** Unspecified injury of greater saphenous vein at lower leg level
- √7ᵗʰ **S85.301** Unspecified injury of greater saphenous vein at lower leg level, right leg ▽
- √7ᵗʰ **S85.302** Unspecified injury of greater saphenous vein at lower leg level, left leg ▽
- √7ᵗʰ **S85.309** Unspecified injury of greater saphenous vein at lower leg level, unspecified leg ▽

√6ᵗʰ **S85.31** Laceration of greater saphenous vein at lower leg level
- √7ᵗʰ **S85.311** Laceration of greater saphenous vein at lower leg level, right leg
- √7ᵗʰ **S85.312** Laceration of greater saphenous vein at lower leg level, left leg
- √7ᵗʰ **S85.319** Laceration of greater saphenous vein at lower leg level, unspecified leg ▽

√6ᵗʰ **S85.39** Other specified injury of greater saphenous vein at lower leg level
- √7ᵗʰ **S85.391** Other specified injury of greater saphenous vein at lower leg level, right leg
- √7ᵗʰ **S85.392** Other specified injury of greater saphenous vein at lower leg level, left leg
- √7ᵗʰ **S85.399** Other specified injury of greater saphenous vein at lower leg level, unspecified leg ▽

√5ᵗʰ **S85.4** Injury of lesser saphenous vein at lower leg level
√6ᵗʰ **S85.40** Unspecified injury of lesser saphenous vein at lower leg level
- √7ᵗʰ **S85.401** Unspecified injury of lesser saphenous vein at lower leg level, right leg ▽
- √7ᵗʰ **S85.402** Unspecified injury of lesser saphenous vein at lower leg level, left leg ▽
- √7ᵗʰ **S85.409** Unspecified injury of lesser saphenous vein at lower leg level, unspecified leg ▽

√6ᵗʰ **S85.41** Laceration of lesser saphenous vein at lower leg level
- √7ᵗʰ **S85.411** Laceration of lesser saphenous vein at lower leg level, right leg
- √7ᵗʰ **S85.412** Laceration of lesser saphenous vein at lower leg level, left leg
- √7ᵗʰ **S85.419** Laceration of lesser saphenous vein at lower leg level, unspecified leg ▽

√6ᵗʰ **S85.49** Other specified injury of lesser saphenous vein at lower leg level
- √7ᵗʰ **S85.491** Other specified injury of lesser saphenous vein at lower leg level, right leg
- √7ᵗʰ **S85.492** Other specified injury of lesser saphenous vein at lower leg level, left leg
- √7ᵗʰ **S85.499** Other specified injury of lesser saphenous vein at lower leg level, unspecified leg ▽

√5ᵗʰ **S85.5** Injury of popliteal vein
√6ᵗʰ **S85.50** Unspecified injury of popliteal vein
- √7ᵗʰ **S85.501** Unspecified injury of popliteal vein, right leg ▽
- √7ᵗʰ **S85.502** Unspecified injury of popliteal vein, left leg ▽
- √7ᵗʰ **S85.509** Unspecified injury of popliteal vein, unspecified leg ▽

√6ᵗʰ **S85.51** Laceration of popliteal vein
- √7ᵗʰ **S85.511** Laceration of popliteal vein, right leg
- √7ᵗʰ **S85.512** Laceration of popliteal vein, left leg
- √7ᵗʰ **S85.519** Laceration of popliteal vein, unspecified leg ▽

√6ᵗʰ **S85.59** Other specified injury of popliteal vein
- √7ᵗʰ **S85.591** Other specified injury of popliteal vein, right leg
- √7ᵗʰ **S85.592** Other specified injury of popliteal vein, left leg
- √7ᵗʰ **S85.599** Other specified injury of popliteal vein, unspecified leg ▽

√5ᵗʰ **S85.8** Injury of other blood vessels at lower leg level
√6ᵗʰ **S85.80** Unspecified injury of other blood vessels at lower leg level
- √7ᵗʰ **S85.801** Unspecified injury of other blood vessels at lower leg level, right leg ▽
- √7ᵗʰ **S85.802** Unspecified injury of other blood vessels at lower leg level, left leg ▽
- √7ᵗʰ **S85.809** Unspecified injury of other blood vessels at lower leg level, unspecified leg ▽

√6ᵗʰ **S85.81** Laceration of other blood vessels at lower leg level
- √7ᵗʰ **S85.811** Laceration of other blood vessels at lower leg level, right leg
- √7ᵗʰ **S85.812** Laceration of other blood vessels at lower leg level, left leg
- √7ᵗʰ **S85.819** Laceration of other blood vessels at lower leg level, unspecified leg ▽

√6ᵗʰ **S85.89** Other specified injury of other blood vessels at lower leg level
- √7ᵗʰ **S85.891** Other specified injury of other blood vessels at lower leg level, right leg
- √7ᵗʰ **S85.892** Other specified injury of other blood vessels at lower leg level, left leg
- √7ᵗʰ **S85.899** Other specified injury of other blood vessels at lower leg level, unspecified leg ▽

EXCLUDES 1 Not coded here   **EXCLUDES 2** Not included here   N Newborn Age: 0   P Pediatric Age: 0-17   M Maternity Age: 12-55   A Adult Age: 15-124

1020   ICD-10-CM 2018

✓5ᵗʰ **S85.9** **Injury of unspecified blood vessel at lower leg level**

   ✓6ᵗʰ **S85.90** **Unspecified injury of unspecified blood vessel at lower leg level**

     ✓7ᵗʰ **S85.901** **Unspecified injury of unspecified blood vessel at lower leg level, right leg** ▽

     ✓7ᵗʰ **S85.902** **Unspecified injury of unspecified blood vessel at lower leg level, left leg** ▽

     ✓7ᵗʰ **S85.909** **Unspecified injury of unspecified blood vessel at lower leg level, unspecified leg** ▽

   ✓6ᵗʰ **S85.91** **Laceration of unspecified blood vessel at lower leg level**

     ✓7ᵗʰ **S85.911** **Laceration of unspecified blood vessel at lower leg level, right leg** ▽

     ✓7ᵗʰ **S85.912** **Laceration of unspecified blood vessel at lower leg level, left leg** ▽

     ✓7ᵗʰ **S85.919** **Laceration of unspecified blood vessel at lower leg level, unspecified leg** ▽

   ✓6ᵗʰ **S85.99** **Other specified injury of unspecified blood vessel at lower leg level**

     ✓7ᵗʰ **S85.991** **Other specified injury of unspecified blood vessel at lower leg level, right leg** ▽

     ✓7ᵗʰ **S85.992** **Other specified injury of unspecified blood vessel at lower leg level, left leg** ▽

     ✓7ᵗʰ **S85.999** **Other specified injury of unspecified blood vessel at lower leg level, unspecified leg** ▽

✓4ᵗʰ **S86** **Injury of muscle, fascia and tendon at lower leg level**

Code also any associated open wound (S81.-)

EXCLUDES 2   *injury of muscle, fascia and tendon at ankle (S96.-)*
                injury of patellar ligament (tendon) (S76.1-)
                sprain of joints and ligaments of knee (S83.-)

TIP: Refer to the Muscle/Tendon table at the beginning of this chapter.

> The appropriate 7th character is to be added to each code from category S86.
> A   initial encounter
> D   subsequent encounter
> S   sequela

  ✓5ᵗʰ **S86.0** **Injury of Achilles tendon**

   ✓6ᵗʰ **S86.00** **Unspecified injury of Achilles tendon**

     ✓7ᵗʰ **S86.001** **Unspecified injury of right Achilles tendon** ▽

     ✓7ᵗʰ **S86.002** **Unspecified injury of left Achilles tendon** ▽

     ✓7ᵗʰ **S86.009** **Unspecified injury of unspecified Achilles tendon** ▽

   ✓6ᵗʰ **S86.01** **Strain of Achilles tendon**

     ✓7ᵗʰ **S86.011** **Strain of right Achilles tendon**

     ✓7ᵗʰ **S86.012** **Strain of left Achilles tendon**

     ✓7ᵗʰ **S86.019** **Strain of unspecified Achilles tendon** ▽

    S86.02 **Laceration of Achilles tendon**

     ✓7ᵗʰ **S86.021** **Laceration of right Achilles tendon**

     ✓7ᵗʰ **S86.022** **Laceration of left Achilles tendon**

     ✓7ᵗʰ **S86.029** **Laceration of unspecified Achilles tendon** ▽

   ✓6ᵗʰ **S86.09** **Other specified injury of Achilles tendon**

     ✓7ᵗʰ **S86.091** **Other specified injury of right Achilles tendon**

     ✓7ᵗʰ **S86.092** **Other specified injury of left Achilles tendon**

     ✓7ᵗʰ **S86.099** **Other specified injury of unspecified Achilles tendon** ▽

  ✓5ᵗʰ **S86.1** **Injury of other muscle(s) and tendon(s) of posterior muscle group at lower leg level**

   ✓6ᵗʰ **S86.10** **Unspecified injury of other muscle(s) and tendon(s) of posterior muscle group at lower leg level**

     ✓7ᵗʰ **S86.101** **Unspecified injury of other muscle(s) and tendon(s) of posterior muscle group at lower leg level, right leg** ▽

     ✓7ᵗʰ **S86.102** **Unspecified injury of other muscle(s) and tendon(s) of posterior muscle group at lower leg level, left leg** ▽

     ✓7ᵗʰ **S86.109** **Unspecified injury of other muscle(s) and tendon(s) of posterior muscle group at lower leg level, unspecified leg** ▽

   ✓6ᵗʰ **S86.11** **Strain of other muscle(s) and tendon(s) of posterior muscle group at lower leg level**

     ✓7ᵗʰ **S86.111** **Strain of other muscle(s) and tendon(s) of posterior muscle group at lower leg level, right leg**

     ✓7ᵗʰ **S86.112** **Strain of other muscle(s) and tendon(s) of posterior muscle group at lower leg level, left leg**

     ✓7ᵗʰ **S86.119** **Strain of other muscle(s) and tendon(s) of posterior muscle group at lower leg level, unspecified leg** ▽

   ✓6ᵗʰ **S86.12** **Laceration of other muscle(s) and tendon(s) of posterior muscle group at lower leg level**

     ✓7ᵗʰ **S86.121** **Laceration of other muscle(s) and tendon(s) of posterior muscle group at lower leg level, right leg**

     ✓7ᵗʰ **S86.122** **Laceration of other muscle(s) and tendon(s) of posterior muscle group at lower leg level, left leg**

     ✓7ᵗʰ **S86.129** **Laceration of other muscle(s) and tendon(s) of posterior muscle group at lower leg level, unspecified leg** ▽

   ✓6ᵗʰ **S86.19** **Other injury of other muscle(s) and tendon(s) of posterior muscle group at lower leg level**

     ✓7ᵗʰ **S86.191** **Other injury of other muscle(s) and tendon(s) of posterior muscle group at lower leg level, right leg**

     ✓7ᵗʰ **S86.192** **Other injury of other muscle(s) and tendon(s) of posterior muscle group at lower leg level, left leg**

     ✓7ᵗʰ **S86.199** **Other injury of other muscle(s) and tendon(s) of posterior muscle group at lower leg level, unspecified leg** ▽

  ✓5ᵗʰ **S86.2** **Injury of muscle(s) and tendon(s) of anterior muscle group at lower leg level**

   ✓6ᵗʰ **S86.20** **Unspecified injury of muscle(s) and tendon(s) of anterior muscle group at lower leg level**

     ✓7ᵗʰ **S86.201** **Unspecified injury of muscle(s) and tendon(s) of anterior muscle group at lower leg level, right leg** ▽

     ✓7ᵗʰ **S86.202** **Unspecified injury of muscle(s) and tendon(s) of anterior muscle group at lower leg level, left leg** ▽

     ✓7ᵗʰ **S86.209** **Unspecified injury of muscle(s) and tendon(s) of anterior muscle group at lower leg level, unspecified leg** ▽

   ✓6ᵗʰ **S86.21** **Strain of muscle(s) and tendon(s) of anterior muscle group at lower leg level**

     ✓7ᵗʰ **S86.211** **Strain of muscle(s) and tendon(s) of anterior muscle group at lower leg level, right leg**

     ✓7ᵗʰ **S86.212** **Strain of muscle(s) and tendon(s) of anterior muscle group at lower leg level, left leg**

     ✓7ᵗʰ **S86.219** **Strain of muscle(s) and tendon(s) of anterior muscle group at lower leg level, unspecified leg** ▽

   ✓6ᵗʰ **S86.22** **Laceration of muscle(s) and tendon(s) of anterior muscle group at lower leg level**

     ✓7ᵗʰ **S86.221** **Laceration of muscle(s) and tendon(s) of anterior muscle group at lower leg level, right leg**

     ✓7ᵗʰ **S86.222** **Laceration of muscle(s) and tendon(s) of anterior muscle group at lower leg level, left leg**

     ✓7ᵗʰ **S86.229** **Laceration of muscle(s) and tendon(s) of anterior muscle group at lower leg level, unspecified leg** ▽

   ✓6ᵗʰ **S86.29** **Other injury of muscle(s) and tendon(s) of anterior muscle group at lower leg level**

     ✓7ᵗʰ **S86.291** **Other injury of muscle(s) and tendon(s) of anterior muscle group at lower leg level, right leg**

     ✓7ᵗʰ **S86.292** **Other injury of muscle(s) and tendon(s) of anterior muscle group at lower leg level, left leg**

✓ Additional Character Req   ✓x7ᵗʰ Placeholder Alert   Manifestation   HCC CMS-HCC Condition   ▽ Unspecified Code   ►◄ Revised Text   ● New Code   ▲ Revised Code Title

    ✓7ᵗʰ **S86.299**   Other injury of muscle(s) and tendon(s) ▽
         of anterior muscle group at lower leg
         level, unspecified leg

✓5ᵗʰ **S86.3**   Injury of muscle(s) and tendon(s) of peroneal muscle group at
     lower leg level

    ✓6ᵗʰ **S86.30**   Unspecified injury of muscle(s) and tendon(s) of
         peroneal muscle group at lower leg level

        ✓7ᵗʰ **S86.301**   Unspecified injury of muscle(s) and ▽
             tendon(s) of peroneal muscle group at
             lower leg level, right leg

        ✓7ᵗʰ **S86.302**   Unspecified injury of muscle(s) and ▽
             tendon(s) of peroneal muscle group at
             lower leg level, left leg

        ✓7ᵗʰ **S86.309**   Unspecified injury of muscle(s) and ▽
             tendon(s) of peroneal muscle group at
             lower leg level, unspecified leg

    ✓6ᵗʰ **S86.31**   Strain of muscle(s) and tendon(s) of peroneal muscle
         group at lower leg level

        ✓7ᵗʰ **S86.311**   Strain of muscle(s) and tendon(s) of
             peroneal muscle group at lower leg level,
             right leg

        ✓7ᵗʰ **S86.312**   Strain of muscle(s) and tendon(s) of
             peroneal muscle group at lower leg level,
             left leg

        ✓7ᵗʰ **S86.319**   Strain of muscle(s) and tendon(s) of ▽
             peroneal muscle group at lower leg
             level, unspecified leg

    ✓6ᵗʰ **S86.32**   Laceration of muscle(s) and tendon(s) of peroneal
         muscle group at lower leg level

        ✓7ᵗʰ **S86.321**   Laceration of muscle(s) and tendon(s) of
             peroneal muscle group at lower leg level,
             right leg

        ✓7ᵗʰ **S86.322**   Laceration of muscle(s) and tendon(s) of
             peroneal muscle group at lower leg level,
             left leg

        ✓7ᵗʰ **S86.329**   Laceration of muscle(s) and tendon(s) ▽
             of peroneal muscle group at lower leg
             level, unspecified leg

    ✓6ᵗʰ **S86.39**   Other injury of muscle(s) and tendon(s) of peroneal
         muscle group at lower leg level

        ✓7ᵗʰ **S86.391**   Other injury of muscle(s) and tendon(s) of
             peroneal muscle group at lower leg level,
             right leg

        ✓7ᵗʰ **S86.392**   Other injury of muscle(s) and tendon(s) of
             peroneal muscle group at lower leg level,
             left leg

        ✓7ᵗʰ **S86.399**   Other injury of muscle(s) and tendon(s) ▽
             of peroneal muscle group at lower leg
             level, unspecified leg

✓5ᵗʰ **S86.8**   Injury of other muscles and tendons at lower leg level

    ✓6ᵗʰ **S86.80**   Unspecified injury of other muscles and tendons at
         lower leg level

        ✓7ᵗʰ **S86.801**   Unspecified injury of other muscle(s) ▽
             and tendon(s) at lower leg level, right leg

        ✓7ᵗʰ **S86.802**   Unspecified injury of other muscle(s) ▽
             and tendon(s) at lower leg level, left leg

        ✓7ᵗʰ **S86.809**   Unspecified injury of other muscle(s) ▽
             and tendon(s) at lower leg level,
             unspecified leg

    ✓6ᵗʰ **S86.81**   Strain of other muscles and tendons at lower leg
         level

        ✓7ᵗʰ **S86.811**   Strain of other muscle(s) and tendon(s) at
             lower leg level, right leg

        ✓7ᵗʰ **S86.812**   Strain of other muscle(s) and tendon(s) at
             lower leg level, left leg

        ✓7ᵗʰ **S86.819**   Strain of other muscle(s) and tendon(s) ▽
             at lower leg level, unspecified leg

    ✓6ᵗʰ **S86.82**   Laceration of other muscles and tendons at lower leg
         level

        ✓7ᵗʰ **S86.821**   Laceration of other muscle(s) and
             tendon(s) at lower leg level, right leg

        ✓7ᵗʰ **S86.822**   Laceration of other muscle(s) and
             tendon(s) at lower leg level, left leg

        ✓7ᵗʰ **S86.829**   Laceration of other muscle(s) and ▽
             tendon(s) at lower leg level,
             unspecified leg

    ✓6ᵗʰ **S86.89**   Other injury of other muscles and tendons at lower
         leg level

        ✓7ᵗʰ **S86.891**   Other injury of other muscle(s) and
             tendon(s) at lower leg level, right leg

        ✓7ᵗʰ **S86.892**   Other injury of other muscle(s) and
             tendon(s) at lower leg level, left leg

        ✓7ᵗʰ **S86.899**   Other injury of other muscle(s) and ▽
             tendon(s) at lower leg level, unspecified
             leg

✓5ᵗʰ **S86.9**   Injury of unspecified muscle and tendon at lower leg level

    ✓6ᵗʰ **S86.90**   Unspecified injury of unspecified muscle and tendon
         at lower leg level

        ✓7ᵗʰ **S86.901**   Unspecified injury of unspecified ▽
             muscle(s) and tendon(s) at lower leg
             level, right leg

        ✓7ᵗʰ **S86.902**   Unspecified injury of unspecified ▽
             muscle(s) and tendon(s) at lower leg
             level, left leg

        ✓7ᵗʰ **S86.909**   Unspecified injury of unspecified ▽
             muscle(s) and tendon(s) at lower leg
             evel, unspecified leg

    ✓6ᵗʰ **S86.91**   Strain of unspecified muscle and tendon at lower leg
         level

        ✓7ᵗʰ **S86.911**   Strain of unspecified muscle(s) and ▽
             tendon(s) at lower leg level, right leg

        ✓7ᵗʰ **S86.912**   Strain of unspecified muscle(s) and ▽
             tendon(s) at lower leg level, left leg

        ✓7ᵗʰ **S86.919**   Strain of unspecified muscle(s) and ▽
             tendon(s) at lower leg level,
             unspecified leg

    ✓6ᵗʰ **S86.92**   Laceration of unspecified muscle and tendon at
         lower leg level

        ✓7ᵗʰ **S86.921**   Laceration of unspecified muscle(s) ▽
             and tendon(s) at lower leg level,
             right leg

        ✓7ᵗʰ **S86.922**   Laceration of unspecified muscle(s) ▽
             and tendon(s) at lower leg level,
             left leg

        ✓7ᵗʰ **S86.929**   Laceration of unspecified muscle(s) ▽
             and tendon(s) at lower leg level,
             unspecified leg

    ✓6ᵗʰ **S86.99**   Other injury of unspecified muscle and tendon at
         lower leg level

        ✓7ᵗʰ **S86.991**   Other injury of unspecified muscle(s) ▽
             and tendon(s) at lower leg level,
             right leg

        ✓7ᵗʰ **S86.992**   Other injury of unspecified muscle(s) ▽
             and tendon(s) at lower leg level,
             left leg

        ✓7ᵗʰ **S86.999**   Other injury of unspecified muscle(s) ▽
             and tendon(s) at lower leg level,
             unspecified leg

✓4ᵗʰ **S87**   **Crushing injury of lower leg**

Use additional code(s) for all associated injuries

EXCLUDES 2   *crushing injury of ankle and foot (S97.-)*

> The appropriate 7th character is to be added to each code from
> category S87.
> A   initial encounter
> D   subsequent encounter
> S   sequela

✓5ᵗʰ **S87.0**   **Crushing injury of knee**

    ✓x7ᵗʰ **S87.00**   Crushing injury of unspecified knee ▽

    ✓x7ᵗʰ **S87.01**   Crushing injury of right knee

    ✓x7ᵗʰ **S87.02**   Crushing injury of left knee

✓5ᵗʰ **S87.8**   **Crushing injury of lower leg**

    ✓x7ᵗʰ **S87.80**   Crushing injury of unspecified lower leg ▽

    ✓x7ᵗʰ **S87.81**   Crushing injury of right lower leg

    ✓x7ᵗʰ **S87.82**   Crushing injury of left lower leg

EXCLUDES 1 Not coded here   **EXCLUDES 2** Not included here   **N** Newborn Age: 0   **P** Pediatric Age: 0-17   **M** Maternity Age: 12-55   **A** Adult Age: 15-124

1022   ICD-10-CM 2018

☑4ᵗʰ S88 Traumatic amputation of lower leg

An amputation not identified as partial or complete should be coded to complete.

EXCLUDES 1   traumatic amputation of ankle and foot (S98.-)

> The appropriate 7th character is to be added to each code from category S88.
> A   initial encounter
> D   subsequent encounter
> S   sequela

☑5ᵗʰ S88.0 Traumatic amputation at knee level

  ☑6ᵗʰ S88.01 Complete traumatic amputation at knee level

    ☑7ᵗʰ **S88.011** Complete traumatic amputation at knee level, right lower leg   HCC

    ☑7ᵗʰ **S88.012** Complete traumatic amputation at knee level, left lower leg   HCC

    ☑7ᵗʰ **S88.019** Complete traumatic amputation at knee level, unspecified lower leg   HCC ▽

  ☑6ᵗʰ S88.02 Partial traumatic amputation at knee level

    ☑7ᵗʰ **S88.021** Partial traumatic amputation at knee level, right lower leg   HCC

    ☑7ᵗʰ **S88.022** Partial traumatic amputation at knee level, left lower leg   HCC

    ☑7ᵗʰ **S88.029** Partial traumatic amputation at knee level, unspecified lower leg   HCC ▽

☑5ᵗʰ S88.1 Traumatic amputation at level between knee and ankle

  ☑6ᵗʰ S88.11 Complete traumatic amputation at level between knee and ankle

    ☑7ᵗʰ **S88.111** Complete traumatic amputation at level between knee and ankle, right lower leg   HCC

    ☑7ᵗʰ **S88.112** Complete traumatic amputation at level between knee and ankle, left lower leg   HCC

    ☑7ᵗʰ **S88.119** Complete traumatic amputation at level between knee and ankle, unspecified lower leg   HCC ▽

  ☑6ᵗʰ S88.12 Partial traumatic amputation at level between knee and ankle

    ☑7ᵗʰ **S88.121** Partial traumatic amputation at level between knee and ankle, right lower leg   HCC

    ☑7ᵗʰ **S88.122** Partial traumatic amputation at level between knee and ankle, left lower leg   HCC

    ☑7ᵗʰ **S88.129** Partial traumatic amputation at level between knee and ankle, unspecified lower leg   HCC ▽

☑5ᵗʰ S88.9 Traumatic amputation of lower leg, level unspecified

  ☑6ᵗʰ S88.91 Complete traumatic amputation of lower leg, level unspecified

    ☑7ᵗʰ **S88.911** Complete traumatic amputation of right lower leg, level unspecified   HCC ▽

    ☑7ᵗʰ **S88.912** Complete traumatic amputation of left lower leg, level unspecified   HCC ▽

    ☑7ᵗʰ **S88.919** Complete traumatic amputation of unspecified lower leg, level unspecified   HCC ▽

  ☑6ᵗʰ S88.92 Partial traumatic amputation of lower leg, level unspecified

    ☑7ᵗʰ **S88.921** Partial traumatic amputation of right lower leg, level unspecified   HCC ▽

    ☑7ᵗʰ **S88.922** Partial traumatic amputation of left lower leg, level unspecified   HCC ▽

    ☑7ᵗʰ **S88.929** Partial traumatic amputation of unspecified lower leg, level unspecified   HCC ▽

☑4ᵗʰ S89 Other and unspecified injuries of lower leg

> **NOTE**   A fracture not indicated as open or closed should be coded to closed.

EXCLUDES 2   other and unspecified injuries of ankle and foot (S99.-)

AHA: 2015, 3Q, 37-39

> The appropriate 7th character is to be added to each code from subcategories S89.0, S89.1, S89.2, and S89.3.
> A   initial encounter for closed fracture
> D   subsequent encounter for fracture with routine healing
> G   subsequent encounter for fracture with delayed healing
> K   subsequent encounter for fracture with nonunion
> P   subsequent encounter for fracture with malunion
> S   sequela

☑5ᵗʰ S89.0 Physeal fracture of upper end of tibia

  ☑6ᵗʰ S89.00 Unspecified physeal fracture of upper end of tibia

    ☑7ᵗʰ **S89.001** Unspecified physeal fracture of upper end of right tibia   ▽

    ☑7ᵗʰ **S89.002** Unspecified physeal fracture of upper end of left tibia   ▽

    ☑7ᵗʰ **S89.009** Unspecified physeal fracture of upper end of unspecified tibia   ▽

  ☑6ᵗʰ S89.01 Salter-Harris Type I physeal fracture of upper end of tibia

    ☑7ᵗʰ **S89.011** Salter-Harris Type I physeal fracture of upper end of right tibia

    ☑7ᵗʰ **S89.012** Salter-Harris Type I physeal fracture of upper end of left tibia

    ☑7ᵗʰ **S89.019** Salter-Harris Type I physeal fracture of upper end of unspecified tibia   ▽

  ☑6ᵗʰ S89.02 Salter-Harris Type II physeal fracture of upper end of tibia

    ☑7ᵗʰ **S89.021** Salter-Harris Type II physeal fracture of upper end of right tibia

    ☑7ᵗʰ **S89.022** Salter-Harris Type II physeal fracture of upper end of left tibia

    ☑7ᵗʰ **S89.029** Salter-Harris Type II physeal fracture of upper end of unspecified tibia   ▽

  ☑6ᵗʰ S89.03 Salter-Harris Type III physeal fracture of upper end of tibia

    ☑7ᵗʰ **S89.031** Salter-Harris Type III physeal fracture of upper end of right tibia

    ☑7ᵗʰ **S89.032** Salter-Harris Type III physeal fracture of upper end of left tibia

    ☑7ᵗʰ **S89.039** Salter-Harris Type III physeal fracture of upper end of unspecified tibia   ▽

  ☑6ᵗʰ S89.04 Salter-Harris Type IV physeal fracture of upper end of tibia

    ☑7ᵗʰ **S89.041** Salter-Harris Type IV physeal fracture of upper end of right tibia

    ☑7ᵗʰ **S89.042** Salter-Harris Type IV physeal fracture of upper end of left tibia

    ☑7ᵗʰ **S89.049** Salter-Harris Type IV physeal fracture of upper end of unspecified tibia   ▽

  ☑6ᵗʰ S89.09 Other physeal fracture of upper end of tibia

    ☑7ᵗʰ **S89.091** Other physeal fracture of upper end of right tibia

    ☑7ᵗʰ **S89.092** Other physeal fracture of upper end of left tibia

    ☑7ᵗʰ **S89.099** Other physeal fracture of upper end of unspecified tibia   ▽

☑5ᵗʰ S89.1 Physeal fracture of lower end of tibia

  ☑6ᵗʰ S89.10 Unspecified physeal fracture of lower end of tibia

    ☑7ᵗʰ **S89.101** Unspecified physeal fracture of lower end of right tibia   ▽

    ☑7ᵗʰ **S89.102** Unspecified physeal fracture of lower end of left tibia   ▽

    ☑7ᵗʰ **S89.109** Unspecified physeal fracture of lower end of unspecified tibia   ▽

  ☑6ᵗʰ S89.11 Salter-Harris Type I physeal fracture of ower end of tibia

    ☑7ᵗʰ **S89.111** Salter-Harris Type I physeal fracture of lower end of right tibia

    ☑7ᵗʰ **S89.112** Salter-Harris Type I physeal fracture of lower end of left tibia

---

☑ Additional Character Req   ☑7ᵗʰ Placeholder Alert   Manifestation   HCC CMS-HCC Condition   ▽ Unspecified Code   ▶◀ Revised Text   ● New Code   ▲ Revised Code Title

√7ᵗʰ **S89.119** Salter-Harris Type I physeal fracture of ▽ lower end of unspecified tibia

√6ᵗʰ **S89.12** Salter-Harris Type II physeal fracture of lower end of tibia

√7ᵗʰ **S89.121** Salter-Harris Type II physeal fracture of lower end of right tibia

√7ᵗʰ **S89.122** Salter-Harris Type II physeal fracture of lower end of left tibia

√7ᵗʰ **S89.129** Salter-Harris Type II physeal fracture of ▽ lower end of unspecified tibia

√6ᵗʰ **S89.13** Salter-Harris Type III physeal fracture of lower end of tibia

> EXCLUDES 1   *fracture of medial malleolus (adult) (S82.5-)*

√7ᵗʰ **S89.131** Salter-Harris Type III physeal fracture of lower end of right tibia

√7ᵗʰ **S89.132** Salter-Harris Type III physeal fracture of lower end of left tibia

√7ᵗʰ **S89.139** Salter-Harris Type III physeal fracture ▽ of lower end of unspecified tibia

√6ᵗʰ **S89.14** Salter-Harris Type IV physeal fracture of lower end of tibia

> EXCLUDES 1   *fracture of medial malleolus (adult) (S82.5-)*

√7ᵗʰ **S89.141** Salter-Harris Type IV physeal fracture of lower end of right tibia

√7ᵗʰ **S89.142** Salter-Harris Type IV physeal fracture of lower end of left tibia

√7ᵗʰ **S89.149** Salter-Harris Type IV physeal fracture ▽ of lower end of unspecified tibia

√6ᵗʰ **S89.19** Other physeal fracture of lower end of tibia

√7ᵗʰ **S89.191** Other physeal fracture of lower end of right tibia

√7ᵗʰ **S89.192** Other physeal fracture of lower end of left tibia

√7ᵗʰ **S89.199** Other physeal fracture of lower end of ▽ unspecified tibia

√5ᵗʰ **S89.2** Physeal fracture of upper end of fibula

√6ᵗʰ **S89.20** Unspecified physeal fracture of upper end of fibula

√7ᵗʰ **S89.201** Unspecified physeal fracture of upper ▽ end of right fibula

√7ᵗʰ **S89.202** Unspecified physeal fracture of upper ▽ end of left fibula

√7ᵗʰ **S89.209** Unspecified physeal fracture of upper ▽ end of unspecified fibula

√6ᵗʰ **S89.21** Salter-Harris Type I physeal fracture of upper end of fibula

√7ᵗʰ **S89.211** Salter-Harris Type I physeal fracture of upper end of right fibula

√7ᵗʰ **S89.212** Salter-Harris Type I physeal fracture of upper end of left fibula

√7ᵗʰ **S89.219** Salter-Harris Type I physeal fracture of ▽ upper end of unspecified fibula

√6ᵗʰ **S89.22** Salter-Harris Type II physeal fracture of upper end of fibula

√7ᵗʰ **S89.221** Salter-Harris Type II physeal fracture of upper end of right fibula

√7ᵗʰ **S89.222** Salter-Harris Type II physeal fracture of upper end of left fibula

√7ᵗʰ **S89.229** Salter-Harris Type II physeal fracture of ▽ upper end of unspecified fibula

√6ᵗʰ **S89.29** Other physeal fracture of upper end of fibula

√7ᵗʰ **S89.291** Other physeal fracture of upper end of right fibula

√7ᵗʰ **S89.292** Other physeal fracture of upper end of left fibula

√7ᵗʰ **S89.299** Other physeal fracture of upper end of ▽ unspecified fibula

√5ᵗʰ **S89.3** Physeal fracture of lower end of fibula

√6ᵗʰ **S89.30** Unspecified physeal fracture of lower end of fibula

√7ᵗʰ **S89.301** Unspecified physeal fracture of lower ▽ end of right fibula

√7ᵗʰ **S89.302** Unspecified physeal fracture of lower ▽ end of left fibula

√7ᵗʰ **S89.309** Unspecified physeal fracture of lower ▽ end of unspecified fibula

√6ᵗʰ **S89.31** Salter-Harris Type I physeal fracture of lower end of fibula

√7ᵗʰ **S89.311** Salter-Harris Type I physeal fracture of lower end of right fibula

√7ᵗʰ **S89.312** Salter-Harris Type I physeal fracture of lower end of left fibula

√7ᵗʰ **S89.319** Salter-Harris Type I physeal fracture of ▽ lower end of unspecified fibula

√6ᵗʰ **S89.32** Salter-Harris Type II physeal fracture of lower end of fibula

√7ᵗʰ **S89.321** Salter-Harris Type II physeal fracture of lower end of right fibula

√7ᵗʰ **S89.322** Salter-Harris Type II physeal fracture of lower end of left fibula

√7ᵗʰ **S89.329** Salter-Harris Type II physeal fracture ▽ of lower end of unspecified fibula

√6ᵗʰ **S89.39** Other physeal fracture of lower end of fibula

√7ᵗʰ **S89.391** Other physeal fracture of lower end of right fibula

√7ᵗʰ **S89.392** Other physeal fracture of lower end of left fibula

√7ᵗʰ **S89.399** Other physeal fracture of lower end of ▽ unspecified fibula

√5ᵗʰ **S89.8** Other specified injuries of lower leg

> The appropriate 7th character is to be added to each code in subcategory S89.8.
> A   initial encounter
> D   subsequent encounter
> S   sequela

√x7ᵗʰ **S89.80** Other specified injuries of unspecified lower leg ▽

√x7ᵗʰ **S89.81** Other specified injuries of right lower leg

√x7ᵗʰ **S89.82** Other specified injuries of left lower leg

√5ᵗʰ **S89.9** Unspecified injury of lower leg

> The appropriate 7th character is to be added to each code in subcategory S89.9.
> A   initial encounter
> D   subsequent encounter
> S   sequela

√x7ᵗʰ **S89.90** Unspecified injury of unspecified lower leg ▽

S89.91 Unspecified injury of right lower leg ▽

√x7ᵗʰ **S89.92** Unspecified injury of left lower leg ▽

Injuries to the ankle and foot (S90-S99)

> EXCLUDES 2   *burns and corrosions (T20-T32)*
> *fracture of ankle and malleolus (S82.-)*
> *frostbite (T33-T34)*
> *insect bite or sting, venomous (T63.4)*

√4ᵗʰ **S90** Superficial injury of ankle, foot and toes

> The appropriate 7th character is to be added to each code from category S90.
> A   initial encounter
> D   subsequent encounter
> S   sequela

√5ᵗʰ **S90.0** Contusion of ankle

√x7ᵗʰ **S90.00** Contusion of unspecified ankle ▽

√x7ᵗʰ **S90.01** Contusion of right ankle

√x7ᵗʰ **S90.02** Contusion of left ankle

√5ᵗʰ **S90.1** Contusion of toe without damage to nail

√6ᵗʰ **S90.11** Contusion of great toe without damage to nail

√7ᵗʰ **S90.111** Contusion of right great toe without damage to nail

√7ᵗʰ **S90.112** Contusion of left great toe without damage to nail

√7ᵗʰ **S90.119** Contusion of unspecified great toe ▽ without damage to nail

√6ᵗʰ **S90.12** Contusion of lesser toe without damage to nail

√7ᵗʰ **S90.121** Contusion of right lesser toe(s) without damage to nail

√7ᵗʰ **S90.122** Contusion of left lesser toe(s) without damage to nail

EXCLUDES 1 Not coded here   EXCLUDES 2 Not included here   N Newborn Age: 0   P Pediatric Age: 0-17   M Maternity Age: 12-55   A Adult Age: 15-124

1024   ICD-10-CM 2018

√7ᵗʰ **S90.129**   Contusion of unspecified lesser toe(s) ▽
without damage to nail
Contusion of toe NOS

√5ᵗʰ **S90.2**   **Contusion of toe with damage to nail**

√6ᵗʰ **S90.21**   **Contusion of great toe with damage to nail**

√7ᵗʰ **S90.211**   Contusion of right great toe with damage
to nail

√7ᵗʰ **S90.212**   Contusion of left great toe with damage to
nail

√7ᵗʰ **S90.219**   Contusion of unspecified great toe with ▽
damage to nail

√6ᵗʰ **S90.22**   **Contusion of lesser toe with damage to nail**

√7ᵗʰ **S90.221**   Contusion of right lesser toe(s) with
damage to nail

√7ᵗʰ **S90.222**   Contusion of left lesser toe(s) with
damage to nail

√7ᵗʰ **S90.229**   Contusion of unspecified lesser toe(s) ▽
with damage to nail

√5ᵗʰ **S90.3**   **Contusion of foot**
EXCLUDES 2   *contusion of toes (S90.1-, S90.2-)*

√x7ᵗʰ **S90.30**   Contusion of unspecified foot ▽
Contusion of foot NOS

√x7ᵗʰ **S90.31**   Contusion of right foot

√x7ᵗʰ **S90.32**   Contusion of left foot

√5ᵗʰ **S90.4**   **Other superficial injuries of toe**

√6ᵗʰ **S90.41**   **Abrasion of toe**

√7ᵗʰ **S90.411**   Abrasion, right great toe

√7ᵗʰ **S90.412**   Abrasion, left great toe

√7ᵗʰ **S90.413**   Abrasion, unspecified great toe ▽

√7ᵗʰ **S90.414**   Abrasion, right lesser toe(s)

√7ᵗʰ **S90.415**   Abrasion, left lesser toe(s)

√7ᵗʰ **S90.416**   Abrasion, unspecified lesser toe(s) ▽

√6ᵗʰ **S90.42**   **Blister (nonthermal) of toe**

√7ᵗʰ **S90.421**   Blister (nonthermal), right great toe

√7ᵗʰ **S90.422**   Blister (nonthermal), left great toe

√7ᵗʰ **S90.423**   Blister (nonthermal), unspecified great ▽
toe

√7ᵗʰ **S90.424**   Blister (nonthermal), right lesser toe(s)

√7ᵗʰ **S90.425**   Blister (nonthermal), left lesser toe(s)

√7ᵗʰ **S90.426**   Blister (nonthermal), unspecified lesser ▽
toe(s)

√6ᵗʰ **S90.44**   **External constriction of toe**
Hair tourniquet syndrome of toe

√7ᵗʰ **S90.441**   External constriction, right great toe

√7ᵗʰ **S90.442**   External constriction, left great toe

√7ᵗʰ **S90.443**   External constriction, unspecified ▽
great toe

√7ᵗʰ **S90.444**   External constriction, right lesser toe(s)

√7ᵗʰ **S90.445**   External constriction, left lesser toe(s)

√7ᵗʰ **S90.446**   External constriction, unspecified ▽
lesser toe(s)

√6ᵗʰ **S90.45**   **Superficial foreign body of toe**
Splinter in the toe

√7ᵗʰ **S90.451**   Superficial foreign body, right great toe

√7ᵗʰ **S90.452**   Superficial foreign body, left great toe

√7ᵗʰ **S90.453**   Superficial foreign body, unspecified ▽
great toe

√7ᵗʰ **S90.454**   Superficial foreign body, right lesser toe(s)

√7ᵗʰ **S90.455**   Superficial foreign body, left lesser toe(s)

√7ᵗʰ **S90.456**   Superficial foreign body, unspecified ▽
lesser toe(s)

√6ᵗʰ **S90.46**   **Insect bite (nonvenomous) of toe**

√7ᵗʰ **S90.461**   Insect bite (nonvenomous), right great toe

√7ᵗʰ **S90.462**   Insect bite (nonvenomous), left great toe

√7ᵗʰ **S90.463**   Insect bite (nonvenomous), unspecified ▽
great toe

√7ᵗʰ **S90.464**   Insect bite (nonvenomous), right lesser
toe(s)

√7ᵗʰ **S90.465**   Insect bite (nonvenomous), left lesser
toe(s)

√7ᵗʰ **S90.466**   Insect bite (nonvenomous), unspecified ▽
lesser toe(s)

√6ᵗʰ **S90.47**   **Other superficial bite of toe**
EXCLUDES 1   *open bite of toe (S91.15-, S91.25-)*

√7ᵗʰ **S90.471**   Other superficial bite of right great toe

√7ᵗʰ **S90.472**   Other superficial bite of left great toe

√7ᵗʰ **S90.473**   Other superficial bite of unspecified ▽
great toe

√7ᵗʰ **S90.474**   Other superficial bite of right lesser toe(s)

√7ᵗʰ **S90.475**   Other superficial bite of left lesser toe(s)

√7ᵗʰ **S90.476**   Other superficial bite of unspecified ▽
lesser toe(s)

√5ᵗʰ **S90.5**   **Other superficial injuries of ankle**

√6ᵗʰ **S90.51**   **Abrasion of ankle**

√7ᵗʰ **S90.511**   Abrasion, right ankle

√7ᵗʰ **S90.512**   Abrasion, left ankle

√7ᵗʰ **S90.519**   Abrasion, unspecified ankle ▽

√6ᵗʰ **S90.52**   **Blister (nonthermal) of ankle**

√7ᵗʰ **S90.521**   Blister (nonthermal), right ankle

√7ᵗʰ **S90.522**   Blister (nonthermal), left ankle

√7ᵗʰ **S90.529**   Blister (nonthermal), unspecified ankle ▽

√6ᵗʰ **S90.54**   **External constriction of ankle**

√7ᵗʰ **S90.541**   External constriction, right ankle

√7ᵗʰ **S90.542**   External constriction, left ankle

√7ᵗʰ **S90.549**   External constriction, unspecified ankle ▽

√6ᵗʰ **S90.55**   **Superficial foreign body of ankle**
Splinter in the ankle

√7ᵗʰ **S90.551**   Superficial foreign body, right ankle

√7ᵗʰ **S90.552**   Superficial foreign body, left ankle

√7ᵗʰ **S90.559**   Superficial foreign body, unspecified ▽
ankle

√6ᵗʰ **S90.56**   **Insect bite (nonvenomous) of ankle**

√7ᵗʰ **S90.561**   Insect bite (nonvenomous), right ankle

√7ᵗʰ **S90.562**   Insect bite (nonvenomous), left ankle

√7ᵗʰ **S90.569**   Insect bite (nonvenomous), unspecified ▽
ankle

√6ᵗʰ **S90.57**   **Other superficial bite of ankle**
EXCLUDES 1   *open bite of ankle (S91.05-)*

√7ᵗʰ **S90.571**   Other superficial bite of ankle, right ankle

√7ᵗʰ **S90.572**   Other superficial bite of ankle, left ankle

√7ᵗʰ **S90.579**   Other superficial bite of ankle, ▽
unspecified ankle

√5ᵗʰ **S90.8**   **Other superficial injuries of foot**

√6ᵗʰ **S90.81**   **Abrasion of foot**

√7ᵗʰ **S90.811**   Abrasion, right foot

√7ᵗʰ **S90.812**   Abrasion, left foot

√7ᵗʰ **S90.819**   Abrasion, unspecified foot ▽

√6ᵗʰ **S90.82**   **Blister (nonthermal) of foot**

√7ᵗʰ **S90.821**   Blister (nonthermal), right foot

√7ᵗʰ **S90.822**   Blister (nonthermal), left foot

√7ᵗʰ **S90.829**   Blister (nonthermal), unspecified foot ▽

√6ᵗʰ **S90.84**   **External constriction of foot**

√7ᵗʰ **S90.841**   External constriction, right foot

√7ᵗʰ **S90.842**   External constriction, left foot

√7ᵗʰ **S90.849**   External constriction, unspecified foot ▽

√6ᵗʰ **S90.85**   **Superficial foreign body of foot**
Splinter in the foot

√7ᵗʰ **S90.851**   Superficial foreign body, right foot

√7ᵗʰ **S90.852**   Superficial foreign body, left foot

√7ᵗʰ **S90.859**   Superficial foreign body, unspecified ▽
foot

√6ᵗʰ **S90.86**   **Insect bite (nonvenomous) of foot**

√7ᵗʰ **S90.861**   Insect bite (nonvenomous), right foot

√7ᵗʰ **S90.862**   Insect bite (nonvenomous), left foot

√7ᵗʰ **S90.869**   Insect bite (nonvenomous), unspecified ▽
foot

√6ᵗʰ **S90.87**   **Other superficial bite of foot**
EXCLUDES 1   *open bite of foot (S91.35-)*

√7ᵗʰ **S90.871**   Other superficial bite of right foot

☑ Additional Character Req   √x7ᵗʰ Placeholder Alert   Manifestation   HCC CMS-HCC Condition   ▽ Unspecified Code   ►◄ Revised Text   ● New Code   ▲ Revised Code Title

ICD-10-CM 2018   **1025**

✓7ᵗʰ **S90.872** Other superficial bite of left foot

✓7ᵗʰ **S90.879** Other superficial bite of unspecified foot ▽

✓5ᵗʰ **S90.9 Unspecified superficial injury of ankle, foot and toe**

✓6ᵗʰ **S90.91 Unspecified superficial injury of ankle**

✓7ᵗʰ **S90.911** Unspecified superficial injury of right ankle ▽

✓7ᵗʰ **S90.912** Unspecified superficial injury of left ankle ▽

✓7ᵗʰ **S90.919** Unspecified superficial injury of unspecified ankle ▽

✓6ᵗʰ **S90.92 Unspecified superficial injury of foot**

✓7ᵗʰ **S90.921** Unspecified superficial injury of right foot ▽

✓7ᵗʰ **S90.922** Unspecified superficial injury of left foot ▽

✓7ᵗʰ **S90.929** Unspecified superficial injury of unspecified foot ▽

✓6ᵗʰ **S90.93 Unspecified superficial injury of toes**

✓7ᵗʰ **S90.931** Unspecified superficial injury of right great toe ▽

✓7ᵗʰ **S90.932** Unspecified superficial injury of left great toe ▽

✓7ᵗʰ **S90.933** Unspecified superficial injury of unspecified great toe ▽

✓7ᵗʰ **S90.934** Unspecified superficial injury of right lesser toe(s) ▽

✓7ᵗʰ **S90.935** Unspecified superficial injury of left lesser toe(s) ▽

✓7ᵗʰ **S90.936** Unspecified superficial injury of unspecified lesser toe(s) ▽

✓4ᵗʰ **S91 Open wound of ankle, foot and toes**

Code also any associated wound infection

EXCLUDES 1 *open fracture of ankle, foot and toes (S92-with 7th character B)*
traumatic amputation of ankle and foot (S98.-)

The appropriate 7th character is to be added to each code from category S91.
A   initial encounter
D   subsequent encounter
S   sequela

✓5ᵗʰ **S91.0 Open wound of ankle**

✓6ᵗʰ **S91.00 Unspecified open wound of ankle**

✓7ᵗʰ **S91.001** Unspecified open wound, right ankle ▽

S91.002 Unspecified open wound, left ankle ▽

✓7ᵗʰ **S91.009** Unspecified open wound, unspecified ankle ▽

✓6ᵗʰ **S91.01 Laceration without foreign body of ankle**

✓7ᵗʰ **S91.011** Laceration without foreign body, right ankle

✓7ᵗʰ **S91.012** Laceration without foreign body, left ankle

✓7ᵗʰ **S91.019** Laceration without foreign body, unspecified ankle ▽

✓6ᵗʰ **S91.02 Laceration with foreign body of ankle**

✓7ᵗʰ **S91.021** Laceration with foreign body, right ankle

✓7ᵗʰ **S91.022** Laceration with foreign body, left ankle

✓7ᵗʰ **S91.029** Laceration with foreign body, unspecified ankle ▽

✓6ᵗʰ **S91.03 Puncture wound without foreign body of ankle**

✓7ᵗʰ **S91.031** Puncture wound without foreign body, right ankle

✓7ᵗʰ **S91.032** Puncture wound without foreign body, left ankle

✓7ᵗʰ **S91.039** Puncture wound without foreign body, unspecified ankle ▽

✓6ᵗʰ **S91.04 Puncture wound with foreign body of ankle**

✓7ᵗʰ **S91.041** Puncture wound with foreign body, right ankle

✓7ᵗʰ **S91.042** Puncture wound with foreign body, left ankle

✓7ᵗʰ **S91.049** Puncture wound with foreign body, unspecified ankle ▽

✓6ᵗʰ **S91.05 Open bite of ankle**

EXCLUDES 1 *superficial bite of ankle (S90.56-, S90.57-)*

✓7ᵗʰ **S91.051** Open bite, right ankle

✓7ᵗʰ **S91.052** Open bite, left ankle

✓7ᵗʰ **S91.059** Open bite, unspecified ankle ▽

✓5ᵗʰ **S91.1 Open wound of toe without damage to nail**

✓6ᵗʰ **S91.10 Unspecified open wound of toe without damage to nail**

✓7ᵗʰ **S91.101** Unspecified open wound of right great toe without damage to nail ▽

✓7ᵗʰ **S91.102** Unspecified open wound of left great toe without damage to nail ▽

✓7ᵗʰ **S91.103** Unspecified open wound of unspecified great toe without damage to nail ▽

✓7ᵗʰ **S91.104** Unspecified open wound of right lesser toe(s) without damage to nail ▽

✓7ᵗʰ **S91.105** Unspecified open wound of left lesser toe(s) without damage to nail ▽

✓7ᵗʰ **S91.106** Unspecified open wound of unspecified lesser toe(s) without damage to nail ▽

✓7ᵗʰ **S91.109** Unspecified open wound of unspecified toe(s) without damage to nail ▽

✓6ᵗʰ **S91.11 Laceration without foreign body of toe without damage to nail**

✓7ᵗʰ **S91.111** Laceration without foreign body of right great toe without damage to nail

✓7ᵗʰ **S91.112** Laceration without foreign body of left great toe without damage to nail

✓7ᵗʰ **S91.113** Laceration without foreign body of unspecified great toe without damage to nail ▽

✓7ᵗʰ **S91.114** Laceration without foreign body of right lesser toe(s) without damage to nail

✓7ᵗʰ **S91.115** Laceration without foreign body of left lesser toe(s) without damage to nail

✓7ᵗʰ **S91.116** Laceration without foreign body of unspecified lesser toe(s) without damage to nail ▽

✓7ᵗʰ **S91.119** Laceration without foreign body of unspecified toe without damage to nail ▽

✓6ᵗʰ **S91.12 Laceration with foreign body of toe without damage to nail**

✓7ᵗʰ **S91.121** Laceration with foreign body of right great toe without damage to nail

✓7ᵗʰ **S91.122** Laceration with foreign body of left great toe without damage to nail

✓7ᵗʰ **S91.123** Laceration with foreign body of unspecified great toe without damage to nail ▽

✓7ᵗʰ **S91.124** Laceration with foreign body of right lesser toe(s) without damage to nail

✓7ᵗʰ **S91.125** Laceration with foreign body of left lesser toe(s) without damage to nail

✓7ᵗʰ **S91.126** Laceration with foreign body of unspecified lesser toe(s) without damage to nail ▽

✓7ᵗʰ **S91.129** Laceration with foreign body of unspecified toe(s) without damage to nail ▽

✓6ᵗʰ **S91.13 Puncture wound without foreign body of toe without damage to nail**

✓7ᵗʰ **S91.131** Puncture wound without foreign body of right great toe without damage to nail

✓7ᵗʰ **S91.132** Puncture wound without foreign body of left great toe without damage to nail

✓7ᵗʰ **S91.133** Puncture wound without foreign body of unspecified great toe without damage to nail ▽

✓7ᵗʰ **S91.134** Puncture wound without foreign body of right lesser toe(s) without damage to nail

✓7ᵗʰ **S91.135** Puncture wound without foreign body of left lesser toe(s) without damage to nail

EXCLUDES 1 Not coded here   EXCLUDES 2 Not included here   Ⓝ Newborn Age: 0   Ⓟ Pediatric Age: 0-17   Ⓜ Maternity Age: 12-55   Ⓐ Adult Age: 15-124

1026   ICD-10-CM 2018

√7ᵗʰ **S91.136** Puncture wound without foreign body of unspecified lesser toe(s) without damage to nail ▽

√7ᵗʰ **S91.139** Puncture wound without foreign body of unspecified toe(s) without damage to nail ▽

√6ᵗʰ **S91.14** Puncture wound with foreign body of toe without damage to nail

    √7ᵗʰ **S91.141** Puncture wound with foreign body of right great toe without damage to nail

    √7ᵗʰ **S91.142** Puncture wound with foreign body of left great toe without damage to nail

    √7ᵗʰ **S91.143** Puncture wound with foreign body of unspecified great toe without damage to nail ▽

    √7ᵗʰ **S91.144** Puncture wound with foreign body of right lesser toe(s) without damage to nail

    √7ᵗʰ **S91.145** Puncture wound with foreign body of left lesser toe(s) without damage to nail

    √7ᵗʰ **S91.146** Puncture wound with foreign body of unspecified lesser toe(s) without damage to nail ▽

    √7ᵗʰ **S91.149** Puncture wound with foreign body of unspecified toe(s) without damage to nail ▽

√6ᵗʰ **S91.15** Open bite of toe without damage to nail
Bite of toe NOS
EXCLUDES 1   *superficial bite of toe (S90.46-, S90.47-)*

    √7ᵗʰ **S91.151** Open bite of right great toe without damage to nail

    √7ᵗʰ **S91.152** Open bite of left great toe without damage to nail

    √7ᵗʰ **S91.153** Open bite of unspecified great toe without damage to nail ▽

    √7ᵗʰ **S91.154** Open bite of right lesser toe(s) without damage to nail

    √7ᵗʰ **S91.155** Open bite of left lesser toe(s) without damage to nail

    √7ᵗʰ **S91.156** Open bite of unspecified lesser toe(s) without damage to nail ▽

    √7ᵗʰ **S91.159** Open bite of unspecified toe(s) without damage to nail ▽

√5ᵗʰ **S91.2** Open wound of toe with damage to nail

    √6ᵗʰ **S91.20** Unspecified open wound of toe with damage to nail

       √7ᵗʰ **S91.201** Unspecified open wound of right great toe with damage to nail ▽

       √7ᵗʰ **S91.202** Unspecified open wound of left great toe with damage to nail ▽

       √7ᵗʰ **S91.203** Unspecified open wound of unspecified great toe with damage to nail ▽

       √7ᵗʰ **S91.204** Unspecified open wound of right lesser toe(s) with damage to nail ▽

       √7ᵗʰ **S91.205** Unspecified open wound of left lesser toe(s) with damage to nail ▽

       √7ᵗʰ **S91.206** Unspecified open wound of unspecified lesser toe(s) with damage to nail ▽

       √7ᵗʰ **S91.209** Unspecified open wound of unspecified toe(s) with damage to nail ▽

    √6ᵗʰ **S91.21** Laceration without foreign body of toe with damage to nail

       √7ᵗʰ **S91.211** Laceration without foreign body of right great toe with damage to nail

       √7ᵗʰ **S91.212** Laceration without foreign body of left great toe with damage to nail

       √7ᵗʰ **S91.213** Laceration without foreign body of unspecified great toe with damage to nail ▽

       √7ᵗʰ **S91.214** Laceration without foreign body of right lesser toe(s) with damage to nail

       √7ᵗʰ **S91.215** Laceration without foreign body of left lesser toe(s) with damage to nail

       √7ᵗʰ **S91.216** Laceration without foreign body of unspecified lesser toe(s) with damage to nail ▽

       √7ᵗʰ **S91.219** Laceration without foreign body of unspecified toe(s) with damage to nail ▽

√6ᵗʰ **S91.22** Laceration with foreign body of toe with damage to nail

    √7ᵗʰ **S91.221** Laceration with foreign body of right great toe with damage to nail

    √7ᵗʰ **S91.222** Laceration with foreign body of left great toe with damage to nail

    √7ᵗʰ **S91.223** Laceration with foreign body of unspecified great toe with damage to nail ▽

    √7ᵗʰ **S91.224** Laceration with foreign body of right lesser toe(s) with damage to nail

    √7ᵗʰ **S91.225** Laceration with foreign body of left lesser toe(s) with damage to nail

    √7ᵗʰ **S91.226** Laceration with foreign body of unspecified lesser toe(s) with damage to nail ▽

    √7ᵗʰ **S91.229** Laceration with foreign body of unspecified toe(s) with damage to nail ▽

√6ᵗʰ **S91.23** Puncture wound without foreign body of toe with damage to nail

    √7ᵗʰ **S91.231** Puncture wound without foreign body of right great toe with damage to nail

    √7ᵗʰ **S91.232** Puncture wound without foreign body of left great toe with damage to nail

    √7ᵗʰ **S91.233** Puncture wound without foreign body of unspecified great toe with damage to nail ▽

    √7ᵗʰ **S91.234** Puncture wound without foreign body of right lesser toe(s) with damage to nail

    √7ᵗʰ **S91.235** Puncture wound without foreign body of left lesser toe(s) with damage to nail

    √7ᵗʰ **S91.236** Puncture wound without foreign body of unspecified lesser toe(s) with damage to nail ▽

    √7ᵗʰ **S91.239** Puncture wound without foreign body of unspecified toe(s) with damage to nail ▽

√6ᵗʰ **S91.24** Puncture wound with foreign body of toe with damage to nail

    √7ᵗʰ **S91.241** Puncture wound with foreign body of right great toe with damage to nail

    √7ᵗʰ **S91.242** Puncture wound with foreign body of left great toe with damage to nail

    √7ᵗʰ **S91.243** Puncture wound with foreign body of unspecified great toe with damage to nail ▽

    √7ᵗʰ **S91.244** Puncture wound with foreign body of right lesser toe(s) with damage to nail

    √7ᵗʰ **S91.245** Puncture wound with foreign body of left lesser toe(s) with damage to nail

    √7ᵗʰ **S91.246** Puncture wound with foreign body of unspecified lesser toe(s) with damage to nail ▽

    √7ᵗʰ **S91.249** Puncture wound with foreign body of unspecified toe(s) with damage to nail ▽

√6ᵗʰ **S91.25** Open bite of toe with damage to nail
Bite of toe with damage to nail NOS
EXCLUDES 1   *superficial bite of toe (S90.46-, S90.47-)*

    √7ᵗʰ **S91.251** Open bite of right great toe with damage to nail

    √7ᵗʰ **S91.252** Open bite of left great toe with damage to nail

    √7ᵗʰ **S91.253** Open bite of unspecified great toe with damage to nail ▽

    √7ᵗʰ **S91.254** Open bite of right lesser toe(s) with damage to nail

    √7ᵗʰ **S91.255** Open bite of left lesser toe(s) with damage to nail

    √7ᵗʰ **S91.256** Open bite of unspecified lesser toe(s) with damage to nail ▽

    √7ᵗʰ **S91.259** Open bite of unspecified toe(s) with damage to nail ▽

√5ᵗʰ **S91.3** Open wound of foot

    √6ᵗʰ **S91.30** Unspecified open wound of foot

       √7ᵗʰ **S91.301** Unspecified open wound, right foot ▽

       S91.302 Unspecified open wound, left foot ▽

       √7ᵗʰ **S91.309** Unspecified open wound, unspecified foot ▽

✅ Additional Character Req   √xTᵗʰ Placeholder Alert   Manifestation   HCC CMS-HCC Condition   ▽ Unspecified Code   ►◄ Revised Text   ● New Code   ▲ Revised Code Title

✓6th **S91.31   Laceration without foreign body of foot**
   ✓7th **S91.311   Laceration without foreign body, right foot**
   ✓7th **S91.312   Laceration without foreign body, left foot**
   ✓7th **S91.319   Laceration without foreign body, unspecified foot** ▽

✓6th **S91.32   Laceration with foreign body of foot**
   ✓7th **S91.321   Laceration with foreign body, right foot**
   ✓7th **S91.322   Laceration with foreign body, left foot**
   ✓7th **S91.329   Laceration with foreign body, unspecified foot** ▽

✓6th **S91.33   Puncture wound without foreign body of foot**
   ✓7th **S91.331   Puncture wound without foreign body, right foot**
   ✓7th **S91.332   Puncture wound without foreign body, left foot**
   ✓7th **S91.339   Puncture wound without foreign body, unspecified foot** ▽

✓6th **S91.34   Puncture wound with foreign body of foot**
   ✓7th **S91.341   Puncture wound with foreign body, right foot**
   ✓7th **S91.342   Puncture wound with foreign body, left foot**
   ✓7th **S91.349   Puncture wound with foreign body, unspecified foot** ▽

✓6th **S91.35   Open bite of foot**
   EXCLUDES 1   superficial bite of foot (S90.86-, S90.87-)
   ✓7th **S91.351   Open bite, right foot**
   ✓7th **S91.352   Open bite, left foot**
   ✓7th **S91.359   Open bite, unspecified foot** ▽

✓4th **S92   Fracture of foot and toe, except ankle**
   NOTE   A fracture not indicated as displaced or nondisplaced should be coded to displaced.
         A fracture not indicated as open or closed should be coded to closed.
   EXCLUDES 1   traumatic amputation of ankle and foot (S98.-)
   EXCLUDES 2   fracture of ankle (S82.-)
         fracture of malleolus (S82.-)
   AHA: 2015, 3Q, 37-39

> The appropriate 7th character is to be added to each code from category S92.
> A   initial encounter for closed fracture
> B   initial encounter for open fracture
> D   subsequent encounter for fracture with routine healing
> G   subsequent encounter for fracture with delayed healing
> K   subsequent encounter for fracture with nonunion
> P   subsequent encounter for fracture with malunion
> S   sequela

✓5th **S92.0   Fracture of calcaneus**
   Heel bone
   Os calcis
   EXCLUDES 2   physeal fracture of calcaneus (S99.0-)

✓6th **S92.00   Unspecified fracture of calcaneus**
   ✓7th **S92.001   Unspecified fracture of right calcaneus** ▽
   ✓7th **S92.002   Unspecified fracture of left calcaneus** ▽
   S92.009   Unspecified fracture of unspecified calcaneus ▽

✓6th **S92.01   Fracture of body of calcaneus**
   ✓7th **S92.011   Displaced fracture of body of right calcaneus**
   ✓7th **S92.012   Displaced fracture of body of left calcaneus**
   ✓7th **S92.013   Displaced fracture of body of unspecified calcaneus** ▽
   ✓7th **S92.014   Nondisplaced fracture of body of right calcaneus**
   ✓7th **S92.015   Nondisplaced fracture of body of left calcaneus**
   ✓7th **S92.016   Nondisplaced fracture of body of unspecified calcaneus** ▽

✓6th **S92.02   Fracture of anterior process of calcaneus**
   ✓7th **S92.021   Displaced fracture of anterior process of right calcaneus**

✓7th **S92.022   Displaced fracture of anterior process of left calcaneus**
✓7th **S92.023   Displaced fracture of anterior process of unspecified calcaneus** ▽
✓7th **S92.024   Nondisplaced fracture of anterior process of right calcaneus**
✓7th **S92.025   Nondisplaced fracture of anterior process of left calcaneus**
✓7th **S92.026   Nondisplaced fracture of anterior process of unspecified calcaneus** ▽

✓6th **S92.03   Avulsion fracture of tuberosity of calcaneus**
   ✓7th **S92.031   Displaced avulsion fracture of tuberosity of right calcaneus**
   ✓7th **S92.032   Displaced avulsion fracture of tuberosity of left calcaneus**
   ✓7th **S92.033   Displaced avulsion fracture of tuberosity of unspecified calcaneus** ▽
   ✓7th **S92.034   Nondisplaced avulsion fracture of tuberosity of right calcaneus**
   ✓7th **S92.035   Nondisplaced avulsion fracture of tuberosity of left calcaneus**
   ✓7th **S92.036   Nondisplaced avulsion fracture of tuberosity of unspecified calcaneus** ▽

✓6th **S92.04   Other fracture of tuberosity of calcaneus**
   ✓7th **S92.041   Displaced other fracture of tuberosity of right calcaneus**
   ✓7th **S92.042   Displaced other fracture of tuberosity of left calcaneus**
   ✓7th **S92.043   Displaced other fracture of tuberosity of unspecified calcaneus** ▽
   ✓7th **S92.044   Nondisplaced other fracture of tuberosity of right calcaneus**
   ✓7th **S92.045   Nondisplaced other fracture of tuberosity of left calcaneus**
   ✓7th **S92.046   Nondisplaced other fracture of tuberosity of unspecified calcaneus** ▽

✓6th **S92.05   Other extraarticular fracture of calcaneus**
   ✓7th **S92.051   Displaced other extraarticular fracture of right calcaneus**
   ✓7th **S92.052   Displaced other extraarticular fracture of left calcaneus**
   ✓7th **S92.053   Displaced other extraarticular fracture of unspecified calcaneus** ▽
   ✓7th **S92.054   Nondisplaced other extraarticular fracture of right calcaneus**
   ✓7th **S92.055   Nondisplaced other extraarticular fracture of left calcaneus**
   ✓7th **S92.056   Nondisplaced other extraarticular fracture of unspecified calcaneus** ▽

✓6th **S92.06   Intraarticular fracture of calcaneus**
   ✓7th **S92.061   Displaced intraarticular fracture of right calcaneus**
   ✓7th **S92.062   Displaced intraarticular fracture of left calcaneus**
   ✓7th **S92.063   Displaced intraarticular fracture of unspecified calcaneus** ▽
   ✓7th **S92.064   Nondisplaced intraarticular fracture of right calcaneus**
   ✓7th **S92.065   Nondisplaced intraarticular fracture of left calcaneus**
   ✓7th **S92.066   Nondisplaced intraarticular fracture of unspecified calcaneus** ▽

✓5th **S92.1   Fracture of talus**
   Astragalus

✓6th **S92.10   Unspecified fracture of talus**
   ✓7th **S92.101   Unspecified fracture of right talus** ▽
   ✓7th **S92.102   Unspecified fracture of left talus** ▽
   S92.109   Unspecified fracture of unspecified talus ▽

✓6th **S92.11   Fracture of neck of talus**
   ✓7th **S92.111   Displaced fracture of neck of right talus**
   ✓7th **S92.112   Displaced fracture of neck of left talus**
   ✓7th **S92.113   Displaced fracture of neck of unspecified talus** ▽

EXCLUDES 1 Not coded here   *EXCLUDES 2* Not included here   N Newborn Age: 0   P Pediatric Age: 0-17   M Maternity Age: 12-55   A Adult Age: 15-124

1028   ICD-10-CM 2018

✓7ᵗʰ **S92.114** Nondisplaced fracture of neck of right talus

✓7ᵗʰ **S92.115** Nondisplaced fracture of neck of left talus

✓7ᵗʰ **S92.116** Nondisplaced fracture of neck of unspecified talus ▽

✓6ᵗʰ **S92.12** Fracture of body of talus

✓7ᵗʰ **S92.121** Displaced fracture of body of right talus

✓7ᵗʰ **S92.122** Displaced fracture of body of left talus

✓7ᵗʰ **S92.123** Displaced fracture of body of unspecified talus ▽

✓7ᵗʰ **S92.124** Nondisplaced fracture of body of right talus

✓7ᵗʰ **S92.125** Nondisplaced fracture of body of left talus

✓7ᵗʰ **S92.126** Nondisplaced fracture of body of unspecified talus ▽

✓6ᵗʰ **S92.13** Fracture of posterior process of talus

✓7ᵗʰ **S92.131** Displaced fracture of posterior process of right talus

✓7ᵗʰ **S92.132** Displaced fracture of posterior process of left talus

✓7ᵗʰ **S92.133** Displaced fracture of posterior process of unspecified talus ▽

✓7ᵗʰ **S92.134** Nondisplaced fracture of posterior process of right talus

✓7ᵗʰ **S92.135** Nondisplaced fracture of posterior process of left talus

✓7ᵗʰ **S92.136** Nondisplaced fracture of posterior process of unspecified talus ▽

✓6ᵗʰ **S92.14** Dome fracture of talus
　　　EXCLUDES 1　*osteochondritis dissecans (M93.2)*

✓7ᵗʰ **S92.141** Displaced dome fracture of right talus

✓7ᵗʰ **S92.142** Displaced dome fracture of left talus

✓7ᵗʰ **S92.143** Displaced dome fracture of unspecified talus ▽

✓7ᵗʰ **S92.144** Nondisplaced dome fracture of right talus

✓7ᵗʰ **S92.145** Nondisplaced dome fracture of left talus

✓7ᵗʰ **S92.146** Nondisplaced dome fracture of unspecified talus ▽

✓6ᵗʰ **S92.15** Avulsion fracture (chip fracture) of talus

✓7ᵗʰ **S92.151** Displaced avulsion fracture (chip fracture) of right talus

✓7ᵗʰ **S92.152** Displaced avulsion fracture (chip fracture) of left talus

✓7ᵗʰ **S92.153** Displaced avulsion fracture (chip fracture) of unspecified talus ▽

✓7ᵗʰ **S92.154** Nondisplaced avulsion fracture (chip fracture) of right talus

✓7ᵗʰ **S92.155** Nondisplaced avulsion fracture (chip fracture) of left talus

✓7ᵗʰ **S92.156** Nondisplaced avulsion fracture (chip fracture) of unspecified talus ▽

✓6ᵗʰ **S92.19** Other fracture of talus

✓7ᵗʰ **S92.191** Other fracture of right talus

✓7ᵗʰ **S92.192** Other fracture of left talus

✓7ᵗʰ **S92.199** Other fracture of unspecified talus ▽

✓5ᵗʰ **S92.2** Fracture of other and unspecified tarsal bone(s)

✓6ᵗʰ **S92.20** Fracture of unspecified tarsal bone(s)

✓7ᵗʰ **S92.201** Fracture of unspecified tarsal bone(s) of right foot ▽

✓7ᵗʰ **S92.202** Fracture of unspecified tarsal bone(s) of left foot ▽

✓7ᵗʰ **S92.209** Fracture of unspecified tarsal bone(s) of unspecified foot ▽

✓6ᵗʰ **S92.21** Fracture of cuboid bone

✓7ᵗʰ **S92.211** Displaced fracture of cuboid bone of right foot

✓7ᵗʰ **S92.212** Displaced fracture of cuboid bone of left foot

✓7ᵗʰ **S92.213** Displaced fracture of cuboid bone of unspecified foot ▽

✓7ᵗʰ **S92.214** Nondisplaced fracture of cuboid bone of right foot

✓7ᵗʰ **S92.215** Nondisplaced fracture of cuboid bone of left foot

✓7ᵗʰ **S92.216** Nondisplaced fracture of cuboid bone of unspecified foot ▽

✓6ᵗʰ **S92.22** Fracture of lateral cuneiform

✓7ᵗʰ **S92.221** Displaced fracture of lateral cuneiform of right foot

✓7ᵗʰ **S92.222** Displaced fracture of lateral cuneiform of left foot

✓7ᵗʰ **S92.223** Displaced fracture of lateral cuneiform of unspecified foot ▽

✓7ᵗʰ **S92.224** Nondisplaced fracture of lateral cuneiform of right foot

✓7ᵗʰ **S92.225** Nondisplaced fracture of lateral cuneiform of left foot

✓7ᵗʰ **S92.226** Nondisplaced fracture of lateral cuneiform of unspecified foot ▽

✓6ᵗʰ **S92.23** Fracture of intermediate cuneiform

✓7ᵗʰ **S92.231** Displaced fracture of intermediate cuneiform of right foot

✓7ᵗʰ **S92.232** Displaced fracture of intermediate cuneiform of left foot

✓7ᵗʰ **S92.233** Displaced fracture of intermediate cuneiform of unspecified foot ▽

✓7ᵗʰ **S92.234** Nondisplaced fracture of intermediate cuneiform of right foot

✓7ᵗʰ **S92.235** Nondisplaced fracture of intermediate cuneiform of left foot

✓7ᵗʰ **S92.236** Nondisplaced fracture of intermediate cuneiform of unspecified foot ▽

✓6ᵗʰ **S92.24** Fracture of medial cuneiform

✓7ᵗʰ **S92.241** Displaced fracture of medial cuneiform of right foot

✓7ᵗʰ **S92.242** Displaced fracture of medial cuneiform of left foot

✓7ᵗʰ **S92.243** Displaced fracture of medial cuneiform of unspecified foot ▽

✓7ᵗʰ **S92.244** Nondisplaced fracture of medial cuneiform of right foot

✓7ᵗʰ **S92.245** Nondisplaced fracture of medial cuneiform of left foot

✓7ᵗʰ **S92.246** Nondisplaced fracture of medial cuneiform of unspecified foot ▽

✓6ᵗʰ **S92.25** Fracture of navicular [scaphoid] of foot

✓7ᵗʰ **S92.251** Displaced fracture of navicular [scaphoid] of right foot

✓7ᵗʰ **S92.252** Displaced fracture of navicular [scaphoid] of left foot

✓7ᵗʰ **S92.253** Displaced fracture of navicular [scaphoid] of unspecified foot ▽

✓7ᵗʰ **S92.254** Nondisplaced fracture of navicular [scaphoid] of right foot

✓7ᵗʰ **S92.255** Nondisplaced fracture of navicular [scaphoid] of left foot

✓7ᵗʰ **S92.256** Nondisplaced fracture of navicular [scaphoid] of unspecified foot ▽

✓5ᵗʰ **S92.3** Fracture of metatarsal bone(s)
　　　EXCLUDES 2　*physeal fracture of metatarsal (S99.1-)*

✓6ᵗʰ **S92.30** Fracture of unspecified metatarsal bone(s)

✓7ᵗʰ **S92.301** Fracture of unspecified metatarsal bone(s), right foot ▽

✓7ᵗʰ **S92.302** Fracture of unspecified metatarsal bone(s), left foot ▽

✓7ᵗʰ **S92.309** Fracture of unspecified metatarsal bone(s), unspecified foot ▽

✓6ᵗʰ **S92.31** Fracture of first metatarsal bone

✓7ᵗʰ **S92.311** Displaced fracture of first metatarsal bone, right foot

✓7ᵗʰ **S92.312** Displaced fracture of first metatarsal bone, left foot

✓7ᵗʰ **S92.313** Displaced fracture of first metatarsal bone, unspecified foot ▽

✓7ᵗʰ **S92.314** Nondisplaced fracture of first metatarsal bone, right foot

✔ Additional Character Req　　✔x7ᵗʰ Placeholder Alert　　Manifestation　　HCC CMS-HCC Condition　　▽ Unspecified Code　　▶◀ Revised Text　　● New Code　　▲ Revised Code Title

ICD-10-CM 2018　　1029

Chapter 19. Injury, Poisoning, and Certain Other Consequences of External Causes

S92.114–S92.314

√7ᵗʰ   S92.315   Nondisplaced fracture of first metatarsal bone, left foot

√7ᵗʰ   S92.316   Nondisplaced fracture of first metatarsal bone, unspecified foot   ▽

√6ᵗʰ S92.32   Fracture of second metatarsal bone

√7ᵗʰ   S92.321   Displaced fracture of second metatarsal bone, right foot

√7ᵗʰ   S92.322   Displaced fracture of second metatarsal bone, left foot

√7ᵗʰ   S92.323   Displaced fracture of second metatarsal bone, unspecified foot   ▽

√7ᵗʰ   S92.324   Nondisplaced fracture of second metatarsal bone, right foot

√7ᵗʰ   S92.325   Nondisplaced fracture of second metatarsal bone, left foot

√7ᵗʰ   S92.326   Nondisplaced fracture of second metatarsal bone, unspecified foot   ▽

√6ᵗʰ S92.33   Fracture of third metatarsal bone

√7ᵗʰ   S92.331   Displaced fracture of third metatarsal bone, right foot

√7ᵗʰ   S92.332   Displaced fracture of third metatarsal bone, left foot

√7ᵗʰ   S92.333   Displaced fracture of third metatarsal bone, unspecified foot   ▽

√7ᵗʰ   S92.334   Nondisplaced fracture of third metatarsal bone, right foot

√7ᵗʰ   S92.335   Nondisplaced fracture of third metatarsal bone, left foot

√7ᵗʰ   S92.336   Nondisplaced fracture of third metatarsal bone, unspecified foot   ▽

√6ᵗʰ S92.34   Fracture of fourth metatarsal bone

√7ᵗʰ   S92.341   Displaced fracture of fourth metatarsal bone, right foot

√7ᵗʰ   S92.342   Displaced fracture of fourth metatarsal bone, left foot

√7ᵗʰ   S92.343   Displaced fracture of fourth metatarsal bone, unspecified foot   ▽

√7ᵗʰ   S92.344   Nondisplaced fracture of fourth metatarsal bone, right foot

√7ᵗʰ   S92.345   Nondisplaced fracture of fourth metatarsal bone, left foot

√7ᵗʰ   S92.346   Nondisplaced fracture of fourth metatarsal bone, unspecified foot   ▽

√6ᵗʰ S92.35   Fracture of fifth metatarsal bone

√7ᵗʰ   S92.351   Displaced fracture of fifth metatarsal bone, right foot

√7ᵗʰ   S92.352   Displaced fracture of fifth metatarsal bone, left foot

√7ᵗʰ   S92.353   Displaced fracture of fifth metatarsal bone, unspecified foot   ▽

√7ᵗʰ   S92.354   Nondisplaced fracture of fifth metatarsal bone, right foot

√7ᵗʰ   S92.355   Nondisplaced fracture of fifth metatarsal bone, left foot

√7ᵗʰ   S92.356   Nondisplaced fracture of fifth metatarsal bone, unspecified foot   ▽

√5ᵗʰ S92.4   Fracture of great toe   ▲

EXCLUDES 2   physeal fracture of phalanx of toe (S99.2-)   ▲

√6ᵗʰ S92.40   Unspecified fracture of great toe   ▲

√7ᵗʰ   S92.401   Displaced unspecified fracture of right great toe   ▽   ▲

√7ᵗʰ   S92.402   Displaced unspecified fracture of left great toe   ▽   ▲

√7ᵗʰ   S92.403   Displaced unspecified fracture of unspecified great toe   ▽   ▲

√7ᵗʰ   S92.404   Nondisplaced unspecified fracture of right great toe   ▽   ▲

√7ᵗʰ   S92.405   Nondisplaced unspecified fracture of left great toe   ▽

√7ᵗʰ   S92.406   Nondisplaced unspecified fracture of unspecified great toe   ▽

√6ᵗʰ S92.41   Fracture of proximal phalanx of great toe

√7ᵗʰ   S92.411   Displaced fracture of proximal phalanx of right great toe

√7ᵗʰ   S92.412   Displaced fracture of proximal phalanx of left great toe

√7ᵗʰ   S92.413   Displaced fracture of proximal phalanx of unspecified great toe   ▽

√7ᵗʰ   S92.414   Nondisplaced fracture of proximal phalanx of right great toe

√7ᵗʰ   S92.415   Nondisplaced fracture of proximal phalanx of left great toe

√7ᵗʰ   S92.416   Nondisplaced fracture of proximal phalanx of unspecified great toe   ▽

√6ᵗʰ S92.42   Fracture of distal phalanx of great toe

√7ᵗʰ   S92.421   Displaced fracture of distal phalanx of right great toe

√7ᵗʰ   S92.422   Displaced fracture of distal phalanx of left great toe

√7ᵗʰ   S92.423   Displaced fracture of distal phalanx of unspecified great toe   ▽

√7ᵗʰ   S92.424   Nondisplaced fracture of distal phalanx of right great toe

√7ᵗʰ   S92.425   Nondisplaced fracture of distal phalanx of left great toe

√7ᵗʰ   S92.426   Nondisplaced fracture of distal phalanx of unspecified great toe   ▽

√6ᵗʰ S92.49   Other fracture of great toe

√7ᵗʰ   S92.491   Other fracture of right great toe

√7ᵗʰ   S92.492   Other fracture of left great toe

√7ᵗʰ   S92.499   Other fracture of unspecified great toe   ▽

S92.5   Fracture of lesser toe(s)

EXCLUDES 2   physeal fracture of phalanx of toe (S99.2-)

√6ᵗʰ S92.50   Unspecified fracture of lesser toe(s)

√7ᵗʰ   S92.501   Displaced unspecified fracture of right lesser toe(s)   ▽

√7ᵗʰ   S92.502   Displaced unspecified fracture of left lesser toe(s)   ▽

√7ᵗʰ   S92.503   Displaced unspecified fracture of unspecified lesser toe(s)   ▽

√7ᵗʰ   S92.504   Nondisplaced unspecified fracture of right lesser toe(s)   ▽

√7ᵗʰ   S92.505   Nondisplaced unspecified fracture of left lesser toe(s)   ▽

√7ᵗʰ   S92.506   Nondisplaced unspecified fracture of unspecified lesser toe(s)   ▽

√6ᵗʰ S92.51   Fracture of proximal phalanx of lesser toe(s)

√7ᵗʰ   S92.511   Displaced fracture of proximal phalanx of right lesser toe(s)

√7ᵗʰ   S92.512   Displaced fracture of proximal phalanx of left lesser toe(s)

√7ᵗʰ   S92.513   Displaced fracture of proximal phalanx of unspecified lesser toe(s)   ▽

√7ᵗʰ   S92.514   Nondisplaced fracture of proximal phalanx of right lesser toe(s)

√7ᵗʰ   S92.515   Nondisplaced fracture of proximal phalanx of left lesser toe(s)

√7ᵗʰ   S92.516   Nondisplaced fracture of proximal phalanx of unspecified lesser toe(s)   ▽

√6ᵗʰ S92.52   Fracture of middle phalanx of lesser toe(s)

√7ᵗʰ   S92.521   Displaced fracture of middle phalanx of right lesser toe(s)

√7ᵗʰ   S92.522   Displaced fracture of middle phalanx of left lesser toe(s)

√7ᵗʰ   S92.523   Displaced fracture of middle phalanx of unspecified lesser toe(s)   ▽

√7ᵗʰ   S92.524   Nondisplaced fracture of middle phalanx of right lesser toe(s)

√7ᵗʰ   S92.525   Nondisplaced fracture of middle phalanx of left lesser toe(s)

√7ᵗʰ   S92.526   Nondisplaced fracture of middle phalanx of unspecified lesser toe(s)   ▽

√6ᵗʰ S92.53   Fracture of distal phalanx of lesser toe(s)

√7ᵗʰ   S92.531   Displaced fracture of distal phalanx of right lesser toe(s)

√7ᵗʰ   S92.532   Displaced fracture of distal phalanx of left lesser toe(s)

EXCLUDES 1 Not coded here   EXCLUDES 2 Not included here   N Newborn Age: 0   P Pediatric Age: 0-17   M Maternity Age: 12-55   A Adult Age: 15-124

1030   ICD-10-CM 2018

√7ᵗʰ **S92.533** **Displaced fracture of distal phalanx of** ▽
unspecified lesser toe(s)

√7ᵗʰ **S92.534** **Nondisplaced fracture of distal phalanx of
right lesser toe(s)**

√7ᵗʰ **S92.535** **Nondisplaced fracture of distal phalanx of
left lesser toe(s)**

√7ᵗʰ **S92.536** **Nondisplaced fracture of distal phalanx** ▽
of unspecified lesser toe(s)

√6ᵗʰ **S92.59** **Other fracture of lesser toe(s)**

√7ᵗʰ **S92.591** **Other fracture of right lesser toe(s)**

√7ᵗʰ **S92.592** **Other fracture of left lesser toe(s)**

√7ᵗʰ **S92.599** **Other fracture of unspecified lesser** ▽
toe(s)

√5ᵗʰ **S92.8** **Other fracture of foot, except ankle**

√6ᵗʰ **S92.81** **Other fracture of foot**
Sesamoid fracture of foot

√7ᵗʰ **S92.811** **Other fracture of right foot**

√7ᵗʰ **S92.812** **Other fracture of left foot**

√7ᵗʰ **S92.819** **Other fracture of unspecified foot** ▽

√5ᵗʰ **S92.9** **Unspecified fracture of foot and toe**

√6ᵗʰ **S92.90** **Unspecified fracture of foot**

√7ᵗʰ **S92.901** **Unspecified fracture of right foot** ▽

√7ᵗʰ **S92.902** **Unspecified fracture of left foot** ▽

√7ᵗʰ **S92.909** **Unspecified fracture of unspecified** ▽
foot

√6ᵗʰ **S92.91** **Unspecified fracture of toe**

√7ᵗʰ **S92.911** **Unspecified fracture of right toe(s)** ▽

√7ᵗʰ **S92.912** **Unspecified fracture of left toe(s)** ▽

√7ᵗʰ **S92.919** **Unspecified fracture of unspecified** ▽
toe(s)

√4ᵗʰ **S93** **Dislocation and sprain of joints and ligaments at ankle, foot and
toe level**
INCLUDES   avulsion of joint or ligament of ankle, foot and toe
laceration of cartilage, joint or ligament of ankle, foot and toe
sprain of cartilage, joint or ligament of ankle, foot and toe
traumatic hemarthrosis of joint or ligament of ankle, foot and
toe
traumatic rupture of joint or ligament of ankle, foot and toe
traumatic subluxation of joint or ligament of ankle, foot and
toe
traumatic tear of joint or ligament of ankle, foot and toe
Code also any associated open wound
EXCLUDES 2   *strain of muscle and tendon of ankle and foot (S96.-)*

The appropriate 7th character is to be added to each code from
category S93.
A   initial encounter
D   subsequent encounter
S   sequela

√5ᵗʰ **S93.0** **Subluxation and dislocation of ankle joint**
Subluxation and dislocation of astragalus
Subluxation and dislocation of fibula, lower end
Subluxation and dislocation of talus
Subluxation and dislocation of tibia, lower end

√x7ᵗʰ **S93.01** **Subluxation of right ankle joint**

√x7ᵗʰ **S93.02** **Subluxation of left ankle joint**

√x7ᵗʰ **S93.03** **Subluxation of unspecified ankle joint** ▽

√x7ᵗʰ **S93.04** **Dislocation of right ankle joint**

√x7ᵗʰ **S93.05** **Dislocation of left ankle joint**

√x7ᵗʰ **S93.06** **Dislocation of unspecified ankle joint** ▽

√5ᵗʰ **S93.1** **Subluxation and dislocation of toe**

√6ᵗʰ **S93.10** **Unspecified subluxation and dislocation of toe**
Dislocation of toe NOS
Subluxation of toe NOS

√7ᵗʰ **S93.101** **Unspecified subluxation of right toe(s)** ▽

√7ᵗʰ **S93.102** **Unspecified subluxation of left toe(s)** ▽

√7ᵗʰ **S93.103** **Unspecified subluxation of unspecified** ▽
toe(s)

√7ᵗʰ **S93.104** **Unspecified dislocation of right toe(s)** ▽

√7ᵗʰ **S93.105** **Unspecified dislocation of left toe(s)** ▽

√7ᵗʰ **S93.106** **Unspecified dislocation of unspecified** ▽
toe(s)

√6ᵗʰ **S93.11** **Dislocation of interphalangeal joint**

√7ᵗʰ **S93.111** **Dislocation of interphalangeal joint of
right great toe**

√7ᵗʰ **S93.112** **Dislocation of interphalangeal joint of left
great toe**

√7ᵗʰ **S93.113** **Dislocation of interphalangeal joint of** ▽
unspecified great toe

√7ᵗʰ **S93.114** **Dislocation of interphalangeal joint of
right lesser toe(s)**

√7ᵗʰ **S93.115** **Dislocation of interphalangeal joint of left
lesser toe(s)**

√7ᵗʰ **S93.116** **Dislocation of interphalangeal joint of** ▽
unspecified lesser toe(s)

√7ᵗʰ **S93.119** **Dislocation of interphalangeal joint of** ▽
unspecified toe(s)

√6ᵗʰ **S93.12** **Dislocation of metatarsophalangeal joint**

√7ᵗʰ **S93.121** **Dislocation of metatarsophalangeal joint
of right great toe**

√7ᵗʰ **S93.122** **Dislocation of metatarsophalangeal joint
of left great toe**

√7ᵗʰ **S93.123** **Dislocation of metatarsophalangeal** ▽
joint of unspecified great toe

√7ᵗʰ **S93.124** **Dislocation of metatarsophalangeal joint
of right lesser toe(s)**

√7ᵗʰ **S93.125** **Dislocation of metatarsophalangeal joint
of left lesser toe(s)**

√7ᵗʰ **S93.126** **Dislocation of metatarsophalangeal** ▽
joint of unspecified lesser toe(s)

√7ᵗʰ **S93.129** **Dislocation of metatarsophalangeal** ▽
joint of unspecified toe(s)

√6ᵗʰ **S93.13** **Subluxation of interphalangeal joint**

√7ᵗʰ **S93.131** **Subluxation of interphalangeal joint of
right great toe**

√7ᵗʰ **S93.132** **Subluxation of interphalangeal joint of
left great toe**

√7ᵗʰ **S93.133** **Subluxation of interphalangeal joint of** ▽
unspecified great toe

√7ᵗʰ **S93.134** **Subluxation of interphalangeal joint of
right lesser toe(s)**

√7ᵗʰ **S93.135** **Subluxation of interphalangeal joint of
left lesser toe(s)**

√7ᵗʰ **S93.136** **Subluxation of interphalangeal joint of** ▽
unspecified lesser toe(s)

√7ᵗʰ **S93.139** **Subluxation of interphalangeal joint of** ▽
unspecified toe(s)

√6ᵗʰ **S93.14** **Subluxation of metatarsophalangeal joint**

√7ᵗʰ **S93.141** **Subluxation of metatarsophalangeal joint
of right great toe**

√7ᵗʰ **S93.142** **Subluxation of metatarsophalangeal joint
of left great toe**

√7ᵗʰ **S93.143** **Subluxation of metatarsophalangeal** ▽
joint of unspecified great toe

√7ᵗʰ **S93.144** **Subluxation of metatarsophalangeal joint
of right lesser toe(s)**

√7ᵗʰ **S93.145** **Subluxation of metatarsophalangeal joint
of left lesser toe(s)**

√7ᵗʰ **S93.146** **Subluxation of metatarsophalangeal** ▽
joint of unspecified lesser toe(s)

√7ᵗʰ **S93.149** **Subluxation of metatarsophalangeal** ▽
joint of unspecified toe(s)

√5ᵗʰ **S93.3** **Subluxation and dislocation of foot**
EXCLUDES 2   *dislocation of toe (S93.1-)*

√6ᵗʰ **S93.30** **Unspecified subluxation and dislocation of foot**
Dislocation of foot NOS
Subluxation of foot NOS

√7ᵗʰ **S93.301** **Unspecified subluxation of right foot** ▽

√7ᵗʰ **S93.302** **Unspecified subluxation of left foot** ▽

√7ᵗʰ **S93.303** **Unspecified subluxation of unspecified** ▽
foot

√7ᵗʰ **S93.304** **Unspecified dislocation of right foot** ▽

√7ᵗʰ **S93.305** **Unspecified dislocation of left foot** ▽

√7ᵗʰ **S93.306** **Unspecified dislocation of unspecified** ▽
foot

☑ Additional Character Req   √x7ᵗʰ Placeholder Alert   Manifestation   HCC CMS-HCC Condition   ▽ Unspecified Code   ▶◀ Revised Text   ● New Code   ▲ Revised Code Title

ICD-10-CM 2018   1031

Chapter 19. Injury, Poisoning, and Certain Other Consequences of External Causes

√6ᵗʰ **S93.31** **Subluxation and dislocation of tarsal joint**
- √7ᵗʰ **S93.311** **Subluxation of tarsal joint of right foot**
- √7ᵗʰ **S93.312** **Subluxation of tarsal joint of left foot**
- √7ᵗʰ **S93.313** **Subluxation of tarsal joint of unspecified foot** ▽
- √7ᵗʰ **S93.314** **Dislocation of tarsal joint of right foot**
- √7ᵗʰ **S93.315** **Dislocation of tarsal joint of left foot**
- √7ᵗʰ **S93.316** **Dislocation of tarsal joint of unspecified foot** ▽

√6ᵗʰ **S93.32** **Subluxation and dislocation of tarsometatarsal joint**
- √7ᵗʰ **S93.321** **Subluxation of tarsometatarsal joint of right foot**
- √7ᵗʰ **S93.322** **Subluxation of tarsometatarsal joint of left foot**
- √7ᵗʰ **S93.323** **Subluxation of tarsometatarsal joint of unspecified** ▽
- √7ᵗʰ **S93.324** **Dislocation of tarsometatarsal joint of right foot**
- √7ᵗʰ **S93.325** **Dislocation of tarsometatarsal joint of left foot**
- √7ᵗʰ **S93.326** **Dislocation of tarsometatarsal joint of unspecified foot** ▽

√6ᵗʰ **S93.33** **Other subluxation and dislocation of foot**
- √7ᵗʰ **S93.331** **Other subluxation of right foot**
- √7ᵗʰ **S93.332** **Other subluxation of left foot**
- √7ᵗʰ **S93.333** **Other subluxation of unspecified foot** ▽
- √7ᵗʰ **S93.334** **Other dislocation of right foot**
- √7ᵗʰ **S93.335** **Other dislocation of left foot**
- √7ᵗʰ **S93.336** **Other dislocation of unspecified foot** ▽

√5ᵗʰ **S93.4** **Sprain of ankle**
- *EXCLUDES 2*   injury of Achilles tendon (S86.0-)
- √6ᵗʰ **S93.40** **Sprain of unspecified ligament of ankle**
  Sprain of ankle NOS
  Sprained ankle NOS
  - √7ᵗʰ **S93.401** **Sprain of unspecified ligament of right ankle** ▽
  - √7ᵗʰ **S93.402** **Sprain of unspecified ligament of left ankle** ▽
  - √7ᵗʰ **S93.409** **Sprain of unspecified ligament of unspecified ankle** ▽
- √6ᵗʰ **S93.41** **Sprain of calcaneofibular ligament**
  - √7ᵗʰ **S93.411** **Sprain of calcaneofibular ligament of right ankle**
  - √7ᵗʰ **S93.412** **Sprain of calcaneofibular ligament of left ankle**
  - √7ᵗʰ **S93.419** **Sprain of calcaneofibular ligament of unspecified ankle** ▽
- √6ᵗʰ **S93.42** **Sprain of deltoid ligament**
  - √7ᵗʰ **S93.421** **Sprain of deltoid ligament of right ankle**
  - √7ᵗʰ **S93.422** **Sprain of deltoid ligament of left ankle**
  - √7ᵗʰ **S93.429** **Sprain of deltoid ligament of unspecified ankle** ▽
- √6ᵗʰ **S93.43** **Sprain of tibiofibular ligament**
  - √7ᵗʰ **S93.431** **Sprain of tibiofibular ligament of right ankle**
  - √7ᵗʰ **S93.432** **Sprain of tibiofibular ligament of left ankle**
  - √7ᵗʰ **S93.439** **Sprain of tibiofibular ligament of unspecified ankle** ▽
- √6ᵗʰ **S93.49** **Sprain of other ligament of ankle**
  Sprain of internal collateral ligament
  Sprain of talofibular ligament
  - √7ᵗʰ **S93.491** **Sprain of other ligament of right ankle**
  - √7ᵗʰ **S93.492** **Sprain of other ligament of left ankle**
  - √7ᵗʰ **S93.499** **Sprain of other ligament of unspecified ankle** ▽

√5ᵗʰ **S93.5** **Sprain of toe**
- √6ᵗʰ **S93.50** **Unspecified sprain of toe**
  - √7ᵗʰ **S93.501** **Unspecified sprain of right great toe** ▽
  - √7ᵗʰ **S93.502** **Unspecified sprain of left great toe** ▽
  - √7ᵗʰ **S93.503** **Unspecified sprain of unspecified great toe** ▽

- √7ᵗʰ **S93.504** **Unspecified sprain of right lesser toe(s)** ▽
- √7ᵗʰ **S93.505** **Unspecified sprain of left lesser toe(s)** ▽
- √7ᵗʰ **S93.506** **Unspecified sprain of unspecified lesser toe(s)** ▽
- √7ᵗʰ **S93.509** **Unspecified sprain of unspecified toe(s)** ▽

√6ᵗʰ **S93.51** **Sprain of interphalangeal joint of toe**
- √7ᵗʰ **S93.511** **Sprain of interphalangeal joint of right great toe**
- √7ᵗʰ **S93.512** **Sprain of interphalangeal joint of left great toe**
- √7ᵗʰ **S93.513** **Sprain of interphalangeal joint of unspecified great toe** ▽
- √7ᵗʰ **S93.514** **Sprain of interphalangeal joint of right lesser toe(s)**
- √7ᵗʰ **S93.515** **Sprain of interphalangeal joint of left lesser toe(s)**
- √7ᵗʰ **S93.516** **Sprain of interphalangeal joint of unspecified lesser toe(s)** ▽
- √7ᵗʰ **S93.519** **Sprain of interphalangeal joint of unspecified toe(s)** ▽

√6ᵗʰ **S93.52** **Sprain of metatarsophalangeal joint of toe**
- √7ᵗʰ **S93.521** **Sprain of metatarsophalangeal joint of right great toe**
- √7ᵗʰ **S93.522** **Sprain of metatarsophalangeal joint of left great toe**
- √7ᵗʰ **S93.523** **Sprain of metatarsophalangeal joint of unspecified great toe** ▽
- √7ᵗʰ **S93.524** **Sprain of metatarsophalangeal joint of right lesser toe(s)**
- √7ᵗʰ **S93.525** **Sprain of metatarsophalangeal joint of left lesser toe(s)**
- √7ᵗʰ **S93.526** **Sprain of metatarsophalangeal joint of unspecified lesser toe(s)** ▽
- √7ᵗʰ **S93.529** **Sprain of metatarsophalangeal joint of unspecified toe(s)** ▽

√5ᵗʰ **S93.6** **Sprain of foot**
- *EXCLUDES 2*   sprain of metatarsophalangeal joint of toe (S93.52-)
  sprain of toe (S93.5-)
- √6ᵗʰ **S93.60** **Unspecified sprain of foot**
  - √7ᵗʰ **S93.601** **Unspecified sprain of right foot** ▽
  - √7ᵗʰ **S93.602** **Unspecified sprain of left foot** ▽
  - √7ᵗʰ **S93.609** **Unspecified sprain of unspecified foot** ▽
- √6ᵗʰ **S93.61** **Sprain of tarsal ligament of foot**
  - √7ᵗʰ **S93.611** **Sprain of tarsal ligament of right foot**
  - √7ᵗʰ **S93.612** **Sprain of tarsal ligament of left foot**
  - √7ᵗʰ **S93.619** **Sprain of tarsal ligament of unspecified foot** ▽
- √6ᵗʰ **S93.62** **Sprain of tarsometatarsal ligament of foot**
  - √7ᵗʰ **S93.621** **Sprain of tarsometatarsal ligament of right foot**
  - √7ᵗʰ **S93.622** **Sprain of tarsometatarsal ligament of left foot**
  - √7ᵗʰ **S93.629** **Sprain of tarsometatarsal ligament of unspecified foot** ▽
- √6ᵗʰ **S93.69** **Other sprain of foot**
  - √7ᵗʰ **S93.691** **Other sprain of right foot**
  - √7ᵗʰ **S93.692** **Other sprain of left foot**
  - √7ᵗʰ **S93.699** **Other sprain of unspecified foot** ▽

√4ᵗʰ **S94** **Injury of nerves at ankle and foot level**
Code also any associated open wound (S91.-)

> The appropriate 7th character is to be added to each code from category S94.
> A   initial encounter
> D   subsequent encounter
> S   sequela

√5ᵗʰ **S94.0** **Injury of lateral plantar nerve**
- √x7ᵗʰ **S94.00** **Injury of lateral plantar nerve, unspecified leg** ▽
- √x7ᵗʰ **S94.01** **Injury of lateral plantar nerve, right leg**
- √x7ᵗʰ **S94.02** **Injury of lateral plantar nerve, left leg**

√5ᵗʰ **S94.1** **Injury of medial plantar nerve**
- √x7ᵗʰ **S94.10** **Injury of medial plantar nerve, unspecified leg** ▽

EXCLUDES 1 Not coded here   *EXCLUDES 2* Not included here   N Newborn Age: 0   P Pediatric Age: 0-17   M Maternity Age: 12-55   A Adult Age: 15-124

1032   ICD-10-CM 2018

√x7ᵗʰ **S94.11** Injury of medial plantar nerve, **right leg**
√x7ᵗʰ **S94.12** Injury of medial plantar nerve, **left leg**

√5ᵗʰ **S94.2** **Injury of deep peroneal nerve at ankle and foot level**
　　Injury of terminal, lateral branch of deep peroneal nerve

√x7ᵗʰ **S94.20** **Injury of deep peroneal nerve at ankle and foot level, unspecified leg** ▽

√x7ᵗʰ **S94.21** **Injury of deep peroneal nerve at ankle and foot level, right leg**

√x7ᵗʰ **S94.22** **Injury of deep peroneal nerve at ankle and foot level, left leg**

√5ᵗʰ **S94.3** **Injury of cutaneous sensory nerve at ankle and foot level**

√x7ᵗʰ **S94.30** **Injury of cutaneous sensory nerve at ankle and foot level, unspecified leg** ▽

√x7ᵗʰ **S94.31** **Injury of cutaneous sensory nerve at ankle and foot level, right leg**

√x7ᵗʰ **S94.32** **Injury of cutaneous sensory nerve at ankle and foot level, left leg**

√5ᵗʰ **S94.8** **Injury of other nerves at ankle and foot level**

√6ᵗʰ **S94.8X** **Injury of other nerves at ankle and foot level**

√7ᵗʰ **S94.8X1** **Injury of other nerves at ankle and foot level, right leg**

√7ᵗʰ **S94.8X2** **Injury of other nerves at ankle and foot level, left leg**

√7ᵗʰ **S94.8X9** **Injury of other nerves at ankle and foot level, unspecified leg** ▽

√5ᵗʰ **S94.9** **Injury of unspecified nerve at ankle and foot level**

√x7ᵗʰ **S94.90** **Injury of unspecified nerve at ankle and foot level, unspecified leg** ▽

√x7ᵗʰ **S94.91** **Injury of unspecified nerve at ankle and foot level, right leg** ▽

√x7ᵗʰ **S94.92** **Injury of unspecified nerve at ankle and foot level, left leg** ▽

√4ᵗʰ **S95** **Injury of blood vessels at ankle and foot level**
　　Code also any associated open wound (S91.-)
　　EXCLUDES 2　injury of posterior tibial artery and vein (S85.1-, S85.8-)

> The appropriate 7th character is to be added to each code from category S95.
> A　initial encounter
> D　subsequent encounter
> S　sequela

√5ᵗʰ **S95.0** **Injury of dorsal artery of foot**

√6ᵗʰ **S95.00** **Unspecified injury of dorsal artery of foot**

√7ᵗʰ **S95.001** **Unspecified injury of dorsal artery of right foot** ▽

√7ᵗʰ **S95.002** **Unspecified injury of dorsal artery of left foot** ▽

√7ᵗʰ **S95.009** **Unspecified injury of dorsal artery of unspecified foot** ▽

√6ᵗʰ **S95.01** **Laceration of dorsal artery of foot**

√7ᵗʰ **S95.011** Laceration of dorsal artery of right foot
√7ᵗʰ **S95.012** Laceration of dorsal artery of left foot
√7ᵗʰ **S95.019** Laceration of dorsal artery of unspecified foot ▽

√6ᵗʰ **S95.09** **Other specified injury of dorsal artery of foot**

√7ᵗʰ **S95.091** **Other specified injury of dorsal artery of right foot**

√7ᵗʰ **S95.092** **Other specified injury of dorsal artery of left foot**

√7ᵗʰ **S95.099** **Other specified injury of dorsal artery of unspecified foot** ▽

√5ᵗʰ **S95.1** **Injury of plantar artery of foot**

√6ᵗʰ **S95.10** **Unspecified injury of plantar artery of foot**

√7ᵗʰ **S95.101** **Unspecified injury of plantar artery of right foot** ▽

√7ᵗʰ **S95.102** **Unspecified injury of plantar artery of left foot** ▽

√7ᵗʰ **S95.109** **Unspecified injury of plantar artery of unspecified foot** ▽

√6ᵗʰ **S95.11** **Laceration of plantar artery of foot**

√7ᵗʰ **S95.111** Laceration of plantar artery of right foot
√7ᵗʰ **S95.112** Laceration of plantar artery of left foot

√7ᵗʰ **S95.119** **Laceration of plantar artery of unspecified foot** ▽

√6ᵗʰ **S95.19** **Other specified injury of plantar artery of foot**

√7ᵗʰ **S95.191** **Other specified injury of plantar artery of right foot**

√7ᵗʰ **S95.192** **Other specified injury of plantar artery of left foot**

√7ᵗʰ **S95.199** **Other specified injury of plantar artery of unspecified foot** ▽

√5ᵗʰ **S95.2** **Injury of dorsal vein of foot**

√6ᵗʰ **S95.20** **Unspecified injury of dorsal vein of foot**

√7ᵗʰ **S95.201** **Unspecified injury of dorsal vein of right foot** ▽

√7ᵗʰ **S95.202** **Unspecified injury of dorsal vein of left foot** ▽

√7ᵗʰ **S95.209** **Unspecified injury of dorsal vein of unspecified foot** ▽

√6ᵗʰ **S95.21** **Laceration of dorsal vein of foot**

√7ᵗʰ **S95.211** Laceration of dorsal vein of right foot
√7ᵗʰ **S95.212** Laceration of dorsal vein of left foot
√7ᵗʰ **S95.219** Laceration of dorsal vein of unspecified foot ▽

√6ᵗʰ **S95.29** **Other specified injury of dorsal vein of foot**

√7ᵗʰ **S95.291** **Other specified injury of dorsal vein of right foot**

√7ᵗʰ **S95.292** **Other specified injury of dorsal vein of left foot**

√7ᵗʰ **S95.299** **Other specified injury of dorsal vein of unspecified foot** ▽

√5ᵗʰ **S95.8** **Injury of other blood vessels at ankle and foot level**

√6ᵗʰ **S95.80** **Unspecified injury of other blood vessels at ankle and foot level**

√7ᵗʰ **S95.801** **Unspecified injury of other blood vessels at ankle and foot level, right leg** ▽

√7ᵗʰ **S95.802** **Unspecified injury of other blood vessels at ankle and foot level, left leg** ▽

√7ᵗʰ **S95.809** **Unspecified injury of other blood vessels at ankle and foot level, unspecified leg** ▽

√6ᵗʰ **S95.81** **Laceration of other blood vessels at ankle and foot level**

√7ᵗʰ **S95.811** **Laceration of other blood vessels at ankle and foot level, right leg**

√7ᵗʰ **S95.812** **Laceration of other blood vessels at ankle and foot level, left leg**

√7ᵗʰ **S95.819** **Laceration of other blood vessels at ankle and foot level, unspecified leg** ▽

√6ᵗʰ **S95.89** **Other specified injury of other blood vessels at ankle and foot level**

√7ᵗʰ **S95.891** **Other specified injury of other blood vessels at ankle and foot level, right leg**

√7ᵗʰ **S95.892** **Other specified injury of other blood vessels at ankle and foot level, left leg**

√7ᵗʰ **S95.899** **Other specified injury of other blood vessels at ankle and foot level, unspecified leg** ▽

√5ᵗʰ **S95.9** **Injury of unspecified blood vessel at ankle and foot level**

√6ᵗʰ **S95.90** **Unspecified injury of unspecified blood vessel at ankle and foot level**

√7ᵗʰ **S95.901** **Unspecified injury of unspecified blood vessel at ankle and foot level, right leg** ▽

√7ᵗʰ **S95.902** **Unspecified injury of unspecified blood vessel at ankle and foot level, left leg** ▽

√7ᵗʰ **S95.909** **Unspecified injury of unspecified blood vessel at ankle and foot level, unspecified leg** ▽

√6ᵗʰ **S95.91** **Laceration of unspecified blood vessel at ankle and foot level**

√7ᵗʰ **S95.911** **Laceration of unspecified blood vessel at ankle and foot level, right leg** ▽

√7ᵗʰ **S95.912** **Laceration of unspecified blood vessel at ankle and foot level, left leg** ▽

✓ Additional Character Req　　√x7ᵗʰ Placeholder Alert　　Manifestation　　HCC CMS-HCC Condition　　▽ Unspecified Code　　▶◀ Revised Text　　● New Code　　▲ Revised Code Title

✓7ᵗʰ **S95.919** Laceration of unspecified blood vessel at ankle and foot level, unspecified leg ▽

✓6ᵗʰ **S95.99** Other specified injury of unspecified blood vessel at ankle and foot level

✓7ᵗʰ **S95.991** Other specified injury of unspecified blood vessel at ankle and foot level, right leg ▽

✓7ᵗʰ **S95.992** Other specified injury of unspecified blood vessel at ankle and foot level, left leg ▽

✓7ᵗʰ **S95.999** Other specified injury of unspecified blood vessel at ankle and foot level, unspecified leg ▽

✓4ᵗʰ **S96 Injury of muscle and tendon at ankle and foot level**
Code also any associated open wound (S91.-)
EXCLUDES 2 *injury of Achilles tendon (S86.0-)*
sprain of joints and ligaments of ankle and foot (S93.-)
TIP: Refer to the Muscle/Tendon table at the beginning of this chapter.

The appropriate 7th character is to be added to each code from category S96.
A   initial encounter
D   subsequent encounter
S   sequela

✓5ᵗʰ **S96.0** Injury of muscle and tendon of long flexor muscle of toe at ankle and foot level

✓6ᵗʰ **S96.00** Unspecified injury of muscle and tendon of long flexor muscle of toe at ankle and foot level

✓7ᵗʰ **S96.001** Unspecified injury of muscle and tendon of long flexor muscle of toe at ankle and foot level, right foot ▽

✓7ᵗʰ **S96.002** Unspecified injury of muscle and tendon of long flexor muscle of toe at ankle and foot level, left foot ▽

✓7ᵗʰ **S96.009** Unspecified injury of muscle and tendon of long flexor muscle of toe at ankle and foot level, unspecified foot ▽

✓6ᵗʰ **S96.01** Strain of muscle and tendon of long flexor muscle of toe at ankle and foot level

✓7ᵗʰ **S96.011** Strain of muscle and tendon of long flexor muscle of toe at ankle and foot level, right foot

✓7ᵗʰ **S96.012** Strain of muscle and tendon of long flexor muscle of toe at ankle and foot level, left foot

✓7ᵗʰ **S96.019** Strain of muscle and tendon of long flexor muscle of toe at ankle and foot level, unspecified foot ▽

✓6ᵗʰ **S96.02** Laceration of muscle and tendon of long flexor muscle of toe at ankle and foot level

✓7ᵗʰ **S96.021** Laceration of muscle and tendon of long flexor muscle of toe at ankle and foot level, right foot

✓7ᵗʰ **S96.022** Laceration of muscle and tendon of long flexor muscle of toe at ankle and foot level, left foot

✓7ᵗʰ **S96.029** Laceration of muscle and tendon of long flexor muscle of toe at ankle and foot level, unspecified foot ▽

✓6ᵗʰ **S96.09** Other injury of muscle and tendon of long flexor muscle of toe at ankle and foot level

✓7ᵗʰ **S96.091** Other injury of muscle and tendon of long flexor muscle of toe at ankle and foot level, right foot

✓7ᵗʰ **S96.092** Other injury of muscle and tendon of long flexor muscle of toe at ankle and foot level, left foot

✓7ᵗʰ **S96.099** Other injury of muscle and tendon of long flexor muscle of toe at ankle and foot level, unspecified foot ▽

✓5ᵗʰ **S96.1** Injury of muscle and tendon of long extensor muscle of toe at ankle and foot level

✓6ᵗʰ **S96.10** Unspecified injury of muscle and tendon of long extensor muscle of toe at ankle and foot level

✓7ᵗʰ **S96.101** Unspecified injury of muscle and tendon of long extensor muscle of toe at ankle and foot level, right foot ▽

✓7ᵗʰ **S96.102** Unspecified injury of muscle and tendon of long extensor muscle of toe at ankle and foot level, left foot ▽

✓7ᵗʰ **S96.109** Unspecified injury of muscle and tendon of long extensor muscle of toe at ankle and foot level, unspecified foot ▽

✓6ᵗʰ **S96.11** Strain of muscle and tendon of long extensor muscle of toe at ankle and foot level

✓7ᵗʰ **S96.111** Strain of muscle and tendon of long extensor muscle of toe at ankle and foot level, right foot

✓7ᵗʰ **S96.112** Strain of muscle and tendon of long extensor muscle of toe at ankle and foot level, left foot

✓7ᵗʰ **S96.119** Strain of muscle and tendon of long extensor muscle of toe at ankle and foot level, unspecified foot ▽

✓6ᵗʰ **S96.12** Laceration of muscle and tendon of long extensor muscle of toe at ankle and foot level

✓7ᵗʰ **S96.121** Laceration of muscle and tendon of long extensor muscle of toe at ankle and foot level, right foot

✓7ᵗʰ **S96.122** Laceration of muscle and tendon of long extensor muscle of toe at ankle and foot level, left foot

✓7ᵗʰ **S96.129** Laceration of muscle and tendon of long extensor muscle of toe at ankle and foot level, unspecified foot ▽

✓6ᵗʰ **S96.19** Other specified injury of muscle and tendon of long extensor muscle of toe at ankle and foot level

✓7ᵗʰ **S96.191** Other specified injury of muscle and tendon of long extensor muscle of toe at ankle and foot level, right foot

✓7ᵗʰ **S96.192** Other specified injury of muscle and tendon of long extensor muscle of toe at ankle and foot level, left foot

✓7ᵗʰ **S96.199** Other specified injury of muscle and tendon of long extensor muscle of toe at ankle and foot level, unspecified foot ▽

✓5ᵗʰ **S96.2** Injury of intrinsic muscle and tendon at ankle and foot level

✓6ᵗʰ **S96.20** Unspecified injury of intrinsic muscle and tendon at ankle and foot level

✓7ᵗʰ **S96.201** Unspecified injury of intrinsic muscle and tendon at ankle and foot level, right foot ▽

✓7ᵗʰ **S96.202** Unspecified injury of intrinsic muscle and tendon at ankle and foot level, left foot ▽

✓7ᵗʰ **S96.209** Unspecified injury of intrinsic muscle and tendon at ankle and foot level, unspecified foot ▽

✓6ᵗʰ **S96.21** Strain of intrinsic muscle and tendon at ankle and foot level

✓7ᵗʰ **S96.211** Strain of intrinsic muscle and tendon at ankle and foot level, right foot

✓7ᵗʰ **S96.212** Strain of intrinsic muscle and tendon at ankle and foot level, left foot

✓7ᵗʰ **S96.219** Strain of intrinsic muscle and tendon at ankle and foot level, unspecified foot ▽

✓6ᵗʰ **S96.22** Laceration of intrinsic muscle and tendon at ankle and foot level

✓7ᵗʰ **S96.221** Laceration of intrinsic muscle and tendon at ankle and foot level, right foot

✓7ᵗʰ **S96.222** Laceration of intrinsic muscle and tendon at ankle and foot level, left foot

✓7ᵗʰ **S96.229** Laceration of intrinsic muscle and tendon at ankle and foot level, unspecified foot ▽

✓6ᵗʰ **S96.29** Other specified injury of intrinsic muscle and tendon at ankle and foot level

✓7ᵗʰ **S96.291** Other specified injury of intrinsic muscle and tendon at ankle and foot level, right foot

✓7ᵗʰ **S96.292** Other specified injury of intrinsic muscle and tendon at ankle and foot level, left foot

√7ᵗʰ **S96.299** Other specified injury of intrinsic muscle and tendon at ankle and foot level, unspecified foot ▽

√5ᵗʰ **S96.8** Injury of other specified muscles and tendons at ankle and foot level

  √6ᵗʰ **S96.80** Unspecified injury of other specified muscles and tendons at ankle and foot level

    √7ᵗʰ **S96.801** Unspecified injury of other specified muscles and tendons at ankle and foot level, right foot ▽

    √7ᵗʰ **S96.802** Unspecified injury of other specified muscles and tendons at ankle and foot level, left foot ▽

    √7ᵗʰ **S96.809** Unspecified injury of other specified muscles and tendons at ankle and foot level, unspecified foot ▽

  √6ᵗʰ **S96.81** Strain of other specified muscles and tendons at ankle and foot level

    √7ᵗʰ **S96.811** Strain of other specified muscles and tendons at ankle and foot level, right foot

    √7ᵗʰ **S96.812** Strain of other specified muscles and tendons at ankle and foot level, left foot

    √7ᵗʰ **S96.819** Strain of other specified muscles and tendons at ankle and foot level, unspecified foot ▽

  √6ᵗʰ **S96.82** Laceration of other specified muscles and tendons at ankle and foot level

    √7ᵗʰ **S96.821** Laceration of other specified muscles and tendons at ankle and foot level, right foot

    √7ᵗʰ **S96.822** Laceration of other specified muscles and tendons at ankle and foot level, left foot

    √7ᵗʰ **S96.829** Laceration of other specified muscles and tendons at ankle and foot level, unspecified foot ▽

  √6ᵗʰ **S96.89** Other specified injury of other specified muscles and tendons at ankle and foot level

    √7ᵗʰ **S96.891** Other specified injury of other specified muscles and tendons at ankle and foot level, right foot

    √7ᵗʰ **S96.892** Other specified injury of other specified muscles and tendons at ankle and foot level, left foot

    √7ᵗʰ **S96.899** Other specified injury of other specified muscles and tendons at ankle and foot level, unspecified foot ▽

√5ᵗʰ **S96.9** Injury of unspecified muscle and tendon at ankle and foot level

  √6ᵗʰ **S96.90** Unspecified injury of unspecified muscle and tendon at ankle and foot level

    √7ᵗʰ **S96.901** Unspecified injury of unspecified muscle and tendon at ankle and foot level, right foot ▽

    √7ᵗʰ **S96.902** Unspecified injury of unspecified muscle and tendon at ankle and foot level, left foot ▽

    √7ᵗʰ **S96.909** Unspecified injury of unspecified muscle and tendon at ankle and foot level, unspecified foot ▽

  √6ᵗʰ **S96.91** Strain of unspecified muscle and tendon at ankle and foot level

    √7ᵗʰ **S96.911** Strain of unspecified muscle and tendon at ankle and foot level, right foot ▽

    √7ᵗʰ **S96.912** Strain of unspecified muscle and tendon at ankle and foot level, left foot ▽

    √7ᵗʰ **S96.919** Strain of unspecified muscle and tendon at ankle and foot level, unspecified foot ▽

  √6ᵗʰ **S96.92** Laceration of unspecified muscle and tendon at ankle and foot level

    √7ᵗʰ **S96.921** Laceration of unspecified muscle and tendon at ankle and foot level, right foot ▽

    √7ᵗʰ **S96.922** Laceration of unspecified muscle and tendon at ankle and foot level, left foot ▽

    √7ᵗʰ **S96.929** Laceration of unspecified muscle and tendon at ankle and foot level, unspecified foot ▽

  √6ᵗʰ **S96.99** Other specified injury of unspecified muscle and tendon at ankle and foot level

    √7ᵗʰ **S96.991** Other specified injury of unspecified muscle and tendon at ankle and foot level, right foot ▽

    √7ᵗʰ **S96.992** Other specified injury of unspecified muscle and tendon at ankle and foot level, left foot ▽

    √7ᵗʰ **S96.999** Other specified injury of unspecified muscle and tendon at ankle and foot level, unspecified foot ▽

√4ᵗʰ **S97 Crushing injury of ankle and foot**
Use additional code(s) for all associated injuries

> The appropriate 7th character is to be added to each code from category S97.
> A   initial encounter
> D   subsequent encounter
> S   sequela

√5ᵗʰ **S97.0** Crushing injury of ankle

  √x7ᵗʰ **S97.00** Crushing injury of unspecified ankle ▽

  √x7ᵗʰ **S97.01** Crushing injury of right ankle

  √x7ᵗʰ **S97.02** Crushing injury of left ankle

√5ᵗʰ **S97.1** Crushing injury of toe

  √6ᵗʰ **S97.10** Crushing injury of unspecified toe(s)

    √7ᵗʰ **S97.101** Crushing injury of unspecified right toe(s) ▽

    √7ᵗʰ **S97.102** Crushing injury of unspecified left toe(s) ▽

    √7ᵗʰ **S97.109** Crushing injury of unspecified toe(s) ▽
Crushing injury of toe NOS

  √6ᵗʰ **S97.11** Crushing injury of great toe

    √7ᵗʰ **S97.111** Crushing injury of right great toe

    √7ᵗʰ **S97.112** Crushing injury of left great toe

    √7ᵗʰ **S97.119** Crushing injury of unspecified great toe ▽

  √6ᵗʰ **S97.12** Crushing injury of lesser toe(s)

    √7ᵗʰ **S97.121** Crushing injury of right lesser toe(s)

    √7ᵗʰ **S97.122** Crushing injury of left lesser toe(s)

    √7ᵗʰ **S97.129** Crushing injury of unspecified lesser toe(s) ▽

√5ᵗʰ **S97.8** Crushing injury of foot

  √x7ᵗʰ **S97.80** Crushing injury of unspecified foot ▽
Crushing injury of foot NOS

  √x7ᵗʰ **S97.81** Crushing injury of right foot

  √x7ᵗʰ **S97.82** Crushing injury of left foot

√4ᵗʰ **S98 Traumatic amputation of ankle and foot**
An amputation not identified as partial or complete should be coded to complete

> The appropriate 7th character is to be added to each code from category S98.
> A   initial encounter
> D   subsequent encounter
> S   sequela

√5ᵗʰ **S98.0** Traumatic amputation of foot at ankle level

  √6ᵗʰ **S98.01** Complete traumatic amputation of foot at ankle level

    √7ᵗʰ **S98.011** Complete traumatic amputation of right foot at ankle level   HCC

    √7ᵗʰ **S98.012** Complete traumatic amputation of left foot at ankle level   HCC

    √7ᵗʰ **S98.019** Complete traumatic amputation of unspecified foot at ankle level   HCC ▽

  √6ᵗʰ **S98.02** Partial traumatic amputation of foot at ankle level

    √7ᵗʰ **S98.021** Partial traumatic amputation of right foot at ankle level   HCC

    √7ᵗʰ **S98.022** Partial traumatic amputation of left foot at ankle level   HCC

    √7ᵗʰ **S98.029** Partial traumatic amputation of unspecified foot at ankle level   HCC ▽

☑ Additional Character Req   √x7ᵗʰ Placeholder Alert   Manifestation   HCC CMS-HCC Condition   ▽ Unspecified Code   ►◄ Revised Text   ● New Code   ▲ Revised Code Title

ICD-10-CM 2018   1035

Chapter 19. Injury, Poisoning, and Certain Other Consequences of External Causes

S96.299–S98.029

☑5th S98.1 Traumatic amputation of one toe

☑6th S98.11 Complete traumatic amputation of great toe

☑7th S98.111 Complete traumatic amputation of right great toe `HCC`

☑7th S98.112 Complete traumatic amputation of left great toe `HCC`

☑7th S98.119 Complete traumatic amputation of unspecified great toe `HCC` ▽

☑6th S98.12 Partial traumatic amputation of great toe

☑7th S98.121 Partial traumatic amputation of right great toe `HCC`

☑7th S98.122 Partial traumatic amputation of left great toe `HCC`

☑7th S98.129 Partial traumatic amputation of unspecified great toe `HCC` ▽

☑6th S98.13 Complete traumatic amputation of one lesser toe
Traumatic amputation of toe NOS

☑7th S98.131 Complete traumatic amputation of one right lesser toe `HCC`

☑7th S98.132 Complete traumatic amputation of one left lesser toe `HCC`

☑7th S98.139 Complete traumatic amputation of one unspecified lesser toe `HCC` ▽

☑6th S98.14 Partial traumatic amputation of one lesser toe

☑7th S98.141 Partial traumatic amputation of one right lesser toe `HCC`

☑7th S98.142 Partial traumatic amputation of one left lesser toe `HCC`

☑7th S98.149 Partial traumatic amputation of one unspecified lesser toe `HCC` ▽

☑5th S98.2 Traumatic amputation of two or more lesser toes

☑6th S98.21 Complete traumatic amputation of two or more lesser toes

☑7th S98.211 Complete traumatic amputation of two or more right lesser toes `HCC`

☑7th S98.212 Complete traumatic amputation of two or more left lesser toes `HCC`

☑7th S98.219 Complete traumatic amputation of two or more unspecified lesser toes `HCC` ▽

☑6th S98.22 Partial traumatic amputation of two or more lesser toes

☑7th S98.221 Partial traumatic amputation of two or more right lesser toes `HCC`

☑7th S98.222 Partial traumatic amputation of two or more left lesser toes `HCC`

☑7th S98.229 Partial traumatic amputation of two or more unspecified lesser toes `HCC` ▽

☑5th S98.3 Traumatic amputation of midfoot

☑6th S98.31 Complete traumatic amputation of midfoot

☑7th S98.311 Complete traumatic amputation of right midfoot `HCC`

☑7th S98.312 Complete traumatic amputation of left midfoot `HCC`

☑7th S98.319 Complete traumatic amputation of unspecified midfoot `HCC` ▽

☑6th S98.32 Partial traumatic amputation of midfoot

☑7th S98.321 Partial traumatic amputation of right midfoot `HCC`

☑7th S98.322 Partial traumatic amputation of left midfoot `HCC`

☑7th S98.329 Partial traumatic amputation of unspecified midfoot `HCC` ▽

☑5th S98.9 Traumatic amputation of foot, level unspecified

☑6th S98.91 Complete traumatic amputation of foot, level unspecified

☑7th S98.911 Complete traumatic amputation of right foot, level unspecified `HCC` ▽

☑7th S98.912 Complete traumatic amputation of left foot, level unspecified `HCC` ▽

☑7th S98.919 Complete traumatic amputation of unspecified foot, level unspecified `HCC` ▽

☑6th S98.92 Partial traumatic amputation of foot, level unspecified

☑7th S98.921 Partial traumatic amputation of right foot, level unspecified `HCC` ▽

☑7th S98.922 Partial traumatic amputation of left foot, level unspecified `HCC` ▽

☑7th S98.929 Partial traumatic amputation of unspecified foot, level unspecified `HCC` ▽

☑4th S99 Other and unspecified injuries of ankle and foot

☑5th S99.0 Physeal fracture of calcaneus

> The appropriate 7th character is to be added to each code from subcategories S99.0.
> A initial encounter for closed fracture
> B initial encounter for open fracture
> D subsequent encounter for fracture with routine healing
> G subsequent encounter for fracture with delayed healing
> K subsequent encounter for fracture with nonunion
> P subsequent encounter for fracture with malunion
> S sequela

☑6th S99.00 Unspecified physeal fracture of calcaneus

☑7th S99.001 Unspecified physeal fracture of right calcaneus ▽

☑7th S99.002 Unspecified physeal fracture of left calcaneus ▽

☑7th S99.009 Unspecified physeal fracture of unspecified calcaneus ▽

☑6th S99.01 Salter-Harris Type I physeal fracture of calcaneus

☑7th S99.011 Salter-Harris Type I physeal fracture of right calcaneus

☑7th S99.012 Salter-Harris Type I physeal fracture of left calcaneus

☑7th S99.019 Salter-Harris Type I physeal fracture of unspecified calcaneus ▽

☑6th S99.02 Salter-Harris Type II physeal fracture of calcaneus

☑7th S99.021 Salter-Harris Type II physeal fracture of right calcaneus

☑7th S99.022 Salter-Harris Type II physeal fracture of left calcaneus

☑7th S99.029 Salter-Harris Type II physeal fracture of unspecified calcaneus ▽

☑6th S99.03 Salter-Harris Type III physeal fracture of calcaneus

☑7th S99.031 Salter-Harris Type III physeal fracture of right calcaneus

☑7th S99.032 Salter-Harris Type III physeal fracture of left calcaneus

☑7th S99.039 Salter-Harris Type III physeal fracture of unspecified calcaneus ▽

☑6th S99.04 Salter-Harris Type IV physeal fracture of calcaneus

☑7th S99.041 Salter-Harris Type IV physeal fracture of right calcaneus

☑7th S99.042 Salter-Harris Type IV physeal fracture of left calcaneus

☑7th S99.049 Salter-Harris Type IV physeal fracture of unspecified calcaneus ▽

☑6th S99.09 Other physeal fracture of calcaneus

☑7th S99.091 Other physeal fracture of right calcaneus

☑7th S99.092 Other physeal fracture of left calcaneus

☑7th S99.099 Other physeal fracture of unspecified calcaneus ▽

☑5th S99.1 Physeal fracture of metatarsal

> The appropriate 7th character is to be added to each code from subcategories S99.1.
> A initial encounter for closed fracture
> B initial encounter for open fracture
> D subsequent encounter for fracture with routine healing
> G subsequent encounter for fracture with delayed healing
> K subsequent encounter for fracture with nonunion
> P subsequent encounter for fracture with malunion
> S sequela

☑6th S99.10 Unspecified physeal fracture of metatarsal

☑7th S99.101 Unspecified physeal fracture of right metatarsal ▽

EXCLUDES 1 Not coded here · **EXCLUDES 2** Not included here · **N** Newborn Age: 0 · **P** Pediatric Age: 0-17 · **M** Maternity Age: 12-55 · **A** Adult Age: 15-124

1036
ICD-10-CM 2018

✓7ᵗʰ **S99.102** Unspecified physeal fracture of left ▽
metatarsal

✓7ᵗʰ **S99.109** Unspecified physeal fracture of ▽
unspecified metatarsal

✓6ᵗʰ **S99.11** Salter-Harris Type I physeal fracture of metatarsal

✓7ᵗʰ **S99.111** Salter-Harris Type I physeal fracture of
right metatarsal

✓7ᵗʰ **S99.112** Salter-Harris Type I physeal fracture of left
metatarsal

✓7ᵗʰ **S99.119** Salter-Harris Type I physeal fracture ▽
of unspecified metatarsal

✓6ᵗʰ **S99.12** Salter-Harris Type II physeal fracture of metatarsal

✓7ᵗʰ **S99.121** Salter-Harris Type II physeal fracture of
right metatarsal

✓7ᵗʰ **S99.122** Salter-Harris Type II physeal fracture of
left metatarsal

✓7ᵗʰ **S99.129** Salter-Harris Type II physeal fracture ▽
of unspecified metatarsal

✓6ᵗʰ **S99.13** Salter-Harris Type III physeal fracture of metatarsal

✓7ᵗʰ **S99.131** Salter-Harris Type III physeal fracture of
right metatarsal

✓7ᵗʰ **S99.132** Salter-Harris Type III physeal fracture of
left metatarsal

✓7ᵗʰ **S99.139** Salter-Harris Type III physeal fracture ▽
of unspecified metatarsal

✓6ᵗʰ **S99.14** Salter-Harris Type IV physeal fracture of metatarsal

✓7ᵗʰ **S99.141** Salter-Harris Type IV physeal fracture of
right metatarsal

✓7ᵗʰ **S99.142** Salter-Harris Type IV physeal fracture of
left metatarsal

✓7ᵗʰ **S99.149** Salter-Harris Type IV physeal fracture ▽
of unspecified metatarsal

✓6ᵗʰ **S99.19** Other physeal fracture of metatarsal

✓7ᵗʰ **S99.191** Other physeal fracture of right metatarsal

✓7ᵗʰ **S99.192** Other physeal fracture of left metatarsal

✓7ᵗʰ **S99.199** Other physeal fracture of unspecified ▽
metatarsal

✓5ᵗʰ **S99.2** Physeal fracture of phalanx of toe

> The appropriate 7th character is to be added to each code
> from subcategories S99.2.
> A initial encounter for closed fracture
> B initial encounter for open fracture
> D subsequent encounter for fracture with routine healing
> G subsequent encounter for fracture with delayed
>   healing
> K subsequent encounter for fracture with nonunion
> P subsequent encounter for fracture with malunion
> S sequela

✓6ᵗʰ **S99.20** Unspecified physeal fracture of phalanx of toe

✓7ᵗʰ **S99.201** Unspecified physeal fracture of ▽
phalanx of right toe

✓7ᵗʰ **S99.202** Unspecified physeal fracture of ▽
phalanx of left toe

✓7ᵗʰ **S99.209** Unspecified physeal fracture of ▽
phalanx of unspecified toe

✓6ᵗʰ **S99.21** Salter-Harris Type I physeal fracture of phalanx of
toe

✓7ᵗʰ **S99.211** Salter-Harris Type I physeal fracture of
phalanx of right toe

✓7ᵗʰ **S99.212** Salter-Harris Type I physeal fracture of
phalanx of left toe

✓7ᵗʰ **S99.219** Salter-Harris Type I physeal fracture ▽
of phalanx of unspecified toe

✓6ᵗʰ **S99.22** Salter-Harris Type II physeal fracture of phalanx of
toe

✓7ᵗʰ **S99.221** Salter-Harris Type II physeal fracture of
phalanx of right toe

✓7ᵗʰ **S99.222** Salter-Harris Type II physeal fracture of
phalanx of left toe

✓7ᵗʰ **S99.229** Salter-Harris Type II physeal fracture ▽
of phalanx of unspecified toe

✓6ᵗʰ **S99.23** Salter-Harris Type III physeal fracture of phalanx of
toe

✓7ᵗʰ **S99.231** Salter-Harris Type III physeal fracture of
phalanx of right toe

✓7ᵗʰ **S99.232** Salter-Harris Type III physeal fracture of
phalanx of left toe

✓7ᵗʰ **S99.239** Salter-Harris Type III physeal fracture ▽
of phalanx of unspecified toe

✓6ᵗʰ **S99.24** Salter-Harris Type IV physeal fracture of phalanx of
toe

✓7ᵗʰ **S99.241** Salter-Harris Type IV physeal fracture of
phalanx of right toe

✓7ᵗʰ **S99.242** Salter-Harris Type IV physeal fracture of
phalanx of left toe

✓7ᵗʰ **S99.249** Salter-Harris Type IV physeal fracture ▽
of phalanx of unspecified toe

✓6ᵗʰ **S99.29** Other physeal fracture of phalanx of toe

✓7ᵗʰ **S99.291** Other physeal fracture of phalanx of right
toe

✓7ᵗʰ **S99.292** Other physeal fracture of phalanx of left
toe

✓7ᵗʰ **S99.299** Other physeal fracture of phalanx of ▽
unspecified toe

✓5ᵗʰ **S99.8** Other specified injuries of ankle and foot

> The appropriate 7th character is to be added to each code
> from subcategory S99.8.
> A initial encounter
> D subsequent encounter
> S sequela

✓6ᵗʰ **S99.81** Other specified injuries of ankle

✓7ᵗʰ **S99.811** Other specified injuries of right ankle

✓7ᵗʰ **S99.812** Other specified injuries of left ankle

✓7ᵗʰ **S99.819** Other specified injuries of unspecified ▽
ankle

✓6ᵗʰ **S99.82** Other specified injuries of foot

✓7ᵗʰ **S99.821** Other specified injuries of right foot

✓7ᵗʰ **S99.822** Other specified injuries of left foot

✓7ᵗʰ **S99.829** Other specified injuries of unspecified ▽
foot

✓5ᵗʰ **S99.9** Unspecified injury of ankle and foot

> The appropriate 7th character is to be added to each code
> from subcategory S99.9.
> A initial encounter
> D subsequent encounter
> S sequela

✓6ᵗʰ **S99.91** Unspecified injury of ankle

✓7ᵗʰ **S99.911** Unspecified injury of right ankle ▽

✓7ᵗʰ **S99.912** Unspecified injury of left ankle ▽

✓7ᵗʰ **S99.919** Unspecified injury of unspecified ankle ▽

✓6ᵗʰ **S99.92** Unspecified injury of foot

✓7ᵗʰ **S99.921** Unspecified injury of right foot ▽

✓7ᵗʰ **S99.922** Unspecified injury of left foot ▽

✓7ᵗʰ **S99.929** Unspecified injury of unspecified foot ▽

Injury, Poisoning And Certain Other Consequences Of External Causes (T07-T88)

Injuries involving multiple body regions (T07)

EXCLUDES 1   burns and corrosions (T20-T32)
frostbite (T33-T34)
insect bite or sting, venomous (T63.4)
sunburn (L55.-)

✓x7ᵗʰ **T07** **Unspecified multiple injuries** ▽
EXCLUDES 1   injury NOS ▶(T14.90)◀

> The appropriate 7th character is to be added to code T07.
> A initial encounter
> D subsequent encounter
> S sequela

Injury of unspecified body region (T14)

✓4ᵗʰ T14   Injury of unspecified body region
> EXCLUDES 1   *multiple unspecified injuries (T07)*
>
> The appropriate 7th character is to be added to each code from category T14.
> A   initial encounter
> D   subsequent encounter
> S   sequela

    ✓x7ᵗʰ T14.8   Other injury of unspecified body region
         Abrasion NOS
         Contusion NOS
         Crush injury NOS
         Fracture NOS
         Skin injury NOS
         Vascular injury NOS
         ▶Wound NOS◀

    ✓5ᵗʰ T14.9   Unspecified injury

       ✓x7ᵗʰ T14.90   Injury, unspecified   ▽
            Injury NOS

       ✓x7ᵗʰ T14.91   Suicide attempt   **HCC**
            Attempted suicide NOS

Effects of foreign body entering through natural orifice (T15-T19)

> EXCLUDES 2   *foreign body accidentally left in operation wound (T81.5-)*
> *foreign body in penetrating wound—See open wound by body region*
> *residual foreign body in soft tissue (M79.5)*
> *splinter, without open wound—See superficial injury by body region*

✓4ᵗʰ T15   Foreign body on external eye
> EXCLUDES 2   *foreign body in penetrating wound of orbit and eye ball (S05.4-, S05.5-)*
> *open wound of eyelid and periocular area (S01.1-)*
> *retained foreign body in eyelid (H02.8-)*
> *retained (old) foreign body in penetrating wound of orbit and eye ball (H05.5-, H44.6-, H44.7-)*
> *superficial foreign body of eyelid and periocular area (S00.25-)*

> The appropriate 7th character is to be added to each code from category T15.
> A   initial encounter
> D   subsequent encounter
> S   sequela

    ✓5ᵗʰ T15.0   Foreign body in cornea
       ✓x7ᵗʰ T15.00   Foreign body in cornea, unspecified eye   ▽
       ✓x7ᵗʰ T15.01   Foreign body in cornea, right eye
       ✓x7ᵗʰ T15.02   Foreign body in cornea, left eye

    ✓5ᵗʰ T15.1   Foreign body in conjunctival sac
       ✓x7ᵗʰ T15.10   Foreign body in conjunctival sac, unspecified eye ▽
       ✓x7ᵗʰ T15.11   Foreign body in conjunctival sac, right eye
       ✓x7ᵗʰ T15.12   Foreign body in conjunctival sac, left eye

    ✓5ᵗʰ T15.8   Foreign body in other and multiple parts of external eye
         Foreign body in lacrimal punctum
       ✓x7ᵗʰ T15.80   Foreign body in other and multiple parts of external eye, unspecified eye   ▽
       ✓x7ᵗʰ T15.81   Foreign body in other and multiple parts of external eye, right eye
       ✓x7ᵗʰ T15.82   Foreign body in other and multiple parts of external eye, left eye

    ✓5ᵗʰ T15.9   Foreign body on external eye, part unspecified
       ✓x7ᵗʰ T15.90   Foreign body on external eye, part unspecified, unspecified eye   ▽
       ✓x7ᵗʰ T15.91   Foreign body on external eye, part unspecified, right eye   ▽
       ✓x7ᵗʰ T15.92   Foreign body on external eye, part unspecified, left eye   ▽

✓4ᵗʰ T16   Foreign body in ear
> INCLUDES   foreign body in auditory canal
>
> The appropriate 7th character is to be added to each code from category T16.
> A   initial encounter
> D   subsequent encounter
> S   sequela

    ✓x7ᵗʰ T16.1   Foreign body in right ear
    ✓x7ᵗʰ T16.2   Foreign body in left ear
    ✓x7ᵗʰ T16.9   Foreign body in ear, unspecified ear   ▽

✓4ᵗʰ T17   Foreign body in respiratory tract

> The appropriate 7th character is to be added to each code from category T17.
> A   initial encounter
> D   subsequent encounter
> S   sequela

    ✓x7ᵗʰ T17.0   Foreign body in nasal sinus
    ✓x7ᵗʰ T17.1   Foreign body in nostril
         Foreign body in nose NOS

    ✓5ᵗʰ T17.2   Foreign body in pharynx
         Foreign body in nasopharynx
         Foreign body in throat NOS

       ✓6ᵗʰ T17.20   Unspecified foreign body in pharynx
          ✓7ᵗʰ T17.200   Unspecified foreign body in pharynx causing asphyxiation   ▽
          ✓7ᵗʰ T17.208   Unspecified foreign body in pharynx causing other injury   ▽

       ✓6ᵗʰ T17.21   Gastric contents in pharynx
          Aspiration of gastric contents into pharynx
          Vomitus in pharynx
          ✓7ᵗʰ T17.210   Gastric contents in pharynx causing asphyxiation
          ✓7ᵗʰ T17.218   Gastric contents in pharynx causing other injury

       ✓6ᵗʰ T17.22   Food in pharynx
          Bones in pharynx
          Seeds in pharynx
          ✓7ᵗʰ T17.220   Food in pharynx causing asphyxiation
          ✓7ᵗʰ T17.228   Food in pharynx causing other injury

       ✓6ᵗʰ T17.29   Other foreign object in pharynx
          ✓7ᵗʰ T17.290   Other foreign object in pharynx causing asphyxiation
          ✓7ᵗʰ T17.298   Other foreign object in pharynx causing other injury

    ✓5ᵗʰ T17.3   Foreign body in larynx
       ✓6ᵗʰ T17.30   Unspecified foreign body in larynx
          ✓7ᵗʰ T17.300   Unspecified foreign body in larynx causing asphyxiation   ▽
          ✓7ᵗʰ T17.308   Unspecified foreign body in larynx causing other injury   ▽

       ✓6ᵗʰ T17.31   Gastric contents in larynx
          Aspiration of gastric contents into larynx
          Vomitus in larynx
          ✓7ᵗʰ T17.310   Gastric contents in larynx causing asphyxiation
          ✓7ᵗʰ T17.318   Gastric contents in larynx causing other injury

       ✓6ᵗʰ T17.32   Food in larynx
          Bones in larynx
          Seeds in larynx
          ✓7ᵗʰ T17.320   Food in larynx causing asphyxiation
          ✓7ᵗʰ T17.328   Food in larynx causing other injury

       ✓6ᵗʰ T17.39   Other foreign object in larynx
          ✓7ᵗʰ T17.390   Other foreign object in larynx causing asphyxiation
          ✓7ᵗʰ T17.398   Other foreign object in larynx causing other injury

    ✓5ᵗʰ T17.4   Foreign body in trachea
       ✓6ᵗʰ T17.40   Unspecified foreign body in trachea
          ✓7ᵗʰ T17.400   Unspecified foreign body in trachea causing asphyxiation   ▽
          ✓7ᵗʰ T17.408   Unspecified foreign body in trachea causing other injury   ▽

       ✓6ᵗʰ T17.41   Gastric contents in trachea
          Aspiration of gastric contents into trachea
          Vomitus in trachea
          ✓7ᵗʰ T17.410   Gastric contents in trachea causing asphyxiation
          ✓7ᵗʰ T17.418   Gastric contents in trachea causing other injury

---

EXCLUDES 1   Not coded here   EXCLUDES 2   Not included here   **N** Newborn Age: 0   **P** Pediatric Age: 0-17   **M** Maternity Age: 12-55   **A** Adult Age: 15-124

√6ᵗʰ **T17.42　Food in trachea**
　　Bones in trachea
　　Seeds in trachea

　　√7ᵗʰ **T17.420　Food in trachea causing asphyxiation**

　　√7ᵗʰ **T17.428　Food in trachea causing other injury**

√6ᵗʰ **T17.49　Other foreign object in trachea**

　　√7ᵗʰ **T17.490　Other foreign object in trachea causing asphyxiation**

　　√7ᵗʰ **T17.498　Other foreign object in trachea causing other injury**

√5ᵗʰ **T17.5　Foreign body in bronchus**

√6ᵗʰ **T17.50　Unspecified foreign body in bronchus**

　　√7ᵗʰ **T17.500　Unspecified foreign body in bronchus causing asphyxiation** ▽

　　√7ᵗʰ **T17.508　Unspecified foreign body in bronchus causing other injury** ▽

√6ᵗʰ **T17.51　Gastric contents in bronchus**
　　Aspiration of gastric contents into bronchus
　　Vomitus in bronchus

　　√7ᵗʰ **T17.510　Gastric contents in bronchus causing asphyxiation**

　　√7ᵗʰ **T17.518　Gastric contents in bronchus causing other injury**

√6ᵗʰ **T17.52　Food in bronchus**
　　Bones in bronchus
　　Seeds in bronchus

　　√7ᵗʰ **T17.520　Food in bronchus causing asphyxiation**

　　√7ᵗʰ **T17.528　Food in bronchus causing other injury**

√6ᵗʰ **T17.59　Other foreign object in bronchus**

　　√7ᵗʰ **T17.590　Other foreign object in bronchus causing asphyxiation**

　　√7ᵗʰ **T17.598　Other foreign object in bronchus causing other injury**

√5ᵗʰ **T17.8　Foreign body in other parts of respiratory tract**
　　Foreign body in bronchioles
　　Foreign body in lung

√6ᵗʰ **T17.80　Unspecified foreign body in other parts of respiratory tract**

　　√7ᵗʰ **T17.800　Unspecified foreign body in other parts of respiratory tract causing asphyxiation** ▽

　　√7ᵗʰ **T17.808　Unspecified foreign body in other parts of respiratory tract causing other injury** ▽

√6ᵗʰ **T17.81　Gastric contents in other parts of respiratory tract**
　　Aspiration of gastric contents into other parts of respiratory tract
　　Vomitus in other parts of respiratory tract

　　√7ᵗʰ **T17.810　Gastric contents in other parts of respiratory tract causing asphyxiation**

　　√7ᵗʰ **T17.818　Gastric contents in other parts of respiratory tract causing other injury**

√6ᵗʰ **T17.82　Food in other parts of respiratory tract**
　　Bones in other parts of respiratory tract
　　Seeds in other parts of respiratory tract

　　√7ᵗʰ **T17.820　Food in other parts of respiratory tract causing asphyxiation**

　　√7ᵗʰ **T17.828　Food in other parts of respiratory tract causing other injury**

√6ᵗʰ **T17.89　Other foreign object in other parts of respiratory tract**

　　√7ᵗʰ **T17.890　Other foreign object in other parts of respiratory tract causing asphyxiation**

　　√7ᵗʰ **T17.898　Other foreign object in other parts of respiratory tract causing other injury**

√5ᵗʰ **T17.9　Foreign body in respiratory tract, part unspecified**

√6ᵗʰ **T17.90　Unspecified foreign body in respiratory tract, part unspecified**

　　√7ᵗʰ **T17.900　Unspecified foreign body in respiratory tract, part unspecified causing asphyxiation** ▽

　　√7ᵗʰ **T17.908　Unspecified foreign body in respiratory tract, part unspecified causing other injury** ▽

√6ᵗʰ **T17.91　Gastric contents in respiratory tract, part unspecified**
　　Aspiration of gastric contents into respiratory tract, part unspecified
　　Vomitus in trachea respiratory tract, part unspecified

　　√7ᵗʰ **T17.910　Gastric contents in respiratory tract, part unspecified causing asphyxiation** ▽

　　√7ᵗʰ **T17.918　Gastric contents in respiratory tract, part unspecified causing other injury** ▽

√6ᵗʰ **T17.92　Food in respiratory tract, part unspecified**
　　Bones in respiratory tract, part unspecified
　　Seeds in respiratory tract, part unspecified

　　√7ᵗʰ **T17.920　Food in respiratory tract, part unspecified causing asphyxiation** ▽

　　√7ᵗʰ **T17.928　Food in respiratory tract, part unspecified causing other injury** ▽

√6ᵗʰ **T17.99　Other foreign object in respiratory tract, part unspecified**

　　√7ᵗʰ **T17.990　Other foreign object in respiratory tract, part unspecified in causing asphyxiation** ▽

　　√7ᵗʰ **T17.998　Other foreign object in respiratory tract, part unspecified causing other injury** ▽

√4ᵗʰ **T18　Foreign body in alimentary tract**
　EXCLUDES 2　*foreign body in pharynx (T17.2-)*

> The appropriate 7th character is to be added to each code from category T18.
> A　initial encounter
> D　subsequent encounter
> S　sequela

√×7ᵗʰ **T18.0　Foreign body in mouth**

√5ᵗʰ **T18.1　Foreign body in esophagus**
　EXCLUDES 2　*foreign body in respiratory tract (T17.-)*

√6ᵗʰ **T18.10　Unspecified foreign body in esophagus**

　　√7ᵗʰ **T18.100　Unspecified foreign body in esophagus causing compression of trachea** ▽
　　　　Unspecified foreign body in esophagus causing obstruction of respiration

　　√7ᵗʰ **T18.108　Unspecified foreign body in esophagus causing other injury** ▽

√6ᵗʰ **T18.11　Gastric contents in esophagus**
　　Vomitus in esophagus

　　√7ᵗʰ **T18.110　Gastric contents in esophagus causing compression of trachea**
　　　　Gastric contents in esophagus causing obstruction of respiration

　　√7ᵗʰ **T18.118　Gastric contents in esophagus causing other injury**

√6ᵗʰ **T18.12　Food in esophagus**
　　Bones in esophagus
　　Seeds in esophagus

　　√7ᵗʰ **T18.120　Food in esophagus causing compression of trachea**
　　　　Food in esophagus causing obstruction of respiration

　　√7ᵗʰ **T18.128　Food in esophagus causing other injury**

√6ᵗʰ **T18.19　Other foreign object in esophagus**
　　AHA: 2015, 1Q, 23

　　√7ᵗʰ **T18.190　Other foreign object in esophagus causing compression of trachea**
　　　　Other foreign body in esophagus causing obstruction of respiration

　　√7ᵗʰ **T18.198　Other foreign object in esophagus causing other injury**

√×7ᵗʰ **T18.2　Foreign body in stomach**

√×7ᵗʰ **T18.3　Foreign body in small intestine**

√×7ᵗʰ **T18.4　Foreign body in colon**

√×7ᵗʰ **T18.5　Foreign body in anus and rectum**
　　Foreign body in rectosigmoid (junction)

√×7ᵗʰ **T18.8　Foreign body in other parts of alimentary tract**

√×7ᵗʰ **T18.9　Foreign body of alimentary tract, part unspecified** ▽
　　Foreign body in digestive system NOS
　　Swallowed foreign body NOS

☑ Additional Character Req　√×7ᵗʰ Placeholder Alert　Manifestation　HCC CMS-HCC Condition　▽ Unspecified Code　▶◀ Revised Text　● New Code　▲ Revised Code Title

✓4ᵗʰ **T19**   **Foreign body in genitourinary tract**
> EXCLUDES 2   complications due to implanted mesh (T83.7-)
> mechanical complications of contraceptive device (intrauterine) (vaginal) (T83.3-)
> presence of contraceptive device (intrauterine) (vaginal) (Z97.5)

> The appropriate 7th character is to be added to each code from category T19.
> A   initial encounter
> D   subsequent encounter
> S   sequela

✓x7ᵗʰ **T19.0**   **Foreign body in urethra**
✓x7ᵗʰ **T19.1**   **Foreign body in bladder**
✓x7ᵗʰ **T19.2**   **Foreign body in vulva and vagina**   ♀
✓x7ᵗʰ **T19.3**   **Foreign body in uterus**   ♀
✓x7ᵗʰ **T19.4**   **Foreign body in penis**   ♂
✓x7ᵗʰ **T19.8**   **Foreign body in other parts of genitourinary tract**
✓x7ᵗʰ **T19.9**   **Foreign body in genitourinary tract, part unspecified**   ▽

Burns and corrosions (T20-T32)

> INCLUDES   burns (thermal) from electrical heating appliances
> burns (thermal) from electricity
> burns (thermal) from flame
> burns (thermal) from friction
> burns (thermal) from hot air and hot gases
> burns (thermal) from hot objects
> burns (thermal) from lightning
> burns (thermal) from radiation
> chemical burn [corrosion] (external) (internal)
> scalds
> EXCLUDES 2   erythema [dermatitis] ab igne (L59.0)
> radiation-related disorders of the skin and subcutaneous tissue (L55-L59)
> sunburn (L55.-)
> AHA: 2016, 2Q, 4

Burns and corrosions of external body surface, specified by site (T20-T25)

> INCLUDES   burns and corrosions of first degree [erythema]
> burns and corrosions of second degree [blisters] [epidermal loss]
> burns and corrosions of third degree [deep necrosis of underlying tissue] [full-thickness skin loss]
> Use additional code from category T31 or T32 to identify extent of body surface involved

✓4ᵗʰ **T20**   **Burn and corrosion of head, face, and neck**
> EXCLUDES 2   burn and corrosion of ear drum (T28.41, T28.91)
> burn and corrosion of eye and adnexa (T26.-)
> burn and corrosion of mouth and pharynx (T28.0)
> AHA: 2015, 1Q, 18-19

> The appropriate 7th character is to be added to each code from category T20.
> A   initial encounter
> D   subsequent encounter
> S   sequela

✓5ᵗʰ **T20.0**   **Burn of unspecified degree of head, face, and neck**
> Use additional external cause code to identify the source, place and intent of the burn (X00-X19, X75-X77, X96-X98, Y92)

   ✓x7ᵗʰ **T20.00**   **Burn of unspecified degree of head, face, and neck, unspecified site**   ▽

   ✓6ᵗʰ **T20.01**   **Burn of unspecified degree of ear [any part, except ear drum]**
> EXCLUDES 2   burn of ear drum (T28.41-)

     ✓7ᵗʰ **T20.011**   **Burn of unspecified degree of right ear [any part, except ear drum]**   ▽

     ✓7ᵗʰ **T20.012**   **Burn of unspecified degree of left ear [any part, except ear drum]**   ▽

     ✓7ᵗʰ **T20.019**   **Burn of unspecified degree of unspecified ear [any part, except ear drum]**   ▽

   ✓x7ᵗʰ **T20.02**   **Burn of unspecified degree of lip(s)**   ▽

   ✓x7ᵗʰ **T20.03**   **Burn of unspecified degree of chin**   ▽

Rule of Nines Estimation of Total Body Surface Burned

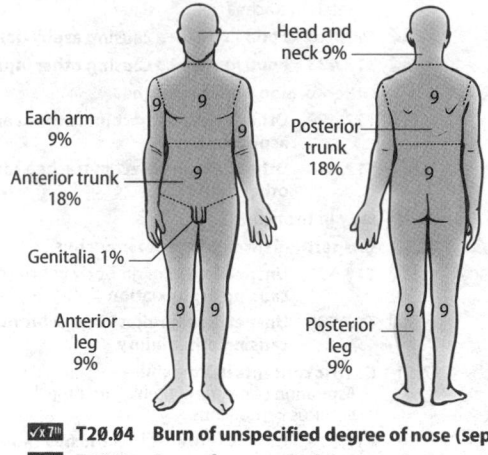

Head and neck 9%
Each arm 9%
Posterior trunk 18%
Anterior trunk 18%
Genitalia 1%
Anterior leg 9%
Posterior leg 9%

✓x7ᵗʰ **T20.04**   **Burn of unspecified degree of nose (septum)**   ▽
✓x7ᵗʰ **T20.05**   **Burn of unspecified degree of scalp [any part]**   ▽
✓x7ᵗʰ **T20.06**   **Burn of unspecified degree of forehead and cheek**   ▽
✓x7ᵗʰ **T20.07**   **Burn of unspecified degree of neck**   ▽
✓x7ᵗʰ **T20.09**   **Burn of unspecified degree of multiple sites of head, face, and neck**   ▽

✓5ᵗʰ **T20.1**   **Burn of first degree of head, face, and neck**
> Use additional external cause code to identify the source, place and intent of the burn (X00-X19, X75-X77, X96-X98, Y92)

   ✓x7ᵗʰ **T20.10**   **Burn of first degree of head, face, and neck, unspecified site**   ▽

   ✓6ᵗʰ **T20.11**   **Burn of first degree of ear [any part, except ear drum]**
> EXCLUDES 2   burn of ear drum (T28.41-)

     ✓7ᵗʰ **T20.111**   **Burn of first degree of right ear [any part, except ear drum]**

     ✓7ᵗʰ **T20.112**   **Burn of first degree of left ear [any part, except ear drum]**

     ✓7ᵗʰ **T20.119**   **Burn of first degree of unspecified ear [any part, except ear drum]**   ▽

   ✓x7ᵗʰ **T20.12**   **Burn of first degree of lip(s)**
   ✓x7ᵗʰ **T20.13**   **Burn of first degree of chin**
   ✓x7ᵗʰ **T20.14**   **Burn of first degree of nose (septum)**
   ✓x7ᵗʰ **T20.15**   **Burn of first degree of scalp [any part]**
   ✓x7ᵗʰ **T20.16**   **Burn of first degree of forehead and cheek**
   ✓x7ᵗʰ **T20.17**   **Burn of first degree of neck**
   ✓x7ᵗʰ **T20.19**   **Burn of first degree of multiple sites of head, face, and neck**

Degree of Burns

Epidermis
Dermis
Subcutaneous

Normal   First Degree Burn

Epidermis
Dermis
Subcutaneous

Second Degree Burn   Third Degree Burn

✓5ᵗʰ **T20.2** **Burn of second degree of head, face, and neck**
Use additional external cause code to identify the source, place and intent of the burn (X00-X19, X75-X77, X96-X98, Y92)

✓x7ᵗʰ **T20.20** **Burn of second degree of head, face, and neck, unspecified site** ▽

✓6ᵗʰ **T20.21** **Burn of second degree of ear [any part, except ear drum]**
EXCLUDES 2   *burn of ear drum (T28.41-)*

✓7ᵗʰ **T20.211** **Burn of second degree of right ear [any part, except ear drum]**

✓7ᵗʰ **T20.212** **Burn of second degree of left ear [any part, except ear drum]**

✓7ᵗʰ **T20.219** **Burn of second degree of unspecified ear [any part, except ear drum]** ▽

✓x7ᵗʰ **T20.22** **Burn of second degree of lip(s)**

✓x7ᵗʰ **T20.23** **Burn of second degree of chin**

✓x7ᵗʰ **T20.24** **Burn of second degree of nose (septum)**

✓x7ᵗʰ **T20.25** **Burn of second degree of scalp [any part]**

✓x7ᵗʰ **T20.26** **Burn of second degree of forehead and cheek**

✓x7ᵗʰ **T20.27** **Burn of second degree of neck**

✓x7ᵗʰ **T20.29** **Burn of second degree of multiple sites of head, face, and neck**

✓5ᵗʰ **T20.3** **Burn of third degree of head, face, and neck**
Use additional external cause code to identify the source, place and intent of the burn (X00-X19, X75-X77, X96-X98, Y92)

✓x7ᵗʰ **T20.30** **Burn of third degree of head, face, and neck, unspecified site** ▽

✓6ᵗʰ **T20.31** **Burn of third degree of ear [any part, except ear drum]**
EXCLUDES 2   *burn of ear drum (T28.41-)*
AHA: 2015, 1Q, 18

✓7ᵗʰ **T20.311** **Burn of third degree of right ear [any part, except ear drum]**

✓7ᵗʰ **T20.312** **Burn of third degree of left ear [any part, except ear drum]**

✓7ᵗʰ **T20.319** **Burn of third degree of unspecified ear [any part, except ear drum]** ▽

✓x7ᵗʰ **T20.32** **Burn of third degree of lip(s)**

✓x7ᵗʰ **T20.33** **Burn of third degree of chin**

✓x7ᵗʰ **T20.34** **Burn of third degree of nose (septum)**

✓x7ᵗʰ **T20.35** **Burn of third degree of scalp [any part]**

✓x7ᵗʰ **T20.36** **Burn of third degree of forehead and cheek**

✓x7ᵗʰ **T20.37** **Burn of third degree of neck**

✓x7ᵗʰ **T20.39** **Burn of third degree of multiple sites of head, face, and neck**

✓5ᵗʰ **T20.4** **Corrosion of unspecified degree of head, face, and neck**
Code first (T51-T65) to identify chemical and intent
Use additional external cause code to identify place (Y92)

✓x7ᵗʰ **T20.40** **Corrosion of unspecified degree of head, face, and neck, unspecified site** ▽

✓6ᵗʰ **T20.41** **Corrosion of unspecified degree of ear [any part, except ear drum]**
EXCLUDES 2   *corrosion of ear drum (T28.91-)*

✓7ᵗʰ **T20.411** **Corrosion of unspecified degree of right ear [any part, except ear drum]** ▽

✓7ᵗʰ **T20.412** **Corrosion of unspecified degree of left ear [any part, except ear drum]** ▽

✓7ᵗʰ **T20.419** **Corrosion of unspecified degree of unspecified ear [any part, except ear drum]** ▽

✓x7ᵗʰ **T20.42** **Corrosion of unspecified degree of lip(s)** ▽

✓x7ᵗʰ **T20.43** **Corrosion of unspecified degree of chin** ▽

✓x7ᵗʰ **T20.44** **Corrosion of unspecified degree of nose (septum)** ▽

✓x7ᵗʰ **T20.45** **Corrosion of unspecified degree of scalp [any part]** ▽

✓x7ᵗʰ **T20.46** **Corrosion of unspecified degree of forehead and cheek** ▽

✓x7ᵗʰ **T20.47** **Corrosion of unspecified degree of neck** ▽

✓x7ᵗʰ **T20.49** **Corrosion of unspecified degree of multiple sites of head, face, and neck** ▽

✓5ᵗʰ **T20.5** **Corrosion of first degree of head, face, and neck**
Code first (T51-T65) to identify chemical and intent
Use additional external cause code to identify place (Y92)

✓x7ᵗʰ **T20.50** **Corrosion of first degree of head, face, and neck, unspecified site** ▽

✓6ᵗʰ **T20.51** **Corrosion of first degree of ear [any part, except ear drum]**
EXCLUDES 2   *corrosion of ear drum (T28.91-)*

✓7ᵗʰ **T20.511** **Corrosion of first degree of right ear [any part, except ear drum]**

✓7ᵗʰ **T20.512** **Corrosion of first degree of left ear [any part, except ear drum]**

✓7ᵗʰ **T20.519** **Corrosion of first degree of unspecified ear [any part, except ear drum]** ▽

✓x7ᵗʰ **T20.52** **Corrosion of first degree of lip(s)**

✓x7ᵗʰ **T20.53** **Corrosion of first degree of chin**

✓x7ᵗʰ **T20.54** **Corrosion of first degree of nose (septum)**

✓x7ᵗʰ **T20.55** **Corrosion of first degree of scalp [any part]**

✓x7ᵗʰ **T20.56** **Corrosion of first degree of forehead and cheek**

✓x7ᵗʰ **T20.57** **Corrosion of first degree of neck**

✓x7ᵗʰ **T20.59** **Corrosion of first degree of multiple sites of head, face, and neck**

✓5ᵗʰ **T20.6** **Corrosion of second degree of head, face, and neck**
Code first (T51-T65) to identify chemical and intent
Use additional external cause code to identify place (Y92)

✓x7ᵗʰ **T20.60** **Corrosion of second degree of head, face, and neck, unspecified site** ▽

✓6ᵗʰ **T20.61** **Corrosion of second degree of ear [any part, except ear drum]**
EXCLUDES 2   *corrosion of ear drum (T28.91-)*

✓7ᵗʰ **T20.611** **Corrosion of second degree of right ear [any part, except ear drum]**

✓7ᵗʰ **T20.612** **Corrosion of second degree of left ear [any part, except ear drum]**

✓7ᵗʰ **T20.619** **Corrosion of second degree of unspecified ear [any part, except ear drum]** ▽

✓x7ᵗʰ **T20.62** **Corrosion of second degree of lip(s)**

✓x7ᵗʰ **T20.63** **Corrosion of second degree of chin**

✓x7ᵗʰ **T20.64** **Corrosion of second degree of nose (septum)**

✓x7ᵗʰ **T20.65** **Corrosion of second degree of scalp [any part]**

✓x7ᵗʰ **T20.66** **Corrosion of second degree of forehead and cheek**

✓x7ᵗʰ **T20.67** **Corrosion of second degree of neck**

✓x7ᵗʰ **T20.69** **Corrosion of second degree of multiple sites of head, face, and neck**

✓5ᵗʰ **T20.7** **Corrosion of third degree of head, face, and neck**
Code first (T51-T65) to identify chemical and intent
Use additional external cause code to identify place (Y92)

✓x7ᵗʰ **T20.70** **Corrosion of third degree of head, face, and neck, unspecified site** ▽

✓6ᵗʰ **T20.71** **Corrosion of third degree of ear [any part, except ear drum]**
EXCLUDES 2   *corrosion of ear drum (T28.91-)*

✓7ᵗʰ **T20.711** **Corrosion of third degree of right ear [any part, except ear drum]**

✓7ᵗʰ **T20.712** **Corrosion of third degree of left ear [any part, except ear drum]**

✓7ᵗʰ **T20.719** **Corrosion of third degree of unspecified ear [any part, except ear drum]** ▽

✓x7ᵗʰ **T20.72** **Corrosion of third degree of lip(s)**

✓x7ᵗʰ **T20.73** **Corrosion of third degree of chin**

✓x7ᵗʰ **T20.74** **Corrosion of third degree of nose (septum)**

✓x7ᵗʰ **T20.75** **Corrosion of third degree of scalp [any part]**

✓x7ᵗʰ **T20.76** **Corrosion of third degree of forehead and cheek**

✓x7ᵗʰ **T20.77** **Corrosion of third degree of neck**

✓x7ᵗʰ **T20.79** **Corrosion of third degree of multiple sites of head, face, and neck**

✓ Additional Character Req   ✓x7ᵗʰ Placeholder Alert   Manifestation   HCC CMS-HCC Condition   ▽ Unspecified Code   ▶◀ Revised Text   ● New Code   ▲ Revised Code Title

✓4ᵗʰ **T21 Burn and corrosion of trunk**
> **INCLUDES** burns and corrosion of hip region
> **EXCLUDES 2** *burns and corrosion of axilla (T22.- with fifth character 4)*
> *burns and corrosion of scapular region (T22.- with fifth character 6)*
> *burns and corrosion of shoulder (T22.- with fifth character 5)*

> The appropriate 7th character is to be added to each code from category T21.
> A   initial encounter
> D   subsequent encounter
> S   sequela

✓5ᵗʰ **T21.0 Burn of unspecified degree of trunk**
> Use additional external cause code to identify the source, place and intent of the burn (X00-X19, X75-X77, X96-X98, Y92)

✓x7ᵗʰ **T21.00 Burn of unspecified degree of trunk, unspecified site** ▽

✓x7ᵗʰ **T21.01 Burn of unspecified degree of chest wall** ▽
> Burn of of unspecified degree of breast

✓x7ᵗʰ **T21.02 Burn of unspecified degree of abdominal wall** ▽
> Burn of unspecified degree of flank
> Burn of unspecified degree of groin

✓x7ᵗʰ **T21.03 Burn of unspecified degree of upper back** ▽
> Burn of unspecified degree of interscapular region

✓x7ᵗʰ **T21.04 Burn of unspecified degree of lower back** ▽

✓x7ᵗʰ **T21.05 Burn of unspecified degree of buttock** ▽
> Burn of unspecified degree of anus

✓x7ᵗʰ **T21.06 Burn of unspecified degree of male genital region** ♂▽
> Burn of unspecified degree of penis
> Burn of unspecified degree of scrotum
> Burn of unspecified degree of testis

✓x7ᵗʰ **T21.07 Burn of unspecified degree of female genital region** ♀▽
> Burn of unspecified degree of labium (majus) (minus)
> Burn of unspecified degree of perineum
> Burn of unspecified degree of vulva
> **EXCLUDES 2** *burn of vagina (T28.3)*

✓x7ᵗʰ **T21.09 Burn of unspecified degree of other site of trunk** ▽

✓5ᵗʰ **T21.1 Burn of first degree of trunk**
> Use additional external cause code to identify the source, place and intent of the burn (X00-X19, X75-X77, X96-X98, Y92)

✓x7ᵗʰ **T21.10 Burn of first degree of trunk, unspecified site** ▽

✓x7ᵗʰ **T21.11 Burn of first degree of chest wall**
> Burn of first degree of breast

✓x7ᵗʰ **T21.12 Burn of first degree of abdominal wall**
> Burn of first degree of flank
> Burn of first degree of groin

✓x7ᵗʰ **T21.13 Burn of first degree of upper back**
> Burn of first degree of interscapular region

✓x7ᵗʰ **T21.14 Burn of first degree of lower back**

✓x7ᵗʰ **T21.15 Burn of first degree of buttock**
> Burn of first degree of anus

✓x7ᵗʰ **T21.16 Burn of first degree of male genital region** ♂
> Burn of first degree of penis
> Burn of first degree of scrotum
> Burn of first degree of testis

✓x7ᵗʰ **T21.17 Burn of first degree of female genital region** ♀
> Burn of first degree of labium (majus) (minus)
> Burn of first degree of perineum
> Burn of first degree of vulva
> **EXCLUDES 2** *burn of vagina (T28.3)*

✓x7ᵗʰ **T21.19 Burn of first degree of other site of trunk**

✓5ᵗʰ **T21.2 Burn of second degree of trunk**
> Use additional external cause code to identify the source, place and intent of the burn (X00-X19, X75-X77, X96-X98, Y92)

✓x7ᵗʰ **T21.20 Burn of second degree of trunk, unspecified site** ▽

✓x7ᵗʰ **T21.21 Burn of second degree of chest wall**
> Burn of second degree of breast

✓x7ᵗʰ **T21.22 Burn of second degree of abdominal wall**
> Burn of second degree of flank
> Burn of second degree of groin

✓x7ᵗʰ **T21.23 Burn of second degree of upper back**
> Burn of second degree of interscapular region

✓x7ᵗʰ **T21.24 Burn of second degree of lower back**

✓x7ᵗʰ **T21.25 Burn of second degree of buttock**
> Burn of second degree of anus

✓x7ᵗʰ **T21.26 Burn of second degree of male genital region** ♂
> Burn of second degree of penis
> Burn of second degree of scrotum
> Burn of second degree of testis

✓x7ᵗʰ **T21.27 Burn of second degree of female genital region** ♀
> Burn of second degree of labium (majus) (minus)
> Burn of second degree of perineum
> Burn of second degree of vulva
> **EXCLUDES 2** *burn of vagina (T28.3)*

✓x7ᵗʰ **T21.29 Burn of second degree of other site of trunk**

✓5ᵗʰ **T21.3 Burn of third degree of trunk**
> Use additional external cause code to identify the source, place and intent of the burn (X00-X19, X75-X77, X96-X98, Y92)

✓x7ᵗʰ **T21.30 Burn of third degree of trunk, unspecified site** ▽

✓x7ᵗʰ **T21.31 Burn of third degree of chest wall**
> Burn of third degree of breast
> **AHA:** 2016, 2Q, 5

✓x7ᵗʰ **T21.32 Burn of third degree of abdominal wall**
> Burn of third degree of flank
> Burn of third degree of groin

✓x7ᵗʰ **T21.33 Burn of third degree of upper back**
> Burn of third degree of interscapular region

✓x7ᵗʰ **T21.34 Burn of third degree of lower back**

✓x7ᵗʰ **T21.35 Burn of third degree of buttock**
> Burn of third degree of anus

✓x7ᵗʰ **T21.36 Burn of third degree of male genital region** ♂
> Burn of third degree of penis
> Burn of third degree of scrotum
> Burn of third degree of testis

✓x7ᵗʰ **T21.37 Burn of third degree of female genital region** ♀
> Burn of third degree of labium (majus) (minus)
> Burn of third degree of perineum
> Burn of third degree of vulva
> **EXCLUDES 2** *burn of vagina (T28.3)*

✓x7ᵗʰ **T21.39 Burn of third degree of other site of trunk**

✓5ᵗʰ **T21.4 Corrosion of unspecified degree of trunk**
> Code first (T51-T65) to identify chemical and intent
> Use additional external cause code to identify place (Y92)

✓x7ᵗʰ **T21.40 Corrosion of unspecified degree of trunk, unspecified site** ▽

✓x7ᵗʰ **T21.41 Corrosion of unspecified degree of chest wall** ▽
> Corrosion of unspecified degree of breast

✓x7ᵗʰ **T21.42 Corrosion of unspecified degree of abdominal wall** ▽
> Corrosion of unspecified degree of flank
> Corrosion of unspecified degree of groin

✓x7ᵗʰ **T21.43 Corrosion of unspecified degree of upper back** ▽
> Corrosion of unspecified degree of interscapular region

✓x7ᵗʰ **T21.44 Corrosion of unspecified degree of lower back** ▽

✓x7ᵗʰ **T21.45 Corrosion of unspecified degree of buttock** ▽
> Corrosion of unspecified degree of anus

✓x7ᵗʰ **T21.46 Corrosion of unspecified degree of male genital region** ♂▽
> Corrosion of unspecified degree of penis
> Corrosion of unspecified degree of scrotum
> Corrosion of unspecified degree of testis

✓x7ᵗʰ **T21.47 Corrosion of unspecified degree of female genital region** ♀▽
> Corrosion of unspecified degree of labium (majus) (minus)
> Corrosion of unspecified degree of perineum
> Corrosion of unspecified degree of vulva
> **EXCLUDES 2** *corrosion of vagina (T28.8)*

✓x7ᵗʰ **T21.49 Corrosion of unspecified degree of other site of trunk** ▽

✓5ᵗʰ **T21.5 Corrosion of first degree of trunk**
> Code first (T51-T65) to identify chemical and intent
> Use additional external cause code to identify place (Y92)

✓x7ᵗʰ **T21.50 Corrosion of first degree of trunk, unspecified site** ▽

✓x7ᵗʰ **T21.51 Corrosion of first degree of chest wall**
> Corrosion of first degree of breast

✓x7ᵗʰ **T21.52 Corrosion of first degree of abdominal wall**
> Corrosion of first degree of flank
> Corrosion of first degree of groin

EXCLUDES 1 Not coded here   **EXCLUDES 2** Not included here   **N** Newborn Age: 0   **P** Pediatric Age: 0-17   **M** Maternity Age: 12-55   **A** Adult Age: 15-124

1042   ICD-10-CM 2018

☑x7ᵗʰ **T21.53 Corrosion of first degree of upper back**
Corrosion of first degree of interscapular region

☑x7ᵗʰ **T21.54 Corrosion of first degree of lower back**

☑x7ᵗʰ **T21.55 Corrosion of first degree of buttock**
Corrosion of first degree of anus

☑x7ᵗʰ **T21.56 Corrosion of first degree of male genital region** ♂
Corrosion of first degree of penis
Corrosion of first degree of scrotum
Corrosion of first degree of testis

☑x7ᵗʰ **T21.57 Corrosion of first degree of female genital region** ♀
Corrosion of first degree of labium (majus) (minus)
Corrosion of first degree of perineum
Corrosion of first degree of vulva
EXCLUDES 2   *corrosion of vagina (T28.8)*

☑x7ᵗʰ **T21.59 Corrosion of first degree of other site of trunk**

☑5ᵗʰ **T21.6 Corrosion of second degree of trunk**
Code first (T51-T65) to identify chemical and intent
Use additional external cause code to identify place (Y92)

☑x7ᵗʰ **T21.60 Corrosion of second degree of trunk, unspecified** ▽
site

☑x7ᵗʰ **T21.61 Corrosion of second degree of chest wall**
Corrosion of second degree of breast

☑x7ᵗʰ **T21.62 Corrosion of second degree of abdominal wall**
Corrosion of second degree of flank
Corrosion of second degree of groin

☑x7ᵗʰ **T21.63 Corrosion of second degree of upper back**
Corrosion of second degree of interscapular region

☑x7ᵗʰ **T21.64 Corrosion of second degree of lower back**

☑x7ᵗʰ **T21.65 Corrosion of second degree of buttock**
Corrosion of second degree of anus

☑x7ᵗʰ **T21.66 Corrosion of second degree of male genital region** ♂
Corrosion of second degree of penis
Corrosion of second degree of scrotum
Corrosion of second degree of testis

☑x7ᵗʰ **T21.67 Corrosion of second degree of female genital** ♀
region
Corrosion of second degree of labium (majus) (minus)
Corrosion of second degree of perineum
Corrosion of second degree of vulva
EXCLUDES 2   *corrosion of vagina (T28.8)*

☑x7ᵗʰ **T21.69 Corrosion of second degree of other site of trunk**

☑5ᵗʰ **T21.7 Corrosion of third degree of trunk**
Code first (T51-T65) to identify chemical and intent
Use additional external cause code to identify place (Y92)

☑x7ᵗʰ **T21.70 Corrosion of third degree of trunk, unspecified** ▽
site

☑x7ᵗʰ **T21.71 Corrosion of third degree of chest wall**
Corrosion of third degree of breast

☑x7ᵗʰ **T21.72 Corrosion of third degree of abdominal wall**
Corrosion of third degree of flank
Corrosion of third degree of groin

☑x7ᵗʰ **T21.73 Corrosion of third degree of upper back**
Corrosion of third degree of interscapular region

☑x7ᵗʰ **T21.74 Corrosion of third degree of lower back**

☑x7ᵗʰ **T21.75 Corrosion of third degree of buttock**
Corrosion of third degree of anus

☑x7ᵗʰ **T21.76 Corrosion of third degree of male genital region** ♂
Corrosion of third degree of penis
Corrosion of third degree of scrotum
Corrosion of third degree of testis

☑x7ᵗʰ **T21.77 Corrosion of third degree of female genital region** ♀
Corrosion of third degree of labium (majus) (minus)
Corrosion of third degree of perineum
Corrosion of third degree of vulva
EXCLUDES 2   *corrosion of vagina (T28.8)*

☑x7ᵗʰ **T21.79 Corrosion of third degree of other site of trunk**

☑4ᵗʰ **T22 Burn and corrosion of shoulder and upper limb, except wrist and hand**
EXCLUDES 2   *burn and corrosion of interscapular region (T21.-)*
burn and corrosion of wrist and hand (T23.-)

The appropriate 7th character is to be added to each code from
category T22.
A   initial encounter
D   subsequent encounter
S   sequela

☑5ᵗʰ **T22.0 Burn of unspecified degree of shoulder and upper limb, except wrist and hand**
Use additional external cause code to identify the source, place
and intent of the burn (X00-X19, X75-X77, X96-X98, Y92)

☑x7ᵗʰ **T22.00 Burn of unspecified degree of shoulder and** ▽
upper limb, except wrist and hand, unspecified site

☑6ᵗʰ **T22.01 Burn of unspecified degree of forearm**

☑7ᵗʰ **T22.011 Burn of unspecified degree of right** ▽
forearm

☑7ᵗʰ **T22.012 Burn of unspecified degree of left** ▽
forearm

☑7ᵗʰ **T22.019 Burn of unspecified degree of** ▽
unspecified forearm

☑6ᵗʰ **T22.02 Burn of unspecified degree of elbow**

☑7ᵗʰ **T22.021 Burn of unspecified degree of right** ▽
elbow

☑7ᵗʰ **T22.022 Burn of unspecified degree of left** ▽
elbow

☑7ᵗʰ **T22.029 Burn of unspecified degree of** ▽
unspecified elbow

☑6ᵗʰ **T22.03 Burn of unspecified degree of upper arm**

☑7ᵗʰ **T22.031 Burn of unspecified degree of** ▽
right upper arm

☑7ᵗʰ **T22.032 Burn of unspecified degree of** ▽
left upper arm

☑7ᵗʰ **T22.039 Burn of unspecified degree of** ▽
unspecified upper arm

☑6ᵗʰ **T22.04 Burn of unspecified degree of axilla**

☑7ᵗʰ **T22.041 Burn of unspecified degree of** ▽
right axilla

☑7ᵗʰ **T22.042 Burn of unspecified degree of** ▽
left axilla

☑7ᵗʰ **T22.049 Burn of unspecified degree of** ▽
unspecified axilla

☑6ᵗʰ **T22.05 Burn of unspecified degree of shoulder**

☑7ᵗʰ **T22.051 Burn of unspecified degree of right** ▽
shoulder

☑7ᵗʰ **T22.052 Burn of unspecified degree of left** ▽
shoulder

☑7ᵗʰ **T22.059 Burn of unspecified degree of** ▽
unspecified shoulder

☑6ᵗʰ **T22.06 Burn of unspecified degree of scapular region**

☑7ᵗʰ **T22.061 Burn of unspecified degree of right** ▽
scapular region

☑7ᵗʰ **T22.062 Burn of unspecified degree of left** ▽
scapular region

☑7ᵗʰ **T22.069 Burn of unspecified degree of** ▽
unspecified scapular region

☑6ᵗʰ **T22.09 Burn of unspecified degree of multiple sites of shoulder and upper limb, except wrist and hand**

☑7ᵗʰ **T22.091 Burn of unspecified degree of multiple** ▽
sites of right shoulder and upper limb, except wrist and hand

☑7ᵗʰ **T22.092 Burn of unspecified degree of multiple** ▽
sites of left shoulder and upper limb, except wrist and hand

☑7ᵗʰ **T22.099 Burn of unspecified degree of multiple** ▽
sites of unspecified shoulder and upper limb, except wrist and hand

☑5ᵗʰ **T22.1 Burn of first degree of shoulder and upper limb, except wrist and hand**
Use additional external cause code to identify the source, place
and intent of the burn (X00-X19, X75-X77, X96-X98, Y92)

☑x7ᵗʰ **T22.10 Burn of first degree of shoulder and upper limb,** ▽
except wrist and hand, unspecified site

☑ Additional Character Req   ☑x7ᵗʰ Placeholder Alert   Manifestation   HCC CMS-HCC Condition   ▽ Unspecified Code   ►◄ Revised Text   ● New Code   ▲ Revised Code Title

ICD-10-CM 2018   1043

√6ᵗʰ **T22.11** **Burn of first degree of forearm**
     √7ᵗʰ **T22.111** **Burn of first degree of right forearm**
     √7ᵗʰ **T22.112** **Burn of first degree of left forearm**
     √7ᵗʰ **T22.119** **Burn of first degree of unspecified forearm** ▽

√6ᵗʰ **T22.12** **Burn of first degree of elbow**
     √7ᵗʰ **T22.121** **Burn of first degree of right elbow**
     √7ᵗʰ **T22.122** **Burn of first degree of left elbow**
     √7ᵗʰ **T22.129** **Burn of first degree of unspecified elbow** ▽

√6ᵗʰ **T22.13** **Burn of first degree of upper arm**
     √7ᵗʰ **T22.131** **Burn of first degree of right upper arm**
     √7ᵗʰ **T22.132** **Burn of first degree of left upper arm**
     √7ᵗʰ **T22.139** **Burn of first degree of unspecified upper arm** ▽

√6ᵗʰ **T22.14** **Burn of first degree of axilla**
     √7ᵗʰ **T22.141** **Burn of first degree of right axilla**
     √7ᵗʰ **T22.142** **Burn of first degree of left axilla**
     √7ᵗʰ **T22.149** **Burn of first degree of unspecified axilla** ▽

√6ᵗʰ **T22.15** **Burn of first degree of shoulder**
     √7ᵗʰ **T22.151** **Burn of first degree of right shoulder**
     √7ᵗʰ **T22.152** **Burn of first degree of left shoulder**
     √7ᵗʰ **T22.159** **Burn of first degree of unspecified shoulder** ▽

√6ᵗʰ **T22.16** **Burn of first degree of scapular region**
     √7ᵗʰ **T22.161** **Burn of first degree of right scapular region**
     √7ᵗʰ **T22.162** **Burn of first degree of left scapular region**
     √7ᵗʰ **T22.169** **Burn of first degree of unspecified scapular region** ▽

√6ᵗʰ **T22.19** **Burn of first degree of multiple sites of shoulder and upper limb, except wrist and hand**
     √7ᵗʰ **T22.191** **Burn of first degree of multiple sites of right shoulder and upper limb, except wrist and hand**
     √7ᵗʰ **T22.192** **Burn of first degree of multiple sites of left shoulder and upper limb, except wrist and hand**
     √7ᵗʰ **T22.199** **Burn of first degree of multiple sites of unspecified shoulder and upper limb, except wrist and hand** ▽

√5ᵗʰ **T22.2** **Burn of second degree of shoulder and upper limb, except wrist and hand**
Use additional external cause code to identify the source, place and intent of the burn (X00-X19, X75-X77, X96-X98, Y92)

√×7ᵗʰ **T22.20** **Burn of second degree of shoulder and upper limb, except wrist and hand, unspecified site** ▽

√6ᵗʰ **T22.21** **Burn of second degree of forearm**
     √7ᵗʰ **T22.211** **Burn of second degree of right forearm**
     √7ᵗʰ **T22.212** **Burn of second degree of left forearm**
     √7ᵗʰ **T22.219** **Burn of second degree of unspecified forearm** ▽

√6ᵗʰ **T22.22** **Burn of second degree of elbow**
     √7ᵗʰ **T22.221** **Burn of second degree of right elbow**
     √7ᵗʰ **T22.222** **Burn of second degree of left elbow**
     √7ᵗʰ **T22.229** **Burn of second degree of unspecified elbow** ▽

√6ᵗʰ **T22.23** **Burn of second degree of upper arm**
     √7ᵗʰ **T22.231** **Burn of second degree of right upper arm**
     √7ᵗʰ **T22.232** **Burn of second degree of left upper arm**
     √7ᵗʰ **T22.239** **Burn of second degree of unspecified upper arm** ▽

√6ᵗʰ **T22.24** **Burn of second degree of axilla**
     √7ᵗʰ **T22.241** **Burn of second degree of right axilla**
     √7ᵗʰ **T22.242** **Burn of second degree of left axilla**
     √7ᵗʰ **T22.249** **Burn of second degree of unspecified axilla** ▽

√6ᵗʰ **T22.25** **Burn of second degree of shoulder**
     √7ᵗʰ **T22.251** **Burn of second degree of right shoulder**
     √7ᵗʰ **T22.252** **Burn of second degree of left shoulder**

     √7ᵗʰ **T22.259** **Burn of second degree of unspecified shoulder** ▽

√6ᵗʰ **T22.26** **Burn of second degree of scapular region**
     √7ᵗʰ **T22.261** **Burn of second degree of right scapular region**
     √7ᵗʰ **T22.262** **Burn of second degree of left scapular region**
     √7ᵗʰ **T22.269** **Burn of second degree of unspecified scapular region** ▽

√6ᵗʰ **T22.29** **Burn of second degree of multiple sites of shoulder and upper limb, except wrist and hand**
     √7ᵗʰ **T22.291** **Burn of second degree of multiple sites of right shoulder and upper limb, except wrist and hand**
     √7ᵗʰ **T22.292** **Burn of second degree of multiple sites of left shoulder and upper limb, except wrist and hand**
     √7ᵗʰ **T22.299** **Burn of second degree of multiple sites of unspecified shoulder and upper limb, except wrist and hand** ▽

√5ᵗʰ **T22.3** **Burn of third degree of shoulder and upper limb, except wrist and hand**
Use additional external cause code to identify the source, place and intent of the burn (X00-X19, X75-X77, X96-X98, Y92)

√×7ᵗʰ **T22.30** **Burn of third degree of shoulder and upper limb, except wrist and hand, unspecified site** ▽

√6ᵗʰ **T22.31** **Burn of third degree of forearm**
     √7ᵗʰ **T22.311** **Burn of third degree of right forearm**
     √7ᵗʰ **T22.312** **Burn of third degree of left forearm**
     √7ᵗʰ **T22.319** **Burn of third degree of unspecified forearm** ▽

√6ᵗʰ **T22.32** **Burn of third degree of elbow**
     √7ᵗʰ **T22.321** **Burn of third degree of right elbow**
     √7ᵗʰ **T22.322** **Burn of third degree of left elbow**
     √7ᵗʰ **T22.329** **Burn of third degree of unspecified elbow** ▽

√6ᵗʰ **T22.33** **Burn of third degree of upper arm**
     √7ᵗʰ **T22.331** **Burn of third degree of right upper arm**
     √7ᵗʰ **T22.332** **Burn of third degree of left upper arm**
     √7ᵗʰ **T22.339** **Burn of third degree of unspecified upper arm** ▽

√6ᵗʰ **T22.34** **Burn of third degree of axilla**
     √7ᵗʰ **T22.341** **Burn of third degree of right axilla**
     √7ᵗʰ **T22.342** **Burn of third degree of left axilla**
     √7ᵗʰ **T22.349** **Burn of third degree of unspecified axilla** ▽

√6ᵗʰ **T22.35** **Burn of third degree of shoulder**
     √7ᵗʰ **T22.351** **Burn of third degree of right shoulder**
     √7ᵗʰ **T22.352** **Burn of third degree of left shoulder**
     √7ᵗʰ **T22.359** **Burn of third degree of unspecified shoulder** ▽

√6ᵗʰ **T22.36** **Burn of third degree of scapular region**
     √7ᵗʰ **T22.361** **Burn of third degree of right scapular region**
     √7ᵗʰ **T22.362** **Burn of third degree of left scapular region**
     √7ᵗʰ **T22.369** **Burn of third degree of unspecified scapular region** ▽

√6ᵗʰ **T22.39** **Burn of third degree of multiple sites of shoulder and upper limb, except wrist and hand**
     √7ᵗʰ **T22.391** **Burn of third degree of multiple sites of right shoulder and upper limb, except wrist and hand**
     √7ᵗʰ **T22.392** **Burn of third degree of multiple sites of left shoulder and upper limb, except wrist and hand**
     √7ᵗʰ **T22.399** **Burn of third degree of multiple sites of unspecified shoulder and upper limb, except wrist and hand** ▽

EXCLUDES 1 Not coded here   **EXCLUDES 2** Not included here   **N** Newborn Age: 0   **P** Pediatric Age: 0-17   **M** Maternity Age: 12-55   **A** Adult Age: 15-124

1044   ICD-10-CM 2018

☑5ᵗʰ **T22.4** **Corrosion of unspecified degree of shoulder and upper limb, except wrist and hand**
　　　Code first (T51-T65) to identify chemical and intent
　　　Use additional external cause code to identify place (Y92)

☑x7ᵗʰ　**T22.40** **Corrosion of unspecified degree of shoulder and upper limb, except wrist and hand, unspecified site** ▽

☑6ᵗʰ　**T22.41** **Corrosion of unspecified degree of forearm**

☑7ᵗʰ　　**T22.411** **Corrosion of unspecified degree of right forearm** ▽

☑7ᵗʰ　　**T22.412** **Corrosion of unspecified degree of left forearm** ▽

☑7ᵗʰ　　**T22.419** **Corrosion of unspecified degree of unspecified forearm** ▽

☑6ᵗʰ　**T22.42** **Corrosion of unspecified degree of elbow**

☑7ᵗʰ　　**T22.421** **Corrosion of unspecified degree of right elbow** ▽

☑7ᵗʰ　　**T22.422** **Corrosion of unspecified degree of left elbow** ▽

☑7ᵗʰ　　**T22.429** **Corrosion of unspecified degree of unspecified elbow** ▽

☑6ᵗʰ　**T22.43** **Corrosion of unspecified degree of upper arm**

☑7ᵗʰ　　**T22.431** **Corrosion of unspecified degree of right upper arm** ▽

☑7ᵗʰ　　**T22.432** **Corrosion of unspecified degree of left upper arm** ▽

☑7ᵗʰ　　**T22.439** **Corrosion of unspecified degree of unspecified upper arm** ▽

☑6ᵗʰ　**T22.44** **Corrosion of unspecified degree of axilla**

☑7ᵗʰ　　**T22.441** **Corrosion of unspecified degree of right axilla** ▽

☑7ᵗʰ　　**T22.442** **Corrosion of unspecified degree of left axilla** ▽

☑7ᵗʰ　　**T22.449** **Corrosion of unspecified degree of unspecified axilla** ▽

☑6ᵗʰ　**T22.45** **Corrosion of unspecified degree of shoulder**

☑7ᵗʰ　　**T22.451** **Corrosion of unspecified degree of right shoulder** ▽

☑7ᵗʰ　　**T22.452** **Corrosion of unspecified degree of left shoulder** ▽

☑7ᵗʰ　　**T22.459** **Corrosion of unspecified degree of unspecified shoulder** ▽

☑6ᵗʰ　**T22.46** **Corrosion of unspecified degree of scapular region**

☑7ᵗʰ　　**T22.461** **Corrosion of unspecified degree of right scapular region** ▽

☑7ᵗʰ　　**T22.462** **Corrosion of unspecified degree of left scapular region** ▽

☑7ᵗʰ　　**T22.469** **Corrosion of unspecified degree of unspecified scapular region** ▽

☑6ᵗʰ　**T22.49** **Corrosion of unspecified degree of multiple sites of shoulder and upper limb, except wrist and hand**

☑7ᵗʰ　　**T22.491** **Corrosion of unspecified degree of multiple sites of right shoulder and upper limb, except wrist and hand** ▽

☑7ᵗʰ　　**T22.492** **Corrosion of unspecified degree of multiple sites of left shoulder and upper limb, except wrist and hand** ▽

☑7ᵗʰ　　**T22.499** **Corrosion of unspecified degree of multiple sites of unspecified shoulder and upper limb, except wrist and hand** ▽

☑5ᵗʰ **T22.5** **Corrosion of first degree of shoulder and upper limb, except wrist and hand**
　　　Code first (T51-T65) to identify chemical and intent
　　　Use additional external cause code to identify place (Y92)

☑x7ᵗʰ　**T22.50** **Corrosion of first degree of shoulder and upper limb, except wrist and hand unspecified site** ▽

☑6ᵗʰ　**T22.51** **Corrosion of first degree of forearm**

☑7ᵗʰ　　**T22.511** **Corrosion of first degree of right forearm**

☑7ᵗʰ　　**T22.512** **Corrosion of first degree of left forearm**

☑7ᵗʰ　　**T22.519** **Corrosion of first degree of unspecified forearm** ▽

☑6ᵗʰ　**T22.52** **Corrosion of first degree of elbow**

☑7ᵗʰ　　**T22.521** **Corrosion of first degree of right elbow**

☑7ᵗʰ　　**T22.522** **Corrosion of first degree of left elbow**

☑7ᵗʰ　　**T22.529** **Corrosion of first degree of unspecified elbow** ▽

☑6ᵗʰ　**T22.53** **Corrosion of first degree of upper arm**

☑7ᵗʰ　　**T22.531** **Corrosion of first degree of right upper arm**

☑7ᵗʰ　　**T22.532** **Corrosion of first degree of left upper arm**

☑7ᵗʰ　　**T22.539** **Corrosion of first degree of unspecified upper arm** ▽

☑6ᵗʰ　**T22.54** **Corrosion of first degree of axilla**

☑7ᵗʰ　　**T22.541** **Corrosion of first degree of right axilla**

☑7ᵗʰ　　**T22.542** **Corrosion of first degree of left axilla**

☑7ᵗʰ　　**T22.549** **Corrosion of first degree of unspecified axilla** ▽

☑6ᵗʰ　**T22.55** **Corrosion of first degree of shoulder**

☑7ᵗʰ　　**T22.551** **Corrosion of first degree of right shoulder**

☑7ᵗʰ　　**T22.552** **Corrosion of first degree of left shoulder**

☑7ᵗʰ　　**T22.559** **Corrosion of first degree of unspecified shoulder** ▽

☑6ᵗʰ　**T22.56** **Corrosion of first degree of scapular region**

☑7ᵗʰ　　**T22.561** **Corrosion of first degree of right scapular region**

☑7ᵗʰ　　**T22.562** **Corrosion of first degree of left scapular region**

☑7ᵗʰ　　**T22.569** **Corrosion of first degree of unspecified scapular region** ▽

☑6ᵗʰ　**T22.59** **Corrosion of first degree of multiple sites of shoulder and upper limb, except wrist and hand**

☑7ᵗʰ　　**T22.591** **Corrosion of first degree of multiple sites of right shoulder and upper limb, except wrist and hand**

☑7ᵗʰ　　**T22.592** **Corrosion of first degree of multiple sites of left shoulder and upper limb, except wrist and hand**

☑7ᵗʰ　　**T22.599** **Corrosion of first degree of multiple sites of unspecified shoulder and upper limb, except wrist and hand** ▽

☑5ᵗʰ **T22.6** **Corrosion of second degree of shoulder and upper limb, except wrist and hand**
　　　Code first (T51-T65) to identify chemical and intent
　　　Use additional external cause code to identify place (Y92)

☑x7ᵗʰ　**T22.60** **Corrosion of second degree of shoulder and upper limb, except wrist and hand, unspecified site** ▽

☑6ᵗʰ　**T22.61** **Corrosion of second degree of forearm**

☑7ᵗʰ　　**T22.611** **Corrosion of second degree of right forearm**

☑7ᵗʰ　　**T22.612** **Corrosion of second degree of left forearm**

☑7ᵗʰ　　**T22.619** **Corrosion of second degree of unspecified forearm** ▽

☑6ᵗʰ　**T22.62** **Corrosion of second degree of elbow**

☑7ᵗʰ　　**T22.621** **Corrosion of second degree of right elbow**

☑7ᵗʰ　　**T22.622** **Corrosion of second degree of left elbow**

☑7ᵗʰ　　**T22.629** **Corrosion of second degree of unspecified elbow** ▽

☑6ᵗʰ　**T22.63** **Corrosion of second degree of upper arm**

☑7ᵗʰ　　**T22.631** **Corrosion of second degree of right upper arm**

☑7ᵗʰ　　**T22.632** **Corrosion of second degree of left upper arm**

☑7ᵗʰ　　**T22.639** **Corrosion of second degree of unspecified upper arm** ▽

☑6ᵗʰ　**T22.64** **Corrosion of second degree of axilla**

☑7ᵗʰ　　**T22.641** **Corrosion of second degree of right axilla**

☑7ᵗʰ　　**T22.642** **Corrosion of second degree of left axilla**

☑7ᵗʰ　　**T22.649** **Corrosion of second degree of unspecified axilla** ▽

☑6ᵗʰ　**T22.65** **Corrosion of second degree of shoulder**

☑7ᵗʰ　　**T22.651** **Corrosion of second degree of right shoulder**

☑7ᵗʰ　　**T22.652** **Corrosion of second degree of left shoulder**

☑7ᵗʰ　　**T22.659** **Corrosion of second degree of unspecified shoulder** ▽

☑ Additional Character Req　　☑x7ᵗʰ Placeholder Alert　　Manifestation　　ᴴᶜᶜ CMS-HCC Condition　　▽ Unspecified Code　　▶◀ Revised Text　　● New Code　　▲ Revised Code Title

√6ᵗʰ **T22.66** **Corrosion of second degree of scapular region**

     √7ᵗʰ **T22.661** **Corrosion of second degree of right scapular region**

     √7ᵗʰ **T22.662** **Corrosion of second degree of left scapular region**

     √7ᵗʰ **T22.669** **Corrosion of second degree of unspecified scapular region** ▽

√6ᵗʰ **T22.69** **Corrosion of second degree of multiple sites of shoulder and upper limb, except wrist and hand**

     √7ᵗʰ **T22.691** **Corrosion of second degree of multiple sites of right shoulder and upper limb, except wrist and hand**

     √7ᵗʰ **T22.692** **Corrosion of second degree of multiple sites of left shoulder and upper limb, except wrist and hand**

     √7ᵗʰ **T22.699** **Corrosion of second degree of multiple sites of unspecified shoulder and upper limb, except wrist and hand** ▽

√5ᵗʰ **T22.7** **Corrosion of third degree of shoulder and upper limb, except wrist and hand**

     Code first (T51-T65) to identify chemical and intent
     Use additional external cause code to identify.place (Y92)

√x7ᵗʰ **T22.70** **Corrosion of third degree of shoulder and upper limb, except wrist and hand, unspecified site** ▽

√6ᵗʰ **T22.71** **Corrosion of third degree of forearm**

     √7ᵗʰ **T22.711** **Corrosion of third degree of right forearm**

     √7ᵗʰ **T22.712** **Corrosion of third degree of left forearm**

     √7ᵗʰ **T22.719** **Corrosion of third degree of unspecified forearm** ▽

√6ᵗʰ **T22.72** **Corrosion of third degree of elbow**

     √7ᵗʰ **T22.721** **Corrosion of third degree of right elbow**

     √7ᵗʰ **T22.722** **Corrosion of third degree of left elbow**

     √7ᵗʰ **T22.729** **Corrosion of third degree of unspecified elbow** ▽

√6ᵗʰ **T22.73** **Corrosion of third degree of upper arm**

     √7ᵗʰ **T22.731** **Corrosion of third degree of right upper arm**

     √7ᵗʰ **T22.732** **Corrosion of third degree of left upper arm**

     √7ᵗʰ **T22.739** **Corrosion of third degree of unspecified upper arm** ▽

√6ᵗʰ **T22.74** **Corrosion of third degree of axilla**

     √7ᵗʰ **T22.741** **Corrosion of third degree of right axilla**

     √7ᵗʰ **T22.742** **Corrosion of third degree of left axilla**

     √7ᵗʰ **T22.749** **Corrosion of third degree of unspecified axilla** ▽

√6ᵗʰ **T22.75** **Corrosion of third degree of shoulder**

     √7ᵗʰ **T22.751** **Corrosion of third degree of right shoulder**

     √7ᵗʰ **T22.752** **Corrosion of third degree of left shoulder**

     √7ᵗʰ **T22.759** **Corrosion of third degree of unspecified shoulder** ▽

√6ᵗʰ **T22.76** **Corrosion of third degree of scapular region**

     √7ᵗʰ **T22.761** **Corrosion of third degree of right scapular region**

     √7ᵗʰ **T22.762** **Corrosion of third degree of left scapular region**

     √7ᵗʰ **T22.769** **Corrosion of third degree of unspecified scapular region** ▽

√6ᵗʰ **T22.79** **Corrosion of third degree of multiple sites of shoulder and upper limb, except wrist and hand**

     √7ᵗʰ **T22.791** **Corrosion of third degree of multiple sites of right shoulder and upper limb, except wrist and hand**

     √7ᵗʰ **T22.792** **Corrosion of third degree of multiple sites of left shoulder and upper limb, except wrist and hand**

     √7ᵗʰ **T22.799** **Corrosion of third degree of multiple sites of unspecified shoulder and upper limb, except wrist and hand** ▽

√4ᵗʰ **T23** **Burn and corrosion of wrist and hand**
     AHA: 2015, 1Q, 19

The appropriate 7th character is to be added to each code from category T23.
A   initial encounter
D   subsequent encounter
S   sequela

√5ᵗʰ **T23.0** **Burn of unspecified degree of wrist and hand**
     Use additional external cause code to identify the source, place and intent of the burn (X00-X19, X75-X77, X96-X98, Y92)

√6ᵗʰ **T23.00** **Burn of unspecified degree of hand, unspecified site**

     √7ᵗʰ **T23.001** **Burn of unspecified degree of right hand, unspecified site** ▽

     √7ᵗʰ **T23.002** **Burn of unspecified degree of left hand, unspecified site** ▽

     √7ᵗʰ **T23.009** **Burn of unspecified degree of unspecified hand, unspecified site** ▽

√6ᵗʰ **T23.01** **Burn of unspecified degree of thumb (nail)**

     √7ᵗʰ **T23.011** **Burn of unspecified degree of right thumb (nail)** ▽

     √7ᵗʰ **T23.012** **Burn of unspecified degree of left thumb (nail)** ▽

     √7ᵗʰ **T23.019** **Burn of unspecified degree of unspecified thumb (nail)** ▽

√6ᵗʰ **T23.02** **Burn of unspecified degree of single finger (nail) except thumb**

     √7ᵗʰ **T23.021** **Burn of unspecified degree of single right finger (nail) except thumb** ▽

     √7ᵗʰ **T23.022** **Burn of unspecified degree of single left finger (nail) except thumb** ▽

     √7ᵗʰ **T23.029** **Burn of unspecified degree of unspecified single finger (nail) except thumb** ▽

√6ᵗʰ **T23.03** **Burn of unspecified degree of multiple fingers (nail), not including thumb**

     √7ᵗʰ **T23.031** **Burn of unspecified degree of multiple right fingers (nail), not including thumb** ▽

     √7ᵗʰ **T23.032** **Burn of unspecified degree of multiple left fingers (nail), not including thumb** ▽

     √7ᵗʰ **T23.039** **Burn of unspecified degree of unspecified multiple fingers (nail), not including thumb** ▽

√6ᵗʰ **T23.04** **Burn of unspecified degree of multiple fingers (nail), including thumb**

     √7ᵗʰ **T23.041** **Burn of unspecified degree of multiple right fingers (nail), including thumb** ▽

     √7ᵗʰ **T23.042** **Burn of unspecified degree of multiple left fingers (nail), including thumb** ▽

     √7ᵗʰ **T23.049** **Burn of unspecified degree of unspecified multiple fingers (nail), including thumb** ▽

√6ᵗʰ **T23.05** **Burn of unspecified degree of palm**

     √7ᵗʰ **T23.051** **Burn of unspecified degree of right palm** ▽

     √7ᵗʰ **T23.052** **Burn of unspecified degree of left palm** ▽

     √7ᵗʰ **T23.059** **Burn of unspecified degree of unspecified palm** ▽

√6ᵗʰ **T23.06** **Burn of unspecified degree of back of hand**

     √7ᵗʰ **T23.061** **Burn of unspecified degree of back of right hand** ▽

     √7ᵗʰ **T23.062** **Burn of unspecified degree of back of left hand** ▽

     √7ᵗʰ **T23.069** **Burn of unspecified degree of back of unspecified hand** ▽

√6ᵗʰ **T23.07** **Burn of unspecified degree of wrist**

     √7ᵗʰ **T23.071** **Burn of unspecified degree of right wrist** ▽

     √7ᵗʰ **T23.072** **Burn of unspecified degree of left wrist** ▽

     √7ᵗʰ **T23.079** **Burn of unspecified degree of unspecified wrist** ▽

EXCLUDES 1 Not coded here   EXCLUDES 2 Not included here   N Newborn Age: 0   P Pediatric Age: 0-17   M Maternity Age: 12-55   A Adult Age: 15-124

1046   ICD-10-CM 2018

☑6ᵗʰ **T23.09** **Burn of unspecified degree of multiple sites of wrist and hand**

    ☑7ᵗʰ **T23.091** Burn of unspecified degree of multiple sites of right wrist and hand ▽

    ☑7ᵗʰ **T23.092** Burn of unspecified degree of multiple sites of left wrist and hand ▽

    ☑7ᵗʰ **T23.099** Burn of unspecified degree of multiple sites of unspecified wrist and hand

☑5ᵗʰ **T23.1** **Burn of first degree of wrist and hand**

    Use additional external cause code to identify the source, place and intent of the burn (X00-X19, X75-X77, X96-X98, Y92)

  ☑6ᵗʰ **T23.10** **Burn of first degree of hand, unspecified site**

    ☑7ᵗʰ **T23.101** Burn of first degree of right hand, unspecified site ▽

    ☑7ᵗʰ **T23.102** Burn of first degree of left hand, unspecified site ▽

    ☑7ᵗʰ **T23.109** Burn of first degree of unspecified hand, unspecified site ▽

  ☑6ᵗʰ **T23.11** **Burn of first degree of thumb (nail)**

    ☑7ᵗʰ **T23.111** Burn of first degree of right thumb (nail)

    ☑7ᵗʰ **T23.112** Burn of first degree of left thumb (nail)

    ☑7ᵗʰ **T23.119** Burn of first degree of unspecified thumb (nail) ▽

  ☑6ᵗʰ **T23.12** **Burn of first degree of single finger (nail) except thumb**

    ☑7ᵗʰ **T23.121** Burn of first degree of single right finger (nail) except thumb

    ☑7ᵗʰ **T23.122** Burn of first degree of single left finger (nail) except thumb

    ☑7ᵗʰ **T23.129** Burn of first degree of unspecified single finger (nail) except thumb ▽

  ☑6ᵗʰ **T23.13** **Burn of first degree of multiple fingers (nail), not including thumb**

    ☑7ᵗʰ **T23.131** Burn of first degree of multiple right fingers (nail), not including thumb

    ☑7ᵗʰ **T23.132** Burn of first degree of multiple left fingers (nail), not including thumb

    ☑7ᵗʰ **T23.139** Burn of first degree of unspecified multiple fingers (nail), not including thumb ▽

  ☑6ᵗʰ **T23.14** **Burn of first degree of multiple fingers (nail), including thumb**

    ☑7ᵗʰ **T23.141** Burn of first degree of multiple right fingers (nail), including thumb

    ☑7ᵗʰ **T23.142** Burn of first degree of multiple left fingers (nail), including thumb

    ☑7ᵗʰ **T23.149** Burn of first degree of unspecified multiple fingers (nail), including thumb ▽

  ☑6ᵗʰ **T23.15** **Burn of first degree of palm**

    ☑7ᵗʰ **T23.151** Burn of first degree of right palm

    ☑7ᵗʰ **T23.152** Burn of first degree of left palm

    ☑7ᵗʰ **T23.159** Burn of first degree of unspecified palm ▽

  ☑6ᵗʰ **T23.16** **Burn of first degree of back of hand**

    ☑7ᵗʰ **T23.161** Burn of first degree of back of right hand

    ☑7ᵗʰ **T23.162** Burn of first degree of back of left hand

    ☑7ᵗʰ **T23.169** Burn of first degree of back of unspecified hand ▽

  ☑6ᵗʰ **T23.17** **Burn of first degree of wrist**

    ☑7ᵗʰ **T23.171** Burn of first degree of right wrist

    ☑7ᵗʰ **T23.172** Burn of first degree of left wrist

    ☑7ᵗʰ **T23.179** Burn of first degree of unspecified wrist ▽

  ☑6ᵗʰ **T23.19** **Burn of first degree of multiple sites of wrist and hand**

    ☑7ᵗʰ **T23.191** Burn of first degree of multiple sites of right wrist and hand

    ☑7ᵗʰ **T23.192** Burn of first degree of multiple sites of left wrist and hand

    ☑7ᵗʰ **T23.199** Burn of first degree of multiple sites of unspecified wrist and hand ▽

☑5ᵗʰ **T23.2** **Burn of second degree of wrist and hand**

    Use additional external cause code to identify the source, place and intent of the burn (X00-X19, X75-X77, X96-X98, Y92)

  ☑6ᵗʰ **T23.20** **Burn of second degree of hand, unspecified site**

    ☑7ᵗʰ **T23.201** Burn of second degree of right hand, unspecified site ▽

    ☑7ᵗʰ **T23.202** Burn of second degree of left hand, unspecified site ▽

    ☑7ᵗʰ **T23.209** Burn of second degree of unspecified hand, unspecified site ▽

  ☑6ᵗʰ **T23.21** **Burn of second degree of thumb (nail)**

    ☑7ᵗʰ **T23.211** Burn of second degree of right thumb (nail)

    ☑7ᵗʰ **T23.212** Burn of second degree of left thumb (nail)

    ☑7ᵗʰ **T23.219** Burn of second degree of unspecified thumb (nail) ▽

  ☑6ᵗʰ **T23.22** **Burn of second degree of single finger (nail) except thumb**

    ☑7ᵗʰ **T23.221** Burn of second degree of single right finger (nail) except thumb

    ☑7ᵗʰ **T23.222** Burn of second degree of single left finger (nail) except thumb

    ☑7ᵗʰ **T23.229** Burn of second degree of unspecified single finger (nail) except thumb ▽

  ☑6ᵗʰ **T23.23** **Burn of second degree of multiple fingers (nail), not including thumb**

    ☑7ᵗʰ **T23.231** Burn of second degree of multiple right fingers (nail), not including thumb

    ☑7ᵗʰ **T23.232** Burn of second degree of multiple left fingers (nail), not including thumb

    ☑7ᵗʰ **T23.239** Burn of second degree of unspecified multiple fingers (nail), not including thumb ▽

  ☑6ᵗʰ **T23.24** **Burn of second degree of multiple fingers (nail), including thumb**

    ☑7ᵗʰ **T23.241** Burn of second degree of multiple right fingers (nail), including thumb

    ☑7ᵗʰ **T23.242** Burn of second degree of multiple left fingers (nail), including thumb

    ☑7ᵗʰ **T23.249** Burn of second degree of unspecified multiple fingers (nail), including thumb ▽

  ☑6ᵗʰ **T23.25** **Burn of second degree of palm**

    ☑7ᵗʰ **T23.251** Burn of second degree of right palm

    ☑7ᵗʰ **T23.252** Burn of second degree of left palm

    ☑7ᵗʰ **T23.259** Burn of second degree of unspecified palm ▽

  ☑6ᵗʰ **T23.26** **Burn of second degree of back of hand**

    ☑7ᵗʰ **T23.261** Burn of second degree of back of right hand

    ☑7ᵗʰ **T23.262** Burn of second degree of back of left hand

    ☑7ᵗʰ **T23.269** Burn of second degree of back of unspecified hand ▽

  ☑6ᵗʰ **T23.27** **Burn of second degree of wrist**

    ☑7ᵗʰ **T23.271** Burn of second degree of right wrist

    ☑7ᵗʰ **T23.272** Burn of second degree of left wrist

    ☑7ᵗʰ **T23.279** Burn of second degree of unspecified wrist ▽

  ☑6ᵗʰ **T23.29** **Burn of second degree of multiple sites of wrist and hand**

    ☑7ᵗʰ **T23.291** Burn of second degree of multiple sites of right wrist and hand

    ☑7ᵗʰ **T23.292** Burn of second degree of multiple sites of left wrist and hand

    ☑7ᵗʰ **T23.299** Burn of second degree of multiple sites of unspecified wrist and hand ▽

☑5ᵗʰ **T23.3** **Burn of third degree of wrist and hand**

    Use additional external cause code to identify the source, place and intent of the burn (X00-X19, X75-X77, X96-X98, Y92)

  ☑6ᵗʰ **T23.30** **Burn of third degree of hand, unspecified site**
      AHA: 2016, 2Q, 5

    ☑7ᵗʰ **T23.301** Burn of third degree of right hand, unspecified site ▽

☑ Additional Character Req   ☑7ᵗʰ Placeholder Alert   <u>Manifestation</u>   **HCC** CMS-HCC Condition   ▽ Unspecified Code   ►◄ Revised Text   ● New Code   ▲ Revised Code Title

√7ᵗʰ **T23.302** Burn of third degree of **left hand,** unspecified site ▽

√7ᵗʰ **T23.309** Burn of third degree of unspecified hand, unspecified site ▽

√6ᵗʰ **T23.31** Burn of third degree of thumb (nail)

√7ᵗʰ **T23.311** Burn of third degree of **right** thumb (nail)

√7ᵗʰ **T23.312** Burn of third degree of **left** thumb (nail)

√7ᵗʰ **T23.319** Burn of third degree of unspecified thumb (nail) ▽

√6ᵗʰ **T23.32** Burn of third degree of **single finger** (nail) except thumb

√7ᵗʰ **T23.321** Burn of third degree of single right finger (nail) except thumb

√7ᵗʰ **T23.322** Burn of third degree of single left finger (nail) except thumb

√7ᵗʰ **T23.329** Burn of third degree of unspecified single finger (nail) except thumb ▽

√6ᵗʰ **T23.33** Burn of third degree of **multiple fingers** (nail), not including thumb

√7ᵗʰ **T23.331** Burn of third degree of multiple right fingers (nail), not including thumb

√7ᵗʰ **T23.332** Burn of third degree of multiple left fingers (nail), not including thumb

√7ᵗʰ **T23.339** Burn of third degree of unspecified multiple fingers (nail), not including thumb ▽

√6ᵗʰ **T23.34** Burn of third degree of **multiple fingers** (nail), including thumb

√7ᵗʰ **T23.341** Burn of third degree of multiple right fingers (nail), including thumb

√7ᵗʰ **T23.342** Burn of third degree of multiple left fingers (nail), including thumb

√7ᵗʰ **T23.349** Burn of third degree of unspecified multiple fingers (nail), including thumb ▽

√6ᵗʰ **T23.35** Burn of third degree of **palm**

√7ᵗʰ **T23.351** Burn of third degree of **right** palm

√7ᵗʰ **T23.352** Burn of third degree of **left** palm

√7ᵗʰ **T23.359** Burn of third degree of unspecified palm ▽

√6ᵗʰ **T23.36** Burn of third degree of **back of hand**

√7ᵗʰ **T23.361** Burn of third degree of back of **right** hand

√7ᵗʰ **T23.362** Burn of third degree of back of **left** hand

√7ᵗʰ **T23.369** Burn of third degree of back of unspecified hand ▽

√6ᵗʰ **T23.37** Burn of third degree of **wrist**

√7ᵗʰ **T23.371** Burn of third degree of **right** wrist

√7ᵗʰ **T23.372** Burn of third degree of **left** wrist

√7ᵗʰ **T23.379** Burn of third degree of unspecified wrist ▽

√6ᵗʰ **T23.39** Burn of third degree of **multiple sites** of wrist and hand

√7ᵗʰ **T23.391** Burn of third degree of multiple sites of **right** wrist and hand

√7ᵗʰ **T23.392** Burn of third degree of multiple sites of **left** wrist and hand

√7ᵗʰ **T23.399** Burn of third degree of multiple sites of unspecified wrist and hand ▽

√5ᵗʰ **T23.4** **Corrosion of unspecified degree of wrist and hand**

Code first (T51-T65) to identify chemical and intent

Use additional external cause code to identify place (Y92)

√6ᵗʰ **T23.40** Corrosion of unspecified degree of hand, unspecified site

√7ᵗʰ **T23.401** Corrosion of unspecified degree of **right** hand, unspecified site ▽

√7ᵗʰ **T23.402** Corrosion of unspecified degree of **left** hand, unspecified site ▽

√7ᵗʰ **T23.409** Corrosion of unspecified degree of unspecified hand, unspecified site ▽

√6ᵗʰ **T23.41** Corrosion of unspecified degree of **thumb** (nail)

√7ᵗʰ **T23.411** Corrosion of unspecified degree of **right** thumb (nail) ▽

√7ᵗʰ **T23.412** Corrosion of unspecified degree of **left** thumb (nail) ▽

√7ᵗʰ **T23.419** Corrosion of unspecified degree of unspecified thumb (nail) ▽

√6ᵗʰ **T23.42** Corrosion of unspecified degree of **single finger** (nail) except thumb

√7ᵗʰ **T23.421** Corrosion of unspecified degree of single **right** finger (nail) except thumb ▽

√7ᵗʰ **T23.422** Corrosion of unspecified degree of single **left** finger (nail) except thumb ▽

√7ᵗʰ **T23.429** Corrosion of unspecified degree of unspecified single finger (nail) except thumb ▽

√6ᵗʰ **T23.43** Corrosion of unspecified degree of **multiple fingers** (nail), not including thumb

√7ᵗʰ **T23.431** Corrosion of unspecified degree of multiple **right** fingers (nail), not including thumb ▽

√7ᵗʰ **T23.432** Corrosion of unspecified degree of multiple **left** fingers (nail), not including thumb ▽

√7ᵗʰ **T23.439** Corrosion of unspecified degree of unspecified multiple fingers (nail), not including thumb ▽

√6ᵗʰ **T23.44** Corrosion of unspecified degree of **multiple fingers** (nail), including thumb

√7ᵗʰ **T23.441** Corrosion of unspecified degree of multiple **right** fingers (nail), including thumb ▽

√7ᵗʰ **T23.442** Corrosion of unspecified degree of multiple **left** fingers (nail), including thumb ▽

√7ᵗʰ **T23.449** Corrosion of unspecified degree of unspecified multiple fingers (nail), including thumb ▽

√6ᵗʰ **T23.45** Corrosion of unspecified degree of **palm**

√7ᵗʰ **T23.451** Corrosion of unspecified degree of **right** palm ▽

√7ᵗʰ **T23.452** Corrosion of unspecified degree of **left** palm ▽

√7ᵗʰ **T23.459** Corrosion of unspecified degree of unspecified palm ▽

√6ᵗʰ **T23.46** Corrosion of unspecified degree of **back of hand**

√7ᵗʰ **T23.461** Corrosion of unspecified degree of back of **right** hand ▽

√7ᵗʰ **T23.462** Corrosion of unspecified degree of back of **left** hand ▽

√7ᵗʰ **T23.469** Corrosion of unspecified degree of back of unspecified hand ▽

√6ᵗʰ **T23.47** Corrosion of unspecified degree of **wrist**

√7ᵗʰ **T23.471** Corrosion of unspecified degree of **right** wrist ▽

√7ᵗʰ **T23.472** Corrosion of unspecified degree of **left** wrist ▽

√7ᵗʰ **T23.479** Corrosion of unspecified degree of unspecified wrist ▽

√6ᵗʰ **T23.49** Corrosion of unspecified degree of **multiple sites** of wrist and hand

√7ᵗʰ **T23.491** Corrosion of unspecified degree of multiple sites of **right** wrist and hand ▽

√7ᵗʰ **T23.492** Corrosion of unspecified degree of multiple sites of **left** wrist and hand ▽

√7ᵗʰ **T23.499** Corrosion of unspecified degree of multiple sites of unspecified wrist and hand ▽

√5ᵗʰ **T23.5** **Corrosion of first degree of wrist and hand**

Code first (T51-T65) to identify chemical and intent

Use additional external cause code to identify place (Y92)

√6ᵗʰ **T23.50** Corrosion of first degree of hand, unspecified site

√7ᵗʰ **T23.501** Corrosion of first degree of **right** hand, unspecified site ▽

√7ᵗʰ **T23.502** Corrosion of first degree of **left** hand, unspecified site ▽

√7ᵗʰ **T23.509** Corrosion of first degree of unspecified hand, unspecified site ▽

√6ᵗʰ **T23.51** Corrosion of first degree of **thumb** (nail)

√7ᵗʰ **T23.511** Corrosion of first degree of **right** thumb (nail) ▽

EXCLUDES 1 Not coded here   EXCLUDES 2 Not included here   N Newborn Age: 0   P Pediatric Age: 0-17   M Maternity Age: 12-55   A Adult Age: 15-124

1048   ICD-10-CM 2018

√7ᵗʰ **T23.512** Corrosion of first degree of left thumb (nail)

√7ᵗʰ **T23.519** Corrosion of first degree of unspecified ▽ thumb (nail)

√6ᵗʰ **T23.52** Corrosion of first degree of single finger (nail) except thumb

　√7ᵗʰ **T23.521** Corrosion of first degree of single right finger (nail) except thumb

　√7ᵗʰ **T23.522** Corrosion of first degree of single left finger (nail) except thumb

　√7ᵗʰ **T23.529** Corrosion of first degree of unspecified ▽ single finger (nail) except thumb

√6ᵗʰ **T23.53** Corrosion of first degree of multiple fingers (nail), not including thumb

　√7ᵗʰ **T23.531** Corrosion of first degree of multiple right fingers (nail), not including thumb

　√7ᵗʰ **T23.532** Corrosion of first degree of multiple left fingers (nail), not including thumb

　√7ᵗʰ **T23.539** Corrosion of first degree of unspecified ▽ multiple fingers (nail), not including thumb

√6ᵗʰ **T23.54** Corrosion of first degree of multiple fingers (nail), including thumb

　√7ᵗʰ **T23.541** Corrosion of first degree of multiple right fingers (nail), including thumb

　√7ᵗʰ **T23.542** Corrosion of first degree of multiple left fingers (nail), including thumb

　√7ᵗʰ **T23.549** Corrosion of first degree of unspecified ▽ multiple fingers (nail), including thumb

√6ᵗʰ **T23.55** Corrosion of first degree of palm

　√7ᵗʰ **T23.551** Corrosion of first degree of right palm

　√7ᵗʰ **T23.552** Corrosion of first degree of left palm

　√7ᵗʰ **T23.559** Corrosion of first degree of unspecified ▽ palm

√6ᵗʰ **T23.56** Corrosion of first degree of back of hand

　√7ᵗʰ **T23.561** Corrosion of first degree of back of right hand

　√7ᵗʰ **T23.562** Corrosion of first degree of back of left hand

　√7ᵗʰ **T23.569** Corrosion of first degree of back of ▽ unspecified hand

√6ᵗʰ **T23.57** Corrosion of first degree of wrist

　√7ᵗʰ **T23.571** Corrosion of first degree of right wrist

　√7ᵗʰ **T23.572** Corrosion of first degree of left wrist

　√7ᵗʰ **T23.579** Corrosion of first degree of unspecified ▽ wrist

√6ᵗʰ **T23.59** Corrosion of first degree of multiple sites of wrist and hand

　√7ᵗʰ **T23.591** Corrosion of first degree of multiple sites of right wrist and hand

　√7ᵗʰ **T23.592** Corrosion of first degree of multiple sites of left wrist and hand

　√7ᵗʰ **T23.599** Corrosion of first degree of multiple ▽ sites of unspecified wrist and hand

√5ᵗʰ **T23.6** Corrosion of second degree of wrist and hand

Code first (T51-T65) to identify chemical and intent

Use additional external cause code to identify place (Y92)

√6ᵗʰ **T23.60** Corrosion of second degree of hand, unspecified site

　√7ᵗʰ **T23.601** Corrosion of second degree of right ▽ hand, unspecified site

　√7ᵗʰ **T23.602** Corrosion of second degree of left ▽ hand, unspecified site

　√7ᵗʰ **T23.609** Corrosion of second degree of ▽ unspecified hand, unspecified site

√6ᵗʰ **T23.61** Corrosion of second degree of thumb (nail)

　√7ᵗʰ **T23.611** Corrosion of second degree of right thumb (nail)

　√7ᵗʰ **T23.612** Corrosion of second degree of left thumb (nail)

　√7ᵗʰ **T23.619** Corrosion of second degree of ▽ unspecified thumb (nail)

√6ᵗʰ **T23.62** Corrosion of second degree of single finger (nail) except thumb

　√7ᵗʰ **T23.621** Corrosion of second degree of single right finger (nail) except thumb

　√7ᵗʰ **T23.622** Corrosion of second degree of single left finger (nail) except thumb

　√7ᵗʰ **T23.629** Corrosion of second degree of ▽ unspecified single finger (nail) except thumb

√6ᵗʰ **T23.63** Corrosion of second degree of multiple fingers (nail), not including thumb

　√7ᵗʰ **T23.631** Corrosion of second degree of multiple right fingers (nail), not including thumb

　√7ᵗʰ **T23.632** Corrosion of second degree of multiple left fingers (nail), not including thumb

　√7ᵗʰ **T23.639** Corrosion of second degree of ▽ unspecified multiple fingers (nail), not including thumb

√6ᵗʰ **T23.64** Corrosion of second degree of multiple fingers (nail), including thumb

　√7ᵗʰ **T23.641** Corrosion of second degree of multiple right fingers (nail), including thumb

　√7ᵗʰ **T23.642** Corrosion of second degree of multiple left fingers (nail), including thumb

　√7ᵗʰ **T23.649** Corrosion of second degree of ▽ unspecified multiple fingers (nail), including thumb

√6ᵗʰ **T23.65** Corrosion of second degree of palm

　√7ᵗʰ **T23.651** Corrosion of second degree of right palm

　√7ᵗʰ **T23.652** Corrosion of second degree of left palm

　√7ᵗʰ **T23.659** Corrosion of second degree of ▽ unspecified palm

√6ᵗʰ **T23.66** Corrosion of second degree of back of hand

　√7ᵗʰ **T23.661** Corrosion of second degree back of right hand

　√7ᵗʰ **T23.662** Corrosion of second degree back of left hand

　√7ᵗʰ **T23.669** Corrosion of second degree back of ▽ unspecified hand

√6ᵗʰ **T23.67** Corrosion of second degree of wrist

　√7ᵗʰ **T23.671** Corrosion of second degree of right wrist

　√7ᵗʰ **T23.672** Corrosion of second degree of left wrist

　√7ᵗʰ **T23.679** Corrosion of second degree of ▽ unspecified wrist

√6ᵗʰ **T23.69** Corrosion of second degree of multiple sites of wrist and hand

　√7ᵗʰ **T23.691** Corrosion of second degree of multiple sites of right wrist and hand

　√7ᵗʰ **T23.692** Corrosion of second degree of multiple sites of left wrist and hand

　√7ᵗʰ **T23.699** Corrosion of second degree of multiple ▽ sites of unspecified wrist and hand

√5ᵗʰ **T23.7** Corrosion of third degree of wrist and hand

Code first (T51-T65) to identify chemical and intent

Use additional external cause code to identify place (Y92)

√6ᵗʰ **T23.70** Corrosion of third degree of hand, unspecified site

　√7ᵗʰ **T23.701** Corrosion of third degree of right hand, ▽ unspecified site

　√7ᵗʰ **T23.702** Corrosion of third degree of left hand, ▽ unspecified site

　√7ᵗʰ **T23.709** Corrosion of third degree of ▽ unspecified hand, unspecified site

√6ᵗʰ **T23.71** Corrosion of third degree of thumb (nail)

　√7ᵗʰ **T23.711** Corrosion of third degree of right thumb (nail)

　√7ᵗʰ **T23.712** Corrosion of third degree of left thumb (nail)

　√7ᵗʰ **T23.719** Corrosion of third degree of ▽ unspecified thumb (nail)

√6ᵗʰ **T23.72** Corrosion of third degree of single finger (nail) except thumb

　√7ᵗʰ **T23.721** Corrosion of third degree of single right finger (nail) except thumb

---

☑ Additional Character Req　　√x7ᵗʰ Placeholder Alert　　Manifestation　　HCC CMS-HCC Condition　　▽ Unspecified Code　　►◄ Revised Text　　● New Code　　▲ Revised Code Title

ICD-10-CM 2018

1049

√7th **T23.722** Corrosion of third degree of single left finger (nail) except thumb

√7th **T23.729** Corrosion of third degree of unspecified single finger (nail) except thumb ▽

√6th **T23.73** Corrosion of third degree of multiple fingers (nail), not including thumb

√7th **T23.731** Corrosion of third degree of multiple right fingers (nail), not including thumb

√7th **T23.732** Corrosion of third degree of multiple left fingers (nail), not including thumb

√7th **T23.739** Corrosion of third degree of unspecified multiple fingers (nail), not including thumb ▽

√6th **T23.74** Corrosion of third degree of multiple fingers (nail), including thumb

√7th **T23.741** Corrosion of third degree of multiple right fingers (nail), including thumb

√7th **T23.742** Corrosion of third degree of multiple left fingers (nail), including thumb

√7th **T23.749** Corrosion of third degree of unspecified multiple fingers (nail), including thumb ▽

√6th **T23.75** Corrosion of third degree of palm

√7th **T23.751** Corrosion of third degree of right palm

√7th **T23.752** Corrosion of third degree of left palm

√7th **T23.759** Corrosion of third degree of unspecified palm ▽

√6th **T23.76** Corrosion of third degree of back of hand

√7th **T23.761** Corrosion of third degree of back of right hand

√7th **T23.762** Corrosion of third degree of back of left hand

√7th **T23.769** Corrosion of third degree back of unspecified hand ▽

√6th **T23.77** Corrosion of third degree of wrist

√7th **T23.771** Corrosion of third degree of right wrist

√7th **T23.772** Corrosion of third degree of left wrist

√7th **T23.779** Corrosion of third degree of unspecified wrist ▽

√6th **T23.79** Corrosion of third degree of multiple sites of wrist and hand

√7th **T23.791** Corrosion of third degree of multiple sites of right wrist and hand

√7th **T23.792** Corrosion of third degree of multiple sites of left wrist and hand

√7th **T23.799** Corrosion of third degree of multiple sites of unspecified wrist and hand ▽

√4th **T24** Burn and corrosion of lower limb, except ankle and foot

> EXCLUDES 2   burn and corrosion of ankle and foot (T25.-)
> burn and corrosion of hip region (T21.-)

> The appropriate 7th character is to be added to each code from category T24.
> A   initial encounter
> D   subsequent encounter
> S   sequela

√5th **T24.0** Burn of unspecified degree of lower limb, except ankle and foot

> Use additional external cause code to identify the source, place and intent of the burn (X00-X19, X75-X77, X96-X98, Y92)

√6th **T24.00** Burn of unspecified degree of unspecified site of lower limb, except ankle and foot

√7th **T24.001** Burn of unspecified degree of unspecified site of right lower limb, except ankle and foot ▽

√7th **T24.002** Burn of unspecified degree of unspecified site of left lower limb, except ankle and foot ▽

√7th **T24.009** Burn of unspecified degree of unspecified site of unspecified lower limb, except ankle and foot ▽

√6th **T24.01** Burn of unspecified degree of thigh

√7th **T24.011** Burn of unspecified degree of right thigh ▽

√7th **T24.012** Burn of unspecified degree of left thigh ▽

√7th **T24.019** Burn of unspecified degree of unspecified thigh ▽

√6th **T24.02** Burn of unspecified degree of knee

√7th **T24.021** Burn of unspecified degree of right knee ▽

√7th **T24.022** Burn of unspecified degree of left knee ▽

√7th **T24.029** Burn of unspecified degree of unspecified knee ▽

√6th **T24.03** Burn of unspecified degree of lower leg

√7th **T24.031** Burn of unspecified degree of right lower leg ▽

√7th **T24.032** Burn of unspecified degree of left lower leg ▽

√7th **T24.039** Burn of unspecified degree of unspecified lower leg ▽

√6th **T24.09** Burn of unspecified degree of multiple sites of lower limb, except ankle and foot

√7th **T24.091** Burn of unspecified degree of multiple sites of right lower limb, except ankle and foot ▽

√7th **T24.092** Burn of unspecified degree of multiple sites of left lower limb, except ankle and foot ▽

√7th **T24.099** Burn of unspecified degree of multiple sites of unspecified lower limb, except ankle and foot ▽

√5th **T24.1** Burn of first degree of lower limb, except ankle and foot

> Use additional external cause code to identify the source, place and intent of the burn (X00-X19, X75-X77, X96-X98, Y92)

√6th **T24.10** Burn of first degree of unspecified site of lower limb, except ankle and foot

√7th **T24.101** Burn of first degree of unspecified site of right lower limb, except ankle and foot ▽

√7th **T24.102** Burn of first degree of unspecified site of left lower limb, except ankle and foot ▽

√7th **T24.109** Burn of first degree of unspecified site of unspecified lower limb, except ankle and foot ▽

√6th **T24.11** Burn of first degree of thigh

√7th **T24.111** Burn of first degree of right thigh

√7th **T24.112** Burn of first degree of left thigh

√7th **T24.119** Burn of first degree of unspecified thigh ▽

√6th **T24.12** Burn of first degree of knee

√7th **T24.121** Burn of first degree of right knee

√7th **T24.122** Burn of first degree of left knee

√7th **T24.129** Burn of first degree of unspecified knee ▽

√6th **T24.13** Burn of first degree of lower leg

√7th **T24.131** Burn of first degree of right lower leg

√7th **T24.132** Burn of first degree of left lower leg

√7th **T24.139** Burn of first degree of unspecified lower leg ▽

√6th **T24.19** Burn of first degree of multiple sites of lower limb, except ankle and foot

√7th **T24.191** Burn of first degree of multiple sites of right lower limb, except ankle and foot

√7th **T24.192** Burn of first degree of multiple sites of left lower limb, except ankle and foot

√7th **T24.199** Burn of first degree of multiple sites of unspecified lower limb, except ankle and foot ▽

√5th **T24.2** Burn of second degree of lower limb, except ankle and foot

> Use additional external cause code to identify the source, place and intent of the burn (X00-X19, X75-X77, X96-X98, Y92)

√6th **T24.20** Burn of second degree of unspecified site of lower limb, except ankle and foot

√7th **T24.201** Burn of second degree of unspecified site of right lower limb, except ankle and foot ▽

EXCLUDES 1 Not coded here   EXCLUDES 2 Not included here   N Newborn Age: 0   P Pediatric Age: 0-17   M Maternity Age: 12-55   A Adult Age: 15-124

1050   ICD-10-CM 2018

☑7ᵗʰ **T24.202** Burn of second degree of unspecified site of **left** lower limb, except ankle and foot ▽

☑7ᵗʰ **T24.209** Burn of second degree of unspecified site of unspecified lower limb, except ankle and foot ▽

☑6ᵗʰ **T24.21** Burn of second degree of thigh

     ☑7ᵗʰ **T24.211** Burn of second degree of right thigh

     ☑7ᵗʰ **T24.212** Burn of second degree of left thigh

     ☑7ᵗʰ **T24.219** Burn of second degree of unspecified thigh ▽

☑6ᵗʰ **T24.22** Burn of second degree of knee

     ☑7ᵗʰ **T24.221** Burn of second degree of right knee

     ☑7ᵗʰ **T24.222** Burn of second degree of left knee

     ☑7ᵗʰ **T24.229** Burn of second degree of unspecified knee ▽

☑6ᵗʰ **T24.23** Burn of second degree of lower leg

     ☑7ᵗʰ **T24.231** Burn of second degree of right lower leg

     ☑7ᵗʰ **T24.232** Burn of second degree of left lower leg

     ☑7ᵗʰ **T24.239** Burn of second degree of unspecified lower leg ▽

☑6ᵗʰ **T24.29** Burn of second degree of multiple sites of lower limb, except ankle and foot

     ☑7ᵗʰ **T24.291** Burn of second degree of multiple sites of right lower limb, except ankle and foot

     ☑7ᵗʰ **T24.292** Burn of second degree of multiple sites of left lower limb, except ankle and foot

     ☑7ᵗʰ **T24.299** Burn of second degree of multiple sites of unspecified lower limb, except ankle and foot ▽

☑5ᵗʰ **T24.3** Burn of third degree of lower limb, except ankle and foot
     Use additional external cause code to identify the source, place and intent of the burn (X00-X19, X75-X77, X96-X98, Y92)

☑6ᵗʰ **T24.30** Burn of third degree of unspecified site of lower limb, except ankle and foot

     ☑7ᵗʰ **T24.301** Burn of third degree of unspecified site of right lower limb, except ankle and foot ▽

     ☑7ᵗʰ **T24.302** Burn of third degree of unspecified site of **left** lower limb, except ankle and foot ▽

     ☑7ᵗʰ **T24.309** Burn of third degree of unspecified site of unspecified lower limb, except ankle and foot ▽

☑6ᵗʰ **T24.31** Burn of third degree of thigh

     ☑7ᵗʰ **T24.311** Burn of third degree of right thigh

     ☑7ᵗʰ **T24.312** Burn of third degree of left thigh

     ☑7ᵗʰ **T24.319** Burn of third degree of unspecified thigh ▽

☑6ᵗʰ **T24.32** Burn of third degree of knee

     ☑7ᵗʰ **T24.321** Burn of third degree of right knee

     ☑7ᵗʰ **T24.322** Burn of third degree of left knee

     ☑7ᵗʰ **T24.329** Burn of third degree of unspecified knee ▽

☑6ᵗʰ **T24.33** Burn of third degree of lower leg

     ☑7ᵗʰ **T24.331** Burn of third degree of right lower leg

     ☑7ᵗʰ **T24.332** Burn of third degree of left lower leg

     ☑7ᵗʰ **T24.339** Burn of third degree of unspecified lower leg ▽

☑6ᵗʰ **T24.39** Burn of third degree of multiple sites of lower limb, except ankle and foot
     AHA: 2016, 2Q, 4

     ☑7ᵗʰ **T24.391** Burn of third degree of multiple sites of right lower limb, except ankle and foot

     ☑7ᵗʰ **T24.392** Burn of third degree of multiple sites of left lower limb, except ankle and foot

     ☑7ᵗʰ **T24.399** Burn of third degree of multiple sites of unspecified lower limb, except ankle and foot ▽

☑5ᵗʰ **T24.4** Corrosion of unspecified degree of lower limb, except ankle and foot
     Code first (T51-T65) to identify chemical and intent
     Use additional external cause code to identify place (Y92)

☑6ᵗʰ **T24.40** Corrosion of unspecified degree of unspecified site of lower limb, except ankle and foot

     ☑7ᵗʰ **T24.401** Corrosion of unspecified degree of unspecified site of right lower limb, except ankle and foot ▽

     ☑7ᵗʰ **T24.402** Corrosion of unspecified degree of unspecified site of left lower limb, except ankle and foot ▽

     ☑7ᵗʰ **T24.409** Corrosion of unspecified degree of unspecified site of unspecified lower limb, except ankle and foot ▽

☑6ᵗʰ **T24.41** Corrosion of unspecified degree of thigh

     ☑7ᵗʰ **T24.411** Corrosion of unspecified degree of right thigh ▽

     ☑7ᵗʰ **T24.412** Corrosion of unspecified degree of left thigh ▽

     ☑7ᵗʰ **T24.419** Corrosion of unspecified degree of unspecified thigh ▽

☑6ᵗʰ **T24.42** Corrosion of unspecified degree of knee

     ☑7ᵗʰ **T24.421** Corrosion of unspecified degree of right knee ▽

     ☑7ᵗʰ **T24.422** Corrosion of unspecified degree of left knee ▽

     ☑7ᵗʰ **T24.429** Corrosion of unspecified degree of unspecified knee ▽

☑6ᵗʰ **T24.43** Corrosion of unspecified degree of lower leg

     ☑7ᵗʰ **T24.431** Corrosion of unspecified degree of right lower leg ▽

     ☑7ᵗʰ **T24.432** Corrosion of unspecified degree of left lower leg ▽

     ☑7ᵗʰ **T24.439** Corrosion of unspecified degree of unspecified lower leg ▽

☑6ᵗʰ **T24.49** Corrosion of unspecified degree of multiple sites of lower limb, except ankle and foot

     ☑7ᵗʰ **T24.491** Corrosion of unspecified degree of multiple sites of right lower limb, except ankle and foot ▽

     ☑7ᵗʰ **T24.492** Corrosion of unspecified degree of multiple sites of left lower limb, except ankle and foot ▽

     ☑7ᵗʰ **T24.499** Corrosion of unspecified degree of multiple sites of unspecified lower limb, except ankle and foot ▽

☑5ᵗʰ **T24.5** Corrosion of first degree of lower limb, except ankle and foot
     Code first (T51-T65) to identify chemical and intent
     Use additional external cause code to identify place (Y92)

☑6ᵗʰ **T24.50** Corrosion of first degree of unspecified site of lower limb, except ankle and foot

     ☑7ᵗʰ **T24.501** Corrosion of first degree of unspecified site of right lower limb, except ankle and foot ▽

     ☑7ᵗʰ **T24.502** Corrosion of first degree of unspecified site of left lower limb, except ankle and foot ▽

     ☑7ᵗʰ **T24.509** Corrosion of first degree of unspecified site of unspecified lower limb, except ankle and foot ▽

☑6ᵗʰ **T24.51** Corrosion of first degree of thigh

     ☑7ᵗʰ **T24.511** Corrosion of first degree of right thigh

     ☑7ᵗʰ **T24.512** Corrosion of first degree of left thigh

     ☑7ᵗʰ **T24.519** Corrosion of first degree of unspecified thigh ▽

☑6ᵗʰ **T24.52** Corrosion of first degree of knee

     ☑7ᵗʰ **T24.521** Corrosion of first degree of right knee

     ☑7ᵗʰ **T24.522** Corrosion of first degree of left knee

     ☑7ᵗʰ **T24.529** Corrosion of first degree of unspecified knee ▽

☑6ᵗʰ **T24.53** Corrosion of first degree of lower leg

     ☑7ᵗʰ **T24.531** Corrosion of first degree of right lower leg

     ☑7ᵗʰ **T24.532** Corrosion of first degree of left lower leg

☑ Additional Character Req   ☑7ᵗʰ Placeholder Alert   Manifestation   HCC CMS-HCC Condition   ▽ Unspecified Code   ►◄ Revised Text   ● New Code   ▲ Revised Code Title

ICD-10-CM 2018   **1051**

Chapter 19. Injury, Poisoning, and Certain Other Consequences of External Causes

T24.202–T24.532

√6ᵗʰ **T24.539** Corrosion of first degree of unspecified ▽
lower leg

√6ᵗʰ **T24.59** Corrosion of first degree of multiple sites of lower
limb, except ankle and foot

√7ᵗʰ **T24.591** Corrosion of first degree of multiple sites
of right lower limb, except ankle and foot

√7ᵗʰ **T24.592** Corrosion of first degree of multiple sites
of left lower limb, except ankle and foot

√7ᵗʰ **T24.599** Corrosion of first degree of multiple ▽
sites of unspecified lower limb, except
ankle and foot

√5ᵗʰ **T24.6** Corrosion of second degree of lower limb, except ankle and
foot
Code first (T51-T65) to identify chemical and intent
Use additional external cause code to identify place (Y92)

√6ᵗʰ **T24.60** Corrosion of second degree of unspecified site of
lower limb, except ankle and foot

√7ᵗʰ **T24.601** Corrosion of second degree of ▽
unspecified site of right lower limb,
except ankle and foot

√7ᵗʰ **T24.602** Corrosion of second degree of ▽
unspecified site of left lower limb,
except ankle and foot

√7ᵗʰ **T24.609** Corrosion of second degree of ▽
unspecified site of unspecified lower
limb, except ankle and foot

√6ᵗʰ **T24.61** Corrosion of second degree of thigh

√7ᵗʰ **T24.611** Corrosion of second degree of right thigh

√7ᵗʰ **T24.612** Corrosion of second degree of left thigh

√7ᵗʰ **T24.619** Corrosion of second degree of ▽
unspecified thigh

√6ᵗʰ **T24.62** Corrosion of second degree of knee

√7ᵗʰ **T24.621** Corrosion of second degree of right knee

√7ᵗʰ **T24.622** Corrosion of second degree of left knee

√7ᵗʰ **T24.629** Corrosion of second degree of ▽
unspecified knee

√6ᵗʰ **T24.63** Corrosion of second degree of lower leg

√7ᵗʰ **T24.631** Corrosion of second degree of right lower
leg

√7ᵗʰ **T24.632** Corrosion of second degree of left lower
leg

√7ᵗʰ **T24.639** Corrosion of second degree of ▽
unspecified lower leg

√6ᵗʰ **T24.69** Corrosion of second degree of multiple sites of lower
limb, except ankle and foot

√7ᵗʰ **T24.691** Corrosion of second degree of multiple
sites of right lower limb, except ankle and
foot

√7ᵗʰ **T24.692** Corrosion of second degree of multiple
sites of left lower limb, except ankle and
foot

√7ᵗʰ **T24.699** Corrosion of second degree of multiple ▽
sites of unspecified lower limb, except
ankle and foot

√5ᵗʰ **T24.7** Corrosion of third degree of lower limb, except ankle and foot
Code first (T51-T65) to identify chemical and intent
Use additional external cause code to identify place (Y92)

√6ᵗʰ **T24.70** Corrosion of third degree of unspecified site of lower
limb, except ankle and foot

√7ᵗʰ **T24.701** Corrosion of third degree of ▽
unspecified site of right lower limb,
except ankle and foot

√7ᵗʰ **T24.702** Corrosion of third degree of ▽
unspecified site of left lower limb,
except ankle and foot

√7ᵗʰ **T24.709** Corrosion of third degree of ▽
unspecified site of unspecified lower
limb, except ankle and foot

√6ᵗʰ **T24.71** Corrosion of third degree of thigh

√7ᵗʰ **T24.711** Corrosion of third degree of right thigh

√7ᵗʰ **T24.712** Corrosion of third degree of left thigh

√7ᵗʰ **T24.719** Corrosion of third degree of ▽
unspecified thigh

√6ᵗʰ **T24.72** Corrosion of third degree of knee

√7ᵗʰ **T24.721** Corrosion of third degree of right knee

√7ᵗʰ **T24.722** Corrosion of third degree of left knee

√7ᵗʰ **T24.729** Corrosion of third degree of ▽
unspecified knee

√6ᵗʰ **T24.73** Corrosion of third degree of lower leg

√7ᵗʰ **T24.731** Corrosion of third degree of right lower
leg

√7ᵗʰ **T24.732** Corrosion of third degree of left lower leg

√7ᵗʰ **T24.739** Corrosion of third degree of ▽
unspecified lower leg

√6ᵗʰ **T24.79** Corrosion of third degree of multiple sites of lower
limb, except ankle and foot

√7ᵗʰ **T24.791** Corrosion of third degree of multiple sites
of right lower limb, except ankle and foot

√7ᵗʰ **T24.792** Corrosion of third degree of multiple sites
of left lower limb, except ankle and foot

√7ᵗʰ **T24.799** Corrosion of third degree of multiple ▽
sites of unspecified lower limb, except
ankle and foot

√4ᵗʰ **T25** **Burn and corrosion of ankle and foot**

> The appropriate 7th character is to be added to each code from
> category T25.
> A   initial encounter
> D   subsequent encounter
> S   sequela

√5ᵗʰ **T25.0** Burn of unspecified degree of ankle and foot
Use additional external cause code to identify the source, place
and intent of the burn (X00-X19, X75-X77, X96-X98, Y92)

√6ᵗʰ **T25.01** Burn of unspecified degree of ankle

√7ᵗʰ **T25.011** Burn of unspecified degree of right ▽
ankle

√7ᵗʰ **T25.012** Burn of unspecified degree of left ▽
ankle

√7ᵗʰ **T25.019** Burn of unspecified degree of ▽
unspecified ankle

√6ᵗʰ **T25.02** Burn of unspecified degree of foot
EXCLUDES 2   burn of unspecified degree of toe(s) (nail)
(T25.03-)

√7ᵗʰ **T25.021** Burn of unspecified degree of right ▽
foot

√7ᵗʰ **T25.022** Burn of unspecified degree of left ▽
foot

√7ᵗʰ **T25.029** Burn of unspecified degree of ▽
unspecified foot

√6ᵗʰ **T25.03** Burn of unspecified degree of toe(s) (nail)

√7ᵗʰ **T25.031** Burn of unspecified degree of right ▽
toe(s) (nail)

√7ᵗʰ **T25.032** Burn of unspecified degree of left ▽
toe(s) (nail)

√7ᵗʰ **T25.039** Burn of unspecified degree of ▽
unspecified toe(s) (nail)

√6ᵗʰ **T25.09** Burn of unspecified degree of multiple sites of ankle
and foot

√7ᵗʰ **T25.091** Burn of unspecified degree of ▽
multiple sites of right ankle and foot

√7ᵗʰ **T25.092** Burn of unspecified degree of ▽
multiple sites of left ankle and foot

√7ᵗʰ **T25.099** Burn of unspecified degree of ▽
multiple sites of unspecified ankle
and foot

√5ᵗʰ **T25.1** Burn of first degree of ankle and foot
Use additional external cause code to identify the source, place
and intent of the burn (X00-X19, X75-X77, X96-X98, Y92)

√6ᵗʰ **T25.11** Burn of first degree of ankle

√7ᵗʰ **T25.111** Burn of first degree of right ankle

√7ᵗʰ **T25.112** Burn of first degree of left ankle

√7ᵗʰ **T25.119** Burn of first degree of unspecified ▽
ankle

√6ᵗʰ **T25.12** Burn of first degree of foot
EXCLUDES 2   burn of first degree of toe(s) (nail) (T25.13-)

√7ᵗʰ **T25.121** Burn of first degree of right foot

√7ᵗʰ **T25.122** Burn of first degree of left foot

Chapter 19. Injury, Poisoning, and Certain Other Consequences of External Causes

✓7ᵗʰ **T25.129** Burn of first degree of unspecified ▽
foot

✓6ᵗʰ **T25.13** Burn of first degree of toe(s) (nail)

   ✓7ᵗʰ **T25.131** Burn of first degree of right toe(s) (nail)

   ✓7ᵗʰ **T25.132** Burn of first degree of left toe(s) (nail)

   ✓7ᵗʰ **T25.139** Burn of first degree of unspecified ▽
toe(s) (nail)

✓6ᵗʰ **T25.19** Burn of first degree of multiple sites of ankle and
foot

   ✓7ᵗʰ **T25.191** Burn of first degree of multiple sites of
right ankle and foot

   ✓7ᵗʰ **T25.192** Burn of first degree of multiple sites of left
ankle and foot

   ✓7ᵗʰ **T25.199** Burn of first degree of multiple sites ▽
of unspecified ankle and foot

✓5ᵗʰ **T25.2** Burn of second degree of ankle and foot
Use additional external cause code to identify the source, place
and intent of the burn (X00-X19, X75-X77, X96-X98, Y92)

✓6ᵗʰ **T25.21** Burn of second degree of ankle

   ✓7ᵗʰ **T25.211** Burn of second degree of right ankle

   ✓7ᵗʰ **T25.212** Burn of second degree of left ankle

   ✓7ᵗʰ **T25.219** Burn of second degree of unspecified ▽
ankle

✓6ᵗʰ **T25.22** Burn of second degree of foot
EXCLUDES 2   burn of second degree of toe(s) (nail)
(T25.23-)

   ✓7ᵗʰ **T25.221** Burn of second degree of right foot

   ✓7ᵗʰ **T25.222** Burn of second degree of left foot

   ✓7ᵗʰ **T25.229** Burn of second degree of unspecified ▽
foot

✓6ᵗʰ **T25.23** Burn of second degree of toe(s) (nail)

   ✓7ᵗʰ **T25.231** Burn of second degree of right toe(s) (nail)

   ✓7ᵗʰ **T25.232** Burn of second degree of left toe(s) (nail)

   ✓7ᵗʰ **T25.239** Burn of second degree of unspecified ▽
toe(s) (nail)

✓6ᵗʰ **T25.29** Burn of second degree of multiple sites of ankle and
foot

   ✓7ᵗʰ **T25.291** Burn of second degree of multiple sites of
right ankle and foot

   ✓7ᵗʰ **T25.292** Burn of second degree of multiple sites of
left ankle and foot

   ✓7ᵗʰ **T25.299** Burn of second degree of multiple sites ▽
of unspecified ankle and foot

✓5ᵗʰ **T25.3** Burn of third degree of ankle and foot
Use additional external cause code to identify the source, place
and intent of the burn (X00-X19, X75-X77, X96-X98, Y92)

✓6ᵗʰ **T25.31** Burn of third degree of ankle

   ✓7ᵗʰ **T25.311** Burn of third degree of right ankle

   ✓7ᵗʰ **T25.312** Burn of third degree of left ankle

   ✓7ᵗʰ **T25.319** Burn of third degree of unspecified ▽
ankle

✓6ᵗʰ **T25.32** Burn of third degree of foot
EXCLUDES 2   burn of third degree of toe(s) (nail) (T25.33-)

   ✓7ᵗʰ **T25.321** Burn of third degree of right foot

   ✓7ᵗʰ **T25.322** Burn of third degree of left foot

   ✓7ᵗʰ **T25.329** Burn of third degree of unspecified ▽
foot

✓6ᵗʰ **T25.33** Burn of third degree of toe(s) (nail)

   ✓7ᵗʰ **T25.331** Burn of third degree of right toe(s) (nail)

   ✓7ᵗʰ **T25.332** Burn of third degree of left toe(s) (nail)

   ✓7ᵗʰ **T25.339** Burn of third degree of unspecified ▽
toe(s) (nail)

✓6ᵗʰ **T25.39** Burn of third degree of multiple sites of ankle and
foot

   ✓7ᵗʰ **T25.391** Burn of third degree of multiple sites of
right ankle and foot

   ✓7ᵗʰ **T25.392** Burn of third degree of multiple sites of
left ankle and foot

   ✓7ᵗʰ **T25.399** Burn of third degree of multiple sites ▽
of unspecified ankle and foot

✓5ᵗʰ **T25.4** Corrosion of unspecified degree of ankle and foot
Code first (T51-T65) to identify chemical and intent
Use additional external cause code to identify place (Y92)

✓6ᵗʰ **T25.41** Corrosion of unspecified degree of ankle

   ✓7ᵗʰ **T25.411** Corrosion of unspecified degree of ▽
right ankle

   ✓7ᵗʰ **T25.412** Corrosion of unspecified degree of ▽
left ankle

   ✓7ᵗʰ **T25.419** Corrosion of unspecified degree of ▽
unspecified ankle

✓6ᵗʰ **T25.42** Corrosion of unspecified degree of foot
EXCLUDES 2   corrosion of unspecified degree of toe(s)
(nail) (T25.43-)

   ✓7ᵗʰ **T25.421** Corrosion of unspecified degree of ▽
right foot

   ✓7ᵗʰ **T25.422** Corrosion of unspecified degree of ▽
left foot

   ✓7ᵗʰ **T25.429** Corrosion of unspecified degree of ▽
unspecified foot

✓6ᵗʰ **T25.43** Corrosion of unspecified degree of toe(s) (nail)

   ✓7ᵗʰ **T25.431** Corrosion of unspecified degree of ▽
right toe(s) (nail)

   ✓7ᵗʰ **T25.432** Corrosion of unspecified degree of ▽
left toe(s) (nail)

   ✓7ᵗʰ **T25.439** Corrosion of unspecified degree of ▽
unspecified toe(s) (nail)

✓6ᵗʰ **T25.49** Corrosion of unspecified degree of multiple sites of
ankle and foot

   ✓7ᵗʰ **T25.491** Corrosion of unspecified degree of ▽
multiple sites of right ankle and foot

   ✓7ᵗʰ **T25.492** Corrosion of unspecified degree of ▽
multiple sites of left ankle and foot

   ✓7ᵗʰ **T25.499** Corrosion of unspecified degree of ▽
multiple sites of unspecified ankle and
foot

✓5ᵗʰ **T25.5** Corrosion of first degree of ankle and foot
Code first (T51-T65) to identify chemical and intent
Use additional external cause code to identify place (Y92)

✓6ᵗʰ **T25.51** Corrosion of first degree of ankle

   ✓7ᵗʰ **T25.511** Corrosion of first degree of right ankle

   ✓7ᵗʰ **T25.512** Corrosion of first degree of left ankle

   ✓7ᵗʰ **T25.519** Corrosion of first degree of unspecified ▽
ankle

✓6ᵗʰ **T25.52** Corrosion of first degree of foot
EXCLUDES 2   corrosion of first degree of toe(s) (nail)
(T25.53-)

   ✓7ᵗʰ **T25.521** Corrosion of first degree of right foot

   ✓7ᵗʰ **T25.522** Corrosion of first degree of left foot

   ✓7ᵗʰ **T25.529** Corrosion of first degree of unspecified ▽
foot

✓6ᵗʰ **T25.53** Corrosion of first degree of toe(s) (nail)

   ✓7ᵗʰ **T25.531** Corrosion of first degree of right toe(s)
(nail)

   ✓7ᵗʰ **T25.532** Corrosion of first degree of left toe(s) (nail)

   ✓7ᵗʰ **T25.539** Corrosion of first degree of unspecified ▽
toe(s) (nail)

✓6ᵗʰ **T25.59** Corrosion of first degree of multiple sites of ankle
and foot

   ✓7ᵗʰ **T25.591** Corrosion of first degree of multiple sites
of right ankle and foot

   ✓7ᵗʰ **T25.592** Corrosion of first degree of multiple sites
of left ankle and foot

   ✓7ᵗʰ **T25.599** Corrosion of first degree of multiple ▽
sites of unspecified ankle and foot

✓5ᵗʰ **T25.6** Corrosion of second degree of ankle and foot
Code first (T51-T65) to identify chemical and intent
Use additional external cause code to identify place (Y92)

✓6ᵗʰ **T25.61** Corrosion of second degree of ankle

   ✓7ᵗʰ **T25.611** Corrosion of second degree of right ankle

   ✓7ᵗʰ **T25.612** Corrosion of second degree of left ankle

   ✓7ᵗʰ **T25.619** Corrosion of second degree of ▽
unspecified ankle

T25.129–T25.619

☑ Additional Character Req   ✓7ᵗʰ Placeholder Alert   Manifestation   HCC CMS-HCC Condition   ▽ Unspecified Code   ►◄ Revised Text   ● New Code   ▲ Revised Code Title

ICD-10-CM 2018   1053

✓6ᵗʰ **T25.62 Corrosion of second degree of foot**
EXCLUDES 2 *corrosion of second degree of toe(s) (nail) (T25.63-)*

    ✓7ᵗʰ **T25.621 Corrosion of second degree of right foot**

    ✓7ᵗʰ **T25.622 Corrosion of second degree of left foot**

    ✓7ᵗʰ **T25.629 Corrosion of second degree of unspecified foot** ▽

✓6ᵗʰ **T25.63 Corrosion of second degree of toe(s) (nail)**

    ✓7ᵗʰ **T25.631 Corrosion of second degree of right toe(s) (nail)**

    ✓7ᵗʰ **T25.632 Corrosion of second degree of left toe(s) (nail)**

    ✓7ᵗʰ **T25.639 Corrosion of second degree of unspecified toe(s) (nail)** ▽

✓6ᵗʰ **T25.69 Corrosion of second degree of multiple sites of ankle and foot**

    ✓7ᵗʰ **T25.691 Corrosion of second degree of right ankle and foot**

    ✓7ᵗʰ **T25.692 Corrosion of second degree of left ankle and foot**

    ✓7ᵗʰ **T25.699 Corrosion of second degree of unspecified ankle and foot** ▽

✓5ᵗʰ **T25.7 Corrosion of third degree of ankle and foot**
Code first (T51-T65) to identify chemical and intent
Use additional external cause code to identify place (Y92)

  ✓6ᵗʰ **T25.71 Corrosion of third degree of ankle**

    ✓7ᵗʰ **T25.711 Corrosion of third degree of right ankle**

    ✓7ᵗʰ **T25.712 Corrosion of third degree of left ankle**

    ✓7ᵗʰ **T25.719 Corrosion of third degree of unspecified ankle** ▽

  ✓6ᵗʰ **T25.72 Corrosion of third degree of foot**
EXCLUDES 2 *corrosion of third degree of toe(s) (nail) (T25.73-)*

    ✓7ᵗʰ **T25.721 Corrosion of third degree of right foot**

    ✓7ᵗʰ **T25.722 Corrosion of third degree of left foot**

    ✓7ᵗʰ **T25.729 Corrosion of third degree of unspecified foot** ▽

  ✓6ᵗʰ **T25.73 Corrosion of third degree of toe(s) (nail)**

    ✓7ᵗʰ **T25.731 Corrosion of third degree of right toe(s) (nail)**

    ✓7ᵗʰ **T25.732 Corrosion of third degree of left toe(s) (nail)**

    ✓7ᵗʰ **T25.739 Corrosion of third degree of unspecified toe(s) (nail)** ▽

  ✓6ᵗʰ **T25.79 Corrosion of third degree of multiple sites of ankle and foot**

    ✓7ᵗʰ **T25.791 Corrosion of third degree of multiple sites of right ankle and foot**

    ✓7ᵗʰ **T25.792 Corrosion of third degree of multiple sites of left ankle and foot**

    ✓7ᵗʰ **T25.799 Corrosion of third degree of multiple sites of unspecified ankle and foot** ▽

Burns and corrosions confined to eye and internal organs (T26-T28)

✓4ᵗʰ **T26 Burn and corrosion confined to eye and adnexa**

> The appropriate 7th character is to be added to each code from category T26.
> A   initial encounter
> D   subsequent encounter
> S   sequela

✓5ᵗʰ **T26.0 Burn of eyelid and periocular area**
Use additional external cause code to identify the source, place and intent of the burn (X00-X19, X75-X77, X96-X98, Y92)

  ✓x7ᵗʰ **T26.00 Burn of unspecified eyelid and periocular area** ▽

  ✓x7ᵗʰ **T26.01 Burn of right eyelid and periocular area**

  ✓x7ᵗʰ **T26.02 Burn of left eyelid and periocular area**

✓5ᵗʰ **T26.1 Burn of cornea and conjunctival sac**
Use additional external cause code to identify the source, place and intent of the burn (X00-X19, X75-X77, X96-X98, Y92)

  ✓x7ᵗʰ **T26.10 Burn of cornea and conjunctival sac, unspecified eye** ▽

  ✓x7ᵗʰ **T26.11 Burn of cornea and conjunctival sac, right eye**

  ✓x7ᵗʰ **T26.12 Burn of cornea and conjunctival sac, left eye**

✓5ᵗʰ **T26.2 Burn with resulting rupture and destruction of eyeball**
Use additional external cause code to identify the source, place and intent of the burn (X00-X19, X75-X77, X96-X98, Y92)

  ✓x7ᵗʰ **T26.20 Burn with resulting rupture and destruction of unspecified eyeball** ▽

  ✓x7ᵗʰ **T26.21 Burn with resulting rupture and destruction of right eyeball**

  ✓x7ᵗʰ **T26.22 Burn with resulting rupture and destruction of left eyeball**

✓5ᵗʰ **T26.3 Burns of other specified parts of eye and adnexa**
Use additional external cause code to identify the source, place and intent of the burn (X00-X19, X75-X77, X96-X98, Y92)

  ✓x7ᵗʰ **T26.30 Burns of other specified parts of unspecified eye and adnexa** ▽

  ✓x7ᵗʰ **T26.31 Burns of other specified parts of right eye and adnexa**

  ✓x7ᵗʰ **T26.32 Burns of other specified parts of left eye and adnexa**

✓5ᵗʰ **T26.4 Burn of eye and adnexa, part unspecified**
Use additional external cause code to identify the source, place and intent of the burn (X00-X19, X75-X77, X96-X98, Y92)

  ✓x7ᵗʰ **T26.40 Burn of unspecified eye and adnexa, part unspecified** ▽

  ✓x7ᵗʰ **T26.41 Burn of right eye and adnexa, part unspecified** ▽

  ✓x7ᵗʰ **T26.42 Burn of left eye and adnexa, part unspecified** ▽

✓5ᵗʰ **T26.5 Corrosion of eyelid and periocular area**
Code first (T51-T65) to identify chemical and intent
Use additional external cause code to identify place (Y92)

  ✓x7ᵗʰ **T26.50 Corrosion of unspecified eyelid and periocular area** ▽

  ✓x7ᵗʰ **T26.51 Corrosion of right eyelid and periocular area**

  ✓x7ᵗʰ **T26.52 Corrosion of left eyelid and periocular area**

✓5ᵗʰ **T26.6 Corrosion of cornea and conjunctival sac**
Code first (T51-T65) to identify chemical and intent
Use additional external cause code to identify place (Y92)

  ✓x7ᵗʰ **T26.60 Corrosion of cornea and conjunctival sac, unspecified eye** ▽

  ✓x7ᵗʰ **T26.61 Corrosion of cornea and conjunctival sac, right eye**

  ✓x7ᵗʰ **T26.62 Corrosion of cornea and conjunctival sac, left eye**

✓5ᵗʰ **T26.7 Corrosion with resulting rupture and destruction of eyeball**
Code first (T51-T65) to identify chemical and intent
Use additional external cause code to identify place (Y92)

  ✓x7ᵗʰ **T26.70 Corrosion with resulting rupture and destruction of unspecified eyeball** ▽

  ✓x7ᵗʰ **T26.71 Corrosion with resulting rupture and destruction of right eyeball**

  ✓x7ᵗʰ **T26.72 Corrosion with resulting rupture and destruction of left eyeball**

✓5ᵗʰ **T26.8 Corrosions of other specified parts of eye and adnexa**
Code first (T51-T65) to identify chemical and intent
Use additional external cause code to identify place (Y92)

  ✓x7ᵗʰ **T26.80 Corrosions of other specified parts of unspecified eye and adnexa** ▽

  ✓x7ᵗʰ **T26.81 Corrosions of other specified parts of right eye and adnexa**

  ✓x7ᵗʰ **T26.82 Corrosions of other specified parts of left eye and adnexa**

✓5ᵗʰ **T26.9 Corrosion of eye and adnexa, part unspecified**
Code first (T51-T65) to identify chemical and intent
Use additional external cause code to identify place (Y92)

  ✓x7ᵗʰ **T26.90 Corrosion of unspecified eye and adnexa, part unspecified** ▽

  ✓x7ᵗʰ **T26.91 Corrosion of right eye and adnexa, part unspecified** ▽

  ✓x7ᵗʰ **T26.92 Corrosion of left eye and adnexa, part unspecified** ▽

EXCLUDES 1 Not coded here   EXCLUDES 2 Not included here   N Newborn Age: 0   P Pediatric Age: 0-17   M Maternity Age: 12-55   A Adult Age: 15-124

1054   ICD-10-CM 2018

☑4ᵗʰ **T27 Burn and corrosion of respiratory tract**
　　　Use additional external cause code to identify the source and intent of
　　　the burn (X00-X19, X75-X77, X96-X98)
　　　Use additional external cause code to identify place (Y92)

> The appropriate 7th character is to be added to each code from
> category T27.
> A　　initial encounter
> D　　subsequent encounter
> S　　sequela

☑x7ᵗʰ **T27.0 Burn of larynx and trachea**
☑x7ᵗʰ **T27.1 Burn involving larynx and trachea with lung**
☑x7ᵗʰ **T27.2 Burn of other parts of respiratory tract**
　　　Burn of thoracic cavity
☑x7ᵗʰ **T27.3 Burn of respiratory tract, part unspecified**　　▽
　　　~~Code first (T51-T65) to identify chemical and intent for codes~~
　　　~~T27.4-T27.7~~
☑x7ᵗʰ **T27.4 Corrosion of larynx and trachea**
　　　►Code first (T51-T65) to identify chemical and intent◄
☑x7ᵗʰ **T27.5 Corrosion involving larynx and trachea with lung**
☑x7ᵗʰ **T27.6 Corrosion of other parts of respiratory tract**
　　　►Code first (T51-T65) to identify chemical and intent◄
☑x7ᵗʰ **T27.7 Corrosion of respiratory tract, part unspecified**　　▽
　　　►Code first (T51-T65) to identify chemical and intent◄

☑4ᵗʰ **T28 Burn and corrosion of other internal organs**
　　　Use additional external cause code to identify the source and intent of
　　　the burn (X00- X19, X75-X77, X96-X98)
　　　Use additional external cause code to identify place (Y92)

> The appropriate 7th character is to be added to each code from
> category T28.
> A　　initial encounter
> D　　subsequent encounter
> S　　sequela

☑x7ᵗʰ **T28.0 Burn of mouth and pharynx**
☑x7ᵗʰ **T28.1 Burn of esophagus**
☑x7ᵗʰ **T28.2 Burn of other parts of alimentary tract**
☑x7ᵗʰ **T28.3 Burn of internal genitourinary organs**
☑5ᵗʰ **T28.4 Burns of other and unspecified internal organs**
　　　►Code first (T51-T65) to identify chemical and intent◄
　　☑x7ᵗʰ **T28.40 Burn of unspecified internal organ**　　▽
　　☑6ᵗʰ **T28.41 Burn of ear drum**
　　　　☑7ᵗʰ **T28.411 Burn of right ear drum**
　　　　☑7ᵗʰ **T28.412 Burn of left ear drum**
　　　　☑7ᵗʰ **T28.419 Burn of unspecified ear drum**　　▽
　　☑x7ᵗʰ **T28.49 Burn of other internal organ**
　　　　　~~Code first (T51-T65) to identify chemical and intent~~
　　　　　~~for T28.5-T28.9~~
☑x7ᵗʰ **T28.5 Corrosion of mouth and pharynx**
　　　►Code first (T51-T65) to identify chemical and intent◄
☑x7ᵗʰ **T28.6 Corrosion of esophagus**
　　　►Code first (T51-T65) to identify chemical and intent◄
☑x7ᵗʰ **T28.7 Corrosion of other parts of alimentary tract**
　　　►Code first (T51-T65) to identify chemical and intent◄
☑x7ᵗʰ **T28.8 Corrosion of internal genitourinary organs**
　　　►Code first (T51-T65) to identify chemical and intent◄
☑5ᵗʰ **T28.9 Corrosions of other and unspecified internal organs**
　　　►Code first (T51-T65) to identify chemical and intent◄
　　☑x7ᵗʰ **T28.90 Corrosions of unspecified internal organs**　　▽
　　☑6ᵗʰ **T28.91 Corrosions of ear drum**
　　　　☑7ᵗʰ **T28.911 Corrosions of right ear drum**
　　　　☑7ᵗʰ **T28.912 Corrosions of left ear drum**
　　　　☑7ᵗʰ **T28.919 Corrosions of unspecified ear drum**　　▽
　　☑x7ᵗʰ **T28.99 Corrosions of other internal organs**

Burns and corrosions of multiple and unspecified body regions (T30-T32)

☑4ᵗʰ **T30 Burn and corrosion, body region unspecified**
　　T30.0 Burn of unspecified body region, unspecified degree　　▽
　　　This code is not for inpatient use. Code to specified site and
　　　degree of burns.
　　　Burn NOS
　　　Multiple burns NOS
　　T30.4 Corrosion of unspecified body region, unspecified degree　　▽
　　　This code is not for inpatient use. Code to specified site and
　　　degree of corrosion.
　　　Corrosion NOS
　　　Multiple corrosion NOS

☑4ᵗʰ **T31 Burns classified according to extent of body surface involved**
　　NOTE　　This category is to be used as the primary code only when the
　　　site of the burn is unspecified. It should be used as a
　　　supplementary code with categories T20-T25 when the site is
　　　specified.
　　T31.0 Burns involving less than 10% of body surface
☑5ᵗʰ **T31.1 Burns involving 10-19% of body surface**
　　　**T31.10 Burns involving 10-19% of body surface with 0% to
　　　　　　9% third degree burns**
　　　　　Burns involving 10-19% of body surface NOS
　　　T31.11 Burns involving 10-19% of body surface with　　HCC
　　　　　　10-19% third degree burns
☑5ᵗʰ **T31.2 Burns involving 20-29% of body surface**
　　　**T31.20 Burns involving 20-29% of body surface with
　　　　　　0% to 9% third degree burns**
　　　　　Burns involving 20-29% of body surface NOS
　　　T31.21 Burns involving 20-29% of body surface with　　HCC
　　　　　　10-19% third degree burns
　　　T31.22 Burns involving 20-29% of body surface with　　HCC
　　　　　　20-29% third degree burns
☑5ᵗʰ **T31.3 Burns involving 30-39% of body surface**
　　　**T31.30 Burns involving 30-39% of body surface with
　　　　　　0% to 9% third degree burns**
　　　　　Burns involving 30-39% of body surface NOS
　　　T31.31 Burns involving 30-39% of body surface with　　HCC
　　　　　　10-19% third degree burns
　　　T31.32 Burns involving 30-39% of body surface with　　HCC
　　　　　　20-29% third degree burns
　　　T31.33 Burns involving 30-39% of body surface with　　HCC
　　　　　　30-39% third degree burns
☑5ᵗʰ **T31.4 Burns involving 40-49% of body surface**
　　　**T31.40 Burns involving 40-49% of body surface with
　　　　　　0% to 9% third degree burns**
　　　　　Burns involving 40-49% of body surface NOS
　　　T31.41 Burns involving 40-49% of body surface with　　HCC
　　　　　　10-19% third degree burns
　　　T31.42 Burns involving 40-49% of body surface with　　HCC
　　　　　　20-29% third degree burns
　　　T31.43 Burns involving 40-49% of body surface with　　HCC
　　　　　　30-39% third degree burns
　　　T31.44 Burns involving 40-49% of body surface with　　HCC
　　　　　　40-49% third degree burns
☑5ᵗʰ **T31.5 Burns involving 50-59% of body surface**
　　　**T31.50 Burns involving 50-59% of body surface with
　　　　　　0% to 9% third degree burns**
　　　　　Burns involving 50-59% of body surface NOS
　　　T31.51 Burns involving 50-59% of body surface with　　HCC
　　　　　　10-19% third degree burns
　　　T31.52 Burns involving 50-59% of body surface with　　HCC
　　　　　　20-29% third degree burns
　　　T31.53 Burns involving 50-59% of body surface with　　HCC
　　　　　　30-39% third degree burns
　　　T31.54 Burns involving 50-59% of body surface with　　HCC
　　　　　　40-49% third degree burns
　　　T31.55 Burns involving 50-59% of body surface with　　HCC
　　　　　　50-59% third degree burns
☑5ᵗʰ **T31.6 Burns involving 60-69% of body surface**
　　　**T31.60 Burns involving 60-69% of body surface with
　　　　　　0% to 9% third degree burns**
　　　　　Burns involving 60-69% of body surface NOS
　　　T31.61 Burns involving 60-69% of body surface with　　HCC
　　　　　　10-19% third degree burns

☑ Additional Character Req　　☑x7ᵗʰ Placeholder Alert　　Manifestation　　HCC CMS-HCC Condition　　▽ Unspecified Code　　►◄ Revised Text　　● New Code　　▲ Revised Code Title

T31.62　Burns involving 60-69% of body surface with 20-29% third degree burns `HCC`

T31.63　Burns involving 60-69% of body surface with 30-39% third degree burns `HCC`

T31.64　Burns involving 60-69% of body surface with 40-49% third degree burns `HCC`

T31.65　Burns involving 60-69% of body surface with 50-59% third degree burns `HCC`

T31.66　Burns involving 60-69% of body surface with 60-69% third degree burns `HCC`

✓5th **T31.7　Burns involving 70-79% of body surface**

T31.70　Burns involving 70-79% of body surface with 0% to 9% third degree burns
　　　　Burns involving 70-79% of body surface NOS

T31.71　Burns involving 70-79% of body surface with 10-19% third degree burns `HCC`

T31.72　Burns involving 70-79% of body surface with 20-29% third degree burns `HCC`

T31.73　Burns involving 70-79% of body surface with 30-39% third degree burns `HCC`

T31.74　Burns involving 70-79% of body surface with 40-49% third degree burns `HCC`

T31.75　Burns involving 70-79% of body surface with 50-59% third degree burns `HCC`

T31.76　Burns involving 70-79% of body surface with 60-69% third degree burns `HCC`

T31.77　Burns involving 70-79% of body surface with 70-79% third degree burns `HCC`

✓5th **T31.8　Burns involving 80-89% of body surface**

T31.80　Burns involving 80-89% of body surface with 0% to 9% third degree burns
　　　　Burns involving 80-89% of body surface NOS

T31.81　Burns involving 80-89% of body surface with 10-19% third degree burns `HCC`

T31.82　Burns involving 80-89% of body surface with 20-29% third degree burns `HCC`

T31.83　Burns involving 80-89% of body surface with 30-39% third degree burns `HCC`

T31.84　Burns involving 80-89% of body surface with 40-49% third degree burns `HCC`

T31.85　Burns involving 80-89% of body surface with 50-59% third degree burns `HCC`

T31.86　Burns involving 80-89% of body surface with 60-69% third degree burns `HCC`

T31.87　Burns involving 80-89% of body surface with 70-79% third degree burns `HCC`

T31.88　Burns involving 80-89% of body surface with 80-89% third degree burns `HCC`

✓5th **T31.9　Burns involving 90% or more of body surface**

T31.90　Burns involving 90% or more of body surface with 0% to 9% third degree burns
　　　　Burns involving 90% or more of body surface NOS

T31.91　Burns involving 90% or more of body surface with 10-19% third degree burns `HCC`

T31.92　Burns involving 90% or more of body surface with 20-29% third degree burns `HCC`

T31.93　Burns involving 90% or more of body surface with 30-39% third degree burns `HCC`

T31.94　Burns involving 90% or more of body surface with 40-49% third degree burns `HCC`

T31.95　Burns involving 90% or more of body surface with 50-59% third degree burns `HCC`

T31.96　Burns involving 90% or more of body surface with 60-69% third degree burns `HCC`

T31.97　Burns involving 90% or more of body surface with 70-79% third degree burns `HCC`

T31.98　Burns involving 90% or more of body surface with 80-89% third degree burns `HCC`

T31.99　Burns involving 90% or more of body surface with 90% or more third degree burns `HCC`

✓4th **T32　Corrosions classified according to extent of body surface involved**

> **NOTE**　This category is to be used as the primary code only when the site of the corrosion is unspecified. It may be used as a supplementary code with categories T20-T25 when the site is specified.

T32.0　Corrosions involving less than 10% of body surface

✓5th **T32.1　Corrosions involving 10-19% of body surface**

T32.10　Corrosions involving 10-19% of body surface with 0% to 9% third degree corrosion
　　　　Corrosions involving 10-19% of body surface NOS

T32.11　Corrosions involving 10-19% of body surface with 10-19% third degree corrosion `HCC`

✓5th **T32.2　Corrosions involving 20-29% of body surface**

T32.20　Corrosions involving 20-29% of body surface with 0% to 9% third degree corrosion

T32.21　Corrosions involving 20-29% of body surface with 10-19% third degree corrosion `HCC`

T32.22　Corrosions involving 20-29% of body surface with 20-29% third degree corrosion `HCC`

✓5th **T32.3　Corrosions involving 30-39% of body surface**

T32.30　Corrosions involving 30-39% of body surface with 0% to 9% third degree corrosion

T32.31　Corrosions involving 30-39% of body surface with 10-19% third degree corrosion `HCC`

T32.32　Corrosions involving 30-39% of body surface with 20-29% third degree corrosion `HCC`

T32.33　Corrosions involving 30-39% of body surface with 30-39% third degree corrosion `HCC`

✓5th **T32.4　Corrosions involving 40-49% of body surface**

T32.40　Corrosions involving 40-49% of body surface with 0% to 9% third degree corrosion

T32.41　Corrosions involving 40-49% of body surface with 10-19% third degree corrosion

T32.42　Corrosions involving 40-49% of body surface with 20-29% third degree corrosion `HCC`

T32.43　Corrosions involving 40-49% of body surface with 30-39% third degree corrosion `HCC`

T32.44　Corrosions involving 40-49% of body surface with 40-49% third degree corrosion `HCC`

✓5th **T32.5　Corrosions involving 50-59% of body surface**

T32.50　Corrosions involving 50-59% of body surface with 0% to 9% third degree corrosion

T32.51　Corrosions involving 50-59% of body surface with 10-19% third degree corrosion `HCC`

T32.52　Corrosions involving 50-59% of body surface with 20-29% third degree corrosion `HCC`

T32.53　Corrosions involving 50-59% of body surface with 30-39% third degree corrosion `HCC`

T32.54　Corrosions involving 50-59% of body surface with 40-49% third degree corrosion `HCC`

T32.55　Corrosions involving 50-59% of body surface with 50-59% third degree corrosion `HCC`

✓5th **T32.6　Corrosions involving 60-69% of body surface**

T32.60　Corrosions involving 60-69% of body surface with 0% to 9% third degree corrosion

T32.61　Corrosions involving 60-69% of body surface with 10-19% third degree corrosion `HCC`

T32.62　Corrosions involving 60-69% of body surface with 20-29% third degree corrosion `HCC`

T32.63　Corrosions involving 60-69% of body surface with 30-39% third degree corrosion `HCC`

T32.64　Corrosions involving 60-69% of body surface with 40-49% third degree corrosion `HCC`

T32.65　Corrosions involving 60-69% of body surface with 50-59% third degree corrosion `HCC`

T32.66　Corrosions involving 60-69% of body surface with 60-69% third degree corrosion `HCC`

✓5th **T32.7　Corrosions involving 70-79% of body surface**

T32.70　Corrosions involving 70-79% of body surface with 0% to 9% third degree corrosion

T32.71　Corrosions involving 70-79% of body surface with 10-19% third degree corrosion `HCC`

T32.72　Corrosions involving 70-79% of body surface with 20-29% third degree corrosion `HCC`

	T32.73	Corrosions involving 70-79% of body surface with 30-39% third degree corrosion	HCC
	T32.74	Corrosions involving 70-79% of body surface with 40-49% third degree corrosion	HCC
	T32.75	Corrosions involving 70-79% of body surface with 50-59% third degree corrosion	HCC
	T32.76	Corrosions involving 70-79% of body surface with 60-69% third degree corrosion	HCC
	T32.77	Corrosions involving 70-79% of body surface with 70-79% third degree corrosion	HCC

√5th **T32.8** Corrosions involving 80-89% of body surface

	T32.80	Corrosions involving 80-89% of body surface with 0% to 9% third degree corrosion	
	T32.81	Corrosions involving 80-89% of body surface with 10-19% third degree corrosion	HCC
	T32.82	Corrosions involving 80-89% of body surface with 20-29% third degree corrosion	HCC
	T32.83	Corrosions involving 80-89% of body surface with 30-39% third degree corrosion	HCC
	T32.84	Corrosions involving 80-89% of body surface with 40-49% third degree corrosion	HCC
	T32.85	Corrosions involving 80-89% of body surface with 50-59% third degree corrosion	HCC
	T32.86	Corrosions involving 80-89% of body surface with 60-69% third degree corrosion	HCC
	T32.87	Corrosions involving 80-89% of body surface with 70-79% third degree corrosion	HCC
	T32.88	Corrosions involving 80-89% of body surface with 80-89% third degree corrosion	HCC

√5th **T32.9** Corrosions involving 90% or more of body surface

	T32.90	Corrosions involving 90% or more of body surface with 0% to 9% third degree corrosion	
	T32.91	Corrosions involving 90% or more of body surface with 10-19% third degree corrosion	HCC
	T32.92	Corrosions involving 90% or more of body surface with 20-29% third degree corrosion	HCC
	T32.93	Corrosions involving 90% or more of body surface with 30-39% third degree corrosion	HCC
	T32.94	Corrosions involving 90% or more of body surface with 40-49% third degree corrosion	HCC
	T32.95	Corrosions involving 90% or more of body surface with 50-59% third degree corrosion	HCC
	T32.96	Corrosions involving 90% or more of body surface with 60-69% third degree corrosion	HCC
	T32.97	Corrosions involving 90% or more of body surface with 70-79% third degree corrosion	HCC
	T32.98	Corrosions involving 90% or more of body surface with 80-89% third degree corrosion	HCC
	T32.99	Corrosions involving 90% or more of body surface with 90% or more third degree corrosion	HCC

Frostbite (T33-T34)

EXCLUDES 2   *hypothermia and other effects of reduced temperature (T68, T69-)*

√4th **T33** **Superficial frostbite**

INCLUDES   frostbite with partial thickness skin loss

> The appropriate 7th character is to be added to each code from category T33.
> A   initial encounter
> D   subsequent encounter
> S   sequela

√5th **T33.0** Superficial frostbite of head

√6th   **T33.01**   Superficial frostbite of ear

    √7th   **T33.011**   Superficial frostbite of right ear

    √7th   **T33.012**   Superficial frostbite of left ear

    √7th   **T33.019**   Superficial frostbite of unspecified ear   ▽

√x7th   **T33.02**   Superficial frostbite of nose

√x7th   **T33.09**   Superficial frostbite of other part of head

√x7th   **T33.1**   Superficial frostbite of neck

√x7th   **T33.2**   Superficial frostbite of thorax

√x7th   **T33.3**   Superficial frostbite of abdominal wall, lower back and pelvis

√5th **T33.4** Superficial frostbite of arm

EXCLUDES 2   *superficial frostbite of wrist and hand (T33.5-)*

√x7th   **T33.40**   Superficial frostbite of unspecified arm   ▽

√x7th   **T33.41**   Superficial frostbite of right arm

√x7th   **T33.42**   Superficial frostbite of left arm

√5th **T33.5** Superficial frostbite of wrist, hand, and fingers

√6th   **T33.51**   Superficial frostbite of wrist

    √7th   **T33.511**   Superficial frostbite of right wrist

    √7th   **T33.512**   Superficial frostbite of left wrist

    √7th   **T33.519**   Superficial frostbite of unspecified wrist   ▽

√6th   **T33.52**   Superficial frostbite of hand

    EXCLUDES 2   *superficial frostbite of fingers (T33.53-)*

    √7th   **T33.521**   Superficial frostbite of right hand

    √7th   **T33.522**   Superficial frostbite of left hand

    √7th   **T33.529**   Superficial frostbite of unspecified hand   ▽

√6th   **T33.53**   Superficial frostbite of finger(s)

    √7th   **T33.531**   Superficial frostbite of right finger(s)

    √7th   **T33.532**   Superficial frostbite of left finger(s)

    √7th   **T33.539**   Superficial frostbite of unspecified finger(s)   ▽

√5th **T33.6** Superficial frostbite of hip and thigh

√x7th   **T33.60**   Superficial frostbite of unspecified hip and thigh   ▽

√x7th   **T33.61**   Superficial frostbite of right hip and thigh

√x7th   **T33.62**   Superficial frostbite of left hip and thigh

√5th **T33.7** Superficial frostbite of knee and lower leg

EXCLUDES 2   *superficial frostbite of ankle and foot (T33.8-)*

√x7th   **T33.70**   Superficial frostbite of unspecified knee and lower leg   ▽

√x7th   **T33.71**   Superficial frostbite of right knee and lower leg

√x7th   **T33.72**   Superficial frostbite of left knee and lower leg

√5th **T33.8** Superficial frostbite of ankle, foot, and toe(s)

√6th   **T33.81**   Superficial frostbite of ankle

    √7th   **T33.811**   Superficial frostbite of right ankle

    √7th   **T33.812**   Superficial frostbite of left ankle

    √7th   **T33.819**   Superficial frostbite of unspecified ankle   ▽

√6th   **T33.82**   Superficial frostbite of foot

    √7th   **T33.821**   Superficial frostbite of right foot

    √7th   **T33.822**   Superficial frostbite of left foot

    √7th   **T33.829**   Superficial frostbite of unspecified foot   ▽

√6th   **T33.83**   Superficial frostbite of toe(s)

    √7th   **T33.831**   Superficial frostbite of right toe(s)

    √7th   **T33.832**   Superficial frostbite of left toe(s)

    √7th   **T33.839**   Superficial frostbite of unspecified toe(s)   ▽

√5th **T33.9** Superficial frostbite of other and unspecified sites

√x7th   **T33.90**   Superficial frostbite of unspecified sites   ▽
Superficial frostbite NOS

√x7th   **T33.99**   Superficial frostbite of other sites
Superficial frostbite of leg NOS
Superficial frostbite of trunk NOS

√4th **T34** **Frostbite with tissue necrosis**

> The appropriate 7th character is to be added to each code from category T34.
> A   initial encounter
> D   subsequent encounter
> S   sequela

√5th **T34.0** Frostbite with tissue necrosis of head

√6th   **T34.01**   Frostbite with tissue necrosis of ear

    √7th   **T34.011**   Frostbite with tissue necrosis of right ear

    √7th   **T34.012**   Frostbite with tissue necrosis of left ear

    √7th   **T34.019**   Frostbite with tissue necrosis of unspecified ear   ▽

√x7th   **T34.02**   Frostbite with tissue necrosis of nose

√x7th   **T34.09**   Frostbite with tissue necrosis of other part of head

√x7th   **T34.1**   Frostbite with tissue necrosis of neck

√x7th   **T34.2**   Frostbite with tissue necrosis of thorax

√x7th   **T34.3**   Frostbite with tissue necrosis of abdominal wall, lower back and pelvis

---

☑ Additional Character Req   √x7th Placeholder Alert   Manifestation   HCC CMS-HCC Condition   ▽ Unspecified Code   ►◄ Revised Text   ● New Code   ▲ Revised Code Title

✓5ᵗʰ **T34.4**   **Frostbite with tissue necrosis of arm**
    EXCLUDES 2   *frostbite with tissue necrosis of wrist and hand (T34.5-)*

✓x7ᵗʰ **T34.40**   **Frostbite with tissue necrosis of unspecified arm** ▽

✓x7ᵗʰ **T34.41**   **Frostbite with tissue necrosis of right arm**

✓x7ᵗʰ **T34.42**   **Frostbite with tissue necrosis of left arm**

✓5ᵗʰ **T34.5**   **Frostbite with tissue necrosis of wrist, hand, and finger(s)**

✓6ᵗʰ **T34.51**   **Frostbite with tissue necrosis of wrist**

✓7ᵗʰ **T34.511**   **Frostbite with tissue necrosis of right wrist**

✓7ᵗʰ **T34.512**   **Frostbite with tissue necrosis of left wrist**

✓7ᵗʰ **T34.519**   **Frostbite with tissue necrosis of unspecified wrist** ▽

✓6ᵗʰ **T34.52**   **Frostbite with tissue necrosis of hand**
    EXCLUDES 2   *frostbite with tissue necrosis of finger(s) (T34.53-)*

✓7ᵗʰ **T34.521**   **Frostbite with tissue necrosis of right hand**

✓7ᵗʰ **T34.522**   **Frostbite with tissue necrosis of left hand**

✓7ᵗʰ **T34.529**   **Frostbite with tissue necrosis of unspecified hand** ▽

✓6ᵗʰ **T34.53**   **Frostbite with tissue necrosis of finger(s)**

✓7ᵗʰ **T34.531**   **Frostbite with tissue necrosis of right finger(s)**

✓7ᵗʰ **T34.532**   **Frostbite with tissue necrosis of left finger(s)**

✓7ᵗʰ **T34.539**   **Frostbite with tissue necrosis of unspecified finger(s)** ▽

✓5ᵗʰ **T34.6**   **Frostbite with tissue necrosis of hip and thigh**

✓x7ᵗʰ **T34.60**   **Frostbite with tissue necrosis of unspecified hip and thigh** ▽

✓x7ᵗʰ **T34.61**   **Frostbite with tissue necrosis of right hip and thigh**

✓x7ᵗʰ **T34.62**   **Frostbite with tissue necrosis of left hip and thigh**

✓5ᵗʰ **T34.7**   **Frostbite with tissue necrosis of knee and lower leg**
    EXCLUDES 2   *frostbite with tissue necrosis of ankle and foot (T34.8-)*

✓x7ᵗʰ **T34.70**   **Frostbite with tissue necrosis of unspecified knee and lower leg** ▽

✓x7ᵗʰ **T34.71**   **Frostbite with tissue necrosis of right knee and lower leg**

✓x7ᵗʰ **T34.72**   **Frostbite with tissue necrosis of left knee and lower leg**

✓5ᵗʰ **T34.8**   **Frostbite with tissue necrosis of ankle, foot, and toe(s)**

✓6ᵗʰ **T34.81**   **Frostbite with tissue necrosis of ankle**

✓7ᵗʰ **T34.811**   **Frostbite with tissue necrosis of right ankle**

✓7ᵗʰ **T34.812**   **Frostbite with tissue necrosis of left ankle**

✓7ᵗʰ **T34.819**   **Frostbite with tissue necrosis of unspecified ankle** ▽

✓6ᵗʰ **T34.82**   **Frostbite with tissue necrosis of foot**

✓7ᵗʰ **T34.821**   **Frostbite with tissue necrosis of right foot**

✓7ᵗʰ **T34.822**   **Frostbite with tissue necrosis of left foot**

✓7ᵗʰ **T34.829**   **Frostbite with tissue necrosis of unspecified foot** ▽

✓6ᵗʰ **T34.83**   **Frostbite with tissue necrosis of toe(s)**

✓7ᵗʰ **T34.831**   **Frostbite with tissue necrosis of right toe(s)**

✓7ᵗʰ **T34.832**   **Frostbite with tissue necrosis of left toe(s)**

✓7ᵗʰ **T34.839**   **Frostbite with tissue necrosis of unspecified toe(s)** ▽

✓5ᵗʰ **T34.9**   **Frostbite with tissue necrosis of other and unspecified sites**

✓x7ᵗʰ **T34.90**   **Frostbite with tissue necrosis of unspecified sites** ▽
    Frostbite with tissue necrosis NOS

✓x7ᵗʰ **T34.99**   **Frostbite with tissue necrosis of other sites**
    Frostbite with tissue necrosis of leg NOS
    Frostbite with tissue necrosis of trunk NOS

Poisoning by, adverse effects of and underdosing of drugs, medicaments and biological substances (T36-T50)

INCLUDES   adverse effect of correct substance properly administered
    poisoning by overdose of substance
    poisoning by wrong substance given or taken in error
    underdosing by (inadvertently) (deliberately) taking less substance than prescribed or instructed

Code first, for adverse effects, the nature of the adverse effect, such as:
    adverse effect NOS (T88.7)
    aspirin gastritis (K29.-)
    blood disorders (D56-D76)
    contact dermatitis (L23-L25)
    dermatitis due to substances taken internally (L27.-)
    nephropathy (N14.0-N14.2)

NOTE   The drug giving rise to the adverse effect should be identified by use of codes from categories T36-T50 with fifth or sixth character 5.

Use additional code(s) to specify:
    manifestations of poisoning
    underdosing or failure in dosage during medical and surgical care (Y63.6, Y63.8-Y63.9)
    underdosing of medication regimen (Z91.12-, Z91.13-)

EXCLUDES 1   *toxic reaction to local anesthesia in pregnancy (O29.3-)*

EXCLUDES 2   *abuse and dependence of psychoactive substances (F10-F19)*
    abuse of non-dependence-producing substances (F55.-)
    drug reaction and poisoning affecting newborn (P00-P96)
    pathological drug intoxication (inebriation) (F10-F19)

AHA: 2016, 2Q, 8; 2015, 3Q, 22

✓4ᵗʰ **T36**   **Poisoning by, adverse effect of and underdosing of systemic antibiotics**

    EXCLUDES 1   *antineoplastic antibiotics (T45.1-)*
    locally applied antibiotic NEC (T49.0)
    topically used antibiotic for ear, nose and throat (T49.6)
    topically used antibiotic for eye (T49.5)

> The appropriate 7th character is to be added to each code from category T36.
> A   initial encounter
> D   subsequent encounter
> S   sequela

✓5ᵗʰ **T36.0**   **Poisoning by, adverse effect of and underdosing of penicillins**

✓6ᵗʰ **T36.0X**   **Poisoning by, adverse effect of and underdosing of penicillins**

✓7ᵗʰ **T36.0X1**   **Poisoning by penicillins, accidental (unintentional)**
    Poisoning by penicillins NOS

² ✓7ᵗʰ **T36.0X2**   **Poisoning by penicillins, intentional self-harm**   HCC

✓7ᵗʰ **T36.0X3**   **Poisoning by penicillins, assault**

✓7ᵗʰ **T36.0X4**   **Poisoning by penicillins, undetermined**

✓7ᵗʰ **T36.0X5**   **Adverse effect of penicillins**

✓7ᵗʰ **T36.0X6**   **Underdosing of penicillins**

✓5ᵗʰ **T36.1**   **Poisoning by, adverse effect of and underdosing of cephalosporins and other beta-lactam antibiotics**

✓6ᵗʰ **T36.1X**   **Poisoning by, adverse effect of and underdosing of cephalosporins and other beta-lactam antibiotics**

✓7ᵗʰ **T36.1X1**   **Poisoning by cephalosporins and other beta-lactam antibiotics, accidental (unintentional)**
    Poisoning by cephalosporins and other beta-lactam antibiotics NOS

² ✓7ᵗʰ **T36.1X2**   **Poisoning by cephalosporins and other beta-lactam antibiotics, intentional self-harm**   HCC

✓7ᵗʰ **T36.1X3**   **Poisoning by cephalosporins and other beta-lactam antibiotics, assault**

✓7ᵗʰ **T36.1X4**   **Poisoning by cephalosporins and other beta-lactam antibiotics, undetermined**

✓7ᵗʰ **T36.1X5**   **Adverse effect of cephalosporins and other beta-lactam antibiotics**

✓7ᵗʰ **T36.1X6**   **Underdosing of cephalosporins and other beta-lactam antibiotics**

²   HCC with 7th character indicating initial encounter (A or B - specific to category) OR sequela.

EXCLUDES 1   Not coded here   EXCLUDES 2   Not included here   N Newborn Age: 0   P Pediatric Age: 0-17   M Maternity Age: 12-55   A Adult Age: 15-124

1058   ICD-10-CM 2018

✓5ᵗʰ **T36.2 Poisoning by, adverse effect of and underdosing of chloramphenicol group**

  ✓6ᵗʰ **T36.2X Poisoning by, adverse effect of and underdosing of chloramphenicol group**

    ✓7ᵗʰ **T36.2X1 Poisoning by chloramphenicol group, accidental (unintentional)**
        Poisoning by chloramphenicol group NOS

    2 ✓7ᵗʰ **T36.2X2 Poisoning by chloramphenicol group, intentional self-harm** HCC

    ✓7ᵗʰ **T36.2X3 Poisoning by chloramphenicol group, assault**

    ✓7ᵗʰ **T36.2X4 Poisoning by chloramphenicol group, undetermined**

    ✓7ᵗʰ **T36.2X5 Adverse effect of chloramphenicol group**

    ✓7ᵗʰ **T36.2X6 Underdosing of chloramphenicol group**

✓5ᵗʰ **T36.3 Poisoning by, adverse effect of and underdosing of macrolides**

  ✓6ᵗʰ **T36.3X Poisoning by, adverse effect of and underdosing of macrolides**

    ✓7ᵗʰ **T36.3X1 Poisoning by macrolides, accidental (unintentional)**
        Poisoning by macrolides NOS

    2 ✓7ᵗʰ **T36.3X2 Poisoning by macrolides, intentional self-harm** HCC

    ✓7ᵗʰ **T36.3X3 Poisoning by macrolides, assault**

    ✓7ᵗʰ **T36.3X4 Poisoning by macrolides, undetermined**

    ✓7ᵗʰ **T36.3X5 Adverse effect of macrolides**

    ✓7ᵗʰ **T36.3X6 Underdosing of macrolides**

✓5ᵗʰ **T36.4 Poisoning by, adverse effect of and underdosing of tetracyclines**

  ✓6ᵗʰ **T36.4X Poisoning by, adverse effect of and underdosing of tetracyclines**

    ✓7ᵗʰ **T36.4X1 Poisoning by tetracyclines, accidental (unintentional)**
        Poisoning by tetracyclines NOS

    2 ✓7ᵗʰ **T36.4X2 Poisoning by tetracyclines, intentional self-harm** HCC

    ✓7ᵗʰ **T36.4X3 Poisoning by tetracyclines, assault**

    ✓7ᵗʰ **T36.4X4 Poisoning by tetracyclines, undetermined**

    ✓7ᵗʰ **T36.4X5 Adverse effect of tetracyclines**

    ✓7ᵗʰ **T36.4X6 Underdosing of tetracyclines**

✓5ᵗʰ **T36.5 Poisoning by, adverse effect of and underdosing of aminoglycosides**
    Poisoning by, adverse effect of and underdosing of streptomycin

  ✓6ᵗʰ **T36.5X Poisoning by, adverse effect of and underdosing of aminoglycosides**

    ✓7ᵗʰ **T36.5X1 Poisoning by aminoglycosides, accidental (unintentional)**
        Poisoning by aminoglycosides NOS

    2 ✓7ᵗʰ **T36.5X2 Poisoning by aminoglycosides, intentional self-harm** HCC

    ✓7ᵗʰ **T36.5X3 Poisoning by aminoglycosides, assault**

    ✓7ᵗʰ **T36.5X4 Poisoning by aminoglycosides, undetermined**

    ✓7ᵗʰ **T36.5X5 Adverse effect of aminoglycosides**

    ✓7ᵗʰ **T36.5X6 Underdosing of aminoglycosides**

✓5ᵗʰ **T36.6 Poisoning by, adverse effect of and underdosing of rifampicins**

  ✓6ᵗʰ **T36.6X Poisoning by, adverse effect of and underdosing of rifampicins**

    ✓7ᵗʰ **T36.6X1 Poisoning by rifampicins, accidental (unintentional)**
        Poisoning by rifampicins NOS

    2 ✓7ᵗʰ **T36.6X2 Poisoning by rifampicins, intentional self-harm** HCC

    ✓7ᵗʰ **T36.6X3 Poisoning by rifampicins, assault**

    ✓7ᵗʰ **T36.6X4 Poisoning by rifampicins, undetermined**

    ✓7ᵗʰ **T36.6X5 Adverse effect of rifampicins**

    ✓7ᵗʰ **T36.6X6 Underdosing of rifampicins**

✓5ᵗʰ **T36.7 Poisoning by, adverse effect of and underdosing of antifungal antibiotics, systemically used**

  ✓6ᵗʰ **T36.7X Poisoning by, adverse effect of and underdosing of antifungal antibiotics, systemically used**

    ✓7ᵗʰ **T36.7X1 Poisoning by antifungal antibiotics, systemically used, accidental (unintentional)**
        Poisoning by antifungal antibiotics, systemically used NOS

    2 ✓7ᵗʰ **T36.7X2 Poisoning by antifungal antibiotics, systemically used, intentional self-harm** HCC

    ✓7ᵗʰ **T36.7X3 Poisoning by antifungal antibiotics, systemically used, assault**

    ✓7ᵗʰ **T36.7X4 Poisoning by antifungal antibiotics, systemically used, undetermined**

    ✓7ᵗʰ **T36.7X5 Adverse effect of antifungal antibiotics, systemically used**

    ✓7ᵗʰ **T36.7X6 Underdosing of antifungal antibiotics, systemically used**

✓5ᵗʰ **T36.8 Poisoning by, adverse effect of and underdosing of other systemic antibiotics**

  ✓6ᵗʰ **T36.8X Poisoning by, adverse effect of and underdosing of other systemic antibiotics**
    AHA: 2017, 1Q, 39

    ✓7ᵗʰ **T36.8X1 Poisoning by other systemic antibiotics, accidental (unintentional)**
        Poisoning by other systemic antibiotics NOS

    2 ✓7ᵗʰ **T36.8X2 Poisoning by other systemic antibiotics, intentional self-harm** HCC

    ✓7ᵗʰ **T36.8X3 Poisoning by other systemic antibiotics, assault**

    ✓7ᵗʰ **T36.8X4 Poisoning by other systemic antibiotics, undetermined**

    ✓7ᵗʰ **T36.8X5 Adverse effect of other systemic antibiotics**

    ✓7ᵗʰ **T36.8X6 Underdosing of other systemic antibiotics**

✓5ᵗʰ **T36.9 Poisoning by, adverse effect of and underdosing of unspecified systemic antibiotic**

  ✓×7ᵗʰ **T36.91 Poisoning by unspecified systemic antibiotic, accidental (unintentional)** ▽
    Poisoning by systemic antibiotic NOS

  2 ✓×7ᵗʰ **T36.92 Poisoning by unspecified systemic antibiotic, intentional self-harm** HCC ▽

  ✓×7ᵗʰ **T36.93 Poisoning by unspecified systemic antibiotic, assault** ▽

  ✓×7ᵗʰ **T36.94 Poisoning by unspecified systemic antibiotic, undetermined** ▽

  ✓×7ᵗʰ **T36.95 Adverse effect of unspecified systemic antibiotic** ▽

  ✓×7ᵗʰ **T36.96 Underdosing of unspecified systemic antibiotic** ▽

✓4ᵗʰ **T37 Poisoning by, adverse effect of and underdosing of other systemic anti-infectives and antiparasitics**

  EXCLUDES 1 *anti-infectives topically used for ear, nose and throat (T49.6-)*
  anti-infectives topically used for eye (T49.5-)
  locally applied anti-infectives NEC (T49.Ø-)

> The appropriate 7th character is to be added to each code from category T37.
> A   initial encounter
> D   subsequent encounter
> S   sequela

✓5ᵗʰ **T37.Ø Poisoning by, adverse effect of and underdosing of sulfonamides**

  ✓6ᵗʰ **T37.ØX Poisoning by, adverse effect of and underdosing of sulfonamides**

    ✓7ᵗʰ **T37.ØX1 Poisoning by sulfonamides, accidental (unintentional)**
        Poisoning by sulfonamides NOS

    2 ✓7ᵗʰ **T37.ØX2 Poisoning by sulfonamides, intentional self-harm** HCC

    ✓7ᵗʰ **T37.ØX3 Poisoning by sulfonamides, assault**

    ✓7ᵗʰ **T37.ØX4 Poisoning by sulfonamides, undetermined**

---

2   HCC with 7th character indicating initial encounter (A or B - specific to category) OR sequela.

✓ Additional Character Req   ✓×7ᵗʰ Placeholder Alert   Manifestation   HCC CMS-HCC Condition   ▽ Unspecified Code   ►◄ Revised Text   ● New Code   ▲ Revised Code Title

√7ᵗʰ **T37.0X5** **Adverse effect of sulfonamides**

√7ᵗʰ **T37.0X6** **Underdosing of sulfonamides**

√5ᵗʰ **T37.1** **Poisoning by, adverse effect of and underdosing of antimycobacterial drugs**
> EXCLUDES 1   *rifampicins (T36.6-)*
> *streptomycin (T36.5-)*

√6ᵗʰ **T37.1X** **Poisoning by, adverse effect of and underdosing of antimycobacterial drugs**

√7ᵗʰ **T37.1X1** **Poisoning by antimycobacterial drugs, accidental (unintentional)**
> Poisoning by antimycobacterial drugs NOS

2 √7ᵗʰ **T37.1X2** **Poisoning by antimycobacterial drugs, intentional self-harm**   HCC

√7ᵗʰ **T37.1X3** **Poisoning by antimycobacterial drugs, assault**

√7ᵗʰ **T37.1X4** **Poisoning by antimycobacterial drugs, undetermined**

√7ᵗʰ **T37.1X5** **Adverse effect of antimycobacterial drugs**

√7ᵗʰ **T37.1X6** **Underdosing of antimycobacterial drugs**

√5ᵗʰ **T37.2** **Poisoning by, adverse effect of and underdosing of antimalarials and drugs acting on other blood protozoa**
> EXCLUDES 1   *hydroxyquinoline derivatives (T37.8-)*

√6ᵗʰ **T37.2X** **Poisoning by, adverse effect of and underdosing of antimalarials and drugs acting on other blood protozoa**

√7ᵗʰ **T37.2X1** **Poisoning by antimalarials and drugs acting on other blood protozoa, accidental (unintentional)**
> Poisoning by antimalarials and drugs acting on other blood protozoa NOS

2 √7ᵗʰ **T37.2X2** **Poisoning by antimalarials and drugs acting on other blood protozoa, intentional self-harm**   HCC

√7ᵗʰ **T37.2X3** **Poisoning by antimalarials and drugs acting on other blood protozoa, assault**

√7ᵗʰ **T37.2X4** **Poisoning by antimalarials and drugs acting on other blood protozoa, undetermined**

√7ᵗʰ **T37.2X5** **Adverse effect of antimalarials and drugs acting on other blood protozoa**

√7ᵗʰ **T37.2X6** **Underdosing of antimalarials and drugs acting on other blood protozoa**

√5ᵗʰ **T37.3** **Poisoning by, adverse effect of and underdosing of other antiprotozoal drugs**

√6ᵗʰ **T37.3X** **Poisoning by, adverse effect of and underdosing of other antiprotozoal drugs**

√7ᵗʰ **T37.3X1** **Poisoning by other antiprotozoal drugs, accidental (unintentional)**
> Poisoning by other antiprotozoal drugs NOS

2 √7ᵗʰ **T37.3X2** **Poisoning by other antiprotozoal drugs, intentional self-harm**   HCC

√7ᵗʰ **T37.3X3** **Poisoning by other antiprotozoal drugs, assault**

√7ᵗʰ **T37.3X4** **Poisoning by other antiprotozoal drugs, undetermined**

√7ᵗʰ **T37.3X5** **Adverse effect of other antiprotozoal drugs**

√7ᵗʰ **T37.3X6** **Underdosing of other antiprotozoal drugs**

√5ᵗʰ **T37.4** **Poisoning by, adverse effect of and underdosing of anthelminthics**

√6ᵗʰ **T37.4X** **Poisoning by, adverse effect of and underdosing of anthelminthics**

√7ᵗʰ **T37.4X1** **Poisoning by anthelminthics, accidental (unintentional)**
> Poisoning by anthelminthics NOS

2 √7ᵗʰ **T37.4X2** **Poisoning by anthelminthics, intentional self-harm**   HCC

√7ᵗʰ **T37.4X3** **Poisoning by anthelminthics, assault**

√7ᵗʰ **T37.4X4** **Poisoning by anthelminthics, undetermined**

√7ᵗʰ **T37.4X5** **Adverse effect of anthelminthics**

√7ᵗʰ **T37.4X6** **Underdosing of anthelminthics**

√5ᵗʰ **T37.5** **Poisoning by, adverse effect of and underdosing of antiviral drugs**
> EXCLUDES 1   *amantadine (T42.8-)*
> *cytarabine (T45.1-)*

√6ᵗʰ **T37.5X** **Poisoning by, adverse effect of and underdosing of antiviral drugs**

√7ᵗʰ **T37.5X1** **Poisoning by antiviral drugs, accidental (unintentional)**
> Poisoning by antiviral drugs NOS

2 √7ᵗʰ **T37.5X2** **Poisoning by antiviral drugs, intentional self-harm**   HCC

√7ᵗʰ **T37.5X3** **Poisoning by antiviral drugs, assault**

√7ᵗʰ **T37.5X4** **Poisoning by antiviral drugs, undetermined**

√7ᵗʰ **T37.5X5** **Adverse effect of antiviral drugs**

√7ᵗʰ **T37.5X6** **Underdosing of antiviral drugs**

√5ᵗʰ **T37.8** **Poisoning by, adverse effect of and underdosing of other specified systemic anti-infectives and antiparasitics**
> Poisoning by, adverse effect of and underdosing of hydroxyquinoline derivatives
> EXCLUDES 1   *antimalarial drugs (T37.2-)*

√6ᵗʰ **T37.8X** **Poisoning by, adverse effect of and underdosing of other specified systemic anti-infectives and antiparasitics**

√7ᵗʰ **T37.8X1** **Poisoning by other specified systemic anti-infectives and antiparasitics, accidental (unintentional)**
> Poisoning by other specified systemic anti-infectives and antiparasitics NOS

2 √7ᵗʰ **T37.8X2** **Poisoning by other specified systemic anti-infectives and antiparasitics, intentional self-harm**   HCC

√7ᵗʰ **T37.8X3** **Poisoning by other specified systemic anti-infectives and antiparasitics, assault**

√7ᵗʰ **T37.8X4** **Poisoning by other specified systemic anti-infectives and antiparasitics, undetermined**

√7ᵗʰ **T37.8X5** **Adverse effect of other specified systemic anti-infectives and antiparasitics**

√7ᵗʰ **T37.8X6** **Underdosing of other specified systemic anti-infectives and antiparasitics**

√5ᵗʰ **T37.9** **Poisoning by, adverse effect of and underdosing of unspecified systemic anti-infective and antiparasitics**

√x7ᵗʰ **T37.91** **Poisoning by unspecified systemic anti-infective and antiparasitics, accidental (unintentional)** ▽
> Poisoning by, adverse effect of and underdosing of systemic anti-infective and antiparasitics NOS

2 √x7ᵗʰ **T37.92** **Poisoning by unspecified systemic anti-infective and antiparasitics, intentional self-harm**   HCC ▽

√x7ᵗʰ **T37.93** **Poisoning by unspecified systemic anti-infective and antiparasitics, assault** ▽

√x7ᵗʰ **T37.94** **Poisoning by unspecified systemic anti-infective and antiparasitics, undetermined** ▽

√x7ᵗʰ **T37.95** **Adverse effect of unspecified systemic anti-infective and antiparasitic** ▽

√x7ᵗʰ **T37.96** **Underdosing of unspecified systemic anti-infectives and antiparasitics** ▽

---

2   HCC with 7th character indicating initial encounter (A or B - specific to category) OR sequela.

EXCLUDES 1 Not coded here   EXCLUDES 2 Not included here   N Newborn Age: 0   P Pediatric Age: 0-17   M Maternity Age: 12-55   A Adult Age: 15-124

1060   ICD-10-CM 2018

✓4th **T38**   **Poisoning by, adverse effect of and underdosing of hormones and their synthetic substitutes and antagonists, not elsewhere classified**

EXCLUDES 1   *mineralocorticoids and their antagonists (T50.0-)*
oxytocic hormones (T48.0-)
parathyroid hormones and derivatives (T50.9-)

> The appropriate 7th character is to be added to each code from category T38.
> A   initial encounter
> D   subsequent encounter
> S   sequela

✓5th **T38.0**   **Poisoning by, adverse effect of and underdosing of glucocorticoids and synthetic analogues**

EXCLUDES 1   *glucocorticoids, topically used (T49.-)*

✓6th **T38.0X**   **Poisoning by, adverse effect of and underdosing of glucocorticoids and synthetic analogues**

✓7th **T38.0X1**   **Poisoning by glucocorticoids and synthetic analogues, accidental (unintentional)**
Poisoning by glucocorticoids and synthetic analogues NOS

2 ✓7th **T38.0X2**   **Poisoning by glucocorticoids and synthetic analogues, intentional self-harm**   HCC

✓7th **T38.0X3**   **Poisoning by glucocorticoids and synthetic analogues, assault**

✓7th **T38.0X4**   **Poisoning by glucocorticoids and synthetic analogues, undetermined**

✓7th **T38.0X5**   **Adverse effect of glucocorticoids and synthetic analogues**

✓7th **T38.0X6**   **Underdosing of glucocorticoids and synthetic analogues**

✓5th **T38.1**   **Poisoning by, adverse effect of and underdosing of thyroid hormones and substitutes**

✓6th **T38.1X**   **Poisoning by, adverse effect of and underdosing of thyroid hormones and substitutes**

✓7th **T38.1X1**   **Poisoning by thyroid hormones and substitutes, accidental (unintentional)**
Poisoning by thyroid hormones and substitutes NOS

2 ✓7th **T38.1X2**   **Poisoning by thyroid hormones and substitutes, intentional self-harm**   HCC

✓7th **T38.1X3**   **Poisoning by thyroid hormones and substitutes, assault**

✓7th **T38.1X4**   **Poisoning by thyroid hormones and substitutes, undetermined**

✓7th **T38.1X5**   **Adverse effect of thyroid hormones and substitutes**

✓7th **T38.1X6**   **Underdosing of thyroid hormones and substitutes**

✓5th **T38.2**   **Poisoning by, adverse effect of and underdosing of antithyroid drugs**

✓6th **T38.2X**   **Poisoning by, adverse effect of and underdosing of antithyroid drugs**

✓7th **T38.2X1**   **Poisoning by antithyroid drugs, accidental (unintentional)**
Poisoning by antithyroid drugs NOS

2 ✓7th **T38.2X2**   **Poisoning by antithyroid drugs, intentional self-harm**   HCC

✓7th **T38.2X3**   **Poisoning by antithyroid drugs, assault**

✓7th **T38.2X4**   **Poisoning by antithyroid drugs, undetermined**

✓7th **T38.2X5**   **Adverse effect of antithyroid drugs**

✓7th **T38.2X6**   **Underdosing of antithyroid drugs**

✓5th **T38.3**   **Poisoning by, adverse effect of and underdosing of insulin and oral hypoglycemic [antidiabetic] drugs**

✓6th **T38.3X**   **Poisoning by, adverse effect of and underdosing of insulin and oral hypoglycemic [antidiabetic] drugs**

✓7th **T38.3X1**   **Poisoning by insulin and oral hypoglycemic [antidiabetic] drugs, accidental (unintentional)**
Poisoning by insulin and oral hypoglycemic [antidiabetic] drugs NOS

2 ✓7th **T38.3X2**   **Poisoning by insulin and oral hypoglycemic [antidiabetic] drugs, intentional self-harm**   HCC

✓7th **T38.3X3**   **Poisoning by insulin and oral hypoglycemic [antidiabetic] drugs, assault**

✓7th **T38.3X4**   **Poisoning by insulin and oral hypoglycemic [antidiabetic] drugs, undetermined**

✓7th **T38.3X5**   **Adverse effect of insulin and oral hypoglycemic [antidiabetic] drugs**

✓7th **T38.3X6**   **Underdosing of insulin and oral hypoglycemic [antidiabetic] drugs**

✓5th **T38.4**   **Poisoning by, adverse effect of and underdosing of oral contraceptives**
Poisoning by, adverse effect of and underdosing of multiple- and single-ingredient oral contraceptive preparations

✓6th **T38.4X**   **Poisoning by, adverse effect of and underdosing of oral contraceptives**

✓7th **T38.4X1**   **Poisoning by oral contraceptives, accidental (unintentional)**
Poisoning by oral contraceptives NOS

2 ✓7th **T38.4X2**   **Poisoning by oral contraceptives, intentional self-harm**   HCC

✓7th **T38.4X3**   **Poisoning by oral contraceptives, assault**

✓7th **T38.4X4**   **Poisoning by oral contraceptives, undetermined**

✓7th **T38.4X5**   **Adverse effect of oral contraceptives**

✓7th **T38.4X6**   **Underdosing of oral contraceptives**

✓5th **T38.5**   **Poisoning by, adverse effect of and underdosing of other estrogens and progestogens**
Poisoning by, adverse effect of and underdosing of estrogens and progestogens mixtures and substitutes

✓6th **T38.5X**   **Poisoning by, adverse effect of and underdosing of other estrogens and progestogens**

✓7th **T38.5X1**   **Poisoning by other estrogens and progestogens, accidental (unintentional)**
Poisoning by other estrogens and progestogens NOS

2 ✓7th **T38.5X2**   **Poisoning by other estrogens and progestogens, intentional self-harm**   HCC

✓7th **T38.5X3**   **Poisoning by other estrogens and progestogens, assault**

✓7th **T38.5X4**   **Poisoning by other estrogens and progestogens, undetermined**

✓7th **T38.5X5**   **Adverse effect of other estrogens and progestogens**

✓7th **T38.5X6**   **Underdosing of other estrogens and progestogens**

✓5th **T38.6**   **Poisoning by, adverse effect of and underdosing of antigonadotrophins, antiestrogens, antiandrogens, not elsewhere classified**
Poisoning by, adverse effect of and underdosing of tamoxifen

✓6th **T38.6X**   **Poisoning by, adverse effect of and underdosing of antigonadotrophins, antiestrogens, antiandrogens, not elsewhere classified**

✓7th **T38.6X1**   **Poisoning by antigonadotrophins, antiestrogens, antiandrogens, not elsewhere classified, accidental (unintentional)**
Poisoning by antigonadotrophins, antiestrogens, antiandrogens, not elsewhere classified NOS

2 ✓7th **T38.6X2**   **Poisoning by antigonadotrophins, antiestrogens, antiandrogens, not elsewhere classified, intentional self-harm**   HCC

✓7th **T38.6X3**   **Poisoning by antigonadotrophins, antiestrogens, antiandrogens, not elsewhere classified, assault**

✓7th **T38.6X4**   **Poisoning by antigonadotrophins, antiestrogens, antiandrogens, not elsewhere classified, undetermined**

✓7th **T38.6X5**   **Adverse effect of antigonadotrophins, antiestrogens, antiandrogens, not elsewhere classified**

✓7th **T38.6X6**   **Underdosing of antigonadotrophins, antiestrogens, antiandrogens, not elsewhere classified**

---

2   HCC with 7th character indicating initial encounter (A or B - specific to category) OR sequela.

✔ Additional Character Req   ✔x7th Placeholder Alert   Manifestation   HCC CMS-HCC Condition   ▽ Unspecified Code   ▶◀ Revised Text   ● New Code   ▲ Revised Code Title

✓5th **T38.7** **Poisoning by, adverse effect of and underdosing of androgens and anabolic congeners**

    ✓6th **T38.7X** **Poisoning by, adverse effect of and underdosing of androgens and anabolic congeners**

        ✓7th **T38.7X1** **Poisoning by androgens and anabolic congeners, accidental (unintentional)**
            Poisoning by androgens and anabolic congeners NOS

        2 ✓7th **T38.7X2** **Poisoning by androgens and anabolic** HCC **congeners, intentional self-harm**

        ✓7th **T38.7X3** **Poisoning by androgens and anabolic congeners, assault**

        ✓7th **T38.7X4** **Poisoning by androgens and anabolic congeners, undetermined**

        ✓7th **T38.7X5** **Adverse effect of androgens and anabolic congeners**

        ✓7th **T38.7X6** **Underdosing of androgens and anabolic congeners**

✓5th **T38.8** **Poisoning by, adverse effect of and underdosing of other and unspecified hormones and synthetic substitutes**

    ✓6th **T38.80** **Poisoning by, adverse effect of and underdosing of unspecified hormones and synthetic substitutes**

        ✓7th **T38.801** **Poisoning by unspecified hormones** ▽ **and synthetic substitutes, accidental (unintentional)**
            Poisoning by unspecified hormones and synthetic substitutes NOS

        2 ✓7th **T38.802** **Poisoning by unspecified hormones** HCC ▽ **and synthetic substitutes, intentional self-harm**

        ✓7th **T38.803** **Poisoning by unspecified hormones** ▽ **and synthetic substitutes, assault**

        ✓7th **T38.804** **Poisoning by unspecified hormones** ▽ **and synthetic substitutes, undetermined**

        ✓7th **T38.805** **Adverse effect of unspecified** ▽ **hormones and synthetic substitutes**

        ✓7th **T38.806** **Underdosing of unspecified hormones** ▽ **and synthetic substitutes**

    ✓6th **T38.81** **Poisoning by, adverse effect of and underdosing of anterior pituitary [adenohypophyseal] hormones**

        ✓7th **T38.811** **Poisoning by anterior pituitary [adenohypophyseal] hormones, accidental (unintentional)**
            Poisoning by anterior pituitary [adenohypophyseal] hormones NOS

        2 ✓7th **T38.812** **Poisoning by anterior pituitary** HCC **[adenohypophyseal] hormones, intentional self-harm**

        ✓7th **T38.813** **Poisoning by anterior pituitary [adenohypophyseal] hormones, assault**

        ✓7th **T38.814** **Poisoning by anterior pituitary [adenohypophyseal] hormones, undetermined**

        ✓7th **T38.815** **Adverse effect of anterior pituitary [adenohypophyseal] hormones**

        ✓7th **T38.816** **Underdosing of anterior pituitary [adenohypophyseal] hormones**

    ✓6th **T38.89** **Poisoning by, adverse effect of and underdosing of other hormones and synthetic substitutes**

        ✓7th **T38.891** **Poisoning by other hormones and synthetic substitutes, accidental (unintentional)**
            Poisoning by other hormones and synthetic substitutes NOS

        2 ✓7th **T38.892** **Poisoning by other hormones and** HCC **synthetic substitutes, intentional self-harm**

        ✓7th **T38.893** **Poisoning by other hormones and synthetic substitutes, assault**

        ✓7th **T38.894** **Poisoning by other hormones and synthetic substitutes, undetermined**

        ✓7th **T38.895** **Adverse effect of other hormones and synthetic substitutes**

        ✓7th **T38.896** **Underdosing of other hormones and synthetic substitutes**

✓5th **T38.9** **Poisoning by, adverse effect of and underdosing of other and unspecified hormone antagonists**

    ✓6th **T38.90** **Poisoning by, adverse effect of and underdosing of unspecified hormone antagonists**

        ✓7th **T38.901** **Poisoning by unspecified hormone** ▽ **antagonists, accidental (unintentional)**
            Poisoning by unspecified hormone antagonists NOS

        2 ✓7th **T38.902** **Poisoning by unspecified hormone** HCC ▽ **antagonists, intentional self-harm**

        ✓7th **T38.903** **Poisoning by unspecified hormone** ▽ **antagonists, assault**

        ✓7th **T38.904** **Poisoning by unspecified hormone** ▽ **antagonists, undetermined**

        ✓7th **T38.905** **Adverse effect of unspecified hormone** ▽ **antagonists**

        ✓7th **T38.906** **Underdosing of unspecified hormone** ▽ **antagonists**

    ✓6th **T38.99** **Poisoning by, adverse effect of and underdosing of other hormone antagonists**

        ✓7th **T38.991** **Poisoning by other hormone antagonists, accidental (unintentional)**
            Poisoning by other hormone antagonists NOS

        2 ✓7th **T38.992** **Poisoning by other hormone** HCC **antagonists, intentional self-harm**

        ✓7th **T38.993** **Poisoning by other hormone antagonists, assault**

        ✓7th **T38.994** **Poisoning by other hormone antagonists, undetermined**

        ✓7th **T38.995** **Adverse effect of other hormone antagonists**

        ✓7th **T38.996** **Underdosing of other hormone antagonists**

✓4th **T39** **Poisoning by, adverse effect of and underdosing of nonopioid analgesics, antipyretics and antirheumatics**

> The appropriate 7th character is to be added to each code from category T39.
> A   initial encounter
> D   subsequent encounter
> S   sequela

    ✓5th **T39.0** **Poisoning by, adverse effect of and underdosing of salicylates**

        ✓6th **T39.01** **Poisoning by, adverse effect of and underdosing of aspirin**
            Poisoning by, adverse effect of and underdosing of acetylsalicylic acid

            ✓7th **T39.011** **Poisoning by aspirin, accidental (unintentional)**

            2 ✓7th **T39.012** **Poisoning by aspirin, intentional** HCC **self-harm**

            ✓7th **T39.013** **Poisoning by aspirin, assault**

            ✓7th **T39.014** **Poisoning by aspirin, undetermined**

            ✓7th **T39.015** **Adverse effect of aspirin**
                AHA: 2016, 1Q, 15

            ✓7th **T39.016** **Underdosing of aspirin**

        ✓6th **T39.09** **Poisoning by, adverse effect of and underdosing of other salicylates**

            ✓7th **T39.091** **Poisoning by salicylates, accidental (unintentional)**
                Poisoning by salicylates NOS

            2 ✓7th **T39.092** **Poisoning by salicylates, intentional** HCC **self-harm**

            ✓7th **T39.093** **Poisoning by salicylates, assault**

            ✓7th **T39.094** **Poisoning by salicylates, undetermined**

            ✓7th **T39.095** **Adverse effect of salicylates**

            ✓7th **T39.096** **Underdosing of salicylates**

    ✓5th **T39.1** **Poisoning by, adverse effect of and underdosing of 4-Aminophenol derivatives**

        ✓6th **T39.1X** **Poisoning by, adverse effect of and underdosing of 4-Aminophenol derivatives**

            ✓7th **T39.1X1** **Poisoning by 4-Aminophenol derivatives, accidental (unintentional)**
                Poisoning by 4-Aminophenol derivatives NOS

---

2   HCC with 7th character indicating initial encounter (A or B - specific to category) OR sequela.

EXCLUDES 1 Not coded here   EXCLUDES 2 Not included here   N Newborn Age: 0   P Pediatric Age: 0-17   M Maternity Age: 12-55   A Adult Age: 15-124

1062   ICD-10-CM 2018

2 ✓7th **T39.1X2 Poisoning by 4-Aminophenol derivatives, intentional self-harm** HCC

✓7th **T39.1X3 Poisoning by 4-Aminophenol derivatives, assault**

✓7th **T39.1X4 Poisoning by 4-Aminophenol derivatives, undetermined**

✓7th **T39.1X5 Adverse effect of 4-Aminophenol derivatives**

✓7th **T39.1X6 Underdosing of 4-Aminophenol derivatives**

✓5th **T39.2 Poisoning by, adverse effect of and underdosing of pyrazolone derivatives**

✓6th **T39.2X Poisoning by, adverse effect of and underdosing of pyrazolone derivatives**

✓7th **T39.2X1 Poisoning by pyrazolone derivatives, accidental (unintentional)**
Poisoning by pyrazolone derivatives NOS

2 ✓7th **T39.2X2 Poisoning by pyrazolone derivatives, intentional self-harm** HCC

✓7th **T39.2X3 Poisoning by pyrazolone derivatives, assault**

✓7th **T39.2X4 Poisoning by pyrazolone derivatives, undetermined**

✓7th **T39.2X5 Adverse effect of pyrazolone derivatives**

✓7th **T39.2X6 Underdosing of pyrazolone derivatives**

✓5th **T39.3 Poisoning by, adverse effect of and underdosing of other nonsteroidal anti-inflammatory drugs [NSAID]**

✓6th **T39.31 Poisoning by, adverse effect of and underdosing of propionic acid derivatives**
Poisoning by, adverse effect of and underdosing of fenoprofen
Poisoning by, adverse effect of and underdosing of flurbiprofen
Poisoning by, adverse effect of and underdosing of ibuprofen
Poisoning by, adverse effect of and underdosing of ketoprofen
Poisoning by, adverse effect of and underdosing of naproxen
Poisoning by, adverse effect of and underdosing of oxaprozin

✓7th **T39.311 Poisoning by propionic acid derivatives, accidental (unintentional)**

2 ✓7th **T39.312 Poisoning by propionic acid derivatives, intentional self-harm** HCC

✓7th **T39.313 Poisoning by propionic acid derivatives, assault**

✓7th **T39.314 Poisoning by propionic acid derivatives, undetermined**

✓7th **T39.315 Adverse effect of propionic acid derivatives**

✓7th **T39.316 Underdosing of propionic acid derivatives**

✓6th **T39.39 Poisoning by, adverse effect of and underdosing of other nonsteroidal anti-inflammatory drugs [NSAID]**

✓7th **T39.391 Poisoning by other nonsteroidal anti-inflammatory drugs [NSAID], accidental (unintentional)**
Poisoning by other nonsteroidal anti-inflammatory drugs NOS

2 ✓7th **T39.392 Poisoning by other nonsteroidal anti-inflammatory drugs [NSAID], intentional self-harm** HCC

✓7th **T39.393 Poisoning by other nonsteroidal anti-inflammatory drugs [NSAID], assault**

✓7th **T39.394 Poisoning by other nonsteroidal anti-inflammatory drugs [NSAID], undetermined**

✓7th **T39.395 Adverse effect of other nonsteroidal anti-inflammatory drugs [NSAID]**

✓7th **T39.396 Underdosing of other nonsteroidal anti-inflammatory drugs [NSAID]**

✓5th **T39.4 Poisoning by, adverse effect of and underdosing of antirheumatics, not elsewhere classified**

EXCLUDES 1   *poisoning by, adverse effect of and underdosing of glucocorticoids (T38.0-)*
poisoning by, adverse effect of and underdosing of salicylates (T39.0-)

✓6th **T39.4X Poisoning by, adverse effect of and underdosing of antirheumatics, not elsewhere classified**

✓7th **T39.4X1 Poisoning by antirheumatics, not elsewhere classified, accidental (unintentional)**
Poisoning by antirheumatics, not elsewhere classified NOS

2 ✓7th **T39.4X2 Poisoning by antirheumatics, not elsewhere classified, intentional self-harm** HCC

✓7th **T39.4X3 Poisoning by antirheumatics, not elsewhere classified, assault**

✓7th **T39.4X4 Poisoning by antirheumatics, not elsewhere classified, undetermined**

✓7th **T39.4X5 Adverse effect of antirheumatics, not elsewhere classified**

✓7th **T39.4X6 Underdosing of antirheumatics, not elsewhere classified**

✓5th **T39.8 Poisoning by, adverse effect of and underdosing of other nonopioid analgesics and antipyretics, not elsewhere classified**

✓6th **T39.8X Poisoning by, adverse effect of and underdosing of other nonopioid analgesics and antipyretics, not elsewhere classified**

✓7th **T39.8X1 Poisoning by other nonopioid analgesics and antipyretics, not elsewhere classified, accidental (unintentional)**
Poisoning by other nonopioid analgesics and antipyretics, not elsewhere classified NOS

2 ✓7th **T39.8X2 Poisoning by other nonopioid analgesics and antipyretics, not elsewhere classified, intentional self-harm** HCC

✓7th **T39.8X3 Poisoning by other nonopioid analgesics and antipyretics, not elsewhere classified, assault**

✓7th **T39.8X4 Poisoning by other nonopioid analgesics and antipyretics, not elsewhere classified, undetermined**

✓7th **T39.8X5 Adverse effect of other nonopioid analgesics and antipyretics, not elsewhere classified**

✓7th **T39.8X6 Underdosing of other nonopioid analgesics and antipyretics, not elsewhere classified**

✓5th **T39.9 Poisoning by, adverse effect of and underdosing of unspecified nonopioid analgesic, antipyretic and antirheumatic**

✓x7th **T39.91 Poisoning by unspecified nonopioid analgesic, antipyretic and antirheumatic, accidental (unintentional)** ▽
Poisoning by nonopioid analgesic, antipyretic and antirheumatic NOS

2 ✓x7th **T39.92 Poisoning by unspecified nonopioid analgesic, antipyretic and antirheumatic, intentional self-harm** HCC ▽

✓x7th **T39.93 Poisoning by unspecified nonopioid analgesic, antipyretic and antirheumatic, assault** ▽

✓x7th **T39.94 Poisoning by unspecified nonopioid analgesic, antipyretic and antirheumatic, undetermined** ▽

✓x7th **T39.95 Adverse effect of unspecified nonopioid analgesic, antipyretic and antirheumatic** ▽

✓x7th **T39.96 Underdosing of unspecified nonopioid analgesic, antipyretic and antirheumatic** ▽

---

2   HCC with 7th character indicating initial encounter (A or B - specific to category) OR sequela.

✓ Additional Character Req   ✓x7th Placeholder Alert   Manifestation   HCC CMS-HCC Condition   ▽ Unspecified Code   ▶◀ Revised Text   ● New Code   ▲ Revised Code Title

ICD-10-CM 2018   1063

✓4th **T40** **Poisoning by, adverse effect of and underdosing of narcotics and psychodysleptics [hallucinogens]**

EXCLUDES 2 *drug dependence and related mental and behavioral disorders due to psychoactive substance use (F10-F19-)*

> The appropriate 7th character is to be added to each code from category T40.
> A   initial encounter
> D   subsequent encounter
> S   sequela

✓5th **T40.0** **Poisoning by, adverse effect of and underdosing of opium**

   ✓6th **T40.0X** **Poisoning by, adverse effect of and underdosing of opium**

     ✓7th **T40.0X1** **Poisoning by opium, accidental (unintentional)**
       Poisoning by opium NOS

     2 ✓7th **T40.0X2** **Poisoning by opium, intentional self-harm** HCC

     ✓7th **T40.0X3** **Poisoning by opium, assault**

     ✓7th **T40.0X4** **Poisoning by opium, undetermined**

     ✓7th **T40.0X5** **Adverse effect of opium**

     ✓7th **T40.0X6** **Underdosing of opium**

✓5th **T40.1** **Poisoning by and adverse effect of heroin**

   ✓6th **T40.1X** **Poisoning by and adverse effect of heroin**

     ✓7th **T40.1X1** **Poisoning by heroin, accidental (unintentional)**
       Poisoning by heroin NOS

     2 ✓7th **T40.1X2** **Poisoning by heroin, intentional self-harm** HCC

     ✓7th **T40.1X3** **Poisoning by heroin, assault**

     ✓7th **T40.1X4** **Poisoning by heroin, undetermined**

✓5th **T40.2** **Poisoning by, adverse effect of and underdosing of other opioids**

   ✓6th **T40.2X** **Poisoning by, adverse effect of and underdosing of other opioids**

     ✓7th **T40.2X1** **Poisoning by other opioids, accidental (unintentional)**
       Poisoning by other opioids NOS

     2 ✓7th **T40.2X2** **Poisoning by other opioids, intentional self-harm** HCC

     ✓7th **T40.2X3** **Poisoning by other opioids, assault**

     ✓7th **T40.2X4** **Poisoning by other opioids, undetermined**

     ✓7th **T40.2X5** **Adverse effect of other opioids**

     ✓7th **T40.2X6** **Underdosing of other opioids**

✓5th **T40.3** **Poisoning by, adverse effect of and underdosing of methadone**

   ✓6th **T40.3X** **Poisoning by, adverse effect of and underdosing of methadone**

     ✓7th **T40.3X1** **Poisoning by methadone, accidental (unintentional)**
       Poisoning by methadone NOS

     2 ✓7th **T40.3X2** **Poisoning by methadone, intentional self-harm** HCC

     ✓7th **T40.3X3** **Poisoning by methadone, assault**

     ✓7th **T40.3X4** **Poisoning by methadone, undetermined**

     ✓7th **T40.3X5** **Adverse effect of methadone**

     ✓7th **T40.3X6** **Underdosing of methadone**

✓5th **T40.4** **Poisoning by, adverse effect of and underdosing of other synthetic narcotics**

   ✓6th **T40.4X** **Poisoning by, adverse effect of and underdosing of other synthetic narcotics**

     ✓7th **T40.4X1** **Poisoning by other synthetic narcotics, accidental (unintentional)**
       Poisoning by other synthetic narcotics NOS

     2 ✓7th **T40.4X2** **Poisoning by other synthetic narcotics, intentional self-harm** HCC

     ✓7th **T40.4X3** **Poisoning by other synthetic narcotics, assault**

     ✓7th **T40.4X4** **Poisoning by other synthetic narcotics, undetermined**

     ✓7th **T40.4X5** **Adverse effect of other synthetic narcotics**

     ✓7th **T40.4X6** **Underdosing of other synthetic narcotics**

✓5th **T40.5** **Poisoning by, adverse effect of and underdosing of cocaine**

   ✓6th **T40.5X** **Poisoning by, adverse effect of and underdosing of cocaine**

     ✓7th **T40.5X1** **Poisoning by cocaine, accidental (unintentional)**
       Poisoning by cocaine NOS
       AHA: 2016, 2Q, 8

     2 ✓7th **T40.5X2** **Poisoning by cocaine, intentional self-harm** HCC

     ✓7th **T40.5X3** **Poisoning by cocaine, assault**

     ✓7th **T40.5X4** **Poisoning by cocaine, undetermined**

     ✓7th **T40.5X5** **Adverse effect of cocaine**

     ✓7th **T40.5X6** **Underdosing of cocaine**

✓5th **T40.6** **Poisoning by, adverse effect of and underdosing of other and unspecified narcotics**

   ✓6th **T40.60** **Poisoning by, adverse effect of and underdosing of unspecified narcotics**

     ✓7th **T40.601** **Poisoning by unspecified narcotics, accidental (unintentional)** ▽
       Poisoning by narcotics NOS

     2 ✓7th **T40.602** **Poisoning by unspecified narcotics, intentional self-harm** HCC ▽

     ✓7th **T40.603** **Poisoning by unspecified narcotics, assault** ▽

     ✓7th **T40.604** **Poisoning by unspecified narcotics, undetermined** ▽

     ✓7th **T40.605** **Adverse effect of unspecified narcotics** ▽

     ✓7th **T40.606** **Underdosing of unspecified narcotics** ▽

   ✓6th **T40.69** **Poisoning by, adverse effect of and underdosing of other narcotics**

     ✓7th **T40.691** **Poisoning by other narcotics, accidental (unintentional)**
       Poisoning by other narcotics NOS

     2 ✓7th **T40.692** **Poisoning by other narcotics, intentional self-harm** HCC

     ✓7th **T40.693** **Poisoning by other narcotics, assault**

     ✓7th **T40.694** **Poisoning by other narcotics, undetermined**

     ✓7th **T40.695** **Adverse effect of other narcotics**

     ✓7th **T40.696** **Underdosing of other narcotics**

✓5th **T40.7** **Poisoning by, adverse effect of and underdosing of cannabis (derivatives)**

   ✓6th **T40.7X** **Poisoning by, adverse effect of and underdosing of cannabis (derivatives)**

     ✓7th **T40.7X1** **Poisoning by cannabis (derivatives), accidental (unintentional)**
       Poisoning by cannabis NOS

     2 ✓7th **T40.7X2** **Poisoning by cannabis (derivatives), intentional self-harm** HCC

     ✓7th **T40.7X3** **Poisoning by cannabis (derivatives), assault**

     ✓7th **T40.7X4** **Poisoning by cannabis (derivatives), undetermined**

     ✓7th **T40.7X5** **Adverse effect of cannabis (derivatives)**

     ✓7th **T40.7X6** **Underdosing of cannabis (derivatives)**

✓5th **T40.8** **Poisoning by and adverse effect of lysergide [LSD]**

   ✓6th **T40.8X** **Poisoning by and adverse effect of lysergide [LSD]**

     ✓7th **T40.8X1** **Poisoning by lysergide [LSD], accidental (unintentional)**
       Poisoning by lysergide [LSD]NOS

     2 ✓7th **T40.8X2** **Poisoning by lysergide [LSD], intentional self-harm** HCC

     ✓7th **T40.8X3** **Poisoning by lysergide [LSD], assault**

     ✓7th **T40.8X4** **Poisoning by lysergide [LSD], undetermined**

✓5th **T40.9** **Poisoning by, adverse effect of and underdosing of other and unspecified psychodysleptics [hallucinogens]**

   ✓6th **T40.90** **Poisoning by, adverse effect of and underdosing of unspecified psychodysleptics [hallucinogens]**

     ✓7th **T40.901** **Poisoning by unspecified psychodysleptics [hallucinogens], accidental (unintentional)** ▽

---

2 HCC with 7th character indicating initial encounter (A or B - specific to category) OR sequela.

EXCLUDES 1 Not coded here   EXCLUDES 2 Not included here   N Newborn Age: 0   P Pediatric Age: 0-17   M Maternity Age: 12-55   A Adult Age: 15-124

2 ☑7th **T40.902** **Poisoning by unspecified** HCC ▽
psychodysleptics [hallucinogens],
intentional self-harm

☑7th **T40.903** **Poisoning by unspecified** ▽
psychodysleptics [hallucinogens],
assault

☑7th **T40.904** **Poisoning by unspecified** ▽
psychodysleptics [hallucinogens],
undetermined

☑7th **T40.905** **Adverse effect of unspecified** ▽
psychodysleptics [hallucinogens]

☑7th **T40.906** **Underdosing of unspecified** ▽
psychodysleptics

☑6th **T40.99** **Poisoning by, adverse effect of and underdosing of**
other psychodysleptics [hallucinogens]

☑7th **T40.991** **Poisoning by other psychodysleptics**
[hallucinogens], accidental
(unintentional)
Poisoning by other psychodysleptics
[hallucinogens] NOS

2 ☑7th **T40.992** **Poisoning by other psychodysleptics** HCC
[hallucinogens], intentional self-harm

☑7th **T40.993** **Poisoning by other psychodysleptics**
[hallucinogens], assault

☑7th **T40.994** **Poisoning by other psychodysleptics**
[hallucinogens], undetermined

☑7th **T40.995** **Adverse effect of other psychodysleptics**
[hallucinogens]

☑7th **T40.996** **Underdosing of other psychodysleptics**

☑4th **T41** **Poisoning by, adverse effect of and underdosing of anesthetics**
and therapeutic gases
EXCLUDES 1   benzodiazepines (T42.4-)
cocaine (T40.5-)
complications of anesthesia during labor and delivery (O74.-)
complications of anesthesia during pregnancy (O29.-)
complications of anesthesia during the puerperium (O89.-)
opioids (T40.0-T40.2-)

The appropriate 7th character is to be added to each code from
category T41.
A   initial encounter
D   subsequent encounter
S   sequela

☑5th **T41.0** **Poisoning by, adverse effect of and underdosing of inhaled**
anesthetics
EXCLUDES 1   oxygen (T41.5-)

☑6th **T41.0X** **Poisoning by, adverse effect of and underdosing of**
inhaled anesthetics

☑7th **T41.0X1** **Poisoning by inhaled anesthetics,**
accidental (unintentional)
Poisoning by inhaled anesthetics NOS

2 ☑7th **T41.0X2** **Poisoning by inhaled anesthetics,** HCC
intentional self-harm

☑7th **T41.0X3** **Poisoning by inhaled anesthetics, assault**

☑7th **T41.0X4** **Poisoning by inhaled anesthetics,**
undetermined

☑7th **T41.0X5** **Adverse effect of inhaled anesthetics**

☑7th **T41.0X6** **Underdosing of inhaled anesthetics**

☑5th **T41.1** **Poisoning by, adverse effect of and underdosing of**
intravenous anesthetics
Poisoning by, adverse effect of and underdosing of
thiobarbiturates

☑6th **T41.1X** **Poisoning by, adverse effect of and underdosing of**
intravenous anesthetics

☑7th **T41.1X1** **Poisoning by intravenous anesthetics,**
accidental (unintentional)
Poisoning by intravenous anesthetics NOS

2 ☑7th **T41.1X2** **Poisoning by intravenous anesthetics,** HCC
intentional self-harm

☑7th **T41.1X3** **Poisoning by intravenous anesthetics,**
assault

☑7th **T41.1X4** **Poisoning by intravenous anesthetics,**
undetermined

☑7th **T41.1X5** **Adverse effect of intravenous anesthetics**

☑7th **T41.1X6** **Underdosing of intravenous anesthetics**

☑5th **T41.2** **Poisoning by, adverse effect of and underdosing of other and**
unspecified general anesthetics

☑6th **T41.20** **Poisoning by, adverse effect of and underdosing of**
unspecified general anesthetics

☑7th **T41.201** **Poisoning by unspecified general** ▽
anesthetics, accidental (unintentional)
Poisoning by general anesthetics NOS

2 ☑7th **T41.202** **Poisoning by unspecified general** HCC ▽
anesthetics, intentional self-harm

☑7th **T41.203** **Poisoning by unspecified general** ▽
anesthetics, assault

☑7th **T41.204** **Poisoning by unspecified general** ▽
anesthetics, undetermined

☑7th **T41.205** **Adverse effect of unspecified general** ▽
anesthetics

☑7th **T41.206** **Underdosing of unspecified general** ▽
anesthetics

☑6th **T41.29** **Poisoning by, adverse effect of and underdosing of**
other general anesthetics

☑7th **T41.291** **Poisoning by other general anesthetics,**
accidental (unintentional)
Poisoning by other general anesthetics
NOS

2 ☑7th **T41.292** **Poisoning by other general** HCC
anesthetics, intentional self-harm

☑7th **T41.293** **Poisoning by other general**
anesthetics, assault

☑7th **T41.294** **Poisoning by other general**
anesthetics, undetermined

☑7th **T41.295** **Adverse effect of other general**
anesthetics

☑7th **T41.296** **Underdosing of other general anesthetics**

☑5th **T41.3** **Poisoning by, adverse effect of and underdosing of local**
anesthetics
Cocaine (topical)
EXCLUDES 2   poisoning by cocaine used as a central nervous system
stimulant (T40.5X1-T40.5X4)

☑6th **T41.3X** **Poisoning by, adverse effect of and underdosing of**
local anesthetics

☑7th **T41.3X1** **Poisoning by local anesthetics, accidental**
(unintentional)
Poisoning by local anesthetics NOS

2 ☑7th **T41.3X2** **Poisoning by local anesthetics,** HCC
intentional self-harm

☑7th **T41.3X3** **Poisoning by local anesthetics, assault**

☑7th **T41.3X4** **Poisoning by local anesthetics,**
undetermined

☑7th **T41.3X5** **Adverse effect of local anesthetics**

☑7th **T41.3X6** **Underdosing of local anesthetics**

☑5th **T41.4** **Poisoning by, adverse effect of and underdosing of**
unspecified anesthetic

☑x7th **T41.41** **Poisoning by unspecified anesthetic, accidental** ▽
(unintentional)
Poisoning by anesthetic NOS

2 ☑x7th **T41.42** **Poisoning by unspecified anesthetic,** HCC ▽
intentional self-harm

☑x7th **T41.43** **Poisoning by unspecified anesthetic, assault** ▽

☑x7th **T41.44** **Poisoning by unspecified anesthetic,** ▽
undetermined

☑x7th **T41.45** **Adverse effect of unspecified anesthetic** ▽

☑x7th **T41.46** **Underdosing of unspecified anesthetics** ▽

☑5th **T41.5** **Poisoning by, adverse effect of and underdosing of**
therapeutic gases

☑6th **T41.5X** **Poisoning by, adverse effect of and underdosing of**
therapeutic gases

☑7th **T41.5X1** **Poisoning by therapeutic gases,**
accidental (unintentional)
Poisoning by therapeutic gases NOS

2 ☑7th **T41.5X2** **Poisoning by therapeutic gases,** HCC
intentional self-harm

☑7th **T41.5X3** **Poisoning by therapeutic gases, assault**

☑7th **T41.5X4** **Poisoning by therapeutic gases,**
undetermined

☑7th **T41.5X5** **Adverse effect of therapeutic gases**

☑ Additional Character Req   ☑x7th Placeholder Alert   Manifestation   HCC CMS-HCC Condition   ▽ Unspecified Code   ▶◀ Revised Text   ● New Code   ▲ Revised Code Title

Chapter 19. Injury, Poisoning, and Certain Other Consequences of External Causes

✓7th **T41.5X6**   **Underdosing of therapeutic gases**

✓4th **T42**   **Poisoning by, adverse effect of and underdosing of antiepileptic, sedative- hypnotic and antiparkinsonism drugs**

> EXCLUDES 2   drug dependence and related mental and behavioral disorders due to psychoactive substance use (F10.- -F19.-)

The appropriate 7th character is to be added to each code from category T42.
A   initial encounter
D   subsequent encounter
S   sequela

✓5th **T42.0**   **Poisoning by, adverse effect of and underdosing of hydantoin derivatives**

    ✓6th **T42.0X**   **Poisoning by, adverse effect of and underdosing of hydantoin derivatives**

       ✓7th **T42.0X1**   **Poisoning by hydantoin derivatives, accidental (unintentional)**
          Poisoning by hydantoin derivatives NOS

       2 ✓7th **T42.0X2**   **Poisoning by hydantoin derivatives, intentional self-harm**   HCC

       ✓7th **T42.0X3**   **Poisoning by hydantoin derivatives, assault**

       ✓7th **T42.0X4**   **Poisoning by hydantoin derivatives, undetermined**

       ✓7th **T42.0X5**   **Adverse effect of hydantoin derivatives**

       ✓7th **T42.0X6**   **Underdosing of hydantoin derivatives**

✓5th **T42.1**   **Poisoning by, adverse effect of and underdosing of iminostilbenes**
     Poisoning by, adverse effect of and underdosing of carbamazepine

    ✓6th **T42.1X**   **Poisoning by, adverse effect of and underdosing of iminostilbenes**

       ✓7th **T42.1X1**   **Poisoning by iminostilbenes, accidental (unintentional)**
          Poisoning by iminostilbenes NOS

       2 ✓7th **T42.1X2**   **Poisoning by iminostilbenes, intentional self-harm**   HCC

       ✓7th **T42.1X3**   **Poisoning by iminostilbenes, assault**

       ✓7th **T42.1X4**   **Poisoning by iminostilbenes, undetermined**

       ✓7th **T42.1X5**   **Adverse effect of iminostilbenes**

       ✓7th **T42.1X6**   **Underdosing of iminostilbenes**

✓5th **T42.2**   **Poisoning by, adverse effect of and underdosing of succinimides and oxazolidinediones**

    ✓6th **T42.2X**   **Poisoning by, adverse effect of and underdosing of succinimides and oxazolidinediones**

       ✓7th **T42.2X1**   **Poisoning by succinimides and oxazolidinediones, accidental (unintentional)**
          Poisoning by succinimides and oxazolidinediones NOS

       2 ✓7th **T42.2X2**   **Poisoning by succinimides and oxazolidinediones, intentional self-harm**   HCC

       ✓7th **T42.2X3**   **Poisoning by succinimides and oxazolidinediones, assault**

       ✓7th **T42.2X4**   **Poisoning by succinimides and oxazolidinediones, undetermined**

       ✓7th **T42.2X5**   **Adverse effect of succinimides and oxazolidinediones**

       ✓7th **T42.2X6**   **Underdosing of succinimides and oxazolidinediones**

✓5th **T42.3**   **Poisoning by, adverse effect of and underdosing of barbiturates**

> EXCLUDES 1   poisoning by, adverse effect of and underdosing of thiobarbiturates (T41.1-)

    ✓6th **T42.3X**   **Poisoning by, adverse effect of and underdosing of barbiturates**

       ✓7th **T42.3X1**   **Poisoning by barbiturates, accidental (unintentional)**
          Poisoning by barbiturates NOS

       2 ✓7th **T42.3X2**   **Poisoning by barbiturates, intentional self-harm**   HCC

       ✓7th **T42.3X3**   **Poisoning by barbiturates, assault**

       ✓7th **T42.3X4**   **Poisoning by barbiturates, undetermined**

       ✓7th **T42.3X5**   **Adverse effect of barbiturates**

✓7th **T42.3X6**   **Underdosing of barbiturates**

✓5th **T42.4**   **Poisoning by, adverse effect of and underdosing of benzodiazepines**

    ✓6th **T42.4X**   **Poisoning by, adverse effect of and underdosing of benzodiazepines**

       ✓7th **T42.4X1**   **Poisoning by benzodiazepines, accidental (unintentional)**
          Poisoning by benzodiazepines NOS

       2 ✓7th **T42.4X2**   **Poisoning by benzodiazepines, intentional self-harm**   HCC

       ✓7th **T42.4X3**   **Poisoning by benzodiazepines, assault**

       ✓7th **T42.4X4**   **Poisoning by benzodiazepines, undetermined**

       ✓7th **T42.4X5**   **Adverse effect of benzodiazepines**

       ✓7th **T42.4X6**   **Underdosing of benzodiazepines**

✓5th **T42.5**   **Poisoning by, adverse effect of and underdosing of mixed antiepileptics**

    ✓6th **T42.5X**   **Poisoning by, adverse effect of and underdosing of antiepileptics**

       ✓7th **T42.5X1**   **Poisoning by mixed antiepileptics, accidental (unintentional)**
          Poisoning by mixed antiepileptics NOS

       2 ✓7th **T42.5X2**   **Poisoning by mixed antiepileptics, intentional self-harm**   HCC

       ✓7th **T42.5X3**   **Poisoning by mixed antiepileptics, assault**

       ✓7th **T42.5X4**   **Poisoning by mixed antiepileptics, undetermined**

       ✓7th **T42.5X5**   **Adverse effect of mixed antiepileptics**

       ✓7th **T42.5X6**   **Underdosing of mixed antiepileptics**

✓5th **T42.6**   **Poisoning by, adverse effect of and underdosing of other antiepileptic and sedative-hypnotic drugs**
     Poisoning by, adverse effect of and underdosing of methaqualone
     Poisoning by, adverse effect of and underdosing of valproic acid

> EXCLUDES 1   poisoning by, adverse effect of and underdosing of carbamazepine (T42.1-)

    ✓6th **T42.6X**   **Poisoning by, adverse effect of and underdosing of other antiepileptic and sedative-hypnotic drugs**

       ✓7th **T42.6X1**   **Poisoning by other antiepileptic and sedative-hypnotic drugs, accidental (unintentional)**
          Poisoning by other antiepileptic and sedative-hypnotic drugs NOS

       2 ✓7th **T42.6X2**   **Poisoning by other antiepileptic and sedative-hypnotic drugs, intentional self-harm**   HCC

       ✓7th **T42.6X3**   **Poisoning by other antiepileptic and sedative-hypnotic drugs, assault**

       ✓7th **T42.6X4**   **Poisoning by other antiepileptic and sedative-hypnotic drugs, undetermined**

       ✓7th **T42.6X5**   **Adverse effect of other antiepileptic and sedative-hypnotic drugs**

       ✓7th **T42.6X6**   **Underdosing of other antiepileptic and sedative-hypnotic drugs**

✓5th **T42.7**   **Poisoning by, adverse effect of and underdosing of unspecified antiepileptic and sedative-hypnotic drugs**

    ✓x7th **T42.71**   **Poisoning by unspecified antiepileptic and sedative-hypnotic drugs, accidental (unintentional)** ▽
       Poisoning by antiepileptic and sedative-hypnotic drugs NOS

    2 ✓x7th **T42.72**   **Poisoning by unspecified antiepileptic and sedative-hypnotic drugs, intentional self-harm**   HCC ▽

    ✓x7th **T42.73**   **Poisoning by unspecified antiepileptic and sedative-hypnotic drugs, assault** ▽

    ✓x7th **T42.74**   **Poisoning by unspecified antiepileptic and sedative-hypnotic drugs, undetermined** ▽

    ✓x7th **T42.75**   **Adverse effect of unspecified antiepileptic and sedative-hypnotic drugs** ▽

    ✓x7th **T42.76**   **Underdosing of unspecified antiepileptic and sedative-hypnotic drugs** ▽

2   HCC with 7th character indicating initial encounter (A or B - specific to category) OR sequela.

EXCLUDES 1 Not coded here   EXCLUDES 2 Not included here   N Newborn Age: 0   P Pediatric Age: 0-17   M Maternity Age: 12-55   A Adult Age: 15-124

1066   ICD-10-CM 2018

√5ᵗʰ **T42.8** **Poisoning by, adverse effect of and underdosing of antiparkinsonism drugs and other central muscle-tone depressants**
Poisoning by, adverse effect of and underdosing of amantadine

√6ᵗʰ **T42.8X** **Poisoning by, adverse effect of and underdosing of antiparkinsonism drugs and other central muscle-tone depressants**

√7ᵗʰ **T42.8X1** **Poisoning by antiparkinsonism drugs and other central muscle-tone depressants, accidental (unintentional)**
Poisoning by antiparkinsonism drugs and other central muscle-tone depressants NOS

2 √7ᵗʰ **T42.8X2** **Poisoning by antiparkinsonism drugs and other central muscle-tone depressants, intentional self-harm** HCC

√7ᵗʰ **T42.8X3** **Poisoning by antiparkinsonism drugs and other central muscle-tone depressants, assault**

√7ᵗʰ **T42.8X4** **Poisoning by antiparkinsonism drugs and other central muscle-tone depressants, undetermined**

√7ᵗʰ **T42.8X5** **Adverse effect of antiparkinsonism drugs and other central muscle-tone depressants**

√7ᵗʰ **T42.8X6** **Underdosing of antiparkinsonism drugs and other central muscle-tone depressants**

√4ᵗʰ **T43** **Poisoning by, adverse effect of and underdosing of psychotropic drugs, not elsewhere classified**
EXCLUDES 1   appetite depressants (T50.5-)
    barbiturates (T42.3-)
    benzodiazepines (T42.4-)
    methaqualone (T42.6-)
    psychodysleptics [hallucinogens] (T40.7-T40.9-)
EXCLUDES 2   drug dependence and related mental and behavioral disorders due to psychoactive substance use (F10.- -F19.-)

The appropriate 7th character is to be added to each code from category T43.
A   initial encounter
D   subsequent encounter
S   sequela

√5ᵗʰ **T43.0** **Poisoning by, adverse effect of and underdosing of tricyclic and tetracyclic antidepressants**

√6ᵗʰ **T43.01** **Poisoning by, adverse effect of and underdosing of tricyclic antidepressants**

√7ᵗʰ **T43.011** **Poisoning by tricyclic antidepressants, accidental (unintentional)**
Poisoning by tricyclic antidepressants NOS

2 √7ᵗʰ **T43.012** **Poisoning by tricyclic antidepressants, intentional self-harm** HCC

√7ᵗʰ **T43.013** **Poisoning by tricyclic antidepressants, assault**

√7ᵗʰ **T43.014** **Poisoning by tricyclic antidepressants, undetermined**

√7ᵗʰ **T43.015** **Adverse effect of tricyclic antidepressants**

√7ᵗʰ **T43.016** **Underdosing of tricyclic antidepressants**

√6ᵗʰ **T43.02** **Poisoning by, adverse effect of and underdosing of tetracyclic antidepressants**

√7ᵗʰ **T43.021** **Poisoning by tetracyclic antidepressants, accidental (unintentional)**
Poisoning by tetracyclic antidepressants NOS

2 √7ᵗʰ **T43.022** **Poisoning by tetracyclic antidepressants, intentional self-harm** HCC

√7ᵗʰ **T43.023** **Poisoning by tetracyclic antidepressants, assault**

√7ᵗʰ **T43.024** **Poisoning by tetracyclic antidepressants, undetermined**

√7ᵗʰ **T43.025** **Adverse effect of tetracyclic antidepressants**

√7ᵗʰ **T43.026** **Underdosing of tetracyclic antidepressants**

√5ᵗʰ **T43.1** **Poisoning by, adverse effect of and underdosing of monoamine-oxidase-inhibitor antidepressants**

√6ᵗʰ **T43.1X** **Poisoning by, adverse effect of and underdosing of monoamine-oxidase-inhibitor antidepressants**

√7ᵗʰ **T43.1X1** **Poisoning by monoamine-oxidase-inhibitor antidepressants, accidental (unintentional)**
Poisoning by monoamine-oxidase-inhibitor antidepressants NOS

2 √7ᵗʰ **T43.1X2** **Poisoning by monoamine-oxidase-inhibitor antidepressants, intentional self-harm** HCC

√7ᵗʰ **T43.1X3** **Poisoning by monoamine-oxidase-inhibitor antidepressants, assault**

√7ᵗʰ **T43.1X4** **Poisoning by monoamine-oxidase-inhibitor antidepressants, undetermined**

√7ᵗʰ **T43.1X5** **Adverse effect of monoamine-oxidase-inhibitor antidepressants**

√7ᵗʰ **T43.1X6** **Underdosing of monoamine-oxidase-inhibitor antidepressants**

√5ᵗʰ **T43.2** **Poisoning by, adverse effect of and underdosing of other and unspecified antidepressants**

√6ᵗʰ **T43.20** **Poisoning by, adverse effect of and underdosing of unspecified antidepressants**

√7ᵗʰ **T43.201** **Poisoning by unspecified antidepressants, accidental (unintentional)** ▽
Poisoning by antidepressants NOS

2 √7ᵗʰ **T43.202** **Poisoning by unspecified antidepressants, intentional self-harm** HCC ▽

√7ᵗʰ **T43.203** **Poisoning by unspecified antidepressants, assault** ▽

√7ᵗʰ **T43.204** **Poisoning by unspecified antidepressants, undetermined** ▽

√7ᵗʰ **T43.205** **Adverse effect of unspecified antidepressants** ▽
►Antidepressant discontinuation syndrome◄

√7ᵗʰ **T43.206** **Underdosing of unspecified antidepressants** ▽

√6ᵗʰ **T43.21** **Poisoning by, adverse effect of and underdosing of selective serotonin and norepinephrine reuptake inhibitors**
Poisoning by, adverse effect of and underdosing of SSNRI antidepressants

√7ᵗʰ **T43.211** **Poisoning by selective serotonin and norepinephrine reuptake inhibitors, accidental (unintentional)**

2 √7ᵗʰ **T43.212** **Poisoning by selective serotonin and norepinephrine reuptake inhibitors, intentional self-harm** HCC

√7ᵗʰ **T43.213** **Poisoning by selective serotonin and norepinephrine reuptake inhibitors, assault**

√7ᵗʰ **T43.214** **Poisoning by selective serotonin and norepinephrine reuptake inhibitors, undetermined**

√7ᵗʰ **T43.215** **Adverse effect of selective serotonin and norepinephrine reuptake inhibitors**

√7ᵗʰ **T43.216** **Underdosing of selective serotonin and norepinephrine reuptake inhibitors**

√6ᵗʰ **T43.22** **Poisoning by, adverse effect of and underdosing of selective serotonin reuptake inhibitors**
Poisoning by, adverse effect of and underdosing of SSRI antidepressants

√7ᵗʰ **T43.221** **Poisoning by selective serotonin reuptake inhibitors, accidental (unintentional)**

2 √7ᵗʰ **T43.222** **Poisoning by selective serotonin reuptake inhibitors, intentional self-harm** HCC

√7ᵗʰ **T43.223** **Poisoning by selective serotonin reuptake inhibitors, assault**

√7ᵗʰ **T43.224** **Poisoning by selective serotonin reuptake inhibitors, undetermined**

√7ᵗʰ **T43.225** **Adverse effect of selective serotonin reuptake inhibitors**

√7ᵗʰ **T43.226** **Underdosing of selective serotonin reuptake inhibitors**

---

2   HCC with 7th character indicating initial encounter (A or B - specific to category) OR sequela.

☑ Additional Character Req   ☑x7ᵗʰ Placeholder Alert   Manifestation   HCC CMS-HCC Condition   ▽ Unspecified Code   ►◄ Revised Text   ● New Code   ▲ Revised Code Title

Chapter 19. Injury, Poisoning, and Certain Other Consequences of External Causes

√6ᵗʰ **T43.29** **Poisoning by, adverse effect of and underdosing of other antidepressants**

   √7ᵗʰ **T43.291** **Poisoning by other antidepressants, accidental (unintentional)**
        Poisoning by other antidepressants NOS

  2 √7ᵗʰ **T43.292** **Poisoning by other antidepressants, intentional self-harm** HCC

   √7ᵗʰ **T43.293** **Poisoning by other antidepressants, assault**

   √7ᵗʰ **T43.294** **Poisoning by other antidepressants, undetermined**

   √7ᵗʰ **T43.295** **Adverse effect of other antidepressants**

   √7ᵗʰ **T43.296** **Underdosing of other antidepressants**

√5ᵗʰ **T43.3** **Poisoning by, adverse effect of and underdosing of phenothiazine antipsychotics and neuroleptics**

 √6ᵗʰ **T43.3X** **Poisoning by, adverse effect of and underdosing of phenothiazine antipsychotics and neuroleptics**

   √7ᵗʰ **T43.3X1** **Poisoning by phenothiazine antipsychotics and neuroleptics, accidental (unintentional)**
        Poisoning by phenothiazine antipsychotics and neuroleptics NOS

  2 √7ᵗʰ **T43.3X2** **Poisoning by phenothiazine antipsychotics and neuroleptics, intentional self-harm** HCC

   √7ᵗʰ **T43.3X3** **Poisoning by phenothiazine antipsychotics and neuroleptics, assault**

   √7ᵗʰ **T43.3X4** **Poisoning by phenothiazine antipsychotics and neuroleptics, undetermined**

   √7ᵗʰ **T43.3X5** **Adverse effect of phenothiazine antipsychotics and neuroleptics**

   √7ᵗʰ **T43.3X6** **Underdosing of phenothiazine antipsychotics and neuroleptics**

√5ᵗʰ **T43.4** **Poisoning by, adverse effect of and underdosing of butyrophenone and thiothixene neuroleptics**

 √6ᵗʰ **T43.4X** **Poisoning by, adverse effect of and underdosing of butyrophenone and thiothixene neuroleptics**

   √7ᵗʰ **T43.4X1** **Poisoning by butyrophenone and thiothixene neuroleptics, accidental (unintentional)**
        Poisoning by butyrophenone and thiothixene neuroleptics NOS

  2 √7ᵗʰ **T43.4X2** **Poisoning by butyrophenone and thiothixene neuroleptics, intentional self-harm** HCC

   √7ᵗʰ **T43.4X3** **Poisoning by butyrophenone and thiothixene neuroleptics, assault**

   √7ᵗʰ **T43.4X4** **Poisoning by butyrophenone and thiothixene neuroleptics, undetermined**

   √7ᵗʰ **T43.4X5** **Adverse effect of butyrophenone and thiothixene neuroleptics**

   √7ᵗʰ **T43.4X6** **Underdosing of butyrophenone and thiothixene neuroleptics**

√5ᵗʰ **T43.5** **Poisoning by, adverse effect of and underdosing of other and unspecified antipsychotics and neuroleptics**

    EXCLUDES 1   poisoning by, adverse effect of and underdosing of rauwolfia (T46.5-)

 √6ᵗʰ **T43.50** **Poisoning by, adverse effect of and underdosing of unspecified antipsychotics and neuroleptics**

   √7ᵗʰ **T43.501** **Poisoning by unspecified anti-psychotics and neuroleptics, accidental (unintentional)** ▽
        Poisoning by antipsychotics and neuroleptics NOS

  2 √7ᵗʰ **T43.502** **Poisoning by unspecified anti-psychotics and neuroleptics, intentional self-harm** HCC ▽

   √7ᵗʰ **T43.503** **Poisoning by unspecified anti-psychotics and neuroleptics, assault** ▽

   √7ᵗʰ **T43.504** **Poisoning by unspecified anti-psychotics and neuroleptics, undetermined** ▽

   √7ᵗʰ **T43.505** **Adverse effect of unspecified antipsychotics and neuroleptics** ▽

   √7ᵗʰ **T43.506** **Underdosing of unspecified antipsychotics and neuroleptics** ▽

 √6ᵗʰ **T43.59** **Poisoning by, adverse effect of and underdosing of other antipsychotics and neuroleptics**
    AHA: 2017, 1Q, 40

   √7ᵗʰ **T43.591** **Poisoning by other antipsychotics and neuroleptics, accidental (unintentional)**
        Poisoning by other antisychotics and neuroleptics NOS

  2 √7ᵗʰ **T43.592** **Poisoning by other antipsychotics and neuroleptics, intentional self-harm** HCC

   √7ᵗʰ **T43.593** **Poisoning by other antipsychotics and neuroleptics, assault**

   √7ᵗʰ **T43.594** **Poisoning by other antipsychotics and neuroleptics, undetermined**

   √7ᵗʰ **T43.595** **Adverse effect of other antipsychotics and neuroleptics**

   √7ᵗʰ **T43.596** **Underdosing of other antipsychotics and neuroleptics**

√5ᵗʰ **T43.6** **Poisoning by, adverse effect of and underdosing of psychostimulants**

    EXCLUDES 1   poisoning by, adverse effect of and underdosing of cocaine (T40.5-)

 √6ᵗʰ **T43.60** **Poisoning by, adverse effect of and underdosing of unspecified psychostimulant**

   √7ᵗʰ **T43.601** **Poisoning by unspecified psychostimulants, accidental (unintentional)** ▽
        Poisoning by psychostimulants NOS

  2 √7ᵗʰ **T43.602** **Poisoning by unspecified psychostimulants, intentional self-harm** HCC ▽

   √7ᵗʰ **T43.603** **Poisoning by unspecified psychostimulants, assault** ▽

   √7ᵗʰ **T43.604** **Poisoning by unspecified psychostimulants, undetermined** ▽

   √7ᵗʰ **T43.605** **Adverse effect of unspecified psychostimulants** ▽

   √7ᵗʰ **T43.606** **Underdosing of unspecified psychostimulants** ▽

 √6ᵗʰ **T43.61** **Poisoning by, adverse effect of and underdosing of caffeine**

   √7ᵗʰ **T43.611** **Poisoning by caffeine, accidental (unintentional)**
        Poisoning by caffeine NOS

  2 √7ᵗʰ **T43.612** **Poisoning by caffeine, intentional self-harm** HCC

   √7ᵗʰ **T43.613** **Poisoning by caffeine, assault**

   √7ᵗʰ **T43.614** **Poisoning by caffeine, undetermined**

   √7ᵗʰ **T43.615** **Adverse effect of caffeine**

   √7ᵗʰ **T43.616** **Underdosing of caffeine**

 √6ᵗʰ **T43.62** **Poisoning by, adverse effect of and underdosing of amphetamines**
    Poisoning by, adverse effect of and underdosing of methamphetamines

   √7ᵗʰ **T43.621** **Poisoning by amphetamines, accidental (unintentional)**
        Poisoning by amphetamines NOS

  2 √7ᵗʰ **T43.622** **Poisoning by amphetamines, intentional self-harm** HCC

   √7ᵗʰ **T43.623** **Poisoning by amphetamines, assault**

   √7ᵗʰ **T43.624** **Poisoning by amphetamines, undetermined**

   √7ᵗʰ **T43.625** **Adverse effect of amphetamines**

   √7ᵗʰ **T43.626** **Underdosing of amphetamines**

 √6ᵗʰ **T43.63** **Poisoning by, adverse effect of and underdosing of methylphenidate**

   √7ᵗʰ **T43.631** **Poisoning by methylphenidate, accidental (unintentional)**
        Poisoning by methylphenidate NOS

  2 √7ᵗʰ **T43.632** **Poisoning by methylphenidate, intentional self-harm** HCC

   √7ᵗʰ **T43.633** **Poisoning by methylphenidate, assault**

   √7ᵗʰ **T43.634** **Poisoning by methylphenidate, undetermined**

   √7ᵗʰ **T43.635** **Adverse effect of methylphenidate**

---

2   HCC with 7th character indicating initial encounter (A or B - specific to category) OR sequela.

EXCLUDES 1 Not coded here   EXCLUDES 2 Not included here   N Newborn Age: 0   P Pediatric Age: 0-17   M Maternity Age: 12-55   A Adult Age: 15-124

1068   ICD-10-CM 2018

√7ᵗʰ **T43.636** Underdosing of methylphenidate

√6ᵗʰ **T43.69** Poisoning by, adverse effect of and underdosing of other psychostimulants

     √7ᵗʰ **T43.691** Poisoning by other psychostimulants, accidental (unintentional)
         Poisoning by other psychostimulants NOS

     ² √7ᵗʰ **T43.692** Poisoning by other psychostimulants, **HCC** intentional self-harm

     √7ᵗʰ **T43.693** Poisoning by other psychostimulants, assault

     √7ᵗʰ **T43.694** Poisoning by other psychostimulants, undetermined

     √7ᵗʰ **T43.695** Adverse effect of other psychostimulants

     √7ᵗʰ **T43.696** Underdosing of other psychostimulants

√5ᵗʰ **T43.8** Poisoning by, adverse effect of and underdosing of other psychotropic drugs

   √6ᵗʰ **T43.8X** Poisoning by, adverse effect of and underdosing of other psychotropic drugs

     √7ᵗʰ **T43.8X1** Poisoning by other psychotropic drugs, accidental (unintentional)
         Poisoning by other psychotropic drugs NOS

     ² √7ᵗʰ **T43.8X2** Poisoning by other psychotropic **HCC** drugs, intentional self-harm

     √7ᵗʰ **T43.8X3** Poisoning by other psychotropic drugs, assault

     √7ᵗʰ **T43.8X4** Poisoning by other psychotropic drugs, undetermined

     √7ᵗʰ **T43.8X5** Adverse effect of other psychotropic drugs

     √7ᵗʰ **T43.8X6** Underdosing of other psychotropic drugs

√5ᵗʰ **T43.9** Poisoning by, adverse effect of and underdosing of unspecified psychotropic drug

   √x7ᵗʰ **T43.91** Poisoning by unspecified psychotropic drug, accidental (unintentional) ▽
         Poisoning by psychotropic drug NOS

   ² √x7ᵗʰ **T43.92** Poisoning by unspecified psychotropic drug, **HCC** ▽ intentional self-harm

   √x7ᵗʰ **T43.93** Poisoning by unspecified psychotropic drug, assault ▽

   √x7ᵗʰ **T43.94** Poisoning by unspecified psychotropic drug, undetermined ▽

   √x7ᵗʰ **T43.95** Adverse effect of unspecified psychotropic drug ▽

   √x7ᵗʰ **T43.96** Underdosing of unspecified psychotropic drug ▽

√4ᵗʰ **T44** Poisoning by, adverse effect of and underdosing of drugs primarily affecting the autonomic nervous system

> The appropriate 7th character is to be added to each code from category T44.
> A   initial encounter
> D   subsequent encounter
> S   sequela

√5ᵗʰ **T44.0** Poisoning by, adverse effect of and underdosing of anticholinesterase agents

   √6ᵗʰ **T44.0X** Poisoning by, adverse effect of and underdosing of anticholinesterase agents

     √7ᵗʰ **T44.0X1** Poisoning by anticholinesterase agents, accidental (unintentional)
         Poisoning by anticholinesterase agents NOS

     ² √7ᵗʰ **T44.0X2** Poisoning by anticholinesterase **HCC** agents, intentional self-harm

     √7ᵗʰ **T44.0X3** Poisoning by anticholinesterase agents, assault

     √7ᵗʰ **T44.0X4** Poisoning by anticholinesterase agents, undetermined

     √7ᵗʰ **T44.0X5** Adverse effect of anticholinesterase agents

     √7ᵗʰ **T44.0X6** Underdosing of anticholinesterase agents

√5ᵗʰ **T44.1** Poisoning by, adverse effect of and underdosing of other parasympathomimetics [cholinergics]

   √6ᵗʰ **T44.1X** Poisoning by, adverse effect of and underdosing of other parasympathomimetics [cholinergics]

     √7ᵗʰ **T44.1X1** Poisoning by other parasympathomimetics [cholinergics], accidental (unintentional)
         Poisoning by other parasympathomimetics [cholinergics] NOS

     ² √7ᵗʰ **T44.1X2** Poisoning by other **HCC** parasympathomimetics [cholinergics], intentional self-harm

     √7ᵗʰ **T44.1X3** Poisoning by other parasympathomimetics [cholinergics], assault

     √7ᵗʰ **T44.1X4** Poisoning by other parasympathomimetics [cholinergics], undetermined

     √7ᵗʰ **T44.1X5** Adverse effect of other parasympathomimetics [cholinergics]

     √7ᵗʰ **T44.1X6** Underdosing of other parasympathomimetics

√5ᵗʰ **T44.2** Poisoning by, adverse effect of and underdosing of ganglionic blocking drugs

   √6ᵗʰ **T44.2X** Poisoning by, adverse effect of and underdosing of ganglionic blocking drugs

     √7ᵗʰ **T44.2X1** Poisoning by ganglionic blocking drugs, accidental (unintentional)
         Poisoning by ganglionic blocking drugs NOS

     ² √7ᵗʰ **T44.2X2** Poisoning by ganglionic blocking **HCC** drugs, intentional self-harm

     √7ᵗʰ **T44.2X3** Poisoning by ganglionic blocking drugs, assault

     √7ᵗʰ **T44.2X4** Poisoning by ganglionic blocking drugs, undetermined

     √7ᵗʰ **T44.2X5** Adverse effect of ganglionic blocking drugs

     √7ᵗʰ **T44.2X6** Underdosing of ganglionic blocking drugs

√5ᵗʰ **T44.3** Poisoning by, adverse effect of and underdosing of other parasympatholytics [anticholinergics and antimuscarinics] and spasmolytics
     Poisoning by, adverse effect of and underdosing of papaverine

   √6ᵗʰ **T44.3X** Poisoning by, adverse effect of and underdosing of other parasympatholytics [anticholinergics and antimuscarinics] and spasmolytics

     √7ᵗʰ **T44.3X1** Poisoning by other parasympatholytics [anticholinergics and antimuscarinics] and spasmolytics, accidental (unintentional)
         Poisoning by other parasympatholytics [anticholinergics and antimuscarinics] and spasmolytics NOS

     ² √7ᵗʰ **T44.3X2** Poisoning by other para- **HCC** sympatholytics [anticholinergics and antimuscarinics] and spasmolytics, intentional self-harm

     √7ᵗʰ **T44.3X3** Poisoning by other parasympatholytics [anticholinergics and antimuscarinics] and spasmolytics, assault

     √7ᵗʰ **T44.3X4** Poisoning by other parasympatholytics [anticholinergics and antimuscarinics] and spasmolytics, undetermined

     √7ᵗʰ **T44.3X5** Adverse effect of other parasympatholytics [anticholinergics and antimuscarinics] and spasmolytics

     √7ᵗʰ **T44.3X6** Underdosing of other parasympatholytics [anticholinergics and antimuscarinics] and spasmolytics

---

² HCC with 7th character indicating initial encounter (A or B - specific to category) OR sequela.

☑ Additional Character Req   √x7ᵗʰ Placeholder Alert   Manifestation   **HCC** CMS-HCC Condition   ▽ Unspecified Code   ►◄ Revised Text   ● New Code   ▲ Revised Code Title

Chapter 19. Injury, Poisoning, and Certain Other Consequences of External Causes

☑5th T44.4 Poisoning by, adverse effect of and underdosing of predominantly alpha-adrenoreceptor agonists
Poisoning by, adverse effect of and underdosing of metaraminol

☑6th T44.4X Poisoning by, adverse effect of and underdosing of predominantly alpha-adrenoreceptor agonists

☑7th **T44.4X1 Poisoning by predominantly alpha-adrenoreceptor agonists, accidental (unintentional)**
Poisoning by predominantly alpha-adrenoreceptor agonists NOS

2 ☑7th **T44.4X2 Poisoning by predominantly alpha adrenoreceptor agonists, intentional self-harm** HCC

☑7th **T44.4X3 Poisoning by predominantly alpha-adrenoreceptor agonists, assault**

☑7th **T44.4X4 Poisoning by predominantly alpha-adrenoreceptor agonists, undetermined**

☑7th **T44.4X5 Adverse effect of predominantly alpha-adrenoreceptor agonists**

☑7th **T44.4X6 Underdosing of predominantly alpha-adrenoreceptor agonists**

☑5th T44.5 Poisoning by, adverse effect of and underdosing of predominantly beta-adrenoreceptor agonists
EXCLUDES 1 *poisoning by, adverse effect of and underdosing of beta-adrenoreceptor agonists used in asthma therapy (T48.6-)*

☑6th T44.5X Poisoning by, adverse effect of and underdosing of predominantly beta-adrenoreceptor agonists

☑7th **T44.5X1 Poisoning by predominantly beta-adrenoreceptor agonists, accidental (unintentional)**
Poisoning by predominantly beta-adrenoreceptor agonists NOS

2 ☑7th **T44.5X2 Poisoning by predominantly beta-adrenoreceptor agonists, intentional self-harm** HCC

☑7th **T44.5X3 Poisoning by predominantly beta-adrenoreceptor agonists, assault**

☑7th **T44.5X4 Poisoning by predominantly beta-adrenoreceptor agonists, undetermined**

☑7th **T44.5X5 Adverse effect of predominantly beta-adrenoreceptor agonists**

☑7th **T44.5X6 Underdosing of predominantly beta-adrenoreceptor agonists**

☑5th T44.6 Poisoning by, adverse effect of and underdosing of alpha-adrenoreceptor antagonists
EXCLUDES 1 *poisoning by, adverse effect of and underdosing of ergot alkaloids (T48.0)*

☑6th T44.6X Poisoning by, adverse effect of and underdosing of alpha-adrenoreceptor antagonists

☑7th **T44.6X1 Poisoning by alpha-adrenoreceptor antagonists, accidental (unintentional)**
Poisoning by alpha-adrenoreceptor antagonists NOS

2 ☑7th **T44.6X2 Poisoning by alpha-adrenoreceptor antagonists, intentional self-harm** HCC

☑7th **T44.6X3 Poisoning by alpha-adrenoreceptor antagonists, assault**

☑7th **T44.6X4 Poisoning by alpha-adrenoreceptor antagonists, undetermined**

☑7th **T44.6X5 Adverse effect of alpha-adrenoreceptor antagonists**

☑7th **T44.6X6 Underdosing of alpha-adrenoreceptor antagonists**

☑5th T44.7 Poisoning by, adverse effect of and underdosing of beta-adrenoreceptor antagonists

☑6th T44.7X Poisoning by, adverse effect of and underdosing of beta-adrenoreceptor antagonists

☑7th **T44.7X1 Poisoning by beta-adrenoreceptor antagonists, accidental (unintentional)**
Poisoning by beta-adrenoreceptor antagonists NOS

2 ☑7th **T44.7X2 Poisoning by beta-adrenoreceptor antagonists, intentional self-harm** HCC

☑7th **T44.7X3 Poisoning by beta-adrenoreceptor antagonists, assault**

☑7th **T44.7X4 Poisoning by beta-adrenoreceptor antagonists, undetermined**

☑7th **T44.7X5 Adverse effect of beta-adrenoreceptor antagonists**

☑7th **T44.7X6 Underdosing of beta-adrenoreceptor antagonists**

☑5th T44.8 Poisoning by, adverse effect of and underdosing of centrally-acting and adrenergic-neuron- blocking agents
EXCLUDES 1 *poisoning by, adverse effect of and underdosing of clonidine (T46.5)*
poisoning by, adverse effect of and underdosing of guanethidine (T46.5)

☑6th T44.8X Poisoning by, adverse effect of and underdosing of centrally-acting and adrenergic-neuron-blocking agents

☑7th **T44.8X1 Poisoning by centrally-acting and adrenergic-neuron-blocking agents, accidental (unintentional)**
Poisoning by centrally-acting and adrenergic-neuron-blocking agents NOS

2 ☑7th **T44.8X2 Poisoning by centrally-acting and adrenergic-neuron-blocking agents, intentional self-harm** HCC

☑7th **T44.8X3 Poisoning by centrally-acting and adrenergic-neuron-blocking agents, assault**

☑7th **T44.8X4 Poisoning by centrally-acting and adrenergic-neuron-blocking agents, undetermined**

☑7th **T44.8X5 Adverse effect of centrally-acting and adrenergic-neuron-blocking agents**

☑7th **T44.8X6 Underdosing of centrally-acting and adrenergic-neuron-blocking agents**

☑5th T44.9 Poisoning by, adverse effect of and underdosing of other and unspecified drugs primarily affecting the autonomic nervous system
Poisoning by, adverse effect of and underdosing of drug stimulating both alpha and beta-adrenoreceptors

☑6th T44.90 Poisoning by, adverse effect of and underdosing of unspecified drugs primarily affecting the autonomic nervous system

☑7th **T44.901 Poisoning by unspecified drugs primarily affecting the autonomic nervous system, accidental (unintentional)** ▽
Poisoning by unspecified drugs primarily affecting the autonomic nervous system NOS

2 ☑7th **T44.902 Poisoning by unspecified drugs primarily affecting the autonomic nervous system, intentional self-harm** HCC ▽

☑7th **T44.903 Poisoning by unspecified drugs primarily affecting the autonomic nervous system, assault** ▽

☑7th **T44.904 Poisoning by unspecified drugs primarily affecting the autonomic nervous system, undetermined** ▽

☑7th **T44.905 Adverse effect of unspecified drugs primarily affecting the autonomic nervous system** ▽

☑7th **T44.906 Underdosing of unspecified drugs primarily affecting the autonomic nervous system** ▽

☑6th T44.99 Poisoning by, adverse effect of and underdosing of other drugs primarily affecting the autonomic nervous system

☑7th **T44.991 Poisoning by other drug primarily affecting the autonomic nervous system, accidental (unintentional)**
Poisoning by other drugs primarily affecting the autonomic nervous system NOS

2 ☑7th **T44.992 Poisoning by other drug primarily affecting the autonomic nervous system, intentional self-harm** HCC

---

2 HCC with 7th character indicating initial encounter (A or B - specific to category) OR sequela.

√7ᵗʰ **T44.993** **Poisoning by other drug primarily affecting the autonomic nervous system, assault**

√7ᵗʰ **T44.994** **Poisoning by other drug primarily affecting the autonomic nervous system, undetermined**

√7ᵗʰ **T44.995** **Adverse effect of other drug primarily affecting the autonomic nervous system**

√7ᵗʰ **T44.996** **Underdosing of other drug primarily affecting the autonomic nervous system**

√4ᵗʰ **T45** **Poisoning by, adverse effect of and underdosing of primarily systemic and hematological agents, not elsewhere classified**

> The appropriate 7th character is to be added to each code from category T45.
> A   initial encounter
> D   subsequent encounter
> S   sequela

√5ᵗʰ **T45.0** **Poisoning by, adverse effect of and underdosing of antiallergic and antiemetic drugs**
> EXCLUDES 1   poisoning by, adverse effect of and underdosing of phenothiazine-based neuroleptics (T43.3)

√6ᵗʰ **T45.0X** **Poisoning by, adverse effect of and underdosing of antiallergic and antiemetic drugs**

√7ᵗʰ **T45.0X1** **Poisoning by antiallergic and antiemetic drugs, accidental (unintentional)**
> Poisoning by antiallergic and antiemetic drugs NOS

2 √7ᵗʰ **T45.0X2** **Poisoning by antiallergic and antiemetic drugs, intentional self-harm** HCC

√7ᵗʰ **T45.0X3** **Poisoning by antiallergic and antiemetic drugs, assault**

√7ᵗʰ **T45.0X4** **Poisoning by antiallergic and antiemetic drugs, undetermined**

√7ᵗʰ **T45.0X5** **Adverse effect of antiallergic and antiemetic drugs**

√7ᵗʰ **T45.0X6** **Underdosing of antiallergic and antiemetic drugs**

√5ᵗʰ **T45.1** **Poisoning by, adverse effect of and underdosing of antineoplastic and immunosuppressive drugs**
> EXCLUDES 1   poisoning by, adverse effect of and underdosing of tamoxifen (T38.6)
> **AHA:** 2014, 4Q, 22

√6ᵗʰ **T45.1X** **Poisoning by, adverse effect of and underdosing of antineoplastic and immunosuppressive drugs**

√7ᵗʰ **T45.1X1** **Poisoning by antineoplastic and immunosuppressive drugs, accidental (unintentional)**
> Poisoning by antineoplastic and immunosuppressive drugs NOS

2 √7ᵗʰ **T45.1X2** **Poisoning by antineoplastic and immunosuppressive drugs, intentional self-harm** HCC

√7ᵗʰ **T45.1X3** **Poisoning by antineoplastic and immunosuppressive drugs, assault**

√7ᵗʰ **T45.1X4** **Poisoning by antineoplastic and immunosuppressive drugs, undetermined**

√7ᵗʰ **T45.1X5** **Adverse effect of antineoplastic and immunosuppressive drugs**

√7ᵗʰ **T45.1X6** **Underdosing of antineoplastic and immunosuppressive drugs**

√5ᵗʰ **T45.2** **Poisoning by, adverse effect of and underdosing of vitamins**
> EXCLUDES 2   poisoning by, adverse effect of and underdosing of iron (T45.4)
> poisoning by, adverse effect of and underdosing of nicotinic acid (derivatives) (T46.7)
> poisoning by, adverse effect of and underdosing of vitamin K (T45.7)

√6ᵗʰ **T45.2X** **Poisoning by, adverse effect of and underdosing of vitamins**

√7ᵗʰ **T45.2X1** **Poisoning by vitamins, accidental (unintentional)**
> Poisoning by vitamins NOS

2 √7ᵗʰ **T45.2X2** **Poisoning by vitamins, intentional self-harm** HCC

√7ᵗʰ **T45.2X3** **Poisoning by vitamins, assault**

√7ᵗʰ **T45.2X4** **Poisoning by vitamins, undetermined**

√7ᵗʰ **T45.2X5** **Adverse effect of vitamins**

√7ᵗʰ **T45.2X6** **Underdosing of vitamins**
> EXCLUDES 1   vitamin deficiencies (E50-E56)

√5ᵗʰ **T45.3** **Poisoning by, adverse effect of and underdosing of enzymes**

√6ᵗʰ **T45.3X** **Poisoning by, adverse effect of and underdosing of enzymes**

√7ᵗʰ **T45.3X1** **Poisoning by enzymes, accidental (unintentional)**
> Poisoning by enzymes NOS

2 √7ᵗʰ **T45.3X2** **Poisoning by enzymes, intentional self-harm** HCC

√7ᵗʰ **T45.3X3** **Poisoning by enzymes, assault**

√7ᵗʰ **T45.3X4** **Poisoning by enzymes, undetermined**

√7ᵗʰ **T45.3X5** **Adverse effect of enzymes**

√7ᵗʰ **T45.3X6** **Underdosing of enzymes**

√5ᵗʰ **T45.4** **Poisoning by, adverse effect of and underdosing of iron and its compounds**

√6ᵗʰ **T45.4X** **Poisoning by, adverse effect of and underdosing of iron and its compounds**

√7ᵗʰ **T45.4X1** **Poisoning by iron and its compounds, accidental (unintentional)**
> Poisoning by iron and its compounds NOS

2 √7ᵗʰ **T45.4X2** **Poisoning by iron and its compounds, intentional self-harm** HCC

√7ᵗʰ **T45.4X3** **Poisoning by iron and its compounds, assault**

√7ᵗʰ **T45.4X4** **Poisoning by iron and its compounds, undetermined**

√7ᵗʰ **T45.4X5** **Adverse effect of iron and its compounds**

√7ᵗʰ **T45.4X6** **Underdosing of iron and its compounds**
> EXCLUDES 1   iron deficiency (E61.1)

√5ᵗʰ **T45.5** **Poisoning by, adverse effect of and underdosing of anticoagulants and antithrombotic drugs**

√6ᵗʰ **T45.51** **Poisoning by, adverse effect of and underdosing of anticoagulants**

√7ᵗʰ **T45.511** **Poisoning by anticoagulants, accidental (unintentional)**
> Poisoning by anticoagulants NOS

2 √7ᵗʰ **T45.512** **Poisoning by anticoagulants, intentional self-harm** HCC

√7ᵗʰ **T45.513** **Poisoning by anticoagulants, assault**

√7ᵗʰ **T45.514** **Poisoning by anticoagulants, undetermined**

√7ᵗʰ **T45.515** **Adverse effect of anticoagulants**
> **AHA:** 2016, 1Q, 14; 2013, 2Q, 34

√7ᵗʰ **T45.516** **Underdosing of anticoagulants**

√6ᵗʰ **T45.52** **Poisoning by, adverse effect of and underdosing of antithrombotic drugs**
> Poisoning by, adverse effect of and underdosing of antiplatelet drugs
> EXCLUDES 2   poisoning by, adverse effect of and underdosing of aspirin (T39.01-)
> poisoning by, adverse effect of and underdosing of acetylsalicylic acid (T39.01-)

√7ᵗʰ **T45.521** **Poisoning by antithrombotic drugs, accidental (unintentional)**
> Poisoning by antithrombotic drug NOS

2 √7ᵗʰ **T45.522** **Poisoning by antithrombotic drugs, intentional self-harm** HCC

√7ᵗʰ **T45.523** **Poisoning by antithrombotic drugs, assault**

√7ᵗʰ **T45.524** **Poisoning by antithrombotic drugs, undetermined**

√7ᵗʰ **T45.525** **Adverse effect of antithrombotic drugs**
> **AHA:** 2016, 1Q, 15

√7ᵗʰ **T45.526** **Underdosing of antithrombotic drugs**

√5ᵗʰ **T45.6** **Poisoning by, adverse effect of and underdosing of fibrinolysis-affecting drugs**

√6ᵗʰ **T45.60** **Poisoning by, adverse effect of and underdosing of unspecified fibrinolysis-affecting drugs**

√7ᵗʰ **T45.601** **Poisoning by unspecified fibrinolysis-affecting drugs, accidental (unintentional)** ▽
> Poisoning by fibrinolysis-affecting drug NOS

---

2   HCC with 7th character indicating initial encounter (A or B - specific to category) OR sequela.

☑ Additional Character Req   √x7ᵗʰ Placeholder Alert   Manifestation   HCC CMS-HCC Condition   ▽ Unspecified Code   ►◄ Revised Text   ● New Code   ▲ Revised Code Title

2 ✓7ᵗʰ **T45.602** **Poisoning by unspecified** HCC ▽
fibrinolysis-affecting drugs,
intentional self-harm

✓7ᵗʰ **T45.603** **Poisoning by unspecified fibrinolysis-** ▽
affecting drugs, assault

✓7ᵗʰ **T45.604** **Poisoning by unspecified fibrinolysis-** ▽
affecting drugs, undetermined

✓7ᵗʰ **T45.605** **Adverse effect of unspecified fibrino-** ▽
lysis- affecting drugs

✓7ᵗʰ **T45.606** **Underdosing of unspecified fibrino-** ▽
lysis- affecting drugs

✓6ᵗʰ **T45.61** **Poisoning by, adverse effect of and underdosing of**
thrombolytic drugs

✓7ᵗʰ **T45.611** **Poisoning by thrombolytic drug,**
accidental (unintentional)
Poisoning by thrombolytic drug NOS

2 ✓7ᵗʰ **T45.612** **Poisoning by thrombolytic drug,** HCC
intentional self-harm

✓7ᵗʰ **T45.613** **Poisoning by thrombolytic drug, assault**

✓7ᵗʰ **T45.614** **Poisoning by thrombolytic drug,**
undetermined

✓7ᵗʰ **T45.615** **Adverse effect of thrombolytic drugs**
AHA: 2017, 2Q, 9

✓7ᵗʰ **T45.616** **Underdosing of thrombolytic drugs**

✓6ᵗʰ **T45.62** **Poisoning by, adverse effect of and underdosing of**
hemostatic drugs

✓7ᵗʰ **T45.621** **Poisoning by hemostatic drug, accidental**
(unintentional)
Poisoning by hemostatic drug NOS

2 ✓7ᵗʰ **T45.622** **Poisoning by hemostatic drug,** HCC
intentional self-harm

✓7ᵗʰ **T45.623** **Poisoning by hemostatic drug, assault**

✓7ᵗʰ **T45.624** **Poisoning by hemostatic drug,**
undetermined

✓7ᵗʰ **T45.625** **Adverse effect of hemostatic drug**

✓7ᵗʰ **T45.626** **Underdosing of hemostatic drugs**

✓6ᵗʰ **T45.69** **Poisoning by, adverse effect of and underdosing of**
other fibrinolysis-affecting drugs

✓7ᵗʰ **T45.691** **Poisoning by other fibrinolysis-affecting**
drugs, accidental (unintentional)
Poisoning by other fibrinolysis-affecting
drug NOS

2 ✓7ᵗʰ **T45.692** **Poisoning by other fibrinolysis-** HCC
affecting drugs, intentional self-harm

✓7ᵗʰ **T45.693** **Poisoning by other fibrinolysis-affecting**
drugs, assault

✓7ᵗʰ **T45.694** **Poisoning by other fibrinolysis-affecting**
drugs, undetermined

✓7ᵗʰ **T45.695** **Adverse effect of other fibrinolysis-**
affecting drugs

✓7ᵗʰ **T45.696** **Underdosing of other fibrinolysis-**
affecting drugs

✓5ᵗʰ **T45.7** **Poisoning by, adverse effect of and underdosing of**
anticoagulant antagonists, vitamin K and other coagulants

✓6ᵗʰ **T45.7X** **Poisoning by, adverse effect of and underdosing of**
anticoagulant antagonists, vitamin K and other
coagulants

✓7ᵗʰ **T45.7X1** **Poisoning by anticoagulant antagonists,**
vitamin K and other coagulants,
accidental (unintentional)
Poisoning by anticoagulant antagonists,
vitamin K and other coagulants NOS

2 ✓7ᵗʰ **T45.7X2** **Poisoning by anticoagulant** HCC
antagonists, vitamin K and other
coagulants, intentional self-harm

✓7ᵗʰ **T45.7X3** **Poisoning by anticoagulant antagonists,**
vitamin K and other coagulants, assault

✓7ᵗʰ **T45.7X4** **Poisoning by anticoagulant antagonists,**
vitamin K and other coagulants,
undetermined

✓7ᵗʰ **T45.7X5** **Adverse effect of anticoagulant**
antagonists, vitamin K and other
coagulants

✓7ᵗʰ **T45.7X6** **Underdosing of anticoagulant antagonist,**
vitamin K and other coagulants
EXCLUDES 1 *vitamin K deficiency (E56.1)*

✓5ᵗʰ **T45.8** **Poisoning by, adverse effect of and underdosing of other**
primarily systemic and hematological agents
Poisoning by, adverse effect of and underdosing of liver
preparations and other antianemic agents
Poisoning by, adverse effect of and underdosing of natural
blood and blood products
Poisoning by, adverse effect of and underdosing of plasma
substitute
EXCLUDES 2 *poisoning by, adverse effect of and underdosing of*
immunoglobulin (T50.Z1)
poisoning by, adverse effect of and underdosing of iron
(T45.4)
transfusion reactions (T80.-)

✓6ᵗʰ **T45.8X** **Poisoning by, adverse effect of and underdosing of**
other primarily systemic and hematological agents

✓7ᵗʰ **T45.8X1** **Poisoning by other primarily systemic and**
hematological agents, accidental
(unintentional)
Poisoning by other primarily systemic and
hematological agents NOS

2 ✓7ᵗʰ **T45.8X2** **Poisoning by other primarily systemic** HCC
and hematological agents, intentional
self-harm

✓7ᵗʰ **T45.8X3** **Poisoning by other primarily systemic and**
hematological agents, assault

✓7ᵗʰ **T45.8X4** **Poisoning by other primarily systemic and**
hematological agents, undetermined

✓7ᵗʰ **T45.8X5** **Adverse effect of other primarily systemic**
and hematological agents

✓7ᵗʰ **T45.8X6** **Underdosing of other primarily systemic**
and hematological agents

✓5ᵗʰ **T45.9** **Poisoning by, adverse effect of and underdosing of**
unspecified primarily systemic and hematological agent

✓×7ᵗʰ **T45.91** **Poisoning by unspecified primarily systemic and** ▽
hematological agent, accidental (unintentional)
Poisoning by primarily systemic and hematological
agent NOS

2 ✓×7ᵗʰ **T45.92** **Poisoning by unspecified primarily systemic** HCC ▽
and hematological agent, intentional self-harm

✓×7ᵗʰ **T45.93** **Poisoning by unspecified primarily systemic and** ▽
hematological agent, assault

✓×7ᵗʰ **T45.94** **Poisoning by unspecified primarily systemic and** ▽
hematological agent, undetermined

✓×7ᵗʰ **T45.95** **Adverse effect of unspecified primarily systemic** ▽
and hematological agent

✓×7ᵗʰ **T45.96** **Underdosing of unspecified primarily systemic** ▽
and hematological agent

✓4ᵗʰ **T46** **Poisoning by, adverse effect of and underdosing of agents**
primarily affecting the cardiovascular system
EXCLUDES 1 *poisoning by, adverse effect of and underdosing of metaraminol*
(T44.4)

The appropriate 7th character is to be added to each code from
category T46.
A   initial encounter
D   subsequent encounter
S   sequela

✓5ᵗʰ **T46.0** **Poisoning by, adverse effect of and underdosing of cardiac-**
stimulant glycosides and drugs of similar action

✓6ᵗʰ **T46.0X** **Poisoning by, adverse effect of and underdosing of**
cardiac-stimulant glycosides and drugs of similar
action

✓7ᵗʰ **T46.0X1** **Poisoning by cardiac-stimulant**
glycosides and drugs of similar action,
accidental (unintentional)
Poisoning by cardiac-stimulant glycosides
and drugs of similar action NOS

2 ✓7ᵗʰ **T46.0X2** **Poisoning by cardiac-stimulant** HCC
glycosides and drugs of similar action,
intentional self-harm

✓7ᵗʰ **T46.0X3** **Poisoning by cardiac-stimulant**
glycosides and drugs of similar action,
assault

2   HCC with 7th character indicating initial encounter (A or B - specific to category) OR sequela.

EXCLUDES 1 Not coded here   EXCLUDES 2 Not included here   N Newborn Age: 0   P Pediatric Age: 0-17   M Maternity Age: 12-55   A Adult Age: 15-124

1072

ICD-10-CM 2018

√7ᵗʰ **T46.0X4** Poisoning by cardiac-stimulant glycosides and drugs of similar action, **undetermined**

√7ᵗʰ **T46.0X5** **Adverse effect** of cardiac-stimulant glycosides and drugs of similar action

√7ᵗʰ **T46.0X6** **Underdosing** of cardiac-stimulant glycosides and drugs of similar action

√5ᵗʰ **T46.1** Poisoning by, adverse effect of and underdosing of calcium-channel blockers

√6ᵗʰ **T46.1X** Poisoning by, adverse effect of and underdosing of **calcium-channel blockers**

√7ᵗʰ **T46.1X1** Poisoning by calcium-channel blockers, **accidental** (unintentional)
Poisoning by calcium-channel blockers NOS

2 √7ᵗʰ **T46.1X2** Poisoning by calcium-channel blockers, **intentional self-harm** `HCC`

√7ᵗʰ **T46.1X3** Poisoning by calcium-channel blockers, **assault**

√7ᵗʰ **T46.1X4** Poisoning by calcium-channel blockers, **undetermined**

√7ᵗʰ **T46.1X5** **Adverse effect** of calcium-channel blockers

√7ᵗʰ **T46.1X6** **Underdosing** of calcium-channel blockers

√5ᵗʰ **T46.2** Poisoning by, adverse effect of and underdosing of other antidysrhythmic drugs, not elsewhere classified
EXCLUDES 1 *poisoning by, adverse effect of and underdosing of beta-adrenoreceptor antagonists (T44.7-)*

√6ᵗʰ **T46.2X** Poisoning by, adverse effect of and underdosing of other antidysrhythmic drugs

√7ᵗʰ **T46.2X1** Poisoning by other antidysrhythmic drugs, **accidental** (unintentional)
Poisoning by other antidysrhythmic drugs NOS

2 √7ᵗʰ **T46.2X2** Poisoning by other antidysrhythmic drugs, **intentional self-harm** `HCC`

√7ᵗʰ **T46.2X3** Poisoning by other antidysrhythmic drugs, **assault**

√7ᵗʰ **T46.2X4** Poisoning by other antidysrhythmic drugs, **undetermined**

√7ᵗʰ **T46.2X5** **Adverse effect** of other antidysrhythmic drugs

√7ᵗʰ **T46.2X6** **Underdosing** of other antidysrhythmic drugs

√5ᵗʰ **T46.3** Poisoning by, adverse effect of and underdosing of coronary vasodilators
Poisoning by, adverse effect of and underdosing of dipyridamole
EXCLUDES 1 *poisoning by, adverse effect of and underdosing of calcium-channel blockers (T46.1)*

√6ᵗʰ **T46.3X** Poisoning by, adverse effect of and underdosing of **coronary vasodilators**

√7ᵗʰ **T46.3X1** Poisoning by coronary vasodilators, **accidental** (unintentional)
Poisoning by coronary vasodilators NOS

2 √7ᵗʰ **T46.3X2** Poisoning by coronary vasodilators, **intentional self-harm** `HCC`

√7ᵗʰ **T46.3X3** Poisoning by coronary vasodilators, **assault**

√7ᵗʰ **T46.3X4** Poisoning by coronary vasodilators, **undetermined**

√7ᵗʰ **T46.3X5** **Adverse effect** of coronary vasodilators

√7ᵗʰ **T46.3X6** **Underdosing** of coronary vasodilators

√5ᵗʰ **T46.4** Poisoning by, adverse effect of and underdosing of angiotensin-converting-enzyme inhibitors

√6ᵗʰ **T46.4X** Poisoning by, adverse effect of and underdosing of **angiotensin-converting-enzyme inhibitors**

√7ᵗʰ **T46.4X1** Poisoning by angiotensin-converting-enzyme inhibitors, **accidental** (unintentional)
Poisoning by angiotensin-converting-enzyme inhibitors NOS

2 √7ᵗʰ **T46.4X2** Poisoning by angiotensin-converting- enzyme inhibitors, **intentional self-harm** `HCC`

√7ᵗʰ **T46.4X3** Poisoning by angiotensin-converting-enzyme inhibitors, **assault**

√7ᵗʰ **T46.4X4** Poisoning by angiotensin-converting-enzyme inhibitors, **undetermined**

√7ᵗʰ **T46.4X5** **Adverse effect** of angiotensin-converting-enzyme inhibitors

√7ᵗʰ **T46.4X6** **Underdosing** of angiotensin-converting-enzyme inhibitors

√5ᵗʰ **T46.5** Poisoning by, adverse effect of and underdosing of other antihypertensive drugs
EXCLUDES 2 *poisoning by, adverse effect of and underdosing of beta-adrenoreceptor antagonists (T44.7)*
poisoning by, adverse effect of and underdosing of calcium-channel blockers (T46.1)
poisoning by, adverse effect of and underdosing of diuretics (T50.0-T50.2)

√6ᵗʰ **T46.5X** Poisoning by, adverse effect of and underdosing of other antihypertensive drugs

√7ᵗʰ **T46.5X1** Poisoning by other antihypertensive drugs, **accidental** (unintentional)
Poisoning by other antihypertensive drugs NOS

2 √7ᵗʰ **T46.5X2** Poisoning by other antihypertensive drugs, **intentional self-harm** `HCC`

√7ᵗʰ **T46.5X3** Poisoning by other antihypertensive drugs, **assault**

√7ᵗʰ **T46.5X4** Poisoning by other antihypertensive drugs, **undetermined**

√7ᵗʰ **T46.5X5** **Adverse effect** of other antihypertensive drugs

√7ᵗʰ **T46.5X6** **Underdosing** of other antihypertensive drugs

√5ᵗʰ **T46.6** Poisoning by, adverse effect of and underdosing of antihyperlipidemic and antiarteriosclerotic drugs

√6ᵗʰ **T46.6X** Poisoning by, adverse effect of and underdosing of **antihyperlipidemic and antiarteriosclerotic** drugs

√7ᵗʰ **T46.6X1** Poisoning by antihyperlipidemic and antiarteriosclerotic drugs, **accidental** (unintentional)
Poisoning by antihyperlipidemic and antiarteriosclerotic drugs NOS

2 √7ᵗʰ **T46.6X2** Poisoning by antihyperlipidemic and antiarteriosclerotic drugs, **intentional self-harm** `HCC`

√7ᵗʰ **T46.6X3** Poisoning by antihyperlipidemic and antiarteriosclerotic drugs, **assault**

√7ᵗʰ **T46.6X4** Poisoning by antihyperlipidemic and antiarteriosclerotic drugs, **undetermined**

√7ᵗʰ **T46.6X5** **Adverse effect** of antihyperlipidemic and antiarteriosclerotic drugs

√7ᵗʰ **T46.6X6** **Underdosing** of antihyperlipidemic and antiarteriosclerotic drugs

√5ᵗʰ **T46.7** Poisoning by, adverse effect of and underdosing of peripheral vasodilators
Poisoning by, adverse effect of and underdosing of nicotinic acid (derivatives)
EXCLUDES 1 *poisoning by, adverse effect of and underdosing of papaverine (T44.3)*

√6ᵗʰ **T46.7X** Poisoning by, adverse effect of and underdosing of **peripheral vasodilators**

√7ᵗʰ **T46.7X1** Poisoning by peripheral vasodilators, **accidental** (unintentional)
Poisoning by peripheral vasodilators NOS

2 √7ᵗʰ **T46.7X2** Poisoning by peripheral vasodilators, **intentional self-harm** `HCC`

√7ᵗʰ **T46.7X3** Poisoning by peripheral vasodilators, **assault**

√7ᵗʰ **T46.7X4** Poisoning by peripheral vasodilators, **undetermined**

√7ᵗʰ **T46.7X5** **Adverse effect** of peripheral vasodilators

√7ᵗʰ **T46.7X6** **Underdosing** of peripheral vasodilators

---

2   HCC with 7th character indicating initial encounter (A or B - specific to category) OR sequela.

☑ Additional Character Req   √x7ᵗʰ Placeholder Alert   Manifestation   `HCC` CMS-HCC Condition   ▽ Unspecified Code   ►◄ Revised Text   ● New Code   ▲ Revised Code Title

✓5ᵗʰ **T46.8** **Poisoning by, adverse effect of and underdosing of antivaricose drugs, including sclerosing agents**

  ✓6ᵗʰ **T46.8X** **Poisoning by, adverse effect of and underdosing of antivaricose drugs, including sclerosing agents**

    ✓7ᵗʰ **T46.8X1** **Poisoning by antivaricose drugs, including sclerosing agents, accidental (unintentional)**
        Poisoning by antivaricose drugs, including sclerosing agents NOS

    2 ✓7ᵗʰ **T46.8X2** **Poisoning by antivaricose drugs, including sclerosing agents, intentional self-harm** HCC

    ✓7ᵗʰ **T46.8X3** **Poisoning by antivaricose drugs, including sclerosing agents, assault**

    ✓7ᵗʰ **T46.8X4** **Poisoning by antivaricose drugs, including sclerosing agents, undetermined**

    ✓7ᵗʰ **T46.8X5** **Adverse effect of antivaricose drugs, including sclerosing agents**

    ✓7ᵗʰ **T46.8X6** **Underdosing of antivaricose drugs, including sclerosing agents**

✓5ᵗʰ **T46.9** **Poisoning by, adverse effect of and underdosing of other and unspecified agents primarily affecting the cardiovascular system**

  ✓6ᵗʰ **T46.90** **Poisoning by, adverse effect of and underdosing of unspecified agents primarily affecting the cardiovascular system**

    ✓7ᵗʰ **T46.901** **Poisoning by unspecified agents primarily affecting the cardiovascular system, accidental (unintentional)** ▽

    2 ✓7ᵗʰ **T46.902** **Poisoning by unspecified agents primarily affecting the cardiovascular system, intentional self-harm** HCC ▽

    ✓7ᵗʰ **T46.903** **Poisoning by unspecified agents primarily affecting the cardiovascular system, assault** ▽

    ✓7ᵗʰ **T46.904** **Poisoning by unspecified agents primarily affecting the cardiovascular system, undetermined** ▽

    ✓7ᵗʰ **T46.905** **Adverse effect of unspecified agents primarily affecting the cardiovascular system** ▽

    ✓7ᵗʰ **T46.906** **Underdosing of unspecified agents primarily affecting the cardiovascular system** ▽

  ✓6ᵗʰ **T46.99** **Poisoning by, adverse effect of and underdosing of other agents primarily affecting the cardiovascular system**

    ✓7ᵗʰ **T46.991** **Poisoning by other agents primarily affecting the cardiovascular system, accidental (unintentional)**

    2 ✓7ᵗʰ **T46.992** **Poisoning by other agents primarily affecting the cardiovascular system, intentional self-harm** HCC

    ✓7ᵗʰ **T46.993** **Poisoning by other agents primarily affecting the cardiovascular system, assault**

    ✓7ᵗʰ **T46.994** **Poisoning by other agents primarily affecting the cardiovascular system, undetermined**

    ✓7ᵗʰ **T46.995** **Adverse effect of other agents primarily affecting the cardiovascular system**

    ✓7ᵗʰ **T46.996** **Underdosing of other agents primarily affecting the cardiovascular system**

✓4ᵗʰ **T47** **Poisoning by, adverse effect of and underdosing of agents primarily affecting the gastrointestinal system**

> The appropriate 7th character is to be added to each code from category T47.
> A   initial encounter
> D   subsequent encounter
> S   sequela

✓5ᵗʰ **T47.0** **Poisoning by, adverse effect of and underdosing of histamine H2-receptor blockers**

  ✓6ᵗʰ **T47.0X** **Poisoning by, adverse effect of and underdosing of histamine H2-receptor blockers**

    ✓7ᵗʰ **T47.0X1** **Poisoning by histamine H2-receptor blockers, accidental (unintentional)**
        Poisoning by histamine H2-receptor blockers NOS

    2 ✓7ᵗʰ **T47.0X2** **Poisoning by histamine H2-receptor blockers, intentional self-harm** HCC

    ✓7ᵗʰ **T47.0X3** **Poisoning by histamine H2-receptor blockers, assault**

    ✓7ᵗʰ **T47.0X4** **Poisoning by histamine H2-receptor blockers, undetermined**

    ✓7ᵗʰ **T47.0X5** **Adverse effect of histamine H2-receptor blockers**

    ✓7ᵗʰ **T47.0X6** **Underdosing of histamine H2-receptor blockers**

✓5ᵗʰ **T47.1** **Poisoning by, adverse effect of and underdosing of other antacids and anti-gastric-secretion drugs**

  ✓6ᵗʰ **T47.1X** **Poisoning by, adverse effect of and underdosing of other antacids and anti-gastric-secretion drugs**

    ✓7ᵗʰ **T47.1X1** **Poisoning by other antacids and anti-gastric-secretion drugs, accidental (unintentional)**
        Poisoning by other antacids and anti-gastric-secretion drugs NOS

    2 ✓7ᵗʰ **T47.1X2** **Poisoning by other antacids and anti-gastric-secretion drugs, intentional self-harm** HCC

    ✓7ᵗʰ **T47.1X3** **Poisoning by other antacids and anti-gastric-secretion drugs, assault**

    ✓7ᵗʰ **T47.1X4** **Poisoning by other antacids and anti-gastric-secretion drugs, undetermined**

    ✓7ᵗʰ **T47.1X5** **Adverse effect of other antacids and anti-gastric-secretion drugs**

    ✓7ᵗʰ **T47.1X6** **Underdosing of other antacids and anti-gastric-secretion drugs**

✓5ᵗʰ **T47.2** **Poisoning by, adverse effect of and underdosing of stimulant laxatives**

  ✓6ᵗʰ **T47.2X** **Poisoning by, adverse effect of and underdosing of stimulant laxatives**

    ✓7ᵗʰ **T47.2X1** **Poisoning by stimulant laxatives, accidental (unintentional)**
        Poisoning by stimulant laxatives NOS

    2 ✓7ᵗʰ **T47.2X2** **Poisoning by stimulant laxatives, intentional self-harm** HCC

    ✓7ᵗʰ **T47.2X3** **Poisoning by stimulant laxatives, assault**

    ✓7ᵗʰ **T47.2X4** **Poisoning by stimulant laxatives, undetermined**

    ✓7ᵗʰ **T47.2X5** **Adverse effect of stimulant laxatives**

    ✓7ᵗʰ **T47.2X6** **Underdosing of stimulant laxatives**

✓5ᵗʰ **T47.3** **Poisoning by, adverse effect of and underdosing of saline and osmotic laxatives**

  ✓6ᵗʰ **T47.3X** **Poisoning by and adverse effect of saline and osmotic laxatives**

    ✓7ᵗʰ **T47.3X1** **Poisoning by saline and osmotic laxatives, accidental (unintentional)**
        Poisoning by saline and osmotic laxatives NOS

    2 ✓7ᵗʰ **T47.3X2** **Poisoning by saline and osmotic laxatives, intentional self-harm** HCC

    ✓7ᵗʰ **T47.3X3** **Poisoning by saline and osmotic laxatives, assault**

    ✓7ᵗʰ **T47.3X4** **Poisoning by saline and osmotic laxatives, undetermined**

    ✓7ᵗʰ **T47.3X5** **Adverse effect of saline and osmotic laxatives**

---

2   HCC with 7th character indicating initial encounter (A or B - specific to category) OR sequela.

EXCLUDES 1 Not coded here   EXCLUDES 2 Not included here   N Newborn Age: 0   P Pediatric Age: 0-17   M Maternity Age: 12-55   A Adult Age: 15-124

1074   ICD-10-CM 2018

☑7th **T47.3X6 Underdosing of saline and osmotic laxatives**

☑5th **T47.4 Poisoning by, adverse effect of and underdosing of other laxatives**

☑6th **T47.4X Poisoning by, adverse effect of and underdosing of other laxatives**

☑7th **T47.4X1 Poisoning by other laxatives, accidental (unintentional)**
Poisoning by other laxatives NOS

2 ☑7th **T47.4X2 Poisoning by other laxatives, intentional self-harm** HCC

☑7th **T47.4X3 Poisoning by other laxatives, assault**

☑7th **T47.4X4 Poisoning by other laxatives, undetermined**

☑7th **T47.4X5 Adverse effect of other laxatives**

☑7th **T47.4X6 Underdosing of other laxatives**

☑5th **T47.5 Poisoning by, adverse effect of and underdosing of digestants**

☑6th **T47.5X Poisoning by, adverse effect of and underdosing of digestants**

☑7th **T47.5X1 Poisoning by digestants, accidental (unintentional)**
Poisoning by digestants NOS

2 ☑7th **T47.5X2 Poisoning by digestants, intentional self-harm** HCC

☑7th **T47.5X3 Poisoning by digestants, assault**

☑7th **T47.5X4 Poisoning by digestants, undetermined**

☑7th **T47.5X5 Adverse effect of digestants**

☑7th **T47.5X6 Underdosing of digestants**

☑5th **T47.6 Poisoning by, adverse effect of and underdosing of antidiarrheal drugs**

EXCLUDES 2   *poisoning by, adverse effect of and underdosing of systemic antibiotics and other anti-infectives (T36-T37)*

☑6th **T47.6X Poisoning by, adverse effect of and underdosing of antidiarrheal drugs**

☑7th **T47.6X1 Poisoning by antidiarrheal drugs, accidental (unintentional)**
Poisoning by antidiarrheal drugs NOS

2 ☑7th **T47.6X2 Poisoning by antidiarrheal drugs, intentional self-harm** HCC

☑7th **T47.6X3 Poisoning by antidiarrheal drugs, assault**

☑7th **T47.6X4 Poisoning by antidiarrheal drugs, undetermined**

☑7th **T47.6X5 Adverse effect of antidiarrheal drugs**

☑7th **T47.6X6 Underdosing of antidiarrheal drugs**

☑5th **T47.7 Poisoning by, adverse effect of and underdosing of emetics**

☑6th **T47.7X Poisoning by, adverse effect of and underdosing of emetics**

☑7th **T47.7X1 Poisoning by emetics, accidental (unintentional)**
Poisoning by emetics NOS

2 ☑7th **T47.7X2 Poisoning by emetics, intentional self-harm** HCC

☑7th **T47.7X3 Poisoning by emetics, assault**

☑7th **T47.7X4 Poisoning by emetics, undetermined**

☑7th **T47.7X5 Adverse effect of emetics**

☑7th **T47.7X6 Underdosing of emetics**

☑5th **T47.8 Poisoning by, adverse effect of and underdosing of other agents primarily affecting gastrointestinal system**

☑6th **T47.8X Poisoning by, adverse effect of and underdosing of other agents primarily affecting gastrointestinal system**

☑7th **T47.8X1 Poisoning by other agents primarily affecting gastrointestinal system, accidental (unintentional)**
Poisoning by other agents primarily affecting gastrointestinal system NOS

2 ☑7th **T47.8X2 Poisoning by other agents primarily affecting gastrointestinal system, intentional self-harm** HCC

☑7th **T47.8X3 Poisoning by other agents primarily affecting gastrointestinal system, assault**

☑7th **T47.8X4 Poisoning by other agents primarily affecting gastrointestinal system, undetermined**

☑7th **T47.8X5 Adverse effect of other agents primarily affecting gastrointestinal system**

☑7th **T47.8X6 Underdosing of other agents primarily affecting gastrointestinal system**

☑5th **T47.9 Poisoning by, adverse effect of and underdosing of unspecified agents primarily affecting the gastrointestinal system**

☑x7th **T47.91 Poisoning by unspecified agents primarily affecting the gastrointestinal system, accidental (unintentional)** ▽
Poisoning by agents primarily affecting the gastrointestinal system NOS

2 ☑x7th **T47.92 Poisoning by unspecified agents primarily affecting the gastrointestinal system, intentional self-harm** HCC ▽

☑x7th **T47.93 Poisoning by unspecified agents primarily affecting the gastrointestinal system, assault** ▽

☑x7th **T47.94 Poisoning by unspecified agents primarily affecting the gastrointestinal system, undetermined** ▽

☑x7th **T47.95 Adverse effect of unspecified agents primarily affecting the gastrointestinal system** ▽

☑x7th **T47.96 Underdosing of unspecified agents primarily affecting the gastrointestinal system** ▽

☑4th **T48 Poisoning by, adverse effect of and underdosing of agents primarily acting on smooth and skeletal muscles and the respiratory system**

> The appropriate 7th character is to be added to each code from category T48.
> A   initial encounter
> D   subsequent encounter
> S   sequela

☑5th **T48.0 Poisoning by, adverse effect of and underdosing of oxytocic drugs**

EXCLUDES 1   *poisoning by, adverse effect of and underdosing of estrogens, progestogens and antagonists (T38.4-T38.6)*

☑6th **T48.0X Poisoning by, adverse effect of and underdosing of oxytocic drugs**

☑7th **T48.0X1 Poisoning by oxytocic drugs, accidental (unintentional)**
Poisoning by oxytocic drugs NOS

2 ☑7th **T48.0X2 Poisoning by oxytocic drugs, intentional self-harm** HCC

☑7th **T48.0X3 Poisoning by oxytocic drugs, assault**

☑7th **T48.0X4 Poisoning by oxytocic drugs, undetermined**

☑7th **T48.0X5 Adverse effect of oxytocic drugs**

☑7th **T48.0X6 Underdosing of oxytocic drugs**

☑5th **T48.1 Poisoning by, adverse effect of and underdosing of skeletal muscle relaxants [neuromuscular blocking agents]**

☑6th **T48.1X Poisoning by, adverse effect of and underdosing of skeletal muscle relaxants [neuromuscular blocking agents]**

☑7th **T48.1X1 Poisoning by skeletal muscle relaxants [neuromuscular blocking agents], accidental (unintentional)**
Poisoning by skeletal muscle relaxants [neuromuscular blocking agents] NOS

2 ☑7th **T48.1X2 Poisoning by skeletal muscle relaxants [neuromuscular blocking agents], intentional self-harm** HCC

☑7th **T48.1X3 Poisoning by skeletal muscle relaxants [neuromuscular blocking agents], assault**

☑7th **T48.1X4 Poisoning by skeletal muscle relaxants [neuromuscular blocking agents], undetermined**

☑7th **T48.1X5 Adverse effect of skeletal muscle relaxants [neuromuscular blocking agents]**

☑7th **T48.1X6 Underdosing of skeletal muscle relaxants [neuromuscular blocking agents]**

---

2   HCC with 7th character indicating initial encounter (A or B - specific to category) OR sequela.

☑ Additional Character Req   ☑x7th Placeholder Alert   Manifestation   HCC CMS-HCC Condition   ▽ Unspecified Code   ►◄ Revised Text   ● New Code   ▲ Revised Code Title

Chapter 19. Injury, Poisoning, and Certain Other Consequences of External Causes

√5ᵗʰ **T48.2** **Poisoning by, adverse effect of and underdosing of other and unspecified drugs acting on muscles**

√6ᵗʰ **T48.20** **Poisoning by, adverse effect of and underdosing of unspecified drugs acting on muscles**

√7ᵗʰ **T48.201** **Poisoning by unspecified drugs acting on muscles, accidental (unintentional)** ▽
Poisoning by unspecified drugs acting on muscles NOS

2 √7ᵗʰ **T48.202** **Poisoning by unspecified drugs acting on muscles, intentional self-harm** HCC ▽

√7ᵗʰ **T48.203** **Poisoning by unspecified drugs acting on muscles, assault** ▽

√7ᵗʰ **T48.204** **Poisoning by unspecified drugs acting on muscles, undetermined** ▽

√7ᵗʰ **T48.205** **Adverse effect of unspecified drugs acting on muscles** ▽

√7ᵗʰ **T48.206** **Underdosing of unspecified drugs acting on muscles** ▽

√6ᵗʰ **T48.29** **Poisoning by, adverse effect of and underdosing of other drugs acting on muscles**

√7ᵗʰ **T48.291** **Poisoning by other drugs acting on muscles, accidental (unintentional)**
Poisoning by other drugs acting on muscles NOS

2 √7ᵗʰ **T48.292** **Poisoning by other drugs acting on muscles, intentional self-harm** HCC

√7ᵗʰ **T48.293** **Poisoning by other drugs acting on muscles, assault**

√7ᵗʰ **T48.294** **Poisoning by other drugs acting on muscles, undetermined**

√7ᵗʰ **T48.295** **Adverse effect of other drugs acting on muscles**

√7ᵗʰ **T48.296** **Underdosing of other drugs acting on muscles**

√5ᵗʰ **T48.3** **Poisoning by, adverse effect of and underdosing of antitussives**

√6ᵗʰ **T48.3X** **Poisoning by, adverse effect of and underdosing of antitussives**

√7ᵗʰ **T48.3X1** **Poisoning by antitussives, accidental (unintentional)**
Poisoning by antitussives NOS

2 √7ᵗʰ **T48.3X2** **Poisoning by antitussives, intentional self-harm** HCC

√7ᵗʰ **T48.3X3** **Poisoning by antitussives, assault**

√7ᵗʰ **T48.3X4** **Poisoning by antitussives, undetermined**

√7ᵗʰ **T48.3X5** **Adverse effect of antitussives**

√7ᵗʰ **T48.3X6** **Underdosing of antitussives**

√5ᵗʰ **T48.4** **Poisoning by, adverse effect of and underdosing of expectorants**

√6ᵗʰ **T48.4X** **Poisoning by, adverse effect of and underdosing of expectorants**

√7ᵗʰ **T48.4X1** **Poisoning by expectorants, accidental (unintentional)**
Poisoning by expectorants NOS

2 √7ᵗʰ **T48.4X2** **Poisoning by expectorants, intentional self-harm** HCC

√7ᵗʰ **T48.4X3** **Poisoning by expectorants, assault**

√7ᵗʰ **T48.4X4** **Poisoning by expectorants, undetermined**

√7ᵗʰ **T48.4X5** **Adverse effect of expectorants**

√7ᵗʰ **T48.4X6** **Underdosing of expectorants**

√5ᵗʰ **T48.5** **Poisoning by, adverse effect of and underdosing of other anti-common-cold drugs**
Poisoning by, adverse effect of and underdosing of decongestants

EXCLUDES 2   *poisoning by, adverse effect of and underdosing of antipyretics, NEC (T39.9-)*
poisoning by, adverse effect of and underdosing of non-steroidal antiinflammatory drugs (T39.3-)
poisoning by, adverse effect of and underdosing of salicylates (T39.0-)

√6ᵗʰ **T48.5X** **Poisoning by, adverse effect of and underdosing of other anti-common-cold drugs**

√7ᵗʰ **T48.5X1** **Poisoning by other anti-common-cold drugs, accidental (unintentional)**
Poisoning by other anti-common-cold drugs NOS

2 √7ᵗʰ **T48.5X2** **Poisoning by other anti-common-cold drugs, intentional self-harm** HCC

√7ᵗʰ **T48.5X3** **Poisoning by other anti-common-cold drugs, assault**

√7ᵗʰ **T48.5X4** **Poisoning by other anti-common-cold drugs, undetermined**

√7ᵗʰ **T48.5X5** **Adverse effect of other anti-common-cold drugs**

√7ᵗʰ **T48.5X6** **Underdosing of other anti-common-cold drugs**

√5ᵗʰ **T48.6** **Poisoning by, adverse effect of and underdosing of antiasthmatics, not elsewhere classified**
Poisoning by, adverse effect of and underdosing of beta-adrenoreceptor agonists used in asthma therapy

EXCLUDES 1   *poisoning by, adverse effect of and underdosing of anterior pituitary [adenohypophyseal] hormones (T38.8)*
poisoning by, adverse effect of and underdosing of beta-adrenoreceptor agonists not used in asthma therapy (T44.5)

√6ᵗʰ **T48.6X** **Poisoning by, adverse effect of and underdosing of antiasthmatics**

√7ᵗʰ **T48.6X1** **Poisoning by antiasthmatics, accidental (unintentional)**
Poisoning by antiasthmatics NOS

2 √7ᵗʰ **T48.6X2** **Poisoning by antiasthmatics, intentional self-harm** HCC

√7ᵗʰ **T48.6X3** **Poisoning by antiasthmatics, assault**

√7ᵗʰ **T48.6X4** **Poisoning by antiasthmatics, undetermined**

√7ᵗʰ **T48.6X5** **Adverse effect of antiasthmatics**

√7ᵗʰ **T48.6X6** **Underdosing of antiasthmatics**

√5ᵗʰ **T48.9** **Poisoning by, adverse effect of and underdosing of other and unspecified agents primarily acting on the respiratory system**

√6ᵗʰ **T48.90** **Poisoning by, adverse effect of and underdosing of unspecified agents primarily acting on the respiratory system**

√7ᵗʰ **T48.901** **Poisoning by unspecified agents primarily acting on the respiratory system, accidental (unintentional)** ▽

2 √7ᵗʰ **T48.902** **Poisoning by unspecified agents primarily acting on the respiratory system, intentional self-harm** HCC ▽

√7ᵗʰ **T48.903** **Poisoning by unspecified agents primarily acting on the respiratory system, assault** ▽

√7ᵗʰ **T48.904** **Poisoning by unspecified agents primarily acting on the respiratory system, undetermined** ▽

√7ᵗʰ **T48.905** **Adverse effect of unspecified agents primarily acting on the respiratory system** ▽

√7ᵗʰ **T48.906** **Underdosing of unspecified agents primarily acting on the respiratory system** ▽

√6ᵗʰ **T48.99** **Poisoning by, adverse effect of and underdosing of other agents primarily acting on the respiratory system**

√7ᵗʰ **T48.991** **Poisoning by other agents primarily acting on the respiratory system, accidental (unintentional)**

---

2   HCC with 7th character indicating initial encounter (A or B - specific to category) OR sequela.

EXCLUDES 1 Not coded here   EXCLUDES 2 Not included here   N Newborn Age: 0   P Pediatric Age: 0-17   M Maternity Age: 12-55   A Adult Age: 15-124

1076   ICD-10-CM 2018

2 ✓7th **T48.992** **Poisoning by other agents primarily acting on the respiratory system, intentional self-harm** HCC

✓7th **T48.993** **Poisoning by other agents primarily acting on the respiratory system, assault**

✓7th **T48.994** **Poisoning by other agents primarily acting on the respiratory system, undetermined**

✓7th **T48.995** **Adverse effect of other agents primarily acting on the respiratory system**

✓7th **T48.996** **Underdosing of other agents primarily acting on the respiratory system**

✓4th **T49** **Poisoning by, adverse effect of and underdosing of topical agents primarily affecting skin and mucous membrane and by ophthalmological, otorhinolaryngological and dental drugs**

INCLUDES poisoning by, adverse effect of and underdosing of glucocorticoids, topically used

The appropriate 7th character is to be added to each code from category T49.
A   initial encounter
D   subsequent encounter
S   sequela

✓5th **T49.0** **Poisoning by, adverse effect of and underdosing of local antifungal, anti-infective and anti-inflammatory drugs**

✓6th **T49.0X** **Poisoning by, adverse effect of and underdosing of local antifungal, anti-infective and anti-inflammatory drugs**

✓7th **T49.0X1** **Poisoning by local antifungal, anti-infective and anti-inflammatory drugs, accidental (unintentional)**
Poisoning by local antifungal, anti-infective and anti-inflammatory drugs NOS

2 ✓7th **T49.0X2** **Poisoning by local antifungal, anti-infective and anti-inflammatory drugs, intentional self-harm** HCC

✓7th **T49.0X3** **Poisoning by local antifungal, anti-infective and anti-inflammatory drugs, assault**

✓7th **T49.0X4** **Poisoning by local antifungal, anti-infective and anti-inflammatory drugs, undetermined**

✓7th **T49.0X5** **Adverse effect of local antifungal, anti-infective and anti-inflammatory drugs**

✓7th **T49.0X6** **Underdosing of local antifungal, anti-infective and anti-inflammatory drugs**

✓5th **T49.1** **Poisoning by, adverse effect of and underdosing of antipruritics**

✓6th **T49.1X** **Poisoning by, adverse effect of and underdosing of antipruritics**

✓7th **T49.1X1** **Poisoning by antipruritics, accidental (unintentional)**
Poisoning by antipruritics NOS

2 ✓7th **T49.1X2** **Poisoning by antipruritics, intentional self-harm** HCC

✓7th **T49.1X3** **Poisoning by antipruritics, assault**

✓7th **T49.1X4** **Poisoning by antipruritics, undetermined**

✓7th **T49.1X5** **Adverse effect of antipruritics**

✓7th **T49.1X6** **Underdosing of antipruritics**

✓5th **T49.2** **Poisoning by, adverse effect of and underdosing of local astringents and local detergents**

✓6th **T49.2X** **Poisoning by, adverse effect of and underdosing of local astringents and local detergents**

✓7th **T49.2X1** **Poisoning by local astringents and local detergents, accidental (unintentional)**
Poisoning by local astringents and local detergents NOS

2 ✓7th **T49.2X2** **Poisoning by local astringents and local detergents, intentional self-harm** HCC

✓7th **T49.2X3** **Poisoning by local astringents and local detergents, assault**

✓7th **T49.2X4** **Poisoning by local astringents and local detergents, undetermined**

✓7th **T49.2X5** **Adverse effect of local astringents and local detergents**

✓7th **T49.2X6** **Underdosing of local astringents and local detergents**

✓5th **T49.3** **Poisoning by, adverse effect of and underdosing of emollients, demulcents and protectants**

✓6th **T49.3X** **Poisoning by, adverse effect of and underdosing of emollients, demulcents and protectants**

✓7th **T49.3X1** **Poisoning by emollients, demulcents and protectants, accidental (unintentional)**
Poisoning by emollients, demulcents and protectants NOS

2 ✓7th **T49.3X2** **Poisoning by emollients, demulcents and protectants, intentional self-harm** HCC

✓7th **T49.3X3** **Poisoning by emollients, demulcents and protectants, assault**

✓7th **T49.3X4** **Poisoning by emollients, demulcents and protectants, undetermined**

✓7th **T49.3X5** **Adverse effect of emollients, demulcents and protectants**

✓7th **T49.3X6** **Underdosing of emollients, demulcents and protectants**

✓5th **T49.4** **Poisoning by, adverse effect of and underdosing of keratolytics, keratoplastics, and other hair treatment drugs and preparations**

✓6th **T49.4X** **Poisoning by, adverse effect of and underdosing of keratolytics, keratoplastics, and other hair treatment drugs and preparations**

✓7th **T49.4X1** **Poisoning by keratolytics, keratoplastics, and other hair treatment drugs and preparations, accidental (unintentional)**
Poisoning by keratolytics, keratoplastics, and other hair treatment drugs and preparations NOS

2 ✓7th **T49.4X2** **Poisoning by keratolytics, keratoplastics, and other hair treatment drugs and preparations, intentional self-harm** HCC

✓7th **T49.4X3** **Poisoning by keratolytics, keratoplastics, and other hair treatment drugs and preparations, assault**

✓7th **T49.4X4** **Poisoning by keratolytics, keratoplastics, and other hair treatment drugs and preparations, undetermined**

✓7th **T49.4X5** **Adverse effect of keratolytics, keratoplastics, and other hair treatment drugs and preparations**

✓7th **T49.4X6** **Underdosing of keratolytics, keratoplastics, and other hair treatment drugs and preparations**

✓5th **T49.5** **Poisoning by, adverse effect of and underdosing of ophthalmological drugs and preparations**

✓6th **T49.5X** **Poisoning by, adverse effect of and underdosing of ophthalmological drugs and preparations**

✓7th **T49.5X1** **Poisoning by ophthalmological drugs and preparations, accidental (unintentional)**
Poisoning by ophthalmological drugs and preparations NOS

2 ✓7th **T49.5X2** **Poisoning by ophthalmological drugs and preparations, intentional self-harm** HCC

✓7th **T49.5X3** **Poisoning by ophthalmological drugs and preparations, assault**

✓7th **T49.5X4** **Poisoning by ophthalmological drugs and preparations, undetermined**

✓7th **T49.5X5** **Adverse effect of ophthalmological drugs and preparations**

✓7th **T49.5X6** **Underdosing of ophthalmological drugs and preparations**

✓5th **T49.6** **Poisoning by, adverse effect of and underdosing of otorhinolaryngological drugs and preparations**

✓6th **T49.6X** **Poisoning by, adverse effect of and underdosing of otorhinolaryngological drugs and preparations**

✓7th **T49.6X1** **Poisoning by otorhinolaryngological drugs and preparations, accidental (unintentional)**
Poisoning by otorhinolaryngological drugs and preparations NOS

2 HCC with 7th character indicating initial encounter (A or B - specific to category) OR sequela.

☑ Additional Character Req   ✓x7th Placeholder Alert   Manifestation   HCC CMS-HCC Condition   ▽ Unspecified Code   ▶◀ Revised Text   ● New Code   ▲ Revised Code Title

2 ✓7ᵗʰ **T49.6X2** **Poisoning by otorhinolaryngological drugs and preparations, intentional self-harm** ᴴᶜᶜ

  ✓7ᵗʰ **T49.6X3** **Poisoning by otorhinolaryngological drugs and preparations, assault**

  ✓7ᵗʰ **T49.6X4** **Poisoning by otorhinolaryngological drugs and preparations, undetermined**

  ✓7ᵗʰ **T49.6X5** **Adverse effect of otorhinolaryngological drugs and preparations**

  ✓7ᵗʰ **T49.6X6** **Underdosing of otorhinolaryngological drugs and preparations**

✓5ᵗʰ **T49.7** **Poisoning by, adverse effect of and underdosing of dental drugs, topically applied**

  ✓6ᵗʰ **T49.7X** **Poisoning by, adverse effect of and underdosing of dental drugs, topically applied**

    ✓7ᵗʰ **T49.7X1** **Poisoning by dental drugs, topically applied, accidental (unintentional)**
       Poisoning by dental drugs, topically applied NOS

    2 ✓7ᵗʰ **T49.7X2** **Poisoning by dental drugs, topically applied, intentional self-harm** ᴴᶜᶜ

    ✓7ᵗʰ **T49.7X3** **Poisoning by dental drugs, topically applied, assault**

    ✓7ᵗʰ **T49.7X4** **Poisoning by dental drugs, topically applied, undetermined**

    ✓7ᵗʰ **T49.7X5** **Adverse effect of dental drugs, topically applied**

    ✓7ᵗʰ **T49.7X6** **Underdosing of dental drugs, topically applied**

✓5ᵗʰ **T49.8** **Poisoning by, adverse effect of and underdosing of other topical agents**
   Poisoning by, adverse effect of and underdosing of spermicides

  ✓6ᵗʰ **T49.8X** **Poisoning by, adverse effect of and underdosing of other topical agents**

    ✓7ᵗʰ **T49.8X1** **Poisoning by other topical agents, accidental (unintentional)**
       Poisoning by other topical agents NOS

    2 ✓7ᵗʰ **T49.8X2** **Poisoning by other topical agents, intentional self-harm** ᴴᶜᶜ

    ✓7ᵗʰ **T49.8X3** **Poisoning by other topical agents, assault**

    ✓7ᵗʰ **T49.8X4** **Poisoning by other topical agents, undetermined**

    ✓7ᵗʰ **T49.8X5** **Adverse effect of other topical agents**

    ✓7ᵗʰ **T49.8X6** **Underdosing of other topical agents**

✓5ᵗʰ **T49.9** **Poisoning by, adverse effect of and underdosing of unspecified topical agent**

  ✓x7ᵗʰ **T49.91** **Poisoning by unspecified topical agent, accidental (unintentional)** ▽

  2 ✓x7ᵗʰ **T49.92** **Poisoning by unspecified topical agent, intentional self-harm** ᴴᶜᶜ ▽

  ✓x7ᵗʰ **T49.93** **Poisoning by unspecified topical agent, assault** ▽

  ✓x7ᵗʰ **T49.94** **Poisoning by unspecified topical agent, undetermined** ▽

  ✓x7ᵗʰ **T49.95** **Adverse effect of unspecified topical agent** ▽

  ✓x7ᵗʰ **T49.96** **Underdosing of unspecified topical agent** ▽

✓4ᵗʰ **T50** **Poisoning by, adverse effect of and underdosing of diuretics and other and unspecified drugs, medicaments and biological substances**

> The appropriate 7th character is to be added to each code from category T50.
> A   initial encounter
> D   subsequent encounter
> S   sequela

✓5ᵗʰ **T50.0** **Poisoning by, adverse effect of and underdosing of mineralocorticoids and their antagonists**

  ✓6ᵗʰ **T50.0X** **Poisoning by, adverse effect of and underdosing of mineralocorticoids and their antagonists**

    ✓7ᵗʰ **T50.0X1** **Poisoning by mineralocorticoids and their antagonists, accidental (unintentional)**
       Poisoning by mineralocorticoids and their antagonists NOS

    2 ✓7ᵗʰ **T50.0X2** **Poisoning by mineralocorticoids and their antagonists, intentional self-harm** ᴴᶜᶜ

    ✓7ᵗʰ **T50.0X3** **Poisoning by mineralocorticoids and their antagonists, assault**

    ✓7ᵗʰ **T50.0X4** **Poisoning by mineralocorticoids and their antagonists, undetermined**

    ✓7ᵗʰ **T50.0X5** **Adverse effect of mineralocorticoids and their antagonists**

    ✓7ᵗʰ **T50.0X6** **Underdosing of mineralocorticoids and their antagonists**

✓5ᵗʰ **T50.1** **Poisoning by, adverse effect of and underdosing of loop [high-ceiling] diuretics**

  ✓6ᵗʰ **T50.1X** **Poisoning by, adverse effect of and underdosing of loop [high-ceiling] diuretics**

    ✓7ᵗʰ **T50.1X1** **Poisoning by loop [high-ceiling] diuretics, accidental (unintentional)**
       Poisoning by loop [high-ceiling] diuretics NOS

    2 ✓7ᵗʰ **T50.1X2** **Poisoning by loop [high-ceiling] diuretics, intentional self-harm** ᴴᶜᶜ

    ✓7ᵗʰ **T50.1X3** **Poisoning by loop [high-ceiling] diuretics, assault**

    ✓7ᵗʰ **T50.1X4** **Poisoning by loop [high-ceiling] diuretics, undetermined**

    ✓7ᵗʰ **T50.1X5** **Adverse effect of loop [high-ceiling] diuretics**

    ✓7ᵗʰ **T50.1X6** **Underdosing of loop [high-ceiling] diuretics**

✓5ᵗʰ **T50.2** **Poisoning by, adverse effect of and underdosing of carbonic-anhydrase inhibitors, benzothiadiazides and other diuretics**
   Poisoning by, adverse effect of and underdosing of acetazolamide

  ✓6ᵗʰ **T50.2X** **Poisoning by, adverse effect of and underdosing of carbonic-anhydrase inhibitors, benzothiadiazides and other diuretics**

    ✓7ᵗʰ **T50.2X1** **Poisoning by carbonic-anhydrase inhibitors, benzothiadiazides and other diuretics, accidental (unintentional)**
       Poisoning by carbonic-anhydrase inhibitors, benzothiadiazides and other diuretics NOS

    2 ✓7ᵗʰ **T50.2X2** **Poisoning by carbonic-anhydrase inhibitors, benzothiadiazides and other diuretics, intentional self-harm** ᴴᶜᶜ

    ✓7ᵗʰ **T50.2X3** **Poisoning by carbonic-anhydrase inhibitors, benzothiadiazides and other diuretics, assault**

    ✓7ᵗʰ **T50.2X4** **Poisoning by carbonic-anhydrase inhibitors, benzothiadiazides and other diuretics, undetermined**

    ✓7ᵗʰ **T50.2X5** **Adverse effect of carbonic-anhydrase inhibitors, benzothiadiazides and other diuretics**

    ✓7ᵗʰ **T50.2X6** **Underdosing of carbonic-anhydrase inhibitors, benzothiadiazides and other diuretics**

✓5ᵗʰ **T50.3** **Poisoning by, adverse effect of and underdosing of electrolytic, caloric and water-balance agents**
   Poisoning by, adverse effect of and underdosing of oral rehydration salts

  ✓6ᵗʰ **T50.3X** **Poisoning by, adverse effect of and underdosing of electrolytic, caloric and water-balance agents**

    ✓7ᵗʰ **T50.3X1** **Poisoning by electrolytic, caloric and water-balance agents, accidental (unintentional)**
       Poisoning by electrolytic, caloric and water-balance agents NOS

    2 ✓7ᵗʰ **T50.3X2** **Poisoning by electrolytic, caloric and water-balance agents, intentional self-harm** ᴴᶜᶜ

    ✓7ᵗʰ **T50.3X3** **Poisoning by electrolytic, caloric and water-balance agents, assault**

    ✓7ᵗʰ **T50.3X4** **Poisoning by electrolytic, caloric and water-balance agents, undetermined**

    ✓7ᵗʰ **T50.3X5** **Adverse effect of electrolytic, caloric and water-balance agents**

    ✓7ᵗʰ **T50.3X6** **Underdosing of electrolytic, caloric and water-balance agents**

---

2   HCC with 7th character indicating initial encounter (A or B - specific to category) OR sequela.

EXCLUDES1 Not coded here   **EXCLUDES2** Not included here   **N** Newborn Age: 0   **P** Pediatric Age: 0-17   **M** Maternity Age: 12-55   **A** Adult Age: 15-124

1078   ICD-10-CM 2018

✓5ᵗʰ **T50.4** Poisoning by, adverse effect of and underdosing of drugs affecting uric acid metabolism

    ✓6ᵗʰ **T50.4X** Poisoning by, adverse effect of and underdosing of drugs affecting uric acid metabolism

      ✓7ᵗʰ **T50.4X1** Poisoning by drugs affecting uric acid metabolism, accidental (unintentional)
        Poisoning by drugs affecting uric acid metabolism NOS

      2 ✓7ᵗʰ **T50.4X2** Poisoning by drugs affecting uric acid metabolism, intentional self-harm   HCC

      ✓7ᵗʰ **T50.4X3** Poisoning by drugs affecting uric acid metabolism, assault

      ✓7ᵗʰ **T50.4X4** Poisoning by drugs affecting uric acid metabolism, undetermined

      ✓7ᵗʰ **T50.4X5** Adverse effect of drugs affecting uric acid metabolism

      ✓7ᵗʰ **T50.4X6** Underdosing of drugs affecting uric acid metabolism

✓5ᵗʰ **T50.5** Poisoning by, adverse effect of and underdosing of appetite depressants

    ✓6ᵗʰ **T50.5X** Poisoning by, adverse effect of and underdosing of appetite depressants

      ✓7ᵗʰ **T50.5X1** Poisoning by appetite depressants, accidental (unintentional)
        Poisoning by appetite depressants NOS

      2 ✓7ᵗʰ **T50.5X2** Poisoning by appetite depressants, intentional self-harm   HCC

      ✓7ᵗʰ **T50.5X3** Poisoning by appetite depressants, assault

      ✓7ᵗʰ **T50.5X4** Poisoning by appetite depressants, undetermined

      ✓7ᵗʰ **T50.5X5** Adverse effect of appetite depressants

      ✓7ᵗʰ **T50.5X6** Underdosing of appetite depressants

✓5ᵗʰ **T50.6** Poisoning by, adverse effect of and underdosing of antidotes and chelating agents
    Poisoning by, adverse effect of and underdosing of alcohol deterrents

    ✓6ᵗʰ **T50.6X** Poisoning by, adverse effect of and underdosing of antidotes and chelating agents

      ✓7ᵗʰ **T50.6X1** Poisoning by antidotes and chelating agents, accidental (unintentional)
        Poisoning by antidotes and chelating agents NOS

      2 ✓7ᵗʰ **T50.6X2** Poisoning by antidotes and chelating agents, intentional self-harm   HCC

      ✓7ᵗʰ **T50.6X3** Poisoning by antidotes and chelating agents, assault

      ✓7ᵗʰ **T50.6X4** Poisoning by antidotes and chelating agents, undetermined

      ✓7ᵗʰ **T50.6X5** Adverse effect of antidotes and chelating agents

      ✓7ᵗʰ **T50.6X6** Underdosing of antidotes and chelating agents

✓5ᵗʰ **T50.7** Poisoning by, adverse effect of and underdosing of analeptics and opioid receptor antagonists

    ✓6ᵗʰ **T50.7X** Poisoning by, adverse effect of and underdosing of analeptics and opioid receptor antagonists

      ✓7ᵗʰ **T50.7X1** Poisoning by analeptics and opioid receptor antagonists, accidental (unintentional)
        Poisoning by analeptics and opioid receptor antagonists NOS

      2 ✓7ᵗʰ **T50.7X2** Poisoning by analeptics and opioid receptor antagonists, intentional self-harm   HCC

      ✓7ᵗʰ **T50.7X3** Poisoning by analeptics and opioid receptor antagonists, assault

      ✓7ᵗʰ **T50.7X4** Poisoning by analeptics and opioid receptor antagonists, undetermined

      ✓7ᵗʰ **T50.7X5** Adverse effect of analeptics and opioid receptor antagonists

      ✓7ᵗʰ **T50.7X6** Underdosing of analeptics and opioid receptor antagonists

✓5ᵗʰ **T50.8** Poisoning by, adverse effect of and underdosing of diagnostic agents

    ✓6ᵗʰ **T50.8X** Poisoning by, adverse effect of and underdosing of diagnostic agents

      ✓7ᵗʰ **T50.8X1** Poisoning by diagnostic agents, accidental (unintentional)
        Poisoning by diagnostic agents NOS

      2 ✓7ᵗʰ **T50.8X2** Poisoning by diagnostic agents, intentional self-harm   HCC

      ✓7ᵗʰ **T50.8X3** Poisoning by diagnostic agents, assault

      ✓7ᵗʰ **T50.8X4** Poisoning by diagnostic agents, undetermined

      ✓7ᵗʰ **T50.8X5** Adverse effect of diagnostic agents

      ✓7ᵗʰ **T50.8X6** Underdosing of diagnostic agents

✓5ᵗʰ **T50.A** Poisoning by, adverse effect of and underdosing of bacterial vaccines

    ✓6ᵗʰ **T50.A1** Poisoning by, adverse effect of and underdosing of pertussis vaccine, including combinations with a pertussis component

      ✓7ᵗʰ **T50.A11** Poisoning by pertussis vaccine, including combinations with a pertussis component, accidental (unintentional)

      2 ✓7ᵗʰ **T50.A12** Poisoning by pertussis vaccine, including combinations with a pertussis component, intentional self-harm   HCC

      ✓7ᵗʰ **T50.A13** Poisoning by pertussis vaccine, including combinations with a pertussis component, assault

      ✓7ᵗʰ **T50.A14** Poisoning by pertussis vaccine, including combinations with a pertussis component, undetermined

      ✓7ᵗʰ **T50.A15** Adverse effect of pertussis vaccine, including combinations with a pertussis component

      ✓7ᵗʰ **T50.A16** Underdosing of pertussis vaccine, including combinations with a pertussis component

    ✓6ᵗʰ **T50.A2** Poisoning by, adverse effect of and underdosing of mixed bacterial vaccines without a pertussis component

      ✓7ᵗʰ **T50.A21** Poisoning by mixed bacterial vaccines without a pertussis component, accidental (unintentional)

      2 ✓7ᵗʰ **T50.A22** Poisoning by mixed bacterial vaccines without a pertussis component, intentional self-harm   HCC

      ✓7ᵗʰ **T50.A23** Poisoning by mixed bacterial vaccines without a pertussis component, assault

      ✓7ᵗʰ **T50.A24** Poisoning by mixed bacterial vaccines without a pertussis component, undetermined

      ✓7ᵗʰ **T50.A25** Adverse effect of mixed bacterial vaccines without a pertussis component

      ✓7ᵗʰ **T50.A26** Underdosing of mixed bacterial vaccines without a pertussis component

    ✓6ᵗʰ **T50.A9** Poisoning by, adverse effect of and underdosing of other bacterial vaccines

      ✓7ᵗʰ **T50.A91** Poisoning by other bacterial vaccines, accidental (unintentional)

      2 ✓7ᵗʰ **T50.A92** Poisoning by other bacterial vaccines, intentional self-harm   HCC

      ✓7ᵗʰ **T50.A93** Poisoning by other bacterial vaccines, assault

      ✓7ᵗʰ **T50.A94** Poisoning by other bacterial vaccines, undetermined

      ✓7ᵗʰ **T50.A95** Adverse effect of other bacterial vaccines

      ✓7ᵗʰ **T50.A96** Underdosing of other bacterial vaccines

✓5ᵗʰ **T50.B** Poisoning by, adverse effect of and underdosing of viral vaccines

    ✓6ᵗʰ **T50.B1** Poisoning by, adverse effect of and underdosing of smallpox vaccines

      ✓7ᵗʰ **T50.B11** Poisoning by smallpox vaccines, accidental (unintentional)

      2 ✓7ᵗʰ **T50.B12** Poisoning by smallpox vaccines, intentional self-harm   HCC

---

2   HCC with 7th character indicating initial encounter (A or B - specific to category) OR sequela.

✓ Additional Character Req   ✓x7ᵗʰ Placeholder Alert   Manifestation   HCC CMS-HCC Condition   ▽ Unspecified Code   ►◄ Revised Text   ● New Code   ▲ Revised Code Title

Chapter 19. Injury, Poisoning, and Certain Other Consequences of External Causes

T50.B13–T51.3X4

☑7th **T50.B13**   Poisoning by smallpox vaccines, **assault**

☑7th **T50.B14**   Poisoning by smallpox vaccines, **undetermined**

☑7th **T50.B15**   **Adverse effect** of smallpox vaccines

☑7th **T50.B16**   **Underdosing** of smallpox vaccines

☑6th **T50.B9**   Poisoning by, adverse effect of and underdosing of other viral vaccines

     ☑7th **T50.B91**   Poisoning by other viral vaccines, **accidental (unintentional)**

     2 ☑7th **T50.B92**   Poisoning by other viral vaccines, **intentional self-harm**   HCC

     ☑7th **T50.B93**   Poisoning by other viral vaccines, **assault**

     ☑7th **T50.B94**   Poisoning by other viral vaccines, **undetermined**

     ☑7th **T50.B95**   **Adverse effect** of other viral vaccines

     ☑7th **T50.B96**   **Underdosing** of other viral vaccines

☑5th **T50.Z**   Poisoning by, adverse effect of and underdosing of other vaccines and biological substances

     ☑6th **T50.Z1**   Poisoning by, adverse effect of and underdosing of **immunoglobulin**

         ☑7th **T50.Z11**   Poisoning by immunoglobulin, **accidental (unintentional)**

         2 ☑7th **T50.Z12**   Poisoning by immunoglobulin, **intentional self-harm**   HCC

         ☑7th **T50.Z13**   Poisoning by immunoglobulin, **assault**

         ☑7th **T50.Z14**   Poisoning by immunoglobulin, **undetermined**

         ☑7th **T50.Z15**   **Adverse effect** of immunoglobulin

         ☑7th **T50.Z16**   **Underdosing** of immunoglobulin

     ☑6th **T50.Z9**   Poisoning by, adverse effect of and underdosing of other vaccines and biological substances

         ☑7th **T50.Z91**   Poisoning by other vaccines and biological substances, **accidental (unintentional)**

         2 ☑7th **T50.Z92**   Poisoning by other vaccines and biological substances, **intentional self-harm**   HCC

         ☑7th **T50.Z93**   Poisoning by other vaccines and biological substances, **assault**

         ☑7th **T50.Z94**   Poisoning by other vaccines and biological substances, **undetermined**

         ☑7th **T50.Z95**   **Adverse effect** of other vaccines and biological substances

         ☑7th **T50.Z96**   **Underdosing** of other vaccines and biological substances

☑5th **T50.9**   Poisoning by, adverse effect of and underdosing of other and unspecified drugs, medicaments and biological substances

     AHA: 2016, 1Q, 38; 2015, 1Q, 21

     ☑6th **T50.90**   Poisoning by, adverse effect of and underdosing of unspecified drugs, medicaments and biological substances

         ☑7th **T50.901**   Poisoning by unspecified drugs, medicaments and biological substances, **accidental (unintentional)**   ▽

         2 ☑7th **T50.902**   Poisoning by unspecified drugs, medicaments and biological substances, **intentional self-harm**   HCC ▽

         ☑7th **T50.903**   Poisoning by unspecified drugs, medicaments and biological substances, **assault**   ▽

         ☑7th **T50.904**   Poisoning by unspecified drugs, medicaments and biological substances, **undetermined**   ▽

         ☑7th **T50.905**   **Adverse effect** of unspecified drugs, medicaments and biological substances   ▽

         ☑7th **T50.906**   **Underdosing** of unspecified drugs, medicaments and biological substances   ▽

     ☑6th **T50.99**   Poisoning by, adverse effect of and underdosing of other drugs, medicaments and biological substances

         ☑7th **T50.991**   Poisoning by other drugs, medicaments and biological substances, **accidental (unintentional)**

         2 ☑7th **T50.992**   Poisoning by other drugs, medicaments and biological substances, **intentional self-harm**   HCC

☑7th **T50.993**   Poisoning by other drugs, medicaments and biological substances, **assault**

☑7th **T50.994**   Poisoning by other drugs, medicaments and biological substances, **undetermined**

☑7th **T50.995**   **Adverse effect** of other drugs, medicaments and biological substances

☑7th **T50.996**   **Underdosing** of other drugs, medicaments and biological substances

Toxic effects of substances chiefly nonmedicinal as to source (T51-T65)

NOTE   When no intent is indicated code to accidental. Undetermined intent is only for use when there is specific documentation in the record that the intent of the toxic effect cannot be determined.

Use additional code(s) for all associated manifestations of toxic effect, such as:
     personal history of foreign body fully removed (Z87.821)
     respiratory conditions due to external agents (J60-J70)
     to identify any retained foreign body, if applicable (Z18.-)

EXCLUDES 1   contact with and (suspected) exposure to toxic substances (Z77.-)

AHA: 2017, 1Q, 39-40

☑4th **T51**   **Toxic effect of alcohol**

> The appropriate 7th character is to be added to each code from category T51.
> A   initial encounter
> D   subsequent encounter
> S   sequela

☑5th **T51.0**   **Toxic effect of ethanol**
     Toxic effect of ethyl alcohol
     EXCLUDES 2   *acute alcohol intoxication or 'hangover' effects (F10.129, F10.229, F10.929)*
         drunkenness (F10.129, F10.229, F10.929)
         pathological alcohol intoxication (F10.129, F10.229, F10.929)

     ☑6th **T51.0X**   **Toxic effect of ethanol**

         ☑7th **T51.0X1**   **Toxic effect of ethanol, accidental (unintentional)**
             Toxic effect of ethanol NOS

         2 ☑7th **T51.0X2**   **Toxic effect of ethanol, intentional self-harm**   HCC

         ☑7th **T51.0X3**   **Toxic effect of ethanol, assault**

         ☑7th **T51.0X4**   **Toxic effect of ethanol, undetermined**

☑5th **T51.1**   **Toxic effect of methanol**
     Toxic effect of methyl alcohol

     ☑6th **T51.1X**   **Toxic effect of methanol**

         ☑7th **T51.1X1**   **Toxic effect of methanol, accidental (unintentional)**
             Toxic effect of methanol NOS

         2 ☑7th **T51.1X2**   **Toxic effect of methanol, intentional self-harm**   HCC

         ☑7th **T51.1X3**   **Toxic effect of methanol, assault**

         ☑7th **T51.1X4**   **Toxic effect of methanol, undetermined**

☑5th **T51.2**   **Toxic effect of 2-Propanol**
     Toxic effect of isopropyl alcohol

     ☑6th **T51.2X**   **Toxic effect of 2-Propanol**

         ☑7th **T51.2X1**   **Toxic effect of 2-Propanol, accidental (unintentional)**
             Toxic effect of 2-Propanol NOS

         2 ☑7th **T51.2X2**   **Toxic effect of 2-Propanol, intentional self-harm**   HCC

         ☑7th **T51.2X3**   **Toxic effect of 2-Propanol, assault**

         ☑7th **T51.2X4**   **Toxic effect of 2-Propanol, undetermined**

☑5th **T51.3**   **Toxic effect of fusel oil**
     Toxic effect of amyl alcohol
     Toxic effect of butyl [1-butanol] alcohol
     Toxic effect of propyl [1-propanol] alcohol

     ☑6th **T51.3X**   **Toxic effect of fusel oil**

         ☑7th **T51.3X1**   **Toxic effect of fusel oil, accidental (unintentional)**
             Toxic effect of fusel oil NOS

         2 ☑7th **T51.3X2**   **Toxic effect of fusel oil, intentional self-harm**   HCC

         ☑7th **T51.3X3**   **Toxic effect of fusel oil, assault**

         ☑7th **T51.3X4**   **Toxic effect of fusel oil, undetermined**

---

2   HCC with 7th character indicating initial encounter (A or B - specific to category) OR sequela.

EXCLUDES 1 Not coded here   **EXCLUDES 2** Not included here   **N** Newborn Age: 0   **P** Pediatric Age: 0-17   **M** Maternity Age: 12-55   **A** Adult Age: 15-124

1080   ICD-10-CM 2018

☑5th **T51.8** **Toxic effect of other alcohols**

   ☑6th **T51.8X** **Toxic effect of other alcohols**

      ☑7th **T51.8X1** **Toxic effect of other alcohols, accidental (unintentional)**
         Toxic effect of other alcohols NOS

     2 ☑7th **T51.8X2** **Toxic effect of other alcohols, intentional self-harm** HCC

      ☑7th **T51.8X3** **Toxic effect of other alcohols, assault**

      ☑7th **T51.8X4** **Toxic effect of other alcohols, undetermined**

☑5th **T51.9** **Toxic effect of unspecified alcohol**

   ☑x7th **T51.91** **Toxic effect of unspecified alcohol, accidental (unintentional)** ▽

   2 ☑x7th **T51.92** **Toxic effect of unspecified alcohol, intentional self-harm** HCC ▽

   ☑x7th **T51.93** **Toxic effect of unspecified alcohol, assault** ▽

   ☑x7th **T51.94** **Toxic effect of unspecified alcohol, undetermined** ▽

☑4th **T52** **Toxic effect of organic solvents**

   EXCLUDES 1   *halogen derivatives of aliphatic and aromatic hydrocarbons (T53.-)*

   The appropriate 7th character is to be added to each code from category T52.
   A   initial encounter
   D   subsequent encounter
   S   sequela

☑5th **T52.0** **Toxic effects of petroleum products**
   Toxic effects of ether petroleum
   Toxic effects of gasoline [petrol]
   Toxic effects of kerosene [paraffin oil]
   Toxic effects of naphtha petroleum
   Toxic effects of paraffin wax
   Toxic effects of spirit petroleum

   ☑6th **T52.0X** **Toxic effects of petroleum products**

      ☑7th **T52.0X1** **Toxic effect of petroleum products, accidental (unintentional)**
         Toxic effects of petroleum products NOS

     2 ☑7th **T52.0X2** **Toxic effect of petroleum products, intentional self-harm** HCC

      ☑7th **T52.0X3** **Toxic effect of petroleum products, assault**

      ☑7th **T52.0X4** **Toxic effect of petroleum products, undetermined**

☑5th **T52.1** **Toxic effects of benzene**

   EXCLUDES 1   *homologues of benzene (T52.2)*
               nitroderivatives and aminoderivatives of benzene and its homologues (T65.3)

   ☑6th **T52.1X** **Toxic effects of benzene**

      ☑7th **T52.1X1** **Toxic effect of benzene, accidental (unintentional)**
         Toxic effects of benzene NOS

     2 ☑7th **T52.1X2** **Toxic effect of benzene, intentional self-harm** HCC

      ☑7th **T52.1X3** **Toxic effect of benzene, assault**

      ☑7th **T52.1X4** **Toxic effect of benzene, undetermined**

☑5th **T52.2** **Toxic effects of homologues of benzene**
   Toxic effects of toluene [methylbenzene]
   Toxic effects of xylene [dimethylbenzene]

   ☑6th **T52.2X** **Toxic effects of homologues of benzene**

      ☑7th **T52.2X1** **Toxic effect of homologues of benzene, accidental (unintentional)**
         Toxic effects of homologues of benzene NOS

     2 ☑7th **T52.2X2** **Toxic effect of homologues of benzene, intentional self-harm** HCC

      ☑7th **T52.2X3** **Toxic effect of homologues of benzene, assault**

      ☑7th **T52.2X4** **Toxic effect of homologues of benzene, undetermined**

☑5th **T52.3** **Toxic effects of glycols**

   ☑6th **T52.3X** **Toxic effects of glycols**

      ☑7th **T52.3X1** **Toxic effect of glycols, accidental (unintentional)**
         Toxic effects of glycols NOS

---

     2 ☑7th **T52.3X2** **Toxic effect of glycols, intentional self-harm** HCC

      ☑7th **T52.3X3** **Toxic effect of glycols, assault**

      ☑7th **T52.3X4** **Toxic effect of glycols, undetermined**

☑5th **T52.4** **Toxic effects of ketones**

   ☑6th **T52.4X** **Toxic effects of ketones**

      ☑7th **T52.4X1** **Toxic effect of ketones, accidental (unintentional)**
         Toxic effects of ketones NOS

     2 ☑7th **T52.4X2** **Toxic effect of ketones, intentional self-harm** HCC

      ☑7th **T52.4X3** **Toxic effect of ketones, assault**

      ☑7th **T52.4X4** **Toxic effect of ketones, undetermined**

☑5th **T52.8** **Toxic effects of other organic solvents**

   ☑6th **T52.8X** **Toxic effects of other organic solvents**

      ☑7th **T52.8X1** **Toxic effect of other organic solvents, accidental (unintentional)**
         Toxic effects of other organic solvents NOS

     2 ☑7th **T52.8X2** **Toxic effect of other organic solvents, intentional self-harm** HCC

      ☑7th **T52.8X3** **Toxic effect of other organic solvents, assault**

      ☑7th **T52.8X4** **Toxic effect of other organic solvents, undetermined**

☑5th **T52.9** **Toxic effects of unspecified organic solvent**

   ☑x7th **T52.91** **Toxic effect of unspecified organic solvent, accidental (unintentional)** ▽

   2 ☑x7th **T52.92** **Toxic effect of unspecified organic solvent, intentional self-harm** HCC ▽

   ☑x7th **T52.93** **Toxic effect of unspecified organic solvent, assault** ▽

   ☑x7th **T52.94** **Toxic effect of unspecified organic solvent, undetermined** ▽

☑4th **T53** **Toxic effect of halogen derivatives of aliphatic and aromatic hydrocarbons**

   The appropriate 7th character is to be added to each code from category T53.
   A   initial encounter
   D   subsequent encounter
   S   sequela

☑5th **T53.0** **Toxic effects of carbon tetrachloride**
   Toxic effects of tetrachloromethane

   ☑6th **T53.0X** **Toxic effects of carbon tetrachloride**

      ☑7th **T53.0X1** **Toxic effect of carbon tetrachloride, accidental (unintentional)**
         Toxic effects of carbon tetrachloride NOS

     2 ☑7th **T53.0X2** **Toxic effect of carbon tetrachloride, intentional self-harm** HCC

      ☑7th **T53.0X3** **Toxic effect of carbon tetrachloride, assault**

      ☑7th **T53.0X4** **Toxic effect of carbon tetrachloride, undetermined**

☑5th **T53.1** **Toxic effects of chloroform**
   Toxic effects of trichloromethane

   ☑6th **T53.1X** **Toxic effects of chloroform**

      ☑7th **T53.1X1** **Toxic effect of chloroform, accidental (unintentional)**
         Toxic effects of chloroform NOS

     2 ☑7th **T53.1X2** **Toxic effect of chloroform, intentional self-harm** HCC

      ☑7th **T53.1X3** **Toxic effect of chloroform, assault**

      ☑7th **T53.1X4** **Toxic effect of chloroform, undetermined**

☑5th **T53.2** **Toxic effects of trichloroethylene**
   Toxic effects of trichloroethene

   ☑6th **T53.2X** **Toxic effects of trichloroethylene**

      ☑7th **T53.2X1** **Toxic effect of trichloroethylene, accidental (unintentional)**
         Toxic effects of trichloroethylene NOS

     2 ☑7th **T53.2X2** **Toxic effect of trichloroethylene, intentional self-harm** HCC

      ☑7th **T53.2X3** **Toxic effect of trichloroethylene, assault**

---

2   HCC with 7th character indicating initial encounter (A or B - specific to category) OR sequela.

☑ Additional Character Req   ☑x7th Placeholder Alert   Manifestation   HCC CMS-HCC Condition   ▽ Unspecified Code   ►◄ Revised Text   ● New Code   ▲ Revised Code Title

√7th T53.2X4 Toxic effect of trichloroethylene, undetermined

√5th T53.3 Toxic effects of tetrachloroethylene
Toxic effects of perchloroethylene
Toxic effect of tetrachloroethene

    √6th T53.3X Toxic effects of tetrachloroethylene

      √7th T53.3X1 Toxic effect of tetrachloroethylene, accidental (unintentional)
Toxic effects of tetrachloroethylene NOS

      2 √7th T53.3X2 Toxic effect of tetrachloroethylene, intentional self-harm HCC

      √7th T53.3X3 Toxic effect of tetrachloroethylene, assault

      √7th T53.3X4 Toxic effect of tetrachloroethylene, undetermined

√5th T53.4 Toxic effects of dichloromethane
Toxic effects of methylene chloride

    √6th T53.4X Toxic effects of dichloromethane

      √7th T53.4X1 Toxic effect of dichloromethane, accidental (unintentional)
Toxic effects of dichloromethane NOS

      2 √7th T53.4X2 Toxic effect of dichloromethane, intentional self-harm HCC

      √7th T53.4X3 Toxic effect of dichloromethane, assault

      √7th T53.4X4 Toxic effect of dichloromethane, undetermined

√5th T53.5 Toxic effects of chlorofluorocarbons

    √6th T53.5X Toxic effects of chlorofluorocarbons

      √7th T53.5X1 Toxic effect of chlorofluorocarbons, accidental (unintentional)
Toxic effects of chlorofluorocarbons NOS

      2 √7th T53.5X2 Toxic effect of chlorofluorocarbons, intentional self-harm HCC

      √7th T53.5X3 Toxic effect of chlorofluorocarbons, assault

      √7th T53.5X4 Toxic effect of chlorofluorocarbons, undetermined

√5th T53.6 Toxic effects of other halogen derivatives of aliphatic hydrocarbons

    √6th T53.6X Toxic effects of other halogen derivatives of aliphatic hydrocarbons

      √7th T53.6X1 Toxic effect of other halogen derivatives of aliphatic hydrocarbons, accidental (unintentional)
Toxic effects of other halogen derivatives of aliphatic hydrocarbons NOS

      2 √7th T53.6X2 Toxic effect of other halogen derivatives of aliphatic hydrocarbons, intentional self-harm HCC

      √7th T53.6X3 Toxic effect of other halogen derivatives of aliphatic hydrocarbons, assault

      √7th T53.6X4 Toxic effect of other halogen derivatives of aliphatic hydrocarbons, undetermined

√5th T53.7 Toxic effects of other halogen derivatives of aromatic hydrocarbons

    √6th T53.7X Toxic effects of other halogen derivatives of aromatic hydrocarbons

      √7th T53.7X1 Toxic effect of other halogen derivatives of aromatic hydrocarbons, accidental (unintentional)
Toxic effects of other halogen derivatives of aromatic hydrocarbons NOS

      2 √7th T53.7X2 Toxic effect of other halogen derivatives of aromatic hydrocarbons, intentional self-harm HCC

      √7th T53.7X3 Toxic effect of other halogen derivatives of aromatic hydrocarbons, assault

      √7th T53.7X4 Toxic effect of other halogen derivatives of aromatic hydrocarbons, undetermined

√5th T53.9 Toxic effects of unspecified halogen derivatives of aliphatic and aromatic hydrocarbons

    √x7th T53.91 Toxic effect of unspecified halogen derivatives of aliphatic and aromatic hydrocarbons, accidental (unintentional) ▽

2 √x7th T53.92 Toxic effect of unspecified halogen derivatives of aliphatic and aromatic hydrocarbons, intentional self-harm HCC ▽

√x7th T53.93 Toxic effect of unspecified halogen derivatives of aliphatic and aromatic hydrocarbons, assault ▽

√x7th T53.94 Toxic effect of unspecified halogen derivatives of aliphatic and aromatic hydrocarbons, undetermined ▽

√4th T54 Toxic effect of corrosive substances

> The appropriate 7th character is to be added to each code from category T54.
> A   initial encounter
> D   subsequent encounter
> S   sequela

√5th T54.0 Toxic effects of phenol and phenol homologues

    √6th T54.0X Toxic effects of phenol and phenol homologues

      √7th T54.0X1 Toxic effect of phenol and phenol homologues, accidental (unintentional)
Toxic effects of phenol and phenol homologues NOS

      2 √7th T54.0X2 Toxic effect of phenol and phenol homologues, intentional self-harm HCC

      √7th T54.0X3 Toxic effect of phenol and phenol homologues, assault

      √7th T54.0X4 Toxic effect of phenol and phenol homologues, undetermined

√5th T54.1 Toxic effects of other corrosive organic compounds

    √6th T54.1X Toxic effects of other corrosive organic compounds

      √7th T54.1X1 Toxic effect of other corrosive organic compounds, accidental (unintentional)
Toxic effects of other corrosive organic compounds NOS

      2 √7th T54.1X2 Toxic effect of other corrosive organic compounds, intentional self-harm HCC

      √7th T54.1X3 Toxic effect of other corrosive organic compounds, assault

      √7th T54.1X4 Toxic effect of other corrosive organic compounds, undetermined

√5th T54.2 Toxic effects of corrosive acids and acid-like substances
Toxic effects of hydrochloric acid
Toxic effects of sulfuric acid

    √6th T54.2X Toxic effects of corrosive acids and acid-like substances

      √7th T54.2X1 Toxic effect of corrosive acids and acid-like substances, accidental (unintentional)
Toxic effects of corrosive acids and acid-like substances NOS

      2 √7th T54.2X2 Toxic effect of corrosive acids and acid-like substances, intentional self-harm HCC

      √7th T54.2X3 Toxic effect of corrosive acids and acid-like substances, assault

      √7th T54.2X4 Toxic effect of corrosive acids and acid-like substances, undetermined

√5th T54.3 Toxic effects of corrosive alkalis and alkali-like substances
Toxic effects of potassium hydroxide
Toxic effects of sodium hydroxide

    √6th T54.3X Toxic effects of corrosive alkalis and alkali-like substances

      √7th T54.3X1 Toxic effect of corrosive alkalis and alkali-like substances, accidental (unintentional)
Toxic effects of corrosive alkalis and alkali-like substances NOS

      2 √7th T54.3X2 Toxic effect of corrosive alkalis and alkali-like substances, intentional self-harm HCC

      √7th T54.3X3 Toxic effect of corrosive alkalis and alkali-like substances, assault

      √7th T54.3X4 Toxic effect of corrosive alkalis and alkali-like substances, undetermined

√5th T54.9 Toxic effects of unspecified corrosive substance

    √x7th T54.91 Toxic effect of unspecified corrosive substance, accidental (unintentional) ▽

---

2 HCC with 7th character indicating initial encounter (A or B - specific to category) OR sequela.

2 ✓x7ᵗʰ **T54.92** **Toxic effect of unspecified corrosive substance, intentional self-harm** HCC ▽

✓x7ᵗʰ **T54.93** **Toxic effect of unspecified corrosive substance, assault** ▽

✓x7ᵗʰ **T54.94** **Toxic effect of unspecified corrosive substance, undetermined** ▽

✓4ᵗʰ **T55** **Toxic effect of soaps and detergents**

> The appropriate 7th character is to be added to each code from category T55.
> A   initial encounter
> D   subsequent encounter
> S   sequela

✓5ᵗʰ **T55.0** **Toxic effect of soaps**

✓6ᵗʰ **T55.0X** **Toxic effect of soaps**

✓7ᵗʰ **T55.0X1** **Toxic effect of soaps, accidental (unintentional)**
Toxic effect of soaps NOS

2 ✓7ᵗʰ **T55.0X2** **Toxic effect of soaps, intentional self-harm** HCC

✓7ᵗʰ **T55.0X3** **Toxic effect of soaps, assault**

✓7ᵗʰ **T55.0X4** **Toxic effect of soaps, undetermined**

✓5ᵗʰ **T55.1** **Toxic effect of detergents**

✓6ᵗʰ **T55.1X** **Toxic effect of detergents**

✓7ᵗʰ **T55.1X1** **Toxic effect of detergents, accidental (unintentional)**
Toxic effect of detergents NOS

2 ✓7ᵗʰ **T55.1X2** **Toxic effect of detergents, intentional self-harm** HCC

✓7ᵗʰ **T55.1X3** **Toxic effect of detergents, assault**

✓7ᵗʰ **T55.1X4** **Toxic effect of detergents, undetermined**

✓4ᵗʰ **T56** **Toxic effect of metals**
INCLUDES   toxic effects of fumes and vapors of metals
toxic effects of metals from all sources, except medicinal substances
Use additional code to identify any retained metal foreign body, if applicable (Z18.0-, T18.1-)
EXCLUDES 1   arsenic and its compounds (T57.0)
manganese and its compounds (T57.2)

> The appropriate 7th character is to be added to each code from category T56.
> A   initial encounter
> D   subsequent encounter
> S   sequela

✓5ᵗʰ **T56.0** **Toxic effects of lead and its compounds**

✓6ᵗʰ **T56.0X** **Toxic effects of lead and its compounds**

✓7ᵗʰ **T56.0X1** **Toxic effect of lead and its compounds, accidental (unintentional)**
Toxic effects of lead and its compounds NOS

2 ✓7ᵗʰ **T56.0X2** **Toxic effect of lead and its compounds, intentional self-harm** HCC

✓7ᵗʰ **T56.0X3** **Toxic effect of lead and its compounds, assault**

✓7ᵗʰ **T56.0X4** **Toxic effect of lead and its compounds, undetermined**

✓5ᵗʰ **T56.1** **Toxic effects of mercury and its compounds**

✓6ᵗʰ **T56.1X** **Toxic effects of mercury and its compounds**

✓7ᵗʰ **T56.1X1** **Toxic effect of mercury and its compounds, accidental (unintentional)**
Toxic effects of mercury and its compounds NOS

2 ✓7ᵗʰ **T56.1X2** **Toxic effect of mercury and its compounds, intentional self-harm** HCC

✓7ᵗʰ **T56.1X3** **Toxic effect of mercury and its compounds, assault**

✓7ᵗʰ **T56.1X4** **Toxic effect of mercury and its compounds, undetermined**

✓5ᵗʰ **T56.2** **Toxic effects of chromium and its compounds**

✓6ᵗʰ **T56.2X** **Toxic effects of chromium and its compounds**

✓7ᵗʰ **T56.2X1** **Toxic effect of chromium and its compounds, accidental (unintentional)**
Toxic effects of chromium and its compounds NOS

2 ✓7ᵗʰ **T56.2X2** **Toxic effect of chromium and its compounds, intentional self-harm** HCC

✓7ᵗʰ **T56.2X3** **Toxic effect of chromium and its compounds, assault**

✓7ᵗʰ **T56.2X4** **Toxic effect of chromium and its compounds, undetermined**

✓5ᵗʰ **T56.3** **Toxic effects of cadmium and its compounds**

✓6ᵗʰ **T56.3X** **Toxic effects of cadmium and its compounds**

✓7ᵗʰ **T56.3X1** **Toxic effect of cadmium and its compounds, accidental (unintentional)**
Toxic effects of cadmium and its compounds NOS

2 ✓7ᵗʰ **T56.3X2** **Toxic effect of cadmium and its compounds, intentional self-harm** HCC

✓7ᵗʰ **T56.3X3** **Toxic effect of cadmium and its compounds, assault**

✓7ᵗʰ **T56.3X4** **Toxic effect of cadmium and its compounds, undetermined**

✓5ᵗʰ **T56.4** **Toxic effects of copper and its compounds**

✓6ᵗʰ **T56.4X** **Toxic effects of copper and its compounds**

✓7ᵗʰ **T56.4X1** **Toxic effect of copper and its compounds, accidental (unintentional)**
Toxic effects of copper and its compounds NOS

2 ✓7ᵗʰ **T56.4X2** **Toxic effect of copper and its compounds, intentional self-harm** HCC

✓7ᵗʰ **T56.4X3** **Toxic effect of copper and its compounds, assault**

✓7ᵗʰ **T56.4X4** **Toxic effect of copper and its compounds, undetermined**

✓5ᵗʰ **T56.5** **Toxic effects of zinc and its compounds**

✓6ᵗʰ **T56.5X** **Toxic effects of zinc and its compounds**

✓7ᵗʰ **T56.5X1** **Toxic effect of zinc and its compounds, accidental (unintentional)**
Toxic effects of zinc and its compounds NOS

2 ✓7ᵗʰ **T56.5X2** **Toxic effect of zinc and its compounds, intentional self-harm** HCC

✓7ᵗʰ **T56.5X3** **Toxic effect of zinc and its compounds, assault**

✓7ᵗʰ **T56.5X4** **Toxic effect of zinc and its compounds, undetermined**

✓5ᵗʰ **T56.6** **Toxic effects of tin and its compounds**

✓6ᵗʰ **T56.6X** **Toxic effects of tin and its compounds**

✓7ᵗʰ **T56.6X1** **Toxic effect of tin and its compounds, accidental (unintentional)**
Toxic effects of tin and its compounds NOS

2 ✓7ᵗʰ **T56.6X2** **Toxic effect of tin and its compounds, intentional self-harm** HCC

✓7ᵗʰ **T56.6X3** **Toxic effect of tin and its compounds, assault**

✓7ᵗʰ **T56.6X4** **Toxic effect of tin and its compounds, undetermined**

✓5ᵗʰ **T56.7** **Toxic effects of beryllium and its compounds**

✓6ᵗʰ **T56.7X** **Toxic effects of beryllium and its compounds**

✓7ᵗʰ **T56.7X1** **Toxic effect of beryllium and its compounds, accidental (unintentional)**
Toxic effects of beryllium and its compounds NOS

2 ✓7ᵗʰ **T56.7X2** **Toxic effect of beryllium and its compounds, intentional self-harm** HCC

✓7ᵗʰ **T56.7X3** **Toxic effect of beryllium and its compounds, assault**

✓7ᵗʰ **T56.7X4** **Toxic effect of beryllium and its compounds, undetermined**

✓5ᵗʰ **T56.8** **Toxic effects of other metals**

✓6ᵗʰ **T56.81** **Toxic effect of thallium**

✓7ᵗʰ **T56.811** **Toxic effect of thallium, accidental (unintentional)**
Toxic effect of thallium NOS

2 ✓7ᵗʰ **T56.812** **Toxic effect of thallium, intentional self-harm** HCC

✓7ᵗʰ **T56.813** **Toxic effect of thallium, assault**

✓7ᵗʰ **T56.814** **Toxic effect of thallium, undetermined**

---

2   HCC with 7th character indicating initial encounter (A or B - specific to category) OR sequela.

✓ Additional Character Req   ✓x7ᵗʰ Placeholder Alert   Manifestation   HCC CMS-HCC Condition   ▽ Unspecified Code   ▶◀ Revised Text   ● New Code   ▲ Revised Code Title

√6ᵗʰ **T56.89**   **Toxic effects of other metals**

     √7ᵗʰ **T56.891**   **Toxic effect of other metals, accidental (unintentional)**
         Toxic effects of other metals NOS

   2   √7ᵗʰ **T56.892**   **Toxic effect of other metals, intentional self-harm**   HCC

     √7ᵗʰ **T56.893**   **Toxic effect of other metals, assault**

     √7ᵗʰ **T56.894**   **Toxic effect of other metals, undetermined**

√5ᵗʰ **T56.9**   **Toxic effects of unspecified metal**

     √7ᵗʰ **T56.91**   **Toxic effect of unspecified metal, accidental (unintentional)**   ▽

   2   √×7ᵗʰ **T56.92**   **Toxic effect of unspecified metal, intentional self-harm**   HCC ▽

     √×7ᵗʰ **T56.93**   **Toxic effect of unspecified metal, assault**   ▽

     √×7ᵗʰ **T56.94**   **Toxic effect of unspecified metal, undetermined**   ▽

√4ᵗʰ **T57**   **Toxic effect of other inorganic substances**

> The appropriate 7th character is to be added to each code from category T57.
> A   initial encounter
> D   subsequent encounter
> S   sequela

√5ᵗʰ **T57.0**   **Toxic effect of arsenic and its compounds**

     √6ᵗʰ **T57.0X**   **Toxic effect of arsenic and its compounds**

         √7ᵗʰ **T57.0X1**   **Toxic effect of arsenic and its compounds, accidental (unintentional)**
            Toxic effect of arsenic and its compounds NOS

     2   √7ᵗʰ **T57.0X2**   **Toxic effect of arsenic and its compounds, intentional self-harm**   HCC

         √7ᵗʰ **T57.0X3**   **Toxic effect of arsenic and its compounds, assault**

         √7ᵗʰ **T57.0X4**   **Toxic effect of arsenic and its compounds, undetermined**

√5ᵗʰ **T57.1**   **Toxic effect of phosphorus and its compounds**
     EXCLUDES 1   *organophosphate insecticides (T60.0)*

     √6ᵗʰ **T57.1X**   **Toxic effect of phosphorus and its compounds**

         √7ᵗʰ **T57.1X1**   **Toxic effect of phosphorus and its compounds, accidental (unintentional)**
            Toxic effect of phosphorus and its compounds NOS

     2   √7ᵗʰ **T57.1X2**   **Toxic effect of phosphorus and its compounds, intentional self-harm**   HCC

         √7ᵗʰ **T57.1X3**   **Toxic effect of phosphorus and its compounds, assault**

         √7ᵗʰ **T57.1X4**   **Toxic effect of phosphorus and its compounds, undetermined**

√5ᵗʰ **T57.2**   **Toxic effect of manganese and its compounds**

     √6ᵗʰ **T57.2X**   **Toxic effect of manganese and its compounds**

         √7ᵗʰ **T57.2X1**   **Toxic effect of manganese and its compounds, accidental (unintentional)**
            Toxic effect of manganese and its compounds NOS

     2   √7ᵗʰ **T57.2X2**   **Toxic effect of manganese and its compounds, intentional self-harm**   HCC

         √7ᵗʰ **T57.2X3**   **Toxic effect of manganese and its compounds, assault**

         √7ᵗʰ **T57.2X4**   **Toxic effect of manganese and its compounds, undetermined**

√5ᵗʰ **T57.3**   **Toxic effect of hydrogen cyanide**

     √6ᵗʰ **T57.3X**   **Toxic effect of hydrogen cyanide**

         √7ᵗʰ **T57.3X1**   **Toxic effect of hydrogen cyanide, accidental (unintentional)**
            Toxic effect of hydrogen cyanide NOS

     2   √7ᵗʰ **T57.3X2**   **Toxic effect of hydrogen cyanide, intentional self-harm**   HCC

         √7ᵗʰ **T57.3X3**   **Toxic effect of hydrogen cyanide, assault**

         √7ᵗʰ **T57.3X4**   **Toxic effect of hydrogen cyanide, undetermined**

√5ᵗʰ **T57.8**   **Toxic effect of other specified inorganic substances**

     √6ᵗʰ **T57.8X**   **Toxic effect of other specified inorganic substances**

         √7ᵗʰ **T57.8X1**   **Toxic effect of other specified inorganic substances, accidental (unintentional)**
            Toxic effect of other specified inorganic substances NOS

     2   √7ᵗʰ **T57.8X2**   **Toxic effect of other specified inorganic substances, intentional self-harm**   HCC

         √7ᵗʰ **T57.8X3**   **Toxic effect of other specified inorganic substances, assault**

         √7ᵗʰ **T57.8X4**   **Toxic effect of other specified inorganic substances, undetermined**

√5ᵗʰ **T57.9**   **Toxic effect of unspecified inorganic substance**

     √×7ᵗʰ **T57.91**   **Toxic effect of unspecified inorganic substance, accidental (unintentional)**   ▽

     2   √×7ᵗʰ **T57.92**   **Toxic effect of unspecified inorganic substance, intentional self-harm**   HCC ▽

     √×7ᵗʰ **T57.93**   **Toxic effect of unspecified inorganic substance, assault**   ▽

     √×7ᵗʰ **T57.94**   **Toxic effect of unspecified inorganic substance, undetermined**   ▽

√4ᵗʰ **T58**   **Toxic effect of carbon monoxide**
     INCLUDES   asphyxiation from carbon monoxide
                toxic effect of carbon monoxide from all sources

> The appropriate 7th character is to be added to each code from category T58.
> A   initial encounter
> D   subsequent encounter
> S   sequela

√5ᵗʰ **T58.0**   **Toxic effect of carbon monoxide from motor vehicle exhaust**
     Toxic effect of exhaust gas from gas engine
     Toxic effect of exhaust gas from motor pump

     √×7ᵗʰ **T58.01**   **Toxic effect of carbon monoxide from motor vehicle exhaust, accidental (unintentional)**

     2   √×7ᵗʰ **T58.02**   **Toxic effect of carbon monoxide from motor vehicle exhaust, intentional self-harm**   HCC

     √×7ᵗʰ **T58.03**   **Toxic effect of carbon monoxide from motor vehicle exhaust, assault**

     √×7ᵗʰ **T58.04**   **Toxic effect of carbon monoxide from motor vehicle exhaust, undetermined**

√5ᵗʰ **T58.1**   **Toxic effect of carbon monoxide from utility gas**
     Toxic effect of acetylene
     Toxic effect of gas NOS used for lighting, heating, cooking
     Toxic effect of water gas

     √×7ᵗʰ **T58.11**   **Toxic effect of carbon monoxide from utility gas, accidental (unintentional)**

     2   √×7ᵗʰ **T58.12**   **Toxic effect of carbon monoxide from utility gas, intentional self-harm**   HCC

     √×7ᵗʰ **T58.13**   **Toxic effect of carbon monoxide from utility gas, assault**

     √×7ᵗʰ **T58.14**   **Toxic effect of carbon monoxide from utility gas, undetermined**

√5ᵗʰ **T58.2**   **Toxic effect of carbon monoxide from incomplete combustion of other domestic fuels**
     Toxic effect of carbon monoxide from incomplete combustion of coal, coke, kerosene, wood

     √6ᵗʰ **T58.2X**   **Toxic effect of carbon monoxide from incomplete combustion of other domestic fuels**

         √7ᵗʰ **T58.2X1**   **Toxic effect of carbon monoxide from incomplete combustion of other domestic fuels, accidental (unintentional)**

     2   √7ᵗʰ **T58.2X2**   **Toxic effect of carbon monoxide from incomplete combustion of other domestic fuels, intentional self-harm**   HCC

         √7ᵗʰ **T58.2X3**   **Toxic effect of carbon monoxide from incomplete combustion of other domestic fuels, assault**

         √7ᵗʰ **T58.2X4**   **Toxic effect of carbon monoxide from incomplete combustion of other domestic fuels, undetermined**

---

2   HCC with 7th character indicating initial encounter (A or B - specific to category) OR sequela.

EXCLUDES 1 Not coded here   EXCLUDES 2 Not included here   N Newborn Age: 0   P Pediatric Age: 0-17   M Maternity Age: 12-55   A Adult Age: 15-124

1084   ICD-10-CM 2018

√5th **T58.8** **Toxic effect of carbon monoxide from other source**
Toxic effect of carbon monoxide from blast furnace gas
Toxic effect of carbon monoxide from fuels in industrial use
Toxic effect of carbon monoxide from kiln vapor

     √6th **T58.8X** **Toxic effect of carbon monoxide from other source**

         √7th **T58.8X1** **Toxic effect of carbon monoxide from other source, accidental (unintentional)**

         2 √7th **T58.8X2** **Toxic effect of carbon monoxide from** HCC **other source, intentional self-harm**

         √7th **T58.8X3** **Toxic effect of carbon monoxide from other source, assault**

         √7th **T58.8X4** **Toxic effect of carbon monoxide from other source, undetermined**

√5th **T58.9** **Toxic effect of carbon monoxide from unspecified source**

     √x7th **T58.91** **Toxic effect of carbon monoxide from unspecified source, accidental (unintentional)** ▽

     2 √x7th **T58.92** **Toxic effect of carbon monoxide from unspecified source, intentional self-harm** HCC ▽

     √x7th **T58.93** **Toxic effect of carbon monoxide from unspecified source, assault** ▽

     √x7th **T58.94** **Toxic effect of carbon monoxide from unspecified source, undetermined** ▽

√4th **T59** **Toxic effect of other gases, fumes and vapors**
     INCLUDES   aerosol propellants
     EXCLUDES 1   *chlorofluorocarbons (T53.5)*

> The appropriate 7th character is to be added to each code from category T59.
> A   initial encounter
> D   subsequent encounter
> S   sequela

√5th **T59.0** **Toxic effect of nitrogen oxides**

     √6th **T59.0X** **Toxic effect of nitrogen oxides**

         √7th **T59.0X1** **Toxic effect of nitrogen oxides, accidental (unintentional)**
Toxic effect of nitrogen oxides NOS

         2 √7th **T59.0X2** **Toxic effect of nitrogen oxides,** HCC **intentional self-harm**

         √7th **T59.0X3** **Toxic effect of nitrogen oxides, assault**

         √7th **T59.0X4** **Toxic effect of nitrogen oxides, undetermined**

√5th **T59.1** **Toxic effect of sulfur dioxide**

     √6th **T59.1X** **Toxic effect of sulfur dioxide**

         √7th **T59.1X1** **Toxic effect of sulfur dioxide, accidental (unintentional)**
Toxic effect of sulfur dioxide NOS

         2 √7th **T59.1X2** **Toxic effect of sulfur dioxide,** HCC **intentional self-harm**

         √7th **T59.1X3** **Toxic effect of sulfur dioxide, assault**

         √7th **T59.1X4** **Toxic effect of sulfur dioxide, undetermined**

√5th **T59.2** **Toxic effect of formaldehyde**

     √6th **T59.2X** **Toxic effect of formaldehyde**

         √7th **T59.2X1** **Toxic effect of formaldehyde, accidental (unintentional)**
Toxic effect of formaldehyde NOS

         2 √7th **T59.2X2** **Toxic effect of formaldehyde,** HCC **intentional self-harm**

         √7th **T59.2X3** **Toxic effect of formaldehyde, assault**

         √7th **T59.2X4** **Toxic effect of formaldehyde, undetermined**

√5th **T59.3** **Toxic effect of lacrimogenic gas**
Toxic effect of tear gas

     √6th **T59.3X** **Toxic effect of lacrimogenic gas**

         √7th **T59.3X1** **Toxic effect of lacrimogenic gas, accidental (unintentional)**
Toxic effect of lacrimogenic gas NOS

         2 √7th **T59.3X2** **Toxic effect of lacrimogenic gas,** HCC **intentional self-harm**

         √7th **T59.3X3** **Toxic effect of lacrimogenic gas, assault**

         √7th **T59.3X4** **Toxic effect of lacrimogenic gas, undetermined**

√5th **T59.4** **Toxic effect of chlorine gas**

     √6th **T59.4X** **Toxic effect of chlorine gas**

         √7th **T59.4X1** **Toxic effect of chlorine gas, accidental (unintentional)**
Toxic effect of chlorine gas NOS

         2 √7th **T59.4X2** **Toxic effect of chlorine gas,** HCC **intentional self-harm**

         √7th **T59.4X3** **Toxic effect of chlorine gas, assault**

         √7th **T59.4X4** **Toxic effect of chlorine gas, undetermined**

√5th **T59.5** **Toxic effect of fluorine gas and hydrogen fluoride**

     √6th **T59.5X** **Toxic effect of fluorine gas and hydrogen fluoride**

         √7th **T59.5X1** **Toxic effect of fluorine gas and hydrogen fluoride, accidental (unintentional)**
Toxic effect of fluorine gas and hydrogen fluoride NOS

         2 √7th **T59.5X2** **Toxic effect of fluorine gas and** HCC **hydrogen fluoride, intentional self-harm**

         √7th **T59.5X3** **Toxic effect of fluorine gas and hydrogen fluoride, assault**

         √7th **T59.5X4** **Toxic effect of fluorine gas and hydrogen fluoride, undetermined**

√5th **T59.6** **Toxic effect of hydrogen sulfide**

     √6th **T59.6X** **Toxic effect of hydrogen sulfide**

         √7th **T59.6X1** **Toxic effect of hydrogen sulfide, accidental (unintentional)**
Toxic effect of hydrogen sulfide NOS

         2 √7th **T59.6X2** **Toxic effect of hydrogen sulfide,** HCC **intentional self-harm**

         √7th **T59.6X3** **Toxic effect of hydrogen sulfide, assault**

         √7th **T59.6X4** **Toxic effect of hydrogen sulfide, undetermined**

√5th **T59.7** **Toxic effect of carbon dioxide**

     √6th **T59.7X** **Toxic effect of carbon dioxide**

         √7th **T59.7X1** **Toxic effect of carbon dioxide, accidental (unintentional)**
Toxic effect of carbon dioxide NOS

         2 √7th **T59.7X2** **Toxic effect of carbon dioxide,** HCC **intentional self-harm**

         √7th **T59.7X3** **Toxic effect of carbon dioxide, assault**

         √7th **T59.7X4** **Toxic effect of carbon dioxide, undetermined**

√5th **T59.8** **Toxic effect of other specified gases, fumes and vapors**

     √6th **T59.81** **Toxic effect of smoke**
Smoke inhalation
     EXCLUDES 2   *toxic effect of cigarette (tobacco) smoke (T65.22-)*

         √7th **T59.811** **Toxic effect of smoke, accidental (unintentional)**
Toxic effect of smoke NOS
AHA: 2013, 4Q, 121

         2 √7th **T59.812** **Toxic effect of smoke, intentional** HCC **self-harm**

         √7th **T59.813** **Toxic effect of smoke, assault**

         √7th **T59.814** **Toxic effect of smoke, undetermined**

     √6th **T59.89** **Toxic effect of other specified gases, fumes and vapors**

         √7th **T59.891** **Toxic effect of other specified gases, fumes and vapors, accidental (unintentional)**

         2 √7th **T59.892** **Toxic effect of other specified gases,** HCC **fumes and vapors, intentional self-harm**

         √7th **T59.893** **Toxic effect of other specified gases, fumes and vapors, assault**

         √7th **T59.894** **Toxic effect of other specified gases, fumes and vapors, undetermined**

√5th **T59.9** **Toxic effect of unspecified gases, fumes and vapors**

     √x7th **T59.91** **Toxic effect of unspecified gases, fumes and vapors, accidental (unintentional)** ▽

     2 √x7th **T59.92** **Toxic effect of unspecified gases, fumes and vapors, intentional self-harm** HCC ▽

     √x7th **T59.93** **Toxic effect of unspecified gases, fumes and vapors, assault** ▽

---

2   HCC with 7th character indicating initial encounter (A or B - specific to category) OR sequela.

√ Additional Character Req   √x7th Placeholder Alert   Manifestation   HCC CMS-HCC Condition   ▽ Unspecified Code   ►◄ Revised Text   ● New Code   ▲ Revised Code Title

✓x7ᵗʰ **T59.94** Toxic effect of unspecified gases, fumes and ▽
vapors, **undetermined**

✓4ᵗʰ **T60** **Toxic effect of pesticides**
INCLUDES toxic effect of wood preservatives

> The appropriate 7th character is to be added to each code from
> category T60.
> A   initial encounter
> D   subsequent encounter
> S   sequela

✓5ᵗʰ **T60.0** Toxic effect of organophosphate and carbamate insecticides
✓6ᵗʰ **T60.0X** Toxic effect of **organophosphate and carbamate
insecticides**
✓7ᵗʰ **T60.0X1** Toxic effect of organophosphate and
carbamate insecticides, **accidental
(unintentional)**
Toxic effect of organophosphate and
carbamate insecticides NOS
2 ✓7ᵗʰ **T60.0X2** Toxic effect of organophosphate HCC
and carbamate insecticides,
intentional self-harm
✓7ᵗʰ **T60.0X3** Toxic effect of organophosphate and
carbamate insecticides, **assault**
✓7ᵗʰ **T60.0X4** Toxic effect of organophosphate and
carbamate insecticides, **undetermined**

✓5ᵗʰ **T60.1** Toxic effect of halogenated insecticides
EXCLUDES 1 chlorinated hydrocarbon (T53.-)
✓6ᵗʰ **T60.1X** Toxic effect of **halogenated insecticides**
✓7ᵗʰ **T60.1X1** Toxic effect of halogenated insecticides,
accidental (unintentional)
Toxic effect of halogenated insecticides
NOS
2 ✓7ᵗʰ **T60.1X2** Toxic effect of halogenated HCC
insecticides, **intentional self-harm**
✓7ᵗʰ **T60.1X3** Toxic effect of halogenated
insecticides, **assault**
✓7ᵗʰ **T60.1X4** Toxic effect of halogenated
insecticides, **undetermined**

✓5ᵗʰ **T60.2** Toxic effect of other insecticides
✓6ᵗʰ **T60.2X** Toxic effect of other insecticides
✓7ᵗʰ **T60.2X1** Toxic effect of other insecticides,
accidental (unintentional)
Toxic effect of other insecticides NOS
2 ✓7ᵗʰ **T60.2X2** Toxic effect of other insecticides, HCC
intentional self-harm
✓7ᵗʰ **T60.2X3** Toxic effect of other insecticides, **assault**
✓7ᵗʰ **T60.2X4** Toxic effect of other insecticides,
undetermined

✓5ᵗʰ **T60.3** Toxic effect of herbicides and fungicides
✓6ᵗʰ **T60.3X** Toxic effect of **herbicides and fungicides**
✓7ᵗʰ **T60.3X1** Toxic effect of herbicides and fungicides,
accidental (unintentional)
Toxic effect of herbicides and fungicides
NOS
2 ✓7ᵗʰ **T60.3X2** Toxic effect of herbicides and HCC
fungicides, **intentional self-harm**
✓7ᵗʰ **T60.3X3** Toxic effect of herbicides and
fungicides, **assault**
✓7ᵗʰ **T60.3X4** Toxic effect of herbicides and
fungicides, **undetermined**

✓5ᵗʰ **T60.4** Toxic effect of rodenticides
EXCLUDES 1 strychnine and its salts (T65.1)
thallium (T56.81-)
✓6ᵗʰ **T60.4X** Toxic effect of **rodenticides**
✓7ᵗʰ **T60.4X1** Toxic effect of rodenticides, **accidental
(unintentional)**
Toxic effect of rodenticides NOS
2 ✓7ᵗʰ **T60.4X2** Toxic effect of rodenticides, HCC
intentional self-harm
✓7ᵗʰ **T60.4X3** Toxic effect of rodenticides, **assault**
✓7ᵗʰ **T60.4X4** Toxic effect of rodenticides,
undetermined

✓5ᵗʰ **T60.8** Toxic effect of other pesticides
✓6ᵗʰ **T60.8X** Toxic effect of other pesticides
✓7ᵗʰ **T60.8X1** Toxic effect of other pesticides, **accidental
(unintentional)**
Toxic effect of other pesticides NOS
2 ✓7ᵗʰ **T60.8X2** Toxic effect of other pesticides, HCC
intentional self-harm
✓7ᵗʰ **T60.8X3** Toxic effect of other pesticides, **assault**
✓7ᵗʰ **T60.8X4** Toxic effect of other pesticides,
undetermined

✓5ᵗʰ **T60.9** Toxic effect of unspecified pesticide
✓x7ᵗʰ **T60.91** Toxic effect of unspecified pesticide, **accidental** ▽
(unintentional)
2 ✓x7ᵗʰ **T60.92** Toxic effect of unspecified pesticide, HCC ▽
intentional self-harm
✓x7ᵗʰ **T60.93** Toxic effect of unspecified pesticide, **assault** ▽
✓x7ᵗʰ **T60.94** Toxic effect of unspecified pesticide, ▽
undetermined

✓4ᵗʰ **T61** **Toxic effect of noxious substances eaten as seafood**
EXCLUDES 1 allergic reaction to food, such as:
anaphylactic reaction or shock due to adverse food reaction
(T78.0-)
bacterial foodborne intoxications (A05.-)
dermatitis (L23.6, L25.4, L27.2)
food protein-induced enterocolitis syndrome (K52.21)
food protein-induced enteropathy (K52.22)
gastroenteritis (noninfective) (K52.29)
toxic effect of aflatoxin and other mycotoxins (T64)
toxic effect of cyanides (T65.0-)
toxic effect of harmful algae bloom (T65.82-)
toxic effect of hydrogen cyanide (T57.3-)
toxic effect of mercury (T56.1-)
toxic effect of red tide (T65.82-)

> The appropriate 7th character is to be added to each code from
> category T61.
> A   initial encounter
> D   subsequent encounter
> S   sequela

✓5ᵗʰ **T61.0** **Ciguatera fish** poisoning
✓x7ᵗʰ **T61.01** Ciguatera fish poisoning, **accidental** (unintentional)
2 ✓x7ᵗʰ **T61.02** Ciguatera fish poisoning, **intentional self-harm** HCC
✓x7ᵗʰ **T61.03** Ciguatera fish poisoning, **assault**
✓x7ᵗʰ **T61.04** Ciguatera fish poisoning, **undetermined**

✓5ᵗʰ **T61.1** **Scombroid fish** poisoning
Histamine-like syndrome
✓x7ᵗʰ **T61.11** Scombroid fish poisoning, **accidental** (unintentional)
2 ✓x7ᵗʰ **T61.12** Scombroid fish poisoning, **intentional self-harm** HCC
✓x7ᵗʰ **T61.13** Scombroid fish poisoning, **assault**
✓x7ᵗʰ **T61.14** Scombroid fish poisoning, **undetermined**

✓5ᵗʰ **T61.7** Other fish and shellfish poisoning
✓6ᵗʰ **T61.77** Other **fish** poisoning
✓7ᵗʰ **T61.771** Other fish poisoning, **accidental**
(unintentional)
2 ✓7ᵗʰ **T61.772** Other fish poisoning, **intentional** HCC
self-harm
✓7ᵗʰ **T61.773** Other fish poisoning, **assault**
✓7ᵗʰ **T61.774** Other fish poisoning, **undetermined**
✓6ᵗʰ **T61.78** Other **shellfish** poisoning
✓7ᵗʰ **T61.781** Other shellfish poisoning, **accidental**
(unintentional)
2 ✓7ᵗʰ **T61.782** Other shellfish poisoning, **intentional** HCC
self-harm
✓7ᵗʰ **T61.783** Other shellfish poisoning, **assault**
✓7ᵗʰ **T61.784** Other shellfish poisoning, **undetermined**

✓5ᵗʰ **T61.8** Toxic effect of other seafood
✓6ᵗʰ **T61.8X** Toxic effect of other seafood
✓7ᵗʰ **T61.8X1** Toxic effect of other seafood, **accidental**
(unintentional)
2 ✓7ᵗʰ **T61.8X2** Toxic effect of other seafood, HCC
intentional self-harm
✓7ᵗʰ **T61.8X3** Toxic effect of other seafood, **assault**

---

2 HCC with 7th character indicating initial encounter (A or B - specific to category) OR sequela.

☑7ᵗʰ **T61.8X4** **Toxic effect of other seafood, undetermined**

☑5ᵗʰ **T61.9** **Toxic effect of unspecified seafood**

   ☑x7ᵗʰ **T61.91** **Toxic effect of unspecified seafood, accidental (unintentional)** ▽

   2 ☑x7ᵗʰ **T61.92** **Toxic effect of unspecified seafood, intentional self-harm** HCC ▽

   ☑x7ᵗʰ **T61.93** **Toxic effect of unspecified seafood, assault** ▽

   ☑x7ᵗʰ **T61.94** **Toxic effect of unspecified seafood, undetermined** ▽

☑4ᵗʰ **T62** **Toxic effect of other noxious substances eaten as food**

   EXCLUDES 1   *allergic reaction to food, such as:*
      anaphylactic shock (reaction) due to adverse food reaction (T78.0-)
      bacterial food borne intoxications (A05.-)
      dermatitis (L23.6, L25.4, L27.2)
      food protein-induced enterocolitis syndrome (K52.21)
      food protein-induced enteropathy (K52.22)
      gastroenteritis (noninfective) (K52.29)
   toxic effect of aflatoxin and other mycotoxins (T64)
   toxic effect of cyanides (T65.0-)
   toxic effect of hydrogen cyanide (T57.3-)
   toxic effect of mercury (T56.1-)

> The appropriate 7th character is to be added to each code from category T62.
> A   initial encounter
> D   subsequent encounter
> S   sequela

☑5ᵗʰ **T62.0** **Toxic effect of ingested mushrooms**

   ☑6ᵗʰ **T62.0X** **Toxic effect of ingested mushrooms**

      ☑7ᵗʰ **T62.0X1** **Toxic effect of ingested mushrooms, accidental (unintentional)**
           Toxic effect of ingested mushrooms NOS

      2 ☑7ᵗʰ **T62.0X2** **Toxic effect of ingested mushrooms, intentional self-harm** HCC

      ☑7ᵗʰ **T62.0X3** **Toxic effect of ingested mushrooms, assault**

      ☑7ᵗʰ **T62.0X4** **Toxic effect of ingested mushrooms, undetermined**

☑5ᵗʰ **T62.1** **Toxic effect of ingested berries**

   ☑6ᵗʰ **T62.1X** **Toxic effect of ingested berries**

      ☑7ᵗʰ **T62.1X1** **Toxic effect of ingested berries, accidental (unintentional)**
           Toxic effect of ingested berries NOS

      2 ☑7ᵗʰ **T62.1X2** **Toxic effect of ingested berries, intentional self-harm** HCC

      ☑7ᵗʰ **T62.1X3** **Toxic effect of ingested berries, assault**

      ☑7ᵗʰ **T62.1X4** **Toxic effect of ingested berries, undetermined**

☑5ᵗʰ **T62.2** **Toxic effect of other ingested (parts of) plant(s)**

   ☑6ᵗʰ **T62.2X** **Toxic effect of other ingested (parts of) plant(s)**

      ☑7ᵗʰ **T62.2X1** **Toxic effect of other ingested (parts of) plant(s), accidental (unintentional)**
           Toxic effect of other ingested (parts of) plant(s) NOS

      2 ☑7ᵗʰ **T62.2X2** **Toxic effect of other ingested (parts of) plant(s), intentional self-harm** HCC

      ☑7ᵗʰ **T62.2X3** **Toxic effect of other ingested (parts of) plant(s), assault**

      ☑7ᵗʰ **T62.2X4** **Toxic effect of other ingested (parts of) plant(s), undetermined**

☑5ᵗʰ **T62.8** **Toxic effect of other specified noxious substances eaten as food**

   ☑6ᵗʰ **T62.8X** **Toxic effect of other specified noxious substances eaten as food**

      ☑7ᵗʰ **T62.8X1** **Toxic effect of other specified noxious substances eaten as food, accidental (unintentional)**
           Toxic effect of other specified noxious substances eaten as food NOS

      2 ☑7ᵗʰ **T62.8X2** **Toxic effect of other specified noxious substances eaten as food, intentional self-harm** HCC

      ☑7ᵗʰ **T62.8X3** **Toxic effect of other specified noxious substances eaten as food, assault**

      ☑7ᵗʰ **T62.8X4** **Toxic effect of other specified noxious substances eaten as food, undetermined**

☑5ᵗʰ **T62.9** **Toxic effect of unspecified noxious substance eaten as food**

   ☑x7ᵗʰ **T62.91** **Toxic effect of unspecified noxious substance eaten as food, accidental (unintentional)** ▽
       Toxic effect of unspecified noxious substance eaten as food NOS

   2 ☑x7ᵗʰ **T62.92** **Toxic effect of unspecified noxious substance eaten as food, intentional self-harm** HCC ▽

   ☑x7ᵗʰ **T62.93** **Toxic effect of unspecified noxious substance eaten as food, assault** ▽

   ☑x7ᵗʰ **T62.94** **Toxic effect of unspecified noxious substance eaten as food, undetermined** ▽

☑4ᵗʰ **T63** **Toxic effect of contact with venomous animals and plants**

   INCLUDES   bite or touch of venomous animal
               pricked or stuck by thorn or leaf
   EXCLUDES 2   *ingestion of toxic animal or plant (T61.-, T62.-)*

> The appropriate 7th character is to be added to each code from category T63.
> A   initial encounter
> D   subsequent encounter
> S   sequela

☑5ᵗʰ **T63.0** **Toxic effect of snake venom**

   ☑6ᵗʰ **T63.00** **Toxic effect of unspecified snake venom**

      ☑7ᵗʰ **T63.001** **Toxic effect of unspecified snake venom, accidental (unintentional)** ▽
           Toxic effect of unspecified snake venom NOS

      2 ☑7ᵗʰ **T63.002** **Toxic effect of unspecified snake venom, intentional self-harm** HCC ▽

      ☑7ᵗʰ **T63.003** **Toxic effect of unspecified snake venom, assault** ▽

      ☑7ᵗʰ **T63.004** **Toxic effect of unspecified snake venom, undetermined** ▽

   ☑6ᵗʰ **T63.01** **Toxic effect of rattlesnake venom**

      ☑7ᵗʰ **T63.011** **Toxic effect of rattlesnake venom, accidental (unintentional)**
           Toxic effect of rattlesnake venom NOS

      2 ☑7ᵗʰ **T63.012** **Toxic effect of rattlesnake venom, intentional self-harm** HCC

      ☑7ᵗʰ **T63.013** **Toxic effect of rattlesnake venom, assault**

      ☑7ᵗʰ **T63.014** **Toxic effect of rattlesnake venom, undetermined**

   ☑6ᵗʰ **T63.02** **Toxic effect of coral snake venom**

      ☑7ᵗʰ **T63.021** **Toxic effect of coral snake venom, accidental (unintentional)**
           Toxic effect of coral snake venom NOS

      2 ☑7ᵗʰ **T63.022** **Toxic effect of coral snake venom, intentional self-harm** HCC

      ☑7ᵗʰ **T63.023** **Toxic effect of coral snake venom, assault**

      ☑7ᵗʰ **T63.024** **Toxic effect of coral snake venom, undetermined**

   ☑6ᵗʰ **T63.03** **Toxic effect of taipan venom**

      ☑7ᵗʰ **T63.031** **Toxic effect of taipan venom, accidental (unintentional)**
           Toxic effect of taipan venom NOS

      2 ☑7ᵗʰ **T63.032** **Toxic effect of taipan venom, intentional self-harm** HCC

      ☑7ᵗʰ **T63.033** **Toxic effect of taipan venom, assault**

      ☑7ᵗʰ **T63.034** **Toxic effect of taipan venom, undetermined**

   ☑6ᵗʰ **T63.04** **Toxic effect of cobra venom**

      ☑7ᵗʰ **T63.041** **Toxic effect of cobra venom, accidental (unintentional)**
           Toxic effect of cobra venom NOS

      2 ☑7ᵗʰ **T63.042** **Toxic effect of cobra venom, intentional self-harm** HCC

      ☑7ᵗʰ **T63.043** **Toxic effect of cobra venom, assault**

      ☑7ᵗʰ **T63.044** **Toxic effect of cobra venom, undetermined**

---

2   HCC with 7th character indicating initial encounter (A or B - specific to category) OR sequela.

☑ Additional Character Req   ☑x7ᵗʰ Placeholder Alert   Manifestation   HCC CMS-HCC Condition   ▽ Unspecified Code   ▶◀ Revised Text   ● New Code   ▲ Revised Code Title

✓6ᵗʰ **T63.06**   **Toxic effect of venom of other North and South American snake**

    ✓7ᵗʰ **T63.061**   **Toxic effect of venom of other North and South American snake, accidental (unintentional)**
       Toxic effect of venom of other North and South American snake NOS

    2 ✓7ᵗʰ **T63.062**   **Toxic effect of venom of other North and South American snake, intentional self-harm** HCC

    ✓7ᵗʰ **T63.063**   **Toxic effect of venom of other North and South American snake, assault**

    ✓7ᵗʰ **T63.064**   **Toxic effect of venom of other North and South American snake, undetermined**

✓6ᵗʰ **T63.07**   **Toxic effect of venom of other Australian snake**

    ✓7ᵗʰ **T63.071**   **Toxic effect of venom of other Australian snake, accidental (unintentional)**
       Toxic effect of venom of other Australian snake NOS

    2 ✓7ᵗʰ **T63.072**   **Toxic effect of venom of other Australian snake, intentional self-harm** HCC

    ✓7ᵗʰ **T63.073**   **Toxic effect of venom of other Australian snake, assault**

    ✓7ᵗʰ **T63.074**   **Toxic effect of venom of other Australian snake, undetermined**

✓6ᵗʰ **T63.08**   **Toxic effect of venom of other African and Asian snake**

    ✓7ᵗʰ **T63.081**   **Toxic effect of venom of other African and Asian snake, accidental (unintentional)**
       Toxic effect of venom of other African and Asian snake NOS

    2 ✓7ᵗʰ **T63.082**   **Toxic effect of venom of other African and Asian snake, intentional self-harm** HCC

    ✓7ᵗʰ **T63.083**   **Toxic effect of venom of other African and Asian snake, assault**

    ✓7ᵗʰ **T63.084**   **Toxic effect of venom of other African and Asian snake, undetermined**

✓6ᵗʰ **T63.09**   **Toxic effect of venom of other snake**

    ✓7ᵗʰ **T63.091**   **Toxic effect of venom of other snake, accidental (unintentional)**
       Toxic effect of venom of other snake NOS

    2 ✓7ᵗʰ **T63.092**   **Toxic effect of venom of other snake, intentional self-harm** HCC

    ✓7ᵗʰ **T63.093**   **Toxic effect of venom of other snake, assault**

    ✓7ᵗʰ **T63.094**   **Toxic effect of venom of other snake, undetermined**

✓5ᵗʰ **T63.1**   **Toxic effect of venom of other reptiles**

   ✓6ᵗʰ **T63.11**   **Toxic effect of venom of gila monster**

    ✓7ᵗʰ **T63.111**   **Toxic effect of venom of gila monster, accidental (unintentional)**
       Toxic effect of venom of gila monster NOS

    2 ✓7ᵗʰ **T63.112**   **Toxic effect of venom of gila monster, intentional self-harm** HCC

    ✓7ᵗʰ **T63.113**   **Toxic effect of venom of gila monster, assault**

    ✓7ᵗʰ **T63.114**   **Toxic effect of venom of gila monster, undetermined**

   ✓6ᵗʰ **T63.12**   **Toxic effect of venom of other venomous lizard**

    ✓7ᵗʰ **T63.121**   **Toxic effect of venom of other venomous lizard, accidental (unintentional)**
       Toxic effect of venom of other venomous lizard NOS

    2 ✓7ᵗʰ **T63.122**   **Toxic effect of venom of other venomous lizard, intentional self-harm** HCC

    ✓7ᵗʰ **T63.123**   **Toxic effect of venom of other venomous lizard, assault**

    ✓7ᵗʰ **T63.124**   **Toxic effect of venom of other venomous lizard, undetermined**

   ✓6ᵗʰ **T63.19**   **Toxic effect of venom of other reptiles**

    ✓7ᵗʰ **T63.191**   **Toxic effect of venom of other reptiles, accidental (unintentional)**
       Toxic effect of venom of other reptiles NOS

    2 ✓7ᵗʰ **T63.192**   **Toxic effect of venom of other reptiles, intentional self-harm** HCC

    ✓7ᵗʰ **T63.193**   **Toxic effect of venom of other reptiles, assault**

    ✓7ᵗʰ **T63.194**   **Toxic effect of venom of other reptiles, undetermined**

✓5ᵗʰ **T63.2**   **Toxic effect of venom of scorpion**

   ✓6ᵗʰ **T63.2X**   **Toxic effect of venom of scorpion**

    ✓7ᵗʰ **T63.2X1**   **Toxic effect of venom of scorpion, accidental (unintentional)**
       Toxic effect of venom of scorpion NOS

    2 ✓7ᵗʰ **T63.2X2**   **Toxic effect of venom of scorpion, intentional self-harm** HCC

    ✓7ᵗʰ **T63.2X3**   **Toxic effect of venom of scorpion, assault**

    ✓7ᵗʰ **T63.2X4**   **Toxic effect of venom of scorpion, undetermined**

✓5ᵗʰ **T63.3**   **Toxic effect of venom of spider**

   ✓6ᵗʰ **T63.30**   **Toxic effect of unspecified spider venom**

    ✓7ᵗʰ **T63.301**   **Toxic effect of unspecified spider venom, accidental (unintentional)** ▽

    2 ✓7ᵗʰ **T63.302**   **Toxic effect of unspecified spider venom, intentional self-harm** HCC ▽

    ✓7ᵗʰ **T63.303**   **Toxic effect of unspecified spider venom, assault** ▽

    ✓7ᵗʰ **T63.304**   **Toxic effect of unspecified spider venom, undetermined** ▽

   ✓6ᵗʰ **T63.31**   **Toxic effect of venom of black widow spider**

    ✓7ᵗʰ **T63.311**   **Toxic effect of venom of black widow spider, accidental (unintentional)**

    2 ✓7ᵗʰ **T63.312**   **Toxic effect of venom of black widow spider, intentional self-harm** HCC

    ✓7ᵗʰ **T63.313**   **Toxic effect of venom of black widow spider, assault**

    ✓7ᵗʰ **T63.314**   **Toxic effect of venom of black widow spider, undetermined**

   ✓6ᵗʰ **T63.32**   **Toxic effect of venom of tarantula**

    ✓7ᵗʰ **T63.321**   **Toxic effect of venom of tarantula, accidental (unintentional)**

    2 ✓7ᵗʰ **T63.322**   **Toxic effect of venom of tarantula, intentional self-harm** HCC

    ✓7ᵗʰ **T63.323**   **Toxic effect of venom of tarantula, assault**

    ✓7ᵗʰ **T63.324**   **Toxic effect of venom of tarantula, undetermined**

   ✓6ᵗʰ **T63.33**   **Toxic effect of venom of brown recluse spider**

    ✓7ᵗʰ **T63.331**   **Toxic effect of venom of brown recluse spider, accidental (unintentional)**

    2 ✓7ᵗʰ **T63.332**   **Toxic effect of venom of brown recluse spider, intentional self-harm** HCC

    ✓7ᵗʰ **T63.333**   **Toxic effect of venom of brown recluse spider, assault**

    ✓7ᵗʰ **T63.334**   **Toxic effect of venom of brown recluse spider, undetermined**

   ✓6ᵗʰ **T63.39**   **Toxic effect of venom of other spider**

    ✓7ᵗʰ **T63.391**   **Toxic effect of venom of other spider, accidental (unintentional)**

    2 ✓7ᵗʰ **T63.392**   **Toxic effect of venom of other spider, intentional self-harm** HCC

    ✓7ᵗʰ **T63.393**   **Toxic effect of venom of other spider, assault**

    ✓7ᵗʰ **T63.394**   **Toxic effect of venom of other spider, undetermined**

✓5ᵗʰ **T63.4**   **Toxic effect of venom of other arthropods**

   ✓6ᵗʰ **T63.41**   **Toxic effect of venom of centipedes and venomous millipedes**

    ✓7ᵗʰ **T63.411**   **Toxic effect of venom of centipedes and venomous millipedes, accidental (unintentional)**

    2 ✓7ᵗʰ **T63.412**   **Toxic effect of venom of centipedes and venomous millipedes, intentional self-harm** HCC

    ✓7ᵗʰ **T63.413**   **Toxic effect of venom of centipedes and venomous millipedes, assault**

---

2   HCC with 7th character indicating initial encounter (A or B - specific to category) OR sequela.

EXCLUDES 1 Not coded here   **EXCLUDES 2** Not included here   **N** Newborn Age: 0   **P** Pediatric Age: 0-17   **M** Maternity Age: 12-55   **A** Adult Age: 15-124

1088   ICD-10-CM 2018

√7ᵗʰ **T63.414** **Toxic effect of venom of centipedes and venomous millipedes, undetermined**

√6ᵗʰ **T63.42** **Toxic effect of venom of ants**

√7ᵗʰ **T63.421** **Toxic effect of venom of ants, accidental (unintentional)**

2 √7ᵗʰ **T63.422** **Toxic effect of venom of ants, intentional self-harm** `HCC`

√7ᵗʰ **T63.423** **Toxic effect of venom of ants, assault**

√7ᵗʰ **T63.424** **Toxic effect of venom of ants, undetermined**

√6ᵗʰ **T63.43** **Toxic effect of venom of caterpillars**

√7ᵗʰ **T63.431** **Toxic effect of venom of caterpillars, accidental (unintentional)**

2 √7ᵗʰ **T63.432** **Toxic effect of venom of caterpillars, intentional self-harm** `HCC`

√7ᵗʰ **T63.433** **Toxic effect of venom of caterpillars, assault**

√7ᵗʰ **T63.434** **Toxic effect of venom of caterpillars, undetermined**

√6ᵗʰ **T63.44** **Toxic effect of venom of bees**

√7ᵗʰ **T63.441** **Toxic effect of venom of bees, accidental (unintentional)**

2 √7ᵗʰ **T63.442** **Toxic effect of venom of bees, intentional self-harm** `HCC`

√7ᵗʰ **T63.443** **Toxic effect of venom of bees, assault**

√7ᵗʰ **T63.444** **Toxic effect of venom of bees, undetermined**

√6ᵗʰ **T63.45** **Toxic effect of venom of hornets**

√7ᵗʰ **T63.451** **Toxic effect of venom of hornets, accidental (unintentional)**

2 √7ᵗʰ **T63.452** **Toxic effect of venom of hornets, intentional self-harm** `HCC`

√7ᵗʰ **T63.453** **Toxic effect of venom of hornets, assault**

√7ᵗʰ **T63.454** **Toxic effect of venom of hornets, undetermined**

√6ᵗʰ **T63.46** **Toxic effect of venom of wasps**
Toxic effect of yellow jacket

√7ᵗʰ **T63.461** **Toxic effect of venom of wasps, accidental (unintentional)**

2 √7ᵗʰ **T63.462** **Toxic effect of venom of wasps, intentional self-harm** `HCC`

√7ᵗʰ **T63.463** **Toxic effect of venom of wasps, assault**

√7ᵗʰ **T63.464** **Toxic effect of venom of wasps, undetermined**

√6ᵗʰ **T63.48** **Toxic effect of venom of other arthropod**

√7ᵗʰ **T63.481** **Toxic effect of venom of other arthropod, accidental (unintentional)**

2 √7ᵗʰ **T63.482** **Toxic effect of venom of other arthropod, intentional self-harm** `HCC`

√7ᵗʰ **T63.483** **Toxic effect of venom of other arthropod, assault**

√7ᵗʰ **T63.484** **Toxic effect of venom of other arthropod, undetermined**

√5ᵗʰ **T63.5** **Toxic effect of contact with venomous fish**
EXCLUDES 2   *poisoning by ingestion of fish (T61.-)*

√6ᵗʰ **T63.51** **Toxic effect of contact with stingray**

√7ᵗʰ **T63.511** **Toxic effect of contact with stingray, accidental (unintentional)**

2 √7ᵗʰ **T63.512** **Toxic effect of contact with stingray, intentional self-harm** `HCC`

√7ᵗʰ **T63.513** **Toxic effect of contact with stingray, assault**

√7ᵗʰ **T63.514** **Toxic effect of contact with stingray, undetermined**

√6ᵗʰ **T63.59** **Toxic effect of contact with other venomous fish**

√7ᵗʰ **T63.591** **Toxic effect of contact with other venomous fish, accidental (unintentional)**

2 √7ᵗʰ **T63.592** **Toxic effect of contact with other venomous fish, intentional self-harm** `HCC`

√7ᵗʰ **T63.593** **Toxic effect of contact with other venomous fish, assault**

√7ᵗʰ **T63.594** **Toxic effect of contact with other venomous fish, undetermined**

√5ᵗʰ **T63.6** **Toxic effect of contact with other venomous marine animals**
EXCLUDES 1   *sea-snake venom (T63.09)*
EXCLUDES 2   *poisoning by ingestion of shellfish (T61.78-)*

√6ᵗʰ **T63.61** **Toxic effect of contact with Portugese Man-o-war**
Toxic effect of contact with bluebottle

√7ᵗʰ **T63.611** **Toxic effect of contact with Portugese Man-o-war, accidental (unintentional)**

2 √7ᵗʰ **T63.612** **Toxic effect of contact with Portugese Man-o-war, intentional self-harm** `HCC`

√7ᵗʰ **T63.613** **Toxic effect of contact with Portugese Man-o-war, assault**

√7ᵗʰ **T63.614** **Toxic effect of contact with Portugese Man-o-war, undetermined**

√6ᵗʰ **T63.62** **Toxic effect of contact with other jellyfish**

√7ᵗʰ **T63.621** **Toxic effect of contact with other jellyfish, accidental (unintentional)**

2 √7ᵗʰ **T63.622** **Toxic effect of contact with other jellyfish, intentional self-harm** `HCC`

√7ᵗʰ **T63.623** **Toxic effect of contact with other jellyfish, assault**

√7ᵗʰ **T63.624** **Toxic effect of contact with other jellyfish, undetermined**

√6ᵗʰ **T63.63** **Toxic effect of contact with sea anemone**

√7ᵗʰ **T63.631** **Toxic effect of contact with sea anemone, accidental (unintentional)**

2 √7ᵗʰ **T63.632** **Toxic effect of contact with sea anemone, intentional self-harm** `HCC`

√7ᵗʰ **T63.633** **Toxic effect of contact with sea anemone, assault**

√7ᵗʰ **T63.634** **Toxic effect of contact with sea anemone, undetermined**

√6ᵗʰ **T63.69** **Toxic effect of contact with other venomous marine animals**

√7ᵗʰ **T63.691** **Toxic effect of contact with other venomous marine animals, accidental (unintentional)**

2 √7ᵗʰ **T63.692** **Toxic effect of contact with other venomous marine animals, intentional self-harm** `HCC`

√7ᵗʰ **T63.693** **Toxic effect of contact with other venomous marine animals, assault**

√7ᵗʰ **T63.694** **Toxic effect of contact with other venomous marine animals, undetermined**

√5ᵗʰ **T63.7** **Toxic effect of contact with venomous plant**

√6ᵗʰ **T63.71** **Toxic effect of contact with venomous marine plant**

√7ᵗʰ **T63.711** **Toxic effect of contact with venomous marine plant, accidental (unintentional)**

2 √7ᵗʰ **T63.712** **Toxic effect of contact with venomous marine plant, intentional self-harm** `HCC`

√7ᵗʰ **T63.713** **Toxic effect of contact with venomous marine plant, assault**

√7ᵗʰ **T63.714** **Toxic effect of contact with venomous marine plant, undetermined**

√6ᵗʰ **T63.79** **Toxic effect of contact with other venomous plant**

√7ᵗʰ **T63.791** **Toxic effect of contact with other venomous plant, accidental (unintentional)**

2 √7ᵗʰ **T63.792** **Toxic effect of contact with other venomous plant, intentional self-harm** `HCC`

√7ᵗʰ **T63.793** **Toxic effect of contact with other venomous plant, assault**

√7ᵗʰ **T63.794** **Toxic effect of contact with other venomous plant, undetermined**

√5ᵗʰ **T63.8** **Toxic effect of contact with other venomous animals**

√6ᵗʰ **T63.81** **Toxic effect of contact with venomous frog**
EXCLUDES 1   *contact with nonvenomous frog (W62.0)*

√7ᵗʰ **T63.811** **Toxic effect of contact with venomous frog, accidental (unintentional)**

2 √7ᵗʰ **T63.812** **Toxic effect of contact with venomous frog, intentional self-harm** `HCC`

√7ᵗʰ **T63.813** **Toxic effect of contact with venomous frog, assault**

√7ᵗʰ **T63.814** **Toxic effect of contact with venomous frog, undetermined**

---

2   HCC with 7th character indicating initial encounter (A or B - specific to category) OR sequela.

☑ Additional Character Req   √ₓ7ᵗʰ Placeholder Alert   Manifestation   `HCC` CMS-HCC Condition   ▽ Unspecified Code   ►◄ Revised Text   ● New Code   ▲ Revised Code Title

ICD-10-CM 2018   1089

Chapter 19. Injury, Poisoning, and Certain Other Consequences of External Causes

T63.414-T63.814

√6ᵗʰ **T63.82**   **Toxic effect of contact with venomous toad**
> EXCLUDES 1   contact with nonvenomous toad (W62.1)

    √7ᵗʰ **T63.821**   **Toxic effect of contact with venomous toad, accidental (unintentional)**

    2 √7ᵗʰ **T63.822**   **Toxic effect of contact with venomous toad, intentional self-harm**   HCC

    √7ᵗʰ **T63.823**   **Toxic effect of contact with venomous toad, assault**

    √7ᵗʰ **T63.824**   **Toxic effect of contact with venomous toad, undetermined**

√6ᵗʰ **T63.83**   **Toxic effect of contact with other venomous amphibian**
> EXCLUDES 1   contact with nonvenomous amphibian (W62.9)

    √7ᵗʰ **T63.831**   **Toxic effect of contact with other venomous amphibian, accidental (unintentional)**

    2 √7ᵗʰ **T63.832**   **Toxic effect of contact with other venomous amphibian, intentional self-harm**   HCC

    √7ᵗʰ **T63.833**   **Toxic effect of contact with other venomous amphibian, assault**

    √7ᵗʰ **T63.834**   **Toxic effect of contact with other venomous amphibian, undetermined**

√6ᵗʰ **T63.89**   **Toxic effect of contact with other venomous animals**

    √7ᵗʰ **T63.891**   **Toxic effect of contact with other venomous animals, accidental (unintentional)**

    2 √7ᵗʰ **T63.892**   **Toxic effect of contact with other venomous animals, intentional self-harm**   HCC

    √7ᵗʰ **T63.893**   **Toxic effect of contact with other venomous animals, assault**

    √7ᵗʰ **T63.894**   **Toxic effect of contact with other venomous animals, undetermined**

√5ᵗʰ **T63.9**   **Toxic effect of contact with unspecified venomous animal**

    √x7ᵗʰ **T63.91**   **Toxic effect of contact with unspecified venomous animal, accidental (unintentional)** ▽

    2 √x7ᵗʰ **T63.92**   **Toxic effect of contact with unspecified venomous animal, intentional self-harm**   IICC ▽

    √x7ᵗʰ **T63.93**   **Toxic effect of contact with unspecified venomous animal, assault** ▽

    √x7ᵗʰ **T63.94**   **Toxic effect of contact with unspecified venomous animal, undetermined** ▽

√4ᵗʰ **T64**   **Toxic effect of aflatoxin and other mycotoxin food contaminants**

> The appropriate 7th character is to be added to each code from category T64.
> A   initial encounter
> D   subsequent encounter
> S   sequela

√5ᵗʰ **T64.0**   **Toxic effect of aflatoxin**

    √x7ᵗʰ **T64.01**   **Toxic effect of aflatoxin, accidental (unintentional)**

    2 √x7ᵗʰ **T64.02**   **Toxic effect of aflatoxin, intentional self-harm**   HCC

    √x7ᵗʰ **T64.03**   **Toxic effect of aflatoxin, assault**

    √x7ᵗʰ **T64.04**   **Toxic effect of aflatoxin, undetermined**

√5ᵗʰ **T64.8**   **Toxic effect of other mycotoxin food contaminants**

    √x7ᵗʰ **T64.81**   **Toxic effect of other mycotoxin food contaminants, accidental (unintentional)**

    2 √x7ᵗʰ **T64.82**   **Toxic effect of other mycotoxin food contaminants, intentional self-harm**   HCC

    √x7ᵗʰ **T64.83**   **Toxic effect of other mycotoxin food contaminants, assault**

    √x7ᵗʰ **T64.84**   **Toxic effect of other mycotoxin food contaminants, undetermined**

√4ᵗʰ **T65**   **Toxic effect of other and unspecified substances**

> The appropriate 7th character is to be added to each code from category T65.
> A   initial encounter
> D   subsequent encounter
> S   sequela

√5ᵗʰ **T65.0**   **Toxic effect of cyanides**
> EXCLUDES 1   hydrogen cyanide (T57.3-)

    √6ᵗʰ **T65.0X**   **Toxic effect of cyanides**

      √7ᵗʰ **T65.0X1**   **Toxic effect of cyanides, accidental (unintentional)**
       Toxic effect of cyanides NOS

      2 √7ᵗʰ **T65.0X2**   **Toxic effect of cyanides, intentional self-harm**   HCC

      √7ᵗʰ **T65.0X3**   **Toxic effect of cyanides, assault**

      √7ᵗʰ **T65.0X4**   **Toxic effect of cyanides, undetermined**

√5ᵗʰ **T65.1**   **Toxic effect of strychnine and its salts**

    √6ᵗʰ **T65.1X**   **Toxic effect of strychnine and its salts**

      √7ᵗʰ **T65.1X1**   **Toxic effect of strychnine and its salts, accidental (unintentional)**
       Toxic effect of strychnine and its salts NOS

      2 √7ᵗʰ **T65.1X2**   **Toxic effect of strychnine and its salts, intentional self-harm**   HCC

      √7ᵗʰ **T65.1X3**   **Toxic effect of strychnine and its salts, assault**

      √7ᵗʰ **T65.1X4**   **Toxic effect of strychnine and its salts, undetermined**

√5ᵗʰ **T65.2**   **Toxic effect of tobacco and nicotine**
> EXCLUDES 2   nicotine dependence (F17.-)

    √6ᵗʰ **T65.21**   **Toxic effect of chewing tobacco**

      √7ᵗʰ **T65.211**   **Toxic effect of chewing tobacco, accidental (unintentional)**
       Toxic effect of chewing tobacco NOS

      2 √7ᵗʰ **T65.212**   **Toxic effect of chewing tobacco, intentional self-harm**   HCC

      √7ᵗʰ **T65.213**   **Toxic effect of chewing tobacco, assault**

      √7ᵗʰ **T65.214**   **Toxic effect of chewing tobacco, undetermined**

    √6ᵗʰ **T65.22**   **Toxic effect of tobacco cigarettes**
      Toxic effect of tobacco smoke
      Use additional code for exposure to second hand tobacco smoke (Z57.31, Z77.22)

      √7ᵗʰ **T65.221**   **Toxic effect of tobacco cigarettes, accidental (unintentional)**
       Toxic effect of tobacco cigarettes NOS

      2 √7ᵗʰ **T65.222**   **Toxic effect of tobacco cigarettes, intentional self-harm**   HCC

      √7ᵗʰ **T65.223**   **Toxic effect of tobacco cigarettes, assault**

      √7ᵗʰ **T65.224**   **Toxic effect of tobacco cigarettes, undetermined**

    √6ᵗʰ **T65.29**   **Toxic effect of other tobacco and nicotine**

      √7ᵗʰ **T65.291**   **Toxic effect of other tobacco and nicotine, accidental (unintentional)**
       Toxic effect of other tobacco and nicotine NOS

      2 √7ᵗʰ **T65.292**   **Toxic effect of other tobacco and nicotine, intentional self-harm**   HCC

      √7ᵗʰ **T65.293**   **Toxic effect of other tobacco and nicotine, assault**

      √7ᵗʰ **T65.294**   **Toxic effect of other tobacco and nicotine, undetermined**

√5ᵗʰ **T65.3**   **Toxic effect of nitroderivatives and aminoderivatives of benzene and its homologues**
    Toxic effect of anilin [benzenamine]
    Toxic effect of nitrobenzene
    Toxic effect of trinitrotoluene

    √6ᵗʰ **T65.3X**   **Toxic effect of nitroderivatives and aminoderivatives of benzene and its homologues**

      √7ᵗʰ **T65.3X1**   **Toxic effect of nitroderivatives and aminoderivatives of benzene and its homologues, accidental (unintentional)**
       Toxic effect of nitroderivatives and aminoderivatives of benzene and its homologues NOS

---

2   HCC with 7th character indicating initial encounter (A or B - specific to category) OR sequela.

EXCLUDES 1 Not coded here   EXCLUDES 2 Not included here   N Newborn Age: 0   P Pediatric Age: 0-17   M Maternity Age: 12-55   A Adult Age: 15-124

1090   ICD-10-CM 2018

2 ☑7ᵗʰ **T65.3X2 Toxic effect of nitroderivatives and** HCC
aminoderivatives of benzene and its
homologues, intentional self-harm

☑7ᵗʰ **T65.3X3 Toxic effect of nitroderivatives and**
aminoderivatives of benzene and its
homologues, assault

☑7ᵗʰ **T65.3X4 Toxic effect of nitroderivatives and**
aminoderivatives of benzene and its
homologues, undetermined

☑5ᵗʰ **T65.4 Toxic effect of carbon disulfide**

 ☑6ᵗʰ **T65.4X Toxic effect of carbon disulfide**

  ☑7ᵗʰ **T65.4X1 Toxic effect of carbon disulfide, accidental**
(unintentional)
Toxic effect of carbon disulfide NOS

  2 ☑7ᵗʰ **T65.4X2 Toxic effect of carbon disulfide,** HCC
intentional self-harm

  ☑7ᵗʰ **T65.4X3 Toxic effect of carbon disulfide, assault**

  ☑7ᵗʰ **T65.4X4 Toxic effect of carbon disulfide,**
undetermined

☑5ᵗʰ **T65.5 Toxic effect of nitroglycerin and other nitric acids and esters**
Toxic effect of 1,2,3-Propanetriol trinitrate

 ☑6ᵗʰ **T65.5X Toxic effect of nitroglycerin and other nitric acids**
and esters

  ☑7ᵗʰ **T65.5X1 Toxic effect of nitroglycerin and other**
nitric acids and esters, accidental
(unintentional)
Toxic effect of nitroglycerin and other nitric
acids and esters NOS

  2 ☑7ᵗʰ **T65.5X2 Toxic effect of nitroglycerin and** HCC
other nitric acids and esters,
intentional self-harm

  ☑7ᵗʰ **T65.5X3 Toxic effect of nitroglycerin and other**
nitric acids and esters, assault

  ☑7ᵗʰ **T65.5X4 Toxic effect of nitroglycerin and other**
nitric acids and esters, undetermined

☑5ᵗʰ **T65.6 Toxic effect of paints and dyes, not elsewhere classified**

 ☑6ᵗʰ **T65.6X Toxic effect of paints and dyes, not elsewhere**
classified

  ☑7ᵗʰ **T65.6X1 Toxic effect of paints and dyes, not**
elsewhere classified, accidental
(unintentional)
Toxic effect of paints and dyes NOS

  2 ☑7ᵗʰ **T65.6X2 Toxic effect of paints and dyes, not** HCC
elsewhere classified, intentional self-harm

  ☑7ᵗʰ **T65.6X3 Toxic effect of paints and dyes, not**
elsewhere classified, assault

  ☑7ᵗʰ **T65.6X4 Toxic effect of paints and dyes, not**
elsewhere classified, undetermined

☑5ᵗʰ **T65.8 Toxic effect of other specified substances**

 ☑6ᵗʰ **T65.81 Toxic effect of latex**

  ☑7ᵗʰ **T65.811 Toxic effect of latex, accidental**
(unintentional)
Toxic effect of latex NOS

  2 ☑7ᵗʰ **T65.812 Toxic effect of latex, intentional** HCC
self-harm

  ☑7ᵗʰ **T65.813 Toxic effect of latex, assault**

  ☑7ᵗʰ **T65.814 Toxic effect of latex, undetermined**

 ☑6ᵗʰ **T65.82 Toxic effect of harmful algae and algae toxins**
Toxic effect of (harmful) algae bloom NOS
Toxic effect of blue-green algae bloom
Toxic effect of brown tide
Toxic effect of cyanobacteria bloom
Toxic effect of Florida red tide
Toxic effect of pfiesteria piscicida
Toxic effect of red tide

  ☑7ᵗʰ **T65.821 Toxic effect of harmful algae and algae**
toxins, accidental (unintentional)
Toxic effect of harmful algae and algae
toxins NOS

  2 ☑7ᵗʰ **T65.822 Toxic effect of harmful algae and** HCC
algae toxins, intentional self-harm

  ☑7ᵗʰ **T65.823 Toxic effect of harmful algae and**
algae toxins, assault

  ☑7ᵗʰ **T65.824 Toxic effect of harmful algae and**
algae toxins, undetermined

☑6ᵗʰ **T65.83 Toxic effect of fiberglass**

 ☑7ᵗʰ **T65.831 Toxic effect of fiberglass, accidental**
(unintentional)
Toxic effect of fiberglass NOS

 2 ☑7ᵗʰ **T65.832 Toxic effect of fiberglass, intentional** HCC
self-harm

 ☑7ᵗʰ **T65.833 Toxic effect of fiberglass, assault**

 ☑7ᵗʰ **T65.834 Toxic effect of fiberglass, undetermined**

☑6ᵗʰ **T65.89 Toxic effect of other specified substances**

 ☑7ᵗʰ **T65.891 Toxic effect of other specified substances,**
accidental (unintentional)
Toxic effect of other specified substances
NOS

 2 ☑7ᵗʰ **T65.892 Toxic effect of other specified** HCC
substances, intentional self-harm

 ☑7ᵗʰ **T65.893 Toxic effect of other specified**
substances, assault

 ☑7ᵗʰ **T65.894 Toxic effect of other specified**
substances, undetermined

☑5ᵗʰ **T65.9 Toxic effect of unspecified substance**

 ☑7ᵗʰ **T65.91 Toxic effect of unspecified substance,** ▽
accidental (unintentional)
Poisoning NOS

 2 ☑7ᵗʰ **T65.92 Toxic effect of unspecified substance,** HCC ▽
intentional self-harm

 ☑7ᵗʰ **T65.93 Toxic effect of unspecified substance, assault** ▽

 ☑7ᵗʰ **T65.94 Toxic effect of unspecified substance,** ▽
undetermined

Other and unspecified effects of external causes (T66-T78)

☑7ᵗʰ **T66 Radiation sickness, unspecified** ▽
EXCLUDES 1 *specified adverse effects of radiation, such as:*
burns (T20-T31)
leukemia (C91-C95)
radiation gastroenteritis and colitis (K52.0)
radiation pneumonitis (J70.0)
radiation related disorders of the skin and subcutaneous tissue
(L55-L59)
radiation sunburn (L55.-)

The appropriate 7th character is to be added to code T66.
A initial encounter
D subsequent encounter
S sequela

☑4ᵗʰ **T67 Effects of heat and light**
EXCLUDES 1 *erythema [dermatitis] ab igne (L59.0)*
malignant hyperpyrexia due to anesthesia (T88.3)
radiation-related disorders of the skin and subcutaneous tissue
(L55-L59)
EXCLUDES 2 *burns (T20-T31)*
sunburn (L55.-)
sweat disorder due to heat (L74-L75)

The appropriate 7th character is to be added to each code from
category T67.
A initial encounter
D subsequent encounter
S sequela

☑7ᵗʰ **T67.0 Heatstroke and sunstroke**
Heat apoplexy Siriasis
Heat pyrexia Thermoplegia
Use additional code(s) to identify any associated complications
of heatstroke, such as:
coma and stupor (R40.-)
systemic inflammatory response syndrome (R65.1-)
DEF: Headache, vertigo, cramps, and elevated body temperature
due to prolonged exposure to high environmental temperatures;
requires emergency intervention.

☑7ᵗʰ **T67.1 Heat syncope**
Heat collapse

☑7ᵗʰ **T67.2 Heat cramp**

☑7ᵗʰ **T67.3 Heat exhaustion, anhydrotic**
Heat prostration due to water depletion
EXCLUDES 1 *heat exhaustion due to salt depletion (T67.4)*

☑7ᵗʰ **T67.4 Heat exhaustion due to salt depletion**
Heat prostration due to salt (and water) depletion

2 HCC with 7th character indicating initial encounter (A or B - specific to category) OR sequela.

☑ Additional Character Req ☑7ᵗʰ Placeholder Alert Manifestation HCC CMS-HCC Condition ▽ Unspecified Code ►◄ Revised Text ● New Code ▲ Revised Code Title
ICD-10-CM 2018 1091

(left margin) **Chapter 19. Injury, Poisoning, and Certain Other Consequences of External Causes**   **T67.5–T71.151**

√x7ᵗʰ **T67.5 Heat exhaustion, unspecified** ▽
Heat prostration NOS

√x7ᵗʰ **T67.6 Heat fatigue, transient**

√x7ᵗʰ **T67.7 Heat edema**

√x7ᵗʰ **T67.8 Other effects of heat and light**

√x7ᵗʰ **T67.9 Effect of heat and light, unspecified** ▽

√x7ᵗʰ **T68 Hypothermia**
Accidental hypothermia
Hypothermia NOS
Use additional code to identify source of exposure:
    exposure to excessive cold of man-made origin (W93)
    exposure to excessive cold of natural origin (X31)
    EXCLUDES 1 *hypothermia following anesthesia (T88.51)*
        hypothermia not associated with low environmental
          temperature (R68.0)
        hypothermia of newborn (P80.-)
    EXCLUDES 2 *frostbite (T33-T34)*

> The appropriate 7th character is to be added to code T68.
> A   initial encounter
> D   subsequent encounter
> S   sequela

√4ᵗʰ **T69 Other effects of reduced temperature**
Use additional code to identify source of exposure:
    exposure to excessive cold of man-made origin (W93)
    exposure to excessive cold of natural origin (X31)
    EXCLUDES 2 *frostbite (T33-T34)*

> The appropriate 7th character is to be added to each code from category T69.
> A   initial encounter
> D   subsequent encounter
> S   sequela

√5ᵗʰ **T69.0 Immersion hand and foot**

√6ᵗʰ **T69.01 Immersion hand**

√7ᵗʰ **T69.011 Immersion hand, right hand**

√7ᵗʰ **T69.012 Immersion hand, left hand**

√7ᵗʰ **T69.019 Immersion hand, unspecified hand** ▽

√6ᵗʰ **T69.02 Immersion foot**
Trench foot

√7ᵗʰ **T69.021 Immersion foot, right foot**

√7ᵗʰ **T69.022 Immersion foot, left foot**

√7ᵗʰ **T69.029 Immersion foot, unspecified foot** ▽

√x7ᵗʰ **T69.1 Chilblains**
DEF: Red, swollen, itchy skin primarily affecting the fingers and toes, nose and ears, and legs; follows damp-cold exposure; can also be associated with pruritus and a burning feeling.

√x7ᵗʰ **T69.8 Other specified effects of reduced temperature**

√x7ᵗʰ **T69.9 Effect of reduced temperature, unspecified** ▽

√4ᵗʰ **T70 Effects of air pressure and water pressure**

> The appropriate 7th character is to be added to each code from category T70.
> A   initial encounter
> D   subsequent encounter
> S   sequela

√x7ᵗʰ **T70.0 Otitic barotrauma**
Aero-otitis media
Effects of change in ambient atmospheric pressure or water pressure on ears

√x7ᵗʰ **T70.1 Sinus barotrauma**
Aerosinusitis
Effects of change in ambient atmospheric pressure on sinuses

√5ᵗʰ **T70.2 Other and unspecified effects of high altitude**
    EXCLUDES 2 *polycythemia due to high altitude (D75.1)*

√x7ᵗʰ **T70.20 Unspecified effects of high altitude** ▽

√x7ᵗʰ **T70.29 Other effects of high altitude**
Alpine sickness
Anoxia due to high altitude
Barotrauma NOS
Hypobaropathy
Mountain sickness

√x7ᵗʰ **T70.3 Caisson disease [decompression sickness]**
Compressed-air disease
Diver's palsy or paralysis
DEF: Rapid reduction in air pressure while breathing compressed air; symptoms include skin lesions, joint pains, and respiratory and neurological problems.

√x7ᵗʰ **T70.4 Effects of high-pressure fluids**
Hydraulic jet injection (industrial)
Pneumatic jet injection (industrial)
Traumatic jet injection (industrial)

√x7ᵗʰ **T70.8 Other effects of air pressure and water pressure**

√x7ᵗʰ **T70.9 Effect of air pressure and water pressure, unspecified** ▽

√4ᵗʰ **T71 Asphyxiation**
Mechanical suffocation
Traumatic suffocation
    EXCLUDES 1 *acute respiratory distress (syndrome) (J80)*
        anoxia due to high altitude (T70.2)
        asphyxia NOS (R09.01)
        asphyxia from carbon monoxide (T58.-)
        asphyxia from inhalation of food or foreign body (T17.-)
        asphyxia from other gases, fumes and vapors (T59.-)
        respiratory distress (syndrome) in newborn (P22.-)

> The appropriate 7th character is to be added to each code from category T71.
> A   initial encounter
> D   subsequent encounter
> S   sequela

√5ᵗʰ **T71.1 Asphyxiation due to mechanical threat to breathing**
Suffocation due to mechanical threat to breathing

√6ᵗʰ **T71.11 Asphyxiation due to smothering under pillow**

√7ᵗʰ **T71.111 Asphyxiation due to smothering under pillow, accidental**
Asphyxiation due to smothering under pillow NOS

2 √7ᵗʰ **T71.112 Asphyxiation due to smothering under pillow, intentional self-harm** HCC

√7ᵗʰ **T71.113 Asphyxiation due to smothering under pillow, assault**

√7ᵗʰ **T71.114 Asphyxiation due to smothering under pillow, undetermined**

√6ᵗʰ **T71.12 Asphyxiation due to plastic bag**

√7ᵗʰ **T71.121 Asphyxiation due to plastic bag, accidental**
Asphyxiation due to plastic bag NOS

2 √7ᵗʰ **T71.122 Asphyxiation due to plastic bag, intentional self-harm** HCC

√7ᵗʰ **T71.123 Asphyxiation due to plastic bag, assault**

√7ᵗʰ **T71.124 Asphyxiation due to plastic bag, undetermined**

√6ᵗʰ **T71.13 Asphyxiation due to being trapped in bed linens**

√7ᵗʰ **T71.131 Asphyxiation due to being trapped in bed linens, accidental**
Asphyxiation due to being trapped in bed linens NOS

2 √7ᵗʰ **T71.132 Asphyxiation due to being trapped in bed linens, intentional self-harm** HCC

√7ᵗʰ **T71.133 Asphyxiation due to being trapped in bed linens, assault**

√7ᵗʰ **T71.134 Asphyxiation due to being trapped in bed linens, undetermined**

√6ᵗʰ **T71.14 Asphyxiation due to smothering under another person's body (in bed)**

√7ᵗʰ **T71.141 Asphyxiation due to smothering under another person's body (in bed), accidental**
Asphyxiation due to smothering under another person's body (in bed) NOS

√7ᵗʰ **T71.143 Asphyxiation due to smothering under another person's body (in bed), assault**

√7ᵗʰ **T71.144 Asphyxiation due to smothering under another person's body (in bed), undetermined**

√6ᵗʰ **T71.15 Asphyxiation due to smothering in furniture**

√7ᵗʰ **T71.151 Asphyxiation due to smothering in furniture, accidental**
Asphyxiation due to smothering in furniture NOS

---

2   HCC with 7th character indicating initial encounter (A or B - specific to category) OR sequela.

EXCLUDES 1 Not coded here   **EXCLUDES 2** Not included here   N Newborn Age: 0   P Pediatric Age: 0-17   M Maternity Age: 12-55   A Adult Age: 15-124

2 ✓7ᵗʰ **T71.152** **Asphyxiation due to smothering in furniture, intentional self-harm** `HCC`

✓7ᵗʰ **T71.153** **Asphyxiation due to smothering in furniture, assault**

✓7ᵗʰ **T71.154** **Asphyxiation due to smothering in furniture, undetermined**

✓6ᵗʰ **T71.16** **Asphyxiation due to hanging**
Hanging by window shade cord
Use additional code for any associated injuries, such as:
    crushing injury of neck (S17.-)
    fracture of cervical vertebrae (S12.0-S12.2-)
    open wound of neck (S11.-)

✓7ᵗʰ **T71.161** **Asphyxiation due to hanging, accidental**
Asphyxiation due to hanging NOS
Hanging NOS

2 ✓7ᵗʰ **T71.162** **Asphyxiation due to hanging, intentional self-harm** `HCC`

✓7ᵗʰ **T71.163** **Asphyxiation due to hanging, assault**

✓7ᵗʰ **T71.164** **Asphyxiation due to hanging, undetermined**

✓6ᵗʰ **T71.19** **Asphyxiation due to mechanical threat to breathing due to other causes**

✓7ᵗʰ **T71.191** **Asphyxiation due to mechanical threat to breathing due to other causes, accidental**
Asphyxiation due to other causes NOS

2 ✓7ᵗʰ **T71.192** **Asphyxiation due to mechanical threat to breathing due to other causes, intentional self-harm** `HCC`

✓7ᵗʰ **T71.193** **Asphyxiation due to mechanical threat to breathing due to other causes, assault**

✓7ᵗʰ **T71.194** **Asphyxiation due to mechanical threat to breathing due to other causes, undetermined**

✓5ᵗʰ **T71.2** **Asphyxiation due to systemic oxygen deficiency due to low oxygen content in ambient air**
Suffocation due to systemic oxygen deficiency due to low oxygen content in ambient air

✓x7ᵗʰ **T71.20** **Asphyxiation due to systemic oxygen deficiency due to low oxygen content in ambient air due to unspecified cause** ▽

✓x7ᵗʰ **T71.21** **Asphyxiation due to cave-in or falling earth**
Use additional code for any associated cataclysm (X34-X38)

✓6ᵗʰ **T71.22** **Asphyxiation due to being trapped in a car trunk**

✓7ᵗʰ **T71.221** **Asphyxiation due to being trapped in a car trunk, accidental**

2 ✓7ᵗʰ **T71.222** **Asphyxiation due to being trapped in a car trunk, intentional self-harm** `HCC`

✓7ᵗʰ **T71.223** **Asphyxiation due to being trapped in a car trunk, assault**

✓7ᵗʰ **T71.224** **Asphyxiation due to being trapped in a car trunk, undetermined**

✓6ᵗʰ **T71.23** **Asphyxiation due to being trapped in a (discarded) refrigerator**

✓7ᵗʰ **T71.231** **Asphyxiation due to being trapped in a (discarded) refrigerator, accidental**

2 ✓7ᵗʰ **T71.232** **Asphyxiation due to being trapped in a (discarded) refrigerator, intentional self-harm** `HCC`

✓7ᵗʰ **T71.233** **Asphyxiation due to being trapped in a (discarded) refrigerator, assault**

✓7ᵗʰ **T71.234** **Asphyxiation due to being trapped in a (discarded) refrigerator, undetermined**

✓x7ᵗʰ **T71.29** **Asphyxiation due to being trapped in other low oxygen environment**

✓x7ᵗʰ **T71.9** **Asphyxiation due to unspecified cause** ▽
Suffocation (by strangulation) due to unspecified cause
Suffocation NOS
Systemic oxygen deficiency due to low oxygen content in ambient air due to unspecified cause
Systemic oxygen deficiency due to mechanical threat to breathing due to unspecified cause
Traumatic asphyxia NOS

✓4ᵗʰ **T73** **Effects of other deprivation**

The appropriate 7th character is to be added to each code from category T73.
A   initial encounter
D   subsequent encounter
S   sequela

✓x7ᵗʰ **T73.0** **Starvation**
Deprivation of food

✓x7ᵗʰ **T73.1** **Deprivation of water**

✓x7ᵗʰ **T73.2** **Exhaustion due to exposure**

✓x7ᵗʰ **T73.3** **Exhaustion due to excessive exertion**
Exhaustion due to overexertion

✓x7ᵗʰ **T73.8** **Other effects of deprivation**

✓x7ᵗʰ **T73.9** **Effect of deprivation, unspecified** ▽

✓4ᵗʰ **T74** **Adult and child abuse, neglect and other maltreatment, confirmed**
Use additional code, if applicable, to identify any associated current injury
Use additional external cause code to identify perpetrator, if known (Y07.-)
EXCLUDES 1   *abuse and maltreatment in pregnancy (O9A.3-, O9A.4-, O9A.5-)*
      adult and child maltreatment, suspected (T76.-)

The appropriate 7th character is to be added to each code from category T74.
A   initial encounter
D   subsequent encounter
S   sequela

✓5ᵗʰ **T74.0** **Neglect or abandonment, confirmed**

✓x7ᵗʰ **T74.01** **Adult neglect or abandonment, confirmed** `A`

✓x7ᵗʰ **T74.02** **Child neglect or abandonment, confirmed** `P`

✓5ᵗʰ **T74.1** **Physical abuse, confirmed**
EXCLUDES 2   *sexual abuse (T74.2-)*

✓x7ᵗʰ **T74.11** **Adult physical abuse, confirmed** `A`

✓x7ᵗʰ **T74.12** **Child physical abuse, confirmed** `P`
EXCLUDES 2   *shaken infant syndrome (T74.4)*

✓5ᵗʰ **T74.2** **Sexual abuse, confirmed**
Rape, confirmed
Sexual assault, confirmed

✓x7ᵗʰ **T74.21** **Adult sexual abuse, confirmed** `A`

✓x7ᵗʰ **T74.22** **Child sexual abuse, confirmed** `P`

✓5ᵗʰ **T74.3** **Psychological abuse, confirmed**

✓x7ᵗʰ **T74.31** **Adult psychological abuse, confirmed** `A`

✓x7ᵗʰ **T74.32** **Child psychological abuse, confirmed** `P`

✓x7ᵗʰ **T74.4** **Shaken infant syndrome** `P`

✓5ᵗʰ **T74.9** **Unspecified maltreatment, confirmed**

✓x7ᵗʰ **T74.91** **Unspecified adult maltreatment, confirmed** `A` ▽

✓x7ᵗʰ **T74.92** **Unspecified child maltreatment, confirmed** `P` ▽

✓4ᵗʰ **T75** **Other and unspecified effects of other external causes**
EXCLUDES 1   *adverse effects NEC (T78.-)*
EXCLUDES 2   *burns (electric) (T20-T31)*

The appropriate 7th character is to be added to each code from category T75.
A   initial encounter
D   subsequent encounter
S   sequela

✓5ᵗʰ **T75.0** **Effects of lightning**
Struck by lightning

✓x7ᵗʰ **T75.00** **Unspecified effects of lightning** ▽
Struck by lightning NOS

✓x7ᵗʰ **T75.01** **Shock due to being struck by lightning**

✓x7ᵗʰ **T75.09** **Other effects of lightning**
Use additional code for other effects of lightning

✓x7ᵗʰ **T75.1** **Unspecified effects of drowning and nonfatal submersion** ▽
Immersion
EXCLUDES 1   *specified effects of drowning—code to effects*

✓5ᵗʰ **T75.2** **Effects of vibration**

✓x7ᵗʰ **T75.20** **Unspecified effects of vibration** ▽

✓x7ᵗʰ **T75.21** **Pneumatic hammer syndrome**

✓x7ᵗʰ **T75.22** **Traumatic vasospastic syndrome**

---

2 HCC with 7th character indicating initial encounter (A or B - specific to category) OR sequela.

☑ Additional Character Req   ✓x7ᵗʰ Placeholder Alert   Manifestation   `HCC` CMS-HCC Condition   ▽ Unspecified Code   ▶◀ Revised Text   ● New Code   ▲ Revised Code Title

ICD-10-CM 2018   1093

√x7th T75.23 Vertigo from infrasound
> EXCLUDES 1   *vertigo NOS (R42)*

√x7th T75.29 Other effects of vibration

√x7th T75.3 Motion sickness
Airsickness
Seasickness
Travel sickness
Use additional external cause code to identify vehicle or type of motion (Y92.81-, Y93.5-)

√x7th T75.4 Electrocution
Shock from electric current
Shock from electroshock gun (taser)

√5th T75.8 Other specified effects of external causes

√x7th T75.81 Effects of abnormal gravitation [G] forces

√x7th T75.82 Effects of weightlessness

√x7th T75.89 Other specified effects of external causes

√4th T76 Adult and child abuse, neglect and other maltreatment, suspected
Use additional code, if applicable, to identify any associated current injury
> EXCLUDES 1   *adult and child maltreatment, confirmed (T74.-)*
> *suspected abuse and maltreatment in pregnancy (O9A.3-, O9A.4-, O9A.5-)*
> *suspected adult physical abuse, ruled out (Z04.71)*
> *suspected adult sexual abuse, ruled out (Z04.41)*
> *suspected child physical abuse, ruled out (Z04.72)*
> *suspected child sexual abuse, ruled out (Z04.42)*

The appropriate 7th character is to be added to each code from category T76.
A   initial encounter
D   subsequent encounter
S   sequela

√5th T76.Ø Neglect or abandonment, suspected

√x7th T76.01 Adult neglect or abandonment, suspected   A

√x7th T76.02 Child neglect or abandonment, suspected   P

√5th T76.1 Physical abuse, suspected

√x7th T76.11 Adult physical abuse, suspected   A

√x7th T76.12 Child physical abuse, suspected   P

√5th T76.2 Sexual abuse, suspected
Rape, suspected
~~Sexual abuse, suspected~~
> EXCLUDES 1   *alleged abuse, ruled out (Z04.7)*

√x7th T76.21 Adult sexual abuse, suspected   A

√x7th T76.22 Child sexual abuse, suspected   P

√5th T76.3 Psychological abuse, suspected

√x7th T76.31 Adult psychological abuse, suspected   A

√x7th T76.32 Child psychological abuse, suspected   P

√5th T76.9 Unspecified maltreatment, suspected

√x7th T76.91 Unspecified adult maltreatment, suspected   A ▽

√x7th T76.92 Unspecified child maltreatment, suspected   P ▽

√4th T78 Adverse effects, not elsewhere classified
> EXCLUDES 2   *complications of surgical and medical care NEC (T80-T88)*

The appropriate 7th character is to be added to each code from category T78.
A   initial encounter
D   subsequent encounter
S   sequela

√5th T78.Ø Anaphylactic reaction due to food
Anaphylactic reaction due to adverse food reaction
Anaphylactic shock or reaction due to nonpoisonous foods
Anaphylactoid reaction due to food

√x7th T78.00 Anaphylactic reaction due to unspecified food   ▽

√x7th T78.01 Anaphylactic reaction due to peanuts

√x7th T78.02 Anaphylactic reaction due to shellfish (crustaceans)

√x7th T78.03 Anaphylactic reaction due to other fish

√x7th T78.04 Anaphylactic reaction due to fruits and vegetables

√x7th T78.05 Anaphylactic reaction due to tree nuts and seeds
> EXCLUDES 2   *anaphylactic reaction due to peanuts (T78.01)*

√x7th T78.06 Anaphylactic reaction due to food additives

√x7th T78.07 Anaphylactic reaction due to milk and dairy products

√x7th T78.08 Anaphylactic reaction due to eggs

√x7th T78.09 Anaphylactic reaction due to other food products

√x7th T78.1 Other adverse food reactions, not elsewhere classified
Use additional code to identify the type of reaction, if applicable
> EXCLUDES 1   *anaphylactic reaction or shock due to adverse food reaction (T78.Ø-)*
> *anaphylactic reaction due to food (T78.Ø-)*
> *bacterial food borne intoxications (A05.-)*
> EXCLUDES 2   *allergic and dietetic gastroenteritis and colitis (K52.29)*
> *allergic rhinitis due to food (J30.5)*
> *dermatitis due to food in contact with skin (L23.6, L24.6, L25.4)*
> *dermatitis due to ingested food (L27.2)*
> *food protein-induced enterocolitis syndrome (K52.21)*
> *food protein-induced enteropathy (K52.22)*

√x7th T78.2 Anaphylactic shock, unspecified   ▽
Allergic shock
Anaphylactic reaction
Anaphylaxis
> EXCLUDES 1   *anaphylactic reaction or shock due to adverse effect of correct medicinal substance properly administered (T88.6)*
> *anaphylactic reaction or shock due to adverse food reaction (T78.Ø-)*
> *anaphylactic reaction or shock due to serum (T80.5-)*

√x7th T78.3 Angioneurotic edema
Allergic angioedema
Giant urticaria
Quincke's edema
> EXCLUDES 1   *serum urticaria (T80.6-)*
> *urticaria (L50.-)*

√5th T78.4 Other and unspecified allergy
> EXCLUDES 1   *specified types of allergic reaction such as:*
> *allergic diarrhea (K52.29)*
> *allergic gastroenteritis and colitis (K52.29)*
> *dermatitis (L23-L25, L27-)*
> *food protein-induced enterocolitis syndrome (K52.21)*
> *food protein-induced enteropathy (K52.22)*
> *hay fever (J30.1)*

√x7th T78.40 Allergy, unspecified   ▽
Allergic reaction NOS
Hypersensitivity NOS

√x7th T78.41 Arthus phenomenon
Arthus reaction

√x7th T78.49 Other allergy

√x7th T78.8 Other adverse effects, not elsewhere classified

Certain early complications of trauma (T79)

√4th T79 Certain early complications of trauma, not elsewhere classified
> EXCLUDES 2   *acute respiratory distress syndrome (J80)*
> *complications occurring during or following medical procedures (T80-T88)*
> *complications of surgical and medical care NEC (T80-T88)*
> *newborn respiratory distress syndrome (P22.0)*

The appropriate 7th character is to be added to each code from category T79.
A   initial encounter
D   subsequent encounter
S   sequela

[1] **√x7th T79.Ø Air embolism (traumatic)**   HCC
> EXCLUDES 1   *air embolism complicating abortion or ectopic or molar pregnancy (O00-O07, O08.2)*
> *air embolism complicating pregnancy, childbirth and the puerperium (O88.0)*
> *air embolism following infusion, transfusion, and therapeutic injection (T80.0)*
> *air embolism following procedure NEC (T81.7-)*
> **DEF:** Arterial or venous obstruction due to introduction of air bubbles into the blood vessels following surgery or trauma.

---

[1] HCC with 7th character indicating initial encounter (A, B or C - specific to category).

EXCLUDES 1 Not coded here   EXCLUDES 2 Not included here   N Newborn Age: 0   P Pediatric Age: 0-17   M Maternity Age: 12-55   A Adult Age: 15-124

1094   ICD-10-CM 2018

[1] ✓x7ᵗʰ **T79.1 Fat embolism (traumatic)**   HCC
> *EXCLUDES 1*   *fat embolism complicating:*
>> *abortion or ectopic or molar pregnancy (O00-O07, O08.2)*
>> *pregnancy, childbirth and the puerperium (O88.8)*
>
> **DEF:** Arterial blockage due to the entrance of fat into the circulatory system after fracture of large bones or administration of corticosteroids.

[1] ✓x7ᵗʰ **T79.2 Traumatic secondary and recurrent hemorrhage and seroma**   HCC

[1] ✓x7ᵗʰ **T79.4 Traumatic shock**   HCC
> Shock (immediate) (delayed) following injury
> *EXCLUDES 1*   *anaphylactic shock due to adverse food reaction (T78.0-)*
>> *anaphylactic shock due to correct medicinal substance properly administered (T88.6)*
>> *anaphylactic shock due to serum (T80.5-)*
>> *anaphylactic shock NOS (T78.2)*
>> *anesthetic shock (T88.2)*
>> *electric shock (T75.4)*
>> *nontraumatic shock NEC (R57.-)*
>> *obstetric shock (O75.1)*
>> *postprocedural shock (T81.1-)*
>> *septic shock (R65.21)*
>> *shock complicating abortion or ectopic or molar pregnancy (O00-O07, O08.3)*
>> *shock due to lightning (T75.01)*
>> *shock NOS (R57.9)*

[1] ✓x7ᵗʰ **T79.5 Traumatic anuria**   HCC
> Crush syndrome
> Renal failure following crushing

[1] ✓x7ᵗʰ **T79.6 Traumatic ischemia of muscle**   HCC
> Traumatic rhabdomyolysis
> Volkmann's ischemic contracture
> *EXCLUDES 2*   *anterior tibial syndrome (M76.8)*
>> *compartment syndrome (traumatic) (T79.A-)*
>> *nontraumatic ischemia of muscle (M62.2-)*

[1] ✓x7ᵗʰ **T79.7 Traumatic subcutaneous emphysema**   HCC
> *EXCLUDES 1*   *emphysema NOS (J43)*
>> *emphysema (subcutaneous) resulting from a procedure (T81.82)*

✓5ᵗʰ **T79.A Traumatic compartment syndrome**
> *EXCLUDES 1*   *fibromyalgia (M79.7)*
>> *nontraumatic compartment syndrome (M79.A-)*
>> *traumatic ischemic infarction of muscle (T79.6)*
>
> **DEF:** Compression of nerves and blood vessels within an enclosed muscle space due to previous trauma, which leads to impaired blood flow and muscle and nerve damage.

[1] ✓x7ᵗʰ **T79.A0 Compartment syndrome, unspecified**   HCC ▽
> Compartment syndrome NOS

✓6ᵗʰ **T79.A1 Traumatic compartment syndrome of upper extremity**
> Traumatic compartment syndrome of shoulder, arm, forearm, wrist, hand, and fingers

[1] ✓7ᵗʰ **T79.A11 Traumatic compartment syndrome of right upper extremity**   HCC

[1] ✓7ᵗʰ **T79.A12 Traumatic compartment syndrome of left upper extremity**   HCC

[1] ✓7ᵗʰ **T79.A19 Traumatic compartment syndrome of unspecified upper extremity**   HCC ▽

✓6ᵗʰ **T79.A2 Traumatic compartment syndrome of lower extremity**
> Traumatic compartment syndrome of hip, buttock, thigh, leg, foot, and toes

[1] ✓7ᵗʰ **T79.A21 Traumatic compartment syndrome of right lower extremity**   HCC

[1] ✓7ᵗʰ **T79.A22 Traumatic compartment syndrome of left lower extremity**   HCC

[1] ✓7ᵗʰ **79.A29 Traumatic compartment syndrome of unspecified lower extremity**   HCC ▽

[1] ✓x7ᵗʰ **T79.A3 Traumatic compartment syndrome of abdomen**   HCC

[1] ✓x7ᵗʰ **T79.A9 Traumatic compartment syndrome of other sites**   HCC

[1] ✓x7ᵗʰ **T79.8 Other early complications of trauma**   HCC

[1] ✓x7ᵗʰ **T79.9 Unspecified early complication of trauma**   HCC ▽

Complications of surgical and medical care, not elsewhere classified (T80-T88)

Use additional code for adverse effect, if applicable, to identify drug (T36-T50 with fifth or sixth character 5)

Use additional code(s) to identify the specified condition resulting from the complication

Use additional code to identify devices involved and details of circumstances (Y62-Y82)
> *EXCLUDES 2*   *any encounters with medical care for postprocedural conditions in which no complications are present, such as:*
>> *artificial opening status (Z93.-)*
>> *closure of external stoma (Z43.-)*
>> *fitting and adjustment of external prosthetic device (Z44.-)*
>
>> *burns and corrosions from local applications and irradiation (T20-T32)*
>> *complications of surgical procedures during pregnancy, childbirth and the puerperium (O00-O9A)*
>> *mechanical complication of respirator [ventilator] (J95.850)*
>> *poisoning and toxic effects of drugs and chemicals (T36-T65 with fifth or sixth character 1-4 or 6)*
>> *postprocedural fever (R50.82)*
>> *specified complications classified elsewhere, such as:*
>>> *cerebrospinal fluid leak from spinal puncture (G97.0)*
>>> *colostomy malfunction (K94.0-)*
>>> *disorders of fluid and electrolyte imbalance (E86-E87)*
>>> *functional disturbances following cardiac surgery (I97.0-I97.1)*
>>> *intraoperative and postprocedural complications of specified body systems (D78.-, E36.-, E89.-, G97.3-, G97.4, H59.3-, H59.-, H95.2-, H95.3, I97.4-, I97.5, J95.6-, J95.7, K91.6-, L76.-, M96.-, N99.-)*
>>> *ostomy complications (J95.0-, K94.-, N99.5-)*
>>> *postgastric surgery syndromes (K91.1)*
>>> *postlaminectomy syndrome NEC (M96.1)*
>>> *postmastectomy lymphedema syndrome (I97.2)*
>>> *postsurgical blind-loop syndrome (K91.2)*
>>> *ventilator associated pneumonia (J95.851)*

AHA: 2015, 1Q, 15

✓4ᵗʰ **T80 Complications following infusion, transfusion and therapeutic injection**
> **INCLUDES**   complications following perfusion
> *EXCLUDES 2*   *bone marrow transplant rejection (T86.01)*
>> *febrile nonhemolytic transfusion reaction (R50.84)*
>> *fluid overload due to transfusion (E87.71)*
>> *posttransfusion purpura (D69.51)*
>> *transfusion associated circulatory overload (TACO) (E87.71)*
>> *transfusion (red blood cell) associated hemochromatosis (E83.111)*
>> *transfusion related acute lung injury (TRALI) (J95.84)*

> The appropriate 7th character is to be added to each code from category T80.
> A   initial encounter
> D   subsequent encounter
> S   sequela

✓x7ᵗʰ **T80.0 Air embolism following infusion, transfusion and therapeutic injection**

✓x7ᵗʰ **T80.1 Vascular complications following infusion, transfusion and therapeutic injection**
> Use additional code to identify the vascular complication
> *EXCLUDES 2*   *extravasation of vesicant agent (T80.81-)*
>> *infiltration of vesicant agent (T80.81-)*
>> *postprocedural vascular complications (T81.7-)*
>> *vascular complications specified as due to prosthetic devices, implants and grafts (T82.8-, T83.8-, T84.8-, T85.8-)*

---

[1]   HCC with 7th character indicating initial encounter (A, B or C - specific to category).

☑ Additional Character Req   ✓x7ᵗʰ Placeholder Alert   Manifestation   HCC CMS-HCC Condition   ▽ Unspecified Code   ▶◀ Revised Text   ● New Code   ▲ Revised Code Title

✓5ᵗʰ **T80.2** **Infections** following infusion, transfusion and therapeutic injection

Use additional code to identify the specific infection, such as: sepsis (A41.9)

Use additional code (R65.2-) to identify severe sepsis, if applicable

EXCLUDES 2   *infections specified as due to prosthetic devices, implants and grafts (T82.6-T82.7, T83.5-T83.6, T84.5-T84.7, T85.7)*
postprocedural infections (T81.4-)

✓6ᵗʰ **T80.21** **Infection** due to central venous catheter

Infection due to pulmonary artery catheter (Swan-Ganz catheter)

✓7ᵗʰ **T80.211** **Bloodstream infection** due to central venous catheter

Catheter-related bloodstream infection (CRBSI) NOS

Central line-associated bloodstream infection (CLABSI)

Bloodstream infection due to Hickman catheter

Bloodstream infection due to peripherally inserted central catheter (PICC)

Bloodstream infection due to portacath (port-a-cath)

Bloodstream infection due to pulmonary artery catheter

Bloodstream infection due to triple lumen catheter

Bloodstream infection due to umbilical venous catheter

✓7ᵗʰ **T80.212** **Local infection** due to central venous catheter

Exit or insertion site infection

Local infection due to Hickman catheter

Local infection due to peripherally inserted central catheter (PICC)

Local infection due to portacath (port-a-cath)

Local infection due to pulmonary artery catheter

Local infection due to triple lumen catheter

Local infection due to umbilical venous catheter

Port or reservoir infection

Tunnel infection

✓7ᵗʰ **T80.218** **Other infection** due to central venous catheter

Other central line-associated infection

Other infection due to Hickman catheter

Other infection due to peripherally inserted central catheter (PICC)

Other infection due to portacath (port-a-cath)

Other infection due to pulmonary artery catheter

Other infection due to triple lumen catheter

Other infection due to umbilical venous catheter

✓7ᵗʰ **T80.219** **Unspecified infection** due to central   ▽ venous catheter

Central line-associated infection NOS

Unspecified infection due to Hickman catheter

Unspecified infection due to peripherally inserted central catheter (PICC)

Unspecified infection due to portacath (port-a-cath)

Unspecified infection due to pulmonary artery catheter

Unspecified infection due to triple lumen catheter

Unspecified infection due to umbilical venous catheter

✓x7ᵗʰ **T80.22** **Acute infection** following transfusion, infusion, or injection of blood and blood products

✓x7ᵗʰ **T80.29** **Infection** following other infusion, transfusion and therapeutic injection

✓5ᵗʰ **T80.3** **ABO incompatibility** reaction due to transfusion of blood or blood products

EXCLUDES 1   *minor blood group antigens reactions (Duffy) (E) (K(ell)) (Kidd) (Lewis) (M) (N) (P) (S) (T80.A)*

✓x7ᵗʰ **T80.30** **ABO incompatibility** reaction due to transfusion   ▽ of blood or blood products, unspecified

ABO incompatibility blood transfusion NOS

Reaction to ABO incompatibility from transfusion NOS

✓6ᵗʰ **T80.31** **ABO incompatibility** with hemolytic transfusion reaction

✓7ᵗʰ **T80.310** **ABO incompatibility** with acute hemolytic transfusion reaction

ABO incompatibility with hemolytic transfusion reaction less than 24 hours after transfusion

Acute hemolytic transfusion reaction (AHTR) due to ABO incompatibility

✓7ᵗʰ **T80.311** **ABO incompatibility** with delayed hemolytic transfusion reaction

ABO incompatibility with hemolytic transfusion reaction 24 hours or more after transfusion

Delayed hemolytic transfusion reaction (DHTR) due to ABO incompatibility

✓7ᵗʰ **T80.319** **ABO incompatibility** with hemolytic   ▽ transfusion reaction, unspecified

ABO incompatibility with hemolytic transfusion reaction at unspecified time after transfusion

Hemolytic transfusion reaction (HTR) due to ABO incompatibility NOS

✓x7ᵗʰ **T80.39** **Other ABO incompatibility** reaction due to transfusion of blood or blood products

Delayed serologic transfusion reaction (DSTR) from ABO incompatibility

Other ABO incompatible blood transfusion

Other reaction to ABO incompatible blood transfusion

✓5ᵗʰ **T80.4** **Rh incompatibility** reaction due to transfusion of blood or blood products

Reaction due to incompatibility of Rh antigens (C) (c) (D) (E) (e)

✓x7ᵗʰ **T80.40** **Rh incompatibility** reaction due to transfusion   ▽ of blood or blood products, unspecified

Reaction due to Rh factor in transfusion NOS

Rh incompatible blood transfusion NOS

✓6ᵗʰ **T80.41** **Rh incompatibility** with hemolytic transfusion reaction

✓7ᵗʰ **T80.410** **Rh incompatibility** with acute hemolytic transfusion reaction

Acute hemolytic transfusion reaction (AHTR) due to Rh incompatibility

Rh incompatibility with hemolytic transfusion reaction less than 24 hours after transfusion

✓7ᵗʰ **T80.411** **Rh incompatibility** with delayed hemolytic transfusion reaction

Delayed hemolytic transfusion reaction (DHTR) due to Rh incompatibility

Rh incompatibility with hemolytic transfusion reaction 24 hours or more after transfusion

✓7ᵗʰ **T80.419** **Rh incompatibility** with hemolytic   ▽ transfusion reaction, unspecified

Hemolytic transfusion reaction (HTR) due to Rh incompatibility NOS

Rh incompatibility with hemolytic transfusion reaction at unspecified time after transfusion

✓x7ᵗʰ **T80.49** **Other Rh incompatibility** reaction due to transfusion of blood or blood products

Delayed serologic transfusion reaction (DSTR) from Rh incompatibility

Other reaction to Rh incompatible blood transfusion

✓5ᵗʰ **T80.A** **Non-ABO incompatibility** reaction due to transfusion of blood or blood products

Reaction due to incompatibility of minor antigens (Duffy) (Kell) (Kidd) (Lewis) (M) (N) (P) (S)

✓x7ᵗʰ **T80.A0** **Non-ABO incompatibility** reaction due to   ▽ transfusion of blood or blood products, unspecified

Non-ABO antigen incompatibility reaction from transfusion NOS

EXCLUDES 1 Not coded here   *EXCLUDES 2* Not included here   **N** Newborn Age: 0   **P** Pediatric Age: 0-17   **M** Maternity Age: 12-55   **A** Adult Age: 15-124

1096   ICD-10-CM 2018

√6ᵗʰ **T80.A1** **Non-ABO incompatibility with hemolytic transfusion reaction**

√7ᵗʰ **T80.A10** **Non-ABO incompatibility with acute hemolytic transfusion reaction**
Acute hemolytic transfusion reaction (AHTR) due to non-ABO incompatibility
Non-ABO incompatibility with hemolytic transfusion reaction less than 24 hours after transfusion

√7ᵗʰ **T80.A11** **Non-ABO incompatibility with delayed hemolytic transfusion reaction**
Delayed hemolytic transfusion reaction (DHTR) due to non-ABO incompatibility
Non-ABO incompatibility with hemolytic transfusion reaction 24 or more hours after transfusion

√7ᵗʰ **T80.A19** **Non-ABO incompatibility with hemolytic transfusion reaction, unspecified** ▽
Hemolytic transfusion reaction (HTR) due to non-ABO incompatibility NOS
Non-ABO incompatibility with hemolytic transfusion reaction at unspecified time after transfusion

√x7ᵗʰ **T80.A9** **Other non-ABO incompatibility reaction due to transfusion of blood or blood products**
Delayed serologic transfusion reaction (DSTR) from non-ABO incompatibility
Other reaction to non-ABO incompatible blood transfusion

√5ᵗʰ **T80.5** **Anaphylactic reaction due to serum**
Allergic shock due to serum
Anaphylactic shock due to serum
Anaphylactoid reaction due to serum
Anaphylaxis due to serum
EXCLUDES 1   *ABO incompatibility reaction due to transfusion of blood or blood products (T80.3-)*
allergic reaction or shock NOS (T78.2)
anaphylactic reaction or shock NOS (T78.2)
anaphylactic reaction or shock due to adverse effect of correct medicinal substance properly administered (T88.6)
other serum reaction (T80.6-)
DEF: Life-threatening hypersensitivity to foreign serum; causes respiratory distress, vascular collapse, and shock.

√x7ᵗʰ **T80.51** **Anaphylactic reaction due to administration of blood and blood products**

√x7ᵗʰ **T80.52** **Anaphylactic reaction due to vaccination**

√x7ᵗʰ **T80.59** **Anaphylactic reaction due to other serum**

√5ᵗʰ **T80.6** **Other serum reactions**
Intoxication by serum
Protein sickness
Serum rash
Serum sickness
Serum urticaria
EXCLUDES 2   *serum hepatitis (B16-B19)*
DEF: Serum sickness: Hypersensitivity to foreign serum; causes fever, hives, swelling, and lymphadenopathy.

√x7ᵗʰ **T80.61** **Other serum reaction due to administration of blood and blood products**

√x7ᵗʰ **T80.62** **Other serum reaction due to vaccination**

√x7ᵗʰ **T80.69** **Other serum reaction due to other serum**
▶Code also, if applicable, arthropathy in hypersensitivity reactions classified elsewhere (M36.4)◀

√5ᵗʰ **T80.8** **Other complications following infusion, transfusion and therapeutic injection**

√6ᵗʰ **T80.81** **Extravasation of vesicant agent**
Infiltration of vesicant agent

√7ᵗʰ **T80.810** **Extravasation of vesicant antineoplastic chemotherapy**
Infiltration of vesicant antineoplastic chemotherapy

√7ᵗʰ **T80.818** **Extravasation of other vesicant agent**
Infiltration of other vesicant agent

√x7ᵗʰ **T80.89** **Other complications following infusion, transfusion and therapeutic injection**
Delayed serologic transfusion reaction (DSTR), unspecified incompatibility
Use additional code to identify graft-versus-host reaction, if applicable, (D89.81-)

√5ᵗʰ **T80.9** **Unspecified complication following infusion, transfusion and therapeutic injection**

√x7ᵗʰ **T80.90** **Unspecified complication following infusion and therapeutic injection** ▽

√6ᵗʰ **T80.91** **Hemolytic transfusion reaction, unspecified incompatibility**
EXCLUDES 1   *ABO incompatibility with hemolytic transfusion reaction (T80.31-)*
Non-ABO incompatibility with hemolytic transfusion reaction (T80.A1-)
Rh incompatibility with hemolytic transfusion reaction (T80.41-)

√7ᵗʰ **T80.910** **Acute hemolytic transfusion reaction, unspecified incompatibility** ▽

√7ᵗʰ **T80.911** **Delayed hemolytic transfusion reaction,▽ unspecified incompatibility**

√7ᵗʰ **T80.919** **Hemolytic transfusion reaction, unspecified incompatibility, unspecified as acute or delayed** ▽
Hemolytic transfusion reaction NOS

√x7ᵗʰ **T80.92** **Unspecified transfusion reaction** ▽
Transfusion reaction NOS

√4ᵗʰ **T81** **Complications of procedures, not elsewhere classified**
Use additional code for adverse effect, if applicable, to identify drug (T36-T50 with fifth or sixth character 5)
EXCLUDES 2   *complications following immunization (T88.0-T88.1)*
complications following infusion, transfusion and therapeutic injection (T80.-)
complications of transplanted organs and tissue (T86.-)
specified complications classified elsewhere, such as:
complication of prosthetic devices, implants and grafts (T82-T85)
dermatitis due to drugs and medicaments (L23.3, L24.4, L25.1, L27.0-L27.1)
endosseous dental implant failure (M27.6-)
floppy iris syndrome (IFIS) (intraoperative) (H21.81)
intraoperative and postprocedural complications of specific body system (D78.-, E36.-, E89.-, G97.3-, G97.4, H59.3-, H59.-, H95.2-, H95.3, I97.4-, I97.5, J95, K91.-, L76.-, M96.-, N99.-)
ostomy complications (J95.0-, K94.-, N99.5-)
plateau iris syndrome (post-iridectomy) (postprocedural) (H21.82)
poisoning and toxic effects of drugs and chemicals (T36-T65 with fifth or sixth character 1-4 or 6)

The appropriate 7th character is to be added to each code from category T81.
A   initial encounter
D   subsequent encounter
S   sequela

√5ᵗʰ **T81.1** **Postprocedural shock**
Shock during or resulting from a procedure, not elsewhere classified
EXCLUDES 1   *anaphylactic shock due to correct substance properly administered (T88.6)*
anaphylactic shock due to serum (T80.5-)
anaphylactic shock NOS (T78.2)
anesthetic shock (T88.2)
electric shock (T75.4)
obstetric shock (O75.1)
septic shock (R65.21)
shock following abortion or ectopic or molar pregnancy (O00-O07, O08.3)
traumatic shock (T79.4)

√x7ᵗʰ **T81.10** **Postprocedural shock unspecified** ▽
Collapse NOS during or resulting from a procedure, not elsewhere classified
Postprocedural failure of peripheral circulation
Postprocedural shock NOS

¹ √x7ᵗʰ **T81.11** **Postprocedural cardiogenic shock** [HCC]

---

¹ HCC with 7th character indicating initial encounter (A, B or C - specific to category).

☑ Additional Character Req   √x7ᵗʰ Placeholder Alert   Manifestation   [HCC] CMS-HCC Condition   ▽ Unspecified Code   ▶◀ Revised Text   ● New Code   ▲ Revised Code Title

[1] ✓x7ᵗʰ **T81.12 Postprocedural septic shock**   `HCC`
     Postprocedural endotoxic shock resulting from a procedure, not elsewhere classified
     Postprocedural gram-negative shock resulting from a procedure, not elsewhere classified
     Code first underlying infection
     Use additional code, to identify any associated acute organ dysfunction, if applicable

✓x7ᵗʰ **T81.19 Other postprocedural shock**
     Postprocedural hypovolemic shock

✓5ᵗʰ **T81.3 Disruption of wound, not elsewhere classified**
     Disruption of any suture materials or other closure methods
     EXCLUDES 1   breakdown (mechanical) of permanent sutures (T85.612)
          displacement of permanent sutures (T85.622)
          disruption of cesarean delivery wound (O90.0)
          disruption of perineal obstetric wound (O90.1)
          mechanical complication of permanent sutures NEC (T85.692)
     AHA: 2014, 1Q, 23

✓x7ᵗʰ **T81.30 Disruption of wound, unspecified**   ▽
     Disruption of wound NOS

✓x7ᵗʰ **T81.31 Disruption of external operation (surgical) wound, not elsewhere classified**
     Dehiscence of operation wound NOS
     Disruption of operation wound NOS
     Disruption or dehiscence of closure of cornea
     Disruption or dehiscence of closure of mucosa
     Disruption or dehiscence of closure of skin and subcutaneous tissue
     Full-thickness skin disruption or dehiscence
     Superficial disruption or dehiscence of operation wound
     EXCLUDES 1   dehiscence of amputation stump (T87.81)

✓x7ᵗʰ **T81.32 Disruption of internal operation (surgical) wound, not elsewhere classified**
     Deep disruption or dehiscence of operation wound NOS
     Disruption or dehiscence of closure of internal organ or other internal tissue
     Disruption or dehiscence of closure of muscle or muscle flap
     Disruption or dehiscence of closure of ribs or rib cage
     Disruption or dehiscence of closure of skull or craniotomy
     Disruption or dehiscence of closure of sternum or sternotomy
     Disruption or dehiscence of closure of tendon or ligament
     Disruption or dehiscence of closure of superficial or muscular fascia

✓x7ᵗʰ **T81.33 Disruption of traumatic injury wound repair**
     Disruption or dehiscence of closure of traumatic laceration (external) (internal)

✓x7ᵗʰ **T81.4 Infection following a procedure**
     Intra-abdominal abscess following a procedure
     Postprocedural infection, not elsewhere classified
     Sepsis following a procedure
     Stitch abscess following a procedure
     Subphrenic abscess following a procedure
     Wound abscess following a procedure
     Use additional code to identify infection
     Use additional code (R65.2-) to identify severe sepsis, if applicable
     EXCLUDES 1   obstetric surgical wound infection (O86.0)
          postprocedural fever NOS (R50.82)
          postprocedural retroperitoneal abscess (K68.11)
     EXCLUDES 2   bleb associated endophthalmitis (H59.4-)
          infection due to infusion, transfusion and therapeutic injection (T80.2-)
          infection due to prosthetic devices, implants and grafts (T82.6-T82.7, T83.5-T83.6, T84.5-T84.7, T85.7)
     AHA: 2014, 1Q, 23

✓5ᵗʰ **T81.5 Complications of foreign body accidentally left in body following procedure**
     AHA: 2014, 4Q, 24

✓6ᵗʰ **T81.50 Unspecified complication of foreign body accidentally left in body following procedure**

✓7ᵗʰ **T81.500 Unspecified complication of foreign body accidentally left in body following surgical operation**   ▽

✓7ᵗʰ **T81.501 Unspecified complication of foreign body accidentally left in body following infusion or transfusion**   ▽

✓7ᵗʰ **T81.502 Unspecified complication of foreign body accidentally left in body following kidney dialysis**   `HCC` ▽

✓7ᵗʰ **T81.503 Unspecified complication of foreign body accidentally left in body following injection or immunization**   ▽

✓7ᵗʰ **T81.504 Unspecified complication of foreign body accidentally left in body following endoscopic examination**   ▽

✓7ᵗʰ **T81.505 Unspecified complication of foreign body accidentally left in body following heart catheterization**   ▽

✓7ᵗʰ **T81.506 Unspecified complication of foreign body accidentally left in body following aspiration, puncture or other catheterization**   ▽

✓7ᵗʰ **T81.507 Unspecified complication of foreign body accidentally left in body following removal of catheter or packing**   ▽

✓7ᵗʰ **T81.508 Unspecified complication of foreign body accidentally left in body following other procedure**   ▽

✓7ᵗʰ **T81.509 Unspecified complication of foreign body accidentally left in body following unspecified procedure**   ▽

✓6ᵗʰ **T81.51 Adhesions due to foreign body accidentally left in body following procedure**

✓7ᵗʰ **T81.510 Adhesions due to foreign body accidentally left in body following surgical operation**

✓7ᵗʰ **T81.511 Adhesions due to foreign body accidentally left in body following infusion or transfusion**

✓7ᵗʰ **T81.512 Adhesions due to foreign body accidentally left in body following kidney dialysis**   `HCC`

✓7ᵗʰ **T81.513 Adhesions due to foreign body accidentally left in body following injection or immunization**

✓7ᵗʰ **T81.514 Adhesions due to foreign body accidentally left in body following endoscopic examination**

✓7ᵗʰ **T81.515 Adhesions due to foreign body accidentally left in body following heart catheterization**

✓7ᵗʰ **T81.516 Adhesions due to foreign body accidentally left in body following aspiration, puncture or other catheterization**

✓7ᵗʰ **T81.517 Adhesions due to foreign body accidentally left in body following removal of catheter or packing**

✓7ᵗʰ **T81.518 Adhesions due to foreign body accidentally left in body following other procedure**

✓7ᵗʰ **T81.519 Adhesions due to foreign body accidentally left in body following unspecified procedure**   ▽

✓6ᵗʰ **T81.52 Obstruction due to foreign body accidentally left in body following procedure**

✓7ᵗʰ **T81.520 Obstruction due to foreign body accidentally left in body following surgical operation**

✓7ᵗʰ **T81.521 Obstruction due to foreign body accidentally left in body following infusion or transfusion**

✓7ᵗʰ **T81.522 Obstruction due to foreign body accidentally left in body following kidney dialysis**   `HCC`

✓7ᵗʰ **T81.523 Obstruction due to foreign body accidentally left in body following injection or immunization**

✓7ᵗʰ **T81.524 Obstruction due to foreign body accidentally left in body following endoscopic examination**

---

[1]   HCC with 7th character indicating initial encounter (A, B or C - specific to category).

EXCLUDES 1 Not coded here   *EXCLUDES 2* Not included here   N Newborn Age: 0   P Pediatric Age: 0-17   M Maternity Age: 12-55   A Adult Age: 15-124

1098   ICD-10-CM 2018

√7ᵗʰ **T81.525 Obstruction due to foreign body accidentally left in body following heart catheterization**

√7ᵗʰ **T81.526 Obstruction due to foreign body accidentally left in body following aspiration, puncture or other catheterization**

√7ᵗʰ **T81.527 Obstruction due to foreign body accidentally left in body following removal of catheter or packing**

√7ᵗʰ **T81.528 Obstruction due to foreign body accidentally left in body following other procedure**

√7ᵗʰ **T81.529 Obstruction due to foreign body accidentally left in body following unspecified procedure** ▽

√6ᵗʰ **T81.53 Perforation due to foreign body accidentally left in body following procedure**

√7ᵗʰ **T81.530 Perforation due to foreign body accidentally left in body following surgical operation**

√7ᵗʰ **T81.531 Perforation due to foreign body accidentally left in body following infusion or transfusion**

√7ᵗʰ **T81.532 Perforation due to foreign body accidentally left in body following kidney dialysis** HCC

√7ᵗʰ **T81.533 Perforation due to foreign body accidentally left in body following injection or immunization**

√7ᵗʰ **T81.534 Perforation due to foreign body accidentally left in body following endoscopic examination**

√7ᵗʰ **T81.535 Perforation due to foreign body accidentally left in body following heart catheterization**

√7ᵗʰ **T81.536 Perforation due to foreign body accidentally left in body following aspiration, puncture or other catheterization**

√7ᵗʰ **T81.537 Perforation due to foreign body accidentally left in body following removal of catheter or packing**

√7ᵗʰ **T81.538 Perforation due to foreign body accidentally left in body following other procedure**

√7ᵗʰ **T81.539 Perforation due to foreign body accidentally left in body following unspecified procedure** ▽

√6ᵗʰ **T81.59 Other complications of foreign body accidentally left in body following procedure**

EXCLUDES 2   *obstruction or perforation due to prosthetic devices and implants intentionally left in body (T82.0-T82.5, T83.0-T83.4, T83.7, T84.0-T84.4, T85.0-T85.6)*

√7ᵗʰ **T81.590 Other complications of foreign body accidentally left in body following surgical operation**

√7ᵗʰ **T81.591 Other complications of foreign body accidentally left in body following infusion or transfusion**

√7ᵗʰ **T81.592 Other complications of foreign body accidentally left in body following kidney dialysis** HCC

√7ᵗʰ **T81.593 Other complications of foreign body accidentally left in body following injection or immunization**

√7ᵗʰ **T81.594 Other complications of foreign body accidentally left in body following endoscopic examination**

√7ᵗʰ **T81.595 Other complications of foreign body accidentally left in body following heart catheterization**

√7ᵗʰ **T81.596 Other complications of foreign body accidentally left in body following aspiration, puncture or other catheterization**

√7ᵗʰ **T81.597 Other complications of foreign body accidentally left in body following removal of catheter or packing**

√7ᵗʰ **T81.598 Other complications of foreign body accidentally left in body following other procedure**

√7ᵗʰ **T81.599 Other complications of foreign body accidentally left in body following unspecified procedure** ▽

√5ᵗʰ **T81.6 Acute reaction to foreign substance accidentally left during a procedure**

EXCLUDES 2   *complications of foreign body accidentally left in body cavity or operation wound following procedure (T81.5-)*

√x7ᵗʰ **T81.60 Unspecified acute reaction to foreign substance accidentally left during a procedure** ▽

√x7ᵗʰ **T81.61 Aseptic peritonitis due to foreign substance accidentally left during a procedure**
Chemical peritonitis

√x7ᵗʰ **T81.69 Other acute reaction to foreign substance accidentally left during a procedure**

√5ᵗʰ **T81.7 Vascular complications following a procedure, not elsewhere classified**
Air embolism following procedure NEC
Phlebitis or thrombophlebitis resulting from a procedure

EXCLUDES 1   *embolism complicating abortion or ectopic or molar pregnancy (O00-O07, O08.2)*
embolism complicating pregnancy, childbirth and the puerperium (O88.-)
traumatic embolism (T79.0)

EXCLUDES 2   *embolism due to prosthetic devices, implants and grafts (T82.8-, T83.81, T84.8-, T85.81-)*
embolism following infusion, transfusion and therapeutic injection (T80.0)

√6ᵗʰ **T81.71 Complication of artery following a procedure, not elsewhere classified**

√7ᵗʰ **T81.710 Complication of mesenteric artery following a procedure, not elsewhere classified**

√7ᵗʰ **T81.711 Complication of renal artery following a procedure, not elsewhere classified**

√7ᵗʰ **T81.718 Complication of other artery following a procedure, not elsewhere classified**

√7ᵗʰ **T81.719 Complication of unspecified artery following a procedure, not elsewhere classified** ▽

√x7ᵗʰ **T81.72 Complication of vein following a procedure, not elsewhere classified**

√5ᵗʰ **T81.8 Other complications of procedures, not elsewhere classified**

EXCLUDES 2   *hypothermia following anesthesia (T88.51)*
malignant hyperpyrexia due to anesthesia (T88.3)

√x7ᵗʰ **T81.81 Complication of inhalation therapy**

√x7ᵗʰ **T81.82 Emphysema (subcutaneous) resulting from a procedure**

√x7ᵗʰ **T81.83 Persistent postprocedural fistula**

√x7ᵗʰ **T81.89 Other complications of procedures, not elsewhere classified**
Use additional code to specify complication, such as:
postprocedural delirium (F05)
AHA: 2014, 1Q, 23

√x7ᵗʰ **T81.9 Unspecified complication of procedure** ▽

√4ᵗʰ **T82 Complications of cardiac and vascular prosthetic devices, implants and grafts**

EXCLUDES 2   *failure and rejection of transplanted organs and tissue (T86.-)*

The appropriate 7th character is to be added to each code from category T82.
A   initial encounter
D   subsequent encounter
S   sequela

√5ᵗʰ **T82.0 Mechanical complication of heart valve prosthesis**
Mechanical complication of artificial heart valve

EXCLUDES 1   *mechanical complication of biological heart valve graft (T82.22-)*

√x7ᵗʰ **T82.01 Breakdown (mechanical) of heart valve prosthesis**

√x7ᵗʰ **T82.02 Displacement of heart valve prosthesis**
Malposition of heart valve prosthesis

√x7ᵗʰ **T82.03 Leakage of heart valve prosthesis**

√ Additional Character Req   √x7ᵗʰ Placeholder Alert   Manifestation   HCC CMS-HCC Condition   ▽ Unspecified Code   ►◄ Revised Text   ● New Code   ▲ Revised Code Title

√x7ᵗʰ **T82.09 Other mechanical complication of heart valve prosthesis**
Obstruction (mechanical) of heart valve prosthesis
Perforation of heart valve prosthesis
Protrusion of heart valve prosthesis

√5ᵗʰ **T82.1 Mechanical complication of cardiac electronic device**

√6ᵗʰ **T82.11 Breakdown (mechanical) of cardiac electronic device**

√7ᵗʰ **T82.110 Breakdown (mechanical) of cardiac electrode**

√7ᵗʰ **T82.111 Breakdown (mechanical) of cardiac pulse generator (battery)**

√7ᵗʰ **T82.118 Breakdown (mechanical) of other cardiac electronic device**

√7ᵗʰ **T82.119 Breakdown (mechanical) of unspecified ▽ cardiac electronic device**

√6ᵗʰ **T82.12 Displacement of cardiac electronic device**
Malposition of cardiac electronic device

√7ᵗʰ **T82.120 Displacement of cardiac electrode**

√7ᵗʰ **T82.121 Displacement of cardiac pulse generator (battery)**

√7ᵗʰ **T82.128 Displacement of other cardiac electronic device**

√7ᵗʰ **T82.129 Displacement of unspecified cardiac ▽ electronic device**

√6ᵗʰ **T82.19 Other mechanical complication of cardiac electronic device**
Leakage of cardiac electronic device
Obstruction of cardiac electronic device
Perforation of cardiac electronic device
Protrusion of cardiac electronic device

√7ᵗʰ **T82.190 Other mechanical complication of cardiac electrode**

√7ᵗʰ **T82.191 Other mechanical complication of cardiac pulse generator (battery)**

√7ᵗʰ **T82.198 Other mechanical complication of other cardiac electronic device**

√7ᵗʰ **T82.199 Other mechanical complication of ▽ unspecified cardiac device**

√5ᵗʰ **T82.2 Mechanical complication of coronary artery bypass graft and biological heart valve graft**
EXCLUDES 1 *mechanical complication of artificial heart valve prosthesis (T82.0-)*

√6ᵗʰ **T82.21 Mechanical complication of coronary artery bypass graft**

√7ᵗʰ **T82.211 Breakdown (mechanical) of coronary artery bypass graft**

√7ᵗʰ **T82.212 Displacement of coronary artery bypass graft**
Malposition of coronary artery bypass graft

√7ᵗʰ **T82.213 Leakage of coronary artery bypass graft**

√7ᵗʰ **T82.218 Other mechanical complication of coronary artery bypass graft**
Obstruction, mechanical of coronary artery bypass graft
Perforation of coronary artery bypass graft
Protrusion of coronary artery bypass graft

√6ᵗʰ **T82.22 Mechanical complication of biological heart valve graft**

√7ᵗʰ **T82.221 Breakdown (mechanical) of biological heart valve graft**

√7ᵗʰ **T82.222 Displacement of biological heart valve graft**
Malposition of biological heart valve graft

√7ᵗʰ **T82.223 Leakage of biological heart valve graft**

√7ᵗʰ **T82.228 Other mechanical complication of biological heart valve graft**
Obstruction of biological heart valve graft
Perforation of biological heart valve graft
Protrusion of biological heart valve graft

√5ᵗʰ **T82.3 Mechanical complication of other vascular grafts**

√6ᵗʰ **T82.31 Breakdown (mechanical) of other vascular grafts**

1 √7ᵗʰ **T82.310 Breakdown (mechanical) of aortic (bifurcation) graft (replacement)** HCC

1 √7ᵗʰ **T82.311 Breakdown (mechanical) of carotid arterial graft (bypass)** HCC

1 √7ᵗʰ **T82.312 Breakdown (mechanical) of femoral arterial graft (bypass)** HCC

1 √7ᵗʰ **T82.318 Breakdown (mechanical) of other vascular grafts** HCC

1 √7ᵗʰ **T82.319 Breakdown (mechanical) of unspecified vascular grafts** HCC ▽

√6ᵗʰ **T82.32 Displacement of other vascular grafts**
Malposition of other vascular grafts

1 √7ᵗʰ **T82.320 Displacement of aortic (bifurcation) graft (replacement)** HCC

1 √7ᵗʰ **T82.321 Displacement of carotid arterial graft (bypass)** HCC

1 √7ᵗʰ **T82.322 Displacement of femoral arterial graft (bypass)** HCC

1 √7ᵗʰ **T82.328 Displacement of other vascular grafts** HCC

1 √7ᵗʰ **T82.329 Displacement of unspecified vascular grafts** HCC ▽

√6ᵗʰ **T82.33 Leakage of other vascular grafts**

1 √7ᵗʰ **T82.330 Leakage of aortic (bifurcation) graft (replacement)** HCC

1 √7ᵗʰ **T82.331 Leakage of carotid arterial graft (bypass)** HCC

1 √7ᵗʰ **T82.332 Leakage of femoral arterial graft (bypass)** HCC

1 √7ᵗʰ **T82.338 Leakage of other vascular grafts** HCC

1 √7ᵗʰ **T82.339 Leakage of unspecified vascular graft** HCC ▽

√6ᵗʰ **T82.39 Other mechanical complication of other vascular grafts**
Obstruction (mechanical) of other vascular grafts
Perforation of other vascular grafts
Protrusion of other vascular grafts

1 √7ᵗʰ **T82.390 Other mechanical complication of aortic (bifurcation) graft (replacement)** HCC

1 √7ᵗʰ **T82.391 Other mechanical complication of carotid arterial graft (bypass)** HCC

1 √7ᵗʰ **T82.392 Other mechanical complication of femoral arterial graft (bypass)** HCC

1 √7ᵗʰ **T82.398 Other mechanical complication of other vascular grafts** HCC

1 √7ᵗʰ **T82.399 Other mechanical complication of unspecified vascular grafts** HCC ▽

√5ᵗʰ **T82.4 Mechanical complication of vascular dialysis catheter**
Mechanical complication of hemodialysis catheter
EXCLUDES 1 *mechanical complication of intraperitoneal dialysis catheter (T85.62)*

√x7ᵗʰ **T82.41 Breakdown (mechanical) of vascular dialysis catheter** HCC

√x7ᵗʰ **T82.42 Displacement of vascular dialysis catheter** HCC
Malposition of vascular dialysis catheter

√x7ᵗʰ **T82.43 Leakage of vascular dialysis catheter** HCC

√x7ᵗʰ **T82.49 Other complication of vascular dialysis catheter** HCC
Obstruction (mechanical) of vascular dialysis catheter
Perforation of vascular dialysis catheter
Protrusion of vascular dialysis catheter

√5ᵗʰ **T82.5 Mechanical complication of other cardiac and vascular devices and implants**
EXCLUDES 2 *mechanical complication of epidural and subdural infusion catheter (T85.61)*

√6ᵗʰ **T82.51 Breakdown (mechanical) of other cardiac and vascular devices and implants**

1 √7ᵗʰ **T82.510 Breakdown (mechanical) of surgically created arteriovenous fistula** HCC

1 √7ᵗʰ **T82.511 Breakdown (mechanical) of surgically created arteriovenous shunt** HCC

√7ᵗʰ **T82.512 Breakdown (mechanical) of artificial heart**

1 √7ᵗʰ **T82.513 Breakdown (mechanical) of balloon (counterpulsation) device** HCC

1 √7ᵗʰ **T82.514 Breakdown (mechanical) of infusion catheter** HCC

1 √7ᵗʰ **T82.515 Breakdown (mechanical) of umbrella device** HCC

---

1 HCC with 7th character indicating initial encounter (A, B or C - specific to category).

1 ✓7ᵗʰ T82.518 **Breakdown (mechanical) of other** HCC
cardiac and vascular devices and implants

✓7ᵗʰ T82.519 **Breakdown (mechanical) of** ▽
unspecified cardiac and vascular
devices and implants

✓6ᵗʰ T82.52 **Displacement of other cardiac and vascular devices**
and implants
Malposition of other cardiac and vascular devices and
implants

1 ✓7ᵗʰ T82.520 **Displacement of surgically created** HCC
arteriovenous fistula

1 ✓7ᵗʰ T82.521 **Displacement of surgically created** HCC
arteriovenous shunt

✓7ᵗʰ T82.522 **Displacement of artificial heart**

1 ✓7ᵗʰ T82.523 **Displacement of balloon** HCC
(counterpulsation) device

1 ✓7ᵗʰ T82.524 **Displacement of infusion catheter** HCC

1 ✓7ᵗʰ T82.525 **Displacement of umbrella device** HCC

1 ✓7ᵗʰ T82.528 **Displacement of other cardiac and** HCC
vascular devices and implants

✓7ᵗʰ T82.529 **Displacement of unspecified cardiac** ▽
and vascular devices and implants

✓6ᵗʰ T82.53 **Leakage of other cardiac and vascular devices and**
implants

1 ✓7ᵗʰ T82.530 **Leakage of surgically created** HCC
arteriovenous fistula

1 ✓7ᵗʰ T82.531 **Leakage of surgically created** HCC
arteriovenous shunt

✓7ᵗʰ T82.532 **Leakage of artificial heart**

1 ✓7ᵗʰ T82.533 **Leakage of balloon (counterpulsation)** HCC
device

1 ✓7ᵗʰ T82.534 **Leakage of infusion catheter** HCC

1 ✓7ᵗʰ T82.535 **Leakage of umbrella device** HCC

1 ✓7ᵗʰ T82.538 **Leakage of other cardiac and** HCC
vascular devices and implants

✓7ᵗʰ T82.539 **Leakage of unspecified cardiac and** ▽
vascular devices and implants

✓6ᵗʰ T82.59 **Other mechanical complication of other cardiac and**
vascular devices and implants
Obstruction (mechanical) of other cardiac and vascular
devices and implants
Perforation of other cardiac and vascular devices and
implants
Protrusion of other cardiac and vascular devices and
implants

1 ✓7ᵗʰ T82.590 **Other mechanical complication of** HCC
surgically created arteriovenous fistula

1 ✓7ᵗʰ T82.591 **Other mechanical complication of** HCC
surgically created arteriovenous shunt

✓7ᵗʰ T82.592 **Other mechanical complication of artificial**
heart

1 ✓7ᵗʰ T82.593 **Other mechanical complication of** HCC
balloon (counterpulsation) device

1 ✓7ᵗʰ T82.594 **Other mechanical complication of** HCC
infusion catheter

1 ✓7ᵗʰ T82.595 **Other mechanical complication of** HCC
umbrella device

1 ✓7ᵗʰ T82.598 **Other mechanical complication of** HCC
other cardiac and vascular devices
and implants

✓7ᵗʰ T82.599 **Other mechanical complication of** ▽
unspecified cardiac and vascular
devices and implants

1 ✓x7ᵗʰ T82.6 **Infection and inflammatory reaction due to cardiac** HCC
valve prosthesis
Use additional code to identify infection

1 ✓x7ᵗʰ T82.7 **Infection and inflammatory reaction due to other** HCC
cardiac and vascular devices, implants and grafts
Use additional code to identify infection

✓5ᵗʰ T82.8 **Other specified complications of cardiac and vascular**
prosthetic devices, implants and grafts

✓6ᵗʰ T82.81 **Embolism due to cardiac and vascular prosthetic**
devices, implants and grafts

✓7ᵗʰ T82.817 **Embolism due to cardiac prosthetic**
devices, implants and grafts

✓7ᵗʰ T82.818 **Embolism due to vascular prosthetic** HCC
devices, implants and grafts

✓6ᵗʰ T82.82 **Fibrosis due to cardiac and vascular prosthetic**
devices, implants and grafts

✓7ᵗʰ T82.827 **Fibrosis due to cardiac prosthetic devices,**
implants and grafts

1 ✓7ᵗʰ T82.828 **Fibrosis due to vascular prosthetic** HCC
devices, implants and grafts

✓6ᵗʰ T82.83 **Hemorrhage due to cardiac and vascular prosthetic**
devices, implants and grafts

✓7ᵗʰ T82.837 **Hemorrhage due to cardiac prosthetic**
devices, implants and grafts

1 ✓7ᵗʰ T82.838 **Hemorrhage due to vascular** HCC
prosthetic devices, implants and grafts

✓6ᵗʰ T82.84 **Pain due to cardiac and vascular prosthetic devices,**
implants and grafts

✓7ᵗʰ T82.847 **Pain due to cardiac prosthetic devices,**
implants and grafts

1 ✓7ᵗʰ T82.848 **Pain due to vascular prosthetic** HCC
devices, implants and grafts

✓6ᵗʰ T82.85 **Stenosis due to cardiac and vascular prosthetic**
devices, implants and grafts

✓7ᵗʰ T82.855 **Stenosis of coronary artery stent**
In-stent stenosis (restenosis) of coronary
artery stent
Restenosis of coronary artery stent

1 ✓7ᵗʰ T82.856 **Stenosis of peripheral vascular stent** HCC
In-stent stenosis (restenosis) of peripheral
vascular stent
Restenosis of peripheral vascular stent

✓7ᵗʰ T82.857 **Stenosis of other cardiac prosthetic**
devices, implants and grafts

1 ✓7ᵗʰ T82.858 **Stenosis of other vascular prosthetic** HCC
devices, implants and grafts

✓6ᵗʰ T82.86 **Thrombosis of cardiac and vascular prosthetic**
devices, implants and grafts

✓7ᵗʰ T82.867 **Thrombosis due to cardiac prosthetic**
devices, implants and grafts

1 ✓7ᵗʰ T82.868 **Thrombosis due to vascular prosthetic** HCC
devices, implants and grafts

✓6ᵗʰ T82.89 **Other specified complication of cardiac and vascular**
prosthetic devices, implants and grafts

✓7ᵗʰ T82.897 **Other specified complication of**
cardiac prosthetic devices, implants
and grafts

1 ✓7ᵗʰ T82.898 **Other specified complication of** HCC
vascular prosthetic devices, implants
and grafts

✓x7ᵗʰ T82.9 **Unspecified complication of cardiac and vascular** ▽
prosthetic device, implant and graft

✓4ᵗʰ T83 **Complications of genitourinary prosthetic devices, implants and**
grafts
EXCLUDES 2 *failure and rejection of transplanted organs and tissue (T86.-)*

> The appropriate 7th character is to be added to each code from
> category T83.
> A   initial encounter
> D   subsequent encounter
> S   sequela

✓5ᵗʰ T83.0 **Mechanical complication of** urinary catheter
EXCLUDES 2 *complications of stoma of urinary tract (N99.5-)*

✓6ᵗʰ T83.01 **Breakdown (mechanical) of urinary catheter**

1 ✓7ᵗʰ T83.010 **Breakdown (mechanical) of** HCC
cystostomy catheter

1 ✓7ᵗʰ T83.011 **Breakdown (mechanical) of** HCC
indwelling urethral catheter

1 ✓7ᵗʰ T83.012 **Breakdown (mechanical) of** HCC
nephrostomy catheter

1 ✓7ᵗʰ T83.018 **Breakdown (mechanical) of other** HCC
urinary catheter
Breakdown (mechanical) of Hopkins
catheter
Breakdown (mechanical) of ileostomy
catheter
Breakdown (mechanical) urostomy
catheter

---

1 HCC with 7th character indicating initial encounter (A, B or C - specific to category).

✓ Additional Character Req   ✓x7ᵗʰ Placeholder Alert   Manifestation   HCC CMS-HCC Condition   ▽ Unspecified Code   ▶◀ Revised Text   ● New Code   ▲ Revised Code Title

ICD-10-CM 2018   1101

√6ᵗʰ **T83.02 Displacement of urinary catheter**
Malposition of urinary catheter

1 √7ᵗʰ **T83.020 Displacement of cystostomy catheter** HCC

1 √7ᵗʰ **T83.021 Displacement of indwelling urethral catheter** HCC

1 √7ᵗʰ **T83.022 Displacement of nephrostomy catheter** HCC

1 √7ᵗʰ **T83.028 Displacement of other urinary catheter** HCC
Displacement of Hopkins catheter
Displacement of ileostomy catheter
Displacement of urostomy catheter

√6ᵗʰ **T83.03 Leakage of urinary catheter**

1 √7ᵗʰ **T83.030 Leakage of cystostomy catheter** HCC

1 √7ᵗʰ **T83.031 Leakage of indwelling urethral catheter** HCC

1 √7ᵗʰ **T83.032 Leakage of nephrostomy catheter** HCC

1 √7ᵗʰ **T83.038 Leakage of other urinary catheter** HCC
Leakage of Hopkins catheter
Leakage of ileostomy catheter
Leakage of urostomy catheter

√6ᵗʰ **T83.09 Other mechanical complication of urinary catheter**
Obstruction (mechanical) of urinary catheter
Perforation of urinary catheter
Protrusion of urinary catheter

1 √7ᵗʰ **T83.090 Other mechanical complication of cystostomy catheter** HCC

1 √7ᵗʰ **T83.091 Other mechanical complication of indwelling urethral catheter** HCC

1 √7ᵗʰ **T83.092 Other mechanical complication of nephrostomy catheter** HCC

1 √7ᵗʰ **T83.098 Other mechanical complication of other urinary catheter** HCC
Other mechanical complication of Hopkins catheter
Other mechanical complication of ileostomy catheter
Other mechanical complication of urostomy catheter

√5ᵗʰ **T83.1 Mechanical complication of other urinary devices and implants**

√6ᵗʰ **T83.11 Breakdown (mechanical) of other urinary devices and implants**

1 √7ᵗʰ **T83.110 Breakdown (mechanical) of urinary electronic stimulator device** HCC
EXCLUDES 2 *breakdown (mechanical) of electrode (lead) for sacral nerve neurostimulator (T85.111)*
breakdown (mechanical) of implanted electronic sacral neurostimulator, pulse generator or receiver (T85.113)

1 √7ᵗʰ **T83.111 Breakdown (mechanical) of implanted urinary sphincter** HCC

1 √7ᵗʰ **T83.112 Breakdown (mechanical) of indwelling ureteral stent** HCC

1 √7ᵗʰ **T83.113 Breakdown (mechanical) of other urinary stents** HCC
Breakdown (mechanical) of ileal conduit stent
Breakdown (mechanical) of nephroureteral stent

1 √7ᵗʰ **T83.118 Breakdown (mechanical) of other urinary devices and implants** HCC

√6ᵗʰ **T83.12 Displacement of other urinary devices and implants**
Malposition of other urinary devices and implants

1 √7ᵗʰ **T83.120 Displacement of urinary electronic stimulator device** HCC
EXCLUDES 2 *displacement of electrode (lead) for sacral nerve neurostimulator (T85.121)*
displacement of implanted electronic sacral neurostimulator, pulse generator or receiver (T85.123/0

1 √7ᵗʰ **T83.121 Displacement of implanted urinary sphincter** HCC

1 √7ᵗʰ **T83.122 Displacement of indwelling ureteral stent** HCC

1 √7ᵗʰ **T83.123 Displacement of other urinary stents** HCC
Displacement of ileal conduit stent
Displacement of nephroureteral stent

1 √7ᵗʰ **T83.128 Displacement of other urinary devices and implants** HCC

√6ᵗʰ **T83.19 Other mechanical complication of other urinary devices and implants**
Leakage of other urinary devices and implants
Obstruction (mechanical) of other urinary devices and implants
Perforation of other urinary devices and implants
Protrusion of other urinary devices and implants

1 √7ᵗʰ **T83.190 Other mechanical complication of urinary electronic stimulator device** HCC
EXCLUDES 2 *other mechanical complication of electrode (lead) for sacral nerve neurostimulator (T85.191)*
other mechanical complication of implanted electronic sacral neurostimulator, pulse generator or receiver (T85.193)

1 √7ᵗʰ **T83.191 Other mechanical complication of implanted urinary sphincter** HCC

1 √7ᵗʰ **T83.192 Other mechanical complication of indwelling ureteral stent** HCC

1 √7ᵗʰ **T83.193 Other mechanical complication of other urinary stent** HCC
Other mechanical complication of ileal conduit stent
Other mechanical complication of nephroureteral stent

1 √7ᵗʰ **T83.198 Other mechanical complication of other urinary devices and implants** HCC

√5ᵗʰ **T83.2 Mechanical complication of graft of urinary organ**

1 √x7ᵗʰ **T83.21 Breakdown (mechanical) of graft of urinary organ** HCC

1 √x7ᵗʰ **T83.22 Displacement of graft of urinary organ** HCC
Malposition of graft of urinary organ

1 √x7ᵗʰ **T83.23 Leakage of graft of urinary organ** HCC

1 √x7ᵗʰ **T83.24 Erosion of graft of urinary organ** HCC

1 √x7ᵗʰ **T83.25 Exposure of graft of urinary organ** HCC

1 √x7ᵗʰ **T83.29 Other mechanical complication of graft of urinary organ** HCC
Obstruction (mechanical) of graft of urinary organ
Perforation of graft of urinary organ
Protrusion of graft of urinary organ

√5ᵗʰ **T83.3 Mechanical complication of intrauterine contraceptive device**

√x7ᵗʰ **T83.31 Breakdown (mechanical) of intrauterine contraceptive device** ♀

√x7ᵗʰ **T83.32 Displacement of intrauterine contraceptive device** ♀
Malposition of intrauterine contraceptive device
Missing string of intrauterine contraceptive device

√x7ᵗʰ **T83.39 Other mechanical complication of intrauterine contraceptive device** ♀
Leakage of intrauterine contraceptive device
Obstruction (mechanical) of intrauterine contraceptive device
Perforation of intrauterine contraceptive device
Protrusion of intrauterine contraceptive device

√5ᵗʰ **T83.4 Mechanical complication of other prosthetic devices, implants and grafts of genital tract**

√6ᵗʰ **T83.41 Breakdown (mechanical) of other prosthetic devices, implants and grafts of genital tract**

1 √7ᵗʰ **T83.410 Breakdown (mechanical) of implanted penile prosthesis** HCC♂
Breakdown (mechanical) of penile prosthesis cylinder
Breakdown (mechanical) of penile prosthesis pump
Breakdown (mechanical) of penile prosthesis reservoir

1 √7ᵗʰ **T83.411 Breakdown (mechanical) of implanted testicular prosthesis** HCC

1 HCC with 7th character indicating initial encounter (A, B or C - specific to category).

1 ✓7ᵗʰ **T83.418 Breakdown (mechanical) of other** HCC
prosthetic devices, implants and
grafts of genital tract

✓6ᵗʰ **T83.42 Displacement of other prosthetic devices, implants**
and grafts of genital tract
Malposition of other prosthetic devices, implants and
grafts of genital tract

1 ✓7ᵗʰ **T83.420 Displacement of implanted penile** HCC ♂
prosthesis
Displacement of penile prosthesis cylinder
Displacement of penile prosthesis pump
Displacement of penile prosthesis reservoir

1 ✓7ᵗʰ **T83.421 Displacement of implanted testicular** HCC
prosthesis

1 ✓7ᵗʰ **T83.428 Displacement of other prosthetic** HCC
devices, implants and grafts of
genital tract

✓6ᵗʰ **T83.49 Other mechanical complication of other prosthetic**
devices, implants and grafts of genital tract
Leakage of other prosthetic devices, implants and
grafts of genital tract
Obstruction, mechanical of other prosthetic devices,
implants and grafts of genital tract
Perforation of other prosthetic devices, implants and
grafts of genital tract
Protrusion of other prosthetic devices, implants and
grafts of genital tract

1 ✓7ᵗʰ **T83.490 Other mechanical complication of** HCC ♂
implanted penile prosthesis
Other mechanical complication of penile
prosthesis cylinder
Other mechanical complication of penile
prosthesis pump
Other mechanical complication of penile
prosthesis reservoir

1 ✓7ᵗʰ **T83.491 Other mechanical complication of** HCC
implanted testicular prosthesis

1 ✓7ᵗʰ **T83.498 Other mechanical complication of** HCC
other prosthetic devices, implants
and grafts of genital tract

✓5ᵗʰ **T83.5 Infection and inflammatory reaction due to prosthetic device,**
implant and graft in urinary system
Use additional code to identify infection

✓6ᵗʰ **T83.51 Infection and inflammatory reaction due to urinary**
catheter
EXCLUDES 2   *complications of stoma of urinary tract*
(N99.5-)

1 ✓7ᵗʰ **T83.510 Infection and inflammatory reaction** HCC
due to cystostomy catheter

1 ✓7ᵗʰ **T83.511 Infection and inflammatory reaction** HCC
due to indwelling urethral catheter

1 ✓7ᵗʰ **T83.512 Infection and inflammatory reaction** HCC
due to nephrostomy catheter

1 ✓7ᵗʰ **T83.518 Infection and inflammatory reaction** HCC
due to other urinary catheter
Infection and inflammatory reaction due to
Hopkins catheter
Infection and inflammatory reaction due to
ileostomy catheter
Infection and inflammatory reaction due to
urostomy catheter

✓6ᵗʰ **T83.59 Infection and inflammatory reaction due to**
prosthetic device, implant and graft in urinary
system

1 ✓7ᵗʰ **T83.590 Infection and inflammatory reaction** HCC
due to implanted urinary
neurostimulation device
EXCLUDES 2   *infection and inflammatory*
reaction due to electrode
lead of sacral nerve
neurostimulator (T85.732)
infection and inflammatory reac-
tion due to pulse generator
or receiver of sacral nerve
neurostimulator (T85.734)

1 ✓7ᵗʰ **T83.591 Infection and inflammatory reaction** HCC
due to implanted urinary sphincter

1 ✓7ᵗʰ **T83.592 Infection and inflammatory reaction** HCC
due to indwelling ureteral stent

1 ✓7ᵗʰ **T83.593 Infection and inflammatory reaction** HCC
due to other urinary stents
Infection and inflammatory reaction due to
ileal conduit stents
Infection and inflammatory reaction due to
nephroureteral stent

1 ✓7ᵗʰ **T83.598 Infection and inflammatory reaction** HCC
due to other prosthetic device, implant
and graft in urinary system

✓5ᵗʰ **T83.6 Infection and inflammatory reaction due to prosthetic device,**
implant and graft in genital tract
Use additional code to identify infection

1 ✓x7ᵗʰ **T83.61 Infection and inflammatory reaction due to** HCC
implanted penile prosthesis
Infection and inflammatory reaction due to penile
prosthesis cylinder
Infection and inflammatory reaction due to penile
prosthesis pump
Infection and inflammatory reaction due to penile
prosthesis reservoir

1 ✓x7ᵗʰ **T83.62 Infection and inflammatory reaction due to** HCC
implanted testicular prosthesis

1 ✓x7ᵗʰ **T83.69 Infection and inflammatory reaction due to** HCC
other prosthetic device, implant and graft in
genital tract

✓5ᵗʰ **T83.7 Complications due to implanted mesh and other prosthetic**
materials

✓6ᵗʰ **T83.71 Erosion of implanted mesh and other prosthetic**
materials to surrounding organ or tissue

1 ✓7ᵗʰ **T83.711 Erosion of implanted vaginal mesh** HCC ♀
to surrounding organ or tissue
Erosion of implanted vaginal mesh into
pelvic floor muscles

1 ✓7ᵗʰ **T83.712 Erosion of implanted urethral mesh** HCC
to surrounding organ or tissue
Erosion of implanted female urethral sling
Erosion of implanted male urethral sling
Erosion of implanted urethral mesh into
pelvic floor muscles

1 ✓7ᵗʰ **T83.713 Erosion of implanted urethral bulking** HCC
agent to surrounding organ or tissue

1 ✓7ᵗʰ **T83.714 Erosion of implanted ureteral bulking** HCC
agent to surrounding organ or tissue

1 ✓7ᵗʰ **T83.718 Erosion of other implanted mesh to** HCC
organ or tissue

1 ✓7ᵗʰ **T83.719 Erosion of other prosthetic materials** HCC
to surrounding organ or tissue

✓6ᵗʰ **T83.72 Exposure of implanted mesh and other prosthetic**
materials into surrounding organ or tissue
Extrusion of implanted mesh

1 ✓7ᵗʰ **T83.721 Exposure of implanted vaginal** HCC ♀
mesh into vagina
Exposure of implanted vaginal mesh
through vaginal wall

1 ✓7ᵗʰ **T83.722 Exposure of implanted urethral** HCC
mesh into urethra
Exposure of implanted female urethral
sling
Exposure of implanted male urethral sling
Exposure of implanted urethral mesh
through urethral wall

1 ✓7ᵗʰ **T83.723 Exposure of implanted urethral** HCC
bulking agent into urethra

1 ✓7ᵗʰ **T83.724 Exposure of implanted ureteral** HCC
bulking agent into ureter

1 ✓7ᵗʰ **T83.728 Exposure of other implanted mesh** HCC
into organ or tissue

1 ✓7ᵗʰ **T83.729 Exposure of other prosthetic** HCC
materials into organ or tissue

1 ✓x7ᵗʰ **T83.79 Other specified complications due to other** HCC
genitourinary prosthetic materials

✓5ᵗʰ **T83.8 Other specified complications of genitourinary prosthetic**
devices, implants and grafts

1 ✓x7ᵗʰ **T83.81 Embolism due to genitourinary prosthetic** HCC
devices, implants and grafts

1 ✓x7ᵗʰ **T83.82 Fibrosis due to genitourinary prosthetic** HCC
devices, implants and grafts

---

1 HCC with 7th character indicating initial encounter (A, B or C - specific to category).

✓ Additional Character Req   ✓x7ᵗʰ Placeholder Alert   Manifestation   HCC CMS-HCC Condition   ▽ Unspecified Code   ▶◀ Revised Text   ● New Code   ▲ Revised Code Title

Chapter 19. Injury, Poisoning, and Certain Other Consequences of External Causes

¹ ✓x7ᵗʰ **T83.83** **Hemorrhage due to genitourinary prosthetic devices, implants and grafts** `HCC`

¹ ✓x7ᵗʰ **T83.84** **Pain due to genitourinary prosthetic devices, implants and grafts** `HCC`

¹ ✓x7ᵗʰ **T83.85** **Stenosis due to genitourinary prosthetic devices, implants and grafts** `HCC`

¹ ✓x7ᵗʰ **T83.86** **Thrombosis due to genitourinary prosthetic devices, implants and grafts** `HCC`

¹ ✓x7ᵗʰ **T83.89** **Other specified complication of genitourinary prosthetic devices, implants and grafts** `HCC`

¹ ✓x7ᵗʰ **T83.9** **Unspecified complication of genitourinary prosthetic device, implant and graft** `HCC` ▽

✓4ᵗʰ **T84** **Complications of internal orthopedic prosthetic devices, implants and grafts**

     EXCLUDES 2   *failure and rejection of transplanted organs and tissues (T86.-)*
               fracture of bone following insertion of orthopedic implant, joint prosthesis or bone plate (M96.6)

> The appropriate 7th character is to be added to each code from category T84.
> A   initial encounter
> D   subsequent encounter
> S   sequela

✓5ᵗʰ **T84.0** **Mechanical complication of internal joint prosthesis**

   ✓6ᵗʰ **T84.01** **Broken internal joint prosthesis**
         Breakage (fracture) of prosthetic joint
         Broken prosthetic joint implant
          EXCLUDES 1   *periprosthetic joint implant fracture ►(M97-)◄*

     ¹ ✓7ᵗʰ **T84.010** Broken internal **right hip** prosthesis `HCC`
     ¹ ✓7ᵗʰ **T84.011** Broken internal **left hip** prosthesis `HCC`
     ¹ ✓7ᵗʰ **T84.012** Broken internal **right knee** prosthesis `HCC`
     ¹ ✓7ᵗʰ **T84.013** Broken internal **left knee** prosthesis `HCC`
     ¹ ✓7ᵗʰ **T84.018** Broken internal joint prosthesis, **other site** `HCC`
           Use additional code to identify the joint (Z96.6-)
     ✓7ᵗʰ **T84.019** Broken internal joint prosthesis, **unspecified site** `HCC` ▽

   ✓6ᵗʰ **T84.02** **Dislocation of internal joint prosthesis**
         Instability of internal joint prosthesis
         Subluxation of internal joint prosthesis

     ¹ ✓7ᵗʰ **T84.020** Dislocation of internal **right hip** prosthesis `HCC`
     ¹ ✓7ᵗʰ **T84.021** Dislocation of internal **left hip** prosthesis `HCC`
     ¹ ✓7ᵗʰ **T84.022** Instability of internal **right knee** prosthesis `HCC`
     ¹ ✓7ᵗʰ **T84.023** Instability of internal **left knee** prosthesis `HCC`
     ¹ ✓7ᵗʰ **T84.028** Dislocation of other internal joint prosthesis `HCC`
           Use additional code to identify the joint (Z96.6-)
     ¹ ✓7ᵗʰ **T84.029** Dislocation of unspecified internal joint prosthesis `HCC` ▽

   ✓6ᵗʰ **T84.03** **Mechanical loosening of internal prosthetic joint**
         Aseptic loosening of prosthetic joint

     ¹ ✓7ᵗʰ **T84.030** Mechanical loosening of internal **right hip** prosthetic joint `HCC`
     ¹ ✓7ᵗʰ **T84.031** Mechanical loosening of internal **left hip** prosthetic joint `HCC`
     ¹ ✓7ᵗʰ **T84.032** Mechanical loosening of internal **right knee** prosthetic joint `HCC`
     ¹ ✓7ᵗʰ **T84.033** Mechanical loosening of internal **left knee** prosthetic joint `HCC`
     ¹ ✓7ᵗʰ **T84.038** Mechanical loosening of other internal prosthetic joint `HCC`
           Use additional code to identify the joint (Z96.6-)
     ¹ ✓7ᵗʰ **T84.039** Mechanical loosening of unspecified internal prosthetic joint `HCC` ▽

✓6ᵗʰ **T84.05** **Periprosthetic osteolysis of internal prosthetic joint**
     Use additional code to identify major osseous defect, if applicable (M89.7-)

   ¹ ✓7ᵗʰ **T84.050** Periprosthetic osteolysis of internal prosthetic **right hip joint** `HCC`
   ¹ ✓7ᵗʰ **T84.051** Periprosthetic osteolysis of internal prosthetic **left hip joint** `HCC`
   ¹ ✓7ᵗʰ **T84.052** Periprosthetic osteolysis of internal prosthetic **right knee joint** `HCC`
   ¹ ✓7ᵗʰ **T84.053** Periprosthetic osteolysis of internal prosthetic **left knee joint** `HCC`
   ¹ ✓7ᵗʰ **T84.058** Periprosthetic osteolysis of other internal prosthetic joint `HCC`
        Use additional code to identify the joint (Z96.6-)
   ¹ ✓7ᵗʰ **T84.059** Periprosthetic osteolysis of unspecified internal prosthetic joint `HCC` ▽

✓6ᵗʰ **T84.06** **Wear of articular bearing surface of internal prosthetic joint**

   ¹ ✓7ᵗʰ **T84.060** Wear of articular bearing surface of internal prosthetic **right hip joint** `HCC`
   ¹ ✓7ᵗʰ **T84.061** Wear of articular bearing surface of internal prosthetic **left hip joint** `HCC`
   ¹ ✓7ᵗʰ **T84.062** Wear of articular bearing surface of internal prosthetic **right knee joint** `HCC`
   ¹ ✓7ᵗʰ **T84.063** Wear of articular bearing surface of internal prosthetic **left knee joint** `HCC`
   ¹ ✓7ᵗʰ **T84.068** Wear of articular bearing surface of other internal prosthetic joint `HCC`
        Use additional code to identify the joint (Z96.6-)
   ¹ ✓7ᵗʰ **T84.069** Wear of articular bearing surface of unspecified internal prosthetic joint `HCC` ▽

✓6ᵗʰ **T84.09** **Other mechanical complication of internal joint prosthesis**
     Prosthetic joint implant failure NOS

   ¹ ✓7ᵗʰ **T84.090** Other mechanical complication of **internal right hip prosthesis** `HCC`
   ¹ ✓7ᵗʰ **T84.091** Other mechanical complication of **internal left hip prosthesis** `HCC`
   ¹ ✓7ᵗʰ **T84.092** Other mechanical complication of **internal right knee prosthesis** `HCC`
   ¹ ✓7ᵗʰ **T84.093** Other mechanical complication of **internal left knee prosthesis** `HCC`
   ¹ ✓7ᵗʰ **T84.098** Other mechanical complication of **other internal joint prosthesis** `HCC`
        Use additional code to identify the joint (Z96.6-)
   ¹ ✓7ᵗʰ **T84.099** Other mechanical complication of **unspecified internal joint prosthesis** `HCC` ▽

✓5ᵗʰ **T84.1** **Mechanical complication of internal fixation device of bones of limb**
     EXCLUDES 2   *mechanical complication of internal fixation device of bones of feet (T84.2-)*
            mechanical complication of internal fixation device of bones of fingers (T84.2-)
            mechanical complication of internal fixation device of bones of hands (T84.2-)
            mechanical complication of internal fixation device of bones of toes (T84.2-)

   ✓6ᵗʰ **T84.11** **Breakdown (mechanical) of internal fixation device of bones of limb**

     ¹ ✓7ᵗʰ **T84.110** Breakdown (mechanical) of internal fixation device of **right humerus** `HCC`
     ¹ ✓7ᵗʰ **T84.111** Breakdown (mechanical) of internal fixation device of **left humerus** `HCC`
     ¹ ✓7ᵗʰ **T84.112** Breakdown (mechanical) of internal fixation device of bone of **right forearm** `HCC`
     ¹ ✓7ᵗʰ **T84.113** Breakdown (mechanical) of internal fixation device of bone of **left forearm** `HCC`
     ¹ ✓7ᵗʰ **T84.114** Breakdown (mechanical) of internal fixation device of **right femur** `HCC`
     ¹ ✓7ᵗʰ **T84.115** Breakdown (mechanical) of internal fixation device of **left femur** `HCC`
     ¹ ✓7ᵗʰ **T84.116** Breakdown (mechanical) of internal fixation device of bone of **right lower leg** `HCC`

---

¹   HCC with 7th character indicating initial encounter (A, B or C - specific to category).

EXCLUDES 1 Not coded here   **EXCLUDES 2** Not included here   **N** Newborn Age: 0   **P** Pediatric Age: 0-17   **M** Maternity Age: 12-55   **A** Adult Age: 15-124

1104   ICD-10-CM 2018

T83.83–T84.116

1 ✓7ᵗʰ **T84.117 Breakdown (mechanical) of internal** HCC
fixation device of bone of left lower leg

1 ✓7ᵗʰ **T84.119 Breakdown (mechanical) of** HCC ▽
internal fixation device of
unspecified bone of limb

✓6ᵗʰ **T84.12 Displacement of internal fixation device of bones of**
limb
Malposition of internal fixation device of bones of limb

1 ✓7ᵗʰ **T84.120 Displacement of internal fixation** HCC
device of right humerus

1 ✓7ᵗʰ **T84.121 Displacement of internal fixation** HCC
device of left humerus

1 ✓7ᵗʰ **T84.122 Displacement of internal fixation** HCC
device of bone of right forearm

1 ✓7ᵗʰ **T84.123 Displacement of internal fixation** HCC
device of bone of left forearm

1 ✓7ᵗʰ **T84.124 Displacement of internal fixation** HCC
device of right femur

1 ✓7ᵗʰ **T84.125 Displacement of internal fixation** HCC
device of left femur

1 ✓7ᵗʰ **T84.126 Displacement of internal fixation** HCC
device of bone of right lower leg

1 ✓7ᵗʰ **T84.127 Displacement of internal fixation** HCC
device of bone of left lower leg

1 ✓7ᵗʰ **T84.129 Displacement of internal fixation** HCC ▽
device of unspecified bone of limb

✓6ᵗʰ **T84.19 Other mechanical complication of internal fixation**
device of bones of limb
Obstruction (mechanical) of internal fixation device of
bones of limb
Perforation of internal fixation device of bones of limb
Protrusion of internal fixation device of bones of limb

1 ✓7ᵗʰ **T84.190 Other mechanical complication of** HCC
internal fixation device of right humerus

1 ✓7ᵗʰ **T84.191 Other mechanical complication of** HCC
internal fixation device of left humerus

1 ✓7ᵗʰ **T84.192 Other mechanical complication of** HCC
internal fixation device of bone of right
forearm

1 ✓7ᵗʰ **T84.193 Other mechanical complication of** HCC
internal fixation device of bone of left
forearm

1 ✓7ᵗʰ **T84.194 Other mechanical complication of** HCC
internal fixation device of right femur

1 ✓7ᵗʰ **T84.195 Other mechanical complication of** HCC
internal fixation device of left femur

1 ✓7ᵗʰ **T84.196 Other mechanical complication of** HCC
internal fixation device of bone of right
lower leg

1 ✓7ᵗʰ **T84.197 Other mechanical complication of** HCC
internal fixation device of bone of left
lower leg

1 ✓7ᵗʰ **T84.199 Other mechanical complication of** HCC ▽
internal fixation device of unspecified
bone of limb

✓5ᵗʰ **T84.2 Mechanical complication of internal fixation device of other**
bones

✓6ᵗʰ **T84.21 Breakdown (mechanical) of internal fixation device**
of other bones

1 ✓7ᵗʰ **T84.210 Breakdown (mechanical) of internal** HCC
fixation device of bones of hand and
fingers

1 ✓7ᵗʰ **T84.213 Breakdown (mechanical) of internal** HCC
fixation device of bones of foot and toes

1 ✓7ᵗʰ **T84.216 Breakdown (mechanical) of internal** HCC
fixation device of vertebrae

1 ✓7ᵗʰ **T84.218 Breakdown (mechanical) of internal** HCC
fixation device of other bones

✓6ᵗʰ **T84.22 Displacement of internal fixation device of other**
bones
Malposition of internal fixation device of other bones

1 ✓7ᵗʰ **T84.220 Displacement of internal fixation** HCC
device of bones of hand and fingers

1 ✓7ᵗʰ **T84.223 Displacement of internal fixation** HCC
device of bones of foot and toes

1 ✓7ᵗʰ **T84.226 Displacement of internal fixation** HCC
device of vertebrae

1 ✓7ᵗʰ **T84.228 Displacement of internal fixation** HCC
device of other bones

✓6ᵗʰ **T84.29 Other mechanical complication of internal fixation**
device of other bones
Obstruction (mechanical) of internal fixation device of
other bones
Perforation of internal fixation device of other bones
Protrusion of internal fixation device of other bones

1 ✓7ᵗʰ **T84.290 Other mechanical complication of** HCC
internal fixation device of bones of
hand and fingers

1 ✓7ᵗʰ **T84.293 Other mechanical complication of** HCC
internal fixation device of bones of
foot and toes

1 ✓7ᵗʰ **T84.296 Other mechanical complication of** HCC
internal fixation device of vertebrae

1 ✓7ᵗʰ **T84.298 Other mechanical complication of** HCC
internal fixation device of other bones

✓5ᵗʰ **T84.3 Mechanical complication of other bone devices, implants and**
grafts
EXCLUDES 2   *other complications of bone graft (T86.83-)*

✓6ᵗʰ **T84.31 Breakdown (mechanical) of other bone devices,**
implants and grafts

1 ✓7ᵗʰ **T84.310 Breakdown (mechanical) of** HCC
electronic bone stimulator

1 ✓7ᵗʰ **T84.318 Breakdown (mechanical) of other** HCC
bone devices, implants and grafts

✓6ᵗʰ **T84.32 Displacement of other bone devices, implants and**
grafts
Malposition of other bone devices, implants and grafts

1 ✓7ᵗʰ **T84.320 Displacement of electronic bone** HCC
stimulator

1 ✓7ᵗʰ **T84.328 Displacement of other bone devices,** HCC
implants and grafts
AHA: 2014, 4Q, 28

✓6ᵗʰ **T84.39 Other mechanical complication of other bone**
devices, implants and grafts
Obstruction (mechanical) of other bone devices,
implants and grafts
Perforation of other bone devices, implants and grafts
Protrusion of other bone devices, implants and grafts

1 ✓7ᵗʰ **T84.390 Other mechanical complication of** HCC
electronic bone stimulator

1 ✓7ᵗʰ **T84.398 Other mechanical complication of** HCC
other bone devices, implants and grafts

✓5ᵗʰ **T84.4 Mechanical complication of other internal orthopedic**
devices, implants and grafts

✓6ᵗʰ **T84.41 Breakdown (mechanical) of other internal**
orthopedic devices, implants and grafts

1 ✓7ᵗʰ **T84.410 Breakdown (mechanical) of muscle** HCC
and tendon graft

1 ✓7ᵗʰ **T84.418 Breakdown (mechanical) of other** HCC
internal orthopedic devices, implants
and grafts

✓6ᵗʰ **T84.42 Displacement of other internal orthopedic devices,**
implants and grafts
Malposition of other internal orthopedic devices,
implants and grafts

1 ✓7ᵗʰ **T84.420 Displacement of muscle and tendon** HCC
graft

1 ✓7ᵗʰ **T84.428 Displacement of other internal** HCC
orthopedic devices, implants and grafts

✓6ᵗʰ **T84.49 Other mechanical complication of other internal**
orthopedic devices, implants and grafts
Mechanical complication of other internal orthopedic
devices, implants and grafts NOS
Obstruction (mechanical) of other internal orthopedic
devices, implants and grafts
Perforation of other internal orthopedic devices,
implants and grafts
Protrusion of other internal orthopedic devices,
implants and grafts

1 ✓7ᵗʰ **T84.490 Other mechanical complication of** HCC
muscle and tendon graft

1 ✓7ᵗʰ **T84.498 Other mechanical complication of** HCC
other internal orthopedic devices,
implants and grafts

---

1   HCC with 7th character indicating initial encounter (A, B or C - specific to category).

☑ Additional Character Req   ✓x7ᵗʰ Placeholder Alert   Manifestation   HCC CMS-HCC Condition   ▽ Unspecified Code   ►◄ Revised Text   ● New Code   ▲ Revised Code Title

ICD-10-CM 2018   1105

T84.117–T84.498

√5th **T84.5   Infection and inflammatory reaction due to internal joint prosthesis**
> Use additional code to identify infection
> **AHA:** 2015, 1Q, 16

1 √x7th **T84.50   Infection and inflammatory reaction due to unspecified internal joint prosthesis** HCC ▽

1 √x7th **T84.51   Infection and inflammatory reaction due to internal right hip prosthesis** HCC

1 √x7th **T84.52   Infection and inflammatory reaction due to internal left hip prosthesis** HCC

1 √x7th **T84.53   Infection and inflammatory reaction due to internal right knee prosthesis** HCC

1 √x7th **T84.54   Infection and inflammatory reaction due to internal left knee prosthesis** HCC

1 √x7th **T84.59   Infection and inflammatory reaction due to other internal joint prosthesis** HCC

√5th **T84.6   Infection and inflammatory reaction due to internal fixation device**
> Use additional code to identify infection

1 √x7th **T84.60   Infection and inflammatory reaction due to internal fixation device of unspecified site** HCC ▽

√6th **T84.61   Infection and inflammatory reaction due to internal fixation device of arm**

1 √7th **T84.610   Infection and inflammatory reaction due to internal fixation device of right humerus** HCC

1 √7th **T84.611   Infection and inflammatory reaction due to internal fixation device of left humerus** HCC

1 √7th **T84.612   Infection and inflammatory reaction due to internal fixation device of right radius** HCC

1 √7th **T84.613   Infection and inflammatory reaction due to internal fixation device of left radius** HCC

1 √7th **T84.614   Infection and inflammatory reaction due to internal fixation device of right ulna** HCC

1 √7th **T84.615   Infection and inflammatory reaction due to internal fixation device of left ulna** HCC

1 √7th **T84.619   Infection and inflammatory reaction due to internal fixation device of unspecified bone of arm** HCC ▽

√6th **T84.62   Infection and inflammatory reaction due to internal fixation device of leg**

1 √7th **T84.620   Infection and inflammatory reaction due to internal fixation device of right femur** HCC

1 √7th **T84.621   Infection and inflammatory reaction due to internal fixation device of left femur** HCC

1 √7th **T84.622   Infection and inflammatory reaction due to internal fixation device of right tibia** HCC

1 √7th **T84.623   Infection and inflammatory reaction due to internal fixation device of left tibia** HCC

1 √7th **T84.624   Infection and inflammatory reaction due to internal fixation device of right fibula** HCC

1 √7th **T84.625   Infection and inflammatory reaction due to internal fixation device of left fibula** HCC

1 √7th **T84.629   Infection and inflammatory reaction due to internal fixation device of unspecified bone of leg** HCC ▽

1 √x7th **T84.63   Infection and inflammatory reaction due to internal fixation device of spine** HCC

1 √x7th **T84.69   Infection and inflammatory reaction due to internal fixation device of other site** HCC

1 √x7th **T84.7   Infection and inflammatory reaction due to other internal orthopedic prosthetic devices, implants and grafts** HCC
> Use additional code to identify infection

√5th **T84.8   Other specified complications of internal orthopedic prosthetic devices, implants and grafts**

1 √x7th **T84.81   Embolism due to internal orthopedic prosthetic devices, implants and grafts** HCC

1 √x7th **T84.82   Fibrosis due to internal orthopedic prosthetic devices, implants and grafts** HCC

1 √x7th **T84.83   Hemorrhage due to internal orthopedic prosthetic devices, implants and grafts** HCC

1 √x7th **T84.84   Pain due to internal orthopedic prosthetic devices, implants and grafts** HCC

1 √x7th **T84.85   Stenosis due to internal orthopedic prosthetic devices, implants and grafts** HCC

1 √x7th **T84.86   Thrombosis due to internal orthopedic prosthetic devices, implants and grafts** HCC

1 √x7th **T84.89   Other specified complication of internal orthopedic prosthetic devices, implants and grafts** HCC

1 √x7th **T84.9   Unspecified complication of internal orthopedic prosthetic device, implant and graft** HCC ▽

√4th **T85   Complications of other internal prosthetic devices, implants and grafts**

> EXCLUDES 2   *failure and rejection of transplanted organs and tissue (T86.-)*

> The appropriate 7th character is to be added to each code from category T85.
> A   initial encounter
> D   subsequent encounter
> S   sequela

√5th **T85.0   Mechanical complication of ventricular intracranial (communicating) shunt**

1 √x7th **T85.01   Breakdown (mechanical) of ventricular intracranial (communicating) shunt** HCC

1 √x7th **T85.02   Displacement of ventricular intracranial (communicating) shunt** HCC
> Malposition of ventricular intracranial (communicating) shunt

1 √x7th **T85.03   Leakage of ventricular intracranial (communicating) shunt** HCC

1 √x7th **T85.09   Other mechanical complication of ventricular intracranial (communicating) shunt** HCC
> Obstruction (mechanical) of ventricular intracranial (communicating) shunt
> Perforation of ventricular intracranial (communicating) shunt
> Protrusion of ventricular intracranial (communicating) shunt

√5th **T85.1   Mechanical complication of implanted electronic stimulator of nervous system**

√6th **T85.11   Breakdown (mechanical) of implanted electronic stimulator of nervous system**

1 √7th **T85.110   Breakdown (mechanical) of implanted electronic neurostimulator of brain electrode (lead)** HCC

1 √7th **T85.111   Breakdown (mechanical) of implanted electronic neurostimulator of peripheral nerve electrode (lead)** HCC
> Breakdown of electrode (lead) for cranial nerve neurostimulators
> Breakdown of electrode (lead) for gastric neurostimulator
> Breakdown of electrode (lead) for sacral nerve neurostimulator
> Breakdown of electrode (lead) for vagal nerve neurostimulators

1 √7th **T85.112   Breakdown (mechanical) of implanted electronic neurostimulator of spinal cord electrode (lead)** HCC

1 √7th **T85.113   Breakdown (mechanical) of implanted electronic neurostimulator, generator** HCC
> Breakdown (mechanical) of implanted electronic neurostimuator generator, brain, peripheral, gastric, spinal
> Breakdown (mechanical) of implanted electronic sacral neurostimulator, pulse generator or receiver

---

1   HCC with 7th character indicating initial encounter (A, B or C - specific to category).

EXCLUDES 1 Not coded here   EXCLUDES 2 Not included here   N Newborn Age: 0   P Pediatric Age: 0-17   M Maternity Age: 12-55   A Adult Age: 15-124

1106   ICD-10-CM 2018

[1] ✓7th **T85.118 Breakdown (mechanical) of other implanted electronic stimulator of nervous system** HCC

✓6th **T85.12 Displacement of implanted electronic stimulator of nervous system**
Malposition of implanted electronic stimulator of nervous system

[1] ✓7th **T85.120 Displacement of implanted electronic neurostimulator of brain electrode (lead)** HCC

[1] ✓7th **T85.121 Displacement of implanted electronic neurostimulator of peripheral nerve electrode (lead)** HCC
Displacement of electrode (lead) for cranial nerve neurostimulators
Displacement of electrode (lead) for gastric neurostimulator
Displacement of electrode (lead) for sacral nerve neurostimulator
Displacement of electrode (lead) for vagal nerve neurostimulators

[1] ✓7th **T85.122 Displacement of implanted electronic neurostimulator of spinal cord electrode (lead)** HCC

[1] ✓7th **T85.123 Displacement of implanted electronic neurostimulator, generator** HCC
Displacement of implanted electronic neurostimulator generator, brain, peripheral, gastric, spinal
Displacement of implanted electronic sacral neurostimulator, pulse generator or receiver

[1] ✓7th **T85.128 Displacement of other implanted electronic stimulator of nervous system** HCC

✓6th **T85.19 Other mechanical complication of implanted electronic stimulator of nervous system**
Leakage of implanted electronic stimulator of nervous system
Obstruction (mechanical) of implanted electronic stimulator of nervous system
Perforation of implanted electronic stimulator of nervous system
Protrusion of implanted electronic stimulator of nervous system

[1] ✓7th **T85.190 Other mechanical complication of implanted electronic neurostimulator of brain electrode (lead)** HCC

[1] ✓7th **T85.191 Other mechanical complication of implanted electronic neurostimulator of peripheral nerve electrode (lead)** HCC
Other mechanical complication of electrode (lead) for cranial nerve neurostimulators
Other mechanical complication of electrode (lead) for gastric neurostimulator
Other mechanical complication of electrode (lead) for sacral nerve neurostimulator
Other mechanical complication of electrode (lead) for vagal nerve neurostimulators

[1] ✓7th **T85.192 Other mechanical complication of implanted electronic neurostimulator of spinal cord electrode (lead)** HCC

[1] ✓7th **T85.193 Other mechanical complication of implanted electronic neurostimulator, generator** HCC
Other mechanical complication of implanted electronic neurostimulator generator, brain, peripheral, gastric, spinal
Other mechanical complication of implanted electronic sacral neurostimulator, pulse generator or receiver

[1] ✓7th **T85.199 Other mechanical complication of other implanted electronic stimulator of nervous system** HCC

✓5th **T85.2 Mechanical complication of intraocular lens**

✓x7th **T85.21 Breakdown (mechanical) of intraocular lens**

✓x7th **T85.22 Displacement of intraocular lens**
Malposition of intraocular lens

✓x7th **T85.29 Other mechanical complication of intraocular lens**
Obstruction (mechanical) of intraocular lens
Perforation of intraocular lens
Protrusion of intraocular lens

✓5th **T85.3 Mechanical complication of other ocular prosthetic devices, implants and grafts**
EXCLUDES 2   *other complications of corneal graft (T86.84-)*

✓6th **T85.31 Breakdown (mechanical) of other ocular prosthetic devices, implants and grafts**

✓7th **T85.310 Breakdown (mechanical) of prosthetic orbit of right eye**

✓7th **T85.311 Breakdown (mechanical) of prosthetic orbit of left eye**

✓7th **T85.318 Breakdown (mechanical) of other ocular prosthetic devices, implants and grafts**

✓6th **T85.32 Displacement of other ocular prosthetic devices, implants and grafts**
Malposition of other ocular prosthetic devices, implants and grafts

✓7th **T85.320 Displacement of prosthetic orbit of right eye**

✓7th **T85.321 Displacement of prosthetic orbit of left eye**

✓7th **T85.328 Displacement of other ocular prosthetic devices, implants and grafts**

✓6th **T85.39 Other mechanical complication of other ocular prosthetic devices, implants and grafts**
Obstruction (mechanical) of other ocular prosthetic devices, implants and grafts
Perforation of other ocular prosthetic devices, implants and grafts
Protrusion of other ocular prosthetic devices, implants and grafts

✓7th **T85.390 Other mechanical complication of prosthetic orbit of right eye**

✓7th **T85.391 Other mechanical complication of prosthetic orbit of left eye**

✓7th **T85.398 Other mechanical complication of other ocular prosthetic devices, implants and grafts**

✓5th **T85.4 Mechanical complication of breast prosthesis and implant**

✓x7th **T85.41 Breakdown (mechanical) of breast prosthesis and implant**

✓x7th **T85.42 Displacement of breast prosthesis and implant**
Malposition of breast prosthesis and implant

✓x7th **T85.43 Leakage of breast prosthesis and implant**

✓x7th **T85.44 Capsular contracture of breast implant**

✓x7th **T85.49 Other mechanical complication of breast prosthesis and implant**
Obstruction (mechanical) of breast prosthesis and implant
Perforation of breast prosthesis and implant
Protrusion of breast prosthesis and implant

✓5th **T85.5 Mechanical complication of gastrointestinal prosthetic devices, implants and grafts**

✓6th **T85.51 Breakdown (mechanical) of gastrointestinal prosthetic devices, implants and grafts**

✓7th **T85.510 Breakdown (mechanical) of bile duct prosthesis**

✓7th **T85.511 Breakdown (mechanical) of esophageal anti-reflux device**

✓7th **T85.518 Breakdown (mechanical) of other gastrointestinal prosthetic devices, implants and grafts**

✓6th **T85.52 Displacement of gastrointestinal prosthetic devices, implants and grafts**
Malposition of gastrointestinal prosthetic devices, implants and grafts

✓7th **T85.520 Displacement of bile duct prosthesis**

✓7th **T85.521 Displacement of esophageal anti-reflux device**

✓7th **T85.528 Displacement of other gastrointestinal prosthetic devices, implants and grafts**

---

[1] HCC with 7th character indicating initial encounter (A, B or C - specific to category).

✓ Additional Character Req   ✓x7th Placeholder Alert   Manifestation   HCC CMS-HCC Condition   ▽ Unspecified Code   ▶◀ Revised Text   ● New Code   ▲ Revised Code Title

ICD-10-CM 2018   **1107**

✓6ᵗʰ **T85.59 Other mechanical complication of gastrointestinal prosthetic devices, implants and grafts**
Obstruction, mechanical of gastrointestinal prosthetic devices, implants and grafts
Perforation of gastrointestinal prosthetic devices, implants and grafts
Protrusion of gastrointestinal prosthetic devices, implants and grafts

✓7ᵗʰ **T85.590 Other mechanical complication of bile duct prosthesis**

✓7ᵗʰ **T85.591 Other mechanical complication of esophageal anti-reflux device**

✓7ᵗʰ **T85.598 Other mechanical complication of other gastrointestinal prosthetic devices, implants and grafts**

✓5ᵗʰ **T85.6 Mechanical complication of other specified internal and external prosthetic devices, implants and grafts**

✓6ᵗʰ **T85.61 Breakdown (mechanical) of other specified internal prosthetic devices, implants and grafts**

✓7ᵗʰ **T85.610 Breakdown (mechanical) of cranial or spinal infusion catheter**
Breakdown (mechanical) of epidural infusion catheter
Breakdown (mechanical) of intrathecal infusion catheter
Breakdown (mechanical) of subarachnoid infusion catheter
Breakdown (mechanical) of subdural infusion catheter

✓7ᵗʰ **T85.611 Breakdown (mechanical) of** `HCC`
intraperitoneal dialysis catheter
EXCLUDES 1   mechanical complication of vascular dialysis catheter (T82.4-)

✓7ᵗʰ **T85.612 Breakdown (mechanical) of permanent sutures**
EXCLUDES 1   mechanical complication of permanent (wire) suture used in bone repair (T84.1-T84.2)

✓7ᵗʰ **T85.613 Breakdown (mechanical) of artificial skin graft and decellularized allodermis**
Failure of artificial skin graft and decellularized allodermis
Non-adherence of artificial skin graft and decellularized allodermis
Poor incorporation of artificial skin graft and decellularized allodermis
Shearing of artificial skin graft and decellularized allodermis

✓7ᵗʰ **T85.614 Breakdown (mechanical) of insulin pump**

1 ✓7ᵗʰ **T85.615 Breakdown (mechanical) of other** `HCC`
nervous system device, implant or graft
Breakdown (mechanical) of intrathecal infusion pump

✓7ᵗʰ **T85.618 Breakdown (mechanical) of other specified internal prosthetic devices, implants and grafts**

✓6ᵗʰ **T85.62 Displacement of other specified internal prosthetic devices, implants and grafts**
Malposition of other specified internal prosthetic devices, implants and grafts

✓7ᵗʰ **T85.620 Displacement of cranial or spinal infusion catheter**
Displacement of epidural infusion catheter
Displacement of intrathecal infusion catheter
Displacement of subarachnoid infusion catheter
Displacement of subdural infusion catheter

✓7ᵗʰ **T85.621 Displacement of intraperitoneal** `HCC`
dialysis catheter
EXCLUDES 1   mechanical complication of vascular dialysis catheter (T82.4-)

✓7ᵗʰ **T85.622 Displacement of permanent sutures**
EXCLUDES 1   mechanical complication of permanent (wire) suture used in bone repair (T84.1-T84.2)

✓7ᵗʰ **T85.623 Displacement of artificial skin graft and decellularized allodermis**
Dislodgement of artificial skin graft and decellularized allodermis
~~Displacement of artificial skin graft and decellularized allodermis~~

✓7ᵗʰ **T85.624 Displacement of insulin pump**

1 ✓7ᵗʰ **T85.625 Displacement of other nervous** `HCC`
system device, implant or graft
Displacement of intrathecal infusion pump

✓7ᵗʰ **T85.628 Displacement of other specified internal prosthetic devices, implants and grafts**

✓6ᵗʰ **T85.63 Leakage of other specified internal prosthetic devices, implants and grafts**

✓7ᵗʰ **T85.630 Leakage of cranial or spinal infusion catheter**
Leakage of epidural infusion catheter
Leakage of intrathecal infusion catheter infusion catheter
Leakage of subdural infusion catheter
Leakage of subarachnoid infusion catheter

✓7ᵗʰ **T85.631 Leakage of intraperitoneal dialysis** `HCC`
catheter
EXCLUDES 1   mechanical complication of vascular dialysis catheter (T82.4)

✓7ᵗʰ **T85.633 Leakage of insulin pump**

1 ✓7ᵗʰ **T85.635 Leakage of other nervous system** `HCC`
device, implant or graft
Leakage of intrathecal infusion pump

✓7ᵗʰ **T85.638 Leakage of other specified internal prosthetic devices, implants and grafts**

✓6ᵗʰ **T85.69 Other mechanical complication of other specified internal prosthetic devices, implants and grafts**
Obstruction, mechanical of other specified internal prosthetic devices, implants and grafts
Perforation of other specified internal prosthetic devices, implants and grafts
Protrusion of other specified internal prosthetic devices, implants and grafts

✓7ᵗʰ **T85.690 Other mechanical complication of cranial or spinal infusion catheter**
Other mechanical complication of epidural infusion catheter
Other mechanical complication of intrathecal infusion catheter
Other mechanical complication of subarachnoid infusion catheter
Other mechanical complication of subdural infusion catheter

✓7ᵗʰ **T85.691 Other mechanical complication of** `HCC`
intraperitoneal dialysis catheter
EXCLUDES 1   mechanical complication of vascular dialysis catheter (T82.4)

✓7ᵗʰ **T85.692 Other mechanical complication of permanent sutures**
EXCLUDES 1   mechanical complication of permanent (wire) suture used in bone repair (T84.1-T84.2)

✓7ᵗʰ **T85.693 Other mechanical complication of artificial skin graft and decellularized allodermis**

✓7ᵗʰ **T85.694 Other mechanical complication of insulin pump**

1 ✓7ᵗʰ **T85.695 Other mechanical complication of** `HCC`
other nervous system device, implant or graft
Other mechanical complication of intrathecal infusion pump

✓7ᵗʰ **T85.698 Other mechanical complication of other specified internal prosthetic devices, implants and grafts**
Mechanical complication of nonabsorbable surgical material NOS

---

1   HCC with 7th character indicating initial encounter (A, B or C - specific to category).

EXCLUDES 1 Not coded here   *EXCLUDES 2* Not included here   N Newborn Age: 0   P Pediatric Age: 0-17   M Maternity Age: 12-55   A Adult Age: 15-124

1108   ICD-10-CM 2018

☑5ᵗʰ **T85.7 Infection and inflammatory reaction due to other internal prosthetic devices, implants and grafts**
Use additional code to identify infection

1 ☑x7ᵗʰ **T85.71 Infection and inflammatory reaction due to peritoneal dialysis catheter** HCC

1 ☑x7ᵗʰ **T85.72 Infection and inflammatory reaction due to insulin pump** HCC

☑6ᵗʰ **T85.73 Infection and inflammatory reaction due to nervous system devices, implants and graft**

1 ☑7ᵗʰ **T85.730 Infection and inflammatory reaction due to ventricular intracranial (communicating) shunt** HCC

1 ☑7ᵗʰ **T85.731 Infection and inflammatory reaction due to implanted electronic neurostimulator of brain, electrode (lead)** HCC

1 ☑7ᵗʰ **T85.732 Infection and inflammatory reaction due to implanted electronic neurostimulator of peripheral nerve, electrode (lead)** HCC
Infection and inflammatory reaction due to electrode (lead) for cranial nerve neurostimulators
Infection and inflammatory reaction due to electrode (lead) for gastric neurostimulator
Infection and inflammatory reaction due to electrode (lead) for sacral nerve neurostimulator
Infection and inflammatory reaction due to electrode (lead) for vagal nerve neurostimulators

1 ☑7ᵗʰ **T85.733 Infection and inflammatory reaction due to implanted electronic neurostimulator of spinal cord, electrode (lead)** HCC

1 ☑7ᵗʰ **T85.734 Infection and inflammatory reaction due to implanted electronic neurostimulator, generator** HCC
Generator pocket infection

1 ☑7ᵗʰ **T85.735 Infection and inflammatory reaction due to cranial or spinal infusion catheter** HCC
Infection and inflammatory reaction due to epidural catheter
Infection and inflammatory reaction due to intrathecal infusion catheter
Infection and inflammatory reaction due to subarachnoid catheter
Infection and inflammatory reaction due to subdural catheter

1 ☑7ᵗʰ **T85.738 Infection and inflammatory reaction due to other nervous system device, implant or graft** HCC
Infection and inflammatory reaction due to intrathecal infusion pump

1 ☑x7ᵗʰ **T85.79 Infection and inflammatory reaction due to other internal prosthetic devices, implants and grafts** HCC

☑5ᵗʰ **T85.8 Other specified complications of internal prosthetic devices, implants and grafts, not elsewhere classified**

☑6ᵗʰ **T85.81 Embolism due to internal prosthetic devices, implants and grafts, not elsewhere classified**

1 ☑7ᵗʰ **T85.810 Embolism due to nervous system prosthetic devices, implants and grafts** HCC

☑7ᵗʰ **T85.818 Embolism due to other internal prosthetic devices, implants and grafts**

☑6ᵗʰ **T85.82 Fibrosis due to internal prosthetic devices, implants and grafts, not elsewhere classified**

1 ☑7ᵗʰ **T85.820 Fibrosis due to nervous system prosthetic devices, implants and grafts** HCC

☑7ᵗʰ **T85.828 Fibrosis due to other internal prosthetic devices, implants and grafts**

☑6ᵗʰ **T85.83 Hemorrhage due to internal prosthetic devices, implants and grafts, not elsewhere classified**

1 ☑7ᵗʰ **T85.830 Hemorrhage due to nervous system prosthetic devices, implants and grafts** HCC

☑7ᵗʰ **T85.838 Hemorrhage due to other internal prosthetic devices, implants and grafts**

☑6ᵗʰ **T85.84 Pain due to internal prosthetic devices, implants and grafts, not elsewhere classified**

1 ☑7ᵗʰ **T85.840 Pain due to nervous system prosthetic devices, implants and grafts** HCC

☑7ᵗʰ **T85.848 Pain due to other internal prosthetic devices, implants and grafts**

☑6ᵗʰ **T85.85 Stenosis due to internal prosthetic devices, implants and grafts, not elsewhere classified**

1 ☑7ᵗʰ **T85.850 Stenosis due to nervous system prosthetic devices, implants and grafts** HCC

☑7ᵗʰ **T85.858 Stenosis due to other internal prosthetic devices, implants and grafts**

☑6ᵗʰ **T85.86 Thrombosis due to internal prosthetic devices, implants and grafts, not elsewhere classified**

1 ☑7ᵗʰ **T85.860 Thrombosis due to nervous system prosthetic devices, implants and grafts** HCC

☑7ᵗʰ **T85.868 Thrombosis due to other internal prosthetic devices, implants and grafts**

☑6ᵗʰ **T85.89 Other specified complication of internal prosthetic devices, implants and grafts, not elsewhere classified**
Erosion or breakdown of subcutaneous device pocket

1 ☑7ᵗʰ **T85.890 Other specified complication of nervous system prosthetic devices, implants and grafts** HCC

☑7ᵗʰ **T85.898 Other specified complication of other internal prosthetic devices, implants and grafts**

☑x7ᵗʰ **T85.9 Unspecified complication of internal prosthetic device, implant and graft** ▽
Complication of internal prosthetic device, implant and graft NOS

☑4ᵗʰ **T86 Complications of transplanted organs and tissue**
Use additional code to identify other transplant complications, such as:
graft-versus-host disease (D89.81-)
malignancy associated with organ transplant (C80.2)
post-transplant lymphoproliferative disorders (PTLD) (D47.Z1)

☑5ᵗʰ **T86.0 Complications of bone marrow transplant**

T86.00 Unspecified complication of bone marrow transplant HCC ▽

T86.01 Bone marrow transplant rejection HCC

T86.02 Bone marrow transplant failure HCC

T86.03 Bone marrow transplant infection HCC

T86.09 Other complications of bone marrow transplant HCC

☑5ᵗʰ **T86.1 Complications of kidney transplant**

T86.10 Unspecified complication of kidney transplant ▽

T86.11 Kidney transplant rejection

T86.12 Kidney transplant failure
AHA: 2013, 1Q, 24

T86.13 Kidney transplant infection
Use additional code to specify infection

T86.19 Other complication of kidney transplant

☑5ᵗʰ **T86.2 Complications of heart transplant**
EXCLUDES 1   complication of:
artificial heart device (T82.5)
heart-lung transplant (T86.3)

T86.20 Unspecified complication of heart transplant HCC ▽

T86.21 Heart transplant rejection HCC

T86.22 Heart transplant failure HCC

T86.23 Heart transplant infection HCC
Use additional code to specify infection

☑6ᵗʰ **T86.29 Other complications of heart transplant**

T86.290 Cardiac allograft vasculopathy HCC
EXCLUDES 1   atherosclerosis of coronary arteries (I25.75-, I25.76-, I25.81-)

T86.298 Other complications of heart transplant HCC

☑5ᵗʰ **T86.3 Complications of heart-lung transplant**

T86.30 Unspecified complication of heart-lung transplant HCC ▽

T86.31 Heart-lung transplant rejection HCC

T86.32 Heart-lung transplant failure HCC

---

1   HCC with 7th character indicating initial encounter (A, B or C - specific to category).

Chapter 19. Injury, Poisoning, and Certain Other Consequences of External Causes

T86.33   **Heart-lung transplant infection**   `HCC`
    Use additional code to specify infection

T86.39   **Other complications of heart-lung transplant**   `HCC`

√5th **T86.4**   **Complications of liver transplant**

T86.40   **Unspecified complication of liver transplant**   `HCC` ▽

T86.41   **Liver transplant rejection**   `HCC`

T86.42   **Liver transplant failure**   `HCC`

T86.43   **Liver transplant infection**   `HCC`
    Use additional code to identify infection, such as:
      cytomegalovirus (CMV) infection (B25.-)

T86.49   **Other complications of liver transplant**   `HCC`

T86.5   **Complications of stem cell transplant**   `HCC`
    Complications from stem cells from peripheral blood
    Complications from stem cells from umbilical cord

√5th **T86.8**   **Complications of other transplanted organs and tissues**

√6th **T86.81**   **Complications of lung transplant**
    EXCLUDES 1   complication of heart-lung transplant
      (T86.3-)

T86.810   **Lung transplant rejection**   `HCC`

T86.811   **Lung transplant failure**   `HCC`

T86.812   **Lung transplant infection**   `HCC`
    Use additional code to specify infection

T86.818   **Other complications of lung transplant**   `HCC`

T86.819   **Unspecified complication of lung transplant**   `HCC` ▽

√6th **T86.82**   **Complications of skin graft (allograft) (autograft)**
    EXCLUDES 2   complication of artificial skin graft (T85.693)

T86.820   **Skin graft (allograft) rejection**

T86.821   **Skin graft (allograft) (autograft) failure**

T86.822   **Skin graft (allograft) (autograft) infection**
    Use additional code to specify infection

T86.828   **Other complications of skin graft (allograft) (autograft)**

T86.829   **Unspecified complication of skin graft (allograft) (autograft)**   ▽

√6th **T86.83**   **Complications of bone graft**
    EXCLUDES 2   mechanical complications of bone graft
      (T84.3-)

T86.830   **Bone graft rejection**

T86.831   **Bone graft failure**

T86.832   **Bone graft infection**
    Use additional code to specify infection

T86.838   **Other complications of bone graft**

T86.839   **Unspecified complication of bone graft**   ▽

√6th **T86.84**   **Complications of corneal transplant**
    EXCLUDES 2   mechanical complications of corneal graft
      (T85.3-)

T86.840   **Corneal transplant rejection**

T86.841   **Corneal transplant failure**

T86.842   **Corneal transplant infection**   `HCC`
    Use additional code to specify infection

T86.848   **Other complications of corneal transplant**

T86.849   **Unspecified complication of corneal transplant**   ▽

√6th **T86.85**   **Complication of intestine transplant**

T86.850   **Intestine transplant rejection**   `HCC`

T86.851   **Intestine transplant failure**   `HCC`

T86.852   **Intestine transplant infection**   `HCC`
    Use additional code to specify infection

T86.858   **Other complications of intestine transplant**   `HCC`

T86.859   **Unspecified complication of intestine transplant**   `HCC` ▽

√6th **T86.89**   **Complications of other transplanted tissue**
    Transplant failure or rejection of pancreas

T86.890   **Other transplanted tissue rejection**

T86.891   **Other transplanted tissue failure**

T86.892   **Other transplanted tissue infection**
    Use additional code to specify infection

T86.898   **Other complications of other transplanted tissue**

T86.899   **Unspecified complication of other transplanted tissue**   ▽

√5th **T86.9**   **Complication of unspecified transplanted organ and tissue**

T86.90   **Unspecified complication of unspecified transplanted organ and tissue**   ▽

T86.91   **Unspecified transplanted organ and tissue rejection**   ▽

T86.92   **Unspecified transplanted organ and tissue failure**   ▽

T86.93   **Unspecified transplanted organ and tissue infection**   ▽
    Use additional code to specify infection

T86.99   **Other complications of unspecified transplanted organ and tissue**   ▽

√4th **T87**   **Complications peculiar to reattachment and amputation**

√5th **T87.0**   **Complications of reattached (part of) upper extremity**

√6th **T87.0X**   **Complications of reattached (part of) upper extremity**

T87.0X1   **Complications of reattached (part of) right upper extremity**   `HCC`

T87.0X2   **Complications of reattached (part of) left upper extremity**   `HCC`

T87.0X9   **Complications of reattached (part of) unspecified upper extremity**   `HCC` ▽

√5th **T87.1**   **Complications of reattached (part of) lower extremity**

√6th **T87.1X**   **Complications of reattached (part of) lower extremity**

T87.1X1   **Complications of reattached (part of) right lower extremity**   `HCC`

T87.1X2   **Complications of reattached (part of) left lower extremity**   `HCC`

T87.1X9   **Complications of reattached (part of) unspecified lower extremity**   `HCC` ▽

T87.2   **Complications of other reattached body part**   `HCC`

√5th **T87.3**   **Neuroma of amputation stump**
    DEF: Non-neoplastic tumor generated at the proximal end of severed, partially transected, or injured nerve following amputation.

T87.30   **Neuroma of amputation stump, unspecified extremity**   `HCC` ▽

T87.31   **Neuroma of amputation stump, right upper extremity**   `HCC`

T87.32   **Neuroma of amputation stump, left upper extremity**   `HCC`

T87.33   **Neuroma of amputation stump, right lower extremity**   `HCC`

T87.34   **Neuroma of amputation stump, left lower extremity**   `HCC`

√5th **T87.4**   **Infection of amputation stump**

T87.40   **Infection of amputation stump, unspecified extremity**   `HCC` ▽

T87.41   **Infection of amputation stump, right upper extremity**   `HCC`

T87.42   **Infection of amputation stump, left upper extremity**   `HCC`

T87.43   **Infection of amputation stump, right lower extremity**   `HCC`

T87.44   **Infection of amputation stump, left lower extremity**   `HCC`

√5th **T87.5**   **Necrosis of amputation stump**

T87.50   **Necrosis of amputation stump, unspecified extremity**   `HCC` ▽

T87.51   **Necrosis of amputation stump, right upper extremity**   `HCC`

T87.52   **Necrosis of amputation stump, left upper extremity**   `HCC`

T87.53   **Necrosis of amputation stump, right lower extremity**   `HCC`

T87.54   **Necrosis of amputation stump, left lower extremity**   `HCC`

√5th **T87.8**   **Other complications of amputation stump**

T87.81   **Dehiscence of amputation stump**   `HCC`

EXCLUDES 1 Not coded here   EXCLUDES 2 Not included here   N Newborn Age: 0   P Pediatric Age: 0-17   M Maternity Age: 12-55   A Adult Age: 15-124

1110   ICD-10-CM 2018

T86.33–T87.81

T87.89 **Other complications of amputation stump** HCC
Amputation stump contracture
Amputation stump contracture of next proximal joint
Amputation stump flexion
Amputation stump edema
Amputation stump hematoma
EXCLUDES 2   *phantom limb syndrome (G54.6-G54.7)*

T87.9 **Unspecified complications of amputation stump** HCC ▽

☑4ᵗʰ **T88** **Other complications of surgical and medical care, not elsewhere classified**
EXCLUDES 2   *complication following infusion, transfusion and therapeutic injection (T80.-)*
complication following procedure NEC (T81.-)
complications of anesthesia in labor and delivery (O74.-)
complications of anesthesia in pregnancy (O29.-)
complications of anesthesia in puerperium (O89.-)
complications of devices, implants and grafts (T82-T85)
complications of obstetric surgery and procedure (O75.4)
dermatitis due to drugs and medicaments (L23.3, L24.4, L25.1, L27.0-L27.1)
poisoning and toxic effects of drugs and chemicals (T36-T65 with fifth or sixth character 1-4 or 6)
specified complications classified elsewhere

> The appropriate 7th character is to be added to each code from category T88.
> A   initial encounter
> D   subsequent encounter
> S   sequela

☑ₓ7ᵗʰ **T88.0** **Infection following immunization**
Sepsis following immunization

☑ₓ7ᵗʰ **T88.1** **Other complications following immunization, not elsewhere classified**
Generalized vaccinia
Rash following immunization
EXCLUDES 1   *vaccinia not from vaccine (B08.011)*
EXCLUDES 2   *anaphylactic shock due to serum (T80.5-)*
other serum reactions (T80.6-)
postimmunization arthropathy (M02.2)
postimmunization encephalitis (G04.02)
postimmunization fever (R50.83)

☑ₓ7ᵗʰ **T88.2** **Shock due to anesthesia**
Use additional code for adverse effect, if applicable, to identify drug (T41.- with fifth or sixth character 5)
EXCLUDES 1   *complications of anesthesia (in):*
labor and delivery (O74.-)
postprocedural shock NOS (T81.1-)
pregnancy (O29.-)
puerperium (O89.-)

☑ₓ7ᵗʰ **T88.3** **Malignant hyperthermia due to anesthesia**
Use additional code for adverse effect, if applicable, to identify drug (T41.- with fifth or sixth character 5)

☑ₓ7ᵗʰ **T88.4** **Failed or difficult intubation**

☑5ᵗʰ **T88.5** **Other complications of anesthesia**
Use additional code for adverse effect, if applicable, to identify drug (T41.- with fifth or sixth character 5)

☑ₓ7ᵗʰ **T88.51** **Hypothermia following anesthesia**

☑ₓ7ᵗʰ **T88.52** **Failed moderate sedation during procedure**
Failed conscious sedation during procedure
EXCLUDES 2   *personal history of failed moderate sedation (Z92.83)*

☑ₓ7ᵗʰ **T88.53** **Unintended awareness under general anesthesia during procedure**
EXCLUDES 2   *personal history of unintended awareness under general anesthesia (Z92.84)*

☑ₓ7ᵗʰ **T88.59** **Other complications of anesthesia**

☑ₓ7ᵗʰ **T88.6** **Anaphylactic reaction due to adverse effect of correct drug or medicament properly administered**
Anaphylactic shock due to adverse effect of correct drug or medicament properly administered
Anaphylactoid reaction NOS
Use additional code for adverse effect, if applicable, to identify drug (T36-T50 with fifth or sixth character 5)
EXCLUDES 1   *anaphylactic reaction due to serum (T80.5-)*
anaphylactic shock or reaction due to adverse food reaction (T78.0-)

☑ₓ7ᵗʰ **T88.7** **Unspecified adverse effect of drug or medicament** ▽
Drug hypersensitivity NOS
Drug reaction NOS
Use additional code for adverse effect, if applicable, to identify drug (T36-T50 with fifth or sixth character 5)
EXCLUDES 1   *specified adverse effects of drugs and medicaments (A00-R94 and T80-T88.6, T88.8)*

☑ₓ7ᵗʰ **T88.8** **Other specified complications of surgical and medical care, not elsewhere classified**
Use additional code to identify the complication

☑ₓ7ᵗʰ **T88.9** **Complication of surgical and medical care, unspecified** ▽

Chapter 20. External Causes of Morbidity (V00–Y99)

Chapter Specific Guidelines with Coding Examples

The chapter specific guidelines from the ICD-10-CM Official Guidelines for Coding and Reporting have been provided below. Along with these guidelines are coding examples, contained in the shaded boxes, that have been developed to help illustrate the coding and/or sequencing guidance found in these guidelines.

The external causes of morbidity codes should never be sequenced as the first-listed or principal diagnosis.

External cause codes are intended to provide data for injury research and evaluation of injury prevention strategies. These codes capture how the injury or health condition happened (cause), the intent (unintentional or accidental; or intentional, such as suicide or assault), the place where the event occurred the activity of the patient at the time of the event, and the person's status (e.g., civilian, military).

There is no national requirement for mandatory ICD-10-CM external cause code reporting. Unless a provider is subject to a state-based external cause code reporting mandate or these codes are required by a particular payer, reporting of ICD-10-CM codes in Chapter 20, External Causes of Morbidity, is not required. In the absence of a mandatory reporting requirement, providers are encouraged to voluntarily report external cause codes, as they provide valuable data for injury research and evaluation of injury prevention strategies.

a. General external cause coding guidelines

1) Used with any code in the range of A00.0–T88.9, Z00–Z99

An external cause code may be used with any code in the range of A00.0–T88.9, Z00–Z99, classification that is a health condition due to an external cause. Though they are most applicable to injuries, they are also valid for use with such things as infections or diseases due to an external source, and other health conditions, such as a heart attack that occurs during strenuous physical activity.

> Actinic reticuloid due to tanning bed use
>
> **L57.1**   **Actinic reticuloid**
>
> **W89.1XXA**   **Exposure to tanning bed, initial encounter**
>
> *Explanation:* An external cause code may be used with any code in the range of A00.0–T88.9, Z00–Z99, classifications that describe health conditions due to an external cause. Code W89.1 Exposure to tanning bed requires a seventh character of A to report this initial encounter, with a placeholder X for the fifth and sixth characters.

2) External cause code used for length of treatment

Assign the external cause code, with the appropriate 7th character (initial encounter, subsequent encounter or sequela) for each encounter for which the injury or condition is being treated.

Most categories in chapter 20 have a 7th character requirement for each applicable code. Most categories in this chapter have three 7th character values: A, initial encounter, D, subsequent encounter and S, sequela. While the patient may be seen by a new or different provider over the course of treatment for an injury or condition, assignment of the 7th character for external cause should match the 7th character of the code assigned for the associated injury or condition for the encounter.

3) Use the full range of external cause codes

Use the full range of external cause codes to completely describe the cause, the intent, the place of occurrence, and if applicable, the activity of the patient at the time of the event, and the patient's status, for all injuries, and other health conditions due to an external cause.

4) Assign as many external cause codes as necessary

Assign as many external cause codes as necessary to fully explain each cause. If only one external code can be recorded, assign the code most related to the principal diagnosis.

5) The selection of the appropriate external cause code

The selection of the appropriate external cause code is guided by the Alphabetic Index of External Causes and by Inclusion and Exclusion notes in the Tabular List.

6) External cause code can never be a principal diagnosis

An external cause code can never be a principal (first-listed) diagnosis.

7) Combination external cause codes

Certain of the external cause codes are combination codes that identify sequential events that result in an injury, such as a fall which results in striking against an object. The injury may be due to either event or both.

The combination external cause code used should correspond to the sequence of events regardless of which caused the most serious injury.

> Toddler tripped and fell while walking and struck his head on an end table, sustaining a scalp contusion
>
> **S00.03XA**   **Contusion of scalp, initial encounter**
>
> **W01.190A**   **Fall on same level from slipping, tripping and stumbling with subsequent striking against furniture, initial encounter**
>
> *Explanation:* Combination external cause codes identify sequential events that result in an injury, such as a fall resulting in striking against an object. The injury may be due to either or both events.

8) No external cause code needed in certain circumstances

No external cause code from Chapter 20 is needed if the external cause and intent are included in a code from another chapter (e.g. T36.0X1- Poisoning by penicillins, accidental (unintentional)).

b. Place of occurrence guideline

Codes from category Y92, Place of occurrence of the external cause, are secondary codes for use after other external cause codes to identify the location of the patient at the time of injury or other condition.

Generally, a place of occurrence code is assigned only once, at the initial encounter for treatment. However, in the rare instance that a new injury occurs during hospitalization, an additional place of occurrence code may be assigned. No 7th characters are used for Y92.

Do not use place of occurrence code Y92.9 if the place is not stated or is not applicable.

> A farmer was working in his barn and sustained a foot contusion when the horse stepped on his left foot
>
> **S90.32XA**   **Contusion of left foot, initial encounter**
>
> **W55.19XA**   **Other contact with horse, initial encounter**
>
> **Y92.71**   **Barn as the place of occurrence of the external cause**
>
> *Explanation:* A place-of-occurrence code from category Y92 is assigned at the initial encounter to identify the location of the patient at the time the injury occurred.

c. Activity code

Assign a code from category Y93, Activity code, to describe the activity of the patient at the time the injury or other health condition occurred.

An activity code is used only once, at the initial encounter for treatment. Only one code from Y93 should be recorded on a medical record.

The activity codes are not applicable to poisonings, adverse effects, misadventures or sequela.

Do not assign Y93.9, Unspecified activity, if the activity is not stated.

A code from category Y93 is appropriate for use with external cause and intent codes if identifying the activity provides additional information about the event.

> Ranch hand who was grooming a horse sustained a foot contusion when the horse stepped on his left foot
>
> **S90.32XA**   **Contusion of left foot, initial encounter**
>
> **W55.19XA**   **Other contact with horse, initial encounter**
>
> **Y93.K3**   **Activity, grooming and shearing an animal**
>
> *Explanation:* One activity code from category Y93 is assigned at the initial encounter only to describe the activity of the patient at the time the injury occurred.

d. Place of occurrence, activity, and status codes used with other external cause code

When applicable, place of occurrence, activity, and external cause status codes are sequenced after the main external cause code(s). Regardless of the number of external cause codes assigned, generally there should be only one place of occurrence code, one activity code, and one external cause status code assigned to an encounter. However, in the rare instance that a new injury occurs during hospitalization, an additional place of occurrence code may be assigned.

Chapter 20. External Causes of Morbidity

e. If the reporting format limits the number of external cause codes

If the reporting format limits the number of external cause codes that can be used in reporting clinical data, report the code for the cause/intent most related to the principal diagnosis. If the format permits capture of additional external cause codes, the cause/intent, including medical misadventures, of the additional events should be reported rather than the codes for place, activity, or external status.

f. Multiple external cause coding guidelines

More than one external cause code is required to fully describe the external cause of an illness or injury. The assignment of external cause codes should be sequenced in the following priority:

If two or more events cause separate injuries, an external cause code should be assigned for each cause. The first-listed external cause code will be selected in the following order:

External codes for child and adult abuse take priority over all other external cause codes.

See Section I.C.19., Child and Adult abuse guidelines.

External cause codes for terrorism events take priority over all other external cause codes except child and adult abuse.

External cause codes for cataclysmic events take priority over all other external cause codes except child and adult abuse and terrorism.

External cause codes for transport accidents take priority over all other external cause codes except cataclysmic events, child and adult abuse and terrorism.

Activity and external cause status codes are assigned following all causal (intent) external cause codes.

The first-listed external cause code should correspond to the cause of the most serious diagnosis due to an assault, accident, or self-harm, following the order of hierarchy listed above..

> 30-year-old man accidentally discharged his hunting rifle, sustaining an open gunshot wound, with no retained bullet fragments, to the right thigh, which caused him to fall down the stairs, resulting in closed displaced comminuted fracture of his left radial shaft
>
> | | |
> |---|---|
> | **S71.131A** | **Puncture wound without foreign body, right thigh, initial encounter** |
> | **S52.352A** | **Displaced comminuted fracture of shaft of radius, left arm, initial encounter for closed fracture** |
> | **W33.02XA** | **Accidental discharge of hunting rifle, initial encounter** |
> | **W10.9XXA** | **Fall (on) (from) unspecified stairs and steps, initial encounter** |
>
> *Explanation:* If two or more events cause separate injuries, an external cause code should be assigned for each cause.

g. Child and adult abuse guideline

Adult and child abuse, neglect and maltreatment are classified as assault. Any of the assault codes may be used to indicate the external cause of any injury resulting from the confirmed abuse.

For confirmed cases of abuse, neglect and maltreatment, when the perpetrator is known, a code from Y07, Perpetrator of maltreatment and neglect, should accompany any other assault codes.

See Section I.C.19. Adult and child abuse, neglect and other maltreatment

h. Unknown or undetermined intent guideline

If the intent (accident, self-harm, assault) of the cause of an injury or other condition is unknown or unspecified, code the intent as accidental intent. All transport accident categories assume accidental intent.

1) Use of undetermined intent

External cause codes for events of undetermined intent are only for use if the documentation in the record specifies that the intent cannot be determined.

i. Sequelae (late effects) of external cause guidelines

1) Sequelae external cause codes

Sequela are reported using the external cause code with the 7th character "S" for sequela. These codes should be used with any report of a late effect or sequela resulting from a previous injury.

See Section I.B.10 Sequela (Late Effects)

2) Sequela external cause code with a related current injury

A sequela external cause code should never be used with a related current nature of injury code.

3) Use of sequela external cause codes for subsequent visits

Use a late effect external cause code for subsequent visits when a late effect of the initial injury is being treated. Do not use a late effect external cause code for subsequent visits for follow-up care (e.g., to assess healing, to receive rehabilitative therapy) of the injury when no late effect of the injury has been documented.

j. Terrorism guidelines

1) Cause of injury identified by the Federal Government (FBI) as terrorism

When the cause of an injury is identified by the Federal Government (FBI) as terrorism, the first-listed external cause code should be a code from category Y38, Terrorism. The definition of terrorism employed by the FBI is found at the inclusion note at the beginning of category Y38. Use additional code for place of occurrence (Y92.-). More than one Y38 code may be assigned if the injury is the result of more than one mechanism of terrorism.

2) Cause of an injury is suspected to be the result of terrorism

When the cause of an injury is suspected to be the result of terrorism a code from category Y38 should not be assigned. Suspected cases should be classified as assault.

3) Code Y38.9, Terrorism, secondary effects

Assign code Y38.9, Terrorism, secondary effects, for conditions occurring subsequent to the terrorist event. This code should not be assigned for conditions that are due to the initial terrorist act.

It is acceptable to assign code Y38.9 with another code from Y38 if there is an injury due to the initial terrorist event and an injury that is a subsequent result of the terrorist event.

k. External cause status

A code from category Y99, External cause status, should be assigned whenever any other external cause code is assigned for an encounter, including an Activity code, except for the events noted below. Assign a code from category Y99, External cause status, to indicate the work status of the person at the time the event occurred. The status code indicates whether the event occurred during military activity, whether a non-military person was at work, whether an individual including a student or volunteer was involved in a non-work activity at the time of the causal event.

A code from Y99, External cause status, should be assigned, when applicable, with other external cause codes, such as transport accidents and falls. The external cause status codes are not applicable to poisonings, adverse effects, misadventures or late effects.

Do not assign a code from category Y99 if no other external cause codes (cause, activity) are applicable for the encounter.

An external cause status code is used only once, at the initial encounter for treatment. Only one code from Y99 should be recorded on a medical record.

Do not assign code Y99.9, Unspecified external cause status, if the status is not stated.

Chapter 20. External Causes of Morbidity (V00-Y99)

NOTE   This chapter permits the classification of environmental events and circumstances as the cause of injury, and other adverse effects. Where a code from this section is applicable, it is intended that it shall be used secondary to a code from another chapter of the Classification indicating the nature of the condition. Most often, the condition will be classifiable to Chapter 19, Injury, poisoning and certain other consequences of external causes (S00-T88). Other conditions that may be stated to be due to external causes are classified in Chapters I to XVIII. For these conditions, codes from Chapter 20 should be used to provide additional information as to the cause of the condition.

This chapter contains the following blocks:

V00-X58	Accidents
V00-V99	Transport accidents
V00-V09	Pedestrian injured in transport accident
V10-V19	Pedal cycle rider injured in transport accident
V20-V29	Motorcycle rider injured in transport accident
V30-V39	Occupant of three-wheeled motor vehicle injured in transport accident
V40-V49	Car occupant injured in transport accident
V50-V59	Occupant of pick-up truck or van injured in transport accident
V60-V69	Occupant of heavy transport vehicle injured in transport accident
V70-V79	Bus occupant injured in transport accident
V80-V89	Other land transport accidents
V90-V94	Water transport accidents
V95-V97	Air and space transport accidents
V98-V99	Other and unspecified transport accidents
W00-X58	Other external causes of accidental injury
W00-W19	Slipping, tripping, stumbling and falls
W20-W49	Exposure to inanimate mechanical forces
W50-W64	Exposure to animate mechanical forces
W65-W74	Accidental non-transport drowning and submersion
W85-W99	Exposure to electric current, radiation and extreme ambient air temperature and pressure
X00-X08	Exposure to smoke, fire and flames
X10-X19	Contact with heat and hot substances
X30-X39	Exposure to forces of nature
X50	~~Overexertion and strenuous or repetitive movements~~
X52-X58	Accidental exposure to other specified factors
X71-X83	Intentional self-harm
X92-Y09	Assault
Y21-Y33	Event of undetermined intent
Y35-Y38	Legal intervention, operations of war, military operations, and terrorism
Y62-Y84	Complications of medical and surgical care
Y62-Y69	Misadventures to patients during surgical and medical care
Y70-Y82	Medical devices associated with adverse incidents in diagnostic and therapeutic use
Y83-Y84	Surgical and other medical procedures as the cause of abnormal reaction of the patient, or of later complication, without mention of misadventure at the time of the procedure
Y90-Y99	Supplementary factors related to causes of morbidity classified elsewhere

Accidents (V00-X58)

NOTE   This section is structured in 12 groups. Those relating to land transport accidents (V00-V89) reflect the victim's mode of transport and are subdivided to identify the victim's 'counterpart' or the type of event. The vehicle of which the injured person is an occupant is identified in the first two characters since it is seen as the most important factor to identify for prevention purposes. A transport accident is one in which the vehicle involved must be moving or running or in use for transport purposes at the time of the accident.

Use additional code to identify:
airbag injury (W22.1)
type of street or road (Y92.4-)
use of cellular telephone and other electronic equipment at the time of the transport accident (Y93.C-)

EXCLUDES 1   *agricultural vehicles in stationary use or maintenance (W31.-)*
assault by crashing of motor vehicle (Y03.-)
automobile or motor cycle in stationary use or maintenance—code to type of accident
crashing of motor vehicle, undetermined intent (Y32)
intentional self-harm by crashing of motor vehicle (X82)

EXCLUDES 2   *transport accidents due to cataclysm (X34-X38)*

NOTE   Definitions related to transport accidents:

(a)   A transport accident (V00-V99) is any accident involving a device designed primarily for, or used at the time primarily for, conveying persons or good from one place to another.

(b)   A public highway [trafficway] or street is the entire width between property lines (or other boundary lines) of land open to the public as a matter of right or custom for purposes of moving persons or property from one place to another. A roadway is that part of the public highway designed, improved and customarily used for vehicular traffic.

(c)   A traffic accident is any vehicle accident occurring on the public highway [i.e. originating on, terminating on, or involving a vehicle partially on the highway]. A vehicle accident is assumed to have occurred on the public highway unless another place is specified, except in the case of accidents involving only off-road motor vehicles, which are classified as nontraffic accidents unless the contrary is stated.

(d)   A nontraffic accident is any vehicle accident that occurs entirely in any place other than a public highway.

(e)   A pedestrian is any person involved in an accident who was not at the time of the accident riding in or on a motor vehicle, railway train, streetcar or animal-drawn or other vehicle, or on a pedal cycle or animal. This includes, a person changing a tire, working on a parked car, or a person on foot. It also includes the user of a pedestrian conveyance such as a babystroller, ice-skates, skis, sled, roller skates, a skateboard, nonmotorized or motorized wheelchair, motorized mobility scooter, or nonmotorized scooter.

(f)   A driver is an occupant of a transport vehicle who is operating or intending to operate it.

(g)   A passenger is any occupant of a transport vehicle other than the driver, except a person traveling on the outside of the vehicle.

(h)   A person on the outside of a vehicle is any person being transported by a vehicle but not occupying the space normally reserved for the driver or passengers, or the space intended for the transport of property. This includes a person travelling on the bodywork, bumper, fender, roof, running board or step of a vehicle, as well as, hanging on the outside of the vehicle.

(i)   A pedal cycle is any land transport vehicle operated solely by nonmotorized pedals including a bicycle or tricycle.

(j)   A pedal cyclist is any person riding a pedal cycle or in a sidecar or trailer attached to a pedal cycle.

(k)   A motorcycle is a two-wheeled motor vehicle with one or two riding saddles and sometimes with a third wheel for the support of a sidecar. The sidecar is considered part of the motorcycle. This includes a moped, motor scooter, or motorized bicycle.

(l)   A motorcycle rider is any person riding a motorcycle or in a sidecar or trailer attached to the motorcycle.

(m)   A three-wheeled motor vehicle is a motorized tricycle designed primarily for on-road use. This includes a motor-driven tricycle, a motorized rickshaw, or a three-wheeled motor car.

(n)   A car [automobile] is a four-wheeled motor vehicle designed primarily for carrying up to 7 persons. A trailer being towed by the car is considered part of the car. It does not include a van or minivan - see definition (o).

(o)   A pick-up truck or van is a four or six-wheeled motor vehicle designed for carrying passengers as well as property or cargo weighing less than the local limit for classification as a heavy goods vehicle, and not requiring a special driver's license. This includes a minivan and a sport-utility vehicle (SUV).

(p)   A heavy transport vehicle is a motor vehicle designed primarily for carrying property, meeting local criteria for classification as a heavy goods vehicle in terms of weight and requiring a special driver's license.

(q)   A bus (coach) is a motor vehicle designed or adapted primarily for carrying more than 10 passengers, and requiring a special driver's license.

(r)   A railway train or railway vehicle is any device, with or without freight or passenger cars couple to it, designed for traffic on a railway track. This includes subterranean (subways) or elevated trains.

(s)   A streetcar, is a device designed and used primarily for transporting passengers within a municipality, running on rails, usually subject to normal traffic control signals, and operated principally on a right-of-way that forms part of the roadway. This includes a tram or trolley that runs on rails. A trailer being towed by a streetcar is considered part of the streetcar.

(t)   A special vehicle mainly used on industrial premises is a motor vehicle designed primarily for use within the buildings and premises of industrial or commercial establishments. This includes battery-powered airport passenger vehicles or baggage/mail trucks, forklifts, coal-cars in a coal mine, logging cars and trucks used in mines or quarries.

Chapter 20. External Causes of Morbidity

V00–V00.322

(u)   A special vehicle mainly used in agriculture is a motor vehicle designed specifically for use in farming and agriculture (horticulture), to work the land, tend and harvest crops and transport materials on the farm. This includes harvesters, farm machinery and tractor and trailers.

(v)   A special construction vehicle is a motor vehicle designed specifically for use on construction and demolition sites. This includes bulldozers, diggers, earth levellers, dump trucks. backhoes, front-end loaders, pavers, and mechanical shovels.

(w)   A special all-terrain vehicle is a motor vehicle of special design to enable it to negotiate over rough or soft terrain, snow or sand. Examples of special design are high pressure, special wheels and tires, tracks, and support on a cushion of air. This includes snow mobiles, All-terrain vehicles (ATV), and dune buggies. It does not include passenger vehicle designated as Sport Utility Vehicles. (SUV)

(x)   A watercraft is any device designed for transporting passengers or goods on water. This includes motor or sailboats, ships, and hovercraft.

(y)   An aircraft is any device for transporting passengers or goods in the air. This includes hot-air balloons, gliders, helicopters and airplanes.

(z)   A military vehicle is any motorized vehicle operating on a public roadway owned by the military and being operated by a member of the military

Pedestrian injured in transport accident (V00-V09)

INCLUDES   person changing tire on transport vehicle
person examining engine of vehicle broken down in (on side of) road

EXCLUDES 1   *fall due to non-transport collision with other person (W03)*
pedestrian on foot falling (slipping) on ice and snow (W00.-)
struck or bumped by another person (W51)

> The appropriate 7th character is to be added to each code from categories V00-V09.
> A   initial encounter
> D   subsequent encounter
> S   sequela

✓4th **V00**   **Pedestrian conveyance accident**
Use additional place of occurrence and activity external cause codes, if known (Y92-, Y93-)
EXCLUDES 1   *collision with another person without fall (W51)*
fall due to person on foot colliding with another person on foot (W03)
fall from non-moving wheelchair, nonmotorized scooter and motorized mobility scooter without collision (W05.-)
pedestrian (conveyance) collision with other land transport vehicle (V01-V09)
pedestrian on foot falling (slipping) on ice and snow (W00.-)

✓5th **V00.0**   **Pedestrian on foot injured in collision with pedestrian conveyance**

✓x7th **V00.01**   **Pedestrian on foot injured in collision with roller-skater**

✓x7th **V00.02**   **Pedestrian on foot injured in collision with skateboarder**

✓x7th **V00.09**   **Pedestrian on foot injured in collision with other pedestrian conveyance**

✓5th **V00.1**   **Rolling-type pedestrian conveyance accident**
EXCLUDES 1   *accident with babystroller (V00.82-)*
accident with motorized mobility scooter (V00.83-)
accident with wheelchair (powered) (V00.81-)

✓6th **V00.11**   **In-line roller-skate accident**

✓7th **V00.111**   **Fall from in-line roller-skates**

✓7th **V00.112**   **In-line roller-skater colliding with stationary object**

✓7th **V00.118**   **Other in-line roller-skate accident**
EXCLUDES 1   *roller-skater collision with other land transport vehicle (V01-V09 with 5th character 1)*

✓6th **V00.12**   **Non-in- line roller-skate accident**

✓7th **V00.121**   **Fall from non-in-line roller-skates**

✓7th **V00.122**   **Non-in-line roller-skater colliding with stationary object**

✓7th **V00.128**   **Other non-in-line roller-skating accident**
EXCLUDES 1   *roller-skater collision with other land transport vehicle (V01-V09 with 5th character 1)*

✓6th **V00.13**   **Skateboard accident**

✓7th **V00.131**   **Fall from skateboard**

✓7th **V00.132**   **Skateboarder colliding with stationary object**

✓7th **V00.138**   **Other skateboard accident**
EXCLUDES 1   *skateboarder collision with other land transport vehicle (V01-V09 with 5th character 2)*

✓6th **V00.14**   **Scooter (nonmotorized) accident**
EXCLUDES 1   *motorscooter accident (V20-V29)*

✓7th **V00.141**   **Fall from scooter (nonmotorized)**

✓7th **V00.142**   **Scooter (nonmotorized) colliding with stationary object**

✓7th **V00.148**   **Other scooter (nonmotorized) accident**
EXCLUDES 1   *scooter (nonmotorized) collision with other land transport vehicle (V01-V09 with fifth character 9)*

✓6th **V00.15**   **Heelies accident**
Rolling shoe
Wheeled shoe
Wheelies accident

✓7th **V00.151**   **Fall from heelies**

✓7th **V00.152**   **Heelies colliding with stationary object**

✓7th **V00.158**   **Other heelies accident**

✓6th **V00.18**   **Accident on other rolling-type pedestrian conveyance**

✓7th **V00.181**   **Fall from other rolling-type pedestrian conveyance**

✓7th **V00.182**   **Pedestrian on other rolling-type pedestrian conveyance colliding with stationary object**

✓7th **V00.188**   **Other accident on other rolling-type pedestrian conveyance**

✓5th **V00.2**   **Gliding-type pedestrian conveyance accident**

✓6th **V00.21**   **Ice-skates accident**

✓7th **V00.211**   **Fall from ice-skates**

✓7th **V00.212**   **Ice-skater colliding with stationary object**

✓7th **V00.218**   **Other ice-skates accident**
EXCLUDES 1   *ice-skater collision with other land transport vehicle (V01-V09 with 5th digit 9)*

✓6th **V00.22**   **Sled accident**

✓7th **V00.221**   **Fall from sled**

✓7th **V00.222**   **Sledder colliding with stationary object**

✓7th **V00.228**   **Other sled accident**
EXCLUDES 1   *sled collision with other land transport vehicle (V01-V09 with 5th digit 9)*

✓6th **V00.28**   **Other gliding-type pedestrian conveyance accident**

✓7th **V00.281**   **Fall from other gliding-type pedestrian conveyance**

✓7th **V00.282**   **Pedestrian on other gliding-type pedestrian conveyance colliding with stationary object**

✓7th **V00.288**   **Other accident on other gliding-type pedestrian conveyance**
EXCLUDES 1   *gliding-type pedestrian conveyance collision with other land transport vehicle (V01-V09 with 5th digit 9)*

✓5th **V00.3**   **Flat-bottomed pedestrian conveyance accident**

✓6th **V00.31**   **Snowboard accident**

✓7th **V00.311**   **Fall from snowboard**

✓7th **V00.312**   **Snowboarder colliding with stationary object**

✓7th **V00.318**   **Other snowboard accident**
EXCLUDES 1   *snowboarder collision with other land transport vehicle (V01-V09 with 5th digit 9)*

✓6th **V00.32**   **Snow-ski accident**

✓7th **V00.321**   **Fall from snow-skis**

✓7th **V00.322**   **Snow-skier colliding with stationary object**

EXCLUDES 1 Not coded here   EXCLUDES 2 Not included here   N Newborn Age: 0   P Pediatric Age: 0-17   M Maternity Age: 12-55   A Adult Age: 15-124

1116   ICD-10-CM 2018

✓7th **V00.328 Other snow-ski accident**
> EXCLUDES 1 *snow-skier collision with other land transport vehicle (V01-V09 with 5th digit 9)*

✓6th **V00.38 Other flat-bottomed pedestrian conveyance accident**

✓7th **V00.381 Fall from other flat-bottomed pedestrian conveyance**

✓7th **V00.382 Pedestrian on other flat-bottomed pedestrian conveyance colliding with stationary object**

✓7th **V00.388 Other accident on other flat-bottomed pedestrian conveyance**

✓5th **V00.8 Accident on other pedestrian conveyance**

✓6th **V00.81 Accident with wheelchair (powered)**

✓7th **V00.811 Fall from moving wheelchair (powered)**
> EXCLUDES 1 *fall from non-moving wheelchair (W05.0)*

✓7th **V00.812 Wheelchair (powered) colliding with stationary object**

✓7th **V00.818 Other accident with wheelchair (powered)**

✓6th **V00.82 Accident with babystroller**

✓7th **V00.821 Fall from babystroller**

✓7th **V00.822 Babystroller colliding with stationary object**

✓7th **V00.828 Other accident with babystroller**

✓6th **V00.83 Accident with motorized mobility scooter**

V00.831 Fall from motorized mobility scooter
> EXCLUDES 1 *fall from non-moving motorized mobility scooter (W05.2)*

V00.832 Motorized mobility scooter colliding with stationary object

V00.838 Other accident with motorized mobility scooter

✓6th **V00.89 Accident on other pedestrian conveyance**

✓7th **V00.891 Fall from other pedestrian conveyance**

✓7th **V00.892 Pedestrian on other pedestrian conveyance colliding with stationary object**

✓7th **V00.898 Other accident on other pedestrian conveyance**
> EXCLUDES 1 *other pedestrian (conveyance) collision with other land transport vehicle (V01-V09 with 5th digit 9)*

✓4th **V01 Pedestrian injured in collision with pedal cycle**

✓5th **V01.0 Pedestrian injured in collision with pedal cycle in nontraffic accident**

✓x7th **V01.00 Pedestrian on foot injured in collision with pedal cycle in nontraffic accident**
Pedestrian NOS injured in collision with pedal cycle in nontraffic accident

✓x7th **V01.01 Pedestrian on roller-skates injured in collision with pedal cycle in nontraffic accident**

✓x7th **V01.02 Pedestrian on skateboard injured in collision with pedal cycle in nontraffic accident**

✓x7th **V01.09 Pedestrian with other conveyance injured in collision with pedal cycle in nontraffic accident**
Pedestrian with babystroller injured in collision with pedal cycle in nontraffic accident
Pedestrian on ice-skates injured in collision with pedal cycle in nontraffic accident
Pedestrian on nonmotorized scooter injured in collision with pedal cycle in nontraffic accident
Pedestrian on sled injured in collision with pedal cycle in nontraffic accident
Pedestrian on snowboard injured in collision with pedal cycle in nontraffic accident
Pedestrian on snow-skis injured in collision with pedal cycle in nontraffic accident
Pedestrian in wheelchair (powered) injured in collision with pedal cycle in nontraffic accident
Pedestrian in motorized mobility scooter injured in collision with pedal cycle in nontraffic accident

✓5th **V01.1 Pedestrian injured in collision with pedal cycle in traffic accident**

✓x7th **V01.10 Pedestrian on foot injured in collision with pedal cycle in traffic accident**
Pedestrian NOS injured in collision with pedal cycle in traffic accident

✓x7th **V01.11 Pedestrian on roller-skates injured in collision with pedal cycle in traffic accident**

✓x7th **V01.12 Pedestrian on skateboard injured in collision with pedal cycle in traffic accident**

✓x7th **V01.19 Pedestrian with other conveyance injured in collision with pedal cycle in traffic accident**
Pedestrian with babystroller injured in collision with pedal cycle in traffic accident
Pedestrian on ice-skates injured in collision with pedal cycle in traffic accident
Pedestrian on nonmotorized scooter injured in collision with pedal cycle in traffic accident
Pedestrian on sled injured in collision with pedal cycle in traffic accident
Pedestrian on snowboard injured in collision with pedal cycle in traffic accident
Pedestrian on snow-skis injured in collision with pedal cycle in traffic accident
Pedestrian in wheelchair (powered) injured in collision with pedal cycle in traffic accident
Pedestrian in motorized mobility scooter injured in collision with pedal cycle in traffic accident

✓5th **V01.9 Pedestrian injured in collision with pedal cycle, unspecified whether traffic or nontraffic accident**

✓x7th **V01.90 Pedestrian on foot injured in collision with pedal cycle, unspecified whether traffic or nontraffic accident** ▽
Pedestrian NOS injured in collision with pedal cycle, unspecified whether traffic or nontraffic accident

✓x7th **V01.91 Pedestrian on roller-skates injured in collision with pedal cycle, unspecified whether traffic or nontraffic accident** ▽

✓x7th **V01.92 Pedestrian on skateboard injured in collision with pedal cycle, unspecified whether traffic or nontraffic accident** ▽

✓x7th **V01.99 Pedestrian with other conveyance injured in collision with pedal cycle, unspecified whether traffic or nontraffic accident** ▽
Pedestrian with babystroller injured in collision with pedal cycle, unspecified whether traffic or nontraffic accident
Pedestrian on ice-skates injured in collision with pedal cycle unspecified, whether traffic or nontraffic accident
Pedestrian on nonmotorized scooter injured in collision with pedal cycle, unspecified whether traffic or nontraffic accident
Pedestrian on sled injured in collision with pedal cycle unspecified, whether traffic or nontraffic accident
Pedestrian on snowboard injured in collision with pedal cycle, unspecified whether traffic or nontraffic accident
Pedestrian on snow-skis injured in collision with pedal cycle, unspecified whether traffic or nontraffic accident
Pedestrian in wheelchair (powered) injured in collision with pedal cycle, unspecified whether traffic or nontraffic accident
Pedestrian in motorized mobility scooter injured in collision with pedal cycle, unspecified whether traffic or nontraffic accident

✓4th **V02 Pedestrian injured in collision with two- or three-wheeled motor vehicle**

✓5th **V02.0 Pedestrian injured in collision with two- or three-wheeled motor vehicle in nontraffic accident**

✓x7th **V02.00 Pedestrian on foot injured in collision with two- or three-wheeled motor vehicle in nontraffic accident**
Pedestrian NOS injured in collision with two- or three-wheeled motor vehicle in nontraffic accident

✓x7th **V02.01 Pedestrian on roller-skates injured in collision with two- or three-wheeled motor vehicle in nontraffic accident**

✓ Additional Character Req   ✓x7th Placeholder Alert   Manifestation   HCC CMS-HCC Condition   ▽ Unspecified Code   ►◄ Revised Text   ● New Code   ▲ Revised Code Title

ICD-10-CM 2018   **1117**

✓x7th **V02.02** **Pedestrian on skateboard injured in collision with two- or three-wheeled motor vehicle in nontraffic accident**

✓x7th **V02.09** **Pedestrian with other conveyance injured in collision with two- or three-wheeled motor vehicle in nontraffic accident**
Pedestrian with babystroller injured in collision with two- or three-wheeled motor vehicle in nontraffic accident
Pedestrian on ice-skates injured in collision with two- or three-wheeled motor vehicle in nontraffic accident
Pedestrian on nonmotorized scooter injured in collision with two- or three-wheeled motor vehicle in nontraffic accident
Pedestrian on sled injured in collision with two- or three-wheeled motor vehicle in nontraffic accident
Pedestrian on snowboard injured in collision with two- or three-wheeled motor vehicle in nontraffic accident
Pedestrian on snow-skis injured in collision with two- or three-wheeled motor vehicle in nontraffic accident
Pedestrian in wheelchair (powered) injured in collision with two- or three-wheeled motor vehicle in nontraffic accident
Pedestrian in motorized mobility scooter injured in collision with two- or three-wheeled motor vehicle in nontraffic accident

✓5th **V02.1** **Pedestrian injured in collision with two- or three-wheeled motor vehicle in traffic accident**

✓x7th **V02.10** **Pedestrian on foot injured in collision with two- or three-wheeled motor vehicle in traffic accident**
Pedestrian NOS injured in collision with two- or three-wheeled motor vehicle in traffic accident

✓x7th **V02.11** **Pedestrian on roller-skates injured in collision with two- or three-wheeled motor vehicle in traffic accident**

✓x7th **V02.12** **Pedestrian on skateboard injured in collision with two- or three-wheeled motor vehicle in traffic accident**

✓x7th **V02.19** **Pedestrian with other conveyance injured in collision with two- or three-wheeled motor vehicle in traffic accident**
Pedestrian with babystroller injured in collision with two- or three-wheeled motor vehicle in traffic accident
Pedestrian on ice-skates injured in collision with two- or three-wheeled motor vehicle in traffic accident
Pedestrian on nonmotorized scooter injured in collision with two- or three-wheeled motor vehicle in traffic accident
Pedestrian on sled injured in collision with two- or three-wheeled motor vehicle in traffic accident
Pedestrian on snowboard injured in collision with two- or three-wheeled motor vehicle in traffic accident
Pedestrian on snow-skis injured in collision with two- or three-wheeled motor vehicle in traffic accident
Pedestrian in wheelchair (powered) injured in collision with two- or three-wheeled motor vehicle in traffic accident
Pedestrian in motorized mobility scooter injured in collision with two- or three-wheeled motor vehicle in traffic accident

✓5th **V02.9** **Pedestrian injured in collision with two- or three-wheeled motor vehicle, unspecified whether traffic or nontraffic accident**

✓x7th **V02.90** **Pedestrian on foot injured in collision with two- or three-wheeled motor vehicle, unspecified whether traffic or nontraffic accident** ▽
Pedestrian NOS injured in collision with two- or three-wheeled motor vehicle, unspecified whether traffic or nontraffic accident

✓x7th **V02.91** **Pedestrian on roller-skates injured in collision with two- or three-wheeled motor vehicle, unspecified whether traffic or nontraffic accident** ▽

✓x7th **V02.92** **Pedestrian on skateboard injured in collision with two- or three-wheeled motor vehicle, unspecified whether traffic or nontraffic accident** ▽

✓x7th **V02.99** **Pedestrian with other conveyance injured in collision with two- or three-wheeled motor vehicle, unspecified whether traffic or nontraffic accident** ▽
Pedestrian with babystroller injured in collision with two- or three-wheeled motor vehicle, unspecified whether traffic or nontraffic accident
Pedestrian on ice-skates injured in collision with two- or three-wheeled motor vehicle, unspecified whether traffic or nontraffic accident
Pedestrian on nonmotorized scooter injured in collision with two- or three-wheeled motor vehicle, unspecified whether traffic or nontraffic accident
Pedestrian on sled injured in collision with two- or three-wheeled motor vehicle, unspecified whether traffic or nontraffic accident
Pedestrian on snowboard injured in collision with two- or three-wheeled motor vehicle, unspecified whether traffic or nontraffic accident
Pedestrian on snow-skis injured in collision with two- or three-wheeled motor vehicle, unspecified whether traffic or nontraffic accident
Pedestrian in wheelchair (powered) injured in collision with two- or three-wheeled motor vehicle, unspecified whether traffic or nontraffic accident
Pedestrian in motorized mobility scooter injured in collision with two- or three-wheeled motor vehicle, unspecified whether traffic or nontraffic accident

✓4th **V03** **Pedestrian injured in collision with car, pick-up truck or van**

✓5th **V03.0** **Pedestrian injured in collision with car, pick-up truck or van in nontraffic accident**

✓x7th **V03.00** **Pedestrian on foot injured in collision with car, pick-up truck or van in nontraffic accident**
Pedestrian NOS injured in collision with car, pick-up truck or van in nontraffic accident

✓x7th **V03.01** **Pedestrian on roller-skates injured in collision with car, pick-up truck or van in nontraffic accident**

✓x7th **V03.02** **Pedestrian on skateboard injured in collision with car, pick-up truck or van in nontraffic accident**

✓x7th **V03.09** **Pedestrian with other conveyance injured in collision with car, pick-up truck or van in nontraffic accident**
Pedestrian with babystroller injured in collision with car, pick-up truck or van in nontraffic accident
Pedestrian on ice-skates injured in collision with car, pick-up truck or van in nontraffic accident
Pedestrian on nonmotorized scooter injured in collision with car, pick-up truck or van in nontraffic accident
Pedestrian on sled injured in collision with car, pick-up truck or van in nontraffic accident
Pedestrian on snowboard injured in collision with car, pick-up truck or van in nontraffic accident
Pedestrian on snow-skis injured in collision with car, pick-up truck or van in nontraffic accident
Pedestrian in wheelchair (powered) injured in collision with car, pick-up truck or van in nontraffic accident
Pedestrian in motorized mobility scooter injured in collision with car, pick-up truck or van in nontraffic accident

✓5th **V03.1** **Pedestrian injured in collision with car, pick-up truck or van in traffic accident**

✓x7th **V03.10** **Pedestrian on foot injured in collision with car, pick-up truck or van in traffic accident**
Pedestrian NOS injured in collision with car, pick-up truck or van in traffic accident

✓x7th **V03.11** **Pedestrian on roller-skates injured in collision with car, pick-up truck or van in traffic accident**

✓x7th **V03.12** **Pedestrian on skateboard injured in collision with car, pick-up truck or van in traffic accident**

EXCLUDES 1 Not coded here   EXCLUDES 2 Not included here   N Newborn Age: 0   P Pediatric Age: 0-17   M Maternity Age: 12-55   A Adult Age: 15-124

1118   ICD-10-CM 2018

☑x7ᵗʰ **V03.19 Pedestrian with other conveyance injured in collision with car, pick-up truck or van in traffic accident**
> Pedestrian with babystroller injured in collision with car, pick-up truck or van in traffic accident
> Pedestrian on ice-skates injured in collision with car, pick-up truck or van in traffic accident
> Pedestrian on nonmotorized scooter injured in collision with car, pick-up truck or van in traffic accident
> Pedestrian on sled injured in collision with car, pick-up truck or van in traffic accident
> Pedestrian on snowboard injured in collision with car, pick-up truck or van in traffic accident
> Pedestrian on snow-skis injured in collision with car, pick-up truck or van in traffic accident
> Pedestrian in wheelchair (powered) injured in collision with car, pick-up truck or van in traffic accident
> Pedestrian in motorized mobility scooter injured in collision with car, pick-up truck or van in traffic accident

☑5ᵗʰ **V03.9 Pedestrian injured in collision with car, pick-up truck or van, unspecified whether traffic or nontraffic accident**

    ☑x7ᵗʰ **V03.90 Pedestrian on foot injured in collision with car, pick-up truck or van, unspecified whether traffic or nontraffic accident** ▽
> Pedestrian NOS injured in collision with car, pick-up truck or van, unspecified whether traffic or nontraffic accident

    ☑x7ᵗʰ **V03.91 Pedestrian on roller-skates injured in collision with car, pick-up truck or van, unspecified whether traffic or nontraffic accident** ▽

    ☑x7ᵗʰ **V03.92 Pedestrian on skateboard injured in collision with car, pick-up truck or van, unspecified whether traffic or nontraffic accident** ▽

    ☑x7ᵗʰ **V03.99 Pedestrian with other conveyance injured in collision with car, pick-up truck or van, unspecified whether traffic or nontraffic accident** ▽
> Pedestrian with babystroller injured in collision with car, pick-up truck or van, unspecified whether traffic or nontraffic accident
> Pedestrian on ice-skates injured in collision with car, pick-up truck or van, unspecified whether traffic or nontraffic accident
> Pedestrian on nonmotorized scooter injured in collision with car, pick-up truck or van, unspecified whether traffic or nontraffic accident
> Pedestrian on sled injured in collision with car, pick-up truck or van in nontraffic accident
> Pedestrian on snowboard injured in collision with car, pick-up truck or van, unspecified whether traffic or nontraffic accident
> Pedestrian on snow-skis injured in collision with car, pick-up truck or van, unspecified whether traffic or nontraffic accident
> Pedestrian in wheelchair (powered) injured in collision with car, pick-up truck or van, unspecified whether traffic or nontraffic accident
> Pedestrian in motorized mobility scooter injured in collision with car, pick-up truck or van, unspecified whether traffic or nontraffic accident

☑4ᵗʰ **V04 Pedestrian injured in collision with heavy transport vehicle or bus**
> *EXCLUDES 1*   *pedestrian injured in collision with military vehicle (V09.01, V09.21)*

☑5ᵗʰ **V04.0 Pedestrian injured in collision with heavy transport vehicle or bus in nontraffic accident**

    ☑x7ᵗʰ **V04.00 Pedestrian on foot injured in collision with heavy transport vehicle or bus in nontraffic accident**
> Pedestrian NOS injured in collision with heavy transport vehicle or bus in nontraffic accident

    ☑x7ᵗʰ **V04.01 Pedestrian on roller-skates injured in collision with heavy transport vehicle or bus in nontraffic accident**

    ☑x7ᵗʰ **V04.02 Pedestrian on skateboard injured in collision with heavy transport vehicle or bus in nontraffic accident**

☑x7ᵗʰ **V04.09 Pedestrian with other conveyance injured in collision with heavy transport vehicle or bus in nontraffic accident**
> Pedestrian with babystroller injured in collision with heavy transport vehicle or bus in nontraffic accident
> Pedestrian on ice-skates injured in collision with heavy transport vehicle or bus in nontraffic accident
> Pedestrian on nonmotorized scooter injured in collision with heavy transport vehicle or bus in nontraffic accident
> Pedestrian on sled injured in collision with heavy transport vehicle or bus in nontraffic accident
> Pedestrian on snowboard injured in collision with heavy transport vehicle or bus in nontraffic accident
> Pedestrian on snow-skis injured in collision with heavy transport vehicle or bus in nontraffic accident
> Pedestrian in wheelchair (powered) injured in collision with heavy transport vehicle or bus in nontraffic accident
> Pedestrian in motorized mobility scooter injured in collision with heavy transport vehicle or bus in nontraffic accident

☑5ᵗʰ **V04.1 Pedestrian injured in collision with heavy transport vehicle or bus in traffic accident**

    ☑x7ᵗʰ **V04.10 Pedestrian on foot injured in collision with heavy transport vehicle or bus in traffic accident**
> Pedestrian NOS injured in collision with heavy transport vehicle or bus in traffic accident

    ☑x7ᵗʰ **V04.11 Pedestrian on roller-skates injured in collision with heavy transport vehicle or bus in traffic accident**

    ☑x7ᵗʰ **V04.12 Pedestrian on skateboard injured in collision with heavy transport vehicle or bus in traffic accident**

    ☑x7ᵗʰ **V04.19 Pedestrian with other conveyance injured in collision with heavy transport vehicle or bus in traffic accident**
> Pedestrian with babystroller injured in collision with heavy transport vehicle or bus in traffic accident
> Pedestrian on ice-skates injured in collision with heavy transport vehicle or bus in traffic accident
> Pedestrian on nonmotorized scooter injured in collision with heavy transport vehicle or bus in traffic accident
> Pedestrian on sled injured in collision with heavy transport vehicle or bus in traffic accident
> Pedestrian on snowboard injured in collision with heavy transport vehicle or bus in traffic accident
> Pedestrian on snow-skis injured in collision with heavy transport vehicle or bus in traffic accident
> Pedestrian in wheelchair (powered) injured in collision with heavy transport vehicle or bus in traffic accident
> Pedestrian in motorized mobility scooter injured in collision with heavy transport vehicle or bus in traffic accident

☑5ᵗʰ **V04.9 Pedestrian injured in collision with heavy transport vehicle or bus, unspecified whether traffic or nontraffic accident**

    ☑x7ᵗʰ **V04.90 Pedestrian on foot injured in collision with heavy transport vehicle or bus, unspecified whether traffic or nontraffic accident** ▽
> Pedestrian NOS injured in collision with heavy transport vehicle or bus, unspecified whether traffic or nontraffic accident

    ☑x7ᵗʰ **V04.91 Pedestrian on roller-skates injured in collision with heavy transport vehicle or bus, unspecified whether traffic or nontraffic accident** ▽

    ☑x7ᵗʰ **V04.92 Pedestrian on skateboard injured in collision with heavy transport vehicle or bus, unspecified whether traffic or nontraffic accident** ▽

☑ Additional Character Req   ☑x7ᵗʰ Placeholder Alert   Manifestation   **HCC** CMS-HCC Condition   ▽ Unspecified Code   ►◄ Revised Text   ● New Code   ▲ Revised Code Title

√x7ᵗʰ V04.99 Pedestrian with other conveyance injured in collision with heavy transport vehicle or bus, unspecified whether traffic or nontraffic accident ▽
  Pedestrian with babystroller injured in collision with heavy transport vehicle or bus, unspecified whether traffic or nontraffic accident
  Pedestrian on ice-skates injured in collision with heavy transport vehicle or bus, unspecified whether traffic or nontraffic accident
  Pedestrian on nonmotorized scooter injured in collision with heavy transport vehicle or bus, unspecified whether traffic or nontraffic accident
  Pedestrian on sled injured in collision with heavy transport vehicle or bus, unspecified whether traffic or nontraffic accident
  Pedestrian on snowboard injured in collision with heavy transport vehicle or bus, unspecified whether traffic or nontraffic accident
  Pedestrian on snow-skis injured in collision with heavy transport vehicle or bus, unspecified whether traffic or nontraffic accident
  Pedestrian in wheelchair (powered) injured in collision with heavy transport vehicle or bus, unspecified whether traffic or nontraffic accident
  Pedestrian in motorized mobility scooter injured in collision with heavy transport vehicle or bus, unspecified whether traffic or nontraffic accident

√4ᵗʰ **V05 Pedestrian injured in collision with railway train or railway vehicle**

√5ᵗʰ **V05.0 Pedestrian injured in collision with railway train or railway vehicle in nontraffic accident**

√x7ᵗʰ **V05.00 Pedestrian on foot injured in collision with railway train or railway vehicle in nontraffic accident**
  Pedestrian NOS injured in collision with railway train or railway vehicle in nontraffic accident

√x7ᵗʰ **V05.01 Pedestrian on roller-skates injured in collision with railway train or railway vehicle in nontraffic accident**

√x7ᵗʰ **V05.02 Pedestrian on skateboard injured in collision with railway train or railway vehicle in nontraffic accident**

√x7ᵗʰ **V05.09 Pedestrian with other conveyance injured in collision with railway train or railway vehicle in nontraffic accident**
  Pedestrian with babystroller injured in collision with railway train or railway vehicle in nontraffic accident
  Pedestrian on ice-skates injured in collision with railway train or railway vehicle in nontraffic accident
  Pedestrian on nonmotorized scooter injured in collision with railway train or railway vehicle in nontraffic accident
  Pedestrian on sled injured in collision with railway train or railway vehicle in nontraffic accident
  Pedestrian on snowboard injured in collision with railway train or railway vehicle in nontraffic accident
  Pedestrian on snow-skis injured in collision with railway train or railway vehicle in nontraffic accident
  Pedestrian in wheelchair (powered) injured in collision with railway train or railway vehicle in nontraffic accident
  Pedestrian in motorized mobility scooter injured in collision with railway train or railway vehicle in nontraffic accident

√5ᵗʰ **V05.1 Pedestrian injured in collision with railway train or railway vehicle in traffic accident**

√x7ᵗʰ **V05.10 Pedestrian on foot injured in collision with railway train or railway vehicle in traffic accident**
  Pedestrian NOS injured in collision with railway train or railway vehicle in traffic accident

√x7ᵗʰ **V05.11 Pedestrian on roller-skates injured in collision with railway train or railway vehicle in traffic accident**

√x7ᵗʰ **V05.12 Pedestrian on skateboard injured in collision with railway train or railway vehicle in traffic accident**

√x7ᵗʰ **V05.19 Pedestrian with other conveyance injured in collision with railway train or railway vehicle in traffic accident**
  Pedestrian with babystroller injured in collision with railway train or railway vehicle in traffic accident
  Pedestrian on ice-skates injured in collision with railway train or railway vehicle in traffic accident
  Pedestrian on nonmotorized scooter injured in collision with railway train or railway vehicle in traffic accident
  Pedestrian on sled injured in collision with railway train or railway vehicle in traffic accident
  Pedestrian on snowboard injured in collision with railway train or railway vehicle in traffic accident
  Pedestrian on snow-skis injured in collision with railway train or railway vehicle in traffic accident
  Pedestrian in wheelchair (powered) injured in collision with railway train or railway vehicle in traffic accident
  Pedestrian in motorized mobility scooter injured in collision with railway train or railway vehicle in traffic accident

√5ᵗʰ **V05.9 Pedestrian injured in collision with railway train or railway vehicle, unspecified whether traffic or nontraffic accident**

√x7ᵗʰ **V05.90 Pedestrian on foot injured in collision with railway train or railway vehicle, unspecified whether traffic or nontraffic accident** ▽
  Pedestrian NOS injured in collision with railway train or railway vehicle, unspecified whether traffic or nontraffic accident

√x7ᵗʰ **V05.91 Pedestrian on roller-skates injured in collision with railway train or railway vehicle, unspecified whether traffic or nontraffic accident** ▽

√x7ᵗʰ **V05.92 Pedestrian on skateboard injured in collision with railway train or railway vehicle, unspecified whether traffic or nontraffic accident** ▽

√x7ᵗʰ **V05.99 Pedestrian with other conveyance injured in collision with railway train or railway vehicle, unspecified whether traffic or nontraffic accident** ▽
  Pedestrian with babystroller injured in collision with railway train or railway vehicle, unspecified whether traffic or nontraffic
  Pedestrian on ice-skates injured in collision with railway train or railway vehicle, unspecified whether traffic or nontraffic
  Pedestrian on nonmotorized scooter injured in collision with railway train or railway vehicle, unspecified whether traffic or nontraffic
  Pedestrian on sled injured in collision with railway train or railway vehicle, unspecified whether traffic or nontraffic
  Pedestrian on snowboard injured in collision with railway train or railway vehicle, unspecified whether traffic or nontraffic
  Pedestrian on snow-skis injured in collision with railway train or railway vehicle, unspecified whether traffic or nontraffic
  Pedestrian in wheelchair (powered) injured in collision with railway train or railway vehicle, unspecified whether traffic or nontraffic
  Pedestrian in motorized mobility scooter injured in collision with railway train or railway vehicle, unspecified whether traffic or nontraffic

√4ᵗʰ **V06 Pedestrian injured in collision with other nonmotor vehicle**
  INCLUDES collision with animal-drawn vehicle, animal being ridden, nonpowered streetcar
  EXCLUDES 1 *pedestrian injured in collision with pedestrian conveyance (V00.0-)*

√5ᵗʰ **V06.0 Pedestrian injured in collision with other nonmotor vehicle in nontraffic accident**

√x7ᵗʰ **V06.00 Pedestrian on foot injured in collision with other nonmotor vehicle in nontraffic accident**
  Pedestrian NOS injured in collision with other nonmotor vehicle in nontraffic accident

√x7ᵗʰ **V06.01 Pedestrian on roller-skates injured in collision with other nonmotor vehicle in nontraffic accident**

√x7ᵗʰ **V06.02 Pedestrian on skateboard injured in collision with other nonmotor vehicle in nontraffic accident**

EXCLUDES 1 Not coded here   EXCLUDES 2 Not included here   N Newborn Age: 0   P Pediatric Age: 0-17   M Maternity Age: 12-55   A Adult Age: 15-124

1120   ICD-10-CM 2018

V04.99–V06.02

☑x7ᵗʰ **V06.09 Pedestrian with other conveyance injured in collision with other nonmotor vehicle in nontraffic accident**
Pedestrian with babystroller injured in collision with other nonmotor vehicle in nontraffic accident
Pedestrian on ice-skates injured in collision with other nonmotor vehicle in nontraffic accident
Pedestrian on nonmotorized scooter injured in collision with other nonmotor vehicle in nontraffic accident
Pedestrian on sled injured in collision with other nonmotor vehicle in nontraffic accident
Pedestrian on snowboard injured in collision with other nonmotor vehicle in nontraffic accident
Pedestrian on snow-skis injured in collision with other nonmotor vehicle in nontraffic accident
Pedestrian in wheelchair (powered) injured in collision with other nonmotor vehicle in nontraffic accident
Pedestrian in motorized mobility scooter injured in collision with other nonmotor vehicle in nontraffic accident

☑5ᵗʰ **V06.1 Pedestrian injured in collision with other nonmotor vehicle in traffic accident**

☑x7ᵗʰ **V06.10 Pedestrian on foot injured in collision with other nonmotor vehicle in traffic accident**
Pedestrian NOS injured in collision with other nonmotor vehicle in traffic accident

☑x7ᵗʰ **V06.11 Pedestrian on roller-skates injured in collision with other nonmotor vehicle in traffic accident**

☑x7ᵗʰ **V06.12 Pedestrian on skateboard injured in collision with other nonmotor vehicle in traffic accident**

☑x7ᵗʰ **V06.19 Pedestrian with other conveyance injured in collision with other nonmotor vehicle in traffic accident**
Pedestrian with babystroller injured in collision with other nonmotor vehicle in nontraffic accident
Pedestrian on ice-skates injured in collision with other nonmotor vehicle in traffic accident
Pedestrian on nonmotorized scooter injured in collision with other nonmotor vehicle in traffic accident
Pedestrian on sled injured in collision with other nonmotor vehicle in traffic accident
Pedestrian on snowboard injured in collision with other nonmotor vehicle in traffic accident
Pedestrian on snow-skis injured in collision with other nonmotor vehicle in traffic accident
Pedestrian in wheelchair (powered) injured in collision with other nonmotor vehicle in traffic accident
Pedestrian in motorized mobility scooter injured in collision with other nonmotor vehicle in traffic accident

☑5ᵗʰ **V06.9 Pedestrian injured in collision with other nonmotor vehicle, unspecified whether traffic or nontraffic accident**

☑x7ᵗʰ **V06.90 Pedestrian on foot injured in collision with other nonmotor vehicle, unspecified whether traffic or nontraffic accident** ▽
Pedestrian NOS injured in collision with other nonmotor vehicle, unspecified whether traffic or nontraffic accident

☑x7ᵗʰ **V06.91 Pedestrian on roller-skates injured in collision with other nonmotor vehicle, unspecified whether traffic or nontraffic accident** ▽

☑x7ᵗʰ **V06.92 Pedestrian on skateboard injured in collision with other nonmotor vehicle, unspecified whether traffic or nontraffic accident** ▽

☑x7ᵗʰ **V06.99 Pedestrian with other conveyance injured in collision with other nonmotor vehicle, unspecified whether traffic or nontraffic accident** ▽
Pedestrian with babystroller injured in collision with other nonmotor vehicle, unspecified whether traffic or nontraffic accident
Pedestrian on ice-skates injured in collision with other nonmotor vehicle, unspecified whether traffic or nontraffic accident
Pedestrian on nonmotorized scooter injured in collision with other nonmotor vehicle, unspecified whether traffic or nontraffic accident
Pedestrian on sled injured in collision with other nonmotor vehicle, unspecified whether traffic or nontraffic accident
Pedestrian on snowboard injured in collision with other nonmotor vehicle, unspecified whether traffic or nontraffic accident
Pedestrian on snow-skis injured in collision with other nonmotor vehicle, unspecified whether traffic or nontraffic accident
Pedestrian in wheelchair (powered) injured in collision with other nonmotor vehicle, unspecified whether traffic or nontraffic accident
Pedestrian in motorized mobility scooter injured in collision with other nonmotor vehicle, unspecified whether traffic or nontraffic accident

☑4ᵗʰ **V09 Pedestrian injured in other and unspecified transport accidents**

☑5ᵗʰ **V09.0 Pedestrian injured in nontraffic accident involving other and unspecified motor vehicles**

☑x7ᵗʰ **V09.00 Pedestrian injured in nontraffic accident involving unspecified motor vehicles** ▽

☑x7ᵗʰ **V09.01 Pedestrian injured in nontraffic accident involving military vehicle**

☑x7ᵗʰ **V09.09 Pedestrian injured in nontraffic accident involving other motor vehicles**
Pedestrian injured in nontraffic accident by special vehicle

☑x7ᵗʰ **V09.1 Pedestrian injured in unspecified nontraffic accident** ▽

☑5ᵗʰ **V09.2 Pedestrian injured in traffic accident involving other and unspecified motor vehicles**

☑x7ᵗʰ **V09.20 Pedestrian injured in traffic accident involving unspecified motor vehicles** ▽

☑x7ᵗʰ **V09.21 Pedestrian injured in traffic accident involving military vehicle**

☑x7ᵗʰ **V09.29 Pedestrian injured in traffic accident involving other motor vehicles**

☑x7ᵗʰ **V09.3 Pedestrian injured in unspecified traffic accident** ▽

☑x7ᵗʰ **V09.9 Pedestrian injured in unspecified transport accident** ▽

Pedal cycle rider injured in transport accident (V10-V19)

INCLUDES any non-motorized vehicle, excluding an animal-drawn vehicle, or a sidecar or trailer attached to the pedal cycle

EXCLUDES 2 *rupture of pedal cycle tire (W37.0)*

The appropriate 7th character is to be added to each code from categories V10-V19.
A   initial encounter
D   subsequent encounter
S   sequela

☑4ᵗʰ **V10 Pedal cycle rider injured in collision with pedestrian or animal**
EXCLUDES 1 *pedal cycle rider collision with animal-drawn vehicle or animal being ridden (V16.-)*

☑x7ᵗʰ **V10.0 Pedal cycle driver injured in collision with pedestrian or animal in nontraffic accident**

☑x7ᵗʰ **V10.1 Pedal cycle passenger injured in collision with pedestrian or animal in nontraffic accident**

☑x7ᵗʰ **V10.2 Unspecified pedal cyclist injured in collision with pedestrian or animal in nontraffic accident** ▽

☑x7ᵗʰ **V10.3 Person boarding or alighting a pedal cycle injured in collision with pedestrian or animal**

☑x7ᵗʰ **V10.4 Pedal cycle driver injured in collision with pedestrian or animal in traffic accident**

☑x7ᵗʰ **V10.5 Pedal cycle passenger injured in collision with pedestrian or animal in traffic accident**

☑x7ᵗʰ **V10.9 Unspecified pedal cyclist injured in collision with pedestrian or animal in traffic accident** ▽

√4ᵗʰ **V11 Pedal cycle rider injured in collision with other pedal cycle**

√x7ᵗʰ **V11.0** Pedal cycle **driver** injured in collision with other pedal cycle in **nontraffic accident**

√x7ᵗʰ **V11.1** Pedal cycle **passenger** injured in collision with other pedal cycle in **nontraffic accident**

√x7ᵗʰ **V11.2** Unspecified pedal cyclist injured in collision with other pedal cycle in **nontraffic accident** ▽

√x7ᵗʰ **V11.3** Person boarding or alighting a pedal cycle injured in collision with other pedal cycle

√x7ᵗʰ **V11.4** Pedal cycle **driver** injured in collision with other pedal cycle in **traffic accident**

√x7ᵗʰ **V11.5** Pedal cycle **passenger** injured in collision with other pedal cycle in **traffic accident**

√x7ᵗʰ **V11.9** Unspecified pedal cyclist injured in collision with other pedal cycle in **traffic accident** ▽

√4ᵗʰ **V12 Pedal cycle rider injured in collision with two- or three-wheeled motor vehicle**

√x7ᵗʰ **V12.0** Pedal cycle **driver** injured in collision with two- or three-wheeled motor vehicle in **nontraffic accident**

√x7ᵗʰ **V12.1** Pedal cycle **passenger** injured in collision with two- or three-wheeled motor vehicle in **nontraffic accident**

√x7ᵗʰ **V12.2** Unspecified pedal cyclist injured in collision with two- or three-wheeled motor vehicle in **nontraffic accident** ▽

√x7ᵗʰ **V12.3** Person boarding or alighting a pedal cycle injured in collision with two- or three-wheeled motor vehicle

√x7ᵗʰ **V12.4** Pedal cycle **driver** injured in collision with two- or three-wheeled motor vehicle in **traffic accident**

√x7ᵗʰ **V12.5** Pedal cycle **passenger** injured in collision with two- or three-wheeled motor vehicle in **traffic accident**

√x7ᵗʰ **V12.9** Unspecified pedal cyclist injured in collision with two- or three-wheeled motor vehicle in **traffic accident** ▽

√4ᵗʰ **V13 Pedal cycle rider injured in collision with car, pick-up truck or van**

√x7ᵗʰ **V13.0** Pedal cycle **driver** injured in collision with car, pick-up truck or van in **nontraffic accident**

√x7ᵗʰ **V13.1** Pedal cycle **passenger** injured in collision with car, pick-up truck or van in **nontraffic accident**

√x7ᵗʰ **V13.2** Unspecified pedal cyclist injured in collision with car, pick-up truck or van in **nontraffic accident** ▽

√x7ᵗʰ **V13.3** Person boarding or alighting a pedal cycle injured in collision with car, pick-up truck or van

√x7ᵗʰ **V13.4** Pedal cycle **driver** injured in collision with car, pick-up truck or van in **traffic accident**

√x7ᵗʰ **V13.5** Pedal cycle **passenger** injured in collision with car, pick-up truck or van in **traffic accident**

√x7ᵗʰ **V13.9** Unspecified pedal cyclist injured in collision with car, pick-up truck or van in **traffic accident** ▽

√4ᵗʰ **V14 Pedal cycle rider injured in collision with heavy transport vehicle or bus**

EXCLUDES 1   *pedal cycle rider injured in collision with military vehicle (V19.81)*

√x7ᵗʰ **V14.0** Pedal cycle **driver** injured in collision with heavy transport vehicle or bus in **nontraffic accident**

√x7ᵗʰ **V14.1** Pedal cycle **passenger** injured in collision with heavy transport vehicle or bus in **nontraffic accident**

√x7ᵗʰ **V14.2** Unspecified pedal cyclist injured in collision with heavy transport vehicle or bus in **nontraffic accident** ▽

√x7ᵗʰ **V14.3** Person boarding or alighting a pedal cycle injured in collision with heavy transport vehicle or bus

√x7ᵗʰ **V14.4** Pedal cycle **driver** injured in collision with heavy transport vehicle or bus in **traffic accident**

√x7ᵗʰ **V14.5** Pedal cycle **passenger** injured in collision with heavy transport vehicle or bus in **traffic accident**

√x7ᵗʰ **V14.9** Unspecified pedal cyclist injured in collision with heavy transport vehicle or bus in **traffic accident** ▽

√4ᵗʰ **V15 Pedal cycle rider injured in collision with railway train or railway vehicle**

√x7ᵗʰ **V15.0** Pedal cycle **driver** injured in collision with railway train or railway vehicle in **nontraffic accident**

√x7ᵗʰ **V15.1** Pedal cycle **passenger** injured in collision with railway train or railway vehicle in **nontraffic accident**

√x7ᵗʰ **V15.2** Unspecified pedal cyclist injured in collision with railway train or railway vehicle in **nontraffic accident** ▽

√x7ᵗʰ **V15.3** Person boarding or alighting a pedal cycle injured in collision with railway train or railway vehicle

√x7ᵗʰ **V15.4** Pedal cycle **driver** injured in collision with railway train or railway vehicle in **traffic accident**

√x7ᵗʰ **V15.5** Pedal cycle **passenger** injured in collision with railway train or railway vehicle in **traffic accident**

√x7ᵗʰ **V15.9** Unspecified pedal cyclist injured in collision with railway train or railway vehicle in **traffic accident** ▽

√4ᵗʰ **V16 Pedal cycle rider injured in collision with other nonmotor vehicle**

INCLUDES   collision with animal-drawn vehicle, animal being ridden, streetcar

√x7ᵗʰ **V16.0** Pedal cycle **driver** injured in collision with other nonmotor vehicle in **nontraffic accident**

√x7ᵗʰ **V16.1** Pedal cycle **passenger** injured in collision with other nonmotor vehicle in **nontraffic accident**

√x7ᵗʰ **V16.2** Unspecified pedal cyclist injured in collision with other nonmotor vehicle in **nontraffic accident** ▽

√x7ᵗʰ **V16.3** Person boarding or alighting a pedal cycle injured in collision with other nonmotor vehicle in **nontraffic accident**

√x7ᵗʰ **V16.4** Pedal cycle **driver** injured in collision with other nonmotor vehicle in **traffic accident**

√x7ᵗʰ **V16.5** Pedal cycle **passenger** injured in collision with other nonmotor vehicle in **traffic accident**

√x7ᵗʰ **V16.9** Unspecified pedal cyclist injured in collision with other nonmotor vehicle in **traffic accident** ▽

√4ᵗʰ **V17 Pedal cycle rider injured in collision with fixed or stationary object**

√x7ᵗʰ **V17.0** Pedal cycle **driver** injured in collision with fixed or stationary object in **nontraffic accident**

√x7ᵗʰ **V17.1** Pedal cycle **passenger** injured in collision with fixed or stationary object in **nontraffic accident**

√x7ᵗʰ **V17.2** Unspecified pedal cyclist injured in collision with fixed or stationary object in **nontraffic accident** ▽

√x7ᵗʰ **V17.3** Person boarding or alighting a pedal cycle injured in collision with fixed or stationary object

√x7ᵗʰ **V17.4** Pedal cycle **driver** injured in collision with fixed or stationary object in **traffic accident**

√x7ᵗʰ **V17.5** Pedal cycle **passenger** injured in collision with fixed or stationary object in **traffic accident**

√x7ᵗʰ **V17.9** Unspecified pedal cyclist injured in collision with fixed or stationary object in **traffic accident** ▽

√4ᵗʰ **V18 Pedal cycle rider injured in noncollision transport accident**

INCLUDES   fall or thrown from pedal cycle (without antecedent collision)
overturning pedal cycle NOS
overturning pedal cycle without collision

√x7ᵗʰ **V18.0** Pedal cycle **driver** injured in noncollision transport accident in **nontraffic accident**

√x7ᵗʰ **V18.1** Pedal cycle **passenger** injured in noncollision transport accident in **nontraffic accident**

√x7ᵗʰ **V18.2** Unspecified pedal cyclist injured in noncollision transport accident in **nontraffic accident** ▽

√x7ᵗʰ **V18.3** Person boarding or alighting a pedal cycle injured in noncollision transport accident

√x7ᵗʰ **V18.4** Pedal cycle **driver** injured in noncollision transport accident in **traffic accident**

√x7ᵗʰ **V18.5** Pedal cycle **passenger** injured in noncollision transport accident in **traffic accident**

√x7ᵗʰ **V18.9** Unspecified pedal cyclist injured in noncollision transport accident in **traffic accident** ▽

√4ᵗʰ **V19 Pedal cycle rider injured in other and unspecified transport accidents**

√5ᵗʰ **V19.0** Pedal cycle **driver** injured in collision with other and unspecified motor vehicles in **nontraffic accident**

√x7ᵗʰ **V19.00** Pedal cycle driver injured in collision with unspecified motor vehicles in nontraffic accident ▽

√x7ᵗʰ **V19.09** Pedal cycle driver injured in collision with other motor vehicles in nontraffic accident

√5ᵗʰ **V19.1** Pedal cycle **passenger** injured in collision with other and unspecified motor vehicles in **nontraffic accident**

√x7ᵗʰ **V19.10** Pedal cycle passenger injured in collision with unspecified motor vehicles in nontraffic accident ▽

√x7ᵗʰ **V19.19** Pedal cycle passenger injured in collision with other motor vehicles in nontraffic accident

---

EXCLUDES 1 Not coded here   EXCLUDES 2 Not included here   **N** Newborn Age: 0   **P** Pediatric Age: 0-17   **M** Maternity Age: 12-55   **A** Adult Age: 15-124

√5ᵗʰ V19.2 Unspecified pedal cyclist injured in collision with other and unspecified motor vehicles in nontraffic accident

  √x7ᵗʰ **V19.20 Unspecified pedal cyclist injured in collision with** ▽ **unspecified motor vehicles in nontraffic accident**
       Pedal cycle collision NOS, nontraffic

  √x7ᵗʰ **V19.29 Unspecified pedal cyclist injured in collision with** ▽ **other motor vehicles in nontraffic accident**

√x7ᵗʰ V19.3 Pedal cyclist (driver) (passenger) injured in unspecified ▽ **nontraffic accident**
       Pedal cycle accident NOS, nontraffic
       Pedal cyclist injured in nontraffic accident NOS

√5ᵗʰ V19.4 Pedal cycle driver injured in collision with other and unspecified motor vehicles in traffic accident

  √x7ᵗʰ **V19.40 Pedal cycle driver injured in collision with** ▽ **unspecified motor vehicles in traffic accident**

  √x7ᵗʰ **V19.49 Pedal cycle driver injured in collision with other motor vehicles in traffic accident**

√5ᵗʰ V19.5 Pedal cycle passenger injured in collision with other and unspecified motor vehicles in traffic accident

  √x7ᵗʰ **V19.50 Pedal cycle passenger injured in collision with** ▽ **unspecified motor vehicles in traffic accident**

  √x7ᵗʰ **V19.59 Pedal cycle passenger injured in collision with other motor vehicles in traffic accident**

√5ᵗʰ V19.6 Unspecified pedal cyclist injured in collision with other and unspecified motor vehicles in traffic accident

  √x7ᵗʰ **V19.60 Unspecified pedal cyclist injured in collision with** ▽ **unspecified motor vehicles in traffic accident**
       Pedal cycle collision NOS (traffic)

  √x7ᵗʰ **V19.69 Unspecified pedal cyclist injured in collision with other motor vehicles in traffic accident**

√5ᵗʰ V19.8 Pedal cyclist (driver) (passenger) injured in other specified transport accidents

  √x7ᵗʰ **V19.81 Pedal cyclist (driver) (passenger) injured in transport accident with military vehicle**

  √x7ᵗʰ **V19.88 Pedal cyclist (driver) (passenger) injured in other specified transport accidents**

√x7ᵗʰ V19.9 Pedal cyclist (driver) (passenger) injured in unspecified ▽ **traffic accident**
       Pedal cycle accident NOS

Motorcycle rider injured in transport accident (V20-V29)

INCLUDES   moped
           motorcycle with sidecar
           motorized bicycle
           motor scooter

EXCLUDES 1   *three-wheeled motor vehicle (V30-V39)*

> The appropriate 7th character is to be added to each code from categories V20-V29.
> A   initial encounter
> D   subsequent encounter
> S   sequela

√4ᵗʰ V20 Motorcycle rider injured in collision with pedestrian or animal
     EXCLUDES 1   *motorcycle rider collision with animal-drawn vehicle or animal being ridden (V26.-)*

  √x7ᵗʰ **V20.0 Motorcycle driver injured in collision with pedestrian or animal in nontraffic accident**

  √x7ᵗʰ **V20.1 Motorcycle passenger injured in collision with pedestrian or animal in nontraffic accident**

  √x7ᵗʰ **V20.2 Unspecified motorcycle rider injured in collision with** ▽ **pedestrian or animal in nontraffic accident**

  √x7ᵗʰ **V20.3 Person boarding or alighting a motorcycle injured in collision with pedestrian or animal**

  √x7ᵗʰ **V20.4 Motorcycle driver injured in collision with pedestrian or animal in traffic accident**

  √x7ᵗʰ **V20.5 Motorcycle passenger injured in collision with pedestrian or animal in traffic accident**

  √x7ᵗʰ **V20.9 Unspecified motorcycle rider injured in collision with** ▽ **pedestrian or animal in traffic accident**

√4ᵗʰ V21 Motorcycle rider injured in collision with pedal cycle

  √x7ᵗʰ **V21.0 Motorcycle driver injured in collision with pedal cycle in nontraffic accident**

  √x7ᵗʰ **V21.1 Motorcycle passenger injured in collision with pedal cycle in nontraffic accident**

  √x7ᵗʰ **V21.2 Unspecified motorcycle rider injured in collision with** ▽ **pedal cycle in nontraffic accident**

  √x7ᵗʰ **V21.3 Person boarding or alighting a motorcycle injured in collision with pedal cycle**

  √x7ᵗʰ **V21.4 Motorcycle driver injured in collision with pedal cycle in traffic accident**

  √x7ᵗʰ **V21.5 Motorcycle passenger injured in collision with pedal cycle in traffic accident**

  √x7ᵗʰ **V21.9 Unspecified motorcycle rider injured in collision with** ▽ **pedal cycle in traffic accident**

√4ᵗʰ V22 Motorcycle rider injured in collision with two- or three-wheeled motor vehicle

  √x7ᵗʰ **V22.0 Motorcycle driver injured in collision with two- or three-wheeled motor vehicle in nontraffic accident**

  √x7ᵗʰ **V22.1 Motorcycle passenger injured in collision with two- or three-wheeled motor vehicle in nontraffic accident**

  √x7ᵗʰ **V22.2 Unspecified motorcycle rider injured in collision with two-** ▽ **or three-wheeled motor vehicle in nontraffic accident**

  √x7ᵗʰ **V22.3 Person boarding or alighting a motorcycle injured in collision with two- or three-wheeled motor vehicle**

  √x7ᵗʰ **V22.4 Motorcycle driver injured in collision with two- or three-wheeled motor vehicle in traffic accident**

  √x7ᵗʰ **V22.5 Motorcycle passenger injured in collision with two- or three-wheeled motor vehicle in traffic accident**

  √x7ᵗʰ **V22.9 Unspecified motorcycle rider injured in collision with two-** ▽ **or three-wheeled motor vehicle in traffic accident**

√4ᵗʰ V23 Motorcycle rider injured in collision with car, pick-up truck or van

  √x7ᵗʰ **V23.0 Motorcycle driver injured in collision with car, pick-up truck or van in nontraffic accident**

  √x7ᵗʰ **V23.1 Motorcycle passenger injured in collision with car, pick-up truck or van in nontraffic accident**

  √x7ᵗʰ **V23.2 Unspecified motorcycle rider injured in collision with car,** ▽ **pick-up truck or van in nontraffic accident**

  √x7ᵗʰ **V23.3 Person boarding or alighting a motorcycle injured in collision with car, pick-up truck or van**

  √x7ᵗʰ **V23.4 Motorcycle driver injured in collision with car, pick-up truck or van in traffic accident**

  √x7ᵗʰ **V23.5 Motorcycle passenger injured in collision with car, pick-up truck or van in traffic accident**

  √x7ᵗʰ **V23.9 Unspecified motorcycle rider injured in collision with car,** ▽ **pick-up truck or van in traffic accident**

√4ᵗʰ V24 Motorcycle rider injured in collision with heavy transport vehicle or bus
     EXCLUDES 1   *motorcycle rider injured in collision with military vehicle (V29.81)*

  √x7ᵗʰ **V24.0 Motorcycle driver injured in collision with heavy transport vehicle or bus in nontraffic accident**

  √x7ᵗʰ **V24.1 Motorcycle passenger injured in collision with heavy transport vehicle or bus in nontraffic accident**

  √x7ᵗʰ **V24.2 Unspecified motorcycle rider injured in collision with** ▽ **heavy transport vehicle or bus in nontraffic accident**

  √x7ᵗʰ **V24.3 Person boarding or alighting a motorcycle injured in collision with heavy transport vehicle or bus**

  √x7ᵗʰ **V24.4 Motorcycle driver injured in collision with heavy transport vehicle or bus in traffic accident**

  √x7ᵗʰ **V24.5 Motorcycle passenger injured in collision with heavy transport vehicle or bus in traffic accident**

  √x7ᵗʰ **V24.9 Unspecified motorcycle rider injured in collision with** ▽ **heavy transport vehicle or bus in traffic accident**

√4ᵗʰ V25 Motorcycle rider injured in collision with railway train or railway vehicle

  √x7ᵗʰ **V25.0 Motorcycle driver injured in collision with railway train or railway vehicle in nontraffic accident**

  √x7ᵗʰ **V25.1 Motorcycle passenger injured in collision with railway train or railway vehicle in nontraffic accident**

  √x7ᵗʰ **V25.2 Unspecified motorcycle rider injured in collision with** ▽ **railway train or railway vehicle in nontraffic accident**

  √x7ᵗʰ **V25.3 Person boarding or alighting a motorcycle injured in collision with railway train or railway vehicle**

  √x7ᵗʰ **V25.4 Motorcycle driver injured in collision with railway train or railway vehicle in traffic accident**

  √x7ᵗʰ **V25.5 Motorcycle passenger injured in collision with railway train or railway vehicle in traffic accident**

☑ Additional Character Req   √x7ᵗʰ Placeholder Alert   Manifestation   HCC CMS-HCC Condition   ▽ Unspecified Code   ►◄ Revised Text   ● New Code   ▲ Revised Code Title

Chapter 20. External Causes of Morbidity

√x7ʰ **V25.9 Unspecified motorcycle rider injured in collision with railway train or railway vehicle in traffic accident** ▽

√4ʰ **V26 Motorcycle rider injured in collision with other nonmotor vehicle**
INCLUDES collision with animal-drawn vehicle, animal being ridden, streetcar

√x7ʰ **V26.0 Motorcycle driver injured in collision with other nonmotor vehicle in nontraffic accident**

√x7ʰ **V26.1 Motorcycle passenger injured in collision with other nonmotor vehicle in nontraffic accident**

√x7ʰ **V26.2 Unspecified motorcycle rider injured in collision with other nonmotor vehicle in nontraffic accident** ▽

√x7ʰ **V26.3 Person boarding or alighting a motorcycle injured in collision with other nonmotor vehicle**

√x7ʰ **V26.4 Motorcycle driver injured in collision with other nonmotor vehicle in traffic accident**

√x7ʰ **V26.5 Motorcycle passenger injured in collision with other nonmotor vehicle in traffic accident**

√x7ʰ **V26.9 Unspecified motorcycle rider injured in collision with other nonmotor vehicle in traffic accident** ▽

√4ʰ **V27 Motorcycle rider injured in collision with fixed or stationary object**

√x7ʰ **V27.0 Motorcycle driver injured in collision with fixed or stationary object in nontraffic accident**

√x7ʰ **V27.1 Motorcycle passenger injured in collision with fixed or stationary object in nontraffic accident**

√x7ʰ **V27.2 Unspecified motorcycle rider injured in collision with fixed or stationary object in nontraffic accident** ▽

√x7ʰ **V27.3 Person boarding or alighting a motorcycle injured in collision with fixed or stationary object**

√x7ʰ **V27.4 Motorcycle driver injured in collision with fixed or stationary object in traffic accident**

√x7ʰ **V27.5 Motorcycle passenger injured in collision with fixed or stationary object in traffic accident**

√x7ʰ **V27.9 Unspecified motorcycle rider injured in collision with fixed or stationary object in traffic accident** ▽

√4ʰ **V28 Motorcycle rider injured in noncollision transport accident**
INCLUDES fall or thrown from motorcycle (without antecedent collision)
overturning motorcycle NOS
overturning motorcycle without collision

√x7ʰ **V28.0 Motorcycle driver injured in noncollision transport accident in nontraffic accident**

√x7ʰ **V28.1 Motorcycle passenger injured in noncollision transport accident in nontraffic accident**

√x7ʰ **V28.2 Unspecified motorcycle rider injured in noncollision transport accident in nontraffic accident** ▽

√x7ʰ **V28.3 Person boarding or alighting a motorcycle injured in noncollision transport accident**

√x7ʰ **V28.4 Motorcycle driver injured in noncollision transport accident in traffic accident**

√x7ʰ **V28.5 Motorcycle passenger injured in noncollision transport accident in traffic accident**

√x7ʰ **V28.9 Unspecified motorcycle rider injured in noncollision transport accident in traffic accident** ▽

√4ʰ **V29 Motorcycle rider injured in other and unspecified transport accidents**

√5ʰ **V29.0 Motorcycle driver injured in collision with other and unspecified motor vehicles in nontraffic accident**

√x7ʰ **V29.00 Motorcycle driver injured in collision with unspecified motor vehicles in nontraffic accident** ▽

√x7ʰ **V29.09 Motorcycle driver injured in collision with other motor vehicles in nontraffic accident**

√5ʰ **V29.1 Motorcycle passenger injured in collision with other and unspecified motor vehicles in nontraffic accident**

√x7ʰ **V29.10 Motorcycle passenger injured in collision with unspecified motor vehicles in nontraffic accident** ▽

√x7ʰ **V29.19 Motorcycle passenger injured in collision with other motor vehicles in nontraffic accident**

√5ʰ **V29.2 Unspecified motorcycle rider injured in collision with other and unspecified motor vehicles in nontraffic accident**

√x7ʰ **V29.20 Unspecified motorcycle rider injured in collision with unspecified motor vehicles in nontraffic accident** ▽
Motorcycle collision NOS, nontraffic

√x7ʰ **V29.29 Unspecified motorcycle rider injured in collision with other motor vehicles in nontraffic accident** ▽

√x7ʰ **V29.3 Motorcycle rider (driver) (passenger) injured in unspecified nontraffic accident** ▽
Motorcycle accident NOS, nontraffic
Motorcycle rider injured in nontraffic accident NOS

√5ʰ **V29.4 Motorcycle driver injured in collision with other and unspecified motor vehicles in traffic accident**

√x7ʰ **V29.40 Motorcycle driver injured in collision with unspecified motor vehicles in traffic accident** ▽

√x7ʰ **V29.49 Motorcycle driver injured in collision with other motor vehicles in traffic accident**

√5ʰ **V29.5 Motorcycle passenger injured in collision with other and unspecified motor vehicles in traffic accident**

√x7ʰ **V29.50 Motorcycle passenger injured in collision with unspecified motor vehicles in traffic accident** ▽

√x7ʰ **V29.59 Motorcycle passenger injured in collision with other motor vehicles in traffic accident**

√5ʰ **V29.6 Unspecified motorcycle rider injured in collision with other and unspecified motor vehicles in traffic accident**

√x7ʰ **V29.60 Unspecified motorcycle rider injured in collision with unspecified motor vehicles in traffic accident** ▽
Motorcycle collision NOS (traffic)

√x7ʰ **V29.69 Unspecified motorcycle rider injured in collision with other motor vehicles in traffic accident** ▽

√5ʰ **V29.8 Motorcycle rider (driver) (passenger) injured in other specified transport accidents**

√x7ʰ **V29.81 Motorcycle rider (driver) (passenger) injured in transport accident with military vehicle**

√x7ʰ **V29.88 Motorcycle rider (driver) (passenger) injured in other specified transport accidents**

√x7ʰ **V29.9 Motorcycle rider (driver) (passenger) injured in unspecified traffic accident** ▽
Motorcycle accident NOS

Occupant of three-wheeled motor vehicle injured in transport accident (V30-V39)

INCLUDES motorized rickshaw
motorized tricycle
three-wheeled motor car
EXCLUDES1 all-terrain vehicles (V86.-)
motorcycle with sidecar (V20-V29)
vehicle designed primarily for off-road use (V86.-)

The appropriate 7th character is to be added to each code from categories V30-V39.
A initial encounter
D subsequent encounter
S sequela

√4ʰ **V30 Occupant of three-wheeled motor vehicle injured in collision with pedestrian or animal**
EXCLUDES1 three-wheeled motor vehicle collision with animal-drawn vehicle or animal being ridden (V36.-)

√x7ʰ **V30.0 Driver of three-wheeled motor vehicle injured in collision with pedestrian or animal in nontraffic accident**

√x7ʰ **V30.1 Passenger in three-wheeled motor vehicle injured in collision with pedestrian or animal in nontraffic accident**

√x7ʰ **V30.2 Person on outside of three-wheeled motor vehicle injured in collision with pedestrian or animal in nontraffic accident**

√x7ʰ **V30.3 Unspecified occupant of three-wheeled motor vehicle injured in collision with pedestrian or animal in nontraffic accident** ▽

√x7ʰ **V30.4 Person boarding or alighting a three-wheeled motor vehicle injured in collision with pedestrian or animal**

√x7ʰ **V30.5 Driver of three-wheeled motor vehicle injured in collision with pedestrian or animal in traffic accident**

√x7ʰ **V30.6 Passenger in three-wheeled motor vehicle injured in collision with pedestrian or animal in traffic accident**

√x7ʰ **V30.7 Person on outside of three-wheeled motor vehicle injured in collision with pedestrian or animal in traffic accident**

√x7ʰ **V30.9 Unspecified occupant of three-wheeled motor vehicle injured in collision with pedestrian or animal in traffic accident** ▽

☑4ᵗʰ **V31 Occupant of three-wheeled motor vehicle injured in collision with pedal cycle**

✓x7ᵗʰ **V31.0 Driver of three-wheeled motor vehicle injured in collision with pedal cycle in nontraffic accident**

✓x7ᵗʰ **V31.1 Passenger in three-wheeled motor vehicle injured in collision with pedal cycle in nontraffic accident**

✓x7ᵗʰ **V31.2 Person on outside of three-wheeled motor vehicle injured in collision with pedal cycle in nontraffic accident**

✓x7ᵗʰ **V31.3 Unspecified occupant of three-wheeled motor vehicle injured in collision with pedal cycle in nontraffic accident** ▽

✓x7ᵗʰ **V31.4 Person boarding or alighting a three-wheeled motor vehicle injured in collision with pedal cycle**

✓x7ᵗʰ **V31.5 Driver of three-wheeled motor vehicle injured in collision with pedal cycle in traffic accident**

✓x7ᵗʰ **V31.6 Passenger in three-wheeled motor vehicle injured in collision with pedal cycle in traffic accident**

✓x7ᵗʰ **V31.7 Person on outside of three-wheeled motor vehicle injured in collision with pedal cycle in traffic accident**

✓x7ᵗʰ **V31.9 Unspecified occupant of three-wheeled motor vehicle injured in collision with pedal cycle in traffic accident** ▽

☑4ᵗʰ **V32 Occupant of three-wheeled motor vehicle injured in collision with two- or three-wheeled motor vehicle**

✓x7ᵗʰ **V32.0 Driver of three-wheeled motor vehicle injured in collision with two- or three-wheeled motor vehicle in nontraffic accident**

✓x7ᵗʰ **V32.1 Passenger in three-wheeled motor vehicle injured in collision with two- or three-wheeled motor vehicle in nontraffic accident**

✓x7ᵗʰ **V32.2 Person on outside of three-wheeled motor vehicle injured in collision with two- or three-wheeled motor vehicle in nontraffic accident**

✓x7ᵗʰ **V32.3 Unspecified occupant of three-wheeled motor vehicle injured in collision with two- or three-wheeled motor vehicle in nontraffic accident** ▽

✓x7ᵗʰ **V32.4 Person boarding or alighting a three-wheeled motor vehicle injured in collision with two- or three-wheeled motor vehicle**

✓x7ᵗʰ **V32.5 Driver of three-wheeled motor vehicle injured in collision with two- or three-wheeled motor vehicle in traffic accident**

✓x7ᵗʰ **V32.6 Passenger in three-wheeled motor vehicle injured in collision with two- or three-wheeled motor vehicle in traffic accident**

✓x7ᵗʰ **V32.7 Person on outside of three-wheeled motor vehicle injured in collision with two- or three-wheeled motor vehicle in traffic accident**

✓x7ᵗʰ **V32.9 Unspecified occupant of three-wheeled motor vehicle injured in collision with two- or three-wheeled motor vehicle in traffic accident** ▽

☑4ᵗʰ **V33 Occupant of three-wheeled motor vehicle injured in collision with car, pick-up truck or van**

✓x7ᵗʰ **V33.0 Driver of three-wheeled motor vehicle injured in collision with car, pick-up truck or van in nontraffic accident**

✓x7ᵗʰ **V33.1 Passenger in three-wheeled motor vehicle injured in collision with car, pick-up truck or van in nontraffic accident**

✓x7ᵗʰ **V33.2 Person on outside of three-wheeled motor vehicle injured in collision with car, pick-up truck or van in nontraffic accident**

✓x7ᵗʰ **V33.3 Unspecified occupant of three-wheeled motor vehicle injured in collision with car, pick-up truck or van in nontraffic accident** ▽

✓x7ᵗʰ **V33.4 Person boarding or alighting a three-wheeled motor vehicle injured in collision with car, pick-up truck or van**

✓x7ᵗʰ **V33.5 Driver of three-wheeled motor vehicle injured in collision with car, pick-up truck or van in traffic accident**

✓x7ᵗʰ **V33.6 Passenger in three-wheeled motor vehicle injured in collision with car, pick-up truck or van in traffic accident**

✓x7ᵗʰ **V33.7 Person on outside of three-wheeled motor vehicle injured in collision with car, pick-up truck or van in traffic accident**

✓x7ᵗʰ **V33.9 Unspecified occupant of three-wheeled motor vehicle injured in collision with car, pick-up truck or van in traffic accident** ▽

☑4ᵗʰ **V34 Occupant of three-wheeled motor vehicle injured in collision with heavy transport vehicle or bus**

> EXCLUDES 1 *occupant of three-wheeled motor vehicle injured in collision with military vehicle (V39.81)*

✓x7ᵗʰ **V34.0 Driver of three-wheeled motor vehicle injured in collision with heavy transport vehicle or bus in nontraffic accident**

✓x7ᵗʰ **V34.1 Passenger in three-wheeled motor vehicle injured in collision with heavy transport vehicle or bus in nontraffic accident**

✓x7ᵗʰ **V34.2 Person on outside of three-wheeled motor vehicle injured in collision with heavy transport vehicle or bus in nontraffic accident**

✓x7ᵗʰ **V34.3 Unspecified occupant of three-wheeled motor vehicle injured in collision with heavy transport vehicle or bus in nontraffic accident** ▽

✓x7ᵗʰ **V34.4 Person boarding or alighting a three-wheeled motor vehicle injured in collision with heavy transport vehicle or bus**

✓x7ᵗʰ **V34.5 Driver of three-wheeled motor vehicle injured in collision with heavy transport vehicle or bus in traffic accident**

✓x7ᵗʰ **V34.6 Passenger in three-wheeled motor vehicle injured in collision with heavy transport vehicle or bus in traffic accident**

✓x7ᵗʰ **V34.7 Person on outside of three-wheeled motor vehicle injured in collision with heavy transport vehicle or bus in traffic accident**

✓x7ᵗʰ **V34.9 Unspecified occupant of three-wheeled motor vehicle injured in collision with heavy transport vehicle or bus in traffic accident** ▽

☑4ᵗʰ **V35 Occupant of three-wheeled motor vehicle injured in collision with railway train or railway vehicle**

✓x7ᵗʰ **V35.0 Driver of three-wheeled motor vehicle injured in collision with railway train or railway vehicle in nontraffic accident**

✓x7ᵗʰ **V35.1 Passenger in three-wheeled motor vehicle injured in collision with railway train or railway vehicle in nontraffic accident**

✓x7ᵗʰ **V35.2 Person on outside of three-wheeled motor vehicle injured in collision with railway train or railway vehicle in nontraffic accident**

✓x7ᵗʰ **V35.3 Unspecified occupant of three-wheeled motor vehicle injured in collision with railway train or railway vehicle in nontraffic accident** ▽

✓x7ᵗʰ **V35.4 Person boarding or alighting a three-wheeled motor vehicle injured in collision with railway train or railway vehicle**

✓x7ᵗʰ **V35.5 Driver of three-wheeled motor vehicle injured in collision with railway train or railway vehicle in traffic accident**

✓x7ᵗʰ **V35.6 Passenger in three-wheeled motor vehicle injured in collision with railway train or railway vehicle in traffic accident**

✓x7ᵗʰ **V35.7 Person on outside of three-wheeled motor vehicle injured in collision with railway train or railway vehicle in traffic accident**

✓x7ᵗʰ **V35.9 Unspecified occupant of three-wheeled motor vehicle injured in collision with railway train or railway vehicle in traffic accident** ▽

☑4ᵗʰ **V36 Occupant of three-wheeled motor vehicle injured in collision with other nonmotor vehicle**

> INCLUDES collision with animal-drawn vehicle, animal being ridden, streetcar

✓x7ᵗʰ **V36.0 Driver of three-wheeled motor vehicle injured in collision with other nonmotor vehicle in nontraffic accident**

✓x7ᵗʰ **V36.1 Passenger in three-wheeled motor vehicle injured in collision with other nonmotor vehicle in nontraffic accident**

✓x7ᵗʰ **V36.2 Person on outside of three-wheeled motor vehicle injured in collision with other nonmotor vehicle in nontraffic accident**

✓x7ᵗʰ **V36.3 Unspecified occupant of three-wheeled motor vehicle injured in collision with other nonmotor vehicle in nontraffic accident** ▽

✓x7ᵗʰ **V36.4 Person boarding or alighting a three-wheeled motor vehicle injured in collision with other nonmotor vehicle**

✓x7ᵗʰ **V36.5 Driver of three-wheeled motor vehicle injured in collision with other nonmotor vehicle in traffic accident**

✓x7ᵗʰ **V36.6 Passenger in three-wheeled motor vehicle injured in collision with other nonmotor vehicle in traffic accident**

✓x7ᵗʰ **V36.7 Person on outside of three-wheeled motor vehicle injured in collision with other nonmotor vehicle in traffic accident**

✓x7ᵗʰ **V36.9 Unspecified occupant of three-wheeled motor vehicle injured in collision with other nonmotor vehicle in traffic accident** ▽

☑4ᵗʰ **V37 Occupant of three-wheeled motor vehicle injured in collision with fixed or stationary object**

✓x7ᵗʰ **V37.0 Driver of three-wheeled motor vehicle injured in collision with fixed or stationary object in nontraffic accident**

✓x7ᵗʰ **V37.1 Passenger in three-wheeled motor vehicle injured in collision with fixed or stationary object in nontraffic accident**

☑ Additional Character Req   ✓x7ᵗʰ Placeholder Alert   Manifestation   HCC CMS-HCC Condition   ▽ Unspecified Code   ▶◀ Revised Text   ● New Code   ▲ Revised Code Title

✓x7ᵗʰ **V37.2** **Person on outside of three-wheeled motor vehicle injured in collision with fixed or stationary object in nontraffic accident**

✓x7ᵗʰ **V37.3** **Unspecified occupant of three-wheeled motor vehicle** ▽ **injured in collision with fixed or stationary object in nontraffic accident**

✓x7ᵗʰ **V37.4** **Person boarding or alighting a three-wheeled motor vehicle injured in collision with fixed or stationary object**

✓x7ᵗʰ **V37.5** **Driver of three-wheeled motor vehicle injured in collision with fixed or stationary object in traffic accident**

✓x7ᵗʰ **V37.6** **Passenger in three-wheeled motor vehicle injured in collision with fixed or stationary object in traffic accident**

✓x7ᵗʰ **V37.7** **Person on outside of three-wheeled motor vehicle injured in collision with fixed or stationary object in traffic accident**

✓x7ᵗʰ **V37.9** **Unspecified occupant of three-wheeled motor vehicle** ▽ **injured in collision with fixed or stationary object in traffic accident**

✓4ᵗʰ **V38** **Occupant of three-wheeled motor vehicle injured in noncollision transport accident**

> INCLUDES   fall or thrown from three-wheeled motor vehicle
> overturning of three-wheeled motor vehicle NOS
> overturning of three-wheeled motor vehicle without collision

✓x7ᵗʰ **V38.0** **Driver of three-wheeled motor vehicle injured in noncollision transport accident in nontraffic accident**

✓x7ᵗʰ **V38.1** **Passenger in three-wheeled motor vehicle injured in noncollision transport accident in nontraffic accident**

✓x7ᵗʰ **V38.2** **Person on outside of three-wheeled motor vehicle injured in noncollision transport accident in nontraffic accident**

✓x7ᵗʰ **V38.3** **Unspecified occupant of three-wheeled motor vehicle** ▽ **injured in noncollision transport accident in nontraffic accident**

✓x7ᵗʰ **V38.4** **Person boarding or alighting a three-wheeled motor vehicle injured in noncollision transport accident**

✓x7ᵗʰ **V38.5** **Driver of three-wheeled motor vehicle injured in noncollision transport accident in traffic accident**

✓x7ᵗʰ **V38.6** **Passenger in three-wheeled motor vehicle injured in noncollision transport accident in traffic accident**

✓x7ᵗʰ **V38.7** **Person on outside of three-wheeled motor vehicle injured in noncollision transport accident in traffic accident**

✓x7ᵗʰ **V38.9** **Unspecified occupant of three-wheeled motor vehicle** ▽ **injured in noncollision transport accident in traffic accident**

✓4ᵗʰ **V39** **Occupant of three-wheeled motor vehicle injured in other and unspecified transport accidents**

✓5ᵗʰ **V39.0** **Driver of three-wheeled motor vehicle injured in collision with other and unspecified motor vehicles in nontraffic accident**

✓x7ᵗʰ **V39.00** **Driver of three-wheeled motor vehicle injured** ▽ **in collision with unspecified motor vehicles in nontraffic accident**

✓x7ᵗʰ **V39.09** **Driver of three-wheeled motor vehicle injured in collision with other motor vehicles in nontraffic accident**

✓5ᵗʰ **V39.1** **Passenger in three-wheeled motor vehicle injured in collision with other and unspecified motor vehicles in nontraffic accident**

✓x7ᵗʰ **V39.10** **Passenger in three-wheeled motor vehicle** ▽ **injured in collision with unspecified motor vehicles in nontraffic accident**

✓x7ᵗʰ **V39.19** **Passenger in three-wheeled motor vehicle injured in collision with other motor vehicles in nontraffic accident**

✓5ᵗʰ **V39.2** **Unspecified occupant of three-wheeled motor vehicle injured in collision with other and unspecified motor vehicles in nontraffic accident**

✓x7ᵗʰ **V39.20** **Unspecified occupant of three-wheeled motor** ▽ **vehicle injured in collision with unspecified motor vehicles in nontraffic accident**

> Collision NOS involving three-wheeled motor vehicle, nontraffic

✓x7ᵗʰ **V39.29** **Unspecified occupant of three-wheeled motor** ▽ **vehicle injured in collision with other motor vehicles in nontraffic accident**

✓x7ᵗʰ **V39.3** **Occupant (driver) (passenger) of three-wheeled motor** ▽ **vehicle injured in unspecified nontraffic accident**

> Accident NOS involving three-wheeled motor vehicle, nontraffic
> Occupant of three-wheeled motor vehicle injured in nontraffic accident NOS

✓5ᵗʰ **V39.4** **Driver of three-wheeled motor vehicle injured in collision with other and unspecified motor vehicles in traffic accident**

✓x7ᵗʰ **V39.40** **Driver of three-wheeled motor vehicle injured** ▽ **in collision with unspecified motor vehicles in traffic accident**

✓x7ᵗʰ **V39.49** **Driver of three-wheeled motor vehicle injured in collision with other motor vehicles in traffic accident**

✓5ᵗʰ **V39.5** **Passenger in three-wheeled motor vehicle injured in collision with other and unspecified motor vehicles in traffic accident**

✓x7ᵗʰ **V39.50** **Passenger in three-wheeled motor vehicle** ▽ **injured in collision with unspecified motor vehicles in traffic accident**

✓x7ᵗʰ **V39.59** **Passenger in three-wheeled motor vehicle injured in collision with other motor vehicles in traffic accident**

✓5ᵗʰ **V39.6** **Unspecified occupant of three-wheeled motor vehicle injured in collision with other and unspecified motor vehicles in traffic accident**

✓x7ᵗʰ **V39.60** **Unspecified occupant of three-wheeled motor** ▽ **vehicle injured in collision with unspecified motor vehicles in traffic accident**

> Collision NOS involving three-wheeled motor vehicle (traffic)

✓x7ᵗʰ **V39.69** **Unspecified occupant of three-wheeled motor** ▽ **vehicle injured in collision with other motor vehicles in traffic accident**

✓5ᵗʰ **V39.8** **Occupant (driver) (passenger) of three-wheeled motor vehicle injured in other specified transport accidents**

✓x7ᵗʰ **V39.81** **Occupant (driver) (passenger) of three-wheeled motor vehicle injured in transport accident with military vehicle**

✓x7ᵗʰ **V39.89** **Occupant (driver) (passenger) of three-wheeled motor vehicle injured in other specified transport accidents**

✓x7ᵗʰ **V39.9** **Occupant (driver) (passenger) of three-wheeled motor** ▽ **vehicle injured in unspecified traffic accident**

> Accident NOS involving three-wheeled motor vehicle

Car occupant injured in transport accident (V40-V49)

> INCLUDES   a four-wheeled motor vehicle designed primarily for carrying passengers
> automobile (pulling a trailer or camper)
>
> EXCLUDES 1   bus (V50-V59)
> minibus (V50-V59)
> minivan (V50-V59)
> motorcoach (V70-V79)
> pick-up truck (V50-V59)
> sport utility vehicle (SUV) (V50-V59)

> The appropriate 7th character is to be added to each code from categories V40-V49.
> A   initial encounter
> D   subsequent encounter
> S   sequela

✓4ᵗʰ **V40** **Car occupant injured in collision with pedestrian or animal**

> EXCLUDES 1   car collision with animal-drawn vehicle or animal being ridden (V46.-)

✓x7ᵗʰ **V40.0** **Car driver injured in collision with pedestrian or animal in nontraffic accident**

✓x7ᵗʰ **V40.1** **Car passenger injured in collision with pedestrian or animal in nontraffic accident**

✓x7ᵗʰ **V40.2** **Person on outside of car injured in collision with pedestrian or animal in nontraffic accident**

✓x7ᵗʰ **V40.3** **Unspecified car occupant injured in collision with** ▽ **pedestrian or animal in nontraffic accident**

✓x7ᵗʰ **V40.4** **Person boarding or alighting a car injured in collision with pedestrian or animal**

✓x7ᵗʰ **V40.5** **Car driver injured in collision with pedestrian or animal in traffic accident**

✓x7ᵗʰ **V40.6** **Car passenger injured in collision with pedestrian or animal in traffic accident**

✓x7ᵗʰ **V40.7** **Person on outside of car injured in collision with pedestrian or animal in traffic accident**

EXCLUDES 1 Not coded here   EXCLUDES 2 Not included here   N Newborn Age: 0   P Pediatric Age: 0-17   M Maternity Age: 12-55   A Adult Age: 15-124

1126   ICD-10-CM 2018

√x7ᵗʰ **V40.9** Unspecified car occupant injured in collision with pedestrian or animal **in traffic accident** ▽

√4ᵗʰ **V41 Car occupant injured in collision with pedal cycle**

√x7ᵗʰ **V41.0** Car **driver** injured in collision with pedal cycle **in nontraffic accident**

√x7ᵗʰ **V41.1** Car **passenger** injured in collision with pedal cycle **in nontraffic accident**

√x7ᵗʰ **V41.2** Person on outside of car injured in collision with pedal cycle **in nontraffic accident**

√x7ᵗʰ **V41.3** Unspecified car occupant injured in collision with pedal cycle **in nontraffic accident** ▽

√x7ᵗʰ **V41.4** Person boarding or alighting a car injured in collision with pedal cycle

√x7ᵗʰ **V41.5** Car **driver** injured in collision with pedal cycle **in traffic accident**

√x7ᵗʰ **V41.6** Car **passenger** injured in collision with pedal cycle **in traffic accident**

√x7ᵗʰ **V41.7** Person on outside of car injured in collision with pedal cycle **in traffic accident**

√x7ᵗʰ **V41.9** Unspecified car occupant injured in collision with pedal cycle **in traffic accident** ▽

√4ᵗʰ **V42 Car occupant injured in collision with two- or three-wheeled motor vehicle**

√x7ᵗʰ **V42.0** Car **driver** injured in collision with two- or three-wheeled motor vehicle **in nontraffic accident**

√x7ᵗʰ **V42.1** Car **passenger** injured in collision with two- or three-wheeled motor vehicle **in nontraffic accident**

√x7ᵗʰ **V42.2** Person on outside of car injured in collision with two- or three-wheeled motor vehicle **in nontraffic accident**

√x7ᵗʰ **V42.3** Unspecified car occupant injured in collision with two- or three-wheeled motor vehicle **in nontraffic accident** ▽

√x7ᵗʰ **V42.4** Person boarding or alighting a car injured in collision with two- or three-wheeled motor vehicle

√x7ᵗʰ **V42.5** Car **driver** injured in collision with two- or three-wheeled motor vehicle **in traffic accident**

√x7ᵗʰ **V42.6** Car **passenger** injured in collision with two- or three-wheeled motor vehicle **in traffic accident**

√x7ᵗʰ **V42.7** Person on outside of car injured in collision with two- or three-wheeled motor vehicle **in traffic accident**

√x7ᵗʰ **V42.9** Unspecified car occupant injured in collision with two- or three-wheeled motor vehicle **in traffic accident** ▽

√4ᵗʰ **V43 Car occupant injured in collision with car, pick-up truck or van**

√5ᵗʰ **V43.0** Car **driver** injured in collision with car, pick-up truck or van **in nontraffic accident**

√x7ᵗʰ **V43.01** Car driver injured in collision with **sport utility vehicle** in nontraffic accident

√x7ᵗʰ **V43.02** Car driver injured in collision with other type car in nontraffic accident

√x7ᵗʰ **V43.03** Car driver injured in collision with **pick-up truck** in nontraffic accident

√x7ᵗʰ **V43.04** Car driver injured in collision with **van** in nontraffic accident

√5ᵗʰ **V43.1** Car **passenger** injured in collision with car, pick-up truck or van **in nontraffic accident**

√x7ᵗʰ **V43.11** Car passenger injured in collision with **sport utility vehicle** in nontraffic accident

√x7ᵗʰ **V43.12** Car passenger injured in collision with other type car in nontraffic accident

√x7ᵗʰ **V43.13** Car passenger injured in collision with **pick-up** in nontraffic accident

√x7ᵗʰ **V43.14** Car passenger injured in collision with **van** in nontraffic accident

√5ᵗʰ **V43.2** Person on outside of car injured in collision with car, pick-up truck or van **in nontraffic accident**

√x7ᵗʰ **V43.21** Person on outside of car injured in collision with **sport utility vehicle** in nontraffic accident

√x7ᵗʰ **V43.22** Person on outside of car injured in collision with other type car in nontraffic accident

√x7ᵗʰ **V43.23** Person on outside of car injured in collision with **pick-up truck** in nontraffic accident

√x7ᵗʰ **V43.24** Person on outside of car injured in collision with **van** in nontraffic accident

√5ᵗʰ **V43.3** Unspecified car occupant injured in collision with car, pick-up truck or van **in nontraffic accident**

√x7ᵗʰ **V43.31** Unspecified car occupant injured in collision with **sport utility vehicle** in nontraffic accident ▽

√x7ᵗʰ **V43.32** Unspecified car occupant injured in collision with other type car in nontraffic accident ▽

√x7ᵗʰ **V43.33** Unspecified car occupant injured in collision with **pick-up truck** in nontraffic accident ▽

√x7ᵗʰ **V43.34** Unspecified car occupant injured in collision with **van** in nontraffic accident ▽

√5ᵗʰ **V43.4** Person boarding or alighting a car injured in collision with car, pick-up truck or van

√x7ᵗʰ **V43.41** Person boarding or alighting a car injured in collision with **sport utility vehicle**

√x7ᵗʰ **V43.42** Person boarding or alighting a car injured in collision with other type car

√x7ᵗʰ **V43.43** Person boarding or alighting a car injured in collision with **pick-up truck**

√x7ᵗʰ **V43.44** Person boarding or alighting a car injured in collision with **van**

√5ᵗʰ **V43.5** Car **driver** injured in collision with car, pick-up truck or van **in traffic accident**

√x7ᵗʰ **V43.51** Car driver injured in collision with **sport utility vehicle** in traffic accident

√x7ᵗʰ **V43.52** Car driver injured in collision with other type car in traffic accident

√x7ᵗʰ **V43.53** Car driver injured in collision with **pick-up truck** in traffic accident

√x7ᵗʰ **V43.54** Car driver injured in collision with **van** in traffic accident

√5ᵗʰ **V43.6** Car **passenger** injured in collision with car, pick-up truck or van **in traffic accident**

√x7ᵗʰ **V43.61** Car passenger injured in collision with **sport utility vehicle** in traffic accident

√x7ᵗʰ **V43.62** Car passenger injured in collision with other type car in traffic accident

√x7ᵗʰ **V43.63** Car passenger injured in collision with **pick-up truck** in traffic accident

√x7ᵗʰ **V43.64** Car passenger injured in collision with **van** in traffic accident

√5ᵗʰ **V43.7** Person on outside of car injured in collision with car, pick-up truck or van **in traffic accident**

√x7ᵗʰ **V43.71** Person on outside of car injured in collision with **sport utility vehicle** in traffic accident

√x7ᵗʰ **V43.72** Person on outside of car injured in collision with other type car in traffic accident

√x7ᵗʰ **V43.73** Person on outside of car injured in collision with **pick-up truck** in traffic accident

√x7ᵗʰ **V43.74** Person on outside of car injured in collision with **van** in traffic accident

√5ᵗʰ **V43.9** Unspecified car occupant injured in collision with car, pick-up truck or van **in traffic accident**

√x7ᵗʰ **V43.91** Unspecified car occupant injured in collision with **sport utility vehicle** in traffic accident ▽

√x7ᵗʰ **V43.92** Unspecified car occupant injured in collision with other type car in traffic accident ▽

√x7ᵗʰ **V43.93** Unspecified car occupant injured in collision with **pick-up truck** in traffic accident ▽

√x7ᵗʰ **V43.94** Unspecified car occupant injured in collision with **van** in traffic accident ▽

√4ᵗʰ **V44 Car occupant injured in collision with heavy transport vehicle or bus**

EXCLUDES 1 car occupant injured in collision with military vehicle (V49.81)

√x7ᵗʰ **V44.0** Car **driver** injured in collision with heavy transport vehicle or bus **in nontraffic accident**

√x7ᵗʰ **V44.1** Car **passenger** injured in collision with heavy transport vehicle or bus **in nontraffic accident**

√x7ᵗʰ **V44.2** Person on outside of car injured in collision with heavy transport vehicle or bus **in nontraffic accident**

√x7ᵗʰ **V44.3** Unspecified car occupant injured in collision with heavy transport vehicle or bus **in nontraffic accident** ▽

√x7ᵗʰ **V44.4** Person boarding or alighting a car injured in collision with heavy transport vehicle or bus

---

☑ Additional Character Req √x7ᵗʰ Placeholder Alert Manifestation HCC CMS-HCC Condition ▽ Unspecified Code ►◄ Revised Text ● New Code ▲ Revised Code Title

Chapter 20. External Causes of Morbidity

√x7ᵗʰ **V44.5** Car driver injured in collision with heavy transport vehicle or bus in traffic accident

√x7ᵗʰ **V44.6** Car passenger injured in collision with heavy transport vehicle or bus in traffic accident

√x7ᵗʰ **V44.7** Person on outside of car injured in collision with heavy transport vehicle or bus in traffic accident

√x7ᵗʰ **V44.9** Unspecified car occupant injured in collision with heavy transport vehicle or bus in traffic accident ▽

√4ᵗʰ **V45** Car occupant injured in collision with railway train or railway vehicle

√x7ᵗʰ **V45.0** Car driver injured in collision with railway train or railway vehicle in nontraffic accident

√x7ᵗʰ **V45.1** Car passenger injured in collision with railway train or railway vehicle in nontraffic accident

√x7ᵗʰ **V45.2** Person on outside of car injured in collision with railway train or railway vehicle in nontraffic accident

√x7ᵗʰ **V45.3** Unspecified car occupant injured in collision with railway train or railway vehicle in nontraffic accident ▽

√x7ᵗʰ **V45.4** Person boarding or alighting a car injured in collision with railway train or railway vehicle

√x7ᵗʰ **V45.5** Car driver injured in collision with railway train or railway vehicle in traffic accident

√x7ᵗʰ **V45.6** Car passenger injured in collision with railway train or railway vehicle in traffic accident

√x7ᵗʰ **V45.7** Person on outside of car injured in collision with railway train or railway vehicle in traffic accident

√x7ᵗʰ **V45.9** Unspecified car occupant injured in collision with railway train or railway vehicle in traffic accident ▽

√4ᵗʰ **V46** Car occupant injured in collision with other nonmotor vehicle

INCLUDES   collision with animal-drawn vehicle, animal being ridden, streetcar

√x7ᵗʰ **V46.0** Car driver injured in collision with other nonmotor vehicle in nontraffic accident

√x7ᵗʰ **V46.1** Car passenger injured in collision with other nonmotor vehicle in nontraffic accident

√x7ᵗʰ **V46.2** Person on outside of car injured in collision with other nonmotor vehicle in nontraffic accident

√x7ᵗʰ **V46.3** Unspecified car occupant injured in collision with other nonmotor vehicle in nontraffic accident ▽

√x7ᵗʰ **V46.4** Person boarding or alighting a car injured in collision with other nonmotor vehicle

√x7ᵗʰ **V46.5** Car driver injured in collision with other nonmotor vehicle in traffic accident

√x7ᵗʰ **V46.6** Car passenger injured in collision with other nonmotor vehicle in traffic accident

√x7ᵗʰ **V46.7** Person on outside of car injured in collision with other nonmotor vehicle in traffic accident

√x7ᵗʰ **V46.9** Unspecified car occupant injured in collision with other nonmotor vehicle in traffic accident ▽

√4ᵗʰ **V47** Car occupant injured in collision with fixed or stationary object

√x7ᵗʰ **V47.0** Car driver injured in collision with fixed or stationary object in nontraffic accident

√x7ᵗʰ **V47.1** Car passenger injured in collision with fixed or stationary object in nontraffic accident

√x7ᵗʰ **V47.2** Person on outside of car injured in collision with fixed or stationary object in nontraffic accident

√x7ᵗʰ **V47.3** Unspecified car occupant injured in collision with fixed or stationary object in nontraffic accident ▽

√x7ᵗʰ **V47.4** Person boarding or alighting a car injured in collision with fixed or stationary object

√x7ᵗʰ **V47.5** Car driver injured in collision with fixed or stationary object in traffic accident

√x7ᵗʰ **V47.6** Car passenger injured in collision with fixed or stationary object in traffic accident

√x7ᵗʰ **V47.7** Person on outside of car injured in collision with fixed or stationary object in traffic accident

√x7ᵗʰ **V47.9** Unspecified car occupant injured in collision with fixed or stationary object in traffic accident ▽

√4ᵗʰ **V48** Car occupant injured in noncollision transport accident

INCLUDES   overturning car NOS
         overturning car without collision

√x7ᵗʰ **V48.0** Car driver injured in noncollision transport accident in nontraffic accident

√x7ᵗʰ **V48.1** Car passenger injured in noncollision transport accident in nontraffic accident

√x7ᵗʰ **V48.2** Person on outside of car injured in noncollision transport accident in nontraffic accident

√x7ᵗʰ **V48.3** Unspecified car occupant injured in noncollision transport accident in nontraffic accident ▽

√x7ᵗʰ **V48.4** Person boarding or alighting a car injured in noncollision transport accident

√x7ᵗʰ **V48.5** Car driver injured in noncollision transport accident in traffic accident

√x7ᵗʰ **V48.6** Car passenger injured in noncollision transport accident in traffic accident

√x7ᵗʰ **V48.7** Person on outside of car injured in noncollision transport accident in traffic accident

√x7ᵗʰ **V48.9** Unspecified car occupant injured in noncollision transport accident in traffic accident ▽

√4ᵗʰ **V49** Car occupant injured in other and unspecified transport accidents

√5ᵗʰ **V49.0** Driver injured in collision with other and unspecified motor vehicles in nontraffic accident

√x7ᵗʰ **V49.00** Driver injured in collision with unspecified motor vehicles in nontraffic accident ▽

√x7ᵗʰ **V49.09** Driver injured in collision with other motor vehicles in nontraffic accident

√5ᵗʰ **V49.1** Passenger injured in collision with other and unspecified motor vehicles in nontraffic accident

√x7ᵗʰ **V49.10** Passenger injured in collision with unspecified motor vehicles in nontraffic accident ▽

√x7ᵗʰ **V49.19** Passenger injured in collision with other motor vehicles in nontraffic accident

√5ᵗʰ **V49.2** Unspecified car occupant injured in collision with other and unspecified motor vehicles in nontraffic accident

√x7ᵗʰ **V49.20** Unspecified car occupant injured in collision with unspecified motor vehicles in nontraffic accident ▽
         Car collision NOS, nontraffic

√x7ᵗʰ **V49.29** Unspecified car occupant injured in collision with other motor vehicles in nontraffic accident ▽

√x7ᵗʰ **V49.3** Car occupant (driver) (passenger) injured in unspecified nontraffic accident ▽
         Car accident NOS, nontraffic
         Car occupant injured in nontraffic accident NOS

√5ᵗʰ **V49.4** Driver injured in collision with other and unspecified motor vehicles in traffic accident

√x7ᵗʰ **V49.40** Driver injured in collision with unspecified motor vehicles in traffic accident ▽

√x7ᵗʰ **V49.49** Driver injured in collision with other motor vehicles in traffic accident

√5ᵗʰ **V49.5** Passenger injured in collision with other and unspecified motor vehicles in traffic accident

√x7ᵗʰ **V49.50** Passenger injured in collision with unspecified motor vehicles in traffic accident ▽

√x7ᵗʰ **V49.59** Passenger injured in collision with other motor vehicles in traffic accident

√5ᵗʰ **V49.6** Unspecified car occupant injured in collision with other and unspecified motor vehicles in traffic accident

√x7ᵗʰ **V49.60** Unspecified car occupant injured in collision with unspecified motor vehicles in traffic accident ▽
         Car collision NOS (traffic)

√x7ᵗʰ **V49.69** Unspecified car occupant injured in collision with other motor vehicles in traffic accident ▽

√5ᵗʰ **V49.8** Car occupant (driver) (passenger) injured in other specified transport accidents

√x7ᵗʰ **V49.81** Car occupant (driver) (passenger) injured in transport accident with military vehicle

√x7ᵗʰ **V49.88** Car occupant (driver) (passenger) injured in other specified transport accidents

√x7ᵗʰ **V49.9** Car occupant (driver) (passenger) injured in unspecified traffic accident ▽
         Car accident NOS

EXCLUDES 1 Not coded here   EXCLUDES 2 Not included here   N Newborn Age: 0   P Pediatric Age: 0-17   M Maternity Age: 12-55   A Adult Age: 15-124

1128   ICD-10-CM 2018

Occupant of pick-up truck or van injured in transport accident (V50-V59)

INCLUDES   a four or six wheel motor vehicle designed primarily for carrying passengers and property but weighing less than the local limit for classification as a heavy goods vehicle

     minibus
     minivan
     sport utility vehicle (SUV)
     truck
     van

EXCLUDES 1   heavy transport vehicle (V60-V69)

The appropriate 7th character is to be added to each code from categories V50-V59.
A   initial encounter
D   subsequent encounter
S   sequela

✓4th V50 Occupant of pick-up truck or van injured in collision with pedestrian or animal

EXCLUDES 1   pick-up truck or van collision with animal-drawn vehicle or animal being ridden (V56.-)

√x7th **V50.0** Driver of pick-up truck or van injured in collision with pedestrian or animal in nontraffic accident

√x7th **V50.1** Passenger in pick-up truck or van injured in collision with pedestrian or animal in nontraffic accident

√x7th **V50.2** Person on outside of pick-up truck or van injured in collision with pedestrian or animal in nontraffic accident

√x7th **V50.3** Unspecified occupant of pick-up truck or van injured in collision with pedestrian or animal in nontraffic accident ▽

√x7th **V50.4** Person boarding or alighting a pick-up truck or van injured in collision with pedestrian or animal

√x7th **V50.5** Driver of pick-up truck or van injured in collision with pedestrian or animal in traffic accident

√x7th **V50.6** Passenger in pick-up truck or van injured in collision with pedestrian or animal in traffic accident

√x7th **V50.7** Person on outside of pick-up truck or van injured in collision with pedestrian or animal in traffic accident

√x7th **V50.9** Unspecified occupant of pick-up truck or van injured in collision with pedestrian or animal in traffic accident ▽

✓4th V51 Occupant of pick-up truck or van injured in collision with pedal cycle

√x7th **V51.0** Driver of pick-up truck or van injured in collision with pedal cycle in nontraffic accident

√x7th **V51.1** Passenger in pick-up truck or van injured in collision with pedal cycle in nontraffic accident

√x7th **V51.2** Person on outside of pick-up truck or van injured in collision with pedal cycle in nontraffic accident

√x7th **V51.3** Unspecified occupant of pick-up truck or van injured in collision with pedal cycle in nontraffic accident ▽

√x7th **V51.4** Person boarding or alighting a pick-up truck or van injured in collision with pedal cycle

√x7th **V51.5** Driver of pick-up truck or van injured in collision with pedal cycle in traffic accident

√x7th **V51.6** Passenger in pick-up truck or van injured in collision with pedal cycle in traffic accident

√x7th **V51.7** Person on outside of pick-up truck or van injured in collision with pedal cycle in traffic accident

√x7th **V51.9** Unspecified occupant of pick-up truck or van injured in collision with pedal cycle in traffic accident ▽

✓4th V52 Occupant of pick-up truck or van injured in collision with two- or three-wheeled motor vehicle

√x7th **V52.0** Driver of pick-up truck or van injured in collision with two- or three-wheeled motor vehicle in nontraffic accident

√x7th **V52.1** Passenger in pick-up truck or van injured in collision with two- or three-wheeled motor vehicle in nontraffic accident

√x7th **V52.2** Person on outside of pick-up truck or van injured in collision with two- or three-wheeled motor vehicle in nontraffic accident

√x7th **V52.3** Unspecified occupant of pick-up truck or van injured in collision with two- or three-wheeled motor vehicle in nontraffic accident ▽

√x7th **V52.4** Person boarding or alighting a pick-up truck or van injured in collision with two- or three-wheeled motor vehicle

√x7th **V52.5** Driver of pick-up truck or van injured in collision with two- or three-wheeled motor vehicle in traffic accident

√x7th **V52.6** Passenger in pick-up truck or van injured in collision with two- or three-wheeled motor vehicle in traffic accident

√x7th **V52.7** Person on outside of pick-up truck or van injured in collision with two- or three-wheeled motor vehicle in traffic accident

√x7th **V52.9** Unspecified occupant of pick-up truck or van injured in collision with two- or three-wheeled motor vehicle in traffic accident ▽

✓4th V53 Occupant of pick-up truck or van injured in collision with car, pick-up truck or van

√x7th **V53.0** Driver of pick-up truck or van injured in collision with car, pick-up truck or van in nontraffic accident

√x7th **V53.1** Passenger in pick-up truck or van injured in collision with car, pick-up truck or van in nontraffic accident

√x7th **V53.2** Person on outside of pick-up truck or van injured in collision with car, pick-up truck or van in nontraffic accident

√x7th **V53.3** Unspecified occupant of pick-up truck or van injured in collision with car, pick-up truck or van in nontraffic accident ▽

√x7th **V53.4** Person boarding or alighting a pick-up truck or van injured in collision with car, pick-up truck or van

√x7th **V53.5** Driver of pick-up truck or van injured in collision with car, pick-up truck or van in traffic accident

√x7th **V53.6** Passenger in pick-up truck or van injured in collision with car, pick-up truck or van in traffic accident

√x7th **V53.7** Person on outside of pick-up truck or van injured in collision with car, pick-up truck or van in traffic accident

√x7th **V53.9** Unspecified occupant of pick-up truck or van injured in collision with car, pick-up truck or van in traffic accident ▽

✓4th V54 Occupant of pick-up truck or van injured in collision with heavy transport vehicle or bus

EXCLUDES 1   occupant of pick-up truck or van injured in collision with military vehicle (V59.81)

√x7th **V54.0** Driver of pick-up truck or van injured in collision with heavy transport vehicle or bus in nontraffic accident

√x7th **V54.1** Passenger in pick-up truck or van injured in collision with heavy transport vehicle or bus in nontraffic accident

√x7th **V54.2** Person on outside of pick-up truck or van injured in collision with heavy transport vehicle or bus in nontraffic accident

√x7th **V54.3** Unspecified occupant of pick-up truck or van injured in collision with heavy transport vehicle or bus in nontraffic accident ▽

√x7th **V54.4** Person boarding or alighting a pick-up truck or van injured in collision with heavy transport vehicle or bus

√x7th **V54.5** Driver of pick-up truck or van injured in collision with heavy transport vehicle or bus in traffic accident

√x7th **V54.6** Passenger in pick-up truck or van injured in collision with heavy transport vehicle or bus in traffic accident

√x7th **V54.7** Person on outside of pick-up truck or van injured in collision with heavy transport vehicle or bus in traffic accident

√x7th **V54.9** Unspecified occupant of pick-up truck or van injured in collision with heavy transport vehicle or bus in traffic accident ▽

✓4th V55 Occupant of pick-up truck or van injured in collision with railway train or railway vehicle

√x7th **V55.0** Driver of pick-up truck or van injured in collision with railway train or railway vehicle in nontraffic accident

√x7th **V55.1** Passenger in pick-up truck or van injured in collision with railway train or railway vehicle in nontraffic accident

√x7th **V55.2** Person on outside of pick-up truck or van injured in collision with railway train or railway vehicle in nontraffic accident

√x7th **V55.3** Unspecified occupant of pick-up truck or van injured in collision with railway train or railway vehicle in nontraffic accident ▽

√x7th **V55.4** Person boarding or alighting a pick-up truck or van injured in collision with railway train or railway vehicle

√x7th **V55.5** Driver of pick-up truck or van injured in collision with railway train or railway vehicle in traffic accident

√x7th **V55.6** Passenger in pick-up truck or van injured in collision with railway train or railway vehicle in traffic accident

√x7th **V55.7** Person on outside of pick-up truck or van injured in collision with railway train or railway vehicle in traffic accident

√x7th **V55.9** Unspecified occupant of pick-up truck or van injured in collision with railway train or railway vehicle in traffic accident ▽

☑ Additional Character Req   √x7th Placeholder Alert   Manifestation   HCC CMS-HCC Condition   ▽ Unspecified Code   ►◄ Revised Text   ● New Code   ▲ Revised Code Title

Chapter 20. External Causes of Morbidity

V56–V60.1

✓4ᵗʰ **V56**   **Occupant of pick-up truck or van injured in collision with other nonmotor vehicle**

> **INCLUDES**   collision with animal-drawn vehicle, animal being ridden, streetcar

✓x7ᵗʰ **V56.0**   **Driver of pick-up truck or van injured in collision with other nonmotor vehicle in nontraffic accident**

✓x7ᵗʰ **V56.1**   **Passenger in pick-up truck or van injured in collision with other nonmotor vehicle in nontraffic accident**

✓x7ᵗʰ **V56.2**   **Person on outside of pick-up truck or van injured in collision with other nonmotor vehicle in nontraffic accident**

✓x7ᵗʰ **V56.3**   **Unspecified occupant of pick-up truck or van injured in collision with other nonmotor vehicle in nontraffic accident** ▽

✓x7ᵗʰ **V56.4**   **Person boarding or alighting a pick-up truck or van injured in collision with other nonmotor vehicle**

✓x7ᵗʰ **V56.5**   **Driver of pick-up truck or van injured in collision with other nonmotor vehicle in traffic accident**

✓x7ᵗʰ **V56.6**   **Passenger in pick-up truck or van injured in collision with other nonmotor vehicle in traffic accident**

✓x7ᵗʰ **V56.7**   **Person on outside of pick-up truck or van injured in collision with other nonmotor vehicle in traffic accident**

✓x7ᵗʰ **V56.9**   **Unspecified occupant of pick-up truck or van injured in collision with other nonmotor vehicle in traffic accident** ▽

✓4ᵗʰ **V57**   **Occupant of pick-up truck or van injured in collision with fixed or stationary object**

✓x7ᵗʰ **V57.0**   **Driver of pick-up truck or van injured in collision with fixed or stationary object in nontraffic accident**

✓x7ᵗʰ **V57.1**   **Passenger in pick-up truck or van injured in collision with fixed or stationary object in nontraffic accident**

✓x7ᵗʰ **V57.2**   **Person on outside of pick-up truck or van injured in collision with fixed or stationary object in nontraffic accident**

✓x7ᵗʰ **V57.3**   **Unspecified occupant of pick-up truck or van injured in collision with fixed or stationary object in nontraffic accident** ▽

✓x7ᵗʰ **V57.4**   **Person boarding or alighting a pick-up truck or van injured in collision with fixed or stationary object**

✓x7ᵗʰ **V57.5**   **Driver of pick-up truck or van injured in collision with fixed or stationary object in traffic accident**

✓x7ᵗʰ **V57.6**   **Passenger in pick-up truck or van injured in collision with fixed or stationary object in traffic accident**

✓x7ᵗʰ **V57.7**   **Person on outside of pick-up truck or van injured in collision with fixed or stationary object in traffic accident**

✓x7ᵗʰ **V57.9**   **Unspecified occupant of pick-up truck or van injured in collision with fixed or stationary object in traffic accident** ▽

✓4ᵗʰ **V58**   **Occupant of pick-up truck or van injured in noncollision transport accident**

> **INCLUDES**   overturning pick-up truck or van NOS
> overturning pick-up truck or van without collision

✓x7ᵗʰ **V58.0**   **Driver of pick-up truck or van injured in noncollision transport accident in nontraffic accident**

✓x7ᵗʰ **V58.1**   **Passenger in pick-up truck or van injured in noncollision transport accident in nontraffic accident**

✓x7ᵗʰ **V58.2**   **Person on outside of pick-up truck or van injured in noncollision transport accident in nontraffic accident**

✓x7ᵗʰ **V58.3**   **Unspecified occupant of pick-up truck or van injured in noncollision transport accident in nontraffic accident** ▽

✓x7ᵗʰ **V58.4**   **Person boarding or alighting a pick-up truck or van injured in noncollision transport accident**

✓x7ᵗʰ **V58.5**   **Driver of pick-up truck or van injured in noncollision transport accident in traffic accident**

✓x7ᵗʰ **V58.6**   **Passenger in pick-up truck or van injured in noncollision transport accident in traffic accident**

✓x7ᵗʰ **V58.7**   **Person on outside of pick-up truck or van injured in noncollision transport accident in traffic accident**

✓x7ᵗʰ **V58.9**   **Unspecified occupant of pick-up truck or van injured in noncollision transport accident in traffic accident** ▽

✓4ᵗʰ **V59**   **Occupant of pick-up truck or van injured in other and unspecified transport accidents**

✓5ᵗʰ **V59.0**   **Driver of pick-up truck or van injured in collision with other and unspecified motor vehicles in nontraffic accident**

✓x7ᵗʰ **V59.00**   **Driver of pick-up truck or van injured in collision with unspecified motor vehicles in nontraffic accident** ▽

✓x7ᵗʰ **V59.09**   **Driver of pick-up truck or van injured in collision with other motor vehicles in nontraffic accident**

✓5ᵗʰ **V59.1**   **Passenger in pick-up truck or van injured in collision with other and unspecified motor vehicles in nontraffic accident**

✓x7ᵗʰ **V59.10**   **Passenger in pick-up truck or van injured in collision with unspecified motor vehicles in nontraffic accident** ▽

✓x7ᵗʰ **V59.19**   **Passenger in pick-up truck or van injured in collision with other motor vehicles in nontraffic accident**

✓5ᵗʰ **V59.2**   **Unspecified occupant of pick-up truck or van injured in collision with other and unspecified motor vehicles in nontraffic accident**

✓x7ᵗʰ **V59.20**   **Unspecified occupant of pick-up truck or van injured in collision with unspecified motor vehicles in nontraffic accident** ▽
> Collision NOS involving pick-up truck or van, nontraffic

✓x7ᵗʰ **V59.29**   **Unspecified occupant of pick-up truck or van injured in collision with other motor vehicles in nontraffic accident**

✓5ᵗʰ **V59.3**   **Occupant (driver) (passenger) of pick-up truck or van injured in unspecified nontraffic accident** ▽
> Accident NOS involving pick-up truck or van, nontraffic
> Occupant of pick-up truck or van injured in nontraffic accident NOS

✓5ᵗʰ **V59.4**   **Driver of pick-up truck or van injured in collision with other and unspecified motor vehicles in traffic accident**

✓x7ᵗʰ **V59.40**   **Driver of pick-up truck or van injured in collision with unspecified motor vehicles in traffic accident** ▽

✓x7ᵗʰ **V59.49**   **Driver of pick-up truck or van injured in collision with other motor vehicles in traffic accident**

✓5ᵗʰ **V59.5**   **Passenger in pick-up truck or van injured in collision with other and unspecified motor vehicles in traffic accident**

✓x7ᵗʰ **V59.50**   **Passenger in pick-up truck or van injured in collision with unspecified motor vehicles in traffic accident** ▽

✓x7ᵗʰ **V59.59**   **Passenger in pick-up truck or van injured in collision with other motor vehicles in traffic accident**

✓5ᵗʰ **V59.6**   **Unspecified occupant of pick-up truck or van injured in collision with other and unspecified motor vehicles in traffic accident**

✓x7ᵗʰ **V59.60**   **Unspecified occupant of pick-up truck or van injured in collision with unspecified motor vehicles in traffic accident** ▽
> Collision NOS involving pick-up truck or van (traffic)

✓x7ᵗʰ **V59.69**   **Unspecified occupant of pick-up truck or van injured in collision with other motor vehicles in traffic accident** ▽

✓5ᵗʰ **V59.8**   **Occupant (driver) (passenger) of pick-up truck or van injured in other specified transport accidents**

✓x7ᵗʰ **V59.81**   **Occupant (driver) (passenger) of pick-up truck or van injured in transport accident with military vehicle**

✓x7ᵗʰ **V59.88**   **Occupant (driver) (passenger) of pick-up truck or van injured in other specified transport accidents**

✓5ᵗʰ **V59.9**   **Occupant (driver) (passenger) of pick-up truck or van injured in unspecified traffic accident** ▽
> Accident NOS involving pick-up truck or van

Occupant of heavy transport vehicle injured in transport accident (V60-V69)

> **INCLUDES**   18 wheeler
> armored car
> panel truck
> **EXCLUDES 1**   *bus*
> *motorcoach*

> The appropriate 7th character is to be added to each code from categories V60-V69.
> A   initial encounter
> D   subsequent encounter
> S   sequela

✓4ᵗʰ **V60**   **Occupant of heavy transport vehicle injured in collision with pedestrian or animal**
> **EXCLUDES 1**   *heavy transport vehicle collision with animal-drawn vehicle or animal being ridden (V66.-)*

✓x7ᵗʰ **V60.0**   **Driver of heavy transport vehicle injured in collision with pedestrian or animal in nontraffic accident**

✓x7ᵗʰ **V60.1**   **Passenger in heavy transport vehicle injured in collision with pedestrian or animal in nontraffic accident**

EXCLUDES 1 Not coded here   **EXCLUDES 2** Not included here   **N** Newborn Age: 0   **P** Pediatric Age: 0-17   **M** Maternity Age: 12-55   **A** Adult Age: 15-124

√x7ᵗʰ **V60.2** Person on outside of heavy transport vehicle injured in collision with pedestrian or animal in nontraffic accident

√x7ᵗʰ **V60.3** Unspecified occupant of heavy transport vehicle injured in collision with pedestrian or animal in nontraffic accident ▽

√x7ᵗʰ **V60.4** Person boarding or alighting a heavy transport vehicle injured in collision with pedestrian or animal

√x7ᵗʰ **V60.5** Driver of heavy transport vehicle injured in collision with pedestrian or animal in traffic accident

√x7ᵗʰ **V60.6** Passenger in heavy transport vehicle injured in collision with pedestrian or animal in traffic accident

√x7ᵗʰ **V60.7** Person on outside of heavy transport vehicle injured in collision with pedestrian or animal in traffic accident

√x7ᵗʰ **V60.9** Unspecified occupant of heavy transport vehicle injured in collision with pedestrian or animal in traffic accident ▽

✓4ᵗʰ **V61 Occupant of heavy transport vehicle injured in collision with pedal cycle**

√x7ᵗʰ **V61.0** Driver of heavy transport vehicle injured in collision with pedal cycle in nontraffic accident

√x7ᵗʰ **V61.1** Passenger in heavy transport vehicle injured in collision with pedal cycle in nontraffic accident

√x7ᵗʰ **V61.2** Person on outside of heavy transport vehicle injured in collision with pedal cycle in nontraffic accident

√x7ᵗʰ **V61.3** Unspecified occupant of heavy transport vehicle injured in collision with pedal cycle in nontraffic accident ▽

√x7ᵗʰ **V61.4** Person boarding or alighting a heavy transport vehicle injured in collision with pedal cycle while boarding or alighting

√x7ᵗʰ **V61.5** Driver of heavy transport vehicle injured in collision with pedal cycle in traffic accident

√x7ᵗʰ **V61.6** Passenger in heavy transport vehicle injured in collision with pedal cycle in traffic accident

√x7ᵗʰ **V61.7** Person on outside of heavy transport vehicle injured in collision with pedal cycle in traffic accident

√x7ᵗʰ **V61.9** Unspecified occupant of heavy transport vehicle injured in collision with pedal cycle in traffic accident ▽

✓4ᵗʰ **V62 Occupant of heavy transport vehicle injured in collision with two- or three-wheeled motor vehicle**

√x7ᵗʰ **V62.0** Driver of heavy transport vehicle injured in collision with two- or three-wheeled motor vehicle in nontraffic accident

√x7ᵗʰ **V62.1** Passenger in heavy transport vehicle injured in collision with two- or three-wheeled motor vehicle in nontraffic accident

√x7ᵗʰ **V62.2** Person on outside of heavy transport vehicle injured in collision with two- or three-wheeled motor vehicle in nontraffic accident

√x7ᵗʰ **V62.3** Unspecified occupant of heavy transport vehicle injured in collision with two- or three-wheeled motor vehicle in nontraffic accident ▽

√x7ᵗʰ **V62.4** Person boarding or alighting a heavy transport vehicle injured in collision with two- or three-wheeled motor vehicle

√x7ᵗʰ **V62.5** Driver of heavy transport vehicle injured in collision with two- or three-wheeled motor vehicle in traffic accident

√x7ᵗʰ **V62.6** Passenger in heavy transport vehicle injured in collision with two- or three-wheeled motor vehicle in traffic accident

√x7ᵗʰ **V62.7** Person on outside of heavy transport vehicle injured in collision with two- or three-wheeled motor vehicle in traffic accident

√x7ᵗʰ **V62.9** Unspecified occupant of heavy transport vehicle injured in collision with two- or three-wheeled motor vehicle in traffic accident ▽

✓4ᵗʰ **V63 Occupant of heavy transport vehicle injured in collision with car, pick-up truck or van**

√x7ᵗʰ **V63.0** Driver of heavy transport vehicle injured in collision with car, pick-up truck or van in nontraffic accident

√x7ᵗʰ **V63.1** Passenger in heavy transport vehicle injured in collision with car, pick-up truck or van in nontraffic accident

√x7ᵗʰ **V63.2** Person on outside of heavy transport vehicle injured in collision with car, pick-up truck or van in nontraffic accident

√x7ᵗʰ **V63.3** Unspecified occupant of heavy transport vehicle injured in collision with car, pick-up truck or van in nontraffic accident ▽

√x7ᵗʰ **V63.4** Person boarding or alighting a heavy transport vehicle injured in collision with car, pick-up truck or van

√x7ᵗʰ **V63.5** Driver of heavy transport vehicle injured in collision with car, pick-up truck or van in traffic accident

√x7ᵗʰ **V63.6** Passenger in heavy transport vehicle injured in collision with car, pick-up truck or van in traffic accident

√x7ᵗʰ **V63.7** Person on outside of heavy transport vehicle injured in collision with car, pick-up truck or van in traffic accident

√x7ᵗʰ **V63.9** Unspecified occupant of heavy transport vehicle injured in collision with car, pick-up truck or van in traffic accident ▽

✓4ᵗʰ **V64 Occupant of heavy transport vehicle injured in collision with heavy transport vehicle or bus**

     EXCLUDES 1 *occupant of heavy transport vehicle injured in collision with military vehicle (V69.81)*

√x7ᵗʰ **V64.0** Driver of heavy transport vehicle injured in collision with heavy transport vehicle or bus in nontraffic accident

√x7ᵗʰ **V64.1** Passenger in heavy transport vehicle injured in collision with heavy transport vehicle or bus in nontraffic accident

√x7ᵗʰ **V64.2** Person on outside of heavy transport vehicle injured in collision with heavy transport vehicle or bus in nontraffic accident

√x7ᵗʰ **V64.3** Unspecified occupant of heavy transport vehicle injured in collision with heavy transport vehicle or bus in nontraffic accident ▽

√x7ᵗʰ **V64.4** Person boarding or alighting a heavy transport vehicle injured in collision with heavy transport vehicle or bus while boarding or alighting

√x7ᵗʰ **V64.5** Driver of heavy transport vehicle injured in collision with heavy transport vehicle or bus in traffic accident

√x7ᵗʰ **V64.6** Passenger in heavy transport vehicle injured in collision with heavy transport vehicle or bus in traffic accident

√x7ᵗʰ **V64.7** Person on outside of heavy transport vehicle injured in collision with heavy transport vehicle or bus in traffic accident

√x7ᵗʰ **V64.9** Unspecified occupant of heavy transport vehicle injured in collision with heavy transport vehicle or bus in traffic accident ▽

✓4ᵗʰ **V65 Occupant of heavy transport vehicle injured in collision with railway train or railway vehicle**

√x7ᵗʰ **V65.0** Driver of heavy transport vehicle injured in collision with railway train or railway vehicle in nontraffic accident

√x7ᵗʰ **V65.1** Passenger in heavy transport vehicle injured in collision with railway train or railway vehicle in nontraffic accident

√x7ᵗʰ **V65.2** Person on outside of heavy transport vehicle injured in collision with railway train or railway vehicle in nontraffic accident

√x7ᵗʰ **V65.3** Unspecified occupant of heavy transport vehicle injured in collision with railway train or railway vehicle in nontraffic accident ▽

√x7ᵗʰ **V65.4** Person boarding or alighting a heavy transport vehicle injured in collision with railway train or railway vehicle

√x7ᵗʰ **V65.5** Driver of heavy transport vehicle injured in collision with railway train or railway vehicle in traffic accident

√x7ᵗʰ **V65.6** Passenger in heavy transport vehicle injured in collision with railway train or railway vehicle in traffic accident

√x7ᵗʰ **V65.7** Person on outside of heavy transport vehicle injured in collision with railway train or railway vehicle in traffic accident

√x7ᵗʰ **V65.9** Unspecified occupant of heavy transport vehicle injured in collision with railway train or railway vehicle in traffic accident ▽

✓4ᵗʰ **V66 Occupant of heavy transport vehicle injured in collision with other nonmotor vehicle**

     INCLUDES collision with animal-drawn vehicle, animal being ridden, streetcar

√x7ᵗʰ **V66.0** Driver of heavy transport vehicle injured in collision with other nonmotor vehicle in nontraffic accident

√x7ᵗʰ **V66.1** Passenger in heavy transport vehicle injured in collision with other nonmotor vehicle in nontraffic accident

√x7ᵗʰ **V66.2** Person on outside of heavy transport vehicle injured in collision with other nonmotor vehicle in nontraffic accident

√x7ᵗʰ **V66.3** Unspecified occupant of heavy transport vehicle injured in collision with other nonmotor vehicle in nontraffic accident ▽

✓ Additional Character Req   ✓x7ᵗʰ Placeholder Alert   Manifestation   HCC CMS-HCC Condition   ▽ Unspecified Code   ▶◀ Revised Text   ● New Code   ▲ Revised Code Title

ICD-10-CM 2018   1131

✓x7ᵗʰ **V66.4** Person boarding or alighting a heavy transport vehicle injured in collision with other nonmotor vehicle

✓x7ᵗʰ **V66.5** Driver of heavy transport vehicle injured in collision with other nonmotor vehicle in traffic accident

✓x7ᵗʰ **V66.6** Passenger in heavy transport vehicle injured in collision with other nonmotor vehicle in traffic accident

✓x7ᵗʰ **V66.7** Person on outside of heavy transport vehicle injured in collision with other nonmotor vehicle in traffic accident

✓x7ᵗʰ **V66.9** Unspecified occupant of heavy transport vehicle injured ▽ in collision with other nonmotor vehicle in traffic accident

✓4ᵗʰ **V67 Occupant of heavy transport vehicle injured in collision with fixed or stationary object**

✓x7ᵗʰ **V67.0** Driver of heavy transport vehicle injured in collision with fixed or stationary object in nontraffic accident

✓x7ᵗʰ **V67.1** Passenger in heavy transport vehicle injured in collision with fixed or stationary object in nontraffic accident

✓x7ᵗʰ **V67.2** Person on outside of heavy transport vehicle injured in collision with fixed or stationary object in nontraffic accident

✓x7ᵗʰ **V67.3** Unspecified occupant of heavy transport vehicle injured in ▽ collision with fixed or stationary object in nontraffic accident

✓x7ᵗʰ **V67.4** Person boarding or alighting a heavy transport vehicle injured in collision with fixed or stationary object

✓x7ᵗʰ **V67.5** Driver of heavy transport vehicle injured in collision with fixed or stationary object in traffic accident

✓x7ᵗʰ **V67.6** Passenger in heavy transport vehicle injured in collision with fixed or stationary object in traffic accident

✓x7ᵗʰ **V67.7** Person on outside of heavy transport vehicle injured in collision with fixed or stationary object in traffic accident

✓x7ᵗʰ **V67.9** Unspecified occupant of heavy transport vehicle injured ▽ in collision with fixed or stationary object in traffic accident

✓4ᵗʰ **V68 Occupant of heavy transport vehicle injured in noncollision transport accident**
     INCLUDES overturning heavy transport vehicle NOS
                   overturning heavy transport vehicle without collision

✓x7ᵗʰ **V68.0** Driver of heavy transport vehicle injured in noncollision transport accident in nontraffic accident

✓x7ᵗʰ **V68.1** Passenger in heavy transport vehicle injured in noncollision transport accident in nontraffic accident

✓x7ᵗʰ **V68.2** Person on outside of heavy transport vehicle injured in noncollision transport accident in nontraffic accident

✓x7ᵗʰ **V68.3** Unspecified occupant of heavy transport vehicle injured ▽ in noncollision transport accident in nontraffic accident

✓x7ᵗʰ **V68.4** Person boarding or alighting a heavy transport vehicle injured in noncollision transport accident

✓x7ᵗʰ **V68.5** Driver of heavy transport vehicle injured in noncollision transport accident in traffic accident

✓x7ᵗʰ **V68.6** Passenger in heavy transport vehicle injured in noncollision transport accident in traffic accident

✓x7ᵗʰ **V68.7** Person on outside of heavy transport vehicle injured in noncollision transport accident in traffic accident

✓x7ᵗʰ **V68.9** Unspecified occupant of heavy transport vehicle injured ▽ in noncollision transport accident in traffic accident

✓4ᵗʰ **V69 Occupant of heavy transport vehicle injured in other and unspecified transport accidents**

✓5ᵗʰ **V69.0** Driver of heavy transport vehicle injured in collision with other and unspecified motor vehicles in nontraffic accident

✓x7ᵗʰ **V69.00** Driver of heavy transport vehicle injured in ▽ collision with unspecified motor vehicles in nontraffic accident

✓x7ᵗʰ **V69.09** Driver of heavy transport vehicle injured in collision with other motor vehicles in nontraffic accident

✓5ᵗʰ **V69.1** Passenger in heavy transport vehicle injured in collision with other and unspecified motor vehicles in nontraffic accident

✓x7ᵗʰ **V69.10** Passenger in heavy transport vehicle injured in ▽ collision with unspecified motor vehicles in nontraffic accident

✓x7ᵗʰ **V69.19** Passenger in heavy transport vehicle injured in collision with other motor vehicles in nontraffic accident

✓5ᵗʰ **V69.2** Unspecified occupant of heavy transport vehicle injured in collision with other and unspecified motor vehicles in nontraffic accident

✓x7ᵗʰ **V69.20** Unspecified occupant of heavy transport vehicle ▽ injured in collision with unspecified motor vehicles in nontraffic accident
         Collision NOS involving heavy transport vehicle, nontraffic

✓x7ᵗʰ **V69.29** Unspecified occupant of heavy transport vehicle ▽ injured in collision with other motor vehicles in nontraffic accident

✓x7ᵗʰ **V69.3** Occupant (driver) (passenger) of heavy transport vehicle ▽ injured in unspecified nontraffic accident
         Accident NOS involving heavy transport vehicle, nontraffic
         Occupant of heavy transport vehicle injured in nontraffic accident NOS

✓5ᵗʰ **V69.4** Driver of heavy transport vehicle injured in collision with other and unspecified motor vehicles in traffic accident

✓x7ᵗʰ **V69.40** Driver of heavy transport vehicle injured in ▽ collision with unspecified motor vehicles in traffic accident

✓x7ᵗʰ **V69.49** Driver of heavy transport vehicle injured in collision with other motor vehicles in traffic accident

✓5ᵗʰ **V69.5** Passenger in heavy transport vehicle injured in collision with other and unspecified motor vehicles in traffic accident

✓x7ᵗʰ **V69.50** Passenger in heavy transport vehicle injured in ▽ collision with unspecified motor vehicles in traffic accident

✓x7ᵗʰ **V69.59** Passenger in heavy transport vehicle injured in collision with other motor vehicles in traffic accident

✓5ᵗʰ **V69.6** Unspecified occupant of heavy transport vehicle injured in collision with other and unspecified motor vehicles in traffic accident

✓x7ᵗʰ **V69.60** Unspecified occupant of heavy transport vehicle ▽ injured in collision with unspecified motor vehicles in traffic accident
         Collision NOS involving heavy transport vehicle (traffic)

✓x7ᵗʰ **V69.69** Unspecified occupant of heavy transport vehicle ▽ injured in collision with other motor vehicles in traffic accident

✓5ᵗʰ **V69.8** Occupant (driver) (passenger) of heavy transport vehicle injured in other specified transport accidents

✓x7ᵗʰ **V69.81** Occupant (driver) (passenger) of heavy transport vehicle injured in transport accidents with military vehicle

✓x7ᵗʰ **V69.88** Occupant (driver) (passenger) of heavy transport vehicle injured in other specified transport accidents

✓x7ᵗʰ **V69.9** Occupant (driver) (passenger) of heavy transport vehicle ▽ injured in unspecified traffic accident
         Accident NOS involving heavy transport vehicle

Bus occupant injured in transport accident (V70-V79)

INCLUDES motorcoach
EXCLUDES 1 minibus (V50-V59)

The appropriate 7th character is to be added to each code from categories V70-V79.
A   initial encounter
D   subsequent encounter
S   sequela

✓4ᵗʰ **V70 Bus occupant injured in collision with pedestrian or animal**
     EXCLUDES 1 bus collision with animal-drawn vehicle or animal being ridden (V76.-)

✓x7ᵗʰ **V70.0** Driver of bus injured in collision with pedestrian or animal in nontraffic accident

✓x7ᵗʰ **V70.1** Passenger on bus injured in collision with pedestrian or animal in nontraffic accident

✓x7ᵗʰ **V70.2** Person on outside of bus injured in collision with pedestrian or animal in nontraffic accident

✓x7ᵗʰ **V70.3** Unspecified occupant of bus injured in collision with ▽ pedestrian or animal in nontraffic accident

✓x7ᵗʰ **V70.4** Person boarding or alighting from bus injured in collision with pedestrian or animal

✓x7ᵗʰ **V70.5** Driver of bus injured in collision with pedestrian or animal in traffic accident

---

EXCLUDES 1 Not coded here   **EXCLUDES 2** Not included here   **N** Newborn Age: 0   **P** Pediatric Age: 0-17   **M** Maternity Age: 12-55   **A** Adult Age: 15-124

1132   ICD-10-CM 2018

☑x7ᵗʰ **V70.6** Passenger on bus injured in collision with pedestrian or animal **in traffic accident**

☑x7ᵗʰ **V70.7** Person on outside of bus injured in collision with pedestrian or animal **in traffic accident**

☑x7ᵗʰ **V70.9** Unspecified occupant of bus injured in collision with pedestrian or animal **in traffic accident** ▽

☑4ᵗʰ **V71** Bus occupant injured in collision with pedal cycle

☑x7ᵗʰ **V71.0** Driver of bus injured in collision with pedal cycle **in nontraffic accident**

☑x7ᵗʰ **V71.1** Passenger on bus injured in collision with pedal cycle **in nontraffic accident**

☑x7ᵗʰ **V71.2** Person on outside of bus injured in collision with pedal cycle **in nontraffic accident**

☑x7ᵗʰ **V71.3** Unspecified occupant of bus injured in collision with pedal cycle **in nontraffic accident** ▽

☑x7ᵗʰ **V71.4** Person boarding or alighting from bus injured in collision with pedal cycle

☑x7ᵗʰ **V71.5** Driver of bus injured in collision with pedal cycle **in traffic accident**

☑x7ᵗʰ **V71.6** Passenger on bus injured in collision with pedal cycle **in traffic accident**

☑x7ᵗʰ **V71.7** Person on outside of bus injured in collision with pedal cycle **in traffic accident**

☑x7ᵗʰ **V71.9** Unspecified occupant of bus injured in collision with pedal cycle **in traffic accident** ▽

☑4ᵗʰ **V72** Bus occupant injured in collision with two- or three-wheeled motor vehicle

☑x7ᵗʰ **V72.0** Driver of bus injured in collision with two- or three-wheeled motor vehicle **in nontraffic accident**

☑x7ᵗʰ **V72.1** Passenger on bus injured in collision with two- or three-wheeled motor vehicle **in nontraffic accident**

☑x7ᵗʰ **V72.2** Person on outside of bus injured in collision with two- or three-wheeled motor vehicle **in nontraffic accident**

☑x7ᵗʰ **V72.3** Unspecified occupant of bus injured in collision with two- or three-wheeled motor vehicle **in nontraffic accident** ▽

☑x7ᵗʰ **V72.4** Person boarding or alighting from bus injured in collision with two- or three-wheeled motor vehicle

☑x7ᵗʰ **V72.5** Driver of bus injured in collision with two- or three-wheeled motor vehicle **in traffic accident**

☑x7ᵗʰ **V72.6** Passenger on bus injured in collision with two- or three-wheeled motor vehicle **in traffic accident**

☑x7ᵗʰ **V72.7** Person on outside of bus injured in collision with two- or three-wheeled motor vehicle **in traffic accident**

☑x7ᵗʰ **V72.9** Unspecified occupant of bus injured in collision with two- or three-wheeled motor vehicle **in traffic accident** ▽

☑4ᵗʰ **V73** Bus occupant injured in collision with car, pick-up truck or van

☑x7ᵗʰ **V73.0** Driver of bus injured in collision with car, pick-up truck or van **in nontraffic accident**

☑x7ᵗʰ **V73.1** Passenger on bus injured in collision with car, pick-up truck or van **in nontraffic accident**

☑x7ᵗʰ **V73.2** Person on outside of bus injured in collision with car, pick-up truck or van **in nontraffic accident**

☑x7ᵗʰ **V73.3** Unspecified occupant of bus injured in collision with car, pick-up truck or van **in nontraffic accident** ▽

☑x7ᵗʰ **V73.4** Person boarding or alighting from bus injured in collision with car, pick-up truck or van

☑x7ᵗʰ **V73.5** Driver of bus injured in collision with car, pick-up truck or van **in traffic accident**

☑x7ᵗʰ **V73.6** Passenger on bus injured in collision with car, pick-up truck or van **in traffic accident**

☑x7ᵗʰ **V73.7** Person on outside of bus injured in collision with car, pick-up truck or van **in traffic accident**

☑x7ᵗʰ **V73.9** Unspecified occupant of bus injured in collision with car, pick-up truck or van **in traffic accident** ▽

☑4ᵗʰ **V74** Bus occupant injured in collision with heavy transport vehicle or bus

EXCLUDES 1 *bus occupant injured in collision with military vehicle (V79.81)*

☑x7ᵗʰ **V74.0** Driver of bus injured in collision with heavy transport vehicle or bus **in nontraffic accident**

☑x7ᵗʰ **V74.1** Passenger on bus injured in collision with heavy transport vehicle or bus **in nontraffic accident**

☑x7ᵗʰ **V74.2** Person on outside of bus injured in collision with heavy transport vehicle or bus **in nontraffic accident**

☑x7ᵗʰ **V74.3** Unspecified occupant of bus injured in collision with heavy transport vehicle or bus **in nontraffic accident** ▽

☑x7ᵗʰ **V74.4** Person boarding or alighting from bus injured in collision with heavy transport vehicle or bus

☑x7ᵗʰ **V74.5** Driver of bus injured in collision with heavy transport vehicle or bus **in traffic accident**

☑x7ᵗʰ **V74.6** Passenger on bus injured in collision with heavy transport vehicle or bus **in traffic accident**

☑x7ᵗʰ **V74.7** Person on outside of bus injured in collision with heavy transport vehicle or bus **in traffic accident**

☑x7ᵗʰ **V74.9** Unspecified occupant of bus injured in collision with heavy transport vehicle or bus **in traffic accident** ▽

☑4ᵗʰ **V75** Bus occupant injured in collision with railway train or railway vehicle

☑x7ᵗʰ **V75.0** Driver of bus injured in collision with railway train or railway vehicle **in nontraffic accident**

☑x7ᵗʰ **V75.1** Passenger on bus injured in collision with railway train or railway vehicle **in nontraffic accident**

☑x7ᵗʰ **V75.2** Person on outside of bus injured in collision with railway train or railway vehicle **in nontraffic accident**

☑x7ᵗʰ **V75.3** Unspecified occupant of bus injured in collision with railway train or railway vehicle **in nontraffic accident** ▽

☑x7ᵗʰ **V75.4** Person boarding or alighting from bus injured in collision with railway train or railway vehicle

☑x7ᵗʰ **V75.5** Driver of bus injured in collision with railway train or railway vehicle **in traffic accident**

☑x7ᵗʰ **V75.6** Passenger on bus injured in collision with railway train or railway vehicle **in traffic accident**

☑x7ᵗʰ **V75.7** Person on outside of bus injured in collision with railway train or railway vehicle **in traffic accident**

☑x7ᵗʰ **V75.9** Unspecified occupant of bus injured in collision with railway train or railway vehicle **in traffic accident** ▽

☑4ᵗʰ **V76** Bus occupant injured in collision with other nonmotor vehicle

INCLUDES collision with animal-drawn vehicle, animal being ridden, streetcar

☑x7ᵗʰ **V76.0** Driver of bus injured in collision with other nonmotor vehicle **in nontraffic accident**

☑x7ᵗʰ **V76.1** Passenger on bus injured in collision with other nonmotor vehicle **in nontraffic accident**

☑x7ᵗʰ **V76.2** Person on outside of bus injured in collision with other nonmotor vehicle **in nontraffic accident**

☑x7ᵗʰ **V76.3** Unspecified occupant of bus injured in collision with other nonmotor vehicle **in nontraffic accident** ▽

☑x7ᵗʰ **V76.4** Person boarding or alighting from bus injured in collision with other nonmotor vehicle

☑x7ᵗʰ **V76.5** Driver of bus injured in collision with other nonmotor vehicle **in traffic accident**

☑x7ᵗʰ **V76.6** Passenger on bus injured in collision with other nonmotor vehicle **in traffic accident**

☑x7ᵗʰ **V76.7** Person on outside of bus injured in collision with other nonmotor vehicle **in traffic accident**

☑x7ᵗʰ **V76.9** Unspecified occupant of bus injured in collision with other nonmotor vehicle **in traffic accident** ▽

☑4ᵗʰ **V77** Bus occupant injured in collision with fixed or stationary object

☑x7ᵗʰ **V77.0** Driver of bus injured in collision with fixed or stationary object **in nontraffic accident**

☑x7ᵗʰ **V77.1** Passenger on bus injured in collision with fixed or stationary object **in nontraffic accident**

☑x7ᵗʰ **V77.2** Person on outside of bus injured in collision with fixed or stationary object **in nontraffic accident**

☑x7ᵗʰ **V77.3** Unspecified occupant of bus injured in collision with fixed or stationary object **in nontraffic accident** ▽

☑x7ᵗʰ **V77.4** Person boarding or alighting from bus injured in collision with fixed or stationary object

☑x7ᵗʰ **V77.5** Driver of bus injured in collision with fixed or stationary object **in traffic accident**

☑x7ᵗʰ **V77.6** Passenger on bus injured in collision with fixed or stationary object **in traffic accident**

☑x7ᵗʰ **V77.7** Person on outside of bus injured in collision with fixed or stationary object **in traffic accident**

☑x7ᵗʰ **V77.9** Unspecified occupant of bus injured in collision with fixed or stationary object **in traffic accident** ▽

✓ Additional Character Req   x7ᵗʰ Placeholder Alert   Manifestation   HCC CMS-HCC Condition   ▽ Unspecified Code   ▶◀ Revised Text   ● New Code   ▲ Revised Code Title

Chapter 20. External Causes of Morbidity *(left margin)*

V78–V80.710 *(left margin)*

√4ᵗʰ **V78** **Bus occupant injured in noncollision transport accident**
  INCLUDES   overturning bus NOS
          overturning bus without collision

√x7ᵗʰ **V78.0** **Driver of bus injured in noncollision transport accident in nontraffic accident**

√x7ᵗʰ **V78.1** **Passenger on bus injured in noncollision transport accident in nontraffic accident**

√x7ᵗʰ **V78.2** **Person on outside of bus injured in noncollision transport accident in nontraffic accident**

√x7ᵗʰ **V78.3** **Unspecified occupant of bus injured in noncollision transport accident in nontraffic accident** ▽

√x7ᵗʰ **V78.4** **Person boarding or alighting from bus injured in noncollision transport accident**

√x7ᵗʰ **V78.5** **Driver of bus injured in noncollision transport accident in traffic accident**

√x7ᵗʰ **V78.6** **Passenger on bus injured in noncollision transport accident in traffic accident**

√x7ᵗʰ **V78.7** **Person on outside of bus injured in noncollision transport accident in traffic accident**

√x7ᵗʰ **V78.9** **Unspecified occupant of bus injured in noncollision transport accident in traffic accident** ▽

√4ᵗʰ **V79** **Bus occupant injured in other and unspecified transport accidents**

√5ᵗʰ **V79.0** **Driver of bus injured in collision with other and unspecified motor vehicles in nontraffic accident**

√x7ᵗʰ **V79.00** **Driver of bus injured in collision with unspecified motor vehicles in nontraffic accident** ▽

√x7ᵗʰ **V79.09** **Driver of bus injured in collision with other motor vehicles in nontraffic accident**

√5ᵗʰ **V79.1** **Passenger on bus injured in collision with other and unspecified motor vehicles in nontraffic accident**

√x7ᵗʰ **V79.10** **Passenger on bus injured in collision with unspecified motor vehicles in nontraffic accident** ▽

√x7ᵗʰ **V79.19** **Passenger on bus injured in collision with other motor vehicles in nontraffic accident**

√5ᵗʰ **V79.2** **Unspecified bus occupant injured in collision with other and unspecified motor vehicles in nontraffic accident**

√x7ᵗʰ **V79.20** **Unspecified bus occupant injured in collision with unspecified motor vehicles in nontraffic accident** ▽
     Bus collision NOS, nontraffic

√x7ᵗʰ **V79.29** **Unspecified bus occupant injured in collision with other motor vehicles in nontraffic accident** ▽

√x7ᵗʰ **V79.3** **Bus occupant (driver) (passenger) injured in unspecified nontraffic accident** ▽
     Bus accident NOS, nontraffic
     Bus occupant injured in nontraffic accident NOS

√5ᵗʰ **V79.4** **Driver of bus injured in collision with other and unspecified motor vehicles in traffic accident**

√x7ᵗʰ **V79.40** **Driver of bus injured in collision with unspecified motor vehicles in traffic accident** ▽

√x7ᵗʰ **V79.49** **Driver of bus injured in collision with other motor vehicles in traffic accident**

√5ᵗʰ **V79.5** **Passenger on bus injured in collision with other and unspecified motor vehicles in traffic accident**

√x7ᵗʰ **V79.50** **Passenger on bus injured in collision with unspecified motor vehicles in traffic accident** ▽

√x7ᵗʰ **V79.59** **Passenger on bus injured in collision with other motor vehicles in traffic accident**

√5ᵗʰ **V79.6** **Unspecified bus occupant injured in collision with other and unspecified motor vehicles in traffic accident**

√x7ᵗʰ **V79.60** **Unspecified bus occupant injured in collision with unspecified motor vehicles in traffic accident** ▽
     Bus collision NOS (traffic)

√x7ᵗʰ **V79.69** **Unspecified bus occupant injured in collision with other motor vehicles in traffic accident** ▽

√5ᵗʰ **V79.8** **Bus occupant (driver) (passenger) injured in other specified transport accidents**

√x7ᵗʰ **V79.81** **Bus occupant (driver) (passenger) injured in transport accidents with military vehicle**

√x7ᵗʰ **V79.88** **Bus occupant (driver) (passenger) injured in other specified transport accidents**

√x7ᵗʰ **V79.9** **Bus occupant (driver) (passenger) injured in unspecified traffic accident** ▽
     Bus accident NOS

Other land transport accidents (V80-V89)

The appropriate 7th character is to be added to each code from categories V80-V89.
A   initial encounter
D   subsequent encounter
S   sequela

√4ᵗʰ **V80** **Animal-rider or occupant of animal-drawn vehicle injured in transport accident**

√5ᵗʰ **V80.0** **Animal-rider or occupant of animal drawn vehicle injured by fall from or being thrown from animal or animal-drawn vehicle in noncollision accident**

√6ᵗʰ **V80.01** **Animal-rider injured by fall from or being thrown from animal in noncollision accident**

√7ᵗʰ **V80.010** **Animal-rider injured by fall from or being thrown from horse in noncollision accident**

√7ᵗʰ **V80.018** **Animal-rider injured by fall from or being thrown from other animal in noncollision accident**

√x7ᵗʰ **V80.02** **Occupant of animal-drawn vehicle injured by fall from or being thrown from animal-drawn vehicle in noncollision accident**
     Overturning animal-drawn vehicle NOS
     Overturning animal-drawn vehicle without collision

√5ᵗʰ **V80.1** **Animal-rider or occupant of animal-drawn vehicle injured in collision with pedestrian or animal**
  EXCLUDES 1   animal-rider or animal-drawn vehicle collision with animal-drawn vehicle or animal being ridden (V80.7)

√x7ᵗʰ **V80.11** **Animal-rider injured in collision with pedestrian or animal**

√x7ᵗʰ **V80.12** **Occupant of animal-drawn vehicle injured in collision with pedestrian or animal**

√5ᵗʰ **V80.2** **Animal-rider or occupant of animal-drawn vehicle injured in collision with pedal cycle**

√x7ᵗʰ **V80.21** **Animal-rider injured in collision with pedal cycle**

√x7ᵗʰ **V80.22** **Occupant of animal-drawn vehicle injured in collision with pedal cycle**

√5ᵗʰ **V80.3** **Animal-rider or occupant of animal-drawn vehicle injured in collision with two- or three-wheeled motor vehicle**

√x7ᵗʰ **V80.31** **Animal-rider injured in collision with two- or three-wheeled motor vehicle**

√x7ᵗʰ **V80.32** **Occupant of animal-drawn vehicle injured in collision with two- or three-wheeled motor vehicle**

√5ᵗʰ **V80.4** **Animal-rider or occupant of animal-drawn vehicle injured in collision with car, pick-up truck, van, heavy transport vehicle or bus**
  EXCLUDES 1   animal-rider injured in collision with military vehicle (V80.910)
       occupant of animal-drawn vehicle injured in collision with military vehicle (V80.920)

√x7ᵗʰ **V80.41** **Animal-rider injured in collision with car, pick-up truck, van, heavy transport vehicle or bus**

√x7ᵗʰ **V80.42** **Occupant of animal-drawn vehicle injured in collision with car, pick-up truck, van, heavy transport vehicle or bus**

√5ᵗʰ **V80.5** **Animal-rider or occupant of animal-drawn vehicle injured in collision with other specified motor vehicle**

√x7ᵗʰ **V80.51** **Animal-rider injured in collision with other specified motor vehicle**

√x7ᵗʰ **V80.52** **Occupant of animal-drawn vehicle injured in collision with other specified motor vehicle**

√5ᵗʰ **V80.6** **Animal-rider or occupant of animal-drawn vehicle injured in collision with railway train or railway vehicle**

√x7ᵗʰ **V80.61** **Animal-rider injured in collision with railway train or railway vehicle**

√x7ᵗʰ **V80.62** **Occupant of animal-drawn vehicle injured in collision with railway train or railway vehicle**

√5ᵗʰ **V80.7** **Animal-rider or occupant of animal-drawn vehicle injured in collision with other nonmotor vehicles**

√6ᵗʰ **V80.71** **Animal-rider or occupant of animal-drawn vehicle injured in collision with animal being ridden**

√7ᵗʰ **V80.710** **Animal-rider injured in collision with other animal being ridden**

EXCLUDES 1 Not coded here   EXCLUDES 2 Not included here   N Newborn Age: 0   P Pediatric Age: 0-17   M Maternity Age: 12-55   A Adult Age: 15-124

✓7ᵗʰ **V80.711** Occupant of animal-drawn vehicle injured in collision with animal being ridden

✓6ᵗʰ **V80.72** Animal-rider or occupant of animal-drawn vehicle injured in collision with other animal-drawn vehicle

✓7ᵗʰ **V80.720** Animal-rider injured in collision with animal-drawn vehicle

✓7ᵗʰ **V80.721** Occupant of animal-drawn vehicle injured in collision with other animal-drawn vehicle

✓6ᵗʰ **V80.73** Animal-rider or occupant of animal-drawn vehicle injured in collision with streetcar

✓7ᵗʰ **V80.730** Animal-rider injured in collision with streetcar

✓7ᵗʰ **V80.731** Occupant of animal-drawn vehicle injured in collision with streetcar

✓6ᵗʰ **V80.79** Animal-rider or occupant of animal-drawn vehicle injured in collision with other nonmotor vehicles

✓7ᵗʰ **V80.790** Animal-rider injured in collision with other nonmotor vehicles

✓7ᵗʰ **V80.791** Occupant of animal-drawn vehicle injured in collision with other nonmotor vehicles

✓5ᵗʰ **V80.8** Animal-rider or occupant of animal-drawn vehicle injured in collision with fixed or stationary object

✓x7ᵗʰ **V80.81** Animal-rider injured in collision with fixed or stationary object

✓x7ᵗʰ **V80.82** Occupant of animal-drawn vehicle injured in collision with fixed or stationary object

✓5ᵗʰ **V80.9** Animal-rider or occupant of animal-drawn vehicle injured in other and unspecified transport accidents

✓6ᵗʰ **V80.91** Animal-rider injured in other and unspecified transport accidents

✓7ᵗʰ **V80.910** Animal-rider injured in transport accident with military vehicle

✓7ᵗʰ **V80.918** Animal-rider injured in other transport accident

✓7ᵗʰ **V80.919** Animal-rider injured in unspecified transport accident ▽
Animal rider accident NOS

✓6ᵗʰ **V80.92** Occupant of animal-drawn vehicle injured in other and unspecified transport accidents

✓7ᵗʰ **V80.920** Occupant of animal-drawn vehicle injured in transport accident with military vehicle

✓7ᵗʰ **V80.928** Occupant of animal-drawn vehicle injured in other transport accident

✓7ᵗʰ **V80.929** Occupant of animal-drawn vehicle ▽
injured in unspecified transport accident
Animal-drawn vehicle accident NOS

✓4ᵗʰ **V81** Occupant of railway train or railway vehicle injured in transport accident
INCLUDES   derailment of railway train or railway vehicle
person on outside of train
EXCLUDES 1   streetcar (V82.-)

✓x7ᵗʰ **V81.0** Occupant of railway train or railway vehicle injured in collision with motor vehicle in nontraffic accident
EXCLUDES 1   occupant of railway train or railway vehicle injured due to collision with military vehicle (V81.83)

✓x7ᵗʰ **V81.1** Occupant of railway train or railway vehicle injured in collision with motor vehicle in traffic accident
EXCLUDES 1   occupant of railway train or railway vehicle injured due to collision with military vehicle (V81.83)

✓x7ᵗʰ **V81.2** Occupant of railway train or railway vehicle injured in collision with or hit by rolling stock

✓x7ᵗʰ **V81.3** Occupant of railway train or railway vehicle injured in collision with other object
Railway collision NOS

✓x7ᵗʰ **V81.4** Person injured while boarding or alighting from railway train or railway vehicle

✓x7ᵗʰ **V81.5** Occupant of railway train or railway vehicle injured by fall in railway train or railway vehicle

✓x7ᵗʰ **V81.6** Occupant of railway train or railway vehicle injured by fall from railway train or railway vehicle

✓x7ᵗʰ **V81.7** Occupant of railway train or railway vehicle injured in derailment without antecedent collision

✓5ᵗʰ **V81.8** Occupant of railway train or railway vehicle injured in other specified railway accidents

✓x7ᵗʰ **V81.81** Occupant of railway train or railway vehicle injured due to explosion or fire on train

✓x7ᵗʰ **V81.82** Occupant of railway train or railway vehicle injured due to object falling onto train
Occupant of railway train or railway vehicle injured due to falling earth onto train
Occupant of railway train or railway vehicle injured due to falling rocks onto train
Occupant of railway train or railway vehicle injured due to falling snow onto train
Occupant of railway train or railway vehicle injured due to falling trees onto train

✓x7ᵗʰ **V81.83** Occupant of railway train or railway vehicle injured due to collision with military vehicle

✓x7ᵗʰ **V81.89** Occupant of railway train or railway vehicle injured due to other specified railway accident

✓x7ᵗʰ **V81.9** Occupant of railway train or railway vehicle injured in ▽
unspecified railway accident
Railway accident NOS

✓4ᵗʰ **V82** Occupant of powered streetcar injured in transport accident
INCLUDES   interurban electric car
person on outside of streetcar
tram (car)
trolley (car)
EXCLUDES 1   bus (V70-V79)
motorcoach (V70-V79)
nonpowered streetcar (V76.-)
train (V81.-)

✓x7ᵗʰ **V82.0** Occupant of streetcar injured in collision with motor vehicle in nontraffic accident

✓x7ᵗʰ **V82.1** Occupant of streetcar injured in collision with motor vehicle in traffic accident

✓x7ᵗʰ **V82.2** Occupant of streetcar injured in collision with or hit by rolling stock

✓x7ᵗʰ **V82.3** Occupant of streetcar injured in collision with other object
EXCLUDES 1   collision with animal-drawn vehicle or animal being ridden (V82.8)

✓x7ᵗʰ **V82.4** Person injured while boarding or alighting from streetcar

✓x7ᵗʰ **V82.5** Occupant of streetcar injured by fall in streetcar
EXCLUDES 1   fall in streetcar:
while boarding or alighting (V82.4)
with antecedent collision (V82.0-V82.3)

✓x7ᵗʰ **V82.6** Occupant of streetcar injured by fall from streetcar
EXCLUDES 1   fall from streetcar:
while boarding or alighting (V82.4)
with antecedent collision (V82.0-V82.3)

✓x7ᵗʰ **V82.7** Occupant of streetcar injured in derailment without antecedent collision
EXCLUDES 1   occupant of streetcar injured in derailment with antecedent collision (V82.0-V82.3)

✓x7ᵗʰ **V82.8** Occupant of streetcar injured in other specified transport accidents
Streetcar collision with military vehicle
Streetcar collision with train or nonmotor vehicles

✓x7ᵗʰ **V82.9** Occupant of streetcar injured in unspecified traffic ▽
accident
Streetcar accident NOS

✓4ᵗʰ **V83** Occupant of special vehicle mainly used on industrial premises injured in transport accident
INCLUDES   battery-powered airport passenger vehicle
battery-powered truck (baggage) (mail)
coal-car in mine
forklift (truck)
logging car
self-propelled industrial truck
station baggage truck (powered)
tram, truck, or tub (powered) in mine or quarry
EXCLUDES 1   special construction vehicles (V85.-)
special industrial vehicle in stationary use or maintenance (W31.-)

✓x7ᵗʰ **V83.0** Driver of special industrial vehicle injured in traffic accident

✓x7ᵗʰ **V83.1** Passenger of special industrial vehicle injured in traffic accident

✓x7ᵗʰ **V83.2** Person on outside of special industrial vehicle injured in traffic accident

☑ Additional Character Req   ✓x7ᵗʰ Placeholder Alert   Manifestation   HCC CMS-HCC Condition   ▽ Unspecified Code   ▶◀ Revised Text   ● New Code   ▲ Revised Code Title

ICD-10-CM 2018   1135

√x7ᵗʰ V83.3 Unspecified occupant of special industrial vehicle injured in **traffic accident** ▽

√x7ᵗʰ V83.4 Person injured while **boarding or alighting from** special industrial vehicle

√x7ᵗʰ V83.5 Driver of special industrial vehicle injured **in nontraffic accident**

√x7ᵗʰ V83.6 Passenger of special industrial vehicle injured **in nontraffic accident**

√x7ᵗʰ V83.7 Person on **outside** of special industrial vehicle injured in **nontraffic accident**

√x7ᵗʰ V83.9 Unspecified occupant of special industrial vehicle injured in **nontraffic accident** ▽
Special-industrial-vehicle accident NOS

√4ᵗʰ V84 Occupant of special vehicle mainly used in agriculture injured in transport accident
INCLUDES self-propelled farm machinery
tractor (and trailer)
EXCLUDES 1 *animal-powered farm machinery accident (W30.8-)*
contact with combine harvester (W30.0)
special agricultural vehicle in stationary use or maintenance (W30.-)

√x7ᵗʰ V84.0 Driver of special agricultural vehicle injured in **traffic accident**

√x7ᵗʰ V84.1 Passenger of special agricultural vehicle injured in **traffic accident**

√x7ᵗʰ V84.2 Person on **outside** of special agricultural vehicle injured in **traffic accident**

√x7ᵗʰ V84.3 Unspecified occupant of special agricultural vehicle injured in **traffic accident** ▽

√x7ᵗʰ V84.4 Person injured while **boarding or alighting** from special agricultural vehicle

√x7ᵗʰ V84.5 Driver of special agricultural vehicle injured in **nontraffic accident**

√x7ᵗʰ V84.6 Passenger of special agricultural vehicle injured in **nontraffic accident**

√x7ᵗʰ V84.7 Person on **outside** of special agricultural vehicle injured in **nontraffic accident**

√x7ᵗʰ V84.9 Unspecified occupant of special agricultural vehicle injured in **nontraffic accident** ▽
Special-agricultural vehicle accident NOS

√4ᵗʰ V85 Occupant of special construction vehicle injured in transport accident
INCLUDES bulldozer
digger
dump truck
earth-leveller
mechanical shovel
road-roller
EXCLUDES 1 *special industrial vehicle (V83.-)*
special construction vehicle in stationary use or maintenance (W31.-)

√x7ᵗʰ V85.0 Driver of special construction vehicle injured in **traffic accident**

√x7ᵗʰ V85.1 Passenger of special construction vehicle injured in **traffic accident**

√x7ᵗʰ V85.2 Person on **outside** of special construction vehicle injured in **traffic accident**

√x7ᵗʰ V85.3 Unspecified occupant of special construction vehicle injured in **traffic accident** ▽

√x7ᵗʰ V85.4 Person injured while **boarding or alighting** from special construction vehicle

√x7ᵗʰ V85.5 Driver of special construction vehicle injured in **nontraffic accident**

√x7ᵗʰ V85.6 Passenger of special construction vehicle injured in **nontraffic accident**

√x7ᵗʰ V85.7 Person on **outside** of special construction vehicle injured in **nontraffic accident**

√x7ᵗʰ V85.9 Unspecified occupant of special construction vehicle injured in **nontraffic accident** ▽
Special-construction-vehicle accident NOS

√4ᵗʰ V86 Occupant of special all-terrain or other off-road motor vehicle, injured in transport accident
EXCLUDES 1 *special all-terrain vehicle in stationary use or maintenance (W31.-)*
sport-utility vehicle (V50-V59)
three-wheeled motor vehicle designed for on-road use (V30-V39)

√5ᵗʰ V86.0 Driver of special all-terrain or other off-road motor vehicle injured in **traffic accident**

   √x7ᵗʰ V86.01 Driver of **ambulance** or **fire engine** injured in traffic accident

   √x7ᵗʰ V86.02 Driver of **snowmobile** injured in traffic accident

   √x7ᵗʰ V86.03 Driver of **dune buggy** injured in traffic accident

   √x7ᵗʰ V86.04 Driver of **military vehicle** injured in traffic accident

   ● **√x7ᵗʰ V86.05** Driver of **3- or 4- wheeled all-terrain vehicle (ATV)** injured in traffic accident

   ● **√x7ᵗʰ V86.06** Driver of **dirt bike or motor/cross bike** injured in traffic accident

   √x7ᵗʰ V86.09 Driver of other special all-terrain or other off-road motor vehicle injured in traffic accident
Driver of dirt bike injured in traffic accident
Driver of go cart injured in traffic accident
Driver of golf cart injured in traffic accident

√5ᵗʰ V86.1 Passenger of special all-terrain or other off-road motor vehicle injured in **traffic accident**

   √x7ᵗʰ V86.11 Passenger of **ambulance** or **fire engine** injured in traffic accident

   √x7ᵗʰ V86.12 Passenger of **snowmobile** injured in traffic accident

   √x7ᵗʰ V86.13 Passenger of **dune buggy** injured in traffic accident

   √x7ᵗʰ V86.14 Passenger of **military vehicle** injured in traffic accident

   ● **√x7ᵗʰ V86.15** Passenger of **3- or 4- wheeled all-terrain vehicle (ATV)** injured in traffic accident

   ● **√x7ᵗʰ V86.16** Passenger of **dirt bike or motor/cross bike** injured in traffic accident

   √x7ᵗʰ V86.19 Passenger of other special all-terrain or other off-road motor vehicle injured in traffic accident
Passenger of dirt bike injured in traffic accident
Passenger of go cart injured in traffic accident
Passenger of golf cart injured in traffic accident

√5ᵗʰ V86.2 Person on **outside** of special all-terrain or other off-road motor vehicle injured in **traffic accident**

   √x7ᵗʰ V86.21 Person on outside of **ambulance** or **fire engine** injured in traffic accident

   √x7ᵗʰ V86.22 Person on outside of **snowmobile** injured in traffic accident

   √x7ᵗʰ V86.23 Person on outside of **dune buggy** injured in traffic accident

   √x7ᵗʰ V86.24 Person on outside of **military vehicle** injured in traffic accident

   ● **√x7ᵗʰ V86.25** Person on outside of **3- or 4- wheeled all-terrain vehicle (ATV)** injured in traffic accident

   ● **√x7ᵗʰ V86.26** Person on outside of **dirt bike or motor/cross bike** injured in traffic accident

   √x7ᵗʰ V86.29 Person on outside of other special all-terrain or other off-road motor vehicle injured in traffic accident
Person on outside of dirt bike injured in traffic accident
Person on outside of go cart in traffic accident
Person on outside of golf cart injured in traffic accident

√5ᵗʰ V86.3 Unspecified occupant of special all-terrain or other off-road motor vehicle injured in **traffic accident**

   √x7ᵗʰ V86.31 Unspecified occupant of **ambulance or fire engine** injured in traffic accident ▽

   √x7ᵗʰ V86.32 Unspecified occupant of **snowmobile** injured in traffic accident ▽

   √x7ᵗʰ V86.33 Unspecified occupant of **dune buggy** injured in traffic accident ▽

   √x7ᵗʰ V86.34 Unspecified occupant of **military vehicle** injured in traffic accident ▽

   ● **√x7ᵗʰ V86.35** Unspecified occupant of **3- or 4- wheeled all-terrain vehicle (ATV)** injured in traffic accident ▽

   ● **√x7ᵗʰ V86.36** Unspecified occupant of **dirt bike or motor/cross bike** injured in traffic accident ▽

EXCLUDES 1 Not coded here   **EXCLUDES 2** Not included here   **N** Newborn Age: 0   **P** Pediatric Age: 0-17   **M** Maternity Age: 12-55   **A** Adult Age: 15-124

1136   ICD-10-CM 2018

√x7th **V86.39** **Unspecified occupant of other special all-terrain** ▽
or other off-road motor vehicle injured in traffic
accident
Unspecified occupant of dirt bike injured in traffic
accident
Unspecified occupant of go cart injured in traffic
accident
Unspecified occupant of golf cart injured in traffic
accident

√5th **V86.4** **Person injured while boarding or alighting from special**
all-terrain or other off-road motor vehicle

√x7th **V86.41** **Person injured while boarding or alighting from**
ambulance or fire engine

√x7th **V86.42** **Person injured while boarding or alighting from**
snowmobile

√x7th **V86.43** **Person injured while boarding or alighting from**
dune buggy

√x7th **V86.44** **Person injured while boarding or alighting from**
military vehicle

● √x7th **V86.45** **Person injured while boarding or alighting from a 3-**
or 4- wheeled all-terrain vehicle (ATV)

● √x7th **V86.46** **Person injured while boarding or alighting from a**
dirt bike or motor/cross bike

√x7th **V86.49** **Person injured while boarding or alighting from**
other special all-terrain or other off-road motor
vehicle
Person injured while boarding or alighting from dirt
bike
Person injured while boarding or alighting from go
cart
Person injured while boarding or alighting from golf
cart

√5th **V86.5** **Driver of special all-terrain or other off-road motor vehicle**
injured in nontraffic accident

√x7th **V86.51** **Driver of ambulance or fire engine injured in**
nontraffic accident

√x7th **V86.52** **Driver of snowmobile injured in nontraffic accident**

√x7th **V86.53** **Driver of dune buggy injured in nontraffic accident**

√x7th **V86.54** **Driver of military vehicle injured in nontraffic**
accident

● √x7th **V86.55** **Driver of 3- or 4- wheeled all-terrain vehicle (ATV)**
injured in nontraffic accident

● √x7th **V86.56** **Driver of dirt bike or motor/cross bike injured in**
nontraffic accident

√x7th **V86.59** **Driver of other special all-terrain or other off-road**
motor vehicle injured in nontraffic accident
Driver of dirt bike injured in nontraffic accident
Driver of go cart injured in nontraffic accident
Driver of golf cart injured in nontraffic accident

√5th **V86.6** **Passenger of special all-terrain or other off-road motor**
vehicle injured in nontraffic accident

√x7th **V86.61** **Passenger of ambulance or fire engine injured in**
nontraffic accident

√x7th **V86.62** **Passenger of snowmobile injured in nontraffic**
accident

√x7th **V86.63** **Passenger of dune buggy injured in nontraffic**
accident

√x7th **V86.64** **Passenger of military vehicle injured in nontraffic**
accident

● √x7th **V86.65** **Passenger of 3- or 4- wheeled all-terrain vehicle**
(ATV) injured in nontraffic accident

● √x7th **V86.66** **Passenger of dirt bike or motor/cross bike injured in**
nontraffic accident

√x7th **V86.69** **Passenger of other special all-terrain or other**
off-road motor vehicle injured in nontraffic accident
Passenger of dirt bike injured in nontraffic accident
Passenger of go cart injured in nontraffic accident
Passenger of golf cart injured in nontraffic accident

√5th **V86.7** **Person on outside of special all-terrain or other off-road**
motor vehicle injured in nontraffic accident

√x7th **V86.71** **Person on outside of ambulance or fire engine**
injured in nontraffic accident

√x7th **V86.72** **Person on outside of snowmobile injured in**
nontraffic accident

√x7th **V86.73** **Person on outside of dune buggy injured in**
nontraffic accident

√x7th **V86.74** **Person on outside of military vehicle injured in**
nontraffic accident

● √x7th **V86.75** **Person on outside of 3- or 4- wheeled all-terrain**
vehicle (ATV) injured in nontraffic accident

● √x7th **V86.76** **Person on outside of dirt bike or motor/cross bike**
injured in nontraffic accident

√x7th **V86.79** **Person on outside of other special all-terrain or**
other off-road motor vehicles injured in nontraffic
accident
Person on outside of dirt bike injured in nontraffic
accident
Person on outside of go cart injured in nontraffic
accident
Person on outside of golf cart injured in nontraffic
accident

√5th **V86.9** **Unspecified occupant of special all-terrain or other off-road**
motor vehicle injured in nontraffic accident

√x7th **V86.91** **Unspecified occupant of ambulance or fire** ▽
engine injured in nontraffic accident

√x7th **V86.92** **Unspecified occupant of snowmobile injured in** ▽
nontraffic accident

√x7th **V86.93** **Unspecified occupant of dune buggy injured in** ▽
nontraffic accident

√x7th **V86.94** **Unspecified occupant of military vehicle injured** ▽
in nontraffic accident

● √x7th **V86.95** **Unspecified occupant of 3- or 4- wheeled all-** ▽
terrain vehicle (ATV) injured in nontraffic accident

● √x7th **V86.96** **Unspecified occupant of dirt bike or motor/cross** ▽
bike injured in nontraffic accident

√x7th **V86.99** **Unspecified occupant of other special all-terrain** ▽
or other off-road motor vehicle injured in
nontraffic accident
All-terrain motor-vehicle accident NOS
Off-road motor-vehicle accident NOS
Other motor-vehicle accident NOS
~~Unspecified occupant of dirt bike injured in nontraffic~~
~~accident~~
Unspecified occupant of go cart injured in nontraffic
accident
Unspecified occupant of golf cart injured in nontraffic
accident

√4th **V87** **Traffic accident of specified type but victim's mode of transport**
unknown
EXCLUDES 1   *collision involving:*
pedal cycle (V10-V19)
pedestrian (V01-V09)

√x7th **V87.0** **Person injured in collision between car and two- or**
three-wheeled powered vehicle (traffic)

√x7th **V87.1** **Person injured in collision between other motor vehicle and**
two- or three-wheeled motor vehicle (traffic)

√x7th **V87.2** **Person injured in collision between car and pick-up truck or**
van (traffic)

√x7th **V87.3** **Person injured in collision between car and bus (traffic)**

√x7th **V87.4** **Person injured in collision between car and heavy transport**
vehicle (traffic)

√x7th **V87.5** **Person injured in collision between heavy transport vehicle**
and bus (traffic)

√x7th **V87.6** **Person injured in collision between railway train or railway**
vehicle and car (traffic)

√x7th **V87.7** **Person injured in collision between other specified motor**
vehicles (traffic)

√x7th **V87.8** **Person injured in other specified noncollision transport**
accidents involving motor vehicle (traffic)

√x7th **V87.9** **Person injured in other specified (collision)(noncollision)**
transport accidents involving nonmotor vehicle (traffic)

√4th **V88** **Nontraffic accident of specified type but victim's mode of**
transport unknown
EXCLUDES 1   *collision involving:*
pedal cycle (V10-V19)
pedestrian (V01-V09)

√x7th **V88.0** **Person injured in collision between car and two-or**
three-wheeled motor vehicle, nontraffic

√x7th **V88.1** **Person injured in collision between other motor vehicle and**
two- or three-wheeled motor vehicle, nontraffic

√x7th **V88.2** **Person injured in collision between car and pick-up truck or**
van, nontraffic

√x7th **V88.3** **Person injured in collision between car and bus, nontraffic**

✔ Additional Character Req   √x7th Placeholder Alert   Manifestation   HCC CMS-HCC Condition   ▽ Unspecified Code   ►◄ Revised Text   ● New Code   ▲ Revised Code Title

✓x7ᵗʰ **V88.4** Person injured in collision between **car and heavy transport vehicle, nontraffic**

✓x7ᵗʰ **V88.5** Person injured in collision between **heavy transport vehicle and bus, nontraffic**

✓x7ᵗʰ **V88.6** Person injured in collision between **railway train or railway vehicle and car, nontraffic**

✓x7ᵗʰ **V88.7** Person injured in collision between **other specified motor vehicle, nontraffic**

✓x7ᵗʰ **V88.8** Person injured in **other specified noncollision transport accidents involving motor vehicle, nontraffic**

✓x7ᵗʰ **V88.9** Person injured in **other specified (collision)(noncollision) transport accidents involving nonmotor vehicle, nontraffic**

✓4ᵗʰ **V89 Motor- or nonmotor-vehicle accident, type of vehicle unspecified**

✓x7ᵗʰ **V89.0** Person injured in unspecified **motor-vehicle accident, nontraffic** ▽
        Motor-vehicle accident NOS, nontraffic

✓x7ᵗʰ **V89.1** Person injured in unspecified **nonmotor-vehicle accident, nontraffic** ▽
        Nonmotor-vehicle accident NOS (nontraffic)

✓x7ᵗʰ **V89.2** Person injured in unspecified **motor-vehicle accident, traffic** ▽
        Motor-vehicle accident [MVA] NOS
        Road (traffic) accident [RTA] NOS

✓x7ᵗʰ **V89.3** Person injured in unspecified **nonmotor-vehicle accident, traffic** ▽
        Nonmotor-vehicle traffic accident NOS

✓x7ᵗʰ **V89.9** Person injured in unspecified **vehicle accident** ▽
        Collision NOS

Water transport accidents (V90-V94)

The appropriate 7th character is to be added to each code from categories V90-V94.
A   initial encounter
D   subsequent encounter
S   sequela

✓4ᵗʰ **V90 Drowning and submersion due to accident to watercraft**
        EXCLUDES 1   civilian water transport accident involving military watercraft (V94.81-)
                    fall into water not from watercraft (W16.-)
                    military watercraft accident in military or war operations (Y36.0-, Y37.0-)
                    water-transport-related drowning or submersion without accident to watercraft (V92.-)

✓5ᵗʰ **V90.0 Drowning and submersion due to watercraft overturning**

✓x7ᵗʰ **V90.00** Drowning and submersion due to **merchant ship overturning**

✓x7ᵗʰ **V90.01** Drowning and submersion due to **passenger ship overturning**
            Drowning and submersion due to Ferry-boat overturning
            Drowning and submersion due to Liner overturning

✓x7ᵗʰ **V90.02** Drowning and submersion due to **fishing boat overturning**

✓x7ᵗʰ **V90.03** Drowning and submersion due to other **powered watercraft overturning**
            Drowning and submersion due to Hovercraft (on open water) overturning
            Drowning and submersion due to Jet ski overturning

✓x7ᵗʰ **V90.04** Drowning and submersion due to **sailboat overturning**

✓x7ᵗʰ **V90.05** Drowning and submersion due to **canoe or kayak overturning**

✓x7ᵗʰ **V90.06** Drowning and submersion due to **(nonpowered) inflatable craft overturning**

✓x7ᵗʰ **V90.08** Drowning and submersion due to other **unpowered watercraft overturning**
            Drowning and submersion due to windsurfer overturning

✓x7ᵗʰ **V90.09** Drowning and submersion due to **unspecified watercraft overturning** ▽
            Drowning and submersion due to boat NOS overturning
            Drowning and submersion due to ship NOS overturning
            Drowning and submersion due to watercraft NOS overturning

✓5ᵗʰ **V90.1 Drowning and submersion due to watercraft sinking**

✓x7ᵗʰ **V90.10** Drowning and submersion due to **merchant ship sinking**

✓x7ᵗʰ **V90.11** Drowning and submersion due to **passenger ship sinking**
            Drowning and submersion due to Ferry-boat sinking
            Drowning and submersion due to Liner sinking

✓x7ᵗʰ **V90.12** Drowning and submersion due to **fishing boat sinking**

✓x7ᵗʰ **V90.13** Drowning and submersion due to other **powered watercraft sinking**
            Drowning and submersion due to Hovercraft (on open water) sinking
            Drowning and submersion due to Jet ski sinking

✓x7ᵗʰ **V90.14** Drowning and submersion due to **sailboat sinking**

✓x7ᵗʰ **V90.15** Drowning and submersion due to **canoe or kayak sinking**

✓x7ᵗʰ **V90.16** Drowning and submersion due to **(nonpowered) inflatable craft sinking**

✓x7ᵗʰ **V90.18** Drowning and submersion due to other **unpowered watercraft sinking**

✓x7ᵗʰ **V90.19** Drowning and submersion due to **unspecified watercraft sinking** ▽
            Drowning and submersion due to boat NOS sinking
            Drowning and submersion due to ship NOS sinking
            Drowning and submersion due to watercraft NOS sinking

✓5ᵗʰ **V90.2 Drowning and submersion due to falling or jumping from burning watercraft**

✓x7ᵗʰ **V90.20** Drowning and submersion due to falling or jumping from burning **merchant ship**

✓x7ᵗʰ **V90.21** Drowning and submersion due to falling or jumping from burning **passenger ship**
            Drowning and submersion due to falling or jumping from burning Ferry-boat
            Drowning and submersion due to falling or jumping from burning Liner

✓x7ᵗʰ **V90.22** Drowning and submersion due to falling or jumping from burning **fishing boat**

✓x7ᵗʰ **V90.23** Drowning and submersion due to falling or jumping from other burning **powered** watercraft
            Drowning and submersion due to falling and jumping from burning Hovercraft (on open water)
            Drowning and submersion due to falling and jumping from burning Jet ski

✓x7ᵗʰ **V90.24** Drowning and submersion due to falling or jumping from burning **sailboat**

✓x7ᵗʰ **V90.25** Drowning and submersion due to falling or jumping from burning **canoe or kayak**

✓x7ᵗʰ **V90.26** Drowning and submersion due to falling or jumping from burning **(nonpowered) inflatable craft**

✓x7ᵗʰ **V90.27** Drowning and submersion due to falling or jumping from burning **water-skis**

✓x7ᵗʰ **V90.28** Drowning and submersion due to falling or jumping from other burning **unpowered watercraft**
            Drowning and submersion due to falling and jumping from burning surf-board
            Drowning and submersion due to falling and jumping from burning windsurfer

✓x7ᵗʰ **V90.29** Drowning and submersion due to falling or jumping from unspecified burning watercraft ▽
            Drowning and submersion due to falling or jumping from burning boat NOS
            Drowning and submersion due to falling or jumping from burning ship NOS
            Drowning and submersion due to falling or jumping from burning watercraft NOS

✓5ᵗʰ **V90.3 Drowning and submersion due to falling or jumping from crushed watercraft**

✓x7ᵗʰ **V90.30** Drowning and submersion due to falling or jumping from crushed **merchant ship**

✓x7ᵗʰ **V90.31** Drowning and submersion due to falling or jumping from crushed **passenger ship**
            Drowning and submersion due to falling and jumping from crushed Ferry boat
            Drowning and submersion due to falling and jumping from crushed Liner

√x7ᵗʰ **V90.32** **Drowning and submersion due to falling or jumping from crushed fishing boat**

√x7ᵗʰ **V90.33** **Drowning and submersion due to falling or jumping from other crushed powered watercraft**
Drowning and submersion due to falling and jumping from crushed Hovercraft
Drowning and submersion due to falling and jumping from crushed Jet ski

√x7ᵗʰ **V90.34** **Drowning and submersion due to falling or jumping from crushed sailboat**

√x7ᵗʰ **V90.35** **Drowning and submersion due to falling or jumping from crushed canoe or kayak**

√x7ᵗʰ **V90.36** **Drowning and submersion due to falling or jumping from crushed (nonpowered) inflatable craft**

√x7ᵗʰ **V90.37** **Drowning and submersion due to falling or jumping from crushed water-skis**

√x7ᵗʰ **V90.38** **Drowning and submersion due to falling or jumping from other crushed unpowered watercraft**
Drowning and submersion due to falling and jumping from crushed surf-board
Drowning and submersion due to falling and jumping from crushed windsurfer

√x7ᵗʰ **V90.39** **Drowning and submersion due to falling or jumping from crushed unspecified watercraft** ▽
Drowning and submersion due to falling and jumping from crushed boat NOS
Drowning and submersion due to falling and jumping from crushed ship NOS
Drowning and submersion due to falling and jumping from crushed watercraft NOS

√5ᵗʰ **V90.8** **Drowning and submersion due to other accident to watercraft**

√x7ᵗʰ **V90.80** **Drowning and submersion due to other accident to merchant ship**

√x7ᵗʰ **V90.81** **Drowning and submersion due to other accident to passenger ship**
Drowning and submersion due to other accident to Ferry-boat
Drowning and submersion due to other accident to Liner

√x7ᵗʰ **V90.82** **Drowning and submersion due to other accident to fishing boat**

√x7ᵗʰ **V90.83** **Drowning and submersion due to other accident to other powered watercraft**
Drowning and submersion due to other accident to Hovercraft (on open water)
Drowning and submersion due to other accident to Jet ski

√x7ᵗʰ **V90.84** **Drowning and submersion due to other accident to sailboat**

√x7ᵗʰ **V90.85** **Drowning and submersion due to other accident to canoe or kayak**

√x7ᵗʰ **V90.86** **Drowning and submersion due to other accident to (nonpowered) inflatable craft**

√x7ᵗʰ **V90.87** **Drowning and submersion due to other accident to water-skis**

√x7ᵗʰ **V90.88** **Drowning and submersion due to other accident to other unpowered watercraft**
Drowning and submersion due to other accident to surf-board
Drowning and submersion due to other accident to windsurfer

√x7ᵗʰ **V90.89** **Drowning and submersion due to other accident to unspecified watercraft** ▽
Drowning and submersion due to other accident to boat NOS
Drowning and submersion due to other accident to ship NOS
Drowning and submersion due to other accident to watercraft NOS

√4ᵗʰ **V91** **Other injury due to accident to watercraft**
INCLUDES   any injury except drowning and submersion as a result of an accident to watercraft
EXCLUDES 1   *civilian water transport accident involving military watercraft (V94.81-)*
military watercraft accident in military or war operations (Y36, Y37.-)
EXCLUDES 2   *drowning and submersion due to accident to watercraft (V90.-)*

√5ᵗʰ **V91.0** **Burn due to watercraft on fire**
EXCLUDES 1   *burn from localized fire or explosion on board ship without accident to watercraft (V93.-)*

√x7ᵗʰ **V91.00** **Burn due to merchant ship on fire**

√x7ᵗʰ **V91.01** **Burn due to passenger ship on fire**
Burn due to Ferry-boat on fire
Burn due to Liner on fire

√x7ᵗʰ **V91.02** **Burn due to fishing boat on fire**

√x7ᵗʰ **V91.03** **Burn due to other powered watercraft on fire**
Burn due to Hovercraft (on open water) on fire
Burn due to Jet ski on fire

√x7ᵗʰ **V91.04** **Burn due to sailboat on fire**

√x7ᵗʰ **V91.05** **Burn due to canoe or kayak on fire**

√x7ᵗʰ **V91.06** **Burn due to (nonpowered) inflatable craft on fire**

√x7ᵗʰ **V91.07** **Burn due to water-skis on fire**

√x7ᵗʰ **V91.08** **Burn due to other unpowered watercraft on fire**

√x7ᵗʰ **V91.09** **Burn due to unspecified watercraft on fire** ▽
Burn due to boat NOS on fire
Burn due to ship NOS on fire
Burn due to watercraft NOS on fire

√5ᵗʰ **V91.1** **Crushed between watercraft and other watercraft or other object due to collision**
Crushed by lifeboat after abandoning ship in a collision
NOTE   Select the specified type of watercraft that the victim was on at the time of the collision

√x7ᵗʰ **V91.10** **Crushed between merchant ship and other watercraft or other object due to collision**

√x7ᵗʰ **V91.11** **Crushed between passenger ship and other watercraft or other object due to collision**
Crushed between Ferry-boat and other watercraft or other object due to collision
Crushed between Liner and other watercraft or other object due to collision

√x7ᵗʰ **V91.12** **Crushed between fishing boat and other watercraft or other object due to collision**

√x7ᵗʰ **V91.13** **Crushed between other powered watercraft and other watercraft or other object due to collision**
Crushed between Hovercraft (on open water) and other watercraft or other object due to collision
Crushed between Jet ski and other watercraft or other object due to collision

√x7ᵗʰ **V91.14** **Crushed between sailboat and other watercraft or other object due to collision**

√x7ᵗʰ **V91.15** **Crushed between canoe or kayak and other watercraft or other object due to collision**

√x7ᵗʰ **V91.16** **Crushed between (nonpowered) inflatable craft and other watercraft or other object due to collision**

√x7ᵗʰ **V91.18** **Crushed between other unpowered watercraft and other watercraft or other object due to collision**
Crushed between surfboard and other watercraft or other object due to collision
Crushed between windsurfer and other watercraft or other object due to collision

√x7ᵗʰ **V91.19** **Crushed between unspecified watercraft and other watercraft or other object due to collision** ▽
Crushed between boat NOS and other watercraft or other object due to collision
Crushed between ship NOS and other watercraft or other object due to collision
Crushed between watercraft NOS and other watercraft or other object due to collision

☑ Additional Character Req   √x7ᵗʰ Placeholder Alert   Manifestation   HCC CMS-HCC Condition   ▽ Unspecified Code   ►◄ Revised Text   ● New Code   ▲ Revised Code Title

ICD-10-CM 2018   **1139**

✓5ᵗʰ V91.2 Fall due to collision between watercraft and other watercraft or other object

Fall while remaining on watercraft after collision

> **NOTE** Select the specified type of watercraft that the victim was on at the time of the collision.

> **EXCLUDES 1** crushed between watercraft and other watercraft and other object due to collision (V91.1-)
> drowning and submersion due to falling from crushed watercraft (V90.3-)

✓x7ᵗʰ V91.20 Fall due to collision between merchant ship and other watercraft or other object

✓x7ᵗʰ V91.21 Fall due to collision between passenger ship and other watercraft or other object

Fall due to collision between Ferry-boat and other watercraft or other object

Fall due to collision between Liner and other watercraft or other object

✓x7ᵗʰ V91.22 Fall due to collision between fishing boat and other watercraft or other object

✓x7ᵗʰ V91.23 Fall due to collision between other powered watercraft and other watercraft or other object

Fall due to collision between Hovercraft (on open water) and other watercraft or other object

Fall due to collision between Jet ski and other watercraft or other object

✓x7ᵗʰ V91.24 Fall due to collision between sailboat and other watercraft or other object

✓x7ᵗʰ V91.25 Fall due to collision between canoe or kayak and other watercraft or other object

✓x7ᵗʰ V91.26 Fall due to collision between (nonpowered) inflatable craft and other watercraft or other object

✓x7ᵗʰ V91.29 Fall due to collision between unspecified watercraft and other watercraft or other object ▽

Fall due to collision between boat NOS and other watercraft or other object

Fall due to collision between ship NOS and other watercraft or other object

Fall due to collision between watercraft NOS and other watercraft or other object

✓5ᵗʰ V91.3 Hit or struck by falling object due to accident to watercraft

Hit or struck by falling object (part of damaged watercraft or other object) after falling or jumping from damaged watercraft

> **EXCLUDES 2** drowning or submersion due to fall or jumping from damaged watercraft (V90.2-, V90.3-)

✓x7ᵗʰ V91.30 Hit or struck by falling object due to accident to merchant ship

✓x7ᵗʰ V91.31 Hit or struck by falling object due to accident to passenger ship

Hit or struck by falling object due to accident to Ferry-boat

Hit or struck by falling object due to accident to Liner

✓x7ᵗʰ V91.32 Hit or struck by falling object due to accident to fishing boat

✓x7ᵗʰ V91.33 Hit or struck by falling object due to accident to other powered watercraft

Hit or struck by falling object due to accident to Hovercraft (on open water)

Hit or struck by falling object due to accident to Jet ski

✓x7ᵗʰ V91.34 Hit or struck by falling object due to accident to sailboat

✓x7ᵗʰ V91.35 Hit or struck by falling object due to accident to canoe or kayak

✓x7ᵗʰ V91.36 Hit or struck by falling object due to accident to (nonpowered) inflatable craft

✓x7ᵗʰ V91.37 Hit or struck by falling object due to accident to water-skis

Hit by water-skis after jumping off of waterskis

✓x7ᵗʰ V91.38 Hit or struck by falling object due to accident to other unpowered watercraft

Hit or struck by surf-board after falling off damaged surf-board

Hit or struck by object after falling off damaged windsurfer

✓x7ᵗʰ V91.39 Hit or struck by falling object due to accident to unspecified watercraft ▽

Hit or struck by falling object due to accident to boat NOS

Hit or struck by falling object due to accident to ship NOS

Hit or struck by falling object due to accident to watercraft NOS

✓5ᵗʰ V91.8 Other injury due to other accident to watercraft

✓x7ᵗʰ V91.80 Other injury due to other accident to merchant ship

✓x7ᵗʰ V91.81 Other injury due to other accident to passenger ship

Other injury due to other accident to Ferry-boat

Other injury due to other accident to Liner

✓x7ᵗʰ V91.82 Other injury due to other accident to fishing boat

✓x7ᵗʰ V91.83 Other injury due to other accident to other powered watercraft

Other injury due to other accident to Hovercraft (on open water)

Other injury due to other accident to Jet ski

✓x7ᵗʰ V91.84 Other injury due to other accident to sailboat

✓x7ᵗʰ V91.85 Other injury due to other accident to canoe or kayak

✓x7ᵗʰ V91.86 Other injury due to other accident to (nonpowered) inflatable craft

✓x7ᵗʰ V91.87 Other injury due to other accident to water-skis

✓x7ᵗʰ V91.88 Other injury due to other accident to other unpowered watercraft

Other injury due to other accident to surf-board

Other injury due to other accident to windsurfer

✓x7ᵗʰ V91.89 Other injury due to other accident to unspecified watercraft ▽

Other injury due to other accident to boat NOS

Other injury due to other accident to ship NOS

Other injury due to other accident to watercraft NOS

✓4ᵗʰ V92 Drowning and submersion due to accident on board watercraft, without accident to watercraft

> **EXCLUDES 1** civilian water transport accident involving military watercraft (V94.81-)
> drowning or submersion due to accident to watercraft (V90-V91)
> drowning or submersion of diver who voluntarily jumps from boat not involved in an accident (W16.711, W16.721)
> fall into water without watercraft (W16.-)
> military watercraft accident in military or war operations (Y36, Y37)

✓5ᵗʰ V92.0 Drowning and submersion due to fall off watercraft

Drowning and submersion due to fall from gangplank of watercraft

Drowning and submersion due to fall overboard watercraft

> **EXCLUDES 2** hitting head on object or bottom of body of water due to fall from watercraft (V94.0-)

✓x7ᵗʰ V92.00 Drowning and submersion due to fall off merchant ship

✓x7ᵗʰ V92.01 Drowning and submersion due to fall off passenger ship

Drowning and submersion due to fall off Ferry-boat

Drowning and submersion due to fall off Liner

✓x7ᵗʰ V92.02 Drowning and submersion due to fall off fishing boat

✓x7ᵗʰ V92.03 Drowning and submersion due to fall off other powered watercraft

Drowning and submersion due to fall off Hovercraft (on open water)

Drowning and submersion due to fall off Jet ski

✓x7ᵗʰ V92.04 Drowning and submersion due to fall off sailboat

✓x7ᵗʰ V92.05 Drowning and submersion due to fall off canoe or kayak

✓x7ᵗʰ V92.06 Drowning and submersion due to fall off (nonpowered) inflatable craft

✓x7ᵗʰ V92.07 Drowning and submersion due to fall off water-skis

> **EXCLUDES 1** drowning and submersion due to falling off burning water-skis (V90.27)
> drowning and submersion due to falling off crushed water-skis (V90.37)
> hit by boat while water-skiing NOS (V94.X)

EXCLUDES 1 Not coded here   **EXCLUDES 2** Not included here   **N** Newborn Age: 0   **P** Pediatric Age: 0-17   **M** Maternity Age: 12-55   **A** Adult Age: 15-124

1140   ICD-10-CM 2018

✓x7ᵗʰ V92.08 Drowning and submersion due to fall off other unpowered watercraft
Drowning and submersion due to fall off surf-board
Drowning and submersion due to fall off windsurfer
> **EXCLUDES 1** *drowning and submersion due to fall off burning unpowered watercraft (V90.28)*
> *drowning and submersion due to fall off crushed unpowered watercraft (V90.38)*
> *drowning and submersion due to fall off damaged unpowered watercraft (V90.88)*
> *drowning and submersion due to rider of nonpowered watercraft being hit by other watercraft (V94.-)*
> *other injury due to rider of nonpowered watercraft being hit by other watercraft (V94.-)*

✓x7ᵗʰ V92.09 Drowning and submersion due to fall off unspecified watercraft ▽
Drowning and submersion due to fall off boat NOS
Drowning and submersion due to fall off ship
Drowning and submersion due to fall off watercraft NOS

✓5ᵗʰ V92.1 Drowning and submersion due to being thrown overboard by motion of watercraft
> **EXCLUDES 1** *drowning and submersion due to fall off surf-board (V92.08)*
> *drowning and submersion due to fall off water-skis (V92.07)*
> *drowning and submersion due to fall off windsurfer (V92.08)*

✓x7ᵗʰ V92.10 Drowning and submersion due to being thrown overboard by motion of merchant ship

✓x7ᵗʰ V92.11 Drowning and submersion due to being thrown overboard by motion of passenger ship
Drowning and submersion due to being thrown overboard by motion of Ferry-boat
Drowning and submersion due to being thrown overboard by motion of Liner

✓x7ᵗʰ V92.12 Drowning and submersion due to being thrown overboard by motion of fishing boat

✓x7ᵗʰ V92.13 Drowning and submersion due to being thrown overboard by motion of other powered watercraft
Drowning and submersion due to being thrown overboard by motion of Hovercraft

✓x7ᵗʰ V92.14 Drowning and submersion due to being thrown overboard by motion of sailboat

✓x7ᵗʰ V92.15 Drowning and submersion due to being thrown overboard by motion of canoe or kayak

✓x7ᵗʰ V92.16 Drowning and submersion due to being thrown overboard by motion of (nonpowered) inflatable craft

✓x7ᵗʰ V92.19 Drowning and submersion due to being thrown overboard by motion of unspecified watercraft ▽
Drowning and submersion due to being thrown overboard by motion of boat NOS
Drowning and submersion due to being thrown overboard by motion of ship NOS
Drowning and submersion due to being thrown overboard by motion of watercraft NOS

✓5ᵗʰ V92.2 Drowning and submersion due to being washed overboard from watercraft
Code first any associated cataclysm (X37.0-)

✓x7ᵗʰ V92.20 Drowning and submersion due to being washed overboard from merchant ship

✓x7ᵗʰ V92.21 Drowning and submersion due to being washed overboard from passenger ship
Drowning and submersion due to being washed overboard from Ferry-boat
Drowning and submersion due to being washed overboard from Liner

✓x7ᵗʰ V92.22 Drowning and submersion due to being washed overboard from fishing boat

✓x7ᵗʰ V92.23 Drowning and submersion due to being washed overboard from other powered watercraft
Drowning and submersion due to being washed overboard from Hovercraft (on open water)
Drowning and submersion due to being washed overboard from Jet ski

✓x7ᵗʰ V92.24 Drowning and submersion due to being washed overboard from sailboat

✓x7ᵗʰ V92.25 Drowning and submersion due to being washed overboard from canoe or kayak

✓x7ᵗʰ V92.26 Drowning and submersion due to being washed overboard from (nonpowered) inflatable craft

✓x7ᵗʰ V92.27 Drowning and submersion due to being washed overboard from water-skis
> **EXCLUDES 1** *drowning and submersion due to fall off water-skis (V92.07)*

✓x7ᵗʰ V92.28 Drowning and submersion due to being washed overboard from other unpowered watercraft
Drowning and submersion due to being washed overboard from surf-board
Drowning and submersion due to being washed overboard from windsurfer

✓x7ᵗʰ V92.29 Drowning and submersion due to being washed overboard from unspecified watercraft ▽
Drowning and submersion due to being washed overboard from boat NOS
Drowning and submersion due to being washed overboard from ship NOS
Drowning and submersion due to being washed overboard from watercraft NOS

✓4ᵗʰ V93 Other injury due to accident on board watercraft, without accident to watercraft
> **EXCLUDES 1** *civilian water transport accident involving military watercraft (V94.81-)*
> *other injury due to accident to watercraft (V91.-)*
> *military watercraft accident in military or war operations (Y36, Y37.-)*
> **EXCLUDES 2** *drowning and submersion due to accident on board watercraft, without accident to watercraft (V92.-)*

✓5ᵗʰ V93.0 Burn due to localized fire on board watercraft
> **EXCLUDES 1** *burn due to watercraft on fire (V91.0-)*

✓x7ᵗʰ V93.00 Burn due to localized fire on board merchant vessel

✓x7ᵗʰ V93.01 Burn due to localized fire on board passenger vessel
Burn due to localized fire on board Ferry-boat
Burn due to localized fire on board Liner

✓x7ᵗʰ V93.02 Burn due to localized fire on board fishing boat

✓x7ᵗʰ V93.03 Burn due to localized fire on board other powered watercraft
Burn due to localized fire on board Hovercraft
Burn due to localized fire on board Jet ski

✓x7ᵗʰ V93.04 Burn due to localized fire on board sailboat

✓x7ᵗʰ V93.09 Burn due to localized fire on board unspecified watercraft ▽
Burn due to localized fire on board boat NOS
Burn due to localized fire on board ship NOS
Burn due to localized fire on board watercraft NOS

✓5ᵗʰ V93.1 Other burn on board watercraft
Burn due to source other than fire on board watercraft
> **EXCLUDES 1** *burn due to watercraft on fire (V91.0-)*

✓x7ᵗʰ V93.10 Other burn on board merchant vessel

✓x7ᵗʰ V93.11 Other burn on board passenger vessel
Other burn on board Ferry-boat
Other burn on board Liner

✓x7ᵗʰ V93.12 Other burn on board fishing boat

✓x7ᵗʰ V93.13 Other burn on board other powered watercraft
Other burn on board Hovercraft
Other burn on board Jet ski

✓x7ᵗʰ V93.14 Other burn on board sailboat

✓x7ᵗʰ V93.19 Other burn on board unspecified watercraft ▽
Other burn on board boat NOS
Other burn on board ship NOS
Other burn on board watercraft NOS

✓5ᵗʰ V93.2 Heat exposure on board watercraft
> **EXCLUDES 1** *exposure to man-made heat not aboard watercraft (W92)*
> *exposure to natural heat while on board watercraft (X30)*
> *exposure to sunlight while on board watercraft (X32)*
> **EXCLUDES 2** *burn due to fire on board watercraft (V93.0-)*

✓x7ᵗʰ V93.20 Heat exposure on board merchant ship

✓x7ᵗʰ V93.21 Heat exposure on board passenger ship
Heat exposure on board Ferry-boat
Heat exposure on board Liner

✓x7ᵗʰ V93.22 Heat exposure on board fishing boat

✓ Additional Character Req   ✓x7ᵗʰ Placeholder Alert   Manifestation   HCC CMS-HCC Condition   ▽ Unspecified Code   ►◄ Revised Text   ● New Code   ▲ Revised Code Title

√x7ᵗʰ **V93.23 Heat exposure on board other powered watercraft**
Heat exposure on board hovercraft

√x7ᵗʰ **V93.24 Heat exposure on board sailboat**

√x7ᵗʰ **V93.29 Heat exposure on board unspecified watercraft** ▽
Heat exposure on board boat NOS
Heat exposure on board ship NOS
Heat exposure on board watercraft NOS

√5ᵗʰ **V93.3 Fall on board watercraft**
EXCLUDES 1   *fall due to collision of watercraft (V91.2-)*

√x7ᵗʰ **V93.30 Fall on board merchant ship**

√x7ᵗʰ **V93.31 Fall on board passenger ship**
Fall on board Ferry-boat
Fall on board Liner

√x7ᵗʰ **V93.32 Fall on board fishing boat**

√x7ᵗʰ **V93.33 Fall on board other powered watercraft**
Fall on board Hovercraft (on open water)
Fall on board Jet ski

√x7ᵗʰ **V93.34 Fall on board sailboat**

√x7ᵗʰ **V93.35 Fall on board canoe or kayak**

√x7ᵗʰ **V93.36 Fall on board (nonpowered) inflatable craft**

√x7ᵗʰ **V93.38 Fall on board other unpowered watercraft**

√x7ᵗʰ **V93.39 Fall on board unspecified watercraft** ▽
Fall on board boat NOS
Fall on board ship NOS
Fall on board watercraft NOS

√5ᵗʰ **V93.4 Struck by falling object on board watercraft**
Hit by falling object on board watercraft
EXCLUDES 1   *struck by falling object due to accident to watercraft (V91.3)*

√x7ᵗʰ **V93.40 Struck by falling object on merchant ship**

√x7ᵗʰ **V93.41 Struck by falling object on passenger ship**
Struck by falling object on Ferry-boat
Struck by falling object on Liner

√x7ᵗʰ **V93.42 Struck by falling object on fishing boat**

√x7ᵗʰ **V93.43 Struck by falling object on other powered watercraft**
Struck by falling object on Hovercraft

√x7ᵗʰ **V93.44 Struck by falling object on sailboat**

√x7ᵗʰ **V93.48 Struck by falling object on other unpowered watercraft**

√x7ᵗʰ **V93.49 Struck by falling object on unspecified watercraft** ▽

√5ᵗʰ **V93.5 Explosion on board watercraft**
Boiler explosion on steamship
EXCLUDES 2   *fire on board watercraft (V93.0-)*

√x7ᵗʰ **V93.50 Explosion on board merchant ship**

√x7ᵗʰ **V93.51 Explosion on board passenger ship**
Explosion on board Ferry-boat
Explosion on board Liner

√x7ᵗʰ **V93.52 Explosion on board fishing boat**

√x7ᵗʰ **V93.53 Explosion on board other powered watercraft**
Explosion on board **Hovercraft**
Explosion on board Jet ski

√x7ᵗʰ **V93.54 Explosion on board sailboat**

√x7ᵗʰ **V93.59 Explosion on board unspecified watercraft** ▽
Explosion on board boat NOS
Explosion on board ship NOS
Explosion on board watercraft NOS

√5ᵗʰ **V93.6 Machinery accident on board watercraft**
EXCLUDES 1   *machinery explosion on board watercraft (V93.4-)*
machinery fire on board watercraft (V93.0-)

√x7ᵗʰ **V93.60 Machinery accident on board merchant ship**

√x7ᵗʰ **V93.61 Machinery accident on board passenger ship**
Machinery accident on board Ferry-boat
Machinery accident on board Liner

√x7ᵗʰ **V93.62 Machinery accident on board fishing boat**

√x7ᵗʰ **V93.63 Machinery accident on board other powered watercraft**
Machinery accident on board Hovercraft

√x7ᵗʰ **V93.64 Machinery accident on board sailboat**

√x7ᵗʰ **V93.69 Machinery accident on board unspecified watercraft** ▽
Machinery accident on board boat NOS
Machinery accident on board ship NOS
Machinery accident on board watercraft NOS

√5ᵗʰ **V93.8 Other injury due to other accident on board watercraft**
Accidental poisoning by gases or fumes on watercraft

√x7ᵗʰ **V93.80 Other injury due to other accident on board merchant ship**

√x7ᵗʰ **V93.81 Other injury due to other accident on board passenger ship**
Other injury due to other accident on board Ferry-boat
Other injury due to other accident on board Liner

√x7ᵗʰ **V93.82 Other injury due to other accident on board fishing boat**

√x7ᵗʰ **V93.83 Other injury due to other accident on board other powered watercraft**
Other injury due to other accident on board Hovercraft
Other injury due to other accident on board Jet ski

√x7ᵗʰ **V93.84 Other injury due to other accident on board sailboat**

√x7ᵗʰ **V93.85 Other injury due to other accident on board canoe or kayak**

√x7ᵗʰ **V93.86 Other injury due to other accident on board (nonpowered) inflatable craft**

√x7ᵗʰ **V93.87 Other injury due to other accident on board water-skis**
Hit or struck by object while waterskiing

√x7ᵗʰ **V93.88 Other injury due to other accident on board other unpowered watercraft**
Hit or struck by object while surfing
Hit or struck by object while on board windsurfer

√x7ᵗʰ **V93.89 Other injury due to other accident on board unspecified watercraft** ▽
Other injury due to other accident on board boat NOS
Other injury due to other accident on board ship NOS
Other injury due to other accident on board watercraft NOS

√4ᵗʰ **V94 Other and unspecified water transport accidents**
EXCLUDES 1   *military watercraft accidents in military or war operations (Y36, Y37)*

√x7ᵗʰ **V94.0 Hitting object or bottom of body of water due to fall from watercraft**
EXCLUDES 2   *drowning and submersion due to fall from watercraft (V92.0-)*

√5ᵗʰ **V94.1 Bather struck by watercraft**
Swimmer hit by watercraft

√x7ᵗʰ **V94.11 Bather struck by powered watercraft**

√x7ᵗʰ **V94.12 Bather struck by nonpowered watercraft**

√5ᵗʰ **V94.2 Rider of nonpowered watercraft struck by other watercraft**

√x7ᵗʰ **V94.21 Rider of nonpowered watercraft struck by other nonpowered watercraft**
Canoer hit by other nonpowered watercraft
Surfer hit by other nonpowered watercraft
Windsurfer hit by other nonpowered watercraft

√x7ᵗʰ **V94.22 Rider of nonpowered watercraft struck by powered watercraft**
Canoer hit by motorboat
Surfer hit by motorboat
Windsurfer hit by motorboat

√5ᵗʰ **V94.3 Injury to rider of (inflatable) watercraft being pulled behind other watercraft**

√x7ᵗʰ **V94.31 Injury to rider of (inflatable) recreational watercraft being pulled behind other watercraft**
Injury to rider of inner-tube pulled behind motor boat

√x7ᵗʰ **V94.32 Injury to rider of non-recreational watercraft being pulled behind other watercraft**
Injury to occupant of dingy being pulled behind boat or ship
Injury to occupant of life-raft being pulled behind boat or ship

√x7ᵗʰ **V94.4 Injury to barefoot water-skier**
Injury to person being pulled behind boat or ship

√5ᵗʰ **V94.8 Other water transport accident**

√6ᵗʰ **V94.81 Water transport accident involving military watercraft**

√7ᵗʰ **V94.810 Civilian watercraft involved in water transport accident with military watercraft**
Passenger on civilian watercraft injured due to accident with military watercraft

---

EXCLUDES 1 Not coded here   EXCLUDES 2 Not included here   N Newborn Age: 0   P Pediatric Age: 0-17   M Maternity Age: 12-55   A Adult Age: 15-124

      ✓7ᵗʰ   **V94.811**   **Civilian in water injured by military watercraft**

      ✓7ᵗʰ   **V94.818**   **Other water transport accident involving military watercraft**

   ✓x7ᵗʰ   **V94.89**   **Other water transport accident**

   ✓x7ᵗʰ   **V94.9**   **Unspecified water transport accident** ▽
       Water transport accident NOS

Air and space transport accidents (V95-V97)

EXCLUDES1   *military aircraft accidents in military or war operations (Y36, Y37)*

The appropriate 7th character is to be added to each code from categories V95-V97.
A   initial encounter
D   subsequent encounter
S   sequela

✓4ᵗʰ   **V95**   **Accident to powered aircraft causing injury to occupant**

   ✓5ᵗʰ   **V95.0**   **Helicopter accident injuring occupant**

      ✓x7ᵗʰ   **V95.00**   **Unspecified helicopter accident injuring occupant** ▽

      ✓x7ᵗʰ   **V95.01**   **Helicopter crash injuring occupant**

      ✓x7ᵗʰ   **V95.02**   **Forced landing of helicopter injuring occupant**

      ✓x7ᵗʰ   **V95.03**   **Helicopter collision injuring occupant**
       Helicopter collision with any object, fixed, movable or moving

      ✓x7ᵗʰ   **V95.04**   **Helicopter fire injuring occupant**

      ✓x7ᵗʰ   **V95.05**   **Helicopter explosion injuring occupant**

      ✓x7ᵗʰ   **V95.09**   **Other helicopter accident injuring occupant**

   ✓5ᵗʰ   **V95.1**   **Ultralight, microlight or powered-glider accident injuring occupant**

      ✓x7ᵗʰ   **V95.10**   **Unspecified ultralight, microlight or powered-glider accident injuring occupant** ▽

      ✓x7ᵗʰ   **V95.11**   **Ultralight, microlight or powered-glider crash injuring occupant**

      ✓x7ᵗʰ   **V95.12**   **Forced landing of ultralight, microlight or powered-glider injuring occupant**

      ✓x7ᵗʰ   **V95.13**   **Ultralight, microlight or powered-glider collision injuring occupant**
       Ultralight, microlight or powered-glider collision with any object, fixed, movable or moving

      ✓x7ᵗʰ   **V95.14**   **Ultralight, microlight or powered-glider fire injuring occupant**

      ✓x7ᵗʰ   **V95.15**   **Ultralight, microlight or powered-glider explosion injuring occupant**

      ✓x7ᵗʰ   **V95.19**   **Other ultralight, microlight or powered-glider accident injuring occupant**

   ✓5ᵗʰ   **V95.2**   **Other private fixed-wing aircraft accident injuring occupant**

      ✓x7ᵗʰ   **V95.20**   **Unspecified accident to other private fixed-wing aircraft, injuring occupant** ▽

      ✓x7ᵗʰ   **V95.21**   **Other private fixed-wing aircraft crash injuring occupant**

      ✓x7ᵗʰ   **V95.22**   **Forced landing of other private fixed-wing aircraft injuring occupant**

      ✓x7ᵗʰ   **V95.23**   **Other private fixed-wing aircraft collision injuring occupant**
       Other private fixed-wing aircraft collision with any object, fixed, movable or moving

      ✓x7ᵗʰ   **V95.24**   **Other private fixed-wing aircraft fire injuring occupant**

      ✓x7ᵗʰ   **V95.25**   **Other private fixed-wing aircraft explosion injuring occupant**

      ✓x7ᵗʰ   **V95.29**   **Other accident to other private fixed-wing aircraft injuring occupant**

   ✓5ᵗʰ   **V95.3**   **Commercial fixed-wing aircraft accident injuring occupant**

      ✓x7ᵗʰ   **V95.30**   **Unspecified accident to commercial fixed-wing aircraft injuring occupant** ▽

      ✓x7ᵗʰ   **V95.31**   **Commercial fixed-wing aircraft crash injuring occupant**

      ✓x7ᵗʰ   **V95.32**   **Forced landing of commercial fixed-wing aircraft injuring occupant**

      ✓x7ᵗʰ   **V95.33**   **Commercial fixed-wing aircraft collision injuring occupant**
       Commercial fixed-wing aircraft collision with any object, fixed, movable or moving

      ✓x7ᵗʰ   **V95.34**   **Commercial fixed-wing aircraft fire injuring occupant**

      ✓x7ᵗʰ   **V95.35**   **Commercial fixed-wing aircraft explosion injuring occupant**

      ✓x7ᵗʰ   **V95.39**   **Other accident to commercial fixed-wing aircraft injuring occupant**

   ✓5ᵗʰ   **V95.4**   **Spacecraft accident injuring occupant**

      ✓x7ᵗʰ   **V95.40**   **Unspecified spacecraft accident injuring occupant** ▽

      ✓x7ᵗʰ   **V95.41**   **Spacecraft crash injuring occupant**

      ✓x7ᵗʰ   **V95.42**   **Forced landing of spacecraft injuring occupant**

      ✓x7ᵗʰ   **V95.43**   **Spacecraft collision injuring occupant**
       Spacecraft collision with any object, fixed, moveable or moving

      ✓x7ᵗʰ   **V95.44**   **Spacecraft fire injuring occupant**

      ✓x7ᵗʰ   **V95.45**   **Spacecraft explosion injuring occupant**

      ✓x7ᵗʰ   **V95.49**   **Other spacecraft accident injuring occupant**

   ✓x7ᵗʰ   **V95.8**   **Other powered aircraft accidents injuring occupant**

   ✓x7ᵗʰ   **V95.9**   **Unspecified aircraft accident injuring occupant** ▽
       Aircraft accident NOS
       Air transport accident NOS

✓4ᵗʰ   **V96**   **Accident to nonpowered aircraft causing injury to occupant**

   ✓5ᵗʰ   **V96.0**   **Balloon accident injuring occupant**

      ✓x7ᵗʰ   **V96.00**   **Unspecified balloon accident injuring occupant** ▽

      ✓x7ᵗʰ   **V96.01**   **Balloon crash injuring occupant**

      ✓x7ᵗʰ   **V96.02**   **Forced landing of balloon injuring occupant**

      ✓x7ᵗʰ   **V96.03**   **Balloon collision injuring occupant**
       Balloon collision with any object, fixed, moveable or moving

      ✓x7ᵗʰ   **V96.04**   **Balloon fire injuring occupant**

      ✓x7ᵗʰ   **V96.05**   **Balloon explosion injuring occupant**

      ✓x7ᵗʰ   **V96.09**   **Other balloon accident injuring occupant**

   ✓5ᵗʰ   **V96.1**   **Hang-glider accident injuring occupant**

      ✓x7ᵗʰ   **V96.10**   **Unspecified hang-glider accident injuring occupant** ▽

      ✓x7ᵗʰ   **V96.11**   **Hang-glider crash injuring occupant**

      ✓x7ᵗʰ   **V96.12**   **Forced landing of hang-glider injuring occupant**

      ✓x7ᵗʰ   **V96.13**   **Hang-glider collision injuring occupant**
       Hang-glider collision with any object, fixed, moveable or moving

      ✓x7ᵗʰ   **V96.14**   **Hang-glider fire injuring occupant**

      ✓x7ᵗʰ   **V96.15**   **Hang-glider explosion injuring occupant**

      ✓x7ᵗʰ   **V96.19**   **Other hang-glider accident injuring occupant**

   ✓5ᵗʰ   **V96.2**   **Glider (nonpowered) accident injuring occupant**

      ✓x7ᵗʰ   **V96.20**   **Unspecified glider (nonpowered) accident injuring occupant** ▽

      ✓x7ᵗʰ   **V96.21**   **Glider (nonpowered) crash injuring occupant**

      ✓x7ᵗʰ   **V96.22**   **Forced landing of glider (nonpowered) injuring occupant**

      ✓x7ᵗʰ   **V96.23**   **Glider (nonpowered) collision injuring occupant**
       Glider (nonpowered) collision with any object, fixed, moveable or moving

      ✓x7ᵗʰ   **V96.24**   **Glider (nonpowered) fire injuring occupant**

      ✓x7ᵗʰ   **V96.25**   **Glider (nonpowered) explosion injuring occupant**

      ✓x7ᵗʰ   **V96.29**   **Other glider (nonpowered) accident injuring occupant**

   ✓x7ᵗʰ   **V96.8**   **Other nonpowered-aircraft accidents injuring occupant**
       Kite carrying a person accident injuring occupant

   ✓x7ᵗʰ   **V96.9**   **Unspecified nonpowered-aircraft accident injuring occupant** ▽
       Nonpowered-aircraft accident NOS

✓4ᵗʰ   **V97**   **Other specified air transport accidents**

   ✓x7ᵗʰ   **V97.0**   **Occupant of aircraft injured in other specified air transport accidents**
       Fall in, on or from aircraft in air transport accident
       EXCLUDES1   *accident while boarding or alighting aircraft (V97.1)*

   ✓x7ᵗʰ   **V97.1**   **Person injured while boarding or alighting from aircraft**

   ✓5ᵗʰ   **V97.2**   **Parachutist accident**

      ✓x7ᵗʰ   **V97.21**   **Parachutist entangled in object**
       Parachutist landing in tree

      ✓x7ᵗʰ   **V97.22**   **Parachutist injured on landing**

☑ Additional Character Req   ✓x7ᵗʰ Placeholder Alert   Manifestation   HCC CMS-HCC Condition   ▽ Unspecified Code   ▶◀ Revised Text   ● New Code   ▲ Revised Code Title

√x7ᵗʰ **V97.29 Other parachutist accident**

√5ᵗʰ **V97.3 Person on ground injured in air transport accident**

√x7ᵗʰ **V97.31 Hit by object falling from aircraft**
Hit by crashing aircraft
Injured by aircraft hitting house
Injured by aircraft hitting car

√x7ᵗʰ **V97.32 Injured by rotating propeller**

√x7ᵗʰ **V97.33 Sucked into jet engine**

√x7ᵗʰ **V97.39 Other injury to person on ground due to air transport accident**

√5ᵗʰ **V97.8 Other air transport accidents, not elsewhere classified**
EXCLUDES 1 aircraft accident NOS (V95.9)
exposure to changes in air pressure during ascent or descent (W94.-)

√6ᵗʰ **V97.81 Air transport accident involving military aircraft**

√7ᵗʰ **V97.810 Civilian aircraft involved in air transport accident with military aircraft**
Passenger in civilian aircraft injured due to accident with military aircraft

√7ᵗʰ **V97.811 Civilian injured by military aircraft**

√7ᵗʰ **V97.818 Other air transport accident involving military aircraft**

√x7ᵗʰ **V97.89 Other air transport accidents, not elsewhere classified**
Injury from machinery on aircraft

Other and unspecified transport accidents (V98-V99)
EXCLUDES 1 vehicle accident, type of vehicle unspecified (V89.-)

The appropriate 7th character is to be added to each code from categories V98-V99.
A   initial encounter
D   subsequent encounter
S   sequela

√4ᵗʰ **V98 Other specified transport accidents**

√x7ᵗʰ **V98.0 Accident to, on or involving cable-car, not on rails**
Caught or dragged by cable-car, not on rails
Fall or jump from cable-car, not on rails
Object thrown from or in cable-car, not on rails

√x7ᵗʰ **V98.1 Accident to, on or involving land-yacht**

√x7ᵗʰ **V98.2 Accident to, on or involving ice yacht**

√x7ᵗʰ **V98.3 Accident to, on or involving ski lift**
Accident to, on or involving ski chair-lift
Accident to, on or involving ski-lift with gondola

√x7ᵗʰ **V98.8 Other specified transport accidents**

√x7ᵗʰ **V99 Unspecified transport accident** ▽

OTHER EXTERNAL CAUSES OF ACCIDENTAL INJURY (W00-X58)

Slipping, tripping, stumbling and falls (W00-W19)
EXCLUDES 1 assault involving a fall (Y01-Y02)
fall from animal (V80.-)
fall (in) (from) machinery (in operation) (W28-W31)
fall (in) (from) transport vehicle (V01-V99)
intentional self-harm involving a fall (X80-X81)
EXCLUDES 2 at risk for fall (history of fall) (Z91.81)
fall (in) (from) burning building (X00.-)
fall into fire ▶(X00-X04, X08)◀

The appropriate 7th character is to be added to each code from category W00-W19.
A   initial encounter
D   subsequent encounter
S   sequela

√4ᵗʰ **W00 Fall due to ice and snow**
INCLUDES pedestrian on foot falling (slipping) on ice and snow
EXCLUDES 1 fall on (from) ice and snow involving pedestrian conveyance (V00.-)
fall from stairs and steps not due to ice and snow (W10.-)
AHA: 2016, 2Q, 4

√x7ᵗʰ **W00.0 Fall on same level due to ice and snow**

√x7ᵗʰ **W00.1 Fall from stairs and steps due to ice and snow**

√x7ᵗʰ **W00.2 Other fall from one level to another due to ice and snow**

√x7ᵗʰ **W00.9 Unspecified fall due to ice and snow** ▽

√4ᵗʰ **W01 Fall on same level from slipping, tripping and stumbling**
INCLUDES fall on moving sidewalk
EXCLUDES 1 fall due to bumping (striking) against object (W18.0-)
fall in shower or bathtub (W18.2-)
fall on same level NOS (W18.30)
fall on same level from slipping, tripping and stumbling due to ice or snow (W00.0)
fall off or from toilet (W18.1-)
slipping, tripping and stumbling NOS (W18.40)
slipping, tripping and stumbling without falling (W18.4-)

√x7ᵗʰ **W01.0 Fall on same level from slipping, tripping and stumbling without subsequent striking against object**
Falling over animal

√5ᵗʰ **W01.1 Fall on same level from slipping, tripping and stumbling with subsequent striking against object**

√x7ᵗʰ **W01.10 Fall on same level from slipping, tripping and stumbling with subsequent striking against unspecified object** ▽

√6ᵗʰ **W01.11 Fall on same level from slipping, tripping and stumbling with subsequent striking against sharp object**

√7ᵗʰ **W01.110 Fall on same level from slipping, tripping and stumbling with subsequent striking against sharp glass**

√7ᵗʰ **W01.111 Fall on same level from slipping, tripping and stumbling with subsequent striking against power tool or machine**

√7ᵗʰ **W01.118 Fall on same level from slipping, tripping and stumbling with subsequent striking against other sharp object**

√7ᵗʰ **W01.119 Fall on same level from slipping, tripping and stumbling with subsequent striking against unspecified sharp object** ▽

√6ᵗʰ **W01.19 Fall on same level from slipping, tripping and stumbling with subsequent striking against other object**

√7ᵗʰ **W01.190 Fall on same level from slipping, tripping and stumbling with subsequent striking against furniture**

√7ᵗʰ **W01.198 Fall on same level from slipping, tripping and stumbling with subsequent striking against other object**

√x7ᵗʰ **W03 Other fall on same level due to collision with another person**
Fall due to non-transport collision with other person
EXCLUDES 1 collision with another person without fall (W51)
crushed or pushed by a crowd or human stampede (W52)
fall involving pedestrian conveyance (V00-V09)
fall due to ice or snow (W00)
fall on same level NOS (W18.30)
AHA: 2012, 4Q, 108

√x7ᵗʰ **W04 Fall while being carried or supported by other persons**
Accidentally dropped while being carried

√4ᵗʰ **W05 Fall from non-moving wheelchair, nonmotorized scooter and motorized mobility scooter**
EXCLUDES 1 fall from moving wheelchair (powered) (V00.811)
fall from moving motorized mobility scooter (V00.831)
fall from nonmotorized scooter (V00.141)

√x7ᵗʰ **W05.0 Fall from non-moving wheelchair**

√x7ᵗʰ **W05.1 Fall from non-moving nonmotorized scooter**

√x7ᵗʰ **W05.2 Fall from non-moving motorized mobility scooter**

√x7ᵗʰ **W06 Fall from bed**

√x7ᵗʰ **W07 Fall from chair**

√x7ᵗʰ **W08 Fall from other furniture**

√4ᵗʰ **W09 Fall on and from playground equipment**
EXCLUDES 1 fall involving recreational machinery (W31)g

√x7ᵗʰ **W09.0 Fall on or from playground slide**

√x7ᵗʰ **W09.1 Fall from playground swing**

√x7ᵗʰ **W09.2 Fall on or from jungle gym**

√x7ᵗʰ **W09.8 Fall on or from other playground equipment**

√4ᵗʰ **W10 Fall on and from stairs and steps**
EXCLUDES 1 Fall from stairs and steps due to ice and snow (W00.1)

√x7ᵗʰ **W10.0 Fall (on)(from) escalator**

√x7ᵗʰ **W10.1 Fall (on)(from) sidewalk curb**

√x7ᵗʰ **W10.2 Fall (on)(from) incline**
Fall (on) (from) ramp

EXCLUDES 1 Not coded here   EXCLUDES 2 Not included here   N Newborn Age: 0   P Pediatric Age: 0-17   M Maternity Age: 12-55   A Adult Age: 15-124

☑x7ᵗʰ **W10.8** Fall (on) (from) other stairs and steps

☑x7ᵗʰ **W10.9** Fall (on) (from) unspecified stairs and steps   ▽

☑x7ᵗʰ **W11 Fall on and from ladder**

☑x7ᵗʰ **W12 Fall on and from scaffolding**

☑4ᵗʰ **W13 Fall from, out of or through building or structure**

    ☑x7ᵗʰ **W13.0** Fall from, out of or through balcony
        Fall from, out of or through railing

    ☑x7ᵗʰ **W13.1** Fall from, out of or through bridge

    ☑x7ᵗʰ **W13.2** Fall from, out of or through roof

    ☑x7ᵗʰ **W13.3** Fall through floor

    ☑x7ᵗʰ **W13.4** Fall from, out of or through window
        EXCLUDES 2 *fall with subsequent striking against sharp glass (W01.110)*

    ☑x7ᵗʰ **W13.8** Fall from, out of or through other building or structure
        Fall from, out of or through viaduct
        Fall from, out of or through wall
        Fall from, out of or through flag-pole

    ☑x7ᵗʰ **W13.9** Fall from, out of or through building, not otherwise specified   ▽
        EXCLUDES 1 *collapse of a building or structure (W20.-)*
                  fall or jump from burning building or structure (X00.-)

☑x7ᵗʰ **W14 Fall from tree**

☑x7ᵗʰ **W15 Fall from cliff**

☑4ᵗʰ **W16 Fall, jump or diving into water**
    EXCLUDES 1 *accidental non-watercraft drowning and submersion not involving fall (W65-W74)*
                  effects of air pressure from diving (W94.-)
                  fall into water from watercraft (V90-V94)
                  hitting an object or against bottom when falling from watercraft (V94.0)
    EXCLUDES 2 *striking or hitting diving board (W21.4)*

    ☑5ᵗʰ **W16.0** Fall into swimming pool
        Fall into swimming pool NOS
        EXCLUDES 1 *fall into empty swimming pool (W17.3)*

       ☑6ᵗʰ **W16.01** Fall into swimming pool striking water surface

          ☑7ᵗʰ **W16.011** Fall into swimming pool striking water surface causing drowning and submersion
               EXCLUDES 1 *drowning and submersion while in swimming pool without fall (W67)*

          ☑7ᵗʰ **W16.012** Fall into swimming pool striking water surface causing other injury

       ☑6ᵗʰ **W16.02** Fall into swimming pool striking bottom

          ☑7ᵗʰ **W16.021** Fall into swimming pool striking bottom causing drowning and submersion
               EXCLUDES 1 *drowning and submersion while in swimming pool without fall (W67)*

          ☑7ᵗʰ **W16.022** Fall into swimming pool striking bottom causing other injury

       ☑6ᵗʰ **W16.03** Fall into swimming pool striking wall

          ☑7ᵗʰ **W16.031** Fall into swimming pool striking wall causing drowning and submersion
               EXCLUDES 1 *drowning and submersion while in swimming pool without fall (W67)*

          ☑7ᵗʰ **W16.032** Fall into swimming pool striking wall causing other injury

    ☑5ᵗʰ **W16.1** Fall into natural body of water
        Fall into lake   Fall into river
        Fall into open sea   Fall into stream

       ☑6ᵗʰ **W16.11** Fall into natural body of water striking water surface

          ☑7ᵗʰ **W16.111** Fall into natural body of water striking water surface causing drowning and submersion
               EXCLUDES 1 *drowning and submersion while in natural body of water without fall (W69)*

          ☑7ᵗʰ **W16.112** Fall into natural body of water striking water surface causing other injury

       ☑6ᵗʰ **W16.12** Fall into natural body of water striking bottom

          ☑7ᵗʰ **W16.121** Fall into natural body of water striking bottom causing drowning and submersion
               EXCLUDES 1 *drowning and submersion while in natural body of water without fall (W69)*

          ☑7ᵗʰ **W16.122** Fall into natural body of water striking bottom causing other injury

       ☑6ᵗʰ **W16.13** Fall into natural body of water striking side

          ☑7ᵗʰ **W16.131** Fall into natural body of water striking side causing drowning and submersion
               EXCLUDES 1 *drowning and submersion while in natural body of water without fall (W69)*

          ☑7ᵗʰ **W16.132** Fall into natural body of water striking side causing other injury

    ☑5ᵗʰ **W16.2** Fall in (into) filled bathtub or bucket of water

       ☑6ᵗʰ **W16.21** Fall in (into) filled bathtub
          EXCLUDES 1 *fall into empty bathtub (W18.2)*

          ☑7ᵗʰ **W16.211** Fall in (into) filled bathtub causing drowning and submersion
               EXCLUDES 1 *drowning and submersion while in filled bathtub without fall (W65)*

          ☑7ᵗʰ **W16.212** Fall in (into) filled bathtub causing other injury

       ☑6ᵗʰ **W16.22** Fall in (into) bucket of water

          ☑7ᵗʰ **W16.221** Fall in (into) bucket of water causing drowning and submersion

          ☑7ᵗʰ **W16.222** Fall in (into) bucket of water causing other injury

    ☑5ᵗʰ **W16.3** Fall into other water
        Fall into fountain
        Fall into reservoir

       ☑6ᵗʰ **W16.31** Fall into other water striking water surface

          ☑7ᵗʰ **W16.311** Fall into other water striking water surface causing drowning and submersion
               EXCLUDES 1 *drowning and submersion while in other water without fall (W73)*

          ☑7ᵗʰ **W16.312** Fall into other water striking water surface causing other injury

       ☑6ᵗʰ **W16.32** Fall into other water striking bottom

          ☑7ᵗʰ **W16.321** Fall into other water striking bottom causing drowning and submersion
               EXCLUDES 1 *drowning and submersion while in other water without fall (W73)*

          ☑7ᵗʰ **W16.322** Fall into other water striking bottom causing other injury

       ☑6ᵗʰ **W16.33** Fall into other water striking wall

          ☑7ᵗʰ **W16.331** Fall into other water striking wall causing drowning and submersion
               EXCLUDES 1 *drowning and submersion while in other water without fall (W73)*

          ☑7ᵗʰ **W16.332** Fall into other water striking wall causing other injury

    ☑5ᵗʰ **W16.4** Fall into unspecified water

       ☑x7ᵗʰ **W16.41** Fall into unspecified water causing drowning and submersion   ▽

       ☑x7ᵗʰ **W16.42** Fall into unspecified water causing other injury   ▽

    ☑5ᵗʰ **W16.5** Jumping or diving into swimming pool

       ☑6ᵗʰ **W16.51** Jumping or diving into swimming pool striking water surface

          ☑7ᵗʰ **W16.511** Jumping or diving into swimming pool striking water surface causing drowning and submersion
               EXCLUDES 1 *drowning and submersion while in swimming pool without jumping or diving (W67)*

          ☑7ᵗʰ **W16.512** Jumping or diving into swimming pool striking water surface causing other injury

---

☑ Additional Character Req   ☑x7ᵗʰ Placeholder Alert   Manifestation   HCC CMS-HCC Condition   ▽ Unspecified Code   ▶◀ Revised Text   ● New Code   ▲ Revised Code Title

ICD-10-CM 2018   1145

✓6ᵗʰ **W16.52 Jumping or diving into swimming pool striking bottom**

✓7ᵗʰ **W16.521 Jumping or diving into swimming pool striking bottom causing drowning and submersion**
     EXCLUDES 1 *drowning and submersion while in swimming pool without jumping or diving (W67)*

✓7ᵗʰ **W16.522 Jumping or diving into swimming pool striking bottom causing other injury**

✓6ᵗʰ **W16.53 Jumping or diving into swimming pool striking wall**

✓7ᵗʰ **W16.531 Jumping or diving into swimming pool striking wall causing drowning and submersion**
     EXCLUDES 1 *drowning and submersion while in swimming pool without jumping or diving (W67)*

✓7ᵗʰ **W16.532 Jumping or diving into swimming pool striking wall causing other injury**

✓5ᵗʰ **W16.6 Jumping or diving into natural body of water**
Jumping or diving into lake
Jumping or diving into open sea
Jumping or diving into river
Jumping or diving into stream

✓6ᵗʰ **W16.61 Jumping or diving into natural body of water striking water surface**

✓7ᵗʰ **W16.611 Jumping or diving into natural body of water striking water surface causing drowning and submersion**
     EXCLUDES 1 *drowning and submersion while in natural body of water without jumping or diving (W69)*

✓7ᵗʰ **W16.612 Jumping or diving into natural body of water striking water surface causing other injury**

✓6ᵗʰ **W16.62 Jumping or diving into natural body of water striking bottom**

✓7ᵗʰ **W16.621 Jumping or diving into natural body of water striking bottom causing drowning and submersion**
     EXCLUDES 1 *drowning and submersion while in natural body of water without jumping or diving (W69)*

✓7ᵗʰ **W16.622 Jumping or diving into natural body of water striking bottom causing other injury**

✓5ᵗʰ **W16.7 Jumping or diving from boat**
     EXCLUDES 1 *fall from boat into water—see watercraft accident (V90-V94)*

✓6ᵗʰ **W16.71 Jumping or diving from boat striking water surface**

✓7ᵗʰ **W16.711 Jumping or diving from boat striking water surface causing drowning and submersion**

✓7ᵗʰ **W16.712 Jumping or diving from boat striking water surface causing other injury**

✓6ᵗʰ **W16.72 Jumping or diving from boat striking bottom**

✓7ᵗʰ **W16.721 Jumping or diving from boat striking bottom causing drowning and submersion**

✓7ᵗʰ **W16.722 Jumping or diving from boat striking bottom causing other injury**

✓5ᵗʰ **W16.8 Jumping or diving into other water**
Jumping or diving into fountain
Jumping or diving into reservoir

✓6ᵗʰ **W16.81 Jumping or diving into other water striking water surface**

✓7ᵗʰ **W16.811 Jumping or diving into other water striking water surface causing drowning and submersion**
     EXCLUDES 1 *drowning and submersion while in other water without jumping or diving (W73)*

✓7ᵗʰ **W16.812 Jumping or diving into other water striking water surface causing other injury**

✓6ᵗʰ **W16.82 Jumping or diving into other water striking bottom**

✓7ᵗʰ **W16.821 Jumping or diving into other water striking bottom causing drowning and submersion**
     EXCLUDES 1 *drowning and submersion while in other water without jumping or diving (W73)*

✓7ᵗʰ **W16.822 Jumping or diving into other water striking bottom causing other injury**

✓6ᵗʰ **W16.83 Jumping or diving into other water striking wall**

✓7ᵗʰ **W16.831 Jumping or diving into other water striking wall causing drowning and submersion**
     EXCLUDES 1 *drowning and submersion while in other water without jumping or diving (W73)*

✓7ᵗʰ **W16.832 Jumping or diving into other water striking wall causing other injury**

✓5ᵗʰ **W16.9 Jumping or diving into unspecified water**

✓x7ᵗʰ **W16.91 Jumping or diving into unspecified water causing drowning and submersion** ▽

✓x7ᵗʰ **W16.92 Jumping or diving into unspecified water causing other injury** ▽

✓4ᵗʰ **W17 Other fall from one level to another**

✓x7ᵗʰ **W17.0 Fall into well**

✓x7ᵗʰ **W17.1 Fall into storm drain or manhole**

✓x7ᵗʰ **W17.2 Fall into hole**
Fall into pit

✓x7ᵗʰ **W17.3 Fall into empty swimming pool**
     EXCLUDES 1 *fall into filled swimming pool (W16.0-)*

✓x7ᵗʰ **W17.4 Fall from dock**

✓5ᵗʰ **W17.8 Other fall from one level to another**

✓x7ᵗʰ **W17.81 Fall down embankment (hill)**

✓x7ᵗʰ **W17.82 Fall from (out of) grocery cart**
Fall due to grocery cart tipping over

✓x7ᵗʰ **W17.89 Other fall from one level to another**
Fall from cherry picker
Fall from lifting device
Fall from mobile elevated work platform [MEWP]
Fall from sky lift
AHA: 2015, 2Q, 6

✓4ᵗʰ **W18 Other slipping, tripping and stumbling and falls**

✓5ᵗʰ **W18.0 Fall due to bumping against object**
Striking against object with subsequent fall
     EXCLUDES 1 *fall on same level due to slipping, tripping, or stumbling with subsequent striking against object (W01.1-)*

✓x7ᵗʰ **W18.00 Striking against unspecified object with subsequent fall** ▽

✓x7ᵗʰ **W18.01 Striking against sports equipment with subsequent fall**

✓x7ᵗʰ **W18.02 Striking against glass with subsequent fall**

✓x7ᵗʰ **W18.09 Striking against other object with subsequent fall**

✓5ᵗʰ **W18.1 Fall from or off toilet**

✓x7ᵗʰ **W18.11 Fall from or off toilet without subsequent striking against object**
Fall from (off) toilet NOS

✓x7ᵗʰ **W18.12 Fall from or off toilet with subsequent striking against object**

✓x7ᵗʰ **W18.2 Fall in (into) shower or empty bathtub**
     EXCLUDES 1 *fall in full bathtub causing drowning or submersion (W16.21-)*

✓5ᵗʰ **W18.3 Other and unspecified fall on same level**

✓x7ᵗʰ **W18.30 Fall on same level, unspecified** ▽

✓x7ᵗʰ **W18.31 Fall on same level due to stepping on an object**
Fall on same level due to stepping on an animal
     EXCLUDES 1 *slipping, tripping and stumbling without fall due to stepping on animal (W18.41)*

✓x7ᵗʰ **W18.39 Other fall on same level**

✓5ᵗʰ **W18.4 Slipping, tripping and stumbling without falling**
     EXCLUDES 1 *collision with another person without fall (W51)*

✓x7ᵗʰ **W18.40 Slipping, tripping and stumbling without falling, unspecified** ▽

EXCLUDES 1 Not coded here   **EXCLUDES 2** Not included here   **N** Newborn Age: 0   **P** Pediatric Age: 0-17   **M** Maternity Age: 12-55   **A** Adult Age: 15-124

☑x7ᵗʰ **W18.41** **Slipping, tripping and stumbling without falling due to stepping on object**
> Slipping, tripping and stumbling without falling due to stepping on animal
> **EXCLUDES 1** *slipping, tripping and stumbling with fall due to stepping on animal (W18.31)*

☑x7ᵗʰ **W18.42** **Slipping, tripping and stumbling without falling due to stepping into hole or opening**

☑x7ᵗʰ **W18.43** **Slipping, tripping and stumbling without falling due to stepping from one level to another**

☑x7ᵗʰ **W18.49** **Other slipping, tripping and stumbling without falling**

☑x7ᵗʰ **W19 Unspecified fall** ▽
> Accidental fall NOS
> **AHA:** 2012, 4Q, 95

Exposure to inanimate mechanical forces (W20-W49)

EXCLUDES 1 *assault (X92-Y09)*
> *contact or collision with animals or persons (W50-W64)*
> *exposure to inanimate mechanical forces involving military or war operations (Y36.-, Y37.-)*
> *intentional self-harm (X71-X83)*

> The appropriate 7th character is to be added to each code from categories W20-W49.
> A   initial encounter
> D   subsequent encounter
> S   sequela

☑4ᵗʰ **W20** **Struck by thrown, projected or falling object**
> Code first any associated:
> cataclysm (X34-X39)
> lightning strike (T75.00)
> **EXCLUDES 1** *falling object in machinery accident (W24, W28-W31)*
> *falling object in transport accident (V01-V99)*
> *object set in motion by explosion (W35-W40)*
> *object set in motion by firearm (W32-W34)*
> *struck by thrown sports equipment (W21.-)*

☑x7ᵗʰ **W20.0** **Struck by falling object in cave-in**
> **EXCLUDES 2** *asphyxiation due to cave-in (T71.21)*

☑x7ᵗʰ **W20.1** **Struck by object due to collapse of building**
> **EXCLUDES 1** *struck by object due to collapse of burning building (X00.2, X02.2)*

☑x7ᵗʰ **W20.8** **Other cause of strike by thrown, projected or falling object**
> **EXCLUDES 1** *struck by thrown sports equipment (W21.-)*

☑4ᵗʰ **W21** **Striking against or struck by sports equipment**
> **EXCLUDES 1** *assault with sports equipment (Y08.0-)*
> *striking against or struck by sports equipment with subsequent fall (W18.01)*

☑5ᵗʰ **W21.0** **Struck by hit or thrown ball**
   ☑x7ᵗʰ **W21.00** **Struck by hit or thrown ball, unspecified type** ▽
   ☑x7ᵗʰ **W21.01** **Struck by football**
   ☑x7ᵗʰ **W21.02** **Struck by soccer ball**
   ☑x7ᵗʰ **W21.03** **Struck by baseball**
   ☑x7ᵗʰ **W21.04** **Struck by golf ball**
   ☑x7ᵗʰ **W21.05** **Struck by basketball**
   ☑x7ᵗʰ **W21.06** **Struck by volleyball**
   ☑x7ᵗʰ **W21.07** **Struck by softball**
   ☑x7ᵗʰ **W21.09** **Struck by other hit or thrown ball**

☑5ᵗʰ **W21.1** **Struck by bat, racquet or club**
   ☑x7ᵗʰ **W21.11** **Struck by baseball bat**
   ☑x7ᵗʰ **W21.12** **Struck by tennis racquet**
   ☑x7ᵗʰ **W21.13** **Struck by golf club**
   ☑x7ᵗʰ **W21.19** **Struck by other bat, racquet or club**

☑5ᵗʰ **W21.2** **Struck by hockey stick or puck**
   ☑6ᵗʰ **W21.21** **Struck by hockey stick**
     ☑7ᵗʰ **W21.210** **Struck by ice hockey stick**
     ☑7ᵗʰ **W21.211** **Struck by field hockey stick**
   ☑6ᵗʰ **W21.22** **Struck by hockey puck**
     ☑7ᵗʰ **W21.220** **Struck by ice hockey puck**
     ☑7ᵗʰ **W21.221** **Struck by field hockey puck**

☑5ᵗʰ **W21.3** **Struck by sports foot wear**
   ☑x7ᵗʰ **W21.31** **Struck by shoe cleats**
> Stepped on by shoe cleats

☑x7ᵗʰ **W21.32** **Struck by skate blades**
> Skated over by skate blades

☑x7ᵗʰ **W21.39** **Struck by other sports foot wear**

☑x7ᵗʰ **W21.4** **Striking against diving board**
> Use additional code for subsequent falling into water, if applicable (W16.-)

☑5ᵗʰ **W21.8** **Striking against or struck by other sports equipment**
   ☑x7ᵗʰ **W21.81** **Striking against or struck by football helmet**
   ☑x7ᵗʰ **W21.89** **Striking against or struck by other sports equipment**

☑x7ᵗʰ **W21.9** **Striking against or struck by unspecified sports equipment** ▽

☑4ᵗʰ **W22** **Striking against or struck by other objects**
> **EXCLUDES 1** *striking against or struck by object with subsequent fall (W18.09)*

☑5ᵗʰ **W22.0** **Striking against stationary object**
> **EXCLUDES 1** *striking against stationary sports equipment (W21.8)*

   ☑x7ᵗʰ **W22.01** **Walked into wall**
   ☑x7ᵗʰ **W22.02** **Walked into lamppost**
   ☑x7ᵗʰ **W22.03** **Walked into furniture**
   ☑6ᵗʰ **W22.04** **Striking against wall of swimming pool**
     ☑7ᵗʰ **W22.041** **Striking against wall of swimming pool causing drowning and submersion**
> **EXCLUDES 1** *drowning and submersion while swimming without striking against wall (W67)*
     ☑7ᵗʰ **W22.042** **Striking against wall of swimming pool causing other injury**
   ☑x7ᵗʰ **W22.09** **Striking against other stationary object**

☑5ᵗʰ **W22.1** **Striking against or struck by automobile airbag**
   ☑x7ᵗʰ **W22.10** **Striking against or struck by unspecified automobile airbag** ▽
   ☑x7ᵗʰ **W22.11** **Striking against or struck by driver side automobile airbag**
   ☑x7ᵗʰ **W22.12** **Striking against or struck by front passenger side automobile airbag**
   ☑x7ᵗʰ **W22.19** **Striking against or struck by other automobile airbag**

☑x7ᵗʰ **W22.8** **Striking against or struck by other objects**
> Striking against or struck by object NOS
> **EXCLUDES 1** *struck by thrown, projected or falling object (W20.-)*

☑4ᵗʰ **W23** **Caught, crushed, jammed or pinched in or between objects**
> **EXCLUDES 1** *injury caused by cutting or piercing instruments (W25-W27)*
> *injury caused by firearms malfunction (W32.1, W33.1-, W34.1-)*
> *injury caused by lifting and transmission devices (W24.-)*
> *injury caused by machinery (W28-W31)*
> *injury caused by nonpowered hand tools (W27.-)*
> *injury caused by transport vehicle being used as a means of transportation (V01-V99)*
> *injury caused by struck by thrown, projected or falling object (W20.-)*

☑x7ᵗʰ **W23.0** **Caught, crushed, jammed, or pinched between moving objects**

☑x7ᵗʰ **W23.1** **Caught, crushed, jammed, or pinched between stationary objects**

☑4ᵗʰ **W24** **Contact with lifting and transmission devices, not elsewhere classified**
> **EXCLUDES 1** *transport accidents (V01-V99)*

☑x7ᵗʰ **W24.0** **Contact with lifting devices, not elsewhere classified**
> Contact with chain hoist
> Contact with drive belt
> Contact with pulley (block)

☑x7ᵗʰ **W24.1** **Contact with transmission devices, not elsewhere classified**
> Contact with transmission belt or cable

☑x7ᵗʰ **W25 Contact with sharp glass**
> Code first any associated:
> injury due to flying glass from explosion or firearm discharge (W32-W40)
> transport accident (V00-V99)
> **EXCLUDES 1** *fall on same level due to slipping, tripping and stumbling with subsequent striking against sharp glass (W01.10)*
> *striking against sharp glass with subsequent fall (W18.02)*
> **EXCLUDES 2** *glass embedded in skin (W45)*

☑ Additional Character Req   ☑x7ᵗʰ Placeholder Alert   Manifestation   **HCC** CMS-HCC Condition   ▽ Unspecified Code   ►◄ Revised Text   ● New Code   ▲ Revised Code Title

✓4ᵗʰ **W26 Contact with other sharp objects**
> EXCLUDES 2   *sharp object(s) embedded in skin (W45)*

✓ₓ7ᵗʰ **W26.0 Contact with knife**
> EXCLUDES 1   *contact with electric knife (W29.1)*

✓ₓ7ᵗʰ **W26.1 Contact with sword or dagger**

✓ₓ7ᵗʰ **W26.2 Contact with edge of stiff paper**
> Paper cut

✓ₓ7ᵗʰ **W26.8 Contact with other sharp object(s), not elsewhere classified**
> Contact with tin can lid

✓ₓ7ᵗʰ **W26.9 Contact with unspecified sharp object(s)**   ▽

✓4ᵗʰ **W27 Contact with nonpowered hand tool**

✓ₓ7ᵗʰ **W27.0 Contact with workbench tool**
> Contact with auger
> Contact with axe
> Contact with chisel
> Contact with handsaw
> Contact with screwdriver

✓ₓ7ᵗʰ **W27.1 Contact with garden tool**
> Contact with hoe
> Contact with nonpowered lawn mower
> Contact with pitchfork
> Contact with rake

✓ₓ7ᵗʰ **W27.2 Contact with scissors**

✓ₓ7ᵗʰ **W27.3 Contact with needle (sewing)**
> EXCLUDES 1   *contact with hypodermic needle (W46.-)*

✓ₓ7ᵗʰ **W27.4 Contact with kitchen utensil**
> Contact with fork
> Contact with ice-pick
> Contact with can-opener NOS

✓ₓ7ᵗʰ **W27.5 Contact with paper-cutter**

✓ₓ7ᵗʰ **W27.8 Contact with other nonpowered hand tool**
> Contact with nonpowered sewing machine
> Contact with shovel

✓ₓ7ᵗʰ **W28 Contact with powered lawn mower**
> Powered lawn mower (commercial) (residential)
> EXCLUDES 1   *contact with nonpowered lawn mower (W27.1)*
> EXCLUDES 2   *exposure to electric current (W86.-)*

✓4ᵗʰ **W29 Contact with other powered hand tools and household machinery**
> EXCLUDES 1   *contact with commercial machinery (W31.82)*
>   *contact with hot household appliance (X15)*
>   *contact with nonpowered hand tool (W27.-)*
>   *exposure to electric current (W86)*

✓ₓ7ᵗʰ **W29.0 Contact with powered kitchen appliance**
> Contact with blender
> Contact with can-opener
> Contact with garbage disposal
> Contact with mixer

✓ₓ7ᵗʰ **W29.1 Contact with electric knife**

✓ₓ7ᵗʰ **W29.2 Contact with other powered household machinery**
> Contact with electric fan
> Contact with powered dryer (clothes) (powered) (spin)
> Contact with washing-machine
> Contact with sewing machine

✓ₓ7ᵗʰ **W29.3 Contact with powered garden and outdoor hand tools and machinery**
> Contact with chainsaw
> Contact with edger
> Contact with garden cultivator (tiller)
> Contact with hedge trimmer
> Contact with other powered garden tool
> EXCLUDES 1   *contact with powered lawn mower (W28)*

✓ₓ7ᵗʰ **W29.4 Contact with nail gun**

▲ ✓ₓ7ᵗʰ **W29.8 Contact with other powered hand tools and household machinery**
> Contact with do-it-yourself tool NOS

✓4ᵗʰ **W30 Contact with agricultural machinery**
> INCLUDES   animal-powered farm machine
> EXCLUDES 1   *agricultural transport vehicle accident (V01-V99)*
>   *explosion of grain store (W40.8)*
>   *exposure to electric current (W86.-)*

✓ₓ7ᵗʰ **W30.0 Contact with combine harvester**
> Contact with reaper
> Contact with thresher

✓ₓ7ᵗʰ **W30.1 Contact with power take-off devices (PTO)**

✓ₓ7ᵗʰ **W30.2 Contact with hay derrick**

✓ₓ7ᵗʰ **W30.3 Contact with grain storage elevator**
> EXCLUDES 1   *explosion of grain store (W40.8)*

✓5ᵗʰ **W30.8 Contact with other specified agricultural machinery**

✓ₓ7ᵗʰ **W30.81 Contact with agricultural transport vehicle in stationary use**
> Contact with agricultural transport vehicle under repair, not on public roadway
> EXCLUDES 1   *agricultural transport vehicle accident (V01-V99)*

✓ₓ7ᵗʰ **W30.89 Contact with other specified agricultural machinery**

✓ₓ7ᵗʰ **W30.9 Contact with unspecified agricultural machinery**   ▽
> Contact with farm machinery NOS

✓4ᵗʰ **W31 Contact with other and unspecified machinery**
> EXCLUDES 1   *contact with agricultural machinery (W30.-)*
>   *contact with machinery in transport under own power or being towed by a vehicle (V01-V99)*
>   *exposure to electric current (W86)*

✓ₓ7ᵗʰ **W31.0 Contact with mining and earth-drilling machinery**
> Contact with bore or drill (land) (seabed)
> Contact with shaft hoist
> Contact with shaft lift
> Contact with undercutter

✓ₓ7ᵗʰ **W31.1 Contact with metalworking machines**
> Contact with abrasive wheel
> Contact with forging machine
> Contact with lathe
> Contact with mechanical shears
> Contact with metal drilling machine
> Contact with milling machine
> Contact with power press
> Contact with rolling-mill
> Contact with metal sawing machine

✓ₓ7ᵗʰ **W31.2 Contact with powered woodworking and forming machines**
> Contact with band saw
> Contact with bench saw
> Contact with circular saw
> Contact with molding machine
> Contact with overhead plane
> Contact with powered saw
> Contact with radial saw
> Contact with sander
> EXCLUDES 1   *nonpowered woodworking tools (W27.0)*

✓ₓ7ᵗʰ **W31.3 Contact with prime movers**
> Contact with gas turbine
> Contact with internal combustion engine
> Contact with steam engine
> Contact with water driven turbine

✓5ᵗʰ **W31.8 Contact with other specified machinery**

✓ₓ7ᵗʰ **W31.81 Contact with recreational machinery**
> Contact with roller coaster

✓ₓ7ᵗʰ **W31.82 Contact with other commercial machinery**
> Contact with commercial electric fan
> Contact with commercial kitchen appliances
> Contact with commercial powered dryer (clothes) (powered) (spin)
> Contact with commercial washing-machine
> Contact with commercial sewing machine
> EXCLUDES 1   *contact with household machinery (W29.-)*
>   *contact with powered lawn mower (W28)*

✓ₓ7ᵗʰ **W31.83 Contact with special construction vehicle in stationary use**
> Contact with special construction vehicle under repair, not on public roadway
> EXCLUDES 1   *special construction vehicle accident (V01-V99)*

✓ₓ7ᵗʰ **W31.89 Contact with other specified machinery**

✓ₓ7ᵗʰ **W31.9 Contact with unspecified machinery**   ▽
> Contact with machinery NOS

EXCLUDES 1 Not coded here   EXCLUDES 2 Not included here   **N** Newborn Age: 0   **P** Pediatric Age: 0-17   **M** Maternity Age: 12-55   **A** Adult Age: 15-124

☑4ᵗʰ W32 Accidental handgun discharge and malfunction

INCLUDES   accidental discharge and malfunction of gun for single hand use
accidental discharge and malfunction of pistol
accidental discharge and malfunction of revolver
handgun discharge and malfunction NOS

EXCLUDES 1   *accidental airgun discharge and malfunction (W34.010, W34.110)*
accidental BB gun discharge and malfunction (W34.010, W34.110)
accidental pellet gun discharge and malfunction (W34.010, W34.110)
accidental shotgun discharge and malfunction (W33.01, W33.11)
assault by handgun discharge (X93)
handgun discharge involving legal intervention (Y35.0-)
handgun discharge involving military or war operations (Y36.4-)
intentional self-harm by handgun discharge (X72)
Very pistol discharge and malfunction (W34.09, W34.19)

☑x7ᵗʰ **W32.0 Accidental handgun discharge**

☑x7ᵗʰ **W32.1 Accidental handgun malfunction**
Injury due to explosion of handgun (parts)
Injury due to malfunction of mechanism or component of handgun
Injury due to recoil of handgun
Powder burn from handgun

☑4ᵗʰ W33 Accidental rifle, shotgun and larger firearm discharge and malfunction

INCLUDES   rifle, shotgun and larger firearm discharge and malfunction NOS

EXCLUDES 1   *accidental airgun discharge and malfunction (W34.010, W34.110)*
accidental BB gun discharge and malfunction (W34.010, W34.110)
accidental handgun discharge and malfunction (W32.-)
accidental pellet gun discharge and malfunction (W34.010, W34.110)
assault by rifle, shotgun and larger firearm discharge (X94)
firearm discharge involving legal intervention (Y35.0-)
firearm discharge involving military or war operations (Y36.4-)
intentional self-harm by rifle, shotgun and larger firearm discharge (X73)

☑5ᵗʰ **W33.0 Accidental rifle, shotgun and larger firearm discharge**

☑x7ᵗʰ **W33.00 Accidental discharge of unspecified larger firearm** ▽
Discharge of unspecified larger firearm NOS

☑x7ᵗʰ **W33.01 Accidental discharge of shotgun**
Discharge of shotgun NOS

☑x7ᵗʰ **W33.02 Accidental discharge of hunting rifle**
Discharge of hunting rifle NOS

☑x7ᵗʰ **W33.03 Accidental discharge of machine gun**
Discharge of machine gun NOS

☑x7ᵗʰ **W33.09 Accidental discharge of other larger firearm**
Discharge of other larger firearm NOS

☑5ᵗʰ **W33.1 Accidental rifle, shotgun and larger firearm malfunction**
Injury due to explosion of rifle, shotgun and larger firearm (parts)
Injury due to malfunction of mechanism or component of rifle, shotgun and larger firearm
Injury due to piercing, cutting, crushing or pinching due to (by) slide trigger mechanism, scope or other gun part
Injury due to recoil of rifle, shotgun and larger firearm
Powder burn from rifle, shotgun and larger firearm

☑x7ᵗʰ **W33.10 Accidental malfunction of unspecified larger firearm** ▽
Malfunction of unspecified larger firearm NOS

☑x7ᵗʰ **W33.11 Accidental malfunction of shotgun**
Malfunction of shotgun NOS

☑x7ᵗʰ **W33.12 Accidental malfunction of hunting rifle**
Malfunction of hunting rifle NOS

☑x7ᵗʰ **W33.13 Accidental malfunction of machine gun**
Malfunction of machine gun NOS

☑x7ᵗʰ **W33.19 Accidental malfunction of other larger firearm**
Malfunction of other larger firearm NOS

☑4ᵗʰ W34 Accidental discharge and malfunction from other and unspecified firearms and guns

☑5ᵗʰ **W34.0 Accidental discharge from other and unspecified firearms and guns**

☑x7ᵗʰ **W34.00 Accidental discharge from unspecified firearms or gun** ▽
Discharge from firearm NOS
Gunshot wound NOS
Shot NOS

☑6ᵗʰ **W34.01 Accidental discharge of gas, air or spring-operated guns**

☑7ᵗʰ **W34.010 Accidental discharge of airgun**
Accidental discharge of BB gun
Accidental discharge of pellet gun

☑7ᵗʰ **W34.011 Accidental discharge of paintball gun**
Accidental injury due to paintball discharge

☑7ᵗʰ **W34.018 Accidental discharge of other gas, air or spring-operated gun**

☑x7ᵗʰ **W34.09 Accidental discharge from other specified firearms**
Accidental discharge from Very pistol [flare]

☑5ᵗʰ **W34.1 Accidental malfunction from other and unspecified firearms and guns**

☑x7ᵗʰ **W34.10 Accidental malfunction from unspecified firearms or gun** ▽
Firearm malfunction NOS

☑6ᵗʰ **W34.11 Accidental malfunction of gas, air or spring-operated guns**

☑7ᵗʰ **W34.110 Accidental malfunction of airgun**
Accidental malfunction of BB gun
Accidental malfunction of pellet gun

☑7ᵗʰ **W34.111 Accidental malfunction of paintball gun**
Accidental injury due to paintball gun malfunction

☑7ᵗʰ **W34.118 Accidental malfunction of other gas, air or spring-operated gun**

☑x7ᵗʰ **W34.19 Accidental malfunction from other specified firearms**
Accidental malfunction from Very pistol [flare]

☑x7ᵗʰ **W35 Explosion and rupture of boiler**
EXCLUDES 1   *explosion and rupture of boiler on watercraft (V93.4)*

☑4ᵗʰ W36 Explosion and rupture of gas cylinder

☑x7ᵗʰ **W36.1 Explosion and rupture of aerosol can**

☑x7ᵗʰ **W36.2 Explosion and rupture of air tank**

☑x7ᵗʰ **W36.3 Explosion and rupture of pressurized-gas tank**

☑x7ᵗʰ **W36.8 Explosion and rupture of other gas cylinder**

☑x7ᵗʰ **W36.9 Explosion and rupture of unspecified gas cylinder** ▽

☑4ᵗʰ W37 Explosion and rupture of pressurized tire, pipe or hose

☑x7ᵗʰ **W37.0 Explosion of bicycle tire**

☑x7ᵗʰ **W37.8 Explosion and rupture of other pressurized tire, pipe or hose**

☑x7ᵗʰ **W38 Explosion and rupture of other specified pressurized devices**

☑x7ᵗʰ **W39 Discharge of firework**

☑4ᵗʰ W40 Explosion of other materials
EXCLUDES 1   *assault by explosive material (X96)*
explosion involving legal intervention (Y35.1-)
explosion involving military or war operations (Y36.0-, Y36.2-)
intentional self-harm by explosive material (X75)

☑x7ᵗʰ **W40.0 Explosion of blasting material**
Explosion of blasting cap
Explosion of detonator
Explosion of dynamite
Explosion of explosive (any) used in blasting operations

☑x7ᵗʰ **W40.1 Explosion of explosive gases**
Explosion of acetylene
Explosion of butane
Explosion of coal gas
Explosion in mine NOS
Explosion of explosive gas
Explosion of fire damp
Explosion of gasoline fumes
Explosion of methane
Explosion of propane

☑ Additional Character Req   ☑x7ᵗʰ Placeholder Alert   Manifestation   HCC CMS-HCC Condition   ▽ Unspecified Code   ▶◀ Revised Text   ● New Code   ▲ Revised Code Title

ICD-10-CM 2018   1149

✓x7ᵗʰ **W40.8 Explosion of other specified explosive materials**
Explosion in dump NOS
Explosion in factory NOS
Explosion in grain store
Explosion in munitions
> EXCLUDES 1   *explosion involving legal intervention (Y35.1-)*
> *explosion involving military or war operations (Y36.0-, Y36.2-)*

✓x7ᵗʰ **W40.9 Explosion of unspecified explosive materials** ▽
Explosion NOS

✓4ᵗʰ **W42 Exposure to noise**

✓x7ᵗʰ **W42.0 Exposure to supersonic waves**

✓x7ᵗʰ **W42.9 Exposure to other noise**
Exposure to sound waves NOS

✓4ᵗʰ **W45 Foreign body or object entering through skin**
> INCLUDES   foreign body or object embedded in skin
> nail embedded in skin
> EXCLUDES 2   *contact with hand tools (nonpowered) (powered) (W27-W29)*
> *contact with other sharp object(s) (W26.-)*
> *contact with sharp glass (W25.-)*
> *struck by objects (W20-W22)*

✓x7ᵗʰ **W45.0 Nail entering through skin**

✓x7ᵗʰ **W45.8 Other foreign body or object entering through skin**
Splinter in skin NOS

✓4ᵗʰ **W46 Contact with hypodermic needle**

✓x7ᵗʰ **W46.0 Contact with hypodermic needle**
Hypodermic needle stick NOS

✓x7ᵗʰ **W46.1 Contact with contaminated hypodermic needle**

✓4ᵗʰ **W49 Exposure to other inanimate mechanical forces**
> INCLUDES   exposure to abnormal gravitational [G] forces
> exposure to inanimate mechanical forces NEC
> EXCLUDES 1   *exposure to inanimate mechanical forces involving military or war operations (Y36.-, Y37.-)*

✓5ᵗʰ **W49.0 Item causing external constriction**

✓x7ᵗʰ **W49.01 Hair causing external constriction**

✓x7ᵗʰ **W49.02 String or thread causing external constriction**

✓x7ᵗʰ **W49.03 Rubber band causing external constriction**

✓x7ᵗʰ **W49.04 Ring or other jewelry causing external constriction**

✓x7ᵗʰ **W49.09 Other specified item causing external constriction**

✓x7ᵗʰ **W49.9 Exposure to other inanimate mechanical forces**

Exposure to animate mechanical forces (W50-W64)

> EXCLUDES 1   *Toxic effect of contact with venomous animals and plants (T63.-)*

The appropriate 7th character is to be added to each code from categories W50-W64.
A   initial encounter
D   subsequent encounter
S   sequela

✓4ᵗʰ **W50 Accidental hit, strike, kick, twist, bite or scratch by another person**
> INCLUDES   hit, strike, kick, twist, bite, or scratch by another person NOS
> EXCLUDES 1   *assault by bodily force (Y04)*
> *struck by objects (W20-W22)*

✓x7ᵗʰ **W50.0 Accidental hit or strike by another person**
Hit or strike by another person NOS

✓x7ᵗʰ **W50.1 Accidental kick by another person**
Kick by another person NOS

✓x7ᵗʰ **W50.2 Accidental twist by another person**
Twist by another person NOS

✓x7ᵗʰ **W50.3 Accidental bite by another person**
Human bite
Bite by another person NOS

✓x7ᵗʰ **W50.4 Accidental scratch by another person**
Scratch by another person NOS

✓x7ᵗʰ **W51 Accidental striking against or bumped into by another person**
> EXCLUDES 1   *assault by striking against or bumping into by another person (Y04.2)*
> *fall due to collision with another person (W03)*

✓x7ᵗʰ **W52 Crushed, pushed or stepped on by crowd or human stampede**
Crushed, pushed or stepped on by crowd or human stampede with or without fall

✓4ᵗʰ **W53 Contact with rodent**
> INCLUDES   contact with saliva, feces or urine of rodent

✓5ᵗʰ **W53.0 Contact with mouse**

✓x7ᵗʰ **W53.01 Bitten by mouse**

✓x7ᵗʰ **W53.09 Other contact with mouse**

✓5ᵗʰ **W53.1 Contact with rat**

✓x7ᵗʰ **W53.11 Bitten by rat**

✓x7ᵗʰ **W53.19 Other contact with rat**

✓5ᵗʰ **W53.2 Contact with squirrel**

✓x7ᵗʰ **W53.21 Bitten by squirrel**

✓x7ᵗʰ **W53.29 Other contact with squirrel**

✓5ᵗʰ **W53.8 Contact with other rodent**

✓x7ᵗʰ **W53.81 Bitten by other rodent**

✓x7ᵗʰ **W53.89 Other contact with other rodent**

✓4ᵗʰ **W54 Contact with dog**
> INCLUDES   contact with saliva, feces or urine of dog

✓x7ᵗʰ **W54.0 Bitten by dog**

✓x7ᵗʰ **W54.1 Struck by dog**
Knocked over by dog

✓x7ᵗʰ **W54.8 Other contact with dog**

✓4ᵗʰ **W55 Contact with other mammals**
> INCLUDES   contact with saliva, feces or urine of mammal
> EXCLUDES 1   *animal being ridden—see transport accidents*
> *bitten or struck by dog (W54)*
> *bitten or struck by rodent (W53.-)*
> *contact with marine mammals (W56.-)*

✓5ᵗʰ **W55.0 Contact with cat**

✓x7ᵗʰ **W55.01 Bitten by cat**

✓x7ᵗʰ **W55.03 Scratched by cat**

✓x7ᵗʰ **W55.09 Other contact with cat**

✓5ᵗʰ **W55.1 Contact with horse**

✓x7ᵗʰ **W55.11 Bitten by horse**

✓x7ᵗʰ **W55.12 Struck by horse**

✓x7ᵗʰ **W55.19 Other contact with horse**

✓5ᵗʰ **W55.2 Contact with cow**
Contact with bull

✓x7ᵗʰ **W55.21 Bitten by cow**

✓x7ᵗʰ **W55.22 Struck by cow**
Gored by bull

✓x7ᵗʰ **W55.29 Other contact with cow**

✓5ᵗʰ **W55.3 Contact with other hoof stock**
Contact with goats
Contact with sheep

✓x7ᵗʰ **W55.31 Bitten by other hoof stock**

✓x7ᵗʰ **W55.32 Struck by other hoof stock**
Gored by goat
Gored by ram

✓x7ᵗʰ **W55.39 Other contact with other hoof stock**

✓5ᵗʰ **W55.4 Contact with pig**

✓x7ᵗʰ **W55.41 Bitten by pig**

✓x7ᵗʰ **W55.42 Struck by pig**

✓x7ᵗʰ **W55.49 Other contact with pig**

✓5ᵗʰ **W55.5 Contact with raccoon**

✓x7ᵗʰ **W55.51 Bitten by raccoon**

✓x7ᵗʰ **W55.52 Struck by raccoon**

✓x7ᵗʰ **W55.59 Other contact with raccoon**

✓5ᵗʰ **W55.8 Contact with other mammals**

✓x7ᵗʰ **W55.81 Bitten by other mammals**

✓x7ᵗʰ **W55.82 Struck by other mammals**

✓x7ᵗʰ **W55.89 Other contact with other mammals**

✓4ᵗʰ **W56 Contact with nonvenomous marine animal**
> EXCLUDES 1   *contact with venomous marine animal (T63.-)*

✓5ᵗʰ **W56.0 Contact with dolphin**

✓x7ᵗʰ **W56.01 Bitten by dolphin**

✓x7ᵗʰ **W56.02 Struck by dolphin**

✓x7ᵗʰ **W56.09 Other contact with dolphin**

EXCLUDES 1 Not coded here   EXCLUDES 2 Not included here   N Newborn Age: 0   P Pediatric Age: 0-17   M Maternity Age: 12-55   A Adult Age: 15-124

1150   ICD-10-CM 2018

☑5ᵗʰ **W56.1 Contact with sea lion**
    ✓x7ᵗʰ **W56.11 Bitten by sea lion**
    ✓x7ᵗʰ **W56.12 Struck by sea lion**
    ✓x7ᵗʰ **W56.19 Other contact with sea lion**

☑5ᵗʰ **W56.2 Contact with orca**
    Contact with killer whale
    ✓x7ᵗʰ **W56.21 Bitten by orca**
    ✓x7ᵗʰ **W56.22 Struck by orca**
    ✓x7ᵗʰ **W56.29 Other contact with orca**

☑5ᵗʰ **W56.3 Contact with other marine mammals**
    ✓x7ᵗʰ **W56.31 Bitten by other marine mammals**
    ✓x7ᵗʰ **W56.32 Struck by other marine mammals**
    ✓x7ᵗʰ **W56.39 Other contact with other marine mammals**

☑5ᵗʰ **W56.4 Contact with shark**
    ✓x7ᵗʰ **W56.41 Bitten by shark**
    ✓x7ᵗʰ **W56.42 Struck by shark**
    ✓x7ᵗʰ **W56.49 Other contact with shark**

☑5ᵗʰ **W56.5 Contact with other fish**
    ✓x7ᵗʰ **W56.51 Bitten by other fish**
    ✓x7ᵗʰ **W56.52 Struck by other fish**
    ✓x7ᵗʰ **W56.59 Other contact with other fish**

☑5ᵗʰ **W56.8 Contact with other nonvenomous marine animals**
    ✓x7ᵗʰ **W56.81 Bitten by other nonvenomous marine animals**
    ✓x7ᵗʰ **W56.82 Struck by other nonvenomous marine animals**
    ✓x7ᵗʰ **W56.89 Other contact with other nonvenomous marine animals**

✓x7ᵗʰ **W57 Bitten or stung by nonvenomous insect and other nonvenomous arthropods**
    EXCLUDES 1   *contact with venomous insects and arthropods (T63.2-, T63.3-, T63.4-)*

☑4ᵗʰ **W58 Contact with crocodile or alligator**
☑5ᵗʰ **W58.0 Contact with alligator**
    ✓x7ᵗʰ **W58.01 Bitten by alligator**
    ✓x7ᵗʰ **W58.02 Struck by alligator**
    ✓x7ᵗʰ **W58.03 Crushed by alligator**
    ✓x7ᵗʰ **W58.09 Other contact with alligator**

☑5ᵗʰ **W58.1 Contact with crocodile**
    ✓x7ᵗʰ **W58.11 Bitten by crocodile**
    ✓x7ᵗʰ **W58.12 Struck by crocodile**
    ✓x7ᵗʰ **W58.13 Crushed by crocodile**
    ✓x7ᵗʰ **W58.19 Other contact with crocodile**

☑4ᵗʰ **W59 Contact with other nonvenomous reptiles**
    EXCLUDES 1   *contact with venomous reptile (T63.0-, T63.1-)*

☑5ᵗʰ **W59.0 Contact with nonvenomous lizards**
    ✓x7ᵗʰ **W59.01 Bitten by nonvenomous lizards**
    ✓x7ᵗʰ **W59.02 Struck by nonvenomous lizards**
    ✓x7ᵗʰ **W59.09 Other contact with nonvenomous lizards**
        Exposure to nonvenomous lizards

☑5ᵗʰ **W59.1 Contact with nonvenomous snakes**
    ✓x7ᵗʰ **W59.11 Bitten by nonvenomous snake**
    ✓x7ᵗʰ **W59.12 Struck by nonvenomous snake**
    ✓x7ᵗʰ **W59.13 Crushed by nonvenomous snake**
    ✓x7ᵗʰ **W59.19 Other contact with nonvenomous snake**

☑5ᵗʰ **W59.2 Contact with turtles**
    EXCLUDES 1   *contact with tortoises (W59.8-)*
    ✓x7ᵗʰ **W59.21 Bitten by turtle**
    ✓x7ᵗʰ **W59.22 Struck by turtle**
    ✓x7ᵗʰ **W59.29 Other contact with turtle**
        Exposure to turtles

☑5ᵗʰ **W59.8 Contact with other nonvenomous reptiles**
    ✓x7ᵗʰ **W59.81 Bitten by other nonvenomous reptiles**
    ✓x7ᵗʰ **W59.82 Struck by other nonvenomous reptiles**
    ✓x7ᵗʰ **W59.83 Crushed by other nonvenomous reptiles**
    ✓x7ᵗʰ **W59.89 Other contact with other nonvenomous reptiles**

✓x7ᵗʰ **W60 Contact with nonvenomous plant thorns and spines and sharp leaves**
    EXCLUDES 1   *contact with venomous plants (T63.7-)*

☑4ᵗʰ **W61 Contact with birds (domestic) (wild)**
    INCLUDES   contact with excreta of birds

☑5ᵗʰ **W61.0 Contact with parrot**
    ✓x7ᵗʰ **W61.01 Bitten by parrot**
    ✓x7ᵗʰ **W61.02 Struck by parrot**
    ✓x7ᵗʰ **W61.09 Other contact with parrot**
        Exposure to parrots

☑5ᵗʰ **W61.1 Contact with macaw**
    ✓x7ᵗʰ **W61.11 Bitten by macaw**
    ✓x7ᵗʰ **W61.12 Struck by macaw**
    ✓x7ᵗʰ **W61.19 Other contact with macaw**
        Exposure to macaws

☑5ᵗʰ **W61.2 Contact with other psittacines**
    ✓x7ᵗʰ **W61.21 Bitten by other psittacines**
    ✓x7ᵗʰ **W61.22 Struck by other psittacines**
    ✓x7ᵗʰ **W61.29 Other contact with other psittacines**
        Exposure to other psittacines

☑5ᵗʰ **W61.3 Contact with chicken**
    ✓x7ᵗʰ **W61.32 Struck by chicken**
    ✓x7ᵗʰ **W61.33 Pecked by chicken**
    ✓x7ᵗʰ **W61.39 Other contact with chicken**
        Exposure to chickens

☑5ᵗʰ **W61.4 Contact with turkey**
    ✓x7ᵗʰ **W61.42 Struck by turkey**
    ✓x7ᵗʰ **W61.43 Pecked by turkey**
    ✓x7ᵗʰ **W61.49 Other contact with turkey**

☑5ᵗʰ **W61.5 Contact with goose**
    ✓x7ᵗʰ **W61.51 Bitten by goose**
    ✓x7ᵗʰ **W61.52 Struck by goose**
    ✓x7ᵗʰ **W61.59 Other contact with goose**

☑5ᵗʰ **W61.6 Contact with duck**
    ✓x7ᵗʰ **W61.61 Bitten by duck**
    ✓x7ᵗʰ **W61.62 Struck by duck**
    ✓x7ᵗʰ **W61.69 Other contact with duck**

☑5ᵗʰ **W61.9 Contact with other birds**
    ✓x7ᵗʰ **W61.91 Bitten by other birds**
    ✓x7ᵗʰ **W61.92 Struck by other birds**
    ✓x7ᵗʰ **W61.99 Other contact with other birds**
        Contact with bird NOS

☑4ᵗʰ **W62 Contact with nonvenomous amphibians**
    EXCLUDES 1   *contact with venomous amphibians (T63.81-R63.83)*
    ✓x7ᵗʰ **W62.0 Contact with nonvenomous frogs**
    ✓x7ᵗʰ **W62.1 Contact with nonvenomous toads**
    ✓x7ᵗʰ **W62.9 Contact with other nonvenomous amphibians**

✓x7ᵗʰ **W64 Exposure to other animate mechanical forces**
    INCLUDES   exposure to nonvenomous animal NOS
    EXCLUDES 1   *contact with venomous animal (T63.-)*

Accidental non-transport drowning and submersion (W65-W74)

EXCLUDES 1   *accidental drowning and submersion due to fall into water (W16.-)*
    accidental drowning and submersion due to water transport accident (V90.-, V92.-)
EXCLUDES 2   *accidental drowning and submersion due to cataclysm (X34-X39)*

> The appropriate 7th character is to be added to each code from categories W65-W74.
> A   initial encounter
> D   subsequent encounter
> S   sequela

✓x7ᵗʰ **W65 Accidental drowning and submersion while in bath-tub**
    EXCLUDES 1   *accidental drowning and submersion due to fall in (into) bathtub (W16.211)*

✓x7ᵗʰ **W67 Accidental drowning and submersion while in swimming-pool**
    EXCLUDES 1   *accidental drowning and submersion due to fall into swimming pool (W16.011, W16.021, W16.031)*
    accidental drowning and submersion due to striking into wall of swimming pool (W22.041)

☑ Additional Character Req   ✓x7ᵗʰ Placeholder Alert   Manifestation   HCC CMS-HCC Condition   ▽Unspecified Code   ►◄ Revised Text   ● New Code   ▲ Revised Code Title

ICD-10-CM 2018   1151

√x7ᵗʰ **W69 Accidental drowning and submersion while in natural water**
Accidental drowning and submersion while in lake
Accidental drowning and submersion while in open sea
Accidental drowning and submersion while in river
Accidental drowning and submersion while in stream
EXCLUDES 1   *accidental drowning and submersion due to fall into natural body of water (W16.111, W16.121, W16.131)*

√x7ᵗʰ **W73 Other specified cause of accidental non-transport drowning and submersion**
Accidental drowning and submersion while in quenching tank
Accidental drowning and submersion while in reservoir
EXCLUDES 1   *accidental drowning and submersion due to fall into other water (W16.311, W16.321, W16.331)*

√x7ᵗʰ **W74 Unspecified cause of accidental drowning and submersion** ▽
Drowning NOS

Exposure to electric current, radiation and extreme ambient air temperature and pressure (W85-W99)

EXCLUDES 1   *exposure to:*
failure in dosage of radiation or temperature during surgical and medical care (Y63.2-Y63.5)
lightning (T75.0-)
natural cold (X31)
natural heat (X30)
natural radiation NOS (X39)
radiological procedure and radiotherapy (Y84.2)
sunlight (X32)

The appropriate 7th character is to be added to each code from categories W85-W99.
A   initial encounter
D   subsequent encounter
S   sequela

√x7ᵗʰ **W85 Exposure to electric transmission lines**
Broken power line

√4ᵗʰ **W86 Exposure to other specified electric current**

√x7ᵗʰ **W86.0 Exposure to domestic wiring and appliances**

√x7ᵗʰ **W86.1 Exposure to industrial wiring, appliances and electrical machinery**
Exposure to conductors
Exposure to control apparatus
Exposure to electrical equipment and machinery
Exposure to transformers

√x7ᵗʰ **W86.8 Exposure to other electric current**
Exposure to wiring and appliances in or on farm (not farmhouse)
Exposure to wiring and appliances outdoors
Exposure to wiring and appliances in or on public building
Exposure to wiring and appliances in or on residential institutions
Exposure to wiring and appliances in or on schools

√4ᵗʰ **W88 Exposure to ionizing radiation**
EXCLUDES 1   *exposure to sunlight (X32)*

√x7ᵗʰ **W88.0 Exposure to X-rays**

√x7ᵗʰ **W88.1 Exposure to radioactive isotopes**

√x7ᵗʰ **W88.8 Exposure to other ionizing radiation**

√4ᵗʰ **W89 Exposure to man-made visible and ultraviolet light**
INCLUDES   exposure to welding light (arc)
EXCLUDES 1   *exposure to sunlight (X32)*

√x7ᵗʰ **W89.0 Exposure to welding light (arc)**

√x7ᵗʰ **W89.1 Exposure to tanning bed**

√x7ᵗʰ **W89.8 Exposure to other man-made visible and ultraviolet light**

√x7ᵗʰ **W89.9 Exposure to unspecified man-made visible and ultraviolet light** ▽

√4ᵗʰ **W90 Exposure to other nonionizing radiation**
EXCLUDES 1   *exposure to sunlight (X32)*

√x7ᵗʰ **W90.0 Exposure to radiofrequency**

√x7ᵗʰ **W90.1 Exposure to infrared radiation**

√x7ᵗʰ **W90.2 Exposure to laser radiation**

√x7ᵗʰ **W90.8 Exposure to other nonionizing radiation**

√x7ᵗʰ **W92 Exposure to excessive heat of man-made origin**

√4ᵗʰ **W93 Exposure to excessive cold of man-made origin**

√5ᵗʰ **W93.0 Contact with or inhalation of dry ice**

√x7ᵗʰ **W93.01 Contact with dry ice**

√x7ᵗʰ **W93.02 Inhalation of dry ice**

√5ᵗʰ **W93.1 Contact with or inhalation of liquid air**

√x7ᵗʰ **W93.11 Contact with liquid air**
Contact with liquid hydrogen
Contact with liquid nitrogen

√x7ᵗʰ **W93.12 Inhalation of liquid air**
Inhalation of liquid hydrogen
Inhalation of liquid nitrogen

√x7ᵗʰ **W93.2 Prolonged exposure in deep freeze unit or refrigerator**

√x7ᵗʰ **W93.8 Exposure to other excessive cold of man-made origin**

√4ᵗʰ **W94 Exposure to high and low air pressure and changes in air pressure**

√x7ᵗʰ **W94.0 Exposure to prolonged high air pressure**

√5ᵗʰ **W94.1 Exposure to prolonged low air pressure**

√x7ᵗʰ **W94.11 Exposure to residence or prolonged visit at high altitude**

√x7ᵗʰ **W94.12 Exposure to other prolonged low air pressure**

√5ᵗʰ **W94.2 Exposure to rapid changes in air pressure during ascent**

√x7ᵗʰ **W94.21 Exposure to reduction in atmospheric pressure while surfacing from deep-water diving**

√x7ᵗʰ **W94.22 Exposure to reduction in atmospheric pressure while surfacing from underground**

√x7ᵗʰ **W94.23 Exposure to sudden change in air pressure in aircraft during ascent**

√x7ᵗʰ **W94.29 Exposure to other rapid changes in air pressure during ascent**

√5ᵗʰ **W94.3 Exposure to rapid changes in air pressure during descent**

√x7ᵗʰ **W94.31 Exposure to sudden change in air pressure in aircraft during descent**

√x7ᵗʰ **W94.32 Exposure to high air pressure from rapid descent in water**

√x7ᵗʰ **W94.39 Exposure to other rapid changes in air pressure during descent**

√x7ᵗʰ **W99 Exposure to other man-made environmental factors**

Exposure to smoke, fire and flames (X00-X08)

EXCLUDES 1   *arson (X97)*
EXCLUDES 2   *explosions (W35-W40)*
lightning (T75.0-)
transport accident (V01-V99)

The appropriate 7th character is to be added to each code from categories X00-X08.
A   initial encounter
D   subsequent encounter
S   sequela

√4ᵗʰ **X00 Exposure to uncontrolled fire in building or structure**
INCLUDES   conflagration in building or structure
Code first any associated cataclysm
EXCLUDES 2   *exposure to ignition or melting of nightwear (X05)*
exposure to ignition or melting of other clothing and apparel (X06.-)
exposure to other specified smoke, fire and flames (X08.-)
AHA: 2016, 2Q, 5

√x7ᵗʰ **X00.0 Exposure to flames in uncontrolled fire in building or structure**

√x7ᵗʰ **X00.1 Exposure to smoke in uncontrolled fire in building or structure**

√x7ᵗʰ **X00.2 Injury due to collapse of burning building or structure in uncontrolled fire**
EXCLUDES 1   *injury due to collapse of building not on fire (W20.1)*

√x7ᵗʰ **X00.3 Fall from burning building or structure in uncontrolled fire**

√x7ᵗʰ **X00.4 Hit by object from burning building or structure in uncontrolled fire**

√x7ᵗʰ **X00.5 Jump from burning building or structure in uncontrolled fire**

√x7ᵗʰ **X00.8 Other exposure to uncontrolled fire in building or structure**

√4ᵗʰ **X01 Exposure to uncontrolled fire, not in building or structure**
INCLUDES   exposure to forest fire

√x7ᵗʰ **X01.0 Exposure to flames in uncontrolled fire, not in building or structure**

√x7ᵗʰ **X01.1 Exposure to smoke in uncontrolled fire, not in building or structure**

√x7ᵗʰ **X01.3 Fall due to uncontrolled fire, not in building or structure**

EXCLUDES 1 Not coded here   EXCLUDES 2 Not included here   N Newborn Age: 0   P Pediatric Age: 0-17   M Maternity Age: 12-55   A Adult Age: 15-124

1152   ICD-10-CM 2018

√x7ᵗʰ **X01.4 Hit by object** due to uncontrolled fire, not in building or structure

√x7ᵗʰ **X01.8 Other exposure** to uncontrolled fire, not in building or structure

√4ᵗʰ **X02 Exposure to controlled fire in building or structure**
INCLUDES exposure to fire in fireplace
exposure to fire in stove

√x7ᵗʰ **X02.0 Exposure to flames** in controlled fire in building or structure

√x7ᵗʰ **X02.1 Exposure to smoke** in controlled fire in building or structure

√x7ᵗʰ **X02.2 Injury due to collapse** of burning building or structure in controlled fire
EXCLUDES 1 injury due to collapse of building not on fire (W20.1)

√x7ᵗʰ **X02.3 Fall from** burning building or structure in controlled fire

√x7ᵗʰ **X02.4 Hit by object** from burning building or structure in controlled fire

√x7ᵗʰ **X02.5 Jump from** burning building or structure in controlled fire

√x7ᵗʰ **X02.8 Other exposure** to controlled fire in building or structure

√4ᵗʰ **X03 Exposure to controlled fire, not in building or structure**
INCLUDES exposure to bon fire
exposure to camp-fire
exposure to trash fire

√x7ᵗʰ **X03.0 Exposure to flames** in controlled fire, not in building or structure

√x7ᵗʰ **X03.1 Exposure to smoke** in controlled fire, not in building or structure

√x7ᵗʰ **X03.3 Fall due to** controlled fire, not in building or structure

√x7ᵗʰ **X03.4 Hit by object** due to controlled fire, not in building or structure

√x7ᵗʰ **X03.8 Other exposure** to controlled fire, not in building or structure

√x7ᵗʰ **X04 Exposure to ignition of highly flammable material**
Exposure to ignition of gasoline
Exposure to ignition of kerosene
Exposure to ignition of petrol
EXCLUDES 2 exposure to ignition or melting of nightwear (X05)
exposure to ignition or melting of other clothing and apparel (X06)
AHA: 2016, 2Q, 4

√x7ᵗʰ **X05 Exposure to ignition or melting of nightwear**
EXCLUDES 2 exposure to uncontrolled fire in building or structure (X00.-)
exposure to uncontrolled fire, not in building or structure (X01.-)
exposure to controlled fire in building or structure (X02.-)
exposure to controlled fire, not in building or structure (X03.-)
exposure to ignition of highly flammable materials (X04.-)

√4ᵗʰ **X06 Exposure to ignition or melting of other clothing and apparel**
EXCLUDES 2 exposure to uncontrolled fire in building or structure (X00.-)
exposure to uncontrolled fire, not in building or structure (X01.-)
exposure to controlled fire in building or structure (X02.-)
exposure to controlled fire, not in building or structure (X03.-)
exposure to ignition of highly flammable materials (X04.-)

√x7ᵗʰ **X06.0 Exposure to ignition** of plastic jewelry

√x7ᵗʰ **X06.1 Exposure to melting** of plastic jewelry

√x7ᵗʰ **X06.2 Exposure to ignition** of other clothing and apparel

√x7ᵗʰ **X06.3 Exposure to melting** of other clothing and apparel

√4ᵗʰ **X08 Exposure to other specified smoke, fire and flames**

√5ᵗʰ **X08.0 Exposure to bed fire**
Exposure to mattress fire

√x7ᵗʰ **X08.00 Exposure to bed fire due to unspecified burning material** ▽

√x7ᵗʰ **X08.01 Exposure to bed fire due to burning cigarette**

√x7ᵗʰ **X08.09 Exposure to bed fire due to other burning material**

√5ᵗʰ **X08.1 Exposure to sofa fire**

√x7ᵗʰ **X08.10 Exposure to sofa fire due to unspecified burning material** ▽

√x7ᵗʰ **X08.11 Exposure to sofa fire due to burning cigarette**

√x7ᵗʰ **X08.19 Exposure to sofa fire due to other burning material**

√5ᵗʰ **X08.2 Exposure to other furniture fire**

√x7ᵗʰ **X08.20 Exposure to other furniture fire due to unspecified burning material** ▽

√x7ᵗʰ **X08.21 Exposure to other furniture fire due to burning cigarette**

√x7ᵗʰ **X08.29 Exposure to other furniture fire due to other burning material**

√x7ᵗʰ **X08.8 Exposure to other specified smoke, fire and flames**

Contact with heat and hot substances (X10-X19)
EXCLUDES 1 exposure to excessive natural heat (X30)
exposure to fire and flames ▶(X00-X08)◀

The appropriate 7th character is to be added to each code from categories X10-X19.
A   initial encounter
D   subsequent encounter
S   sequela

√4ᵗʰ **X10 Contact with hot drinks, food, fats and cooking oils**

√x7ᵗʰ **X10.0 Contact with hot drinks**

√x7ᵗʰ **X10.1 Contact with hot food**

√x7ᵗʰ **X10.2 Contact with fats and cooking oils**

√4ᵗʰ **X11 Contact with hot tap-water**
INCLUDES contact with boiling tap-water
contact with boiling water NOS
EXCLUDES 1 contact with water heated on stove (X12)

√x7ᵗʰ **X11.0 Contact with hot water in bath or tub**
EXCLUDES 1 contact with running hot water in bath or tub (X11.1)

√x7ᵗʰ **X11.1 Contact with running hot water**
Contact with hot water running out of hose
Contact with hot water running out of tap

√x7ᵗʰ **X11.8 Contact with other hot tap-water**
Contact with hot water in bucket
Contact with hot tap-water NOS

√x7ᵗʰ **X12 Contact with other hot fluids**
Contact with water heated on stove
EXCLUDES 1 hot (liquid) metals (X18)

√4ᵗʰ **X13 Contact with steam and other hot vapors**

√x7ᵗʰ **X13.0 Inhalation of steam and other hot vapors**

√x7ᵗʰ **X13.1 Other contact with steam and other hot vapors**

√4ᵗʰ **X14 Contact with hot air and other hot gases**

√x7ᵗʰ **X14.0 Inhalation of hot air and gases**

√x7ᵗʰ **X14.1 Other contact with hot air and other hot gases**

√4ᵗʰ **X15 Contact with hot household appliances**
EXCLUDES 1 contact with heating appliances (X16)
contact with powered household appliances (W29.-)
exposure to controlled fire in building or structure due to household appliance (X02.8)
exposure to household appliances electrical current (W86.0)

√x7ᵗʰ **X15.0 Contact with hot stove (kitchen)**

√x7ᵗʰ **X15.1 Contact with hot toaster**

√x7ᵗʰ **X15.2 Contact with hotplate**

√x7ᵗʰ **X15.3 Contact with hot saucepan or skillet**

√x7ᵗʰ **X15.8 Contact with other hot household appliances**
Contact with cooker   Contact with light bulbs
Contact with kettle

√x7ᵗʰ **X16 Contact with hot heating appliances, radiators and pipes**
EXCLUDES 1 contact with powered appliances (W29.-)
exposure to controlled fire in building or structure due to appliance (X02.8)
exposure to industrial appliances electrical current (W86.1)

√x7ᵗʰ **X17 Contact with hot engines, machinery and tools**
EXCLUDES 1 contact with hot heating appliances, radiators and pipes (X16)
contact with hot household appliances (X15)

√x7ᵗʰ **X18 Contact with other hot metals**
Contact with liquid metal

√x7ᵗʰ **X19 Contact with other heat and hot substances**
EXCLUDES 1 objects that are not normally hot, e.g., an object made hot by a house fire ▶(X00-X08)◀

Chapter 20. External Causes of Morbidity *(side tab)*

Exposure to forces of nature (X30-X39)

> The appropriate 7th character is to be added to each code from categories X30-X39.
> A   initial encounter
> D   subsequent encounter
> S   sequela

√x7th **X30   Exposure to excessive natural heat**
    Exposure to excessive heat as the cause of sunstroke
    Exposure to heat NOS
    EXCLUDES 1   *excessive heat of man-made origin (W92)*
                    exposure to man-made radiation (W89)
                    exposure to sunlight (X32)
                    exposure to tanning bed (W89)

√x7th **X31   Exposure to excessive natural cold**
    Excessive cold as the cause of chilblains NOS
    Excessive cold as the cause of immersion foot or hand
    Exposure to cold NOS
    Exposure to weather conditions
    EXCLUDES 1   *cold of man-made origin (W93.-)*
                    contact with or inhalation of dry ice (W93.-)
                    contact with or inhalation of liquefied gas (W93.-)

√x7th **X32   Exposure to sunlight**
    EXCLUDES 1   *man-made radiation (tanning bed) (W89)*
    EXCLUDES 2 ▶*radiation-related disorders of the skin and subcutaneous tissue (L55-L59)*◀

√x7th **X34   Earthquake**
    EXCLUDES 2   *tidal wave (tsunami) due to earthquake (X37.41)*

√x7th **X35   Volcanic eruption**
    EXCLUDES 2   *tidal wave (tsunami) due to volcanic eruption (X37.41)*

√4th **X36   Avalanche, landslide and other earth movements**
    INCLUDES   victim of mudslide of cataclysmic nature
    EXCLUDES 1   *earthquake (X34)*
    EXCLUDES 2   *transport accident involving collision with avalanche or landslide not in motion (V01-V99)*

    √x7th **X36.0   Collapse of dam or man-made structure causing earth movement**

    √x7th **X36.1   Avalanche, landslide, or mudslide**

√4th **X37   Cataclysmic storm**

    √x7th **X37.0   Hurricane**
          Storm surge
          Typhoon

    √x7th **X37.1   Tornado**
          Cyclone
          Twister

    √x7th **X37.2   Blizzard (snow) (ice)**

    √x7th **X37.3   Dust storm**

    √5th **X37.4   Tidalwave**

        √x7th **X37.41   Tidal wave due to earthquake or volcanic eruption**
               Tidal wave NOS
               Tsunami

        √x7th **X37.42   Tidal wave due to storm**

        √x7th **X37.43   Tidal wave due to landslide**

    √x7th **X37.8   Other cataclysmic storms**
          Cloudburst
          Torrential rain
          EXCLUDES 2   *flood (X38)*

    √x7th **X37.9   Unspecified cataclysmic storm**   ▽
          Storm NOS
          EXCLUDES 1   *collapse of dam or man-made structure causing earth movement (X39.0)*

√x7th **X38   Flood**
    Flood arising from remote storm
    Flood of cataclysmic nature arising from melting snow
    Flood resulting directly from storm
    EXCLUDES 1   *collapse of dam or man-made structure causing earth movement (X39.0)*
                    tidal wave NOS (X37.41)
                    tidal wave caused by storm (X37.2)

√4th **X39   Exposure to other forces of nature**

    √5th **X39.0   Exposure to natural radiation**
        EXCLUDES 1   *contact with and (suspected) exposure to radon and other naturally occuring radiation (Z77.123)*
                      exposure to man-made radiation (W88-W90)
                      exposure to sunlight (X32)

        √x7th **X39.01   Exposure to radon**

        √x7th **X39.08   Exposure to other natural radiation**

    √x7th **X39.8   Other exposure to forces of nature**

Overexertion and strenuous or repetitive movements (X50)

√4th **X50   Overexertion and strenuous or repetitive movements**

> The appropriate 7th character is to be added to each code from category X50.
> A   initial encounter
> D   subsequent encounter
> S   sequela

    √x7th **X50.0   Overexertion from strenuous movement or load**
          Lifting heavy objects
          Lifting weights

    √x7th **X50.1   Overexertion from prolonged static or awkward postures**
          Prolonged bending
          Prolonged kneeling
          Prolonged reaching
          Prolonged sitting
          Prolonged standing
          Prolonged twisting
          Static bending
          Static kneeling
          Static reaching
          Static sitting
          Static standing
          Static twisting

    √x7th **X50.3   Overexertion from repetitive movements**
          Use of hand as hammer
          EXCLUDES 2   *overuse from prolonged static or awkward postures (X50.1)*

    √x7th **X50.9   Other and unspecified overexertion or strenuous movements or postures**   ▽
          Contact pressure
          Contact stress

Accidental exposure to other specified factors (X52-X58)

> The appropriate 7th character is to be added to each code from categories X52-X58.
> A   initial encounter
> D   subsequent encounter
> S   sequela

√x7th **X52   Prolonged stay in weightless environment**
    Weightlessness in spacecraft (simulator)

√x7th **X58   Exposure to other specified factors**
    Accident NOS
    Exposure NOS

Intentional self-harm (X71-X83)

Purposely self-inflicted injury
Suicide (attempted)

> The appropriate 7th character is to be added to each code from categories X71-X83.
> A   initial encounter
> D   subsequent encounter
> S   sequela

√4th **X71   Intentional self-harm by drowning and submersion**

    √x7th **X71.0   Intentional self-harm by drowning and submersion while in bathtub**   HCC

    √x7th **X71.1   Intentional self-harm by drowning and submersion while in swimming pool**   HCC

    √x7th **X71.2   Intentional self-harm by drowning and submersion after jump into swimming pool**   HCC

    √x7th **X71.3   Intentional self-harm by drowning and submersion in natural water**   HCC

    √x7th **X71.8   Other intentional self-harm by drowning and submersion**   HCC

    √x7th **X71.9   Intentional self-harm by drowning and submersion, unspecified**   HCC ▽

√x7th **X72   Intentional self-harm by handgun discharge**   HCC
    Intentional self-harm by gun for single hand use
    Intentional self-harm by pistol
    Intentional self-harm by revolver
    EXCLUDES 1   *Very pistol (X74.8)*

EXCLUDES 1 Not coded here   EXCLUDES 2 Not included here   N Newborn Age: 0   P Pediatric Age: 0-17   M Maternity Age: 12-55   A Adult Age: 15-124

1154   **ICD-10-CM 2018**

☑4th **X73** **Intentional self-harm by rifle, shotgun and larger firearm discharge**
    EXCLUDES 1   *airgun (X74.Ø1)*

  ☑x7th **X73.Ø** Intentional self-harm by **shotgun** discharge   HCC

  ☑x7th **X73.1** Intentional self-harm by **hunting rifle** discharge   HCC

  ☑x7th **X73.2** Intentional self-harm by **machine gun** discharge   HCC

  ☑x7th **X73.8** Intentional self-harm by other larger firearm discharge   HCC

  ☑x7th **X73.9** Intentional self-harm by unspecified larger firearm discharge   HCC ▽

☑4th **X74** **Intentional self-harm by other and unspecified firearm and gun discharge**

  ☑5th **X74.Ø** Intentional self-harm by gas, air or spring-operated guns

    ☑x7th **X74.Ø1** **Intentional self-harm by airgun**   HCC
       Intentional self-harm by BB gun discharge
       Intentional self-harm by pellet gun discharge

    ☑x7th **X74.Ø2** **Intentional self-harm by paintball gun**   HCC

    ☑x7th **X74.Ø9** **Intentional self-harm by other gas, air or spring-operated gun**   HCC

  ☑x7th **X74.8** Intentional self-harm by other firearm discharge   HCC
       Intentional self-harm by Very pistol [flare] discharge

  ☑x7th **X74.9** Intentional self-harm by unspecified firearm discharge   HCC ▽

☑x7th **X75** **Intentional self-harm by explosive material**   HCC

☑x7th **X76** **Intentional self-harm by smoke, fire and flames**   HCC

☑4th **X77** **Intentional self-harm by steam, hot vapors and hot objects**

  ☑x7th **X77.Ø** Intentional self-harm by **steam or hot vapors**   HCC

  ☑x7th **X77.1** Intentional self-harm by **hot tap water**   HCC

  ☑x7th **X77.2** Intentional self-harm by **other hot fluids**   HCC

  ☑x7th **X77.3** Intentional self-harm by **hot household appliances**   HCC

  ☑x7th **X77.8** Intentional self-harm by **other hot objects**   HCC

  ☑x7th **X77.9** Intentional self-harm by **unspecified hot objects**   HCC ▽

☑4th **X78** **Intentional self-harm by sharp object**

  ☑x7th **X78.Ø** Intentional self-harm by **sharp glass**   HCC

  ☑x7th **X78.1** Intentional self-harm by **knife**   HCC

  ☑x7th **X78.2** Intentional self-harm by **sword or dagger**   HCC

  ☑x7th **X78.8** Intentional self-harm by **other sharp object**   HCC

  ☑x7th **X78.9** Intentional self-harm by **unspecified sharp object**   HCC ▽

☑x7th **X79** **Intentional self-harm by blunt object**   HCC

☑x7th **X80** **Intentional self-harm by jumping from a high place**   HCC
     Intentional fall from one level to another

☑4th **X81** **Intentional self-harm by jumping or lying in front of moving object**

  ☑x7th **X81.Ø** Intentional self-harm by jumping or lying in front of motor vehicle   HCC

  ☑x7th **X81.1** Intentional self-harm by jumping or lying in front of (subway) train   HCC

  ☑x7th **X81.8** Intentional self-harm by jumping or lying in front of other moving object   HCC

☑4th **X82** **Intentional self-harm by crashing of motor vehicle**

  ☑x7th **X82.Ø** Intentional collision of motor vehicle with other motor vehicle   HCC

  ☑x7th **X82.1** Intentional collision of motor vehicle with train   HCC

  ☑x7th **X82.2** Intentional collision of motor vehicle with tree   HCC

  ☑x7th **X82.8** Other intentional self-harm by crashing of motor vehicle   HCC

☑4th **X83** **Intentional self-harm by other specified means**
    EXCLUDES 1   *intentional self-harm by poisoning or contact with toxic substance—see Table of Drugs and Chemicals*

  ☑x7th **X83.Ø** Intentional self-harm by **crashing of aircraft**   HCC

  ☑x7th **X83.1** Intentional self-harm by **electrocution**   HCC

  ☑x7th **X83.2** Intentional self-harm by **exposure to extremes of cold**   HCC

  ☑x7th **X83.8** Intentional self-harm by **other specified means**   HCC

Assault (X92-Y09)

INCLUDES   homicide
         injuries inflicted by another person with intent to injure or kill, by any means

EXCLUDES 1   *injuries due to legal intervention (Y35.-)*
         injuries due to operations of war (Y36.-)
         injuries due to terrorism (Y38.-)

> The appropriate 7th character is to be added to each code from categories X92-YØ4 and YØ8.
> A   initial encounter
> D   subsequent encounter
> S   sequela

☑4th **X92** **Assault by drowning and submersion**

  ☑x7th **X92.Ø** **Assault by drowning and submersion while in bathtub**

  ☑x7th **X92.1** **Assault by drowning and submersion while in swimming pool**

  ☑x7th **X92.2** **Assault by drowning and submersion after push into swimming pool**

  ☑x7th **X92.3** **Assault by drowning and submersion in natural water**

  ☑x7th **X92.8** **Other assault by drowning and submersion**

  ☑x7th **X92.9** **Assault by drowning and submersion, unspecified**   ▽

☑x7th **X93** **Assault by handgun discharge**
     Assault by discharge of gun for single hand use
     Assault by discharge of pistol
     Assault by discharge of revolver
    EXCLUDES 1   *Very pistol (X95.8)*

☑4th **X94** **Assault by rifle, shotgun and larger firearm discharge**
    EXCLUDES 1   *airgun (X95.Ø1)*

  ☑x7th **X94.Ø** **Assault by shotgun**

  ☑x7th **X94.1** **Assault by hunting rifle**

  ☑x7th **X94.2** **Assault by machine gun**

  ☑x7th **X94.8** **Assault by other larger firearm discharge**

  ☑x7th **X94.9** **Assault by unspecified larger firearm discharge**   ▽

☑4th **X95** **Assault by other and unspecified firearm and gun discharge**

  ☑5th **X95.Ø** **Assault by gas, air or spring-operated guns**

    ☑x7th **X95.Ø1** **Assault by airgun discharge**
       Assault by BB gun discharge
       Assault by pellet gun discharge

    ☑x7th **X95.Ø2** **Assault by paintball gun discharge**

    ☑x7th **X95.Ø9** **Assault by other gas, air or spring-operated gun**

  ☑x7th **X95.8** **Assault by other firearm discharge**
       Assault by Very pistol [flare] discharge

  ☑x7th **X95.9** **Assault by unspecified firearm discharge**   ▽

☑4th **X96** **Assault by explosive material**
    EXCLUDES 1   *incendiary device (X97)*
         terrorism involving explosive material (Y38.2-)

  ☑x7th **X96.Ø** **Assault by antipersonnel bomb**
    EXCLUDES 1   *antipersonnel bomb use in military or war (Y36.2-)*

  ☑x7th **X96.1** **Assault by gasoline bomb**

  ☑x7th **X96.2** **Assault by letter bomb**

  ☑x7th **X96.3** **Assault by fertilizer bomb**

  ☑x7th **X96.4** **Assault by pipe bomb**

  ☑x7th **X96.8** **Assault by other specified explosive**

  ☑x7th **X96.9** **Assault by unspecified explosive**   ▽

☑x7th **X97** **Assault by smoke, fire and flames**
     Assault by arson
     Assault by cigarettes
     Assault by incendiary device

☑4th **X98** **Assault by steam, hot vapors and hot objects**

  ☑x7th **X98.Ø** **Assault by steam or hot vapors**

  ☑x7th **X98.1** **Assault by hot tap water**

  ☑x7th **X98.2** **Assault by hot fluids**

  ☑x7th **X98.3** **Assault by hot household appliances**

  ☑x7th **X98.8** **Assault by other hot objects**

  ☑x7th **X98.9** **Assault by unspecified hot objects**   ▽

☑4th **X99** **Assault by sharp object**
    EXCLUDES 1   *assault by strike by sports equipment (YØ8.Ø-)*

  ☑x7th **X99.Ø** **Assault by sharp glass**

  ☑x7th **X99.1** **Assault by knife**

  ☑x7th **X99.2** **Assault by sword or dagger**

☑ Additional Character Req   ☑x7th Placeholder Alert   Manifestation   HCC CMS-HCC Condition   ▽ Unspecified Code   ►◄ Revised Text   ● New Code   ▲ Revised Code Title

√x7th **X99.8**   **Assault by other sharp object**

√x7th **X99.9**   **Assault by unspecified sharp object** ▽
     Assault by stabbing NOS

√x7th **Y00**   **Assault by blunt object**
     EXCLUDES 1   *assault by strike by sports equipment (Y08.0-)*

√x7th **Y01**   **Assault by pushing from high place**

√4th **Y02**   **Assault by pushing or placing victim in front of moving object**

√x7th **Y02.0**   **Assault by pushing or placing victim in front of motor vehicle**

√x7th **Y02.1**   **Assault by pushing or placing victim in front of (subway) train**

√x7th **Y02.8**   **Assault by pushing or placing victim in front of other moving object**

√4th **Y03**   **Assault by crashing of motor vehicle**

√x7th **Y03.0**   **Assault by being hit or run over by motor vehicle**

√x7th **Y03.8**   **Other assault by crashing of motor vehicle**

√4th **Y04**   **Assault by bodily force**
     EXCLUDES 1   *assault by:*
         submersion (X92.-)
         use of weapon (X93-X95, X99, Y00)

√x7th **Y04.0**   **Assault by unarmed brawl or fight**

√x7th **Y04.1**   **Assault by human bite**

√x7th **Y04.2**   **Assault by strike against or bumped into by another person**

√x7th **Y04.8**   **Assault by other bodily force**
     Assault by bodily force NOS

√4th **Y07**   **Perpetrator of assault, maltreatment and neglect**
     NOTE   Codes from this category are for use only in cases of confirmed abuse (T74.-)
         Selection of the correct perpetrator code is based on the relationship between the perpetrator and the victim
     INCLUDES   perpetrator of abandonment
         perpetrator of emotional neglect
         perpetrator of mental cruelty
         perpetrator of physical abuse
         perpetrator of physical neglect
         perpetrator of sexual abuse
         perpetrator of torture

√5th **Y07.0**   **Spouse or partner, perpetrator of maltreatment and neglect**
     Spouse or partner, perpetrator of maltreatment and neglect against spouse or partner

     Y07.01   **Husband, perpetrator of maltreatment and neglect**

     Y07.02   **Wife, perpetrator of maltreatment and neglect**

     Y07.03   **Male partner, perpetrator of maltreatment and neglect**

     Y07.04   **Female partner, perpetrator of maltreatment and neglect**

√5th **Y07.1**   **Parent (adoptive) (biological), perpetrator of maltreatment and neglect**

     Y07.11   **Biological father, perpetrator of maltreatment and neglect**

     Y07.12   **Biological mother, perpetrator of maltreatment and neglect**

     Y07.13   **Adoptive father, perpetrator of maltreatment and neglect**

     Y07.14   **Adoptive mother, perpetrator of maltreatment and neglect**

√5th **Y07.4**   **Other family member, perpetrator of maltreatment and neglect**

√6th **Y07.41**   **Sibling, perpetrator of maltreatment and neglect**
     EXCLUDES 1   *stepsibling, perpetrator of maltreatment and neglect (Y07.435, Y07.436)*

     Y07.410   **Brother, perpetrator of maltreatment and neglect**

     Y07.411   **Sister, perpetrator of maltreatment and neglect**

√6th **Y07.42**   **Foster parent, perpetrator of maltreatment and neglect**

     Y07.420   **Foster father, perpetrator of maltreatment and neglect**

     Y07.421   **Foster mother, perpetrator of maltreatment and neglect**

√6th **Y07.43**   **Stepparent or stepsibling, perpetrator of maltreatment and neglect**

     Y07.430   **Stepfather, perpetrator of maltreatment and neglect**

     Y07.432   **Male friend of parent (co-residing in household), perpetrator of maltreatment and neglect**

     Y07.433   **Stepmother, perpetrator of maltreatment and neglect**

     Y07.434   **Female friend of parent (co-residing in household), perpetrator of maltreatment and neglect**

     Y07.435   **Stepbrother, perpetrator or maltreatment and neglect**

     Y07.436   **Stepsister, perpetrator of maltreatment and neglect**

√6th **Y07.49**   **Other family member, perpetrator of maltreatment and neglect**

     Y07.490   **Male cousin, perpetrator of maltreatment and neglect**

     Y07.491   **Female cousin, perpetrator of maltreatment and neglect**

     Y07.499   **Other family member, perpetrator of maltreatment and neglect**

√5th **Y07.5**   **Non-family member, perpetrator of maltreatment and neglect**

     Y07.50   **Unspecified non-family member, perpetrator of maltreatment and neglect** ▽

√6th **Y07.51**   **Daycare provider, perpetrator of maltreatment and neglect**

     Y07.510   **At-home childcare provider, perpetrator of maltreatment and neglect**

     Y07.511   **Daycare center childcare provider, perpetrator of maltreatment and neglect**

     Y07.512   **At-home adultcare provider, perpetrator of maltreatment and neglect**

     Y07.513   **Adultcare center provider, perpetrator of maltreatment and neglect**

     Y07.519   **Unspecified daycare provider, perpetrator of maltreatment and neglect** ▽

√6th **Y07.52**   **Healthcare provider, perpetrator of maltreatment and neglect**

     Y07.521   **Mental health provider, perpetrator of maltreatment and neglect**

     Y07.528   **Other therapist or healthcare provider, perpetrator of maltreatment and neglect**
         Nurse, perpetrator of maltreatment and neglect
         Occupational therapist, perpetrator of maltreatment and neglect
         Physical therapist, perpetrator of maltreatment and neglect
         Speech therapist, perpetrator of maltreatment and neglect

     Y07.529   **Unspecified healthcare provider, perpetrator of maltreatment and neglect** ▽

     Y07.53   **Teacher or instructor, perpetrator of maltreatment and neglect**
     Coach, perpetrator of maltreatment and neglect

     Y07.59   **Other non-family member, perpetrator of maltreatment and neglect**

     Y07.9   **Unspecified perpetrator of maltreatment and neglect** ▽

√4th **Y08**   **Assault by other specified means**

√5th **Y08.0**   **Assault by strike by sport equipment**

√x7th **Y08.01**   **Assault by strike by hockey stick**

√x7th **Y08.02**   **Assault by strike by baseball bat**

√x7th **Y08.09**   **Assault by strike by other specified type of sport equipment**

√5th **Y08.8**   **Assault by other specified means**

√x7th **Y08.81**   **Assault by crashing of aircraft**

√x7th **Y08.89**   **Assault by other specified means**

Y09   **Assault by unspecified means** ▽
     Assassination (attempted) NOS
     Homicide (attempted) NOS
     Manslaughter (attempted) NOS
     Murder (attempted) NOS

EXCLUDES 1 Not coded here   EXCLUDES 2 Not included here   N Newborn Age: 0   P Pediatric Age: 0-17   M Maternity Age: 12-55   A Adult Age: 15-124

1156   ICD-10-CM 2018

Event of undetermined intent (Y21-Y33)

Undetermined intent is only for use when there is specific documentation in the record that the intent of the injury cannot be determined. If no such documentation is present, code to accidental (unintentional).

> The appropriate 7th character is to be added to each code from categories Y21-Y33.
> A   initial encounter
> D   subsequent encounter
> S   sequela

✓4th **Y21**   **Drowning and submersion, undetermined intent**

   ✓x7th **Y21.0**   **Drowning and submersion while in bathtub, undetermined intent**

   ✓x7th **Y21.1**   **Drowning and submersion after fall into bathtub, undetermined intent**

   ✓x7th **Y21.2**   **Drowning and submersion while in swimming pool, undetermined intent**

   ✓x7th **Y21.3**   **Drowning and submersion after fall into swimming pool, undetermined intent**

   ✓x7th **Y21.4**   **Drowning and submersion in natural water, undetermined intent**

   ✓x7th **Y21.8**   **Other drowning and submersion, undetermined intent**

   ✓x7th **Y21.9**   **Unspecified drowning and submersion, undetermined intent**   ▽

✓x7th **Y22**   **Handgun discharge, undetermined intent**
     Discharge of gun for single hand use, undetermined intent
     Discharge of pistol, undetermined intent
     Discharge of revolver, undetermined intent
     EXCLUDES 2   *Very pistol (Y24.8)*

✓4th **Y23**   **Rifle, shotgun and larger firearm discharge, undetermined intent**
     EXCLUDES 2   *airgun (Y24.0)*

   ✓x7th **Y23.0**   **Shotgun discharge, undetermined intent**

   ✓x7th **Y23.1**   **Hunting rifle discharge, undetermined intent**

   ✓x7th **Y23.2**   **Military firearm discharge, undetermined intent**

   ✓x7th **Y23.3**   **Machine gun discharge, undetermined intent**

   ✓x7th **Y23.8**   **Other larger firearm discharge, undetermined intent**

   ✓x7th **Y23.9**   **Unspecified larger firearm discharge, undetermined intent** ▽

✓4th **Y24**   **Other and unspecified firearm discharge, undetermined intent**

   ✓x7th **Y24.0**   **Airgun discharge, undetermined intent**
       BB gun discharge, undetermined intent
       Pellet gun discharge, undetermined intent

   ✓x7th **Y24.8**   **Other firearm discharge, undetermined intent**
       Paintball gun discharge, undetermined intent
       Very pistol [flare] discharge, undetermined intent

   ✓x7th **Y24.9**   **Unspecified firearm discharge, undetermined intent**   ▽

✓x7th **Y25**   **Contact with explosive material, undetermined intent**

✓x7th **Y26**   **Exposure to smoke, fire and flames, undetermined intent**

✓4th **Y27**   **Contact with steam, hot vapors and hot objects, undetermined intent**

   ✓x7th **Y27.0**   **Contact with steam and hot vapors, undetermined intent**

   ✓x7th **Y27.1**   **Contact with hot tap water, undetermined intent**

   ✓x7th **Y27.2**   **Contact with hot fluids, undetermined intent**

   ✓x7th **Y27.3**   **Contact with hot household appliance, undetermined intent**

   ✓x7th **Y27.8**   **Contact with other hot objects, undetermined intent**

   ✓x7th **Y27.9**   **Contact with unspecified hot objects, undetermined intent** ▽

✓4th **Y28**   **Contact with sharp object, undetermined intent**

   ✓x7th **Y28.0**   **Contact with sharp glass, undetermined intent**

   ✓x7th **Y28.1**   **Contact with knife, undetermined intent**

   ✓x7th **Y28.2**   **Contact with sword or dagger, undetermined intent**

   ✓x7th **Y28.8**   **Contact with other sharp object, undetermined intent**

   ✓x7th **Y28.9**   **Contact with unspecified hot objects, undetermined intent** ▽

✓x7th **Y29**   **Contact with blunt object, undetermined intent**

✓x7th **Y30**   **Falling, jumping or pushed from a high place, undetermined intent**
     Victim falling from one level to another, undetermined intent

✓x7th **Y31**   **Falling, lying or running before or into moving object, undetermined intent**

✓x7th **Y32**   **Crashing of motor vehicle, undetermined intent**

✓x7th **Y33**   **Other specified events, undetermined intent**

Legal intervention, operations of war, military operations, and terrorism (Y35-Y38)

> The appropriate 7th character is to be added to each code from categories Y35-Y38.
> A   initial encounter
> D   subsequent encounter
> S   sequela

✓4th **Y35**   **Legal intervention**
     INCLUDES   any injury sustained as a result of an encounter with any law enforcement official, serving in any capacity at the time of the encounter, whether on-duty or off-duty. Includes: injury to law enforcement official, suspect and bystander

   ✓5th **Y35.0**   **Legal intervention involving firearm discharge**

     ✓6th **Y35.00**   **Legal intervention involving unspecified firearm discharge**
         Legal intervention involving gunshot wound
         Legal intervention involving shot NOS

       ✓7th **Y35.001**   **Legal intervention involving unspecified firearm discharge, law enforcement official injured** ▽

       ✓7th **Y35.002**   **Legal intervention involving unspecified firearm discharge, bystander injured** ▽

       ✓7th **Y35.003**   **Legal intervention involving unspecified firearm discharge, suspect injured** ▽

     ✓6th **Y35.01**   **Legal intervention involving injury by machine gun**

       ✓7th **Y35.011**   **Legal intervention involving injury by machine gun, law enforcement official injured**

       ✓7th **Y35.012**   **Legal intervention involving injury by machine gun, bystander injured**

       ✓7th **Y35.013**   **Legal intervention involving injury by machine gun, suspect injured**

     ✓6th **Y35.02**   **Legal intervention involving injury by handgun**

       ✓7th **Y35.021**   **Legal intervention involving injury by handgun, law enforcement official injured**

       ✓7th **Y35.022**   **Legal intervention involving injury by handgun, bystander injured**

       ✓7th **Y35.023**   **Legal intervention involving injury by handgun, suspect injured**

     ✓6th **Y35.03**   **Legal intervention involving injury by rifle pellet**

       ✓7th **Y35.031**   **Legal intervention involving injury by rifle pellet, law enforcement official injured**

       ✓7th **Y35.032**   **Legal intervention involving injury by rifle pellet, bystander injured**

       ✓7th **Y35.033**   **Legal intervention involving injury by rifle pellet, suspect injured**

     ✓6th **Y35.04**   **Legal intervention involving injury by rubber bullet**

       ✓7th **Y35.041**   **Legal intervention involving injury by rubber bullet, law enforcement official injured**

       ✓7th **Y35.042**   **Legal intervention involving injury by rubber bullet, bystander injured**

       ✓7th **Y35.043**   **Legal intervention involving injury by rubber bullet, suspect injured**

     ✓6th **Y35.09**   **Legal intervention involving other firearm discharge**

       ✓7th **Y35.091**   **Legal intervention involving other firearm discharge, law enforcement official injured**

       ✓7th **Y35.092**   **Legal intervention involving other firearm discharge, bystander injured**

       ✓7th **Y35.093**   **Legal intervention involving other firearm discharge, suspect injured**

   ✓5th **Y35.1**   **Legal intervention involving explosives**

     ✓6th **Y35.10**   **Legal intervention involving unspecified explosives**

       ✓7th **Y35.101**   **Legal intervention involving unspecified explosives, law enforcement official injured** ▽

✓ Additional Character Req   ✓x7th Placeholder Alert   Manifestation   HCC CMS-HCC Condition   ▽ Unspecified Code   ▶◀ Revised Text   ● New Code   ▲ Revised Code Title

Chapter 20. External Causes of Morbidity

√7ᵗʰ **Y35.102** Legal intervention involving unspecified explosives, **bystander** injured ▽

√7ᵗʰ **Y35.103** Legal intervention involving unspecified explosives, **suspect** injured ▽

√6ᵗʰ **Y35.11** Legal intervention involving injury by **dynamite**

  √7ᵗʰ **Y35.111** Legal intervention involving injury by dynamite, **law enforcement official** injured

  √7ᵗʰ **Y35.112** Legal intervention involving injury by dynamite, **bystander** injured

  √7ᵗʰ **Y35.113** Legal intervention involving injury by dynamite, **suspect** injured

√6ᵗʰ **Y35.12** Legal intervention involving injury by **explosive shell**

  √7ᵗʰ **Y35.121** Legal intervention involving injury by explosive shell, **law enforcement official** injured

  √7ᵗʰ **Y35.122** Legal intervention involving injury by explosive shell, **bystander** injured

  √7ᵗʰ **Y35.123** Legal intervention involving injury by explosive shell, **suspect** injured

√6ᵗʰ **Y35.19** Legal intervention involving other explosives
  Legal intervention involving injury by grenade
  Legal intervention involving injury by mortar bomb

  √7ᵗʰ **Y35.191** Legal intervention involving other explosives, **law enforcement official** injured

  √7ᵗʰ **Y35.192** Legal intervention involving other explosives, **bystander** injured

  √7ᵗʰ **Y35.193** Legal intervention involving other explosives, **suspect** injured

√5ᵗʰ **Y35.2** Legal intervention involving gas
  Legal intervention involving asphyxiation by gas
  Legal intervention involving poisoning by gas

√6ᵗʰ **Y35.20** Legal intervention involving unspecified gas

  √7ᵗʰ **Y35.201** Legal intervention involving unspecified gas, **law enforcement official** injured ▽

  √7ᵗʰ **Y35.202** Legal intervention involving unspecified gas, **bystander** injured ▽

  √7ᵗʰ **Y35.203** Legal intervention involving unspecified gas, **suspect** injured ▽

√6ᵗʰ **Y35.21** Legal intervention involving injury by **tear gas**

  √7ᵗʰ **Y35.211** Legal intervention involving injury by tear gas, **law enforcement official** injured

  √7ᵗʰ **Y35.212** Legal intervention involving injury by tear gas, **bystander** injured

  √7ᵗʰ **Y35.213** Legal intervention involving injury by tear gas, **suspect** injured

√6ᵗʰ **Y35.29** Legal intervention involving other gas

  √7ᵗʰ **Y35.291** Legal intervention involving other gas, **law enforcement official** injured

  √7ᵗʰ **Y35.292** Legal intervention involving other gas, **bystander** injured

  √7ᵗʰ **Y35.293** Legal intervention involving other gas, **suspect** injured

√5ᵗʰ **Y35.3** Legal intervention involving blunt objects
  Legal intervention involving being hit or struck by blunt object

√6ᵗʰ **Y35.30** Legal intervention involving unspecified blunt objects

  √7ᵗʰ **Y35.301** Legal intervention involving unspecified blunt objects, **law enforcement official** injured ▽

  √7ᵗʰ **Y35.302** Legal intervention involving unspecified blunt objects, **bystander** injured ▽

  √7ᵗʰ **Y35.303** Legal intervention involving unspecified blunt objects, **suspect** injured ▽

√6ᵗʰ **Y35.31** Legal intervention involving **baton**

  √7ᵗʰ **Y35.311** Legal intervention involving baton, **law enforcement official** injured

  √7ᵗʰ **Y35.312** Legal intervention involving baton, **bystander** injured

  √7ᵗʰ **Y35.313** Legal intervention involving baton, **suspect** injured

√6ᵗʰ **Y35.39** Legal intervention involving other blunt objects

  √7ᵗʰ **Y35.391** Legal intervention involving other blunt objects, **law enforcement** official injured

  √7ᵗʰ **Y35.392** Legal intervention involving other blunt objects, **bystander** injured

  √7ᵗʰ **Y35.393** Legal intervention involving other blunt objects, **suspect** injured

√5ᵗʰ **Y35.4** Legal intervention involving **sharp objects**
  Legal intervention involving being cut by sharp objects
  Legal intervention involving being stabbed by sharp objects

√6ᵗʰ **Y35.40** Legal intervention involving unspecified sharp objects

  √7ᵗʰ **Y35.401** Legal intervention involving unspecified sharp objects, **law enforcement official** injured ▽

  √7ᵗʰ **Y35.402** Legal intervention involving unspecified sharp objects, **bystander** injured ▽

  √7ᵗʰ **Y35.403** Legal intervention involving unspecified sharp objects, **suspect** injured ▽

√6ᵗʰ **Y35.41** Legal intervention involving **bayonet**

  √7ᵗʰ **Y35.411** Legal intervention involving bayonet, **law enforcement official** injured

  √7ᵗʰ **Y35.412** Legal intervention involving bayonet, **bystander** injured

  √7ᵗʰ **Y35.413** Legal intervention involving bayonet, **suspect** injured

√6ᵗʰ **Y35.49** Legal intervention involving other sharp objects

  √7ᵗʰ **Y35.491** Legal intervention involving other sharp objects, **law enforcement official** injured

  √7ᵗʰ **Y35.492** Legal intervention involving other sharp objects, **bystander** injured

  √7ᵗʰ **Y35.493** Legal intervention involving other sharp objects, **suspect** injured

√5ᵗʰ **Y35.8** Legal intervention involving other specified means

√6ᵗʰ **Y35.81** Legal intervention involving **manhandling**

  √7ᵗʰ **Y35.811** Legal intervention involving manhandling, **law enforcement official** injured

  √7ᵗʰ **Y35.812** Legal intervention involving manhandling, **bystander** injured

  √7ᵗʰ **Y35.813** Legal intervention involving manhandling, **suspect** injured

√6ᵗʰ **Y35.89** Legal intervention involving other specified means

  √7ᵗʰ **Y35.891** Legal intervention involving other specified means, **law enforcement official** injured

  √7ᵗʰ **Y35.892** Legal intervention involving other specified means, **bystander** injured

  √7ᵗʰ **Y35.893** Legal intervention involving other specified means, **suspect** injured

√5ᵗʰ **Y35.9** Legal intervention, means unspecified

  √x7ᵗʰ **Y35.91** Legal intervention, means unspecified, **law enforcement official** injured ▽

  √x7ᵗʰ **Y35.92** Legal intervention, means unspecified, **bystander** injured ▽

  √x7ᵗʰ **Y35.93** Legal intervention, means unspecified, **suspect** injured ▽

√4ᵗʰ **Y36** **Operations of war**
  INCLUDES injuries to military personnel and civilians caused by war, civil insurrection, and peacekeeping missions
  EXCLUDES 1 *injury to military personnel occurring during peacetime military operations (Y37.-)*
    military vehicles involved in transport accidents with non-military vehicle during peacetime (V09.01, V09.21, V19.81, V29.81, V39.81, V49.81, V59.81, V69.81, V79.81)
  AHA: 2014, 3Q, 4

√5ᵗʰ **Y36.0** War operations involving explosion of marine weapons

√6ᵗʰ **Y36.00** War operations involving explosion of unspecified marine weapon
  War operations involving underwater blast NOS

  √7ᵗʰ **Y36.000** War operations involving explosion of unspecified marine weapon, military personnel ▽

EXCLUDES 1 Not coded here   EXCLUDES 2 Not included here   N Newborn Age: 0   P Pediatric Age: 0-17   M Maternity Age: 12-55   A Adult Age: 15-124

1158   ICD-10-CM 2018

Y35.102–Y36.000

☑7ᵗʰ **Y36.001** **War operations involving explosion of unspecified marine weapon, civilian** ▽

☑6ᵗʰ **Y36.01** **War operations involving explosion of depth-charge**

    ☑7ᵗʰ **Y36.010** **War operations involving explosion of depth-charge, military personnel**

    ☑7ᵗʰ **Y36.011** **War operations involving explosion of depth-charge, civilian**

☑6ᵗʰ **Y36.02** **War operations involving explosion of marine mine**

    War operations involving explosion of marine mine, at sea or in harbor

    ☑7ᵗʰ **Y36.020** **War operations involving explosion of marine mine, military personnel**

    ☑7ᵗʰ **Y36.021** **War operations involving explosion of marine mine, civilian**

☑6ᵗʰ **Y36.03** **War operations involving explosion of sea-based artillery shell**

    ☑7ᵗʰ **Y36.030** **War operations involving explosion of sea-based artillery shell, military personnel**

    ☑7ᵗʰ **Y36.031** **War operations involving explosion of sea-based artillery shell, civilian**

☑6ᵗʰ **Y36.04** **War operations involving explosion of torpedo**

    ☑7ᵗʰ **Y36.040** **War operations involving explosion of torpedo, military personnel**

    ☑7ᵗʰ **Y36.041** **War operations involving explosion of torpedo, civilian**

☑6ᵗʰ **Y36.05** **War operations involving accidental detonation of onboard marine weapons**

    ☑7ᵗʰ **Y36.050** **War operations involving accidental detonation of onboard marine weapons, military personnel**

    ☑7ᵗʰ **Y36.051** **War operations involving accidental detonation of onboard marine weapons, civilian**

☑6ᵗʰ **Y36.09** **War operations involving explosion of other marine weapons**

    ☑7ᵗʰ **Y36.090** **War operations involving explosion of other marine weapons, military personnel**

    ☑7ᵗʰ **Y36.091** **War operations involving explosion of other marine weapons, civilian**

☑5ᵗʰ **Y36.1** **War operations involving destruction of aircraft**

☑6ᵗʰ **Y36.10** **War operations involving unspecified destruction of aircraft**

    ☑7ᵗʰ **Y36.100** **War operations involving unspecified destruction of aircraft, military personnel** ▽

    ☑7ᵗʰ **Y36.101** **War operations involving unspecified destruction of aircraft, civilian** ▽

☑6ᵗʰ **Y36.11** **War operations involving destruction of aircraft due to enemy fire or explosives**

    War operations involving destruction of aircraft due to air to air missile

    War operations involving destruction of aircraft due to explosive placed on aircraft

    War operations involving destruction of aircraft due to rocket propelled grenade [RPG]

    War operations involving destruction of aircraft due to small arms fire

    War operations involving destruction of aircraft due to surface to air missile

    ☑7ᵗʰ **Y36.110** **War operations involving destruction of aircraft due to enemy fire or explosives, military personnel**

    ☑7ᵗʰ **Y36.111** **War operations involving destruction of aircraft due to enemy fire or explosives, civilian**

☑6ᵗʰ **Y36.12** **War operations involving destruction of aircraft due to collision with other aircraft**

    ☑7ᵗʰ **Y36.120** **War operations involving destruction of aircraft due to collision with other aircraft, military personnel**

    ☑7ᵗʰ **Y36.121** **War operations involving destruction of aircraft due to collision with other aircraft, civilian**

☑6ᵗʰ **Y36.13** **War operations involving destruction of aircraft due to onboard fire**

    ☑7ᵗʰ **Y36.130** **War operations involving destruction of aircraft due to onboard fire, military personnel**

    ☑7ᵗʰ **Y36.131** **War operations involving destruction of aircraft due to onboard fire, civilian**

☑6ᵗʰ **Y36.14** **War operations involving destruction of aircraft due to accidental detonation of onboard munitions and explosives**

    ☑7ᵗʰ **Y36.140** **War operations involving destruction of aircraft due to accidental detonation of onboard munitions and explosives, military personnel**

    ☑7ᵗʰ **Y36.141** **War operations involving destruction of aircraft due to accidental detonation of onboard munitions and explosives, civilian**

☑6ᵗʰ **Y36.19** **War operations involving other destruction of aircraft**

    ☑7ᵗʰ **Y36.190** **War operations involving other destruction of aircraft, military personnel**

    ☑7ᵗʰ **Y36.191** **War operations involving other destruction of aircraft, civilian**

☑5ᵗʰ **Y36.2** **War operations involving other explosions and fragments**

    EXCLUDES 1 *war operations involving explosion of aircraft (Y36.1-)*

        war operations involving explosion of marine weapons (Y36.0-)

        war operations involving explosion of nuclear weapons (Y36.5-)

        war operations involving explosion occurring after cessation of hostilities (Y36.8-)

☑6ᵗʰ **Y36.20** **War operations involving unspecified explosion and fragments**

    War operations involving air blast NOS

    War operations involving blast NOS

    War operations involving blast fragments NOS

    War operations involving blast wave NOS

    War operations involving blast wind NOS

    War operations involving explosion NOS

    War operations involving explosion of bomb NOS

    ☑7ᵗʰ **Y36.200** **War operations involving unspecified explosion and fragments, military personnel** ▽

    ☑7ᵗʰ **Y36.201** **War operations involving unspecified explosion and fragments, civilian** ▽

☑6ᵗʰ **Y36.21** **War operations involving explosion of aerial bomb**

    ☑7ᵗʰ **Y36.210** **War operations involving explosion of aerial bomb, military personnel**

    ☑7ᵗʰ **Y36.211** **War operations involving explosion of aerial bomb, civilian**

☑6ᵗʰ **Y36.22** **War operations involving explosion of guided missile**

    ☑7ᵗʰ **Y36.220** **War operations involving explosion of guided missile, military personnel**

    ☑7ᵗʰ **Y36.221** **War operations involving explosion of guided missile, civilian**

☑6ᵗʰ **Y36.23** **War operations involving explosion of improvised explosive device [IED]**

    War operations involving explosion of person-borne improvised explosive device [IED]

    War operations involving explosion of vehicle-borne improvised explosive device [IED]

    War operations involving explosion of roadside improvised explosive device [IED]

    ☑7ᵗʰ **Y36.230** **War operations involving explosion of improvised explosive device [IED], military personnel**

    ☑7ᵗʰ **Y36.231** **War operations involving explosion of improvised explosive device [IED], civilian**

☑6ᵗʰ **Y36.24** **War operations involving explosion due to accidental detonation and discharge of own munitions or munitions launch device**

    ☑7ᵗʰ **Y36.240** **War operations involving explosion due to accidental detonation and discharge of own munitions or munitions launch device, military personnel**

    ☑7ᵗʰ **Y36.241** **War operations involving explosion due to accidental detonation and discharge of own munitions or munitions launch device, civilian**

☑ Additional Character Req   ☑ˣ⁷ᵗʰ Placeholder Alert   Manifestation   **HCC** CMS-HCC Condition   ▽ Unspecified Code   ►◄ Revised Text   ● New Code   ▲ Revised Code Title

Chapter 20. External Causes of Morbidity

Y36.25–Y36.51

√6th **Y36.25**   **War operations involving fragments from munitions**

     √7th **Y36.250**   War operations involving fragments from munitions, **military personnel**

     √7th **Y36.251**   War operations involving fragments from munitions, **civilian**

√6th **Y36.26**   **War operations involving fragments of improvised explosive device [IED]**

     War operations involving fragments of person-borne improvised explosive device [IED]

     War operations involving fragments of vehicle-borne improvised explosive device [IED]

     War operations involving fragments of roadside improvised explosive device [IED]

     √7th **Y36.260**   **War operations involving fragments of improvised explosive device [IED], military personnel**

     √7th **Y36.261**   **War operations involving fragments of improvised explosive device [IED], civilian**

√6th **Y36.27**   **War operations involving fragments from weapons**

     √7th **Y36.270**   **War operations involving fragments from weapons, military personnel**

     √7th **Y36.271**   **War operations involving fragments from weapons, civilian**

√6th **Y36.29**   **War operations involving other explosions and fragments**

     War operations involving explosion of grenade

     War operations involving explosions of land mine

     War operations involving shrapnel NOS

     √7th **Y36.290**   **War operations involving other explosions and fragments, military personnel**

     √7th **Y36.291**   **War operations involving other explosions and fragments, civilian**

√5th **Y36.3**   **War operations involving fires, conflagrations and hot substances**

     War operations involving smoke, fumes, and heat from fires, conflagrations and hot substances

     EXCLUDES 1   *war operations involving fires and conflagrations aboard military aircraft (Y36.1-)*

        war operations involving fires and conflagrations aboard military watercraft (Y36.0-)

        war operations involving fires and conflagrations caused indirectly by conventional weapons (Y36.2-)

        war operations involving fires and thermal effects of nuclear weapons (Y36.53-)

√6th **Y36.30**   **War operations involving unspecified fire, conflagration and hot substance**

     √7th **Y36.300**   **War operations involving unspecified fire, conflagration and hot substance, military personnel** ▽

     √7th **Y36.301**   **War operations involving unspecified fire, conflagration and hot substance, civilian** ▽

√6th **Y36.31**   **War operations involving gasoline bomb**

     War operations involving incendiary bomb

     War operations involving petrol bomb

     √7th **Y36.310**   **War operations involving gasoline bomb, military personnel**

     √7th **Y36.311**   **War operations involving gasoline bomb, civilian**

√6th **Y36.32**   **War operations involving incendiary bullet**

     √7th **Y36.320**   **War operations involving incendiary bullet, military personnel**

     √7th **Y36.321**   **War operations involving incendiary bullet, civilian**

√6th **Y36.33**   **War operations involving flamethrower**

     √7th **Y36.330**   **War operations involving flamethrower, military personnel**

     √7th **Y36.331**   **War operations involving flamethrower, civilian**

√6th **Y36.39**   **War operations involving other fires, conflagrations and hot substances**

     √7th **Y36.390**   **War operations involving other fires, conflagrations and hot substances, military personnel**

     √7th **Y36.391**   **War operations involving other fires, conflagrations and hot substances, civilian**

√5th **Y36.4**   **War operations involving firearm discharge and other forms of conventional warfare**

√6th **Y36.41**   **War operations involving rubber bullets**

     √7th **Y36.410**   **War operations involving rubber bullets, military personnel**

     √7th **Y36.411**   **War operations involving rubber bullets, civilian**

√6th **Y36.42**   **War operations involving firearms pellets**

     √7th **Y36.420**   **War operations involving firearms pellets, military personnel**

     √7th **Y36.421**   **War operations involving firearms pellets, civilian**

√6th **Y36.43**   **War operations involving other firearms discharge**

     War operations involving bullets NOS

     EXCLUDES 1   *war operations involving munitions fragments (Y36.25-)*

        war operations involving incendiary bullets (Y36.32-)

     √7th **Y36.430**   **War operations involving other firearms discharge, military personnel**

     √7th **Y36.431**   **War operations involving other firearms discharge, civilian**

√6th **Y36.44**   **War operations involving unarmed hand to hand combat**

     EXCLUDES 1   *war operations involving combat using blunt or piercing object (Y36.45-)*

        war operations involving intentional restriction of air and airway (Y36.46-)

        war operations involving unintentional restriction of air and airway (Y36.47-)

     √7th **Y36.440**   **War operations involving unarmed hand to hand combat, military personnel**

     √7th **Y36.441**   **War operations involving unarmed hand to hand combat, civilian**

√6th **Y36.45**   **War operations involving combat using blunt or piercing object**

     √7th **Y36.450**   **War operations involving combat using blunt or piercing object, military personnel**

     √7th **Y36.451**   **War operations involving combat using blunt or piercing object, civilian**

√6th **Y36.46**   **War operations involving intentional restriction of air and airway**

     √7th **Y36.460**   **War operations involving intentional restriction of air and airway, military personnel**

     √7th **Y36.461**   **War operations involving intentional restriction of air and airway, civilian**

√6th **Y36.47**   **War operations involving unintentional restriction of air and airway**

     √7th **Y36.470**   **War operations involving unintentional restriction of air and airway, military personnel**

     √7th **Y36.471**   **War operations involving unintentional restriction of air and airway, civilian**

√6th **Y36.49**   **War operations involving other forms of conventional warfare**

     √7th **Y36.490**   **War operations involving other forms of conventional warfare, military personnel**

     √7th **Y36.491**   **War operations involving other forms of conventional warfare, civilian**

√5th **Y36.5**   **War operations involving nuclear weapons**

     War operations involving dirty bomb NOS

√6th **Y36.50**   **War operations involving unspecified effect of nuclear weapon**

     √7th **Y36.500**   **War operations involving unspecified effect of nuclear weapon, military personnel** ▽

     √7th **Y36.501**   **War operations involving unspecified effect of nuclear weapon, civilian** ▽

√6th **Y36.51**   **War operations involving direct blast effect of nuclear weapon**

     War operations involving blast pressure of nuclear weapon

---

EXCLUDES 1 Not coded here   EXCLUDES 2 Not included here   **N** Newborn Age: 0   **P** Pediatric Age: 0-17   **M** Maternity Age: 12-55   **A** Adult Age: 15-124

☑7ᵗʰ **Y36.510 War operations involving direct blast effect of nuclear weapon, military personnel**

☑7ᵗʰ **Y36.511 War operations involving direct blast effect of nuclear weapon, civilian**

☑6ᵗʰ **Y36.52 War operations involving indirect blast effect of nuclear weapon**
     War operations involving being thrown by blast of nuclear weapon
     War operations involving being struck or crushed by blast debris of nuclear weapon

☑7ᵗʰ **Y36.520 War operations involving indirect blast effect of nuclear weapon, military personnel**

☑7ᵗʰ **Y36.521 War operations involving indirect blast effect of nuclear weapon, civilian**

☑6ᵗʰ **Y36.53 War operations involving thermal radiation effect of nuclear weapon**
     War operations involving direct heat from nuclear weapon
     War operation involving fireball effects from nuclear weapon

☑7ᵗʰ **Y36.530 War operations involving thermal radiation effect of nuclear weapon, military personnel**

☑7ᵗʰ **Y36.531 War operations involving thermal radiation effect of nuclear weapon, civilian**

☑6ᵗʰ **Y36.54 War operation involving nuclear radiation effects of nuclear weapon**
     War operation involving acute radiation exposure from nuclear weapon
     War operation involving exposure to immediate ionizing radiation from nuclear weapon
     War operation involving fallout exposure from nuclear weapon
     War operation involving secondary effects of nuclear weapons

☑7ᵗʰ **Y36.540 War operation involving nuclear radiation effects of nuclear weapon, military personnel**

☑7ᵗʰ **Y36.541 War operation involving nuclear radiation effects of nuclear weapon, civilian**

☑6ᵗʰ **Y36.59 War operation involving other effects of nuclear weapons**

☑7ᵗʰ **Y36.590 War operation involving other effects of nuclear weapons, military personnel**

☑7ᵗʰ **Y36.591 War operation involving other effects of nuclear weapons, civilian**

☑5ᵗʰ **Y36.6 War operations involving biological weapons**

☑6ᵗʰ **Y36.6X War operations involving biological weapons**

☑7ᵗʰ **Y36.6X0 War operations involving biological weapons, military personnel**

☑7ᵗʰ **Y36.6X1 War operations involving biological weapons, civilian**

☑5ᵗʰ **Y36.7 War operations involving chemical weapons and other forms of unconventional warfare**
     EXCLUDES 1   *war operations involving incendiary devices (Y36.3-, Y36.5-)*

☑6ᵗʰ **Y36.7X War operations involving chemical weapons and other forms of unconventional warfare**

☑7ᵗʰ **Y36.7X0 War operations involving chemical weapons and other forms of unconventional warfare, military personnel**

☑7ᵗʰ **Y36.7X1 War operations involving chemical weapons and other forms of unconventional warfare, civilian**

☑5ᵗʰ **Y36.8 War operations occurring after cessation of hostilities**
     War operations classifiable to categories Y36.0-Y36.8 but occurring after cessation of hostilities

☑6ᵗʰ **Y36.81 Explosion of mine placed during war operations but exploding after cessation of hostilities**

☑7ᵗʰ **Y36.810 Explosion of mine placed during war operations but exploding after cessation of hostilities, military personnel**

☑7ᵗʰ **Y36.811 Explosion of mine placed during war operations but exploding after cessation of hostilities, civilian**

☑6ᵗʰ **Y36.82 Explosion of bomb placed during war operations but exploding after cessation of hostilities**

☑7ᵗʰ **Y36.820 Explosion of bomb placed during war operations but exploding after cessation of hostilities, military personnel**

☑7ᵗʰ **Y36.821 Explosion of bomb placed during war operations but exploding after cessation of hostilities, civilian**

☑6ᵗʰ **Y36.88 Other war operations occurring after cessation of hostilities**

☑7ᵗʰ **Y36.880 Other war operations occurring after cessation of hostilities, military personnel**

☑7ᵗʰ **Y36.881 Other war operations occurring after cessation of hostilities, civilian**

☑6ᵗʰ **Y36.89 Unspecified war operations occurring after cessation of hostilities**

☑7ᵗʰ **Y36.890 Unspecified war operations occurring after cessation of hostilities, military personnel** ▽

☑7ᵗʰ **Y36.891 Unspecified war operations occurring after cessation of hostilities, civilian** ▽

☑5ᵗʰ **Y36.9 Other and unspecified war operations**

☑×7ᵗʰ **Y36.90 War operations, unspecified** ▽

☑×7ᵗʰ **Y36.91 War operations involving unspecified weapon of mass destruction [WMD]** ▽

☑×7ᵗʰ **Y36.92 War operations involving friendly fire**

☑4ᵗʰ **Y37 Military operations**
     INCLUDES   injuries to military personnel and civilians occurring during peacetime on military property and during routine military exercises and operations
     EXCLUDES 1   *military aircraft involved in aircraft accident with civilian aircraft (V97.81-)*
         military vehicles involved in transport accident with civilian vehicle (V09.01, V09.21, V19.81, V29.81, V39.81, V49.81, V59.81, V69.81, V79.81)
         military watercraft involved in water transport accident with civilian watercraft (V94.81-)
         war operations (Y36.-)

☑5ᵗʰ **Y37.0 Military operations involving explosion of marine weapons**

☑6ᵗʰ **Y37.00 Military operations involving explosion of unspecified marine weapon**
     Military operations involving underwater blast NOS

☑7ᵗʰ **Y37.000 Military operations involving explosion ▽ of unspecified marine weapon, military personnel**

☑7ᵗʰ **Y37.001 Military operations involving explosion ▽ of unspecified marine weapon, civilian**

☑6ᵗʰ **Y37.01 Military operations involving explosion of depth-charge**

☑7ᵗʰ **Y37.010 Military operations involving explosion of depth-charge, military personnel**

☑7ᵗʰ **Y37.011 Military operations involving explosion of depth-charge, civilian**

☑6ᵗʰ **Y37.02 Military operations involving explosion of marine mine**
     Military operations involving explosion of marine mine, at sea or in harbor

☑7ᵗʰ **Y37.020 Military operations involving explosion of marine mine, military personnel**

☑7ᵗʰ **Y37.021 Military operations involving explosion of marine mine, civilian**

☑6ᵗʰ **Y37.03 Military operations involving explosion of sea-based artillery shell**

☑7ᵗʰ **Y37.030 Military operations involving explosion of sea-based artillery shell, military personnel**

☑7ᵗʰ **Y37.031 Military operations involving explosion of sea-based artillery shell, civilian**

☑6ᵗʰ **Y37.04 Military operations involving explosion of torpedo**

☑7ᵗʰ **Y37.040 Military operations involving explosion of torpedo, military personnel**

☑7ᵗʰ **Y37.041 Military operations involving explosion of torpedo, civilian**

☑ Additional Character Req   ☑×7ᵗʰ Placeholder Alert   Manifestation   HCC CMS-HCC Condition   ▽ Unspecified Code   ►◄ Revised Text   ● New Code   ▲ Revised Code Title

ICD-10-CM 2018   1161

Chapter 20. External Causes of Morbidity

Y36.510–Y37.041

Chapter 20. External Causes of Morbidity

Y37.05–Y37.261

√6ᵗʰ **Y37.05**   **Military operations involving accidental detonation of onboard marine weapons**

  √7ᵗʰ **Y37.050**   **Military operations involving accidental detonation of onboard marine weapons, military personnel**

  √7ᵗʰ **Y37.051**   **Military operations involving accidental detonation of onboard marine weapons, civilian**

√6ᵗʰ **Y37.09**   **Military operations involving explosion of other marine weapons**

  √7ᵗʰ **Y37.090**   **Military operations involving explosion of other marine weapons, military personnel**

  √7ᵗʰ **Y37.091**   **Military operations involving explosion of other marine weapons, civilian**

√5ᵗʰ **Y37.1**   **Military operations involving destruction of aircraft**

√6ᵗʰ **Y37.10**   **Military operations involving unspecified destruction of aircraft**

  √7ᵗʰ **Y37.100**   **Military operations involving unspecified destruction of aircraft, military personnel**   ▽

  √7ᵗʰ **Y37.101**   **Military operations involving unspecified destruction of aircraft, civilian**   ▽

√6ᵗʰ **Y37.11**   **Military operations involving destruction of aircraft due to enemy fire or explosives**

   Military operations involving destruction of aircraft due to air to air missile

   Military operations involving destruction of aircraft due to explosive placed on aircraft

   Military operations involving destruction of aircraft due to rocket propelled grenade [RPG]

   Military operations involving destruction of aircraft due to small arms fire

   Military operations involving destruction of aircraft due to surface to air missile

  √7ᵗʰ **Y37.110**   **Military operations involving destruction of aircraft due to enemy fire or explosives, military personnel**

  √7ᵗʰ **Y37.111**   **Military operations involving destruction of aircraft due to enemy fire or explosives, civilian**

√6ᵗʰ **Y37.12**   **Military operations involving destruction of aircraft due to collision with other aircraft**

  √7ᵗʰ **Y37.120**   **Military operations involving destruction of aircraft due to collision with other aircraft, military personnel**

  √7ᵗʰ **Y37.121**   **Military operations involving destruction of aircraft due to collision with other aircraft, civilian**

√6ᵗʰ **Y37.13**   **Military operations involving destruction of aircraft due to onboard fire**

  √7ᵗʰ **Y37.130**   **Military operations involving destruction of aircraft due to onboard fire, military personnel**

  √7ᵗʰ **Y37.131**   **Military operations involving destruction of aircraft due to onboard fire, civilian**

√6ᵗʰ **Y37.14**   **Military operations involving destruction of aircraft due to accidental detonation of onboard munitions and explosives**

  √7ᵗʰ **Y37.140**   **Military operations involving destruction of aircraft due to accidental detonation of onboard munitions and explosives, military personnel**

  √7ᵗʰ **Y37.141**   **Military operations involving destruction of aircraft due to accidental detonation of onboard munitions and explosives, civilian**

√6ᵗʰ **Y37.19**   **Military operations involving other destruction of aircraft**

  √7ᵗʰ **Y37.190**   **Military operations involving other destruction of aircraft, military personnel**

  √7ᵗʰ **Y37.191**   **Military operations involving other destruction of aircraft, civilian**

√5ᵗʰ **Y37.2**   **Military operations involving other explosions and fragments**

   EXCLUDES 1   *military operations involving explosion of aircraft (Y37.1-)*

    military operations involving explosion of marine weapons (Y37.0-)

    military operations involving explosion of nuclear weapons (Y37.5-)

√6ᵗʰ **Y37.20**   **Military operations involving unspecified explosion and fragments**

   Military operations involving air blast NOS

   Military operations involving blast NOS

   Military operations involving blast fragments NOS

   Military operations involving blast wave NOS

   Military operations involving blast wind NOS

   Military operations involving explosion NOS

   Military operations involving explosion of bomb NOS

  √7ᵗʰ **Y37.200**   **Military operations involving unspecified explosion and fragments, military personnel**   ▽

  √7ᵗʰ **Y37.201**   **Military operations involving unspecified explosion and fragments, civilian**   ▽

√6ᵗʰ **Y37.21**   **Military operations involving explosion of aerial bomb**

  √7ᵗʰ **Y37.210**   **Military operations involving explosion of aerial bomb, military personnel**

  √7ᵗʰ **Y37.211**   **Military operations involving explosion of aerial bomb, civilian**

√6ᵗʰ **Y37.22**   **Military operations involving explosion of guided missile**

  √7ᵗʰ **Y37.220**   **Military operations involving explosion of guided missile, military personnel**

  √7ᵗʰ **Y37.221**   **Military operations involving explosion of guided missile, civilian**

√6ᵗʰ **Y37.23**   **Military operations involving explosion of improvised explosive device [IED]**

   Military operations involving explosion of person-borne improvised explosive device [IED]

   Military operations involving explosion of vehicle-borne improvised explosive device [IED]

   Military operations involving explosion of roadside improvised explosive device [IED]

  √7ᵗʰ **Y37.230**   **Military operations involving explosion of improvised explosive device [IED], military personnel**

  √7ᵗʰ **Y37.231**   **Military operations involving explosion of improvised explosive device [IED], civilian**

√6ᵗʰ **Y37.24**   **Military operations involving explosion due to accidental detonation and discharge of own munitions or munitions launch device**

  √7ᵗʰ **Y37.240**   **Military operations involving explosion due to accidental detonation and discharge of own munitions or munitions launch device, military personnel**

  √7ᵗʰ **Y37.241**   **Military operations involving explosion due to accidental detonation and discharge of own munitions or munitions launch device, civilian**

√6ᵗʰ **Y37.25**   **Military operations involving fragments from munitions**

  √7ᵗʰ **Y37.250**   **Military operations involving fragments from munitions, military personnel**

  √7ᵗʰ **Y37.251**   **Military operations involving fragments from munitions, civilian**

√6ᵗʰ **Y37.26**   **Military operations involving fragments of improvised explosive device [IED]**

   Military operations involving fragments of person-borne improvised explosive device [IED]

   Military operations involving fragments of vehicle-borne improvised explosive device [IED]

   Military operations involving fragments of roadside improvised explosive device [IED]

  √7ᵗʰ **Y37.260**   **Military operations involving fragments of improvised explosive device [IED], military personnel**

  √7ᵗʰ **Y37.261**   **Military operations involving fragments of improvised explosive device [IED], civilian**

EXCLUDES 1 Not coded here   EXCLUDES 2 Not included here   N Newborn Age: 0   P Pediatric Age: 0-17   M Maternity Age: 12-55   A Adult Age: 15-124

1162   ICD-10-CM 2018

☑6ᵗʰ **Y37.27** Military operations involving **fragments from weapons**

    ☑7ᵗʰ **Y37.270** Military operations involving fragments from weapons, **military personnel**

    ☑7ᵗʰ **Y37.271** Military operations involving fragments from weapons, **civilian**

☑6ᵗʰ **Y37.29** Military operations involving **other explosions and fragments**

    Military operations involving explosion of grenade
    Military operations involving explosions of land mine
    Military operations involving shrapnel NOS

    ☑7ᵗʰ **Y37.290** Military operations involving other explosions and fragments, **military personnel**

    ☑7ᵗʰ **Y37.291** Military operations involving other explosions and fragments, **civilian**

☑5ᵗʰ **Y37.3** Military operations involving **fires, conflagrations and hot substances**

    Military operations involving smoke, fumes, and heat from fires, conflagrations and hot substances

    EXCLUDES 1   *military operations involving fires and conflagrations aboard military aircraft (Y37.1-)*
    military operations involving fires and conflagrations aboard military watercraft (Y37.0-)
    military operations involving fires and conflagrations caused indirectly by conventional weapons (Y37.2-)
    military operations involving fires and thermal effects of nuclear weapons (Y36.53-)

    ☑6ᵗʰ **Y37.30** Military operations involving **unspecified fire, conflagration and hot substance**

        ☑7ᵗʰ **Y37.300** Military operations involving unspecified fire, conflagration and hot substance, **military personnel** ▽

        ☑7ᵗʰ **Y37.301** Military operations involving unspecified fire, conflagration and hot substance, **civilian** ▽

    ☑6ᵗʰ **Y37.31** Military operations involving **gasoline bomb**

        Military operations involving incendiary bomb
        Military operations involving petrol bomb

        ☑7ᵗʰ **Y37.310** Military operations involving gasoline bomb, **military personnel**

        ☑7ᵗʰ **Y37.311** Military operations involving gasoline bomb, **civilian**

    ☑6ᵗʰ **Y37.32** Military operations involving **incendiary bullet**

        ☑7ᵗʰ **Y37.320** Military operations involving incendiary bullet, **military personnel**

        ☑7ᵗʰ **Y37.321** Military operations involving incendiary bullet, **civilian**

    ☑6ᵗʰ **Y37.33** Military operations involving **flamethrower**

        ☑7ᵗʰ **Y37.330** Military operations involving flamethrower, **military personnel**

        ☑7ᵗʰ **Y37.331** Military operations involving flamethrower, **civilian**

    ☑6ᵗʰ **Y37.39** Military operations involving **other fires, conflagrations and hot substances**

        ☑7ᵗʰ **Y37.390** Military operations involving other fires, conflagrations and hot substances, **military personnel**

        ☑7ᵗʰ **Y37.391** Military operations involving other fires, conflagrations and hot substances, **civilian**

☑5ᵗʰ **Y37.4** Military operations involving **firearm discharge and other forms of conventional warfare**

    ☑6ᵗʰ **Y37.41** Military operations involving **rubber bullets**

        ☑7ᵗʰ **Y37.410** Military operations involving rubber bullets, **military personnel**

        ☑7ᵗʰ **Y37.411** Military operations involving rubber bullets, **civilian**

    ☑6ᵗʰ **Y37.42** Military operations involving **firearms pellets**

        ☑7ᵗʰ **Y37.420** Military operations involving firearms pellets, **military personnel**

        ☑7ᵗʰ **Y37.421** Military operations involving firearms pellets, **civilian**

☑6ᵗʰ **Y37.43** Military operations involving **other firearms discharge**

    Military operations involving bullets NOS

    EXCLUDES 1   *military operations involving munitions fragments (Y37.25-)*
    military operations involving incendiary bullets (Y37.32-)

    ☑7ᵗʰ **Y37.430** Military operations involving other firearms discharge, **military personnel**

    ☑7ᵗʰ **Y37.431** Military operations involving other firearms discharge, **civilian**

☑6ᵗʰ **Y37.44** Military operations involving **unarmed hand to hand combat**

    EXCLUDES 1   *military operations involving combat using blunt or piercing object (Y37.45-)*
    military operations involving intentional restriction of air and airway (Y37.46-)
    military operations involving unintentional restriction of air and airway (Y37.47-)

    ☑7ᵗʰ **Y37.440** Military operations involving unarmed hand to hand combat, **military personnel**

    ☑7ᵗʰ **Y37.441** Military operations involving unarmed hand to hand combat, **civilian**

☑6ᵗʰ **Y37.45** Military operations involving **combat using blunt or piercing object**

    ☑7ᵗʰ **Y37.450** Military operations involving combat using blunt or piercing object, **military personnel**

    ☑7ᵗʰ **Y37.451** Military operations involving combat using blunt or piercing object, **civilian**

☑6ᵗʰ **Y37.46** Military operations involving **intentional restriction of air and airway**

    ☑7ᵗʰ **Y37.460** Military operations involving intentional restriction of air and airway, **military personnel**

    ☑7ᵗʰ **Y37.461** Military operations involving intentional restriction of air and airway, **civilian**

☑6ᵗʰ **Y37.47** Military operations involving **unintentional restriction of air and airway**

    ☑7ᵗʰ **Y37.470** Military operations involving unintentional restriction of air and airway, **military personnel**

    ☑7ᵗʰ **Y37.471** Military operations involving unintentional restriction of air and airway, **civilian**

☑6ᵗʰ **Y37.49** Military operations involving **other forms of conventional warfare**

    ☑7ᵗʰ **Y37.490** Military operations involving other forms of conventional warfare, **military personnel**

    ☑7ᵗʰ **Y37.491** Military operations involving other forms of conventional warfare, **civilian**

☑5ᵗʰ **Y37.5** Military operations involving **nuclear weapons**

    Military operation involving dirty bomb NOS

    ☑6ᵗʰ **Y37.50** Military operations involving **unspecified effect of nuclear weapon**

        ☑7ᵗʰ **Y37.500** Military operations involving unspecified effect of nuclear weapon, **military personnel** ▽

        ☑7ᵗʰ **Y37.501** Military operations involving unspecified effect of nuclear weapon, **civilian** ▽

    ☑6ᵗʰ **Y37.51** Military operations involving **direct blast effect of nuclear weapon**

        Military operations involving blast pressure of nuclear weapon

        ☑7ᵗʰ **Y37.510** Military operations involving direct blast effect of nuclear weapon, **military personnel**

        ☑7ᵗʰ **Y37.511** Military operations involving direct blast effect of nuclear weapon, **civilian**

☑ Additional Character Req   ☑x7ᵗʰ Placeholder Alert   Manifestation   HCC CMS-HCC Condition   ▽ Unspecified Code   ►◄ Revised Text   ● New Code   ▲ Revised Code Title

ICD-10-CM 2018   1163

✓6ᵗʰ **Y37.52 Military operations involving indirect blast effect of nuclear weapon**
Military operations involving being thrown by blast of nuclear weapon
Military operations involving being struck or crushed by blast debris of nuclear weapon

     ✓7ᵗʰ **Y37.520 Military operations involving indirect blast effect of nuclear weapon, military personnel**

     ✓7ᵗʰ **Y37.521 Military operations involving indirect blast effect of nuclear weapon, civilian**

✓6ᵗʰ **Y37.53 Military operations involving thermal radiation effect of nuclear weapon**
Military operations involving direct heat from nuclear weapon
Military operation involving fireball effects from nuclear weapon

     ✓7ᵗʰ **Y37.530 Military operations involving thermal radiation effect of nuclear weapon, military personnel**

     ✓7ᵗʰ **Y37.531 Military operations involving thermal radiation effect of nuclear weapon, civilian**

✓6ᵗʰ **Y37.54 Military operation involving nuclear radiation effects of nuclear weapon**
Military operation involving acute radiation exposure from nuclear weapon
Military operation involving exposure to immediate ionizing radiation from nuclear weapon
Military operation involving fallout exposure from nuclear weapon
Military operation involving secondary effects of nuclear weapons

     ✓7ᵗʰ **Y37.540 Military operation involving nuclear radiation effects of nuclear weapon, military personnel**

     ✓7ᵗʰ **Y37.541 Military operation involving nuclear radiation effects of nuclear weapon, civilian**

✓6ᵗʰ **Y37.59 Military operation involving other effects of nuclear weapons**

     ✓7ᵗʰ **Y37.590 Military operation involving other effects of nuclear weapons, military personnel**

     ✓7ᵗʰ **Y37.591 Military operation involving other effects of nuclear weapons, civilian**

✓5ᵗʰ **Y37.6 Military operations involving biological weapons**

     ✓6ᵗʰ **Y37.6X Military operations involving biological weapons**

         ✓7ᵗʰ **Y37.6X0 Military operations involving biological weapons, military personnel**

         ✓7ᵗʰ **Y37.6X1 Military operations involving biological weapons, civilian**

✓5ᵗʰ **Y37.7 Military operations involving chemical weapons and other forms of unconventional warfare**
EXCLUDES 1   *military operations involving incendiary devices (Y36.3-, Y36.5-)*

     ✓6ᵗʰ **Y37.7X Military operations involving chemical weapons and other forms of unconventional warfare**

         ✓7ᵗʰ **Y37.7X0 Military operations involving chemical weapons and other forms of unconventional warfare, military personnel**

         ✓7ᵗʰ **Y37.7X1 Military operations involving chemical weapons and other forms of unconventional warfare, civilian**

✓5ᵗʰ **Y37.9 Other and unspecified military operations**

     ✓x7ᵗʰ **Y37.90 Military operations, unspecified**   ▽

     ✓x7ᵗʰ **Y37.91 Military operations involving unspecified weapon of mass destruction [WMD]**   ▽

     ✓x7ᵗʰ **Y37.92 Military operations involving friendly fire**

✓4ᵗʰ **Y38 Terrorism**
NOTE These codes are for use to identify injuries resulting from the unlawful use of force or violence against persons or property to intimidate or coerce a Government, the civilian population, or any segment thereof, in furtherance of political or social objective.
Use additional code for place of occurrence (Y92.-)

✓5ᵗʰ **Y38.0 Terrorism involving explosion of marine weapons**
Terrorism involving depth-charge
Terrorism involving marine mine
Terrorism involving mine NOS, at sea or in harbor
Terrorism involving sea-based artillery shell
Terrorism involving torpedo
Terrorism involving underwater blast

     ✓6ᵗʰ **Y38.0X Terrorism involving explosion of marine weapons**

         ✓7ᵗʰ **Y38.0X1 Terrorism involving explosion of marine weapons, public safety official injured**

         ✓7ᵗʰ **Y38.0X2 Terrorism involving explosion of marine weapons, civilian injured**

         ✓7ᵗʰ **Y38.0X3 Terrorism involving explosion of marine weapons, terrorist injured**

✓5ᵗʰ **Y38.1 Terrorism involving destruction of aircraft**
Terrorism involving aircraft burned
Terrorism involving aircraft exploded
Terrorism involving aircraft being shot down
Terrorism involving aircraft used as a weapon

     ✓6ᵗʰ **Y38.1X Terrorism involving destruction of aircraft**

         ✓7ᵗʰ **Y38.1X1 Terrorism involving destruction of aircraft, public safety official injured**

         ✓7ᵗʰ **Y38.1X2 Terrorism involving destruction of aircraft, civilian injured**

         ✓7ᵗʰ **Y38.1X3 Terrorism involving destruction of aircraft, terrorist injured**

✓5ᵗʰ **Y38.2 Terrorism involving other explosions and fragments**
Terrorism involving antipersonnel (fragments) bomb
Terrorism involving blast NOS
Terrorism involving explosion NOS
Terrorism involving explosion of breech block
Terrorism involving explosion of cannon block
Terrorism involving explosion (fragments) of artillery shell
Terrorism involving explosion (fragments) of bomb
Terrorism involving explosion (fragments) of grenade
Terrorism involving explosion (fragments) of guided missile
Terrorism involving explosion (fragments) of land mine
Terrorism involving explosion of mortar bomb
Terrorism involving explosion of munitions
Terrorism involving explosion (fragments) of rocket
Terrorism involving explosion (fragments) of shell
Terrorism involving shrapnel
Terrorism involving mine NOS, on land
EXCLUDES 1   *terrorism involving explosion of nuclear weapon (Y38.5)*
             terrorism involving suicide bomber (Y38.81)

     ✓6ᵗʰ **Y38.2X Terrorism involving other explosions and fragments**

         ✓7ᵗʰ **Y38.2X1 Terrorism involving other explosions and fragments, public safety official injured**

         ✓7ᵗʰ **Y38.2X2 Terrorism involving other explosions and fragments, civilian injured**

         ✓7ᵗʰ **Y38.2X3 Terrorism involving other explosions and fragments, terrorist injured**

✓5ᵗʰ **Y38.3 Terrorism involving fires, conflagration and hot substances**
Terrorism involving conflagration NOS
Terrorism involving fire NOS
Terrorism involving petrol bomb
EXCLUDES 1   *terrorism involving fire or heat of nuclear weapon (Y38.5)*

     ✓6ᵗʰ **Y38.3X Terrorism involving fires, conflagration and hot substances**

         ✓7ᵗʰ **Y38.3X1 Terrorism involving fires, conflagration and hot substances, public safety official injured**

         ✓7ᵗʰ **Y38.3X2 Terrorism involving fires, conflagration and hot substances, civilian injured**

         ✓7ᵗʰ **Y38.3X3 Terrorism involving fires, conflagration and hot substances, terrorist injured**

✓5ᵗʰ **Y38.4 Terrorism involving firearms**
Terrorism involving carbine bullet
Terrorism involving machine gun bullet
Terrorism involving pellets (shotgun)
Terrorism involving pistol bullet
Terrorism involving rifle bullet
Terrorism involving rubber (rifle) bullet

✓6ᵗʰ **Y38.4X Terrorism involving firearms**

✓7ᵗʰ **Y38.4X1 Terrorism involving firearms, public safety official injured**

✓7ᵗʰ **Y38.4X2 Terrorism involving firearms, civilian injured**

✓7ᵗʰ **Y38.4X3 Terrorism involving firearms, terrorist injured**

✓5ᵗʰ **Y38.5 Terrorism involving nuclear weapons**
Terrorism involving blast effects of nuclear weapon
Terrorism involving exposure to ionizing radiation from nuclear weapon
Terrorism involving fireball effect of nuclear weapon
Terrorism involving heat from nuclear weapon

✓6ᵗʰ **Y38.5X Terrorism involving nuclear weapons**

✓7ᵗʰ **Y38.5X1 Terrorism involving nuclear weapons, public safety official injured**

✓7ᵗʰ **Y38.5X2 Terrorism involving nuclear weapons, civilian injured**

✓7ᵗʰ **Y38.5X3 Terrorism involving nuclear weapons, terrorist injured**

✓5ᵗʰ **Y38.6 Terrorism involving biological weapons**
Terrorism involving anthrax
Terrorism involving cholera
Terrorism involving smallpox

✓6ᵗʰ **Y38.6X Terrorism involving biological weapons**

✓7ᵗʰ **Y38.6X1 Terrorism involving biological weapons, public safety official injured**

✓7ᵗʰ **Y38.6X2 Terrorism involving biological weapons, civilian injured**

✓7ᵗʰ **Y38.6X3 Terrorism involving biological weapons, terrorist injured**

✓5ᵗʰ **Y38.7 Terrorism involving chemical weapons**
Terrorism involving gases, fumes, chemicals
Terrorism involving hydrogen cyanide
Terrorism involving phosgene
Terrorism involving sarin

✓6ᵗʰ **Y38.7X Terrorism involving chemical weapons**

✓7ᵗʰ **Y38.7X1 Terrorism involving chemical weapons, public safety official injured**

✓7ᵗʰ **Y38.7X2 Terrorism involving chemical weapons, civilian injured**

✓7ᵗʰ **Y38.7X3 Terrorism involving chemical weapons, terrorist injured**

✓5ᵗʰ **Y38.8 Terrorism involving other and unspecified means**

✓✗7ᵗʰ **Y38.80 Terrorism involving unspecified means** ▽
Terrorism NOS

✓6ᵗʰ **Y38.81 Terrorism involving suicide bomber**

✓7ᵗʰ **Y38.811 Terrorism involving suicide bomber, public safety official injured**

✓7ᵗʰ **Y38.812 Terrorism involving suicide bomber, civilian injured**

✓6ᵗʰ **Y38.89 Terrorism involving other means**
Terrorism involving drowning and submersion
Terrorism involving lasers
Terrorism involving piercing or stabbing instruments

✓7ᵗʰ **Y38.891 Terrorism involving other means, public safety official injured**

✓7ᵗʰ **Y38.892 Terrorism involving other means, civilian injured**

✓7ᵗʰ **Y38.893 Terrorism involving other means, terrorist injured**

✓5ᵗʰ **Y38.9 Terrorism, secondary effects**
NOTE This code is for use to identify injuries occurring subsequent to a terrorist attack, not those that are due to the initial terrorist attack.

✓6ᵗʰ **Y38.9X Terrorism, secondary effects**

✓7ᵗʰ **Y38.9X1 Terrorism, secondary effects, public safety official injured**

✓7ᵗʰ **Y38.9X2 Terrorism, secondary effects, civilian injured**

Complications of medical and surgical care (Y62-Y84)

INCLUDES complications of medical devices
surgical and medical procedures as the cause of abnormal reaction of the patient, or of later complication, without mention of misadventure at the time of the procedure

Misadventures to patients during surgical and medical care (Y62-Y69)

EXCLUDES 1 surgical and medical procedures as the cause of abnormal reaction of the patient, without mention of misadventure at the time of the procedure (Y83-Y84)
EXCLUDES 2 breakdown or malfunctioning of medical device (during procedure) (after implantation) (ongoing use) (Y70-Y82)

✓4ᵗʰ **Y62 Failure of sterile precautions during surgical and medical care**

Y62.0 Failure of sterile precautions during surgical operation

Y62.1 Failure of sterile precautions during infusion or transfusion

Y62.2 Failure of sterile precautions during kidney dialysis and other perfusion **HCC**

Y62.3 Failure of sterile precautions during injection or immunization

Y62.4 Failure of sterile precautions during endoscopic examination

Y62.5 Failure of sterile precautions during heart catheterization

Y62.6 Failure of sterile precautions during aspiration, puncture and other catheterization

Y62.8 Failure of sterile precautions during other surgical and medical care

Y62.9 Failure of sterile precautions during unspecified surgical and medical care ▽

✓4ᵗʰ **Y63 Failure in dosage during surgical and medical care**
EXCLUDES 2 accidental overdose of drug or wrong drug given in error (T36-T50)

Y63.0 Excessive amount of blood or other fluid given during transfusion or infusion

Y63.1 Incorrect dilution of fluid used during infusion

Y63.2 Overdose of radiation given during therapy

Y63.3 Inadvertent exposure of patient to radiation during medical care

Y63.4 Failure in dosage in electroshock or insulin-shock therapy

Y63.5 Inappropriate temperature in local application and packing

Y63.6 Underdosing and nonadministration of necessary drug, medicament or biological substance

Y63.8 Failure in dosage during other surgical and medical care

Y63.9 Failure in dosage during unspecified surgical and medical care ▽

✓4ᵗʰ **Y64 Contaminated medical or biological substances**

Y64.0 Contaminated medical or biological substance, transfused or infused

Y64.1 Contaminated medical or biological substance, injected or used for immunization

Y64.8 Contaminated medical or biological substance administered by other means

Y64.9 Contaminated medical or biological substance administered by unspecified means ▽
Administered contaminated medical or biological substance NOS

✓4ᵗʰ **Y65 Other misadventures during surgical and medical care**

Y65.0 Mismatched blood in transfusion

Y65.1 Wrong fluid used in infusion

Y65.2 Failure in suture or ligature during surgical operation

Y65.3 Endotracheal tube wrongly placed during anesthetic procedure

Y65.4 Failure to introduce or to remove other tube or instrument

✓5ᵗʰ **Y65.5 Performance of wrong procedure (operation)**

Y65.51 Performance of wrong procedure (operation) on correct patient
Wrong device implanted into correct surgical site
EXCLUDES 1 performance of correct procedure (operation) on wrong side or body part (Y65.53)

✓ Additional Character Req   ✓✗7ᵗʰ Placeholder Alert   Manifestation   **HCC** CMS-HCC Condition   ▽ Unspecified Code   ►◄ Revised Text   ● New Code   ▲ Revised Code Title

Y65.52 Performance of procedure (operation) on patient not scheduled for surgery
Performance of procedure (operation) intended for another patient
Performance of procedure (operation) on wrong patient

Y65.53 Performance of correct procedure (operation) on wrong side or body part
Performance of correct procedure (operation) on wrong side
Performance of correct procedure (operation) on wrong site

Y65.8 Other specified misadventures during surgical and medical care

Y66 Nonadministration of surgical and medical care
Premature cessation of surgical and medical care
EXCLUDES 1   DNR status (Z66)
     palliative care (Z51.5)

Y69 Unspecified misadventure during surgical and medical care ▽

Medical devices associated with adverse incidents in diagnostic and therapeutic use (Y70-Y82)

INCLUDES   breakdown or malfunction of medical devices (during use) (after implantation) (ongoing use)
EXCLUDES 2   breakdown or malfunctioning of medical device (after implantation) (during procedure) (ongoing use) (Y70-Y82)
     later complications following use of medical devices without breakdown or malfunctioning of device (Y83-Y84)
     misadventure to patients during surgical and medical care, classifiable to (Y62-Y69)
     surgical and other medical procedures as the cause of abnormal reaction of the patient, or of later complication, without mention of misadventure at the time of the procedure (Y83-Y84)

✓4ᵗʰ Y70 Anesthesiology devices associated with adverse incidents

Y70.0 Diagnostic and monitoring anesthesiology devices associated with adverse incidents

Y70.1 Therapeutic (nonsurgical) and rehabilitative anesthesiology devices associated with adverse incidents

Y70.2 Prosthetic and other implants, materials and accessory anesthesiology devices associated with adverse incidents

Y70.3 Surgical instruments, materials and anesthesiology devices (including sutures) associated with adverse incidents

Y70.8 Miscellaneous anesthesiology devices associated with adverse incidents, not elsewhere classified

✓4ᵗʰ Y71 Cardiovascular devices associated with adverse incidents

Y71.0 Diagnostic and monitoring cardiovascular devices associated with adverse incidents

Y71.1 Therapeutic (nonsurgical) and rehabilitative cardiovascular devices associated with adverse incidents

Y71.2 Prosthetic and other implants, materials and accessory cardiovascular devices associated with adverse incidents

Y71.3 Surgical instruments, materials and cardiovascular devices (including sutures) associated with adverse incidents

Y71.8 Miscellaneous cardiovascular devices associated with adverse incidents, not elsewhere classified

✓4ᵗʰ Y72 Otorhinolaryngological devices associated with adverse incidents

Y72.0 Diagnostic and monitoring otorhinolaryngological devices associated with adverse incidents

Y72.1 Therapeutic (nonsurgical) and rehabilitative otorhinolaryngological devices associated with adverse incidents

Y72.2 Prosthetic and other implants, materials and accessory otorhinolaryngological devices associated with adverse incidents

Y72.3 Surgical instruments, materials and otorhinolaryngological devices (including sutures) associated with adverse incidents

Y72.8 Miscellaneous otorhinolaryngological devices associated with adverse incidents, not elsewhere classified

✓4ᵗʰ Y73 Gastroenterology and urology devices associated with adverse incidents

Y73.0 Diagnostic and monitoring gastroenterology and urology devices associated with adverse incidents

Y73.1 Therapeutic (nonsurgical) and rehabilitative gastroenterology and urology devices associated with adverse incidents

Y73.2 Prosthetic and other implants, materials and accessory gastroenterology and urology devices associated with adverse incidents

Y73.3 Surgical instruments, materials and gastroenterology and urology devices (including sutures) associated with adverse incidents

Y73.8 Miscellaneous gastroenterology and urology devices associated with adverse incidents, not elsewhere classified

✓4ᵗʰ Y74 General hospital and personal-use devices associated with adverse incidents

Y74.0 Diagnostic and monitoring general hospital and personal-use devices associated with adverse incidents

Y74.1 Therapeutic (nonsurgical) and rehabilitative general hospital and personal-use devices associated with adverse incidents

Y74.2 Prosthetic and other implants, materials and accessory general hospital and personal-use devices associated with adverse incidents

Y74.3 Surgical instruments, materials and general hospital and personal-use devices (including sutures) associated with adverse incidents

Y74.8 Miscellaneous general hospital and personal-use devices associated with adverse incidents, not elsewhere classified

✓4ᵗʰ Y75 Neurological devices associated with adverse incidents

Y75.0 Diagnostic and monitoring neurological devices associated with adverse incidents

Y75.1 Therapeutic (nonsurgical) and rehabilitative neurological devices associated with adverse incidents

Y75.2 Prosthetic and other implants, materials and neurological devices associated with adverse incidents

Y75.3 Surgical instruments, materials and neurological devices (including sutures) associated with adverse incidents

Y75.8 Miscellaneous neurological devices associated with adverse incidents, not elsewhere classified

✓4ᵗʰ Y76 Obstetric and gynecological devices associated with adverse incidents

Y76.0 Diagnostic and monitoring obstetric and gynecological devices associated with adverse incidents ♀

Y76.1 Therapeutic (nonsurgical) and rehabilitative obstetric and gynecological devices associated with adverse incidents ♀

Y76.2 Prosthetic and other implants, materials and accessory obstetric and gynecological devices associated with adverse incidents ♀

Y76.3 Surgical instruments, materials and obstetric and gynecological devices (including sutures) associated with adverse incidents ♀

Y76.8 Miscellaneous obstetric and gynecological devices associated with adverse incidents, not elsewhere classified ♀

✓4ᵗʰ Y77 Ophthalmic devices associated with adverse incidents

Y77.0 Diagnostic and monitoring ophthalmic devices associated with adverse incidents

Y77.1 Therapeutic (nonsurgical) and rehabilitative ophthalmic devices associated with adverse incidents

Y77.2 Prosthetic and other implants, materials and accessory ophthalmic devices associated with adverse incidents

Y77.3 Surgical instruments, materials and ophthalmic devices (including sutures) associated with adverse incidents

Y77.8 Miscellaneous ophthalmic devices associated with adverse incidents, not elsewhere classified

✓4ᵗʰ Y78 Radiological devices associated with adverse incidents

Y78.0 Diagnostic and monitoring radiological devices associated with adverse incidents

Y78.1 Therapeutic (nonsurgical) and rehabilitative radiological devices associated with adverse incidents

Y78.2 Prosthetic and other implants, materials and accessory radiological devices associated with adverse incidents

Y78.3 Surgical instruments, materials and radiological devices (including sutures) associated with adverse incidents

Y78.8 Miscellaneous radiological devices associated with adverse incidents, not elsewhere classified

✓4ᵗʰ Y79 Orthopedic devices associated with adverse incidents

Y79.0 Diagnostic and monitoring orthopedic devices associated with adverse incidents

Y79.1 Therapeutic (nonsurgical) and rehabilitative orthopedic devices associated with adverse incidents

Y79.2 Prosthetic and other implants, materials and accessory orthopedic devices associated with adverse incidents

EXCLUDES 1 Not coded here   *EXCLUDES 2* Not included here   **N** Newborn Age: 0   **P** Pediatric Age: 0-17   **M** Maternity Age: 12-55   **A** Adult Age: 15-124

1166   ICD-10-CM 2018

Y79.3   **Surgical instruments, materials and orthopedic devices** (including sutures) associated with adverse incidents

Y79.8   **Miscellaneous orthopedic devices** associated with adverse incidents, not elsewhere classified

✓4ᵗʰ Y80   Physical medicine devices associated with adverse incidents

Y80.0   **Diagnostic and monitoring** physical medicine devices associated with adverse incidents

Y80.1   **Therapeutic (nonsurgical) and rehabilitative** physical medicine devices associated with adverse incidents

Y80.2   **Prosthetic and other implants,** materials and accessory physical medicine devices associated with adverse incidents

Y80.3   **Surgical instruments, materials** and physical medicine devices (including sutures) associated with adverse incidents

Y80.8   **Miscellaneous physical medicine devices** associated with adverse incidents, not elsewhere classified

✓4ᵗʰ Y81   General- and plastic-surgery devices associated with adverse incidents

Y81.0   **Diagnostic and monitoring** general- and plastic-surgery devices associated with adverse incidents

Y81.1   **Therapeutic (nonsurgical) and rehabilitative** general- and plastic-surgery devices associated with adverse incidents

Y81.2   **Prosthetic and other implants,** materials and accessory general- and plastic-surgery devices associated with adverse incidents

Y81.3   **Surgical instruments, materials** and general- and plastic-surgery devices (including sutures) associated with adverse incidents

Y81.8   **Miscellaneous general- and plastic-surgery devices** associated with adverse incidents, not elsewhere classified

✓4ᵗʰ Y82   Other and unspecified medical devices associated with adverse incidents

Y82.8   **Other medical devices** associated with adverse incidents

Y82.9   **Unspecified medical devices** associated with adverse incidents   ▽

Surgical and other medical procedures as the cause of abnormal reaction of the patient, or of later complication, without mention of misadventure at the time of the procedure (Y83-Y84)

> **EXCLUDES 1**   misadventures to patients during surgical and medical care, classifiable to (Y62-Y69)
>
> **EXCLUDES 2**   breakdown or malfunctioning of medical device (after implantation) (during procedure) (ongoing use) (Y70-Y82)

✓4ᵗʰ Y83   Surgical operation and other surgical procedures as the cause of abnormal reaction of the patient, or of later complication, without mention of misadventure at the time of the procedure

Y83.0   **Surgical operation with transplant of whole organ** as the cause of abnormal reaction of the patient, or of later complication, without mention of misadventure at the time of the procedure

Y83.1   **Surgical operation with implant of artificial internal device** as the cause of abnormal reaction of the patient, or of later complication, without mention of misadventure at the time of the procedure

Y83.2   **Surgical operation with anastomosis, bypass or graft** as the cause of abnormal reaction of the patient, or of later complication, without mention of misadventure at the time of the procedure

Y83.3   **Surgical operation with formation of external stoma** as the cause of abnormal reaction of the patient, or of later complication, without mention of misadventure at the time of the procedure

Y83.4   **Other reconstructive surgery** as the cause of abnormal reaction of the patient, or of later complication, without mention of misadventure at the time of the procedure

Y83.5   **Amputation of limb(s)** as the cause of abnormal reaction of the patient, or of later complication, without mention of misadventure at the time of the procedure

Y83.6   **Removal of other organ (partial) (total)** as the cause of abnormal reaction of the patient, or of later complication, without mention of misadventure at the time of the procedure

Y83.8   **Other surgical procedures** as the cause of abnormal reaction of the patient, or of later complication, without mention of misadventure at the time of the procedure

Y83.9   **Surgical procedure, unspecified** as the cause of abnormal reaction of the patient, or of later complication, without mention of misadventure at the time of the procedure   ▽

✓4ᵗʰ Y84   Other medical procedures as the cause of abnormal reaction of the patient, or of later complication, without mention of misadventure at the time of the procedure

Y84.0   **Cardiac catheterization** as the cause of abnormal reaction of the patient, or of later complication, without mention of misadventure at the time of the procedure

Y84.1   **Kidney dialysis** as the cause of abnormal reaction of the patient, or of later complication, without mention of misadventure at the time of the procedure

Y84.2   **Radiological procedure and radiotherapy** as the cause of abnormal reaction of the patient, or of later complication, without mention of misadventure at the time of the procedure
> **AHA:** 2017, 1Q, 33

Y84.3   **Shock therapy** as the cause of abnormal reaction of the patient, or of later complication, without mention of misadventure at the time of the procedure

Y84.4   **Aspiration of fluid** as the cause of abnormal reaction of the patient, or of later complication, without mention of misadventure at the time of the procedure

Y84.5   **Insertion of gastric or duodenal sound** as the cause of abnormal reaction of the patient, or of later complication, without mention of misadventure at the time of the procedure

Y84.6   **Urinary catheterization** as the cause of abnormal reaction of the patient, or of later complication, without mention of misadventure at the time of the procedure

Y84.7   **Blood-sampling** as the cause of abnormal reaction of the patient, or of later complication, without mention of misadventure at the time of the procedure

Y84.8   **Other medical procedures** as the cause of abnormal reaction of the patient, or of later complication, without mention of misadventure at the time of the procedure
> **AHA:** 2014, 4Q, 24

Y84.9   **Medical procedure, unspecified** as the cause of abnormal reaction of the patient, or of later complication, without mention of misadventure at the time of the procedure   ▽

Supplementary factors related to causes of morbidity classified elsewhere (Y90-Y99)

> **NOTE**   These categories may be used to provide supplementary information concerning causes of morbidity. They are not to be used for single-condition coding.

✓4ᵗʰ Y90   Evidence of alcohol involvement determined by blood alcohol level

Code first any associated alcohol related disorders (F10)

Y90.0   **Blood alcohol level of less than 20 mg/100 ml**

Y90.1   **Blood alcohol level of 20-39 mg/100 ml**

Y90.2   **Blood alcohol level of 40-59 mg/100 ml**

Y90.3   **Blood alcohol level of 60-79 mg/100 ml**

Y90.4   **Blood alcohol level of 80-99 mg/100 ml**

Y90.5   **Blood alcohol level of 100-119 mg/100 ml**

Y90.6   **Blood alcohol level of 120-199 mg/100 ml**

Y90.7   **Blood alcohol level of 200-239 mg/100 ml**

Y90.8   **Blood alcohol level of 240 mg/100 ml or more**

Y90.9   **Presence of alcohol in blood, level not specified**   ▽

✓4ᵗʰ Y92   Place of occurrence of the external cause

The following category is for use, when relevant, to identify the place of occurrence of the external cause. Use in conjunction with an activity code.

Place of occurrence should be recorded only at the initial encounter for treatment

✓5ᵗʰ Y92.0   Non-institutional (private) residence as the place of occurrence of the external cause

> **EXCLUDES 1**   abandoned or derelict house (Y92.89)
> home under construction but not yet occupied (Y92.6-)
> institutional place of residence (Y92.1-)

✓6ᵗʰ Y92.00   Unspecified non-institutional (private) residence as the place of occurrence of the external cause

Y92.000   **Kitchen** of unspecified non-institutional (private) residence as the place of occurrence of the external cause   ▽

Y92.001   **Dining room** of unspecified non-institutional (private) residence as the place of occurrence of the external cause   ▽

☑ Additional Character Req   ✓x7ᵗʰ Placeholder Alert   Manifestation   HCC CMS-HCC Condition   ▽ Unspecified Code   ►◄ Revised Text   ● New Code   ▲ Revised Code Title

ICD-10-CM 2018   1167

Y92.002 Bathroom of unspecified non-institutional (private) residence single-family (private) house as the place of occurrence of the external cause ▽

Y92.003 Bedroom of unspecified non-institutional (private) residence as the place of occurrence of the external cause ▽

Y92.007 Garden or yard of unspecified non-institutional (private) residence as the place of occurrence of the external cause ▽

Y92.008 Other place in unspecified non-institutional (private) residence as the place of occurrence of the external cause ▽

Y92.009 Unspecified place in unspecified non-institutional (private) residence as the place of occurrence of the external cause ▽
  Home (NOS) as the place of occurrence of the external cause

√6ᵗʰ **Y92.01** Single-family non-institutional (private) house as the place of occurrence of the external cause
  Farmhouse as the place of occurrence of the external cause
  EXCLUDES 1   barn (Y92.71)
    chicken coop or hen house (Y92.72)
    farm field (Y92.73)
    orchard (Y92.74)
    single family mobile home or trailer (Y92.02-)
    slaughter house (Y92.86)

Y92.010 Kitchen of single-family (private) house as the place of occurrence of the external cause

Y92.011 Dining room of single-family (private) house as the place of occurrence of the external cause

Y92.012 Bathroom of single-family (private) house as the place of occurrence of the external cause

Y92.013 Bedroom of single-family (private) house as the place of occurrence of the external cause

Y92.014 Private driveway to single-family (private) house as the place of occurrence of the external cause

Y92.015 Private garage of single-family (private) house as the place of occurrence of the external cause

Y92.016 Swimming-pool in single-family (private) house or garden as the place of occurrence of the external cause

Y92.017 Garden or yard in single-family (private) house as the place of occurrence of the external cause

Y92.018 Other place in single-family (private) house as the place of occurrence of the external cause

Y92.019 Unspecified place in single-family (private) house as the place of occurrence of the external cause ▽

√6ᵗʰ **Y92.02** Mobile home as the place of occurrence of the external cause

Y92.020 Kitchen in mobile home as the place of occurrence of the external cause

Y92.021 Dining room in mobile home as the place of occurrence of the external cause

Y92.022 Bathroom in mobile home as the place of occurrence of the external cause

Y92.023 Bedroom in mobile home as the place of occurrence of the external cause

Y92.024 Driveway of mobile home as the place of occurrence of the external cause

Y92.025 Garage of mobile home as the place of occurrence of the external cause

Y92.026 Swimming-pool of mobile home as the place of occurrence of the external cause

Y92.027 Garden or yard of mobile home as the place of occurrence of the external cause

Y92.028 Other place in mobile home as the place of occurrence of the external cause

Y92.029 Unspecified place in mobile home as the place of occurrence of the external cause ▽

√6ᵗʰ **Y92.03** Apartment as the place of occurrence of the external cause
  Condominium as the place of occurrence of the external cause
  Co-op apartment as the place of occurrence of the external cause

Y92.030 Kitchen in apartment as the place of occurrence of the external cause

Y92.031 Bathroom in apartment as the place of occurrence of the external cause

Y92.032 Bedroom in apartment as the place of occurrence of the external cause

Y92.038 Other place in apartment as the place of occurrence of the external cause

Y92.039 Unspecified place in apartment as the place of occurrence of the external cause ▽

√6ᵗʰ **Y92.04** Boarding-house as the place of occurrence of the external cause

Y92.040 Kitchen in boarding-house as the place of occurrence of the external cause

Y92.041 Bathroom in boarding-house as the place of occurrence of the external cause

Y92.042 Bedroom in boarding-house as the place of occurrence of the external cause

Y92.043 Driveway of boarding-house as the place of occurrence of the external cause

Y92.044 Garage of boarding-house as the place of occurrence of the external cause

Y92.045 Swimming-pool of boarding-house as the place of occurrence of the external cause

Y92.046 Garden or yard of boarding-house as the place of occurrence of the external cause

Y92.048 Other place in boarding-house as the place of occurrence of the external cause

Y92.049 Unspecified place in boarding-house as the place of occurrence of the external cause ▽

√6ᵗʰ **Y92.09** Other non-institutional residence as the place of occurrence of the external cause
  AHA: 2017, 2Q, 10

Y92.090 Kitchen in other non-institutional residence as the place of occurrence of the external cause

Y92.091 Bathroom in other non-institutional residence as the place of occurrence of the external cause

Y92.092 Bedroom in other non-institutional residence as the place of occurrence of the external cause

Y92.093 Driveway of other non-institutional residence as the place of occurrence of the external cause

Y92.094 Garage of other non-institutional residence as the place of occurrence of the external cause

Y92.095 Swimming-pool of other non-institutional residence as the place of occurrence of the external cause

Y92.096 Garden or yard of other non-institutional residence as the place of occurrence of the external cause

Y92.098 Other place in other non-institutional residence as the place of occurrence of the external cause

Y92.099 Unspecified place in other non-institutional residence as the place of occurrence of the external cause ▽

√5ᵗʰ **Y92.1** Institutional (nonprivate) residence as the place of occurrence of the external cause

Y92.10 Unspecified residential institution as the place of occurrence of the external cause ▽

√6ᵗʰ **Y92.11** Children's home and orphanage as the place of occurrence of the external cause

Y92.110 Kitchen in children's home and orphanage as the place of occurrence of the external cause

Y92.111 Bathroom in children's home and orphanage as the place of occurrence of the external cause

---

EXCLUDES 1 Not coded here   EXCLUDES 2 Not included here   N Newborn Age: 0   P Pediatric Age: 0-17   M Maternity Age: 12-55   A Adult Age: 15-124

1168   ICD-10-CM 2018

Y92.112 **Bedroom** in children's home and orphanage as the place of occurrence of the external cause

Y92.113 **Driveway** of children's home and orphanage as the place of occurrence of the external cause

Y92.114 **Garage** of children's home and orphanage as the place of occurrence of the external cause

Y92.115 **Swimming-pool** of children's home and orphanage as the place of occurrence of the external cause

Y92.116 **Garden or yard** of children's home and orphanage as the place of occurrence of the external cause

Y92.118 **Other place** in children's home and orphanage as the place of occurrence of the external cause

Y92.119 **Unspecified place** in children's home ▽ and orphanage as the place of occurrence of the external cause

✓6ᵗʰ **Y92.12** **Nursing home** as the place of occurrence of the external cause
Home for the sick as the place of occurrence of the external cause
Hospice as the place of occurrence of the external cause
AHA: 2017, 2Q, 10

Y92.120 **Kitchen** in nursing home as the place of occurrence of the external cause

Y92.121 **Bathroom** in nursing home as the place of occurrence of the external cause

Y92.122 **Bedroom** in nursing home as the place of occurrence of the external cause

Y92.123 **Driveway** of nursing home as the place of occurrence of the external cause

Y92.124 **Garage** of nursing home as the place of occurrence of the external cause

Y92.125 **Swimming-pool** of nursing home as the place of occurrence of the external cause

Y92.126 **Garden or yard** of nursing home as the place of occurrence of the external cause

Y92.128 **Other place** in nursing home as the place of occurrence of the external cause

Y92.129 **Unspecified place** in nursing home as ▽ the place of occurrence of the external cause

✓6ᵗʰ **Y92.13** **Military base** as the place of occurrence of the external cause
EXCLUDES 1 military training grounds (Y92.83)

Y92.130 **Kitchen** on military base as the place of occurrence of the external cause

Y92.131 **Mess hall** on military base as the place of occurrence of the external cause

Y92.133 **Barracks** on military base as the place of occurrence of the external cause

Y92.135 **Garage** on military base as the place of occurrence of the external cause

Y92.136 **Swimming-pool** on military base as the place of occurrence of the external cause

Y92.137 **Garden or yard** on military base as the place of occurrence of the external cause

Y92.138 **Other place** on military base as the place of occurrence of the external cause

Y92.139 **Unspecified place** military base as the ▽ place of occurrence of the external cause

✓6ᵗʰ **Y92.14** **Prison** as the place of occurrence of the external cause

Y92.140 **Kitchen** in prison as the place of occurrence of the external cause

Y92.141 **Dining room** in prison as the place of occurrence of the external cause

Y92.142 **Bathroom** in prison as the place of occurrence of the external cause

Y92.143 **Cell** of prison as the place of occurrence of the external cause

Y92.146 **Swimming-pool** of prison as the place of occurrence of the external cause

Y92.147 **Courtyard** of prison as the place of occurrence of the external cause

Y92.148 **Other place** in prison as the place of occurrence of the external cause

Y92.149 **Unspecified place** in prison as the ▽ place of occurrence of the external cause

✓6ᵗʰ **Y92.15** **Reform school** as the place of occurrence of the external cause

Y92.150 **Kitchen** in reform school as the place of occurrence of the external cause

Y92.151 **Dining room** in reform school as the place of occurrence of the external cause

Y92.152 **Bathroom** in reform school as the place of occurrence of the external cause

Y92.153 **Bedroom** in reform school as the place of occurrence of the external cause

Y92.154 **Driveway** of reform school as the place of occurrence of the external cause

Y92.155 **Garage** of reform school as the place of occurrence of the external cause

Y92.156 **Swimming-pool** of reform school as the place of occurrence of the external cause

Y92.157 **Garden or yard** of reform school as the place of occurrence of the external cause

Y92.158 **Other place** in reform school as the place of occurrence of the external cause

Y92.159 **Unspecified place** in reform school as ▽ the place of occurrence of the external cause

✓6ᵗʰ **Y92.16** **School dormitory** as the place of occurrence of the external cause
EXCLUDES 1 reform school as the place of occurrence of the external cause (Y92.15-)
school buildings and grounds as the place of occurrence of the external cause (Y92.2-)
school sports and athletic areas as the place of occurrence of the external cause (Y92.3-)

Y92.160 **Kitchen** in school dormitory as the place of occurrence of the external cause

Y92.161 **Dining room** in school dormitory as the place of occurrence of the external cause

Y92.162 **Bathroom** in school dormitory as the place of occurrence of the external cause

Y92.163 **Bedroom** in school dormitory as the place of occurrence of the external cause

Y92.168 **Other place** in school dormitory as the place of occurrence of the external cause

Y92.169 **Unspecified place** in school dormitory ▽ as the place of occurrence of the external cause

✓6ᵗʰ **Y92.19** **Other specified residential institution** as the place of occurrence of the external cause
AHA: 2017, 2Q, 10

Y92.190 **Kitchen** in other specified residential institution as the place of occurrence of the external cause

Y92.191 **Dining room** in other specified residential institution as the place of occurrence of the external cause

Y92.192 **Bathroom** in other specified residential institution as the place of occurrence of the external cause

Y92.193 **Bedroom** in other specified residential institution as the place of occurrence of the external cause

Y92.194 **Driveway** of other specified residential institution as the place of occurrence of the external cause

Y92.195 **Garage** of other specified residential institution as the place of occurrence of the external cause

Y92.196 **Pool** of other specified residential institution as the place of occurrence of the external cause

Y92.197 **Garden or yard** of other specified residential institution as the place of occurrence of the external cause

Y92.198 **Other place** in other specified residential institution as the place of occurrence of the external cause

Y92.199   **Unspecified place** in other specified residential institution as the place of occurrence of the external cause   ▽

✓6th **Y92.2**   **School, other institution and public administrative area** as the place of occurrence of the external cause

Building and adjacent grounds used by the general public or by a particular group of the public

EXCLUDES 1   *building under construction as the place of occurrence of the external cause (Y92.6)*

residential institution as the place of occurrence of the external cause (Y92.1)

school dormitory as the place of occurrence of the external cause (Y92.16-)

sports and athletics area of schools as the place of occurrence of the external cause (Y92.3-)

✓6th **Y92.21**   **School (private) (public) (state)** as the place of occurrence of the external cause

Y92.210   **Daycare center** as the place of occurrence of the external cause

Y92.211   **Elementary school** as the place of occurrence of the external cause

Kindergarten as the place of occurrence of the external cause

Y92.212   **Middle school** as the place of occurrence of the external cause

Y92.213   **High school** as the place of occurrence of the external cause

AHA: 2012, 4Q, 108

Y92.214   **College** as the place of occurrence of the external cause

University as the place of occurrence of the external cause

Y92.215   **Trade school** as the place of occurrence of the external cause

Y92.218   **Other school** as the place of occurrence of the external cause

Y92.219   **Unspecified school** as the place of occurrence of the external cause   ▽

Y92.22   **Religious institution** as the place of occurrence of the external cause

Church as the place of occurrence of the external cause

Mosque as the place of occurrence of the external cause

Synagogue as the place of occurrence of the external cause

✓6th **Y92.23**   **Hospital** as the place of occurrence of the external cause

EXCLUDES 1   *ambulatory (outpatient) health services establishments (Y92.53-)*

home for the sick as the place of occurrence of the external cause (Y92.12-)

hospice as the place of occurrence of the external cause (Y92.12-)

nursing home as the place of occurrence of the external cause (Y92.12-)

Y92.230   **Patient room** in hospital as the place of occurrence of the external cause

Y92.231   **Patient bathroom** in hospital as the place of occurrence of the external cause

Y92.232   **Corridor** of hospital as the place of occurrence of the external cause

Y92.233   **Cafeteria** of hospital as the place of occurrence of the external cause

Y92.234   **Operating room** of hospital as the place of occurrence of the external cause

Y92.238   **Other place** in hospital as the place of occurrence of the external cause

Y92.239   **Unspecified place** in hospital as the place of occurrence of the external cause   ▽

✓6th **Y92.24**   **Public administrative building** as the place of occurrence of the external cause

Y92.240   **Courthouse** as the place of occurrence of the external cause

Y92.241   **Library** as the place of occurrence of the external cause

Y92.242   **Post office** as the place of occurrence of the external cause

Y92.243   **City hall** as the place of occurrence of the external cause

Y92.248   **Other public administrative building** as the place of occurrence of the external cause

✓6th **Y92.25**   **Cultural building** as the place of occurrence of the external cause

Y92.250   **Art Gallery** as the place of occurrence of the external cause

Y92.251   **Museum** as the place of occurrence of the external cause

Y92.252   **Music hall** as the place of occurrence of the external cause

Y92.253   **Opera house** as the place of occurrence of the external cause

Y92.254   **Theater (live)** as the place of occurrence of the external cause

Y92.258   **Other cultural public building** as the place of occurrence of the external cause

Y92.26   **Movie house or cinema** as the place of occurrence of the external cause

Y92.29   **Other specified public building** as the place of occurrence of the external cause

Assembly hall as the place of occurrence of the external cause

Clubhouse as the place of occurrence of the external cause

✓5th **Y92.3**   **Sports and athletics area** as the place of occurrence of the external cause

✓6th **Y92.31**   **Athletic court** as the place of occurrence of the external cause

EXCLUDES 1   *tennis court in private home or garden (Y92.09)*

Y92.310   **Basketball court** as the place of occurrence of the external cause

Y92.311   **Squash court** as the place of occurrence of the external cause

Y92.312   **Tennis court** as the place of occurrence of the external cause

Y92.318   **Other athletic court** as the place of occurrence of the external cause

✓6th **Y92.32**   **Athletic field** as the place of occurrence of the external cause

Y92.320   **Baseball field** as the place of occurrence of the external cause

Y92.321   **Football field** as the place of occurrence of the external cause

Y92.322   **Soccer field** as the place of occurrence of the external cause

Y92.328   **Other athletic field** as the place of occurrence of the external cause

Cricket field as the place of occurrence of the external cause

Hockey field as the place of occurrence of the external cause

✓6th **Y92.33**   **Skating rink** as the place of occurrence of the external cause

Y92.330   **Ice skating rink (indoor) (outdoor)** as the place of occurrence of the external cause

Y92.331   **Roller skating rink** as the place of occurrence of the external cause

Y92.34   **Swimming pool (public)** as the place of occurrence of the external cause

EXCLUDES 1   *swimming pool in private home or garden (Y92.016)*

Y92.39   **Other specified sports and athletic area** as the place of occurrence of the external cause

Golf-course as the place of occurrence of the external cause

Gymnasium as the place of occurrence of the external cause

Riding-school as the place of occurrence of the external cause

Stadium as the place of occurrence of the external cause

EXCLUDES 1 Not coded here   EXCLUDES 2 Not included here   N Newborn Age: 0   P Pediatric Age: 0-17   M Maternity Age: 12-55   A Adult Age: 15-124

1170   ICD-10-CM 2018

✓5ᵗʰ Y92.4 Street, highway and other paved roadways as the place of occurrence of the external cause
> EXCLUDES 1   *private driveway of residence (Y92.014, Y92.024, Y92.043, Y92.093, Y92.113, Y92.123, Y92.154, Y92.194)*

✓6ᵗʰ Y92.41 Street and highway as the place of occurrence of the external cause
    Y92.410 Unspecified street and highway as the ▽ place of occurrence of the external cause
         Road NOS as the place of occurrence of the external cause
    Y92.411 Interstate highway as the place of occurrence of the external cause
         Freeway as the place of occurrence of the external cause
         Motorway as the place of occurrence of the external cause
    Y92.412 Parkway as the place of occurrence of the external cause
    Y92.413 State road as the place of occurrence of the external cause
    Y92.414 Local residential or business street as the place of occurrence of the external cause
    Y92.415 Exit ramp or entrance ramp of street or highway as the place of occurrence of the external cause

✓6ᵗʰ Y92.48 Other paved roadways as the place of occurrence of the external cause
    Y92.480 Sidewalk as the place of occurrence of the external cause
    Y92.481 Parking lot as the place of occurrence of the external cause
    Y92.482 Bike path as the place of occurrence of the external cause
    Y92.488 Other paved roadways as the place of occurrence of the external cause

✓5ᵗʰ Y92.5 Trade and service area as the place of occurrence of the external cause
> EXCLUDES 1   *garage in private home (Y92.015)*
> *schools and other public administration buildings (Y92.2-)*

✓6ᵗʰ Y92.51 Private commercial establishments as the place of occurrence of the external cause
    Y92.510 Bank as the place of occurrence of the external cause
    Y92.511 Restaurant or café as the place of occurrence of the external cause
    Y92.512 Supermarket, store or market as the place of occurrence of the external cause
    Y92.513 Shop (commercial) as the place of occurrence of the external cause

✓6ᵗʰ Y92.52 Service areas as the place of occurrence of the external cause
    Y92.520 Airport as the place of occurrence of the external cause
    Y92.521 Bus station as the place of occurrence of the external cause
    Y92.522 Railway station as the place of occurrence of the external cause
    Y92.523 Highway rest stop as the place of occurrence of the external cause
    Y92.524 Gas station as the place of occurrence of the external cause
         Petroleum station as the place of occurrence of the external cause
         Service station as the place of occurrence of the external cause

✓6ᵗʰ Y92.53 Ambulatory health services establishments as the place of occurrence of the external cause
    Y92.530 Ambulatory surgery center as the place of occurrence of the external cause
         Outpatient surgery center, including that connected with a hospital as the place of occurrence of the external cause
         Same day surgery center, including that connected with a hospital as the place of occurrence of the external cause

    Y92.531 Health care provider office as the place of occurrence of the external cause
         Physician office as the place of occurrence of the external cause
    Y92.532 Urgent care center as the place of occurrence of the external cause
    Y92.538 Other ambulatory health services establishments as the place of occurrence of the external cause

Y92.59 Other trade areas as the place of occurrence of the external cause
     Office building as the place of occurrence of the external cause
     Casino as the place of occurrence of the external cause
     Garage (commercial) as the place of occurrence of the external cause
     Hotel as the place of occurrence of the external cause
     Radio or television station as the place of occurrence of the external cause
     Shopping mall as the place of occurrence of the external cause
     Warehouse as the place of occurrence of the external cause

✓5ᵗʰ Y92.6 Industrial and construction area as the place of occurrence of the external cause
    Y92.61 Building [any] under construction as the place of occurrence of the external cause
    Y92.62 Dock or shipyard as the place of occurrence of the external cause
         Dockyard as the place of occurrence of the external cause
         Dry dock as the place of occurrence of the external cause
         Shipyard as the place of occurrence of the external cause
    Y92.63 Factory as the place of occurrence of the external cause
         Factory building as the place of occurrence of the external cause
         Factory premises as the place of occurrence of the external cause
         Industrial yard as the place of occurrence of the external cause
    Y92.64 Mine or pit as the place of occurrence of the external cause
         Mine as the place of occurrence of the external cause
    Y92.65 Oil rig as the place of occurrence of the external cause
         Pit (coal) (gravel) (sand) as the place of occurrence of the external cause
    Y92.69 Other specified industrial and construction area as the place of occurrence of the external cause
         Gasworks as the place of occurrence of the external cause
         Power-station (coal) (nuclear) (oil) as the place of occurrence of the external cause
         Tunnel under construction as the place of occurrence of the external cause
         Workshop as the place of occurrence of the external cause

✓5ᵗʰ Y92.7 Farm as the place of occurrence of the external cause
     Ranch as the place of occurrence of the external cause
> EXCLUDES 1   *farmhouse and home premises of farm (Y92.01-)*

    Y92.71 Barn as the place of occurrence of the external cause
    Y92.72 Chicken coop as the place of occurrence of the external cause
         Hen house as the place of occurrence of the external cause
    Y92.73 Farm field as the place of occurrence of the external cause
    Y92.74 Orchard as the place of occurrence of the external cause
    Y92.79 Other farm location as the place of occurrence of the external cause

✓5ᵗʰ Y92.8 Other places as the place of occurrence of the external cause
    ✓6ᵗʰ Y92.81 Transport vehicle as the place of occurrence of the external cause
> EXCLUDES 1   *transport accidents (V00-V99)*

    Y92.810 Car as the place of occurrence of the external cause

---

✔ Additional Character Req   ✔x7ᵗʰ Placeholder Alert   Manifestation   HCC CMS-HCC Condition   ▽ Unspecified Code   ►◄ Revised Text   ● New Code   ▲ Revised Code Title

Y92.811 Bus as the place of occurrence of the external cause

Y92.812 Truck as the place of occurrence of the external cause

Y92.813 Airplane as the place of occurrence of the external cause

Y92.814 Boat as the place of occurrence of the external cause

Y92.815 Train as the place of occurrence of the external cause

Y92.816 Subway car as the place of occurrence of the external cause

Y92.818 Other transport vehicle as the place of occurrence of the external cause

✓6th **Y92.82 Wilderness area**

Y92.820 Desert as the place of occurrence of the external cause

Y92.821 Forest as the place of occurrence of the external cause

Y92.828 Other wilderness area as the place of occurrence of the external cause
Swamp as the place of occurrence of the external cause
Mountain as the place of occurrence of the external cause
Marsh as the place of occurrence of the external cause
Prairie as the place of occurrence of the external cause

✓6th **Y92.83 Recreation area as the place of occurrence of the external cause**

Y92.830 Public park as the place of occurrence of the external cause

Y92.831 Amusement park as the place of occurrence of the external cause

Y92.832 Beach as the place of occurrence of the external cause
Seashore as the place of occurrence of the external cause

Y92.833 Campsite as the place of occurrence of the external cause

Y92.834 Zoological garden (Zoo) as the place of occurrence of the external cause

Y92.838 Other recreation area as the place of occurrence of the external cause

Y92.84 Military training ground as the place of occurrence of the external cause

Y92.85 Railroad track as the place of occurrence of the external cause

Y92.86 Slaughter house as the place of occurrence of the external cause

Y92.89 Other specified places as the place of occurrence of the external cause
Derelict house as the place of occurrence of the external cause

Y92.9 Unspecified place or not applicable   ▽

✓4th **Y93 Activity codes**

NOTE Category Y93 is provided for use to indicate the activity of the person seeking healthcare for an injury or health condition, such as a heart attack while shoveling snow, which resulted from, or was contributed to, by the activity. These codes are appropriate for use for both acute injuries, such as those from chapter 19, and conditions that are due to the long-term, cumulative effects of an activity, such as those from chapter 13. They are also appropriate for use with external cause codes for cause and intent if identifying the activity provides additional information on the event. These codes should be used in conjunction with codes for external cause status (Y99) and place of occurrence (Y92).

This section contains the following broad activity categories:

Y93.0   Activities involving walking and running
Y93.1   Activities involving water and water craft
Y93.2   Activities involving ice and snow
Y93.3   Activities involving climbing, rappelling, and jumping off
Y93.4   Activities involving dancing and other rhythmic movement
Y93.5   Activities involving other sports and athletics played individually
Y93.6   Activities involving other sports and athletics played as a team or group
Y93.7   Activities involving other specified sports and athletics
Y93.A   Activities involving other cardiorespiratory exercise
Y93.B   Activities involving other muscle strengthening exercises
Y93.C   Activities involving computer technology and electronic devices
Y93.D   Activities involving arts and handcrafts
Y93.E   Activities involving personal hygiene and interior property and clothing maintenance
Y93.F   Activities involving caregiving
Y93.G   Activities involving food preparation, cooking and grilling
Y93.H   Activities involving exterior property and land maintenance, building and construction
Y93.I   Activities involving roller coasters and other types of external motion
Y93.J   Activities involving playing musical instrument
Y93.K   Activities involving animal care
Y93.8   Activities, other specified
Y93.9   Activity, unspecified

✓5th **Y93.0 Activities involving walking and running**
EXCLUDES 1 activity, walking an animal (Y93.K1)
activity, walking or running on a treadmill (Y93.A1)

Y93.01 Activity, walking, marching and hiking
Activity, walking, marching and hiking on level or elevated terrain
EXCLUDES 1 activity, mountain climbing (Y93.31)

Y93.02 Activity, running

✓5th **Y93.1 Activities involving water and water craft**
EXCLUDES 1 activities involving ice (Y93.2-)

Y93.11 Activity, swimming

Y93.12 Activity, springboard and platform diving

Y93.13 Activity, water polo

Y93.14 Activity, water aerobics and water exercise

Y93.15 Activity, underwater diving and snorkeling
Activity, SCUBA diving

Y93.16 Activity, rowing, canoeing, kayaking, rafting and tubing
Activity, canoeing, kayaking, rafting and tubing in calm and turbulent water

Y93.17 Activity, water skiing and wake boarding

Y93.18 Activity, surfing, windsurfing and boogie boarding
Activity, water sliding

Y93.19 Activity, other involving water and watercraft
Activity involving water NOS
Activity, parasailing
Activity, water survival training and testing

✓5th **Y93.2 Activities involving ice and snow**
EXCLUDES 1 activity, shoveling ice and snow (Y93.H1)

Y93.21 Activity, ice skating
Activity, figure skating (singles) (pairs)
Activity, ice dancing
EXCLUDES 1 activity, ice hockey (Y93.22)

Y93.22 Activity, ice hockey

Y93.23 Activity, snow (alpine) (downhill) skiing, snow boarding, sledding, tobogganing and snow tubing
EXCLUDES 1 activity, cross country skiing (Y93.24)

Y93.24 Activity, cross country skiing
Activity, nordic skiing

EXCLUDES 1 Not coded here   **EXCLUDES 2** Not included here   **N** Newborn Age: 0   **P** Pediatric Age: 0-17   **M** Maternity Age: 12-55   **A** Adult Age: 15-124

1172
ICD-10-CM 2018

Y93.29   Activity, other involving ice and snow
Activity involving ice and snow NOS

✓5ᵗʰ **Y93.3   Activities involving climbing, rappelling and jumping off**
EXCLUDES 1   *activity, hiking on level or elevated terrain (Y93.Ø1)*
activity, jumping rope (Y93.56)
activity, trampoline jumping (Y93.44)

Y93.31   Activity, mountain climbing, rock climbing and wall climbing

Y93.32   Activity, rappelling

Y93.33   Activity, BASE jumping
Activity, Building, Antenna, Span, Earth jumping

Y93.34   Activity, bungee jumping

Y93.35   Activity, hang gliding

Y93.39   Activity, other involving climbing, rappelling and jumping off

✓5ᵗʰ **Y93.4   Activities involving dancing and other rhythmic movement**
EXCLUDES 1   *activity, martial arts (Y93.75)*

Y93.41   Activity, dancing
AHA: 2012, 4Q, 108

Y93.42   Activity, yoga

Y93.43   Activity, gymnastics
Activity, rhythmic gymnastics
EXCLUDES 1   *activity, trampolining (Y93.44)*

Y93.44   Activity, trampolining

Y93.45   Activity, cheerleading

Y93.49   Activity, other involving dancing and other rhythmic movements

✓5ᵗʰ **Y93.5   Activities involving other sports and athletics played individually**
EXCLUDES 1   *activity, dancing (Y93.41)*
activity, gymnastic (Y93.43)
activity, trampolining (Y93.44)
activity, yoga (Y93.42)

Y93.51   Activity, roller skating (inline) and skateboarding

Y93.52   Activity, horseback riding

Y93.53   Activity, golf

Y93.54   Activity, bowling

Y93.55   Activity, bike riding

Y93.56   Activity, jumping rope

Y93.57   Activity, non-running track and field events
EXCLUDES 1   *activity, running (any form) (Y93.Ø2)*

Y93.59   Activity, other involving other sports and athletics played individually
EXCLUDES 1   *activities involving climbing, rappelling, and jumping (Y93.3-)*
activities involving ice and snow (Y93.2-)
activities involving walking and running (Y93.Ø-)
activities involving water and watercraft (Y93.1-)

✓5ᵗʰ **Y93.6   Activities involving other sports and athletics played as a team or group**
EXCLUDES 1   *activity, ice hockey (Y93.22)*
activity, water polo (Y93.13)

Y93.61   Activity, American tackle football
Activity, football NOS

Y93.62   Activity, American flag or touch football

Y93.63   Activity, rugby

Y93.64   Activity, baseball
Activity, softball

Y93.65   Activity, lacrosse and field hockey

Y93.66   Activity, soccer

Y93.67   Activity, basketball

Y93.68   Activity, volleyball (beach) (court)

Y93.6A   Activity, physical games generally associated with school recess, summer camp and children
Activity, capture the flag
Activity, dodge ball
Activity, four square
Activity, kickball

Y93.69   Activity, other involving other sports and athletics played as a team or group
Activity, cricket

✓5ᵗʰ **Y93.7   Activities involving other specified sports and athletics**

Y93.71   Activity, boxing

Y93.72   Activity, wrestling

Y93.73   Activity, racquet and hand sports
Activity, handball
Activity, racquetball
Activity, squash
Activity, tennis

Y93.74   Activity, frisbee
Activity, ultimate frisbee

Y93.75   Activity, martial arts
Activity, combatives

Y93.79   Activity, other specified sports and athletics
EXCLUDES 1   *sports and athletics activities specified in categories Y93.Ø-Y93.6*

✓5ᵗʰ **Y93.A   Activities involving other cardiorespiratory exercise**
Activities involving physical training

Y93.A1   Activity, exercise machines primarily for cardiorespiratory conditioning
Activity, elliptical and stepper machines
Activity, stationary bike
Activity, treadmill

Y93.A2   Activity, calisthenics
Activity, jumping jacks
Activity, warm up and cool down

Y93.A3   Activity, aerobic and step exercise

Y93.A4   Activity, circuit training

Y93.A5   Activity, obstacle course
Activity, challenge course
Activity, confidence course

Y93.A6   Activity, grass drills
Activity, guerilla drills

Y93.A9   Activity, other involving cardiorespiratory exercise
EXCLUDES 1   *activities involving cardiorespiratory exercise specified in categories Y93.Ø-Y93.7*

✓5ᵗʰ **Y93.B   Activities involving other muscle strengthening exercises**

Y93.B1   Activity, exercise machines primarily for muscle strengthening

Y93.B2   Activity, push-ups, pull-ups, sit-ups

Y93.B3   Activity, free weights
Activity, barbells
Activity, dumbbells

Y93.B4   Activity, pilates

Y93.B9   Activity, other involving muscle strengthening exercises
EXCLUDES 1   *activities involving muscle strengthening specified in categories Y93.Ø-Y93.A*

✓5ᵗʰ **Y93.C   Activities involving computer technology and electronic devices**
EXCLUDES 1   *activity, electronic musical keyboard or instruments (Y93.J-)*

Y93.C1   Activity, computer keyboarding
Activity, electronic game playing using keyboard or other stationary device

Y93.C2   Activity, hand held interactive electronic device
Activity, cellular telephone and communication device
Activity, electronic game playing using interactive device
EXCLUDES 1   *activity, electronic game playing using keyboard or other stationary device (Y93.C1)*

Y93.C9   Activity, other involving computer technology and electronic devices

✓5ᵗʰ **Y93.D   Activities involving arts and handcrafts**
EXCLUDES 1   *activities involving playing musical instrument (Y93.J-)*

Y93.D1   Activity, knitting and crocheting

Y93.D2   Activity, sewing

Y93.D3   Activity, furniture building and finishing
Activity, furniture repair

Y93.D9   Activity, other involving arts and handcrafts

✓5ᵗʰ **Y93.E   Activities involving personal hygiene and interior property and clothing maintenance**
EXCLUDES 1   *activities involving cooking and grilling (Y93.G-)*
activities involving exterior property and land maintenance, building and construction (Y93.H-)
activities involving caregiving (Y93.F-)
activity, dishwashing (Y93.G1)
activity, food preparation (Y93.G1)
activity, gardening (Y93.H2)

Y93.E1   Activity, personal bathing and showering

Y93.E2   Activity, laundry

☑ Additional Character Req   ✓x7ᵗʰ Placeholder Alert   Manifestation   HCC CMS-HCC Condition   ▽ Unspecified Code   ▶◀ Revised Text   ● New Code   ▲ Revised Code Title

Y93.E3	**Activity, vacuuming**	
Y93.E4	**Activity, ironing**	
Y93.E5	**Activity, floor mopping and cleaning**	
Y93.E6	**Activity, residential relocation**	
	Activity, packing up and unpacking involved in moving to a new residence	
Y93.E8	**Activity, other personal hygiene**	
Y93.E9	**Activity, other interior property and clothing maintenance**	

✓5ᵗʰ **Y93.F**   **Activities involving caregiving**
Activity involving the provider of caregiving

Y93.F1	**Activity, caregiving, bathing**
Y93.F2	**Activity, caregiving, lifting**
Y93.F9	**Activity, other caregiving**

✓5ᵗʰ **Y93.G**   **Activities involving food preparation, cooking and grilling**

Y93.G1	**Activity, food preparation and clean up**
	Activity, dishwashing
Y93.G2	**Activity, grilling and smoking food**
Y93.G3	**Activity, cooking and baking**
	Activity, use of stove, oven and microwave oven
Y93.G9	**Activity, other involving cooking and grilling**

✓5ᵗʰ **Y93.H**   **Activities involving exterior property and land maintenance, building and construction**

Y93.H1	**Activity, digging, shoveling and raking**
	Activity, dirt digging
	Activity, raking leaves
	Activity, snow shoveling
Y93.H2	**Activity, gardening and landscaping**
	Activity, pruning, trimming shrubs, weeding
Y93.H3	**Activity, building and construction**
Y93.H9	**Activity, other involving exterior property and land maintenance, building and construction**

✓5ᵗʰ **Y93.I**   **Activities involving roller coasters and other types of external motion**

Y93.I1	**Activity, rollercoaster riding**
Y93.I9	**Activity, other involving external motion**

✓5ᵗʰ **Y93.J**   **Activities involving playing musical instrument**
Activity involving playing electric musical instrument

Y93.J1	**Activity, piano playing**
	Activity, musical keyboard (electronic) playing
Y93.J2	**Activity, drum and other percussion instrument playing**
Y93.J3	**Activity, string instrument playing**
Y93.J4	**Activity, winds and brass instrument playing**

✓5ᵗʰ **Y93.K**   **Activities involving animal care**
  EXCLUDES 1   *activity, horseback riding (Y93.52)*

Y93.K1	**Activity, walking an animal**
Y93.K2	**Activity, milking an animal**
Y93.K3	**Activity, grooming and shearing an animal**
Y93.K9	**Activity, other involving animal care**

✓5ᵗʰ **Y93.8**   **Activities, other specified**

Y93.81	**Activity, refereeing a sports activity**
Y93.82	**Activity, spectator at an event**
Y93.83	**Activity, rough housing and horseplay**
Y93.84	**Activity, sleeping**
Y93.85	**Activity, choking game**
	Activity, blackout game
	Activity, fainting game
	Activity, pass out game
Y93.89	**Activity, other specified**

Y93.9   **Activity, unspecified**   ▽

Y95   **Nosocomial condition**
    AHA: 2013, 4Q, 119

✓4ᵗʰ **Y99**   **External cause status**
  NOTE   A single code from category Y99 should be used in conjunction with the external cause code(s) assigned to a record to indicate the status of the person at the time the event occurred.

Y99.0   **Civilian activity done for income or pay**
Civilian activity done for financial or other compensation
  EXCLUDES 1   *military activity (Y99.1)*
               volunteer activity (Y99.2)

Y99.1   **Military activity**
  EXCLUDES 1   *activity of off duty military personnel (Y99.8)*

Y99.2   **Volunteer activity**
  EXCLUDES 1   *activity of child or other family member assisting in compensated work of other family member (Y99.8)*

Y99.8   **Other external cause status**
Activity NEC
Activity of child or other family member assisting in compensated work of other family member
Hobby not done for income
Leisure activity
Off-duty activity of military personnel
Recreation or sport not for income or while a student
Student activity
  EXCLUDES 1   *civilian activity done for income or compensation (Y99.0)*
               military activity (Y99.1)
    AHA: 2012, 4Q, 108

Y99.9   **Unspecified external cause status**   ▽

EXCLUDES 1 Not coded here   EXCLUDES 2 Not included here   N Newborn Age: 0   P Pediatric Age: 0-17   M Maternity Age: 12-55   A Adult Age: 15-124

1174   ICD-10-CM 2018

Chapter 21. Factors Influencing Health Status and Contact with Health Services (Z00–Z99)

Chapter Specific Guidelines with Coding Examples

The chapter specific guidelines from the ICD-10-CM Official Guidelines for Coding and Reporting have been provided below. Along with these guidelines are coding examples, contained in the shaded boxes, that have been developed to help illustrate the coding and/or sequencing guidance found in these guidelines.

Note: The chapter specific guidelines provide additional information about the use of Z codes for specified encounters.

a. Use of Z codes in any healthcare setting

Z codes are for use in any healthcare setting. Z codes may be used as either a first-listed (principal diagnosis code in the inpatient setting) or secondary code, depending on the circumstances of the encounter. Certain Z codes may only be used as first-listed or principal diagnosis.

> Patient with middle lobe lung cancer presents for initiation of chemotherapy
>
> **Z51.11**   **Encounter for antineoplastic chemotherapy**
>
> **C34.2**   **Malignant neoplasm of middle lobe, bronchus or lung**
>
> *Explanation:* A Z code can be used as first-listed in this situation based on guidelines in this chapter as well as chapter 2, "Neoplasms."

> Patient has chronic lymphocytic leukemia for which the patient had previous chemotherapy and is now in remission
>
> **C91.11**   **Chronic lymphocytic leukemia of B-cell type in remission**
>
> **Z92.21**   **Personal history of antineoplastic chemotherapy**
>
> *Explanation:*The personal history Z code is used to describe a secondary (supplementary) diagnosis to identify that this patient has had chemotherapy in the past.

b. Z codes indicate a reason for an encounter

Z codes are not procedure codes. A corresponding procedure code must accompany a Z code to describe any procedure performed.

c. Categories of Z codes

1) Contact/exposure

Category Z20 indicates contact with, and suspected exposure to, communicable diseases. These codes are for patients who do not show any sign or symptom of a disease but are suspected to have been exposed to it by close personal contact with an infected individual or are in an area where a disease is epidemic.

Category Z77, Other contact with and (suspected) exposures hazardous to health, indicates contact with and suspected exposures hazardous to health.

Contact/exposure codes may be used as a first-listed code to explain an encounter for testing, or, more commonly, as a secondary code to identify a potential risk.

2) Inoculations and vaccinations

Code Z23 is for encounters for inoculations and vaccinations. It indicates that a patient is being seen to receive a prophylactic inoculation against a disease. Procedure codes are required to identify the actual administration of the injection and the type(s) of immunizations given. Code Z23 may be used as a secondary code if the inoculation is given as a routine part of preventive health care, such as a well-baby visit.

3) Status

Status codes indicate that a patient is either a carrier of a disease or has the sequelae or residual of a past disease or condition. This includes such things as the presence of prosthetic or mechanical devices resulting from past treatment. A status code is informative, because the status may affect the course of treatment and its outcome. A status code is distinct from a history code. The history code indicates that the patient no longer has the condition.

A status code should not be used with a diagnosis code from one of the body system chapters, if the diagnosis code includes the information provided by the status code. For example, code Z94.1, Heart transplant status, should not be used with a code from subcategory T86.2, Complications of heart transplant. The status code does not provide

additional information. The complication code indicates that the patient is a heart transplant patient.

For encounters for weaning from a mechanical ventilator, assign a code from subcategory J96.1, Chronic respiratory failure, followed by code Z99.11, Dependence on respirator [ventilator] status.

The status Z codes/categories are:

Z14   Genetic carrier

Genetic carrier status indicates that a person carries a gene, associated with a particular disease, which may be passed to offspring who may develop that disease. The person does not have the disease and is not at risk of developing the disease.

Z15   Genetic susceptibility to disease

Genetic susceptibility indicates that a person has a gene that increases the risk of that person developing the disease.

Codes from category Z15 should not be used as principal or first-listed codes. If the patient has the condition to which he/she is susceptible, and that condition is the reason for the encounter, the code for the current condition should be sequenced first. If the patient is being seen for follow-up after completed treatment for this condition, and the condition no longer exists, a follow-up code should be sequenced first, followed by the appropriate personal history and genetic susceptibility codes. If the purpose of the encounter is genetic counseling associated with procreative management, code Z31.5, Encounter for genetic counseling, should be assigned as the first-listed code, followed by a code from category Z15. Additional codes should be assigned for any applicable family or personal history.

Z16   Resistance to antimicrobial drugs

This code indicates that a patient has a condition that is resistant to antimicrobial drug treatment. Sequence the infection code first.

Z17   Estrogen receptor status

Z18   Retained foreign body fragments

Z19   Hormone sensitivity malignancy status

Z21   Asymptomatic HIV infection status

This code indicates that a patient has tested positive for HIV but has manifested no signs or symptoms of the disease.

Z22   Carrier of infectious disease

Carrier status indicates that a person harbors the specific organisms of a disease without manifest symptoms and is capable of transmitting the infection.

Z28.3   Underimmunization status

Z33.1   Pregnant state, incidental

This code is a secondary code only for use when the pregnancy is in no way complicating the reason for visit. Otherwise, a code from the obstetric chapter is required.

Z66   Do not resuscitate

This code may be used when it is documented by the provider that a patient is on do not resuscitate status at any time during the stay.

Z67   Blood type

Z68   Body mass index (BMI)

As with all other secondary diagnosis codes, the BMI codes should only be assigned when they meet the definition of a reportable diagnosis (see Section III, Reporting Additional Diagnoses).

Z74.01   Bed confinement status

Z76.82   Awaiting organ transplant status

Z78   Other specified health status

Code Z78.1, Physical restraint status, may be used when it is documented by the provider that a patient has been put in restraints during the current encounter. Please note that this code should not be reported when it is documented by the provider that a patient is temporarily restrained during a procedure.

Z79   Long-term (current) drug therapy

Codes from this category indicate a patient's continuous use of a prescribed drug (including such things as aspirin therapy) for the long-term treatment of a condition or for prophylactic use. It is not for use for patients who have addictions to drugs. This subcategory is not for use of medications for detoxification or maintenance programs to prevent withdrawal symptoms in patients with drug dependence (e.g., methadone maintenance for opiate dependence). Assign the appropriate code for the drug dependence instead.

Assign a code from Z79 if the patient is receiving a medication for an extended period as a prophylactic measure (such as for the prevention of deep vein thrombosis) or as treatment of a chronic condition (such as arthritis) or a disease requiring a lengthy course of treatment (such as cancer). Do not assign a code from category Z79 for medication being administered for a brief period of time to treat an acute illness or injury (such as a course of antibiotics to treat acute bronchitis).

Z88   Allergy status to drugs, medicaments and biological substances

Except: Z88.9, Allergy status to unspecified drugs, medicaments and biological substances status

Z89   Acquired absence of limb

Z90   Acquired absence of organs, not elsewhere classified

Z91.0-   Allergy status, other than to drugs and biological substances

Z92.82   Status post administration of tPA (rtPA) in a different facility within the last 24 hours prior to admission to a current facility

Assign code Z92.82, Status post administration of tPA (rtPA) in a different facility within the last 24 hours prior to admission to current facility, as a secondary diagnosis when a patient is received by transfer into a facility and documentation indicates they were administered tissue plasminogen activator (tPA) within the last 24 hours prior to admission to the current facility.

This guideline applies even if the patient is still receiving the tPA at the time they are received into the current facility.

The appropriate code for the condition for which the tPA was administered (such as cerebrovascular disease or myocardial infarction) should be assigned first.

Code Z92.82 is only applicable to the receiving facility record and not to the transferring facility record.

Z93   Artificial opening status

Z94   Transplanted organ and tissue status

Z95   Presence of cardiac and vascular implants and grafts

Z96   Presence of other functional implants

Z97   Presence of other devices

Z98   Other postprocedural states

Assign code Z98.85, Transplanted organ removal status, to indicate that a transplanted organ has been previously removed. This code should not be assigned for the encounter in which the transplanted organ is removed. The complication necessitating removal of the transplant organ should be assigned for that encounter.

See section I.C19. for information on the coding of organ transplant complications.

Z99   Dependence on enabling machines and devices, not elsewhere classified

Note: Categories Z89-Z90 and Z93-Z99 are for use only if there are no complications or malfunctions of the organ or tissue replaced, the amputation site or the equipment on which the patient is dependent.

4) History (of)

There are two types of history Z codes, personal and family. Personal history codes explain a patient's past medical condition that no longer exists and is not receiving any treatment, but that has the potential for recurrence, and therefore may require continued monitoring.

Family history codes are for use when a patient has a family member(s) who has had a particular disease that causes the patient to be at higher risk of also contracting the disease.

Personal history codes may be used in conjunction with follow-up codes and family history codes may be used in conjunction with screening codes to explain the need for a test or procedure. History codes are also acceptable on any medical record regardless of the reason for visit. A history of an illness, even if no longer present, is important information that may alter the type of treatment ordered.

The history Z code categories are:

Z80   Family history of primary malignant neoplasm

Z81   Family history of mental and behavioral disorders

Z82   Family history of certain disabilities and chronic diseases (leading to disablement)

Z83   Family history of other specific disorders

Z84   Family history of other conditions

Z85   Personal history of malignant neoplasm

Z86   Personal history of certain other diseases

Z87   Personal history of other diseases and conditions

Z91.4-   Personal history of psychological trauma, not elsewhere classified

Z91.5   Personal history of self-harm

Z91.8-   Other specified personal risk factors, not elsewhere classified

Exception: Z91.83, Wandering in diseases classified elsewhere

Z92   Personal history of medical treatment

Except: Z92.0, Personal history of contraception

Except: Z92.82, Status post administration of tPA (rtPA) in a different facility within the last 24 hours prior to admission to a current facility

5) Screening

Screening is the testing for disease or disease precursors in seemingly well individuals so that early detection and treatment can be provided for those who test positive for the disease (e.g., screening mammogram).

The testing of a person to rule out or confirm a suspected diagnosis because the patient has some sign or symptom is a diagnostic examination, not a screening. In these cases, the sign or symptom is used to explain the reason for the test.

A screening code may be a first-listed code if the reason for the visit is specifically the screening exam. It may also be used as an additional code if the screening is done during an office visit for other health problems. A screening code is not necessary if the screening is inherent to a routine examination, such as a pap smear done during a routine pelvic examination.

Should a condition be discovered during the screening then the code for the condition may be assigned as an additional diagnosis.

> Prostate screening of healthy 50-year-old male patient; PSA noted to be elevated but normal digital rectal exam
>
> **Z12.5**   **Encounter for screening for malignant neoplasm of prostate**
>
> **R97.20**   **Elevated prostate specific antigen [PSA]**
>
> *Explanation:* The patient had no signs or symptoms of any prostate-related illness prior to coming in for the screening. The screening code is appropriately used as the first-listed code to signify that this was for routine screening. The elevated PSA is reported as a secondary diagnosis to reflect that an abnormal lab value was found as a result of the screening procedure(s).

The Z code indicates that a screening exam is planned. A procedure code is required to confirm that the screening was performed.

The screening Z codes/categories:

Z11   Encounter for screening for infectious and parasitic diseases

Z12   Encounter for screening for malignant neoplasms

Z13   Encounter for screening for other diseases and disorders

Except: Z13.9, Encounter for screening, unspecified

Z36   Encounter for antenatal screening for mother

6) Observation

There are three observation Z code categories. They are for use in very limited circumstances when a person is being observed for a suspected condition that is ruled out. The observation codes are not for use if an injury or illness or any signs or symptoms related to the suspected condition are present. In such cases the diagnosis/symptom code is used with the corresponding external cause code.

The observation codes are to be used as principal diagnosis only. The only exception to this is when the principal diagnosis is required to be a code from category Z38, Liveborn infants according to place of birth and type of delivery. Then a code from category Z05, Encounter for observation and evaluation of newborn for suspected diseases and conditions ruled out, is sequenced after the Z38 code. Additional codes may be used in addition to the observation code but only if they are unrelated to the suspected condition being observed.

Codes from subcategory Z03.7, Encounter for suspected maternal and fetal conditions ruled out, may either be used as a first-listed or as an additional code assignment depending on the case. They are for use in very limited circumstances on a maternal record when an encounter is for a suspected maternal or fetal condition that is ruled out during that encounter (for example, a maternal or fetal condition may be suspected due to an abnormal test result). These codes should not be used when the condition is confirmed. In those cases, the confirmed condition should be coded. In addition, these codes are not for use if an illness or any signs or symptoms related to the suspected condition or problem are present. In such cases the diagnosis/symptom code is used.

Additional codes may be used in addition to the code from subcategory Z03.7, but only if they are unrelated to the suspected condition being evaluated.

Codes from subcategory Z03.7 may not be used for encounters for antenatal screening of mother. *See Section I.C.21. Screening.*

For encounters for suspected fetal condition that are inconclusive following testing and evaluation, assign the appropriate code from category O35, O36, O40 or O41.

The observation Z code categories:

Z03   Encounter for medical observation for suspected diseases and conditions ruled out

Z04   Encounter for examination and observation for other reasons

      Except: Z04.9, Encounter for examination and observation for unspecified reason

Z05   Encounter for observation and evaluation of newborn for suspected diseases and conditions ruled out

7) Aftercare

Aftercare visit codes cover situations when the initial treatment of a disease has been performed and the patient requires continued care during the healing or recovery phase, or for the long-term consequences of the disease. The aftercare Z code should not be used if treatment is directed at a current, acute disease. The diagnosis code is to be used in these cases. Exceptions to this rule are codes Z51.0, Encounter for antineoplastic radiation therapy, and codes from subcategory Z51.1, Encounter for antineoplastic chemotherapy and immunotherapy. These codes are to be first-listed, followed by the diagnosis code when a patient's encounter is solely to receive radiation therapy, chemotherapy, or immunotherapy for the treatment of a neoplasm. If the reason for the encounter is more than one type of antineoplastic therapy, code Z51.0 and a code from subcategory Z51.1 may be assigned together, in which case one of these codes would be reported as a secondary diagnosis.

The aftercare Z codes should also not be used for aftercare for injuries. For aftercare of an injury, assign the acute injury code with the appropriate 7th character (for subsequent encounter).

The aftercare codes are generally first-listed to explain the specific reason for the encounter. An aftercare code may be used as an additional code when some type of aftercare is provided in addition to the reason for admission and no diagnosis code is applicable. An example of this would be the closure of a colostomy during an encounter for treatment of another condition.

Aftercare codes should be used in conjunction with other aftercare codes or diagnosis codes to provide better detail on the specifics of an aftercare encounter visit, unless otherwise directed by the classification. Should a patient receive multiple types of antineoplastic therapy during the same encounter, code Z51.0, Encounter for antineoplastic radiation therapy, and codes from subcategory Z51.1, Encounter for antineoplastic chemotherapy and immunotherapy, may be used together on a record. The sequencing of multiple aftercare codes depends on the circumstances of the encounter.

Certain aftercare Z code categories need a secondary diagnosis code to describe the resolving condition or sequelae. For others, the condition is included in the code title.

Additional Z code aftercare category terms include fitting and adjustment, and attention to artificial openings.

Status Z codes may be used with aftercare Z codes to indicate the nature of the aftercare. For example code Z95.1, Presence of aortocoronary bypass graft, may be used with code Z48.812, Encounter for surgical aftercare following surgery on the circulatory system, to indicate the surgery for which the aftercare is being performed. A status code should not be used when the aftercare code indicates the type of status, such as using Z43.0, Encounter for attention to tracheostomy, with Z93.0, Tracheostomy status.

The aftercare Z category/codes:

Z42   Encounter for plastic and reconstructive surgery following medical procedure or healed injury

Z43   Encounter for attention to artificial openings

Z44   Encounter for fitting and adjustment of external prosthetic device

Z45   Encounter for adjustment and management of implanted device

Z46   Encounter for fitting and adjustment of other devices

Z47   Orthopedic aftercare

Z48   Encounter for other postprocedural aftercare

Z49   Encounter for care involving renal dialysis

Z51   Encounter for other aftercare and medical care

8) Follow-up

The follow-up codes are used to explain continuing surveillance following completed treatment of a disease, condition, or injury. They imply that the condition has been fully treated and no longer exists. They should not be confused with aftercare codes, or injury codes with a 7th character for subsequent encounter, that explain ongoing care of a healing condition or its sequelae. Follow-up codes may be used in conjunction with history codes to provide the full picture of the healed condition and its treatment. The follow-up code is sequenced first, followed by the history code.

A follow-up code may be used to explain multiple visits. Should a condition be found to have recurred on the follow-up visit, then the diagnosis code for the condition should be assigned in place of the follow-up code.

The follow-up Z code categories:

Z08   Encounter for follow-up examination after completed treatment for malignant neoplasm

Z09   Encounter for follow-up examination after completed treatment for conditions other than malignant neoplasm

Z39   Encounter for maternal postpartum care and examination

Follow-up for patient several months after completing a regime of IV antibiotics for recurrent pneumonia; lungs are clear and pneumonia is resolved

Z09   **Encounter for follow-up examination after completed treatment for conditions other than malignant neoplasm**

Z87.01   **Personal history of pneumonia (recurrent)**

Explanation: Code Z09 identifies the follow-up visit as being unrelated to a malignant neoplasm, and code Z87 describes the condition that has now resolved.

Follow-up for patient several months after completing a regime of IV antibiotics for recurrent pneumonia; pneumonia has recurred, and a new antibiotic regimen has been prescribed

J18.9   **Pneumonia, unspecified organism**

Explanation: Since the follow-up exam for pneumonia determined that the pneumonia was not resolved or recurred, code Z09 Encounter for follow-up examination after completed treatment for conditions other than malignant neoplasm, no longer applies. Instead the first-listed code describes the pneumonia.

---

9) Donor

Codes in category Z52, Donors of organs and tissues, are used for living individuals who are donating blood or other body tissue. These codes are only for individuals donating for others, not for self-donations. They are not used to identify cadaveric donations.

10) Counseling

Counseling Z codes are used when a patient or family member receives assistance in the aftermath of an illness or injury, or when support is required in coping with family or social problems. They are not used in conjunction with a diagnosis code when the counseling component of care is considered integral to standard treatment.

The counseling Z codes/categories:

Z30.0-   Encounter for general counseling and advice on contraception

Z31.5   Encounter for genetic counseling

Z31.6-   Encounter for general counseling and advice on procreation

Z32.2   Encounter for childbirth instruction

Z32.3   Encounter for childcare instruction

Z69   Encounter for mental health services for victim and perpetrator of abuse

Z70   Counseling related to sexual attitude, behavior and orientation

Z71   Persons encountering health services for other counseling and medical advice, not elsewhere classified

Z76.81   Expectant mother prebirth pediatrician visit

11) Encounters for obstetrical and reproductive services

See Section I.C.15. Pregnancy, Childbirth, and the Puerperium, for further instruction on the use of these codes.

Z codes for pregnancy are for use in those circumstances when none of the problems or complications included in the codes from the Obstetrics chapter exist (a routine prenatal visit or postpartum care). Codes in category Z34, Encounter for supervision of normal pregnancy, are always first-listed and are not to be used with any other code from the OB chapter.

Codes in category Z3A, Weeks of gestation, may be assigned to provide additional information about the pregnancy. Category Z3A codes should not be assigned for pregnancies with abortive outcomes (categories O00-O08), elective termination of pregnancy (code Z33.32), nor for postpartum conditions, as category Z3A is not applicable to these conditions. The date of the admission should be used to determine weeks of gestation for inpatient admissions that encompass more than one gestational week.

The outcome of delivery, category Z37, should be included on all maternal delivery records. It is always a secondary code. Codes in category Z37 should not be used on the newborn record.

Z codes for family planning (contraceptive) or procreative management and counseling should be included on an obstetric record either during the pregnancy or the postpartum stage, if applicable.

Z codes/categories for obstetrical and reproductive services:

Z30	Encounter for contraceptive management
Z31	Encounter for procreative management
Z32.2	Encounter for childbirth instruction
Z32.3	Encounter for childcare instruction
Z33	Pregnant state
Z34	Encounter for supervision of normal pregnancy
Z36	Encounter for antenatal screening of mother
Z3A	Weeks of gestation
Z37	Outcome of delivery
Z39	Encounter for maternal postpartum care and examination
Z76.81	Expectant mother prebirth pediatrician visit

12) Newborns and infants

See Section I.C.16. Newborn (Perinatal) Guidelines, for further instruction on the use of these codes.

Newborn Z codes/categories:

Z76.1	Encounter for health supervision and care of foundling
Z00.1-	Encounter for routine child health examination
Z38	Liveborn infants according to place of birth and type of delivery

13) Routine and administrative examinations

The Z codes allow for the description of encounters for routine examinations, such as, a general check-up, or, examinations for administrative purposes, such as, a pre-employment physical. The codes are not to be used if the examination is for diagnosis of a suspected condition or for treatment purposes. In such cases the diagnosis code is used. During a routine exam, should a diagnosis or condition be discovered, it should be coded as an additional code. Pre-existing and chronic conditions and history codes may also be included as additional codes as long as the examination is for administrative purposes and not focused on any particular condition.

Some of the codes for routine health examinations distinguish between "with" and "without" abnormal findings. Code assignment depends on the information that is known at the time the encounter is being coded. For example, if no abnormal findings were found during the examination, but the encounter is being coded before test results are back, it is acceptable to assign the code for "without abnormal findings." When assigning a code for "with abnormal findings," additional code(s) should be assigned to identify the specific abnormal finding(s).

12-month-old boy presented for well-child visit; pediatrician notices some eczema on the child's scalp and back of the knees

Z00.121   **Encounter for routine child health examination with abnormal findings**

L30.9   **Dermatitis, unspecified**

Explanation: The Z code identifying that this is a routine well-child visit is reported first. Because an abnormal finding (eczema) was documented, a code for this condition may also be appended.

Pre-operative examination and pre-procedural laboratory examination Z codes are for use only in those situations when a patient is being cleared for a procedure or surgery and no treatment is given.

The Z codes/categories for routine and administrative examinations:

Z00	Encounter for general examination without complaint, suspected or reported diagnosis
Z01	Encounter for other special examination without complaint, suspected or reported diagnosis
Z02	Encounter for administrative examination
	Except: Z02.9, Encounter for administrative examinations, unspecified
Z32.0-	Encounter for pregnancy test

14) Miscellaneous Z codes

The miscellaneous Z codes capture a number of other health care encounters that do not fall into one of the other categories. Certain of these codes identify the reason for the encounter; others are for use as additional codes that provide useful information on circumstances that may affect a patient's care and treatment.

Prophylactic organ removal

For encounters specifically for prophylactic removal of an organ (such as prophylactic removal of breasts due to a genetic susceptibility to cancer or a family history of cancer), the principal or first-listed code should be a code from category Z40, Encounter for prophylactic surgery, followed by the appropriate codes to identify the associated risk factor (such as genetic susceptibility or family history).

If the patient has a malignancy of one site and is having prophylactic removal at another site to prevent either a new primary malignancy or metastatic disease, a code for the malignancy should also be assigned in addition to a code from subcategory Z40.0, Encounter for prophylactic surgery for risk factors related to malignant neoplasms. A Z40.0 code should not be assigned if the patient is having organ removal for treatment of a malignancy, such as the removal of the testes for the treatment of prostate cancer.

Miscellaneous Z codes/categories:

Z28	Immunization not carried out
	Except: Z28.3, Underimmunization status
Z29	Encounter for other prophylactic measures
Z40	Encounter for prophylactic surgery
Z41	Encounter for procedures for purposes other than remedying health state
	Except: Z41.9, Encounter for procedure for purposes other than remedying health state, unspecified
Z53	Persons encountering health services for specific procedures and treatment, not carried out
Z55	Problems related to education and literacy
Z56	Problems related to employment and unemployment
Z57	Occupational exposure to risk factors
Z58	Problems related to physical environment
Z59	Problems related to housing and economic circumstances
Z60	Problems related to social environment
Z62	Problems related to upbringing
Z63	Other problems related to primary support group, including family circumstances
Z64	Problems related to certain psychosocial circumstances
Z65	Problems related to other psychosocial circumstances
Z72	Problems related to lifestyle
	Note: These codes should be assigned only when the documentation specifies that the patient has an associated problem
Z73	Problems related to life management difficulty
Z74	Problems related to care provider dependency
	Except: Z74.01, Bed confinement status
Z75	Problems related to medical facilities and other health care
Z76.0	Encounter for issue of repeat prescription
Z76.3	Healthy person accompanying sick person
Z76.4	Other boarder to healthcare facility
Z76.5	Malingerer [conscious simulation]
Z91.1-	Patient's noncompliance with medical treatment and regimen
Z91.83	Wandering in diseases classified elsewhere
Z91.89	Other specified personal risk factors, not elsewhere classified

15) Nonspecific Z codes

Certain Z codes are so non-specific, or potentially redundant with other codes in the classification, that there can be little justification for their use in the inpatient setting. Their use in the outpatient setting should be limited to those instances when there is no further documentation to permit more precise coding. Otherwise, any sign or symptom or any other reason for visit that is captured in another code should be used.

Nonspecific Z codes/categories:

Z02.9	Encounter for administrative examinations, unspecified
Z04.9	Encounter for examination and observation for unspecified reason
Z13.9	Encounter for screening, unspecified
Z41.9	Encounter for procedure for purposes other than remedying health state, unspecified
Z52.9	Donor of unspecified organ or tissue
Z86.59	Personal history of other mental and behavioral disorders
Z88.9	Allergy status to unspecified drugs, medicaments and biological substances status
Z92.0	Personal history of contraception

16) Z codes that may only be principal/first-listed diagnosis

The following Z codes/categories may only be reported as the principal/first-listed diagnosis, except when there are multiple encounters on the same day and the medical records for the encounters are combined:

Z00	Encounter for general examination without complaint, suspected or reported diagnosis
	Except: Z00.6
Z01	Encounter for other special examination without complaint, suspected or reported diagnosis
Z02	Encounter for administrative examination
Z03	Encounter for medical observation for suspected diseases and conditions ruled out
Z04	Encounter for examination and observation for other reasons
Z33.2	Encounter for elective termination of pregnancy

Z31.81	Encounter for male factor infertility in female patient
Z31.83	Encounter for assisted reproductive fertility procedure cycle
Z31.84	Encounter for fertility preservation procedure
Z34	Encounter for supervision of normal pregnancy
Z39	Encounter for maternal postpartum care and examination
Z38	Liveborn infants according to place of birth and type of delivery
Z42	Encounter for plastic and reconstructive surgery following medical procedure or healed injury
Z51.0	Encounter for antineoplastic radiation therapy
Z51.1-	Encounter for antineoplastic chemotherapy and immunotherapy
Z52	Donors of organs and tissues
	Except: Z52.9, Donor of unspecified organ or tissue
Z76.1	Encounter for health supervision and care of foundling
Z76.2	Encounter for health supervision and care of other healthy infant and child
Z99.12	Encounter for respirator [ventilator] dependence during power failure

Female patient seen at 32 weeks' gestation to check the progress of her first pregnancy

Z34.03	**Encounter for supervision of normal first pregnancy, third trimester**
Z3A.32	**32 weeks gestation of pregnancy**

Explanation: Category Z34 is appropriate as a first-listed diagnosis. Category Z3A helps to clarify at which point in the pregnancy the patient was provided supervision.

Chapter 21. Factors Influencing Health Status and Contact With Health Services (Z00-Z99)

NOTE Z codes represent reasons for encounters. A corresponding procedure code must accompany a Z code if a procedure is performed. Categories Z00-Z99 are provided for occasions when circumstances other than a disease, injury or external cause classifiable to categories A00-Y89 are recorded as "diagnoses" or "problems". This can arise in two main ways:

(a) When a person who may or may not be sick encounters the health services for some specific purpose, such as to receive limited care or service for a current condition, to donate an organ or tissue, to receive prophylactic vaccination (immunization), or to discuss a problem which is in itself not a disease or injury.

(b) When some circumstance or problem is present which influences the person's health status but is not in itself a current illness or injury.

This chapter contains the following blocks:

Z00-Z13	Persons encountering health services for examinations
Z14-Z15	Genetic carrier and genetic susceptibility to disease
Z16	Resistance to antimicrobial drugs
Z17	Estrogen receptor status
Z18	Retained foreign body fragments
~~Z19~~	~~Hormone sensitivity malignancy status~~
Z20-Z29	Persons with potential health hazards related to communicable diseases
Z30-Z39	Persons encountering health services in circumstances related to reproduction
Z40-Z53	Encounters for other specific health care
Z55-Z65	Persons with potential health hazards related to socioeconomic and psychosocial circumstances
Z66	Do not resuscitate status
Z67	Blood type
Z68	Body mass index (BMI)
Z69-Z76	Persons encountering health services in other circumstances
Z77-Z99	Persons with potential health hazards related to family and personal history and certain conditions influencing health status

Persons encountering health services for examinations (Z00-Z13)

NOTE Nonspecific abnormal findings disclosed at the time of these examinations are classified to categories R70-R94.

EXCLUDES 1 examinations related to pregnancy and reproduction (Z30-Z36, Z39-)

✓4ᵗʰ Z00 Encounter for general examination without complaint, suspected or reported diagnosis
> *EXCLUDES 1* encounter for examination for administrative purposes (Z02.-)
> *EXCLUDES 2* encounter for pre-procedural examinations (Z01.81-)
> special screening examinations (Z11-Z13)

✓5ᵗʰ Z00.0 Encounter for general adult medical examination
> Encounter for adult periodic examination (annual) (physical) and any associated laboratory and radiologic examinations
> *EXCLUDES 1* encounter for examination of sign or symptom—code to sign or symptom
> general health check-up of infant or child (Z00.12-)

Z00.00 Encounter for general adult medical examination without abnormal findings PDx A
> Encounter for adult health check-up NOS
> **AHA:** 2016, 1Q, 36

Z00.01 Encounter for general adult medical examination with abnormal findings PDx A
> Use additional code to identify abnormal findings
> **AHA:** 2016, 1Q, 35-36

✓5ᵗʰ Z00.1 Encounter for newborn, infant and child health examinations

✓6ᵗʰ Z00.11 Newborn health examination
> Health check for child under 29 days old
> Use additional code to identify any abnormal findings
> *EXCLUDES 1* health check for child over 28 days old (Z00.12-)

Z00.110 Health examination for newborn under 8 days old PDx N
> Health check for newborn under 8 days old

Z00.111 Health examination for newborn 8 to 28 days old PDx N
> Health check for newborn 8 to 28 days old
> Newborn weight check

✓6ᵗʰ Z00.12 Encounter for routine child health examination
> Encounter for development testing of infant or child
> Health check (routine) for child over 28 days old
> *EXCLUDES 1* health check for child under 29 days old (Z00.11-)
> health supervision of foundling or other healthy infant or child (Z76.1-Z76.2)
> newborn health examination (Z00.11-)

Z00.121 Encounter for routine child health examination with abnormal findings PDx P
> Use additional code to identify abnormal findings
> **AHA:** 2016, 1Q, 34-35

Z00.129 Encounter for routine child health examination without abnormal findings PDx P
> Encounter for routine child health examination NOS
> **AHA:** 2016, 1Q, 34

Z00.2 Encounter for examination for period of rapid growth in childhood PDx P

Z00.3 Encounter for examination for adolescent development state PDx P
> Encounter for puberty development state

Z00.5 Encounter for examination of potential donor of organ and tissue PDx

Z00.6 Encounter for examination for normal comparison and control in clinical research program
> Examination of participant or control in clinical research program

✓5ᵗʰ Z00.7 Encounter for examination for period of delayed growth in childhood

Z00.70 Encounter for examination for period of delayed growth in childhood without abnormal findings PDx P

Z00.71 Encounter for examination for period of delayed growth in childhood with abnormal findings PDx P
> Use additional code to identify abnormal findings

Z00.8 Encounter for other general examination PDx
> Encounter for health examination in population surveys

✓4ᵗʰ Z01 Encounter for other special examination without complaint, suspected or reported diagnosis
> **INCLUDES** routine examination of specific system
> **NOTE** Codes from category Z01 represent the reason for the encounter. A separate procedure code is required to identify any examinations or procedures performed.
> *EXCLUDES 1* encounter for examination for administrative purposes (Z02.-)
> encounter for examination for suspected conditions, proven not to exist (Z03.-)
> encounter for laboratory and radiologic examinations as a component of general medical examinations (Z00.0-)
> encounter for laboratory, radiologic and imaging examinations for sign(s) and symptom(s)—code to the sign(s) or symptom(s)
> *EXCLUDES 2* screening examinations (Z11-Z13)

✓5ᵗʰ Z01.0 Encounter for examination of eyes and vision
> *EXCLUDES 1* examination for driving license (Z02.4)

Z01.00 Encounter for examination of eyes and vision without abnormal findings PDx
> Encounter for examination of eyes and vision NOS

Z01.01 Encounter for examination of eyes and vision with abnormal findings PDx
> Use additional code to identify abnormal findings

✓5ᵗʰ Z01.1 Encounter for examination of ears and hearing

Z01.10 Encounter for examination of ears and hearing without abnormal findings PDx
> Encounter for examination of ears and hearing NOS
> **AHA:** 2016, 4Q, 24

✓6ᵗʰ Z01.11 Encounter for examination of ears and hearing with abnormal findings PDx
> **AHA:** 2016, 3Q, 17-18

Z01.110 Encounter for hearing examination following failed hearing screening PDx

Z01.118 Encounter for examination of ears and hearing with other abnormal findings PDx
> Use additional code to identify abnormal findings

Z01.12 Encounter for hearing conservation and treatment PDx

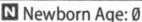

EXCLUDES 1 Not coded here   *EXCLUDES 2* Not included here   **N** Newborn Age: 0   **P** Pediatric Age: 0-17   **M** Maternity Age: 12-55   **A** Adult Age: 15-124   **PDx** Primary Dx

✓5ᵗʰ Z01.2 Encounter for dental examination and cleaning

> **Z01.20 Encounter for dental examination and cleaning without abnormal findings** `PDx`
> > Encounter for dental examination and cleaning NOS
>
> **Z01.21 Encounter for dental examination and cleaning with abnormal findings** `PDx`
> > Use additional code to identify abnormal findings

✓5ᵗʰ Z01.3 Encounter for examination of blood pressure

> **Z01.30 Encounter for examination of blood pressure without abnormal findings** `PDx`
> > Encounter for examination of blood pressure NOS
>
> **Z01.31 Encounter for examination of blood pressure with abnormal findings** `PDx`
> > Use additional code to identify abnormal findings

✓5ᵗʰ Z01.4 Encounter for gynecological examination

> *EXCLUDES 2*   *pregnancy examination or test (Z32.0-)*
> *routine examination for contraceptive maintenance (Z30.4-)*
>
> **✓6ᵗʰ Z01.41 Encounter for routine gynecological examination**
> > Encounter for general gynecological examination with or without cervical smear
> > Encounter for gynecological examination (general) (routine) NOS
> > Encounter for pelvic examination (annual) (periodic)
> > Use additional code:
> > > for screening for human papillomavirus, if applicable, (Z11.51)
> > > for screening vaginal pap smear, if applicable (Z12.72)
> > > to identify acquired absence of uterus, if applicable (Z90.71-)
> >
> > *EXCLUDES 1*   *gynecologic examination status-post hysterectomy for malignant condition (Z08)*
> > *screening cervical pap smear not a part of a routine gynecological examination (Z12.4)*
> >
> > **Z01.411 Encounter for gynecological examination (general) (routine) with abnormal findings** `PDx` ♀
> > > Use additional code to identify abnormal findings
> >
> > **Z01.419 Encounter for gynecological examination (general) (routine) without abnormal findings** `PDx` ♀
>
> **Z01.42 Encounter for cervical smear to confirm findings of recent normal smear following initial abnormal smear** `PDx` ♀

✓5ᵗʰ Z01.8 Encounter for other specified special examinations

> **✓6ᵗʰ Z01.81 Encounter for preprocedural examinations**
> > Encounter for preoperative examinations
> > Encounter for radiological and imaging examinations as part of preprocedural examination
> >
> > **Z01.810 Encounter for preprocedural cardiovascular examination** `PDx`
> >
> > **Z01.811 Encounter for preprocedural respiratory examination** `PDx`
> >
> > **Z01.812 Encounter for preprocedural laboratory examination** `PDx`
> > > Blood and urine tests prior to treatment or procedure
> >
> > **Z01.818 Encounter for other preprocedural examination** `PDx`
> > > Encounter for preprocedural examination NOS
> > > Encounter for examinations prior to antineoplastic chemotherapy
>
> **Z01.82 Encounter for allergy testing** `PDx`
> > *EXCLUDES 1*   *encounter for antibody response examination (Z01.84)*
>
> **Z01.83 Encounter for blood typing** `PDx`
> > Encounter for Rh typing
>
> **Z01.84 Encounter for antibody response examination** `PDx`
> > Encounter for immunity status testing
> > *EXCLUDES 1*   *encounter for allergy testing (Z01.82)*
>
> **Z01.89 Encounter for other specified special examinations** `PDx`

✓4ᵗʰ Z02 Encounter for administrative examination

> **Z02.0 Encounter for examination for admission to educational institution** `PDx`
> > Encounter for examination for admission to preschool (education)
> > Encounter for examination for re-admission to school following illness or medical treatment
>
> **Z02.1 Encounter for pre-employment examination** `PDx`
>
> **Z02.2 Encounter for examination for admission to residential institution** `PDx`
> > *EXCLUDES 1*   *examination for admission to prison (Z02.89)*
>
> **Z02.3 Encounter for examination for recruitment to armed forces** `PDx`
>
> **Z02.4 Encounter for examination for driving license** `PDx`
>
> **Z02.5 Encounter for examination for participation in sport** `PDx`
> > *EXCLUDES 1*   *blood-alcohol and blood-drug test (Z02.83)*
>
> **Z02.6 Encounter for examination for insurance purposes** `PDx`
>
> **✓5ᵗʰ Z02.7 Encounter for issue of medical certificate**
> > *EXCLUDES 1*   *encounter for general medical examination (Z00-Z01, Z02.0-Z02.6, Z02.8-Z02.9)*
> >
> > **Z02.71 Encounter for disability determination** `PDx`
> > > Encounter for issue of medical certificate of incapacity
> > > Encounter for issue of medical certificate of invalidity
> >
> > **Z02.79 Encounter for issue of other medical certificate** `PDx`
>
> **✓5ᵗʰ Z02.8 Encounter for other administrative examinations**
> > **Z02.81 Encounter for paternity testing** `PDx`
> >
> > **Z02.82 Encounter for adoption services** `PDx`
> >
> > **Z02.83 Encounter for blood-alcohol and blood-drug test** `PDx`
> > > Use additional code for findings of alcohol or drugs in blood (R78.-)
> >
> > **Z02.89 Encounter for other administrative examinations** `PDx`
> > > Encounter for examination for admission to prison
> > > Encounter for examination for admission to summer camp
> > > Encounter for immigration examination
> > > Encounter for naturalization examination
> > > Encounter for premarital examination
> > > *EXCLUDES 1*   *health supervision of foundling or other healthy infant or child (Z76.1-Z76.2)*
>
> **Z02.9 Encounter for administrative examinations, unspecified** `PDx` ▽

✓4ᵗʰ Z03 Encounter for medical observation for suspected diseases and conditions ruled out

> *NOTE*   This category is to be used when a person without a diagnosis is suspected of having an abnormal condition, without signs or symptoms, which requires study, but after examination and observation, is ruled out. This category is also for use for administrative and legal observation status.
>
> *EXCLUDES 1*   *contact with and (suspected) exposures hazardous to health (Z77.-)*
> ▶*encounter for observation and evaluation of newborn for suspected diseases and conditions ruled out (Z05.0-)*◀
> ~~*newborn observation for suspected condition, ruled out (P00-P04)*~~
> *person with feared complaint in whom no diagnosis is made (Z71.1)*
> *signs or symptoms under study—code to signs or symptoms*
>
> **Z03.6 Encounter for observation for suspected toxic effect from ingested substance ruled out** `PDx`
> > Encounter for observation for suspected adverse effect from drug
> > Encounter for observation for suspected poisoning
>
> **✓5ᵗʰ Z03.7 Encounter for suspected maternal and fetal conditions ruled out**
> > Encounter for suspected maternal and fetal conditions not found
> > *EXCLUDES 1*   *known or suspected fetal anomalies affecting management of mother, not ruled out (O26-, O35-, O36-, O40-, O41-)*
> >
> > **Z03.71 Encounter for suspected problem with amniotic cavity and membrane ruled out** `PDx` Ⓜ ♀
> > > Encounter for suspected oligohydramnios ruled out
> > > Encounter for suspected polyhydramnios ruled out
> >
> > **Z03.72 Encounter for suspected placental problem ruled out** `PDx` Ⓜ ♀
> >
> > **Z03.73 Encounter for suspected fetal anomaly ruled out** `PDx` Ⓜ ♀

✓ Additional Character Req   ✓⁷ᵗʰ Placeholder Alert   Manifestation   `HCC` CMS-HCC Condition   ▽ Unspecified Code   ▶◀ Revised Text   ● New Code   ▲ Revised Code Title

ICD-10-CM 2018   1181

Chapter 21. Factors Influencing Health Status and Contact with Health Services

Z03.74 Encounter for suspected **problem with fetal growth** ruled out `PDx` `M♀`

Z03.75 Encounter for suspected **cervical shortening** ruled out `PDx` `M♀`

Z03.79 Encounter for other suspected maternal and fetal conditions ruled out `PDx` `M♀`

√5ᵗʰ **Z03.8** Encounter for **observation** for other suspected diseases and conditions ruled out

√6ᵗʰ **Z03.81** Encounter for observation for suspected **exposure to biological agents** ruled out

Z03.810 Encounter for observation for suspected exposure to **anthrax** ruled out `PDx`

Z03.818 Encounter for observation for suspected exposure to other biological agents ruled out `PDx`

Z03.89 Encounter for observation for other suspected diseases and conditions ruled out `PDx`

√4ᵗʰ **Z04** **Encounter for examination and observation for other reasons**
`INCLUDES` encounter for examination for medicolegal reasons
This category is to be used when a person without a diagnosis is suspected of having an abnormal condition, without signs or symptoms, which requires study, but after examination and observation, is ruled-out. This category is also for use for administrative and legal observation status.

Z04.1 Encounter for examination and observation following **transport accident** `PDx`
`EXCLUDES 1` encounter for examination and observation following work accident (Z04.2)

Z04.2 Encounter for examination and observation following **work accident** `PDx`

Z04.3 Encounter for examination and observation following **other accident** `PDx`

√5ᵗʰ **Z04.4** Encounter for examination and observation following **alleged rape**
Encounter for examination and observation of victim following alleged rape
Encounter for examination and observation of victim following alleged sexual abuse

Z04.41 Encounter for examination and observation following alleged **adult rape** `PDx` `A`
Suspected adult rape, ruled out
Suspected adult sexual abuse, ruled out

Z04.42 Encounter for examination and observation following alleged **child rape** `PDx` `P`
Suspected child rape, ruled out
Suspected child sexual abuse, ruled out

Z04.6 Encounter for **general psychiatric examination, requested by authority** `PDx`

√5ᵗʰ **Z04.7** Encounter for examination and observation following **alleged physical abuse**

Z04.71 Encounter for examination and observation following alleged **adult physical abuse** `PDx` `A`
Suspected adult physical abuse, ruled out
`EXCLUDES 1` confirmed case of adult physical abuse (T74.-)
encounter for examination and observation following alleged adult sexual abuse (Z04.41)
suspected case of adult physical abuse, not ruled out (T76.-)

Z04.72 Encounter for examination and observation following alleged **child physical abuse** `PDx` `P`
Suspected child physical abuse, ruled out
`EXCLUDES 1` confirmed case of child physical abuse (T74.-)
encounter for examination and observation following alleged child sexual abuse (Z04.42)
suspected case of child physical abuse, not ruled out (T76.-)

Z04.8 Encounter for examination and observation for other specified reasons `PDx`
Encounter for examination and observation for request for expert evidence

Z04.9 Encounter for examination and observation for unspecified reason `PDx` ▽
Encounter for observation NOS

√4ᵗʰ **Z05** **Encounter for observation of newborn for suspected diseases and conditions ruled out**
▶This category is to be used for newborns, within the neonatal period (the first 28 days of life), who are suspected of having an abnormal condition, but without signs or symptoms, and which, after examination and observation, is ruled out.◀
`EXCLUDES 2` ~~newborn observation for suspected condition, related to exposure from the mother or birth process (P00-P04)~~

Z05.0 Observation and evaluation of newborn for suspected **cardiac** condition ruled out

Z05.1 Observation and evaluation of newborn for suspected **infectious** condition ruled out

Z05.2 Observation and evaluation of newborn for suspected **neurological** condition ruled out

Z05.3 Observation and evaluation of newborn for suspected **respiratory** condition ruled out

√5ᵗʰ **Z05.4** Observation and evaluation of newborn for suspected **genetic, metabolic or immunologic** condition ruled out

Z05.41 Observation and evaluation of newborn for suspected **genetic** condition ruled out

Z05.42 Observation and evaluation of newborn for suspected **metabolic** condition ruled out

Z05.43 Observation and evaluation of newborn for suspected **immunologic** condition ruled out

Z05.5 Observation and evaluation of newborn for suspected **gastrointestinal** condition ruled out

Z05.6 Observation and evaluation of newborn for suspected **genitourinary** condition ruled out

√5ᵗʰ **Z05.7** Observation and evaluation of newborn for suspected **skin, subcutaneous, musculoskeletal and connective tissue** condition ruled out

Z05.71 Observation and evaluation of newborn for suspected **skin and subcutaneous tissue** condition ruled out

Z05.72 Observation and evaluation of newborn for suspected **musculoskeletal** condition ruled out

Z05.73 Observation and evaluation of newborn for suspected **connective tissue** condition ruled out

Z05.8 Observation and evaluation of newborn for other specified suspected condition ruled out

Z05.9 Observation and evaluation of newborn for unspecified suspected condition ruled out ▽

Z08 **Encounter for follow-up examination after completed treatment for malignant neoplasm**
Medical surveillance following completed treatment
Use additional code to identify any acquired absence of organs (Z90.-)
Use additional code to identify the personal history of malignant neoplasm (Z85.-)
`EXCLUDES 1` aftercare following medical care (Z43-Z49, Z51)

Z09 **Encounter for follow-up examination after completed treatment for conditions other than malignant neoplasm**
Medical surveillance following completed treatment
Use additional code to identify any applicable history of disease code (Z86-, Z87-)
`EXCLUDES 1` aftercare following medical care (Z43-Z49, Z51)
surveillance of contraception (Z30.4-)
surveillance of prosthetic and other medical devices (Z44-Z46)
AHA: 2017, 1Q, 9; 2015, 1Q, 8

√4ᵗʰ **Z11** **Encounter for screening for infectious and parasitic diseases**
Screening is the testing for disease or disease precursors in asymptomatic individuals so that early detection and treatment can be provided for those who test positive for the disease.
`EXCLUDES 1` encounter for diagnostic examination—code to sign or symptom

Z11.0 Encounter for screening for **intestinal** infectious diseases

Z11.1 Encounter for screening for **respiratory tuberculosis**

Z11.2 Encounter for screening for other bacterial diseases

Z11.3 Encounter for screening for infections with a **predominantly sexual mode of transmission**
`EXCLUDES 2` encounter for screening for human immunodeficiency virus [HIV] (Z11.4)
encounter for screening for human papillomavirus (Z11.51)

Z11.4 Encounter for screening for **human immunodeficiency virus [HIV]**

☑5ᵗʰ **Z11.5** **Encounter for screening for other viral diseases**
> *EXCLUDES 2* *encounter for screening for viral intestinal disease (Z11.0)*

Z11.51 **Encounter for screening for human papillomavirus (HPV)**

Z11.59 **Encounter for screening for other viral diseases**

Z11.6 **Encounter for screening for other protozoal diseases and helminthiases**
> *EXCLUDES 2* *encounter for screening for protozoal intestinal disease (Z11.0)*

Z11.8 **Encounter for screening for other infectious and parasitic diseases**
> Encounter for screening for chlamydia
> Encounter for screening for rickettsial
> Encounter for screening for spirochetal
> Encounter for screening for mycoses

Z11.9 **Encounter for screening for infectious and parasitic diseases, unspecified** ▽

☑4ᵗʰ **Z12** **Encounter for screening for malignant neoplasms**
> Screening is the testing for disease or disease precursors in asymptomatic individuals so that early detection and treatment can be provided for those who test positive for the disease.
> Use additional code to identify any family history of malignant neoplasm (Z80.-)
> *EXCLUDES 1* *encounter for diagnostic examination—code to sign or symptom*

Z12.0 **Encounter for screening for malignant neoplasm of stomach**

☑5ᵗʰ **Z12.1** **Encounter for screening for malignant neoplasm of intestinal tract**
> **AHA:** 2017, 1Q, 8, 9

Z12.10 **Encounter for screening for malignant neoplasm of intestinal tract, unspecified** ▽

Z12.11 **Encounter for screening for malignant neoplasm of colon**
> Encounter for screening colonoscopy NOS

Z12.12 **Encounter for screening for malignant neoplasm of rectum**

Z12.13 **Encounter for screening for malignant neoplasm of small intestine**

Z12.2 **Encounter for screening for malignant neoplasm of respiratory organs**

☑5ᵗʰ **Z12.3** **Encounter for screening for malignant neoplasm of breast**

Z12.31 **Encounter for screening mammogram for malignant neoplasm of breast**
> *EXCLUDES 1* *inconclusive mammogram (R92.2)*
> **AHA:** 2015, 1Q, 24

Z12.39 **Encounter for other screening for malignant neoplasm of breast**

Z12.4 **Encounter for screening for malignant neoplasm of cervix** ♀
> Encounter for screening pap smear for malignant neoplasm of cervix
> *EXCLUDES 1* *when screening is part of general gynecological examination (Z01.4-)*
> *EXCLUDES 2* *encounter for screening for human papillomavirus (Z11.51)*

Z12.5 **Encounter for screening for malignant neoplasm of prostate** ♂

Z12.6 **Encounter for screening for malignant neoplasm of bladder**

☑5ᵗʰ **Z12.7** **Encounter for screening for malignant neoplasm of other genitourinary organs**

Z12.71 **Encounter for screening for malignant neoplasm of testis** ♂

Z12.72 **Encounter for screening for malignant neoplasm of vagina** ♀
> Vaginal pap smear status-post hysterectomy for non-malignant condition
> Use additional code to identify acquired absence of uterus (Z90.71-)
> *EXCLUDES 1* *vaginal pap smear status-post hysterectomy for malignant conditions (Z08)*

Z12.73 **Encounter for screening for malignant neoplasm of ovary** ♀

Z12.79 **Encounter for screening for malignant neoplasm of other genitourinary organs**

☑5ᵗʰ **Z12.8** **Encounter for screening for malignant neoplasm of other sites**

Z12.81 **Encounter for screening for malignant neoplasm of oral cavity**

Z12.82 **Encounter for screening for malignant neoplasm of nervous system**

Z12.83 **Encounter for screening for malignant neoplasm of skin**

Z12.89 **Encounter for screening for malignant neoplasm of other sites**

Z12.9 **Encounter for screening for malignant neoplasm, site unspecified** ▽

☑4ᵗʰ **Z13** **Encounter for screening for other diseases and disorders**
> Screening is the testing for disease or disease precursors in asymptomatic individuals so that early detection and treatment can be provided for those who test positive for the disease.
> *EXCLUDES 1* *encounter for diagnostic examination—code to sign or symptom*

Z13.0 **Encounter for screening for diseases of the blood and blood-forming organs and certain disorders involving the immune mechanism**

Z13.1 **Encounter for screening for diabetes mellitus**

☑5ᵗʰ **Z13.2** **Encounter for screening for nutritional, metabolic and other endocrine disorders**

Z13.21 **Encounter for screening for nutritional disorder**

☑6ᵗʰ **Z13.22** **Encounter for screening for metabolic disorder**

Z13.220 **Encounter for screening for lipoid disorders**
> Encounter for screening for cholesterol level
> Encounter for screening for hypercholesterolemia
> Encounter for screening for hyperlipidemia

Z13.228 **Encounter for screening for other metabolic disorders**

Z13.29 **Encounter for screening for other suspected endocrine disorder**
> *EXCLUDES 1* *encounter for screening for diabetes mellitus (Z13.1)*

Z13.4 **Encounter for screening for certain developmental disorders in childhood** ℗
> Encounter for screening for developmental handicaps in early childhood
> *EXCLUDES 1* *routine development testing of infant or child (Z00.1-)*

Z13.5 **Encounter for screening for eye and ear disorders**
> *EXCLUDES 2* *encounter for general hearing examination (Z01.1-)*
> *encounter for general vision examination (Z01.0-)*
> **AHA:** 2016, 3Q, 17

Z13.6 **Encounter for screening for cardiovascular disorders**

☑5ᵗʰ **Z13.7** **Encounter for screening for genetic and chromosomal anomalies**
> *EXCLUDES 1* *genetic testing for procreative management (Z31.4-)*

Z13.71 **Encounter for nonprocreative screening for genetic disease carrier status**

Z13.79 **Encounter for other screening for genetic and chromosomal anomalies**

☑5ᵗʰ **Z13.8** **Encounter for screening for other specified diseases and disorders**
> *EXCLUDES 2* *screening for malignant neoplasms (Z12.-)*

☑6ᵗʰ **Z13.81** **Encounter for screening for digestive system disorders**

Z13.810 **Encounter for screening for upper gastrointestinal disorder**

Z13.811 **Encounter for screening for lower gastrointestinal disorder**
> *EXCLUDES 1* *encounter for screening for intestinal infectious disease (Z11.0)*

Z13.818 **Encounter for screening for other digestive system disorders**

☑6ᵗʰ **Z13.82** **Encounter for screening for musculoskeletal disorder**

Z13.820 **Encounter for screening for osteoporosis**

Z13.828 **Encounter for screening for other musculoskeletal disorder**

☑ Additional Character Req   ☑7ᵗʰ Placeholder Alert   Manifestation   ᴴᶜᶜ CMS-HCC Condition   ▽ Unspecified Code   ►◄ Revised Text   ● New Code   ▲ Revised Code Title

ICD-10-CM 2018   1183

Z13.83 Encounter for screening for respiratory disorder NEC
> EXCLUDES 1   *encounter for screening for respiratory tuberculosis (Z11.1)*

Z13.84 Encounter for screening for dental disorders

✓6ᵗʰ **Z13.85 Encounter for screening for nervous system disorders**

> **Z13.850 Encounter for screening for traumatic brain injury**

> **Z13.858 Encounter for screening for other nervous system disorders**

Z13.88 Encounter for screening for disorder due to exposure to contaminants
> EXCLUDES 1   *those exposed to contaminants without suspected disorders (Z57-Z77-)*

Z13.89 Encounter for screening for other disorder
> Encounter for screening for genitourinary disorders

Z13.9 Encounter for screening, unspecified   ▽

Genetic carrier and genetic susceptibility to disease (Z14-Z15)

✓4ᵗʰ **Z14 Genetic carrier**
> DEF: Individuals carrying a gene mutation associated with a certain disease who typically do not develop the disease but are able to pass mutated gene to offspring.

✓5ᵗʰ **Z14.0 Hemophilia A carrier**

> **Z14.01 Asymptomatic hemophilia A carrier**

> **Z14.02 Symptomatic hemophilia A carrier**

Z14.1 Cystic fibrosis carrier

Z14.8 Genetic carrier of other disease

✓4ᵗʰ **Z15 Genetic susceptibility to disease**
> INCLUDES   confirmed abnormal gene
>
> Use additional code, if applicable, for any associated family history of the disease (Z80-Z84)
>
> EXCLUDES 1   *chromosomal anomalies (Q90-Q99)*

✓5ᵗʰ **Z15.0 Genetic susceptibility to malignant neoplasm**
> Code first, if applicable, any current malignant neoplasm (C00-C75, C81-C96)
>
> Use additional code, if applicable, for any personal history of malignant neoplasm (Z85.-)

> **Z15.01 Genetic susceptibility to malignant neoplasm of breast**

> **Z15.02 Genetic susceptibility to malignant neoplasm of ovary**   ♀

> **Z15.03 Genetic susceptibility to malignant neoplasm of prostate**   ♂

> **Z15.04 Genetic susceptibility to malignant neoplasm of endometrium**   ♀

> **Z15.09 Genetic susceptibility to other malignant neoplasm**

✓5ᵗʰ **Z15.8 Genetic susceptibility to other disease**

> **Z15.81 Genetic susceptibility to multiple endocrine neoplasia [MEN]**
> > EXCLUDES 1   *multiple endocrine neoplasia [MEN] syndromes (E31.2-)*

> **Z15.89 Genetic susceptibility to other disease**

Resistance to antimicrobial drugs (Z16)

✓4ᵗʰ **Z16 Resistance to antimicrobial drugs**
> NOTE   The codes in this category are provided for use as additional codes to identify the resistance and non-responsiveness of a condition to antimicrobial drugs.
>
> Code first the infection
>
> EXCLUDES 1   *Methicillin resistant Staphylococcus aureus infection (A49.02)*
> ~~Methicillin resistant Staphylococcus aureus infection in diseases classified elsewhere (B95.62)~~
> *Methicillin resistant Staphylococcus aureus pneumonia (J15.212)*
> *sepsis due to Methicillin resistant Staphylococcus aureus (A41.02)*

✓5ᵗʰ **Z16.1 Resistance to beta lactam antibiotics**

> **Z16.10 Resistance to unspecified beta lactam antibiotics**   ▽

> **Z16.11 Resistance to penicillins**
> > Resistance to amoxicillin
> > Resistance to ampicillin

> **Z16.12 Extended spectrum beta lactamase (ESBL) resistance**
> > EXCLUDES 2 ▶*Methicillin resistant Staphylococcus aureus infection in diseases classified elsewhere (B95.62)*◀

Z16.19 Resistance to other specified beta lactam antibiotics
> Resistance to cephalosporins

✓5ᵗʰ **Z16.2 Resistance to other antibiotics**

> **Z16.20 Resistance to unspecified antibiotic**   ▽
> > Resistance to antibiotics NOS

> **Z16.21 Resistance to vancomycin**

> **Z16.22 Resistance to vancomycin related antibiotics**

> **Z16.23 Resistance to quinolones and fluoroquinolones**

> **Z16.24 Resistance to multiple antibiotics**

> **Z16.29 Resistance to other single specified antibiotic**
> > Resistance to aminoglycosides
> > Resistance to macrolides
> > Resistance to sulfonamides
> > Resistance to tetracyclines

✓5ᵗʰ **Z16.3 Resistance to other antimicrobial drugs**
> EXCLUDES 1   *resistance to antibiotics (Z16.1-, Z16.2-)*

> **Z16.30 Resistance to unspecified antimicrobial drugs**   ▽
> > Drug resistance NOS

> **Z16.31 Resistance to antiparasitic drug(s)**
> > Resistance to quinine and related compounds

> **Z16.32 Resistance to antifungal drug(s)**

> **Z16.33 Resistance to antiviral drug(s)**

> ✓6ᵗʰ **Z16.34 Resistance to antimycobacterial drug(s)**
> > Resistance to tuberculostatics

> > **Z16.341 Resistance to single antimycobacterial drug**
> > > Resistance to antimycobacterial drug NOS

> > **Z16.342 Resistance to multiple antimycobacterial drugs**

> **Z16.35 Resistance to multiple antimicrobial drugs**
> > EXCLUDES 1   *Resistance to multiple antibiotics only (Z16.24)*

> **Z16.39 Resistance to other specified antimicrobial drug**

Estrogen receptor status (Z17)

✓4ᵗʰ **Z17 Estrogen receptor status**
> Code first malignant neoplasm of breast (C50.-)

Z17.0 Estrogen receptor positive status [ER+]

Z17.1 Estrogen receptor negative status [ER-]

Retained foreign body fragment (Z18)

✓4ᵗʰ **Z18 Retained foreign body fragments**
> INCLUDES   embedded fragment (status)
> embedded splinter (status)
> retained foreign body status
>
> EXCLUDES 1   *artificial joint prosthesis status (Z96.6-)*
> *foreign body accidentally left during a procedure (T81.5-)*
> *foreign body entering through orifice (T15-T19)*
> *in situ cardiac device (Z95.-)*
> *organ or tissue replaced by means other than transplant (Z96.-, Z97.-)*
> *organ or tissue replaced by transplant (Z94.-)*
> *personal history of retained foreign body fully removed (Z87.821)*
> *superficial foreign body (non-embedded splinter)—code to superficial foreign body, by site*
>
> DEF: Embedded or retained fragment, splinter, or foreign body; natural or synthetic; can cause infection.

✓5ᵗʰ **Z18.0 Retained radioactive fragments**

> **Z18.01 Retained depleted uranium fragments**

> **Z18.09 Other retained radioactive fragments**
> > Other retained depleted isotope fragments
> > Retained nontherapeutic radioactive fragments

✓5ᵗʰ **Z18.1 Retained metal fragments**
> EXCLUDES 1   *retained radioactive metal fragments (Z18.01-Z18.09)*

> **Z18.10 Retained metal fragments, unspecified**   ▽
> > Retained metal fragment NOS

> **Z18.11 Retained magnetic metal fragments**

> **Z18.12 Retained nonmagnetic metal fragments**

Z18.2 Retained plastic fragments
> Acrylics fragments
> Diethylhexylphthalates fragments
> Isocyanate fragments

✓5ᵗʰ **Z18.3 Retained organic fragments**

> **Z18.31 Retained animal quills or spines**

> **Z18.32 Retained tooth**

EXCLUDES 1 Not coded here   EXCLUDES 2 Not included here   N Newborn Age: 0   P Pediatric Age: 0-17   M Maternity Age: 12-55   A Adult Age: 15-124   PDx Primary Dx

1184   ICD-10-CM 2018

Z18.33   Retained wood fragments

Z18.39   Other retained organic fragments

✓5ᵗʰ **Z18.8   Other specified retained foreign body**

Z18.81   Retained glass fragments

Z18.83   **Retained stone or crystalline fragments**
     Retained concrete or cement fragments

Z18.89   Other specified retained foreign body fragments

Z18.9   Retained foreign body fragments, unspecified material ▽

Hormone sensitivity malignancy status (Z19)

✓4ᵗʰ **Z19   Hormone sensitivity malignancy status**
     Code first malignant neoplasm — see Table of Neoplasms, by site, malignant

Z19.1   Hormone sensitive malignancy status

Z19.2   Hormone resistant malignancy status
     Castrate resistant prostate malignancy status

Persons with potential health hazards related to communicable diseases (Z20-Z29)

✓4ᵗʰ **Z20   Contact with and (suspected) exposure to communicable diseases**
     EXCLUDES 1   *carrier of infectious disease (Z22.-)*
         diagnosed current infectious or parasitic disease—see Alphabetic Index
     EXCLUDES 2   *personal history of infectious and parasitic diseases (Z86.1-)*

✓5ᵗʰ **Z20.0   Contact with and (suspected) exposure to intestinal infectious diseases**

Z20.01   **Contact with and (suspected) exposure to intestinal infectious diseases due to Escherichia coli (E. coli)**

Z20.09   **Contact with and (suspected) exposure to other intestinal infectious diseases**

Z20.1   Contact with and (suspected) exposure to tuberculosis

Z20.2   Contact with and (suspected) exposure to infections with a predominantly sexual mode of transmission

Z20.3   Contact with and (suspected) exposure to rabies

Z20.4   Contact with and (suspected) exposure to rubella

Z20.5   Contact with and (suspected) exposure to viral hepatitis

Z20.6   Contact with and (suspected) exposure to human immunodeficiency virus [HIV]
     EXCLUDES 1   *asymptomatic human immunodeficiency virus [HIV] HIV infection status (Z21)*

Z20.7   Contact with and (suspected) exposure to pediculosis, acariasis and other infestations

✓5ᵗʰ **Z20.8   Contact with and (suspected) exposure to other communicable diseases**

✓6ᵗʰ **Z20.81   Contact with and (suspected) exposure to other bacterial communicable diseases**

Z20.810   **Contact with and (suspected) exposure to anthrax**

Z20.811   **Contact with and (suspected) exposure to meningococcus**

Z20.818   **Contact with and (suspected) exposure to other bacterial communicable diseases**

✓6ᵗʰ **Z20.82   Contact with and (suspected) exposure to other viral communicable diseases**

Z20.820   **Contact with and (suspected) exposure to varicella**

Z20.828   **Contact with and (suspected) exposure to other viral communicable diseases**

Z20.89   **Contact with and (suspected) exposure to other communicable diseases**

Z20.9   Contact with and (suspected) exposure to unspecified communicable disease ▽

Z21   Asymptomatic human immunodeficiency virus [HIV] infection status   HCC
     HIV positive NOS
     Code first human immunodeficiency virus [HIV] disease complicating pregnancy, childbirth and the puerperium, if applicable (O98.7-)
     EXCLUDES 1   *acquired immunodeficiency syndrome (B20)*
         contact with human immunodeficiency virus [HIV] (Z20.6)
         exposure to human immunodeficiency virus [HIV] (Z20.6)
         human immunodeficiency virus [HIV] disease (B20)
         inconclusive laboratory evidence of human immunodeficiency virus [HIV] (R75)
     DEF: Phase of human immunodeficiency virus (HIV) infection with no clinical symptoms; may last for 10 years or more.

✓4ᵗʰ **Z22   Carrier of infectious disease**
     INCLUDES   colonization status
         suspected carrier
     EXCLUDES 2   *carrier of viral hepatitis (B18.-)*

Z22.0   Carrier of typhoid

Z22.1   Carrier of other intestinal infectious diseases

Z22.2   Carrier of diphtheria

✓5ᵗʰ **Z22.3   Carrier of other specified bacterial diseases**

Z22.31   Carrier of bacterial disease due to **meningococci**

✓6ᵗʰ **Z22.32   Carrier of bacterial disease due to staphylococci**

Z22.321   **Carrier or suspected carrier of Methicillin susceptible Staphylococcus aureus**
     MSSA colonization

Z22.322   **Carrier or suspected carrier of Methicillin resistant Staphylococcus aureus**
     MRSA colonization

✓6ᵗʰ **Z22.33   Carrier of bacterial disease due to streptococci**

Z22.330   **Carrier of Group B streptococcus**
     EXCLUDES 1   *carrier of streptococcus group B (GBS) complicating pregnancy, childbirth and the puerperium (O99.82-)*

Z22.338   Carrier of other streptococcus

Z22.39   Carrier of other specified bacterial diseases

Z22.4   Carrier of infections with a predominantly sexual mode of transmission

Z22.6   Carrier of human T-lymphotropic virus type-1 [HTLV-1] infection

Z22.8   Carrier of other infectious diseases

Z22.9   Carrier of infectious disease, unspecified ▽

Z23   Encounter for immunization
     Code first any routine childhood examination
     NOTE   Procedure codes are required to identify the types of immunizations given

✓4ᵗʰ **Z28   Immunization not carried out and underimmunization status**
     INCLUDES   vaccination not carried out

✓5ᵗʰ **Z28.0   Immunization not carried out because of contraindication**

Z28.01   **Immunization not carried out because of acute illness of patient**

Z28.02   **Immunization not carried out because of chronic illness or condition of patient**

Z28.03   **Immunization not carried out because of immune compromised state of patient**

Z28.04   **Immunization not carried out because of patient allergy to vaccine or component**

Z28.09   **Immunization not carried out because of other contraindication**

Z28.1   Immunization not carried out because of patient decision for reasons of belief or group pressure
     Immunization not carried out because of religious belief

✓5ᵗʰ **Z28.2   Immunization not carried out because of patient decision for other and unspecified reason**

Z28.20   **Immunization not carried out because of patient decision for unspecified reason** ▽

Z28.21   **Immunization not carried out because of patient refusal**

Z28.29   **Immunization not carried out because of patient decision for other reason**

Z28.3   Underimmunization status
     Delinquent immunization status
     Lapsed immunization schedule status

✓5ᵗʰ **Z28.8   Immunization not carried out for other reason**

Z28.81   **Immunization not carried out due to patient having had the disease**

Z28.82   **Immunization not carried out because of caregiver refusal**
     Immunization not carried out because of guardian refusal
     Immunization not carried out because of parent refusal
     EXCLUDES 1   *immunization not carried out because of caregiver refusal because of religious belief (Z28.1)*

Z28.89   Immunization not carried out for other reason

Z28.9   Immunization not carried out for unspecified reason ▽

✓ Additional Character Req   ✓x7ᵗʰ Placeholder Alert   Manifestation   HCC CMS-HCC Condition   ▽ Unspecified Code   ►◄ Revised Text   ● New Code   ▲ Revised Code Title

✓4ᵗʰ Z29 Encounter for other prophylactic measures
> **EXCLUDES 1** *desensitization to allergens (Z51.6)*
> *prophylactic surgery (Z40.-)*

✓5ᵗʰ Z29.1 Encounter for prophylactic immunotherapy
Encounter for administration of immunoglobulin

Z29.11 Encounter for prophylactic immunotherapy for respiratory syncytial virus (RSV)

Z29.12 Encounter for prophylactic antivenin

Z29.13 Encounter for prophylactic Rho(D) immune globulin

Z29.14 Encounter for prophylactic rabies immune globin

Z29.3 Encounter for prophylactic fluoride administration

Z29.8 Encounter for other specified prophylactic measures

Z29.9 Encounter for prophylactic measures, unspecified ▽

Persons encountering health services in circumstances related to reproduction (Z30-Z39)

✓4ᵗʰ Z30 Encounter for contraceptive management
> **DEF:** Contraceptive management to prevent pregnancy; methods include oral medications, intrauterine devices, and surgical procedures for males and females (sterilization).

✓5ᵗʰ Z30.0 Encounter for general counseling and advice on contraception

✓6ᵗʰ Z30.01 Encounter for initial prescription of contraceptives
> **EXCLUDES 1** *encounter for surveillance of contraceptives (Z30.4-)*

Z30.011 Encounter for initial prescription of contraceptive pills ♀

Z30.012 Encounter for prescription of emergency contraception ♀
Encounter for postcoital contraception

Z30.013 Encounter for initial prescription of injectable contraceptive ♀

Z30.014 Encounter for initial prescription of intrauterine contraceptive device ♀
> **EXCLUDES 1** *encounter for insertion of intrauterine contraceptive device (Z30.430, Z30.432)*

Z30.015 Encounter for initial prescription of vaginal ring hormonal contraceptive

Z30.016 Encounter for initial prescription of transdermal patch hormonal contraceptive device

Z30.017 Encounter for initial prescription of implantable subdermal contraceptive

Z30.018 Encounter for initial prescription of other contraceptives ♀
Encounter for initial prescription of barrier contraception
Encounter for initial prescription of diaphragm

Z30.019 Encounter for initial prescription of contraceptives, unspecified ♀▽

Z30.02 Counseling and instruction in natural family planning to avoid pregnancy

Z30.09 Encounter for other general counseling and advice on contraception
Encounter for family planning advice NOS

Z30.2 Encounter for sterilization

✓5ᵗʰ Z30.4 Encounter for surveillance of contraceptives

Z30.40 Encounter for surveillance of contraceptives, unspecified ▽

Z30.41 Encounter for surveillance of contraceptive pills ♀
Encounter for repeat prescription for contraceptive pill

Z30.42 Encounter for surveillance of injectable contraceptive ♀

✓6ᵗʰ Z30.43 Encounter for surveillance of intrauterine contraceptive device

Z30.430 Encounter for insertion of intrauterine contraceptive device ♀

Z30.431 Encounter for routine checking of intrauterine contraceptive device ♀

Z30.432 Encounter for removal of intrauterine contraceptive device ♀

Z30.433 Encounter for removal and reinsertion of intrauterine contraceptive device ♀
Encounter for replacement of intrauterine contraceptive device

Z30.44 Encounter for surveillance of vaginal ring hormonal contraceptive device ♀

Z30.45 Encounter for surveillance of transdermal patch hormonal contraceptive device ♀

Z30.46 Encounter for surveillance of implantable subdermal contraceptive ♀
Encounter for checking, reinsertion or removal of implantable subdermal contraceptive

Z30.49 Encounter for surveillance of other contraceptives ♀
Encounter for surveillance of barrier contraception
Encounter for surveillance of diaphragm

Z30.8 Encounter for other contraceptive management
Encounter for postvasectomy sperm count
Encounter for routine examination for contraceptive maintenance
> **EXCLUDES 1** *sperm count following sterilization reversal (Z31.42)*
> *sperm count for fertility testing (Z31.41)*

Z30.9 Encounter for contraceptive management, unspecified ▽

✓4ᵗʰ Z31 Encounter for procreative management
> **EXCLUDES 1** *complications associated with artificial fertilization (N98.-)*
> *female infertility (N97.-)*
> *male infertility (N46.-)*

Z31.0 Encounter for reversal of previous sterilization

✓5ᵗʰ Z31.4 Encounter for procreative investigation and testing
> **EXCLUDES 1** *postvasectomy sperm count (Z30.8)*

Z31.41 Encounter for fertility testing
Encounter for fallopian tube patency testing
Encounter for sperm count for fertility testing

Z31.42 Aftercare following sterilization reversal
Sperm count following sterilization reversal

✓6ᵗʰ Z31.43 Encounter for genetic testing of female for procreative management
Use additional code for recurrent pregnancy loss, if applicable (N96, O26.2-)
> **EXCLUDES 1** *nonprocreative genetic testing (Z13.7-)*

Z31.430 Encounter of female for testing for genetic disease carrier status for procreative management ♀

Z31.438 Encounter for other genetic testing of female for procreative management ♀

✓6ᵗʰ Z31.44 Encounter for genetic testing of male for procreative management
> **EXCLUDES 1** *nonprocreative genetic testing (Z13.7-)*

Z31.440 Encounter of male for testing for genetic disease carrier status for procreative management ♂

Z31.441 Encounter for testing of male partner patient with recurrent pregnancy loss 🅰♂

Z31.448 Encounter for other genetic testing of male for procreative management 🅰♂

Z31.49 Encounter for other procreative investigation and testing

▲ **Z31.5 Encounter for procreative genetic counseling**

✓5ᵗʰ Z31.6 Encounter for general counseling and advice on procreation

Z31.61 Procreative counseling and advice using natural family planning

Z31.62 Encounter for fertility preservation counseling
Encounter for fertility preservation counseling prior to cancer therapy
Encounter for fertility preservation counseling prior to surgical removal of gonads

Z31.69 Encounter for other general counseling and advice on procreation

Z31.7 Encounter for procreative management and counseling for gestational carrier
> **EXCLUDES 1** *pregnant state, gestational carrier (Z33.3)*

✓5ᵗʰ Z31.8 Encounter for other procreative management

Z31.81 Encounter for male factor infertility in female patient 🅿🆇♀

Z31.82 Encounter for Rh incompatibility status
AHA: 2015, 3Q, 40; 2014, 4Q, 17

Z31.83 Encounter for assisted reproductive fertility procedure cycle 🅿🆇♀
Patient undergoing in vitro fertilization cycle
Use additional code to identify the type of infertility
> **EXCLUDES 1** *pre-cycle diagnosis and testing—code to reason for encounter*

EXCLUDES 1 Not coded here   **EXCLUDES 2** Not included here   **N** Newborn Age: 0   **P** Pediatric Age: 0-17   **M** Maternity Age: 12-55   **A** Adult Age: 15-124   **PDx** Primary Dx

1186   ICD-10-CM 2018

Z31.84   **Encounter for fertility preservation procedure**   `PDx`
   Encounter for fertility preservation procedure prior to cancer therapy
   Encounter for fertility preservation procedure prior to surgical removal of gonads

Z31.89   **Encounter for other procreative management**

Z31.9   **Encounter for procreative management, unspecified**   ▽

✓4ᵗʰ **Z32**   **Encounter for pregnancy test and childbirth and childcare instruction**

✓5ᵗʰ   **Z32.0**   **Encounter for pregnancy test**

Z32.00   **Encounter for pregnancy test, result unknown**   ♀
   Encounter for pregnancy test NOS

Z32.01   **Encounter for pregnancy test, result positive**   Ⓜ♀

Z32.02   **Encounter for pregnancy test, result negative**   ♀

Z32.2   **Encounter for childbirth instruction**

Z32.3   **Encounter for childcare instruction**
   Encounter for prenatal or postpartum childcare instruction

✓4ᵗʰ **Z33**   **Pregnant state**

Z33.1   **Pregnant state, incidental**   Ⓜ♀
   Pregnant state NOS
   `EXCLUDES 1`   *complications of pregnancy (O00-O9A)*
      pregnant state, gestational carrier (Z33.3)

Z33.2   **Encounter for elective termination of pregnancy**   `PDx` Ⓜ♀
   `EXCLUDES 1`   *early fetal death with retention of dead fetus (O02.1)*
      late fetal death (O36.4)
      spontaneous abortion (O03)

Z33.3   **Pregnant state, gestational carrier**   Ⓜ♀
   `EXCLUDES 1`   *encounter for procreative management and counseling for gestational carrier (Z31.7)*

✓4ᵗʰ **Z34**   **Encounter for supervision of normal pregnancy**
   `EXCLUDES 1`   *any complication of pregnancy (O00-O9A)*
      encounter for pregnancy test (Z32.0-)
      encounter for supervision of high risk pregnancy (O09.-)
   AHA: 2014, 4Q, 17

✓5ᵗʰ   **Z34.0**   **Encounter for supervision of normal first pregnancy**

Z34.00   **Encounter for supervision of normal first pregnancy, unspecified trimester**   `PDx` Ⓜ♀▽

Z34.01   **Encounter for supervision of normal first pregnancy, first trimester**   `PDx` Ⓜ♀

Z34.02   **Encounter for supervision of normal first pregnancy, second trimester**   `PDx` Ⓜ♀

Z34.03   **Encounter for supervision of normal first pregnancy, third trimester**   `PDx` Ⓜ♀

✓5ᵗʰ   **Z34.8**   **Encounter for supervision of other normal pregnancy**

Z34.80   **Encounter for supervision of other normal pregnancy, unspecified trimester**   `PDx` Ⓜ♀▽

Z34.81   **Encounter for supervision of other normal pregnancy, first trimester**   `PDx` Ⓜ♀

Z34.82   **Encounter for supervision of other normal pregnancy, second trimester**   `PDx` Ⓜ♀

Z34.83   **Encounter for supervision of other normal pregnancy, third trimester**   `PDx` Ⓜ♀

✓5ᵗʰ   **Z34.9**   **Encounter for supervision of normal pregnancy, unspecified**

Z34.90   **Encounter for supervision of normal pregnancy, unspecified, unspecified trimester**   `PDx` Ⓜ♀▽

Z34.91   **Encounter for supervision of normal pregnancy, unspecified, first trimester**   `PDx` Ⓜ♀▽

Z34.92   **Encounter for supervision of normal pregnancy, unspecified, second trimester**   `PDx` Ⓜ♀▽

Z34.93   **Encounter for supervision of normal pregnancy, unspecified, third trimester**   `PDx` Ⓜ♀▽

✓4ᵗʰ **Z36**   **Encounter for antenatal screening of mother**
   `INCLUDES`   ▶encounter for placental sample (taken vaginally)
      screening is the testing for disease or disease precursors in asymptomatic individuals so that early detection and treatment can be provided for those who test positive for the disease◀
   `EXCLUDES 1`   *abnormal findings on antenatal screening of mother (O28.-)*
      diagnostic examination—code to sign or symptom
      encounter for suspected maternal and fetal conditions ruled out (Z03.7-)
      suspected fetal condition affecting management of pregnancy—code to condition in Chapter 15
   `EXCLUDES 2`   ▶*abnormal findings on antenatal screening of mother (O28.-)*◀
      genetic counseling and testing (Z31.43-, Z31.5)
      routine prenatal care (Z34)

●   Z36.0   **Encounter for antenatal screening for chromosomal anomalies**

●   Z36.1   **Encounter for antenatal screening for raised alphafetoprotein level**
   Encounter for antenatal screening for elevated maternal serum alphafetoprotein level

●   Z36.2   **Encounter for other antenatal screening follow-up**
   Non-visualized anatomy on a previous scan

●   Z36.3   **Encounter for antenatal screening for malformations**
   Screening for a suspected anomaly

●   Z36.4   **Encounter for antenatal screening for fetal growth retardation**
   Intrauterine growth restriction (IUGR)/small-for-dates

●   Z36.5   **Encounter for antenatal screening for isoimmunization**

●   ✓5ᵗʰ   **Z36.8**   **Encounter for other antenatal screening**

●   Z36.81   **Encounter for antenatal screening for hydrops fetalis**

●   Z36.82   **Encounter for antenatal screening for nuchal translucency**

●   Z36.83   **Encounter for fetal screening for congenital cardiac abnormalities**

●   Z36.84   **Encounter for antenatal screening for fetal lung maturity**

●   Z36.85   **Encounter for antenatal screening for Streptococcus B**

●   Z36.86   **Encounter for antenatal screening for cervical length**
   Screening for risk of pre-term labor

●   Z36.87   **Encounter for antenatal screening for uncertain dates**

●   Z36.88   **Encounter for antenatal screening for fetal macrosomia**
   Screening for large-for-dates

●   Z36.89   **Encounter for other specified antenatal screening**

●   Z36.8A   **Encounter for antenatal screening for other genetic defects**

●   Z36.9   **Encounter for antenatal screening, unspecified**   ▽

✓4ᵗʰ **Z3A**   **Weeks of gestation**
   `NOTE`   Codes from category Z3A are for use, only on the maternal record, to indicate the weeks of gestation of the pregnancy, if known.
   Code first complications of pregnancy, childbirth and the puerperium ▶(O09-O9A)◀
   AHA: 2016, 2Q, 34; 2014, 3Q, 17; 2014, 2Q, 9; 2013, 2Q, 33

✓5ᵗʰ   **Z3A.0**   **Weeks of gestation of pregnancy, unspecified or less than 10 weeks**

Z3A.00   **Weeks of gestation of pregnancy not specified** Ⓜ♀▽

Z3A.01   **Less than 8 weeks gestation of pregnancy**   Ⓜ♀

Z3A.08   **8 weeks gestation of pregnancy**   Ⓜ♀

Z3A.09   **9 weeks gestation of pregnancy**   Ⓜ♀

✓5ᵗʰ   **Z3A.1**   **Weeks of gestation of pregnancy, weeks 10-19**

Z3A.10   **10 weeks gestation of pregnancy**   Ⓜ♀

Z3A.11   **11 weeks gestation of pregnancy**   Ⓜ♀

Z3A.12   **12 weeks gestation of pregnancy**   Ⓜ♀

Z3A.13   **13 weeks gestation of pregnancy**   Ⓜ♀

Z3A.14   **14 weeks gestation of pregnancy**   Ⓜ♀

Z3A.15   **15 weeks gestation of pregnancy**   Ⓜ♀

Z3A.16   **16 weeks gestation of pregnancy**   Ⓜ♀

Z3A.17   **17 weeks gestation of pregnancy**   Ⓜ♀

Z3A.18   **18 weeks gestation of pregnancy**   Ⓜ♀

Z3A.19   **19 weeks gestation of pregnancy**   Ⓜ♀

✓ Additional Character Req   `✓x7ᵗʰ` Placeholder Alert   Manifestation   `HCC` CMS-HCC Condition   ▽ Unspecified Code   ▶◀ Revised Text   ● New Code   ▲ Revised Code Title

ICD-10-CM 2018   **1187**

√5ᵗʰ **Z3A.2 Weeks of gestation of pregnancy, weeks 20-29**

Z3A.20	20 weeks gestation of pregnancy	M♀
Z3A.21	21 weeks gestation of pregnancy	M♀
Z3A.22	22 weeks gestation of pregnancy	M♀
Z3A.23	23 weeks gestation of pregnancy	M♀
Z3A.24	24 weeks gestation of pregnancy	M♀
Z3A.25	25 weeks gestation of pregnancy	M♀
Z3A.26	26 weeks gestation of pregnancy	M♀
Z3A.27	27 weeks gestation of pregnancy	M♀
Z3A.28	28 weeks gestation of pregnancy	M♀
Z3A.29	29 weeks gestation of pregnancy	M♀

√5ᵗʰ **Z3A.3 Weeks of gestation of pregnancy, weeks 30-39**

Z3A.30	30 weeks gestation of pregnancy	M♀
Z3A.31	31 weeks gestation of pregnancy	M♀
Z3A.32	32 weeks gestation of pregnancy	M♀
Z3A.33	33 weeks gestation of pregnancy	M♀
Z3A.34	34 weeks gestation of pregnancy	M♀
Z3A.35	35 weeks gestation of pregnancy	M♀
Z3A.36	36 weeks gestation of pregnancy	M♀
Z3A.37	37 weeks gestation of pregnancy	M♀
Z3A.38	38 weeks gestation of pregnancy	M♀
Z3A.39	39 weeks gestation of pregnancy	M♀

√5ᵗʰ **Z3A.4 Weeks of gestation of pregnancy, weeks 40 or greater**
     AHA: 2014, 4Q, 23

Z3A.40	40 weeks gestation of pregnancy	M♀
Z3A.41	41 weeks gestation of pregnancy	M♀
Z3A.42	42 weeks gestation of pregnancy	M♀
Z3A.49	Greater than 42 weeks gestation of pregnancy	M♀

√4ᵗʰ **Z37 Outcome of delivery**
     This category is intended for use as an additional code to identify the outcome of delivery on the mother's record. It is not for use on the newborn record.
     EXCLUDES 1   stillbirth (P95)

Z37.0 Single live birth   M♀
     AHA: 2016, 2Q, 34; 2014, 2Q, 9

Z37.1 Single stillbirth   M♀

Z37.2 Twins, both liveborn   M♀

Z37.3 Twins, one liveborn and one stillborn   M♀

Z37.4 Twins, both stillborn   M♀

√5ᵗʰ **Z37.5 Other multiple births, all liveborn**

Z37.50	Multiple births, unspecified, all liveborn	M♀▽
Z37.51	Triplets, all liveborn	M♀
Z37.52	Quadruplets, all liveborn	M♀
Z37.53	Quintuplets, all liveborn	M♀
Z37.54	Sextuplets, all liveborn	M♀
Z37.59	Other multiple births, all liveborn	M♀

√5ᵗʰ **Z37.6 Other multiple births, some liveborn**

Z37.60	Multiple births, unspecified, some liveborn	M♀▽
Z37.61	Triplets, some liveborn	M♀
Z37.62	Quadruplets, some liveborn	M♀
Z37.63	Quintuplets, some liveborn	M♀
Z37.64	Sextuplets, some liveborn	M♀
Z37.69	Other multiple births, some liveborn	M♀

Z37.7 Other multiple births, all stillborn   M♀

Z37.9 Outcome of delivery, unspecified   M♀▽
     Multiple birth NOS
     Single birth NOS

√4ᵗʰ **Z38 Liveborn infants according to place of birth and type of delivery**
     This category is for use as the principal code on the initial record of a newborn baby. It is to be used for the initial birth record only. It is not to be used on the mother's record.
     AHA: 2017, 2Q, 5-7; 2016, 3Q, 18; 2015, 2Q, 15

√5ᵗʰ **Z38.0 Single liveborn infant, born in hospital**
     Single liveborn infant, born in birthing center or other health care facility

Z38.00	Single liveborn infant, delivered vaginally	PDx N
Z38.01	Single liveborn infant, delivered by cesarean	PDx N

Z38.1 Single liveborn infant, born outside hospital   PDx N

Z38.2 Single liveborn infant, unspecified as to place of birth   PDx N ▽
     Single liveborn infant NOS

√5ᵗʰ **Z38.3 Twin liveborn infant, born in hospital**

Z38.30	Twin liveborn infant, delivered vaginally	PDx N
Z38.31	Twin liveborn infant, delivered by cesarean	PDx N

Z38.4 Twin liveborn infant, born outside hospital   PDx N

Z38.5 Twin liveborn infant, unspecified as to place of birth   PDx N ▽

√5ᵗʰ **Z38.6 Other multiple liveborn infant, born in hospital**

Z38.61	Triplet liveborn infant, delivered vaginally	PDx N
Z38.62	Triplet liveborn infant, delivered by cesarean	PDx N
Z38.63	Quadruplet liveborn infant, delivered vaginally	PDx N
Z38.64	Quadruplet liveborn infant, delivered by cesarean	PDx N
Z38.65	Quintuplet liveborn infant, delivered vaginally	PDx N
Z38.66	Quintuplet liveborn infant, delivered by cesarean	PDx N
Z38.68	Other multiple liveborn infant, delivered vaginally	PDx N
Z38.69	Other multiple liveborn infant, delivered by cesarean	PDx N

Z38.7 Other multiple liveborn infant, born outside hospital   PDx N

Z38.8 Other multiple liveborn infant, unspecified as to place of birth   PDx N ▽

√4ᵗʰ **Z39 Encounter for maternal postpartum care and examination**

Z39.0 Encounter for care and examination of mother immediately after delivery   PDx M♀
     Care and observation in uncomplicated cases when the delivery occurs outside a healthcare facility
     EXCLUDES 1   care for postpartum complication—see Alphabetic index

Z39.1 Encounter for care and examination of lactating mother   PDx M♀
     Encounter for supervision of lactation
     EXCLUDES 1   disorders of lactation (O92.-)

Z39.2 Encounter for routine postpartum follow-up   PDx M♀

Encounters for other specific health care (Z40-Z53)

Categories Z40-Z53 are intended for use to indicate a reason for care. They may be used for patients who have already been treated for a disease or injury, but who are receiving aftercare or prophylactic care, or care to consolidate the treatment, or to deal with a residual state.
     EXCLUDES 2   follow-up examination for medical surveillance after treatment (Z08-Z09)

√4ᵗʰ **Z40 Encounter for prophylactic surgery**
     EXCLUDES 1   organ donations (Z52.-)
                  therapeutic organ removal—code to condition

√5ᵗʰ **Z40.0 Encounter for prophylactic surgery for risk factors related to malignant neoplasms**
     Admission for prophylactic organ removal
     Use additional code to identify risk factor

Z40.00	Encounter for prophylactic removal of unspecified organ	▽
Z40.01	Encounter for prophylactic removal of breast	
▲ Z40.02	Encounter for prophylactic removal of ovary(s) ♀ ►Encounter for prophylactic removal of ovary(s) and fallopian tube(s)◄	
● Z40.03	Encounter for prophylactic removal of fallopian tube(s)	
Z40.09	Encounter for prophylactic removal of other organ	

Z40.8 Encounter for other prophylactic surgery

Z40.9 Encounter for prophylactic surgery, unspecified   ▽

√4ᵗʰ **Z41 Encounter for procedures for purposes other than remedying health state**

Z41.1 Encounter for cosmetic surgery
     Encounter for cosmetic breast implant
     Encounter for cosmetic procedure
     EXCLUDES 1   encounter for plastic and reconstructive surgery following medical procedure or healed injury (Z42.-)
                  encounter for post-mastectomy breast implantation (Z42.1)

Z41.2 Encounter for routine and ritual male circumcision   ♂

Z41.3 Encounter for ear piercing

EXCLUDES 1 Not coded here   **EXCLUDES 2** Not included here   N Newborn Age: 0   P Pediatric Age: 0-17   M Maternity Age: 12-55   A Adult Age: 15-124   PDx Primary Dx

1188   ICD-10-CM 2018

Z41.8 Encounter for other procedures for purposes other than remedying health state

Z41.9 Encounter for procedure for purposes other than remedying health state, unspecified ▽

✓4ᵗʰ **Z42 Encounter for plastic and reconstructive surgery following medical procedure or healed injury**

> EXCLUDES 1 *encounter for cosmetic plastic surgery (Z41.1)*
> *encounter for plastic surgery for treatment of current injury—code to relevent injury*

Z42.1 Encounter for breast reconstruction following mastectomy   PDx A

> EXCLUDES 1 *deformity and disproportion of reconstructed breast (N65.1-)*

Z42.8 Encounter for other plastic and reconstructive surgery following medical procedure or healed injury   PDx
   AHA: 2017, 1Q, 42

✓4ᵗʰ **Z43 Encounter for attention to artificial openings**

> INCLUDES closure of artificial openings
> passage of sounds or bougies through artificial openings
> reforming artificial openings
> removal of catheter from artificial openings
> toilet or cleansing of artificial openings
>
> EXCLUDES 1 *artificial opening status only, without need for care (Z93.-)*
> *complications of external stoma (J95.0-, K94.-, N99.5-)*
>
> EXCLUDES 2 *fitting and adjustment of prosthetic and other devices (Z44-Z46)*

Z43.0 Encounter for attention to tracheostomy   HCC

Z43.1 Encounter for attention to gastrostomy   HCC

> EXCLUDES 2 ▶*artificial opening status only, without need for care (Z93.-)*◀

Z43.2 Encounter for attention to ileostomy   HCC

Z43.3 Encounter for attention to colostomy   HCC

Z43.4 Encounter for attention to other artificial openings of digestive tract   HCC

Z43.5 Encounter for attention to cystostomy   HCC

Z43.6 Encounter for attention to other artificial openings of urinary tract   HCC
   Encounter for attention to nephrostomy
   Encounter for attention to ureterostomy
   Encounter for attention to urethrostomy

Z43.7 Encounter for attention to artificial vagina

Z43.8 Encounter for attention to other artificial openings   HCC

Z43.9 Encounter for attention to unspecified artificial opening   HCC ▽

✓4ᵗʰ **Z44 Encounter for fitting and adjustment of external prosthetic device**

> INCLUDES removal or replacement of external prosthetic device
> EXCLUDES 1 *malfunction or other complications of device—see Alphabetical Index*
> *presence of prosthetic device (Z97.-)*

✓5ᵗʰ **Z44.0** Encounter for fitting and adjustment of artificial arm

✓6ᵗʰ **Z44.00** Encounter for fitting and adjustment of unspecified artificial arm

Z44.001 Encounter for fitting and adjustment of unspecified right artificial arm ▽

Z44.002 Encounter for fitting and adjustment of unspecified left artificial arm ▽

Z44.009 Encounter for fitting and adjustment of unspecified artificial arm, unspecified arm ▽

✓6ᵗʰ **Z44.01** Encounter for fitting and adjustment of complete artificial arm

Z44.011 Encounter for fitting and adjustment of complete right artificial arm

Z44.012 Encounter for fitting and adjustment of complete left artificial arm

Z44.019 Encounter for fitting and adjustment of complete artificial arm, unspecified arm ▽

✓6ᵗʰ **Z44.02** Encounter for fitting and adjustment of partial artificial arm

Z44.021 Encounter for fitting and adjustment of partial artificial right arm

Z44.022 Encounter for fitting and adjustment of partial artificial left arm

Z44.029 Encounter for fitting and adjustment of partial artificial arm, unspecified arm ▽

✓5ᵗʰ **Z44.1** Encounter for fitting and adjustment of artificial leg

✓6ᵗʰ **Z44.10** Encounter for fitting and adjustment of unspecified artificial leg

Z44.101 Encounter for fitting and adjustment of unspecified right artificial leg   HCC ▽

Z44.102 Encounter for fitting and adjustment of unspecified left artificial leg   HCC ▽

Z44.109 Encounter for fitting and adjustment of unspecified artificial leg, unspecified leg   HCC ▽

✓6ᵗʰ **Z44.11** Encounter for fitting and adjustment of complete artificial leg

Z44.111 Encounter for fitting and adjustment of complete right artificial leg   HCC

Z44.112 Encounter for fitting and adjustment of complete left artificial leg   HCC

Z44.119 Encounter for fitting and adjustment of complete artificial leg, unspecified leg   HCC ▽

✓6ᵗʰ **Z44.12** Encounter for fitting and adjustment of partial artificial leg

Z44.121 Encounter for fitting and adjustment of partial artificial right leg   HCC

Z44.122 Encounter for fitting and adjustment of partial artificial left leg   HCC

Z44.129 Encounter for fitting and adjustment of partial artificial leg, unspecified leg   HCC ▽

✓5ᵗʰ **Z44.2** Encounter for fitting and adjustment of artificial eye

> EXCLUDES 1 *mechanical complication of ocular prosthesis (T85.3)*

Z44.20 Encounter for fitting and adjustment of artificial eye, unspecified ▽

Z44.21 Encounter for fitting and adjustment of artificial right eye

Z44.22 Encounter for fitting and adjustment of artificial left eye

✓5ᵗʰ **Z44.3** Encounter for fitting and adjustment of external breast prosthesis

> EXCLUDES 1 *complications of breast implant (T85.4-)*
> *encounter for adjustment or removal of breast implant (Z45.81-)*
> *encounter for initial breast implant insertion for cosmetic breast augmentation (Z41.1)*
> *encounter for breast reconstruction following mastectomy (Z42.1)*

Z44.30 Encounter for fitting and adjustment of external breast prosthesis, unspecified breast ▽

Z44.31 Encounter for fitting and adjustment of external right breast prosthesis

Z44.32 Encounter for fitting and adjustment of external left breast prosthesis

Z44.8 Encounter for fitting and adjustment of other external prosthetic devices

Z44.9 Encounter for fitting and adjustment of unspecified external prosthetic device ▽

✓4ᵗʰ **Z45 Encounter for adjustment and management of implanted device**

> INCLUDES removal or replacement of implanted device
> EXCLUDES 1 *malfunction or other complications of device – see Alphabetical Index*
> *presence of prosthetic and other devices (Z95-Z97)*
> EXCLUDES 2 *encounter for fitting and adjustment of non-implanted device (Z46.-)*

✓5ᵗʰ **Z45.0** Encounter for adjustment and management of cardiac device

✓6ᵗʰ **Z45.01** Encounter for adjustment and management of cardiac pacemaker
   Encounter for adjustment and management of cardiac resynchronization therapy pacemaker (CRT-P)

> EXCLUDES 1 *encounter for adjustment and management of automatic implantable cardiac defibrillator with synchronous cardiac pacemaker (Z45.02)*

Z45.010 Encounter for checking and testing of cardiac pacemaker pulse generator [battery]
   Encounter for replacing cardiac pacemaker pulse generator [battery]

Z45.Ø18 **Encounter for adjustment and management of other part of cardiac pacemaker**
EXCLUDES 2 ▶presence of prosthetic and other devices (Z95-Z97)◀

Z45.Ø2 **Encounter for adjustment and management of automatic implantable cardiac defibrillator**
Encounter for adjustment and management of automatic implantable cardiac defibrillator with synchronous cardiac pacemaker
Encounter for adjustment and management of cardiac resynchronization therapy defibrillator (CRT-D)

Z45.Ø9 **Encounter for adjustment and management of other cardiac device**

Z45.1 **Encounter for adjustment and management of infusion pump**

Z45.2 **Encounter for adjustment and management of vascular access device**
Encounter for adjustment and management of vascular catheters
EXCLUDES 1 encounter for adjustment and management of renal dialysis catheter (Z49.Ø1)

✓5th **Z45.3** **Encounter for adjustment and management of implanted devices of the special senses**

Z45.31 **Encounter for adjustment and management of implanted visual substitution device**

✓6th **Z45.32** **Encounter for adjustment and management of implanted hearing device**
EXCLUDES 1 encounter for fitting and adjustment of hearing aide (Z46.1)

Z45.32Ø **Encounter for adjustment and management of bone conduction device**

Z45.321 **Encounter for adjustment and management of cochlear device**

Z45.328 **Encounter for adjustment and management of other implanted hearing device**

✓5th **Z45.4** **Encounter for adjustment and management of implanted nervous system device**

Z45.41 **Encounter for adjustment and management of cerebrospinal fluid drainage device**
Encounter for adjustment and management of cerebral ventricular (communicating) shunt

Z45.42 **Encounter for adjustment and management of neuropacemaker (brain) (peripheral nerve) (spinal cord)**

Z45.49 **Encounter for adjustment and management of other implanted nervous system device**
AHA: 2014, 3Q, 19

✓5th **Z45.8** **Encounter for adjustment and management of other implanted devices**

✓6th **Z45.81** **Encounter for adjustment or removal of breast implant**
Encounter for elective implant exchange (different material) (different size)
Encounter for removal of tissue expander without synchronous insertion of permanent implant
EXCLUDES 1 complications of breast implant (T85.4-)
encounter for initial breast implant insertion for cosmetic breast augmentation (Z41.1)
encounter for breast reconstruction following mastectomy (Z42.1)

Z45.811 **Encounter for adjustment or removal of right breast implant**

Z45.812 **Encounter for adjustment or removal of left breast implant**

Z45.819 **Encounter for adjustment or removal of unspecified breast implant** ▽

Z45.82 **Encounter for adjustment or removal of myringotomy device (stent) (tube)**

Z45.89 **Encounter for adjustment and management of other implanted devices**
AHA: 2014, 4Q, 26-28

Z45.9 **Encounter for adjustment and management of unspecified implanted device** ▽

✓4th **Z46** **Encounter for fitting and adjustment of other devices**
INCLUDES removal or replacement of other device
EXCLUDES 1 malfunction or other complications of device—see Alphabetical Index
EXCLUDES 2 encounter for fitting and management of implanted devices (Z45.-)
issue of repeat prescription only (Z76.Ø)
presence of prosthetic and other devices (Z95-Z97)

Z46.Ø **Encounter for fitting and adjustment of spectacles and contact lenses**

Z46.1 **Encounter for fitting and adjustment of hearing aid**
EXCLUDES 1 encounter for adjustment and management of implanted hearing device (Z45.32-)

Z46.2 **Encounter for fitting and adjustment of other devices related to nervous system and special senses**
EXCLUDES 2 encounter for adjustment and management of implanted nervous system device (Z45.4-)
encounter for adjustment and management of implanted visual substitution device (Z45.31)

Z46.3 **Encounter for fitting and adjustment of dental prosthetic device**
Encounter for fitting and adjustment of dentures

Z46.4 **Encounter for fitting and adjustment of orthodontic device**

✓5th **Z46.5** **Encounter for fitting and adjustment of other gastrointestinal appliance and device**
EXCLUDES 1 encounter for attention to artificial openings of digestive tract (Z43.1-Z43.4)

Z46.51 **Encounter for fitting and adjustment of gastric lap band**

Z46.59 **Encounter for fitting and adjustment of other gastrointestinal appliance and device**

Z46.6 **Encounter for fitting and adjustment of urinary device**
EXCLUDES 2 attention to artificial openings of urinary tract (Z43.5, Z43.6)

✓5th **Z46.8** **Encounter for fitting and adjustment of other specified devices**

Z46.81 **Encounter for fitting and adjustment of insulin pump**
Encounter for insulin pump instruction and training
Encounter for insulin pump titration

Z46.82 **Encounter for fitting and adjustment of non-vascular catheter**

Z46.89 **Encounter for fitting and adjustment of other specified devices**
Encounter for fitting and adjustment of wheelchair

Z46.9 **Encounter for fitting and adjustment of unspecified device** ▽

✓4th **Z47** **Orthopedic aftercare**
EXCLUDES 1 aftercare for healing fracture—code to fracture with 7th character D

Z47.1 **Aftercare following joint replacement surgery**
Use additional code to identify the joint (Z96.6-)

Z47.2 **Encounter for removal of internal fixation device**
EXCLUDES 1 encounter for adjustment of internal fixation device for fracture treatment—code to fracture with appropriate 7th character
encounter for removal of external fixation device—code to fracture with 7th character D
infection or inflammatory reaction to internal fixation device (T84.6-)
mechanical complication of internal fixation device (T84.1-)

✓5th **Z47.3** **Aftercare following explantation of joint prosthesis**
Aftercare following explantation of joint prosthesis, staged procedure
Encounter for joint prosthesis insertion following prior explantation of joint prosthesis
AHA: 2015, 1Q, 16

Z47.31 **Aftercare following explantation of shoulder joint prosthesis**
EXCLUDES 1 acquired absence of shoulder joint following prior explantation of shoulder joint prosthesis (Z89.23-)
shoulder joint prosthesis explantation status (Z89.23-)

EXCLUDES 1 Not coded here   EXCLUDES 2 Not included here   N Newborn Age: Ø   P Pediatric Age: Ø-17   M Maternity Age: 12-55   A Adult Age: 15-124   PDx Primary Dx

Z47.32   **Aftercare following explantation of hip joint prosthesis**
> *EXCLUDES 1*   *acquired absence of hip joint following prior explantation of hip joint prosthesis (Z89.62-)*
> *hip joint prosthesis explantation status (Z89.62-)*

Z47.33   **Aftercare following explantation of knee joint prosthesis**
> *EXCLUDES 1*   *acquired absence of knee joint following prior explantation of knee prosthesis (Z89.52-)*
> *knee joint prosthesis explantation status (Z89.52-)*

✓5ᵗʰ **Z47.8**   **Encounter for other orthopedic aftercare**

Z47.81   **Encounter for orthopedic aftercare following surgical amputation**
> Use additional code to identify the limb amputated (Z89.-)

Z47.82   **Encounter for orthopedic aftercare following scoliosis surgery**

Z47.89   **Encounter for other orthopedic aftercare**
> AHA: 2015, 1Q, 8

✓4ᵗʰ **Z48**   **Encounter for other postprocedural aftercare**
> *EXCLUDES 1* ▶*encounter for aftercare following injury – code to Injury, by site, with appropriate 7th character for subsequent encounter*◀
> *encounter for follow-up examination after completed treatment (Z08-Z09)*
> *EXCLUDES 2*   *encounter for attention to artificial openings (Z43.-)*
> *encounter for fitting and adjustment of prosthetic and other devices (Z44-Z46)*
> AHA: 2015, 4Q, 38; 2015, 1Q, 6-7

✓5ᵗʰ **Z48.0**   **Encounter for attention to dressings, sutures and drains**
> *EXCLUDES 1*   *encounter for planned postprocedural wound closure (Z48.1)*

Z48.00   **Encounter for change or removal of nonsurgical wound dressing**
> Encounter for change or removal of wound dressing NOS

Z48.01   **Encounter for change or removal of surgical wound dressing**

Z48.02   **Encounter for removal of sutures**
> Encounter for removal of staples

Z48.03   **Encounter for change or removal of drains**

Z48.1   **Encounter for planned postprocedural wound closure**
> *EXCLUDES 1*   *encounter for attention to dressings and sutures (Z48.0-)*

✓5ᵗʰ **Z48.2**   **Encounter for aftercare following organ transplant**

Z48.21   **Encounter for aftercare following heart transplant**   HCC

Z48.22   **Encounter for aftercare following kidney transplant**

Z48.23   **Encounter for aftercare following liver transplant**   HCC

Z48.24   **Encounter for aftercare following lung transplant**   HCC

✓6ᵗʰ **Z48.28**   **Encounter for aftercare following multiple organ transplant**

Z48.280   **Encounter for aftercare following heart-lung transplant**   HCC

Z48.288   **Encounter for aftercare following multiple organ transplant**

✓6ᵗʰ **Z48.29**   **Encounter for aftercare following other organ transplant**

Z48.290   **Encounter for aftercare following bone marrow transplant**   HCC

Z48.298   **Encounter for aftercare following other organ transplant**

Z48.3   **Aftercare following surgery for neoplasm**
> Use additional code to identify the neoplasm

✓5ᵗʰ **Z48.8**   **Encounter for other specified postprocedural aftercare**

✓6ᵗʰ **Z48.81**   **Encounter for surgical aftercare following surgery on specified body systems**
> NOTE   These codes identify the body system requiring aftercare. They are for use in conjunction with other aftercare codes to fully explain the aftercare encounter. The condition treated should also be coded if still present.
> *EXCLUDES 1*   *aftercare for injury—code the injury with 7th character D*
> *aftercare following surgery for neoplasm (Z48.3)*
> *EXCLUDES 2*   *aftercare following organ transplant (Z48.2-)*
> *orthopedic aftercare (Z47.-)*
> AHA: 2015, 4Q, 38

Z48.810   **Encounter for surgical aftercare following surgery on the sense organs**

Z48.811   **Encounter for surgical aftercare following surgery on the nervous system**
> *EXCLUDES 2*   *encounter for surgical aftercare following surgery on the sense organs (Z48.810)*

Z48.812   **Encounter for surgical aftercare following surgery on the circulatory system**
> AHA: 2012, 4Q, 96

Z48.813   **Encounter for surgical aftercare following surgery on the respiratory system**

Z48.814   **Encounter for surgical aftercare following surgery on the teeth or oral cavity**

Z48.815   **Encounter for surgical aftercare following surgery on the digestive system**

Z48.816   **Encounter for surgical aftercare following surgery on the genitourinary system**
> *EXCLUDES 1*   *encounter for aftercare following sterilization reversal (Z31.42)*

Z48.817   **Encounter for surgical aftercare following surgery on the skin and subcutaneous tissue**

Z48.89   **Encounter for other specified surgical aftercare**

✓4ᵗʰ **Z49**   **Encounter for care involving renal dialysis**
> Code also associated end stage renal disease (N18.6)

✓5ᵗʰ **Z49.0**   **Preparatory care for renal dialysis**
> Encounter for dialysis instruction and training

Z49.01   **Encounter for fitting and adjustment of extracorporeal dialysis catheter**   HCC
> Removal or replacement of renal dialysis catheter
> Toilet or cleansing of renal dialysis catheter

Z49.02   **Encounter for fitting and adjustment of peritoneal dialysis catheter**   HCC

✓5ᵗʰ **Z49.3**   **Encounter for adequacy testing for dialysis**

Z49.31   **Encounter for adequacy testing for hemodialysis** HCC

Z49.32   **Encounter for adequacy testing for peritoneal dialysis**   HCC
> Encounter for peritoneal equilibration test

✓4ᵗʰ **Z51**   **Encounter for other aftercare and medical care**
> Code also condition requiring care
> *EXCLUDES 1*   *follow-up examination after treatment (Z08-Z09)*

Z51.0   **Encounter for antineoplastic radiation therapy**   PDx

✓5ᵗʰ **Z51.1**   **Encounter for antineoplastic chemotherapy and immunotherapy**
> *EXCLUDES 2*   *encounter for chemotherapy and immunotherapy for nonneoplastic condition—code to condition*

Z51.11   **Encounter for antineoplastic chemotherapy**   PDx
> AHA: 2015, 3Q, 19

Z51.12   **Encounter for antineoplastic immunotherapy**   PDx

Z51.5   **Encounter for palliative care**
> AHA: 2017, 1Q, 48

Z51.6   **Encounter for desensitization to allergens**

☑ Additional Character Req   ✓×7ᵗʰ Placeholder Alert   Manifestation   HCC CMS-HCC Condition   ▽ Unspecified Code   ▶◀ Revised Text   ● New Code   ▲ Revised Code Title

ICD-10-CM 2018   1191

Chapter 21. Factors Influencing Health Status and Contact with Health Services

Z51.8–Z57.9

✓5ᵗʰ **Z51.8 Encounter for other specified aftercare**
EXCLUDES 1   *holiday relief care (Z75.5)*

Z51.81 Encounter for therapeutic drug level monitoring
Code also any long-term (current) drug therapy (Z79.-)
EXCLUDES 1   *encounter for blood-drug test for administrative or medicolegal reasons (Z02.83)*
DEF: Drug monitoring: Measurement of the level of a specific drug in the body or measurement of a specific function to assess effectiveness of a drug.

Z51.89 Encounter for other specified aftercare
AHA: 2012, 4Q, 95-97

✓4ᵗʰ **Z52 Donors of organs and tissues**
INCLUDES   autologous and other living donors
EXCLUDES 1   cadaveric donor—omit code
examination of potential donor (Z00.5)
AHA: 2012, 4Q, 99

✓5ᵗʰ **Z52.0 Blood donor**

   ✓6ᵗʰ **Z52.00 Unspecified blood donor**
     Z52.000 Unspecified donor, whole blood PDx ▽
     Z52.001 Unspecified donor, stem cells PDx ▽
     Z52.008 Unspecified donor, other blood PDx ▽

   ✓6ᵗʰ **Z52.01 Autologous blood donor**
     Z52.010 Autologous donor, whole blood PDx
     Z52.011 Autologous donor, stem cells PDx
     Z52.018 Autologous donor, other blood PDx

   ✓6ᵗʰ **Z52.09 Other blood donor**
     Volunteer donor
     Z52.090 Other blood donor, whole blood PDx
     Z52.091 Other blood donor, stem cells PDx
     Z52.098 Other blood donor, other blood PDx

✓5ᵗʰ **Z52.1 Skin donor**
   Z52.10 Skin donor, unspecified PDx ▽
   Z52.11 Skin donor, autologous PDx
   Z52.19 Skin donor, other PDx

✓5ᵗʰ **Z52.2 Bone donor**
   Z52.20 Bone donor, unspecified PDx ▽
   Z52.21 Bone donor, autologous PDx
   Z52.29 Bone donor, other PDx

Z52.3 Bone marrow donor PDx
Z52.4 Kidney donor PDx
Z52.5 Cornea donor PDx
Z52.6 Liver donor PDx

✓5ᵗʰ **Z52.8 Donor of other specified organs or tissues**

   ✓6ᵗʰ **Z52.81 Egg (Oocyte) donor**
     Z52.810 Egg (Oocyte) donor under age 35, anonymous recipient PDx ♀
      Egg donor under age 35 NOS
     Z52.811 Egg (Oocyte) donor under age 35, designated recipient PDx ♀
     Z52.812 Egg (Oocyte) donor age 35 and over, anonymous recipient PDx ♀
      Egg donor age 35 and over NOS
     Z52.813 Egg (Oocyte) donor age 35 and over, designated recipient PDx ♀
     Z52.819 Egg (Oocyte) donor, unspecified PDx ♀▽

   Z52.89 Donor of other specified organs or tissues PDx

Z52.9 Donor of unspecified organ or tissue ▽
   Donor NOS

✓4ᵗʰ **Z53 Persons encountering health services for specific procedures and treatment, not carried out**

   ✓5ᵗʰ **Z53.0 Procedure and treatment not carried out because of contraindication**
     Z53.01 Procedure and treatment not carried out due to patient smoking
     Z53.09 Procedure and treatment not carried out because of other contraindication

   Z53.1 Procedure and treatment not carried out because of patient's decision for reasons of belief and group pressure

   ✓5ᵗʰ **Z53.2 Procedure and treatment not carried out because of patient's decision for other and unspecified reasons**
     Z53.20 Procedure and treatment not carried out because of patient's decision for unspecified reasons ▽

Z53.21 Procedure and treatment not carried out due to patient leaving prior to being seen by health care provider

Z53.29 Procedure and treatment not carried out because of patient's decision for other reasons

✓5ᵗʰ **Z53.3 Procedure converted to open procedure**
   Z53.31 Laparoscopic surgical procedure converted to open procedure
   Z53.32 Thoracoscopic surgical procedure converted to open procedure
   Z53.33 Arthroscopic surgical procedure converted to open procedure
   Z53.39 Other specified procedure converted to open procedure

Z53.8 Procedure and treatment not carried out for other reasons
Z53.9 Procedure and treatment not carried out, unspecified reason ▽

Persons with potential health hazards related to socioeconomic and psychosocial circumstances (Z55-Z65)

✓4ᵗʰ **Z55 Problems related to education and literacy**
EXCLUDES 1   *disorders of psychological development (F80-F89)*
   Z55.0 Illiteracy and low-level literacy
   Z55.1 Schooling unavailable and unattainable
   Z55.2 Failed school examinations
   Z55.3 Underachievement in school
   Z55.4 Educational maladjustment and discord with teachers and classmates
   Z55.8 Other problems related to education and literacy
     Problems related to inadequate teaching
   Z55.9 Problems related to education and literacy, unspecified ▽
     Academic problems NOS

✓4ᵗʰ **Z56 Problems related to employment and unemployment**
EXCLUDES 2   *occupational exposure to risk factors (Z57.-)*
problems related to housing and economic circumstances (Z59.-)
   Z56.0 Unemployment, unspecified ▽
   Z56.1 Change of job A
   Z56.2 Threat of job loss
   Z56.3 Stressful work schedule
   Z56.4 Discord with boss and workmates
   Z56.5 Uncongenial work environment
     Difficult conditions at work
   Z56.6 Other physical and mental strain related to work
   ✓5ᵗʰ **Z56.8 Other problems related to employment**
     Z56.81 Sexual harassment on the job
     Z56.82 Military deployment status
      Individual (civilian or military) currently deployed in theater or in support of military war, peacekeeping and humanitarian operations
     Z56.89 Other problems related to employment
   Z56.9 Unspecified problems related to employment ▽
     Occupational problems NOS

✓4ᵗʰ **Z57 Occupational exposure to risk factors**
   Z57.0 Occupational exposure to noise
   Z57.1 Occupational exposure to radiation
   Z57.2 Occupational exposure to dust
   ✓5ᵗʰ **Z57.3 Occupational exposure to other air contaminants**
     Z57.31 Occupational exposure to environmental tobacco smoke
      EXCLUDES 2   *exposure to environmental tobacco smoke (Z77.22)*
     Z57.39 Occupational exposure to other air contaminants
   Z57.4 Occupational exposure to toxic agents in agriculture
     Occupational exposure to solids, liquids, gases or vapors in agriculture
   Z57.5 Occupational exposure to toxic agents in other industries
     Occupational exposure to solids, liquids, gases or vapors in other industries
   Z57.6 Occupational exposure to extreme temperature
   Z57.7 Occupational exposure to vibration
   Z57.8 Occupational exposure to other risk factors
   Z57.9 Occupational exposure to unspecified risk factor ▽

☑4ᵗʰ **Z59 Problems related to housing and economic circumstances**
> *EXCLUDES 2* *problems related to upbringing (Z62.-)*

Z59.0 Homelessness

Z59.1 Inadequate housing
Lack of heating
Restriction of space
Technical defects in home preventing adequate care
Unsatisfactory surroundings
> *EXCLUDES 1* *problems related to the natural and physical environment (Z77.1-)*

Z59.2 Discord with neighbors, lodgers and landlord

Z59.3 Problems related to living in residential institution
Boarding-school resident
> *EXCLUDES 1* *institutional upbringing (Z62.2)*

Z59.4 Lack of adequate food and safe drinking water
Inadequate drinking water supply
> *EXCLUDES 1* *effects of hunger (T73.0)*
> *inappropriate diet or eating habits (Z72.4)*
> *malnutrition (E40-E46)*

Z59.5 Extreme poverty

Z59.6 Low income

Z59.7 Insufficient social insurance and welfare support

Z59.8 Other problems related to housing and economic circumstances
Foreclosure on loan
Isolated dwelling
Problems with creditors

Z59.9 Problem related to housing and economic circumstances, unspecified ▽

☑4ᵗʰ **Z60 Problems related to social environment**

Z60.0 Problems of adjustment to life-cycle transitions
Empty nest syndrome
Phase of life problem
Problem with adjustment to retirement [pension]

Z60.2 Problems related to living alone

Z60.3 Acculturation difficulty
Problem with migration
Problem with social transplantation
DEF: A problem in adapting to a different culture or environment not based on any coexisting mental disorder.

Z60.4 Social exclusion and rejection
Exclusion and rejection on the basis of personal characteristics, such as unusual physical appearance, illness or behavior.
> *EXCLUDES 1* *target of adverse discrimination such as for racial or religious reasons (Z60.5)*

Z60.5 Target of (perceived) adverse discrimination and persecution
> *EXCLUDES 1* *social exclusion and rejection (Z60.4)*

Z60.8 Other problems related to social environment

Z60.9 Problem related to social environment, unspecified ▽

☑4ᵗʰ **Z62 Problems related to upbringing**
> *INCLUDES* current and past negative life events in childhood
> current and past problems of a child related to upbringing
> *EXCLUDES 2* *maltreatment syndrome (T74.-)*
> *problems related to housing and economic circumstances (Z59.-)*

Z62.0 Inadequate parental supervision and control

Z62.1 Parental overprotection

☑5ᵗʰ **Z62.2 Upbringing away from parents**
> *EXCLUDES 1* *problems with boarding school (Z59.3)*

Z62.21 Child in welfare custody 🅿
Child in care of non-parental family member
Child in foster care
> *EXCLUDES 2* *problem for parent due to child in welfare custody (Z63.5)*

Z62.22 Institutional upbringing
Child living in orphanage or group home

Z62.29 Other upbringing away from parents

Z62.3 Hostility towards and scapegoating of child 🅿

Z62.6 Inappropriate (excessive) parental pressure

☑5ᵗʰ **Z62.8 Other specified problems related to upbringing**

☑6ᵗʰ **Z62.81 Personal history of abuse in childhood**

Z62.810 Personal history of physical and sexual abuse in childhood
> *EXCLUDES 1* *current child physical abuse (T74.12, T76.12)*
> *current child sexual abuse (T74.22, T76.22)*

Z62.811 Personal history of psychological abuse in childhood
> *EXCLUDES 1* *current child psychological abuse (T74.32, T76.32)*

Z62.812 Personal history of neglect in childhood
> *EXCLUDES 1* *current child neglect (T74.02, T76.02)*

Z62.819 Personal history of unspecified abuse in childhood ▽
> *EXCLUDES 1* *current child abuse NOS (T74.92, T76.92)*

☑6ᵗʰ **Z62.82 Parent-child conflict**

Z62.820 Parent-biological child conflict
Parent-child problem NOS

Z62.821 Parent-adopted child conflict

Z62.822 Parent-foster child conflict

☑6ᵗʰ **Z62.89 Other specified problems related to upbringing**

Z62.890 Parent-child estrangement NEC

Z62.891 Sibling rivalry

Z62.898 Other specified problems related to upbringing

Z62.9 Problem related to upbringing, unspecified ▽

☑4ᵗʰ **Z63 Other problems related to primary support group, including family circumstances**
> *EXCLUDES 2* *maltreatment syndrome (T74-, T76)*
> *parent-child problems (Z62.-)*
> *problems related to negative life events in childhood (Z62.-)*
> *problems related to upbringing (Z62.-)*

Z63.0 Problems in relationship with spouse or partner
▶Relationship distress with spouse or intimate partner◀
> *EXCLUDES 1* *counseling for spousal or partner abuse problems (Z69.1)*
> *counseling related to sexual attitude, behavior, and orientation (Z70.-)*

Z63.1 Problems in relationship with in-laws

☑5ᵗʰ **Z63.3 Absence of family member**
> *EXCLUDES 1* *absence of family member due to disappearance and death (Z63.4)*
> *absence of family member due to separation and divorce (Z63.5)*

Z63.31 Absence of family member due to military deployment
Individual or family affected by other family member being on military deployment
> *EXCLUDES 1* *family disruption due to return of family member from military deployment (Z63.71)*

Z63.32 Other absence of family member

Z63.4 Disappearance and death of family member
Assumed death of family member
Bereavement
AHA: 2014, 1Q, 25

Z63.5 Disruption of family by separation and divorce
Marital estrangement

Z63.6 Dependent relative needing care at home

☑5ᵗʰ **Z63.7 Other stressful life events affecting family and household**

Z63.71 Stress on family due to return of family member from military deployment
Individual or family affected by family member having returned from military deployment (current or past conflict)

Z63.72 Alcoholism and drug addiction in family

Z63.79 Other stressful life events affecting family and household
Anxiety (normal) about sick person in family
Health problems within family
Ill or disturbed family member
Isolated family

Z63.8 Other specified problems related to primary support group
Family discord NOS
Family estrangement NOS
High expressed emotional level within family
Inadequate family support NOS
Inadequate or distorted communication within family

Z63.9 Problem related to primary support group, unspecified ▽
Relationship disorder NOS

☑ Additional Character Req   ☑x7ᵗʰ Placeholder Alert   Manifestation   ᴴᶜᶜ CMS-HCC Condition   ▽ Unspecified Code   ▶◀ Revised Text   ● New Code   ▲ Revised Code Title

✓4ᵗʰ **Z64 Problems related to certain psychosocial circumstances**

    Z64.0 Problems related to unwanted pregnancy ♀

    Z64.1 Problems related to multiparity ♀

    Z64.4 Discord with counselors
        Discord with probation officer
        Discord with social worker

✓4ᵗʰ **Z65 Problems related to other psychosocial circumstances**

    Z65.0 Conviction in civil and criminal proceedings without imprisonment

    Z65.1 Imprisonment and other incarceration

    Z65.2 Problems related to release from prison

    Z65.3 Problems related to other legal circumstances
        Arrest
        Child custody or support proceedings
        Litigation
        Prosecution

    Z65.4 Victim of crime and terrorism
        Victim of torture

    Z65.5 Exposure to disaster, war and other hostilities
        EXCLUDES 1 *target of perceived discrimination or persecution (Z60.5)*

    Z65.8 Other specified problems related to psychosocial circumstances
        ►Religious or spiritual problem◄

    Z65.9 Problem related to unspecified psychosocial circumstances ▽

Do not resuscitate status (Z66)

Z66 Do not resuscitate
    DNR status
    DEF: Medical order written by a physician that instructs others not to perform cardiopulmonary resuscitation (CPR), intubation, or advanced life support (ACLS); prevents unnecessary invasive treatment to prolong life should breathing stop or cardiac arrest occur.

Blood type (Z67)

✓4ᵗʰ **Z67 Blood type**
    AHA: 2015, 3Q, 40

    ✓5ᵗʰ **Z67.1 Type A blood**
        Z67.10 Type A blood, Rh positive
        Z67.11 Type A blood, Rh negative

    ✓5ᵗʰ **Z67.2 Type B blood**
        Z67.20 Type B blood, Rh positive
        Z67.21 Type B blood, Rh negative

    ✓5ᵗʰ **Z67.3 Type AB blood**
        Z67.30 Type AB blood, Rh positive
        Z67.31 Type AB blood, Rh negative

    ✓5ᵗʰ **Z67.4 Type O blood**
        Z67.40 Type O blood, Rh positive
        Z67.41 Type O blood, Rh negative

    ✓5ᵗʰ **Z67.9 Unspecified blood type**
        Z67.90 Unspecified blood type, Rh positive ▽
        Z67.91 Unspecified blood type, Rh negative ▽

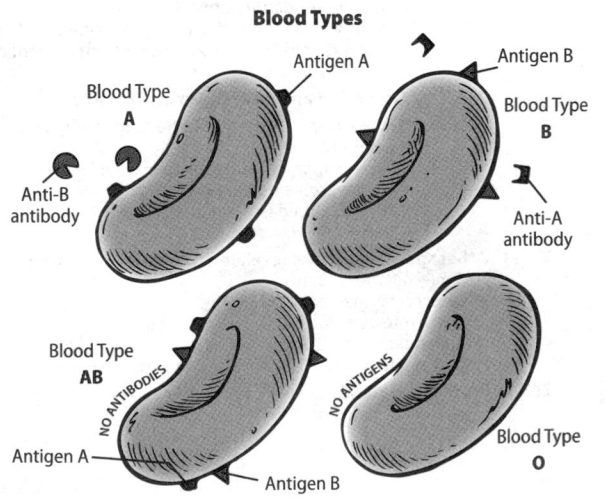

Blood Types

Antigen A

Antigen B

Blood Type **A**

Blood Type **B**

Anti-B antibody

Anti-A antibody

Blood Type **AB**

NO ANTIBODIES

NO ANTIGENS

Antigen A

Antigen B

Blood Type **O**

Body mass index [BMI] (Z68)

✓4ᵗʰ **Z68 Body mass index [BMI]**
    Kilograms per meters squared
    NOTE BMI adult codes are for use for persons 21 years of age or older.
        BMI pediatric codes are for use for persons 2-20 years of age. These percentiles are based on the growth charts published by the Centers for Disease Control and Prevention (CDC).
    AHA: 2017, 1Q, 39
    DEF: Index used to help determine whether an individual is underweight, a healthy weight, overweight, or obese.

▲   **Z68.1 Body mass index [BMI] 19.9 or less, adult** Ⓐ

    ✓5ᵗʰ **Z68.2 Body mass index [BMI] 20-29, adult**
        Z68.20 Body mass index [BMI] 20.0-20.9, adult Ⓐ
        Z68.21 Body mass index [BMI] 21.0-21.9, adult Ⓐ
        Z68.22 Body mass index [BMI] 22.0-22.9, adult Ⓐ
        Z68.23 Body mass index [BMI] 23.0-23.9, adult Ⓐ
        Z68.24 Body mass index [BMI] 24.0-24.9, adult Ⓐ
        Z68.25 Body mass index [BMI] 25.0-25.9, adult Ⓐ
        Z68.26 Body mass index [BMI] 26.0-26.9, adult Ⓐ
        Z68.27 Body mass index [BMI] 27.0-27.9, adult Ⓐ
        Z68.28 Body mass index [BMI] 28.0-28.9, adult Ⓐ
        Z68.29 Body mass index [BMI] 29.0-29.9, adult Ⓐ

    ✓5ᵗʰ **Z68.3 Body mass index [BMI] 30-39, adult**
        Z68.30 Body mass index [BMI] 30.0-30.9, adult Ⓐ
        Z68.31 Body mass index [BMI] 31.0-31.9, adult Ⓐ
        Z68.32 Body mass index [BMI] 32.0-32.9, adult Ⓐ
        Z68.33 Body mass index [BMI] 33.0-33.9, adult Ⓐ
        Z68.34 Body mass index [BMI] 34.0-34.9, adult Ⓐ
        Z68.35 Body mass index [BMI] 35.0-35.9, adult Ⓐ
        Z68.36 Body mass index [BMI] 36.0-36.9, adult Ⓐ
        Z68.37 Body mass index [BMI] 37.0-37.9, adult Ⓐ
        Z68.38 Body mass index [BMI] 38.0-38.9, adult Ⓐ
        Z68.39 Body mass index [BMI] 39.0-39.9, adult Ⓐ

    ✓5ᵗʰ **Z68.4 Body mass index [BMI] 40 or greater, adult**
        Z68.41 Body mass index [BMI] 40.0-44.9, adult HCC Ⓐ
        Z68.42 Body mass index [BMI] 45.0-49.9, adult HCC Ⓐ
        Z68.43 Body mass index [BMI] 50-59.9, adult HCC Ⓐ
        Z68.44 Body mass index [BMI] 60.0-69.9, adult HCC Ⓐ
        Z68.45 Body mass index [BMI] 70 or greater, adult HCC Ⓐ

    ✓5ᵗʰ **Z68.5 Body mass index [BMI] pediatric**
        Z68.51 Body mass index [BMI] pediatric, less than 5th percentile for age
        Z68.52 Body mass index [BMI] pediatric, 5th percentile to less than 85th percentile for age
        Z68.53 Body mass index [BMI] pediatric, 85th percentile to less than 95th percentile for age
        Z68.54 Body mass index [BMI] pediatric, greater than or equal to 95th percentile for age

Persons encountering health services in other circumstances (Z69-Z76)

✓4ᵗʰ **Z69 Encounter for mental health services for victim and perpetrator of abuse**
    INCLUDES counseling for victims and perpetrators of abuse

    ✓5ᵗʰ **Z69.0 Encounter for mental health services for child abuse problems**
        ✓6ᵗʰ **Z69.01 Encounter for mental health services for parental child abuse**
            Z69.010 Encounter for mental health services for victim of parental child abuse Ⓟ
                ►Encounter for mental health services for victim of child abuse by parent
                Encounter for mental health services for victim of child neglect by parent
                Encounter for mental health services for victim of child psychological abuse by parent
                Encounter for mental health services for victim of child sexual abuse by parent◄

Z69.011 **Encounter for mental health services for perpetrator** of parental child abuse
▶Encounter for mental health services for perpetrator of parental child neglect
Encounter for mental health services for perpetrator of parental child psychological abuse
Encounter for mental health services for perpetrator of parental child sexual abuse◄
EXCLUDES 1 encounter for mental health services for non-parental child abuse (Z69.02-)

✓6th **Z69.02** **Encounter for mental health services for non-parental child abuse**

Z69.020 **Encounter for mental health services** [P] **for victim of non-parental child abuse**
▶Encounter for mental health services for victim of non-parental child neglect
Encounter for mental health services for victim of non-parental child psychological abuse
Encounter for mental health services for victim of non-parental child sexual abuse◄

Z69.021 **Encounter for mental health services for perpetrator of non-parental child abuse**
▶Encounter for mental health services for perpetrator of non-parental child neglect
Encounter for mental health services for perpetrator of non-parental child psychological abuse
Encounter for mental health services for perpetrator of non-parental child sexual abuse◄

✓5th **Z69.1** **Encounter for mental health services for spousal or partner abuse problems**

Z69.11 **Encounter for mental health services for victim of spousal or partner abuse**
▶Encounter for mental health services for victim of spouse or partner neglect
Encounter for mental health services for victim of spouse or partner psychological abuse
Encounter for mental health services for victim of spouse or partner violence, physical◄

Z69.12 **Encounter for mental health services for perpetrator of spousal or partner abuse**
▶Encounter for mental health services for perpetrator of spouse or partner neglect
Encounter for mental health services for perpetrator of spouse or partner psychological abuse
Encounter for mental health services for perpetrator of spouse or partner violence, physical
Encounter for mental health services for perpetrator of spouse or partner violence, sexual◄

✓5th **Z69.8** **Encounter for mental health services for victim or perpetrator of other abuse**

Z69.81 **Encounter for mental health services for victim of other abuse**
▶Encounter for mental health services for perpetrator of non-spousal adult abuse
Encounter for mental health services for victim of non-spousal adult abuse
Encounter for mental health services for victim of spouse or partner violence, sexual◄
Encounter for rape victim counseling

Z69.82 **Encounter for mental health services for perpetrator of other abuse**

✓4th **Z70** **Counseling related to sexual attitude, behavior and orientation**
INCLUDES encounter for mental health services for sexual attitude, behavior and orientation
EXCLUDES 2 contraceptive or procreative counseling (Z30-Z31)

Z70.0 **Counseling related to sexual attitude**

Z70.1 **Counseling related to patient's sexual behavior and orientation**
Patient concerned regarding impotence
Patient concerned regarding non-responsiveness
Patient concerned regarding promiscuity
Patient concerned regarding sexual orientation

Z70.2 **Counseling related to sexual behavior and orientation of third party**
Advice sought regarding sexual behavior and orientation of child
Advice sought regarding sexual behavior and orientation of partner
Advice sought regarding sexual behavior and orientation of spouse

Z70.3 **Counseling related to combined concerns regarding sexual attitude, behavior and orientation**

Z70.8 **Other sex counseling**
Encounter for sex education

Z70.9 **Sex counseling, unspecified** ▽

✓4th **Z71** **Persons encountering health services for other counseling and medical advice, not elsewhere classified**
EXCLUDES 2 contraceptive or procreation counseling (Z30-Z31)
sex counseling (Z70.-)

Z71.0 **Person encountering health services to consult on behalf of another person**
Person encountering health services to seek advice or treatment for non-attending third party
EXCLUDES 2 anxiety (normal) about sick person in family (Z63.7)
expectant (adoptive) parent(s) pre-birth pediatrician visit (Z76.81)

Z71.1 **Person with feared health complaint in whom no diagnosis is made**
Person encountering health services with feared condition which was not demonstrated
Person encountering health services in which problem was normal state
"Worried well"
EXCLUDES 1 medical observation for suspected diseases and conditions proven not to exist (Z03.-)

Z71.2 **Person consulting for explanation of examination or test findings**

Z71.3 **Dietary counseling and surveillance**
Use additional code for any associated underlying medical condition
Use additional code to identify body mass index (BMI), if known (Z68.-)

✓5th **Z71.4** **Alcohol abuse counseling and surveillance**
Use additional code for alcohol abuse or dependence (F10.-)

Z71.41 **Alcohol abuse counseling and surveillance of alcoholic**

Z71.42 **Counseling for family member of alcoholic**
Counseling for significant other, partner, or friend of alcoholic

✓5th **Z71.5** **Drug abuse counseling and surveillance**
Use additional code for drug abuse or dependence (F11-F16, F18-F19)

Z71.51 **Drug abuse counseling and surveillance of drug abuser**

Z71.52 **Counseling for family member of drug abuser**
Counseling for significant other, partner, or friend of drug abuser

Z71.6 **Tobacco abuse counseling**
Use additional code for nicotine dependence (F17.-)

Z71.7 **Human immunodeficiency virus [HIV] counseling**

✓5th **Z71.8** **Other specified counseling**
EXCLUDES 2 counseling for contraception (Z30.0-)
~~counseling for genetics (Z31.5)~~
~~counseling for procreative management (Z31.6-)~~

Z71.81 **Spiritual or religious counseling**

Z71.82 **Exercise counseling**

Z71.83 **Encounter for nonprocreative genetic counseling**
EXCLUDES 1 counseling for procreative genetics (Z31.5)
counseling for procreative management (Z31.6)

Z71.89 **Other specified counseling**

Z71.9 **Counseling, unspecified** ▽
Encounter for medical advice NOS

✓ Additional Character Req   ✓x7th Placeholder Alert   Manifestation   HCC CMS-HCC Condition   ▽ Unspecified Code   ▶◄ Revised Text   ● New Code   ▲ Revised Code Title

Chapter 21. Factors Influencing Health Status and Contact with Health Services

Z69.011–Z71.9

✓4th **Z72 Problems related to lifestyle**
    EXCLUDES 2   *problems related to life-management difficulty (Z73.-)*
               problems related to socioeconomic and psychosocial
               circumstances (Z55-Z65)

    Z72.0 Tobacco use
       Tobacco use NOS
       EXCLUDES 1   *history of tobacco dependence (Z87.891)*
               nicotine dependence (F17.2-)
               tobacco dependence (F17.2-)
               tobacco use during pregnancy (O99.33-)

    Z72.3 Lack of physical exercise

    Z72.4 Inappropriate diet and eating habits
       EXCLUDES 1   *behavioral eating disorders of infancy or childhood*
               (F98.2- F98.3)
               eating disorders (F50.-)
               lack of adequate food (Z59.4)
               malnutrition and other nutritional deficiencies
               (E40-E64)

    ✓5th **Z72.5 High risk sexual behavior**
       Promiscuity
       EXCLUDES 1   *paraphilias (F65)*

       Z72.51 High risk heterosexual behavior

       Z72.52 High risk homosexual behavior

       Z72.53 High risk bisexual behavior

    Z72.6 Gambling and betting
       EXCLUDES 1   *compulsive or pathological gambling (F63.0)*

    ✓5th **Z72.8 Other problems related to lifestyle**

       ✓6th **Z72.81 Antisocial behavior**
           EXCLUDES 1   *conduct disorders (F91.-)*

          Z72.810 Child and adolescent antisocial   **P**
                   behavior
                   Antisocial behavior (child) (adolescent)
                      without manifest psychiatric disorder
                   Delinquency NOS
                   Group delinquency
                   Offenses in the context of gang
                      membership
                   Stealing in company with others
                   Truancy from school

          Z72.811 Adult antisocial behavior   **A**
                   Adult antisocial behavior without manifest
                      psychiatric disorder

       ✓6th **Z72.82 Problems related to sleep**

          Z72.820 Sleep deprivation
                   Lack of adequate sleep
             EXCLUDES 1   *insomnia (G47.0-)*

          Z72.821 Inadequate sleep hygiene
                   Bad sleep habits
                   Irregular sleep habits
                   Unhealthy sleep wake schedule
             EXCLUDES 1   *insomnia (F51.0-, G47.0-)*

       Z72.89 Other problems related to lifestyle
          Self-damaging behavior

    Z72.9 Problem related to lifestyle, unspecified   ▽

✓4th **Z73 Problems related to life management difficulty**
    EXCLUDES 2   *problems related to socioeconomic and psychosocial*
               circumstances (Z55-Z65)
    DEF: State of emotional, mental, and physical exhaustion; causing
    difficulties in managing personal, school, or work circumstances; usually
    due to prolonged stress; poor interpersonal relationship skills, or parenting
    skills.

    Z73.0 Burn-out

    Z73.1 Type A behavior pattern

    Z73.2 Lack of relaxation and leisure

    Z73.3 Stress, not elsewhere classified
       Physical and mental strain NOS
       EXCLUDES 1   *stress related to employment or unemployment (Z56.-)*

    Z73.4 Inadequate social skills, not elsewhere classified

    Z73.5 Social role conflict, not elsewhere classified

    Z73.6 Limitation of activities due to disability
       EXCLUDES 1   *care-provider dependency (Z74.-)*

    ✓5th **Z73.8 Other problems related to life management difficulty**

       ✓6th **Z73.81 Behavioral insomnia of childhood**
          DEF: Behaviors on the part of the child or caregivers that
          cause negative compliance with a child's sleep schedule;
          results in lack of adequate sleep.

          Z73.810 Behavioral insomnia of childhood,   **P**
                   sleep-onset association type

          Z73.811 Behavioral insomnia of childhood,   **P**
                   limit setting type

          Z73.812 Behavioral insomnia of childhood,   **P**
                   combined type

          Z73.819 Behavioral insomnia of childhood,   **P** ▽
                   unspecified type

       Z73.82 Dual sensory impairment

       Z73.89 Other problems related to life management
          difficulty

    Z73.9 Problem related to life management difficulty, unspecified ▽

✓4th **Z74 Problems related to care provider dependency**
    EXCLUDES 2   *dependence on enabling machines or devices NEC (Z99.-)*

    ✓5th **Z74.0 Reduced mobility**

       Z74.01 Bed confinement status
          Bedridden

       Z74.09 Other reduced mobility
          Chair ridden
          Reduced mobility NOS
          EXCLUDES 2   *wheelchair dependence (Z99.3)*

    Z74.1 Need for assistance with personal care

    Z74.2 Need for assistance at home and no other household member
       able to render care

    Z74.3 Need for continuous supervision

    Z74.8 Other problems related to care provider dependency

    Z74.9 Problem related to care provider dependency, unspecified ▽

✓4th **Z75 Problems related to medical facilities and other health care**

    Z75.0 Medical services not available in home
       EXCLUDES 1   *no other household member able to render care (Z74.2)*

    Z75.1 Person awaiting admission to adequate facility elsewhere

    Z75.2 Other waiting period for investigation and treatment

    Z75.3 Unavailability and inaccessibility of health-care facilities
       EXCLUDES 1   *bed unavailable (Z75.1)*

    Z75.4 Unavailability and inaccessibility of other helping agencies

    Z75.5 Holiday relief care

    Z75.8 Other problems related to medical facilities and other health
       care

    Z75.9 Unspecified problem related to medical facilities and   ▽
       other health care

✓4th **Z76 Persons encountering health services in other circumstances**

    Z76.0 Encounter for issue of repeat prescription
       Encounter for issue of repeat prescription for appliance
       Encounter for issue of repeat prescription for medicaments
       Encounter for issue of repeat prescription for spectacles
       EXCLUDES 2   *issue of medical certificate (Z02.7)*
               repeat prescription for contraceptive (Z30.4-)

    Z76.1 Encounter for health supervision and care of foundling   **PDx**

    Z76.2 Encounter for health supervision and care of other   **PDx** **P**
       healthy infant and child
       Encounter for medical or nursing care or supervision of healthy
          infant under circumstances such as adverse socioeconomic
          conditions at home
       Encounter for medical or nursing care or supervision of healthy
          infant under circumstances such as awaiting foster or
          adoptive placement
       Encounter for medical or nursing care or supervision of healthy
          infant under circumstances such as maternal illness
       Encounter for medical or nursing care or supervision of healthy
          infant under circumstances such as number of children at
          home preventing or interfering with normal care

    Z76.3 Healthy person accompanying sick person

    Z76.4 Other boarder to healthcare facility
       EXCLUDES 1   *homelessness (Z59.0)*

    Z76.5 Malingerer [conscious simulation]
       Person feigning illness (with obvious motivation)
       EXCLUDES 1   *factitious disorder (F68.1-)*
               peregrinating patient (F68.1-)
       DEF: Act of intentionally exaggerating an illness or disability in
       order to receive personal gain; or to avoid punishment or
       responsibility.

    ✓5th **Z76.8 Persons encountering health services in other specified**
       circumstances

       Z76.81 Expectant parent(s) prebirth pediatrician visit
          Pre-adoption pediatrician visit for adoptive parent(s)

       Z76.82 Awaiting organ transplant status
          Patient waiting for organ availability

EXCLUDES 1 Not coded here   EXCLUDES 2 Not included here   **N** Newborn Age: 0   **P** Pediatric Age: 0-17   **M** Maternity Age: 12-55   **A** Adult Age: 15-124   **PDx** Primary Dx

1196   ICD-10-CM 2018

Z76.89   **Persons encountering health services in other specified circumstances**
Persons encountering health services NOS
AHA: 2014, 2Q, 10

Persons with potential health hazards related to family and personal history and certain conditions influencing health status (Z77-Z99)

Code also any follow-up examination (Z08-Z09)

✓4ᵗʰ **Z77**   **Other contact with and (suspected) exposures hazardous to health**
INCLUDES   contact with and (suspected) exposures to potential hazards to health
EXCLUDES 2   contact with and (suspected) exposure to communicable diseases (Z20.-)
exposure to (parental) (environmental) tobacco smoke in the perinatal period (P96.81)
newborn affected by noxious substances transmitted via placenta or breast milk (P04.-)
occupational exposure to risk factors (Z57.-)
retained foreign body (Z18.-)
retained foreign body fully removed (Z87.821)
toxic effects of substances chiefly nonmedicinal as to source (T51-T65)

✓5ᵗʰ **Z77.0**   **Contact with and (suspected) exposure to hazardous, chiefly nonmedicinal, chemicals**

✓6ᵗʰ **Z77.01**   **Contact with and (suspected) exposure to hazardous metals**

Z77.010   **Contact with and (suspected) exposure to arsenic**

Z77.011   **Contact with and (suspected) exposure to lead**

Z77.012   **Contact with and (suspected) exposure to uranium**
EXCLUDES 1   retained depleted uranium fragments (Z18.01)

Z77.018   **Contact with and (suspected) exposure to other hazardous metals**
Contact with and (suspected) exposure to chromium compounds
Contact with and (suspected) exposure to nickel dust

✓6ᵗʰ **Z77.02**   **Contact with and (suspected) exposure to hazardous aromatic compounds**

Z77.020   **Contact with and (suspected) exposure to aromatic amines**

Z77.021   **Contact with and (suspected) exposure to benzene**

Z77.028   **Contact with and (suspected) exposure to other hazardous aromatic compounds**
Aromatic dyes NOS
Polycyclic aromatic hydrocarbons

✓6ᵗʰ **Z77.09**   **Contact with and (suspected) exposure to other hazardous, chiefly nonmedicinal, chemicals**

Z77.090   **Contact with and (suspected) exposure to asbestos**

Z77.098   **Contact with and (suspected) exposure to other hazardous, chiefly nonmedicinal, chemicals**
Dyes NOS

✓5ᵗʰ **Z77.1**   **Contact with and (suspected) exposure to environmental pollution and hazards in the physical environment**

✓6ᵗʰ **Z77.11**   **Contact with and (suspected) exposure to environmental pollution**

Z77.110   **Contact with and (suspected) exposure to air pollution**

Z77.111   **Contact with and (suspected) exposure to water pollution**

Z77.112   **Contact with and (suspected) exposure to soil pollution**

Z77.118   **Contact with and (suspected) exposure to other environmental pollution**

✓6ᵗʰ **Z77.12**   **Contact with and (suspected) exposure to hazards in the physical environment**

Z77.120   **Contact with and (suspected) exposure to mold (toxic)**

Z77.121   **Contact with and (suspected) exposure to harmful algae and algae toxins**
Contact with and (suspected) exposure to (harmful) algae bloom NOS
Contact with and (suspected) exposure to blue-green algae bloom
Contact with and (suspected) exposure to brown tide
Contact with and (suspected) exposure to cyanobacteria bloom
Contact with and (suspected) exposure to Florida red tide
Contact with and (suspected) exposure to pfiesteria piscicida
Contact with and (suspected) exposure to red tide

Z77.122   **Contact with and (suspected) exposure to noise**

Z77.123   **Contact with and (suspected) exposure to radon and other naturally occuring radiation**
EXCLUDES 2   radiation exposure as the cause of a confirmed condition (W88-W90, X39.0-)
radiation sickness NOS (T66)

Z77.128   **Contact with and (suspected) exposure to other hazards in the physical environment**

✓5ᵗʰ **Z77.2**   **Contact with and (suspected) exposure to other hazardous substances**

Z77.21   **Contact with and (suspected) exposure to potentially hazardous body fluids**

Z77.22   **Contact with and (suspected) exposure to environmental tobacco smoke (acute) (chronic)**
Exposure to second hand tobacco smoke (acute) (chronic)
Passive smoking (acute) (chronic)
EXCLUDES 1   nicotine dependence (F17.-)
tobacco use (Z72.0)
EXCLUDES 2   occupational exposure to environmental tobacco smoke (Z57.31)

Z77.29   **Contact with and (suspected) exposure to other hazardous substances**
AHA: 2016, 2Q, 33

Z77.9   **Other contact with and (suspected) exposures hazardous to health**

✓4ᵗʰ **Z78**   **Other specified health status**
EXCLUDES 2   asymptomatic human immunodeficiency virus [HIV] infection status (Z21)
postprocedural status (Z93- Z99)
sex reassignment status (Z87.890)

Z78.0   **Asymptomatic menopausal state**   Ⓐ♀
Menopausal state NOS
Postmenopausal status NOS
EXCLUDES 2   symptomatic menopausal state (N95.1)

Z78.1   **Physical restraint status**
EXCLUDES 1   physical restraint due to a procedure - omit code
DEF: Application of mechanical restraining devices or manual restraints; used to limit physical mobility of a patient.

Z78.9   **Other specified health status**

✓4ᵗʰ **Z79**   **Long term (current) drug therapy**
INCLUDES   long term (current) drug use for prophylactic purposes
Code also any therapeutic drug level monitoring (Z51.81)
EXCLUDES 2   drug abuse and dependence (F11-F19)
drug use complicating pregnancy, childbirth, and the puerperium (O99.32-)
long term (current) use of oral antidiabetic drugs (Z79.84)
long term (current) use of oral hypoglycemic drugs (Z79.84)

✓5ᵗʰ **Z79.0**   **Long term (current) use of anticoagulants and antithrombotics/antiplatelets**
EXCLUDES 2   long term (current) use of aspirin (Z79.82)

Z79.01   **Long term (current) use of anticoagulants**

Z79.02   **Long term (current) use of antithrombotics/antiplatelets**

Z79.1   **Long term (current) use of non-steroidal anti-inflammatories (NSAID)**
EXCLUDES 2   long term (current) use of aspirin (Z79.82)

Z79.2   **Long term (current) use of antibiotics**

Z79.3   **Long term (current) use of hormonal contraceptives**
Long term (current) use of birth control pill or patch

Z79.4   **Long term (current) use of insulin**   ᴴᶜᶜ

✓ Additional Character Req   ✓7ˣᵗʰ Placeholder Alert   Manifestation   ᴴᶜᶜ CMS-HCC Condition   ▽ Unspecified Code   ►◄ Revised Text   ● New Code   ▲ Revised Code Title

Chapter 21. Factors Influencing Health Status and Contact with Health Services

Z79.5–Z82.8

✓5ᵗʰ Z79.5 Long term (current) use of steroids
    Z79.51 Long term (current) use of inhaled steroids
    Z79.52 Long term (current) use of systemic steroids

✓5ᵗʰ Z79.8 Other long term (current) drug therapy
    ✓6ᵗʰ Z79.81 Long term (current) use of agents affecting estrogen receptors and estrogen levels
        Code first, if applicable:
          malignant neoplasm of breast (C50.-)
          malignant neoplasm of prostate (C61)
        Use additional code, if applicable, to identify:
          estrogen receptor positive status (Z17.0)
          family history of breast cancer (Z80.3)
          genetic susceptibility to malignant neoplasm (cancer) (Z15.0-)
          personal history of breast cancer (Z85.3)
          personal history of prostate cancer (Z85.46)
          postmenopausal status (Z78.0)
        EXCLUDES 1 ▶hormone replacement therapy◀ (Z79.890)

        Z79.810 Long term (current) use of selective estrogen receptor modulators (SERMs)
          Long term (current) use of raloxifene (Evista)
          Long term (current) use of tamoxifen (Nolvadex)
          Long term (current) use of toremifene (Fareston)

        Z79.811 Long term (current) use of aromatase inhibitors
          Long term (current) use of anastrozole (Arimidex)
          Long term (current) use of exemestane (Aromasin)
          Long term (current) use of letrozole (Femara)

        Z79.818 Long term (current) use of other agents affecting estrogen receptors and estrogen levels
          Long term (current) use of estrogen receptor downregulators
          Long term (current) use of fulvestrant (Faslodex)
          Long term (current) use of gonadotropin-releasing hormone (GnRH) agonist
          Long term (current) use of goserelin acetate (Zoladex)
          Long term (current) use of leuprolide acetate (leuprorelin) (Lupron)
          Long term (current) use of megestrol acetate (Megace)

    Z79.82 Long term (current) use of aspirin
    Z79.83 Long term (current) use of bisphosphonates
    Z79.84 Long term (current) use of oral hypoglycemic drugs
        Long term (current) use of oral antidiabetic drugs
        EXCLUDES 2 long term (current) use of insulin (Z79.4)

    ✓6ᵗʰ Z79.89 Other long term (current) drug therapy
        ▲ **Z79.890 Hormone replacement therapy**
        Z79.891 Long term (current) use of opiate analgesic
          Long term (current) use of methadone for pain management
          EXCLUDES 1 methadone use NOS (F11.9-)
                use of methadone for treatment of heroin addiction (F11.2-)
        Z79.899 Other long term (current) drug therapy
          AHA: 2015, 4Q, 34; 2015, 3Q, 21

✓4ᵗʰ Z80 Family history of primary malignant neoplasm
    Z80.0 Family history of malignant neoplasm of digestive organs
        Conditions classifiable to C15-C26
    Z80.1 Family history of malignant neoplasm of trachea, bronchus and lung
        Conditions classifiable to C33-C34
    Z80.2 Family history of malignant neoplasm of other respiratory and intrathoracic organs
        Conditions classifiable to C30-C32, C37-C39
    Z80.3 Family history of malignant neoplasm of breast
        Conditions classifiable to C50-
    ✓5ᵗʰ Z80.4 Family history of malignant neoplasm of genital organs
        Conditions classifiable to C51-C63
        Z80.41 Family history of malignant neoplasm of ovary

        Z80.42 Family history of malignant neoplasm of prostate
        Z80.43 Family history of malignant neoplasm of testis
        Z80.49 Family history of malignant neoplasm of other genital organs

    ✓5ᵗʰ Z80.5 Family history of malignant neoplasm of urinary tract
        Conditions classifiable to C64-C68
        Z80.51 Family history of malignant neoplasm of kidney
        Z80.52 Family history of malignant neoplasm of bladder
        Z80.59 Family history of malignant neoplasm of other urinary tract organ

    Z80.6 Family history of leukemia
        Conditions classifiable to C91-C95
    Z80.7 Family history of other malignant neoplasms of lymphoid, hematopoietic and related tissues
        Conditions classifiable to C81-C90, C96-
    Z80.8 Family history of malignant neoplasm of other organs or systems
        Conditions classifiable to C00-C14, C40-C49, C69-C79
    Z80.9 Family history of malignant neoplasm, unspecified ▽
        Conditions classifiable to C80.1

✓4ᵗʰ Z81 Family history of mental and behavioral disorders
    Z81.0 Family history of intellectual disabilities
        Conditions classifiable to F70-F79
    Z81.1 Family history of alcohol abuse and dependence
        Conditions classifiable to F10-
    Z81.2 Family history of tobacco abuse and dependence
        Conditions classifiable to F17-
    Z81.3 Family history of other psychoactive substance abuse and dependence
        Conditions classifiable to F11-F16, F18-F19
    Z81.4 Family history of other substance abuse and dependence
        Conditions classifiable to F55
    Z81.8 Family history of other mental and behavioral disorders
        Conditions classifiable elsewhere in F01-F99

✓4ᵗʰ Z82 Family history of certain disabilities and chronic diseases (leading to disablement)
    Z82.0 Family history of epilepsy and other diseases of the nervous system
        Conditions classifiable to G00-G99
    Z82.1 Family history of blindness and visual loss
        Conditions classifiable to H54-
    Z82.2 Family history of deafness and hearing loss
        Conditions classifiable to H90-H91
    Z82.3 Family history of stroke
        Conditions classifiable to I60-I64
    ✓5ᵗʰ Z82.4 Family history of ischemic heart disease and other diseases of the circulatory system
        Conditions classifiable to I00-I52, I65-I99
        Z82.41 Family history of sudden cardiac death
        Z82.49 Family history of ischemic heart disease and other diseases of the circulatory system
    Z82.5 Family history of asthma and other chronic lower respiratory diseases
        Conditions classifiable to J40-J47
        EXCLUDES 2 family history of other diseases of the respiratory system (Z83.6)
    ✓5ᵗʰ Z82.6 Family history of arthritis and other diseases of the musculoskeletal system and connective tissue
        Conditions classifiable to M00-M99
        Z82.61 Family history of arthritis
        Z82.62 Family history of osteoporosis
        Z82.69 Family history of other diseases of the musculoskeletal system and connective tissue
    ✓5ᵗʰ Z82.7 Family history of congenital malformations, deformations and chromosomal abnormalities
        Conditions classifiable to Q00-Q99
        Z82.71 Family history of polycystic kidney
        Z82.79 Family history of other congenital malformations, deformations and chromosomal abnormalities
    Z82.8 Family history of other disabilities and chronic diseases leading to disablement, not elsewhere classified

EXCLUDES 1 Not coded here   *EXCLUDES 2* Not included here   **N** Newborn Age: 0   **P** Pediatric Age: 0-17   **M** Maternity Age: 12-55   **A** Adult Age: 15-124   **PDx** Primary Dx

1198   ICD-10-CM 2018

☑️4ᵗʰ **Z83 Family history of other specific disorders**

> *EXCLUDES 2*   *contact with and (suspected) exposure to communicable disease in the family (Z20.-)*

Z83.0 Family history of human immunodeficiency virus [HIV] disease
Conditions classifiable to B20

Z83.1 Family history of other infectious and parasitic diseases
Conditions classifiable to A00-B19, B25-B94, B99

Z83.2 Family history of diseases of the blood and blood-forming organs and certain disorders involving the immune mechanism
Conditions classifiable to D50-D89

Z83.3 Family history of diabetes mellitus
Conditions classifiable to E08-E13

☑️5ᵗʰ **Z83.4 Family history of other endocrine, nutritional and metabolic diseases**
Conditions classifiable to E00-E07, E15-E88

Z83.41 Family history of multiple endocrine neoplasia [MEN] syndrome

Z83.42 Family history of familial hypercholesterolemia

Z83.49 Family history of other endocrine, nutritional and metabolic diseases

☑️5ᵗʰ **Z83.5 Family history of eye and ear disorders**

☑️6ᵗʰ **Z83.51 Family history of eye disorders**
Conditions classifiable to H00-H53, H55-H59
> *EXCLUDES 2* *family history of blindness and visual loss (Z82.1)*

Z83.511 Family history of glaucoma

Z83.518 Family history of other specified eye disorder

Z83.52 Family history of ear disorders
Conditions classifiable to H60-H83, H92-H95
> *EXCLUDES 2* *family history of deafness and hearing loss (Z82.2)*

Z83.6 Family history of other diseases of the respiratory system
Conditions classifiable to J00-J39, J60-J99
> *EXCLUDES 2* *family history of asthma and other chronic lower respiratory diseases (Z82.5)*

☑️5ᵗʰ **Z83.7 Family history of diseases of the digestive system**
Conditions classifiable to K00-K93

Z83.71 Family history of colonic polyps
> *EXCLUDES 1* *family history of malignant neoplasm of digestive organs (Z80.0)*
> *EXCLUDES 2* ▶*family history of malignant neoplasm of digestive organs (Z80.0)*◀

Z83.79 Family history of other diseases of the digestive system

☑️4ᵗʰ **Z84 Family history of other conditions**

Z84.0 Family history of diseases of the skin and subcutaneous tissue
Conditions classifiable to L00-L99

Z84.1 Family history of disorders of kidney and ureter
Conditions classifiable to N00-N29

Z84.2 Family history of other diseases of the genitourinary system
Conditions classifiable to N30-N99

Z84.3 Family history of consanguinity

☑️5ᵗʰ **Z84.8 Family history of other specified conditions**

Z84.81 Family history of carrier of genetic disease

Z84.82 Family history of sudden infant death syndrome
Family history of SIDS

Z84.89 Family history of other specified conditions

☑️4ᵗʰ **Z85 Personal history of malignant neoplasm**
Code first any follow-up examination after treatment of malignant neoplasm (Z08)
Use additional code to identify:
  alcohol use and dependence (F10.-)
  exposure to environmental tobacco smoke (Z77.22)
  history of tobacco dependence (Z87.891)
  occupational exposure to environmental tobacco smoke (Z57.31)
  tobacco dependence (F17.-)
  tobacco use (Z72.0)
> *EXCLUDES 2* *personal history of benign neoplasm (Z86.01-)*
> *personal history of carcinoma-in-situ (Z86.00-)*

☑️5ᵗʰ **Z85.0 Personal history of malignant neoplasm of digestive organs**
AHA: 2017, 1Q, 9

Z85.00 Personal history of malignant neoplasm of unspecified digestive organ ▽

Z85.01 Personal history of malignant neoplasm of esophagus
Conditions classifiable to C15

☑️6ᵗʰ **Z85.02 Personal history of malignant neoplasm of stomach**

Z85.020 Personal history of malignant carcinoid tumor of stomach
Conditions classifiable to C7A.092

Z85.028 Personal history of other malignant neoplasm of stomach
Conditions classifiable to C16

☑️6ᵗʰ **Z85.03 Personal history of malignant neoplasm of large intestine**

Z85.030 Personal history of malignant carcinoid tumor of large intestine
Conditions classifiable to C7A.022-C7A.025, C7A.029

Z85.038 Personal history of other malignant neoplasm of large intestine
Conditions classifiable to C18

☑️6ᵗʰ **Z85.04 Personal history of malignant neoplasm of rectum, rectosigmoid junction, and anus**

Z85.040 Personal history of malignant carcinoid tumor of rectum
Conditions classifiable to C7A.026

Z85.048 Personal history of other malignant neoplasm of rectum, rectosigmoid junction, and anus
Conditions classifiable to C19-C21

Z85.05 Personal history of malignant neoplasm of liver
Conditions classifiable to C22

☑️6ᵗʰ **Z85.06 Personal history of malignant neoplasm of small intestine**

Z85.060 Personal history of malignant carcinoid tumor of small intestine
Conditions classifiable to C7A.01-

Z85.068 Personal history of other malignant neoplasm of small intestine
Conditions classifiable to C17

Z85.07 Personal history of malignant neoplasm of pancreas
Conditions classifiable to C25

Z85.09 Personal history of malignant neoplasm of other digestive organs

☑️5ᵗʰ **Z85.1 Personal history of malignant neoplasm of trachea, bronchus and lung**

☑️6ᵗʰ **Z85.11 Personal history of malignant neoplasm of bronchus and lung**

Z85.110 Personal history of malignant carcinoid tumor of bronchus and lung
Conditions classifiable to C7A.090

Z85.118 Personal history of other malignant neoplasm of bronchus and lung
Conditions classifiable to C34

Z85.12 Personal history of malignant neoplasm of trachea
Conditions classifiable to C33

☑️5ᵗʰ **Z85.2 Personal history of malignant neoplasm of other respiratory and intrathoracic organs**

Z85.20 Personal history of malignant neoplasm of unspecified respiratory organ ▽

Z85.21 Personal history of malignant neoplasm of larynx
Conditions classifiable to C32

Z85.22 Personal history of malignant neoplasm of nasal cavities, middle ear, and accessory sinuses
Conditions classifiable to C30-C31

☑️ Additional Character Req   ☑️7ᵗʰ Placeholder Alert   Manifestation   HCC CMS-HCC Condition   ▽ Unspecified Code   ▶◀ Revised Text   ● New Code   ▲ Revised Code Title

Chapter 21. Factors Influencing Health Status and Contact with Health Services

√6ᵗʰ **Z85.23** **Personal history of malignant neoplasm of thymus**

    Z85.230 **Personal history of malignant carcinoid tumor of thymus**
         Conditions classifiable to C7A.091

    Z85.238 **Personal history of other malignant neoplasm of thymus**
         Conditions classifiable to C37

  Z85.29 **Personal history of malignant neoplasm of other respiratory and intrathoracic organs**

  Z85.3 **Personal history of malignant neoplasm of breast**
     Conditions classifiable to C50.-

√5ᵗʰ **Z85.4** **Personal history of malignant neoplasm of genital organs**
     Conditions classifiable to C51-C63

    Z85.40 **Personal history of malignant neoplasm of unspecified female genital organ** ♀▽

    Z85.41 **Personal history of malignant neoplasm of cervix uteri** ♀

    Z85.42 **Personal history of malignant neoplasm of other parts of uterus** ♀

    Z85.43 **Personal history of malignant neoplasm of ovary** ♀

    Z85.44 **Personal history of malignant neoplasm of other female genital organs** ♀

    Z85.45 **Personal history of malignant neoplasm of unspecified male genital organ** ♂▽

    Z85.46 **Personal history of malignant neoplasm of prostate** ♂

    Z85.47 **Personal history of malignant neoplasm of testis** ♂

    Z85.48 **Personal history of malignant neoplasm of epididymis** ♂

    Z85.49 **Personal history of malignant neoplasm of other male genital organs** ♂

√5ᵗʰ **Z85.5** **Personal history of malignant neoplasm of urinary tract**
     Conditions classifiable to C64-C68

    Z85.50 **Personal history of malignant neoplasm of unspecified urinary tract organ** ▽

    Z85.51 **Personal history of malignant neoplasm of bladder**

√6ᵗʰ **Z85.52** **Personal history of malignant neoplasm of kidney**
     EXCLUDES 1 *personal history of malignant neoplasm of renal pelvis (Z85.53)*

    Z85.520 **Personal history of malignant carcinoid tumor of kidney**
         Conditions classifiable to C7A.093

    Z85.528 **Personal history of other malignant neoplasm of kidney**
         Conditions classifiable to C64

    Z85.53 **Personal history of malignant neoplasm of renal pelvis**

    Z85.54 **Personal history of malignant neoplasm of ureter**

    Z85.59 **Personal history of malignant neoplasm of other urinary tract organ**

  Z85.6 **Personal history of leukemia**
     Conditions classifiable to C91-C95
     EXCLUDES 1 *leukemia in remission C91.0-C95.9 with 5th character 1*

√5ᵗʰ **Z85.7** **Personal history of other malignant neoplasms of lymphoid, hematopoietic and related tissues**

    Z85.71 **Personal history of Hodgkin lymphoma**
         Conditions classifiable to C81

    Z85.72 **Personal history of non-Hodgkin lymphomas**
         Conditions classifiable to C82-C85

    Z85.79 **Personal history of other malignant neoplasms of lymphoid, hematopoietic and related tissues**
         Conditions classifiable to C88-C90, C96
         EXCLUDES 1 *multiple myeloma in remission (C90.01)*
                   plasma cell leukemia in remission (C90.11)
                   plasmacytoma in remission (C90.21)

√5ᵗʰ **Z85.8** **Personal history of malignant neoplasms of other organs and systems**
     Conditions classifiable to C00-C14, C40-C49, C69-C75, C7A.098, C76-C79

√6ᵗʰ **Z85.81** **Personal history of malignant neoplasm of lip, oral cavity, and pharynx**

    Z85.810 **Personal history of malignant neoplasm of tongue**

    Z85.818 **Personal history of malignant neoplasm of other sites of lip, oral cavity, and pharynx**

    Z85.819 **Personal history of malignant neoplasm of unspecified site of lip, oral cavity, and pharynx** ▽

√6ᵗʰ **Z85.82** **Personal history of malignant neoplasm of skin**

    Z85.820 **Personal history of malignant melanoma of skin**
         Conditions classifiable to C43

    Z85.821 **Personal history of Merkel cell carcinoma**
         Conditions classifiable to C4A

    Z85.828 **Personal history of other malignant neoplasm of skin**
         Conditions classifiable to C44

√6ᵗʰ **Z85.83** **Personal history of malignant neoplasm of bone and soft tissue**

    Z85.830 **Personal history of malignant neoplasm of bone**

    Z85.831 **Personal history of malignant neoplasm of soft tissue**
         EXCLUDES 2 *personal history of malignant neoplasm of skin (Z85.82-)*

√6ᵗʰ **Z85.84** **Personal history of malignant neoplasm of eye and nervous tissue**

    Z85.840 **Personal history of malignant neoplasm of eye**

    Z85.841 **Personal history of malignant neoplasm of brain**

    Z85.848 **Personal history of malignant neoplasm of other parts of nervous tissue**

√6ᵗʰ **Z85.85** **Personal history of malignant neoplasm of endocrine glands**

    Z85.850 **Personal history of malignant neoplasm of thyroid**

    Z85.858 **Personal history of malignant neoplasm of other endocrine glands**

  Z85.89 **Personal history of malignant neoplasm of other organs and systems**

  Z85.9 **Personal history of malignant neoplasm, unspecified** ▽
     Conditions classifiable to C7A.00, C80.1

√4ᵗʰ **Z86** **Personal history of certain other diseases**
     Code first any follow-up examination after treatment (Z09)

√5ᵗʰ **Z86.0** **Personal history of in-situ and benign neoplasms and neoplasms of uncertain behavior**
     EXCLUDES 2 *personal history of malignant neoplasms (Z85.-)*
     AHA: 2017, 1Q, 9

√6ᵗʰ **Z86.00** **Personal history of in-situ neoplasm**
     Conditions classifiable to D00-D09

    Z86.000 **Personal history of in-situ neoplasm of breast**
         Personal history of cervical intraepithelial neoplasia III [CIN III]

    Z86.001 **Personal history of in-situ neoplasm of cervix uteri** ♀

    Z86.008 **Personal history of in-situ neoplasm of other site**
         Personal history of vaginal intraepithelial neoplasia III [VAIN III]
         Personal history of vulvar intraepithelial neoplasia III [VIN III]

√6ᵗʰ **Z86.01** **Personal history of benign neoplasm**

    Z86.010 **Personal history of colonic polyps**
         AHA: 2017, 1Q, 14

    Z86.011 **Personal history of benign neoplasm of the brain**

    Z86.012 **Personal history of benign carcinoid tumor**

    Z86.018 **Personal history of other benign neoplasm**
         AHA: 2017, 1Q, 14

  Z86.03 **Personal history of neoplasm of uncertain behavior**

√5ᵗʰ **Z86.1** **Personal history of infectious and parasitic diseases**
     Conditions classifiable to A00-B89, B99
     EXCLUDES 1 *personal history of infectious diseases specific to a body system*
                 sequelae of infectious and parasitic diseases (B90-B94)

  Z86.11 **Personal history of tuberculosis**

  Z86.12 **Personal history of poliomyelitis**

  Z86.13 **Personal history of malaria**

  Z86.14 **Personal history of Methicillin resistant Staphylococcus aureus infection**
     Personal history of MRSA infection

EXCLUDES 1 Not coded here   EXCLUDES 2 Not included here   N Newborn Age: 0   P Pediatric Age: 0-17   M Maternity Age: 12-55   A Adult Age: 15-124   PDx Primary Dx

1200   ICD-10-CM 2018

Z86.19   Personal history of other infectious and parasitic diseases

Z86.2   **Personal history of diseases of the blood and blood-forming organs and certain disorders involving the immune mechanism**
Conditions classifiable to D50-D89

☑5ᵗʰ Z86.3   **Personal history of endocrine, nutritional and metabolic diseases**
Conditions classifiable to E00-E88

Z86.31   Personal history of **diabetic foot ulcer**
EXCLUDES 2   *current diabetic foot ulcer (E08.621, E09.621, E10.621, E11.621, E13.621)*

Z86.32   Personal history of **gestational diabetes**   ♀
Personal history of conditions classifiable to O24.4-
EXCLUDES 1   *gestational diabetes mellitus in current pregnancy (O24.4-)*

Z86.39   Personal history of other endocrine, nutritional and metabolic disease

☑5ᵗʰ Z86.5   **Personal history of mental and behavioral disorders**
Conditions classifiable to F40-F59

Z86.51   Personal history of **combat and operational stress reaction**   Ⓐ

Z86.59   Personal history of other mental and behavioral disorders

☑5ᵗʰ Z86.6   **Personal history of diseases of the nervous system and sense organs**
Conditions classifiable to G00-G99, H00-H95
EXCLUDES 2   *personal history of anaphylactic shock (Z87.892)*

Z86.61   Personal history of **infections of the central nervous system**
Personal history of encephalitis
Personal history of meningitis

Z86.69   Personal history of other diseases of the nervous system and sense organs

☑5ᵗʰ Z86.7   **Personal history of diseases of the circulatory system**
Conditions classifiable to I00-I99
EXCLUDES 2   *old myocardial infarction (I25.2)*
personal history of anaphylactic shock (Z87.892)
postmyocardial infarction syndrome (I24.1)

☑6ᵗʰ Z86.71   Personal history of **venous thrombosis and embolism**
Z86.711   Personal history of **pulmonary** embolism
Z86.718   Personal history of other venous thrombosis and embolism

Z86.72   Personal history of **thrombophlebitis**

Z86.73   Personal history of **transient ischemic attack (TIA), and cerebral infarction without residual deficits**
Personal history of prolonged reversible ischemic neurological deficit (PRIND)
Personal history of stroke NOS without residual deficits
EXCLUDES 1   *personal history of traumatic brain injury (Z87.820)*
sequelae of cerebrovascular disease (I69.-)
AHA: 2012, 4Q, 92

Z86.74   Personal history of **sudden cardiac arrest**
Personal history of sudden cardiac death successfully resuscitated

Z86.79   Personal history of other diseases of the circulatory system

☑4ᵗʰ Z87   **Personal history of other diseases and conditions**
Code first any follow-up examination after treatment (Z09)

☑5ᵗʰ Z87.0   **Personal history of diseases of the respiratory system**
Conditions classifiable to J00-J99

Z87.01   Personal history of **pneumonia** (recurrent)

Z87.09   Personal history of other diseases of the respiratory system

☑5ᵗʰ Z87.1   **Personal history of diseases of the digestive system**
Conditions classifiable to K00-K93

Z87.11   Personal history of **peptic ulcer** disease

Z87.19   Personal history of other diseases of the digestive system
AHA: 2017, 1Q, 14

Z87.2   **Personal history of diseases of the skin and subcutaneous tissue**
Conditions classifiable to L00-L99
EXCLUDES 2   *personal history of diabetic foot ulcer (Z86.31)*

☑5ᵗʰ Z87.3   **Personal history of diseases of the musculoskeletal system and connective tissue**
Conditions classifiable to M00-M99
EXCLUDES 2   *personal history of (healed) traumatic fracture (Z87.81)*

☑6ᵗʰ Z87.31   Personal history of (healed) **nontraumatic fracture**
Z87.310   Personal history of (healed) **osteoporosis fracture**
Personal history of (healed) fragility fracture
Personal history of (healed) collapsed vertebra due to osteoporosis

Z87.311   Personal history of (healed) other **pathological fracture**
Personal history of (healed) collapsed vertebra NOS
EXCLUDES 2   *personal history of osteoporosis fracture (Z87.310)*

Z87.312   Personal history of (healed) **stress fracture**
Personal history of (healed) fatigue fracture

Z87.39   Personal history of other diseases of the musculoskeletal system and connective tissue

☑5ᵗʰ Z87.4   **Personal history of diseases of genitourinary system**
Conditions classifiable to N00-N99

☑6ᵗʰ Z87.41   Personal history of **dysplasia of the female genital tract**
EXCLUDES 1   *personal history of intraepithelial neoplasia III of female genital tract ▶(Z86.001, Z86.008)◀*
personal history of malignant neoplasm of female genital tract (Z85.40-Z85.44)
Z87.410   Personal history of **cervical** dysplasia   ♀
Z87.411   Personal history of **vaginal** dysplasia   ♀
Z87.412   Personal history of **vulvar** dysplasia   ♀

Z87.42   Personal history of other diseases of the **female** genital tract

☑6ᵗʰ Z87.43   Personal history of diseases of the **male genital organs**
Z87.430   Personal history of **prostatic dysplasia**   ♂
EXCLUDES 1   *personal history of malignant neoplasm of prostate (Z85.46)*
Z87.438   Personal history of other diseases of **male** genital organs   ♂

☑6ᵗʰ Z87.44   Personal history of diseases of the **urinary system**
EXCLUDES 1   *personal history of malignant neoplasm of cervix uteri (Z85.41)*
Z87.440   Personal history of **urinary (tract) infections**
Z87.441   Personal history of **nephrotic syndrome**
Z87.442   Personal history of **urinary calculi**
Personal history of kidney stones
Z87.448   Personal history of other diseases of urinary system

☑5ᵗʰ Z87.5   **Personal history of complications of pregnancy, childbirth and the puerperium**
Conditions classifiable to O00-O9A
EXCLUDES 2   *recurrent pregnancy loss (N96)*
Z87.51   Personal history of **pre-term labor**   ♀
EXCLUDES 1   *current pregnancy with history of pre-term labor (O09.21-)*
Z87.59   Personal history of other complications of pregnancy, childbirth and the puerperium   ♀
Personal history of trophoblastic disease

Chapter 21. Factors Influencing Health Status and Contact with Health Services

✓5ᵗʰ **Z87.7** **Personal history of (corrected) congenital malformations**
Conditions classifiable to Q00-Q89 that have been repaired or corrected

> EXCLUDES 1 *congenital malformations that have been partially corrected or repaired but which still require medical treatment—code to condition*
>
> EXCLUDES 2 *other postprocedural states (Z98.-)*
> *personal history of medical treatment (Z92.-)*
> *presence of cardiac and vascular implants and grafts (Z95.-)*
> *presence of other devices (Z97.-)*
> *presence of other functional implants (Z96.-)*
> *transplanted organ and tissue status (Z94.-)*

✓6ᵗʰ **Z87.71** **Personal history of (corrected) congenital malformations of genitourinary system**

  Z87.710 **Personal history of (corrected) hypospadias** ♂

  Z87.718 **Personal history of other specified (corrected) congenital malformations of genitourinary system**

✓6ᵗʰ **Z87.72** **Personal history of (corrected) congenital malformations of nervous system and sense organs**

  Z87.720 **Personal history of (corrected) congenital malformations of eye**

  Z87.721 **Personal history of (corrected) congenital malformations of ear**

  Z87.728 **Personal history of other specified (corrected) congenital malformations of nervous system and sense organs**

✓6ᵗʰ **Z87.73** **Personal history of (corrected) congenital malformations of digestive system**

  Z87.730 **Personal history of (corrected) cleft lip and palate**

  Z87.738 **Personal history of other specified (corrected) congenital malformations of digestive system**

Z87.74 **Personal history of (corrected) congenital malformations of heart and circulatory system**

Z87.75 **Personal history of (corrected) congenital malformations of respiratory system**

Z87.76 **Personal history of (corrected) congenital malformations of integument, limbs and musculoskeletal system**

✓6ᵗʰ **Z87.79** **Personal history of other (corrected) congenital malformations**

  Z87.790 **Personal history of (corrected) congenital malformations of face and neck**

  Z87.798 **Personal history of other (corrected) congenital malformations**

✓5ᵗʰ **Z87.8** **Personal history of other specified conditions**

> EXCLUDES 2 *personal history of self harm (Z91.5)*

Z87.81 **Personal history of (healed) traumatic fracture**

> EXCLUDES 2 *personal history of (healed) nontraumatic fracture (Z87.31-)*

✓6ᵗʰ **Z87.82** **Personal history of other (healed) physical injury and trauma**
Conditions classifiable to S00-T88, except traumatic fractures

  Z87.820 **Personal history of traumatic brain injury**

> EXCLUDES 1 *personal history of transient ischemic attack (TIA), and cerebral infarction without residual deficits (Z86.73)*

  Z87.821 **Personal history of retained foreign body fully removed**

  Z87.828 **Personal history of other (healed) physical injury and trauma**

✓6ᵗʰ **Z87.89** **Personal history of other specified conditions**

  Z87.890 **Personal history of sex reassignment**

  Z87.891 **Personal history of nicotine dependence**

> EXCLUDES 1 *current nicotine dependence (F17.2-)*
>
> AHA: 2017, 2Q, 27

  Z87.892 **Personal history of anaphylaxis**
Code also allergy status such as:
allergy status to drugs, medicaments and biological substances (Z88.-)
allergy status, other than to drugs and biological substances (Z91.0-)

Z87.898 **Personal history of other specified conditions**
AHA: 2013, 1Q, 21

✓4ᵗʰ **Z88** **Allergy status to drugs, medicaments and biological substances**

> EXCLUDES 2 *allergy status, other than to drugs and biological substances (Z91.0-)*
>
> AHA: 2015, 3Q, 23

Z88.0 **Allergy status to penicillin**

Z88.1 **Allergy status to other antibiotic agents status**

Z88.2 **Allergy status to sulfonamides status**

Z88.3 **Allergy status to other anti-infective agents status**

Z88.4 **Allergy status to anesthetic agent status**

Z88.5 **Allergy status to narcotic agent status**

Z88.6 **Allergy status to analgesic agent status**

Z88.7 **Allergy status to serum and vaccine status**

Z88.8 **Allergy status to other drugs, medicaments and biological substances status**

Z88.9 **Allergy status to unspecified drugs, medicaments and biological substances status** ▽

✓4ᵗʰ **Z89** **Acquired absence of limb**

> INCLUDES amputation status
> postprocedural loss of limb
> post-traumatic loss of limb
>
> EXCLUDES 1 *acquired deformities of limbs (M20-M21)*
> *congenital absence of limbs (Q71-Q73)*

✓5ᵗʰ **Z89.0** **Acquired absence of thumb and other finger(s)**

✓6ᵗʰ **Z89.01** **Acquired absence of thumb**

  Z89.011 **Acquired absence of right thumb**

  Z89.012 **Acquired absence of left thumb**

  Z89.019 **Acquired absence of unspecified thumb** ▽

✓6ᵗʰ **Z89.02** **Acquired absence of other finger(s)**

> EXCLUDES 2 *acquired absence of thumb (Z89.01-)*

  Z89.021 **Acquired absence of right finger(s)**

  Z89.022 **Acquired absence of left finger(s)**

  Z89.029 **Acquired absence of unspecified finger(s)** ▽

✓5ᵗʰ **Z89.1** **Acquired absence of hand and wrist**

✓6ᵗʰ **Z89.11** **Acquired absence of hand**

  Z89.111 **Acquired absence of right hand**

  Z89.112 **Acquired absence of left hand**

  Z89.119 **Acquired absence of unspecified hand** ▽

✓6ᵗʰ **Z89.12** **Acquired absence of wrist**
Disarticulation at wrist

  Z89.121 **Acquired absence of right wrist**

  Z89.122 **Acquired absence of left wrist**

  Z89.129 **Acquired absence of unspecified wrist** ▽

✓5ᵗʰ **Z89.2** **Acquired absence of upper limb above wrist**

✓6ᵗʰ **Z89.20** **Acquired absence of upper limb, unspecified level**

  Z89.201 **Acquired absence of right upper limb, unspecified level** ▽

  Z89.202 **Acquired absence of left upper limb, unspecified level** ▽

  Z89.209 **Acquired absence of unspecified upper limb, unspecified level** ▽
Acquired absence of arm NOS

✓6ᵗʰ **Z89.21** **Acquired absence of upper limb below elbow**

  Z89.211 **Acquired absence of right upper limb below elbow**

  Z89.212 **Acquired absence of left upper limb below elbow**

  Z89.219 **Acquired absence of unspecified upper limb below elbow** ▽

✓6ᵗʰ **Z89.22** **Acquired absence of upper limb above elbow**
Disarticulation at elbow

  Z89.221 **Acquired absence of right upper limb above elbow**

  Z89.222 **Acquired absence of left upper limb above elbow**

  Z89.229 **Acquired absence of unspecified upper limb above elbow** ▽

EXCLUDES 1 Not coded here   EXCLUDES 2 Not included here   N Newborn Age: 0   P Pediatric Age: 0-17   M Maternity Age: 12-55   A Adult Age: 15-124   PDx Primary Dx

1202   ICD-10-CM 2018

☑6ᵗʰ **Z89.23** **Acquired absence of shoulder**
Acquired absence of shoulder joint following explantation of shoulder joint prosthesis, with or without presence of antibiotic-impregnated cement spacer

     Z89.231 **Acquired absence of right shoulder**

     Z89.232 **Acquired absence of left shoulder**

     Z89.239 **Acquired absence of unspecified shoulder** ▽

☑5ᵗʰ **Z89.4** **Acquired absence of toe(s), foot, and ankle**

   ☑6ᵗʰ **Z89.41** **Acquired absence of great toe**

     Z89.411 **Acquired absence of right great toe** HCC

     Z89.412 **Acquired absence of left great toe** HCC

     Z89.419 **Acquired absence of unspecified great toe** HCC ▽

   ☑6ᵗʰ **Z89.42** **Acquired absence of other toe(s)**
EXCLUDES 2 *acquired absence of great toe (Z89.41-)*

     Z89.421 **Acquired absence of other right toe(s)** HCC

     Z89.422 **Acquired absence of other left toe(s)** HCC

     Z89.429 **Acquired absence of other toe(s), unspecified side** HCC ▽

   ☑6ᵗʰ **Z89.43** **Acquired absence of foot**

     Z89.431 **Acquired absence of right foot** HCC

     Z89.432 **Acquired absence of left foot** HCC

     Z89.439 **Acquired absence of unspecified foot** HCC ▽

   ☑6ᵗʰ **Z89.44** **Acquired absence of ankle**
Disarticulation of ankle

     Z89.441 **Acquired absence of right ankle** HCC

     Z89.442 **Acquired absence of left ankle** HCC

     Z89.449 **Acquired absence of unspecified ankle** HCC ▽

☑5ᵗʰ **Z89.5** **Acquired absence of leg below knee**

   ☑6ᵗʰ **Z89.51** **Acquired absence of leg below knee**

     Z89.511 **Acquired absence of right leg below knee** HCC

     Z89.512 **Acquired absence of left leg below knee** HCC

     Z89.519 **Acquired absence of unspecified leg below knee** HCC ▽

   ☑6ᵗʰ **Z89.52** **Acquired absence of knee**
Acquired absence of knee joint following explantation of knee joint prosthesis, with or without presence of antibiotic-impregnated cement spacer

     Z89.521 **Acquired absence of right knee**

     Z89.522 **Acquired absence of left knee**

     Z89.529 **Acquired absence of unspecified knee** ▽

☑5ᵗʰ **Z89.6** **Acquired absence of leg above knee**

   ☑6ᵗʰ **Z89.61** **Acquired absence of leg above knee**
Acquired absence of leg NOS
Disarticulation at knee

     Z89.611 **Acquired absence of right leg above knee** HCC

     Z89.612 **Acquired absence of left leg above knee** HCC

     Z89.619 **Acquired absence of unspecified leg above knee** HCC ▽

   ☑6ᵗʰ **Z89.62** **Acquired absence of hip**
Acquired absence of hip joint following explantation of hip joint prosthesis, with or without presence of antibiotic-impregnated cement spacer
Disarticulation at hip

     Z89.621 **Acquired absence of right hip joint**

     Z89.622 **Acquired absence of left hip joint**

     Z89.629 **Acquired absence of unspecified hip joint** ▽

   Z89.9 **Acquired absence of limb, unspecified** ▽

☑4ᵗʰ **Z90** **Acquired absence of organs, not elsewhere classified**
INCLUDES postprocedural or post-traumatic loss of body part NEC
EXCLUDES 1 *congenital absence—see Alphabetical Index*
EXCLUDES 2 *postprocedural absence of endocrine glands (E89.-)*

   ☑5ᵗʰ **Z90.0** **Acquired absence of part of head and neck**

     Z90.01 **Acquired absence of eye**

     Z90.02 **Acquired absence of larynx**

     Z90.09 **Acquired absence of other part of head and neck**
Acquired absence of nose
EXCLUDES 2 *teeth (K08.1)*

   ☑5ᵗʰ **Z90.1** **Acquired absence of breast and nipple**

     Z90.10 **Acquired absence of unspecified breast and nipple** ▽

     Z90.11 **Acquired absence of right breast and nipple**

     Z90.12 **Acquired absence of left breast and nipple**

     Z90.13 **Acquired absence of bilateral breasts and nipples**

   Z90.2 **Acquired absence of lung [part of]**

   Z90.3 **Acquired absence of stomach [part of]**

   ☑5ᵗʰ **Z90.4** **Acquired absence of other specified parts of digestive tract**

   ☑6ᵗʰ **Z90.41** **Acquired absence of pancreas**
Code also exocrine pancreatic insufficiency (K86.81)
Use additional code to identify any associated:
insulin use (Z79.4)
diabetes mellitus, postpancreatectomy (E13.-)

     Z90.410 **Acquired total absence of pancreas**
Acquired absence of pancreas NOS

     Z90.411 **Acquired partial absence of pancreas**

     Z90.49 **Acquired absence of other specified parts of digestive tract**

   Z90.5 **Acquired absence of kidney**

   Z90.6 **Acquired absence of other parts of urinary tract**
Acquired absence of bladder

   ☑5ᵗʰ **Z90.7** **Acquired absence of genital organ(s)**
EXCLUDES 1 *personal history of sex reassignment (Z87.890)*
EXCLUDES 2 *female genital mutilation status (N90.81-)*

   ☑6ᵗʰ **Z90.71** **Acquired absence of cervix and uterus**

     Z90.710 **Acquired absence of both cervix and uterus** ♀
Acquired absence of uterus NOS
Status post total hysterectomy

     Z90.711 **Acquired absence of uterus with remaining cervical stump** ♀
Status post partial hysterectomy with remaining cervical stump

     Z90.712 **Acquired absence of cervix with remaining uterus** ♀

   ☑6ᵗʰ **Z90.72** **Acquired absence of ovaries**

     Z90.721 **Acquired absence of ovaries, unilateral** ♀

     Z90.722 **Acquired absence of ovaries, bilateral** ♀

     Z90.79 **Acquired absence of other genital organ(s)**

   ☑5ᵗʰ **Z90.8** **Acquired absence of other organs**

     Z90.81 **Acquired absence of spleen**

     Z90.89 **Acquired absence of other organs**

☑4ᵗʰ **Z91** **Personal risk factors, not elsewhere classified**
EXCLUDES 2 *contact with and (suspected) exposures hazardous to health (Z77.-)*
exposure to pollution and other problems related to physical environment (Z77.1-)
▶*female genital mutilation status (N90.81-)*◀
personal history of physical injury and trauma (Z87.81, Z87.82-)
occupational exposure to risk factors (Z57.-)

   ☑5ᵗʰ **Z91.0** **Allergy status, other than to drugs and biological substances**
EXCLUDES 2 *allergy status to drugs, medicaments, and biological substances (Z88.-)*

   ☑6ᵗʰ **Z91.01** **Food allergy status**
EXCLUDES 2 *food additives allergy status (Z91.02)*

     Z91.010 **Allergy to peanuts**

     Z91.011 **Allergy to milk products**
EXCLUDES 1 *lactose intolerance (E73.-)*

     Z91.012 **Allergy to eggs**

     Z91.013 **Allergy to seafood**
Allergy to shellfish
Allergy to octopus or squid ink

     Z91.018 **Allergy to other foods**
Allergy to nuts other than peanuts

     Z91.02 **Food additives allergy status**

   ☑6ᵗʰ **Z91.03** **Insect allergy status**

     Z91.030 **Bee allergy status**

     Z91.038 **Other insect allergy status**

☑ Additional Character Req   ✓x7ᵗʰ Placeholder Alert   Manifestation   HCC CMS-HCC Condition   ▽ Unspecified Code   ▶◀ Revised Text   ● New Code   ▲ Revised Code Title

√6th Z91.04 Nonmedicinal substance allergy status

    Z91.040 Latex allergy status
        Latex sensitivity status

    Z91.041 Radiographic dye allergy status
        Allergy status to contrast media used for diagnostic X-ray procedure

    Z91.048 Other nonmedicinal substance allergy status

    Z91.09 Other allergy status, other than to drugs and biological substances

√5th Z91.1 Patient's noncompliance with medical treatment and regimen

    Z91.11 Patient's noncompliance with dietary regimen

    √6th Z91.12 Patient's intentional underdosing of medication regimen
        Code first underdosing of medication (T36-T50) with fifth or sixth character 6
        EXCLUDES 1 *adverse effect of prescribed drug taken as directed—code to adverse effect*
           poisoning (overdose)—code to poisoning

        Z91.120 Patient's intentional underdosing of medication regimen due to financial hardship

        Z91.128 Patient's intentional underdosing of medication regimen for other reason

    √6th Z91.13 Patient's unintentional underdosing of medication regimen
        Code first underdosing of medication (T36-T50) with fifth or sixth character 6
        EXCLUDES 1 *adverse effect of prescribed drug taken as directed—code to adverse effect*
           poisoning (overdose)—code to poisoning

        Z91.130 Patient's unintentional underdosing of medication regimen due to age-related debility

        Z91.138 Patient's unintentional underdosing of medication regimen for other reason

    Z91.14 Patient's other noncompliance with medication regimen
        Patient's underdosing of medication NOS

    Z91.15 Patient's noncompliance with renal dialysis HCC

    Z91.19 Patient's noncompliance with other medical treatment and regimen
        ▶Nonadherence to medical treatment◀

√5th Z91.4 Personal history of psychological trauma, not elsewhere classified

    √6th Z91.41 Personal history of adult abuse
        EXCLUDES 2 *personal history of abuse in childhood (Z62.81-)*

        Z91.410 Personal history of adult physical and sexual abuse A
           EXCLUDES 1 *current adult physical abuse (T74.11, T76.11)*
               current adult sexual abuse (T74.21, T76.11)

        Z91.411 Personal history of adult psychological abuse A

        Z91.412 Personal history of adult neglect A
           EXCLUDES 1 *current adult neglect (T74.01, T76.01)*

        Z91.419 Personal history of unspecified adult abuse A ▽

    Z91.49 Other personal history of psychological trauma, not elsewhere classified

Z91.5 Personal history of self-harm
    Personal history of parasuicide
    Personal history of self-poisoning
    Personal history of suicide attempt

√5th Z91.8 Other specified personal risk factors, not elsewhere classified

    Z91.81 History of falling
        At risk for falling

    Z91.82 Personal history of military deployment A
        Individual (civilian or military) with past history of military war, peacekeeping and humanitarian deployment (current or past conflict)
        Returned from military deployment

Z91.83 *Wandering in diseases classified elsewhere*
    Code first underlying disorder such as:
        Alzheimer's disease (G30.-)
        autism or pervasive developmental disorder (F84.-)
        intellectual disabilities (F70-F79)
        unspecified dementia with behavioral disturbance (F03.9-)

● **√6th Z91.84 Oral health risk factors**
●   **Z91.841 Risk for dental caries, low**
●   **Z91.842 Risk for dental caries, moderate**
●   **Z91.843 Risk for dental caries, high**
●   **Z91.849 Unspecified risk for dental caries** ▽

    Z91.89 Other specified personal risk factors, not elsewhere classified
        AHA: 2017, 1Q, 45

√4th Z92 Personal history of medical treatment
    EXCLUDES 2 *postprocedural states (Z98.-)*

    Z92.0 Personal history of contraception
        EXCLUDES 1 *counseling or management of current contraceptive practices (Z30.-)*
           long term (current) use of contraception (Z79.3)
           presence of (intrauterine) contraceptive device (Z97.5)

    √5th Z92.2 Personal history of drug therapy
        EXCLUDES 2 *long term (current) drug therapy (Z79.-)*

        Z92.21 Personal history of antineoplastic chemotherapy
        Z92.22 Personal history of monoclonal drug therapy
        Z92.23 Personal history of estrogen therapy

        √6th Z92.24 Personal history of steroid therapy
           Z92.240 Personal history of inhaled steroid therapy
           Z92.241 Personal history of systemic steroid therapy
               Personal history of steroid therapy NOS

        Z92.25 Personal history of immunosupression therapy
           EXCLUDES 2 *personal history of steroid therapy (Z92.24)*

        Z92.29 Personal history of other drug therapy

    Z92.3 Personal history of irradiation
        Personal history of exposure to therapeutic radiation
        EXCLUDES 1 *exposure to radiation in the physical environment (Z77.12)*
           occupational exposure to radiation (Z57.1)

    √5th Z92.8 Personal history of other medical treatment

        Z92.81 Personal history of extracorporeal membrane oxygenation (ECMO)

        Z92.82 Status post administration of tPA (rtPA) in a different facility within the last 24 hours prior to admission to current facility
           Code first condition requiring tPA administration, such as:
               acute cerebral infarction (I63.-)
               acute myocardial infarction (I21-, I22-)
           AHA: 2013, 4Q, 124

        Z92.83 Personal history of failed moderate sedation
           Personal history of failed conscious sedation
           EXCLUDES 2 *failed moderate sedation during procedure (T88.52)*

        Z92.84 Personal history of unintended awareness under general anesthesia
           EXCLUDES 2 *unintended awareness under general anesthesia during procedure (T88.53)*

        Z92.89 Personal history of other medical treatment

√4th Z93 Artificial opening status
    EXCLUDES 1 *artificial openings requiring attention or management (Z43.-)*
           complications of external stoma (J95.0-, K94.-, N99.5-)

    Z93.0 Tracheostomy status HCC
        AHA: 2013, 4Q, 129

    Z93.1 Gastrostomy status HCC
    Z93.2 Ileostomy status HCC
    Z93.3 Colostomy status HCC
    Z93.4 Other artificial openings of gastrointestinal tract status HCC

    √5th Z93.5 Cystostomy status
        Z93.50 Unspecified cystostomy status HCC ▽
        Z93.51 Cutaneous-vesicostomy status HCC
        Z93.52 Appendico-vesicostomy status HCC
        Z93.59 Other cystostomy status HCC

EXCLUDES 1 Not coded here   *EXCLUDES 2* Not included here   N Newborn Age: 0   P Pediatric Age: 0-17   M Maternity Age: 12-55   A Adult Age: 15-124   PDx Primary Dx

1204   ICD-10-CM 2018

Z93.6 **Other artificial openings of urinary tract status**   `HCC`
Nephrostomy status
Ureterostomy status
Urethrostomy status

Z93.8 **Other artificial opening status**   `HCC`

Z93.9 **Artificial opening status, unspecified**   `HCC` ▽

✓4th **Z94** **Transplanted organ and tissue status**
     `INCLUDES`   organ or tissue replaced by heterogenous or homogenous transplant
     `EXCLUDES 1`   complications of transplanted organ or tissue—see Alphabetical Index
     `EXCLUDES 2`   presence of vascular grafts (Z95.-)

Z94.0 **Kidney transplant status**

Z94.1 **Heart transplant status**   `HCC`
     `EXCLUDES 1`   artificial heart status (Z95.812)
                heart-valve replacement status (Z95.2-Z95.4)

Z94.2 **Lung transplant status**   `HCC`

Z94.3 **Heart and lungs transplant status**   `HCC`

Z94.4 **Liver transplant status**   `HCC`

Z94.5 **Skin transplant status**
Autogenous skin transplant status

Z94.6 **Bone transplant status**

Z94.7 **Corneal transplant status**

✓5th **Z94.8** **Other transplanted organ and tissue status**

    Z94.81 **Bone marrow transplant status**   `HCC`

    Z94.82 **Intestine transplant status**   `HCC`

    Z94.83 **Pancreas transplant status**   `HCC`

    Z94.84 **Stem cells transplant status**   `HCC`

    Z94.89 **Other transplanted organ and tissue status**

Z94.9 **Transplanted organ and tissue status, unspecified** ▽

✓4th **Z95** **Presence of cardiac and vascular implants and grafts**
     `EXCLUDES 1`   ~~complications of cardiac and vascular devices, implants and grafts (T82.-)~~
     `EXCLUDES 2`   ►complications of cardiac and vascular devices, implants and grafts (T82.-)◄

Z95.0 **Presence of cardiac pacemaker**
Presence of cardiac resynchronization therapy (CRT-P) pacemaker
     `EXCLUDES 1`   adjustment or management of cardiac device (Z45.0-)
                adjustment or management of cardiac pacemaker (Z45.0)
                presence of automatic (implantable) cardiac defibrillator with synchronous cardiac pacemaker (Z95.810)

Z95.1 **Presence of aortocoronary bypass graft**
Presence of coronary artery bypass graft

Z95.2 **Presence of prosthetic heart valve**
Presence of heart valve NOS

Z95.3 **Presence of xenogenic heart valve**

Z95.4 **Presence of other heart-valve replacement**

Z95.5 **Presence of coronary angioplasty implant and graft**
     `EXCLUDES 1`   coronary angioplasty status without implant and graft (Z98.61)

✓5th **Z95.8** **Presence of other cardiac and vascular implants and grafts**

    ✓6th **Z95.81** **Presence of other cardiac implants and grafts**

        Z95.810 **Presence of automatic (implantable) cardiac defibrillator**
Presence of automatic (implantable) cardiac defibrillator with synchronous cardiac pacemaker
Presence of cardiac resynchronization therapy defibrillator (CRT-D)
Presence of cardioverter-defibrillator (ICD)

        Z95.811 **Presence of heart assist device**   `HCC`

        Z95.812 **Presence of fully implantable artificial heart**   `HCC`

        Z95.818 **Presence of other cardiac implants and grafts**

    ✓6th **Z95.82** **Presence of other vascular implants and grafts**

        Z95.820 **Peripheral vascular angioplasty status with implants and grafts**
         `EXCLUDES 1`   peripheral vascular angioplasty without implant and graft (Z98.62)

        Z95.828 **Presence of other vascular implants and grafts**
Presence of intravascular prosthesis NEC

Z95.9 **Presence of cardiac and vascular implant and graft, unspecified** ▽

✓4th **Z96** **Presence of other functional implants**
     `EXCLUDES 2`   complications of internal prosthetic devices, implants and grafts (T82-T85)
                fitting and adjustment of prosthetic and other devices (Z44-Z46)

Z96.0 **Presence of urogenital implants**

Z96.1 **Presence of intraocular lens**
Presence of pseudophakia

✓5th **Z96.2** **Presence of otological and audiological implants**

    Z96.20 **Presence of otological and audiological implant, unspecified** ▽

    Z96.21 **Cochlear implant status**

    Z96.22 **Myringotomy tube(s) status**

    Z96.29 **Presence of other otological and audiological implants**
Presence of bone-conduction hearing device
Presence of eustachian tube stent
Stapes replacement

Z96.3 **Presence of artificial larynx**

✓5th **Z96.4** **Presence of endocrine implants**

    Z96.41 **Presence of insulin pump (external) (internal)**

    Z96.49 **Presence of other endocrine implants**

Z96.5 **Presence of tooth-root and mandibular implants**

✓5th **Z96.6** **Presence of orthopedic joint implants**

    Z96.60 **Presence of unspecified orthopedic joint implant** ▽

    ✓6th **Z96.61** **Presence of artificial shoulder joint**

        Z96.611 **Presence of right artificial shoulder joint**

        Z96.612 **Presence of left artificial shoulder joint**

        Z96.619 **Presence of unspecified artificial shoulder joint** ▽

    ✓6th **Z96.62** **Presence of artificial elbow joint**

        Z96.621 **Presence of right artificial elbow joint**

        Z96.622 **Presence of left artificial elbow joint**

        Z96.629 **Presence of unspecified artificial elbow joint** ▽

    ✓6th **Z96.63** **Presence of artificial wrist joint**

        Z96.631 **Presence of right artificial wrist joint**

        Z96.632 **Presence of left artificial wrist joint**

        Z96.639 **Presence of unspecified artificial wrist joint** ▽

    ✓6th **Z96.64** **Presence of artificial hip joint**
Hip-joint replacement (partial) (total)

        Z96.641 **Presence of right artificial hip joint**

        Z96.642 **Presence of left artificial hip joint**

        Z96.643 **Presence of artificial hip joint, bilateral**

        Z96.649 **Presence of unspecified artificial hip joint** ▽

    ✓6th **Z96.65** **Presence of artificial knee joint**

        Z96.651 **Presence of right artificial knee joint**

        Z96.652 **Presence of left artificial knee joint**

        Z96.653 **Presence of artificial knee joint, bilateral**

        Z96.659 **Presence of unspecified artificial knee joint** ▽

    ✓6th **Z96.66** **Presence of artificial ankle joint**

        Z96.661 **Presence of right artificial ankle joint**

        Z96.662 **Presence of left artificial ankle joint**

        Z96.669 **Presence of unspecified artificial ankle joint** ▽

    ✓6th **Z96.69** **Presence of other orthopedic joint implants**

        Z96.691 **Finger-joint replacement of right hand**

        Z96.692 **Finger-joint replacement of left hand**

        Z96.693 **Finger-joint replacement, bilateral**

        Z96.698 **Presence of other orthopedic joint implants**

✓ Additional Character Req   ✓x7th Placeholder Alert   Manifestation   `HCC` CMS-HCC Condition   ▽ Unspecified Code   ►◄ Revised Text   ● New Code   ▲ Revised Code Title

ICD-10-CM 2018   **1205**

Z96.7   **Presence of other bone and tendon implants**
Presence of skull plate

☑5ᵗʰ **Z96.8**   **Presence of other specified functional implants**

    Z96.81   **Presence of artificial skin**

    Z96.89   **Presence of other specified functional implants**

Z96.9   **Presence of functional implant, unspecified** ▽

☑4ᵗʰ **Z97**   **Presence of other devices**
EXCLUDES 1   *complications of internal prosthetic devices, implants and grafts (T82-T85)*
fitting and adjustment of prosthetic and other devices (Z44-Z46)
EXCLUDES 2   *presence of cerebrospinal fluid drainage device (Z98.2)*

Z97.0   **Presence of artificial eye**

☑5ᵗʰ **Z97.1**   **Presence of artificial limb (complete) (partial)**

    Z97.10   **Presence of artificial limb (complete) (partial), unspecified** ▽

    Z97.11   **Presence of artificial right arm (complete) (partial)**

    Z97.12   **Presence of artificial left arm (complete) (partial)**

    Z97.13   **Presence of artificial right leg (complete) (partial)**

    Z97.14   **Presence of artificial left leg (complete) (partial)**

    Z97.15   **Presence of artificial arms, bilateral (complete) (partial)**

    Z97.16   **Presence of artificial legs, bilateral (complete) (partial)**

Z97.2   **Presence of dental prosthetic device (complete) (partial)**
Presence of dentures (complete) (partial)

Z97.3   **Presence of spectacles and contact lenses**

Z97.4   **Presence of external hearing-aid**

Z97.5   **Presence of (intrauterine) contraceptive device** ♀
EXCLUDES 1   *checking, reinsertion or removal of implantable subdermal contraceptive (Z30.46)*
checking, reinsertion or removal of intrauterine contraceptive device (Z30.43-)

Z97.8   **Presence of other specified devices**

☑4ᵗʰ **Z98**   **Other postprocedural states**
EXCLUDES 2   *aftercare (Z43-Z49, Z51)*
follow-up medical care (Z08- Z09)
postprocedural complication—see Alphabetical Index

Z98.0   **Intestinal bypass and anastomosis status**
EXCLUDES 2   *bariatric surgery status (Z98.84)*
gastric bypass status (Z98.84)
obesity surgery status (Z98.84)

Z98.1   **Arthrodesis status**

Z98.2   **Presence of cerebrospinal fluid drainage device**
Presence of CSF shunt

Z98.3   **Post therapeutic collapse of lung status**
Code first underlying disease

☑5ᵗʰ **Z98.4**   **Cataract extraction status**
Use additional code to identify intraocular lens implant status (Z96.1)
EXCLUDES 1   *aphakia (H27.0)*

    Z98.41   **Cataract extraction status, right eye**

    Z98.42   **Cataract extraction status, left eye**

    Z98.49   **Cataract extraction status, unspecified eye** ▽

☑5ᵗʰ **Z98.5**   **Sterilization status**
EXCLUDES 1   *female infertility (N97.-)*
male infertility (N46.-)

    Z98.51   **Tubal ligation status** ♀

    Z98.52   **Vasectomy status** A♂

☑5ᵗʰ **Z98.6**   **Angioplasty status**

    Z98.61   **Coronary angioplasty status**
EXCLUDES 1   *coronary angioplasty status with implant and graft (Z95.5)*

    Z98.62   **Peripheral vascular angioplasty status**
EXCLUDES 1   *peripheral vascular angioplasty status with implant and graft (Z95.820)*

☑5ᵗʰ **Z98.8**   **Other specified postprocedural states**

☑6ᵗʰ **Z98.81**   **Dental procedure status**

    Z98.810   **Dental sealant status**

    Z98.811   **Dental restoration status**
Dental crown status
Dental fillings status

    Z98.818   **Other dental procedure status**

Z98.82   **Breast implant status**
EXCLUDES 1   *breast implant removal status (Z98.86)*

Z98.83   **Filtering (vitreous) bleb after glaucoma surgery status**
EXCLUDES 1   *inflammation (infection) of postprocedural bleb (H59.4-)*

Z98.84   **Bariatric surgery status**
Gastric banding status
Gastric bypass status for obesity
Obesity surgery status
EXCLUDES 1   *bariatric surgery status complicating pregnancy, childbirth, or the puerperium (O99.84)*
EXCLUDES 2   *intestinal bypass and anastomosis status (Z98.0)*

Z98.85   **Transplanted organ removal status**
Transplanted organ previously removed due to complication, failure, rejection or infection
EXCLUDES 1   *encounter for removal of transplanted organ—code to complication of transplanted organ (T86.-)*

Z98.86   **Personal history of breast implant removal**

☑6ᵗʰ **Z98.87**   **Personal history of in utero procedure**

    Z98.870   **Personal history of in utero procedure during pregnancy** ♀
EXCLUDES 2   *complications from in utero procedure for current pregnancy (O35.7)*
supervision of current pregnancy with history of in utero procedure during previous pregnancy (O09.82-)

    Z98.871   **Personal history of in utero procedure while a fetus**

☑6ᵗʰ **Z98.89**   **Other specified postprocedural states**

    Z98.890   **Other specified postprocedural states**
Personal history of surgery, not elsewhere classified

    Z98.891   **History of uterine scar from previous surgery**
EXCLUDES 1   *maternal care due to uterine scar from previous surgery (O34.2-)*

☑4ᵗʰ **Z99**   **Dependence on enabling machines and devices, not elsewhere classified**
EXCLUDES 1   *cardiac pacemaker status (Z95.0)*

Z99.0   **Dependence on aspirator**

☑5ᵗʰ **Z99.1**   **Dependence on respirator**
Dependence on ventilator

    Z99.11   **Dependence on respirator [ventilator] status** HCC
AHA: 2015, 1Q, 21

    Z99.12   **Encounter for respirator [ventilator] dependence during power failure** HCC PDx
EXCLUDES 1   *mechanical complication of respirator [ventilator] (J95.850)*

Z99.2   **Dependence on renal dialysis** HCC
Hemodialysis status
Peritoneal dialysis status
Presence of arteriovenous shunt for dialysis
Renal dialysis status NOS
EXCLUDES 1   *encounter for fitting and adjustment of dialysis catheter (Z49.0-)*
EXCLUDES 2   *noncompliance with renal dialysis (Z91.15)*
AHA: 2016, 1Q, 12; 2013, 4Q, 125

Z99.3   **Dependence on wheelchair**
Wheelchair confinement status
Code first cause of dependence, such as:
muscular dystrophy (G71.0)
obesity (E66.-)

EXCLUDES 1 Not coded here   EXCLUDES 2 Not included here   N Newborn Age: 0   P Pediatric Age: 0-17   M Maternity Age: 12-55   A Adult Age: 15-124   PDx Primary Dx

1206   ICD-10-CM 2018

☑5ᵗʰ **Z99.8** **Dependence on other enabling machines and devices**

    Z99.81 **Dependence on supplemental oxygen**
        Dependence on long-term oxygen
        AHA: 2013, 4Q, 129

    Z99.89 **Dependence on other enabling machines and devices**
        Dependence on machine or device NOS

☑ Additional Character Req   ✓ˣ⁷ᵗʰ Placeholder Alert   Manifestation   ᴴᶜᶜ CMS-HCC Condition   ▽ Unspecified Code   ▶◀ Revised Text   ● New Code   ▲ Revised Code Title

ICD-10-CM 2018   **1207**

Illustrations

Chapter 3. Diseases of the Blood and Blood-forming Organs and Certain Disorders Involving the Immune Mechanism (D50–D89)

Red Blood Cells

White Blood Cell

Platelet

Coagulation

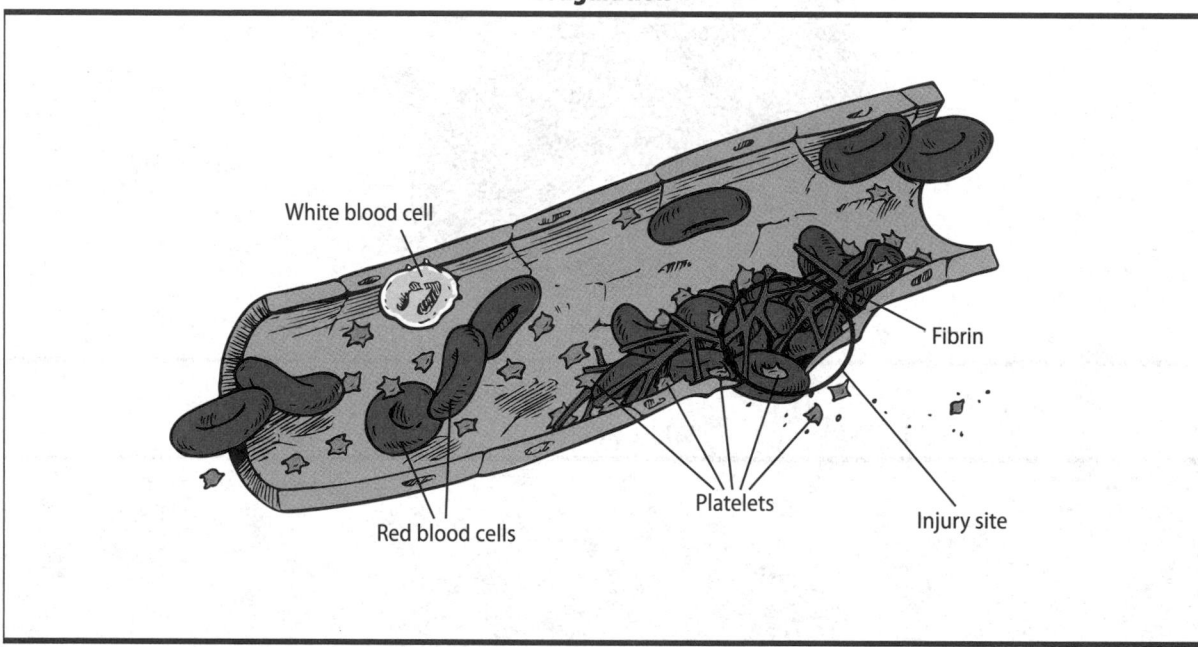

White blood cell

Fibrin

Platelets

Injury site

Red blood cells

Spleen Anatomical Location and External Structures

Spleen Interior Structures

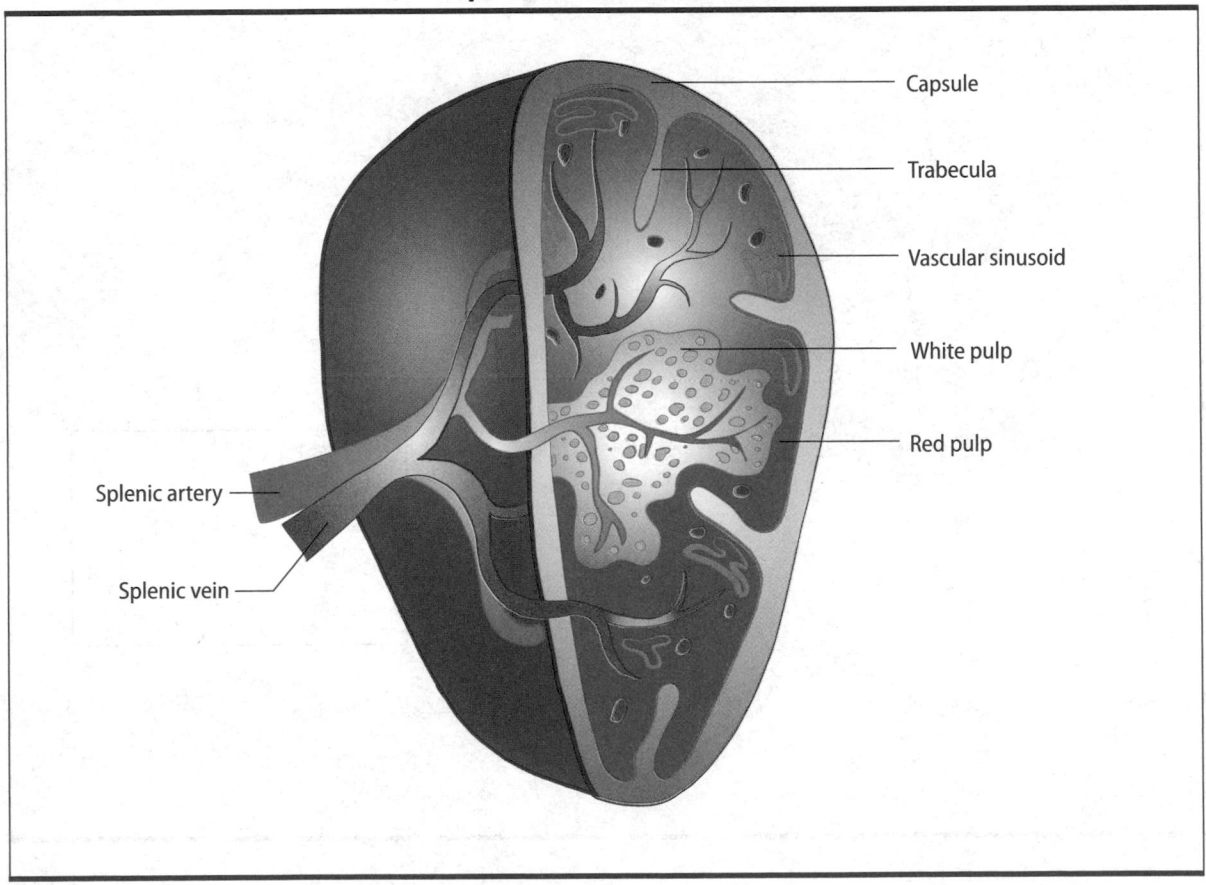

Chapter 4. Endocrine, Nutritional and Metabolic Diseases (EØØ–E89)

Endocrine System

Thyroid

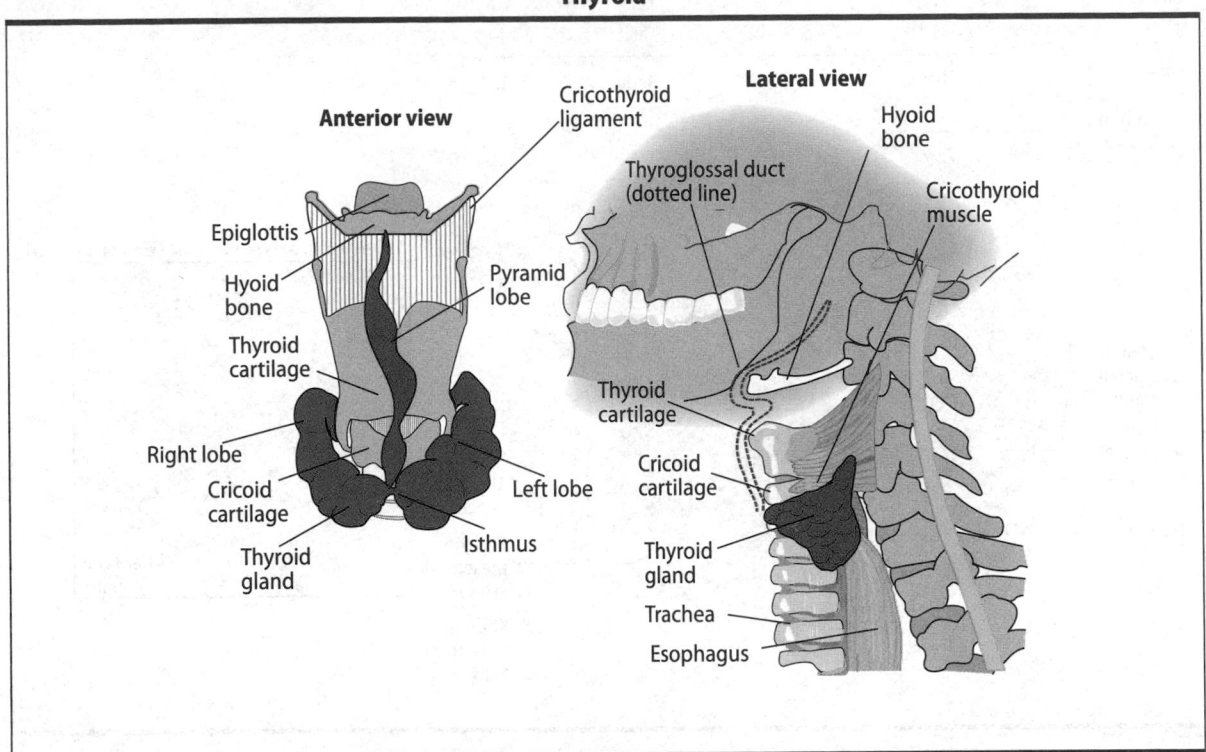

Thyroid and Parathyroid Glands

Pancreas

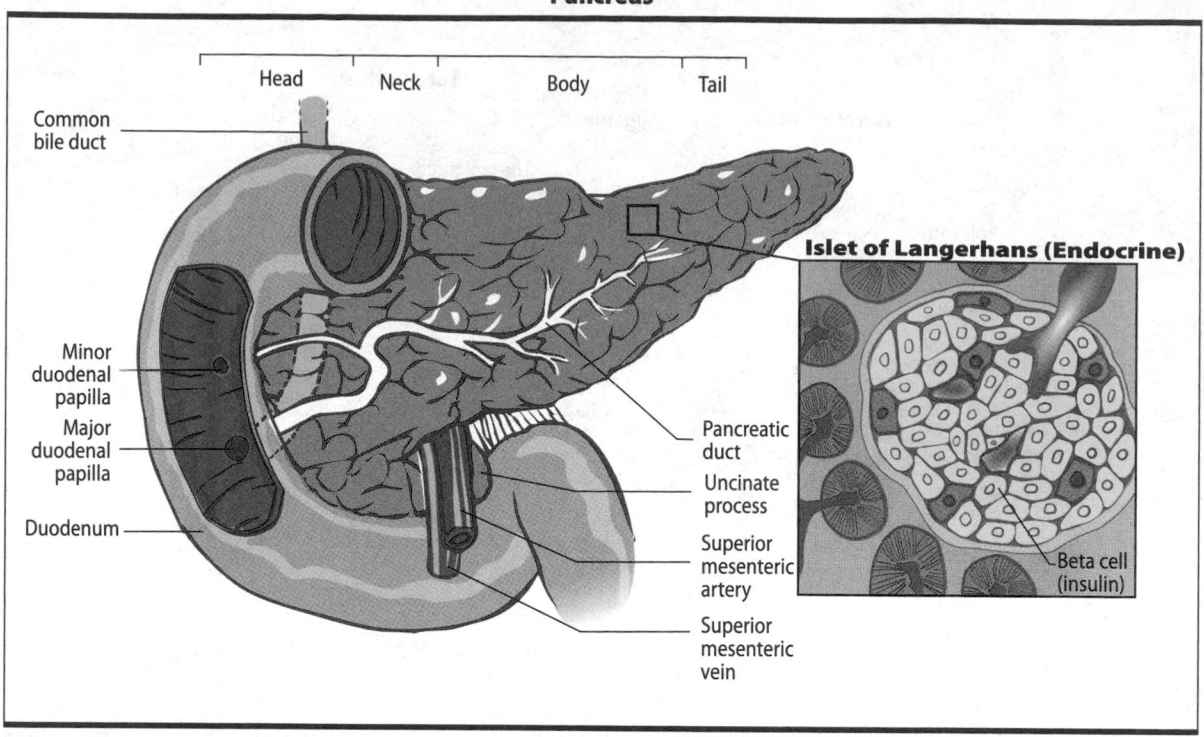

Islet of Langerhans (Endocrine)

Head | Neck | Body | Tail

Common bile duct

Minor duodenal papilla

Major duodenal papilla

Duodenum

Pancreatic duct

Uncinate process

Superior mesenteric artery

Superior mesenteric vein

Beta cell (insulin)

Anatomy of the Adrenal Gland

Adrenal glands

Kidney

Capsule

Cortex

Medulla

Structure of an Ovary

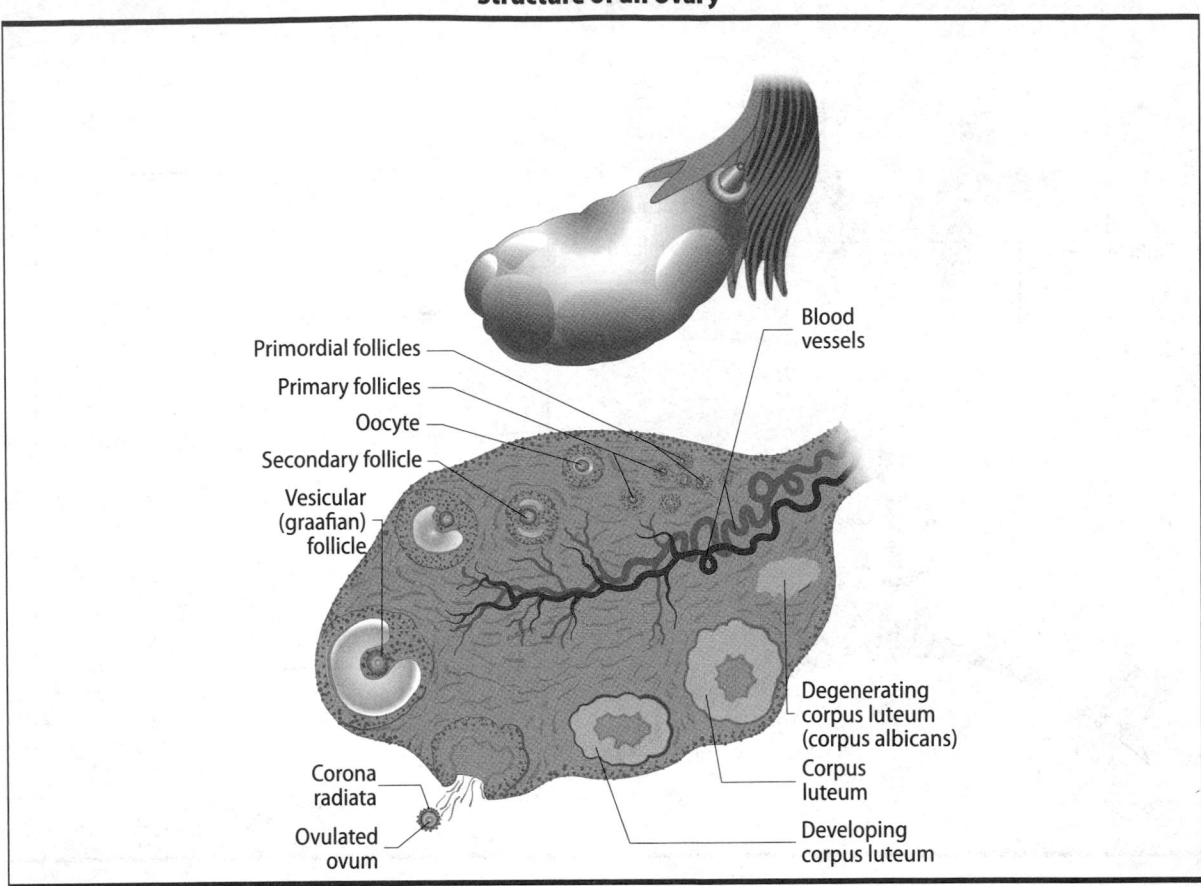

Testis and Associated Structures

Thymus

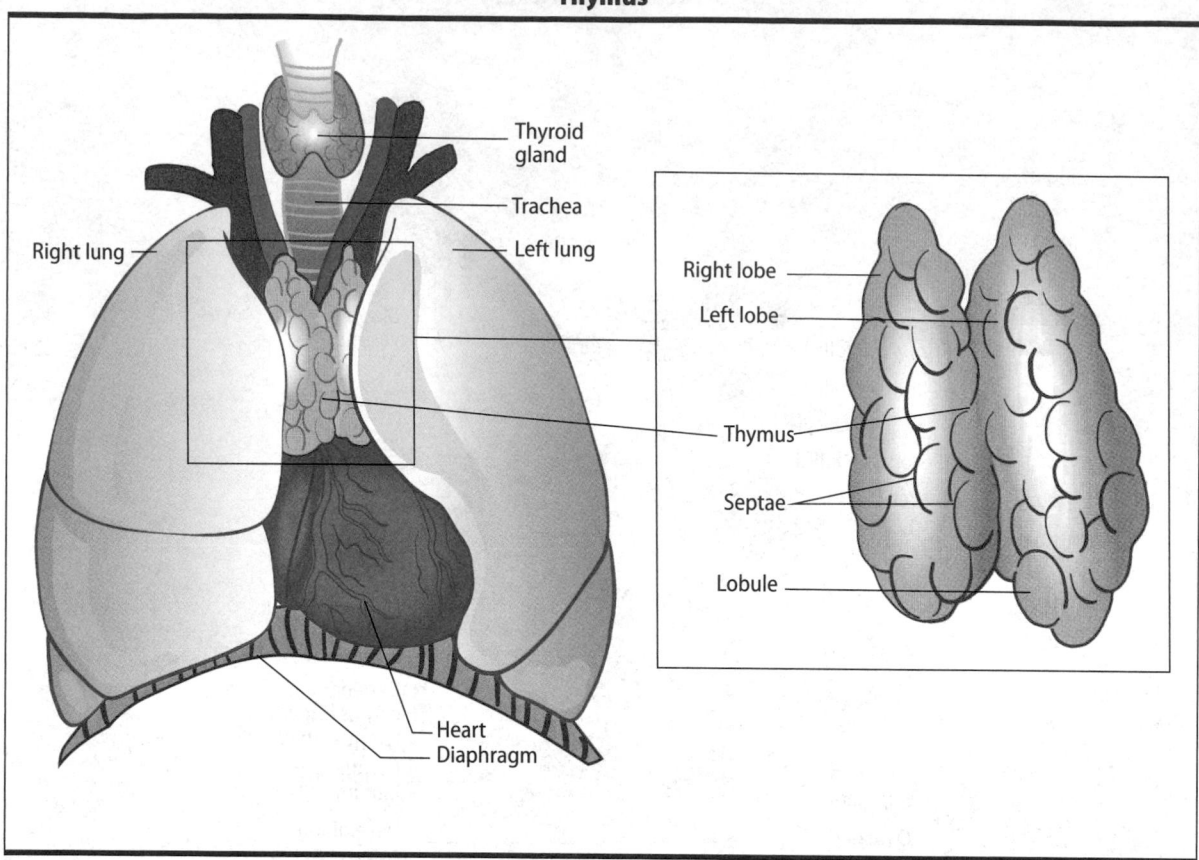

Chapter 6. Diseases of the Nervous System (G00–G99)

Brain

Cranial Nerves

Peripheral Nervous System

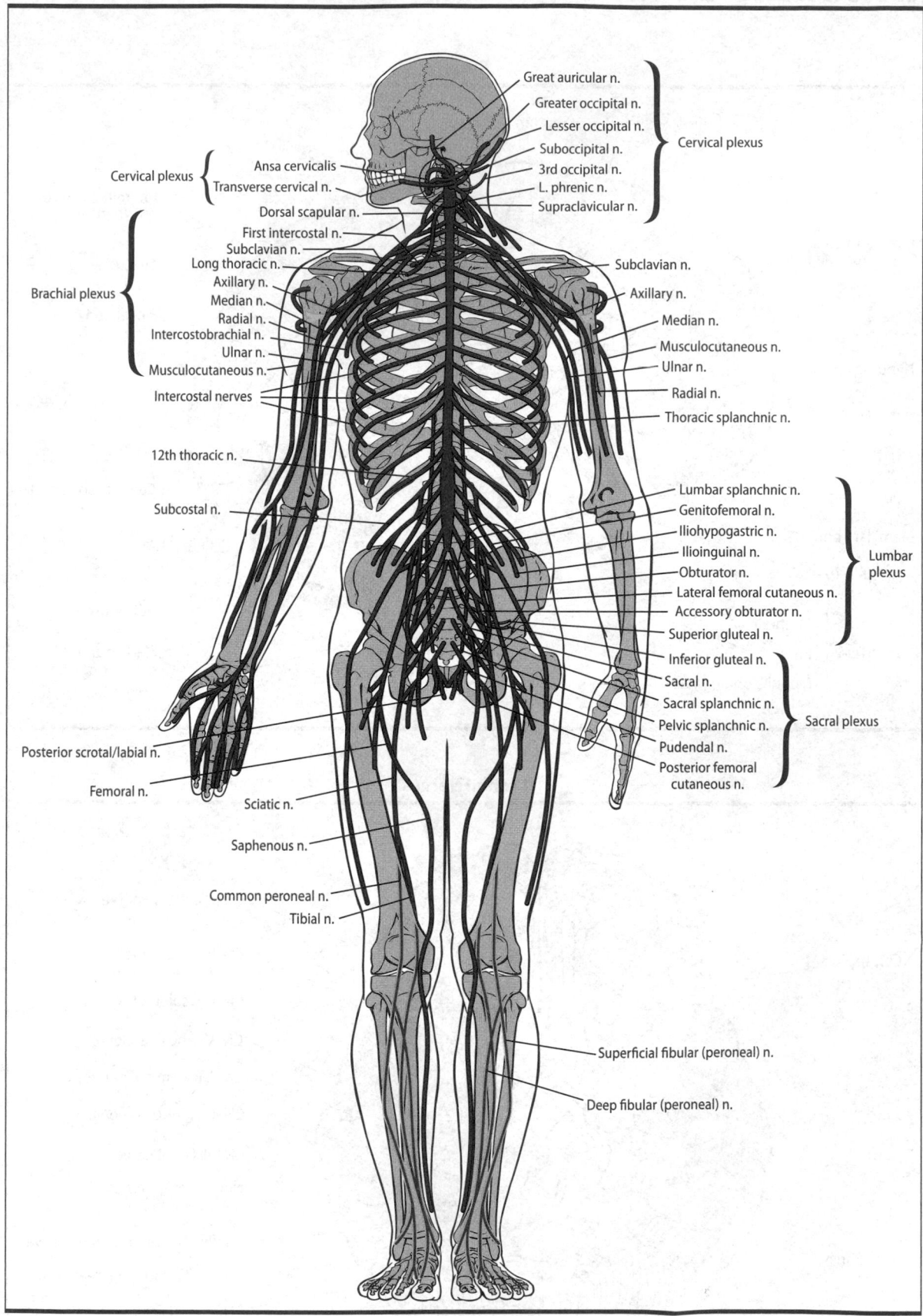

Spinal Cord and Spinal Nerves

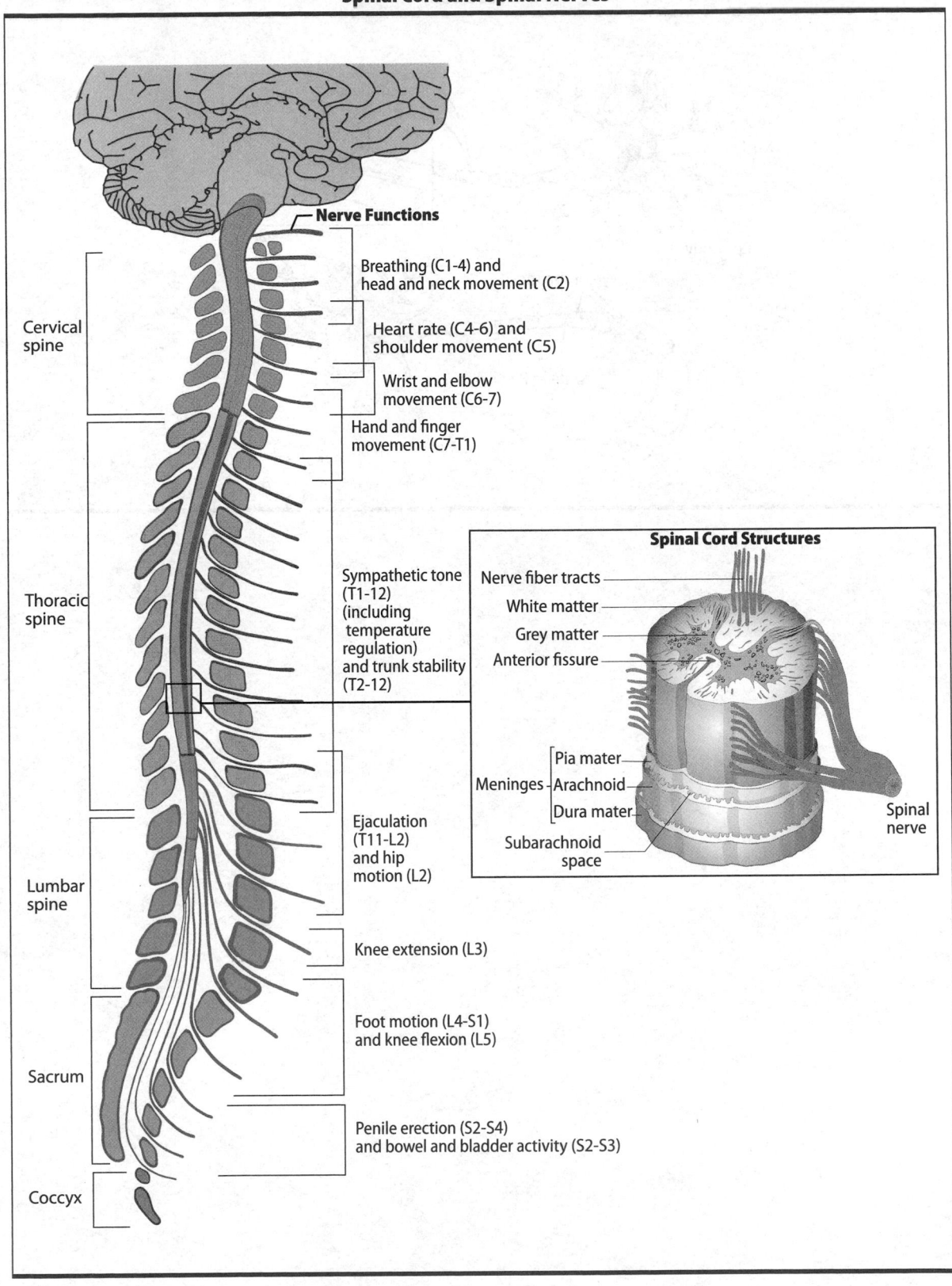

Nerve Functions

Breathing (C1-4) and
head and neck movement (C2)

Heart rate (C4-6) and
shoulder movement (C5)

Wrist and elbow
movement (C6-7)

Hand and finger
movement (C7-T1)

Sympathetic tone
(T1-12)
(including
temperature
regulation)
and trunk stability
(T2-12)

Ejaculation
(T11-L2)
and hip
motion (L2)

Knee extension (L3)

Foot motion (L4-S1)
and knee flexion (L5)

Penile erection (S2-S4)
and bowel and bladder activity (S2-S3)

Cervical
spine

Thoracic
spine

Lumbar
spine

Sacrum

Coccyx

Spinal Cord Structures

Nerve fiber tracts

White matter

Grey matter

Anterior fissure

Pia mater

Meninges — Arachnoid

Dura mater

Subarachnoid
space

Spinal
nerve

Nerve Cell

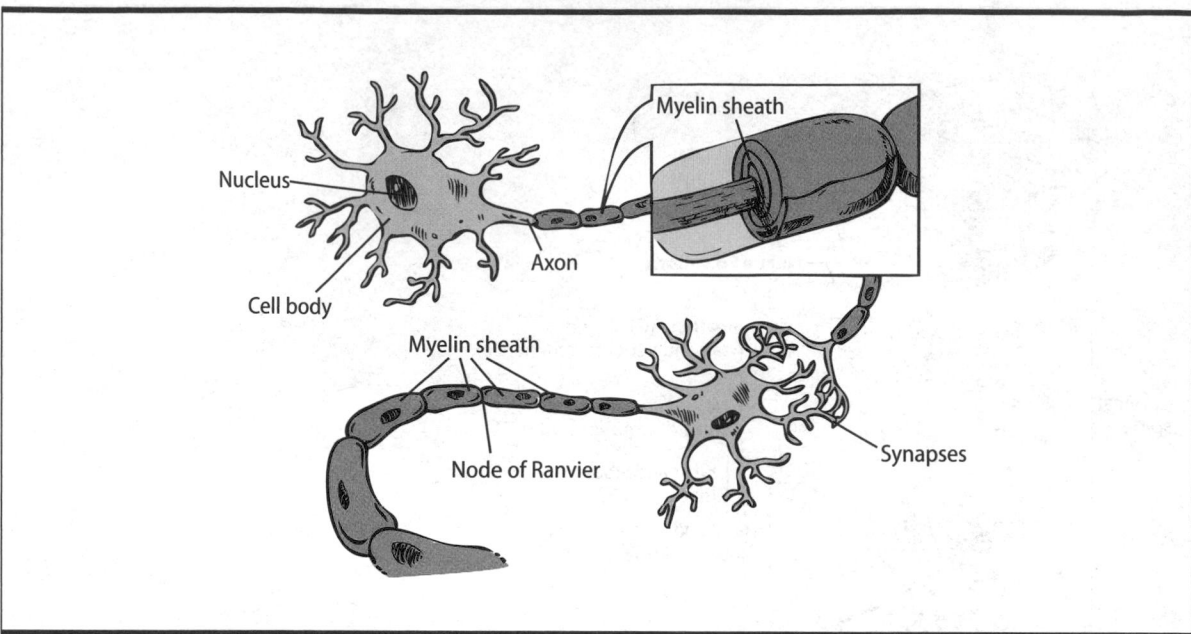

Chapter 7. Diseases of the Eye and Adnexa (H00–H59)

Eye

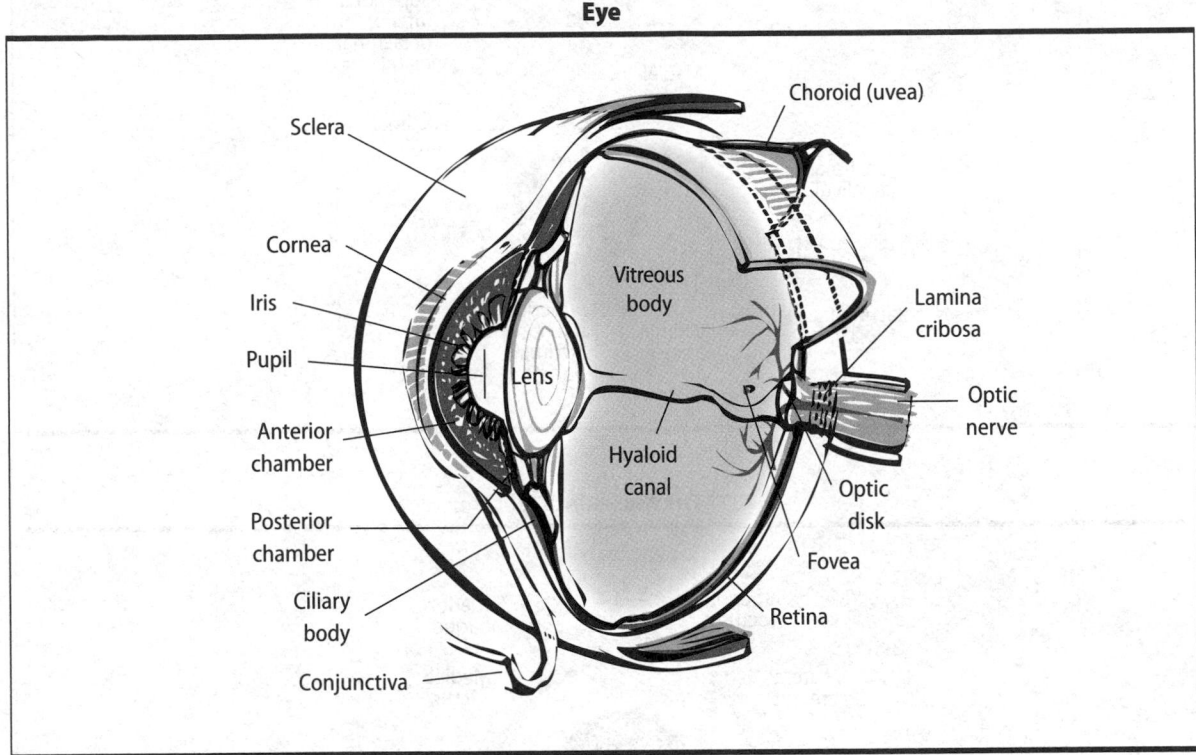

Posterior Pole of Globe/Flow of Aqueous Humor

Lacrimal System

Eye Musculature

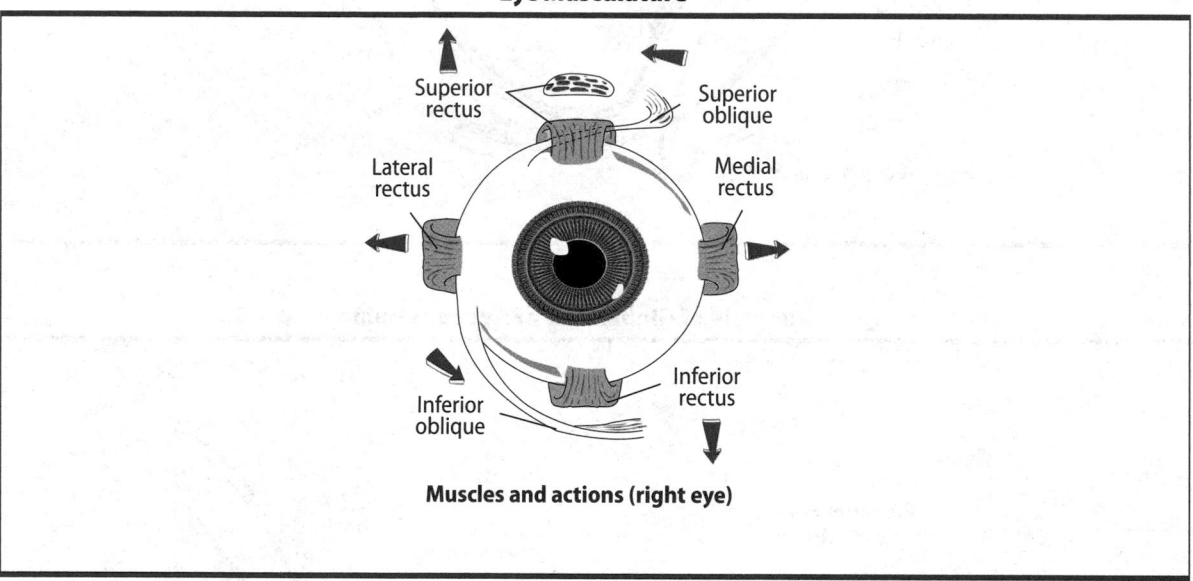

Muscles and actions (right eye)

Eyelid Structures

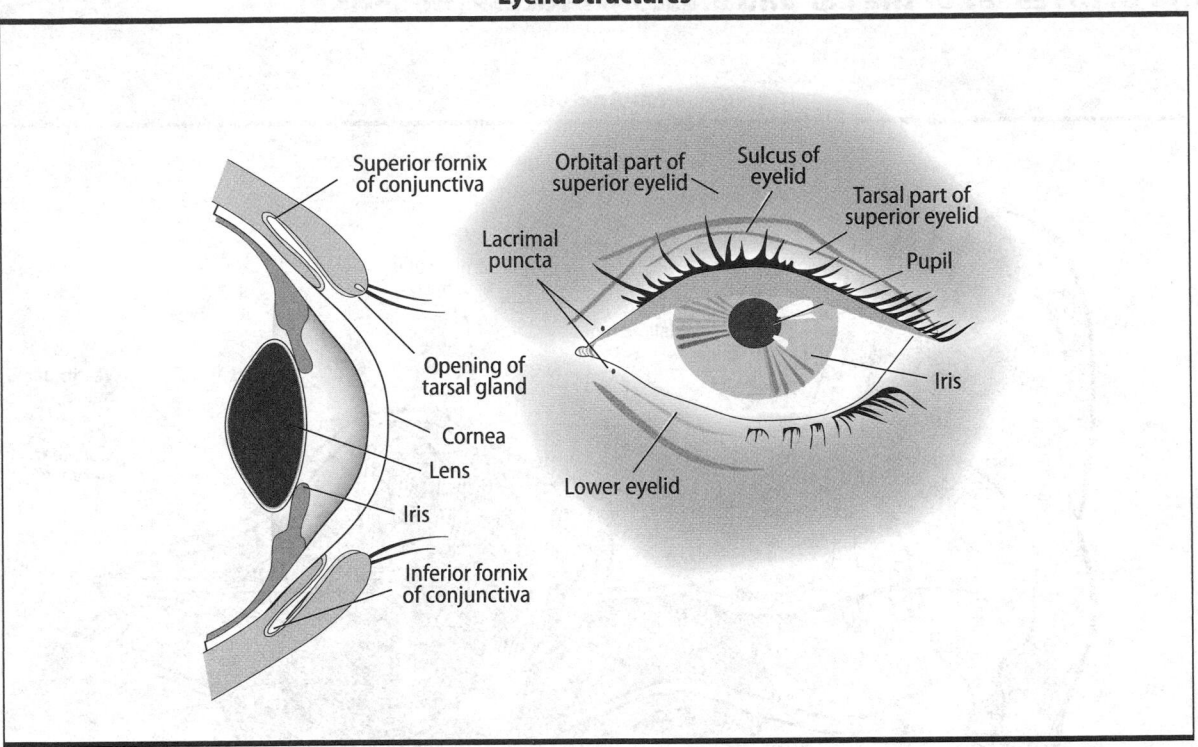

Chapter 8. Diseases of the Ear and Mastoid Process (H60–H95)

Ear Anatomy

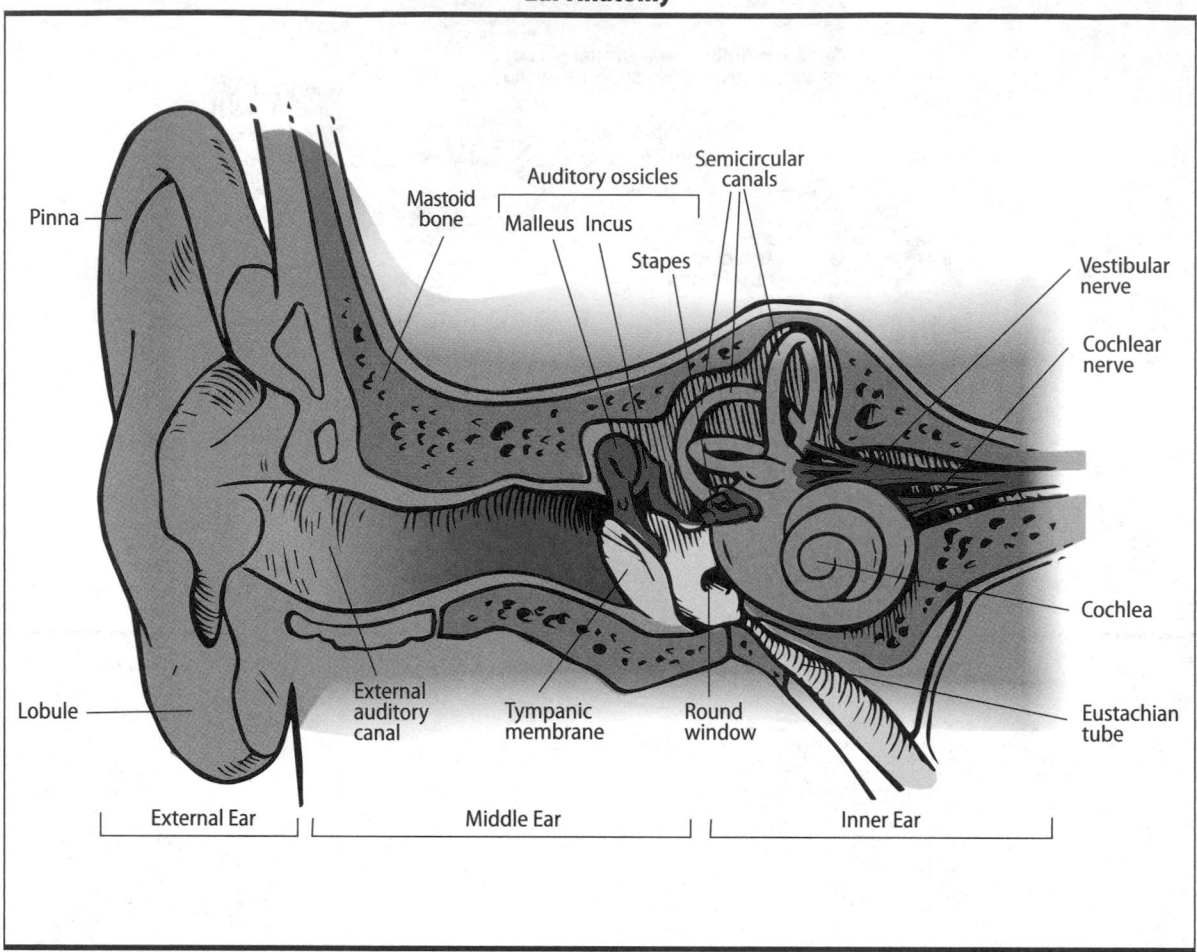

Chapter 9. Diseases of the Circulatory System (I00–I99)

Anatomy of the Heart

Heart Cross Section

Heart Valves

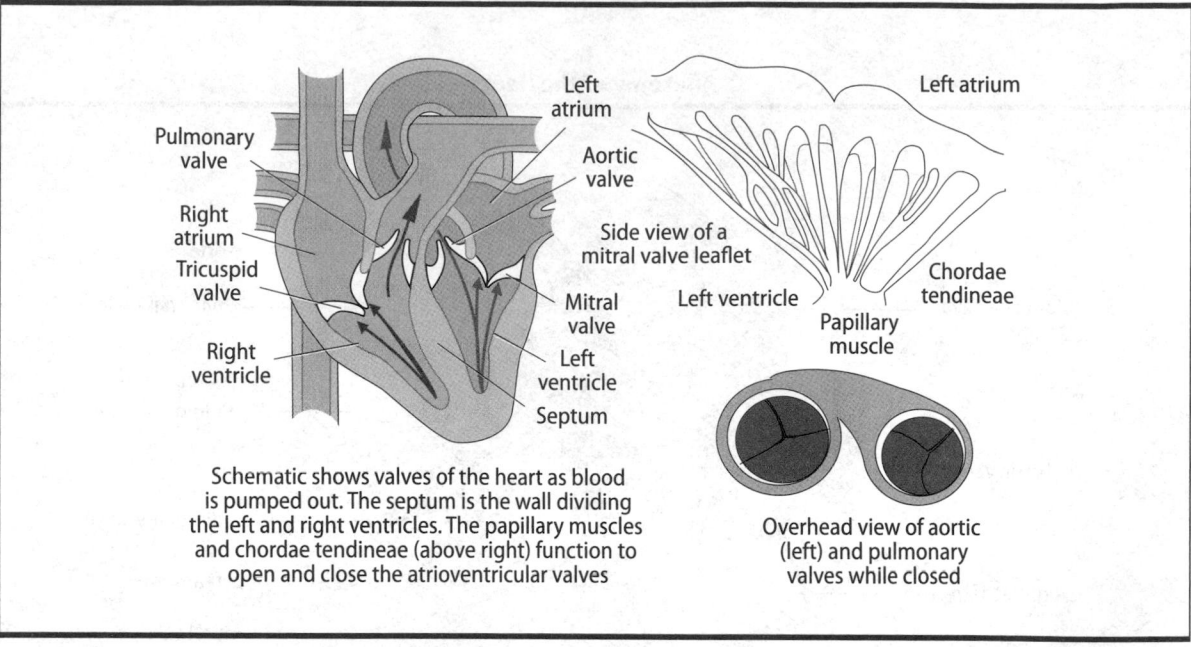

Schematic shows valves of the heart as blood
is pumped out. The septum is the wall dividing
the left and right ventricles. The papillary muscles
and chordae tendineae (above right) function to
open and close the atrioventricular valves

Overhead view of aortic
(left) and pulmonary
valves while closed

Heart Conduction System

Coronary Arteries

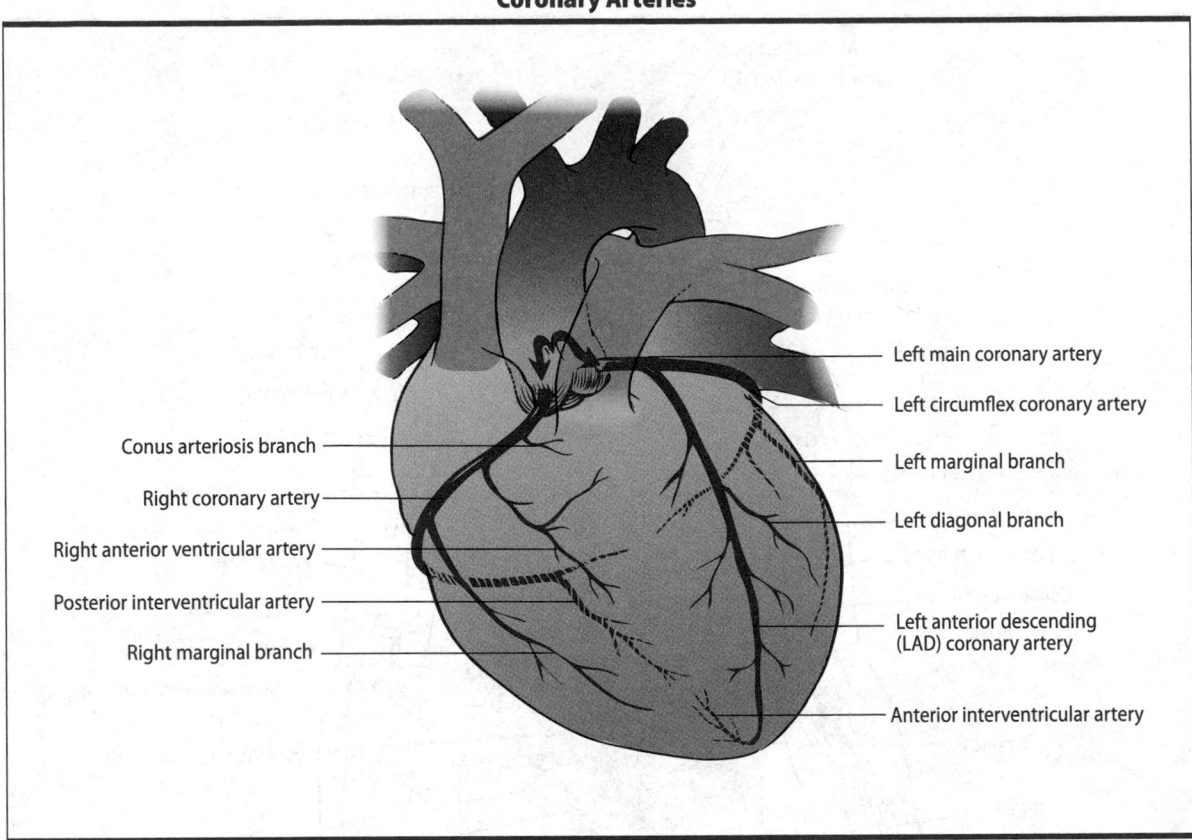

Left main coronary artery

Left circumflex coronary artery

Conus arteriosis branch

Left marginal branch

Right coronary artery

Left diagonal branch

Right anterior ventricular artery

Posterior interventricular artery

Left anterior descending (LAD) coronary artery

Right marginal branch

Anterior interventricular artery

Arteries

Veins

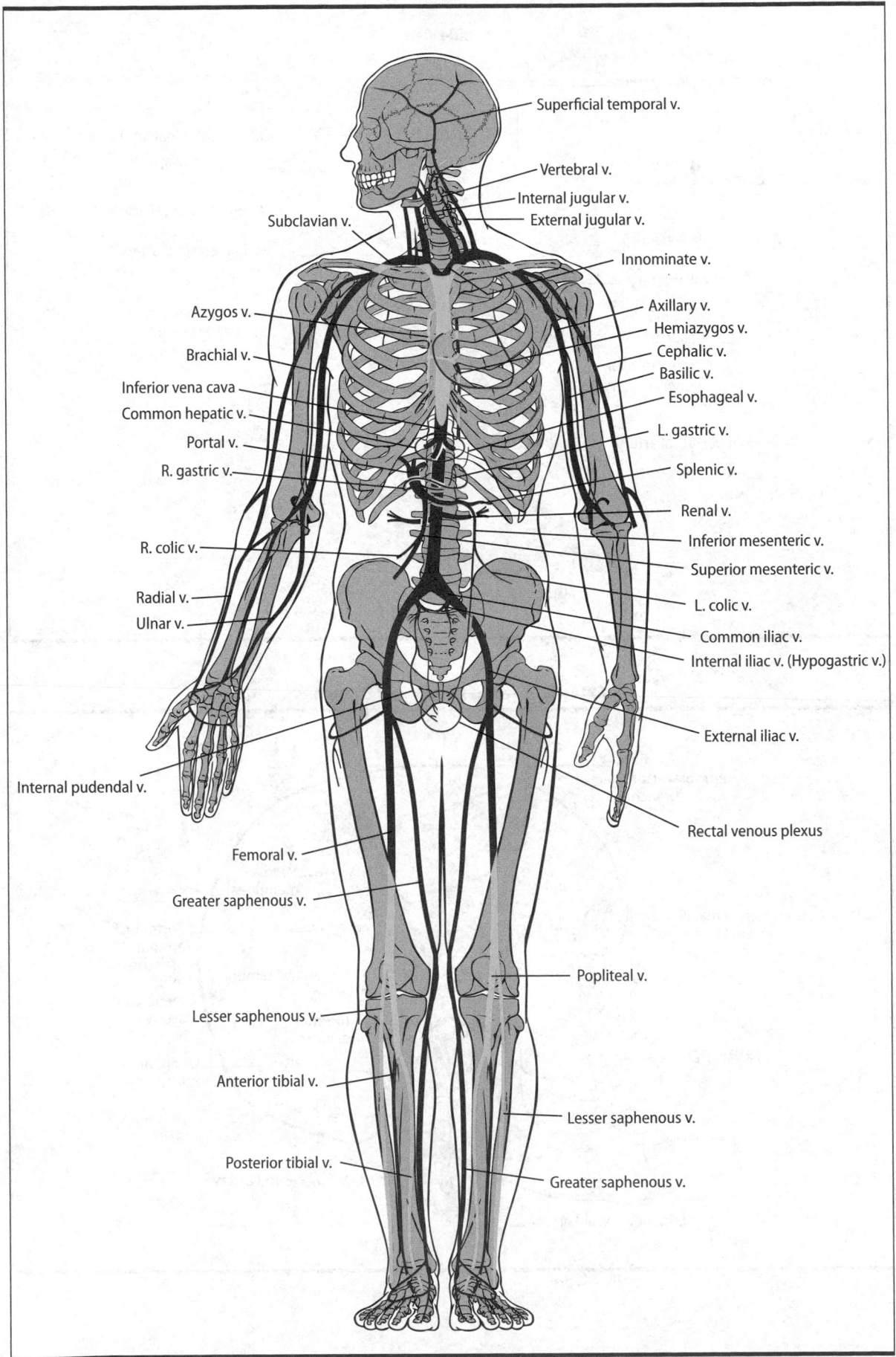

Internal Carotid and Vertebral Arteries and Branches

Side View

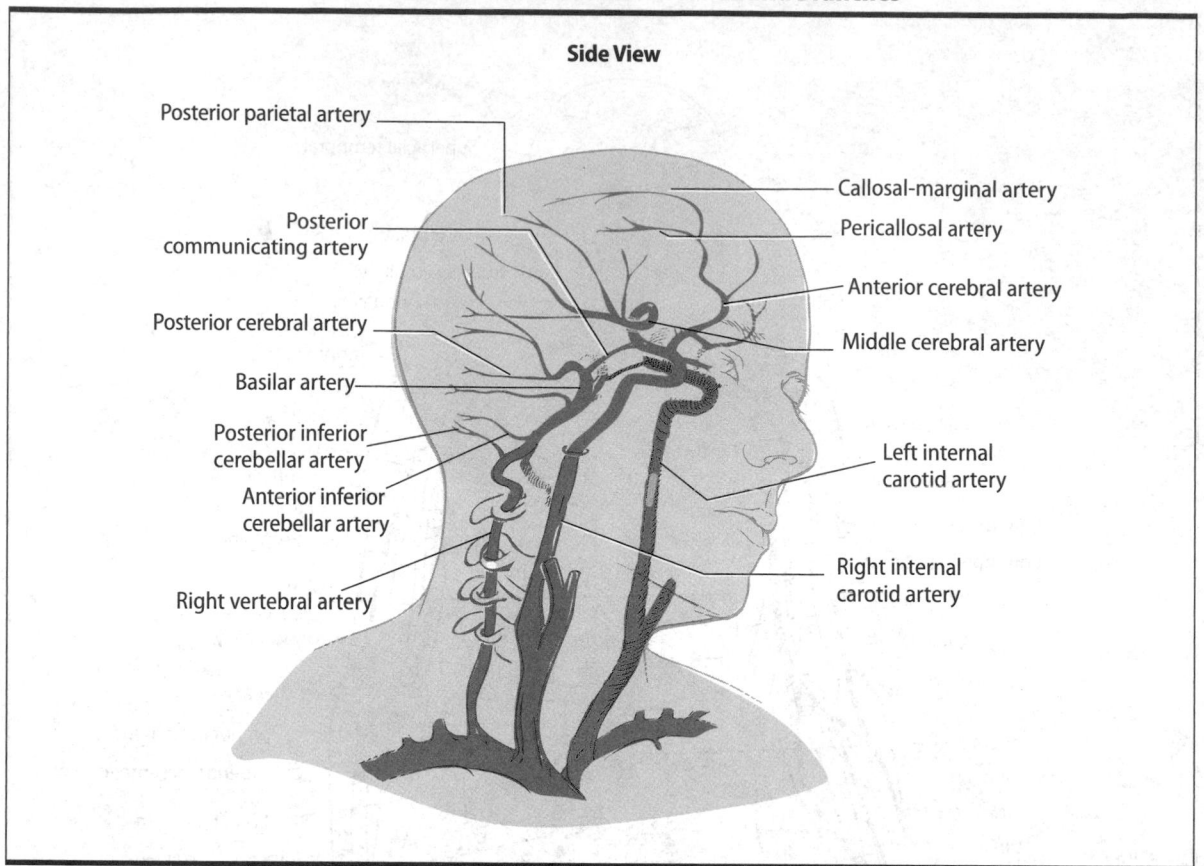

External Carotid Artery and Branches

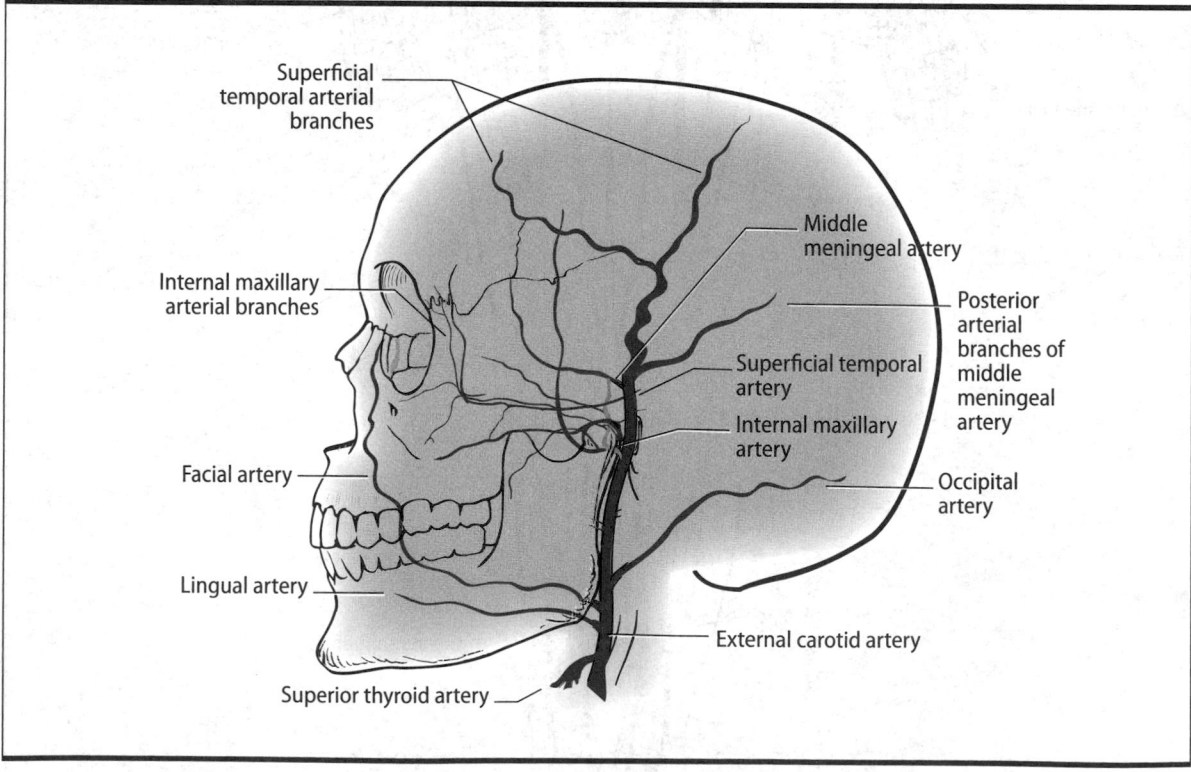

Branches of Abdominal Aorta

Portal Venous Circulation

Lymphatic System

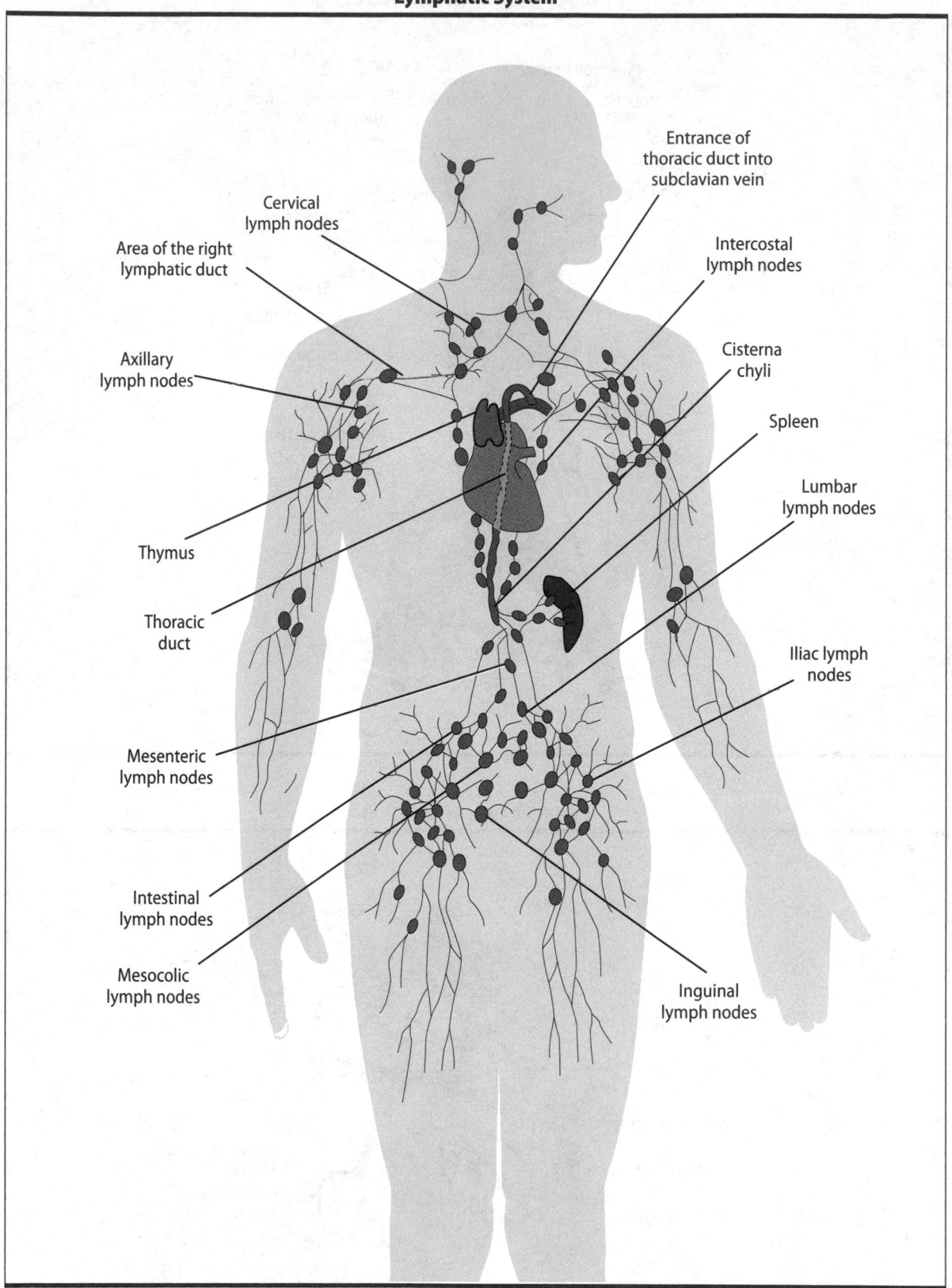

Axillary Lymph Nodes

Sternum

Parasternal nodes

Clavicle

Deltoid muscle

Brachialis muscle

Lateral nodes

Subscapular nodes

Pectoral nodes

Axillary lymph nodes

Central nodes

Latissimus dorsi muscle

Rectus abdominis muscle

Lymphatic System of Head and Neck

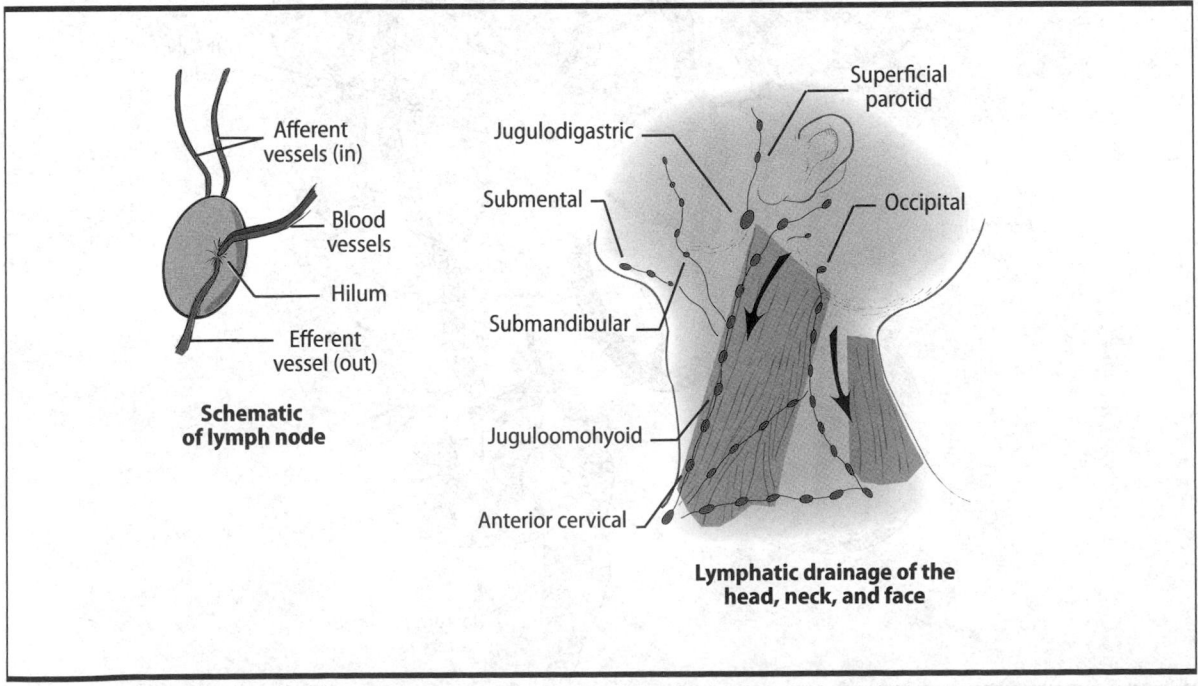

Afferent vessels (in)

Blood vessels

Hilum

Efferent vessel (out)

Schematic of lymph node

Superficial parotid

Jugulodigastric

Submental

Occipital

Submandibular

Juguloomohyoid

Anterior cervical

Lymphatic drainage of the head, neck, and face

Lymphatic Capillaries

Schematic of lymphatic capillaries

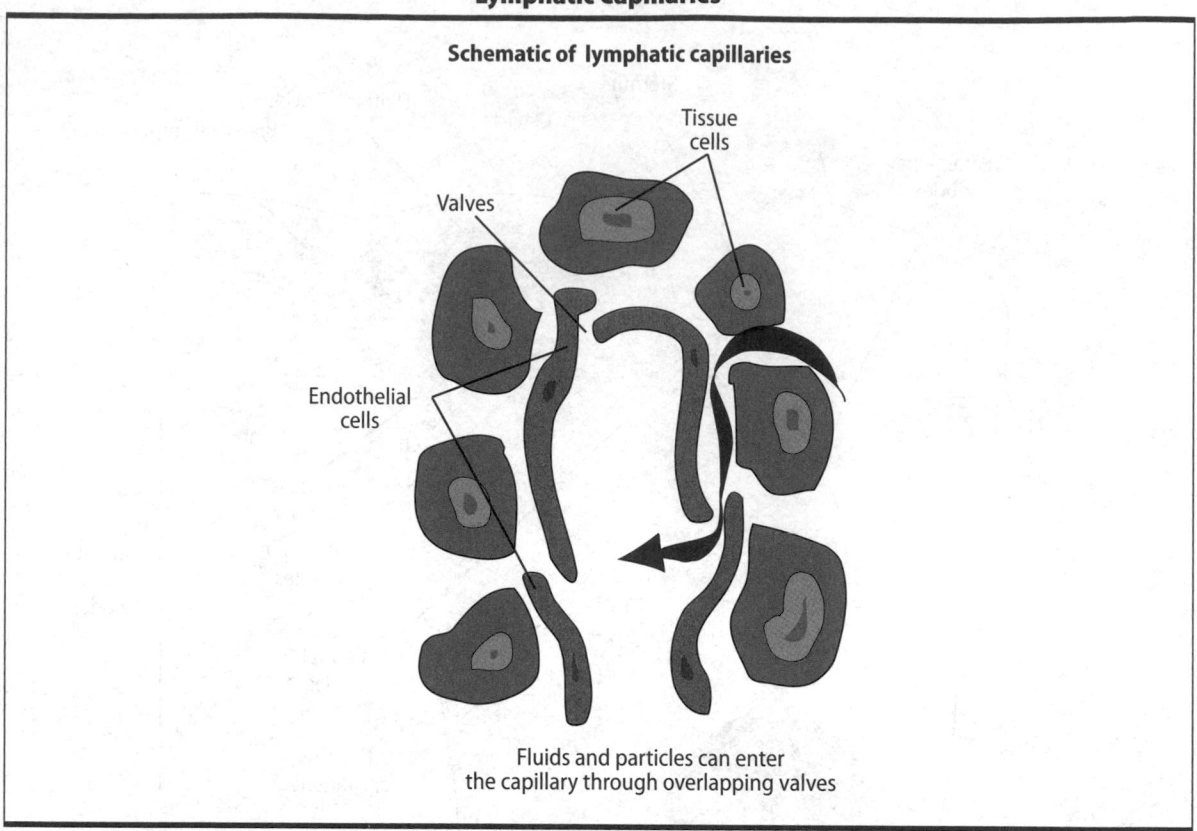

Tissue
cells

Valves

Endothelial
cells

Fluids and particles can enter
the capillary through overlapping valves

Lymphatic Drainage

Lymphatic drainage of the colon follows blood supply

Middle colic
nodes

Paracolic
nodes

Left colic
nodes

Ascending
colon

Cecum

Rectum

Chapter 10. Diseases of the Respiratory System (J00–J99)

Respiratory System

Nasal cavity and paranasal sinuses

Nostril

Oral cavity

Pharynx

Larynx

Trachea

Pleura

Right lung

Left lung

Carina of trachea

Right main / primary bronchus

Left main/ primary bronchus

Secondary (lobar) bronchi

Tertiary (segmental) bronchi

Bronchioles

Alveoli

Diaphragm

Upper Respiratory System

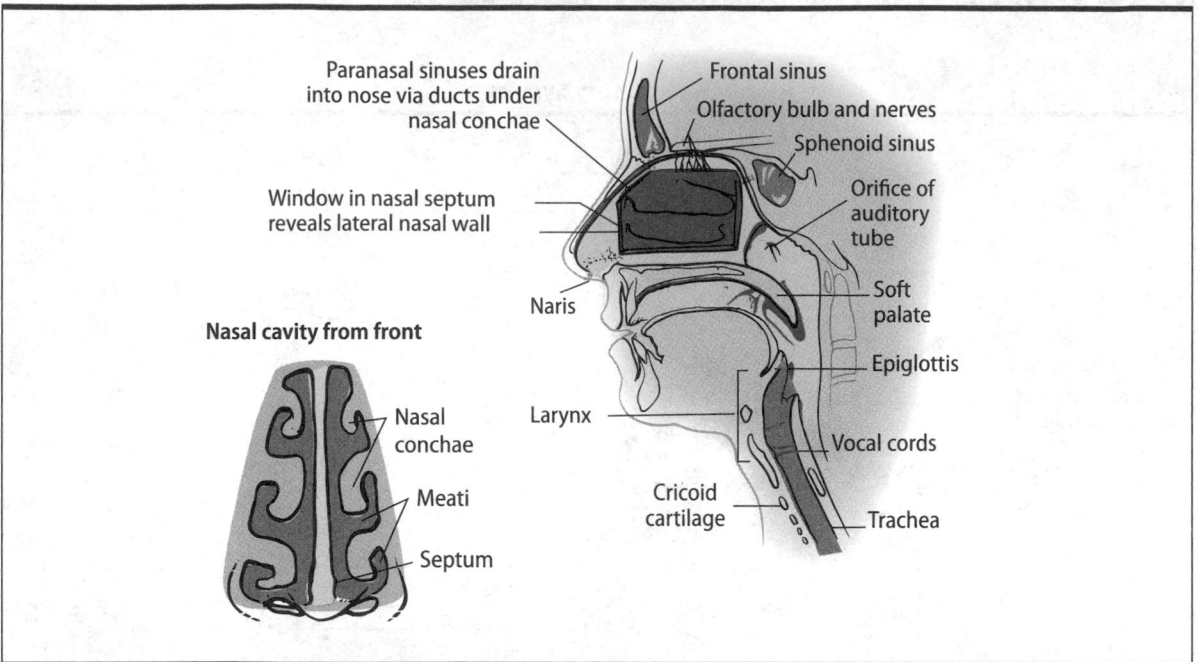

Paranasal sinuses drain into nose via ducts under nasal conchae

Window in nasal septum reveals lateral nasal wall

Nasal cavity from front

Naris

Nasal conchae

Meati

Septum

Frontal sinus

Olfactory bulb and nerves

Sphenoid sinus

Orifice of auditory tube

Soft palate

Epiglottis

Larynx

Vocal cords

Cricoid cartilage

Trachea

Lower Respiratory System

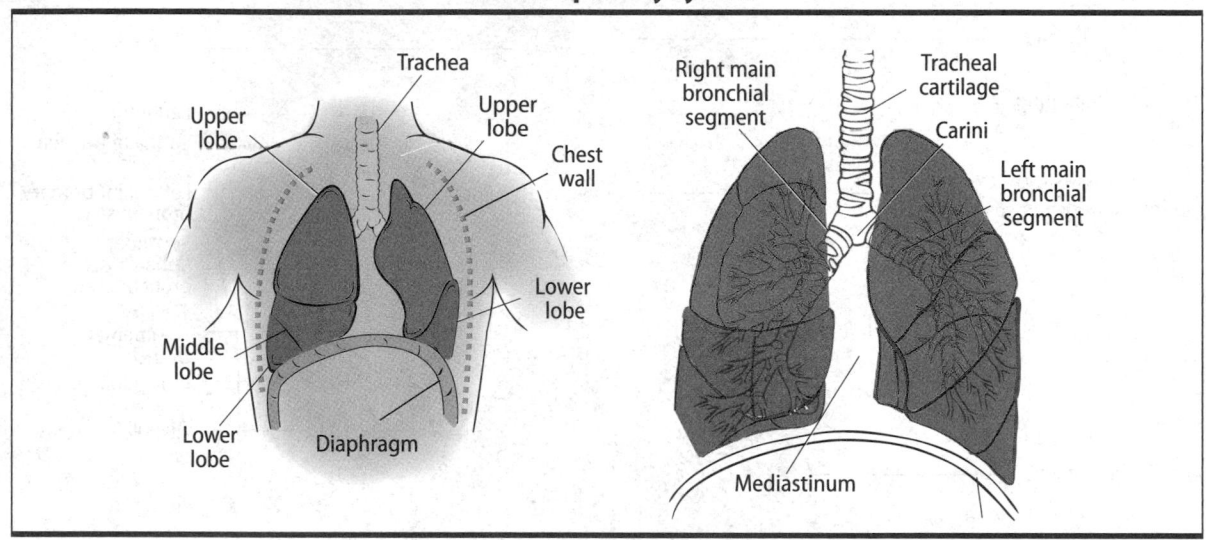

Trachea

Upper lobe

Upper lobe

Chest wall

Lower lobe

Middle lobe

Lower lobe

Diaphragm

Right main bronchial segment

Tracheal cartilage

Carini

Left main bronchial segment

Mediastinum

Paranasal Sinuses

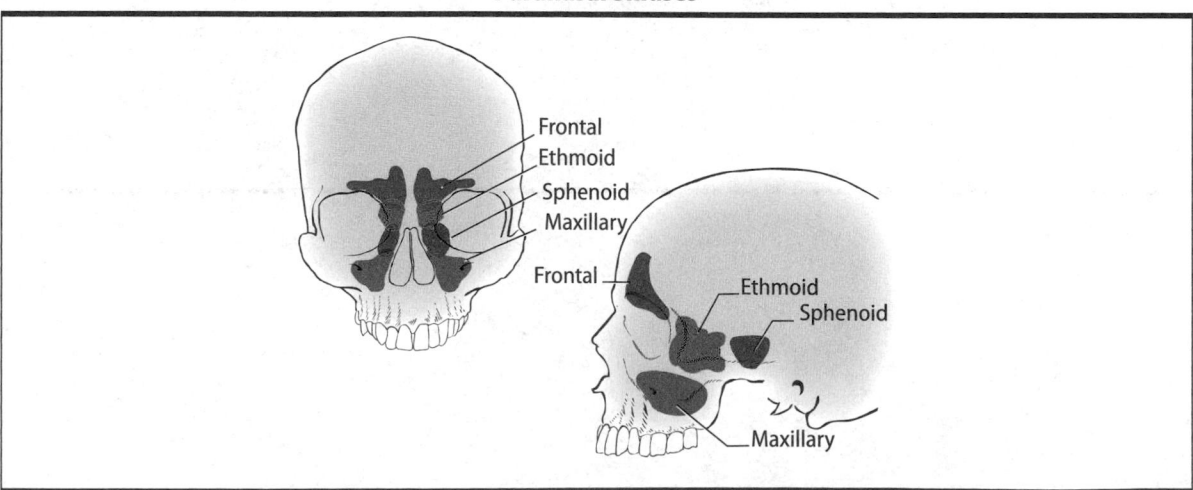

Frontal

Ethmoid

Sphenoid

Maxillary

Frontal

Ethmoid

Sphenoid

Maxillary

Lung Segments

Alveoli

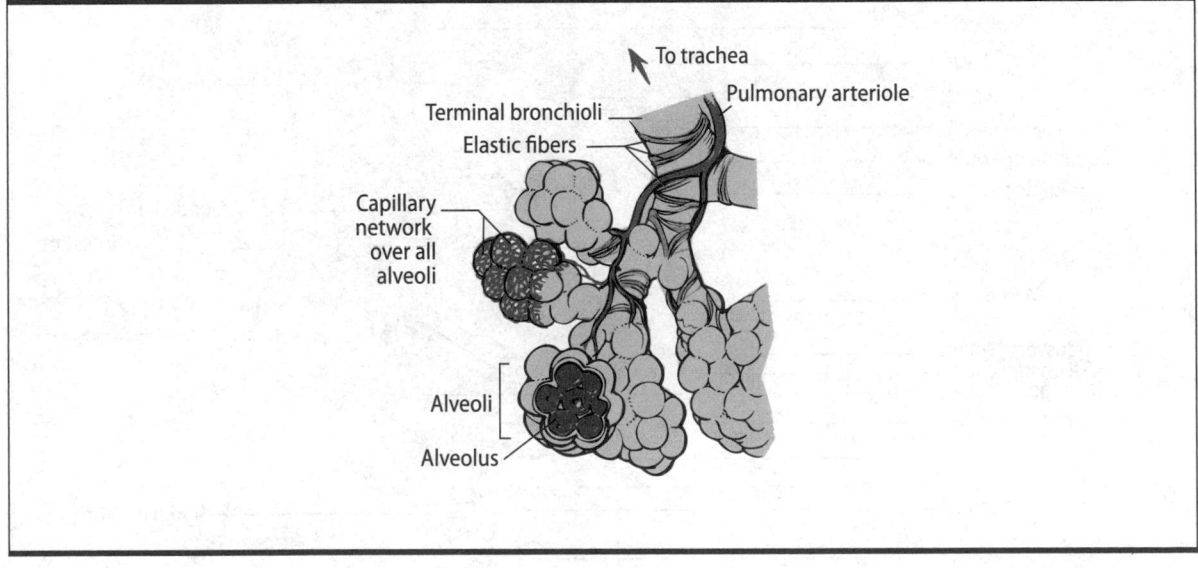

Chapter 11. Diseases of the Digestive System (KØØ–K95)

Digestive System

Omentum and Mesentery

Peritoneum and Retroperitoneum

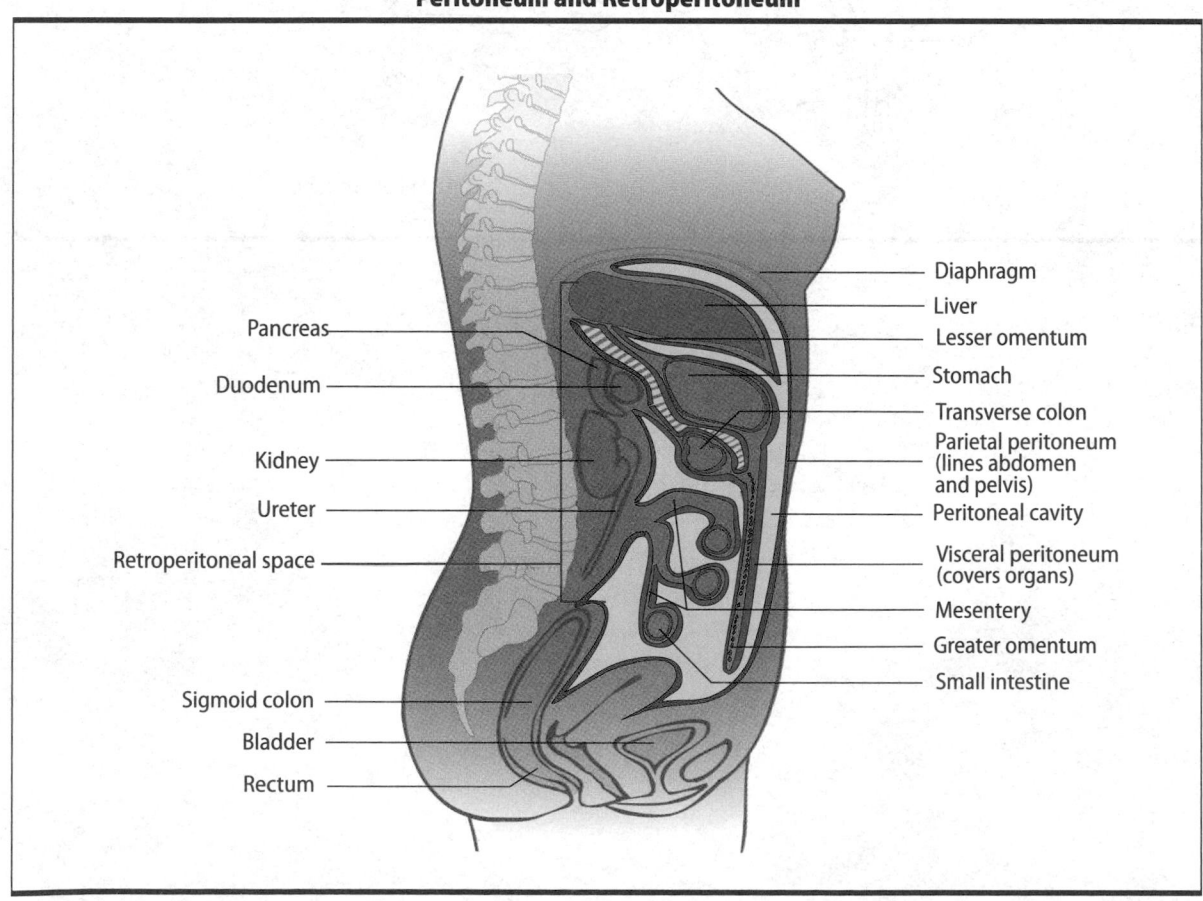

Chapter 12. Diseases of the Skin and Subcutaneous Tissue (LØØ–L99)

Nail Anatomy

Skin and Subcutaneous Tissue

Chapter 13. Diseases of the Musculoskeletal System and Connective Tissue (M00–M99)

Bones and Joints

Shoulder Anterior View

Shoulder Posterior View

Elbow Anterior View

Elbow Posterior View

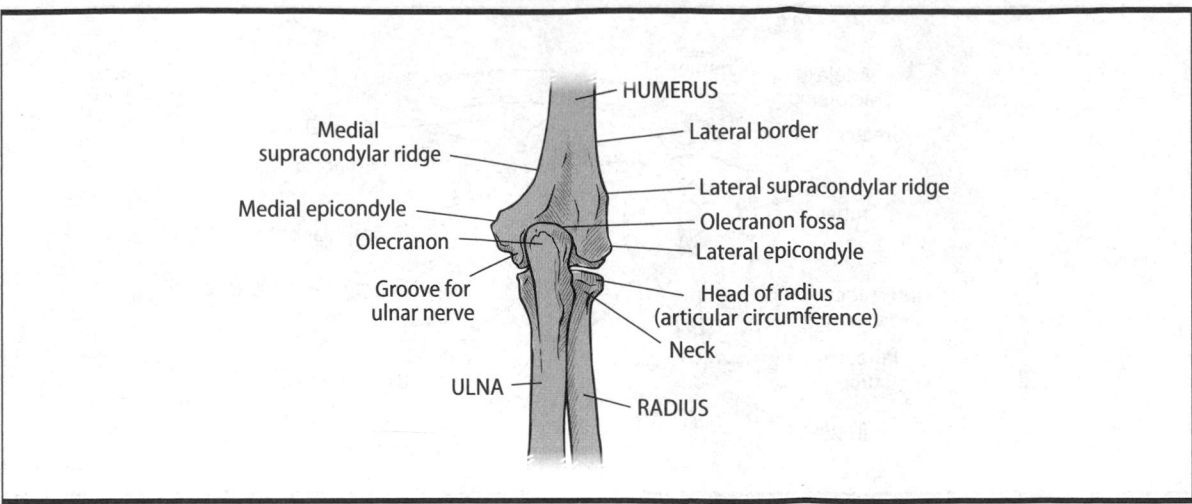

HUMERUS
Medial supracondylar ridge
Lateral border
Lateral supracondylar ridge
Medial epicondyle
Olecranon fossa
Olecranon
Lateral epicondyle
Groove for ulnar nerve
Head of radius (articular circumference)
Neck
ULNA
RADIUS

Hand

Phalanges (digits)

Distal phalanx

Middle phalanx

Interphalangeal joints

Proximal phalanx

Distal phalanx (thumb)

Metacarpophalangeal joint

Metacarpals

Proximal phalanx (thumb)

Carpometacarpal joint

5   4   3   2

1

Hamate

Pisiform

Carpals

Trapezium

Trapezoid

Scaphoid

Triquetral   Lunate   Cuboid

Hip Anterior View

Hip Posterior View

Knee Anterior View

Knee Posterior View

Foot

Muscles

Chapter 14. Diseases of the Genitourinary System (N00–N99)

Urinary System

Male Genitourinary System

Female Internal Genitalia

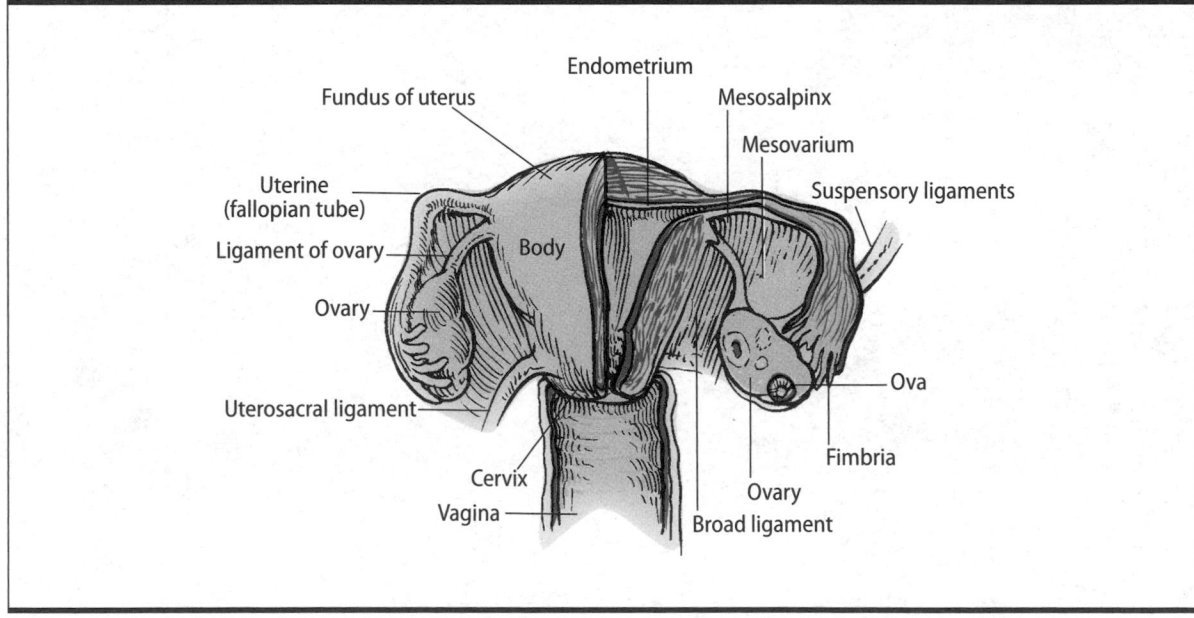

Female Genitourinary Tract Lateral View

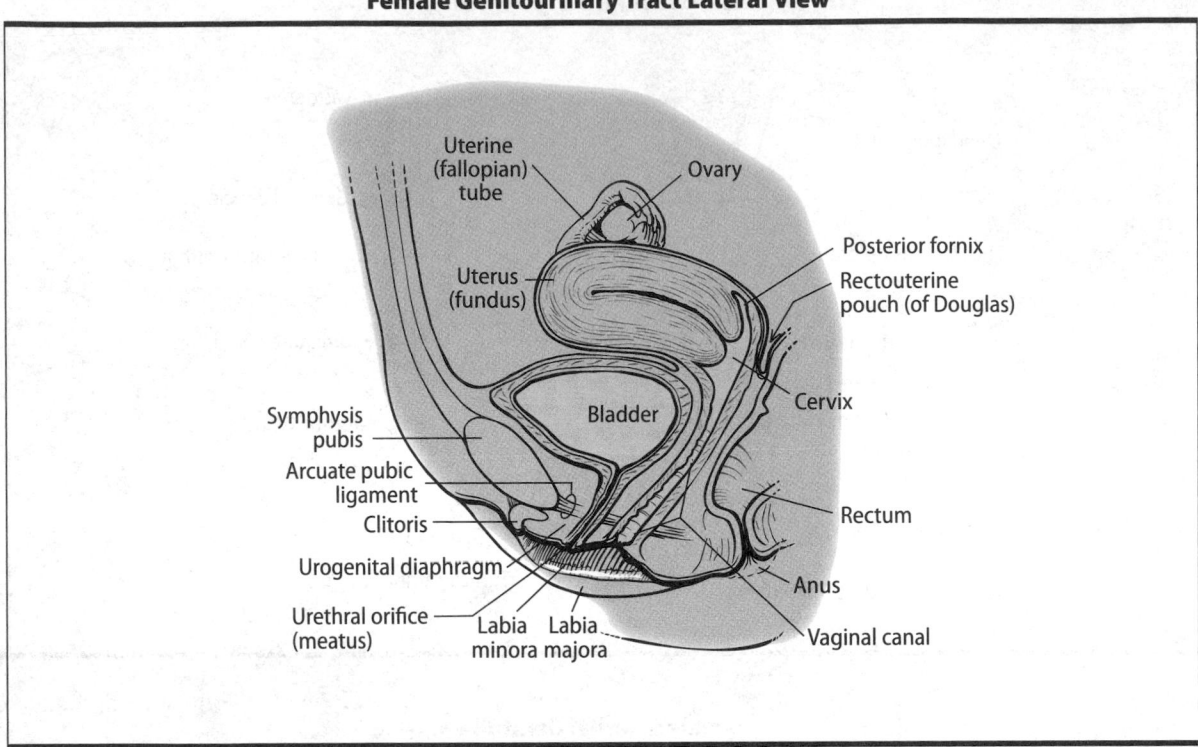

Chapter 15. Pregnancy, Childbirth and the Puerperium (O00–O9A)

Term Pregnancy – Single Gestation

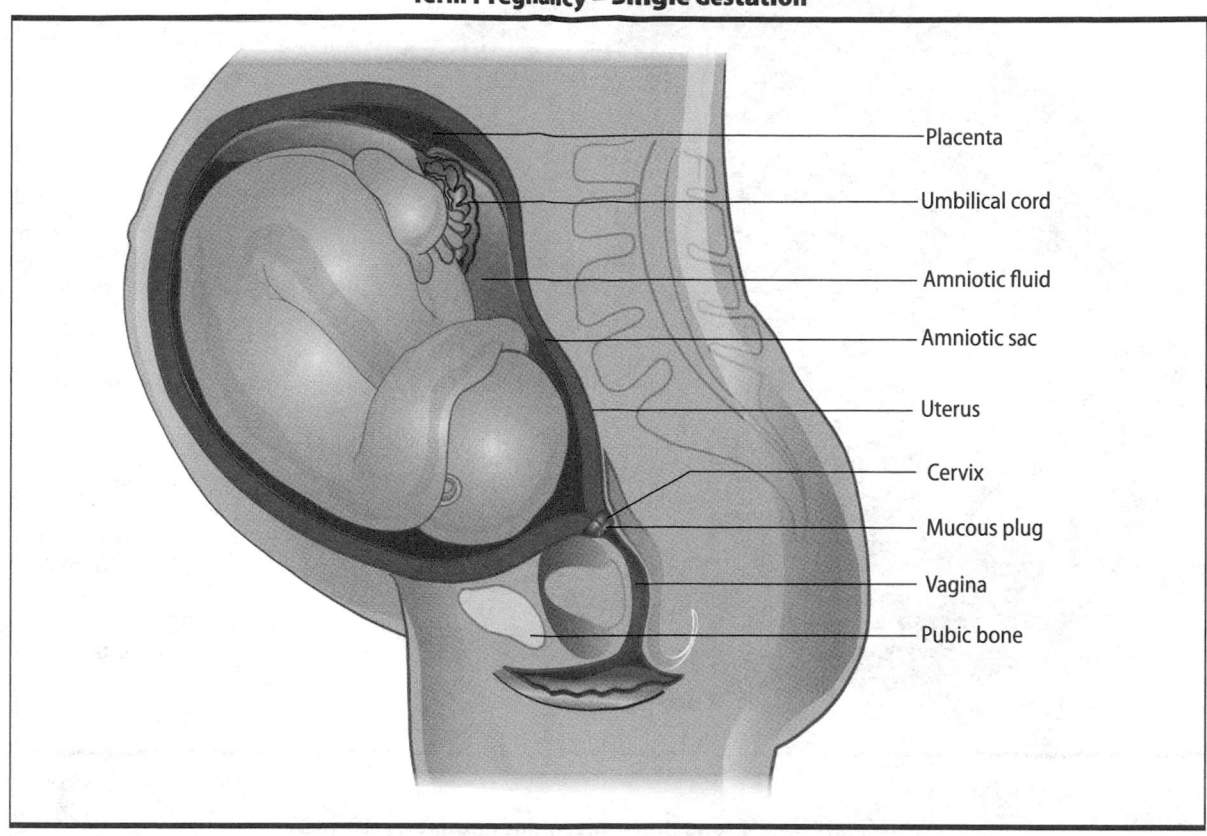

- Placenta
- Umbilical cord
- Amniotic fluid
- Amniotic sac
- Uterus
- Cervix
- Mucous plug
- Vagina
- Pubic bone

Twin Gestation–Dichorionic–Diamniotic (DI-DI)

- 2 Chorionic sacs
- 2 Amniotic sacs
- 2 Fetuses
- 2 Umbilical cords
- 2 Placentas

Twin Gestation–Monochorionic–Diamniotic (MO-DI)

1 Chorionic sac

2 Amniotic sacs

2 Fetuses

2 Umbilical cords

1 Placenta

Twin Gestation–Monochorionic–Monoamniotic (MO-MO)

1 Chorionic sac

1 Amniotic sac

2 Fetuses

2 Umbilical cords

1 Placenta

Chapter 19. Injury, Poisoning and Certain Other Consequences of External Causes (S00–T88)

Types of Fractures

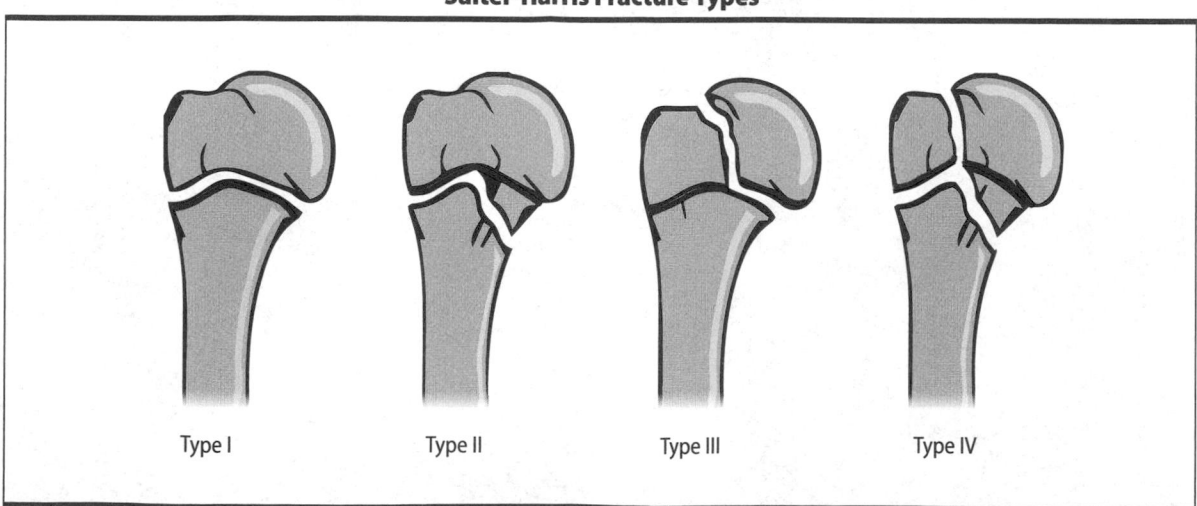

| Normal | Transverse | Open/Compound | Oblique | Oblique displaced |
| Comminuted | Segmental | Avulsed | Spiral | Greenstick |

Salter-Harris Fracture Types

| Type I | Type II | Type III | Type IV |